III. RESPIRATORY GAS TRANSPORT

Oxygen delivery ($\dot{Q}_{O_2}$)	$= \dot{Q}_T \times Ca_{O_2}$
Arterial oxygen content (Ca_{O_2})	$= 1.39 \times Sa_{O_2} \times [Hgb] + .0031 \times Pa_{O_2}$
Mixed venous oxygen content ($C\bar{v}_{O_2}$)	$= 1.39 \times S\bar{v}_{O_2} \times [Hgb] + .0031 \times P\bar{v}_{O_2}$
Arterio-venous oxygen content difference	$= Ca_{O_2} - C\bar{v}_{O_2}$
Oxygen consumption ($\dot{V}_{O_2}$)	$= \dot{Q}_T (Ca_{O_2} - C\bar{v}_{O_2})$
Extraction fraction	$= \dfrac{Ca_{O_2} - C\bar{v}_{O_2}}{Ca_{O_2}}$
Respiratory quotient (RQ)	$= \dfrac{\dot{V}_{CO_2}}{\dot{V}_{O_2}}$
CO_2 production ($\dot{V}_{CO_2}$)	$= f \cdot V_T \cdot F_{E_{CO_2}}$
O_2 consumption ($\dot{V}_{O_2}$)	$= f \cdot V_T \cdot (F_{I_{O_2}} - F_{E_{O_2}})$, when RQ = 1.0

IV. CIRCULATORY PARAMETERS AND CALCULATIONS

Systemic systolic pressure (SP)	100–140 mmHg
Systemic diastolic pressure (DP)	60–90 mmHg
Pulse pressure (SP − DP)	30–50 mmHg
Mean arterial pressure (BP, mmHg)	$\dfrac{(SP + 2DP)}{3}$ at normal heart rate
Heart rate (HR)	60–90/min
Stroke volume (SV)	50–100 mL
Stroke index (SI)	SV/Body surface area (BSA) = 35–50 mL/m^2
Right atrial pressure (Pra)	2–8 mmHg
Pulmonary systolic pressure	16–24 mmHg
Pulmonary diastolic pressure	5–12 mmHg
Pulmonary pulse pressure	8–15 mmHg
Mean pulmonary artery pressure ($P\overline{pa}$)	9–16 mmHg
Mean pulmonary capillary wedge pressure (Ppw)	5–12 mmHg
Cardiac output ($\dot{Q}_T = SV \times HR$)	4–6 L/min
Cardiac index ($CI = \dot{Q}_T/BSA$)	2.5–3 L/min/m^2
Systemic vascular resistance	
$SVR = \dfrac{\overline{BP} - Pra}{\dot{Q}_T}$	10–15 mmHg/L/min (to convert to c.g.s. units, multiply ×80) (900–1200 dyne · s/cm^5)
Pulmonary vascular resistance	
$PVR = \dfrac{Ppa - Ppw}{Q_T}$	1.5–2.5 mmHg/L/min (120–200 dyne · s/cm^5)
Venous return $(VR) = \dfrac{Pms - Pra}{Rvr}$	4–6 L/min
where Pms = mean systemic pressure	10–15 mmHg
Rvr = resistance to venous return	1–2 mmHg/L/min

PRINCIPLES OF CRITICAL CARE

Editors

Jesse B. Hall, M.D.
Director of Critical Care Services
Associate Professor of Medicine and Anesthesia and Critical Care
Section of Pulmonary and Critical Care Medicine
University of Chicago Medical Center
Chicago, Illinois

Gregory A. Schmidt, M.D.
Director of Critical Care Training Program
Associate Professor of Medicine and Anesthesia and Critical Care
Section of Pulmonary and Critical Care Medicine
University of Chicago Medical Center
Chicago, Illinois

Lawrence D.H. Wood, M.D., Ph.D.
Director of Academic Programs
Professor of Medicine and Anesthesia and Critical Care
Section of Pulmonary and Critical Care Medicine
University of Chicago Medical Center
Chicago, Illinois

Associate Editors

Jameel Ali, M.D., Dip. Med. Ed.
Professor of Surgery
Director, Postgraduate Education
Department of Surgery
University of Toronto
Toronto, Ontario, Canada

Charles J. Fisher, Jr., M.D.
Director
Center for Critical Care Research
University Hospital of Cleveland
Cleveland, Ohio

Leonard D. Hudson, M.D.
Professor of Medicine
Head, Division of Pulmonary and Critical Care Medicine
University of Washington School of Medicine
Seattle, Washington

Marguerite R. Kinney, D.N.Sc., R.N.
Professor and Coordinator
Cardiovascular Nursing Graduate Programs
University of Alabama at Birmingham
School of Nursing
Birmingham, Alabama

R. Bruce Light, M.D.
Associate Professor of Medicine
Sections of Infectious Diseases and Critical Care Medicine
University of Manitoba
Winnipeg, Manitoba, Canada

John M. Luce, M.D.
Associate Professor of Medicine and Anesthesia
University of California, San Francisco
Associate Director
Medical-Surgical Intensive Care Unit
San Francisco General Hospital
San Francisco, California

Jacob Iasha Sznajder, M.D.
Associate Professor of Medicine
University of Illinois at Chicago
Director, Pulmonary Medicine Division
Michael Reese Hospital
Chicago, Illinois

Uri Taitelman, M.D.
Director, Poison Information Center
Rambam Medical Center
Haifa, Israel

Jean-Louis Vincent, M.D.
Department of Intensive Care
Erasme University Hospital
Free University of Brussels
Brussels, Belgium

PRINCIPLES OF CRITICAL CARE

Editors

JESSE B. HALL, M.D.
GREGORY A. SCHMIDT, M.D.
LAWRENCE D.H. WOOD, M.D., Ph.D.

Associate Editors

JAMEEL ALI, M.D., Dip. Med. Ed.
CHARLES J. FISHER, Jr., M.D.
LEONARD D. HUDSON, M.D.
MARGUERITE R. KINNEY, D.N.Sc., R.N.
R. BRUCE LIGHT, M.D.
JOHN M. LUCE, M.D.
JACOB IASHA SZNAJDER, M.D.
URI TAITELMAN, M.D.
JEAN-LOUIS VINCENT, M.D.

Silvia M. Jovel
Editorial Assistant

McGRAW-HILL, INC.
Health Professions Division

New York St. Louis San Francisco
Auckland Bogotá Caracas Lisbon London
Madrid Mexico Milan Montreal New Delhi
Paris San Juan Singapore Sydney Tokyo Toronto

Circles: Concerning the symbol on the cover

The three converging circles symbolize the origins and principles of exemplary critical care. Anesthesia, Medicine, and Surgery overlap considerably with each other; the central area in which the unique disciplines most edify the others is critical care. Within this area, the whole circle of providing care for critically ill patients ideally intersects with teaching exemplary care and researching better diagnostic and therapeutic approaches. At a third, concurrent level of human attitudes, the pursuit of excellence in each discipline overlaps productively with the circles of compassion and awe as the intensive care providers practice and are formed by the principles of critical care.

PRINCIPLES OF CRITICAL CARE

ISBN 0-07-071589-0

1234567890 K G P K G P 98765432

This book was set in Palatino by York Graphic Services, Inc.;
its designer was Joan O'Connor;
the editors were J. Dereck Jeffers and Peter McCurdy;
the production supervisor was Roger Kasunic;
the index was prepared by Irving Condé Tullar.
Arcata Graphics/Kingsport was printer and binder.

Library of Congress Cataloging-in-Publication Data

Principles of critical care / Jesse B. Hall, Gregory A. Schmidt, Lawrence D.H. Wood, [editors]; Jameel Ali . . . [et al, associate editors].
p. cm.
Includes bibliographical references.
Includes index.
ISBN 0-07-071589-0
1. Critical care medicine. 2. Intensive care units. I. Hall, Jesse B. II. Wood, Lawrence D. H. III. Schmidt, Gregory A.
[DNLM: 1. Critical Care. 2. Intensive Care Units—organization & administration. WX 218 P9573]
RC86.7.P752 1992
616'.028—dc20
DNLM/DLC
for Library of Congress 92-6364
CIP

To former students, residents, and fellows,
for their inspiration;

Present colleagues, for their ideas and vision;

Aaron, Daniel, and Barbara, for their love; and

My father, for teaching me that valid information
is a necessary starting point, and that some
crises are best treated with a slow hand.

JBH

To Tom and Bev
who got things started;

S. S. and C. P.
who keep them rolling;

and Karen,
who reminds me why.

GAS

To my parents and teachers, for
encouraging me to think;

My children and students, for
enthusiasm and hope;

My colleagues, for companionship in our
shared pursuit of excellence
and compassion; and

Elaine and the Lord of Life, for
delight and awe.

LDHW

CONTENTS

SECTION B
Management of the Intensive Care Unit

SECTION C
Stabilization and Transport of the Critically Ill

PART III
DIAGNOSIS AND MANAGEMENT OF CRITICAL ILLNESS

SECTION A
Complications of Critical Care

SECTION B
Multiple Systems Organ Failure (MSOF)

SECTION H
Infectious Disorders in the Critically Ill

SECTION I
Cardiovascular Disorders in the Critically Ill

SECTION J
Pulmonary Disorders in the Critically Ill

PART IV

PERSPECTIVES ON CRITICAL CARE

CONTRIBUTORS

J.G. ABEL, M.D.
Department of Vascular Surgery
Sunnybrook Medical Centre
North York, Ontario, Canada [16]*

CYRIL ABRAHAMS, M.D.
Director, Surgical Pathology
Professor of Pathology
University of Chicago
Chicago, Illinois [18]

NAOKI AIKAWA, M.D.
Associate Professor, Department of Emergency Medicine
School of Medicine
Keio University
Tokyo, Japan [189D]

RICHARD K. ALBERT, M.D.
Section Head, Division of Pulmonary and Critical Care
Professor of Medicine
University of Washington Medical Center
Seattle, Washington [137]

TIMOTHY E. ALBERTSON, M.D., Ph.D.
Chief, Division of Pulmonary and Critical Care Medicine
University of California, Davis
Sacramento, California [131, 169, 174, 179]

JAMEEL ALI, M.D., Dip. Med. Ed.
Professor of Surgery
Director, Postgraduate Medicine
Department of Surgery
University of Toronto
Toronto, Ontario, Canada [16, 59, 63, 84]

*The numbers in brackets refer to chapters written or co-written by the contributor.

ROBLEE P. ALLEN, M.D
Assistant Clinical Professor
Division of Pulmonary and Critical Care Medicine
University of California, Davis
Sacramento, California [169]

CARROL A. ALVAREZ, R.N.
Clinical Nurse Specialist
Harborview Medical Center
Seattle, Washington [44]

JOHN ALVERDY, M.D.
Department of Surgery
Michael Reese Hospital
Chicago, Illinois [86]

BRIAN T. ANDREWS, M.D.
Department of Neurological Surgery
University of California, San Francisco
San Francisco General Hospital
San Francisco, California [34]

FRED Y. AOKI, M.D.
Professor of Medicine
Head, Section of Clinical Pharmacology
University of Manitoba Health Sciences Center
Winnipeg, Manitoba, Canada [96]

PAUL M. ARNOW, M.D.
Associate Professor of Medicine
Chief, Section of Infectious Diseases
University of Chicago
Chicago, Illinois [43]

HERNAN ARTUCCIO, M.D.
Professor of Intensive Care Medicine
Director, Intensive Care Department
Hospital de Clinicas
School of Medicine, Universidad de la Republica
Montevideo, Uruguay [189F]

JEFFREY ASKANAZI, M.D.
Associate Attending, Division of Nutrition
Department of Anesthesiology/Critical Care
Albert Einstein College of Medicine and Montefiore Medical Center
Bronx, New York [91–95]

JOSEPH J. AUSTIN, M.D.
Ancaster, Ontario, Canada [124]

STEVEN J. BARKER, M.D., Ph.D.
Associate Professor and Acting Chairman of Anesthesia
University of California, Irvine
Orange, California [13]

V. THEODORE BARNETT, M.D.
Instructor, Medicine
University of Illinois at Chicago
College of Medicine
Chicago, Illinois [158]

BEVERLY W. BARON, M.D.
Assistant Professor of Pathology
University of Chicago
Chicago, Illinois [35, 146]

JOSEPH M. BARON, M.D.
Associate Professor of Medicine
Director, Coagulation and Bone Marrow Laboratory
University of Chicago
Chicago, Illinois [35, 146]

JOHN T. BARRON, M.D., Ph.D.
Assistant Professor of Medicine
Section of Cardiology
Rush Presbyterian St. Luke Medical Center
Chicago, Illinois [116]

WALTER G. BARR, M.D.
Associate Professor of Medicine
Chief, Section of Rheumatology
Stritch School of Medicine
Maywood, Illinois [126]

HISHAM S. BASSIOUNY, M.D.
Assistant Professor of Surgery
University of Chicago
Chicago, Illinois [23]

MARA BAUN, R.N., D.N.Sc.
Professor and Director
Niedfelt Nursing Research Center
College of Nursing
University of Nebraska Medical Center
Omaha, Nebraska [187a]

NANCY BERGSTROM, R.N., Ph.D.
Professor, College of Nursing
University of Nebraska Medical Center
Omaha, Nebraska [187F]

J.M.A. BOHNEN, M.D.
Wellesley Hospital
Toronto, Ontario, Canada [85]

E.J. BOW, M.D.
Associate Professor of Medicine and Medical Microbiology
University of Manitoba
St. Boniface General Hospital
Winnipeg, Manitoba, Canada [99]

DAVID G. BRACHMAN, M.D.
Instructor, Radiation Oncology
University of Chicago
Chicago, Illinois [152]

T. STEPHEN BRENNAN, M.D.
Assistant Professor of Medicine
Renal Section
Baylor College of Medicine
Houston, Texas [153, 156]

JEFFREY BRENT, M.D., Ph.D.
Assistant Medical Director
Rocky Mountain Poison and Drug Center
Assistant Professor of Pediatrics and Surgery
University of Colorado Health Sciences Center
Denver, Colorado [178, 181]

STEPHANIE J. BRISTER, M.D.
Cardiovascular Surgeon
Hamilton General Hospital
McMaster Clinic
Hamilton, Ontario, Canada [28]

GERALD BRISTOW, M.D.
Associate Dean and Professor of Anesthesia
Department of Medicine
University of Manitoba
Winnipeg, Manitoba, Canada [73]

JAY B. BRODSKY, M.D.
Professor of Anesthesia
Stanford University Medical Center
Stanford, California [10]

STEVEN D. BROWN, M.D.
Associate in Medicine
Duke University Medical Center
Durham, North Carolina [74]

DAVID S. BRUCE, M.D.
Research Fellow
Section of Transplantation Surgery
University of Chicago
Chicago, Illinois [77]

THOMAS E. BUMP, M.D.
Associate Professor of Medicine
Director, Arrhythmia Service
University of Chicago
Chicago, Illinois [31, 32, 120]

SIMON BURSZTEIN, M.D.
Director, Department of General Intensive Care
Rambam Medical Center
Haifa, Israel [91, 92, 94, 189C]

JOHN BUSE, M.D., Ph.D.
Instructor, Endocrinology
University of Chicago
Chicago, Illinois [159]

THOMAS C. BUTLER, M.D.
Professor of Medicine and Microbiology
Chief, Division of Infectious Diseases
Texas Technical University
Health Sciences Center
Lubbock, Texas [108]

JOHN S. CAPPS, R.R.T.
Manager, Respiratory Care Services
Emanuel Hospital
Portland, Oregon [38]

MARK B. CARR, M.D.
Fellow, Infectious Diseases
University of Alabama at Birmingham
Birmingham, Alabama [101]

JOHN D. CARROLL, M.D.
Associate Professor of Medicine
Director, Hans Hecht Cardiac Catheterization Laboratory
University of Chicago
Chicago, Illinois [26]

FRANK B. CERRA, M.D.
Professor of Surgery
Director, Critical Care and Nutrition
University of Minnesota
University of Minnesota Hospitals and Clinic
Minneapolis, Minnesota [56]

P. JOAN CHESNEY, M.D.
Professor of Pediatrics
University of Tennessee, Memphis
Le BonHeur Children's Medical Center
Memphis, Tennessee [113]

RORY W. CHILDERS, M.D.
Professor of Medicine
Director, Heart Station
University of Chicago
Chicago, Illinois [30]

TERESA CHOU, M.P.H.
Infection Control
Section of Infectious Disease
Department of Medicine
Chicago, Illinois [43]

ANTHONY W. CHOW, M.D.
Professor of Medicine
University of British Columbia and Vancouver General Hospital
Vancouver, British Columbia, Canada [105]

ELIZABETH T. CLARK, M.D.
Chief Resident, Department of Surgery
University of Chicago
Chicago, Illinois [167]

TERRY P. CLEMMER, M.D.
Director, Critical Care Medicine
Latter Day Saints Hospital
Salt Lake City, Utah [40]

JOHN M. CLOCHESY, R.N., M.S., C.S.
Instructor, Acute and Critical Care Nursing
Frances Payne Bolton School of Nursing
Case Western Reserve University
Cleveland, Ohio [187G]

C. GLENN COBBS, M.D.
Professor of Medicine
Division of Infectious Diseases
University of Alabama Medical Center
Birmingham, Alabama [101]

JOHN CONLY, M.D.
Associate Professor of Medicine
Section of Infectious Diseases
University of Saskatchewan
Saskatoon, Saskatchewan, Canada [106]

THOMAS CORBRIDGE, M.D.
Staff Physician, Immunology and Respiratory Medicine
National Jewish Center
Denver, Colorado [132]

JOSEPH P. COYLE, M.D.
Staff Anesthesiologist
Carolina Medical Center
Charlotte, North Carolina [87]

STEVEN W. CRAWFORD, M.D.
Critical Care Director
Fred Hutchinson Cancer Research Center
Clinical Research Division
Seattle, Washington [150]

ROBERT K. CRONE, M.D.
Professor, Anesthesiology and Pediatrics
University of Washington School of Medicine
Director of Anesthesia
Children's Hospital and Medical Center
Seattle, Washington [186]

JOHN P. CULVER, M.D.
Director, Quality Assurance
Harborview Medical Center
Seattle, Washington [42]

RICHARD C. DART, M.D., Ph.D.
Research Director, Emergency Medicine
University of Arizona Medical Center
Tucson, Arizona [182]

NICOLA P. D'ATTELLIS, M.D.
Resident in Anesthesiology
The Albert Einstein College of Medicine
Bronx, New York [94]

SYLVIE ANNE BURSZTEIN-DeMYTTENAERE, M.D.
Head, Intensive Care Unit
Lady Davis Carmel Hospital
Haifa, Israel [95]

ROBERT H. DEMLING, M.D.
Director, Longwood Area Trauma Center
Boston, Massachusetts [68–70]

CHRISTOPHER M. DENNIS, M.D.
Respiratory Physiology Department
Papworth Hospital
Papworth Everard
Cambridge, England [79]

A.R. DOWNS, M.D.
Professor of Surgery
University of Manitoba
Health Sciences Centre
Winnipeg, Manitoba, Canada [65]

KATHLEEN DRACUP, R.N., D.N.Sc.
Professor, School of Nursing
University of California–Los Angeles
Los Angeles, California [187H]

KENNETH A. DRASNER, M.D.
Assistant Professor of Anesthesia
University of California, San Francisco
San Francisco, California [82]

JEFFERY DRAZEN, M.D.
Chief, Combined Pulmonary and Critical Care Division
Beth Israel Hospital and Brigham and Women's Hospital
Boston, Massachusetts [8]

MATTHEW J. ELLENHORN, M.D.
Clinical Professor of Medical Toxicology
Drew/UCLA School of Medicine
Los Angeles, California [168, 170–172]

WILLIAM J. ELLIOTT, M.D., Ph.D.
Assistant Professor of Medicine, Clinical
Pharmacology & Physical Science
University of Chicago
Chicago, Illinois [123, 125]

DAVID H. ELWYN, Ph.D.
Research Scientist
Department of Anesthesiology/Critical Care
The Albert Einstein College of Medicine and Montefiore Medical Center
Bronx, New York [90]

JEAN C. EMOND, M.D.
Assistant Professor of Surgery
Director, Liver Transplantation
University of Chicago
Chicago, Illinois [80]

PHILLIP FACTOR, M.D.
Fellow, Pulmonary and Critical Care Medicine
University of Chicago
Chicago, Illinois [24]

TED FELDMAN, M.D.
Assistant Professor of Medicine
Director, Coronary Care Unit
University of Chicago
Chicago, Illinois [26]

KEVIN L. FERGUSON, M.D.
Fellow, Critical Care Medicine
SUNY Health Science Center
Syracuse, New York [51]

CHARLES J. FISHER, Jr., M.D.
Director, Center for Critical Care Research
University Hospital of Cleveland
Cleveland, Ohio [49]

MALCOLM McD. FISHER, M.D., M.B.Ch.B.
Head, Intensive Therapy Unit
Royal North Shore Hospital
St. Leonards, New South Wales, Australia [189A]

MATTHEW E. FINK, M.D.
Associate Professor and Director of Critical Care Neurology
Neurologic and Critical Care Research
New York, New York [144]

JOHN P. FLAHERTY, M.D.
Assistant Professor of Medicine
University of Chicago
Chicago, Illinois [43]

GINI FLEMING, M.D.
Fellow, Department of Hematology/Oncology
University of Chicago
Chicago, Illinois [151]

DUANE FOLLMAN, M.D.
Assistant Professor of Medicine
University of Chicago
Chicago, Illinois [122]

MARQUIS D. FOREMAN, R.N., Ph.D.
Assistant Professor
Department of Medical-Surgical Nursing
College of Nursing
University of Illinois at Chicago
Chicago, Illinois [187I]

GARRETT E. FOULKE, M.D.
Associate Professor of Clinical Internal Medicine
Division of Pulmonary and Critical Care Medicine
University of California, Davis
Sacramento, California [50, 131, 169]

JOHN C. GALBRAITH, M.D.
Clinical Fellow, Medical Microbiology and Infectious Diseases
University of Alberta
Edmonton, Alberta, Canada [104]

REED M. GARDNER, Ph.D.
Professor of Medical Informatics
Latter Day Saints Hospital
Salt Lake City, Utah [41]

LARRY M. GENTILELLO, M.D.
Assistant Professor of Surgery
University of Washington School of Medicine
Seattle, Washington [27]

EUGENE F. GEPPERT, M.D.
Associate Professor of Medicine
University of Chicago Medical Center
Chicago, Illinois [15, 17, 138, 139]

BRUCE L. GEWERTZ, M.D.
Professor of Surgery
Faculty Dean of Medical Education
University of Chicago
Chicago, Illinois [167]

DAVID M. GILLUM, M.D.
Assistant Professor of Medicine
Western Nephrology and Metabolic Bone Disease Clinic
Lakewood, Colorado [153, 155]

DAYLE HOSEK GLEASON, R.N.
Director, Medical Nursing
Group Health Central Hospital
Seattle, Washington [36]

LAWRENCE TIM GOODNOUGH, M.D.
Associate Professor of Medicine and Pathology
Case Western Reserve University
Director, Component Therapy Center
Associate Director, Blood Bank
University Hospital of Cleveland
Cleveland, Ohio [147]

LAWRENCE J. GOTTLIEB, M.D.
Associate Professor of Clinical Surgery
University of Chicago
Chicago, Illinois [12, 66]

WILLIAM J. GRADISHAR, M.D.
Assistant Professor of Medicine
Northwestern University Medical School
Chicago, Illinois [149]

PERRY GRAY, M.D.
Clinical Fellow, Critical Care Medicine
University of Manitoba
Winnipeg, Manitoba, Canada [110]

DAVID D. GRETLER, M.D.
Fellow in Cardiology
Department of Medicine
University of Chicago
Chicago, Illinois [125]

PAMELA S. GRIM, M.D.
Medical Director, Hyperbaric Oxygen Unit
University of Chicago
Chicago, Illinois [12]

JOHN D. HAIGH, M.D.
Clinical Assistant Professor of Medicine and Anesthesiology
University of Calgary
Foothills Hospital
Calgary, Alberta, Canada [81]

JESSE B. HALL, M.D.
Director of Critical Care Services
Associate Professor of Medicine and Anesthesiology and Critical Care
Section of Pulmonary and Critical Care Medicine
University of Chicago Medical Center
Chicago, Illinois [4, 11, 52, 72, 88, 127–130, 135, 154, 157, 173, 177]

S.M. HAMILTON, M.D.
Assistant Professor of Surgery
University of Alberta
Edmonton, Alberta, Canada [7]

IRA M. HANAN, M.D.
Assistant Professor of Medicine
University of Chicago
Chicago, Illinois [33, 163]

DANIEL F. HANLEY, Jr., M.D.
Department of Neurology
Johns Hopkins Hospital
Baltimore, Maryland [141]

GODFREY K.M. HARDING, M.D., B.Sc.
Professor of Medicine and Medical Microbiology
University of Manitoba
Head, Section of Infectious Diseases
St. Boniface General Hospital
Winnipeg, Manitoba, Canada [107]

THOMAS HEFFRON, M.D.
Assistant Professor of Surgery
Section of Hepatobiliary and Liver Transplant Surgery
University of Chicago
Chicago, Illinois [76]

TIM W. HIGENBOTTAM, B.Sc., M.D.
Consultant Physician
Regional Pulmonary Physiology Laboratory
Papworth Hospital
Papworth Everard, Cambridge, England [79]

THOMAS L. HIGGINS, M.D.
Director, Cardiothoracic Intensive Care Unit
The Cleveland Clinic Foundation
Cleveland, Ohio [87]

PHILIP C. HOFFMAN, M.D.
Associate Professor of Medicine
University of Chicago
Chicago, Illinois [145, 149]

BARBARA HOLTZCLAW, R.N., Ph.D.
School of Nursing
Vanderbilt University
Nashville, Tennessee [187B]

LEONARD D. HUDSON, M.D.
Professor of Medicine
Head, Division of Pulmonary and Critical Care Medicine
University of Washington School of Medicine
Harborview Medical Center
Seattle, Washington [42]

EDWARD INGENITO, M.D., Ph.D.
Assistant Professor
Director, Medical Intensive Care Unit
Brigham and Women's Hospital
Boston, Massachusetts [8]

PHILIP JACOBS, Ph.D.
Health Care Economist
Department of Health Services Administration
University of Alberta
Edmonton, Alberta, Canada [39]

MICHAEL JASTREMSKI, M.D.
Professor and Director
Critical Care and Emergency Medicine
SUNY Health Science Center
Syracuse, New York [51]

GARTH E. JOHNSON, M.D.
Chief, Orthopedic Surgery
Ottawa Civic Hospital
Ottawa, Ontario, Canada [61, 65]

LISA KAPLOWITZ, M.D.
Associate Professor
Department of Medicine
Division of Infectious Diseases
Medical College of Virginia
Virginia Commonwealth University
Richmond, Virginia [111]

MARSHALL B. KAPP, J.D., M.P.H.
Professor, Community Health Director
Office of Geriatric Medicine and Gerontology
School of Medicine, Wright State University
Dayton, Ohio [45]

JEFFREY A. KATZ, M.D.
Associate Professor of Anesthesiology
University of California, San Francisco
San Francisco General Hospital
San Francisco, California [82]

MITCHELL F. KEAMY III, M.D.
Las Vegas, Nevada [6, 72, 83]

E. GARNER KING, M.D.
Chairman and Professor
Department of Medicine
Walter Mackenzie Health Sciences Center
University of Alberta
Edmonton, Alberta, Canada [7, 134]

MARGUERITE R. KINNEY, D.N.Sc., R.N.
Professor and Coordinator, Cardiovascular Nursing Graduate Programs
University of Alabama at Birmingham
School of Nursing
Birmingham, Alabama [187]

WILLIAM A. KNAUS, M.D.
Professor, Anesthesiology
Director, ICU Research Unit
George Washington University Medical Center
Washington, D.C. [46]

STEVEN KOENIG, M.D.
Chief, Pulmonary Section
USAF Medical Center
Scott Air Force Base, Illinois [160]

VIRGINIA KOHLMAN-CARRIERI, R.N., D.N.Sc.
Associate Professor
Department of Physiological Nursing
University of California-San Francisco
San Francisco, California [187D]

STEVEN N. KONSTADT, M.D.
Associate Professor of Anesthesiology
Mt. Sinai Medical Center
New York, New York [21, 22]

RICHARD A. LARSON, M.D.
Associate Professor of Medicine
University of Chicago
Chicago, Illinois [148]

JAMES W. LEATHERMAN, M.D.
Assistant Professor of Medicine
University of Minnesota
Hennepin County Medical Center
Minneapolis, Minnesota [25]

ELEANOR D. LEDERER, M.D.
Associate Professor of Medicine
University of Louisville
Louisville, Kentucky [155, 156]

RAPHAEL LEE, M.D., Sc.D.
Associate Professor of Surgery and Organismal Biology
University of Chicago
Chicago, Illinois [66]

ILO E. LEPPIK, M.D.
Clinical Professor of Neurology and Pharmacy Practice
University of Minnesota
Minneapolis, Minnesota [142]

JERROLD H. LEVY, M.D.
Associate Professor of Anesthesiology
Section of Anesthesiology
Emory University
Atlanta, Georgia [89]

THEODORE H. LEWIS, Jr., M.D.
Assistant Professor of Medicine
University of Chicago
Chicago, Illinois [154, 164]

R. BRUCE LIGHT, M.D.
Associate Professor of Medicine
Sections of Infectious Diseases and Critical Care Medicine
University of Manitoba
St. Boniface Hospital
Winnipeg, Manitoba, Canada [55, 97, 98, 102]

ALEX G. LITTLE, M.D.
Chairman, Department of Surgery
University of Nevada School of Medicine
Las Vegas, Nevada [27]

G. RICHARD LONG, M.D.
Department of Medicine
University of Manitoba
St. Boniface General Hospital
Winnipeg, Manitoba, Canada [109]

ERIC K. LOUIE, M.D.
Associate Professor of Medicine
Loyola University Medical Center
Maywood, Illinois [21]

JOHN M. LUCE, M.D.
Associate Professor of Medicine and Anesthesia
University of California, San Francisco
Associate Director
Medical-Surgical Intensive Care Unit
San Francisco General Hospital
San Francisco, California [143]

JAMES R. MACHO, M.D.
Assistant Professor of Surgery
Department of Surgery
University of California-San Francisco
San Francisco General Hospital
San Francisco, California [67]

HEBER MACMAHON, M.D.
Associate Professor of Radiology
University of Chicago
Chicago, Illinois [19]

SHELLEY MALAN, R.N., M.S., C.C.R.N.
Nursing Administration
Albany Medical Center
Albany, New York [44]

JOHN J. MARINI, M.D.
Professor and Director, Pulmonary and Critical Care Medicine
St. Paul Ramsey Medical Center
St. Paul, Minnesota [14, 25]

GEORGE M. MATUSCHAK, M.D.
Associate Professor of Medicine
St. Louis University Medical Center
St. Louis, Missouri [53]

T.J. MCDONNELL, M.B.
Assistant Professor
Divisions of Pulmonary and Critical Care Medicine
University of Alberta
Edmonton, Alberta, Canada [134]

NORMA MAZZA, M.D.
Associate Professor of Intensive Care Medicine
Intensive Care Department
Hospital de Clinicas
School of Medicine, Universidad de la Republica
Montevideo, Uruguay [189F]

MANFRED MEYER, M.D., D.Sc.
Professor
Clinic of Anesthesiology and Intensive Care
Berlin, Germany [189G]

FREDERICK G. MIHM, M.D.
Associate Professor of Anesthesia
Stanford University Medical Center
Stanford, California [10]

DINIS REIS MIRANDA, M.D.
Intensive Care Division
Academisch Ziekenhuis Groningen
Groningen, The Netherlands [189I]

PAMELA H. MITCHELL, R.N., M.S.
Professor of Physiological Nursing
School of Nursing
University of Washington
Seattle, Washington [37]

R. BRIAN MITCHELL, M.D.
Fellow, Hematology/Oncology
University of Chicago
Chicago, Illinois [145]

T. MICHAEL MOLES, M.B., B.S.
Reader in Anaesthetics
University of Hong Kong
Chief of Anaesthesia, Prince Philip Hospital
Hong Kong [189B]

JULIO SERGIO GONZALEZ MONTANER, M.D.
Director, AIDS Research Program and Infectious Disease Clinic
St. Paul's Hospital/University of British Columbia
Vancouver, British Columbia, Canada [100]

STEVEN M. MONTNER, M.D.
Assistant Professor of Radiology
University of Chicago Medical Center
Chicago, Illinois [19]

ALAN H. MORRIS, M.D.
Director of Research/Pulmonary Division
Professor of Medicine
University of Utah
Latter Day Saints Hospital
Salt Lake City, Utah [29, 41]

DEBRA K. MOSER, R.N., M.N.
School of Nursing
University of California-Los Angeles
Los Angeles, California [187H]

JONATHAN MOSS, M.D.
Professor, Anesthesia and Critical Care
University of Chicago
Chicago, Illinois [89]

RICHARD J. MOULTON, M.D.
St. Michael's Hospital
Toronto, Ontario, Canada [60]

JOHN MURRAY, M.D.
Professor of Medicine
San Francisco Hospital Chest Division
San Francisco, California [188]

R.A. MUSTARD, M.D.
University of Toronto
Wellesley Hospital
Toronto, Ontario, Canada [85]

AVI NAHUM, M.D.
Staff Physician, Pulmonary and Critical Care
Department of Medicine
St. Paul Ramsey Medical Center
St. Paul, Minnesota [58]

THOMAS W. NOSEWORTHY, M.D., M.P.H.
Associate Professor and Associate Director
Faculty Division of Critical Care Medicine
University of Alberta
Alberta, Canada [39]

JAMES F. ORME, Jr., M.D.
Associate Professor of Medicine
University of Utah
Latter Day Saints Hospital
Salt Lake City, Utah [40]

P. PEARL O'ROURKE, M.D.
Assistant Professor of Anesthesiology and Pediatrics
University of Washington
Children's Hospital and Medical Center
Seattle, Washington [186]

EDWARD A. PANACEK, M.D.
Acting Director
Division of Critical Care Emergency
Assistant Professor of Medicine
University Hospitals of Cleveland
Cleveland, Ohio [47, 48, 180]

JOSEPH E. PARRILLO, M.D.
James B. Herrick Professor of Medicine
Chief, Cardiology and Critical Care Medicine
Rush Medical College
Rush Presbyterian St. Luke's Hospital
Chicago, Illinois [116]

LYNN PATEL, M.D.
Associate Professor of Anesthesiology
University of Manitoba
Winnipeg, Manitoba, Canada [73]

PETER PHILLIPS, M.D.
Clinical Assistant Professor
Department of Medicine
St. Paul's Hospital
University of British Columbia
Vancouver, British Columbia, Canada [100]

GIANCARLO PIANO, M.D.
Department of Surgery
Michael Reese Hospital
Chicago, Illinois [86]

CLAUDE A. PIANTADOSI, M.D.
Associate Professor of Medicine
Duke University Medical Center
Durham, North Carolina [74]

DANIEL PICUS, M.D.
Associate Professor of Radiology
Chief, Interventional Radiology
Mallinkrodt Institute of Radiology
Washington University School of Medicine
St. Louis, Missouri [20]

SUSAN PINGLETON, M.D.
Professor of Medicine
University of Kansas
Kansas City, Kansas [52]

LAWRENCE H. PITTS, M.D.
Professor of Neurosurgery
University of California-San Francisco
San Francisco General Hospital
San Francisco, California [34]

KENNETH S. POLONSKY, M.D.
Professor and Section Chief, Endocrinology
University of Chicago
Chicago, Illinois [159]

PETER D. POTGIETER
Respiratory Intensive Care Unit
Groote Schuur Hospital
Capetown, Republic of South Africa [189E]

WILLIAM J. POWERS, M.D.
Associate Professor of Neurology and Radiology
Division of Radiation Sciences
Mallinckrodt Institute of Radiology
Washington University
St. Louis, Missouri [141]

KENNETH PRESBERG, M.D.
Assistant Professor of Medicine
Medical College of Wisconsin
Milwaukee, Wisconsin [117]

KATHLEEN PUNTILLO, R.N., M.S.N.
San Anselmo, California [187E]

THOMAS A. RAFFIN, M.D.
Associate Professor of Medicine
Chief, Pulmonary and Critical Care Medicine
Stanford University
Stanford, California [185]

BIANCA RAIKHLIN-EISENKRAFT, Ph.D.
Israel Poison Information Center
Rambam Medical Center
Haifa, Israel [177]

DAVID D. RALPH, M.D.
Associate Professor of Medicine
University of Washington
Seattle, Washington [36]

SAMUEL REFETOFF, M.D.
Professor of Medicine/Pediatrics
University of Chicago
Chicago, Illinois [161, 162]

RICHARD K. REZNICK, M.D., M.Ed.
Assistant Professor of Surgery
University of Toronto
Toronto Western Hospital
Toronto, Ontario, Canada [166]

JEAN E. RINALDO, M.D.
Associate Professor of Medicine
Chief, Pulmonary and Critical Care Medicine
Vanderbilt University
Center for Lung Research
Nashville, Tennessee [54]

DANIEL ROBERTS, M.D.
Associate Professor of Medicine
University of Manitoba
Director, Medical Intensive Care Unit
Winnipeg, Manitoba, Canada [110]

GARY L. ROBERTSON, M.D.
Professor of Medicine
Northwestern University
Chicago, Illinois [157]

JOHN A. ROBINSON, M.D.
Professor of Medicine
Section of Rheumatology
Stritch School of Medicine
Loyola University of Chicago
Maywood, Illinois [126]

ROBERTO RODRIGUEZ-ROISIN, M.D.
Professor of Medicine
Hospital Clinic
Villarroel, Barcelona, Spain [188]

MICHAEL F. ROIZEN, M.D.
Professor and Chairman, Department of Anesthesia and Critical Care
University of Chicago
Chicago, Illinois [89]

CHARIS ROUSSOS, M.D., Ph.D.
Professor of Medicine
Chairman, Critical Care
University of Athens School of Medicine
Attiki, Greece [133]

BARRY RUMACK, M.D.
Director, Rocky Mountain Poison and Drug Center
Denver, Colorado [178, 181]

FINDLAY E. RUSSELL, M.D., Ph.D.
Professor of Pharmacology and Toxicology
College of Pharmacy
University of Arizona
Tucson, Arizona [182]

JAMES A. RUSSELL, M.D.
Associate Professor of Medicine
Head, Critical Care Medicine
St. Paul's Hospital
University of British Columbia
Vancouver, British Columbia, Canada [100]

WILLIAM F. RUTHERFORD, M.D.
Assistant Professor of Medicine
Case Western Reserve University
Division of Critical Care Medicine
University Hospitals of Cleveland
Cleveland, Ohio [47, 48]

RICHARD W. SAMSEL, M.D.
Assistant Professor of Medicine
University of Chicago
Chicago, Illinois [57]

IAN H. SANTORO, M.D.
Fellow, Cardiology
University of Oklahoma Health Sciences Center
Oklahoma City, Oklahoma [120]

JONATHAN SAUNDERS, M.D.
Department of Surgery
University of Chicago
Chicago, Illinois [66]

ANTHONY SCHAPERA, M.B., Ch.B.
Assistant Professor of Anesthesia
University of California-San Francisco
San Francisco General Hospital
San Francisco, California [82]

W. MICHAEL SCHELD, M.D.
Department of Internal Medicine
University of Virginia School of Medicine
Charlottsville, Virginia [103]

GREGORY A. SCHMIDT, M.D.
Director of Critical Care Training Program
Associate Professor of Medicine and Anesthesiology and Critical Care
Section of Pulmonary and Critical Care Medicine
University of Chicago Medical Center
Chicago, Illinois [3, 5, 20, 71, 118, 119, 129, 158, 160, 164, 173, 175]

KAREN T. SCHMIDT, M.D.
Assistant Professor of Medicine
Stritch School of Medicine
Loyola University of Chicago
Maywood, Illinois [71]

ROBERT B. SCHOENE, M.D.
Associate Professor of Medicine
Harborview Medical Center
Seattle, Washington [75]

B.D. SCHOUTEN, R.N.
Department of Surgery
Wellesley Hospital
University of Toronto
Toronto, Ontario, Canada [85]

PAUL T. SCHUMACKER, Ph.D.
Associate Professor
Section of Pulmonary and Critical Care Medicine
University of Chicago
Chicago, Illinois [57]

LAURENCE SEGIL, M.D.
Assistant Professor of Anesthesia
University of Illinois Hospital
Chicago, Illinois [22]

GERARD J. SHEEHAN, M.D.
Assistant Professor of Medicine
University Hospital
Edmonton, Alberta, Canada [107, 134]

B. WILLIAM SHRAGGE, M.D.
McMaster Clinical Unit
Hamilton General Hospital
Hamilton, Ontario, Canada [28, 124]

PIERRE SINGER, M.D.
Department of Intensive Care
Rambam Medical Center
Technion, Israeli Technical Institute of Science
Haifa, Israel [92]

CARL A. SIRIO, M.D.
Critical Care Medicine
The National Institutes of Health
Bethesda, Maryland [46]

BJÖRN SKEIE, M.D.
Division of Critical Care Medicine
Department of Anesthesiology
Albert Einstein College of Medicine
Bronx, New York
Ullevaal Hospital
University of Oslo
Oslo, Norway [93]

DUDLEY SMITH, M.S.
Administrative Director
University Air Care
Cincinnati, Ohio [49]

JEFFREY S. SOBLE, M.D.
Assistant Professor of Medicine
Associate Director, Medical ICU
Rush Presbyterian St. Lukes Medical Center
Chicago, Illinois [31, 32, 120]

PAUL SOBOTKA, M.D.
Assistant Professor of Medicine
Loyola University Medical Center
Maywood, Illinois [122]

ELDAR SÖREIDE, M.D.
Division of Critical Care Medicine
Department of Anesthesiology
Albert Einstein College of Medicine
Bronx, New York
Ullevaal Hospital
University of Oslo
Oslo, Norway [93]

D. IAN SOUTTER, M.D.
Department of Surgery
University of Toronto
St. Michael's Hospital
Toronto, Ontario, Canada [62]

JOHN F.A. SPANGENBERG
Intensive Care Division
Academisch Liekenhuis Groningen
Groningen, The Netherlands [189I]

JAMES K. STOLLER, M.D.
Head, Section of Respiratory Therapy
Cleveland Clinic Foundation
Cleveland, Ohio [9]

NANCY A. STOTTS, R.N., Ed.D
Associate Professor
University of California-San Francisco
San Francisco, California [187C]

MARY E. STREK, M.D.
Assistant Professor of Medicine
University of Chicago
Chicago, Illinois [88]

KEITH M. SULLIVAN, M.D.
Division of Clinical Research
Fred Hutchinson Cancer Research Center
Seattle, Washington [150]

PETER M. SUTER, M.D.
Division des Soins Intensifs Chirurgie
Department d'Anesthesiologie
Hôpital Cantonal Universitaire de Genève
Geneva, Switzerland [189H]

JACOB IASHA SZNAJDER, M.D.
Associate Professor of Medicine
University of Illinois at Chicago
Director, Pulmonary Medicine Division
Michael Reese Hospital
Chicago, Illinois [24, 29, 58, 136]

URI TAITELMAN, M.D.
Director, Poison Information Center
Rambam Medical Center
Haifa, Israel [168, 175, 176, 183, 184]

BRYCE R. TAYLOR, M.D.
Head, Division of General Surgery
University of Toronto
Toronto General Hospital
Toronto, Ontario, Canada [165]

KERRY TEPLINSKY, M.D.
Anaheim Cardiology Medical Group, Inc.
Anaheim, California [121]

CLARK D. TERRELL, M.D.
Assistant Professor of Psychiatry
University of Texas
Health Science Center of San Antonio
San Antonio, Texas [140]

ROBERT STEVEN THARRATT, M.D.
Section of Pulmonary Medicine
University of California
Davis Medical Center
Sacramento, California [169, 174, 179]

J. RICHARD THISTLETHWAITE, M.D.
Associate Professor of Surgery
University of Chicago
Chicago, Illinois [77]

MARVIN TILE, M.D., B.Sc.
Professor of Surgery
University of Toronto
Sunnybrook Medical Centre
Toronto, Ontario, Canada [64]

THOMAS R.J. TODD, M.D.
Associate Professor of Surgery
University of Toronto
Toronto General Hospital
Toronto, Ontario, Canada [78]

KEVIN K. TREMPER, M.D., Ph.D.
Chairman and Professor
Department of Anesthesia
University of Michigan
Ann Arbor, Michigan [13]

JONATHAN D. TRUWIT, M.D.
Assistant Professor of Medicine
University of Virginia
University of Virginia Health Sciences Center
Charlottesville, Virginia [14]

ALLAN R. TUNKEL, M.D., Ph.D.
Division of Infectious Diseases
University of Virginia School of Medicine
Charlottesville, Virginia [103]

D. LORNE TYRRELL, M.D., Ph.D.
Professor and Chairman
Medical Microbiology and Infectious Diseases
Department of Medicine
Health Sciences Centre
University of Alberta Hospital
Edmonton, Alberta, Canada [104]

ERIC VALLIERES, M.D.
Ottawa Civic Hospital
Ottawa, Ontario, Canada [78]

JEAN-LOUIS VINCENT, M.D.
Department of Intensive Care
Erasme University Hospital
Free University of Brussels
Brussels, Belgium [189]

NICHOLAS VOGELZANG, M.D.
Associate Professor of Medicine
University of Chicago
Chicago, Illinois [151]

CONNIE WALLECK, R.N., M.S.
Senior Associate Director of Nursing
SUNY Health Science Center
Syracuse, New York [51]

DAVID H. WALKER, M.D.
Professor and Chairman
Department of Pathology
University of Texas at Galveston
Galveston, Texas [111]

KEITH R. WALLEY, M.D.
Assistant Professor of Medicine
Associate Director, ICU
St. Paul Hospital
Vancouver, British Columbia, Canada [114, 115]

JOHN WALLWORK, M.B., B.Sc.
Consultant Surgeon
Heart-Lung Transplant Research Unit
Papworth Hospital
Papworth Everard
England [79]

DAVID A. WARRELL, M.A., D.M., D.Sc.
Professor of Tropical Medicine and Infectious Diseases
University of Oxford
Nuffield Department of Clinical Medicine
John Radcliffe Hospital
Headington, Oxford, England [112]

RALPH R. WEICHSELBAUM, M.D.
Harold H. Hines Professor and Chairman
Department of Radiation Oncology
University of Chicago
Chicago, Illinois [152]

ROY E. WEISS, M.D.
Assistant Professor of Medicine
University of Chicago
Chicago, Illinois [161, 162]

MICHAEL G. WISE, M.D.
Chairman, Department of Psychiatry
Oschner Clinic
New Orleans, Louisiana [140]

LAWRENCE D.H. WOOD, M.D., Ph.D.
Director of Academic Programs
Professor of Medicine and Anesthesiology and Critical Care
Section of Pulmonary and Critical Care Medicine
University of Chicago Medical Center
Chicago, Illinois [1, 2, 11, 114, 115, 117, 127, 128, 130, 132]

MARK WYLAM, M.D.
Assistant Professor of Medicine and Pediatrics
University of Chicago
Chicago, Illinois [135]

CHRISTOPHER K. ZARINS, M.D.
Professor of Surgery
Chief, Vascular Surgery
University of Chicago
Chicago, Illinois [86]

AARON ZUCKER, M.D.
Medical Director, Pediatrics ICU
Associate Professor of Pediatrics
University of Chicago
Chicago, Illinois [136]

PREFACE

A definitive text of critical care must achieve two distinctly different goals: the explication of the complex pathophysiology common to all critically ill patients, and the in-depth discussion of procedures, diseases, and issues integral to the care of the critically ill and the management of the modern intensive care unit. In editing this new book we aimed to provide both a basic curriculum for learning critical care and a complete reference text.

Our approach to patient care, teaching, and investigation of critical care is energized fundamentally by our clinical practice. In turn, our practice is informed, animated, and balanced by the information and environment arising from and around learning and research. Clinical excellence is founded in careful history taking, physical examination, and laboratory testing. These data serve to raise questions concerning the mechanisms for the patient's disease, upon which a complete, prioritized differential diagnosis is formulated and treatment plan initiated. The reality, complexity, and limitations apparent daily in the ICU drive our search for better understanding of the pathophysiology of critical care and new, effective therapies.

While teaching and delivering critical care, several pitfalls on the path to exemplary practice have become apparent to us. By its very nature, critical care is exciting and attracts physicians having an inclination to action. Despite its obvious utility in urgent circumstances, this proclivity can replace effective clinical discipline with excessive, unfocused ICU procedures. We believe this common approach inverts the stable pyramid of bedside skills, placing most attention on the least informative source of data while losing the rational foundation for diagnosis and treatment. An associated problem is that ICU procedures become an end in themselves rather than a means to answer thoughtful clinical questions. Too often, these procedures are implemented to provide "monitoring," ignoring that the only alarm resides in the intensivist's intellect. Students of critical care benefit from the dictum: "Don't just do something, stand there—take time to process the gathered data to formulate a working hypothesis concerning the mechanism(s) responsible for each patient's main problem(s) so that the next diagnostic or treatment intervention can best test that possibility." Without this exhortation to thoughtful clinical decision-making, students of critical care are swept away by the burgeoning tools of the ICU toward the unproductive subspecialty of Critical Care Technology.

Thus, this book emphasizes up front the mechanisms of critical illness and the interpretation of ICU procedures. Beyond enhancing the clinical scholarship of critical care, we contend that this approach maximizes another hallowed principle of patient care—"First, Do No Harm." Despite excited opinions to the contrary, we believe that effective critical care is rarely based in brilliant, incisive, dramatic, and innovative interventions, but most often derives from meticulously identifying and titrating each of the patient's multiple problems toward improvement at an urgent but continuous pace. This conservative approach breeds skepticism toward innovative strategies: novel treatments require objective clinical trial before they are implemented and traditional therapies require clarification of goals and adverse effects in each patient before their use can be optimized. Accordingly, we have encouraged our contributors and each other to state cautiously and with experimental support their diagnostic and therapeutic approaches to critical illness, and to acknowledge that each approach has adverse effects in order to define the least intervention required to achieve its stated therapeutic goal.

Our personal appreciation of this approach is magnified and refined by our learning interactions with students of critical care at all levels—from freshman to senior medical students through residents in Anesthesiology, Medicine, and Surgery to Critical Care Fellows and practicing intensivists seeking continuing medical education. In such teaching sessions, these students always question the principles of critical care and how best to impart them, thereby helping direct our own search for better teaching. Accordingly, we conceived this book to help all of these students acquire a scholarly approach to principles of critical care, and to help us continue our quest for defining and teaching these principles. We have organized *Principles of Critical Care* as follows:

I. **Pathophysiology of Critical Illness** Several themes underlie the manifestations of critical illness, almost without regard for the precipitating factors. A conceptual framework for understanding these common derangements facilitates the articulation of a working diagnosis. This clinical hypothesis guides initial therapy, which is then titrated or revised at an urgent, informed pace.

II. **Organization of Critical Care** A disciplined familiarity with "rules" for resuscitation and stabilization provides a window of opportunity to effect more specific diagnostic and treatment plans. We emphasize accurate interpretation of safely conducted ICU procedures in a well-organized unit.

III. **Diagnosis and Management of Critical Illness** This section is an up-to-date, accessible description of the unique presentation, differential diagnosis, and management of specific diseases. This knowledge is harnessed with appropriate skepticism, based in scholarly review of the literature.

IV. **Perspectives on Critical Care** We believe that our own perspectives on adult, largely North American, critical care are enlightened by viewing our specialty from the point of view of pediatricians, nurses, ethicists, clinical investigators, and those practicing critical care elsewhere.

We enjoy teaching principles of critical care! We came to our affection for teaching the diagnosis and treatment of critical illness through Internal Medicine, albeit by different tracks. Two of us (JH, GS) were educated at the University of Chicago's Pritzker School of Medicine and Internal Medicine Residency before serving as chief medical residents in 1981 and 1985, respectively. The other (LW) graduated in medicine from the University of Manitoba in Winnipeg, Canada, completed a Ph.D. Program at McGill University in Montreal in the course of his internal medicine residency, then joined the Critical Care Faculty in Winnipeg in 1975. There, critical care had a long tradition of effective collaboration among anesthesiologists, internists, and surgeons in the ICU and in the research laboratories. When we three began to work together in 1982 at the University of Chicago, our experience in programs emphasizing clinical excellence combined with our questioning, mechanistic approach to patients' problems to help establish a four-part program for teaching critical care that parallels the structure of this text.

We attempted to incorporate this mechanistic questioning approach to critical care as a theme of *Principles of Critical Care* by writing part I and contributing 25 other chapters, and by encouraging this approach in the planning and editorial review of each chapter. Of course, few intensivists have the breadth of expertise or the time to write well about such a scope of critical care problems by themselves, so we recruited colleagues who share our vision concerning academic critical care. In general, we are convinced that clinical scholarship in critical care is conferred by balanced involvement in both management and investigation of critical illness, so we invited nine associate editors who actively deliver intensive care and publish about it. They contributed another 22 chapters and coordinated the recruitment of contributors with a similar scholarly approach encompassing about 80 chapters in 9 sections of this book. Our selection of associate editors having a shared spirit was considerably aided by our having practiced, researched, published, or taught with each. This selection also achieved institutional and geographic diversification by providing an editorial base in many international centers of excellence in critical care.

Dr. Jameel Ali is a Canadian trauma surgeon actively involved in providing and teaching ATLS and Critical Care in North America. His wide range of publications on critical care topics addresses mechanisms in basic science journals like the Journal of Applied Physiology and clinical investigations in the best surgical and medical journals. From this base in surgical critical care and its considerable overlap with Anesthesiology and Medicine, Dr. Ali coordinated most of the thirty chapters aimed at essential surgical aspects of critical care. Dr. Bruce Light is another Canadian intensivist who practices and teaches as a specialist in Infectious Diseases, and who publishes his basic and clinical research on both areas in excellent peer-reviewed journals. Infection and sepsis are such major contributors to critical illness that we were pleased to have an expert in both coordinate the 20 chapters devoted to this area. Dr. Uri Taitelman is an Israeli intensivist and nephrologist who directs the Poison Control Center in Haifa. Beyond coordinating the seventeen chapter section on overdose and poisoning, Dr. Taitelman conferred a Middle Eastern perspective on critical care to ensure expert contributions on other important critical care topics such as the section on Nutrition. In the same way, Dr. Jean-Louis Vincent from Brussels coordinated further international contributions by recruiting experts from around the world to provide their informed perspectives on critical care in Part IV. In this regard, our colleague in Chicago, Dr. Iasha Sznajder, is an academic intensivist with international roots who helped recruit expert contributions from around the world and at home.

The other four of our Associate Editors were born and trained in the United States. Dr. Charles Fisher is an Emergency Medicine specialist and intensivist practicing and publishing from the Department of Emergency and Critical Care Medicine at Case Western Reserve in Cleveland. Dr. Fisher coordinated the important section on stabilization and transport of the critically ill. Dr. Len Hudson is a Critical Care physician in Seattle who organized much of the important section on Management of the Intensive Care Unit. Dr. Marguerite Kinney has contributed much to current Critical Care Nursing scholarship through her research and publications. Dr. Kinney was an important contributor to ensuring physician-nurse teamwork throughout this book. Dr. John Luce is a Pulmonary and Critical Care specialist in San Francisco who organized the Section on Neuropsychiatric Disorders in Critical Illness. In addition to his practice and teaching of critical care, Dr. Luce, like each of the other American Associate Editors, is an active participant in major Scientific Centers of Research (SCOR), Program Project Grants (PPG), or multicenter trials coordinated by the National Institutes of Health to address investigational aspects of critical care.

The research and clinical expertise of all the Associate Editors is much broader than their special focus in this book's organization, so their scholarship was also helpful in providing editorial suggestions on many other chapters through our three stages of review and revision. With their help, our review process was closer to that enforced by excellent peer-reviewed journals than that encountered by most contributors of invited book chapters. We hope the attendant frustrations and revisions of the authors provide a better learning experience for the readers. A key element in this process was to encourage authors to view their topic through their intensivist eyes. It is not practical to review all critical illness in the detail of textbooks of Anesthesiology, Internal Medicine, or Surgery, as would occur if authors wrote about their subspecialty topic in a comprehensive way before proceeding to a discussion of the patient who becomes critically ill. We encouraged our contributors to describe the differential diagnosis and management of each disease as the intensivist sees the patient. We anticipated that this goal would be aided by including a case in each chapter of Part III to illustrate the principles of diagnosis and management. In many instances these cases are real cases with teaching value. Others have been modified (or wholly created) in order to eliminate distractions and clarify important didactic issues. At times the patients in the cases are not managed expeditiously or optimally (as in real life); in these instances we have tried to incorporate suggested improvements in care into the case discussion. Because the intensivist is often seeking information about his patient without the luxury of time, we encouraged our authors to place the essential information as several "Key Points" at the beginning of each chapter. We hope the reader finds these innovations helpful in linking each chapter's scholarship with the clinical reality of critical care.

In addition to our associate editors and individual authors, others too numerous to mention facilitated the completion of this book. We are especially indebted to our own students of Critical Care at the University of Chicago who motivate our teaching—our Critical Care fellows; residents in Anesthesia, Medicine, Neurology, Obstetrics and Gynecology, Pediatrics, and Surgery; and the medical students at the Pritzker School of Medicine. Through his commitment to academic excellence, our Chairman of Medicine, Dr. Arthur Rubenstein, has created a department which fosters clinical scholarship. Dr. Alan Leff, our Section Chief of Pulmonary and Critical Care Medicine, leads a section devoted to the highest ideals of care, teaching, and investigation. Our colleagues in providing critical care within the Section, Dr. Theodore Lewis, Dr. Richard Samsel, and Dr. Paul Schumacker, combine with Dr. Michael Roizen, Head of the Department of Anesthesia and Critical Care, Dr. Thomas Vargish, Head of Surgical Critical Care, and Dr. Aaron Zucker, Head of Pediatric Critical Care, to make our practice of Interdisciplinary Critical Care at the University of Chicago interesting and exciting.

Even with all this help, we could not have completed the organization and editing of this book without the superb efforts of our publisher, McGraw-Hill, especially through the supervision of J. Dereck Jeffers and Peter McCurdy. They have guided this group of academic physicians through the world of publishing to make these ideas and approaches more widely available, and we are thankful for this process.

Finally, the creation of a book such as this one is a birthing process that will not occur simply by the spirit breathed into the project by its senior authors, nor the considerable efforts of many contributors, nor the meticulous work of its publishers. This book's midwife was Ms. Silvia Jovel, our Editorial Assistant, a remarkable colleague who guided all of our efforts through the day-to-day difficulties of writing this text. To this task she brought competence, elan, and humor that delighted and aided all who were fortunate enough to work with her. We especially acknowledge her contributions, without which we would not likely have overcome the innumerable impediments during the three years from imagining to publishing this book.

Jesse B. Hall, M.D.
Gregory A. Schmidt, M.D.
Lawrence D.H. Wood, M.D., Ph.D.

INTRODUCTION
THE ORIGINS AND EVOLUTION OF CRITICAL CARE

Editors' Introduction

Critical care has evolved over the last four decades into a subspecialty of anesthesia, medicine, and surgery requiring this 2470 page book to describe its complexity and scholarship. It is almost humorous to recall our recent, rudimentary origins for the information of a new breed of students of critical care, most of whom were born about the same time as the specialty. To remind us of our roots, it is helpful to relate the development of critical care as it was experienced by those who were there, complete with the details which formed the frontlines of their battle in responding to serious patient problems in innovative ways and in awkward clinical circumstances. Their desire to provide something better for critically ill patients was supported neither by the medical community nor by a complete understanding of pathophysiology or technology. So approaches were developed, sometimes de novo, sometimes by borrowing, and the process was always exciting and arduous.

Accordingly, we have asked Dr. Reuben Cherniack and Dr. Tom Petty to recall how critical care began and where they think it is going. They are regarded by us as founding fathers of critical care in Canada (R.C.) and the United States (T.P.), and each has been the mentor of several generations of intensivists. Ever the raconteur, Tom has elected a personal anecdotal style, while Reuben relates the Canadian evolution with characteristic wonder and skepticism. Taken together, their stories remind us of the seminal role played by pulmonologists in early critical care. Yet their stories also reflect how their own desires to be complete physicians sowed the seeds of the interdepartmental, interdisciplinary, and team approaches which are the foundation of critical care today.

One main reason for story telling is to provide a vision for the future. Even though everything we relate is now taken for granted, the new problems facing critical care in the 1990s are no more or less complex or solvable when contemporary clinician-scientists apply their excellence and compassion to them than were those faced by the pioneers.

Dr. Tom Petty Recalls the Beginnings of Critical Care

Tom graduated from the University of Colorado Medical School in 1958. He had seen a few patients with polio treated in tank respirators, but never had any firsthand experience. Tom interned at Philadelphia General Hospital, which then had approximately 2000 beds and 108 interns. The interns ran the hospital. He took care of all manner of desperately ill individuals, usually without any supervision other than a casual overview from a resident who was sometimes available. Preeclampsia and eclampsia were managed with large doses of magnesium sulfate. Blood replacement in hemorrhagic states was generally available but you might have to wait an hour or two to get cross-matched blood. Metaraminol (Aramine), methoxamine (Vasoxyl), and norepinephrine (Levophed) were the pressors used in shock states. Levophed was always given by cut-downs which would be deftly placed by an intern in a matter of minutes. No one on Levophed ever survived. There was no intensive care unit.

Hypertensive emergencies were treated with phenobarbital, hydralazine, rauwolfia, and veratrum alkaloids. Convulsive states were managed with phenytoin (Dilantin) and phenobarbital. There was no such thing as an arterial blood gas or a mechanical ventilator. Heart failure was treated with infusions of aminophylline, mercurials, and intravenous digoxin.

Tom then moved to Ann Arbor as a first year resident at the University of Michigan. What a demotion! Now residents and fellows were everywhere. In the third month of Tom's residency, a patient was admitted to the hematology service for work-up of polycythemia rubra vera. Even then, Tom recognized this large, overweight, smoking man as a "blue bloater." In order to be "academic," Tom decided that proof of arterial hypoxemia would be wise. He convinced a pediatric lab technician whose job it was to run the Van Slyke (for the manometric measurement of oxygen content) to do an arterial blood gas if Tom would obtain it.

Although he had never considered doing it before, he wondered why a simple glass syringe with a minute amount of heparin and a number 20 needle wouldn't work. He explained to the man that the measurement of blood oxygen in states like his was important. It took only about 3 s to enter a readily palpable radial artery and Tom was pleased to see fairly red blood pumping into the syringe. After it filled with 10 mL, Tom put the needle in a cork, making sure that there was no air bubble, and he had the man apply pressure with an alcohol sponge for 30 min. After one hour of painstaking and precision analysis, the arterial oxygen saturation proved to be 82%, thus indicating that the degree of hypoxemia was substantial. The next day this was reported to the attending physician on morning rounds, who became immediately indignant. Had Tom consulted with the cardiologists, whose job it was to place the indwelling needle? What about bleeding complications in a patient with polycythemia rubra vera? Tom was embarrassed when he was temporarily suspended, only to be reinstated later the next day by the Chairman, the late William Robinson. But Tom always thought that that was the slickest way to get blood out of an artery, compared with the gowning, masking, gloving, and scrubbing for the placement of an indwelling Riley or Cournand needle, which the cardiologists "controlled."

During this year, pneumonias associated with leukemia were managed in oxygen tents, usually without benefit of any blood gas determinations. These patients all died. Status asthmaticus was treated in the emergency room with subcutaneous adrenalin, intravenous corticosteroids, and intravenous aminophylline. These patients all survived. No one gave oxygen to patients with COPD for fear of CO_2 retention. Most of these patients died. There was no evidence of mechanical ventilation during that year, and no intensive care unit.

FELLOWSHIP TRAINING IN CRITICAL CARE!?

After that fascinating year, Tom moved back to Denver. He completed his residency at the University of Colorado Medical Center and in 1962 began his fellowship under the direction of Roger Mitchell and the late Giles Filley. Tom was told that it would be his job to treat anyone—other than neurological emergencies (then the province of the neurologists)—if respiratory failure might complicate their course and they were considered to be salvageable. Tom was concerned that he did not have any significant skills for the management of patients in acute respiratory failure. You can imagine his anxiety when, on July 1, 1962, the first day of the Fellowship, he was asked to take over the care of a huge man, aged 74, who had just arrived at Denver Stapleton Airport and had collapsed while changing planes. He had a "bad cold" which proved to be pneumonia. With the assistance of the Chief Resident, Ed Genten, now of New Orleans, and some help from the late James Stevens, then Head of the Division of Neurology at the University of Colorado, Tom took over the management of this huge man, who he ventilated inside a tank respiratory after a tracheostomy was performed by the surgical staff. This was an almost around-the-clock chore. It was very difficult to get arterial blood gas samples by reaching through the portals of the tank; manipulating a Riley needle into the brachial artery was almost impossible. But Tom made several attempts at this because the cardiologists claimed that this was the only way that arterial blood could be properly drawn. Finally, Tom gave up and used his old syringe technique, which proved much more successful. "What possible difference could the method of entering an artery make?" Tom thought. To make a long story short, this man died 17 days later, following an obstructing volvulus that required surgery. The final event was sepsis. At this time, Tom was thoroughly discouraged about his first experience in the management of a patient with acute respiratory failure who had previously been healthy and who certainly should have had a chance to survive.

Following completion of a single year of pulmonary fellowship training, Tom accepted the invitation of his Chief, Dr. Gordon Micklejohn, to be Chief Resident. During this period, Tom became involved with nine patients who required mechanical ventilation. Most had various stages of chronic obstructive pulmonary disease. All received mechanical ventilation from a pressure-cycled ventilator, i.e., Bennett or Bird, via a tracheostomy. Five patients died in a rudimentary intensive care unit, which did have splendid nursing care. Four patients recovered and left the unit. Two died of their underlying respiratory disease before hospital discharge. Neither was placed back on the ventilator. Two were discharged and left the hospital, but both were dead in less than six months of respiratory failure. Tom, however, felt that progress was being made and he was extremely pleased to be given an opportunity to attend the New York Academy of Sciences' special meeting on respiratory failure, which took place in February 1964.[1] There Tom met David Bates, now of Vancouver, who was the conference co-chairman. David befriended Tom by inviting him to breakfast on arrangement by Giles Filley. Tom also was invited to go to the Royal Victoria Hospital to see Dr. Bates' respiratory care unit after the New York conference. There he met Nick Anthonisen, who, dressed in a white suit, was running a blood gas in an "Astrup machine." Tom saw Nick obtain arterial blood exactly the way he had with an heparinized syringe and disposable needle. Nick said, "everyone does it this way." Tom was impressed with the organization of the Bates' unit and the splendid care that was being received by the number of patients requiring mechanical ventilation usually with a pressure-cycled machine. Some patients were being treated with tank respirators.

AN EARLY RESPIRATORY CARE UNIT

Tom returned to the University of Colorado full of excitement. He accepted the Chairman's offer to join the faculty as Assistant Professor of Medicine in 1964. His charge was to develop a respiratory care service for the Colorado General Hospital. For support, Tom requested his own blood-gas machine and 400 sq. ft. was promised in the new hospital which was under construction and nearing completion. At first, Tom set up his blood gas machine in a renovated storeroom in the old pulmonary function laboratory because it had a sink and a window with a view. With the assistance of Giles Filley and his technician, and the Radiometer salesman, Bill Davis, Tom learned to do blood gases on his own instruments which at that time sold for $2500. Tom was ecstatic when he finally mastered the Astrup carbon dioxide method and oxygen saturation with an American Optical Oximeter. Oximetry and pH was easy; P_{CO_2} determination took more skill. Oxygen tension measurement with a Clark Electrode was still another matter. Care in changing and calibration of the electrode would often take half a day. It is a fair estimate to say that it took Tom the better part of two months to be reasonably adept at blood-gas measurements.

Tom felt that research should be an integral part of his budding programs. Along with two Fellows, Bernie Levine, now of Phoenix, and Boyd Bigelow, still in Denver, blood gas response to controlled low flow oxygen in acutely ill patients with COPD was studied. They found that it was possible to correct hypoxemia without CO_2 retention in most patients.[2] Reuben was conducting similar studies in Winnipeg.[3]

Tom and his group decided that the new respiratory care service should provide mechanical ventilation for all patients in acute respiratory failure. He was immediately joined by Dave Ashbaugh who had been Chief Resident in Surgery at the same time that Tom was Chief Resident in Medicine. This began a long, friendly relationship between Tom and Dave. The first call to ventilate a patient with advanced COPD came in late August 1964. Tom, Bernie, and Boyd were attending a party at Giles Filley's home. When the call came, it was 10:00 PM. Earl, the patient, was 62, with a previously measured FEV_1 of less than 1 L. The surgeons quickly performed a tracheostomy and Boyd and Bernie placed the patient on 100% oxygen delivered by a Bennett PR-2 pressure-cycled ventilator. Tom ran the blood gases: pH 7.19, P_{CO_2} 74 mmHg, and P_{O_2} 245 mmHg. With the machine set on 40% oxygen, the P_{O_2} was 120 mmHg. All blood gases were obtained by simple syringe arterial puncture. The machine was readjusted several times, always guided by arterial blood gas analysis. They were up all night. To make a long story short, Earl recovered after seven days of mechanical ventilation. Tom, Bernie, and Boyd ran all the blood gases. Dave helped on morning rounds. Rounds were at 7:30 AM each day, which would give Dave a chance to scrub on his 8:00 o'clock case.

The new hospital was about to open and Tom was given the promised 400 sq. ft. in an area intended to be a three-bed ward, adjacent to the 12-bed medical intensive care unit. The surgical intensive care unit was one floor below. Louise Nett joined the group on February 1, 1965, as the Respiratory Care Nurse Specialist. She had no previous background in respiratory care and thus the physicians were a full six months ahead of her in experience. She learned rapidly. On February 23, 1965, the old Colorado General Hospital was closed and the team moved across the street to the new facility, now called University Hospital. The blood gas lab was called the "Respiratory Failure Unit." This error was quickly corrected with a sign reading "Respiratory Care Unit." There was usually at least one patient, sometimes on the medical service and on other occasions in the surgical unit below. The two units were considered as modules of the same service. In fact, the budding respiratory care service was unique in its interdisciplinary nature. All patients were ventilated in the intensive care unit. Very shortly thereafter, Tom convinced Giles Filley that he should hire Susie, Giles' technician, as the first blood-gas technician. What a momentous occasion that was! This made blood gases much more available. House staff were taught arterial puncture, and a study establishing the safety and simplicity of arterial puncture was published in 1966.[4] They actually timed residents, fellows, and even faculty for the interval between preparation of a syringe and the securing of an adequate sample corked and ready for the lab. No serious complications were observed during this "study." It seems almost hilarious now that this helped set the stage for the widespread use of arterial blood gases.

ARDS, PEEP AND HYPOXEMIC RESPIRATORY FAILURE

Not too long thereafter, Dave got called about a patient who suffered massive highway trauma. Earlier he had resurrected the old 1954 Engstrom volume-controlled ventilator; after reading the instructions, both Dave and Tom thought that this machine had merit because it had a higher pressure capability than the pressure-cycled machines in current use. It also had the capability of expiratory pressure called "expiratory retard." Dave learned that expiratory retard would greatly improve arterial oxygenation at a given F_{IO_2} in this first patient who died of complications of highway trauma in a matter of days. At that time this method was called continuous positive pressure breathing.[5]

A woman was dying of acute hemorrhagic pancreatitis and a first-year Fellow, Mike Finigan, now of Rochester, New York, put the patient on the Engstrom respirator. This was reserved for the most serious patients. The patient could not be oxygenated with an F_{IO_2} of 1.0. Mike came to get Tom, whose office was then and for several years thereafter in the blood-gas laboratory. This laboratory also was the work place of Louise and it became a training center to be described later. Mike asked Tom what this knob he was told was expiratory retard did. Tom said, "I don't know." He turned it on and gave it a twist to the right. This produced an end expiratory pressure of 10 cmH_2O. They were astonished to see a blue patient turn pink before their eyes![6] Blood pressure, which was being monitored, improved slightly and urine flow, which was nil, increased somewhat. A blood gas was done immediately and the physicians were astonished to see the improvement. Wondering whether there was a true effect of end expiratory pressure, it was discontinued and this woman turned blue in a matter of 30 min. The urine flow decreased and blood pressure became almost unobtainable. PEEP (our new name[6]) was reinstituted with the results shown in Table 1.[7] The woman ultimately died of complications of hemorrhagic pancreatitis but these simple bedside observations on the effectiveness of PEEP in improving arterial oxygen in a critically ill patient dramatically altered the approach of the group.

TABLE 1 Adult Respiratory Distress Syndrome*

	1 PM	1:30 PM 10 cm PEEP	2 PM No PEEP	2:30 PM 10 cm PEEP
P_{IO_2}	560	555	550	560
Pa_{O_2}	44	125	45	135
Pa_{CO_2}	30	32	30	33

*56 year-old female with acute hemorrhagic pancreatitis and shock.

Tom and his associates are probably best known for their characterization of adult respiratory distress syndrome (ARDS). They soon recognized that these patients presented a form of acute respiratory failure distinct from COPD, postoperative problems, poisonings, and patients with neuromuscular forms of acute respiratory failure. Patients with a variety of insults to the lung, or body in general, were found to develop bilateral symmetrical alveolar infiltrates, reduced compliance, and refractory hypoxemia. High inflation pressures were required to maintain ventilation. As both Dave and Tom learned, end expiratory pressure would greatly improve oxygenation. In 1967 they reported their first description and many reports have followed thereafter.[8–10] The choice of the term was due in part to the fact that the pathophysiology and pathology so closely resembled the respiratory distress syndrome of the newborn. While the mechanisms are different, it is possible that these two syndromes share a surfactant abnormality as the common denominator. Of course in ARDS it is an acquired defect and a result rather than the cause of the original lung injury.

The group was extremely enthusiastic about the rediscovery of PEEP. Table 2 lists their formal reporting of the *apparent* effect of PEEP on survival in ARDS. It is perhaps unfortunate that a controlled clinical trial of PEEP was not done at the time of its introduction into wider use. Today we remain convinced that PEEP improves arterial oxygenation, but otherwise have many questions about its effectiveness and impact upon survival in ARDS.

TEACHING CRITICAL CARE

In the early ARDS era, Tom and his colleagues most commonly used the Ohio volume-cycled ventilator for the most severe cases; they almost never ventilated patients with pressure-cycled devices feeling that they should "spread the word" so to speak, about emerging methods of intensive respiratory care (later to be renamed critical care medicine). They organized a one-week training program for both practicing and academic pulmonologists.[11] Ten physicians came and spent an entire day with the group in Denver, making rounds and gaining hands on experience with patients. Often they would draw their first arterial blood gas and even "run it." They would help participate in patient placements on ventilators, making daily rounds and attending a limited number of conferences. One afternoon lab session provided experience in bronchoscopy, chest tube placement, tracheostomy, and resuscitation.[11] Later, these programs were cosponsored by the American College of Chest Physicians under the designation of the National Refresher Course in Pulmonary Medicine. As these programs evolved, they became international in scope, and were limited to 20 physicians for a week's experience. A training program for community hospitals in the Colorado-Wyoming region in methods of intensive and rehabilitative respiratory care was also developed with a grant from the Regional Medical Program in the 1970s. Some of the impact of this community education experience could be documented.[12] On the 10-year anniversary of the beginning of the intensive respiratory care service, the combined experience was reported, showing that nearly 80% of critically ill patients requiring mechanical ventilation could recover from acute respiratory failure in the decade 1964 to 1974 (Tables 3 and 4).[13] Notably, this was before the era of extremely aggressive therapy for malignancies, the widespread acceptance of organ transplantation, or AIDS.

Naturally this group had many unique experiences. A middle-aged woman with Guillain-Barré syndrome was totally paralyzed for 180 days, but was successfully extubated after 267 days of mechanical ventilatory support. At that time, that was the longest recorded period of such

TABLE 2 Mortality From Respiratory Distress Syndrome

	Patients	Deaths from RDS
Intermittent positive-pressure breathing	7	5
Continuous positive-pressure breathing (PEEP)	14	4

TABLE 3 Respiratory Care Unit, 1964–1974: Survival Data by Diagnosis

Principal Diagnosis	Total	Died*	Survived
Chronic airway obstruction	134	27	107(79.8)
Other pulmonary disease (asthma, pneumonia, interstitial pneumonitis, adult respiratory distress syndrome)	116	40	76(65.5)
Surgical problems			
Postoperative†	1,009	170	839(83.1)
Trauma‡	168	69	99(58.9)
Poisonings	145	19	126(86.9)
Neurological emergencies (Guillain-Barre, myasthenia, cerebrovascular catastrophes)	115	50	65(56.5)
Miscellaneous, including cardiac arrest from all causes	200	101	99(49.5)
TOTAL	1,877	466	1,411(75.2)

*Includes deaths from all causes.
†The majority of open heart cases; all with blood gas abnormalities.
‡Includes massive burns and adult respiratory distress syndrome.

TABLE 4 Respiratory Care Unit: Survival Data by Year

	Total Cases	Survival, %
1968–1969	171	62
1969–1970	212	76
1970–1971	256	80
1971–1972	272	79
1972–1973	295	78
1973–1974	257	77

therapy. This patient recovered to leave the hospital. Later a young woman with acute intermittent porphyria and simultaneous hyperparathyroidism, both of which produced a profound neuropathy, was ventilated and then weaned after 14 months.

The approach to weaning from mechanical ventilation was pragmatic and based upon principles established during the polio era. Progressive short periods off the ventilator, followed by rest, were used. This method of alternatively working and resting was successful in patients transferred from other hospitals, who had failed other methods of weaning.[14]

These early experiences were reported in a textbook, *Intensive and Rehabilitive Care,* which achieved three editions (Lea & Febiger, Philadelphia 1971, 1974, 1982). Individual reports of complications of mechanical ventilation[15] and the outcome of endothracheal tube compared with tracheostomy tube ventilation[16] are examples of the prospective accumulation of new data. There were also descriptions of the organization and functioning of this critical care service.[17,18] Fairly early on, there was concern about the fact that many people had their death extended by mechanical ventilation. Several articles dealing with the ethics of resuscitation and mechanical ventilation were written.[19,20]

The critical care movement was developing in the late 1970s and throughout the 1980s. Tom always felt that any qualified physician, with an organized team, could properly provide the details of management of the critically ill. He continued to embrace that philosophy. But as the practice of critical care medicine has evolved, pulmonologists have played a major role in both the provision of service to patients and in the certification process.[21] It has been an interesting era, still unfolding. How to provide the most cost-efficient, humane, cost-effective care is a challenge for all. Selection in the allocation and application of our resources is required. At all times the patient's comfort, dignity, and constitutional right to privacy and self-determination must be embraced. We will learn more as time and experience accumulate.

Dr. Reuben Cherniack Recalls the Origins of Critical Care

This book, which deals with contemporary issues in critical care and is directed at delivery of exemplary care, has appropriate emphasis on the importance of identifying and probing unanswered questions. By laying the groundwork of current concepts of the pathophysiology of the critically ill patient, and then discussing the latest technology for investigation and care of such patients, multisystem failure is properly highlighted. With the logarithmic explosion of interest in investigation and management of the critically ill patient over the past four decades, it is of interest to reflect on the origins and early evolution of critical care and the developments that have taken place over the past four decades.

POLIOMYELITIS, COPD, AND VENTILATORY SUPPORT

The concept of intensive pulmonary care of critically ill patients essentially arose in Scandinavia and North America in the early 1950s as a consequence of a world-wide epidemic of poliomyelitis. In the Scandinavian countries there were inadequate "iron lungs" (tank respirators) to manage these paralyzed patients, and anesthesiologists, along with other physicians and allied health professionals, working in shifts, ventilated patients by applying rhythmic inflation of anesthesia bags through endotracheal tubes and tracheostomies. In Winnipeg alone where this author resided, there were several thousand cases of poliomyelitis, and over 200 patients required mechanical ventilation. Respiratory status was monitored by relatively simple techniques; the vital capacity serving as a guide to the progression of respiratory muscle paralysis. An entire hospital was devoted to the care of poliomyelitis, with separate wards assigned to those requiring ventilators, and "iron lungs" were bought or borrowed from everywhere. These patients were critically ill, requiring detailed attention around the clock, and personnel became highly skilled in respiratory care by on-the-job training. This was also the beginning of interdisciplinary activity as physicians, trained in diverse specialties, collaborated in studies of the underlying mechanisms of disordered function as well as the application of newer therapies.

It was a natural progression to apply these principles of management of respiratory failure to patients with chronic obstructive pulmonary disease who developed acute respiratory failure. This was a time when the administration of oxygen to such patients was considered dangerous because it led to increased hypercapnia and was considered causally related to respiratory arrest. Acute respiratory insufficiency in these patients was relatively common, and a few beds were designated for the management of such patients in our teaching hospital. The congregation of patients with similar problems, in turn, fostered studies which led to improved understanding of the mechanisms of disordered function and major new concepts in management. Studies of the interaction between the work of breathing and control of respiration, and the resulting development of respiratory failure, pointed out the importance of intensive application of measures designed to reduce the work of breathing. The paradox between the dire consequences of severe hypoxemia and the fear of oxygen therapy was alleviated when it was demonstrated that hypoxemia could be corrected without worsening ventilatory function in acutely ill patients with COPD if oxygen therapy was coupled to measures to reduce the work of breathing. It is interesting to note that several decades later, further studies demonstrated that the development of significant hypercapnia following oxygen administration was due to an increase in dead space rather than a reduction in total ventilation.

The development of arterial blood gas electrodes for assessment of gas exchange and acid-base balance was a giant step forward in the further progress of critical care. During the polio epidemic, and early in the management of hypercapnic failure, the adequacy of ventilation was monitored by assessments of the arterial blood gas tensions using the Riley "bubble technique." This was an arduous procedure that required at least 20 min/sample and when this was combined with VanSlyke determinations of oxygen and carbon dioxide content, evaluation of the large number of patients took hours. The development of the Astrup apparatus shortened the time of evaluation somewhat, but this technique only determined the CO_2 tension, and assessment of oxygenation remained difficult. The relatively rapid and noninvasive estimate of the arterial P_{CO_2}, using the CO_2 rebreathing technique, which was developed by Moran Campbell, was an advance, and residents in Winnipeg made regular "rounds" carrying their rebreathing bag and hustling down to the lab to pass the equilibrated gas through a CO_2 meter. However, it was the blood gas electrodes, and latterly, the addition of oximetry, which made assessment of gas exchange infinitely easier, more rapid, and revolutionized intensive care. Easy accessibility of blood gas tensions led to increased recognition of severe hypoxemic failure and awareness of marked alterations in gas exchange in many disorders. Increasingly, blood gas analysis facilitated the synthesis of cardiopulmonary function, including hypoperfused states, as well as characterization of metabolic disturbances. Very early, the ability to assess blood gas tensions enabled recognition of severe hypoxemia following an acute myocardial infarction and low cardiac output, as well as the associated development of hypercapnia in left heart failure or pulmonary edema.

THE ORIGINS OF INTERDISCIPLINARY CRITICAL CARE

Few physicians or hospitals were interested in the concept of critical care in the early days, and internists, on the whole, turned a deaf ear to any presentations dealing with this subject. Indeed, the mere suggestion of the benefit of a respiratory therapy department met with much derision from the rest of the medical staff. It was even suggested that the only difference between patients moved to our special care area and those on the general wards was that those in our unit "died pink." On the other hand, this author found common ground with many anesthesiologists and was invited to be a visiting professor or to participate in so many of their meetings that switching specialties was entertained seriously. Later pulmonologists recognized the validity of the concept of intensive care, and the Denver group, in particular, carried its banner. Their hallmark description of severe hypoxemic failure, which they likened to the respiratory distress syndrome of the newborn, and called the adult respiratory distress syndrome, and their descriptions of the benefit of positive end-expiratory pressure, and the critical parameters that determined the potential for weaning from the ventilator laid the foundations for the discipline and the art of managing ventilated patients.

This book also appropriately devotes a section to the organization and management of specialized units for delivery of intensive care. In the early days, these concepts were difficult to apply, even though experiences in pulmonary disease made it clear that a large segment of the patients in the general hospital who were suffering from respiratory failure, cardiac arrhythmias, circulatory collapse or severe fluid and electrolyte or acid-base imbalance would benefit from similar intensive care. That such patients would be best cared for in a special area where highly trained personnel could provide special attention and care directed at respiratory, cardiac, renal, and neurologic malfunction was emphasized by the chaos and frustration that was often associated with the management of critical situations on the general medical and surgical wards. Nurses and physicians on these wards, with their divided responsibilities, generally had insufficient time and background knowledge to attend to the minute details which often made the difference between life and death. With much urging, it was agreed that only a full time trained nursing staff could provide the technical competence required for the care of these critically ill patients, and also that the physician who was not constantly involved in such care, could not maintain the necessary technical competence and expertise. At the same time, advances in the complexity of surgical techniques resulted in the need for closer titration of perioperative care. With genuine reluctance, centralized intensive care units were allowed to develop in some major institutions.

With the development of these units and the concept of interdisciplinary participation, the specialty of critical care began to grow. Virtually from its inception in Winnipeg, it was recognized that care of the critically ill would be optimal if the disciplines and clinical skills derived from each of the major departments was utilized. Thus, a critical care team was developed, consisting of a pulmonologist, a cardiologist, a surgeon and an anesthesiologist, and they "rounded" together regularly, along with, when indicated, the renal/metabolic group. At the same time, the importance of the bedside team in ensuring ready availability of all resources possible for each critically ill patient was stressed. The investigation and care of the patient was coordinated by the nurse at the bedside, along with full time residents, who were responsible for moment-to-moment care and the activities of physiotherapists, respiratory therapists and dieticians, as well as the participation of occupational therapists and social workers, who played a vital role in rehabilitation of the patients.

It has been interesting to follow the changes in attitude to intensive care and the development of this specialty as it has flourished, from its days as a poor orphan, to that of a self-standing discipline, with its own special academic requirements. In its early stages, it was considered that optimum management of the patient who is prone to multiple organ failure could be provided by any good "questioning" physician who recognized when help was needed from the different disciplines, along with well-trained personnel in a special care unit. However, the complexities of multiple organ failure have made it clear that most have neither the time nor the technical competence and expertise necessary to provide optimal care of the critically ill. Because the management of respiratory failure is often pivotal in the management of the critically ill patient, it is fitting that pulmonologists play a predominant role in the care of such patients. However, it is critical that the attending staff also be able to recognize and manage acute circulatory, neurologic, and acid-base, as well as fluid and electrolyte disturbances. In addition, it must be emphasized that centralized critical care units, in addition to fostering exemplary care, provide an ideal environment for the application of a questioning approach to management and clinical research in critically ill patients. The need for this combination of clinical and investigative skills, which is embodied in the "clinician/scientist," is now being recognized more frequently and is perhaps the most telling argument for the full-time "intensivist."

PAST SUCCESSES AND FUTURE CHALLENGES

Over the past four decades, the activity of intensive care units has changed considerably. Much has been learned about mechanisms of disordered function in hypercapnic respiratory failure, and this, in turn, has led to the application of newer concepts of management. Studies in the early units have moved ventilators a considerable distance from the "iron lungs," and new more efficient volume-cycled ventilators have been developed. It is of interest that virtually simultaneously the Winnipeg group worked with the Puritan-Bennett Company to develop the MA-1 volume cycled ventilator, and the Denver group helped design the Ohio 560 volume cycled ventilator. Both of these ventilators, and their successors, have contributed significantly to the management of acute respiratory failure. In addition, emphasis on early recognition of acute insults in COPD and therapy directed at reducing the work of breathing has led to marked changes in admission patterns to critical care units. The importance of preventive measures has led to programs of ongoing care of patients with COPD outside of the hospital, and the development of rehabilitation and home care programs has virtually eliminated the need for admission of patients with COPD to such units. Experience from the polio epidemic is also reflected in the proliferation of programs providing home ventilation for patients with neuromuscular disorders and with COPD.

On the other hand, advances in knowledge of mechanisms of disturbance in acute hypoxemic failure have been slower. We have learned about the conditions which predispose to the development of the acute respiratory distress syndrome, but the basic alterations leading to the development of the acute lung injury and the cellular events that occur remain mainly conjecture. It is possible that the currently popular use of techniques of cellular and molecular biology may yield some insight into the mechanisms at work in cellular damage, but it still is only in the context of clinical/physiologic investigation that it will be possible to correlate the cellular and molecular events with organ structure and function in critical illness. Unhappily, there has been little progress in the management of acute lung injury and multiorgan failure, and mortality remains high. Many important questions remain to be answered, not the least of which is understanding of the underlying mechanisms of development of ARDS and the interactions of multiple organ failure. Even time-honored PEEP has not been evaluated in a controlled situation and questions remain about its effectiveness and impact upon survival in ARDS.

The ethical problems associated with discontinuation of life support will continue and clear definitions and criteria must be established by the medical profession. What is probably the major challenge for the future will be reduction of the enormous costs of provision of intensive care, and investigation of methods of making it cost-efficient. In particular, this will entail studies directed at delineation, in advance, of those patients who will benefit from intensive care and those who will not. Also, the efficacy of the increased tendency for individual specialty intensive care units with their duplication of equipment and personnel will require scrutiny. This diversification of critical care units in a single institution may militate against provision of optimal care, in that personnel may develop "blinders" and fail to recognize situations outside of their area of expertise. Politics will probably dictate continued separation of these units, and it will behoove the "powers that be" to develop joint training programs dealing with all aspects of critical care for all personnel from the different units, including those in emergency rooms. The problems are obviously international, and it is appropriate that this book acknowledges the interest and important contributions of physicians in other parts of the world to the critical care area, and provides a perspective, and perhaps even a touch of sanity, from outside of North America.

Hopefully, these problems will be solved in the near future. Whatever takes place over the next decade or two, it is important to reiterate that interdisciplinary consultation and research remains essential. Advances in management result from the ability to recognize the unusual or unexplained, and the conduct of investigation directed at testing of hypotheses or answering the clinical questions. This problem solving approach, in turn, leads to improved understanding of the mechanisms underlying disturbed function and the rapid application of new knowledge to the investigation and care of the critically ill patient. The approach adopted in this book follows these principles and the importance of continued clinical investigation is underlined by the perspective on clinical investigation of critical illness provided by Dr. Murray and Dr. Roisin, as well as the case presentations which allow appreciation of the pathophysiologic alterations that are present and the application of therapeutic measures directed at correcting these alterations.

References

1. Nahas GG, Bates DV (eds): Respiratory failure. Ann NY Acad Sci 121:653–958, 1965.
2. Bigelow DV, Petty TL, Levine BE, et al: The effect of oxygen breathing on arterial blood gases in patients with chronic air-

way obstruction living at 5200 feet. Am Rev Respir Dis 96:28–34, 1967.
3. Cherniack RM, Hakimpour H: The rational use of oxygen in chronic respiratory insufficiency. JAMA 199:178–182, 1967.
4. Petty TL, Bigelow DB, Levine BE: The simplicity and safety of arterial puncture. JAMA 195:693–695, 1966.
5. Ashbaugh DG, Petty TL, Bigelow DB, et al: Continuous positive pressure breathing (CPPB) in adult respiratory distress syndrome. J Thoracic Cardiovasc Surg 57:31–41, 1969.
6. Petty TL: PEEP. Chest 61:309–310, 1972.
7. Petty TL, Nett LM, Ashbaugh DG: Improvement in oxygenation in the adult respiratory distress syndrome by positive end expiratory pressure. Resp Care 16:173–176, 1971.
8. Ashbaugh DG, Bigelow DB, Petty TL, et al: Acute respiratory distress in adults. Lancet 2:319–323, 1967.
9. Petty TL, Ashbaugh DG: The adult respiratory distress syndrome: Clinical features, factors influencing prognosis and principles of management. Chest 60:233–239, 1971.
10. Petty TL: Acute respiratory distress syndrome (ARDS). Dis Mon 36:3–58, 1990.
11. Petty TL, Nett LM, Bigelow DB, et al: The management of acute and chronic respiratory insufficiency (a one week training course). Arch Environ Health 17:398–402, 1968.
12. Petty TL, Neff TA, Nett LM, et al: A program for community training in respiratory care. Chest 64:636–640, 1973.
13. Petty TL, Lakshminarayan S, Sahn SA, et al: Intensive respiratory care unit. Review of ten years' experience. JAMA 233:34–37, 1975.
14. Zwillich CW, Pierson DJ, Creagh CE, et al: Complications of assisted ventilation. A prospective study of 354 consecutive episodes. Am J Med 57:161–170, 1974.
15. Stauffer JL, Olson DE, Petty TL: Complications and consequences of endotracheal intubation and tracheotomy. Am J Med 70:65–76, 1981.
16. Petty TL, Bigelow DB, Nett LM: The intensive respiratory care unit. An approach to the care of acute respiratory failure. Calif Med 107:381–384, 1967.
17. Petty TL, Dulfano MJ, Singer M, et al: Essentials of an intensive respiratory care unit. Chest 59:554–556, 1971.
18. Morganroth ML, Morganroth JL, Nett LM, et al: Criteria for weaning from prolonged mechanical ventilation. Arch Intern Med 144:1012–1016, 1987.
19. Nett LM, Petty TL: Reconciling ethical principles and new technology (A commentary on critical care medicine and mechanical ventilation). Resp Care 30:610–620, 1985.
20. Petty TL: Resuscitation decisions. Clin Geriatr Med 2:535–545, 1986.
21. Rogers RM, Petty TL, Hudson LD, et al: Critical care medicine certification and pulmonary disease trainees. Am Rev Respir Dis 142:495–496, 1990.

PRINCIPLES OF CRITICAL CARE

PART I

THE PATHOPHYSIOLOGY OF CRITICAL ILLNESS

EDITORS' INTRODUCTION

In approaching the critically ill patient, it is helpful to have a conceptual framework of the patterns of organ system dysfunction shared by most types of critical illness. Accordingly, this part of the book outlines five areas of organ system physiology as a basis for reviewing the most common disturbances imposed by severe illnesses: **1.** the respiratory system, **2.** the cardiovascular system, **3.** the internal environment, **4.** the central nervous system, and **5.** the digestive system. We believe that readers return to this conceptual framework at the bedside of each new critically ill patient in their care. When we describe the specific diagnostic and management approaches to diverse critical illnesses in Part III, this understanding provides an effective tool common to critical care for each condition. This approach complements the specific etiology and therapy of individual illnesses, because the opportunity for favorably treating many concurrent organ system failures in each patient occurs early in the critical illness, when the specific diagnosis and focused therapy are less important than resuscitation and stabilization according to the following principles.

Critically ill patients present many diagnostic and therapeutic problems to their attending physicians, the consultant intensive care specialist, the resident housestaff and the intensive care nursing staff. Recent advances in intensive care management and monitoring technology facilitate early detection of pathophysiology of vital functions, allowing the potential for prevention and early treatment. However, this greater volume of diagnostic data and possible therapeutic interventions can occasionally create "information overload" for medical attendants, confounding rather than complementing clinical skills. The purpose of this section is to provide students of intensive care with an informed practical approach to integrating established concepts of pathophysiology with conventional clinical skills. This is neither a course in physiology nor a comprehensive review of how to treat critical illness. Rather, it is a response to a need voiced by intensive care personnel for a conceptual framework of physiology relevant to understanding and treating disturbances of vital functions. The approach emphasizes schematic illustrations of essential pathophysiologic models and their utility in approaching disease processes. We pay less attention to citing the experimental observations supporting and correcting the models or to reciting suggestions for detailed care of specific critical illnesses. We stress the conceptual approach, believing that it provides the physician or nurse with a plan for thoughtful continual adjustment, which will enhance the patient's potential for healing and recovery.

Chapter 1
THE RESPIRATORY SYSTEM

L.D.H. WOOD

Gas Transport between the Lungs and Body Tissue

OXYGEN DELIVERY AND CONSUMPTION

Organ systems of the body require a source of energy to perform their function. The respiratory system connects the atmosphere or ventilator to mixed venous blood returning from these organ systems via extensive pulmonary vascular beds in the lung. Oxygen (O_2) is extracted from inspired gas and transferred via the arterial blood flow (cardiac output [$\dot{Q}_T$]), to the body tissues. There, carbon-containing foods combine with O_2 to release energy fueling the organ functions, producing carbon dioxide (CO_2) as an end product. In turn, CO_2 is transferred via mixed venous blood (venous return, VR) to diffuse into the inspired gas and to be expelled in gas expired from the lungs into the atmosphere.

Figure 1-1 depicts this process, and this section reviews the rules and equations governing and describing transport of the respiratory gases between the lungs and the systemic organs in the steady state. By steady state is meant that the volume of O_2 consumed by the tissues per minute ($\dot{V}_{O_2}$) is equal to the O_2 uptake from the lungs; that the CO_2 produced in the tissues ($\dot{V}_{CO_2}$) equals the CO_2 expelled from the lungs; that oxygenation is the sole source of tissue energy (i.e., there is no anaerobic metabolism); and that $\dot{Q}_T$ equals VR. Accordingly, there is no storage or depletion of respiratory gases in the body. In this steady state, there is a fixed ratio ($R = \dot{V}_{CO_2}/\dot{V}_{O_2}$) of CO_2 produced to O_2 consumed in the tissues; and R is set by the types of carbon-containing food being metabolized. For carbohydrates, R is 1.0; for lipids, R is 0.7; and for protein, R is 0.83.

Figure 1-1 also depicts the transport of oxygen ($\dot{Q}_{O_2}$) from the lungs to the tissues by $\dot{Q}_T$. In health, $\dot{Q}_T$ is about 80 mL kg^{-1} min^{-1}, and each 100 ml blood flowing to the tissues contains about 20 mL oxygen (Ca_{O_2}). Accordingly, oxygen transport to the tissues ($\dot{Q}_{O_2} = \dot{Q}_T \times Ca_{O_2}$) is about 16 mL kg^{-1} min^{-1}. The normal resting oxygen consumption extracted by peripheral tissues is about 4 mL kg^{-1} min^{-1}, so that VR from the tissues to the right heart has an oxygen content (Cv_{O_2}) of about 12 mL kg^{-1} min^{-1}. In any patient, $\dot{V}_{O_2}$ can be calculated from the Fick equation: $\dot{V}_{O_2} = \dot{Q}_T(Ca_{O_2} - Cv_{O_2})$. Figure 1-1 also illustrates that $\dot{V}_{O_2}$ can be calculated spirometrically by measuring the difference between inspired oxygen and expired oxygen; then the Fick equation may be rearranged to estimate cardiac output: $\dot{Q}_T = \dot{V}_{O_2}/(Ca_{O_2} - Cv_{O_2})$.

Critical illness often reduces $\dot{Q}_{O_2}$, but $\dot{V}_{O_2}$ is maintained because peripheral tissues extract more oxygen from Ca_{O_2}, so Cv_{O_2} decreases. When the tissue O_2 extraction fraction [$EF = (Ca_{O_2} - Cv_{O_2})/Ca_{O_2}$] doubles as $\dot{Q}_{O_2}$ is halved (see continuous line in Fig. 1-2, lower panel), $\dot{V}_{O_2}$ is independent of $\dot{Q}_{O_2}$ (see continuous line in Fig. 1-2, upper panel). Below a critical value of $\dot{Q}_{O_2}(\dot{Q}_{O_2}c)$, O_2 extraction cannot increase sufficiently to maintain $\dot{V}_{O_2}$, as indicated by the interrupted lines in both panels of Fig. 1-2. Thus, $\dot{Q}_{O_2}c$ marks the onset of supply dependence of O_2 consumption, and the value of EF at $\dot{Q}_{O_2}c$ (EFc) indicates the extraction limit for maintaining aerobic metabolism. Figure 1-3 combines the relationships of both $\dot{V}_{O_2}$ (left ordinate) and EF (right ordinate) with $\dot{Q}_{O_2}$ (abscissa) to review the concept of O_2 extraction limits using typical values for patients with *normal* extraction, and then for patients having extraction defects, or *pathologic* supply dependence of O_2 consumption.

As illustrated by the Xs and horizontal continuous line in Fig. 1-3, $\dot{V}_{O_2}$ is 4 mL^{-1} kg^{-1} min^{-1} independent of changes in $\dot{Q}_{O_2}$ from 32 to 6 mL kg^{-1} min^{-1}. When $\dot{Q}_{O_2}$ is doubled from 16 to 32 mL kg^{-1} min^{-1} by increasing $\dot{Q}_T$ or Ca_{O_2}, EF decreases from 0.25 to 0.125 along the hyperbolic continuous line, as the peripheral tissues take the same required O_2 consumption from a greater delivery. Similarly, when the normal $\dot{Q}_{O_2}$ is reduced to 8 mL kg^{-1} min^{-1}, EF increases to 0.5 as the tissues maintain their normal O_2 consumption by extracting a greater proportion of the reduced O_2 delivery. This horizontal portion of the $\dot{V}_{O_2}/\dot{Q}_{O_2}$ relationship indicates that O_2 consumption is independent from O_2 supply; this is quite different from the relationship observed when

FIGURE 1-1 Schematic illustrating exchange of oxygen (O_2) and carbon dioxide (CO_2) between the lungs (upper balloon) and the body tissues (lower box) by way of the intervening cardiac output ($\dot{Q}_T$) and venous return (VR). The lungs are ventilated with fresh gas ($\dot{V}_I$); the alveolar ventilation ($\dot{V}_A$) equilibrates with alveolar blood, while the dead space ventilation ($\dot{V}_D$) does not, such that the mixed expired ventilation ($\dot{V}_E$) contains less O_2 and more CO_2 than $\dot{V}_I$. This model of steady state gas exchange illustrates spirometric measurements of $\dot{V}_{CO_2}$, $\dot{V}_{O_2}$, and R; concurrent arterial and venous blood gas measurements allow calculations of $\dot{Q}_T$, Q_{O_2}, $\dot{V}_{O_2}$, O_2 extraction fraction (EF), V_D/V_T and $A - a\ D_{O_2}$. For further discussion and definition of symbols, see text.

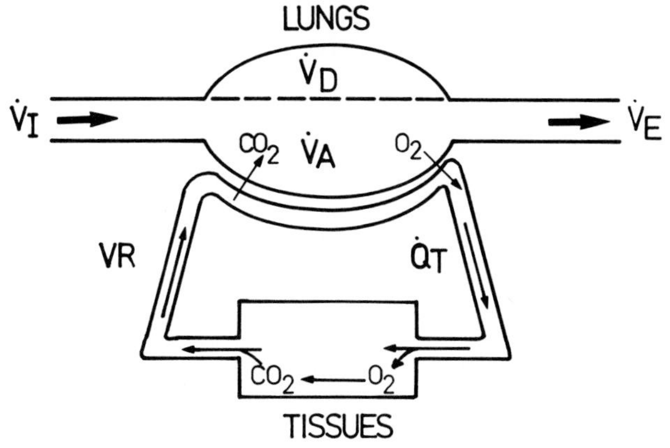

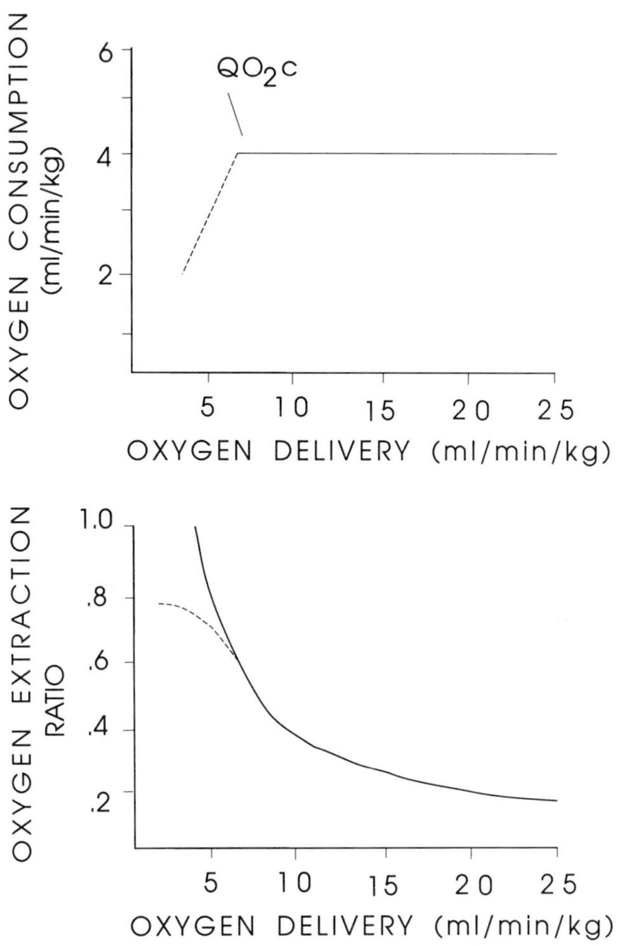

FIGURE 1-2 ***Upper Panel:*** **Oxygen consumption ($\dot{V}_{O_2}$) remains virtually constant at normal or high values of oxygen delivery ($\dot{Q}_{O_2}$), but becomes limited by $\dot{Q}_{O_2}$ below a critical delivery threshold ($\dot{Q}_{O_2}$c). (See interrupted line indicating supply dependent $\dot{V}_{O_2}$).** ***Lower Panel:*** **Oxygen extraction fraction increases as $\dot{Q}_{O_2}$ is reduced, until the critical extraction fraction (EFc) is reached; when delivery is reduced further, oxygen extraction cannot increase sufficiently to maintain the $\dot{V}_{O_2}$ (see interrupted line).**

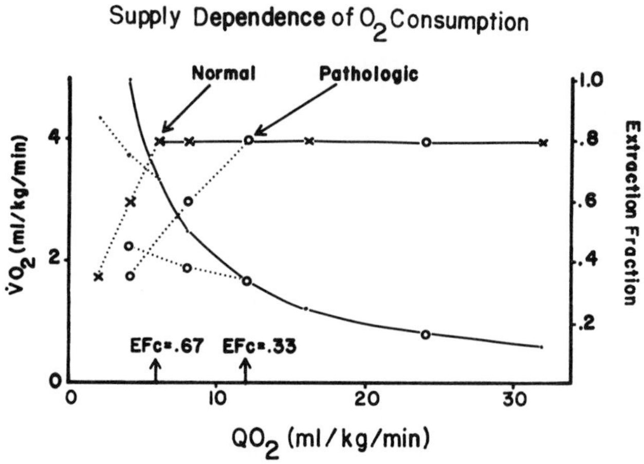

FIGURE 1-3 Oxygen consumption ($\dot{V}_{O_2}$, left ordinate) and oxygen extraction fraction (EF, right ordinate) are plotted against oxygen delivery ($\dot{Q}_{O_2}$, abscissa), to illustrate both normal (EFc = 0.67) and pathologic (EFc = 0.33) supply dependence of O_2 consumption. For further discussion, see text.

$\dot{Q}_{O_2}$ is further reduced to 4 mL kg^{-1} min^{-1}. As indicated by the hyperbolic relationship between extraction fraction and $\dot{Q}_{O_2}$, $\dot{V}_{O_2}$ would be maintained in these circumstances only if the peripheral tissues extracted all of the $\dot{Q}_{O_2}$; that is, EF = 1.0. However, EF does not rise to 1, for in these circumstances depicted in Fig. 1-3, EF increases only to 0.75, so $\dot{V}_{O_2}$ falls from 4 to 3 mL kg^{-1} min^{-1} along the interrupted line relating $\dot{V}_{O_2}$ to $\dot{Q}_{O_2}$. A halving of $\dot{Q}_{O_2}$ to a value of 2 mL kg^{-1} min^{-1} is associated with further increase in extraction fraction to 0.88 as $\dot{V}_{O_2}$ decreases to 1.8 mL kg^{-1} min^{-1}.

Accordingly, the interrupted line through the Xs in Fig. 1-3 denotes a phase of supply dependence of oxygen utilization; that is, O_2 consumption decreases with O_2 delivery, a phenomenon best attributed to tissues becoming limited in their capacity to extract oxygen. Patients, experimental animals, and isolated perfused organs all have oxygen consumptions which become dependent on supply when EF exceeds values of about 0.67. This limit of aerobic metabolism appears to be associated with increased lactic acid production, an increase in the lactic:pyruvate (L:P) ratio, and a decrease in the production of high energy adenosine triphosphate (ATP) bonds, all suggesting the onset of a less efficient oxygen utilization associated with anaerobic metabolism and lactic acidosis. At this limit of aerobic metabolism, mixed venous blood is about 33 percent saturated and the mixed venous P_{O_2} ($P\bar{v}_{O_2}$) is <25 mmHg. That anaerobic metabolism begins when blood exiting the tissues has a P_{O_2} as high as 25 mmHg could be due to diffusion limitation between the end capillary and the tissue cells farthest from that vessel. Yet, cell cultures do not become anaerobic until the P_{O_2} in their bath falls to values as low as 0.5 to 1.0 mmHg, and estimations of the diffusion gradient for oxygen through typical normal tissue cylinders predict values <5 mmHg, all suggesting that diffusion limitation of aerobic metabolism occurs when P_{O_2} exiting capillaries of anaerobic tissues becomes as low as 5 mmHg. The higher $P\bar{v}_{O_2}$ at this limit of aerobic metabolism may be due to arterial admixture via peripheral arteriovenous shunts, to a relatively large variation in the matching of a limited $\dot{Q}_{O_2}$ among peripheral parallel tissues having quite different values of $\dot{V}_{O_2}$, or to countercurrent diffusion of oxygen.

To explain these mechanisms, Fig. 1-4 presents a schematic model of the peripheral circulation; one tissue compartment has a high metabolic rate and $\dot{V}_{O_2}$, while the other has no $\dot{V}_{O_2}$. Neural and metabolic regulation constricts the vessel to the low $\dot{V}_{O_2}$ unit and dilates the vessel to the high $\dot{V}_{O_2}$ unit to match $\dot{Q}_{O_2}$ to $\dot{V}_{O_2}$. In conditions of limited $\dot{Q}_{O_2}$ and optimal $\dot{V}_{O_2}/\dot{Q}_{O_2}$ matching, no flow would perfuse the low $\dot{V}_{O_2}$ unit and all the flow perfuses the high $\dot{V}_{O_2}$ unit, so it stays aerobic until its tissue and venous $P_{O_2} < 5$ mmHg when EF approaches 1.0. Note that if the matching is incomplete such that one-third of the total flow perfused the unit with no $\dot{V}_{O_2}$, the blood will leave that unit with a venous saturation of 100%; meanwhile, the compartment

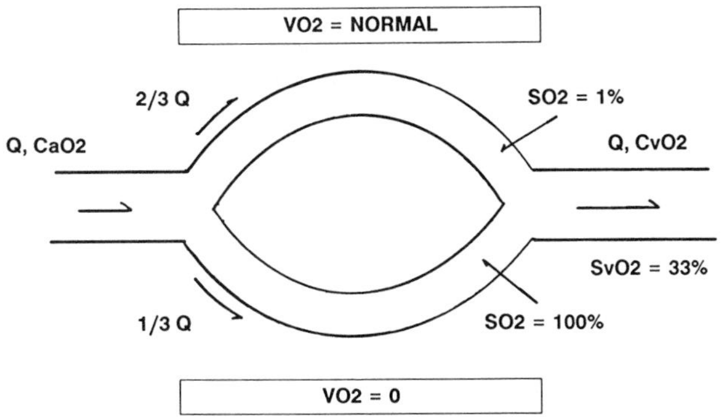

FIGURE 1-4 Schematic of the distribution of a limited $\dot{Q}_{O_2}$ ($\dot{Q}$, Ca_{O_2}) between two compartments having normal $\dot{V}_{O_2}$ (upper) and $\dot{V}_{O_2} = 0$ (lower). To the extent that neural and metabolic control were complete, no blood flow would perfuse the tissue compartment having $\dot{V}_{O_2} = 0$; then the other compartment would maintain aerobic metabolism until $\dot{Q}_{O_2}$ fell to a very low value when nearly all oxygen is extracted ($S_{O_2} = 1\%$) and Pv_{O_2} is very low (less than 5 mmHg). When control of the microcirculation is not complete, one third of the blood flow perfuses the unit with no $\dot{V}_{O_2}$, such that the other unit becomes anaerobic at a higher value of $\dot{Q}_{O_2}$; then the mixed venous blood exiting both units contains more oxygen ($Sv_{O_2} = 33\%$) and the calculated extraction fraction is lower than 1.0 (EFc = 0.67). Note that similar results would occur if $\dot{V}_{O_2}$ in the lower compartment were a finite low value, but $\dot{Q}_{O_2}$ was high with respect to that $\dot{V}_{O_2}$; in either case of peripheral shunt or high $\dot{Q}_{O_2}/\dot{V}_{O_2}$, countercurrent diffusion of oxygen from the lower to the upper unit can contribute to a higher effluent P_{O_2} from the upper anaerobic unit than is in its tissues. Conceivably, factors associated with critical illness further confound this matching of a limited $\dot{Q}_{O_2}$ among tissues having varying $\dot{V}_{O_2}$, such that a greater amount of a limited $\dot{Q}_{O_2}$ is distributed to high $\dot{Q}_{O_2}/\dot{V}_{O_2}$ units, thereby stealing blood from the potentially anaerobic units to raise $\dot{Q}_{O_2}c$ and lower EFc, causing pathologic supply dependence of oxygen consumption.

with a high $\dot{V}_{O_2}$ gets less of the total flow and so becomes anaerobic ($P_{O_2} < 5$ mmHg) at a higher total flow and $\dot{Q}_{O_2}$. Note further that the mixed venous blood draining both compartments will have a higher saturation due to the arterial admixture from the unit with no $\dot{V}_{O_2}$. Now the $\dot{Q}_{O_2}c$ is increased and EFc is about 0.67. As described, this exemplifies a peripheral shunt of 33 percent of the peripheral blood flow, yet anatomic shunts of this magnitude have not been found. A similar outcome is predicted from Fig. 1-4 when the shunted compartment has a finite $\dot{V}_{O_2}$, but its $\dot{Q}_{O_2}$ is large with respect to its $\dot{V}_{O_2}$ when the other unit becomes anaerobic due to its low $\dot{Q}_{O_2}/\dot{V}_{O_2}$ ratio. Then, high O_2 saturation in venous effluent from the high $\dot{Q}_{O_2}/\dot{V}_{O_2}$ unit will increase the mixed venous saturation even when the other unit becomes anaerobic. Conceivably, such peripheral $\dot{Q}_{O_2}/\dot{V}_{O_2}$ variance arises when a range of metabolic activity is not tightly matched to $\dot{Q}_{O_2}$ by the flow-regulating mechanisms of the circulation. In either case of true shunt or $\dot{Q}_{O_2}/\dot{V}_{O_2}$ variance, large P_{O_2} differences may develop across short distances, allowing for O_2 diffusion between the two vessels such that effluent P_{O_2} from the anaerobic unit may considerably exceed 5 mmHg. Since the two compartments in Fig. 1-4 can represent different organs (e.g., adipose tissue and heart) or adjacent tissues within the same organ, these three mechanisms can account for supply dependence of $\dot{V}_{O_2}$ at high values of Pv_{O_2} for both the whole body or within individual organs.

PATHOLOGIC SUPPLY DEPENDENCE OF OXYGEN CONSUMPTION?

These mechanisms responsible for optimal oxygen extraction underlying the normal supply dependence of O_2 consumption may be confounded in critical illness. Patients with adult respiratory distress syndrome (ARDS) or sepsis have oxygen consumptions that appear to depend on oxygen supply at levels of $\dot{Q}_{O_2}$ substantially above the normal aerobic limits ($\dot{Q}_{O_2}c$). As depicted by the open circles in Fig. 1-3, oxygen consumption appears to be maintained as $\dot{Q}_{O_2}$ is reduced from 24 to 12 mL kg^{-1} min^{-1}, but below that delivery, $\dot{V}_{O_2}$ begins to decrease. As indicated by the open circles on the hyperbolic extraction fraction line, oxygen extraction increases to maintain $\dot{V}_{O_2}$ to an EFc of 0.33, but at lower levels of $\dot{Q}_{O_2}$, extraction cannot increase enough to maintain $\dot{V}_{O_2}$. Accordingly, in these circumstances there appears to be a pathologic supply dependence of O_2 consumption signalled by inability to extract oxygen from a limited $\dot{Q}_{O_2}$ at levels well below the normal EFc of 0.67. Such extraction defects observed in bacteremia and in endotoxemia can be attributed to suboptimal distribution of a limited $\dot{Q}_{O_2}$ *among* various organs having different oxygen requirements, but they have also been observed *within* individual organs, such as the gut, suggesting that the O_2 extraction defect of sepsis resides at least in part within individual organs. Presumably, sepsis causes O_2 extraction defects by confounding the regulation of $\dot{Q}_{O_2}/\dot{V}_{O_2}$ variance by the microcirculation in these animal models (see discussion of Fig. 1-4 above).

Although impaired oxygen extraction has been demonstrated in canine models of bacteremia and endotoxemia, evidence for such pathologic supply dependence of $\dot{V}_{O_2}$ in patients is not conclusive. Whether or not extraction defects exist, adequate aerobic metabolism may be enhanced by interventions which reduce $\dot{V}_{O_2}$ as well as increase $\dot{Q}_{O_2}$. Fig. 1-5 illustrates the effects of increased metabolic rate frequently observed in critical illness. The continuous line drawn through the Xs repeats the $\dot{V}_{O_2}/\dot{Q}_{O_2}$ relationship and the EF/$\dot{Q}_{O_2}$ relationship from Fig. 1-3, except for the expanded $\dot{V}_{O_2}$ scale on the left ordinate. A second interrupted $\dot{V}_{O_2}/\dot{Q}_{O_2}$ relationship is drawn through closed circles corresponding to a threefold increase in $\dot{V}_{O_2}$, and the corresponding EF-$\dot{Q}_{O_2}$ relationship is the interrupted hyperbolic curve drawn through the closed circles up and to the right of the normal EF-$\dot{Q}_{O_2}$ relationships. A twofold increase in $\dot{V}_{O_2}$ has been observed in febrile patients having multiple trauma, burns, or sepsis, and a similar increase over basal metabolic rate has been observed and attributed to the increased work of breathing in patients with acute respiratory failure. Even in the absence of oxygen extraction defects, such circumstances require that $\dot{Q}_{O_2}c$ triple in proportion to a threefold increase in $\dot{V}_{O_2}$ to maintain aerobic metabolism.

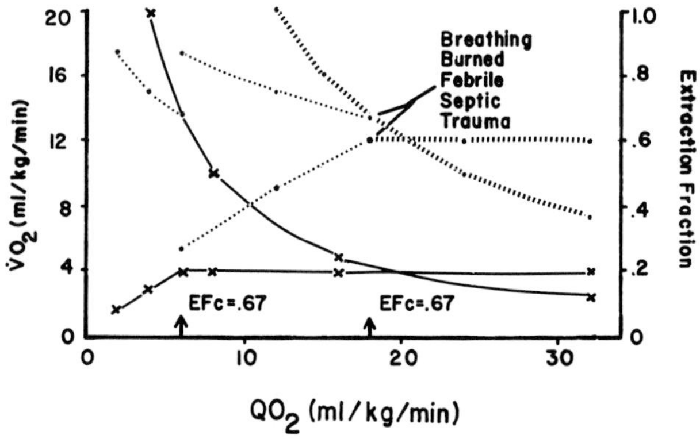

FIGURE 1-5 Axes as for Figure 1-3, except that $\dot{V}_{O_2}$ scale has been expanded to display the $\dot{V}_{O_2}/\dot{Q}_{O_2}$ and EF/$\dot{Q}_{O_2}$ relationships when $\dot{V}_{O_2}$ is increased 3-fold (interrupted lines through closed circles) by several common manifestations of critical illness (work of breathing, burns, fever, sepsis, and trauma), for comparison with the normal relationship (see continuous lines through X's). When $\dot{V}_{O_2}$ is tripled, EF is tripled at every value of $\dot{Q}_{O_2}$, and supply dependence of O_2 consumption begins at a value of $\dot{Q}_{O_2}$ 3 times greater than for the patient with normal $\dot{V}_{O_2}$ despite normal EFc = 0.67. Accordingly, $\dot{Q}_{O_2}$ must increase with $\dot{V}_{O_2}$ to maintain aerobic metabolism, or $\dot{V}_{O_2}$ must be reduced. For further discussion, see text.

Accordingly, measures which reduce the metabolic rate such as muscle relaxation, artificial respiration, and cooling the patient all lessen the demand for oxygen delivery and diminish the tendency to anaerobic metabolism in critical illness.

It follows that lactic acidosis at high levels of oxygen transport does not necessarily signal pathologic supply dependence of oxygen utilization; rather, the high O_2 demands of critical illness may exceed even normal extraction limits from the apparently high but insufficient O_2 transport. Furthermore, the presence of lactic acidosis when $\dot{Q}_{O_2}$ is high does not necessarily indicate anaerobic metabolism. Clinical and experimental studies demonstrate that progressive reduction in $\dot{Q}_{O_2}$ due to hypovolemic or cardiogenic shock is associated with lactic acidemia having a high L:P; yet, in septic shock, the frequently observed lactic acidemia, even at high levels of $\dot{Q}_{O_2}$, is not associated with an increased L:P ratio, for the pyruvate levels have risen in proportion to the lactate levels. These observations raise the possibility that metabolic utilization of tissue protein stores in septic shock produces abundant pyruvate in excess of that required for generation of high energy ATP bonds through aerobic glycolysis; then excess pyruvate circulates in normal equilibrium with excess lactate, and clinicians mistake this lactic acidosis for anaerobic metabolism. To the extent that pathologic supply dependence does not occur in patients and that the lactic acidosis of sepsis is not anaerobic, the common critical care practice of maximizing $\dot{Q}T$ and $\dot{Q}_{O_2}$ confers no benefit on oxygen utilization.

THE OXYHEMOGLOBIN DISSOCIATION CURVE

When pulmonary blood equilibrates with alveolar oxygen tension (PA_{O_2}), the amount of O_2 in physical solution varies linearly with P_{O_2}. Yet the low solubility of O_2 in plasma (0.003 mL/mmHg P_{O_2}/100 mL) allows only 0.3 mL O_2 in 100 mL blood during air breathing (PA_{O_2} = 100 mmHg) and 2.0 mL O_2 in 100 mL blood during O_2 breathing (PA_{O_2} = 650).

Most of the blood content is carried on hemoglobin, the saturation of which varies in a nonlinear manner with P_{O_2} (Fig. 1-6). In conditions of normal pH, P_{CO_2}, and temperature, hemoglobin is 50% saturated at a P_{O_2} value (P50) of about 27 mmHg. Around P50, saturation changes considerably for small changes in P_{O_2}, such that hemoglobin is 75% saturated at the $P\bar{v}_{O_2}$ of 40 mmHg, and is 90% saturated at a P_{O_2} value of about 55 mmHg. As P_{O_2} increases above this value, there can be little further increase in O_2 saturation, which is about 100% at P_{O_2} = 100 mmHg. At this value, each gram of hemoglobin carries about 1.34 mL O_2, so normal blood having a hemoglobin concentration of 15 g/dL carries about 20 mL O_2 in each 100 mL.

At reduced values of P_{CO_2}, hydrogen ion concentration ($[H^+]$), and temperature, the hemoglobin has a greater affinity for O_2, as indicated by greater O_2 saturation at each P_{O_2} value in the upper interrupted oxyhemoglobin dissociation curve in Fig. 1-6. Conversely, increased P_{CO_2}, $[H^+]$, and temperature reduce affinity for O_2, shifting the oxyhemoglobin curve down and to the right. This necessitates correction of P_{O_2} values measured by blood-gas electrodes to those values in the patient. For example, in a febrile patient having a given O_2 content in arterial blood drawn into

FIGURE 1-6 Oxyhemoglobin dissociation curves: O_2 saturation (%) and content (mL O_2 per 100 mL blood) are plotted on the ordinate versus blood partial pressure of oxygen (mmHg) on the abscissa. The continuous curve through closed circles represents normal values of $[H^+]$ concentration (pH 7.40), P_{CO_2} (40), temperature (T = 37°C) and 2,3-DPG levels. The interrupted curve up and to the left shows the greater affinity of hemoglobin for O_2 with reduction in each of these 4 variables. The dotted curve down and to the right shows the opposite effect of increasing levels of these 4 variables. The dashed line close to the abscissa shows the solubility of O_2 in plasma, account for 0.3 mL O_2/100 mL blood during air breathing (P_{O_2} = 100 mmHg), and 2.0 mL O_2/100 mL blood during O_2 breathing (P_{O_2} = 650). For discussion, see text.

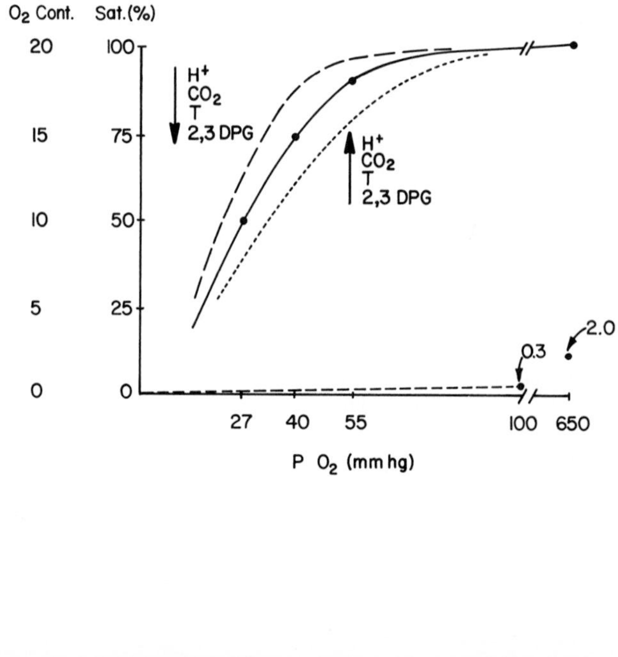

a syringe, Pa_{O_2} falls as blood cools to 37°C (98.6°F) in the measuring electrode because the greater affinity of cooled hemoglobin for O_2 carries the same volume of O_2 in the blood at a lower P_{O_2}. This is like moving from the dotted lower oxyhemoglobin dissociation curve in Fig. 1-6 horizontally (at the same O_2 content) to the continuous curve, so Pa_{O_2} in the body of the febrile patient is underestimated. Conversely, Pa_{O_2} is overestimated in hypothermic patients, and correction of these Pa_{O_2} values must be made to the patients' body temperatures. A similar rationale requires adjustment of blood P_{O_2} for pH and P_{CO_2}, and the estimation of blood O_2 saturation for a given P_{O_2} requires an oxyhemoglobin dissociation curve at the in vivo pH, P_{CO_2}, and temperature. These calculations are often aided by a computer programmed with the shape of the curve (which changes little with these variables), and with its position which varies as the P50 of blood increases systematically with P_{CO_2}, $[H^+]$, and temperature. A fourth variable occasionally influencing P50 is the level of 2,3-diphosphoglycerate (2,3-DPG), which is depleted in stored blood, giving greater oxygen affinity to the blood of critically ill patients having multiple transfusions. Accordingly, it is helpful to measure P50 in such patients for accurate deductions of O_2 saturation or to measure the oxyhemoglobin saturation directly for calculations of blood O_2 contents.

Note from the curves in Fig. 1-6 that these effects of altered hemoglobin affinity are greatest where O_2 saturation can change most, that is, below P_{O_2} values of 55 mmHg. Accordingly, mixed venous values are affected in all patients and arterial values are less affected except in very hypoxemic patients. This leads to erratic and erroneous interpretations of O_2 consumption based on differences in arterial and mixed venous O_2 contents ($a - \bar{v}_{O_2}$) when these are estimated from Pa_{O_2} and Pv_{O_2} measurements without careful corrections. Note further that O_2 saturation and content change considerably between P_{O_2} values of 25 and 45 mmHg, viz., about 1% saturation/mmHg or about 1 mL O_2/100 mL blood/5 mmHg. Accordingly, small errors in blood-gas electrode determinations of P_{O_2} lead to large errors in O_2 saturation and contents, especially for mixed venous blood. In many units caring for the critically ill, arterial and mixed venous blood samples are analyzed and interpreted to give information about O_2 transport. Awareness of these few limitations prevents overinterpretation of blood-gas derivations as well as undue reliance on these measurements when they conflict with clinical assessment.

Figure 1-7 contrasts the normal oxyhemoglobin dissociation curve with that observed in two common disorders. In anemia with half-normal hemoglobin concentration (7.5 g/dL), fully saturated blood carries only 10 mL O_2/100 mL blood as indicated by the lower interrupted line drawn through the closed circles. When $\dot{Q}_T$ is 5.0 L min^{-1}, Cv_{O_2} must fall to 5 mL O_2/100 mL blood to maintain O_2 consumption at 250 mL/min, so Sv_{O_2} is 50% (5/10) and Pv_{O_2} is 27 mmHg (P50), a value approaching tissue hypoxia. Often, $\dot{Q}_T$ is increased in the anemic patient, associated with an increase in Pv_{O_2} and less tissue hypoxia. The upper interrupted curve in Fig. 1-7 represents carbon monoxide (CO) poisoning having a 50% carboxyhemoglobin saturation. As a result, the remaining normal hemoglobin when fully saturated carries 10 mL O_2/100 mL blood, but the P50 is much reduced by the greatly increased affinity for oxygen by the hemoglobin sites not bound by CO. Note on this carboxyhemoglobin dissociation curve that Pv_{O_2} must decrease to about 15 mmHg before Cv_{O_2} falls to 5 mL O_2%. This is one cause of anaerobic metabolism in CO poisoning; the rationale for ventilating such patients with very high fraction inspired oxygen (FI_{O_2}) is not to increase O_2 content but to hasten elimination of CO. Poisoning of mitochondrial electron transfer by CO also contributes to the tissue hypoxia.

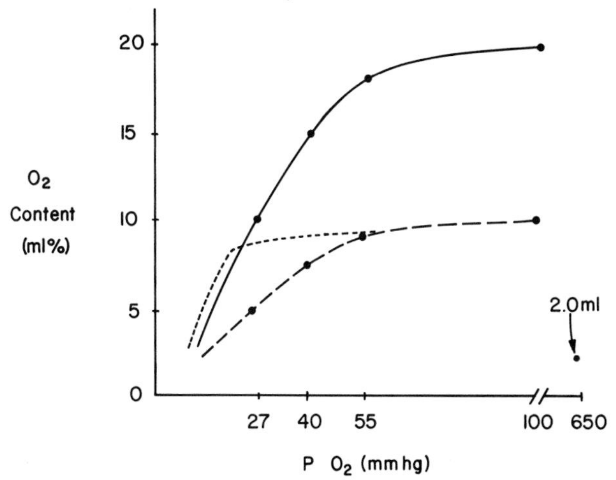

FIGURE 1-7 The normal oxyhemoglobin dissociation curve (continuous line through closed circles) is compared with anemia (7.5 g % Hb—interrupted line through closed circles) and carbon monoxide poisoning (COHb = 50%, dotted line). Axes as for Fig. 1-6. Anemia reduces Pv_{O_2} by reducing Ca_{O_2}; for a given reduction in Ca_{O_2}, CO poisoning reduces Pv_{O_2} much further by increasing the affinity of hemoglobin binding sites for O_2. For discussion, see text.

AN APPROACH TO INADEQUATE BLOOD TRANSPORT OF OXYGEN

During air breathing, arterialized blood leaves the normal alveoli with a Pa_{O_2} of about 100 mmHg. When the hemoglobin concentration is 15 g/dL, the Ca_{O_2} is about 20 mL/100 mL blood on the fully saturated hemoglobin, and about 0.3 mL in physical solution (see Fig. 1-6). Accordingly, a $\dot{Q}_T$ of 5.0 L/min transports 1000 mL/min of O_2 to the tissues. There, tissue metabolism extracts 250 mL/min, so 5.0 L min^{-1} of mixed venous blood returns to the lungs with 750 ml/min of O_2, or a mixed venous O_2 content ($C\bar{v}_{O_2}$) of 15 mL/100 mL blood. Because this O_2 content corresponds to 75% O_2 saturation (15/20), $P\bar{v}_{O_2}$ is 40 mmHg as determined by the oxyhemoglobin dissociation curve for mixed venous pH, P_{CO_2}, and temperature. Note that the corresponding increase in CO_2 content as blood passes through the tissues raises P_{CO_2} and $[H^+]$ to reduce the affinity of hemoglobin for O_2. Accordingly, $P\bar{v}_{O_2}$ is a few mmHg higher after the tissues extract 5 mL O_2 from each 100 mL of blood than it would be at greater hemoglobin affinity for O_2.

In many critically ill patients, the O_2 transport to the tissues is reduced by abnormally low $\dot{Q}_T$, hemoglobin, or O_2 saturation. Consider the effects of acute myocardial injury or hypovolemia which reduces $\dot{Q}_T$ to 2.5 L min^{-1}. To maintain the $\dot{V}_{O_2}$ necessary for aerobic metabolism, the tissues must extract 250 mL/min from half the blood flow, so Cv_{O_2} decreases to 10 mL O_2/100 mL blood. Because this value corresponds to 50% saturation (10/20) of the normal hemoglobin concentrations, $P\bar{v}_{O_2}$ is 27 mmHg. When $\dot{Q}_T$ is returned toward normal with vasoactive drug therapy, $P\bar{v}_{O_2}$ rises again. In another patient with normal $\dot{Q}_T$ (5 L min^{-1}) but severe arterial hypoxemia (Pa_{O_2} = 40, O_2 saturation = 75%, Ca_{O_2} = 15 mL O_2/100 mL blood), $C\bar{v}_{O_2}$ must decrease to 10 mL/100 mL blood to provide the tissues with 250 mL/min of O_2, so $P\bar{v}_{O_2}$ decreases to 27 mmHg. When $\dot{Q}_T$ increases in response to hypoxia, $P\bar{v}_{O_2}$ increases again. In a third patient with normal $\dot{Q}_T$ and Pa_{O_2} but with reduced concentration of normal hemoglobin (7.5 g/100 mL blood), Ca_{O_2} is reduced to 10 mL/100 mL blood (see Fig. 1-7). Accordingly, $C\bar{v}_{O_2}$ and $P\bar{v}_{O_2}$ must decrease to 5 mL/100 mL blood and 27 mmHg, respectively, to maintain aerobic metabolism, and these venous values increase again with greater $\dot{Q}_T$ or hemoglobin concentration.

These considerations illustrate that the end point of reduced O_2 transport in the blood is reduced $P\bar{v}_{O_2}$. Since $P\bar{v}_{O_2}$ approximates the P_{O_2} adjacent to the exchange vessels in the tissues, it is the driving pressure for O_2 diffusion from the capillaries to the metabolizing cells. When $P\bar{v}_{O_2}$ falls too low, insufficient O_2 diffuses to maintain aerobic metabolism, and the cells begin to produce lactic acid as the end point of anaerobic metabolism. Accordingly, reduced $P\bar{v}_{O_2}$ and increased serum lactate (or falling pH with unchanged Pa_{CO_2}) are indications of tissue hypoxia. This improves with therapy increasing Ca_{O_2} (by increasing hemoglobin or O_2 saturation) and increasing $\dot{Q}_T$. In many critically ill patients, two or three of these factors reducing O_2 transport to the tissues coexist, so attention to optimizing all these ($\dot{Q}_T$, hemoglobin concentration, and O_2 saturation) is reasonable in the hypoxic patient.

Of course, optimizing does not mean maximizing, and the end point of each therapeutic approach needs to be selected for the individual patient. Patients with low $\dot{Q}_T$ due to heart disease may not tolerate infusions of packed erythrocytes even though their tissue hypoxia is made worse by concurrent anemia. Yet, thoughtful integration of packed cells within the plasma volume reduction is often helpful in such patients and may prevent anaerobic metabolism at a time when $\dot{Q}_T$ cannot be increased to adequate levels. In other patients with severe arterial hypoxemia and O_2 desaturation due to acute hypoxemic respiratory failure, tissue hypoxia may be relieved by increasing $\dot{Q}_T$ and hematocrit. Yet this is often associated with higher central blood volume and pulmonary vascular pressures which increase pulmonary vascular leak unless vasoactive drugs, diuretics, and fluid restriction are used concurrently. Again, thoughtful integration of the three approaches to therapy of tissue hypoxia provides the optimal level of circulating hemoglobin and $\dot{Q}_T$ while reducing rather than aggravating the pulmonary edema. Some patients with chronic severe anemia (viz., chronic renal failure) become acutely ill with low $\dot{Q}_T$ or hypoxemic respiratory failure. Their tissue hypoxia is often ameliorated by prompt, transient increases in their hemoglobin concentration without circulatory overload, as by plasmapheresis. Yet the institution of this therapy, like the others mentioned above, has complications which must be weighed against the likely benefit in that patient at that time. Accordingly, this approach to therapy of reduced blood O_2 transport implements early each of the three major interventions ($\dot{Q}_T$, hematocrit, Sa_{O_2}) in a combination best suited to the condition of each patient.

Little has been said about dissolved O_2, for it contributes a small amount to $\dot{Q}_{O_2}$. Yet in critical hypoxemia, raising the F_{IO_2} to maximal values may be effective. Consider again the patient with acute myocardial infarction without lung disease in whom low $\dot{Q}_T$ has lowered $P\bar{v}_{O_2}$ to 27 mmHg during air breathing. Even though the hemoglobin is fully saturated, Ca_{O_2} may be increased by 1.7 mL/100 mL blood when Pa_{O_2} is increased to 650 mmHg by ventilation with O_2. Then $C\bar{v}_{O_2}$ increases from 10 to 11.7 mL O_2/100 mL blood, raising mixed venous saturations to 58% and $P\bar{v}_{O_2}$ to about 34 mmHg; of course, if anaerobic metabolism existed before oxygen therapy, $C\bar{v}_{O_2}$ may not increase as much as Ca_{O_2} because $\dot{V}_{O_2}$ increases with oxygen. These changes tend to diminish tissue hypoxia and the adverse consequences of anaerobic metabolism by an amount equivalent to that achieved by a 1 g/dL increase in hemoglobin or a 0.2 L min^{-1} increase in $\dot{Q}_T$, and so complement a combined approach to hypoxia. Increasing F_{IO_2} may be effected by nasal prongs to deliver O_2 at 1 to 5 L min^{-1} (F_{IO_2} = 0.21 to 0.4), by rebreathing masks (F_{IO_2} = 0.21 to 0.6), or by head tent (F_{IO_2} = 0.21 to 0.8). The ranges of F_{IO_2} are to indicate that all methods frequently give no O_2 enrichment due to inadequate delivery to the patient (lower limit) and that the amount of O_2 delivered is often less than expected (upper limit), even when the O_2 delivery system is working properly.

With its attendant risks, tracheal intubation ensures delivery of the highest possible F_{IO_2} and allows another approach to therapy of tissue hypoxia, namely, to reduce $\dot{V}_{O_2}$. Normally, the work of breathing is very low, but in patients with acute hypoxemic respiratory failure and its associated tachypnea and lung stiffness, $\dot{V}_{O_2}$ of the respiratory muscles alone can exceed 500 mL/min. Normally, $\dot{Q}_T$ increases with $\dot{V}_{O_2}$, as in exercise, to keep $C\bar{v}_{O_2}$ and $P\bar{v}_{O_2}$ close to their resting values. Yet, consider the effects of such work of breathing in the common circumstance of cardiogenic pulmonary edema when $\dot{Q}_T$ may not increase much above 5.0 L min^{-1}. Then, $C\bar{v}_{O_2}$ must fall toward 5 mL O_2/100 mL blood to deliver the total $\dot{V}_{O_2}$ of 750 mL/min so $P\bar{v}_{O_2}$ approaches 22 mmHg (see Fig. 1-5) associated with tissue hypoxia and anaerobic metabolism. Relaxation of the respiratory muscles and positive-pressure ventilation reduces $\dot{V}_{O_2}$ to 250 mL/min and raises $P\bar{v}_{O_2}$ to normal with no change in $\dot{Q}_T$.

A less dramatic effect on tissue hypoxemia in patients already ventilated is to reduce $\dot{V}_{O_2}$ by cooling the febrile hypoxic patient. Consider the patient with pneumonia causing Pa_{O_2} of 40 mmHg (Ca_{O_2} = 15 mL/100 mL). Then reduction of $\dot{V}_{O_2}$ from 500 to 250 mL/min by sedation, muscle relaxation, and cooling from 40° to 37°C (104° to 98.6°F) raises $C\overline{v}_{O_2}$ from 5 to 10 mL O_2/100 mL blood. This increase in mixed venous saturation from 25 to 50% would increase $P\overline{v}_{O_2}$ from 22 to 27 mmHg in normothermic blood. The left shift of the oxyhemoglobin dissociation curve (see Fig. 1-6) between 40° and 37°C (104° to 98.6°F) does not limit oxygen extraction in canine studies of the limits of aerobic metabolism, so cooling the febrile patient may be enough to relieve tissue hypoxia in critical situations. A second approach of marginal value in patients with tissue hypoxia due to reduced O_2 saturations in hypoxemic respiratory failure is to shift the oxyhemoglobin curve to the left by hyperventilation. If this is done without further reduction of $\dot{Q}_T$, improved arterial saturation and Ca_{O_2} at the same Pa_{O_2} provides greater O_2 transport to the tissues. Because the leftward shift of the curve is not parallel but is further shifted at higher saturations, $C\overline{v}_{O_2}$ does not increase with respiratory alkalosis as much as Ca_{O_2} does for the same $P\overline{v}_{O_2}$. When this approach relieves tissue hypoxia what probably happens is that $P\overline{v}_{O_2}$ rises slightly to increase the rate-limiting tissue diffusion step of aerobic metabolism, so $\dot{V}_{O_2}$ increases. These last two therapeutic approaches need further study before they can be used confidently.

To illustrate how several clinical interventions have a beneficial effect on tissue hypoxia, this discussion emphasized how $P\overline{v}_{O_2}$ tracks the changes in $\dot{Q}_{O_2}$. Yet reference to the discussion of Fig. 1-4 reveals that the value of $P\overline{v}_{O_2}$ at the onset of anaerobic metabolism might vary widely as a result of the $\dot{Q}_{O_2}/\dot{V}_{O_2}$ variance among peripheral tissues. This is especially true in the septic patient when very high $\dot{Q}_T$ and $\dot{Q}_{O_2}$ are associated with very high values of $P\overline{v}_{O_2}$ and lactic acidosis. To the extent that such lactic acidosis arises from anaerobic metabolism, the rise in $P\overline{v}_{O_2}$ with increased $\dot{Q}_{O_2}$ in the septic patient confounds the utility of $P\overline{v}_{O_2}$ as a marker. Even in the apparent absence of sepsis, the value of $P\overline{v}_{O_2}$ at the onset of anaerobic metabolism varies widely. Accordingly, measuring and following changes in $P\overline{v}_{O_2}$ and venous saturation in conjunction with acid-base status and lactic acid measurements allows deductions concerning the effects of altered $\dot{Q}_{O_2}$ on $\dot{V}_{O_2}$ and aerobic metabolism, but these are nonspecific and subject to errors and uncertainties.

Exchange of Gas in the Lungs

Consider again the schematic illustration in Fig. 1-1 of gas exchange between the atmosphere and body tissues, this time to focus on lung gas exchange. Inspired air flows into the lung at a rate ($\dot{V}_I$) of about 6 L/min. There, O_2 diffuses into mixed venous blood and CO_2 diffuses from mixed venous blood at an equal rate (when R = 1) of about 250 mL/min. Then the same volume of gas is expelled ($\dot{V}_E = \dot{V}_I$) containing a greater expired fraction of CO_2 ($F_{E_{CO_2}}$) and a smaller expired fraction of O_2 ($F_{E_{O_2}}$) than the corresponding fractions in the inspired air ($F_{I_{O_2}}$ = 0.21, $F_{I_{CO_2}}$ = 0).

FRACTIONS AND PARTIAL PRESSURES OF LUNG GASES

As depicted in Fig. 1.1, the O_2 consumed by the tissues ($\dot{V}_{O_2}$ = 240 mL/min) is supplied to venous blood traversing the lungs by inspired gas, and the tissue CO_2 production ($\dot{V}_{CO_2} = \dot{V}_{O_2}$ when R = 1) exits the venous blood in the lungs via the expired ventilation ($\dot{V}_E$ = 6 L/min).

$$\dot{V}_{CO_2} = \dot{V}_E F_{E_{CO_2}} \tag{1-1}$$

$$\dot{V}_{O_2} = \dot{V}_E(F_{I_{O_2}} - F_{E_{O_2}}) \tag{1-2}$$

Using these values, gas expired each minute contains 240 mL CO_2 in 6000 mL, so the $F_{E_{CO_2}}$ is 0.04. Since expired O_2 is 240 mL/min < inspired O_2 (0.21 × 6000 = 1260 mL/min), the $F_{E_{O_2}}$ is 1020/6000 or 0.17.

The total pressure in lung gas spaces is the atmospheric or barometric pressure (P_B). The partial pressure of each gas (P_g) is given by it volume fraction (F_g) in the mixture times P_B. Barometric pressure is about 747 mmHg and water vapor has a relatively constant partial pressure (P_{H_2O} = 47 mmHg) in gas saturated at body temperature, so the respiratory gases share the remaining partial pressure ($P_B - P_{H_2O}$ = 700 mmHg)

$$P_g = F_g(P_B - P_{H_2O}) \tag{1-3}$$

Accordingly, the partial pressures of oxygen in inspired gas ($P_{I_{O_2}}$) and mixed expired gas ($P_{E_{CO_2}}$) are about 147(0.21 × 700) and 119(0.17 × 700) mmHg, respectively, during air breathing and mixed expired P_{CO_2} ($P_{E_{CO_2}}$ = 0.04 × 700) is about 28 mmHg. Note that when R = 1, $P_{I_{O_2}} = P_{E_{O_2}} + P_{E_{CO_2}}$ since the volume of O_2 taken from inspired gas is replaced by an equal volume of CO_2. Note further that the partial pressure of the fourth gas in the lung, nitrogen (N_2), is the same in inspired and expired gas when R = 1 ($P_{I_{N_2}} = P_{E_{N_2}}$ = 0.79 × 700 = 553).

ALVEOLAR EXCHANGE OF CARBON DIOXIDE

Ventilation of lungs occurs by cyclic inflation with a tidal volume (V_T) of 500 mL (6 mL/kg) twelve times per minute. About one-third of each V_T does not contact the pulmonary circulation because it remains in conducting airways or ventilates nonperfused alveoli. Since no gas transfer can occur, this is dead space ventilation (V_D = 2 L/min). The rest of the expired gas is alveolar ventilation ($\dot{V}_A = V_E - V_D$ = 4 L/min), for it ventilates alveoli providing a large exchange surface for transfer of O_2 and CO_2 between inspired gas and mixed venous blood, resulting in the equilibration of gas partial pressures in the alveoli with those in the arterial blood exiting the alveoli. When 240 mL/min of CO_2 diffuses from mixed venous blood into 4.0 L/min of inspired gas ventilating the alveolar space, the alveolar fraction of P_{CO_2} is 240/4000 or 0.06, and the alveolar partial pressure of CO_2 ($P_{A_{CO_2}}$) is 42 ($F_{A_{CO_2}}$ (P_B-47)). Thus, the alveolar equation for CO_2 is:

$$P_{A_{CO_2}} = \dot{V}_{CO_2}/\dot{V}_A \cdot k \tag{1-4}$$

In health, increased $\dot{V}_{CO_2}$ is accompanied by increased $\dot{V}_A$ to keep Pa_{CO_2} within a narrow range. This occurs in large part because increased $[H^+]$ associated with increased Pa_{CO_2} stimulates the drive to breathe, causing increased V_E and $\dot{V}_A$ whenever Pa_{CO_2} rises and vice versa. When a variety of critical illnesses reduce $\dot{V}_A$ by half, $P_{A_{CO_2}}$ doubles according to Eq. 1-4; and when a ventilator is set to provide twice the normal $\dot{V}_A$, Pa_{CO_2} is halved.

Expired gas contains both alveolar ($P_{A_{CO_2}} = 42$) and dead space gas ($P_{I_{CO_2}} = 0$), so $P_{E_{CO_2}}$ will be less than Pa_{CO_2} in proportion to the fraction of dead space to the tidal volume (V_D/V_T).

$$V_D/V_T = (Pa_{CO_2} - P_{E_{CO_2}})/Pa_{CO_2} \qquad (1\text{-}5)$$

Normally when $P_{E_{CO_2}}$ is 28 and Pa_{CO_2} is 42, $V_D/V_T = 0.33$, so we deduce that one-third of $\dot{V}_I$ must appear in the mixed expired gas without contact with the pulmonary circulation. When pulmonary embolism or high alveolar pressure reduce the perfusion of many more air spaces, $P_{E_{CO_2}}$ decreases because a greater proportion of inspired gas is not exposed to the pulmonary circulation, and V_D/V_T increases.

ALVEOLAR EXCHANGE OF OXYGEN

$P_{A_{O_2}}$ is $< P_{I_{O_2}}$ because oxygen diffuses from inspired gas into mixed venous blood until blood and gas tensions are equal at the exchanging surface ($P_{A_{O_2}} = Pa_{O_2}$). When R is 1.0, the amount of O_2 moving from inspired gas to blood equals the amount of CO_2 moving from blood to inspired gas. Since that $\dot{V}_{CO_2}$ raises P_{CO_2} from zero ($P_{I_{CO_2}}$) to 42 ($P_{A_{CO_2}}$) mmHg, the $\dot{V}_{O_2}$ must reduce $P_{I_{O_2}}$ by an identical amount to set the value of $P_{A_{O_2}}$:

$$P_{A_{O_2}} = P_{I_{O_2}} - P_{A_{CO_2}} \qquad (1\text{-}6)$$

This alveolar equation for oxygen shows that variations in ventilation effect $P_{A_{O_2}}$ only indirectly by altering $P_{A_{CO_2}}$ according to Eq. 1-4. Thus, alveolar hypoventilation which raises $P_{A_{CO_2}}$ from 42 to 84 will reduce $P_{A_{O_2}}$ during air breathing (when $P_{I_{O_2}} = 0.21 \times 700 = 147$; see Eq. 1-3) from 105 to 63 mmHg. And alveolar hyperventilation which reduces $P_{A_{CO_2}}$ from 42 to 21 will raise $P_{A_{O_2}}$ from 105 to 126. In a clinical context, these extreme variations in alveolar ventilation and $P_{A_{CO_2}}$ (21 to 84 mmHg) have relatively small effect on $P_{A_{O_2}}$ (63 to 126) compared to the much larger effect on $P_{A_{O_2}}$ effected by increasing $F_{I_{O_2}}$ from 0.21 to 1, when $P_{I_{O_2}}$ increases from 147 to 700. Accordingly, variations in ventilation have a controlling and substantial effect on $P_{A_{CO_2}}$, but have an indirect and minor effect on $P_{A_{O_2}}$; in contrast, varying $F_{I_{O_2}}$ has no effect on $P_{A_{CO_2}}$, but is a major determinant of $P_{A_{O_2}}$.

When $R < 1.0$, the alveolar equation for O_2 is modified to account for the fact that less CO_2 enters the alveoli than the amount of O_2 that enters the blood.

$$P_{A_{O_2}} = P_{I_{O_2}} - P_{A_{CO_2}}/R \qquad (1\text{-}7)$$

Accordingly, $P_{A_{O_2}}$ is reduced from $P_{I_{O_2}}$ by a factor $(R^{-1}) > P_{A_{CO_2}}$ is increased from $P_{I_{CO_2}}$. One consequence is that $P_{A_{N_2}}$ increases above $P_{I_{N_2}}$ even though no nitrogen exchanges across the alveoli, as if the alveolar nitrogen were concentrated when more O_2 is removed than CO_2 is added. A second result is that $\dot{V}_E$ is slightly $< \dot{V}_I$, so $F_{E_{N_2}}$ is slightly $> F_{I_{N_2}}$ when $R < 1.0$. These corrections are important to derivations of more precise equations describing alveolar gas exchange which easily fill chapters in textbooks. Yet adequate understanding of gas exchange in most critical illness is provided by the simpler equations and concepts above.

DO DIFFUSION DEFECTS CONTRIBUTE TO HYPOXEMIA IN CRITICAL ILLNESS?

Note that these considerations of lung gas exchange assume equality between alveolar and arterial values for P_{CO_2} and for P_{O_2}. This is so because there is complete equilibration by diffusion between alveolar gas and pulmonary blood as it traverses the exchange surface. This is depicted in the lower panel of Fig. 1-8, where mixed venous blood enters the gas exchanging portion of the lung at time 0 on the abscissa with a P_{O_2} of 40 mmHg on the ordinate. Long before the blood exits the gas exchanging area at time 1.0 s, the P_{O_2} has risen to equal the P_{O_2} of about 600 mmHg during O_2 breathing in the normal alveolus, depicted as compartment #2 in the lung model at the top of Fig. 1-8. The interrupted line represents a hypothetical very slow diffusion across the alveolar-capillary membranes, such that blood transiting the gas exchange area in 1.0 s has not reached equilibrium with the $P_{A_{O_2}}$, causing a large difference between $P_{A_{O_2}}$ and $Pa_{O_2}(A-aD_{O_2})$.

It was once thought that such incomplete diffusion contributed significantly to $(A - aD_{O_2})$ in many lung diseases, but the multiple inert gas elimination technique (MIGET) has demonstrated that nearly all $(A - aD_{O_2})$ is explained by shunt or other ventilation perfusion ($\dot{V}/\dot{Q}$) mismatch. In pulmonary fibrosis and emphysema, such destruction of the alveolar surface can occur that there may be insufficient time for diffusion equilibration, especially during exercise or other conditions of high pulmonary blood flow and low O_2 saturation in mixed venous blood. The shorter transit time causes a greater $(A - aD_{O_2})$ and more hypoxemia, as depicted by the continuous line in Fig. 1-7 departing the interrupted line at 0.5 s and at a P_{O_2} of 50; a lower $P\bar{v}_{O_2}$ necessitates much greater O_2 diffusion before equilibration occurs with $P_{A_{O_2}}$ in these diseased lungs. Even in these cases, the resulting $(A - aD_{O_2})$ is small and the arterial hypoxemia is corrected with modest increases in $F_{I_{O_2}}$. Accordingly, arterial hypoxemia due to large $(A - aD_{O_2})$ requires another explanation than can be provided by the one-compartment lung model of Fig. 1-1; hence, the two-compartment model at the top of Fig. 1-8 is used to explain the refractory hypoxemia of shunt and the correctable hypoxemia of other $\dot{V}/\dot{Q}$ mismatch.

REFRACTORY HYPOXEMIA DUE TO INTRAPULMONARY SHUNT

In many critical illnesses, alveolar spaces become flooded with pulmonary edema, pus, or blood, as depicted in com-

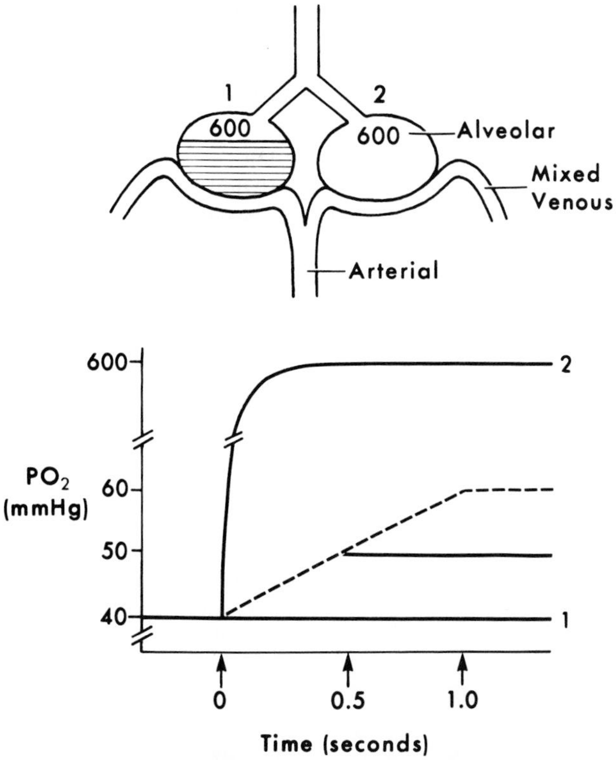

FIGURE 1-8 Schematic of pulmonary oxygen exchange in a two compartment model of the lung ventilated with oxygen (upper); the lower panel shows mixed venous blood ($P\bar{v}_{O_2}$ = 40, ordinate) entering the gas exchange area of each compartment at time zero and exiting each compartment 1 second later (abscissa). P_{O_2} in the ideal alveolus (#2) rises rapidly to equilibrate with the alveolar P_{O_2} ($P_{A_{O_2}}$ = 600); by contrast the P_{O_2} in the flooded alveolus (#1) exits the gas exchange area at $P\bar{v}_{O_2}$ since no oxygen can diffuse through the flooded airspace. Accordingly, mixture of the venous blood exiting #1 with the oxygenated blood from #2 causes arterial desaturation despite O_2 therapy due to the large intrapulmonary shunt ($\dot{Q}_S/\dot{Q}_T$).

The interrupted line in the lower panel represents a hypothetical diffusion defect in which P_{O_2} rises very slowly through the thickened gas exchange area of compartment #1, thereby exiting with a blood P_{O_2} (60 mmHg) very much less than $P_{A_{O_2}}$. To the extent such barriers to complete diffusion equilibration exist in critical illness, they could mimic true $\dot{Q}_S/\dot{Q}_T$, as well as the increase in $\dot{Q}_S/\dot{Q}_T$ observed as $\dot{Q}_T$ increases, when pulmonary transit time decreases to 0.5 seconds (see lower P_{O_2} = 50 mmHg when the blood exits the gas exchange area of compartment #1 at 0.5 seconds). However, most evidence suggests that diffusion defects cause minimal pulmonary oxygen exchange abnormalities in critical illness, so the increase in $\dot{Q}_S/\dot{Q}_T$ with increased $\dot{Q}_T$ requires other explanations. For further discussion, see text.

partment #1 at the top left of Fig. 1-8. To the extent these flooded airspaces are perfused with mixed venous blood, this blood traverses the lung without exchanging gas as if it were shunted directly from the right heart to the left heart, as depicted on the lower panel where the continuous line #1 exits the lung gas exchange area at the same $P\bar{v}_{O_2}$ = 40 as it entered. The fraction of the total pulmonary blood flow which is shunted ($\dot{Q}_S/\dot{Q}_T$) causes arterial hypoxemia when the venous blood with low oxygen content in compartment #1 mixes with well-oxygenated blood coming from nonflooded alveoli of compartment #2. For example, if half the blood flow perfused compartment #1 ($\dot{Q}_S/\dot{Q}_T$ = 0.5) during air breathing ($P_{A_{O_2}}$ = 100 mmHg), arterial blood would be an equal mixture of mixed venous blood having a P_{O_2} of 40 mmHg and blood coming from the ideal or unflooded alveolus having P_{O_2} of 100 mmHg. Reference to Fig. 1-6 reveals that the saturation of these two components is 75 and 100%, respectively, such that the average saturation of the arterial blood is 87.5%, giving a Pa_{O_2} of about 50 mmHg. Accordingly, Pa_{O_2} is much closer to Pv_{O_2} than to $P_{A_{O_2}}$ due to the nonlinear oxyhemoglobin dissociation curve. This effect is much more pronounced when $P_{A_{O_2}}$ is increased to the very high value of 600 mmHg by oxygen therapy (see Fig. 1-8). Now the blood exiting the normal alveoli #2 has a very high P_{O_2}, but this does not change the content of that blood much, because the hemoglobin was already 100% saturated, and the amount added to solution is only about 1.5 mL/100 mL blood (see Fig. 1-6); and the blood exiting the flooded alveoli still has mixed venous saturation for the greater $F_{I_{O_2}}$ cannot gain access to the mixed venous blood through the flooded airspaces. The arterial content rises slightly from 17.5 to 18.25 mL O_2/100 mL blood, so Pa_{O_2} rises slightly to about 60 mmHg.

These calculations illustrate the mechanism whereby the venous admixture of intrapulmonary shunt causes arterial hypoxemia which is refractory to oxygen therapy. The shunt fraction is calculated:

$$\dot{Q}_S/\dot{Q}_T = (Cc_{O_2} - Ca_{O_2})/(Cc_{O_2} - Cv_{O_2}) \qquad (1\text{-}8)$$

where Cc_{O_2} is the oxygen content in blood exiting the ideal or nonflooded alveoli. Several simplifying features of this equation are worth noting. The denominator of the shunt fraction is approximately equal to the arterial to venous O_2 content differences, and so is inversely related to the $\dot{Q}_T$ as indicated by the Fick equation. Accordingly, for a given value of $\dot{Q}_S/\dot{Q}_T$, the arterial content, and so Pa_{O_2}, will increase as $\dot{Q}_T$ increases because the mixed venous oxygen content in blood traversing the flooded alveoli is higher; this lowers the arterial content less when a given fraction of shunted $\dot{Q}_T$ is mixed with well-oxygenated blood traversing unflooded alveoli, so raising $\dot{Q}_T$ and $\dot{Q}_{O_2}$ treats the arterial hypoxemia of shunt, while reducing $\dot{Q}_T$ and $\dot{Q}_{O_2}$ aggravates the arterial hypoxemia. A second feature of the shunt equation is that the numerator is the difference in oxygen content between blood exiting the ideal alveoli and that in arterial blood; when the arterial blood is fully saturated, the difference in these contents must be due to the difference in oxygen dissolved in plasma. In turn, this difference can be calculated from the $(A - aD_{O_2})$ multiplied by 0.003, so an $(A - aD_{O_2})$ of 100 mmHg indicates a 6 percent $\dot{Q}_S/\dot{Q}_T$ when $\dot{Q}_T$ is normal, as calculated from the numerator (100 × 0.003) divided by the normal $(A - v)_{O_2}$ content difference (5 mL O_2/100 mL blood). Note that large intrapulmonary shunts are associated with marked airspace flooding on the chest radiograph, but that right-to-left intracardiac shunts are not; a large value of $\dot{Q}_S/\dot{Q}_T$ without lung infiltrates suggests a patent foramen ovale or other cardiac defect which can be detected by an ultrasonic bubble study or a dye curve. Note further that areas of low $\dot{V}/\dot{Q}$ ratio cause hypoxia and low Ca_{O_2} when $FI_{O_2} < 0.5$, leading to an overestimate of true shunt by Eq. 1-8. Accordingly, $\dot{Q}s/\dot{Q}T$ should be calculated to represent true shunt only when FI_{O_2} is 0.6 or greater, when even very low $\dot{V}/\dot{Q}$ units have values of PA_{O_2} sufficient to saturate fully the blood perfusing them.

Because hypoxemia due to shunt is refractory to O_2 therapy, several adjunctive treatments are helpful to support the hypoxic patient with flooded airspaces. Positive end-expiratory pressure (PEEP) reduces $\dot{Q}s/\dot{Q}T$ in pulmonary edema without reducing the edema. Figure 1-9 summarizes the results of one study of canine oleic acid edema in which split-ventilation applied PEEP to only one lung; $\dot{Q}s/\dot{Q}T$ decreased from 24 to 5 percent with PEEP, while edema as estimated from the wet:dry weight ratio (W:D) was much greater than normal (W:D = 4) but did not change with PEEP (W:D 9.7 versus 10.3). Accordingly, PEEP reduced $\dot{Q}s/\dot{Q}T$ by redistributing the edema, signalled by a reduction in the number of flooded alveoli from 80 to 20 percent. Morphometry found that most of the displaced alveolar liquid was in the lung peribronchovascular interstitial spaces in the PEEP lung. It seems likely that PEEP increases lung volume such that stretched alveolar walls pull on the adventitia surrounding relatively stiff bronchi and vessels, thereby lowering interstitial pressure to drain the alveolar liquid allowing reaeration of the perfused alveoli.

The greater the PEEP, the less the shunt. Yet this beneficial effect is offset in part by associated increases in alveolar pressure which cause pneumothorax and increased VD/VT and by increased pleural pressure which tends to reduce

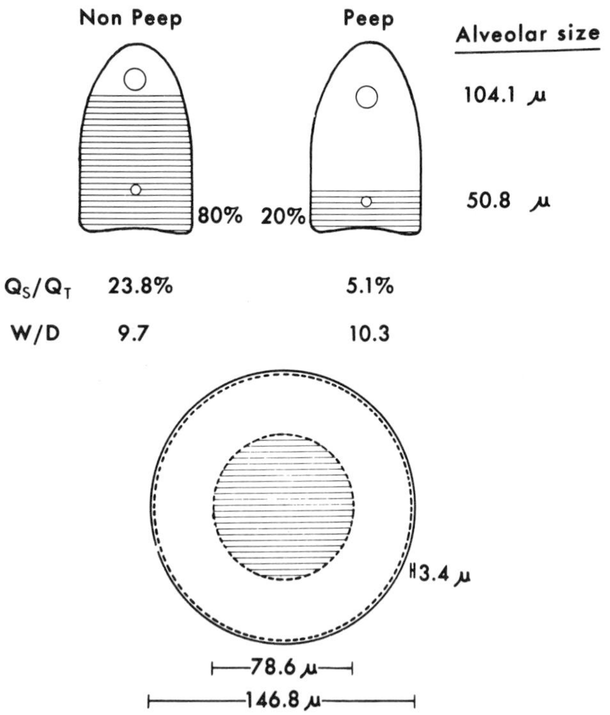

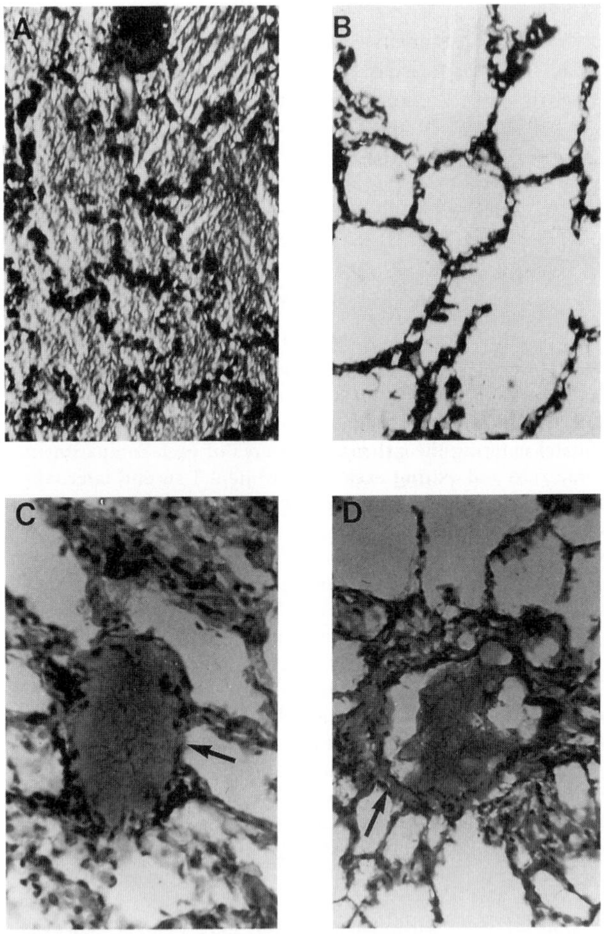

FIGURE 1-9 Effect of PEEP on $\dot{Q}s/\dot{Q}T$ in pulmonary edema. ***Left Panel:*** **Schematic showing that PEEP reduced the fraction of alveoli flooded by pulmonary edema from 80% (left upper lung) to 20% (right upper lung) while reducing $\dot{Q}s/\dot{Q}T$ from 24 to 5% (middle table) without changing the wet to dry weight ratio of the lung (W/D). In both the non-PEEP and PEEP lungs, flooded alveoli were much smaller (mean linear intercept ($L_m = 51\ \mu$) compared to the nonflooded alveoli ($L_m = 104\ \mu$). The relative alveolar sizes are indicated by the open circles in the lungs of the upper panel; these are reproduced in the lower panel, where the flooded alveoli (cross-hatched, small circle) has about 1/2 the diameter of the unflooded alveolus (larger open circle). The interrupted line within the nonflooded alveolar diameter represents the thickness of edema (3.4 μ) which would accommodate all the edema in the flooded alveolus if PEEP redistributed the alveolar edema around the circumference of the larger nonflooded alveolus; this could explain the effect of PEEP in reducing shunt.**

Right Panel: **The more likely explanation of the reduction in $\dot{Q}s/\dot{Q}T$ is that PEEP redistributed the edema from the alveolar space into the peribronchovascular interstitium. Panels A and B compare the histological appearance of the non-PEEP and PEEP lungs, respectively; all the edema displaced from panel B was found in the peribronchovascular tissue of panel D (PEEP lung), while much less edema was found in the interstitium of the non-PEEP lung (panel C). (Reproduced with permission from Malo et al: J Appl Physiol 57:1002, 1984.)**

venous return and $\dot{Q}_T$. As with many critical care interventions, it is helpful to define the goal of PEEP therapy such that the adverse effects are minimized. One approach uses the least PEEP providing 90% saturation of an adequate circulating hemoglobin on nontoxic $F_{I_{O_2}}$; because PEEP raises end-inspired alveolar pressures, volumes and dead space, it is helpful to reduce V_T on PEEP to the lowest value effecting adequate CO_2 elimination.

Note in Fig. 1-9 that the non-PEEP lung had a 24 percent shunt when 80 percent of the alveoli were flooded. This occurs because mechanical distortion and hypoxic pulmonary vasoconstriction (HPV) reduce blood flow to flooded airspaces. Some pulmonary vasoactive drugs (sodium nitroprusside, prostaglandin E) increase shunt by blocking HPV, while other agents or interventions increase $\dot{Q}_T$ and $P\bar{v}_{O_2}$ which may increase shunt by blocking HPV. When airspaces are flooded with more viscous liquids like pus in pneumonia, PEEP cannot redistribute this alveolar liquid; instead, PEEP raises alveolar pressure preferentially in the nonflooded units, redistributing blood flow toward the flooded units, which increases the shunt.

HYPOXEMIA DUE TO INCREASED VENTILATION TO PERFUSION VARIANCE

In many other critical illnesses, it is not uncommon to observe hypoxemia in the absence of airspace flooding. For example, chronic obstructive pulmonary disease (COPD), pulmonary fibrosis, asthma, and acute pulmonary embolism are all associated with arterial hypoxemia which is quite responsive to oxygen therapy. Consideration of the two-compartment lung model in Fig. 1-10 illustrates the similarities and differences between the hypoxemia of intrapulmonary shunt in flooded lungs and the hypoxemia due to $\dot{V}/\dot{Q}$ variance in obstructive and restrictive lung diseases. In the latter group with increased $\dot{V}/\dot{Q}$ variance, compartment #1 is not flooded but is very poorly ventilated. Accordingly, $P_{A_{O_2}}$ in compartment #1 can approach $P\bar{v}_{O_2}$ during air breathing, but even small increments in $F_{I_{O_2}}$ cause large increases in $P_{A_{O_2}}$ and so correct the arterial hypoxemia.

We have considered earlier the condition of alveolar hypoventilation in which arterial hypoxemia develops because excess alveolar CO_2 lowers the alveolar O_2 according to the alveolar air equation (see Eqs. 1-6 and 1-7). To illustrate the effect of hypoventilation more clearly, consider the observation that many patients become hypoxemic during hemodialysis, which removes about half the CO_2 produced by the body. Since Pa_{CO_2} does not decrease, $\dot{V}_A$ must be reduced by 50 percent in these patients, such that mixing of 120 mL/min CO_2 in 2000 mL/min alveolar ventilation keeps $F_{A_{CO_2}}$ at 0.06. Yet, the oxygen uptake from the lungs remains at 240 mL/min, giving a lung ratio of $\dot{V}_{CO_2}/\dot{V}_{O_2}$ of 0.5. Accordingly, $P_{A_{O_2}}$ falls during dialysis from 105 to 63 mmHg because twice as much O_2 is removed from inspired air as CO_2 is added to it. Seen in another way, uptake of 240 mL/min from 4.0 L/min alveolar ventilation before hemodialysis causes the O_2 fraction to decrease from

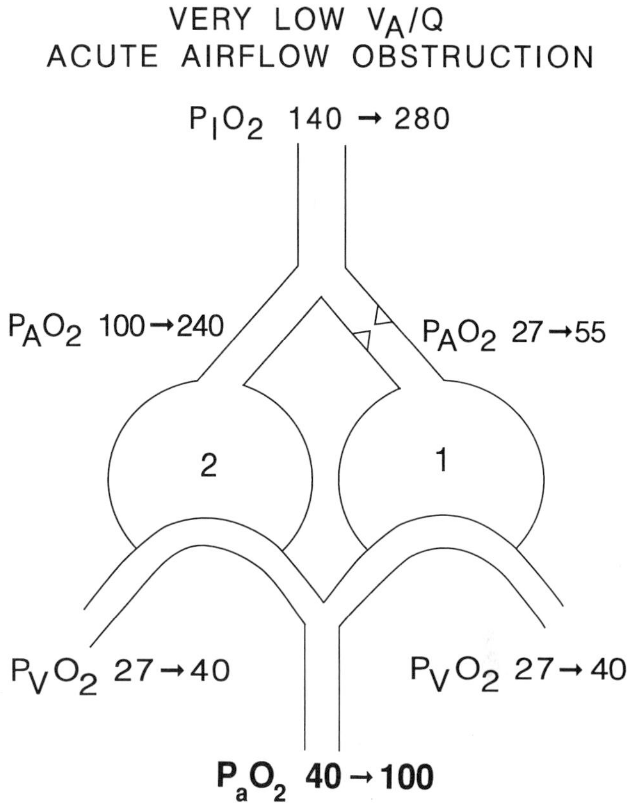

FIGURE 1-10 Effects of very low ventilation in relation to perfusion on arterial hypoxemia during air breathing and during oxygen enrichment ($F_{I_{O_2}}$ = 0.4). Airflow obstruction in compartment 1 reduces the ventilation such that alveolar P_{O_2} approaches $P\bar{v}_{O_2}$ = 27 mmHg. Venous admixture of the effluent from #1 causes arterial hypoxemia (Pa_{O_2} = 40 mmHg). Oxygen enrichment raises $P_{A_{O_2}}$ in #1 to 55 mmHg, a value providing nearly complete saturation of the hemoglobin perfusing #1; then admixture of this blood with that in the ideal alveolus (#2, $P_{A_{O_2}}$ = 240 mmHg when $F_{I_{O_2}}$ = 0.4) corrects the arterial hypoxemia (Pa_{O_2} = 100 mmHg). For further discussion, see text.

0.21 ($F_{I_{O_2}}$) to 0.15 ($F_{A_{O_2}}$); uptake of the same $\dot{V}_{O_2}$ from the reduced $\dot{V}_A$ (2 L/min) during hemodialysis reduced $F_{A_{O_2}}$ to 0.09, and so $P_{A_{O_2}}$ = 63 mmHg. As described above $P_{A_{N_2}}$ increases and $\dot{V}_E$ becomes less than $\dot{V}_I$ when R = 0.5 during hemodialysis. This example illustrates how arterial hypoxemia occurs when $\dot{V}_A$ is reduced without arterial hypercapnia because $\dot{V}_{CO_2}$ is reduced by hemodialysis. We now consider two-compartment models of gas exchange in which the ratio $\dot{V}_{CO_2}/\dot{V}_{O_2}$ in one unit can be considerably <1.0 because the ventilation of that unit ($\dot{V}_A$) is reduced relative to its perfusion ($\dot{Q}$). In such a lung unit, $P_{A_{O_2}}$ can decrease considerably as in the whole lung during hemodialysis.

Such hypoventilation of airspaces receiving half the pulmonary blood flow as in compartment #1 of Fig. 1-10 can account for alveolar gas tensions which approach the mixed venous values; that is, $P_{A_{O_2}}$ = 40 mmHg, $P_{A_{CO_2}}$ = 46 mmHg. Of course, such hypoventilation causes these units to exchange little CO_2 between mixed venous blood and the alveoli while oxygen is still taken up from the alveolar gas to reduce P_{AO_2} toward mixed venous levels. Such units have very low values of R, and since more oxygen is being removed from alveoli than CO_2 is being added to the alveoli, the airspace will tend to collapse unless sufficient gas is drawn past the airflow obstruction. To the extent that the alveoli can maintain their total partial pressure, then P_{AO_2} falls more than P_{ACO_2} rises, and P_{N_2} must increase. Indeed, this nitrogen concentration is the mechanism that maintains airspaces inflated, and allows P_{AO_2} in many perfused but hypoventilated lung units to approach the same mixed venous values to cause similar severe hypoxemia during air breathing as did the large $\dot{Q}s/\dot{Q}_T$ considered above.

The major difference between shunt and $\dot{V}/\dot{Q}$ mismatch occurs when F_{IO_2} is increased. Consider the effect of breathing oxygen on the P_{AO_2} in hypoventilated but not flooded airspaces. Over time, the nitrogen is washed out of the hypoventilated airspaces, when there are only two gases in all alveoli—oxygen and CO_2. The CO_2 cannot rise higher than the $P\overline{v}_{CO_2}$, so P_{AO_2} must rise above 600 mmHg or the alveoli collapse. Indeed, some hypoventilated alveoli perfused by a small fraction of mixed venous blood (up to 0.05 $\dot{Q}_T$) do collapse, creating a small additional shunt during oxygen breathing. Yet, the vast majority of airspaces remain patent with a $P_{AO_2} > 600$ mmHg, and as a result, the Pa_{O_2} rises to approximate that in normal lungs breathing 100% oxygen. This different response to oxygen therapy allows the separation of hypoxemia due to such $\dot{V}/\dot{Q}$ variance from that due to intrapulmonary shunt. Equally important is the implication that modest amounts of O_2 enrichment can correct arterial hypoxemia and tissue hypoxia in most patients with severe obstructive and restrictive lung diseases. In the past, physicians have been cautious with O_2 therapy, especially in patients with COPD, for fear of aggravating hypoventilation by blocking the hypoxic drive to breathe. Recent clinical investigation refutes that hypothetical concern when O_2 therapy is administered under close observation, suggesting that the goal of therapy is to give enough O_2 to relieve hypoxia in those patients. Correctable adverse effects of hypoxia include alveolar hypoxic vasoconstriction, cor pulmonale, sleep disordered breathing, and arrhythmias.

In patients with a wide $\dot{V}/\dot{Q}$ variance, reduction in $\dot{Q}_T$ and P_{VO_2} aggravates hypoxemia. This accounts for much of the arterial desaturation observed during exercise in pulmonary fibrosis, emphysema, and pulmonary hypertension. In each case, $\dot{V}_{O_2}$ increases so P_{VO_2} falls when the right ventricular output is limited by its afterload. Similarly, reduced pulmonary blood flow after pulmonary embolism perfuses intercurrent low $\dot{V}_A/\dot{Q}$ units with very low P_{VO_2} to cause much of the observed hypoxemia. In all these patients, the hypoxemia is quite responsive to O_2 therapy, and is further ameliorated by HPV. Accordingly, intercurrent use of vasoactive drugs which block HPV worsen hypoxia by increasing the blood flow to very low $\dot{V}/\dot{Q}$ units.

Mechanics of the Respiratory System

DYNAMIC AND STATIC RELATIONSHIPS BETWEEN RESPIRATORY PRESSURES AND VOLUMES

Mechanics is the study of the relationship between force applied to an object and the resultant motion of the object. For the respiratory system the force applied is expressed as force per unit area, or applied pressure (ΔP). The resultant motions, usually expressed as linear displacement, are expressed for the respiratory system as the cube of the linear displacement (cm^3) or volume change (ΔV). Likewise, displacement per unit time or velocity is expressed as volume change per unit time, or flow rate ($\dot{V}$), and the rate of change velocity, or acceleration, is expressed as volume acceleration ($\ddot{V}$). Thus the motions of the respiratory system—volume, flow, and acceleration—result from the applied pressure, and the equation of motion states that the applied pressure is opposed by equal forces in the resultant motions:

$$\Delta P = \Delta V \cdot Ers + \dot{V} \cdot Rrs + \ddot{V} \cdot Irs \quad (1\text{-}9)$$

The units of volume, flow, and acceleration can be converted to pressure units by the appropriate constant of proportionality. The pressure cost of a volume change, elastic pressure (Pel), is determined by multiplying the volume change by the elastance of the respiratory system (Ers) having the units cmH_2O/L. Likewise the units of flow are converted to resistant pressure (Pr) by multiplying flow by the resistance of the respiratory system (Rrs) having the units $cmH_2O/L/s$. Finally, volume acceleration is converted to accelerative pressure (Pacc) by multiplying by the inertia of the respiratory system (Irs) having the units $cmH_2O/L/s^2$. For most purposes in the ICU (except during high frequency ventilation), the Pacc is negligible because Irs is very small. Accordingly, the equation of motion for the respiratory system is depicted in Fig. 1-11 and is written: $\Delta P = Pel + Pr$. Since $Pr = \text{flow} \times \text{resistance}$, Pr is zero when flow is zero, simplifying the equation even further. Now, $\Delta P = Pel$ when $\dot{V} = 0$.

One application of the equation of motion for patients on a ventilator is depicted in Fig. 1-12 (upper left panel). Peak pressure on the ventilator is the sum of Pel and Pr. In patients without lung disease, peak pressure rarely exceeds 20 cmH_2O when the V_T is 500 mL and the inspiratory flow rate is 60 L/min or 1 L/s. By adding an inflation hold to the ventilator or by transiently occluding the expiratory line of the ventilator, the lungs and chest wall remain distended by the V_T after inspiratory flow has terminated. In this case, the ventilator pressure dial falls from its peak value of 20 cmH_2O to about 10 cmH_2O. Since flow is O, the applied pressure equals Pel for a volume change of 500 mL. The elastance is calculated as Pel/V_T or 20 cmH_2O/L, the upper limit of normal respiratory elastance. The difference between peak pressure and Pel is the resistive pressure associated with the flow of 1 L/s. Accordingly, resistance is

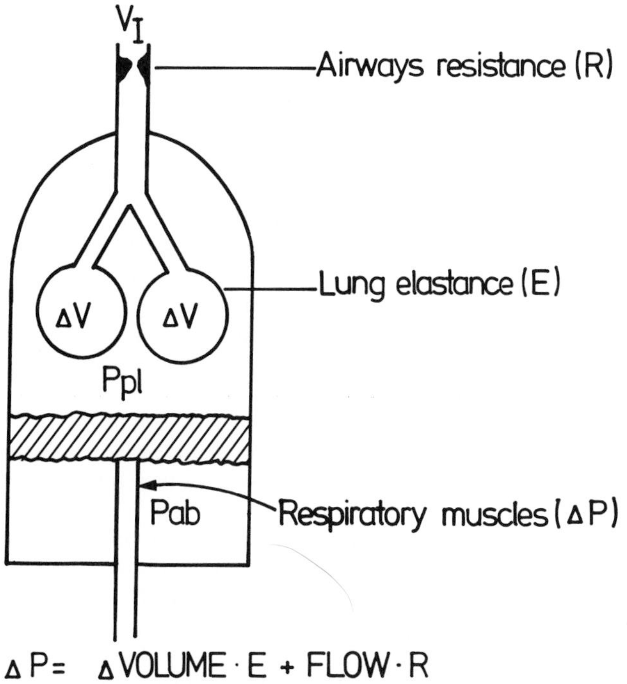

FIGURE 1-11 Schematic of the mechanical characteristics of the respiratory system. Inspiratory flow ($\dot{V}_I$) is delivered through an airway with resistance (R) to a two compartment lung model, the units of which have elastance (E) and are distended by the delivered volume (ΔV). During positive pressure ventilation, lung distention raises the pressure between the lungs and chest wall (Ppl) to increase the volume of the chest wall, in part by pushing the diaphragm downward (see piston at the floor of the thorax) to raise the abdominal pressure (Pab); during a spontaneous breath, the respiratory muscles (ΔP) pull the piston down to lower Ppl and inspire ΔV across R. In either case, ΔP = the elastic pressure (Pel = ΔV × E) + the resistive pressure (Pr = $\dot{V}_I$ × R).

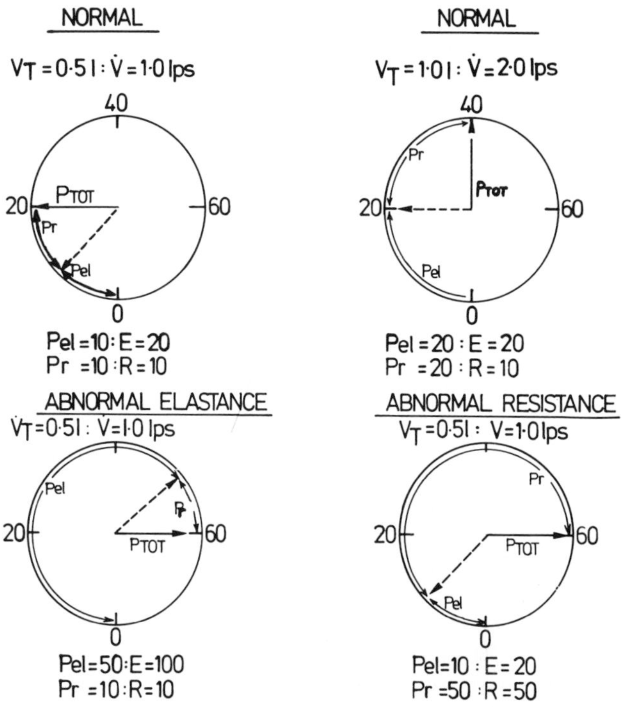

FIGURE 1-12 Schematic of the pressure dial on a mechanical ventilator illustrating the measurement of respiratory elastic pressures (Pel) and resistive pressures (Pr), and a calculation of elastance (E) and resistance (R). The upper panels illustrate normal respiratory mechanics for a normal tidal volume and flow rate (left), and for a large tidal volume and flow rate (right panel). The lower panels illustrate abnormal elastance (left) and abnormal resistance (right panel). For discussion, see text.

10 $cmH_2O/L/s$. With the usual respiratory tubing and a recently inserted size 8 to 9 endotracheal tube there is a resistance of about 6 $cmH_2O/L/s$, and the remaining 4 $cmH_2O/L/s$ represents the upper limit of normal resistance to air flow in the patient's airways. Note that resistance of the same endotracheal tube after 7 days can increase up to 15 to 20 $cmH_2O/L/s$ due to kinks and inspissated secretions. Note further that this evaluation of mechanics in awake patients who are not paralyzed is confounded by erratic respiratory muscle activity which can increase or decrease the peak and/or inflation hold pressures independent from the Ers and Rrs. Accordingly, reliable measurements must be obtained in such patients with careful attention to exclude artifacts of respiratory effort.

In the same patient, if VT were doubled to 1000 mL, the inflation hold pressure would rise to about 20 cmH_2O so respiratory elastance remains at 20 cmH_2O/L; if inspiratory flow were also doubled to 2 L/s, peak pressure will be 40 cmH_2O, elastic pressure will be 20 cmH_2O, and the calculated elastance and resistance will not change significantly from the original values, even though the peak and pause pressures have each doubled (see Fig. 1-12, upper right panel). These considerations assume linear pressure-volume and pressure-flow relationships in the respiratory system, a constant volume-cycled ventilator, and also assume a square wave inspiratory flow pattern on the ventilator, such that the peak airway pressure just prior to end inspiration is measured at a constant flow. Note that changing the flow pattern of the breath will change the actual flow at end inspiration, and so change Pr considerably without any change in the airways resistance. The increasing or decreasing flow profiles for each breath on current volume-cycled ventilators allow the physician assuming constant flow to overestimate or underestimate resistance considerably. Note further that Pel in this case was calculated assuming that end-expired alveolar pressure was zero; when PEEP is added, ΔPel is the pause pressure minus PEEP. In many cases of airflow obstruction, intrinsic PEEP (PEEPi) develops giving a positive alveolar pressure when the pressure at the airway reads zero. These considerations indicate how pressure on the ventilator may be simply recorded and used to calculate respiratory elastance and resistance to diagnose abnormal values and to follow these abnormalities as a result of progression of the disease or its treatment.

A variety of lung diseases increase the Ers or stiffness of the respiratory system (see Fig. 1-12, lower left). For example, acute pulmonary edema floods airspaces and decreases the volume of the lungs into which a constant VT can be delivered. In such patients, peak pressure may rise to 60 cmH_2O and the inflation hold pressure may rise to 50 cmH_2O for a VT of 500 mL. In that case, elastance is 100 cmH_2O/L and resistance is 10 $cmH_2O/L/s$. As a result of diuresis or other therapeutic interventions, edema and elastance may decrease with time as detected by falling Ers if it is measured. Note that much of the apparent stiffness of the respiratory system in diseases like pulmonary edema, ARDS, and pneumonia is due to filling of the airspaces with liquid so that they cannot receive any of the VT. This panel of Fig. 1-12 corresponds to the flooding of 80 percent of the alveoli schematically depicted in the upper left "non-PEEP" lung in Fig. 1-9 responsible for 24 percent shunt. Consider that a VT of 500 mL ventilates only the 20 percent unflooded portion of that lung, markedly overdistending those units just as a normal lung would be overdistended by ventilation with a tidal volume of 2.5 L!

Figure 1-13 illustrates the changes in static volume-pressure (P-V) relationships of the respiratory system induced by pulmonary edema to indicate the mechanical effects of PEEP. When edema floods airspaces, the end-expiratory volume is reduced, ΔPel for constant VT is much increased, and hysteresis of the P-V curve is much increased. As a result, addition of 10 cmH_2O PEEP appears to increase the end-expiratory volume along the inflation limb of the P-V curve much less after edema than it would before edema. Yet, PEEP works to reduce $\dot{Q}s/\dot{Q}T$ by redistributing edema out of alveoli into the lung interstitium, recruiting previously flooded airspaces to accommodate the VT. On the P-V curve, such recruitment is measured as a large increase in lung volume for a small increase in pressure along the steep portion of the inflation limb. Lung units so recruited on inflation do not fill with edema again when PEEP maintains end-expiratory volume, and that volume increases much more on PEEP than would be predicted from the inflation P-V curve before PEEP. Accordingly, PEEP increases lung volume considerably, pushing the chest wall out by a correspondingly larger increase in pleural pressure (Ppl) than would be predicted. One consequence of these mechanical changes is that the increase in Ppl with PEEP is often as great or greater in pulmonary edema as in normal lungs, and the ΔPpl/PEEP fraction varies considerably among patients.

In contrast to diseases which increase elastance, some diseases increase the Rrs without changing elastance significantly (see Fig. 1-12, lower right panel). In acute asthma, peak pressure may rise to 60 cmH_2O when flow rate is 1 L/s and VT is 500 mL. Yet inflation hold pressure may be only 20 cmH_2O, indicating Rrs of 40 $cmH_2O/L/s$ and an increased respiratory elastance of 40 cmH_2O/L. Efficacy of bronchodilation may be followed by the reduction in peak pressure and Pr with no change in Pel. Note that peak pressure can be reduced considerably from 60 cmH_2O by reducing inspiratory flow rate to reduce the Pr drop. The problem caused is that inspiratory time becomes twice as long, thereby shortening the time for the lung to exhale the VT through severely obstructed airways. Such a strategy often leads to dynamic hyperinflation when the next breath is delivered before the last is out. This causes PEEPi, which can be measured by occluding the airway at end-expiration and awaiting equilibration of the alveolar pressure with that at the airway opening (Fig. 1-14). Indeed, most newly

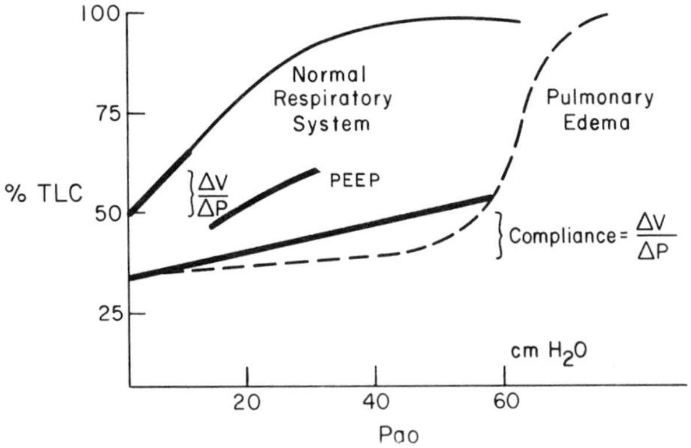

	Before edema	After edema
ΔV(litres) with PEEP (20 cm H_2O)	1.42±0.38	1.39±0.22
ΔPpl (cm H_2O) with PEEP	10.1±2.2	9.7±0.7
Lung Compliance (ml/cm H_2O)	102±28	47±17

FIGURE 1-13 Relationships between lung volume (ordinate, % total lung capacity) and pressure across the respiratory system (abscissa, Pao, cmH_2O). The thin continuous line represents the inflation pressure volume relationship of the normal respiratory system, showing an end expired lung volume (Pao = 0) of 50% TLC, and an inflation compliance (ΔV/ΔP) during a tidal volume of about 10% TLC (thick line). By contrast, the interrupted line shows the inflation PV curve after pulmonary edema floods many lung units, reducing the end expired lung volume to about 30% TLC; then a tidal inflation of the same ΔV causes a much larger increase in ΔPao because there are many fewer airspaces to accommodate the tidal volume. Adding 15 cm of PEEP might be expected to produce a much smaller change in an expired lung volume in edematous lungs than in a normal respiratory system; yet when PEEP is effective in reducing $\dot{Q}s/\dot{Q}T$ by redistributing alveolar edema, the increase in end expired lung volume (and so in Ppl) is as much after pulmonary edema as in the normal respiratory system. (See table at right of graph.) (Reproduced with permission from Hall JB and Wood LDH: Medical Grand Rounds 3:183, 1984; and from Prewitt RM and Wood LDH: Am J Physiol 236:H534, 1979.)

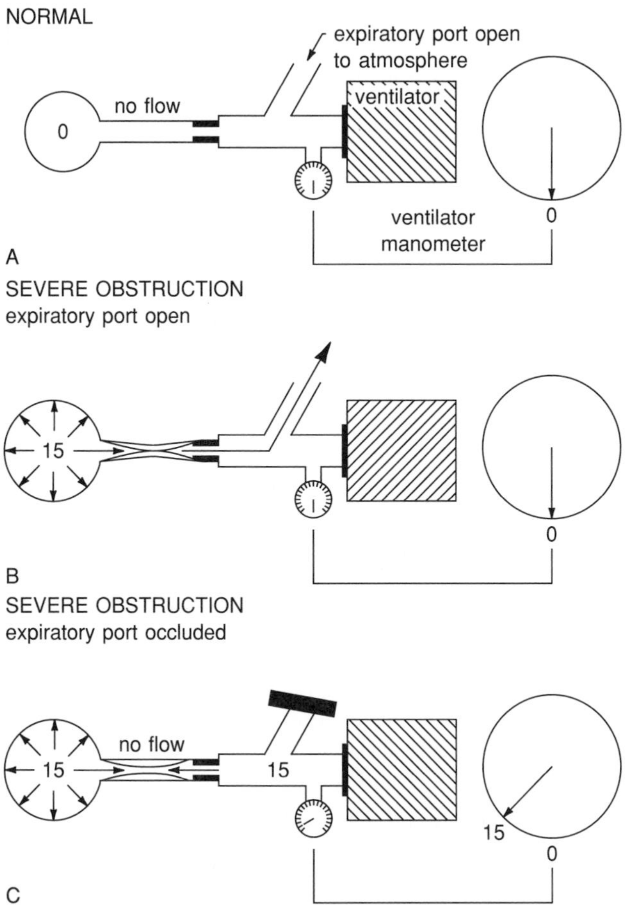

FIGURE 1-14 Measurement of intrinsic PEEP (PEEPi) by expiratory port occlusion. *a*. Normally alveolar pressure is atmospheric at the end of exhalation. *b*. With severe airflow obstruction alveolar pressure remains elevated (in this example at 15 cmH_2O) and slow flow continues, even at the end of the set exhalation period. The ventilator manometer senses negligible pressure because it is opened to the atmosphere through large bore tubing and downstream from the site of flow limitation. *c*. With gas flow stopped by occlusion of the expiratory port at the end of the set exhalation period, pressure equilibrates throughout the lung-ventilator system and is displayed on the ventilator manometer. (Reproduced with permission from Pepe P, Marini JP: Am Rev Resp Dis 126:166, 1982.)

intubated ventilated asthmatic patients have PEEPi of 5 to 15 cmH_2O; when the correct end-expiratory pressure in the example above is PEEPi = 10 cmH_2O, the ΔPel of the respiratory system is only 10 cmH_2O (inflation hold pressure of 20 cmH_2O minus PEEPi) so the correct Ers is normal (20 cmH_2O/L).

To sort which flow to use in severe airflow obstruction, it is also useful to consider the distribution of pressure along the airway between the airway opening (Pao) and the alveoli. When flow is zero the measured pressure is constant along this path and is equal to Pao. The Pel is the largest pressure in the alveoli throughout the respiratory cycle even when peak pressure rises considerably higher than Pel. This is so because Pr is the pressure drop due to flow resistance between Pao and the peripheral airways. In obstructive airways diseases, most of the rise in pressure occurs between the ventilator and the obstructed airways, yet these high airway pressures are thought to cause less barotrauma than correspondingly high pressures in the airspaces because alveoli are more fragile than the robust proximal airways. Accordingly, PEEPi often causes more barotrauma when inspiratory flow is reduced than the high peak pressures cause at high flow and less PEEPi. As an intervention to reduce intrinsic PEEPi, reduction of minute ventilation through either reduced rate or V_T is more effective than increasing flow rate. In the agitated patient with status asthmaticus, this necessitates sedation and muscle relaxation on intubation to prevent rapid triggering of the ventilator and to allow such control of ventilation.

STATIC PRESSURE-VOLUME (P-V) RELATIONSHIPS OF THE LUNG AND CHEST WALL

Figure 1-15 plots pressure in cmH_2O (abscissa) against lung volume (ordinate) as a percent of the total lung capacity (TLC). When the pressure across the total respiratory system is zero (see continuous line), lung volume is approximately 50 percent TLC. Consider a patient lying intubated and relaxed on the operating table. From the end-expired volume, the patient's lungs and chest wall are inflated. As volume increases, the pressure applied to the respiratory system increases in a curvilinear manner, with a small change in pressure per large change in volume at first and then a large change in pressure per small change in volume near TLC. Likewise, if volume is removed from the end-expired lung volume, pressure across the respiratory system becomes negative in a curvilinear manner—a small change in pressure per large change in volume near functional residual capacity (FRC) and then a large change in pressure per small change in volume until no more volume can be removed. This lower limit of volume is the residual volume (RV) trapped behind closed small airways or re-

FIGURE 1-15 Pressure volume relationships of the respiratory system (continuous curve), of the lungs (interrupted curve), and of the chest wall (dotted curve). For discussion, see text.

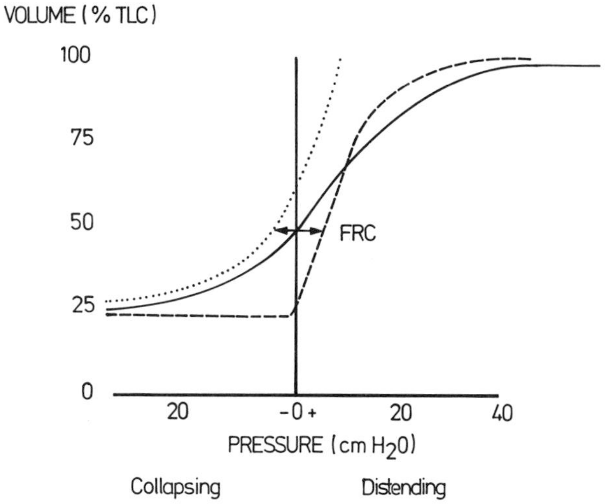

tained because the chest wall will not decrease its volume further. This balance of forces of the chest wall tending to recoil outward and the lungs tending to recoil inward causes the negative pleural pressure between the lungs and the chest wall at FRC. Further reductions in Ppl cause further reductions in chest wall volume, which approximately parallel the P-V relationship of the lung alone. Likewise, increases of Ppl above zero increase the chest wall volume in an essentially linear manner. Accordingly, when the change in pressure across the total respiratory system (ΔPao) is 10 cm/L volume change, ΔPL (across the lungs) and ΔPpl (across the chest wall) are about equal to 5 cmH_2O each.

FRC is decreased when lung elastic recoil is increased. This may occur in pulmonary fibrosis or in pulmonary edema. FRC is increased when lung elastic recoil is decreased as in emphysema, and the PEEPi of severe airflow obstruction raises FRC dynamically even when the static P-V characteristics of the lung are normal. Even more common abnormalities in FRC in the ICU occur due to abnormalities in the P-V relationship of the chest wall. The floor of the chest wall is the diaphragm. In the upright position abdominal contents are hung from the diaphragm tending to pull it down or in an inspiratory position. The supine position causes the weight of the abdominal contents to push up on the diaphragm displacing it in an expiratory direction. Consider an intubated upright patient having a corked endotracheal tube, such that Pao at end expiration is zero. When the patient becomes supine, pressure in the airway rises due to the pressure of abdominal contents on the diaphragm, and Pao rises 3 to 10 cmH_2O. If the cork is pulled, respiratory gas is expired until Pao is zero again. This reduction in FRC in the supine position is due to a shift to the right of the P-V curve of the chest wall. Then the new balance of forces of outward recoil of the chest wall and inward recoil of the lungs occurs at a lower lung volume and less negative Ppl. If the patient is obese, these changes are greater for there is a greater pressure applied to the floor of the chest wall. Likewise, ascites, peritonitis, or upper abdominal surgery increase the pressure of the abdominal contents and decrease FRC further, and inhaled anesthetic agents relax the crural part of the diaphragm to reduce FRC. The consequence of these reductions in FRC on gas exchange will be evident after examining the mechanisms responsible for the distribution of ventilation and perfusion in the lung.

PLEURAL PRESSURE AND THE VERTICAL GRADIENTS OF LUNG VOLUME AND VENTILATION

Until now, we have considered that pressures are applied to the respiratory system in a uniform manner. However, in an upright patient the pressure in a pleural space at the top of the lung is about 7.5 cmH_2O more negative than the pressure in the pleural space at the bottom of the lung. This is analogous to the pressure in a column of water 30 cm high being 30 cmH_2O negative at the top relative to the bottom of the column. The lung may be considered as a column of liquid having a density one-quarter that of water, such that the average lung being 30 cm in distance from top to bottom will have a pressure at the bottom 7.5 cmH_2O (30×0.25) more positive than the pressure at the top. This conforms to the measured gradient of Ppl in upright people at FRC where the pressure at the top of the pleural space is about -10 cmH_2O and the pressure at the bottom of the pleural space is about -2.5 cmH_2O. The relative volumes of airspaces exposed to PL of 10 and 2.5 cmH_2O are given in the P-V curve depicted in Fig. 1-16.

Airspaces near the top of the lung have a volume of about 65 percent of their TLC, whereas airspaces at the bottom of the lung have a volume of about 35 percent of their TLC. Furthermore, the smaller airspaces at the bottom of the lung are located on the steeper part of the lung P-V curve than the larger airspaces at the top of the lung located on the flatter part of the P-V curve. Accordingly, an equal change in Ppl during inspiration of about 5 cmH_2O will cause twice the volume change in the smaller airspaces at the bottom of the lung than in the larger airspaces at the top of the lung. Accordingly, ventilation is much better to lower lung regions than to upper lung regions as depicted in Fig. 1-16, right panel. This is convenient for the perfusion of upper lung regions is less than the perfusion of lower lung regions so that ventilation is matched to perfusion from the top to the bottom of the lung.

AIRWAYS CLOSURE AND ATELECTASIS

Now consider that the reductions in lung volume due to supine position, obesity, upper abdominal surgery, ascites, or peritonitis reduce the transpulmonary pressure of all lung regions as indicated on the left of Fig. 1-16. Ppl in the upper lung regions is now -5 cmH_2O, whereas Ppl in the lower lung regions is $+2.5$ cmH_2O. Thus, the gradient of Ppl from top to bottom of the lung is maintained at 7.5 cmH_2O, but airspaces lie on a different portion of their P-V curve as indicated in Fig. 1-16. Now the lower airspaces lie on the part of the P-V curve in which no change in volume occurs for even large changes of pressure. This occurs because the Ppl exceeds the pressure in the airways and so closes them. Airways closure stops the ventilation of these low lung regions which receive the majority of the blood flow. Thus, lower lung regions in such patients have little ventilation in relation to their large blood flow causing arterial hypoxemia and/or resorption atelectasis. In contrast, the upper regions now lie on the steep part of their P-V curve thereby receiving most the ventilation yet having a small proportion of the pulmonary blood flow.

This phenomenon can be described in another way (Fig. 1-17). Following a full expiration to RV, airspaces at the bottom of the lung are at about 20 percent TLC while airspaces at the top of the lung are at about 60 percent TLC. The nitrogen concentration in each airspace is about 0.8. Following a VC inspiration of pure oxygen, lower lung region nitrogen concentration is reduced to 16%(0.2×0.8) while upper lung region nitrogen concentration is reduced less to 0.48(0.6×0.8) During the subsequent expiration nitrogen concentration is initially zero as the oxygen is washed out

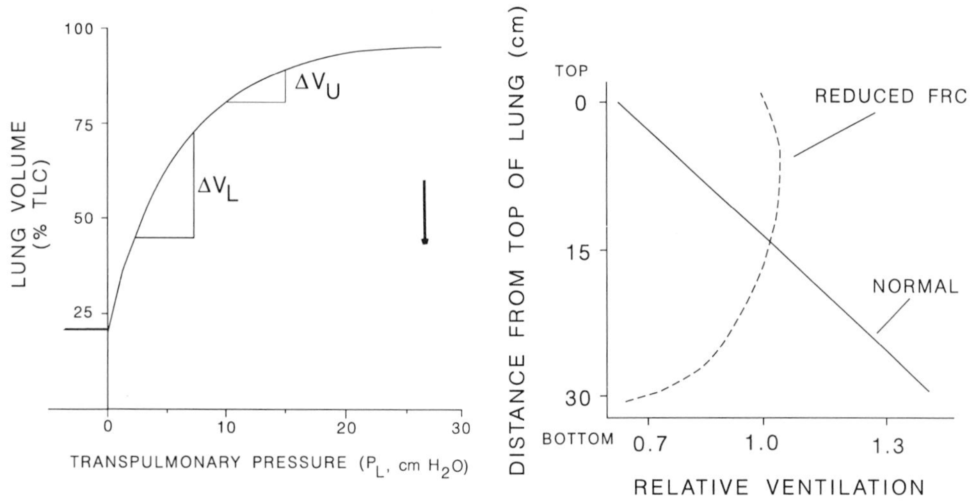

FIGURE 1-16 Schematic illustrating the vertical gradient of pleural pressure and ventilation. The left panel plots lung volume (percent TLC, ordinate) versus transpulmonary pressure (PL, cmH_2O—abscissa). At end expiration, upper lung regions (U) are larger and less compliant than lower lung regions (L) due to the vertical gradient of pleural pressure. Accordingly, a spontaneous breath ($\Delta P_L = 5\ cmH_2O$) causes $\Delta V_L > \Delta V_U$, as depicted by the continuous line in the right panel showing greater ventilation at the bottom of the lung than at the top. By contrast, factors reducing FRC raise the pleural pressure to close airways ventilating lower lung regions ($P_L = -2.5$), so ΔP_L of 5 cmH_2O causes $\Delta V_L < \Delta V_U$, as depicted by the interrupted line in the right panel showing less ventilation to lower lung regions. Such hypoventilation of well perfused lower lung regions causes hypoxemia and reabsorption atelectasis in ventilated patients; other departures from the normal regional distribution of ventilation determined by the static elastic properties of the lung cause insignificant changes in pulmonary gas exchange (i.e., increased flow rate, positive pressure ventilation). Accordingly, most of the abnormalities of ventilation distribution responsible for increased ($A{-}aD_{O_2}$) and V_D/V_T occur within lung regions as a result of abnormalities in resistance and compliance of peripheral lung units.

of the airspaces, and then rises to a value intermediate between the alveolar concentrations in upper and lower regions (about 30%) through most of the expiration (phase III) until the lung volume is reached at which many of the lower airspaces close. Then, all the gas comes from upper lung regions having the higher nitrogen concentration of 0.48, so there is a steep rise of expired nitrogen concentration (phase IV).

FIGURE 1-17 Tracing of expiratory nitrogen concentration during a slow expiration from TLC to RV after a full inspiration of pure O_2. The four phases are indicated.

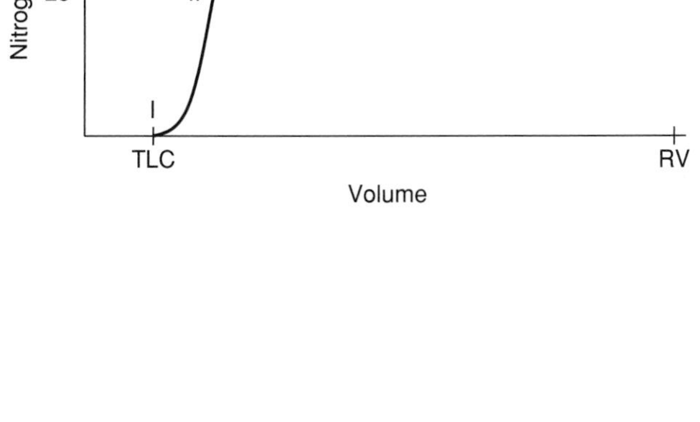

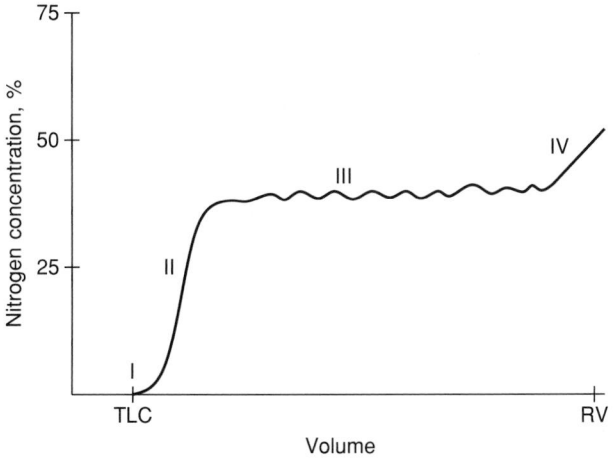

This rise indicates airways closure and is called the closing volume (CV). In healthy young patients, CV is about 30 percent TLC whereas FRC is about 50 percent TLC. As indicated in the Fig. 1-18, normal tidal ventilation occurs at lung volumes above CVs. FRC increases slightly with age and CV more with age so that CV becomes equal to FRC at about 60 years in upright patients. Because FRC decreases in the supine position, CV is equal to FRC in the supine position at about age 45. FRC decreases further in obese patients so that FRC is less than CV, indicating that a portion of the normal ventilation occurs below CV, associated with arterial hypoxemia because the poorly ventilated lung units are well perfused. Upper abdominal surgery, ascites, peritonitis, and obesity reduce FRC further below CV. CV is increased by age, smoking, and overhydration as might occur in the perioperative period. Accordingly, moving from left to right in Fig. 1-18, we arrive at the typical postoperative patient—a supine, elderly, obese, smoker, recently anesthetized for upper abdominal surgery having incisional pain and being overhydrated; the reduced FRC is much below the increased CV, promoting arterial hypoxemia and collapse of dependent airways.

The reason for listing this litany of abnormalities promoting arterial hypoxemia is to provide ways of avoiding that disorder. For example, ventilating patients in the upright position increases FRC. Turning patients regularly shifts the lung region which is dependent and subject to airways closure and hypoventilation. Note, that the degree of hypoventilation was dependent on the gradient of Ppl which is about equal from top to bottom in the lung regardless of

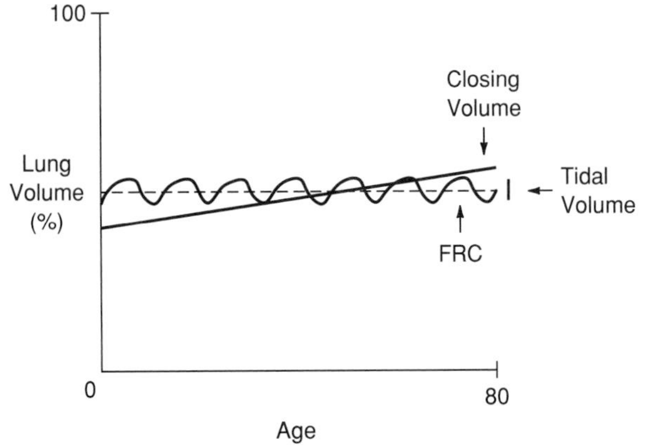

FIGURE 1-18 Schematic showing FRC (interrupted line) and closing volume (CV, continuous line)—each expressed as lung volume (% TLC) on the ordinate—versus age in years on the abscissa. Typical tidal ventilation begins above CV in younger upright patients, but many factors can reduce FRC such that tidal ventilation occurs below CV to promote hypoxemia and atelectasis; other factors increase CV to promote perioperative respiratory failure. The complication of atelectasis is minimized by maneuvers which maintain FRC and reduce CV.

position: upright, lateral decubitus, supine, or prone, all have about the same vertical distance. Efforts to minimize elevations in abdominal pressure due to pain or muscle spasm using analgesics, muscle relaxants, or transcutaneous nerve stimulation all increase FRC in the appropriate patients. PEEP also increases FRC by raising the airway pressure at end expiration and pushing the volume of the lung and chest wall upward along the V-P relationship.

Acute Respiratory Failure

CLASSIFICATION BY MECHANISM

A descriptive survey of patients requiring mechanical ventilation for respiratory failure reveals four patterns of pathophysiology, each having a predominant mechanism (Table 1-1). Failure of oxygenation due to intrapulmonary shunt (↑ $\dot{Q}s/\dot{Q}_T$) causes hypoxemia refractory to O_2 therapy despite hyperventilation and reduced Pa_{CO_2} in type I or acute hypoxemic respiratory failure (AHRF). Primary failure of alveolar ventilation (↓ $\dot{V}_A$) leads to CO_2 retention and arterial hypercapnia associated with reduced Pa_{O_2} which corrects easily with O_2 therapy in type II or hypoventilatory respiratory failure. Beyond their gas exchange abnormalities, these two classical types of respiratory failure have distinctly different clinical presentations and different abnormalities in the mechanics of breathing, while they share mechanisms leading to respiratory muscle dysfunction and fatigue.

The intensive care physician frequently encounters patients in the perioperative period who are unusually susceptible to atelectasis as a primary mechanism causing type III or perioperative respiratory failure. In general, abnormal abdominal mechanics reduce the end-expired lung volume (↓ FRC) below the increased closing volume (↑ CV) in these patients leading to hypoventilation, hypoxia, and progressive collapse of dependent lung units. The end result can be type I AHRF, or type II hypoventilation, or both. Yet, identification of atelectasis as a distinct mechanism leading to a third type of respiratory failure can be harnessed to prevent lung collapse by reducing the adverse effects of common clinical circumstances promoting reduction in FRC and of those conditions promoting increased airways closure. Because many of these mechanisms are shared by patients with type I or type II respiratory failure, implementation of approaches to minimize atelectasis should be a part of the management of all patients with respiratory failure.

A significant number of ventilated patients fall outside the categories of type I, II or III respiratory failure. These are the patients who have been intubated and stabilized with ventilatory support during a hypoperfusion state, so type IV respiratory failure is most commonly due to cardiogenic, hypovolemic, or septic shock without associated pulmonary problems. The appropriate rationale for ventilator therapy in these patients who are frequently tachypneic with erratic respiratory patterns is to stabilize gas exchange and minimize the steal of a limited $\dot{Q}_T$ by the working respiratory muscles until the mechanism for the hypoperfusion state is identified and corrected. Again, the mechanism of this type IV respiratory failure may be shared in part by patients having primary mechanisms for type I, II, or III respiratory failure, so the causes of reduced blood flow, hypotension, anemia, acidosis, and sepsis need identification and correction in each type of acute respiratory failure.

Consider the differences in clinical description of patients with type I AHRF from patients with type II hypoventilatory respiratory failure. In the second type, ↓ $\dot{V}_A$ is caused by reduced drive to breathe (drug overdoses, head injuries) or by reduced coupling of the adequate or increased drive to breathe to the respiratory muscles (myasthenia gravis, Guillain-Barré syndrome, amyotrophic lateral sclerosis [ALS], botulism, muscle-relaxing drugs). Alveolar hypoventilation also occurs commonly in respiratory diseases characterized by airflow obstruction and wasted ventilation; Pa_{CO_2} increases despite increased CNS drive to breathe, adequate neuromuscular coupling, and increased total ventilation (status asthmaticus, acute on chronic respiratory failure of patients with COPD or restrictive pulmonary disease). The clinical presentation of each of these categories of hypoventilating patients contrasts markedly with that of patients presenting with type I AHRF, where cyanosis, tachypnea, and refractory hypoxemia lead to early identification of airspace flooding by physical and radiologic examination. Then the differential diagnosis of the airspace flooding leading to ↑ $\dot{Q}s/\dot{Q}_T$ includes cardiogenic or permeability pulmonary edema, pneumonia, or lung hemorrhage, each having specific etiologies and therapy.

While specific diagnostic and treatment plans are being implemented, supportive therapy for patients with AHRF includes four objectives: **1.** stabilization of the patient on the ventilator with minimal respiratory work, **2.** ventilation with the least V_T providing adequate CO_2 elimination,

TABLE 1-1 Acute Respiratory Failure

Type	I Acute Hypoxemic	II Hypoventilatory	III Perioperative	IV Shock
Mechanism	↑ $\dot{Q}S/\dot{Q}T$	↓ $\dot{V}A$	Atelectasis	Hypoperfusion
Etiology	Airspace flooding	1. ↓ CNS drive 2. ↓ Neuromuscular coupling 3. ↑ Work/deadspace	1. ↓ FRC 2. ↑ CV	1. Cardiogenic 2. Hypovolemic 3. Septic
Clinical Description	1. Pulmonary edema • Cardiogenic • ARDS 2. Pneumonia 3. Lung hemorrhage 4. Chest trauma	1. Overdose/injury 2. Myasthenia gravis Polyradiculitis/ALS Botulism/curare 3. Asthma/COPD Pulmonary fibrosis Kyphoscoliosis	1. Supine/obese Ascites/peritonitis Upper abdominal Incision, anesthesia 2. Age/smoking Fluid overload Bronchospasm Airway secretions	1. Myocardial infarct Pulmonary hypertension 2. Hemorrhage Dehydration Tamponade 3. Bacteremia Endotoxemia

3. addition of the least amount of PEEP effecting 90% saturation of an adequate circulating hemoglobin on a nontoxic F_{IO_2}, and **4.** cardiovascular management to reduce airspace edema by seeking the lowest pulmonary vascular pressures compatible with an adequate $\dot{Q}T$ and oxygen transport to the peripheral tissues (see Chap. 128 for further discussion). Each of these goals of management of type I AHRF differs from the goals of management of type II hypoventilatory respiratory failure, where the patients with depressed CNS drive or reduced neuromuscular coupling receive adequate ventilation and require minimal oxygen supplementation with careful attention to preventing atelectasis and correcting hypoperfusion until the abnormal neurologic condition resolves (see Chap. 143). The patients requiring ventilation for airflow obstruction are supported with bronchodilator therapy and ventilator settings which minimize PEEPi until the airways resistance is reduced sufficiently for the respiratory muscles to achieve adequate ventilation independent from the ventilator (see Chaps. 129, 130, and 132).

RESPIRATORY MUSCLE FUNCTION AND FATIGUE

The respiratory muscles share with other major muscle groups of the body the characteristic that excessive work leads to fatigue. This concept seems to explain why patients with severe airflow obstruction or airspace flooding ultimately stop breathing, and why patients requiring mechanical ventilation for these and other causes of respiratory failure are unable to breathe independent from the ventilator until the load on their respiratory muscles is reduced, or the respiratory muscles become stronger, or both.

Data illustrating this concept for the respiratory muscles are presented in Fig. 1-19. On the ordinate is respiratory muscle effort as a percent of the maximum effort achievable, and the time to respiratory muscle fatigue is on the abscissa. When the respiratory effort exerted (load) is equal to the maximum respiratory effort, the muscles are able to work against that load for only the shortest of time before they fatigue. In contrast, when the respiratory load is less than about one-third of the maximum respiratory strength, the respiratory muscles can perform that load for an infinite period of time. Between these extremes, there is a curvilinear increase in the time to respiratory muscle fatigue as the respiratory load is reduced in relation to the maximum respiratory strength. Since spontaneous ventilation is necessarily a continuous process, i.e., the time to fatigue must be infinite for the patient to continue breathing independent of the ventilator, it is essential that the work of spontaneous ventilation is less than one-third of the maximal respiratory effort achievable. In normal patients, the maximum negative inspiratory force (NIF) measured at FRC exceeds 100 cmH_2O, whereas the work of spontaneous breathing is <10 cmH_2O, providing considerable respiratory muscle reserve before the conditions of fatigue are approached. In contrast, patients with acute respiratory failure frequently have values of NIF <30 cmH_2O while the load on the respi-

FIGURE 1-19 Ratio of diaphragmatic pressure generation (Pdi) achieved by inspiratory resistance loading as fraction of maximal diaphragmatic pressure generation (Pdi_{max}) is plotted against duration of time to fatigue in normal volunteers. As inspiratory load is increased such that breath requires near maximal diaphragm pressure generation, time to fatigue is exceedingly short. As this ratio approaches 40%, time to fatigue approaches infinite value, suggesting that spontaneous ventilation can be sustained. (Reproduced with permission from C Roussos and PT Macklem: J Appl Physiol 43:189, 1977.)

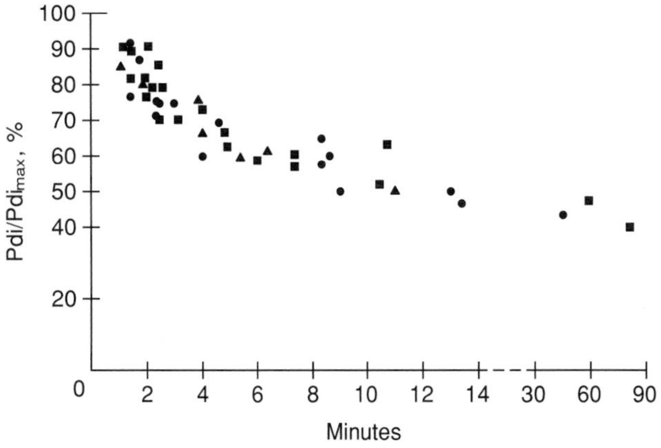

ratory muscles, as measured by the pressure generated by the ventilator during each breath, exceeds 30 cmH_2O. Such values predict that the patient's respiratory muscles will fatigue quickly if spontaneous ventilation were required, an hypothesis easily confirmed in such patients who breathe rapidly and insufficiently when taken off the ventilator.

Another measure of maximum respiratory effort in the conscious patient is VC. As a rough guideline in accord with the concept of Fig. 1-19, when VC is three times the V_T required to maintain eucapnia and normal pH, respiratory muscle fatigue is unlikely. A corresponding alternate measure of respiratory load is the minute ventilation ($\dot{V}_E$) required to maintain normal Pa_{CO_2} and pH. Factors which increase CO_2 production, deadspace, or metabolic acidosis necessarily increase this ventilation and so promote respiratory muscle fatigue. Such fatigue is often signalled by increased respiratory rate (f > 35/min), by paradoxical respiratory motion (the abdomen moves in with inspiration as the fatigued diaphragm is pulled craniad by the negative Ppl), and by the patient's unexplained somnolence or decreased responsiveness. Accordingly, evaluation of the patient's ability to resume spontaneous ventilation includes measurements of NIF, VC, V_T, f, and $\dot{V}_E$, observation of the respiratory motions during a period of spontaneous breathing, and asking the patient whether he or she is "getting enough air."

Respiratory muscle fatigue is thought to occur in many patients with type I AHRF or severe airflow obstruction and may occur to a lesser extent in patients with type III respiratory failure or with neuromuscular diseases. Current evidence and common sense suggest that the treatment for respiratory muscle fatigue is respiratory muscle rest, a strategy which must be balanced in nearly all patients against a thoughtful respiratory exercise program. The timing of the move from respiratory muscle rest to an exercise program is not currently guided by objective criteria identifying fatigue. Accordingly, many physicians who consider this problem develop empirical guidelines as to the likely presence of respiratory muscle fatigue integrated with the type of early ventilator management necessary for the patient's overall condition. For example, the cardiovascular stability and optimal ventilator management of patients with type I AHRF is frequently enhanced by respiratory muscle rest during the first 6 h after elective intubation for severe hypoxemia. During this time, the acutely depleted glycogen stores of the resting respiratory muscle are repleted, and the accumulated lactic acid or other metabolites associated with fatigue are washed out; then the patient is ready to move to a respiratory exercise program. In contrast, the patient with acute on chronic respiratory failure who has developed respiratory muscle fatigue over a longer period of time may require up to 72 h of respiratory muscle rest before resuming an exercise program free from fatigue.

It is important to note that many patients being managed for respiratory muscle rest by mechanical ventilation are actually working as hard or harder than during spontaneous ventilation by breathing actively against the ventilator. This is easily detected by clinical examination coupled with observation of the airway pressure which should rise at the start of each ventilated breath. In many patients, the airway pressure stays at or below zero during inspiration, indicating active inspiration by the patient; the amount and duration of inspiratory effort can often be assessed by the fall in central venous or pulmonary artery pressure with each inspiration. When respiratory rest is indicated, it can be achieved in these circumstances by increasing the inspiratory flow rate, by increasing the $\dot{V}_E$ or, if these measures of eliminating the patient's respiratory effort are inadequate, by sedating and paralyzing the patient to ensure respiratory rest.

VENTILATOR MODE AND RESPIRATORY MUSCLE EXERCISE

As soon as the patient with respiratory failure is stabilized on the ventilator, the physician should make a decision whether to rest the fatigued respiratory muscles or to institute a program of respiratory muscle exercise in those patients where fatigue is neither evident nor expected. The objective of the respiratory exercise program is to increase the tone, power, and coordination of the respiratory muscles. The efficacy of each program in increasing tone and power is evaluated by the daily NIF and VC measurements. Coordination is evaluated by bedside observation of how the patient's respiratory efforts interact with the ventilator and in a manner comfortable to the patient. Here, the goal is to adjust the ventilator such that the patient receives a breath on demand at a volume and frequency within the ranges expected for that patient off the ventilator. Several different modes of ventilation seek to achieve these goals of increased tone, power, and coordination during the liberation process.

Muscles may be strengthened by isometric or isotonic exercise. The simple common mode of *assist/control (A/C) volume-cycled ventilation* can be used for isometric exercise of the respiratory muscles as follows. With the V_T set at 8 to 10 mL/kg, the patient's spontaneous rate of triggering the ventilator at low sensitivity is noted. The control rate is set several breaths below the patient's spontaneous rate so that the patient will trigger all breaths. Then the sensitivity necessary to trigger the ventilator is decreased from the usual −1 to −2 cmH_2O toward a more negative value not to exceed −10 cmH_2O, or one-third of the patient's measured NIF, whichever comes first. The former limit is set because most patients feel uncomfortable with the trigger sensitivity more negative than −10, and the latter limit is set to avoid respiratory muscle fatigue as described above. The rate of progression from −1 toward these limits is titrated according to the patient's tolerance. Successful implementation of this respiratory exercise program is indicated by the patient's triggering every breath without respiratory distress, and its effect is confirmed by a progressively increasing value of NIF. Failure of this mode is indicated by the patient's inability to trigger every breath. This leads to respiratory discoordination and is cause to reduce the pressure needed to initiate a breath until the patient does trigger each breath. A second problem occurs when a patient's inspiratory efforts persist throughout the ventilated breath sufficient to keep the airway pressure below PEEP. Then the patient is actually doing all the work of breathing, including some imposed by the ventilator. This should be detected and corrected as described above before it leads to respiratory muscle fatigue.

A common ventilator mode for isotonic exercise is *synchronized intermittent mandatory ventilation (SIMV).* In this mode, a mandatory rate of about 8 breaths/min delivers a V_T of 8 to 10 mL/kg. Since this provides insufficient alveolar ventilation to eliminate all CO_2 production at a rate slower than patients enjoy, the patient breathes spontaneously between these intermittent mandatory breaths from a ventilator reservoir having the same $F_{I_{O_2}}$ and PEEP. So that the mandatory breath is not stacked on top of the patient's spontaneous breath, the ventilator is programmed to deliver the mandatory breath with the patient's spontaneous respiratory effort. Then the SIMV rate can be progressively reduced as the patient approaches liberation from the ventilator, such that the patient's spontaneous V_T and Vf approach that needed to ventilate independent from the ventilator. Successful SIMV moves progressively from a rate of 8 to a rate of 0 while the patient resumes spontaneous breathing; in the interim, NIF and VC should increase progressively. Failure of SIMV is indicated by an erratic breathing pattern in which the intermittent mandatory breaths have interspersed between them rapid (40 to 60 breaths/min) shallow (<150 mL) breaths confounding the goal of respiratory coordination and delaying liberation of the patient from the ventilator. In critical care units using both common modes of ventilation, it is not uncommon to see physicians attempt to increase patient exercise by reducing the control rate in the A/C mode—an intervention which has no effect on the patient's spontaneous trigger rate or respiratory muscle exercise but places the patient at risk of a low backup or control rate meant to be a safety factor in case the critically ill patient loses respiratory drive for any of a variety of reasons.

A third mode of ventilation which can provide an effective respiratory muscle exercise program is *pressure support.* Consider again the patient having a peak pressure on the ventilator of 30 cmH_2O and an NIF of 30 cmH_2O. As discussed above, this patient can probably generate about 10 cmH_2O with each inspiration without inducing respiratory muscle fatigue, so a pressure support of 20 cmH_2O can be provided such that the patient can generate the required inspiratory effort to maintain an adequate V_T. Here, the initial test of the adequacy of the patient's personal effort is whether the patient maintains the required V_T at an appropriately low respiratory rate. As the NIF increases with time on this mode, the pressure support can be progressively diminished from 20 toward 0 as tolerated within the limits preventing respiratory muscle fatigue and maintaining an acceptable respiratory pattern.

LIBERATION OF THE PATIENT FROM MECHANICAL VENTILATION

Like other emergencies, acute respiratory failure requires urgent resuscitative interventions, including mechanical ventilation. Because these interventions also impose complications, morbidity and mortality, they should be discontinued just as soon as they are no longer indicated. That process of withdrawing mechanical ventilation often proceeds more slowly than its urgent institution as part of the physician's caution to ensure that the patient can do without it. Indeed, the term "weaning" has been applied to connote the cautious withdrawal of a life-sustaining ventilator from a dependent patient. All too often, this subjects that patient to excessive duration of ventilator management with emphasis on a weaning mode (A/C, SIMV, pressure support) as the major intervention aimed to achieve spontaneous breathing. A more aggressive approach attempts to "liberate" the patients as soon as possible from mechanical ventilation by using the mode as an exercise program. Then ventilator mode becomes a thoughtful part of a larger program addressing *about 50 correctable factors* constraining the patient's freedom to breathe (Table 1-2).

This effective approach to liberating patients from the ventilator measures and attempts to increase the values of NIF and VC while simultaneously measuring and reducing the respiratory load. The left-hand column of Table 1-2 lists correctable factors to reduce the respiratory muscle load. As a general rule, these are the abnormal respiratory mechanics associated with the several types of acute respiratory failure. For type I AHRF, seeking the lowest pulmonary wedge pressure (Ppw) compatible with an adequate $\dot{Q}_T$ reduces edema formation. Preliminary evidence suggests that β agonists like terbutaline might enhance the clearance by active transport of pulmonary edema out of airspaces but the significance of this therapy is not yet clear. Appropriate, early antibiotic therapy combines with chest physiotherapy and bedside suctioning to minimize the mechanical load in pneumonia. Occasionally, draining large pleural effusions or stabilizing a flail chest can increase the efficiency of respiratory muscles in patients with AHRF. PEEP reduces elastic work of breathing by redistributing edema out of alveoli into the interstitium, and continual titration to the least PEEP achieving adequate O_2 exchange and the least V_T achieving adequate CO_2 elimination prevents untoward hyperinflation as the edema is cleared (see Chap. 128 for further discussion). In some patients with high alveolar pressures and low pulmonary artery pressure (Ppa), CO_2 retention is occasionally corrected by decreasing V_T and $\dot{V}_E$. This paradoxical effect is likely due to the reduced alveolar deadspace effected by lower alveolar pressure to recruit perfusion of those airspaces.

The left column of Table 1-2 lists the correctable factors of acute-on-chronic respiratory failure which are also relevant to managing the patient with status asthmaticus and may overlap considerably with type I and type III respiratory failure. Of course, the major reduction in resistive load in patients with severe airflow obstruction is effected by bronchodilator therapy (intravenous aminophylline, inhaled β agonists, systemic or inhaled steroids) to reduce the resistive component of the respiratory muscle load. Eliminating hypoxemia by providing adequate oxygen therapy often improves the patient's level of consciousness by increasing systemic oxygen transport, and has an often overlooked

TABLE 1-2 Liberation of the Patient from Mechanical Ventilation

Correctable Factors Decreasing Respiratory Muscle Load	Correctable Factors Increasing Respiratory Muscle Strength
Type I—AHRF	Type IV—Shock
Reduce edema production	Hypoperfusion
Enhance edema clearance	Hypotension
Treat pneumonia	Anemia
Drain pleural effusions	Hypoxia
Stabilize chest wall	Sepsis
"Least" PEEP	Fever
Minimize deadspace	Acidosis
	Electrolytes (K^+, Ca^{2+}, Mg^{2+}, PO_4^{3-})
Type II—Airflow Obstruction	Protein—calorie nutrition
Hypoxemia—give O_2	Aminophylline
Reverse sedation	
Bronchodilation	Common Confounding Conditions
Clear bronchial secretions	Neuromuscular disease
Treat bronchial infection	Muscle relaxing drugs
Pneumothorax—chest tube	Coma, sedation
Fractured ribs—nerve block	Cerebrovascular accident
Decrease PEEPi	Subclinical status epilepticus
Allow HCO_3 accumulation	Hypothyroidism
Reduce CO_2 production	Phrenic nerve paralysis
Type III—Perioperative Respiratory Failure	Respiratory Muscle Fatigue
Posturize and pummel	
Ventilate 45° upright	Respiratory Muscle Exercise Program
Incisional/abdominal pain	Tone
Drain ascites	Power
Reexpand atelectasis early	Coordination
Stop smoking	Animation
Avoid overhydration	

side effect of relieving hypoxic bronchoconstriction. This mechanism is most likely responsible for the observed CO_2 retention despite maintained $\dot{V}_E$ in patients with acute-on-chronic respiratory failure who receive sufficient oxygen therapy. Occasionally, the depressed sensorium may be corrected by reversing or reducing sedative drug effects, i.e., naloxone for opiates, flumazenil for benzodiazapines, or forced alkaline diuresis for phenobarbital. Treatment of the increased airway resistance is enhanced by effective clearing of bronchial secretions through endobronchial suctioning associated with posturizing, pummelling, and vibrating the patient's thorax, all combined with effective antibacterial therapy of endobronchial infections. The early diagnosis and treatment of intercurrent and complicating thoracic abnormalities (pneumothorax, fractured ribs) often increase the breathing efficiency of these patients. In severe airflow obstruction, ventilator settings which allow sufficient expiratory time (small V_T, reduced rate and $\dot{V}_E$, higher inspiratory flow rate), act to decrease PEEPi and lung hyperinflation which causes inefficiency and weakness of respiratory muscles. Furthermore, with PEEPi of 15 cmH_2O, the patient must generate sufficient inspiratory muscle activity to reduce the end-expired alveolar pressure by >15 cmH_2O before the next breath is delivered by the ventilator—an often overlooked component of the respiratory muscle load in patients with severe airflow obstruction. Such strategies to reduce PEEPi often reduce alveolar ventilation associated with CO_2 retention. In patients with acute-on-chronic respiratory failure, the accumulation of bicarbonate corrects the respiratory acidosis; this allows the patient to breathe less to maintain a normal pH, thereby lowering respiratory work. A complementary strategy is to identify and eliminate all factors causing excess CO_2 production (excess carbohydrate nutrition, fever, sepsis, excess respiratory muscle work).

Patients with hypoventilatory respiratory failure due to reduced CNS drive or inadequate neuromuscular coupling do not usually have increased respiratory muscle load. Accordingly, their management on the ventilator aims to prevent the complications of acquired infection and atelectasis. The principles of preventing or reversing type III perioperative respiratory failure are helpful to achieve these goals as listed in Table 1-2. Bedside nurses in the ICU turn the patient every 1 to 2 h from the supine position to the left or right lateral decubitus position; during this time, they provide vigorous chest physiotherapy with pummeling, chest vibration, and endotracheal suction. In patients vulnerable to atelectasis, a fourth position 30° to 45° upright is helpful by reducing the load imposed by the abdomen; also, the addition of sighs and PEEP return the end-expired lung volume to a position above the patient's CV. Special attention to the treatment of incisional or abdominal pain, (epidural anesthesia, transcutaneous nerve stimulation) and to minimize the intraabdominal pressure of ascites or tight bandages helps to prevent atelectasis. When lobe or lung collapse is detected by physical or radiologic examination, an early aggressive approach to reexpansion includes placing the patient in the lateral decubitus position with the collapsed lobe uppermost for vigorous pummelling and suctioning, and then increasing the V_T progressively to a pressure limit of 40 cmH_2O with end-inspiratory pauses. Reexpansion often occurs within 10 min and is signalled by a fall in the ΔPel associated with the normal V_T at the end of the reexpansion manuever; if this reexpansion is not confirmed radiologically, repeating these manuevers after bronchoscopy to clear endobronchial obstruction is indicated. Once reexpansion has occurred, the implementation of increased levels of PEEP or sighs or both often prevents further episodes of atelectasis. Discontinuation of smoking at least 6 weeks prior to elective operations reduces bronchorrhea and atelectasis, and avoiding overhydration in perioperative patients especially vulnerable to atelectasis reduces this problem.

The right column of Table 1-2 lists correctable factors increasing respiratory muscle strength, first in the context of those many disturbances of the circulation or internal environment most common to patients with type IV respiratory failure. Attempting to liberate patients with hypoperfusion states or hypotension is not successful. Correction of these hemodynamic variables complements the correction of anemia, hypoxemia, and acidosis to provide dramatic increases in the objectively measured respiratory muscle strength by NIF and VC. Similarly, attempting to liberate patients who are septic or have body temperatures >38.5°C (101.7°F) is often unsuccessful. While these systemic abnormalities are being corrected, it is also helpful to initiate adequate protein calorie nutrition using protein (1 g/kg) and calories (30 kcal/g protein), of which calories <50 percent should be carbohydrate and the rest are lipid. Elemental malnutrition is corrected by adjustments of serum potassium, calcium, magnesium and phosphate; severe abnormalities of each of these electrolytes are sufficient to cause respiratory muscle fatigue, so that modest abnormalities in the patient already weakened by critical illness may converge to make the patient weaker than necessary. When each of these abnormalities has been corrected, there is some evidence that respiratory muscles may be strengthened by the infusion of aminophylline in doses which achieve serum concentrations associated with effective bronchodilation.

When all other factors are corrected, but the patient remains weak, it is helpful to exclude clinical conditions which occasionally cause reduced respiratory muscle strength. Neuromuscular disease, muscle relaxing drugs, sedatives, coma, and intercurrent cerebral vascular accidents cause obscure reduction in respiratory muscle strength. Often overlooked causes of inadequate respiratory muscle function are subclinical status epilepticus, hypothyroidism, and paralysis of the phrenic nerve on one or both sides after cardiac surgery with cold cardioplegia or other thoracic trauma.

Systematic correction of the 50 abnormalities listed in Table 1-2 hastens the time when the patient's respiratory effort is able to handle the respiratory load without muscle fatigue. As the patient approaches this time, it is helpful for the physician to reevaluate the load at a smaller V_T approaching that with which most patients breathe after coming off the ventilator. Often, this is in the region of 4 to 6 mL/kg, or V_T of 300 to 500 mL, associated with an increase in respiratory rate to 24 to 36/min. Reevaluation of the elastic load of these smaller V_Ts will confirm a proportionately smaller elastic work of breathing. At that time it is also helpful for the physician to review with each patient the reasons for an optimistic prognosis for resuming spontaneous breathing. In this context, a brief (1 h) evaluation of the patient's ability to breathe is conducted by the bedside nurse or physician. Prior assurance to patients that they will be placed back on the ventilator if they are distressed, and that they will be attended closely during this demonstration of spontaneous ventilation anticipates and ameliorates anxiety. At the end of the trial, the NIF and VC may be measured again to indicate early signs of weakness or fatigue, and an arterial blood-gas sample is obtained to confirm the adequacy of alveolar ventilation. If patients feel comfortable, they may proceed soon after this initial trial to a longer period of spontaneous breathing culminating in the removal of the ventilator from the patient's room. Preparation of individual patients for their own breathing pattern and addressing directly the anxiety of resuming spontaneous breathing turns this final step in the liberation process into a confirmation instead of a major hurdle fraught with high incidence of "failure to wean." This latter outcome occurs with progressive tachypnea, diaphoresis, pallor, hypertension, and tachycardia, usually without any deterioration in lung gas exchange before the patient is placed back on the ventilator. This constellation of symptoms and signs is best explained as a sympathetic nervous system response to disordered proprioception of breathing and anxiety.

The timing of this last step in liberating the patient from the ventilator is often influenced by the patient's general demeanor as much as by the objective indicators of respiratory strength and load. A close relationship between the patient and the physician/nurse/respiratory therapy team during this liberation process allows members of the team to anticipate accurately the golden moment when the patient is ready to breathe spontaneously. This moment is often indicated as much by the gleam in the patient's eye as by objective indicators. Throughout this process, a concerted effort is directed to animating the patient. This approach includes physiotherapy, active and passive limb exercises, and timely mobilization of the patient from the bed to chair to ambulation; daytime stimulation by encouraging visitors, interactions with the bedside nurse, patient-selected radio, TV or tapes; and nighttime rest aided by minimal short-acting sedatives and minimal disturbances by unit light and noise. All promote animation of the patient and earlier liberation from mechanical ventilation.

Chapter 2

THE CARDIOVASCULAR SYSTEM

L.D.H. WOOD

A primary role of the cardiovascular system is to deliver energy sources from the gut and liver, and oxygen from the lungs, to all systemic organ systems for their aerobic metabolism; effluent from these tissues removes the waste products of metabolism, delivering them to the lungs, kidney, and liver for excretion. This process is facilitated by return of the whole circulation through the lungs, where CO_2 is eliminated and O_2 is taken up to arterialize the blood. As depicted in Fig. 2-1, this central circulation is located within the thoracic cavity; movement of gas between the atmosphere and the alveolar space is effected by the respiratory muscles—especially the diaphragm, depicted in Fig. 2-1 as a piston at the floor of the thoracic cavity. Beyond effecting ventilation to permit pulmonary gas exchange, spontaneous movement of the piston lowers the pleural pressure (Ppl), which approximates the pressure on the outside of extraalveolar vessels including the right and left heart (depicted as chambers labeled *Pra* and *Pla*); changes in alveolar pressure (PA) affect pressures within alveolar vessels. Once the blood leaves the lung and enters the left heart, the ventricular pumping function ejects blood into the stiff, high-resistance arterial circulation to perfuse the systemic capillary beds, where O_2 is consumed and CO_2 taken up before the venous blood returns to the right heart through the large-volume, very compliant, low-resistance venous circuit.

This chapter reviews the physiology of this circuit as a basis for understanding the many disturbances of circulation associated with critical illness. It begins with a description of left ventricular pumping function, follows with the mechanisms whereby the cardiac output ($\dot{Q}_T$) is controlled by the systemic vessels, and completes the circuit with a discussion of the pulmonary circulation and lung liquid flux. Along the way, common mechanical interactions between respiration and the circulation are highlighted, and diagnostic and management approaches to ventricular dysfunction, shock, pulmonary hypertension, and edema are outlined.

Ventricular Mechanics

VENTRICULAR-VASCULAR COUPLING

Figure 2-2 illustrates the typical events in the two phases of ventricular activity: active contraction (systole) and relaxation (diastole). In Fig. 2-2 (diastole), the left ventricle is filling through the open mitral valve from the left atrium while the aortic valve is closed. Following electrical stimulation and contraction of the left ventricle, in Fig. 2-2 (systole), a stroke volume (SV) is being ejected into the proximal arterial chamber. Because more blood is being ejected than runs off through the peripheral resistance located in the distal arterioles, the arterial walls are distended outward, raising the pressure (P) in inverse proportion to the capacitance ($C = \Delta V/\Delta P$) of the walls of the larger arteries proximal to the resistance vessels. As the ventricle's vol-

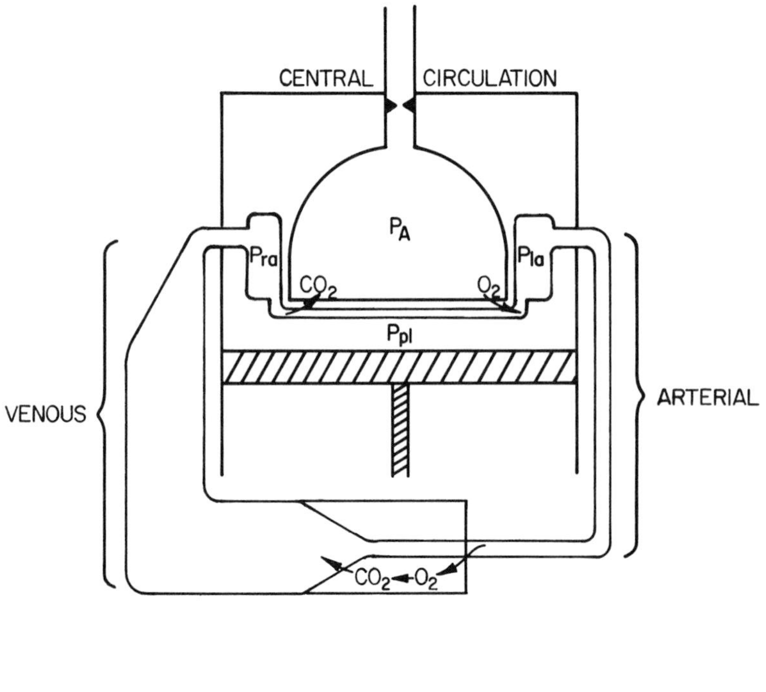

FIGURE 2-1 Schematic representation of the circulation proceeding from the left atrium (where pressure is denoted *Pla*) through a high-pressure arterial system (low volume, low compliance, high resistance) to the peripheral tissues (where O_2 leaves the vessels to produce energy and CO_2, shown entering the vessels), then proceeding through the low-pressure venous system (high volume, high compliance, low resistance), which returns blood to the right atrium (where pressure is denoted *Pra*). The circuit is completed by perfusing the lung back to the left atrium; the pulmonary vessels are shown in close apposition with the alveoli (where pressure is denoted *PA*), facilitating gas exchange. This central circulation is enclosed in the thorax, the floor of which is the diaphragm (indicated by the piston). Between the lungs and the thorax is the pleural space (where pressure is denoted *Ppl*); Ppl approximates the pressure on the outside of all extraalveolar vessels within the central circulation, including the heart, whereas PA is the pressure outside the alveolar vessels. The anatomic arrangement accounts for the many mechanical interactions between respiration and circulation in critical illness described throughout this chapter.

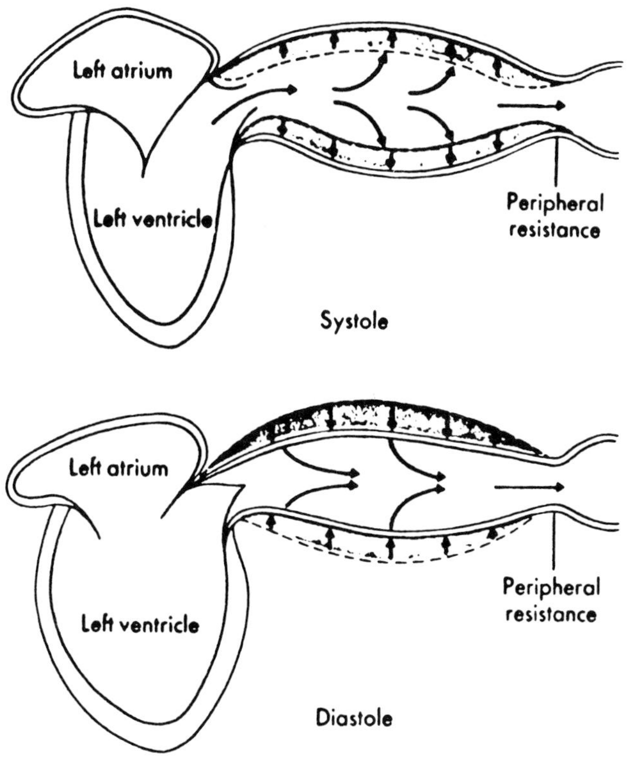

FIGURE 2-2 During ventricular systole the stroke volume ejected by the ventricle results in some forward capillary flow, but most of the ejected volume is stored in the elastic arteries. During ventricular diastole the elastic recoil of the arterial walls maintain capillary flow through the remainder of the cardiac cycle. Accordingly, PP is proportional to SV, and DP increases with peripheral resistance, HR, and vascular capacitance, all of which reduce the diastolic runoff of the ejected volume. (Reproduced, with permission, from Berne RM, Levy MN (eds): *Physiology*. St. Louis, Mosby, 1988, p 487.)

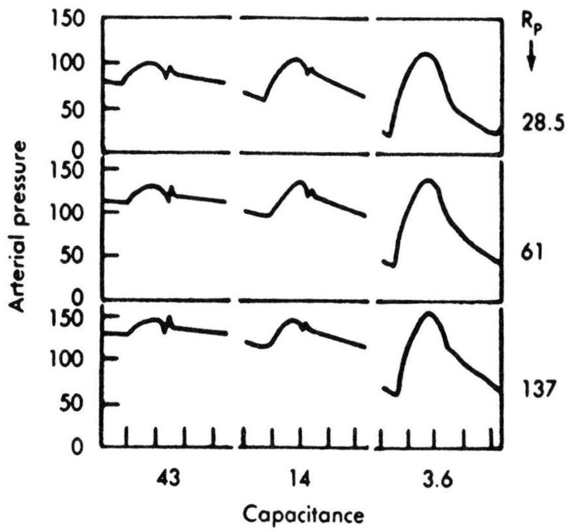

FIGURE 2-3 The changes in aortic pressures with changes in arterial capacitance and peripheral resistance (Rp). (Reproduced, with permission, from Berne RM, and Levy MN (eds): *Physiology*. St. Louis, Mosby, 1988, p 491.)

ume decreases, its ability to generate pressure decreases, as dictated by the mechanical properties of cardiac muscle (see below), until ventricular systolic pressure falls below the simultaneous arterial pressure. Then the aortic valve closes, as indicated by the dicrotic notch on the arterial pressure pulse (see Fig. 2-3). As the ventricle relaxes, the mitral valve opens, and the ventricle fills along its diastolic volume-pressure (V-P) curve; this diastolic filling is aided by atrial contraction and by suction by the ventricle relaxing from its low end-contraction volume. During diastole, the part of the SV stored in the distended arterial bed continues to run off through the peripheral resistance, associated with a progressive fall in the arterial pressure until the next contraction.

This ventricular-vascular coupling acts as a hydraulic filter to convert the intermittent ejection of an SV into a continuous organ flow. It also reduces the work of the heart by allowing some of the energy imparted by the systolic ventricle to the blood to be stored in distention of the arterial chamber and returned to the circulation by continued flow while the ventricle is resting in diastole. The peripheral, or systemic, vascular resistance (SVR) is also essential both to the control of blood pressure (BP = $\dot{Q}_T \times$SVR) and to the distribution of blood flow among, or within, organs according to tissue needs. For example, in conditions of hypovolemic or cardiogenic shock, reflex sympathetic output constricts arterioles, especially in the mesenteric, renal, and skin vascular beds to preserve flow to vital organs like the heart and brain, by maintaining aortic BP; alternatively, during pyrexia and tachypnea, the increased metabolic need demands a high $\dot{Q}_T$ associated with dilatation of the coronary and respiratory muscle vessels induced by accumulation of anaerobic metabolites (adenosine, H^+, K^+) to maintain adequate O_2 flow to these vital pumps.

For a given state of ventricular pumping function, the arterial pulse pressure changes considerably with changes in the mechanical characteristics of the arterial circuit (see Fig. 2-3). The center panel shows a typical arterial pulse wave, having a systolic pressure (SP) of 120 mmHg, a diastolic pressure (DP) of 80 mmHg, and a dicrotic notch (DN) of about 90 mmHg, which approximates the mean BP. In the panel immediately below, the increase in SVR causes DP to increase to 110 mmHg because of reduced peripheral runoff; then, the SV raises SP to a higher value of 140 mmHg. Note that the pulse pressure (PP), at 30 mmHg, is reduced compared to that in the central panel (PP = 40 mmHg) because the SV is slightly reduced by the increased afterload (see below). Conversely, in the panel immediately above the center panel, a reduction in the SVR lowers DP to 50 mmHg, so the mean BP and SP are both reduced, as is typically noted in patients with septic shock. Note that PP is increased because SV is increased, in part because of reduced ventricular afterload (see below). Moving to the right of the center panel, the compliance, or capacitance, of the arterial circuit is much decreased, so that the stiff vessels discharge the stored SV very rapidly through the normal SVR; accordingly, DP is reduced, but

SP is normal or increased because PP is very large in these stiff vessels. Such PP levels account for the systolic hypertension in elderly patients with considerable atherosclerosis stiffening the central arterial chamber. In contrast, the panel to the left of the central panel shows the small PP characteristic of children with large arterial capacitance.

Clinical evaluation of the cardiovascular system in patients with critical illness is much aided by interpretation of the DP, the PP, and indices of SVR—such as the rate of nail bed color return after releasing pressure on the fingernail, and digital temperature. For example, a hypotensive patient with a heart rate (HR) of 110 beats per minute (bpm), an SP/DP of 100/40, and warm extremities with good nail bed return has a high $\dot{Q}_T$ and a low SVR. This is so because the large PP (60 mmHg) signals a large SV, which, when multiplied by increased HR, gives increased $\dot{Q}_T$; and the low DP indicates rapid peripheral runoff through low SVR confirmed by digital examination and low mean BP (60 mmHg) in the face of the high $\dot{Q}_T$. By contrast, a second hypotensive patient with the same HR and mean BP but an SP/DP of 80/65 and cold extremities with very slow nail bed return has a low $\dot{Q}_T$ with increased SVR indicated by the small PP (hence low SV and $\dot{Q}_T$), preserved DP, and constricted digital vessels. Of course, the relationship between PP and SV is not quantitative, because it is proportioned by an unknown constant—the vascular capacitance. Nevertheless, in a given critically ill patient whose vascular capacitance changes minimally in a course of acute interventions, a change in PP is the earliest indicator of a change in SV.

The relationships between the vascular mechanical characteristics and PP is illustrated by comparing systemic (120/80) with pulmonary artery pulse pressure (20/10). Since the SVs from the left and right ventricles are equal, the fourfold difference in PP is due in large part to the much lower capacitance of the thick systemic arteries than that of the thin, distensible, pulmonary arteries. Similarly, the sixfold difference in mean systemic BP (90 mmHg) from mean pulmonary artery blood pressure (Ppa = 15 mmHg) is due to the very much lower pulmonary vascular resistance (PVR), compared to SVR. Because PVR is so low, a substantial portion of the right ventricular SV traverses the pulmonary vascular bed during systole, so much less is stored in the pulmonary vessels during ejection than is stored in the systemic vessels. As a result, the pulmonary vascular distention is less than the systemic vascular distention during systole for a given SV, so pulmonary PP is reduced even further than one would predict for the difference in capacitance between the two vessels. It is not uncommon for physicians to express the relationship between BP and $\dot{Q}_T$ as a single calculated value: $SVR = (BP - Pra)/\dot{Q}_T \times 80$, where "Pra" is right atrial pressure and 80 is a constant correcting the resistance units (mmHg/L/min) to metric units (dyne·s/cm^5). This calculation assumes that Pra is the outflow pressure at the end of the circulation, and implies that changes in SVR signal changes in vascular caliber. Yet the effective outflow pressure is the critical closing pressure (Pc) in collapsible arterioles having vascular tone that can change Pc from 5 to 40 mmHg! Accordingly, in evaluating the vascular resistance it is less misleading to report and relate the important measured variables, BP and $\dot{Q}_T$; subtracting Pra and multiplying by 80 imparts no further information.

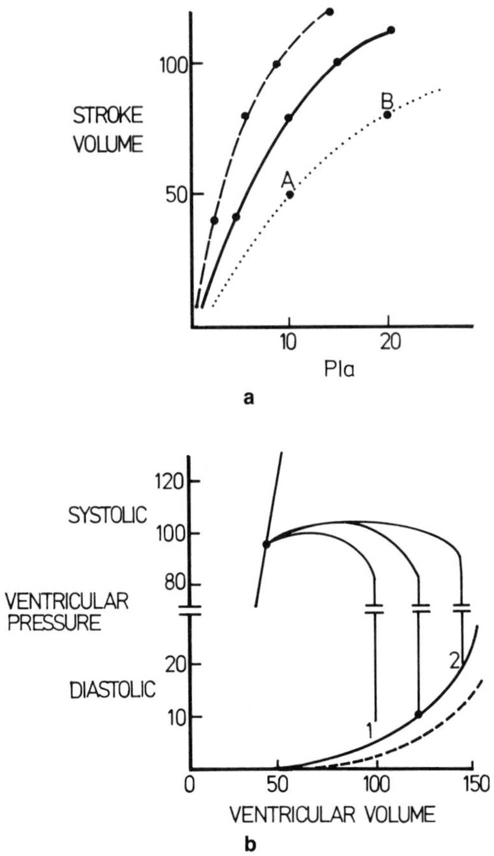

FIGURE 2-4 ***a.*** **Several Starling function curves: SV (ordinate, mL) is plotted against Pla (mmHg) on the abscissa. The middle continuous line depicts a normal Starling function curve for comparison with a depressed curve (dotted line AB), and with a curve depicting enhanced ventricular function (interrupted curve); note that all three curves may have the same systolic function (contractility) if diastolic volume-pressure (V-P) relations or afterload differ from each other.** ***b.*** **The corresponding left ventricular volume (abscissa, mL)–pressure (ordinate, mmHg) relationships; note the break in the ordinate scale to emphasize the normal diastolic V-P curve (continuous line 1,2) and the end-systolic V-P relationship (continuous line up and to the left). For discussion of the three V-P loops originating from the diastolic curve, see text. The interrupted diastolic V-P curve depicts a more compliant chamber such as the right ventricle, where there is less diastolic pressure for each volume.**

THE STARLING CURVE OF THE HEART

Figure 2-4*a* presents Starling relationships of the heart. On the abscissa is plotted left atrial pressure (Pla), which approximates the filling pressure of the left ventricle. On the ordinate is plotted SV (mL); this volume ejected per beat of the heart is one measure of ventricular output. It can be expressed as another measure of output by multiplying by the pressure developed during each beat to obtain stroke work ($SW = SV \times (BP - Pla)$). As filling pressure of the heart increases, the ejected volume and the work done by the heart increase in a curvilinear manner; at higher filling pressures there is less increase in SV per increase in Pla than at lower values of Pla. On the continuous Starling curve in Fig. 2.4*a*, the normal Pla (10 mmHg) is associated with a normal SV (75 mL) calculated from $\dot{Q}_T$ (6.0 L/min) divided by HR (80 bpm). When hypovolemia lowers Pla to 5 mmHg, SV falls to 40 mL, lowering $\dot{Q}_T$; if therapeutic expansion of the circulating volume raises Pla to 20 mmHg, SV increases to 100 mL, raising $\dot{Q}_T$ above normal.

These relationships are a common framework for understanding ventricular function in critical illness. A shift up and to the left of the Starling curve generally indicates enhanced ventricular function, with greater SV for a given filling pressure (see interrupted curve). Note that the interrupted curve would also represent right ventricular function if Pra were plotted against SV, because the filling pressure of the thin right ventricle is less than that of the thick left ventricle. Note further that if both right ventricle and left ventricle curves were expressed as SW, the Starling curve for the right ventricle would now lie down and to the right of the left ventricle curve, because the pressure developed by the right ventricle (Ppa − Pra) is only one-sixth that generated by the left ventricle (BP-Pla). Conversely, a shift down and to the right, with reduced SV at a given filling pressure (see dotted Starling curve through A, B), indicates depressed ventricular function. Of course, the lower SV for Pla of 10 mmHg at A could be due to reduced contractility, to increased BP allowing the same SW to eject a smaller SV at A, or to a stiffer ventricle allowing a smaller left ventricular end diastolic volume (LVEDV) at Pla = 10 mmHg. This variety of mechanisms to explain the same data is a limitation of the analysis of hemodynamics by the Starling curve, so a more complete description of ventricular function is helpful.

The ventricular function revealed by the Starling relationship is based on the mechanical properties of the relaxed (diastolic) and the contracting (systolic) volume-pressure relationships of the ventricle. This section reviews the factors that influence the diastolic and systolic mechanics in health and disease, and relates these mechanics to the corresponding Starling function curves of the heart. In Fig. 2-4*b*, left ventricular pressures at end-diastole and end-systole (LVEDP, LVESP) are plotted against the corresponding volumes (LVEDV, LVESV). The continuous end-diastolic V-P curve is marked with a dot at LVEDP 10 mmHg, where the normal LVEDV is 120 mL. When the ventricle contracts, pressure rises at the same volume until the aortic valve is opened, and blood is ejected until the valve closes again at LVESV = 45 mL. The stroke volume (LVEDV − LVESV) is 75 mL, as plotted on the continuous Starling curve in Fig. 2-4*a*. When hypovolemia reduces LVEDV (marked "1" in Fig. 2-4*b*), both LVEDP and SV decrease along the Starling curve above; if volume expansion increases LVEDV to the level marked "2," both SV and LVEDP increase along the Starling curve. The interrupted diastolic V-P curve in the lower panel plots the normal RV curve, where a smaller end-diastolic pressure (EDP) is associated with each end-diastolic volume (EDV). Hence, the corresponding interrupted RV Starling curve in the upper panel is shifted up and to the left of the continuous LV curve.

Note that the intracardiac pressures, such as Pla, are measured with respect to atmospheric pressure, so they do not represent true transmural, or filling, pressures of the heart chamber when the pressure on the outside of the heart is not atmospheric. Pericardial pressure is most often equal to pleural pressure (Ppl), which is subatmospheric during spontaneous breathing (−3 to −10 mmHg), and can become very negative in airflow obstruction or very positive with mechanical ventilation and positive end-expiratory pressure (PEEP). For convenience, the following discussion refers to the intravascular pressures as transmural or filling pressures, and any cause for altered pericardial pressure is noted.

THE DIASTOLIC VOLUME-PRESSURE (V-P) CURVE AND VENTRICULAR FILLING DISORDERS

FIgure 2-4*b* plots left ventricular diastolic volume against left ventricular diastolic pressure. As ventricular volume increases from zero, the transmural pressure of the ventricle does not exceed zero until about 50 mL (the unstressed volume) is added. Then LVEDP increases in a curvilinear manner with ventricular volume (the stressed volume); at first there is a large change in volume for a small change in pressure, and then a small change in volume for a large change in pressure. If the pericardium is removed, these V-P characteristics are more linear, so that the large change in LVEDP at higher values of LVEDV is no longer evident. Thus the pericardium acts like a membrane with a large unstressed volume surrounding the heart loosely up to a given ventricular volume, but at greater LVEDV it becomes very stiff. At higher heart volumes, most of the pressure across the heart is across the pericardium, accounting for the very steep rise in the diastolic V-P relationship. In the presence of the pericardial effusion, the volume at which the pericardium becomes a limiting membrane is reduced by the volume of the effusion. When the effusion is large enough, reduced end-diastolic volumes are associated with quite large end-diastolic pressures. In turn, these pressures reduce venous return (VR) by raising Pra, keeping both end-diastolic volume and $\dot{Q}_T$ abnormally low. Tension pneumothorax, massive pleural effusions, high levels of PEEP, and greatly increased abdominal pressures can all act to raise pressure outside the heart (Ppl), and so reduce LVEDV and SV despite high values of LVEDP.

Several other abnormalities in critical illness can impair the diastolic filling of the ventricle. Table 2-1 lists these conditions associated with high left atrial or pulmonary artery occlusion pressures (Ppw) and low LVEDV. Intercurrent left ventricular hypertrophy or infiltrative diseases (amyloidosis) occasionally stiffen the relaxed ventricle so that high filling pressures are needed to maintain an adequate SV, and inadequate filling time or poorly coordinated atrial contraction impairs ventricular filling. A right-to-left shift of the interventricular septum can also restrict diastolic filling, as depicted in Fig. 2-5. The normal diastolic V-P relation-

TABLE 2-1 Common Causes of Diastolic Dysfunction in Critically Ill Patients Signaled by High Left Atrial Pressure (Pla) and Low Left Ventricular End-Diastolic Volume (LVEDV)

External compression
Pericardial effusion or constriction
Positive-pressure ventilation with PEEP
Tension pneumothorax, massive pleural effusions
Greatly increased abdominal pressure
Myocardial stiffness
Left ventricular hypertrophy—aortic stenosis, systemic hypertension
Infiltrative diseases—amyloidosis
Ischemic heart disease
Ventricular interdependence and right-to-left septal shift
Pulmonary hypertension
Right ventricular infarction
High levels of PEEP
Intraventricular filling defects
Tumor
Clot
Rhythm or valvular impediments to filling
Tachycardia
Heart block
Atrial fibrillation or flutter
Mitral stenosis

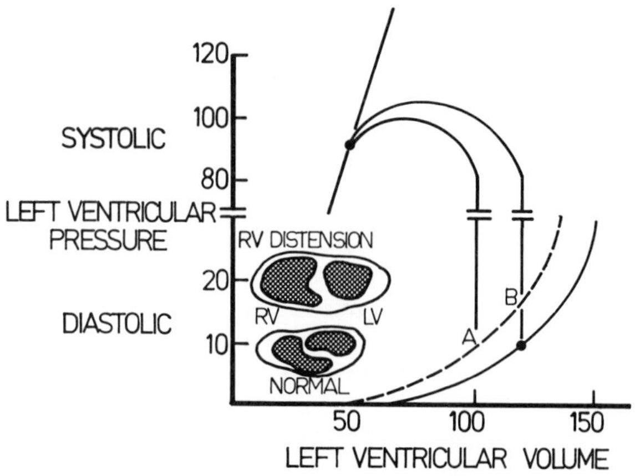

FIGURE 2-5 Ventricular interdependence affects the diastolic V-P relationship. The axes are labeled as in Fig. 2-4, and the continuous diastolic and systolic V-P relationships are as measured in the normal heart, which fills the right ventricle (RV) and left ventricle (LV) homogeneously (as depicted in the lower inset cross section of a normal heart). In contrast, right ventricular distention (upper inset) displaces the septum from right to left and encroaches on the volume of LV, causing the end-diastolic V-P curve to shift up and to the left (interrupted curve AB).

ship is measured during synchronous filling of the left and right ventricles, and these relationships are quite similar to those measured in the excised heart. In the excised heart, the effects of unequal filling of the two ventricles have been shown to cause a shift in the diastolic V-P curve on account of ventricular interdependence, as follows: Beginning at the unstressed volumes of each ventricle, equal volumes are added to each ventricle and the corresponding pressures are measured along the continuous end-diastolic V-P curve (Fig. 2-5); the lower inset shows a cross section of the heart with homogeneous filling of the two ventricles separated by a normal interventricular septum. At the upper limits of ventricular volume, the left ventricle alone is emptied and then filled again while the right ventricle remains distended, as in the upper inset in Fig. 2-5. The new diastolic curve is associated with a corresponding increased LVEDP at each left ventricular volume (see interrupted diastolic V-P curve in Fig. 2-5). Presumably, the distention of the right ventricle causes the interventricular septum to bulge from right to left, thereby reducing the unstressed volume and compliance of the left ventricle. This effect of ventricular interdependence is much less marked when the pericardium is removed, perhaps because the limiting membrane of the pericardium restricts freedom of motion of the left ventricle, making it more vulnerable to displacements of the septum.

Accordingly, conditions in which the right ventricle is abnormally loaded (e.g., acute pulmonary embolism, acute-on-chronic respiratory failure due to obstructive or restrictive lung disease), may impede the emptying of the right ventricle, causing it to work at a higher end-diastolic volume. Then left ventricular filling pressures will be higher than expected for the end-diastolic volume. This provides one possible explanation for why PEEP is often associated with increased filling pressure to maintain a normal stroke volume even when LVEDP is corrected to the true filling pressure by subtracting the increase in Ppl (ΔPpl) measured when PEEP is applied. For example, the SV of 75 mL at LVEDP of 10 mmHg depicted by the contraction beginning from the dot in Fig. 2-5 would be related to an LVEDP of 17 mmHg at B on the interrupted V-P curve during PEEP; and at the same LVEDP of 10 mmHg, SV is reduced by PEEP when LVEDV is reduced to A in Fig. 2-5. Note that these results are observed with no change in the end-systolic V-P curve; note further that the values of LVEDP have been corrected for observed effects of PEEP on Ppl and pericardial pressure, so the true transmural filling pressures are plotted.

Acute myocardial ischemia also displaces the diastolic V-P curve of the left ventricle upward and to the left. It is conceivable that the myocardial injury alters the elastic properties of the relaxed ventricle. Then, a higher ventricular filling pressure is required at each end-diastolic volume. This accounts for the oft-noted observation that patients with acute myocardial injury need values of LVEDP as high as 20 mmHg to maintain adequate $\dot{Q}_T$, while normal patients need filling pressures less than 10 mmHg. Some therapeutic agents (e.g., sodium nitroprusside) used in the management of acute myocardial injury actually return the diastolic V-P relationships toward normal. This effect may be advantageous if it reduces myocardial oxygen consumption by reducing diastolic wall stress without reducing the end-diastolic volume responsible for the subsequent SV. Plotted in terms of Starling relationships, the effects of these agents are to reduce filling pressure without changing SV—an observation suggesting improved pumping func-

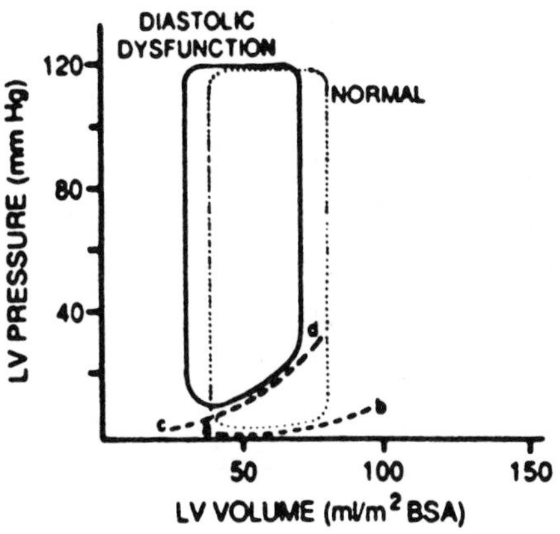

	NORMAL	DIASTOLIC DYSFUNCTION
END DIASTOLIC VOLUME (ml/m^2)	80	70
END SYSTOLIC VOLUME (ml/m^2)	40	30
STROKE VOLUME (ml/m^2)	40	40
EJECTION FRACTION (%)	50	56
END DIASTOLIC PRESSURE (mm Hg)	10	25
MEAN DIASTOLIC PRESSURE (mm Hg)	5	18

a

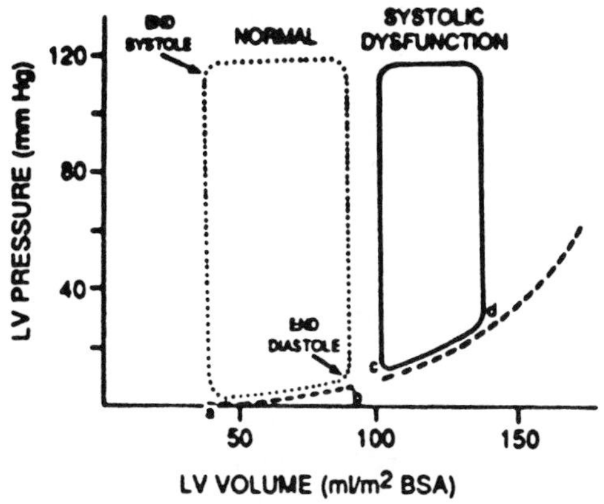

	NORMAL	SYSTOLIC DYSFUNCTION
END DIASTOLIC VOLUME (ml/m^2)	80	135
END SYSTOLIC VOLUME (ml/m^2)	40	105
STROKE VOLUME (ml/m^2)	40	30
EJECTION FRACTION (%)	50	20
END DIASTOLIC PRESSURE (mm Hg)	10	25

b

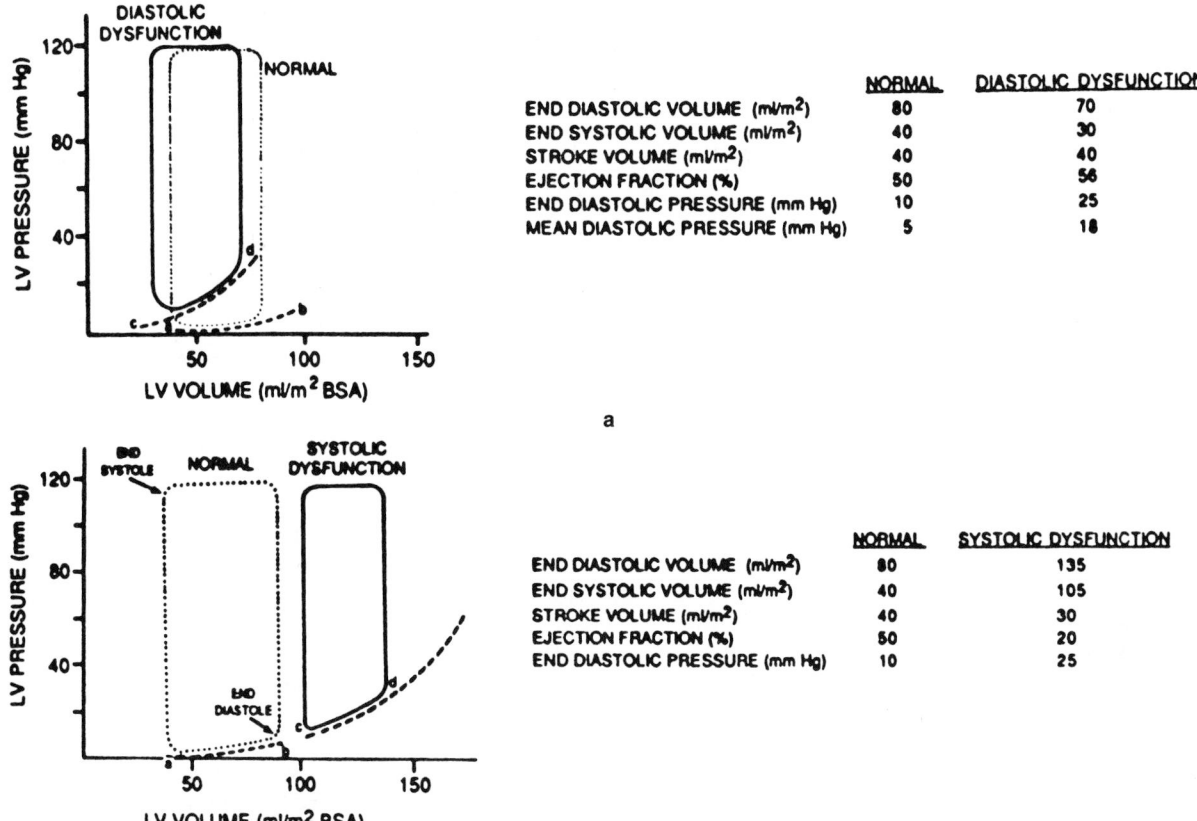

FIGURE 2-6 ***a.*** **Schematic diagram of a V-P loop from a normal subject (dotted line) and one with diastolic dysfunction (solid line). Interrupted lines represent the diastolic V-P relations. Isolated diastolic dysfunction is characterized by a leftward shift of the V-P loop. Contractile performance is normal (normal or increased ejection fraction; normal or decreased SV). However, left ventricular pressures throughout diastole are increased; at a common diastolic volume equal to 70 mL/m^2, left ventricular diastolic pressure is 25 mmHg in the patient with diastolic failure, compared with 5 mmHg in a normal subject.** ***b.*** **Schematic diagram of the V-P loop from a normal subject (dotted line) and one with systolic dysfunction (solid line). The interrupted line represents the diastolic pressure-volume relation. Systolic dysfunction is characterized by a displacement of the pressure-volume loop to the right. Despite compensatory dilation, SV and ejection fraction remains low. Left ventricular diastolic pressures are increased as a result of large left ventricular volume. (Reproduced, with permission, from Zile MR: Diastolic dysfunction. Mod Concepts Cardiovasc Dis 59:1, 1990.)**

tion of the left ventricle. Yet, nitroprusside does not enhance the systolic characteristics of the left ventricle. Conversely, the effects of PEEP on Starling relationships are to depress the SV at a given filling pressure, suggesting reduced ventricular contractility. Again, this conclusion is misleading, for the ventricular pumping function has not been changed; only the diastolic V-P relationship has been. This distinction is illustrated by comparison of the abnormalities in V-P loops and corresponding hemodynamic measurements between a patient with diastolic dysfunction (Fig. 2-6*a*) and one with systolic dysfunction (Fig. 2-6*b*).

THE END-SYSTOLIC V-P CURVE AND CONTRACTILITY

We now turn to the systolic mechanics. Figure 2-7 plots left ventricular volume, on the abscissa, against left ventricular pressure, on the ordinate. The normal diastolic relationship is drawn in the lower right-hand portion of each panel. Consider the left panel, in which a ventricle during systole contracts without ejecting any blood. A large pressure (A) is generated during this isovolumic contraction from a normal LVEDV (marked "I"). When LVEDV is reduced to the level marked "2," the pressure generated during a similar isovolumic contraction is much less (B), as a manifestation of the force-length characteristics of the myocardium. That is, the less the muscle is stretched, the less force it can generate. The units of force in the hollow sphere of myocardium are the units of pressure, or force per unit area. When end-diastolic volume is decreased to the level marked "3," isovolumic pressure decreases further (C), so that a line connecting the end-systolic pressure volume points (ABC) is linear and extrapolates toward the origin.

Now consider a different experimental situation, in which the ventricle can eject against a pressure afterload that is controlled. When the pressure afterload is set at B, the ventricle shortens from "I" to an LVESV lying on the end-systolic V-P curve at B (see interrupted SV line). If

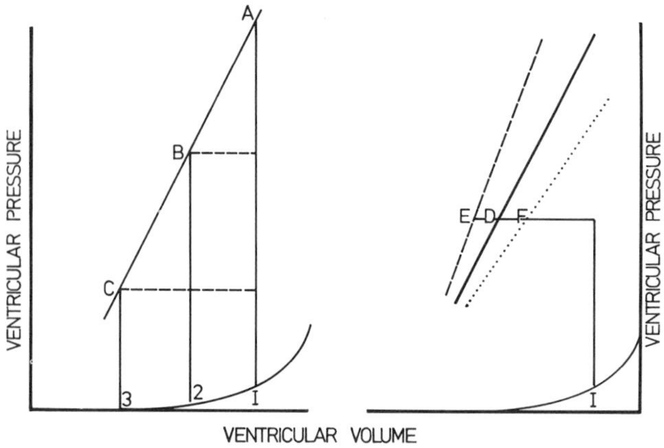

FIGURE 2-7 An operational index of contractility in critical illness—the end-systolic V-P curve. Ventricular pressure (ordinates) is plotted against ventricular volume (abscissa). ***left panel:*** **Isovolumetric contractions of the ventricles from three end-diastolic volumes (I, 2, 3) generate descending maximum pressures (A, B, C) to produce the end-systolic V-P line (ABC). At end-diastolic volume 1, reduction of the pressure afterload from B to C allows the ventricle to eject further, thereby increasing SV (for further discussion, see text).** ***right panel:*** **Compared to the normal end-systolic V-P relationship (D), infusion of epinephrine or other inotropic agents enhances contractility by shifting the end-systolic V-P curve upward and to the left (interrupted curve), so that SV increases from the same end-diastolic volume (labeled I) and the same end-systolic pressure afterload by enabling ejection to a smaller end-systolic volume (labeled E). By contrast, propranolol or other negative inotropic intervention depresses contractility, as indicated by the dotted end-systolic V-P curve shifted downward and to the right, so that SV is reduced at the same end-diastolic volume (I) and end-systolic pressure afterload by impairing ejection to a larger end-systolic volume (F) (for further discussion, see text).**

LVESP is reduced to C, the ventricle shortens further from the same LVEDP ("1") to the smaller LVESV, so the interrupted SV line is increased. Note that the contracting ventricle was able to shorten against the afterload pressure B until its volume reached "2"; at that lower volume, the maximum pressure that can be generated is equal to the afterload (B) pressure, so the aortic valve closes and ejection is over. Similarly, when afterload pressure decreases from B to C, the ventricle can eject further, to "3," where the maximum generated pressure equals the afterload and the aortic valve is closed at the combination of LVESP and LVESV marked "C."

The line ABC, connecting all measured end-systolic V-P points, is an indicator of the pumping function, or contractility, of the heart; for this line defines the volume to which the ventricle can shorten against each afterload for a given contractile state. In the right panel of Fig. 2-7, line ABC is replotted as the continuous line D, and the typical V-P loop is drawn schematically from LVEDV "1." Agents that enhance contractility (epinephrine, calcium, dobutamine, dopamine) shift the end systolic V-P relationship upward and to the left, as indicated by the interrupted line (E). Then the ventricle can shorten to a smaller end-systolic volume (marked "E") for each afterload, thereby increasing SV at a given LVEDV and LVEDP. Conversely, negative inotropes (like propranolol) and myocardial ischemia move the end-systolic V-P relationship downward and to the right, as indicated by the dotted line (F). Then end-systolic volume is increased for a given pressure afterload (marked "F"), reducing the SV at a given filling pressure. Such a reduction in contractility is another cause for the depressed Starling curve AB in Fig. 2-4*a*; its effect on the V-P loop and corresponding hemodynamic measurements are illustrated in Fig. 2-6*b*.

AN APPROACH TO ACUTE VENTRICULAR DYSFUNCTION

These concepts provide a framework for understanding the pathophysiology and therapy of acute myocardial infarction. Figure 2-8 depicts normal diastolic and systolic V-P relationships and indicates a normal systolic ejection *(continuous lines)*. From LVEDV = 120 mL and LVEDP = 10 mmHg, the ventricle contracts isovolumically until the aortic valve opens at DP = 80 mmHg. Blood is then ejected as SP rises to 110 and falls again toward LVESP = 90 mmHg and LVESV = 50 mL, when the aortic valve closes to generate the dicrotic notch on the arterial pressure trace. Accordingly, SV is 70 mL at Pla = 10 and $\dot{Q}_T$ is 5.6 L/min when HR = 80 bpm. Acute myocardial infarction depresses the end-systolic V-P relationship so that the end-systolic volume is increased to 90 mL at a reduced LVESP = 75 mmHg *(interrupted line)*. At the same time, the end-diastolic volume is increased to 130 mL to accommodate the VR, and end-diastolic pressure is increased even more than expected (LVEDP = 30 mmHg) because of the shift upward and to the left of the end-diastolic V-P relationship *(interrupted line)*. Thus stroke volume (40 mL) and $\dot{Q}_T$ (4.4 L/min)

FIGURE 2-8 Schematic representation of left ventricular end-diastolic and end-systolic V-P relations before (continuous curves) and after (interrupted curves) acute myocardial infarction. The myocardial injury depresses the contractility to increase end-systolic volume despite the fall in pressure afterload; accordingly, LVEDV increases to accommodate venous return, while LVEDP increases even more on account of the diastolic dysfunction of the myocardial injury. Accordingly, left ventricular dysfunction is signaled by reduced SV and $\dot{Q}_T$ despite a large elevation in LVEDP; therapy aims to reduce preload, enhance contractility, and reduce afterload (for further discussion, see text).

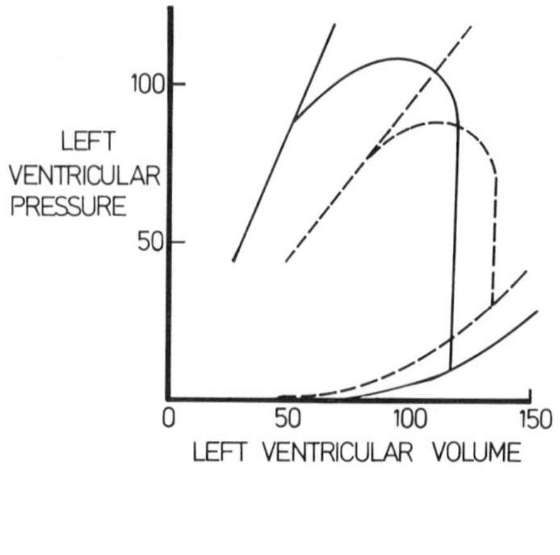

are reduced despite reflex tachycardia (HR 110 bpm) at an increased left ventricular filling pressure, and BP is reduced (SP/DP = 90/70) despite reflex increase in SVR.

Conventional therapy consists of preload reduction, inotropic agents, and afterload reduction. Interventions like morphine, furosemide, nitroglycerin, and rotating tourniquets reduce VR by dilating venous capacitance beds to increase the unstressed volume and reduce mean systemic pressure (Pms—see below). In turn, this reduces LVEDV and LVEDP. The reduction in end-diastolic volume tends to reduce SV along the steep diastolic V-P curve, so there is a large reduction in LVEDP for a small reduction in LVEDV and SV. Furthermore, the potential adverse effect of reduced SV is often offset by increased contractility and reduced afterload when myocardial wall stress is reduced by the reduction in LVEDV and LVEDP. Reduced afterload and reduced myocardial O_2 consumption improve ventricular pumping function by shifting the end-systolic V-P relationship upward and to the left, so LVESV decreases and SV increases. Further, the reduced end-diastolic pressure reduces the complication of cardiogenic pulmonary edema.

Positive inotropic agents, like dopamine and dobutamine, act directly on the myocardium to reduce end-systolic volume at a given end-systolic pressure, thereby increasing SV. Afterload-reducing agents, like nitroprusside, dilate peripheral arteries to lower end-systolic pressure and afterload; in turn, end-systolic volume decreases along the depressed end-systolic V-P relationship to increase SV. Nitroprusside also reduces end-diastolic pressure without changing end-diastolic volume; this effect appears to enhance ventricular function viewed on the Starling relationship, as discussed above. The reduction in LVEDP reduces pulmonary edema, and may also reduce the myocardial oxygen demands by reducing ventricular wall stress. To the extent that it does the latter, end-systolic V-P relations may shift to the left, because of enhanced contractility. In some patients with cardiogenic shock, vasodilator therapy appears to increase SV and $\dot{Q}_T$ without decreasing, or even increasing, arterial BP; that is, arterial dilation appears to reduce end-systolic volume at a given end-systolic pressure as if contractility were enhanced.

Other critical illnesses cause ventricular dysfunction characterized by reduced SV at increased Pla. Arterial hypoxemia and acidemia both depress the end-systolic V-P curve and increase diastolic stiffness, as shown by the interrupted curves in Fig. 2-8. Acute arterial hypertension raises the pressure afterload from C to B in Fig. 2-7 (left panel), so SV decreases from I minus C to I minus B. Then LVEDV increases to accommodate VR, so LVEDP increases, often more than expected, because of diastolic stiffness—in turn due to chronic left ventricular hypertrophy. Accordingly, pulmonary edema is a common complication, and it responds to vasodilator therapy when BP is reduced. In some or all of these conditions, diastolic dysfunction merits special management. Where acute or acute-on-chronic congestive heart failure is present, reduction of LVEDP and LVEDV, maintaining atrial contraction, increasing the duration of diastole, and minimizing myocardial ischemia are helpful. Each of these therapeutic measures is also helpful in managing hypoperfusion states associated with diastolic dysfunction.

Valvular dysfunction mimics systolic and diastolic dysfunction so that LVEDV is much increased and the forward SV is reduced, causing the LVESV (LVEDV − SV) to increase even though the left ventricle empties with each beat. Consider the effects on an absent aortic valve in Fig. 2.2. After a vigorous systolic ejection, aortic blood runs off both forward and backward in diastole, so that LVEDP and arterial DP become equal at 40 mmHg. The large LVEDV then ejects a large SV to raise SP to 120 mmHg, causing a bounding pulse pressure of 80 mmHg, but the aortic regurgitation reduces forward SV and $\dot{Q}_T$ to a low value. Consider also mitral valve incompetence in Fig. 2-2. During systole, a large fraction of the blood ejected from the ventricle regurgitates to the left atrium, reducing forward SV and $\dot{Q}_T$ but raising LVEDV and LVEDP when the left atrium fills the ventricle in diastole. In this circumstance, PP and BP are reduced. In both cases the ventricular mechanics resemble the interrupted curves in Fig. 2-8 and improve toward the normal continuous curves when forward flow is increased by vasodilator therapy, which lowers SVR to allow more peripheral runoff and less regurgitant flow.

Control of $\dot{Q}_T$ by the Systemic Vessels

Ventricular pumping function generates the flow in the circulation, but control of the $\dot{Q}_T$ resides in the systemic vessels. Indeed, the heart is best regarded as a mechanical pump having diastolic and systolic mechanical properties that determine how it accommodates the venous return. This section reviews the mechanical characteristics of the systemic vessels as a basis for understanding control of the VR in health and in critical illness.

A simplified model of the cardiovascular system is depicted in Fig. 2-1. Two muscle pumps are arranged in series. The right atrium and the right ventricle receive blood from the systemic venous reservoirs and pump it through the lungs and into the left atrium and ventricle, which in turn pumps blood out into the systemic arterial system. This central circulation is enclosed in the thoracic cavity and is exposed to pressures on the outside of the vessels, which are equal either to the pleural pressure or to pleural pressure modified by forces exerted by the lungs on the intrapulmonary vessels. The rest of the circuit, the systemic circulation, is separated into two compartments in series. The arterial compartment has high resistance, low compliance, and high pressure. The venous compartment has high compliance, low resistance, and low pressure. There is a progressive drop in pressure within the systemic circuit from the highest value, at the outlet of the left ventricle, to the lowest value, in the right atrium.

THE VASCULAR V-P RELATIONSHIP OF THE SYSTEMIC VESSELS

Consider the distribution of vascular pressure and volumes when the heart has stopped beating. Then the pressure throughout the vascular system is the same, and it is called the *mean systemic pressure* (Pms). This pressure is much lower than the arterial pressure and is closer to the right atrial pressure (Pra). When flow stops, blood drains from the high-pressure, low-volume arterial system into the large-volume, low-pressure venous system, which accommodates the displaced volume with little change in pressure. Now consider starting the two pumps in series. On the first beat the left heart pumps blood from the central circulation into the systemic circuit, raising the pressure there. At the same time the right heart pumps blood into the lungs, thereby lowering its pressure (Pra) with respect to Pms, so blood flows from the venous reservoir to the right atrium. The pressure on the venous side falls slightly below Pms, while the pressure on the arterial side rises considerably above Pms with succeeding beats of the heart. This continues until a steady state is reached, where arterial pressure has risen enough to drive the whole SV of each succeeding heartbeat through the high arterial resistance into the venous reservoir. Pms does not change between the state of no flow and the new state of steady flow, because neither the vascular volume nor the compliance of the vessels has changed. All that has changed is the distribution of the vascular volume from the compliant veins to the stiff arteries; this volume shift creates the pressure difference driving flow through the circuit.

The V-P characteristics of the vascular system are displayed in Fig. 2-9. On the abscissa is Pms, and on the ordinate is the volume of the systemic vessels. Beginning from low vascular volume in Fig. 2-9*a*, it is possible to add increments of volume to the circuit without increasing the transmural pressure of the vessels. This is analogous to the V-P characteristics of an empty meteorologic balloon having a pressure on the inside of zero relative to the pressure on the outside; unfolding the balloon fills its with a large volume without changing its transmural pressure. Further volume can be added to the balloon, or the vessels, until sufficient volume stresses the walls. Then, additional increments of volume are associated with an increase in transmural pressure; this volume range is the *stressed volume* of the vascular system. The volume range not associated with a positive change in transmural pressure is the *unstressed volume*. The slope of the relationship between the change in stressed volume and the change in Pms is the compliance ($\Delta V/\Delta P$) of the vascular system. At each stressed volume, vascular compliance determines Pms according to this V-P relationship.

Pms is the driving pressure for venous return to the right atrium when circulation resumes. It can be increased in order to increase venous return in three ways (see Fig. 2-9). Additional vascular volume may be infused into the system (Fig. 2-9*b*), the unstressed volume may be reduced (Fig. 2-9*c*), or the compliance may be reduced without changing the unstressed volume (Fig. 2-9*d*). The latter two mechanisms are mediated by vascular reflexes (see below) responding to the need for increased VR and $\dot{Q}_T$; they usually occur together. The unstressed volume may also be reduced by redistribution of vascular volume from unstressed regions into the stressed volume of the circulation. Raising the legs of a supine patient with inadequate $\dot{Q}_T$ returns a portion of the unstressed vascular volume from the large veins in the legs to the stressed volume, thereby increasing Pms and VR; so does a military antishock trousers (MAST) suit. When the heart has either an improvement in inotropic state or a reduction in afterload, blood is shifted from the central compartment to the stressed volume of the systemic circuit, raising Pms and VR.

THE VENOUS RETURN AND CARDIAC FUNCTION CURVES

Before the heart was started in the discussion above, Pra was equal to the pressure throughout the vascular system (Pms). With each succeeding heartbeat Pra decreases below

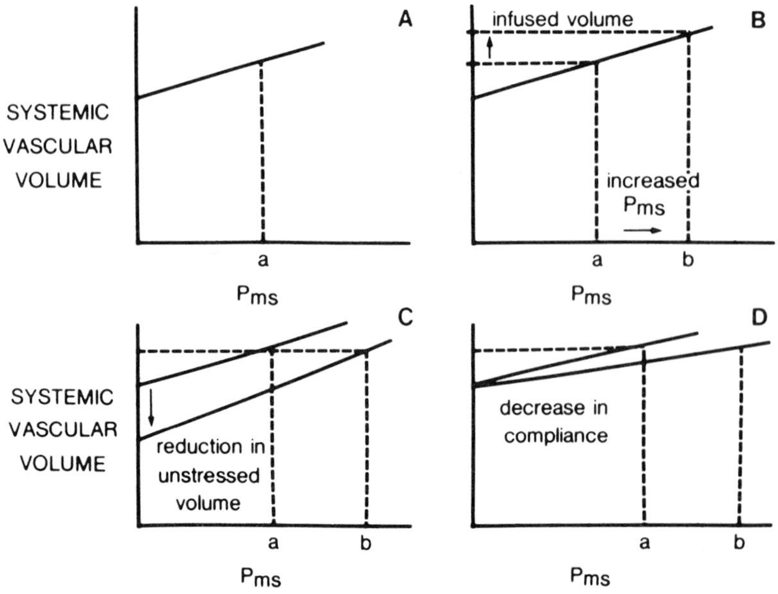

FIGURE 2-9 Mean systemic pressure (Pms) can be increased by the addition of stressed volume to the systemic vascular circuit (*a*). This can occur in three ways: *b*, an infusion of volume into the systemic vasculature; *c*, a reduction in the unstressed volume of the vasculature at constant intravascular volume, which occurs with baroreceptor reflexes, hypoxemia, elevation of the legs, or use of MAST trousers; *d*, a decrease in systemic vascular compliance, which often accompanies baroreceptor reflexes. (Reproduced, with permission, from Goldberg H, and Rabson J: Control of the cardiac output by the systemic vessels. Am J Cardiol 47:696, 1981.)

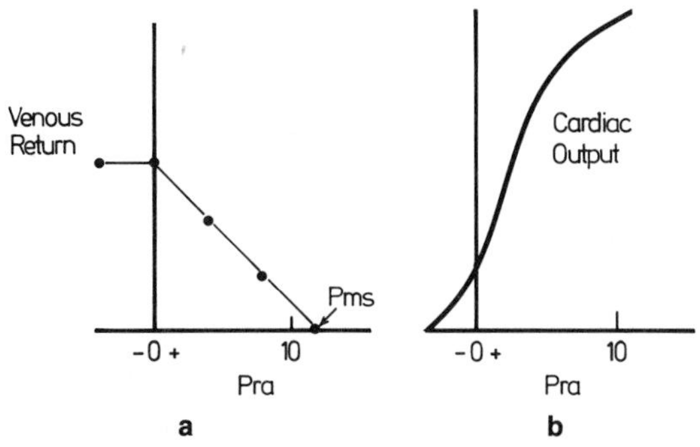

FIGURE 2-10 Relationships between Pra (abscissa) and: *a*, VR; and *b*, Q̇T. In *a*, VR is 0 when Pra is equal to Pms; as Pra is decreased progressively, VR *increases* until Pra equals 0 along the VR curve, the slope of which is 1/RVR. At lower values of Pra, VR does not increase further, because of flow limitation in the collapsible great veins as they enter the thorax. In contrast, *b* shows that Q̇T *decreases* as Pra decreases along the cardiac function curve, because end-diastolic volume decreases.

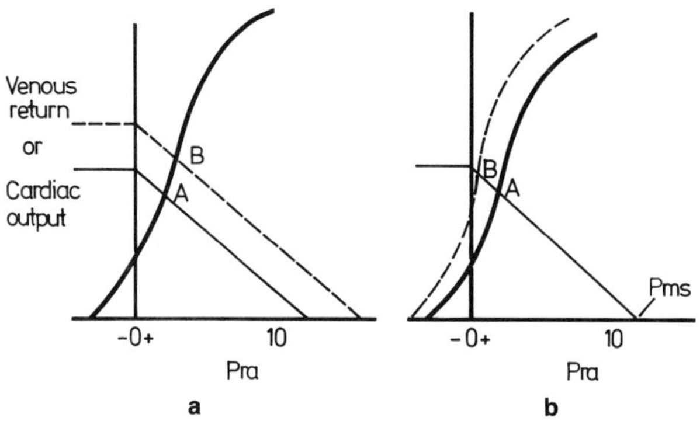

FIGURE 2-11 Mechanisms increasing VR. The VR and Q̇T curves from Fig. 2-10 are replotted on the same axes (see continuous lines intersecting at point A). This intersection marks the unique value of Pra where VR equals Q̇T in both Fig. 2-11*a* and *b*. When this value of Q̇T is insufficient, VR can be increased by increasing Pms without changing RVR, indicated by the interrupted VR curve intersecting the unchanged Q̇T curve at a higher Q̇T and Pra (see B in Fig. 2-11*a*). In Fig. 2-11*b*, VR is increased from A to B by increased cardiac function (see interrupted cardiac function curve intersecting the original VR curve at B). Accordingly, inotropic agents that increase contractility can produce modest increases in VR by lowering Pra, but further increases are limited by compression of the great veins at lower values of Pra (see Fig. 2-11*b*); note that such enhanced cardiac function displaces central blood volume into the peripheral circulation, tending to increase Pms and so promote further increases in VR, as depicted in Fig. 2-11*a*. Often such inotropic agents (dopamine, epinephrine) also raise Pms by venoconstriction.

Pms and VR increases. This sequence was repeated in a more controlled steady state by replacing the heart with a pump set to keep Pra at a given value while VR was measured. Typical data are plotted in Fig. 2-10*a*. As Pra is reduced from 12, to 8, to 4, to 0 mmHg (indicated by the closed circles), VR increases progressively with the driving pressure (Pms − Pra). The slope of the relationship between VR and Pms − Pra is the resistance of venous return (RVR = Δ(Pms − Pra)/ΔPra). Note that when right atrial pressure falls below 0, VR does not increase further because flow becomes limited entering the thorax. This occurs when the pressure in these collapsible great veins falls below the atmospheric pressure outside the veins. Then further reductions in Pra and central venous pressure are associated with progressive collapse of the veins rather than increase in VR.

For a given stressed vascular volume and compliance, Pms is set and RVR is relatively constant. In the absence of pulmonary hypertension or right heart dysfunction, left ventricular function will determine Pra and so determine VR to the right heart, which must equal the Q̇T from the left heart. Output from the heart is described by the cardiac function curve, drawn as the relationship between Pra *(abscissa)* and Q̇T *(ordinate)* in Fig. 2.10*b*. As discussed, the heart is able to eject a larger SV and Q̇T when the DP is greater, because more distended ventricles eject to about the same end-systolic volume as less distended ventricles do. Accordingly, as Pra decreases, Q̇T falls along the cardiac function curve in Fig. 2-10*b*. Yet, VR increases as Pra falls, until VR = Q̇T at a unique value of Pra indicated by the intersection of the cardiac function and VR curves, as replotted on the same abscissa in Fig. 2-11. (See point A in both Fig. 2-11*a* and Fig. 2-11*b*.)

When this Q̇T is insufficient, VR can be increased in several ways. A new steady state of increased VR is achieved by increasing Pms with no change in RVR, indicated by the interrupted VR curve in Fig. 2-11*a*. This new VR curve intersects the same cardiac function curve at a higher value of Q̇T, at point B. Note that this method of increasing VR is associated with a rise in Pra. Because of the steep slope of the cardiac function curve in normal hearts, large increases in VR occur with only small increases of Pra. Alternatively, VR can be increased by enhanced cardiac function by way of increasing contractility or decreasing afterload of the heart. This is depicted as an upward shift of the cardiac function curve, as in Fig. 2-11*b*, so that greater Q̇T occurs at each Pra. Note that the increase on each VR curve by this mechanism is associated with a reduction in Pra. Note further that in the normal heart, only a small change in VR is possible (from A to B in Fig. 2-11*b*), and greater reductions in Pra do not increase Q̇T further, since VR becomes flow-limited as Pra falls below zero. This explains why inotropic agents that enhance contractility are ineffective in hypovolemic shock.

When cardiac pumping function is depressed, as depicted by the interrupted line in Fig. 2-12, VR is reduced from A to B for the same value of Pms as Pra increases. Then the patient must retain fluid or initiate cardiac reflexes to increase Pms toward the new value required to maintain adequate cardiac output, as in chronic congestive heart failure. This is associated with a large increase in Pra from B to C, which in turn causes jugular venous distention, hepatomegaly, and peripheral edema. Diuretic reduction of vascular volumes will correct these cosmetic abnormalities at the expense of reducing Pms and VR. By contrast, inotropic and vasodilator drugs, which improve the depressed cardiac function by shifting the interrupted cardiac function curve upward, increase Q̇T and lower Pra more effectively than in patients with normal cardiac function.

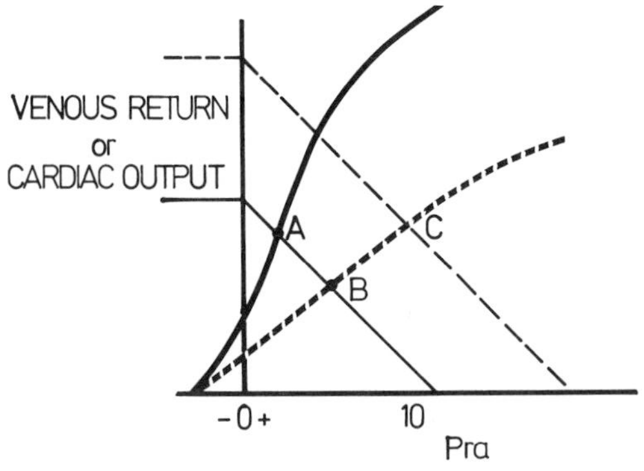

FIGURE 2-12 Reduced cardiac function (interrupted curve BC) reduces the steady-state VR from A to B, because Pra increases along the normal VR curve (continuous line AB). In response, baroreceptor reflexes and/or vascular volume retention increases Pms so that the new interrupted VR curve intersects the depressed cardiac function curve at C, whereby $\dot{Q}_T$ has returned to normal at increased Pra. Note that the new steady state can be produced by systolic or diastolic dysfunction of either the left or right ventricle (for further discussion, see text).

Although strong evidence supports the efficacy of positive inotropic agents in improving reduced $\dot{Q}_T$ due to depressed left ventricular function, their therapeutic effect on right ventricular dysfunction is much less evident. Indeed, conditions of increased load on the right ventricle (e.g., acute pulmonary embolism, primary pulmonary hypertension, high levels of PEEP) are probably not associated with depressed cardiac function curves, so reduced VR is less likely to be corrected by inotropic agents. Insufficiency of the tricuspid valve is another condition in which elevated Pms and the associated signs of right heart "failure"—e.g., peripheral edema, hepatomegaly, and jugular venous distention—are required to maintain VR because Pra is increased. Yet right ventricular pumping function is normal in the sense that further increase in Pra causes similar increase in $\dot{Q}_T$ as at lower values of RVEDV.

Accordingly, in hypoperfused states due to pulmonary hypertension, providing an adequate volume challenge while minimizing reversible vasoconstriction with oxygen and pulmonary vasodilators is the first approach to therapy. Yet, recent evidence suggests that the distended right ventricle may begin to function poorly with further volume infusion, in part because of its high wall tension and low perfusion pressure. Then, raising the systemic arterial pressure with α-agonists (e.g., phenylephrine) may improve the secondary ischemic and hypoxic dysfunction of the right ventricle by preserving its coronary blood flow. Similarly, the function of the infarcted right ventricle may be enhanced by agents known to enhance left ventricular contractility (e.g., dobutamine), in part through the systolic interdependence of the two ventricles; that is, the more vigorous contraction of the left ventricle aids the shortening of the injured right ventricle, to which it is attached.

RESISTANCE TO VR

At a given Pms and Pra, VR might be increased by reduced RVR. The RVR is an average of all the regional resistances from the systemic circuit back to the right atrium. Each regional resistance (R) is weighted by its contribution to the entire systemic vascular compliance (C/CT) and to the fraction of the cardiac output draining from that region (F/FT):

$$RVR = R_1(C_1/CT)(F_1/FT) + R_2(C_2/CT)(F_2/FT) + \cdots R_n(C_n/CT)(F_n/FT) \quad (2\text{-}1)$$

In most conditions, RVR remains relatively constant, increasing only slightly with large adrenergic stimulation; even then the increase in regional resistances is offset by redistribution of blood flow to peripheral beds having low resistance and/or compliance. One illustration of this effect is the opening of an abdominal arteriovenous fistula, between the aorta and the inferior vena cava, which doubles VR at the same values of Pms and Pra (Fig. 2-13). Consider aliquots of blood leaving the left heart simultaneously; the aliquot traversing the fistula returns to the right heart before the aliquot perfusing the lower body returns. When a greater fraction of the $\dot{Q}_T$ traverses the opened fistula having very low compliance and resistance, more blood returns to the heart because RVR decreases. This manifestation of reduced RVR may account for poorly explained hemodynamic changes in septic shock, when high $\dot{Q}_T$ is associated with increased blood flow to skeletal muscle, mimicking in part the hemodynamics of exercise; that is, some metabolic stimulus increases the fraction of $\dot{Q}_T$ perfusing the low-resistance and low-compliance skeletal muscle bed, thereby reducing RVR and increasing VR, which the heart accommodates with increased LVEDV and SV despite septic depression in contractility. Hypoxia, hypercapnea, acidosis,

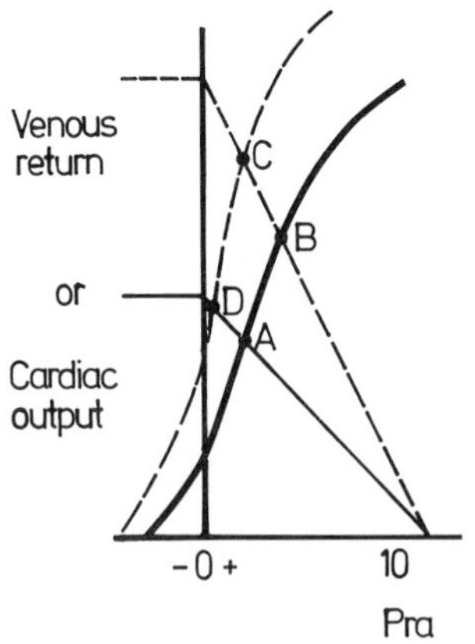

FIGURE 2-13 A reduction in RVR (interrupted VR curve BC) increases cardiac output from A to B at the same value of Pms, compared to that observed with normal RVR (continuous VR curve AD), even when cardiac function is not changed (continuous cardiac function curve AB). These data schematically depict the effects of opening a large arteriovenous fistula, with the exception that $\dot{Q}_T$ increases even more (from A to C), because opening the fistula reduces the afterload on the left ventricle to improve cardiac function (see interrupted cardiac function curve DC). Conceivably, minor variations of RVR due to effects of critical illness (sepsis, hypoxemia, acidemia), or the use of vasoactive drugs in critical illness, account for substantial increases in VR (for further discussion see text).

and peripheral effects of vasoactive or inotropic drugs can alter RVR by causing nonuniform changes in regional vascular resistance and compliance, but these effects have not yet received much study in critical illness.

Note, in Fig. 2-13, that increased venous return from A to B is associated with increased Pra when RVR is reduced without changing the cardiac function curve. In fact, Pra does not increase, and VR actually increases from A to C, as if arteriovenous shunting improved cardiac function from the continuous to the interrupted cardiac function curve shown in the figure. One explanation is that reduced SVR associated with arteriovenous shunting lowers the afterload on the left ventricle to improve cardiac function.

In cardiogenic shock, infusions of vasoactive drugs (e.g., dopamine, dobutamine) increase $\dot{Q}_T$ and reduce Pra. This is attributed to positive inotropic effects returning the cardiac function curve toward normal, as depicted in Fig. 2-12. Critically ill patients without abnormal heart function also respond to these drugs with increased $\dot{Q}_T$. If the only effects of these drugs were the inotropic effects, indicated by the interrupted cardiac function curve in Fig. 2-13, VR would increase slightly from A to D, in association with reduced Pra. Yet cardiac output often increases considerably during vasoactive drug infusions in these patients, in association with no change or an increase in Pra, as from A to C or from A to B in Fig. 2-13. It is conceivable that the inotropic drugs also have peripheral vasoactive effects on RVR (or on Pms), accounting for part of the increase in cardiac output.

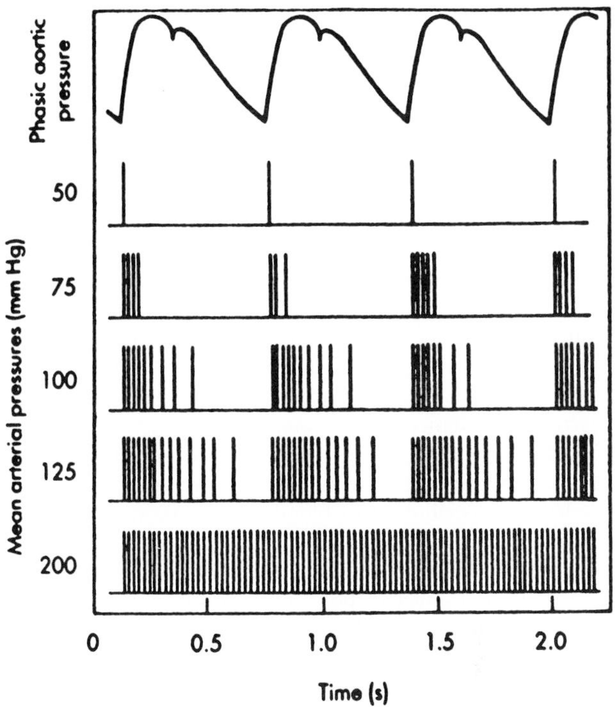

FIGURE 2-14 Relationship of aortic blood pressure in the firing of a single afferent nerve fiber from the carotid sinus at different levels of mean arterial pressure (Reproduced, with permission, from Berne RM, Levy MN (eds): *Physiology*. St. Louis, Mosby, 1988. p 519).

NEURAL AND METABOLIC CONTROL OF VR

The cardiovascular system is well designed to maintain BP within a relatively narrow range and to distribute blood flow according to metabolic needs. The principle regulator of BP is the baroreceptor reflex. The pressure receptors reside in the carotid sinus, at the bifurcation of the common carotid artery. When arterial BP is very high, the baroreceptors fire continuously, and when the BP is very low there is very little activity arising from the carotid sinus (see Fig. 2-14). Impulses from the carotid sinus travel via the sinus and glossopharyngeal nerves to the cardioregulatory center in the medulla. This afferent traffic suppresses the inherent tonic efferent output from the regulatory center via the sympathetic nerves to four major target organs:

1. The sympathetic nerves release norepinephrine to constrict arteriolar smooth muscle. The result is increased SVR, with a consequent increase in mean BP. For a given BP, the blood flow drops to the organs where arteriolar vasoconstriction is greatest. This is especially evident in the mesenteric vasculature, the skin, and the renal cortex, while sympathetically induced vasoconstriction is virtually absent in the coronary and cerebral circulation. Accordingly, flow to these vital organs is preserved at the expense of a redistribution away from the skin, kidneys, and gut.
2. Increased sympathetic activity to the heart is associated with reflex inhibition of vagal output from the cardioregulatory center to increase heart rate and contractility. To the extent that VR has not increased, increased rate and contractility act to decrease end-diastolic and end-systolic volume of both ventricles. The consequent reduction in Pra produces a modest increase in VR and $\dot{Q}_T$.
3. Sympathetic innervation of the venular smooth muscle releases norepinephrine to constrict the venous capacitance vessels. This has very little effect on SVR but increases VR and $\dot{Q}_T$ by raising Pms through reduction of the compliance and unstressed volume of the veins.
4. Efferent sympathetic outflow from the cardioregulatory center stimulates release of epinephrine from the adrenal medulla. The net effect of the humoral output is to augment the venous constriction and raise Pms while reducing the SVR through arteriolar smooth muscle dilatation. Of course, the circulating epinephrine also enhances the rate and contractility of the heart, so that the increased VR is accommodated without excessive increases in the end-diastolic volume.

Consider the following typical results of an oft-repeated, complex canine experiment to illustrate how baroreceptor reflexes initiated by hypotension actually increase $\dot{Q}_T$. This description is meant to convey an insight into the ways in which vasoactive drugs used in critically ill patients increase $\dot{Q}_T$. For simplicity, an infusion of a known concentration of epinephrine represents the output from the cardioregulatory center. During the infusion, $\dot{Q}_T$ increases from 4.3 to 10.3 L/min and HR increases from 120 to 160 bpm, so SV increases from 35 to 65 mL when pulmonary artery wedge pressure decreases from 8.5 to 7.5 mmHg and Pra decreases from 3 to 2 mmHg; systemic blood pressure decreases from 140/110 to 130/70. One common interpretation of these results is that epinephrine enhances the inotropic and chronotropic states of the heart so that SV and HR increase to increase $\dot{Q}_T$.

When this experiment was repeated after the heart was replaced by a mechanical pump controlled to keep Pra constant, the infusion of epinephrine was associated with an identical increase in VR. Of course, the mechanical pump had no adrenergic receptors; the increase in VR was effected by a measured decrease in unstressed volume and in vascular compliance, which caused a large increase in Pms. The effects of the epinephrine infusion on arteriolar and venular smooth muscle would have increased RVR, were it not for a redistribution of blood to the fast time-constant components of the peripheral circulation (see Fig. 2-15). The measured RVR did not change, so the increase in Pms at the same Pra effected the increase in VR; presumably the epinephrine increased Pms and VR when the heart was present in the first experiment, so the increased $\dot{Q}_T$ was associated with, but not due to, the positive inotropic and chronotropic effects of epinephrine. By this alternate explanation of the increase in $\dot{Q}_T$ in the first experiment, the adrenergic increase in HR and contractility helps the left ventricle to accommodate the increase in VR at a lower LVEDV.

FIGURE 2-15 Relationship between flow ($\dot{Q}$) and right atrial pressure (Pra) before and during epinephrine infusion calculated for isovolemic conditions. The broken line represents the effect of epinephrine on the elastic and resistive properties alone (increased RVR), so redistribution of $\dot{Q}$ to the rapid regions returns RVR to the normal ("before") value. (Reproduced, with permission, from Caldini P et al: Effect of epinephrine on pressure, flow, and volume relationships in the systemic circulation of dogs. Circ Res 34:606, 1974.)

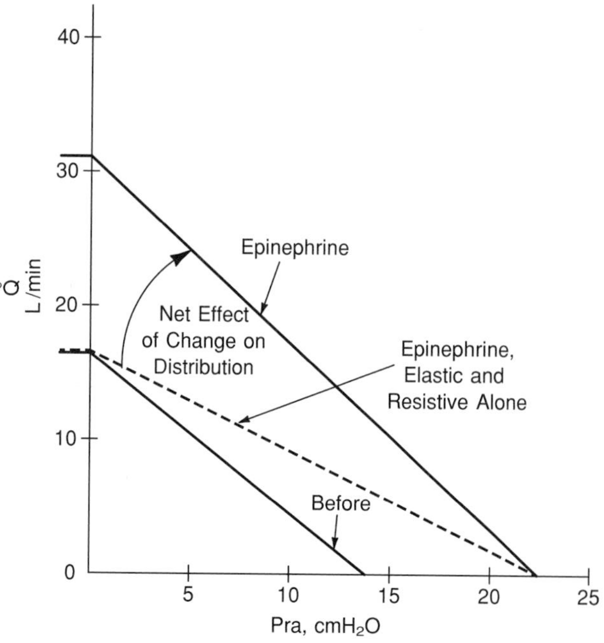

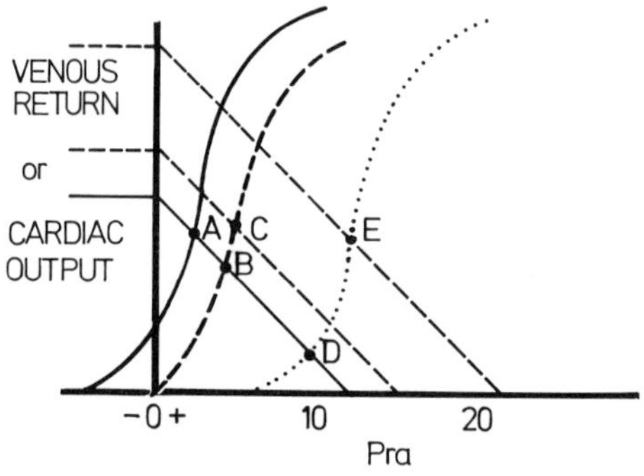

FIGURE 2-16 Effects of increased pleural pressure (Ppl) on VR and $\dot{Q}_T$. Compared to the normal steady state (continuous VR and cardiac function curves), increasing Ppl and Pra by 4 mmHg shifts the normal cardiac function curves to the right (interrupted cardiac function curve BC), so that VR decreases from A to B. This accounts for the fall in $\dot{Q}_T$ when thoracotomy exposes the right atrium to atmospheric pressure; similarly, the increase in Ppl and Pra when PEEP is applied to a patient with an intact thorax decreases $\dot{Q}_T$. In both cases, baroreceptor reflexes or iatrogenic expansion of vascular volume increases Pms to allow the new interrupted VR curve to intersect the displaced cardiac function curve at C, returning $\dot{Q}_T$ to normal. A much larger increase in PEEP raises Ppl and Pra even more, so that the displaced normal cardiac function curve (dotted curve DE) intersects the normal VR curves at a very low value of $\dot{Q}_T$ (D). Then returning $\dot{Q}_T$ to a normal value (E) requires a larger increase in Pms to allow the new interrupted VR curve to intersect the dotted function curve at E (for further discussion, see text).

PLEURAL PRESSURE (Ppl)

In preceding illustrations and discussions, values of Pms and Pra were expressed relative to atmospheric pressure; yet the transmural pressure of the right atrium exceeds Pra by the subatmospheric value (about −4 mmHg) of the Ppl surrounding the heart. Consider the effect of opening the thorax, which raises Ppl from −4 to 0 mmHg; then VR decreases (from A to B in Fig. 2-16), because Pra increases. This is indicated by the interrupted cardiac function curve, which is shifted to the right by the increase in pressure outside the heart but is parallel to the normal cardiac function curve (the continuous line passing through point A in Fig. 2-16). Normal VR can be restored (from B to C in Fig. 2-16) by increasing Pms by an amount equal to the rise in Ppl and Pra induced by the thoracotomy. Then transmural Pra will be the same as in condition A in Fig. 2-16, and Pra will have increased from A to C (also in Fig. 2-16) at the same $\dot{Q}_T$.

This mechanism for the fall in $\dot{Q}_T$ with thoracotomy also explains the fall in cardiac output with PEEP. Ppl within an intact thorax rises with positive-pressure ventilation, raising Pra and reducing VR. When PEEP increases end-expired lung volume, the inflated lungs push the thorax to an increased volume via a greater Ppl. Because the increase in volume of edematous lungs with PEEP is as large as in normal lungs, the increase in Ppl is also large; similarly, Ppl increases equally with each positive-pressure breath whether lungs are edematous or normal. When 8 mmHg PEEP (10 cmH_2O) is added to the ventilator, the end-expiratory value of Ppl rises by about half that amount—e.g., from −4 to 0 mmHg. Accordingly, VR decreases with PEEP from A to B in Fig 2-16, with no change in cardiac function or Pms. $\dot{Q}_T$ is returned to normal by volume infusion or vascular reflexes, which raise Pms by an amount equal to the increase in Ppl and Pra. Of course, greater PEEP (20 cmH_2O as in dotted line DE, Fig. 2-16) reduces VR further (from A to D) and requires larger increases in Pms to return VR to normal (D to E).

Note that $\dot{Q}_T$ is much less susceptible to the deleterious effects of PEEP when Pms is high. In patients with reduced circulatory volume, vascular reflexes are already operating to maintain VR and Pms by reducing unstressed volume and/or vascular compliance. Such patients have little vascular reflex reserve and do not tolerate intubation and positive-pressure ventilation well without considerable intravenous infusion to increase vascular stressed volume. In contrast, well- or overhydrated patients may tolerate even large amounts of PEEP with no reduction in $\dot{Q}_T$, for their previously inactive vascular reflexes can increase Pms in well-filled systemic vessels by the same amount by which Ppl increases with PEEP. These considerations allow the physician to anticipate and treat the hypotension induced by ventilatory therapy; the concept should not be interpreted as an indication for maintaining high circulatory volume in critically ill patients on ventilators, for this often increases lung edema without correcting a problem.

An Approach to Hypoperfusion States

A hypoperfusion state, or shock, is almost always signaled by systemic hypotension; commonly associated clinical features are prerenal oliguria (urine flow <20 mL/h, urine $Na^+ < 20$ meq/L, urine $K^+ > 20$ meq/L, urine specific gravity >1.020), abnormalities of mentation and consciousness, and metabolic acidosis. The mean BP is determined by the product of $\dot{Q}_T$ and SVR. A conceptual framework for the initial diagnosis and management of hypotensive patients is outlined in Table 2-2. In this approach one aims to categorize the patient according to the three common causes of shock (septic, cardiogenic, and hypovolemic) and to initiate early appropriate therapy of the presumed diagnosis. Response to the therapeutic intervention tests the accuracy of the initial diagnosis, so the hemodynamic response is reevaluated within 30 min. The diagnostic decision is aided by collating clinical data from the history, the physical examination, and routine laboratory tests to answer three questions in sequence.

TABLE 2-2 Initial Approach to the Diagnosis and Management of the Hypotensive Patient

Blood pressure (BP) = Cardiac output ($\dot{Q}_T$) × Systemic vascular resistance (SVR)

	IS $\dot{Q}_T$ REDUCED?	
	Yes	No
BP	90/70	90/40
Skin	Cool, blue	Warm, pink
Nail bed return	Slow	Rapid
Heart sounds	Muffled	Crisp
History/lab	Hypovolemic or Cardiogenic etiology	↓ or ↑ WBC and/or temperature Source of infection Immune compromise Severe liver disease
Working diagnosis	See next question	**Septic shock/endotoxemia**
	IS THE HEART TOO FULL?	
	Yes	No
Presentation	Angina, dyspnea	Hemorrhage, dehydration
Signs	Cardiomegaly Extra heart sounds ↑ JVP	Dry mucous membranes ↓ tissue turgor Stool, gastric blood
Lab	ECG, x-ray Echocardiogram	↓ hematocrit ↑ BUN/creatinine
Working diagnosis	**Cardiogenic shock**	**Hypovolemic shock**
	WHAT DOES NOT FIT?	
	Cardiac tamponade Acute pulmonary hypertension Right ventricular infarction	Anaphylaxis Spinal shock Adrenal insufficiency
	Overlapping multiple etiologies	

SEPTIC SHOCK

Is the BP reduced because $\dot{Q}_T$ is reduced, or not? If not, SVR must be reduced—a requirement almost always related to septicemia (abnormally increased or decreased WBC and temperature, source of infection, compromise of the immune system) or to sterile endotoxemia associated with severe liver disease. As indicated in Table 2-2, the low BP is often characterized by a large PP because the SV is large, and by a very low DP because each SV has a rapid peripheral runoff through dilated peripheral arterioles. This gives warm, pink skin with rapid nail bed return and crisp heart sounds. As in the other types of shock, tachycardia is evident, in part because of baroreceptor reflex response to hypotension, but the arterial vasoconstriction response to reflex sympathetic tone is blocked by a monokine (tumor necrosis factor, cachectin) or endothelial-derived relaxing factor (EDRF, or nitric oxide). The combination of tachycardia and large PP signals a large $\dot{Q}_T$, which is almost always present early, unless concurrent hypovolemia or myocardial dysfunction precludes the hyperdynamic circulatory state of sepsis.

Initial therapy starts with appropriate broad-spectrum antibiotics, and expands the circulating volume by intravenous infusion of colloid and crystalloid to exclude associated hypovolemia. The end point of volume infusion is obscure, because $\dot{Q}_T$ is already increased; and though $\dot{Q}_T$ usually increases further with intravenous infusions, the BP rarely increases much with increased $\dot{Q}_T$. Furthermore, the need for even greater $\dot{Q}_T$ to increase O_2 delivery is questionable, because the lactic acidosis of septic shock may not be due to anaerobic metabolism (see Chaps. 1, 56, 57). On the other hand, pulmonary vascular pressures always rise with volume infusion, increasing the pulmonary edema when the septic process increases the permeability of lung vessels. Much evidence suggests that the septic myocardium does not function normally, but this dysfunction is often associated with values of SV above 100 mL at normal values of LVEDP. Accordingly, it seems unlikely that systolic dysfunction contributes to the shock, so infusions of inotropic agents are unlikely to treat shock, even though dobutamine does raise $\dot{Q}_T$ more for a given LVEDP. Vasoconstricting agents (norepinephrine, phenylephrine) are often ineffective in raising BP, because of the arteriolar smooth muscle paralysis of sepsis; yet their use is often associated with untoward local vasoconstriction (ischemic digits and kidneys), so a slow hand in raising systolic pressures above 80 mmHg seems to do less harm. Tachypnea and respiratory distress may be severe, so initial supportive therapy includes consideration of early intubation and mechanical ventilation; this prevents catastrophic respiratory muscle fatigue, respiratory acidosis, and the complications of emergent intubation.

CARDIOGENIC SHOCK

By contrast with septic shock, a low $\dot{Q}_T$ is signaled by a low PP (indicating a low stroke volume), signs of increased SVR (cold, blue, damp extremities; poor nail bed return), and a history or presentation including features suggesting cardiogenic or hypovolemic etiology of hypotension. If $\dot{Q}_T$ is reduced, a second question is asked of the hypotensive patient: is the heart too full, or not? (See Table 2-2).

A positive answer is often signaled by symptoms of ischemic heart disease or arrhythmia, signs of cardiomegaly, the third and fourth sounds or gallop rhythm of heart failure, new murmurs of valvular dysfunction, increased jugular or central venous pressure, and laboratory tests suggesting ischemia (ECG, CPK) or ventricular dysfunction (chest x-ray suggesting cardiomegaly, venous distention or cardiogenic edema; echocardiogram showing regional or global systolic dyskinesia). The most common cause of hypotension associated with a circulation that is too full on initial evaluation is cardiogenic shock due to myocardial ischemia. Initial therapy treats this presumptive diagnosis with inotropic drug therapy (dobutamine, 3 to 10 μg/kg per min) to assist the ejecting function of the ischemic heart, and dopamine (2 to 5 μg/kg per min) to redistribute the reduced $\dot{Q}_T$ toward the renal cortex to preserve kidney function. Such therapy does not address directly the coronary insufficiency and may increase the myocardial O_2 demand (MvO_2). Concurrent sublingual, dermal, or intravenous nitroglycerin ameliorates elements of coronary vasospasm to increase blood flow and reduces preload to reduce MvO_2. Morphine also reduces pain, anxiety, and preload.

In this situation, even a cautious volume challenge (250 mL NaCl over 20 min) is relatively contraindicated before right heart catheterization, because ventricular function and $\dot{Q}_T$ are reduced as often as they are improved by this intervention, and the risk of pulmonary edema is increased. Indeed, when signs of pulmonary edema are present on clinical and radiologic exam of the thorax, diuretics, morphine, and nitroglycerin often reduce preload by relaxing the capacitance veins, in association with an increase in left ventricular systolic performance. On the other hand, about 10 percent of patients with myocardial ischemia present with significant hypovolemia. Accordingly, the clinical assessment of hemodynamics should be supplemented as early as possible with right heart catheterization to confirm the hemodynamic diagnosis and the response to vasoactive agents—i.e., an increase in $\dot{Q}_T$ and BP without excessively high or low pulmonary wedge pressure (Ppw); then appropriate volume infusion or reduction can be titrated using the measured responses of Ppw and $\dot{Q}_T$. When these measures are addressed adequately but the hypoperfusion state persists, early movement toward arteriolar vasodilator therapy or a balloon-assist device is indicated. Note that these latter interventions are not relegated to last-resort status, but are considered early in this initial stabilization of cardiogenic shock.

HYPOVOLEMIC SHOCK

Beyond the absence of clinical features suggesting that the heart is too full, hypovolemic shock is distinguished from cardiogenic shock by several positive clinical features. Often there is an obvious source of external bleeding (multiple trauma, hemoptysis, hematemesis, hematochezia, or melena); internal bleeding is often signaled by blood aspirated from the nasal gastric tube or found on rectal examination; by increasing abdominal girth; or by clinical and radiologic examination of the thoracic cavity for pleural, alveolar, or periaortic blood. Each of these is often associated with a new reduction in the hematocrit. Patients with nonhemorrhagic hypovolemia often present with recognizable excess gastrointestinal fluid losses (vomiting, diarrhea, suctioning, and stomas), excess renal losses (osmotic or drug diuresis, diabetes insipidus), or third space losses (as in extensive burns). Physical examination reveals dry mucous membranes with decreased tissue turgor; the routine laboratory tests often reveal an increased blood urea nitrogen (BUN) level out of proportion to a relatively normal creatinine level, and an increased hematocrit due to hemoconcentration.

The essential initial management of patients with presumed hypovolemic shock necessitates early intravenous access with two large-bore (#14 gauge) catheters for rapid infusion of blood, colloid, and crystalloid solutions for hemorrhagic shock, and the appropriate crystalloid solution for dehydration. An immediate response of increased BP and pulse volume supports the presumed diagnosis, whereas the absence of improvement in these hemodynamics necessitates emergent repair of the site of the blood loss or a reevaluation of the working diagnosis.

WHAT DOES NOT FIT?

The purpose of this initial schema is to formulate a working diagnosis from among the most common presentations of shock so that early and rapid therapy may be initiated. Then the response to the initial therapy either confirms or questions the working diagnosis. When features of the initial clinical presentation or the patient's response to appropriate management question the working diagnosis, early acquisition of more objective hemodynamic data is appropriate. In the interim, other features of the clinical presentation often suggest an etiology of shock that falls outside this simplistic schema; or the possibility of overlapping or concurrent etiologies becomes larger. This section reviews briefly several important differential diagnostic conditions. Their typical hemodynamic results are summarized in Table 2-3 for comparison with corresponding results in septic, cardiogenic, or hypovolemic shock; the interested reader may get the most out of this table by explaining, for each condition, the departures of each measurement from the normal values and from those of the other diagnoses.

CARDIAC TAMPONADE

Pericardial effusion is often suggested early by the clinical setting (renal failure, malignancy, chest pain), by physical examination (elevated neck veins, systolic blood pressure falling more than 10 mmHg on inspiration, distant heart sounds), and/or routine investigations (chest radiograph with "water bottle" heart, low voltage on the ECG). Such a constellation of clinical data requires early echocardiographic confirmation of pericardial effusion. Tamponade is signaled by right ventricular and right atrial collapse—worse on inspiration—with a relatively small left ventricle. Tamponade requires urgent pericardiocentesis or operative drainage via a pericardial window. While awaiting the definitive treatment, intravenous expansion of the circulating volume may produce small increases in BP; reductions in circulating volume (caused by diuretics, nitroglycerin, morphine, or intercurrent hemodialysis) are often associated with a catastrophic reduction in $\dot{Q}_T$ that occurs through reduction of the venous tone and volume necessary to maintain the Pms required to drive VR back to the high Pra.

Right heart catheterization typically reveals a Pra increased to about 16 to 20 mmHg and equal to both the pulmonary artery diastolic pressure and the pulmonary artery wedge pressure; $\dot{Q}_T$ and SV are much reduced. This hemodynamic subset resembles that of cardiogenic shock (high Ppw, low SV). Yet, in the case of pericardial tamponade, Ppw is increased because pericardial pressure is increased, so the transmural pressure of the left ventricle approaches zero, a value consistent with the very low LVEDV accounting for the low SV. Other etiologies of hypotension associated with high cardiac pressures and small ventricular

TABLE 2-3 Typical Hemodynamic Measurements during Right Heart Catheterization for the Initial Diagnosis and Management of Shock

Diagnosis	BP (mmHg)	$\dot{Q}_T$ (L/min)	HR (bpm)	SV (mL)	Ppw (mmHg)	Ppa (mmHg)	Pra (mmHg)
Normal	120/80	5.6	80	70	10	25/10	5
Septic	90/40	9.6	120	80	5	25/10	0
Cardiogenic (LV infarction)	90/70	3.6	120	30	25	35/25	15
RV infarction	90/70	3.6	120	30	10	20/15	15
Pulmonary hypertension	90/70	3.6	120	30	10	80/30	15
Tamponade	90/70	3.6	120	30	20	30/20	20
Hypovolemic	90/70	3.6	120	30	5	15/5	0
Anaphylactic	90/60	4.8	120	40	5	15/5	0
Neurogenic	90/50	4.8	80	60	5	15/5	0
Adrenal insufficiency	90/60	4.8	120	40	5	15/5	0

volumes include constrictive pericarditis, tension pneumothorax, massive pleural effusion, positive-pressure ventilation with high PEEP, and very high intraabdominal pressure.

RIGHT VENTRICULAR OVERLOAD AND INFARCTION

Another clinical presentation that may fall outside the scheme presented in Table 2-2 is the hypotension associated with acute or acute-on-chronic pulmonary hypertension. Shock following acute pulmonary embolism (PE) is often signaled by the clinical setting including risk factors (perioperative period, immobilized patient, hypercoagulable patient, prior PEs); symptoms of acute dyspnea, chest pain, or hemoptysis; physical examination revealing a loud P_2 with a widened and fixed split of S_2; new hypoxia without obvious radiologic explanation; and acute right heart strain on the ECG. Noninvasive Doppler studies of the veins in the lower extremities, ventilation perfusion scans, and pulmonary angiography confirm the diagnosis. Heparin or placement of a filter in the inferior vena cava reduces the incidence of subsequent emboli; some success occurs with thrombolytic therapy (or, in some centers, surgical removal of the embolus) in patients with shock due to pulmonary embolism. Acute-on-chronic pulmonary hypertension causes shock in the setting of prior primary pulmonary hypertension, recurrent pulmonary emboli, progression of collagen vascular disease, or chronic respiratory failure (COPD, pulmonary fibrosis) aggravated in part by hypoxic pulmonary vasoconstriction. In these circumstances, O_2 therapy and pulmonary vasodilator therapy (sodium nitroprusside, prostacyclin) combine to reduce pulmonary hypertension and increase $\dot{Q}_T$ in a small but significant proportion of patients.

Of course, right heart catheterization reveals a unique hemodynamic subset: a very high mean pulmonary artery pressure, a pulmonary artery diastolic pressure considerably greater than the wedge pressure, and reduced $\dot{Q}_T$ and SV. Not uncommonly, the pulmonary artery wedge pressure is normal or increased despite a small LVEDV on echocardiographic examination, which also reveals right-to-left shift of the interventricular septum; presumably this causes stiffening of the diastolic V-P curve of the left ventricle. A complication of pulmonary vasodilator therapy is hypotension due to the systemic arterial dilatation unaccompanied by increased right heart output. Such effects aggravate the hypoperfusion state, perhaps by reducing coronary blood flow to the hypertrophied, dilated, right ventricle. Some evidence suggests that shock associated with pulmonary hypertension is ameliorated by α-agonist therapy (norepinephrine, phenylephrine), which acts as a predominant systemic arteriolar constrictor to raise BP sufficiently to maintain right ventricular perfusion.

Right ventricular infarction causes low pulmonary artery pressures and normal left ventricular filling pressures as the dilated, injured right ventricle is unable to maintain adequate flow to the left heart. Elevated neck veins and Pra tend to decrease with dobutamine infusion, perhaps because the enhanced contractility of the left ventricle improves systolic function of the mechanically interdependent right ventricle. Again, volume expansion often aggravates right ventricular dysfunction, and systemic vasoconstriction may preserve right ventricular perfusion.

ANAPHYLACTIC, NEUROGENIC, AND ADRENAL SHOCK

Other etiologies of shock having unique clinical presentations that usually lead to early diagnosis are anaphylactic shock and neurogenic shock. Beyond identifying the etiology early (through the association of these conditions with intravenous drug infusions and trauma, respectively) the physician should note that the pathophysiologic basis of each is a dilated venous bed with greatly increased unstressed volume of the circulation, leading to hypovolemic shock. Accordingly, the mainstay of therapy for both conditions is adequate volume infusion. Adjunctive therapy for anaphylaxis includes antihistamines, steroids, and epinephrine to antagonize the mediators released in the anaphylactic reaction; a careful search for sources of blood loss and hemorrhagic shock is part of the early resuscitation of a traumatized patient with spinal shock.

Not uncommonly, the presentation of patients with nonhemorrhagic hypovolemic shock raises the question of acute adrenal cortical insufficiency. When that possibility is not obviously excluded it is appropriate to measure the serum cortisol level, provide adequate circulating steroids with dexamethasone, and conduct an ACTH stimulation test to confirm or refute the diagnosis. Characteristically, the hypotension and hypoperfusion in such patients will not respond to adequate vascular volume expansion until the dexamethasone is administered.

MULTIPLE ETIOLOGIES OF SHOCK

With this differential diagnosis and management evaluation in mind, the initial approach to patients with hypoperfusion states should be completed in less time than it takes to read about it. The target is to distinguish between patients with septic shock, cardiogenic shock, and hypovolemic shock, and to initiate an appropriate therapeutic challenge—antibiotics, inotropic agents, and/or a volume challenge within 30 min of presentation. By the response, the diagnosis is confirmed or questioned with special regard to equivocal responses to therapy or to several other diagnostic categories of shock. The next stage of diagnosis and management may be aided by right heart catheterization, to confirm objectively the relationship between wedge pressure and $\dot{Q}_T$ or to exclude errors in the initial diagnosis and management. For example, a 70-year-old woman becomes hypotensive in the immediate postoperative period after internal fixation of a recent fracture of the femur. Vague chest discomfort and ischemic changes in the ECG suggest cardiogenic shock, so dobutamine and dopamine are initiated, but there is no improvement in the hemodynamic status. A right heart catheter is inserted and reveals a cardiac output of 2.5 L/min with a wedge pressure of 3 mmHg. An intravenous infusion of 1 L of saline solution raises the blood pressure 10 mmHg without raising the wedge pressure much; the patient responds to continued transfusions of 6 U of whole blood while an unusually large hemorrhage at the operative site is drained and packed. This clinical vignette is characteristic of the overlapping clinical presentations posed by the major diagnostic categories of shock. Sorting out the primary etiology of the hypoperfusion state often requires considerable additional data. Indeed, this process is rendered more complex by concurrent etiologies contributing to the shock—e.g., the patient with septic shock in whom it is not possible to increase $\dot{Q}_T$ because of intercurrent myocardial dysfunction, the patient with acute myocardial infarction who is hypovolemic, or the patient with hemorrhagic shock who becomes septic. Other combinations of these major categories overlap with confounding effects of tamponade, positive-pressure ventilation, pneumothorax, and pulmonary hypertension—all to challenge the ongoing diagnostic and management approaches (see Chaps. 114 to 126 for further discussion). Nonetheless, complete interpretation of data from right heart catheterization (see Chap. 25) and echocardiography (see Chaps. 21 and 22) complements the changing physical examination findings to allow an early move toward the correct diagnosis and management of shock.

The Pulmonary Circulation

PRESSURES, FLOW, AND RESISTANCE IN PULMONARY VESSELS

In the steady state, $\dot{Q}_T$ from the left heart is equal to VR to the right heart. Accordingly, all the $\dot{Q}_T$ traverses the pulmonary circulation in pulsatile fashion. These pulmonary hemodynamics are depicted in the upper panel of Fig. 2-17. The pulmonary circulation is enclosed in the thorax, so the pressure on the outside of extraalveolar vessels is Ppl, while P_A impinges on the smaller alveolar vessels. The right ventricle ejects blood into the pulmonary artery, raising its pressure (Ppa). This pressure head drives flow through a branching arteriolar system into the lung parenchyma, where a network of very small alveolar septal vessels, or capillaries, pass between the air spaces of the lung to effect pulmonary gas exchange. These septal vessels converge into pulmonary veins, which empty into the left atrium. Pla is often regarded as the outflow pressure of the pulmonary circulation. When this pressure gradient across the pulmonary circulation (Ppa − Pla) is divided by the pulmonary blood flow (Q), the pulmonary vascular resistance (PVR) is calculated (mmHg/L per min); sometimes it is converted to metric units (dyne·s/cm^5) by multiplying by 80.

By this analysis, increasing blood flow from one level to another is associated with increasing pressure drop across the pulmonary circulation (Ppa − Pla) along a unique pressure/flow relationship given by the continuous line in the lower panel of Fig. 2-17. Resistance to pulmonary blood flow may be increased by smooth muscle constriction within the pulmonary arterioles, by compression of the alveolar septal vessels by elevated alveolar pressure, or by obliteration of many of the parallel vascular channels as they traverse the lung (so that the same blood flow must

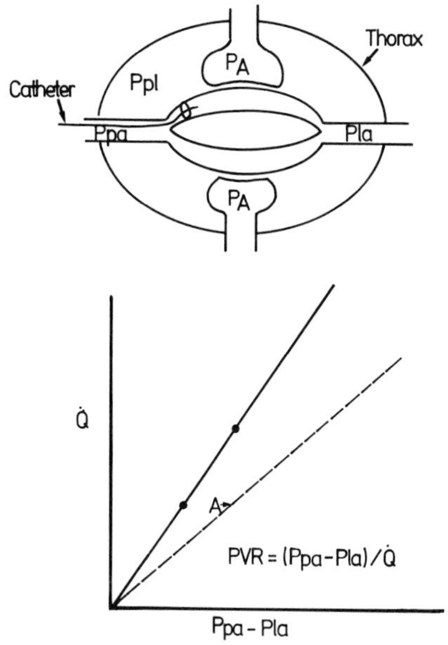

FIGURE 2-17 Schematic of the pulmonary circulation (upper panel) illustrating a simple view of pulmonary vascular resistance (PVR, lower panel). Pulmonary blood flows from the pulmonary arteries (Ppa) through branching vessels to the left atrium (Pla). This central circulation is enclosed by the thorax, which contains air spaces (P_A) that abut alveolar vessels. Between the air spaces and thorax is the pleural space, so Ppl approximates the pressure outside extraalveolar vessels, including the heart. A balloon-tipped catheter is occluding the upper branch of the pulmonary artery so that the catheter tip sits in a stagnant column of blood, continuous with Pla, to provide an estimate of pressure (Ppw)—unless P_A exceeds Pla, when the occlusion pressure exceeds Pla because P_A closes the alveolar vessels; in either case, when the balloon is deflated the catheter tip measures Ppa, and a thermistor near the tip can measure pulmonary blood flow ($\dot{Q}$) by thermodilution technique. The lower panel plots $\dot{Q}$ (ordinate) against Ppa − Pla (abcissa); the inverse of the slope of the continuous line drawn through the two $P\dot{Q}$ points is PVR; for a given $\dot{Q}$ at the lower point, Ppa − Pla increases to A on the interrupted $P\dot{Q}$ line, indicating increased PVR.

flow through fewer channels). Such an increase in pulmonary vascular resistance would be calculated as at point A on the interrupted line in Fig. 2-17, where the pressure difference across the lung (Ppa − Pla) has increased for the same amount of pulmonary blood flow.

Figure 2-17 depicts one way to make these measurements. A catheter with an end hole is passed, via systemic veins, into the thorax. When a small balloon near its tip is inflated, the balloon passes with the VR into the right atrium, right ventricle, and pulmonary artery until it wedges in a pulmonary artery branch, obstructing the flow there. Since there is no flow, the hole in the catheter tip is open to a stagnant column of blood extending through the pulmonary vessels to the left atrium. Accordingly, this pressure (Ppw) approximates left atrial pressure. When the balloon is deflated and flow resumes through that vessel, the pressure there is equal to Ppa. A sensitive thermistor at the tip of the catheter may be used to detect temperature changes following the injection of a bolus of cold saline solution into the right atrium, allowing the estimation of pulmonary blood flow from the resulting thermodilution curve. Note that the pulmonary artery and the left atrium are surrounded by Ppl, so the absolute values of Ppa and Pla change with respiration. When spontaneous active inspiration lowers Ppl, both Ppa and Pla decrease, but the driving pressure of blood flow across the lung stays the same (Ppa − Pla); when positive-pressure inflation raises Ppl, both Ppa and Pla increase. Accordingly, it is helpful to record pulmonary vascular measurements at end-expiration when the mode of ventilation has minimally different effects.

This relatively simple analysis describes the pulmonary circulation as if it were a flow through pipes having rigid walls, the diameter of which can change with arteriolar muscle tone or obliteration of some of the channels. This description is adequate for an overview of the pulmonary circulation, but a more complete understanding of the pulmonary circulation requires consideration of the pressure/flow relationships in collapsible vessels with tone exposed to PA.

FLOW IN COLLAPSIBLE VESSELS WITH TONE

Figure 2-18 depicts a schematic model of flow from the left-hand cylinder (pulmonary artery) through the intervening tube to the right-hand cylinder (left atrium). The hydrostatic pressure in each of the cylinders is represented by the height of the liquid; it is 20 cmH_2O in the left-hand cylinder (Ppa) and 10 cmH_2O in the right-hand cylinder (Pla). This pressure difference drives flow through the intervening tube so that the flow (Q) being poured into the pulmonary artery exactly equals the flow exiting the left atrium.

The pressure/flow relationships for this schematic model are depicted in Fig. 2-19. On the *x* axis is Ppa − Pla, plotted against flow on the *y* axis. The first data point represents the conditions under discussion, where Ppa − Pla is 10 cmH_2O, giving the corresponding flow value. When Pla

FIGURE 2-18 Schematic diagram of flow ($\dot{Q}$) through a collapsible thin-walled tube connecting the left-hand cylinder (Ppa) to the right-hand cylinder (Pla) when the collapsible vessel is exposed to the pressure (PA) greater than that outside Ppa and Pla (Ppl) (for further discussion, see text and Fig. 2.19).

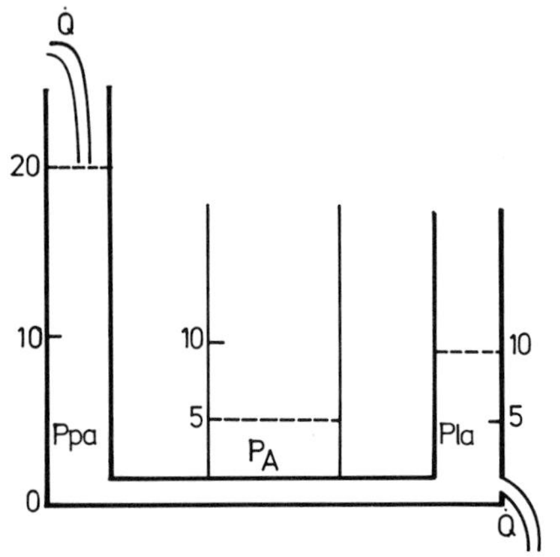

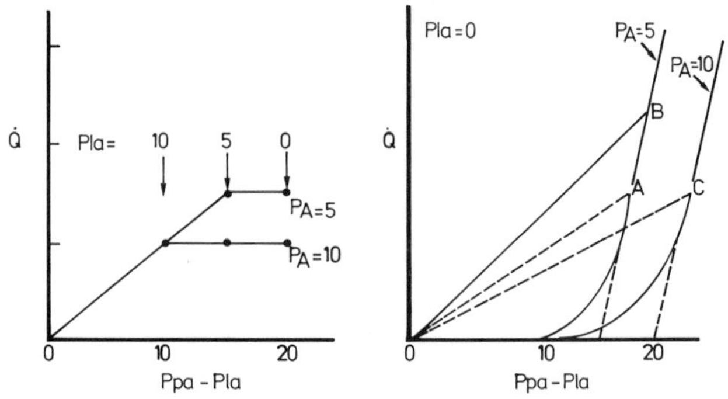

FIGURE 2-19 ***Left panel:*** **Relationships between $\dot{Q}$ and (Ppa − Pla) from the model in Fig. 2-18 (all pressures are in cmH_2O). When PA=5, Ppa = 20 and Pla = 10, flow proceeds through the collapsible vessel; $\dot{Q}$ increases when Pla is reduced to 5, because Ppa − Pla has increased from 10 to 15. But further reduction of Pla to 0 is not associated with further increases in $\dot{Q}$, because the collapsible vessel exposed to PA=5 becomes flow-limited; that is, further reductions in the downstream Pla no longer influence flow through the system, since the effective outflow pressure is PA and the effective driving pressure is Ppa − PA. In this condition (Ppa > PA>Pla), the value of Ppa when $\dot{Q}$ is stopped—the critical closing pressure (Pc)—is equal to PA=5. When PA is increased to 10 at Ppa = 20 and Pla = 10, $\dot{Q}$ is at the leftmost data point, just as it was for PA=5; but further reductions in Pla, to 5 and 0, are not associated with increased values of $\dot{Q}$ because the collapsible vessel exposed to PA=10 limits $\dot{Q}$ when PA>Pla; then, Pc = PA=10. Note that $\dot{Q}$ became limited when PA first exceeded Pla in this model, implying that the collapsible vessel had neither intrinsic stability to resist collapse nor active tone in its wall to promote collapse; yet measured relationships between $\dot{Q}$ and (Ppa − Pla) in real lung suggest that the collapsible vessels have active tone causing them to limit pulmonary blood flow when the inflow Ppa is much greater than the surrounding PA (see right panel).** ***Right panel:*** **Schematic of data obtained from isolated perfused lungs having Pla = 0 and PA=5 or 10. At PA=5, as $\dot{Q}$ is progressively reduced from B to A, Ppa falls along a relatively linear P$\dot{Q}$ plot, which extrapolates along the interrupted line to a Ppa value at $\dot{Q}$ = 0 (Pc) of 15. When PA is increased to 10, progressive reduction in $\dot{Q}$ reduces Ppa along the line parallel to BA but passing through C and extrapolating along the interrupted line to a value of Pc = Ppa = 20. Accordingly, the increase in Pc is equal to the increase in PA, suggesting that critical closure occurs in vessels exposed to PA; yet the value of Pc exceeded PA by 10 in each case, suggesting that these alveolar vessels have active tone. Other experiments in which PA was kept constant at 5 (line BA), but alveoli were exposed to hypoxic gas mixtures, produced P$\dot{Q}$ relationships similar to that through line C; that is, a parallel shift of the P$\dot{Q}$ relationship with an increase in Pc, suggesting that at least part of hypoxic pulmonary vasoconstriction is due to an increase in the tone of alveolar vessels. For discussion of the three lines drawn from the origin to A, B, or C, see text.**

is lowered to 5 cmH_2O in the right-hand cylinder of Fig. 2-18, Ppa − Pla becomes 15 cmH_2O, and flow increases as depicted in Fig. 2-19. When Pla is decreased further to 0 cmH_2O, Ppa − Pla becomes 20 cmH_2O, and flow should increase further. Yet flow does not increase in this model (see Fig. 2-19), because the tube connecting the pulmonary artery with the left atrium is collapsible and is exposed to

P_A, as depicted by the middle cylinder in Fig. 2-18. When Pla decreases below P_A, flow does not increase, because the tube is compressed. This flow limitation phenomenon is analogous to flow over a waterfall: lowering the level at the bottom of the waterfall does not increase the rate of flow.

Now consider the condition when P_A is increased to 10 cmH_2O. When Pla is 10 cmH_2O, Ppa − Pla becomes 10 cmH_2O, and the flow is the same as in the first case. Yet lowering Pla from 10 to 5 cmH_2O does not increase flow, even though Ppa − Pla becomes 15 cmH_2O, as depicted in Fig. 2-19; again, when Pla is lowered to zero, flow does not increase. The principle being illustrated at both values of P_A is that the driving pressure for flow in collapsible tubes is Ppa − P_A, when Pla is less than the pressure around the collapsible tube (P_A). A consequence of this principle of flow in collapsible tubes is that raising P_A can reduce flow in the pulmonary vessels when Ppa and Pla are unchanged.

When Pla is 0 cmH_2O and P_A is 5 cmH_2O, flow will decrease as Ppa is lowered from 20 to 5 cmH_2O; finally the flow will be zero even though Ppa exceeds Pla, because the collapsible tube between the pulmonary artery and the left atrium is closed by P_A. In this example, the closing pressure (Pc) equals P_A. Note that Pc could be less than P_A if the walls of the collapsible tube resisted closure, and could exceed P_A if active constricting tone were exerted by the walls of the collapsible tube. When Pla is less than P_A, Pc can be determined by progressively lowering Q and extrapolating the Ppa − Q plot to Q = 0 when Ppa is equal to Pc. Typical results obtained in isolated perfused lungs are depicted in the right panel of Fig. 2-19, for conditions where Ppa = 5 and Pla = 0 (see line AB). As Ppa is reduced, Q decreases in a linear manner along BA, which extrapolates to zero flow at Ppa = 15 cmH_2O. This is taken to be the average value of Pc, and it exceeds P_A by 10 cmH_2O, suggesting that the collapsible vessels have sufficient tone to increase the closing pressure by 10 cmH_2O above the surrounding pressure.

When P_A is increased to 10 cmH_2O and Ppa is progressively lowered, Q decreases linearly with Ppa along line C, which extrapolates to Q = 0 at Ppa = 20 cmH_2O. Accordingly, the average value of Pc again exceeds P_A by 10 cmH_2O because of vascular tone; and Pc increases by 5 cmH_2O when P_A increases by 5 cmH_2O, suggesting that the collapsible vessels are exposed to alveolar pressures. Raising P_A from 5 to 10 cmH_2O does not change the slope of the pressure/flow relationship, but does increase the pressure difference, Ppa − Pla, at the same flow rate from A to C. This increase is the increase in Pc imposed by the higher P_A on the collapsible alveolar vessels.

Note that the continuous lines in Fig. 2-19 (right panel) depicting real data become curvilinear as Ppa is reduced below the average value of Pc at P_A = 5 cmH_2O and P_A =10 cmH_2O. This suggests that lung vessels have a range of closing pressures, so that they progressively close, or *derecruit,* as their Ppa becomes less than their Pc. Accordingly, vascular resistance rises as Ppa falls, because there are fewer channels for blood flow; this is the main cause of reduced blood flow to upper lung regions (see below), and is a physical basis for increased PVR as pulmonary blood flow

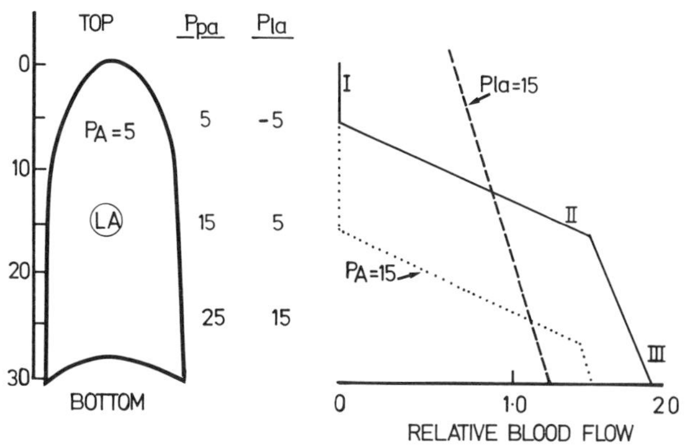

FIGURE 2-20 Schematic diagram depicting the vertical distribution of pulmonary perfusion. On the left is a typical lung measuring 30 cm from top to bottom, having P_A=5 cmH_2O > Ppl (pressure at the lung surface). The middle scale shows typical values of Ppa and Pla measured by a transducer centered at the level of the left atrium (circled "LA"), where Ppa = 15 and Pla = 5. Because of the weight of the column of blood, these vascular pressures decrease toward the top of the lung and increase toward the bottom of the lung. The consequence of the vertical distribution of vascular pressure on relative blood flow (a uniform distribution would give a vertical line at flow = 1.0) is shown on the right by the continuous line labeled I, II, III; the effects of increased Pla (interrupted line of blood flow distribution) and increased P_A (dotted line of distribution) are shown (for discussion, see text).

and Ppa fall to very low values. A more common artifactual increase in PVR as Ppa and Q decrease in the physiologic range is also illustrated in Fig. 2-19 (right panel). Calculated PVR at P_A = 5 cmH_2O (depicted by the line from origin to A) is less than the PVR at P_A = 10 cmH_2O (depicted by the line from origin to C). Accordingly, calculated PVR is increased by increasing the P_A, because Pc has increased. Note further that the PVR decreases from A to B, as depicted by the solid line connecting the origin to B, compared to the interrupted line. This means that merely increasing the flow rate through the pulmonary circulation causes a reduction in the calculated PVR; for example, an infusion of fluid dopamine or dobutamine might increase Q from A to B in association with a large reduction in PVR. Inference that any of these interventions is a pulmonary vasodilator is erroneous!

VERTICAL DISTRIBUTION OF PULMONARY BLOOD FLOW

The left-hand panel of Fig. 2-20 depicts a lung in the upright position with a scale, in centimeters, from the top to the bottom of the lung, which has an average length of 30 cm at end-expiration—i.e., at functional residual capacity (FRC); for simplicity, FRC is set by letting P_A equal 5 cmH_2O and Ppl equals 0 cmH_2O (as in an open thorax). Vascular pressures within the lung are referenced to the left atrium, which is halfway down the lung—i.e., 15 cm from the top. At that level the Ppa is measured to be 15 cmH_2O, and the Pla is measured to be 5 cmH_2O. Blood in vessels extending toward the top or toward the bottom of the lung has a specific gravity approximately equal to that of water. Accordingly, pressure in pulmonary arteries 10 cm above the left atrium is 5 cmH_2O; and 10 cm below the left atrium, Ppa is 25 cmH_2O. After the blood passes through alveolar vessels, it drains into veins having hydrostatic pressures greater than the Pla toward the bottom of the lung (15 cmH_2O at 10 cm distance below the left atrium), and less than the Pla in lung regions above the left atrium (−5 cmH_2O 10 cm above the left atrial level). The lung itself has PA that is 5 cmH_2O greater than the Ppl at end-expiration, and PA is the same from top to bottom within the air spaces of the lung.

In the right panel of Fig. 2-20, relative blood flow is plotted (on the x axis) against vertical distance from top to bottom of the lung (on the y axis). Consider first the continuous line: from the top of the lung to a distance 5 cm below the top of the lung, Ppa increases from 0 to 5 cmH_2O. Because all these values of Ppa are less than PA, there is no low, because the alveolar vessels are closed. This region, where Ppa is less than PA, denotes Zone I.

As distance from the top of the lung increases from 5 to 15 cm, Ppa increases from 5 to 15 cmH_2O, and venular pressure (designated Pla) increases from −5 to 5 cmH_2O. In this Zone II of the lung, Ppa is greater than PA, which is greater than Pla; as discussed in the section above, the driving pressure for blood flow through these lung regions is Ppa − PA, and this value increases with distance down Zone II of the lung. Accordingly, relative blood flow increases with distance down the lung in this zone.

As distance from the top of the lung increases from 15 to 30 cm, Ppa increases from 15 to 30 cmH_2O and Pla increases from 5 to 20 cmH_2O. Note that Pla exceeds PA throughout this lung region, so Ppa is greater than Pla, which is greater than PA (Zone III). The driving pressure (Ppa − Pla) does not change from 15 to 30 cm from the top of the lung, so relative blood flow should not change unless PVR has changed. Yet relative blood flow does increase with vertical distance from the top of the lung in Zone III, indicating that the PVR must decrease toward the bottom of the lung.

There are two possible mechanisms accounting for this reduction in PVR through Zone III. The higher pressures in the pulmonary arteries and veins may distend the vessels at the bottom of the lung, thereby decreasing their resistance to flow by increasing the radius of vessels. Alternatively, the higher pressure within the arteries may recruit more lung vessels by exceeding their critical Pc. This would allow a greater number of vessels to conduct pulmonary blood flow toward the bottom of the lung, and so reduce the resistance to pulmonary blood flow. Vascular recruitment and distention occur in Zone II as well, accounting for part of the increase in relative blood flow with vertical distance from the top of the lung in that region.

Now consider the interrupted line labeled "Pla = 15" (Fig. 2-20, right panel). This represents the vertical distribution of relative blood flow in conditions of volume overload or congestive heart failure when Pla is high. Then the pressure in pulmonary veins 10 cm above the left atrium would be 5 cmH_2O—i.e., equal to the PA, so that Zone III would begin 5 cm from the top of the lung. Of course, to maintain blood flow through the lung, the Ppa must increase as the Pla; for example, Ppa at the level of the left atrium is 25 cmH_2O. Thus, the gradient for pulmonary blood flow (Ppa − Pla) would be 10 cmH_2O from the region near the top of the lung to the bottom of the lung, and blood flow would increase slightly because of recruitment or distention of vessels through Zone III. Note that there is a much more uniform distribution of blood flow when the Pla is increased, compared to the continuous line in the normal conditions where Pla is 5 cmH_2O; this accounts for the chest-radiologic sign of increased Pla—increased flow and distention of upper lobe vessels.

Consider also the condition depicted by the dotted line (Fig. 2-20), where PA is increased to 15 cmH_2O. If there were no change in Ppa and Pla associated with this inflation of the lung, Zone I would now extend to 15 cm from the top of the lung, where Ppa first equals PA. Zone II would extend from here to 25 cm from top of the lung, where Pla first equals PA, and there would be a small Zone III in the bottom 5 cm of the lung. This dotted line illustrates the effect of high values of PA and lung inflation to increase the zone of the lung receiving no pulmonary blood flow. One often-overlooked adverse effect of positive-pressure ventilation with high PEEP or high tidal volume (VT) is the large increase in dead space (VD/VT) caused by the high PA; not infrequently, alveolar ventilation can actually increase when VT is reduced in these conditions, causing a paradoxical fall in Pa_{CO_2}.

As described above, this same phenomenon could occur when PA remains at 5 cmH_2O, but the tone around alveolar vessels is increased by 10 cmH_2O, thereby raising Pc by 10 cmH_2O and increasing Zone I. This latter mechanism may be how alveolar hypoxia reduces the perfusion of hypoxic lung units. Alveolar hypoxic vasoconstriction improves pulmonary O_2 exchange by reducing the perfusion to lung regions having low ventilation and low O_2 tensions. This matching of perfusion to ventilation improves pulmonary gas exchange and is associated with an increase in Ppa. A conventional view is that hypoxic vasoconstriction occurs in pulmonary arterioles perfusing hypoxic regions; for example, in Fig. 2-17, hypoventilation and hypoxia in the upper alveolus would cause constriction of the upper branch of the pulmonary artery rather than compression of the alveolar vessels, where little smooth muscle can be found. However, compelling evidence exists that alveolar hypoxia increases Pc without changing the slope of the pulmonary P-Q relationship; for example, in the right panel of Fig. 2-19, alveolar hypoxia shifts the P-Q data from line BA to line C in the absence of a change in PA. Conceivably, interstitial contractile elements in the septa respond to hypoxia by increasing Pc. Such a mechanism would confer a tighter control on $\dot{V}/\dot{Q}$ matching by localizing the constricting effect of alveolar hypoxia at a more peripheral circulatory site than pulmonary arterioles. Note that PA_{O_2} during air breathing does not approach values low enough to cause hypoxic pulmonary vasoconstriction (HPV) (PA_{O_2} <50 mmHg) until $\dot{V}/Q$ approaches 0.1. Such $\dot{V}/\dot{Q}$ values are not observed in normal lungs, so increased F_{IO_2} does not reduce Ppa or PVR because there is no HPV to block. Note further that the vertical gradient of perfusion is in the same direction as the vertical gradient of ventilation, so that in the normal lung the lower values of $\dot{V}/\dot{Q}$ are at the base of the lung and approach 0.5; because the P_{AO_2} in such lung units does not fall below 70 mmHg, the effluent blood is fully saturated, so there is minimal defect in pulmonary gas exchange associated with the vertical gradients of perfusion—unless ventilation of dependent regions is impaired by abnormal airway closure and/or breathing at low lung volumes, as described in Chap. 1.

PULMONARY HYPERTENSION

Several conditions cause or complicate critical illness by obstructing such a large fraction of the pulmonary vascular bed that the right ventricle cannot maintain adequate output against the high Ppa. In acute pulmonary hypertension following a large pulmonary embolus, a hypoperfusion state is often observed when Ppa increases from a normal value of less than 20 mmHg to a value greater than 40 mmHg. Chronic or acute-on-chronic pulmonary hypertension develops in chronic obstructive pulmonary disease (COPD), sleep-disordered breathing (SDB), and pulmonary fibrosis of diverse etiologies, in part because of HPV. Alveolar hypoxia is the main cause of HPV, which is relieved by modest increases in F_{IO_2}, but HPV also causes most of the increase in Ppa during acute hypoxemic respiratory failure, when HPV is ameliorated by increasing mixed venous P_{O_2} ($P_{\bar{V}O_2}$). Another part of the vascular obstruction is due to obliteration of vascular bed by the disease process (emphysematous destruction of alveolar septa, or disordered healing with collagen scarring to occlude small vessels—as in the proliferative phase of adult respiratory distress syndrome [ARDS]). These pathologic processes may aggravate the loss of vascular bed due to the intraluminal or intramural obstruction in less common conditions of primary pulmonary hypertension, collagen vascular diseases, pneumonectomy, and recurrent pulmonary embolic disease. Because all these causes of increased PVR are compounded by external compression of a limited alveolar vascular bed by positive-pressure ventilation with PEEP or high values of V_T, it is not uncommon for the hypoperfused, hypotensive state in such patients to be aggravated by ventilator therapy implemented to stabilize their shock.

Therapies designed to reduce PVR (O_2, pulmonary vasodilators, thrombolytic agents) should include considerations to reduce P_A (reduce PEEP, V_T, ventilator rate), all in concert with inotropic agents (dobutamine) and a titration of circulating volume, informed by the possibility that increasing volume may impair right ventricular function. Early use of α-adrenergic drugs (e.g., phenylephrine) for systemic vasoconstriction may raise BP to improve right ventricular perfusion with minimal effects on PVR, because of the sparse α-receptor distribution in the pulmonary circulation; accordingly, it is not irrational to combine phenylephrine with a pulmonary vasodilator to "buy time" for amelioration of the underlying conditions. Of course, these medical therapies are temporizing and are marginally effective, so the long-term outcome of these conditions has been improved dramatically by the current surgical and immunosuppressive techniques of heart-lung transplantation; in some centers pulmonary thrombectomy is an option for acute or recurrent pulmonary embolism, which is life-threatening.

Several common hemodynamic and gas exchange manifestations of the pathophysiology of pulmonary hypertension merit explanation. Note in Table 2-3 that the pulmonary pulse pressure is large (80/30) even though SV is abnormally low (30 mL). Unlike the systemic circulation, where much of the SV is stored during systolic ejection in proximal elastic arteries and discharged during diastole, the normal pulmonary circulation has such a low PVR that most of the ejected SV traverses the lung during systole, and there is no diastolic flow; accordingly, the diastolic Ppa is often equal to the Ppw. Yet when PVR is increased sufficiently to cause Ppa to exceed 40 mmHg, much of the right ventricular SV is stored in large elastic pulmonary arteries during systole for subsequent diastolic flow through the lung; pulmonary pulse pressure is increased in proportion to the greater systolic distention. Furthermore, diastolic Ppa exceeds Ppw because of the resistive pressure drop of diastolic flow through a high PVR. Indeed, pulmonary hypertension is one of a few conditions where even Ppw can exceed LVEDP because of the resistive pressure drop caused by blood flow through the pulmonary veins between the vascular segment occluded by the inflated balloon and the left atrium (other rare conditions are mitral stenosis, left atrial myxoma, and pulmonary venoocclusive disease).

In the normal pulmonary circulation, blood flow can increase threefold (from 5 to 15 L/min), as during heavy exercise, with only a small increase in Ppa (from 15 to 20 mmHg) and no change in Ppw; as a result PVR decreases as $\dot{Q}_T$ increases, in part because of recruitment and distention of vessels. In early pulmonary hypertension, the resting Ppa and PVR are often minimally elevated, but modest increases in $\dot{Q}_T$, as in light exercise, cause large increase in Ppa, in part because the disease has obliterated recruitable pulmonary vessels. One consequence of this exercise-induced acute exacerbation of pulmonary hypertension is that the right ventricle is not able to maintain the $\dot{Q}_T$ required to meet the metabolic demands of exercise (because of the increased afterload and resultant increased Pra, which impedes VR); hence $P_{\bar{V}O_2}$ falls. Perfusion of the lung with blood having low $P_{\bar{V}O_2}$ is the major cause of exercise-induced arterial desaturation in emphysema and pulmonary fibrosis. That is, the diseased lungs of these patients have a wide V/Q variance, including a large fraction of the total perfusion to lung units with V/Q below 0.1, but this rarely reduces Pa_{O_2} below 70 mmHg until $P_{\bar{V}O_2}$ is reduced during exercise. Similarly, the abnormal V/Q variance induced by pulmonary embolism is insufficient to reduce Pa_{O_2} much unless $\dot{Q}_T$, and so $P_{\bar{V}O_2}$, is reduced; significant perfusion of units having low V/Q by blood with low $P_{\bar{V}O_2}$ is the cause of most of the hypoxemia following pulmonary embolus. As discussed in Chap. 1, such hypoxemia is quite responsive to modest O_2 enrichment of inspired air; this explains the efficacy of long-term O_2 therapy in ameliorating the pulmonary hypertension of COPD, SDB, and pulmonary fibrosis, and the ease of correcting Pa_{O_2} in acute pulmonary embolism and in other etiologies of acute-on-chronic pulmonary hypertension—with the exception of acute hypoxemic respiratory failure.

Indeed, when full arterial saturation requires an FI_{O_2} greater than 0.4, a search for causes of true shunt should begin. Not infrequently this reveals intercurrent airspace-filling disease (pulmonary edema, pneumonia) or atelectasis, both of which have been documented as causes of additional refractory hypoxemia in pulmonary embolism. Less often, intracardiac right-to-left shunts are detected by dye or bubble echocardiography through an incomplete atrial septum or patent foramen ovale; presumably the shunt is induced by the underlying pulmonary hypertension. The distinction between intrapulmonary and intracardiac shunt in pulmonary hypertension influences the approach to therapy for the hypoxemia. PEEP often reduces intrapulmonary shunt but increases intracardiac shunt; and pulmonary edema is reduced by lowering Ppw, while treatment of intracardiac shunt requires lowering of Pra with respect to Pla (pulmonary vasodilators and/or systemic vasoconstrictors). Whenever shunt-induced arterial hypoxemia confounds management of pulmonary hypertension, both the hypoxemia and the PVR may be reduced by raising Pv_{O_2} through measures that increase O_2 delivery (cardiac output, hematocrit, and arterial saturation via transient increases in FI_{O_2} to very high levels), and through concurrent measures to reduce O_2 consumption (ventilator therapy with respiratory muscle rest, treatment of fever with antipyretics, cooling blanket with muscle relaxation, early effective treatment of sepsis). Several controversial questions about further management of pulmonary hypertension are best answered by titration in each patient. For example, reducing a hematocrit greater than 60 lowers PVR by reducing blood viscosity, and raising a hematocrit less than 30 increases Pv_{O_2}; between these extremes, titration for best effect on PVR and on the patient's improvement is indicated. Respiratory and metabolic acidemia have been implicated in aggravating pulmonary hypertension, but their effects are small. The benefits of correcting these abnormalities must be weighed against potential adverse effects; that is, increasing tidal volume and ventilator rate to correct acidemia may actually increase PVR and Ppa via alveolar vascular compression.

PULMONARY EDEMA

In health, the interstitial spaces of all systemic organs and of the lungs are protected from accumulation of excess extravascular liquid, or edema. Critical illness introduces several abnormalities to overwhelm these defenses, and edema regularly spills from the pulmonary interstitium into the alveoli to cause intrapulmonary shunt, tachypnea, and increased work of breathing. Edema production can be reduced by lowering pulmonary vascular pressure, if this intervention does not cause inadequate $\dot{Q}_T$ and insufficient oxygen transport ($\dot{Q}_{O_2}$). Judicious use of vasoactive drugs (dobutamine, dopamine, nitroprusside) can maintain adequate $\dot{Q}_T$ and $\dot{Q}_{O_2}$ at reduced Ppw at the risk of increasing shunt and hypoxemia. Since the hypoxemia of pulmonary edema is refractory to O_2 therapy, and because high FI_{O_2} causes further lung injury and edema, PEEP is particularly helpful in redistributing edema out of the airspaces into the peribronchovascular interstitium to reduce shunt; yet excess PEEP increases Ppl to reduce VR and $\dot{Q}_{O_2}$. This section reviews the mechanisms responsible for pulmonary edema formation and clearance, how these are adversely affected in critical illness, and an approach to prevention and management of edema and its adverse effects.

Figure 2-21 is a schematic diagram depicting the circulatory factors governing the movement of edema ($\dot{Q}_E$) between the pulmonary vessels and the lung interstitial tissues; the Starling equation describing lung liquid flux is written beneath the figure. On the left-hand end is the pulmonary artery coming from the right ventricle (not shown), which branches out into very small vessels, one of which is shown here, passing between two alveolar walls. At the other end is a pulmonary vein, which empties into the left atrium and has about the same pressure as the left ventricle at end-diastole (LVEDP). The hydrostatic pressure in the microvessels of the lung (Pmv, about 12 mmHg) lies about halfway between Ppa (normally about 15 mmHg) and LVEDP (normally about 10 mmHg). The small vessels have a massive surface area (S), which is necessary for gas exchange; however, an adverse effect of the large S is that it also provides much area for liquid to leak out of the vessels into the perimicrovascular or septal interstitium. Hydrostatic pressure in the septal interstitial space (Pis, about −4 mmHg) is subatmospheric, in part because it drains into the peribronchovascular interstitium, which has a more negative pressure (see below) and in part because lymph vessels—valved, like veins, for unidirectional flow—actively remove liquid from the interstitial spaces, which have intrinsic structural stability to resist collapse. Accordingly, there is a positive hydrostatic pressure (Pmv − Pis, about 16 mmHg) driving edema across the microvascular endothelium to the lung septal interstitium. Like any membrane, the vascular wall presents a barrier to this bulk flow

FIGURE 2-21 Schematic representation of Starling forces governing the flux of lung liquid from intravascular to extravascular space (for discussion and definition of symbols, see text). (From Hall JB, Wood LDH: Acute hypoxemic respiratory failure. Med Grand Rounds 3:184, 1984. By permission of Plenum Press.)

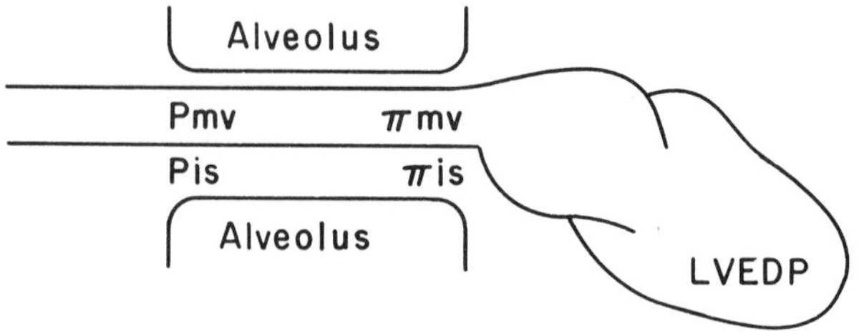

$$\text{Edema Flow} = [(\text{Pmv}-\text{Pis}) - (\pi\text{mv}-\pi\text{is})\,\sigma]\,\text{Kf}$$

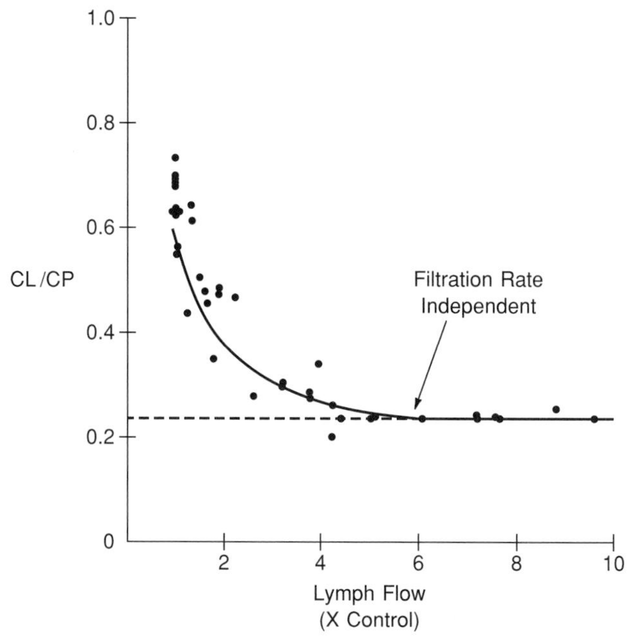

FIGURE 2-22 Lymph-to-plasma concentration ratios (CL/CP, ordinate) as a function of lymph flow from data obtained in unanesthetized sheep. (Reproduced with permission, from Taylor et al: Interstitial spaces and lymphatics, in AP Fishman and AB Fisher (eds): *Handbook of Physiology. The Respiratory System, Circulation and Non-Respiratory Functions.* Bethesda, MD, Am Physiol Soc, 1984, Volume I, Section 3, Chap. 4, pp. 167–230.)

of liquid characterized by its permeability to water (Kf, expressed in mL edema/min per mmHg); Kf includes S, and so is heavily weighted by the characteristics of the alveolar vessels where so much of S resides.

The microvascular membrane is also characterized by its permeability to circulating proteins, dominated by albumin and globulin; this property is the reflection coefficient, σ. If these plasma proteins were completely reflected ($\sigma = 1$), no protein would pass from lung blood to interstitium; in contrast, if the microvascular membrane were freely permeable ($\sigma = 0$), interstitial protein concentration as indicated by lung lymph (CL) would equal that of plasma proteins (CP). As shown in Fig. 2-22, CL/CP is about 0.6 in the normal steady-state edema flow in most mammals; when $\dot{Q}_E$ as estimated from lung lymph flow (QL) is progressively increased by elevating Pmv, CL/CP falls to a plateau value of about 0.3. This plateau value indicates the microvascular protein reflection coefficient ($\sigma = 1 - CL/CP = 0.7$) measured in conditions of high $\dot{Q}_E$; at lower $\dot{Q}_E$, water diffuses from interstitium to blood along the concentration gradient for water established by CP's being greater than CL.

Accordingly, two simultaneous processes govern water movement between blood and interstitium: bulk flow from blood to interstitium [$\dot{Q}_E = (Pmv - Pis)Kf$], and diffusion of water from interstitium to blood driven by the hydrostatic equivalent [$(\pi mv - \pi is)\sigma$] of the concentration difference for water, where π is the colloid osmotic pressure. This value has been measured for plasma (πmv about 20 mmHg) and for lung lymph ($\pi$is about 12 mmHg) by placing either liquid on one side of a pressure-transducing membrane permeable to 0.9% NaCl but impermeable to protein ($\sigma = 1$); on the other side of the membrane is saline solution, which diffuses along its water concentration gradient across the membrane into the plasma (or lymph) chamber. Then the membrane is bent toward the saline by the measured hydrostatic pressure (π) equivalent of the difference in water concentration produced by the difference in colloid concentration between the chambers. Note that only part of the concentration difference between CP and CL acts across the microvascular membrane, because it is permeable to protein ($\sigma = 0.7$). These considerations explain why the oncotic pressure term $(\pi mv - \pi is)\sigma$, normally about 6 mmHg, is subtracted from the hydrostatic pressure term (Pmv − Pis) in the Starling equation for lung liquid flux as written beneath Fig. 2-21; normally this equation gives a value of $QE = \Delta PKf$, where ΔP is about 10 mmHg. Accordingly, Kf can be measured by methods measuring $\dot{Q}_E$ and ΔP; for example, when lymph flow (QL) is assumed equal to QE as in Fig. 2-22, then $Kf = \dot{Q}_L/\Delta P$.

When $\dot{Q}_E$ is increased by increasing Pmv, several factors act to keep the lungs from collecting excess liquid. First, lymphatic flow increases. Second, increased $\dot{Q}_E$ reduces CL/CP to increase the oncotic term and so reduce $\dot{Q}_E$. Third, if $\dot{Q}_L$ is less than $\dot{Q}_E$, edema accumulates in the tight alveolar septal interstitium, raising Pis from −4 mmHg to a value a little above 0 mmHg; this decreases ΔP and so decreases $\dot{Q}_E$. During edema accumulation, the increased septal Pis drives edema through tissue planes toward intraparenchymal peribronchovascular interstitium, where Pis is rendered even more subatmospheric (−10 mmHg) by the outward pull of alveolar walls on the adventitia surrounding the relatively stiff bronchi and vessels. This adventitial pull renders Pis even more negative with each inspiration, creating a cyclic suction to move edema from the alveolar septa toward the hilum of the lung, where peribronchovascular interstitial pressures are most negative, where the tissues have the largest capacity to accommodate the edema, and where the densest accumulation of lymphatics is arranged to clear the edema to the systemic veins. This accounts for the Kerley lines, the bronchial cuffing, and the perihilar "butterfly" distribution of interstitial cardiogenic pulmonary edema on the chest radiograph. When edemagenesis continues to fill these interstitial reservoirs, Pis rises at the alveolar septa, disrupting tight junctions between alveolar type I epithelium to flood the air spaces. Histologic morphometry of edematous lungs reveals that flooded alveoli have about one-eighth the volume of unflooded alveoli, indicating that a relatively small volume of alveolar edema floods eight times that volume of airspace; for example, in a patient with an end-expired lung gas volume of 4 L, 250 mL of alveolar edema fills half the air spaces (8×250 mL $= 2$ L), accounting for a large intrapulmonary shunt and for a large reduction in lung compliance, because only half the lung is ventilated.

By contrast with this distribution of cardiogenic edema, a greater proportion of noncardiogenic edema accumulates in air spaces. Because interstitial edema causes little impairment of lung gas exchange, noncardiogenic edema—as develops in the early exudative stage of ARDS—has a much greater shunt per edema volume than cardiogenic edema. Presumably, this different distribution of edema occurs because the lung injury, which increases Kf and decreases σ, also damages the alveolar epithelial barrier, so increased $\dot{Q}_E$ has access to a low-resistance pathway to a very large reservoir for edema—the air spaces of the lung. Often, the hydrostatic pressure driving edema from vessels to airspace is normal or reduced; as $\dot{Q}_E$ increases at normal Pmv (increased Kf) following an acute lung injury, CL/CP does not decrease as in cardiogenic edema (see Fig. 2-22), but increases slightly to a value of about 0.8, so that the reflection coefficient decreases ($\sigma = 1 - CL/CP = 0.2$).

Although cardiogenic or noncardiogenic edema often floods airspaces in a short time (hours) to increase shunt and work of breathing, the clearance of alveolar edema usually takes days even when the process increasing edema formation has been reversed. Alveolar edema is cleared very slowly from noninjured lungs by active transport of sodium; water follows the osmotic gradient through an intact alveolar membrane, and this clearance is impaired by the oncotic pressure of any protein in the alveolar liquid. Little is known about mechanisms of clearance in injured lungs. Accordingly, treatments of the adverse effects of alveolar edema focus on reducing edema or redistributing it. PEEP increases end-expired lung volume to lower Pis and increase capacity in the peribronchovascular interstitium; in turn, this redistributes much of the alveolar edema into this interstitial reservoir, in association with the aeration of flooded air spaces at a much increased alveolar volume to reduce shunt and to increase lung compliance without altering the amount of edema. Because lung volume increases greatly when PEEP is effective in redistributing edema, Ppl must increase to push the chest wall to an equivalently higher volume. This raises Pra to reduce VR and BP unless the patient's baroreceptor reflexes, or iatrogenic infusions of fluid or vasoactive drugs, maintain Pms and $\dot{Q}_T$. Since the aim of PEEP therapy is to maintain arterial saturation (above 90%) of an adequate circulating hemoglobin (above 12 g%) on a nontoxic F_{IO_2} (below 0.6)—all to effect adequate $\dot{Q}_{O_2}$ without aggravating the lung injury with O_2 toxicity—it is helpful to use the least PEEP possible to achieve these goals so as not to reduce $\dot{Q}_T$. Because PEEP already increases end-expired lung volume, superimposed large values of V_T cause pulmonary barotrauma and further reduce VR; using the least V_T effecting adequate CO_2 elimination minimizes these complications. It is remarkable how rapidly PEEP redistributes edema to reduce hypoxemia (minutes), and how rapidly the shunt returns when PEEP is removed. Accordingly, the informed intensivist can implement an effective, tolerable estimate of least PEEP in less than 5 min in a ventilated patient in whom BP and pulse oximetry are being monitored continuously. When PEEP is effective, plans to prevent its inadvertent removal—as during routine bedside suctioning—can prevent sudden hypoxemic cardiovascular catastrophe.

Whereas ventilator management redistributes edema, thereby stabilizing gas exchange and its effects on $\dot{Q}_{O_2}$ cardiovascular management of both cardiogenic and noncardiogenic edema aims to reduce edema formation and accu-

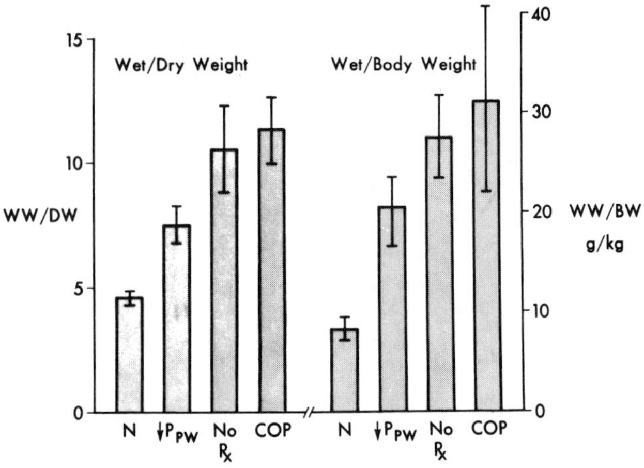

FIGURE 2-23 The treatment of noncardiogenic pulmonary edema. Gravimetric estimates of pulmonary edema in excised lungs (mean ± SD) from four groups of anesthetized dogs: "N" are the values from normal noninjured lungs, for comparison with the three other groups receiving intravenous oleic acid (OA) to cause pulmonary vascular leak for 5 h; "No Rx" denotes a group where Ppw is 10 mmHg and πmv is 16 mmHg—edema increased by about 6 mL per g of lung dry weight compared to the uninjured group. In contrast, reduction of Ppw from 10 to 5 mmHg 1 h after OA ("↓ Ppw" group) reduced the edema accumulation to half that amount; raising πmv by 5 mmHg without changing Pmv in the fourth group ("COP") had no significant effect on edema. (Collated and reproduced, with permission, from Prewitt et al: Treatment of acute low pressure pulmonary edema in dogs: Relative effects of hydrostatic and oncotic pressure, Nitroprusside and PEEP. J Clin Invest 67:409, 1981.)

mulation, thereby reducing the duration and complications of intensive care. Cardiogenic edema is caused by high Pmv, often related to acute or acute-on-chronic left ventricular dysfunction, which increases LVEDP. Reducing the central blood volume by venodilating agents (morphine, furosemide, nitroglycerin) or procedures (rotating tourniquets, phlebotomy, diuresis) reduces LVEDP and edemagenesis; but excess preload reduction will adversely reduce $\dot{Q}_T$ from a poorly functioning ventricle, which often requires a higher LVEDP (16 to 24 mmHg) than normal (8 to 12 mmHg). Where indicated, vasoactive drugs to enhance systolic function (dobutamine, amrinone, nitroglycerine, O_2) or to reduce afterload (calcium channel blockers, nitroprusside), and measures to correct diastolic dysfunction (prolong filling time, maintain coordinated atrial contraction, correct myocardial hypoxemia and ischemia) all act to reduce the LVEDP required for adequate $\dot{Q}_T$ and so reduce cardiogenic edema formation as predicted by the Starling equation. Increasing πmv by colloid infusion also reduces edema formation, provided that Pmv is not increased; note that an albumin infusion that raises πmv from 15 to 20 mmHg and Pmv from 25 to 30 mmHg causes more $\dot{Q}_E$, because σ is 0.7.

Colloid infusion is even less helpful in reducing noncardiogenic edema, where σ is much reduced. In one study of oleic acid–induced noncardiogenic edema in dogs, raising πmv by 5 mmHg had no effect on edema when Pmv was not allowed to change, but lowering Pmv by 5 mmHg (when πmv did not change) reduced edema by 50 percent over the same 4 h of treatment (see Fig. 2-23). Compelling evidence in other animal and clinical studies of acute lung injury supports the therapeutic effect of reducing pulmonary vascular pressures in reducing pulmonary edema. When noncardiogenic occurs at normal or low Pmv, the reduction of LVEDP by only 5 mmHg reduces LVEDV, SV, and $\dot{Q}_T$ by as much as a 20-mmHg reduction in LVEDP in cardiogenic edema (see Fig. 2-24). Accordingly, in reducing the measured Ppw in a patient with acute lung injury one must avoid causing an inadequate $\dot{Q}_T$ and $\dot{Q}_{O_2}$. Just as in cardiogenic edema, Ppw can be reduced considerably without evidence of inadequate output and $\dot{Q}_{O_2}$; and vasoactive drugs and increased hematocrit are effective in restoring adequacy of $\dot{Q}_{O_2}$ at low Ppw when indicated. This approach constantly seeks the least Ppw associated with an adequate $\dot{Q}_T$ and $\dot{Q}_{O_2}$ during the early stage of edema formation in ARDS. Of course, this is only symptomatic treatment, for there are as yet no specific therapies for the acute lung injury that correct an increased Kf and a reduced σ. The aim is to minimize the edema consequence of the vascular injury, thereby shortening the duration of ventilation therapy and ICU care.

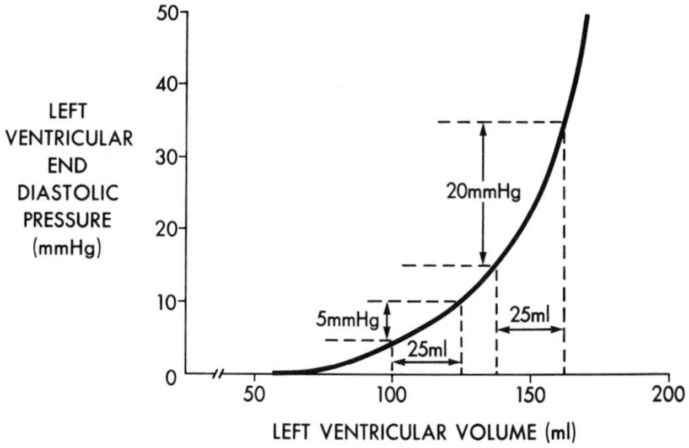

FIGURE 2-24 **Schematic diagram showing the diastolic volume (abcissa)–pressure (ordinate) relationship for the left ventricle. When LVEDV is reduced by 25 mL, LVEDP decreases by 20 mmHg in cardiogenic edema and by 5 mmHg in noncardiogenic edema. Both reductions have large and similar effects to reduce pulmonary edema, but vasoactive drugs and transfusion with packed red blood cells may be necessary to maintain $\dot{Q}O_2$ at the reduced preload. (Reproduced, with permission, from Ali J et al: The effect of furosemide in canine low pressure pulmonary edema. J Clin Invest 64:1494, 1979.)**

Chapter 3

ACID-BASE AND ELECTROLYTE HOMEOSTASIS

GREGORY A. SCHMIDT

Acid-base and electrolyte abnormalities frequently accompany serious illness. In many cases, these derangements compound the illness or threaten life and demand urgent correction. In others, a result merely reflects the devastation of illness; attempted treatment may be detrimental rather than beneficial. In some, the significance of the abnormal laboratory test remains controversial. The following sections review the homeostatic mechanisms which maintain normal hydrogen ion and electrolyte concentrations in health. The factors which perturb the normal balance are discussed, as well as the significance of these abnormalities. Finally, while specific treatment measures are generally left to later chapters, a conceptual approach to therapy is given.

Acid-Base Physiology

Hydrogen ion concentration ($[H^+]$) is one of the most precisely controlled parameters of the internal milieu. Normally, $[H^+]$ is maintained between 36 nanoequivalents per liter (neq/L) (pH = 7.44) and 43 neq/L (pH = 7.36), a difference of only 7 neq/L. Even in the most critically ill patient it is exceedingly rare to see arterial pH fall below 6.8 ($[H^+]$ = 160 neq/L), or rise above 7.8 ($[H^+]$ = 16 neq/L). This chapter reviews acid-base physiology from the conventional perspective and begins with a discussion of the basic chemistry and biochemistry of the hydrogen ion. The normal homeostatic mechanisms which work to preserve $[H^+]$ are presented, followed by an analysis of their derangements. This section concludes with a brief introduction to an alternative approach to understanding acid-base physiology, utilizing the concept of the strong ion difference (SID).

When considering derangements of acid-base homeostasis, the focus is on the intracellular $[H^+]$ and its effects on cellular function. Proteins, which constitute the enzymatic machinery of cells and perform necessary structural and regulatory functions, contain many charged moieties which are sensitive to $[H^+]$. Even a very small change in $[H^+]$ has the capacity to alter the ratio of positively and negatively charged groups, and thereby compromise the role of the protein in cellular function. A dramatic example of such an effect of $[H^+]$ on enzymatic function is the sensitivity of phosphofructokinase to pH. The activity of this important regulator of cellular glycolysis falls by 90 percent as pH is lowered only 0.1 pH unit.

Cellular homeostasis is aimed at defending the ionic charge of proteins, not the cellular $[H^+]$ per se. Evidence for this comes from the effect of changes in temperature on cellular $[H^+]$ and protein charge. As temperature rises or falls, $[H^+]$ moves in a parallel manner (pH varies inversely). Despite this, the ratio of positively charged groups to negatively charged ones on cellular proteins remains unchanged, obviously a useful quality if enzymatic activity is to remain unaffected. At any given temperature and ionic strength, however, control of $[H^+]$ is equivalent to constant protein charge. This justifies the practical focus on $[H^+]$ as the best available measure of cellular protein charge.

An important limitation in applying acid-base chemistry to clinical situations is that our window on cellular $[H^+]$ is through the pH of blood. Since the metabolic flux of CO_2 is from the cytoplasm to the blood, one would guess that the $[H^+]$ progressively lessens along this route. Therefore, intracellular $[H^+]$ and blood $[H^+]$ would be quite different, a fact confirmed by measurement of $[H^+]$.* For example, as measured by nuclear magnetic resonance spectroscopy, intracellular pH in human muscle is normally about 7.0, whereas extracellular pH is 7.4. One obvious example in which it is important to distinguish between the $[H^+]$ of blood and that of the cells is in the use of alkalinizing solutions in the treatment of metabolic acidosis. When sodium bicarbonate is infused into the blood, one expects the blood to become more alkaline (lower $[H^+]$). However, since CO_2 (the P_{CO_2} of a bicarbonate solution exceeds 200 mmHg) rapidly diffuses into cells, while HCO_3^- does not, the immediate effect on the cell is an abrupt worsening of acidosis (higher $[H^+]$). Although the clinical relevance of this effect is vigorously debated and remains unsettled, it points out the risks of making the overly simplistic assumption that changes in blood $[H^+]$ mirror changes in the cell.

The controversy regarding the definition of respiratory acidosis when the Pv_{CO_2} and the Pa_{CO_2} differ substantially is another arena which calls attention to the difference between the $[H^+]$ of blood and that of the cell. This topic has been particularly debated in the setting of cardiopulmonary arrest during resuscitation. Some have asked whether ventilation is truly adequate when the Pa_{CO_2} is normal yet the Pv_{CO_2} is abnormally high.

The Fick principle is typically applied to oxygen transport, but pertains to CO_2 transport as well. This principle relates the difference between arterial and venous oxygen contents to oxygen consumption and the cardiac output ($\dot{Q}_T$) in the steady state:

$$\dot{V}_{O_2} = \dot{Q}_T \times (Ca_{O_2} - C\bar{v}_{O_2}) \qquad (3\text{-}1)$$

where $\dot{V}_{O_2}$ is oxygen consumption, $\dot{Q}_T$ is cardiac output, Ca_{O_2} is arterial oxygen content and $C\bar{v}_{O_2}$ is mixed venous oxygen content.

*This assumes that there is not an overwhelming, energy-requiring process of cellular acid extrusion. There is an important mechanism for cellular acid extrusion; however, it does not outweigh the effect of cellular metabolic and respiratory acid production. Such mechanisms probably do account for the much higher pH in mitochondria (pH = 7.5), where CO_2 is generated, than in the cell.

This relationship must also apply to CO_2 transport. Thus:

$$\dot{V}_{CO_2} = \dot{Q}T \times (Ca_{CO_2} - C\overline{v}_{CO_2}) \qquad (3\text{-}2)$$

where Ca_{CO_2} is arterial CO_2 content and $C\overline{v}_{CO_2}$ is venous CO_2 content.

The important point is that when the $\dot{Q}T$ is abnormally low, the $(a\text{-}v)_{CO_2}$ will widen just as the oxygen content widens. In practice, P_{CO_2} is measured rather than CO_2 content, but the principle holds. A discrepancy between Pa_{CO_2} and Pv_{CO_2} is therefore predictable during states of impaired $\dot{Q}T$. The implications of this for assessing the degree of ventilation in hypoperfusion states are unclear. What the clinician seeks is neither the Pa_{CO_2} nor Pv_{CO_2}, but the cellular $[H^+]$ (or, equivalently, the net protein charge). Until there are better ways to assess cellular acid-base status in vivo, it will be hard to advocate an approach to therapy based on the Pv_{CO_2}. The development of practical methods of measuring cellular $[H^+]$ may provide insights regarding how best to ventilate the hypoperfused patient. More generally, in all states of deranged acid-base homeostasis, clinical medicine would benefit from a knowledge of cellular $[H^+]$ and its response to therapeutic interventions. However, minimally invasive methods of determining cellular $[H^+]$ in critically ill patients are many years away. For now, blood $[H^+]$ and P_{CO_2} must suffice, but their limitations should be kept in mind.

Basic Concepts

THE CHEMISTRY OF $[H^+]$

Pure water (H_2O) ionizes slightly at body temperature to form minute quantities of hydrogen ion (H^+) and hydroxide ion (OH^-). At equilibrium, this dissociation is described by the equation:

$$\frac{[H^+][OH^-]}{[H_2O]} = K_{H_2O} \qquad (3\text{-}3)$$

where K_{H_2O} is the dissociation constant of water and the quantities in brackets indicate concentrations in equivalents per liter (eq/L).

The K_{H_2O} at body temperature is 4.3×10^{-16} eq/L, but since the concentration of water ($[H_2O]$) is itself constant at 55.3 mol/L, it is usually incorporated into the dissociation constant. This forms a new term, the ion product for water (K'_{H_2O}) whose value is 2.4×10^{-14} eq/L:

$$K'_{H_2O} = [H^+] \times [OH^-] \qquad (3\text{-}4)$$

Since electroneutrality demands that $[H^+] = [OH^-]$, the $[H^+]$ can be calculated to be 1.55×10^{-7} eq/L, or 155 neq/L. The pH of pure water at body temperature, defined as the negative of the base 10 logarithm of $[H^+]$, is therefore 6.8.

THE CARBON DIOXIDE/BICARBONATE BUFFER SYSTEM

In vivo, the addition of weak acids and weak bases complicates the calculation of $[H^+]$ greatly. Dissolved CO_2 reacts with water to form carbonic acid (H_2CO_3). This hydration proceeds rapidly in the presence of carbonic anhydrase, an enzyme present in red blood cells (RBCs) and renal tubular cells. Reversible dissociation of carbonic acid yields equal numbers of H^+ and bicarbonate (HCO_3^-) ions. Therefore:

$$\frac{[H^+][HCO_3^-]}{[H_2CO_3]} = K'_{H_2CO_3} \qquad (3\text{-}5)$$

However, carbonic acid is present only in small amounts and is not directly measured. Rather, P_{CO_2} is the clinically determined parameter (See Chap. 13). By Henry's law, dissolved CO_2 is proportional to P_{CO_2}:

$$[CO_{2_{dis}}] = k \times P_{CO_2} \qquad (3\text{-}6)$$

where $k = 0.03$ meq/L/mmHg

Further, since only a tiny amount of dissolved CO_2 forms carbonic acid, use of $[CO_{2_{dis}}]$, or P_{CO_2} in place of $[H_2CO_3]$, greatly overestimates the resulting $[H^+]$. This problem is solved by using an apparent dissociation constant for H_2CO_3 (K'_a), rather than the true dissociation constant (K'). This allows a rewriting of the equation for the dissociation of carbonic acid as follows:

$$\frac{[H^+][HCO_3^-]}{P_{CO_2} \times 0.03} = K'_a \qquad (3\text{-}7)$$

or, rearranging and taking the base 10 logarithm of both sides:

$$pH = pK'_a + \log \frac{[HCO_3^-]}{P_{CO_2} \times 0.03} \qquad (3\text{-}8)$$

where $pK'_a = 6.1$.

This is the familiar Henderson-Hasselbalch equation which describes the effect of changes in $[HCO_3^-]$ or P_{CO_2} on pH. Alternatively, this can be expressed as the equivalent, but simpler, Henderson equation:

$$[H^+] = 24 \times P_{CO_2}/[HCO_3^-] \qquad (3\text{-}9)$$

where $[H^+]$ is expressed in neq/L.

With the normal P_{CO_2} of 40 and HCO_3^- of 24, the pH is calculated to be 7.40 ($[H^+] = 24 \times 40/24 = 40$ neq/L).

Acid-Base Homeostasis

The body is remarkably adept at maintaining a normal $[H^+]$ in the face of acidic challenges. For example, the normal production of CO_2 is about 15,000 meq/day. Since the entire range of $[H^+]$ which is compatible with life is only 140 neq/L (or 0.006 meq in a 70-kg adult), the metabolic produc-

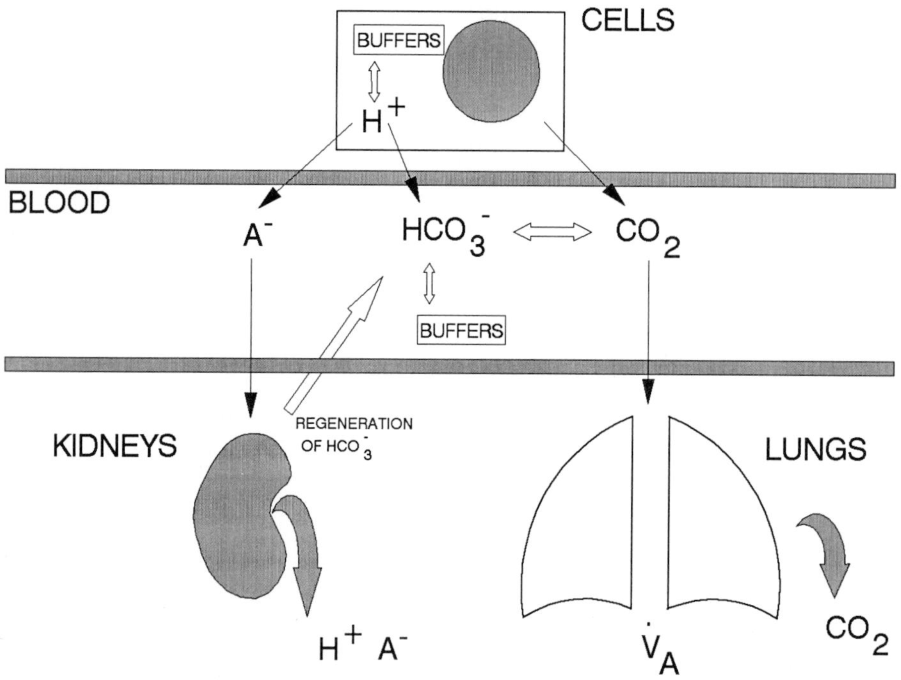

FIGURE 3-1 Acid-base homeostasis depends on buffering, renal function, and elimination of CO_2 by the lungs. Cells produce volatile acid (CO_2), which enters the bloodstream where it is transported as CO_2 and, through buffering by hemoglobin, as bicarbonate. CO_2 is then eliminated by the lungs through $\dot{V}_A$. Hydrogen ions are buffered intracellularly, as well as in the blood, and must be eliminated with their nonvolatile acid anions in the kidney. Excretion of acid is linked to regeneration of bicarbonate which returns to the blood.

tion of CO_2 (volatile acid) is a huge acid load. Clearly, buffering has an important role in reducing the impact of an acid (or base) challenge on the resulting plasma $[H^+]$. Secondly, the lungs are able to excrete an equal amount of CO_2 via the alveolar ventilation ($\dot{V}_A$), thereby maintaining P_{CO_2}.

A much smaller, but equally important, acid load is derived from the normal catabolism of food and cellular constituents. This nonvolatile acid production amounts to only 1 meq/kg/day, but it cannot be eliminated through the lungs. The anions of these nonvolatile acids must be excreted though the kidneys while bicarbonate is regenerated. In critically ill patients, nonvolatile acid production can increase dramatically. For example, starvation entails a shift to stored fats as an energy source, with a concommitant increment in ketoacid production. This alone can result in mild metabolic acidosis. However, burns, major

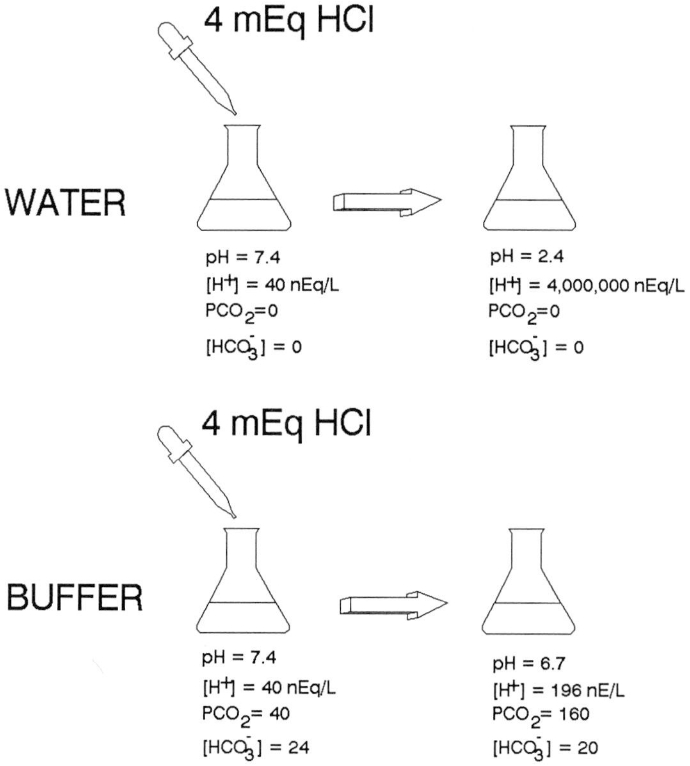

FIGURE 3-2 Buffers have a dramatic effect to ameliorate the $[H^+]$ of pH change due to addition of acid (or base). Compare the effect of adding equal amounts of hydrochloric acid to water (slightly alkalinized to make the $[H^+]$ physiologic) or to a buffered solution. Note the large increment in $[H^+]$ in water and the much smaller change in the buffer.

trauma, and sepsis will further increase nonvolatile acid production.

The defense against changes in [H^+] includes extracellular and intracellular buffering, control of P_{CO_2}, and modulation of [HCO_3^-] (Fig. 3-1). The following sections describe the roles of buffering, control of P_{CO_2} (by the lungs), and maintenance of [HCO_3^-] (by the kidneys and cellular metabolism) in day-to-day homeostasis. Subsequent sections will then expand on this foundation by describing clinically significant derangements of acid-base physiology.

BUFFERING

The P_{CO_2}/HCO_3^- acid-base pair is the most important buffer system in the body. Compare the dramatic difference when acid is added to water or, alternatively, to a solution containing physiologic concentrations of sodium bicarbonate and CO_2 (Fig. 3-2).

A buffer is most effective in defending against acid or base challenges when the pH of the solution is near the p*K* of the buffer. Despite the fact that the pK'_a of the CO_2/HCO_3 pair (6.1) is far from the physiologic pH (7.4), this buffer is important because of the independent control which can be exerted over the acid form (CO_2), and the base form (HCO_3^-) by the lung and kidney, respectively. For example, compare the effect of adding acid to a volume of blood when nothing operates to control P_{CO_2} (as in Fig. 3-2), with the effect when the acid is added but the P_{CO_2} of the blood is held constant at 40 mmHg (Fig. 3-3).

The most important nonbicarbonate buffer in blood is the hemoglobin molecule. Hemoglobin contains large amounts of the amino acid histidine, with its neutrophilic imidazole moiety. At least some of the histidine groups have a pK_a which is near the physiologic pH, but dependent on the saturation of hemoglobin with oxygen. This accounts for a remarkable property of hemoglobin. When hemoglobin releases its oxygen to the tissues, the pK_a changes and hemoglobin is able to buffer more acid. This is useful, since at the same time CO_2 is entering the blood, thereby raising [H^+]. As the H^+ ions are buffered, HCO_3^- is released into the RBC. The rising intracellular [HCO_3^-] leads to passive diffusion out of the RBC into the plasma. Electroneutrality is preserved by inward movement of chloride (the "chloride shift") from the plasma. This arrangement, whereby CO_2 (an acid) is transported to the lungs as bicarbonate (a base) via buffering by hemoglobin is illustrated in Figs. 3-4 and 3-5. If this mechanism were not available, then CO_2 would have to be transported as dissolved CO_2 rather than as bicarbonate. To return CO_2 generated in the tissues ($\dot{V}_{CO_2}$) solely as dissolved CO_2 would require P_{CO_2} dramatically higher than is physiologic (P_{CO_2} of roughly 130) or, alternatively, a much higher $\dot{Q}$T. The packaging of large concentrations of hemoglobin with carbonic anhydrase within red blood cells is a truly elegant solution to the acid challenge of metabolically produced carbon dioxide.

Other important buffers include cellular proteins, intracellular organic phosphates, and plasma proteins, especially albumin. During renal failure, carbonates and phosphates of bone provide a huge buffer pool from which to limit the inexorable depletion of bicarbonate by ongoing daily nonvolatile acid production.

MAINTAINING A NORMAL P_{CO_2}

The P_{CO_2} is determined by the ratio of carbon dioxide production ($\dot{V}_{CO_2}$) and $\dot{V}$A. $\dot{V}_{CO_2}$ follows the minute-to-minute

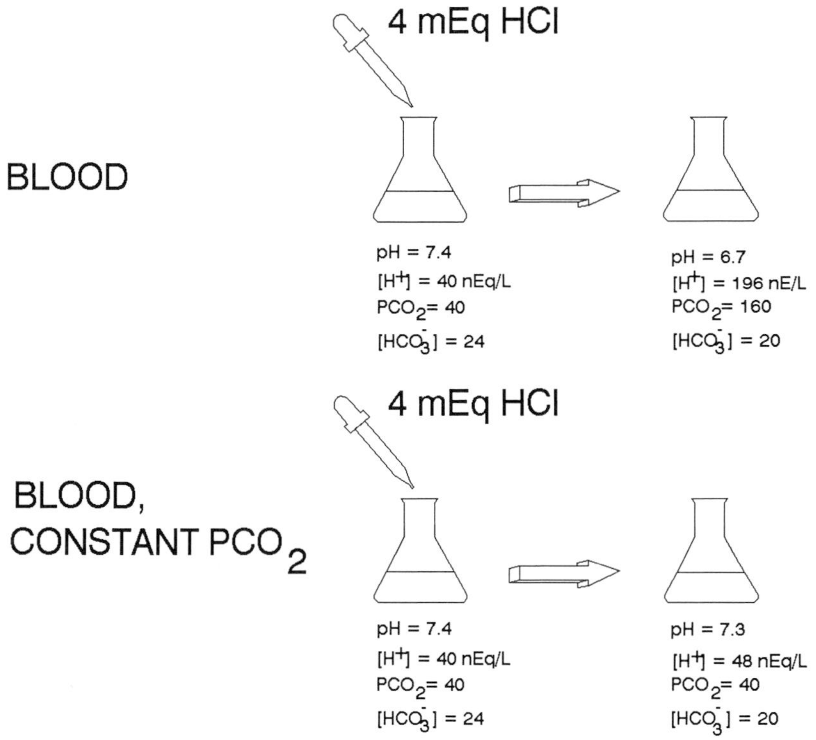

FIGURE 3-3 The P_{CO_2}/HCO_3 buffer system is particularly powerful due to the ability of the lungs and kidneys to alter the concentrations of both the acid and base forms of the buffer. Compare the effect of adding acid to blood when the P_{CO_2} is allowed to rise versus the effect when the P_{CO_2} is kept constant (as by $\dot{V}$A). Note the minimal impact of the acid load on blood pH in the second case.

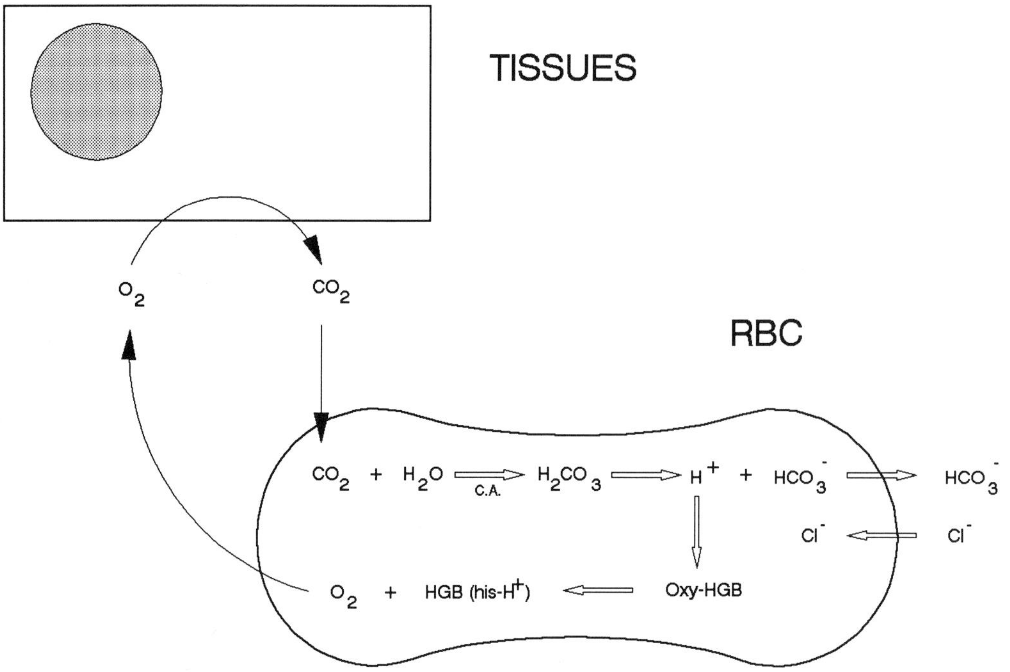

FIGURE 3-4 Tissues produce CO_2 which enters the RBC. There, it combines with water to form carbonic acid in a reaction facilitated by carbonic anhydrase. Carbonic acid dissociates, the hydrogen ion is buffered by hemoglobin, and intra-RBC $[HCO_3]$ rises. Bicarbonate diffuses out of the cells while electroneutrality is maintained by movement of chloride. Thus, through the buffering of hemoglobin, CO_2 is transported as bicarbonate. At the same time, addition of the hydrogen ion to hemoglobin shifts the oxyhemoglobin dissociation curve, which facilitates release of oxygen to the metabolizing tissues. {HGB(his-H^+) indicates that histidine groups of hemoglobin are acidified.}

changes in metabolic rate. Central chemoreceptors, which are sensitive to tiny changes in P_{CO_2}, quickly adjust $\dot{V}_A$ to maintain P_{CO_2} in the normal range of about 40 mmHg. Thus, P_{CO_2} is an indicator of the adequacy of ventilation.

Additional inputs into the level of ventilation include $[H^+]$ through effects on the central chemoreceptors, cortical influences (e.g., voluntary hyperventilation, anxiety), sensory inputs from the chest wall, and information from peripheral chemoreceptors in the carotid arteries and the aorta (which respond not only to P_{CO_2}, but to P_{O_2}). When these stimuli raise ventilation beyond that necessary to maintain a normal P_{CO_2}, hyperventilation, also called respiratory alkalosis, results. Alternatively, when $\dot{V}_A$ is not maintained at a level sufficient to preserve a normal P_{CO_2}, hypoventilation with respiratory acidosis results. Respiratory acidosis is equivalent to type II respiratory failure (see Chap. 1).

MAINTAINING A NORMAL $[HCO_3^-]$

RENAL FACTORS

Control of the $[HCO_3^-]$ is largely a function of the kidneys (Fig. 3-6). Since the plasma $[HCO_3^-]$ is 24 meq/L, and the glomerular filtration rate (GFR) is 120 mL/min (173 L/day), 4.2 equivalents (or about three-fourths of a pound) of sodium bicarbonate is filtered into renal tubular fluid every day. To maintain plasma $[HCO_3^-]$, the kidneys must resorb all this filtered bicarbonate (reclamation). The proximal tubule performs most of this task.

Once the filtered bicarbonate has been reclaimed, further secretion of hydrogen ions by the distal nephron is necessary to recoup the bicarbonate titrated by the daily nonvolatile acid production (regeneration). For each hydrogen ion excreted, one bicarbonate is returned to the plasma. The distal nephron can maximally lower the urine pH only to 4.5. In the absence of any urinary buffer, this corresponds to a $[H^+]$ of only 32,000 neq/L (0.03 meq/L). Since approximately 100 meq/day of nonvolatile acid must be excreted, prohibitively high urine volumes would be required if only 0.03 meq hydrogen ions could be excreted per liter. Urinary phosphate excretion and, more importantly, renal ammonia production provide urinary buffers to aid acid excretion. These substances react with the secreted hydrogen ion to blunt the effect on pH. Thus, far greater amounts of acid can be excreted in a small volume of urine. Renal synthesis of ammonia is augmented by acidosis. It is this mechanism which accounts for most of the increase in urinary acid excretion in metabolic acidosis.

Thus, the body depends on carefully balanced hydrogen ion secretion to maintain acid-base balance. The precise mechanisms which control hydrogen ion secretion are not conclusively delineated. Pa_{CO_2} appears to play a role, since hypocapnia decreases renal hydrogen ion secretion, while hypercapnia augments it, regardless of serum pH. Alterations in intravascular volume affect hydrogen ion secretion,

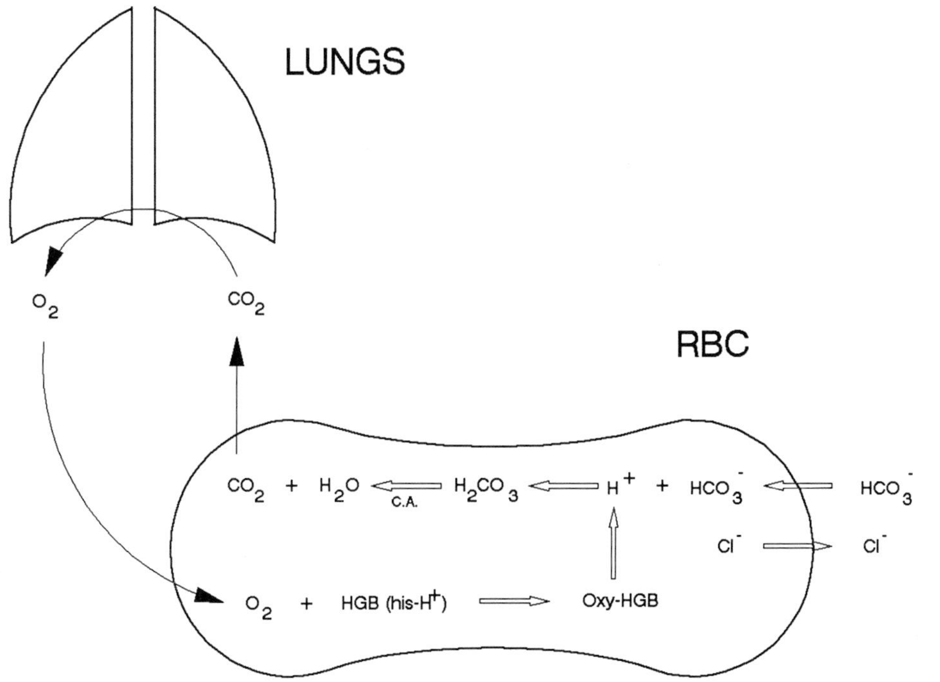

FIGURE 3-5 The process described in Fig. 3-4 is reversed in the lungs. CO_2 is eliminated by $\dot{V}_A$, lowering the intracellular bicarbonate concentration, leading to intracellular movement of HCO_3. The concommitant fall in [H^+] facilitates the release of hydrogen ions from hemoglobin. This shifts the oxyhemoglobin dissociation curve, favoring onloading of oxygen in the lungs. {HGB(his-H^+) indicates that histidine groups of hemoglobin are acidified.}

since sodium and hydrogen ion handling in the kidney are linked (vide infra).

The result of normal nutritional intake and tissue catabolism is to produce excess hydrogen ions, especially during critical illness. Therefore, the renal tasks of reclaiming and regenerating bicarbonate are particularly important. Of course, there are situations in which the role of the kidneys is to lose bicarbonate. For example, hydrogen ions may be leaving the body by a nonrenal route, such as the gastrointestinal tract. During vomiting and nasogastric suctioning, as long as euvolemia is ensured, acid-base balance is usually maintained through excretion of bicarbonate.

Alternatively, there may be exogenous administration of bicarbonate or a substance equivalent to bicarbonate. Intravenously or orally administered bicarbonate, citrate, acetate, or lactate will consume hydrogen ions during their metabolism. Common sources of these substances in the ICU include parenteral nutrition formulas, massive blood product administration, plasmapheresis, and sodium bicarbonate given during resuscitation. To preserve a normal [H^+], either the administered ion or bicarbonate must be excreted.

LACTATE HOMEOSTASIS

While the *net* daily nonvolatile acid production is only about 100 meq/day, a substantial metabolic flux entails the generation and consumption of large amounts of acid. Most tissues are capable only of producing and not consuming lactate. Some (i.e., RBCs) are obliged to produce lactate, since they lack mitochondria, and thus, lack the capacity for oxidative metabolism. The liver and kidney alone have the capacity to consume significant amounts of lactate (under unusual circumstances a few other tissues can consume lactate as well, but their contribution is dwarfed by the liver and kidney). The producers and consumers cooperate through the cyclic utilization of lactate in the Cori cycle (Fig. 3-7). At rest, nearly 1500 meq lactate is produced and consumed each day. During critical illness, this amount can increase dramatically.

Lactate is formed only from pyruvate in a reaction catalyzed by lactate dehydrogenase (LDH). In the process reduced NAD (NADH) is converted to nicotinamide-adenine dinucleotide (NAD), and a hydrogen ion is generated. The fate of lactate is simply to be converted back to pyruvate (only trivial amounts are excreted in the urine), a reaction which requires NAD.

$$\text{Pyruvate} + \text{NADH} + \text{H}^+ \xleftrightarrow{\text{LDH}} \text{Lactate} + \text{NAD} \quad (3\text{-}10)$$

Therefore, to understand the role of lactate in normal metabolism, it is necessary to analyze the biochemistry of pyruvate. Pyruvate is the key intermediate at the nexus of glycolysis, gluconeogenesis, and the tricarboxylic acid cycle (Fig. 3-8).

GLYCOLYSIS. Glucose is catabolized to pyruvate in an irreversible set of reactions called glycolysis. All cells are capable of glycolysis, but certain organs are particularly well equipped with the cellular machinery to create pyruvate (and thereby lactate) in this way. In particular, muscle, brain, skin, RBCs, and intestine have large amounts of glycolytic enzymes.

GLUCONEOGENESIS. Pyruvate can be converted back to glucose, through oxaloacetate, by a series of reactions termed gluconeogenesis. It is through these steps that the Cori cycling of lactate back to glucose is achieved. Gluconeogenesis is not simply the reverse of glycolysis, however,

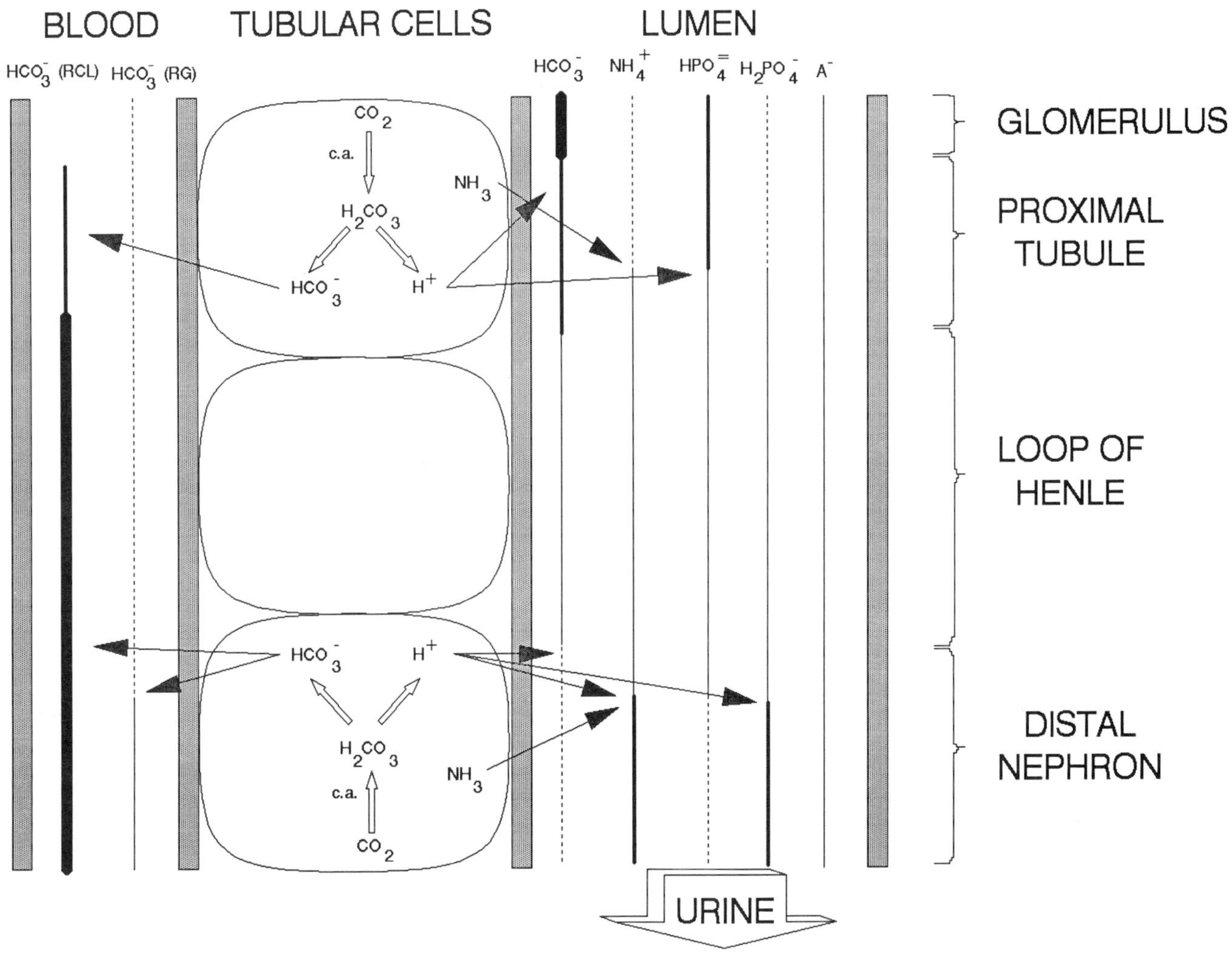

FIGURE 3-6 A simplified view of renal acid-base homeostasis demonstrates reclamation of filtered bicarbonate and regeneration of titrated bicarbonate. At the right is a schematic tubular lumen, on the left is the renal microcirculation, and interposed between them are the renal tubular cells. Relative amounts of ions are indicated by the width of the line under each heading. Reclamation is largely due to hydrogen ion secretion in the proximal tubule. This substantially reduces the amount of bicarbonate in the tubule, while restoring the blood bicarbonate to near normal, since for each hydrogen ion secreted, a bicarbonate is returned to the blood. Reclaimed bicarbonate is indicated under the heading HCO_3^-(RCL). Hydrogen ion secretion beyond that needed to reclaim filtered bicarbonate is used to titrate ammonia (produced from glutamine by renal tubular cells) and inorganic phosphate. Note the rising amounts of ammonium (NH_4^+) and acidified phosphate ($H_2PO_4^-$) in the distal nephron. The bicarbonate formed by the secretion of hydrogen ions by the distal nephron is added to the blood as regenerated bicarbonate, HCO_3^-(RG). (c.a. indicates carbonic anhydrase, A^- acid anions.)

since several of the reactions in each pathway proceed irreversibly. Rather, it requires a unique enzymatic capacity found chiefly in the liver and kidney.

The pyruvate required for gluconeogenesis can alternatively be derived from catabolism of protein, and in particular, from the liberation of alanine from muscle. Finally, fatty acids and ketone bodies contribute to pyruvate through their breakdown to acetylcoenzyme A (acetyl-CoA).

TRICARBOXYLIC ACID CYCLE. The quantitatively most important fate of pyruvate is oxidation to carbon dioxide and water in the mitochondria. This process requires aerobic conditions, so that one consequence of anoxia is a buildup of pyruvate, and consequently, lactate (vide infra). The first step of this path is conversion of pyruvate to acetyl-CoA by pyruvate dehydrogenase (PDH). The activity of this enzyme is modified by several factors, including insulin and dichloroacetate. Acetyl-CoA can be fully oxidized through the electron transport chain but, alternatively, can be used to make fatty acids, ketone bodies, or cholesterol.

Derangements of Acid-Base Homeostasis

Despite the mechanisms for maintenance of $[H^+]$ by buffering, regulation of P_{CO_2}, and control of bicarbonate by the kidneys and the Cori cycle, clinical disturbances of the acid-base milieu are common. The following section reviews

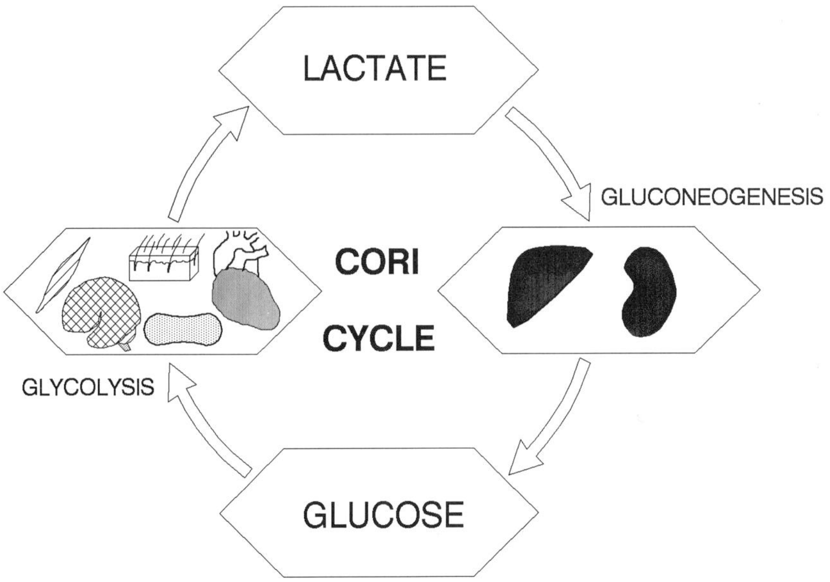

FIGURE 3-7 Glucose is metabolized to lactic acid (via glycolysis) by muscle, central nervous system (CNS), skin, RBCs, and heart, which is transported in the circulation as lactate. Lactate is consumed by the liver and kidney and utilized to produce glucose (gluconeogenesis). This cycling of glucose and lactate is referred to as the Cori cycle.

FIGURE 3-8 The interrelationship of glycolysis, gluconeogenesis, the tricarboxylic acid cycle, and oxidative metabolism are indicated. The tricarboxylic acid cycle and oxidative metabolism take place only within the mitochondria. PEP, phosphoenolpyruvate; LDH, lactate dehydrogenase; PDH, pyruvate dehydrogenase; FFA, free fatty acids; TCA, tricarboxylic acid. Dichloroacetate stimulates PHD activity while insulin lack decreases it.

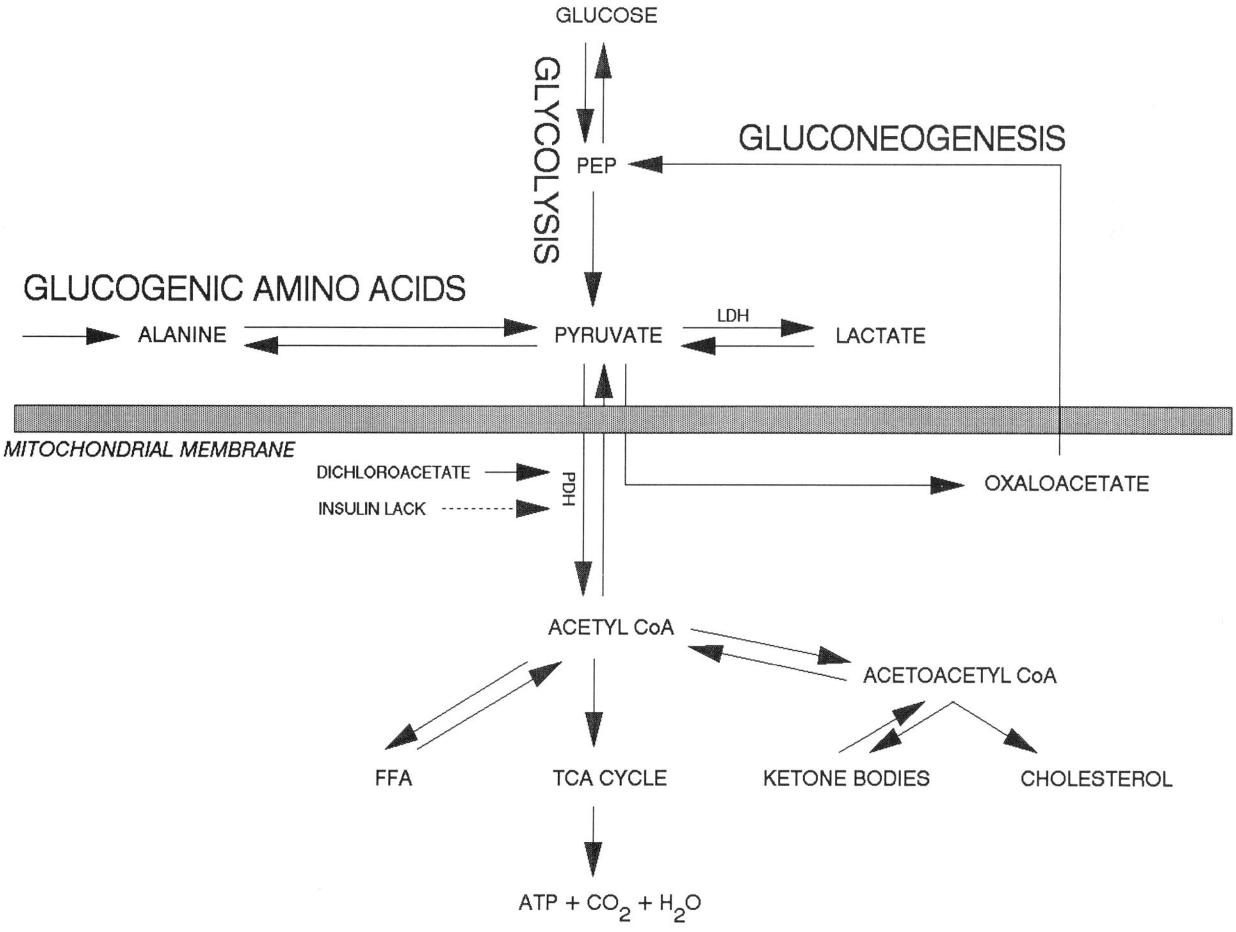

failures of P_{CO_2} control (respiratory alkalosis and acidosis), and then of $[HCO_3^-]$ control (metabolic alkalosis and acidosis). Finally, for each of the four primary acid-base derangements, the body's attempt to return $[H^+]$ toward normal (compensation) is discussed.

DEFINITION OF TERMS

Acidemia is an abnormally low pH (or equivalently, a high blood $[H^+]$) defined as a pH below 7.36. Acidemia is brought about by one of many pathologic processes, collectively called *acidoses*. Therefore, the presence of acidemia implies an underlying acidosis. However, while acidosis usually leads to acidemia, it doesn't always (since there may be a concomitant alkalosis of greater magnitude). Conversely, *alkalemia* is present when the pH is above 7.44 (or $[H^+]$ below 36 neq/L). Alkalemia is caused by an underlying *alkalosis*. When an acidosis and an alkalosis operate simultaneously, there can only be one resulting plasma $[H^+]$. The consequent $[H^+]$ may be high, low, or even normal. Therefore, it is important to distinguish between the -emia (the blood pH), and the -osis (the underlying pathologic process).

Analyzing the innumerable acid-base pairs in the body in terms of the HCO_3^-/P_{CO_2} system has immense clinical utility. By the Henderson equation (vide supra), a rise in $[H^+]$ above normal must be due to a rise in P_{CO_2} or a fall in $[HCO_3^-]$ (or both). In the case of the former, the primary physiologic derangement is inadequate elimination of CO_2 through the lungs (respiratory acidosis). In contrast, a rise in $[H^+]$ due to a fall in $[HCO_3^-]$ is called metabolic acidosis.

Similarly, respiratory alkalosis is the excessive elimination of CO_2, while metabolic alkalosis is a rise in $[HCO_3^-]$. Each of the primary disorders of respiratory alkalosis, respiratory acidosis, metabolic alkalosis, and metabolic acidosis engenders an attempt by the body to restore the pH of the body toward normal. These responses are termed *compensatory* or *secondary alkaloses* or *acidoses*.

CONSEQUENCES OF ACIDEMIA AND ALKALEMIA

The physiologic effects of acidemia and alkalemia are thoroughly detailed in Chap. 158. In overview, each detrimentally affects cellular performance, presumably by altering protein charge, thereby affecting structure or function. The most relevant consequence of acidemia in critically ill patients is depression of muscular contractility, especially in the heart and diaphragm. Acidemia is more prevalent in the ICU than alkalemia, which may account for physicians' greater fears of low pH than high pH. However, alkalemia has important detrimental effects as well, including life-threatening arrhythmias, neuromuscular irritability, ionized hypocalcemia, hypoventilation, and impaired pulmonary gas exchange.

RESPIRATORY ALKALOSIS

Conceptually, respiratory alkalosis can result either from excessive excretion of CO_2 (elevated $\dot{V}_A$, hyperventilation) or from decreased CO_2 production. In most clinical situations this second possibility is ignored since any reduction in $\dot{V}_{CO_2}$ should simply cause a reduction in ventilation, not respiratory alkalosis. However, in the ICU, ventilation may be controlled by the physician, rather than the patient. If $\dot{V}_{CO_2}$ falls and the physician fails to reduce ventilation in a ventilated and pharmacologically paralyzed (or heavily sedated) patient, alkalosis will result. An example of this is a patient who is on a ventilator but septic, febrile, agitated, and in respiratory distress, who is then given a paralytic drug and treated with antipyretics. $\dot{V}_{CO_2}$ may fall to less than half its original value. If the ventilator is not adjusted accordingly, alkalosis ensues.

More commonly, respiratory alkalosis is due to excessive ventilation, rather than low $\dot{V}_{CO_2}$. Again, the physician may be responsible for this by inappropriate or intentional ventilator settings. Alternatively, the patient may be driving his own ventilation in response to cortical, chemoreceptor, chest wall, or other stimuli. Especially common causes in the ICU include sepsis, acidemia, pain, and CNS, liver, or pulmonary disease (see Chap. 158). When the stimulus to hyperventilation is metabolic acidosis, the resulting respiratory alkalosis is called compensatory alkalosis.

An acute reduction in P_{CO_2} leads to a predictable change in $[H^+]$. For a fall in P_{CO_2} of 10 mmHg, the pH rises by 0.08 units. Alternatively:

$$\Delta[H^+] = 0.8 \times \Delta P_{CO_2} \qquad (3\text{-}11)$$

RESPIRATORY ACIDOSIS

The pathophysiology of respiratory acidosis is excessive $\dot{V}_{CO_2}$ or inadequate $\dot{V}_A$. Since $\dot{V}_A$ should easily rise to meet the demand of increased $\dot{V}_{CO_2}$, respiratory acidosis implies failure of ventilation (type 2 respiratory failure). Once again, however, in the mechanically ventilated patient, a rise in $\dot{V}_{CO_2}$ (e.g., due to fever or sepsis) will result in new respiratory acidosis until ventilation is adjusted. The pathophysiology of respiratory failure is beyond the scope of this chapter but can be broadly categorized into insufficient drive, inadequate neuromuscular competence, or excessive load (or some combination—see Chap. 1).

The acute effect on pH or $[H^+]$ of respiratory acidosis is of the same magnitude as in respiratory alkalosis. For each 10 mmHg rise in P_{CO_2}, the pH falls by 0.08 units. As for respiratory alkalosis:

$$\Delta[H^+] = 0.8 \times \Delta P_{CO_2} \qquad (3\text{-}12)$$

METABOLIC ALKALOSIS

INITIATION PHASE

When metabolic alkalosis is present (the $[HCO_3^-]$ is high), the inciting cause should be distinguished from the factors which contribute to its maintenance. Metabolic alkalemia can be initiated by excessive production (or administration) of bicarbonate or by loss of hydrogen ions.

EXCESSIVE BICARBONATE PRODUCTION. Metabolic alkalosis is typically caused by excessive renal bicarbonate generation (acid excretion). Hydrogen ion secretion into the urine is governed by the delivery of sodium, chloride, and bicarbonate to the distal nephron, as well as by the rate of secretion of hydrogen ions (thereby involving aldosterone, potassium, and CO_2). Mineralocorticoid excess, as in hyperaldosteronism or steroid administration, directly stimulates distal nephron acidification. While mineralocorticoid excess is an uncommon cause of alkalosis in critically ill patients, it contributes to the pathogenesis in many of them. For example, diuretic administration causes volume depletion, which stimulates aldosterone release, which promotes hydrogen ion secretion.

Similarly, vomiting and nasogastric suction initiate alkalosis partly through loss of acid, but also because of renal mechanisms. Chloride and volume are lost in gastric fluid in addition to hydrogen ions. This provokes secondary hyperaldosteronism and consequent renal acidification. Further, hypovolemia stimulates renal sodium avidity in an attempt to maintain arterial filling. To prevent sodium loss, the tubule augments sodium-hydrogen exchange. This increment in hydrogen ion secretion accelerates bicarbonate resorption. Thus, the apparently simple generation of alkalosis through loss of stomach acid is, in fact, a complex interaction of acid loss, secondary mineralocorticoid excess, and volume contraction.

A simple cause of metabolic alkalosis is posthypercapneic alkalosis. In the setting of chronic respiratory acidosis, the kidneys generate excess bicarbonate in an attempt to restore $[H^+]$. If P_{CO_2} is subsequently reduced by mechanical ventilation or by a response to bronchodilator therapy, the excess bicarbonate will cause alkalosis until it can be excreted.

ALKALI ADMINISTRATION. It is obvious that administration of large amounts of bicarbonate will lead to alkalosis. Nevertheless, this is not an uncommon cause of alkalosis in the ICU. This occurs because bicarbonate is often given inappropriately, for example, to treat the acidosis of respiratory failure (although such use may be appropriate when the respiratory failure cannot be reversed, as in severe status asthmaticus). Alternatively, it may be given in a setting in which a metabolic acid anion (such as lactate or ketoacid anions) remains in the circulation, then is converted back to bicarbonate when the underlying disease is treated.

Less obvious are situations in which substances equivalent to bicarbonate are given, such as acetate, lactate, or citrate. Therefore, metabolic alkalosis may be initiated by parenteral nutrition (acetate), plasmapheresis, blood product administration, or liver transplantation (citrate).

LOSS OF HYDROGEN IONS. Renal loss of hydrogen ions is equivalent to renal production of bicarbonate, discussed above. Hydrogen ions can also be lost from the gastrointestinal tract. Vomiting and nasogastric suction involve direct loss of hydrogen ions from the body. Since gastric acid production involves reciprocal bicarbonate generation in gastric blood, alkalosis results. These conditions are described above, since, in addition to acid loss, they also entail renal mechanisms. A final cause of nonrenal acid loss is in rare patients with chloride-losing diarrheas. Although most patients with diarrhea lose bicarbonate in the stool and become acidemic, rarely, hydrogen ions are secreted, leading to alkalosis. Examples include occasional patients with villous adenomas and those with the pancreatic cholera syndrome.

MAINTENANCE PHASE

Whatever the precipitant of a metabolic alkalemia, the kidneys should promptly increase bicarbonate excretion, restoring pH. For example, oral administration of 100 meq/day of sodium bicarbonate for several weeks fails to cause alkalemia. Therefore, sustained alkalosis implies an impairment of renal excretion of bicarbonate, nearly always due to pathologically avid reclamation of filtered bicarbonate, or to failure to deliver enough glomerular filtrate to the tubules. The important factors which may contribute to maintenance of alkalosis in individual patients include volume depletion, hypochloremia (although whether chloride has an effect independent of volume depletion is controversial), mineralocorticoid excess, and a reduced (or absent) GFR.

The most common cause of persistent metabolic alkalosis in critically ill patients is hypovolemia. This is particularly common in postsurgical patients who are often intravascularly volume depleted despite receiving substantial intravenous fluids and in patients receiving diuretics. Drug therapies, including blood products and nutritional fluids, should be reviewed as well, since they may contribute to a sustained alkalosis. In the rare patient in whom consideration of these factors does not lead to diagnosis or correction of alkalosis, the possibility of mineralocorticoid excess should be considered. The urinary chloride may be useful in this context, being very low in the chloride-responsive alkaloses (e.g., hypovolemia), and not low in the chloride-resistant alkaloses (e.g., mineralocorticoid excess).

METABOLIC ACIDOSIS

Metabolic acidosis is the most complex of the acid-base disorders. To understand a fall in $[HCO_3^-]$, it is essential to consider renal bicarbonate handling, gastrointestinal bicarbonate losses, exogenously administered acids or acid-generating substances, and tissue metabolism.

RENAL FACTORS

Failure of the kidney to accurately reclaim or regenerate bicarbonate leads to derangements in plasma $[H^+]$, as in the renal tubular acidoses (RTAs) and renal failure.

PROXIMAL (TYPE 2) RENAL TUBULAR ACIDOSIS. In these disorders, proximal reclamation of filtered bicarbonate is impaired with consequent delivery of large amounts to the distal nephron. Initially, the distal nephron is overwhelmed and bicarbonate is lost into the urine. As the plasma bicarbonate falls, the filtered load falls as well. Thus, as acidosis develops, the proximal tubule eventually becomes able to reclaim the entire (albeit reduced) filtered load. Then bicarbonate is no longer delivered distally, and the healthy distal nephron can acidify the urine normally. Typically, the plasma bicarbonate stabilizes at about 15 meq/L.

Causes of proximal RTA seen in the ICU include drugs (especially acetazolamide, mafenide acetate), amyloidosis, heavy-metal poisoning, and myeloma (see Chap. 158). Most adults have associated dysfunction of the proximal tubule including aminoaciduria, phosphaturia, and glycosuria. The clinical picture may be dominated by these associated problems, especially when hypophosphatemia is severe. If treatment of proximal RTA with bicarbonate is attempted, the filtered load simply increases, and the bicarbonate is lost in the urine. Even large amounts of bicarbonate fail to maintain a normal pH. A potentially devastating outcome of this approach is life-threatening hypokalemia. Shohl's solution (potassium citrate) is a preferred approach since potassium is provided, while the citrate is metabolized to bicarbonate.

DISTAL (TYPE 1) RENAL TUBULAR ACIDOSIS. As noted above, the distal nephron must secrete hydrogen and titrate urinary phosphate and ammonia (titratable acidity) to regenerate enough bicarbonate to compensate for daily nonvolatile acid production. If the distal nephron is dysfunctional, bicarbonate stores will be gradually but inexorably consumed. The urine can never be maximally acidified, so that failure of urine pH to fall below 6.0 in the face of systemic acidosis should suggest this diagnosis. Typically, distal RTA is not severe, but it can result in life-threatening acidemia, especially during superimposed critical illness. Concomitant hypokalemia can cause muscle weakness, impede respiratory compensation, and further contribute to the life-threatening nature of the acidemia.

Distal RTA is common in the ICU, since it accompanies many systemic disorders (e.g., sickle cell disease, chronic active hepatitis, hypercalcemia), renal diseases (e.g., renal transplant rejection, obstructive uropathy, nephrocalcinosis), and drug therapies (e.g., amphotericin B, lithium, drug-induced acute interstitial nephritis). In most adults with distal RTA, since filtered bicarbonate is successfully reclaimed by the proximal tubule, it does not appear in the urine. Therefore, only small amounts of sodium bicarbonate (or equivalent) are necessary to prevent acidemia from developing (about 100 meq/day, the nonvolatile acid production).

RENAL FAILURE. If renal failure is complete, there is no filtered bicarbonate and no need for its reclamation. However, the lack of capacity for regeneration of bicarbonate lost to nonvolatile acid production leads to acidosis. The anion gap is increased (vide infra) due to the coincident inability to excrete unmeasured anions such as sulfate, due to the reduction in GFR. In chronic renal failure, plasma bicarbonate is maintained above 14 meq/L by virtue of the huge buffering capacity of bone. During critical illness, however, acute increases in acid production may lead to life-threatening acidemia, necessitating treatment.

GASTROINTESTINAL BICARBONATE LOSSES

In health, the gastrointestinal tract loses only about 35 meq/day of alkali (equivalent to gaining 35 meq acid), accounting for about one-third of daily nonvolatile acid production. However, several gastrointestinal tract secretions contain substantial amounts of bicarbonate, including pancreatic juice, bile, and small intestinal fluid. Therefore, loss of large volumes of these secretions, for example through diarrhea or fistulas, can cause metabolic acidosis. In most circumstances, the kidneys can simply regenerate an equal amount of bicarbonate so that acidosis is not sustained. However, when renal perfusion is compromised by severe dehydration, there is renal disease, or bicarbonate losses are great (e.g., cholera), severe acidosis may result.

EXOGENOUS ACIDS AND ACID-GENERATING SUBSTANCES

It is obvious that an infusion of hydrochloric acid will lead to metabolic acidosis by titrating bicarbonate. What is less apparent is that several substances generate the equivalent of hydrochloric acid during their metabolism. For example, ammonium chloride is metabolized to hydrogen ions and urea. This fact is occasionally exploited as a means to treat patients with severe metabolic alkalosis. In addition, the amino acids lysine, arginine, and histidine produce hydrogen ions when they are catabolized. Arginine hydrochloride has also been used to treat metabolic alkalosis (although the risk of life-threatening hyperkalemia has prompted a shift to other therapies). More relevant for the intensivist, solutions of amino acids used in parenteral nutrition contain large amounts of these acidogenic amino acids and are capable of causing mild metabolic acidosis.

Severe metabolic acidoses can result from several acid-generating toxins. Ingestions of ethylene glycol or methanol produce potentially fatal CNS toxicity and metabolic acidosis. Ethylene glycol is metabolized to glycolic acid (as well as to glyoxalic and oxalic acids), which appears to be responsible for the acidosis. Methanol is also metabolized to an acid (formic acid), but poisoning with this alcohol is complicated by an additional mechanism. Formic acid and formaldehyde, an intermediate product, are both highly toxic compounds which interfere with the electron transport chain. By disrupting oxidative metabolism, they cause lactic acidosis, which contributes to the metabolic acidosis of methanol intoxication.

DERANGED TISSUE METABOLISM

During normal metabolism, many acids, most notably lactic acid and ketoacids, are both generated and consumed. In health, these acids have a minimal impact on $[H^+]$. The pathologic states of lactic acidosis and ketoacidosis, however, are two of the most dramatic and life-threatening acidoses encountered in the ICU.

LACTIC ACIDOSIS. As discussed above, lactic acidosis can be thought of as a derangement of the Cori cycle. Surpluses of lactic acid can result not only from overproduction (usually by muscle or intestine), but also by underconsumption (by the liver) (see Fig. 3-7).

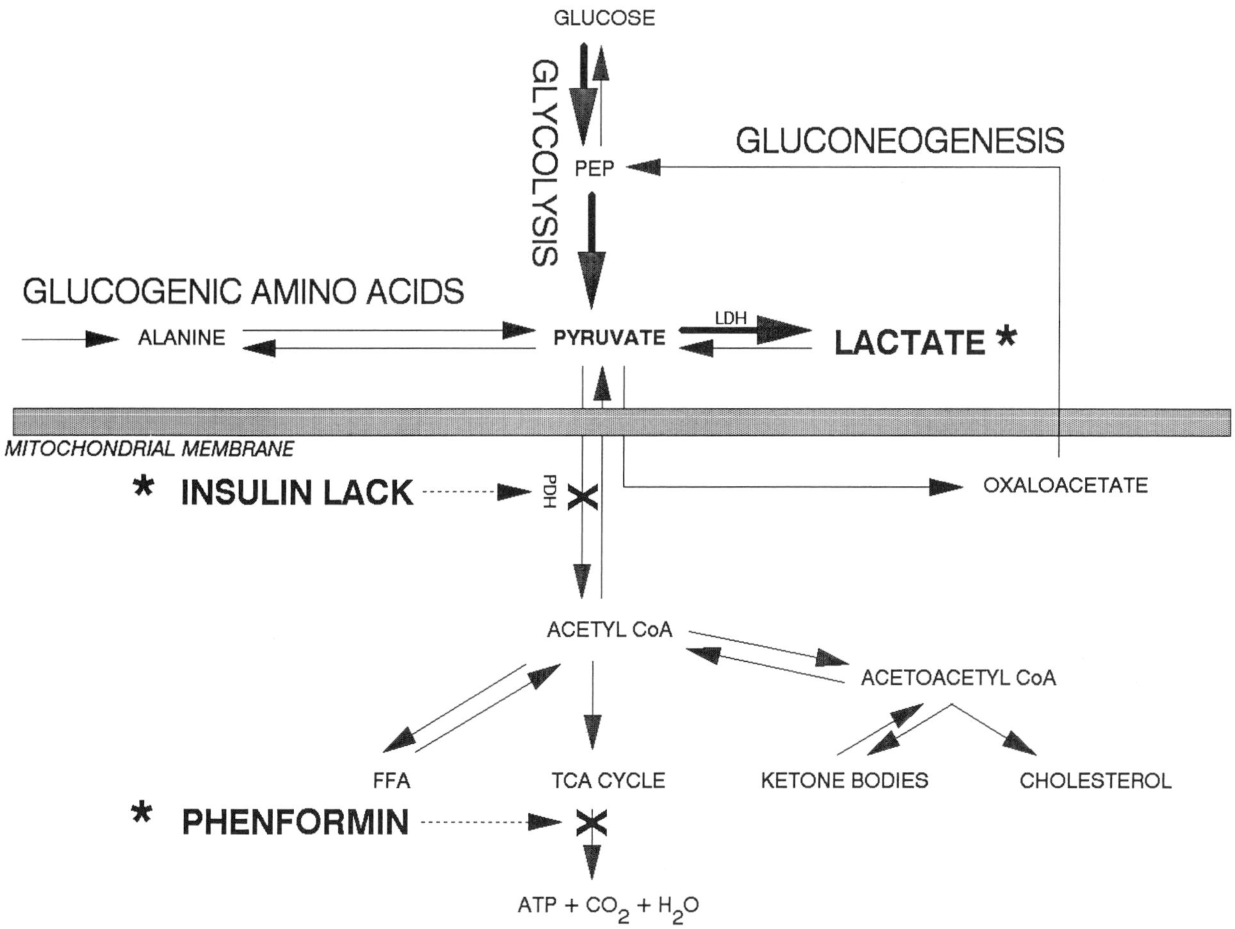

FIGURE 3-9 The propensity for diabetics taking phenformin to develop lactic acidosis may by due to the combined effects of insulin lack (which decreases PDH activity) and poisoning of oxidative metabolism (by phenformin). Since the cell is unable to derive sufficient ATP through oxidative metabolism, glycolysis is stimulated. This produces large amounts of pyruvate, and consequently, lactate. PEP, phosphoenolpyruvate; LDH, lactate dehydrogenase; PDH, pyruvate dehydrogenase; FFA, free fatty acids; TCA, tricarboxylic acid.

Overproduction of lactic acid implies overproduction or underutilization of pyruvate (see Fig. 3-8). Some pyruvate is derived from alanine as proteins are catabolized. It is therefore possible that excessive muscle breakdown, especially during critical illness, may contribute to lactic acidosis. However, overproduction of pyruvate in glycolytic tissues is the usual source of excess lactate. This is typically the result of an impairment in oxidative metabolism. If pyruvate cannot enter the tricarboxylic acid cycle (via acetyl-CoA) to be converted to CO_2, then glycolysis is stimulated in an attempt to provide adenosine triphosphate (ATP) for cellular function. Large amounts of pyruvate are formed, then converted to lactate to recoup NAD for further glycolysis.

Several distinct mechanisms of impaired oxidative metabolism lead to lactic acidosis. Failure of adequate oxygen delivery to individual tissues (e.g., ischemia of bowel or leg) or to all organs (e.g., hypoxemia, cardiogenic shock, severe anemia) is a common mechanism in the ICU. Similarly, oxygen delivery which is normal, yet insufficient for unusual activity (exercise, seizures) has the same effect. On the other hand, failure of cellular oxygen utilization, in the face of adequate oxygen delivery, also results in lactic acidosis. Examples include poisoning with cyanide, carbon monoxide, salicylate, and methanol. Sepsis was long considered an example of cellular impairment of oxygen consumption, although more likely it is another instance of failure of perfusion (on a microvascular level).

Underconsumption of lactate is also an important mechanism of lactic acidosis. Failure of the liver to cooperate in its half of the Cori cycle leads to severe acidosis, even if lactate production is normal. This can explain the acidosis of hepatic failure even without invoking concurrent endotoxemia. However, underconsumption of lactate by the liver may play a contributing role in many patients with lactic acidosis. In view of the remarkable capacity for the normal liver to increase lactate extraction and metabolism, it would be surprising if some component of impaired hepatic uptake did not accompany most forms of lactic acidosis. Dichloroacetate, a potential therapy for lactic acidosis, has shown promising results in animal and human experiments. It appears to work by stimulating PDH, the enzyme

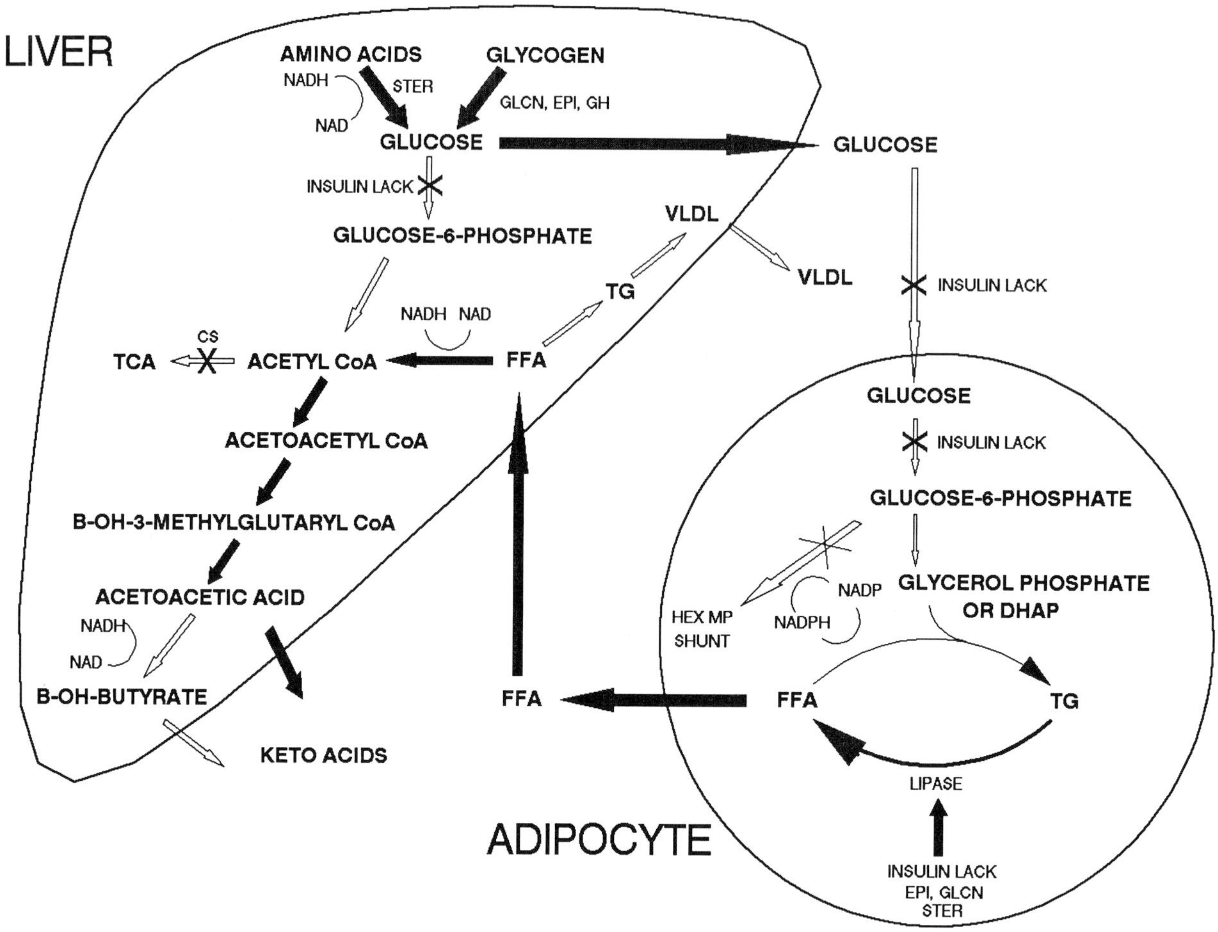

FIGURE 3-10 Diabetic ketoacidosis (DKA). Biochemical pathways in the liver are illustrated on the left, while those in the adipocytes are indicated on the right. Insulin lack leads to impaired entry of glucose into glycolysis, and blood levels rise. In the adipocyte, this has the added effect of impeding triglyceride synthesis, since glycerol phosphate and DHAP are unavailable for reacting with free fatty acids. In addition, reduced flux through the hexose monophosphate shunt generates insufficient NADPH, a necessary cofactor in triglyceride synthesis. At the same time, insulin lack stimulates lipase, leading to release of free fatty acids, and blood levels rise dramatically. Free fatty acid uptake by the liver is essentially unlimited, and results in generation of acetyl-CoA. Citrate synthetase activity is impaired in DKA, leading to redirection of much of acetyl-CoA toward keto acid synthesis. NAD, nicotinamide adenine dinucleotide; NADH, reduced nicotinamide adenine dinucleotide; STER, corticosteroids; GLCN, glucagon; EPI, epinephrine; GH, growth hormone; CS, citrate synthetase; TCA, tricarboxylic acid cycle; FFA, free fatty acids; TG, triglyceride; VLDL, very low density lipoprotein; HEX MP SHUNT, hexose monophosphate shunt.

which limits entry of pyruvate into the tricarboxylic acid cycle. In this way it augments hepatic metabolism of lactate, thereby consuming hydrogen ions. Insulin lack has the opposite effect on PDH, which may explain the tendency of diabetics to develop lactic acidosis. It also helps to account for fatal cases of lactic acidosis when phenformin therapy (vide infra) was used for the treatment of diabetes (Fig. 3-9).

Several factors can cause the liver to shift from its usual role as lactate consumer to lactate producer. A fall in hepatic blood flow appears to be one such stimulus. This provides an explanation for hepatic lactate production in shock states. Another example is the reduced hepatic blood flow induced by respiratory alkalosis. There is experimental evidence that prolonged hyperventilation causes normal hepatic lactate uptake to cease and lactate production to begin. This may contribute to the lactic acidosis of salicylate intoxication (since respiratory alkalosis is a regular finding), independent of the salicylate effect of cellular oxidative metabolism. In other situations, a rise in hepatocyte [H^+] leads to hepatic lactate production. Since liver cell [H^+] has been shown to paradoxically rise following bicarbonate infusion in animal models of lactic acidosis (probably due to diffusion of CO_2 into cells), this may explain part of the increment in lactic acid production which follows this therapy. Another example of the effect of increasing liver cell [H^+] on lactate production is administration of phenformin, a hypoglycemic drug. Phenformin appears to block hepatic gluconeogenesis by inhibiting pyruvate carboxylase. Such inhibition lowers intracellular pH, and in animal models, leads to lactate production by the liver.

KETOACIDOSIS. Both diabetic ketoacidosis (DKA) and alcoholic ketoacidosis (AKA) lead to severe illness. The cause of DKA is insulin deficiency. The consequences of insulin deficiency include impaired lipogenesis and augmented lipolysis, compounded by release of catecholamines, glucagon and cortisol, which lead to striking mobilization of free fatty acids (Fig. 3-10). Hepatic uptake of free fatty acids is virtually limitless. Once within the hepatocyte, fatty acids are reconverted into triglycerides or are converted to acetyl-CoA. Since entry of acetyl-CoA into the tricarboxylic acid cycle is blunted in DKA, acetoacetyl-CoA is preferentially formed. This is converted to acetoacetic acid which is released into the circulation. Since the synthesis of this ketoacid outstrips its catabolism, acidosis ensues. Fatty acids which are resynthesized into triglycerides during ketoacidosis account for both the fatty liver of DKA and the hyperlipoproteinemia.

AKA resembles DKA. Free fatty acid concentrations are very high and insulin is barely detectable. Once again, hepatic synthesis of ketoacids (both directly from ethanol metabolism and from fatty acid breakdown) exceeds peripheral utilization, resulting in acidosis. Why this only occurs in rare alcoholics is unknown, but there may be undiscovered factors which predispose certain individuals to its development. In contrast to DKA, the ratio of β-hydroxybutyrate to acetoacetate is very high in AKA. This is the result of the high NADH:NAD ratio related to the metabolism of ethanol (Fig. 3-11).

COMPENSATION

Any deviation in $[H^+]$ from 40 neq/L prompts an attempt by the body to restore $[H^+]$ toward normal. If the primary derangement is respiratory, then the compensation will be by the kidneys (metabolic). Primary metabolic disturbances engender changes in $\dot{V}_A$ to alter P_{CO_2}. In all cases, the compensatory response is predictable and serves to repair the $[H^+]$ toward, but never to, normal. Therefore, the impact

FIGURE 3-11 Alcoholic ketoacidosis (AKA). Insulin lack, due to low blood glucose levels, leads to impaired synthesis of triglycerides, and release of free fatty acids as in DKA. Free fatty acids are similarly metabolized to keto acids. However, catabolism of ethanol generates excessive amounts of NADH. The resulting increase in the NADH:NAD ratio facilitates the conversion of acetoacetate to β-hydroxy-butyrate, explaining the observed pattern of keto acids in the blood. NAD, nicotinamide adenine dinucleotide; NADH, reduced nicotinamide adenine dinucleotide; STER, corticosteroids; GLCN, glucagon; EPI, epinephrine; GH, growth hormone; CS, citrate synthetase; TCA, tricarboxylic acid cycle; FFA, free fatty acids; TG, triglyceride; HEX MP SHUNT, hexose monophosphate shunt.

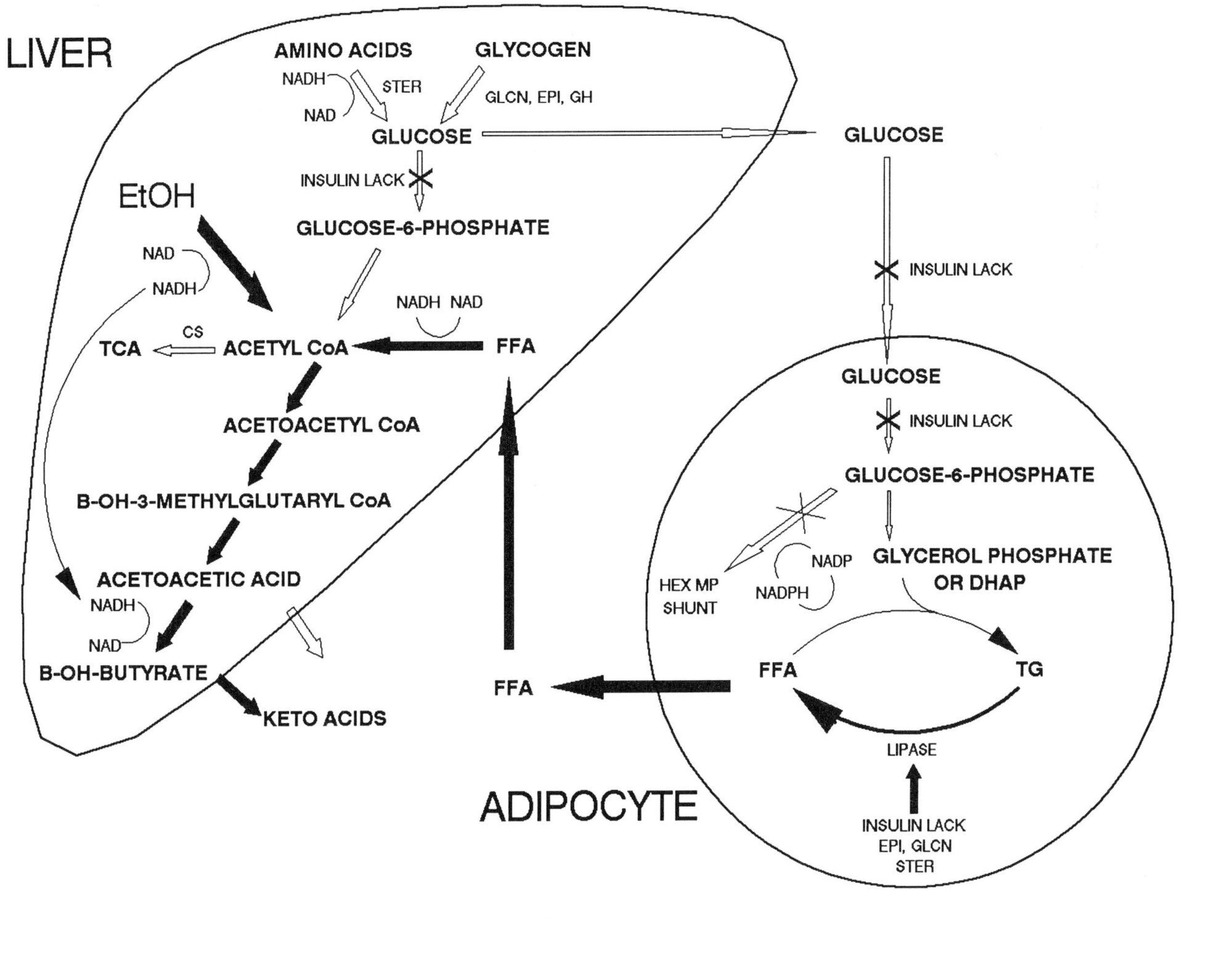

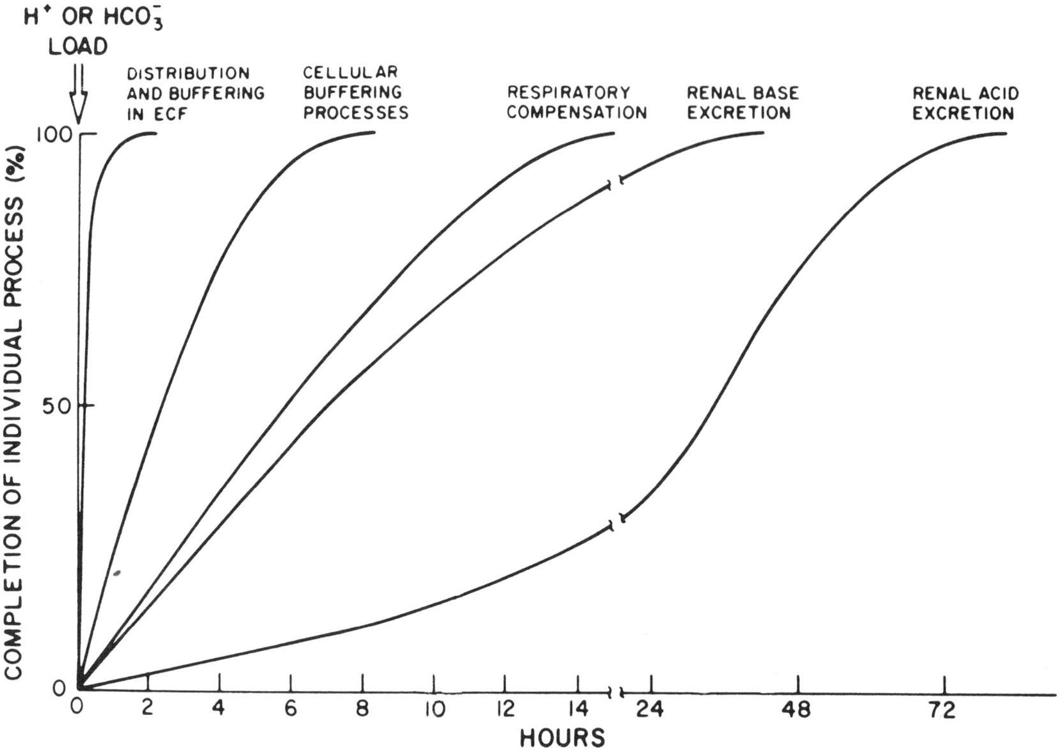

FIGURE 3-12 Evolution of the compensatory response to acid-base disturbances is illustrated as a function of time. (Reprinted with permission from Cogan MG, Rector FC: Acid-base disorders, in Brenner BM, Rector FC (eds): *The Kidney*, Philadelphia, Saunders, 1986, pp. 457–517.)

on $[H^+]$ of a sudden derangement in acid-base status is maximal immediately following onset of the derangement. With time, as compensation evolves, the expected deviation of the $[H^+]$ from normal lessens. The time course of each is characteristic, assuming that the compensatory system is not diseased (Fig. 3-12). The magnitude of impact on $[H^+]$ for both the acute derangement, as well as following complete compensation is summarized in Fig. 3-13. All formulas for predicted compensation make assumptions about the patient which rarely hold in critically ill patients. For example, acid-base derangements occur and evolve rapidly and often prompt therapeutic intervention. Since full compensation takes 12 to 100 h, it is the exceptional patient who has the opportunity to demonstrate his compensatory capacity. Moreover, compensation requires intact function of the compensatory system, as well as cardiovascular stability and, sometimes, neuromuscular competence. Thus, a patient with a metabolic acidosis must have the ability to increase alveolar ventilation and sustain it. This assumption rarely holds in sepsis, the most common important cause of metabolic (lactic) acidosis in the ICU. Similarly, renal compensation requires intact renal function and renal perfusion, which are all too often lacking in sick patients.

For these reasons, equations and graphs describing predicted responses to acid-base derangements are of limited utility in the ICU. Nevertheless, since they provide insight into normal physiology, they may aid the clinician seeking to understand pathophysiology.

COMPENSATION FOR METABOLIC ACIDOSIS

Central chemoreceptors, sensitive to changes in $[H^+]$, respond to metabolic acidosis by increasing $\dot{V}_A$. In patients with established metabolic acidosis, the magnitude of compensation can be estimated from the following equation:

$$\text{Predicted } P_{CO_2} = 1.5 \times [HCO_3^-] + 8 \pm 2 \qquad (3\text{-}13)$$

Coincident or evolving respiratory failure will prevent full compensation. The increased respiratory workload necessitated by persistent metabolic acidosis can itself precipitate respiratory failure. In many patients with severe acidosis, especially if hemodynamic instability is present, it is prudent to take over the work of breathing by instituting mechanical ventilation, rather than wait for the patient to prove his ability to compensate.

COMPENSATION FOR METABOLIC ALKALOSIS

Evidence to support the notion that hypoventilation occurs in response to metabolic alkalosis is now convincing. The expected compensation is calculated from:

$$\text{Predicted } P_{CO_2} = 0.73 \times [HCO_3^-] + 20 \pm 2 \qquad (3\text{-}14)$$

As a patient hypoventilates to allow P_{CO_2} to rise, the P_{O_2} will fall. It is fairly common for the P_{O_2} to fall even into the 50s or 40s in response to severe alkalemia. Failure to understand these points can lead to errors in management. For

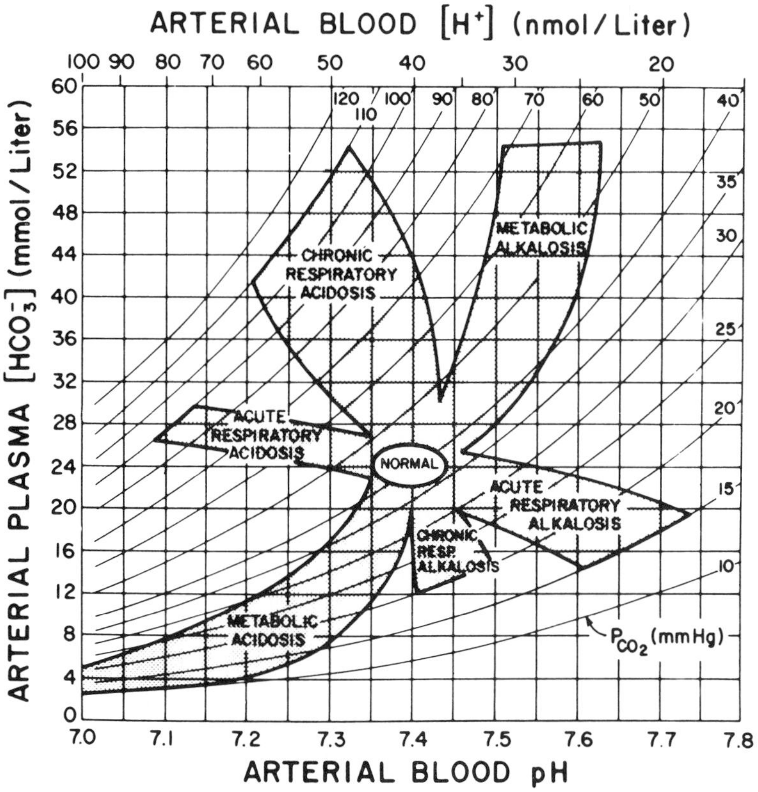

FIGURE 3-13 Acid-base nomogram. This figure outlines the 95 percent confidence limits for the normal compensatory responses to acid-base derangements. (Reprinted with permission from Cogan MG, Rector FC: Acid-base disorders, in Brenner BM, Rector FC (eds): *The Kidney*, Philadelphia, Saunders, 1986, pp. 457–517.)

example, a common situation is a patient on a ventilator with severe metabolic alkalosis and a P_{CO_2} of 50. Physicians frequently interpret the P_{CO_2} to indicate that the patient is not yet ready to come off the ventilator. If they understood this to be a normal response to alkalemia, they would proceed with liberation from the ventilator while addressing the cause of the underlying alkalosis. It is commonly stated that metabolic alkalosis prolongs the need for mechanical ventilation by reducing the drive to breathe. While alkalosis does decrease the drive to breathe, it is not clear that this is bad. The elevated $[HCO_3^-]$ helps the patient maintain an acceptable $[H^+]$ while he hypoventilates. Drive to breathe is less because less is needed. This should decrease respiratory workload and facilitate the transition to spontaneous breathing. All of this assumes that the elevated P_{CO_2} itself does not have important detrimental effects, an assumption which is probably accurate within limits. It is possible that the severe volume depletion, which likely underlies the alkalosis, might impede liberation from the ventilator on hemodynamic grounds. What seems most likely in this circumstance, however, is that metabolic alkalosis itself does not prolong mechanical ventilation, the physician does.

COMPENSATION FOR RESPIRATORY ACIDOSIS

Immediately following a decrement in ventilation, renal hydrogen ion secretion and urinary excretion of ammonium increase. These increases lead to a sustained increase in plasma bicarbonate concentration. The expected chronic compensation can be found from:

$$\text{Predicted } [H^+] = 0.24 \times P_{CO_2} + 27 \qquad (3\text{-}15)$$

or, alternatively,

$$\text{Predicted } [HCO_3^-] = (P_{CO_2} - 40) \times 0.3 + 24 \qquad (3\text{-}16)$$

COMPENSATION FOR RESPIRATORY ALKALOSIS

Minutes following an increase in $\dot{V}_A$, bicarbonate excretion and urinary pH increase. Similarly, titratable acidity (urinary ammonium and phosphate) falls. The consequence is a falling plasma $[HCO_3^-]$ and a return of the $[H^+]$ toward normal. Following complete compensation, the expected $[H^+]$ is found from:

$$\text{Predicted } [H^+] = (40 - P_{CO_2}) \times 0.17 + 40 \qquad (3\text{-}17)$$

An Alternative View: The Strong Ion Difference

In the conventional approach to acid-base physiology of biologic systems, the focus is on $[H^+]$ as the determinant of acidity. A consequence of this view is that it leads to the mistaken notion that the only way to make a solution more acidic is to add hydrogen ions. This leads to confusion when the student of acid-base physiology tries to understand aspects in which the relevant changing ion is chloride, for example, rather than the hydrogen ion.

In an alternative approach, largely developed by Peter Stewart, $[H^+]$ is not an independent variable and the determinant of acidity. Rather, $[H^+]$ is a dependent variable which changes in response to three independent variables: the P_{CO_2}, the total concentration of nonvolatile weak acids (plasma proteins and, less importantly, phosphate), and the SID (vide infra). This approach is attractive because it is more fundamentally correct than the conventional approach, it is amenable to quantitative analysis, and it provides insight into biologic mechanisms. It suffers from being less familiar and somewhat mathematically daunting. Nevertheless, it is receiving increasing recognition in medical journals and texts. Anyone who studies acid-base physiology should become familiar with this approach. An overview will be given here but the interested reader should pursue one of the available thorough reviews.

DEFINITIONS

Strong electrolytes are those which are fully dissociated in aqueous solution. For example, sodium is a strong cation and chloride is a strong anion. When sodium chloride is dissolved in water, the solution contains water, hydrogen ions, hydroxide ions, sodium ions, and chloride ions, but no undissociated sodium chloride. Other biologically relevant strong ions include K^+, Mg^{++}, Ca^{++}, $SO_4^=$, lactate, and ketoacid anions.

Weak electrolytes dissociate incompletely in aqueous solution. In contrast to strong electrolytes, the concentrations of weak electrolytes change in response to alterations in other variables. For example, take a weak acid HA which dissociates incompletely to H^+ and A^-. At equilibrium,

$$\frac{[H^+][A^-]}{[HA]} = K_a \qquad (3\text{-}18)$$

where K_a is the dissociation constant for HA.

If HCl is added to a solution of HA, the concentration of A^- will decrease while the concentration of HA will increase. This is strikingly different from what happens when HCl is added to a solution of Na^+ and Cl^-. Nevertheless, the total concentration of all forms of A (A^- and HA, or A_{TOT}) does not change; merely the degree of dissociation changes.

DETERMINANTS OF $[H^+]$

SOLUTIONS OF STRONG IONS. In a solution made by adding measured quantities of NaOH and HCl, the final concentrations of Na^+ and Cl^- are easily calculable. Although the derivation is beyond the scope of this chapter, the $[H^+]$ can also be found and depends only on the $[Na^+]$, $[Cl^-]$, and the dissociation constant of water:

$$[H^+] = \{K'_{H_2O} + ([Na^+] - [Cl^-])^2/4\}^{1/2} - ([Na^+] - [Cl^-])/2 \qquad (3\text{-}19)$$

Where K'_{H_2O} is the dissociation constant for water

A similar equation can be derived for the $[OH^-]$. In these equations, the $[Na^+]$ and $[Cl^-]$ always appear as the *difference* between them, $[Na^+] - [Cl^-]$. Because all strong ions dissociate fully and are not involved in any chemical reactions, the particular ion in solution is unimportant. All that matters is the charge of the ion and its amount. Therefore, in more complex solutions of strong ions containing K^+, Mg^{++}, and others, the term $[Na^+] - [Cl^-]$ can be expanded to:

$$[Na^+] + [K^+] + [Mg^{++}] + [Ca^{++}] - [Cl^-] - [SO_4^=], \text{ etc.} \qquad (3\text{-}20)$$

It is convenient in all such equations to replace this long list of ion concentrations with the equivalent term [SID], the strong ion difference. The SID is the sum of the concentrations of the strong base cations, less the sum of the concentrations of the strong acid anions. Now the equation for $[H^+]$ becomes:

$$[H^+] = \{K'_{H_2O} + ([SID]/2)^2\}^{1/2} - [SID]/2 \qquad (3\text{-}21)$$

The important point is that in solutions of strong ions, an observation of a change in $[H^+]$ (or pH) means that the [SID] has changed. In these simple solutions, the $[H^+]$ is a dependent quantity, inseparable from the concentrations of strong ions in the solution. Biologic solutions are more complicated since they contain weak acids and CO_2, but the [SID] remains a critically important determinant of $[H^+]$. In biologic fluids, the [SID] is nearly always positive, and typically has a value of about 40 meq/L. As the [SID] increases, $[H^+]$ falls (pH rises). Conversely, as [SID] decreases, $[H^+]$ rises.

SOLUTIONS CONTAINING STRONG IONS AND WEAK ACIDS. Biologically relevant fluids contain many weak acids, each with its own dissociation constant, K_a. Fortunately, little accuracy is lost in lumping them all together and using a single value of K_a and a total concentration of weak acid, $[A_{TOT}]$. If only strong ions and weak acids are present in a solution, the $[H^+]$ is determined by the [SID] and how its magnitude compares with $[A_{TOT}]$. Quantitatively, the calculation of $[H^+]$ is unwieldy without the aid of computers (but easily performed with them). However, since $[A_{TOT}]$ largely consists of proteins whose concentrations do not normally change rapidly with time, qualitatively most changes in $[H^+]$ are still due to changes in [SID].

SOLUTIONS CONTAINING STRONG IONS, WEAK ACIDS, AND CARBON DIOXIDE. These more complex solutions resemble biologically relevant fluids. Since CO_2 reacts rapidly with water (in the presence of carbonic anhydrase) to produce carbonic acid, it has a major effect on $[H^+]$. P_{CO_2} in body fluids is determined by the ratio of CO_2 production and CO_2 elimination and cannot be controlled by individual cells. Thus, P_{CO_2} and [SID] are the two most important independent variables which determine $[H^+]$, with $[A_{TOT}]$ a less important third determinant in blood, intracellular fluid, and extracellular fluids. Given the independent variables [SID], $[A_{TOT}]$, and P_{CO_2}, it is possible to quantitatively solve for the dependent variables $[H^+]$, $[OH^-]$, and $[HCO_3^-]$.

THE REVISED VIEW

In contrast to the conventional approach which focuses on $[H^+]$ and $[HCO_3^-]$ as the important determinants of the acid-base state of fluids, in this alternative view the $[H^+]$ and $[HCO_3^-]$ are merely responding to [SID], $[A_{TOT}]$, and P_{CO_2}. Changes in pH must result from changes in one or more of these quantities. Modulation of [SID] is largely effected by the kidneys. Lesser changes result from strong ion absorption or secretion in the gastrointestinal tract (although this may be critically important in diseases such as cholera). In pathologic states, large amounts of lactate (a strong anion) can be generated by cells. The P_{CO_2} is determined by $\dot{V}_{CO_2}$ and $\dot{V}_A$. $[A_{TOT}]$, which mostly reflects protein concentrations, only varies when large amounts of protein are lost (e.g., in massive burns). Nevertheless, hypoproteinemia causes a clinically relevant metabolic alkalosis by itself and without invoking a renal mechanism. This is one example in which the conventional approach to acid-base simply fails to explain the clinical observation.

Another advantage over the conventional approach is that this concept makes it easy to understand why gastrointestinal loss of chloride leads to alkalosis, a common sticking point in the teaching of acid-base medicine. Loss of chloride in excess of loss of strong cations increases [SID], the prime determinant of $[H^+]$.

Compensation is conceptually simple in this approach as well. When $[H^+]$ changes due to abnormalities of P_{CO_2}, the kidneys act to shift [SID] by the differential reabsorption of Na^+ and Cl^-, in a way which restores $[H^+]$ toward normal. Similarly, when $[H^+]$ is abnormal due to alterations in [SID], $\dot{V}_A$ is modified to change P_{CO_2}, thereby restoring $[H^+]$.

PRACTICAL APPLICATION

Analysis of any acid-base derangement begins with assessment of the $[H^+]$ and the P_{CO_2}. These should be plotted on the plasma $[H^+]$-P_{CO_2} diagram (Fig. 3-14), yielding the [SID]. From the position on the plot, the major respiratory (P_{CO_2}) or metabolic (SID) abnormality is determined. For example, if a patient has an $[H^+]$ of 28 neq/L (pH = 7.55) and a P_{CO_2} of 49, the [SID] is 64 meq/L (from Fig. 3-14). This indicates a nonrespiratory alkalosis, since the [SID] is elevated well above the normal value of 40 meq/L. The next step is to consider the potential causes of the elevated [SID]. In the example of metabolic alkalosis, this typically is

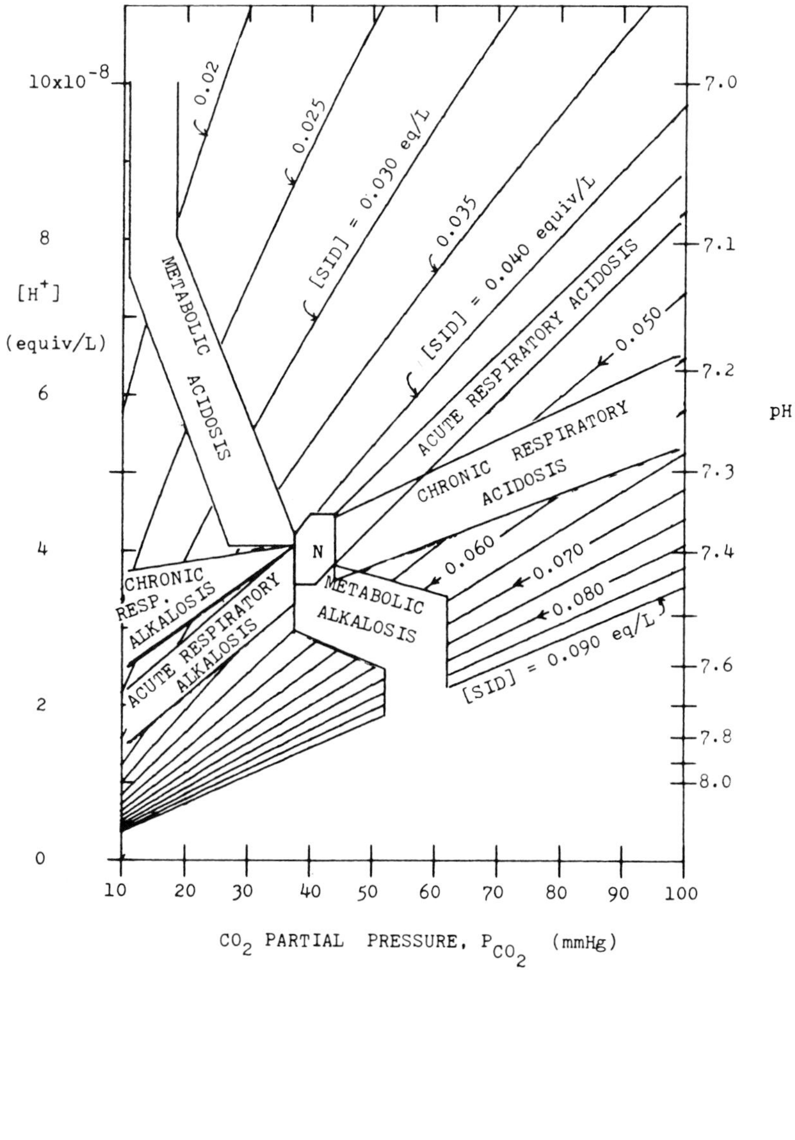

FIGURE 3-14 Acid-base nomogram. Plotting the $[H^+]$ and P_{CO_2} gives the [SID] and indicates the nature of the major underlying acid-base derangement. (Reprinted with permission from Stewart PA: *How to Understand Acid-Base: A Quantitative Acid-Base Primer for Biology and Medicine.* New York, Elsevier, 1981.)

a gain in sodium in excess of chloride, as with administration of sodium bicarbonate or sodium acetate (since acetate is metabolized to CO_2), or loss of chloride in excess of sodium in the gastrointestinal tract or in the urine (e.g., diuretic therapy or chloride-losing diarrhea). The approach to therapy in this example is to restore the [SID] toward normal by administering more strong anions than strong cations. The most direct way of accomplishing this is to give hydrochloric acid, which contains the strong anion, chloride, but no strong cation. Alternatively, one can infuse normal saline. Since normal saline has an [SID] of 0, adding it to plasma will lower the [SID] of the mixture toward the normal value of 40. Further, since the task of maintaining a normal plasma [SID] falls primarily to the kidneys, the clinician must search for the apparent renal dysfunction (e.g., hypovolemia, hyperaldosteronism).

IMPLICATIONS

This approach has some important implications for understanding acid-base physiology and pathophysiology. If, for example, the kidneys excrete more chloride than sodium, the [SID] of blood increases, and therefore, the $[H^+]$ decreases (or pH rises). For the kidneys to raise blood pH, they *must* excrete more chloride (the only available strong anion) than sodium (the most available strong cation). In attempting to understand how the kidneys achieve net acid excretion, the relevant question to ask is, "how do the kidneys excrete chloride?" It is meaningless to wonder whether the kidneys actually secrete hydrogen ions, absorb hydroxide ions, or absorb bicarbonate ions. These are not strong ions; therefore, transporting them across membranes cannot affect the [SID]. Paradoxical as it sounds, excretion of hydrogen ions alone by the kidneys, without excretion of a strong anion (chloride), simply cannot affect pH.

Electrolyte Disorders

Electrolyte disorders confront the intensivist daily. They are consequences of critical illness and its therapy, and cause their own superimposed morbidity and mortality. Yet, chapters devoted to specific diseases rarely provide an approach to common electrolyte complications. This section presents a conceptual framework which can be applied to electrolyte derangements, regardless of the specific primary disease.

MAGNESIUM

Disorders of this cation are exceedingly common in critically ill patients. In one series, hypomagnesemia was found in 65 percent of patients in a medical ICU. Yet hypomagnesemia is both underrecognized and underappreciated in many ICUs. In contrast, hypermagnesemia is uncommon, typically iatrogenic, and of little clinical relevance.

MAGNESIUM HOMEOSTASIS

Magnesium enters the body through the diet, drugs, and magnesium-containing infusions. Many patients in the ICU have preexisting dietary lack because of chronic illness, gastrointestinal disease (especially esophageal disease), or alcoholism. Magnesium deficiency is exacerbated by critical illness itself since the patient depends solely on the physician for its provision. Because the total body store of magnesium is so high (about 2000 meq), dietary lack alone rarely causes hypomagnesemia. It will hasten development of significant hypomagnesemia, however.

Intake which exceeds demand is excreted by the kidney, which serves as the dominant controller of magnesium homeostasis. When dietary supply is reduced, as is typical in the ICU, renal resorption increases and urinary losses fall to very small values. Nevertheless, during critical illness, many factors conspire to create hypomagnesemia.

CAUSES OF HYPOMAGNESEMIA

Loss of magnesium ion typically occurs through the gastrointestinal tract or the kidney. Rarely, magnesium is lost from the skin or redistributed internally in a way that leads to serum hypomagnesemia.

GASTROINTESTINAL LOSS OF MAGNESIUM. Many conditions of malabsorption and diarrhea lead to magnesium deficiency. Mucosal diseases such as Crohn's disease, sprue, radiation enteritis, short gut syndrome, jejunoileal bypass, and Whipple's disease lead to failure of absorption of magnesium. Cholestatic liver disease and pancreatic insufficiency (including cystic fibrosis) lead to stool loss of magnesium in much the same way as loss of calcium. More directly, patients with biliary drainage or fistulas can lose up to 15 meq magnesium/L fluid. Smaller amounts are lost through nasogastric suction and in diarrheal stools.

RENAL LOSS OF MAGNESIUM. More commonly, magnesium is lost through the urine. Renal reabsorption shares a common pathway with that of sodium and calcium. Thus, increased flux of sodium or calcium through the nephron leads to magnesium loss. Patients receiving intravenous hydration as part of their management risk developing hypomagnesemia. Similarly, hyperaldosteronism, through its effect on distal sodium delivery, increases urinary magnesium wasting. Many drugs given in the ICU impair renal reabsorption of magnesium. These include aminoglycosides, loop diuretics (but also including osmotic diuretics such as glucose and mannitol), amphotericin B, cisplatin, and cyclosporin. Hypophosphatemia, another common electrolyte abnormality in critically ill patients, causes magnesuria. Finally, renal diseases themselves, such as interstitial nephritis, acute tubular necrosis, and postobstructive states, lead to urinary loss of magnesium.

SKIN LOSS AND INTERNAL REDISTRIBUTION. Burned patients often develop hypomagnesemia, probably through loss of magnesium in the burn wound. In several conditions, magnesium is not lost from the body but is sequestered in an unusable site. Magnesium can be complexed by infused citrate in a manner analagous to calcium chelation, making it unavailable for cellular utilization. In an unusual syndrome, seen in patients with bone disease due to hyperparathyroidism or hyperthyroidism who then have their underlying disease treated, large amounts of magnesium are rapidly deposited into bone ("hungry bone syndrome"), leading to hypomagnesemia. Another example of internal redistribution occurs in patients with severely catabolic states who then undergo refeeding. Infusion of glucose and amino acids with stimulation or administration of insulin causes avid cellular uptake of magnesium. Treatment of DKA is one such setting in which hypomagnesemia is predictable.

CONSEQUENCES OF MAGNESIUM DEFICIENCY

Magnesium is the second most abundant cation in the intracellular milieu (next to potassium). It is a required cofactor in all biochemical processes utilizing ATP. Metabolism of protein, carbohydrate, fat, and nucleic acids depends on it. Magnesium is necessary for neuromuscular transmission, contractile protein regulation, and maintenance of cellular membrane integrity.

The clinical consequences of magnesium deficiency are largely cardiovascular and neuromuscular. Most patients remain asymptomatic. Nevertheless, magnesium deficiency can be life-threatening. Cardiovascular manifestations include ventricular and supraventricular tachyarrhythmias, torsades de pointes, ventricular fibrillation, and susceptibility to the toxic effects of digoxin. Some arrhythmias are refractory to standard antiarrhythmic therapy, only abating when magnesium is given. Hypomagnesemia has also been implicated in cardiomyopathy, coronary spasm, and even atherogenesis. Neuromuscular consequences include muscle weakness, seizures, psychiatric manifestations, myoclonus, and movement disorders (such as chorea and asterixis). Other than serious arrhythmias, respiratory muscle weakness is probably the most important effect of hypomagnesemia and can contribute to prolonged mechanical ventilation. On occasion, gastrointestinal dysmotility and anemia have been attributed to magnesium deficiency as well. Finally, hypomagnesemia can cause refractory hypocalcemia (by impairing parathyroid hormone [PTH] release and function) and hypokalemia (by impairing renal reabsorption).

SIGNIFICANCE OF HYPOMAGNESEMIA

Like calcium, magnesium is partly bound to albumin in the blood so that low total magnesium levels do not necessarily reflect ionized hypomagnesemia. Ionized magnesium determinations are not yet practical in most hospitals. Even when ionized hypomagnesemia is present, its significance in the critically ill is unknown. Clearly, some patients suffer serious consequences of magnesium deficiency. However, whether serum hypomagnesemia needs to be treated in all patients is not known. A further complexity is that a normal serum magnesium level may cloak cellular magnesium deficiency, as has been demonstrated in studies of intracellular magnesium and parenteral magnesium tolerance testing. Some patients with arrhythmias or renal potassium wasting have been shown to have normomagnesemic magnesium deficiency.

TREATMENT

Given that treatment of magnesium deficiency is safe and simple, it seems preferable to search for and treat hypomagnesemia until further studies are concluded. All critically ill patients should be screened for hypomagnesemia on admission. In subgroups of patients, such as those with prolonged ventilator dependence, multisystem organ failure, and predictable ongoing renal losses of magnesium, the serum magnesium level should be rechecked at 3-day intervals. All patients with refractory hypokalemia or hypocalcemia should also be considered potentially magnesium deficient. Finally, patients with intractable arrhythmias should have the serum magnesium level determined and possibly even receive empirical infusion of magnesium sulfate.

Treatment of hypomagnesemia in the ICU is usually by the intravenous route, since oral repletion is often impractical. Initially, 8 to 16 meq can be given as magnesium sulfate (1 to 2 g 50% $MgSO_4$). It is important to remember that a bolus of magnesium will briefly restore the serum magnesium level, but body stores will remain seriously depleted. Therefore, maintenance therapy should be initiated, such as 8 meq/day intravenously, for at least several days. This should be continued for as long as oral magnesium intake is limited or ongoing losses persist. Any excess magnesium will be excreted by the kidneys. If renal dysfunction is present, any maintenance therapy should be at a lower dose, and serum levels should be reassessed daily to avoid hypermagnesemia.

HYPERMAGNESEMIA

Mild and asymptomatic hypermagnesemia is occasionally seen in critically ill patients, especially those with renal failure. Symptoms do not appear until the serum level exceeds 4 mg/dL. Serious hypermagnesemia, which results in neuromuscular depression, hypotension, and asystole, is rare and nearly always iatrogenic. Obvious settings include the administration of magnesium intravenously, as in the treatment of eclampsia or of magnesium deficiency (usually in the setting of renal insufficiency). Less apparent sources of magnesium include magnesium-containing antacids and enemas. Treatment typically requires only discontinuation of the source of magnesium. Calcium antagonizes the effects of hypermagnesemia and should be given intravenously in severe instances. Dialysis is effective in life-threatening cases.

CALCIUM

Calcium disorders have long been recognized in critically ill patients. It is only in the past several years, however, that the frequency with which hypocalcemia is present has been appreciated. As many as 70 percent of patients in one series had ionized hypocalcemia at the time of admission to the ICU. More commonly, an incidence of about 25 percent is reported, but this depends significantly on the characteristics of the patient population. With the increased recognition of the incidence of hypocalcemia has come a realization of the complexity of its interpretation and management. Hypercalcemia, on the other hand, is far less common, and better understood.

CALCIUM HOMEOSTASIS

Serum calcium is derived from gastrointestinal absorption, parenteral administration, and bone storage sites. It is lost from the body through the feces and urine. Calcium is present in blood as ionized calcium (the physiologically active form), protein-bound calcium, and chelated calcium. Since about 40 percent of calcium is protein (largely albumin)-bound, abnormalities of protein concentration will affect the total serum calcium concentration. Total calcium levels may be low even though the ionized, physiologically relevant form is normal. Conversely, since only about half of calcium is in the ionized form, it is possible for a normal total calcium level to mask ionized hypocalcemia. Further, the blood $[H^+]$ and level of free fatty acids affect the degree of protein binding, so that two patients with the same total calcium and albumin levels can have importantly different ionized calcium concentrations. Finally, several chelating substances, including phosphate, affect the ionized calcium level without reducing the total. For all of these reasons, it is important to measure ionized calcium, rather than total calcium content, in many clinical situations. In contrast to magnesium, regulation of ionized calcium concentration depends little on intake and renal handling, but rather on serum phosphate concentration, hormonal influences, and the tremendous skeletal reservoir of calcium. Vitamin D and PTH play essential roles in the homeostasis of calcium.

THE ROLE OF PHOSPHATE. Inorganic phosphate has the ability to complex with calcium, causing it to be deposited in tissues. It was formerly believed that there was an inverse relationship between phosphate and calcium based on a presumed equilibrium between bone and the extracellular fluid. However, this is now known to be incorrect; an acute rise in serum phosphate concentration will cause the serum calcium level to fall importantly, but this is only true in pathologic conditions of hyperphosphatemia, not as part of normal calcium regulation.

THE ROLES OF VITAMIN D, PARATHYROID HORMONE, AND CALCITONIN. The main source of vitamin D activity is from the conversion of 7-dehydrocholesterol in the skin to vitamin D_3 (cholecalciferol) by ultraviolet irradiation. A lesser amount comes from fortified milk which contains vitamin D_2. Vitamin D_3 is metabolized to 25-hydroxy-D_3 in the liver. Further metabolism to 1,25-dihydroxy-D_3, the active vitamin, occurs in the kidney. This conversion is augmented by PTH, providing a mechanism for the restitution of the serum calcium concentration. Since these metabolic steps are required for biologic activity of vitamin D, it is apparent that hepatic and renal disease have the capacity to cause hypocalcemia. Acidemia and high levels of inorganic phosphate inhibit the renal production of 1,25-dihydroxy-D_3. Vitamin D stimulates intestinal absorption of calcium and phosphorus, permits mobilization of calcium and phosphorus from bone by PTH, and enhances tubular resorption of phosphate.

The function of PTH is to maintain serum calcium concentration. Ionized hypocalcemia stimulates production of PTH which, in turn, stimulates osteoclastic bone resorption and release of calcium and phosphorus (as long as vitamin D is present). In addition, PTH causes phosphaturia but increases renal resorption of calcium. Calcitonin, which is a potent hypocalcemic and hypophosphatemic peptide, has no clear role in normal homeostasis, but is useful therapeutically.

CAUSES OF HYPOCALCEMIA

This foundation provides a starting point for the differential diagnosis of ionized hypocalcemia. Classically, this has included vitamin D deficiency, hypoparathyroidism, chelators, drugs, and pancreatitis. Of historical interest, pathologic investigations led to a belief that pancreatitis causes hypocalcemia by saponification of retroperitoneal fat. It was later discovered that only minor amounts of calcium were actually deposited as soaps, leading to consideration of alternate mechanisms of hypocalcemia in these patients. These mechanisms are of tremendous interest to intensivists because it now seems that a similar pathophysiology underlies the hypocalcemia of many diverse critical illnesses. Of the many ICU patients with ionized hypocalcemia, less than half will have one of the classically known causes.

VITAMIN D DEFICIENCY. Vitamin D deficiency leads to hypocalcemia because of both impaired gastrointestinal absorption and interference with PTH-mediated mobilization of calcium from bone. Vitamin D deficiency can result from a fat-deficient diet, malabsorption (including pancreatic insufficiency, biliary cirrhosis, sprue, gastrectomy, and jejunoileal bypass), or altered metabolism (such as hepatic or renal insufficiency). It is being increasingly recognized in critically ill patients, probably since so many patients in ICUs suffer from preexisting chronic illness and malnutrition.

HYPOPARATHYROIDISM. The most common cause of hypoparathyroidism is surgical, usually related to thyroidectomy. However, during neck surgical procedures, even when the parathyroid glands are not removed, there is often a temporary, postoperative hypoparathyroid state. In nonsurgical settings, functional hypoparathyroidism can result from magnesium deficiency, since this cation is necessary for PTH secretion. In patients with refractory hypocalcemia with no identifiable cause, magnesium therapy usually results in improvement in the serum calcium concentration. Some drugs (such as cytotoxic agents) appear to have a toxic effect on the glands, leading to hypoparathyroidism. Finally, hypoparathyroidism may be part of the spectrum of polyglandular autoimmune failure. Therefore, this diagnosis should be considered in hypocalcemic patients with other autoimmune endocrine deficiencies.

CHELATORS AND DRUGS. Several substances bind calcium when they are administered and thereby reduce ionized (but not total) calcium. These include albumin, citrate (during massive blood transfusion), radiocontrast dye, protamine, bicarbonate, and phosphate. Ionized hypocalcemia following the intravenous infusion of sodium bicarbonate has been implicated in the detrimental hemodynamic effects of this therapy in human lactic acidosis. It is important to be vigilant for occult sources of hyperphosphatemia as a cause of hypocalcemia. These include the tumor lysis syndrome, rhabdomyolysis, and renal failure. Even iatrogenic administration of phosphate can be unrecognized. In one case, continuous use of phosphate enemas led to hypocalcemic cardiac arrest. Finally, cisplatin can lead to renal calcium wasting.

HYPOCALCEMIA OF CRITICAL ILLNESS. Patients with gram-negative sepsis, pancreatitis, and toxic shock syndrome frequently develop hypocalcemia. There are few studies in which the mechanisms are addressed, and some of these are contradictory. Conceptually, hypocalcemia should result from hypoparathyroidism, hypovitaminosis D, or tissue resistance to these hormones (or some combination). In the best analysis of septic, hypocalcemic patients, a multifactorial origin was described. Most patients had either parathyroid insufficiency, or renal 1-α-hydroxylase deficiency. Those with 1-α-hydroxylase deficiency typically had renal failure. Vitamin D deficiency and acquired vitamin D resistance were discovered in fewer patients. The etiology of hypocalcemia in critically ill patients clearly bears further study.

CONSEQUENCES OF HYPOCALCEMIA

Calcium is a necessary element for the function of all cells. It is required for membrane integrity, enzyme activity, and cellular division. Muscle contraction (including cardiac muscle), neuronal conduction, endocrine and exocrine gland secretion, immune responses, complement activation, and the coagulation cascade all depend on its presence.

The clinical consequences of ionized hypocalcemia range from cardiac arrest to no symptoms whatever. Of particular interest to the intensivist are hypotension, cardiac systolic dysfunction, arrhythmias, tetany, seizures, muscle weakness, and laryngospasm. We have been impressed with the complete lack of hypocalcemic symptoms in some patients with the hypocalcemia of critical illness (e.g., rhabdomyolysis and sepsis). This has been confirmed in a series of 60 critically ill patients, 12 of whom were hypocalcemic. These patients had no increased incidence of classic hypocalcemic signs.

SIGNIFICANCE OF HYPOCALCEMIA

Hypocalcemia has been correlated with increased mortality in critically ill patients. It seems unlikely that this is cause and effect, but rather, that hypocalcemia is a marker for severity of illness. Regardless, it is not a given that hypocalcemia in the critically ill patient is physiologically similar to the hypocalcemia of hypoparathyroidism. By analogy with the effect of critical illness on thyroid hormone levels, hypocalcemia may be of little direct clinical significance. Further, treatment aimed at restoring "normality" might not be necessary and could even be counterproductive.

It is important to consider the possibility that the concentration of ionized calcium in the serum does not accurately reflect intracellular calcium. Cellular calcium is partitioned by several membrane systems, including the cell membrane, the endoplasmic reticulum, and the inner mitochondrial membrane. Energy-requiring processes maintain cytosolic calcium at a level that is tremendously lower than the level found in the endoplasmic reticulum or in the extracellular fluid. Thus, while the total intracellular calcium concentration is about 1.0 mmol, that calcium is not distributed homogenously; free cytosolic calcium is only 0.1 μmol, four orders of magnitude lower. Presumably, it is this relatively low cytosolic calcium concentration which confers on calcium its role as a regulator ion.

In states of cellular injury, such as sepsis, it appears that intracellular calcium regulation breaks down, allowing a rise in free cytosolic calcium concentration. This can occur even in the setting of serum ionized hypocalcemia. Inappropriate elevations of intracellular calcium set loose vicious cascades which can lead to cell death. Proteases, nucleases, some ATPases, and phospholipases can be activated. Calcium-mediated phospholipase activation can generate fatty acids which have the capacity to damage membranes and generate toxic oxygen free radicals. In addition, excitation-contraction coupling is stimulated and oxidative phosphorylation derailed. Elevated intracellular calcium content has also been implicated in the "no-reflow" phenomenon, in which restoration of perfusion pressure to blood vessels following an ischemic insult fails to completely (sometimes even partially) restore blood flow. These points have important implications for the management of patients with ionized hypocalcemia who might also have cellular injury or ischemia.

TREATMENT

In patients with symptomatic hypocalcemia due, for example, to vitamin D deficiency or to hypoparathyroidism, there is no controversy regarding treatment. Calcium is clearly indicated and beneficial. Subsequently, it is usually important to diagnose and treat the specific underlying disease which led to hypocalcemia. However, to assume that patients with hypocalcemia of critical illness will similarly benefit from treatment with calcium is a potential oversimplification.

In patients who develop tetany, seizures, or arrhythmias attributable to hypocalcemia, treatment should probably be given (e.g., 1 g calcium chloride intravenously). However, since arrhythmias and seizures are so common in critically ill patients, especially those sick enough to develop severe ionized hypocalcemia, it is rarely clear that hypocalcemia is the culprit. Some investigators have noted a threshold for malignant ventricular arrhythmias at an ionized calcium of 2.5 mg/dL and have therefore recommended empirical therapy at or near this level. Whether this is of any benefit remains to be established.

Much has been made of the hypotension and resistance to vasoactive drugs in patients with ionized hypocalcemia due to sepsis. Theoretically, improvement in cardiac contractility or in vasomotor tone or responsiveness might confer a survival benefit in these hypoperfused patients. In patients on chronic hemodialysis, even modest increments in blood ionized calcium improve cardiac contractility. Moreover, most intensivists have given calcium to a critically ill patient and subsequently seen an impressive rise in the blood pressure.

It is not clear, however, that administration of calcium is beneficial in hypoperfused patients. In animals with endotoxic shock, calcium therapy is associated with increased mortality (despite an improvement in mean arterial pressure). These data and the concerns noted above regarding the detrimental effects of uncontrolled elevations of cytosolic calcium have prompted caution. For example, calcium is no longer routinely recommended in the setting of cardiopulmonary resuscitation. In fact, the use of calcium channel blockers has been advocated as a potential strategy in various types of shock. In animal models of endotoxic and hemorrhagic shock, calcium channel blockers have been beneficial in preserving cellular integrity and improving survival.

Of course, it is too early to recommend calcium channel blockers to hypoperfused patients based only on animal data and theoretical concerns. The further depression of myocardial contractility and blood pressure makes such drugs potentially dangerous. However, it seems similarly unwise to administer calcium routinely. Not only are supportive human studies lacking, but animal data suggest a detriment. Further evaluation of these treatments, based on valid clinical protocols, is necessary before either can be advocated.

HYPERCALCEMIA

Hypercalcemia is much less common in critically ill patients than hypocalcemia. Nevertheless, it was reported in as many as 15 percent of patients in a surgical ICU. In most instances, however, hypercalcemia is mild and of little clinical consequence. The hypercalcemia of malignancy occasionally requires treatment in an ICU, and this subject is fully covered in Chap. 149.

Clinical signs related to hypercalcemia include nephrogenic diabetes insipidus, muscular (including diaphragm) weakness, arrhythmias, coma, and seizures. The most common causes of hypercalcemia in the ICU are the humoral hypercalcemia of malignancy, hyperparathyroidism, iatrogenic hypercalcemia due to calcium administration, and recovery from acute renal failure. A hypothesis has been advanced that there may be, in addition, a syndrome of rebound hypercalcemia which follows the hypocalcemia of critical illness described above.

General treatment measures include assurance of adequate hydration, correction of coincident electrolyte disturbances, and therapy for the underlying cause. Specific therapies are discussed elsewhere in this text.

PHOSPHATE

Hypophosphatemia is common in patients at risk of becoming critically ill. Moreover, it often develops as a consequence of critical illness or its treatment. Depletion of phosphate clearly contributes to morbidity and, further, is potentially lethal. Hyperphosphatemia is less common and of less interest. Although it can cause serious hypocalcemia and metastatic calcification, hyperphosphatemia per se has no known adverse effects.

PHOSPHATE HOMEOSTASIS

The sources of phosphate include the gastrointestinal tract, bone stores, and parenteral administration. Phosphorus is generally well absorbed from the gastrointestinal tract, but this can be impeded by substances which bind it, such as magnesium-, calcium, and aluminum hydroxide-containing antacids. In the serum, phosphorus occurs primarily as the inorganic phosphate ion but also as a component of protein-bound phospholipids. The serum level of phosphate is not directly feedback regulated but depends instead on intake, urinary loss, and the hormonal responses directed at maintaining a normal serum calcium concentration. Vitamin D acts to increase both gastrointestinal absorption and tubular reabsorption of phosphorus and to mobilize it from bone. PTH releases phosphate (with calcium) from bone, but promotes its loss in the urine. Because the serum phosphate concentration is not directly regulated, it varies more widely than most electrolytes. When serum phosphate is grossly elevated, large amounts form colloidal complexes with calcium and are deposited into the tissues.

CAUSES OF HYPOPHOSPHATEMIA

The numerous causes of hypophosphatemia can be divided into deficient intake, intracellular shift, and excessive urinary excretion. In any given patient, two or more of these factors often combine to produce severe, clinically important hypophosphatemia.

DEFICIENT INTAKE. Failure to supply adequate phosphate (through enteral or parenteral nutrition or phosphate supplementation) to a critically ill patient is the most obvious cause for deficient intake and can lead to hypophosphatemia during protracted illness. Less apparently, many patients present to intensivists already severely phosphate depleted. For example, patients with preexisting starvation, malnutrition, malabsorption, alcoholism, vitamin D deficiency, or on chronic therapy with phosphate-binding antacids can be severely phosphate depleted despite normal admission values for serum phosphate. Only subsequently does their severe deficiency become evident.

INTRACELLULAR SHIFT. The most common reason for substantial amounts of phosphate to shift into cells is stimulation of glycolysis. Hypophosphatemia related to enhanced glycolysis is typically seen in response to either carbohydrate administration or respiratory alkalosis. Administration of glucose, especially after starvation, draws phosphate into the production of phosphorylated intermediates and high-energy phosphates as glycolysis resumes. Hypophosphatemia due to this mechanism is particularly common following the institution of hyperalimentation, but can also be seen following enteral refeeding of patients with alcoholism, anorexia nervosa, and esophageal or head and neck cancer. Intracellular movement of phosphate is particularly exaggerated during insulin treatment of DKA, in which insulin-stimulated hexokinase activity combines with rapid glucose entry to drive glycolysis. This is compounded by the renal phosphate losses typical of DKA (vide infra). Finally, refeeding-induced hypophosphatemia has been implicated in the syndrome of anasarca and death seen in some prisoners following World War II.

Respiratory alkalosis is also capable of causing hypophosphatemia, occasionally of severe degree. The mechanism is probably related to stimulation of glycolysis as well. The reduction in Pa_{CO_2} leads to rapid diffusion of CO_2 from cells, resulting in intracellular alkalosis. This directly stimulates PDH, the important rate-limiting enzyme which regulates pyruvate concentration, thereby facilitating glycolysis. Therefore, the many critical illnesses which cause hyperventilation, such as sepsis, hepatic failure, withdrawal, and CNS injury place patients at risk for hypophosphatemia. Even iatrogenic respiratory alkalosis due to intentional or inadvertent overventilation can lead to hypophosphatemia.

RENAL PHOSPHATE LOSSES. Several conditions can precipitate hypophosphatemia related to excessive urinary losses. Phosphate resorption is impaired by volume expansion and diuretic therapy. Osmotic diuresis has this effect as well, and for this reason, patients with DKA who tolerate prolonged polyuria before seeking medical attention become severely phosphate depleted. Magnesium deficiency leads to impaired conservation of phosphate and consequently its deficiency as well. This likely contributes to the hypophosphatemia seen in alcoholics. Some disorders of the proximal tubule are associated with renal phosphate wasting such as that seen in drug toxicity, multiple myeloma, amyloidosis, and following renal transplantation. Burned patients develop hypophosphatemia as well, in part due to fluid administration and the solute diuresis that is typical of burns. Defects in tubular function have been additionally proposed. Finally, since PTH is phosphaturic, hyperparathyroidism leads to hypophosphatemia.

CONSEQUENCES

Phosphate is an essential component of every cell and participates in innumerable cellular processes. Its most crucial role is in the storage of energy, as exemplified in the high-energy bonds of ATP. Without this, there would be no muscular contraction, nerve conduction, active transport of nutrients, and so on. However, it is also necessary as a structural element in cell membranes, nucleic acids, and phosphoproteins. Phosphate is involved in the metabolism of fats, proteins, and most notably, carbohydrates. It also modulates the synthesis of red blood cell 2,3-diphosphoglycerate (2,3-DPG), which affects the oxygen-carrying capacity of hemoglobin. Since phosphate is crucial for the function of every cell and organ, the clinical expression of severe hypophosphatemia is broad.

The clinical manifestations of hypophosphatemia include red cell, white cell, and platelet dysfunction. Of these, the most important is probably the depression of chemotaxis and phagocytosis in white cells. Thus, hypophosphatemia may contribute to the risk of life-threatening infection in critically ill patients. Weakness of the respiratory muscles (including respiratory failure) and heart (congestive cardiomyopathy) can lead to prolonged ICU stay and death. Metabolic encephalopathy, even to the point of coma or seizures, is a CNS consequence of severe hypophosphatemia. Finally, rhabdomyolysis may result from phosphate depletion, especially in alcoholics who are refed.

TREATMENT

Given the frequency of hypophosphatemia in critically ill patients, its serious consequences, and the ease of treatment, serum phosphate levels should be routinely checked following ICU admission. In patients at risk of developing hypophosphatemia, such as those with alcoholism, DKA, or burns, phosphate should be assayed serially. Further, in any patient with unexplained heart failure, this disorder should be excluded since it is a truly reversible cause of cardiomyopathy. Similarly, the patient who is having difficulty coming off of the ventilator may have a component of muscle weakness secondary to hypophosphatemia. In patients with respiratory failure who have superimposed moderate hypophosphatemia, intravenous phosphate repletion results in prompt and dramatic improvements in respiratory muscle strength.

In occasional situations it may be appropriate to give phosphate by the oral route. Several preparations are available for this purpose, but they are unpredictably absorbed and often provoke diarrhea. Therefore, it is more common to give intravenous potassium phosphate. In severe hypophosphatemia, 0.08 mmol/kg body weight, given over 6 h, is the usual dose. In all cases, sources of ongoing loss of phosphate should be sought, and maintenance phosphate should be added to enteral formulas or parenteral fluids.

VOLUME

Accurate regulation of volume is crucial for survival. As discussed in Chap. 2, insufficient volume leads to impairment of ventricular filling, depression of $\dot{Q}_T$, and hypoperfusion of critical organs. On the other hand, excessive volume causes pulmonary vascular congestion, pulmonary edema, and hypoxemia. In health, the volume status is exquisitely controlled. During critical illness, however, derangements of volume regulation are the rule. In the ICU, the physician frequently becomes responsible for this aspect of homeostasis.

The conceptual framework adopted here will equate volume homeostasis to sodium homeostasis. Thus, if sodium is added to the body, it is assumed that water will be added as well or retained in response to the added sodium. In this way, adding sodium is equivalent to adding sodium and water or volume. Similarly, if sodium is lost from the body, it is assumed that water is lost in concert or will be lost in response to the loss of sodium. Loss of sodium is then equivalent to loss of sodium plus water or loss of volume. Disorders in which sodium and water do not move in step will be considered as disorders of free water homeostasis and are discussed subsequently.

A second conceptual point relates to consideration of the edematous states. Much of the literature dealing with the clinical assessment of volume status considers the edematous states as forms of hypervolemia. In this chapter, volume status will be determined solely in terms of arterial filling (vide infra). This simplification leads to better prediction of the neurohumoral responses seen in hypovolemia, including most edematous states. Moreover, it focuses attention on the relevant parameter in critically ill patients—the ability to perfuse vital organs. Most of the edematous disorders are characterized by arterial underfilling or hypovolemia. While total body sodium and water are in excess, this fluid is not available to maintain organ perfusion. Therefore, the presence of edema fluid is largely irrelevant in the assessment of volume status.

VOLUME HOMEOSTASIS

In its control of volume, the body primarily attempts to regulate arterial filling, rather than venous filling or some other parameter. More subtle adjustments based on venous filling or atrial pressure (e.g., atrial natriuretic peptide) are only of secondary importance. The high pressure, low compliance, arterial bed contains less than 2 percent of the intravascular volume. It is thus poised to detect the slightest of changes in volume. Further, it makes sense that volume control is geared largely toward defense of arterial filling, since it is the arterial circulation which is responsible for maintaining tissue perfusion.

Two factors appear to determine whether arterial filling is adequate or not—$\dot{Q}_T$ and peripheral vascular resistance. Arterial overfilling occurs when either $\dot{Q}_T$ or peripheral vascular resistance is abnormally high. Conversely, arterial underfilling is present when $\dot{Q}_T$ or peripheral vascular resistance is abnormally low. The manner in which the body detects changes in these parameters has not been fully defined. The baroreceptors in the aortic arch and carotid artery are the best known potential sensors of arterial filling, but additional receptors are found in the afferent renal arteriole, and the left ventricle. It is more puzzling to consider how the body could monitor systemic vascular resistance (SVR). There is some evidence that arterial baroreceptors have the capacity to sense pulse pressure, which, of course, is related to $\dot{Q}_T$. In this way, the body could integrate absolute pressure and pressure waveform to gauge SVR. An additional possibility is that the peripheral microcirculation is able to convey information to the CNS regarding adequacy of perfusion as a measure of arterial filling.

Once the body detects an abnormality of arterial filling, it effects a homeostatic response via sympathetic nerves, modulation of the renin-angiotensin-aldosterone system, and nonosmotic release of antidiuretic hormone (ADH). The response to arterial underfilling includes a stereotyped neurohumoral profile. Plasma renin activity, aldosterone secretion, and plasma norepinephrine and ADH levels all increase. Moreover, there is extensive direct adrenergic innervation of the afferent and efferent glomerular arterioles, the juxtaglomerular apparatus, and much of the nephron itself. In the face of arterial underfilling, whether due to

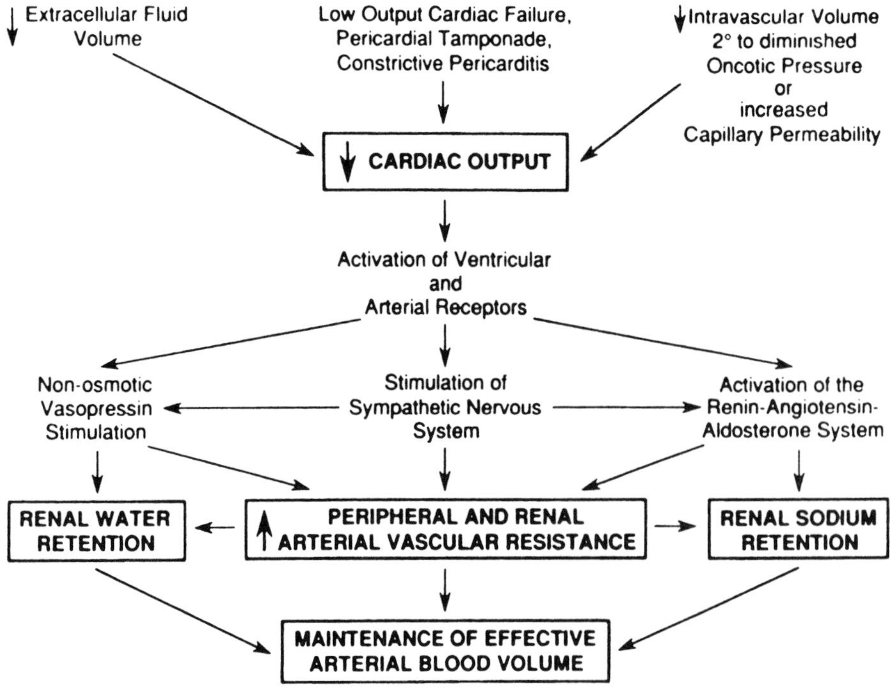

FIGURE 3-15 Pathophysiology of renal sodium and water retention initiated by reduced $\dot{Q}_T$. (Reprinted with permission from Schrier RW: Body fluid volume regulation in health and disease: A unifying hypothesis. Ann Intern Med 113:155–9, 1990.)

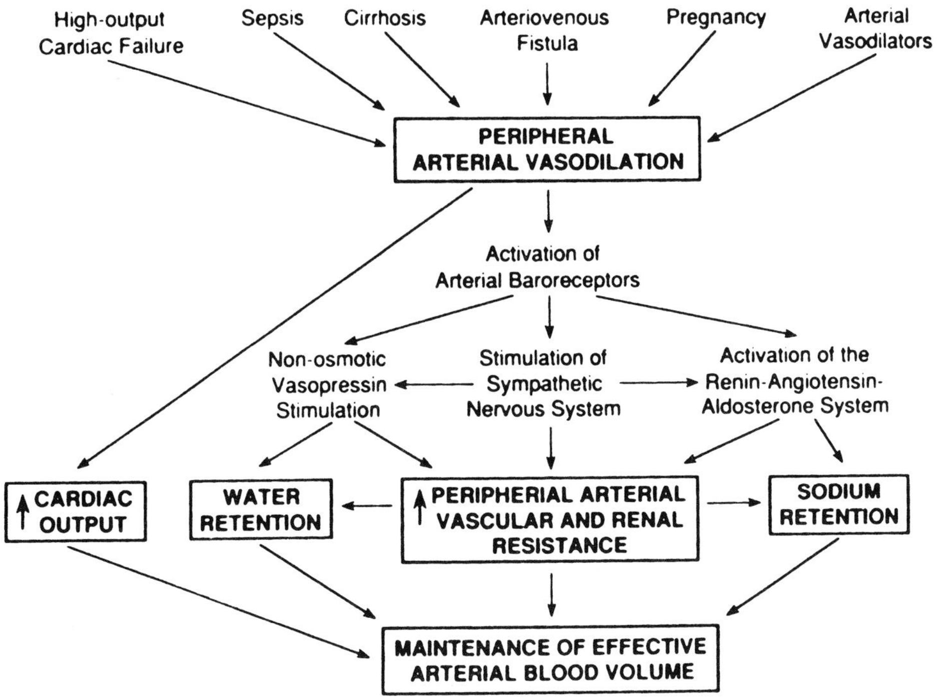

FIGURE 3-16 Pathophysiology of renal sodium and water retention initiated by peripheral arterial vasodilation. (Reprinted from Schrier RW: Body fluid volume regulation in health and disease: A unifying hypothesis. Ann Intern Med 113:155–9, 1990.)

decreased $\dot{Q}_T$ or to peripheral arterial vasodilation, the normal response of the kidney is to retain sodium and water (Figs. 3-15 and 3-16). This gradually restores volume, eventually resulting in adequate arterial filling. In contrast, in arterial overfilling, plasma renin activity and release of renin, norepinephrine, and ADH are suppressed. This leads to excretion of sodium and water in the urine, with normalization of arterial filling. Therefore, the body is provided with a mechanism for counteracting any change in volume status and restoring the normal state.

In health, adequate arterial filling is equivalent to adequate filling of the venous compartment, as well as the interstitial and intracellular compartments. Therefore, control of the small arterial compartment amply controls total body volume. This is not true in several disease states. Arterial filling can become dissociated from the intracellular volume in the disorders of free water, discussed later. Alternatively, pump failure (e.g., left ventricular failure, pulmonary hypertension, cardiac tamponade) leads to venous and interstitial overfilling while the arterial circuit is underfilled. Therefore, these diseases are associated with the formation of edema. Finally, in states of pathologically reduced SVR, the extravascular compartment may be overfilled while the arterial compartment remains underfilled, also resulting in the formation of edema.

HYPOVOLEMIA

In the broadest sense, hypovolemia can be considered to include all causes of low $\dot{Q}_T$ and low SVR. This approach is useful in understanding the physiologic responses to each of these, such as tachycardia and renal sodium and water retention. However, the mechanisms governing $\dot{Q}_T$ are covered in Chap. 2. This discussion will be limited to low $\dot{Q}_T$ due to loss of volume from the intravascular compartment and to a brief analysis of edemagenesis in the low SVR states.

CAUSES OF INTRAVASCULAR HYPOVOLEMIA. Intravascular hypovolemia results from inadequate intake of sodium and water or excessive losses. Sources of volume include the gastrointestinal tract and parenteral routes, usually a vein. Because the kidney is adept at conserving volume in the face of decreased intake, clinically important hypovolemia nearly always implies excessive loss. Nevertheless, a protracted period of poor intake can precede critical illness and therefore contribute to hypovolemia.

More usually, intravascular hypovolemia is the result of loss of sodium and water through the kidney, the gastrointestinal tract, the respiratory tract, the skin, wounds, drainage procedures (e.g., paracentesis, thoracentesis), or directly from the vasculature. Renal losses are often due to diuretic drugs or to osmotic diuresis. Common culprits include glycosuria and administration of mannitol. Osmotically active solutes are occasionally occult, for example, as seen following massive burns when destroyed tissue is catabolized. The gastrointestinal tract is the site of volume loss during severe vomiting or diarrhea or when there is an abnormal fistula or drain. Skin losses can be extensive during exertion or hyperthermia and when skin integrity is compromised because of burns, wounds, or severe dermatologic illness. Vascular losses include bleeding and capillary leakage. Bleeding is not always evident. For example, in the setting of trauma, a rather small scalp wound can bleed extensively. This may not be evident by the time the patient reaches the doctor. Even when bleeding occurs in the hospital, it may be occult. Several liters of blood in the gastrointestinal tract, thigh, pelvis, or retroperitoneum can easily escape notice. Capillary leakage is a regular feature of critical illness and can lead to hypovolemia. Examples include sepsis, toxic shock syndrome, pancreatitis, cirrhosis, and necrotizing fasciitis. Skin and respiratory fluid loss are commonly lumped together as "insensible losses." In critically ill patients, however, many additional types of loss are "insensible," and often of great magnitude.

EDEMAGENESIS IN THE LOW SYSTEMIC VASCULAR RESISTANCE STATES. Edema formation in the low SVR states (e.g., cirrhosis, pregnancy, sepsis, arteriovenous fistula) depends on a change in the microvasculature. Arteriolar vasodilation recruits capillary surface area and increases capillary hydrostatic pressure. Recent evidence suggests that it increases interstitial compliance as well, thereby minimizing the effect of small amounts of edema to inhibit further edemagenesis. These factors join to generate edema, which in turn perpetuates arterial underfilling and leads to further sodium and water retention. This explains the well-recognized difficulty in attempting to replete the arterial circulation in cirrhosis and similar circumstances.

CONSEQUENCES, DIAGNOSIS AND TREATMENT OF HYPOVOLEMIA. The compensatory response to hypovolemia, as discussed above, includes tachycardia and renal retention of sodium and water. The more direct consequences relate to the difficulty in achieving ventricular filling, with inadequate cardiac output. Because this directly threatens organ function, hypovolemia should always be excluded in hypoperfusion states and treated when found. As an additional consequence, the severely hypovolemic patient may become severely hyponatremic due to nonosmotic release of ADH (vide infra). Early detection or prevention of hypovolemia relies heavily on following the daily weight and the intake-output records. Physical examination may reveal decreased skin turgor, orthostatic hypotension, low venous pressures, or a source of volume loss. When there is time, urinary volumes or sodium concentration may provide clues to volume status. Unfortunately, in critically ill patients, the examination is often unhelpful or impractical, and normal renal function is a luxury. Therefore, invasive measures of volume, such as central venous and pulmonary capillary wedge pressures, are often essential. Ideally, such invasive monitors will be supplanted by newer methods, such as echocardiography, as technology improves.

Treatment includes control of any sources of ongoing volume loss, and restitution of volume using saline, blood or colloid. It is important to remember that hypovolemia only becomes evident when 10 to 20 percent of intravascular volume has been lost. A patient in acute hypovolemic shock has probably lost nearly 40 percent of his intravascular volume. When hypovolemia has developed over a longer time, such as in DKA, huge volumes are sometimes necessary to restore euvolemia.

HYPERVOLEMIA

Intravascular hypervolemia is a consequence of taking in more sodium and water than is lost. From a practical standpoint, the renal capacity for water excretion is great. Therefore, hypervolemia nearly always implies a defect in renal excretion of water (although the mechanism of that defect may not be intrinsically renal, as in cardiac pump failure). Volume is typically gained through the gastrointestinal tract and intravascular lines. Mobilization of previously sequestered fluid is an additional important and occult cause of hypervolemia. For example, the patient with septic shock is often given large volumes of fluid in an often futile attempt to restore arterial filling. When sepsis resolves, fluid can be rapidly resorbed from "third spaces," resulting in hypervolemia. A different, dramatic example is pulmonary edema following relief of cardiac tamponade. As tamponade progresses, fluid is retained in response to arterial underfilling (often with a few additional liters provided intravenously by the physician). While tamponade is clearly detrimental, it does impede venous return, thereby protecting the lungs from high filling pressures. Following the reduction in pericardial pressure, fluid previously sequestered in the veins and tissues streams back to the lungs, leading to high pressure pulmonary edema.

When hypervolemia is present, the kidneys respond by wasting sodium and water. Since renal capacity for volume excretion is so prodigious, hypervolemia usually implies impaired renal function. Even without "excessive" volume administration, impairment of renal sodium excretion will promptly lead to hypervolemia. A conceptually similar type of hypervolemia is that which occurs when any large source of volume loss is controlled. For example, if large volume diarrhea is being treated with equal volume infusion, but then becomes controlled, the kidneys will be presented with a substantial challenge. In this instance, no increment in volume intake occurs, yet hypervolemia results.

The most important consequence of hypervolemia is pulmonary edema leading to hypoxemia and increased work of breathing. Volume accumulation in other tissues is largely a cosmetic problem, but can precipitate skin breakdown or infection, and may contribute to other organ dysfunction.

Treatment of hypervolemia involves reducing sources of fluid intake while facilitating losses. While diuretic agents are usually sufficient, low dose dopamine may hasten diuresis. In rare circumstances, phlebotomy or ultrafiltration may be needed. In some patients, it is prudent to use continuous arteriovenous hemofiltration before catastrophic volume overload occurs.

FREE WATER

The osmotic pressure of plasma is narrowly controlled. When free water is retained in excess of sodium, hyponatremia (hypoosmolarity) results. In contrast, free water losses which exceed sodium losses lead to hypernatremia (hyperosmolarity). Each of these common conditions has serious consequences for cellular function. Both are associated with substantial morbidity and mortality.

OSMOLAR HOMEOSTASIS

Regulation of plasma osmolarity depends on the renal handling of water and the thirst mechanism. Thirst (or access to free water) is generally blunted in critically ill patients, so this aspect of free water homeostasis will not be discussed further. Hypotonic plasma provokes free water excretion (the creation of dilute urine). Hypertonicity stimulates concentration of urine as free water is retained. Urinary concentration (free water retention) requires that the collecting duct be permeable to water, which requires the presence of ADH. Urinary dilution necessitates impermeable collecting ducts and, therefore, the absence of ADH. Thus, while adequate renal function is essential for free water regulation, it is ADH which controls water homeostasis. ADH is produced by both osmotic and nonosmotic stimuli. Osmotic release of ADH is responsible for control of plasma osmolarity. Nonosmotic release of ADH requires a pathologic stimulus which becomes important in disease, but is not a normal homeostatic mechanism.

A group of "osmoreceptor" cells in the hypothalamus is exquisitely sensitive to changes in plasma osmolarity. These cells can detect a change in osmolarity of less than 1 percent. A drop in plasma osmolarity causes prompt reduction in the release of ADH from the posterior pituitary gland. On the other hand, when osmolarity rises slightly, ADH is secreted. In this way, minute abnormalities in plasma osmolarity lead to rapid compensatory changes in renal water handling.

HYPEROSMOLARITY

CAUSES OF HYPEROSMOLARITY. Hyperosmolarity results either when excess free water is lost from the body or excess sodium is added. This discussion will be simplified by considering hyperosmolarity and hypernatremia to be equivalent. While it is possible to have hyperosmolarity initially without hypernatremia (due to hyperglycemia or mannitol), the osmotic diuresis typically soon causes water loss and hypernatremia as well.

Free water can be lost through the skin, the lungs, or the kidneys. If losses from burns, sweating, or dermatitis are not replaced, hyperosmolarity results. Insensible water losses through skin and lung are increased in febrile patients, sometimes dramatically. Renal water losses occur during osmotic diuresis or when the collecting ducts remain impermeable to water. In addition, osmotically active solutes in the urine (e.g., glucose, mannitol) can prevent resorption of the water they are dissolved in, despite maximally permeable collecting ducts. Collecting duct impermeability (diabetes insipidus) implies a lack of ADH or a lack of ADH effect. Absence of ADH is termed *neurogenic diabetes insipidus*. Causes include destruction of the hypothalamus or pituitary gland (e.g., stroke, trauma, pituitary surgery). Renal insensitivity to circulating ADH constitutes *nephrogenic diabetes insipidus*. This may be due to underlying renal disease, hypercalcemia, hypokalemia, sickle cell disease, or drugs (e.g., lithium, amphotericin). In the complete absence of ADH, a staggering output of dilute urine ensues (as much as 50 L/day).

The addition of excess sodium is nearly always iatrogenic. One of the most common causes of mild hyperosmolarity in critically ill patients is massive resuscitation with normal saline solution, which is slightly, but definitely, hyperosmolar (155 mmol Na/L). Infusion of markedly hypertonic fluids is a less common but more dramatic cause of hypernatremia. Sodium bicarbonate is occasionally given in massive amounts to acidemic patients and can rapidly raise osmolarity to dangerous levels. Hypertonic saline, which is used to treat hyponatremia, only leads to hyperosmolarity when there is a therapeutic error.

CONSEQUENCES OF HYPEROSMOLARITY. Excessively osmolar plasma draws water from within cells. This is particularly important in the CNS. The brain shrinks initially as water is lost from brain cells. Over days, the cells generate osmotically active substances ("idiogenic osmoles") which tend to restore cellular volume despite ongoing plasma hypertonicity. This has important implications for treatment. Cellular dehydration seems particularly detrimental to neurons. This is clinically manifest as lethargy, hyperreflexia, seizures, and coma. Gross shrinkage in the brain causes anatomic deformity with rupture of cerebral vessels, compounding injury.

TREATMENT OF HYPEROSMOLARITY. The first concern should be to treat the underlying cause of water loss or sodium addition. Rare patients who have become hyperosmolar due to addition of sodium may repair their osmolarity given just time and adequate renal function. Sodium losses can be hastened with a diuretic, which also facilitates administration of free water. In the great majority of hypernatremic patients who are also volume depleted, free water should be given to restore the deficit. Total body water is 60 percent of body weight. Therefore, the free water required to normalize serum sodium can be calculated from the following formula:

$$\text{Deficit} = (\text{Na}^+ - 140)/140 \times \text{body weight (kg)} \times 0.6 \quad (3\text{-}22)$$

This amount of free water will correct the serum sodium concentration, but does not take into account whether the patient is total body sodium depleted (usual) or overloaded (rare). Therefore, sodium may need to be given in addition to free water. Generally, free water should be restored over several days to reduce osmolarity no faster than 2 mO/h. Faster correction risks excessive movement of water into cells which have generated idiogenic osmoles, which can lead to cerebral edema. More gradual correction allows resolution of intracellular osmoles, preventing cellular swelling.

HYPOOSMOLARITY

CAUSES OF HYPOOSMOLARITY. Conceptually, hypoosmolarity can be due to excessive sodium loss or to excessive retention of free water. In practice, sodium is not lost out of proportion to water. However, in the face of sodium and water losses, continued free water intake leads to a situation analogous to isolated sodium loss. The resulting hyponatremia turns off the signal for osmotic release of ADH. However, significant hypovolemia is a powerful stimulus for the nonosmotic secretion of ADH, and it overrides the effect of osmolarity. Therefore, in the presence of significant hypovolemia, continued release of ADH leads to retention of free water, despite hyponatremia. Any condition which leads to ongoing losses of sodium and water can therefore cause hyponatremia. Common etiologies include gastrointestinal fluid losses (vomiting, diarrhea), renal wasting (diuretics, osmotic diuresis, mineralocorticoid deficiency), and third space sequestration. A similar pathophysiology underlies the hyponatremia of the edematous states, conditions in which there is arterial underfilling, or effective hypovolemia.

Inappropriate retention of free water occurs when the kidneys are unable to excrete a free water load or when ADH is inappropriately present. Renal free water excretion requires adequate renal, thyroid, and adrenal function. Therefore, screening for endocrine disease is usually part of the evaluation of hyponatremia. Various drugs impair free water excretion by several mechanisms, including release of ADH and suppression of medullary prostaglandins. Cyclophosphamide, carbamazepine, clofibrate, chlorpropamide, vincristine, nonsteroidal anti-inflammatory drugs, and morphine all have an antidiuretic effect and have been implicated in hyponatremia.

Persistent secretion of ADH despite hyponatremia may be due to hypovolemia or drugs, as described above, or to pain. Finally, ADH release may be "inappropriate," leading to the syndrome of inappropriate ADH (SIADH). This syndrome is frequently considered among the possible causes of hyponatremia in critically ill patients, but is rather uncommon. The diagnosis can only be made after excluding hypovolemia, edematous disorders, hypothyroidism, adrenal insufficiency, renal failure, and drugs. Disorders implicated in the causation of SIADH include carcinoma (lung, pancreas), lung disease (tuberculosis, pneumonia, aspergillosis, lung abscess), and CNS disorders (head trauma, cerebrovascular accident, meningitis, encephalitis, brain abscess, tumors).

The coalescence of several hyponatremia-causing factors in the postoperative period puts surgical patients at risk for hyponatremia. The combination of pain, morphine, and free water administration occasionally provides the ingredients for a postoperative disaster. In one series of 15 previously healthy patients undergoing elective surgical procedures, hyponatremia led to a stereotyped clinical picture. At about 48 h postoperatively, patients complained of severe headache and nausea, seized, and developed focal or generalized neurologic signs. Nearly all of the patients were women. In the hours following the acute deterioration, the diagnosis was typically obscure, despite the availability of the serum sodium (average $[Na^+] = 108$) in the medical record. Delay until hyponatremia was recognized as the problem and treated averaged 16 h. In the meanwhile, 42 consultations were requested and numerous tests performed. Fifteen patients underwent 15 computed tomography scans, 9 lumbar punctures, 7 angiograms, 9 electroencephalograms and 2 brain biopsies. The outcome was devastating. Most of these previously healthy patients died or remained permanently vegetative, while a few suffered other, permanent neurologic disability. This experience highlights the seriousness of hyponatremia and the lack of familiarity many clinicians have with its development postoperatively.

CONSEQUENCES OF HYPONATREMIA. Hyponatremia leads to cellular uptake of water with swelling. In severe cases, there is cerebral edema, occasionally leading to herniation. The remarkable clinical effects relate to disturbed CNS function. Headache, depression of consciousness, seizures, coma, and death may result. As noted above, patients often suffer permanent neurologic disability.

TREATMENT OF HYPONATREMIA. The approach to the treatment of hyponatremia is controversial and is fully discussed in Chap. 156. Here, only a conceptual framework is provided. First, the underlying disorder (e.g., hypovolemia, adrenal insufficiency) should be discerned, since it may have adverse consequences beyond hyponatremia. The hyponatremia itself can be corrected by encouraging the loss of free water or by adding sodium to the body. In the edematous disorders, renal failure, endocrinopathies, and SIADH, it may be appropriate simply to restrict free water, while allowing insensible losses to continue. This may require changing maintenance intravenous infusions, as well as dissolving drugs in saline rather than dextrose.

When hyponatremia is severe, correction with saline solution is required. In most situations, isotonic saline solution will allow restoration of a normal serum sodium level as long as the kidneys can create a dilute urine. When hyponatremia is severe or symptomatic, hypertonic saline solution may become necessary.

POTASSIUM

Potassium is the most prevalent cation in the body and is essential for the function of all cells. Both hyperkalemia and hypokalemia are common during critical illness, and both cause substantial morbidity. Despite the widespread appreciation of the importance of potassium disorders, these remain important causes of ICU mortality.

POTASSIUM HOMEOSTASIS

Potassium is provided largely through the gastrointestinal tract and intravenous infusions. However, during critical illness, the huge intracellular pool of potassium may be a source for redistribution to the serum. Potassium exits the bloodstream primarily through the kidneys. In chronic renal failure, substantial fecal losses aid homeostasis. Finally, potassium can shift into cells in a few circumstances, such as during intensive bronchodilator therapy with β agonists.

Control of the serum K^+ is exerted by hormonal responses and renal potassium handling. Aldosterone secretion is stimulated by a rise in serum potassium concentration, prompting increased renal excretion. Similarly, hyperkalemia leads to insulin release, which aids potassium movement into cells. In part because they lack insulin, diabetics are especially liable to develop hyperkalemia. Cellular uptake is further facilitated by epinephrine, which is released by the adrenal glands as $[K^+]$ rises (Fig. 3-17).

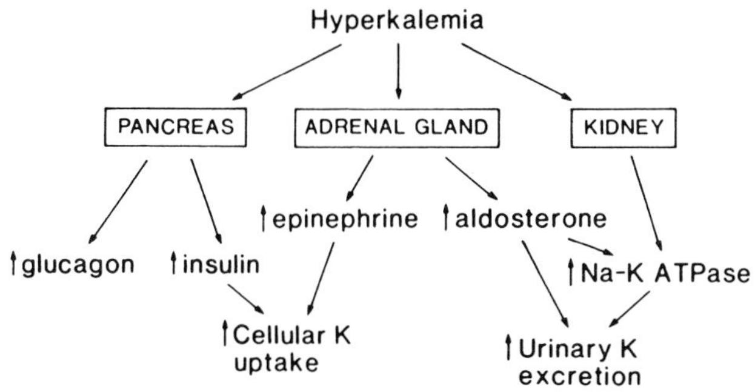

FIGURE 3-17 The body's adaptive response to hyperkalemia is illustrated. (Reprinted with permission from Gabow PA, Peterson LN: Disorders of potassium metabolism, in Schrier RW (ed): *Renal and Electrolyte Disorders.* Boston, Little, Brown, 1980, pp. 183–221.)

The serum $[K^+]$ is a poor indicator of the total body stores of potassium. Since the serum $[K^+]$ is so low, only about 60 meq is found extracellularly in a healthy adult. In contrast, nearly 3500 meq is contained within the cells. For this reason, even moderate hypokalemia is a sign of a severe deficit of total body potassium (Fig. 3-18). It is also for this reason that attempted repletion of potassium is so dangerous. Even a small fraction of the potassium required to replete a deficit can be lethal if acutely added to the tiny serum pool.

CAUSES OF HYPERKALEMIA

It is first important to realize that there are several causes of factitious hyperkalemia. Most notable is the apparent hyperkalemia related to hemolysis of the blood sample. A similar mechanism underlies the false hyperkalemia in some patients with gross elevations of leukocyte or platelet count. Both leukocytes and platelets are rich in potassium, which can be released as the blood clots. Prolonged tourniquet application is a final example. An electrocardiogram (ECG) can be helpful in distinguishing true hyperkalemia from factitious hyperkalemia (see Chap. 30).

Three mechanisms can produce hyperkalemia—excessive intake, extracellular shift, and impaired excretion. In most healthy adults, the renal capacity for potassium excretion in the face of augmented intake is so large that excessive intake simply cannot cause hyperkalemia. This is of little reassurance in critically ill patients since renal potassium handling is so often impaired, even when gross renal function appears normal. The only important external route for potassium intake is through intravascular infusions. The usual source is potassium intentionally given to correct hypokalemia or added to maintenance fluids and parenteral nutrition solutions. Other, less obvious sources are occasionally important, such as large doses of potassium penicillin.

Shift of potassium from the cells into the serum is related to massive cellular destruction, acidemia, or other rare causes. Cell lysis sufficient to cause hyperkalemia can complicate the cytotoxic therapy of malignancies or even spontaneous tumor lysis. Crush injuries and nontraumatic rhabdomyolysis release potassium from the muscles, one of the largest pools of cellular potassium. Similarly, gangrene, some snake bites, and brisk hemolysis provide a potassium

FIGURE 3-18 The relationship of serum $[K^+]$ and total body potassium is exponential. Therefore, similar increments in total body potassium have little effect on serum $[K^+]$ when the level is low, but a much greater impact when the $[K^+]$ is high.

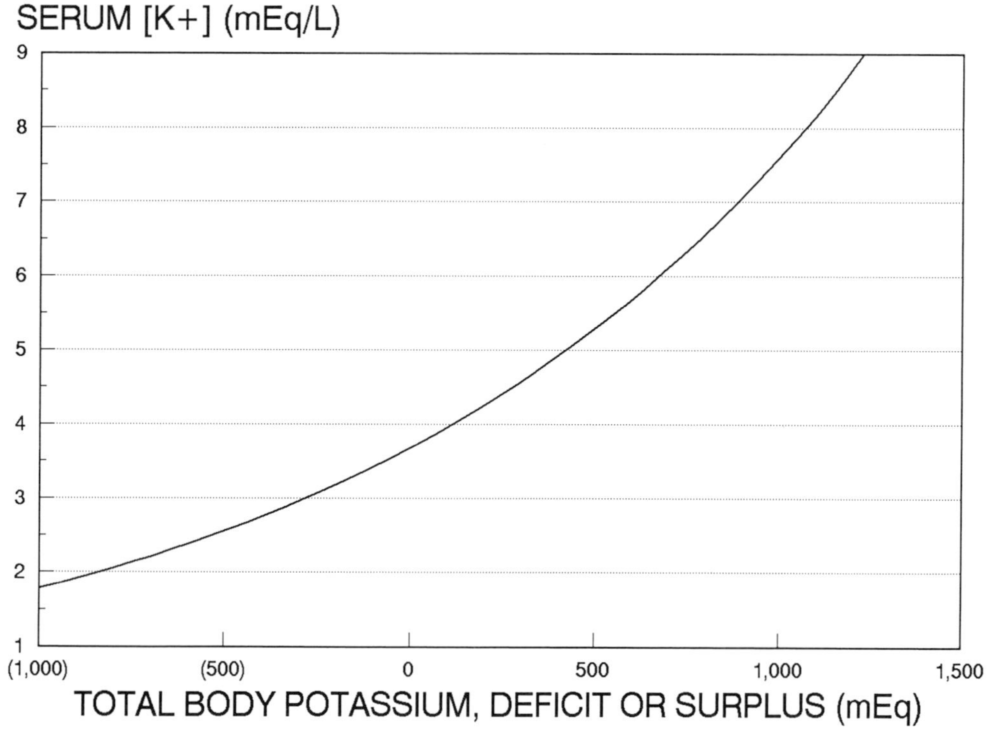

load. Acidemia causes a shift of potassium out of cells, apparently in response to an inward shift of hydrogen ions. This is seen in both respiratory and metabolic acidosis, although its magnitude is related to factors besides the [H^+], such as the acid anion. Far more unusual etiologies for massive shifts of potassium out of cells are digitalis intoxication and hyperkalemic familial periodic paralysis.

In the majority of patients, hyperkalemia is the result of impaired renal excretion of potassium. Factors influencing renal handling of potassium include renal function, delivery of solute to the distal tubule, aldosterone, and diuretic drugs. Acute renal failure directly impairs renal K^+ secretion, commonly causing hyperkalemia. In chronic renal failure, compensation by remaining nephrons preserves potassium homeostasis until creatinine clearance is well below 10 mL/min. Nevertheless, the margin for handling incremental potassium loads is small, so that any excess intake or extracellular shift precipitates hyperkalemia. Potassium excretion depends on adequate delivery of solute to the distal tubule, so that hypovolemia and hypoperfusion states put patients at risk for hyperkalemia. Aldosterone deficiency may result from adrenal insufficiency, which leads to hyperkalemia. Unexplained hyperkalemia should prompt consideration of a diagnosis of adrenal insufficiency, especially if other signs are present (see Chap. 160). A more common cause of aldosterone lack is hyporeninemic hypoaldosteronism (type IV RTA). In this condition, seen in diabetics and patients with interstitial nephritis, renin release by the juxtaglomerular apparatus is impaired. Disordered renal function also underlies the tendency of patients with sickle cell disease to develop hyperkalemia. Finally, potassium-sparing diuretics are readily implicated as a cause for hyperkalemia as long as the medication list is reviewed.

In many critically ill patients, more than one component of increased intake, extracellular shift, or impaired excretion is present. One dramatic, recurring example occurs in patients with hematologic malignancies. It is a common scenario for such patients to be neutropenic and septic, requiring numerous drug infusions. Renal potassium wasting due to amphotericin and aminoglycosides develops, initially causing hypokalemia. Potassium is given intravenously with little impact on the serum level, due to ongoing renal wasting. Potassium infusion is increased to the maximum permitted by nursing policy, but fails to raise the serum level above 3.0. Sometimes, a potassium-sparing diuretic is added in an attempt to halt ongoing losses. Tissue damage, possibly with systemic acidemia, may shift some potassium out of cells and into the serum. In the meanwhile, a combination of sepsis, drug toxicity, and hypotension takes its toll on renal function, although urine output and serum creatinine concentration remain grossly normal. Finally, the [K^+] creeps over 3.2 in what appears to be a victory for the physicians. Six hours later, a wide complex rhythm is noted, and the patient suffers a cardiac arrest. The [K^+] is found to be 8.0. In this example, a large total body potassium deficit combines with ongoing renal losses to create refractory hypokalemia. Large intravenous infusions of potassium, sometimes in excess of 300 meq/day, are given initially just to maintain a constant, low [K^+]. In this situation, where the entire amount of extracellular (including serum) potassium is only 60 meq, a minor decrement in renal potassium wasting provides a substrate for disaster.

CONSEQUENCE OF HYPERKALEMIA

The clinically relevant consequences of acute hyperkalemia relate to its effects on membrane excitability. Both cardiac and peripheral neuromuscular tissues demonstrate important detrimental responses. The ECG manifestations are discussed in detail in Chap. 30 but culminate in cardiac arrest. This complication of hyperkalemia makes potassium one of the leading causes of iatrogenic drug deaths. Because of this, we have implemented a system by which a serum [K^+] is routinely assayed as part of arterial blood-gas analysis in all patients with cardiac arrest. Both increased and decreased neuromuscular excitability can be seen with hyperkalemia. Most important in the ICU is severe muscle weakness which can lead to respiratory failure.

TREATMENT OF HYPERKALEMIA

This topic is fully covered in Chap. 156. The general strategies include limitation of intake (discontinue infusions), encouragement of intracellular shifting of potassium (insulin, glucose, bicarbonate), antagonism of the membrane effects (calcium), and hastened excretion (diuresis, ion exchange resins, dialysis).

CAUSES OF HYPOKALEMIA

Hypokalemia generally implies gastrointestinal or renal loss of potassium. Since potassium is normally well conserved by the kidneys, dietary potassium deficiency requires prolonged near-starvation. Nevertheless, in some chronically ill patients, alcoholics, and women with anorexia nervosa, severe hypokalemia may be a function of dietary lack. Rarely, hypokalemia results from intracellular shift of potassium, as in the initiation of hyperalimentation, the administration of β agonists, or the rare condition of familial hypokalemic periodic paralysis.

Potassium can be lost from the gastrointestinal tract in patients with diarrhea. Thus, patients with acute diseases such as gastroenteritis, as well as chronic illnesses such as malabsorption, may be hypokalemic. Villous adenomas can secrete a high potassium fluid, making this type of colonic tumor an important cause of hypokalemia. Upper gastrointestinal tract fluids contain little potassium so that vomiting, for example, leads to little direct loss of the ion. However, indirect potassium wasting is prominent, making vomiting an important renal cause of hypokalemia.

In several conditions, failure of renal conservation of potassium leads to hypokalemia. Vomiting causes metabolic alkalosis with bicarbonaturia. This enhances urinary losses of potassium. In addition, the hypovolemia of vomiting stimulates release of aldosterone, which magnifies the loss. Other causes of hyperaldosteronism also lead to renal potassium wasting, such as the edematous states (e.g., cirrhosis, congestive heart failure) and exogenous steroid administration. As noted previously, RTA (both proximal and distal) and hypomagnesemia can both cause renal potassium losses. All causes of increased distal tubular flow augment potassium wasting, including diuretic drugs and osmotic diuresis. Finally, urinary potassium losses are related to lysozymuria in some patients with acute leukemia.

CONSEQUENCES OF HYPOKALEMIA

Many different organ systems are affected by hypokalemia. The common thread seems to be the effect of serum hypokalemia on transmembrane electrical potential. Cardiac effects include increased supraventricular and ventricular arrhythmias, especially in patients on cardiac glycosides. Extreme hypokalemia in experimental animals provokes ventricular fibrillation. The impact of hypokalemia on the heart is readily seen in a routine ECG (see Chap. 30). Nevertheless, in critically ill patients not on digoxin, whether or not moderate hypokalemia truly contributes to clinically relevant arrhythmias is questionable.

Since hypokalemia decreases neuromuscular excitability, skeletal muscle weakness (including the diaphragm) and smooth muscle weakness can follow. Muscle weakness can be severe, even to the point of flaccid quadriplegia. Ileus is a common consequence of the effect of hypokalemia on smooth muscle. Paradoxically, hypokalemia causes constriction in the vasculature. This vasoconstriction may contribute to the causation of rhabdomyolysis in potassium deficient patients. Renal consequences of hypokalemia include nephrogenic diabetes insipidus and renal phosphate wasting (with hypophosphatemia). Finally, hepatic encephalopathy may be exacerbated by hypokalemia.

TREATMENT OF HYPOKALEMIA

Since hypokalemia has numerous detrimental effects which can further complicate or prolong critical illness, potassium repletion is generally appropriate. Hypokalemia is rarely life-threatening, however, so that therapy should generally be gradual and judicious. Patients dying a potassium-related death nearly always die of hyperkalemia, not hypokalemia, often as an iatrogenic complication. This is because large amounts of potassium must pass through a very small extracellular compartment to replace the intracellular deficiency. Therefore, oral repletion of potassium should be used if this route is practical. Sources of ongoing loss should be corrected, if possible. Potassium should be added to maintenance fluids, such as 40 meq KCl/L. When it is necessary to more rapidly reverse a potassium deficit, KCl can be given at a rate of 10 meq/h intravenously. In extreme circumstances, and with ECG monitoring, this can be increased for brief periods to as high as 40 meq/h. Finally, the addition of potassium-sparing diuretics may make management simpler, but risks abrupt hyperkalemia.

Chapter 4

THE CENTRAL NERVOUS SYSTEM

JESSE HALL

The understanding of central nervous system (CNS) pathophysiology in the critical care setting is daunting yet crucial, since neuropsychiatric abnormalities are ubiquitous and often determine the patient's ultimate course. The intensivist may be called on to manage patients with prior insult, such as head trauma or ischemic injury, or may be required to evaluate CNS dysfunction arising in the course of diverse illnesses. The infections, polypharmaceutical drug requirements, metabolic derangements, and perfusion abnormalities during critical illness result in a remarkably high incidence of encephalopathy. In addition, neurosurgical and cardiopulmonary bypass procedures carry a high incidence of perioperative CNS complications. The degree of neurologic dysfunction may be profound and obvious, but often is subtle and masked by the impaired communication with and difficult examination of the critically ill. Virtually any physiologic or biochemical abnormality arising from critical illness or any intervention made to support organ function carries the potential for adverse consequences on brain function and viability. Finally, continued support of patients with deep coma and minimal neurologic function is warranted if brain dysfunction is reversible (e.g., drug overdose or hepatic encephalopathy awaiting liver transplantation) but inappropriate if recovery is impossible. Such issues of prognosis in widely disparate patient groups arise routinely. As for many aspects of critical care, the intensivist is required to achieve extraordinary balance; this balance is one between the adverse and beneficial effects of interventions on all organ systems, and the balance of judgments applied to the individual patient in light of information derived from large albeit slightly different patient groups.

Both the management of the patient and the approach to new information arising from basic and clinical investigations is best accomplished within a framework of understanding that incorporates a broad overview of organ system pathophysiology. This chapter begins with a discussion of acute brain failure, most often signaled in the ICU by abnormalities in level of consciousness, and a problem encountered routinely in surgical and medical patients. The approach to diagnosis and nature of specific encephalopathies are described. Within this context, communication with the patient and the psychiatric impact of critical illness and ICU stay are described. Discussion then turns to a number of pathophysiologic considerations that are most often highlighted in neuroanesthesia and the management of patients with brain ischemia and head injury—brain metabolism, determinants of cerebral blood flow (CBF) and tissue perfusion, contributions to abnormal elevations of intracranial pressure (ICP), and characteristics of hypoxic injury. Of course, these principles apply to many patients with critical illness, but our ability to monitor pathophysiologic changes and intervene in a rational way is often limited. A review of the various interventions used to prevent and minimize brain dysfunction are described, including both an overview of standard supportive measures as well as an appropriately skeptical summary of potential future interventions. Finally, prognosis following serious CNS dysfunction is discussed.

Acute, Reversible Brain Failure Associated with Critical Illness

The range of CNS abnormalities encountered in the management of critical illness is extraordinarily wide. Focal injuries such as thrombotic stroke or subarachnoid hemorrhage (SAH) may precipitate critical illness or arise in the midst of other disease processes. Ischemic injury may be caused by focal vascular events or may be global following cardiopulmonary arrest. Drug effects on the CNS are common given the polypharmacy necessarily practiced in the ICU. During mechanical ventilation and management of hypoperfused states, the adequacy of CBF is always in question. Certain complications of supportive therapy, such as air embolus related to positive-pressure ventilation, which are extraordinarily rare outside of this care environment, may be more common than is usually appreciated. Encephalopathic states are frequent and psychiatric consequences of acute illness mount as duration of stay in the ICU increases. Indeed, as more than one organ failure develops in patients with critical illness, some degree of abnormal CNS function is nearly universally present.

In fact, the critical care physician must be familiar with nearly the entire differential diagnoses of neurologic, neurosurgical, and psychiatric disease. This task can be overwhelming, and some operational approach is necessary. Plum and Posner have generated a now classic formulation for assessment of the comatose patient. Based on considerable experimental and clinical evidence, consciousness is viewed as arising when structures lying within the brain stem and termed collectively the ascending reticular activating system (ARAS) produce a generalized nonspecific activation of the cerebral cortex. Consciousness is impaired by structural lesions of the ARAS, supratentorial mass lesions or elevated ICP causing secondary compression and dysfunction of the brain stem, or global depression of cortical (and potentially brain stem) neuronal function (e.g., seizures, drug or metabolic disturbances, globally diminished flow, or infection). This construct classifies etiologies of coma as supratentorial, subtentorial, and multifocal-diffuse, with use of the history, physical examination, and directed laboratory tests to arrive at rapid, specific diagnosis. Although these principles are indispensable in the critically ill patient, some shift in emphasis and approach is appropriate.

RECOGNITION OF ACUTE BRAIN FAILURE

The entry point to evaluation of the CNS in critical illness is most often mental status changes and often changes not as profound as coma. Just as each organ system has readily identified manifestations of failure in critical illness—oliguria and creatinine elevation in renal failure, hypoxemia and hypoventilation in respiratory failure—abnormalities in mental status usually constitute the earliest evidence for brain failure. These behavioral and mental status changes defining acute brain failure include confusion, delirium, agitation, lethargy, stupor, and coma (Table 4-1).

A number of conditions of critical illness can confound recognition and assessment of acute brain failure. The high incidence of abnormalities in mental status can lull nursing and medical staff into accepting their existence and failing to recognize subtle changes in a patient's course. Technologies such as mechanical ventilation can mask neurologic change, impair communication with the patient, and make physical examination difficult. It should be emphasized that *every change in mental status must be interpreted as possibly signaling a new pathophysiologic process and that ongoing serial neurologic examinations are the key to determining the course of brain dysfunction.*

FACILITATING COMMUNICATION IN THE ICU

As in cases of abnormal mentation encountered elsewhere, altered mental status in the ICU in and of itself impairs communication with the patient, confounding efforts to collect information to achieve definitive diagnosis and to treat the patient effectively and compassionately. Many aspects of critical illness further compound these difficulties. As mentioned, life-support interventions including indwelling catheters, dialysis machines, and mechanical ventilators make even bedside access to the patient difficult, much less detailed examination. Sedation and analgesia are frequently required for the critically ill patient, and on occasion muscle relaxation is necessary as well. The multitude of abnormalities routinely documented in the course of monitoring these patients (e.g., fever, leukocytosis, electrolyte disturbances, hypotension) often point to multiple potential etiologies for a diminished level of consciousness. Finally, some patients exhibit worsening of a prior abnormal neurologic status with new features raising the difficult question of when earlier neurologic evaluation must be repeated.

TABLE 4-1 Features of Acute Brain Failure

- Early signs include fluctuating mental status, sleep-wake disturbances, emotional lability, inappropriate behavior, decreased attention span
- Confusional states
- Delirium, characterized by floridly abnormal mentation with disorientation, agitation, irritability, misperception of reality, and hallucinations
- Lethargy and stupor, with blunted mentation and decreasing responsiveness to the environment and other stimuli
- Coma, a sleeplike state from which the patient is unarousable

TABLE 4-2 Facilitating Communication with the Critically Ill Patient

Collateral history
- From family
- From nursing staff

Communication with the alert patient
- Lip reading
- Letter pads
- Electronic spelling devices
- "Talking" tracheostomy

Limited use of sedatives and hypnotics
Periodic discontinuation of sedation and muscle relaxation
Daily review of all drugs administered

Clinical decision-making, patient evaluation, and effective treatment are difficult in this environment. Several recommendations can be made to facilitate communication and evaluation of new CNS processes (Table 4-2). Approaches to exchange of information with alert patients undergoing mechanical ventilation include lip reading, writing, word/letter pads, and electronic spelling devices. "Talking" tracheostomy tubes which provide for airflow through the larynx can be useful in selected patients. Collateral history should be sought at all times from nursing, family members, and respiratory therapists. This group can often help frame the extent of prior neurologic dysfunction (if any), signal early subtle changes difficult for the physician to appreciate, and help define the nature of a fluctuating mental status. Sedatives, analgesics, and muscle relaxants must be used only when the clinician is willing to accept the confounding problem of a murky neurologic status. The impact of these medications can be minimized by intermittent withdrawal (a drug "holiday" at which time careful neurologic examination is performed). This is recommended on a daily basis for patients undergoing full sedation and muscle relaxation. Finally, it is necessary to incorporate a full review of drug administration to each patient on a daily basis, particularly in conjunction with assessment of CNS function.

KEY FEATURES OF THE PHYSICAL EXAMINATION

All components of the neurologic examination are useful in assessing abnormal mental status, but several are so important that they should be determined and recorded at least daily (and more frequently in a patient with changing status) once acute brain failure is suspected (Table 4-3). Description of the level of consciousness should be simple and consistent between observers using the information. One reasonable schema describes patients as alert, lethargic (responsive to voice and capable of following the simplest command, but incapable of sustained attention), stuporous (aroused only with significant stimulation and then too briefly to follow commands), and comatose (unresponsive and in a sleeplike state). Pupillary responses to light and accommodation as well as size should be determined, with special attention to asymmetries. Corneal reflexes should be determined. Eye movements should be determined by

TABLE 4-3 Key Features of the Neurologic Examination in Assessment of Acute Brain Failure

Level of consciousness
Alert
Lethargic
Stuporous
Comatose
Pupils
Light response
Accommodation
Size
Symmetry
Ocular movements
Eyelid position and tone
Corneal reflex
Oculocephalic reflex
Oculovestibular reflex
Nystagmus
Conjugate gaze
Respiratory rate and pattern
Motor function
Tone
Spontaneous
Purposeful
Symmetry
Posturing

observing the resting position of gaze, the presence of roving eye movements (and whether conjugate or not), and the presence of nystagmus. In patients without purposeful gaze or full conjugate spontaneous eye movements, further testing is in order by either moving the head (oculocephalic reflex, not to be performed if there is a suspicion of an unstable spine injury) or by oculocaloric testing (to be performed only if the tympanic membrane is intact). Respiratory rate and pattern should be noted but have so many influences in the setting of critical illness that results other than frank ataxic breathing (a completely irregular pattern with deep and shallow breaths occurring randomly, characteristic of severe brain stem dysfunction) are more often than not difficult to interpret. Finally, motor function should be determined, including whether movement is spontaneous, is in response to painful stimulation, is purposeful, or is symmetric. If flexor (decorticate) or extensor (decerebrate) posturing occurs, it should be noted.

EXCLUDING FOCAL INJURY, ISCHEMIA, AND INFECTION

The first task in the assessment of the deeply obtunded or unconscious patient is the determination of whether or not focal injury is present. Focal neurologic abnormalities are the sine qua non to identify structural lesions early, but frequently imaging of the CNS will be necessary regardless of findings (see Chap. 141). If collateral laboratory information or the setting warrant lumbar puncture, this should be accomplished early in the course of evaluation (see Chap. 103).

EXCLUDING STATUS EPILEPTICUS

The vast majority of patients with seizures complicating acute brain failure manifest generalized convulsions which are obvious on observation. Rarely patients may exhibit generalized or complex partial seizures causing significant changes in mental status but without major motor manifestations. Unusual but problematic are the patients with generalized subclinical seizures or whose clonic motor activity is masked by coincident muscle relaxation, traumatic CNS or spinal cord injury, or partial treatment with antiepileptics or sedatives. In these patients, intermittent generalized seizures and postictal state may combine to yield prolonged coma. Since sustained epileptic activity appears to cause neuronal injury and because identification of seizures will permit prompt therapy and avoidance of confounding searches for other causes of coma, it is advisable to be vigilant for clinical signs suggesting seizures and to consider early electroencephalographic (EEG) evaluation in appropriate patients.

A number of factors operative during critical illness increase the likelihood of seizure disorders. Of course traumatic, infectious, or ischemic processes may result in neuronal injury and may create epileptigenic foci. Disruption of the blood-brain barrier (vide infra) may promote high concentrations of certain drugs in the CNS with the potential for induction of seizures. This phenomenon is seen with high-dose penicillin therapy used to treat meningitis. Determining if seizures are resulting from infection or its treatment can be singularly difficult. A number of drugs routinely used in critical care (lidocaine, theophylline) are notorious for causing seizures. Finally, a number of consequences of (hyperthermia) and drugs used in (steroids) critical illness may lower seizure threshold and worsen any underlying seizure disorder.

SPECIFIC ENCEPHALOPATHIES

SEPSIS

The incidence of neurologic abnormalities in patients with blood culture positive sepsis or the "sepsis syndrome" (fever, hyperdynamic circulation, and infectious focus in the absence of documented bacteremia) is very high. A number of clinical studies have indicated that septic encephalopathy is associated with a poor outcome, perhaps more so than any other single organ dysfunction in sepsis. Direct CNS involvement by the infecting organisms is not thought to be common in sepsis, and hence mechanisms causing "remote" CNS dysfunction are often invoked. This judgment regarding direct CNS involvement is necessarily based on absence of physical findings of abscess or meningoencephalitis, noninflammatory and culture negative CSF findings, and absence of anatomic lesions on computed tomography (CT) scan or magnetic resonance imaging (MRI). Some careful postmortem evaluations have documented the presence of CNS microabscesses in patients with septic foci elsewhere (most prominently pneumonia), which suggests that the precise role of CNS-penetrating antibiotics in the management of "septic encephalopathy" and the true incidence of primary CNS involvement may as yet be unclear.

Metabolic and circulatory abnormalities associated with sepsis could produce or contribute to brain failure. In animal models and human studies of sepsis, increased plasma concentrations of aromatic and sulfur-containing amino acids are seen, in association with a relative decrease in concentrations of branched chain amino acids. Brain phenylalanine and glutamine concentrations are increased, and at least in animal models, marked alterations are seen in the rate of transport of particular amino acids into the CNS. These changes in amino acid metabolism promote increased levels of the neurotransmitters serotonin and 5-hydroxyindoleacetic acid and decreases in norepinephrine, gross neurobiochemical changes associated with inhibition of behavior, motor activity, and level of consciousness. In addition, these metabolic derangements may result in increased γ-aminobutyric acid (GABA) receptor stimulation, an inhibitory system that could diminish level of consciousness. These amino acid and neurotransmitter changes are strikingly similar to those seen in severe liver failure with hepatic encephalopathy, and some have suggested a parallel set of mechanisms causing CNS dysfunction. However, while branched chain amino acid administration has been shown to have some beneficial effects in hepatic encephalopathy, this intervention has not reversed neurotransmitter changes in animal models of sepsis.

Reduction in total CBF or maldistribution of flow may result in an ischemic contribution to septic encephalopathy. Investigations in a number of animal models have documented reduced CBF in sepsis, but these are the very models that fail to recreate the hyperdynamic circulation typical of human sepsis. In the limited data collected in human beings, CBF does appear to be reduced and not solely as a result of mean arterial pressures (MAP) falling below a lower autoregulatory threshold (vide infra), since CBF is not correlated to MAP. Interestingly, alterations in flow in association with changes in Pa_{CO_2} in septic patients are similar to those found in normal patients. To the extent that CBF is reduced in sepsis, reductions in Pa_{CO_2} that are common during sepsis-driven hyperventilation may further compromise brain perfusion.

OSMOTIC INJURY

Rapid changes in serum osmolarity are common in critical illness. Analysis of contributions to hyperosmolar states is aided by the following formulation: serum osmolality (mO/kg) = 2 (Na + K) + (glucose/18) + (BUN/2.8) + exogenous solutes, where sodium and potassium concentrations are expressed as meq/L and glucose and blood urea nitrogen (BUN) are expressed as mg/dL. Exogenous solutes include certain toxic ingestions (ethanol, salicylates, methanol, ethylene glycol, although the osmolar injury may be overshadowed by other toxic effects of these agents), antibiotics in very high concentration, highly osmotic nutritional preparations, and osmotic drugs such as mannitol. Hyperosmolar states that may emerge during critical illness include renal failure, hyperglycemia including nonketotic hyperosmolar coma, and hypernatremia resulting from diabetes insipidus.

The mechanisms producing CNS dysfunction as a result of hyperosmolarity are not clear. Changes in transmembrane ionic gradients and hence cell electrophysiologic performance are likely. Hypernatremia in the range of 160 to 170 meq/L is often associated with some degree of lethargy while levels above 180 meq/L are associated with some degree of confusion and obtundation.

Virtually all instances of severe hyposmolarity are hyponatremic states associated with disordered water metabolism. This is rather common in critical illness since inappropriate secretion of antidiuretic hormone is associated with CNS trauma and infection, pulmonary disease and mechanical ventilation, a wide variety of malignancies, and the postoperative state. Mild hyponatremia typifies certain disorders with reduction (diuretic excess, salt-losing nephritis, mineralocorticoid deficiency, diarrhea, vomiting, fluid "third spacing") and expansion (congestive heart failure and cirrhosis) of extracellular fluid. In addition, too rapid a correction of hyperosmolar states can result in a picture similar to severe hypoosmolarity.

The mechanisms by which brain dysfunction and injury are produced by hypoosmolar states are not well established. Brain edema is likely important, particularly when injury is seen during too rapid correction of hyperosmolarity. This is seen most often when chronic or compensated hyperosmolar states are treated with massive infusions of water. It is said that osmolar factors elaborated within the CNS during long-standing hyperosmolarity (so-called idiogenic osms) are incapable of crossing the blood-brain barrier at a rapid rate, resulting in significant brain edema during correction of serum osmolarity. In hyponatremic states brain water content seems to be of paramount importance in determining level of consciousness, and the return to the alert state parallels reduction in brain water. Hyponatremia-associated changes in intra- and extracellular ion concentrations and hence membrane potential may be important factors determining neuronal excitability.

Both the rate of development and degree of hyponatremia are important in determining CNS manifestations. Data from patients with moderate to severe (serum Na $<$ 128 meq/L) hyponatremia are shown in Fig. 4-1, with data grouped for acute and chronic states. When convulsions or coma were present, it was usually in patients with a serum Na concentration of 95 to 110 meq/L. Convulsions were never seen with serum Na concentrations above 121 meq/L. As indicated in Fig. 4-2, rapid evolution of hyponatremia is associated with large increases in brain water and adverse consequences of brain edema; this increase in brain water is substantially less when hyponatremia evolves over days to weeks.

An interesting disorder, described primarily in alcoholics with hyponatremia, is central pontine myelinolysis, characterized by destruction of the myelin sheaths in the central basis pontis. When these lesions are large, neurologic abnormalities including ocular and pupillary paralysis, dysarthria, quadriparesis, and incontinence are seen. This lesion has been ascribed to too rapid correction of hyponatremia

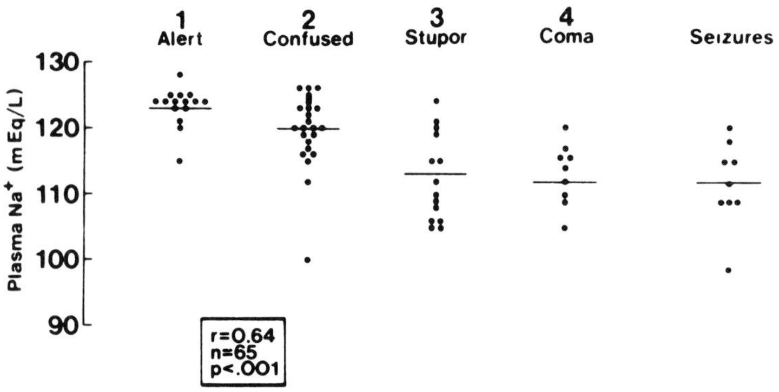

FIGURE 4-1 Disturbances in level of consciousness related to plasma sodium concentration in 65 patients with a plasma Na^+ of 128 meq/L or less. There is a high degree of correlation but overlap exists between groups. All patients manifesting seizures had a plasma $Na^+ \leq 121$ meq/L. (With permission from Arieff AI, Llach F, Massry SG: Neurologic manifestations and morbidity of hyponatremia: Correlation with brain water and electrolytes. Medicine 55:121, 1976)

but this relationship is not clear and has been called into question by some authors.

HEPATIC ENCEPHALOPATHY

Liver failure is characterized by a host of metabolic abnormalities as well as frequent encephalopathy. Much evidence now suggests that altered levels of amino acids, particularly aromatic compounds, occur in liver failure, and that these amino acids are transported into the CNS in abnormally large quantities. According to this hypothesis, this altered CNS metabolism results in activation of inhibitory GABA neurotransmitter systems. Supporting this are the observations that nutritional manipulations to reduce aromatic amino acid levels (usually by substituting branched chain acids) ameliorate symptoms in these patients. Interestingly, benzodiazepine receptors may play a significant role in this encephalopathy, since some improvement in the syndrome can be achieved with receptor antagonists such as flumazenil.

Severe hepatic encephalopathy may be complicated at any point by cerebral edema; this is particularly frequent in patients with fulminant hepatic failure (see Chap. 164). The etiology of this complication is unclear, but may be related to either interruption of the blood-brain barrier or interference with membrane pumps which maintain transmembrane ionic gradients. With advanced cerebral edema, ICP rises and cerebral perfusion pressure (CPP) falls, with the potential for ischemic injury. At this point, monitoring and therapy must be directed at the edema and elevated ICP, by analogy to patients with similar complications following head trauma (vide infra).

FIGURE 4-2 Brain water in normal rabbits and with decreases in serum sodium over varying periods of time. Note that the acute decrease in serum sodium over 2 h caused brain water to increase 17 percent, while an equivalent but more gradual change over 3.5 or 16 days increased brain water by only 7 percent. (With permission from Arieff AI, Guisado R: Effects on the central nervous system of hypernatremic and hyponatremic states. Kidney Int 10:104, 1976)

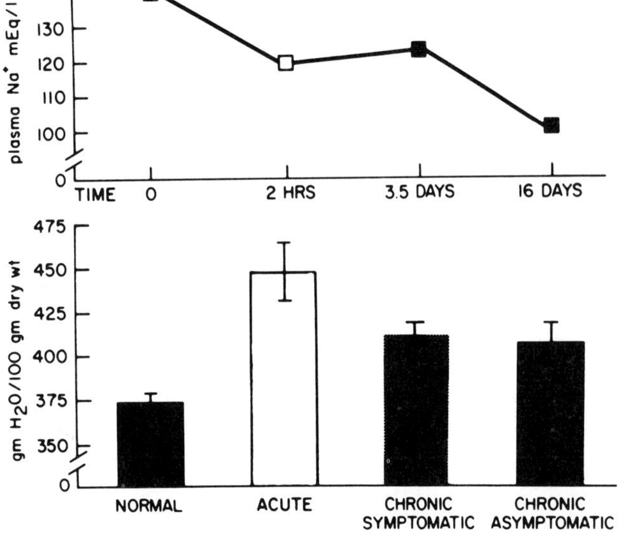

HYPOGLYCEMIA

Since glucose is the major carbohydrate substrate used during neuronal oxidative phosphorylation, one formulation of hypoglycemic brain injury postulated an "energy failure" mechanism akin to hypoxia or ischemia. Much evidence suggests that this is not the case. After pure hypoglycemic insult even severely damaged brains show selective neuronal necrosis rather than infarction histopathologically. While brain pH is decreased during ischemic insult due to anaerobic metabolism, it actually increases during hypoglycemia, an effect attributed to deamination of amino acids, consumption of metabolic acids, and failure of lactic acid production. Depression of cerebral oxygen consumption during experimental hypoglycemia is less than predicted by the usual stoichiometric relationship between glucose and oxygen, suggesting alternative fuels are used during this insult.

One of the important metabolic adjustments during hypoglycemia appears to be altered amino acid metabolism, with a rise in brain aspartate levels. Since transmembrane ion gradients do change during hypoglycemia, leading to increased permeability, extracellular (and eventually cerebrospinal fluid [CSF]) aspartate levels likely rise. This raises the possibility that aspartate, known to act as an excitatory neurotransmitter (vide infra), could act as a neurotoxin, similar to various hypotheses concerning neuronal injury during hypoxia or status epilepticus.

Regardless of mechanism, hypoglycemia is a cause of global CNS depression that is encountered in patients presenting de novo as well as in those evolving abnormalities in the course of critical illness. *Potentially reversible and potentially capable of devastating CNS injury if left untreated, hypoglycemia must be considered in all patients.* Mental status changes are rarely seen at serum glucose levels above 50 mg/dL, and permanent brain damage is usually associated with substantially lower levels producing coma sustained for an hour or more. Clinical symptoms and signs are dominated by the effects of hypoglycemia on the brain and the sympathetic discharge accompanying a low blood sugar. The former most typically results in depression of consciousness with or without seizures, although agitation and focal neurologic signs are not rare. The sympathetic activation results in sweating, tremor, tachycardia, and anxiety. Common causes of hypoglycemia in the ICU are severe liver dysfunction, excessive insulin administration, inadequate or inadvertent discontinuation of calorie support, uremia, and septic shock.

COFACTOR DEFICIENCY

While a number of vitamin B deficiencies are associated with mild to moderate derangements of cognition, coma appears limited to thiamine deficiency. The symptom complex associated with this deficiency, termed Wernicke's disease, results from neuronal damage of gray matter surrounding the third and fourth ventricles. Clinical manifestations include markedly impaired memory with confusion or obtundation that may progress to coma. A diagnosis of thiamine deficiency in a comatose patient can only be made with certainty if there is accompanying nystagmus and oculomotor paralysis which responds to replacement therapy. Nonetheless, thiamine administration is appropriate in all cases of coma of unknown etiology. The source of thiamine deficiency is dietary lack, usually in alcoholics, and on occasion precipitated by vitamin-free calorie administration to malnourished individuals.

PSYCHIATRIC DISORDERS

The term *ICU psychosis* is often applied to transient neuropsychiatric disorders associated with ICU admission. Typical manifestations are inappropriate behavior and delirium, often worse at night, that begin after 3 to 5 days of ICU stay and worsen over time if not treated and if underlying illnesses progress. Many have objected to this term as a diagnostic "catchall" and admittedly, too ready an invocation of this explanation for unusual patient behavior has no doubt delayed appropriate diagnosis and management. Accordingly, since the manifestations of this disorder overlap entirely with the full range of organic encephalopathies, it should only be applied to patients who have all other etiologies considered and excluded.

THE DILEMMA OF MULTIFACTORIAL BRAIN FAILURE

When the thoughtful and thorough clinician has completed the assessment of the critically ill patient with abnormal mental status, the information base often points to multiple factors contributing to CNS dysfunction. The patient with questionable prior anoxic insult, treated but ongoing sepsis, mild hyponatremia and hypoosmolarity, liver dysfunction and elevated serum ammonia level, and receiving multiple drugs affecting level of consciousness is much more common than the patient with severe hypoglycemia identified and, once treated, returned to normal function. Nonetheless, the exercise remains one of search for such rapidly correctable abnormalities, and then more gradual correction of the multiple possible etiologies of brain failure, including the underlying disease(s).

Metabolism and Physiology of the Central Nervous System and Response to Injury

OXYGEN AND SUBSTRATE REQUIREMENTS

Like all other organ systems of the body, the CNS requires an energy source to perform its functions. Under nonpathologic conditions approximately one-half of this energy is expended in processes relating to basic cellular function, and one-half is expended in the electrophysiologic work performed by interconnected neurons. Like other tissues, this energy is generated when carbon-containing foods combine with oxygen in the course of cellular respiration.

Unlike many other tissues, the brain under normal conditions utilizes glucose almost exclusively as the substrate for energy production. Anaerobic utilization of glucose via glycolysis is a relatively inefficient means of energy generation:

$$\text{glucose} + 2\text{ADP} + 2\text{PO}_4 \rightarrow 2\ \text{lactate} + 2\text{ATP} \quad (4\text{-}1)$$

as compared to energy generation by respiration under aerobic conditions:

$$\text{glucose} + 6\text{O}_2 + 38\text{ADP} \rightarrow 6\text{CO}_2 + 6\text{H}_2\text{O} + 38\text{ATP} \quad (4\text{-}2)$$

Since brain energy requirements are high and the capacity for the cytoplasmic enzyme system responsible for glycolysis limited, the brain depends on high and nearly constant glucose and oxygen delivery to support cellular respiration. The typical CNS glucose uptake is 5 to 6 mg/100 g tissue/min, which is associated with an oxygen consumption of 3.5 mL/100 g tissue/min. The 1200 to 1400 g adult brain, constituting approximately 2 percent of total body mass, consumes 42 to 49 mL oxygen/min, or about 20 percent of the body's total oxygen consumption ($\dot{V}_{O_2}$).

Interestingly, the rate of glucose consumption by the CNS is approximately equal to the total rate of gluconeogenesis by the liver under fasting conditions, underlining the importance of this metabolic link in sustaining cerebral function during food deprivation. Glucose moves rapidly from the blood to the CNS via diffusion and facilitated transport that is not energy dependent. While in vitro brain slices are capable of metabolizing a number of substrates, including fatty acids, the inability of these substances to readily traverse the blood-brain barrier may limit their significance as energy sources in vivo. Nonetheless many substances likely do cross this barrier in small quantities, since a large number of transport systems for proteins and lipids have been identified in recent years. During starvation and some phases of critical illness the brain is able to utilize various ketone bodies as an energy source, but it cannot function without glucose as a major substrate, and ketone bodies never supply a majority of the brain's fuel. Nonetheless, this contribution is significant since in starvation CNS glucose requirements may exceed hepatic synthetic capacity, particularly if liver function is impaired.

Not all glucose taken up by the brain is immediately combusted. Only about one-third of glucose removed from the blood is metabolized immediately to CO_2, while the rest is converted to cell proteins, amino acids, and lipids. Thus there appears to be an internal cycling of various energy sources, while the net energetics is such that glucose uptake accounts for virtually all energy supply to the brain under normal conditions. Glucose reserves in the forms of free glucose and glycogen are small, and it has been estimated that they would be exhausted *under aerobic* conditions in 2 to 3 min if all blood supply was halted. If both glucose and oxygen supplies were terminated, as in circulatory arrest, then under anaerobic conditions glycolysis could provide brain energy requirements for only 10 to 20 s. Nonetheless, some recent experimental evidence has shown that some capacity to generate energy intermediates exists even with complete ischemia, suggesting metabolic failure alone does not fully explain ischemic injury (vide infra).

INFLUENCES UPON CEREBRAL METABOLIC RATE O_2

As the heart increases its oxygen consumption in relation to increases in contractility, rate, and loading, regional cerebral metabolic rate for O_2 ($CMRO_2$) relates to local electrophysiologic activity in the brain. Tasks such as spatial reasoning, semantic classification, verbal problem solving, and recall can all be used to elicit hemispheric and regional increases in CBF and $CMRO_2$. Total brain $CMRO_2$, however, does not vary widely in health. Interestingly, $CMRO_2$ during sleep is similar to or slightly higher than that measured in the waking state, belying older notions that this was a metabolically inert period for the CNS. By contrast, most studies evaluating comatose states have demonstrated that $CMRO_2$ falls.

Conditions that increase or decrease global electrophysiologic activity can alter $CMRO_2$ substantially. Thus, status epilepticus causes both oxygen and glucose requirements to increase significantly. In contrast, cessation of electrical activity, such as occurs very shortly after the onset of global brain ischemia (vide infra), can reduce $CMRO_2$ by approximately 50 percent. It is likely that various pharmacologic agents such as barbiturates which diminish brain oxygen and glucose requirements do so by reducing or terminating electrophysiologic activity.

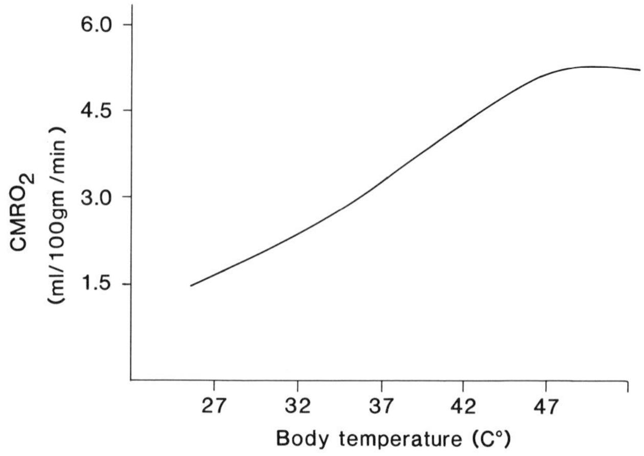

FIGURE 4-3 The relationship of cerebral oxygen consumption ($CMRO_2$) to body temperature. Note the linear increase in $CMRO_2$ over a wide range of body temperatures. $CMRO_2$ plateaus above approximately 42 to 43°C (107.6 to 109.4°F) and this plateau is associated with evolution of coma.

Temperature exerts a potent effect upon $CMRO_2$ (Fig. 4-3). A decline of approximately 10°C (from 37° to 27°C, 98.6 to 80.6°F) will halve oxygen requirement. This mechanism has been invoked to explain the clinical observation of functional preservation after prolonged ischemia in cold water near-drowning. Above normal body temeprature $CMRO_2$ rises sharply until approximately 42° or 43°C (107.6° or 109.4°F), above which metabolic rate does not increase and may actually fall. These extremes of hyperthermia are associated with slowing of the EEG and the evolution of coma. Thus, diminished electrophysiologic activity may in part explain the upper limits of temperature-driven hypermetabolism. Limitation to glucose transport or intracellular utilization may also be important.

REGULATION OF CEREBRAL BLOOD FLOW

INFLUENCE OF CEREBRAL METABOLIC RATE O_2

Oxygen delivery to the CNS is a product of CBF and arterial oxygen content. Since brain metabolic rate is high and oxygen and substrate reserves are minimal, the CNS relies on a generous blood flow to support normal function. Oxygen extraction by the brain is slightly greater than that of the whole body at rest, as reflected by an arteriovenous oxygen content difference ($AVDO_2$) across the brain of 5 to 7 vol %, as opposed to 3 to 5 vol % for the body. This high extraction ratio is the consequence of $CMRO_2$ being increased more than CBF, which is approximately 50 mL/100 g tissue/min, or a total of 600 to 700 mL/min, approximately 12 to 14 percent of total cardiac output.

CBF is tightly linked to $CMRO_2$ over a wide range. Increased neuronal metabolic activity usually accompanies increased neurotransmission. Increased neurotransmission is associated with increased frequency of action potentials with release of potassium from the nerve cell and consequent increases in extracellular potassium concentration. This is particularly true in the CNS since the extracellular space is small and the intra-extracellular potassium gradient large. Elevation of extracellular potassium concentration to a sufficient degree will result in dilation of cerebral resistance vessels, causing increased blood flow to closely track local increases in synaptic transmission.

While extracellular potassium accumulation may be a mechanism linking blood flow to neuronal electrophysiologic work, flow is also likely linked to metabolic events, and likely controlled in part by end products of cellular metabolism. To the extent that glucose and oxygen deliveries are inadequate to meet metabolic needs, tissues produce hydrogen ions and adenosine in increased amounts which accumulate in the extravascular space. These substances too have been demonstrated to cause vasodilation in most arterial beds, including the cerebrovasculature. Indeed, much evidence points to adenosine as a primary mediator of vascular tone and a controller of the matching of blood flow to metabolic need.

Drugs inhibiting the action of adenosine (theophylline, caffeine, other phosphodiesterase inhibitors) uncouple CBF from $CMRO_2$, whereas drugs which inhibit adenosine reuptake (dipyridamole, papaverine) appear to potentiate $CMRO_2$-driven increases in CBF. Some of these drug effects may be significant clinically. Theophylline has been shown to reduce CBF in patients with chronic obstructive pulmonary disease (COPD). In addition, theophylline has been shown to decrease CBF during both normoxia and hypoxemia in normal human beings, but does not prevent the increase in CBF during hypoxemia that maintains oxygen delivery.

FIGURE 4-4 The relationship of CBF to Pa_{O_2}, Pa_{CO_2}, and mean aortic pressure (P_{ao}). Note that CBF rises sharply as Pa_{O_2} falls below 60 mmHg, a point at which small decrements in Pa_{O_2} are associated with large decreases in hemoglobin saturation and arterial oxygen content, due to the steep shape of the oxygen-hemoglobin dissociation curve. Note that decreases of Pa_{CO_2} from 40 to 20 to 25 mmHg are associated with an approximately 50 percent decrease in CBF. Finally, CBF remains constant over a wide range of P_{ao}, a phenomenon attributed to vascular autoregulation.

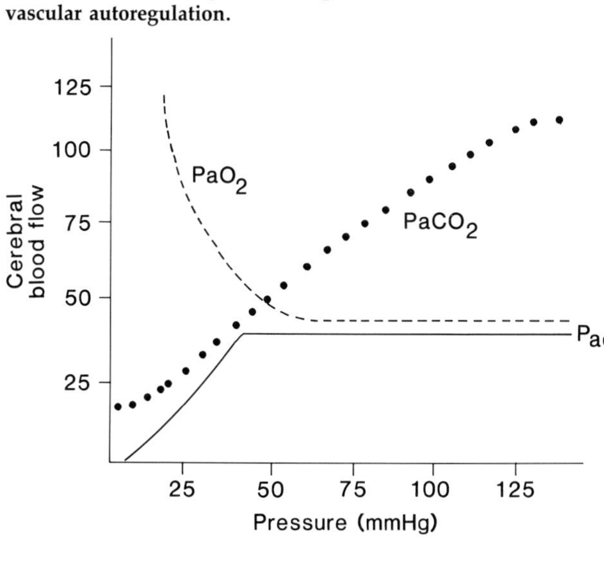

Cerebral Blood Flow and Arterial Oxygen Content

CBF tends to rise in circumstances of diminished arterial oxygen content and thus oxygen delivery is maintained. This is likely achieved by the same mechanisms that facilitate a matching of oxygen delivery to uptake as $CMRO_2$ varies. Mild to moderate degrees of hypoxemia do not significantly alter CBF (Fig. 4-4), in accord with the relatively minor contribution of dissolved oxygen to arterial oxygen content. At a normal Pa_{CO_2} and blood pressure, Pa_{O_2} values below 60 mmHg are associated with a sharp and progressive increase in CBF (see Fig. 4-4). This is explained by the shape of the oxygen-hemoglobin saturation curve, with small decrements in Pa_{O_2} below 60 mmHg associated with relatively large decrements in hemoglobin saturation. Similarly, changes in arterial oxygen content resulting from alterations in hemoglobin concentration are accompanied by opposing changes in CBF which maintain oxygen delivery to the brain. In Fig. 4-5, the inverse linear relationship between arterial oxygen content and CBF in patients whose chronic hemoglobin concentrations varied over a wide range due to hematologic diseases (polycythemia vera, hemolytic anemia, etc.) is shown. With acute changes in hemoglobin concentration the precise CBF adjustments are less clear, but it is likely that flow increases somewhat less for a decrement in arterial oxygen content in the acute circumstance. Despite the reduction in arterial oxygen content and hence delivery associated with acute anemia, CBF increases to maintain tissue oxygen delivery may be less than those required to maintain total oxygen delivery because of increased efficiency of oxygen distribution by the microcirculation resulting from blood rheologic effects of hemodilution (vide infra). The lower acceptable limit of oxygen delivery to the brain is not likely exceeded in most instances of uncomplicated anemia, since normal CNS function is seen with hematocrits as low as 7 to 10 percent. Of course this presumes normal saturation and circulatory compensation to maintain acceptable oxygen delivery. Any degree of superimposed hypoxemia, circulatory inadequacy, or diminished local control of blood flow could reduce oxygen availability to inadequate levels.

Cerebral Blood Flow and Pa_{CO_2}

Pa_{CO_2} has a significant effect on cerebral vascular resistance and hence CBF. As shown in Fig. 4-4, over most of the range of physiologic Pa_{CO_2} (20 to 80 mmHg), CBF increases linearly and nearly one-to-one with increasing Pa_{CO_2}. This effect of Pa_{CO_2} to regulate CBF is likely mediated by changes in brain extracellular hydrogen ion concentration. If Pa_{CO_2} is abruptly lowered and maintained, as occurs during intentional hyperventilation of the brain injured patient (vide infra), CBF acutely falls and then gradually returns to baseline over 24 to 48 h, consistent with the time course for restoration of extracellular pH. Of course, abrupt return to the former Pa_{CO_2} will be associated with extracellular acidosis and a potentially large increase in CBF. This may have adverse effects on ICP (vide infra).

Autoregulation

Autoregulation is defined as the ability of a vasculature to maintain constant flow over a wide range of mean aortic

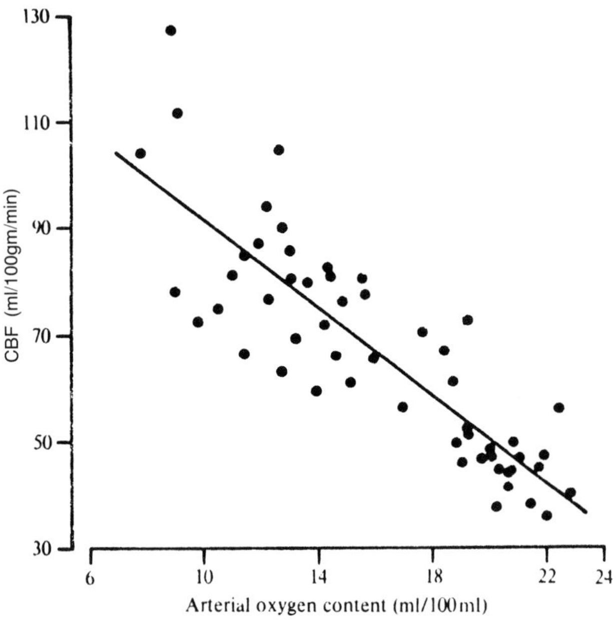

FIGURE 4-5 The relationship of CBF to arterial oxygen content in patients with widely different hemoglobin concentrations due to a variety of hematologic disorders. Note that oxygen delivery is maintained by increases in CBF in compensation for diminished arterial oxygen content.

pressures (MAP) (see Fig. 4-4). It is a property of many tissue beds but the cerebrovasculature is remarkable for the range of MAPs over which flow is maintained nearly constant. Many favor a "myogenic" hypothesis to explain this behavior, which postulates that increase in tension within the vessel wall associated with increase in blood pressure is a signal which results in increased smooth muscle tone. Data from a number of animal models support this general hypothesis. Interestingly, however, when arterial pressure is increased by increasing the cerebral venous pressure, arterial vasoconstriction is not seen, the expected result if increased wall tension directly increases smooth muscle tone. Metabolic events may also play a role, although the magnitude and time course of extravascular potassium, hydrogen ion, and adenosine concentration changes suggest they are not dominant influences on vascular tone under conditions of changing aortic pressure.

Whatever the mechanism(s), the cerebrovasculature dilates in response to decreases in blood pressure and constricts in response to elevations in blood pressure. The time course for this response is at least seconds to at least as long as minutes for a complete response, so that very acute changes in blood pressure are accompanied by an early parallel change in flow. For the fully compensated state (and with a normal Pa_{O_2} and Pa_{CO_2}), CBF remains constant until a mean blood pressure of 50 to 60 mmHg, at which point it falls nearly linearly with further decrements in flow. At flows below 20 mL/100 g tissue/min cerebral insufficiency is seen. Above 125 to 150 mmHg, CBF increases with increments in pressure, partly explaining the increase in ICP associated with malignant hypertension.

A number of conditions appear to influence the lower and upper limits of autoregulation (Fig. 4-6). Chronic hypertension shifts the autoregulatory curve rightward as shown, explaining the ability of patients with severe chronic hypertension to tolerate extremes of blood pressure without central nervous dysfunction, as well as explaining the manifestations of cerebrovascular insufficiency seen in chronic hypertension if blood pressure is lowered excessively, even to only modest levels of hypotension. Although these explanations are often invoked to explain patient responses to spontaneous or iatrogenic changes in blood pressure, it should be noted that the data for autoregulation in human beings is somewhat scant, due to the difficulty in obtaining reliable flow estimates under conditions of extreme blood pressure alteration which would serve to define the upper and lower thresholds of autoregulation.

Hemorrhagic shock and head trauma shift the lower limit of autoregulation rightward and the upper limit leftward (Fig. 4-7) at least in animal models. The range of effective autoregulation is thus narrow, and even modest hypotension may result in initiation or potentiation of CNS injury, while excessive elevations of blood pressure carry the potential for increased perfusion and consequent cerebral edema (vide infra).

Neurohumoral Regulation of Blood Flow

Aside from influences on the mean aortic pressure, which would secondarily only affect CBF if blood pressure fluctuated outside the bounds of autoregulation, neurohumoral mechanisms are not thought to substantially directly affect CBF under normal conditions. Some influences, however, may be of consequence in critical illness. Sympathomimetic noradrenergic stimulation in a number of models results in

FIGURE 4-6 Changes in the pattern of autoregulation with chronic hypertension. Note that there is a rightward shift of the curve in patients with chronic hypertension (interrupted line). This implies that "breakthrough" from autoregulation occurs at a higher pressure, and that decreases in CBF occur at higher mean aortic pressures as well. This implies that patients with chronic hypertension may tolerate higher aortic pressures without development of adverse CNS consequences, though they might also become symptomatic from diminished CBF if blood pressure is reduced acutely, even to a "normal" range.

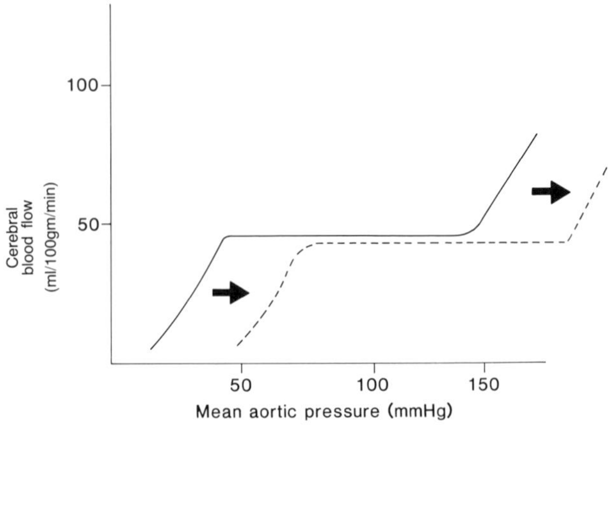

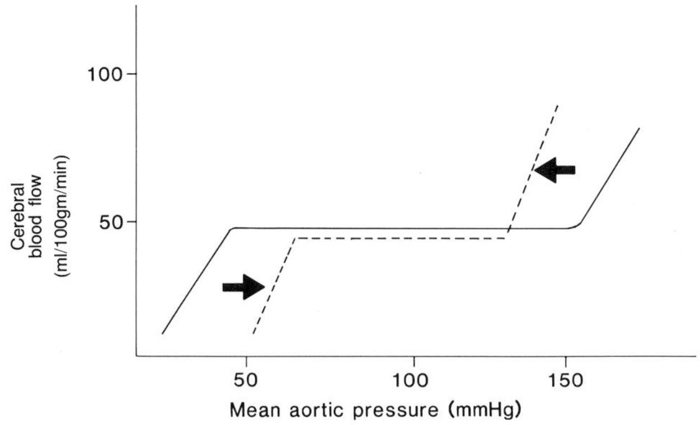

FIGURE 4-7 Perturbations in autoregulation following head trauma or hemorrhagic shock (interrupted line). Note that these patients regulate flow over a narrower range of mean aortic pressures, suggesting they are more vulnerable to a fall in CBF with even modest hypotension, and would be subject to excessive cerebral perfusion with systemic hypertension.

a modest reduction in blood flow, diminished cerebral blood volume due to a constriction of cerebral veins, and a decrease in the rate of production of CSF (vide infra). The effects of large doses of exogenous catecholamines and sympathomimetic amines, such as occurs during support of the circulation in critical illness, are not well studied. Peptidergic innervation of cerebral vessels has been demonstrated although data concerning the effect of neurotransmitters such as vasoactive intestinal polypeptide are conflicting.

Humoral factors which may be of significance in regulating cerebrovascular resistance include prostaglandins (PGs) and histamine. Prostacyclin (PGI_2) and PGE_2 have been shown to dilate resistance vessels. The results from studies using interventions with agents such as indomethacin which inhibit cyclooxygenase and PG synthesis suggest that PG modulation of vascular tone is of minor consequence under normal conditions, but may be of greater significance under conditions associated with interruption of the blood-brain barrier.

Hemorrheologic Considerations

Rheology is the study of the flow and deformation of matter, and the rheologic properties of blood are significant in determining flow in the microcirculation. Simple fluids such as water, plasma, and hemoglobin solution exhibit mechanical behavior such that the plot of stress versus strain for the fluid is linear. Since the viscosity of the fluid is defined as the slope of the stress versus strain relationship, it is constant over a wide range of dynamic conditions. Such fluids are termed Newtonian as regards this property. Blood does not behave in this fashion, and stress does not vary linearly with strain. It might be helpful intuitively to state that blood can support a stress at rest, a property more typical of solids than most liquids. Thus, blood viscosity varies with the dynamics of flow.

The factors influencing blood viscosity are shear rate (stress), red cell deformability, red cell aggregation, plasma viscosity, and hematocrit. While the non-Newtonian properties of blood do not significantly influence flow characteristics in the central circulation or large vessels, they may be important in determining characteristics of capillary flow under pathologic conditions. In several disease states, such as polycythemia and hyperviscosity syndromes (multiple myeloma, Waldenstrom's macroglobulinemia), red cell aggregates increase markedly with consequent increases in viscosity and vascular resistance. In low flow states, shear rates fall and viscosity increases with the potential for worsening the low flow state. If hypoperfused portions of a tissue bed become acidotic, red cell aggregation is promoted with the potential for worsened hypoperfusion.

Some rheologic manipulations of blood have been clearly demonstrated to improve CNS function. Plasmapheresis of patients with hyperviscosity caused by abnormal serum protein elevations or phlebotomy with hemodilution of patients with polycythemia often dramatically improves neurologic function. Benefits to be derived from such interventions in patients with prior or ongoing hypoxic injury and normal blood viscosity are as yet undefined. On the one hand hemodilution might improve microcirculatory distribution of blood flow and hence oxygen delivery; on the other hand, reduction of hemoglobin concentration could reduce oxygen delivery if compensatory increase in flow or improvement in its distribution did not occur. To date, clinical studies of hemodilution in patients with focal ischemic insult (stroke) have been equivocal in the results obtained. It is difficult to make recommendations other than to treat hyperviscosity syndromes specifically.

DETERMINANTS OF CEREBRAL PERFUSION PRESSURE

CBF is determined by the CPP of the CNS and the resistance of the cerebral vessels to flow:

$$CBF = \frac{(MAP - ICP)}{R} \qquad (4\text{-}3)$$

where MAP is mean arterial pressure, ICP is intracranial pressure, and R is cerebral vascular resistance. Under normal circumstances ICP is low (typically <10 mmHg), and MAP varies over a considerable range. Autoregulation of the vascular circuit, by varying R, achieves nearly constant CBF, as described above. Under pathologic conditions, ICP may rise dramatically and to a level that impairs CBF. Many purported therapies of acute brain injury are directed at elevations of ICP. Accordingly, a discussion of the influences on ICP is appropriate.

Intracranial Pressure and Intracranial Hypertension

The CNS may be viewed as residing within a fixed volume container, the cranium, and consisting of the brain substance, blood volume, and CSF compartments. With a change in the volume of any single compartment, as in the evolution of cerebral edema, there must be a compensatory decrease in the volume of another compartment. As individual compartments reach mechanical limits, volume shifts fail to compensate for pathologic processes. As these compensatory mechanisms are exhausted, small incremental volume changes cause large pressure changes. With increased ICP, the compliance of the CNS tends to decrease. Significant regional pressure differences within the system likely occur, and indeed following injury are responsible for catastrophic complications such as herniation. Nonetheless clinical ICP monitoring relies on determining CSF pressure, assuming that reflects ICP generally.

THE CEREBROSPINAL FLUID COMPARTMENT. CSF is produced largely in the choroid plexus, most prominently in the walls of the lateral ventricles and the roofs of the third and fourth ventricles. Lesser contributions of fluid are from the ependymal lining and the perivascular spaces. Fluid produced within the ventricles flows to the basal cisterns through the foramina of Luschka and Magendie in the caudal fourth ventricle. From here CSF migrates over the convexities, where it is taken up by the arachnoid granulations projecting into the dural venous sinuses. In adults the total volume of CSF is approximately 120 to 150 mL with a daily production of approximately 450 to 600 mL, resulting in turnover of this compartment four to six times daily. Because of the relatively high rate of production, any acute disparity between formation and absorption can drastically increase ICP.

While the rate of formation of CSF, approximately 0.35 mL/min, remains constant over a wide range of CSF pressures (0 to 220 mmH_2O), absorption is minimal until a pressure of 70 mmH_2O (point A, Fig. 4-8) is reached. Absorption increases with increasing pressure such that above a pressure of approximately 110 mmH_2O absorption exceeds formation (point B, Fig. 4-8), resulting in a net decrease in the volume of this compartment. This then is a compensatory (albeit acting over hours to days) mechanism for controlling ICP elevations, with absorption exceeding production and net CSF volume decreasing.

FIGURE 4-8 Relationship of CSF flow to CSF pressure. Formation of CSF remains constant over a wide range. Above a pressure of approximately 60 mmH_2O (point A) absorption begins and increases linearly such that at pressures over 110 mmH_2O (point B), absorption exceeds formation and CSF volume falls, acting to reduce CSF pressure.

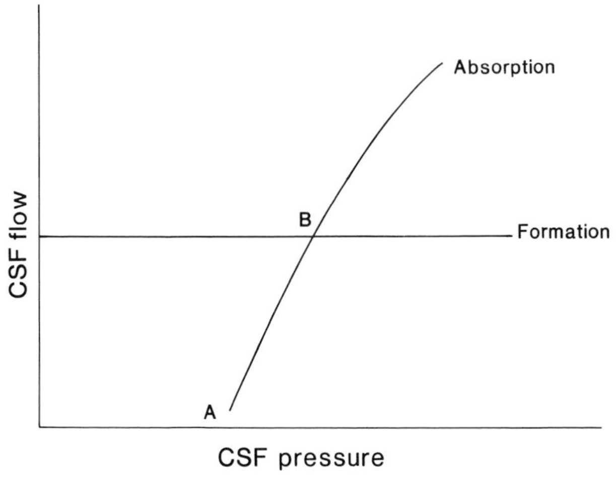

THE VASCULAR COMPARTMENT. As noted above, intracranial blood volume may vary with changes in CBF mediated via autoregulation, the effects of Pa_{CO_2}, or local vasodilation in response to $CMRO_2$. Alternatively, venous blood volume may increase in the setting of obstruction, such as the superior vena cava syndrome or with sinus thrombosis. A number of conditions could result in relatively acute vascular changes with adverse consequences for ICP. During hypertensive crisis, the upper limits of autoregulation may be exceeded, with elevation of ICP. Acute hypercapnia may similarly increase intracranial blood volume and ICP. Finally, conditions which drive a high $CMRO_2$ (hyperthermia, status epilepticus) could have similar effects.

THE TISSUE COMPARTMENT. The major cause of an increase in the volume of the brain parenchyma and hence an increase in the ICP is tissue edema. In general, the extravascular space of the CNS is protected from ingress of fluid and solutes. It has long been recognized that blood constituents have impaired transport into the brain substance, a phenomenon termed the *blood-brain barrier*. Teleologically this barrier provides a protected environment for synaptic transmission, serving as a barrier to entry of substances that might act as neurotransmitters or block transmission, as well as to changes in milieu (e.g., alterations in electrolyte concentrations or pH) that could interfere with transmission. Most of the capillary endothelium of the CNS exhibits tight junctions, an anatomic substrate of this diffusion barrier between the intra- and extravascular spaces (although these tight junctions are notably absent in certain regions of the brain, including portions of the hypothalamus, area postrema, and subcommissural organs). The functional basis of this barrier is not only anatomic, however, and endothelial cell enzymes have been described which metabolize acetylcholine, GABA, dopamine, and enkephalins, thus blocking entrance of these substances into the extravascular space.

In general, the rate of transfer of solutes into the CNS is inversely proportional to their molecular weight. Since a major component of the blood-brain barrier is the two-layer lipid membrane of the brain endothelial cell, lipid solubility is a major determinant of the uptake of a substance into the brain. Protein-bound substances are usually poorly transported, although if they are highly lipophilic there may be a sufficient movement into the brain parenchyma to still result in a high uptake even during a single pass through the cerebral circulation. Hydrophilic substances necessary for brain function tend to be transported by facilitated diffusion or active mechanisms.

A number of conditions may impair this barrier and facilitate transport into the brain parenchyma. Inflammation, such as occurs with meningitis, interrupts endothelial anatomy permitting antibiotics that usually do not appreciably enter the CNS to achieve high CSF and tissue concentrations. Tight junctions may be interrupted by physical injury or osmotic changes. Repeated seizures, acute elevation of blood pressure, global ischemia, and hyperosmolar loads have all been described to increase the movement of blood constituents across the blood-brain barrier. All of these forms of endothelial cell injury may be associated with excess fluid passage into the extravascular space, a phenomenon termed *vasogenic edema.*

Processes causing failure of cell metabolism within the CNS, such as ischemia or exposure to toxins, will cause neurons to accumulate intracellular water and swell, a phenomenon termed *cytotoxic edema.* Most often insults to the CNS produce both vasogenic and cytotoxic edema. The net result is an increase in the volume of the tissue compartment with an associated increase in ICP.

Cerebrospinal Fluid Pressure and Compliance Characteristics

As mentioned above, it is often the CSF compartment pressure that is monitored clinically. When measured via lumbar puncture in the lateral decubitus position, normal CSF pressures range from 5 to 15 mmHg or 65 to 195 mmH_2O. CSF pressure normally decreases during inspiration and increases with expiration, changes attributed to respiratory cycle fluctuations in venous flow. Systemic arterial pressure pulsations may be noted during continuous monitoring of the CSF pressure.

During pathologic elevation of the ICP intermittent acute increases in pressure may be seen, often with a waveform described as *plateau waves.* These transient (usually 5 to 20 min) pressure elevations may reach levels of 50 to 100 mmHg. On many occasions this worsened intracranial hypertension is preceded by increased systemic blood pressure, hypercapnia, painful stimuli, or increased activity, but there may be no premonitory signs or abnormalities.

FIGURE 4-9 Relationship of CSF volume to CSF pressure. Initial increases in volume do not increase pressure greatly since compression of the venous system provides a "protective" factor preventing intracranial hypertension (zone 1). When this mechanism is no longer operative, further increases in CSF volume cause large increases in pressure (zone 2), until pressure rises above diastolic blood pressure. Further pressure rises are somewhat blunted by diminished arterial flow and blood volume (zone 3). Finally, as all vascular compartments have been maximally compressed, further increases in CSF volume cause very large increases in pressure (zone 4).

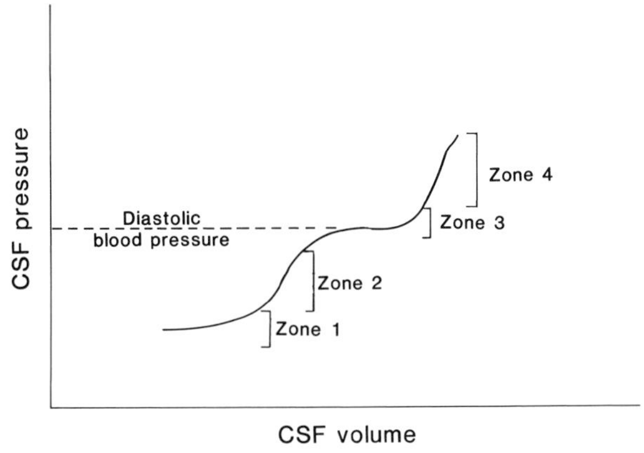

Angiograms during spontaneous plateau waves have shown arteriolar dilation, an observation supporting the notion that these waveforms arise from disordered autoregulation with transient increases in cerebral blood volume. Plateau waves per se are not indicative of significant CNS pathology, since they are seen during REM sleep in normal individuals.

Pressure-volume relationships for the CSF have been described, but the applicability of data from animal models or normal human beings to human disease states remains controversial. A schematized relationship of pressure and volume is shown in Fig. 4-9. As shown, small increases in CSF volume may not be associated with large pressure changes, as compensation occurs by compression of the intracranial venous system (zone 1). As this compensatory mechanism is exhausted, pressure rises sharply with further increases in volume (zone 2) until a second plateau (zone 3) is reached, thought to be associated with ICP exceeding diastolic blood pressure with a resulting decrease in arterial blood volume. Following exhaustion of this compensatory mechanism, ICP rises sharply with further volume increase in any intracranial compartment (zone 4).

Central Venous Effects on Intracranial Pressure and Cerebral Blood Flow

Normally central venous pressure (CVP) is slightly less than ICP, both are low, and neither significantly influences CBF. Under these normal conditions and to a first approximation, CPP is determined solely by MAP. If ICP is abnormally high, CPP will be lower at any given MAP (vide supra). As CVP increases, as in right heart failure or during mechanical ventilation with positive pressure, or as local venous obstruction occurs, as with tracheostomy or endotracheal tube taping or in superior vena cava syndrome or with vasculitis and venoocclusion in meningitis, CVP increases ICP and CPP, and CBF may be adversely affected. This would be particularly true if MAP were low or brain autoregulation impaired. In addition, elevations of venous pressure constitute hydrostatic forces increasing any tendency toward tissue edema. Finally, high venous pressure and venous engorgement of the CNS can reduce the distensibility of this compartment, making it less capable of volume reduction in compensation for tissue edema or increases in arterial blood volume.

Positive-End Expiratory Pressure and Intracranial Pressure

The behavior of elevations of CVP and ICP described above suggests a mechanism of a Starling resistor regulating cerebral venous outflow. To the extent this were true, excessive amounts of positive end-expiratory pressure (PEEP) could increase CVP, reduce CPP, and initiate or perpetuate ischemic injury to the brain. In practice this is not commonly encountered for two reasons. First, in most brain-injured patients, ICP greatly exceeds CVP. More importantly, when PEEP is utilized to treat intrapulmonary shunt, a gas exchange failure arising typically from alveolar flooding which produces concomitant decreases in lung compliance, the effect of PEEP to elevate CVP is minimal. Nonetheless, this possible adverse consequence of positive-pressure ventilation and PEEP must be considered in all patients at risk for brain hypoperfusion. If PEEP is used in excessive amounts or inappropriately in patients with minimal intrapulmonary shunt and near normal lung compliance, the possibility of CVP elevations impairing CVP arises. Additionally, misuse of PEEP in just these ways will cause diminished venous return, diminished cardiac output, and potentially arterial hypotension, causing CPP to fall even further.

The Systemic Circulatory Response to Increased Intracranial Pressure

The classic Cushing response of bradycardia and hypertension was originally described in a number of animal models characterized by extreme increase in ICP with immediate and devastating brain injury. It is rarely encountered clinically, and then in similar catastrophes such as brain herniation. More typically, patients with brain injury manifest increased sympathetic tone with tachycardia, hypertension, and increased cardiac output. In a number of animal models, the best predictor for the onset and magnitude of this response is a decrease in $CMRO_2$, and the increase in blood pressure that is seen appears to blunt the fall in CPP and CBF that would otherwise occur under conditions of elevated ICP and disordered autoregulation. The relative unresponsiveness of the cerebrovasculature to α-receptor stimulation during this response, unlike many other tissue beds, may permit preferential shunting of flow to the brain. Recognition of this phenomenon is important clinically, since hypertensive states following brain injury may be beneficial in maintaining CBF. Of course, a number of brain injuries are initiated by extremes of blood pressure elevation, and the distinction between homeostatic response and initiating event can be difficult (vide infra).

Hypoxic Central Nervous System Injury

Brain hypoxia usually arises as a result of a failure of oxygen delivery. This may be caused by diminished hemoglobin (anemic hypoxia), arterial desaturation (hypoxic hypoxia) or decreased flow (stagnant hypoxia or ischemia). If a high flow to the CNS is maintained, injury on the basis of anemia or hypoxemia alone is unlikely. CNS injury is virtually unheard of even in severe anemia, and patients are routinely encountered who tolerate brief periods of severe hypoxemia, with Pa_{O_2} of 20 to 40 mmHg. Cessation of flow, however, is very poorly tolerated. Following global ischemia, such as follows cardiac arrest, brain electrical activity ceases within 5 to 10 s. Within 15 to 30 s oxygen stores are depleted and oxidative phosphorylation ceases. At this point anaerobic glycolysis continues to supply energy to the cell, but glucose and glycogen stores are soon exhausted and within 4 to 7 min tissue adenosine triphosphate (ATP) levels fall. Without adequate energy supplies, ionic gradients across cell membranes decay and biochemical events are initiated which are followed shortly by ultrastructural changes and irreversible cell injury. Thus, most identifiable CNS injury arises from either diminished flow or combinations of reduction in hemoglobin, Pa_{O_2} and flow.

When considering ischemic injury, either in the context of evaluating experimental results or treating patients, it is useful to distinguish between *focal injury* (such as stroke) and *global injury* (such as postcardiac arrest). In focal injury, it is likely that the area of maximal ischemic injury is surrounded by a *penumbra zone,* defined as marginally perfused tissue with no or reversible neuronal injury. Preservation or augmentation of flow to this area might carry the potential to limit the extent of ischemic injury. In focal injuries, the effect of any intervention on regional distributions of flow could be of paramount importance, since any "steal" of flow from the penumbra region could theoretically extend ultimate ischemic injury and increase neurologic dysfunction. Having made this distinction, it should be noted that even in global ischemia regional differences in extent of injury are very common. This selective regional vulnerability is due, in part, to differences in susceptibility to ischemic injury and anatomic differences in the microcirculation ("watershed" regions of the brain).

FLOW THRESHOLDS FOR CEREBRAL ISCHEMIA

Varying levels of CBF have been associated with varying degrees of CNS dysfunction. This notion of threshold for various components of ischemic injury is likely important, since in critical illness the whole brain is not likely always subject to "all-or-none" conditions of perfusion. While normal CBF is approximately 50 mL/100 g tissue/min, electrical failure (defined as attenuation of EEG signal) occurs when flow is reduced to 15 to 20 mL/100 g tissue/min. At flows of approximately 10 mL/100 g tissue/min, a number of metabolic and biochemical abnormalities develop. ATP depletion occurs and free fatty acids are liberated with generation of intracellular acidosis. Extracellular potassium and cytoplasmic calcium concentrations increase and brain water content begins to increase. Unlike conditions of complete global ischemia—known to cause neuronal cell death over minutes—the duration of time that these low flow conditions may be tolerated without sustaining irreversible injury is not determined. Nonetheless, some investigations suggest that continuation of the events described during low flow for more than several hours is likely to result in irreversible cell injury.

INJURY DURING THE ISCHEMIC PHASE

Much interest has focused on the role of calcium as a mediator of injury following prolonged ischemia. The multiple mechanisms controlling intracellular calcium concentration—cell membrane ATP-dependent calcium translocase, cell membrane Na^+/Ca^{++} exchange pump, Ca^{++} uptake by the endoplasmic reticulum, and mitochondrial Ca^{++} uptake—are all energy-dependent processes. As energy sources are depleted following the onset of ischemia, massive influx of calcium into the cell occurs. This has a number of consequences (Fig. 4-10). Mitochondrial accumulation of calcium has the potential to uncouple oxidative phosphor-

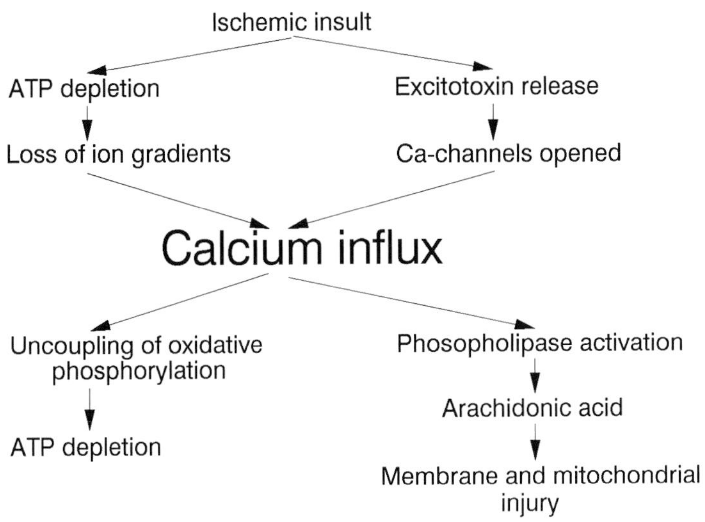

FIGURE 4-10 The central role of neuronal calcium influx in ischemic injury. Ischemic insult can cause both cellular energy "failure" (with ATP depletion and loss of transmembrane ion gradients) and release of excitatory neurotransmitters, both of which cause intracellular calcium concentrations to rise. This results in uncoupling of oxidative phosphorylation (with further ATP depletion) as well as increased arachidonic production, with consequent membrane and mitochondrial injury via a number of pathways.

ylation and impair any existing ATP synthesis. High intracellular calcium concentrations favor proteolysis, with consequent damage to cell and mitochondrial membranes. Activation of phospholipase A_2 results in hydrolysis of phospholipids within membranes, resulting in physical disruption of the membrane.

Membrane phospholipid hydrolysis releases a number of free fatty acids, most prominently arachidonic acid (Fig. 4-11). Under normal conditions free fatty acid metabolism is predominantly to acetyl-CoA with entry into the tricarboxylic acid cycle. This metabolic route is energy dependent, however, and under conditions of ischemia with ATP depletion and high calcium concentrations, arachidonic acid concentrations rise. This elevation of arachidonic acid concentration has been noted following hypoxia, ischemia, trauma, convulsions, and severe hypoglycemia. In the presence of oxygen following reperfusion (vide infra), PG synthesis is stimulated (see Fig. 4-11). The cascade of PGs produced has a number of effects which could modulate further tissue injury, including platelet aggregation, altered microvascular permeability, vasodilation, and vasoconstriction.

INJURY MEDIATED BY EXCITATORY NEUROTRANSMITTERS

Some ischemic injury may be modified by biochemical alterations operative at the synapse. The brain contains a large number of receptors for amino acids, and specific amino acids appear to play a major role as excitatory neurotransmitters. At least four receptor subsets have been described: **1.** the *N*-methyl-D-aspartate (NMDA) receptor (agonists include NMDA, aspartate, and ibotenate); **2.** the quisqualate receptor (agonists include α-amino-3-hydroxy-5-methyl-4-isoxazolepropionate [AMPA], quisqualate, and L-glutamate); **3.** the kainate receptor (agonists include kainate, domoate, and L-glutamate); and **4.** the L-2-amino-4-phosphonobutyrate receptor. When agonists of these receptors achieve high local concentrations, focal neuronal degeneration occurs. This has led to the notion of these substances acting as "excitotoxins" in a number of pathologic states. The NMDA receptor is linked to an ion channel and excessive excitation resulting from high concentrations of glutamate can result in influx of sodium and water into cells. Some data suggest that one mechanism of injury related to these excitotoxins is excessive membrane depolarization with massive chloride entry into the cell and eventual osmotic cell lysis. In addition to this mechanism of early cell injury, a delayed injury has been described that can require up to a day to occur if the offending amino acid neurotransmitter is removed after exposure of the cell. This delayed injury appears related to calcium entry into the cell, since removal of extracellular calcium is protective. Calcium flux into the cell is related to extracellular glutamate concentration in at least two ways. Cell depolarization

FIGURE 4-11 Increased calcium levels facilitate the action of phospholipase to convert membrane phospholipids to arachidonic acid. Under anaerobic conditions, entry of arachidonic acid into the Kreb's cycle is limited and concentrations increase. When reperfusion occurs and aerobic metabolism is reestablished, these high levels of arachidonic acid result in generation of endoperoxides and leukotrienes, pathways of prostaglandin synthesis that could have diverse effects on tissue and cellular function.

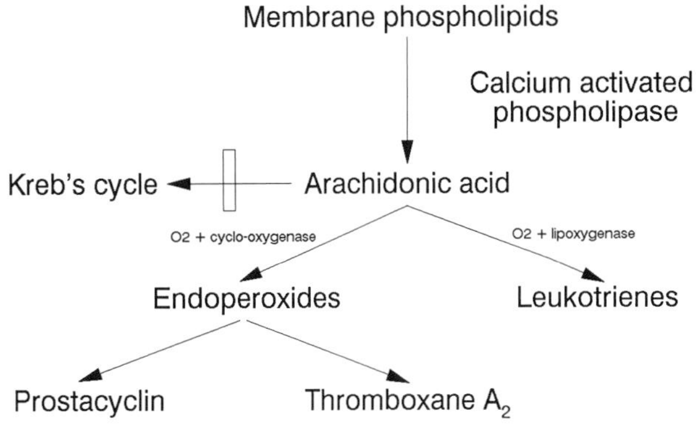

by stimulation of the NMDA receptor could cause calcium influx via voltage-sensitive calcium channels. In addition, glutamate is one of a number of agonists that appear to result in calcium influx by gating the activity of agonist-operated calcium channels.

Thus, ischemic or hypoxic neuronal injury could occur or be extended by these mechanisms somewhat apart from the metabolic insult causing anaerobic cell death. Anaerobic metabolism under conditions of ischemia has been shown to cause release of glutamate, as well as other amino acid neurotransmitters. If extracellular concentrations were to achieve critical levels, the immediate and delayed injuries described above could represent nonmetabolic pathways to cell death. The density of NMDA receptors appears to be high in those areas of the brain (hippocampus, Purkinje cell layers of the cerebellum, thalamus, and layers five and six of the cerebral cortex) that show particular vulnerability to ischemic injury. In some models of focal ischemia, blockade with competitive antagonists at the NMDA receptor ameliorates the extent of brain damage.

PERFUSION ABNORMALITIES FOLLOWING ISCHEMIA

Rarely, flow following transient ischemic injury such as cardiac arrest is markedly reduced even after establishment of a stable circulation. This phenomenon has been termed *no-reflow* and has been ascribed to platelet aggregation, increased viscosity, vascular compression by tissue edema, and disseminated intravascular coagulation (DIC).

More commonly, global CNS ischemia is followed by a hyperemic response when circulation is restored (Fig. 4-12). It is likely that this increased flow is related to diminished vascular tone developing during the ischemic period. Following the hyperemic period, it is common to find a sustained period of diminished flow, which may be one-half or less of normal CBF despite a return of $CMRO_2$ to near normal. Some have invoked this mechanism to explain the watershed distribution of neuronal injury noted after circulatory arrest, a condition of no flow that would otherwise be expected to yield randomly but homogeneously distributed injury.

FIGURE 4-12 The pattern of CBF following incomplete ischemic injury. Following ischemia, there is usually a hyperemic response which diminishes over hours to a reduced CBF approximately 50 percent of base line, which is sustained for a prolonged period of time.

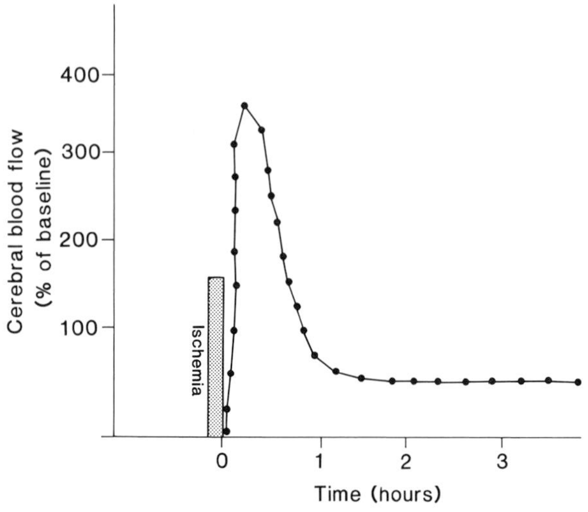

Following induction of global ischemia in various models, postischemic hypoperfusion can be present for hours to days. Precapillary constriction appears to play a role in this process and may be mediated by calcium-dependent activation of the contractile apparatus of specialized endothelial cells. Calcium channel blockade and inhibition of PG synthesis may represent pharmacologic interventions that could ameliorate or reverse this process.

OTHER VASCULAR EVENTS MODULATING ISCHEMIC INJURY

While microvascular changes likely result in hypoperfusion following recovery from global ischemia, macrovascular events often result in potentiation of injury following hemorrhage into the subarachnoid space. Cerebral vasospasm is a well-recognized complication of SAH that can result in ischemic injury. Angiographic evidence of vasospasm can be seen in a majority of patients following SAH, and clinical manifestations of this process will be present in as many as one-third. The incidence and severity of spasm is greatest approximately a week following initial hemorrhage, although it may be encountered as early as days after injury and may persist for weeks.

The presence of blood in the subarachnoid space is likely important in the pathogenesis since the degree of vasospasm is related to the amount of hemorrhage and removal of blood in some models blunts the degree of vasospasm. Arterial narrowing results from both structural and functional changes. Pathologically, arteries are narrowed and exhibit intraluminal platelet aggregates, intimal swelling and proliferation, endothelial cell injury, infiltration of the media by inflammatory cells, and manifestations of vessel denervation. A number of mediators of vasospasm including serotonin, bradykinin, PGs, and oxygen-free radicals have been identified. Clot lysis occurring approximately a week after hemorrhage may initiate free radical production, as oxyhemoglobin is released and converted to methemoglobin and superoxide anion. Via the modified Fenton reaction, superoxide anion in the presence of ferric ion will produce the hydroxyl radical which is capable of lipid peroxidation and initiation of cascades that result in tissue inflammation and injury. Biochemical markers of free radical generation have been identified following SAH, and some investigations have demonstrated benefit from free radical scavengers.

The consequences of the morphologic and functional vessel changes are several. Frank ischemia may result if flow is inadequate to meet tissue oxygen requirements. Cell and vessel endothelial injury may result in cytotoxic and vasogenic edema, with elevation of ICP and further compromise of perfusion. Finally, these vascular abnormalities

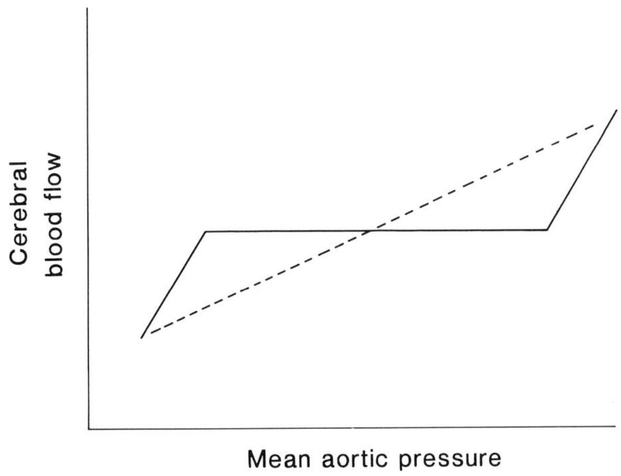

FIGURE 4-13 Loss of autoregulation over the entire range of aortic pressures (interrupted line). Such disordered regulation of flow may exist in peri-infarct regions, following trauma, or even in some diffuse brain injuries. Adequate CBF then becomes dependent on maintenance of a critical aortic pressure.

may result in loss of autoregulation over a wide range of systemic blood pressures (Fig. 4-13). The tissue segment subserved by the injured and dysfunctional vasculature then becomes highly dependent on systemic blood pressure for maintenance of perfusion, and conditions of hypotension, such as is sought during surgery with aneurysm clipping, could result in further ischemic insult.

REPERFUSION INJURY

As noted above (see Fig. 4-10), ischemic conditions can result in intracellular calcium accumulation which promotes phospholipase A_2 activity. The arachidonic acid produced during degradation of membrane phospholipids can, in the presence of oxygen, result in the generation of a number of leukotrienes, endoperoxides, hydroperoxy acids, and PGs which have detrimental tissue effects. Thus reperfusion, by restoration of oxygen supply, may complete or potentiate tissue injury.

Reperfusion may similarly have adverse consequences because of generation of oxygen free radicals. These molecular species contain an unpaired electron in the outer orbital ring and are highly reactive, capable of oxidizing a large number of biologically important compounds and initiating cascades with widespread effects. Free radicals produced during aerobic conditions of oxidative phosphorylation remain tightly bound within the mitochondrial membrane with little potential for cell injury. During ischemia, utilization of existing ATP stores results in production of hypoxanthine. The intracellular enzyme xanthine oxidase is activated and converts hypoxanthine to xanthine, a reaction resulting in the reduction of oxygen to superoxide anion. Superoxide anion is itself capable of reaction with cell proteins and lipids, but production of this free radical during complete ischemia is limited. During reperfusion, however, superoxide production increases. More importantly, the presence of increased quantities of oxygen, in the presence of iron, promotes generation of hydroxyl radicals, a much more reactive species.

To the extent that these mechanisms are operative during reperfusion, the management of ischemia may be confounded by this paradoxical response to restoration of blood flow. Should such reperfusion-initiated events be proven to be substantial following human ischemic injury, a number of strategies could be used to modify their course. Reperfusion could be initiated under anoxic conditions with free radical scavengers such as superoxide dismutase, catalase, or vitamin E. Such scavengers could also be of benefit if given early in ischemia, in anticipation of restoration of flow. Since ionic iron is required to catalyze the modified Fenton reaction, metal chelators such as deferoxamine may find clinical applications. Finally, xanthine oxidase inhibitors such as allopurinol may be of use to limit xanthine production and generation of superoxide radical.

PARTIAL VERSUS COMPLETE ISCHEMIA

Via the mechanisms of arachidonic acid cascade and free radical generation, brain tissue with partial ischemia or fluctuating levels of perfusion could sustain injury, as described above. Other mechanisms of injury may be important in the setting of partial ischemia. High intracellular hydrogen ion concentration, specifically acidosis to a pH of 5.5 or less, results in cell death caused by protein and membrane denaturation. Ischemia results in lactic acidosis as tissue glucose stores are metabolized anaerobically. The modest glucose stores of CNS tissue limit the degree of lactic acidosis following ischemic injury. Under conditions of partial ischemia, glucose supply may continue and be sufficient to drive intracellular lactate production with consequent acidosis.

A number of observations support this mechanism of injury. In animal models, induction of hyperglycemia prior to ischemic injury increases intracellular lactate levels, and intracellular lactate achieves a higher concentration during partial ischemia than complete ischemia of equal duration. If animals are made hyperglycemic prior to induction of global ischemia, intracellular pH reaches a lower nadir during reperfusion than in normoglycemic animals. This has been attributed to a period of anaerobic metabolism fueled by glucose delivery prior to restoration of oxidative phosphorylation.

Limited data exist for human ischemic injuries. Assessing the global ischemia sustained during cardiac arrest, one retrospective study has found that lower serum glucose levels are associated with more rapid resolution of coma and recovery of greater neurologic function. In focal ischemia, correlations have been established between recovery from stroke and lower serum glucose levels at the time of initial evaluation.

It is difficult to generate specific guidelines for manipulation of glucose levels from the available information. Since hypoglycemia is a common and serious cause of metabolic coma with the potential to cause irreversible injury, it should be carefully avoided. Benefits to be derived from

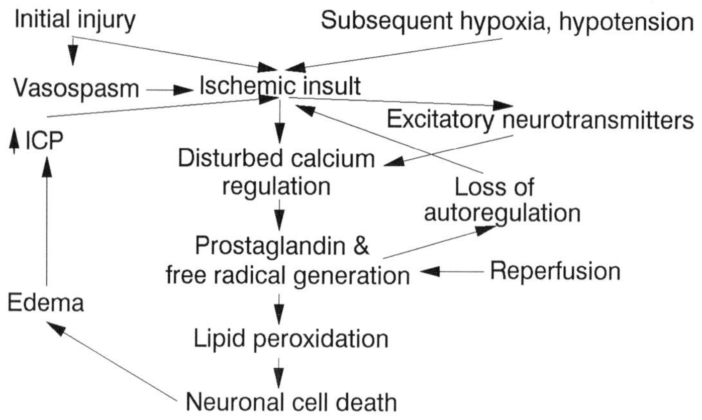

FIGURE 4-14 Pathways for potentiation or perpetuation of injury. Following the initial injury (and worsened by any associated hypoxia or hypotension), disturbed calcium regulation results in prostaglandin and free radical generation. To the extent these phenomena cause loss of autoregulation of CBF, further ischemic injury may occur. In addition, the initial insult may result in excessive release of excitatory neurotransmitters which potentiate influx of calcium into cells. Vasospasm may complicate ischemia following the initial insult. Finally, neuronal death and vascular events result in edemagenesis, with elevation in ICP and further ischemia.

"tight" regulation of hyperglycemia are not yet validated. Indeed, control of hyperglycemia in critical illness is extraordinarily difficult, given the relative insulin resistance of the hypermetabolic state.

PERPETUATION OF ISCHEMIC INJURY

Ischemic injury as described might be self-perpetuating in a number of different ways (Fig. 4-14). Vascular injury or humoral factors generated during ischemia could cause microvascular obstruction to flow or large vessel spasm that impairs perfusion even after restoration of a failed circulation. Cell death and vascular injury promote tissue edema, with elevation of ICP, diminished CPP, and potential hypoperfusion. Loss of autoregulation may make peri-ischemic regions of the brain particularly liable to further injury. Restoration of flow may have adverse effects, initiating further cell injury. Finally, even after the injury related to the "self-catabolism" of ischemia is complete, potential mechanisms of ongoing neuronal damage such as release of excitotoxins exist.

Hypertensive Brain Injury

A number of mechanisms operate to cause CNS damage during hypertensive crises. As seen in Fig. 4-6, extreme elevations in MAP will result in "breakthrough" from autoregulation with high cerebral blood volumes contributing to elevations in ICP. CSF pressures are typically above 150 mmH_2O in patients with hypertensive encephalopathy and may be as high as 300 to 400 mmH_2O. Patients with chronic hypertension will exhibit a shift of the autoregulation curve to the right, thus often tolerating MAPs as high as 175 mmHg.

These extreme elevations of MAP are also associated with multifocal vasoconstriction with fibrinoid necrosis of arterioles and diffuse parenchymal brain injury including microinfarcts and hemorrhage. It is not clear if all of these changes are initiated by high intravascular pressures, but subsequent injury is likely mediated by inflammatory response and activation of complement and coagulation cascades in the microcirculation. It is interesting that similar pathologic changes may be seen in sickle cell anemia, cryoglobulinemia, bacterial endocarditis, fat embolism, toxemia of pregnancy, DIC, and various vasculitic disorders. Finally, extreme blood pressure elevations result in significant brain edema, further contributing to elevation of ICP and further compromising brain perfusion. The combination of diffuse cerebral edema and increased ICP yields the typical findings of headache, global decrease in cortical function to the point of coma, and papilledema. The focal vascular abnormalities with consequent ischemia yield a number of focal findings including seizures and often transient focal abnormalities on the neurologic examination such as asymmetric myoclonus or a unilateral Babinski sign. Since the underlying focal lesions are microvascular, the expected deficits should be minor, and indeed deficits such as hemiparesis or cranial nerve dysfunctions should prompt consideration of hemorrhage or infarction complicating hypertension, or a hypertensive response to cerebrovascular disease.

Cerebral Resuscitation and Preservation

Based on limited understanding of the pathophysiology of brain injury during critical illness, a number of strategies have been suggested to restore brain function following insult and to prevent further damage. Although each has hypothetical benefits, clear demonstration of clinical utility is lacking for most interventions, and application of many of these approaches can be difficult and even overtly dangerous. Rather than prescribing specific methods or agents to achieve "brain resuscitation" we hope to provide the student of critical care with an understanding of principles that apply to the management of all critically ill patients, including those who have sustained certain ischemic injury (focal or global) as well as those who manifest more nonspecific neurologic dysfunction intercurrent with critical illness such as shock or multiorgan failure. In many regards optimal management of CNS dysfunction is the balancing of opposing potential threats to CNS viability. By way of example, controlled hyperventilation is often used to reduce CBF and thus reduce elevated ICP. This potential benefit must be weighed against the effects of diminished perfusion and elevation of intrathoracic and hence cerebral venous pressure, consequences of this intervention which could conspire to reduce perfusion to a point resulting in further ischemic injury. Similarly, use of vasoactive drugs which reduce vasospasm and its attendant ischemia could result in a shunting of blood flow away from regions of marginal perfusion with undesirable results. In this regard, the balancing of goals in the management of the CNS is identical to most interventions in critical care.

ROUTINE SUPPORTIVE THERAPY

In clinical series the incidence of secondary brain insult following catastrophic injury is high and at least in retrospect often preventable. Hypoxemia and anemia clearly should be avoided in patients who have any actual or potential for CNS hypoperfusion. Optimal circulatory function is particularly important following trauma, shock, or CNS ischemia because of alterations in brain autoregulation of CBF. Ventilatory failure resulting in hypercapnia is particularly disastrous in these patients because of the increased CBF and intracranial hypertension induced by this metabolic derangement.

A number of observations concerning intracranial hypertension will be made below, but several aspects of routine care should be stressed. The need for intubation and mechanical ventilation is often high within the priorities of the clinician in brain-injured patients, due to their depressed level of consciousness and the need to avoid hypoxemia or hypercapnia superimposed on prior injury. Manipulation of the airway, however, can be a powerful stimulus to further increases in ICP and stimulation should be minimized. Barbiturates are preferred sedatives as adjuncts to intubation, and they minimize ICP rise. Intravenous lidocaine blunts increase in ICP during laryngoscopy and is useful in this setting. Narcotics and benzodiazepines are also acceptable adjuncts to intubation. Succinyl choline has been reported to have adverse effects and increase ICP, which is unfortunate since it is in other regards an ideal agent for rapid induction of patients during intubation with short duration of paralysis. Nondepolarizing muscle agents, which cause histamine release, are relatively contraindicated since histamine release is associated with increased ICP.

Positive-pressure ventilation, particularly when coupled with PEEP, will increase intrathoracic pressure. If CVP exceeds ICP, then it will be the downstream pressure in the equation determining CBF ($CBF = (MAP - CVP)/R$ when $CVP > ICP$). Under conditions of low mean aortic pressure, cerebral hypoperfusion could result. Efforts in this setting should be directed at minimizing elevation of intrathoracic pressure, with small tidal volumes, short inspiratory times, least PEEP, and treatment of any component of airflow obstruction to minimize dynamic hyperinflation and intrinsic PEEP (see Chaps. 129 and 130).

As noted earlier in this chapter, seizure activity dramatically elevates $CMRO_2$, with the potential for demand to exceed delivery with potentiation of ischemic injury. In addition, even with abundant oxygen and substrate delivery, sustained seizures may result in neuronal injury, perhaps via mechanisms involving amino acid excitotoxins discussed above. The management of status epilepticus in the critically ill is confounded by difficulties in recognizing this state and the frequent requirement for multiple antiepileptics. Motor activity accompanying status epilepticus may be masked by muscle relaxants, and even without such agents status epilepticus without tonic-clonic movements may occur. We advocate early diagnostic evaluation with EEG in comatose critically ill patients, with a low threshold to repeat this test if CNS function remains unclear. Once identified, seizures should be treated promptly, with rapid titration of medications to high therapeutic serum levels and addition of other agents if repeat studies do not confirm seizure control (see Chap. 142).

The mounting evidence suggesting even modest hyperglycemia can result in worsened intracellular acidosis in ischemic brain injury would suggest that "tight" control of serum glucose be instituted for most critically ill patients with CNS dysfunction. This is often difficult, since insulin resistance and elevations of blood glucose levels to 150 to 250 mg/dL is common in the critically ill, even without preexisting disorders of glucose metabolism. Continuous insulin infusion titrated against calorie load and metabolic state and informed by frequent monitoring of serum glucose should permit control of this parameter to approximately 140 mg/dL in the majority of patients, without causing undesirable levels of hypoglycemia.

BARBITURATE COMA

The ability of barbiturates to lower $CMRO_2$ has been known for many years, an effect likely related to cessation of electrophysiologic activity. It is not surprising, therefore, that the notion that deep barbiturate coma could benefit patients with ischemic brain injury arose. After publication of rather preliminary animal studies likely overinterpreted to indicate a benefit, this intervention found widespread uncontrolled application to patients with diverse CNS injuries, including postarrest, near drowning, head injury, Reye's syndrome, and hepatic encephalopathy. This occurred despite some data suggesting that decreases in $CMRO_2$ were accompanied by parallel decreases in CBF, suggesting no benefit in terms of oxygen balance.

When prospective clinical trials were conducted in patients with global ischemia, no benefit could be documented. Indeed, when some basic investigations in animal models were repeated, earlier reported benefits could not be confirmed. The failure of this intervention to confer benefit may be related to the failure to achieve improvement in oxygen or other substrate balance; alternatively, adverse circulatory consequences resulting from induction of barbiturate coma may outweigh any limited metabolic benefits to the CNS function. The lesson to be learned from this experience is simple: mechanistically appealing interventions cannot be applied to patient management without clearcut demonstration of benefit. At the present time barbiturates may have a role in decreasing abnormally elevated ICP (vide infra) and perhaps in specific settings including anesthetic management during controlled hypoperfusion. Their routine use in the setting of global cerebral ischemia however is unwarranted.

HYPOTHERMIA

Hypothermia, by analogy to barbiturate coma, could reduce the extent of ischemic injury if imbalances in oxygen supply relative to delivery were addressed by reduction of total oxygen consumption. This mechanism has been invoked to explain the recovery of neurologic function after sustained cold water immersion and in the setting of circulatory arrest during surgery. The use of this intervention in diverse forms of CNS injury encountered in the ICU has not been evaluated, and the technical difficulties in maintaining such temperature control, as well as the potential adverse effects on other organ systems make it unlikely to be of major benefit. Treatment of hyperthermia, however, does seem warranted, and critically ill patients with demonstrable or potential CNS dysfunction should be promptly returned to normothermia (see Chap. 73).

CALCIUM CHANNEL BLOCKERS

Rapidly expanding knowledge of the role of calcium as a membrane charge carrier, intracellular message transducer, and regulator of multiple metabolic pathways has, not surprisingly, caused much attention to focus on the role of calcium in a number of CNS injuries. Pharmacologic agents which affect calcium channels could have brain protective actions via a number of general mechanisms. By limiting the increase in intracellular calcium following ischemic injury, many of the cascades causing irreversible damage to membranes and cytoskeletal components might be prevented. Calcium channel blocking drugs might also have beneficial effects on brain perfusion by restoring the diminished flow that typically follows the hyperemic phase of reperfusion after ischemic insult, or by preventing vasospasm after focal injur'es such as SAH. Also, mechanisms of neuronal injury that relate to pathologic stimulation of receptors by excitatory amino acids, such as the NMDA receptor (vide supra), might also be prevented by calcium channel blockade, since calcium influx characterizes this situation as well.

While a large number of investigations have been conducted to evaluate the efficacy of calcium channel blocking as agents to prevent or minimize brain injury, it should be stated at the outset that the central hypothesis of calcium-mediated cell death is supported by largely circumstantial evidence. In some models, anoxic cell injury appears to occur without a significant change in intracellular calcium concentration. Interestingly, in some models of ischemia in which calcium channel blocking agents appear to be protective, elevations of intracellular calcium concentration are not prevented. It remains to be determined how central to ischemic injury calcium influx is, as opposed to being an epiphenomenon of cell injury by other means. It is possible that ATP depletion or intracellular acidosis related to tissue hypoxia are the events that lead to both calcium influx and cell injury. Of course, multiple complementary pathways to cell death may exist.

This cautionary and appropriately skeptical tone not withstanding, some overview of the burgeoning literature of calcium channel blockade in CNS injury is appropriate. The first observation to be made is that these studies involve multiple models (several animal species and man), injuries (both focal and global ischemia), end points of improved function (survival, EEG criteria, neurologic performance, histopathology, etc.), and agents (verapamil, nimodipine, nicardipine, flunarizine, lidoflazine, and s-emopamil, among others).

Global Ischemia

The evidence for benefit from these agents following global ischemic injury is entirely from animal models and is weak, and indeed suggests that any benefits are likely related to events other than prevention of the initial massive influx of calcium into injured neurons after ischemic insult. Among the various agents tested, flunarizine and nicardipine are perhaps the most promising, although present information does not strongly support clinical trials in human beings.

Focal Ischemia

Focal lesions such as stroke may represent a more hopeful lesion for preservation of neuronal viability and function, since a penumbral region at risk may be salvageable. Results obtained in animal models suggest that delay of treatment even a few hours after focal ischemic insult markedly reduces the efficacy of this intervention. Even with early treatment, data for clear limit in infarct size are conflicting. In those experiments that investigated mechanism of benefit, calcium channel blockers appeared to prevent the fall in cellular pH in the penumbra zone and in a few but not all studies increased blood flow to the peri-infarct regions. Of the calcium antagonists tested in multiple animal models, isradipine and s-emopamil are likely most efficacious to reduce infarct size. Prospective double-blind, randomized clinical trials have been limited to nimodipine. In all trials the drug was begun 24 to 48 h following the onset of acute ischemic stroke. In one investigation in 60 patients neurologic function, defined as level of consciousness and general disability, at 4 weeks postevent was improved in the group receiving nimodipine. In a second study of 186 patients mortality at 4 weeks was reduced in the nimopidine group but did not clearly relate to neurologic status. In a third study no significant differences were noted. These clinical results suggest further testing of these agents in the setting of focal ischemic injury is appropriate, although their use should not be generalized and should be restricted to settings of clinical investigation.

Subarachnoid Hemorrhage

The clinical investigations concerning the use of calcium channel blockers following SAH are remarkably consistent in the clear findings of reduction of subsequent neurologic deficits. Prospectively, a number of investigators anticipated such a result based on the high incidence of vascular spasm following SAH and the observation that cerebral arterial spasm probably originates from mechanisms similar to coronary artery spasm and is responsive to manipulation of intracellular calcium concentration. Interestingly, in some clinical investigations the incidence of spasm, at least as angiographically defined, is not reduced by nimodipine, despite a reduced incidence of infarction and improved outcome. If calcium channel blockers do not confer benefit by alleviating spasm, it is possible that they improve nutritional blood flow or propitiously influence intracellular metabolism. The present information would strongly support the use of calcium channel blockade following SAH, with most of the clinical data available concerning use of nimodipine and nicardipine.

N-METHYL-D-ASPARTATE-RECEPTOR BLOCKERS

Both competitive and noncompetitive antagonists for the NMDA receptor have been described but use of these agents to limit ischemic injury has been confounded by the fact that most cross the blood-brain barrier poorly, and it is difficult to achieve effective concentrations at the sites of action. In addition, in general naturally occurring excitatory neurotransmitters appear rapidly after onset of ischemia and then their concentration falls rapidly during reperfusion, suggesting the window of opportunity for use of antagonists may be quite narrow.

Not surprisingly, benefits from the use of these agents in various animal models of global ischemia are not impressive. A single agent ((+)-5-methyl-10,11-dihydro-5H-debenzo(a,d)cyclohepten-5,10-imine maleate) has been described which achieves significant brain concentrations when given intravascularly, although the study of this agent is limited largely to models of status epilepticus. Should other agents become available, they may find application in some ischemic injuries, particularly focal and ongoing ischemia. It is also possible such agents could be used prior to ischemic insult during the anesthetic management of patients during cardiac, vascular, or neurosurgical procedures.

HEMODILUTION AND OTHER MANIPULATIONS OF BLOOD RHEOLOGY

As discussed earlier in this chapter, manipulation of blood rheology in theory could improve tissue perfusion and hence oxygen delivery. This notion has most often been raised in the context of focal ischemic injury, a circumstance in which improved perfusion of the penumbra zone could result in limitation of the extent of injury and ultimate neurologic compromise. The manipulations that have been evaluated most often in experimental models or clinical trials are hemodilution or use of agents (particularly pentoxifylline) that increase red blood cell deformability. Of course, if hemodilution did not improve peri-infarct perfusion and instead critically lowered oxygen-carrying capacity, potentiation of ischemic injury could occur.

In both animal and human studies, CBF has been demonstrated to increase with hemodilution, an expected response, and in some animal models of ischemic injury regional flow to the penumbra region is preferentially increased. Some but not all prospective clinical studies have demonstrated greater early recovery of neurologic function in patients undergoing normovolemic hemodilution following acute stroke, but the majority of studies fail to demonstrate substantial differences in survival or ultimate functional level which is attained. At present, manipulation of blood rheology must be viewed as experimental, with benefits and patient selection to be yet defined. Clearly such an intervention should not be considered in patients with inadequate total CBF or hypoxemia.

MANIPULATION OF CEREBRAL PERFUSION PRESSURE

Certainly patients having experienced head trauma or hypovolemic shock must be maintained at a generous aortic pressure following resuscitation, given the disordered autoregulation manifested in the wake of these insults. This can usually be achieved by adequate volume resuscitation, correction of complicating factors such as tension pneumothorax or cardiac tamponade, and correction of ventricular dysfunction with inotropes.

More problematic are patients with high flow shock and marked reductions in blood pressure, such as occurs during sepsis or rarely with neurogenic shock following spinal cord or massive CNS damage. We have certainly encountered many patients with systolic blood pressures of 60 mmHg and remarkable preservation of neurologic function, and when direct observation indicates minimal or no CNS dysfunction, attempts to raise blood pressure with infusions of sympathomimetic amines are not warranted. Even when CNS abnormalities are apparent by examination, it is not clear that maneuvers which raise blood pressure will preferentially improve CNS perfusion or outcome. Serial CBF studies would be of interest in this setting but are not routinely available. Without more specific information, it is difficult to make recommendations for interventions with selective benefit for CNS function, and we suggest that the usual parameters of perfusion dictate therapy (see Chap. 114).

Since local autoregulation of CBF is lost in focal ischemic injury, vasopressor drugs might cause a beneficial increase in flow to the ischemic region by increasing CPP. Despite this appealing rationale and the fact that such an approach has been anecdotally reported to be useful for the treatment of ischemic complications of angiography, in the limited number of clinical trials no benefit was seen in patients with acute stroke. Although manipulation of the blood pressure upward is not likely to be of general benefit, it is important to stress (vide supra) that perfusion pressures following acute stroke should be generous and the clinician should not be overzealous in the control of mild to moderate degrees of hypertension.

MANIPULATION OF INTRACRANIAL PRESSURE

ICP can be reduced by removing CSF volume, by reducing tissue volume (i.e., reduction of cerebral edema), or by reducing blood volume. Indeed, each of these interventions has been used in the management of patients with elevated ICP.

MONITORING INTRACRANIAL PRESSURE

ICP may be directly measured during puncture of the spinal canal or ventricles or indirectly by measurement of tension at the dural surface. Inference of elevation of ICP is on occasion possible by physical examination (e.g., the patient with hepatic encephalopathy manifesting coma and posturing or the patient with a focal ischemic injury undergoing neurologic deterioration with signs of uncal herniation) or by imaging techniques (e.g., brain CT scan indicating cerebral edema with midline shift). However, these findings are often late and difficult to use to titrate ongoing therapy. Continuous monitoring, particularly of patients at risk for deterioration, would seem desirable. Though the widest clinical experience with ICP monitoring has evolved in patients with head trauma and Reye's syndrome, in no patient group has consistent benefit in terms of neurologic outcome or survival been demonstrated. This circumstance is rather akin to invasive hemodynamic monitoring, another invasive technology used routinely in critical care to titrate therapy routinely that has not been demonstrated to benefit patients in broad clinical trials. At the present time monitoring of ICP remains an institutional and patient-by-patient decision.

Practically, monitoring is accomplished by intraventricular catheter or epidural or subdural bolt. The former carries a risk of more catastrophic outcome from nosocomial infection although it does permit removal of CSF as an intervention to reduce ICP. If this is undertaken, it is useful to create a compliance curve of volume change against pressure, to determine patient response and the general characteristics of the cranial contents. If extensive measures are undertaken to manipulate ICP (vide infra), it would seem that invasive monitoring is warranted, since most of these interventions carry the risk of untoward side effects and should only be implemented if the ICP is elevated and responds to the given intervention.

CORTICOSTEROIDS

Corticosteroids have the theoretical benefits of reducing inflammation and stabilizing membrane function, two properties which could benefit patients with diffuse or focal brain injury. They have no role, however, in global or focal ischemia. Their use should be restricted to a few circumstances of marked inflammation accompanying chronic or subacute lesions, including metastatic tumors of the CNS, brain abscess, and perhaps meningitis with marked basilar meningeal inflammation.

OSMOTIC AGENTS AND OTHER DIURETICS

Osmotic agents such as mannitol or glycerol are potent agents to reduce cerebral edema and if this contributes significantly to elevated ICP are useful in its control. Mannitol is most frequently used for this indication and is administered in a dose of 0.25 to 1 g/kg and typically causes a reduction in ICP in 15 to 30 min. Infusions may be continued for a prolonged period of time until underlying causes of elevated ICP subside and brain compliance returns to normal. Mannitol is cleared by the kidneys, acts as an osmotic diuretic, and places the patient at risk for hypovolemia and electrolyte disturbances. Following injury the brain is not impermeable to mannitol and after prolonged use equilibration across the blood-brain barrier may diminish response. Patients must be followed closely for the hyperosmolarity induced by this agent. Serum osmolarity is best maintained between 300 to 310 mO and should not be allowed to increase above 320 mO.

Loop diuretics such as furosemide and carbonic anhydrase inhibitors such as acetazolamide can also be used, either alone or in combination with osmotic diuretics. The onset of action with these agents is generally slower than with mannitol but they may be preferred for the long-term (over weeks) management of patients, because they avoid the problem of movement of the osmotic agent into brain tissue with the potential for rebound cerebral edema and elevation of ICP when hydration is undertaken.

BARBITURATES

As noted above, high dose barbiturate administration is not justified in global ischemic brain injury. However, the reduction in $CMRO_2$ and accompanying fall in CBF associated with barbiturates can be used to reduce ICP, particularly in those patients not responding to other interventions. Pentobarbital has been used most frequently and will induce coma with a silent EEG and maximally reduced $CMRO_2$ when serum levels of 30 to 40 mg/L are achieved. Patients undergoing this therapy can manifest marked circulatory instability, and invasive hemodynamic monitoring during the initiation of therapy is probably wise. Serum levels of the drug and EEG recordings should be obtained regularly. Like other forms of extreme sedation during critical illness, this intervention eliminates the neurologic examination from patient assessment.

HYPERVENTILATION

Controlled hyperventilation to a Pa_{CO_2} of 25 mmHg will raise tissue pH, increase cerebrovascular resistance, decrease CBF, and thus reduce ICP. Of course this intervention risks further ischemic injury and the benefits of decreasing ICP must be weighed against this. One approach to help in this assessment is to cannulate the jugular bulb and determine $AVDO_2$ across the circulation. An $AVDO_2$ of >5–7 vol % suggests CBF is inadequate and should not be further reduced.

Once hypocapnia has resulted in diminished CBF, tissue pH returns toward normal by increasing bicarbonate concentration. This results in a gradual return in CBF to previous levels. This restoration of flow begins in 6 to 8 h and is usually complete in 24 to 48 h. This suggests that hyperventilation is most effective as an initial intervention to manage elevated ICP. When other measures have been instituted to manage the ICP, Pa_{CO_2} should be allowed to gradually return to normal so that hyperventilation can again be instituted for unanticipated increases in ICP. Whenever Pa_{CO_2} is allowed to rise, the patient must be monitored closely for untoward increases in ICP related to increases in CBF.

Prognosis

It would be invaluable to have tools for prognosis that allowed early and certain determination of level of recovery for individual patients with brain injury or dysfunction during critical illness. Such information would inform compassionate care of the individual and appropriate utilization of resources. Unfortunately, all studies of coma prognosis are limited by methodologic problems that diminish the utility of the criteria analyzed and certainly limit the application of such criteria to the individual patient. Thus, while judgments are necessarily made on a daily basis concerning patients in ICUs around the world, we caution that the science of prognostication is rudimentary and certainly in need of further investigation and validation.

Outside the setting of drug overdose, coma generally portends a poor outcome for ICU patients. In one evaluation of more than 500 patients in two general medical-surgical ICUs, mortality was best predicted by the occurrence of coma, cardiopulmonary resuscitation, and shock. Coma of >48 h duration was associated with mortality rate of 77 percent as compared to 11 percent mortality without coma. The coexistence of coma and shock predicted a 95 percent ICU mortality. This and many other investigations have highlighted the power of multiple organ failures in predicting for poor outcome. Interestingly, however, even this "clinical saw" has broken down in some analyses. For example, the concurrence of renal failure with coma has actually predicted for improved outcome over coma alone, perhaps because the component of metabolic encephalopathy in renal failure is treatable. This points to the limitations of generalizing information (e.g., the poor prognosis demonstrated by respiratory failure patients who have other organ failures) to other patient groups (e.g., the comatose patient).

Other investigations of prognosis after the onset of coma have tended to distinguish between nontraumatic and traumatic etiologies. In one of the largest series of patients with nontraumatic coma of diverse etiologies, including 500 subjects, only 16 percent led an independent life at some point within the first year; the remainder either died without recovery from coma (61 percent), never improved beyond the vegetative state (12 percent), or regained consciousness but required assistance for day-to-day functioning (11 percent). If a patient lacked two of the three brain stem reflexes tested (corneal, pupillary, and oculovesticular), even within hours of the onset of coma, the likelihood of recovery of independent function was remote (1 of 120). The etiology of nontraumatic coma also appeared to have prognostic significance, with the worst prognosis for patients with structural lesions (SAH or other cerebrovascular disease), intermediate for hypoxic encephalopathy, and best for hepatic encephalopathy. In our own experience, even profound coma with brain stem dysfunction in the setting of hepatic encephalopathy is reversible, as is seen in patients undergoing liver transplantation for fulminant hepatic failure. However, the concurrence of hepatic encephalopathy with coma and acute respiratory failure has been reported to markedly worsen prognosis (in fact, making survival almost unprecedented), again highlighting the need to consider subsets of patients with multiple organ dysfunctions when attempting to gauge outcome.

Depth of coma has also been used as a predictor of outcome in traumatic brain injury. In one large series of 1311 head injured patients, the Glasgow coma score (GCS, Table 4-4) correlated with survival. A GCS of 3 was associated with 83 percent mortality, 4 to 5 with 49 percent mortality, 6 to 7 with 24 percent mortality, and >8 with 0.3 percent mortality. By analogy to nontraumatic coma, the specific etiology of brain dysfunction following head injury likely influences outcome. In one series of more than 1000 patients with head injury and a GCS of <8, recovery rate appeared strongly correlated to the underlying anatomic lesion. Patients who sustained acute subdural hematoma and exhibited a GCS of 3 to 5 had only a 25 percent survival, with an incidence of recovery to the point of independent functioning of <10 percent. By contrast, patients with diffuse neuronal injury (with brain contusions or hematomata

TABLE 4-4 Glasgow Coma Score

Eyes	Open	Spontaneously	4
		To verbal command	3
		To pain	2
	No response		1
Best motor response		Obeys verbal command	6
	To pain	Localizes	5
		Flexion-withdrawal	4
		Decorticates	3
		Decerebrates	2
		No response (flaccid)	1
Best verbal response		Oriented and converses	5
		Disoriented/converses	4
		Inappropriate words	3
		Incomprehensible sounds	2
		No response	1
Total Score			3–15

excluded by CT imaging) and GCS scores of 6 to 8 had greater than 90 percent survival and two-thirds recovered substantial neurologic function.

Such relatively large series have helped inform judgments (albeit cautious and limited in scope) on outcome after derangements in CNS function based on etiology, concurrence of other organ failures, and most importantly, the serial neurologic examinations. Regarding the significance of recovery or lack thereof over time, one investigation of patients surviving cardiopulmonary resuscitation demonstrated that approximately 25 percent lacked pupillary light reflexes at the time of the initial examination; none of these patients recovered independent daily function. The presence of this reflex along with conjugate eye movements and response to pain identified a subset of patients with an approximately 40 percent chance of complete recovery. If the physical examination 24 h later improved in terms of eye opening responses and localization of pain response, the incidence of complete recovery was almost two-thirds. On the other hand, if the examination 24 h later was characterized by absent motor responses (excepting posturing) and eye movements that were neither orienting or conjugate, the incidence of complete recovery was <1 percent.

At the present, prognosis relies almost entirely on direct bedside observation and examination. Physiologic abnormalities as determined by evoked potentials or EEG or biochemical markers of neuronal injury determined by technology such as MRI may offer additional information for prognosis in the future. As discussed earlier in this chapter, abnormalities of CBF are frequent after diverse brain injuries, and hypoperfusion may result in further ischemic injury. Global and regional brain blood flow can be assessed clinically using nonradioactive xenon-enhanced CT scanning. Since certain flow thresholds have been identified that result in irreversible neuronal injury (vide supra), this technology is particularly promising as a prognostic tool.

Irreversible Cessation of Brain Function

A recent governmental commission has issued guidelines for the determination of death that has now been widely accepted throughout the United States. These guidelines state that an individual who has sustained either irreversible cessation of circulatory and respiratory functions or irreversible cessation of all functions of the entire brain, including the brain stem, is dead. Although brain death is almost invariably followed by failure of the circulation, this may require weeks to develop. Since maintenance of brain dead patients with full supportive measures places an undue emotional strain on families and staff, critical care resources are often scarce and must be directed to patients with the potential for recovery, and transplant programs require the donation of healthy organs, it is important that patients with brain death be identified early.

A number of authoritative groups and institutions have issued criteria for brain death that concur in their essentials, although there are many differences in the suggested duration of time over which a diagnosis of brain death is made and the recommended correlative laboratory testing. Since legal guidelines also pertain to this clinical problem, the clinician should be aware that there are different recommendations on a state-by-state basis in the United States.

The judgment of brain death should be made by a physician experienced in this assessment. The patient should have coma of established cause, and confounding factors of hypothermia (core temperature <30°C, 86°F), drug overdose (including therapeutic agents such as barbiturates and muscle relaxants), and shock must not be present, since these conditions may mimic the clinical picture of brain death. With these conditions excluded, the patient should then undergo physical examination which demonstrates (Table 4-5) no cerebral function, and absence of all brain stem reflexes.

A number of observations should be made concerning details of the physical examination. Seizure activity and posturing (either decorticate or decerebrate) are inconsistent with a diagnosis of brain death. Purely spinal cord reflexes (including a ciliospinal reflex) may be present and do not exclude the diagnosis of brain death. The pupils must be fixed to light but need not be fully dilated nor equal. There should be no ocular movements in response to head turning or caloric irrigation of the ears. Apnea must be confirmed. There are many recommendations for performing this test. Most guidelines suggest a particular increase in the Pa_{CO_2} as the measure of the signal driving ventilation; of course, the exact change in brain stem pH is not known to the clinician, and prior hyperventilation or acid-base disturbances may cloud interpretation of an apnea test. We suggest that the patient have some stable state of ventilation for several hours prior to the test. The patient should then be placed on an F_{IO_2} of 1.0 with 2 breaths/min. This will prevent hypoxemia from developing during hypoventilation. Under these conditions, the Pa_{CO_2} will rise 3 to 6 mmHg/min. The patient should be hypoventilated until the Pa_{CO_2} rises 15 to 20 mmHg, an increment which constitutes a significant drive to breathe if brain stem function is intact. During this period of time, pulse oximetry can be performed to exclude arterial desaturation, which is unlikely with this approach unless pulmonary gas exchange is markedly abnormal.

TABLE 4-5 Clinical Testing for Brain Death

- Conditions which may mimic brain death (e.g., hypothermia, drug overdose) must be excluded.
- Spinal reflexes are not tested and may be present.
- Decorticate and decerebrate posturing must be absent, but can be difficult to distinguish on occasion from complex spinal reflexes.
- Pupils must be light fixed but need not be dilated or symmetric.
- Corneal reflex must be absent.
- Oculovestibular reflex must be absent.
- Apnea must be confirmed.
- Ciliospinal, jaw, and snout reflexes, as well as plantar response, may continue in brain death and should not be tested.

This information, gathered by history and physical examination, is the data base on which the clinical diagnosis of brain death is made. Most authors recommend that the findings on examination be prolonged and thus confirmed on at least two assessments. We feel that examinations 12 h apart almost invariably satisfy this criterion, although some authors recommend examinations separated by 24 h or more. In addition, many published guidelines suggest auxiliary laboratory testing to confirm the clinical impression (Table 4-6). Most recommendations are for either EEG or some assessment of blood flow to the brain. These tests are certainly useful, but they clearly do not replace bedside criteria, which are mandatory in making the diagnosis of brain death. In addition, a number of cautions regarding interpretation should be made. In several series, patients have been identified with persistence of EEG activity despite meeting all clinical criteria for brain death. When these patients are maintained with supportive care, eventual progression to circulatory collapse and asystole occurred, and pathologic findings of brain necrosis were present. This suggests that a requirement for an isoelectric EEG may unnecessarily delay diagnosis in some patients. Also, since standard EEG recordings primarily reflect cerebral and cortical electrical activity, patients have been reported with an isoelectric EEG but preservation of brain stem reflexes, although this is very rare. Similarly, brain flow studies are not a perfect test for diagnosis of brain death. When flow has completely ceased, angiography, or radioisotope angiography offer compelling evidence of tissue death. Equivocal results may be present, however, in patients with unequivocal clinical evidence of brain death, at least soon after lethal brain injury.

TABLE 4-6 Auxiliary Laboratory Testing in Brain Death

- EEG
- Evoked potentials
- Angiography
- Radioisotope angiography

Chapter 5

GUT DYSFUNCTION AND NUTRITION

GREGORY A. SCHMIDT

The gut has long been underappreciated in critically ill patients. Following abdominal surgery, major trauma, serious infections, and shock, the gut appears quiescent on the surface. Bowel sounds frequently cease and oral feeding is limited or impossible. Nevertheless, it is now clear that the gut serves important metabolic functions in critical illness and exhibits accelerated metabolic activity despite the lack of enteral feeding.

Further, the abdomen is a frequent source of difficulty for the patient and physician. Distention, pain, diarrhea, and interference with nutrition are regularly encountered in the ICU. In addition, the mucosal barrier function of the bowel can be compromised by severe illness. Bacterial products, and even bacteria themselves, may traverse the mucosa and gain access to the portal circulation. Far from being inert, the gut thus becomes a threat to survival by augmenting or perpetuating systemic injury. This chapter provides a condensed review of gastrointestinal physiology, followed by a discussion of common, nonhemorrhagic abnormalities of gut function seen in critically ill patients. It concludes with an overview of nutritional principles applicable to critically ill patients. Gastrointestinal bleeding and stress ulceration are thoroughly covered in Chap. 163, while gastrointestinal infections are discussed in Chap. 108.

Normal Physiology

It is convenient to discuss motility, digestion, and absorption separately, but important to remember that they are intertwined. Motor activity serves to mix nutrients with digestive enzymes, as well as to promote contact of the chyme with mucosal absorptive cells. In addition, absorption of various substances affects hormonal secretion and, in part, determines the pattern of motor activity of the gut.

MOTILITY

STOMACH MOTOR FUNCTION. Normal gastrointestinal motility depends on intrinsic neural control, extrinsic innervation, and hormonal influences. Cells in the distal half of the stomach exhibit discrete, cyclic changes in membrane potential. These periodic, partial depolarizations (slow waves) are characteristic of gastric smooth muscle cells, and are seen whether or not there are corresponding mechanical contractions (Fig. 5-1). These constitute the basic electrical rhythm (BER) of the stomach. Superimposed on some slow waves are electrical spikes; these result in contraction of gastric smooth muscle. A phase lag in the slow waves as they propogate from mid stomach to pylorus provides a mechanism for the superimposed mechanical contractions to result in coordinated, directional peristalsis. Spikes are seen only during slow wave depolarizations, although all slow waves do not exhibit spikes (and therefore are not associated with contraction). Although the slow waves do not, in themselves, result in contraction of muscle, they coordinate it by setting the pattern on which spikes occur. The frequency of the BER at rest is approximately 3 cycles/min, and can be modified by neural and hormonal influences. Similarly, the occurrence of spike bursts, and therefore the rate of peristalsis, is modulated by neurohumoral control. Spike activity is depressed by sympathetic stimulation and catecholamines, a factor relevant in patients with trauma, surgery, and shock. Gastric emptying is extremely complex and is affected by intrinsic and extrinsic nerves, release of several gastrointestinal hormones, contents of the stomach, and pharmacologic therapies.

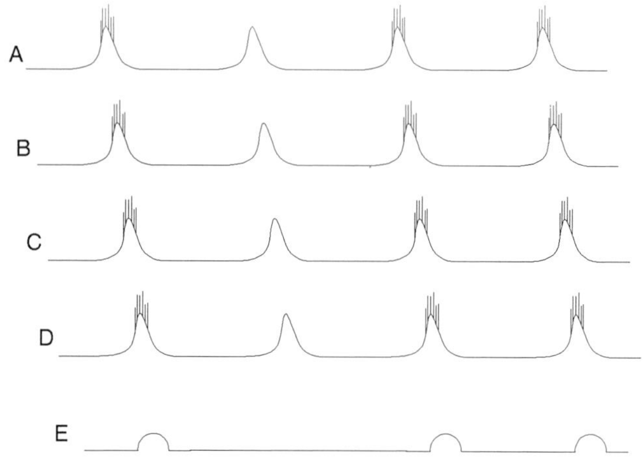

FIGURE 5-1 Slow waves. Graphs A through D represent the transmembrane potential of groups of muscle cells progressively more distal in the stomach. Note that most, but not all, of the slow wave depolarizations show superimposed spike potentials. Graph E demonstrates the mechanical activity at one point in the stomach muscle; contraction only follows slow waves when there are superimposed spike potentials.

SMALL BOWEL MOTILITY. An area near the sphincter of Oddi initiates the BER of the intestine, and peristalsis proceeds from the duodenum toward the ileum. The frequency of slow waves is about 12 cycles/min in the duodenum. Again, superimposed spike bursts determine whether muscular contraction occurs. Control of motility in the small bowel is predominantly effected by intrinsic and extrinsic neural inputs (where sympathetic stimulation is inhibitory), but is influenced by humoral substances as well.

A reflex, termed the *intestinointestinal inhibitory reflex*, has important implications for seriously ill patients. Abnormal distention of a segment of bowel reflexly inhibits tone and motility of the entire small bowel. The reflex arc is centered in the spinal cord and is effected through sympathetic pathways. The longer the segment of distended bowel, the less the intraluminal pressure needs to be to trigger the reflex. Understanding this reflex provides a rationale for cessation of enteral feeding and institution of bowel decompression in states of impaired motility.

COLONIC MOTION. The muscular structure of the colon is unusual in that it lacks the usual continuous layer of longitudinal smooth muscle, but instead consists of bands called teniae coli. This is reflected in the lack of typical peristalsis in most of the colon, and the resulting prolonged storage time of colonic contents. Once or twice per day, a process called *mass movement* pushes a bolus of fecal material toward the sigmoid. In healthy persons, mass movement is often instigated by eating (the *gastrocolic reflex*), a phenomenon probably mediated by gastrin. Mass movement is inhibited by sympathetic activity. The rectosigmoid does exhibit peristalsis and serves to propel the fecal bolus out of the body. This activity is neurally coordinated.

DIGESTION AND ABSORPTION

Digestion is the process by which dietary substances are broken down into more elemental nutrients. Thus, carbohydrates are digested to monosaccharides and disaccharides, fats to fatty acids and monoglycerides, and proteins to peptides and amino acids. Once digested, nutrients are then absorbed through, or between, intestinal cells, and finally transported to the portal blood or lymphatics. To some extent, critically ill patients are relieved of the necessity for digestion when enteral nutrition is provided in the form of partially predigested formulas. Absorption remains necessary, however, unless nutrition is given parenterally. Carbohydrates, fats, and proteins are each digested and absorbed by distinct pathways.

CARBOHYDRATES. Since only monosaccharides are readily transported across the mucosa, disaccharides and starches must be digested before they can be absorbed. Starch is broken down by pancreatic amylase into oligosaccharides, then to disaccharides. Disaccharidases, on or within the intestinal microvilli, further digest disaccharides into their component monosaccharides. These sugars are then actively transported into the mucosal cells. This process involves cotransport with sodium, and requires energy expenditure. Lactose digestion differs from that of other disaccharides since the rate of hydrolysis by brush border enzymes is significantly slower. In states of mucosal dysfunction, lactose maldigestion will become apparent before that of other sugars. This is potentially relevant in critically ill patients, since several enteral formulas contain lactose. Nevertheless, these lactose-containing supplements have not generally been shown to cause more problems with diarrhea than nonlactose-containing ones.

FATS. Fats are provided largely as long-chain triglycerides. Digestion involves hydrolysis to fatty acids and monoglycerides. This is achieved in a complex process involving pancreatic lipase, colipase, and bile salts. Entry of fat into the duodenum provokes the secretion of gut hormones (secretin and cholecystokinin-pancreozymin) which stimulate the secretion of bile and pancreatic juice. The surface-active properties of bile salts permit lipase to gain access to the water-insoluble fat. Colipase, a pancreatic protein, facilitates the binding of lipase to triglyceride. Lipase hydrolyzes triglyceride to fatty acids and monoglycerides, which then diffuse from the fat-enzyme-bile salt complex toward the intestinal mucosa. Thus, disorders of pancreatic function, hepatic synthesis, biliary patency, enterohepatic circulation of bile salts, and gut endocrine coordination can all potentially lead to maldigestion of triglycerides.

Bile salts are synthesized in the liver, secreted in conjugated form in the bile, and eventually resorbed in the terminal ileum. Since ileal absorption is normally quite efficient (90 percent complete), hepatic synthesis easily compensates for stool losses of bile salts. Fecal losses can be magnified by chelation of bile salts by drugs (e.g., cholestyramine) or by disturbed ileal resorption (e.g., terminal ileitis). The conjugated form of bile salts is necessary for normal fat digestion because the deconjugated forms are poorly soluble at the ambient enteric pH. When there is stasis of bowel contents (or a blind loop), a common occurrence in the ICU, bacterial overgrowth leads to deconjugation of bile salts. Since deconjugated bile salts function poorly, maldigestion results.

Bile salts are essential, not only for digestion of fat, but for absorption as well. At the concentration present in intestinal contents, conjugated bile acids aggregate to form micelles. As monoglycerides and fatty acids are released from triglyceride, they are emulsified by these bile salts, forming mixed micelles. Mixed micelles then approximate the surface of mucosal cells and allow their contents to diffuse into the cells. Lipid components which have been derived from long-chain triglycerides are reesterified by the endoplasmic reticulum in gut mucosal cells. The resulting triglyceride is incorporated into chylomicrons and very low density lipoprotein by merging with apolipoproteins, cholesterol, and phospholipid. Finally, these lipoproteins are secreted into the lacteals and enter the lymph. In contrast, medium-chain fatty acids are not reincorporated into triglyceride. These fatty acids directly enter the portal blood and are transported as free fatty acids.

PROTEINS. Proteins are digested by gastric, pancreatic, and enteric hydrolytic enzymes, leading to dipeptides and amino acids. Amino acids are absorbed by several distinct transport mechanisms, each of which requires energy expenditure, and probably cotransport with sodium as well. Dipeptides are even more readily absorbed than amino acids, apparently through a different transport system. Dipeptidases within the cytoplasm complete the digestion to component amino acids. Intact proteins are also directly absorbed in small quantities by endocytosis, but this seems of little importance in the critically ill.

WATER AND ELECTROLYTES. Water is actively absorbed throughout the bowel. Fluid and electrolytes can pass directly through mucosal cells (transcellular transport) or between cells (paracellular pathway). This occurs through several mechanisms, incompletely delineated, each requiring energy. In some instances, hormonal influences direct absorption of electrolytes, as in the vitamin D^3-mediated transport of calcium.

REVERSE ABSORPTION. The tremendous surface area and rich vasculature of the bowel, so useful for the absorption of nutrients, also comprises a huge membrane for the loss of substances into the bowel lumen. In several instances, this characteristic of the gut is used for therapeutic purposes. For example, activated charcoal administration is useful in theophylline intoxication. This is so even when the drug has been given intravenously. The mechanism of increased theophylline clearance is "dialysis" across the gut mucosa, with adsorption of the drug to charcoal. Another example is the use of Kayexelate, orally or rectally, for removing potassium in patients with renal failure.

Less advantageous to physicians is the effect of excessive osmoles in the gut lumen. When enteral feedings are incompletely digested or absorbed, they contribute to an osmotic gradient favoring fluid movement from the gut microcirculation to the lumen. Diarrhea results when fluid losses cannot be compensated by increased distal absorption. Even more dramatically, infection by *Vibrio cholerae* produces an enterotoxin which stimulates adenylate cyclase, raising the intracellular cyclic adenosine monophosphate level (cAMP). This leads to dramatic secretion of an isotonic fluid by all portions of the small intestine, causing tremendous fluid and electrolyte losses.

METABOLISM

BLOOD FLOW. Approximately 30 percent of the cardiac output is directed to the gut through the celiac, superior mesenteric (SMA), and inferior mesenteric arteries (IMA). At a cellular level, the majority of the blood (75 percent) is distributed to the mucosa, supporting its high level of metabolic activity. Blood supply to most of the gut is redundant so that occlusion of any vessel does not result in ischemia. An important exception is the midportion of the small intestine, supplied only through the SMA. While celiac or IMA occlusion is often well tolerated, obstruction to SMA flow typically causes lethal intestinal infarction. Gut perfusion depends on systemic factors such as cardiac output and aortic pressure, but is also subject to local neural and humoral factors.

The splanchnic circulation is substantially influenced by the autonomic nervous system. Within 1 min of acute hemorrhage, the sympathetic innervation acts to redistribute 1 L blood away from the splanchnic circulation to sustain critical organ perfusion. Despite this, microcirculatory mechanisms act to maintain gut tissue flow. In fact, such autoregulatory compensation can significantly ameliorate the impact of a reduction in perfusion pressure, so that intestinal flow can be sustained despite a 70 percent drop in arterial pressure. This phenomenon, termed *escape*, also

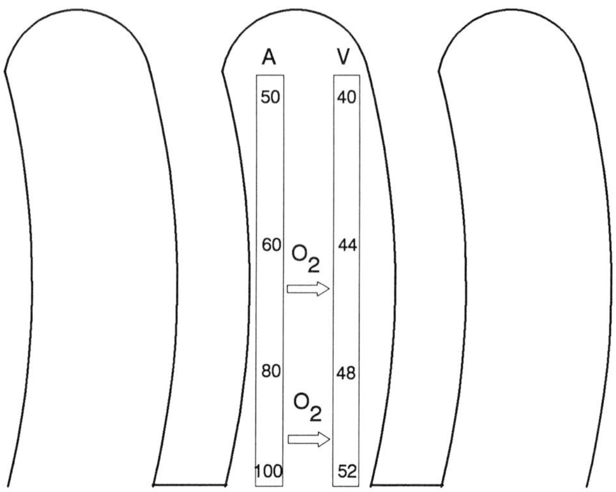

FIGURE 5-2 Countercurrent oxygen flux in intestinal villi. Some oxygen diffuses directly from the incoming arteriole to the outgoing venule, limiting the oxygen delivered to the tip of the villus. This potentially detrimental flux of oxygen is aided by low blood flow. Numbers are P_{O_2} in mmHg. A, arteriolar inflow; V, venous outflow.

comes into play during continuous infusion of vasoconstricting drugs. One of the consequences of sympathetic stimulation, however, is a redistribution of flow from the mucosa to the submucosa. Thus, the mucosa may be critically hypoperfused, despite nearly normal overall gut flow. The existence of countercurrent exchange of oxygen at the base of villi, from arteriolar inflow to venular outflow, steals some oxygen delivery from the villus tips (Fig. 5-2). This effect is facilitated by slow blood flow, so that when gut perfusion is severely compromised, necrosis of villus tips ensues.

Parasympathetic stimulation (e.g., feeding, organophosphate poisoning) increases mesenteric blood flow, although indirectly. This occurs because parasympathetic activity stimulates gut secretion and motility, activities which generate vasodilating metabolites and hormones.

Humoral substances, as well as neural influences, affect blood flow. Enteral feeding stimulates an increase in gut flow, in part, due to release of vasodilating hormones (e.g., cholecystokinin), and local vasodilators (e.g., serotonin, histamine). Of particular relevance in the ICU are drug therapies which activate the receptors of endogenous hormones. Infusions of epinephrine, norepinephrine, vasopressin, and moderate or high dose dopamine all decrease blood flow, while low dose dopamine augments flow.

GLUCOSE. The gut is one of the tissues which is rich in glycolytic enzymes, but less suited to oxidative metabolism. Therefore, substantial amounts of glucose are taken up by the mucosa, but only metabolized as far as lactate. Lactate then enters the portal blood, proceeds to the liver, and is reconverted to glucose (gluconeogenesis). During times of severe stress, glucose is spared for those organs which are obligate users, and glutamine uptake by the gut is augmented for energy needs. In addition, some of the glutamine is metabolized to alanine which can then be used for additional glucose synthesis in the liver.

GLUTAMINE. Glutamine metabolism plays two important roles in the gut response to critical illness. First, it is a path by which carbon sources for hepatic gluconeogenesis are processed. During severe stress, glutamine is released from muscle and lung. As noted above, glutamine replaces glucose as an energy source for the gut and provides a substrate for hepatic gluconeogenesis (after conversion to alanine by the intestinal mucosa). The ammonia released in this process contributes to hepatic urea synthesis and accounts for much of the loss of nitrogen during catabolic periods.

The second important role of glutamine is that it appears necessary for the normal mucosal barrier function. It has long been known that full nutritional support can be delivered through a central vein. However, the gut promptly atrophies if concomitant enteral feeding is not provided. Glutamine is not included in typical central formulas because it is classified as a nonessential amino acid, it represents an ammonia load, and it is poorly soluble. There is accumulating evidence, however, that glutamine is an essential nutrient for the gut. According to this hypothesis, gut atrophy during parenteral feeding may be due to a critical lack of glutamine. Mucosal atrophy may allow translocation of bacteria from the lumen to the lymphatics and the circulation. Once bacteria are not adequately contained, they may contribute to systemic inflammation, perpetuating multisystem organ failure (MSOF) (vide infra).

MUCOSAL INTEGRITY

NORMAL FLORA. Large numbers of bacteria are found in the gastrointestinal tract. The flora remains relatively constant in any given individual, but can rapidly fluctuate in response to illness, environment, or drugs. Few organisms are seen in the proximal gut, but their quantity increases with distance from the stomach. In the colon, nearly one-third of the dry weight of the feces consists of bacteria. Typical isolates in the colon include *Bacteroides*, *Bifidobacterium*, *Eubacterium*, and *Peptostreptococcus*. Despite the exposure of a tremendous surface area of the gut to this hostile microbial environment, the mucosa is a highly effective barrier preventing access of organisms and toxins.

DEFENSE AGAINST TRANSLOCATION. Movement of bacteria or yeast across the intestinal mucosa is termed *translocation*. The defense against translocation requires a healthy gut and depends on physical barriers (gastric acid, epithelial mucus layer, tight junctions), motility, phagocytic cells, and the gut-associated lymphoid tissue (GALT). Interference with gastric acidity, a routine part of preventive critical care, causes colonization of the normally sterile stomach and may contribute to nosocomial pneumonia. Normal motility is clearly important in limiting the proliferation of microorganisms as well. Peristalsis tends to roll bacteria up into intestinal mucus, then sends them toward the rectum. The relevance of this mechanism is evidenced by the effect on bacterial overgrowth in patients with chronic motility disorders or anatomic causes of stasis. For example, patients with small bowel diverticuli or stasis due to scleroderma routinely have bacterial overgrowth, often associated with diarrhea. Phagocytic cells must participate in the normal ecology of the bowel since chemotherapy-induced neutropenia renders the bowel susceptible to invasion. The GALT is responsible for secreting antigen-specific IgA into the lumen. T and B lymphocytes in the lamina propria are geographically well poised to defend against invasion. Glutamine is essential for gut metabolism during critical illness (vide supra), and apparently for normal structure and function as well, particularly during illness. How all of these factors interact to limit translocation is not fully known.

Disordered Motility

CLINICAL SYNDROMES

GASTRIC ATONY. Disordered gastric emptying is relatively uncommon in critically ill patients. Causes include drugs (e.g., narcotics), diabetes mellitus, severe electrolyte imbalances, respiratory failure, acidemia, trauma, and central nervous system diseases. Gastric atony may present insidiously, with mild abdominal distention or increased gastric residuals following feeding, or catastrophically, with massive pulmonary aspiration. Occasionally, the diagnosis is made from routine chest radiographs.

ILEUS. Motility disorders of the small bowel frequently complicate critical illness and are routine following laparotomy. Abdominal processes, acute infections, drugs, hypokalemia, and trauma lead the list of possible etiologies (Table 5-1). It is known that postoperative ileus is due to overwhelming sympathetic outflow from the splanchnic nerves. It seems likely that many other types of ileus, such as that following trauma and shock, are similarly mediated. Electrolyte disturbances might directly impair intrinsic muscle cell rhythmicity and alter the slow wave pattern (BER). Alternatively, disturbed smooth muscle cell electrical potentials might prevent the superimposed spike bursts necessary for peristalsis or directly impede smooth muscle contraction. Drugs have many direct and indirect effects on the gut. The most direct examples of this involve interaction of drug with gut receptor sites, as exemplified by the action of narcotics.

Ileus typically presents as abdominal distention. Additionally, vomiting, aspiration, pain, or respiratory failure may herald its onset. Ileus can be differentiated from other causes of abdominal distention (ascites, hemorrhage) by physical examination, abdominal radiograph, or ultrasound. Excluding mechanical obstruction is more difficult, and relies on the examination, x-ray findings, clinical setting, and evolution over time.

COLONIC PSEUDOOBSTRUCTION. Acute dilation of the colon not due to mechanical obstruction is an uncommon,

TABLE 5-1 Causes of Ileus

Abdominal Diseases
Peritonitis
Pancreatitis
Surgery and abdominal trauma
Retroperitoneal hemorrhage
Unrelieved mechanical obstruction
Infections
Sepsis
Pneumonia
Pyelonephritis
Drugs and Poisonings
Narotics
Anticholinergics
Cyclic antidepressants and phenothiazines
Calcium channel blockers
Ganglionic blockers
Mushroom poisoning
Electrolyte Derangements
Hypokalemia
Hypomagnesemia
Hypercalcemia
Miscellaneous
Shock and intestinal ischemia
Myocardial infarction
Rib or vertebral fracture
Scleroderma
Vasculitis
Parkinson's disease

but potentially devastating, occurrence in critically ill patients. Precipitants include sepsis, cardiogenic shock, major trauma, electrolyte derangements (hypokalemia, hypomagnesemia), drugs (narcotics, clonidine, phenothiazines, cyclic antidepressants, ganglion blockers, antiparkinsonian agents), abdominal disease (cholecystitis, pancreatitis, laparotomy), hepatic failure, uremia, metastatic cancer, hypothyroidism, and *Amanita* poisoning. Underlying diseases which seem to predispose to colonic pseudoobstruction include neurologic diseases (parkinsonism, multiple sclerosis, stroke, brain tumor, spinal cord transection), muscle disorders, pregnancy, and alcoholism. The typical patient presents with abdominal distention, often with preserved bowel sounds. Alternatively, massive colonic distention is detected on routine chest radiography or on an abdominal film. Usually the right colon is disproportionately dilated. The normal cecal diameter is 3.5 to 8.5 cm and is $<$7.5 cm in most normal persons. In pseudoobstruction, the diameter often exceeds 12 cm, above which the risk of perforation becomes significant. Colonoscopy serves to exclude obstruction and is usually therapeutic as well (vide infra).

CLINICAL CONSEQUENCES

Gastric atony, ileus, and colonic pseudoobstruction share several consequences which will be discussed in common. Most notable are elevated intraabdominal pressure, heightened risk of pulmonary aspiration, interference with nutrition, and impaired drug absorption.

ELEVATED INTRAABDOMINAL PRESSURE. Dilation of the stomach, small bowel, or colon raises intraabdominal pressure and thereby reduces functional residual capacity (FRC). Most critically ill patients already have a reduced FRC related to the supine position, muscular weakness, abdominal pain, ascites, or pulmonary edema. In addition, their closing volume (CV) may be simultaneously increased, due to advanced age, smoking, or airway disease. These two factors, reduced FRC and increased CV, lead to closure of airways during tidal breathing, thus causing atelectasis (see Chaps. 1 and 84). By further lowering FRC, abdominal distention exacerbates the tendency of the critically ill patient to develop atelectasis and respiratory failure.

A second feature of abdominal distention is that the work of breathing is related, in part, to the pressure that the diaphragm is required to generate with each breath. When abdominal pressure rises, the diaphragm has to work harder to maintain ventilation. By this mechanism, gut dysmotility may precipitate respiratory failure or prolong the need for mechanical ventilation.

RISK OF ASPIRATION. A further effect of increased intraabdominal (and therefore, intragastric) pressures is a tendency for regurgitation of gastric contents into the pharynx. Since many critically ill patients have depressed consciousness or impaired airway protection, pulmonary aspiration is a real risk, with consequences of acute hypoxemic respiratory failure or nosocomial pneumonia (see Chap. 136). Patients with disordered gastrointestinal motility are also susceptible to bacterial overgrowth, which potentially magnifies the effects of aspiration. Cuffed endotracheal tubes may limit, but do not prevent, pulmonary aspiration, and so are little insurance against this potentially lethal complication.

INTERFERENCE WITH NUTRITION. In one series of patients with acute respiratory failure, nearly half the patients developed abdominal distention during their ICU stay. Abdominal distention typically interrupts enteral feeding. At worst, attempts at nutrition are put on hold indefinitely. At best, parenteral nutrition, with its much higher risk and expense, is substituted. In some patients with postoperative ileus, needle catheter jejunostomy may be safe and successful.

DISORDERED DRUG ABSORPTION. Impaired gastric emptying leads to unpredictable effects on delivery of drugs to the intestine and varying rates of absorption. Bacterial overgrowth in the small bowel reduces drug uptake for several reasons—steatorrhea, drug metabolism by bacteria, and mucosal cell damage. Malabsorption of fat-soluble preparations is particularly likely.

TREATMENT

Several general measures apply to all causes of abdominal distention. First, mechanical causes of obstruction, such as peptic ulcer disease, adhesions, and tumors, must be excluded. Then, precipitants of disordered motility (especially drugs and electrolyte disturbances) should be sought and aggressively corrected. When narcotics are implicated, naloxone may bring about remarkable improvement. In most instances, enteral feeding should be discontinued, or at least reduced, to lessen the risk of aspiration. In patients with gastric atony, it may be possible to place a nasoenteric tube into the duodenum, bypassing the area of stasis. In the more common conditions of ileus and colonic pseudoobstruction, however, cessation of feeding and institution of nasogastric suction are necessary. Nasogastric suction does more than simply remove air and secretions. By decompressing a segment of bowel, it interrupts the intestinointestinal inhibitory reflex (vide supra), thereby contributing to recovery of bowel not directly decompressed.

To reduce the tendency to atelectasis, patients should be turned frequently and moved to the sitting position if at all possible. This will also reduce the work of breathing for those breathing spontaneously. For patients on mechanical ventilation, the addition of continuous positive airway pressure (CPAP) or positive end-expiratory pressure (PEEP) to restore FRC toward normal will further guard against atelectasis and hypoxemia.

GASTRIC ATONY AND ILEUS. Other than the general measures described above, there is little in the way of specific treatment for these disorders. Prokinetic agents have not been extensively studied but may be of some utility. Metaclopramide (10 mg intravenously) has been used with occasional benefit in patients with postoperative gastric atony and ileus. The newer prokinetic agents, domperidone and cisapride (4 mg intravenously), may have a role as well.

COLONIC PSEUDOOBSTRUCTION. In addition to the general measures detailed above, specific attempts to relieve colonic dilation may be necessary. As the cecal diameter exceeds 12 cm, perforation becomes progressively likely. Simple placement of a rectal tube may suffice, but the standard approach should be to perform colonoscopy. This procedure serves to rule out obstruction as well as to remove colonic gas. A long tube can be left in the colon to facilitate continued decompression. Care must be taken to carry out the examination without insufflating more gas into the colon. In some patients, repeat colonoscopy may be necessary for recurrent dilation, but the procedure is successful in about three-fourths of cases. Several days are required for full resolution of the syndrome, even after decompression. Therefore, prompt refeeding usually results in recurrence. If colonoscopic decompression cannot be accomplished, percutaneous cecostomy or laparotomy may be necessary.

Diarrhea and Malabsorption

Diarrhea is the most common expression of gastrointestinal dysfunction in critically ill patients. It is seen in approximately 50 percent of those who are enterally fed. While not usually a cause of mortality, diarrhea contributes substantially to morbidity and to demands on nursing time. Its greatest significance is that it provides an indicator of gastrointestinal dysfunction and should prompt the intensivist to pursue the underlying cause.

ETIOLOGY

In some patients, the cause is an obvious, preexisting condition such as sprue or inflammatory bowel disease. Many chronic illnesses are associated with intestinal bacterial overgrowth (Table 5-2), which causes diarrhea through interference with normal bile salt function (intraluminal deconjugation by bacteria as well as impaired micellar function). Bacterial overgrowth is known to occur acutely as well, especially in patients treated with antacids or histamine-blocking drugs. In other patients, the diarrhea is directly related to the reason for critical illness, such as intestinal infection or massive bowel resection for infarction. In a larger group of patients, a drug is the culprit. For example, antacids and cimetidine are frequently implicated in patients with diarrhea. Even more commonly, antibiotics are deemed the cause. It is particularly important to exclude pseudomembranous colitis in critically ill patients, since failure to make the diagnosis is a potentially devastating management error.

DIARRHEA OF CRITICAL ILLNESS

Evidence indicates that there is a diarrhea of critical illness, distinct from these specific causes. Even after considering all of the above etiologies of diarrhea, the critical care physician is frequently left without an explanation in a given patient. In the typical case, liquid stools begin with institution of enteral feeding and cease when feedings are held, suggesting an osmotic diarrhea. Rarely, a lactose-containing formula is responsible in a patient who is lactose intolerant. In most patients, however, diarrhea persists despite lactose-free feedings. Lactose-free, isotonic formulas do not cause diarrhea in normal volunteers or in patients with can-

TABLE 5-2 Intestinal Bacterial Overgrowth

Motility Disorders
Ileus and gastroparesis
Vagotomy
Autonomic neuropathy (including diabetes)
Drugs
Hypothyroidism
Scleroderma, amyloidosis
Anatomic Derangements
Strictures
Diverticula
Partial mechanical obstruction
Postsurgical
Fistulous tracts
Miscellaneous
Antacid regimens
Pancreatic insufficiency

cer who are hypoalbuminemic, but not critically ill, even when started at full strength. Therefore, the enteral formula itself is not to blame. Several potential alternative mechanisms include decreased plasma oncotic pressure, excessive mucosal capillary permeability, and protein calorie malnutrition.

DECREASED PLASMA ONCOTIC PRESSURE. The diarrhea of critical illness has been related to serum hypoalbuminemia. In one study, all patients who became rapidly hypoalbuminemic (<2.5 g/dL) developed diarrhea, whereas no patient with albumin level >2.6 g/dL did. One explanation for the association with serum albumin concentration depends on the importance of albumin in maintaining the normal balance of oncotic and hydrostatic forces affecting fluid flux across the extensive vasculature of the gut. By this mechanism, a marked drop in plasma oncotic pressure leads to fluid leakage into the interstitium of the bowel, overwhelming the ability of lymphatic drainage to return the fluid to the circulation. However, this hypothesis must not be complete, because it fails to explain the lack of diarrhea in some patients with extreme hypoalbuminemia as well as its occurrence in patients with a normal serum albumin level.

EXCESSIVE MUCOSAL CAPILLARY PERMEABILITY. In critically ill patients, a number of mediators are released which have the potential to cause a leaky microcirculation. Interleukin-1 (IL-1), tumor necrosis factor (TNF), bradykinin, and some prostaglandins facilitate fluid movement across capillaries. Especially when superimposed on the fall in plasma oncotic pressure due to concomitant hypoalbuminemia, this mechanism may be relevant. An apparent association between acute respiratory failure and diarrhea is intriguing in that it supports the notion of a systemic alteration in vascular permeability.

PROTEIN-CALORIE MALNUTRITION. Critically ill patients often develop protein-calorie malnutrition and are typically in negative nitrogen balance. In children who suffer acute protein-calorie malnutrition due primarily to protein deficiency (kwashiorkor), diarrhea is common, although incompletely understood. In both settings, several contributors to diarrhea can be identified. Abnormalities of protein synthesis contribute to reduced intestinal villous height, which results in a reduced surface area for absorption. In addition, activity of brush border disaccharidases and peptidases is reduced. Such a deficiency would lead to malabsorption of carbohydrates and proteins, which would then act to cause osmotic water loss from the bowel. Impaired pancreatic enzyme secretion, another consequence of protein-calorie malnutrition, contributes to malabsorption of fats. As malabsorption of nutrients progresses, malnutrition worsens, and a downward spiral is initiated.

IMPLICATIONS FOR THERAPY

The distress of patients and nurses is reason enough to search for treatments for the diarrhea of critically ill patients. In addition, there is evidence that patients who manifest diarrhea have excess mortality. In one study, this association was noted even when patients were stratified according to severity of illness. It may be that gastrointestinal dysfunction, as revealed by intolerance of feedings, is a subtle indicator of a sicker patient than indicated by standard scores of severity of illness. Alternatively, patients who cannot tolerate enteral feeding may develop early malnutrition, gut atrophy, and bacterial translocation (vide infra). By this mechanism, diarrhea may actually have a detrimental impact on survival.

If hypoalbuminemia is a major contributor to diarrhea, then albumin infusion may lead to improvement, and some evidence supports this. On the other hand, if protein-calorie malnutrition is the predominant cause of diarrhea, then prompt institution of nutrition is essential. Since gut atrophy and bacterial translocation occur within hours of acute illness, trauma, or burns, one group of investigators has worried that an attempt to use the enteral route (which often fails) simply wastes time. They have suggested that immediate parenteral nutrition may be a superior approach, but this has never been investigated. Finally, there has been some success reported with the use of formulas containing small molecular weight peptides, rather than the standard protein-based solutions. Possibly, this form of protein is easier to digest and absorb, reversing protein malnutrition, resulting in improved mucosal function, and thereby restoring normal absorptive capacity. In a group of critically ill, hypoalbuminemic patients, use of peptide-based enteral feedings was associated with dramatic improvement in serum albumin concentration. It seems that there is further room for investigation of the causes and treatments of the diarrhea of critical illness.

Translocation and Gut-Related Sepsis

ETIOLOGY OF GUT BARRIER FAILURE

The normal barrier function of the gut may be compromised by local injury to the gut as well as by severe systemic illness. These include such local insults to the bowel as intestinal infection, radiation enteritis, chemotherapy-induced mucositis, inflammatory bowel diseases, and ischemic injury. Systemic disorders are important as well, such as sepsis, massive trauma, severe malnutrition, and all hypoperfusion states. It is easy to understand how local bowel injury allows bacteria or their products to enter the circulation; the pathogenesis in systemic disorders is more cryptic. Nevertheless, fatal systemic infections with gut-related bacteria, with no infective focus found at autopsy despite intensive searching, are major problems in patients with trauma, burns, and MSOF.

PATHOPHYSIOLOGY OF TRANSLOCATION

Systemic illness probably facilitates bacterial translocation by generating local gut injury. In experimental models, hemorrhagic shock induces mucosal damage in a dose-dependent fashion. Some of this injury may be mediated by oxygen-free radicals, since it is ameliorated by xanthine oxidase inhibition. Excessive mucosal leakiness can be demonstrated as early as 2 h after a defined stimulus, with bacteria found in the mesenteric lymph nodes. From there, bacteria can enter the systemic circulation causing sepsis. In addition, bacteria or bacterial products may affect the liver via the portal blood. This could result in direct hepatic injury (e.g., the cholestatis of sepsis) or indirectly stimulate the release of monokines from hepatic mononuclear cells. Release of IL-1, interleukin-6, and TNF then provokes the sepsis syndrome. It is even possible that bacteria liberated through translocation due to systemic illness, if not contained, can induce further mucosal derangement, perpetuating the septic state. Although this sequence of events has not been conclusively demonstrated in patients, substantial circumstantial evidence indicates that it contributes significantly to morbidity and mortality.

THE ROLE OF NUTRITION

Nutritional modulation alone, even without a local gut or systemic injury, can produce bacterial translocation. In one study, two-thirds of healthy animals given no oral nutrition, but fed with a standard parenteral nutrition formula, developed translocation. While similar information has not been obtained for human beings, in patients on total parenteral nutrition (TPN), villous atrophy can be demonstrated, a feature which may indicate a less than healthy gut barrier.

THE IMPORTANCE OF ENTERAL FEEDING. When injury is superimposed, the impact of nutrition is even more striking. One day following burn injury, experimental animals which are fed only lactated Ringer's solution demonstrate a 50 percent reduction in jejunal mucosal weight (also, in thickness and DNA content). In contrast, similar animals which are given enteral feeding immediately postburn show no significant reduction in mucosal weight.

In addition, prompt enteral feeding can ameliorate the hypermetabolic response typical of injury. When enteral feeding is delayed for several days, a hypermetabolic response is seen with a rise in energy expenditure of nearly 200 percent. Immediate feeding inhibits this increase by 80 percent. Similar salutary effects can be shown on serum cortisol levels and adrenal weight. These findings suggest that bacterial translocation is occurring in animals not enterally fed and is prevented (or lessened) when food is given.

THE ROLE OF GLUTAMINE. The specifics of nutrition are relevant as well. As noted above, animals given only TPN develop translocation. If the same TPN solution is given enterally, translocation is significantly reduced, although not eliminated. Standard enteral feeding, however, prevents translocation. There is accumulating evidence that glutamine is a critical factor in the gut response to nutrition and a major determinant of translocation. Glutamine, which is essential for normal bowel integrity, is not provided in standard TPN formulas. It is, however, a component of enteral feedings. In this hypothesis, glutamine is necessary for the normal gut barrier function, and its deficiency leads to translocation. In fact, glutamine-enriched diets diminish bowel injury and translocation in animals treated with chemotherapy or radiation. Of further interest, sepsis and endotoxemia have been shown to impair gut mucosal utilization of glutamine. This information provides a potential pathophysiologic mechanism for sepsis-induced mucosal permeability. Thus, sepsis leads to intestinal mucosal deficiency of glutamine. Glutamine depletion leads to impaired synthesis of purines and pyrimidines (since glutamine is the nitrogen donor for these reactions), thereby impairing cell replication. In addition, since glutamine is the principal fuel of the gut, energy generation may be compromised. Finally, since glutamine is essential for lymphocyte function, its deficiency may impair the GALT. Some combination of these factors eventuates in a disordered gut barrier, and bacteria enter the circulation.

THE IMPACT OF DIETARY LIPID. In burn injury, the lipid constituents of enteral feedings appear important as well. Animals fed with linoleic acid were compared with those given fish oil (one-third of which consisted of omega-3 fatty acids). Animals given fish oil had significantly greater body weight, but significantly lower adrenal weight, than those fed with linoleic acid. Several measures of lymphocyte-mediated immune function showed impairment in animals given linoleic acid, a result which was partly blocked by concomitant indomethacin administration. These findings suggest a possible role for nutritionally derived cyclooxygenase metabolites in burn-related immune suppression. A prospective trial in burned patients using a diet based on these findings revealed a reduction in wound infection and mortality in those given the special diet.

IMPLICATIONS FOR THERAPY

Provision of nutrition clearly affects outcome in critically ill patients. The enteral route is preferred because of safety, ease, and cost. In addition, the enteral route is probably superior in the prevention of bacterial translocation, and therefore, is likely to be beneficial in limiting the occurrence of MSOF. This may be due, in part, to the important role of glutamine in maintaining a healthy gut barrier, since this amino acid is not contained in standard TPN solutions. Because the enteral route is not always practical, there is a role for parenteral formulas which incorporate glutamine or contain dipeptides which include glutamine. The principle of early enteral feeding likely underlies the impressive historical improvement in burn survival noted in the early 1970s. With further study, we may learn even better how to save patients with massive trauma, septic shock, and hemorrhage, by perfecting our approach to nutrition.

Nonobstructive Cholestasis

Many critically ill patients develop elevations of serum bilirubin associated with normal synthetic function and no evidence of hepatic necrosis. Serious infection is the most common predisposing factor, but multiple trauma and the postoperative state are also associated. This finding typically prompts an investigation for biliary obstruction, hepatitis, and drug toxicity, usually with no definite cause found.

In experimental animals, endotoxin infusion results in cholestasis, suggesting a role for this substance in the pathogenesis of cholestasis. However, gram-positive infections commonly underlie the cholestasis of sepsis as well. In particular, severe pneumococcal pneumonia and staphylococcal endocarditis precipitate this syndrome. Recently, lipoteichoic acid, derived from *Staphylococcus aureus*, has been shown to cause defective hepatic excretory function. Yet, it seems likely that there is a mechanism common to both gram-positive and gram-negative sepsis as well as other forms of nonobstructive jaundice.

A clue has been suggested from the treatment of patients with malignancy using interleukin-2 (IL-2). These patients develop profound cholestasis, without hepatocellular injury or necrosis, which resolves within a few days of discontinuation of IL-2. IL-2 may directly affect bile secretion or it may induce other cytokines (e.g., TNF) which then cause hepatic dysfunction. Hepatocytes are not known to have IL-2 receptors, but the many lymphoid cells in the liver might mediate the effect. Since both gram-positive and gram-negative bacteria have the capacity to induce cytokine production, this may provide a mechanism for hyperbilirubinemia.

A similar pathophysiology may pertain in patients without sepsis, but with bowel-related translocation. Stimulation by bacterial products of cytokines from liver-associated mononuclear cells could explain postoperative and trauma-related jaundice in some patients. A clearer picture of nonobstructive cholestasis is likely to emerge soon in this rapidly evolving field.

Nutrition

Until the past 30 years, feeding critically ill patients was impossible. The detrimental effects of starvation were added to the injury of critical illness, compounding morbidity and mortality. The current availability of a broad array of enteral and parenteral formulas makes nourishment of any severely ill patient possible. It is now appropriate to devise a plan for nutrition in all patients admitted to the ICU, once initial resuscitation is accomplished. Reassessment of the goals and methods of nutritional support should be part of the daily care of critically ill patients.

This chapter includes an overview of the neuroendocrine response to injury, the detrimental consequences of failure to provide nutrition, and recommendations for feeding critically ill patients. Each of these topics is more fully elaborated in Chaps. 90 to 95.

The nutritional needs of patients in the ICU are largely of two types. One group of patients is hypercatabolic due to injury (e.g., septic shock, multiple trauma), is resistant to protein administration, and demonstrates a high caloric need. A smaller group consists of patients who are predominantly malnourished, rather than acutely injured (e.g., acute on chronic respiratory failure). These patients are protein avid and require fewer calories. It is important to realize that nutritional needs evolve in a dynamic way over time. For example, the patient who is markedly hypermetabolic 3 days following multiple trauma may not be hypermetabolic a month later, although he may still be in the ICU on a ventilator. In fact, if nutritional needs have not been fully met during the early, hypermetabolic phase, after a month the patient may be predominantly malnourished. There is even substantial variation in energy expenditure from day to day in a given patient, making accurate assessment of nutritional needs even more difficult. These points highlight the need to periodically reassess the metabolic status of patients in the ICU and to reevaluate each patient's nutritional plan on an ongoing basis.

THE RESPONSE TO INJURY

Patients admitted to the ICU have suffered a wide assortment of insults, ranging from minor surgical procedures to massive burns. Although there are significant quantitative differences in the physiologic responses to trauma, surgery, sepsis, and burns, the substantial qualitative similarities can be termed the *stress response*. Each of these injuries provokes a realignment of metabolic homeostasis (hypermetabolism), the purpose of which is to subserve repair of damaged tissue.

NEUROENDOCRINE MEDIATION. Hypermetabolism is mediated by neural and humoral pathways. Pain receptors and other nerve endings at the site of injury transmit signals to the hypothalamus, where they are integrated with various physiologic and psychologic inputs. The hypothalamus subsequently activates the sympathetic nervous system, stimulates the adrenal medulla, and spurs the pituitary gland to produce growth hormone and ACTH. In addition, inflammatory cells recruited to areas of tissue damage secrete polypeptides, such as IL-1 and TNF. These substances amplify the hypothalamic inputs, but have further direct effects on liver, muscles, and the reticuloendothelial system. Finally, gut translocation (vide supra) may independently activate the injury response, compounding and propagating hypermetabolism (Fig. 5-3).

METABOLIC CONSEQUENCES. The outcome of the neuroendocrine response to injury is a set of stereotyped metabolic derangements. The fundamental purpose of these changes can only be guessed at, but the likely goals are wound repair and control of infection. For example, wounds consume tremendous quantities of glucose and may benefit from the typical hyperglycemia of injury. The importance of glutamine for white blood cell production and gut mucosal integrity has previously been discussed; ensuring sufficient amounts may necessitate muscle protein catabolism. Meeting these and other goals necessitates the readjustment of normal carbohydrate, protein, and fat metabolism.

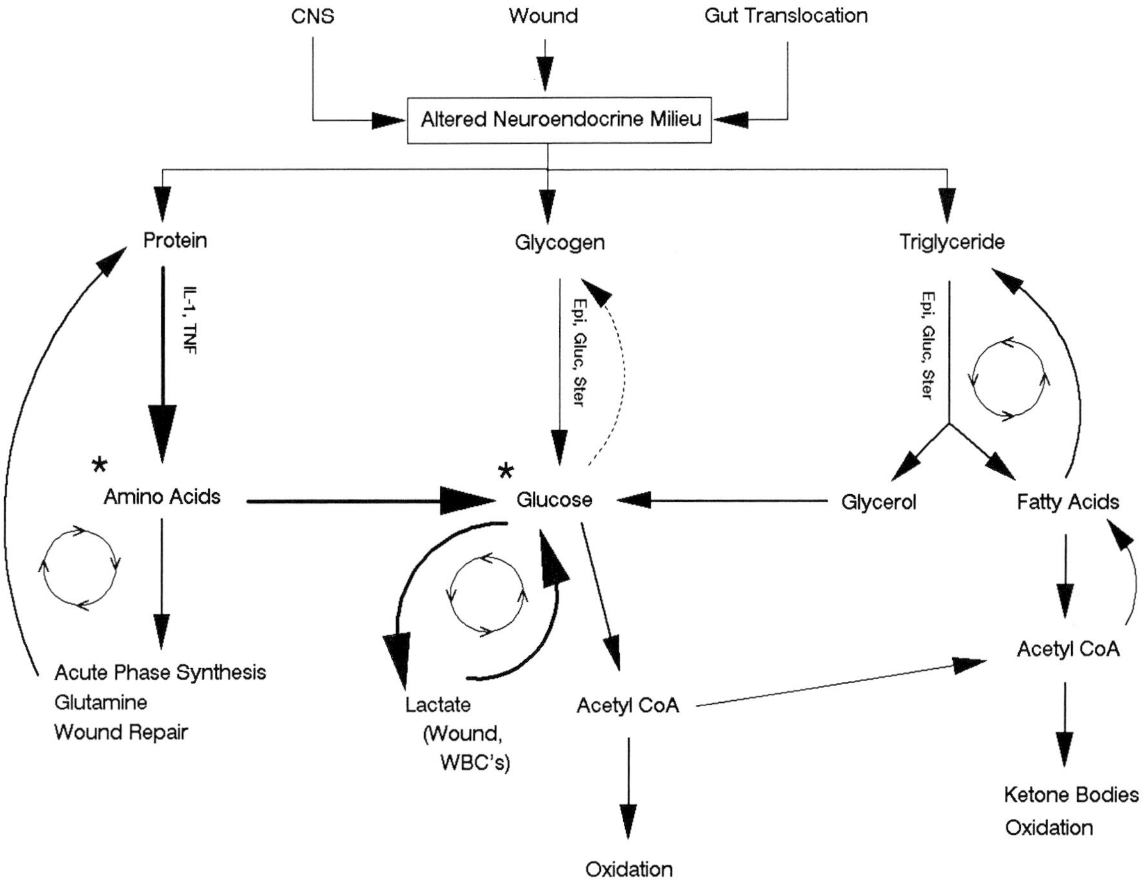

FIGURE 5-3 Hypermetabolism in critical illness. The goals of the neuroendocrine alterations seen in critically ill patients seem to be to provide adequate glucose for wound repair and sufficient amino acids for new protein synthesis. Glutamine appears to be particularly important in maintaining the integrity of rapidly dividing tissues such as immune cells, bone marrow cells, and the gut mucosa. The arrowed circles indicate substrate cycles in which energy is consumed with no net production of structural or metabolic materials. Epi, epinephrine; Gluc, glucagon; Ster, corticosteroids; IL-1, interleukin 1; TNF, tumor necrosis factor.

Carbohydrate Metabolism. Both glucose and insulin levels are increased following injury. Thus, part of the stress response includes insulin resistance, attributable to the pronounced release of counterregulatory hormones (glucagon, cortisol, epinephrine). Nevertheless, hyperglycemia is a result of increased synthesis rather than decreased consumption of glucose. Glucose is derived from amino acids and the glycerol component of fat through gluconeogenesis in addition to that given enterally or intravenously. The amount produced more than compensates for the increased oxidation of glucose in injured patients. Glucose turnover is augmented even more than glucose oxidation, with large amounts being glycolized to lactate in damaged tissues, then back to glucose in the liver. Although such cycling does not result in net consumption of glucose, large quantities of energy are lost and heat generated.

Protein Metabolism. Protein synthesis is elevated for the production of acute phase reactants, wound repair, and synthesis of inflammatory cells. However, protein breakdown (largely in muscle) greatly exceeds synthesis, leading to net catabolism (negative nitrogen balance). Some of this protein is broken down to provide amino acids required for new synthesis. However, most is converted to glucose to supply the brain, wound, and white blood cells. In severe injury, nitrogen loss can be as high as 30 g/day, corresponding to 180 g protein daily.

Fat Metabolism. Oxidation of fat is increased in hypermetabolic patients to provide energy. However, mobilization of triglyceride from fat stores greatly exceeds the amount oxidized. Most of the liberated fatty acids are simply reesterified to fat in an energy-consuming "substrate cycle." Plasma glycerol levels rise, providing for gluconeogenesis. Ketogenesis is inhibited by the elevated insulin levels, so that ketone body concentrations are not elevated.

THE RATIONALE FOR NUTRITION

During starvation, raw materials for new synthesis, as well as energy for maintaining all life processes, must be derived from within the body. While small stores of energy are present as muscle and liver glycogen, these are depleted in the first hours to days of starvation. Much larger adipose deposits may be available to contribute to caloric needs, but they cannot meet the demand for glucose and essential amino acids. The response to starvation includes the breakdown of protein to provide these building blocks. Only the nervous system is spared this internal cannibalism, while muscles suffer the most.

The detrimental impact of protein breakdown is reflected in the morbidity and mortality of patients who are starved, compared with those who are fed, especially as demonstrated in infectious complications and delayed wound healing. Respiratory failure is another consequence of nutritional deprivation, because the respiratory muscles are not shielded from structural protein loss. Even healthy subjects who are starved demonstrate reductions in respiratory muscle function and spirometric values. Conversely, adequate nutrition is of demonstrated benefit to ventilator-dependent patients.

NUTRITIONAL GUIDELINES

The goal of nutrition is largely to prevent catabolism of protein. Simply infusing glucose reduces protein breakdown, but substantial losses continue, especially in the most seriously ill patients. The protein-sparing effect of glucose increases with the amount infused, but even when enough is given to meet the energy expenditure, nitrogen losses continue. Protein losses can be further limited by providing nitrogen (as amino acid infusions or enteral protein hydrolysates). Severely ill patients are resistant to nitrogen intake, however, and increasing benefits are seen only up to about 200 mg nitrogen/kg/day. Above this amount, no additional nitrogen sparing is apparent.

Zero nitrogen balance can be achieved, even in the sickest patients, but only by giving glucose or lipid in amounts greatly exceeding energy requirements. Unfortunately, giving this much energy has negative consequences. Excess parenteral lipid is tolerated poorly, with rising triglyceride levels, hyperlipidemia, and consequences for pulmonary gas exchange. Even enteral lipid seems harmful when given in large quantities and may be immunosuppressive. Carbohydrate excess leads to fat deposition (lipogenesis), which greatly increases CO_2 production. Thus, while the primary goal of nutrition is to limit protein catabolism, this must be tempered by the negative consequences of reaching zero nitrogen balance. The best compromise for the critically ill patient is not known.

ENERGY EXPENDITURE. Nutritional guidelines are necessarily arbitrary and will remain so until large numbers of patients are studied comparing various approaches. It makes sense that nutritional supplementation should match the energy needs of each individual patient. However, measuring energy needs remains impractical in most ICUs. The resting energy expenditure (REE) can be estimated from the Harris-Benedict equation, which takes into account age, sex, height, and weight. This is often modified by a factor to account for the severity of illness and the degree of malnutrition, for example using the data of Kinney. However, these estimations only poorly predict the actual measured energy expenditure in critically ill patients. In fact, simply choosing an average value for REE (e.g., 1850 kcal) is as accurate as using formulas in predicting the measured value in an individual patient. Since complicated equations do so poorly, their use is probably not justified. If REE is not measured, it is simpler and as accurate to use a fixed value for determining caloric needs. Hopefully, future developments in metabolic assessment will allow the widespread use of accurate, inexpensive methods to determine nutritional needs, leading to a rational, individualized plan for each patient.

SPECIFIC GUIDELINES. A reasonable set of guidelines is to give critically ill adults 40 kcal/kg/day, with a ratio of 150 calories/g nitrogen. For a 70-kg patient, this corresponds to 2800 kcal and 19 g nitrogen (about 118 g protein) a day. For patients who are malnourished, but not severely stressed (e.g., exacerbation of chronic obstructive pulmonary disease), fewer calories are necessary. Such patients should be given 32.5 kcal/day with a ratio of 100 calories/g nitrogen. For a 60-kg malnourished patient, this corresponds to 1950 kcal and 19.5 g nitrogen (122 g protein) a day (Table 5-3). Nonprotein calories can be given as lipid or carbohydrate, and the particular amount of each is probably not important (but vide infra). Most often, nonprotein calories are given as 70 percent carbohydrate and 30 percent fat.

Ideally, nutrition can be given enterally, since this route is cheaper, safer, and may reduce bacterial translocation. When the enteral route is not available, parenteral nutrition should be considered. In patients who are relatively healthy, and who are expected to resume eating in short order, dextrose-containing fluids may suffice. However, in most critically ill patients, it is important to institute nutrition on admission, even if this requires the parenteral route.

SPECIAL SITUATIONS. It is occasionally necessary to adjust the nutritional goals because of complicating illness, such as hepatic failure. In the future, nutrition may become even more tailored to the specific patient, with different formulas for patients who are burned, septic, encephalopathic, or in

TABLE 5-3 Nutritional Guidelines

1. Patients who are minimally injured and likely to resume eating in 3 days or less can be given dextrose-containing fluids alone.
2. Seriously injured or septic patients should receive 40 kcal/kg/day, with a ratio of 150 calories/g nitrogen. Carbohydrate should contribute 50–70% of nonprotein calories.
3. Malnourished patients who are not septic or seriously injured should receive 32.5 kcal/day with a ratio of 100 calories/g nitrogen. Carbohydrate should contribute 50–70% of nonprotein calories.
4. The enteral route should be used whenever possible, with a commercially available polymeric preparation.
5. The amount of CO_2 produced per calorie can be reduced by increasing the proportion of lipid. This may be appropriate in rare situations where a decrement in CO_2 production may facilitate successful spontaneous ventilation.

respiratory failure. Given the current state of knowledge, only a few particular conditions require adjustment of nutrition.

Hepatic Failure. Protein restriction is often necessary in the patient with impaired hepatic function. In patients who are comatose, complete avoidance of enteral protein is appropriate. In those who are only mildly encephalopathic, initial restriction to 20 to 40 g protein daily may suffice. The rate of protein administration may be increased if it is tolerated without worsening mental function. The use of parenteral formulas which contain high concentrations of branched-chain amino acids may allow the provision of protein without a deterioration in mentation, but the utility of these solutions remains controversial (see Chap. 93).

Renal Failure. In patients with uremia, it is appropriate to reduce the nitrogen load of enteral or parenteral feedings. Restriction of protein intake to 40 to 60 g/day will ameliorate the rise in blood urea nitrogen (BUN). Once renal recovery begins, or dialysis becomes necessary, dietary protein should be increased to a more usual amount. In the patient who develops renal failure as a complication of sepsis or multiple trauma, it may be preferable to give full nutrition while instituting early dialysis.

Chronic Obstructive Pulmonary Disease. The amount of CO_2 produced per calorie consumed differs among carbohydrate, fat, and protein. This is generally expressed as the ratio of moles of CO_2 produced per moles of oxygen consumed ($\dot{V}_{CO_2}/\dot{V}_{O_2}$), called the respiratory quotient (RQ). The value of RQ for carbohydrate is 1.0, for fat 0.7, and for protein, 0.8. Thus it is possible to adjust (slightly) the amount of CO_2 produced in any patient by altering the constituents of the nutritional formula. Most commonly this is applied in patients with limited ability to excrete CO_2, in whom a greater fraction of the calories is given as fat.

PART II

THE ORGANIZATION OF CRITICAL CARE

EDITORS' INTRODUCTION

This part of the text is divided into "Procedures and Technology in the ICU," "Management of the ICU," and "Stabilization and Transport of the Critically Ill." In "Procedures and Technology," the technical aspects which underlie the practice of critical care medicine are described. In each chapter, the indications, contraindications, technique, and complications of essential procedures are reviewed. Some procedures (such as thoracentesis) are well established in medicine, and their indications are generally agreed upon. The place of others (such as extracorporeal membrane oxygenation or hyperbaric oxygenation) in critical care is yet to be completely defined, and their indications are vigorously debated. In covering these controversial topics we attempt to place the subject in perspective to inform the practicing intensivist. Our goal is to facilitate the application of new technology where it contributes to patient care. On the other hand, we urge restraint when "high tech" is requested simply because it is new.

In each of these procedural chapters, the emphasis is on thoughtful interpretation of the results, instead of technical expertise. While technical competence is essential, it is not sufficient. This is consonant with our belief that critical care is not defined by the technology of the ICU. Rather, technology is employed to aid the physician in his or her attempt to discern and synthesize the pathophysiology of critical illness. Procedures should be instituted with discrete physiologic goals or to answer a specific question. In this way, technology contributes to care instead of confounding it.

In "Management of the ICU," several issues crucial to the efficient functioning of the modern, multidisciplinary ICU are described. The ICU is no longer simply a room in which ventilators are used. Instead, in the well-functioning ICU, the physical plant and technology are planned to facilitate the delivery of care while also responding to new opportunities in this rapidly evolving field. The physician director, the nursing manager, and the respiratory therapist must build a mutually supportive environment conducive to teaching, learning, and care. Intensivists must be aware of economic and legal concerns as ICUs capture the interest of politicians, ethicists, and the courts. Finally, the managers of ICUs can build on experience. Quality assurance, triage and severity scoring, and infection surveillance are essential to the continued smooth running of ICUs and, indeed, to their improvement over time.

The final component of this part of the text, "Stabilization and Transport of the Critically Ill,'' is intended to guide the resuscitation of seriously ill patients in order for them to benefit from critical care, and to provide for their safety when the controlled environs of the ICU must temporarily be left behind. It closes with the concepts underlying successful disaster planning. Of course, the approaches to resuscitation described here form the basis for the initial therapy of many critical illnesses described in Part III. We place the discussion of this topic here to complete ''The Organization of Critical Care'' in the belief that the timely stabilization of critically ill patients depends on the prior organization of structures and personnel to efficiently implement the concepts of pathophysiology discussed in Part I.

SECTION A

PROCEDURES AND TECHNOLOGY IN THE ICU

Chapter 6

AIRWAY MANAGEMENT AND INTUBATION

MITCHELL KEAMY

TABLE 6-1 Indications for Intubation

Cardiopulmonary arrest
Airway support
- Mechanical airway obstruction (e.g., edema, pharyngeal mass)
- Pharyngeal instability (facial fractures)
- Depressed level of consciousness with absent gag reflex, absent cough, or inability to maintain airway with head in flexion
- Bulbar or generalized motor weakness

Respiratory failure
- Arterial blood gases with P_{O_2} <50 torr or arterial hemoglobin saturation <85% on F_{IO_2} >0.6
- Severe respiratory acidosis or severe uncompensated metabolic acidosis without an obviously reversible etiology
- Tachypnea >35 breaths/min with accessory muscle recruitment and signs of patient distress (i.e., diaphoresis, tachy- or bradydysrhythmias, severe dyspnea, clammy cyanosis)

Miscellaneous
- Frequent recurrent nonperfusing dysrhythmias
- Hemodynamically compromising sepsis

Endotracheal intubation is a highly invasive intervention that deprives the patient of speech and inflicts severe physical and emotional discomfort. The performance of endotracheal intubation is frequently attended by a dramatic stabilization of a critical situation; less frequently, but more memorably, a mismanaged intubation can disrupt an otherwise controlled situation, and in the extreme can precipitate death. Moreover, such calamity may not simply be the result of failure to establish an appropriate prosthetic airway, but may be the result of secondary neurologic and cardiovascular stresses associated with the introduction and manipulation of a foreign body in the pharynx and trachea.

Most commonly, the endotracheal tube (ETT) is placed to provide a convenient gastight coupling to a mechanical ventilator or to provide a reliable conduit to deliver inhalation or positive-pressure therapy. It is used to ensure an adequate low resistance pathway for pulmonary gas flow in patients who for neurologic or mechanical reasons cannot sustain the complex pharyngeal coordination required to maintain a patent airway. Least reliably, it is used as a means to protect the lungs from aspiration of pharyngeal and other gastrointestinal secretions.[1]

Assessing the Need for Intubation

The need for intubation can be obvious and immediate (cardiopulmonary arrest), emergent (hypoventilation, respiratory acidosis with obtundation), or subtle (depressed level of consciousness with impaired airway protective reflexes). Initial evaluation must proceed rapidly (Table 6-1). In a patient who is spontaneously breathing, high flow oxygen at maximal fraction inspired oxygen (F_{IO_2}) should be administered and the cardiac rhythm, blood pressure, and arterial blood gases obtained. Pulse oximetry allows continuous visible and audible assessment of oxygen saturation and is advisable. While the evaluation is underway, helpers should gather the equipment necessary to support immediate intubation.

Obtundation, stupor, or coma may be caused by hypoxia and possibly hypercapnia. If changes in mental status are the result of hypoxia, ventilation and intubation are urgent, because even brief periods of hypoxia may result in irreversible cerebral injury. Also, hypoxia sufficient to depress the level of consciousness often leads to precipitous cardiovascular collapse. In contrast, hypercapnia and concomitant acidosis are well tolerated in patients without intercurrent intracranial pathology, with the primary consequence being cardiac dysrhythmias. On occasion, patients with adequate blood gases but extreme respiratory distress will involute, becoming oblivious to external stimulation as they focus on respiration. Following intubation and assisted ventilation, such patients will become alert to their surroundings and will interact appropriately. Thus, need for intubation is often determined independent of blood gas results.

Depressed consciousness is a relative indication for intubation. Absent gag reflex or cough on suctioning suggests absent airway protective reflexes. If the cervical spine is stable, the head should be flexed. Airway obstruction on flexion demonstrates the patient's inability to maintain a patent airway and is an indication for elective intubation. Patients who require appliances or special attention to maintain airway patency (e.g., oral airway in a stuporous patient) should be prophylactically intubated; experience suggests that such situations are unstable and can unexpectedly result in vomiting with aspiration or sudden unrecognized obstruction with respiratory arrest. Patients with depressed level of consciousness should be assessed when they are asleep and otherwise undisturbed, because at that time the risk of obstruction and aspiration is greatest.

Cyanosis is an unreliable sign of hypoxemia. It is detected when at least 5 g/dL hemoglobin are desaturated.

Therefore, cyanosis may be absent in anemia in the presence of dangerous hypoxemia. Conversely, polycythemic patients or patients with venous plethora (e.g., superior vena cava syndrome) may manifest cyanosis with adequate arterial saturation. Fortunately, the increasing availability of pulse oximetry has made the unreliable visual assessment of cyanosis less clinically pertinent. Cyanosis with cold diaphoretic skin suggests intense autonomic stress and circulatory failure and is usually accompanied by tachycardia. If the patient is bradycardic, full arrest is imminent, and intubation and resuscitation should be performed immediately.

Respiratory efforts should be noted. Slow deep respirations (<10/min) suggest pharmacologic, metabolic, or neurologic respiratory depression. This sense is reinforced if the patient exhibits no distress in the face of uncompensated hypercapnia. Tachypnea (>30/min) is a nonspecific finding that may indicate respiratory load disorders such as decreased compliance from pulmonary edema or pneumonia, increased resistance in asthma or chronic obstructive pulmonary disease (COPD), weakened or fatigued muscles of respiration, or increased minute volume requirements due to increased dead space or increased metabolic rate. It is also a common finding in pulmonary embolus. Tachypnea itself is not an indication for intubation, but a respiratory rate >35 breaths/min associated with the use of the accessory muscles of respiration suggests a mechanical respiratory load that the patient will not be able to sustain.

Respiratory motions should be examined for symmetry. Side-to-side asymmetry is present with pneumothorax, splinting, massive unilateral consolidation, or bronchial obstruction. Flail chest will present with paradoxical motion of the affected segment. With airway obstruction, patients demonstrate a characteristic rocking motion, as diaphragm inspiratory effort causes the upper chest to paradoxically retract. During the evaluation, respiratory flow should be assessed by placing a hand in front of the patient's mouth and nose. If flow is absent with visible respiratory efforts, the airway should be opened by head extension and advancement of the mandible.

By the end of this brief examination, the need for immediate intubation will have been established. During this evaluation, an arterial sample for blood gas should be drawn and sent to the laboratory. A Pa_{O_2} <50 mmHg or an arterial hemoglobin saturation <85 percent on >60 percent O_2 by mask is a commonly held marker of the need for intubation. This is in part because it is virtually impossible to maintain an inspired oxygen concentration >60 percent by any available mask delivery system. In addition, intubation is likely to be necessary to facilitate therapy with positive end-expiratory pressure (PEEP), although selected patients may benefit from continuous positive pressure (CPAP) by mask.[2]

An arterial pH <7.30, either from respiratory acidosis or uncompensated metabolic acidosis, reflects inability of the respiratory system to maintain acid-base homeostasis. If the patient remains stable, such acidosis may be tolerated while specific therapy is instituted (e.g., acute bronchodilator therapy, reversal of residual pharmacologic neuromuscular block, treatment of narcotic overdose or diabetic ketoacidosis) provided that the physician remains at hand to initiate intubation and ventilatory support should the therapy be unsuccessful.

Normal arterial blood gases should not engender a false sense of security in a patient with subjective respiratory distress. Impending mechanical respiratory failure is often preceded by a period of hyperventilation and alkalosis. Simple clinical guidelines include an assessment of the patient's ability to talk. The inability to converse in full phrases suggests an absence of respiratory reserve.

In equivocal situations, sequential measurement of respiratory rate, arterial blood gases, and forced vital capacity (FVC) will provide data on which to base the need for intubation. FVC >15 ml/kg body weight, when associated with an acceptable arterial blood gas value, is a predictor of adequate mechanical respiratory capacity. FVC <12 ml/kg should alert the clinician to the potential need for airway support; such low capacity is insufficient to power cough and promote the sighs necessary to clear airways and avoid progressive atelectasis.

Equipment and Initial Preparation

Ideally, securing the airway should be accomplished with minimal risk and with no negative perturbations in hemo-

TABLE 6-2 Equipment List for Intubation

Cardiac Arrest
Laryngoscope with functioning light
ETTs 7.5, 8.0, 8.5
Suction with Yankauer tip
Malleable metal stylet
10-ml syringe for cuff inflation
Oxygen supply with bag and mask ventilation system
Stethoscope
Gloves
Eye protection
Urgent and Elective Intubation
Functioning IV line
Monitors:
- ECG
- Blood pressure system
- Pulse oximeter

Suction catheters
Resuscitation cart
Adjuvant drugs:
- Atropine
- IV lidocaine
- Ephedrine
- Paralytics (succinylcholine, vecuronium)
- Sedatives/hypnotics/narcotics
- Topical anesthetics

Tape
Magill forceps
Fiberoptic scope
Cricothyrotomy
Scalpel
Kelly clamp
6.0 cuffed ETT

dynamics or blood gases. During intubation, circumstances change rapidly. Factors that may complicate the procedure (e.g., vomiting or anatomic irregularities) should be anticipated. To this end, appropriate monitoring, tools, and drugs should be assembled prior to attempting intubation (Table 6-2). In cardiopulmonary arrest, intubation must be accomplished immediately. In this situation, minimum required equipment is an ETT (with a functioning cuff), stylet, laryngoscope, oxygen bag-mask, and suction. Patients in less immediate need of intubation can be supported with bag-mask assistance coordinated with their spontaneous respiratory efforts, while appropriate preparations are made. Table 6-2 contains a list of equipment which should be available to support intubation in the ICU.

While preparation is made for the intubation, a further patient evaluation should be undertaken to survey for potential impediments and risks (Table 6-3). The airway anatomy should be evaluated. Micrognathia, short neck, temporomandibular joint disease, or cervical spine immobility may make direct laryngoscopy problematic. The time of last gastric ingestion orally or from gavage should be ascertained to evaluate the potential for regurgitation and pulmonary aspiration. Cardiovascular and neurologic status should be reviewed, since intubation can provoke intracranial hypertension, systemic arterial hypertension, and tachycardia. Coagulopathy, thrombocytopenia, and immunocompromise are contraindications to nasal intubation. Medication allergies should be checked, and any readily available historical information from anesthetic records or previous intubation notes should be gathered. The intravenous lines should be checked for adequate flow and position, and if available, the chest radiograph should be reviewed at the bedside.

Monitoring should include electrocardiogram, frequent blood pressure measurement (preferably automatic), and a pulse oximeter. In particular, the pulse oximeter is a more specific guide to the need for return to bag-mask ventilation than the rule of 15 s per intubation attempt.

TABLE 6-3 Evaluation for Intubation

Airway anatomy
Micrognathia, small oropharynx, "bull neck," temporomandibular joint dysfunction, cervical spine immobility, nasal deformity
Medication allergies
Aspiration risk
Time to last oral intake or gastric feed, upper gastrointestinal bleeding, bowel obstruction, vomiting
Cardiovascular status
Angina, ischemia, myocardial infarction, cardiomyopathy, dysrhythmias
Neurologic status
Increased intracranial pressure, ischemic symptoms, intracranial aneurysm or hemorrhage, cervical spine pathology
Musculoskeletal
Recent cord denervation injuries, crush injuries, burns
Coagulation
Thrombocytopenia, anticoagulant therapy, or coagulopathy
Past intubation problems
Availability of an adequate IV
Chest radiograph

Intubation and the Risk of Aspiration

It is prudent to assume that all patients in need of urgent intubation have large gastric volumes that greatly enhance the likelihood of regurgitation, either passive (in the case of the paralyzed patient) or secondary to retching induced by the presence of instruments in the posterior pharynx. The presence of vomitus in the pharynx greatly complicates the attempt to intubate by obscuring the view, while simultaneously presenting the risk of aspiration, and placing an obstruction to ongoing respiration in a patient who is already compromised. The pulmonary consequences of aspiration are a function of the volume of aspirant, its acidity, and the presence of particulates.[3]

It is difficult to predict the rate of gastric emptying in critically ill patients. Most severe disease states delay gastric emptying, and the luxury of being able to delay intubation is not typically available in the ICU. Nasogastric suction is not reliable in ensuring an empty stomach, but may decrease gastric contents. If indwelling, the nasogastric tube should be placed on suction and then removed so as not to mechanically interfere with intubation. A nasogastric tube may also act as a wick for passive regurgitation. If not in place, and if the patient is sufficiently stable, a nasogastric tube should be temporarily passed for partial gastric evacuation prior to intubation. Although it enhances gastric emptying, metoclopramide is impractical in the ICU because it requires 90 min to work.

Like metoclopramide, H_2 blockers, though frequently advocated before surgery for raising gastric pH, are too slow to be of practical benefit in the ICU. Particulate antacids (e.g., milk of magnesia and aluminum sulfates) provoke severe pneumonia on aspiration and are contraindicated. Clear antacids such as magnesium citrate are useful in reducing acidity at the expense of a larger residual gastric volume. Patients in need of intubation are not usually able to drink fluids, but if a nasogastric tube is in place, magnesium citrate can be instilled and suctioned out after 5 min.

It is imperative that adequate suction be available, with a suitable large bore rigid tip (Yankauer tip) to facilitate removal of foreign matter. In particular, the suction port of a bronchoscope cannot be relied on to provide adequate suction power in this setting and must be supplemented. Cricoid pressure (Sellick maneuver) prior to intubation provides relative protection against the risk of aspiration by physically occluding the esophagus. This is accomplished by placing the thumb and middle fingers over the cricoid cartilage, with the index finger resting on the thyroid cartilage. Firm pressure, sufficient to occlude the esophagus, is applied. The pressure should be maintained until tube position is confirmed by auscultation of the lung fields and epigastrium. Its use is standard for intubation in all patients with suspected gastric contents.

Procedures for Intubation

There is no reason, other than tradition, that dictates the choice of direct laryngoscopy as the preferred technique for placement of an ETT. In fact, many anesthesiologists now routinely use the fiberoptic bronchoscope for tube placement in difficult airways. In this section, specific consideration will be given to the techniques of oral intubation with direct laryngoscopy, blind nasal intubation, intubation with the flexible bronchoscope, and cricothyrotomy.

GENERAL CONSIDERATIONS

Compared to the operating room environment, arterial oxygen desaturation proceeds quite rapidly following discontinuation of spontaneous or mechanical ventilation in the patient with impending respiratory failure, for the obvious reasons of diminished functional residual capacity, increased metabolic rate, and impaired gas exchange. For this reason, all intubations in the ICU should be preceded by ventilation with 100% oxygen for 1 to 2 min if possible. Intubation under difficult circumstances requires concentration, which typically causes even the experienced operator to lose sight of both the overall patient condition and the passage of time. Thus, it is imperative that when intubation is problematic, another individual signal the need to return to bag-mask ventilation.

Ideally, three people are involved in a controlled ICU intubation: the operator; an assistant who applies cricoid pressure, helps to suction, insufflates oxygen during intubation attempts, stabilizes the head in awake patients or patients with suspected neck injuries, and supervises the nonoperative field; and a second assistant who watches the monitors and administers drugs as directed by the operator.

No matter what technique is chosen, initial preparations must be made to facilitate safe intubation. While equipment is gathered and pertinent history is elicited, the bed should be moved away from the wall and the headboard removed. If possible, the bed should be raised so that the mattress surface is approximately waist high. If the headboard is fixed, the patient should be placed diagonally in bed to provide access to the pharynx. Ventilation should be assisted with 100% oxygen by mask and hand-bag, carefully synchronized with the patient's spontaneous inspiratory efforts; the clinician should attempt to augment each inspiration by 200 to 300 ml. This frequently has a calming effect on the patient, who gradually has a decrease in air hunger. This in turn may allow lowering of the head of the bed to the required flat position, a position which may otherwise be uncomfortable for the dyspneic patient.

OROTRACHEAL INTUBATION

Orotracheal intubation is performed with direct laryngoscopy. Its advantages are minimal equipment needs, and it is the best technique in apneic patients. Its disadvantages include the necessity for suitable pharyngeal anatomy, the risk of cervical spine motion in patients with cervical spine abnormalities, and the common requirement for sedation and paralysis to allow direct laryngoscopy.

An 8.0 or 8.5 ETT should be chosen for adults; this is large enough to accommodate a flexible fiberoptic bronchoscope and to provide a low resistance conduit for spontaneous respiration. The cuff integrity should be confirmed by injection and withdrawal of 10 cc air, and a malleable stylet should be inserted to provide a 50 to 60° anterior bend approximately 5 cm from the tube tip. The stylet must be bent at the back, to ensure that the stylet tip does not extend beyond the tube tip; fatal esophageal and tracheal tears have occurred from protruding stylets. A Macintosh 3 or 4 blade is most commonly used for adult intubations; the light should be checked and suction should be available. Gloves should be donned. Following sedation, block, or paralysis, should these be indicated, the head is placed in the "modified sniffing position" unless contraindicated by preexisting cervical spine abnormalities. As the name suggests, this is the position taken when actively sniffing and is attained with the head neutral (neither extended nor flexed) and advanced forward. This provides the best position for viewing the larynx in patients with normal anatomy.

Following preoxygenation and application of cricoid pressure, the patient is sedated, and if necessary, paralyzed. The laryngoscope is held in the left hand, close to the junction of the blade and handle. The right thumb and index finger are used to open the mouth; they are crossed, with the thumb on the lower incisors and the index finger on the upper incisors. An exaggeration of the crossed finger position will force the pharynx open, and the laryngoscope blade is inserted in the right side of the mouth. The scope blade is passed as far as possible without resistance into the pharynx, following the natural curve of the blade and tongue, and keeping the tongue to the left side of the mouth. After insertion, the blade is moved anteriorly and to the midline, the flange on the blade serving to push the tongue to the patient's left and out of the field of vision. If the epiglottis and larynx are not visualized, the blade and handle are lifted anteriorly along the long axis of the handle, without twisting or levering (Fig. 6-1, *top*). If cord structures cannot be seen, the scope should be gently withdrawn until the epiglottis drops into view. The blade is then advanced into the vallecula and lifted to expose the larynx.

Once the cords are visualized (Fig. 6-2), the ETT is passed into the pharynx with the right hand from the right side of the mouth, and the tip is passed through the cords without resistance. The tube cuff should be seen to pass between the vocal cords and anterior to the arytenoid cartilages. If a stylet is in place, it should be removed by an assistant while tube position is observed.

Inability to see the cord structures may occur for a number of reasons. If the epiglottis is in the way, additional lift along the axis of the laryngoscope handle should be applied to open the airway. Rotational leverage should be avoided (Fig. 6-1, *bottom*), damage to the teeth will result, and visualization will be impaired by the narrower oral opening that will be achieved. The person applying cricoid pressure can be instructed to manipulate the glottis externally, if it will be of benefit in enhancing the view. If poor visibility is due to oral secretions or vomitus, the obvious solution is suctioning. Most commonly for neophytes, the scope is passed too deeply, showing esophagus, or too shallowly, exposing the base of the tongue. Difficulty arises when the patient has anatomic irregularities that complicate the procedure. Common problems include micrognathia, temporomandibular joint immobility, or limitations in neck flexion/extension. Laryngeal anatomy may be deep or anteriorly displaced as normal anatomic variants or may be obscured or displaced by pathology of the pharynx and neck. In such cases, direct visualization of the larynx may be problematic. If the mask airway is adequate to maintain arterial saturation and the risk of aspiration is low, other techniques can be considered. Alternate approaches include the application of steep flexion to the head, the use of a Miller straight blade, and the application of pressure to the thyroid cartilage by an assistant to manipulate the larynx into view. As mentioned above, it is easy to become preoccupied with laryngeal exposure, forgetting the need for intermittent ventilation; brief attempts to secure the airway should be punctuated by bouts of bag-mask ventilation to maintain arterial saturation.

As a last resort, if the epiglottis is seen but the cords cannot be visualized, the tube can be passed blindly. This is accomplished by exaggerating the bend in the stylet and passing the tube tip along the posterior surface of the epiglottis, advancing the tube off the stylet in the hopes it will pass through the cords. The risk of esophageal intubation is high in any technique where the tube is not seen to pass through the cords. Once the tube is placed, the cuff should be inflated with sufficient air to provide a seal against inspiratory gas leakage. Following tube placement, no matter what technique, ETT position must be verified by the auscultation of bilateral breath sounds, by the absence of epigastric sounds which would indicate gastric insufflation, by the presence of inspiratory chest rise, and by end tidal CO_2 elimination if a monitor is available. During the bronchoscopic intubation, visualization of tracheal cartilages is obviously an appropriate substitute, although auscultation should be performed to rule out mainstem intubation.

The tube should be fixed in position with a hand resting on the face, while hand-bag breaths are administered with 100% oxygen. Any uncertainty regarding tube position should be resolved by auscultation, and if necessary, repeat laryngoscopy with an assistant holding the ETT in position to confirm tracheal placement. Various methods are commonly used to fasten the tube. In general, it is best to defer to the nursing staff, who routinely maintain the appliance. In cases where the face will not support tape or circumferential head fasteners (e.g., severe facial burns) the tube can be wired with stainless steel to firmly rooted teeth. A chest radiograph should be obtained immediately following intubation, and a detailed note should be written including technique, anatomic findings, any difficulties encountered, and the depth of the tube at the teeth.

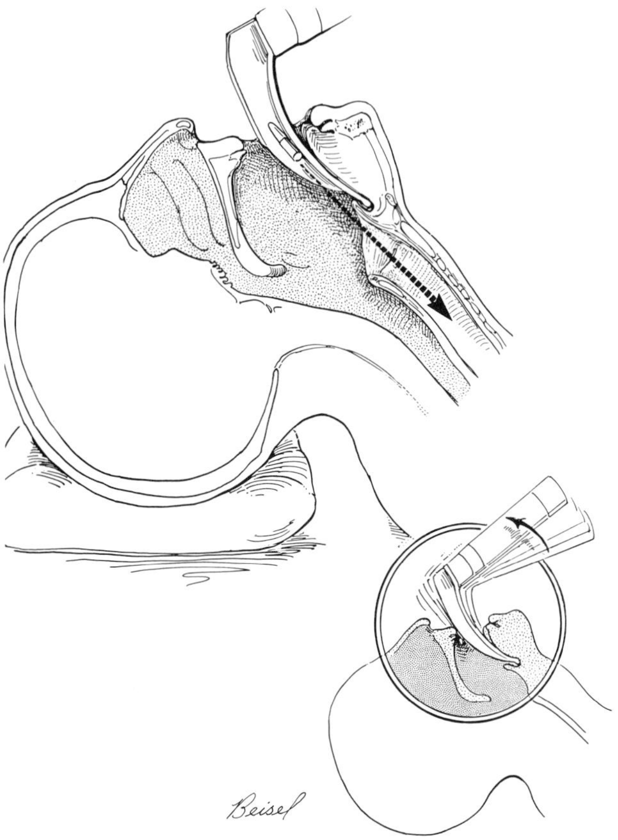

FIGURE 6-1 ***(Top)*** **Correct position of head and laryngoscope for direct laryngoscopy.** ***(Bottom)*** **Rotational leverage obscures the view and causes dental trauma. (Reprinted by permission of Little Brown & Co., copyright 1986.)**

FIGURE 6-2 Full direct laryngoscopic view of glottis. (Reprinted by permission of Little Brown & Co., copyright 1986.)

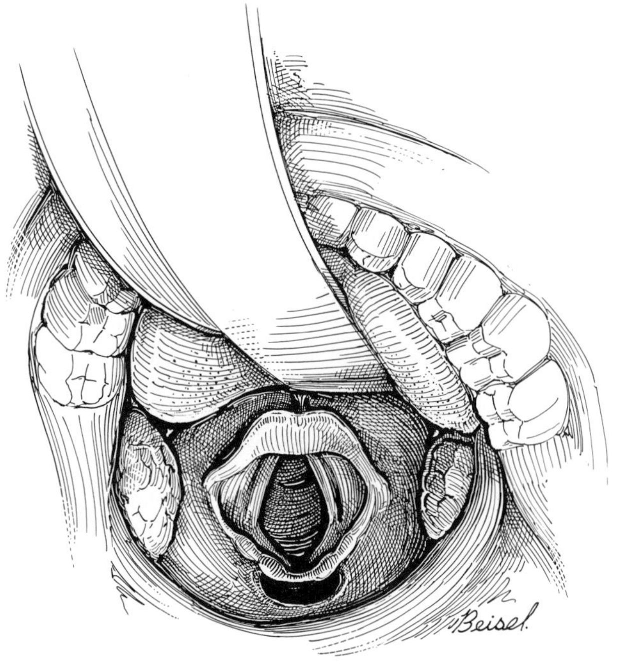

NASOTRACHEAL INTUBATION

Nasotracheal intubation has the advantage of allowing free access to the mouth for oral hygiene and allows lip-reading for communication. It is easier to fasten and likely to be positionally more stable than an oral ETT. Blind or fiberoptic nasal intubation has the advantage of not requiring head extension or mandibular mobility. Disadvantages include a high incidence of purulent and serous otitis and sinusitis and the risk of damage to turbinates and nares. Contraindications to nasal intubation include immunocompromise and acute facial or cerebral trauma, where the integrity of the cribriform plate is not known. Patients on full therapeutic anticoagulation or those with coagulopathy should not undergo nasal intubation. Platelet count <80,000 or platelet dysfunction due to renal failure or drugs is also a contraindication because of the risk of nasal hemorrhage, which may complicate intubation as well as being difficult to control. Placement can be performed blindly, guided by tube-transmitted breath sounds, fiberoptically, or by direct laryngoscopy. Blind or fiberoptic nasotracheal intubation requires a spontaneously respiring patient and for fiberoptic placement, preferably one who can swallow secretions.

Nasal intubation requires first that the nasal mucous membranes be vasoconstricted to decrease hemorrhage and lubricated to facilitate tube passage. Traditionally, 4% cocaine was used in this role; concerns about hypertension and the decreased availability of cocaine in the ICU make the combination of 0.5% phenylephrine, lidocaine spray, and lidocaine jelly the preferred choice. The phenylephrine is best applied in aerosol spray, while the nasal septum is assessed for obvious deviation. Lidocaine jelly may be applied to the nostril with a jelly-coated suction catheter or rubber nasal trumpet airway. A lubricated 7.0 or 7.5 ETT is passed posteriorly into the nose; this should be aimed straight back to the occiput, like a nasogastric tube. Usually, there is resistance to passage, which may be overcome by steady continuous pressure. There is a risk of burrowing under the mucosa of the nose, resulting in dramatic hemorrhage. To avoid this risk, a No. 18 French suction catheter should first be passed through the tube and then into the nose to act as a guide for the ETT to follow. Once the tube has passed into the pharynx, the suction catheter is withdrawn. Breath sounds should be clearly audible through the tube. The tube is slowly advanced on inspiration; loss of breath sounds indicates passage into the esophagus, while coughing and loss of phonation follow successful tracheal cannulation. If the tube is not passing on repeated attempts, the tube should be withdrawn 3 or 4 cm and manipulated to provoke a cough. Coughing is followed by a deep inspiration, which will sometimes serve to suck the tube into the trachea. Head position may be altered to flexion or to one side. Alternatively, a tube with a ring manipulator (Endotrol) can be used; retracting the finger ring brings the tube tip forward, facilitating tracheal passage of the tube. If a nasogastric tube is in place, it should be removed before blind nasal intubation to avoid channeling of the ETT by the nasogastric tube.

If direct laryngoscopy is preferred, the tube can be passed to the posterior pharynx and the tube advanced through the trachea as in orotracheal intubation. Magill forceps are used to control the tip. They are available in most intubation sets, and their application is intuitive. The nasal turbinates are sharp, and damage to the ETT cuff can occur with nasal passage. If the tube passes successfully, but the cuff will not hold air and seal, a tube change will be required. In the interim, the pharynx can be packed with an abdominal lap pad or large gauze if the patient will tolerate it, which will effectively seal the tube. This allows time to stabilize the patient prior to the tube change.

With fiberoptic intubation, the tube is passed into the posterior pharynx as before. A larger tube (7.5 or 8.0) is required. The scope is lubricated and passed through the nasotracheal tube. It is important that a tube of sufficient size be selected and that the scope be well lubricated. The consequence of neglecting this detail will be a degloved scope, which will require expensive factory repair. Once in the pharynx, the tip of the scope is guided through the cords, and the shaft of the scope is used as a guide as the ETT is advanced over the scope into the trachea. Tongue retraction anteriorly is frequently helpful. Retraction can be accomplished by gauze wrapping the tongue or by the use of a tongue retractor or simple tongue blade. This technique requires facility with the fiberoptic bronchoscope. In addition, a backup suction unit is required, because the scope suction channel is typically not sufficient to clear pharyngeal secretions. This technique can be used orally as well, but the acute angle from oropharynx to glottis makes passage more difficult. Whenever the fiberoptic scope is passed orally, a bite-block should be used.

CRICOTHYROTOMY

On occasion, even the experienced airway clinician is confronted with a situation where endotracheal intubation cannot be accomplished. If bag-mask ventilation can be effectively administered, and regurgitation is not impending, an emergency does not exist, and the clinician can carefully consider alternate positions, approaches, or instruments to aid in securing the airway. If ventilation is problematic, a true emergency exists and must be addressed immediately. Current strategy in such situations calls for the performance of a cricothyrotomy. In addition, cricothyrotomy is an appropriate first-line airway approach in patients with frankly unstable necks in need of urgent intubation. It requires a scalpel and a blunt dissecting instrument, such as a hemostat. The cricothyroid notch is localized, and the skin and subcutaneous tissues are incised until the membrane is punctured (Fig. 6-3). The clamp is used to bluntly expand the membrane opening, and a small tracheostomy tube (5 or 6) or ETT (6.0) is passed into the trachea. The use of a 12- or 14-gauge angiocatheter has been advocated by some as an alternative technique. This is effective if a high pressure insufflation valve is available, since hand-bag pressure will not be sufficient to force gas through such a narrow lumen. In addition, when insufflating through an angiocatheter,

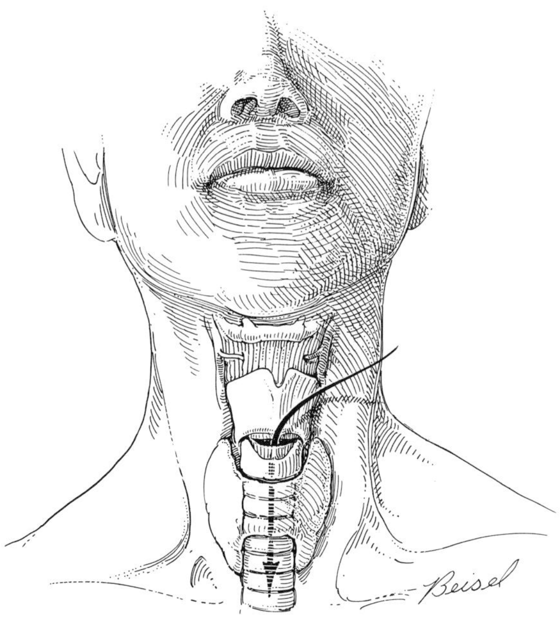

FIGURE 6-3 Cricothyroid membrane. A small (6.0) ETT provides a suitable emergency cricothyroid airway. (Reprinted by permission of Little Brown & Co., copyright 1986.)

the larynx and pharynx must be unobstructed to allow passive exhalation, since thoracic cage recoil is not sufficient to propel gas flow through a 12-gauge orifice.

Many of the older style cricothyrotomy kits contain sharp metal tracheal cannulae. Their use should be avoided due to the risk of tracheal laceration. Tracheostomy, which is performed lower in the neck, is not suitable as an emergency procedure because of the risk of severe hemorrhage.

Intubation and Intercurrent Diseases

Conscious patients in severe respiratory distress who are intubated unsedated (if they will tolerate this) exhibit a typical physiologic response. Initially, they will become hypertensive and tachycardic, if not already maximally stressed by preexisting hypoxia and hypercapnia. The larynx is exquisitely sensitive to the presence of a foreign body, becoming less so only after minutes to hours of continued exposure. This sensitivity and the sensitivity of the tongue to the pressure induced by laryngoscopy are the sources of the extreme hypertension and tachycardia that can accompany intubation. Once the tube is secured and mechanical ventilation instituted, a period of hypotension frequently ensues, which can be quite severe. The shift from negative to positive intrathoracic pressure resulting from mechanical ventilation and PEEP can provoke hypotension, especially in patients who are relatively hypovolemic from hemorrhage, pharmacologic diuresis, or sepsis. This phenomenon is most prominent in patients with airflow obstruction and air trapping and in those patients quickly placed on high levels of PEEP. Such patients may require a period of gentle bag ventilation while volume is infused intravenously. Direct laryngoscopy provokes histamine release, which may also explain the hypotension. This hypotension responds to intravenous volume administration. Bradycardia should be treated with an anticholinergic such as 0.4 mg atropine or 0.2 mg glycopyrrolate. Ephedrine, 5 mg, is another appropriate choice to provide brief (3 to 5 min) inotropy, chronotropy, and increased vascular tone while volume is administered.

The hypertension/tachycardia and following hypotension both represent significant stresses to the cardiovascular system. Patients with ischemic myocardium can infarct from the stress of intubation. Cardiomyopathy also sensitizes patients to the cardiac and neurodepressant effects of sedatives and narcotics. This is presumably due to greater distribution of intravenously administered drugs to the brain, heart, and lungs relative to other tissues in patients with low cardiac output. The result is a greatly decreased requirement for sedating drugs.

Patients with intracranial aneurysm or recent intracranial hemorrhage require careful blood pressure control to avoid exacerbation of the bleeding or aneurysm rupture. In the days following rupture, patients may develop cerebral arterial vasospasm. As in cerebral artery or carotid stenosis, hypotension is likely to result in ischemia in these patients with vasospasm, since normal autoregulatory mechanisms are impaired.

Patients with intracranial lesions predisposing to cerebral edema present a clinically significant challenge, because laryngotracheal stimulation is a potent stimulus to intracranial hypertension with consequent risk of herniation or ischemia. Lidocaine, 1.5 mg/kg, administered intravenously at least 3 min prior to intubation, tube manipulation, or suctioning will ameliorate, but not entirely eliminate, the rise in intracranial pressure (ICP). Pentothal is also beneficial. A full dose is 5 to 6 mg/kg, administered as an intravenous bolus. Most ICU patients, however, will not tolerate the resulting myocardial depression and vasodilation. The mechanism of the ICP rise is not strictly vascular in that it will occur despite adequate blood pressure control. It will also be seen despite paralysis. Nevertheless, straining or coughing and systemic hypertension will exacerbate intracranial hypertension and its associated pathology and are to be carefully avoided during intubation.

Patients with severe facial trauma or closed head injury should not be intubated nasally because undiagnosed basilar skull and cribriform plate fractures provide a path for the passage of the tube into the cranium. Such patients also present a risk for oral intubation until cervical spine instability is ruled out. In patients who present for intubation following acute head and neck trauma, the choices are orotracheal intubation with in-line stabilization of the head, fiberoptic intubation, or cricothyrotomy. Fiberoptic intubation is frequently hindered by oral hemorrhage. If oral intubation is elected, an associate should provide 15 to 20 lb traction on the head, and the position should be carefully maintained during laryngoscopy to avoid flexion. With attention to neck immobilization, an unstable cervical spine is not a contraindication to oral intubation and does not increase the incidence of spinal cord injury.[4]

The intubation of patients with pharyngeal or upper gastrointestinal bleeding is most safely accomplished by awake oral laryngoscopy, augmented with light sedation. In this setting, paralysis or heavy sedation frequently results in blood aspiration and difficulty with visualization of the glottis. In severe cases, an extra suction system should be available to aid in maintaining a clear field.

Patients who are immunocompromised require special attention to minimize tracheal soiling during intubation. The consequences of aspiration can be particularly dire in this population, and nasal intubation is avoided due to the risk of carriage of nasal flora into the trachea and the ongoing risk of sinusitis.

Bronchospastic disease is exacerbated by tracheal intubation as a direct result of the noxious pharyngeal and tracheal stimulation. In this population, intubation is best accomplished with heavy sedation and paralysis either before or immediately following intubation. Aerosol lidocaine provokes bronchospasm and is not typically used as an intubation anesthetic in patients with bronchospastic airway disease.

Pharmacologic Aid to Intubation

Drug therapy during intubation has three goals: to establish a situation most favorable for safe intubation (sedation, paralysis), to provide relief from the discomfort associated with the procedure, and to decrease hormonal, neurologic, and cardiovascular stress. Of course, in patients who are being intubated in the context of full cardiopulmonary arrest, these are moot issues. By contrast, patients who are still conscious prior to intubation will benefit from some combination of amnesia, analgesia, hypnosis, muscle paralysis, and autonomic stabilization.

Local anesthesia is one reasonable approach to alleviating the pain and stress of intubation. Many anesthesiologists use a combination of topical oral anesthesia, transtracheal anesthesia, and superior laryngeal nerve blocks. This is probably excessively complex, and an excellent substitute is 4% lidocaine in a pressure nebulizer, delivered by mask as one would deliver any inhalation therapy. Lidocaine is rapidly absorbed systemically through the mucosa, so the dose should be carefully titrated so that no more than 4 mg/kg is administered. Cases of massive aspiration following such anesthesia are known, since airway protection relies in part on intact sensation in the hypopharynx and glottis. Alternate topical anesthesia can be provided with any of the commercially available aerosol ester anesthetic sprays (benzocaine, cetacaine), bearing in mind that these are not metered, and toxic reactions can occur.

In patients who are agitated, disoriented, combative, or uncooperative, systemic sedation and sometimes paralysis are indicated. The current sedative of choice is midazolam. It is water soluble and is a potent anxiolytic, amnestic, and hypnotic. It will occasionally cause a fall in blood pressure, usually secondary to its anxiolysis. A dose of 1 mg intravenously is an appropriate starting point; sudden apnea, a rare but reported side effect of midazolam, is obviously less a concern in the setting of impending intubation, although vigilance is key. Narcotic adjuncts to intubation are appropriate to blunt the response to laryngoscopy and intubation. The pain of laryngoscopic tongue retraction and passage of a foreign body into the trachea is effectively alleviated by narcosis. Any narcotic is appropriate here, although Demerol and the newer synthetics (Alfentanil, Fentanyl) are most rapid in onset and provoke less hypotension than morphine. Demerol has other neuropsychologic effects as well, which, though making it less useful as a chronic analgesic, probably enhance the amnestic effect of the benzodiazepines when used in combination.

Strategically, paralysis must be considered a last resort intervention in ICU intubation. It provokes respiratory arrest, which depending on the drug used, dose used, and patient condition, will persist from 5 min to hours. Obviously, any doubt about the ability to secure an airway should preclude the use of a paralytic. Succinylcholine (1.2 mg/kg) and vecuronium (0.1 mg/kg) are the most commonly administered paralytics for intubation. The use of pharmacologic paralysis is discussed in Chap. 83.

In the patient for whom gradual sedation is unfeasible or in whom wide hemodynamic alteration is to be stringently avoided, appropriate drugs to augment and antagonize the catecholamine levels should be available. In anesthesia, peri-intubation hypertension is typically controlled with pentothal (potent, rapidly acting hypnotic, myocardial depressant, and vasodilator, brief duration) esmolol, nitroprusside, or labetalol. Catecholamine augmentation is usually accomplished with dopamine infusion or ephedrine bolus (5 to 10 mg). These drugs are titrated to individual patient needs, with the recognition that hemodynamic states swing rapidly in the time surrounding intubation and the initiation of mechanical ventilation.

Changing the ETT

Like initial intubation, tube changes can be a critical episode in the ICU course. Unlike vascular catheters, there is no reason to prophylactically change ETTs. Appropriate indications include tube cuff failure, change in size of tube to allow bronchoscopy or to decrease airway resistance, or a change from oral to nasal position. The use of stiff tube changers alone should be discouraged; displacing the changer while the tube is out or difficulty sliding the new tube over the changer does occur and can provoke a true emergency.

Uncomplicated tube changes should be approached much as initial intubation. The same set of preparations should be made, including ensuring the availability of a full set of intubation equipment. If possible, the change should be delayed until the stomach is empty. The actual change should be preceded by a brief period of ventilation with 100% oxygen. Sedation and paralysis are usually easily administered in this setting because of the presence of an

ETT. Direct laryngoscopy is usually the technique of choice because of the difficulty inherent in trying to locate the glottis fiberoptically with a tube already in place. While an assistant holds the old tube in position, direct laryngoscopy is performed, and the glottis is identified. The new tube is inserted into the pharynx and its tip brought to the glottis next to the old tube. The assistant then deflates the cuff on the old tube and withdraws it, as the new tube is advanced into the trachea. The cuff is inflated and the position checked. It is imperative that the old tube not be withdrawn until the operator can confidently define the anatomy and maintain the view once the old tube is withdrawn. Usually, haste is not necessary in tube changes, and sedation should be liberally administered unless contraindicated by hemodynamic considerations.

In the most difficult airways, changers or a bronchoscope may be used in conjunction with simultaneous direct laryngoscopy to add control. For instance, in burn patients with severe pharyngeal mucosal edema, it may require three people to manage a tube change. With the patient sedated and paralyzed, one person will perform direct laryngoscopy and identify the passage of the current ETT as best as possible. The second person will direct a fiberoptic bronchoscope with the new ETT mounted to the first operator, who in turn directs the fiberoptic scope into the trachea next to the current tube. When the fiberoptic bronchoscopist identifies tracheal cartilages and carina, the third operator effects the change by withdrawing the old tube and sliding the new tube over the scope. All the while, the direct laryngoscopist continues to observe the hypopharynx and if possible, the cords, to stabilize the process. Such management is unusual, but demonstrates that every reasonable effort must be made to ensure a controlled airway.

Physiologic Effects of Intubation

The presence of a well-positioned ETT alters pulmonary mechanics and dynamics in a predictable fashion. In normal subjects, functional residual capacity, total lung volume, and vital capacity (VC) are not diminished by the presence of an ETT. Anatomic dead space is reduced by the substitution of an ETT for the nasopharynx.[5] The cross-sectional area of an 8.0 ETT is similar to that of the normal adult glottis; however, resistance to flow is somewhat higher because the tube presents a much longer flow conduit than the glottis. In normal experimental subjects, peak flow is diminished about 20 percent by an 8.0 ETT. The tubes limit cough performance, both by blunting peak flow rate and by blocking the normal tracheal collapse and reexpansion which helps to propel mucus to the mouth. In the range of gas flows encountered during adult spontaneous ventilation, ETT size dramatically affects resistance to flow; a 9.0 tube offers one-third the resistance of an 8.0, whereas a 7.0 tube offers twice the resistance of an 8.0 tube. In addition, in vitro resistance measurements underestimate the in vivo resistance offered by chronic endotracheal intubation. This high resistance is probably the result of partial tube kinking and inspissated secretions.[6] In normal subjects, intubation provokes increased distal airway resistance consistent with bronchospasm.[7] Young adults also occasionally exhibit dramatic decreases in VC and negative inspiratory pressure, which seem to be effort related and may lead to an underestimation of the patient's mechanical capacity to sustain spontaneous ventilation.

Care of the Intubated Patient

The endotracheal appliance requires frequent inspection and maintenance to minimize complications. Nurses and respiratory therapists should routinely check cuff pressure, maintaining pressure <25 cmH2O. Cuff pressure can be measured using any one of a number of commercially available manometers. Nurses and therapists should be instructed to suction carefully and to apply positive pressure by bag to the ETT during cuff manipulations to avoid aspiration of intratracheal material from above the cuff as it is deflated.

Daily physicians' working rounds should include a systematic evaluation of the ETT. The tube fastening site should be examined for tissue irritation or necrosis, and hand-bag ventilation should be briefly performed with simultaneous auscultation to evaluate patency, position, and leak. The tube fastening system should be inspected to ensure an adequate grip on the face and tube with minimal play. Tube depth markings should correspond to the charted depth, and the cuff pilot balloon should be palpated. A stiff balloon is overinflated; the balloon should be full but soft. If high pressures are required to maintain a seal, consideration should be given to changing to a foam cuff appliance. Sinusitis is common with nasal intubation, and patients with nonlocalized fever or obvious maxillary tenderness should be examined with computed tomography (CT) scan, Water's radiograph, or transillumination.

The daily chest radiograph is useful in verifying tube position and cuff-induced tracheal pathology. ETTs are manufactured with a molded barium strip to facilitate radiographic visualization of the tip position. Optimally, the tip should lie in the midtrachea, 4 cm above the carina. Head position alters tube depth; flexion advances the tube 1 to 3 cm toward the carina, and extension or lateral rotation will retract the tube up to 2 cm toward the pharynx. Day-to-day comparison of cuff diameter will offer an early warning of tracheal dilation and impending tracheal rupture or tracheomalacia. Widening silhouette is associated with a progressive increase in cuff volume and pressure requirements to maintain a seal and will alert the intensivist to the need for changing appliance type or position.

Bronchoscopy is indicated for assessing tracheal trauma in patients with signs of airway pathology such as widening silhouette or bleeding. In patients who have undergone conversion of prolonged endotracheal intubation to tracheotomy, the glottis should be visualized either directly with a laryngoscope or with a fiberoptic scope to assess the degree of residual and progressive damage. This can be accomplished safely with the patient sedated. The presence of identifiable cord injury should prompt consultation by a laryngologist for evaluation and early intervention. Fiberoptic laryngoscopy may also be indicated to assess cord function during extubation from prolonged intubation.

Complications of Intubation

Complications of endotracheal intubation may be acute or chronic and are typically the result of mechanical trauma to the delicate cord structures and airway mucosa (Table 6-4). In recent decades, the incidence of injury appears to have decreased due to the substitution of softer materials and highly compliant high volume cuffs for the hard rubber tubes.

The most acute and potentially lethal complication of endotracheal intubation is an obstructed tube. This can occur because of biting, kinking of the tube, or luminal obstruction with mucus, vomitus (which has leaked past the cuff and is coughed retrograde into the tube), or clot. The first response of any physician evaluating an ETT problem should be to disconnect the ventilator and provide handbag ventilation. This simultaneously isolates a likely problem source (the mechanical ventilator) and provides a much better sense of the mechanical situation than auscultation alone. Problems such as cuff leak, displaced ETT, patient discoordination and "bucking," or tube obstruction are immediately apparent. The addition of auscultation will inform the examiner of bronchospasm and mainstem intubation. An obstructed tube is an emergency situation. If the patient is aggressively bucking, has paroxysmal coughing, or is biting the tube, rapid paralysis will relieve the immediate obstruction and facilitate further assessment. A suction catheter should pass freely down the tube. If the catheter cannot be passed and no remediable kinking is obvious, the tube must be immediately replaced, or removed to allow bag-mask ventilation.

TABLE 6-4 Complications of Intubation

Peri-Intubation
Right mainstem intubation
Esophageal intubation
Gastric aspiration
Dental injury, tooth aspiration
Tracheal or esophageal tear
Hypertension/tachycardia with secondary cardiac or CNS injury
Hypotension
Temporomandibular joint dislocation
Vocal cord tear or arytenoid dislocation
Bronchospasm
Epistaxis
Nasopharyngeal mucosal tear
Avulsed nasal turbinate
Cardiac dysrhythmias
Pain
Acute
Obstructed ETT
Right mainstem intubation
Cuff leak
Aspiration
Chronic
Serous or purulent otitis
Sinusitis, sepsis
Nose or lip necrosis
Tracheal mucosal injury
Tracheomalacia
Laryngeal stricture, secondary to:
  Posterior cricoarytenoid muscle edema, scarring
  Vocal cord synechiae
  Tracheal stenosis

Pharyngeal, laryngeal, and tracheal trauma can be precipitated by intubation. Mandibular dislocation can occur and if unrecognized, becomes very difficult to correct. Dental trauma is common; dislodged teeth, if rapidly reimplanted, will usually maintain vitality. Arytenoid dislocation or vocal cord tear are rare and are associated with excessively forceful intubation or the use of a protruding metal stylet. Stylet use may also cause esophageal or tracheal perforation, which can initiate a fatal mediastinitis. Right mainstem intubation or esophageal intubation, although occurring relatively frequently, should be immediately recognized by auscultation of both lung fields and the epigastrium following intubation. These will present no harmful sequelae if rapidly corrected. Obviously, unrecognized esophageal intubation presents the threat of asphyxiation. Mainstem intubation will result in hypoxia due to pulmonary shunt, and, by exposing the ventilated lung to relatively large tidal volumes, may promote barotrauma. Pulmonary aspiration of gastric contents may provoke bronchospasm, as may the presence of the ETT in the trachea. Epistaxis during attempted nasal intubation can be quite severe, on occasion requiring surgical intervention for its control.

Chronic complications of endotracheal intubation are listed in Table 6-4. Although specific data implicating tracheal appliances in the promotion of pneumonia are lacking, the presence of an ETT alters normal pharyngeal and tracheal function. The inflated cuff will retard tracheal mucociliary clearance.[8] Coordinated swallowing is hindered by the presence of an ETT or tracheostomy tube, resulting in the pooling of pharyngeal secretions above the tracheal tube cuff. ETT cuffs are relatively ineffective in blocking tracheal aspiration,[9] and it is likely that the majority of intubated patients aspirate small volumes of oral secretions during routine appliance care. To some extent, this can be decreased by the application of modest levels of PEEP (5 cmH_2O). This presumably acts to provide a constant upward pressure on the appliance cuff and trachea, thus retarding the gravitational flow of supraglottic materials. Oral hygiene is hindered by the presence of the appliance, which is likely to enhance the already high incidence of pharyngeal colonization in these bedridden, chronically hospitalized patients.[10–12]

Purulent and serous otitis have been reported as consequences of tracheal intubation, and serous otitis may persist following appliance removal. Purulent sinusitis has been variously reported in 2 to 26 percent of patients who are chronically nasally intubated[13,14] and can lead to fatal sepsis. Immunocompromised patients are particularly disposed to this complication.

Tracheal mucosal injury results from lateral pressure exerted against the mucosa by the inflated tube cuff, inhibiting capillary flow. Over time, this results in scarring, which may interrupt mucociliary transport, and in the extreme, can result in stricture.[15] Stricture, however, is less likely from simple mucosal injury than from tracheal cartilage disruption, which occurs as a necessary consequence of tracheotomy or from tracheomalacia.

Tracheomalacia is usually the consequence of extremely high lateral cuff pressures, either inadvertent, or out of the necessity to maintain a gas seal in patients requiring high ventilatory pressures. Management of tracheomalacia is directed at relieving pressure on the malacic segment. This is best accomplished with a locking collar tracheostomy appliance, which uses a wire-wound ("armored") ETT as a tracheostomy tube with adjustable depth. A tracheostomy placed in this fashion is less likely to alter its position with head movement, allowing precise cuff positioning guided by chest radiograph and bronchoscopy.

Laryngeal injury is directly related to the duration of intubation. Short-term intubation (2 to 5 days) may provoke arytenoid and posterior commissure edema which will present as postextubation stridor. Longer periods of intubation (> 10 days) are associated with a 10 to 12 percent incidence of laryngotracheal stenosis due to scarring of the posterior commissure, immobilizing the arytenoid cartilages which are responsible for vocal cord abduction.[16–20] This stenosis may occur late. Occasionally, bilaterally denuded vocal cords may develop granulation tissue which evolves into bridging scar tissue causing glottic obstruction. This is amenable to surgical correction.

Extubation of the Critically Ill Patient

Extubation following more than 2 or 3 days of intubation should be approached cautiously. In addition to the obvious necessity for adequate VC and respiratory drive, the patient should be assessed for level of consciousness and the ability to generate sufficient pharyngeal muscle tone to support the upper airway. It is important to keep in mind that level of consciousness may fluctuate, with the nadir occurring most often at night. Gavage nutrition should be stopped for 6 to 8 h prior to extubation to minimize gastric residual volume. Prior to extubation, the patient should be suctioned and the means for bag-mask ventilation should be available. Airway equipment should be inspected for normal functioning and should be immediately available. The intubation note should be reviewed to assess for the difficulty of reintubation should problems occur. If the intubation was difficult, a clinician with suitable reintubation skills should be identified and asked to stand-by. If intubation has been chronic (>6 days), it is prudent to view the cords for injury and motion. This is most simply accomplished by passing a small diameter fiberoptic scope to the tip of the ETT and observing cord function and anatomy as the tube is withdrawn past the glottis. Typically, coughing immediately follows extubation, which allows a quick assessment of cord position and mobility.

Patients with failed prior extubation and subsequent reintubation, those with facial burns or infections, or those with severe anatomic impediments to intubation benefit from a more deliberate approach to extubation. The ETT cuff should be deflated and the leak past the tube into the pharynx on hand-bag ventilation assessed. The absence of a leak suggests significant tracheal or glottic edema that may warrant a delay in extubation. Direct laryngoscopy should be performed to examine supraglottic anatomy and to evaluate the possibility of oral reintubation. Finally, the patient can be extubated over the fiberoptic scope, with the scope left in position long enough to ensure initial respiration and to allow cord assessment. Usually, the period of intubation will have desensitized the larynx sufficiently that the scope will be easily tolerated, and its presence provides a ready path for rapid reintubation.

Inspiratory stridor or frank inspiratory obstruction occurs in <5 percent of chronically intubated patients. Retained secretions on the vocal cords may provoke laryngospasm, although this is distinctly uncommon in patients who have had their vocal cords desensitized by the presence of an ETT for a long time. More common is posterior commissure edema. The posterior commissure, the mucosa-covered muscular bridge between the arytenoid cartilages, makes up the most posterior component of the glottic opening. The posterior cricoarytenoid muscles, of which the posterior commissure is comprised, abduct the vocal cords through a lever action on the arytenoids. With the head in a neutral position, an orotracheal tube must maintain an acute curve in passing from the lips to the trachea. This curve causes the tube to wedge into the posterior glottis, applying force to the posterior commissure. Over a period of days, especially with tube movement, the muscles become edematous or frankly fibrotic. When this occurs, cord abduction is compromised, resulting in obstruction and stridor.

The initial management of postextubation stridor includes bag-mask ventilation, carefully synchronized to augment the patient's inspiratory efforts. If mask CPAP is available or can be provided by a skilled hand on a Jackson-Reese style collapsing bag circuit, it will aid gas flow by dilating the hypopharynx and providing a slightly larger glottic opening. Racemic epinephrine should be used by nebulizer to minimize the degree of reversible mucosal edema that may be contributing to airway narrowing. If conservative therapy fails, as evidenced by persisting stridor, patient agitation, or deteriorating blood gases, the patient should be reintubated. The usual approach is to use a small ETT (6.0 or 6.5) preferably passed nasally to minimize the force applied to the posterior commissure. The patient should be treated with 4 mg dexamethasone every 6 h for 2 days, and a laryngologist should be consulted.

Occasionally, a helium-oxygen (heliox) gas mixture can be used therapeutically in patients with upper airway stridor.[21,22] The lesser kinematic viscosity of helium allows smooth laminar gas flow through narrowed orifices at flow rates which would provoke turbulence with oxygen and nitrogen. It is provided as a mixture of 80% helium and 20% oxygen, which can then be blended with O_2 to provide the appropriate FI_{O_2} through a mask or ventilator. Below a helium concentration of 60 percent, the mixture loses most of its clinical benefit. It should be warmed and humidified, since the high specific heat of helium will result in patient hypothermia if cold bottled gas is administered. The patient should be monitored closely. Progression of stridor may be masked by heliox until the larynx is critically narrowed. Heliox is probably most useful in aiding ventilation and spontaneous respiration through a small ETT placed for stridor.

Immediately following extubation, patients will be hoarse and will have poor airway protective reflexes. If phonation difficulties persist past 24 h, indirect fiberoptic laryngoscopy should be performed to assess cord function. Oral intake should be delayed 24 h in all recently extubated chronically intubated patients to allow the return of normal airway sensation and protective reflexes.

References

1. Keamy MF: Airway management, in Kofke, Levy: *Postoperative Critical Care Procedures of The Massachusetts General Hospital.* Little Brown, 1986, pp 1–31.
2. Covelli HD, Weled BJ, Beekman JF: Efficacy of continuous positive airway pressure administered by face mask. Chest 81(2):147, 1982.
3. Wynne JW, Modell JH: Respiratory aspiration of stomach contents. Ann Intern Med 87:466, 1977.
4. Holley J, Jorden R: Airway management in patients with unstable cervical spine fractures. Ann Emerg Med 18(11):1237, 1989.
5. Gal TJ: Pulmonary mechanics in normal subjects following endotracheal intubation. Anesthesiology 52:27, 1980.
6. Wright PE, Marini JJ, Bernard GR: In vitro versus in vivo comparison of endotracheal airflow resistance, Am Rev Respir Dis 140:10, 1989.
7. Gal TJ: Effects of endotracheal intubation on normal cough performance. Anesthesiology 52:324, 1980.
8. Sackner MA, Hirsch J, Epstein S: Effect of cuffed endotracheal tubes on tracheal mucous velocity. Chest 68:774, 1975.
9. Seegobin RD, van Hasselt GL: Aspiration beyond endotracheal cuffs. Can Anaesth Soc J 33(3):273, 1986.
10. Johanson SG, Pierce AK, Sanford JP: Changing pharyngeal bacterial flora of hospitalized patients. N Engl J Med 281:1137, 1969.
11. Valenti WM, Trudell RG, Bentley DW: Factors predisposing to oropharyngeal colonization with gram-negative bacilli in the aged. N Engl J Med 298:1108, 1978.
12. Bryant LR, Trinkle JK, Mobin-Uddin K et al: Bacterial colonization profile with tracheal intubation and mechanical ventilation. Arch Surg 104:647, 1972.
13. Pope TL, Sterling CB, Leitner YB: Maxillary sinusitis after nasotracheal intubation. South Med J 74:610, 1981.
14. O'Reilly MJ, Reddick EJ, Black W et al: Sepsis from sinusitis in nasotracheally intubated patients. A diagnostic dilemma. Am J Surg 147:601, 1984.
15. Belson TP: Cuff induced tracheal injury in dogs following prolonged intubation. Laryngoscope 93:549, 1983.
16. Kastanos N, Estopa Miro R, Marin Perez A et al: Laryngotracheal injury due to endotracheal intubation: Incidence, evolution, and predisposing factors. A prospective long-term study. Crit Care Med 11(5):362, 1983.
17. Bishop MJ, Weymuller EA, Fink BR: Laryngeal effects of prolonged intubation. Anesth Analg 63:335, 1984.
18. Whited RE: A prospective study of laryngotracheal sequelae in long term intubation. Laryngoscope 94:367, 1984.
19. Whited RE: Posterior commissure stenosis post long-term intubation. Laryngoscope 93:1314, 1983.
20. Dubich MN, Wright BD: Comparison of laryngeal pathology following long-term oral and nasal endotracheal intubations. Anesth Analg 57:663, 1978.
21. Orr JB: Helium-oxygen gas mixtures in the management of patients with airway obstruction. Ear Nose Throat J 67(12):866, 1988.
22. Houck JR, Keamy MF, McDonough JM: Effect of helium concentration on experimental upper airway obstruction. Ann Otol Rhinol Laryngol 99:556, 1990.

Chapter 7

TRACHEOSTOMY

E.G. KING
S.M. HAMILTON

Tracheostomy (used interchangeably with the term *tracheotomy*) is an important adjunctive measure in respiratory care. For some patients, it may be lifesaving, either for acute upper airway obstruction or for the longer term needs of tracheobronchial toilet and successful weaning from mechanical ventilation. It should be an integral part of the coordinated care of the critically ill patient and not treated as an isolated surgical procedure. With proper performance of the procedure and thoughtful subsequent management, using the principle of *controlling the airway* at all times, tracheostomy-related disasters should not befall any patient.

Indications for Tracheostomy

There are three fundamental indications for establishment of a tracheostomy:[1,2] **1.** to overcome upper airway obstruction; **2.** to provide airway access for maintenance of tracheobronchial toilet or long-term assisted mechanical ventilation; and **3.** to facilitate weaning from mechanical to spontaneous ventilation. Although there are no arguments about the first indication, lively debates are waged between critical care and other interested physicians and surgeons over the second and third indications. The arguments center around "when," "where," "by whom," and "how." Although there are no clear-cut answers to all of these issues, the following represents the authors' view of the literature and the accumulated experience and bias of 20 years and in excess of 1500 tracheostomies in the practice of critical care.

WHEN

There is little doubt that it is much easier to maintain tracheobronchial toilet through a tracheostomy than an endotracheal tube (ETT). Not only is the tracheostomy a shorter and more direct route to the lower airway, but usually a half or full size larger tube can be used to preserve a tracheostomy. In contrast to a translaryngeal ETT, tracheostomy is more comfortable, because the patient, if awake, may eat and swallow, and with the appropriate tracheostomy tube or communication-assist device, is able to interact more effectively with the care-giving team. The tracheostomy tube is more stable, less likely to be dislodged, and allows maintenance of reasonable oral hygiene.[2]

Despite these obvious advantages to tracheostomy, there has been a progressive tendency in common critical care practice to leave translaryngeal ETTs in place for longer and longer periods. The reasons relate in part to ease of access, a reluctance to do an operation that brings with it some hazards, a neck scar as a reminder of the serious illness, and the favorable experience with relatively few complications in most patients, even with prolonged intubation. In fact, it is commonplace for ETTs to be in place for weeks without any untoward effects being evident on extubation. The major hazard to prolonged endotracheal intubation relates to the potential for laryngeal damage with resultant scarring and postextubation upper airway obstruction or dysphonia.[3–8] Although the precise pathogenesis of laryngeal injury is uncertain, factors producing ETT-related morbidity include insertion trauma, time of tube in situ, abrasion and movement, and pressure. Unfortunately, these injuries, although relatively uncommon, are serious. Satisfactory means of dealing with them are not available. Injuries consist of pressure- or abrasion-related mucosal denudation and perichondritis leading to posterior commissural stenosis, posterior cordal synechiae, arytenoid fixation (or displacement with traumatic intubations), and subglottic (cricoid) stenosis. The serious nature of these injuries is not recognized until after extubation, and it is only with prospective follow-ups of intubated patients that we have begun to develop an appreciation for the frequency and severity of the problems.

How long should an ETT be left in place before a tracheostomy is performed? In truth, we do not know the answer to this question at the moment. There is agreement that for patients who are restless, moving about, swallowing and gagging frequently, with a fetid oral cavity, who have large amounts of tracheobronchial secretions that are difficult to clear, and who have an underlying condition that will not be resolved in 7 to 10 days, an early tracheotomy is a reasonable course to take. In contrast, the patient who is quiet, has a clean mouth and clean airways and has an underlying condition likely to resolve in a few days, will likely do well with an ETT alone. Between these extremes are a great number of patients for whom the decision regarding timing of tracheostomy will be a function of the critical care physician's judgment, experience, and bias. Our experience suggests that females and patients with diabetes mellitus, purulent pneumonias, rheumatoid arthritis, or ankylosing spondylitis, as well as those who are keloid formers, are at special risk for developing postextubation laryngeal complications; these patients might be considered for early tracheostomy. Patients who are suspected of having had direct laryngeal trauma at the time of injury or who had known traumatic intubations could also be considered for early tracheostomy, largely to minimize ongoing laryngeal injury and to allow proper inspection and necessary treatment of a damaged larynx while at the same time maintaining tracheobronchial access.

In addition to the ETT-associated problems of oral hygiene, effectiveness of tracheobronchial toilet, and laryngeal injury must be added postextubation laryngeal dysfunction (motor and sensory)[7] and difficulty in weaning from assisted mechanical ventilation for those patients whose spontaneous ventilatory capability is marginal. The nonelastic load imposed on the respiratory system by a tube is related to length and diameter: for many patients struggling to breathe on their own, weaning from mechanical ventilation with a tracheostomy is clearly easier than with an ETT.[9]

In summary, despite newer ETTs and stabilization devices for them, for any patient requiring tracheobronchial access for a period exceeding a few days, a tracheostomy offers many advantages. The physician must weigh the risks and benefits of the procedure for any given patient against the convenience of the ETT's insertion and apparent short-term success for most patients.

WHERE AND BY WHOM

Unless the patient is going to the operating room from the ICU for some other procedure, tracheostomy should be performed in the ICU. ICUs should have appropriate lights, stretcher beds, equipment, and personnel to carry out this usually straightforward procedure. The operation should seldom, if ever, be carried out under general anesthesia, and the elective procedure should always be preceded by translaryngeal endotracheal intubation. It makes little sense to transport a critically ill patient, usually with multiple tubes, lines, and support devices to the operating room: if surgeons only feel at ease in operating rooms, it is unlikely that they understand the affairs of the ICU well enough to be doing the tracheotomies. Ideally, the person who does the tracheotomy should be the one who subsequently looks after both it and the patient. Setting aside this ideal, in the usual ICU circumstance, the job should be done by a surgeon who does many of them and is intimately familiar not only with the procedure itself but also with the usual ICU routines for respiratory care and the subsequent management of the tracheostomy.

HOW

PREOPERATIVE CHECK LIST

The patient should be hemodynamically stable and all correctable biochemical parameters should be normalized. Tube feeds must be stopped at least 4 h before the procedure and the stomach aspirated. The patient whose respiratory condition is unstable or deteriorating is not a candidate for the procedure until the situation has stabilized. Generally, tracheostomy is postponed if the fraction inspired oxygen (F_{IO_2}) is >0.6, if the positive end-expiratory pressure (PEEP) requirement is >10 cmH_2O, or if the peak airway pressure is >65 cmH_2O. Heparin infusions are stopped 6 h prior to surgery and resumed 12 h postoperatively. Thrombocytopenia of <50,000 and prothrombin time prolongation of greater than 20 percent beyond control are corrected with platelet, plasma, or cryoprecipitate transfusions. The uremic patient may pose special problems with respect to coagulation and electrolyte status. These are usually rectified by carefully timed dialysis and use of DDAVP or cryoprecipitate or both.

PREMEDICATION

All patients should receive an intravenous analgesic and hypnotic/amnestic. Morphine (0.1 to 0.25 mg/kg) can unmask hypotension but provides effective analgesia and sedation. Fentanyl (3.5 to 15 μg/kg) may also be used; in this dose range it rarely causes hypotension and produces excellent analgesia and sedation. It is slowly infused in 50 to 100 μg aliquots until the desired effect is achieved; the dose may be supplemented during the procedure as necessary. A vagus-blocking intravenous dose of atropine (0.015 mg/kg) should be administered, because manipulation of the trachea and the use of opioid analgesics may produce bradycardia. In elderly patients with ischemic heart disease and a resting pulse rate >110/min, it is not necessary to use atropine if bradycardia does not occur during initial positioning and manipulation of the patient.

ANALGESIA

Pain control is established and maintained with local anesthesia in the form of 1% Xylocaine without epinephrine. It is important to surgically control bleeding, and epinephrine may mask bleeders, particularly in patients with coagulopathy. Skin and deeper tissues are thoroughly infiltrated to produce a complete field block.

THE PROCEDURE

Table 7-1 outlines the usual surgical implements required for performance of a tracheostomy, and Figure 7-1 demonstrates a typical tray. Whenever possible, the patient's shoulders should be elevated on folded towels or a sandbag and the head centered with sandbags or an occipital "donut." This extends the neck, bringing the trachea into a more superficial position, elevates the larynx above the sternal notch, and ensures that the trachea remains centered.

After wide skin preparation with a bacteriocidal agent (e.g., povidone-iodine) the area around the operative field

TABLE 7-1 Surgical Equipment Necessary for Tracheostomy

Positioning and Draping
Sandbags
Towels
Limb drape
Cautery ground pad
Light source
Instruments
Scalpel: #15 and #20 blades
Electrocautery
Syringe 10 cc: 25-gauge needle
Mosquito clamps: 4
Shallow retractors (Sens): 2
Deep retractors (Pole): 2
Straight scissors
Metzenbaum scissors
Mixter clamps: 2
Suction catheter: #10
Ligature: 3–0 silk, tapered needle
Gauze: 2 × 2 and 4 × 4
Tracheostomy tube: have selection of sizes available
Medication
Prep solution
Xylocaine 1%

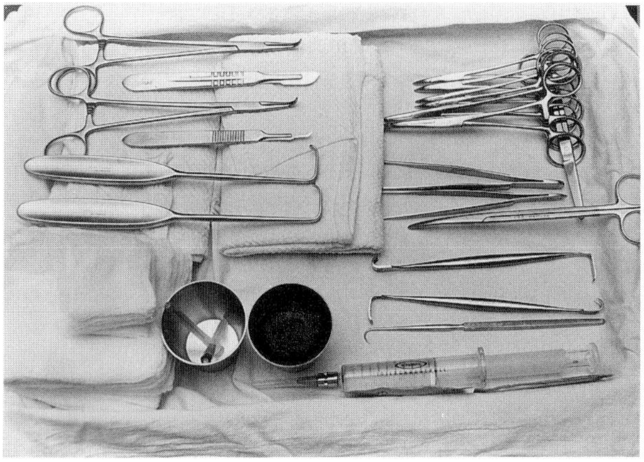

FIGURE 7-1 Surgical instruments required for tracheostomy (see Table 7-1).

is draped, leaving head and ETT access to those supervising the airway.

The skin incision is made as a gentle upward ellipse 1 cm below the lower border of the palpated cricoid. Bleeding is controlled either with mosquito hemostat-plain gut ligature or electrocautery. The skin incision is carried on through the platysma to expose the longitudinal strap muscles of the neck. Dissection is then switched to sharp-blunt, using Metzenbaum scissors and appropriate retraction. Anterior communicating veins may be encountered in this plane and should be controlled. Great care is taken at all stages of the operation to stay precisely in the midline. This avoids unnecessary bleeding, keeps the operator out of the vital structures lateral to the trachea, and ensures that the tracheal incision will be in the anterior and not in the lateral tracheal wall. The strap muscles are retracted to the side, thereby exposing the pretracheal fascia, which is attached superiorly to the cricoid, splits to ensheath the thyroid gland, and then courses caudad into the superior mediastinum. As a general rule, it is not necessary to divide the thyroid isthmus. By exerting gentle caudad pressure on the thyroid isthmus, the pretracheal fascia can be entered, allowing downward displacement of the thyroid and exposure of the anterior tracheal wall. Alternatively, the trachea can be approached from below the thyroid isthmus. When this tracheal approach is used, it is imperative that the vessels coursing along the inferior margin of the isthmus be isolated, ligated, and divided before cephalad retraction is placed on the thyroid gland. Occasionally, the thyroid isthmus will be particularly large, extending beneath the manubrium as a pyramidal lobe, or the gland will be peculiarly high in position. The thyroid may also be adherent to the underlying trachea (usually in association with old thyroiditis) and under these circumstances, it is often necessary to divide and suture-ligate (3–0 silk) the isthmus, thereby exposing the trachea.

Once exposed, the anterior wall of the trachea is carefully infiltrated with local anesthetic and 5 to 10 mL is directly introduced into the tracheal lumen, care being taken not to damage the ETT cuff. The tracheal hook, placed gently under the first ring, is used to bring the trachea into a more superficial position in the wound. A small scalpel (#15 blade) is used to incise the second or third tracheal ring and the adjacent intercartilaginous membrane precisely in the midline, the incision being carried caudad through the third and fourth rings as necessary with Metzenbaum scissors. Pole retractors are then inserted into the tracheal lumen, opening the resultant anterior vertical tracheal incision and exposing the underlying ETT.

The ETT is slowly removed and when the tip is at the upper margin of the new tracheal stoma, the catheter over which the tracheostomy tube is to be inserted is quickly introduced into the airway followed by the tracheostomy tube itself, which is threaded over the catheter (Figs. 7-2 and 7-3). The tracheostomy tube cuff is then inflated to the "just leak" level, and the ventilator tubing is switched from the ETT to tracheostomy tube. It is to be emphasized that the tracheostomy tube is inserted from the side and then rotated into position with a gentle screwing motion and that care must be taken to not damage the posterior tracheal wall with the tracheostomy tube tip. The ETT is left taped in place until it is ascertained that the tracheostomy tube is appropriately positioned and that ventilation is adequate. Once airway security is ensured, the ETT can be removed.

When the tracheostomy tube insertion is completed, towels or sandbags beneath the shoulders are carefully removed and only then should the tracheostomy tube ties be firmly secured with the neck in a neutral position. Dislodgement commonly occurs if the ties are secured while the neck is extended, because they will loosen when the head and neck are returned to their usual alignment.

Checks of appropriate placement include: unchanged or lower peak airway pressures as measured on the ventilator,

FIGURE 7-2 Tracheostomy tube with guide catheter. In a modification of the Seldinger technique, a No. 10 suction catheter is used as the "guide wire."

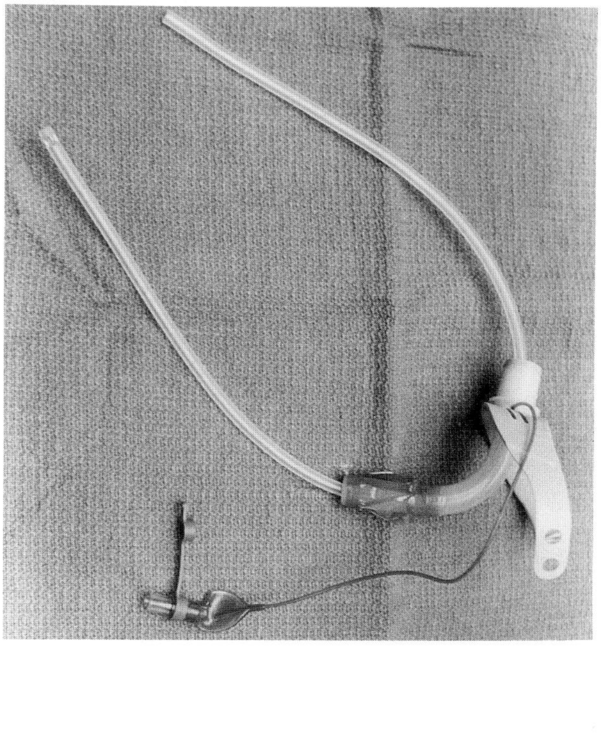

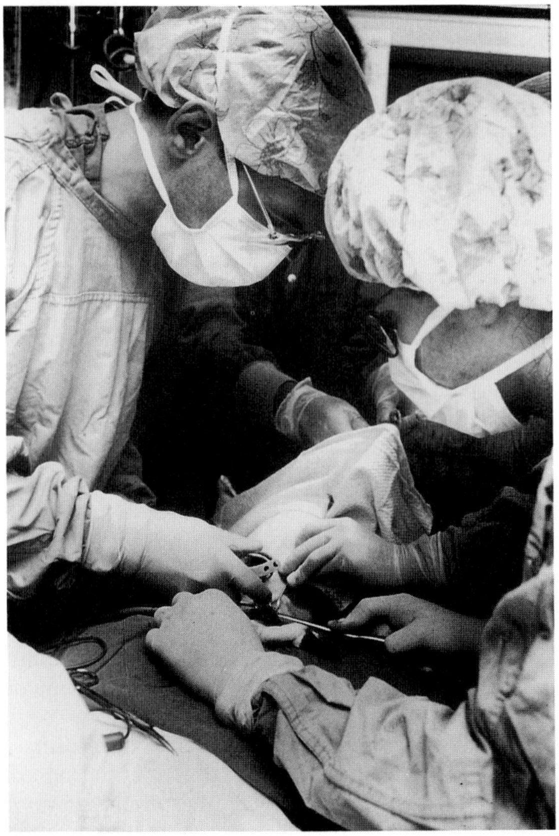

FIGURE 7-3 Introducing the tracheostomy tube into the airway. The suction catheter is introduced into the tracheostomy as the "guide." With gentle pressure and a 90° twist from the side, the cuffed tracheostomy tube is introduced into the trachea over the suction catheter, which is promptly removed.

equal air entry bilaterally on auscultation, a forceful expiratory blast with tracheostomy tube placement, fiberoptic bronchoscopic direct view through the tracheostomy tube, and finally, a posttracheostomy chest x-ray. If the tracheostomy tube has been misplaced or become dislodged, the tube should be removed immediately, the ETT pushed back into place, and the cuff reinflated to reestablish adequate ventilation.

The tracheostomy wound should not be sutured because this is or rapidly becomes a dirty wound that is best left exposed. All that is required is a simple dry dressing.

Scrupulous attention must be directed toward ligating vessels that might potentially bleed later, including those in the skin edges and within the platysma, the anterior jugular vein and, if the inferior isthmus or pyramidal lobe of the thyroid is mobilized, the thyroidea ima artery. Bleeding from the thyroid gland is best controlled by suture ligatures.

The Emergency Airway

Emergency access to the airway is required only for catastrophic airway obstruction. Inability to achieve translaryngeal intubation in an asphyxiating patient is the major indication for resorting to rapid surgical access. Needle cricothyroidostomy using a large bore needle (≥14 gauge) may be used as a temporizing measure. When connected to oxygen flowing at 15 L/min, using a Y connector in line to pulse the flow, adequate oxygenation may be maintained for a short period. This technique does not, however, permit adequate ventilation.

The definitive surgical procedure to provide emergency airway control is the cricothyroidostomy.[10,11] Using a midline vertical incision, the cricoid membrane is exposed. In the traumatized patient with a laryngeal injury, the cricoid is palpated by working cephalad from the sternal notch. A generous incision may be needed. Once the cricoid is identified, the membrane is split with a scalpel or mosquito clamp, and the airway is secured using a 5 to 6 mm internal diameter noncuffed tracheostomy tube in the adult patient. The cricothyroidostomy can be converted to tracheostomy on an elective basis later under more controlled circumstances.

The emergency tracheotomy is not essentially different from the elective variety—just done with more dispatch. No attention is paid to bleeders until the airway has been secured. The asphyxiating patient usually has grossly engorged neck veins, and therefore the procedure is daunting as blood seemingly spurts after every move of the operator. Once the airway has been entered and secured, however, bleeding rapidly subsides and any persisting bleeders are easily identified and tied off.

Complications of Tracheostomy[2,8,12–14]

Table 7-2 lists the postoperative complications of tracheostomy.

HEMORRHAGE

Hemorrhage in the early postoperative period generally appears within a few hours of tracheotomy and is usually due to improperly tied ligatures or vessels that, while in

TABLE 7-2 Postoperative Complications of Tracheostomy

Early
Hemorrhage
Subcutaneous vessels
Anterior neck veins
Thyroid vessels
Thyroid gland
Coagulopathy
Malpositioning or dislodgement of the tracheostomy tube
Pneumothorax/pneumomediastinum
Late
Hemorrhage
Innominate artery
Infection of lower respiratory tract
Tracheoesophageal fistula
Postdecannulation tracheal stenosis

spasm at the time of operation, dilate once the neurohumoral effects of operative trauma wear off. Occasionally, a severe ooze may arise from an injured thyroid or a late major bleed from a torn thyroidea ima artery. Persistent large volume bleeding should lead one to suspect that dissection was inadvertently carried laterally in the neck.

Although the site of bleeding can usually be ascertained with good lights, retraction, walling-off sponging, and assistance leaving the tracheostomy tube in place, the operator may have to resort to controlling the airway by reinserting the ETT from above, removing the tracheostomy tube, and carefully reexploring the wound.

Although rare, late hemorrhage may be related to tube erosion into the innominate artery. This occurs with a low-lying tracheostomy and should be considered if the tracheostomy tube is pulsatile or there are brief bright red "sentinel" bleeds. Management is by ventilation via a small ETT or tracheostomy tube and by compression of the bleeding fistula by the operator's little finger within the tracheostomy stoma, directed anteriorly. Proper control requires operative access with oversewing of the artery and repositioning of the tracheostomy tube higher in the neck via second and third rings. This complication is almost always a disaster and has a high mortality rate.

MALPOSITION AND DISLODGEMENT

Malpositioned or dislodged tracheostomy tubes are potentially lethal complications that usually occur within a short time of tracheotomy. They may be recognized by the ventilator high pressure alarming or "pressuring-off," development of subcutaneous emphysema, or the absence of any of the signs of a properly placed tube (vide supra). Even suspicion that malplacement or dislodgement has occurred demands urgent and prompt attention. No attempt should be made to reinsert a tube in a fresh tracheostomy without first regaining control of the airway by per os endotracheal intubation. After ETT intubation, the patient is once again placed on shoulder sandbags and with proper equipment, lights, and assistance, the wound is reexplored to identify the tracheostomy stoma and then reinsert the tracheostomy tube over a guide catheter or fiberoptic bronchoscope.

LATERAL DISSECTION MISADVENTURES

Pneumothorax occurring immediately after tracheostomy is usually due to inadvertent invasion of the pleural space by lateral and caudad dissection in those patients whose lung apices protrude into the lower neck. Tube thoracostomy drainage ensures that further leak will be evacuated. With lateral neck dissection, not only may lung apices be injured, but the great vessels of the neck and the recurrent laryngeal nerves are also at risk. In fact, the tracheostomy stoma may even be mistakenly created in the lateral tracheal wall leading to tracheostomy dislodgement and obstruction as well as extensive pressure-related cartilaginous necrosis. These lateral surgical wanderings are usually due to overly enthusiastic retraction on the part of an assistant and may be prevented by scrupulous attention to midline dissection.

TRACHEAL STENOSIS

Tracheal stenosis after tracheostomy most commonly occurs at the stomal site, and an appreciation for the events associated with the normal healing of a tracheal stoma is necessary to understand the evolution of this complication.[12,14]

A tracheal stoma gradually closes and heals by so-called tertiary intention, leaving a small fistulous tract for a considerable time after apparent closure. There is medial collapse of the severed cartilages to create the A-frame deformity seen commonly at endoscopic follow-up. The presence of exuberant granulation tissue at the stomal site or the presence of a suprastomal bar (thought to be related to above-cuff pooling of infected oropharyngeal secretions) often presages the development of a stenotic lesion as progressive cicatrization follows the granulation tissue. Cuff site stenosis is now rare, but tube angulation may be associated with tube tip-induced tracheal wall injury that eventuates in localized airway compromise at this level.

As with ETT complications, certain predispositions to tracheal stomal stenosis include female gender, duration of antecedent endotracheal intubation, rheumatoid arthritis, diabetes mellitus, tendency to keloid formation, and suppurative pneumonias. It has been suggested that prolonged ETT intubation preceding tracheotomy may predispose to tracheal stenosis.[8] Other influences include size and mobility of the tube. Interestingly, the duration that the tube is in situ seems to be an inconstant predictor of the subsequent development of stenosis. Cartilage has no intrinsic blood supply, receiving its vascular support from a segmental system of fine vessels. The cartilage is therefore exquisitely sensitive to pressure and readily undergoes pressure necrosis—thus, the larger the tube or the more mobile it is, the greater the resultant defect that must be closed by tertiary intention. Similarly, the more of the anterior tracheal wall that is removed or "picked clean" during dissection, the greater is the jeopardy to cartilaginous integrity.

Management of tracheal stomal stenosis is by resection of the involved area with primary reanastomosis. This may require mobilization of the trachea with "release" at the hyothyroid end and dissection of the right lung hilum. Gaps of up to 5 cm can be successfully bridged by reanastomosis. This surgery requires careful planning by surgeon and anesthetist and should not be undertaken by those inexperienced in this form of repair.

Tracheostomy Tubes

Tracheostomy tubes come in numerous shapes, sizes, and lengths and are made of several different materials. Least reactive and traumatic tubes are made from Silastic, but they are often hardest to place and somewhat more difficult to suction through. Ideally the tracheostomy tube should be about three-fourths the diameter of the tracheal lumen. For most adult males this is an 8 or 8.5 mm tube with about one size smaller for women. Special tracheostomy tubes have other smaller molded catheters that exit just above the

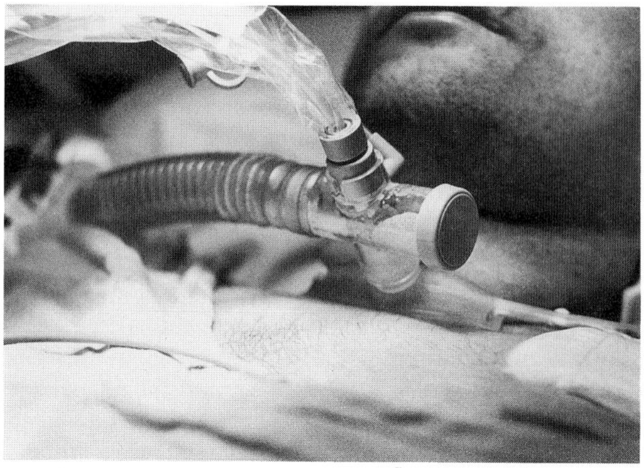

FIGURE 7-4 A swivel adapter should be used to reduce tension on the tracheostomy tube.

cuff either for purposes of communication (the "speaking trach") or suctioning of the suprastomal areas. There is evidence that the "laziness" of the laryngeal mechanism commonly associated with tracheostomy may lead to decannulation difficulties and that the postdecannulation swallowing and aspiration problems can be obviated by blowing air upward through the glottic chink. This serves to keep the above-cuff area of the tracheostomy stoma clear of secretions, allows the patient to talk, and seems to keep the laryngeal mechanism "tuned up" for eventual decannulation. An important feature for all tracheostomy tubes is the presence of some sort of swivel adapter so that tension on the tube by the weight of large bore connecting tubing and accidental tugs can be minimized (Fig. 7-4). To reduce the chance of pressure-induced cartilaginous necrosis, mobility and movement of the tracheostomy tube must be minimized. Many types of tracheostomy tubes are currently available. Virtually all have large volume, compliant cuffs. Every effort should be made to inflate cuffs to the "just leak" level rather than "just seal," and if seal occurs, the cuff pressure should not exceed 15 mmHg at any phase of the respiratory cycle. Unfortunately, a measured cuff pressure of 15 mmHg or less is no guarantee that lateral wall pressure (the key and unmeasured parameter) is not compromising mucosal and perichondrial blood supply, particularly at peak airway pressure when intratracheal pressures are high and hydraulic influences transmit these pressures to the tracheal wall from the cuff at points of contact.

Decannulation

Decannulation may be considered when the tracheostomy is no longer needed, i.e., when the original reasons for its placement have been remedied or resolved. Although there are a number of approaches to decannulation, they are usually intertwined with the issues of weaning from mechanical ventilation. The major reason, however, to leave a tube or obturator of some sort within the tracheal stoma is to keep the fistula open in case ongoing access for either tracheobronchial toilet or assisted ventilation is required. This preservation of the fistula as a safety factor may be achieved by way of insertion of progressively smaller tracheostomy tubes, the use of "buttons," the use of fenestrated tracheostomy tubes, or the use of obturators ("dummy trachs"). Problems with fenestrated tracheostomy tubes include the fact that the fenestration is usually in the wrong place to provide good airway continuity when "plugged" (this can usually be corrected with some "plastic surgery" on the fenestration with a #11 scalpel blade), the presence of a gas-flow resistive structure within the airway, and the flanges and irregularities of the system that tend to accumulate secretions. Granulation tissue uncommonly grows into the fenestration and bleeds with tracheostomy tube movement. Simple plugging of tracheostomy tubes produces many of these same problems and is not a good decannulation ploy. Several types of fistula-maintenance "buttons" are available but may be coughed out (or aspirated!) by some patients. "Dummy tracheostomy" tubes made of dental prosthetic material work extremely well, can readily be customized, do not obstruct the airway, are nonreactive, can be cleaned, and may be used to maintain the tracheal stoma indefinitely.

Permanent Tracheostomy

A permanent tracheostomy can be made by creating a U-shaped (Bjork) flap in the anterior tracheal wall and suturing this to the undermined lower margin of the skin wound. Healing generally takes about 2 weeks and interestingly, there is gradual stratification and squamification of tracheal mucosa adjacent to the stoma. The only reason that this might be carried out is to maintain a patent fistula in patients without a cannula.

Management of the Tracheostomy

Emphasis has already been laid on the importance of controlling and limiting mobility of the tracheostomy tube within the stoma to reduce pressure-induced cartilaginous necrosis. Swivel connectors, support of ventilator flex tubing, and minimization of patient movement of the head and neck are important in contributing to tube-stoma immobility.

Humidification of inspired gases prevents drying and crusting of secretions. Occasionally it may be necessary to instill warmed normal saline directly into a tracheal tube to assist in the clearance and mobilization of sticky or drying mucus or pus.

Suctioning of tracheostomies should be carried out on an "as necessary" basis rather than a clock-dictated schedule. Experienced attendants can readily tell when a patient requires suctioning.

It is the authors' opinion that the routine changing of tracheostomy tubes is unnecessary. Our practice has been to use a firm polyvinyl chloride (PVC) tube until fistulization is established (these tubes are easier to insert through a fresh tracheal stoma) and then at 5 to 7 days change the tube for a Silastic tube with a self-inflating foam cuff. Because Silastic tubes are harder to suction through, PVC tubes are retained in patients with major tracheobronchial toilet needs.

Communication for patients with tracheostomies is often difficult and frustrating but can be satisfactorily achieved by patients and considerate care givers. Writing pads, alphabet and phrase boards, speaking tracheostomy tubes (e.g., the "Pitt trach"), nasopharyngeal catheter vibrators, and external pharyngeal vibrators ("quackers") can be used with varying degrees of success by most patients. Many patients find the high retrograde gas flows necessary to use the speaking tracheostomy tubes irritating, but these tubes are very effective for short-term use. They may offer the added advantage of keeping the vocal cords "tuned up" and responsive to sensory stimulation.

References

1. Heffner JE: Medical indications for tracheostomy. Chest 96(1):186, 1989.
2. Heffner JE, Miller KS, Sahn SA: Tracheostomy in the intensive care unit: Part I. Indications, technique, management. Part II. Complications. Chest 90(3):169, 430, 1986.
3. Whited RE: Laryngeal dysfunction following prolonged intubation. Ann Otol Rhinol Laryngol 88:474, 1979.
4. Whited RE: A prospective study of laryngotracheal sequelae in long term intubation. Laryngoscope 94:367, 1984.
5. Whited RE: Posterior commissure stenosis post long-term intubation. Laryngoscope 93:1314, 1983.
6. Gaynor EB, Greenberg SB: Untoward sequelae of prolonged intubation. Laryngoscope 95:1461, 1985.
7. Colice GL, Stukel TA, Dain B: Laryngeal complications of prolonged intubation. Chest 96(4):877, 1989.
8. Stauffer JL, Olson DE, Petty TL: Complications and consequences of endotracheal intubation and tracheostomy. Am J Med 70:65, 1981.
9. Wright PE, Marini JJ, Bernard GR: In vitro versus in vivo comparison of endotracheal tube airway resistance. Am Rev Respir Dis 140:10, 1989.
10. Kress T, Balasubramaniam S: Cricothyroidotomy. Ann Emerg Med 11(11):197, 1982.
11. Boyd AD, Romita MC, Conlan AA: The clinical evaluation of cricothyroidotomy. Surg Gynecol Obstet 149:365, 1979.
12. Dane TEB, King EG: A prospective study of complications after tracheostomy for assisted ventilation. Chest 67(4):398, 1975.
13. Stock CM, Woodward CG, Shapiro BA et al: Perioperative complications of elective tracheostomy in critically ill patients. Crit Care Med 14(10):861, 1986.
14. Andrews MJ, Pearson FG: Incidence and pathogenesis of tracheal injury following cuffed tube tracheostomy with assisted ventilation: Analysis of a two year prospective study. Ann Surg 173:249, 1979.

Chapter 8

MECHANICAL VENTILATORS

EDWARD P. INGENITO
JEFFREY DRAZEN

Ventilator support is used in caring for many of the patients in medical and surgical ICUs. Management of the ventilated patient requires an understanding of how ventilators and the human respiratory system interact in health and specific disease states, as well as what types of ventilators and modes of ventilator operation are available. This chapter provides an introduction to ventilator management and includes a description of the types of ventilators most commonly encountered, conventional and nonconventional modes of ventilation currently available, and physiologic responses to ventilator application in specific clinical settings.

Indications for Mechanical Ventilation

Although "respiratory failure" is commonly cited as the major indication for initiation of ventilator support, this term has no universally accepted definition. In addition to being imprecise, this diagnosis fails to convey any specific information about the underlying process for which mechanical ventilation is being initiated. A more useful classification of syndromes best managed using mechanical ventilation is one based on underlying pathophysiology. This scheme provides a starting point for formulating a differential diagnosis and for directing therapy. One such classification scheme groups disease processes into four categories: **1.** those such as adult respiratory distress syndrome (ARDS), pulmonary edema, pulmonary hemorrhage, and severe infectious pneumonia which cause hypoxemia unresponsive to supplemental oxygen and in which shunt physiology predominates; **2.** those such as obstructive airways disease with respiratory muscle fatigue, acute and chronic neuromuscular disorders, respiratory depressant effects of medicinal and recreational drugs, or severe endocrinopathies which result in hypercapnia due to alveolar hypoventilation; **3.** those rendering the patient unable to protect and maintain patent airways either because of a decrease in level of consciousness or increase in airway or gastrointestinal secretions; and **4.** acute medical and postsurgical cardiovascular syndromes wherein mechanical ventilation is used as adjunctive therapy to decrease work of breathing.

The application of mechanical ventilation allows the physician to temporarily reverse respiratory failure and thus sustain life. The supportive nature of this intervention should be stressed since only rarely will mechanical ventilator support have a direct therapeutic effect. During the period of ventilator support, specific treatment is generally required to reverse the causes of respiratory failure and return the patient to the premorbid status. The intensivist must choose one from among the many types of available ventilator support modes which will be of greatest benefit in a given case. Despite the wide choice of approaches, the available interventions for the most part are limited and include changing tidal volume, frequency, inspiratory-to-expiratory (I:E) ratios, inspired gas concentrations, the orientation of the patient's body in the gravitational field, and end expired pressures.

General Classes of Ventilators

Mechanical ventilators are specialized pumps which perform the task usually done by the respiratory muscles, i.e., provide an external source of energy to move gases into the lung and allow for passive exhalation. This permits both oxygenation and ventilation (CO_2 elimination). No classification of mechanical ventilators includes all current and potential future systems. Our discussion classifies ventilators based on whether gas is pumped into and out of the lungs using positive pressure applied at the airway opening (i.e., positive-pressure ventilation) or negative pressure applied at the chest wall (i.e., negative-pressure ventilation).

POSITIVE-PRESSURE VENTILATORS

Ventilators of this type produce respiratory flows by generating time-varying positive pressures at the airway opening. There are two major subtypes of positive-pressure ventilators. Pressure-cycled ventilators are those which generate a predetermined pressure versus time profile and terminate inspiration when that predetermined airway pressure has been reached. The physician specifies the peak pressure and pressure waveform, while flow rate and tidal volume are determined by the impedance of the patient's respiratory system. This type of ventilator does not provide stable minute ventilations since a patient's respiratory mechanics change. Therefore, pressure-cycled ventilators are used infrequently in adults. They are more commonly used in neonatal ICUs where unanticipated changes in lung mechanics are smaller in magnitude and less likely to significantly alter minute ventilation.

Volume-cycled ventilators deliver a predetermined tidal volume at a specified inspiratory flow rate and terminate inspiration when that volume has been delivered. Airway pressures are determined by respiratory system impedance. This type of ventilator ensures delivery of a known minute ventilation independent of changes in lung mechanics. Theoretically, an increased risk of barotrauma exists compared to pressure-cycled ventilation since peak airway pressures increase proportionally to respiratory impedance. To ensure patient safety, volume-cycled machines are equipped with a pressure release valve and a high pressure alarm. This alerts the operator to the existence of a problem that can then be evaluated and corrected.

NEGATIVE-PRESSURE VENTILATORS

This class of ventilators includes the "iron lung" and certain types of cuirass ventilators. They produce cyclic pressure gradients across the respiratory system by generating negative pressures at the chest wall surface while the airway opening remains at constant atmospheric pressure. Negative-pressure ventilators are pressure-cycled, allowing the operator to specify the transrespiratory system pressure, while tidal volume and inspiratory and expiratory flows are determined by respiratory system impedance. In theory, these ventilators can be used for managing any respiratory failure patient. However, their generally cumbersome mechanical structure, lack of both availability and familiarity to most ICU physicians, and pressure rather than volume control characteristics make them less desirable than positive-pressure ventilators.

Modes of Mechanical Ventilation

The pattern of machine-determined pressure or volume cycling used to drive gas flows during mechanical ventilation characterizes the *mode* of ventilator operation. In many cases, one class of ventilator can function in any of several different modes. The major differences among the modes are the control and sensing functions used by the ventilator to initiate and terminate breaths. This section describes conventional and nonconventional modes of operation for standard ventilators, including high frequency ventilation.

CONTROL MODE VENTILATION

DESCRIPTION. Volume-cycled control mode ventilation (CMV) is one of the most basic modes of mechanical ventilator support. The ventilator provides a full tidal volume breath at a rate specified by the user. This ventilatory pattern is continued independent of patient effort, and between ventilator breaths, the inspiratory valve is closed to the patient such that no additional breaths can be taken. An example of airway pressure versus time during CMV is shown in Fig. 8-1.

INDICATIONS. Volume-cycled CMV is generally used to support patients without spontaneous respiratory efforts. It ensures that the patient will receive the specified number of breaths at a designated tidal volume independent of spontaneous efforts. Appropriate patients include those unable to ventilate secondary to drug intoxication, those suffering from central and peripheral neurologic disorders that affect respiratory neuromuscular function, and those who are pharmacologically paralyzed.

LIMITATIONS. In the patient without respiratory efforts, this mode of ventilation is usually safe and effective. However, difficulties may arise when the patient is capable of spontaneous respiratory efforts since this can lead to patient-ventilator dysynchrony.[1] This occurs when the patient's breathing cycle is out of phase with that of the ventilator. For example, the patient may try to exhale during the ventilator inspiratory cycle. Because the ventilator will abort any breath for which proximal airway pressure exceeds a preset limit, dysynchrony can result in a significant number of aborted ventilator cycles, which in turn causes hypercapnia. Once the patient can generate spontaneous respiratory efforts, it is best to use one of the modes of ventilation outlined below.

INITIAL SETTINGS. The operator sets inspired oxygen concentration, tidal volume, inspiratory flow rate, end expiratory pressure, and ventilator pressure and volume alarms during ventilator support using control mode. A tidal volume of 10 to 15 mL/kg, rate of 12 breaths/min, and inspired oxygen fraction ($F_{I_{O_2}}$) of 1.0 are common initial settings. Initial peak flow rate is generally set at about 60 L/min with

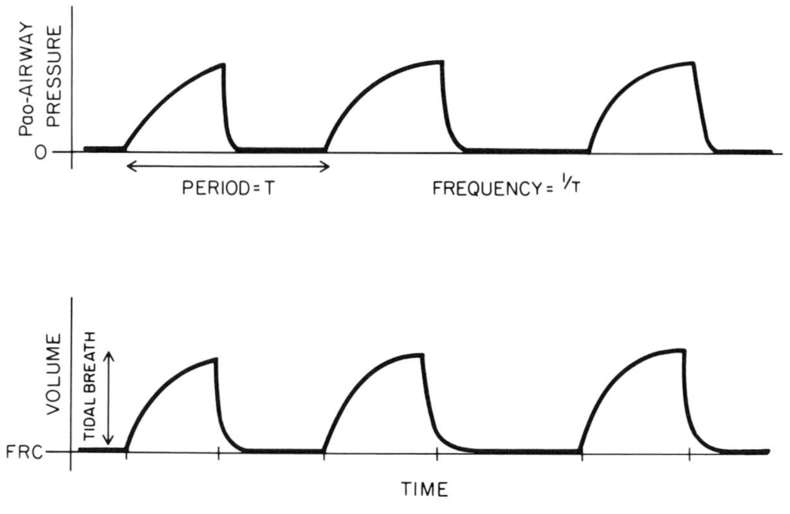

FIGURE 8-1 Airway pressure (Pao) and tidal volume versus time profiles for positive pressure *volume-cycled control mode ventilation.* Fixed tidal volume breaths are delivered at a preset rate. Expiration is passive.

a decreasing ramp waveform such that flow rate and resistive pressures are low when lung volume and elastic pressures are high. The rate, tidal volume, and FI_{O_2} are adjusted as needed to achieve adequate gas exchange. Flow rate may require modification in certain clinical circumstances such as chronic obstructive pulmonary disease (COPD) or asthma, where higher flow rates are often used to allow for increased expiratory times, improved gas distribution, and diminished gas trapping.[2] The same principles outlined here for initial settings apply equally well to other volume-controlled modes of ventilation such as assist-control (A/C), intermittent mandatory ventilation (IMV), and synchronized intermittent mandatory ventilation (SIMV).

ASSIST-CONTROL MODE VENTILATION

DESCRIPTION. The "assist" part of A/C ventilation refers to ventilator supplementation of patient-initiated breaths during the ventilator cycle. This occurs as a consequence of a sensing device within the system which detects patient-initiated breaths as a fall in airway pressure below a specific threshold pressure. When this occurs, the ventilator provides a full tidal volume breath synchronized to patient effort. In assist mode ventilation without "backup," a patient who fails to initiate a spontaneous breath will not receive any ventilator-driven breaths, and thus, changes in respiratory drive affect minute ventilation. Most modern ventilators do not function in simple assist mode, but rather have a combined A/C mode. The "control" part of A/C ventilation refers to the user-specified backup ventilation rate operational during A/C ventilation. Any patient who fails to initiate a spontaneous breath within a predetermined cycle period will receive a ventilator breath. If the spontaneous respiratory rate of the patient exceeds the control rate, then no control breaths are delivered, and the machine functions completely in assist mode. If the patient's spontaneous rate does not exceed the control backup rate, then volume-cycled control breaths will be provided at appropriate intervals as shown in Fig. 8-2.

INDICATIONS. This is a commonly used mode for providing ventilator support. It allows for better synchrony between patient and machine while providing safe volume-cycled ventilator support. It can be applied to awake, moderately sedated, or fully paralyzed patients. It is often chosen as the mode of ventilator support immediately post-intubation or postoperatively when it may initially provide CMV until the patient regains consciousness and begins spontaneous breathing. It is also used to rest patients following T-piece weaning trials and in patients with increased metabolic demands or weakened respiratory muscles who are unable to eliminate carbon dioxide and maintain a normal pH. Examples include worsening metabolic acidosis and hypermetabolism with increased carbon dioxide production due to infection, burns, multisystem organ failure, or carbohydrate loading.[3] Finally, A/C ventilation can be used directly for respiratory muscle strengthening and weaning. A/C requires that a specified inspiratory pressure threshold be exceeded to trigger an assisted breath. To achieve this threshold pressure, the respiratory muscles must work to decompress gas within the lungs. By gradually increasing threshold pressure, a graded exercise program for the respiratory muscles can be provided.[4]

LIMITATIONS. Patient-ventilator dysynchrony can still occur since spontaneous breaths initiated immediately prior to timed breaths will fail to synchronize with the ventilator, leading to "stacking." Rapid changes in blood pH can also result from ventilator-assisted hyperventilation causing respiratory alkalosis. This occurs when A/C ventilation is used in patients who have an increased respiratory drive related to factors other than hypercapnia or hypoxemia (i.e., degree of agitation or lung irritant receptors). COPD patients who are tachypneic may develop auto-positive end expiratory pressure (auto-PEEP) on A/C ventilation with potential for barotrauma.[5] When using the graded threshold approach for weaning, A/C ventilation is associated with two potential problems: **1.** exercise is in part isometric (at least during breath initiation) and exercises performed in this nonphysiologic way may be less

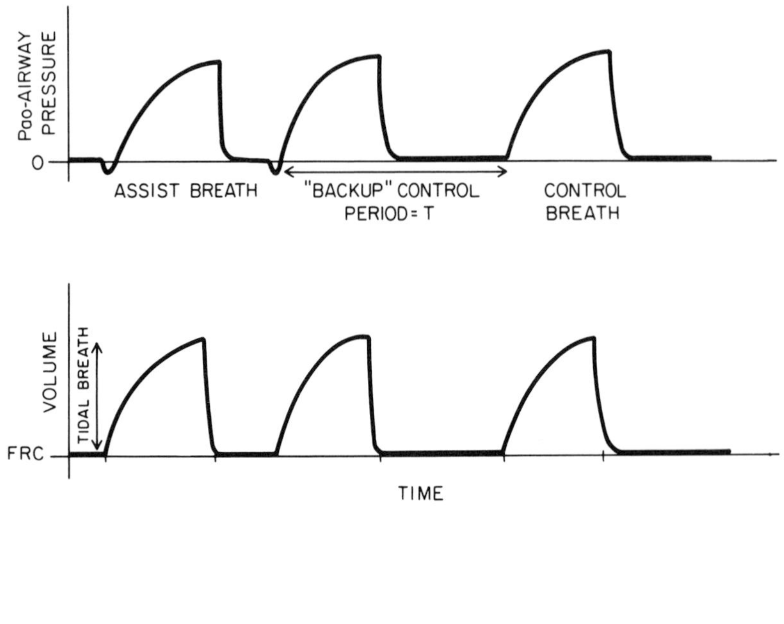

FIGURE 8-2 Airway pressure (Pao) and tidal volume versus time profiles for *assist-control ventilation*. Inspiratory effort by the patient is detected by the machine as a drop in airway pressure below a specific threshold. When this occurs, a full positive pressure tidal volume is delivered in synchrony with the patient's effort. If the patient fails to initiate a breath during the user-specified "backup" period, a positive pressure breath is delivered by the machine.

beneficial than more standard exercise regimens; and **2.** the physician may overestimate a patient's ability to lower intrathoracic pressure, or the patient may tire and become unable to generate adequate negative threshold pressures with time. This could represent a serious hazard if control backup were insufficient since assisted breaths would no longer be provided.

INITIAL SETTINGS. Initial settings for A/C mode ventilation are similar to those for standard control ventilation. Following initiation of ventilator support, patients must be observed for ventilator-assisted hyperpnea and auto-PEEP. The operator should note that decreasing the backup rate during A/C ventilation only affects minute ventilation if the patient's spontaneous rate is less than ventilator backup. If this is not the case, then decreasing the A/C rate will be ineffective in reducing ventilator-related hyperpnea or auto-PEEP.

IMV AND SIMV MODE VENTILATION

DESCRIPTION. Intermittent mandatory ventilation (IMV) and synchronized intermittent mandatory ventilation (SIMV) are similar in mode of operation, indications for use, and limitations. Therefore, they are presented together in this section.

IMV is similar to CMV in that patients receive a predetermined number of time-cycled ventilator breaths independent of their spontaneous respiratory efforts. The difference between IMV and simple CMV is that in IMV, between ventilator breaths, the breathing circuit is open and fresh gas is available for the patient to breathe spontaneously. Frequency and tidal volume of spontaneous breaths are determined by the patient and supplement mandatory breaths by the ventilator. In effect, IMV represents a blend of control and spontaneous ventilation. A profile of airway opening pressure versus time during IMV is presented in Fig. 8-3.

As IMV is to CMV, so is SIMV to A/C mode. During SIMV, the operator sets a backup rate, along with other standard ventilator parameters. Mandatory breaths are delivered at specified intervals. Between them, the patient is able to breathe spontaneously. When a ventilator breath is programmed to occur, the ventilator waits a predetermined trigger period. Any breath initiated during this trigger period will be supplemented by the ventilator such that the patient receives a full assisted tidal breath. If no patient-initiated breath occurs during the trigger period, the ventilator delivers a full unassisted tidal breath. Thus, SIMV represents a combination of A/C with spontaneous ventilation. A profile of airway opening pressure versus time during SIMV is displayed in Fig. 8-4.

INDICATIONS. IMV and SIMV can be used as primary modes of ventilator support in postoperative or newly intubated patients who display minimal spontaneous respiratory efforts because both provide backup ventilation. However, the major design advantage of IMV-SIMV over A/C mode is the opening of the inspiratory valve between ventilator breaths, which allows for spontaneous patient breathing, and theoretically, for respiratory muscle conditioning in the form of pressure-tidal volume work. For this reason, IMV and SIMV are generally thought of as specifically useful for ventilator weaning.[6]

LIMITATIONS. During IMV, patient ventilator dysynchrony is a possibility since mandatory breaths are time-cycled and independent of patient effort. Thus, a patient who is being underventilated by the machine and is breathing spontaneously at a high rate may attempt to expire during mandatory breaths and not receive effective ventilation. This most commonly occurs when weaning proceeds too rapidly in a given patient, resulting in agitation, tachycardia, tachypnea, and diaphoresis. It usually responds to an increase in the IMV rate and mild sedation.

A second theoretical limitation of both IMV and SIMV mode ventilation is that they may delay extubation in some patients because of the "nonphysiologic" way in which respiratory muscle conditioning occurs—exercise during normal spontaneous breaths results from low pressure-high

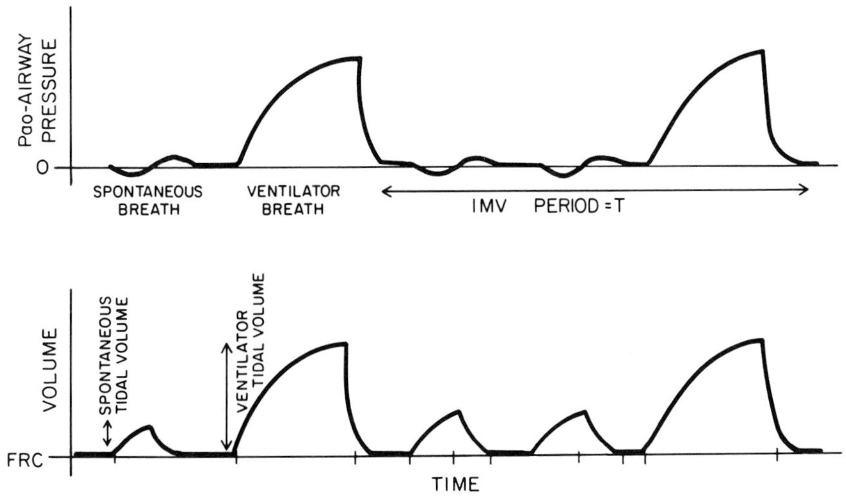

FIGURE 8-3 Airway pressure and tidal volume versus time profiles for *intermittent mandatory ventilation.* Positive pressure volume-cycled breaths are delivered at a preset rate similar to control mode ventilation, except that between breaths, the inspiratory valve to the patient is open, allowing for spontaneous breathing.

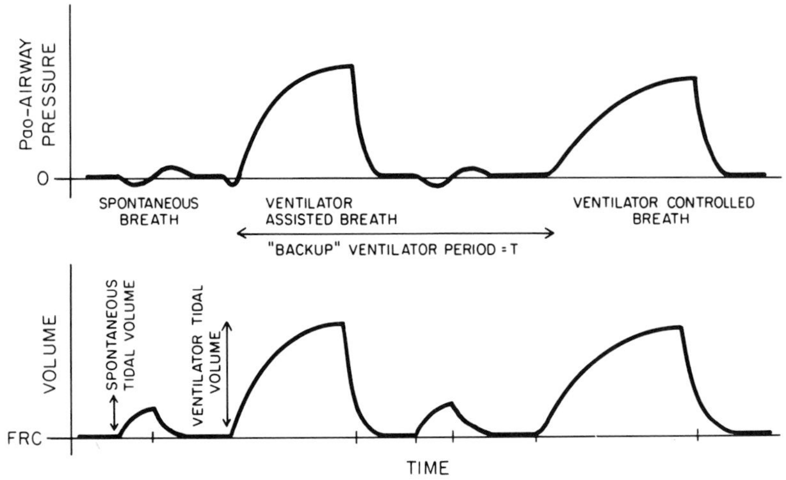

FIGURE 8-4 Airway pressure and tidal volume versus time profiles for *synchronized intermittent mandatory ventilation.* The ventilator "waits" a preset time for the patient to initiate a breath, detected as a decrease in airway pressure below a preset trigger value, similar to assist control ventilation. Full tidal volume positive pressure breaths are then delivered in synchrony with the patient's effort. If no attempt is made to initiate a breath during the backup period, a positive pressure breath is delivered by the machine. Between full tidal breaths, the inspiratory valve to the patient is open, allowing for spontaneous breathing.

volume work cycles, whereas during spontaneous IMV-SIMV breaths, work cycles tend to be high pressure and low volume. This also contrasts with respiratory muscle work during A/C and pressure support (vide infra) modes. This kind of work may affect muscle energy expenditure adversely and may provide less conditioning than low pressure-high volume work cycles.

INITIAL SETTINGS. Initial settings for IMV-SIMV are similar to those used in CMV and A/C ventilation.

PRESSURE SUPPORT VENTILATION

DESCRIPTION. Pressure support ventilation (PSV) is patient triggered, flow-cycled pressure ventilation where each inspiratory effort is augmented by an operator-specified amount (most ventilators allow levels between 1 and 100 cmH_2O) of positive pressure (not tidal volume) at the airway opening. Expiration is passive, and respiratory rate and tidal volume are determined by patient effort and respiratory system impedance, respectively. Pressure support is terminated when inspiratory flow falls below a minimum trigger value sensed by the machine (in general, the operator does not have control of this threshold value). Parameters set by the operator are inspiratory pressure level, FI_{O_2}, and end expired pressure.[7] Profiles of airway pressure and lung volume versus time during PSV at a level of 25 cmH_2O are presented in Fig. 8-5. Example A represents a patient with normal respiratory resistance and compliance, example B a patient with decreased lung compliance, for example fibrotic lung disease, kyphoscoliosis, or fibrothorax, and example C a patient with increased lung resistance, for example, COPD or asthma. The figure demonstrates that different lung volumes and minute ventilations can result from application of the same level of pressure support to patients with different intrinsic lung diseases. This underscores the point that during pressure support ventilation, tidal volume is a function of respiratory system mechanics and patient effort.

INDICATIONS AND LIMITATIONS. PSV is not used as a primary mode of ventilation, but rather to wean patients from ventilator support. Two advantages of PSV over conventional IMV-SIMV weaning have been proposed, although verification of clinical benefit in terms of decreased weaning time has not been demonstrated. The first is a reduction in

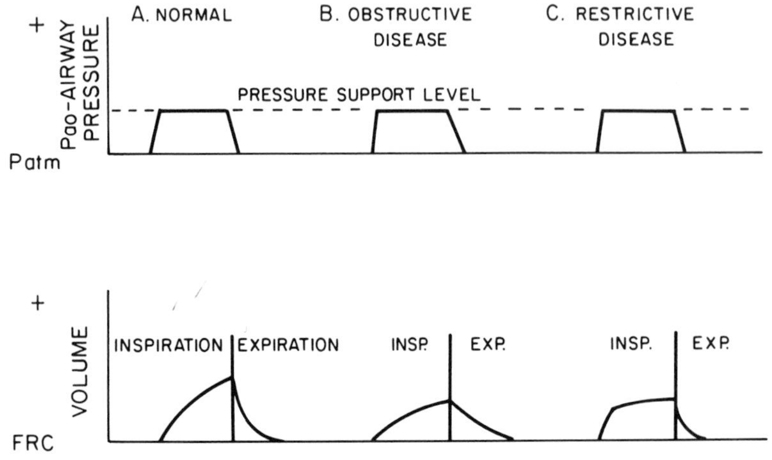

FIGURE 8-5 This figure demonstrates how differences in lung impedance influence tidal volume profiles during pressure support ventilation. Example A depicts airway pressure and tidal volume in a patient with normal airway resistance and lung compliance. Examples B and C depict how airway obstruction and decreased lung compliance affect tidal volume delivered when the airway pressure profile remains the same.

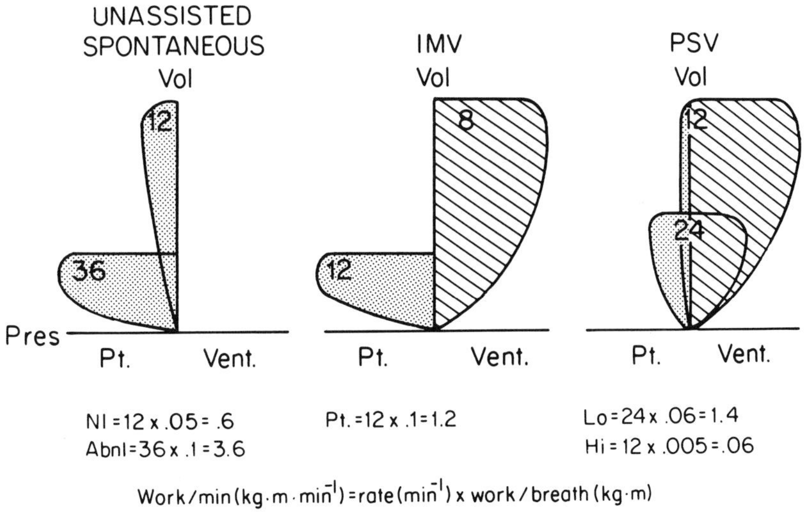

FIGURE 8-6 A comparison of work of breathing during spontaneous respiration, intermittent mandatory ventilation (IMV), and pressure support ventilation (PSV) at fixed minute ventilation. The work per breath with normal lung impedance is depicted as the area within the pressure-volume loop labeled "12" in the left-hand figure. The total work per minute is shown as the work per breath multiplied by the number of breaths per minute. The loop labeled "36" depicts respiratory pressure-volume profiles during spontaneous breathing when lung impedance is abnormally high. The work per breath is twice normal and the tidal volume one-third normal. To maintain the same minute ventilation, six-fold more work must be done by the respiratory system. The middle figure depicts pressure-volume work loads during IMV ventilation in a patient with abnormally high respiratory impedance. Patient work of breathing, represented by the area in the pressure-volume loop labeled "12," is twice normal although the ventilator is providing the majority of the minute ventilation. Spontaneous breaths are low volume–high pressure unlike spontaneous breaths in the normal lung. The right-hand figure illustrates distribution of work between patient and machine during pressure support ventilation under similar conditions. The machine "pressure-assists" each patient-initiated breath. At a low level of pressure support, 24 breaths per minute are required to maintain an adequate minute ventilation. Patient work is the same as during IMV ventilation, about twice that during normal spontaneous breathing. With a high level of pressure support, large tidal volumes can be delivered synchronously with patient-triggered breaths, with the patient work load reduced to a fraction of baseline. This theoretically allows for physiologic pressure volume endurance exercising of respiratory muscles at a time when the respiratory system is unable to perform the work of breathing because of an abnormally high respiratory system impedance. (Figure from McIntyre NR: Pressure support ventilation: Effects on ventilatory reflexes and ventilatory-muscle workloads. Respir Care 32:447, 1987, with permission.)

dyspnea attributed to improved patient-ventilator synchrony, and reduction in afferent signals from chest wall and lung parenchymal mechanoreceptors to the medullary respiratory center. The second is "more physiologic" conditioning of respiratory muscles during weaning. Mechanical ventilation for 72 h or more can cause respiratory muscle deconditioning. The mode of ventilation used during weaning should allow for respiratory muscle conditioning. Studies suggest that work performed by the respiratory muscles during PSV is low pressure-high volume work similar to that of spontaneous breathing and optimal for respiratory muscle conditioning. During IMV-SIMV weaning, respiratory muscles work only during spontaneous, unassisted breaths between mandatory ventilator breaths. Respiratory muscle work performed during unassisted breaths is low volume–high pressure work, in theory less suited for conditioning respiratory muscles. Examples of respiratory muscle pressure-volume workloads during spontaneous, SIMV, and PSV ventilation are shown in Fig. 8-6, contrasting the high pressure–low volume work of spontaneous SIMV breaths to low pressure–high volume work of PSV and normal breaths.

INITIAL SETTINGS. PSV is usually initiated at a pressure level sufficient to provide full tidal volumes (10 to 15 mL/kg), which is designated as *PSVmax.* The level of pressure support is then gradually withdrawn, requiring that the patient's respiratory muscles perform increasing amounts of respiratory work to maintain minute ventilation. Available data suggest that patients weaned using PSV increase their respiratory rate which, in turn, increases the rate of triggering the ventilator as the magnitude of airway pressure support is decreased. Initially, the ventilator performs all the work of breathing as rate increases and tidal volume decreases. When the level of pressure support is no longer sufficient to provide a tidal volume at which the tidal volume-rate product (i.e., minute ventilation) satisfies the patient's respiratory needs (a level of pressure support, usually between 40 and 60 percent of PSVmax), patients begin to actively generate negative pleural pressures and increase tidal volume to maintain minute ventilation. Pressure support is then gradually decreased as tolerated. When adequate gas exchange is achieved with pressure support of about 5 cmH_2O, extubation can usually be attempted.[8]

PRESSURE CONTROL VENTILATION

DESCRIPTION. Pressure control ventilation (PCV) in its most basic form refers to time cycling of a pressure wave at the airway opening, independent of patient respiratory effort. Tidal volume, and thus minute ventilation, are determined by respiratory system impedance; exhalation occurs passively. To avoid patient-ventilator dysynchrony, PCV would require a patient to be either well synchronized with the ventilator or sedated and without spontaneous respiratory efforts. Furthermore, since minute ventilation depends on intrinsic mechanical properties of the respiratory system, PCV would have to be used cautiously in patients with unstable reactive airways disease since changes in respiratory mechanics could have an adverse effect on ventilation.

PCV has limited clinical utility when applied according to this strict definition. A "modified" PCV is used clinically in both adult and pediatric medicine, however, combining patient triggering and pressure cycling or flow cycling with pressure or volume control backup. When a patient initiates a breath, a preset positive pressure is supplied by the ventilator to the airway opening, effectively providing pressure support for the triggered breath. Exhalation is passive. Tidal volume and minute ventilation are determined by the intrinsic impedance of the patient's respiratory system.

INDICATIONS. PCV with backup has been used as a primary mode of ventilation in both medical and surgical ICU patients. It has several theoretical advantages over volume-controlled ventilation. Flow during PCV is decelerating. Thus, peak airway pressure due to flow resistance occurs early in the inspiration, while that due to elastic recoil occurs at end inspiration. This produces lower and less variable peak airway pressures than during equivalent volume-cycled ventilation. A second potential benefit of positive-pressure ventilation using decelerating flow is that peak ventilator flow coincides with the patient's maximal inspiratory effort. This improves patient-ventilatory synchrony and decreases mechanoreceptor stimulation, which may act to stimulate sensations of dyspnea.

LIMITATIONS. The major limitation of PCV is that of pressure-cycled ventilation in general: minute ventilation which depends on the intrinsic impedance of the respiratory system. Patients with unstable lung mechanics therefore require careful observation to ensure adequate ventilation. The theoretical advantages of PCV over conventional volume-controlled ventilation have never been proven, and since most clinicians have less experience with pressure-cycled than volume-cycled ventilation, PCV is not as commonly used in ICU medicine as A/C ventilation and IMV-SIMV.

INITIAL SETTINGS. The clinician must set $F_{I_{O_2}}$, airway pressure level (as with PSV), and end-expiratory pressure, as well as backup mode and rate during PCV. Airway pressure is maintained at PSVmax as defined for PSV, and tidal volume recorded to ensure adequate minute ventilation. Backup rate is chosen to provide adequate minute ventilation in the event of decreased intrinsic respiratory drive and may be supplied either in pressure control or IMV-SIMV mode.

INVERSE RATIO VENTILATION

DESCRIPTION. Inverse ratio ventilation (IRV) refers to mechanical ventilation in which the I:E ratio is set greater than one. This is accomplished using any of three approaches: **1.** pressure-cycled breaths during which the ventilator delivers a preset airway pressure for a fixed period of time at a preset I:E ratio of greater than one; **2.** volume-cycled breaths during which the inspiratory time is prolonged by slowing the inspiratory flow rate, and the I:E ratio is greater than one; and **3.** volume-cycled breaths during which the inspiratory flow rate is not altered, but the inspiratory time is prolonged by adding a pause of preset duration to end inspiration, such that inspiratory plus pause time is greater than expiratory time.

Although each of these approaches will produce a unique flow and airway pressure profile, each will also produce the physiology thought to be beneficial during IRV: **1.** a prolonged inflation cycle to allow for opening of alveolar units with "long opening time constants" which can then participate in gas exchange; and **2.** increased time for gas diffusion across damaged lung regions with decreased diffusion capacity[9] (Fig. 8-7).

To date, no direct measurements of lung volumes or tidal volume distribution have been made during IRV, however. It is therefore possible that IRV improves gas exchange in part or entirely by increasing auto-PEEP.

INDICATIONS. The best-studied clinical indication for considering use of IRV is diffuse lung injury with hypoxemia, where it would be applied as an alternative to conventional A/C ventilation or IMV-SIMV with PEEP. It has been suggested that IRV can provide equivalent oxygenation at lower peak airway and mean airway pressures than CMV or IMV with PEEP.[10] In theory, this would reduce the risk of barotrauma and the potential for hemodynamic compromise.

The majority of clinical trials to date have used IRV in pressure control mode in neonates with respiratory distress syndrome. Descriptions of its use in adult ICU medicine are limited to case reports of patients with diffuse lung injury doing poorly on conventional SIMV-PEEP support, who show improvement or stabilization in hemodynamics, respiratory mechanics, and oxygenation following initiation of IRV. Others have reported survival in critically ill patients managed with IRV following an initial poor clinical response to conventional ventilator support. These successes suggest that IRV may be clinically useful in certain patients with diffuse lung injury when conventional ventilatory support is failing.

LIMITATIONS. Because of limited experience with IRV, the full spectrum of potential limitations associated with its use is probably not yet appreciated. One significant limitation is

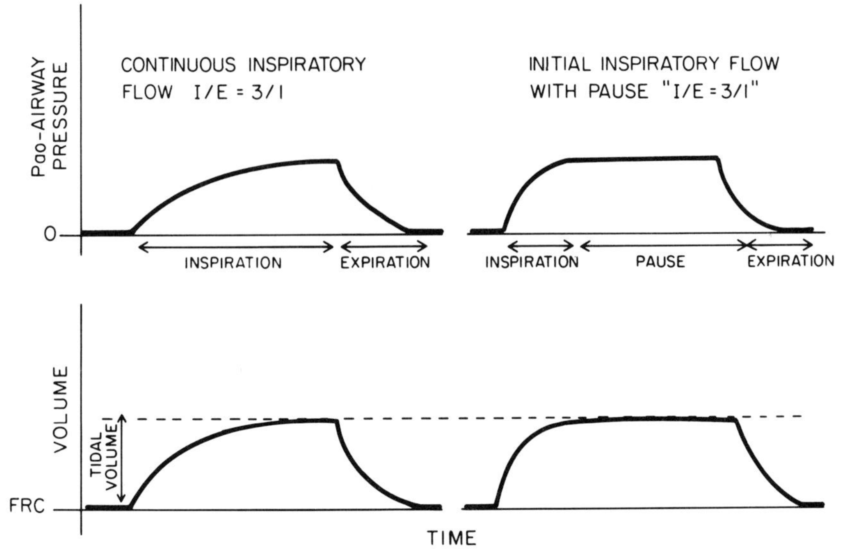

FIGURE 8-7 Airway pressure and tidal volume profiles during *inverse ratio ventilation* achieved in either of two ways. In the first panel, a tidal breath with I/E of 3/1 is provided with continuous inspiratory flow at a slower than normal rate, while expiration occurs passively. In the second panel, a tidal breath with I/E of 3/1 is provided by delivering inflation at a normal flow rate, and including a pause at end-inspiration to achieve an I/E of 3/1.

that IRV requires heavy sedation, often with paralysis, because of the nonphysiologic character of tidal volume cycling. Inadequate sedation could result in pronounced patient-ventilator dysynchrony with deterioration in gas exchange and potential barotrauma. Based on available data, it seems that IRV may prove useful for managing certain patients with diffuse lung injury when they are failing conventional supportive care. Benefits remain unproven, however, and because of the need for paralysis and the potential for hemodynamic compromise and barotrauma, this mode of ventilation must be considered experimental and used with caution.

INITIAL SETTINGS. IRV has been applied to clinical practice almost solely in pressure-cycled mode and settings for application in this manner will be described. As with other types of pressure-cycled ventilation, the operator must specify the airway pressure profile and F_{IO_2}; tidal volume and flow profile are determined by the patient's respiratory system impedance. It is common to start with an I:E ratio of 2:1, although ratios as high as 4:1 have been used with success. Initial settings are 25 to 40 cmH_2O for peak inspiratory pressure, 14 to 20 breaths/min for rate, and 100 percent for F_{IO_2}. Tidal volume, hemodynamics, and blood gases must be monitored, and adjustments made as indicated.

AIRWAY PRESSURE RELEASE VENTILATION

DESCRIPTION. Airway pressure release ventilation (APRV) combines features of continuous positive airway pressure (CPAP) and PCV . Gas exchange is achieved by decreasing pressure at the airway opening below some constant baseline inflation pressure which maintains resting lung volume above functional residual capacity (FRC). The inspiratory flow valve is open throughout the ventilatory cycle such that the patient is able to breathe spontaneously in a manner similar to CPAP. However, at preset intervals, ventilator support is superimposed on spontaneous respirations by releasing the positive pressure at the airway opening and allowing the lungs to deflate either to FRC with airway opening pressure equal to ambient, or to some volume above FRC determined by a preset end expiratory pressure. APRV airway pressure versus time appears as the "inverse" of an IMV profile as depicted in Fig. 8-8.[11]

INDICATIONS. The primary clinical indication for APRV is refractory hypoxemia as a result of diffuse lung injury. The proposed benefits of APRV over conventional ventilator support are that airway and alveolar patency are maintained by continuous positive pressures independent of whether alveolar time constants for opening are long or short, since "peak" positive pressure is maintained between all pressure release breaths. It has been suggested that APRV can achieve adequate blood oxygenation at a lower peak and mean airway pressure than is possible using conventional ventilation. It has also been argued that by allowing for spontaneous respirations, respiratory muscle conditioning can be maintained even in the setting of serious lung injury, because heavy sedation with paralysis has not been required in clinical practice.

LIMITATIONS. Like IRV, APRV has been used infrequently in clinical practice, and it is likely that the full spectrum of potential complications associated with its use is not yet known. In addition, the theoretical benefits of APRV described above have not clearly been demonstrated in patients with diffuse lung injury nor have any trials shown an improvement in clinical outcome among patients treated with APRV compared to conventional support. Theoretical limitations are those associated with other pressure-cycled modes of ventilator support. These include patient-ventilator dysynchrony, inadequate tidal volumes, hemodynamic compromise, and barotrauma.

INITIAL SETTINGS. The operator is responsible for setting airway maintenance pressure (peak airway pressure), air-

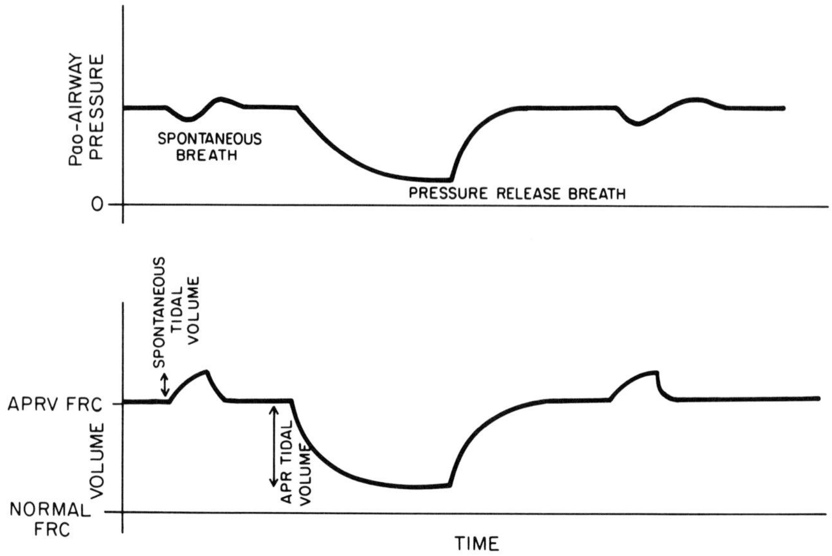

FIGURE 8-8 Airway pressure and tidal volume profiles during *airway pressure release ventilation.* Airway pressure release resting lung volume is significantly higher than normal functional residual capacity. Machine breaths are delivered by decreasing airway pressure, such that the lung deflates from its resting volume to provide tidal ventilation. Delivered tidal volume is controlled by lung impedance, since the user specifies resting and pressure-release pressures. Between tidal breaths, the inspiratory valve to the patient is open, allowing for spontaneous breathing.

way pressure release level, ventilator rate, and F_{IO_2}. Tidal volume and flow rate are determined by the impedance of the patient's respiratory system. Initial settings for airway maintenance pressure range between 20 and 35 cmH_2O, and for airway pressure release level between 2 and 10 cmH_2O. Other settings are as previously described for conventional pressure-cycled ventilation. Careful monitoring of gas exchange, tidal volumes, and hemodynamics is required, and appropriate adjustments must be made as needed.

HIGH FREQUENCY VENTILATION

DESCRIPTION. High frequency ventilation (HFV) is a nonconventional mode of mechanical ventilation during which tidal volumes are equal to or less than dead space volume, and respiratory frequencies vary between 60 and 3600 breaths/min. Gas exchange during HFV does not occur by convection alone as during conventional ventilation, but is thought to involve several processes including: **1.** bulk flow; **2.** net gas flux resulting from asymmetry of inspiratory and expiratory gas concentration profiles due to secondary currents established at airway branch points; **3.** Taylor diffusion; **4.** nonconvective mixing due to pressure fluctuations from cardiac pulsations; and **5.** molecular diffusion.[12] Three types of HFV have been studied for clinical use, including high frequency positive-pressure ventilation (HFPPV), high frequency oscillation (HFO), and high frequency jet ventilation (HFJV). The latter has been used most extensively in human clinical studies. The three types of HFV probably achieve gas exchange by similar mechanisms, although their modes of application are quite different. HFPPV consists of an oscillating positive-pressure wave applied at the airway opening by using a compressed gas source and solenoid valve. F_{IO_2} is varied by adjusting a bias flow of oxygen supplied through a side port and positioned at an angle to the jet's main axis. Gas from the bias flow is entrained into the main axial jet. Exhalation occurs passively through the same side port out a separate arm of an attached Y connector. HFO uses a piston pump that actively pulses gas both into and out of the airways. Fresh gas is continuously supplied to the piston chamber and pumped into the airways, while gas entering the chamber during the reverse or exhalation stroke is vented. HFJV uses a nozzle-shaped jet centered at the endotracheal tube orifice with an angled side port for administering bias flow and allowing for passive exhalation.

INDICATIONS. Indications for HFV as a primary mode of ventilator support include hypoxemia secondary to diffuse lung injury (with or without associated barotrauma) and persistent bronchopleural fistulae. Theoretical benefits of HFV over conventional ventilation include more uniform distribution of ventilation and reduction in ventilation perfusion ($\dot{V}/\dot{Q}$) mismatching, allowing for decreased F_{IO_2} requirements, and lower peak airway pressures with decreased risk of barotrauma and potential for hemodynamic compromise. Its use as a primary mode of ventilation has been studied most extensively in infantile respiratory distress syndrome where it had been used with some success. A recent multicenter controlled clinical trial to more fully assess its clinical utility in this setting had to be stopped because of a high incidence of complications.[13] HFV has also been tried as a primary mode of ventilation in patients with ARDS and in patients with significant barotrauma with the rationale of reducing tidal volume-associated strain in damaged lung tissue, while simultaneously providing needed ventilator support. Unfortunately, it has proven not very useful. Three controlled clinical trials of HFV in ARDS patients have failed to demonstrate any benefit in the ability to oxygenate, decrease ICU hospital time, or improve survival compared to support with conventional ventilation. The anticipated advantages of decreased barotrauma and improved hemodynamics have not been seen. More recent clinical studies have shown that to achieve a level of oxygenation during HFV equivalent to that provided by conventional ventilation with PEEP, similar mean airway pressures are needed. Therefore, although HFV remains an interesting and potentially useful mode of ventilation in certain patients, no data demonstrate decreased morbidity or mortality among ARDS or barotrauma patients treated with HFV when compared to those treated with conventional volume-controlled ventilation.

LIMITATIONS. Two potential complications associated with HFV have been recognized in animal model and human clinical trials: **1.** gas trapping and secondary barotrauma from the high driving pressures needed to create the requisite flow accelerations; and **2.** necrotizing tracheobronchitis immediately downstream of the jet nozzle.

The mechanistic basis for gas trapping in this setting is thought to be flow limitation during a shortened expiratory cycle. When expiratory time shortens to a critical value such that the velocity required to eliminate the HFV-supplied tidal breath exceeds wave speed, then progressive gas trapping will occur, leading rapidly to hyperinflation and barotrauma. It is thus necessary to continuously monitor and attend to airway opening or esophageal pressure measurements or both, and decrease either tidal volume or frequency when sudden increases are noted.

Necrotizing tracheobronchitis is not unique to HFV although some data suggest that it may occur more frequently in this setting and more distal than when observed during conventional ventilation. Its cause is not known, but may be related to high velocity impaction of water microdroplets from the needle valve humidifier system used in HFV.

INITIAL SETTINGS. Clinical application of high frequency ventilation involves two steps: **1.** determining whether a patient is an appropriate candidate; and **2.** deciding on appropriate initial settings. The basic principles underlying the use of HFV are similar to those for conventional mechanical ventilation. Alveolar ventilation is directly proportional to the product of frequency and tidal volume, and thus increasing either of these parameters will decrease Pa_{CO_2}. Pa_{O_2} is proportional to lung volume (by direct application of PEEP or modification of factors affecting auto-PEEP) and to FI_{O_2}, and can be manipulated by altering either of these parameters. These basic concepts are embodied in the practical algorithm developed by Standiford and Morganroth for implementing HFJV, which is taken from their recent review of this topic and is presented in Fig. 8-9.[14]

OTHER MODES OF NONCONVENTIONAL VENTILATION

A variety of additional modes for moving gas into and out of the lungs have been developed including rocking bed

FIGURE 8-9 Guidelines for initiating and adjusting high frequency jet ventilation based on blood-gas results. (Figure from Standiford TJ, Morganroth ML: High frequency ventilation. Chest 96:1380, 1989, with permission.)

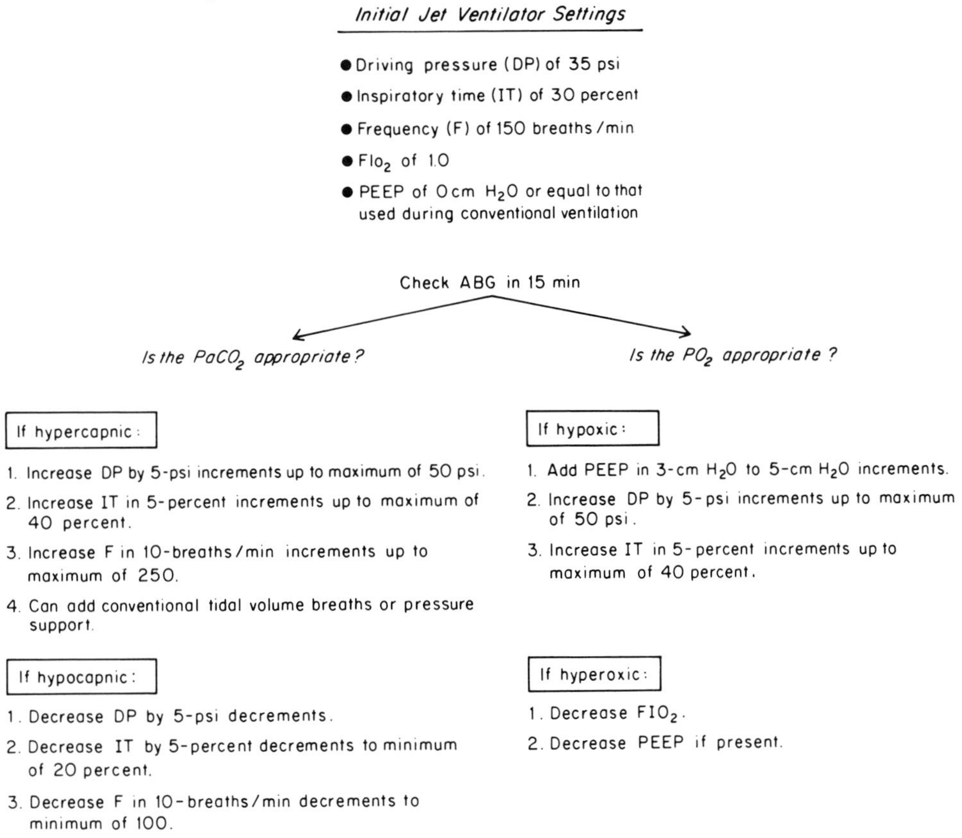
Initial Jet Ventilator Settings
Driving pressure (DP) of 35 psi
Inspiratory time (IT) of 30 percent
Frequency (F) of 150 breaths/min
FIO2 of 1.0
PEEP of 0 cm H2O or equal to that used during conventional ventilation
Check ABG in 15 min
Is the PaCO2 appropriate?
Is the PO2 appropriate?
If hypercapnic:
1. Increase DP by 5-psi increments up to maximum of 50 psi.
2. Increase IT in 5-percent increments up to maximum of 40 percent.
3. Increase F in 10-breaths/min increments up to maximum of 250.
4. Can add conventional tidal volume breaths or pressure support.
If hypoxic:
1. Add PEEP in 3-cm H2O to 5-cm H2O increments.
2. Increase DP by 5-psi increments up to maximum of 50 psi.
3. Increase IT in 5-percent increments up to maximum of 40 percent.
If hypocapnic:
1. Decrease DP by 5-psi decrements.
2. Decrease IT by 5-percent decrements to minimum of 20 percent.
3. Decrease F in 10-breaths/min decrements to minimum of 100.
If hyperoxic:
1. Decrease FIO2.
2. Decrease PEEP if present.

ventilation, constant flow ventilation, extracorporeal membrane oxygenation (ECMO), and low frequency positive-pressure ventilation with extracorporeal carbon dioxide removal (LFPPV-$ECCO_2R$). These latter two modes of ventilation are described in detail in Chap. 29. Although studies of the mechanisms of gas exchange during nonconventional modes of ventilation have provided insight into flow patterns and mass transport within the human respiratory tract, none has definite advantages over conventional ventilation in the critically ill ICU patient.[15]

Another new mode of ventilation which does not require intubation is intermittent positive-pressure ventilation by facemask (IPPVF). IPPVF has been used in two clinical settings: **1.** as a way to circumvent intubation, and its associated morbidity, in a patient with impending respiratory failure who might otherwise require intubation and mechanical ventilator support; and **2.** as an outpatient supplement to respiratory muscle function in patients with chronic lung disease and associated respiratory muscle compromise instead of more conventional negative-pressure ventilator support. Utilization of IPPVF in both these settings has been limited to individual cases, and more careful studies of its potential for general use and benefit are awaited.

PEEP and CPAP

DESCRIPTION. PEEP and CPAP are not separate modes of ventilation per se since they do not provide ventilation. Rather, they are used together with other modes of ventilation or during spontaneous breathing to improve oxygenation. PEEP specifically refers to the application of a fixed amount of positive pressure to a mechanical ventilation cycle during which spontaneous breathing is not present. CPAP, or continuous positive-pressure breathing (CPPB), specifically refers to addition of a fixed amount of positive airway pressure to spontaneous breathing. When both spontaneous and mechanical breaths are superimposed on a fixed positive airway pressure, as might occur during IMV, various terms are used, including IMV with PEEP and IMV with CPAP. The distinction is in many ways artificial since both PEEP and CPAP act by similar physiologic mechanisms, are used for similar clinical indications, and can be implemented using similar mechanical devices (i.e., a Venturi valve, spring-loaded valve, water column, or water-weighted diaphragm). Positive pressure either as PEEP or CPAP for use with other modes of ventilator support, both conventional and nonconventional, is available on most positive-pressure ventilators currently in use.

The benefits of applying positive airway pressure result from its potential ability to open closed alveolar units, which increases lung compliance and tends to make regional impedances to ventilation more homogeneous. Therefore, when used correctly, peak airway pressures may be significantly less than predicted simply from the sum of peak end-inspiratory pressure measured prior to application and positive airway pressure applied. If positive airway pressure is applied in a situation where additional alveolar recruitment cannot or does not occur, then it can have detrimental effects on both hemodynamics and lung mechanics. Peak airway pressures may be significantly higher than predicted from the sum of PEEP and peak pressures measured prior to its application, resulting in decreased venous return and increased risk of barotrauma.[16]

INDICATIONS. The primary indication for use of PEEP is hypoxemia secondary to diffuse lung injury such as occurs in ARDS, alveolar hemorrhage syndromes, and interstitial pneumonitis. PEEP can be added to any of the volume- or pressure-cycled modes of ventilation described previously to help improve oxygenation in this setting. Physiologically, PEEP improves ventilation perfusion matching by opening previously closed gas-exchanging regions, reducing the percentage of lung with zero $\dot{V}/\dot{Q}$ (shunt), and lowering F_{IO_2} requirements below the potentially toxic range. Therefore, PEEP is generally not indicated in the management of patients who are oxygenating adequately or who can be oxygenated with inspired F_{IO_2} below 0.5.

Positive airway pressure can be administered in the nonintubated patient in the form of CPAP using an airtight mask which fits either over both the nose and mouth or just over the nose (i.e., nasal CPAP). The indications for and risks associated with the use of nasal CPAP are different from PEEP and facemask CPAP, and therefore will not be discussed here. The use of CPAP by facemask is limited to those situations in which hypoxemia due to shunt is present, and treatment of the underlying pathologic process is expected to produce rapid improvement and independence from positive airway pressure requirements. The risks of administering CPAP by facemask are identical to those associated with the use of PEEP or CPAP in the ventilated patient described below. The masks are uncomfortable to wear, which makes patient compliance a potential problem. In addition, leaks around the mask can significantly decrease the level of positive pressure administered. CPAP by facemask should therefore be used with the same close observation as any primary mechanical ventilator support mode.

LIMITATIONS. The two most serious and frequent potential complications associated with the use of positive airway pressure applied either as PEEP or CPAP are barotrauma (interstitial emphysema, pneumomediastinum, subcutaneous emphysema, and pneumothorax), and altered hemodynamics. The addition of positive airway pressure generally causes an initial increase in mean and peak airway pressures. If PEEP is functioning to open closed gas-exchanging units, however, a new steady state can be anticipated in which peak airway pressures are similar to or even lower than those measured before addition of PEEP, and lung compliance is either the same or increased. The improvement in mechanics is usually accompanied by an improvement in oxygenation. A decrease in lung compliance with addition of PEEP indicates that additional gas exchanging units are not being recruited and that PEEP is unlikely to be of clinical benefit. The increase in peak and mean airway pressures serves only to decrease venous return, which decreases cardiac output, and to increase the risk of barotrauma, the incidence of which rises sharply with peak airway pressures above 50 cmH_2O. When addition of PEEP results in an improvement in lung compliance and oxygenation, but a decrease in cardiac output, it may be that intravascular volume depletion is present; checking the response to a fluid bolus is often beneficial. Since tissue oxygen delivery depends both on cardiac output and arterial oxygen content (i.e., equal to the product of the two), both must be monitored when adding PEEP for management of hypoxemia. It is often necessary to titrate PEEP to optimize oxygen delivery.

Other potential limitations of PEEP include increased intracranial pressure, decreased renal perfusion (from increased renal vein pressure), hepatic congestion (from increased hepatic vein pressure), and worsening of intracardiac shunts.

INITIAL SETTINGS. PEEP and CPAP are best used in the patient in whom hemodynamic monitoring is available, since blood oxygen level alone is not an adequate indicator of therapeutically appropriate PEEP, and systemic arterial pressure may not be a sensitive enough indicator of hemodynamic status in the critically ill patient. Right- and left-sided pressures and cardiac output should be recorded. It is also useful to measure airway resistance and respiratory system compliance prior to initiating positive airway pressure. Additional positive pressure should be added in small increments, 2.5 to 5.0 cmH_2O at a time, for a trial period of 10 to 15 min while careful observation is maintained looking for evidence of hemodynamic compromise or barotrauma. Respiratory and hemodynamic parameters can then be remeasured after an equilibration period of about 30 to 45 min, and documentation of improvement in oxygen delivery can be obtained. Additional positive pressure can be added and a second trial performed, with the goal of identifying the optimal level of positive pressure as reflected in maximal overall oxygen delivery.

Potential Complications of Mechanical Ventilation

Potential complications associated with the application of mechanical ventilation can be divided into three general categories: **1.** those due to malfunction of or inappropriate use of technology or equipment; **2.** those due to pathologic conditions related to the application of mechanical ventilation; and **3.** those which represent a normal or exaggerated physiologic response to changes in intrathoracic pressures secondary to application of mechanical ventilation. Commonly encountered problems are discussed below.[17]

The most common ventilator-related issues requiring attention by nursing, respiratory therapy, and physician staff in the ICU relate to equipment malfunction or to ventilator settings that require adjustment. Although these are not "complications" strictly speaking, they can result in significant morbidity and even mortality if they are not attended to promptly. These include valve malfunctions, tubing leaks or disconnections, faulty alarms, inappropriate F_{IO_2}, flow rate, alarm, or PEEP settings, endotracheal tube cuff leak, and humidifier malfunctions. Frequent careful recording of ventilator settings, respiratory mechanics, cuff pressure, clinical status, and blood gases can help prevent unrecognized problems of this kind and avoid serious complications.

Other common problems associated with application of mechanical ventilation due to actual pathology include barotrauma, nosocomial pneumonia, aspiration (despite a cuffed endotracheal tube), pulmonary embolus, and gastrointestinal bleeding. The first three have been linked directly to intubation or mechanical ventilation itself, while the last two are associated with the overall state of most patients requiring mechanical ventilation. The clinician must be alert for early signs of barotrauma (interstitial emphysema, subcutaneous or mediastinal air) and clinical changes that might herald the evolution of pneumothorax, requiring chest tube placement. Early recognition of, diagnostic evaluation of, and therapy for nosocomial pneumonia should be pursued, especially in patients with diffuse lung injury who are particularly predisposed to such infections and in whom diagnosis is often difficult. Despite the use of high volume–low pressure cuffed endotracheal tubes, aspiration of gastric and oropharyngeal contents can still occur, and recurrent documented episodes related to tube feedings may require jejunal feeding tube placement. Prophylactic subcutaneous heparin has been shown to reduce the risk of pulmonary embolus in ventilated ICU patients without increasing the incidence of significant bleeding and should be considered in all such patients. Stress-related gastritis in ICU patients can be reduced with H_2 blockers, frequent antacids, or sucralfate and should also be considered in all patients.

Common and potentially important physiologic responses to mechanical ventilation that may require the attention of the clinician include hemodynamic dysfunction and renal dysfunction. Hemodynamic compromise is usually due to increased intrathoracic pressure reducing venous return. In some instances, intravascular volume depletion may contribute to such a response and can be managed with fluid administration. Ventilator adjustment may also be required to lower mean airway and intrathoracic pressures. Renal dysfunction usually manifests itself as hyponatremia with total body sodium excess, as a result of decreased free water and sodium clearance. This response to mechanical ventilation appears to be due to several factors including increased antidiuretic hormone, decreased circulating atrial naturetic factors, and intrarenal shunting of blood from cortical to juxtamedullary nephrons, all contributing to increased efficiency of sodium and fluid resorption. Clinical response in terms of increased urine output and resolution of hyponatremia has been reported with administration of low dose dopamine.

References

1. Marini JJ, Capps JS, and Culver BH: The inspiratory work of breathing during assisted mechanical ventilation. Chest 87:612, 1985.
2. Felton CR, Montenegro HD, and Saidel GM: Inspiratory flow effects on mechanically ventilated patients: Lung volume, inhomogeneity, and arterial oxygenation. Intensive Care Med 10:281, 1984.
3. Pierson DJ: Indications for mechanical ventilation in acute respiratory failure. Respir Care 28:570, 1983.
4. Sahn SA, Lakshminarayan S, and Petty TL: Weaning from mechanical ventilation. JAMA 235:2208, 1976.
5. Pepe PE and Marini JJ: Occult positive end-expiratory pressure in mechanically ventilated patients with airflow obstruction: The auto-PEEP effect. Am Rev Respir Dis 126:166, 1982.
6. Downs JB, Klein EF, Desautels D, et al: Intermittent mandatory ventilation: A new approach to weaning patients from mechanical ventilators. Chest 64:331, 1973.
7. MacIntyre NR: Pressure support ventilation: Effects on ventilatory reflexes and ventilatory-muscle workloads. Respir Care 32:447, 1987.
8. MacIntyre NR: Respiratory function during pressure support ventilation. Chest 89:677, 1986.
9. MacIntyre NR: New forms of mechanical ventilation in adults. Clin Chest Med 9:47, 1988.
10. Gurevitch MJ, Dyke JV, Young ES, et al: Improved oxygenation and lower peak airway pressure in severe adult respiratory distress syndrome: Treatment with inverse ratio ventilation. Chest 89:211, 1986.
11. Stock MC, Downs JB: Airway pressure release ventilation: A new approach to ventilatory support during acute lung injury. Respir Care 32:517, 1987.
12. Froese AB, Bryan AC: High frequency ventilation. Am Rev Respir Dis 135:1363, 1987.
13. HIFI Study Group: High-frequency oscillatory ventilation compared with conventional mechanical ventilation in the treatment of respiratory failure in preterm infants. N Engl J Med 320:88, 1989.
14. Standiford TJ, Morganroth ML: High frequency ventilation. Chest 96:1380, 1989.
15. Slutsky AS: Nonconventional methods of ventilation. Am Rev Respir Dis 138:175, 1988.
16. Maunder RJ, Rice CL, Benson MS, et al: Managing positive end-expiratory pressure (PEEP): The Harborview approach. Respir Care 31:1059, 1986.
17. Streiter RM, Lynch JP: Complications in the ventilated patient. Clin Chest Med 9:127, 1988.

Chapter 9

CURRENT CONTROVERSIES IN APPLYING SPECIFIC MODES OF MECHANICAL VENTILATION

JAMES K. STOLLER

Current ventilator technology offers the intensivist a wide range of choices in managing patients with respiratory failure, both during the acute illness and during weaning from mechanical ventilation. This broad spectrum of ventilatory strategies challenges the present-day intensivist to understand critically these choices and to apply different strategies to optimize patient care. To focus the relative advantages and disadvantages of available ventilatory modes, this chapter reviews current information regarding several controversies in strategies of mechanical ventilation. Specific issues addressed include

1. Does intermittent mandatory ventilation (IMV) accelerate weaning from mechanical ventilation?
2. What information supports the benefits of pressure support ventilation (PSV)?
3. What is the role of inverse ratio ventilation (IRV) in managing respiratory failure from acute lung injury?

Growing ventilator technology and the relative ease with which manufacturers can modify ventilators promise a steady flow of new ventilator features and strategies with which to manage critically ill patients. As will be discussed, PSV and IRV are important newer modes that complement existing strategies. At the same time, the occasional gap between the availability of a new ventilator mode and evidence to support it requires vigilance against fads and novel but unsupported claims. Thoughtful analysis of the available literature and an ongoing demand for studies that directly address clinical needs are the ways intensivists will master available strategies and help resolve existing and future controversies.

Does Intermittent Mandatory Ventilation Accelerate Weaning from Mechanical Ventilation?

After its introduction in 1973, IMV was promoted as an alternative strategy for weaning patients, a claim that enjoyed early anecdotal support.[1] Based on the fact that IMV permits greater patient autonomy than assist-control mode (by allowing the patient to determine the tidal volume of nonmachine breaths), weaning by progressively decreasing the IMV backup rate is an appealing way to allow patients to assume more spontaneous breathing until weaning is complete. More recent reviews[2] continue to suggest that putative advantages of IMV over assist-control ventilation include

1. The avoidance of respiratory alkalosis (because the patient exercises greater control over minute ventilation than with assist-control)
2. Less need for sedation to achieve ventilator synchrony
3. Lower mean airway pressure (because the patient generates negative intrathoracic pressures with spontaneous breaths)
4. Less concern about disuse atrophy of respiratory muscles
5. More rapid weaning from mechanical ventilation

Bolstered by the putative benefits of IMV weaning, most respiratory care practitioners have chosen IMV as the primary weaning mode. Results of a national survey of weaning methods reflecting responses from 132 responding technical directors of respiratory therapy departments show that IMV was employed by 90.2 percent of respondents, usually in a progression to a T-piece trial.[3] An alternative strategy of weaning by alternating assist-controlled periods with intervals of spontaneous breathing through a T-piece was preferred by only 7.8 percent of respondents in this survey.

In view of this preference for IMV as a weaning strategy, it is fair to ask whether controlled data exist to support this practice. The author is aware of three studies which compare the efficacy and duration of weaning with IMV vs. assist-control, none of which establishes the superiority of IMV as a weaning strategy.[4–6] In the earliest report, the duration of mechanical ventilation in patients on IMV vs. non-IMV modes was compared retrospectively for the years 1975 and 1976, shortly after the introduction of IMV.[4] Patients managed by IMV were slower to wean in this study, though the retrospective study design fails to assure the similarity of patients at base line or the similarity of other comaneuvers that might impact on weaning time. Despite these potential shortcomings of the retrospectively designed study, both subsequent controlled trials also failed to show that IMV accelerates weaning.[5,6] In another investigation 30 patients with chronic obstructive pulmonary disease (COPD) were randomly allocated to wean either by IMV or by serial T-piece trials.[3] This preliminary report suggests that compared groups were similar at base line for inspiratory force and spirometry measurements. Identical proportions of patients failed to wean in both groups (2/15), and the mean times to wean on IMV vs. T-piece were similar (10.9 vs. 8.9 days) and not statistically significantly different.

In the most recent available trial, 165 patients satisfying standard weaning criteria were randomized to an IMV wean vs. serial T-piece trials.[6] With successful weaning defined as cessation of mechanical ventilation for at least 48 h, no difference was observed between the compared groups with respect to total time spent on the ventilator (mean 115 h for the IMV group vs. 67 h in the T-piece group, $p > 0.05$) or weaning time (mean 5.8 h in the IMV group vs. 5.9 h in the T-piece group).[6]

In summary, despite initial promise and claims, available experience fails to substantiate the superiority of an IMV strategy over T-piece or assist-control strategies in weaning patients from mechanical ventilation. In the absence of clear-cut evidence that one strategy is favored, clinicians will systematically exercise one approach, only to try a different strategy should the patient fail. The appeal of IMV is based on its providing an easier patient-ventilator interface, allowing the patient to have greater autonomy over ventilation. Yet, with the advent of PSV, even greater patient autonomy and a more comfortable patient-ventilator interface may be available.

Pressure Support Ventilation: Current Status

Pressure support ventilation is a newer mode of mechanical ventilation in which the patient's inspiration is augmented by a ventilator-delivered, preselected positive pressure.[7–9] This positive pressure is servo-controlled to be constant during inspiration. Cessation of a pressure supported breath is determined by a decline in the patient's inspiratory flow demands, and expiratory triggers vary among ventilators providing this mode (Table 9-1). Most commonly, delivery of positive pressure is ended when the patient's inspiratory flow demands fall to 25 percent of the peak inspiratory flow rate. Less common expiratory triggers include inspiratory flow rates from 2 to 6 L/min.

Table 9-2 summarizes the key features of PSV responsible for its current appeal in intensive care management. These include

1. Maximizing patient control of inspiration, thereby enhancing patient comfort on the ventilator[7,9]

TABLE 9-2 Features of Pressure Support Ventilation

Maximize patient control of inspiration
Optimize patient-ventilator synchrony and patient comfort
V_T determined by length and flow of patient's inspiratory effort and by respiratory impedance
Can overcome imposed work of breathing (e.g., endotracheal tube, ventilator circuit)
Allows adjustment of imposed work of breathing (e.g., with decreasing levels of pressure support)
Preferred mode for weaning from mechanical ventilation?
Lower work of breathing than continuous flow, demand valve IMV, and flow-by systems

2. Overcoming the work of breathing imposed by endotracheal tubes and ventilator circuitry[7]
3. Allowing adjustment of the imposed work of breathing[10–12]
4. Providing an alternative mode of weaning from mechanical ventilation[9,10,12]

The sections that follow examine the available evidence on which these impressions are based. Because the patient determines tidal volume by the length and flow of inspiration, PSV has been preferred as an especially comfortable mode of mechanical ventilation. In an early series of 15 stable patients on mechanical ventilation changed from synchronized intermittent mandatory ventilation (SIMV) to PSV, eight of nine patient respondents preferred PSV to SIMV.[9] When the level of pressure support simulated the tidal volume provided on SIMV (so-called PSV_{max}), patients breathed more slowly and comfortably, an experience which has also been reported in other studies.[12,13]

In addition to enhanced patient comfort, much of the current appeal of PSV is based on its ability to minimize the imposed work of breathing for mechanically ventilated patients. It is evident that as the level of pressure support is lowered, the degree of unloading of the patient's respiratory muscles diminishes, and the work of breathing that must be expended by the patient increases. Perhaps the greatest appeal of PSV is that the work of breathing imposed seems to be lower than with alternative modes of

TABLE 9-1 Summary of Functional Characteristics of Ventilators Providing Pressure Support (PS)

		INSPIRATORY TRIGGER		EXPIRATORY TRIGGER	
	PS range, cmH_2O	Flow, L/min	Pressure, cmH_2O	Flow, L/min	Pressure, cmH_2O
Siemens Servo 900C	1–100	—	Adjustable	25% peak	3.0 > PS
Puritan-Bennett 7200a	1–70	—	Adjustable	5	1.5 > PS
Engstrom Erica	1–30	Adjustable	—	6	10.0 > PS
Ohmeda CPU-1	1–30	2	—	2	
Intermed Bear 5	1–72	—	Adjustable	25% peak	
Hamilton Veolar	1–50	—	Adjustable	25% peak	
Bird 6400 ST	1–50	—	Adjustable	25% peak	
Sechrist Model 2200	1–10	—	Adjustable	—	Set PS level

SOURCE: RM Kacmarek, with permission.[7]

mechanical ventilation, i.e., continuous flow or demand valve spontaneous ventilation.[11,12] In a study of eight patients recovering from respiratory failure, the work of breathing using pressure support (at a fixed level of 10 cmH_2O) was compared to demand valve spontaneous ventilation and continuous flow spontaneous ventilation, all modes delivered by a Servo 900C ventilator.[11] Compared with the other ventilatory modes, patients' tidal volumes were higher and respiratory rates were lower with pressure support. In addition, in switching from controlled mechanical ventilation, the decrement in Pa_{O_2} and the rise in Pa_{CO_2} was lowest with PSV. Finally, there was a trend toward lower transdiaphragmatic pressures with pressure support, and the lowest pressure-time index (mean $P_{di} \times T_i/T_{tot}$) was observed with pressure support at 10 cmH_2O. In an extension of this study, the same investigators evaluated PSV in eight patients previously unable to wean from mechanical ventilation[12] who were ventilated on four decreasing levels of pressure support (for 20 min each): 20, 15, 10, and 0 cmH_2O. As the level of pressure support increased to 20 cmH_2O, tidal volume increased and respiratory rates declined, preserving minute ventilation; transdiaphragmatic pressure declined, as did the arterial carbon dioxide tension and the work of breathing. On the basis of this report, the authors suggested that pressure support could successfully decrease the imposed work of breathing and that respiratory muscle fatigue could be averted while preserving gas exchange. For clinical purposes, the optimal level of pressure support was said to be recognizable as the pressure below which contractile activity of the sternocleidomastoid could be observed.

Despite these promising aspects of PSV, claims that it is a preferred strategy for weaning patients from mechanical ventilation lack available proof. The author is aware of a single report in which pressure support is compared to "conventional" ventilation (otherwise unspecified) for weaning patients recovering from coronary artery bypass graft surgery.[14] Weaning from mechanical ventilation was more rapid in recipients of pressure support than in those on conventional ventilation (≤3 h vs. ≤6 h, respectively), although this study did not address the key issue of difficult-to-wean patients. Overall, at the current writing, PSV remains a promising weaning strategy, but further study will be required before this can be clinically endorsed. In the interim, PSV remains one of several attractive ventilatory strategies at the intensivist's disposal in the attempt to wean difficult patients.

Somewhat offsetting the substantial appeal of PSV are the precautions which must be observed in its use.[8,15] First, because the patient determines minute ventilation, PSV is best limited to patients who breathe spontaneously and who are consistently alert. Patients with unreliable inspiratory efforts may receive widely varying and sometimes inadequate ventilation with this mode.

A second potential hazard associated with pressure support is the possibility that development of a circuit leak can cause persistent inspiratory pressure to be delivered. Specifically, because the expiratory trigger is a specified decline in the inspiratory flow rate, circuit leaks that permit continuous circuit flow exceeding this expiratory trigger will cause continuous delivery of airway pressure. This circumstance has been reported to lead to hemodynamic compromise.[15]

Finally, other potential hazards associated with PSV include the development of atelectasis due to smaller tidal volumes in patients with brief inspiratory times and high respiratory impedance, autocycling caused by a circuit leak that allows inspiration to be triggered, and high mean airway pressures associated with high levels of pressure support.[8]

Along with the remaining issue of clinical efficacy as a weaning strategy, the impact of technical differences in the way pressure support is delivered by available ventilators requires further study. Specifically, as shown in Fig. 9-1, some of the available ventilators achieve the specified level of pressure support only late in the inspiratory cycle while others achieve the targeted level of pressure much earlier.[7] While variation in the pressure-volume curve creates the possibility that volume delivery could be customized to the patient's inspiratory pattern, mismatching of the ventilator with the patient's inspiratory pattern runs the risk of increasing the imposed work of breathing. Currently, except for the Siemens 900C, none of the available ventilators allows the respiratory care practitioner to vary the peak flow rate during pressure support, so the appeal of customizing the inspiratory pattern cannot yet be achieved. In addition, further study will be required to clarify the true clinical consequences of variation in the pressure-volume loops from ventilator to ventilator.

Overall, PSV remains a promising mode of mechanical ventilation, with putative advantages in ventilating patients with acute lung injury and mild abnormalities in ex-

FIGURE 9-1 Representative pressure-volume curves during spontaneous breathing via a lung model with 10 cmH_2O pressure support generated by ventilators studied. *(From RM Kacmarek, with permission.*[7]*)*

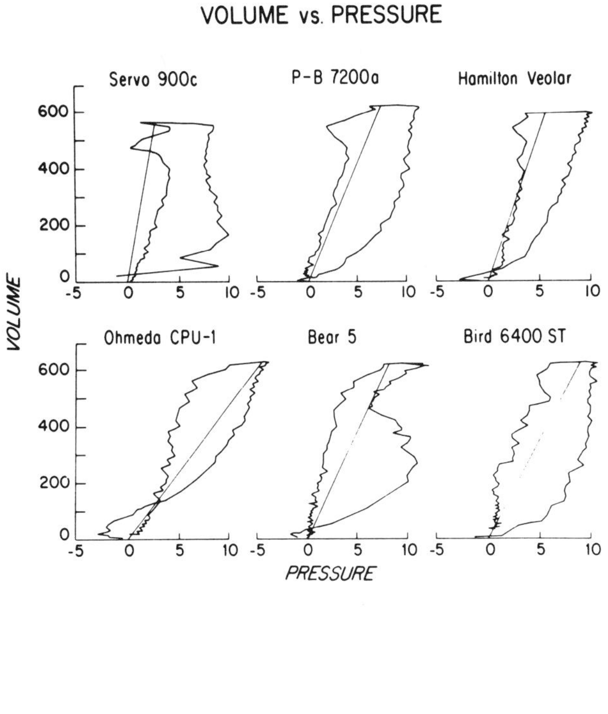

travascular lung water,[16,17] patients in whom the imposed work of breathing is irremediably high (e.g., patients with small endotracheal tubes), and patients who are difficult to wean. However, gaps in the available literature preclude a clear-cut endorsement of PSV at this time, and pending further information, it will remain a useful alternative in the management of patients with respiratory failure.

Inverse Ratio Ventilation: A Strategy for Salvaging Oxygenation in Acute Lung Injury?

When hypoxemia persists despite using high levels of positive end-expiratory pressure (PEEP) for acute lung injury, strategies to salvage oxygenation include extracorporeal techniques (including membrane oxygenation and extracorporeal CO_2 removal–low frequency positive-pressure ventilation), prone posture, and IRV.

Based on its widespread availability with commercial ventilators, IRV seems to be an especially popular strategy to salvage oxygenation. IRV is a ventilatory strategy in which the inspiratory:expiratory (I:E) ratio is adjusted to exceed 1. Differing from conventional mechanical ventilation (in which inspiration is briefer than expiration), IRV can be achieved by one of two strategies: by slowing the rate of inspiratory gas flow during volume-cycled ventilation or increasing the fraction of inspiration during pressure-controlled ventilation.

Several studies in patients with acute lung injury suggest that IRV can improve oxygenation after conventional I:E ratios and/or explicit PEEP have proved unsuccessful. As an example of the efficacy of IRV, Fig. 9-2 depicts the oxygenation course of a young patient with bilateral pneumonia switched from conventional ventilation to IRV (with I:E ratios from 1.5:1 to 4:1).[18] Oxygenation improved as the I:E ratio increased and subsequently deteriorated on returning

FIGURE 9-2 Changes in oxygenation with inverse-ratio ventilation in a patient with acute respiratory failure and bilateral infiltrates. ***(From MJ Gurevitch, with permission.[18])***

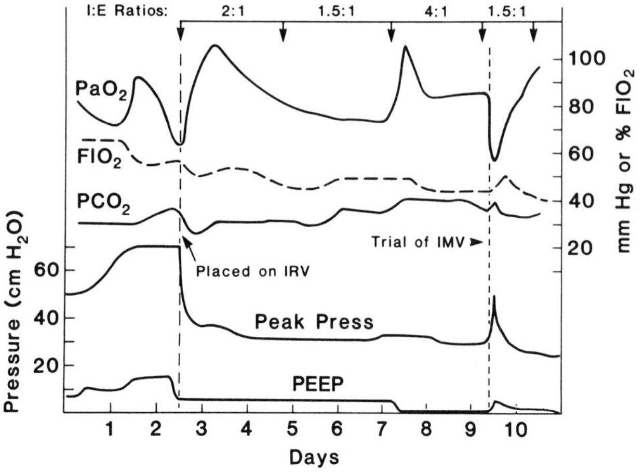

to conventional I:E ratios. Similar experiences from larger series support the observation that IRV can enhance oxygenation in some patients with acute lung injury.[19–21] Although IRV can clearly enhance oxygenation in some patients with acute lung injury, it is equally clear that not all patients will experience benefit and that reliable prediction of those whose oxygenation will improve is not currently possible.[19,21]

Another challenge is to understand the mechanism by which IRV enhances oxygenation. As with explicit PEEP, it is widely held that IRV is associated with enhanced alveolar recruitment, such that intrapulmonary shunt is corrected in acute lung injury. Though proposed mechanisms of improved oxygenation with IRV include a decelerating inspiratory flow pattern and the extended gas mixing time associated with a prolonged inspiration, current debate focuses on whether IRV acts by creating occult or auto-PEEP.

As described by Pepe and Marini,[22] auto-PEEP is end-expiratory pressure in alveoli which can exercise the same hemodynamic and gas-exchange effects of explicit PEEP (i.e., PEEP which is "dialed in"), but which is not routinely measured at the proximal airway. Circumstances fostering auto-PEEP include airflow obstruction and rapid ventilatory rates (with decreased time for gas emptying), such that the lung is not completely emptied prior to the delivery of the next ventilator breath.

Ample studies suggest that IRV can produce auto-PEEP and that the magnitude of auto-PEEP increases as the degree of I:E ratio reversal progresses.[23] I:E reversal (to 4:1) in patients with acute lung injury causes moderate degrees of auto-PEEP (i.e., 10 to 15 cmH_2O) over and above explicit PEEP levels.[24] That the oxygenation effects of IRV are mediated by auto-PEEP has been suggested by one study in which 10 patients with acute respiratory failure were randomly allocated to either IRV (I:E = 4:1) or continuous positive-pressure ventilation (I:E = 1:1.9) and PEEP titrated to preserve the same end-expiratory volume that was created with IRV.[25] When end-expiratory lung volume was preserved (as measured by respiratory impedance plethysmography), IRV and conventional positive-pressure ventilation with explicit PEEP produced comparable decreases in shunt fraction and oxygenation improvement. These observations suggest that IRV and conventional strategies produce similar improvements when similar degrees of alveolar recruitment are ensured, buttressing the argument that IRV creates "PEEP in disguise."[26,27]

Until further clarification is available, the author's view is that IRV should be reserved for circumstances when hypoxemia persists at high levels of PEEP (i.e., above 15 cmH_2O) but should be accompanied by close respiratory and hemodynamic monitoring to detect the presence of auto-PEEP and its consequences.

References

1. Downs JB, Klein EF Jr., Desautels D: Intermittent mandatory ventilation. A new approach to weaning patients from mechanical ventilation. Chest 64:331, 1973.

2. Weisman IM, Rinaldo JE, Rogers RM, et al: State of the art: Intermittent mandatory ventilation. Am Rev Respir Dis 127:641, 1983.
3. Venus B, Smith RA, Mathru M: National survey of methods and criteria used for weaning from mechanical ventilation. Crit Care Med 15:530, 1987.
4. Schachter EN, Tucker D, Beck GJ: Does intermittent mandatory ventilation accelerate weaning? JAMA 246:1210, 1981.
5. Muir JF, Defouilloy C, Pawlicki JP, et al: Acute respiratory failure (ARF) in COPD patients: IMV vs. non-IMV (NIMV) weaning. Am Rev Respir Dis 131:A130, 1985.
6. Tomlinson JR, Miller KS, Lorch DG, et al: A prospective comparison of IMV and T-piece weaning from mechanical ventilation. Chest 96:348, 1989.
7. Kacmarek RM: The role of pressure support ventilation in reducing work of breathing. Respir Care 33:99, 1988.
8. MacIntyre N, Nishimura M, Usada Y, et al: The Nagoya Conference on system design and patient-ventilator interactions during pressure support ventilation. Chest 97:1463, 1990.
9. MacIntyre NR: Respiratory function during pressure support ventilation. Chest 89:677, 1986.
10. MacIntyre NR: Pressure support ventilation: Effects on ventilatory reflexes and ventilatory muscle work load. Respir Care 32:447, 1987.
11. Brochard L, Pluskwa F, Lemaire F: Improved efficacy of spontaneous breathing with inspiratory pressure support. Am Rev Respir Dis 136:411, 1987.
12. Brochard L, Harf A, Lorino H, et al: Inspiratory pressure support prevents diaphragmatic fatigue during weaning from mechanical ventilation. Am Rev Respir Dis 139:513, 1989.
13. Tokioka H, Saito S, Kosaka F: Effect of pressure support ventilation on breathing patterns and respiratory work. Intensive Care Med 15:491, 1989.
14. Prakash O, Meij S: Cardiopulmonary response to inspiratory pressure support during spontaneous ventilation vs. conventional ventilation. Chest 88:403, 1985.
15. Black JW, Grover BS: A hazard of pressure support ventilation. Chest 93:333, 1988.
16. Zeravik J, Borg V, Pfeiffer VJ: Efficacy of pressure support ventilation dependent on extravascular lung water. 97:1412, 1990.
17. McGough EK, Banner MJ, Boysen PG: Pressure support and flow-cycled, assisted mechanical ventilation in acute lung injury. Chest 98:458, 1990.
18. Gurevitch MJ, Van Dyke J, Young ES, et al: Improved oxygenation and lower peak airway pressure in severe adult respiratory distress syndrome. Treatment with inverse ratio ventilation. Chest 89:211, 1986.
19. Tharratt RS, Allen RP, Albertson TE: Pressure-controlled inverse ratio ventilation in severe adult respiratory failure. Chest 94:755, 1988.
20. Ravizza AF, Carugo D, Cerchiari EL, et al: Inversed ratio and conventional ventilations: Comparison of the respiratory effects. Anesthesiology 59:A523, 1983.
21. Lain DC, DiBenedetto R, Morris SL, et al: Pressure control inverse ratio ventilation as a method to reduce peak inspiratory pressure and provide adequate ventilation and oxygenation. Chest 95:1081, 1982.
22. Pepe PE, Marini JJ: Occult positive end expiratory pressure in mechanically ventilated patients with airflow obstruction. Am Rev Respir Dis 126:166, 1982.
23. Hess D, Ruppert T, Kemp T: A bench evaluation of pressure-controlled ventilation. Respir Care 34:1045, 1989.
24. Conoscenti C, Menasha P, Meduri GV, et al: Intrinsic PEEP during inverse-ratio ventilation. Am Rev Respir Dis 135:A55, 1987.
25. Cole AGH, Weller SF, Sykes MK: Inverse ratio ventilation compared with PEEP in adult respiratory failure. Intensive Care Med 10:227, 1984.
26. Duncan SR, Rizk NW, Raffin TA: Inverse ratio ventilation: PEEP in disguise? Chest 92:390, 1987.
27. Kacmarek RM, Hess D: Pressure-controlled inverse-ratio ventilation: Panacea or auto-PEEP? Respir Care 35:945, 1990.

Chapter 10

SPLIT-LUNG VENTILATION

JAY B. BRODSKY
FREDERICK G. MIHM

To facilitate thoracic surgery, techniques for either independent two-lung split ventilation or selective one-lung ventilation were developed.[1] These approaches have been extended to small subsets of critically ill patients in the ICU, often in acute lifesaving situations or in circumstances where established ventilatory techniques are deemed unsuccessful. This chapter describes these techniques and their complications so that the intensivist can use them effectively. Our more difficult task is to describe their indications (Table 10-1). As with many lifesaving interventions in the ICU, anecdotal literature abounds, with the certainty that unsuccessful attempts go unreported. Further, when more conventional therapy has failed, the skeptical intensivist may find it difficult to distinguish between what innovative therapy works versus what the critically ill patient can tolerate. Accordingly, we attempt to cite the established indications for split-lung ventilation and studies providing explanations of mechanisms and results in less obvious uses.

Indications for Split-Lung Ventilation in the ICU

Bronchopleural fistula (BPF) is a serious complication of acute lung disease, trauma, surgery, and positive-pressure ventilation. Although patients with large BPF and severe respiratory acidosis who cannot be adequately ventilated by conventional means are rare, these are the patients who benefit most from split-lung ventilation.[2] Alveolar ventilation can be maintained to only the healthy lung while allowing closure of the BPF and healing of the damaged lung. Alternative therapies, such as high frequency jet ventilation (HFJV) to both lungs, have also been used with variable results, especially in patients with poor lung compliance.[3]

Often patients with severe unilateral lung disease do not respond to conventional ventilatory support. Positive-pressure ventilation to both lungs, with or without continuous positive airway pressure (CPAP) or positive end-expiratory pressure (PEEP) may actually worsen ventilation/perfusion ($\dot{V}/\dot{Q}$) mismatch.[4] By allowing independent selection of tidal volumes and PEEP, split-lung ventilation improves oxygenation in patients with pulmonary contusion, pulmonary edema, aspiration, and pneumonia.[5]

Total unilateral atelectasis usually does not respond to conservative measures (deep breathing, coughing, tracheal suctioning, chest physiotherapy). When aggressive therapies (bronchoscopy, positive-pressure ventilation) fail, split-lung ventilation may be appropriate. Isolation of the lungs allows application of sufficient unilateral CPAP or PEEP to reverse the atelectasis in the affected lung without causing barotrauma to the healthy lung.[6]

Patients with bilateral lung disease (pneumonia, aspiration, pulmonary edema, adult respiratory distress syndrome [ARDS]) have also demonstrated improved pulmonary gas exchange after institution of split-lung ventilation.[4,7,8] In several studies, selective PEEP applied to the dependent lung with the patient in the lateral decubitus position produced a significant reduction in venous admixture without the reduction in cardiac output seen when PEEP was applied in the same patients during conventional two-lung ventilation in the supine position.[4,7,8] Similar encouraging results in patients with ARDS suggest the need for further careful evaluation of split-lung ventilation on morbidity and mortality in these conditions.[8]

Immediate lung separation during acute airway hemorrhage may be lifesaving. A bronchial blocker, a double-lumen tube (DLT), or an uncut endotracheal tube (ETT) advanced into the main bronchus opposite the bleeding site are temporizing measures used until the lesion is identified and appropriate corrective treatment instituted.[9]

TABLE 10-1 Indications for Split-Lung Ventilation

Operating Room	ICU
Protection from contamination	Bronchopleural fistula
Bronchopleural fistula	Unilateral lung disease
Bronchopulmonary lavage	Bilateral lung disease
Drainage of communicating empyema	Airway hemorrhage
Thoracoscopy	
Improved operating conditions	
Pulmonary surgery	
Hiatal hernia repair	
Esophageal surgery	
Transthoracic gastric stapling	
Vertebral column surgery	

Methods to Separate the Lungs

ENDOBRONCHIAL BLOCKADE

The bronchus of a lobe or whole lung can be intentionally obstructed with a gauze tampon, cuffed rubber bronchial blockers, embolectomy balloons, or pulmonary artery or urinary catheters, or by specially designed plastic tubes. Lung tissue distal to the obstruction collapses due to continued absorption of alveolar gas *(absorption atelectasis)*.

The Fogarty embolectomy catheter is the most popular bronchial blocker.[10] For adults No. 8 to 14 French and for children No. 3 to 5 French catheters are used. The styletted distal tip is angled approximately 30° to help direct it into the appropriate mainstem bronchus. After the catheter is passed into the lower trachea, the patient is intubated with a standard ETT. Then, a fiberoptic bronchoscope is passed through or alongside the ETT, and the catheter is advanced until the balloon is in the bronchus to be blocked. The stylet is then removed and balloon position is again verified by observation through the bronchoscope. Whenever lung collapse or isolation is required, the balloon is inflated with air until total occlusion of the bronchus occurs.

The Univent tube consists of a conventional ETT with an additional small anterior lumen in its body containing a thin (2 mm internal diameter) tube with a distal low pressure-high volume balloon that when inflated serves as a blocker.[11] (Fig. 10-1). The blocker tube can be advanced up to 8 cm beyond the tip of the ETT. Before intubation, the bronchial cuff is deflated and the blocker is retracted into the smaller lumen. After tracheal intubation, the tube is twisted 90° toward the bronchus to be occluded, and the blocker is advanced. Blocker placement can be "blind," although positioning is more successfully accomplished with a fiberoptic bronchoscope.[11]

The same Univent tube can be used for either right or left lung blockade. By inflating the balloon a segment, lobe, or entire lung can be isolated and collapsed. Intraoperative displacement frequently occurs with other blockers, often causing unintentional airway obstruction and contamination of the healthy lung. Since the Univent blocker is attached to the main tube, displacement is less likely. The blocker also contains an axial lumen through which suctioning, pulmonary lavage, oxygen insufflation, or even HFJV can be provided. Two-lung ventilation can be reinstituted at any time by deflating the balloon and withdrawing the blocker into the main tube, so the patient need not be reintubated if ventilation is necessary following surgery.

ENDOBRONCHIAL DLTs

With most bronchial blockers, lung tissue distal to the obstruction cannot be suctioned, examined by fiberoptic bronchoscopy, or reexpanded while the blocker is in place. By contrast, DLTs allow each lung to be ventilated independently, collapsed, and reexpanded or examined at any time. During one-lung ventilation with a DLT, CPAP can be applied to the nonventilated lung to improve oxygenation.

FIGURE 10-1 The Univent tube (Fuji Systems Corp., Tokyo, Japan) is a conventional ETT with an additional small anterior lumen containing a thinner tube with a distal endobronchial blocker balloon that can be advanced up to 8 cm beyond the tip of the larger tube.

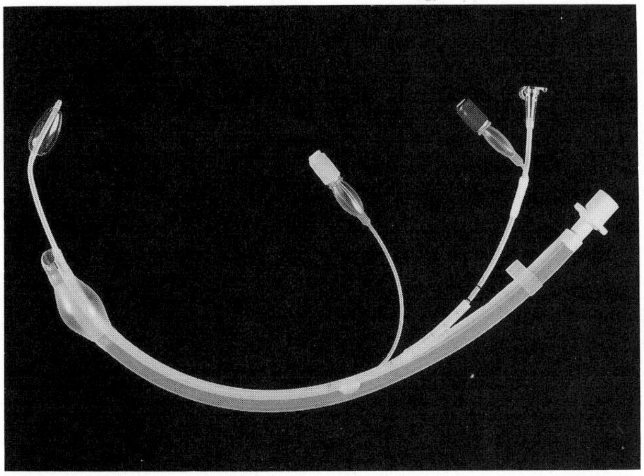

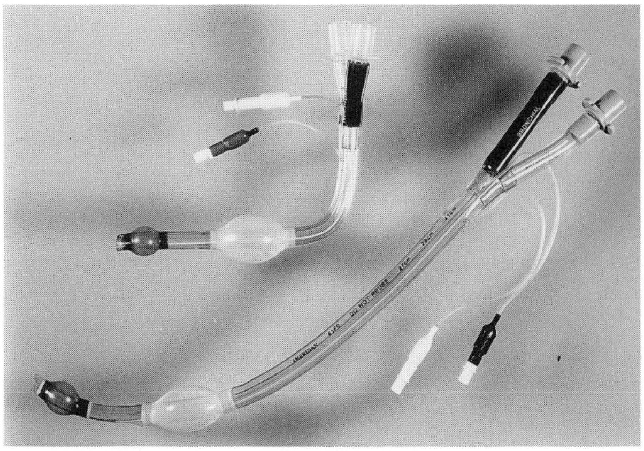

FIGURE 10-2 A standard Robertshaw-style PVC DLT (Broncho-Trach, Sheridan, Argyle, NY) and a shortened Sheridan PVC DLT for patients with tracheostomies.

The original Carlens "bronchial divider" was intended for left lung intubation only. Similar tubes were introduced with fenestrated right endobronchial lumens for right lung intubation. These DLTs have a hook which engages the carina to aid in positioning, but makes passage through the glottis difficult. Robertshaw and others designed DLTs without hooks. These tubes have thinner walls and larger internal lumens with less resistance to airflow than comparably sized Carlens tubes. Modern disposable polyvinylchloride (PVC) DLTs are usually Robertshaw style, although plastic tubes are now available with optional carinal hooks (Carlens style).

All DLTs have two pilot balloons connected to tracheal and bronchial cuffs (Fig. 10-2). Leakage of gas during positive-pressure ventilation is prevented by the proximal tracheal cuff located just above the opening of the shorter, tracheal lumen. Separation of gas flow to each lung and protection from contralateral aspiration is achieved by the distal cuff placed on the longer (endobronchial) lumen. In tubes designed for the right bronchus, the bronchial cuff is fenestrated to allow gas exchange with the right upper lobe bronchus.

A connector at the proximal end of the two lumens permits inspired gas to be delivered into either or both lumens. Each lumen can be opened to the atmosphere independently, so that gas may escape from the unventilated lung, allowing it to collapse while ventilation to the other lung continues. Many PVC DLTs have a diaphragm on each lumen which allows the introduction of suction, insufflation or HFJV catheters, or a fiberoptic bronchoscope into either bronchus without creating a leak which would otherwise lead to lung collapse.

Previously all DLTs were made of red rubber. Although reusable, rubber DLTs have a limited shelf life and are easily damaged during cleaning and resterilization. They become frayed with frequent use so the risk of airway injury may be increased using these tubes. PVC DLTs have generally replaced rubber DLTs. They are available in four sizes (Nos. 35, 37, 39, and 41 French) with corresponding external circumferences of 38, 40, 44, and 45 mm and internal lumen diameters of approximately 5.0, 5.5, 6.0, and 6.5 mm.[12] Their thin tube walls with large internal diameters relative to their external circumference means there is less resistance to airflow compared to equivalent size rubber DLTs. Larger lumens facilitate independent suctioning or passage of a fiberoptic bronchoscope. The clear PVC material allows continuous observation of moisture during ventilation, as well as the presence of secretions or blood coming from either lung.

In contrast to the low volume-high pressure cuffs of rubber DLTs, PVC DLT cuffs have high volume–low pressure properties. The endobronchial cuff is dyed blue so it is easily visualized by fiberoptic bronchoscopy. PVC DLTs have valves for Luer-Lok syringes to prevent accidental deflation of the endobronchial or tracheal cuffs. Both lumens are clearly identified at their proximal ends, and the distal ends have radiopaque markings visible radiologically.

CHOICE OF TUBE

The largest DLT that can atraumatically pass through the glottis should be chosen. For men a No. 41 French tube is usually used, for women a No. 39 French tube.[1] Smaller tubes require greater volumes of air to seal the bronchus, increasing the danger of airway trauma or cuff herniation into the carina. Smaller tubes can be advanced further into the bronchus increasing the risk of obstructing the upper lobe bronchus.[13] There is more resistance to gas flow during one-lung ventilation through the lumen of a smaller tube. If a larger DLT cannot be passed through the larynx or be advanced past the carina, or if there is intrinsic or extrinsic obstruction of the main bronchus, a smaller tube is indicated.

Rubber DLTs small enough to fit through a tracheostomy have too narrow an internal lumen for adequate ventilation. Thinner PVC DLTs can be used safely. For example, a No. 41 French PVC DLT has an external circumference of 45 mm compared to a circumference of 55 mm in a comparable (large) rubber Robertshaw tube. The length of conventional PVC DLTs makes long-term intubation of patients with tracheostomies awkward. Special shortened DLTs are now available for these patients (Fig. 10-2).

RIGHT OR LEFT TUBE

The anatomy of the respiratory tree differs between the right and the left lung; the right main bronchus is only 2 cm long, whereas the left main bronchus is 4 to 5 cm. Whenever a right DLT is used there is a high risk that the distal cuff will obstruct the right upper lobe or carina. The "margin of safety" with a left DLT is greater.[14] A left DLT should be used in virtually all situations except when pathologic abnormalities such as endobronchial obstruction, stenosis, or deviation prevent its passage.

Positioning DLTs

Prior to intubation patients should breathe 100% oxygen, and an adequate level of anesthesia or sedation should be achieved. The tip of the DLT is advanced just past the vocal cords, and the stylet in the endobronchial lumen is removed. As the tube is advanced, it is rotated 90° toward the bronchus to be intubated. Since a left-DLT is preferred, the steps for left bronchial intubation are described (Fig. 10-3).[15]

FIGURE 10-3 The steps for positioning left DLTs. First, both the tracheal (right) and endobronchial (left) cuffs are inflated with air, and the right lumen is occluded. *a*. If breath sounds are present only over the right lung while ventilating through the left lumen, a right-sided intubation has occurred. *b*. Once the DLT is in the left bronchus, the left lumen is occluded and breath sounds should be present only over the right lung. If it is difficult to ventilate through the right lumen, the left cuff is deflated. *c*. If the tube is not far enough into the left bronchus, breath sounds will now be present over both lungs while ventilating through the right lumen. *d*. If the tube is too deep, breath sounds will now be present only over the left lung. The left cuff may be past the orifice of the upper lobe bronchus. *e*. Occluding the left lumen and ventilating through the right will produce breath sounds over the entire right lung and the left upper lung. The left lower lobe will not be ventilated. The left cuff may be obstructing the left upper lobe bronchus. *f*. Ventilating through the left with the right lumen occluded will require very high inspiratory pressures and breath sounds will be present only over the left lower lung. Deflating the left cuff allows the left upper lobe to immediately reexpand. (Redrawn from references 13 and 15. Reproduced with permission.)

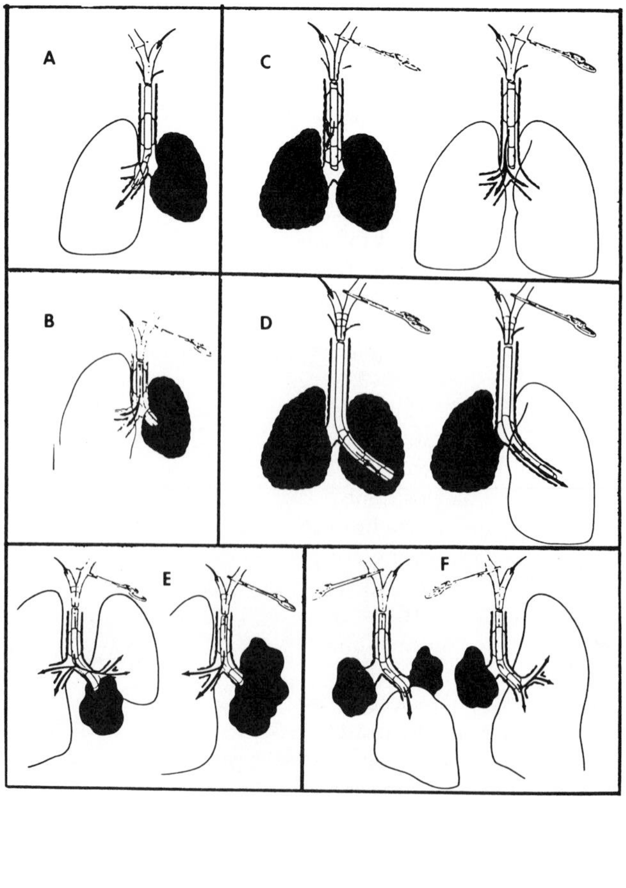

The tube is advanced until moderate resistance to further passage is encountered, usually at a depth of 28 to 30 cm in adults. *Both* the tracheal and endobronchial cuffs are inflated with air. The bronchial cuff should require 1 to 2 mL if an appropriate (large) DLT has been chosen.[16] If greater volumes are needed to seal the airway, one should suspect a cuff leak or herniation of the bronchial cuff above the carina.

Moisture should appear in both lumens with ventilation, and bilateral breath sounds and chest wall movement should be present unless the patient has marked unilateral lung disease.

After listening to the chest, the intensivist clamps the tracheal lumen. Breath sounds should now be present only over the intubated (left) lung. Continued presence of bilateral breath sounds means that the endobronchial cuff is not sealing the bronchus or the tube is not deep enough into the bronchus. Breath sounds only over the right lung means the right bronchus has been intubated (Fig. 10-3*a*).

If a right endobronchial intubation has occurred, both cuffs are deflated and the tip of the tube withdrawn above the carina, rerotated to the left, and advanced. It helps to turn the patient's head and neck to the right (the side opposite the bronchus to be intubated) before readvancing the tube. Both cuffs should be reinflated.

Once the DLT is in the left bronchus, the left lumen is clamped and the patient is ventilated through the tracheal lumen. Breath sounds should now be heard only over the right lung (Fig. 10-3*b*). At this point if there is marked difficulty with ventilation, deflate *only* the endobronchial cuff while continuing to ventilate the tracheal lumen. If the tube is still not deep enough into the bronchus, bilateral breath sounds will now be present (Fig 10-3*c*). If the tube is too deep, breath sounds will be heard only over the left lung (Fig 10-3*d*).

The entire lung must be carefully auscultated. The tube may be so deep that the bronchial cuff is below the orifice of the upper lobe bronchus. In this situation, clamping the left lumen and ventilating through the tracheal lumen will produce breath sounds over the entire right *and* the left upper lung. The left lower lobe will not be ventilated (Fig 10-3*e*).

More commonly, the inflated endobronchial cuff will obstruct the upper lobe bronchus.[13] Ventilating the left side with the tracheal lumen clamped will require high inspiratory pressures, and breath sounds will be present only over the left lower lobe. By deflating the bronchial cuff, the left upper lobe will reexpand and breath sounds will appear over the upper chest (Fig. 10-3*f*).

After it is first positioned, the tube can be withdrawn a few millimeters. If the bronchial seal maintains its competence without requiring additional air, the tube should be readvanced the initial distance back down the bronchus. This maneuver ensures some margin against accidental movement and herniation of the bronchial cuff into the carina.[17]

Cuffs can be displaced by turning the patient, by surgical manipulation, and by head flexion or extension. A pediatric fiberoptic bronchoscope or chest radiograph should be used in the critical care setting to visually confirm cuff position, because in the presence of severe unilateral lung disease, auscultation alone may not be adequate. In the ICU, changes in the peak inspiratory pressure, end tidal CO_2, and mediastinal movement during inspiration cannot be closely monitored as in the patient with an open chest during surgery. The DLT will be in optimal position when there is an unobstructed view down the tracheal lumen of the blue bronchial cuff just below the carina in the appropriate bronchus. Photographs obtained during bronchoscopy through DLTs in correct and incorrect positions are available for identifying problems.[18]

Fiberoptic bronchoscopy has also been used to position larger (No. 39 or 41 French) DLTs.[19] The bronchoscope is placed through the tracheal lumen after the tracheal cuff is beyond the vocal cords. The trachea and carina are inspected as the DLT is advanced into the appropriate bronchus. This may reduce the risk of trauma from "blind" rotation and allows direct visualization of anatomic abnormalities that could hinder placement. If a stylet is needed, a small fiberoptic bronchoscope can be placed in the endobronchial lumen, and the tube can be advanced over it into the appropriate bronchus. As with conventional ETTs, a DLT can be placed over a bronchoscope for tracheal (and bronchial) intubation when visualization of the glottis by direct laryngoscopy is not possible.[20] In this situation, the proximal ends of both lumens should be cut to accommodate the short pediatric fiberoptic bronchoscope.

Complications of DLTs

Clinical experience with DLTs has come from their short-term use during surgery. The most frequently seen problem is malposition. Common positioning problems are not passing the tube sufficiently far into the bronchus, intubating the wrong bronchus, and passing the tube too deep into the appropriate bronchus.[17] Correct position is absolutely essential in certain situations; for example, if the airway to a BPF cannot be isolated from the ventilated normal lung, leakage around the tube could prevent adequate ventilation or cause a tension pneumothorax.

Although anatomic alterations such as deviation of the trachea are often present, a preintubation chest x-ray was not useful in predicting intubation or positioning difficulties.[17] Bronchoscopy immediately prior to intubation may be helpful.[19] Unfamiliarity with placement techniques or the use of small tubes increases the chances of malposition.[21]

DLTs, especially those with carinal hooks, can injure the airway during intubation and extubation. Airway trauma ranges from ecchymosis of the mucous membranes to arytenoid dislocation and torn vocal cords. Laryngeal, tracheal, and distal airway trauma is uncommon with PVC DLTs.[12] There are case reports of PVC DLTs left in place for up to 10 days without evidence of even minor tracheal or bronchial trauma.

Serious injuries are very rare. Tracheobronchial rupture occurred five times in 2700 procedures using Carlens DLTs.[22] Overdistention of the cuffs causing pressure damage or uneven cuff distention pushing the distal lumen tip into the bronchial wall is the cause. Even high volume–low pressure PVC DLT bronchial cuffs develop dangerous high pressures when distended with larger volumes than needed.[16] Airway damage can present with air leak, subcutaneous emphysema, hemorrhage, or cardiovascular instability from tension pneumothorax.

To decrease the chances of injury, the bronchial cuff should be deflated before the patient is moved. However, underinflation of the bronchial cuff can result in a cross-leak and ventilation of the operated lung or contamination of the dependent lung.

Ventilatory Techniques

Once the decision to perform split-lung ventilation has been made, a variety of ventilatory techniques can be used.

During most surgical procedures, the nonoperated dependent lung is ventilated with conventional positive-pressure ventilation while the "up-lung" is allowed to completely collapse. Hypoxemia is unpredictable. PEEP applied to the dependent ventilated lung, CPAP applied to the nonventilated lung, temporary reexpansion of the lung, occlusion of the pulmonary artery to the collapsed lung, and other methods have been used to maximize oxygenation.[23]

In the ICU, independent conventional positive-pressure ventilation to both lungs with selective separate tidal volumes and PEEP has been the most commonly used split-lung ventilation technique. Initially synchronized ventilation of both lungs was performed, but now evidence indicates that asynchronous ventilation of the lungs is hemodynamically better tolerated by many patients.[5,24,25]

Placing the patient in the lateral decubitus rather than the supine position can further improve gas exchange with selective PEEP, while minimizing undesirable hemodynamic effects.[7] There may be limitations to providing adequate nursing care for the patient in the lateral position so this technique may not be practical in certain situations.

References

1. Brodsky JB: Complications of double-lumen tracheal tubes. Chapter: Consequences of endotracheal intubation, in Bishop MJ (ed): *Problems in Anesthesia*, Vol 2, Philadelphia, JB Lippincott, 1988, pp 292–306.
2. Pierson DJ, Horton CA, Bates PW: Persistent bronchopleural air leak during mechanical ventilation: A review of 39 cases. Chest 90:321, 1986.
3. Bishop MJ, Benson MS, Sato P et al: Comparison of high-frequency jet ventilation with conventional mechanical ventilation for bronchopleural fistula. Anesth Analg 66:833, 1987.
4. Hedenstierna G, Baehrendtz S, Klingstedt C et al: Ventilation and perfusion of each lung during differential ventilation with selective PEEP. Anesthesiology 61:369, 1984.
5. Stow PJ, Grant I: Asynchronous independent lung ventilation: Its use in the treatment of acute unilateral lung disease. Anaesthesia 40:163, 1985.
6. Murray JF: Treatment of acute total atelectasis. Anaesthesia 40:158, 1985.
7. Baehrendtz S, Hedenstierna G: Differential ventilation and selective positive end-expiratory pressure: Effects on patients with acute bilateral lung disease. Anesthesiology 61:511, 1984.
8. Siegel JH, Stoklosa JC, Borg U et al: Quantification of symmetric lung pathophysiology as a guide to the use of simultaneous independent lung ventilation in posttraumatic and septic adult respiratory distress syndrome. Ann Surg 202:425, 1985.
9. Garzon AA, Cerrut MM, Golding ME: Exsanguinating hemoptysis. J Thorac Cardiovasc Surg 84:829, 1982.
10. Ginsberg RJ: New technique for one-lung anesthesia using an endobronchial blocker. J Thorac Cardiovasc Surg 82:542, 1981.
11. Karande SV: A new tube for single lung ventilation. Chest 92: 761, 1987.
12. Burton NA, Watson DC, Brodsky JB et al: Advantages of a new polyvinyl chloride double-lumen tube in thoracic surgery. Ann Thorac Surg 36:78, 1983.
13. Brodsky JB, Shulman MS, Mark JBD: Malposition of left-sided double-lumen endobronchial tubes. Anesthesiology 62:667, 1985.
14. Benumof JL, Partridge BL, Salvatierra C et al: Margin of safety in positioning modern double-lumen endotracheal tubes. Anesthesiology 67:729, 1987.
15. Brodsky JB, Mark JBD: A simple technique for accurate placement of double-lumen endobronchial tubes. Anesth Rev 10:26, 1983.
16. Brodsky JB, Adkins MO, Gaba D: Bronchial cuff pressures of double-lumen tubes. Anesth Analg 69:608, 1989.
17. Black AMS, Harrison GA: Difficulties with positioning Robertshaw double lumen tubes. Anaesth Intensive Care 3:299, 1975.
18. Slinger PD: Fiberoptic bronchoscopic positioning of double-lumen tubes. J Cardiothorac Anesth 3:486, 1989.
19. Matthew EB, Hirschmann RA: Placing double-lumen tubes with a fiberoptic bronchoscope. Anesthesiology 65:118, 1986.
20. Shulman MS, Brodsky JB, Levesque PR: Fiberoptic bronchoscopy for tracheal and endobronchial intubation of double-lumen tubes. Can J Anaesth 34:172, 1987.
21. Smith GB, Hirsch NP, Ehrenwerth J: Placement of double-lumen endobronchial tubes. Correlation between clinical impressions and bronchoscopic findings. Br J Anaesth 58:1317, 1986.
22. Guernelli N, Bragaglia RB, Briccoli A et al: Tracheobronchial ruptures due to cuffed Carlens tubes. Ann Thorac Surg 28:66, 1979.
23. Benumof JL: One-lung ventilation: Which lung should be PEEPed? Anesthesiology 56:161, 1982.
24. Doods CP, Hillman KM: Management of massive air leak with asynchronous independent lung ventilation. Intensive Care Med 8:287, 1982.
25. Hillman KM, Barber JD: Asynchronous independent lung ventilation (AILV). Crit Care Med 8:390, 1980.

Chapter 11

OXYGEN THERAPY IN THE CRITICALLY ILL PATIENT

JESSE HALL
L.D.H. WOOD

From the greater strength and vivacity of the flame of a candle, in this pure air, it may be conjectured, that it might be peculiarly salutary to the lungs in certain morbid cases. . . . pure dephlogisticated air might be very useful as a *medicine*. (Joseph Priestley)

Priestley, independent codiscoverer with Carl Wihelm Steele of oxygen in the latter portion of the eighteenth century, almost immediately speculated on the medicinal applications of this substance, which he termed "pure air." However, it was not until this century that Dr. Alvan Barach routinely administered oxygen to hospitalized patients with acute and chronic lung disease, observing that supplemental oxygen relieved dyspnea, improved function, and resolved peripheral edema. Since that time, considerable information has been generated in the investigation of the physiology of oxygen transport, the mechanisms of hypoxemia, and the effects of oxygen therapy. This chapter will update our previous review[1] of the current scientific basis for our understanding of the rationales and benefits of oxygen therapy, with a special focus on the critically ill patient. We begin by brief description of the goals and techniques of oxygen therapy and follow with methods of monitoring its effects. We then detail clinical applications in critical illness, emphasizing oxygen therapy in acute airflow obstruction and in acute hypoxemic respiratory failure (AHRF). Oxygen therapy for carbon monoxide intoxication is discussed in Chap. 175.

Objectives and Techniques for Oxygen Therapy

GOALS OF OXYGEN THERAPY

Enrichment of the oxygen fraction in inspired air ($F_{I_{O_2}}$) is a potential treatment for disorders induced by both alveolar hypoxia and by tissue hypoxia. Alveolar hypoxia (low $P_{A_{O_2}}$) occurs most commonly in obstructive lung diseases in which large numbers of airspaces are poorly ventilated in relation to their perfusion (see Chap. 1). Air inspired with a $P_{I_{O_2}}$ of about 140 mmHg into alveoli with low $\dot{V}_A/\dot{Q}$ has sufficient oxygen removed to approach the mixed venous P_{O_2} of 40 mmHg, while less CO_2 is added to the alveolar gas as it approaches mixed venous P_{CO_2} of 50 mmHg (Fig. 11-1). Low $P_{A_{O_2}}$ stimulates hypoxic pulmonary vasoconstriction (HPV), leading to a reversible component of pulmonary hypertension, right heart dysfunction, and reduced cardiac output ($\dot{Q}_T$). Alveolar hypoxia also causes incomplete saturation of arterial hemoglobin (Sa_{O_2}), thereby reducing arterial O_2 content (Ca_{O_2}) and oxygen delivery ($\dot{Q}_{O_2} = Ca_{O_2} \times \dot{Q}_T$) to systemic organs which may cause tissue hypoxia. As illustrated in Fig. 11-1, increasing $F_{I_{O_2}}$ from 0.2 to 0.4 raises $P_{I_{O_2}}$ to 280 mmHg and virtually eliminates alveolar hypoxia and desaturation in all but the very low $\dot{V}_A/\dot{Q}$ units. Accordingly, one effective, achievable goal for O_2 therapy in exacerbations of these chronic lung diseases provides sufficient O_2 enrichment to ensure $Sa_{O_2} > 90\%$, usually at a Pa_{O_2} of 65 to 70 mmHg, in a reliable, convenient manner.[2]

Oxygen therapy improves tissue hypoxia and minimizes HPV with very few side effects except in AHRF, a constellation of diseases in which airspaces become filled with liquid or cellular elements from the circulation (pulmonary edema, pneumonia, lung hemorrhage). As illustrated in Fig. 11-1, even large and toxic increases in $F_{I_{O_2}}$ are ineffective in increasing Pa_{O_2} and Ca_{O_2} because the inspired oxygen is excluded from the pulmonary blood perfusing the flooded airspaces causing intrapulmonary shunt ($\dot{Q}_S/\dot{Q}_T$). Acute hypoxia seems less well tolerated than the hypoxia of chronic lung diseases, and the acute lung injury which led to AHRF may be more vulnerable to further toxicity from the high $F_{I_{O_2}}$. As a result, effective oxygen therapy requires several adjuncts which seek to minimize the toxic $F_{I_{O_2}}$ required to maintain aerobic tissue metabolism. For example, positive end-expiratory pressure (PEEP) redistributes alveolar edema into the lung interstitium to reduce shunt, and reduced pulmonary artery wedge pressure (Ppw) reduces edema and $\dot{Q}_S/\dot{Q}_T$; yet both interventions tend to decrease $\dot{Q}_T$ unless vasoactive drugs or red blood cell transfusions maintain or raise $\dot{Q}_{O_2}$.[3] Because each adjunctive therapy interacts with O_2 enrichment and each other to relieve or to aggravate tissue hypoxia, the goals or end points of O_2 therapy in AHRF must be integrated. One formulation seeks the least PEEP providing 90% saturation of an adequate circulating hemoglobin on a nontoxic $F_{I_{O_2}}$ and seeks the lowest Ppw compatible with adequate $\dot{Q}_T$ and $\dot{Q}_{O_2}$.[3]

OXYGEN ADMINISTRATION AND MONITORING

PROVIDING OXYGEN TO THE NONINTUBATED PATIENT. The ubiquitous need for oxygen in the modern acute care hospital requires these facilities to have bulk storage with oxygen piped to all patient care areas. The important therapeutic benefits conferred by long-term oxygen therapy (LTOT) have stimulated the development of a variety of other systems for delivering oxygen in the outpatient setting; these include liquid O_2, concentrators and conservation devices as recently reviewed.[1]

Oxygen therapy is most often administered through nasal cannulas or prongs which minimally interfere with speech and eating.[1] Flow rates of 6 L/min of pure oxygen result in approximately a doubling of the $F_{I_{O_2}}$ with little

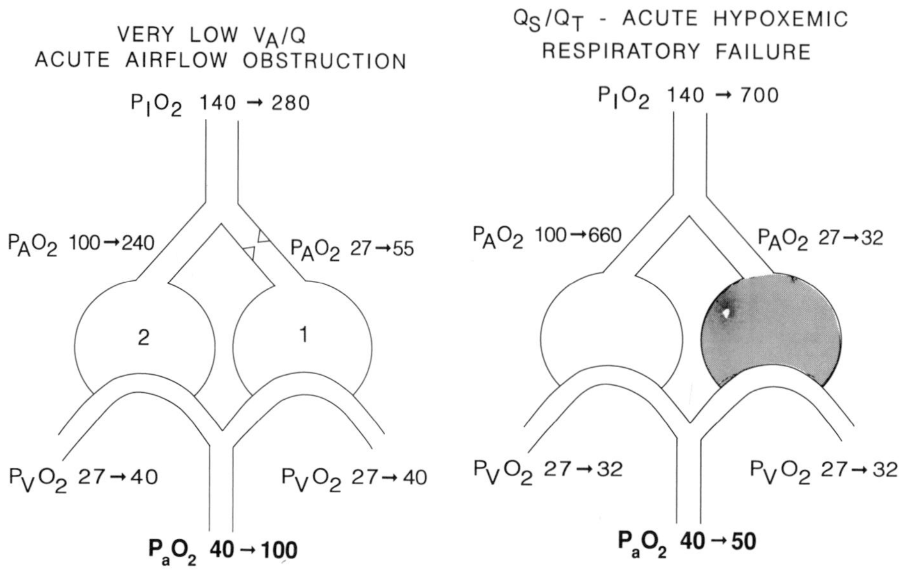

FIGURE 11-1 Effects of oxygen therapy on Pa_{O_2} in acute airflow obstruction (left panel) and in airspace flooding diseases (AHRF, right panel). Each panel depicts a two-compartment lung in which each airspace is perfused by half the mixed venous blood ($P\bar{v}_{O_2}$ = 27 mmHg when FI_{O_2} = 0.21). Acute airflow obstruction causes severe hypoxemia which is relatively easily corrected by oxygen therapy, but hypoxemia in AHRF is refractory to O_2 therapy and so requires adjunctive therapies.

Left Panel. **The obstructed airspace is very poorly ventilated, so alveolar gas tensions approach mixed venous values (PA_{O_2} falls from PI_{O_2} of 140 toward 27 mmHg as all the inspired O_2 is absorbed). By contrast, PA_{O_2} in the ideal alveolus is 100 mmHg ($PI_{O_2} - Pa_{CO_2}/R$), so its pulmonary venous blood becomes fully saturated (S_{O_2} = 100%); when it mixes with an equal amount of mixed venous blood from the obstructed unit (S_{O_2} = 50%), the arterial blood (Sa_{O_2} = 75%) has Pa_{O_2} = 40 mmHg. Raising FI_{O_2} to 0.4 increases the amount of oxygen ventilating the obstructed unit even when ventilation and perfusion do not change, so PA_{O_2} there (55 mmHg) does not become equal to $P\bar{v}_{O_2}$ when the same amount of oxygen is absorbed from the higher PI_{O_2} (280 mmHg). Accordingly, pulmonary venous blood exits the obstructed airspace at S_{O_2} = 90%, and mixes with fully saturated blood from the ideal alveolus carrying more dissolved O_2, causing Sa_{O_2} to approach 100% and Pa_{O_2} to approach 100 mmHg. Note that this increased arterial O_2 transport is associated with increased $P\bar{v}_{O_2}$ (27 to 40 mmHg).**

Right Panel. **During air breathing, all O_2 exchange is as described in the left panel, because half the mixed venous blood traverses the flooded airspace without absorbing any oxygen; accordingly, Pa_{O_2} is 40 mmHg and $P\bar{v}_{O_2}$ is 27 mmHg. Raising FI_{O_2} to 1.0 increases the dissolved O_2 content in the fully saturated blood exiting the ideal alveolus by about 2 mL % (PA_{O_2} increases from 100 to 660), but no O_2 can be absorbed through the flooded airspace. Accordingly, Pa_{O_2} increases slightly (40 to 50 mmHg), so the increased O_2 delivery allows $P\bar{v}_{O_2}$ to increase slightly (27 to 32 mmHg).**

increase at higher flow rates, but variability is great and flow rate should be titrated against some monitor of arterial hemoglobin saturation (vide infra). Mask systems are classified as low flow, in which oxygen is supplied at flow rates that are less than the patient's inspiratory demand, and high flow systems which meet inspiratory demand by a combination of high oxygen flow rates and entrainment of ambient air. The FI_{O_2} may be increased by the addition of a reservoir bag to either a low or high flow system. Partial rebreathing masks allow mixing of expired gas with this reservoir while nonrebreathing masks avoid this by an exhalation valve system.[1]

Continuous transtracheal delivery of oxygen at low flow rates corrects hypoxemia in patients with chronic lung disease, and this approach has now gained wide popularity. This technology reduces oxygen requirements substantially, decreases costs, and is tolerated by most patients with an acceptable incidence of complications.[1,4] Transtracheal delivery of oxygen may be the preferred route for patients who cannot be adequately saturated on high flow nasal cannula therapy. Of interest has been the marked decrease in dyspnea and increased exercise tolerance noted by several investigators.[1,5] Transtracheal gas flow caused a decrease in inspired minute ventilation in patients with chronic obstructive (COPD) and restrictive lung disease.[5] This decrease in inspired ventilation reached levels of 50 percent at flows of 6 L/min, was achieved by reduction in tidal volume (V_T) with respiratory rate remaining constant, and was independent of oxygen delivery or arterial hemoglobin saturation since transtracheal air administration resulted in similar effects. These findings are consistent with the notion that patients receiving transtracheal oxygen therapy have decreased inspiratory work as a mechanism explaining improved dyspnea and exercise capacity and alert clinicians to the possibility that benefits derived from oxygen therapy may be due in some cases to effects apart from correction of hypoxemia.

The use of a low flow oxygen system necessarily results in entrainment of ambient air to meet inspiratory flow demand. The development of high flow mask systems was propelled not only by a desire to achieve a high F_{IO_2}, but also to have entrainment occur in a predictable fashion such that F_{IO_2} could be determined by the clinician, so-called Venturi masks. This would permit "controlled" oxygen therapy in patients who might have adverse consequences from even small increments in F_{IO_2}, a concept which has been questioned (vide infra). Additionally, a known F_{IO_2} would permit calculation of the alveolar-arterial oxygen difference $(A - a)_{O_2}$ and thus facilitate the clinical assessment of lung pathology and associated gas exchange abnormalities. While the concentration of oxygen achieved by many of these devices can vary considerably when tested on simulators, even more striking is the deviation from predicted F_{IO_2} (Table 11-1) when tracheal oxygen concentrations are measured in volunteers with hyperventilatory breathing patterns.[6] Not shown in Table 11-1 is the prevalence of $F_{IO_2} = 0.21$ which occurs on each delivery system when it is not worn correctly, e.g., masks on the forehead, nasal prongs in obstructed nares.

It is not uncommon to hear evaluations of improvement or deterioration in respiratory status based on changes in Pa_{O_2} in nonintubated patients; this practice should be resisted since the conclusions depend on an unknown variable, the F_{IO_2}. While it appears true that high flow systems with rebreathing reservoirs tend to achieve the highest F_{IO_2} in the nonintubated patient, three principles facilitate effective O_2 therapy for typical clinical conditions in patients with respiratory distress: **1.** F_{IO_2} cannot be accurately determined and lung gas exchange efficiency cannot be assessed unless the patient is breathing room air or has undergone tracheal intubation; **2.** it is not necessary to know F_{IO_2} for prevention of depressed drive to breathe, rather give enough oxygen to saturate arterial hemoglobin; and **3.** F_{IO_2} will be considerably <1.0 despite the use of reservoir systems due to mask leaks so monitoring the effect of the delivery system on Sa_{O_2} is important.

MONITORING OXYGEN THERAPY. To the extent that the end point of oxygen therapy is resolution of hypoxemia, direct measurement of P_{O_2} or hemoglobin saturation would provide the most reasonable monitors of efficacy. Although arterial blood-gas analysis has become routine and is useful in the setting of critical illness in view of the information regarding ventilatory and acid-base status that it additionally provides, it is invasive, costly, and does not provide continuous information concerning gas exchange. This last point is important in several settings of oxygen therapy, particularly during exercise or sleep in patients with chronic lung disease and in ICU patients where O_2 exchange may deteriorate quickly. Note that arterial blood-gas analysis in the ICU is not a monitored variable, in that no alarms signal deterioration except for the attentiveness of the bedside nurse-physician team to the results.

The development of pulse oximetry in the past decade has improved the ability to assess saturation on an ongoing basis. By analyzing the pulsatile component of the absorbance of hemoglobin in red and infrared light, these devices avoid much of the difficulty in calibration and operation of the older generation oximeters, and measurements compare favorably with direct arterial oximetry.[7] Errors in measurement of saturation will occur in the presence of elevated bilirubin levels, carboxyhemoglobinemia, or methemoglobinemia although in clinical practice light and motion artifact are the most commonly encountered problems.[1] Since patients with chronic lung disease commonly exhibit significant fluctuations in arterial oxygen saturation, particularly during sleep, these devices are likely to find increasing clinical application, particularly prototypes which allow continuous monitoring in the ambulatory patient. We anticipate growing use of this technology in formal exercise and polysomnographic testing as well as in titrating LTOT in chronic lung disease.[1] The associated improvement in accuracy and reliability makes these devices increasingly helpful in monitoring oxygenation of patients in the ICU. Note, however, that simultaneous monitoring of an index of blood CO_2 is needed before arterial blood-gas analysis is replaced; end-tidal CO_2 monitoring has been helpful for this purpose.

TABLE 11-1

Oxygen Delivery System	'Intended' F_{IO_2}	TRACHEAL O_2 CONCENTRATION Quiet Breathing	Hyperventilating
Nasal Prongs			
3 L/min		22.4	22.7
10 L/min		46.2	30.5
15 L/min		60.9	36.2
Face Mask			
10 L/min	60	53.4	41.0
15 L/min	100	68.1	50.2
Venturi Mask			
4 L/min	28	24.2	21.4
8 L/min	40	36.4	29.4

SOURCE: Modified and reprinted with permission from Reference 6.

Indications and Efficacy of Oxygen Therapy in Critical Illness

OXYGEN THERAPY IN ACUTE AIRFLOW OBSTRUCTION

ACUTE ON CHRONIC RESPIRATORY FAILURE. Patients with COPD often experience acute deteriorations characterized by worsened hypoxemia and hypoventilation, a phenomenon termed acute on chronic respiratory failure (ACRF). As in chronic stable lung disease, much of this hypoxemia is due to $\dot{V}/\dot{Q}$ mismatching and is thus amenable to correction with modest oxygen enrichment of inspired air. While it has been generally accepted that supplemental oxygen is safe when administered long-term to patients with COPD and does not cause worsened hypoventilation,[1] many authors have cautioned that excessive oxygen administration in the more acute setting could precipitate a need for mechanical ventilatory support since patients with COPD might rely on a hypoxic drive to breathe (see Chap. 129). This notion became pervasive with little supportive data; to the contrary, available information from studies in these patients suggests another formulation.

While a further increase in Pa_{CO_2} is almost always seen in COPD patients at the initiation of oxygen therapy, this increment in hypercapnia is not explained on the basis of worsened hypoventilation, and the commonest pattern of breathing after oxygen therapy is an early fall in minute ventilation followed by return to base line. This early fall and then recovery in minute ventilation was confirmed in acutely ill patients with COPD given oxygen.[8,9] Consistent with earlier studies, a large component of the observed elevation in Pa_{CO_2} appeared to be due to increased dead space, a $\dot{V}/\dot{Q}$ alteration that could occur as a result of oxygen-mediated relaxation of airways.[9] Of note, drive to breathe measured by mouth occlusion pressure (P 0.1) was three times normal despite abolition of hypoxic drive by oxygen therapy.[8]

These observations are consistent with a view that the primary determinants of respiratory failure in ACRF are associated with respiratory muscle fatigue as opposed to abnormalities of central drive.[2] Unwarranted reluctance to provide oxygen might actually contribute to ventilatory failure by adverse effects on the patient's muscle function or consciousness. Our own approach is to use sufficient amounts of supplemental oxygen to achieve 90% arterial saturation, recognizing that these patients are in delicate balance as regards ventilatory function, require careful monitoring, and may progress to ventilatory failure requiring mechanical support despite correction of hypoxemia and other abnormalities.[2] This can be accomplished in the vast majority of patients with oxygen by nasal cannula at 3 to 5 L/min. Of course, precise FI_{O_2} is unknown and likely varying over time despite a constant flow, but this is unimportant as the goal is simply adequate arterial saturation.

ACUTE ASTHMA. Asthma is a disease of episodic reversible bronchospasm ranging in severity from a chronic asymptomatic state through episodes necessitating mechanical ventilation. Arterial hypoxemia is a feature of the whole range of severity of the asthmatic episode and is almost entirely attributable to a large fraction of the pulmonary blood flow going to low $\dot{V}A/\dot{Q}$ units in the absence of much true shunt. As a result, modest enrichment of the inspired air corrects the hypoxemia even in patients intubated and mechanically ventilated with status asthmaticus. In eight such patients, Pa_{O_2} was 95 ± 20 mmHg during ventilation with FI_{O_2} ranging from 0.3 to 0.5; the large (A − a)P_{O_2} was due to 17 percent venous admixture, of which only 1.5 percent was due to true shunt. Most of the hypoxemia could be attributed to 28 percent of the pulmonary blood flow perfusing units with $\dot{V}A/\dot{Q} < 0.1$.[10] On the other hand, asymptomatic asthmatics having forced expiratory volume in 1 s (FEV_1) values about 80 percent of predicted demonstrated values of Pa_{O_2} ranging from 70 to 100 mmHg, and hypoxemia when present was attributable to increased perfusion to units with low $\dot{V}A/\dot{Q}$.[11]

Between these extremes, blood-gas determinations in patients during acute bronchospasm showed Pa_{O_2} of 70 ± 10 mmHg and P_{CO_2} of 34 ± 4 mmHg; in these 101 patients, hypoxemia correlated with the severity of airflow obstruction as measured by FEV_1, and the hypoxemia was easily corrected with oxygen therapy because all values of $\dot{Q}S/\dot{Q}T$ were <10 percent.[11] In 10 other asthmatics hospitalized for treatment of their acute severe asthma, Pa_{O_2} was 51 ± 3 mmHg, this hypoxemia was again due to perfusion of a large number of units with low $\dot{V}A/\dot{Q}$, and it did not correlate with the degree of spirometric abnormality until quite late in the course of resolution of the acute asthmatic attack.[11] Taken together, these results suggest that arterial hypoxemia is a marker of the severity of chronic asymptomatic asthma, but it does not warrant oxygen therapy unless associated with other abnormalities such as nocturnal desaturation. In asthmatic patients with acute worsening of bronchospasm, arterial hypoxemia is easily corrected with enriched oxygen, but the severity of hypoxemia contributes little further to the many other symptomatic and objective evaluations of airflow obstruction contributing to the prediction of their need for hospitalization.[11] Accordingly, patients sufficiently ill with status asthmaticus to require ICU admission will usually require supplemental oxygen. This can be delivered by nasal cannula but the need for concurrent nebulized bronchodilator therapy makes a mask delivery system most reasonable during therapy in the first day (see Chap. 131).

UPPER AIRWAY OBSTRUCTION. An uncommon cause of respiratory distress requiring urgent therapy is obstruction of the upper airway. Patients with upper airway obstruction complain of dyspnea with obvious respiratory distress and use of the accessory muscles of respiration; frequently inspiratory stridor is evident. When this problem is severe enough to progress to respiratory failure, arterial blood-gas determinations confirm acute respiratory acidosis, usually without hypoxemia in patients breathing oxygen-enriched gas.[12] Several reports indicate immediate diminution of the signs and symptoms within minutes of breathing heliox, a gas consisting of 21% oxygen in helium. Despite these reports indicating utility, the availability of heliox to emergency rooms or inpatient services is sporadic.[12] Accordingly, it is mentioned here as a variant of oxygen therapy, for the provision of emergency oxygen supplies in health institutions should include the provision of this special gas for this unique condition and therapy. The mechanism for this beneficial effect resides in the density dependence of the flow-related pressure drop across the upper airway. When tumor or other upper airway masses narrow the cross-sectional area of the upper airway, the pressure drop across the orifice increases sufficiently to cause respiratory distress even in the patient with normal inspiratory muscle function.[1] This very large pressure drop is reduced by a factor of three in accord with the reduced gas density when heliox is substituted, accounting for the dramatic and sustained relief in patients with upper airway obstruction.

Heliox has no beneficial effect in the much more common lower airways obstruction because the resistance to airflow is much less dependent on gas density beyond the lobar bronchi where chronic airflow obstruction resides.[1] Yet, a recent study demonstrated marked immediate reduction in airways resistance and Pa_{CO_2} in patients ventilated with heliox for status asthmaticus.[13] Since upper airway obstruction does not disturb $\dot{V}/\dot{Q}$ relationships, patients with no coincident lung disease can be treated with 80:20 helium:oxygen mixtures and no supplemental oxygen. Indeed, increasing the fraction of oxygen diminishes the benefit sought by increasing the density of the gas mixture. Of course, many patients with upper airway obstruction have concurrent lung disease with $\dot{V}/\dot{Q}$ abnormalities (e.g., the patient with COPD and a tumor involving the central airways). In these circumstances, it may be desirable to use heliox mixtures with an $FI_{O_2} > 0.20$. Since it can be confusing for staff to recalibrate and adjust valves as necessary for mixing from heliox and oxygen tanks, we advocate giving the standard heliox mixture (80:20 He:O_2) by mask and additional oxygen by nasal cannula titrated to an adequate arterial saturation.

LONG-TERM OXYGEN THERAPY. In patients with COPD, LTOT corrected erythrocytosis in most if not all patients and reduced pulmonary artery pressure and resistance in many patients with as little as 12 to 15 h of oxygen daily.[1] These early uncontrolled series also demonstrated that LTOT decreased admission to hospital for exacerbations characterized by cor pulmonale and improved central nervous system (CNS) function.[1] These and other clinical observations suggesting improved function and possibly survival caused frequent use of LTOT, despite the expense of this therapy and the frequency of COPD. The Medical Research Council of the United Kingdom and the National Institutes of Health in the United States then sponsored prospective randomized trials to determine long-term benefit of LTOT.[1] It is now clear from these studies that oxygen improves survival in hypoxemic patients with COPD. Several explanations for this effect are possible. Pulmonary hypertension with cor pulmonale confers a mortality rate in excess of 65 percent over 4 years. Conceivably, oxygen therapy relieves or prevents the progression of pulmonary hypertension with associated right heart failure. Alternatively, improved oxygen delivery to peripheral tissues may explain the improved survival.[14]

The use of LTOT must be considered by the intensivist in managing patients with both acute lung disease and ACRF. Patients admitted to the ICU with acute exacerbations of COPD (vide supra) often have been receiving home oxygen therapy; this is a useful marker for the existence of gas exchange abnormalities and pulmonary hypertension with cor pulmonale. Such patients almost invariably require a return to at least the same level of supplemental oxygen and on occasion more at the time of discharge from the ICU and hospital. A reasonable guiding principle is to supply sufficient oxygen by nasal cannula, transtracheal device, or oxygen-conserving device to maintain arterial saturation at >90%. Formal studies with pulse oximetry are useful to define need for increased oxygen during exercise.

Less information exists to guide therapy of patients with restrictive lung diseases. Some of these patients present with acute insults (e.g., pneumonia) superimposed on chronic impairment (e.g., pulmonary fibrosis, kyphoscoliosis). Alternatively, previously healthy patients may sustain diffuse acute lung injury such as adult respiratory distress syndrome (ARDS) which can progress to disordered lung healing and fibrosis over weeks. Recovery may extend well beyond the period of mechanical ventilatory support and even for months following hospital discharge. Both groups of patients should be assessed for the need for continuous oxygen therapy, using criteria similar to patients with COPD.[15,16]

OXYGEN THERAPY IN ACUTE HYPOXEMIC RESPIRATORY FAILURE

LIMITS ON OXYGEN THERAPY AND ROLES FOR ADJUNCTIVE THERAPY. AHRF describes a variety of clinical conditions characterized by relatively acute filling of airspaces with elements of the pulmonary blood such that inspired oxygen is completely excluded from usual uptake by the pulmonary blood perfusing the flooded lung units (see Chap. 1). As a result, an excess fraction of the mixed venous blood passes through the lungs into the left atrium without oxygen uptake to cause arterial hypoxemia as a consequence of the intrapulmonary shunt ($\dot{Q}s/\dot{Q}_T$). In turn, desaturation of the circulating hemoglobin concentration causes reduced delivery of oxygen to the peripheral tissues ($\dot{Q}_{O_2}$) and tissue hypoxia characterized by reduced oxygen consumption ($\dot{V}_{O_2}$) and anaerobic metabolism when the limits of oxygen extraction from desaturated blood are exceeded. Accordingly, arterial and tissue hypoxia are cardinal features of AHRF, yet oxygen therapy provides only limited relief because even 100% oxygen is excluded from the pulmonary blood flow by airspace liquid while nonflooded alveoli are perfused with blood which is nearly completely saturated even during air breathing. This is illustrated in the left panel of Fig. 11-2, where a small increase in FI_{O_2} increases Pa_{O_2} considerably when the shunt is small, yet when $\dot{Q}s/\dot{Q}_T$ is 50 percent changing the inspired gas from air to oxygen only raises the Pa_{O_2} from 38 to 48 mmHg.[17] The right panel of Fig. 11-2 illustrates an often overlooked feature of this small increase in P_{O_2} in AHRF—the arterial oxygen content increased more between an FI_{O_2} of 0.21 and 1.0 when the shunt was 50 percent, than when $\dot{Q}s/\dot{Q}_T$ was 10 percent. At the higher value of $\dot{Q}s/\dot{Q}_T$, the largest part of the increment occurred between 20 and 50% inspired oxygen, all as a consequence of the shape of the oxyhemoglobin dissociation curve.[17]

In general, these consequences of shunt lung disease encourage physicians to use very high FI_{O_2} because the limits of hypoxia for vital organs are not yet well defined and the consequences of excessive hypoxia seem quick and irreversible. For example, one recent evaluation of canine cardiac dysfunction during progressive hypoxemia demonstrated that ventricular contractility first became significantly depressed at Pa_{O_2} values of about 40 mmHg

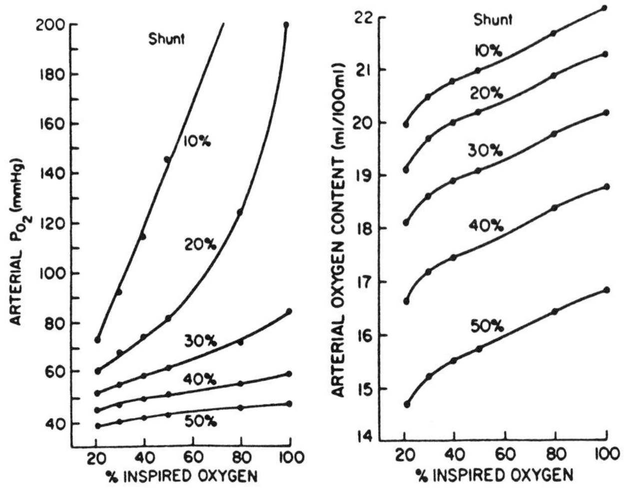

FIGURE 11-2 Pa_{O_2} as a function of inspired oxygen percentage at various degrees of shunt (*left panel*) and increase in arterial oxygen content with increased percent of inspired oxygen at various degrees of shunt (*right panel*). See text for further details. (Reprinted with permission from Reference 17).

and saturation values of about 70%.[18] Relatively minor further reductions in Pa_{O_2} (36 mmHg) and saturation (63%) were associated with progressive anaerobic myocardial metabolism, dilated cardiomyopathy, bradycardia, shock, and death. Such data lend support to the inclination of physicians to keep the Fi_{O_2} of patients with large $\dot{Q}s/\dot{Q}T$ near 1.0 in an attempt to maintain arterial saturation close to 90%. The argument here is that >90% saturation achieves little further Sa_{O_2} and $\dot{Q}_{O_2}$ along the relatively flat slope of the oxyhemoglobin dissociation curve (see Fig. 1-6), while <90% saturation exposes the patient to larger drops in $\dot{Q}_{O_2}$ along the steeper portion of the dissociation curve.[17]

If oxygen therapy for AHRF has a relatively small effect on tissue hypoxia, diverse interventions may be thought of as adjuncts to oxygen therapy designed to maximize beneficial effects while minimizing the toxic effects of oxygen. Of course, each intervention has its own adverse effects so a recurring theme of oxygen therapy in AHRF is to use the least adjunctive therapy achieving a predefined end point so as not to tip the therapeutic balance in the direction of complications.[3] A partial list of adjunctive oxygen therapies includes PEEP, increased circulating hemoglobin concentration, increased $\dot{Q}T$, reduced oxygen consumption, avoiding or treating defects in peripheral oxygen extraction, avoiding interventions which block HPV, preventing secondary lung damage or reduced venous return by using optimal ventilator settings, avoiding atelectasis, and positioning the patient for optimal O_2 exchange (see Chap. 128).

The relative importance of each of these adjunctive measures varies with the causes of airspace filling. One common cause of AHRF is ARDS, which may present different challenges to oxygen therapy between the acute exudative stage dominated by increased $\dot{Q}s/\dot{Q}T$, and the later proliferative phase dominated by fibrosis and a potential for large numbers of very low $\dot{V}A/\dot{Q}$ units which may themselves be more responsive to altered Fi_{O_2} than is large $\dot{Q}s/\dot{Q}T$.[1,15] Other causes of homogeneous airspace filling are cardiogenic pulmonary edema due to left ventricular dysfunction or fluid overload, while inhomogeneous airspace filling occurs in pneumonia, lung contusion with or without flail chest, and atelectasis of dependent lung regions associated with obesity, the supine position, and intraabdominal pathology (see Chap. 84). Each of these specific pulmonary diseases is described elsewhere in this book, so our goal here is to describe how the pathophysiology of lung or peripheral O_2 exchange in AHRF impacts on oxygen therapy and its adjunctive supports.

POSITIVE END-EXPIRATORY PRESSURE. By far the most effective adjunctive support for oxygen therapy in homogeneous airspace filling diseases is PEEP. As airspaces flood with crystalloid or plasma, the VT is delivered to the aerated spaces only, overdistending them as indicated by the very large excursions of transpulmonary pressure. PEEP redistributes the alveolar edema to the peribronchovascular interstitium, thereby reducing the shunt and the tidal pressure excursions by recruiting perfused airspaces to accommodate the delivered volume.[19] It is not uncommon for PEEP < 15 cmH_2O to reduce $\dot{Q}s/\dot{Q}T$ from 50 to 30 percent.[20,21] As indicated by the left panel of Fig. 11-2, such an outcome allows the Fi_{O_2} to be reduced from 100 to 50% while increasing the Pa_{O_2} from 40 to 60 mmHg, associated with an increase in Ca_{O_2} from 16.8 to 19 vol % (see Fig. 11-2, right panel).

This redistribution of edema and airspace recruitment increases the end-expired lung volume much more than would be predicted from a modest increase in PEEP along the pre-PEEP inflation pressure-volume curve of the respiratory system. The chest wall is pushed to a correspondingly higher volume by an increase in pleural pressure (Ppl) which is also larger than one might predict. Increased Ppl raises right atrial pressure to decrease venous return especially in relatively hypovolemic patients whose sympathetic reflexes are already fully utilized to maintain venous return. Accordingly, a progressive rise in PEEP causes a progressive reduction in shunt, but at some point the fall in venous return tips the balance in terms of reducing $\dot{Q}_{O_2}$ despite a progressive rise in arterial oxygen content. Consideration of Fig. 11-2 reveals that when $\dot{Q}s/\dot{Q}T$ is >50 percent, PEEP may be beneficial to high levels in terms of increasing Ca_{O_2}, and so $\dot{Q}_{O_2}$, even if venous return begins to fall; yet where $\dot{Q}s/\dot{Q}T$ is <30 percent even small amounts of PEEP may allow full saturation of the circulating hemoglobin when further increments of PEEP can do little to $\dot{Q}_{O_2}$ except drop the venous return.

One effective, achievable integration of these effects of PEEP applicable to each patient with AHRF is to implement the least PEEP achieving 90% saturation of an adequate circulating hemoglobin on a nontoxic Fi_{O_2}; if this condition is achieved at the cost of reduced venous return and $\dot{Q}T$, a clinical evaluation of the adequacy of the reduced $\dot{Q}T$ and $\dot{Q}_{O_2}$ is essential, for not all reductions in $\dot{Q}T$ cause inadequate organ perfusion or oxygenation. When $\dot{Q}T$ is deemed inadequate, two approaches should be considered. Reduction of the VT to the lowest level effecting adequate CO_2 elimination will help minimize positive pressure-related decrements in venous return. The clinician should also consider expansion of the circulating volume (preferably with packed red blood cells to raise circulating hemoglobin) to the lowest level compatible with adequate $\dot{Q}T$ and $\dot{Q}_{O_2}$ enhanced at low Ppw with vasoactive drugs.[3] The reduction in VT still effecting CO_2 elimination is often associated with a dramatic fall in mean Ppl and a corresponding increase in venous return. This probably occurs because reduced VT on PEEP is associated with reduced alveolar dead space as a consequence of the fall in mean alveolar pressure allowing better perfusion of many alveoli.[20] The application of continuous positive airway pressure (CPAP) probably effects the redistribution of pulmonary edema and consequent reduction in shunt arguably without as much fall in venous return because active inspiration keeps the mean Ppl lower than during positive-pressure ventilation with PEEP.[21] Accordingly, if the patient is both alert and strong, CPAP is an alternative adjunct to O_2 therapy under conditions of careful patient monitoring; this may spare the patient intubation and positive-pressure ventilation long enough for the edema to clear, but at the risk of sudden cardiopulmonary decompensation.[21]

CARDIAC OUTPUT, VASOACTIVE DRUGS, AND SHUNT. In most patients with AHRF, $\dot{Q}T$ tends to be normal or increased,[3,20,22] associated with a normal circulating volume as deduced from the measured pulmonary capillary wedge pressure (Ppw) of about 12 ± 3 mmHg.[22] Yet in the prior discussion, we emphasized seeking the lowest Ppw compatible with an adequate $\dot{Q}T$ and $\dot{Q}_{O_2}$ to minimize the accumulation of pulmonary edema. Such preload reduction is central to the cardiovascular management of cardiogenic pulmonary edema, and this approach has been used to reduce edema in canine models of pulmonary vascular leak.[23] In cardiogenic pulmonary edema, reduction of Ppw from the very high levels producing the edema is often associated with unchanged or increased $\dot{Q}T$, but excessive volume reduction can produce a hypoperfusion state. In acute lung injury when pulmonary vascular leak occurs at normal values of Ppw, reduction of Ppw invariably reduces $\dot{Q}T$, but it is remarkable that many patients with AHRF can have their normal values of Ppw reduced by >10 mmHg without inducing signs of a hypoperfusion state.[22] With this background in mind, it is not uncommon in either type of pulmonary edema to implement vasoactive drug therapy to prevent a hypoperfusion state when Ppw is reduced.[3,22]

Occasionally, these drugs or their associated increase in $\dot{Q}T$ increase the calculated $\dot{Q}S/\dot{Q}T$ in a way inconsequential to the oxygen therapy of AHRF except for the confusion it imparts if the end points of therapy are not clear. For example, it is now clear that increased pulmonary blood flow increases intrapulmonary shunt in patients and in animal models of AHRF.[3,24] These results are best explained by preferential redistribution of the increased blood or hemoglobin flow to the flooded airspaces; blocking of HPV in flooded lung units by the vasoactive drugs or by the associated increase in mixed venous O_2 is one possible mechanism for this redistribution. Whatever the explanation, the effect on Pa_{O_2} and Ca_{O_2} when increased $\dot{Q}T$ increases the shunt of mixed venous blood having higher mixed venous O_2 content is relatively small. Accordingly, in terms of oxygen transport, the goal of vasoactive drug therapy to maintain $\dot{Q}T$ at reduced Ppw is not confounded by the increase in shunt. A minor exception of clinical relevance applies to the use of pulmonary vasodilating drugs to lower pulmonary artery pressure with little change in $\dot{Q}T$ or $P\bar{v}_{O_2}$. Diltiazem and prostaglandin E increased $\dot{Q}S/\dot{Q}T$ by 5 and 10 percent, respectively and so reduced Pa_{O_2} by 7 and 22 mmHg in patients with ARDS; such a use of these vasoactive drugs may necessitate more O_2 therapy, whereas almitrine potentiated HPV in ARDS to reduce $\dot{Q}S/\dot{Q}T$ and to increase Pa_{O_2}.[25,26]

LOWERING OXYGEN CONSUMPTION AND CORRECTING OXYGEN EXTRACTION DEFECTS. In patients with AHRF, $\dot{Q}_{O_2}$ may be reduced by arterial desaturation, anemia, inadequate $\dot{Q}T$, or a combination of these. Several features commonly increase the basal $\dot{V}_{O_2}$ in patients with AHRF, including multiple trauma, burns, sepsis, fever, and the increased work of breathing associated with tachypnea and reduced respiratory compliance. When oxygen consumption is increased threefold by any or all of these factors from a basal level of 280 mL/min to 840 mL/min or about 12 mL/kg/min, the value of $\dot{Q}_{O_2}$ required to maintain aerobic metabolism increases from 420 mL/min to 1250 mL/min assuming no change in the ability of tissues to extract oxygen. To just meet the critical $\dot{Q}_{O_2}$ of 1250 mL/min, $\dot{Q}T$ must be about 10 L/min. This tremendous burden on the oxygen delivery system of patients with AHRF can hardly be handled by some combination of increased $\dot{Q}T$, increased hemoglobin concentration, and increased arterial saturation effected by higher levels of PEEP and FI_{O_2}, so measures to reduce $\dot{V}_{O_2}$ are essential adjuncts to the oxygen therapy of patients with AHRF. One important intervention is elective intubation associated with adequate sedation and muscle relaxation if necessary to eliminate the work of breathing. This intervention facilitates temperature control with antipyretics and cooling blankets by eliminating shivering so the corresponding reduction in $\dot{V}_{O_2}$ reduces the $\dot{Q}_{O_2}$ required.[27] An additional maneuver to improve lung uptake of O_2 is to hyperventilate the patient to shift the oxyhemoglobin dissociation curve to the left; this does not impair O_2 extracted by the peripheral tissues.[28]

A vigorous search for sources of sepsis associated with early effective antibacterial therapy can further reduce $\dot{V}_{O_2}$ and the needs for oxygen therapy. This latter intervention has a special role in eliminating one of the complicating features of AHRF associated with sepsis; that is, a pathologic supply dependence of O_2 utilization in which patients with ARDS or sepsis appear unable to maintain $\dot{V}_{O_2}$ when their peripheral O_2 extraction increases beyond about 0.5 (see Chap. 57). Until the mechanism for this O_2 extraction defect is discovered, there are few other effective therapies than to detect and eliminate the commonest associated diagnosis, septicemia.

OXYGEN THERAPY IN NONHOMOGENEOUS AIRSPACE CONSOLIDATION. A variation on these mechanisms occurs in acute bacterial pneumonia, where mortality in the first 48 h has not changed with the advent of antibiotics perhaps due to complications of severe hypoxia. Much of our detailed understanding of hypoxemia in pneumonia comes from animal models. Canine pneumococcal pneumonia is not associated with reduced lobar blood flow, likely because inflammatory mediators block HPV.[29] Accordingly, hypoxemia can be severe because the blood flow to the consolidated lobe is increased and because that lobe is a metabolic organ consuming oxygen from the mixed venous blood perfusing it. As a result, the lobar venous blood has even less oxygen than mixed venous blood leading to a calculated $\dot{Q}_S/\dot{Q}_T$ much larger than the lobar blood flow's fraction of total pulmonary blood flow. Infusions of indomethacin and aspirin have been associated with a marked reduction in lobar blood flow and $\dot{Q}_S/\dot{Q}_T$[30] and treatment with penicillin and time does likewise.[31] A major reduction in $\dot{Q}_S/\dot{Q}_T$ and increase in arterial oxygen content is effected by positioning the patient with the consolidated lobe in the uppermost position; that is, a patient with a severe right middle and lower lobe pneumonia has a marked reduction in shunt when lying in the left lateral decubitus position as opposed to the right lateral decubitus position.[1] Patients with pneumonia are frequently febrile, and as a result their total body $\dot{V}_{O_2}$ is increased; return of the $\dot{V}_{O_2}$ toward normal by antipyretics reduces the $\dot{Q}_{O_2}$ required to maintain aerobic metabolism.[27] In patients ventilated for severe pneumonia, muscle relaxation and positive-pressure ventilation can also reduce the work of breathing sufficiently to reduce $\dot{V}_{O_2}$ by a factor of two or three. Each of these adjunctive interventions may be particularly helpful in lobar pneumonia, where PEEP tends to be ineffective, likely because it redistributes the pulmonary blood flow toward the consolidated lobe.[32]

In less severe pneumonia, especially after antibacterial therapy has reduced the blood flow to the consolidated lobe, persistent hypoxemia is often alleviated by relatively small increments in the F_{IO_2}.[29] This occurs because $\dot{Q}_S/\dot{Q}_T$ accounts for about half the hypoxemia during air breathing; the other half is due to low $\dot{V}_A/\dot{Q}$ units arising from mechanical interdependence of the consolidated regions with the surrounding lung causing them to hypoventilate in relation to their perfusion. A second condition in which this mechanism for hypoxia is common is pulmonary contusion either with or without associated flail chest. The contusion essentially stops the blood flow to the consolidated hemorrhagic region probably by mechanical distortion or obliteration of the vessels.[33] As a result the shunt in pulmonary contusion is very small but the hypoxia can be quite profound due to the mechanical interdependence of the contused regions with the surrounding lung leading to large numbers of low $\dot{V}_A/\dot{Q}$ units there. This is important to oxygen therapy, for hypoxemic patients with large lung contusions often become well oxygenated with modest amounts of supplemental oxygen by nasal prongs or mask in clinical circumstances where the associated pain or other injuries might lead the prudent physician to believe that intubation and stabilization on a ventilator is imperative for the presumed shunt lung disease. The not infrequent concurrence of flail chest with lung contusion impacts little on the already small shunt, but adds to the hypoventilation of associated regions having very low $\dot{V}_A/\dot{Q}$ leading to severe hypoxemia. Yet measures which enhance ventilation like pain control and mechanical stabilization of the flail often allow simple oxygen supplementation to correct the hypoxemia[34] and spare the patient intubation and positive-pressure ventilation. This has a special advantage in lung contusion where positive-pressure ventilation especially with PEEP is associated with an increase in the underlying lung contusion.[33]

OXYGEN THERAPY DURING ALTERNATIVE MODES OF MECHANICAL VENTILATION. Oxygen therapy may also have a role in some alternative modes of ventilation. For example, during apnea oxygenation is maintained either by prior ventilation with oxygen-enriched mixtures or with continued tracheal insufflation of oxygen at low flow rates;[35] of course CO_2 accumulates at a rate of about 5 to 6 mmHg/min in the first instance and at a slightly lower rate during continuous tracheal flow which effects some alveolar washout of CO_2. Such modes of oxygenation are occasionally useful during bronchoscopy or for brief periods during thoracic surgery to permit better surgical exposure and a motionless operating field, and these periods might be prolonged if constant flow ventilation (CFV) effected adequate CO_2 elimination in patients with normal lungs.[36] In the dog, CFV at rates of 1 to 3 L/kg/min does effect adequate CO_2 elimination and maintains eucapnia associated with moderate arterial hypoxemia in turn due to perfusion of a large number of very low $\dot{V}_A/\dot{Q}$ units.[37] About half the hypoxia during ventilation with air is due to $\dot{V}/\dot{Q}$ variance among lobes, while the other half is due to $\dot{V}_A/\dot{Q}$ variance within lobes; all the hypoxia is corrected by a modest increase in F_{IO_2} from 0.21 to 0.40 with Pa_{O_2} increasing from 60 to 120 mmHg.[38] Of note, the large $\dot{V}_A/\dot{Q}$ variance was associated with, and probably due to, an inhomogeneity of alveolar pressures predictable from the momentum exchange between the inflow jet and the alveolar gas in this unusual mode of ventilation,[38] and the inhomogeneity of alveolar pressures as well as the associated lung hyperinflation were ameliorated by ventilation with heliox.[39] Conceivably, the mechanisms elucidated in these canine studies will facilitate development of better CFV systems to overcome inadequate CO_2 elimination in patients undergoing elective surgery, when modest oxygen enrichment of the inflow jet of air will correct hypoxemia.

In AHRF, even greater benefits of alternative modes of ventilation with very small V_T is anticipated on the basis of reduced barotrauma. For example, CFV with $F_{IO_2} = 0.5$ might achieve adequate oxygenation in patients with large shunts by the usual PEEP effects at high mean airway pressure, without the adverse effects of reduced venous return and increased pneumothorax associated with the usual V_T excursions; in turn, this may reduce pulmonary edema.[40] High frequency oscillatory ventilation (HFOV) may confer a similar advantage during ventilation with 2 to 4 mL/kg V_T at

4 to 20 Hz. HFOV effects adequate CO_2 elimination in patients and in dogs with severe pulmonary edema while CO_2 elimination and lung oxygen exchange seem quite dependent on the main airway pressure via the PEEP effects described above.[41] Note that both CFV and HFOV cause pressure at the airway opening to underestimate the alveolar pressure, so some of the therapeutic effect of these alternative modes on shunt is due to undetected high levels of PEEP.[38,41] Other modes like inverse ratio ventilation improve oxygenation in AHRF by a similar mechanism, i.e., a short expiratory time allows delivery of the next breath before the last breath is out, causing occult intrinsic PEEP. Conceivably, alternative modes of ventilation such as CFV or HFOV will facilitate more effective oxygen therapy of AHRF in the future, but the prudent intensivist will have a slow hand in implementing these new tricks before their benefits and complications are clarified.

References

1. Hall JB, Wood LDH: Oxygen therapy, in West JB, Crystal RG (eds): *The Lung; Scientific Foundation*. New York, Raven Press, 1990, pp 2143–2154.
2. Schmidt GA, Hall JB: Acute on chronic respiratory failure. Assessment and management of patients with COPD in the emergent setting. JAMA 261:3444, 1989.
3. Wood LDH, Prewitt RM: Cardiovascular management in acute hypoxemic respiratory failure. Am J Cardiol 47:963, 1981.
4. McCarty DC, Goodman JR, Petty TL: A program for transtracheal oxygen delivery: Assessment of safety and efficacy. Ann Intern Med 107:802, 1987.
5. Couser JI, Jr, Make BJ: Transtracheal oxygen decreases inspired minute ventilation. Am Rev Respir Dis 139:627, 1989.
6. Gibson RL, Comer PB, Beckham RW, et al: Actual tracheal oxygen concentrations with commonly used oxygen equipment. Anesthesiology 44(1):71, 1976.
7. Nickerson BG, Sarkisian C, Tremper K: Bias and precision of pulse oximeters and arterial oximeters. Chest 93:515, 1988.
8. Aubier M, Murciano D, Fournier M, et al: Central respiratory drive in acute respiratory failure of patients with chronic obstructive pulmonary disease. Am Rev Respir Dis 122:191, 1980.
9. Aubier M, Murciano D, Milic-Emili J, et al: Effects of administration of O_2 on ventilation and blood gases in patients with chronic obstructive pulmonary disease during acute respiratory failure. Am Rev Respir Dis 122:147, 1980.
10. Rodriguez-Roisin R, Ballester E, Roca J, et al: Mechanisms of hypoxemia in patients with status asthmaticus requiring mechanical ventilation. Am Rev Respir Dis 139:732, 1989.
11. Hall JB, Wood LDH: Management of the critically ill asthmatic patient, in Dosman JA, Cockcroft DW (eds): *Obstructive Lung Disease*. Med Clin North Am, 74(3):799, 1990.
12. Curtis JL, Mahlmeister M, Fink JB, et al: Helium oxygen gas therapy: Use and availability for the emergency treatment of inoperable airway obstruction. Chest 90:455, 1986.
13. Gluck EH, Onorato DJ, Castriottu R: Helium-oxygen mixtures in intubated patients with status asthmaticus and respiratory acidosis. Chest 98:693, 1990.
14. Macnee W, Wathen CG, Flenley DC, et al: The effects of controlled oxygen therapy on ventricular function in patients with stable and decompensated cor pulmonale. Am Rev Respir Dis 137:1289, 1988.
15. Agusti A, Roca J, Gea J, et al: Mechanisms of gas exchange impairment in idiopathic pulmonary fibrosis. Am Rev Respir Dis 143:219, 1991.
16. Midgren B, Hansson L, Eriksson L, et al: Oxygen desaturation during sleep and exercise in patients with interstitial lung disease. Thorax 42:353, 1987.
17. Dantzker RM: Gas exchange in the adult respiratory distress syndrome. Clin Chest Med 3:57, 1982.
18. Walley KR, Becker CJ, Hogan RA, et al: Progressive hypoxemia limits oxygen consumption and left ventricular contractility. Circ Res 63:849, 1988.
19. Malo J, Ali J, Wood LDH: How does positive end expiratory pressure reduce intrapulmonary shunt in canine pulmonary edema? J Appl Physiol 57:1002, 1984.
20. Ralph DB, Robertson HT, Weaver LJ, et al: Distribution of ventilation and perfusion during positive end expiratory pressure in the adult respiratory distress syndrome. Am Rev Respir Dis 131:54, 1985.
21. Shelhame JH, Natanson C, Parillo JE: Positive end expiratory pressure in adults. JAMA 251:2692, 1984.
22. Humphrey H, Hall J, Sznajder JI, et al: Improved survival following pulmonary capillary wedge pressure reduction in patients with ARDS. Chest 97:1176, 1990.
23. Long GR, Breen PH, Meyers I, et al: Treatment of canine aspiration pneumonitis: Fluid volume reduction vs. fluid volume expansion. J Appl Physiol 65:1736, 1988.
24. Breen PH, Schumacker PT, Hedenstierna G, et al: How does increased cardiac output increase shunt in pulmonary edema? J Appl Physiol 53:1273, 1982.
25. Melot C, Lejeune P, Leeman M, et al: Prostaglandin E_1 in the adult respiratory distress syndrome. Am Rev Respir Dis 139:106, 1989.
26. Reyes A, Roca J, Rodriguez-Roisin R, et al: Effect of almitrine on ventilation-perfusion distribution in adult respiratory distress syndrome. Am Rev Respir Dis 137:106, 1988.
27. Schumacker PT, Roland J, Saltz S, et al: Effects of hyperthermia and hypothermia on the limit of oxygen extraction by tissues. J Appl Physiol 63:1246, 1987.
28. Schumacker PT, Long GR, Wood LDH: Tissue oxygen extraction during hypovolemia: Role of hemoglobin P50. J Appl Physiol 62:1801, 1987.
29. Light RB, Mink SN, Wood LDH: The pathophysiology of gas exchange and pulmonary perfusion in pneumococcal lobar pneumonia in dogs. J Appl Physiol 50:524, 1981.
30. Light RB: Indomethacin and acetylsalicylic acid reduce intrapulmonary shunt in experimental pneumococcal pneumonia. Am Rev Respir Dis 134:520, 1986.
31. Light RB, Cooligan T, Mink SN, et al: The pathophysiology of recovery in experimental lobar pneumonia. Clin Invest Med 6:147, 1983.
32. Mink SN, Light RB, Cooligan T, et al: The effect of PEEP on gas exchange and pulmonary perfusion in canine lobar pneumonia. J Appl Physiol 50:517, 1981.
33. Craven KD, Oppenheimer L, Wood LDH: Effects of lung contusion and flail chest on pulmonary perfusion and oxygen exchange. J Appl Physiol 47:729, 1979.
34. Mackersie RC, Shackford SR, Hoyt DP: Continuous epidural fentanyl analgesia: Ventilatory function improvement with routine use in treatment of blunt chest injury. J Trauma 27:1207, 1987.
35. Babinski MF, Sierra OG, Smith RB, et al: Clinical application of continuous flow apneic ventilation. Acta Anaesthesiol Scand 29:750, 1985.

36. Breen PH, Sznajder J, Morrison P, et al: Constant flow ventilation in anesthetized patients: Efficacy and safety. Anesth Analg 65:1161, 1986.
37. Schumacker PT, Sznajder J, Nahum A, et al: Ventilation perfusion inequality during constant flow ventilation. J Appl Physiol 62:1255, 1987.
38. Sznajder J, Nahum A, Crawford G, et al: Alveolar pressure inhomogeneity and gas exchange during constant flow ventilation in dogs. J Appl Physiol 67:1489, 1989.
39. Schumacker PT, Samsel RW, Sznajder JI, et al: Gas density dependence of regional VAV and VAQ inequality during constant flow ventilation. J Appl Physiol 66:1722, 1989.
40. Corbridge T, Wood LDH, Crawford G, et al: Adverse effects of large tidal volumes and low peep in canine acid aspiration. Am Rev Respir Dis 141:311, 1990.
41. Breen PH, Ali J, Wood LDH: High frequency ventilation in lung edema: Effects on gas exchange and perfusion. J Appl Physiol 56:187, 1984.

Chapter 12

HYPERBARIC MEDICINE IN CRITICAL CARE

PAMELA S. GRIM
LAWRENCE J. GOTTLIEB

Hyperbaric oxygen (HBO) therapy involves inhalation of 100% O_2 under a pressure greater than 1 atmosphere. Critically ill patients undergoing HBO therapy may require the full gamut of intensive care support, including intubation, respiratory support, central cardiac monitoring, and antiarrhythmic therapy. Although the technical aspects of a hyperbaric chamber's operation are usually directed by a hyperbaric physician, an intensivist may be asked to manage a critically ill patient undergoing HBO therapy. Familiarity with the working of an HBO chamber and awareness of the pitfalls will facilitate collaborative patient care. This chapter updates our previous review of HBO[1] with a special focus on administration, indications, and complications of HBO in the critically ill. Ultimately, more clinical research will need to be done with HBO therapy in acute illness in order to address crucial clinical issues.[2] Although firm physiologic and clinical evidence demonstrates the effectiveness of HBO therapy in decompression sickness (DCS) and air embolism, other common indications, such as carbon monoxide (CO) poisoning and clostridial myonecrosis, rest on a small number of in vitro and in vivo experiments and few clinical trials. As Jacobson et al[3] stated long ago, "If this form of therapy is to achieve a worthwhile and lasting place in the medical armamentarium, it can only do so on a firm basis of accurate physiological data on the effects of both pressure and oxygen obtained in experiments as well controlled as clinical medicine will permit."

Methods of Administration

The administration of HBO therapy requires the construction of a specially designed chamber that can deliver both increased O_2 and high ambient pressure. Considerations in chamber design and operation include pressure integrity, gas delivery and administration, fire prevention, and electrical safety.[1] Bodies that have produced governing codes and standards for hyperbaric chambers include the National Fire Protection Association and the American Society of Mechanical Engineers. Hyperbaric chamber operation is extremely safe. Only one chamber-associated fire occurred between 1970 and 1984.[4] However, chamber operation is a complex process, and it is important that any facility be managed by a physician specially trained in HBO system operation and maintenance. HBO is usually delivered in one of two ways: via a monoplace chamber, which permits only a single patient to be pressurized, or via a multiplace chamber, which can hold two or more patients. Some of the latter type have been built large enough to contain an entire operating suite.

MONOPLACE CHAMBERS IN INTENSIVE CARE

The monoplace chamber allows a single patient to lie supine within a pressure-resistant shell (Fig. 12-1). Many chambers feature a clear acrylic dome that allows the patient to be viewed easily and also allows the patient to observe his or her surroundings. The chamber is ventilated with 100% O_2 with an overhead "dump," which maintains a pure oxygen environment within. The flammable nature of this environment requires that no electronic equipment be maintained within the chamber itself; only specially designed mechanical devices may be used. A monoplace chamber can be pressurized to 3 ATA, a pressure sufficient for most, but not all, patients requiring HBO therapy.[5] The problems of electronic monitoring and the isolation of the patient from attendants present special challenges in caring for a critically ill patient.

FLUID SUPPORT AND MONITORING

Simple matters, such as administering fluid and drugs, become complex when the patient is in a monoplace chamber. In order to overcome the pressurized environment, intravenous lines are attached to electronic pumps that remain external to the chamber. The pressure, which must be overcome by the pumps, can limit the amount of fluid that can be rapidly administered. Intravenous lines are placed in a passthrough that penetrates the hull and is then connected to the patient. Backcheck valves within the chamber prevent rapid exsanguination, which might occur should lines external to the chamber be disrupted; but they cannot be used if venous sampling is desired. Drugs can be administrated through a Y-connector.

Electronic monitoring of chamber patients depends on the resources available to the particular unit. Most monoplace chambers have the capability of monitoring heart rhythm via electric cables that are attached to the

FIGURE 12-1 A monoplace chamber.

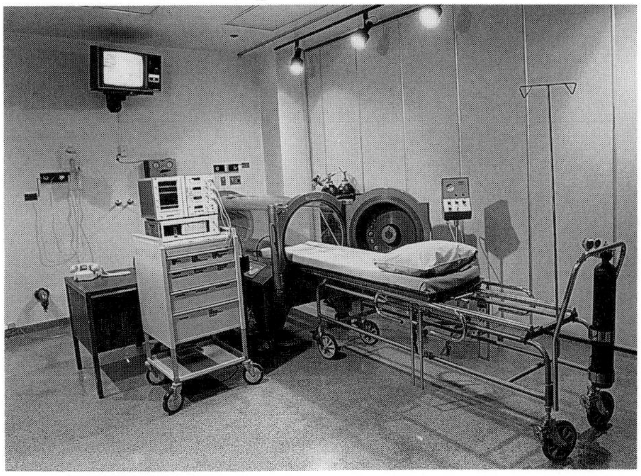

chamber's electric connector. No electronic monitor can be placed inside the chamber. Other monitoring lines can also be used if appropriate signal adapters are available, allowing measurement of blood pressure, central venous pressure, arterial pressure, and pulmonary artery pressures.[6]

RESPIRATORY SUPPORT

Patients in monoplace chambers can be mechanically ventilated using specially designed ventilators. The commonly used Sechrist model, designed for the Sechrist chamber only, is a pressure- rather than volume-cycled ventilator, similar to those now used to ventilate premature infants. The electronic portion of the ventilator remains outside the chamber and is connected via cables to the manifold located within the chamber. A special servo mechanism allows the inner baffle to sense ambient pressure and adjust the delivered pressure so that it remains constant, even with variation in the chamber's ambient pressure. These ventilators are limited in their ability to deliver adequate ventilation of a patient with a very large or very small tidal volume (V_T) requirement or with low lung compliance; this limits the ability of such to treat certain extremely ill patients and some infants.

Endotracheal tube (ET) cuffs require special care during HBO treatments. Increased ambient pressure in the chamber will reduce cuff size and allow a gas leak around the tube. Decreasing the chamber pressure will expand the cuff, occasionally causing it to rupture. Intubated patients receiving HBO should either have the air removed and the ET tube cuff filled with water or be intubated with a special ET tube with a sponge-filled cuff (e.g., the Buvona tube—Fig. 12-2) that will expand and contract passively with pressure changes.

Pneumothorax occurring while a patient is under pressure is fortunately a rare event, but can be difficult to diagnose and treat. Pneumothorax should be suspected in patients appearing to experience worsening respiratory distress during decompression. If a trial of recompression improves respiratory status, the clinical diagnosis has been confirmed. The pneumothorax will enlarge as the chamber pressure is lowered to atmospheric pressure, in accordance

FIGURE 12-2 The Buvona tube.

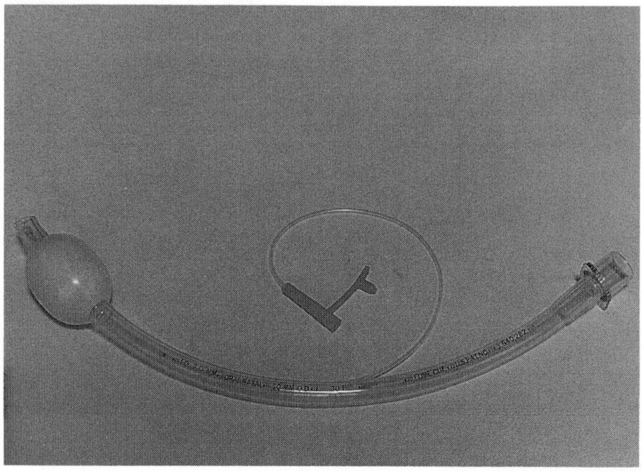

with Boyle's law. Therefore, provisions should be made for immediate thoracostomy once the patient has been evacuated from the chamber.

URGENT DECOMPRESSION

The chief concern in treating critically ill patients is the isolation of the care giver from the patient. Most monoplace units have an emergency vent system by means of which the patient can be returned to atmospheric pressure within 30 s; but in patients with a closed glottis, such as those having seizures, rapid decompression can produce severe pulmonary barotrauma and arterial air embolism. No patient should be decompressed while undergoing the tonic phase of a seizure, or when in any condition in which exhalation may be impeded.

Patients requiring resuscitation with defibrillation also present a special problem. Rapid decompression is necessary. In addition, as a patient is being removed from the chamber, the pure O_2 environment of the chamber is swept into the room, presenting a potential fire hazard with the use of a defibrillator. The patient should be pulled well away from the chamber, and, since O_2-saturated fabrics can ignite easily, the hyperbaric gown should be removed before defibrillation is administered.

MULTIPLACE CHAMBERS IN INTENSIVE CARE

Multiplace chambers are large units that allow treatment of up to six patients at a time. Unlike monoplace chambers, most multiplace chambers are built to achieve 6 to 7 ATA pressure, so that diseases requiring high pressure during treatment, such as diver's decompression sickness and air embolism, can be treated effectively.[7] The multiplace chamber is pressurized with air having no more than 23% O_2; patients breathe 100% O_2 through a mask, headhood, or endotracheal tube. Patients can then take breaks breathing chamber air in which inspired gas has a much lower P_{O_2}. These air breaks permit treatment times to be prolonged with less risk of O_2 toxicity.[8] Multiplace chambers contain an independent pressure unit in which attendants can lock in and out and, thus, have unlimited access to the patient. This access allows almost any procedure performed at the bedside to be performed under pressure. The placement of chest tubes, central lines, and endotracheal tubes is possible within a multiplace chamber.

Care of the critically ill patient is much easier in a multiplace chamber, since an intensivist can personally be present at the bedside and can monitor, and intervene, during the course of therapy. In order to be effective the intensivist should already be familiar with the chamber environment before attempting to "dive" with a patient. Functioning within a noisy, crowded chamber, and at the same time being potentially subjected to nitrogen narcosis, is a unique experience that requires training and experience.

MONITORING

The modern hyperbaric unit has monitoring capabilities similar to those of the intensive care unit (ICU) setting, including on-line electric (cardiac rhythm) monitoring and pressure (intracranial and cardiovascular) monitoring. Transducers are mounted within the chamber and coupled to electronic displays, which must remain outside the chamber because of fire hazard. However, since the multiplace chamber is compressed with air, the risk of fire is less, allowing certain solid-state monitors to be placed within the chamber.

Monitoring oxygenation can be difficult within a multiplace chamber. Blood gas measurements may be rendered unreliable, since "offgassing" of O_2 may occur once the sample leaves the chamber. With appropriate precautions to limit the fire hazard, blood gas analysis may be performed in the multiplace chamber. Skin monitors of O_2 saturation (pulse oximetry) are a fire hazard and cannot be used in the hyperbaric environment. Clinical observation with frequent examinations remains the most reliable method to detect hypoxemia.

RESPIRATORY AND FLUID SUPPORT

Critically ill patients can receive well-controlled support within the multiplace chamber. The presence of an attendant allows hands-on evaluation of the patient's status and easier diagnosis of pulmonary problems than is possible in a monoplace chamber. Endotracheal cuffs need not be filled with water, but must be deflated before the beginning of "descent" or "ascent" and carefully reinflated at the end of pressure changes.

Options for ventilators are also broader. Because of the reduced risk of fire in a multiplace chamber, the Siemens 900B or 900C ventilator, which uses solid-state circuitry, can be used in the multiplace environment without modification. Its adaptability and widespread use make it an excellent ventilator for use in multiplace chambers. The Penlon Oxford ventilator is very popular and is commonly used by HBO physicians because of its small size, ease of use, and reliability. However, it does not have the range of functions and alarms contained in the Siemens, and will require orientation for someone unfamiliar with its use. Time-cycled, pressure-dependent ventilators can also be used, but require careful observation during chamber pressure changes and, in general, are not optimal given other available choices.[9]

Administration of fluid is relatively uncomplicated in a multiplace chamber. Fluid to be administered is maintained within the chamber. Bagged fluids are preferable, since there is little volume change with change of pressures. Glass bottles, in which increasing and decreasing pressure can cause decrease or increase in the volume of air, should be vented to prevent changes in flow rates.

Indications for Hyperbaric Oxygen (HBO) That Arise in Intensive Care Therapy

The indications regarded as standard by the Undersea and Hyperbaric Medical Society that may be seen in the critical care setting are shown in Table 12-1.[1] The mechanism of both the therapeutic and toxic effects of HBO results from two features of treatment: the mechanical effects of increased ambient pressure and the physiologic effects of hyperoxia. Each of the indications described below responds to either or both of these effects during the course of therapy.

TABLE 12-1 Indications for Hyperbaric Oxygen Therapy

Air or gas embolism
Carbon monoxide and/or cyanide poisoning; smoke inhalation
Acute traumatic ischemias such as compartment syndrome and crush injury
Decompression sickness
Enhancement of healing in selected problem wounds
Exceptional blood loss
Clostridial gangrene
Necrotizing soft-tissue infection
Osteomyelitis (refractory)
Radiation necrosis
Osteoradionecrosis and soft-tissue radionecrosis
Caries in radiated bones
Skin grafts or flaps (compromised)

AIR EMBOLISM

Any penetrating wound of the chest or abdomen, or any medical procedure in which an artery or vein comes in contact with the patient's external environment, can result in life-threatening air embolism. Iatrogenic air embolism is frequently undiagnosed; as the signs and symptoms of embolism go unrecognized and untreated, patients may suffer irreversible neurologic deficit or death if the appropriate diagnosis and therapy has not been considered (see Chap. 118). In a hospital setting, diagnosis of air embolism can be made when sudden neurologic or cardiovascular deterioration occurs following air entry into the vascular system in awake patients. The diagnosis is frequently overlooked, however, in anesthetized patients in whom the occurrence of the embolism is substantially separated from the time when the patient can first be examined neurologically (i.e., post-anesthesia). Air embolism must be suspected in *all* patients with penetrating chest injury who deteriorate suddenly after intubation. Air embolism has occurred during cardiovascular surgery, lung biopsy, hemodialysis, central line placement, use of pump oxygenators, and intubation in patients with penetrating lung injury, and even in simple intravenous infusions.[1] Air embolism is also a risk associated with diving. In divers who ascend with their glottis closed, lung volume expands as ambient pressure falls. Rupture of alveoli with dissection into a pulmonary vein can result in arterial air embolism (see Chap. 74). Air embolism into the venous system can be catastrophic when bubbles either obstruct the pulmonary outflow tract or pass through a patent foramen ovale or through the pulmonary capillary system into the arterial system where cardiac and central nervous system embolism can occur.

Initial treatment involves placing the patient head-down in the left lateral decubitus position and administering

100% O_2. ACLS protocols should be used, if necessary, and the patient should be transported to a hyperbaric unit. If a helicopter or nonpressurized aircraft is involved in transport, an altitude of between 500 and 800 ft should be maintained. It should be emphasized that, although delay worsens prognosis, severely affected patients have been treated more than 10 h after the initial embolic event with full recovery.

The optimal method for treatment of air embolism is still controversial among hyperbaric physicians; standard therapy involves U.S. Navy Dive Table 6A in a multiplace chamber. This involves an initial dive to 165 ft (6 ATA) where the patient breaths gas of 50% O_2 and 50% N_2 for 30 min and then undergoes staged ascent breathing 100% O_2 interspersed with air breaks. The ideal treatment of patients with air embolism includes an intensivist accompanying the hyperbaric physician to assist with resuscitation. In addition to recompression and O_2, patients need appropriate fluid administration. Dexamethasone and mannitol should be considered to reduce cerebral edema. Lidocaine has been shown to substantially enhance central nervous system (CNS) recovery in cats after cerebral air embolism.[10] Standard antiarrhythmic doses with a maintenance infusion have been recommended.

Recent work in animals has suggested that the initial deep dive that is a part of U.S. Navy Dive Table 6A may not be necessary, that compression beyond 2.8 ATA with 100% O_2 does not improve cerebral blood flow, and that breathing air at 6 ATA may actually increase intracranial pressure.[11] This has led to the use of monoplace chambers when a multiplace chamber was not available. Treatment with pressure and O_2, even if at less than optimal pressures, has been demonstrated to be beneficial and probably lifesaving.[12]

If the hyperbaric physician has little experience dealing with air embolism he or she should establish telephone contact with experienced personnel. The Divers Alert Network at Duke University maintains a 24-hour hot line, and is staffed by hyperbaric physicians who can offer emergency consultation. The number is 919–684–8111.

DECOMPRESSION SICKNESS (DCS)

While symptoms resulting from decompression can occur with a sudden elevation from sea level to altitudes greater than 18,500 ft, most cases involve diving or other underwater exposure to high atmospheric pressure (e.g., tunnels, caissons, and hyperbaric chambers). Rapid ascent with tissues highly saturated with N_2 will create a high N_2 pressure gradient ultimately causing N_2 gas bubbles large enough and prevalent enough to cause symptoms of decompression sickness (DCS). Two pathologic processes take place: mechanical deformation of tissue by bubbles, and phase interaction between the surface of the gas bubble and plasma components potentially causing disruption of the intravascular coagulation system (see Chap. 74). Fifty percent of DCS symptoms occur within 1 h, and 90 percent within 6 h, after surfacing from a dive. Symptom onset is generally (though not always) less precipitous than air embolism, which usually presents immediately upon surfacing.

Clinical manifestations can be divided into two major types. Type I DCS is defined as "pain only" and involves deep throbbing pain within the joints, usually the large joints of the upper extremities in divers. The origin of symptoms probably involves the mechanical deformation of tendons, ligaments, and other connective tissue.[13] DCS can present purely as a skin manifestation. Typically this is an erythematous mottling of the skin associated with pruritus and a sensation of burning. The rash is generally distributed over fatty tissue and rapidly disappears with chamber recompression. Type II DCS symptoms involve the CNS in either subtle or overt ways and occur in 10 to 25 percent of all cases of DCS in U.S. Navy divers.[14] Subtle changes include changes in mood and personality; more overt symptoms include those of cerebral embolism, spinal cord lesions, peripheral nerve lesions, and otololgic/vestibular manifestations. It has been hypothesized that major symptoms of type II DCS are due to N_2 bubble embolization; however, this does not explain the predominance of spinal cord lesions (approximately 75 percent of cases of type II DCS) over cerebral manifestations. Spinal cord lesions, in fact, probably occur secondary to formation of N_2 gas bubbles within the valveless, low-pressure vertebral venous plexus, with subsequent venous and lymphatic obstruction.[15] Development of type I decompression sickness does not preclude progression to type II symptoms (see Chap. 74). Approximately 1 percent of DCS patients will present with pulmonary symptoms, or the "chokes," usually after very rapid decompression such as that seen with aviators.[16]

Initial treatment in all cases of DCS is administration of O_2 and rapid transport to the nearest HBO facility. Shock should be treated with volume expanders, intubation if necessary, and corticosteroids if CNS involvement is suspected. The single largest cause of treatment failure is failure to diagnose and treat DCS in a timely fashion. Evacuation to a hyperbaric chamber of any kind, despite substantial delays in treatment time, is always the preferred course of action.[17] Definitive treatment of both type I and type II DCS involves HBO therapy (see Chap. 74). Multiplace chambers are preferable because greater pressure can be achieved during treatment; however, DCS has been successfully treated in a monoplace chamber.[12] Treatment schedules involve the use of U.S. Navy tables, which govern depth, timing, and gas mixture during treatment.[11] The hyperbaric physician should act as team leader during treatment of DCS, with the intensivist acting as support staff and consultant.

CARBON MONOXIDE (CO) POISONING

Carbon monoxide (CO) is a product of incomplete combustion of carbonaceous material. Sources of CO poisoning include automobile exhaust, faulty heating systems, and smoke inhalation. It is a common but unpredictable poison that has been studied extensively but remains incompletely understood. CO has an affinity for hemoglobin that is 200 to 250 times that of O_2, so small amounts in inspired air can rapidly produce high levels of carboxyhemoglobin (COHb). In addition to this reduction in effective hemoglobin concentration, CO binding to one or more of the four hemoglobin binding sites increases the affinity of the remaining binding sites for O_2; this shifts the oxyhemoglobin dissociation curve to the left, decreasing O_2 dissociation at the tissue level.[18] Thus CO is thought to produce its toxic effect by producing systemic anoxia. However, in human beings, COHb levels correspond poorly with degree of toxicity and clinical status. A patient presenting with a COHb level of 30 percent may have no neurologic deficit, or may be comatose.[19] This inconsistency in clinical findings has led researchers to propose that CO acts at a tissue level by binding to other heme proteins, particularly cytochrome oxidase, so that toxicity would correspond to tissue concentration rather than COHb concentration.[20] This is compatible with the hypothesis that the length of exposure is a major factor in degree of toxicity. However, data concerning this hypothesis are conflicting, in part because there is no method available to measure tissue levels of CO.

The half-life of COHb is 4 to 5 h in patients breathing room air. Inspiration of 100% O_2 decreases the half-life to 80 min; treatment with 100% O_2 at 2 atmospheres further reduces the half-life to 23 min.[1] Therefore, the initial and most crucial form of therapy for toxic exposure to CO is administration of 100% O_2 via tightly fitted mask or endotracheal tube. HBO therapy ameliorates CO poisoning by displacing CO from hemoglobin, and from the cytochrome system. Despite these advantages, the few controlled clinical trials that have compared HBO therapy with 100% O_2 at 1 atmosphere have been inconclusive.[21,22] Conceivably, subtle effects of CO on cognitive functioning may have been overlooked in evaluating treatment outcomes.[23] Some clinicians have argued that HBO therapy is unnecessary for most exposures when a chamber is not readily available, since 2 h of 100% O_2 frequently brings the level of COHb into a nontoxic range. However, some patients with severe symptoms on exposure that do not resolve with several hours of 100% O_2 will suddenly and dramatically improve during the first, or even second, hyperbaric treatment despite a COHb level of less than 5 percent. Until these anecdotes are refuted, there remains the possibility that subtle CNS sequelae of CO poisonings require HBO therapy, with its attendant complications and impediments to critical care.

CLOSTRIDIAL MYONECROSIS

Gas gangrene, once a common disease of war, is a catastrophic infectious cascade that occurs when a hypoxic environment within a necrotic wound allows clostridial spores to convert to active organisms. Exotoxins produced by these organisms destroy blood cells, abolish host defenses, and cause widespread tissue necrosis.[24] The most injurious of the exotoxins is alpha toxin, which destroys cell membranes and alters capillary permeability.

Basic therapy of clostridial myonecrosis involves wound debridement and antibiotic therapy. Results of in vitro and in vivo studies have suggested that HBO therapy may provide additional benefit by oxygenating compromised tissue, inhibiting alpha toxin production, and possibly inhibiting clostridial reproduction.[1,25] In a dog model of clostridial myonecrosis, no treatment, or treatment with surgery or HBO alone, resulted in a 100 percent mortality rate. Treatment with antibiotics alone resulted in a 50 percent mortality rate; antibiotics and surgery resulted in a 30 percent mortality rate, and the addition of HBO to this regimen reduced mortality to 5 percent.[26] Several uncontrolled series involving patients with clostridial infection have incorporated HBO into the therapeutic regimen.[1,27,28] HBO therapy seems to assist in demarking viable versus nonviable tissue and in stabilizing the overall clinical status of the patient, apparently by inhibiting further production of alpha toxin. In a series of 133 patients a mortality rate of 25 percent was documented in 89 patients who received HBO therapy, versus 45 percent mortality in the 44 patients who did not.[28] To date, however, no controlled clinical trials have been published.

Contraindications and Complications

The only absolute contraindication to HBO therapy is an untreated pneumothorax. Adequate venting with a chest tube should allow a patient to receive treatment safely. The remaining contraindications are relative and should be weighed against the potential benefits of therapy.

The usual complications of HBO are a result of either ambient pressure changes or oxygen toxicity (Table 12-2). The most frequent complications are also the most benign. These generally involve air-filled cavities of the head. Typically, the middle ear or one of the sinuses cannot equalize the internal pressure with the ambient pressure of the chamber. Most sinus and ear problems can be symptomatically treated with antihistamines. Inability to equalize the middle ear may cause damage to the tympanic membrane and inner mucous membranes, resulting in serous otitis, blood within the middle ear, or ruptured tympanic membrane. This complication can be avoided with placement of myringotomy tubes.[29] Similarly, small pockets of air under the filling of a tooth may cause tooth pain.

TABLE 12-2 Major Complications of Hyperbaric Therapy

Barotrauma
Ear or sinus trauma
Tympanic membrane rupture
Pneumothorax
Air embolism
Oxygen toxicity
Central nervous system toxic reactions
Pulmonary toxic reactions
Other
Fire
Reversible visual changes
Claustrophobia

Pneumothorax may occur under the same principles of pressure disequilibrium. Air trapping and volume expansion, especially in a diseased lung, may result in a ruptured bleb and pleural tear.[29] Typically, pneumothoraces develop during decompression. Diagnosis and management, particularly in a monoplace chamber, is discussed under Monoplace Chambers in Intensive Care, above.

Over time, high O_2 levels are toxic to all tissues. CNS toxicity is of greatest concern during HBO therapy, since neural tissue is very sensitive to high concentrations of O_2. Seizure, the most serious neurologic complication, is rare (1.3 cases per 10,000 in one series)[29,30] and usually results in minimal, if any, long-term sequelae. A patient with a history of seizures or high fever may have an increased risk of seizures during HBO treatments. However, most neurologic effects of hyperoxia are seen with pressures of O_2 much higher, and durations much longer, than those used in standard HBO treatments.

While neural toxicity develops under conditions of high concentration of O_2 under pressure and rarely occurs under 2 ATA, pulmonary toxicity, familiar to all intensivists, can occur with sufficient exposure to O_2 under pressures less than 1 ATA. Generally, CNS toxicity occurs earlier at higher pressures, and pulmonary toxicity occurs later at lower pressures.[30] Initial symptoms of pulmonary toxicity include substernal burning, cough, and dyspnea. Continued exposure may result in the development of acute lung injury, manifesting as the adult respiratory distress syndrome (ARDS). In treatment regimens that require long treatment schedules, such as those for air embolism, toxicity is avoided by use of frequent "air breaks," where the patient breaths air for 5- to 15-min breaks. This seems to prolong the patient's ability to tolerate long HBO treatments. Intercurrent use of several uncommon therapies (doxorubicin [Adriamycin], disulfiram [Antabuse], cisplatin) may potentiate O_2 toxicity and should be avoided in patients during HBO therapy.

References

1. Grim PS, Gottlieb LJ, Boddie A, et al: Hyperbaric Oxygen Therapy. JAMA 263:2216, 1990.
2. Gobb G, Robin ED: Hyperbaric oxygen: A therapy in search of diseases. Chest 92:1074, 1987.
3. Jacobson JH, Morsch HC, Rendell-Baker L: Historical perspective of hyperbaric therapy. Ann N Y Acad Sci 117:651, 1965.
4. Reimers SD: Operational safety in clinical hyperbaric chambers. HBO Review 4:113, 1983.
5. Hamilton RW Jr, Sheffield PJ: Hyperbaric chamber safety, in David JC, Hunt TK (eds): *Hyperbaric Oxygen Therapy*. Bethesda, MD, Hyperbaric Medical Society, 1977, p. 41.
6. Grim PS, Gottlieb LJ, Samsel RW, et al: Invasive physiologic monitoring in a monoplace hyperbaric chamber. Undersea Biomedical Research (in press).
7. Sheffield PJ, David JC, Bell GC, Gallagher TJ: Hyperbaric chamber clinical support: Multiplace, in Davis JC, Hunt TK (eds): *Hyperbaric Therapy*. Bethesda, MD, Hyperbaric Medical Society, 1977, p. 25.
8. Hendricks PL, Hall DA, Hunter WH Jr, et al: Extension of pulmonary oxygen tolerance in man at 2 ATA by intermittent oxygen exposure. J Appl Physiol 42:593, 1977.
9. Gallagher TJ, Smith RA, Bell GC: Evaluation of mechanical ventilators in a hyperbaric environment. Aviat Space Environ Med 49:375, 1978.
10. Evans DE, Kobrine A, LeGrys DC, Bradley ME: Protective effect of lidocaine in acute cerebral ischemia induced by air embolism. J Neurosurg 60:257, 1984.
11. Green RD, Leitch DR: Twenty years of treating decompression sickness. Aviat Space Environ Med 58:931, 1987.
12. Hart GB, Strauss MB, Lennon PA: The treatment of decompression sickness and air embolism in a monoplace chamber. J Hyperbar Med 1:1, 1986.
13. Vann RO, Clark HG: Bubble growth and mechanical properties of tissue in decompression. Undersea Biomed Res 2:185, 1975.
14. Rivera JC: Decompression sickness among divers: An analysis of 935 cases. Milit Med 129:314, 1964.
15. Elliott DH, Hallenbeck JM, Bove AA: Acute decompression sickness. Lancet 2:1193, 1974.
16. Neuman TR, Spragg HR, Moser: Cardiopulmonary consequences of decompression stress. Am Rev Respir Dis 117:162, 1978.
17. Kizer KW: Delayed treatment of dysbarism: A retrospective review of 50 cases. JAMA 247:2555, 1982.
18. Roughton FJW, Darling RJ: The effect of carbon monoxide on the oxyhemoglobin dissociation curve. Am J Physiol 141:17, 1940.
19. Norbook DM, Kirkpatrick JN: Treatment of acute carbon monoxide poisoning with hyperbaric oxygen: A review of 115 cases. Ann Emerg Med 14:1168, 1985.
20. Halebain P, Robinson N, Barie P, et al: Whole body oxygen utilization during acute carbon monoxide poisoning and isocapneic nitrogen hypoxia. J Trauma 26:110, 1986.
21. Raphael JC, Elkharrat D, Jars-Guincestre MC, et al: Trial of normobaric and hyperbaric oxygen for acute carbon monoxide intoxication. Lancet 2:414, 1989.
22. Goulan M, Barois A, Rapin M, et al: Carbon monoxide poisoning and acute anoxia. J Hyperbar Med 1:23, 1986.
23. Choi IS: Delayed neurologic sequelae in carbon monoxide intoxication. Ann Neurol 40:433, 1983.
24. Weinstein L, Barza MA: Gas gangrene. N Engl J Med 289:1129, 1973.
25. Holland JA, Hill GB, Wolfe WG, et al: Experimental and clinical experience with hyperbaric oxygen in the treatment of clostridial myonecrosis. Surgery 77:75, 1975.
26. Demello FJ, Hashimoto T, Hitchcock CR: Comparative study of experimental Clostridium perfringens infection in dogs treated with antibiotics, surgery, and hyperbaric oxygen. Surgery 73:936, 1973.
27. Hart GH, Lamb RC, Strauss MB: Gas gangrene: II. A 15-year experience with hyperbaric oxygen. J Trauma 23:995, 1983.
28. Hitchcock CR, Demello FJ, Haglin JJ: Gangrene infection. Surg Clin North Am 55:403, 1975.
29. Bassett BE, Bennett PB: Introduction to the physician and physiological basis of hyperbaric therapy, in David JC, Hunt TM (eds): *Hyperbaric Oxygen Therapy*. Bethesda, MD, Undersea Medical Society, 1977, p. 11.
30. Davis JC, Dunn JM, Heimbach RD: Hyperbaric medicine: Patient selection, treatment procedures, and side effects, in Davis JC, Hunt EK (eds): *Problem Wounds: The Role of Oxygen*. New York, Elsevier, 1988, p. 225.

Chapter 13
BLOOD-GAS ANALYSIS

KEVIN K. TREMPER
STEVEN J. BARKER

The measurement and analysis of blood-gas data have been crucial aspects of critical care medicine since the development of the first practical blood-gas analyzer in 1958. With the more recent advent of in vivo measurement of blood-gas tensions, hemoglobin saturation, expired gas concentrations, and other related variables, science has made the transition from testing to monitoring. We are no longer limited to drawing intermittent blood samples for analysis at remote locations; we can now benefit from continuous, "real-time" data provided at the bedside. In this chapter we shall discuss currently available blood-gas monitoring techniques from the viewpoint of the intensivist. The emphasis will be on the interpretation and clinical use of the data from these devices rather than the details of their function. However, the operating principles of the monitors will be described to the extent that their knowledge is important in the interpretation of the data. If we simply regard monitors as "black boxes," we will be ignorant of situations in which they are likely to present erroneous or misleading results.

The term blood-gas monitoring is interpreted in a broad sense here. We shall discuss monitors that function at four different levels of the gas transport chain: respired gases, arterial blood, tissue, and venous blood. Techniques described at each of these levels will include capnography, pulse oximetry and intraarterial sensors, transcutaneous O_2 and CO_2, and pulmonary artery oximetry. We begin with a review of intermittent in vitro blood-gas analysis, stressing how to obtain the maximum useful information from blood-gas data in the least amount of time. Because entire books have been written on the acid-base aspects of blood-gas analysis,[1,2] and this subject is also discussed in Chaps. 3 and 158 of this text, our coverage here will be concise.

Interpretation of Blood-Gas Data

ACID-BASE STATUS: pH AND P_{CO_2}

Although it is traditional to interpret pH and P_{CO_2} as separate and distinct from P_{O_2}, we should remember that all three variables are linked. Prolonged hypoxia will obviously affect the acid-base status, and a change in pH will shift the oxyhemoglobin dissociation curve and thereby affect oxygenation. Nevertheless, we shall consider the analysis of pH, P_{CO_2}, and acid-base status as separate from that of Pa_{O_2}.

Hydrogen is one of the least plentiful ions in the extracellular fluid (ECF); at 40 nanoequivalents per liter (40×10^{-9} eq/L), it is about three million times less concentrated than sodium. Despite its low concentration, the small size of the hydrogen ion makes it highly reactive with enzymes and other proteins, and the body must regulate $[H^+]$ (square brackets indicate concentrations in mol/L) within rather narrow limits to maintain homeostasis. The pH, defined as $-\log[H^+]$, is normally held between 7.35 and 7.45. If the pH of the ECF is outside this range, the patient has acidemia (low pH) or alkalemia (high pH). We use the term *acidemia* to denote low extracellular pH; *acidosis* refers to a process which tends to reduce pH. The terms *alkalemia* and *alkalosis* are used in the same manner.

Given the consequences of pH derangements discussed in Chap. 158, we shall briefly review the body's defenses against such changes, an understanding of which is crucial to the interpretation of blood-gas data. Acids, which are hydrogen ion donors, are produced in the body in two ways. Carbon dioxide from oxidative metabolism is hydrated to produce carbonic acid:

$$CO_2 + H_2O \rightleftharpoons H_2CO_3 \rightleftharpoons H^+ + HCO_3^- \qquad (13\text{-}1)$$

This reaction, catalyzed by the cytoplasmic enzyme carbonic anhydrase, has an equilibrium heavily shifted to the left: for every H^+ ion there are 800 molecules of CO_2 and H_2CO_3 and 800,000 molecules of CO_2 and H_2O. Noncarbonic acids are also produced by both aerobic and anaerobic metabolism. These "metabolic" acids include phosphoric, sulfuric, lactic, and other acids. Carbonic acid is excreted by the lung in the form of CO_2. Metabolic acids are further metabolized and excreted by the kidneys, which normally remove about 50 mM of metabolic acid per day. Healthy kidneys can acidify the urine to a pH as low as 4.5 (900 times the H^+ concentration of the blood), and can thereby excrete up to 500 mM of acid per day. The lungs and the kidneys are two of the key elements of the body's defenses against pH changes.

The third element of pH control, the body's system of buffers, is discussed elsewhere in this text. We shall briefly review the bicarbonate buffer system, because of its importance in acid-base regulation and in the interpretation of blood-gas data. Recall the Henderson-Hasselbalch equation:

$$pH = pK + \log \frac{[A^-]}{[HA]} \qquad (13\text{-}2)$$

The pK of carbonic acid is 6.1, and the Henderson-Hasselbalch equation for this buffer system is

$$pH = 6.1 + \log \left\{ \frac{[HCO_3^-]}{0.03\ Pa_{CO_2}} \right\} \qquad (13\text{-}3)$$

We have replaced $[H_2CO_3]$, the carbonic acid concentration, by the CO_2 tension (in mmHg) times the solubility coefficient at 37°C (98.6°F), which equals 0.03. This equation implies that at a normal pH of 7.4 and a Pa_{CO_2} of 40 mmHg, the bicarbonate concentration will be 24 mM/L. Given any two of the quantities pH, Pa_{CO_2}, and $[HCO_3^-]$, the third is determined by (Eq. 13-3). As we vary the P_{CO_2}, the change in $[HCO_3^-]$ per unit change in pH is called the *buffer value* (BV):

$$BV = \frac{-\Delta[HCO_3^-]}{\Delta(pH)} \quad (13\text{-}4)$$

The in vivo buffer value for human beings at 37°C (98.6°F) is 10 to 12 mM/L/pH unit. The unit of BV (mM/L/pH) is called the *slyke* (sl). Values of BV measured in vivo will be less than whole blood values by roughly a factor of three, because hemoglobin has a higher concentration in blood than in the ECF. Hemoglobin is the primary noncarbonic buffer, and BV is a measure of the noncarbonic buffer power.

The pH-bicarbonate diagram of Fig. 13-1 illustrates the significance of BV as well as some other aspects of acid-base balance. The nearly straight buffer line passing through the origin (pH = 7.40, $[HCO_3^-]$ = 24) with a slope of −11 sl is the path followed by titrating P_{CO_2} up and down with no change in metabolic acid or base. The isobars, or lines of constant P_{CO_2}, are solutions to the Henderson-Hasselbalch equation (see Eq. 13-3) for the given P_{CO_2} values. A purely respiratory disturbance with no metabolic compensation will fall on the −11 sl buffer line, while a pure metabolic disturbance without respiratory compensation will fall on the P_{CO_2} = 40 mmHg isobar. We shall discuss partial compensation of primary acid-base disturbances and acute versus chronic disturbances after defining some important concepts.

FIGURE 13-1 Bicarbonate versus pH diagram showing primary acid-base imbalances and regions of compensation. The 10 sl buffer line represents pure respiratory disturbances without metabolic compensation. The Pa_{CO_2} = 40 mmHg line represents pure metabolic disturbances without respiratory compensation. Respiratory disturbances with metabolic compensation (acute and chronic) are indicated by the stippled areas; metabolic disturbances with respiratory compensation usually fall within the shaded areas. (Adapted from Goldberg, et al: JAMA 223:269, 1973.)

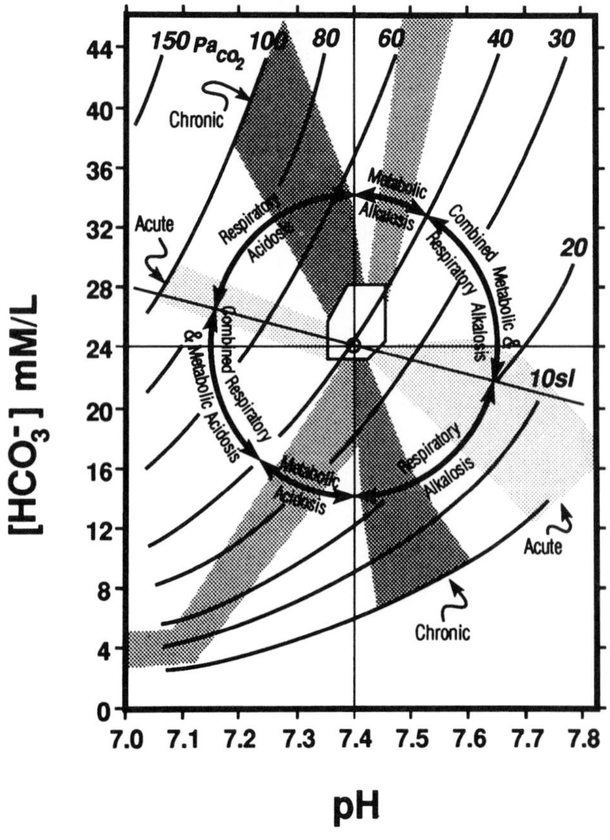

The ECF base excess (BE_e) is a means of quantifying the in vivo metabolic disturbance in the presence of both carbonic and noncarbonic buffer systems. Conceptually, the base excess is found by titrating the system (i.e., the patient) back to a pH of 7.4 by altering P_{CO_2}. BE_e is simply the difference between the patient's actual $[HCO_3^-]$ at pH = 7.4 and the normal value of 24 mM/L. BE_e represents the amount of metabolic acid or base present per liter of ECF. Rather than actually manipulate the patient's P_{CO_2} to achieve a pH of 7.4 (which may not be well tolerated), we can calculate BE_e from Fig. 13-1 or the Siggaard-Anderson nomogram shown in Fig. 13-2. Note that in finding BE_e on Fig. 13-2, we must use the average hemoglobin of the ECF, 3 to 5 g/dL, rather than whole blood values.

If we assume a BV of 10 sl, we can hand-calculate the BE_e as follows. Suppose a patient has a pH of 7.10 and a Pa_{CO_2} of 60 mmHg. From Eq. 13-3, his $[HCO_3^-]$ is 18 mM/L. To raise pH to 7.4 by lowering Pa_{CO_2}, we will follow a line parallel to the 10 sl buffer line until we reach pH = 7.4. Since $-\Delta[HCO_3^-]/\Delta(pH)$ = 10 sl, the change in $[HCO_3^-]$ will be 10 times the change in pH. As pH increases by 0.3, $[HCO_3^-]$ will decrease by 3.0, reaching a new value of 18 − 3 = 15 mM/L. The base excess is the difference between this value and 24 mM/L, or BE_e = 15 − 24 = −9 mM/L. We say that this patient has a BE_e of −9 or a *base deficit* of 9 mM/L. Although our assumed BV of 10 sl is slightly lower than actual measured values, this approximation of BE_e is accurate enough for clinical use. BE_e should always be calculated from 37°C (98.6°F) values of pH and Pa_{CO_2}.

A related concept is the *standard bicarbonate,* whereby we equilibrate whole blood in vitro to a P_{CO_2} of 40 mmHg and then determine the $[HCO_3^-]$. The normal standard bicarbonate is 24 mM/L, and the difference between 24 and the actual standard bicarbonate is a reflection of the metabolic imbalance. Since standard bicarbonate measures only the status of the CO_2-bicarbonate buffer system, this difference is typically about 75 percent of the base deficit. The *buffer base* refers to the total buffering capacity of whole blood, i.e., the sum of the buffer anion concentrations. The normal value of the buffer base is 45 to 50 meq/L, and it is another reflection of metabolic disturbances.

The ratio of bicarbonate : Pa_{CO_2} determines the arterial pH (see Eq. 13-3). When a primary acid-base disturbance alters pH by changing either the numerator or denominator of this ratio, the body will attempt to compensate by changing the other term in the same direction to preserve the ratio. For example, in a primary respiratory acidosis inadequate ventilation causes Pa_{CO_2} to rise, and the kidneys will compensate by retaining $[HCO_3^-]$ and increasing their excretion of H^+. Renal compensation is slow, requiring several days

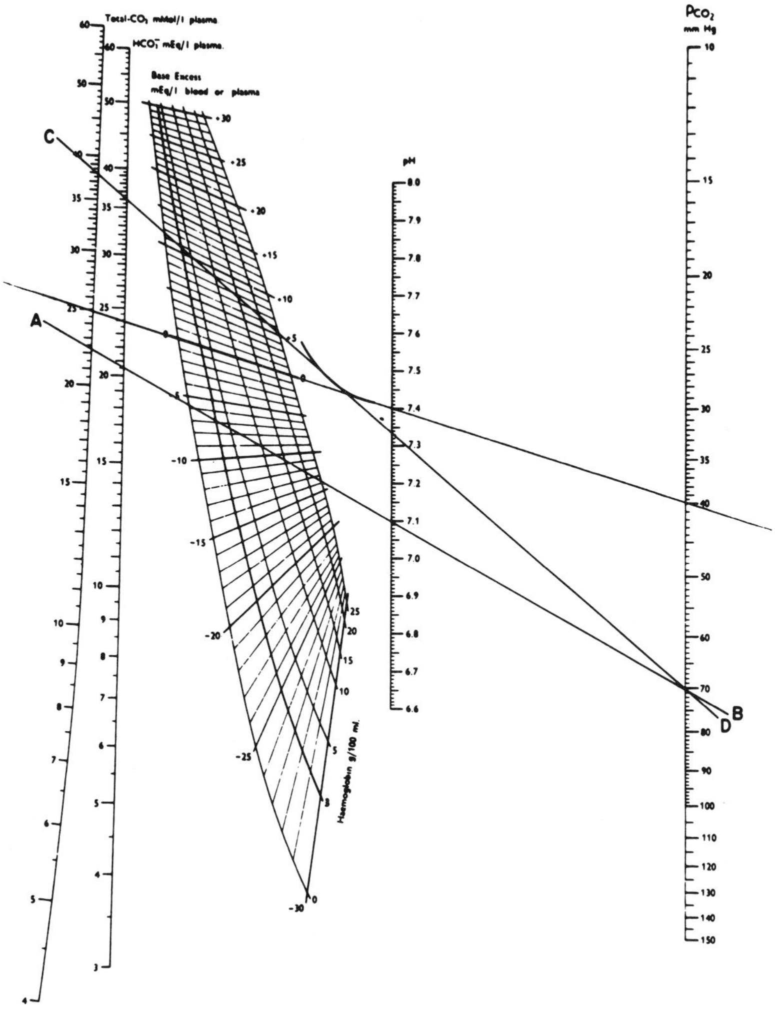

FIGURE 13-2 The Siggaard-Anderson acid-base nomogram. A straight line connecting any two measured values determines the other acid-base parameters shown in the figure at 37°C (98.6°F). To calculate BE_e we must use an average value of hemoglobin for the ECF. The 3-g hemoglobin line, added by Severinghaus, is appropriate for calculating BE_e in most situations. Therefore, a patient with a P_{CO_2} of 70 mmHg and a pH of 7.1 (line AB) will have a BE_e of 7 and an $[HCO_3^-]$ of 20.5 meq/L. For chronic respiratory acidosis, a line drawn from the actual Pa_{CO_2} tangent to the arc located between the pH axis and the BE_e axis (line CD) will indicate the state of maximum compensation. (Modified from Hornbein TF: Acid-base balance; in Miller RD: *Anesthesia.* 2d ed. New York, Churchill Livingstone, 1986, p 1301.)

to reach its maximum, but it can be very effective. This is illustrated by the large pH difference between the acute and chronic respiratory acidosis regions of Fig. 13-1. Such compensation is never complete, i.e., the pH never returns to 7.4 until the primary disturbance itself is corrected.

Given the ability of the body to compensate for primary respiratory disturbances by adjusting $[HCO_3^-]$, it is convenient to establish rules of thumb for predicting the $[HCO_3^-]$ values during acute or chronic imbalances. The most common of these is:

1. Acute disturbance
   a. For every 10 mmHg rise in Pa_{CO_2} above 40 mmHg, $[HCO_3^-]$ rises 1 mM/L.
   b. For every 10 mmHg fall in Pa_{CO_2} below 40 mmHg, $[HCO_3^-]$ falls 2 mM/L.

2. Chronic disturbance
   a. For every 10 mmHg rise in Pa_{CO_2} above 40 mmHg, $[HCO_3^-]$ rises 4 mM/L.
   b. For every 10 mmHg fall in Pa_{CO_2} below 40 mmHg, $[HCO_3^-]$ falls 3 mM/L.

Primary metabolic disturbances are partially compensated by changes in alveolar ventilation. Metabolic acidosis is compensated by hyperventilation, which often reduces the change in pH by 50 percent. A rule of thumb for predicting Pa_{CO_2} during such compensation is:[3]

$$Pa_{CO_2} = 1.5 \times [HCO_3^-] + 8 \qquad (13\text{-}5)$$

Hence, a patient with compensated metabolic acidosis and $[HCO_3^-] = 12$ mM/L would be expected to have a Pa_{CO_2} of 26 mmHg and a pH of 7.29. In primary metabolic alkalosis, the respiratory compensation consists of hypoventilation and an increase in Pa_{CO_2}. However, severely reduced ventilation on room air will decrease PA_{O_2}, and the resulting hypoxemia will stimulate respiratory drive and thus limit the compensation. The rule of thumb for predicting Pa_{CO_2} during compensated metabolic alkalosis is:[3]

$$Pa_{CO_2} = 0.7 \times [HCO_3^-] + 20 \qquad (13\text{-}6)$$

Many protocols have been recommended for evaluating acid-base status from blood-gas data. Our suggestion here is a summary of the discussion above.

1. Evaluate the arterial pH. A pH above 7.45 is alkalemia; a pH below 7.35 is acidemia.

2. Evaluate the Pa_{CO_2}. If it is >45, respiratory acidosis is present; if it is <35, respiratory alkalosis is present.
3. Find the BE_e from a nomogram or by the 10 sl approximation. If BE_e is > +2, metabolic alkalosis is present; if it is more negative than −2, metabolic acidosis is present.
4. Calculate the predicted value of the variable not involved in the primary disturbance to evaluate the degree of compensation. With rare exceptions, the primary disturbance is the one in the direction of the actual change in pH. For a primary respiratory disturbance find predicted $[HCO_3^-]$ and for a primary metabolic disturbance find predicted Pa_{CO_2} (Eqs. 13-5 and 13-6).

OXYGENATION AND Pa_{O_2}

In vitro blood-gas analysis provides us with the arterial oxygen tension or Pa_{O_2}, and it is tempting to equate an adequate Pa_{O_2} with the state of being "well oxygenated." By the latter we mean that the O_2 supply and demand in the tissues are well matched. An adequate Pa_{O_2} is only the first step in this oxygen transport process. Pa_{O_2} is related to arterial hemoglobin saturation by the oxyhemoglobin dissociation curve shown in Fig. 13-3. For the normal position of this curve, a Pa_{O_2} of 40 mmHg corresponds to an arterial saturation (Sa_{O_2}) of 75%, while a Pa_{O_2} of 60 mmHg yields an Sa_{O_2} of 90%. The curve is shifted to the right by decreases in pH or increases in Pa_{CO_2} (Bohr effect) and by increases in 2,3-diphosphoglycerate (2,3-DPG) or temperature. A right shift yields a lower saturation at a given Pa_{O_2} (see Fig. 13-3), i.e., a lower affinity of hemoglobin for oxygen. This will improve "unloading" of oxygen in the capillaries at venous P_{O_2} values, but it also requires higher Pa_{O_2} to achieve high Sa_{O_2} values.

Arterial hemoglobin saturation, Sa_{O_2}, is related to arterial oxygen content, Ca_{O_2}, by:

$$Ca_{O_2} = 1.38(Hb)\,(Sa_{O_2}/100) + 0.003(Pa_{O_2}) \qquad (13\text{-}7)$$

The first term on the right represents hemoglobin-bound oxygen, and the second term is oxygen dissolved in plasma. If Hb = 15g/dL and Pa_{O_2} = 100 mmHg, then Ca_{O_2} = 20.7 + 0.3 = 21 mL/dL. That is, each 100 mL arterial blood will contain 21 mL oxygen, 20.7 mL of which is bound to hemoglobin. To find the normal venous oxygen content, we assume in Eq. (13-7) a venous saturation (Sv_{O_2}) of 75%, and a venous O_2 tension (Pv_{O_2}) of 40 mmHg: Cv_{O_2} = 15.5 + 0.1 = 15.6 mL/dL. The amount of oxygen extracted from each 100 mL blood by the tissues is the difference between the arterial and venous O_2 contents: $Ca_{O_2} - Cv_{O_2}$ = 5.4 mL/dL.

Finally, the quantity of oxygen delivered to tissues is the product of Ca_{O_2} and cardiac output ($\dot{Q}_T$):

$$\begin{aligned} O_2(\text{del}) &= \dot{Q}_T \times Ca_{O_2} \qquad (13\text{-}8)\\ &= 5\ \text{L/min} \times 21\ \text{mL/dL} \times 10\ \text{dL/L} \\ &= 1050\ \text{mL/min} \end{aligned}$$

We have multiplied the result by 10 dL/L since $\dot{Q}_T$ is measured in L/min while Ca_{O_2} is measured in mL/dL. The oxygen consumed per minute, V_{O_2}, is simply the difference between arterial O_2 delivery and venous O_2 return:

$$\begin{aligned} V_{O_2} &= O_2(\text{del}) - O_2(\text{ret}) \qquad (13\text{-}9)\\ &= \dot{Q}_T \times (Ca_{O_2} - Cv_{O_2}) \\ &= \dot{Q}_T \times [1.38(Hb)(Sa_{O_2} - Sv_{O_2})/100] \times 10 \\ V_{O_2} &= 13.8(Hb)(\dot{Q}_T)(Sa_{O_2} - Sv_{O_2})/100 \end{aligned}$$

In substituting for Ca_{O_2} and Cv_{O_2} from (Eq. 13-7), we have neglected the small contribution of plasma-dissolved O_2. Again, using normal values in this Fick equation for O_2 consumption we obtain:

$$V_{O_2} = 13.8(15)(5.0)(100 - 75)/100 = 259\ \text{mL/min}$$

This equation and its normal values should be kept in mind when interpreting Pa_{O_2} values from blood-gas analysis.

We have seen how Pa_{O_2} relates to but does not solely determine the adequacy of tissue oxygenation. Now let us review its use in the evaluation of lung function. The simplest measure of lung function in oxygen uptake is the alveolar-arterial oxygen difference, often called $(A - a)_{O_2}$ or A − a gradient. We find alveolar oxygen tension $P_{A_{O_2}}$ from the alveolar gas equation:[4]

$$P_{A_{O_2}} = F_{I_{O_2}}(P_B - 47) - Pa_{CO_2} \times F \qquad (13\text{-}10)$$

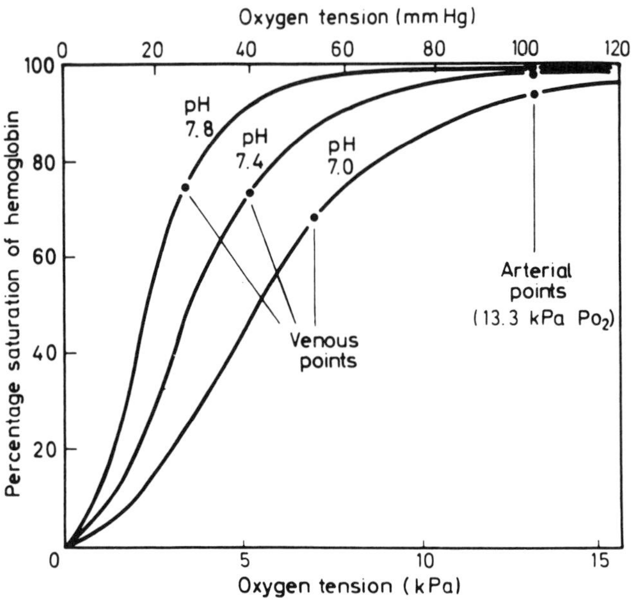

FIGURE 13-3 The oxyhemoglobin dissociation curve, showing percentage saturation and oxygen content of hemoglobin versus oxygen tension in mmHg and kPa. The three curves show the effect of pH (the Bohr effect). Typical arterial and venous values are marked on all three curves. Acidosis reduces hemoglobin's affinity for oxygen, thus facilitating "unloading" of oxygen in the tissues. Alkalosis causes oxygen to be more tightly bound to hemoglobin, facilitating the uptake of oxygen in the lungs when $P_{A_{O_2}}$ is below normal. (Adapted from Nunn JF: *Applied Respiratory Physiology*. 2d ed. London, Butterworth, 1977.)

In this equation, F_{IO_2} is inspired oxygen fraction; P_B is barometric pressure in mmHg; 47 mmHg is the vapor pressure of water at an assumed body temperature of 37°C (98.6°F); Pa_{CO_2} is used to approximate P_{ACO_2} (P_{ACO_2} and Pa_{CO_2} are usually within 2 mmHg); and F is a correction factor reflecting the fact that CO_2 production does not equal O_2 uptake. For $F_{IO_2} < 0.5$, F is roughly the reciprocal of the respiratory quotient R (the ratio of CO_2 produced to O_2 consumed), and is therefore near 1.2.

P_{AO_2} is a function of P_B, F_{IO_2}, and Pa_{CO_2}. For $F_{IO_2} = 0.21$ and $Pa_{CO_2} = 40$ mmHg, the P_{AO_2} at sea level is about 102 mmHg; at Denver (elevation 1600 m) it is 76 mmHg; and at 4000 m (13,100 ft) it is 43 mmHg. As Pa_{CO_2} rises to 60 mmHg at sea level, P_{AO_2} falls to 78 mmHg, and at Pa_{CO_2} = 80 mmHg it reaches 54 mmHg. Hypoventilation can clearly result in hypoxemia when breathing room air. The combination of CO_2 retention and high altitude is particularly dangerous; e.g., for Pa_{CO_2} = 80 mmHg at Denver, we have P_{AO_2} = 27.5 mmHg.

The problem with using $(A - a)_{O_2}$ to evaluate lung function is that the normal range of values depends on both P_B and F_{IO_2}. At sea level for $F_{IO_2} = 0.21$, the normal gradient is 5 to 10 mmHg. For $F_{IO_2} = 1.0$, the normal gradient may range up to 100 mmHg. The arterial:alveolar ratio, $Pa_{O_2}/:P_{AO_2}$, is an alternative parameter that is less dependent on F_{IO_2}. This ratio is normally >0.7 in healthy individuals at any F_{IO_2}, although it may be less during general anesthesia. There are also several "rules of thumb" for evaluating lung function based on room air Pa_{O_2} and age, such as:

$$\text{Normal } Pa_{O_2} = 100 - 0.3 \times \text{age(years)} \qquad (13\text{-}11)$$

Such formulas ignore the effects of P_B and Pa_{CO_2}, either of which may prevent a patient from achieving "normal" Pa_{O_2} values.

Arterial hypoxemia can be caused by alveolar hypoxia (low P_{AO_2}), anatomic right-to-left shunt, ventilation/perfusion ($\dot{V}/\dot{Q}$) mismatch, or pulmonary diffusion barrier. Once we have ruled out low P_{AO_2}, $\dot{V}/\dot{Q}$ mismatch is by far the most common cause in the ICU setting. This is also called intrapulmonary shunt or venous admixture to emphasize the mechanism, namely, venous blood passing through the pulmonary capillaries without becoming oxygenated. Intrapulmonary shunt may be "absolute" with a $\dot{V}/\dot{Q}$ ratio of zero, or "relative" with a $\dot{V}/\dot{Q}$ ratio <1. The total or physiologic shunt can be found from the shunt equation:

$$\frac{Q_S}{Q_T} = \frac{Cc'_{O_2} - Ca_{O_2}}{Cc'_{O_2} - C\bar{v}_{O_2}} \qquad (13\text{-}12)$$

In this equation Q_S is the flow through the shunt, Q_T is total cardiac output, $Cc'O_2$ is the ideal pulmonary capillary O_2 content (determined by assuming $Pc'O_2 = P_{AO_2}$), and Ca_{O_2} and $C\bar{v}_{O_2}$ are the arterial and mixed venous O_2 content, respectively. For a given shunt fraction (Q_S/Q_T) and $C\bar{v}_{O_2}$ value, this equation can be used to predict the behavior of Pa_{O_2} with F_{IO_2} as shown in Fig. 13-4. Note that at high shunt fraction (e.g., $Q_S/Q_T = 0.5$) the Pa_{O_2} becomes relatively unresponsive to increases in F_{IO_2}. The shunt equation also implies that in the presence of fixed shunt, a fall in $C\bar{v}_{O_2}$ will cause a fall in Ca_{O_2}. That is, if the venous blood being admixed with the pulmonary capillary blood has a lower saturation, the resulting arterial blood will also have a lower saturation. By this mechanism, an increased metabolic rate (higher $\dot{V}_{O_2}$) can worsen hypoxemia in the presence of a fixed shunt.

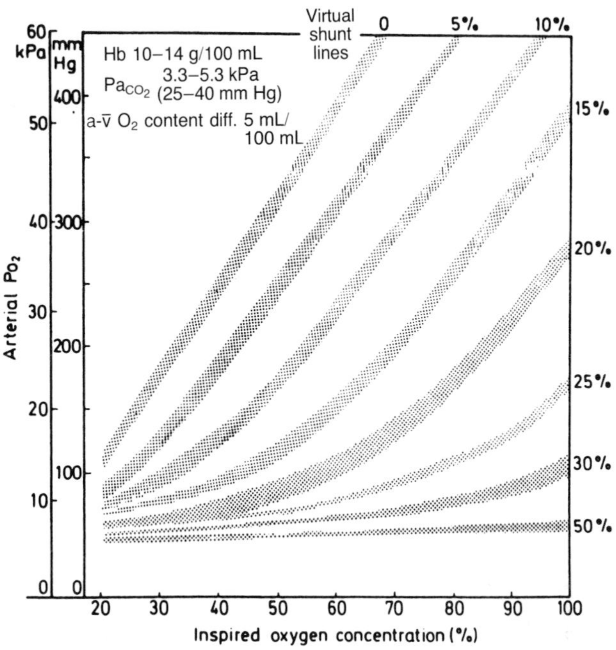

FIGURE 13-4 The isoshunt diagram, showing Pa_{O_2} versus inspired oxygen concentration for different values of shunt Q_S/Q_T. These curves are valid for Hb = 10 to 14 g/dL, Pa_{CO_2} = 25 to 40 mmHg, and $(A - \bar{V})_{O_2}$ = 5 mL/dL. For values of shunt >30 percent, the Pa_{O_2} becomes almost independent of F_{IO_2}. (Adapted from Nunn JF: *Applied Respiratory Physiology.* 2d ed. London, Butterworth, 1977.)

TEMPERATURE CORRECTION

The electrodes in every laboratory blood-gas analyzer are maintained at a constant 37°C (98.6°F), and the pH, P_{CO_2}, and P_{O_2} values are determined at this temperature. If the same blood sample is analyzed at the patient's temperature, different values are obtained. In a patient whose temperature is below 37°C, the temperature-corrected P_{CO_2} and P_{O_2} are lower than the 37°C values, due to the increase in solubility of O_2 and CO_2 with falling temperature. The temperature-corrected pH is higher than the 37°C value, because water is less dissociated into H^+ and OH^- at lower temperatures. The question, then, is which values should we use to treat the patient, uncorrected (37°C) or corrected to patient temperature?

If we cool an in vitro blood sample anaerobically (maintaining constant CO_2 content), the pH of the sample will rise with a slope of −0.015 pH/°C. Recall that the pH of pure water is 7.0 only at 25°C (77°F). As temperature is lowered, less water is dissociated into H^+ and OH^-, so that pH

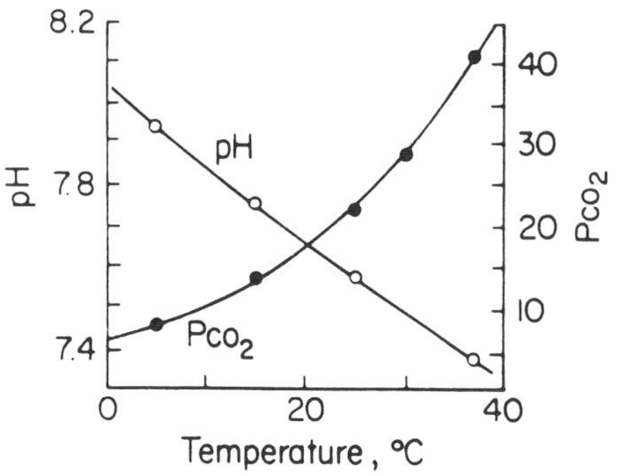

FIGURE 13-5 pH and P_{CO_2} versus temperature for in vitro human arterial blood at constant CO_2 content. The pH falls by 0.015 unit/°C temperature increase. The P_{CO_2} increases by 4.5 percent/°C increase. Ectothermic invertebrates exchanging gases with their environment exhibit a similar dependence of pH on temperature. (From White FN: Acid base homeostasis and temperature, in Marcelleth C, Anderson RH, Becker A, et al: *Pediatric Cardiology*, New York, Churchill Livingstone, 1986, pp 31–38.)

rises. However, the ratio of $[OH^-]/:[H^+]$ remains constant. If we compare the pH of blood with that of the neutral point of water (pNH_2O), we find that blood maintains a constant alkalinity with respect to neutral water across the temperature spectrum. That is, the ratio $[OH^-]/:[H^+]$ is preserved as the blood is cooled.

Given the presence of CO_2 in the blood and not in pure water, researchers deduced that a protein buffer must be responsible for the constant alkalinity of blood relative to water with varying temperature. The only plentiful protein moeity that satisfies the temperature-dependent requirements of this buffer is the imidazole (Im) group of histidine. In vitro experiments have shown that Im is indeed responsible for the pH/temperature slope of whole blood. As temperature varies in our anaerobic blood sample with constant CO_2 content, the fractional dissociation (α) of Im remains constant at about 0.8. Since this is a dominant intracellular protein buffer, the state of charge of all proteins is maintained under these "alphastat" conditions. On the other hand, if we were to maintain normothermic pH during temperature changes (called "pH-stat"), the net charge of intracellular proteins would be variable.

The implication of the alphastat hypothesis is that arterial pH should be allowed to rise with a slope of −0.015 pH/°C as temperature decreases, and that Pa_{CO_2} should be allowed to fall in such a way as to maintain constant CO_2 content. In other words, we should use 37°C (uncorrected) blood-gas data and attempt to maintain these at normal values. This means that the hypothermic patient's actual pH will be higher than 7.40 and his Pa_{CO_2} will be lower than 40 mmHg, as shown in Fig. 13-5. Alphastat regulation maintains constant protein charge state and CO_2 content as stated above. It also allows most enzymes to function near their optimal pH at all temperatures, in contrast to pH-stat. As further supporting evidence, ectotherms such as frogs, turtles, and fish have been found to use alphastat regulation over a wide range of temperatures. That is, their pH varies with about the same temperature slope as in vitro human blood even though they are exchanging gases with their environment at varying metabolic rates. An excellent review of the evidence in favor of alphastat and the use of 37°C blood-gas values has been written by F. White.[5]

SOURCES OF ERROR

In vitro blood-gas analysis is subject to errors in sampling technique and errors inherent in the analyzer itself. The latter are difficult to detect due to the unavailability of a uniformly accepted laboratory standard. In fact, the blood-gas analyzer is generally used as the "gold standard" for other monitoring techniques. Nevertheless, laboratory analyzers can be in error, particularly if the electrodes are not maintained at 37 ± 1°C. Recall that pH changes by 0.015, P_{CO_2} by 4.5 percent, and P_{O_2} by 7 percent for each 1°C temperature change. Electrode contamination by protein deposits may also cause significant errors, which can be avoided by careful sample heparinization and frequent cleaning. Gas calibration should be done as often as recommended by the manufacturer—in most newer clinical laboratory analyzers this is done automatically at fixed time intervals.[6]

Despite a perfectly functioning blood-gas analyzer, serious errors often result from poor sampling technique. Blood should be withdrawn slowly and without significant negative pressure to avoid air bubbles or "foaming" in the sample. CO_2 will diffuse from the sample into the bubbles, resulting in a lower P_{CO_2} and a higher pH reading. The effect of bubbles on P_{O_2} depends on the relationship of the blood P_{O_2} to that of room air (159 mmHg at sea level). Blood P_{O_2} values higher than room air P_{O_2} will be reduced, and those lower will be increased.

Blood samples should be analyzed immediately or stored on ice if they cannot be analyzed within 15 min. Continued metabolism in the blood gradually reduces P_{O_2} and pH while it increases P_{CO_2}. Normally, the rates of change due to metabolism are about 0.001 unit/min for pH and 0.1 mmHg/min for P_{CO_2}. P_{O_2} values will fall faster for fully saturated blood than for venous blood. However, these rates of change are proportional to leukocyte count (leukocytes are metabolically active) and may be much higher in patients with leukocytosis.[7]

Proper heparinization is perhaps the most important aspect of sampling technique. As mentioned above, inadequate heparin will result in protein deposits on the electrodes. On the other hand, excess heparin will affect results in two ways. Heparin itself is an acid and as such will tend to lower the pH of the sample. However, the heparin solution contains no CO_2 and thus lowers the sample P_{CO_2} by dilution, thereby raising pH. Excess heparin will consistently lower P_{CO_2} and calculated $[HCO_3^-]$, but may affect pH in either direction depending on the amount added.[8]

Finally, when a blood sample is drawn from an indwelling arterial cannula connected to a pressure transducer, it is important to avoid contamination of the sample with the flush solution in the connecting tubing. To ensure this, aspirate at least three times the amount of fluid present in the tubing between the cannula and the sampling port and discard this prior to drawing the blood sample. Flush contamination will again reduce P_{CO_2} and alter P_{O_2} toward the room air value.

Pulse Oximetry

TECHNICAL BACKGROUND OF OXIMETRY

Oximetry, a form of spectrophotometry, makes use of the fact that different hemoglobin species absorb differing amounts of light at various wavelengths. Oximeters determine hemoglobin species concentrations by measuring light absorbance either in solutions of lysed red blood cells (RBCs) or in living tissue, as described below. The absorbance of light in dilute solutions is described by the Lambert-Beer law, which states that

$$I_{trans} = I_{in} \times e^{-DC\epsilon} \qquad (13\text{-}13)$$

In this equation, I_{trans} is the intensity of the transmitted light; I_{in} is the intensity of the incident light; D is the distance of transmission through the solution; C is concentration of the solute (hemoglobin); and ϵ is the extinction coefficient, which is a constant for a given hemoglobin species at a specified wavelength. The extinction coefficients of the four most common hemoglobin species are plotted versus wavelength in Fig. 13-6. If more than one hemoglobin species is present in the solution, then the exponent in (Eq. 13-13) will be a summation of similar terms for each species. If the light transmitted through a known thickness of such a solution is measured, then by using the extinction coefficients of Fig. 13-6 the concentrations of each species in the solution can be calculated. This is the principle of spectrophotometry, and it is used by all oximeters which measure

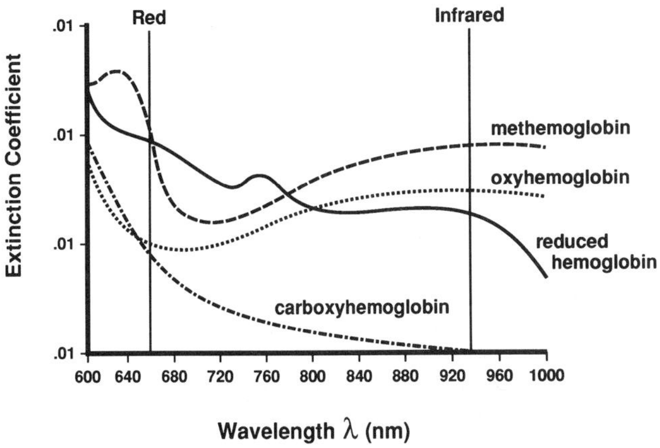

FIGURE 13-6 Light extinction coefficients versus wavelength for four hemoglobin species: oxyhemoglobin, reduced hemoglobin, carboxyhemoglobin, and methemoglobin. Vertical dashed lines indicate light-emitting diode wavelengths used by pulse oximetry. (From Barker SJ, Tremper KK: Pulse oximetry: Applications and limitations, in *Advances in Oxygen Monitoring,* International Anesthesiology Clinics, Boston, Little, Brown, 1987, pp 155–175.)

hemoglobin concentrations both in vitro and in vivo. Clearly such instruments must use at least as many wavelengths of light as there are different hemoglobin species in the solution. If an oximeter is to measure the concentrations of all four hemoglobin species shown in Fig. 13-6, then it must use at least four wavelengths of light.

Laboratory cooximeters determine hemoglobin concentrations by measuring the absorbance of light passing through a hemoglobin suspension in a small quartz cuvette. The "wet" section of the cooximeter aspirates a small sample of heparinized whole blood (typically 1 μL) into the cuvette, where it is hemolyzed ultrasonically to produce a suspension of free hemoglobin. The optical section generates light beams at several wavelengths which pass through the cuvette and then to a series of photodetectors. The earliest cooximeters, developed in the mid 1960s, used only two wavelengths of light and could therefore measure only oxyhemoglobin (O_2Hb) and reduced hemoglobin (RHb). Modern cooximeters use four or more wavelengths and can independently determine the concentrations of O_2Hb, RHb, carboxyhemoglobin (COHb), and methemoglobin (MetHb). Some cooximeters can measure the concentration of fetal hemoglobin (HbF) as well as that of adult hemoglobin (HbA). Since the absorption spectrum of HbF is only slightly different from that of HbA, the HbF determination must generally be made on a well-oxygenated blood sample. MetHb and COHb are measured independently by the modern cooximeter, so that these dyshemoglobins do not cause errors in the determination of O_2Hb and RHb. However, other dyshemoglobins such as sulfhemoglobin (SHb) are not measured or accounted for and can cause errors in readings of the other species.

The electronics section of the cooximeter contains a microcomputer which solves a system of simultaneous equations in the form of (Eq. 13-13), one equation for each light wavelength used. Since the number of equations is equal to the number of wavelengths, the number of unknown hemoglobin species must not be greater than this or errors will occur. Errors will also result from any other undesired light absorbers within the cuvette, most commonly fibrin deposits or impurities within the sample. Therefore, the cuvette must be cleaned periodically and standardized control solutions should be run through the cooximeter to verify accuracy.

The cooximeter determines oxygen saturation by direct measurement of the concentrations of O_2Hb and the other hemoglobin species present. On the other hand, the blood-gas analyzer calculates oxygen saturation from the measured oxygen tension, using an assumed O_2Hb dissociation curve such as that shown in Fig. 13-3. This distinction is especially important in the measurement of $S\bar{v}_{O_2}$. Due to the steepness of the O_2Hb dissociation curve at venous values, a small error in measured P_{O_2} or a small displacement of the curve itself can cause a large error in calculated saturation (see Fig. 13-3). The cooximeter measures saturation without reference to oxygen tension and is therefore not subject to errors of this type.

The pulse oximeter is a two-wavelength in vivo oximeter in which a pulsatile tissue bed is placed between the light

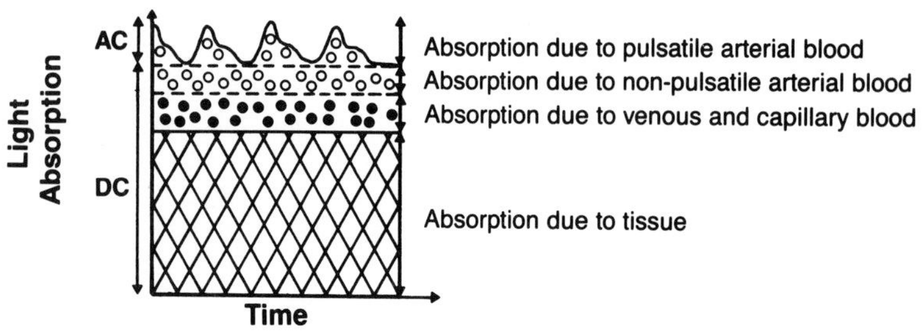

FIGURE 13-7 The light absorbance of living tissue plotted versus time. The absorption of the arterial blood has a pulsatile component, while all other absorbers between the light source and detector are fixed. [From Tremper KK, Barker SJ: Pulse oximetry: Review article. *Anesthesiology* 70 (1):98, 1989.]

source and detector. This is not a simple dilute solution of hemoglobin as in the case of the in vitro cooximeter, for the pulse oximeter must deal with several unwanted absorbances as shown in Fig. 13-7. Pulse oximetry is made possible by the fact that the only pulsating absorbance between the light source and detector is that of the pulsatile arterial blood (see Fig. 13-7). The base-line or DC component of the absorbance results from other absorbers in the tissue bed, including venous blood, capillary blood, solid tissues, and nonpulsatile arterial blood.

Commercially available pulse oximeters use two wavelengths of light, usually 660 nm (red) and 940 nm (near infrared). The pulse oximeter measures the pulsatile or AC component of the absorbance at each wavelength and divides this by the corresponding DC component. This yields a "pulse-added" absorbance that is independent of the incident light intensity. The oximeter then calculates the ratio (R) of the two pulse-added absorbances, which is empirically related to arterial hemoglobin saturation:

$$\frac{AC_{660}/DC_{660}}{AC_{940}/DC_{940}} \qquad (13\text{-}14)$$

The built-in calibration algorithm which relates R to pulse oximeter saturation (Sp_{O_2}) is based on experimental studies in human volunteers. When the ratio R equals 1, the corresponding Sp_{O_2} value is 85%. This fact has clinical implications to be discussed below.

Sa_{O_2} PHYSIOLOGY AND DEFINITIONS

Almost 99 percent of the oxygen content of arterial blood is in the form of hemoglobin-bound oxygen, as shown earlier by (Eq. 13-7). The normal relationship between Sa_{O_2} and Pa_{O_2} is nonlinear, as shown in Fig. 13-3. Three convenient points to remember are $Pa_{O_2} = 27$ mmHg, $Sa_{O_2} = 50\%$; $Pa_{O_2} = 40$ mmHg, $Sa_{O_2} = 75\%$, and $Pa_{O_2} = 60$ mmHg; $Sa_{O_2} = 90\%$. At Pa_{O_2} values above 100 mmHg, Sa_{O_2} is nearly 100% and becomes virtually independent of Pa_{O_2}. Sa_{O_2} monitoring will therefore not show early trends of worsening oxygenation if the initial Pa_{O_2} values are >100 mmHg. A recent animal experiment has shown that endobronchial intubations at Fi_{O_2} values >30% are usually undetected by the pulse oximeter.[9]

Further confusion stems from the two definitions of arterial hemoglobin saturation in common use today. *Fractional saturation* (Sa_{O_2}) is given by:

$$\frac{O_2Hb}{\text{total Hb}} \times 100 = \frac{O_2Hb}{Hb + O_2Hb + MetHb + COHb} \times 100 \qquad (13\text{-}15)$$

where Hb is reduced hemoglobin and MetHb and COHb are methemoglobin and carboxyhemoglobin. *Functional saturation* (FSa_{O_2}) is defined as:

$$\frac{O_2Hb}{Hb + O_2Hb} \times 100 = \frac{O_2Hb}{\text{total Hb} - MetHb - COHb} \times 100 \qquad (13\text{-}16)$$

Note that it is fractional arterial hemoglobin saturation, Sa_{O_2}, that determines the oxygen content in (Eq. 13-7).

SOURCES OF ERROR

The pulse oximeter uses only two wavelengths of light and therefore can distinguish only two unknown hemoglobin species: RHb and O_2Hb. If COHb or MetHb is present, then the pulse oximeter is analogous to a system with fewer equations than unknowns, and it will be unable to determine any of the species concentrations. Two recent animal experiments have characterized pulse oximeter behavior during dyshemoglobinemias. In one of these, dogs were exposed to carbon monoxide over a 3- to 4-h period.[10] At a COHb level of about 70% (i.e., COHb/total Hb = 0.7), pulse oximeter Sp_{O_2} values were approximately 90%. The actual Sa_{O_2} under these conditions was 30%, while the FSa_{O_2} was 100%. The pulse oximeter effectively "sees" COHb as being composed mostly of O_2Hb. In a similar experiment, MetHb levels as high as 60% were induced in dogs by intratracheal aerosolized benzocaine.[11] As MetHb levels increased slowly while the animals breathed 100% oxygen, Sp_{O_2} values trended toward 85%. When the Fi_{O_2} was reduced stepwise at fixed MetHb levels, the three pulse oximeters failed to measure either FSa_{O_2} or Sa_{O_2}. MetHb has a high extinction coefficient at both pulse oximeter wavelengths (see Fig. 13-6). This added absorbance increases both the numerator and denominator of the ratio R, defined by (Eq. 13-14). This tends to force the value of R toward unity, and an R value of 1.0 corresponds to an Sp_{O_2} of 85%, as stated above.

Another hemoglobin species commonly encountered in clinical practice is HbF. HbF has a much higher affinity for oxygen than normal HbA, evidenced by the fact that the P50 (P_{O_2} at which saturation is 50%) of HbF is 17 mmHg while that of HbA is 27 mmHg. Nevertheless, at the two pulse oximeter wavelengths HbF absorbs light similarly to HbA, and it therefore introduces no clinically significant error in pulse oximeter accuracy.[12]

Any substance in the blood that absorbs light at 660 or 940 nm can affect pulse oximeter accuracy. This is illustrated by dyes that are commonly injected into the circulation for diagnostic purposes. The best example of this is intravenous methylene blue, which can cause false Sp_{O_2} readings of near 65% in healthy, normoxemic subjects.[13]

The pulse oximeter is cleverly designed to operate over a wide range of pulse-added absorbances. When the amplitude of the pulsatile signal decreases, the pulse oximeter automatically increases its electronic gain to compensate. However, as amplification is increased, background noise is amplified along with the desired signal. The amplitude of this noise is added to both the numerator and denominator of the ratio R, again forcing its value toward unity. The pulse oximeter therefore has a preselected signal:noise ratio requirement, and once this is no longer met the device will not display an Sp_{O_2} value. Clinical studies in the ICU have shown that a higher incidence of pulse oximeter loss of signal is associated with low $\dot{Q}_T$ states, extremes in systemic vascular resistance, and hypothermia.[14] In most of these clinical situations the pulsatile flow in the distal extremities is reduced. Therefore, if a finger probe fails to function consistently, alternate probe sites should be tried. Ear probes have been used not only on the ear lobe, but also on the nasal septum, the lips, and across the cheek. The recent development of reflection pulse oximetry will make it possible to place sensors on flat tissue surfaces such as the forehead.

Patient motion creates a high amplitude fluctuating absorbance that can be difficult to eliminate. Motion artifact is a serious problem in the recovery room, where patients often shiver as they emerge from anesthesia. In the ICU, the pulse oximeter may fail to function in patients who are either agitated or shivering. The advent of reflection pulse oximetry may also improve performance in these situations.

Other sources of pulse oximeter error are usually less important in the ICU setting. These include errors due to venous blood pulsations, light absorbance by nail polish, errors in light-emitting-diode wavelength, and ambient room light reaching the photodetector. The user must be aware of these sources of error and maintain a high index of suspicion in situations where they are likely to occur. Despite the errors and physiologic limitations discussed above, the pulse oximeter is the most important advance in noninvasive oxygen monitoring in recent years. We strongly recommend continuous pulse oximetry on all ventilator-dependent patients, as well as all other patients whose cardiopulmonary status is potentially unstable.

Capnometry

Capnometry derives from the Greek word "capnos" or smoke, carbon dioxide being the "smoke" of cellular metabolism. The shape and physiologic significance of the

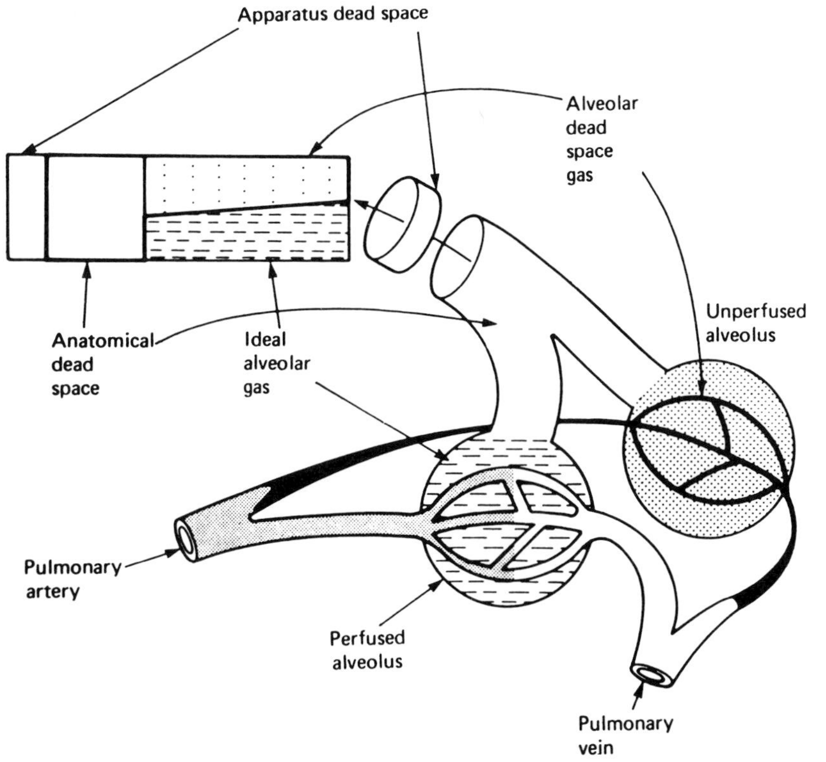

FIGURE 13-8 A schematic illustration of the relationships of the various components of dead space and the alveolar gas. During expiration, the apparatus and anatomic dead space gases are expired sequentially ahead of the alveolar gas, and are therefore called series dead space. Following these gases, the ideal alveolar gas is expired at the same time as the alveolar dead space gas, which is therefore called parallel dead space. The plateau phase of the capnogram results from this mixture of alveolar dead space and ideal alveolar gas. The value of $P_{ET_{CO_2}}$ will depend on the ratio of these last two volumes. (Reprinted with permission from Nunn JF: *Applied Respiratory Physiology.* 3d ed. London, Butterworth, 1987.)

capnogram or expired CO_2 waveform were appreciated as early as 1928. However, the clinical application of this knowledge to respiratory monitoring had to await the development of rapidly responding CO_2 analyzers.[15]

Most capnometers use infrared detection systems, although mass spectrometry and Raman scattering spectrometry are also used for this purpose. Infrared devices detect CO_2 using light absorption spectroscopy, the same technology used in oximetry. Since nitrous oxide absorbs infrared light in the same wavelength range as carbon dioxide, infrared capnometers used in the operating room require a correction factor when nitrous oxide is present. Typically, respiratory gas is aspirated from the breathing circuit as close to the patient as possible through a small diameter tube.[16] The capnometer's response time will be related to the internal volume of the sampling tubing and measurement chamber and the sample aspiration rate. The usual sampling rate is 150 mL/min. Slower sampling rates not only produce delayed data but may distort the waveform due to diffusion along the tubing. Faster sampling rates also cause errors by aspirating not only expired gas but also fresh gas from the ventilator circuit.[16] Because expired gas is normally saturated with water vapor, water condensation in the sampling tube is a common problem with aspirating capnometers. This problem is ameliorated by using water traps, filters, and water absorbing sample tubing.

Aspirating capnometers such as those described above are called "sidestream" devices. Using miniaturized infrared technology, it is also possible to measure CO_2 concentration by means of an optical adapter placed directly in the patient's airway. In this case, all the respired gas passes through the optical measurement chamber, and these instruments are thus called "mainstream" analyzers. Mainstream capnometers have a very fast time response and are not subject to problems caused by clogged sampling tubing or water traps, nor errors caused by high or low gas sampling rates. The relative disadvantages of mainstream capnometers include the size and weight of the airway adapter which is placed on the proximal end of the endotracheal tube, as well as the cost and delicate nature of the miniaturized optical detector.

To properly use capnography, it is essential to understand the fundamental concepts of dead space ventilation. Physiological dead space (VDS) is defined as any part of the tidal volume (VT) which does not participate in gas exchange with the blood. The portion of the VT ventilating well-perfused alveoli is called alveolar volume (VALV); therefore:[17]

$$V_T = V_{DS} + V_{ALV} \quad (13\text{-}17)$$

The physiologic VDS is divided into three components: apparatus, anatomic, and alveolar dead space. The apparatus dead space is the volume contained within the rebreathed segments of the breathing apparatus. This includes the volume contained within the endotracheal tube or breathing mask, and, for a circle breathing system, any connectors or tubing on the patient's side of the Y connector. The anatomic dead space is the volume within the trachea and the conducting airways. In a nonintubated patient, it also includes the volume of the oropharynx and nasopharynx. The alveolar dead space is that portion of the VT ventilating alveoli which are not perfused and do not participate in gas exchange. Figure 13-8 shows the sequence in which these various volumes reach the airway during expiration. The first gas detected is that left within the breathing apparatus at the end of inspiration, the apparatus dead space. This gas has the CO_2 concentration of the inspired gas, which is usually zero. After the apparatus dead space, the next gas to reach the detector is from the anatomic dead space, which also contains little or no CO_2. Finally, gas from the alveoli is detected, including both ideal VALV and alveolar dead space gas. These two gases mix and the measured CO_2 concentration in the airway is the resultant of this mixture. The P_{CO_2} of the alveolar dead space gas is near zero and the P_{CO_2} of the ideal alveolar gas roughly equals PaC_{O_2}. When this gas mixture reaches the detector, the measured P_{CO_2} rapidly rises to the "alveolar plateau" as shown in Fig. 13-8. When inspiration begins, the measured airway P_{CO_2} rapidly drops to zero.

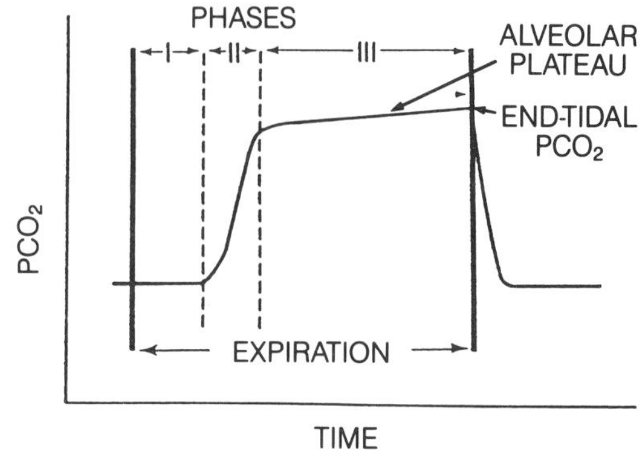

FIGURE 13-9 Expired P_{CO_2} versus time, illustrating the three phases of the normal capnogram. Phase I of the expiratory capnogram results from the apparatus and anatomic dead spaces. The phase II, or rapidly rising, portion represents a mixture of anatomic dead space gas, alveolar dead space gas, and ideal alveolar gas. The phase III portion or alveolar plateau results from a mixture ideal alveolar gas and alveolar dead space gas. (Reproduced from Gravenstein JS, Paulus DA, Hayes TJ: *Capnography in Clinical Practice.* Boston, Butterworth, 1989.)

If there were no alveolar dead space, then the alveolar plateau expired P_{CO_2} value would nearly equal Pa_{CO_2}. On the other hand, if half the VT were alveolar dead space and the other half ideal alveolar volume, then the expired P_{CO_2} plateau value would equal one-half of the Pa_{CO_2}. The difference between Pa_{CO_2} and the end-tidal CO_2 tension (PET_{CO_2}) depends on the ratio of alveolar dead space volume to VT. Figure 13-9 illustrates a normal capnogram, that is, a plot of P_{CO_2} in the airway as a function of time. During early expiration, as the apparatus and anatomic dead space gas is expired, the P_{CO_2} is zero. This is denoted as phase I of the capnogram. When a mixture of alveolar gas and dead space gas reaches the detector, the P_{CO_2} value rapidly rises to reach the alveolar plateau. This rapidly rising portion is called phase II of the capnogram. The alveolar plateau or phase III of the capnogram represents a mixture of ideal alveolar gas and alveolar dead space gas. We have assumed here that all alveoli are either well-perfused ($PA_{CO_2} = Pa_{CO_2}$) or they are unperfused and constitute alveolar dead space containing no CO_2. In reality the lung is composed of units having a continuum of $\dot{V}/\dot{Q}$ ratios. Apparatus and anatomic dead space are also referred to as series dead space because they are expired sequentially, ahead of the alveolar gas. Alveolar dead space is called parallel dead space because it is expired at the same time as the ideal alveolar gas, as shown in Fig. 13-8.

The presence of a normal capnogram implies metabolism to produce CO_2, circulation to transport CO_2 from the tissues to the lungs, and ventilation of the lungs. Continuous capnography therefore monitors all three of these vital functions noninvasively, making it very valuable for intensive care. Deviations from the normal size and shape of the capnogram waveform should be immediately investigated. A depressed or absent capnogram may represent a ventilator disconnect, a cardiac arrest, pulmonary embolism, or a dislodged, misplaced, or obstructed endotracheal tube. Increases in the $Pa_{CO_2} - PET_{CO_2}$ gap can be caused by any factor that increases alveolar dead space. For example, hypotension increases alveolar dead space by increasing the high $\dot{V}/\dot{Q}$ region (West's zone I) of the lung. In this context, the height of the capnogram has also been used to assess the adequacy of cardiopulmonary resuscitation, and it has a strong correlation with patient outcome.[18] Increases in the PET_{CO_2} value can be caused by increased metabolism (sepsis), inadequate ventilation, or the addition of CO_2 to the circulation as in the buffering of metabolic acids. Carbon dioxide rebreathing can be detected by nonzero base-line P_{CO_2} during the inspiratory phase of the capnogram (phase I). Since capnography can detect serious ventilatory and circulatory problems on a breath-by-breath basis, it is rapidly becoming a standard of care for all patients who require mechanical ventilation.[19,20]

Continuous Invasive Blood-Gas Monitoring

INTRAARTERIAL SENSORS

Intermittent arterial sampling and in vitro blood-gas analysis does not provide continuous data and is subject to variable delays between sampling and receiving results. The fact that many ICU patients have indwelling arterial cannulas provides a strong incentive to develop miniaturized sensors to fit through these cannulas and continuously monitor blood-gas values. The first approach to this problem was the development of invasive electrodes based on the same principles as the in vitro blood-gas analyzer. Miniaturized versions of Leland Clark's polarographic oxygen electrode have been inserted through arterial cannulas by several investigators.[21–23] Clinical studies of intraarterial Clark electrodes have reported accuracies ranging from mediocre to good. Reported complications include thrombus formation, embolism, vascular perforation, infarction, lower extremity ischemia (for umbilical artery electrodes),

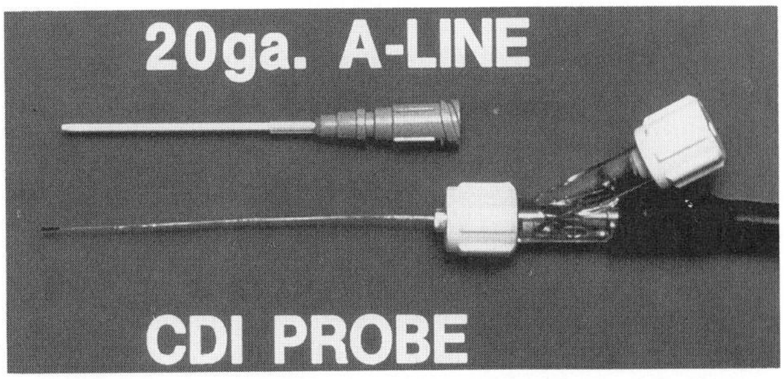

FIGURE 13-10 Photograph of a three-component fiberoptic optode intraarterial blood-gas sensor. Twenty gauge arterial cannula is shown for size comparison. (Reproduced by courtesy of 3M-Cardiovascular Devices, Inc., Irvine, CA.)

hemorrhage, and infection. The relatively large diameter of the Clark electrodes has also caused difficulty in withdrawing blood samples through the arterial cannula and dampening of arterial pressure waveforms. Time-dependent systematic error or "drift" has been frequently reported. This may be related to the formation of platelet aggregates or fibrin deposits on the surface of the oxygen-consuming electrode.

A competing technology for intraarterial monitoring involves the phenomenon of fluorescence quenching, which has been known since the 1930s. Electrons of a fluorescent dye are excited to a higher energy level by an incident photon. These excited electrons can return to lower energy states either by emitting a photon of a wavelength different from the excitation light or by interacting with a specific quenching molecule such as oxygen. Lubbers and Opitz[24] developed the first fluorescence quenching probe that measured both P_{O_2} and P_{CO_2} in gases or liquids. They coined the term "optode" for these fiberoptic blood-gas sensors. The oxygen optode was first miniaturized for intraarterial use in animals in 1984.[25] After further refinement and experimental use in animals, intraarterial optodes have been used in several clinical trials.[26–29] Two of these studies used three-channel optodes which measured pHa, Pa_{CO_2}, and Pa_{O_2}. This three-component optode is approximately 0.5 mm in diameter and passes easily through a 20 gauge radial artery cannula, as shown in Fig. 13-10.

When the optode is tested in vitro, its accuracy is comparable to that of conventional blood-gas analyzers. However, when placed in the artery the optode has been less accurate and reliable. The reasons for this are not entirely clear, but may be related to the formation of platelet aggregates or fibrin deposits on the sensor. When these problems with in vivo performance are overcome, the optode will represent a significant advance in the state-of-the-art of critical patient care. Blood-gas data will be displayed at the patient's bedside continuously, with a time response that can be measured in seconds. The delays and inconveniences of intermittent arterial blood-gas sampling and in vitro analysis will be eliminated.

MIXED VENOUS OXIMETRY

Mixed venous oxygen saturation ($S\bar{v}_{O_2}$) can now be continuously monitored by pulmonary artery oximetry. These fiberoptic $S\bar{v}_{O_2}$ catheters use the technology of reflectance spectrophotometry, which is similar to the oximetry principles discussed above for the pulse oximeter. By measuring the light reflectance of blood at two or more wavelengths, we can calculate the relative proportions of RHb and O_2Hb if these are the only two hemoglobin species present. Modern $S\bar{v}_{O_2}$ catheters use fiberoptic bundles to transmit and receive light to and from the catheter tip. They use light-emitting diodes similar to those of the pulse oximeter to provide monochromatic light at two or three discrete wavelengths. In a two-wavelength mixed venous oximeter, the ratio of the reflectances at both wavelengths is calculated to yield a single number, R. This ratio is then related to a specific value of venous saturation by an empirical algorithm. A disadvantage of the two-wavelength system is that other variables including pH, hematocrit, and blood flow velocity can affect the apparent color of the blood and thus change the relationship between R and $S\bar{v}_{O_2}$. This dependence on other variables is reduced by using three wavelengths and calculating two ratios: $R_1 = I_1/I_2$ and $R_3 = I_3/I_2$. The oximeter algorithm now calculates $S\bar{v}_{O_2}$ as a function of both R_1 and R_3. A comparison of these two systems in dogs showed that the three-wavelength system gives better agreement with in vitro cooximeter $S\bar{v}_{O_2}$ values.[30]

Another problem common to the earlier $S\bar{v}_{O_2}$ catheters was "wall artifact," whereby reflection of light from the pulmonary artery wall could produce a signal that was interpreted as an $S\bar{v}_{O_2}$ value of 85 to 90%. This problem has been reduced by the addition of digital filtering to the signal processor, which effectively edits out any sudden, steplike increases in $S\bar{v}_{O_2}$. The accuracy of three-wavelength pulmonary artery oximetry when compared with intermittent pulmonary venous blood-gas analysis is within acceptable clinical limits.

In our earlier discussion of Pa_{O_2} interpretation, we described oxygen transport through the blood and derived an equation relating oxygen consumption (V_{O_2}) to total hemoglobin, $\dot{Q}_T$, and arterial and venous hemoglobin saturation (Eq. 13-9). We showed that substituting normal values into this Fick equation for O_2 consumption yielded a V_{O_2} of 259 mL/min for a 70-kg adult. During maximal exercise, a healthy individual can increase both $\dot{Q}_T$ and the arterial-venous saturation difference by a factor of three, yielding

$$\begin{aligned} V_{O_2(max)} &= 13.8 \times Hb \times Q_T \times (Sa_{O_2} - S\bar{v}_{O_2})/100 \\ &= 13.8 \times 15 \times 15 \times (0.97 - 0.31) \\ &= 2049 \text{ mL/min} \end{aligned} \qquad (13\text{-}18)$$

That is, he can increase his V_{O_2} by a factor of nine. Note that $S\bar{v}_{O_2}$ has fallen to 31% in this stressed, well-conditioned subject, representing maximal oxygen uptake by tissue.

When oxygen demand exceeds supply, lactic acidosis will result, eventually leading to death if the problem is not corrected. We consider now some common situations in which this occurs. Although it is theoretically possible to achieve an $S\bar{v}_{O_2}$ as low as 31% in compensation for reduced oxygen delivery, values this low will never be tolerated by intensive care patients. Therefore, in the following examples of anemia, hypoxemia, and shock, we assume that maximum compensation occurs at $S\bar{v}_{O_2} = 50\%$. Below this value, lactic acidosis will ensue in most clinical settings.

1. Anemia: If the patient can make full use of compensation from increased $\dot{Q}_T$ (15 L/min) and maximal O_2 uptake, he can achieve a normal V_{O_2} with a hemoglobin as low as 2.5 g/dL:

$$V_{O_2}(\text{anemia}) = 13.8 \times 2.5 \times 15 \times (0.97 - 0.50) = 243 \text{ mL/min}$$

Only if the hemoglobin is <2.5 do we have obligatory acidosis! Patients with hemoglobin in the 5 to 7 g/dL range are thus well within the range of compensation.

2. Hypoxemia: With a normal hemoglobin and maximum $\dot{Q}_T$ but decreased Sa_{O_2}, normal V_{O_2} can occur even with an arterial saturation of 58% (i.e., a Pa_{O_2} of 32 mmHg):

$$V_{O_2}(\text{hypoxemia}) = 13.8 \times 15 \times 15 \times (0.58 - 0.50) = 248 \text{ mL/min}$$

Hypoxemia alone does not necessarily produce lactic acidosis unless compensation is limited by other disease. Note that compensation in these first two examples includes an increase in $\dot{Q}_T$ to 15 L/min combined with a decrease in $S\bar{v}_{O_2}$ to 50%.

3. Shock: If $\dot{Q}_T$ is reduced, we remove one of the compensatory mechanisms used in the above examples, and V_{O_2} must begin to fall when $\dot{Q}_T$ decreases below about 2.5 L/min:

$$V_{O_2}(\text{shock}) = 13.8 \times 15 \times 2.5 \times (0.97 - 0.50) = 243 \text{ mL/min}$$

When maximum compensation is used, we can thus maintain a normal V_{O_2} value despite a sixfold reduction in hemoglobin, a threefold reduction in $Sa_{O_2} - S\bar{v}_{O_2}$, but only a twofold reduction in $\dot{Q}_T$. Beyond these limits, obligatory lactic acidosis occurs. Many patients cannot fully invoke the compensation used in these examples—in particular a maximum $\dot{Q}_T$ of 15 L/min.

We have examined three causes of reduced O_2 delivery that result in decreased $S\bar{v}_{O_2}$: decreased hemoglobin, Sa_{O_2}, or $\dot{Q}_T$. Other causes of decreased $S\bar{v}_{O_2}$ include processes that increase oxygen demand, such as fever, malignant hyperthermia, thyroid storm, exercise, agitation, labored breathing, and shivering. A fall in $S\bar{v}_{O_2}$ may thus represent decreased O_2 supply, increased O_2 demand, or both. When $S\bar{v}_{O_2}$ falls below 50%, most patients will exhibit lactic acidosis; below 30% most will be comatose; and values near 20% are associated with irreversible cellular damage.

What causes $S\bar{v}_{O_2}$ to rise above its normal range of 68 to 77%? In general, high $S\bar{v}_{O_2}$ values result from decreased O_2 uptake by tissue, peripheral arteriovenous (left-to-right) shunting, and inappropriate increases in $\dot{Q}_T$. Clinical conditions which can produce elevated $S\bar{v}_{O_2}$ values include sepsis, Paget's disease of bone, cell poisoning, excessive use of inotropes or vasodilators, liver disease, and hypothermia. A wedged pulmonary artery catheter will cause an

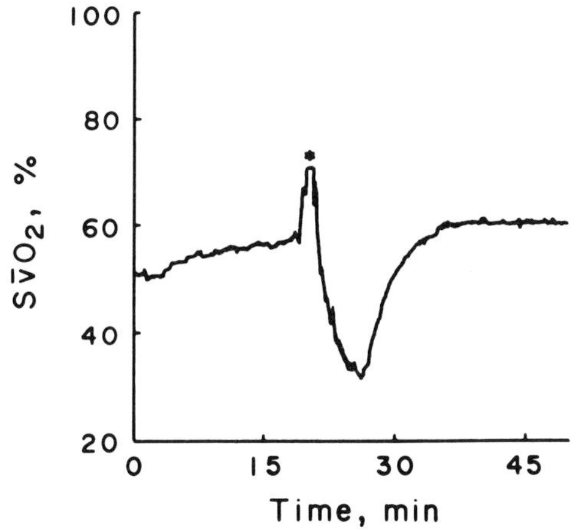

FIGURE 13-11 $S\bar{v}_{O_2}$ **versus time for ventilator-dependent patient with high PEEP. Asterisk indicates wedging of pulmonary artery catheter and disconnection of ventilator. After 30 s the catheter balloon was deflated and the ventilator reconnected.** $S\bar{v}_{O_2}$ **fell precipitously due to arterial hypoxemia resulting from temporary discontinuation of PEEP. (McMichan JC: Continuous monitoring of mixed venous oxygen saturation, theory applied to practice, in Schweiss JF (ed):** ***Continuous Measurement of Blood Oxygen Saturation in the High Risk Patient.*** **Vol 1. San Diego, Beach International, 1982).**

artifactual high $S\bar{v}_{O_2}$ reading, but in this case the monitor is not accurately measuring mixed venous saturation.

We now consider some clinical examples of continuous $S\bar{v}_{O_2}$ monitoring in the intensive care setting. In the interpretation of $S\bar{v}_{O_2}$, we make use of the Fick equation, which from (Eq. 13-9) can be solved for $S\bar{v}_{O_2}$:

$$S\bar{v}_{O_2} = Sa_{O_2} - 100(V_{O_2})/\{13.8 \times Hb \times \dot{Q}_T\} \quad (13\text{-}19)$$

Whenever $S\bar{v}_{O_2}$ changes, the clinician must determine which term(s) in (Eq. 13-19) are responsible. In the operating room, the terms most likely to change significantly are $\dot{Q}_T$ and hemoglobin. However, in the ICU this is not the case. Patients in respiratory failure have varying degrees of arterial desaturation. Equation 13-19 shows that if Sa_{O_2} decreases by 20% and all other terms remain constant, $S\bar{v}_{O_2}$ will also fall by 20% (e.g., from 75 to 55%). In addition, ICU patients have frequent changes in V_{O_2}, which can be increased in this setting by agitation, shivering, coughing, breathing, fever, pain, seizures, defecation, or eating.

FIGURE 13-12 $S\bar{v}_{O_2}$ **versus time in a patient with low** $\dot{Q}_T$**. A gradual decrease in** $S\bar{v}_{O_2}$ **was followed by cardiac arrest at the time indicated by the arrow. (McMichan JC: Continuous monitoring of mixed venous oxygen saturation, theory applied to practice, in Schweiss JF (ed):** ***Continuous Measurement of Blood Oxygen Saturation in the High Risk Patient.*** **Vol 1. San Diego, Beach International, 1982.)**

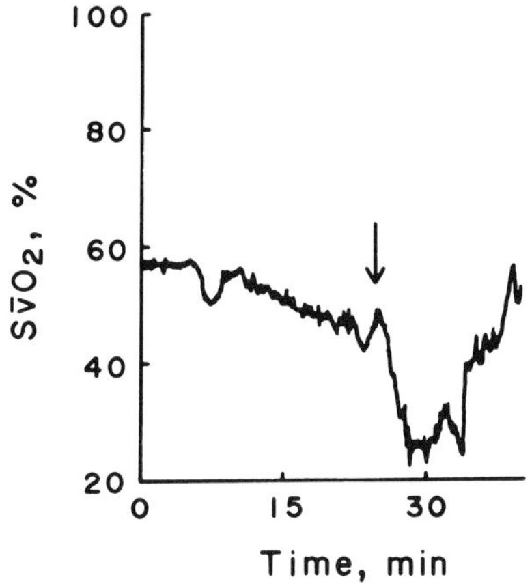

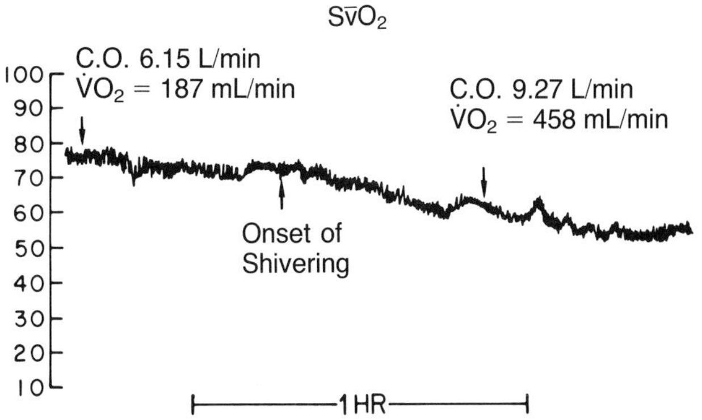

FIGURE 13-13 $S\bar{v}_{O_2}$ **versus time in a patient who began to shiver at the time indicated by the arrow.** $S\bar{v}_{O_2}$ **fell rapidly due to a large increase in** V_{O_2}**, despite an increase in** $\dot{Q}_T$**. The increase in** O_2 **demand exceeded the increase in supply, resulting in decreased** $S\bar{v}_{O_2}$ **(Eq. 13-19). (Hoyt JW, et al: Continuous** $S\bar{v}_{O_2}$ **as predictor of changes in cardiac output: Clinical observations, In Schweiss JF (ed):** ***Continuous Measurement of Blood Oxygen Saturation in the High Risk Patient.*** **Vol 1. San Diego, Beach International, 1982.)**

Figure 13-11 is a continuous plot of $S\bar{v}_{O_2}$ versus time for a patient on mechanical ventilation with a high positive end-expiratory pressure (PEEP) value. At the time indicated by the asterisk, the pulmonary artery catheter balloon was inflated and the ventilator was disconnected. The sudden increase in $S\bar{v}_{O_2}$ demonstrates the artifactual effect of a wedged catheter. After 30 s the balloon was deflated and the ventilator reconnected, followed by a marked decrease in both arterial and mixed venous saturation as shown. In this case the sudden fall in $S\bar{v}_{O_2}$ reflected a corresponding fall in Sa_{O_2} caused by the temporary discontinuation of PEEP. This illustrates the danger of even briefly interrupting PEEP in some ventilator-dependent patients.

Figure 13-12 shows a gradual decrease in $S\bar{v}_{O_2}$ leading to a cardiac arrest, which is accompanied by a more drastic decrease. The initial gradual $S\bar{v}_{O_2}$ decline was associated with a diminishing $\dot{Q}_T$ and could serve as a warning of the impending disaster. Note that even the base-line value of 58% is below the normal range of $S\bar{v}_{O_2}$.

Figure 13-13 illustrates the effect of increased oxygen consumption on $S\bar{v}_{O_2}$. In this trace the patient initially had a $\dot{Q}_T$ of 6 L/min, a calculated V_{O_2} of 187 mL/min, and a normal $S\bar{v}_{O_2}$ value. As indicated on the figure, $S\bar{v}_{O_2}$ began to decline with the onset of shivering. This decline was not accompanied by a decrease in Sa_{O_2}. However, the next thermodilution measurement revealed a $\dot{Q}_T$ >9 L/min and a V_{O_2} of 458 mL/min. This is a good example of a patient who has

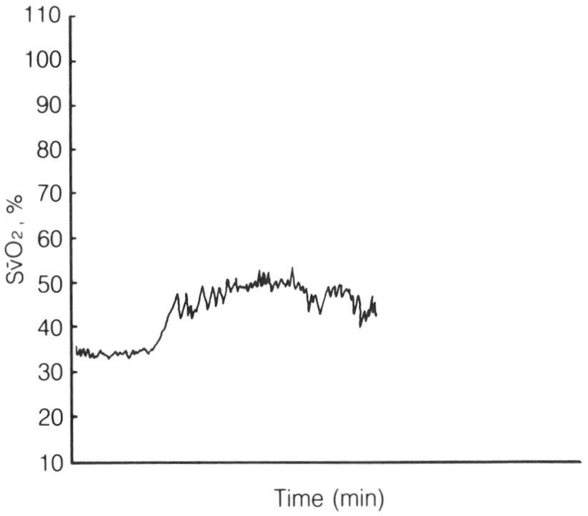

FIGURE 13-14 **$S\bar{v}_{O_2}$ versus time for a patient in cardiogenic shock with an initial $S\bar{v}_{O_2}$ value of 35%. The increase in $S\bar{v}_{O_2}$ to 50% was caused by the onset of sepsis in this patient. In this case an increase in $S\bar{v}_{O_2}$ toward normal values did not herald a favorable prognosis for the patient, who soon died. (Gore JM: Use of continuous monitoring of mixed venous oxygen saturation in the coronary care unit, in Fahey PJ (ed):** ***Continuous Measurement of Blood Oxygen Saturation in the High Risk Patient.*** **Vol 2. San Diego, Beach International, 1985.)**

a compromised circulation even though his $\dot{Q}_T$ has increased over base line. The increase in O_2 demand has outpaced that of O_2 supply, and among the standard monitors this imbalance would be indicated only by $S\bar{v}_{O_2}$.

Not all increases in $S\bar{v}_{O_2}$ herald a good prognosis for the patient. This is shown in Fig. 13-14, the tracing of a patient in cardiogenic shock with an $S\bar{v}_{O_2}$ value of 35%. The sudden increase of $S\bar{v}_{O_2}$ to about 50% could be interpreted as a significant improvement if no other data were considered. However, soon after this the patient spiked a high fever and was found to be septic. In this case, an increase in $S\bar{v}_{O_2}$ toward the normal range was caused by an additional disease process. This situation illustrates a limitation of $S\bar{v}_{O_2}$ monitoring. Since some pathophysiologic changes cause $S\bar{v}_{O_2}$ to decrease and others cause it to increase, it is possible to have two simultaneous opposing clinical changes that result in no change in $S\bar{v}_{O_2}$. For example, a patient could become hypoxemic and septic at the same time. As with any other monitor, the clinician must integrate $S\bar{v}_{O_2}$ with all other available data in assessing the patient.

Continuous $S\bar{v}_{O_2}$ monitoring is also a valuable adjunct in the management of ventilator-dependent patients. For example, as PEEP is slowly increased to improve oxygenation in a patient with pulmonary edema, Sa_{O_2} will generally increase but $\dot{Q}_T$ must eventually decrease as venous return is compromised. At this point, oxygen delivery may begin to fall even though Sa_{O_2} is still rising. $S\bar{v}_{O_2}$ will fall in this case, reflecting the decreased O_2 delivery to tissue. $S\bar{v}_{O_2}$ monitoring thus provides a way of optimizing PEEP with far fewer arterial blood-gas and $\dot{Q}_T$ measurements.

Transcutaneous Gas Measurement

TRANSCUTANEOUS OXYGEN

Transcutaneous oxygen tension (Ptc_{O_2}) is measured by a heated Clark electrode placed on the surface of the skin. In the first reported measurements in 1972, Ptc_{O_2} provided a close approximation of Pa_{O_2} in neonates.[31] Later studies have shown that the relationship between Ptc_{O_2} and Pa_{O_2} depends on both age and hemodynamic conditions. The transcutaneous index is defined as the ratio of $Ptc_{O_2}:Pa_{O_2}$. Table 13-1 illustrates the dependence of Ptc_{O_2} index on both age and $\dot{Q}_T$. While the average Ptc_{O_2} index is 1.0 in term newborns, it is only 0.8 in healthy adults and 0.7 in the elderly. In adult ICU patients, the Ptc_{O_2} index falls below its normal value of 0.8 whenever the cardiac index falls below 2.2 L/min/m^2.[31]

The Ptc_{O_2} index values of Table 13-1 were obtained from sensors on central body locations. Transcutaneous electrodes placed on the extremities will yield a lower Ptc_{O_2} index even in the absence of peripheral vascular disease. If vascular disease is present, transcutaneous index values will be much lower (e.g., 0.1). Ptc_{O_2} can thus be used to assess the degree of peripheral vascular impairment. A recent study has shown that the transcutaneous index is also decreased by acute hypocapnia, especially for peripheral sensor locations.[32] Because of its sensitivity to perfusion, Ptc_{O_2} index is a useful variable in following the progress of resuscitation of adult ICU patients.[33]

Ptc_{O_2} indicates delivery of oxygen to peripheral tissues, and therefore follows trends of Pa_{O_2} only in the absence of perfusion abnormalities. Because of its dependence on perfusion and age as well as on Pa_{O_2}, Ptc_{O_2} monitoring is most frequently used in the neonatal ICU. The lack of widespread clinical application of Ptc_{O_2} in adult ICU medicine is also related to the technical requirements of the technique. These include calibration of the instrument prior to each use, a 10- to 15-min warm-up time after sensor placement on the skin, and the necessity of changing the sensor location at 6-h intervals to prevent skin burns. In addition, the

TABLE 13-1 Changes in Ptc_{O_2} Index with Age and Cardiac Output

Ptc_{O_2} Index[a] (Ptc_{O_2}/Pa_{O_2})	Age Group
1.1	Premature infants
1.0	Newborn
0.84	Pediatric
0.8	Adult
0.7	Older adult (65 years)
$\approx Ptc_{O_2}$ Index[b]	Cardiac Index L/min/m^2
0.8	>2.2
0.5	1.5 to 2.2
0.1	<1.5

[a] All these Ptc_{O_2} index values have a standard deviation of approximately 0.1.
[b] These data are from adult patients.

Clark polarographic electrode of the transcutaneous sensor is a sophisticated device requiring routine maintenance. Newer instruments minimize some of these difficulties by providing easy room air calibration and disposable membrane kits. If the electrode temperature is maintained at 44°C (111.2°F) or less, it can be safely left on the skin of an adult for 8 h or more without changing locations.

Although pulse oximetry is easier to use and interpret, it does not provide the same oxygen transport data as Ptc_{O_2}. Pulse oximetry will not show early downward trends in Pa_{O_2} when the values of the latter are greater than about 80 mmHg, whereas Ptc_{O_2} will consistently reflect such changes. Ptc_{O_2} is the oxygen tension on the surface of heated, hyperemic skin. As such, it follows changes in Pa_{O_2} when perfusion is adequate but decreases dramatically relative to Pa_{O_2} when perfusion is impaired.

TRANSCUTANEOUS CARBON DIOXIDE

The measurement of transcutaneous carbon dioxide (Ptc_{CO_2}) was introduced in the early 1970s shortly after transcutaneous oxygen. The Ptc_{CO_2} sensor contains the same Severinghaus-Stow electrode found in the in vitro blood-gas analyzer. Since this electrode is heated to between 42°C (107.6°F) and 44°C (111.2°F), the CO_2 tension that it measures is generally higher than Pa_{CO_2}. In fact, the first measurements of Ptc_{CO_2} on healthy awake volunteers yielded values of approximately 60 mmHg.[34,35] Several methods have been proposed to adjust Ptc_{CO_2} values to provide a closer estimate of Pa_{CO_2}. The most common method of correction, proposed by Severinghaus, is to divide the measured Ptc_{CO_2} value by 1.33 and subtract 3 mmHg.[34] Clinical studies have shown that Ptc_{CO_2} corrected by this method estimates Pa_{CO_2} to within ± 10 percent.[36]

As in the case of transcutaneous oxygen, Ptc_{CO_2} monitoring has been most extensively used in neonatal intensive care. In contrast to transcutaneous oxygen, Ptc_{CO_2} values appear to be relatively insensitive to local perfusion and do not change significantly with age. Therefore, the interpretation of Ptc_{CO_2} is much easier than that of transcutaneous oxygen. Like any electrochemical measurement, the Ptc_{CO_2} sensor requires calibration before each use. This consists of a two-point calibration using standardized gas mixtures. As in the case of transcutaneous oxygen, the Ptc_{CO_2} electrode requires routine membrane changes and periodic maintenance. Transcutaneous CO_2 is currently an underutilized technique which will probably see more widespread intensive care application in the near future.

Conclusion

Future developments in blood-gas monitoring will include instruments which determine the well-being of specific organs or systems. For example, near infrared spectroscopy may someday be a useful noninvasive monitor of cerebral oxygenation. Routine in vitro blood-gas analysis may be replaced by continuous techniques such as the optode, described above. Eventually, we should hope to monitor all blood-gas variables noninvasively, so that any patient can benefit from this monitoring without considerations of risk versus benefit.

References

1. Cohen JJ, Kassirer JP: *Acid-Base.* Boston, Little, Brown, 1982.
2. Davenport HW: *The ABC of Acid-Base Chemistry.* Chicago, University of Chicago Press, 1974.
3. Bernards WC: Practical management of acid-base disorders: Metabolic component. ASA 1987 Annual Meeting Refresher Course Lectures 124B, American Society of Anesthesiologists, 1987.
4. Nunn JF: *Applied Respiratory Physiology.* London, Butterworth, 1987.
5. White FN: Temperature and acid-base regulation, in Stoelting RK, Barash PG, Gallagher JT (eds): *Advances in Anesthesia.* Vol 6. Chicago, Year Book Medical Publishers, 1989.
6. Minty BD, Barrett AM: Accuracy of an automated blood-gas analyzer operated by untrained staff. Br J Anaesth 50:1031, 1978.
7. Fox MJ, Brody JS, Weintraub LR, et al: Leukocyte larceny: A case of spurious hypoxemia. Am J Med 67:742, 1979.
8. Durbin CG: Monitoring arterial blood gases and acid-base balance, in Lake CL (ed): *Clinical Monitoring.* Philadelphia, Saunders, 1990.
9. Barker SJ, Tremper KK, Hyatt J, et al: Comparison of three oxygen monitors in detecting endobronchial intubation. J Clin Monitoring 4(4):240, 1988.
10. Barker SJ, Tremper KK: The effect of carbon monoxide inhalation on pulse oximetry and transcutaneous PO_2. Anesthesiology 70(1):677, 1987.
11. Barker SJ, Tremper KK, Hyatt J: Effects of methemoglobinemia on pulse oximetry and mixed venous oximetry. Anesthesiology 70(1):112, 1989.
12. Pologe JA, Raley DM: Effects of fetal hemoglobin on pulse oximetry. J Perinatol 7:324, 1987.
13. Scheller MS, Unger RJ, Kelner MJ: Effects of intravenously administered dyes on pulse oximetry readings. Anesthesiology 65:550, 1986.
14. Tremper KK, Hufstedler S, Barker SJ, et al: Accuracy of a pulse oximeter in the critically ill adult: Effect of temperature and hemodynamics. Anesthesiology 63:A175, 1975.
15. Ward SA: The capnogram: Scope and limitations. Semin Anesth 6:216, 1987.
16. Gravenstein JS, Paulus DA, Hayes TJ: *Capnography in Clinical Practice.* Boston, Butterworth, 1989.
17. Nunn JF: *Applied Respiratory Physiology.* 3d ed. London, Butterworth, 1987.
18. Trevino RP, Bisera J, Weil MH, et al: End-tidal CO_2 as a guide to successful cardiopulmonary resuscitation; a preliminary report. Crit Care Med 13:910, 1985.
19. Carlon GC, Ray C, Miodownik S, et al: Capnography in mechanically ventilated patients. Crit Care Med 16:550, 1988.
20. Health Facilities Evaluation and Licensing, Hospital Licensing Standards, Anesthesia Care, Subchapter 18 (Anesthesiology, 8:43B-18.7(D)), New Jersey Register 21, 504, February 21, 1989.
21. Conway M, Durbin GM, Ingram D, et al: Continuous monitoring of arterial oxygen tension using a catheter-tip polarographic electrode in infants. Pediatrics 82(6):929, 1973.

22. Rithalia SVS, Bennett PJ, Tinker J: The performance characteristics of an intraarterial oxygen electrode. Intensive Care Med 7:305, 1981.
23. Bratanow N, Polk K, Bland R, et al: Continuous polarographic monitoring of intraarterial oxygen in the perioperative period. Crit Care Med 13(10):859, 1985.
24. Lubbers DW, Opitz N: Die pCO_2/pO_2-Optode: eine neue pCO_2 bzw. pO_2-Messonde zur Messung des pCO_2 oder pO_2 von Gasen und Flussigkeiten. Z Naturforsch [C] 30:532, 1975.
25. Peterson J, Fitzgerald R, Buckhold D: Fiberoptic probe for in vivo measurement of oxygen partial pressure. Anal Chem 56:62, 1984.
26. Barker SJ, Tremper KK, Hyatt J, et al: Continuous fiberoptic arterial oxygen tension measurements in dogs. J Clin Monitor 3(1):48, 1987.
27. Gehrich JL, Lubbers DW, Opitz N, et al: Optical fluorescence and its application to an intravascular blood gas monitoring system. IEEE Trans Biomed Eng 33:117, 1986.
28. Shapiro BA, Cane RD, Chomka CM, et al: Evaluation of a new intraarterial blood gas system in dogs and humans. Anesthesiology 67(3A):A640, 1987.
29. Barker SJ, Hyatt J, Tremper KK, et al: Fiberoptic intraarterial pHa, PaO_2, and $PaCO_2$ in the operating room. Anesth Analg 68:S16, 1989.
30. Gettinger A, DeTraglia MC, Glass DD: In vivo comparison of two mixed venous saturation catheters. Anesthesiology 66(3):373, 1989
31. Tremper KK: Transcutaneous PO_2 measurement. Can J Anaesth 31:644, 1984.
32. Barker SJ, Tremper KK, Hyatt J: The effect of arterial carbon dioxide tension on transcutaneous oxygen. Anesthesiology 69(3A):A280, 1988.
33. Shoemaker WC, Appel PL, Kram HB: Incidence, physiologic description, compensatory mechanisms, and therapeutic implications of monitored events. Crit Care Med 17:1277, 1989.
34. Severinghaus JW, Stafford M, Bradley AF: $tcPCO_2$ electrode design calibration and temperature gradient problem. Acta Anesthesiol Scand 68 (suppl): 118, 1978.
35. Glenski JA, Kucchiara RF: Transcutaneous O_2 and CO_2 monitoring of neurosurgical patients: Detection of air emboli. Anesthesiology 64:546, 1986.
36. Palmirano B, Severinghaus JW: Transcutaneous PcO_2 and PO_2: A multicenter study of accuracy. J Clin Monit, 1990 (In press).

Chapter 14

MONITORING THE RESPIRATORY SYSTEM

JOHN J. MARINI
JONATHAN TRUWIT

In the intensive care setting, data relevant to the output, efficiency, and reserve of the cardiorespiratory system alert the clinician to sudden untoward events, aid in diagnosis, help guide management decisions, facilitate prognosis, and enable assessment of therapeutic response. This chapter reviews selected aspects of monitoring the respiratory system, emphasizing those most relevant to the critically ill patient receiving ventilatory support. Some of the techniques discussed are now in current practice; others are just emerging from the physiology laboratory as candidates for the clinical setting (Table 14-1).

Monitoring techniques can be classified into those pertaining to the outcome of the respiratory process (as reflected in gas exchange) and those characterizing the load and capacity of the ventilatory system. Indices of gas exchange test either "end-point" variables (for example, Pa_{O_2}, oxygen saturation, Pa_{CO_2}, and pH) or the efficiency of the gas exchange process itself. The mechanical properties of the respiratory system, in conjunction with the minute ventilation requirement ($\dot{V}E$), determine the load placed on the ventilatory pump. The patient's ability to undertake this load is monitored by indices that reflect the neural output of the respiratory center (neural drive indices and breathing pattern) and by measures of muscle strength and reserve.

Monitoring Gas Exchange

END-POINT VARIABLES: BLOOD OXYGENATION AND CO_2 ELIMINATION

Ideally, the adequacy of gas exchange would be monitored directly by assessing metabolic processes in vital tissues. Although recent technologic advances, such as those involving magnetic resonance imaging, have brought this possibility closer to practicality,[1,2] we are currently limited to analyzing the input and output ends of the tissue gas exchange process.

ARTERIAL BLOOD-GAS ANALYSIS

Arterial blood-gas analysis is fundamental to the scientific management of the critically ill patient—a technique familiar to most practitioners of intensive care medicine. The many details of sampling technique, analysis, and interpretation are too numerous to detail here and have been comprehensively reviewed in a recent monograph[3] (see Chapter 13). It is worth noting, however, that reliable and cost-effective on-line measurements of blood pH and gas tensions via fine gauge, optode sensing, fiberoptic arterial catheters may soon be available to facilitate clinical management.[4]

BLOOD OXIMETRY

Perhaps the most useful recent innovation in gas exchange monitoring has been the application of oximetry to the online assessment of arterial and mixed venous oxygen saturation. Although intimately related, O_2 saturation (Sa_{O_2}) and O_2 tension (Pa_{O_2}) provide complementary clinical data. Pa_{O_2} reflects the maximal tension driving oxygen to its mitochondrial sites of utilization. Percentage saturation, interpreted in conjunction with hemoglobin concentration, determines the quantity of oxygen contained in each unit volume of blood.

Transmission (Arterial) Oximetry

In the technique of transmission photometric oximetry, the absorptive properties of oxygenated and deoxygenated hemoglobin are exploited to determine the Sa_{O_2} of arterial blood. Transcutaneous oximetry reflects Sa_{O_2}, enabling rapid adjustment of fractional inspired oxygen (FI_{O_2}), positive end-expiratory pressure (PEEP), and ventilator settings, and warning of arterial desaturation during spontaneous breathing or weaning attempts.

Lightweight probes direct filtered light onto the surface of the earlobe or nailbed. With *ear oximetry*, heat-dilated capillaries suffuse the earlobe with more arterial blood than metabolic processes require. Light of two or three specific wavelengths in the red and infrared ranges shines on this "arterialized" blood specimen, which absorbs or transmits radiant energy in proportion to Sa_{O_2}.[5] The relative absorption of these beams is continuously monitored and displayed as percentage saturation. With modern instruments, output stabilization requires <1 min after probe attachment. Once initial probe stabilization is achieved, fewer than 10 s elapse before a step change in Sa_{O_2} culminates in an appropriate final readout.[6] *Pulse oximeter* probes do not require tissue heating because phasic changes in blood volume and optical density cue the computer to the arterial component of the blood contained in the nailbed of finger or toe. The amount of light received by the photodetector fluctuates with the volume of pulsatile flow. Most units provide pulse rate as well as saturation, and some display a pulse amplitude waveform. Response time to step changes in saturation is somewhat more sluggish for finger than for ear probes.

Instruments currently available are highly accurate (1 to 4 percent) in their upper range (i.e., at saturations >75 to 80 percent). However, most units tend to overestimate the true value at lower saturations. Sensitivity to changes in oxygen exchange is inherently impaired when Sa_{O_2} nears full saturation. Taking instrument accuracy into account, small fluctuations in Sa_{O_2} may correspond to a very wide

TABLE 14-1 Monitoring Techniques in Mechanical Ventilation[a]

GAS EXCHANGE		WORK LOAD		CAPABILITY			
End-Point Variables	Efficiency	Measures of Metabolic Activity	Measures of External Load and Performance	Strength	Breathing Pattern	Ventilatory Drive	Reserve
Arterial blood gases	$P(A - a)_{O_2}$	Oxygen consumption	Minute ventilation ($\dot{V}_E$)	Vital capacity	Frequency	$\dot{V}_E$	EMG power spectrum
Arterial oximetry	$\dot{Q}_S/\dot{Q}_T$	Gas analysis	Work of breathing	MIP	V_T	V_T/ti	Tension-time index
Transmission	Pa_{O_2}/FI_{O_2}	Fick's method	Pressure-time product	P_{Di}-max	ti/ttot	$P_{0.1}$	∫ EMG/P
Pulse	Pa_{O_2}/PA_{O_2}	Volumetric	Transdiaphragmatic pressure (P_{Di})			∫ EMG	Signs of stress
Mixed venous oximetry	V_D/V_T	CO_2 production	Mechanics			Breathing pattern	Paradox
Transcutaneous P_{O_2}		∫ EMG	Airway manometry			Frequency	Alternans
Transconjunctival P_{O_2}			Esophageal manometry			V_T	Tachypnea
Transcutaneous P_{CO_2}			Compliance			ti/ttot	Accessory muscle use
			Lung				f/V_T ratio
			Chest wall				CO_2 drive response
			Resistance				
			Inspiratory				
			Expiratory				
			Inflation impedance				

[a] For abbreviations, see text.

range of Pa_{O_2} values. Many oximeters tend to provide falsely low values of Sa_{O_2} in the setting of hypoperfusion, deep pigmentation, or carboxyhemoglobinemia.[5,7] ("Low perfusion" alarms usually alert the clinician to the inadequacy of photoelectric flux.) Interference from such sources as fluorescent lights and sunlight can be overcome with adequate shielding of the photodetector.[8] Proper fit of the probe onto the finger or ear avoids the problem of "optical shunting" around the tissue. When optical shunting occurs, a portion of the light beam bypasses the skin, causing the default value (81 to 85 percent) to admix with the true saturation. Methemoglobinemia can produce either falsely high or low saturation values, and other dyshemoglobinemias also interfere.[3]

Reflectance Oximetry

TECHNIQUE. Reflectance oximetry is used when a fiberoptic Swan-Ganz catheter continuously samples mixed venous oxygen saturation ($S\bar{v}_{O_2}$) in the pulmonary arterial bloodstream.[9] Light transmitted through a fiberoptic bundle shines onto blood coursing past the distal tip. As in tissue, the extinction and reflection of this filtered light depend on the wavelength of the incident beam and on the oxygen carriage of hemoglobin (Hgb). A computer evaluates the relative absorption of the incident beams and reports saturation. In the pulmonary artery, the oxyhemoglobin dissociation curve is sufficiently linear that oximeter sensitivity and accuracy are rather uniform throughout the clinical range. Saturation values correlate well with values derived by cooximetry, when the catheter tip lies free within the lumen and remains unoccluded by clot, debris, or vessel wall.[9]

Blood withdrawn through the distal port of a pulmonary artery catheter provides "spot" samples that can also help to determine the adequacy of oxygen delivery. Such specimens must be obtained carefully. To avoid contamination with postcapillary blood or with flush solution, one must position the catheter tip in the proximal pulmonary artery, adequately clear the catheter dead space (3 to 5 mL), and gently withdraw the sample over 15 to 20 s.[10]

INTERPRETATION. Reduced $S\bar{v}_{O_2}$ may help explain arterial hypoxemia in the setting of increased venous admixture, especially if desaturation is caused by a regional disorder (e.g., atelectasis). However, any single value of $S\bar{v}_{O_2}$ has no unique implication; it must be interpreted with knowledge of its multiple determinants and the exact clinical setting. As rearrangement of the Fick equation illustrates, $S\bar{v}_{O_2}$ is influenced directly by Sa_{O_2} and the ratio of oxygen consumption to delivery:

$$S\bar{v}_{O_2} \approx Sa_{O_2} - \frac{\dot{V}_{O_2}}{(\dot{Q} \cdot \text{Hgb} \cdot 1.34)} \qquad (14\text{-}1)$$

Mixed venous oxygen tension ($P\bar{v}_{O_2}$) and $S\bar{v}_{O_2}$ tend to decline when Sa_{O_2} falls or when an increased oxygen consumption or decreased Hgb concentration is undercompensated by a parallel increase in cardiac output ($\dot{Q}_T$).[11]

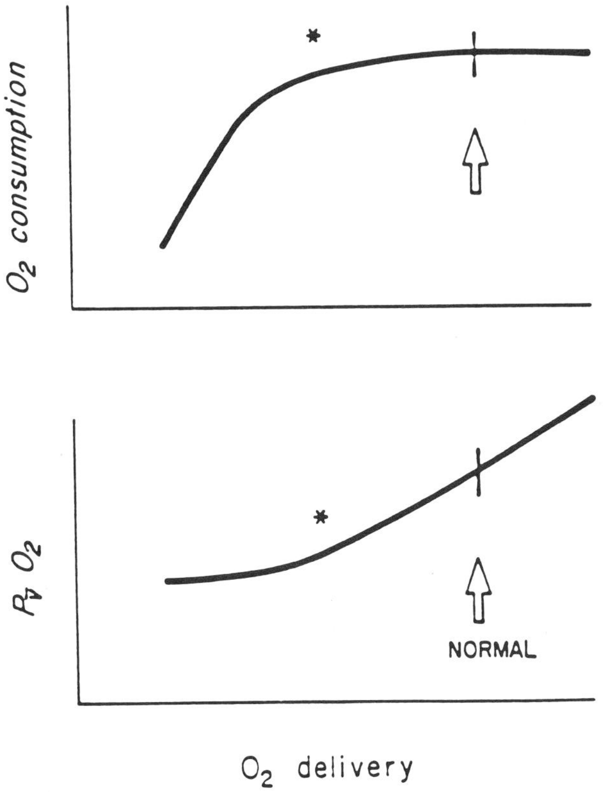

FIGURE 14-1 Relationship of oxygen delivery to oxygen consumption ($\dot{V}_{O_2}$) and mixed venous oxygen tension ($P\bar{v}_{O_2}$). As delivery is reduced from its normal value by reductions in $\dot{Q}_T$, increased oxygen extraction tends to preserve $\dot{V}_{O_2}$ at the expense of a falling $P\bar{v}_{O_2}$. Beyond some critical point (*), however, the limits of extraction are reached, $\dot{V}_{O_2}$ becomes delivery dependent, and $P\bar{v}_{O_2}$ reaches a plateau. The $P\bar{v}_{O_2}$ and $S\bar{v}_{O_2}$ are relatively insensitive in this lower range. (From Marini JJ: Monitoring during mechanical ventilation. Clin Chest Med 9(1):73, 1988, with permission.)

Conversely, $S\bar{v}_{O_2}$ may be misleadingly normal despite inadequate tissue oxygenation in the setting of disordered vasomotor control (e.g., sepsis, cirrhosis).

Monitoring of $S\bar{v}_{O_2}$ should be considered a nonspecific diagnostic aid. An abnormally high value warns that the catheter tip could be in a "permanently wedged" position, sensing fully oxygenated, postcapillary blood. A low value should prompt careful reassessment, especially if it is part of a quickly changing trend. Assuming stable $\dot{V}_{O_2}$, $S\bar{v}_{O_2}$ parallels oxygen delivery over a fairly wide range. $S\bar{v}_{O_2}$ may lose sensitivity, however, when oxygen delivery falls below the critical value that defines the brink of delivery dependence of oxygen consumption (Fig. 14-1).

Although $S\bar{v}_{O_2}$ can be a useful monitor of hemodynamic change in any individual patient, the reliability of $S\bar{v}_{O_2}$ as a hemodynamic or prognostic index tends to vary with the type of disease process. $S\bar{v}_{O_2}$ correlates with prognosis in cardiogenic shock and with response to resuscitation efforts.[12,13] Furthermore, an index that incorporates the $S\bar{v}_{O_2}$, the *oxygen extraction ratio*— (Ca_{O_2} − $C\bar{v}_{O_2}$)/Ca_{O_2}—tends to correlate with outcome; septic patients able to extract oxygen on metabolic demand fare better than those who cannot.[14]

TRANSCUTANEOUS MONITORING OF RESPIRATORY GASES

Oxygen

Unlike oximetry, monitoring of transcutaneous oxygen tension (Ptc_{O_2}) remains sensitive to changes in O_2 exchange when Pa_{O_2} exceeds 60 mmHg, the knee of the oxyhemoglobin dissociation curve. Using a membrane-covered polarographic electrode, transcutaneous oxygen monitoring measures the oxygen concentration in gas equilibrated above a warmed patch of skin.[8,15] Heating to 42°C to 44°C (107.6°F to 111.2°F) aids equilibration of Ptc_{O_2} with Pa_{O_2} by increasing the permeability of the epidermis and by enhancing cutaneous blood flow. In addition, warmed hemoglobin binds less avidly to O_2, boosting the measured pressure toward the arterial value. Transcutaneous oxygen monitoring requires lengthy calibration and stabilization time, careful skin and electrode preparation, and frequent site changes to avoid burning. Response time is longer than for oximetric techniques.

When all technical factors determining Ptc_{O_2} are optimal, changes in Ptc_{O_2} and Pa_{O_2} are closely parallel. This technique is successful in neonatology, in which perfusional crises are infrequent and the poorly cornified skin is well suffused by subsurface capillaries.[8,16] Unfortunately, transcutaneous oxygen monitoring proves less satisfactory in adult medicine.[17] Although Ptc_{O_2} correlates well with Pa_{O_2} during hemodynamic stability, it variably underestimates the arterial value. Ptc_{O_2} also equilibrates slowly with changes in Pa_{O_2}. Finally, during hemodynamic crises, the Ptc_{O_2} appears to track skin perfusion rather than Pa_{O_2}, especially when the cardiac index falls below 1.5 L/min/m^2.[18] Conceivably, this property could prove useful; an abrupt reduction in Ptc_{O_2} without a corroborating change in Pa_{O_2} might warn of an impending perfusion crisis.

Carbon Dioxide

Unlike oxygen, transcutaneous CO_2 is generated in the tissue itself, close to the probe. Local heating improves gaseous diffusion but increases CO_2 production. The transcutaneous P_{CO_2} (Ptc_{CO_2}) monitor invariably reports a value higher than Pa_{CO_2}, usually a difference of 5 to 20 mmHg. In patients with adequate cardiovascular function, the correlation between the arterial and transcutaneous values for P_{CO_2} is somewhat better than for oxygen.[8,19] The Ptc_{CO_2} also appears somewhat less sensitive to changes in hemodynamic status. Furthermore, although its response is sluggish, the Ptc_{CO_2} responds to step changes in gas tension faster than its Ptc_{O_2} counterpart, possibly because CO_2 diffuses more easily through the skin. For these reasons, transcutaneous CO_2 monitoring may be more applicable to an adult population.[20]

OTHER GAS TENSION MEASURING TECHNIQUES

Transconjunctival (Tcj_{O_2}) and transcutaneous oxygen monitoring share a similar operating principle. Perfused by the ophthalmic branch of the internal carotid artery,[21,22] conjunctival capillaries lie in close proximity to the Clark electrode, improving response time in a tissue bed served by a cerebral vessel. Unfortunately, currently available probes require appreciable skill and set-up time to insert and are uncomfortable for conscious patients. Tcj_{O_2}, therefore, finds its greatest usage during coma and in surgical applications.[8]

Implantable tissue oxygen electrodes have been evolving for many years. Even in their current form, however, these probes are invasive and reflect only the oxygen tension in the specific tissue sampled. Thus, despite expanding options, adequacy of tissue oxygenation and perfusion is still best monitored by clinical indices of vital organ function (e.g., urine flow, mental status, heart rhythm, and lactate production.)

OXYGEN CONSUMPTION

Techniques for Analysis

Total body oxygen consumption ($\dot{V}_{O_2}$) is surprisingly difficult to measure accurately at the bedside. Two primary methods are in general use: direct analysis of inspired and expired gases and Fick's method: computation of $\dot{V}_{O_2}$ from the product of cardiac output ($\dot{Q}_T$) and the difference in oxygen content between samples of arterial and mixed venous blood ($Ca_{O_2} - C\bar{v}_{O_2}$). Neither method is accurate when the patient is not in a metabolic steady state at the time of data collection.

EXPIRED GAS ANALYSIS. Critically ill patients are often exposed to high FI_{O_2} and require large minute volumes to achieve effective alveolar ventilation. These characteristics cause such large volumes of oxygen to flush through the lungs (often >15 L/min) that analyses of gas tensions and measurements of $\dot{V}_E$ must be very precise to distinguish the small oxygen deficits (100 to 350 mL/min) that correspond to total body $\dot{V}_{O_2}$. Problems of measurement accuracy become overwhelming when attempts are made to monitor the much smaller changes in $\dot{V}_{O_2}$ that correspond to respiratory effort. In addition, the inspired gas mixture must also be thoroughly blended and invariant in composition.[23] Several bedside methods for accurate measurement of oxygen tension have become available, some with the requisite accuracy for clinical application to critically ill patients. However, although fuel cell and polarographic technologies have recently made impressive advances, precise measurement of $\dot{V}_{O_2}$ in patients receiving high levels of inspired oxygen remains a challenge.

FICK'S METHOD. In Fick's method, the difference in oxygen content between arterial and mixed venous samples is multiplied by the $\dot{Q}_T$ to determine the rate of oxygen consumption. Unfortunately, this determination is greatly influenced by small changes in either the activity of the patient or the $\dot{Q}_T$ over the period of data collection, causing unreliability in the resulting estimate. Furthermore, blood oxygen content must be determined directly by cooximeter. Technical errors in blood analysis and $\dot{Q}_T$ determination are multiplicative.

VOLUMETRIC ANALYSIS. A method of estimating $\dot{V}_{O_2}$ recently introduced to intensive care uses a closed circuit that absorbs CO_2 while continuously metering in the oxygen necessary to keep the total volume of the system in equilibrium.[24] This technique obviates the analytical problems presented by elevated $F_{I_{O_2}}$ but requires manipulation of the breathing circuit to insert the apparatus. Resistance to spontaneous breathing is appreciable, and as currently configured, this system does not appear appropriate for patients with high $\dot{V}_E$ requirements.

Applications of $\dot{V}_{O_2}$ Measurement

Oxygen consumption may be helpful when determining nutritional requirements. However, in other settings its clinical utility is more open to question. Assuming a stable tissue need for oxygen, measurements of $\dot{V}_{O_2}$ may help to gauge the hemodynamic response to therapeutic measures. In theory, an increasing $\dot{V}_{O_2}$ should suggest improvement, whereas failure of $\dot{V}_{O_2}$ to change following intervention implies that output was initially adequate or that the therapeutic intervention was unsuccessful. Unfortunately, however, $\dot{V}_{O_2}$ measurements are not highly reproducible and, as already noted, are subject to sudden changes in underlying metabolic status; they do not serve well as end points for therapeutic intervention. For similar reasons, differences in $\dot{V}_{O_2}$ are unreliable in assessing the breathing effort associated with ventilatory stress, particularly when the patient receives high $F_{I_{O_2}}$.

CO_2 PRODUCTION

The CO_2 excretion rate can be of value in metabolic studies, in computations of wasted ventilation (vide infra), and in gathering information relative to the etiology of hyperpnea. Free from constraints relative to inspired gas concentration, measurements of CO_2 production can be accurate if the sample is collected with adequate care in the steady state over adequate time. The rate of CO_2 elimination is the product of the expired fraction of CO_2 ($F_{E_{CO_2}}$) and the total volume of all gas expelled over the measurement interval. Accurate estimation of CO_2 excretion requires timely gas collection and a sample that is adequately mixed and analyzed. However, whether this value reflects metabolic CO_2 production will depend on the stability of the patient during the period of gas collection, not only with regard to $\dot{V}_{O_2}$ but also in terms of acid-base homeostasis, perfusion, and ventilation. During acute hyperventilation or rapidly developing metabolic acidosis, the rate of CO_2 excretion overestimates the metabolic output until surplus body stores of CO_2 are washed out or bicarbonate stores reach equilibrium. The opposite obtains during hypoventilation.

EFFICIENCY OF O_2 AND CO_2 EXCHANGE

EFFICIENCY OF O_2 EXCHANGE ACROSS THE LUNG

Computing Alveolar Oxygen Tension

To judge the efficiency of gas exchange, mean alveolar oxygen tension ($P_{A_{O_2}}$) must first be computed. For a healthy lung, the ideal $P_{A_{O_2}}$ is obtained from the alveolar gas equation:

$$P_{A_{O_2}} = P_{I_{O_2}} - \frac{Pa_{CO_2}}{R} + [Pa_{CO_2} \cdot F_{I_{O_2}} \cdot \frac{(1 - R)}{R}] \quad (14\text{-}2)$$

where R is the respiratory exchange ratio.[25] Because of its small value, the bracketed righthand term can be neglected for most clinical applications. Under steady-state conditions, R normally varies from ≈0.7 to 1.0, depending on the nature of the metabolic fuel. (When the same patient is being monitored over time, R is generally assumed to be 0.8 or neglected entirely.) At sea level with the patient breathing room air the equation can be simplified to $P_{A_{O_2}} = 147 - 1.25\ Pa_{CO_2}$.

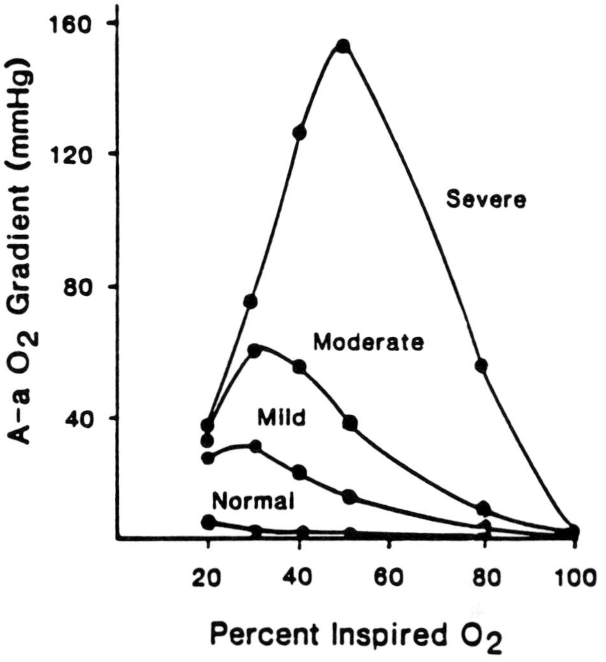

FIGURE 14-2 Relationship of $P(A - a)_{O_2}$ gradient to inspired oxygen percentage under conditions of normal to severe ventilation-perfusion inequality. (From Reference 25, with permission.)

Alveolar to Arterial Oxygen Tension Difference

The difference between alveolar and arterial oxygen tensions, $P(A - a)_{O_2}$, provides a means of eliminating hypoventilation and hypercapnia from consideration as the sole cause of hypoxemia. However, a single value of $P(A - a)_{O_2}$ does not characterize the efficiency of gas exchange across all $F_{I_{O_2}}$ values, even in normal subjects.[26] The $P(A - a)_{O_2}$ difference normally ranges from <10 mmHg on room air to <100 mmHg at an $F_{I_{O_2}}$ of 1.0, increasing modestly with age. Moreover, $P(A - a)_{O_2}$ changes linearly with $F_{I_{O_2}}$ as the extent of $\dot{V}/\dot{Q}$ mismatching increases (Fig. 14-2). Thus, when the $\dot{V}/\dot{Q}$ abnormality is severe and inhomogeneously distributed among gas exchange units, the Pa_{O_2} may vary little with $F_{I_{O_2}}$ until high fractions of inspired oxygen are given. Dramatic improvement may then occur with further increments in F_{IO_2} as very low $\dot{V}/\dot{Q}$ units cease to contribute to the (A − a) difference.[25,26] Given the variability of the Pa_{O_2}/F_{IO_2} ratio, whenever possible it is best to conduct trials of PEEP at an F_{IO_2} appropriate to ongoing management (≤0.60).

Venous Admixture and Shunt

The ability of the fiberoptic Swan-Ganz catheter to provide accurate on-line measurements of $S\bar{v}_{O_2}$ enables *venous admixture* ($\dot{Q}s/\dot{Q}T$) to be estimated with relative ease. In the steady state:

$$\frac{\dot{Q}s}{\dot{Q}T} = \frac{(CA_{O_2} - Ca_{O_2})}{(CA_{O_2} - C\bar{v}_{O_2})} \qquad (14\text{-}3)$$

where oxygen content (expressed in mL O_2 per 100 mL blood) equals the product: $(0.003 \cdot P_{O_2} + 1.34 \cdot S_{O_2} \cdot \text{Hgb})$. Like $P(A - a)_{O_2}$, $\dot{Q}s/\dot{Q}T$ is also influenced by $\dot{V}/\dot{Q}$ inequality at $F_{IO_2} < 1.0$. If the alveoli are patent, the calculated percentage of admixture will diminish toward the normal upper (physiologic) value of ≈5 to 10 percent as F_{IO_2} increases. Conversely, if venous admixture is due entirely to a true right-to-left shunt (blood flowing through completely unventilated tissue, through intrapulmonary venoarterial communications, or through an intracardiac defect), there will be no change in $\dot{Q}s/\dot{Q}T$ as F_{IO_2} increases.

Simplified Measures of Oxygen Exchange

Several approaches have been undertaken to simplify bedside assessment of oxygen exchange efficiency, as well as to obviate the dependence of traditional indices of oxygen exchange on F_{IO_2}. One is to quantitate $P(A - a)_{O_2}$ during the administration of pure oxygen. After a suitable "wash-in" time (5 to 15 min, depending on severity of disease), pure shunt accounts for the entire difference between alveolar and arterial gas tensions. Furthermore, if hemoglobin is fully saturated with oxygen, dividing the $P(A - a)_{O_2}$ by 20 approximates shunt percentage at $F_{IO_2} = 1.0$. The administration of pure oxygen replaces alveolar nitrogen and may cause some poorly ventilated units to collapse as oxygen is absorbed faster than replaced (absorption atelectasis). Nonetheless, determining shunt fraction is worthwhile because refractory hypoxemia alerts the clinician to consider nonparenchymal causes of arterial desaturation (arteriovenous malformation, intracardiac shunting). Furthermore, because Pa_{O_2} shows little response to variations in F_{IO_2} at shunt fractions that exceed 25 percent, the clinician may be encouraged to reduce toxic and marginally effective concentrations of oxygen.

The Pa_{O_2}/F_{IO_2} (P/F) ratio is a convenient and widely used bedside index of oxygen exchange that attempts to adjust for fluctuating F_{IO_2}. Although simple to calculate and useful when $\dot{V}/\dot{Q}$ mismatching is the primary cause for hypoxemia, this ratio does not remain equally sensitive across the entire range of F_{IO_2}, especially when shunt is a major cause for admixture.[27] Another easily calculated index of oxygen exchange efficiency, the arterial to alveolar O_2 tension ratio (Pa_{O_2}/PA_{O_2}), offers similar advantages and disadvantages as F_{IO_2} is varied. Like the P/F ratio, it is a useful bedside index that does not require blood sampling from the central circulation, but it loses reliability in proportion to the degree of shunting.[27,28] Furthermore, in common with all measures that calculate an ideal PA_{O_2}, even the a/A ratio can be misleading when fluctuations occur in the primary determinants of $P\bar{v}_{O_2}$ (Hgb and the balance between oxygen consumption and delivery).

EFFICIENCY OF CO_2 EXCHANGE

Changes in Pa_{CO_2}

Pa_{CO_2} alone is insufficient to track the gas-exchanging properties of the lung and must be interpreted in conjunction with $\dot{V}E$. Pa_{CO_2} may be forced to rise when diminished respiratory drive or marked neuromuscular weakness impairs total ventilation and CO_2 excretion, even if the lung tissue itself remains unaffected. Increased CO_2 production may accentuate this tendency.

Because of the buffering characteristics of the body, arterial CO_2 concentrations respond exponentially after step changes in ventilation, with a half-time ($T_{\frac{1}{2}}$) of ≈3 min during hyperventilation but a slower 16-min $T_{\frac{1}{2}}$ during CO_2 accumulation.[29] These differing time courses should be taken into account when sampling blood-gases after making therapeutic changes or ventilator adjustments. Many vagaries of CO_2 flux can be eliminated in the ventilated patient by controlling the elimination rate and metabolic output of CO_2 with deep sedation/paralysis.

The Dead Space Fraction

The physiologic dead space (VD), the sum of anatomic and alveolar components, quantifies the tidal gas failing to participate in CO_2 elimination. The dead space: tidal volume ratio (VD/VT) reflects the ability of the lung to transfer carbon dioxide from the pulmonary artery to the alveolus. The fraction of wasted ventilation can be estimated from analyzed specimens of arterial blood and mixed expired gas: $V_D/V_T = (Pa_{CO_2} - P\bar{E}_{CO_2})/Pa_{CO_2}$.[30] In collecting the expired gas sample during pressurized ventilator cycles, one should take care to adjust for the volume of gas stored transiently in the compressible portions of the ventilator circuit, failing to gain exposure to the patient. [This value, the circuit compression factor (CF), usually averages 2 to 3 mL/cmH_2O of peak cycling pressure.] In healthy persons, the normal dead space fraction during spontaneous breathing varies from ≈0.35 to 0.15, depending on the vigor of respiration, the depth of the tidal breath, and the $\dot{Q}T$.[31] In the setting of critical illness, however, it is not uncommon for VD/VT to rise to values that exceed 0.7, especially during shallow breathing.[32] Indeed, increased VD often accounts for the majority of the $\dot{V}E$ requirement and CO_2 retention that occur in the terminal phase of acute hypoxemic respiratory failure.

Pathologic processes that increase dead space can be classified as those that diminish aerated alveolar volume (e.g., cyst formation, parenchymal infiltration, fibrosis) and those that interrupt vascular flow (e.g., capillary obliteration, pulmonary embolism, hypotension). In most diseases requiring mechanical ventilation, regional compliance and ventilation time constants vary markedly, so that some alveolar units receive disproportionate ventilation when a common pressure is applied to the airway. Overexpansion of compliant units by high cycling pressure redirects blood flow to more compromised regions, increasing VD/VT. This phenomenon is often apparent when progressive levels of PEEP are applied to support oxygenation. Examination of the airway pressure curve under conditions of controlled, square-wave ventilation may reveal a threshold end-expiratory pressure or VT associated with end-inspiratory overdistention, accelerated dead space formation, and escalating risk of barotrauma.[33,34] Small reductions in PEEP or VT may then reduce peak cycling pressure dramatically.

Capnography

Capnography analyzes the CO_2 concentration of the exhaled airstream. Once anatomic dead space has been cleared, the CO_2 tension at mechanical equilibrium ("end exhalation") tracks the mean alveolar value ($P_{A_{CO_2}}$).[32] Furthermore, when ventilation and perfusion are evenly distributed, $P_{A_{CO_2}}$ closely approximates Pa_{CO_2}. End-tidal P_{CO_2} ($P_{ET_{CO_2}}$) normally underestimates Pa_{CO_2} by 1 to 3 mmHg. Although the correlation between $P_{ET_{CO_2}}$ and Pa_{CO_2} is excellent for patients with normal lungs breathing at low frequencies, the difference between them (ΔP_{CO_2}) widens when ventilation and perfusion are suboptimally matched or frequency rises dramatically.

FIGURE 14-3 Tidal capnography. ***Top.*** **The expiratory phase of normal capnogram consists of a base-line (dead space) segment, a segment in which dead space and tidal gas are mixed (FG), a segment during which gas is primarily from the alveolar compartment (GH), and an inspiratory segment (HI).** ***Middle.*** **Capnogram of patient recovering from neuromuscular paralysis. The notch in the plateau indicates the patient's attempt to inspire.** ***Bottom.*** **Deformed capnographic tracing of patient with airflow obstruction. Note that in this latter instance, end-tidal CO_2 gas tensions will vary with breathing frequency. (Adapted from Stock MC: Noninvasive carbon dioxide monitoring. Crit Care Clin 4(3):511, 1988, with permission.)**

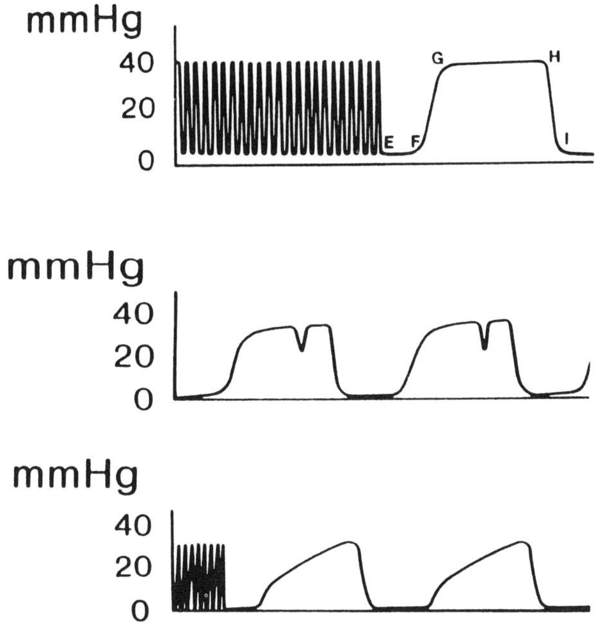

$P_{ET_{CO_2}}$ can be continuously monitored by mass spectroscopy or infrared (IR) absorption spectrophotometry.[8,32] Mass spectroscopy is an expensive technology usually applied sequentially to a number of patients served by the same instrument. Relatively few of these instruments are in clinical use. On the other hand, infrared analyzers are portable, less expensive, and more common. IR probes can be mainstream or sidestream. The main advantages of sidestream analyzers are their lack of imposed dead space and lighter weight. Unfortunately, such units draw continuously from the exhaled gas stream and impose a time delay by requiring the analyzer to be placed at a site remote from the airway. Furthermore, moisture accumulated within the tubing can invalidate the recorded values. Newer, lighter, mainstream probes impose negligible resistance and dead space and are less subject to measurement errors.

As with other monitoring techniques, $P_{ET_{CO_2}}$ must be interpreted cautiously. The normal capnogram is composed of a base line, an ascending portion, a plateau, and a descending portion (Fig. 14-3).[35] The shape of the expired CO_2 curve can give important clues to the etiology for a $Pa_{CO_2} - P_{ET_{CO_2}}$ discrepancy.[32,35] $P_{ET_{CO_2}}$ gives a low range estimate of Pa_{CO_2} in virtually all clinical circumstances. (Therefore, a high value for $P_{ET_{CO_2}}$ strongly suggests hypoventilation.) Abrupt changes in $P_{ET_{CO_2}}$ may reflect such acute processes as aspiration or pulmonary embolism. Although breath-to-breath fluctuations in $P_{ET_{CO_2}}$ can be extreme, the trend of $P_{ET_{CO_2}}$ over time can help to identify gradual changes in CO_2 exchange.

More than with most monitoring methods, technique is crucial to interpretation. It is essential to record and examine the entire tracing, not relying on the digital readout for the end-tidal value. Breathing pattern can be as influential as pathology, especially when gas flow is inhomogeneously distributed, as in airflow obstruction. Failure of the $P_{ET_{CO_2}}$ tracing to achieve a true plateau can occur because sampling technique is inappropriate, because exhalation is too brief (or VT too small), or because ventilation is inhomogeneously distributed (see Fig. 14-3). Thus ΔP_{CO_2} may widen for a variety of reasons, not all of which imply changes in lung disease.[36]

The ΔP_{CO_2} should be minimal when perfused alveoli are maximally recruited. On this basis, ($Pa_{CO_2} - P_{ET_{CO_2}}$) has been suggested as useful when attempting to identify the level of best PEEP (defined as the value of end-expiratory pressure that maximally recruits functional alveoli without overdistending those already open).[31] Indeed, this may be true for patients in whom a clear inflection point on the ascending limb of the airway pressure tracing demonstrates recruitable volume.[33]

Monitoring Lung and Chest Wall Mechanics

Gas flows to and from the alveoli driven by differences in pressure. When a mechanical ventilator provides the entire

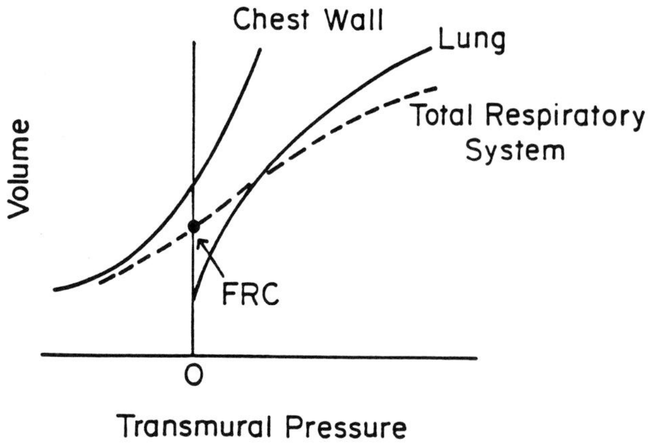

FIGURE 14-4 Static pressure-volume relationships of the lung, relaxed chest wall, and total respiratory system. Transmural pressures of the lung, chest wall, and total respiratory system are (Palv − Ppl), (Ppl), and (Palv), respectively. Functional residual capacity (FRC) defines the equilibrium volume at which the opposing recoil forces of lung and chest wall are balanced. (Adapted from Marini JJ: *Respiratory Medicine for the House-officer,* 2nd ed. Baltimore, Williams Wilkins, 1987, p 4, with permission.)

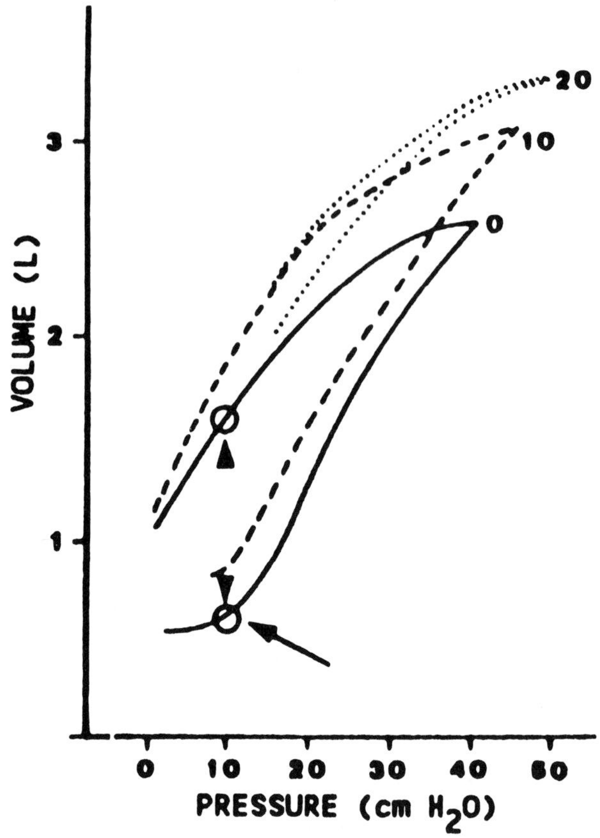

FIGURE 14-5 Static pressure-volume curve for a patient with ARDS at 0, 10, and 20 cmH_2O end-expiratory pressure. Without PEEP applied, the pressure-volume curve of the acutely edematous respiratory system often demonstrates marked hysteresis (arrowheads) and an inflection point (Pflex) on the inflation limb (arrow, right). At the higher levels of PEEP, Pflex and hysteresis diminish and the pressure-volume curve assumes a monotonic, flattened profile. (Adapted from Benito S, LeMaire F: Pulmonary pressure-volume relationship in acute respiratory distress syndrome in adults: Role of positive end-expiratory pressure. J Crit Care 5:27, 1990, with permission.)

inflation work of breathing, the difference between airway and atmospheric pressures can be accounted for in two primary ways:[21] to drive gas between the airway opening and the alveolus,[9] and to expand the alveoli against the combined elastic recoil of the lung and chest wall.[37]

STATIC PRESSURE-VOLUME RELATIONSHIPS

The pressure (ΔP_L) required to expand the lung by a certain volume (ΔV) is the corresponding change in transpulmonary pressure (P_L = alveolar pressure, Palv, minus pleural pressure, Ppl) (Fig. 14-4). The lung compliance ($C_L = \Delta V/\Delta P_L$) defines the pressure required per unit change in lung volume. Under passive conditions, the pressure needed to expand the chest wall by ΔV is given by the average change in intrathoracic pressure (ΔPpl), usually sampled in the esophagus. The distensibility of the relaxed chest wall is characterized by chest wall compliance ($C_W = \Delta V/\Delta Ppl$). Thus, the slope of the pressure-volume relationship for the total respiratory system (C_{RS}) is $\Delta V/\Delta Palv$. In ventilator-derived calculations of compliance, ΔV must be measured at the inlet of the endotracheal tube, or expired volume must be adjusted for the volume stored in compressible circuit elements.

Compliance measurements may have therapeutic and prognostic value in patients with failure of arterial oxygenation (Fig. 14-5). When PEEP is applied incrementally, the static compliance tends to reach its highest value coincident with maximal recruitment of lung units, reduction in shunt fraction, and improvement in oxygen delivery.[33,38] Although this guideline does not always apply, it is a good general rule not to use values of end-expiratory pressure or V_T that depress thoracic compliance, unless safe pressures can be used and there is objective evidence of improved O_2 delivery.[39] Excessive pressures risk barotrauma and hemodynamic compromise without tangible benefit.

Serial changes in the respiratory pressure-volume curve and computed static compliance tend to reflect the course of acute lung injury.[40,41] Maximal depression of lung compliance in adult respiratory distress syndrome (ARDS) often requires 1 to 2 weeks to develop. Severe disease is implied when compliance falls to <25 mL/cmH_2O.

Caution must be exercised when attempting to use C_{RS} as an indicator of underlying tissue elastance. When one interprets the compliance value, both the number of aerated alveoli and the relative position on the pressure-

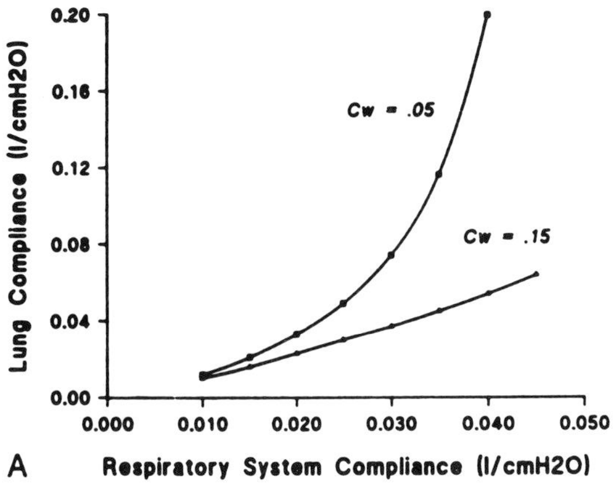

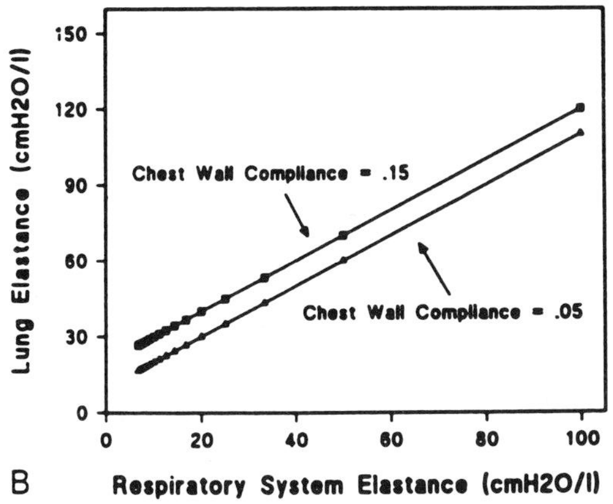

FIGURE 14-6 Mathematical comparison of elastances and compliances of the lung and integrated respiratory system for two fixed values of chest wall (Cw) compliance (0.05 and 0.15 L/cmH_2O). *a.* Because lung and chest wall compliances add in parallel, values for respiratory system compliance may differ considerably (and in curvilinear fashion) from the compliance of the lung, depending on the flexibility of the chest wall. *b.* Unlike compliance, elastances add in series, accounting for the linear relationship between EL and ERS. (From Marini JJ: Lung mechanics in ARDS: Recent conceptual advances and implications for management. Clin Chest Med 11(4):673, 1990, with permission.)

volume curve are important to consider. Ideally, compliance would be referenced to a measure of absolute lung volume (Vabs) [such as FRC or total lung capacity (TLC)] to produce a "specific compliance" CRS/Vabs.[42] (For example, identical pressures drive greatly different volumes into the normal lungs of children and adults. CL is influenced by this volume difference; CL/Vabs is not.) Yet, even in the same individual, CRS may change greatly at the extremes of the vital capacity (VC) range. Thus, most patients with hyperinflated lungs who are ventilated for acute exacerbations of asthma or chronic obstructive pulmonary disease (COPD) exhibit a depressed CRS, despite supernormal tissue distensibility in a lower volume range. This reduction is due, in part, to lung overdistention and, in part, to enhanced chest wall recoil.

CRS may also be depressed at the lower extreme of lung volume if substantial recruitment occurs in the initial portion of tidal inflation, as during pulmonary edema.[43] Thus, as the chest expands, the number of recruited alveoli increases and CRS improves toward its normal value. (A reverse phenomenon, derecruitment, occurs during lung deflation, causing pressure-volume hysteresis.) Thus, CL and CRS may appear to vary with increasing VT, improving until alveolar units are fully recruited or tissue elastic limits are approached. It has been convincingly argued that the demonstrated presence of an inflection point of compliance change (Pflex) during acute respiratory failure indicates the need for additional PEEP.[41,44]

As Katz and colleagues have pointed out, thoracic elastance (ERS), the reciprocal of CRS, has certain advantages for clinical usage.[45] Elastances of the lung (EL) and chest wall (Ew) add in series:

$$\mathrm{E_{RS}} = \mathrm{E_L} + \mathrm{E_W} \qquad (14\text{-}4)$$

On the other hand, compliances add in parallel:

$$\frac{1}{\mathrm{C_{RS}}} = \frac{1}{\mathrm{C_L}} + \frac{1}{\mathrm{C_W}} \qquad (14\text{-}5)$$

Although CRS is often used to track the elastic properties of the lung, the relationship of CRS to CL is not straightforward (see Fig. 14-5):

$$\mathrm{C_{RS}} = \frac{\mathrm{C_L C_W}}{(\mathrm{C_W} + \mathrm{C_L})} \qquad (14\text{-}6)$$

In critically ill patients, chest wall distensibility may be disturbed by abdominal distention, effusions, increased muscular tone, recent surgery, position, soft tissue injury, and so on. Such changes in Cw are important to consider, in that they influence the interpretation of hemodynamic data (e.g., the pulmonary artery occlusion pressure, Pw) as well as the calculations of chest mechanics data. The interpretation of elastance is considerably more straightforward (Fig. 14-6). For example, the CRS should be used to calculate the effect of PEEP on lung volume. However, a given peak airway pressure has different hemodynamic and prognostic significance, depending on whether the lung or chest wall accounts for the stiffness. The fraction of end-expiratory airway pressure (Pawex) transmitted to the pleural space depends on the relative compliances of the lungs and chest wall:[43,46]

$$\Delta \mathrm{V_L} = \mathrm{C_L}\,(\Delta(\mathrm{Pawex} - \mathrm{Ppl})) \qquad (14\text{-}7)$$

$$\Delta \mathrm{V_W} = \mathrm{C_W}\,(\Delta(\mathrm{Ppl})) \qquad (14\text{-}8)$$

and since $\Delta \mathrm{V_L} = \Delta \mathrm{V_W}$,

$$\Delta \mathrm{Ppl} = \Delta \mathrm{Pawex} \left(\frac{\mathrm{C_L}}{(\mathrm{C_L} + \mathrm{C_W})} \right) \qquad (14\text{-}9)$$

Relative stiffness of the lungs and chest wall determines the effect of PEEP on hemodynamics and measured Pw. Normally, $C_L \approx C_W$ over the V_T range, so that $\Delta Ppl \approx \frac{1}{2}\Delta Pawex$. Therefore, about half of a given PEEP increment is normally reflected in the Ppl. With stiff lungs this fraction falls to a lower value, and with a stiff chest wall it rises to a higher value.

USE OF THE AIRWAY PRESSURE TRACING TO CALCULATE EFFECTIVE COMPLIANCE AND RESISTANCE OF THE RESPIRATORY SYSTEM

INSPIRATORY RESISTANCE AND THORACIC COMPLIANCE

Digital technology has greatly expanded the monitoring capability of modern ventilators. During passive inflation, some systems can provide breath-to-breath estimates of R and C_{RS} as well as tracings of flow and airway pressure. Although not always elegantly presented or continuously displayed, all ventilators monitor pressure in the external airway. When a mechanical ventilator expands the chest of a passive subject, calculations of total system compliance and resistance can be made from airway pressure alone. (During active efforts, Paw must be supplemented by esophageal pressure to make the relevant calculations for the lung.)

Airway pressure overcomes the frictional and elastic forces characterized by resistance and compliance.[47] These characteristics of the system can be gauged in several ways. When flow is transiently stopped at end-inspiration, Paw falls to its final value. The difference between this end-inspiratory "stop flow," "plateau," or "peak static" (Ps) pressure and end-expiratory alveolar pressure (Pex, the sum of PEEP and auto-PEEP), determines the component of end-inspiratory inflation pressure necessary to overcome the elastic forces of tidal inflation (Fig. 14-7). When V_T (adjusted for gas compression) is divided by (Ps − Pex), static effective compliance (Ceff) can be computed as:[48]

$$\text{Ceff} = \frac{V_T - [(Ps - PEEP)\,(CF)]}{(Ps - Pex)} \qquad (14\text{-}10)$$

Although the V_T stored in the compressible circuit elements during dynamic cycling is the product of (P_D − PEEP) and CF (where P_D is the peak dynamic pressure), Ps should be substituted for P_D to obtain the appropriate volume correction for static conditions. In clinical practice it is wise to determine the relationship of Ceff to V_T to avoid hyperinflation. At a minimum, the inspiratory dynamic airway pressure tracing should be inspected for signs of overdistention. During constant flow, time is a direct analog of delivered volume, so that the slope of the airway pressure tracing reflects dynamic elastance ($1/C_{RS}$) (Fig. 14-8). Unfortunately, it is not always possible to draw a single tangent to the inflation curve that characterizes the entire inspiratory period.

The maximal pressure achieved just prior to the cessation of gas delivery, P_D, is the total system pressure needed to drive gas to the alveolar level at the set flow rate and to expand the lungs and chest wall by the full V_T. Under passive conditions of constant flow, the difference between P_D and Ps approximates the pressure gradient driving gas flow at end-inspiration and varies with the resistance of the lungs, chest wall, and endotracheal tube. The term "resistance" usually refers to the ratio between the pressure necessary to drive flow (P_R) and flow itself. However, P_R is a nonlinear function of flow, so that R is not constant across all flow rates: $P_R \approx k\dot{V}^{\epsilon}\ (1 \leq \epsilon \leq 2)$. Thus, computed resistance usually rises as flow increases, especially if flow is turbulent.

When corrected for the compression volume of the external circuit, the ratio of delivered volume to (P_D − PEEP), the "dynamic characteristic,"[49] provides an index of the

FIGURE 14-7 Schematic of the airway pressure-time profile during passive ventilation at two rates of constant flow (heavy solid and dashed lines). An end-inspirator pause (segment 2) is interposed between inflation (segment 1) and deflation (segment 3). Airway pressure is outlined in a heavy solid line and alveolar pressure in a fine solid line enclosing shaded and crosshatched areas. Under these constant flow conditions, the length of the inspiratory period reflects the V_I, and the slope of the airway pressure tracing [(Ps − Pex)/V_T] indicates the elastance of the respiratory system. (Note that Pex > PEEP in this instance, the difference being auto-PEEP.)

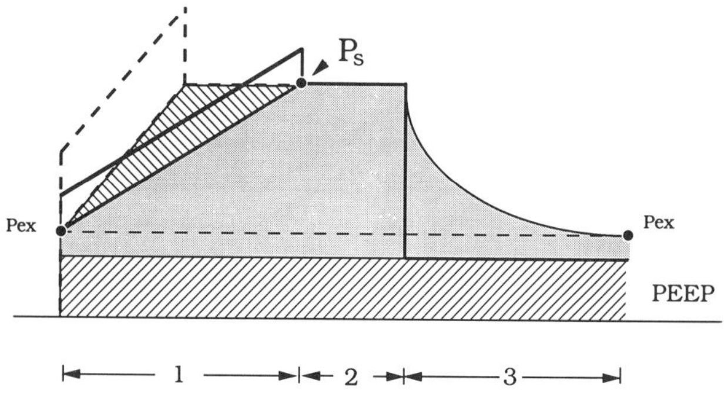

FIGURE 14-8 Volume dependence of compliance during constant flow ventilation under passive conditions. Note that tissue elastance (the tangent to alveolar pressure) varies during the first portion of inspiration. (Adapted from Marini JJ: Monitoring during mechanical ventilation. Clin Chest Med 9(1):73, 1988, with permission.)

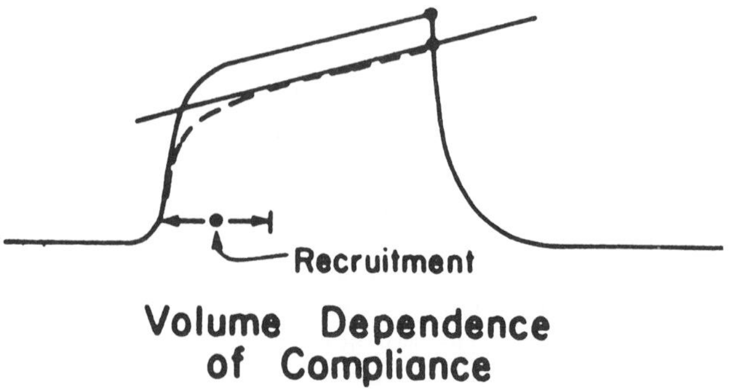

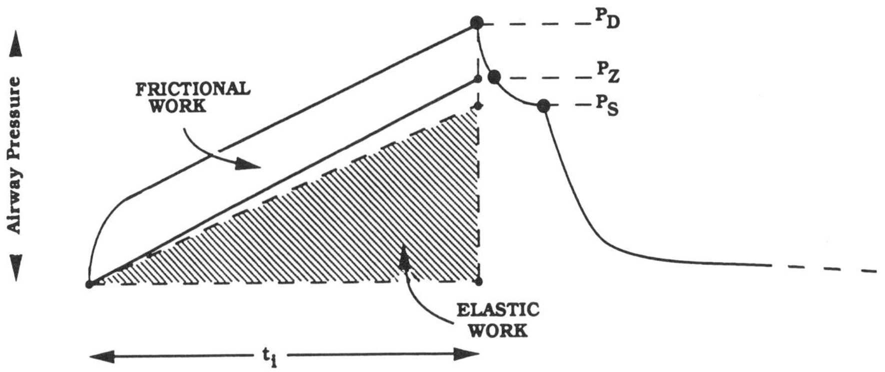

FIGURE 14-9 Partitioning of frictional and elastic impedance during passive inflation at a constant rate of inspiratory flow with end-inspiratory pause applied. Calculations using the first point of zero flow (Pz) will yield lower estimates of resistance and higher estimates of elastance (lower compliance) than will using the end-inspiratory pause or peak static pressure (Ps). PD = peak dynamic pressure. (Adapted from Marini JJ: Lung mechanics in ARDS: Recent conceptual advances and implications for management. Clin Chest Med 11(4):673, 1990, with permission.)

overall difficulty of chest expansion, provided VT and inspiratory flow rate are unchanged and that inflation occurs passively. (Note that this is not a true dynamic compliance value because of the kinetic nature of the measurement.) Because PD is influenced by both the frictional and elastic properties of the thorax, it may be a simple yet valuable indicator of bronchodilator response.[50] During effective bronchodilation, PD reflects not only the decline in frictional work but also any changes that may have occurred in $\dot{V}$E or dynamic hyperinflation.

Because PD decays exponentially to Ps, the exact value assigned to Ps will depend on the duration of flow interruption. (Fig. 14-9). The first point of inspiratory flow cessation (zero flow, ZF) invariably occurs before the plateau is fully achieved, so that the PD − Ps difference (Rmax) usually exceeds the PD − PZF difference (Rmin) by 10 to 20 percent. Therefore, values for end-inspiratory resistance computed using PD − PZF are smaller than those computed with the full PD − Ps value, which includes pressure components related to volume redistribution and stress relaxation. The VT/(PZF − Pex) quotient yields an estimate of (inspiratory) dynamic compliance (Cdyn), a value invariably less than that commonly computed from the VT/(Ps − Pex) ratio. In normal subjects, Rmin, a value influenced by tissue resistance as well as airway resistance, tends to remain stable or fall as flow rate increases, provided that airway opening pressure is measured beyond the tip of an endotracheal tube.[51] In patients with airflow obstruction, however, both Rmin and Rmax demonstrate the expected rise with flow increases.[52]

EXPIRATORY RESISTANCE

In obstructive disorders of the lung, expiratory resistance (Rex) exceeds inspiratory resistance, varies more widely during the tidal cycle, and has great relevance to air trapping.[53,54] Although seldom computed, Rex may be determined during passive exhalation from simultaneous recordings of exhaled airflow and VT (Fig. 14-10). A representative volume (V) is selected (e.g., V = 0.5 VT) and the corresponding flow ($\dot{V}$) recorded. From the estimated upstream alveolar pressure at volume V (Palv(v) ≈ P − V/CRS), expiratory flow resistance, the quotient of alveolar minus airway opening pressure (Pao) and flow, can be approximated at that point from the expression:

$$\text{Rex} = (\text{Palv(v)} - \text{Pao})/\dot{V} \quad \text{or}$$
$$\text{Rex} = [\text{Ps} - (\text{V/C}_{\text{RS}} + \text{Pao})]/\dot{V} \quad (14\text{-}11)$$

In theory, this method should provide a representative estimate of Rex. However, no study is currently available to test its validity against an alternative (plethysmographic or flow interruptive) method.

Once the static (inflation hold) pressure (Ps) is known and the corresponding CRS value has been computed, expiratory resistance can also be estimated from the observed "time constant" of passive deflation. Ideally, the passive respiratory system deflates as a single compartment, and alveolar pressure decays in exponential fashion from its starting value (Ps) (see Fig. 14-10). Alveolar pressure in excess of PEEP, P(t), at any time t after deflation begins can be used to compute Rex.

$$P(t) \approx (\text{Ps} - \text{PEEP})e^{-kt} \quad (14\text{-}12)$$

where e is the base of natural logarithms (2.718), and k is the reciprocal of the product of resistance (Rex) and compliance (C)—a value determined by the impedance of the respiratory system and known as the time constant (τ). When one time constant (τ = RC sec) has elapsed since the onset of deflation, 1/e = 1/2.718 or 37 percent of the starting volume (above PEEP) remains to be expelled. After three time constants, only 5 percent remains. If both CRS and the time constant (measured from a volume-time plot) are available, average expiratory resistance can be computed from their quotient (Rex = τ/C).

In theory, this method for computing Rex provides information unavailable from the inspiratory pressure data commonly used. However, the assumptions on which such estimates are based are often questionable. The lungs and chest wall rarely deflate as an ideal one-compartment system, and the expiratory pathway includes the external apparatus extending from endotracheal tube to the expiratory port as well as the patient's airway. For these and other reasons, expiratory resistance values calculated from the τ/C ratio must be considered crude estimates, at best.

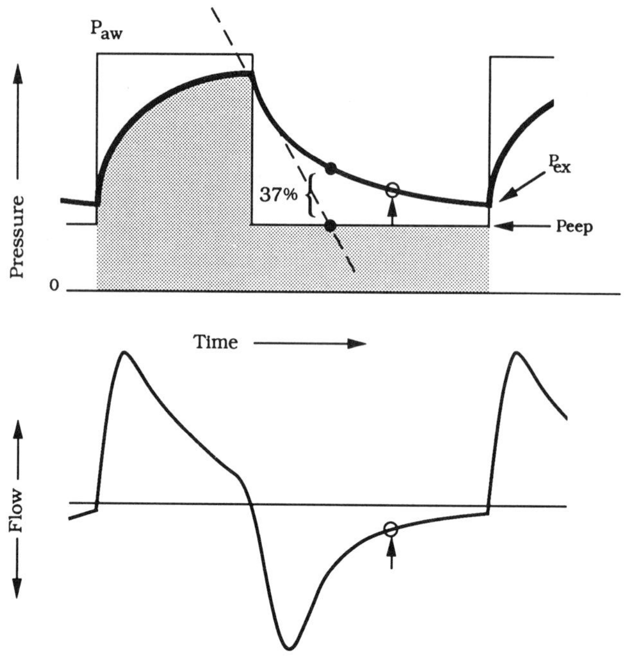

FIGURE 14-10 Airway pressure (fine line), alveolar pressure (heavy line), and airflow during passive inflation with constant pressure (pressure control). *Expiratory* resistance is the quotient $P_R/\dot{V}$, where P_R (the flow-resistive pressure) is the difference between Palv and PEEP, and $\dot{V}$ is the flow that corresponds to the chosen time point (open circle). If the lung deflates as a single compartment, as depicted here, expiratory resistance can be estimated as the quotient of the deflation time constant (τ = RC) and compliance. A tangent drawn to the alveolar pressure curve at deflation onset intersects the PEEP level s seconds later, when 37 percent of the alveolar pressure difference (P_S − PEEP) remains.

Flow Interruption Technique

Repeated interruption of expiratory airflow has recently been adapted by Gottfried and coworkers to determine the mechanics of the respiratory system in acutely ill patients receiving mechanical ventilation.[55] Following end-inspiratory airway occlusion, a series of brief (≈0.2 s) interruptions of expiratory flow is performed during passive deflation (Fig. 14-11). Multiple postinterruption plateaus of airway pressure are thereby created, yielding alveolar pressure estimates that can be used in conjunction with flow and volume tracings to compute Rex and C_{RS}. The interrupter method can be applied to paralyzed or anesthetized patients, either manually or by using a highly responsive solenoid valve system. It is not practical to apply to patients with high $\dot{V}_E$ requirements or to those who respond to flow interruption by muscular contraction.

Although a postinterruption plateau is achieved almost immediately in most normal subjects and in patients with restrictive disease, patients with severe airflow obstruction exhibit a substantial delay before equilibration is achieved. Interestingly, those with expiratory flow limitation demonstrate high flow transients immediately after occlusion release. This observation may have clinical relevance in that expiratory airflow limitation during passive deflation indicates dynamic hyperinflation and may portend both a beneficial response to added PEEP and continued ventilator dependence.[50,56]

ENDOTRACHEAL TUBE RESISTANCE

The endotracheal tube often contributes greatly to airflow resistance.[55,57] Depending on the nature, length, diameter, patency, and angulation of the endotracheal tube, computed values for R may be dominated by the resistive properties of the artificial airway. In vivo, tube resistance may be much higher than that of the same tube prior to insertion,[58] a fact of particular importance for patients with copious airway secretions. Marked flow dependence of calculated resistance may also be demonstrated in certain patients, a phenomenon usually ascribed to turbulence developing in a narrow or partially occluded tube.[55] If endogenous (bronchial) resistance must be monitored precisely, airway pressure should be sensed beyond the carinal tip of the endotracheal tube. This can be done with an intraluminal catheter or by using a tube specially designed for measuring pressure at this site during jet ventilation.

THE AUTO-PEEP (INTRINSIC PEEP, PEEPi) EFFECT

Dynamic hyperinflation and the auto-PEEP phenomenon occur when insufficient time elapses between inflation cycles to reestablish the equilibrium position of the respiratory system.[54,59] When a mechanical ventilator powers inflation, alveolar pressure remains continuously positive through both phases of the ventilatory cycle. Airflow does not cease at end exhalation but continues very slowly as alveolar pressure decompresses through critically narrowed airways (Fig. 14-12). An auto-PEEP effect may be seen in virtually any circumstance causing a high demand for ventilation, even in patients without severe airflow obstruction. Indeed, an auto-PEEP phenomenon has been well described during high-frequency ventilation.[60] Active muscular effort often contributes to the expiratory driving force and may cause alveolar pressure to remain positive at end exhalation, even without notable hyperinflation (Fig. 14-13).

The auto-PEEP effect has numerous hemodynamic and mechanical consequences. Barotrauma is an obvious risk. Furthermore, the hemodynamic consequences of the auto-PEEP effect may be more severe than those incurred with PEEP of a similar level because obstructive lung disease enhances and restrictive disease impairs transmission of airway pressure to the pleural space. Auto-PEEP also adds to the work of breathing, presenting an increased threshold load to spontaneous inspiration and depressing the effective triggering sensitivity of the ventilator.[7,61,62] The addition of counterbalancing PEEP or continuous positive airway pressure (CPAP) to patients with quantifiable auto-PEEP and expiratory flow limitation may improve subject comfort and work of breathing without marked increases in lung volume or peak cycling pressure.[62]

At the bedside, auto-PEEP is suspected when significant flow persists to the very end of exhalation. During passive inflation, auto-PEEP can be quantified by occluding the expiratory port of the ventilator at the end of the period

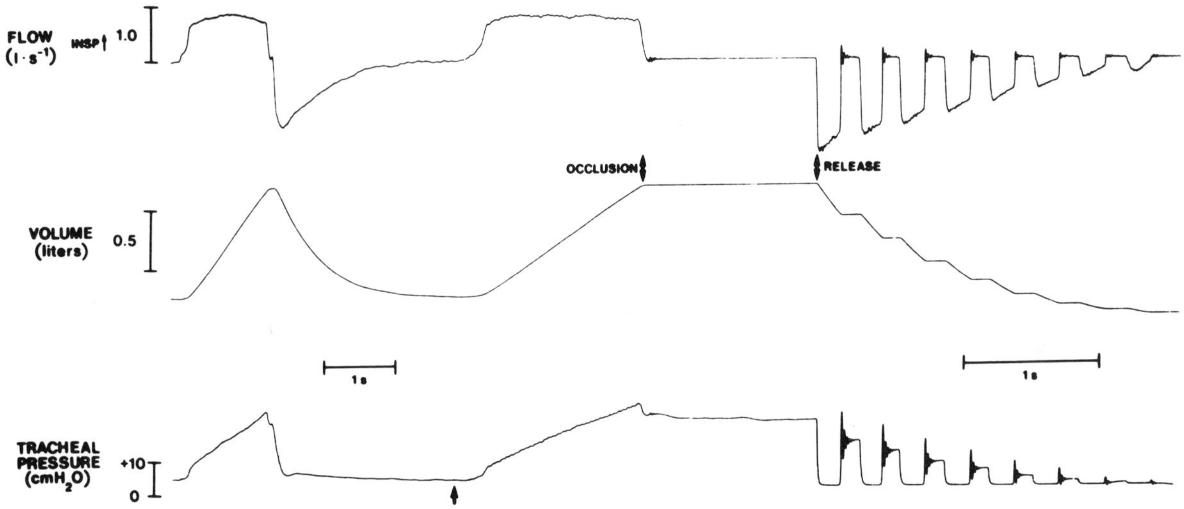

FIGURE 14-11 Interrupter technique for determination of respiratory system mechanics during passive ventilation with constant flow. Here, a series of airway opening occlusions of 0.1 to 0.2 s is performed during exhalation, allowing point-wise computation of resistance and compliance from the recorded pressures, flows, and volumes. With flow transiently stopped, airway (tracheal) pressure reflects alveolar pressure. (From Reference 55, with permission.)

allowed for exhalation between mechanical breaths [the end-expiratory port occlusion method (see Fig. 14-12)].[59] Several currently available ventilators allow prolongation of the exhalation phase with closure of the exhalation valve at the end of the set expiratory time, simplifying the measurement. For accuracy, occlusion must occur just prior to the next ventilator-delivered breath and persist for 0.5 s or longer, timing that is easiest to achieve during controlled ventilation. Auto-PEEP is also the difference between end-inspiratory static pressure and the sum of V_T/C and PEEP. Alternative methods to quantify auto-PEEP require specialized sensing equipment and displays. During controlled inflation, auto-PEEP can theoretically be measured by noting the airway pressure at which inspiratory flow begins.[54] During spontaneous efforts, the deflection of esophageal pressure needed to initiate inspiratory flow can be used to quantify the pressure needed to counterbalance the expiratory action of elastic recoil. This counterbalancing pressure, however, tends to be lower than auto-PEEP measured under passive conditions, possibly because it does not account for the contribution to auto-PEEP made by chest wall recoil.

FIGURE 14-12 The auto-PEEP effect and its measurement by the end-expiratory port occlusion maneuver. Just before the next ventilator inflation cycle, alveolar pressure remains markedly positive (15 cmH_2O) as flow continues through critically narrowed airways. The ventilator manometer approximates auto-PEEP only when pressures equilibrate following occlusion of the expiratory port at end exhalation (*b*). (Adapted from Reference 59, with permission.)

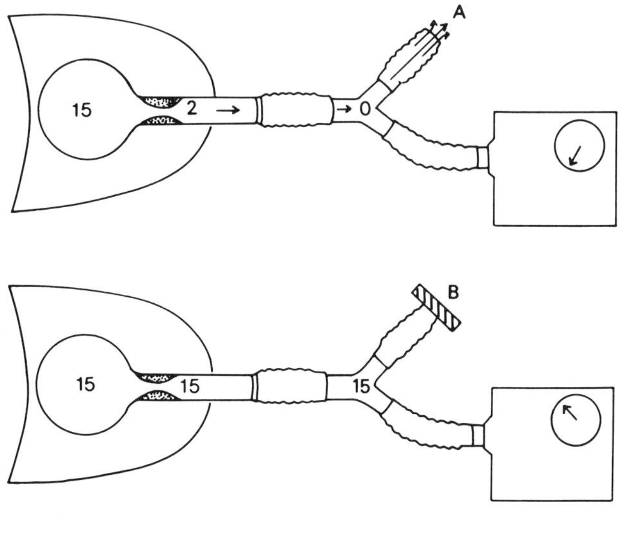

MEASURING ESOPHAGEAL PRESSURE

Fluctuations of global endothoracic pressure can be estimated by a well-positioned esophageal balloon. Esophageal pressure (Pes) enables estimation of force generation during spontaneous breathing and facilitates partitioning of transthoracic pressure into its lung and chest wall components during passive inflation.

TECHNIQUE

In the laboratory setting, the esophageal pressure is measured with a latex balloon (10 cm long) affixed to a multiperforated catheter stent and positioned in the lower or middle third of the esophagus.[63] The 10-cm length samples an adequate portion of the esophagus while minimizing the chance for artifact. (A shorter balloon can be influenced by regional pressure distortions near the heart and posterior mediastinum. A longer balloon may extend into the upper esophagus, a region that poorly reflects changes in global intrapleural pressure.[63,64]) A balloon volume of 0.2 to 0.5 mL transmits changes in intrathoracic pressure accurately during spontaneous cycles. Larger balloon volumes may stimulate esophageal contractions. However, to maintain sensitivity during positive-pressure breathing cycles, a

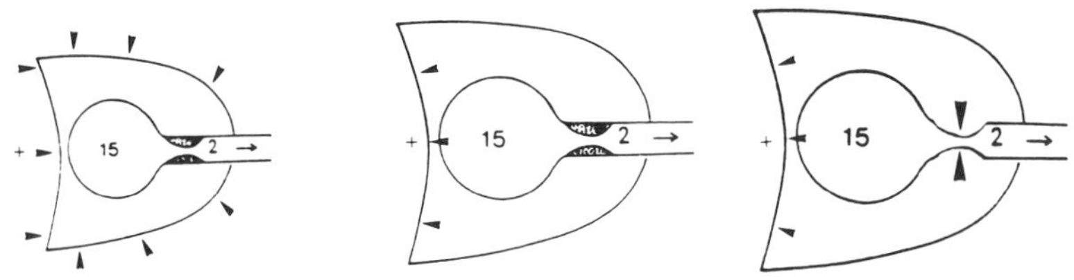

FIGURE 14-13 Three forms of auto-PEEP. Positive alveolar pressure at end exhalation may be due (in total or in part) to forceful expiratory muscle activity (left), to airflow obstruction without limitation to airflow during tidal breathing (middle), or to flow-limiting obstruction with dynamic airway collapse (right). Different mechanisms may coexist within different parts of the lung. Dynamic hyperinflation may or may not be significant when auto-PEEP develops in the setting of active muscular activity.

relatively large balloon volume (0.5 to 1.0 mL) is usually required. A larger volume prevents the balloon from collapsing against the catheter stent, damping the pressure signal. In the upright position, Pes reflects the absolute value of global intrathoracic pressure with acceptable accuracy, but Pes overestimates resting intrathoracic pressure in the supine posture. The weight of the mediastinal contents on the sensing balloon produces this artifact, which may be reduced or obviated by the lateral decubitus position.[65] Although Pes overestimates average Ppl in recumbent positions, *changes* in intrathoracic pressure are tracked well by a balloon in appropriate position.[66] Although the impact of a coexisting nasogastric tube or feeding tube on the accuracy of Pes has not been well studied, experiments in our laboratory suggest that a multiperforated esophageal balloon catheter continues to reflect changes in intrathoracic pressure with acceptable accuracy.

To position the esophageal balloon, one must first pass it into the stomach, a site identified by positive-pressure deflections during forceful inspiratory efforts (sniff test). The balloon is then withdrawn gradually until negative pressure deflections first appear, signaling the emergence of the uppermost hole of the balloon-enveloped portion of the catheter into the intrathoracic compartment. (The multiperforated catheter tends to transmit the most negative pressure to which the balloon is exposed.) The catheter is then withdrawn a distance equivalent to the balloon length ($\approx$10 cm) to ensure that the entire balloon rests in the lower and mid esophagus.[63] Appropriate position can be confirmed by measuring airway and esophageal pressure deflections simultaneously during efforts against an occluded airway.[67] When airway occlusion prevents air from flowing into the lungs, no pressure can dissipate against resistance during breathing efforts and lung volume remains unchanged. It then follows that, on average, no pressure gradient should develop between the occluded airway opening and the pleural space. Therefore, nearly equivalent deflections of airway and esophageal pressure indicate that the balloon is appropriately positioned (Fig. 14-14). Deflections of airway and Pes should agree within 10 percent. Precise balloon placement is much more difficult in the absence of spontaneous efforts. Under passive conditions, the balloon tip is advanced approximately 40 cm from the nostril. A combined nasogastric tube and esophageal balloon that serves a dual clinical purpose has been commercially available. This catheter appears to parallel changes in intrathoracic pressure quite well while simultaneously providing a channel for aspirating stomach contents or administering tube feedings.[68]

USES OF ESOPHAGEAL PRESSURE

Measurements of intrathoracic pressure can provide valuable clinical data. For example, ΔPes offers useful information when interpreting the end-expiratory wedge pressure under conditions of vigorous hyperpnea or elevated alveolar pressure (PEEP, auto-PEEP).[11] The Pes tracing allows calculation of lung compliance and airway resistance during spontaneous breathing and partitions total chest impedance into lung and chest wall components. ΔPes reflects the magnitude of patient effort during spontaneous or machine-aided breathing cycles. Although seldom used for this purpose, ΔPes can be used to compute the work of breathing across the lung and external circuit or to calculate the product of developed pressure and the duration of inspiratory effort (the pressure-time product). Fluctuations in central venous pressure can be used for a similar purpose,[69] but the vascular pressure tracing is variably damped and yields a low-range estimate of effort.

TRANSDIAPHRAGMATIC PRESSURE

Transdiaphragmatic pressure (Pdi), the difference between Pes and gastric pressure (Pga), is generated by a single inspiratory muscle (the diaphragm) and is used primarily in the research setting to quantify its effective contractile force.[70] Although Pdi is seldom used clinically, it is occasionally used in conjunction with phrenic nerve stimulation

FIGURE 14-14 Deflections of airway (Paw) and esophageal pressure (Pes) before and after airway occlusion. Note the nearly equal deflections of Paw and the pressure recorded from this well-placed catheter.

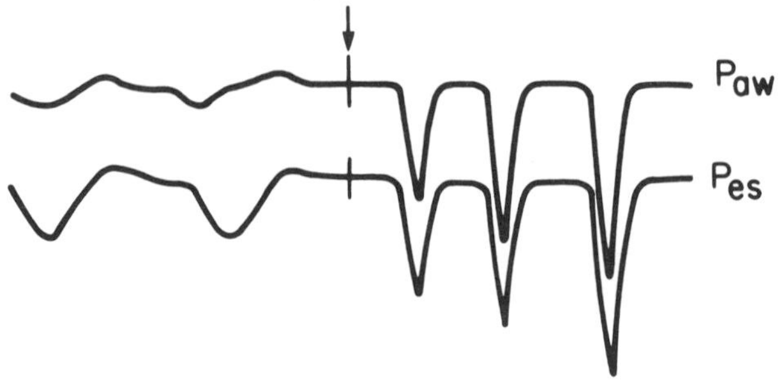

or voluntary effort (e.g., inspiration to TLC, Müeller maneuver, forceful sniffing) to investigate diaphragmatic paralysis.

INFLATION IMPEDANCE: VALUE OF CONTINUOUSLY MONITORING AIRWAY PRESSURE

A continuous tracing of Paw provides useful information commonly neglected at the bedside. Paw can be monitored using the transducer and display equipment normally used for measuring pressures in the pulmonary vasculature. A dedicated transducer must be used for this purpose, however, to avoid the risk of air embolism. Apart from enabling the estimation of R and C_{RS}, the waveform of inspiratory airway pressure traced during a controlled machine cycle provides a graphic representation of the inflation work performed by the ventilator at the particular combination of V_T and flow settings used (Fig.14-15). When inflation occurs passively during constant flow conditions, time and volume are linear analogs of one another. Therefore, the area under the pressure-time curve is proportionate to the pressure-volume work performed by the machine.[47] The mean inflation pressure ($\overline{Pi}$) is the work per liter of ventilation for the particular V_T and flow setting combination used. Provided that flow and V_T do not change, $\overline{Pi}$ indexes the average impedance to chest inflation. {Under passive, constant flow conditions, $\overline{Pi}$ can also be estimated from P_D and Ps without recording the pressure tracing by using the approximation $Pinsp = P_D - \frac{1}{2}[Ps - (PEEP + auto\text{-}PEEP)]$}. Mean Paw for the *entire breathing cycle*, a value correlated with gas exchange efficiency, hemodynamic compromise, and barotrauma, can be estimated as the product of $\overline{Pi}$ and the inspiratory time fraction, adjusted for the effect of applied PEEP:

$$\overline{Paw} = \overline{Pi}(ti/ttot) + PEEP(1 - ti/ttot). \quad (14\text{-}13)$$

Mean Palv deviates from mean Paw only when expiratory (Rex) and inspiratory (Ri) resistances significantly differ:

$$\overline{Palv} = \overline{Paw} + (\dot{V}_E/60)(Rex - Ri). \quad (14\text{-}14)$$

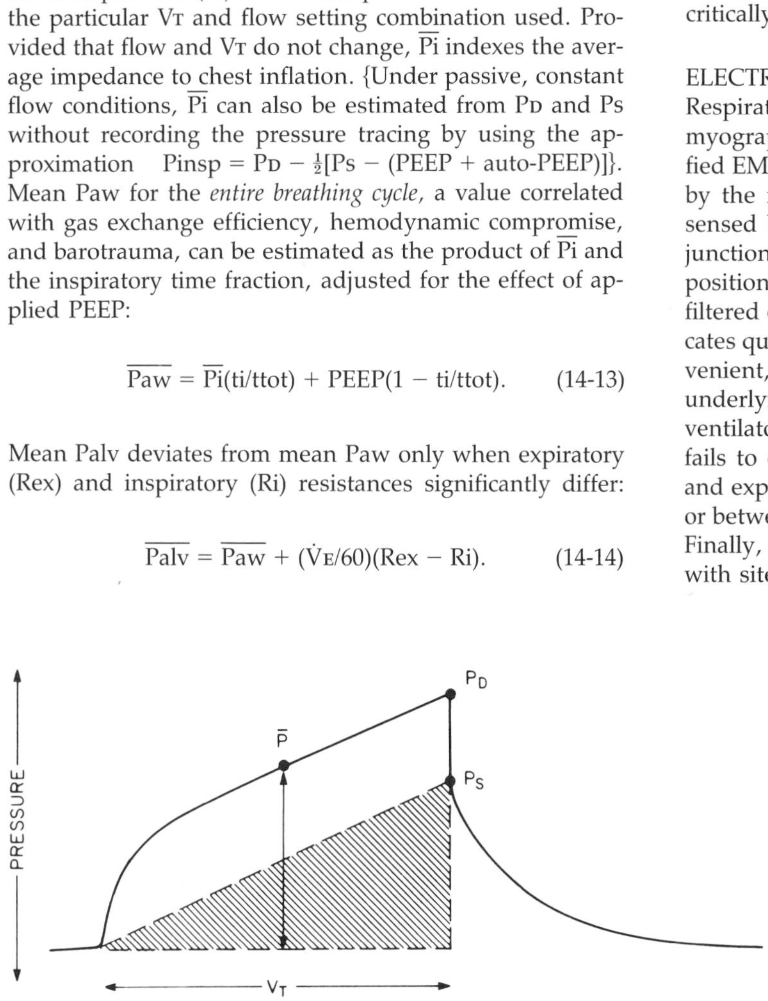

FIGURE 14-15 Tracing of airway pressure against inspired volume during controlled inflation of a passive subject under constant flow conditions. Designated points refer to the pressure that correspond to peak dynamic (P_D), peak static (Ps), and mean inspiratory ($\overline{P}$) values. $\overline{P}$ reflects the work done per liter of ventilation. The shaded area corresponds to inspiratory work done against elastic impedance of the lung and chest wall, whereas the unshaded area reflects work done against frictional impedance. (From Marini JJ: Work of breathing, in Kacmarek RM (ed): *Current Respiratory Care.* Philadelphia, Decker, 1988, pp 188–194, with permission.)

Monitoring Breathing Effort

MEASURES OF RESPIRATORY MUSCLE ACTIVITY

OXYGEN CONSUMPTION OF THE RESPIRATORY SYSTEM ($\dot{V}_{O_2}R$)

Measuring the oxygen consumed by the ventilatory pump ($\dot{V}_{O_2}R$) estimates effort at it most basic level, the level of cellular metabolism. In theory, $\dot{V}_{O_2}R$ accounts for all factors that tax the respiratory muscles, integrating the external workload ($\dot{W}$) and the efficiency (E) of the conversion mechanism: $\dot{V}_{O_2}R = \dot{W}/E$.[71] Two patients with different chest configurations, patterns of muscle activation, or degrees of coordination between the muscles of inspiration and expiration may perform identical external work but consume vastly different amounts of oxygen in the process. Because $\dot{V}_{O_2}R$ cannot be measured directly, total body oxygen consumption ($\dot{V}_{O_2}$) is tracked as ventilatory stresses (e.g., resistance or CO_2 inhalation) are imposed or relieved, perturbing the respiratory system. Without question, there is considerable "noise-to-signal" in such computations, and for reasons outlined earlier, $\dot{V}_{O_2}$ does not lend itself easily to the assessment of breathing effort in the quasi-stable, critically ill patient.

ELECTROMYOGRAPHY

Respiratory muscle activity can also be assessed by electromyography (EMG). The amplitude of an integrated, rectified EMG signal varies directly with the tension developed by the muscle it monitors.[72] Diaphragmatic EMG is best sensed by an electrode anchored at the gastroesophageal junction.[73] Unfortunately, such electrodes are difficult to position and cannot be left in place. Furthermore, unless filtered out, the amplitude of the ECG signal often complicates quantitative interpretation. Surface EMG is more convenient, but specificity of the probe for the small area of underlying muscle limits its utility as a global measure of ventilatory effort. Furthermore, the integrated *surface* EMG fails to discriminate between the activation of inspiratory and expiratory muscles, between tonic and phasic activity, or between respiratory and nonrespiratory muscle activity. Finally, because the amplitude of the EMG varies widely with site preparation, electrode location, and patient anatomy, no absolute standards exist for comparing breathing effort across patients.[73] Like $\dot{V}_{O_2}R$, the EMG is limited to tracking *relative* changes in the activity of the ventilatory system. Despite these drawbacks, EMG of the sternocleidomastoid muscle may offer a practical means of monitoring extrathoracic ventilatory effort.[74] In current ICU practice, transcutaneous nerve stimulation and EMG recording appears most useful in monitoring the depth of pharmacologic paralysis during mechanical ventilation.

DIRECT MEASURES OF EXTERNAL MECHANICAL OUTPUT

Work of Breathing

As already noted, the mechanical work of breathing and breathing effort are not synonymous. If breathing is inefficient, great effort can be expended without accomplishing measurable external work. Nonetheless, mechanical measures of pressure and volume are precisely measurable, and for the same patient tend to fluctuate in the same direction as breathing effort.

QUANTIFYING TOTAL WORK OF CHEST INFLATION. Mechanical work is performed when volume is inspired by a pressure gradient. At any volume (V) above the equilibrium position, a pressure difference is distributed in accordance with the simplified "equation of motion" of the respiratory system:[37]

$$\bar{P} = R(\dot{V}) + \frac{V}{C} \qquad (14\text{-}15)$$

The average pressure ($\bar{P}$) for tidal inflation can be approximated:

$$\bar{P} = R\left(\frac{V_T}{ti}\right) + \frac{V_T}{2C} + Pex \qquad (14\text{-}16)$$

where Pex is the end expiratory alveolar pressure, ti and V_T are inspiratory time and tidal volume, and $\bar{P}$ is numerically equivalent to the work per liter of ventilation.[75] Thus, if R, C, ti, and V_T are known for the spontaneously breathing subject, the *external* work rate can be easily estimated. Work per tidal breath (W_B) can be quantified from the area enclosed within a plot of transmural inflation pressure (P) against inspired volume or from the integrated product of P and $\dot{V}$ (Fig. 14-16):

$$W = \int P\dot{V}\, dt \qquad (14\text{-}17)$$

Total inspiratory mechanical work per minute (power) is the product of P and $\dot{V}_E$ or of W_B and *f*, the breathing frequency. With pressures and volumes expressed in their customary units, a convenient work unit is the joule (or watt-second) ≈10 (cmH_2O liters). One kilogram meter (kgM), another work unit, equals about 10 joules.

In the clinical setting, the objective is to define P, the total transstructural inflation pressure. When the ventilator per-

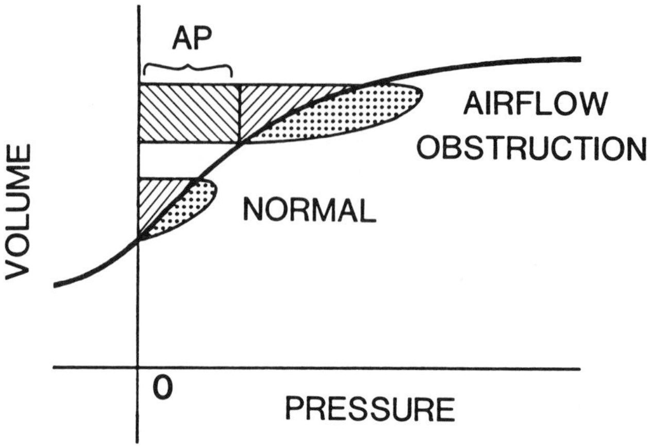

FIGURE 14-16 Plot of volume against transmural inflation pressure during spontaneous breathing for a normal subject and for a patient with severe airflow obstruction. The mechanical work of breathing, composed of frictional (stippled) and elastic (crosshatched) components, is quantified by the relevant pressure-volume areas. When present, auto-PEEP (AP) often contributes greatly to the elastic workload. (From Marini JJ: Ventilatory management of chronic obstructive pulmonary disease, in Cherniack NS (ed): *Chronic Obstructive Pulmonary Disease.* Philadelphia, Saunders, 1990, pp 495–506, with permission.)

forms the entire workload for a passive patient, inspiratory P is simply central airway pressure (referenced to atmospheric pressure). During constant flow conditions volume and time are linear analogs, so that the pressure tracing alone mimics the pressure-volume curve. If inflation is achieved with constant flow, $\bar{P}$ is approximated by the inflation pressure at midcycle (see Fig. 14-15).

To accurately estimate the work rate of spontaneous breathing, flow delivery during passive inflation must approximate the mean inspiratory flow rate of spontaneous breathing, the V_T delivered must be similar, and no inflation effort must occur. Unfortunately, such preconditions often cannot be accomplished without deep sedation or paralysis.

Patient Work During Spontaneous and Machine-Aided Cycles

TRIGGERED VOLUME-LIMITED MACHINE CYCLES. During volume-controlled ventilation, patient effort has generally been assumed negligible whenever the machine aids the breathing cycle. This assumption is undoubtedly correct during controlled ventilation, but recent data indicate that it is often invalid during patient-triggered, machine-assisted inflation.[76,77] Relaxation does not occur abruptly once the machine cycle begins. Rather, effort continues in proportion to respiratory drive and muscle strength.[77] Assuming that similar external work is required to inflate the chest under passive and active conditions, the external work performed by the patient can be quantified from the difference in machine work under passive and active conditions (constant flow and V_T) (Fig. 14-17). When the ventilation requirement or sense of dyspnea is high, or when the

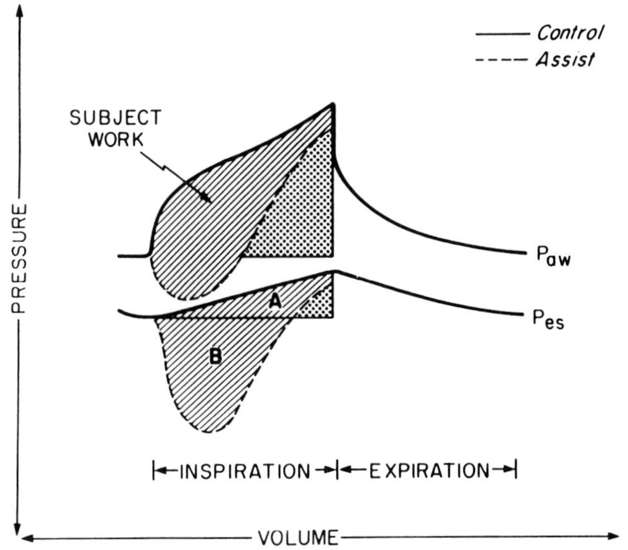

FIGURE 14-17 Active work performed by the patient during triggered volume-limited machine cycles. Because all patient effort originates in muscular contraction of the chest wall, either Paw or Pes can be used as the reference pressure. The hatched areas represent subject work. The stippled areas correspond to machine work. Area A is subject work performed in moving the chest wall. Area B is subject work done in moving the lung. (From Marini JJ: Monitoring during mechanical ventilation. Clin Chest Med 9(1):73, 1988, with permission.)

ventilator is poorly adjusted, exertion levels may approach those of unsupported breathing. Interestingly, the impedance characteristics of the chest (R and C) do not influence the patient's effort significantly, provided that the ventilator satisfies the patient's demand for inspiratory flow.

Any factor that amplifies respiratory drive adds to the patient's work of breathing during triggered machine cycles. Trigger sensitivity, peak flow setting, V_T, and end-expiratory pressure are the key physician-controlled variables. Clues to patient exertion during triggered machine cycles are available from inspection of the deformed and variable airway pressure tracing (Fig. 14-18). When an airway pressure tracing is not used, the only hint of vigorous inspiratory effort may be the stuttering rise of the manometer needle to its peak value. P_D itself may not be far different from the expected value, as patient effort weakens as lung volume increases toward the end of the inflation cycle.

FIGURE 14-18 Continuous airway pressure tracings during patient-triggered, machine-assisted breathing (assist control, constant flow). Uniformity of pressure contours and peak pressures (arrows) suggests synchrony between patient and machine. Asynchrony and excessive breathing workload are indicated by deformation of the normal configuration and variation of peak pressures due to inspiratory (A) or expiratory (B) effort during inflation. (From Reference 75, with permission.)

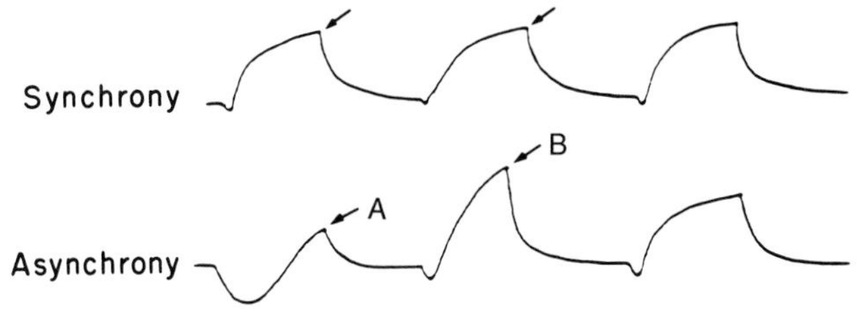

SPONTANEOUS BREATHING CYCLES. Although the work of breathing can be estimated using the equation of motion (see Eq. 14-16), an esophageal balloon is required to directly measure work during spontaneous or pressure-supported breathing cycles. The fluctuation in the segment of Ppl tracing which spans inspiration tracks patient effort against the impedance of the lung and external circuit. Care must be taken to include any component attributable to auto-PEEP. (When PEEP or CPAP is used, fluctuations of pressure should be referenced to the elevated base-line value of Pes.) Inspiratory work can be quantified by electronically integrating the product of Pes and flow or by measuring the area within a plot of Pes against inspired volume. The work done in expanding the chest wall cannot be directly measured during active breathing and must be estimated from published values of chest wall compliance or preferably from the inflation characteristic of the chest wall (Pes × V) traced during controlled (relaxed) inflation. The pressure required to inflate the passive chest wall is largely independent of the flow profile.

PRESSURE-SUPPORTED CYCLES. During ventilation with pressure-support (PSV), the flow profile varies. Consequently Paw tracks only machine work and cannot be used directly in assessing patient effort. The patient's component of the total inspiratory work of breathing can be gauged, nonetheless, using plots of Pes and inspired volume during passive and pressure-supported inflations. The patient's work during the pressure-supported breath can be roughly estimated as the difference between the total work required (gauged from the equation of motion) and the amount of work provided by the machine $\approx$Ps × V_T.

PRESSURE-TIME PRODUCT (PTP) AND PRESSURE-TIME INDEX (PTI)

Isometric components of muscle tension (which consume oxygen without contributing to volume change) fail to register as externally measured work, accounting in large part for the lack of agreement between $\dot{V}_{O_2}R$ and W_B.[78] A pressure-time product (PTP = P × ti) parallels effort and $\dot{V}_{O_2}R$ more closely than W_B because it includes the "isometric" component of muscle pressure and is less influenced by the impedance to contraction.[79] When P is referenced to the maximal isometric pressure that can be generated at FRC (Pmax) and inspiratory time is expressed as a fraction of total cycle length (ttot), a useful effort index is derived:[67]

$$PTI = \bar{P}/Pmax \times ti/ttot \qquad (14\text{-}18)$$

Values of PTI that exceed $\approx$0.15 identify highly stressful breathing workloads that may induce fatigue (see Chap. 133).

INFLUENCE OF AUTO-PEEP ON WB

Because pressure sufficient to counterbalance auto-PEEP must be applied before flow can be initiated, auto-PEEP imposes an inspiratory threshold load. Furthermore, a "block" of external work with the dimensions of auto-PEEP and inspired volume (Vt) forms an important part of the total pressure-volume work described by the equation of motion (Eq. 14-16):

$$W_B = \overline{P} \times Vt \qquad (14\text{-}19)$$

$$W_B = R\left(\frac{Vt^2}{ti}\right) + \left(\frac{Vt^2}{2C}\right) + (\text{auto-PEEP})\,(Vt) \qquad (14\text{-}20)$$

(During work calculations of triggered machine cycles, the additional work imposed by auto-PEEP is accounted for in the proportional elevation of the base-line control curve.) The threshold load imposed by auto-PEEP effectively reduces the trigger sensitivity of the machine to a value equal to the sum of auto-PEEP and the set value. Recent experimental work indicates that judicious use of low levels of CPAP or PEEP can help restore trigger sensitivity and reduce the work of breathing.[61,62,80]

Monitoring Ventilatory Drive and Breathing Pattern

Apart from measuring the components of $\dot{V}_E$ and inspecting the accessory muscles of respiration, few clinicians attempt to assess the magnitude of respiratory drive and breathing pattern on a routine basis. Yet, assessment of respiratory control may be considered central to scientific ventilator management.

IMPORTANCE OF ASSESSING VENTILATORY DRIVE

Considering that ventilatory drive is a primary correlate of dyspnea and the ability to ventilate, it is remarkable that so little clinical attention has previously been paid to drive measurement. Heightened ventilatory drive may signal important perturbations of the cardiopulmonary system. Furthermore, during machine-assisted breathing cycles, ventilatory drive plays a more important role in determining the energy expenditure of the patient than any indicator of ventilatory mechanics, provided the inspiratory flow delivered by the machine exceeds spontaneous flow demand.[77] Derangements in ventilatory drive may also furnish clues regarding the ability of the patient to wean from ventilatory support. Several recent clinical studies demonstrate that most patients who fail to wean from mechanical ventilation have elevated drives to breathe.[81] Interestingly, however, although the base-line levels of drive are high, the increase in ventilatory drive expected in response to CO_2 stimulation fails to occur in patients who cannot be removed from machine support[81] (Fig. 14-19).

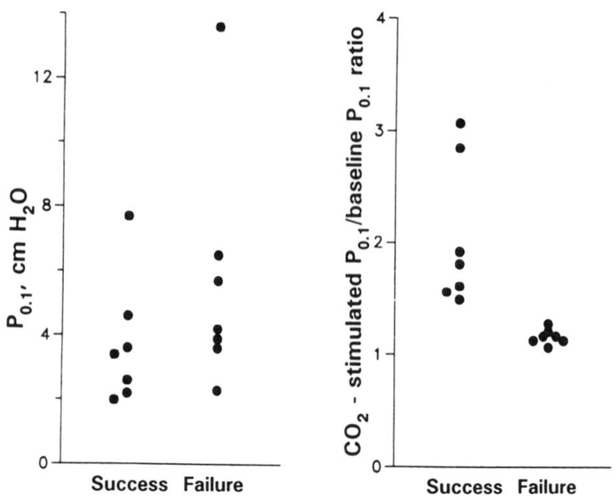

FIGURE 14-19 Airway occlusion pressure ($P_{0.1}$) responses in patients being weaned from mechanical ventilation. *Left.* Note the overlap in values between the patients who were successfully weaned and those who failed the weaning trial. *Right.* The ratio of CO_2-stimulated $P_{0.1}$ to base-line $P_{0.1}$ in the same patients. Note the excellent correspondence of weaning success to response to CO_2 inhalation. (From Reference 92, which is based on data from Reference 81, with permission.)

INDICES OF DRIVE

FLOW-BASED MEASURES: $\dot{V}_E$ AND MEAN INSPIRATORY FLOW

Several methods can be used to index drive during critical illness. When respiratory mechanics and strength reserves are normal, the spontaneous $\dot{V}_E$ directly parallels the output of the ventilatory center. Unfortunately, these conditions are seldom met in the clinical setting. Mean inspiratory flow (Vt/ti), another good indicator of drive in the normal subject, also depends on the mechanical properties of the ventilatory system. Vt/ti is therefore of limited utility, unless used to compare two conditions over time in the same individual whose chest mechanics and muscle strength neither deteriorate nor improve.

AIRWAY OCCLUSION PRESSURE AT 100 MSEC ($P_{0.1}$)

Although influenced to some degree by muscle strength (and therefore by lung volume), the inspiratory pressure developed in the first 100 msec of surreptitious airway occlusion ($P_{0.1}$) is not affected by chest impedance because it is an isometric measurement. Furthermore, the $P_{0.1}$ is measured prior to conscious recognition or reflex response to occlusion, so that the corresponding outflow from the respiratory center reflects the unimpeded cycles that precede it. In the laboratory setting, determinations of $P_{0.1}$ require special apparatus to enable surreptitious interruption of the inspiratory circuit, and the average of three to five measurements is used to minimize the effect of inherent breath-to-breath variation. This type of occlusion maneuver is feasible to conduct at the bedside using a sensitive airway pressure transducer, a phase-adjusted flow transducer, and a calibrated strip chart recorder running at rapid speed. It is, however, inconvenient and time-consuming. Furthermore, the ventilator circuit must be modified to enable noiseless occlusion by a balloon or shutter valve.

The delay imposed by the demand valve systems of certain ventilators in common use provides a quasi-occlusion period long enough to allow close estimation of $P_{0.1}$.[77,82] In normal subjects, this value for $P_{0.1}$ correlates very well with the formal occlusion technique across a wide range of ventilation requirements. Either airway or esophageal pressure can be used for this purpose. The advantage of this method is that every recorded breath potentially provides an estimate of $P_{0.1}$, without the need for circuit modification, technical expertise, time investment, or interruption of the breathing rhythm. $P_{0.1}$ is ideally measured from the onset of inspiratory effort, which generally begins a very short time before flow reversal occurs. If a simultaneous flow tracing is available, either the inflection point of effort onset or the point of ZF can be precisely measured. For clinical purposes, however, the point of ZF usually coincides with the departure of Paw from the end-expiratory pressure base line, obviating the need for flow measurement. What's more, the slope of the Paw tracing during the first 0.1 to 0.25 s of occlusion is usually constant, facilitating $P_{0.1}$ estimation.

Monitoring Strength and Muscle Reserve

The output demanded of the ventilatory muscles is dictated by the product of $\dot{V}_E$ and the work or oxygen cost per liter of ventilation (vide supra). However, the ability of the patient to sustain independent breathing must not be judged on the basis of any absolute value for workload, but rather on workload interpreted against the background of muscular strength and endurance.

STRENGTH MEASURES

Without full patient cooperation it is questionable that any measure of strength can reflect the full capability for pressure development. The two measures of respiratory muscle strength most commonly used in the clinical setting are the vital capacity (VC) and the maximum inspiratory pressure (MIP) generated against an occluded airway.[57]

VITAL CAPACITY

In *acute* disorders of neuromuscular function, VC tends to be preserved relative to MIP for two primary reasons. First, the pressure-volume relationship of the thorax is convex to the volume axis. Second, whereas many seriously ill patients can generate brief spikes of inspiratory pressure, few can or will sustain inspiratory effort long enough to achieve the plateau of their volume curve. Depending on the information desired from the VC, a "stacked" VC may be useful in this setting (Fig. 14-20).[83] This technique measures volume on the inspiratory limb and uses a one-way valve to enable the patient to rest at an elevated volume between

ALTERNATIVE METHOD FOR VITAL CAPACITY ESTIMATION

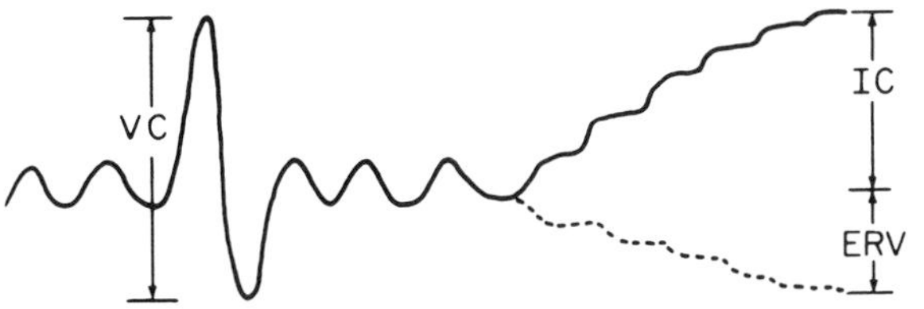

FIGURE 14-20 Spirometric tracing during conventional (VC) maneuver and during "stacked" VC maneuver, conducted by using one-way valves to obtain inspiratory capcity (IC) and expiratory reserve volume (ERV). (From Reference 83, with permission.)

inspiratory efforts. The patient need not cooperate fully with testing—the naturally escalating inspiratory drive to breathe evokes forceful effort. For the same achieved volume, the peak Pes developed during breath stacking and during the standard inspiratory capacity (IC) maneuver are similar. Use of the breath-stacking technique may allow more effective incentive spirometry, particularly with respect to the duration of hyperinflation.[84] A large discrepancy between the conventional and stacked VC may be seen in patients too weak, too uncooperative, or too air-hungry to sustain a single inspiratory effort. Although a stacked VC may reflect the elastic properties of the lungs and chest wall more accurately than a conventional VC maneuver, its ability to accurately reflect strength has yet to be determined.

As the supine position is assumed, VC falls by <20 percent in normal individuals and only slightly more in patients with unilateral diaphragmatic dysfunction. A positioned change in VC >30 percent suggests bilateral diaphragmatic dysfunction or paralysis, particularly if paradoxical abdominal motion and orthopnea are observed. Although fluoroscopy can be helpful in detecting *unilateral* diaphragmatic paralysis, there are many false negative tests. Fluoroscopy is even more unreliable when both leaves of the diaphragm are dysfunctional. When suspected, diaphragmatic dysfunction can be confirmed using esophageal and gastric pressure measurements.

MAXIMAL INSPIRATORY PRESSURE

Assuming full cooperation, a symmetrical reduction in inspiratory and expiratory maximal respiratory pressures strongly suggests generalized muscle weakness. (Although maximal expiratory pressures are seldom measured in critically ill patients, a good *qualitative* indication of expiratory muscle strength can sometimes be observed in the vigor of the coughing effort.) When recording the MIP, lung volume should be trapped in the range between residual volume (RV) and FRC to optimize the mechanical advantage of the inspiratory muscles.[85–87] In poorly cooperative subjects, it is equally important to wait sufficient time to elicit a near maximal increase in respiratory drive. Approximately 20 s or 10 breathing efforts are required to elicit the maximal pressure response from a poorly cooperative patient.[88] The patient must not be overventilated nor overstressed before data recording, and occlusion of the airway must occur at FRC or lesser volume. Introducing a one-way valve that selectively permits expiration ensures that inspiratory efforts initiated late in the series occur at a volume between FRC and residual volume. With each breathing effort, additional air is pumped from the thorax, improving the mechanical advantage of the inspiratory muscles and amplifying respiratory drive.[85,89] Measured in this way, the MIP of most patients on mechanical ventilation exceeds −40 mmHg (−52 cmH_2O), even as they remain ventilator dependent.[88] (Although outward recoil of the chest wall can contribute to the MIP at volumes below the equilibrium point, expiratory reserve volume and outward chest wall recoil is seldom very large in the recumbent position.)

MEASURES OF ENDURANCE

BREATHING PATTERN: FREQUENCY, TIDAL VOLUME, AND INSPIRATORY TIME FRACTION

The breathing pattern provides valuable information often underutilized in the clinical setting. As $\dot{V}_E$ increases during normal exercise, frequency and V_T tend to rise in parallel until V_T approaches a certain fraction of the VC, generally in the range of 50 to 60 percent.[90] At that point, V_T plateaus and frequency accelerates to meet further increases in the ventilation requirement. For the same $\dot{V}_E$, large V_T's require more pressure development than small ones. However, increased V_{DS} is the cost of increasing the breathing frequency (f) while limiting the elastic work expenditure of each individual breath. Thus, although work per breath (W_B) is controlled by limiting V_T, total work (the product of f and W_B) and force output per minute tend to increase beyond some optimal value of f. A continuously rising frequency (to rates exceeding 30 breaths/min) is generally accepted as a warning sign of ventilatory muscle decompensation, especially if f rises as V_T falls.[39] As recently demonstrated by Yang and Tobin, a frequency: V_T ratio >100 breaths · min^{-1}/L may indicate impending fatigue[91] (Fig. 14-21). It should be noted, however, that some patients can increase breathing frequency to a stable 35 or 40 breaths/min and remain well compensated, and even comfortable. At moderate workloads (as during exercise), the breathing rhythm actually becomes more regular with respect to V_T and cycle length. The fatiguing ventilatory system tends to demonstrate breathing patterns that are arrhythmic, disorganized, or frankly chaotic.[92]

As the ventilatory muscles fatigue, the fraction of the breathing cycle spent in inspiration also changes. Under a breathing stress, the ratio between inspiratory time (ti) and the total time available for the breath (ttot) normally increases from ≈0.35 to a value in the range of 0.4 to 0.5. A longer ti taxes the inspiratory muscles by augmenting the tension-time index ($\bar{P}/Pmax \times ti/ttot$).[67,79,93] At the limits of compensation the ti/ttot fails to increase with further stress and may actually decline.

At times of maximal effort, noteworthy alterations may be observed in the pattern of activation and coordination of the ventilatory muscle groups.[94–96] Although normally passive, expiratory muscles may be called into play during expiratory airflow obstruction, when high levels of PEEP or CPAP are used, when the patient is anxious, when machine delivered inspiratory duration is excessive, and when the inspiratory muscles face a stressful burden in relation to their capability.[97] Visible use of the accessory muscles, especially the sternocleidomastoid group, may also signal the approach to the limits of ventilatory compensation.[98]

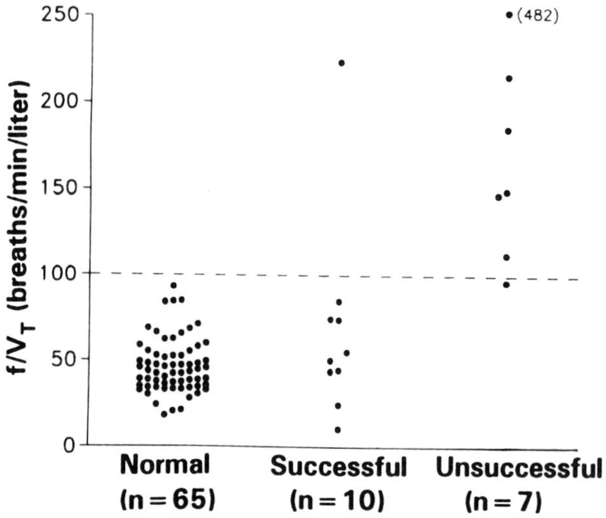

FIGURE 14-21 The ratio of respiratory frequency: tidal volume (f/V_T, breaths/min/L), an index of rapid shallow breathing, in healthy subjects, and in patients being weaned from mechanical ventilation. All but one of the patients who failed the weaning trial had a ratio of ≥100, indicating rapid shallow breathing, whereas 90 percent of the patients in the "success" group had a ratio of <100. (From Tobin MJ, Yang K. Respiratory muscle dysfunction in patients being weaned from mechanical ventilation, in Tobin MJ (ed): *Problems in Critical Care.* Philadelphia, Lippincott, 1990, pp 423–443, which is based on data from Tobin MJ, Chadha TS, Jenouri G, et al: Breathing patterns: 1. Normal subjects. Chest 84:202, 1983, and Reference 96, with permission.)

Two indices once thought to indicate diaphragmatic dysfunction or fatigue—asynchrony between the peak excursions of chest and abdominal compartments and paradoxical inward movement of the abdomen on inspiration—may simply reflect the response to a system under extraordinary stress (Fig. 14-22).[96,99] Asynchrony between the excursions of rib cage and abdomen may be a stage in the development of full-blown abdominal paradox. Respiratory alternans, another reported pattern of fatigue in which the muscles of the chest cage and diaphragm alternate primary responsibility for achieving ventilation,[94] is much less commonly observed. Certain of these patterns appear to be more common in specific types of loading, but the question is not well studied.

Inductance (impedance) plethysmography provides a noninvasive means of monitoring the ventilatory frequency, V_T, ti fraction, and respiratory muscle coordination. With this technique, loose elastic bands are placed about the chest and abdomen. Changes in compartmental volume create proportional changes in the cross-sectional

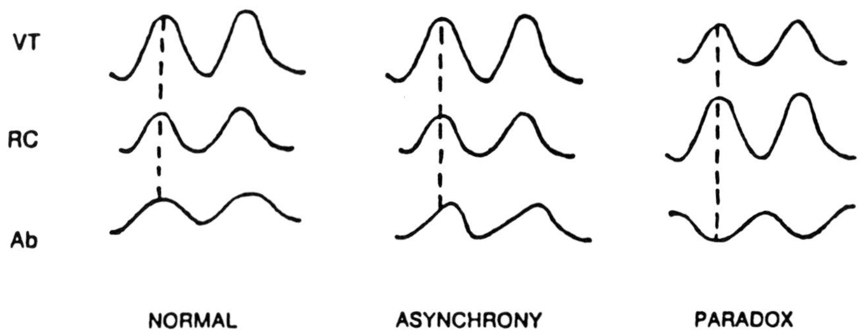

FIGURE 14-22 Inductance plethysmographic tracings of the movements of the rib cage (RC), the abdomen (Ab) and their sum (VT) against time under three levels of stress. Dashed lines are drawn at the time of maximal inspiratory volume achieved by the respiratory system. (From Dantzker DR, Tobin MJ: Monitoring respiratory muscle function. Respir Care 30:422, 1985, with permission.)

areas of electrical inductance loops. Resulting signal fluctuations track compartmental motion and can be summed to estimate overall VT changes. The ratio of total compartmental excursion (amplitude):tidal volume (the MCA/VT ratio) may be a useful indicator of ventilatory distress and provides tangible evidence of mechanically inefficient neuromuscular coupling.[96]

MECHANICAL RESERVE

Such simple indices of ventilatory power reserve as the ratio of $\dot{V}$E:maximum minute ventilation, and the VT/VC have been used for many years to predict the outcome of machine withdrawal. Both on theoretical[93] and on empirical grounds it has been suggested that neither ratio should exceed 50 percent.[57]

ELECTROMYOGRAPHY

The myriad of frequencies that comprise the EMG signal can be filtered for high frequency (50 to 100 Hz) and low frequency (0 to 25 Hz) content. A falling H/L ratio is a sensitive indicator of ventilatory stress and may be a sensitive but nonspecific indicator of developing fatigue.[100] Unfortunately, technically satisfactory EMG is not easily achieved in the ICU, and advanced signal conditioning is required to compute the H/L ratio.

PRESSURE-TIME INDEX

Measured accurately, the MIP can theoretically be used in conjunction with an estimate of the mean inspiratory pressure per spontaneous breath ($\bar{P}$, calculated from the equation of motion) to judge endurance and the likelihood of success when attempting to withdraw mechanical ventilation. In the laboratory setting a $\bar{P}$/Pmax ratio for the diaphragm exceeding 40 percent (with ti/ttot = 0.40) or a pressure-time index (PTI = $\bar{P}$/Pmax × ti/ttot) exceeding 0.15 predicts the inability to sustain a target load.[101] The appropriate ratio for the Pes is not known, but may well be higher. Although no confirmatory data are yet available for the specific clinical setting of the weaning trial, Milic-Emili has recently suggested that data available from the current literature are consistent with these guidelines.[102]

SEQUENTIAL DRIVE INDICES

A practical indication of power reserve may also be provided in a comparison of sequential drive indices, such as the $P_{0.1}$. The $P_{0.1}$ tends to be unusually high at the onset of a failed weaning trial.[81,103] From recent work, it appears that patients who fail to wean from mechanical ventilation do not amplify $P_{0.1}$ appropriately as the Pa_{CO_2} rises.[81] On the other hand, successful candidates demonstrate a significant increment in $P_{0.1}$ when challenged with inspired CO_2. Final judgment on the value of the $P_{0.1}$ as an indicator of ventilatory reserve must await more detailed study.

Acknowledgement

I thank Lisa Scherer for invaluable assistance in preparation of the typescript.

References

1. Cady EB, Costello A, Dawson MJ, et al: Noninvasive investigation of cerebral metabolism in newborn infants by phosphorus nuclear magnetic resonance spectroscopy. Lancet 1:1059, 1983.
2. Hands LJ, Bore PJ, Galloway G, et al: Muscle metabolism in patients with peripheral vascular disease investigated by ^{31}P nuclear magnetic resonance spectroscopy. Clin Sci 71:283, 1986.
3. Malley WJ. *Clinical Blood Gases*. Philadelphia, Saunders. 1990.
4. Shapiro BA, Cane RD, Chomka CM, et al: Preliminary evaluation of an intra-arterial blood gas system in dogs and humans. Crit Care Med 17:455, 1989.
5. Chaudhary BA, Burki NK: Ear oximetry in clinical practice. Am Rev Respir Dis 117:173, 1978.
6. Taylor MB, Whitwam JG: The current status of pulse oximetry. Anesthesia 41:943, 1986.
7. Fleury B, Murciano C, Talamo C, et al: Work of breathing in patients with chronic obstructive pulmonary disease in acute respiratory failure. Am Rev Respir Dis 131:822, 1985.
8. Harris K: Noninvasive monitoring of gas exchange. Respir Care 32:544, 1987.
9. Armstrong RF, Andrew D, Cohen SL, et al: Continuous monitoring of mixed venous oxygen tension $P\bar{v}_{O_2}$ in cardiorespiratory disorders. Lancet 1:632, 1978.
10. Suter PM, Lindauer JM, Fairley HB, et al: Errors in data derived from pulmonary artery blood gas values. Crit Care Med 3:175, 1975.
11. Marini JJ: Hemodynamic monitoring using the pulmonary artery catheter. Crit Care Clin 2(3):551, 1986.

12. Kandel G, Aberman A: Mixed venous oxygen saturation. Its role in the assessment of the critically ill patient. Arch Intern Med 143:1400, 1983.
13. Kasmitz P, Druger GI, Yorra F, et al: Mixed venous oxygen tension and hyperlactatemia survival in severe cardiopulmonary disease. JAMA 236:570, 1976.
14. Heiselman D, Jones J, Cannon L: Continuous monitoring of mixed venous oxygen saturation in septic shock. J Clin Monit 2:237, 1986.
15. Severinghaus JW: Transcutaneous blood gas analysis. Respir Care 27:152, 1982.
16. Yahav J, Mindorrf C, Levison H: The validity of the transcutaneous oxygen tension method in infants and children with cardiorespiratory problems. Am Rev Respir Dis 124:586, 1981.
17. Eberhard P, Mindt W, Schafer R: Cutaneous blood gas monitoring in the adult. Crit Care Med 9:702, 1981.
18. Tremper KK, Shoemaker WC. Transcutaneous oxygen monitoring of critically ill adults with and without low-flow shock. Crit Care Med 9:706, 1981.
19. Tremper KK, Shoemaker WC, Shippy CR, et al: Transcutaneous P_{CO_2} monitoring on adult patients in the ICU and operating room. Crit Care Med 9:752, 1981.
20. McLellan PA, Goldstein RS, Rebuck AS: Transcutaneous carbon dioxide monitoring. Am Rev Respir Dis 124:199, 1981.
21. Abraham E, Smith M, Silver L: Conjunctival and transcutaneous oxygen monitoring during cardiac arrest and cardiopulmonary resuscitation. Crit Care Med 12:419, 1984.
22. Isenberg SJ, Shoemaker WC: The transconjunctival oxygen monitor. Am J Ophthalmol 95:803, 1984.
23. Browning JA, Linberg SE, Turney SZ, et al: The effects of fluctuating $F_{I_{O_2}}$ on metabolic measurements in mechanically ventilated patients. Crit Care Med 10:82, 1982.
24. Bartlett RH, Dechert RE, Mault JR, et al: Measurement of metabolism in multiple organ failure. Surgery 92:771, 1982.
25. Dantzker DR: Mechanisms of hypoxemia and hypercapnia, in Bone RC (ed): *Critical Care: A Comprehensive Approach.* Park Ridge, IL, American College of Chest Physicians, 1984, pp 1–14.
26. West JB: Ventilation perfusion relationships. Am Rev Respir Dis 116:919, 1977.
27. Hess D, Maxwell C: Which is the best index of oxygenation: $P(A - a)_{O_2}$, Pa_{O_2}/PA_{O_2} or $Pa_{O_2}/F_{I_{O_2}}$? Respir Care 30:961, 1985.
28. Gilbert R, Keighley JF: The arterial/alveolar oxygen tension ratio: An index of gas exchange applicable to varying oxygen concentrations. Am Rev Respir Dis 109:142, 1974.
29. Nunn JF: *Applied Respiratory Physiology.* 2d ed. Boston, Butterworths, 1977, pp 354–357.
30. Murray JF: *The Normal Lung.* 2nd ed. Philadelphia, Saunders, 1986, pp 199–200.
31. Murray IP, Modell JH, Gallagher TJ, et al: Titration of PEEP by arterial minus end-tidal carbon dioxide gradient. Chest 85:100, 1984.
32. Fallat RJ: Respiratory monitoring, in Bone RC (ed): *Critical Care: A Comprehensive Approach.* Park Ridge, IL, American College of Chest Physicians, 1984, pp 189–205.
33. Blanch L, Fernandez R, Benito S, et al: Effect of PEEP on the arterial end-tidal carbon dioxide gradient. Chest 92:451, 1987.
34. Milic-Emili J, Polysongsang Y: Respiratory mechanics in the adult respiratory distress syndrome. Crit Care Med 2:573, 1986.
35. Osborn JJ: Use of end-tidal P_{CO_2} in monitoring. Pract Cardiol 8(7):85, 1982.
36. Bakow E: A limitation of capnography. Respir Care 27:167, 1982.
37. Otis AB, Fenn WO, Rahn H: Mechanics of breathing in man. J Appl Physiol 2:592, 1950.
38. Suter PM, Fairley HB, Isenberg MD: Optimum end-expiratory pressure in patients with acute pulmonary failure. N Engl J Med 292:284, 1975.
39. Suter PM: Appropriate lung distention for gas exchange in ARDS. Chest 85:4, 1984.
40. Lamy M, Fallat RJ, Koeniger E, et al: Pathologic features and mechanics of hypoxemia in adult respiratory distress syndrome. Am Rev Respir Dis 114:267, 1976.
41. Matamis D, LeMaire F, Harf A, et al: Total respiratory pressure volume curves in the adult respiratory distress syndrome. Chest 86:58, 1984.
42. Comroe JH: *Physiology of Respiration.* 2d ed. Chicago, Year Book Medical Publishers, 1974, pp 104–105.
43. O'Quin R, Marini JJ, Culver BH, Butler J: Transmission of airway pressure to the pleural space during lung edema and chest wall restriction. J Appl Physiol: Respirat, Environ Exercise Physiol 59(4):1171, 1985.
44. Benito S, Lemaire F: Pulmonary pressure-volume relationship in acute respiratory distress syndrome in adults: Risk of positive end-expiratory pressure. J Crit Care 5(1):27, 1990.
45. Katz JA, Zinn SE, Ozanne GM, et al: Pulmonary, chest wall, and lung-thorax elastances in acute respiratory failure. Chest 80:304, 1981.
46. Chapin JC, Downs JB, Douglas ME, et al: Lung expansion, airway pressure transmission and positive end-expiratory pressure. Arch Surg 114:1193, 1979.
47. Marini JJ, Rodriguez RM, Lamb VJ: Bedside estimation of the inspiratory work of breathing during mechanical ventilation. Chest 89(1):56, 1986.
48. Capps JS, Hicks GH: Monitoring non-gas respiratory variables during mechanical ventilation. Respir Care 32:558, 1987.
49. Bone RC: Monitoring ventilatory mechanics in acute respiratory failure. Respir Care 28:597, 1983.
50. Gay PC, Rodarte JR, Tayyab M, et al: Evaluation of bronchodilator responsiveness in mechanically ventilated patients. Am Rev Respir Dis 136:880, 1987.
51. Bates JHT, Rossi A, Milic-Emili J: Analysis of the behavior of the respiratory system with constant inspiratory flow. J Appl Physiol 58(6):1840, 1985.
52. Gottfried SB, Rossi A, Higgs BD, et al: Noninvasive determination of respiratory system mechanics during mechanical ventilation for acute respiratory failure. Am Rev Respir Dis 131:672, 1985.
53. Rossi A, Gottfried SB, Higgs BD, et al: Respiratory mechanics in mechanically ventilated patients with respiratory failure. J Appl Physiol 58:1849, 1985.
54. Rossi A, Gottfried SB, Zocchi L, et al: Measurement of static compliance of the total respiratory system in patients with acute respiratory failure during mechanical ventilation. The effect of "intrinsic PEEP." Am Rev Respir Dis 131:672, 1985.
55. Gottfried SB, Rossi A, Higgs BD, et al: Noninvasive determination of respiratory system mechanics during mechanical ventilation for acute respiratory failure. Am Rev Respir Dis 131:414, 1985.
56. Kimball WR, Leith DE, Robins AG: Dynamic hyperinflation and ventilator dependence in chronic obstructive pulmonary disease. Am Rev Respir Dis 126:991, 1982.
57. Sahn SA, Lakshminarayan S, Petty TL: Weaning from mechanical ventilation. JAMA 235:2208, 1976.
58. Wright PW, Marini JJ, Bernard GR: In vitro versus in vivo comparison of endotracheal tube airflow resistance. Am Rev Respir Dis 140(1):10, 1989.

59. Pepe PE, Marini JJ: Occult positive end-expiratory pressure in mechanically ventilated patients with airflow obstruction: The auto-PEEP effect. Am Rev Respir Dis 126:166, 1982.
60. Simon BA, Weinmann C, Mitzner W: Mean airway pressure and alveolar pressure during high frequency ventilation. J Appl Physiol 57:1069, 1984.
61. Smith TC, Marini JJ, Lamb VJ: The effect of PEEP on auto-PEEP. Abstract. Chest 89(suppl):443S, 1986.
62. Smith TC, Marini JJ, Lamb VJ: The inspiratory threshold load resulting from airtrapping during mechanical ventilation. Abstract. Am Rev Respir Dis 135:A52, 1987.
63. Macklem PT: *Procedures for Standardized Measurements of Lung Mechanics.* Bethesda, National Heart Institute, 1974.
64. Knowles JH, Hony SK, Rahn H: Possible errors using esophageal balloon in determination of pressure volume characteristics of the lung and thoracic cage. J Appl Physiol 14:525, 1959.
65. Craven KD, Wood LDH: Extrapericardial and esophageal pressures with positive end-expiratory pressure in dogs. J Appl Physiol 51:798, 1981.
66. Baydur A, Behrakis PK, Zin WA, et al: A simple method for assessing the validity of the esophageal balloon technique. Am Rev Respir Dis 126:788, 1982.
67. Bellemare F, Grassino A: Effect of pressure and timing of contraction on human diaphragm fatigue. J Appl Physiol 53:1190, 1982.
68. Gillespie DJ: Comparison of intraesophageal pressure measurements with a nasogastric esophageal balloon system in volunteers. Am Rev Respir Dis 126:583, 1982.
69. Smiseth OA, Refsum H, Tyberg JV: Pericardial pressure assessed by right atrial pressure. A basis for calculation of left ventricular transmural pressure. Am Heart J 108:603, 1984.
70. Nunn JF: *Applied Respiratory Physiology.* 2d ed. Boston, Butterworths, 1977, pp 464–469.
71. Roussos C, Campbell EJM: Respiratory muscle energetics, in Fishman AP, Macklem PT, Mead J (eds): *Handbook of Physiology.* Bethesda, American Physiological Society, 1986, pp 481–510.
72. Bigland B, Lippold OCJ: The relation between force, velocity and integrated electrical activity in human muscles. J Physiol (London) 123:214, 1954.
73. Loring SH, Bruce EW: Methods for study of the chest wall, in Fishman AP, Macklem PT, Mead J (eds): *Handbook of Physiology.* Bethesda, American Physiological Society, 1986, pp 415–428.
74. Moxham J, Niles CM, Newham D, et al: Sternocleidomastoid function and fatigue in man. Clin Sci Mol Med 59:463, 1980.
75. Marini JJ: The role of the inspiratory circuit in the work of breathing during mechanical ventilation. Respir Care 32(6):419, 1987.
76. Marini JJ, Capps JS, Culver BH: The inspiratory work of breathing during assisted mechanical venilation. Chest 87(5):612, 1985.
77. Marini JJ, Rodriguez RM, Lamb VJ: The inspiratory workload of patient-initiated mechanical ventilation. Am Rev Respir Dis 134:902, 1986.
78. McGregor M, Becklake M: The relationship of oxygen costs of breathing to respiratory mechanical work and respiratory force. J Clin Invest 40:971, 1961.
79. Roussos C: Energetics, in Roussos C, Macklem PT (eds): *The Thorax.* New York, Marcel Dekker, 1985, pp 437–492.
80. Simkovitz P, Brown K, Goldberg P, et al: Interaction between intrinsic and externally applied PEEP during mechanical ventilation. Abstract. Am Rev Respir Dis 135:A202, 1987.
81. Montgomery AB, Holle RHO, Neagley SR, et al: Prediction of successful ventilator weaning using airway occlusion pressure and hypercapnic challenge. Chest 4:496, 1987.
82. Taylor RF, Marini JJ, Smith TC, et al: Bedside estimation of respiratory drive during machine-assisted ventilation. Abstract. Am Rev Respir Dis 135:A51, 1987.
83. Marini JJ, Rodriguez RM, Lamb VJ: Involuntary breath stacking. An alternative method for vital capcity estimation in poorly cooperative subjects. Am Rev Respir Dis 134:694, 1986.
84. Baker WL, Lamb VJ, Marini JJ: Breath stacking increases the depth and duration of chest expansion by incentive spirometry. Am Rev Respir Dis 141:343, 1990.
85. Black LF, Hyatt RE: Maximal respiratory pressures. Normal values and relationship to age and sex. Am Rev Respir Dis 99:696, 1969.
86. Black LF, Hyatt RE: Maximal static respiratory pressure in generalized neuromuscular disease. Am Rev Respir Dis 103:641, 1971.
87. Byrd RB, Hyatt RE: Maximal static respiratory pressures in chronic obstructive lung disease. Am Rev Respir Dis 98:848, 1968.
88. Marini JJ, Smith TC, Lamb VJ: Estimation of inspiratory muscle strength in mechanically ventilated patients: The measurement of maximal inspiratory pressure. J Crit Care 1(1):32, 1986.
89. Godfrey S, Campbell EJM: The control of breath holding. Respir Physiol 4:385, 1968.
90. Jensen JI, Lyager S, Pederson OF: The relationship between maximal ventilation, breathing pattern and mechanical limitation of ventilation. J Physiol 309:521, 1980.
91. Yang KL, Tobin MJ: Decision analysis of parameters used to predict outcome of a trial of weaning from mechanical ventilation. Abstract. Am Rev Respir Dis 139:A98, 1989.
92. Tobin MJ, Yang K: Weaning from mechanical ventilation. Crit Care Clin 6:725, 1990.
93. Roussos C, Macklem PT: Inspiratory muscle fatigue, in Fishman AP, Macklem PT, Mead J (eds): *Handbook of Physiology.* Bethesda, American Physiological Society, 1986, pp 511–527.
94. Cohen C, Zagelbaum D, Gross D, et al: Clinical manifestations of inspiratory muscle fatigue. Am J Med 73:308, 1982.
95. Roussos C, Fixley M, Gross D et al: Fatigue of inspiratory muscles and their synergic behaviour. J Appl Physiol 46:897, 1979.
96. Tobin MJ, Perez W, Guenther SM, et al: The pattern of breathing during successful and unsuccessful trials of weaning from mechanical ventilation. Am Rev Respir Dis 134:1111, 1986.
97. DeTroyer A, Loring SH: Action of respiratory muscles, in Fishman AP, Macklem PT, Mead J (eds): *Handbook of Physiology.* Bethesda, American Physiological Society, 1986, pp 443–462.
98. Pardee NE, Winterbauer RH, Allen JD: Bedside evaluation of respiratory distress. Chest 85:203, 1984.
99. Tobin MJ, Perez W, Guenther SM, et al: Does ribcage abdominal paradox signify respiratory muscle fatigue? J Appl Physiol 63(2):851, 1987.
100. Gross D, Grassino A, Ross WRD, et al: Electromyogram pattern of diaphragmatic fatigue. J Appl Physiol 46:1, 1979.
101. Grassino A, Macklem PT: Respiratory muscle fatigue and ventilatory failure. Annu Rev Med 35:625, 1984.
102. Milic-Emili J: Is weaning an art or a science? Am Rev Respir Dis 134:1107, 1986.
103. Sassoon CSH, Te TT, Mahutte CK, et al: Airway occlusion pressure. An important indicator for successful weaning in patients with chronic obstructive pulmonary disease. Am Rev Respir Dis 135:107, 1987.

Chapter 15
THORACENTESIS AND PLEURAL BIOPSY

EUGENE F. GEPPERT

Thoracentesis is the removal of pleural fluid performed either to analyze the fluid in an effort to diagnose its cause or to decrease a patient's discomfort by removing a pleural effusion that is causing pain, dyspnea, or difficulty with mechanical ventilation. *Closed pleural biopsy* is a bedside technique often performed by intensivists in an attempt to diagnose a pleural abnormality through examination of histopathology or culture of the pleural tissue removed. In the ICU it is usually most appropriate to begin the diagnostic investigation of a pleural effusion by performing thoracentesis. Pleural biopsy is usually done as a later, second-stage procedure when thoracentesis together with other studies (see Chap. 138) fail to make a definitive diagnosis. Pleural biopsy is especially useful when infectious diseases, such as pleural tuberculosis or pleural coccidioidomycosis, are considered likely or when pleural malignancy needs to be diagnosed.

Indications for Thoracentesis

Therapeutic thoracentesis is often performed on critically ill patients when the intensivist judges that a very large pleural effusion is likely to be a major contributing cause of the patient's sensation of dyspnea; in this case a therapeutic thoracentesis may palliate the patient's suffering. The mechanism by which a thoracentesis relieves dyspnea in patients with pleural effusion is that the removal of fluid permits reduction in size of the thoracic cage.[1]

Thoracentesis is indicated to diagnose most newly discovered pleural effusions.[2] It is especially important to perform thoracentesis on patients with fever, because empyema is a possible source of infection. Only occasionally is it permissible not to perform thoracentesis on a patient with pleural effusion; this is allowable when the pleural effusion is small, its cause is obvious from what is known about the patient, and the risk of thoracentesis outweighs the advantage of being certain of the contents of the pleural cavity. An example of the foregoing would be a patient with known congestive heart failure who has small bilateral pleural effusions and who is being mechanically ventilated with positive end-expiratory pressure. The most common indications for thoracentesis in the ICU are listed in Table 15-1.

TABLE 15-1 Indications for Thoracentesis in ICU

Newly discovered pleural effusion
Reduction of patient's dyspnea (therapeutic)
Fever in patient with pleural effusion

Preprocedure Considerations

Important preliminary tests before performing thoracentesis include tests of blood coagulation (prothrombin time, activated partial thromboplastin time, platelet count or estimation), and often it is useful to have a lateral decubitus chest film (which may be done as a portable film in many critically ill patients). A lateral decubitus chest film may sometimes reveal the presence of a pleural effusion that was not detected in a portable anteroposterior chest roentgenogram (Fig. 15-1). Coagulation tests help the intensivist estimate the risk of bleeding from the procedure. No strict guidelines exist for what elevations of the prothrombin time or the activated partial thromboplastin time are associated with an unacceptable risk of bleeding. Most physicians attempt to correct any abnormalities of the prothrombin time with vitamin K or administration of fresh frozen plasma prior to the performance of thoracentesis. Abnormalities of activated partial thromboplastin time should be corrected with fresh frozen plasma. We often perform thoracentesis on patients with slight elevation of prothrombin time (prothrombin time up to 15 s with control of about 12 s) in patients who do not have any other apparent coagulopathy. A platelet count of $<20,000$ is a contraindication to thoracentesis, and platelet infusions should be given immediately before performing thoracentesis. If the patient is uremic with a blood urea nitrogen value (BUN) of >60, platelet function may be impaired, and it is useful in such a case to perform thoracentesis after dialysis has lowered the BUN. In some cases it is reasonable to administer DDAVP to patients with renal failure who have a BUN >60 since this agent partially reverses uremic thrombocytopathy (see Chap. 157).

Choosing a site on the chest wall for needle insertion makes use of physical diagnosis (mainly percussion of the area of dullness), roentgenography, and ultrasonography. Pleural effusion discovered by chest percussion should always be confirmed by a chest roentgenogram. The usefulness of the lateral decubitus film is that it demonstrates whether or not the pleural fluid is freely moving within the hemithorax, and it gives some indication of the difficulty of fluid localization. For small or loculated collections, ultrasonography will be important[3] (Fig. 15-2). As a generality, pleural effusions that are large enough to make a lateral stripe of fluid 1 cm thick in the lateral decubitus position can be tapped without particular difficulty.[4] Smaller effusions may require special patient positioning or the help of bedside ultrasonic pictures of the fluid collection. Patients who are intubated on a mechanical ventilator are especially challenging, and the procedure is probably best performed with ultrasonic guidance in most cases. The difficulties and risks involved in performing thoracentesis on a patient who

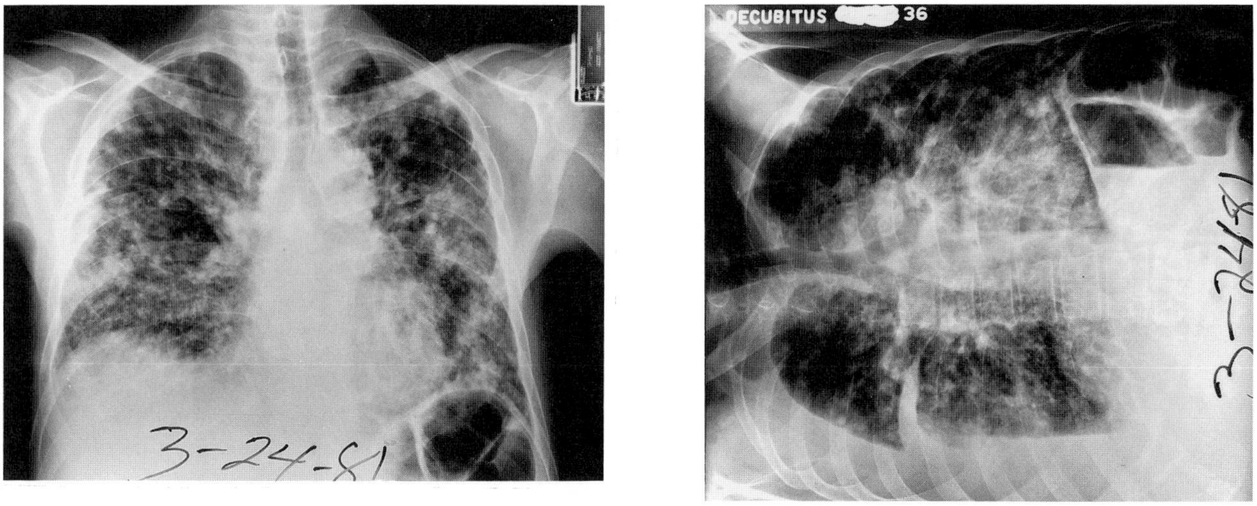

FIGURE 15-1 *a*. Portable chest radiograph reveals diffuse lung infiltrates and a suggestion of right pleural effusion, although no clear meniscus is seen. *b*. With lateral decubitus imaging, a clear fluid level is seen along the dependent chest wall and tracking into the minor fissure.

is being mechanically ventilated are serious enough that the procedure requires special justification. The possibility of empyema is one of the main reasons for going ahead with thoracentesis in this group of patients.

Method

It is not important to put a patient in the sitting position for thoracentesis. Many critically ill patients can have the procedure done while they are supine with the upper body elevated at a slight angle (Fig. 15-3). The operator who performs the procedure should position the patient next to the edge of the mattress and should raise the bed to a level that is comfortable. The patient's arm on the side of the effusion should be held out of the operating field by an assistant. If the patient is a woman with a large breast, tape should be applied to the outer side of the breast to maintain the breast on top of the thorax and out of the midaxillary line. An exposure site that often works well in the very ill is in the midaxillary line, high enough toward the axilla to decrease the likelihood of inadvertant splenic rupture or hepatic laceration. When an ultrasonographer is assisting, the best site will be dictated by the thickest layer of pleural fluid that is not close to the liver or spleen (seen as the diaphragm on ultrasound). Thoracentesis should be done as a two-stage procedure with local anesthesia as the first stage and needle aspiration of fluid as the second stage. The skin should be cleaned with antiseptic solution and local anesthetic should be infiltrated into the skin, the periosteum of nearby ribs (always avoiding the lower margin of the rib since the neurovascular bundle is located there and may be lacerated by the needle), and into the parietal pleura. The parietal pleura can be localized during anesthetic administration by first entering the pleural space (confirmed by aspiration of pleural fluid into the syringe after pulling back on the plunger) and then pulling the needle back until just after the point has been reached in which pleural fluid stops entering the syringe; this is very close to the pain-sensitive parietal pleura. A total of 200 mg 1% lidocaine (20 ml 1% solution) may be used in infiltrating all the pain-sensitive tissues. The local anesthetic should be given enough time to work, about 10 min. At the end of this time it is best to collect the pleural fluid sample for pH and P_{CO_2} in a separate 5 mL heparinized syringe, which allows it to be collected and transferred to the laboratory without ever being exposed to air (air exposure ruins the determination by allowing car-

FIGURE 15-2 Demonstration of ultrasonographic localization of pleural fluid collection. A thin strip of fluid (arrows) is seen accompanying a pneumonic infiltrate (i) with abscess (a) formation. Such localization can be used to guide thoracentesis when physical findings and chest radiograph are ambiguous. (Reprinted with permission from Reference 3.)

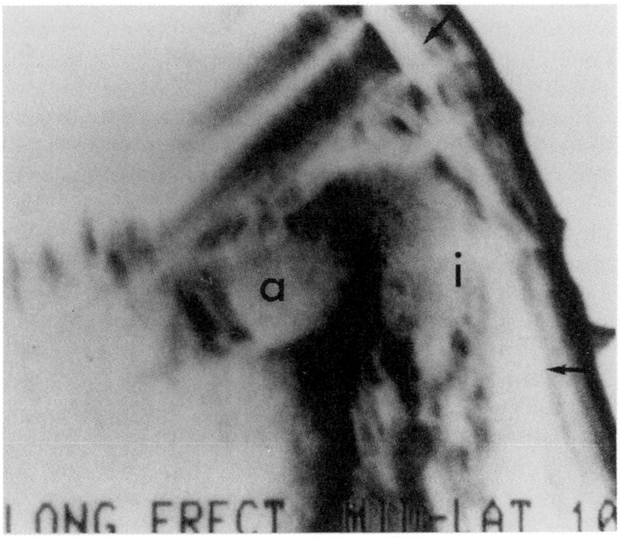

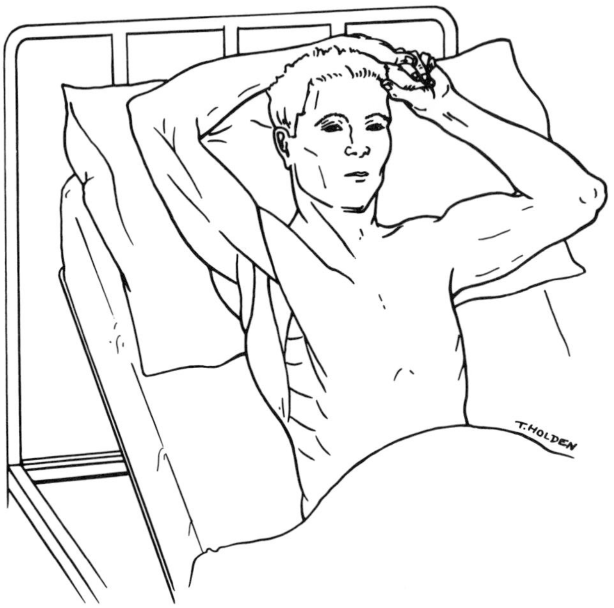

FIGURE 15-3 Patient positioned supine with upper body elevated for thoracentesis. Percussion or ultrasonography is used to locate fluid in the midaxillary line. (Reprinted with permission from Zimmerman CE, *Techniques of Patient Care,* Little Brown, Boston, 1970.)

bon dioxide to diffuse out of the poorly buffered pleural fluid and gives an artificially high pH value).[5] Following collection of the small (2 mL) sample for pH and P_{CO_2}, the intensivist should prepare for the main pleural fluid collection by first adding heparin to all instruments and receptacles that will come into contact with pleural fluid: syringe, needle, plastic tubing, collection bag, plastic tubes for samples, etc. The exact site chosen for entry of the needle should be determined by considering the following: **1.** choose an area overlying or only slightly above a point of dullness to percussion; **2.** the site should always be slightly above a rib to avoid the neurovascular bundle that runs under each rib; **3.** the depth of needle penetration that will be necessary is highly variable since the thickness of the chest wall varies so much among different patients. In some large muscular men, a spinal needle is needed to penetrate to the pleural space.

Once the entry point is chosen, the operator pierces the skin with the needle (or needle catheter assembly if this is preferred) and guides the needle in such a way as to avoid the neurovascular bundle that is located just below each rib. When pleural fluid is aspirated, the operator can collect the sample either by syringe suction or by gravity flow into a collection bag. Table 15-2 presents a checklist of steps in the performance of thoracentesis in the ICU.

TABLE 15-2 Checklist for Thoracentesis in ICU

1. Position patient for comfortable access to fluid collection.
2. Localize the fluid collection (percussion, chest film, ultrasound).
3. Instill local anesthetic and withdraw pleural fluid for determination of pH and respiratory gases.
4. Insert the needle or needle catheter assembly and withdraw fluid.
5. Order portable chest x-ray to check for pneumothorax or hemothorax as a complication.

Complications

The complications experienced during and after thoracentesis in the ICU are similar to those seen in patients who are less ill.[6,7] Generally, less than 1.5 L pleural fluid should be collected in the spontaneously breathing patient to avoid the complication of postthoracentesis pulmonary edema (reexpansion pulmonary edema).[8,9] When the pleural fluid layer is thin at the start of the procedure or if it becomes thin in the course of the procedure, the danger increases that the needle will enter the lung and cause hemoptysis or pneumothorax. In the ICU, a pneumothorax in a mechanically ventilated patient is a much more serious matter than pneumothorax in a spontaneously breathing patient. For this reason, it is prudent to have tube thoracostomy equipment available at the bedside for an emergency tube thoracostomy in case the patient should develop tension pneumothorax or life-threatening hypoxemia as a complication of the procedure. Rarely, air embolism has complicated thoracentesis, and this complication should be suspected if the patient develops a fall in P_{O_2} together with new onset of a stroke immediately after the procedure. Severe hemorrhage has also complicated thoracentesis on unusual occasions. Inadvertent puncture of a diaphragmatic artery or a tortuous intercostal artery has been reported; some patients with malignant pleural effusions have a tendency to bleed heavily even in the absence of laceration of a major blood vessel. Severe bleeding after thoracentesis usually requires thoracotomy to identify the bleeding site and electrocoagulate it. Similarly, inadvertent passage of the thoracentesis needle into the liver or spleen may cause severe abdominal hemorrhage and require laparotomy for repair. Some patients (approximately 2 to 3 percent) exhibit bradycardia and hypotension when the thoracentesis needle enters the pleura. Premedication with atropine should be considered to avoid this complication. The most common complications of thoracentesis in ICU patients are listed in Table 15-3.

Pleural fluid samples should always be sent for protein, lactate dehydrogenase, white blood cell count and differential, and red blood cell count. In most patients, a number of other determinations should also be ordered. These include pH and P_{CO_2}, glucose, amylase, samples for aerobic and anaerobic bacterial culture, acid fast and fungal stains and

TABLE 15-3 Complications of Thoracentesis in ICU

Postthoracentesis pulmonary edema (reexpansion)
Pneumothorax
Intrapleural hemorrhage
Venous air embolism
Hemoptysis
Laceration of liver or spleen
Bradycardia and hypotension

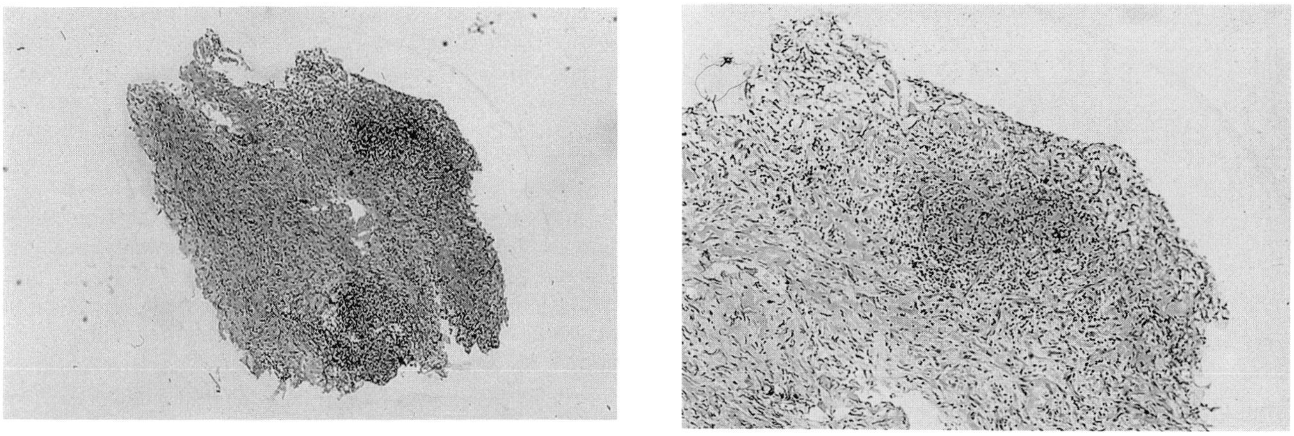

FIGURE 15-4 Pleural biopsy at low *(left)* and high *(right)* power magnification reveals epithelioid granulomas typical of pleural tuberculosis. Cultures were positive for *Mycobacteria tuberculosis.* (See Plate 1.)

cultures, cryptococcal antigen determination, sample for cytologic examination, hematocrit determination for grossly bloody pleural fluid, and other special studies dictated by the particular patient's known diseases and risk factors (see Chap. 138).

Closed Pleural Biopsy

Closed pleural biopsy is a procedure for which there are no emergency indications. The place of closed pleural biopsy in the ICU is in the patient who is hemodynamically stable and in whom it becomes important to document the presence of tuberculosis or coccidioidomycosis of the pleura without delay. Under these conditions, the performance of a pleural biopsy can often provide the diagnosis on histopathologic examination within 24 h. The general indications and contraindications to pleural biopsy are similar to those of thoracentesis; the procedure differs in that the needle used is large, and the risks of bleeding and pneumothorax may be greater.

The method for performing closed pleural biopsy with an Abrams needle is as follows. First the operator chooses two sites on the chest wall for needle entry. These are chosen below the level of dullness determined by chest percussion, and it is advisable to stay as far away from the liver or spleen as possible. The skin, rib periosteum, and parietal pleura are infiltrated with generous amounts of lidocaine (about 200 mg total or 20 mL 1% solution). After waiting 10 min for the anesthetic to have its effect, a scalpel is used to create an introduction wound for the Abrams needle by piercing the skin and the intercostal tissue. The Abrams needle is then introduced into the pleural space by means of a twisting, boring motion. After the needle has perforated the parietal pleura, pleural fluid is aspirated back into a heparinized syringe attached to it. With the operator taking care to avoid the neurovascular bundle below each rib, the Abrams needle is opened so that its cutting trough can be pulled back, and it "catches" the parietal pleura in the trough. The operator then cuts the pleura by a twisting motion on the needle and sucks the tissue into the syringe along with pleural fluid. Three biopsies are taken from each of the two sites for a total of six pieces. The biopsies are then placed in either saline (for culture) or formalin (for histopathology).

Diagnoses that have been made by pleural biopsy include tuberculosis, cancer, coccidioidomycosis, rheumatoid arthritis pleurisy, and others only rarely. An example of a pleural biopsy that proved a diagnosis of tuberculosis of the pleura is shown in Fig. 15-4 (Plate 1). The overall diagnostic rate of closed pleural biopsy is low, probably about 30 percent. A pleural effusion is necessary to perform the procedure, and in some patients it is reasonable to perform closed pleural biopsy at the same time as initial thoracentesis to save valuable time in making a diagnosis. There is rarely any justification for performing pleural biopsy on a patient on mechanical ventilation or in one who is hemodynamically unstable.

References

1. Estenne M, Yernault JC, De Troyer A: Mechanism of relief of dyspnea after thoracocentesis in patients with large pleural effusions. Am J Med 74:813, 1983.
2. Sokolowski JH Jr, Burgher LW, Jones FL et al: Guidelines for thoracentesis and needle biopsy of the pleura. Am Rev Respir Dis 140:257, 1989.
3. Matalon TA, Neiman HL, Mintzer RA: Noncardiac chest sonography, the state of the art. Chest 83(4):675, 1983.
4. Light RW: *Pleural Diseases*. Philadelphia, Lea & Febiger, 1983, p 229.
5. Good JT, Taryle DA, Maulitz RM et al: The diagnostic value of pleural fluid pH. Chest 78:55, 1980.
6. Seneff MG, Corwin RW, Gold LH et al: Complications associated with thoracocentesis. Chest 90:97,1986.
7. Collins TR, Sahn SA: Thoracocentesis: clinical value, complications, technical problems, and patient experience. Chest 91:817, 1987.
8. Trapnell DH, Thurston JGB: Unilateral pulmonary oedema after pleural aspiration. Lancet 1:1367, 1970.
9. Marland AM, Glauser FL: Hemodynamic and pulmonary edema protein measurements in a case of reexpansion pulmonary edema. Chest 81:250, 1982.

Chapter 16
TUBE THORACOSTOMY AND PLEURODESIS

J.G. ABEL
J. ALI

Tube thoracostomy is a lifesaving measure frequently required in the critically ill patient. This technique, combined with the development of techniques of endotracheal intubation and positive-pressure ventilation, has permitted major strides in thoracic surgery and successful management of acute and chronic respiratory failure. The intensivist must therefore be familiar with the indications, technique, and complications of tube thoracostomy. These features of tube thoracostomy as well as the principles of pleurodesis are discussed in this chapter.

Pathophysiology

The pleural space between the visceral and parietal pleura normally contains 0.1 to 0.2 ml/kg fluid.[1] Apposition of the lung to the chest wall is determined by the balance of the outward elastic recoil of the chest wall, the inward elastic recoil of the lung, and the process of gas and fluid removal from the pleural space. The gradient between gas pressure in the pleural space (-1 to 2 cmH_2O) and that at the venous end of the capillaries (-70 cmH_2O) promotes gas resorption at the venous end.[2]

Pleural blood flow has been estimated at 300 ml/h, and pleural fluid flows from the high pressure systemic capillaries of the parietal pleura to the parietal pleural lymphatics at the estimated rate of 5 to 10 L/day.[1] Pleural effusion results when the rate of pleural fluid formation exceeds that of removal. The balance between parietal and visceral pleural hydrostatic pressure and colloid osmotic pressures and those in the pleural space liquid favors the net formation of pleural fluid. The lymphatics absorb fluid across a hydrostatic gradient with an increase in protein content relative to interstitial fluid, thus favoring pleural fluid absorption. As pleural fluid decreases, its pressure becomes less, thus promoting the apposition of the lung and chest wall.

Disturbances in the mechanical forces in the pleural space, including the Starling forces in the capillaries, result in transudative pleural effusions, whereas abnormalities of the pleura itself, such as increased permeability, cause *exudative* effusions. *Malignant* pleural effusions result from obstruction of parietal lymphatic drainage with a decrease in protein clearance and an increase in the osmotic pressure of the pleural fluid.

Tube thoracostomy is indicated when there is actual or potential abnormal accumulation of gas or fluid in the pleural space, which compromises respiratory or circulatory stability. Tension pneumothorax raises right atrial pressure and decreases venous return. A very large pleural effusion may do likewise. The pulmonary gas exchange consequences of pneumothorax and effusion depend on the preexisting pulmonary pathology, and the ventilation/perfusion ($\dot{V}/\dot{Q}$) mismatch resulting from the pleural pathology. The effects of tube thoracostomy on $\dot{V}/\dot{Q}$ relationships cannot be predicted with certainty. In general, $\dot{V}/\dot{Q}$ matching in simple acute pneumothorax and hemothorax should be improved. In most chronic effusions or pneumothorax, expansion of the lung may improve perfusion rapidly, but a transient increase in shunt may exist because of a relative delay in reexpansion of atelectatic lung. Drainage of large effusions is often accompanied by relief of dyspnea, hypercapnia, and hypoxia.

Tube Thoracostomy

INDICATIONS

Indications for tube thoracostomy may be classified as prophylactic or therapeutic, the latter being subclassified into emergent or elective (3–5) (Table 16-1). Although controversial, the potential benefits of prophylactic tube thoracostomy in the critical care setting outweigh any risks. We prefer insertion of prophylactic chest tubes when positive-pressure ventilation is required in patients with multiple rib fractures and underlying large areas of lung contusion or

TABLE 16-1 Indications for Tube Thoracostomy

A. **Prophylactic**
   Multiple rib fractures and large pulmonary contusion in patients requiring mechanical ventilation and PEEP in excess of 20 cmH_2O.
B. **Therapeutic**
   1. Emergent
      a. Traumatic
         1) Pneumothorax
            a) Open
            b) Closed
               1) Simple
               2) Tension
         2) Hemothorax
         3) Hemopneumothorax
         4) Crash protocols
         5) Electromechanical dissociation
      b. Nontraumatic
         1) Spontaneous pneumothorax
            a) Simple
            b) Tension
   2. Elective
      a. Pleural effusion
         1) Nonneoplastic
         2) Neoplastic
      b. Empyema
      c. Chylothorax

flail chest. This is particularly important when positive end-expiratory pressure (PEEP) in excess of 20 cmH_2O is required to correct severe hypoxemia or when a general anesthetic is necessary for surgical procedures. This approach prevents a tension pneumothorax, which may be confused with other primary causes of hemodynamic instability. The emergent use of bilateral chest tubes in crash protocols and electromechanical dissociation is indicated for similar reasons.

TECHNIQUE

All tubes for drainage of the entire pleural space or evacuation of a nonloculated pneumothorax should be placed posteriorly and directed toward the apex. This is because all pneumothoraces, due to the disturbance of pleural fluid dynamics, are accompanied by the formation of pleural fluid, which will accumulate dependently, hence posteriorly in the chest. Also the presence of the chest tube itself causes the formation of 50 to 100 ml of serous fluid per day. Specific loculated effusions or pneumothoraces require precise localization, often under ultrasound or computed tomography (CT) scan control.

Once the insertion site is selected (usually the fifth intercostal space just anterior to the midaxillary line), the chest is prepared and draped widely. The overlying skin, intercostal muscles, and pleura are infiltrated with approximately 10 to 20 ml 1% lidocaine without epinephrine. If the amount of subcutaneous tissue is generous or rapid access is necessary, the skin incision may be made immediately over the desired interspace of entry, but in thin or cachectic persons, a skin incision 2 cm lower than the interspace provides a water and airtight seal around the tube (Fig. 16-1). The skin incision is parallel to the ribs and long enough to admit a finger into the chest. The subcutaneous and intercostal muscles are dissected bluntly with a Kelly clamp or a scalpel when rapid access is required. The plane of dissection is immediately above the upper border of the lower rib of the interspace to avoid the intercostal neurovascular bundle of the rib above. Intermittent palpation with the finger assists in determining the depth of dissection and avoids cardiac injury or puncture of the lung, leading to an air leak which may close slowly in ventilated patients. Puncture of the pleura is best accomplished with the Kelly clamp, rather than the finger, since the finger may elevate the parietal pleura from the chest wall and predispose to extrapleural tube placement. Complicated and subpulmonic collections are best drained following ultrasound or CT localization. The pleural space should be briefly examined digitally, ensuring correct location and the absence of local adhesions to the lungs or heart.

The diameter of the tube is important. In general, in an averaged-sized patient with a simple pneumothorax, no tube smaller than No. 28 French should be used. More narrow tubes have an unacceptably high resistance, which may limit the rate of evacuation of air if a substantial leak is present.[6,7] Smaller tubes may become blocked with fibrinous exudate. If the indication for tube thoracostomy is a hemothorax, larger No. 32 to 40 French tubes are required.

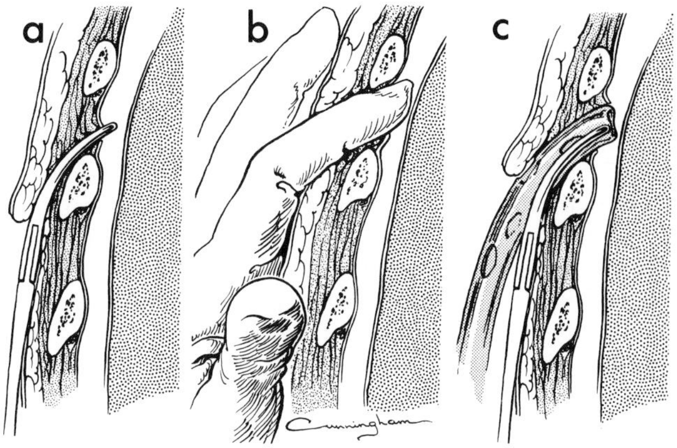

FIGURE 16-1 Technique of chest tube insertion. The incision is made 2 cm below the chosen interspace and the clamp *(a)* followed by the finger *(b)* is inserted into the pleural space above the upper border of the rib. The tube is inserted and directed with the Kelly clamp *(c)*. The tube is then gently directed posteriorly and toward the apex.

The use of chest tubes mounted in trocars is to be avoided, because of the risk of pulmonary, cardiac, diaphragmatic, and abdominal visceral perforations. Some authors advocate catheter aspiration for simple pneumothorax[8] or the use of smaller caliber tubes.[6] These techniques, however, are associated with a 5 to 20 percent failure rate. In the ICU, definitive tube thoracostomy should be the rule.

The actual insertion of the chest tube is accomplished using a curved Kelly clamp. The tube is placed along the convex side of the clamp with the tip closed in its jaws (Fig. 16-1). This allows the accurate guidance of the initial track of the tube within the pleural space. A common mistake with lateral tubes is the placement within the major oblique fissure, which lies close to the fifth intercostal space laterally. This results in early loculation of the chest tube from the pleural cavity and incomplete air and liquid evacuation. All tubes should be placed posteriorly and directed to the apex of the lung. Most tubes now have continuous markings or distance in centimeters from the last drainage site hole to guide in intrathoracic placement. The tube may be marked with a silk ligature or clamp at the approximate skin position to estimate the intrathoracic length of catheter needed to reach the apex. In no instance should force be used to make the tube reach this position, however. Once inserted, the catheter is attached to underwater seal drainage or suction. Suction is required whenever the underwater seal system alone does not maintain evacuation of the pleural space. Once suction has been applied, this may be decreased or discontinued as the fluid or air accumulation in the pleural space disappears. Failure to reexpand the lung despite an adequately functioning chest tube with suction is an indication for insertion of a second chest tube and if despite two adequately functioning large bore chest tubes with suction a continuous air leak persists, a major bronchial tear or bronchopleural fistula should be suspected. Wherever possible, this large airway injury should be treated surgically. However, in many instances this may not be possible, particularly in the presence of gross sepsis.

Until the sepsis is controlled and surgical correction of the bronchopleural fistula is possible, other techniques such as high frequency jet ventilation may be required to maintain adequate gas exchange.[9] In many instances such techniques maintain gas exchange in otherwise critically ill patients until the bronchopleural fisutula heals spontaneously or until it can be corrected surgically. Failure to expand the lung may also result from large clotted hemothoraces and if despite large bore chest tubes the pleural space cannot be evacuated, then these patients should be considered for thoracotomy with surgical evacuation of the clotted hemothorax to allow lung reexpansion. In the past this procedure was used only when there was a mature peel after organization of the clotted hemothorax. More recently, however, evacuation of the pleural space is accomplished on an acute basis without any increase in morbidity or mortality. Occasionally the rapid draining of massive (>1000 ml) effusion or hemothorax and subacute pneumothorax may be associated with reexpansion pulmonary edema.[10,11] To avoid this, the drainage tube may be clamped after drainage of the first 1000 ml and the patient response assessed. The skin around the chest tube is snugly approximated with a large #2 silk or polypropylene purse string suture. This becomes important in trouble-shooting for possible air leaks. The ends of this same suture are used to anchor the tube in position and should indent the tube to prevent migration. Petrolatum gauze dressing is applied to the incision site, and the proximal tube is anchored to the skin to prevent painful excessive movement. All chest tube connections are taped securely.

The chest tube may be attached to the traditional one-to-three bottle underwater seal-suction system (Fig. 16-2) or to a number of commercially available chest drainage collection systems that allow adjustment of the degree of suction and visualization of air leak and that have attachable modules for autotransfusion. Regardless of the drainage system used, the drainage tubes from the chest must be connected to an underwater seal before exposure to the atmosphere or suction. An intermittent or continuous air leak mandates complete examination of the chest tube drainage circuit to ensure it is airtight. Transient clamping of the chest tube will abolish an air leak if it is intrathoracic or from the thoracostomy site, whereas a continuing leak denotes a connector or system leak. As a general principle, chest tubes should never be clamped except for brief diagnostics at the bedside or the staged evacuation of a massive effusion to prevent reexpansion pulmonary edema. Avoidance of chest tube clamping prevents the development of a life threatening tension pneumothorax.

FIGURE 16-2 Chest drainage collection systems. The underwater seal is provided before exposure to the atmosphere or to suction.

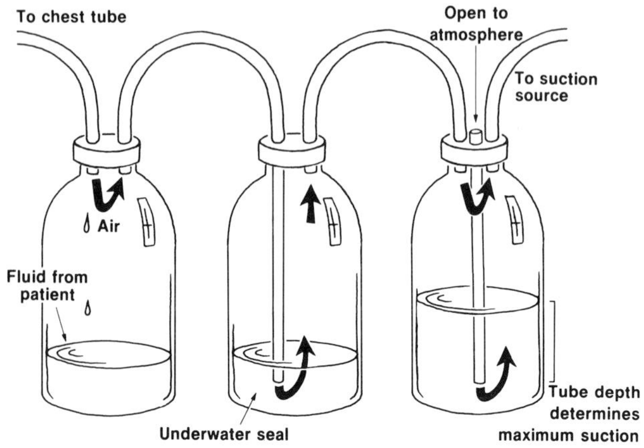

The use of prophylactic antibiotics in tube thoracostomy has been controversial,[12–15] with some studies showing a reduction in the incidence of empyema, and others, no benefit. We do not advocate the routine use of prophylactic antibiotics in either emergent or elective tube thoracostomy.

CHEST TUBE REMOVAL

The technique of chest tube removal is important. As a general rule, the chest tube is removed when the original indication for its use no longer exists. When an air leak has stopped on continuous suction, a chest x-ray with suction removed or underwater seal will confirm that a pneumothorax has not recurred, and the tube may be removed 24 h later. When the tube is inserted for draining a hydrothorax or hemothorax, it may be removed if drainage decreases to less than 100 cc/24 h in the presence of an adequately functioning chest tube as evidenced by movement of the fluid column within the tube with respiration. Although a chest tube may be partially withdrawn provided the drainage holes are not exposed, it should not be advanced into the pleural cavity after the initial insertion. New tubes require new insertion sites. The tube must be removed at a time when positive intrapleural pressure exists. In the ventilated patient, pleural pressure is maximal during the inspiratory phase of an assisted breath. By use of the inspiratory hold mode on the ventilator, positive pleural pressure may be maintained during chest tube withdrawal. In a patient breathing spontaneously, a full inspiration to total lung capacity (TLC), with an accompanying Valsalva maneuver at TLC, maximizes pleural pressure and minimizes the chance of pneumothorax during tube removal. An airtight seal of skin and subcutaneous tissue is important and in thin patients a purse string suture placed around the tube at the time of insertion, or just prior to removal, facilitates this.

COMPLICATIONS OF TUBE THORACOSTOMY

The incidence of complications of tube thoracostomy ranges from 5 to 25 percent.[13] They may be classified as those related to therapeutic failure (incomplete evacuation of air or fluid) and iatrogenic complications of the tube itself (perforation of lung, diaphragm, heart, solid or hollow viscus, injury of a major vessel, chylothorax, pneumothorax on removal). Strict adherence to proper technique avoids most of these complications.

Early therapeutic failure may be related to incorrect tube placement or may signal endotracheal, pneumonic, or pleural pathology preventing complete lung expansion. Bronchoscopy, and if negative, thoracoscopy are indicated. Inability to reexpand a lobe of lung following the evacuation of a malignant pleural effusion is a common problem. An empyema may result if the tube is left in. When this situation is recognized, the chest tube should be removed immediately to allow a sterile exudate to fill the pleural space. Tetracycline instillation (20 mg/kg) may be used to aid in sterilization.

Bleeding as a result of tube thoracostomy is frequently caused by a laceration of an intercostal or internal mammary artery. Proper technique avoids this complication, but persistent bleeding may require thoracotomy.

Persistent pneumothorax in the presence of properly functioning large bore chest tubes should suggest the presence of a bronchopleural fistula, which may require open thoracotomy for closure.

Reported incidence of pleural space infection following tube thoracostomy is variable[14,15] but is usually less than 5 percent. The associated pathologic condition is a major predisposing factor but proper sterile technique is an essential preventive measure. Specific antibiotics and drainage are required for identified infection.

Pleurodesis

In most instances abnormal gas or fluid accumulation in the pleural space responds to tube thoracostomy. However, obliteration of the pleural space, or *pleurodesis,* should be considered in pneumothorax and certain pleural effusions. Pleurodesis may be achieved surgically or chemically.

SURGICAL PLEURODESIS

The indications for surgical pleurodesis are presented in Table 16-2. A single recurrence of an ipsilateral pneumothorax is now accepted as an indication because of the greater than 50 percent incidence of a third event. Bilateral pneumothoraces, regardless of timing, are an absolute indication. Bilateral surgical pleurodesis is performed in staged procedures 10 days apart. A persistent air leak in a good-risk patient mandates surgical pleurodesis, as does failure to evacuate a pneumothorax completely, with incomplete lung reexpansion. When chemical pleurodesis for either benign or malignant disease fails in patients who are good operative risks, surgical pleurodesis may be undertaken if the long-term prognosis is favorable.

TABLE 16-2 Indications for Surgical Pleurodesis

1. Recurrent unilateral spontaneous pneumothorax
2. Synchronous or metachronous bilateral pneumothorax
3. Persistent air leak or pneumothorax
4. Failure of chemical pleurodesis with favorable long-term prognosis

The two techniques of surgical pleurodesis are *pleural abrasion* and *partial pleurectomy.* The choice of procedure is dictated by the underlying pathology and clinical criteria. These have been used most frequently for spontaneous pneumothorax in young men and are usually combined with apical bullectomy. Transaxillary apical bullectomy is performed with the hemithorax turned 20° up from the horizontal and the arm elevated over the head. A short incision parallel to the third intercostal space is made and through this limited exposure apical bullae can be excised with a stapler. The parietal pleura in the area is then either abraded with a gauze sponge or formally removed. In pleurectomy, the parietal pleura is bluntly elevated from the endothoracic fascia beginning at the incision and extending over the apex of the chest wall. The mediastinal pleura is not dissected to avoid damage to the phrenic, vagus, and recurrent laryngeal nerves and the stellate ganglion. The pleural space is drained with a single chest tube, and hospitalization time is generally about 6 days. The recurrence rate of pneumothorax is 0.6 percent.[17] Pleurectomy limited to the apex is said to have the advantage of a more facile second formal thoracotomy, should this be required. Pleural abrasion/apical bullectomy also has a recurrence rate of less than 1 percent,[18,19] but is usually performed through a more formal fourth or fifth intercostal space thoracotomy, with its attendant morbidity.

Formal posterolateral thoractomy is preferred for so-called secondary pneumothoraces occurring with preexisting lung pathology, usually chronic obstructive pulmonary disease. The indication often is for pneumothorax with diffuse bullous disease requiring bullectomy, and excellent exposure of the entire thorax is required. Pleurectomy may be limited to the apex or generalized, but the diaphragmatic and mediastinal pleura is again avoided.[20]

In malignant effusions when the prognosis for survival is at least 6 months, formal thoracotomy and subtotal parietal pleurectomy may be performed, although they often are reserved for failure of chemical pleurodesis.[21] If trapped lung exists, decortication may be performed. This procedure has major associated morbidity and mortality. The best results have been obtained in carcinoma of the breast or melanoma. However, mortality has been up to 10 percent and morbidity 20 percent.[22]

CHEMICAL PLEURODESIS

The indications for chemical pleurodesis are presented in Table 16-3. The most common indication is malignant pleural effusion.[23] Pleurodesis should be reserved for symptomatic effusions with a demonstrated benefit from thoracentesis.[24] Primary therapy for the tumor will often have failed to control pleural effusion. Metastatic pneumothorax requires pleurodesis at presentation.[25] Some authors advocate routine pleuroscopy in spontaneous pneumothorax.[26] If lung blebs are <2 cm in diameter, there is a zero recurrence rate of pneumothorax following tetracycline instillation at pleuroscopy, without concomitant bleb resection.[26]

TABLE 16-3 Indications for Chemical Pleurodesis

1. Malignant pleural effusion with good therapeutic result following thoracentesis
2. Failure of response to standard tumor therapy and (1)
3. Metastatic pneumothorax
4. Pulmonary blebs less than 2 cm at pleuroscopy for spontaneous pneumothorax
5. Pneumothorax or persistent air leak in poor operative risk patients

Blebs >2 cm should be resected. Conservative management of secondary pneumothoraces with tube thoracostomy alone may have a higher failure rate than primary pneumothoraces, and chemical or surgical pleurodesis should be considered early. High-risk patients with pneumothorax or persistent air leak merit an initial trial of chemical pleurodesis.[27,28]

Many agents have been used to achieve control of pleural effusion and pleural symphysis.[24,29] Effective drainage of the pleural space by tube thoracostomy is essential to allow reexpansion of the lung and apposition of the parietal and visceral pleura. Loculations form rapidly around the tube within 24 to 48 h of insertion; therefore, early pleurodesis should be performed once lung expansion has been confirmed. If the lung fails to expand due to entrapment or a proximal bronchial obstruction, pleurodesis will not be successful, and other modalities such as decortication or pleuroperitoneal shunting may be considered.

Tetracycline, 20 mg/kg is dissolved in 100 ml sterile water to which lidocaine hydrochloride, 2.5 mg/kg is added. This solution is injected using a fine bore needle and sterile technique into the self-sealing portion of the chest tubing and is drained dependently into the thorax. Talc suspension or bleomycin may be used in tetracycline allergy. The chest tube is clamped close to the thorax for 3 h. If an air leak is present, the chest tubing is suspended 60 cm above the thorax to allow the continued egress of air, yet retain the sclerosant.[28] Changes in patient position may facilitate distribution of the sclerosant if loculations are present. However, rapid and uniform distribution throughout the contiguous pleural space occurs without changes in position.[30] Lidocaine is absorbed systemically, and 2.5 mg/kg has been suggested as the maximum dose based on the measurement of peak plasma drug levels.[31] Two recent reports[32,33] have suggested that this procedure can be performed effectively using small bore catheters. Talc or tetracycline may also be instilled directly at pleuroscopy if indicated.

After 3 h of contact the chest tube is attached to standard suction drainage. Drainage may increase transiently in the next 24 to 48 h as an exudative reaction to the sclerosant but will then decrease, and the tube is removed when drainage is less than 150 ml/24 h. Pleurodesis may be repeated if the effusion recurs.

Efficacy following chemical pleurodesis has been shown to correlate with pleural fluid glucose and pH levels.[34,35] Low pH and glucose levels are thought to reflect extensive involvement of the pleura by malignancy. Survival following pleurodesis was only 2.1 months in a low pH group compared to 9.8 months in those patients with high pleural fluid pH.[34] Tumor type also determines effectiveness. Carcinoma of the breast is the best responder, while Kaposi's sarcoma in acquired immunodeficiency syndrome (AIDS) is uniformly unsuccessful.[36] Tetracycline, talc suspension, and bleomycin are more than 80 percent effective.[24,29] Since tetracycline and bleomycin have equal efficacy, tetracycline is recommended as more cost-effective. Talc poudrage under general anesthetic is effective 70 percent of the time. Side effects of all the agents are similar (pain, fever, and morbidity of hospitalization).

Malignant effusions refractory to a second pleurodesis may be considered for pleuroperitoneal shunting.[37] A one-way valved conduit is placed through an intercostal space into the pleural cavity and tunnelled subcutaneously to the hypochondrium, where it is inserted intraperitoneally through a small incision. The conduit has a pumping chamber which requires manual compression approximately four times per day to overcome the small abdominal-pleural pressure gradient. The shunt is also useful in nonmalignant conditions such as chylothorax. Success rates of 80 percent are reported.

References

1. Staub NC, Wiener-Kronish JP, Albertine KH: Transport through the pleura, in Chretien J, Bignon J, Hirsch A: *The Pleura in Health and Disease.* New York, Marcel Dekker, 1985, p 170.
2. Agostoni E: Mechanical coupling between lung and chest wall, in: Chretien J, Bignon J, Hirsch A: *The Pleura in Health and Disease.* New York, Marcel Dekker, 1985, p 141.
3. Dalbec AL, Kromer RL: Thoracostomy. Emerg Med Clin North Am 4:441, 1986.
4. Miller KS, Sahn SA: Chest tubes. Indications, technique, management and complications. Chest 91:259, 1987.
5. Symbas PN. Chest drainage tubes. Surg Clin North Am 69:41, 1989.
6. Conces DJ, Tarver RD, Gray WC, Pearcy EA: Treatment of pneumothoraces utilizing small caliber chest tubes. Chest 94:55, 1988.
7. Fuhrman BP, Landrum BG, Ferrara TB et al: Pleural drainage using modified pigtail catheters. Crit Care Med 14:575, 1986.
8. Delius RE, Farouck NO, Horst HM et al: Catheter aspiration for simple pneumothorax. Arch Surg 124:833, 1989.
9. Powner DJ, Grenvik A: Ventilatory management of life threatening bronchopleural fistulae: A summary. Crit Care Med 9:54, 1981.
10. Bernstein A: Reexpansion pulmonary edema. Chest 77:708, 1980.
11. Light RW, Jenkinson SG, Minh VD et al: Observations on pleural fluid pressures as fluid is withdrawn during thoracentesis. Am Rev Respir Dis 121:799, 1980.
12. Eddy CA, Luna GK, Copass M: Empyema thoracic in patients undergoing emergent closed tube thoracostomy for thoracic trauma. Am J Surg 157:494, 1989.
13. Caplan ES, Hoyt NJ, Rodriguez A et al: Empyema occuring in the multiply traumatized patient. J Trauma 24:785, 1984.
14. Leblanc CA, Tucker WY: Prophylactic antibiotics and closed tube thoracostomy. Surg Gynecol Obstet 160:259, 1985.

15. LoCurto JJ, Tischler CD, Swan KG et al: Tube thoracostomy and trauma-antibiotics or not? J Trauma 26:1067, 1986.
16. Daly RC, Mucha P, Pairolero PC et al: The risk of percutaneous thoracostomy for blunt thoracic trauma. Ann Emerg Med 14:865, 1985.
17. Deslauriers J, Beaulieu M, Despres JP et al: Transaxillary pleurectomy for treatment of spontaneous pneumothorax. Ann Thorac Surg 30:569, 1980.
18. Getz SB, Beasley WE: Spontaneous pneumothorax: Am J Surg 145:823, 1983.
19. Granke K, Fischer CR, Gago O et al: The efficacy and timing of operative intervention for spontaneous pneumothorax. Ann Thorac Surg 42:540, 1986.
20. Beattie EJ Jr: The treatment of malignant pleural effusions by partial pleurectomy. Surg Clin North Am 43:99, 1963.
21. Martini M, Bains MS, Beattie EJ: Indications for pleurectomy in malignant effusion. Cancer 35:734, 1975.
22. Shields TW: Technique of pleurectomy, in Shields TW (ed): General Thoracic Surgery, 3rd ed. Philadelphia, Lea & Febiger, 1989, p 622.
23. Sahn SA: Pleural effusion in lung cancer. Clin Chest Med 3:443, 1982.
24. Austin EH, Flye MW: The treatment of recurrent malignant pleural effusion. Ann Thorac Surg 28:190, 1979.
25. Rammohan G, Bonacini M, Dwek JH et al: Pleurodesis in metastatic pneumothorax. Chest 90:918, 1986.
26. Wied U, Halkier E, Hoeier-Madsen K et al: Tetracycline versus silver nitrate pleurodesis in spontaneous pneumothorax. J Thorac Cardiovasc Surg 86:591, 1983.
27. Fleisher AG, McElvaney G, Lawson L et al: Surgical management of spontaneous pneumothorax in patients with acquired immunodeficiency syndrome. Ann Thorac Surg 45:21, 1988.
28. Almassi GH, Haasler GB: Chemical pleurodesis in the presence of persistent air leak. Ann Thorac Surg 47:786, 1989.
29. Ruckdeschel JC: Management of malignant pleural effusion: An overview. Semin Oncol 15:24, 1988.
30. Lorch DG, Gordon L, Wooten S et al: Effect of patient positioning on distribution of tetracycline in the pleural space during pleurodesis. Chest 93:527, 1988.
31. Wooten SA, Strange C, Barbarash R et al: Pharmacokinetics of tetracycline and xylocaine following intrapleural instillation. Am Rev Respir Dis 135:A245, 1987.
32. Parker LA, Charnock GC, Delaney DJ: Small bore catheter drainage and sclerotherapy for malignant pleural effusion. Cancer 64:1218, 1989.
33. Walsh FW, Alberts WM, Solomon DA et al: Malignant pleural effusions: Pleurodesis using a small bore percutaneous catheter. South Med J 82:963, 1989.
34. Sahn SA, Good JT: Pleural fluid pH in malignant effusions. Ann Intern Med 108:345, 1988.
35. Rodriguez-Panadero F, Mejias JL: Low glucose and pH levels in malignant pleural effusions. Am Rev Respir Dis 139:663, 1989.
36. O'Brien RF, Cohn DL: Serosanguineous pleural effusions in AIDS-associated Kaposi's sarcoma. Chest 96:460, 1989.
37. Little AG, Kadowaki MH, Ferguson MD et al: Pleuroperitoneal shunting. Ann Surg 208:443, 1988.

Chapter 17

BRONCHOSCOPY

EUGENE F. GEPPERT

The technique of fiberoptic bronchoscopy has a special role within the ICU. In several ways, the performance of fiberoptic bronchoscopy is fundamentally different from routine diagnostic bronchoscopy, and many of the indications and risks are also distinct.

Indications

Fiberoptic bronchoscopy is the use of a flexible fiberoptic instrument to enter the trachea and mainstem, lobar, and segmental bronchi for a variety of purposes including inspection, therapeutic maneuvers, or the obtaining of diagnostic specimens. The indications for bronchoscopy in the ICU include: **1.** examining the placement site of the endotracheal tube (ETT) in a patient who is being mechanically ventilated, **2.** investigating the cause of lung collapse, **3.** extracting a foreign body, **4.** determining the site of bleeding in the patient who has hemoptysis, **5.** obtaining reliable bacterial cultures from the lungs of patients with pneumonia by means of a protected brush, **6.** searching for possible tracheal or bronchial lacerations in victims of penetrating or blunt trauma, **7.** examining the tracheal lumen for evidence of stenosis, and **8.** detecting the extent and severity of inhalational airways injury. On occasion the fiberoptic bronchoscope may be used as a tool for intubating the trachea of a patient who could not easily be intubated by other methods. Patients who are critically ill with tracheal or carinal obstruction from tumor should be treated with laser bronchoscopy in the operating room to temporarily reopen the airway lumen and thus prevent precipitous suffocation. Table 17-1 lists the most common indications for fiberoptic bronchoscopy in the ICU.

TABLE 17-1 Indications for Bronchoscopy in the ICU

Determination of ETT position
Removal of endobronchial plug causing lung collapse
Extraction of endobronchial foreign body
Determination of bleeding site in hemoptysis
Obtaining of material for cultures or special stains
Search for tracheobronchial lacerations in trauma
Confirmation of suspected tracheal stenosis
Evaluation of the extent and severity of inhalational injury of airways
Placement of an ETT
Examination of tracheal injury related to intubation
Aid in extubation of patient at high risk for immediate extubation failure

Prebronchoscopy Considerations

Patients who could benefit from bronchoscopy should first be examined to determine whether they have any contraindications or conditions of increased risk. Many critically ill patients who could benefit from bronchoscopy are also endotracheally intubated, and it is very helpful to keep in mind at the time of intubation that an ETT with an internal lumen size of at least 8 mm will be needed so that the patient can be adequately ventilated during bronchoscopy. Various fiberoptic bronchoscopes are available, and many of these have been specially designed for unusual circumstances (e.g., those capable of an exaggerated angle of bend for getting the instrument into difficult locations such as the posterior upper lobes). The instrument should be chosen from those available with the specific purpose of the procedure in mind. We usually favor the use of a bronchoscope with the largest possible side channel, because this allows vigorous suctioning and large biopsy forceps. Laser bronchoscopy requires highly specialized equipment that is not used in routine procedures. If the patient is a child or very small adult, it may be most prudent to use a specially designed pediatric bronchoscope with the narrowest possible diameter. Using an instrument with a relatively small suction channel diameter is a disadvantage in that reduced suction can interfere with the clarity of the view of the airways. Small suction channels may also be inadequate for removing blood from the airways of patients with gross hemoptysis.

Some patients require special consideration at the time of bronchoscopy. For example, some special prebronchoscopy preparations are required in the patient who has a potentially serious neck fracture. The initial passage of the bronchoscope may cause great difficulty for this type of patient. Some patients with cervical fracture can safely undergo fiberoptic bronchoscopy if the fracture is well stabilized, but the alternative method of performing the procedure in the operating room with general anesthesia is more prudent in most cases because it avoids the inevitable neck movements associated with coughing. Other patients requiring careful preparation are those with posterior nosebleeds or acute epiglottitis. Patients with recent active posterior nosebleeds should have bronchoscopy done through the transoral route to avoid recurrent bleeding. In patients suspected of having epiglottitis, the opening to the upper airway may be so perilously narrow that the edema induced by an unsuccessful attempt to pass the fiberoptic bronchoscope through it might cause asphyxiation. Tracheostomy or controlled endotracheal intubation done in the operating room is a safer way to ensure airway patency in these patients.

Contraindications

A number of other contraindications may be encountered in the ICU. A patient with unstable angina pectoris or a patient who may be having an acute myocardial infarction, or who has had one within the past 6 weeks, should not have fiberoptic bronchoscopy. Patients with dangerous dysrhythmias such as ventricular tachycardia should not have the procedure until a stable rhythm is ensured. Since fiberoptic bronchscopy often induces a fall in arterial P_{O_2}, it should not be done in patients who cannot maintain their hemoglobin saturation at 90% or above with supplemental oxygen. Even patients who are being mechanically ventilated for the adult respiratory distress syndrome can safely undergo fiberoptic bronchoscopy as long as their oxygen saturation is continuously monitored during the procedure with a pulse oximeter and the saturation can be maintained at 90% or above by making use of 100% oxygen. Patients who are hypotensive or in shock are too ill to undergo bronchoscopy unless a strong potential benefit of bronchoscopy outweighs the risks of the procedure. If bronchial brushing or biopsy is contemplated as part of the procedure, the patient should not have these done unless clotting function is adequate. In general, the blood urea nitrogen (BUN) level should be <60 (to avoid bleeding from platelet dysfunction), the platelet count should be >50,000, and the prothrombin time and activated partial thromboplastin time should be normal or corrected to normal with fresh frozen plasma administration. If only airway inspection is performed, these clotting variables need not be normal.

Method

In critically ill patients, fiberoptic bronchoscopy is a bedside procedure that must be set up with the equipment specially needed for this type of patient. The example used for purposes of illustration is a bronchoscopy performed in a patient who is endotracheally intubated through the mouth and who is being mechanically ventilated. During set up of the bronchoscopy, the patient is informed about what is about to happen even if already informed earlier at the time consent was obtained. The purpose of this is to keep the patient from becoming unduly anxious during the procedure. To help keep the patient calm during the bronchoscopy we use midazolam in doses of 1 mg administered intravenously. In especially agitated patients, up to 3 mg midazolam may be needed (only 1 mg at a time). The respiratory therapist assists the bronchoscopist and informs the operator of changes in setting on the mechanical ventilator during the procedure. Often it is necessary to adjust the tidal volume, respiratory rate, or inspiratory flow : expiratory flow (I : E) ratio to ensure an adequate minute ventilation during the procedure, since the bronchoscopy causes incomplete obstruction of the airway and also often causes a leak of tidal volume. A pulse oximeter is applied to the patient's finger. At the very outset of bronchoscopy, it is advisable to increase the inspired fraction of oxygen (F_{IO_2}) to avoid any desaturation during the procedure; for many patients, 100% oxygen is appropriate for this short period of time. The bronchoscopist then briefly disconnects the ventilator tubing from the ETT so that an "elbow" can be attached that contains a rubber diaphragm through which the bronchoscope will be passed. It is important to note that when the bronchoscope penetrates this diaphragm to enter the ETT, a large leak is almost always introduced into the ventilator circuit. To overcome this leak with enough extra inspired air to give the patient an adequate tidal volume, the ventilator setting for tidal volume must usually be increased a great deal; how much is enough inspired tidal volume can be determined by monitoring the exhaled tidal volume on the ventilator. The leak is the difference between the inspiratory tidal volume that has been set for delivery and the exhaled tidal volume. During the procedure, inspiratory tidal volume can be increased as necessary to account for variable air leaks and to maintain adequate minute ventilation. The respiratory therapist should continue to watch the exhaled tidal volume readouts during the bronchoscopy. Immediately before inserting the fiberoptic bronchoscope into the ETT, the operator squeezes 5 to 10 ml of viscous lidocaine into it to allow passage of the instrument; without it the bronchoscope cannot slide through the ETT. If the ETT is oral, a bite-block should be placed between the patient's teeth and taped in place. This helps prevent the patient from biting the bronchoscope within the ETT, which is a common impulse in a distressed patient. Once the bronchoscope has been passed, all motions should be unusually gentle to avoid tearing the outer sheath of the instrument on the hard distal tip of the ETT. The bronchial tree is then inspected; the patient's hemoglobin saturation and exhaled tidal volumes are watched closely. Following inspection of the airways, the first sample to be taken should be the passage of a protected-lumen catheter for obtaining bacterial cultures. Following this, other procedures such as bronchial brushing for tumor cells, biopsies, and bronchoalveolar lavage can be done in any order. At the end of the procedure, the ventilator is returned to the previous tidal volume and F_{IO_2} at the moment that the leaky diaphragm is removed and the ETT/ventilator tube is reconnected. A checklist for use in performing bronchoscopy on a critically ill patient is given in Table 17-2.

TABLE 17-2 Steps in Performance of Bronchoscopy in the ICU

1. Explain to patient and obtain consent.
2. In mechanically ventilated patients, prepare the ventilator and place an elbow adapter with a diaphragm between the ETT and the Y connector from the ventilator.
3. For patients intubated with an oral ETT and for patients in whom the approach to bronchoscopy will be through the mouth, place a bite-block and tape it to the patient's skin.
4. Anesthetize the trachea with lidocaine.
5. Pass the fiberoptic bronchoscope through the ETT and immediately reassess exhaled minute volume and oxygenation.
6. Obtain samples: cultures, brushings, biopsies, bronchoalveolar lavage.

Specific Indications

ATELECTASIS

In the ICU, the collapse of a single lobe of the lung is not usually an indication for fiberoptic bronchoscopy when the collapse is seen after several days of critical illness. When lobar collapse is seen immediately following trauma or after an episode of aspiration, bronchoscopy is recommended to look for removable obstructing material. Lobar collapse, especially collapse of the left lower lobe, is extremely common in postoperative patients and in patients with neuromuscular weakness. In general, these lobar collapse incidents are not associated with substantially worsened hypoxemia or patient discomfort, and maneuvers other than bronchoscopy are effective in reinflating these lobes in a matter of a few days. Such maneuvers include incentive spirometry in awake, nonintubated patients, the use of large tidal volumes, or sighs, or positive end-expiratory pressure (PEEP) for a few minutes in intubated, mechanically ventilated patients. Marini has studied the use of bronchoscopy in patients with lobar collapse and shown that bronchoscopy is not more effective than respiratory therapy in the treatment of acute lobar atelectasis.[1] In contrast, it is important to point out that collapse of an entire lung is another matter, typically requiring bronchoscopy. Total lung collapse often means that there is obstruction of a mainstem bronchus. Other causes of lobar collapse in the ICU include obstruction of the mainstem bronchus by inspissated airway secretions, clotted blood, aspirated tooth broken off during intubation, aspiration of large food particles, and previously undiagnosed bronchogenic carcinoma located in a mainstem bronchus. Bronchoscopy should only be done after vigorous efforts at suctioning have failed to remove the obstruction. Because the left main bronchus takes off at an angle that makes it difficult to suction with an ordinary straight suction catheter, specially constructed catheters that can be guided toward the left should be used. When bronchoscopy is necessary, lobar obstruction in the form of mucus or blood can usually be dislodged with infusions of saline together with vigorous suctioning and the use of biopsy forceps to help to mechanically dislodge any clumps of mucus. Tooth fragments or other foreign bodies require special foreign body forceps for their removal. In the patient with cystic fibrosis in the ICU, acetylcysteine can be added to the lavage fluid to help break up the inspissated mucus plugs associated with this condition. In most other patients, acetylcysteine solutions are too irritating to the bronchial mucosa to be recommended.

ENDOTRACHEAL INTUBATION

Bronchoscopy may be used in the ICU to intubate the patient, to inspect the position of an ETT or to inspect the condition of the trachea at sites of potential injury induced by the ETT. In general, bronchoscopy is a good method for passing ETTs transnasally or transorally, but it is usually too slow a procedure to be useful during rapid intubation done for respiratory arrest. In less emergent situations, the patient is instructed on what is about to happen, and the nose is prepared with topical application of cocaine solution and then viscous lidocaine solution as a lubricant. The operator then prepositions the ETT inside the nose and nasopharynx without passing the tube into the larynx. The tip of the fiberoptic bronchoscope is passed through the ETT and then into the larynx and from there into the trachea. Once the tip of the bronchoscope is several centimeters above the carina, the operator slides the ETT until it is securely within the mid trachea. The bronchoscope is then slowly and carefully removed, and the patient is given insufflations of oxygen-rich air by means of an ambu bag prior to connection to the mechanical ventilator.

In addition to passing the ETT over the fiberoptic bronchoscope, the scope may be used at any time to inspect the position of an ETT. If the tube is in good position within the trachea, the operator should be able to see the whole carina just as the bronchoscope exits the tip of the ETT. In those cases in which bronchoscopy is being performed to inspect the trachea of an intubated patient, the maneuver is best done if the patient's ETT is used to guide the bronchoscope into the airways and then, after the balloon cuff around the ETT is deflated, the tube is moved up higher in the airway. This allows inspection of the tracheal mucosa that may have been damaged at the previous site of the tube tip or balloon cuff. In patients who have tracheostomy tubes in place, the tracheal mucosa can be inspected for damage by passing the bronchoscope down from above (nose or mouth) and then deflating the cuff.

FOREIGN BODIES

The use of the fiberoptic bronchoscope to retrieve foreign bodies (e.g., teeth broken off during traumatic endotracheal intubation) from the tracheobronchial tree requires the use of a special foreign body snare that envelopes the fragment and allows it to be removed from the patient as the entire bronchoscope is being removed. Large food particles deposited in the tracheobronchial tree during aspiration of stomach contents may be worth removing by means of bronchial suction; so far, no study exists to guide the judgment of the intensivist in the use of fiberoptic bronchoscopy for this condition.

HEMOPTYSIS

Hemoptysis is an indication for fiberoptic bronchoscopy in the ICU. Modern large channel bronchoscopes together with strong suction make it both possible and preferable to use fiberoptic instruments in most patients with gross hemoptysis; in a minority of cases, rigid bronchoscopy will be preferable when the patient has not been intubated and the hemorrhage is truly massive. The purpose of performing fiberoptic bronchoscopy in a patient with gross hemoptysis (i.e., >200 mL/24 h) is to find the cause of the hemorrhage, or, failing this, to at least localize the site of bleeding to a particular lobe so that if an emergency thoracotomy is needed to save the patient from suffocation, the operative approach to the site of bleeding will be correct. The approach to bronchoscopy in the patient with gross hemoptysis involves a preliminary judgment about the pace of hemorrhage. If the patient has already lost more than 2 U blood (900 ml), then the ICU is not the proper place to perform bronchoscopy; instead, the procedure should be done in the operating room with the thoracic surgeon prepared to operate immediately to remove the bleeding lobe or lung. If the pace of bleeding is less than 2 U in a 24-h period, and the patient is hemodynamically stable with blood transfusions, the procedure may be carried out in the ICU.

Most alert patients with gross hemoptysis are frightened, and the patient should be reassured before the procedure. If the patient has marginal oxygen saturation of arterial blood, it is best to perform fiberoptic bronchoscopy by way of a large diameter (8.0 mm or larger) ETT so that a high F_{IO_2} can be delivered during the procedure; if the patient is not in respiratory failure, the ETT can then be removed at the end of the procedure. The timing of fiberoptic bronchoscopy in patients with hemoptysis is different in different clinical situations. Gross hemoptysis with a rapid pace is an emergency that requires bronchoscopy and emergency surgery without delay. Gross hemoptysis with a slower pace of bleeding in a hemodynamically stable patient is not emergent and should be timed for maximum advantage, i.e., the procedure should be done during the day when maximum resources for help are available. It has been shown by Gong and Salvatierra that in patients with hemoptysis and a slow rate of bleeding, the diagnostic yield is not higher if the procedure is timed to take place during active expectoration of blood.[2] However, if the goal of the bronchoscopy is not diagnosis but rather the localization of the bleeding site, it makes sense to try to time the procedure so that it is done during active bleeding. The performance of fiberoptic bronchoscopy in patients with gross hemoptysis is somewhat different from the routine procedure. Usually, vigorous suction is required together with infusion of large amounts of saline to wash the bronchial tree clean for best visibility. Blood clots lying within the bronchial tree tend to look pink through the fiberoptic bronchoscope and may be mistaken for tumor or other endobronchial pathologic lesions; the differentiation of clots from tumor can often be made only by dislodging the clots with aliquots of saline. Another pitfall is that endobronchial blood tends to pool by gravity in the bronchi of the dependent lobes. If, after washing the bronchial segmental orifices clean with saline, the operator can identify a new stream of blood flowing from a particular segmental or subsegmental bronchus, then the bleeding site has been identified. The identification of segmental origin of the bleeding is of great utility to the surgeon in planning possible surgery; even when angiography and embolization of the bronchial artery is the planned approach, the bronchoscopic identification of the bleeding site is helpful. In addition to its usefulness in diagnosing the cause of hemoptysis and localizing the site of bleeding, bronchoscopy has also been used to control lung bleeding. In some cases, the segmental bronchus can be occluded with a balloon catheter placed in the bronchus by a fiberoptic bronchoscope. For short periods of time, the bronchoscope itself can protect the patient from rapid asphyxiation by remaining lodged in a segmental bronchus to prevent blood from spilling into the general tracheobronchial tree.

DIAGNOSTIC SAMPLING

Diagnostic sampling done in ICU patients includes bronchoalveolar lavage, various types of bronchial brushing, endobronchial biopsy and transbronchial biopsy.

BRONCHOALVEOLAR LAVAGE

To perform bronchoalveolar lavage the fiberoptic bronchoscope is advanced into a segmental bronchus until it is wedged in place, and then about 100 to 150 ml of physiologic salt solution is injected through the suction channel and then immediately suctioned back through the bronchoscope and collected. The result is a sample of bronchoalveolar lavage fluid that contains a mixture of cells, microbes, surfactant, proteins, and debris. The greatest utility of bronchoalveolar lavage in ICU patients is its abililty to detect the presence of malignancy, tuberculosis, fungal infection, and *Pneumocystis carinii* (Fig. 17-1). Viral pneumonia can sometimes be diagnosed from ballooning degeneration seen in lavaged cells that are examined with cytologic techniques, by finding viral inclusion bodies or by the use of direct fluorescent antibodies to particular viruses. Viral cultures may also be done on bronchoalveolar lavage fluid. Bronchoalveolar lavage is normally contaminated with small numbers of bacteria from the upper airway and should only be used for aerobic or anaerobic bacterial culture if quantitative cultures are performed. More than 10,000 colony-forming units per milliliter of wash can be used to indicate the presence of pneumonia.[3–6] The antimicrobial sensitivities of the organisms recovered from bronchoalveolar lavage should be used to guide therapy. In the future, immunologic studies done on cells retrieved from the peripheral lung may be helpful in making diagnoses of various infiltrative lung diseases such as hypersensitivity

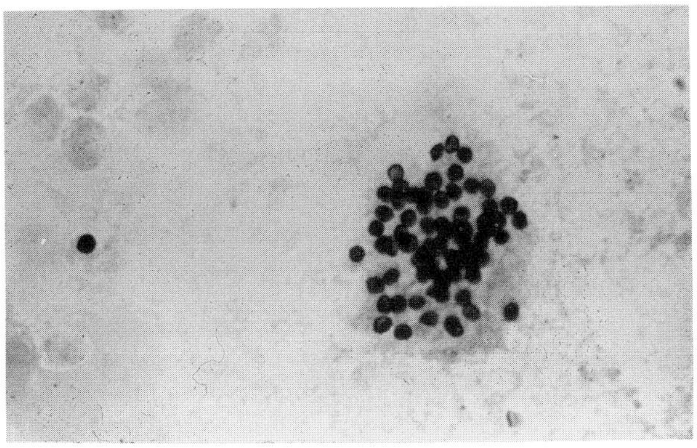

FIGURE 17-1 Silver stain of bronchoalveolar lavage specimen demonstrates 'grape-like cluster' of *P. carinii* organisms. (Reproduced with permission from Science Image Communications, Burbank, CA.) (See also Fig. 18-3, Plate 4.)

pneumonitis. At the present time, these methods are not yet a fully developed clinical tool for these diseases.

BRONCHIAL BRUSHING

Bronchial brushing can be done in ICU patients either by passing brushes through the inner channel of a fiberoptic bronchoscope or by passing naked bronchial brushes through the ETT of an intubated patient. When bronchial brushes are inserted through an ETT without a bronchoscope, care should be taken not to advance the brush too far or pneumothorax may result. One of the most important uses of bronchial brushing in critically ill patients is the technique of sterile sample collection by means of a telescoping plugged catheter/brush assembly. With this tool, uncontaminated samples of airways secretions can be obtained that are very useful in the diagnosis of pneumonia when quantitative cultures are performed. The culture criterion for pneumonia is the growth of more than 1000 colony-forming units per milliliter of brush fluid, prepared by aseptically placing the brush, after its removal from the patient's lung, in a volume of 1 mL physiologic nonbacteriostatic salt solution which should then be promptly delivered to the microbiology laboratory for quantitative culture.[6] Ideally, critically ill patients who have pneumonia should have this procedure done prior to the institution of empirical antimicrobial drugs, but as a practical matter, the procedure is often done on patients who are already being treated with broad-spectrum drugs. An ordinary bronchial brush may be passed through the fiberoptic bronchoscope or ETT when the goal is to collect samples that are not usually affected by contamination from the upper airway, such as tuberculosis, fungal organisms, *P. carinii,* or malignant cells.

BIOPSIES

Endobronchial biopsies are taken under direct vision from lesions inside the bronchi. Most often, these are done to diagnose bronchogenic carcinoma. Transbronchial biopsies are taken by pushing the metal forceps through the wall of a small bronchus and sampling a piece of parenchymal lung tissue. When transbronchial biopsies are performed in critically ill patients, bedside fluoroscopy should be used to help guide the operator so that the forceps do not extend out too far from the hilum and increase the danger of pneumothorax caused by tearing of the visceral pleura. Generally speaking, transbronchial biopsy may be done on critically ill patients if, in the judgment of the intensivist, the patient would be able to tolerate a simple pneumothorax or hemorrhage that might happen as a complication of the procedure. Only one lung is ever biopsied during a single fiberoptic bronchoscopy, a caution intended to prevent the disastrous complication of bilateral pneumothorax. Although several studies have been done in which patients who were on mechanical ventilation with PEEP were subjected to transbronchial biopsy,[7,8] it is best to try to avoid this procedure whenever a good alternative is available. It is preferable to take these patients to the operating room for open lung biopsy since the extra control over bleeding and pneumothorax in the operating room greatly lessens the risk of catastrophic complications. The complication most feared in doing a transbronchial biopsy on a patient who is breathing with the help of a mechanical ventilator is tension pneumothorax. The most plausible indications for transbronchial biopsy in critically ill patients are infectious diseases that have important implications for the treatment regimen. These include diseases such as miliary tuberculosis, miliary coccidioidomycosis, disseminated histoplasmosis, and certain noninfectious diseases such as alveolar proteinosis. In some cases, transbronchial biopsy may be done not to find a treatable diagnosis, but to find a nontreatable disease with important implications for the patient's general prognosis, such as alveolar amyloid or lymphangitic cancer. In every case, the benefits and risks of transbronchial biopsy must be weighed carefully because the danger of tension pneumothorax, air embolism, or bleeding is higher in critically ill patients than in non-critically ill patients.

LASER BRONCHOSCOPY

The use of laser technology in specially constructed bronchoscopes allows for the palliation of upper airway obstruction due to malignancy in the trachea, main carina, or mainstem bronchi. Before treatment, a patient who has critical narrowing of the upper airway has stridor, accessory muscle use, and respiratory distress. Without some form of therapy, these patients suffer from a constant sense of impending suffocation, and they eventually become exhausted from the increased work of breathing. Laser bronchoscopy is a procedure done in the operating room in which a special bronchoscope with quartz fibers transmits laser energy capable of burning and evaporating small bits of living tissue; in this way, the operator is able to widen the lumen of the patient's upper airway by removing bits of obstructing tumor in a "piecemeal" fashion. Once the lumen has been widened beyond the critical orifice size (about 6 mm), the procedure can be stopped and stridor or respiratory distress is usually relieved.

Complications

The complications of fiberoptic bronchoscopy in critically ill patients are listed in Table 17-3. Pneumothorax may result either from a tear in the outer surface of the lung caused by a bronchial brush or forceps, or it may result from barotrauma if very high alveolar pressures caused by coughing or by the mechanical ventilator during the procedure. Underventilation with resultant acute respiratory acidosis may complicate bronchoscopy if the intensivist is not careful to

TABLE 17-3 Complications of Bronchoscopy in the ICU

Pneumothorax: simple or tension
Underventilation of patient
Worsening of hypoxemia
Hemorrhage

observe the minute volume during the bronchoscopy of a patient who is breathing with the aid of a mechanical ventilator. Hypoxemia is another complication that should be actively watched for with an oxygen saturation meter; severe hypoxemia should cause the intensivist to immediately discontinue the bronchoscopy so that all attention can be turned to reversing this severe problem. Excessive or even life-threatening hemorrhage can complicate fiberoptic bronchoscopy, especially if instruments such as bronchial brushes and forceps are passed into the lung.

References

1. Marini JJ, Pierson DJ, Hudson LD: Acute lobar atelectasis: A prospective comparison of fiberoptic bronchoscopy and respiratory therapy. Am Rev Respir Dis 119:971, 1979.
2. Gong H Jr, Salvatierra C: Clinical efficacy of early and delayed fiberoptic bronchoscopy in patients with hemoptysis. Am Rev Respir Dis 124:221, 1981.
3. Brandstetter RD: Flexible fiberoptic bronchoscopy in the intensive care unit. J Intensive Care Med 4:248, 1989.
4. Olopade CO, Prakash UBS: Bronchoscopy in the critical-care unit. Mayo Clin Proc 64:1255, 1989.
5. Helmers RA, Hunninghake GW: Bronchoalveolar lavage in the nonimmunocompromised patient. Chest 96:1184, 1989.
6. Meduri GU: Ventilator-associated pneumonia in patients with respiratory failure: A diagnostic approach. Chest 97:1208, 1990.
7. Papin TA, Grum CM, Weg JG: Transbronchial biopsy during mechanical ventilation. Chest 89:168, 1986.
8. Pincus PS, Kallenbach JM, Hurwitz MD: Transbronchial biopsy during mechanical ventilation. Crit Care Med 15:1136, 1987.

Chapter 18

PATHOLOGIC EXAMINATION OF BODY TISSUES

CYRIL ABRAHAMS

One of the major reasons for the admission of patients to the intensive care unit (ICU) is worsening respiratory function associated with pulmonary infiltration, the cause of which presents a diagnostic and therapeutic dilemma. Arriving at an exact diagnosis is made difficult by the frequent nonspecific nature of the clinical and radiologic findings. The causes of these pulmonary problems include infection, recurrence of a previous malignancy such as a carcinoma or lymphoma, the effect of chemotherapy on the lung, hemorrhage into the lung, or severe diffuse alveolar damage which is associated with the clinical condition of adult respiratory distress syndrome. The best and most accurate method of making a diagnosis is to obtain tissue. This may not always be easy as the severity of the illness may preclude aggressive invasive surgical procedures and the clinician may have to resort to closed procedures such as bronchoalveolar lavage (BAL). It is, of course, important to reach a definitive diagnosis as soon as possible so that adequate and correct therapy can be provided. The pathologist plays an important role, in consultation with the clinician, in helping to diagnose these conditions.

Obtaining a Diagnostic Specimen

There are a number of ways of obtaining tissue for diagnosis. Some, such as the cutting needle biopsy and high-speed trephine biopsy, although useful in diagnosing lung tumors, have unacceptable complication rates in other settings.[1,2,3] Others, such as fine-needle aspiration, have a low complication rate. However, other than in the diagnosis of a solitary mass or neoplasm (or some lung infections), this technique produces an amount of tissue that is too small for investigation of diffuse lung shadowing.[1,4] Transtracheal aspiration may show common bacterial pathogens but usually does not help in the diagnosis of opportunistic infections and is contraindicated in thrombocytopenic patients.[5] In this chapter the use of induced sputum specimens, BAL, transbronchial biopsy (TBB), and open lung biopsy will be discussed.

SPUTUM

Recently, particularly in patients with acquired immunodeficiency syndrome (AIDS), induced sputum specimens are being used for the diagnosis of *Pneumocystis carinii* infections.[6,7] The sputum is induced by having the patient inhale 5% saline administered by an ultrasonic nebulizer over a 10- to 20-min period. During this time, patients are encouraged to cough, but chest physiotherapy is not employed. The specimen must contain alveolar macrophages to be adequate (Fig. 18-1). Squamous epithelial cells alone indicate a specimen derived from the mouth or oropharynx. To make the diagnosis of potentially harmful fungal infection, fungi must be intermingled with alveolar macrophages. Results indicate that although there is a much greater likelihood of diagnosing pneumocystis pneumonia by TBB, induced sputum specimen examination as a first diagnostic step in AIDS patients may obviate the need for bronchoscopy. A negative induced sputum does not exclude a diagnosis of pneumocystis pneumonia. More recently, monoclonal antibodies that react specifically with *P. carinii* were shown to be as sensitive as conventional staining of BAL specimens.[8] Results indicated a high degree of sensitivity. However, the investigators warned that false-positive results will inevitably occur if this technique becomes widely used by less experienced persons.

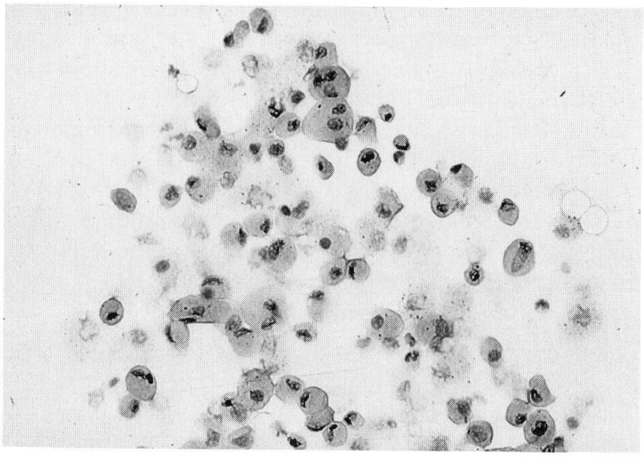

FIGURE 18-1 Adequate induced sputum specimen showing alveolar macrophages [hematoxylin and eosin (H&E) ×100]. (See Plate 2.)

BRONCHOALVEOLAR LAVAGE

BAL is relatively safe, rapid, and a helpful diagnostic aid in critically ill patients with pulmonary infiltrates, particularly in the immunosuppressed patient. It allows sampling of cells and secretions from the lower respiratory tract. There are no complications directly attributable to the procedure such as hemorrhage or pneumothorax.[9] There is usually a slight transient fever the evening after the procedure is performed, occurring in half the patients.[10] There is also a transient increase in pulmonary infiltration roentgenographically. This can be expected to resolve in most patients in 24 h. Even in thrombocytopenic patients (platelets < 70,000 per mm^3) and those requiring mechanical ventilatory support, complications are rare. The highest yields are obtained in immunocompromised patients, and in some series the yield for *Pneumocystis* organisms is 82 percent (Figs.

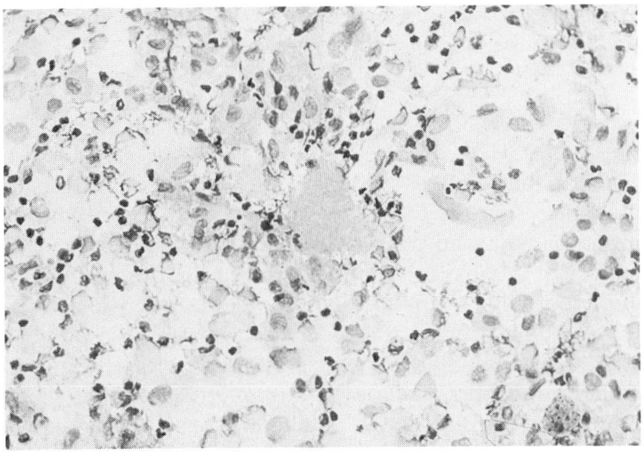

FIGURE 18-2 BAL specimen showing characteristic granular material found in pneumocystis pneumonia infection (H&E ×100). (See Plate 3.)

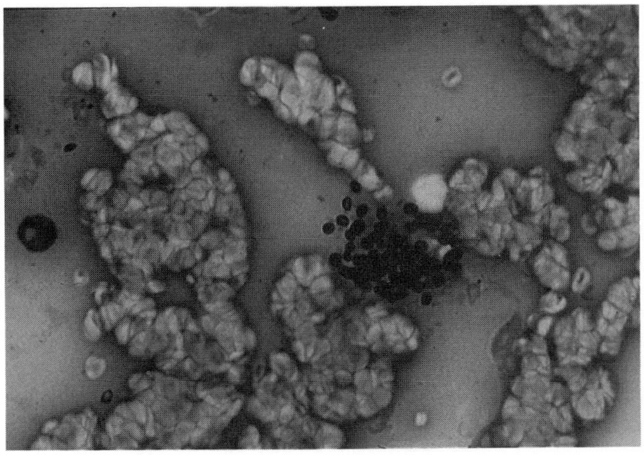

FIGURE 18-3 Cup-and-saucer–shaped *Pneumocystis* organisms seen on BAL (GMS ×100). (See Plate 4.)

18-2 and 18-3).[5,10] In regard to the diagnosis of viral infections, and cytomegalovirus (CMV) in particular, BAL is also useful, in some series with a positivity rate of 83 percent.[5] In fact, the first invasive procedure in the diagnosis of pulmonary infiltrates in AIDS patients is BAL.[6,11] It is not only in the field of infectious disease that BAL may be helpful but also in other conditions. The presence of atypical epithelial cells and alveolar lining epithelial cells suggests drug toxicity, particularly in the appropriate clinical setting. The findings of atypical cells, however, may also be found with viral infections and therefore must be viewed with caution. Confirmation by open lung biopsy may be necessary.[5] The presence of many hemosiderin-laden macrophages indicates intra-alveolar hemorrhage as the primary cause of the pulmonary insufficiency. This may occur particularly in the thrombocytopenic immunocompromised patient where the cause of diffuse pulmonary infiltrates is commonly the result of massive intra-alveolar bleeding.[12] However, pulmonary hemorrhage may be associated with other conditions such as CMV infections.

TECHNIQUE

To perform BAL, the tip of the flexible bronchoscope is wedged into a subsegmental bronchus or into an area of pulmonary infiltration seen on the radiograph (see Chap. 17). Aliquots of 50 to 60 mL of 0.9% NaCl (sterile solution) are injected through the biopsy channel of the bronchoscope, and saline is then aspirated into a sterile sputum trap. The total amount of sterile saline used for each lavage ranges from 70 to 150 mL with a variable yield of between 40 and 70 percent of the volume instilled. For a successful lavage there should be at least 50 mL of fluid. If less than this is obtained, then it is probably not an adequate specimen. Half the specimen is sent to the microbiology laboratory where it is stained with Gram and Ziehl-Neelsen stains and for legionella antigen by direct fluorescent antibody technique. The specimen is also cultured for bacteria (aerobic and anaerobic), fungi, mycobacteria, mycoplasma, and viruses (CMV, herpes simplex, and varicella zoster). The other half of the specimen is submitted to the pathology laboratory where it is mixed with an equal amount of 50% alcohol and centrifuged in safety carriers at 2500 r/min for 20 min. Processing in the pathology laboratory should be done in a laminar flow safety cabinet, and gloves and goggles should be worn throughout the procedure. The sediment is smeared onto albuminized slides. Care must be taken to spread the material out enough to result in a thin preparation. The slides are air dried for a minute, fixed in 95% alcohol for 15 min, and then stained with hematoxylin and eosin, Gomori methenamine-silver stain (GMS), and Ziehl-Neelsen. If pulmonary hemorrhage is suspected, the slides should be stained with the Prussian blue stain for iron. The slides are examined for pneumocystis cysts, fungi, intranuclear and intracytoplasmic inclusions, malignant cells, hemosiderin-laden macrophages, and atypical bronchial epithelial and alveolar lining cells.

DIAGNOSTIC YIELD

In severely immune compromised patients in respiratory failure, BAL is useful in making the correct diagnosis of infections.[1,13] In AIDS patients in particular, *P. carinii* is frequently found. Candida fungus presents as a mixture of yeast cells (blastoconidia) and filamentous elements which may be true hyphae or pseudohyphae. The spores bud off at points of constriction on the filaments which is characteristic. Aspergillus fungus on the other hand has dichotomous branching and septate hyphae (Fig. 18-4). It is not possible to identify the exact species or genus by morphology alone, so a culture of the fungus is required. Unfortunately, not only do fungi grow slowly, they frequently do not grow at all despite their presence in the BAL. The identification of a fungus is, however, adequate for appropriate treatment to be instituted provided there is evidence on the smears that the fungi are derived from the lower respiratory tract.[8] *P. carinii* is the most frequently diagnosed agent responsible for pulmonary failure in the critically ill immunosuppressed patient.[10] The fact that the diagnosis of pneumocystis pneumonia can be made early by BAL is extremely helpful as trimethoprim-sulfamethoxazole in patients with AIDS can be toxic and produces morbidity due

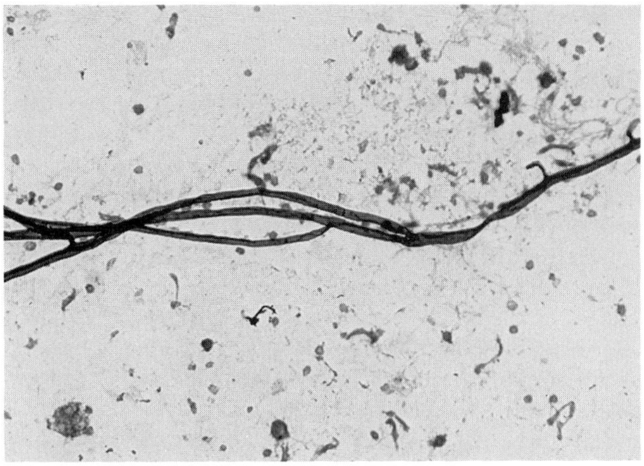

FIGURE 18-4 Hyphae of aspergillus seen on BAL preparation (GMS ×100). (See Plate 5.)

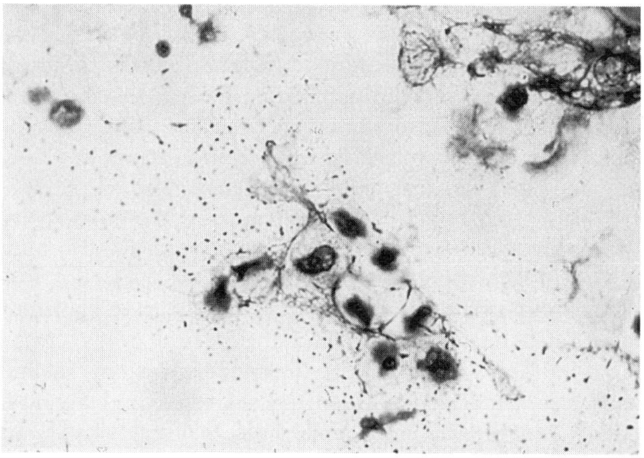

FIGURE 18-5 Mycobacterium tuberculosis seen in bronchoalveolar lavage specimen (Ziehl-Neelsen stain ×100). (See Plate 6.)

to rash, leukopenia, and fever in an already immunocompromised host. Thus accurate, rapid diagnosis of *P. carinii* pneumonia is important to obviate harmful empiric therapy.[10] The presence of CMV may be detected in a number of ways. Cytologic evidence of the virus may be found on microscopic examination of a smear, monoclonal antibody stains for the CMV antigen may be determined on the lavage fluid, and the virus can be cultured, although this takes 5 to 10 days. It is important to realize that the presence of the virus alone does not mean pneumonia is present. Healthy persons are known to shed the virus in the absence of pneumonia. Only if the inclusions are seen in the pulmonary epithelial cells can a pathogenetic role for the virus be established. For these reasons when the suspicion is high, open lung biopsy may be necessary to establish the diagnosis. The same may be said about herpes simplex virus.[14] Although mycobacterium tuberculosis is usually diagnosed by culture of the lavage fluid, it may occasionally be seen on examination of the Ziehl-Neelsen stain of the lavage specimen (Fig. 18-5). This is very helpful as culture may take weeks and the early diagnosis allows therapy to be started with beneficial effects.

TRANSBRONCHIAL BIOPSY

TBB has an excellent record of use in the spontaneously breathing immunocompromised or nonimmunocompromised patient who presents with a pulmonary infiltrate.[15] However, in the diagnosis and management of the critically ill patient with respiratory failure due to pulmonary infiltrates, TBB is problematic. Since these patients are likely to require mechanical ventilation, the risk of barotrauma is high. Many critical care physicians are, therefore, reluctant to perform a TBB[16] and recommend open lung biopsy to obtain tissue. However, there are a few reports dealing with the feasibility, efficacy, and safety of TBB in patients with respiratory failure who are undergoing mechanical ventilation.[17,18] In a recent study, a number of cases were reported where the procedure was performed in the bronchoscopy room or in the ICU.[17] In such patients the TBB was found to be useful in the diagnosis of pulmonary infiltration especially in patients with various opportunistic infections. A definitive diagnosis was made from the TBB in 46 percent of patients, and in others the diagnosis was highly suggestive and enabled the institution of appropriate therapy.[17] In some cases, fungal pneumonia was strongly considered clinically and amphotericin B had been started. TBB excluded fungal infections, and dangerous empiric antifungal chemotherapy was withheld or discontinued.[17] The diagnostic yield in these patients varied. In one series of 15 cases, TBB revealed diagnostic information in only five patients (33 percent).[18] This rose to 47 percent with the use of BAL. This is lower than the 60 to 80 percent diagnostic yield in autonomously breathing patients.[16] TBB may be used in younger patients and in those too ill for open lung biopsy. TBB may be of value in disorders that infiltrate the pulmonary parenchyma along the bronchovascular bundles such as tuberculosis or malignancy. In leukemic patients with a pulmonary infiltrate the cause

FIGURE 18-6 Transbronchial biopsy showing recurrence of leukemia in the lung (H&E ×100). (See Plate 7.)

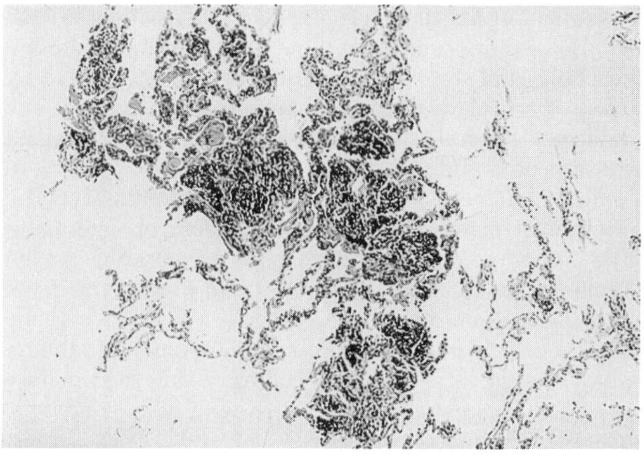

may be recurrence of the original disease (Fig. 18-6), hemorrhage, or pneumocystis pneumonia. In addition to the problems with ventilation, thrombocytopenia or a bleeding disorder is often present and patients are likely to bleed from the procedure. Since hemorrhage and pneumothorax are the two major complications of TBB, this procedure may be life threatening in the critically ill patient.

OPEN LUNG BIOPSY

Despite claims to the contrary, open lung biopsy is still the gold standard for diagnosing the cause of pulmonary infiltrates in critically ill patients with pulmonary insufficiency, whether they are immunocompromised or not. In fact, it is the most accurate diagnostic procedure available with greater than 90 percent accuracy[15,19,20] and a diagnostic yield of 65 percent.[5,21,22] The management of acute respiratory failure due to progressive pulmonary infiltrates presents a common dilemma to the intensive care physician, namely, whether to proceed with an invasive diagnostic procedure. However, once mechanical ventilation is established the traditional approach to invasive diagnosis is open lung biopsy particularly in those patients whose pulmonary process is progressing rapidly. Open lung biopsy is preferred over TBB in patients with severe hypoxemia and coagulation abnormalities as well. The direct control of bleeding in these patients makes it a preferential way to obtain tissue.[23] Specimen size, diagnostic yield, and low morbidity have made open lung biopsy the standard in these situations. There are, however, certain drawbacks in that general anesthesia is required and the standard thoracotomy tube creates the potential for bronchopleural fistula and pleural space infection. Nevertheless open lung biopsy is regarded as being safe, and it has not been proved to be responsible for the demise of critically ill patients, although it may add to their stress.[21]

CHOOSING THE BIOPSY SITE

Most ICU patients who require open lung biopsy have pulmonary disease that progresses with devastating rapidity. The site of biopsy is determined by the extent of the involvement of the lung by the disease process as shown on the radiography, by surgical inspection at thoracotomy, and by the patient's condition. Biopsy of the lingula is easily performed, and hence this segment is frequently chosen.[22] However, it is well known that the lingula is normally subjected to more fibrosis, inflammation, and vasculopathy. It, therefore, may not be representative of a diffuse disease process and is often avoided.[22] This may hold for the diagnosis of chronic diffuse interstitial lung disease but not for the diagnosis of the acutely critically ill patient with respiratory problems. Studies have shown that the lingula is not inherently inferior in giving a diagnostic yield than biopsies removed from other lobes of the lung in this group of patients.[24] In fact the procedure can be performed expeditiously and successfully in the majority of hemodynamically compromised and severely ill patients and is relatively innocuous.[24]

HANDLING THE SPECIMEN

Diagnostic and therapeutic efforts must be highly organized, comprehensive, and expeditious,[25] and the pathologist plays a central role. There should be organizational guidelines available to assure a consistent and thorough approach to the problem. The biopsy is frequently done at the end of the day's operating list and often on a Friday afternoon. This presents problems as the biopsy requires special attention and needs to be handled in a special way. A pathologist or assistant must be available at all times of the day and night so that the specimens can be handled and processed correctly and so that maximum information can be obtained as soon as possible. The laboratory may have to be kept open late and be open at times when it is normally closed such as on weekends and public holidays. At all times the pathologist must be in contact with the surgeon and the intensive care physician so that necessary arrangements for delivery and receipt of the specimen can be made.

When the biopsy is ready, the surgeon, the infectious disease physician, or critical care physician should be responsible for informing the pathologist on call. The surgeon should divide the specimen in half and make certain that the specimen is amply cultured. Samples should be submitted rapidly to the microbiology laboratory with a request for culture of aerobic and anaerobic organisms, virus, and fungi as well as indirect stain by immunofluorescence for *Legionella* organisms. The attending physician or designee, who should be present at the biopsy, must accept the responsibility of hand-carrying the other half of the specimen to the pathology laboratory. Specimens are best transported in capped, sterile, wide-mouth bottles.[25] The pathologist then divides the biopsy specimen. Part is fixed in glutaraldehyde for electron microscopy. A frozen section is prepared for a rapid diagnosis with hematoxylin and eosin; GMS and Ziehl-Neelsen stains should be done routinely. In addition, touch preparations (imprints) or scrimps (scrape and imprint) (Fig. 18-7)[26] of the freshly cut surface should be prepared and examined immediately

FIGURE 18-7 Scrimp preparation of open lung biopsy showing characteristic intranuclear and intracytoplasmic inclusions of CMV (H&E ×100). (See Plate 8.)

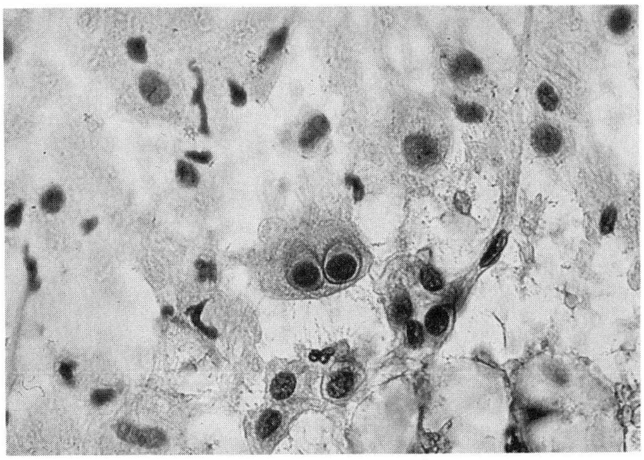

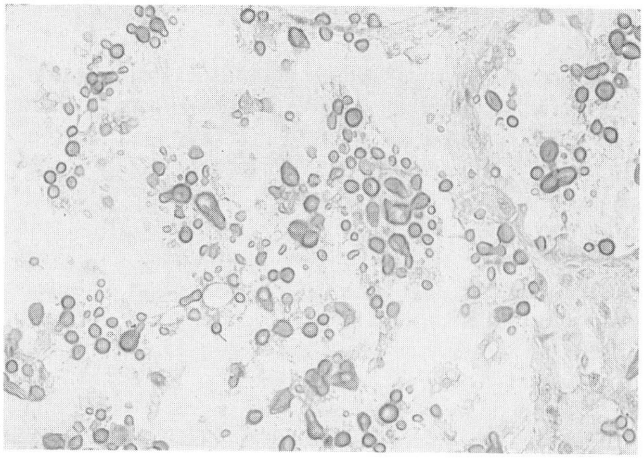

FIGURE 18-8 Budding yeasts showing mucin positive capsule characteristic of cryptococcosis (mucicarmine stain ×100). (See Plate 9.)

with hematoxylin and eosin, Gram, GMS, and Ziehl-Neelsen stains. The remaining specimen is fixed in formalin and processed for routine paraffin sections which must be available the next day (repeating the same stains). In addition, the Prussian blue stain may reveal hemosiderin in macrophages. This is seen in the presence of hemorrhage and is present in excessive quantities in Goodpasture's disease. If fungi are present (particularly yeasts), a mucin stain for cryptococcosis should be done (Fig. 18-8). If clinically or pathologically indicated, immunofluorescent stain for *Legionella* organisms should be added. In addition, it is important to perform connective tissue stains to determine the state of the alveolar walls in regard to presence or absence of fibrosis as well as the nature of any pathologic changes in the blood vessels. The presence of organizing fibroblastic material in alveolar spaces is important since it may indicate that the patient has an organizing pneumonia.

The clinician should be kept informed by the pathologist at all stages of the examination of the tissue so that if a definitive or nondefinitive diagnosis is made, corrective therapy can be started. Time is of the essence for many of these critically ill patients. Pneumocystis cysts can be difficult to find. A helpful feature is the presence of foamy exudate in which the cystic forms are found (Fig. 18-9). The cysts that are seen on the GMS stain are helmet or cup-and-saucer shaped and contain a basophilic dotlike structure in the center that corresponds to the nuclei of sporozoites. It is important to always use *P. carinii* and not fungi as the positive control when staining for the presence of *Pneumocystis* organisms. These organisms require longer staining than fungi, and false negatives may result. Recently, immunohistochemical staining with monoclonal antibodies to *P. carinii* has been utilized in paraffin sections as well as in BAL (Fig. 18-10).[27,28] However, it has been shown that staining for the 2G2 and 6B8 antigens of *P. carinii* does not provide any diagnostic advantage over routine silver staining. It is more time-consuming and is less sensitive than the silver stain when few organisms are present. Silver stains have an added advantage in that they may detect fungi as well. Viral pneumonias are at times difficult to distinguish from one another. Many of the pathogenic viruses affecting the lung parenchyma in these critically ill patients have intranuclear inclusions. In CMV, intracytoplasmic inclusions are also present (Fig. 18-7). These viral intranuclear inclusions are eosinophilic with a surrounding clear halo. It is important not to mistake a large nucleolus in an enlarged type 2 cell or macrophage as a CMV inclusion as these patients may be incorrectly diagnosed as having CMV pneumonia and treated unnecessarily. If there is any uncertainty, confirmation from monoclonal antibody studies by immunoperoxidase techniques (Fig. 18-11) or by electron microscopy should be undertaken. In herpes simplex and varicella infection, "ground glass" nuclei and cell fusion and multinucleation and molding are consistently found. These are not a feature of CMV. In adenovirus, basophilic inclusions are associated with "smudge" cells which are not seen in CMV. Antibodies to adenovirus, respiratory syncytial virus, herpes simple 1 and 2, and herpes zoster make for a more rapid diagnosis of these viruses on fixed, frozen, or freshly smeared tissue samples.[29] Furthermore, in situ hybridization methods, which identify specific viral

FIGURE 18-9 Characteristic foamy honeycomb material seen in alveolar spaces in pneumocystis pneumonia (H&E ×100). (See Plate 10.)

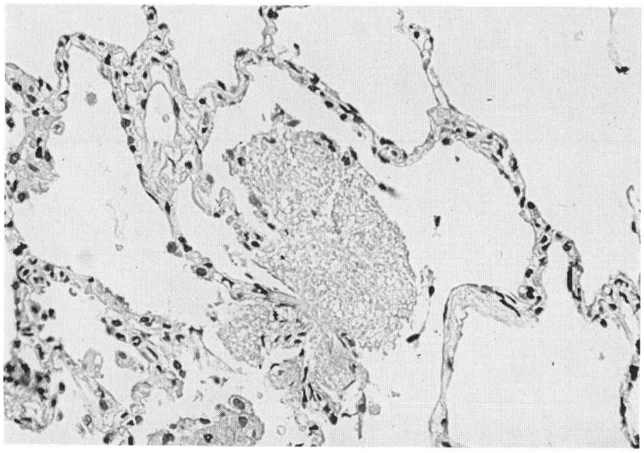

FIGURE 18-10 Monoclonal antibody staining of *P. carinii* (immunohistochemical staining ×100). (See Plate 11.)

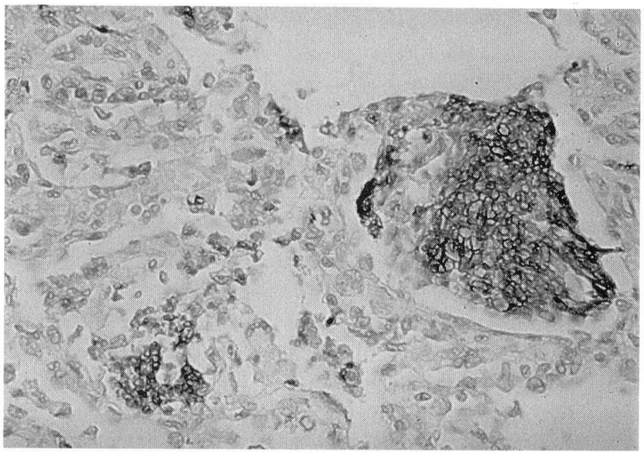

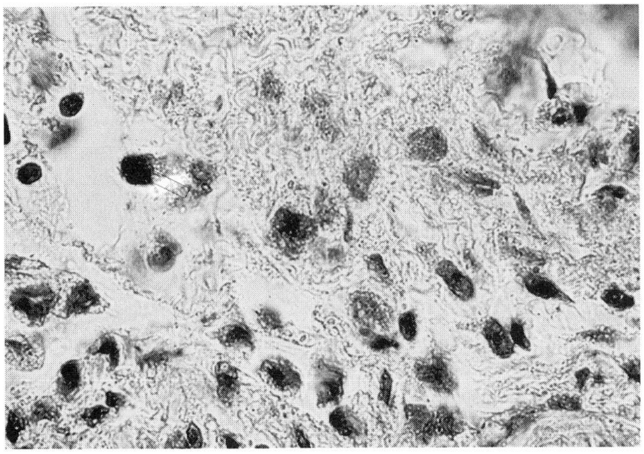

FIGURE 18-11 Monoclonal antibody staining of CMV (immunohistochemical stain ×100). (See Plate 12.)

DNA genomic sequences even in paraffin embedded sections, may help in the diagnosis of acute infection as well as latent chronic infection.[30] Electron microscopy of cells for virus may be helpful.

IMPACT OF OBTAINING AN OPEN LUNG BIOPSY

There are two major issues in assessing the utility of an open lung biopsy in this group of critically ill patients. These include diagnostic yield and improved survival. Although the biopsy results may lead to a change in treatment, the most significant issue is patient outcome. There is no point in subjecting a desperately ill patient to an operation just to make a specific diagnosis so as to give the correct therapy (or to avoid empiric toxic therapy) if survival is unaffected. However, these patients present a diagnostic and therapeutic dilemma, and diagnosis is not possible without obtaining a tissue sample. A central issue which requires elucidation is the benefit likely to accrue to a patient if a specific diagnosis is made by open lung biopsy. In two reports of immunocompromised patients, no significant difference in mortality rate was noted between patients with a specific diagnosis and those without.[25,31] Similarly, there was no difference between those whose treatment was altered because of the diagnosis and those with no treatment changes.

These data, however, do not indicate that open lung biopsy is without value. It is possible that those with specific diagnoses constituted a higher risk group, and the mortality rate in this group may have been even higher had no diagnosis been made.[31] Furthermore, patients with nondiagnostic biopsies were spared further exposure to potentially toxic antimicrobials that have deleterious side effects. It is possible that those patients with nonspecific interstitial pneumonitis may be preselected for survival by the nature of their pulmonary condition in that these patients do not have an overwhelming bacterial infection, deep fungal infection, *P. carinii* pneumonia, or diffuse neoplastic infiltration (all conditions associated with a significant mortality even with specific treatment).[25] The survival statistics for the critically ill immunocompromised patient with pulmonary infiltrate is poor, but high mortality due to untreated underlying disease is substantial, and hence, open lung biopsy should be undertaken on an individualized basis predicated on the total clinical situation.[31] One can argue that in these critically ill patients with pulmonary failure, high mortality is the nature of the beast: nevertheless, knowing the diagnosis allows for optimum treatment and maximizes the chance of survival even if this is small. Because overall prognosis of patients with malignancy has improved and effective treatment is available for many respiratory diseases, accurate diagnosis and prompt treatment of life-threatening pulmonary disorders in this group of critically ill patients is important.[5]

INTERPRETATION OF FINDINGS

The findings on open lung biopsy may be divided into those that are diagnostic and those that are nondiagnostic. They are regarded as diagnostic if an infectious organism is identified histopathologically or recovered in culture; if a specific malignancy is present such as leukemia or if the histopathology is highly suggestive of a specific cause such as bleomycin effect on the lung and the clinical features of the case are compatible with that entity. If the clinical picture is consistent with pneumocystis pneumonia and no organisms are found on the first cuts, it is important to prepare additional sections from the original biopsy specimen. These should be examined by more than one pathologist and by the clinicians.

Nondiagnostic biopsies include interstitial pneumonitis associated with infiltration by mononuclear cells and alveolar thickening, alveolar hemorrhage, and organizing intraalveolar exudate. In immunocompromised patients with pulmonary infiltrates, nondiagnostic findings consisting of nonspecific interstitial pneumonitis are found mainly in those patients who have received bleomycin and total body irradiation.[32] It is generally not possible to accurately predict the cases that are likely to have a diagnostic biopsy. Nondiagnostic biopsies are more likely to be seen in those patients with no prior immunosuppressive therapy, in those who have myeloproliferative rather than lymphoproliferative disease, or in those with a nonhematologic underlying disease and who have granulocytopenia of less than 100 per cubic millimeter at the time of biopsy.[25] In critically ill nonimmunocompromised hosts, bacterial pneumonias are more likely to be the cause of pulmonary infiltrates, whereas in immunocompromised patients the most likely diagnostic findings are *P. carinii* or fungal infections. In this group, biopsy findings are likely to differ depending upon whether the patient has a solid neoplasm, a hematologic malignancy, or AIDS. It is of interest that although CMV and *P. carinii* infections are the most commonly seen in AIDS, in those AIDS patients with a history of drug abuse, CMV is the most common infection.[33]

Autopsy

Many critically ill patients do not survive despite excellent medical care. The autopsy is a useful and only means of accurately determining the cause of death. Recent reviews of discrepancy between clinical and autopsy diagnoses reveal that there is a 20 to 30 percent incidence of missed diagnoses. Some of these may be of a major type: had the correct diagnosis been made, corrective therapy may have changed the course of the disease. Furthermore, in this group of patients it may be of value to determine the effects of chemotherapy, drug regimens, and other treatments. In this way information garnered from the autopsy may help in the treatment of future cases. A case in point would be culture of fungi present in the lung at autopsy. This allows determination of the exact genus of a fungus. This may indicate the success (or otherwise) of the laminar flow rooms in which many of these patients are held. It is also not possible to determine the nature of a pulmonary infiltrate with certainty, except by doing an open lung biopsy. Unfortunately some patients are too ill to undergo this procedure, and the autopsy is the only means of attempting to explain the cause of the infiltrate. If autopsies are not performed in these patients, a golden opportunity to learn is lost.

References

1. Macfarlane J: Lung biopsy. Brit Med J 290:97, 1985.
2. Harrison BDW, Thorpe RS, Kitchener PG, et al. Percutaneous Tru-Cut lung biopsy in the diagnosis of localized pulmonary lesions. Thorax 39:493, 1984.
3. Cunningham JH, Zavala DC, Carry RJ, et al. Trephine air drill, bronchial brush, and fiberoptic transbronchial lung biopsies in immunosuppressed patients. Am Rev Respir Dis 115:213, 1977.
4. Gibney RTN, Man GCW, King EG, et al. Aspiration biopsy in the diagnosis of pulmonary disease. Chest 80:300, 1981.
5. Stover DE, Zaman MB, Hajdu SI, et al. Bronchoalveolar lavage in the diagnosis of pulmonary infiltrates in the immunosuppressed host. Ann Intern Med 101:1, 1984.
6. Bigby T, Margolskee D, Curtis JL, et al. The usefulness of induced sputum in the diagnosis of *Pneumocystis carinii* pneumonia in patients with the acquired immunodeficiency syndrome. Am Rev Respir Dis 133:515, 1986.
7. Ng VL, Gartner I, Weymouth LA, et al. The use of mucolysed sputum for the identification of pulmonary pathogens associated with human immunodeficiency virus infection. Arch Pathol Lab Med 113:488, 1989.
8. Kovacks JA, Ng VL, Masur H, et al. Diagnosis of *Pneumocystis carinii* pneumonia: improved detection in sputum with use of monoclonal antibodies. N Engl J Med 318:558, 1988.
9. Strumpf IJ, Field MK, Cornelius MJ, et al. Safety of fiberoptic bronchoalveolar lavage in evaluation of interstitial lung disease. Chest 80:268, 1982.
10. Ognibene P, Schelhamer J, Gill V, et al. The diagnosis of *Pneumocystis carinii* pneumonia in patients with the acquired immunodeficiency syndrome using subsegmental bronchoalveolar lavage. Am Rev Respir Dis 129:929, 1984.
11. Mann J, Altus C, Webber C, et al. Nonbronchoscopic lung lavage for diagnosis of opportunistic infection in AIDS. Chest 91:319, 1987.
12. Drew WL, Finley TN, Golde DW. Diagnostic lavage and occult pulmonary hemorrhage in thrombocytopenic immunocompromised patients. Am Rev Respir Dis 116:215, 1977.
13. Hopkin JM, Turney JH, Young JA, et al. Rapid diagnosis of obscure pneumonia in immunosuppressed renal patients by cytology of alveolar lavage fluid. Lancet ii:299, 1983.
14. Goldstein RA, Rohatgi PK, Bergofsky EH, et al. Clinical role of bronchoalveolar lavage in adults with pulmonary disease. Am Rev Respir Dis 142:481, 1990.
15. Katzenstein AL. Transbronchial lung biopsy, in Katzenstein AL, Askin FB (eds): *Surgical Pathology of Non-neoplastic Lung Disease,* 2d ed. Philadelphia, WB Saunders, 1990, pp 564–587.
16. Fulkerson WJ. Fiberoptic bronchoscopy: current concepts. N Engl J Med 311:511, 1984.
17. Pincus PS, Kallenbach JM, Hurwitz MD, et al. Transbronchial biopsy during mechanical ventilation. Crit Care Med 15:1136, 1987.
18. Papin TA, Grun CM, Weg JG. Transbronchial biopsy during mechanical ventilation. Chest 89:168, 1986.
19. Burt ME, Flye MW, Webber BL, et al. Prospective evaluation of aspiration needle biopsy, cutting needle, transbronchial and open lung biopsy in patients with pulmonary infiltrates. Ann Thorac Surg 32:146, 1981.
20. Toledo-Pereyra LH, DeMeester TR, Kinealey A, et al. The benefits of open lung biopsy in patients with non-diagnostic transbronchial lung biopsy. A guide to appropriate therapy. Chest 77:647, 1980.
21. Greenman RL, Goodall PT, King D. Lung biopsy in immunocompromised hosts. Am J Med 59:488, 1975.
22. Gaensler EA. Open and closed lung biopsy, in Sacker MA (ed): *Diagnostic Techniques in Pulmonary Disease, Part II.* New York, Marcel Dekker, 1980, pp. 579–622.
23. Singer C, Armstrong D, Rose PP, et al. Diffuse pulmonary infiltrates in immunosuppressed patients: prospective study of 80 cases. Am J Med 66:110, 1979.
24. Wetstein L. Sensitivity and specificity of lingular segmental biopsies of the lung. Chest 90:383, 1986.
25. Jaffe JP, Maki DG. Lung biopsy in immunocompromised patients: One institution's experience and an approach to management of pulmonary disease in the compromised host. Cancer 48:1144, 1981.
26. Abrahams C. The scrimp technique—a method for the rapid diagnosis of surgical pathology specimens. Histopathology 2:225, 1975.
27. Ghali VS, Garcia RL, Skolom J. Fluorescence of *Pneumocystis carinii* in Papanicolau smears. Hum Pathol 15:907, 1984.
28. Travis WD, Pittaluga S, Lipschik GY, et al. Atypical pathologic manifestations of *Pneumocystis carinii* pneumonia in the acquired immune deficiency syndrome: review of 123 lung biopsies from 76 patients with emphasis on cysts, vascular invasion, vasculitis and granulomas. Am J Surg Pathol 14:615, 1990.
29. Hackman RC. Immunohistology for the rapid diagnosis of viral infections. West J Med 145:373, 1986.
30. Sale GE. Infections in transplant recipients, in GE Sale (ed): *Pathology of Organ Transplantation.* Boston, Butterworth, 1990, pp 271–284.
31. Rossiter SJ, Miller DC, Churg AM, et al. Open lung biopsy in the immunosuppressed patient. Is it really beneficial? J Thorac Cardiovasc Surg 77:338, 1979.
32. Pennington JE, Feldman NT. Pulmonary infiltrates and fever in patients with hematologic malignancy. Am J Med 62:581, 1977.
33. Ambrose RA, Lee E-Y, Sharer LR, et al. The acquired immunodeficiency syndrome in intravenous drug abusers and patients with a sexual risk: clinical and postmortem comparisons. Hum Pathol 18:1109, 1987.

Chapter 19

CHEST RADIOLOGY IN THE ICU

HEBER MACMAHON
STEVEN M. MONTNER

Chest radiology plays an important role in the diagnosis and management of patients in the ICU, and increasing numbers of bedside chest x-ray examinations are being performed in hospitals in recent years. This trend is attributed to a combination of factors, including an increase in the numbers of cardiac surgical procedures and transplant operations, as well as more widespread use of assisted ventilation and hemodynamic monitoring systems. Such apparatus tends to make the patient less mobile, and many of the devices themselves require periodic monitoring by radiography. In several large medical centers in the United States, approximately 50 percent of all chest x-ray examinations are now "portables," that is, performed at the bedside with mobile equipment. Although this proportion might suggest overutilization, recent studies have documented the high diagnostic yield of portable radiography in the ICU and have suggested that frequent usage of portable chest radiography is not inappropriate in this situation.[1–3]

Technical Aspects of Bedside Radiography

The full diagnostic potential of bedside radiography is often not realized due to poor image quality. Despite dramatic advances in other areas of medical imaging, the technique of bedside radiography has remained largely unchanged for many years, and physicians and radiologists who interpret ICU portable chest radiographs commonly accept inferior image quality as inevitable. This is usually attributed to intrinsic limitations of mobile equipment, but the problem is primarily one of poor contrast, and the cause is scattered radiation. When x-rays pass through a patient, a proportion continue directly to the film and contribute to the image. However, a significant fraction of the radiation beam scatters at random angles from the patient's body. Some of the scattered radiation reaches the film and appears as diffuse gray density ("fog"), which impairs the image. With fixed equipment in the x-ray department, an antiscatter grid, composed of fine lead strips, in a manner analogous to a venetian window blind, is interposed between the patient and the film to intercept scattered radiation. The grid must be accurately aligned with the x-ray beam, and such precision is difficult to achieve consistently with conventional bedside techniques. Mainly for this reason, antiscatter grids are not used routinely in most hospitals for portable chest radiography. However, when used correctly, a carefully aligned grid can markedly improve the image quality and diagnostic content of portable radiographs[4] (see Plate 52).

Day-to-day variations in image density can be a major problem, especially when the principle function of the examination is to evaluate interval change. These variations can be due to use of different settings on the x-ray machine, changes in source-to-image detector distance (SID), variations in grid alignment, variations in processing conditions, and use of different screen/film combinations. It is important to standardize both kilovoltage (kV) and SID for all adult cases, and to alter milliampere-seconds according to patient size. This reduces the number of variables to a minimum. When a grid is used in combination with a wide latitude film and appropriate kV level, it is not necessary to overpenetrate the lungs to demonstrate catheter or endotracheal tube location in the mediastinum. One approach to standardizing film density involves use of a photo timing device, which is placed behind the film cassette and which terminates the x-ray exposure automatically when the optimal amount of radiation has passed through.[5] Similar systems are widely used in nonportable applications. A second solution involves use of a digital radiography system, which has a photostimulable phosphor plate, instead of film, to record the image.[6] The plate, which is placed in a conventional x-ray cassette and exposed in the usual way, is subsequently scanned by a fine laser beam, which causes it to release energy in the form of light, proportional to the amount of x-ray energy absorbed. The emitted light is measured and recorded, pixel by pixel, to form a digital image. A practical advantage of this type of system is the ability of the computer to modify the density and contrast of the image before it is printed on film for interpretation. Thus, the density of the final image is independent of the x-ray exposure. However, reducing exposure significantly below the conventional range causes a noticeable increase in "noise" (mottle, which is perceived as a grainy appearance). Image processing can also be performed to enhance the visibility of fine detail such as a catheter or pneumothorax (see Plate 53).[7] Digital imaging provides other potential advantages, such as the capacity to select and display clinical images in the ICU or other remote locations on video monitors.[8] Digital systems are currently being used at several medical centers and will almost certainly become more widely used in the future. The main constraints for digital imaging systems at present are cost, image quality, and practical aspects of using video displays for diagnosis.[9]

Interpreting Portable Radiographs

In addition to image quality, some important differences are apparent between portable chest radiographs and those obtained in the radiology department. These variables directly affect interpretation and are important to consider when making comparisons between portable and standard radiographs. These are summarized in Table 19-1.

TABLE 19-1 Comparison between Portable and Standard Radiographs

	Standard Chest X-Ray	Portable Chest X-Ray	Comment
Position	Standing Posterior-anterior projection	Erect, sitting, semierect, or supine Anterior-posterior projection	Increased cardiac magnification and limited pulmonary expansion on portable exam
Beam angle	Horizontal	Variable	Nonhorizontal beam limits ability to detect free air, air-fluid levels, pleural effusions and pneumothorax
Beam energy	kV: 120–140 Exposure time < 1/10 sec	kV: 80–100 Exposure time often > 1/10 sec	Motion blurring more likely with portable technique
X-ray source	72 inches	40–72 inches	Shorter distances contribute to cardiac magnification
Image quality	Superior	Inferior	Mainly due to uncontrolled scattered radiation

The most obvious differences between standard and portable chest radiographs are due to projection. The anteroposterior (AP) projection, combined with a shorter distance, combine to increase cardiac magnification on portable radiographs. The mediastinum also tends to appear wider. If the patient is not fully erect, the vascular pedicle may be distended, and blood flow to the upper lobes may be increased. The patient's actual position can be estimated from several clues: **1.** in many x-ray departments opaque inclinometers are used to indicate the approximate patient angle; **2.** the appearance of the gastric air bubble (air collects in the fundus when erect, in the antrum when supine); and **3.** the breast position in women.

Value and Limitations of ICU Radiography

Certain patterns or combinations of x-ray findings are sufficiently suggestive that a confident diagnosis can be made. However, because the lungs have a limited range of response to disease, the radiographic abnormalities are often nonspecific. In such cases, correlation of the x-ray findings with clinical and laboratory data allow the differential diagnosis to be reduced to a limited number of options.

In the evaluation of sequential chest radiographs in ICU patients, the major considerations are evaluation of the cardiopulmonary status, particularly in terms of interval change; evaluation of the positions of the various tubes, catheters, and monitoring devices, and detection of related problems; and detection of complications of therapy, such as abnormal air collections in patients receiving assisted ventilation. These subjects will be discussed in further detail elsewhere in this chapter. In the case of interval change detection, some general considerations should be borne in mind. In the typical case, the finding of interest consists of localized or diffuse pulmonary infiltrates. An infiltrate is perceived mainly as an area of increased density (i.e., whiteness) in the lung, though details such as air bronchograms or septal lines may also be visible. Increased exudation or edema will increase the density, but less air due to decreased lung inflation will produce a similar effect. Although physicians and radiologists are aware of this basic fact, there is tendency to underestimate the effects of lung inflation when comparing sequential radiographs. When decreased pulmonary inflation is combined with decreased x-ray penetration, the tendency to diagnose worsening infiltrates becomes very strong. In the same way, improved pulmonary inflation and increased x-ray penetration tend to be interpreted as improvement. To compound the problem, pulmonary expansion often decreases in patients with worsening lung disease such as pulmonary edema. No simple guideline eliminates this problem other than awareness of the factors involved and use of caution in diagnosing change based on a single comparison radiograph. In cases being followed with serial x-ray examinations over many days, it is helpful to view several sequential radiographs side by side, to distinguish real from artifactual changes.

Ideally, all bedside x-ray examinations would be performed and interpreted immediately. In practice, because of financial constraints limiting the numbers of technologists and units of equipment, together with fluctuations in the workload throughout the day, various delays are inevitable. To ensure that urgent cases receive prompt attention, some form of prioritization is necessary. At the University of Chicago Hospitals, we use a system requiring that the level of urgency be specified at the time that the request for a portable x-ray examination is made. Levels of urgency vary from category A which requires an immediate response and is reserved for cases with actual or impending cardiac or respiratory arrest, to the least urgent cases which are classified as "routine." Though this type of system is open to abuse by the requesting physician, retrospective review of examinations classified as urgent in our institution indicates that, in general, the categories have been used appropriately.

It is important that ICU radiographs be readily accessible, 24 h a day, to both clinical staff and radiologists. This can be achieved most readily by mounting all ICU radiographs on dedicated motorized film viewers, so that a sequence of recent radiographs is displayed and regularly updated for each ICU patient. To alleviate problems with lost radiographs and delayed reporting that may occur when the original radiographs are maintained in the ICU, a policy of routinely duplicating all ICU radiographs has been in place in our institution for several years. This has virtually eliminated film losses and significant delays in reporting, but the disadvantages of this approach include considerable expense, as well as some losses of image quality that occur with conventional duplication. The long-term solution to this problem lies in digital imaging, whether by digitization of conventional radiographs or by use of other media such as storage phosphor computed radiography. Film digitization allows duplication with essentially no loss of quality, and in fact, considerable improvements in quality can be achieved in cases that have been significantly over- or underexposed. The cost can also be significantly lower than with conventional duplication techniques. Digital images can also be transmitted between the radiology department and the ICU for display on video monitors.

Role of Computed Tomography and Ultrasound

Ultrasound examination is widely available and is versatile in that it can be used at the bedside. In general, ultrasound waves are transmitted through fluid and soft tissues, and ultrasound images are generated from the reflections that occur at tissue interfaces. Ultrasound waves are not well transmitted by air or bone, and this limits its utility in some anatomic areas. One of the most useful applications of ultrasound in the ICU is in localizing fluid collections such as loculated pleural effusions. Accurate determination of the location and size of a fluid collection by ultrasound can increase the yield of thoracentesis in cases with small effusions.[10] It is important to scan the patient in the same position in which thoracentesis will be performed when determining the location of pleural fluid and the optimal point for needle insertion. Even if the pleural fluid is highly loculated, its relationship to the skin may change if the position of the shoulder girdle is altered. It is possible to visualize the fluid and the aspirating needle simultaneously during the procedure for maximum accuracy, though this is rarely necessary for thoracentesis alone.

Computed tomography (CT) has important advantages over plain radiography, particularly in the evaluation of mediastinal and pleural disease.[11] Unlike radiography and ultrasound, the CT scanner cannot be brought to the bedside, and moving a critically ill patient to the x-ray department is potentially difficult. However, a CT scan can provide unique information and is appropriate for ICU patients when used selectively.[12]

The advantage of CT over plain radiography is its ability to display anatomy in discrete axial planes with highly accurate contrast resolution. As a result, CT is considerably more sensitive than plain radiography for detection of fluid collections such as pleural effusions, empyemas, or lung abscesses[13–15] (Fig. 19-1). CT may also reveal an unsuspected loculated pneumothorax, especially in cases where lateral radiographs have not been obtained.[16,17] CT has also

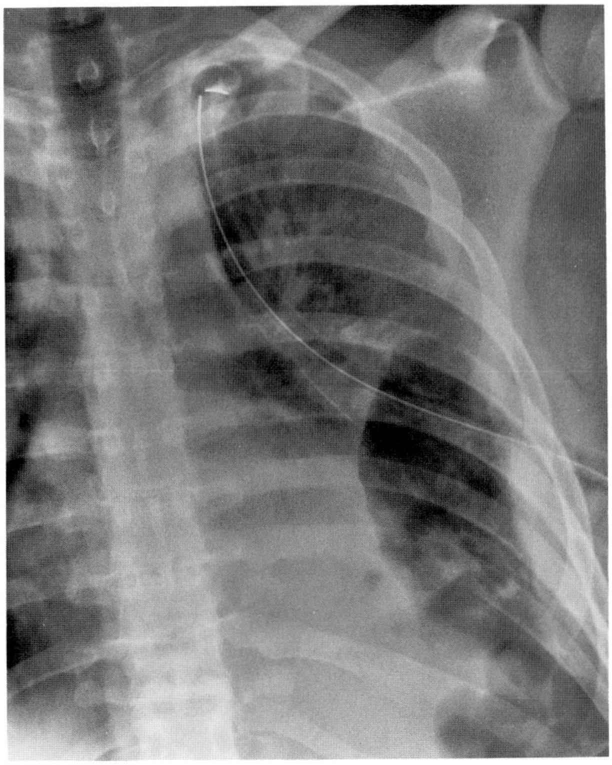

a

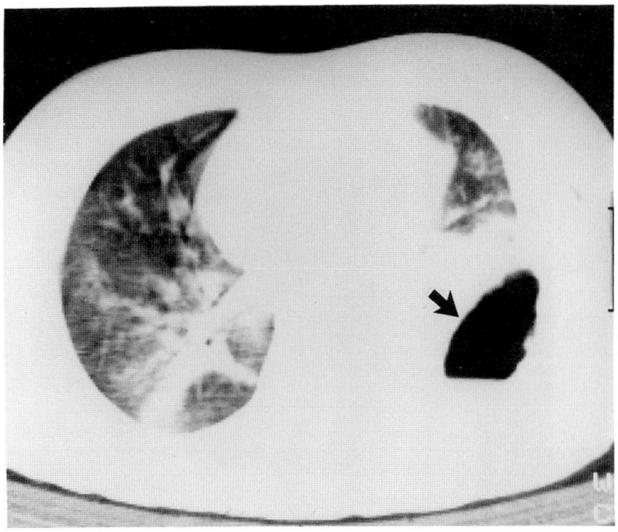

b

FIGURE 19-1 Posteriorly loculated pleural fluid collection and pneumothorax. ***A:*** **An AP view of the chest suggests a loculated air and fluid collection near the left base despite a pleural drain, with consolidation medially.** ***B:*** **A loculated posterolateral hydropneumothorax (arrow), with adjacent consolidation, is better delineated by a CT scan.**

TABLE 19-2 Comparative Costs and Doses for ICU Radiography

Examination	Cost ($)[a]	Radiation Dose (total body equivalent millirems)[b]
Standard chest radiograph (PA and lateral)	100	24
Portable chest radiograph (AP)	150	8
Chest CT scan	750	200–600[c]
Ultrasound examination	250	0

[a] Approximate average total charge.
[b] Average environmental background radiation = 300 millirems/year.
[c] Actual dose may vary widely.

been useful in identifying malpositioned or occluded chest tubes,[18] and it can provide unique information in cases of mediastinal disease, such as hematoma or mediastinitis. In one series, thoracic CT was considered to have added important information in 70 percent of 87 critically ill trauma patients.[13] Therefore, it is appropriate to use CT when certain such specific abnormalities are suspected. In view of the practical difficulties and risks of transporting ICU patients to the scanner and because of the greater expense involved, the use of additional radiographic views or ultrasound examination should be considered first (Table 19-2).

Abnormal Air Collections

Most abnormal air collections in ICU patients are iatrogenic in origin, and detecting them is one of the important functions of the chest radiograph. Unlike pulmonary infiltrates, the appearance of an abnormal air collection is usually specific in terms of location and significance. Detection can be difficult, however, especially when radiographic technique is not optimal.

The common abnormal air collections are pneumothorax, pneumomediastinum, subcutaneous air, and free intraperitoneal air. Pneumothorax is a common complication of attempted central venous catheter placement or thoracentesis, and therefore, it is advisable to obtain a chest radiograph after these procedures.[19] Spontaneous pneumothorax may also occur in patients who are mechanically ventilated, and many of these pneumothoraces will enlarge rapidly with resulting hemodynamic and respiratory compromise.[20,21] In a patient without pleural adhesions, a pneumothorax will tend to rise to the highest part of the pleural space. If the patient is erect, the air will accumulate

FIGURE 19-2 Anteriorly loculated pneumothorax. ***A:*** **Increased volume and haziness of the right hemithorax suggests an anteriorly loculated pneumothorax despite bilateral pleural drains.** ***B:*** **Following insertion of a second chest tube anteriorly on the right, air was immediately expelled under pressure. The mediastinum has moved back towards the midline, consistent with decompression of an anteriorly loculated pneumothorax.**

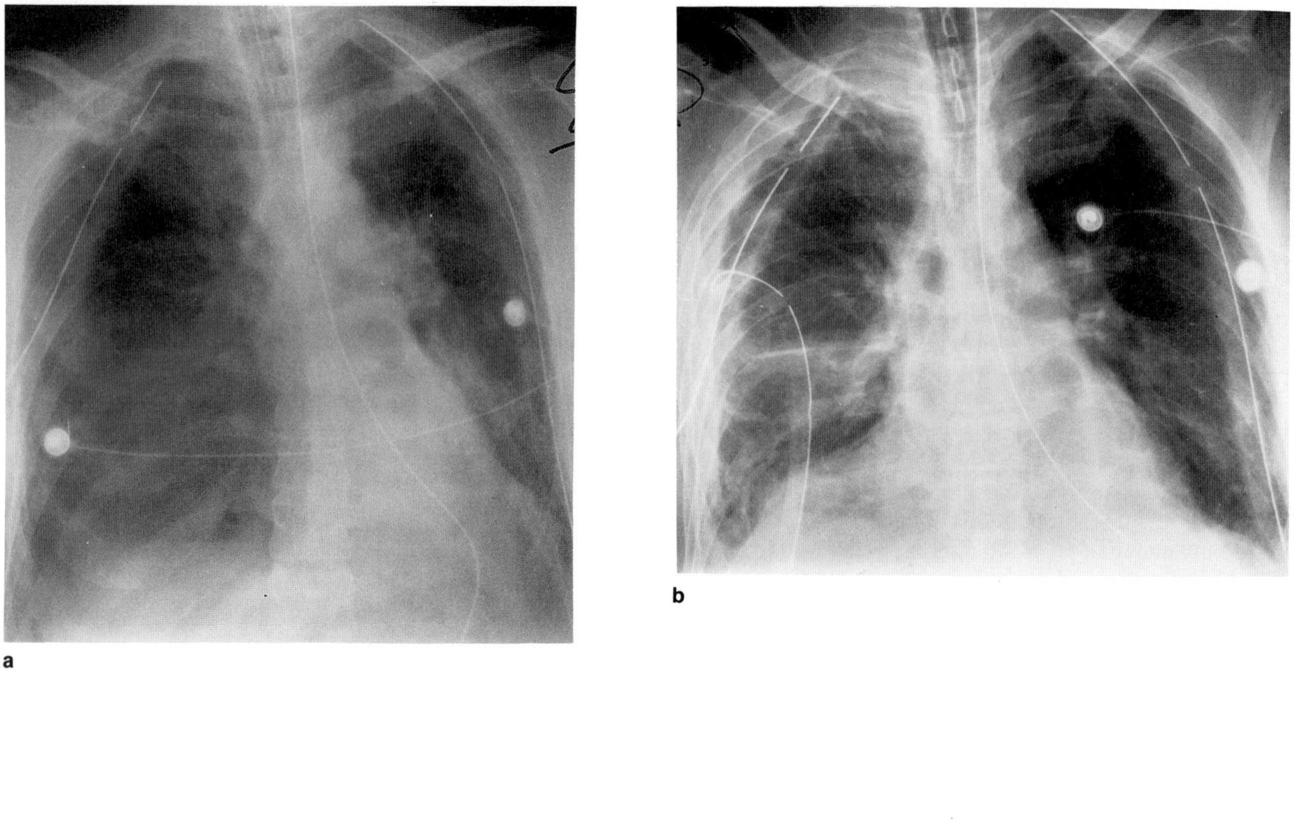

a

b

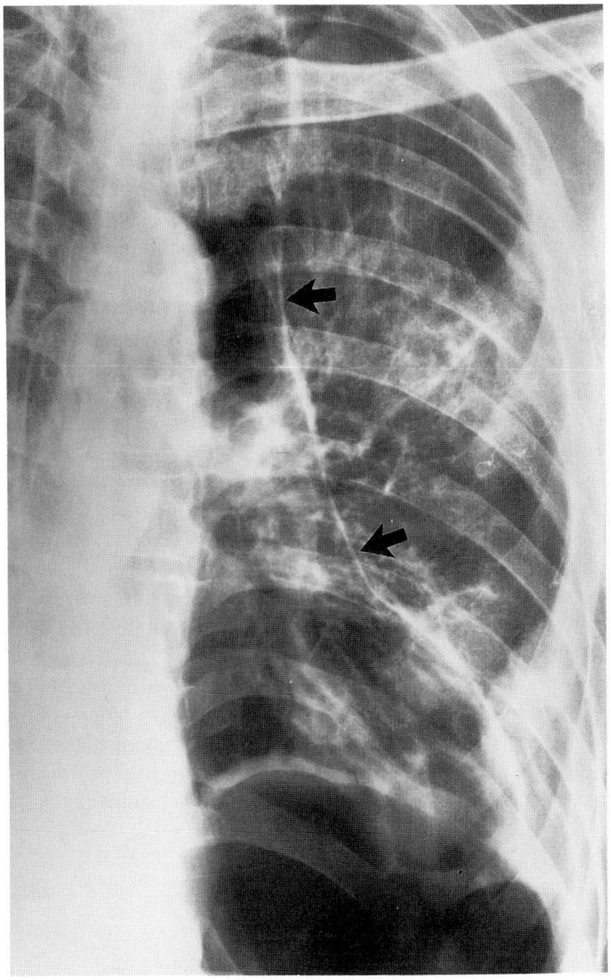

FIGURE 19-3 A medially loculated pneumothorax is present (arrows). Note evidence of a previous thoracotomy with resulting pleural adhesions laterally.

at the apex; if supine, over the anterior surface of the lung. For this reason a small pneumothorax may be difficult to detect on the AP supine chest radiograph. A radiograph taken on expiration often renders a pneumothorax more obvious, though it is not necessary to obtain an expiration view routinely when pneumothorax is suspected. When pleural adhesions are present because of previous surgery or inflammatory disease, a pneumothorax is likely to assume an atypical configuration. For instance, if the pleural surfaces are tethered laterally and superiorly, pneumothorax may present as hazy lucency over the lung with associated signs of increased volume in the affected hemithorax (Fig. 19-2). In some cases the air collection may appear medially or inferiorly to the lung (Fig. 19-3).[22,23] Because bedside portable examinations are generally obtained with a single frontal projection only, such atypical pneumothoraces are easily overlooked. When they are suspected, a portable erect or decubitus lateral radiograph may be necessary to confirm the nature of the problem (Fig. 19-4).

Skin folds on a patient's back can create curvilinear shadows over the lungs, which may closely mimic a pneumo-

a

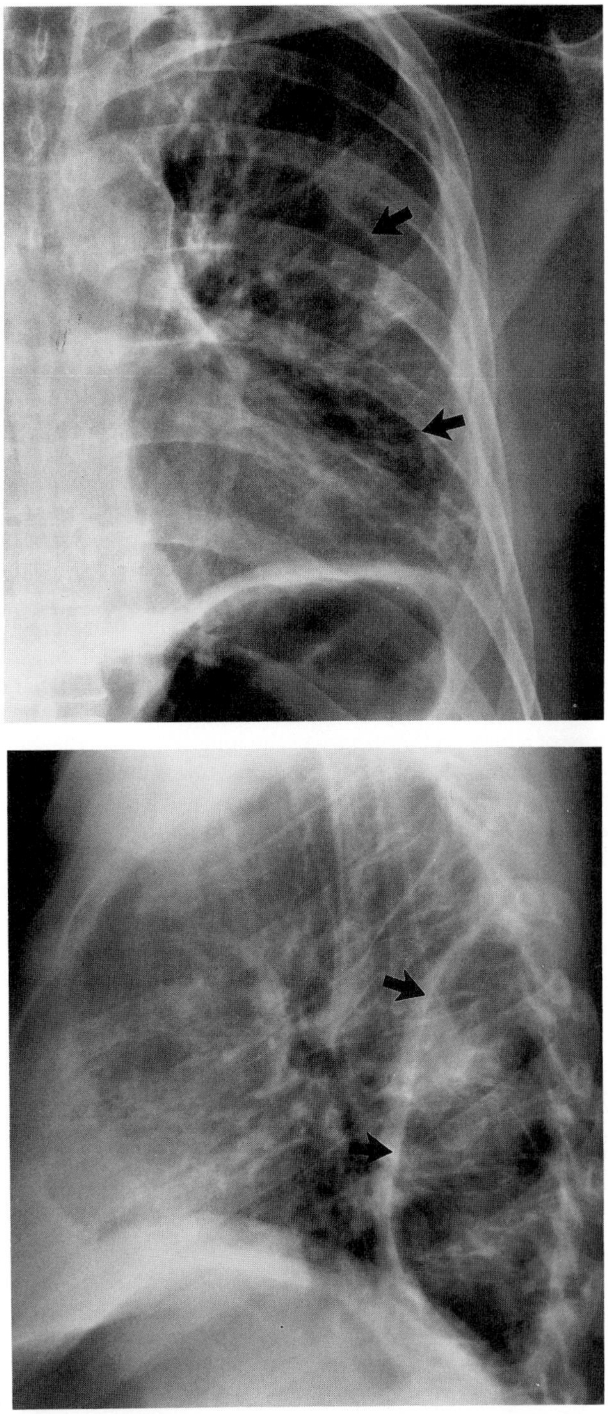

b

FIGURE 19-4 Posteriorly loculated pneumothorax. *A:* The frontal radiograph shows a sharply demarcated lucent area over the medial portion of the left lung (arrows). *B:* A lateral radiograph confirms a posteriorly loculated pneumothorax (arrows).

thorax (see Plate 54*a*). However, with experience, a skin fold can almost always be distinguished from a pneumothorax. Distinguishing characteristics of skins folds include the following: **1.** A skin fold is visualized on a radiograph as a clearly defined change in density (light to dark from medial to lateral) rather than as a sharp line per se. The line which defines a true pneumothorax is the visceral pleura, which is seen as a very fine linear density similar to a pleural fissure (see Plate 54*b*). **2.** Skin folds commonly extend beyond the confines of the thorax. **3.** Skin folds are often multiple and bilateral. **4.** Lung markings are often visible lateral to a skin fold, but absence of lung markings is an unreliable criterion for distinguishing pneumothorax from skin folds. Many cases of skin folds do not show definite lung markings peripherally, especially in older patients with decreased pulmonary perfusion or when radiographic technique is poor. **5.** Skin folds, which may mimic pneumothorax in part of their course, rarely follow the entire outline of the suspected pneumothorax. **6.** Finally, skin folds are usually not reproducible from one examination to the next. Therefore, repeating the x-ray examination usually clarifies the issue.

Pneumomediastinum may occur spontaneously in patients with asthma or those requiring mechanically assisted ventilation, especially if high pressures are used.[21,24] The presumed mechanism is initial rupture of an alveolus and leakage of air via the bronchovascular sheath to the mediastinum. In adults, mediastinal air will usually track superiorly into the neck and thence to the chest wall. One of the important implications of mediastinal emphysema is that it may be followed by pneumothorax, probably due to a rupture of a bleb on the surface of the lung. When mediastinal air surrounds the heart, it can mimic pneumopericardium. However, a true pneumopericardium will be confined by the upper extent of the pericardium at the root of the great vessels (Fig. 19-5). It is also important to be aware that spontaneous pneumopericardium is virtually unknown in adults.[25] Pneumopericardium is most commonly seen after cardiac surgery, penetrating trauma, pericardiocentesis, or other invasive procedures. Mediastinal air may also track inferiorly into the retroperitoneal tissue planes.[26]

FIGURE 19-5 Pneumopericardium (arrows) secondary to intrapericardial pneumonectomy. Note that the air collection does not extend to or above the aortic arch, unlike mediastinal emphysema.

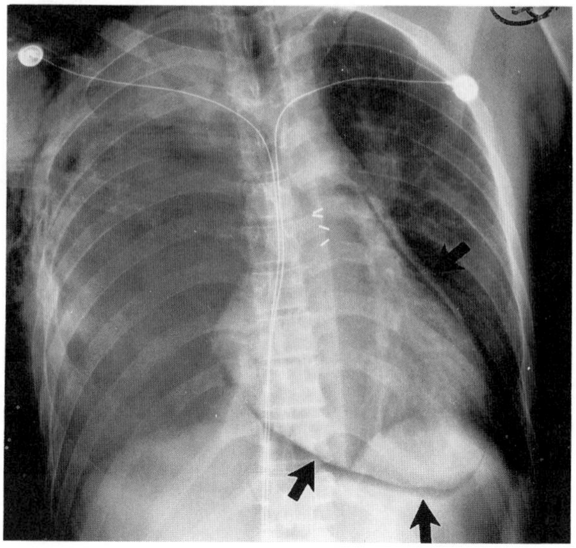

In the absence of recent surgery, free intraperitoneal air usually indicates perforation of the GI tract. Identification of free air can be quite difficult on a portable chest radiograph. This problem is usually related to the angle of the x-ray beam relative to the air collection rather than to the position of the patient. Patients with abdominal pain and distention tend to resist being placed in a completely erect sitting position for a portable chest radiograph. Therefore, the "erect portable chest x-ray" is usually obtained with the patient in a semierect position. To obtain a reasonably undistorted projection of the thorax, the x-ray technologist will generally angle the x-ray beam downward so that it is at approximately 90° to the film. As a result, a small or even a moderately large amount of air which has accumulated beneath the diaphragm may not be obvious, because the beam is traversing it partly en face (Fig. 19-6). When free air is suspected, a left side down lateral decubitus view of the upper abdomen, using a horizontal x-ray beam, is the most sensitive bedside x-ray examination. Any abnormal air collection will be visible over the lateral surface of the liver, where it is unlikely to be confused with bowel gas.

Pneumatoceles can occur in the lungs of patients with pneumonia, particularly in cases due to *Staphylococcus aureus* infection. Their walls are typically smooth and thin, as distinct from necrotic cavities which tend to be thick walled and irregular. Occasionally, when large, they may be difficult to distinguish from loculated pneumothorax. Their relatively spherical configuration and highly localized nature are distinguishing features.

Thoracic Trauma

BLUNT TRAUMA

Patients with blunt thoracic trauma are usually admitted through the emergency room, where a portable supine or semierect chest radiograph is obtained. This may reveal rib fractures, pneumothorax, hemothorax, pulmonary contusion or laceration, or airway injury.

Pulmonary contusion appears as a nonsegmental area of air space infiltrate in typical cases. Rib fractures are usually absent, and the radiographic findings can be more impressive than the clinical picture. The infiltrates appear immediately after trauma and should start to resolve within 48 h. Onset of infiltrates after 72 h or failure to resolve promptly should raise the question of other processes such as infection.[27]

Pulmonary laceration and hematoma may also be seen in blunt chest trauma. A multiloculated cystic cavity is commonly present with air-fluid levels. A pulmonary hematoma may also appear as a discrete nodule, which usually resolves spontaneously, leaving a small scar.[27] Traumatic rupture of alveoli with dissection of air into the pulmonary ligament can cause a focal air collection referred to as a *paramediastinal air cyst.*

Bronchial rupture is a very uncommon consequence of blunt trauma. Characteristic findings include fractures of the upper three ribs, pneumothorax, pneumomediastinum, and a collapsed and abnormally positioned lung, due to

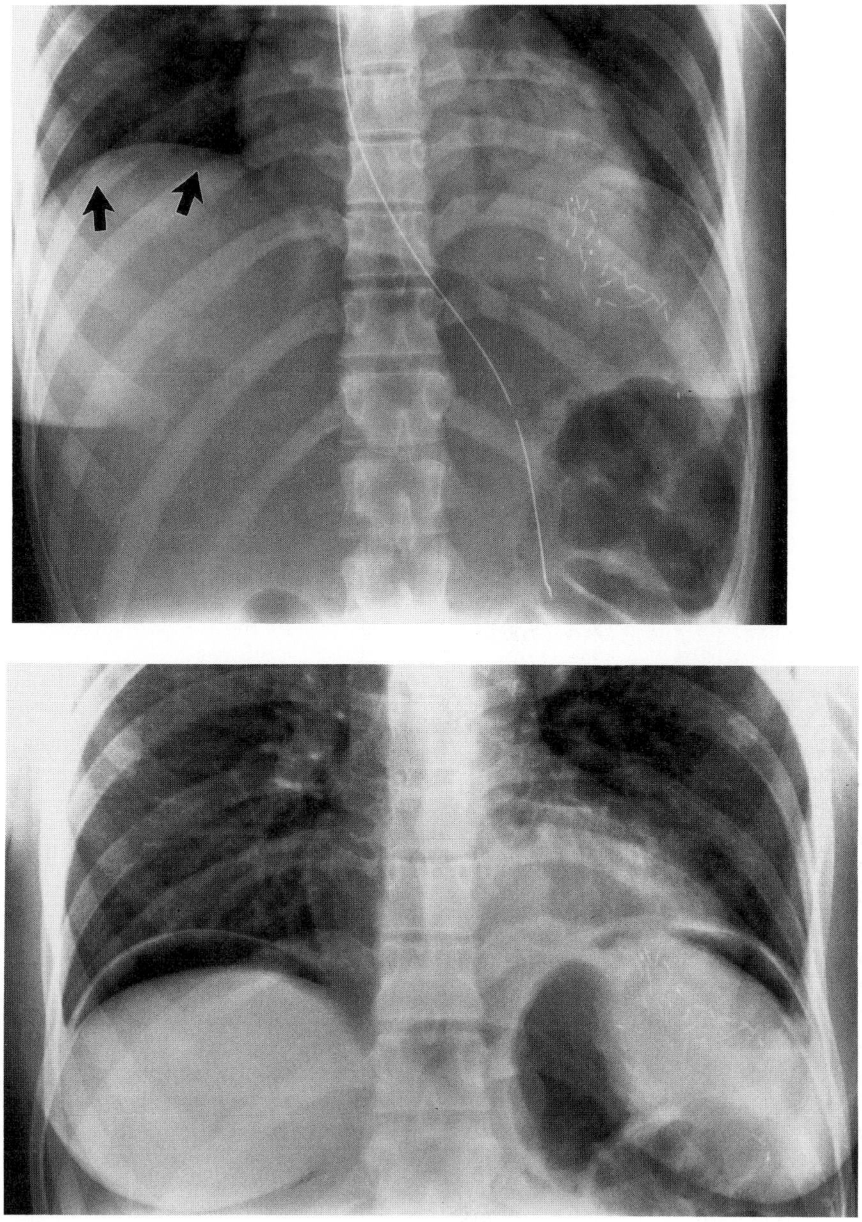

FIGURE 19-6 Pneumoperitoneum (free intraperitoneal air). *A:* A "semierect" radiograph shows abnormal lucency over the liver, with definition of the inferior surface of the right hemidiaphragm (arrows). *B:* An erect view clearly shows a large pneumoperitoneum.

avulsion at the hilum.[28,29] In deceleration injuries, rupture of the aorta or its branches is a common concern. When the initial chest radiograph has been performed in a semisupine position, distention of the great veins combined with magnification due to the AP projection can be misinterpreted as abnormal mediastinal widening (Fig. 19-7). This is particularly common when the patient has a tortuous aorta which may be exaggerated by rotation. Poor image quality due to nongrid technique compounds the diagnostic problem. However, a mediastinal hematoma due to significant vascular injury tends to show certain characteristic features[30] (Fig. 19-8). Important findings in positive cases include loss of definition of the aortic knob, abnormal density superior to the aortic knob extending over the apex of the left lung, widening of the right paratracheal stripe, deviation of the nasogastric tube away from the aorta at the level of the arch, and displacement of the left paraspinous line.[31] In equivocal cases, an upright chest radiograph should be obtained if possible.

When further studies are deemed necessary, the choice between CT and angiography is somewhat controversial.[31] Some authorities recommend obtaining CT of the chest in virtually every case of significant thoracic trauma. Others recommend reserving CT for certain limited indications and favor using angiography in the first instance when there is a suspicion of vascular injury. It is our policy to perform CT of the chest when clinical suspicion for vascular injury is low, but there is a question regarding mediastinal widening on the chest radiograph. In such cases, a CT scan which demonstrates that the apparent mediastinal widening is due to fat deposition or tortuous vessels obviates the need for further investigation. On the other hand, if mediastinal

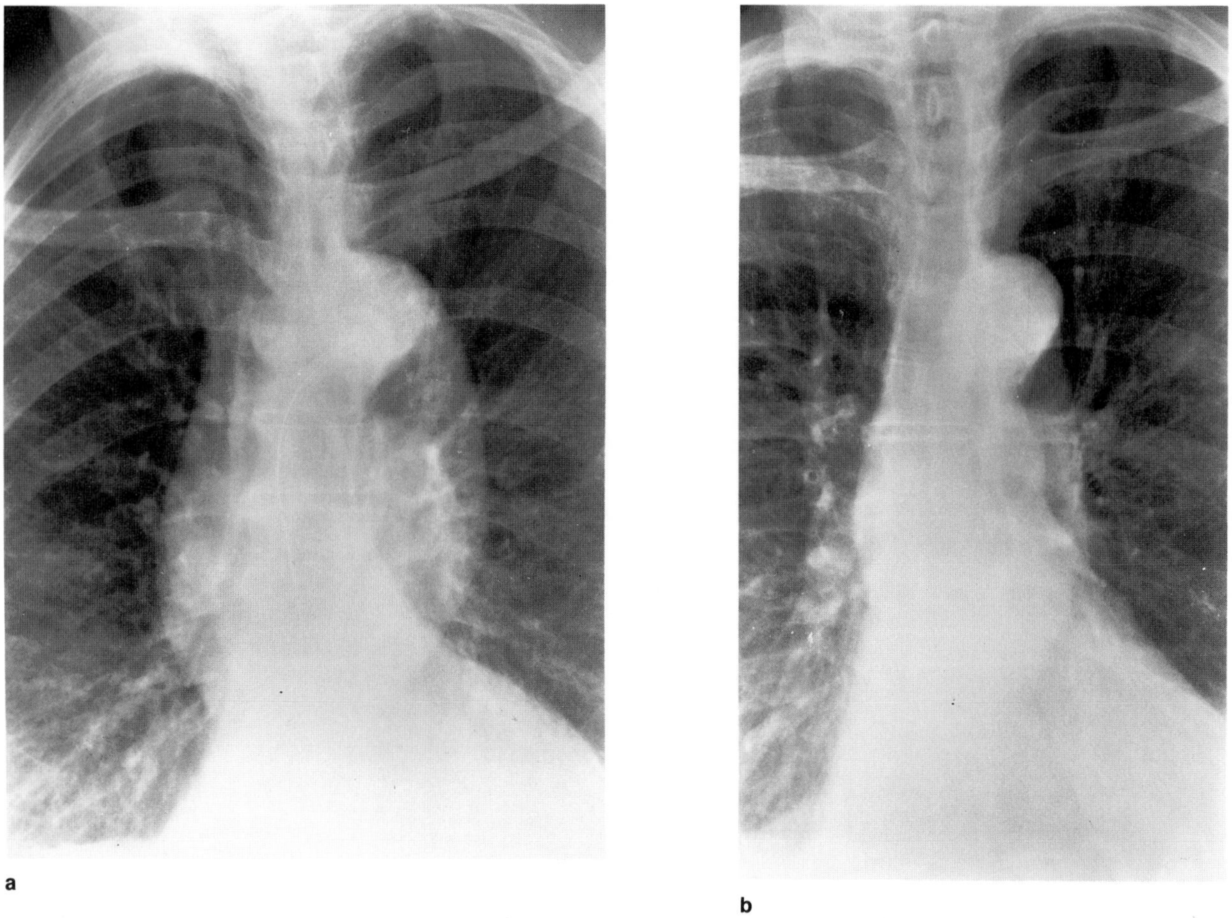

FIGURE 19-7 Spurious mediastinal widening due to a tortuous aorta. ***A:*** **A rotated AP view of the chest shows apparent mediastinal widening at the level of the aortic arch. Note that the widening does not extend cephalad to the aortic arch, which is clearly defined.** ***B:*** **Second, unrotated radiograph of the same patient reveals only a tortuous aorta.**

hematoma seems likely based on the nature of the injury and the appearance of the chest radiograph, we perform aortography immediately. This policy is based on the assumption that an abnormal CT scan showing a mediastinal hematoma will not provide sufficiently specific information to determine the necessity for surgery (many such hematomas are due to venous bleeding) and aortography will still need to be performed.

PENETRATING INJURIES

Penetrating injuries are usually caused by stabbing or gunshot wounds. In either case, pneumothorax, hemothorax, pulmonary laceration, or pulmonary hematoma may result. Injury to the heart, great vessels, or esophagus must also be considered, depending on the site of the injury. In the case of stab wounds, the external puncture wound provides some basis for estimating what internal organs may have been injured. In the case of bullet wounds, the internal course of the projectile and its fragments is notoriously unpredictable. The chest radiograph can provide important clues in the form of a trail of small lead fragments typically shed by unjacketed bullets following impact with a bone.[32] When mediastinal injury is suspected, a CT scan can provide important negative information. If a mediastinal hematoma is confirmed, angiography may be necessary to define the source of bleeding. Unexplained mediastinal emphysema suggests esophageal perforation.[33] If esophageal injury is suspected, a contrast study or esophagoscopy should be performed. Delayed recognition of a esophageal perforation can be an important source of mortality due to acute mediastinitis. A portable AP chest radiograph taken immediately following ingestion of water-soluble contrast material can detect major esophageal leaks though this technique may not provide adequate detail, especially when no grid is used and the patient is large. Fluoroscopic examination with use of multiple views is the recommended technique for excluding perforation. Water-soluble contrast may be used initially, but if no perforation is detected, barium should be substituted in view of its higher density, which provides greater sensitivity for small leaks.

Pleural Effusions

Large free pleural effusions are easily diagnosed by chest radiography, but small or loculated effusions can be overlooked or misinterpreted. On a typical semierect AP chest

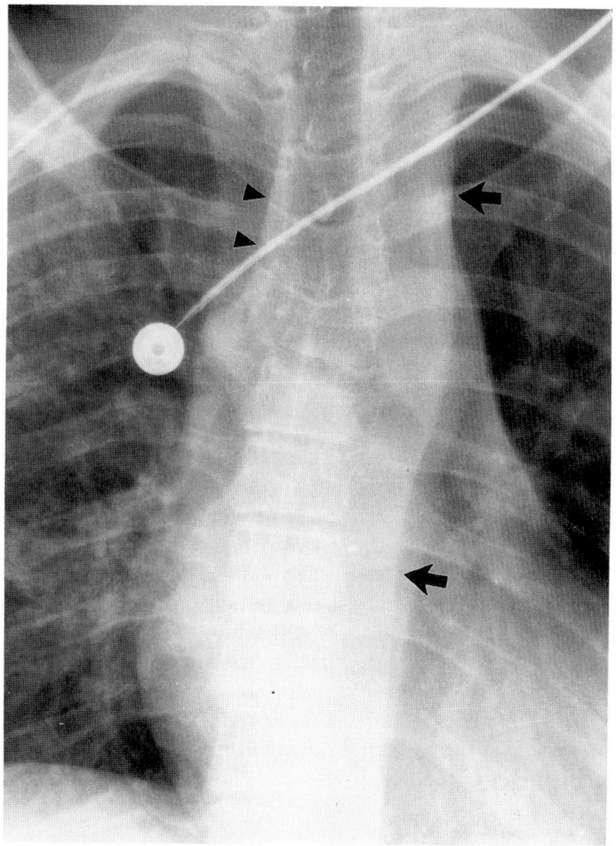

FIGURE 19-8 Mediastinal hematoma due to trauma. Note loss of definition of the aortic knob, with abnormal density extending superiorly and inferiorly from the aortic knob (arrows), and widening of the right paratracheal stripe (arrowheads). Vertebral deformities due to compression fractures are also present.

radiograph, small effusions will tend to collect in the posterior costophrenic angles, which represent the most dependent portions of the pleural cavities. On the AP view this will produce increased density behind the domes of the hemidiaphragms, but blunting of the lateral costophrenic angles may be absent (Fig. 19-9). As the effusions become larger or as the patient assumes a more erect position, blunting of the lateral costophrenic angles will be seen. Blunting of these angles per se is not a specific sign of pleural effusion and may occur due to pulmonary consolidation or scarring. In general, pleural fluid tends to produce homogeneous density and usually tracks superiorly, producing separation of the lung from the chest wall (Fig. 19-10). On a supine chest radiograph, pleural fluid layers out posteriorly to the lungs, initially producing only hazy density.[34] As the amount of fluid increases, it will appear laterally and superiorly to the lung margins, separating the lungs from the chest wall (Fig. 19-11).

Loculation of pleural fluid can take many forms. One of the more common configurations is that of a subpulmonic effusion in which most of the fluid is located between the

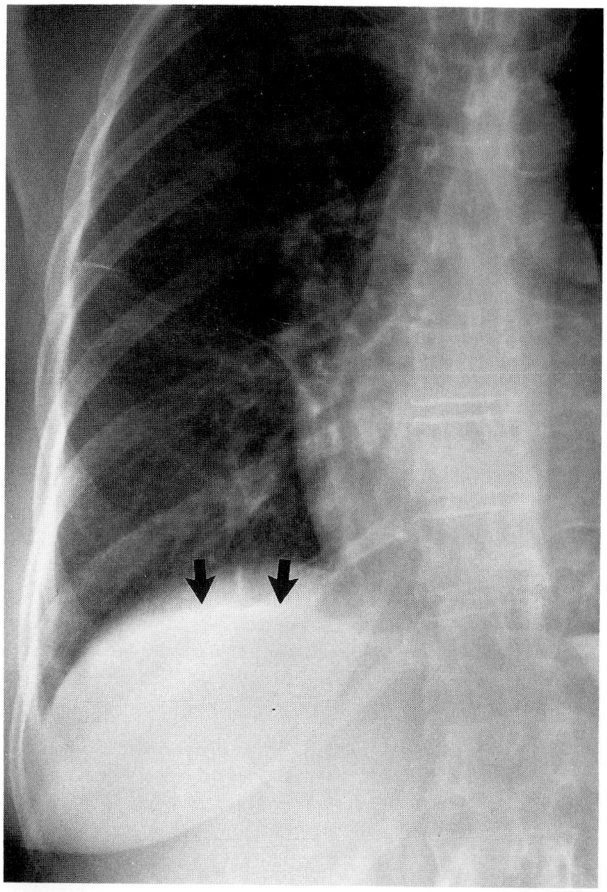

a

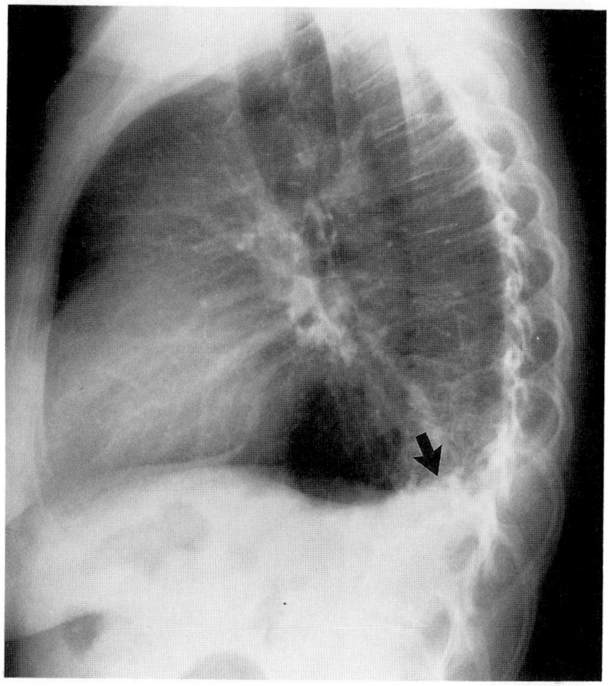

b

FIGURE 19-9 Pleural effusion. ***A:*** **A moderate pleural effusion can present with merely increased density behind the dome of the hemidiaphragm (arrows). There is no significant blunting of the lateral costophrenic angle in this case.** ***B:*** **A lateral view confirms bilateral pleural effusion with several hundred cc's of fluid (arrow).**

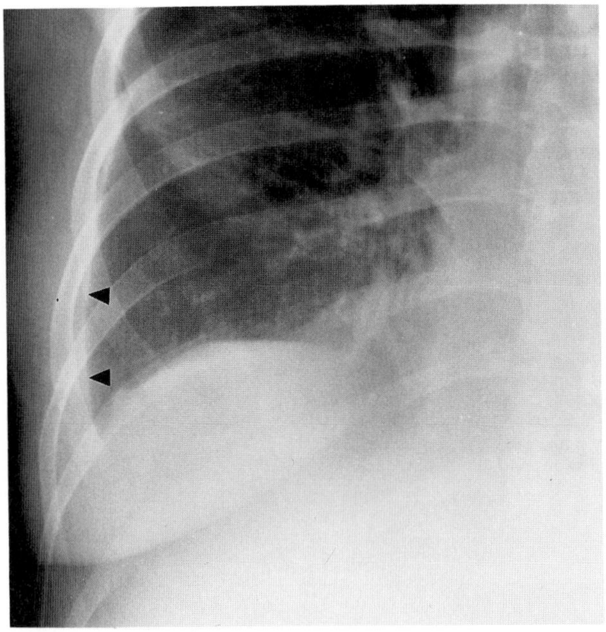

FIGURE 19-10 A typical small pleural effusion shown on a semierect radiograph, tracking laterally with resulting separation of the lung from the chest wall (arrowheads).

FIGURE 19-11 A large pleural effusion layering out posteriorly on a supine radiograph. This produces diffusely increased density in the affected hemithorax, as well as separation of the lung from the chest wall (arrows).

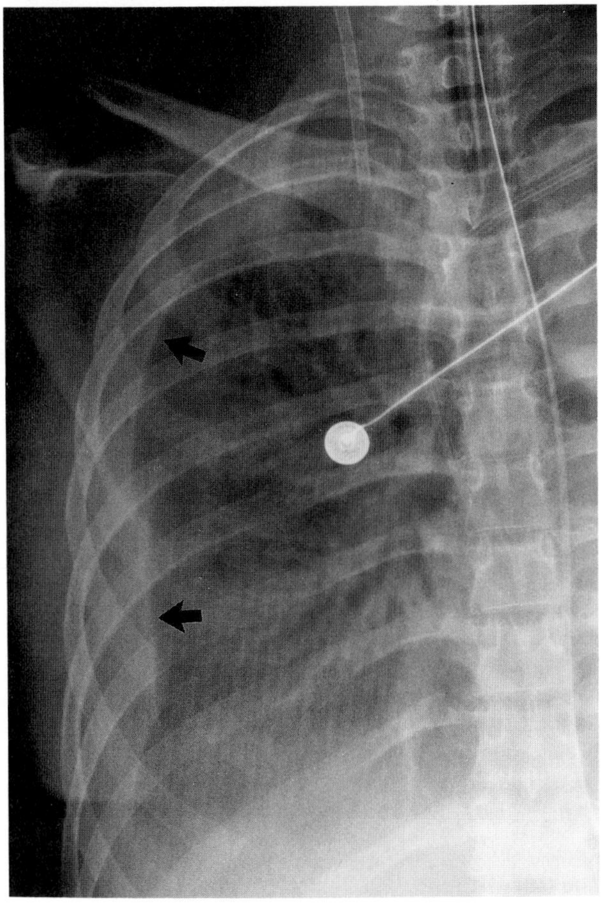

base of the lung and the hemidiaphragm. The appearance can be mistaken for elevation of the hemidiaphragm itself. Usually there is some evidence of pleural fluid laterally or posteriorly and the apparent outline of the hemidiaphragm, which is actually caused by subpulmonic fluid, tends to have a characteristic contour.[35] On the left side, excessive separation of the lung base from the gastric air bubble can be a clue to the presence of subpulmonic effusion.

Pleural effusions commonly extend into the pleural fissures to a variable extent. Pleural fluid located in an incomplete major fissure produces a characteristic appearance, which can be mistaken for cavitation[36] (Fig. 19-12). The area of relative lucency in such cases represents the incomplete portion of the fissure where fluid is unable to enter and which thus appears radiolucent. Pleural fluid may become loculated in the fissures to produce a masslike density, known as a *pseudo tumor* and can be a source of confusion (Fig. 19-13). This finding is most likely to occur as a large effusion is resolving, rather than at the initial presentation. A lateral view of the chest can be helpful to clarify the nature of such loculated fluid collections.

An extremely large pleural effusion can produce complete opacification of a hemithorax. In such cases the underlying lung is collapsed due to compression by the fluid. The mediastinum is shifted away from the affected side and the hemidiaphragm is depressed. However, in the ICU set-

FIGURE 19-12 A right pleural effusion extending into an incomplete major fissure. This is a characteristic appearance which can be mistaken for cavitation. The lucency represents the fused portion of the fissure (arrows), which limits the extension of the fluid.

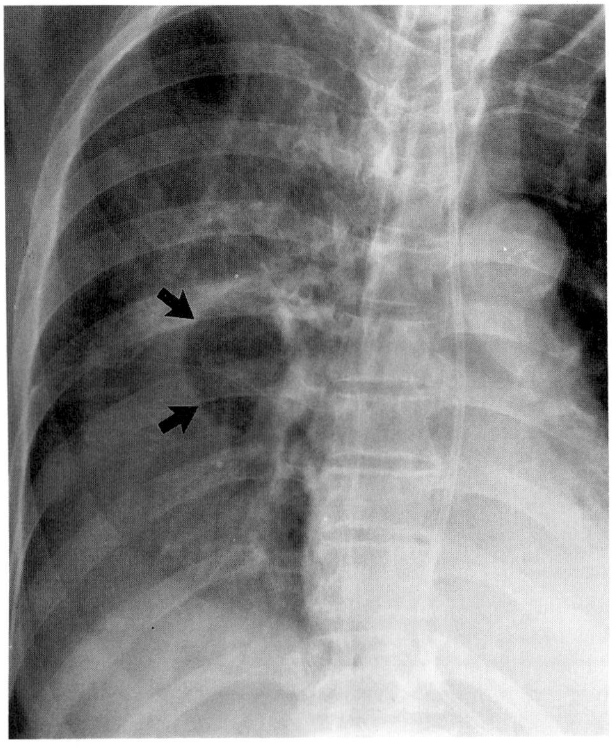

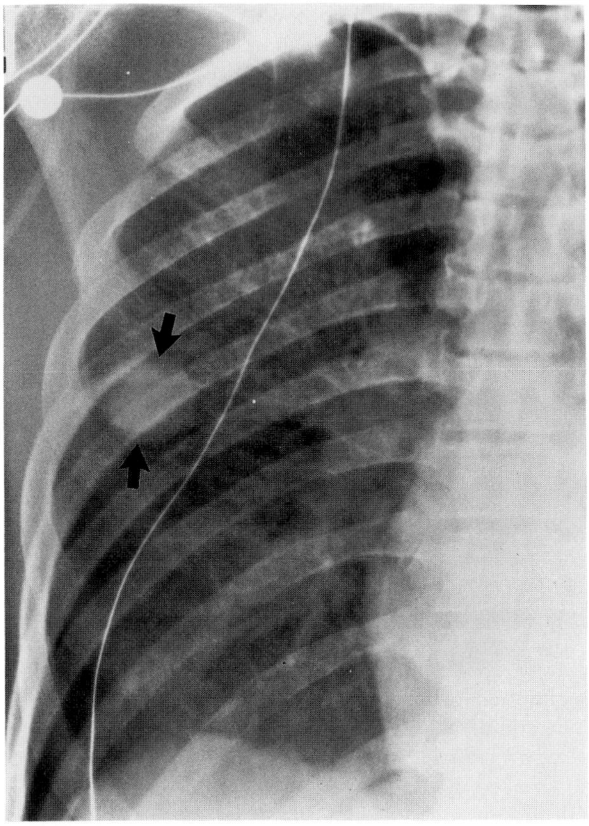

FIGURE 19-13 Pleural fluid loculated in the minor fissure (arrows), producing a mass-like density ("pseudotumor"), which can be mistaken for a tumor nodule.

ting, acute opacification of one hemithorax is more commonly due to total pulmonary atelectasis than pleural effusion. Since both may coexist, it is important to determine which is the primary problem in a given case. A distinction can almost always be made by carefully evaluating the volume of the opacified hemithorax in relation to the opposite side and by comparing to recent previous radiographs. Loss of volume favors atelectasis as the primary etiology. Note that the patient tends to rotate toward the side of the collapsed lung on a AP portable examination, probably because of recoil of the ribs on the affected side. This sometimes leads to misinterpretation of the mediastinal shift as being due to rotation alone (Fig. 19-14).

A common misconception exists concerning the significance of "infiltrate" in association with pleural effusion. When the patient is in an erect or semierect position, pleural effusion tends to accumulate about the lung base. If it is a substantial effusion, the fluid will compress or displace the lung, which normally occupies the same space. This invariably leads to some degree of compression atelectasis.[37] In patients who also have cardiac failure and interstitial pulmonary edema, the tendency to produce consolidation at the lung bases is more marked by virtue of both the increased amount of pulmonary fluid and also, especially in the left lower lobe, by compression by the enlarged heart. In this situation air bronchograms are commonly identified in the basilar portions of the lungs. In the presence of pleural effusions, especially in association with cardiomegaly and pulmonary edema, this finding should not be interpreted as indicating pneumonia. On the other hand, when the extent of pulmonary consolidation is disproportionate

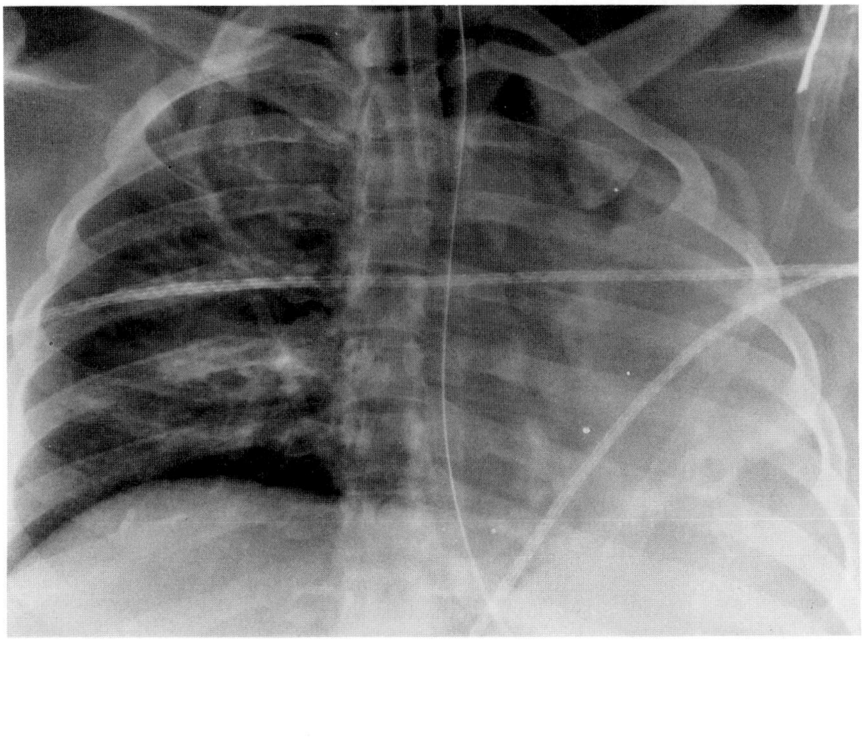

FIGURE 19-14 Extensive atelectasis of the left lung. In addition to mediastinal shift towards the affected hemithorax, the patient is considerably rotated towards the affected side, which makes evaluation of mediastinal position more difficult.

in relation to the volume of pleural fluid, pneumonia and other etiologies should be considered.

Adult Respiratory Distress Syndrome (ARDS)

ARDS is a frequent result of a major systemic insult such as trauma or sepsis. The radiographic findings are not specific, though certain features are sufficiently characteristic to suggest the diagnosis.[38] Pulmonary abnormalities develop typically after 24 to 36 h in the form of bilateral diffuse patchy infiltrates, which tend to become more severe over the next 24 to 48 h. The appearance can be indistinguishable from pulmonary edema from other causes, though the heart does not enlarge and pleural effusions are not a feature of ARDS (Fig. 19-15). One of the most suggestive features is the impressively stable appearance of the infiltrates over many days or even weeks, unlike other types of edema or infection, which tend to progress or regress from day to day. In cases of ARDS, after the infiltrates have stabilized, focal changes are usually due to superimposed pathology such as pneumonia or atelectasis.

Aspiration

The term aspiration is commonly applied to several rather different phenomena that may occur in ICU patients. The first, which is the more common, relates to aspiration of nasal-pharyngeal secretions. This probably occurs to some extent in all intubated patients, though it is not limited to this group.[39] This type of aspiration contributes to the nonspecific basilar infiltrates and atelectasis frequently seen in ICU patients. Aspiration of food and fluids during deglutition may also produce acute air-space infiltrates. Aspiration of acidic gastric contents (Mendelsohn's syndrome) produces a severe pulmonary reaction, typically with acute bilateral air-space infiltrates due to edema. The appearance may be indistinguishable from other causes of acute pulmonary edema.

In general, aspiration should be suspected in patients with impaired consciousness or problems with deglutition who suddenly develop air-space infiltrates in dependent regions of the lungs[39] (Fig. 19-16). The superior segments of the lower lobes are commonly involved in patients who aspirate when supine. In patients who are more nearly erect, the basilar segments of the lower lobes are likely to be affected, especially on the right side. Aspiration pneumonitis due to bland fluids may resolve rapidly unless infection supervenes, in which case the term *aspiration pneumonia* can be used.

Endotracheal and Tracheostomy Tubes

A chest radiograph should be obtained after placement of an endotracheal (ET) tube to verify correct position and exclude complications. The distal end of the tube should be above the carina and the cuff should be completely distal to the vocal cords. Because the position of the tube tip varies with flexion and extension of the neck over a range of approximately 4 cm, some margin is desirable. Thus, depending on the patient's size, the tip of an ET tube should be approximately 5 to 7 cm above the carina with the head in a neutral position.[40] If the tube is advanced too far distally, it tends to enter the right mainstem bronchus. Intubation of the right mainstem bronchus or bronchus intermedius re-

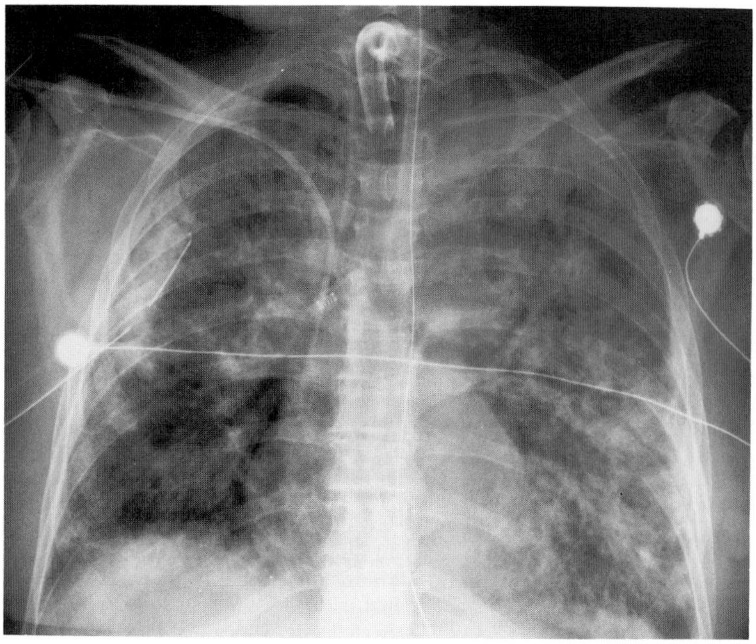

FIGURE 19-15 Adult respiratory distress syndrome (ARDS). Bilateral diffuse patchy infiltrates may be indistinguishable from pulmonary edema due to other causes. Lack of change on sequential radiographs tends to be a feature of these cases.

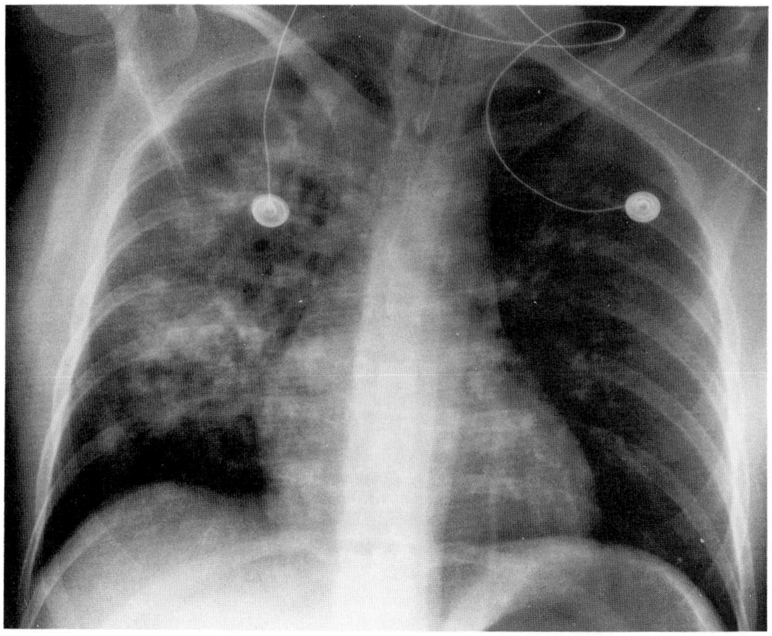

FIGURE 19-16 A typical aspiration pneumonia, developing as an acute airspace infiltrate involving the portions of the right lung that are dependent in a supine patient.

sults in impaired ventilation, and potentially atelectasis of the left lung. At the same time, delivery of excessive volumes to the right lung may cause pneumothorax. Therefore, incorrect placement of an ET tube must be remedied as a matter of urgency. When the tip is located at or immediately above the carina, irritation and ulceration of the mucosa can result. Suction catheters may aggravate this problem. When the tube is located too far proximally, the cuff may impinge on the vocal cords causing local edema as well as an air leak. When the cuff is completely above the cords, there is likely to be a large air leak with resulting aerophagia and gastric distention (Fig. 19-17). In either situation, the patient is at risk for aspiration. Accidental extubation can also occur. Perforation of the hypopharynx or esophagus has been reported as a relatively rare complication of intubation, which can produce mediastinal or subcutaneous emphysema.[41] The inflated cuff should remain in intimate contact with the tracheal mucosa but should not deform the wall of the trachea appreciably. Persistent overinflation of the cuff can lead to mucosal ulceration and eventual stenosis.

After tracheostomy tube placement, it is common to see small amounts of air in the subcutaneous tissues of the neck. Large amounts of subcutaneous air or air dissecting inferiorly into the mediastinum are abnormal findings and suggest a significant air leak. This can result occasionally from perforation of the posterior tracheal membrane or even placement of the tube in the paratracheal soft tissues. Pneumothorax is a rare complication of tracheostomy caused by direct injury to the lung apex. Optimally, the tip of the tracheostomy tube should be one-half to two-thirds of the distance between the stoma and the carina. If the tip of the tracheostomy tube projects above the level of the clavicles on the AP film, partial extubation should be suspected. In this situation, the cuff may be located in the soft tissues anterior to the trachea. If the tube is persistently angulated relative to the trachea, it may erode the mucosa with resulting ulceration. Low placement and angulation of the tube can lead to erosion of the tip through the tracheal wall with formation of a tracheal-innominate artery fistula.[42]

Venous Catheters

Placement of a central venous line can be complicated by pneumothorax, mediastinal hematoma, or hemothorax. A chest radiograph should be obtained to verify correct location and to exclude complications.[43–45] The tip of a central catheter should be located in the innominate veins or superior vena cava but not in the right atrium. A catheter located in the atrium can cause cardiac perforation and may incite arrhythmias.[43,46] If a catheter hangs up at a vascular junction as it is being advanced, a loop may develop. Though it may function normally, a looped catheter is more prone to thrombosis and should be replaced. Local bleeding with resulting mediastinal hematoma is a surprisingly common complication of central catheter placement, though, fortunately, the patient usually remains asymptomatic. Chest pain after catheter insertion may be related to pneumothorax or hematoma. If the course of a catheter is atypical, it may have entered a minor vessel or the venous anatomy may be abnormal (i.e., persistent left-sided superior vena cava). Accidental arterial cannulation or an extraluminal location should also be considered.[45] Hand injection of contrast material through a catheter can be useful to clarify the location of a catheter tip relative to the vascular anatomy. Accurate timing of the x-ray exposure and use of correct exposure technique are critically important. It is necessary to inject a few milliliters initially to opacify the lumen of the catheter. The x-ray exposure should be made during injec-

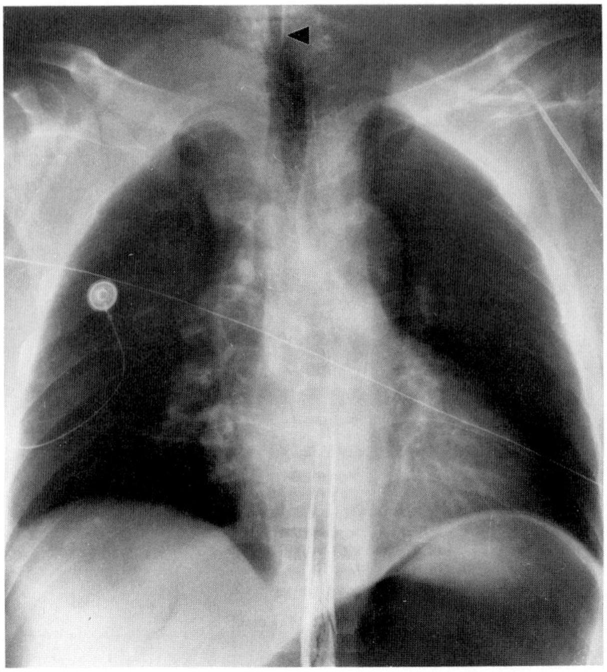

FIGURE 19-17 High ET tube with gastric dilatation. The tip of the endotracheal tube is barely distal to the voice cords (arrowheads) with the cuff presumably in the hypopharynx. Note marked gastric distention, secondary to leakage of air around the ET tube.

tion of a bolus of contrast material to visualize the vascular anatomy in the area of the catheter tip.

The most commonly seen complications of pulmonary artery catheter placement are formation of a loop within the heart, particularly the right atrium, and an excessively distal location indicative of persistent wedging of the catheter (see Plate 55). The ideal resting position for the catheter tip is in the area of the central pulmonary arteries such as a proximal lobar branch. The danger of a persistently wedged catheter is that pulmonary infarction may result.[47] In the absence of persistent wedging, thrombosis may occur, apparently due to intimal erosion by the catheter tip. This is a further potential cause of pulmonary infarction, which usually appears as a focal pleural-based density which resolves in 7 to 14 days. Infarcts are most apt to occur in patients with pulmonary venous hypertension due to cardiac failure.[47]

Aortic counterpulsation balloon catheters can be identified by a radiopaque marker at the catheter tip. The balloon should be located in the descending aorta with the tip distal to the take-off of the left subclavian artery. Excessively proximal placement may compromise blood flow to the major aortic branches while excessively distal placement will reduce its effectiveness. These catheters can also be accidentally placed in a subintimal location with resulting dissection.[48]

Nasogastric or feeding tubes may accidentally enter the trachea during insertion, particularly in patients with impaired consciousness. The new small caliber, flexible tip,

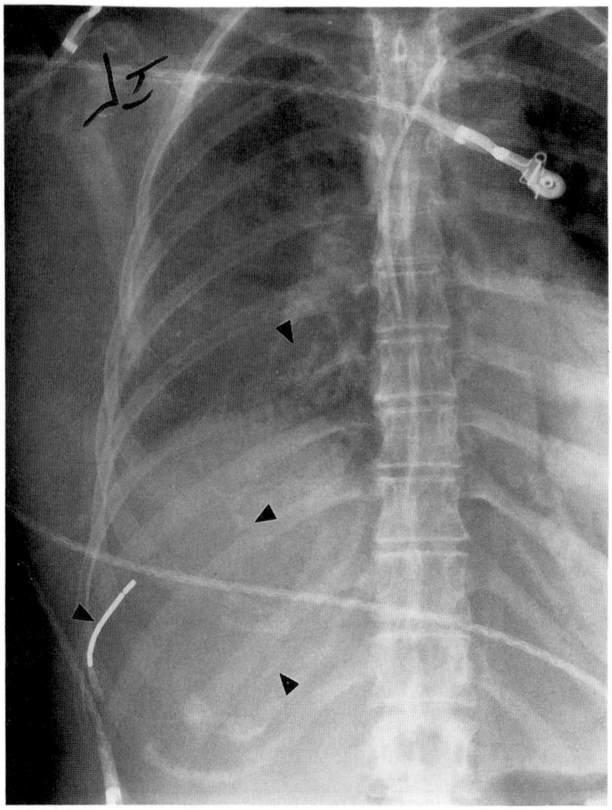

FIGURE 19-18 A feeding tube (arrowheads) has entered the right main stem bronchus, penetrated the visceral pleural, and coiled within the pleural space in the right posterior costophrenic sulcus. A right effusion has resulted, and the effusion is partly subpulmonic in location, contributing to the impression that the tube is in the abdomen.

feeding tubes may pass through the small bronchi and reach the visceral pleura without any perceptible resistance being encountered.[49] If advanced further, the tube will penetrate the pleura and form a loop in the pleural cavity (Fig. 19-18). Because the posterior costophrenic angles considerably overlap the upper abdomen, a feeding tube in the pleural space can be mistaken for one that is in the abdomen. This error is most likely to occur when the position of the tube is verified by an abdominal radiograph. Particular care should be exercised when inserting feeding tubes in patients with impaired consciousness, and radiographs should be obtained to verify the tube position prior to infusion of nutrient materials.

Transvenous Pacemakers

Incorrect placement of transvenous pacemaker electrodes can be identified on a portable AP radiograph, and certain specific appearances should arouse suspicion.[50] One of the more common complications consists of perforation of the right ventricular apex by the electrode, which subsequently advances into the pericardial cavity (Fig. 19-19). The ap-

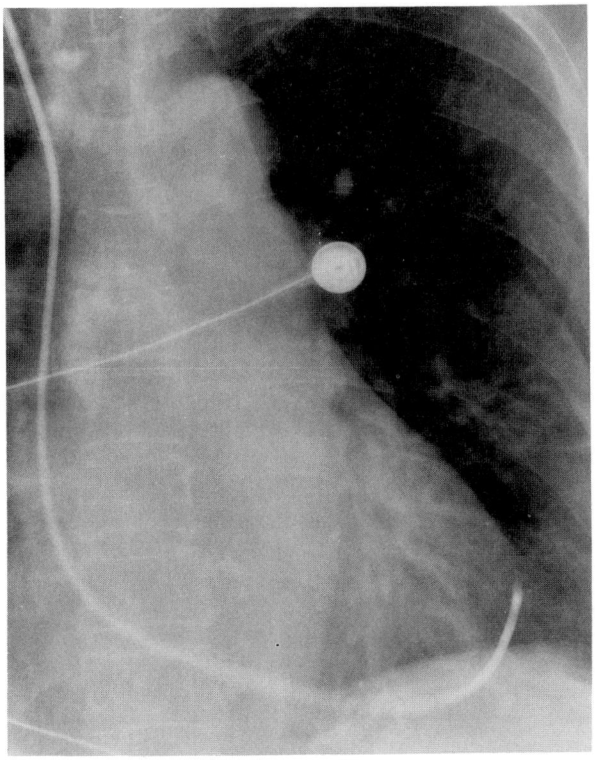

FIGURE 19-19 A pacemaker lead has perforated the right ventricular apex, and advanced into the pericardial space. This complication should be suspected when the electrode terminates to the left of the expected location of the right ventricular apex, and turns upward near its tip.

pearance in such cases is often quite characteristic, with the electrode located excessively far to the left and typically directed slightly cephalad. If the lead is advanced sufficiently far, it will be seen coursing posteriorly over the left ventricular apex. The extreme proximity of the pacemaker lead to the adjacent lung is often a clue to its extracardiac location. A lead that is directed superiorly and to the left in a more central location may have entered the coronary sinus, and this can be confirmed by a lateral chest radiograph. Fracture of the pacemaker lead is less commonly seen than in the past due to use of improved alloy materials. Dislodgement of the electrode is a more common complication, which usually occurs during the first few weeks after insertion.[51]

Radiology of Common Cardiovascular Abnormalities in the ICU

Fluid overload and congestive heart failure are common in ICU patients. Because of pulmonary underinflation and cardiac magnification on portable radiographs, mild cardiomegaly or early interstitial edema may be difficult to detect. Also, because the patient is usually radiographed in a semierect or supine position, the significance of vascular redistribution and distention of the venous pedicle is sometimes uncertain. Small pleural effusions, which can be easily detected on an erect lateral chest radiograph, tend to be concealed on the AP view. However, development of septal lines (Kerley "B" lines) and thickening of the minor fissure due to subpleural edema, can be useful indicators of early edema. Indistinctness of perihilar pulmonary vessels alone, especially in underinflated lungs, is a considerably less reliable finding. Gross cardiomegaly can be diagnosed with confidence, though mild increases in heart size are less readily detected due to variations in patient position, magnification, and lung inflation. The cardiothoracic ratio, which can be used as an approximate yardstick for measuring cardiac size on erect posteroanterior (PA) radiographs, cannot be applied to portable examinations unless the projection is standardized, and a correction factor applied.[52] Distinction between cardiogenic and noncardiogenic edema has not been reproducibly demonstrated by radiographic criteria on portable radiographs. Obviously, the presence of cardiomegaly suggests a cardiac etiology.

In distinguishing edema from other causes of pulmonary infiltrate, the radiographic pattern and chronicity can be helpful. In general, severe bilateral air-space infiltrates which develop suddenly are likely to be due to acute edema or aspiration. Pulmonary edema tends to be symmetrical. Asymmetry can be caused by underlying lung disease, such as bullous emphysema or pulmonary embolism, or may be due to gravitational effects if the patient has been lying on one side for some time prior to the radiograph. In patients with interstitial edema, areas of air space consolidation frequently develop at the lung bases, especially in the lower lobes medially. This finding does not necessarily indicate pneumonia or aspiration, but rather a tendency toward greater edema in the dependent portions of the lungs. Cardiomegaly and pleural effusions may cause compression atelectasis. All of these factors contribute to decreased aeration and a tendency for the lung to consolidate at the bases.

Atelectasis

Atelectasis is one of the more common pulmonary abnormalities in ICU patients. Acute atelectasis is usually caused by bronchial obstruction, such as due to mucous plugging, or compression of the lung, as in cases with pleural effusion. Intubated patients are particularly prone to atelectasis because the presence of a tube in the trachea interferes with their ability to clear secretions by coughing and impairs ciliary clearance of mucus. High concentrations of oxygen also predispose to atelectasis.

When acute bronchial obstruction occurs, air distal to the obstruction is reabsorbed and the involved segment of the lung tends to collapse. The obstructed segment usually does not collapse completely due to accumulation of secretions and transudate within the air spaces. Complete atelectasis of one lung can occur in intubated patients when the endotracheal tube is advanced beyond the carina and the cuff obstructs the contralateral bronchus. Acute atelectasis of an entire lung is indicated by a newly opacified hemithorax with associated volume loss. This is associated with mediastinal shift toward the affected side, approximation of the ipsilateral ribs, and elevation of the ipsilateral hemidiaphragm. Accumulated secretions may fill the bronchi and produce an apparent bronchial "cut off" proximally, and this does not necessarily indicate the presence of an obstructing mass. On a portable radiograph, the patient will usually be rotated toward the affected side, probably due to recoil of the rib cage. The presence of such rotation makes mediastinal shift more difficult to evaluate and sometimes causes the presence of such shift to be overlooked. Atelectasis of a lobe tends to have a more or less characteristic radiographic configuration depending on the lobe involved (Fig. 19-20). Subsegmental atelectasis typically has a linear appearance and commonly occurs at the lung bases of postoperative patients and those with abdominal distention. Rapidity of onset and clearing are common features of atelectasis that help distinguish it from infections and other causes of infiltrate. In many cases, however, a confident distinction between atelectasis and inflammatory infiltrate cannot be made on the basis of a single radiograph.

FIGURE 19-20 Typical, complete left lower lobe atelectasis, presenting as a wedge-shaped area of increased density (arrows) in the retrocardiac region, with volume loss in the left hemithorax.

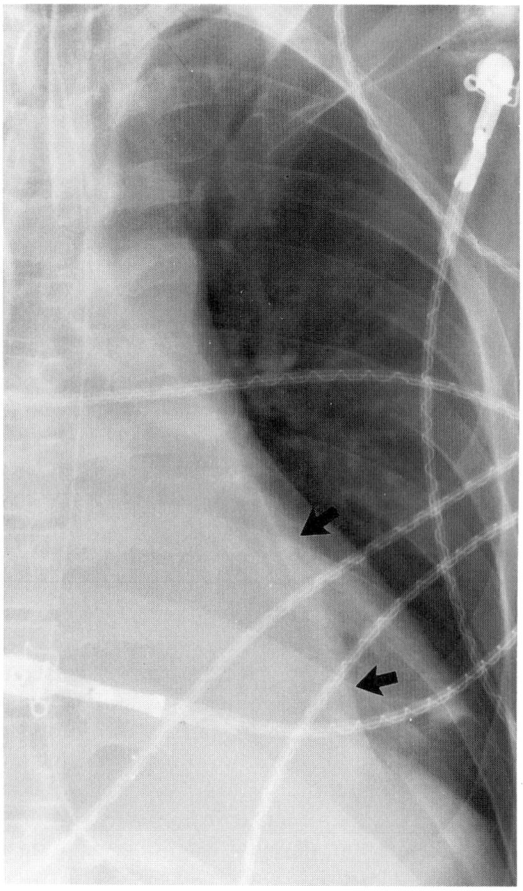

Pneumonia

Noninfectious pulmonary infiltrates are common in ICU patients, and the chest radiograph does not allow a specific diagnosis of pneumonia in most cases. Some evidence indicates that pneumonia is overdiagnosed in the ICU setting, particularly in instances where infiltrates are caused by atelectasis, atypical edema, or pulmonary embolism.[53] Serial chest radiographs can be helpful in monitoring the course of pneumonia and in detecting complications, such as abscess formation and empyema or bronchopleural fistula formation.[54] Focal areas of air trapping or preexisting bullae may mimic cavitation. Actual necrotic lung cavities usually have irregular margins and tend to become more clearly defined as they evolve, so that sequential radiographs are diagnostic. For reasons described earlier, air-fluid levels in the pleural space or pulmonary cavities may not be visualized on portable radiographs (Fig. 19-21). Distinction between pneumonia and pulmonary edema is not always possible, especially in immunosuppressed patients. In such cases, infectious infiltrates are commonly diffuse and bilateral. In patients with normal immunity, most infectious agents produce focal or patchy infiltrates. Pseudomonas pneumonia, however, is commonly bilateral and diffuse. Therefore, a diagnosis of pneumonia must be made on the basis of clinical as well as radiographic findings.

Artifacts

Various types of artifacts may overlie the lungs of ICU patients and can be mistaken for pathology. For instance, the external portion of central catheters, ET tubes and nasogastric tubes can cause confusion when these positions coincide fortuitously with underlying anatomy. A particularly troublesome artifact is caused by certain electrocardiographic (EKG) skin contacts which contain collections of silver nitrate gel approximately 1 cm in diameter (see Plate 56). These gel collections create nodular densities which can be indistinguishable from noncalcified pulmonary nodules. Their true nature can be suspected from their close and constant relationship to the opaque metallic portion of the ECG contact.[55]

References

1. Janower ML, Jennas-Nocera Z, Mukai J: Utility and efficacy of portable chest radiographs. AJR, 142:265, 1984.
2. Eisenberg RL, Akin JR, Hedgcock MW: Optimal use of portable and stat examination. AJR 134:523, 1980.
3. Bekemeyer WB, Crapo RO, Calhoon S, et al: Efficacy of chest radiography in a respiratory intensive care unit: A prospective study. Chest 88:691, 1985.
4. MacMahon H, Yasillo NJ, Carlin M: High-quality radiography with a new laser alignment system. Presented at the Radiological Society of North America, Chicago, November, 1990.
5. Fisher MR, Mintzer RA, Rogers LF, et al: Evaluation of a new mobile automatic exposure control device. AJR 139:1055, 1982.

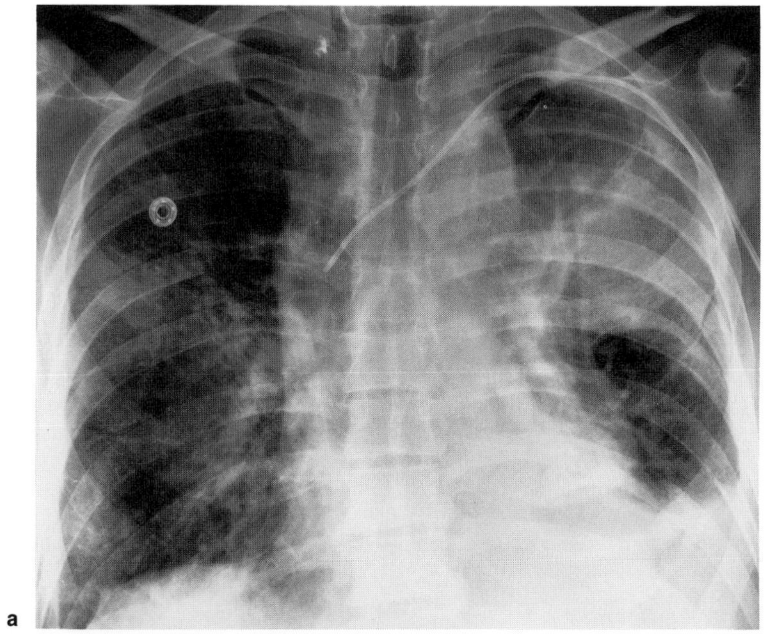

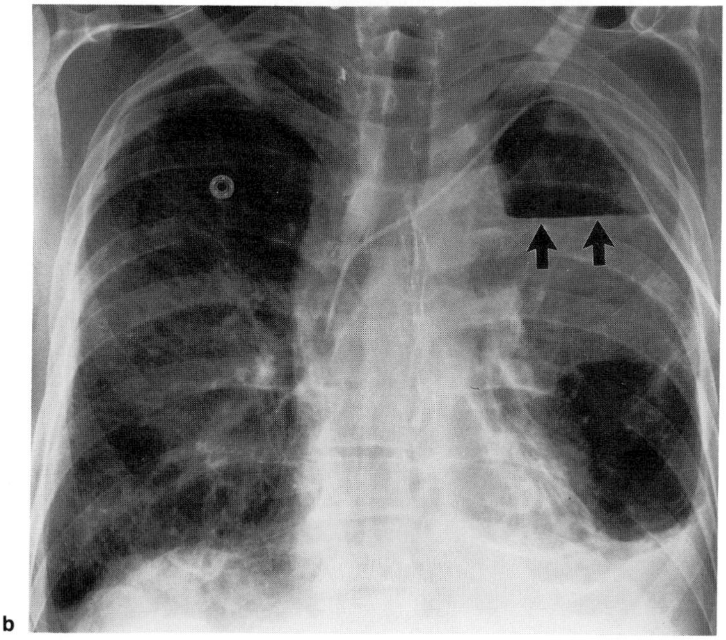

FIGURE 19-21 Detection of air-fluid levels. *A:* A semierect portable radiograph shows hazy density in the left upper lung zone, as well as consolidation and pleural effusion at the left base. *B:* An erect view taken with a horizontal x-ray beam on the same day demonstrates an air fluid level (arrows) due to a large loculated anterior hydropneumothorax.

6. Sonoda M, Takano M, Miyahara J, Kato H: Computed radiography utilizing scanning laser stimulated luminescence. Radiology 148:833, 1983.
7. MacMahon H, Vyborny CJ, Sabeti V, Metz CE, Doi K: The effect of unsharp masking on the detectability of interstitial infiltrates and pneumothoraces. Proc SPIE 555:246, 1985.
8. Merritt CRB, Matthews CC, Scheinhorn D, Balter S: Digital imaging of the chest. J Thorac Imag 1(1):1, 1985.
9. MacMahon H, Metz CE, Doi K, et al: Digital chest radiography: Effect of diagnostic accuracy of hard copy, conventional video, and reversed gray scale video display formats. Radiology 168:669, 1988.
10. Kohan RH, Poe RH, Israel RH, et al. Value of chest ultrasonography versus decubitus roentgenography for thoracentesis. Am Rev Respir Dis 133:1124, 1986.
11. Godwin DJ (ed): *Computed Tomography of the Chest.* Philadelphia, Lippincott, 1984.
12. Peruzzi W, Garner W, Bools J, Rasanen J, Mueller CF, Reilley T: Portable chest roentgenography and computed tomography in critically ill patients. Chest 93(4):722, 1988.
13. Mirvis SE, Tobin KD, Kostrubiak I, Belzberg H: Thoracic CT in detecting occult disease in critically ill patients. AJR 148:685, 1987.
14. Mirvis SE, Rodriguez A, Whitley NO, Tarr RJ: CT evaluation of thoracic infections after major trauma. AJR 144:1183, 1985.
15. Stark DD, Federle MP, Goodman PC, Podrasky AE, Webb WR: Differentiating lung abscess and empyema: Radiology and computed tomography. AJR 141:163, 1983.
16. Tocino IM, Miller MH, Frederick PR. Thomas E: CT detection of occult pneumothorax in head trauma. AJR 143:987, 1984.

17. Wall S, Federle M, Jeffrey R, Brett C: CT diagnosis of unsuspected pneumothorax after blunt abdominal trauma. AJR 143:919, 1983.
18. Stark DD, Federle MP, Goodman PC: CT and radiographic assessment of tube thoracostomy. AJR 141:253, 1983.
19. Mitchell SE, Clark RA: Complications of central venous catheterization. AJR 133:467, 1979.
20. Rohlfing BM, Webb WR, Schlobohn RM: Ventilator-related extra-alveolar air in adults. Radiology 121:25, 1976.
21. Zwillich CW, Pierson DJ, Creach CE, et al: Complications of assisted ventilation. Am J Med 57:161, 1974.
22. Moskowitz PS, Griscom NT: The medial pneumothorax. Radiology 120:143, 1976.
23. Rhea JT, VanSonnenberg E, McLoud TC: Basilar pneumothorax in the supine adult. Radiology 133:593, 1979.
24. McLoud TC, Barash PG, Ravin CE: PEEP: Radiographic features and associated complications. AJR 129:209, 1977.
25. Cimmino CV: Some radio-diagnostic notes on pneumomediastinum, pneumothorax, and pneumopericardium. Va Med Month 94:205, 1967.
26. Kleinman PK, Brill PW, Whalen JP: Anterior pathway for transdiaphragmatic extension of pneumomediastinum. AJR 131:271, 1978.
27. Maltby JD: The post-trauma chest film. CRC Crit Rev Diagn Imag 14:1, 1980.
28. Harvey-Smith W, Bush W, Northrop C: Traumatic bronchial rupture. AJR 134:1189, 1980.
29. Unger JM, Schuchmann GG, Grossman JE, Pellett JR: Tears of the trachea and main bronchi caused by blunt trauma: radiologic findings. AJR 153:1175, 1989.
30. Sefczek DM, Sefczek RJ, Deeb ZL: Radiographic signs of acute traumatic rupture of the thoracic aorta. AJR 141:1259, 1983.
31. Godwin JD, Tolentino CS: Thoracic cardiovascular trauma. J Thorac Imag 2(3):32, 1987.
32. Hollerman JJ, Fackler ML, Coldwell DM, Ben-Menachem Y: Gunshot wounds: 1. Bullets, ballistics, and mechanisms of injury. AJR 155:685, 1990.
33. Love L, Berkow AE: Trauma to the esophagus. Gastrointest Radiol 2:305, 1978.
34. Ruskin JA, Gurney JW, Thorsen MK, Goodman LR: Detection of pleural effusions on supine chest radiographs. AJR 148:681, 1987.
35. Bryk D: Infrapulmonary effusion: Effect of expiration on the pseudodiaphragmatic contour. Radiology 120:33, 1976.
36. Raasch BN, Carsky EW, Lane EJ, et al: Pleural effusion: Explanation of some typical appearances. AJR 139:899, 1982.
37. Paling MR, Griffin GK: Lower lobe collapse due to pleural effusion/A CT analysis J Comput Assist Tomogr 9(6):1079, 1985.
38. Greene RE: Acute respiratory failure and the adult respiratory distress syndrome, in *Radiology 1, Diagnosis-Imaging-Intervention*. Philadelphia, Lippincott, 1988, Chap. 51.
39. Barlett JG, Gorbach SL: The triple threat of aspiration pneumonia. Chest 68:4, 560, 1975.
40. Goodman LR, Conrardy PA, Laing F, Singer MM: Radiographic evaluation of endotracheal tube position. AJR 127:433, 1976.
41. Hirsch M, Abramowitz HB, Shapira S, Barki Y: Hypopharyngeal injury as a result of attempted endotracheal intubation. Radiology 128:37, 1978.
42. Cooper JD: Tracheo-innominate artery fistula—Successful management in three consecutive cases. Ann Thorac Surg 24:439, 1977.
43. Dunbar RD, Mitchell R, Lavine M: Aberrant location of central venous catheters. Lancet 1:711, 1981.
44. Langston CS: The aberrant central venous catheter and its complications. Radiology 100:55, 1971.
45. Deitel M, McIntyre JA: Radiographic confirmation of site of central venous pressure catheters. Can J Surg 14:42, 1971.
46. Hunt R, Hunter TB: Cardiac tamponade and death from perforation of the right atrium by a central venous catheter. AJR 151:1250, 1988.
47. McLoud TC, Putman CE: Radiology of the swan-ganz catheter and associated pulmonary complications. Radiology 116:19, 1975.
48. Hyson EA, Ravin CE, Kelley MJ, Curtis AM: Intraaortic counterpulsation balloon/radiographic considerations. AJR 128:915, 1977.
49. Woodall BH, Winfield DF, Bisset III GS: Inadvertent tracheobronchial placement of feeding tubes. Radiology 165:727, 1987.
50. Hewitt MJ, Chen JTT, Ravin CE, et al: Coronary sinus atrial pacing: Radiographic considerations. AJR 136:323, 1981.
51. Steiner RM, Tegtmeyer CJ: The radiology of cardiac pacemakers, in Morse D, Steiner RM, Parsonnet V (eds): *A Guide to Cardiac Pacemakers*. Philadelphia, Davis, 1983.
52. Milne ENC, Burnett K, Aufrichtig D, McMillan J, Imray T: Assessment of cardiac size on portable chest films. J Thorac Imag 3(2):64, 1988.
53. Bryant LR, Mobin-Uddin K, Dillon ML, Griffen WO: Misdiagnosis of pneumonia in patients needing mechanical respiration. Arch Surg 106:286, 1973.
54. Goodman LR, Goren RA, Teplick SK: The radiographic evaluation of pulmonary infection. Med Clin North Am 64:553, 1980.
55. Kim T, Messersmith RN, MacMahon H: Lung nodule mimicked by EKG lead artifact. Chest 95:237, 1989.

Chapter 20

INTERVENTIONAL RADIOLOGY IN THE INTENSIVE CARE UNIT PATIENT

DANIEL PICUS
GREGORY A. SCHMIDT

Interventional radiology encompasses a wide variety of procedures having in common the placement of needles or catheters or both through the skin under radiologic guidance. The specific type of radiographic guidance varies with the particular circumstance, but includes fluoroscopy, ultrasound, or computed tomography (CT). These procedures often are performed as an alternative or adjunct to surgical intervention. In contrast to surgery, interventional radiology procedures usually are carried out under local anesthesia and do not require an incision. Thus, these procedures generally carry a lower morbidity and mortality than the surgical alternative. This is particularly important in the critically ill ICU patient, in whom all procedures have a higher than average risk.

When and Where to Perform the Procedure

ICU patients are critically ill. Although it is generally preferable to work with a "stable" patient, this is not always possible. Often, the longer one waits for a patient to stabilize, the more the patient's condition deteriorates, and eventually the patient is too sick to benefit. In some cases, stabilization is even counterproductive. For example, patients bleeding from the gastrointestinal tract should undergo immediate angiography while they are bleeding in an effort to localize the source. It makes little sense to wait to perform the examination until the patient is stable (i.e., not bleeding). On the other hand, prior to moving the patient to the special procedures area, appropriate lines should be in place, fluids and blood components available, and oxygen delivery adequate. Deciding when to perform an interventional radiology procedure is often difficult and requires close communication between the intensivist and interventional radiologist, who should be consulted early so there is adequate time for a meaningful exchange.

Just as the decision ***when*** to perform an interventional radiology procedure requires close communication and cooperation, the decision ***where*** to perform the procedure requires joint evaluation by the critical care and interventional radiology staffs. One of the advantages of some interventional radiology procedures is that they may be performed at the bedside. Portable examinations generally are guided by ultrasound. Ultrasound units are mobile, inexpensive, and allow cross-sectional imaging. Ultrasound guidance is useful for a variety of procedures, including percutaneous fluid aspiration, percutaneous biopsy, percutaneous cholecystostomy, and percutaneous abscess drainage. Limitations of ultrasound guidance include the need for direct contact between the ultrasound transducer and the skin. This limits its usefulness in patients with surgical dressings or open wounds.

Many interventional radiology biopsy and drainage procedures are best guided by CT, which provides a detailed display of the relationship of surrounding structures and allows precise planning of a percutaneous access route. CT easily images bowel, bone, and visceral organs, as well as orally and intravenously administered contrast agents. Compared to ultrasound, CT is unhindered by overlying dressings, wounds, or ostomy devices. But CT is not portable—the patient must be transported to the CT scanning suite.

Although CT and ultrasound guidance are useful for some nonvascular procedures, fluoroscopic guidance is required for all vascular interventional procedures and many nonvascular procedures as well. Portable fluoroscopy units are available in most ICUs, but they have several disadvantages. Portable fluroscopy units are cumbersome to use, have no radiographic shielding, and allow imaging of only a small area of the body. In addition, they have no method for recording images and no ability to do digital subtraction angiography. Modern fluoroscopy equipment for interventional radiology includes a large field of view, multiangle orientation, and digital subtraction angiography capability.

The risk in complex interventional procedures is minimized and the success enhanced when the patient is brought to the special procedures suite. But this must be weighed against the increased risk of transporting a critically ill patient. Again, close communication and cooperation between the intensivist and interventional radiologist is crucial to provide the best possible patient care.

Monitoring the Patient in Interventional Radiology

Most interventional radiology procedures should be performed in the radiology department. Therefore, as closely as possible, the ICU environment should be reproduced in the radiology special procedures suite.

EQUIPMENT

All interventional radiology suites should be equipped with basic patient monitoring equipment, including electrocardiography (ECG), noninvasive blood pressure (preferably automated), and pulse oximetry devices. Pulse oximetry units generally are inexpensive and extremely useful for monitoring the patient's base-line respiratory status and the effects of narcotic analgesics used to sedate the patient. The ability to record invasive hemodynamic data is useful also.

A standard emergency "crash" cart should be available, along with a defibrillator and backboard for cardiopulmonary resuscitation. All special procedure suites should also be equipped with a reliable source of oxygen and suction.

PERSONNEL

ICU patients require constant nursing care while in the interventional radiology suite. Most interventional radiology departments employ nurses who are specially trained to care for patients during radiology special procedures. However, the ICU patient generally has special needs, and a nurse from the ICU should accompany the patient to radiology. The ICU nurse is responsible for monitoring and recording vital signs and for administering medications.

Generally, an ICU physician need not accompany patients to the interventional radiology suite. However, this decision must be made case by case, taking into consideration the condition of the patient and the complexity of the procedure.

Nonvascular Interventional Radiology Procedures

PERCUTANEOUS ABSCESS DRAINAGE (PAD)

INDICATIONS AND PATIENT SELECTION

The febrile patient is common in the ICU. A frequent cause, particularly in postsurgical patients, is an abscess. The traditional surgical treatment is incision, removal of the purulent material, and subsequent drainage. In the last 10 to 15 years, PAD has all but replaced surgical drainage as the treatment of choice for abscesses and other abnormal fluid collections (e.g., biloma, urinoma).[1] PAD is less invasive, maintains the integrity of surrounding structures, and can be done at the time of initial diagnosis, saving time and expense. PAD also makes nursing care easier because of the closed drainage system.

PAD is most successful when the fluid collection is well defined, unilocular, and free flowing (Fig. 20-1). These characteristics are found in more than 90 percent of intraabdominal collections. PAD may also be helpful in less favorable situations (e.g., multilocular, necrotic debris), particularly when the patient is a high surgical risk. In such less optimal circumstances, PAD may improve the patient's condition so that more definitive surgical drainage can be performed. The only absolute contraindication to PAD is lack of a safe access route, but this rarely is a problem with CT guidance.

TECHNIQUE

The most important step in PAD is planning the access route. This is done following review of all the pertinent imaging studies. In general, the shortest, straightest tract is best, always taking care to avoid the bowel, pleura, and major blood vessels.

Diagnostic aspiration is performed first, usually with a 22 gauge needle. The position of the needle is confirmed with ultrasound or CT, and fluid is aspirated for diagnosis. If a decision is made to drain the collection, a guidewire is passed through the needle into the collection. Then the tract is dilated and a drainage catheter placed. The catheter is fixed to the skin with a single Prolene suture, allowing easy access for local skin care.

When the catheter is in place, the collection is aspirated as completely as possible. Follow-up imaging should be performed immediately to be certain that all the fluid has been drained. If additional catheters are necessary, they are placed in the same way. Percutaneous catheters are left to drain by gravity, although occasionally they may be connected to low suction.

IMMEDIATE POSTPROCEDURE CARE

The output of the drainage catheter should be monitored carefully. The catheter is left in place as long as it continues to drain, which usually requires 3 to 10 days. Intravenous antibiotics are an essential adjunct to any abscess drainage procedure. Appropriate coverage should be provided based on the culture results.

We usually do not irrigate drainage catheters. Only rarely is the material too viscous to drain. When necessary, irrigation should be done with *small,* 5 to 10 mL aliquots of sterile saline. The irrigation fluid should be injected into the catheter and then allowed to drain on its own. Vigorous suction generally draws debris back into the catheter, causing it to occlude. If the catheter does occlude or fails to drain easily, it should be exchanged for a larger one. This is a relatively simple procedure, but does require fluoroscopic guidance.

Once effective drainage has been established, the patient's condition should improve within 24 to 48 h. Incomplete drainage should be suspected when the patient remains febrile or the white blood cell count remains persistently elevated. In these cases, follow-up CT should be obtained promptly and additional drainage catheters placed as needed. If the drainage first tapers and then abruptly increases, a fistula may be the cause. Injection of contrast media with fluoroscopic guidance usually demonstrates the communication. When a fistula is present, PAD still can be successful, but it may require extended drainage with complete bowel rest.

RESULTS AND COMPLICATIONS

PAD compares favorably with surgical treatment in terms of overall success, duration of drainage, and recurrence rate.[2] Success rates of 80 to 90 percent are reported consistently. These highly favorable results are related to the liberal use of CT, which facilitates accurate delineation of the entire collection, as well as detection and drainage of residual collections. Failure of PAD is most often due to failure to recognize fistulae or undrained collections, premature withdrawal of the catheter, or an attempt to drain a relatively solid collection (e.g., necrotic tumor, pancreatic phlegmon).

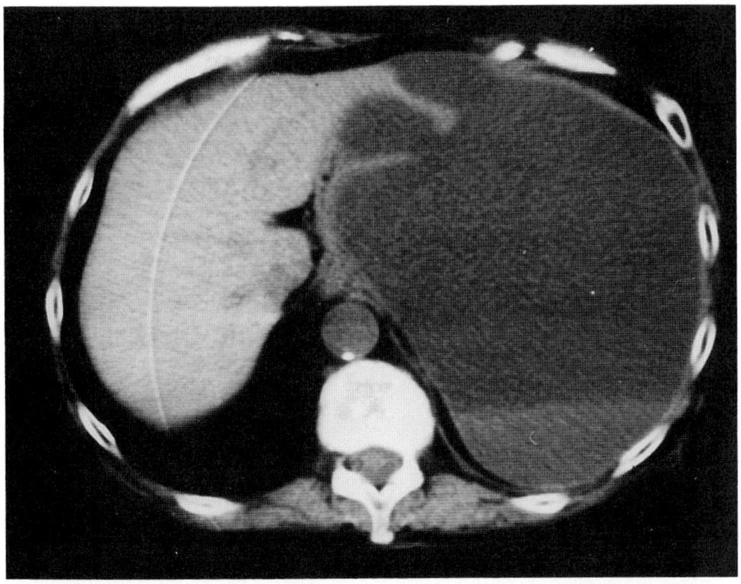
a

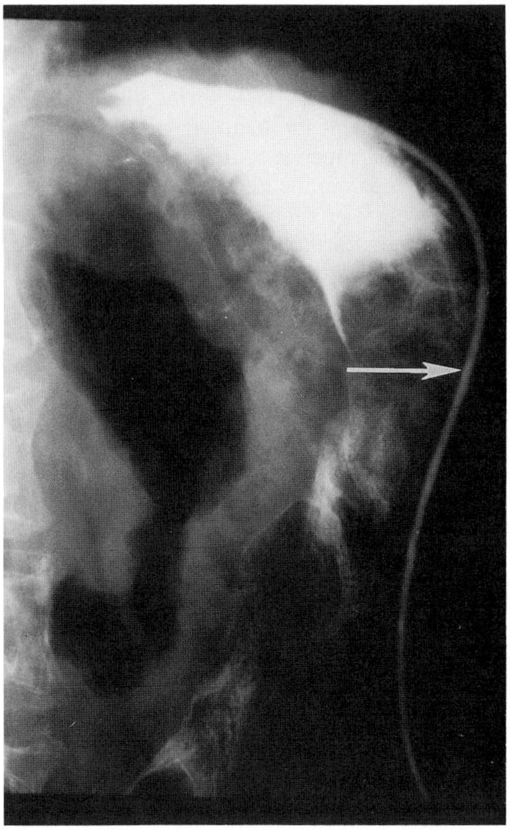
b

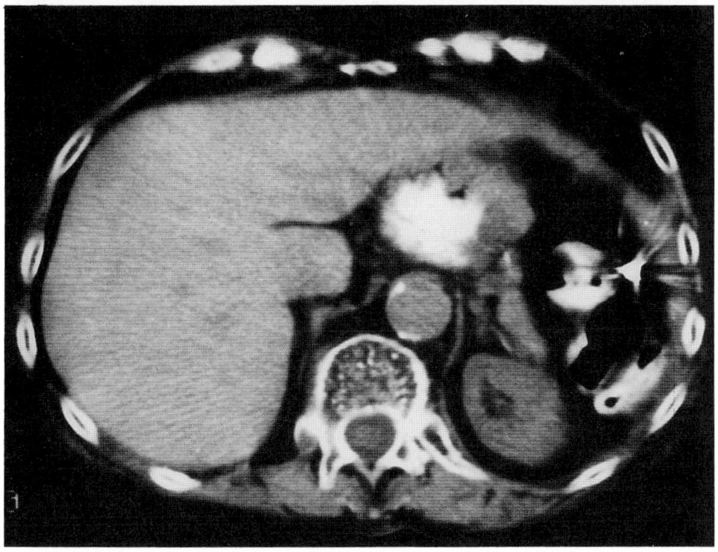
c

FIGURE 20-1 Patient status after splenectomy with fever and an elevated white blood cell count. *a.* CT shows large left upper quadrant fluid collection. *b.* Percutaneous drainage catheter (arrow) was placed under CT guidance. Contrast injection confirms the position of the catheter. *c.* Follow-up CT shows complete resolution of the abscess. The patient's symptoms had resolved.

Complication rates for PAD range from 10 to 15 percent and serious complications are reported in less than 5 percent of cases.[2] Minor complications include transient bacteremia, skin infection, and minor bleeding. Major complications include hemorrhage, sepsis, and bowel perforation. The recurrence rate following PAD is approximately 5 percent. These figures compare favorably with surgical series, which report mortality rates of 10 to 20 percent, and recurrence rates of 15 to 30 percent.

PERCUTANEOUS CHOLECYSTOSTOMY

INDICATIONS AND PATIENT SELECTION

Elective cholecystectomy in an otherwise healthy patient is a safe procedure with an operative mortality rate of < 0.5 percent. However, the morbidity and mortality rates increase dramatically in patients with multiorgan compromise, as is typical in the ICU patient. Historically, critically ill patients have been treated with operative cholecystostomy to temporize until their medical condition stabilizes. At that time a safer, elective cholecystectomy is performed.

Recently, percutaneous cholecystostomy has emerged as an alternative to standard surgical therapy. One advantage of the percutaneous approach is the fact that it can be done at the patient's bedside, with no incision and only local anesthesia.

Indications for percutaneous cholecystostomy include acute calculous or acalculous cholecystitis in a patient too ill for cholecystectomy. In calculous disease, the gallbladder can be removed electively when the patient's condition stabilizes. As an alternative, the stones can be managed without surgical treatment by percutaneous removal or dissolution therapy.[3]

Acute acalculous cholecystitis is being recognized more often as a problem in the ICU (see Chap. 85). However, acute acalculous cholecystitis is difficult to diagnose.[4] Ultrasound is extremely accurate for diagnosing cholelithiasis but is less reliable for diagnosing acute acalculous cholecystitis, with accuracy rates of 50 to 60 percent generally reported. Hepatoiminodiacetic acid (HIDA) scans can diagnose patency of the cystic duct. However, false-positive examinations can occur at a rate of up to 25 to 30 percent. This is particularly true in the ICU patient who has multiple factors leading to false-positive HIDA scans, including total parenteral nutrition, fasting, sepsis, and underlying liver disease.

In patients with acalculous cholecystitis, percutaneous cholecystostomy can provide the correct diagnosis and definitive therapy. Decompression of the gallbladder by percutaneous cholecystostomy can bring dramatic relief of symptoms. Typically, the cystic duct eventually opens, allowing tube removal without requiring a formal cholecystectomy.

TECHNIQUE

Percutaneous cholecystostomy can be done at the patient's bedside with portable ultrasound guidance. Transhepatic access to the gallbladder is preferred to decrease the risk of bile spillage into the peritoneal cavity. A 22 gauge needle is advanced into the gallbladder, and bile is aspirated. Though Gram stain and culture of the bile are helpful, their sensitivity for cholecystitis is low—30 to 50 percent. Neither a negative Gram stain nor a negative culture excludes the diagnosis of acute cholecystitis.[5] Therefore, we prefer to place a cholecystostomy tube immediately rather than wait for analysis of the bile. A guidewire is passed through the needle and coiled in the gallbladder fundus. The tract is dilated and a retention pigtail catheter placed. If the procedure is guided by fluoroscopy, an injection of contrast media is helpful to confirm the position of the catheter. Care should be taken not to over distend an acutely inflamed gallbladder.

IMMEDIATE POSTPROCEDURE CARE

Catheters are left to drain by gravity. When the cystic duct is obstructed, the gallbladder normally produces 50 to 70 mL of clear mucus daily. Larger volumes of bilious drainage indicate cystic duct patency.

When the patient's condition stabilizes, the cholecystostomy tube is injected under fluoroscopic guidance to evaluate for stones in the gallbladder, cystic duct, or common bile duct (Fig. 20-2). If no stones are seen and contrast material flows freely into the duodenum, the tube can be capped. The cholecystostomy tube can be removed 10 to 14 days following placement when a tract has formed.

RESULTS AND COMPLICATIONS

Percutaneous cholecystostomy is successful in more than 95 percent of cases.[6] Interestingly, up to 20 to 30 percent of patients will not have acute cholecystitis. This confirms the difficulty in diagnosing acute cholecystitis in critically ill patients. Percutaneous cholecystostomy still is helpful in these patients because it excludes the diagnosis of acute cholecystitis and avoids unnecessary surgery.

With proper technique, complications are few. Bile peritonitis is avoided by rapidly decompressing the gallbladder and by carefully performing cholangiography with fluoroscopic guidance. Sepsis, hemobilia, and vagal reactions have all been reported in < 5 percent of cases.

Vascular Interventional Radiology Procedures

GASTROINTESTINAL BLEEDING: DIAGNOSIS AND TREATMENT

Interventional radiology plays an important role in the diagnosis and treatment of gastrointestinal bleeding. The overall management of gastrointestinal hemorrhage is discussed elsewhere (see Chap. 163). This section will focus on angiographic localization and treatment of upper and lower gastrointestinal bleeding.

INDICATIONS AND PATIENT SELECTION

Angiography is best performed when the patient is actively bleeding. Frequently this is difficult to determine because by nature, gastrointestinal bleeding is intermittent. In addition, upper and lower gastrointestinal bleeding can result in the accumulation of massive quantities of blood in the bowel lumen; this blood is slowly expelled over the next several hours. The widespread use of endoscopy and nuclear medicine bleeding studies has improved our ability to document active bleeding and localize the site, helping to guide subsequent intervention.

In an effort to locate the bleeding lesion in upper gastrointestinal bleeding, endoscopy always should be performed before angiography. Even if endoscopy cannot determine the specific site of bleeding, active bleeding usually can be confirmed.

Nuclear medicine bleeding studies with technetium-labeled red blood cells are most useful in patients with bleeding distal to the ligament of Treitz. Finding the bleeding site in patients with lower gastrointestinal hemorrhage is a frustrating problem because of its intermittent nature. The advantage of the radionuclide study is the fact that extravasation of the radiopharmaceutical can be monitored over the course of 12 to 24 h because the agent is persistent in the bloodstream. Locating bleeding with angiography, on the other hand, requires active bleeding during the 10 s that the angiographic contrast material is injected into the artery feeding the bleeding segment of bowel. Additional advantages of the radionuclide study are that it can be done portably and it is noninvasive.

TECHNIQUE

Once it is determined that the patient is actively bleeding and will benefit from angiography, the patient must be transported to the special procedures suite. Angiography

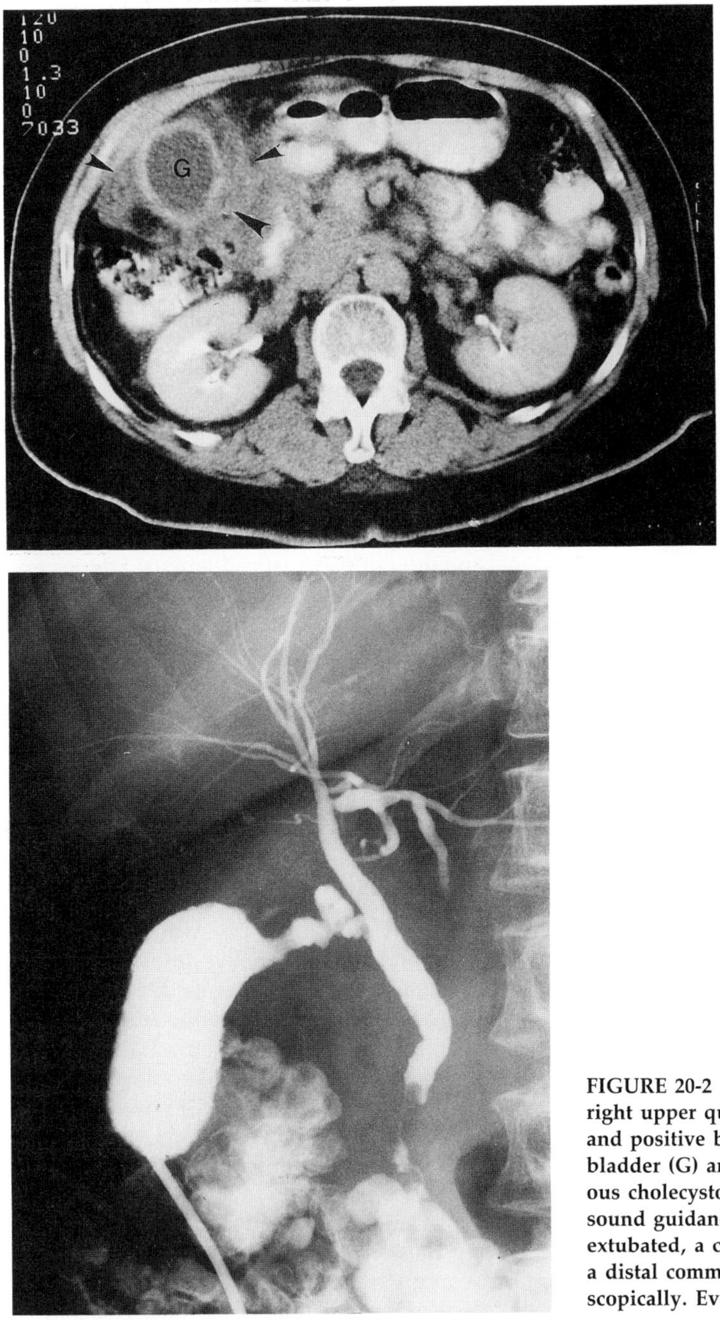

a

b

FIGURE 20-2 Intubated patient with several day history of right upper quadrant pain, elevated white blood cell count, and positive blood cultures. ***a.*** **CT shows a thick-walled gallbladder (G) and pericholecystic fluid (arrowheads). Percutaneous cholecystostomy was performed at the bedside with ultrasound guidance.** ***b.*** **Several days later, when the patient was extubated, a cholangiogram was performed. This demonstrated a distal common bile duct calculus, which was extracted endoscopically. Eventually, the cholecystostomy tube was removed.**

cannot be performed with portable fluoroscopy equipment.

In patients with documented upper gastrointestinal bleeding, the celiac artery is the first vessel injected. Usually this is followed by selective injections of the left gastric artery and gastroduodenal artery. In lower gastrointestinal bleeding, both the superior mesenteric artery and inferior mesenteric artery must be studied. A positive nuclear medicine study is invaluable to direct the subsequent arteriogram.

Acute bleeding is identified by extravasation of contrast media into the lumen of the bowel (Fig. 20-3). A bleeding rate of at least 0.5 mL/min is needed for angiographic visualization. Oblique views often are helpful to project the bowel lumen away from overlying structures such as the spine or contrast-filled bladder.

If a bleeding site is identified, it may be controlled with interventional radiology techniques—either transcatheter embolization or selective vasoconstrictor infusion. The decision to proceed with these therapies should be individualized for each patient. Factors to be considered include the patient's overall medical condition, the cause and location of bleeding, and the local experience.

For lower gastrointestinal bleeding, the nonoperative therapy of choice is *selective vasoconstrictor infusion.* Embolotherapy is valuable in upper gastrointestinal bleeding, but is rarely used to treat patients with lower gastrointesti-

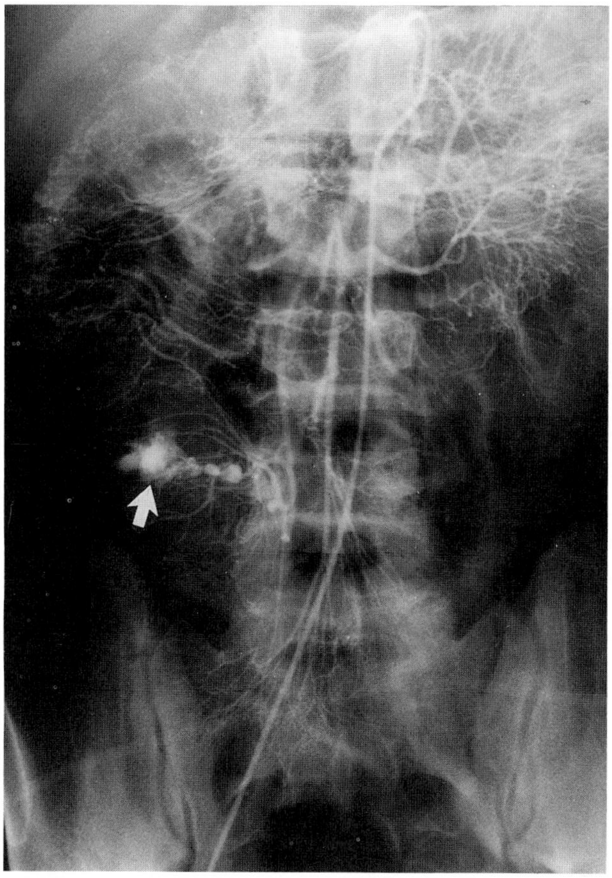

FIGURE 20-3 Superior mesenteric arteriogram shows extravasation from the right colic artery (arrow). Surgery—cecal diverticular bleed.

nal bleeding. This is because of the more tenuous collateral blood supply of the small bowel and colon (vide infra).

The vasoconstrictive agent of choice is vasopressin. It is the pressor component of the active hormone of the posterior pituitary gland. The action of vasopressin is due to both constriction of the splanchnic vascular bed and contraction of the smooth muscle of the gut itself. Direct intra-arterial injection of vasopressin results in fewer systemic side effects than intravenous administration. Infusion of vasopressin produces the best results in patients with a normal coagulation mechanism because control of bleeding depends on the formation of a stable clot at the bleeding site.

Vasopressin infusion is begun immediately following selective angiography. Vasopressin is infused directly into the major artery that feeds the bleeding site. In an area with a dual blood supply (e.g., duodenum), vasopressin must be infused through both vascular beds (celiac and superior mesenteric artery) and is much less effective. The infusion generally is begun at 0.1 to 0.4 U/min with angiography repeated in 20 min to assess the vasoconstrictive effect. If the bleeding stops, the patient is returned to the ICU with the infusion continuing.

If bleeding persists, the vasopressin infusion is increased. Generally, an infusion of >0.4 U/min results in significantly more systemic side effects. If bleeding is not controlled at 0.4 U/min, alternative therapies should be considered.

The vasopressin infusion is continued for 12 to 24 h and then gradually tapered over the next 24 to 48 h while the patient's condition is carefully monitored. An infusion of saline for the final 12 to 24 h is helpful to evaluate for rebleeding. If rebleeding does occur, repeat vasopressin infusion can be helpful.

Transcatheter embolotherapy is an alternative to vasopressin infusion, particularly for the control of upper gastrointestinal hemorrhage. Embolotherapy is most helpful in areas with rich collateral arterial networks (i.e., esophagus, stomach, duodenum, and rectum) where multiple blood supplies minimize the risk of ischemic injury. Bleeding from mucosal lesions in the distal esophagus and gastric fundus (e.g., Mallory-Weiss tear, esophagitis, gastritis) typically are well controlled with embolization of the left gastric artery. Likewise, superselective embolization of the gastroduodenal and inferior pancreaticoduodenal arteries may be effective therapy for bleeding duodenal ulcers.

The best material for embolotherapy of the gastrointestinal tract is Gelfoam—surgical gelatin. Gelfoam can be cut into strips and pledgets and injected directly into the bleeding vessel. Gelfoam is a resorbable agent that provides temporary occlusion for 5 to 10 days, allowing the lesion to heal. Occasionally, if endoscopy has suggested a bleeding site near the gastroesophageal junction, the left gastric artery can be embolized even when no active extravasation is seen. The morbidity of this approach is extremely low, and the method decreases rebleeding.[7]

IMMEDIATE POSTPROCEDURE CARE

Embolotherapy and vasoconstrictive infusions both work by decreasing the pulse pressure at the bleeding site. This allows hemostasis and healing of the bleeding lesion. This approach requires a functioning hemostatic mechanism. Frequently, patients with massive gastrointestinal bleeding have multisystem organ failure (MSOF) or sepsis or have received many units of transfused blood. Any of these can result in an underlying coagulopathy, which should be corrected as rapidly as possible.

Patients on vasopressin infusion must be monitored carefully. During the initial stages, many patients experience abdominal cramps because of vasopressin's effect on the smooth muscle of the gastrointestinal tract. This may result in a dramatic emptying of accumulated blood from the gastrointestinal tract. If the cramps fail to subside in 30 to 60 min or if the cramps recur, significant gut ischemia may be present. The vasopressin dose should be decreased slowly until the pain is relieved. Patients on vasopressin infusion should be monitored carefully for signs of myocardial and peripheral ischemia, arrhythmia, and hyponatremia secondary to the antidiuretic effect of vasopressin. Hyponatremia and decreased urine output are usually treated easily with diuretics.

RESULTS AND COMPLICATIONS

Results with transcatheter therapy for acute gastrointestinal bleeding are highly variable depending on several factors, including the underlying medical condition of the patient, the cause of bleeding, and the particular bleeding site. In our experience, patients with extensive MSOF and gastrointestinal bleeding rarely benefit from intervention. However, as is usually the case, it is difficult to determine beforehand which individual patient may benefit.

In patients without MSOF, control of upper gastrointestinal bleeding with embolotherapy usually is successful in 70 to 80 percent.[8] Likewise, in lower gastrointestinal bleeding, vasopressin infusion is effective in 80 to 90 percent of patients, particularly those with bleeding colonic diverticuli. However, bleeding can recur in up to 30 percent of patients. Even in patients in whom rebleeding occurs, however, temporary control of bleeding can allow elective surgical intervention under more favorable conditions.

Complications of embolotherapy are rare.[9] The rich collateral network around the stomach and duodenum protect against infarction. However, care must be taken in postsurgical patients, in whom collateral vessels are ligated. Backflow of embolic material into the liver and spleen occasionally occurs and is generally well tolerated. Clinically significant hepatic or splenic infarctions are rare.

A relative contraindication to vasopressin infusion is significant coronary, peripheral, or cerebrovascular disease. Complications of vasopressin treatment are typically related to diffuse vasoconstriction, which results in significant ischemia to the heart or extremities. Other complications include arrhythmia and hyponatremia. Thrombosis of the femoral or visceral arteries may result from prolonged placement of the intra-arterial catheter. Significant complications related to catheter-directed vasopressin therapy are infrequent, generally < 10 percent.[10]

FOREIGN BODY RETRIEVAL

INDICATIONS AND PATIENT SELECTION

ICU patients have a multitude of intravascular catheters for infusion and monitoring. Occasionally, a catheter fragment may become dislodged in the vascular system—usually the central veins, heart, or pulmonary arteries. Generally, this occurs during catheter introduction or repositioning. Rarely, no cause is found and detachment may be related to defects in material.

The presence of an intravascular foreign body is usually an indication for its removal. Complications have been reported in up to 70 percent of patients in whom catheter fragments were left in place.[11] Major complications of a retained catheter fragment include vascular perforation, sepsis, arrhythmia, and pulmonary embolism. The medicolegal implications are obvious.

TECHNIQUE

Percutaneous retrieval of the intravascular foreign body is the treatment of choice. Percutaneous removal generally can be accomplished without an incision or general anesthesia. The alternative is a major surgical procedure.

An initial venogram is performed to confirm the intravascular position of the fragment and to find a suitable site for grasping. The most common tool for retrieval is a snare made of very thin guidewire. The wire is passed through a nontapered catheter, which is positioned next to the fragment. The wire is advanced to form a large loop to snare the fragment. After the fragment is snared, the wire is pulled taut to trap it securely at the tip of the catheter (Fig. 20-4). Usually, a slow backward pull on the catheter will fold the fragment over itself, allowing it to be removed through the percutaneous puncture site in the femoral vein. Rarely, a surgical cutdown is necessary if the fragment is too large or nonpliable.

Various other tools are available for percutaneous foreign body removal. These include baskets, graspers, and balloon catheters. Every patient is different, and the particular system must be tailored to the individual problem.

RESULTS AND COMPLICATIONS

The success rate for percutaneous foreign body retrieval is high, although few large series have been reported. Success rates range from 80 to 95 percent.[12] When failure occurs, it is generally due to extravascular fragments or lack of a free end to grasp.

Complications of percutaneous retrieval are rare. Transient arrhythmia may occur when fragments are manipulated or pulled through the heart. Continual ECG monitoring is critical. If the foreign body is firmly adherent to the endothelium, endocardium, or cardiac valve, traction must be applied gently to avoid vascular damage.

PERCUTANEOUS CAVAL FILTER PLACEMENT

INDICATIONS AND PATIENT SELECTION

Pulmonary embolism is an extremely common cause of morbidity and mortality in the ICU patient. Usually, anticoagulation will provide adequate therapy. But in many critically ill patients, anticoagulants are either contraindicated or ineffective. This has led to the development of a number of mechanical devices to "filter" emboli from the lower extremities.[13]

Up until the mid-1980s, these devices were placed by a surgical cutdown in the internal jugular vein. More recently, percutaneous introduction by interventional radiologists has become commonplace.[14] Percutaneous introduction is more convenient because it can be done at the same time as pulmonary angiography. It can be done under local anesthesia, sparing the expense of the anesthesiologist and the operating room. Because an inferior vena cavagram can be done with high quality fluoroscopy, misplacement may be less common.

As placement techniques evolved over the past 10 years, many new devices were developed. Some are well tested and widely available, whereas others are still undergoing clinical trials. Several excellent reviews of caval filters are available.[15,16] Currently, two devices are in widespread clinical use: the No. 24 French Greenfield filter and the Bird's Nest vena caval filter (Fig. 20-5).

Indications for caval filter placement generally fall into three categories: **1.** contraindication to or complication of

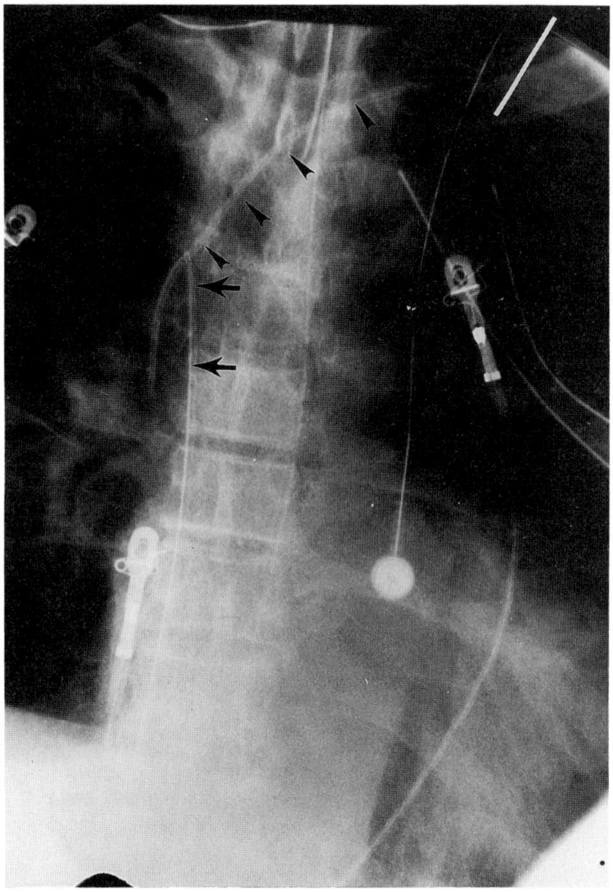

a

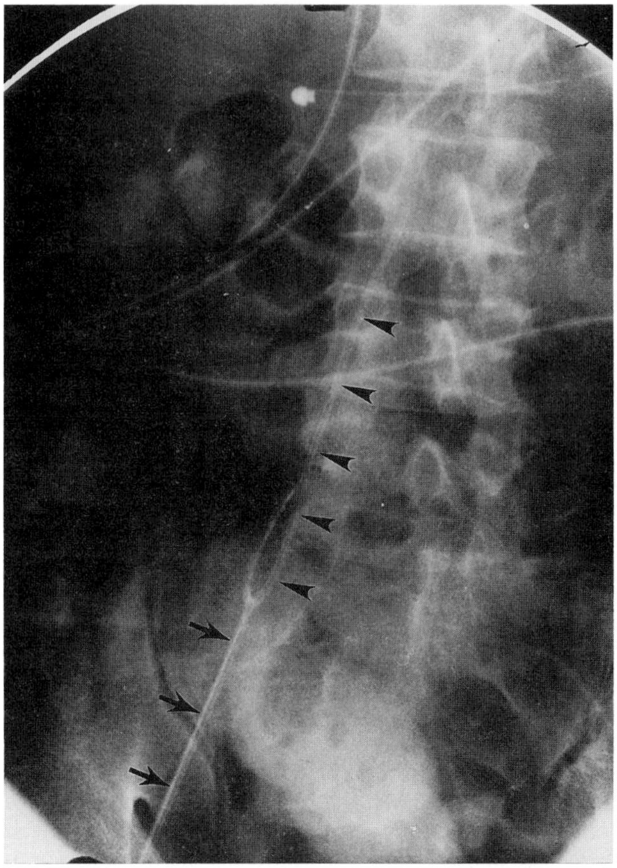

b

FIGURE 20-4 Sheared off triple-lumen catheter. Fragment in the innominate vein and superior vena cava. *a.* Catheter fragment (arrowheads) is snared (arrows) and *b.* pulled out through the percutaneous puncture site in the femoral vein.

anticoagulation in a patient with documented pulmonary emboli, **2.** recurrent pulmonary embolism despite anticoagulation, and **3.** prophylaxis. Although the first two are well-accepted indications, prophylaxis is more controversial.[13,17] Indications for prophylactic vena caval interruption have become more liberal as the procedure has become simpler and safer. Nevertheless, many physicians remain unfamiliar with filter placement or consider it too invasive for common use. We believe that caval interruption is greatly underutilized in the management of critically ill patients.

We advocate prophylactic filter placement (in addition to heparin therapy) in patients with proven venous thromboembolism and cardiovascular compromise or severe chronic obstructive pulmonary disease, as well as in all patients with free-floating pelvic thrombi. In addition, prophylactic caval filter placement should be considered in certain high-risk surgical (orthopedic, trauma, neurosurgical) and oncology patients. If retrievable filters become widely available in the future, prophylactic indications should expand even further.

TECHNIQUE

Inferior vena caval filter placement generally requires the patient to be transported to the interventional radiology suite. Rarely, in highly unstable patients, filter placement may be done at the bedside with portable fluoroscopy equipment. However, this makes the performance of an adequate inferior vena cavagram difficult (vide infra).

The femoral approach is generally preferred for percutaneous caval filter placement because it is easily accessible. The internal jugular approach may have advantages in patients with extensive pelvic and caval thrombosis, tortuous iliac veins, or multiple femoral lines.

An inferior vena cavagram should be performed before the filter is placed. The cavagram is done to demonstrate the level of the renal veins, the presence of thrombus in the inferior vena cava, and the diameter of the inferior vena cava (Fig. 20-6). After the inferior vena cavagram is performed, the puncture site is dilated to a suitable size and a sheath placed. The standard Greenfield filter requires a No. 24 French sheath, whereas the Bird's Nest filter is placed through a No. 12 French sheath. The filter is introduced through the sheath and discharged in the appropriate location. A follow-up cavagram is useful to document filter placement.

The filter should be placed directly below the level of the renal veins. That way, the renal veins retain patency, even if the cava thromboses below the filter. The Greenfield and

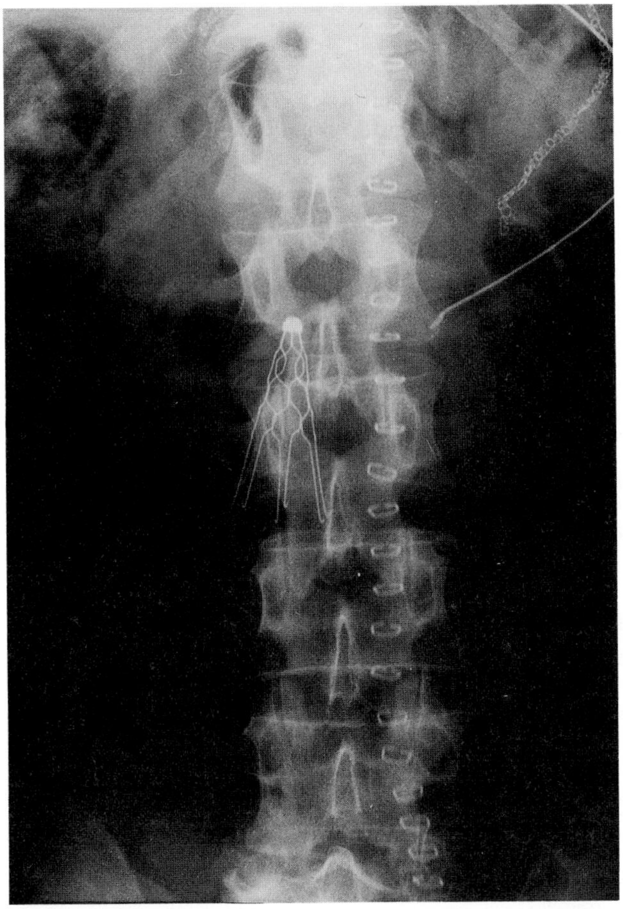

a

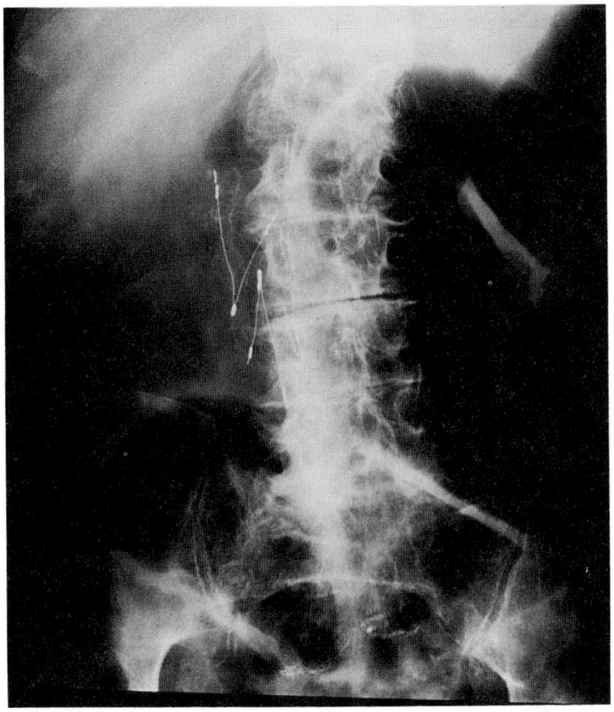

b

FIGURE 20-5 *a.* **Greenfield caval filter.** *b.* **Bird's Nest caval filter.**

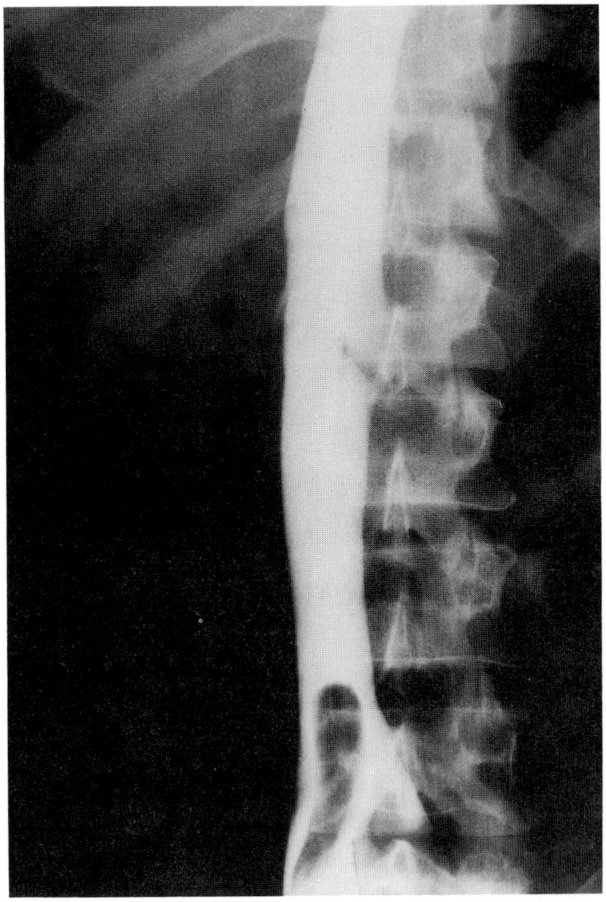

FIGURE 20-6 Inferior vena cavagram prior to filter placement demonstrates a large free-floating caval thrombus.

the Bird's Nest filters both have very low rates of caval thrombosis (vide infra). Therefore, if clot in the inferior vena cava does extend to the level of the renal veins, suprarenal placement may be used.[18]

Even with dilatation of the puncture site to No. 24 French, local hemostasis usually is not a problem. Gentle compression at the puncture site almost always controls bleeding within 5 to 10 min.

IMMEDIATE POSTPROCEDURE CARE

The patient should be kept at bed rest with close observation of the puncture site for 4 to 6 h. If indicated, heparin can be reinstituted immediately after local hemostasis is obtained. Continued heparin therapy can be helpful to prevent extension of the thrombus in the legs.

A plain abdominal radiograph should be obtained to serve as a base line 24 to 36 h after filter placement. For long-term follow-up, plain radiographs are the best way to detect problems such as migration and loss of structural integrity.

RESULTS AND COMPLICATIONS

The No. 24 French Greenfield filter is the gold standard for caval filters. The reported rate of recurrent pulmonary emboli in patients with the Greenfield filter is approximately 2 percent.[19] With the Bird's Nest filter, the recurrence rate is also about 2 percent.[20] In most cases, however, documentation of recurrent pulmonary emboli is extremely difficult to obtain.

Complications of inferior vena cava filter placement include caval thrombosis, filter migration, and trauma at the insertion site. Caval thrombosis with both the Greenfield filter and the Bird's Nest filter is rare—2 to 5 percent. Migration with the Greenfield filter occurred in 28 percent of patients in Greenfield's series.[21] But in most cases the degree of migration was < 1 cm. Following an initial design modification, there have been no reported cases of migration of the Bird's Nest filter.[20]

A potential complication with the percutaneous approach is puncture site thrombosis. Clinically insignificant femoral vein thrombosis has been reported in as many as 30 percent of patients undergoing percutaneous placement of the No. 24 French Greenfield filter. Clinical symptoms, however, are seen in less than 5 percent of patients.[14] Percutaneous placement of the Bird's Nest filter requires dilatation of the puncture site to only No. 12 French. This has significantly decreased the incidence of femoral vein thrombosis (symptomatic and asymptomatic) to less than 2 percent.[22]

CATHETER-DIRECTED FIBRINOLYTIC THERAPY

Local catheter-directed fibrinolytic therapy is an important addition to the nonsurgical treatment of acute and subacute arterial occlusion. The advantage of the catheter-directed technique over systemic therapy is that the fibrinolytic agent's action can be maximized at the site of the vascular occlusion. This permits lower doses and minimizes systemic side effects. Because the method requires maintenance of an intra-arterial catheter for the infusion, these patients routinely are placed in the ICU during the therapy.

INDICATIONS AND PATIENT SELECTION

Catheter-directed fibrinolytic therapy works best in patients with acute thrombosis. Therefore, the best indication is thrombosis that occurs during angiography or angioplasty. The arterial catheter already is in place, and the clot is fresh.

Fibrinolytic therapy also is beneficial in native artery and bypass graft occlusion. Thrombosis in these cases usually is a manifestation of underlying stenotic disease. Frequently, these stenoses can be treated with interventional radiology techniques, sparing the patient a surgical bypass. Best results are seen with occlusions that are less than 6 to 10 weeks old. But the exact age of the clot can be difficult to determine.

Another indication for fibrinolytic therapy is embolic occlusion. In large vessel emboli (e.g., femoral or brachial artery), a Fogarty embolectomy is extremely effective. For small vessel emboli, however, catheter-directed fibrinolytic therapy frequently is the best treatment available, because it is extremely difficult to mechanically remove emboli from these small vessels.

TECHNIQUE

In catheter-directed fibrinolytic therapy, the key is to deliver the agent directly into the thrombus, because then it is possible to directly activate plasminogen bound to the fibrin clot, without activating significant amounts of circulating plasminogen. Various coaxial catheters and multisidehole catheters are available to allow maximum permeation of fibrinolytic agent into the thrombus.

After a complete diagnostic arteriogram, the appropriate catheter is embedded into the thrombus and the infusion begun. Urokinase is our agent of choice. Urokinase is not neutralized by circulating antibodies as is streptokinase. Additionally, systemic side effects, particularly significant bleeding, occur much less often with urokinase than with streptokinase.[23]

No standard dose of urokinase has been agreed on. Our protocol is to lace the clot with 250,000 U urokinase and then begin the infusion with 250,000 U/h for 2 h. After the initial high dose infusion, the dose is decreased to 80,000 to 100,000 U/h for the duration of the therapy.

IMMEDIATE POSTPROCEDURE CARE

Patients undergoing catheter-directed fibrinolytic infusions are placed in the ICU. Here the puncture site and the status of the affected extremity are monitored, as are the patient's bleeding parameters. Patients are kept at strict bed rest, with frequent Doppler examinations of the ischemic extremity.

We usually begin patients on low dose intravenous heparin (500 to 800 U/h) to decrease the incidence of pericatheter thrombosis (see below). Anticoagulation with heparin also is helpful to prevent rebound thrombosis after the fibrinolytic infusion is completed.

Laboratory monitoring tests should include base-line fibrinogen, partial thromboplastin time, prothrombin time, and hematocrit. Every 4 h, the fibrinogen level should be checked to monitor for systemic effects of the fibrinolytic agent. If the fibrinogen level falls below 100 mg/dL, the infusion should be slowed or discontinued. Experience has shown that a fibrinogen level below 100 mg/dL is associated with a significantly increased incidence of remote bleeding.[24] However, fibrinogen levels rarely fall this low during catheter-directed urokinase infusions.

Periodic angiographic follow-up is essential and must be performed in the angiographic suite. High quality fluoroscopic observation is necessary to evaluate progression of lysis. Frequently, the position of the catheter must be changed to keep it embedded in clot.

Successful lysis is generally achieved after 12 to 18 h of infusion. At that point, underlying stenotic lesions are dilated, and the catheter is removed. If no progress is noted over 6 to 12 h, the infusion is stopped. It is critical that all decisions regarding institution of fibrinolytic therapy, continuation of the therapy, and termination of the infusion are made in conjunction with the vascular surgeon caring for the patient.

RESULTS AND COMPLICATIONS

A successful fibrinolytic infusion is generally one that yields either complete lysis or lysis with significant clinical improvement. Success rates reported in the literature vary from 40 to 90 percent, with an average of 60 to 70 percent.[25,26] Comparison of various series is extremely difficult because of heterogeneous patient populations. Generally, success correlates best with age of the thrombus and status of the distal runoff vessels. In addition, urokinase has higher success rates and less morbidity than streptokinase.[24]

Complications are primarily related to bleeding. Most bleeding occurs at arterial puncture sites and is relatively minor. But life-threatening bleeding at remote sites (intracranial, gastrointestinal, retroperitoneal) also has been reported. When serious bleeding occurs, therapy should be discontinued unless the bleeding can be controlled by manual compression. Fresh frozen plasma can be given to replace coagulation factors. Significant bleeding is generally reported in 10 to 12 percent of patients. The risk of bleeding increases with the length of infusion, so the duration of the infusion should be limited to less than 24 h, if possible. Bleeding also can be minimized by maintaining a fibrinogen level of $>$ 100 mg/dL. The use of systemic heparin adds to the risk of bleeding. Therefore, the partial thromboplastin time should be monitored carefully when concomitant heparin therapy is given.

Patients may experience dramatic worsening of their ischemic symptoms during the fibrinolytic infusion. Generally, the symptoms will rapidly resolve by simply continuing the fibrinolytic therapy and treating the patient with narcotic analgesia. The transient worsening of the ischemia in the limb is usually caused by embolization of thrombus into the distal small vessels. Surgery is usually ineffective for such embolization. However, if significant clinical deterioration persists longer than an hour, angiography should be repeated and emergent surgery should be considered.

Pericatheter thrombosis is an occasional problem that is usually caused by poor blood flow along the path of the catheter. To prevent this, the intravascular length of catheter must be kept to a minimum. In addition, the smallest possible catheter system should be used. The incidence of pericatheter thrombosis also can be minimized by using low dose systemic heparin.

References

1. vanSonnenberg E, Mueller PR, Ferrucci JT: Percutaneous drainage of 250 abdominal abscesses and fluid collections. Radiology 151:337, 1984.
2. Gerzof SG, Johnson WC, Robbins AH et al: Expanded criteria for percutaneous abscess drainage. Arch Surg 120:227, 1985.
3. vanSonnenberg E, D'Agostino HB, Casola G et al: Interventional radiology in the gallbladder: Diagnosis, drainage, dissolution, and management of stones, Radiology 174:1, 1990.
4. Werbel GB, Nahrwold DL, Joehl RJ et al: Percutaneous cholecystostomy in the diagnosis and treatment of acute cholecystitis in the high-risk patient. Arch Surg 124:782, 1989.
5. McGahan JP, Lindfors KK: Acute cholecystitis: Diagnostic accuracy of percutaneous aspiration of the gallbladder. Radiology 167:669, 1988.
6. McGahan JP, Lindfors KK: Percutaneous cholecystostomy: An alternative to surgical cholecystostomy for acute cholecystitis. Radiology 173:481, 1989.
7. Lang EV, Picus D, Marx MV et al: Utility of prophylactic left gastric artery embolization. (In press).
8. Keller FS: Nonoperative management of gastrointestinal hemorrhage, in Seminars in Interventional Radiology. New York, Thieme Medical Publishers, 1988.
9. Goldman ML, Land WC, Bradley EL et al: Transcatheter therapeutic embolization in the management of massive upper gastrointestinal bleeding. Radiology 120:513, 1976.
10. Walker TG, Waltman AC: Vasoconstrictive infusion therapy for management of arterial gastrointestinal hemorrhage. Semin Intervent Radiol 5:18, 1988.
11. Fisher RG, Ferreyro R: Evaluation of current techniques for nonsurgical removal of intravascular iatrogenic foreign bodies. Am J Roentgenol 130:541, 1978.
12. Uflacker R, Lima S, Melichar AC: Intravascular foreign bodies: Percutaneous retrieval. Radiology 160:731, 1986.
13. Schmidt GA, Hall JB. Pulmonary embolism: Beyond anticoagulation. Intensive Crit Care Dig 8:3–4, 1989.
14. Pais SO, Tobin KD, Austin CB et al: Percutaneous insertion of the Greenfield inferior vena cava filter: Experience with ninety-six patients. J Vasc Surg 8:460, 1988.
15. Katsamouris AA, Waltman AC, Delichatsios MA et al: Inferior vena cava filters: In vitro comparison of clot trapping and flow dynamics. Radiology 166:361, 1988.
16. Coleman CC: Overview of interruption of the inferior vena cava. Semin Intervent Radiol 3:175, 1986.
17. Tobin KD, Pais SO, Austin CB: Reevaluation of indications for percutaneous placement of the Greenfield filter. Invest Radiol 24:115, 1989.
18. Orsini RA, Jarrell BE: Suprarenal placement of vena caval filters: Indications, techniques, and results. J Vasc Surg 1:124, 1984.
19. Greenfield LJ, Michna BA: Twelve-year clinical experience with the Greenfield vena caval filter. Surgery 104:706, 1988.
20. Roehm JOF, Johnsrude IS, Barth MH et al: The bird's nest inferior vena cava filter: Progress report. Radiology 168:745, 1988.
21. Messmer JM, Greenfield LJ: Greenfield caval filters: Long-term radiographic follow-up study. Radiology 156:613, 1985.
22. Hicks ME, Middleton WD, Picus D et al: Incidence of local venous thrombosis following Bird's Nest IVC filter placement. J Vasc Interv Rad. 1:63–8, 1990.
23. van Breda A, Katzen BT, Deutsch AS: Urokinase versus streptokinase in local thrombolysis. Radiology 165:109, 1987.
24. Marder VJ, Sherry S: Thrombolytic therapy: Current status. N Engl J Med 318:1512, 1585, 1988.
25. Durham JD, Geller SC, Abbott WM et al: Regional infusion of urokinase into occluded lower-extremity bypass grafts: Long-term clinical results. Radiology 172:83, 1989.
26. Klatte EC, Becker GJ, Holden RE et al: Fibrinolytic therapy. Radiology 159:619, 1986.

Chapter 21

DOPPLER ECHOCARDIOGRAPHY: DIAGNOSTIC APPLICATIONS IN THE INTENSIVE CARE UNIT

ERIC K. LOUIE
STEVEN N. KONSTADT

The critically ill patient poses unique challenges to cardiovascular diagnosis. Of great importance is the distinction of cardiac from noncardiac mechanisms of systemic hypoperfusion and hypotension. In addition, many of the patients present with or develop hypoxemic respiratory failure which may be of cardiac or noncardiac origin. Finally acute intrinsic cardiac illness [e.g., ventricular septal rupture following myocardial infarction (MI)], secondary involvement of the heart structures by noncardiac illness (e.g., intracardiac obstruction by intravascular extension of malignant tumors), and indirect effects of noncardiac disease (e.g., right ventricular failure due to pulmonary embolism) need to be distinguished and diagnosed by the characteristic perturbations of cardiac structure and function which they cause. These unstable acutely ill patients often cannot tolerate lengthy complex diagnostic procedures that might require removal from the ICU. Doppler echocardiography is a relatively rapid, noninvasive, bedside imaging procedure that provides detailed structural and physiologic information about cardiac function. Serial examination is relatively inexpensive and poses no significant hazards to the patient, providing a means for monitoring and tracking a patient's condition and the progression of disease. Optimal patient evaluation requires the availability of an experienced echocardiographic technician, who not only is skilled in acquiring high quality cardiac images but who also has a sufficient understanding of cardiac pathophysiology to focus the echocardiographic study on those aspects relevant to the intensivist. Similarly, the echocardiographer must have a detailed understanding of the clinical questions posed by the intensivist so the technician's study may be redirected and amplified to those aspects germane to the patient's care.

Precise echocardiographic diagnosis requires high resolution images, which depend on patient cooperation, flexible patient positioning, and the absence of anatomic or extrinsic obstruction of the ultrasound beam. Unfortunately, these conditions frequently cannot be met in the critically ill patient and, in particular, positive-pressure ventilation with a relatively high functional residual capacity creates a barrier (the inflated lungs) to ultrasound interrogation of the heart from a transducer positioned on the chest wall. Recent advances in transesophageal echocardiography (see Chap. 22) provide a relatively unobstructed ultrasound window to most of the cardiovascular structures imaged by transthoracic echocardiography and better access to the left atrial appendage and the descending aorta. The relative proximity of the esophagus to the left atrium and posterior left ventricle allows the use of higher frequency transducers with superior spatial resolution. Currently available transesophageal echocardiographic technology in the United States permits only limited orientation of the imaging plane and does not implement continuous wave Doppler. It is anticipated that these technical limitations will be circumvented in the future and that transesophageal echocardiography will expand the application of Doppler echocardiographic diagnosis to the majority of critically ill patients who cannot be imaged currently by transthoracic techniques. Subject to these technologic limitations, the principles of Doppler echocardiographic diagnosis discussed in this chapter apply to both transesophageal and transthoracic echocardiography.[1]

Structural and Functional Information Derived by Doppler Echocardiography

TWO-DIMENSIONAL SECTOR SCANNING

Two-dimensional echocardiography uses reflected ultrasound to provide an on-line wide-angle sector tomographic image of cardiac structures moving in real time, which is recorded on video tape or other magnetic storage medium for subsequent off-line playback and frame-by-frame analysis. The power of the technique lies in the inherent spatial orientation of the imaged cardiac structures within the two-dimensional imaging plane and the potential for defining three-dimensional relationships by interrogating a structure with multiple tomographic planes. The weakness of the approach derives from the fact that at least with conventional equipment, absolute coordinates for the tomographic planes are unknown and standardization and reproducibility of tomographic planes depend on internally imaged landmarks. In addition, the sensitivity of the technique for imaging small objects depends on the number of different tomographic planes used by the technician (which depends on operator skill and perseverance). Within these limitations two-dimensional echocardiography provides accurate anatomic information and defines spatial relationships (Figs. 21-1 and 21-2). Because the cavity boundaries and myocardial walls are imaged in real time, functional information (changes in ventricular volume, ejection fraction, etc.) can be derived by comparing end-diastolic and end-systolic images.[2–5] The amplitude of reflected ultrasound signals depends on the changes in acoustic impedance at each reflecting interface. With conventional equipment, qualitative differentiation of highly echo-dense materials (calcified tissue, metallic prostheses, etc.) from

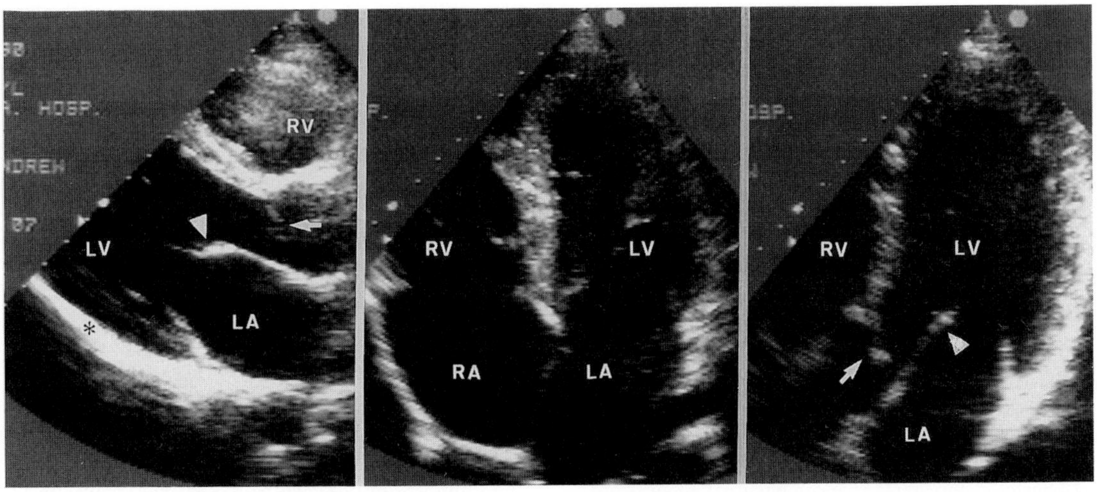

FIGURE 21-1 Diastolic stop frame two-dimensional echocardiographic images of the heart from a normal subject. ***Left.*** **This long axis view of the left atrium (LA) and left ventricle (LV) was obtained from the left parasternal echocardiograhic window with the sector aligned parallel to the left ventricular inflow tract. The anterior leaflet of the mitral valve (solid triangle) and two of the cusps of the aortic valve (small arrow) are seen. Posterior to the left ventricular free wall the bright linear echodensity (asterisk) represents the interface between the pericardium and the epicardium. If a pericardial effusion were present, an echo-free space would be present between those two structures. The left ventricle and right ventricle (RV) are separated by the anterior interventricular septum (top = anterior, bottom = posterior, left = apical, right = basal).** ***Center.*** **This four chamber view of the heart was obtained from the apical echocardiograhic window with the transducer near the point of maximal impulse and the sector angled up toward the subject's right shoulder. This tomographic plane simultaneously images the left ventricle (LV), left atrium (LA), right ventricle (RV), and right atrium (RA) and passes through the crux of the heart (top = apical, bottom = basal, left = subject's right, right = subject's left).** ***Right.*** **This four chamber view of the heart and left ventricular outflow tract was obtained from the same echocardiographic window as the image in the center panel; however, the transducer was angled more anteriorly (more superficially relative to the anterior thorax) to image the aortic valve (small arrow) and aorta as it arises from the left ventricle. The fibrous continuty between the anterior mitral valve (solid triangle), aortic valve, and posterior aortic root is easily demonstrated. The right ventricle (RV) and left atrium (LA) are also imaged in this view (top = apical, bottom = basal, left = subject's right, right = subject's left). Calibrations are 1.0 cm apart.**

normal myocardium and the blood pool is possible, but the absolute amplitude of the signal is a function of the operator's adjustment of signal gain to achieve a "normal" ultrasound signal from adjacent tissues presumed to be uninvolved by pathologic processes. Thus, the apparent echogenicity of cardiac structures depends on appropriate adjustment of receiver gain, transmitted power, and wall filter settings.

ONE-DIMENSIONAL M-MODE SCANNING

M-mode echocardiography provides a record of reflected ultrasound along one ray of the two-dimensional echocardiographic sector. The record format is an X–Y plot with the Y axis representing distance from the transducer to the cardiac structure reflecting ultrasound and the X axis representing elapsed time. Thus, the M-mode tracing depicts the motion of cardiac structures along one spatial dimension (the interrogating ray) as a function of time (Fig. 21-3). The concurrently acquired two-dimensional echocardiogram permits targeting of that interrogating ray through regions of clinical interest (compare Figs. 21-2 and 21-3). The M-mode echocardiogram sacrifices the spatial orientation inherent to the two-dimensional echocardiogram but provides greater spatial resolution in the axial dimension (permitting more precise linear measurements along the interrogating ray) and greater temporal resolution. Used in conjunction with the two-dimensional echocardiogram, the M-mode echocardiogram can provide precise measurements of selected axes of the cardiac chambers and can assist in the precise timing (relative to other physiologic traces such as the ECG) of normal and abnormal motion of cardiac structures.[6]

DOPPLER TECHNIQUES

Doppler techniques[7] used in conjunction with echocardiographic imaging measure the Doppler frequency shift (Δf) of the ultrasound signal reflected off moving ultrasound scatterers (roughly speaking the formed cellular elements in blood) which is proportional to the velocity of their motion (v):

$$\Delta f = \frac{2 f_0 v \cos \theta}{c} \qquad (21\text{-}1)$$

where f_0 is the carrier frequency of the ultrasound transducer, c is the average speed of ultrasound in biologic tis-

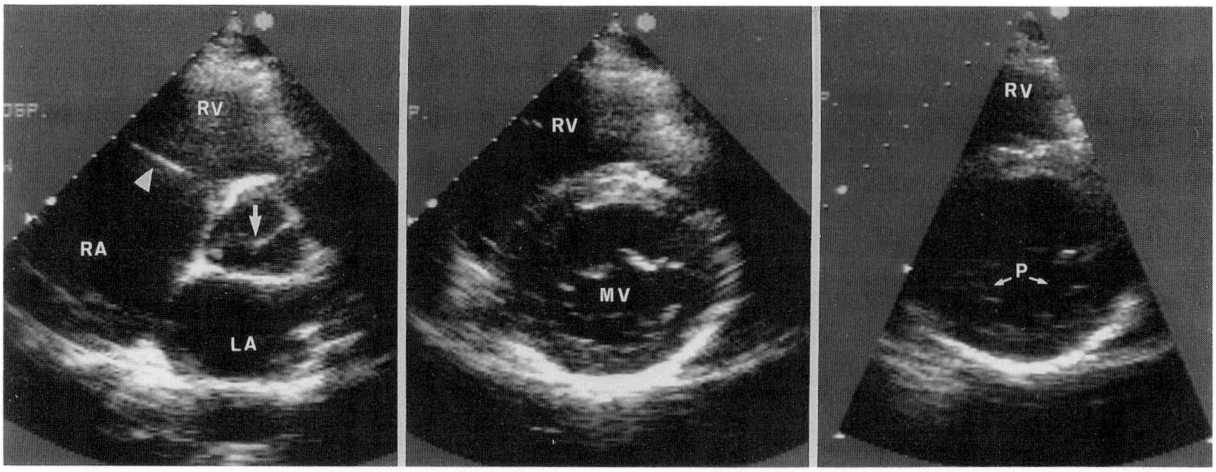

FIGURE 21-2 Diastolic stop frame two-dimensional echocardiographic images of the heart from a normal subject. All three images were obtained from the left parasternal window with the transducer orthogonal to the long axis of the left ventricle. By varying the caudad to cephalad angulation of the transducer, these short axis imaging planes from three separate levels of the heart were obtained (compare to the long axis view of the left ventricle demonstrated in Fig. 21-1, left panel). *Left.* With cephalad angulation of the imaging plane, a short axis image of the base of the heart is obtained with right ventricular (RV) outflow tract anterior and left atrium (LA) posterior. Between these two structures lies the circular cross section of the aortic root with the Y-shaped coaptation lines of the closed aortic valve (small arrow) leaflets. Next to the left atrium lies the right atrium (RA) which is separated from the right ventricle by the tricuspid valve (solid triangle) (top = anterior, bottom = posterior, left = subject's right, right = subject's left). *Center.* With the transducer directed toward the subject's back (neither cephalad nor caudad angulation), the short axis image of the mitral valve (MV) leaflets within the circular left ventricular cavity is obtained. Anterior to the left ventricle lies the right ventricle (RV) (top = anterior, bottom = posterior, left = subject's right, right = subject's left). *Right.* With the transducer angulated caudad, the short axis image of the circular left ventricular cavity at the level of the papillary muscles (P) is seen. The right ventricle (RV) lies anterior to the left ventricle. (Top = anterior, bottom = posterior, left = subject's right, right = subject's left). Calibrations are 1.0 cm apart.

sues (1560 m/s) and θ is the angle between the path of the interrogating Doppler beam and the direction of blood flow. Assuming the interrogating Doppler beam can be aligned parallel to blood flow ($\cos \theta = 1$) then blood flow velocity, v, can be derived from the Doppler frequency shift, Δf, because f_0 and c are constants. The detection and quantitation by Doppler techniques of flow velocities within the cardiovascular system are used in three ways: **1.** to measure bulk flow (e.g., cardiac output in the aorta) through an unrestrictive conduit, **2.** to measure pressure differentials across restrictive orifices (e.g., the mean systolic pressure gradient in aortic stenosis), and **3.** to detect abnormal flow velocities in what should be relatively quiescent regions of the cardiovascular system (e.g., valvular regurgitation, shunt flow, etc.). Bulk flow, Q, through a conduit is measured by estimating flow cross-sectional area with the echocardiographically determined anatomic cross-sectional area of the conduit, A, and assuming that the Doppler-determined velocity of blood flow, v, is constant across that cross section:

$$Q = A \cdot v \tag{21-2}$$

The pressure differential (Δp) across a stenotic orifice is estimated by application of the modified Bernoulli equation which neglects viscous frictional losses and inertial losses due to acceleration and deceleration of blood in a pulsatile system:

$$\Delta p = \tfrac{1}{2}\rho(v_2^2 - v_1^2) \tag{21-3}$$

where ρ is the density of blood and v_2 and v_1 are the flow velocity downstream and upstream of the orifice, respectively. For significantly stenotic orifices, v_2 is much greater than v_1 so that v_1 can be neglected and $\Delta p = 4v_2^2$ (where Δp is expressed in mmHg and v_2 is expressed in m/s). Abnormal flow velocities of valvular regurgitation are identified by the Doppler detection of flow velocities in regions of the cardiovascular system which should be quiescent during specified portions of the cardiac cycle (e.g., for mitral regurgitation the demonstration in systole of flow velocities within the left atrium directed away from the mitral valve).

The magnitude, direction, and localization of flow velocities within the cardiovascular system are determined by two different but complementary Doppler systems: pulsed wave and continuous wave Doppler. *Pulsed wave Doppler* uses discrete pulses of ultrasound transmitted at a pulse repetition frequency set sufficiently low that the returning signal reaches the transducer before the next pulse is transmitted. This permits precise determination of the location from which the velocity measurement was made *(spatial localization)* but results in too slow a sampling rate to unambiguously quantitate high velocities *(velocity ambiguity)*. The

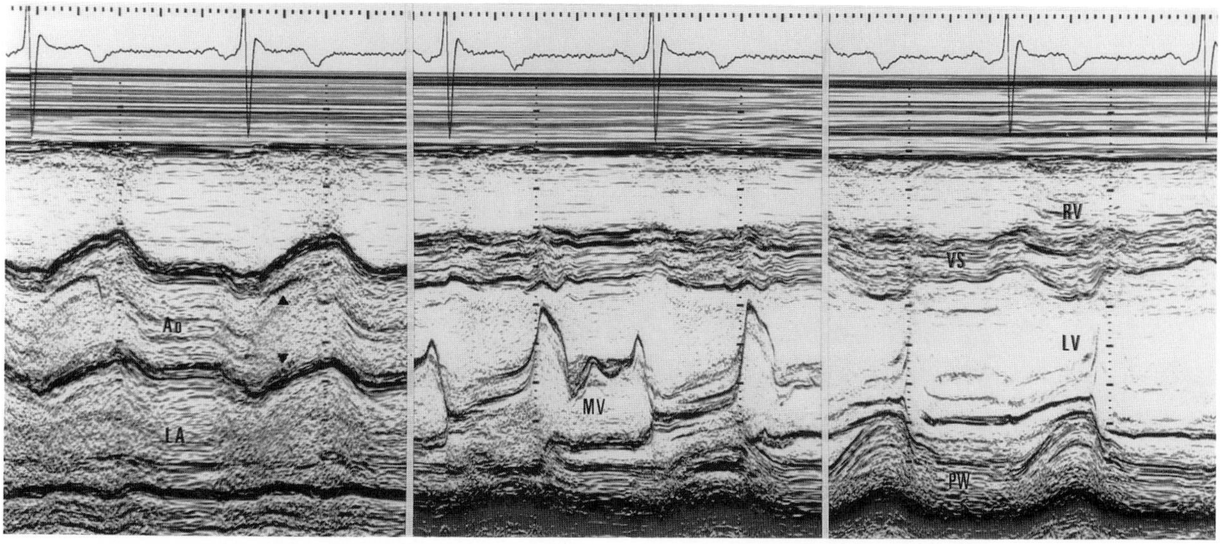

FIGURE 21-3 M-Mode echocardiograms with limb lead II ECG (physiologic trace at top) obtained by directing the M-mode ultrasound beam anteroposteriorly through each of the short axis two-dimensional echocardiographic images in Fig. 21-2. From left to right M-mode echocardiograms at the aortic valve, mitral valve, and distal left ventricular levels were obtained from their respective two-dimensional echocardiographic images illustrated in Fig. 21-2. In each panel the parallel horizontal lines at the top of the figure are the artifacts generated by the interface between the transducer and the thorax of the subject. Anterior structures are on top while posterior structures are on bottom. Time elapses from left to right (see ECG for timing of the phases of the cardiac cycle). Major divisions of the vertical calibrations are 1.0 cm apart. Major divisions of the horizontal calibrations are 200 ms apart. *Left.* The most anterior echo-free cavity is the right ventricular outflow tract with the aortic root (Ao) lying behind it. In systole (following the QRS of the ECG) two of the aortic valve leaflets are imaged at their maximal separation (two solid triangles). The left atrium (LA) is posterior to the aortic root and expands in transverse dimension in systole. *Center.* The most anterior echo-free cavity is the right ventricle which is separated from the left ventricle by the ventricular septum. The motion of the mitral valve (MV) leaflets within the left ventricle is clearly depicted. The anterior mitral leaflet appears to move anteriorly three times in diastole. The first (and largest) leaflet excursion occurs during early rapid ventricular filling while the final leaflet reopening reflects the atrial contribution to left ventricular filling and follows the P wave on the ECG. *Right.* The most anterior echo-free cavity is the right ventricle (RV) which is separated from the more posterior left ventricle (LV) by the ventricular septum (VS). The posterior left ventricular wall (PW) lies just anterior to the pericardium. Note how the left ventricular walls move inward and thicken in systole.

location of the velocity measurement is specified by the sample volume location on a cursor representing the Doppler beam which is superimposed on the two-dimensional echocardiographic image. *Continuous wave Doppler* sends and receives an ongoing stream of ultrasound signals such that frequency shifts are measured all along the interrogating beam without determination of the depth of the location of any particular velocity measurement *(spatial ambiguity)*; however, the high sampling rates achieved permit the precise quantification of very high velocities *(velocity specificity)*. Thus, pulsed Doppler techniques are used to localize velocity measurements of interest; however, when high velocities are encountered (generally in regions of disturbed flow due to valvular regurgitation or stenosis), the pulsed Doppler technique is not capable of unambiguously defining the magnitude and direction of blood flow velocity. The continuous wave Doppler beam is then directed through the region of interest to measure those high velocities.

Data from either technique are portrayed as a time-velocity plot with flow velocity (Doppler frequency shift spectra) on the Y axis and time on the X axis along with the ECG or other physiologic traces for timing purposes (Figs. 21-4 and 21-5). Conventionally, velocities above the X axis represent flow toward the Doppler probe, whereas velocities below the X axis represent flow away from the probe. Pulsed Doppler data can be presented in a two-dimensional format *(color flow Doppler)* with color encoding of velocities in a manner somewhat analogous to the two-dimensional echocardiographic representation of M-mode echocardiographic data. The velocity measured from a given sample volume is assigned a color defined by: **1.** its hue for the direction of flow (e.g., red for flow toward the transducer, blue for flow away from the transducer) **2.** its intensity corresponding roughly to the magnitude of the average velocity within the sample volume (e.g., brighter colors for higher velocities), and **3.** the admixture of a third color (e.g., yellow) to indicate the degree of heterogeneity or variance of velocity measurements within the sample volume. Thus, a high velocity regurgitant stream of blood directed toward the transducer would be represented in bright red with an admixture of yellow (resulting in an orange color) to signify the disordered flow in the regurgitant stream. The color flow Doppler echocardiograph rapidly samples blood flow velocities throughout a two-dimensional echocardiographic sector by multigate pulsed Doppler techniques, assigns col-

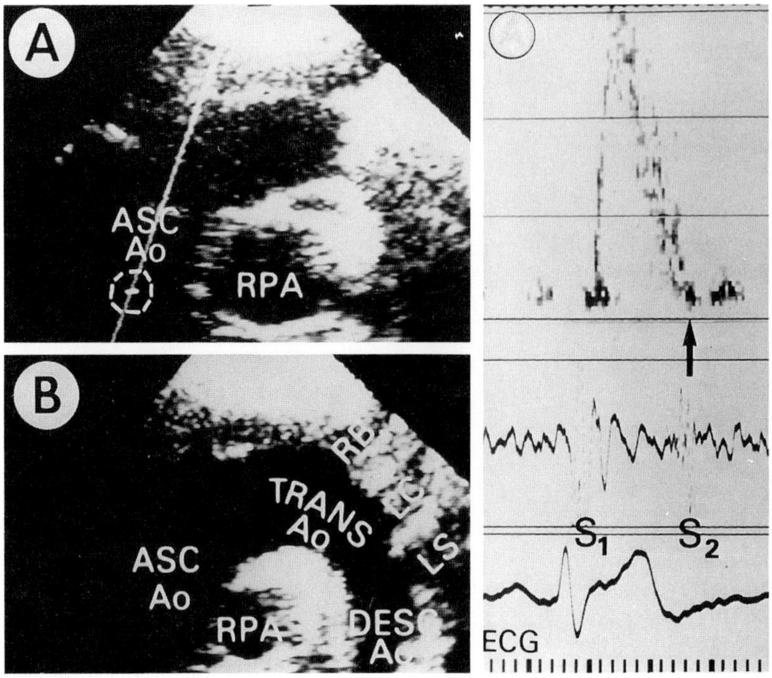

FIGURE 21-4 Pulsed wave Doppler measurement of aortic flow velocities from the suprasternal notch. ***Left.*** **Stop frame two-dimensional echocardiographic images of the ascending (ASC), transverse (TRANS), and descending (DES) aorta (Ao) in relation to the right pulmonary artery (RPA) as viewed from a tansducer positioned in the suprasternal notch. In (A) the position of the pulsed Doppler cursor (dotted line aligned parallel to blood flow in the ascending aorta) and its sample volume (dotted circle in the ascending aorta just above the aortic valve) in relation to the echocardiographic image of the aorta is demonstrated. In (B), identification of the transverse aorta is facilitated by identification of the arch vessels (RB = right brachiocephalic artery, LC = left carotid artery, LS = left subclavian artery).** ***Right.*** **From top to bottom the aortic flow velocity pulsed Doppler spectrum, phonocardiogram (S_1 = first heart sound, S_2 = second heart sound), and electrocardiogram (ECG) are displayed. The common time line is calibrated at 200 ms/major division. The ordinate of the Doppler spectrum is calibrated at increments of 30 cm/s with positive Doppler shifts above the zero base line representing flow toward the transducer positioned in the suprasternal notch. The normal aortic flow velocity profile is characterized by a sharp acceleration beginning shortly after the QRS of the ECG and the S_1 of the phonocardiogram, reaching a peak velocity in early systole followed by a more gradual deceleration phase with flow velocities returning to the zero base line (arrow) simultaneous with the S_2 of the phonocardiogram. From such spectra the acceleration of flow (upstroke slope), peak flow velocity, and flow velocity integral (area under the curve) can be measured. (Adapted and reproduced from Louie EK et al: Am J Cardiol 58:821–826, 1986, with the permission of the publisher.)**

ors to these velocities, and then maps these colors onto the two-dimensional echocardiographic image of the underlying cardiac anatomy. The current implementation of this technology does not permit a precise quantitative representation of blood flow velocity (and it suffers from the problem of velocity ambiguity inherent to pulsed Doppler techniques), but it exploits the spatial localization achieved by pulsed Doppler techniques to provide a real-time color map of blood flow velocities superimposed on the simultaneously acquired two-dimensional echocardiographic image. This representation of the Doppler data is extremely useful in providing spatial orientation for the abnormal flow patterns within the tomographic anatomy and in providing an estimate of the extent of a flow velocity disturbance relative to cardiac chamber size.

CONTRAST ECHOCARDIOGRAPHY

Intravenous echocardiographic contrast agents can be used to improve the definition of endocardial borders, delineate intracavitary masses, detect bidirectional flow (e.g. tricuspid regurgitation), demonstrate intracardiac shunting, and amplify weak spectral Doppler signals. A number of synthetic intravascular agents are under development that use uniform, stable ultrasound scatterers suitable for quantitative analysis of bulk flow and tissue perfusion. In addition, some of these agents are capable of passing through the pulmonary capillaries so that intravenous injection results in delivery of intravascular ultrasonic contrast material to the left side of the heart. In clinical practice outside of the research environment, agitated 0.9% NaCl solutions provide a convenient and safe intravascular ultrasound contrast agent. Brisk exchange of 10 mL 0.9% NaCl between two syringes connected by a stopcock creates microbubbles within the solution, which are invisible to the naked eye, inhomogeneous in size distribution, and too large to cross the pulmonary capillary network. Rapid bolus injection of this solution into either the venous or arterial system produces good ultrasonic intravascular contrast, results in no hemodynamic perturbations, and has not been associated

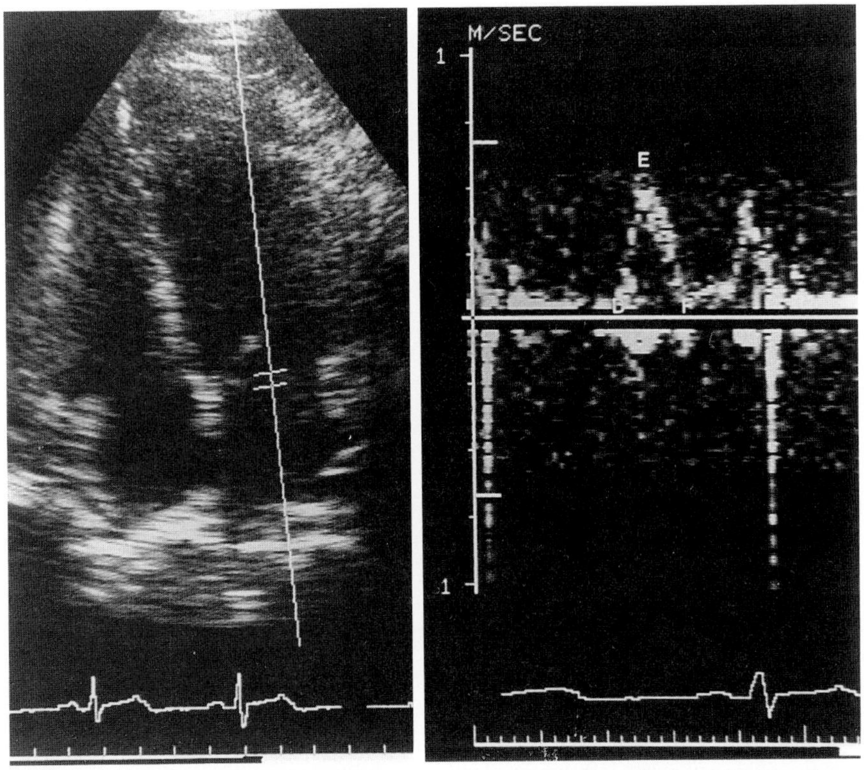

FIGURE 21-5 Pulsed wave Doppler measurement of transmitral flow velocities from the cardiac apex. ***Left.*** **Stop frame two-dimensional echocardiographic image of the apical four chamber view of the heart with the pulsed Doppler cursor (line) positioned in the left ventricular inflow tract parallel to transmitral flow. The cursor runs from the apex of the left ventricle through the left atrium and the Doppler sample volume (double crosshatch) is positioned at the level of the mitral annulus just proximal to the mitral valve leaflets.** ***Right.*** **The pulsed Doppler spectrum of transmitral flow velocities (above) and the ECG (below) are displayed simultaneously with a common time line (calibration: 200 ms/major division). Full scale calibration of the ordinate of the Doppler spectrum is ±1.0 m/s about the zero base line, positive velocities representing flow toward the transducer positioned at the left ventricular apex. In normal sinus rhythm, diastolic filling is characterized by two phases: early rapid filling (D, E, F) and late atrial systolic filling (just preceding the QRS of the ECG). The relative contributions of early and late diastolic filling to total left ventricular filling can be characterized by the peak velocities of each of those two phases or the fractional flow velocity integrals (areas under the curves) of these two phases. (Adapted and reproduced from Louie EK et al: Am J Cardiol 61:1085–1091, 1988, with the permission of the publisher.)**

with adverse sequelae. A typical application of this technique is the detection of small interatrial communications, which may elude anatomic characterization by two-dimensional echocardiography and be associated with too small a transseptal pressure difference to produce easily detected Doppler signals of shunt flow. Bolus injection of 10 mL saline contrast into an antecubital vein results in opacification of the right atrial cavity. If mean right atrial pressure exceeds mean left atrial pressure and an atrial septal defect is present, saline contrast will appear in the left atrium within three cardiac cycles of its appearance in the right atrium. If mean right atrial pressure is somewhat less than mean left atrial pressure, transseptal passage of saline contrast may still occur following maneuvers (coughing, Valsalva release), which abruptly alter intrathoracic pressures resulting in transient elevation of right atrial pressure above left atrial pressure. Of note, the mere presence of transseptal passage of saline contrast does not indicate that a hemodynamically significant atrial septal defect is present. The technique is so sensitive that transseptal passage of saline contrast during respiratory maneuvers can occur through a patent foramen ovale.

Assessment of Systolic and Diastolic Cardiac Function

EJECTION PHASE INDICES OF SYSTOLIC PERFORMANCE

Direct assessment of myocardial fiber shortening and other ejection phase indices of left ventricular systolic function can be achieved by quantitative echocardiographic analysis of end-diastolic and end-systolic left ventricular endocardial contours.[3,8] Given high quality two-dimensional echocardiographic images with clear endocardial resolution one can use simplifying geometric algorithms to calculate left ventricular volumes and hence ejection fraction, [3,9] resulting in reasonable correlations with cineangiographic or radionuclide techniques ($r = 0.75 - 0.78$, standard error of the estimate (SEE) 0.09 − 0.10 for ejection fraction).[9] Although this level of precision is adequate for the clinical evaluation of left ventricular systolic performance, the application of such techniques requires image quality not easily obtained in critically ill patients and dedicated off-line data analysis which is generally not practical in the ICU. Nonetheless, it is often possible to provide a qualitative description of global left ventricular systolic function ("normal," "depressed," "severely depressed," etc.) from the on-line review of multiple tomographic images of the heart contracting in real time. In addition, the heterogeneity or regionality of segmental wall motion abnormalities, such as occurs following myocardial infarction (MI), can also be judged by assessing whether individual myocardial segments thicken and move inward normally or in a depressed fashion.[3] A similar approach has been used to characterize right ventricular systolic performance. The unusual shape of the right ventricle precludes simplifying assumptions and requires the acquisition of multiple tomographic images to adequately characterize its three-dimensional geometry.

To obviate the technical limitations of an anatomic approach (two-dimensional echocardiography) to assessing systolic function, complementary data can be obtained by assessing systemic perfusion using Doppler techniques. In the absence of aortic regurgitation or stenosis, Doppler techniques that measure flow velocity in the left ventricular outflow tract or aorta may be used to characterize left ventricular ejection and to measure cardiac output[8,10–13] (Fig. 21-4). Using continuous wave Doppler interrogation of left ventricular outflow from the suprasternal notch, peak acceleration of blood flow (the maximal slope of the upstroke of the flow velocity profile) has been shown to correlate well with left ventricular ejection fraction ($r = 0.90$).[11] Although the absolute values of various aortic flow velocity parameters may vary from patient to patient and be influenced by physiologic conditions extrinsic to the systolic function of the heart, in a given patient acute changes in systemic vascular resistance can be tracked by the percent change in peak flow velocity (the peak of the flow velocity profile), and acute changes in stroke volume are paralleled by corresponding fractional changes in the flow velocity integral (area under the flow velocity profile).[12] The intensivist is accustomed to assessing left ventricular systolic performance by measuring cardiac output as an index of the efficacy of systemic perfusion. As developed above, mean systolic flow rates, Q, across the aortic valve can be derived from estimates of the spatial-temporal mean systolic velocity in the left ventricular outflow tract and anatomic estimates of the effective flow cross-sectional area, A, [Eq. (21-2)]. Stroke volume is simply the product of Q and left ventricular ejection time (approximated from an arterial pulse tracing, echocardiographic timing of aortic valve motion, or the S_1 to S_2 time interval on a phonocardiogram), and cardiac output is calculated from stroke volume and heart rate. Obviously these measurements depend on a quasi steady state and will not be possible if erratic fluctuations in hemodynamic stability or cardiac rhythm occur.

In addition, two major technical limitations to the application of this approach to noninvasive measurement of cardiac output are: **1.** errors incurred by estimating flow cross-sectional area by the (echocardiographically defined) anatomic boundaries of the left ventricular outflow tract and **2.** failure to achieve alignment of the Doppler beam parallel to aortic blood flow. To address these technical problems a dual beam pulsed wave Doppler system (Vital Science, Quantascope) using an annular array transducer which transmits and receives two concentric ultrasound beams has been adapted for cardiac output measurement from the suprasternal notch window.[13] By comparing the power return of the wide beam (which insonates the total projected cross-sectional area of the ascending aorta) to the power of the narrow beam (which insonates a precalibrated area within the ascending aorta), the flow cross-sectional area of the ascending aorta is determined, and adjustment for the angle of insonation relative to the long axis of the ascending aorta is made. Thus, two-dimensional echocardiographic imaging of the aortic cross section is not required, and angle correction for the direction of blood flow velocity is incorporated in the measurements assuming that flow is axially symmetric. Applying such techniques in the critical care setting one group of investigators has obtained technically adequate studies in 91 percent of patients and excellent linear correlations with simultaneously measured thermodilution cardiac outputs ($r = 0.96$, SEE = 0.55 L/min).[13] This technique is not applicable to patients with disease of the left ventricular outflow tract (e.g., aortic valve disease) and may be difficult to perform in patients with a limited ultrasound window from the suprasternal notch. Even in experienced hands some studies required 30 to 40 min to be performed,[13] seriously limiting its applicability in serial monitoring tasks.

PATTERNS OF DIASTOLIC VENTRICULAR FILLING

Characterization of left ventricular diastolic function and patterns of filling is possible by Doppler echocardiographic techniques although the correlations with patients' symptoms, clinical course, and disease progression have proven somewhat elusive. At least in theory the sequence of left ventricular volumetric changes during diastole can be characterized using frame-by-frame digitization of ventricular endocardial contours.[8] In general, two-dimensional echocardiographic studies in the clinical setting lack sufficient spatial and temporal resolution to permit the estimation of left ventricular filling rates from such data. Assuming the one-dimensional changes along the M-mode echocardiographic beam are representative of the three-dimensional changes of the left ventricular volume (which requires uniformly symmetric left ventricular wall motion), some investigators have digitized M-mode echocardiograms of the left ventricle to quantitate rates of diastolic minor axis lengthening.[8] These techniques require labor intensive off-line analysis largely confined to research settings and not generally applicable to diagnosis in the ICU environment.

Recent research has explored the use of pulsed Doppler echocardiography to characterize left ventricular filling patterns from the diastolic transmitral flow velocity profile (Fig. 21-5).[14] As illustrated in Fig. 21-5, the flow velocity profile is biphasic with the first peak representing the rapid filling phase of early diastolic filling and the second peak representing the atrial contribution to late diastolic filling. The time varying course of transmitral flow velocities is influenced by many factors, including the transmitral pressure differential, the chamber compliance characteristics of the atrium and ventricle, the mitral valve impedance, and external constraints to left ventricular filling (e.g., the pericardium, interactions between left and right ventricles, etc.).[15] Thus, even in the patient with normal mitral valve function, the transmitral flow velocity profile is not a simple reflection of left ventricular diastolic properties and, in particular, exhibits an important dependence on left atrial pressure. Notwithstanding these limitations, an accurate quantitative description of the pattern of left ventricular filling can be obtained by applying Eq. (21-2) where v is measured from the transmitral flow velocity profile at the mitral annulus and A is estimated by the cross-sectional area of the mitral annulus determined by two-dimensional echocardiography. Peak left ventricular filling rates derived by these techniques compare favorably with measurements obtained by quantitative left ventriculography or by high resolution radionuclide time activity curves.[14] One practical application of such measurements is the comparison of the late and early diastolic contributions to left ventricular filling during sinus rhythm to predict the relative change in cardiac output resulting from the loss of atrial systole during ventricular pacing.[16] Patients with a greater dependence on the atrial contribution to diastolic filling (relatively increased late diastolic peak filling rates and velocities) would be expected to have a more favorable response to dual chamber pacing, which preserves the atrial systolic contribution to left ventricular filling.[16]

LIMITATIONS TO THE ASSESSMENT OF SYSTOLIC AND DIASTOLIC FUNCTION

A major limitation of these Doppler echocardiographic assessments of systolic and diastolic ventricular function is that they characterize *ejection performance* and *chamber filling* and do not measure intrinsic myocardial *contractility* and *relaxation/compliance*. As such they are importantly influenced by ventricular loading conditions. Systolic ejection performance can be scaled for loading conditions by the measurement of end-systolic pressure-dimension and wall stress-myocardial fiber shortening relations over a range of afterloads. These relationships are relatively preload independent, afterload scaled reflections of myocardial contractile state.[8,17] In patients without segmental left ventricular systolic dysfunction, the M-mode echocardiogram recorded simultaneously with the intra-arterial pressure can be used to measure left ventricular cavity dimension and wall thickness, while afterload is manipulated pharmacologically to obtain end-systolic pressure-dimension and wall stress-shortening relationships. A calibrated carotid pulse tracing provides an alternative to intra-arterial pres-

FIGURE 21-6 Stop frame two-dimensional echocardiographic images of the four chambers of the heart from the subcostal view in a patient experiencing cardiac tamponade. *Left.* A large pericardial effusion (PE) is represented by the echo-free space adjacent to the free walls of the right ventricle (RV) and right atrium (RA). There is evidence for pericardial fluid adjacent to the free walls of the left ventricle (LV) and left atrium (LA) as well. In this stop frame image from early diastole, the right atrial free wall is convex with respect to the pericardial space and is not compressed. *Right.* By contrast this early systolic stop frame image from the same patient (same image orientation as in left panel) demonstrates marked indentation of the right atrial free wall (arrow) resulting in right atrial collapse, an early sign of cardiac tamponade. In late diastole and early systole, right atrial pressure and volume reach a minimum (following emptying of the right atrium into the right ventricle) and thus the elevated intrapericardial pressure (characteristic of pericardial tamponade) results in inward deflection of the right atrial free wall and compression of the right atrium.

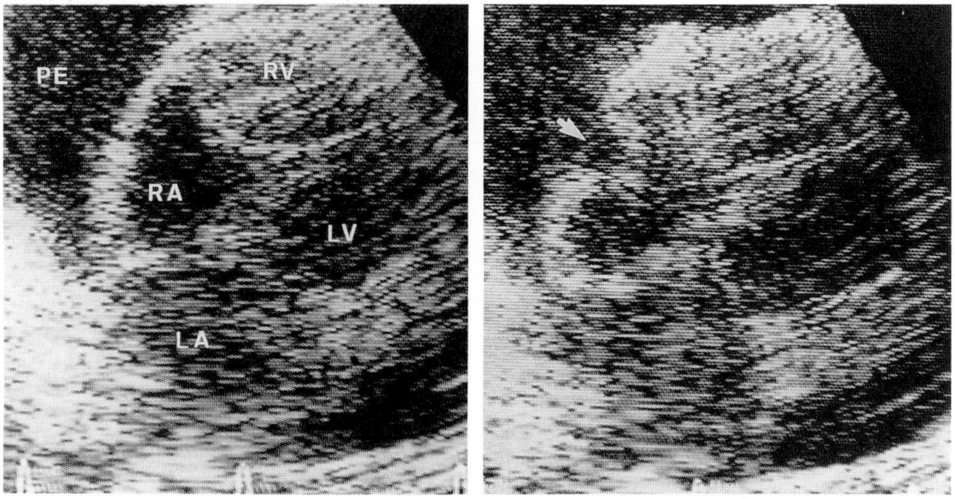

sure monitoring. These measurements require high quality tracings under well-controlled physiologic conditions and considerable off-line analysis so they are not practical for widespread application in the critical care setting. Nonetheless, they illustrate the potential for obtaining detailed physiologic data that more precisely addresses pathophysiologic questions.

Ventricular Interdependence and the Role of the Pericardium

Systemic hypoperfusion need not be a reflection of intrinsic left ventricular systolic or diastolic dysfunction but instead may be a consequence of factors extrinsic to the left ventricle. Cardiac tamponade provides an excellent example of this phenomenon. One of the earliest applications of echocardiography was the diagnosis of pericardial effusion detected as an abnormal relatively echo-free space surrounding the free walls of the heart (Fig. 21-6). In patients with structurally normal cardiac chambers the position of the free walls of the heart between the pericardial space and the intracardiac blood pool is a reflection of the *transmural pressure differential* (difference between intracavitary pressure and intrapericardial pressure). As fluid accumulates within the relatively inelastic confines of the pericardial space, the intrapericardial pressure rises. When intrapericardial pressure rises in excess of right-sided filling pressures (assuming they are lower than left-sided filling pressures and hence represent the threshold for tamponade), filling of the right heart is impeded as the pericardial space compresses the right heart. Cardiac output declines despite normal intrinsic left ventricular systolic function because preload to the left heart is reduced. These phenomena are graphically portrayed by two-dimensional echocardiography. Early in the progression of hemodynamic deterioration, late diastolic and early systolic collapse of the right atrial free wall is noted (Fig. 21-6). Subsequently, early diastolic collapse of the right ventricle is detected as cardiac output falls prior to the onset of systemic hypotension (Fig. 21-7). On pericardiocentesis, reversal of right ventricular collapse precedes resolution of right atrial collapse.[18] In one detailed echocardiographic-hemodynamic study, right ventricular early diastolic collapse was both sensitive (92 percent) and specific (100 percent) for the diagnosis of cardiac tamponade.[18] Because of the technical difficulties of adequately imaging the right atrial free wall, right atrial collapse was a less sensitive (64 percent) though specific (100 percent) sign of cardiac tamponade.[18] As with any clinical condition, the diagnosis of tamponade should take into consideration all available data and not rest solely on echocardiographic findings. Inadequate image quality, failure to examine right ventricular structures from multiple views (Figs. 21-7 and 21-8), and inability to precisely time wall motion in a tachycardic patient can lead to errors in interpretation. The superior temporal resolution of M-mode echocardiography and the dimension versus time format can assist considerably in identifying the early diastolic right ventricular compression

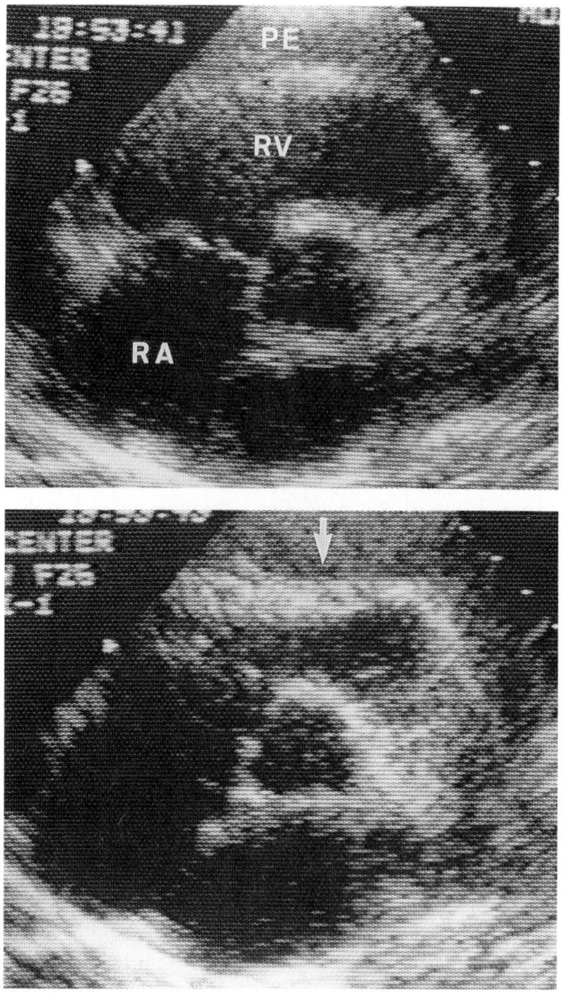

FIGURE 21-7 Stop frame two-dimensional echocardiographic images of the short axis view of the base of the heart imaged from the left parasternal window in a patient experiencing cardiac tamponade. *Top.* A large pericardial effusion (PE) is represented by the echo-free space anterior to the free wall of the right ventricular (RV) outflow tract. No pericardial effusion is imaged posterior to the cardiac structures because the tomographic plane is cephalad to the left ventricle and transects the right (RA) and left atria. Normally the posterior pericardial reflection does not extend this far cephalad. In this early systolic image the right ventricular free wall is convex with respect to the pericardial space, and right ventricular compression is not evident. *Bottom.* By contrast, this early diastolic stop frame image from the same patient (same image orientation as in the top panel) exhibits inward deflection of the right ventricular free wall (arrow) resulting in right ventricular compression, a sign of cardiac tamponade which develops after the onset of right atrial collapse (see Fig. 21-6) but at a time when tamponade physiology may be manifested by reduced cardiac output with preserved systemic pressures. In early diastole, right ventricular pressures reach a nadir before substantial filling has occurred and thus the elevated intrapericardial pressure, characteristic of tamponade physiology, displaces the right ventricular free wall inward.

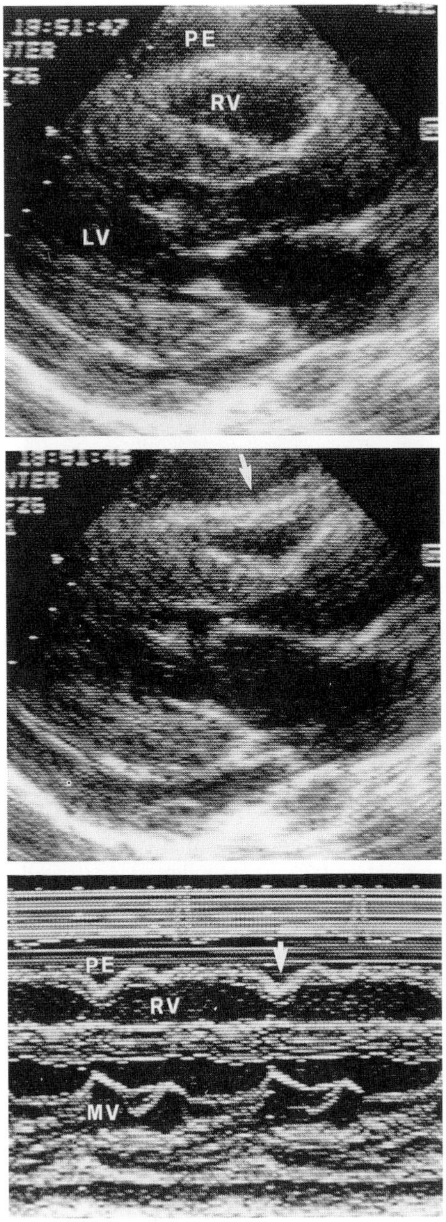

FIGURE 21-8 Stop frame two-dimensional echocardiographic images of the long axis of the left ventricle (top and center panels) and accompanying M-mode echocardiographic recording from the mitral valve level (bottom panel) obtained from the left parasternal window in a patient with cardiac tamponade. *Top.* A large pericardial effusion (PE) is represented by the echo-free space anterior to the free wall of the right ventricle (RV). The fluid extends circumferentially around the heart and is detected as an echo-free space posterior to the free wall of the left ventricle (LV) as well. In this late diastolic image the free wall of the right ventricle is convex with respect to the pericardial space, and right ventricular collapse is not evident. *Center.* By contrast this early diastolic stop frame image from the same patient (same image orientation as in the top panel) demonstrates right ventricular compression (arrow). The detection of right ventricular or right atrial collapse in patients with cardiac tamponade requires examination of the cardiac structures from multiple views (see also Figs. 21-6 and 21-7) to obtain images of sufficient resolution for accurate analysis. *Bottom.* The M-mode echocardiogram obtained with the ultrasound beam directed through the anterior pericardial effusion (PE), right ventricular cavity (RV), and mitral valve (MV) permits accurate timing of right ventricular free wall motion, even in the tachycardic patient experiencing cardiac tamponade. The ECG overlies the upper portion of the M-mode echocardiogram and the QRS complex provides a marker for the end of diastole. The mitral valve exhibits two opening motions equivalent to the early rapid filling phase (the MV symbol is superimposed on the early rapid filling motion of the mitral valve in this figure) and late atrial systolic phases of left ventricular filling. Abnormal inward motion of the right ventricular free wall (arrow) signifying intrapericardial pressures in excess of early diastolic right ventricular pressures occurs in early diastole simultaneously with the early rapid filling phase movement of the mitral valve.

of cardiac tamponade and distinguishing it from the normal inward motion of the right ventricular free wall during systole (Fig. 21-8). The right heart chamber wall motion will only be a reliable indicator of elevated intrapericardial pressure if right heart pressures are relatively normal. For instance, in a patient with severe pulmonary hypertension and right ventricular hypertrophy, the right heart filling pressures may exceed left heart filling pressures such that intrapericardial pressures may rise sufficiently to compromise left heart filling before right atrial or ventricular collapse is evident. Alternatively, loculated pericardial effusions, such as occur following cardiac surgery or in patients with malignant effusions, may result in isolated tamponade of selected chambers of the heart without causing right atrial or ventricular collapse.

In the normal left ventricle, diastolic geometry and filling can be altered indirectly by abnormal loading of the right ventricle, since the two ventricles function in parallel with a common ventricular septum and share the same potentially limiting pericardial space. Doppler echocardiographic identification of predominant or isolated right ventricular dysfunction with secondary indirect derangement of left ventricular function is of the utmost importance as it redirects the intensivist's attention toward potentially reversible pulmonary or pulmonary vascular diseases which may be responsible for apparent cardiovascular collapse. Pure pressure overload of the right ventricle in patients free of left ventricular disease such as occurs in primary pulmonary hypertension,[19] acute massive pulmonary embolism,[20] chronic thromboembolic pulmonary disease,[21] and pulmo-

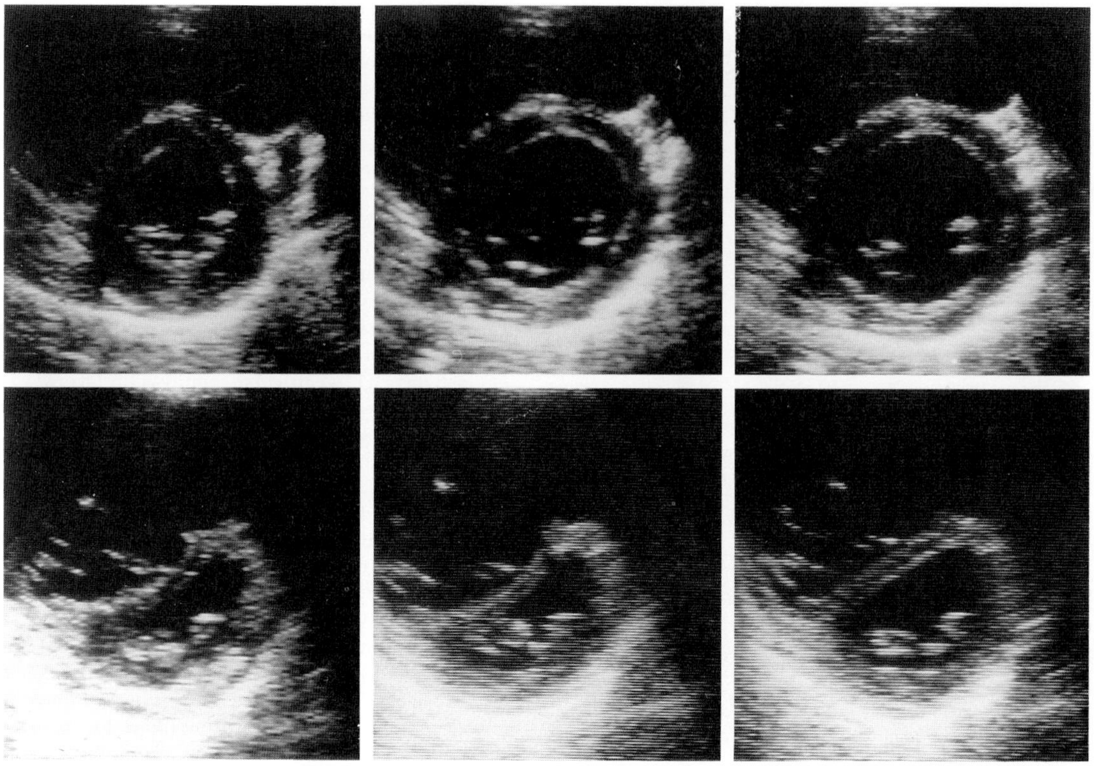

FIGURE 21-9 Stop frame two-dimensional echocardiographic images of the left ventricle in short axis cross section at the level of the chordae tendineae in a normal subject (top row) and in a patient with right ventricular pressure overload due to primary pulmonary hypertension (bottom row). In the normal subject, sequential images of the left ventricular cavity from end systole to end diastole reveal a relatively circular profile which enlarges progressively with left ventricular filling. In the patient with right ventricular pressure overload the transventricular septal pressure differential is reduced (or reversed), and the interventricular septum is deflected leftward toward the center of the left ventricle. This compression of the left ventricle into a D-shaped cross-sectional profile is most marked at end systole. Incomplete restoration toward a more normal left ventricular shape occurs by end diastole. (Adapted and reproduced from Louie EK et al: J Am Coll Cardiol 8:1298–1306, 1986, with the permission of the publisher.)

nary parenchymal diseases which secondarily compromise the pulmonary circulation[22] results in right ventricular enlargement and secondary compression of the left ventricle by displacement of the interventricular septum. The reduction in transventricular septal pressure differential due to right ventricular systolic hypertension results in flattening of the normally circular left ventricular cavity (imaged in the short axis two-dimensional echocardiographic plane) due to leftward shift of the ventricular septum (Fig. 21-9). Echocardiographic imaging throughout the cardiac cycle demonstrates that left ventricular deformation is most marked at end systole and early diastole with partial to complete restoration of left ventricular geometry at end diastole. The magnitude of this end-systolic leftward ventricular septal shift (quantified as normalized septal radius of curvature by two-dimensional echocardiographic techniques) correlates with the ratio of right-to-left ventricular systolic pressures ($r = 0.86$).[23]

These alterations in left ventricular geometry profoundly influence left ventricular diastolic filling. Pulsed Doppler echocardiographic measurement of transmitral flow velocities in patients with primary pulmonary hypertension demonstrates that the early diastolic left ventricular compression impedes early left ventricular filling and results in a greater dependence on atrial systolic filling.[19] Relief of right ventricular systolic hypertension such as occurs during the resolution phase of pulmonary embolism[20] or following thromboendarterectomy for chronic thromboembolic pulmonary hypertension[20,24] results in reversal of the left ventricular compression and improvement in early diastolic left ventricular filling. Often right ventricular *pressure* overload is accompanied by right ventricular *volume* overload due to intracardiac shunting (e.g., atrial septal defect) or tricuspid regurgitation. In isolation, right ventricular *volume* overload results in maximal leftward ventricular septal shift at end diastole. Thus, there is relative impairment of atrial systolic filling and not early diastolic filling.[25,26] Patients having a mixture of right ventricular pressure and volume overload exhibit some combination of these patterns of geometric distortion of the left ventricle. These Doppler and echocardiographic abnormalities are not routinely observed in patients with right ventricular pressure/volume overload secondary to left ventricular systolic dysfunction, because under these circumstances ventricular interaction through the septum is not governed solely by abnormal right ventricular loading but rather by the interplay of abnormal loading on both sides of the ventricular septum.

Characterization of Disorders of the Myocardium, Valvular Structures, and Great Vessels

MYOCARDIAL DISEASES

Echocardiographic techniques can be useful in the rapid identification of myocardial disease as the etiology for passive pulmonary congestion or reduced systemic perfusion.[8] For instance, congestive heart failure may result from impaired left ventricular systolic function (dilated cardiomyopathies) or abnormal left ventricular diastolic filling (restrictive and hypertrophic cardiomyopathies), conditions readily distinguished by echocardiographic imaging (Fig. 21-10). In addition, a variety of reversible insults to myocardial systolic and diastolic function (ischemia, electrolyte derangements, myocardial depression during sepsis) can mimic the functional derangements of intrinsic myocardial disease. Dilated cardiomyopathies are characterized by a hypokinetic enlarged left ventricle without significant increase in left ventricular wall thickness to radius ratio. The left atrium is dilated in proportion to the left ventricular enlargement, and the left ventricular outflow tract is enlarged as a result of ventricular dilation. In striking contrast, restrictive cardiomyopathies are typified by a normal to small left ventricle with preserved systolic function. If the restrictive process results from myocardial infiltration (amyloid), the myocardial walls will be increased in thickness relative to cavity size (increased left ventricular wall thickness to radius ratio) and the texture of the imaged myocardium may reveal characteristic bright specular echoes (see Fig. 21-10, right panel). The markedly increased left ventricular filling pressures, which these patients experience, are reflected in atrial enlargement disproportionate to the ventricular cavity size, and the infiltrative process may result in abnormal thickening of the interatrial septum and atrioventricular valves. Hypertrophic cardiomyopathies, whether acquired as a result of increased left ventricular afterload (e.g., systemic hypertension) or idiopathic, demonstrate normal to small left ventricular cavity size with marked increases in left ventricular wall thickness resulting in an increased wall thickness to radius ratio.[27] The pattern of ventricular hypertrophy in idiopathic hypertrophic cardiomyopathy is usually nonuniform[28] in contradistinction to the symmetric increase in left ventricular wall thickness observed in hypertensive heart disease. Until late in the disease left ventricular systolic function is normal if not hyperdynamic. As is the case with restrictive cardiomyopathies, the increased left ventricular filling pressure

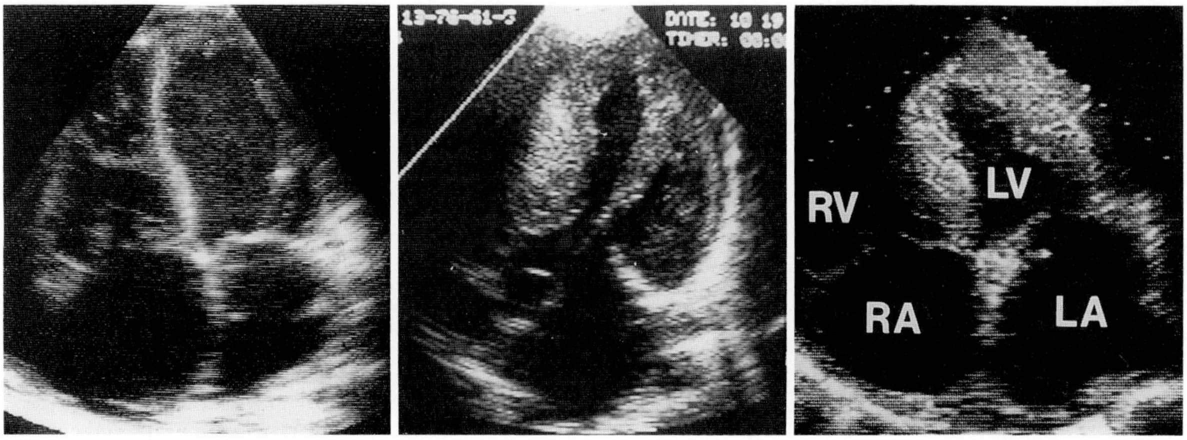

FIGURE 21-10 Stop frame two-dimensional echocardiographic images of the four chambers of the heart from three different patients obtained with the transducer at the left ventricular apex. The image orientation is similar in all three panels. In the right and left panels the left ventricle (LV), right ventricle (RV), left atrium (LA), and right atrium (RA) are simultaneously imaged in a tomographic plane through the crux of the heart and the atrioventricular valves. In the center panel, the transducer has been angled anteriorly such that the left ventricular outflow tract and aortic valve are imaged arising from the left ventricle. *Left. Dilated cardiomyopathy*—All four cardiac chambers are enlarged, and the walls of the left ventricle are normal in thickness. In real-time playback the left ventricular wall motion was diffusely hypokinetic. *Center. Hypertrophic cardiomyopathy*—The left ventricular walls are markedly hypertrophied, and the left ventricular cavity is small. Relative to the left ventricular cavity size the left atrium is enlarged. In real-time playback the left ventricular wall motion was hyperkinetic resulting in cavity obliteration during systole. *Right. Restrictive cardiomyopathy*—Infiltration of the left ventricular myocardium with amyloid in this patient resulted in thickening of the left ventricular walls and abnormally bright specular echoes from the tissue. The left ventricular cavity is relatively normal in size but the left atrium is markedly dilated, and the right heart chambers are enlarged. In real-time playback the inward motion of the left ventricular walls in systole was normal. Occasionally abnormalities of left ventricular cavity expansion in diastole can be appreciated in patients with restrictive cardiomyopathies. (Adapted and reproduced from Louie EK: Echocardiography 4:119–140, 1987, with the permission of the publisher).

found in hypertrophied ventricles results in left atrial enlargement disproportionate to the left ventricular cavity size. In that unique subset of patients in whom the hypertrophic process is particularly marked in the left ventricular outflow tract, dynamic subvalvular left ventricular outflow tract obstruction may develop,[27] which is reflected in systolic anterior motion of the mitral valve and mitral-ventricular septal contact in systole. It is important to realize, however, that the development of subaortic obstruction is *not* a prerequisite for the diagnosis of idiopathic hypertrophic cardiomyopathy, and significant functional disability and cardiovascular morbidity may result from the nonobstructive variants of hypertrophic cardiomyopathy.[28]

In the Western world ischemic cardiomyopathy (dilated cardiomyopathy resulting from loss of functioning myocardium following MI) is still the cause for impaired left ventricular systolic function in the majority of patients. In the final stages, the left ventricle may be so impaired that it is indistinguishable from the diffusely hypocontractile chamber seen in idiopathic dilated cardiomyopathies.[8,29] Often, however, the presence of regional nonuniformity or temporal nonuniformity in left ventricular systolic function will suggest the diagnosis of ischemic cardiomyopathy. Chronically infarcted segments may appear abnormally echo dense and fail to exhibit normal systolic wall thickening. The accompanying endocardial wall motion may be hypokinetic (decreased inward motion toward the ventricular center of mass), akinetic (immobile), or dyskinetic (paradoxic outward systolic motion). Of equal diagnostic importance is the identification of normal myocardial segments remote from the infarction which may exhibit compensatory hyperdynamic systolic function. Of note, in most circumstances echocardiographic measures of abnormal segmental *mechanical* function cannot determine the nature of the underlying pathophysiologic process. Thus, reversible ischemic myocardial dysfunction, acute MI, and old healed MI are not always easily distinguished. In addition, some cardiomyopathic processes will impair regional left ventricular systolic function in a selective manner mimicking ischemic myocardial disease.[8] Hopefully, progress in digital signal processing will foster tissue characterization to address these diagnostic issues.

Doppler echocardiographic techniques are also useful for identifying mechanical complications of ischemic myocardial disease.[30] Acute disruption of necrotic infarcting muscle resulting in left ventricular free wall rupture with pseudoaneurysm formation, ventricular septal perforation, or mitral regurgitation due to a flail mitral valve can all be diagnosed echocardiographically. Often the primary defects can be imaged directly or their consequences (e.g., pericardial effusion following free wall rupture, mitral leaflet malcoaptation following infarction of the subvalvular apparatus) depicted. Doppler echocardiographic evidence for abnormal interventricular shunting or mitral regurgitation can provide physiologic data to complement the anatomic evidence. For example, the Doppler echocardiogram (Plate 13) of a patient with acute mitral regurgitation following inferoposterior wall MI illustrates the complementary roles of anatomic (two-dimensional echocardiographic) and physiologic (Doppler echocardiographic) data. At one end of the spectrum infarction in the vicinity of a papillary muscle may result in ischemic dysfunction of the papillary muscle such that it fails to contract properly, resulting in malcoaptation of the mitral leaflets. At the other end of the spectrum, as illustrated in Plate 13, necrotic disruption of a portion or the tip of the papillary muscle may result in avulsion of the chordae to a portion of the mitral leaflets such that in systole the flail segment prolapses deep into the left atrium. The accompanying color Doppler depiction of the mitral regurgitant jet past the flail posterior mitral leaflet demonstrates a characteristic orientation toward the anterior and superior aspects of the left atrium.

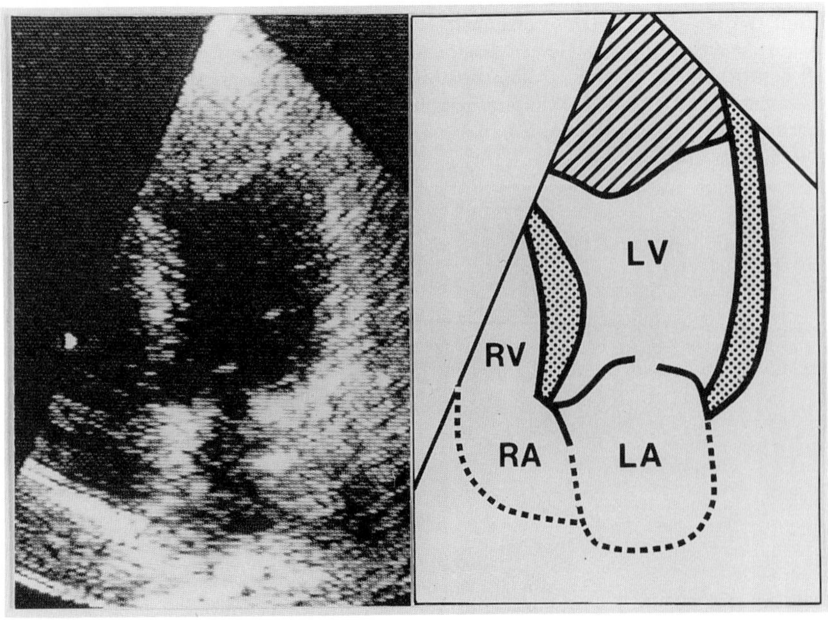

FIGURE 21-11 Stop frame two-dimensional echocardiogram of the four chambers of the heart as imaged from the left ventricular apex along with accompanying schematic diagram. This patient suffered a large anteroapical MI resulting in apical aneurysm formation and thrombus desposition. The left ventricle (LV), left atrium (LA), right ventricle (RV), and right atrium (RA) are imaged simultaneously. In real-time playback a large dyskinetic thin-walled left ventricular apical aneurysm filled with thrombus (crosshatch) was imaged. Protrusion of the thrombus into the left ventricular cavity and mobility of its surface may be predictors of the potential for systemic embolization.

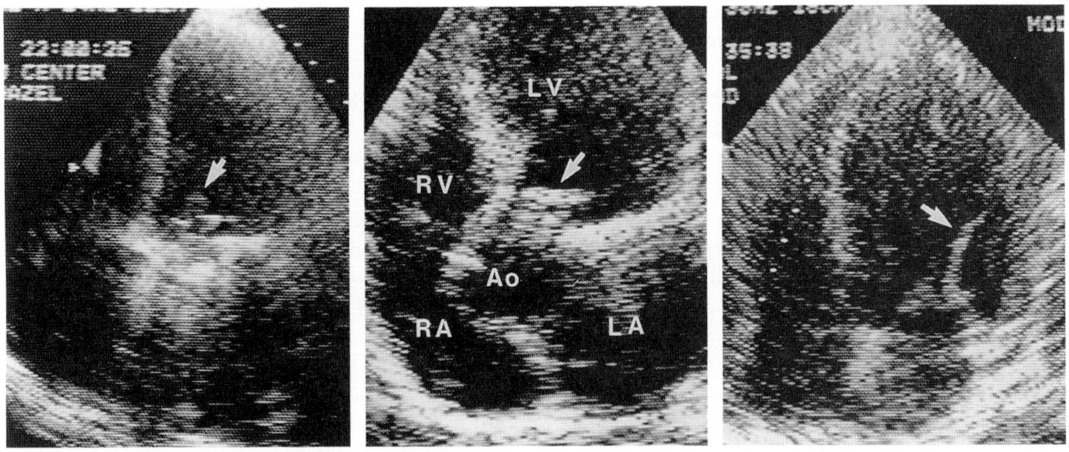

FIGURE 21-12 Stop frame two-dimensional echocardiographic images of the four chambers of the heart imaged from the left ventricular apex. In these three patients the echocardiographic studies focused on the definition of valve-related intracardiac masses. In the center panel the left ventricle (LV), left atrium (LA), right ventricle (RV), right atrium (RA), and proximal aorta (Ao) are imaged simultaneously. In the right and left panels the four cardiac chambers are imaged simultaneously, but the tomographic plane is directed more posteriorly so that the imaging plane passes through the cardiac crux, and the left ventricular outflow tract is not imaged. *Left.* This patient presented with congestive heart failure and hypotension referrable to obstruction of his mechanical prosthetic mitral valve. A "soft" echo density (arrow) representing occlusive thrombus confirmed at surgery protrudes from the mechanical prosthesis (two bright echo densities on the left ventricular side of the mitral annulus). Note that the bright echo densities in the left atrium proximal to the prosthetic mitral valve are reverberation artifacts which obscure potential left atrial extension of the thrombus. *Center.* This patient had calcific aortic stenosis and a remote history of infective endocarditis. The relatively echo-dense and well-circumscribed mass (arrow) in the left ventricular outflow tract proximal to the aortic valve is consistent with a healed vegetation. Note that the aortic valve itself (echo densities distal to the vegetation and just above the Ao symbol) is echo-dense and thick. The vegetation (arrow) was distinguished from the deformed valve on real-time playback by its motion as it prolapsed into the left ventricular outflow tract in diastole. *Right.* This patient had a history of intravenous drug abuse and presented with symptoms and signs of acute infective endocarditis. Real-time playback demonstrated the whip-like motion of a long bulky vegetation (arrow) only a portion of which is captured in this stop frame image. Distinction of the vegetation from the mitral valve and submitral apparatus was obvious because the underlying valvular anatomy was normal.

Another important complication of acute MI (particularly anterior wall infarction) is the development of infarct thinning, infarct expansion, and subsequent left ventricular aneurysm formation.[30] As demonstrated in Fig. 21-11, not only can the abnormal protruding diastolic contour of the left ventricular aneurysm be appreciated by two-dimensional echocardiography, but the presence of associated intracavitary thrombus can also be detected. Intracavitary thrombi which are mobile and protrude into the left ventricular cavity may have a particular proclivity for systemic embolization during the acute phase of MI.[8,30] Such echo-dense intracavitary masses are most commonly seen following anterior wall infarction and in patients with severe depression of global left ventricular systolic function. In the absence of a definite segmental wall motion abnormality, it is quite uncommon for intracavitary thrombi to be detected echocardiographically. Although detailed research studies have suggested that the echocardiogram is highly sensitive and specific for the detection of left ventricular thrombi, in the critical care setting often the transthoracic echocardiogram will be of insufficient quality to produce an exhaustive search for intracavitary thrombi; however, useful information concerning global and regional left ventricular systolic function may still be obtained. In patients with severe reduction in left ventricular systolic dysfunction, mitral valve disease, or atrial fibrillation, the left atrium may also be a source for systemic emboli. Complete interrogation of the left atrium and, in particular, the left atrial appendage is often not achieved by transthoracic echocardiography even under the most favorable circumstances. Transesophageal echocardiography (see Chap. 22) provides the optimal imaging approach to these structures.[1]

VALVULAR ABNORMALITIES

Two-dimensional and Doppler echocardiography have made their greatest impact on the diagnosis and characterization of valvular heart disease.[31,32] The leaflet structure, tissue characteristics, and motion can all be directly visualized in real time by echocardiographic techniques. Congenital malformation of the valves (e.g., bicuspid aortic valve), inflammatory and degenerative changes in the leaflet tissue (e.g., rheumatic mitral valve disease, sclerotic aortic valve disease), and pathologic derangements of the surrounding tissues (e.g., mitral annular calcification) can all be accurately characterized by echocardiography. Of particular interest to the intensivist is the characterization of valve-related intracardiac masses which may explain systemic embolization, constitutional symptoms of endocarditis, sudden onset of valvular obstruction, or progressive valvular regurgitation (Fig. 21-12). Detection of such masses on prosthetic valves or chronically deformed (and calcified) native valves poses special challenges because the echodense prosthetic materials or calcified tissues produce extraneous signals and artifacts which may mimic ectopic masses or obscure pathologic anatomy (see the artifacts in the left atrium generated by the prosthetic valve in Fig. 21-12). In addition, such materials if sufficiently echo dense, prevent the passage of ultrasound and hence acoustically shadow structures lying behind them away from the transducer. This is particularly a problem for transthoracic imaging of the left atrial side of prosthetic valves and represents an important indication for transesophageal echocardiographic imaging (see Chap. 22).

In the left panel of Fig. 21-12, a thrombosed mechanical prosthetic mitral valve is imaged. In real time particular attention was directed toward assessing the seating of the prosthetic valve annulus (to exclude paravalvular dehiscence) and the excursion of the central disc occluder. In this particular patient, occluder motion was limited, signifying potential valvular obstruction. A "soft" echodensity (arrow) protruding beyond the struts and occluder represents the obstructing thrombus which was confirmed at emergency surgery. In the center panel of Fig. 21-12, a healed vegetation of infective endocarditis (arrow) is imaged prolapsing into the left ventricular outflow tract proximal to a calcified and deformed aortic valve. The erratic motion of this echo-dense vegetation distinguished it from other echo densities emanating from the aortic valve which moved in synchrony with valve cusp motion and were thus attributed to degenerative changes in the valve. It should be evident that in the absence of such a large, echo-dense, and abnormally moving structure attached to the valve, it would be impossible to exclude the presence of a small vegetation within the multiple extraneous echoes emanating from the sclerotic aortic valve. Thus, while the echocardiographic detection of vegetations is extremely useful in the diagnosis and management of infective endocarditis, the threshold for detection will be most favorable if the underlying valve tissue is normal (e.g., acute endocarditis in intravenous drug abusers), the pathogenic organism produces bulky vegetations (e.g., fungal endocarditis), and the untreated phase is prolonged (so that the vegetations become large). Although it is commonly observed that with successful treatment, infectious vegetations may become more circumscribed, less mobile, and more echo dense (as in the patient illustrated in the center panel of Fig. 21-12), in general it is speculative to attempt to predict the "age" of a vegetation. In the right panel of Fig. 21-12, a mobile "whiplike" vegetation attached to the previously normal mitral valve of an intravenous drug abuser with acute bacterial endocarditis is imaged. Here the vegetation was easy to identify because of its size, abnormal motion, and the presence of otherwise normal valvular architecture. Echocardiographic diagnosis of infective endocarditis of the tricuspid valve is particularly helpful as the clinical findings may be subtle and the presentation nonspecific. Usually it occurs in the setting of intravenous drug abuse, affects an intrinsically normal tricuspid valve, and goes undetected on clinical grounds for prolonged periods of time (allowing the vegetations to become quite large)—all conditions which favor echocardiographic diagnosis of this otherwise elusive condition.

Doppler echocardiography has contributed significantly in characterizing the hemodynamic alterations resulting from valvular heart disease.[32] Although it is possible to estimate the severity of aortic stenosis by examining cusp motion[33] and to assess inflow obstruction at the mitral valve by planimeterizing the apparent orifice,[34] these echocardiographic methods are time consuming, not applicable in all patients, and relatively crude. Doppler techniques now permit the measurement of peak velocities within the jet of blood passing through a stenotic orifice from which transvalvular pressure gradients can be derived by application of the Bernoulli equation (Fig. 21-13). In a detailed study of simultaneous determination of mean aortic valve systolic gradients by continuous wave Doppler and direct hemodynamic measurement, the agreement between the two techniques was excellent ($r = 0.93$, SEE 10 mmHg).[35] Since the transvalvular pressure gradient depends not only on the severity of stenosis but also on the transvalvular flow rate, investigators have used Doppler techniques to estimate aortic valve area using Eq. (21-2) and the continuity principle. As applied to the cardiovascular system the *continuity principle* states that average flow rates through successive flow cross sections in the heart must be equal. Thus, the bulk rate of transfer of blood through the left ventricular outflow tract (LVOT) must equal the bulk rate of transfer of blood across the aortic valve (AV). Thus, applying Eq. (21-2):

$$Q_{\mathrm{LVOT}} = A_{\mathrm{LVOT}} \cdot V_{\mathrm{LVOT}} = Q_{\mathrm{AV}} = A_{\mathrm{AV}} \cdot V_{\mathrm{AV}}$$

or

$$A_{\mathrm{AV}} = \frac{A_{\mathrm{LVOT}} \cdot V_{\mathrm{LVOT}}}{V_{\mathrm{AV}}} \tag{21-4}$$

If Q in Eq. (21-4) is expressed as blood flow/beat (stroke volume) then V represents the area under the flow velocity profile. Thus, aortic valve area (A_{AV}) can be determined from the cross-sectional area of the left ventricular outflow tract (A_{LVOT}) measured by two-dimensional echocardiography, the velocity of blood flow in the left ventricular outflow tract (V_{LVOT}) measured by pulsed wave Doppler and the velocity of blood flow in the stenotic orifice jet (V_{AV}) measured by continuous wave Doppler. Using such techniques, good agreement has been achieved by comparison to aortic valve area estimates from catheterization derived data using the Gorlin equation ($r = 0.83$, SEE = 0.19 cm).[36] The use of the continuity principle in conjunction with Doppler measurement techniques corrects the estimate of aortic valve area for the increased transvalvular flow due to any associated aortic regurgitation.

Mean transmitral diastolic pressure gradients can be measured in a fashion analogous to the measurement of mean systolic aortic valve gradients (Fig. 21-13). For the ste-

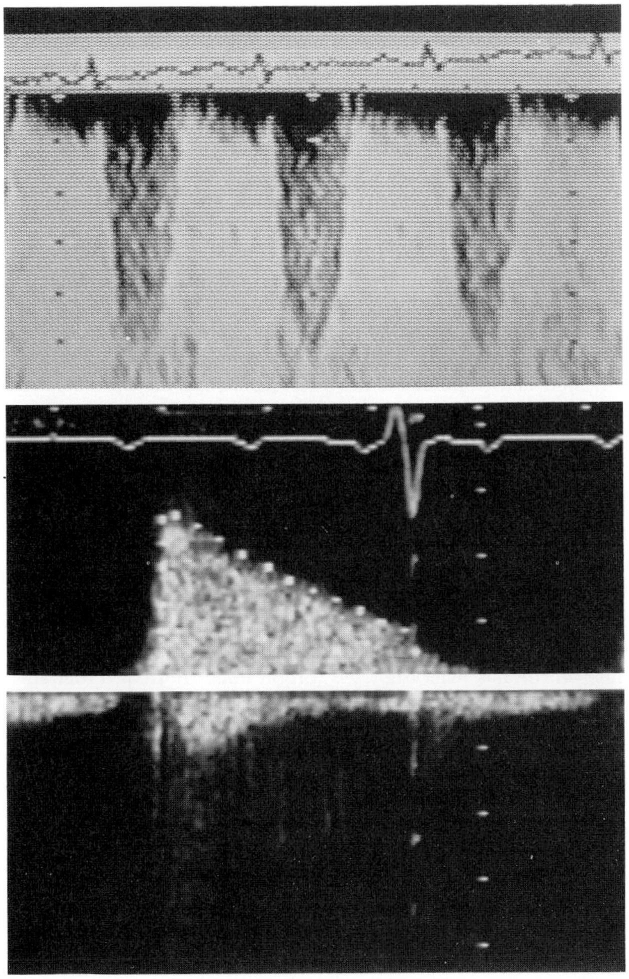

FIGURE 21-13 Continuous wave Doppler spectra obtained from a transducer positioned at the left ventricular apex to measure peak velocities in two patients, one with aortic stenosis (top panel) and one with mitral stenosis (bottom panel). In both panels the ECG is displayed above the Doppler flow velocity spectrum for timing purposes. Time marks along the abscissa are at 200-ms intervals, and dots along the ordinate are at velocity increments of 1.0 m/s. *Top.* All systolic Doppler signals are recorded below the zero base line representing transaortic flow velocities out the aorta and away from the transducer positioned at the left ventricular apex. Whereas normal left ventricular outflow tract velocities peak at approximately 1.0 to 1.7 m/s, the velocities in this patient peak at 5.0 m/s. Using Eq. (21-3) this is equivalent to a peak instantaneous transaortic gradient of 100 mmHg which signifies the presence of severe aortic stenosis (assuming a normal cardiac output). *Bottom.* All diastolic Doppler signals are recorded above the zero base line representing transmitral flow velocities into the left ventricle and toward the transducer positioned at the left ventricular apex. This spectrum does not have the normal biphasic contour seen in sinus rhythm (see Fig. 21-5) because the patient's rhythm is atrial flutter. Whereas normal left ventricular inflow tract velocities peak at 0.6 to 1.3 m/s, this patient with significant mitral stenosis has peak inflow velocities of 2.7 m/s which is equivalent to a peak instantaneous transmitral gradient of 29 mmHg [using Eq. (21-3)]. The envelope of the spectrum has been digitized (bright dots along limits of spectrum) to illustrate the computation of the mean transmitral gradient. In clinical application, measurement of such mean transvalvular gradients by continuous wave Doppler provides excellent estimates of the mean transvalvular gradients measured at cardiac catheterization.

notic mitral orifice, the decay in instantaneous transmitral gradient (and hence the decay in instantaneous transmitral flow velocity) is approximately inversely proportional to the severity of stenosis. Thus, transmitral flow velocities in late diastole fall off rapidly in patients with mild mitral stenosis and fall off slowly in patients with severe mitral stenosis (Fig. 21-13). To use this relationship the pressure half time (t) of the continuous wave transmitral flow velocity envelope (defined as the interval between peak transmitral velocity and velocity/$\sqrt{2}$) is measured as an index of the rate of decay of transmitral flow velocities. From the pressure half time (t) measured in milliseconds an empiric relationship to mitral valve area (A_{MV}) measured in cm^2 has been established:

$$A_{MV} = \frac{220}{t} \qquad (21\text{-}5)$$

Using Eq. (21-5) reasonable correlations ($r = 0.85$, SEE = 0.22 cm) between Doppler and catheterization-determined mitral valve area have been obtained.[34]

Transprosthetic valve mean gradients can also be measured by continuous wave Doppler techniques similar to those used for native valves. Interpretation of the results depends on the state of ventricular systolic function (estimated from the two-dimensional echocardiogram) and the characteristics of the particular prosthesis. Results in a given patient can be compared serially (assuming constant cardiac output) or compared to reference values in the literature stratified for prosthesis type and size.[37,38]

The detection and quantitation of valvular regurgitation and its hemodynamic sequelae have been greatly facilitated by the application of Doppler echocardiographic techniques. In Plate 14 color flow Doppler is used to map the systolic regurgitation in the left atrium (left panel) and the diastolic flow disturbance of aortic regurgitation in the left ventricular outflow tract (right panel). Timing of these abnormal Doppler signals is performed by freeze framing the playback relative to specific portions of the cardiac cycle (determined from the accompanying ECG or the motion of cardiac structures on the two-dimensional echocardiogram). The origin of the flow disturbance can be localized

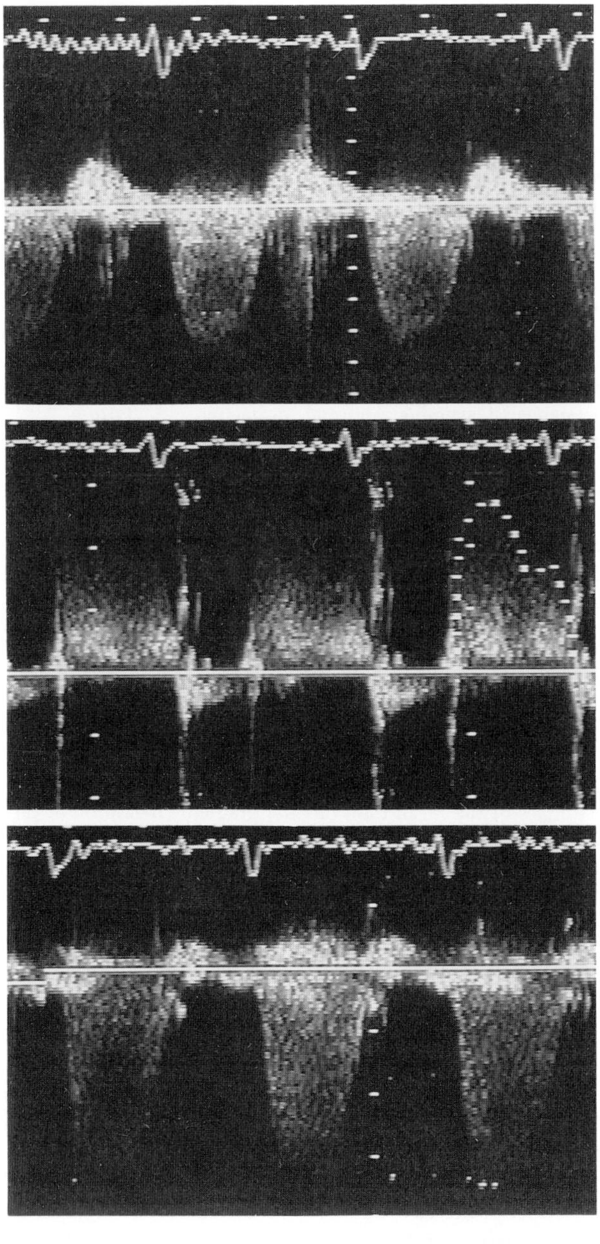

FIGURE 21-14 Continuous wave Doppler spectra of mitral regurgitation (top panel), pulmonic regurgitation (center panel), and tricuspid regurgitation (bottom panel) from the patient whose color flow Doppler echocardiogram is illustrated in Plate 15. Although color flow Doppler provides information concerning the spatial extent of the regurgitant flow velocity disturbance, continuous wave Doppler quantifies the peak velocities in the flow velocity disturbance, which can be related to the peak instantaneous transvalvular pressure differential. The accompanying text explains how these measurements are used to estimate pulmonary artery systolic and diastolic pressures, parameters reflecting the hemodynamic burden of the patient's mitral regurgitation. In each panel the ECG is recorded above the Doppler spectrum. Along the abscissa, time division marks are at 200-ms intervals. Along the ordinate, velocity division marks above and below the zero base line are in increments of 1.0 m/s. *Top.* From an apical transducer position with the Doppler beam directed toward the mitral orifice, peak systolic mitral regurgitation velocities of 4.3 m/s are recorded below the zero base line. *Center.* From a parasternal transducer position with the Doppler beam directed through the pulmonic valve and out the right ventricular outflow tract end-diastolic maximal pulmonic regurgitation velocities of 1.5 m/s are recorded above the zero base line. To better delineate the pulmonic regurgitation spectrum, the envelope of the last profile has been digitized (bright dots). *Bottom.* From an apical transducer position with the Doppler beam directed toward the tricuspid orifice, peak systolic tricuspid regurgitation velocities of approximately 3.0 m/s are recorded below the zero base line.

by examining the relationship of the map of the color flow disturbance in relation to the imaged valvular structures. The disordered flow disturbance of the regurgitant stream and its interaction with the surrounding blood pool is identified by the "speckled" or "mosaic" pattern of bright colors mapped onto the cardiac chambers. Quantitation of such regurgitant lesions is performed by comparing the spatial distribution of the flow disturbance (its volume in three dimensions) to the volume of the receiving chamber.[39–43] When applied to the clinical assessment of mitral regurgitation, the maximal area of the color flow Doppler signal relative to the cross-sectional area of the left atrium permits distinction between angiographic grades of mitral regurgitation and correlates with catheterization estimates of regurgitant fraction ($r = 0.78$).[44] Similarly, the volume of the left ventricular outflow tract occupied by the flow disturbance of aortic regurgitation is related to the volumetric severity of the valvular insufficiency.[41,42] Thus, color flow Doppler estimates of the percentage of the cross-sectional area of the left ventricular outflow tract occupied by the abnormal color Doppler signals or the width of the flow disturbance relative to the diameter of the outflow tract provide practical indices for predicting the angiographic severity of aortic regurgitation.[45]

While two-dimensional echocardiography can measure the effects of valvular regurgitation on left ventricular and atrial chamber size and function, Doppler echocardiography can be used to quantify pulmonary hypertension and right-sided valvular regurgitation resulting from left heart valvular disease. In Plate 15, a patient with moderate to severe mitral regurgitation and secondary tricuspid regurgitation is illustrated. Continuous wave Doppler directed through these regurgitant jets can measure the maximal regurgitant velocities which by application of Eq. (21-3) permits the calculation of the peak pressure difference across the regurgitant valve. For instance, Fig. 21-14 illustrates the continuous wave Doppler spectra obtained with Doppler cursors directed across the mitral valve (top), pulmonic valve (center), and tricuspid valve (bottom) of the same patient illustrated in Plate 15. In the top panel, forward transmitral flow during diastole is recorded above the base line (toward the transducer) and retrograde mitral regurgitation below the base line (away from the transducer). In the center panel, pulmonary regurgitation secondary to pulmonary hypertension is detected as Doppler spectral shifts in diastole above the base line with normal systolic forward flow depicted below the base line. At the end of diastole, the maximal pulmonary regurgitation velocity is 1.5 m/s which corresponds to an end-diastolic pulmonary artery to right ventricle maximal instantaneous pressure differential of 9 mmHg [by application of Eq. (21-3)]. Similarly in the bottom panel, abnormal systolic Doppler frequency shifts representing tricuspid regurgitation are seen below the base line and normal forward transtricuspid flow in diastole is depicted above the base line. The maximal velocities in the tricuspid regurgitation jet are approximately 3.0 m/s, corresponding to a peak systolic right ventricle to right atrium pressure differential of 36 mmHg [by application of Eq. (21-3)]. Simultaneous clinical inspection of the central venous pressure from the jugular veins suggested that the right atrial pressure was approximately 12 mmHg. In the absence of tricuspid or pulmonic stenosis, the right atrial and right ventricular diastolic pressures will be roughly equal, and the right ventricular systolic and pulmonary artery systolic pressures will be equal. Thus, the right atrial pressure (12 mmHg) added to the right ventricular to right atrial systolic pressure differential (36 mmHg) will provide an estimate of peak right ventricular and pulmonary artery systolic pressure (48 mmHg in this patient). The right ventricular diastolic pressure (estimated from the right atrial pressure to be 12 mmHg) added to the pulmonary artery to right ventricular end-diastolic pressure differential (9 mmHg) will provide an estimate of pulmonary artery diastolic pressure (21 mmHg in this patient). The validity of these techniques for estimating the severity of pulmonary hypertension from Doppler-derived tricuspid regurgitation velocities and clinical assessment of the jugular venous pulse has been confirmed in several studies which have shown excellent correlations ($r = 0.93$)[46] between Doppler and hemodynamic measurements of peak pulmonary artery systolic pressure.[46,47] Such analysis of tricuspid regurgitation velocities is not limited to patients with audible murmurs of tricuspid regurgitation or severe pulmonary hypertension. The Doppler echocardiographic techniques available for detecting tricuspid regurgitation are highly sensitive such that in *normal volunteers* minimal degrees of tricuspid regurgitation (presumably "physiologic") can be detected in 44 to 50 percent[48,49] of patients, and spectral envelopes of quality sufficient for measuring peak velocities may be obtained in as many as 32 percent of subjects.[49] As would be expected in patients with significant pulmonary hypertension (pulmonary artery systolic pressure exceeding 35 mmHg) a much higher percentage (80 percent) of patients have tricuspid regurgitation which can be measured by continuous wave Doppler techniques.

Occasionally the wedding of anatomic information from the two-dimensional echocardiogram and physiologic data from the Doppler echocardiographic study provides new insights into pathophysiologic mechanisms of valvular regurgitation which are pivotal to clinical management and not demonstrated by other imaging techniques (angiography, ultrafast computed tomography, cine magnetic resonance imaging) or physiologic measurements (cardiac catheterization). Plate 16 illustrates significant paravalvular regurgitation about a malfunctioning tilting disc mechanical valve in the aortic position. The color flow Doppler map clearly depicts two separate regurgitation streams (upper left panel) passing around the prosthetic valve annulus. The simultaneously acquired two-dimensional echocardiographic image (upper right panel) illustrates the center of the prosthesis (solid triangle) and a separate echo-lucent channel passing anterior to the annulus of the prosthesis (small arrow) which represents the partial dehiscence of the prosthetic valve. In real time an abnormal rocking motion of the prosthesis could be appreciated reflecting the disrupted seating of the valve. The superior time resolution of the M-mode echocardiographic format with superimposed color Doppler overlay (bottom panel) confirms the diastolic timing of the aortic regurgitation depicted by the abnormal color Doppler signal anterior to the anterior mitral leaflet. In the image orthogonal to this view, a short axis cross section of the prosthesis and surrounding tissues (Plate 17) reveals a crescent-shaped paravalvular channel (from 11:00 to 5:00) filled with color Doppler signals of aortic regurgitant flow (left panel). The two streams of paravalvular regurgitation seen in Plate 16 represent the transection of this crescent-shaped color flow Doppler signal in its anterior and posterior limbs. In real time the motion of the central occluder within the prosthetic annulus defining the major and minor orifices for normal transprosthetic flow were appreciated (solid triangle) and distinguished from the prosthetic annular dehiscence (small arrow, right panel). Although echocardiographic artifacts from the prosthesis and postsurgical alteration of the anatomy may render interpretation of these images difficult, significant anatomic and functional information can be obtained from the Doppler echocardiographic study.[50] Transesophageal echocardiography (see Chap. 22) should be particularly helpful in the Doppler echocardiographic evaluation of prosthetic valves particularly in the mitral position where the esophageal window obviates the problems of acoustic shadowing and reverberations which obscure the left atrial side of the prosthesis during transthoracic imaging.[1]

DISEASE OF THE GREAT VESSELS

Assessment of the great vessels in their proximal portions can be achieved by transthoracic echocardiography. Of particular concern to the intensivist is the diagnosis of aortic dissection in the patient with chest pain, unexplained hypotension, or compromised visceral perfusion. Although transthoracic echocardiography has the capability to diagnose the complications related to proximal extension of an aortic dissection (aortic regurgitation, pericardial effusion/tamponade, new left ventricular regional wall motion abnormalities signifying coronary occlusion) and occasionally can be useful in distinguishing valvular from paravalvular aortic regurgitation in this setting,[51] larger portions of the aorta (the arch and descending aorta) are often inaccessible to transthoracic interrogation. Recent studies suggest that transesophageal imaging (see Chap. 22) will greatly expand the application of Doppler echocardiographic techniques to imaging of the great vessels and the diagnosis of aortic dissection.[52,53]

Conclusions

Echocardiographic imaging of cardiac morphology and Doppler characterization and quantitation of intracardiac blood flow can answer diagnostic questions concerning the cardiovascular system which are of great importance to the intensivist. This noninvasive, portable, rapidly performed diagnostic test provides a practical tool for evaluating critically ill patients and tracking their progress. The data obtained is complementary to conventional angiographic and hemodynamic measurements and under certain circumstances may provide reasonable estimates of invasively measured parameters. Under some circumstances the unique combination of anatomic and blood flow information answers clinical questions not approachable by other techniques. Poor image quality and echocardiographic artifacts are common in studies performed in critically ill patients who are immobile, cannot cooperate for the study, and have anatomic or mechanical reasons for poor ultrasound penetration of the thorax. The transesophageal window for Doppler echocardiographic imaging discussed in Chap. 22 should provide solutions to many of these shortcomings of transthoracic echocardiography and permit the application of these principles to a much larger proportion of critically ill patients.

References

1. Seward JB, Khandheria BJ, Oh JK et al: Transesophageal echocardiography: Technique, anatomic correlations, implementation, and clinical applications. Mayo Clin Proc 63:649, 1988.
2. Bansal RC, Tajik AJ, Seward JB et al: Feasibility of detailed two-dimensional echocardiographic examination in adults. Prospective study of 200 patients. Mayo Clin Proc 55:291, 1980.
3. Schiller NB, Shah PM, Crawford M et al: Recommendations for quantitation of the left ventricle by two-dimensional echocardiography. J Am Soc Echocard 2:358, 1989.
4. Pearlman JD, Triulzi MD, King ME et al: Limits of normal left ventricular dimension in growth and development: Analysis of dimensions and variance in the two-dimensional echocardiograms of 268 normal healthy subjects. J Am Cell Cardiol 12:1432, 1988.
5. Schnittger I, Gordon EP, Fitzgerald PJ et al: Standardized intracardiac measurements of two-dimensional echocardiography. J Am Coll Cardiol 2:934, 1983.
6. Henry WL, Gardin JM, Ware JH: Echocardiographic measurements in normal subjects from infancy to old age. Circulation 62:1054, 1980.
7. Nishimura RA, Miller FA Jr, Callahan MJ et al: Doppler echocardiography: Theory, instrumentation, technique and application. Mayo Clin Proc 60:321, 1985.
8. Louie EK: Congestive cardiomyopathy: Doppler echocardiographic assessment of structure and function. Echocardiography 4:119, 1987.
9. Folland ED, Parisi AF, Moynihan PF et al: Assessment of left ventricular ejection fraction and volumes by real-time, two-dimensional echocardiography. Circulation 60:760, 1979.
10. Louie EK, Maron BJ, Green KJ: Variations in flow-velocity waveforms obtained by pulsed Doppler echocardiography in the normal human aorta. Am J Cardiol 58:821, 1986.
11. Sabbah HN, Khaja F, Brymer JF et al: Noninvasive evaluation of left ventricular performance based on peak aortic blood acceleration measured with a continuous-wave Doppler velocity meter. Circulation 74:323, 1986.
12. Elkayam U, Gardin JM, Berkley R et al: The use of Doppler flow velocity measurement to assess the hemodynamic response to vasodilators in patients with heart failure. Circulation 67:377, 1983.
13. Looyenga DS, Liebson PR, Bone RC et al: Determination of cardiac output in critically ill patients by dual beam echocardiography. J Am Coll Cardiol 13:340, 1989.
14. Spirito D, Maron BJ: Doppler echocardiography for assessing left ventricular diastolic function. Ann Intern Med 109:122, 1988.
15. Thomas JD, Weyman AE: Fluid dynamics model of mitral valve flow: description with in vitro validation. J Am Coll Cardiol 13:221, 1989.
16. Konstadt SN, Reich DL, Thys DM et al: Contribution of atrial systole to ventricular filling assessed by transesophageal echocardiography. Anesthesiology 72:971, 1990.
17. Borow KM, Neumann A, Wynne J: Sensitivity of end-systolic pressure-dimension and pressure-volume relations to the inotropic state in humans. Circulation 65:988, 1982.
18. Singh S, Wann LS, Schuchard GH et al: Right ventricular and right atrial collapse in patients with cardiac tamponade—A combined echocardiographic and hemodynamic study. Circulation 70:966, 1984.
19. Louie EK, Rich S, Brundage BH: Doppler echocardiographic assessment of impaired left ventricular filling in patients with right ventricular pressure overload due to primary pulmonary hypertension. J Am Coll Cardiol 8:1298, 1986.
20. Jardin F, Dubourg O, Gueret P et al: Quantitative two-dimensional echocardiography in massive pulmonary embolism: Emphasis on ventricular interdependence and leftward septal displacement. J Am Coll Cardiol 10:1201, 1987.
21. Dittrich HC, Nicod PH, Chow LC et al: Early changes of right heart geometry after pulmonary thromboendarterectomy. J Am Coll Cardiol 11:937, 1988.
22. Jardin F, Gueret P, Prost JF et al: Two-dimensional echocardiographic assessment of left ventricular function in chronic obstructive pulmonary disease. Am Rev Respir Dis 129:135, 1984.
23. King ME, Braun H, Goldblatt A et al: Interventricular septal configuration as a predictor of right ventricular systolic hypertension in children: A cross-sectional echocardiographic study. Circulation 68:68, 1983.

24. Dittrich HC, Chow LC, Nicod PH: Early improvement in left ventricular diastolic function after relief of chronic right ventricular pressure overload. Circulation 80:823, 1989.
25. Louie EK, Bieniarz T, Moore AM et al: Reduced atrial contribution to left ventricular filling in patients with severe tricuspid regurgitation after tricuspid valvulectomy: A Doppler echocardiographic study. J Am Coll Cardiol 16:1617–1624, 1990.
26. Louie EK, Rich S, Levitsky S et al: Differential effects of right ventricular pressure and volume loading on left ventricular filling assessed by Doppler echocardiography. J Am Coll Cardiol 13:196A, 1989.
27. Louie EK, Maron BJ: Hypertrophic cardiomyopathy with extreme increase in left ventricular wall thickness: Functional and morphologic features and clinical significance. J Am Coll Cardiol 8:57, 1986.
28. Louie EK, Maron BJ: Apical hypertrophic cardiomyopathy: Clinical and two-dimensional echocardiographic assessment. Ann Intern Med 106:663, 1987.
29. Reeder GS, Seward JB, Tajik AJ: The role of two-dimensional echocardiography in coronary artery disease. A critical appraisal. Mayo Clin Proc 57:247, 1982.
30. Louie EK, Rich S: Acute myocardial infarction, in Dantzker (ed): *Cardiopulmonary Critical Care,* 2d ed. Philadelphia, WB Saunders (in press).
31. Louie EK: Echocardiographic evaluation of valvular heart disease, in Brundage BH (ed): *Comparative Cardiac Imaging: Function, Flow, Anatomy, Quantitation.* Rockville, MD, Aspen Publishers, 1990, pp. 293–309.
32. Louie EK: Doppler echocardiographic evaluation of valvular heart disease, in Brundage BH (ed): *Comparative Cardiac Imaging: Function, Flow, Anatomy, Quantitation.* Rockville, MD, Aspen Publishers, 1990, pp. 311–328.
33. DeMaria AN, Bommer W, Joye J et al: Value and limitations of cross-sectional echocardiography of the aortic valve in the diagnosis and quantification of valvular aortic stenosis. Circulation 62:304, 1980.
34. Smith MD, Handshoe R, Handshoe S et al: Comparative accuracy of two-dimensional echocardiography and Doppler pressure half-time methods in assessing severity of mitral stenosis in patients with and without prior commissurotomy. Circulation 73:100, 1986.
35. Currie PJ, Seward JB, Reeder GS et al: Continuous wave Doppler echocardiographic assessment of severity of calcific aortic stenosis: A simultaneous Doppler-catheter correlative study in 100 adult patients. Circulation 71:1162, 1985.
36. Oh JK, Taliercio CP, Holmes DR et al: Prediction of the severity of aortic stenosis by Doppler aortic valve area determination: Prospective Doppler-catheterization correlation in 100 patients. J Am Coll Cardiol 11:1227, 1988.
37. Sagar KB, Wann LS, Paulsen WHJ et al: Doppler echocardiographic evaluation of Hancock and Bjork-Shiley prosthetic valves. J Am Coll Cardiol 7:681, 1986.
38. Panidis IP, Rose J, Mintz GS: Normal and abnormal prosthetic valve function as assessed by Doppler echocardiography. J Am Coll Cardiol 8:317, 1986.
39. Louie EK, Louie DS: Doppler echocardiographic detection, characterization and quantification of valvular regurgitation. Am J Card Imaging 3:229, 1989.
40. Yoganathan AP, Cape EG, Sung HW et al: Review of hydrodynamic principles for the cardiologist: Applications to the study of blood flow and jets by imaging techniques. J Am Coll Cardiol 12:1344, 1988.
41. Louie EK, Krukenkamp I, Hariman RJ et al: Quantitative assessment of aortic insufficiency by color flow Doppler in an open chest canine model. Cardiovasc Res 22:145, 1989.
42. Louie EK, Louie DS: Color flow Doppler mapping of aortic regurgitation: Physical principles and clinical application. Am J Card Imaging 2:322, 1988.
43. Sahn DJ: Instrumentation and physical factors related to visualizaton of stenotic and regurgitant jets by Doppler color flow mapping. J Am Coll Cardiol 12:1354, 1988.
44. Helmcke F, Nanda NC, Hsiung MC et al: Color Doppler assessment of mitral regurgitation with orthogonal planes. Circulation 75:175, 1987.
45. Perry GJ, Helmcke F, Nanda NC et al: Evaluation of aortic insufficiency by Doppler color flow mapping. J Am Coll Cardiol 9:952, 1987.
46. Yock PG, Popp RL: Noninvasive estimation of right ventricular systolic pressure by Doppler ultrasound in patients with tricuspid regurgitation. Circulation 70:657, 1984.
47. Berger M, Haimowitz A, Van Tosh A et al: Quantitative assessment of pulmonary hypertension in patients with tricuspid regurgitation using continuous wave Doppler ultrasound. J Am Coll Cardiol 6:359, 1985.
48. Kostucki W, Vandenbossche JL, Friart A et al: Pulsed Doppler regurgitant flow patterns of normal valves. Am J Cardiol 58:309, 1986.
49. Berger M, Hecht SR, Van Tosh A et al: Pulsed and continuous wave Doppler echocardiographic assessment of valvular regurgitation in normal subjects. J Am Coll Cardiol 13:1540, 1989.
50. Kapur KK, Fan P, Nanda NC et al: Doppler color flow mapping in the evaluation of prosthetic mitral and aortic valve function. J Am Coll Cardiol 13:1561, 1989.
51. Liu MW, Louie EK, Levitsky S: Color flow Doppler assessment of aortic regurgitation complicated by aneurysmal dilation and dissection of the ascending aorta in the Marfan syndrome. Am Heart J 115:1118, 1988.
52. Hashimoto S, Kumada T, Osakada G et al: Assessment of transesophageal Doppler echography in dissecting aortic aneurysm. J Am Coll Cardial 14:1253, 1989.
53. Erbel R, Daniel W, Visser C et al: Echocardiography in diagnosis of aortic dissection. Lancet 1:457, 1989.

Chapter 22

PERIOPERATIVE TRANSESOPHAGEAL ECHOCARDIOGRAPHY

LAURENCE SEGIL
STEVEN KONSTADT

Conventional echocardiographic technology is an excellent and established modality for the noninvasive assessment of the structure and function of the heart.[1] In recent years, echocardiography has found increasing application in critical care. As detailed in Chap. 21, echocardiography yields important diagnostic information in a rapid noninvasive fashion. Transesophageal echocardiography (TEE) is a technique that exploits the proximity of the esophagus to the heart to obtain anatomic and physiologic information that may not be possible with precordial imaging. TEE has proven to be very useful in several different settings. TEE is widely used to monitor cardiovascular function in the anesthetized patient during surgery. Since much information is available on this use, this review will comment on operating room applications. In the awake, nonanesthetized patient TEE has proved to be a valuable adjunct in those patients who are difficult to image from the precordium and has assumed primacy over precordial imaging for evaluation of prosthetic valves and intracardiac masses and shunts. TEE has been applied in the critical care unit to both supplement precordial imaging and monitor therapy or disease progression. TEE can be used to gather the same information as conventional echocardiography, but has the advantages of an unobstructed window for ultrasound and a stable transducer position that does not interfere with a surgical procedure. In the ICU, the unobstructed view afforded by the esophageal location of the probe is very important. Positive-pressure ventilation, especially with end-expiratory pressure, frequently makes precordial imaging difficult. Chest wall trauma, abdominal or thoracic surgery, burns, or dressings may interfere with precordial imaging. Therefore, TEE has come to assume an importance in critical care that will likely expand with time.

Physical Basis of Sonographic Imaging

All echocardiography is based on the same physical principles. A steered beam of focused, high frequency (typically >1 MHz) sound is broadcast into a tissue over a several millisecond time interval. When the transducer is not transmitting, it serves as a detector for the ultrasound reflected back from the tissues. Reflection occurs in any tissue or at any tissue interface which alters the speed of sound. The time from the transmission of the signal until it is returned is related to the distance of the echogenic site from the transducer and the speed of sound in the intervening tissues. For practical purposes, this transmission speed is constant for the human body, and the delay between the transmission and the receipt of the ultrasound signal is a direct measure of distance, or depth, of the imaged target from the transducer.

The energy returned to the transducer by any tissue depends on many different factors, but differences in echogenicity are displayed as differences in levels of gray on the echo images created. Therefore, the displayed echo image contains information concerning the distance and angular location of a tissue from the transducer, as well as some measure of tissue echogenicity. Since the ultrasound transmit-receive cycle is repeated many times a second, the display also shows how the structures change over time. The images are reconstructed and displayed to show the two-dimensional structure of the imaged object, as well as a gray scale measure of returned energy. M-mode ultrasonography alternatively displays a plot of distance from the transducer versus time, enabling the measurement of repetitive changes in structure over time. If the imaged structure is in motion in a direction which has any component parallel to the direction of travel of the ultrasound beam, then the frequency of the reflected ultrasound beam will be changed in proportion to the parallel velocity of the imaged structure. This Doppler shifting of the ultrasound beam can also be detected by the receiving transducer and is the physical basis behind Doppler echocardiography. The shift in the ultrasound frequency can be color encoded and displayed over a two-dimensional representation of the imaged structure. Typically, Doppler echocardiography uses red blood cells as the reflectors and therefore provides information on blood velocity which can be superimposed on an image of cardiac structures.

Most currently available TEE probes are phased array transducers fitted on the tip of a standard gastrointestinal endoscope. Other probe technologies, such as mechanical and annular array, are available. The biplane steering controls of the endoscope are left intact for maneuvering the probe tip. The actual ultrasound machine is typically a standard diagnostic cardiology machine with minimal modifications for the TEE probe. Several companies offer biplane transducers that will enable multiple views or simultaneous views without repositioning the probe. Transducers built on 5-mm endoscopes for pediatric use are also available.

Indications for Transesophageal Echocardiography

There are several advantages to esophageal echocardiography in the perioperative period (Table 22-1). During surgery, the anesthesiologist usually has access to the head, while frequently the areas of the chest required for conventional echocardiography are included in the surgical field. A probe located in the esophagus rarely interferes with sur-

TABLE 22-1 Indications for Transesophageal Echocardiography

Monitoring Uses
Chamber volume
Contractility
Ischemia
Valvular function
Intracardiac air or other emboli
Diagnostic Uses
Inadequate precordial images (commonly due to lung or chest wall pathology)
Evaluation or prosthetic valve function
Intracardiac masses
Evaluation of the interatrial septum
Detection of probe-patent foramen ovale
Acute right heart failure

gery. Additionally, the esophagus provides a stable location for the transducer, which enables continuous observation from a fixed location. It is actually very difficult to achieve this with a precordial probe. Bone and air-filled lungs are poor transmitters of ultrasound and frequently interfere with images obtained from the precordium. However, the esophagus lies immediately behind the heart and interference from other structures is minimal. This is particularly useful in patients with pulmonary disease or on positive-pressure ventilation, when increased lung volumes cause difficulty in precordial imaging. The esophageal position of the probe is also excellent for imaging the left atrium and mitral valve. This has proven very useful in the assessment of valve repairs during cardiac surgery.

Technique

The anatomy of the esophagus and stomach limits the positioning of an esophageal probe to a lesser number of imaging locations than are available from the precordium. Except for a few transgastric views, the transducer is restricted to a position in the midline directly behind the heart. Rotation and biplane steering of the probe tip enables limited angulation of the ultrasound beam to change the area imaged, but different views are obtained primarily by varying the depth to which the probe is placed within the esophagus (Fig. 22-1). As the probe is advanced from a proximal position, the examiner is able to view the great vessels, then the root of the aorta along with the surrounding atrial structures, followed by the aortic valve, left ventricular outflow tract, mitral and tricuspid valves, then both ventricles in a long axis view, followed finally by short axis views of the left ventricle at varying levels (Figs. 22-2 through 22-6). The three views used most commonly are a short axis view of the valvular and atrial structures of the base of the heart, the long axis view of both ventricles and atrioventricular (AV) valves, and the short axis view of the left ventricle. Special maneuvers with the probe enable specific examination of the left atrial appendage (Fig. 22-7), interatrial septum, pulmonary veins, venae cavae, and proximal coronary arteries (see Plate 18).

Monitoring with TEE during surgery is usually begun shortly after the patient is anesthetized and intubated. The probe is easy to insert and can usually be placed in less than a minute with imaging beginning immediately. Obviously, it is not a useful monitor during induction. The probe can be left in place throughout a surgical procedure for continuous or intermittent imaging. It appears to be a safe modality even in the presence of anticoagulation. Esophageal pathology such as varices, strictures, tumors, or scleroderma mandate that caution be used, but TEE has been performed even during liver transplantation without untoward complications. The probe can be removed at the conclusion of the anesthetic or left in place for postoperative monitoring in the ICU if the patient is to remain intubated. It is usually possible to place a nasogastric tube along with the TEE probe if the patient's condition necessitates. TEE examinations can be performed in the ICU on intubated patients with supplementary sedation and topical anesthesia or on awake nonintubated patients if adequate topical anesthesia is provided.

From a technical viewpoint, TEE in the awake patient is very similar to upper gastrointestinal endoscopy. In our institution, we have found a set protocol to be useful. Available personnel include the physician performing the examination, an ultrasonographer, and a nurse familiar with anesthesia and the critical care environment. All patients are monitored with an electrocardiogram (ECG), pulse oximeter, and a blood pressure cuff, and have been NPO prior to the examination. Nasal cannula oxygen is available if indicated. Intravenous access is obtained for drug administration. Resuscitation and airway equipment must be available. Suction is critical for patient comfort during the examination. Pretreatment with an antisialogogue such as glycopyrrolate is very helpful, although it does not eliminate the need for suction. Midazolam or another sedative may help an anxious patient tolerate the procedure. Appropriate antibiotics are given in patients with prosthetic valves. We anesthetize the pharynx initially by having the patient gargle with and then swallow a viscous lidocaine preparation. The pharynx is further anesthetized by directly spraying a topical anesthetic on the tongue, hard and soft palate, uvula, and deeper pharyngeal structures. The examiner ought to be able to insert his fingers or a tongue blade to the posterior pharynx without causing the patient any discomfort. The patient is placed in the left lateral decubitus position and given control of a Yankauer suction catheter for secretions. A bite-block is inserted, followed by the TEE probe with the biplane controls unlocked. The probe is gently advanced to the posterior pharynx. If the patient is gagging or uncomfortable, the topical anesthesia is supplemented, or superior laryngeal nerve blocks can be performed. When the probe is near the cricopharyngeus, we ask the patient to swallow while constant gentle pressure is maintained on the probe. Once the probe tip is in the esophagus, it advances easily, can be manipulated to perform the examination, and the patient is usually comfortable and only requires suctioning of the pharynx. At the conclusion of the examination, we observe patients until the effects of any administered sedation have abated and

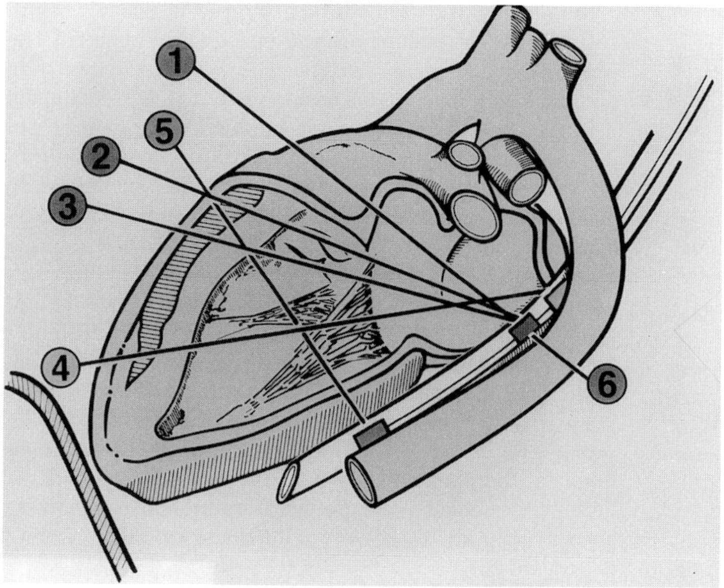

FIGURE 22-1 Positions of the tip of the TEE probe within the esophagus to obtain the standard TEE images. The numbered angles correspond to Figs. 22-2 through 22-7. (Diagram courtesy of Hewlett-Packard, Andover, MA.)

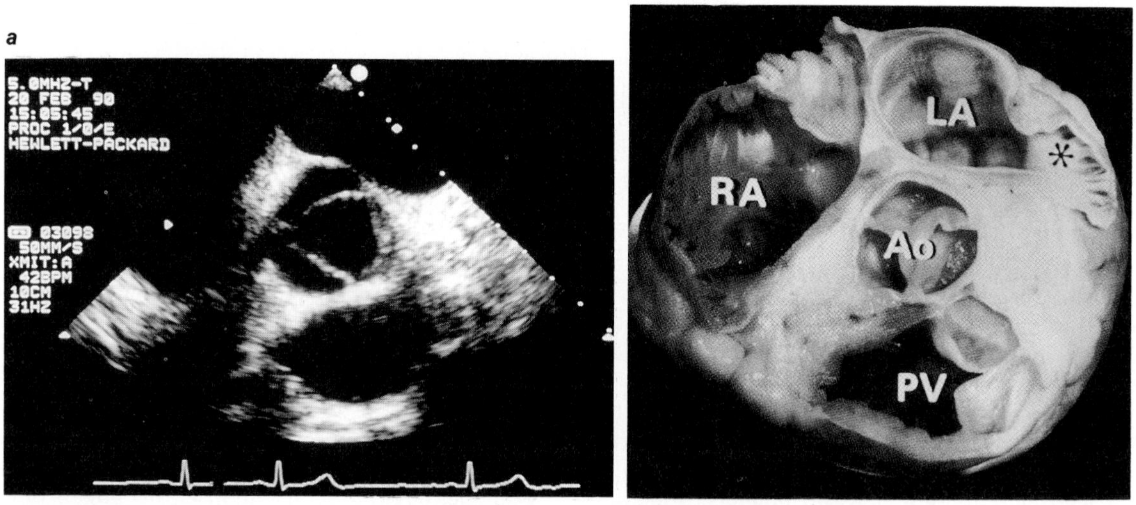

FIGURE 22-2 ***a.*** **Basal short axis view. The left atrium (LA) and its appendage, the aortic valve (Ao), the interatrial septum, the right atrium (RA), the right ventricular outflow tract, and pulmonic valve (PV) can be examined at this depth. Rotation of the probe permits examination of the fossa ovalis, angulation brings in the left atrial appendage.** ***b.*** **Corresponding anatomic section demonstrates visualized structures. (Figure courtesy of Hewlett-Packard, Andover, MA.)**

counsel them to not eat or drink until normal sensation has returned to the pharynx.

Interpretation

To be useful, a monitor must provide easily interpreted data relevant to a patient's clinical condition in a timely fashion. During surgery, the anesthesiologist must rapidly assess the patient's hemodynamic and myocardial status in the face of rapidly changing clinical conditions, such as termination of cardiopulmonary bypass, aortic cross-clamping, or life-threatening hemorrhage. TEE can provide instantaneous, understandable visual information concerning volume status, myocardial contractility and ischemia, and acute changes in valvular or ventricular function. Studies from both Duke Medical Center and the Mayo Clinic have shown that postoperative interpretation by different observers of intraoperative echocardiographic studies are consistent.[2,3] Of note, a study to demonstrate reproa

b

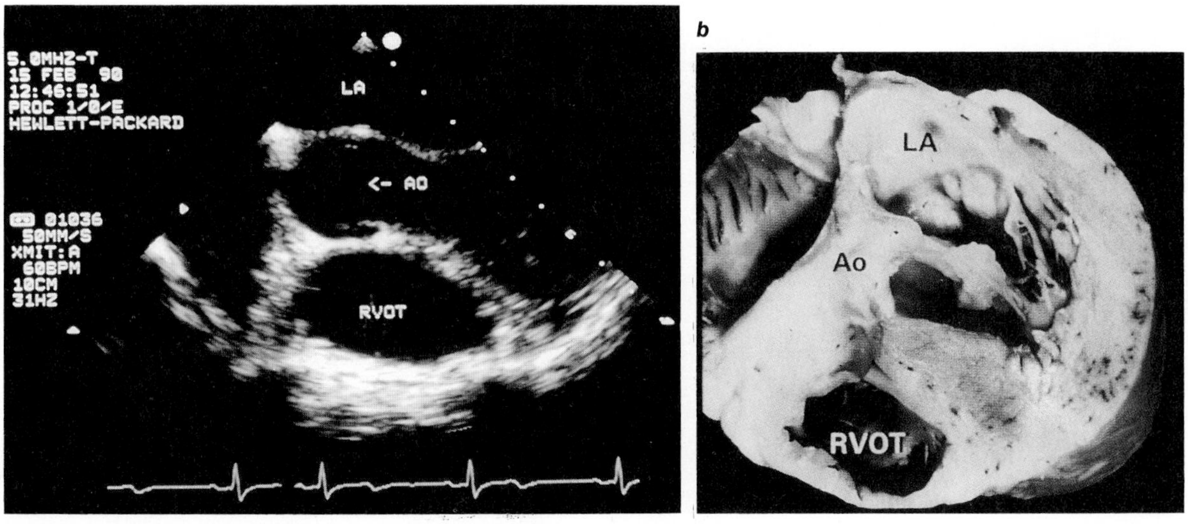

FIGURE 22-3 *a.* **Oblique two chamber view. The left and right ventricular outflow tracts (RVOT), aortic valve (Ao) and aortic root, and the left atrium (LA) can be seen.** *b.* **Corresponding anatomic section. (Figure courtesy of Hewlett-Packard, Andover, MA.)**

a

b

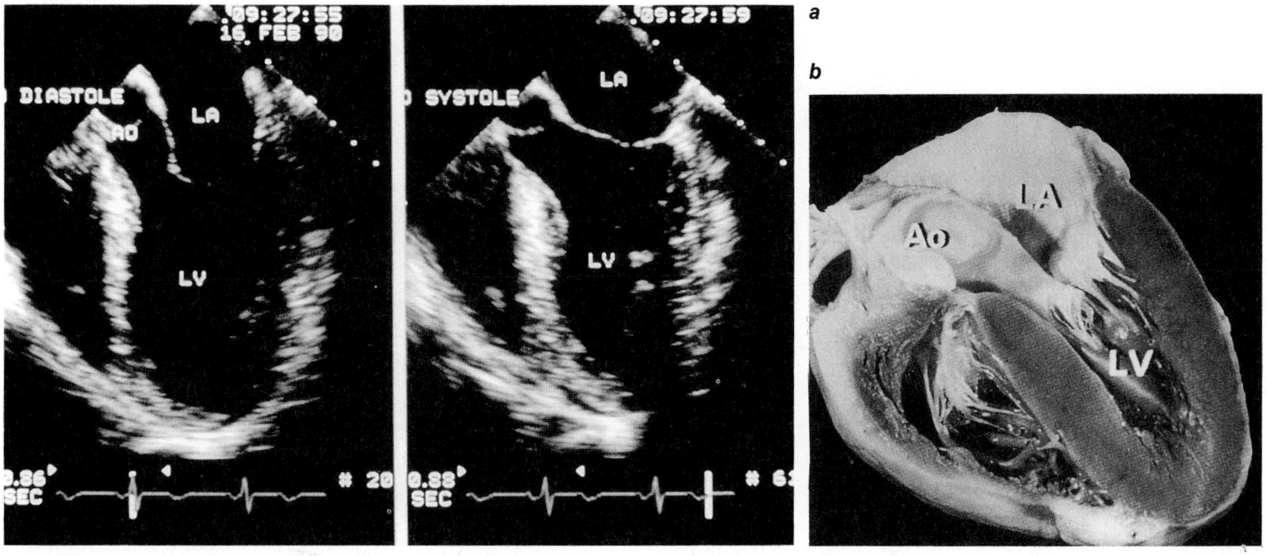

FIGURE 22-4 *a.* **Two chamber long axis view. This provides the best two-dimensional view and appropriate angle for Doppler interrogation of the mitral valve, as well as imaging the left ventricular outflow tract (Ao) and long axis view of the intraventricular septum and free wall of the left ventricle (LV). Systolic ventricular performance can be evaluated from this view. At this level upward angulation usually enables visualization of the pulmonary veins entering the left atrium (LA).** *b.* **Corresponding anatomic section. (Figure courtesy of Hewlett-Packard, Andover, MA.)**

ducibility of interpretations during surgery has not been done. However, TEE appears to fulfill the requirements of a clinically useful monitor.

DETERMINATION OF VENTRICULAR FILLING AND GLOBAL FUNCTION

Continuous observation of the short axis of the left ventricle yields information on ventricular chamber size, wall thickness, and systolic thickening. A rapid qualitative assessment of cardiac function can be made by visual analysis of the extent of systolic left ventricular emptying. Normal contraction results in all segments of the myocardium moving toward the center of the cavity. In poorly contracting hearts, the motion is decreased in some or all of the segments. In addition to these qualitative evaluations, quantitative measurements of left ventricular ejection fraction can also be made. Ideally, the echocardiographic evaluation of

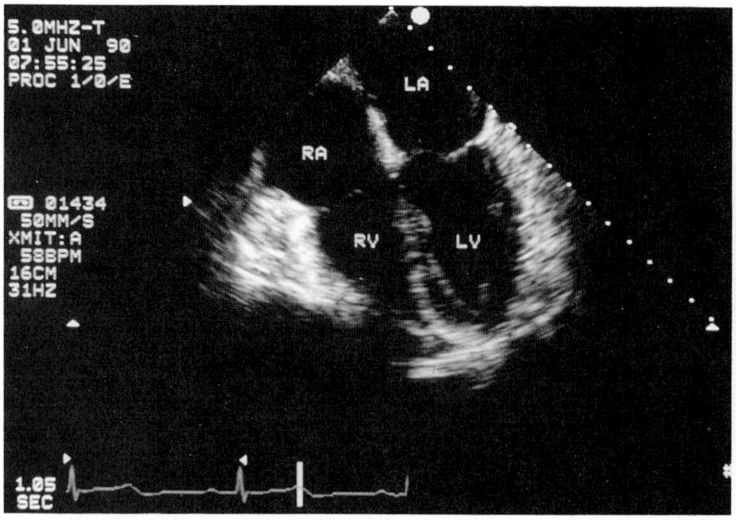

a

b

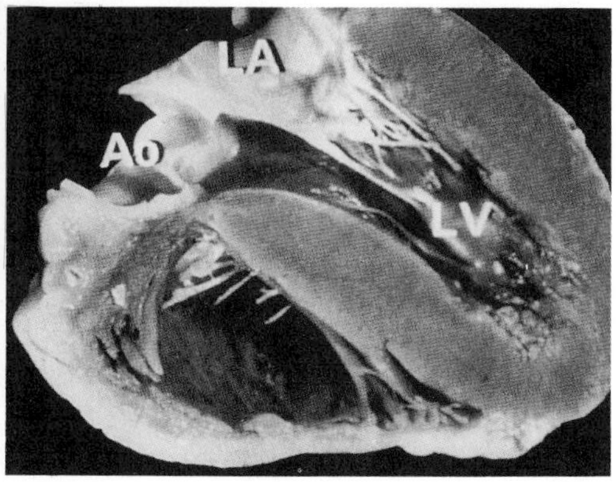

FIGURE 22-5 *a.* **Four chamber view. Allows examination of all four chambers (LA, RA, LV, RV), AV valves, interatrial and interventricular septa. Doppler interrogation of both atria and mitral and tricuspid valves can be performed at this level. Aortic valve regurgitation jets may be seen along the interventricular septum.** *b.* **Corresponding anatomic section. (Figure courtesy of Hewlett-Packard, Andover, MA.)**

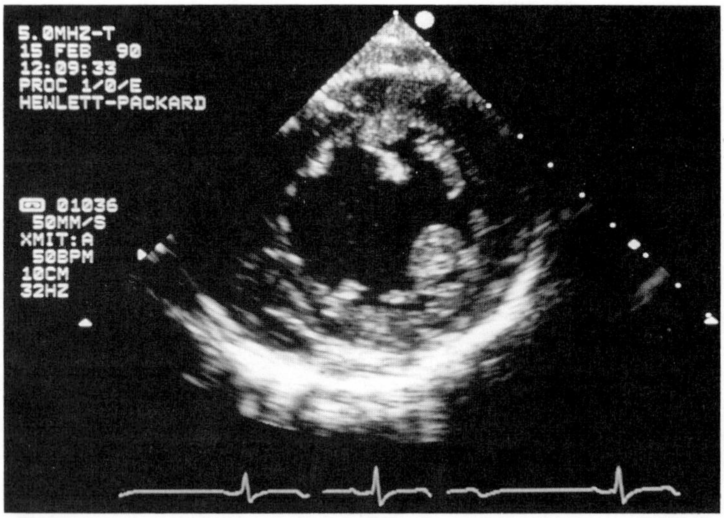

a

b

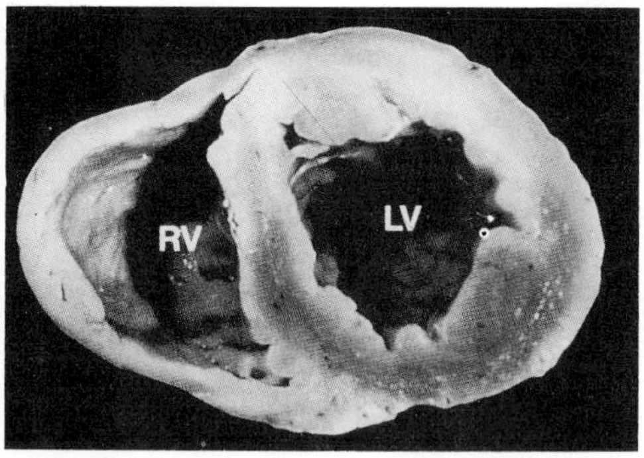

FIGURE 22-6 *a.* **Short axis view of the left ventricle (LV). This is the view most commonly used for intraoperative monitoring. Systolic function can be evaluated, and regional wall motion abnormalities are most easily seen. A portion of the perfusion bed of each of the three main coronary arteries is visible at this level.** *b.* **Corresponding anatomic section. (Figure courtesy of Hewlett-Packard, Andover, MA.)**

global left ventricular function should be performed by the combination of multiple short axis views and a long axis view of the heart. Because of practical considerations in most clinical situations only one plane is imaged and measured. In ventricles with significant heterogeneity in regional wall function the possibility for error is large. The advent of suitable automatic edge detection algorithms and multiplane echocardiographic probes may overcome this limitation.

The determination of chamber size in the monitoring of cardiovascular performance is paramount. Although chamber size is not exactly analogous to preload, certainly chamber size plays a large role in determining myocardial fiber length. Diastolic compliance of either ventricle can change acutely, rendering pressure measurements as a correlate of diastolic chamber size difficult to interpret. The lack of correlation of pulmonary capillary wedge pressure to left ventricular end-diastolic volume and stroke volume has been demonstrated using intraoperative epicardial echocardiography.[4] Echocardiography can potentially display a picture of any of the cardiac chambers directly, allowing immediate measurement of chamber dimensions.[5] Recent work with three-dimensional echocardiography has produced excellent measurements of ventricular volumes.[6]

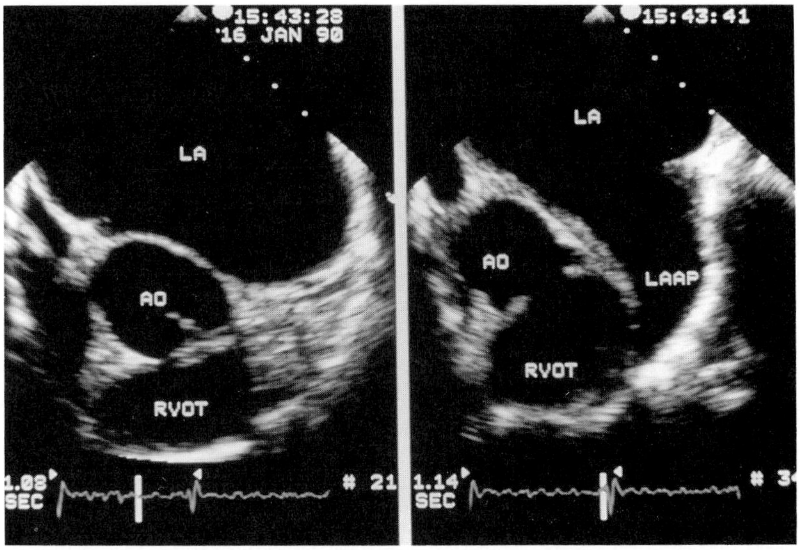

FIGURE 22-7 A markedly dilated left atrium and left atrial appendage (LAAP) as seen by TEE. Note the clear anatomy and the absence of any echogenic clot within the atrium and appendage. (Figure courtesy of Hewlett-Packard, Andover, MA.)

TEE can also be used to assess global left ventricular function. Among the earliest published uses of TEE in the operating room was a series of patients in which conventional invasive hemodynamic measurements did not enable the clinicians to find a cause for hypotension during weaning from cardiopulmonary bypass.[7] TEE demonstrated that two patients had depressed ejection fractions and responded to inotropic support, whereas the remainder had either decreased intravascular volume or low systemic vascular resistance and normal contractility by TEE. This group responded to volume and pressors, respectively. Several studies have confirmed that global ejection fraction measurements made using the short axis view of the left ventricle are reliable. Comparisons have been made with both epicardial echocardiography[4,5] and radionuclide angiography.[8,9] Other measures of global ventricular function which can be calculated include fractional shortening velocity and wall stress,[10] although these assume that there are no regional wall motion abnormalities.

DETECTION OF MYOCARDIAL ISCHEMIA

TEE can immediately observe any change in regional wall motion within the area scanned and therefore has potential as a monitor for acute ischemia. A portion of the perfusion beds of each of the three major coronary arteries can be monitored with the short axis view of the left ventricle. Conversely, TEE can document an acute improvement in segmental wall motion following coronary artery bypass grafting (CABG).[11,12] TEE detection of new regional wall motion abnormalities (RWMA) has been compared to ECG incidence of ischemia (ST segment depression) during vascular and cardiac surgery.[13] In 24 patients with new RWMA by TEE only 6 had episodes of ST segment changes. All patients with ST segment changes had RWMA, and RWMA by TEE occurred prior to or simultaneous with ECG changes. Three patients with a new RWMA that persisted to the conclusion of surgery and monitoring had myocardial infarction; only one had intraoperative ST segment changes. The authors concluded that TEE was more sensitive than 12-lead ECG monitoring for the detection of intraoperative ischemia. The issue of the specificity of RWMA by TEE for ischemia was not addressed. The same investigators confirmed greater sensitivity of TEE versus 7-lead ECG in a series of 60 patients undergoing carotid endarterectomy,[10] using both new RWMA and a calculated measure of wall stress as indicators of myocardial ischemia or risk of its development.

The importance of intraoperative and early postoperative RWMA and ECG changes has also been studied.[14] The prognostic significance of prebypass and postbypass ischemic episodes as assessed by TEE or ECG was evaluated in 50 patients undergoing CABG. TEE had 100 percent sensitivity (52 to 100 percent confidence) for detection of adverse postoperative outcomes (myocardial infarction, congestive heart failure, or cardiac death) if the new RWMA occurred either intraoperatively after cessation of cardiopulmonary bypass or in the ICU postoperatively. Prebypass RWMA did not correlate with an adverse outcome. A 2-lead ECG system was not sensitive or specific in predicting adverse outcomes. In 18 patients with postpump TEE changes, 6 had an adverse outcome. The positive predictive value of a new RWMA in the postpump or early ICU period was 33 percent (95 percent confidence interval 14 to 57 percent), while the negative predictive value was 100 percent (87 to 100 percent). Five patients had ECG changes (2-lead system) in the same time period without concomitant RWMA, none with an adverse outcome. The authors concluded that TEE was more sensitive and specific as a predictor of adverse outcomes than ECG. The study was limited by the use of retrospective analysis (although blinded) of the echo tapes, the small number of adverse events, and the 2-lead ECG system.

In the past, some investigators have claimed that an acute rise in the pulmonary capillary wedge pressure

(PCWP) is a marker for ischemia. This indicator has been compared to TEE detection of ischemia.[15] Although there was a statistically significant rise in the PCWP associated with new RWMA, the magnitude of the rise was too small to make it a clinically useful monitor (3.5 ± 4.8 mmHg). The sensitivity and positive predictive value of a 3 mmHg rise in the PCWP were quite low, 25 and 15 percent respectively. The authors concluded that wedge pressure changes are not a reliable way to monitor for myocardial ischemia, particularly when compared with the sensitivity of RWMA detected by TEE.

MONITORING FOR AIR EMBOLUS

TEE is the most sensitive technique for monitoring for intracardiac air or other embolic material. Intracardiac air is thought to be a major cause of neurologic morbidity following open heart surgery and hemodynamic instability during neurosurgery in the sitting position. An air-blood interface is a superb reflector of ultrasound, enabling TEE to detect as little as 0.2 mL/kg/min of air infused intravenously.[16] TEE is more sensitive than other available ways of detecting venous air embolism, particularly precordial Doppler. An additional benefit is the ability of TEE to distinguish which chambers of the heart contain air. In one series of 20 patients in the sitting position during neurosurgery, 3 exhibited right-to-left atrial shunting of air, presumably due to a probe patent foramen ovale.[17] No other technique for monitoring for air embolism can detect this potentially very dangerous problem.

In another series, intracardiac air was identified in 11 of 15 patients undergoing open cardiotomy but in only 2 of 18 patients in a contemporaneous group of patients undergoing CABG without cardiotomy.[18] The finding of intracardiac air led the clinicians to perform vigorous maneuvers to remove the air. Three patients had postoperative neurologic deficits, all had intracardiac air; none of the patients without air had postoperative deficits. Similar results were obtained in a series of 79 patients in which the incidence of intracardiac air was 67 percent after valve surgery, but only 14 percent after CABG.[19] No adverse neurologic sequelae were reported. Reduction of morbidity from systemic air emboli remains to be proven, but TEE is promising in this regard.

ASSESSMENT OF VALVE FUNCTION

The function of the AV valves following valve repair or replacement is assessed quickly and accurately by color flow mapping using TEE (see Plate 19). After valve repair, the accurate assessment of the presence of residual regurgitation or stenosis is critical to management. The location of the esophageal probe directly behind the left atrium enables TEE to interrogate both AV valves. Many investigators have published their experiences using intraoperative TEE or epicardial echocardiography to facilitate evaluation of surgical correction of complex congenital defects and valve repairs.[20–22] The largest published series on valvular surgery from Duke Medical Center showed that intraoperative assessment of valve function by TEE altered surgical management in 41 of 154 patients and particularly in 42 percent of patients having mitral valve surgery.[20] Although the placement of the probe is not as ideal for the assessment of aortic valve function, it is possible to detect residual regurgitation using either color flow mapping or injection of microbubbles into the aortic root. Because valvular function is easily assessed by TEE without interfering in the surgical field as the patient is being weaned from cardiopulmonary bypass, the technique is now widely used.

DIASTOLIC FUNCTION

Diastolic characteristics of the heart can be successfully investigated with TEE. Again, the favorable view of the mitral valve has been used. A recording of blood velocity over time entering the left ventricle is obtained by placing a Doppler sample volume in the inflow tract. Mitral flow is biphasic; there is an early diastolic phase that is a measure of passive relaxation of the left ventricle, and a late phase caused by atrial systole. Usually passive filling predominates, but as the left ventricle becomes stiff and less compliant, atrial systole becomes more important. TEE Doppler has been used to assess the relative contribution of atrial systole to total left ventricular filling, and it has been found that those patients with a larger component of late diastolic filling drop their stroke volume when ventricular pacing is initiated.[23] In another study, patients with a high central venous pressure (CVP), probably corresponding to elevated intrapericardial pressure, had a greater constraint to early left ventricular filling and were more dependent on atrial systole. After opening the pericardium, early diastolic filling increased in patients with a high CVP.[24]

Other investigators have used the transmitral flow-velocity integral to measure cardiac output. Assuming the diameter of the mitral annulus is constant, cardiac output is directly proportional to the transmitral flow velocity which is readily measured by TEE Doppler. Correlation coefficients as high as $R = 0.98$ compared with thermodilution measurements have been reported, although in some studies there is considerably more scatter.[25]

ATRIAL AND VENTRICULAR THROMBUS

Because of the proximate location of the probe to the left atrium, TEE is more sensitive than precordial echo for the detection of intracardiac thrombi or masses (Fig. 22-8). The superior resolution can permit the distinction between tumor, thrombus, or vegetation in most cases. Some clinicians now consider TEE to be a standard part of the work-up of patients with suspected systemic emboli. It is also useful in assessing patients prior to mitral valvuloplasty, because the morphology of the mitral valve, fossa ovalis, and left atrial appendage can be clearly imaged. Patency of the fossa ovalis can be assessed with the venous injection of microbubbles and observation of their passage across the fossa.

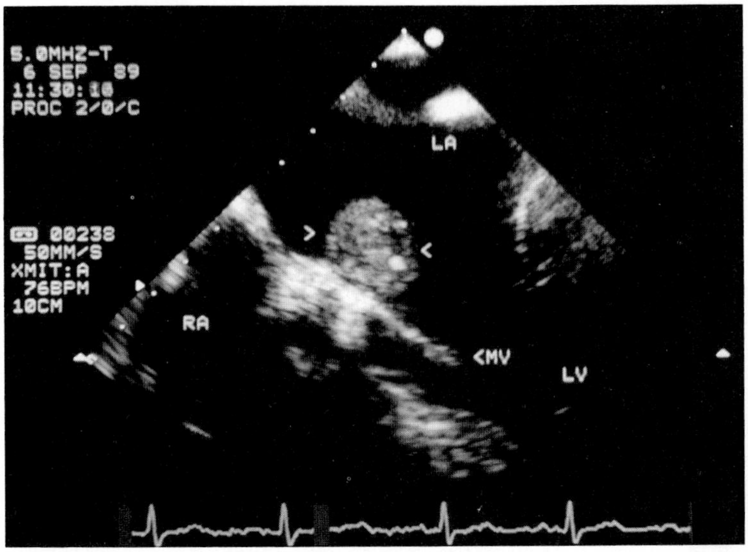

FIGURE 22-8 A large tumor can be seen adherent to the septal attachment of the anterior leaflet of the mitral valve within the left atrium. In patients with mitral or aortic valvular calcification, this location may be difficult to image from the precordium. (Figure courtesy of Hewlett-Packard, Andover, MA.)

APPLICATIONS OF TRANSESOPHAGEAL CONTRAST ECHOCARDIOGRAPHY

One very provocative experimental application of TEE involves new advances in contrast echocardiography. An ultrasound contrast agent consists of microbubbles which create an air-blood interface. Depending on manufacturing technique, they range in size from 2 to 50 μm. The microbubbles follow blood flow and offer the possibility of assessing regional myocardial perfusion with echocardiography. Imaging of coronary perfusion beds in human beings with sonicated Renografin before and after CABG surgery has been accomplished,[26] and the same technique can verify the adequacy of saphenous vein bypass graft anastomoses prior to weaning from cardiopulmonary bypass.[27] Newer contrast agents are being manufactured which can transit the lungs after an intravenous injection (Albunex, Molecular Biosystems). The new small microbubbles offer the intriguing possibility of repeatable noninvasive assessment of myocardial perfusion with echocardiography.[28–30] Contrast echocardiography is also the most sensitive method for detecting intracardiac right-to-left shunts, particularly probe patent foramen ovale.[31]

ASSESSMENT OF RIGHT VENTRICULAR FUNCTION

Frequently, patients on positive-pressure ventilation have inadequate precordial echo examinations because of interference from the lungs and inadequate positioning. TEE can be performed safely and easily in the intubated patient. Invasive hemodynamic measurements are occasionally difficult to interpret in the face of positive end-expiratory pressure (PEEP), and the relative role of right versus left ventricular failure is sometimes hard to judge. TEE has confirmed the observation that PEEP interferes with left ventricular filling by reducing venous return to the right heart and therefore decreases right ventricular preload.[32]

TEE is helpful to identify patients with normal left ventricular systolic function and dilated hypocontractile right ventricles (Fig. 22-9). These patients have high wedge pressures, probably due to ventricular interdependence, and low stroke volumes. The diagnosis of right heart failure made by TEE enables one to optimize their hemodynamic management. It is also possible to diagnose right ventricular failure secondary to acute pulmonary vascular events, at a time when the ECG is suggestive of inferior wall left ventricular ischemia. After making the appropriate diagnosis, one is able to treat the patient by raising the systemic pressure, thereby improving right ventricular perfusion and right ventricular systolic performance. The diagnosis of acute right ventricular infarction after cardiopulmonary bypass when the hemodynamic data suggest pericardial tamponade can also be achieved.

Complications

Despite widespread use, few complications of TEE have been reported in the literature. Some potential complications of TEE are listed in Table 22-2, although not all have been reported. Two cases of transient vocal cord paralysis were reported following monitoring for air embolism in patients undergoing craniotomy in the sitting position.[33] The early TEE probe used in both patients was thicker and stiffer than current probes, and since the introduction of the newer probes, no further incidents have been reported.

There has been one report of a small bowel obstruction caused by the undetected passage of an esophageal stethoscope into a patient's stomach during TEE probe manipulation under general anesthesia.[34] Any object in the pharynx could theoretically be forced into the stomach during probe insertion, and care must be taken to avoid such mishaps.

Despite the size and stiffness of the TEE probe there are few reports of direct esophageal trauma. One elderly woman undergoing cardiac surgery developed a Mallory-Weiss tear thought to be secondary to TEE monitoring.[35]

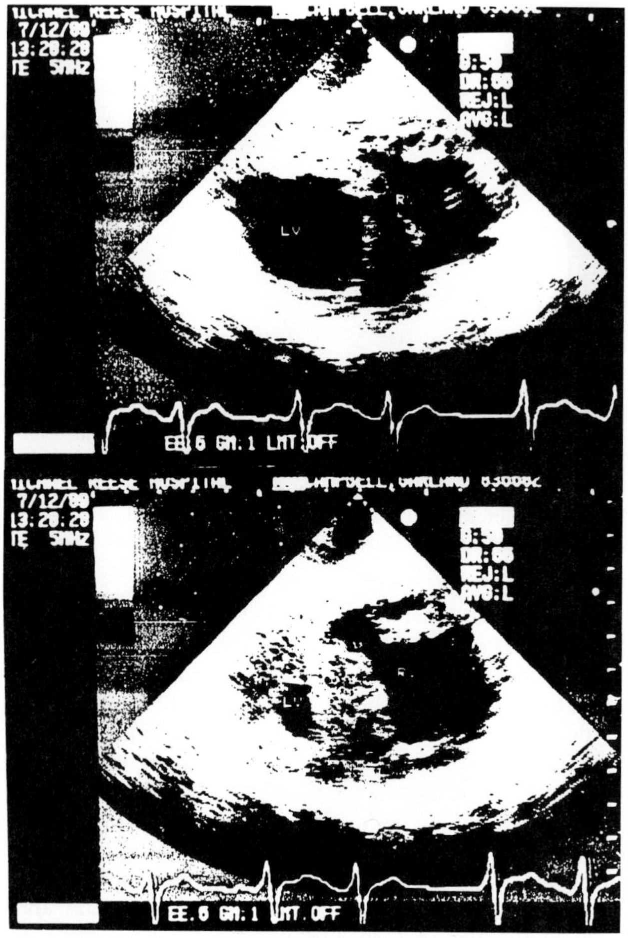

FIGURE 22-9 Right ventricular failure with a hypercontractile left ventricle. The right ventricular cavity (RV) is very dilated and without any apparent contraction in systole, while the left ventricular cavity (LV) is almost completely effaced during systole.

TABLE 22-2 Complications of Transesophageal Echocardiography

Esophageal Injury
Perforation
Tears
Burns
Upper Airway Injury
Laryngeal trauma
Dental and oropharyngeal trauma
Insertion of foreign bodies into stomach
Tracheal insertion of probe
Aspiration
Cardiac Injury
Arrhythmias
Hypertension
Endocarditis
Bacteremia

One death secondary to esophageal perforation in a patient with an undiagnosed esophageal cancer has been reported.

One study examined the pressures produced in the esophagus of anesthetized dogs by the flexion of the TEE probe tip used to maintain monitoring position in the operating room.[36] The investigators found that pressures generated in a balloon manometer attached to the probe were <10 mmHg. Six human beings were studied acutely, five had pressures <17 mmHg, but in one patient pressures of 60 mmHg were observed without sequelae. The authors concluded from a small sample that some patients may be at risk of injury related to high pressures on the esophageal mucosa.

Bacteremia can occur with pharyngeal and esophageal probe insertions. To date, there has been one report of endocarditis occurring within 2 weeks of a TEE examination.[37] The studies to identify the incidence of bacteremia are conflicting. One group of investigators found a 7 percent occurrence of positive blood cultures.[38] Another series reported 17 percent incidence,[39] yet another study reported no new bacteremia in a sample of 85 patients, suggesting a likelihood of bacteremia of under 3 percent.[40] None of the patients in these reported series developed clinical endocarditis. Extrapolating from the literature on bacteremia from upper gastrointestinal endoscopy, one expects a 4 to 8 percent incidence. Therefore, most clinicians recommend antibiotic prophylaxis for patients at risk of endocarditis prior to undergoing TEE examinations.

Other anecdotal reports of mishaps include supraventricular arrhythmias from mechanical stimulation of the left atrium by the probe, bradycardia from undetected hypoxia from oversedation of an awake patient, inadvertent tracheal insertion of the probe, and accidental endotracheal tube disconnections during probe manipulation in anesthetized patients. Interestingly, despite the concern for esophageal burns from heat production by the transducer, no burns have ever been documented even with the use of early probes without tip thermistors.

References

1. Feigenbaum, H: *Echocardiography*. Philadelphia, Lea & Febiger, 1986.
2. Abel MD, Neshimura RA, Callahan MJ, et al: Evaluation of intraoperative transesophageal two-dimensional echocardiography. Anesthesiology 66:64, 1987.
3. Clements FM, Hill R, Kisslo J, Orchard R: How easily can we learn to recognize regional wall motion abnormalities with 2D-transesophageal echocardiography? Proc Soc Cardiovasc Anesthesiol, 7th Annual Meeting, Montreal, 1986.
4. Thys D, Hillel Z, Goldman ME, et al: A comparison of hemodynamic indices derived by invasive monitoring and two-dimensional echocardiography. Anesthesiology 67:630, 1987.
5. Konstadt SN, Thys D, Mindich BP, et al: Validation of quantitative intraoperative transesophageal echocardiography. Anesthesiology 65:418, 1986.
6. Martin RW, Bashein G: Measurement of stroke volume with three-dimensional transesophageal ultrasonic scanning. Anesthesiology 70:470, 1989.

7. Topol EJ, Humphrey LS, Blanck TJJ, et al: Characterization of post-cardiopulmonary bypass hypotension with intraoperative transesophageal echocardiography. Anesthesiology 59:A2, 1983.
8. Martin RW, Graham M, Kao R, Bashein G: Measurement of left ventricular ejection fraction and volumes with three-dimensional reconstructed transesophageal ultrasound scans: Comparison to radionuclide and thermal dilution measurements. J Cardiothorac Anesth 3:260, 1989.
9. Urbanowicz JH, Shaaban MJ, Cohen NH, et al: Comparison of transesophageal echocardiographic and scintigraphic estimates of left ventricular end-diastolic volume index and ejection fraction in patients following coronary artery bypass grafting. Anesthesiology 72:607, 1990.
10. Smith JS, Roizen MF, Cahalan MK, et al: Does anesthetic technique make a difference? Augmentation of systolic blood pressure during carotid endarterectomy: Effects of phenylephrine versus light anesthesia and of isoflurane versus halothane on the incidence of myocardial ischemia. Anesthesiology 69:846, 1988.
11. Topol EJ, Weiss J, Guzman PM, et al: Immediate improvement of dysfunctional myocardial segments after coronary revascularization: Detection by intraoperative transesophageal echocardiography. J Am Coll Cardiol 4(6):1123, 1984.
12. Koolen JJ, Visser Ca, van Wezel HB, et al: Influence of coronary artery bypass surgery on regional left ventricular wall motion: An intraoperative two-dimensional transesophageal echocardiographic study. J Cardiothorac Anesth 1(4):276, 1987.
13. Smith JM, Cahalan MK, Benefiel DJ, et al: Intraoperative detection of myocardial ischemia in high-risk patients: Electrocardiography versus two-dimensional transesophageal echocardiography. Circulation 72(5):1015, 1985.
14. Leung JM, O'Kelly B, Browner WS, et al: Prognostic importance of postbypass regional wall-motion abnormalities in patients undergoing coronary artery bypass graft surgery. Anesthesiology 71:16, 1989.
15. van Daele ME, Sutherland GR, Mitchell MM, et al: Do changes in pulmonary capillary wedge pressure adequately reflect myocardial ischemia during anesthesia? Circulation 81:865, 1990.
16. Glenski JA, Cucchiara RF, Michebfelder JD: Transesophageal echocardiography and transcutaneous O_2 and CO_2 monitoring for detection of venous air embolism. Anesthesiology 64(5):541, 1986.
17. Cucchiara RF, Seward JB, Nishimura RA, et al: Identification of patent foramen ovale during sitting position craniotomy by transesophageal echocardiography with positive airway pressure. Anesthesiology 63(1):107, 1985.
18. Oka Y, Moriwaki KM, Hong Y, et al: Detection of air emboli in the left heart by M-mode transesophageal echocardiography following cardiopulmonary bypass. Anesthesiology 63(1):109, 1985.
19. Rodigas PC, Meyer FJ, Haasler GB, et al: Intraoperative 2-dimensional cardiography: Ejection of microbubbles from the left ventricle after cardiac surgery. Am J Cardiol 50:1130, 1982.
20. Koolen JJ, Visser CA, Wever E, et al: Transesophageal two-dimensional echocardiographic evaluation of biventricular function during positive end-expiratory pressure ventilation after coronary artery bypass grafting. Am J Cardiol 59:1047, 1987.
21. Susanne MK, Kupferwasser I, Raimund E, et al: Regurgitant flow in apparently normal valve prostheses: Improved detection and semiquantitative analysis by transesophageal two-dimensional color-coded Doppler echocardiography. J Am Soc Echocardiog 3(3):187, 1990.
22. Zaharia H, Daniel T, Ritter S, et al: Two-dimensional color flow Doppler echocardiography for the intraoperative monitoring of cardiac shunt flows in patients with congenital heart disease. J Cardiothorac Anesth 1(1):42, 1987.
23. Konstadt SN, Reich DL, Thys DM, et al: Importance of atrial systole to ventricular filling predicted by transesophageal echocardiography. Anesthesiology 72(6):971, 1990.
24. Reynertson SI, Konstadt SK, Louie EK, et al: Impact of pericardiotomy on trans-mitral left ventricular filling: An intra-operative transesophageal pulsed Doppler study. Circulation 82(4):749, 1990.
25. Ellis JE, Runyon-Hass A, Lichtor JL, et al: Can Doppler ultrasound, targeted by two dimensional transesophageal echocardiography, be used to measure cardiac output? Anesthesiology 67(3A):A638, 1987.
26. Smith JS, Feinstein SB, Kapelanski D, et al: Intraoperative determination of myocardial perfusion using contrast echocardiography. Anesthesiology 65(3A):A27, 1986.
27. Kabas JS, Kisslo J, Flick CL, et al: Intraoperative perfusion contrast echocardiography: A method to evaluate the effectiveness of coronary artery bypass grafting. J Thorac Cardiovasc Surg 99:536, 1990.
28. Segil LJ, Dick C, Feinstein SB, Silberman P: Contrast echocardiography—A new technique for intraoperative quantitation of myocardial perfusion. Anesthesiology 57(3A):A100, 1987.
29. Segil LJ, Harper PV, Metz CE, Feinstein SB: Calculation of regional blood flow and volume using an intravascular indicator with an external detector. FASEB J 2(4):A514, 1988.
30. Feinstein SB, Voci P, Segil LJ, Harper PV: Contrast echocardiography (Ch 27) in Marcus ML, Skorton DJ, Schelbert HR, Wolf GL (eds): *Cardiac Imaging—A Companion to Braunwald's* Heart Disease. Saunders, Philadelphia, 1991, pp 557–574.
31. Konstadt SK, Louie E, Kanuri D, et al: Improved intraoperative detection of interatrial shunts by transesophageal echocardiography. Anesthesiology 73:A1209, 1990.
32. Chilkanori T, Masaaki U, Sugimoto H, et al: Transesophageal echocardiographic dimensional analysis of four cardiac chambers during positive end-expiratory pressure. Anesthesiology 63:640, 1985.
33. Cucchiara RF, Nugent M, Seward JB, Messick JM: Air embolism in upright neurosurgical patients: Detection and localization by two-dimensional transesophageal echocardiography. Anesthesiology 60:353, 1984.
34. Humphrey LS: Esophageal stethoscope loss complicating transesophageal echocardiography. J Cardiothorac Anesth 2(3):356, 1988.
35. Dewhirst WE, Stragand MD, Fleming BM. Mallory-Weiss tear complicating intraoperative transesophageal echocardiography in a patient undergoing aortic valve replacement. Anesthesiology 73:777, 1990.
36. Urbanowicz JH, Kernoff RS, Oppenheim G, et al: Transesophageal echocardiography and its potential for esophageal damage. Anesthesiology 72:40, 1990.
37. Foster E, Kusumoto FM, Sobol SM, Shiller NB: Streptococcal endocarditis temporally related to transesophageal echocardiography. J Am Soc Echocardiog 3:424, 1990.
38. Dennig K, Sedlmayr V, Selig B, Rudolph W: Bacteremia with transesophageal echocardiography. Circulation 80:II473, 1989.
39. Gorge G, Erbel R, Henrichs KJ, et al: Positive blood cultures during transesophageal echocardiography. Am J Cardiol 65:1404, 1990.
40. Chandrasekaran K, Bansal RC, Minz GS, et al: Impact of transesophageal color flow Doppler echocardiography in current cardiology practice. Echocardiography 7:115, 1990.

Chapter 23

EVALUATION OF THE PATIENT WITH PERIPHERAL VASCULAR DISEASE

HISHAM S. BASSIOUNY

During the past decade, notable advances in the noninvasive diagnosis of peripheral vascular disorders and their hemodynamic sequelae have been achieved. Duplex ultrasonography has emerged as a safe, accurate, and expedient noninvasive diagnostic modality with numerous applications in patients with arterial and venous disorders. In the critical care setting, noninvasive vascular testing can be particularly valuable since the clinical evaluation is frequently compromised and invasive diagnostic procedures such as contrast angiography are less desirable. This chapter will focus on the evaluation of the most common vascular disorders and complications that may be encountered in the critical care setting with particular emphasis on noninvasive testing. The indications, principles of instrumentation, and limitations are reviewed.

Historical Perspective

In 1847, J.C. Doppler described a physical phenomenon that underlies the basic principles of ultrasound instrumentation. He demonstrated that light or acoustic frequency is perceived to be higher if the observer moves toward the source and vice versa. This principle was applied to blood flow, and in 1959, the first Doppler flow detector was developed.[1] Clinical application of this device was initiated in the early 1960s. Arterial flow mapping (ultrasonic arteriography) evolved, but its limitations were recognized, namely the inability to accurately represent blood flow in calcific vessels and the lack of real-time vascular imaging. In the early 1970s the first duplex ultrasound prototype was introduced and combined two capabilities: a real-time brightness (B) mode image and pulsed Doppler ultrasound. Thus, real-time information regarding the structural characteristics of the vessel wall and the associated flow parameters could be displayed simultaneously. Since the introduction of duplex ultrasonography, technological advancements have improved image resolution and depth of ultrasound penetration and have allowed for color coding of blood flow direction and velocity.

Acute Arterial Insufficiency

Acute upper or lower extremity arterial insufficiency is frequently encountered in the critical care setting, particularly in patients with disseminated atherosclerosis and concomitant cardiac insufficiency. It is important to discriminate between manifestations secondary to arterial insufficiency and those due to a diminished cardiac output since management will vary considerably. Distal embolization of a cardiac thrombus, in situ thrombosis, complicating a preexisting atherosclerotic plaque, and arterial cannulation with thrombosis are common causes of acute arterial ischemia. Acute limb ischemia is recognized by the presence of one or more of the six p's (pain, pallor, paraesthesia, paralysis, poikilothesia, and pulselessness). In most instances, the presentation is unilateral but could be bilateral if abdominal aortic iliac thrombosis or aortic bifurcation saddle embolization is present. Distal hypoperfusion associated with pump failure may mimic acute embolic or thrombotic arterial occlusion; however, involvement of multiple extremities and other organ systems is invariably present. In these instances, noninvasive testing can objectively assess the arterial circulation and provide pertinent information regarding the etiology of ischemia.

CONTINUOUS WAVE DOPPLER

This simple instrument consists of a Doppler pencil probe with an operating frequency of 5 to 10 MHz. The audible signal retrieved provides a subjective analysis of arterial flow but can be analog transformed to a hard copy print of the velocity waveforms. Normal upper and lower extremity waveforms are triphasic. With arterial insufficiency the waveform configuration deteriorates to a biphasic and eventually to a monophasic configuration (Fig. 23-1).[2] The level of occlusion or stenosis can be identified by segmental extremity velocity waveform analysis. For example, hemodynamically significant aortoiliac occlusive disease is represented by biphasic or monophasic waveforms in the femoral artery although a femoral pulse can be occasionally palpated. In acute arterial occlusion there is inadequate collateralization and, hence, the Doppler signal is usually absent distal to the occlusion. The continuous wave (CW) Doppler can also be used to measure segmental extremity blood pressures which provide a quantitative measure of arterial perfusion.[3] Factitiously elevated pressures are frequently found in patients with end stage renal disease and diabetes due to calcific, incompressible vessels. In these instances arterial velocity waveform analysis is more reliable. In patients with compressible arteries, the ankle: brachial pressure index can be used to assess the severity of extremity arterial insufficiency. In general, limb viability is threatened if the ankle index is less than 0.4 with rest pain and tissue loss being common manifestations.[4] Segmental limb pressure measurements should be avoided in patients with distal tibial bypasses as cuff occlusion can impede graft flow and result in graft thrombosis.

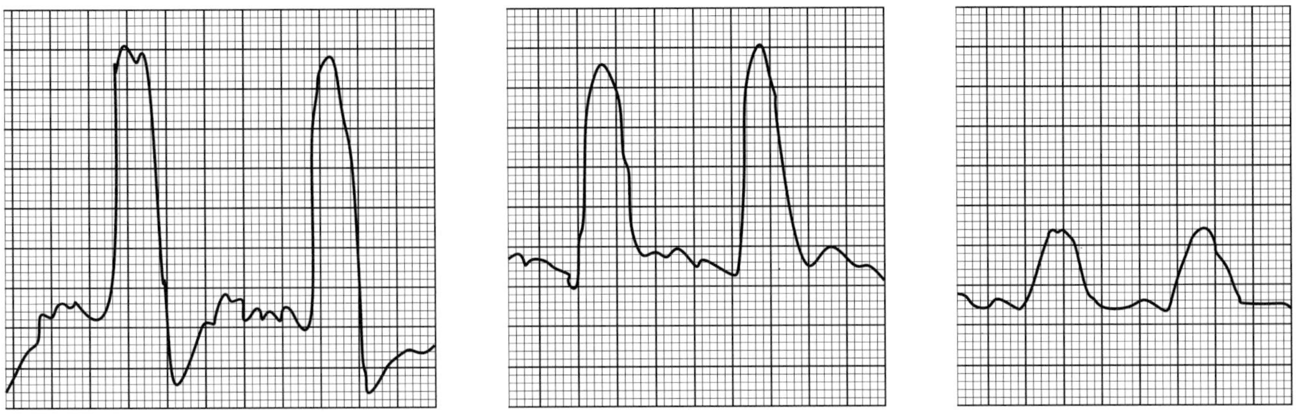

FIGURE 23-1 Waveform configuration: (*A*) triphasic, (*B*) biphasic, and (*C*) monophasic.

DUPLEX ULTRASONOGRAPHY

Better definition of the etiology and precise location of extremity arterial occlusion can be accomplished by duplex ultrasonography. The B-mode image is used to direct the pulsed Doppler sample volume to specific locations within the lumen such that centerline or near-wall flow patterns can be examined. Normal lower extremity arterial velocity parameters are now well characterized in the aortoiliac and femoropopliteal segments. Different degrees of arterial stenoses can be classified according to the various velocity spectral changes (see Plate 20). When compared to angiography, the sensitivity and specificity of duplex ultrasonography in identifying greater than 50 percent luminal diameter reduction of the aortoiliac system is 90 to 100 percent and of the femoropopliteal segment is 65 to 90 percent.[5]

Color coding of blood flow aids in rapid identification of these arteries and any associated flow disturbances. Atherosclerotic plaques are recognized by the presence of calcification, echogenicity, and lumen stenosis. Necrotic or hemorrhagic regions in an atherosclerotic plaque or intraluminal thrombus can be of similar echogenicity and are therefore difficult to discern from luminal blood flow using grey scale B-mode imaging. Color coding of blood flow, however, provides better definition of the arterial wall–blood flow interface.

Deep Venous Thrombosis

The prevalence of deep venous thrombosis (DVT) is probably highest in the intensive care setting where a host of predisposing factors such as prolonged immobility, deficient calf pump muscle action, and malignant and postoperative states coexist, leading to venous stasis and hypercoagulability.

The clinical diagnosis of DVT is unfortunately nonspecific and is accurate at best in only 50 percent of cases.[6] Moreover, a significant number of pulmonary emboli originate from clinically silent lower extremity DVTs. For these reasons, the current diagnosis of DVT has relied on noninvasive testing and a high index of clinical suspicion. Although the lower extremity venous system is most commonly involved, central and upper extremity venous thromboses are not infrequently encountered in the critical care setting because of the use of central venous catheters. These sites can be a source of pulmonary emboli and significant upper extremity morbidity.

NONINVASIVE DIAGNOSIS OF DVT

A number of noninvasive methods are currently available for the diagnosis of DVT. These include continuous wave Doppler ultrasound, plethysmographic techniques, and B-mode ultrasonography alone or with the added capability of pulsed Doppler spectral analysis (duplex) and color flow imaging.

CONTINUOUS WAVE DOPPLER

Using this portable instrument the Doppler probe is applied transcutaneously and the audible signal is subjectively interpreted with and without calf compression distal to the insonated vein. Absent or diminished spontaneous respiratory variation of flow and reduced flow augmentation by distal compression are indicative of DVT. Both upper and lower extremity veins can be examined with this device including the brachial, axillary, subclavian, femoropopliteal, and tibial veins. While simple to operate, it requires examiner skill and experience. Compared to phlebography, CW Doppler has a sensitivity rate ranging from 31 to 96 percent and a specificity rate of 85 to 100 percent in detecting above-the-knee DVTs.[7] The variability of results reported likely reflects the expertise needed to perform the study and interpret the findings. Another drawback is the inability to identify partially occlusive or calf thrombi. Despite these limitations this device can be extremely helpful in experienced hands.

PLETHYSMOGRAPHY

A number of plethysmographic methods are available including impedance air and strain gauge. The most commonly used is impedance plethysmography which relies on variation in the electric resistance across the limb secondary to blood volume changes. With DVT leg venous capacitance decreases with thigh cuff occlusion, and venous outflow is reduced with cuff deflation. Although this technique is extremely accurate in ambulatory patients with iliac and femoropopliteal thrombi,[8] it should be used with caution in patients with congestive heart failure or on ventilatory assistance as hypervolemic states may produce false-positive results. Again this noninvasive test is insensitive to calf and partially occlusive major deep vein thrombi. It also fails to discriminate between acute and chronic venous occlusions.

DUPLEX ULTRASONOGRAPHY

Real-time B-mode ultrasound of the venous system provides a direct assessment of the morphologic changes in the venous wall and lumen. Recent duplex scanners are complemented by color coding of the flow patterns. This permits rapid identification of the vascular segment in question and its patency. In most cases a 5- or 7.5-MHz probe is used. Acute venous thrombosis is diagnosed by vessel incompressibility, clot visualization, and abnormal flow patterns. With improved resolution and edge enhancement, superficial venous segments and the majority of the deep venous segments can be examined. In a prospective study of 220 patients, 66 were found to have no compressible femoral or popliteal veins by duplex scan.[9] All these patients had abnormal venograms (specificity of 100 percent).

It should be recognized that vein incompressibility is not diagnostic of venous thrombosis as certain venous segments are noncompressible by virtue of their anatomic location. These include the vena cava, the iliac and deep femoral veins, and the superficial femoral vein in the adductor canal.[10] In these segments the absence of visualized thrombi and normal flow signals safely exclude the diagnosis of DVT. A unique advantage of real-time ultrasonography is the potential capability of discriminating between acute and chronic thrombi. This can be helpful in selecting appropriate therapy. Spongy, mobile, homogeneous thrombi are usually acute, while firm, heterogeneous, irregular, echogenic, fixed, or recanalized thrombi in the presence of collateral channels indicate chronic thrombosis.[11]

In some reports, DVT was diagnosed by duplex ultrasonography in spite of normal contrast phlebographic study. This may occur if a double femoral or popliteal venous system is present when the channel harboring the thrombus fails to be visualized by the phlebogram.[12]

At the University of Chicago venous duplex ultrasonography is employed routinely for the noninvasive diagnosis of DVT. Ascending contrast phlebography is only performed if the duplex ultrasonographic findings are negative or equivocal in the face of substantial clinical evidence of DVT. If calf vein thrombi are detected, treatment is usually unnecessary unless proximal extension to the popliteal vein occurs or if the patient suffers from pulmonary thromboembolism.

Extracranial Carotid Occlusive Disease

It is estimated that approximately 50 percent of ischemic strokes are related to extracranial carotid occlusive disease. Unfortunately, a significant number of patients will initially present with permanent neurologic impairment without warning symptoms.[22] In general, patients with risk factors for atherosclerosis including diabetes, hypertension, smoking, and hypercholesterolemia, or those who have evidence of coronary or arterial occlusive disease elsewhere should be suspected of having carotid occlusive disease. Patients who present with cervical bruits, TIAs, RINDs, or completed strokes should undergo further diagnostic assessment of the carotid arteries to determine whether hemodynamically significant carotid occlusive disease (75 percent or more luminal area reduction) exists. In the critical care setting, screening for carotid bifurcation disease with arteriography can be hazardous because of hemodynamic instability and renal insufficiency. Alternatively, noninvasive testing with duplex ultrasonography provides a safe and accurate assessment of the extracranial carotid arteries.

DUPLEX ULTRASONOGRAPHY OF THE CAROTID ARTERIES

Using a 5- or 7.5-MHz probe the common, internal, and external carotid arteries as well as the proximal segments of the vertebral arteries can be examined. Occlusive atherosclerotic lesions are imaged in the longitudinal and cross-sectional planes. The severity of stenosis is determined by measuring lesion width, lumen, and arterial diameters. High-resolution ultrasound can characterize plaque morphology and identify echodense (fibrosis or calcification) or echolucent regions in the plaque indicative of plaque necrosis or hemorrhage.[13] Pulsed Doppler spectral analysis additionally provides a quantitative measure of the flow velocity patterns within the normal and diseased segments of the carotid arteries. Peak systolic internal carotid artery velocities greater than 125 cm/s are usually indicative of hemodynamically significant stenoses. The sensitivity and specificity rates for detecting hemodynamically significant stenoses by duplex ultrasonography range from 85 to 90 percent when compared to angiography.[14] Duplex ultrasonography is therefore invaluable in the selection of patients in need of further arteriography and interventional procedures.

Densely calcified plaques with acoustic shadowing of the carotid bifurcation, a high bifurcation, tortuosity, and difficulty in discriminating between preocclusive stenosis and total occlusion of the internal carotid artery remain the major pitfalls of carotid duplex ultrasonography. Color flow imaging alleviates some of these drawbacks and can readily differentiate between a total occlusion and a preocclusive stenosis.

Mesenteric Vascular Disease

Acute occlusion of the celiac and superior mesenteric arteries can result in catastrophic sequelae. The diagnosis can be challenging particularly since most patients present with symptoms out of proportion of physical findings. Once occlusion is suspected, visceral arteriography is necessary to confirm the diagnosis. To date, noninvasive testing of the mesenteric arteries can be accomplished using duplex ultrasonography to visualize and assess flow in the celiac and superior arteries pre- and postprandially, following pharmacologic manipulation, and for the postoperative surveillance of mesenteric revascularization procedures.[15] Under these elective circumstances the proximal segments of mesenteric arteries can be evaluated because of their predictable ventral origin from the abdominal aorta and the preponderance of ostial lesions (see Plate 21). In the acute setting duplex ultrasonography can assess proximal mesenteric arterial patency and thus help differentiate between nonocclusive mesenteric ischemia or vasospasm (associated with generalized hypoperfusion or digitalis toxicity) and mesenteric arterial thrombosis or embolism. The results should be interpreted cautiously since in the majority of cases ileus and dilation of intestinal loops preclude a complete study.

Renal Vascular Disease

RENAL ARTERIAL STENOSIS

Hypertension secondary to renovascular disease is rare and accounts for about 3 percent of the hypertensive patient population. Patients with malignant hypertension, exacerbation of preexisting hypertension, at-risk fibromuscular dysplasia, and hypertension combined with renal insufficiency should be suspected of renovascular arterial occlusive disease. While a number of screening methods such as hypertensive pyelography and radionuclide scanning have been used, they are accompanied by a relatively high false-positive and false-negative rate. Angiographic techniques are invasive and pose the risk of contrast nephropathy and worsening of preexisting renal insufficiency. Duplex ultrasonography is evolving as the most suitable screening procedure for this patient population. The objective of such evaluation is to identify hemodynamically significant stenoses, measure kidney size, and evaluate intraparenchymal flow patterns.

Renal studies require that the patient fast overnight to minimize bowel gas interference. A low-frequency probe is usually used (2 to 3 MHz). The peak systolic velocity in the juxtarenal aorta and along the course of the renal artery is measured (at least five times). A renal aortic peak systolic velocity ratio of 3.5 or more is indicative of hemodynamically significant renal stenosis (greater than 60 percent). Using these criteria duplex ultrasonography carries a specificity rate of 93 to 97 percent and a sensitivity rate of 83 to 90 percent when compared to angiography.[16]

Because of the deep location of the renal arteries real-time visualization of occlusive lesions is difficult, and therefore quantitation of the degree of stenosis depends on multiple velocity measurements along the renal artery from the aortic origin to the hilum of the kidney, rather than real-time B-mode imaging. Velocity spectral analysis can also provide information regarding renal parenchymal vascular resistance and disease.[17] Characteristically, the kidney is a low-resistance end organ, and hence renal arterial flow is anterograde throughout all phases of the cardiac cycle with substantial diastolic flow. Reduced diastolic flow is suggestive of intraparenchymal vascular disease or fibrosis. Limitations include occasional difficulty in locating the left renal artery because of overlying gas and identifying multiple renal polar arteries. The examination requires considerable technical expertise and proper patient preparation.

The role of color flow imaging in this vascular territory remains to be evaluated. This modality appears to expedite localization of the juxtarenal aorta, the left renal vein, and the origin of the renal arteries. Its value in identifying renal arterial stenosis remains to be determined.

RENAL VEIN THROMBOSIS

This is a rare condition which is more frequently encountered in neonates with gastrointestinal tract disturbance, fluid sequestration, and sepsis. Adults with nephrotic syndrome secondary to membranous or membranoproliferative glomerulonephritis are particularly suspectable to renal vein thrombosis due to selective filtration of naturally occurring anticoagulants such as antithrombin 3 and plasma plasminogen activator with the retention of larger-molecular-weight proteins such as fibrinogen and other coagulation factors. The condition should be suspected in neonates who present with severe dehydration and hematuria and in adults with nephrotic syndrome who develop sudden deterioration of renal function, pulmonary embolism, or caval thrombosis.

Although intravenous pyelography is usually the initial test performed, it often provides limited information because of the patient's impaired renal function and inadequate opacification of the patient's kidney. Duplex ultrasonography is now considered the investigation of choice, particularly in children. Renal enlargement without hydronephrosis, decreased echogenicity, and an enlarged renal vein are suggestive of renal vein thrombosis in the acute phase. Intraluminal thrombi or defects can be visualized in the renal vein and vena cava. Using the pulsed Doppler, renal venous flow can be directly assessed. If the noninvasive findings are equivocal, inferior venacavography and selective renal vein injections should be performed.[18]

RENAL TRANSPLANTATION

Acute renal transplant dysfunction in the immediate postoperative period is not unusual. Whether the underlying cause is rejection, acute tubular necrosis (ATN), perigraft infection, ureteric obstruction, or vasculogenic, a specific cause must be determined so that appropriate therapy can be instituted. A number of noninvasive studies are available to study transplant function and vascular integrity. These include magnetic resonance imaging (MRI), renal scintigraphy, and duplex ultrasonography. MRI in the immediate postoperative period is often difficult to perform, while radionuclide scintigraphy fails to adequately assess the perirenal space and vasculature, and its role in differentiating rejection from ATN is controversial.[19] Duplex ultrasonography offers the capability of evaluating allograft arterial inflow, venous outflow, ureteric obstruction, and perinephric fluid collections. Renal arterial velocity spectral analysis provides insight regarding the cause of renal dysfunction and may help in discriminating between parenchymal dysfunction due to rejection, ATN, or cyclosporine toxicity.

In evaluating renal allograft arterial flow, a ratio comparing the peak systolic velocities in the renal and iliac arteries is used to identify hemodynamically significant anastomotic stenoses.[20] A ratio greater than 3 is indicative of a hemodynamically significant stenosis (60 percent or greater). Arteriovenous fistulae or anastomotic pseudoaneurysms exhibit machinery or to-and-fro flow in a space-occupying lesion. Color flow imaging is useful in locating the intra and extrarenal vessels (see Plate 22).

If renal vein thrombosis occurs, there is absent or markedly diminished flow in the allograft, renal, arcuate, and interlobar veins. The graft appears globular and hyperechoic. As a result of venous outflow obstruction, there is increased intrarenal vascular resistance and loss of the diastolic flow component in the arterial velocity waveform.[21]

External compression from lymphocele, hematoma, urinoma, or abscess can be identified and treated under ultrasonographic guidance if necessary.[22] Hydronephrosis secondary to ureteric obstruction can be easily identified.

Although several investigators have attempted to differentiate between acute rejection and ATN using renal arterial hemodynamic parameters such as the diastolic to systolic ratio or resistive and pulsatility indexes,[23,24] there is considerable overlap of the test results in these two forms of renal dysfunction. Normal arterial flow patterns associated with renal allograft dysfunction are suggestive of cyclosporine toxicity since these kidneys have a normal intrarenal vascular resistance[25] in contrast to grafts with acute rejection or ATN.

Iatrogenic Injuries

Peripheral arterial and central venous line placements are common procedures in the intensive care unit. Complications include perivascular hemorrhage, localized hematoma, venous thrombosis, pseudoaneurysmal formation (sterile or infected), and arteriovenous fistulas. Arteriovenous fistulas commonly occur after transfixion of an artery and neighboring vein by the introducing cannula thereby establishing a false communication.

In most instances it is difficult to discern between transmitted arterial pulsations through a hematoma and an actual pseudoaneurysm by physical examinations. A thrill is usually felt and a continuous bruit is heard when a femoral or carotid arteriovenous fistula is present. Accurate diagnosis is easily accomplished with duplex ultrasonography; a pseudoaneurysm appears contiguous with the arterial wall with characteristic swirling to-and-fro flow patterns clearly represented by color flow (see Plate 23). With arteriovenous fistulas, there is continuous pulsatile venous flow and the communication is occasionally visualized. In most instances, diagnostic angiography is unnecessary prior to vascular repair.

Compartment Syndromes

A compartment syndrome develops whenever pressure within a confined compartment exceeds arterial inflow pressure thereby compromising nutrient blood supply to the enclosed neuromuscular structures. The most commonly involved compartments include the volar in the upper extremity and the anterior, lateral, and deep posterior compartments in the lower extremity. Nerve tissue is particularly sensitive to ischemia. Neurologic deficits can appear within minutes, and permanent damage occurs within 12 h. Myonecrosis sets in at 4 h, and contractures can develop as early as 12 h after the ischemic insult. Clinically, early manifestations include diminished motor and sensory function, tightness, and pain in the region of the compartment. Distal pulses and Doppler signals are poor indicators of compartmental pressure and do not correlate with the extent of neuromuscular damage; anterior compartment myonecrosis may occur in face of palpable pedal pulses.

When the clinical diagnosis is equivocal, compartmental pressures can be measured by a number of techniques. In the most widely used, an 18 gauge needle is connected to a water manometer and syringe with a three-way stopcock, and is slowly advanced.[26] Intracompartmental pressure is exceeded when an air bubble or air meniscus moves toward the compartment being examined. Factitiously high pressures can result if the needle is obstructed by edematous muscle. Other measurement techniques include the wick catheter method.[27]

In general, if the compartment pressure rises to 40 mmHg a fasciotomy (incision of deep fascia, skin, and subcutaneous tissues) should be performed to release intracompartmental pressure and allow the swollen muscle to herniate and "breathe." Unfortunately, reliance on an absolute cutoff pressure can misguide therapy as it varies considerably, particularly if generalized hypotension and local vasoconstriction are present. Fasciotomy should therefore be performed once the diagnosis of a compartment syndrome is clinically suspected regardless of compartment pressure measurements.

References

1. Satomura S: Study of flow patterns in peripheral arteries by ultrasonics. J Acoust Soc Jpn 15:151, 1959.

2. Strandness DE, Jr: The use of ultrasound in the evaluation of peripheral vascular disease. Prog Cardiovasc Dis 20:403, 1978.
3. Yao JST, Takaki HS: Techniques of measuring lower limb arterial pressures, in Bernstein EF (ed): *Noninvasive Diagnostic Techniques in Vascular Disease.* St. Louis, CV Mosby Co., 1978.
4. Yao JST, Hobbs JT, Irvine WT: Ankle systolic pressure measurements in arterial disease affecting the lower extremities. Br J Surg 56:376, 1969.
5. Kohler TR, Nance DR, Cramer MM, et al.: Duplex scanning for diagnosis of aortoiliac and femoropopliteal disease: A prospective study. Circulation 76:1074, 1987.
6. Cranley JJ, Canos AJ, Sull WJ: The diagnosis of deep venous thrombosis: Fallibility of clinical signs and symptoms. Arch Surg 111:34, 1976.
7. Sumner DS, Lambeth A: Reliability of Doppler ultrasound in the diagnosis of acute venous thrombosis both above and below the knee. Am J Surg 183:205, 1979.
8. Wheeler HB, O'Donnell JA, Anderson FA, et al.: Occlusive impedance phlebography: A diagnostic procedure for venous thrombosis and pulmonary embolism. Prog Cardiovasc Dis 17:199, 1974.
9. Lensing AWA, Prandoni P, Brandjes D: Detection of deep vein thrombosis by real-time B-mode ultrasonography. N Engl J Med 320:342, 1989.
10. Wright DJ, Shepard AD, McPharlin M, et al.: Pitfalls in lower extremity venous duplex scanning. J Vasc Surg 11(5):675, May 1990.
11. Fronek A: The venous system of the lower extremities. In Fronek A (ed): *Noninvasive Diagnostics in Vascular Surgery.* New York, McGraw-Hill Book Co, 1989.
12. Barnes RW, Nix L, Barnes CL, et al.: Perioperative asymptomatic venous thrombosis: role of duplex scanning versus venography. J Vasc Surg 9:251, 1989.
13. O'Donnell TF, Jr, Erdoes L, Mackey WC, et al.: Correlation of B-mode ultrasound imaging and arteriography with pathologic findings at carotid endarterectomy. Arch Surg 120:443, 1985.
14. Comerota AJ, Cranley JJ, Katz ML, et al.: Real-time B-mode carotid imaging: A three-year multicenter experience. J Vasc Surg 1:84, 1984.
15. Lilly MP, Harward TRS, Flinn WR, et al.: Duplex ultrasound measurement of changes in mesenteric flow velocity with pharmacologic and physiologic alteration of intestinal blood flow in man. J Vasc Surg 9:18, 1989.
16. Hansen KJ, Tribble R, Reavis SW, et al.: Renal duplex sonography: Evaluation of clinical utility. J Vasc Surg 12(3):227, September 1990.
17. Norris CS, Barnes RW: Renal artery flow velocity analysis: a sensitive measure of experimental and clinical renovascular resistance. J Surg Res 36:230, 1984.
18. Shepard AD: Renal vein thrombosis. In Ernst CB and Stanley J (eds): *Current Therapy in Vascular Surgery.* Philadelphia, BC Decker, Inc., 1987.
19. Oh KH, Kupin W, Madrazo B, et al.: Evaluation of the renal allograft by quantitative Duplex sonography and radioisotope renogram. Transplant Proc 21:1917, 1989.
20. Snider JF, Hunter DW, Moradia GP, et al.: Transplant renal artery stenosis: Evaluation with Duplex sonography. Radiology 172:1027, 1989.
21. Reuther G, Wanjura D, Bauer H: Acute renal vein thrombosis in renal allografts: Detection with duplex Doppler US. Radiology 170:557, 1989.
22. Silver TM, Campbell D, Wicks JD, et al.: Peritransplant fluid collections: Ultrasound evaluation and clinical significance. Radiology 138:145, 1981.
23. Don S, Kopecky KK, Filo RS, et al.: Duplex Doppler US of renal allografts: Causes of elevated resistive index. Radiology 171:709, 1989.
24. Rigsby CM, Burns PN, Weltin GG, et al.: Doppler signal quantitation in renal allografts: Comparison in normal and rejecting transplants, with pathologic correlation. Radiology 162:39, 1987.
25. Buckley A, Cooperberg PL, Reeve C, et al.: The distinction between acute renal transplant rejection and cyclosporin nephrotoxicity: Value of Duplex sonography. AJR 149:521, 1987.
26. Whitesides TE, Haney TC, Morimoto K, et a.l: Tissue pressure measurement as a determinant for the need for fasciotomy. Clin Orthop 113:43, 1975.
27. Mubarak SJ, Owen CA, Hargens AR, et al.: Acute compartment syndromes: diagnosis and treatment with the aid of a wick catheter. J Bone Joint Surg (Am) 60:1091, 1978.

Chapter 24
VASCULAR CANNULATION

PHILLIP FACTOR
JACOB IASHA SZNAJDER

Peripheral Venous Cannulation

More than 80 percent of hospitalized patients have one or more of their peripheral veins cannulated during their hospitalization.[1] Peripheral veins are usually the first choice of access in hemodynamically stable patients who require intravenous therapy such as fluids, blood products, medications, or nutrition. These veins are readily accessible in most patients and can often accommodate large bore catheters (intravenous) that may rival central lines in their fluid delivery rates (Table 24-1).[2] Peripheral intravenous catheters can deliver large volumes of fluid to the venous circulation. In the setting of hemodynamic compromise the time from delivery to arrival to the right atrium is unpredictable. Hypertonic infusions and large bore catheters may prove irritating to the venous endothelium thereby leading to the development of infusion phlebitis, patient discomfort, and increased risk of catheter-related infection. Central venous access may be preferable in these settings.

Central Venous Cannulation

Central venous access is preferred over peripheral cannulation for the indications listed in Table 24-2. Contraindications (Table 24-3) to central venous cannulation are not as easily delineated as are the indications. Situations will arise where significant contraindications exist in a patient who nonetheless requires central venous access. Thus, no absolute contraindication to establishing a central line can be identified. Table 24-4 lists the merits and drawbacks for each central venous route. The risk-benefit ratio must be weighed for each patient prior to attempting placement of a central line. Other than coagulopathy or recent fibrinolytic therapy, contraindications are site specific. In general, the operator should use the method that he or she is most familiar and comfortable with.

TABLE 24-1 Nonpressurized Flow Rates of Various Catheters

Catheter Size (Length, in)	Flow Rate, mL/min
8.5F (3.5)	160
14ga (2)	93
16ga (2)	75
16ga (5.25)	64
18ga (2)	62
18ga (8)	13
20ga (2)	42
24ga (3/4)	14

SOURCE: Adapted from Reference 2.

TABLE 24-2 Indications for Central Venous Access

Inadequate peripheral veins
Central venous pressure monitoring (CVP and PA catheters)
Administration of phlebitic medications (potassium, chemotherapy)
Extremely rapid fluid administration
Cardiopulmonary resuscitation
Intracardiac pacing
Frequent phlebotomies
Long-term intravenous therapy (antibiotics, chemotherapy)
Hemodialysis
Hyperalimentation
Administration of vasoactive drugs

TABLE 24-3 Relative Contraindications to Central Venous Cannulation

General
Physician inexperience
Coagulopathy
Recent fibrinolytic therapy
Severe thrombocytopenia
Inability to identify pertinent landmarks
Infection or burn at planned catheter entry site
Uncooperative patient
Subclavian Vein
SVC thrombosis
Upper thoracic trauma
Compromised pulmonary function (COPD, asthma)
High levels of PEEP
Coagulopathy
Internal Jugular Vein
SVC thrombosis
COPD, high levels of PEEP
Tracheostomy and excessive pulmonary secretions
Femoral Vein
Vena caval compromise: clot, extrinsic compression, IVC filter
Local infection at intended insertion site
Absent femoral pulse
Penetrating abdominal trauma
Cardiac arrest or low flow states
Requirements for patient mobility

GENERAL CONSIDERATIONS REGARDING CENTRAL VENOUS CATHETERIZATION

Regardless of the site or method chosen the patient must be well informed and appropriate consent obtained whenever possible. A cooperative patient who understands what is

TABLE 24-4 Advantages and Disadvantages of Various Central Vein Approaches

Approach	Advantages	Disadvantages
External jugular vein	Part of surface anatomy Coagulopathy not prohibitive Low pneumothorax rate Head-of-table access Prominent in elderly	High failure rate Not ideal for prolonged central venous access Uncomfortable Dressing and maintenance are difficult Poor landmarks in obese patients High malposition rate Difficult approach for threading central catheters
Internal jugular	Pneumothorax uncommon High success rate Head-of-table access Control of bleeding is easier Right IJ straight path to SVC (easier to pass catheters; less malposition) Less failure with inexperienced operator	Not ideal for prolonged central venous access (e.g., TPN) Carotid artery puncture relatively frequent Uncomfortable Dressings and catheter difficult to maintain Left internal jugular increases risk of thoracic duct injury Poor landmarks in obese or edematous patients Not ideal for temporary hemodialysis Difficult access with tracheostomies Contraindicated with intracranial HTN Vein more prone to collapse with hypovolemia Difficult access during emergencies when airway control is being established
Supraclavicular	Low incidence of pneumothorax High success rate Easier to pass catheters Accessible from head of table Good landmarks No interference with chest compression Anatomic landmarks constant Short path from skin to vein	Control of bleeding difficult Pneumothorax possible Not ideal for prolonged venous access More uncomfortable Dressings and catheter maintenance difficult Thoracic duct puncture possible Not ideal for temporary hemodialysis Not ideal approach when airway control is necessary
Infraclavicular	Easier to maintain dressings and more comfortable for patient Better landmarks in obesity Large vein less collapsible during volume depletion or shock Better access when airway control is being established Multiple catheter insertions easier when massive volume resuscitation needed	Higher risk of pneumothorax Compression of bleeding site difficult Decreased success rate with inexperience Long pass from skin to vein Catheter malposition common Inaccessible from head of table Interference with chest compressions during CPR
Femoral	Fast, easy access; high success rate Does not interfere with chest compressions Does not interfere with airway management No risk of pneumothorax Supine or head-down position not necessary during insertion	Delayed circulation of drugs during CPR Higher risk of complications in patients with abdominal pathology Prevents patient mobilization Difficult to keep the site sterile Difficult for pulmonary artery catheter insertion
Axillary	Good for burn patients Easily located Low risk for pneumothorax Good for PA catheterization Accurate CVP measurement	Uncomfortable Malposition common
Long arm brachial	Low risk of pneumothorax Coagulopathy not prohibitive Can be used to measure CVP	High malposition rate Thrombosis common Frequent catheter tip displacement with arm movement

SOURCE: Adapted from Reference 11.

occurring will increase the success rate of any procedure.

The appropriate equipment should be prepared and calibrated and the patient correctly positioned. In the absence of elevated intracranial pressure, externalized cerebral ventricular drains, or incipient respiratory failure, most patients can tolerate a few moments of Trendelenburg positioning. Supplemental oxygen should be used to prevent arterial desaturation, especially in a patient who has lower lobe pneumonia or will have a sterile drape placed across his or her face.

Antisepsis should include scrubbing with an iodine-based solution (preferably tincture of iodine) that is allowed to dry prior to skin penetration. Isopropyl alcohol solutions are an acceptable alternative.[3] Sterile technique is required with the placement of any central line. While there are no clear studies to indicate that drapes, masks, gowns, and headware reduce the incidence of line-related infectious complications, their use seems prudent especially when prolonged use of the catheter is intended or a guidewire is used for placement. Inexperienced operators should be closely supervised. Selection of sedated, mechanically ventilated patients should be considered for physicians in training.[4]

Critically ill patients who require central venous cannulation are frequently confused or uncooperative and may require sedation. Extreme caution must be exercised when parenteral sedation is used, especially in patients with compromised cardiopulmonary and neurologic function since uncontrolled general anesthesia may result. When necessary, we recommend using short-acting parenteral benzodiazepines or sedating antihistamines. All patients should be assessed for the need for an artificial airway. In some cases elective intubation may be required prior to catheter placement.

After completion of catheter placement, the presence of good blood flow should always be reconfirmed. A chest x-ray should be obtained to confirm location of the catheter tip. Catheter tips should optimally be placed approximately 2 to 4 cm above the junction of the right atrium and superior vena cava. Catheters placed into the right ventricle or atrium predispose patients to arrhythmias and endocardial or valvular damage. Other signs of correct placement, such as respiratory fluctuations, are not reliable enough to supplant the need for radiographic confirmation.

The overall success rate for cannulation of the first site selected on the first attempt is approximately 60 percent. The likelihood of successful vessel localization diminishes with each successive needle pass. If entry is not achieved by the fifth pass, successful cannulation is unlikely. The risk of complications increases with the number of needle passes.[5,6]

CHOICE OF CATHETERS

Catheter-through-needle devices should be avoided. These cannulation devices require utilization of a larger than necessary needle to allow advancement of a catheter through the lumen of a needle. Additionally, they increase the risk of catheter embolism if the catheter is inadvertently withdrawn through the needle. Readily available catheter-over-needle devices and prepared guidewire kits make this method unnecessary, even in emergency situations. It is also useful for the clinician to be aware of the various measures of catheter size. Tubes, catheters, and needles are generally specified according to internal diameter (usually reported in millimeters), size French (the external circumference in millimeters), or gauge (ga). The relationship of gauge to diameter in centimeters is given in Fig. 24-1.

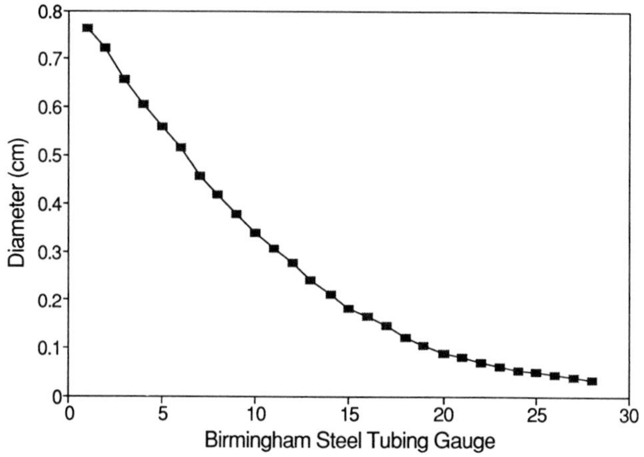

FIGURE 24-1 Relationship of gauge to diameter (in centimeters) for hypodermic tubing.

LONG ARM CATHETERS

Long arm catheters are placed via antecubital veins and advanced into the central venous circulation. Because of their peripheral insertion site, they avoid many of the complications of more central approaches. The ability to readily control bleeding at the entry site makes these catheters reasonable choices for patients with coagulopathies. Successful passage to the intrathoracic veins is variable, and malposition occurs frequently (>50 percent). Placement can be enhanced by placing the arm in an abducted (90°) and slightly flexed position. Use of highly thrombogenic polyethylene catheters has been associated with increased incidences of superior vena cava syndrome, pulmonary emboli, and catheter-related infection. The relatively large diameter of these catheters can occupy the entire lumen of an antecubital vein thereby leading to venous stasis, endothelial injury, and thrombophlebitis. Silicone rubber catheters should be used when possible. Strict aseptic technique has resulted in reduced infection rates.[3]

TUNNELED CATHETERS

The requirement for long-term indwelling central venous catheters has been met with the development of barium impregnated silicone rubber (Silastic) catheters (Hickman, Gorshong, Quinton, Broviac). These pliable catheters are tunneled beneath the skin and inserted into a central vein, usually the subclavian. However, their use in the cephalic, external and internal jugular, saphenous, and femoral veins has been reported. A small Dacron cuff is positioned subcutaneously on the catheter approximately 30 cm from the injection port. The patient's fibroblasts infiltrate the cuff producing a fibrous barrier to migration of bacteria along the catheter into the vascular system.

These indwelling devices allow for long-term central hyperalimentation and facilitate long courses of antibiotics (often in outpatient settings). The management of oncology patients frequently includes use of these catheters since the nature of their disease and the use of vesicant chemotherapeutic agents mandate central venous cannulation.

These catheters require high levels of attention. Entry sites should be cleaned and dressed daily, and catheters should be manipulated using sterile technique. Unused lumens should be flushed with heparinized solutions twice daily and after each use. Most patients and their families can be taught to care for these catheters, allowing for increased independence from hospitals.

The use of these catheters has not been without complication. Multilumen Hickman catheters have been associated with increased risk of infection as compared to single-lumen catheters.[7] Subclavian and superior vena caval thrombosis, malposition, and bleeding complications have been reported. Pneumothorax is uncommon when the catheter is placed by cutdown. Thrombotic occlusion of these catheters is not uncommon. Flushing with pressurized solutions or passage of guidewires through the catheters is not advised because of the risk of catheter perforation. Administration of streptokinase may be successful (see Chap. 119) in clearing catheter clot. Catheter thrombosis increases the risk of central venous catheter infection. Slowed infusion rates or inability to withdraw blood from a chronic indwelling catheter should suggest catheter thrombosis.

TOTALLY IMPLANTABLE CATHETER DEVICES

Totally implantable venous access systems have been developed to obviate some of the complications associated with tunneled catheters. These devices consist of a stainless-steel or plastic portal with a self-sealing diaphragm that is placed subcutaneously, usually over the ribs on the anterior chest. The portal is connected to a silicon rubber catheter that is tunneled subcutaneously and inserted into a central vein. The system is accessed using a Huber needle to avoid damaging the portal diaphragm.

The subcutaneous placement of these devices eliminates the need for daily dressing changes. They are reasonable alternatives for patients who are either noncompliant or cannot be taught to manage Hickman-type catheters. Reported infection rates of 0 to 0.1 infections per 100 days are approximately one-third that of externalized catheters. The system is flushed when not in use to prevent catheter occlusion. Mechanical problems such as occlusion and secondary malposition occur in 10 to 25 percent of catheters.

Improper placement or accidental misplacement of the Huber needle can lead to subcutaneous infusion of fluids. Hence, blood return should be documented, when possible, prior to instillation of vesicants or other tissue-toxic medications. Reservoir infections are extremely difficult to treat and should prompt removal of the device.

DIALYSIS CATHETERS

The requirement for immediate dialysis in the absence of other vascular access (arteriovenous fistula, graft, or Scribner shunt) is an indication for central venous cannulation. The high flows required for dialysis mandate placement of large bore, double-lumen catheters into large veins. The catheters initially used were rigid devices that were associated with significant incidences of venous and myocardial perforation as well as subclavian vein and superior vena caval thrombosis. As a result of these problems short-term femoral vein cannulation was often the access route of choice. Many of these problems have been eliminated with the development of flexible, less thrombogenic, silicone rubber catheters with subcutaneously placed Dacron cuffs (Quinton Permacath). Several centers have also reported their experiences using Hickman catheters in this setting. These catheters can remain in place for several weeks while an arteriovenous fistula matures. Utilization of the subclavian or internal jugular vein allows for the preservation of the vessels of the extremities for future vascular access. The incidence of complications, including infection, has been variably reported to be better than or the same as with other central venous catheters. Catheter management should be similar to that of other central lines.[7]

MULTIPLE-LUMEN CATHETERS

Multilumen catheters have recently supplanted the need for multiple central venous lines. They allow for simultaneous infusions and venous blood sampling. In many medical centers these catheters have become the most frequently placed central venous catheter. However, the use of these catheters has preceded adequate study of their risks, costs, and complications.[7] Conflicting results regarding infection rates have been published. The majority of published reports indicate increased infection rates with these catheters. A recent prospective, nonrandomized study demonstrated no significant difference in infection or colonization rates when triple-lumen catheters were compared to single-lumen polyurethane catheters in patients with similar degrees of illness.[8] The same authors also noted an increased incidence of catheter-related sepsis when catheterization exceeded 6 days.

Pending further study several recommendations regarding the use of these catheters can be made:[7]

1. They should be used only when multiple lines of access are required in patients whose peripheral veins are inadequate to support planned therapy.
2. The subclavian route is the preferred site for these catheters, especially when long-term cannulation is anticipated. Placement should not be through pulmonary artery sheath introducers.
3. A hospital-wide protocol designating specific uses for each port should be established (e.g., proximal port: blood sampling; middle port: total parenteral nutrition (TPN); distal port: fluid and medication infusion). Manipulations of the catheter should be minimized. Unused ports should be flushed with a heparinized solution twice each day.

No specific recommendations can be made regarding duration of catheterization. Routine catheter changes every 5 to 7 days have been documented to reduce the incidence of catheter-related sepsis; however, the incidence of insertion-related complications rises with frequent replacement. Multilumen catheters should be changed using the guidelines discussed below for any central line. In the absence of additional data cannulation beyond 4 weeks is not recommended.

CATHETER SHEATH INTRODUCERS

Catheter sheath introducers are large bore catheters (8.5 F) that were developed to allow placement of pulmonary artery catheters. These devices are typically Teflon-coated short-length (3.5 in.) catheters with a side port for simultaneous infusions while the catheter is in place. They can also be used for rapid volume administration (see below). Several caveats apply when using these devices.

1. The stiffness of these catheters has been associated with perforation of the superior vena cava and innominate veins. Sheath introducers should not be left in place after restoration of intravascular volume or removal of a pulmonary artery (PA) catheter.
2. Air embolization has been associated with this catheter. This has occurred after removal of PA catheters with malfunctioning of the self-sealing valve, replacement of PA catheters with smaller gauge catheters, and with accidental disconnection of the side port from the catheter. This problem can be avoided by replacing sheath introducers with appropriately sized central lines by guidewire exchange at the time of PA catheter removal. If the catheter must remain in place after perforation of the diaphragm, then an obturator should be inserted into the catheter. At no time should a smaller catheter be replaced into the sheath.
3. Infusion of hyperalimentation solutions through these catheters has been associated with increased risks of catheter-related sepsis. Placement beyond 3 days cannot be recommended pending availability of additional data.

A short (3.5 in. to prevent kinking) 8.5 F pulmonary artery catheter introducer placed into a subclavian, internal jugular, or femoral vein can allow for pressurized infusion rates of 1428 mL/min via the side port (using a pressure bag and large bore, urologic tubing.[9] If a 6-in. 14 ga catheter is inserted through the introducer and fluids are infused via both the side port and the 14 ga catheter, the flow rates can be further increased because of production of a venturi effect at the tip of the sheath introducer.[10] Catheters larger than 14 ga limit flow via the side port. It must be kept in mind that in these settings intravenous tubing diameter will be the limiting step. Hence, the use of large bore "trauma" tubing or urologic irrigation tubing is required. Alternatively, blood infusion tubing or short-length standard intravenous tubing can be used.

THE SELDINGER TECHNIQUE[11]

The skin should be cleansed, sterilely draped, and then anesthetized with 1% lidocaine subcutaneously. The puncture site and surrounding 1 to 2 cm should be anesthetized using a minimum amount of anesthetic in order to prevent distortion of superficial landmarks. The cannulating needle (typically 16 to 18 ga) with an attached syringe is then advanced into the skin (with the bevel facing up) and toward the chosen vessel, while at the same time gentle traction is applied to the syringe plunger. The use of a small-gauge finder needle to locate a vessel increases the number of skin penetrations and the risk of complications and is not recommended.

Persistent blood return will confirm penetration of the vessel. The needle can then be redirected to more approximate the course of the vessel. Blood return should be reconfirmed. The syringe is then removed while the needle is held firmly. At no time should the hub of the needle be left open to air since excessive blood loss and/or air embolism may result. Placing the patient in a head-down position and having him exhale or Valsalva will increase intrathoracic pressure and diminish the risk of air embolism.

A guidewire is then advanced through the needle into the vein. The wire should have a flexible, bent tip (J wire) to reduce the risk of vessel wall perforation. It should be advanced 5 to 10 cm. If resistance is encountered, force should not be applied; rather, the wire should be carefully withdrawn through the needle and blood return confirmed with a syringe. If resistance to withdrawal is met, the needle and guide wire should be removed simultaneously to prevent guide wire embolization. The needle should be redirected or the bevel rotated toward the right atrium prior to reinsertion. Altering the patient's position or intrathoracic pressures (Valsalva maneuver, inspiratory pause on ventilated patients, leg elevation) or having the patient turn her head may facilitate guidewire advancement by distending intrathoracic vessels. Force should *never* be used to advance a guidewire (or catheter). If difficulty persists, an alternate site should be selected.

Patients should be monitored for the development of cardiac arrhythmias during central line placement. The appearance of sustained arrhythmias should prompt immediate withdrawal of the guidewire. Subsequent treatment is usually unnecessary.[12] While holding the guidewire with one hand, the needle can be removed by sliding it off the wire. Control of the guidewire should be maintained throughout the procedure. Guidewire migration and emboli have been reported, and their removal can present a challenging problem. Using a straight scalpel blade, a small incision is made through the skin at the insertion site. This is best accomplished by inverting the blade and running the dull edge of the blade along the guidewire. If a plastic dilator is required to create a track for the catheter, it can be advanced over the guidewire into the vessel. Advancement of the dilator frequently requires a small amount of firm pressure and rotation. Once the track has been enlarged the catheter can then be advanced into the vein. Most catheter placement kits require that the dilator be removed prior to placement of the catheter; however, large bore catheter-sheath introducers require that the dilator remain within the catheter during advancement into the vein.

The catheter can now be advanced over the guidewire into the vein (or artery). Advancement should be without significant resistance, although rotating the catheter about the guidewire may facilitate its passage through the skin. Once the catheter has been advanced to its intended distance the guidewire can be withdrawn through the catheter. Blood return should be reconfirmed. Pressure readings or blood gas measurements should then be made to rule out inadvertent arterial cannulation. The catheter should then be fixed to the skin by suture and the appropriate dressing placed. Confirmation of catheter tip location (chest x-ray) and monitoring for side effects should begin immediately.

INTERNAL JUGULAR VEIN CANNULATION

The internal jugular vein runs nearly parallel to the carotid artery. The right internal jugular vein (IJ) runs a nearly straight course into the brachiocephalic vessel and right atrium, making it the preferred route when right heart catheterization is intended. The IJ is an excellent choice of central venous access, and for the experienced operator it has less risk of pneumothorax than do subclavian approaches. Reported successful cannulation rates vary between 58 and 99 percent.[12] The absence of surrounding bony structures makes it a reasonable choice for patients with coagulopathies, since direct pressure can be applied in the event of a bleeding complication.

The internal jugular approach should be reconsidered in patients who are obese (difficulty delineating landmarks), in patients with tracheostomies (secondary to a higher incidence of line-related infections due to contamination by pulmonary secretions), and also in patients who will require prolonged catheterization (reduced neck range of motion, difficult local care and dressing application). Ultrasonic guidance should be considered when landmarks cannot be clearly delineated. This methodology facilitates catheter placement with fewer needle passes and thus potentially fewer complications.[6]

There are three commonly practiced approaches to the internal jugular vein. The method chosen should reflect operator experience and judgment based on the clinical situation.[4] The techniques described below utilize the Seldinger technique (vide supra).

MEDIAN APPROACH (Fig. 24-2)

This approach is good for inexperienced operators since the landmarks are easily identifiable. With the patient supine or in Trendelenburg position and the head turned slightly to the contralateral side, a needle with attached syringe is advanced into the skin at the junction of the sternal and clavicular heads of the sternocleidomastoid muscle. The needle should be held approximately 30° above the skin and directed toward the ipsilateral nipple. The needle should be advanced slowly and the vessel reached within 2 to 3 cm. Injudicious advancement of the needle beyond 2 to 3 cm can result in pneumothorax. If the first pass is unsuccessful, the needle should be completely withdrawn and the angle of the needle reduced by 10 to 15° to the skin. If four to five attempts at locating the vein are unsuccessful, an alternative, ipsilateral site should be selected.[4,13] Evaluation of the patient, including chest x-ray, is required prior to contralateral attempts at cannulation.

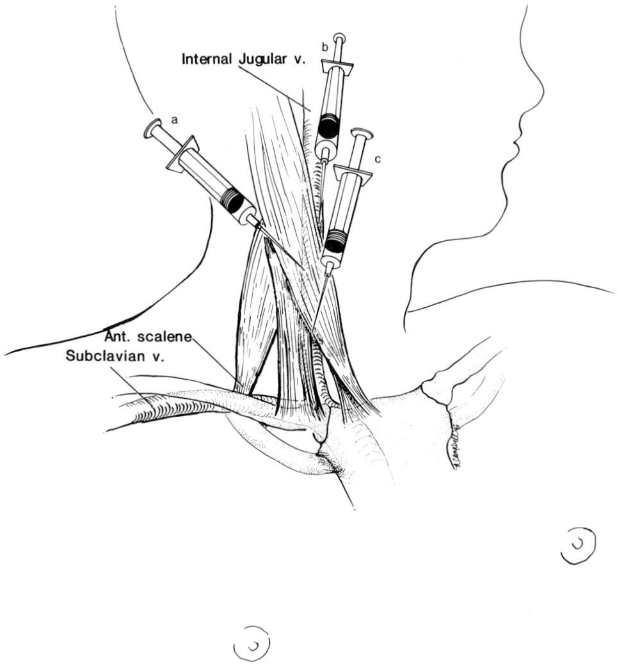

FIGURE 24-2 Internal jugular vein cannulation. ***a.*** **Lateral approach.** ***b.*** **Anterior approach.** ***c.*** **Median approach.**

ANTERIOR APPROACH (Fig. 24-2)

The skin is punctured lateral to the carotid pulse, along the medial border of the sternocleidomastoid muscle, at the level of the inferior margin of the thyroid cartilage. Pressure placed over the carotid artery has been demonstrated by ultrasound analysis to reduce the cross-sectional area of the internal jugular vein and should not be used. Rotation of the head beyond 45° changes the shape of the vessel from rhomboid to round, reducing cannulation success rates, especially in hypovolemic patients.[13] With the needle held approximately 30° over the skin it should be advanced no more than 3 cm toward the ipsilateral nipple. Traction on the skin, at the insertion site, in a direction opposite to the insertion of the needle will help maintain vessel luminal size, leaving the operator with a larger target (the "pull technique").[13] If unsuccessful, the angle between the syringe and skin may be reduced.

LATERAL APPROACH (Fig. 24-2)

The needle is inserted through the skin at the posterior lateral margin of the sternocleidomastoid muscle approximately 4 cm above the sternoclavicular junction, near the point at which the external jugular vein crosses the posterior margin of the sternocleidomastoid muscle. The needle is advanced a maximum of 3 to 4 cm in an inferomedial direction toward the contralateral nipple. The syringe is held at a shallower angle to the skin than the previously described methods, approximately 10 to 15°. This approach has an increased risk of carotid artery puncture; however, the distance from the apex of the lung reduces the risk of pneumothorax.

SUBCLAVIAN VEIN CATHETERIZATION

The reliable anatomy of the subclavian vein has led to the development of easily reproducible techniques for its cannulation. Complication rates for this technique are similar to those for internal jugular techniques.[4] Its location allows for catheter placement at a reasonable distance away from oropharyngeal or tracheal secretions. Subclavian catheters do not limit patient mobility and are better tolerated by awake patients. Surrounding anatomic structures allow for maintenance of vein caliber when patients are hypovolemic. Finally, catheter fixation and dressing are easily accomplished.

The attributes of this approach are counterbalanced by the risks of pneumothorax (0.1 to 7.7 percent incidence) and uncontrolled hematoma formation (0 to 5.0 percent incidence). The risk of pneumothorax is especially increased in patients who are uncooperative, morbidly obese, have chronic obstructive pulmonary disease (COPD), barrel chests, kyphosis, or cachexia, and in emergency settings.[12,14] Alternate approaches should be considered in these patients. Catheter malposition, into the ipsilateral internal jugular or contralateral subclavian vein, occurs in approximately 10 percent of patients when an infraclavicular approach is chosen. Malposition via supraclavicular approaches has been reported to occur in less than 1 percent of patients.[14,15]

The subclavian vein runs from the lateral margins of the first rib to the base of the neck where it joins the internal jugular vein immediately posterior to the sternoclavicular joint. Initially running anterior and inferior to the lateral portions of the subclavian artery, it travels above the first rib where it is separated from the artery by the anterior scalene muscle.

Two approaches are available for cannulation of this vessel: supraclavicular and infraclavicular. We suggest that the operator choose his site based on past experience and training. The methods described below are examples of these approaches; multiple variations have been documented in the medical literature.[12]

Proper positioning of the patient optimizes the success rates of these procedures. Placement of a rolled-up towel or sandbag between the patient's scapulae allows the shoulders to fall posteriorly, pulling the humeral head out of the way, opening up the sternoclavicular region. Rotation of the head may be of assistance if difficulty advancing the guidewire is encountered. Gentle posterior traction on the upper arm can further diminish interference by the humerus.

SUPRACLAVICULAR APPROACHES

Three sites for cutaneous penetration have been described; junctional, anterior scalene, and clavicular notch. Successful cannulation rates range from 85 to 98 percent. All require Trendelenburg positioning to increase central venous pressure. Slight rotation of the head to the contralateral side opens up the intended puncture site and facilitates identification of landmarks. The overall complication rate for this approach varies between 0 to 6 percent.[16] The risk of pneumothorax has been reported to be 1 to 5 percent in the hands of experienced operators[4,17] but is increased with lung disease or with high levels of positive end-expiratory pressure (PEEP). This approach is a reasonable choice for most patients since landmarks are rarely obscured even in morbidly obese patients. Dressing and catheter security are good, and patient mobility limitations are modest.[18]

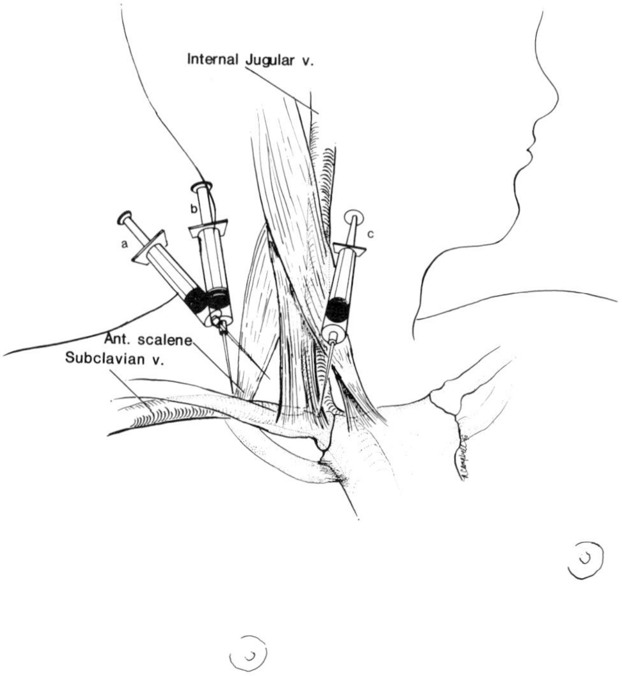

FIGURE 24-3 Supraclavicular subclavian vein cannulation. *a.* Junctional approach. *b.* Anterior scalene approach. *c.* Clavicular notch approach.

Junctional Approach (Fig. 24-3)

Venous entry is at the junction of the subclavian and internal jugular veins. Skin entry is immediately lateral to the clavicular head of the sternocleidomastoid muscle, 1 to 2 cm above the superior margin of the clavicle. The syringe or needle should be elevated approximately 15 to 20° above the skin and advanced in a direction that bisects the angle formed between the lateral margin of the sternocleidomastoid and the superior aspect of the clavicle (toward the contralateral nipple). Penetration depth should be less than 2 cm. This approach allows the needle to remain anterior to the apex of the lung.

Anterior Scalene Approach (Fig. 24-3)

The insertion of the anterior scalene muscle into the first rib can be identified by palpation immediately behind and slightly lateral to the clavicular head of the sternocleidomastoid muscle. The needle is advanced through the skin at the lateral margin of the scalene tubercle and over the first rib in a plane parallel to the anterior chest. It is held at a shallow angle and directed toward the feet. Penetration into the subclavian vein should occur within 1 to 2 cm.

Clavicular Notch Approach (Fig. 24-3)
The clavicular notch can be palpated as a smooth concave surface on the superior margin of the clavicle, slightly lateral to the suprasternal notch. With the neck slightly extended, the needle is advanced through the skin, 1 cm above the clavicular notch, and directed parallel to the long axis of the body, toward the feet. The syringe is held approximately 30° above the skin and advanced no more than 2 to 3 cm. Needle direction is parallel to the brachiocephalic vessels; therefore, redirection after obtaining blood flow may not be necessary prior to advancement of a guidewire.

INFRACLAVICULAR APPROACHES
Many physicians consider this approach the most practical solution for long-term central venous access. Several variations of this approach based on the degree of lateral placement of the cannulating needle are described below. Success rates for this approach vary between 70 and 99 percent.[12]

Medial Approach (Fig. 24-4)
Venous cannulation is begun by entering the skin 1 cm inferior to the clavicle at the junction of the medial one-third and distal two-thirds of the clavicle. The syringe should be elevated 15° from the skin and advanced toward the suprasternal notch. Difficulty advancing the needle under the clavicle is often encountered. Rather than increasing the angle of the needle to the skin, pressure is applied to the needle at the insertion site in a posteriorly directed fashion while continuing to advance the needle. The needle is advanced parallel to the chest wall, thereby reducing posterior displacement of the needle into the apex of the lung. If unsuccessful, slight superior and inferior redirections of the needle may prove rewarding. After venous entry, rotation of the needle bevel toward the right atrium may facilitate guidewire placement and reduce the risk of catheter malposition.

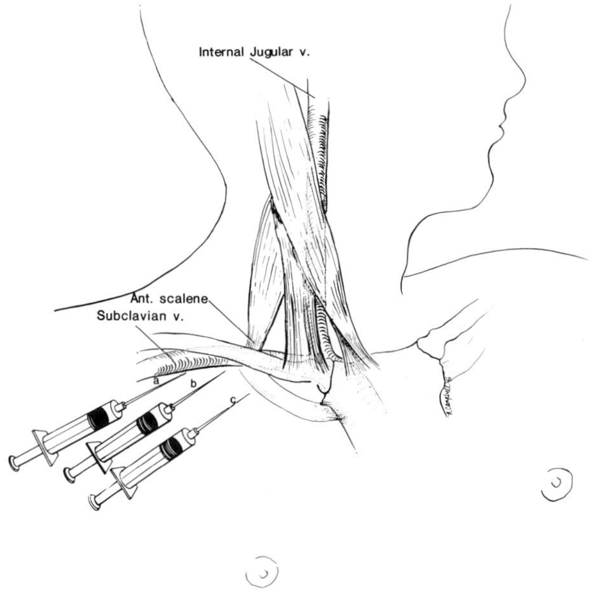

FIGURE 24-4 Infraclavicular subclavian vein cannulation. *a.* Lateral approach. *b.* Middle approach. *c.* Medial approach.

Lateral Approach (Fig. 24-4)
Skin entry occurs at the juncture of the lateral one-third and proximal two-thirds of the clavicle and is otherwise similar to the medial approach. However, the risks of subclavian artery perforation and brachial plexus injury are more significant with this route. This may be a better choice for patients with very narrow sternoclavicular angles since such angles limit medial approaches.

Middle Approach (Fig. 24-4)
The site of needle entry is midway between the medial and lateral approaches. The technique is otherwise the same as described above.

AXILLARY VEIN

This uncommon site can be used to access the central circulation, especially when pulmonary artery catheterization is planned. The axilla is often the only area of normal skin in severely burned patients through which cannulation may be attempted. Its location decreases the incidence of pneumothorax and does not significantly limit patient mobility. Its remote location from pulmonary secretions is associated with a low (2.7 percent) infection rate.[19] Cannulation is achieved by inserting a needle inferior to the axillary artery in the apex of the axilla and advancing it in a direction parallel to the course of the artery. Cephalad catheter tip malpositioning may be diminished by turning the patient's head toward the entry site.

FEMORAL VEIN CANNULATION

The extrathoracic location of this vein makes it an excellent choice for central venous cannulation in patients at extreme risk for pneumothorax. Hemostasis can be attained with direct pressure making this vein a good choice in the face of coagulopathies. It can be used for pressure monitoring if the catheter tip can be advanced above the diaphragm and into the thorax. The disadvantages of this route are listed in Table 24-3. It is frequently used in patients requiring temporary central venous access for hemodialysis. Utilization of soft catheters with low thrombosis potential, combined with short durations of catheterization, has reduced infection rates for femoral catheters. The risk of complications and infection for short-term catheterization equals that of other central routes[20] although increased bacterial colonization rates have been reported.[21] Vigilant evaluation of the catheter site and dressings should be included in caring for femoral vein catheters. If catheter-related sepsis is being considered in a patient with a femoral line, empiric antibi-

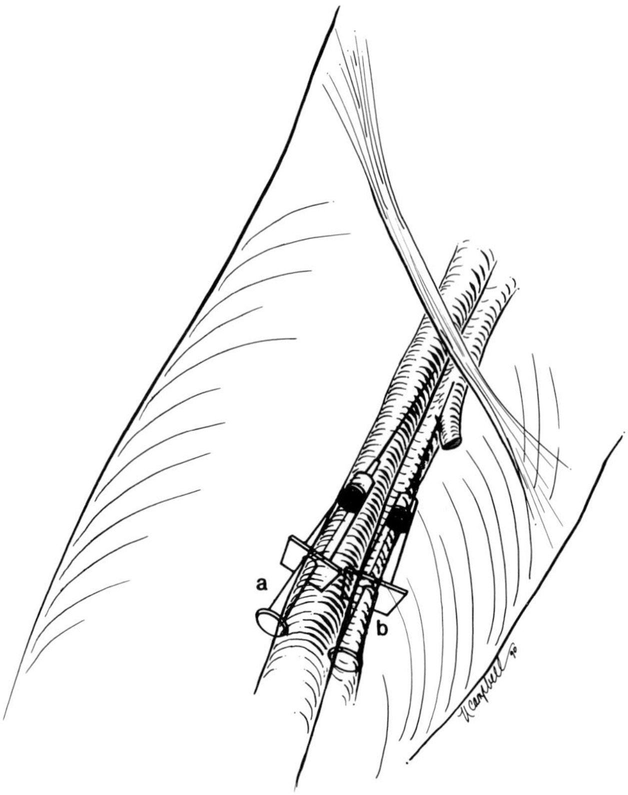

FIGURE 24-5 Femoral artery *(a)* and vein *(b)* cannulation.

otic therapy should include coverage for enteric and urinary organisms.[21]

The lack of interference with cardiopulmonary resuscitation (CPR) makes this vessel a good site for cannulation during cardiac arrests. However, delivery of medications to the right atrium during low flow states is unreliable. It should be used only when central access cannot be attained in the upper portions of the body. Since the presence of this catheter just below the inguinal ligament limits flexion of the hip, alternate sites should be considered in patients whose care and rehabilitation require mobility.

Insertion of a catheter into the femoral vein is similar to the other vessels described above (Fig. 24-5). We recommend the Seldinger technique although appropriate sized catheter-over-needle and peel-away needle devices are also used. The reliable anatomic position of this vein, immediately medial to the femoral artery, allows for successful cannulation rates of 95 to 99 percent.[12] The use of topical locating tricks (e.g., undertaker's rule) in the absence of a femoral pulse is not reliable and cannot be recommended. The absence of a femoral pulse should lead to the selection of an alternate site.

Cannulation of this vessel should be planned 1 to 3 cm below the inguinal ligament. Site selection above the inguinal ligament presents several problems with regard to the anatomic relationship of this vein with other pelvic vessels (e.g., inferior epigastric arteries) and the possibility of peritoneal perforation. In the event of a bleeding complication, hemostasis by application of direct pressure may not be possible above the inguinal ligament.

EXTERNAL JUGULAR VEIN

Although the external jugular vein is not truly a central vein, its junction with the subclavian vein can allow for access to the central venous circulation. Its tortuous course, valves, and lateral position are associated with reduced success rates as compared to more direct central venous cannulation (<75 percent vs. >90 percent). Reliable cannulation rates have been reported by authors who use this vein regularly.[22] There is minimal risk for pneumothorax and carotid artery puncture. Furthermore, it is an excellent choice for patients with coagulopathies.

The location of this vein on the lateral aspect of the neck predisposes to catheter malposition into the ipsilateral subclavian vein. The occasional presence of a venous plexus behind the clavicle can also limit access to the central vasculature. Overall success rates of less than 75 percent and malposition rates of 20 to 30 percent have been reported.[14] Utilization of a flexible J wire may improve central access rates and diminish malposition.[22]

COMPLICATIONS OF CENTRAL VENOUS CANNULATION

PNEUMOTHORAX

The complications associated with central venous catheterization are listed in Table 24-5. Pneumothoraces that occur during central vein cannulation often do not require tube thoracostomy. Patients with respiratory or hemodynamic compromise (tension pneumothorax) or nonresolving pneumothorax require chest tubes. Uncomplicated pneumothorax can be treated with small-diameter, percutaneously placed, catheter-through-needle chest tubes with one-way valves. In the event of unresolved pneumothorax, contralateral central venous cannulation should not be attempted.

TABLE 24-5 Complications of Central Venous Cannulation

Pneumothorax
Catheter or guidewire embolism
Catheter knotting
Air embolism
Central vein thrombosis
Arrhythmias
Myocardial or central vein perforation
Pericardial tamponade
Infection (local or systemic)
Hydrothorax
Hematoma
Phrenic nerve, brachial plexus damage
Subcutaneous emphysema or fluid infiltration
Arterial puncture and/or laceration
Catheter malposition
Thoracic duct laceration

CATHETER EMBOLIZATION
Catheter embolization occurs primarily with the use of catheter-through-needle devices, when the catheter is inadvertently withdrawn through the needle. Removal of these emboli is clinically challenging. Snares directed to the embolus under fluoroscopic guidance should be attempted first. Otherwise, surgical alternatives should be sought. Catheter knotting is frequently a complication of excessive advancement of pulmonary artery catheters. Removal usually requires a cutdown to the involved vessel.

AIR EMBOLIZATION
Air embolism is an underdiagnosed problem of central venous catheterization. The potential for this problem to occur with *any* form of intravascular cannulation exists. Air can reach the venous system via intravenous tubing, malfunctioning sheath introducers, the catheter tract, and the inserting needle. Maintenance of positive venous pressure during insertion should help in preventing this problem. In the event of clinically significant air embolization, anxiety, hypotension, mental status changes, and livedo reticularis may be noted. Patients should be placed in a left lateral decubitus position with the head down. Successful aspiration of air via large bore catheters placed into the right ventricle has been reported (see Chap. 118).

THROMBOSIS
Asymptomatic thrombosis of the central veins occurs in 20 to 70 percent of central veins chronically cannulated. Symptomatic presentations occur in 3 to 5 percent of patients. Diagnosis of catheter-related thrombosis can be difficult but should be based on clinical findings of diminished catheter flow and signs of venous obstruction. When necessary, venography is the diagnostic procedure of choice. Doppler ultrasonography and ^{131}I fibrinogen scanning are less reliable. Management of central vein thrombosis should include removal of the catheter. Administration of thrombolytic agents may be useful in symptomatic patients, although no large studies of its use in this setting are available. Rarely, surgical thrombectomy may be required. Pulmonary embolization can occur when thrombi are sheared off of catheter tips as they are being removed.

Thrombosis results from venous stasis, endothelial injury, and activation of the coagulation cascade. Prevention of this problem requires that each of these factors be addressed. The use of appropriate sized catheters reduces venous stasis. The development of soft, pliable catheters should reduce endothelial injury. Catheter materials that have reduced thrombogenicity, such as silicone rubber and polyurethane, are associated with reduced incidences of thrombus formation. Polyurethane-and Teflon-coated catheters have smooth surfaces which limit platelet adhesion and subsequent thrombus formation. Teflon catheters tend to be stiff and may enhance endothelial injury. Polyurethane appears to be the most reasonable choice for short-term central venous access. Extremely compliant silicone catheters ordinarily require placement by cutdown; as such, they are not readily applicable to most patients in acute settings. The administration of anticoagulants, either through the catheter or orally has clearly been shown to diminish the risk of catheter-related thrombosis. Heparin-coated devices are effective for short-term use only, since the heparin coating either dissolves or is washed off shortly after placement.

ARRHYTHMIAS
Ventricular arrhythmias occur frequently with the passage of a catheter or guidewire into the right ventricle. The potential for injury to the right bundle branch of the myocardial conducting system exists during catheterization. Thus, patients with preexisting left bundle branch blocks may be at risk for the development of complete heart block, especially during right heart and pulmonary artery catheterization. However, this risk has been demonstrated to be very low, so a pacemaker need not be placed prophylactically (see Chapter 32); rather an emergency transcutaneous or transvenous pacemaker should be available.

VASCULAR PERFORATION
Central venous and right ventricular perforation are unusual but not rare complications of central venous cannulation. These complications result from the utilization of stiff catheters that are usually placed too far into the central circulation. Depending on the entry site, patient movement can produce unanticipated advancement of a catheter of 3 (subclavian) to 10 cm (antecubital), depending on the entry site. If perforation through a vessel occurs above the pericardium, the diagnosis will be suggested by the development of a new pleural fluid collection (blood or intravenous fluids) or mediastinal hematoma. If perforation of the thin-walled superior vena cava (SVC) or right ventricle should occur, diagnosis may be delayed until signs of cardiac tamponade develop. Mortality rates of up to 95 percent have been reported in this setting. To reduce this risk, soft catheters (Silastic or polyurethane) that are clearly placed 2 cm or more above the right atrium should be used. The distal portion of the catheter should be parallel to the cannulated vessel, not under tension perpendicular to its wall.

INFECTION
Thirty percent of nosocomial bacteremias are infusion therapy related and are either due to contaminated infusate or, more commonly, catheter infection. Current evidence suggests that catheter infection occurs primarily because of migration of bacteria from the skin, along the catheter tract, to the catheter tip. Infection of the catheter hub can also result in catheter-related infection.[23] Bacteria then adhere either directly to the catheter or to the fibrin sheath that forms around most catheters.[3] An attachable, subcutaneous cuff composed of collagen impregnated with silver ions (Vitacuff) is now available. This device has been demonstrated to significantly reduce the rate of central venous catheter-related infection by preventing bacterial migration along the catheter tract.[24] Catheter infection and catheter-related sepsis have been previously defined[25] based on semiquantitative culture techniques. Studies using these definitions have led to several recommendations. If catheter-related sepsis is suspected in the absence of entry-site

TABLE 24-6 Definition of Catheter-Related Infections*

Catheter colonization	<15 colonies
Catheter infection	≥15 colonies
Catheter-related sepsis	≥15 colonies and positive blood cultures of the same organism

*Assumes growth within 72 h.

cellulitis, the catheter may be changed over a guidewire pending the results of blood and quantitative catheter tip cultures. If the catheter and blood cultures display significant growth (Table 24-6) of the same organism, then catheter-related sepsis is likely. Positive catheter tip culture in the face of negative blood cultures suggests catheter infection. Catheter-related sepsis and catheter infection require replacement of the catheter to an entirely new site. The use of guidewire exchanges continues to be investigated. A single unconfirmed study indicated that serial exchanges, occurring at weekly intervals, reduced the incidence of catheter infection.[26] Other studies demonstrate trends toward catheter-related sepsis when guidewire exchanges are used (especially with multiple-lumen catheters).[27] (See Chaps. 43 and 101.)

While peripheral catheter infection rates in oncology patients have been reported as high as 27.7 infective episodes per 1000 days, the infection rate of tunneled catheters is low (1.37 infections per 1000 days). Short-term central venous catheterization devices such as pulmonary artery catheters and sheath introducers have intermediate infection rates of 3.35 infections per 1000 days. When infection does occur in tunneled catheters, coagulase negative staphylococci are most commonly isolated.[28]

The diagnosis of tunneled-catheter-related infection is difficult. Removal of all chronic indwelling devices with each fever spike of unknown origin is impractical, especially since many catheter infections can be treated with antibiotics. Pour plate culture techniques of cultures drawn through the catheter can be useful. A ratio of colony counts from centrally drawn versus peripherally drawn blood cultures of 10:1 or greater is supportive of central-venous-catheter-related infection in the absence of catheter tip cultures.

Many cases of tunneled-catheter-related bacteremias can be treated medically with high-dose parenteral antibiotics administered via the catheter for at least 4 weeks. Removal of the catheter has been recommended only if the bloodstream cannot be sterilized, signs of septicemia persist after 3 to 5 days of appropriate antibiotic therapy, septic emboli appear, or the catheter tunnel is grossly infected.[3] Successful medical treatment of fungal catheter infections is unlikely and should prompt removal of the catheter. Entry-site infection, defined as inflammation within 2 cm of skin entry, is not an indication for catheter removal. Catheter-related septic central vein thrombosis (CR-SCVT) is defined as persistent bacteremia after catheter removal, in the presence of documented central vein thrombosis. CR-SCVT can be treated medically with antibiotics and anticoagulation.

Arterial Catheterization

Arterial pressure monitoring has become commonplace in critical care settings due to improvements in the function and availability of bedside pressure monitoring devices and the increased use of arterial blood gases. Arterial lines can be used for infusion of fluids and nonvasoactive medications in emergency settings. Because of its peripheral and accessible location, the radial artery is the first choice for arterial cannulation for most patients. The axillary and femoral arteries are less frequently used, though when appropriately selected for a given patient they have similar overall complication rates as radial artery cannulation.

RADIAL ARTERY CANNULATION

Other than the absence of ulnar collateral flow to the hand, no clear contraindications to the cannulation of this vessel can be identified. Patients with Raynaud's phenomenon, and perhaps those with Berger's disease or large vessel angiopathies (vasculitis), should be considered carefully prior to radial artery cannulation.

Fifteen to twenty percent of patients have inadequate collateral circulation to the hand. In the absence of bedside ultrasonic imaging of arterial flow, Allen's test should be performed. This is done by simultaneously occluding both the radial and ulnar arteries immediately proximal to the palmar crease while the wrist is held in a neutral or slightly flexed position. The patient is then instructed to open and close her hand to produce blanching of the hand and digits. Pressure over the ulnar artery is then relinquished and the time for return to normal color is recorded. Color return within 7 s is considered normal, from 7 to 14 s is considered indeterminate, and longer than 14 s is definitely abnormal. This classic bedside maneuver is difficult to perform in patients who are unconscious or uncooperative, jaundiced, vasoconstricted, or have no peripheral pulse secondary to previous catheterizations. False-positive results may occur if the wrist is hyperextended. Fourteen percent of patients with a normal Allen's test had inadequate arterial supply by ultrasonographic evaluation.[29]

As shown in Fig. 24-6, the patient is prepared by mildly dorsiflexing the wrist over a rolled-up towel or roll of gauze, and gently taping the fingers down to prevent motion of the area. After adequate skin preparation and draping, the skin is anesthetized with 0.5 to 1.0 mL of 1% lidocaine without epinephrine. Once the arterial pulsation is clearly felt, the needle (20 to 22 ga) can be advanced through the anesthetized area at a 45° angle into the arterial lumen. The catheter angle should be reduced to 15 to 20° above the skin and advanced 1 to 2 mm further to ensure placement of the entire needle bevel and the distal portion of the plastic catheter into the arterial lumen. Blood return should be reconfirmed. The hub of the needle should be held firmly while the plastic catheter is advanced over the needle and into the artery or a guidewire is advanced into the lumen if using the Seldinger technique (see above). Flush solution should not be administered in an effort to

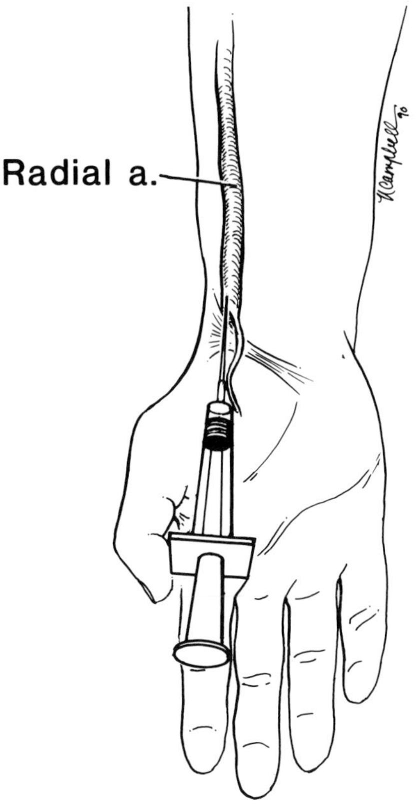

FIGURE 24-6 Radial artery cannulation.

"float" the catheter into place. Penetration of both sides of the vessel is not uncommon. In this instance blood return may not be noted until the catheter is withdrawn 1 to 2 mm. Hence, the catheter should be withdrawn slowly, observing for blood return even when removing the catheter prior to a planned reattempt. At no time should the position of the catheter be changed while the tip of the needle is beneath the skin. Significant alterations in needle position can lacerate the vessel. No more than two to three attempts at cannulating at a given site should be made, and at no time should a needle be reinserted into a plastic catheter that lies beneath the skin.

Catheter placement into the vessel lumen is confirmed by the return of pressurized blood. At this point, a short length (<6 cm) of heparin flushed noncompliant tubing, previously connected to a calibrated pressure transducer (preferably disposable), should be connected to the catheter. The catheter should then be sutured to the skin.

FEMORAL ARTERY CANNULATION

Cannulation of this vessel is similar to the technique of radial artery cannulation, although a larger catheter (18 ga) can be used. The size of this vessel makes it more amenable to use of the Seldinger technique. The vessel should be approached 1 to 3 cm below the inguinal ligament (Fig. 24-5) to prevent perforation of either the peritoneum or one of the smaller branches of the iliac artery. Contraindications include the presence of significant atherosclerosis at the intended entry site or in the aorta, or the absence of pulsations.[30] As with the femoral vein, the use of superficial anatomical locating tricks cannot be recommended.

DORSALIS PEDIS ARTERY CANNULATION

This superficial artery is often the only available site for peripheral arterial cannulation and is a reasonable alternative to radial artery cannulation.[31] Intact collateral circulation can be assessed by simultaneously compressing both the posterior tibial and dorsalis pedis arteries. The patient then wiggles the toes to produce blanching, and the posterior tibial artery is released. The duration to return of normal color is recorded, with normal being less than 10 s. The utility of this test has not been established.

Cannulation of this artery is similar to that of the radial artery. The distance of this vessel from the central circulation, especially in those patients with significant vasoconstriction or on vasoconstrictors, may make this an unreliable source for intraarterial pressure monitoring. Pressure determinations from this artery reflect the sum of the intravascular distending pressure and the reflected waveforms that are created by vessel wall recoil. As such, systolic pressures may be 15 to 20 mmHg greater than cuff pressures. Mean pressures should be similar. Cannulation of this vessel is associated with an increased rate of thrombosis as compared to other sites of cannulation.[31]

AXILLARY ARTERY CANNULATION

While this vessel can be difficult to access, it has a significant collateral circulation, a proximal location, and a large lumen. Like the axillary vein, this artery may be the only available artery for percutaneous cannulation, particularly in severely burned patients. The large lumen of this proximal vessel produces accurate estimates of aortic blood pressure that frequently correlate with cuff pressures. The large lumen to catheter diameter ratio reduces the risk of thrombosis and luminal obliteration. Catheterization of this vessel is based on identification of the axillary pulse and advancement of a catheter (18 ga, nontapered) in a parallel direction.[32] In some medical centers this is the preferred site for arterial monitoring.

Retrograde flow into the cerebral circulation with excessive use of pressurized flushing systems is a greater possibility with this vessel than for the radial artery, especially with cannulation of the right axillary artery. This can lead to cerebral arterial embolism and potentially to brain abscess.

COMPLICATIONS OF ARTERIAL CANNULATION

The overall complication rate of arterial catheterization is difficult to determine but appears to rise with underlying peripheral vascular disease, concomitant coagulopathy, hypotension, duration of catheterization, placement by cutdown, wrist circumference, number of cannulation attempts,[33] and catheter to artery diameter ratio.

The three primary complications of note are bleeding,

distal limb ischemia, and infection. Other less frequent complications are site related and include peripheral nerve damage (especially the radial nerve), arteriovenous fistulas, pseudoaneurysm formation, air embolism, cerebral embolism, retroperitoneal hemorrhage, and peritoneal perforation.

BLEEDING

Bleeding occurs more frequently than with venous cannulation due to the blood pressure of the arterial system. Fortunately, most episodes of blood loss occur in superficial locations where direct pressure can be applied. The femoral artery is a notable exception since significant volumes of blood may accumulate subclinically in the abdomen or subcutaneous tissues of the groin. Coagulopathy is only a relative contraindication to arterial cannulation. Extreme hypertension (systolic blood pressures > 200 mmHg) is not considered a contraindication to arterial cannulation, although site selection (e.g., avoidance of the femoral artery) may be affected.

LIMB-THREATENING ISCHEMIA

Limb-threatening ischemia distal to the insertion site is a rare complication that must be anticipated in any patient, regardless of the presence or absence of peripheral vascular disease. Partial to complete arterial obstruction at the cannulation site occurs in 20 to 48 percent of patients within the first 24 h after cannulation. Distal ischemia occurs either because of luminal obliteration caused by improper catheter size or because of distal embolization from shedding of a clot from the catheter tip.

Inappropriately larger catheters that obliterate the lumen of an artery are associated with higher rates of arterial thrombosis and/or obstruction due to stasis of blood distally. Nontapered, 20 ga catheters have lower morbidity rates in radial arteries than 18 ga catheters. Impairment of flow after catheter removal is inversely related to plasma prothrombin times.[31] Percutaneously placed catheters, as opposed to those placed by cutdown, are associated with decreased rates of radial artery ischemia.

Arterial embolization (fluid or air) can occur after flushing catheters with pressurized anticoagulant solutions. Cerebral embolization has been attributed to excess flushing. The utilization of continuous flushing systems (3 mL/h) may decrease the incidence of catheter-related thrombosis. However, these infusion systems can produce significant degrees of anticoagulation in patients who are unable to adequately clear heparin.

The most significant risk factor for limb-threatening ischemia is the use of end arteries. This applies in particular to brachial artery cannulation. We do not recommend its routine use because of the lack of collateral circulation to the hand. Success with this technique may reflect placement of small gauge catheters into a large-diameter artery.

Permanent ischemic damage is extremely rare, occurring in 0.5 percent of all cannulated arteries. This complication is best avoided by careful site selection and by frequent bedside monitoring of the cannulated extremity.

INFECTION

Arterial catheters provide a portal of bacterial entry into the vascular system. This is readily demonstrated by the recovery of staphylococcal and streptococcal species from catheter cultures. The incidence of arterial-catheter-related infection is equal to that of central venous lines and pulmonary artery catheters (2 to 8 percent).[34] Superficial colonization and infections are more common than are episodes of catheter-related sepsis. Heparinized flush solutions frequently become stagnant columns of dextrose-containing solutions that provide an excellent environment for bacterial growth. The use of saline-based continuous flushing systems and routine changing of these solutions may limit this problem. Disposable pressure transducers have reduced the incidence of arterial-catheter-related infections in certain settings such as cardiac intensive care units. The infusion tubing and flush solution should be changed at 48 h or less intervals.

Minimizing stopcock manipulations and blood withdrawal may reduce the incidence of arterial-line-related infections. Reduction of arterial-catheter-related infections may be achieved by the establishment of protocols that mandate catheter changes at intervals of 96 h or less, replacement of stopcock caps with diaphragms that are regularly changed (after every 20 punctures), and limited tubing system manipulation (blood sampling). Blood withdrawn from catheter systems should not be reinjected.

Alternatives to Venous Cannulation

CORPORA CAVERNOSA

The extensive venous channels within the corpora cavernosa of the penis have led to recommendations for its use as a short-term, high-volume venous access site in hypovolemic patients. The extensive venous communications between the corpora allow insertion of a single needle (18 to 20 ga) through the tough tunica albuginea into either corpus cavernosum. Drainage rates averaging 13.4 mL/s have been reported.[35] No studies reporting clinical use of this technique in emergency settings are available; thus use of the penis should be considered untested.

BONE MARROW

The bone marrow is an alternative site when venous access is limited. The marrow of the ribs or sternum in adults and the proximal tibia, iliac crest, or distal femur of children have long been utilized as alternative vascular access sites for placement of a steel needle (e.g., 18 ga spinal, 16 to 19 ga butterfly, Illinois needle).[36] The noncollapsible intramedullary capillary network within the marrow allows for effective absorption of a variety of fluids and medications such as saline, blood, antibiotics, sodium bicarbonate, and sympathomimetic amines.[37] Hypertonic or strongly alkaline substances should be avoided. Infusion rates in excess of 100 mL/h have been reported in infants. Sterile technique should be employed to lessen the risk of osteomyeli-

TABLE 24-7 Drugs That Can Be Administered Endotracheally

Valium
Atropine
Lidocaine
Isoproterenol
Epinephrine
Naloxone
Terbutaline

tis. The needle should be inserted directly into the marrow. Entry is confirmed by loss of resistance to advancement of the needle, aspiration of marrow, and free forward flow of fluid. Intraosseous lines should be discontinued immediately after intravenous access is secured. The theoretical risks of fat or cortical bone emboli have not been substantiated by clinical reports.

SUBCUTANEOUS

Subcutaneous infusions of small amounts of fluids and medications can be used when other routes are unavailable. Excessive delivery of fluids can result in impairment of blood supply to the skin and subsequent necrosis and sloughing. Subcutaneous administration of medications (e.g., epinephrine, terbutaline, insulin, heparin) has long been used and is well documented to be safe. In patients with circulatory collapse, subcutaneous absorption may be prolonged and unreliable because of peripheral vasoconstriction.

ENDOTRACHEAL

In emergency situations, certain drugs can be administered via an endotracheal tube or into the peritoneum (Table 24-7) prior to or in the absence of intravascular access. The doses require modification (e.g., double the usual epinephrine dose) to counterbalance reduced and delayed absorption. These medications should be diluted into large volumes (10 mL), and instillation should be followed by several forced ventilations to ensure delivery to the peripheral airways. Instillation via a catheter or tube placed at the end of the endotracheal tube may facilitate delivery to the airways.

Venous Cutdown

The utilization of cutdowns for establishment of vascular access has diminished and now occurs primarily in the setting of severe coagulopathies, hypovolemic emergencies, and with the placement of permanent access devices such as the Hickman and Broviac catheters. Cutdowns are otherwise reserved for only the most difficult access patients. Pediatric peripheral cutdowns performed in ideal settings, by experienced surgeons, require an average of 11 min.[38] Given the availability of large bore catheters that can be placed centrally in 2 to 3 min, cutdowns do not seem appropriate first line access in emergency settings.

Catheters placed in this manner are associated with an increased risk of infection and require frequent changing. Ideally they should be placed in sterile settings (operating rooms). Cutdown sites include nearly every superficial (and some deeper) vein in the body.

References

1. Tager IE, Ginsberg MB, Ellis SE, et al. and The Rhode Island nosocomial infection consortium: An epidemiologic study of the risks associated with peripheral intravenous catheters. Am J Epidemio. 118:839, 1983.
2. Rosen KR, Rosen DA: Comparative flow rates for small bore peripheral catheters. Pediatr Emerg Care 2:153, 1986.
3. Maki GG: Infections due to infusion therapy, in Bennet JV, Brachman PS (eds): *Hospital Infections*, 2d ed. Boston, Little Brown, 1986, p 561.
4. Sznajder JI, Zveibel FR, Bitterman H, et al: Central venous catheterization. Failure and complication rates by three percutaneous approaches. Arch Intern Med 146:259, 1986.
5. Mallory DL, McGee WT, Shawtzer T, et al.: Internal jugular vein anatomic freatures can be modified during cannulation attempts. Crit Care Med 16:864, 1988.
6. Mallory DL, McGee WT, Shawtzer T, et al.: Ultrasound guidance improves the success rate of internal jugular vein cannulation. A prospective randomized trial. Chest 98:157, 1990.
7. Farber BF: The multi-lumen catheter: proposed guidelines for its use. Infect Control Hosp Epidemiol 9:206, 1988.
8. Gil RT, Kruse JA, Thill-Baharozian MC, et al.: Triple- vs single-lumen central venous catheters. Arch Intern Med 149:1139, 1989.
9. Miliken SJ, Cain TL, Hansbrough J: Rapid volume replacement for hypovolemic shock: a comparison of techniques and equipment. J Trauma 24:428, 1984.
10. Brown C: Cordis introducers: CVP measurement with fluid infusion. Anesthesiology 55:485, 1981.
11. Seldinger SI: Catheter replacement of the needle in percutaneous arteriography. Acta Radiol 39:368, 1953.
12. Novak RA, Venus B: Clavicular approaches for central vein cannulation, in Venus B, Mallory DL (eds): *Problems in Critical Care: Vascular Cannulation*. Philadelphia, J.B. Lippincott, vol 2, 1988, p. 242.
13. McGee WT, Mallory DL: Cannulation of the internal and external jugular veins, in Venus B, Mallory DL (eds): *Problems in Critical Care: Vascular Cannulation*. Philadelphia, J.B. Lippincott, vol 2, 1988, p 217.
14. Putterman C: Central venous catheterization: Indications, techniques, complications, management. Acute Care 12:219, 1986.
15. Sterner S: A comparison of the supraclavicular approach and the infraclavicular approach for subclavian vein catheterization. Ann Emerg Med 15:421, 1986.
16. Brahos GJ, Cohen MJ: Supraclavicular central venous catheterization: Technique and experience in 250 cases. Wisc Med J 80:36, 1981.
17. Haapaniemi L, Slatis P: Supraclavicular subclavian venipuncture of the superior vena cava. Acta Anaesthesiol Scand 18:12, 1974.
18. Helmkamp BF, Sanko SR: Supraclavicular central venous catheterization. Am J Obstet Gynecol 153:751, 1985.
19. Gouin F, Martin C, Saux P: Central venous catheterization via the axillary vein. Acta Anaesthesiol Scand 81 (suppl):27, 1985.
20. Dailey RH: Femoral vein cannulation: A review. J Emerg Med 2:367, 1985.

21. Tribett D, Brenner M: Peripheral and femoral vein cannulation, in Venus B, Mallory DL (eds): *Problems in Critical Care: Vascular Cannulation*. Philadelphia, J.B. Lippincott, vol 2 1988, p 266.
22. Blitt CD, Wright WA, Petty WC, et al.: Central venus catheterization via the external jugular vein: A technique employing the J-wire. JAMA 229:817, 1979.
23. Cercenado E, Ena J, Rodriguez-Creixems M, et al.: A conservative procedure for the diagnosis of catheter-related infections. Arch Intern Med 150:1417, 1990.
24. Flowers RH, Schwenzer KJ, Kopel RF, et al.: Efficacy of an attachable subcutaneous cuff for the prevention of intravascular catheter-related infection. A randomized trial JAMA 261:878, 1989.
25. Maki DG, Weise CE, Sarafin AW: A semiquantitative culture method for identifying intravenous-catheter-related infection. N Engl J Med 296:1305, 1977.
26. Bozzetti F, Terno G, Bonfanti G, et al.: Prevention and treatment of central venous catheter sepsis by exchange via a guidewire. A prospective controlled trial. Ann Surg 198:48, 1983.
27. Hilton E, Haslett TM, Borentstein MT, et al.: Central catheter infections: single- versus triple-lumen catheters. Influence of guidewires on infection rates when used for replacement of catheters. Am J Med 84:667, 1988.
28. Clarke DE, Raffin TA: Infectious complications of indwelling long-term central venous catheters. Chest 97:966, 1990.
29. Clarke W, Freund PR, Wasse J, et al.: Assessment of adequacy of ulnar arterial flow prior to radial artery catheterization. Anesthesiology 55:A38, 1982.
30. Gurman GA, Kriemernman S: Cannulation of big arteries in critically ill patients. Crit Care Med 13:217, 1985.
31. Naguib M, Hassan M, Farag, H, et al.: Cannulation of the radial and dorsalis pedis arteries. Br J Anaesth 59:482, 1987.
32. Bryan-Brown CW, Kwun KB, Lumb PD, et al: The axillary artery catheter. Heart Lung 12:492, 1983.
33. Wilkins RG: Radial artery cannulation and ischaemic damage. A review. Anaesthesia 40:896, 1985.
34. Veremakis C, Halloran T: The technique of arterial cannulation. J Crit Ill 63:381, 1989.
35. Godec CJ: The penis—A possible alternative emergency fluid access for males? Ann Emerg Med 11:266, 1982.
36. Fiser DH: Intraosseous infusion. N Engl J Med 322:1579, 1990.
37. Harte FA, Chalmers PC, Walsh RF, et al.: Intraosseous fluid administration: a parenteral alternative in pediatric resuscitation. Anesth Analg 66:687, 1987.
38. Iserson KV, Criss EA: Pediatric venous cutdowns: utility in emergency situations. Pediatr Emerg Care 2:231, 1986.

Chapter 25

CLINICAL USE OF THE PULMONARY ARTERY CATHETER

JAMES W. LEATHERMAN
JOHN MARINI

Introduction

Few technological advances of the past two decades have changed the practice of intensive care medicine as much as bedside pulmonary artery (PA) catheterization. Initially used as a tool for guiding therapy of complicated acute myocardial infarction, the balloon-flotation PA catheter is currently used in a variety of other situations. Conditions for which bedside PA catheterization has been advocated include pulmonary edema of unclear etiology, the adult respiratory distress syndrome (ARDS) requiring moderate to high levels of positive end-expiratory pressure (PEEP), septic shock, and high-risk cardiac and noncardiac surgery. It was estimated in 1984 that over two million PA catheters had been inserted since their introduction into clinical medicine.[1] Despite this widespread use, controversy remains regarding the actual impact on patient management and outcome. One extreme position has called for an outright ban on use of the PA catheter, on the grounds that no beneficial effect of this invasive technology has been convincingly demonstrated and that its use may actually increase mortality.[2] A more moderate view, to which we subscribe, contends that the procedural risks of PA catheterization are actually very small and that the hemodynamic information supplied can be of enormous value in guiding therapy of critically ill patients, especially when empirical therapeutic trials have proven unsuccessful or are deemed to be potentially hazardous. Implicit in this latter view, however, is that the physician using the catheter fully understands the fundamental principles of hemodynamic monitoring and is aware of both the potential limitations of the catheter and the common pitfalls associated with interpreting the data. Faulty clinical decisions based on inaccurate or misleading data are likely of greater risk to the patient than are the risks of the procedure itself. This chapter will review use of the PA catheter in the ICU with particular emphasis on the principles and common pitfalls of data acquisition, recording, and application.

Indications

The primary conditions for which bedside PA catheterization is used as a diagnostic or management tool are listed in Table 25-1. In deciding whether to proceed with invasive hemodynamic monitoring, the clinician must consider a number of factors other than the immediate diagnostic and management issues. Procedural risk must be considered, focusing on concerns (e.g., coagulopathy) that might increase risk. The anticipated clinical course over the ensuing days is also important, with a projected unstable and variable hemodynamic pattern favoring invasive monitoring. Potential hazards of empirical therapy must be addressed. Often, the PA catheter is inserted only after empirical management with volume infusion or diuresis has been unsuccessful. In certain instances, however, the potential consequences of empirical management on gas exchange, blood pressure, or renal function are sufficiently worrisome that more precise definition of the underlying physiology is required from the outset. Another consideration is that the physician who knows the patient best may not be the one who is asked to make critical decisions in the middle of the night. For cross-covering physicians, knowledge of the hemodynamic data available from a PA catheter can be of enormous benefit and may result in more rational clinical decision-making. Finally, some of the diagnostic informa-

TABLE 25-1 Clinical Uses of Bedside Pulmonary Artery Catheterization

DIAGNOSTIC USES	Primary Data Sought
Pulmonary edema	Ppw
Shock	$\dot{Q}_T$ and SVR; Ppw; $S\bar{v}_{O_2}$
Oliguric renal failure	Ppw, $\dot{Q}_T$
Perplexing lactic acidemia	$\dot{Q}_T$, $S\bar{v}_{O_2}$
Pulmonary hypertension	Ppa, Ppad, Ppw
Cardiac disorders	
Acute mitral insufficiency	V wave
Ventricular septal defect	ΔO_2 saturation RA → PA
RV infarction	Pra, RVEDP, Ppw
Pericardial tamponade	Pra, RVEDP, Ppad, Ppw
Narrow complex tachyarrhythmia	RA waveform (flutter waves)
Wide complex tachyarrhythmia	RA waveform (cannon A waves)
Lymphatic carcinoma	Aspiration cytology
Microvascular thrombi (ARDS)	Angiography
MONITORING USES	
Assess adequacy of intravascular volume	
Hypotension	
Oliguria	
High-risk surgical patient	
Assess effect of change in Ppw on pulmonary edema	
Assess therapy for shock	
Cardiogenic (vasodilator, inotrope)	
Septic (volume, vasopressor, inotrope)	
Hypovolemic (volume)	
Assess effects of PEEP on D_{O_2} in ARDS	

Ppw, pulmonary wedge pressure; $\dot{Q}_T$, cardiac output; SVR, systemic vascular resistance; $S\bar{v}_{O_2}$, mixed venous oxygen saturation; Ppa, pulmonary artery pressure; Ppad, pulmonary artery diastolic pressure; Pra, right atrial pressure; RVEDP, right ventricular end-diastolic pressure; D_{O_2}, oxygen delivery; RV, right ventricle; RA, right atrium.

TABLE 25-2 Complications of Pulmonary Artery Catheterization

Complications related to central vein cannulation (see Chap. 24)
Complications related to insertion and use of the PA catheter
- Tachyarrhythmias
- Right bundle branch block
- Complete heart block (preexisting left bundle branch block)
- Cardiac perforation
- Thrombosis and embolism
- Pulmonary infarction due to persistent wedging
- Catheter-related sepsis
- PA rupture
- Knotting of the catheter
- Endocarditis, bland and infective
- Pulmonic valve insufficiency
- Balloon fragmentation and embolization

tion available from the PA catheter can also be obtained noninvasively with two-dimensional Doppler echocardiography. For example, pericardial tamponade and certain complications of acute myocardial infarction [ventricular septal defect (VSD), acute mitral regurgitation, right ventricular (RV) infarction] can be accurately diagnosed by echocardiography. The decision to place a PA catheter to diagnose these conditions will clearly be influenced by the availability of high quality echocardiography and by the projected need for ongoing invasive monitoring after a diagnosis has been established. Thus, many variables may influence the decision to insert a PA catheter, and experienced clinicians may disagree on the need for invasive monitoring in individual cases. As such, the disease processes listed in Table 25-1 should perhaps not be considered as *indications* for PA catheterization, but rather as conditions for which insertion of a PA catheter may in certain instances provide enough useful information so as to outweigh the procedure's risk.

Complications

Complications of PA catheter insertion include those that are related to achieving vascular access and those that are due to the catheter itself (Table 25-2). The former are considered elsewhere (see Chap. 24) and only catheter-related complications will be considered here.

ARRHYTHMIA

Both atrial and ventricular tachyarrhythmias can develop as a result of catheter insertion.[3–6] The reported incidence of ventricular ectopy during passage through the RV is highly variable, ranging from 11 to 68 percent in different series.[4] One report documented ventricular tachycardia (VT), defined as three or more consecutive ventricular premature beats, in 53 percent of catheter insertions in the ICU setting.[5] However, a much lower rate of this complication has been reported by others.[4] The incidence of VT is higher in critically ill patients than in those undergoing elective right heart catheterization. This is likely because critically ill patients in the ICU often possess one or more factors that enhance arrhythmia risk (active ischemia, shock, hypoxemia, electrolyte disturbances, acidosis, or high endogenous catecholamine levels). Fortunately, VT that occurs during passage through the RV usually terminates as soon as the catheter tip is advanced beyond the pulmonic valve and thus does not require treatment. In two large series, only 1.3 and 1.5 percent of patients required antiarrhythmic therapy, chest thump, or cardioversion for VT that occurred during PA catheterization.[3,6] Catheter-induced ventricular fibrillation has been reported but is quite rare. Some clinicians recommend prophylactic lidocaine before catheter insertions, but this approach is not widely agreed on. Certainly, lidocaine should be considered if an initial attempt at catheter passage is unsuccessful and has resulted in transient VT. To reduce the risk of VT during catheter insertion, it is advisable to attempt to correct all arrhythmogenic conditions before catheter insertion, to use the full 1.5 mL of air to inflate the balloon, and to keep catheterization time to a minimum.

BUNDLE BRANCH BLOCK

Transient right bundle branch block (RBBB) has been reported to occur in 0.05 to 5 percent of catheterizations.[4] Generally of little consequence, even transient RBBB is obviously of major concern if the patient has preexisting left bundle branch block (LBBB). A recent study of 82 PA catheterizations in the setting of LBBB found no episodes of complete heart block related to catheter insertion and only two episodes of complete heart block while the catheters were in place.[7] (The latter were ascribed to the underlying disease rather than to the catheter per se.) Thus, rather than routinely inserting a prophylactic transvenous pacemaker insertion prior to PA catheterization in the setting of LBBB, a reasonable alternative might be to have an external pacemaker available in the unlikely event of complete heart block.

THROMBOSIS

Although almost always clinically silent, some degree of thrombosis at the site of insertion in the internal jugular vein has been detected by venography or autopsy in the majority of patients undergoing PA catheterization.[8] Thrombi may also develop within the heart and PA.[3] These thrombi can lead to clinically apparent pulmonary embolism but rarely do so. The catheter itself can cause pulmonary infarction from vascular obstruction, usually in the setting of a peripherally placed catheter that is at least partly wedged with the balloon deflated. Although an early study found a 7 percent incidence of pulmonary infarction,[9] more recent series have reported a far lower incidence of this complication (0 to 1.4 percent).[4] Even when infarction does occur, it may be evidenced only by a new radiographic abnormality beyond the catheter tip, without apparent clinical deterioration. Thus, some degree of thrombosis commonly accompanies PA catheterization, but clinically significant thromboembolic events are infrequent. Although heparin bonding of the catheter clearly reduces thrombus formation,[10] it is less certain that this translates into a clinically relevant reduction in risk.

PULMONARY ARTERY RUPTURE

The most serious complication of catheterization, PA rupture, is typically manifested by sudden brisk hemoptysis, from which approximately 50 percent of patients will die.[4] Fortunately, this complication is quite rare, being observed in 0.06 percent and 0.2 percent of catheterizations in two large series.[3,6] Pulmonary hypertension, cardiopulmonary bypass, and anticoagulation place the patient at increased risk for morbidity and mortality due to PA rupture.[4] In a number of reported cases rupture has occurred with the first reinflation of the catheter after initial wedging. It has been suggested that the catheter tip may advance distally with balloon deflation, then subsequent reinflation with the same balloon volume causes rupture.[11]

MISCELLANEOUS COMPLICATIONS

A number of other complications related to PA catheterization have been described (see Table 25-2). A recent review of nine large series indicates that major complications of PA catheterization are uncommon.[4] A different "complication" associated with use of the PA catheter, erroneous recording and interpretation of hemodynamic data that leads to poor clinical decisions and adverse patient outcome, may be much more frequent than these procedural risks. The remainder of this chapter will focus on the principles of data acquisition and their physiologic relevance to caring for the critically ill.

Pressure Monitoring

PRESSURE MONITORING SYSTEM (THE PLUMBING)

Essential system components required for pressure monitoring include a fluid-filled catheter and connecting tubing, a transducer to convert the mechanical energy from the pressure wave into an electrical signal, and a signal processing unit that conditions and amplifies this electrical signal for display (Fig. 25-1). Problems can occur with each of these three components.

Intrathoracic vascular pressures vary dynamically with the cardiac and respiratory cycles. The dynamic pressure waveform can be viewed as comprised of numerous sinusoidal components, mixed in varying proportions.[12] To reproduce this complex pressure signal without significant distortion, the monitoring system must respond faithfully to frequencies at least tenfold greater than that of the resultant waveform. Because human heart rates seldom exceed 150 beats/min (2.5 Hz), a system that responds well to 25

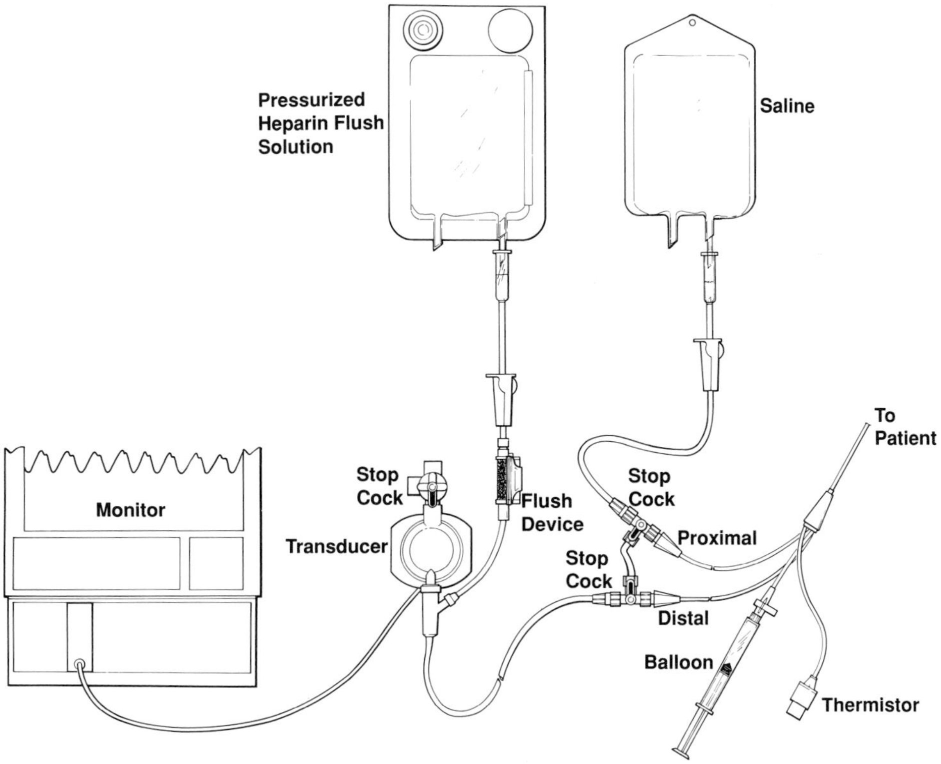

FIGURE 25-1 Standard four-lumen PA catheter with pressure tubing, heparinized flush, transducer, and signal processing unit (monitor). PA or RA pressure can be displayed by stopcock adjustment.

Hz suffices for routine clinical pressure recording. When optimally tuned, modern units generally exceed this requirement.

Two primary features of the pressure monitoring system determine its dynamic response properties: natural resonant frequency and damping.[12,13] Once perturbed, each catheter-transducer system tends to oscillate at a unique (natural resonant) frequency, determined by the elasticity and capacitance of its deformable elements. An undamped system responds well to the low frequency components of a complex wave form, but exaggerates the amplitude of components near the resonant value. Modest damping is desirable for optimal fidelity and to suppress unwanted high frequency vibration ("noise"); however, excessive damping smooths the tracing unnaturally and eliminates important frequency components of the pressure wave form. Overdamping primarily affects systolic and diastolic pressures, but if extreme can sometimes affect mean values (Fig. 25-2). Air bubbles in the monitoring system are the most common cause of overdamping, others being clot, fibrin, or a kinked or partially occluded catheter. Air bubbles produce excessive damping because air is compressible whereas fluid is not, so that mechanical energy is lost in compression and decompression of the bubble.[13] A simple bedside test for overdamping is the "rapid flush" test.[14] Because of the length and small gauge of the catheter, very high pressures are generated near the transducer when the flush device is pinched open, connecting the high pressure flush system to the transducer. An appropriately damped system will show a rapid fall in pressure with an "overshoot" and prompt return to a crisp PA tracing on sudden closure of the flush device. In contrast, an overdamped system will give a tracing that demonstrates a gradual return to the baseline pressure, without an overshoot (Fig. 25-3).

For the hydraulic monitoring system to display accurate pressures, it is essential that the system be opened to atmosphere at the hydrostatic level of interest (left atrium, LA) during calibration. The system is "zeroed" (balanced) by first isolating the catheter from the transducer with the twist of a stopcock. Then the stopcock connected to the transducer is opened to atmosphere and its air-fluid interface is placed at the LA level (midaxillary line, fourth intercostal space). The body angle is not crucial, so that one can zero the transducer with the orthopneic patient upright or semiupright. Once the transducer has been zeroed, however, movement of the transducer above or below the level of the LA will cause the recorded pressure to underestimate or overestimate, respectively, the true value (Fig. 25-4). Because the pulmonary circuit is a low pressure vascular bed, small errors in transducer position may be clinically

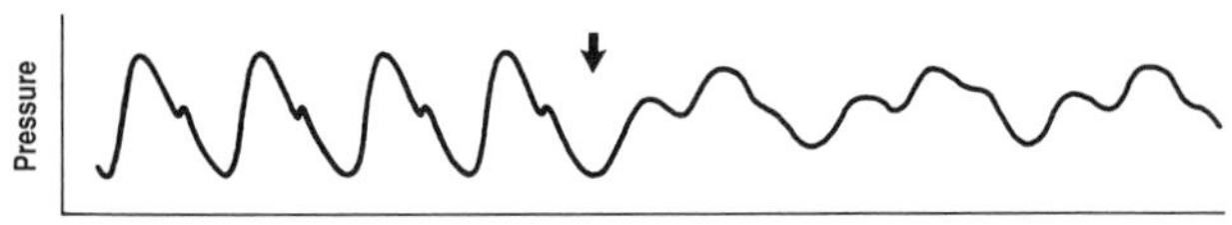

FIGURE 25-2 Effect of overdamping on PA tracing. Arrow indicates onset of damping. (Adapted from Reference 21 with permission.)

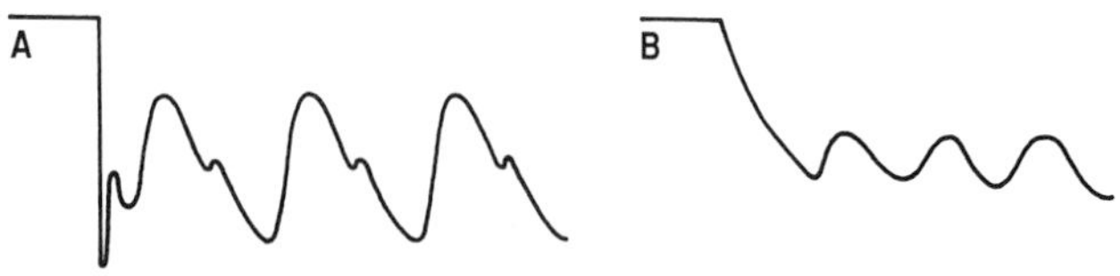

FIGURE 25-3 Rapid-flush test. Appropriately damped system (*a*); overdamped system (*b*).

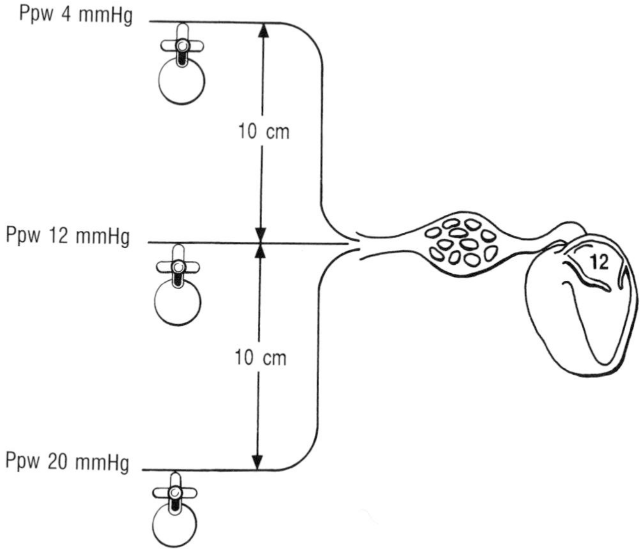

FIGURE 25-4 Effect of transducer malposition on pressure measurement. In this example, LA and wedge pressures (Ppw) are 12 mmHg. Once the transducer has been "zeroed" at LA level (see text), movement of the transducer above or below the LA plane will result in erroneous pressure measurement (10 $cmH_2O \cong 8$ mmHg).

significant. Accuracy is not affected by the position of the tip of the catheter within the chest, so long as the pressure in the subserved capillary bed exceeds local alveolar pressure (see discussion of zone 3, vide infra).

The transducer converts mechanical energy from the fluid-filled tubing into an electrical signal that is then amplified and displayed. Most transducers produce an electrical signal of 50 μV on application of 10 mmHg pressure to the transducer diaphragm.[13] The amplifying portion of the monitor increases this signal five- to tenfold to produce a visible tracing on the screen. Calibration of most modern systems is done internally, but can also be achieved by applying a known amount of static pressure to the transducer by use of a fluid-filled column of water or a three-way stopcock, syringe, and a mercury manometer. This manual method, although tedious, should be undertaken whenever a question arises regarding system accuracy. As with transducer malposition, improper calibration can introduce serious errors into data acquisition.

CATHETER INSERTION

Essential steps in insertion of the PA catheter include site selection for vascular access, insertion of the introducer, assembly and testing of the pressure monitoring system, attachment of the pressure monitoring system to the catheter via fluid-filled tubing, and, finally, insertion of the catheter under guidance of the displayed pressure waveform recorded from the distal port. This section gives only a brief summary of the technique of catheter insertion, including a few common pitfalls. More detailed descriptions of catheter insertion have been published elsewhere.[13]

Access to the right atrium (RA) can be achieved from several sites. The preferred sites for PA catheterization in the ICU are the internal jugular and subclavian veins, because of the relative ease of cannulation and advancement of the catheter across the tricuspid valve, and because catheters inserted from these sites are easily cared for. The choice of vascular access is largely one of personal preference. Some clinicians prefer the left over the right subclavian approach because in the latter approach there are potential problems with catheter kinking as it exits the introducer. The femoral vein is also suitable for catheter insertion, but passage of the catheter through the tricuspid valve is less reliably achieved without fluoroscopy. Caring for catheters inserted from the groin may be more difficult, especially in obese individuals. The antecubital approach is another alternative, but is less suitable for prolonged (i.e., days) use of the catheter. Despite these limitations, a femoral or antecubital approach should be considered when coagulopathy, lung hyperinflation, or other factors increase the risk of cannulation via the internal jugular or subclavian vein.

The PA catheter is inserted through an introducer that has side arm and safety seal features (see Chap. 24). An 8.5 F introducer is adequate for passage of either a 7.0 or 7.5 F catheter. The standard 7.0 F catheter is equipped with four lumens (proximal, distal, balloon, and thermistor). A variety of modifications of the standard four-lumen catheter have been developed. These include an additional lumen for fluid infusion, fiberoptic bundles for continuous measurement of mixed venous oxygen saturation ($S\bar{v}_{O_2}$), a special rapid-response thermistor that allows measurement of RV ejection fraction, an RV port for measurement of RV pressure or for pacing, and a special multipurpose catheter for recording atrial and ventricular electrical activity and for pacing.

Before insertion of the catheter, the pressure monitoring system is assembled and calibrated, and any air bubbles are cleared from the transducer and pressure tubing. Next, the balloon is inflated with 1.5 mL air to ensure its integrity. The proximal and distal lumens are then connected to the appropriate pressure tubing and are well flushed. The proximal and distal ports can be hooked up so as to permit display of both pressures, using separate transducers and separate tubing. Alternatively, a single transducer with pressure tubing can be connected to the distal port while the proximal port is connected to a separate infusion (see Fig. 25-1). Use of a "bridge" and stopcocks then permits monitoring of proximal (RA) pressure when desired. If the latter hookup is used, the stopcocks must be turned so that the distal pressure is displayed during catheter insertion. Mistakenly displaying the pressure signal from the proximal lumen will result in an unexpectedly long length of catheter being inserted without achieving an RV pressure recording. This pitfall should also be suspected if there is ventricular ectopy (tip in RV) while the displayed waveform is still RA.

Just before catheter insertion, the catheter tip is jiggled to ensure an expected response on the monitoring screen. After the catheter is inserted 15 to 20 cm, the rapid-flush test is performed to exclude an overdamped system.[14] (Attempts to pass the catheter under pressure monitoring with an overdamped system are usually frustrating and result in unnecessarily prolonged catheterization time.) The balloon is then inflated with 1.5 mL air, and the catheter gradually advanced until an RV tracing appears on the screen. The RV is usually reached within 30 to 35 cm from the entry sites of the internal jugular or subclavian vein. Once an RV tracing is achieved, it is not usually necessary to advance more than 15 cm of catheter before arriving in the PA. Feeding excessive catheter promotes coiling and possible knotting within the RV. The length of catheter that has been inserted at the time an RV tracing is first seen should be carefully noted. If an additional 15 cm is advanced without achieving a PA tracing, the balloon should be deflated and the catheter withdrawn to the RA. Tricks for encouraging passage from the RV into the PA include turning the patient to one side, elevating the head of the bed, and twisting the catheter in a clockwise direction to enhance entry into the anteriorly located pulmonary outflow tract. Repeated difficulty in passing the catheter through the RV is an indication for fluoroscopy. The PA tracing is recognized by a rise in diastolic pressure and by the appearance of a dicrotic notch due to pulmonic valve closure (Fig. 25-5). Once in the PA, the catheter is gradually advanced until the balloon obstructs forward flow in the artery, recognizable by a change to an atrial waveform and by a fall in mean pressure (see Fig. 25-5). After it is observed that balloon deflation is followed by a transition back to the PA waveform, and that reinflation of the balloon with 1.0 to 1.5 mL air yields a reliable PA occlusion (wedge) pressure (Ppw), the sterile sleeve can be attached to the introducer. Finally, a chest radiograph is obtained to corroborate proper placement.

Two major criteria—an atrial pressure waveform and a fall in mean pressure—are routinely used in the clinical setting to confirm a Ppw tracing. Although the Ppw tracing should have the appearance of an atrial pressure recording, it may not be possible to discern clear-cut a, c, and v waves, because of loss of fidelity in recording waveforms through the dampening caused by the vascular bed, catheter, and pressure tubing. It is crucial that a fall in mean pressure be

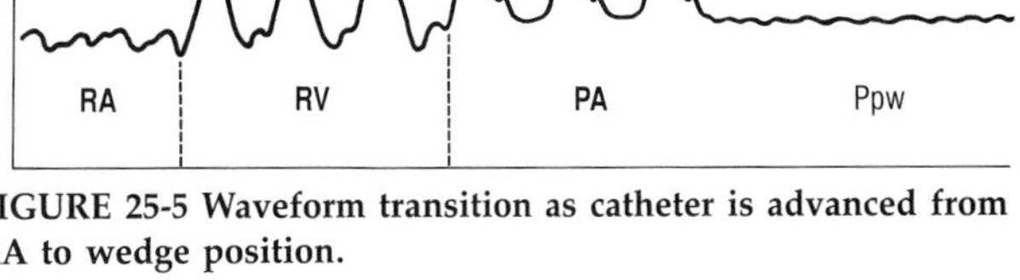

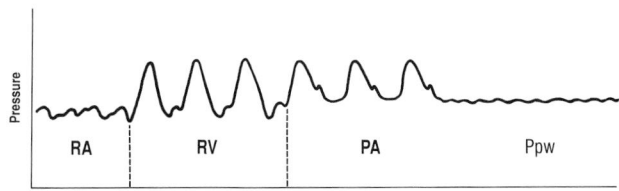

FIGURE 25-5 Waveform transition as catheter is advanced from RA to wedge position.

observed upon balloon inflation in order to define "wedging." With damping of the PA tracing, the tracing may appear atrial in character, but the mean pressure will not fall (see Fig. 25-2). Recording an erroneously high value from a damped PA tracing as the (much lower) Ppw can lead to serious errors. Also, if a damped PA tracing is misinterpreted as a Ppw tracing with the balloon deflated, a properly positioned catheter may be unnecessarily withdrawn in the belief that the tip has migrated too far distally. The rapid-flush test and a chest radiograph to define catheter position will allow differentiation of an appropriately placed catheter with a damped PA tracing versus distal migration of the uninflated catheter into a wedged position.

Two additional criteria (besides the atrial waveform and fall in mean pressure) have been proposed to establish validity of the Ppw tracing.[15,16] One is that highly oxygenated blood be aspirated when the catheter is in the Ppw position.[15,17] This criterion is not uniformly agreed on because in some instances the catheter appears to clearly be wedged and yet there is no convincing change in O_2 saturation in blood withdrawn with the catheter deflated and inflated. Catheter position in a vessel whose capillary bed supplies an area of markedly reduced alveolar ventilation could result in failure to obtain highly oxygenated blood in the Ppw position.[12,18] Also, an estimated 15 to 40 mL PA "dead space" blood could lie between the catheter tip and the capillary bed.[18] When confirmation of the Ppw position is sought by assessing O_2 saturation of aspirated blood, it is recommended that an initial 15 to 20 mL blood be withdrawn and discarded before the sample is obtained. This may reduce the likelihood of getting a false-negative result when the inflated catheter has truly wedged.[18] A false-positive result (i.e., high O_2 saturation in aspirated blood when the catheter is not wedged) could occur if the sample is aspirated too quickly. It is recommended that the sample be aspirated no faster than 3 mL/min.[18]

Another proposed criterion for the Ppw position is that free flow at the tip be present when the catheter is wedged, as evidenced by the ability to withdraw blood easily with suction and by the absence of an "overwedged" tracing.[16] Overwedging, recognizable by a characteristic tracing (Fig. 25-6), occurs when the catheter tip is closed off from the vessel by balloon herniation over the tip or because the tip is positioned against the vessel wall. In either case, the continuing flow from the flush system results in a steady buildup in pressure until an equilibrium is reached between the rates of fluid ingress and egress from the trapped pocket. Overwedging requires repositioning of the catheter until a suitable tracing is obtained.

On occasion, the appearance of an *apparent* Ppw tracing can be seen as the catheter exits from the RV (Fig. 25-7). The cause of this phenomenon is not clear, and when it has been observed in our units we have unfortunately not had fluoroscopy present to clarify catheter position. Perhaps the cather tip lodges beneath the pulmonic valve or in a trabecular pocket. In any event, experienced clinicians should not be fooled, since a convincing PA tracing does not precede the "Ppw" tracing. A second defense against this pitfall is that the "pseudowedge" pressure usually exceeds the

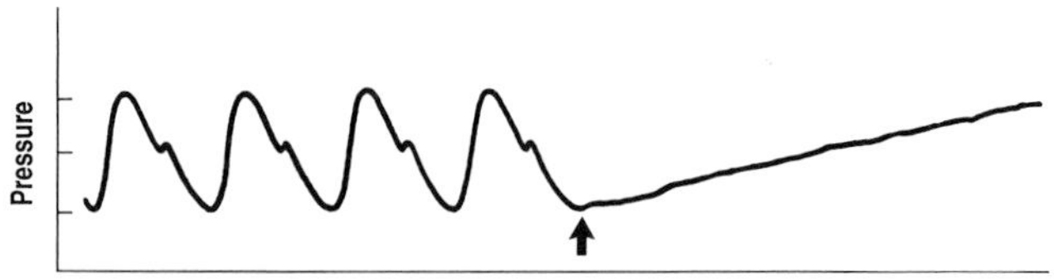

FIGURE 25-6 Overwedging. Arrow indicates time of balloon inflation.

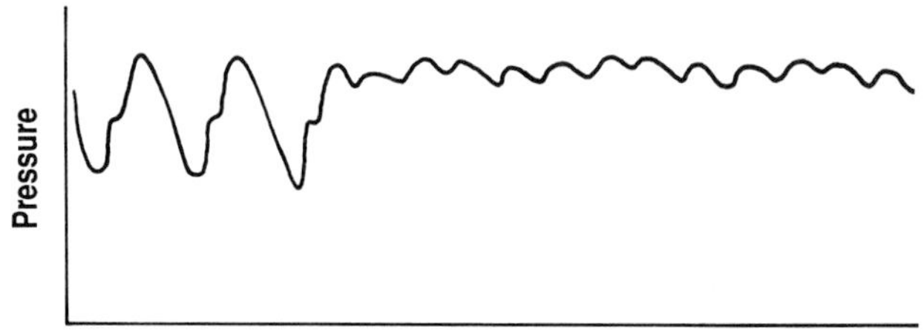

FIGURE 25-7 "Pseudowedge" tracing. Latter part of the tracing has an appearance consistent with an atrial waveform, while the earlier RV tracing could be mistaken for a PA waveform. However, the "wedge pressure" would exceed mean "PA" pressure, which would not be physiologically possible. Such a tracing could result from lodging of the catheter tip in a trabecular pocket or perhaps under the pulmonic valve.

"pseudo-PA" (RV) mean pressure, a condition that would imply absent or reversed flow with the lung. A pseudowedge tracing can also occur if the catheter tip enters the coronary sinus. Avoidance of these and other pitfalls is aided by recording a continuous strip during catheter insertion to ensure that the expected transition in waveform from RA → RV → PA → Ppw can be identified (see Fig. 25).

A number of different clinical conditions can lead to difficulty in recognizing the characteristic waveforms during insertion of the PA catheter. Hypovolemia with reduced stroke volume (SV) will result in diminished pulse pressure and a narrowing of the differences between the diastolic pressures of the RV (RVEDP) and PA (Ppad) and the mean pressure of the PA ($P\overline{pa}$) and the pulmonary vein (Ppw). As a result, the expected transitions in waveforms are less readily appreciated. The transition from RV to PA may also be more difficult to appreciate when RVEDP approaches Ppad as a result of pericardial tamponade, RV infarction, or overt RV failure (Fig. 25-8).[19] Fluoroscopy should be used as an aid to catheter placement when there is uncertainty about catheter position.

Exaggerated excursions in the pressure tracing can result from catheter whip, a problem unique to the PA catheter that results from shocks and mechanical forces transmitted directly to the catheter during ventricular contraction (Fig. 25-9). When measuring the Ppad, it is appropriate to record the value at the plateau just before the systolic rise to avoid whip-induced undershoot of diastolic pressure. For this and other reasons, pressures should be recorded from a visually inspected strip chart rather than by digital scan (vide infra).

The V wave is due to filling of the LA during ventricular systole. Large V waves are often due to mitral regurgita-

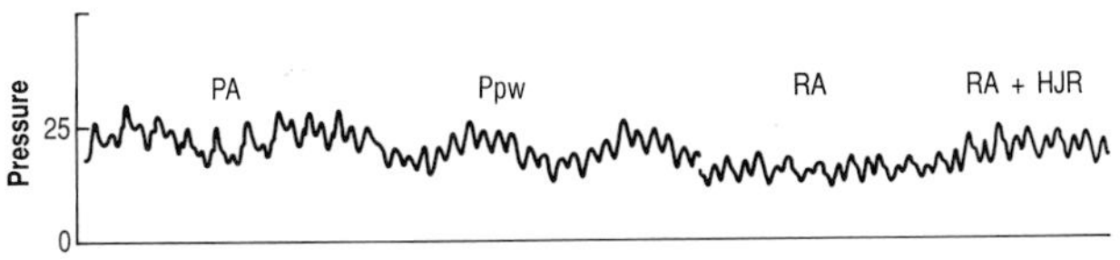

FIGURE 25-8 Right ventricular infarction. Note similarity of tracings from different chambers. Fluoroscopy may be required during insertion to confirm catheter position. (From Reference 19 with permission.)

tion, but may be seen in the absence of mitral regurgitation when the LA is distended and noncompliant, or in the presence of an acute VSD.[19,20] A large V wave may cause the Ppw tracing to resemble the PA waveform, and the mean Ppw may approximate $\overline{Ppa}$ (Fig. 25-10). Thus, it may appear as if the catheter has failed to wedge. In the presence of a V wave, transition from a PA to Ppw tracing is best defined by change in waveform and by noting that the peak of the V wave occurs later in the cardiac cycle than the PA systolic wave.[19] The V wave can usually be detected in the PA waveform, resulting in a bifid PA tracing. As the catheter is wedged, the PA systolic wave disappears but the V wave remains (see Fig. 25-10). The PA systolic wave usually occurs at the time of the T wave of the electrocardiogram (ECG), while the V wave occurs after the T wave. Simultaneous recording of the ECG and pressure tracing with a dual channel recorder is very helpful to confirm the presence of a V wave.

Detection of a V wave may prove to be clinically important for several reasons. In some cases, an intermittent V wave may be the only evidence for episodic myocardial ischemia. In addition to influencing therapy, detection of the intermittent V wave may help clarify the mechanism of ongoing pulmonary edema. Silent ischemia of the papillary muscle may lead to marked elevations in Ppw with alveolar flooding, but between episodes of ischemia the Ppw may be normal. If the intermittent V wave is not appreciated, pulmonary edema may be mistakenly attributed to increased capillary permeability. Finally, if the V wave is mistaken for the PA systolic wave, the catheter could be left in a wedged position with the balloon deflated. This could lead to pulmonary infarction or, of even greater concern, to PA rupture during subsequent balloon inflation.

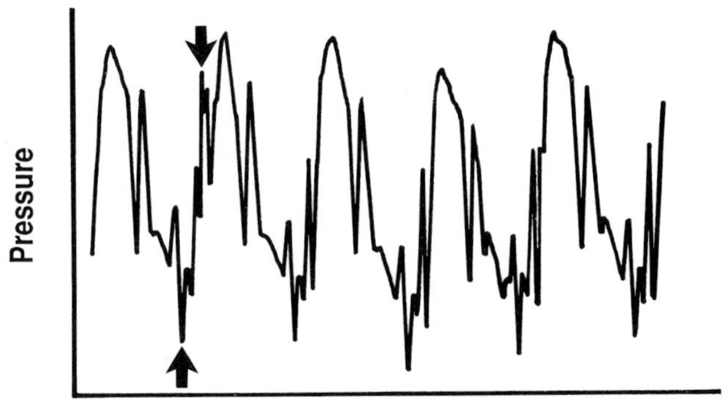

FIGURE 25-9 Catheter whip. Arrow denotes artifactual "shock" transients.

Large swings in intrathoracic pressure may greatly hinder the ability to recognize the expected transition in waveforms during catheter insertion. Large respiratory-related fluctuations in pressure may even be mistaken for systolic-diastolic excursions (Fig. 25-11).[21] (However, respiratory frequency will not match the heart rate.) If large respiratory fluctuations pose a problem during mechanical ventilation, sedation or temporary paralysis may aid delineation of waveforms and will enhance reliability of the measurements obtained.[22]

PULMONARY ARTERY PRESSURE: CLINICAL ASPECTS

Pressure in the PA is a function of the flow generated by RV contraction, resistance within the vascular network, and downstream pressure. The normal pulmonary vascular network is a low-resistance circuit with enormous reserve, so that large (fivefold) increases in cardiac output ($\dot{Q}_T$) do not result in a significant rise in pressure. This large capillary reserve normally offers such minimal resistance to runoff during diastole that Ppad approximates Ppw (unless marked tachycardia shortens diastole and curtails diastolic runoff, increasing the Ppad − Ppw gradient). Factors that increase pulmonary vascular resistance (PVR) (clot, hypoxia, fibrosis, sepsis, acidosis, drugs) will cause the Ppad to exceed Ppw and will increase the driving pressure required to sustain flow across the pulmonary circuit. Indeed, a Ppad − Ppw gradient $>$ 5 mmHg is highly characteristic of ARDS, sepsis, excessive PEEP, and other conditions that increase PVR.[23] In contrast, pulmonary hypertension due solely to increased downstream (LA) pressure is characterized by preservation of the normal Ppad − Ppw gradient.

An increased $\dot{Q}_T$ alone will not cause pulmonary hypertension. However, in the setting of increased vascular resistance, or increased Pla, the degree to which $\overline{Ppa}$ increases will be influenced by the $\dot{Q}_T$. For example, pulmonary hypertension may result from the combination of only a modest increase in vascular resistance and a major increase in $\dot{Q}_T$ due to sepsis, cirrhosis, or other factors. The relative contribution of $\dot{Q}_T$ and increased resistance to the increase in $\overline{Ppa}$ can be assessed by measuring the $\dot{Q}_T$ by thermodilution and calculating PVR. [The PVR is calculated as ($\overline{Ppa}$ − Ppw)/$\dot{Q}_T$.] It should be appreciated, however, that clinical interpretation of the PVR is confounded by the fact that the pulmonary vascular bed behaves like a Starling (variable) resistor; resistance increases as flow ($\dot{Q}_T$) decreases.[24] Thus, the calculated PVR must be interpreted with respect to the $\dot{Q}_T$ at the time the measurement is made.[24] A fall in $\dot{Q}_T$ due to hemorrhage, for example, may result in a rise in the calculated PVR, even though the pulmonary vascular bed has not been directly affected. The PVR may then "normalize," once the $\dot{Q}_T$ is restored to its baseline value.

PULMONARY ARTERY WEDGE PRESSURE

The Ppw is obtained by inflating the catheter balloon with 1 to 1.5 mL air, thus allowing the catheter tip to advance until it obstructs forward flow within a branch of the PA. This

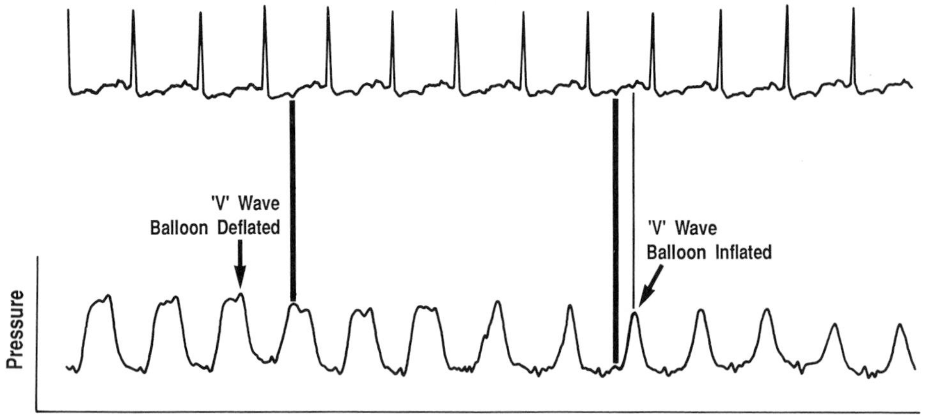

FIGURE 25-10 Effect of V wave on PA and wedge tracings. Note that the V wave occurs later in the cardiac cycle than the PA systolic wave, which is synchronous with the T wave of the ECG (*top*). Heavy line indicates timing of PA systolic wave in cardiac cycle.

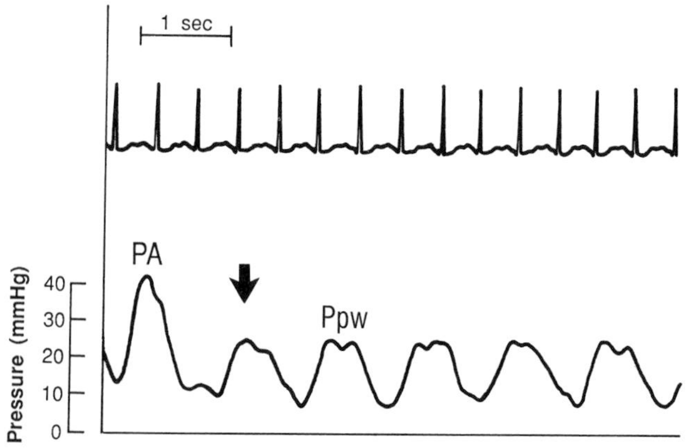

FIGURE 25-11 At rapid ventilatory frequencies, large respiratory fluctuations in the wedge tracing could be mistaken for systolic-diastolic excursions, unless lack of correlation with heart rate is appreciated. The ECG is shown above pressure tracing. Arrow denotes balloon inflation. (From Reference 21 with permission.)

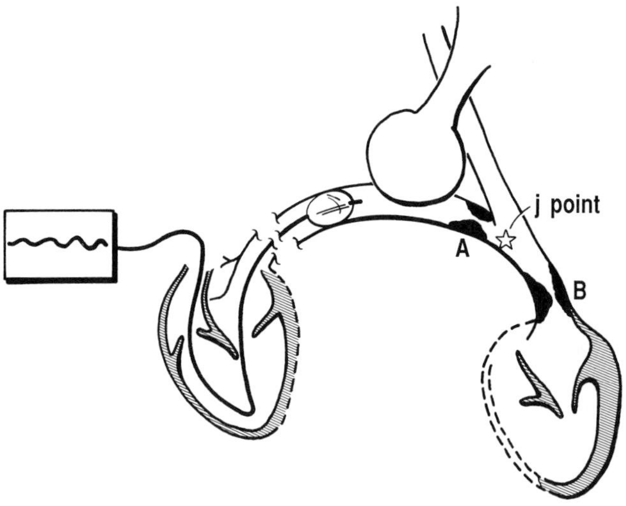

FIGURE 25-12 Principle of the wedge pressure (Ppw) measurement. When the inflated balloon obstructs arterial inflow, the catheter will record the pressure at the junction of the static and flowing venous channels, the j point. An obstruction distal (B) to the j point will cause the Ppw to overestimate Pla. With obstruction proximal (A) to the j point, (e.g., venoocclusive disease), the Ppw accurately reflects Pla, but greatly underestimates P cap. (Adapted from Reference 12 with permission.)

creates a static column of fluid distal to the tip of the catheter. The pressure recorded at the catheter tip (Ppw) is equivalent to the pressure in the occluded pulmonary vein at the point (junction, or j point) where it intersects with blood flow from uninterrupted vessels (Fig. 25-12). The Ppw will approximate Pla as long as there is no obstruction to flow downstream from the j point. The Ppw is used clinically as an estimate of hydrostatic pressure in the pulmonary capillaries (Pcap) and as a measure of the mean Pla in order to assess left ventricular (LV) preload. As such, critical manipulations of intravascular volume and vasoactive drugs are based on the recorded Ppw. Unfortunately, problems with acquisition and use of the Ppw are common and the resultant errors in clinical decision-making may be significant.[16] Earlier, certain problems with obtaining a valid Ppw tracing were discussed (see Catheter Insertion, vide supra). Additional problem areas in using the Ppw include use of the digital scan rather than a strip recording to obtain the Ppw, failure to account for raised intrathoracic pressure on transvascular pressures, and overreliance on the Ppw number per se in diagnosis and management of pulmonary edema and preload assessment.

The recorded Ppw should be obtained at end expiration from a strip recording, rather than by the digital estimate. Although only intravascular pressure is routinely measured, it is the transmural pressure (intravascular minus pleural, Ppw − Ppl) that is of interest. At the end of passive deflation, the lung usually returns to its relaxed volume and intrathoracic pressure to its baseline value. Measurement of Ppw (an intravascular pressure) at other points in the respiratory cycle will be influenced by the tidal variations in the intrathoracic pressure that surrounds the heart and pulmonary vasculature. Digital displays can over- or underestimate the transmural pressure, depending on the sampling interval, the selection algorithm, and the positivity or negativity of intrathoracic pressure during the time of sampling (Fig. 25-13).[12,25] End-expiratory Ppw can be accu-

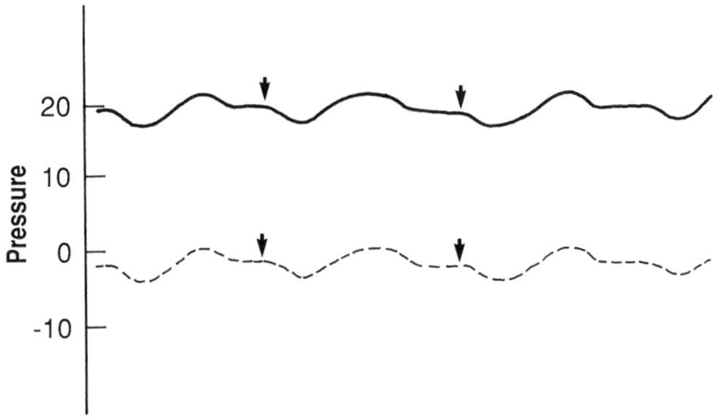

FIGURE 25-13 Effect of varying intrathoracic pressure on the Ppw. Top is Ppw tracing and bottom is Ppl. In this example the patient is receiving assisted mechanical ventilation. Arrows indicate end-expiratory pressures. Negative deflections in intrapleural and Ppw pressures result from inspiratory muscle activity, and subsequent positive deflections represent lung inflation by the ventilator. At end expiration (arrow) the respiratory system has returned to its relaxed state and Ppl is back to baseline (−2 cmH_2O). Transmural Ppw remains approximately constant throughout the ventilating cycle. Since Ppl is not usually measured simultaneously with Ppw, however, it is necessary that the Ppw be recorded at a point where Ppl can be reliably estimated (i.e., end exhalation, assuming no active expiratory muscle activity). A digital scan may under- or overestimate transmural pressure, depending on whether the pressure is sampled during a period of negative or positive change in Ppl.

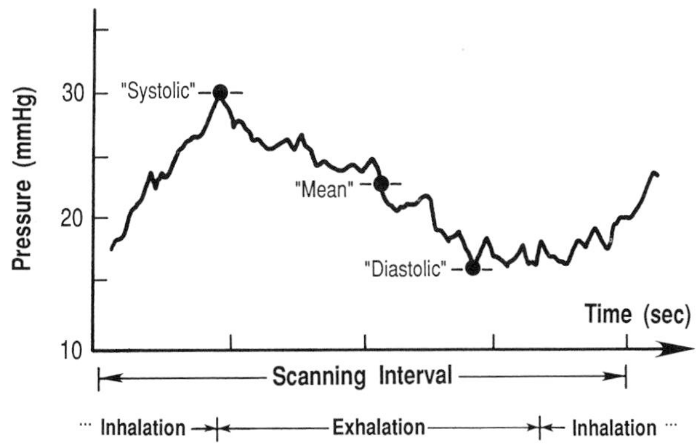

FIGURE 25-14 End-expiratory Ppw is approximated by the "diastolic" digital scan reading during controlled (unassisted) positive-pressure ventilation (shown here) and by the "systolic" digital scan reading during quiet spontaneous breathing. (From Reference 12 with permission.)

rately measured by the "systolic" pressure on the digital scan during quiet spontaneous breathing and by the "diastolic" pressure during controlled (unassisted) positive-pressure ventilation (Fig. 25-14).[12] However, to avoid potential problems with changing breathing pattern, it is best to routinely measure Ppw from a strip recording. A simultaneously recorded pressure from the central airway can help define end expiration more precisely.

A Ppw recorded at end expiration will overestimate the transmural pressure (Ppw − Ppl) if intrathoracic pressure

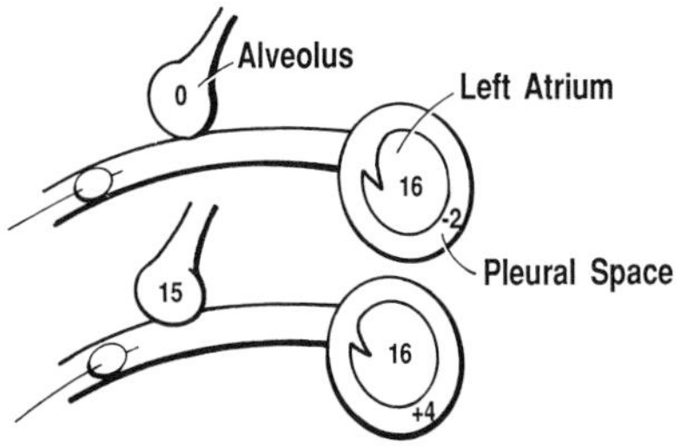

PEEP $cm\ H_2O$	Pleural Pressure mmHg	Intracardiac Pressure mmHg	Transmural Pressure mmHg
0	-2	16	18
15	+4	16	12

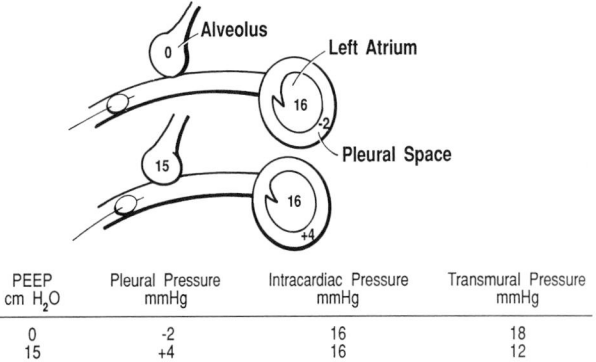

FIGURE 25-15 The effect of PEEP on transmural pressure. In this example, 50 percent of PEEP is transmitted to the juxtacardiac space (15 $cmH_2O \cong 12$ mmHg). The same Ppw of 16 mmHg corresponds to greatly different effective "transmural" filling pressures.

is positive at end expiration (Fig. 25-15). Positive juxtacardiac pressure at end expiration may occur with an increase in lung volume (applied PEEP, auto-PEEP) or without an increase in lung volume (active exhalation). In either case, the presence of increased juxtacardiac pressure must be recognized and taken into account when Ppw is used in clinical decision-making. With relaxed respiratory muscles, the only determinants of Ppl in response to PEEP are the chest wall compliance (Cw) and change in lung volume.[26] The latter is a function of the amount of PEEP and lung compliance (CL). The formula $\Delta Ppl = PEEP \times CL/CL + Cw$ predicts that 50 percent of a given amount of PEEP will be transmitted to the pleural space in normal individuals, because CL and Cw are roughly equal over the tidal volume range.[12] A stiff chest wall enhances the fraction of PEEP transmitted to the pleural space, whereas with stiff lungs, the reduced CL blunts PEEP transmission. One study found that in ARDS the percentage of PEEP transmitted to the pleural space (as measured with an esophageal balloon) varied from 24 to 37 percent.[27] However, esophageal pressure may underestimate the actual juxtacardiac pressure when the heart and lungs are both expanded.[28,29] This variation in Δ Ppl at different sites within the pleural space in response to PEEP might be accentuated by inhomogeneity of lung involvement in ARDS.[30] Thus, in individual patients it is not possible to determine the actual juxtacardiac pressure at a given level of PEEP. Removal of PEEP to measure Ppw is not advisable, because the resultant increase in venous return, and perhaps an acute reduction in RV afterload, creates a different hemodynamic state than existed when PEEP was present. Also, sudden PEEP withdrawal can lead to worsening oxygenation that may not be quickly reversed when PEEP is reinstituted. Recently, it has been shown that Ppw measured within one or two cardiac cycles after PEEP withdrawal (before the Ppw reflects increased venous return) closely predicted actual transmural pressures measured on PEEP.[31,32] With respect to gas exchange, such brief episodes of PEEP withdrawal should be tolerated. Although measuring Ppw by this technique may yield a more accurate estimate of transmural pressure, it is not certain to what extent such refinements contribute to patient management. In most types of clinical decision-making, use of the Ppw should not focus solely on the absolute number per se (unless the transmural Ppw is very high or very low). Rather, *changes* in the Ppw with therapeutic interventions and their correlation with relevant end points (e.g., blood pressure, Pa_{O_2}, $\dot{Q}T$, urine output) are most important and can be assessed as easily with PEEP present as with PEEP withdrawn.

An uncommon but potentially serious problem in obtaining a valid Ppw occurs when the pressure measured on balloon inflation is actually alveolar pressure rather than pulmonary venous pressure. The lung can be divided into three physiologic "zones" on the basis of the relationship of pressures in the pulmonary artery ($P\overline{pa}$), alveolus (Palv), and pulmonary vein (Ppv) (Fig. 25-16).[12] For the Ppw to be reliable, the catheter tip must lie in zone 3 ($P\overline{pa}$ > Ppv > Palv) at end expiration. If Palv is > Ppv (zones 1 and 2) through the entirety of the breathing cycle, then the collapsible alveolar capillaries will pinch closed and the wedged catheter will reflect Palv. Since Ppw is recorded at end expiration, non-zone 3 conditions would be possible only when PEEP is present and PEEP exceeds Pla. (For a non-zone 3 condition to be present when PEEP is < Pla, the catheter tip would have to lie above the level of the LA so that the downstream Ppv was < Pla.) Fortunately, the flow-directed catheter tip tends to place itself at or below the level of the LA, since most blood flows to dependent areas.[33] In addition, even when the catheter lies at the level of the LA there may still be a branch of the occluded artery that lies below the LA in zone 3, and this will prevent the wedged catheter from recording Palv (Fig. 25-17). Finally, damaged lungs may not transmit applied PEEP as fully to the capillary bed as normal lungs, thereby

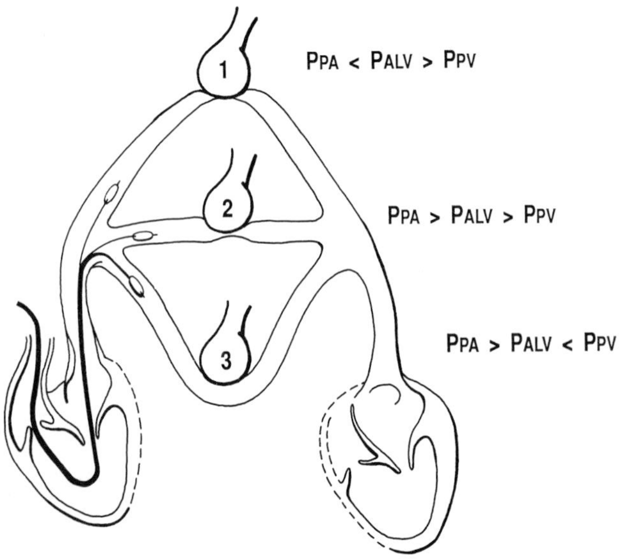

FIGURE 25-16 Physiologic lung "zones," based on the relationship between pressures in the pulmonary artery ($P\overline{pa}$), alveolus (Palv), and pulmonary vein (Ppv). (Adapted from Reference 12 with permission.)

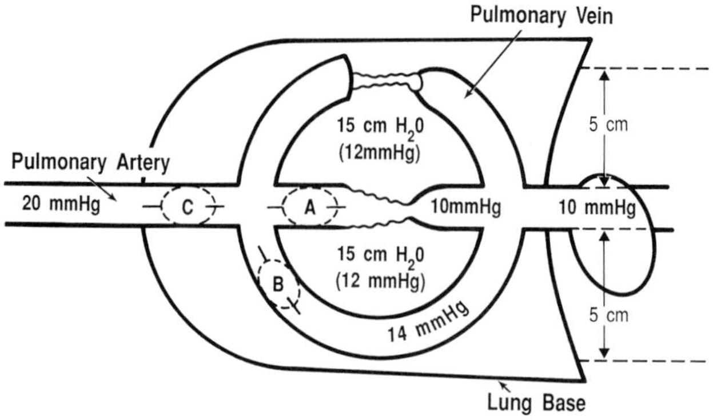

FIGURE 25-17 Reliability of the end-expiratory wedge pressure (Ppw) as a measure of pulmonary venous pressure (Ppv) during application of PEEP. With the balloon inflated, forward flow into the vessel is interrupted and the catheter will record the higher of the two downstream pressures, Ppv or Palv. In this example, Ppv at LA level is <Palv. In catheter position A, the downstream Ppv is <Palv and the latter will be recorded. In position B, the catheter is below the LA and local Ppv in this channel exceeds Palv, preserving vascular patency. Thus, a reliable Ppw (10 mmHg) will be recorded. In position C, the catheter is located at LA level but is situated more proximally than in A. As a branch of the occluded vascular segment remains patent, an accurate Ppw (10 mmHg) will be recorded.

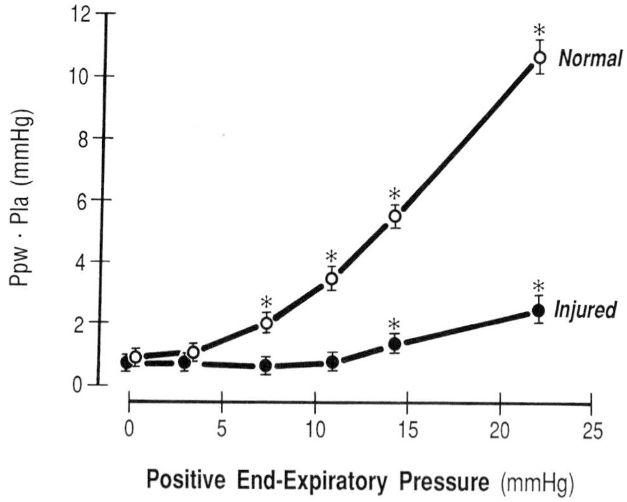

FIGURE 25-18 Effect of lung injury on accuracy of Ppw as an estimate of Pla. At high levels of PEEP, Ppw overestimates Pla in the uninjured lung but accurately predicts Pla in the injured lung. Thus, lung injury favors a zone 3 condition, even though PEEP may significantly exceed Pla. (Adapted from Reference 34 with permission).

protecting against non-zone 3 conditions. In a dog model of unilateral acid injury to the lung, it was shown that the agreement between Ppw and directly measured Pla was excellent up to PEEP of 20 cmH_2O.[34] In contrast, Ppw measured in the uninjured lung overestimated Pla and tracked with Palv at PEEP > 10 cmH_2O (Fig. 25-18).[34] Thus, in the setting of ARDS, a zone 3 condition is very likely to be present at end expiration unless PEEP is very high, and

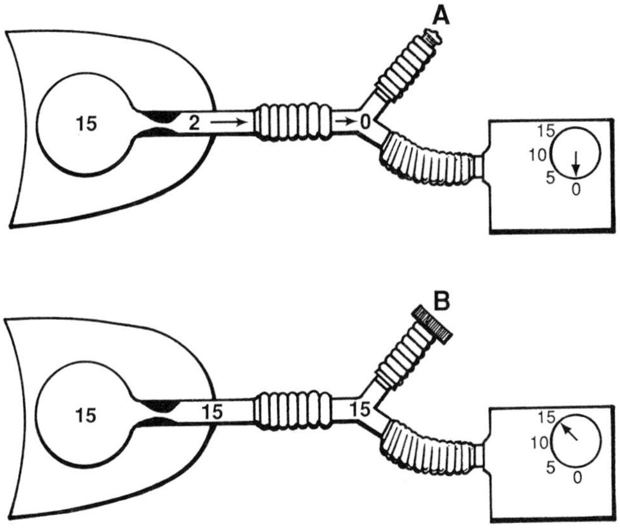

FIGURE 25-19 Estimation of auto-PEEP by the end-expiratory airway occlusion technique. (From Reference 35 with permission.)

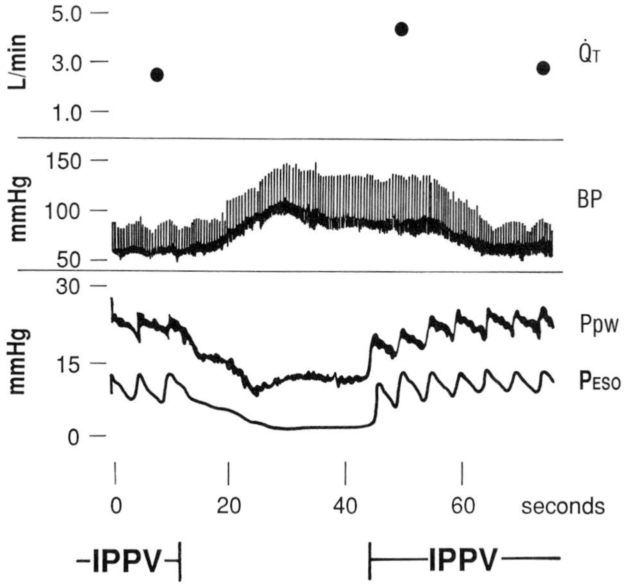

FIGURE 25-20 Effect of auto-PEEP on blood pressure, cardiac output ($\dot{Q}_T$), wedge pressure (Ppw), and esophageal pressure (Peso) is demonstrated by a brief interruption in positive-pressure ventilation (IPPV). (From Reference 35 with permission).

there is either significant hypovolemia or a lateral chest film shows the catheter tip positioned above the level of the LA. A non-zone 3 condition should be suspected if there is a near 1:1 change in Ppw and PEEP on PEEP reduction (i.e., Δ Ppw of 4 mmHg for Δ PEEP of 5 cmH_2O).

Auto-PEEP caused by dynamic hyperinflation may create greater difficulties in use of the Ppw than applied PEEP for several reasons. First, hemodynamically significant auto-PEEP may be occult and thus lead to serious errors in clinical decision-making.[35] Second, auto-PEEP often occurs in the setting of increased C_L and hyperinflation so that a relatively large component of the Palv may be transmitted to the juxtacardiac space. Finally, the compliant lungs may permit the emergence of zone 2 conditions at a level of PEEP that would otherwise result in a zone 3 state in the setting of ARDS. In the absence of respiratory muscle activity, auto-PEEP can be estimated at the bedside by the end-expiratory airway occlusion technique (Fig. 25-19).[35] With respiratory muscle activity present, auto-PEEP is not easily determined. Whether or not the respiratory muscles are active, a brief (20 to 30 s) interruption in positive-pressure ventilation may be useful in assessing the hemodynamic significance of auto-PEEP by observing the change in blood pressure, $\dot{Q}_T$, and Ppw. The presence of hemodynamically significant auto-PEEP is evidenced by an increase in blood pressure and $\dot{Q}_T$ and a reduction in Ppw following the pause (Fig. 25-20).[35] (An unchanged Ppw during the disconnection period does not entirely exclude auto-PEEP, however, since an increase in venous return may offset the reduction in juxtacardiac pressure so that the net result is a stable Ppw, albeit a more favorable $\dot{Q}_T$.) Although auto-PEEP is most often suspected in the setting of airflow obstruction, it is important to realize that it can also occur in patients with ARDS if minute ventilation is very high.[36]

Large errors may be introduced into measurement of the Ppw when patients continue to actively expire at end exhalation, as the end-expiratory Ppw overestimates the transmural pressure that influences LV preload and edema formation (Fig. 25-21). This problem is not limited to patients with obstructive lung disease. One study found that the amount of respiratory excursion in the Ppw tracing from expiration to inspiration correlated with the degree to

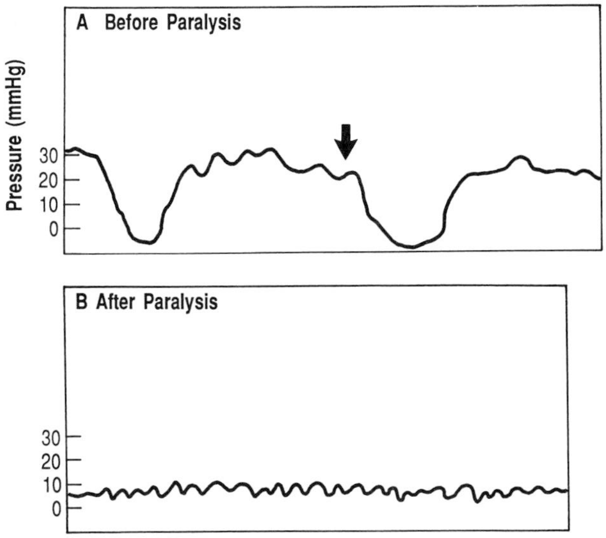

FIGURE 25-21 Effect of vigorous respiratory muscle activity on end-expiratory Ppw. *a.* Patient on mechanical ventilation is observed at the bedside to be making vigorous inspiratory and expiratory efforts. The Ppw measured at end exhalation (arrow) is 25 mmHg. *b.* To obtain a reliable Ppw, respiratory muscle activity is temporarily eliminated with a short-acting paralyzing agent. The Ppw is now measured at 8 mmHg.

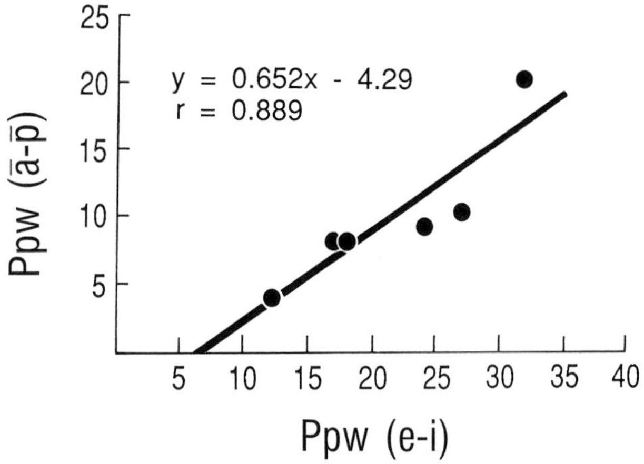

FIGURE 25-22 The difference between the Ppw before (p) and after (a) paralysis correlates with the degree of respiratory excursion in the Ppw from expiration to inspiration (Ppw, e − i) before paralysis. (Adapted from Reference 22 with permission.)

which the measured end-expiratory Ppw overestimated the "true" Ppw recorded postparalysis (Fig. 25-22).[22] A respiration-related Ppw excursion of $\geq$ 10 to 15 mmHg suggests that the end-expiratory Ppw overestimates the true transmural pressure. Unless it can be confirmed by physical examination that all of the respiratory excursion is due to inspiratory muscle activity and that exhalation is truly passive, use of sedation or paralysis in the mechanically ventilated patient may be required to obtain a reliable reading. If the patient is not intubated and cannot be encouraged to breathe quietly long enough to obtain a Ppw tracing without large respiratory excursions, the mean Ppw should be recorded, as this value will more closely approximate the transmural Ppw than will the end-expiratory value.[37,38] (Recording the Ppw while the patient sips through a straw may help eliminate large respiratory fluctuations.) An esophageal balloon can also be used to better define transmural pressure.

CLINICAL USE OF Ppw

The Ppw is used clinically for two primary purposes: an estimate of hydrostatic filtration pressure (Pcap) in the fluid-exchanging pulmonary capillaries and as a measure of LV preload. It is important to realize that the Ppw is not equivalent to Pcap, nor does it define the degree of preload. Nonetheless, when assessed in relationship to other clinical data, measurement of Ppw can be of enormous utility in managing patients with serious cardiorespiratory disorders, especially when changes in Ppw after therapeutic interventions are correlated with relevant clinical parameters, such as gas exchange, blood pressure, $\dot{Q}_T$, and urine output.

The Ppw is used as an estimate of Pcap to aid in the diagnosis of pulmonary edema and in manipulation of intravascular volume. An isolated Ppw reading does not reliably predict whether pulmonary edema occurred on the basis of increased Pcap alone or on the basis of altered permeability, especially if recorded after a therapeutic intervention. Frequently, acute hydrostatic pulmonary edema occurs despite normal intravascular volume on the basis of altered LV compliance (diastolic dysfunction) due to ischemia or accelerated hypertension. By the time a PA catheter is placed, the acute process has often resolved, resulting in a normal or even reduced Ppw, depending in part on what type of therapy (diuretics, vasodilators) has been given. Clarification of the mechanism of pulmonary edema may therefore require a period of clinical observation. The expected Ppw threshold for hydrostatic pulmonary edema, assuming normal permeability, is approximately 22 to 25 mmHg. (A higher threshold is common if the Ppw has been chronically elevated.) Maintaining the Ppw $\leq$ 18 mmHg should lead to marked improvement in clinical and radiographic evidence of pulmonary edema within 24 h if permeability is normal. However, hydrostatic pulmonary edema may persist or worsen if there are intermittent elevations in Ppw due to myocardial ischemia. Such elevations may be very transient and not easily detected by intermittent recording of Ppw. Also, low plasma oncotic pressure could allow pulmonary edema to occur at a Ppw $\leq$ 18 mmHg. The precise role of an isolated reduction in plasma colloid oncotic pressure (Pcosm) in the development of pulmonary edema has not been fully elucidated. The Starling equation predicts that a subnormal ratio of plasma : interstitial protein concentration would permit pulmonary edema to form at a lower transvascular Ppw. The reported observation that acute, but not sustained (> 24 h), reductions in Pcosm allow pulmonary edema to develop at a low Ppw may be explained by a fairly rapid partial equilibration between plasma and interstitial protein concentrations.[39] Because most causes of low Pcosm encountered in the clinical setting occur chronically, it is uncertain to what extent chronic hypoproteinemia increases the risk of hydrostatic pulmonary edema. It is conceivable, however, that rapid reductions in Pcosm and the plasma : interstitial protein concentration (as might occur with large volume crystalloid infusion) would contribute to pulmonary edema.

The pressure in a large pulmonary vein, Ppw, represents a very low-end estimate of the average pressure across the fluid-permeable vascular bed. Normally, about 40 percent of the resistance across the pulmonary vascular bed resides in the small veins (Figure 25-23).[40] When pulmonary arterial (Ra) and venous (Rv) resistance are normally distributed, the Gaar equation predicts Pcap by the formula: $\text{Pcap} = \text{Ppw} + 0.4\,(\overline{\text{Ppa}} - \text{Ppw})$.[40] Since the driving pressure ($\overline{\text{Ppa}} - \text{Ppw}$) across the vascular bed is normally very low, the Pcap will be only a few mmHg above Ppw. However, a significant pressure drop from Pcap to Ppw could occur under conditions of increased Rv, increased $\dot{Q}_T$, or both. For example, in pulmonary venoocclusive disease there is often clinical evidence of increased Pcap (pulmonary edema, Kerley B lines) despite a normal Ppw (see Fig. 25-12).[41] Other conditions that might increase Rv are not yet well defined, but experimental data have shown that certain pharmacologic agents can increase Rv and thus widen the discrepancy between Pcap and Ppw.[42]

At the bedside it has been difficult to determine the relative proportion of PVR due to Ra and to Rv. The clinical setting in which this has greatest relevance is ARDS. In

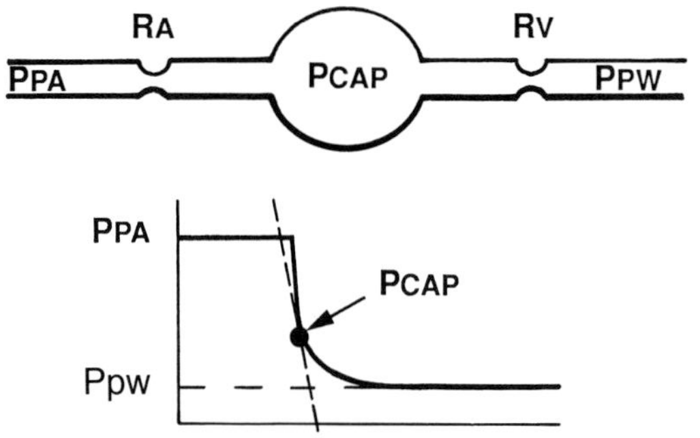

FIGURE 25-23 Pulmonary vascular resistance (PVR) is due to precapillary arteriolar resistance (Ra) and postcapillary venous resistance (Rv). Normally, it is estimated that 60 percent of total PVR is due to Ra and 40 percent is due to Rv. The inflection point during decay from the PA (mean) to the wedge tracing approximates Pcap.

ARDS, the $\overline{\text{Ppa}}$ − Ppw gradient is increased as a result of increased PVR and sometimes increased $\dot{Q}_T$. A large discrepancy between Pcap and Ppw could exist if some of the increased PVR were due to increased Rv. This could be clinically important because of the major impact of small changes in Pcap on lung water in the face of increased permeability.[43] A technique for determining Pcap at the bedside has recently been described.[42,44,45] Careful inspection of the decay in the PA pressure waveform during balloon occlusion may reveal an initial rapid decay and a subsequent slower decay (see Fig. 25-23). It is believed that the rapid decay is due to Ra and the slower decay to Rv. In experimental animals, the inflection point between the rapid and slow components has been shown to predict fairly accurately Pcap as measured by isogravimetric or double occlusion (arterial and venous) techniques.[42,44] The inflection point estimate of Pcap has also been used in human beings, with and without electronic meaning of the PA pressure tracing.[44,45] With a slight modification in the way Pcap was defined, this technique was applied to a group of patients with ARDS and it was found that the estimated Pcap was on average 7 to 8 mmHg higher than the measured Ppw.[45] Interestingly, in this study the estimated Pcap and the calculated Pcap by the Gaar equation were highly correlated.[45] If this bedside estimate of Pcap is indeed accurate, these findings would suggest that the increased PVR in ARDS is due to increases in both Ra and Rv. It should be appreciated, however, that it may be difficult to confidently determine the Pcap by inspection of the pressure tracing following balloon occlusion.[46] While this method of determining Pcap is of interest and may prove to have clinical relevance, at the present time it is not sufficiently well validated to warrant widespread acceptance for bedside use. The important clinical point is that Ppw is a low-range estimate of Pcap; the true value of the latter lies somewhere between $\overline{\text{Ppa}}$ and Ppw. As with other hemodynamic data obtained from the PA catheter, use of the Ppw in diagnosis and management of pulmonary edema should always be interpreted in the context of the entire clinical picture.

Pcap is a major determinant of lung water in permeability pulmonary edema. Reducing Ppw by diuresis, ultrafiltration, or dialysis may markedly benefit gas exchange.[43] There is no minimum value for Ppw below which removal of intravascular volume is contraindicated, provided that $\dot{Q}_T$ is adequate. If the clinical problem is severely impaired gas exchange requiring high fraction inspired oxygen (F_{IO_2}) or high PEEP, then a trial of Ppw reduction is reasonable, so long as $\dot{Q}_T$ and blood pressure remain within acceptable limits. As with all therapeutic manipulations, a measurable and clinically relevant end point (i.e., Pa_{O_2}) should be assessed before and after Ppw reduction.

The second major clinical use of the Ppw is as an indicator of Pla and the adequacy of LV preload. When afterload and intrinsic contractility are held constant, the forcefulness of ventricular contraction is determined by end-diastolic fiber length (preload).[47] Acute changes in fiber length correlate with changes in LV end-diastolic volume (LVEDV), a function of myocardial compliance and transmural filling pressure (LVEDP − Ppl). The reliability of Ppw as an estimate of LVEDP requires that there is neither mitral valve obstruction nor very high filling pressures (> 15 mmHg).[12] High filling pressures may cause the Ppw to underestimate pLVEDP because atrial systole will force LVEDP to rise above mean Pla. Even when Ppw can be relied on as a faithful measure of LVEDP, the relationship between Ppw and LVEDV is affected by conditions that might alter LV compliance (hypertrophy, ischemia, high doses of pressors) or change juxtacardiac pressure (Fig. 25-24). It is not surprising, therefore, that in different patients an equivalent LVEDV may be associated with widely varying Ppw.[48] Accordingly, it is not possible to state what Ppw optimizes preload without defining the relationship between Ppw and $\dot{Q}_T$.

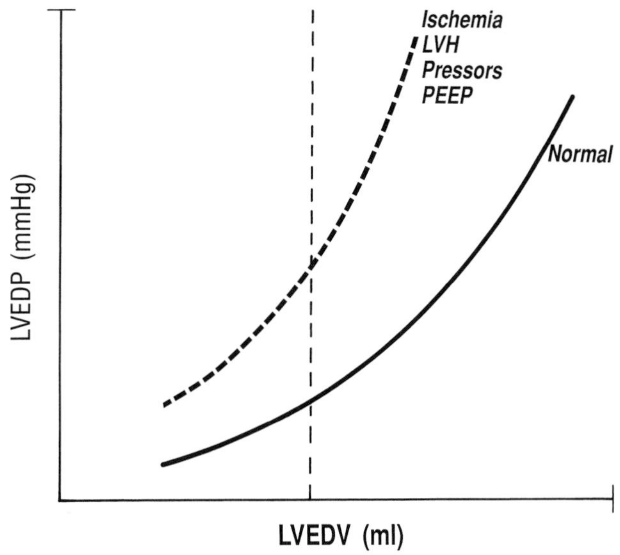

FIGURE 25-24 Pressure-volume (compliance) relationship of the LV. Ischemia, LV hypertrophy (LVH), and high doses of pressors may decrease LV compliance. PEEP increases juxtacardiac pressure and may increase ventricular interdependence due to increased RV afterload. These factors result in a lower LVEDV at a given LVEDP, necessitating a higher LVEDP (and thus a higher Ppw) to achieve optimal preload (as compared to normals).

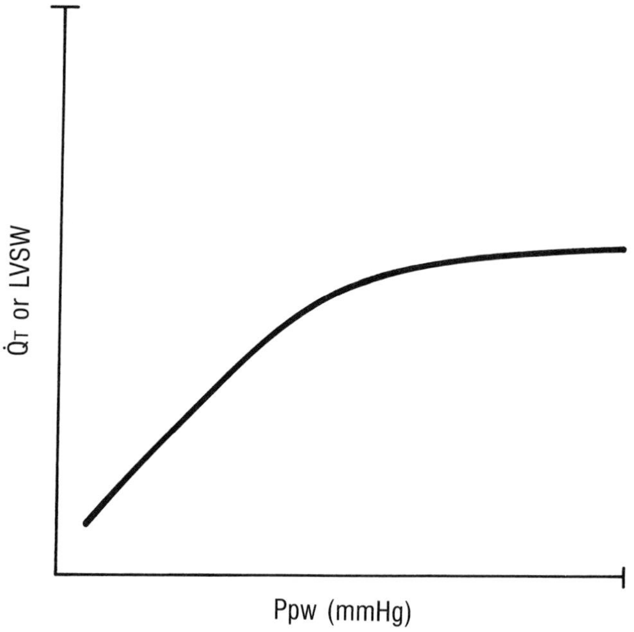

FIGURE 25-25 Relationship between Q̇T or LVSW and wedge pressure (Ppw). Above a certain Ppw, Q̇T and LVSW increase little with further increments in the Ppw. This Ppw value that gives near-optimal volume loading of the left ventricle varies greatly and must be individualized by use of acute volume challenges or diuresis.

Optimal Ppw for preload can be defined as that Ppw above which further increases result in little if any rise in Q̇T, stroke volume (SV), or LV stroke work (LVSW = SV × Pa − Ppw × .0136, where Pa is mean arterial pressure) (Fig. 25-25). In normal individuals, LVSW usually reaches a plateau at a LVEDP of approximately 10 to 12 mmHg range.[49] Likewise, during volume resuscitation from hypovolemic and septic shock, it has been found that optimal Ppw usually lies between 10 and 14 mmHg.[50] In contrast, with acute myocardial infarction, or at high levels of PEEP, a Ppw ≥ 18 mmHg may yield optimal Q̇T.[51] Similarly, following empirical resuscitation from shock, a Ppw of 14 to 18 mmHg could in certain cases represent ongoing hypovolemia because of high doses of pressors or endogenous catecholamines that might reduce effective LV compliance. Because numerous individual factors can affect the relationships among Ppw and LVEDV, it is necessary to define these relationships in individual patients through use of acute volume challenges. After measuring Ppw and Q̇T, and with confounding factors such as PEEP and vasoactive drug therapy held constant, acute volume challenges are given until either the desired clinical result (e.g., reversal of hypotension) is achieved or Ppw rises by 3 to 5 mmHg, at which point Q̇T is again measured. Maintaining a Ppw higher than necessary to achieve optimal Q̇T may be detrimental in patients who are at high risk for ARDS or who have already shown evidence of central vascular overload or edema on chest x-ray. As a rule, the Ppw in this setting should be kept at the lowest level consistent with near-optimal Q̇T, especially early in the disease process, when edema predominates as a cause for impaired gas exchange. Conversely, in the individual whose major problem is hypotension or impaired tissue perfusion, the Ppw should be increased with acute volume infusions until it has been clearly demonstrated that no further improvement in Q̇T can be achieved by fluid resuscitation. Again, the importance of tailoring hemodynamic interventions to the specific clinical problems at hand cannot be overemphasized.

Cardiac Output Measurement

PRINCIPLES OF MEASUREMENT

The thermodilution technique for measuring output (Q̇Ttd) is an indicator dilution method in which the indicator is thermal depression ("cold").[52] Cold fluid is injected through the proximal lumen of the PA catheter into the RA and, after mixing thoroughly in the RV with venous blood returning from the periphery, passes into the PA, where a thermistor at the tip of the catheter senses dynamic changes in temperature. The Stewart-Hamilton formula relates Q̇T to temperature change over time:

$$\dot{Q}_T = \frac{V(TB - TI) \times K1 \times K2}{\int TB(t)dt} \tag{25-1}$$

where V = injected volume; TB = blood temperature; TI = injectate temperature; TB(t)dt = change in blood temperature as a function of time; and *K*1 and *K*2 are computational constants. The numerator contains known constants or measured values, while the denominator is the area beneath the time-temperature curve derived by computer integration of the thermistor signal. Although it would seem that chilling the injectate on ice should enhance Q̇Ttd accuracy and reproducibility by enhancing the strength of the signal, studies have shown that iced and room temperature injectates are usually comparable, as long as careful attention to technique is used.[53]

Properly performed, Q̇Ttd compares favorably with output values obtained by Fick or dye dilution methods. However, given the numerous coefficients in the Stewart-Hamilton formula, it is not surprising that technical errors often produce inaccurate data. Errors may occur if the volume or recorded temperature of the injectate are incorrect or if the wrong computational constant for the catheter in use and injectate temperature is entered into the computer. Warming of iced injectate from the nominal value (0°C) can occur with delays after removing the syringe from the ice bath, prolonged handling of the syringe, or inadequate in-bath thermal equilibration time. Systems that measure the injectate temperature at the site of injection avoid this problem and also permit Q̇Ttd to be measured rapidly on a change in clinical status, without the need for prior cooling of the injectate. In addition to ensuring accuracy of volume, temperature, and computational constants, it is good practice to observe the temperature-time curve as it evolves during injection, to be certain that it is without significant

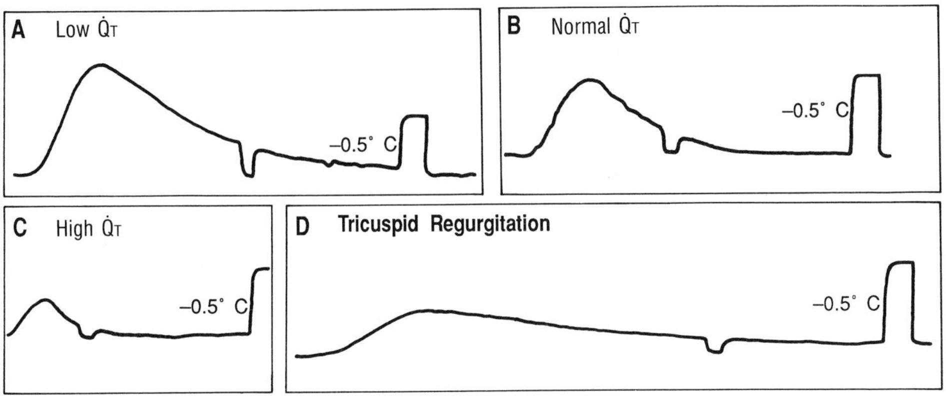

FIGURE 25-26 Thermodilution curves in patients with low, normal, and high cardiac output, and tricuspid regurgitation. The notch on each curve represents the end of data processing. The remainder of the curve is extrapolated. (From Reference 19 with permission.)

irregularity. A valid curve shows a rapid early ascent to a peak value, then smoothly returns to the thermal baseline within 10 to 15 s of injection (Fig. 25-26). Distorted curves may result from inadequate blending of injectate with blood, prolonged (>4 s) or uneven injection, thermistor contact with the vessel wall, respiratory irregularities, or abrupt changes in heart rate and hence SV. Data obtained from irregular curves should be discarded.

Even with careful attention to technique, certain conditions can render $\dot{Q}_{Ttd}$ an unreliable estimate of net systemic output. In essence, $\dot{Q}_{Ttd}$ measures right-sided output over a few cardiac cycles. Major irregularities in cardiac rhythm (e.g., ectopy, atrial fibrillation, paced beats) during the period of injection can therefore affect both the reproducibility of $\dot{Q}_{Ttd}$ determinations and the extent to which $\dot{Q}_{Ttd}$ reflects the output average over a longer period. Left-to-right shunts (atrial septal defect, VSD) increase the ratio of pulmonary : systemic output, causing $\dot{Q}_{Ttd}$ to seriously overestimate systemic output. For example, a patient with an acute ventricular septal perforation after myocardial infarction might be in advanced shock but have a normal $\dot{Q}_{Ttd}$. Tricuspid regurgitation also renders $\dot{Q}_{Ttd}$ unreliable, usually resulting in underestimation of true (forward) output.[54] Significant tricuspid regurgitation can be detected by observing the characteristically attenuated time-temperature curve (see Fig. 25-26).

The measured $\dot{Q}_{Ttd}$ may vary significantly, depending on the phase of the respiratory cycle at which the injection is begun.[55,56] Synchronizing the start of injection to the same point in the respiratory cycle will reduce variability among $\dot{Q}_{Ttd}$ measurements and therefore might be advocated if one is assessing the $\dot{Q}_{Ttd}$ response to a specific intervention. However, the average of multiple, randomly spaced injections tends to give the most accurate individual assessment. Timing of injection may be less important when the respiratory rate is high, because the duration of injection will span the entire respiratory cycle.

Combining assessment of $\dot{Q}_{Ttd}$ with measurement of systemic and pulmonary pressures allows calculation of vascular resistances: $SVR = (\overline{BP} - Pra)/\dot{Q}_T$; $PVR = (\overline{Ppa} - Ppw)/\dot{Q}_T$. To assess the appropriateness of $\dot{Q}_T$ to body mass, $\dot{Q}_{Ttd}$ is referenced to body surface area (BSA) by calculating the cardiac index ($CI = \dot{Q}_T/BSA$). Unlike flow ($\dot{Q}_T$), pulmonary and systemic pressures are not size dependent. Therefore, to avoid misinterpretation due to variation in body mass, it is appropriate to compute indices of systemic (SVRI) and pulmonary (PVRI) vascular resistance by using CI rather than $\dot{Q}_T$ in the resistance calculations.

Measurement of $\dot{Q}_{Ttd}$ can be extremely helpful in the diagnosis and management of critical illness. Knowledge of $\dot{Q}_{Ttd}$ and derived indices of vascular resistance often provides useful information regarding likely mechanisms for hypotension, oliguria, pulmonary hypertension, and unexplained lactic acidosis. Measurement of $\dot{Q}_T$ is of particular value in the management of septic shock and sepsis syndrome. Multiple factors can contribute to septic hypotension. A low SVR due to arterial vasodilation is considered a hallmark of sepsis, but reduced venous return (due to increased venous capacitance) and myocardial dysfunction often contribute to the hemodynamic derangement. The relative contributions of reduced output and reduced SVR in causing hypotension may be difficult to determine by simple clinical assessment. By assessing $\dot{Q}_T$, SVR, and Ppw, the clinician can more rationally apply fluid, pressor, and inotropic therapy for sepsis (see Chap. 114).

Measurement of $\dot{Q}_{Ttd}$ and SVR is also valuable in evaluating the hypotensive patient with ARDS. In ARDS, significant reductions in blood pressure from the baseline value are common and might occur through a number of different mechanisms that call for distinctly different interventions. A fall in blood pressure resulting from a drop in $\dot{Q}_T$ might be the result of hypovolemia, LV dysfunction, pneumothorax, pulmonary emboli, increasing PVR from ARDS, a change in applied PEEP, or gas trapping. Evaluation would consist of measurement of intravascular pressures, airway pressures, and perhaps a chest x-ray, ECG, or echocardiogram. On the other hand, these conditions would be of little concern if it were known that the fall in blood pressure was due to reduced SVR and that $\dot{Q}_T$ was stable or increased. The latter would suggest developing sepsis, but the pharmacologic influence of sedatives and adrenal insufficiency could cause a similar pattern and would need to be considered.[57,58]

A final issue regarding clinical use of the $\dot{Q}_{Ttd}$ relates to the complex interplay between output and Pa_{O_2}. Changes in output can affect Pa_{O_2} in several ways. A fall in $\dot{Q}_T$ may result in a fall in $S\bar{v}_{O_2}$. The latter may contribute to hypoxemia if the percentage of venous admixture remains constant. However, changes in $\dot{Q}_T$ can also effect the amount of intrapulmonary shunting. A decrease in $\dot{Q}_T$ may reduce the shunt fraction and, conversely, an increase in $\dot{Q}_T$ may increase shunt fraction.[59] According to this second mechanism, a fall in $\dot{Q}_T$ could actually improve arterial oxygenation. Finally, it has recently been demonstrated that an increase in $\dot{Q}_T$ will increase lung water in the setting of ARDS, even when pulmonary vascular pressures remain constant.[60] This latter effect may be due to recruitment of fluid-exchanging capillary beds at a higher $\dot{Q}_T$.[60] In an individual patient, therefore, the impact of $\dot{Q}_T$ on Pa_{O_2} will depend on the relative effects of a change in $\dot{Q}_T$ on $S\bar{v}_{O_2}$, intrapulmonary shunt, and lung water. For example, a patient with cardiogenic shock and moderate pulmonary edema might experience an increase in Pa_{O_2} after output is doubled by inotropes, if there is a large increase in $S\bar{v}_{O_2}$ yet minimal change in intrapulmonary shunt and lung water. On the other hand, a patient with ARDS and sepsis may experience no change in $S\bar{v}_{O_2}$ as $\dot{Q}_T$ is increased (vide infra), while an increase in shunt and lung water could lead to worsening oxygenation. Still a third possible outcome is a counterbalancing of improved $S\bar{v}_{O_2}$ and increased shunt fraction, with no net change in Pa_{O_2}. Because of these complex relationships, the effect of a change in $\dot{Q}_T$ on Pa_{O_2} in individual patients is not easily predicted and must be determined empirically by direct measurements of Pa_{O_2} at different $\dot{Q}_T$ values.

Mixed Venous Oxygen Saturation

Measurement of $S\bar{v}_{O_2}$ allows an assessment of the relationship between O_2 delivery (D_{O_2}) and tissue O_2 consumption ($\dot{V}_{O_2}$).[61] D_{O_2} is the product of $\dot{Q}_T$ and arterial O_2 content (Ca_{O_2}), the latter being determined by the hemoglobin and arterial O_2 saturation (Sa_{O_2}). Under normal conditions, $\dot{V}_{O_2}$ is independent of D_{O_2} and is determined by the underlying metabolic activity of tissues.[61] When D_{O_2} is insufficient to meet tissue requirements for aerobic metabolism, as with a reduction in $\dot{Q}_T$ or Sa_{O_2}, the result is a decrease in $S\bar{v}_{O_2}$ (Fig. 25-27).

To reliably assess $S\bar{v}_{O_2}$, it is necessary to measure O_2 saturation in the PA after venous blood from various organs has been thoroughly mixed in the RA and RV. Ordinarily, $S\bar{v}_{O_2}$ is lower in the superior vena cava than in the inferior vena cava, whereas the reverse tends to be true in shock.[62] Thus, venous blood obtained from a central venous catheter may not be a reliable indicator of $S\bar{v}_{O_2}$. The $S\bar{v}_{O_2}$ can be measured intermittently by withdrawing a sample of blood from the distal port of the unwedged PA catheter, or continuously with a fiberoptic PA catheter that measures O_2 saturation by reflectance oximetry. With either method, certain technical aspects of the measurement are crucial to obtaining reliable data.

Intermittent sampling of $S\bar{v}_{O_2}$ is accomplished by discarding the initial 3 mL of blood, then withdrawing a sample very slowly so as to avoid contamination with capillary blood.[18] The $S\bar{v}_{O_2}$ should be measured directly by co-

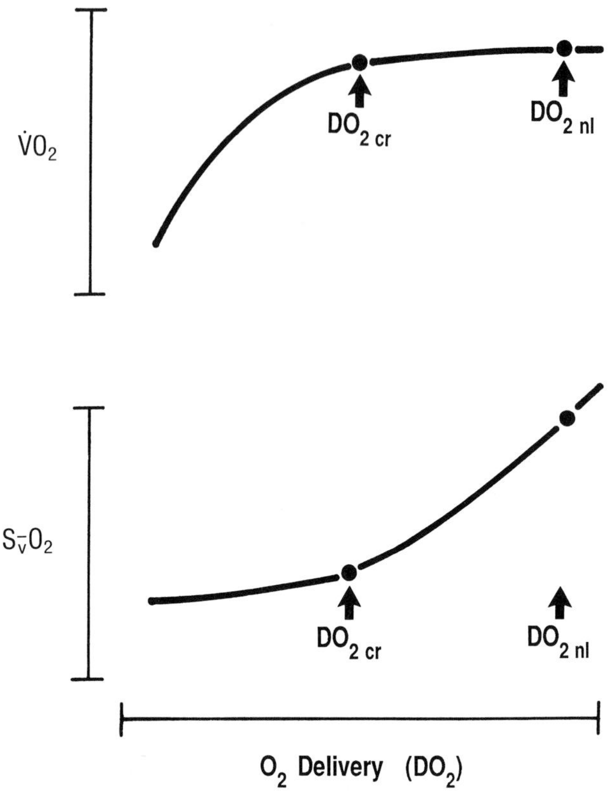

FIGURE 25-27 ***Upper panel:*** **Relationship between oxygen delivery (D_{O_2}) and oxygen consumption ($\dot{V}_{O_2}$).** ***Lower panel:*** **Relationship between D_{O_2} and mixed venous O_2 saturation ($S\bar{v}_{O_2}$). Normally, $\dot{V}_{O_2}$ is independent of D_{O_2} until D_{O_2} falls to a critical value ($D_{O_{2cr}}$), at which point further reductions in D_{O_2} lead to reduced $\dot{V}_{O_2}$. Above $D_{O_{2cr}}$, the $S\bar{v}_{O_2}$ and D_{O_2} are linearly related, but below $D_{O_{2cr}}$ the $S\bar{v}_{O_2}$ does not change markedly as D_{O_2} falls (as long as Sa_{O_2} does not change).**

oximetry. Estimation of the $S\bar{v}_{O_2}$ from measurement of the $P\bar{v}_{O_2}$, pH, and temperature is subject to potentially significant errors, because the steep slope of the O_2 dissociation curve in the venous range dictates that small errors in measurement of $P\bar{v}_{O_2}$ may result in rather large errors in calculation of $S\bar{v}_{O_2}$. The technique of reflectance oximetry for measuring $S\bar{v}_{O_2}$ depends on a progressive change in the absorbance characteristics of hemoglobin as its O_2 saturation decreases.[63] This method has been shown to measure $S\bar{v}_{O_2}$ accurately and reliably. It is necessary that the system be calibrated ex vivo before insertion and that an appropriate level of light intensity be present. Also, periodic comparison of the displayed $S\bar{v}_{O_2}$ with the $S\bar{v}_{O_2}$ measured by cooximetry is advisable to assess the need for recalibration.

In the ICU, the $S\bar{v}_{O_2}$ is used primarily as a way to assess the adequacy and stability of $\dot{Q}_T$ as it relates to tissue aerobic metabolism, or $\dot{V}_{O_2}$. Under normal conditions, the $Sa_{O_2} - S\bar{v}_{O_2}$ difference is approximately 20 to 25%, yielding an $S\bar{v}_{O_2}$ of 65 to 75% when arterial blood is well oxygenated. An $S\bar{v}_{O_2}$ in the normal range may be associated with very different levels of $\dot{Q}_T$, depending on underlying aerobic metabolism. A normal $S\bar{v}_{O_2}$ may be present in one patient who has an increased $\dot{Q}_T$ as a result of fever or agitation, and in another patient who has an appropriately low $\dot{Q}_T$ as a consequence of malnutrition and hypometabolism. For example, an elderly malnourished patient may be found to have a low $\dot{Q}_T$ (e.g., 3.0 L/min). If the $Sa_{O_2} - S\bar{v}_{O_2}$ gradient were normal, this would suggest that the low $\dot{Q}_T$ is appropriate for the underlying metabolic activity. However, if the $Sa_{O_2} - S\bar{v}_{O_2}$ gradient were increased, this would suggest that either intravascular volume or LV function were inadequate.

As long as $\dot{V}_{O_2}$ remains independent of D_{O_2}, a fall in $\dot{Q}_T$ from baseline will result in increased tissue O_2 extraction and a proportional reduction in the $S\bar{v}_{O_2}$ (see Fig. 25-27). At a critically low level of $\dot{Q}_T$, however, tissues will no longer be able to meet their O_2 demands by increased extraction, and the $\dot{V}_{O_2}$ will then become flow dependent. When $\dot{V}_{O_2}$ is flow dependent, the $S\bar{v}_{O_2}$ remains unchanged despite further reductions in $\dot{Q}_T$ (see Fig. 25-27). Therefore, with flow-dependent $\dot{V}_{O_2}$, the $S\bar{v}_{O_2}$ is no longer a reliable indicator of the adequacy or stability of $\dot{Q}_T$. Flow dependency is seen at levels of D_{O_2} that are at or above normal values in certain types of critical illness (see Chap. 57).[61,64]

The primary rationale for continuous measurement of $S\bar{v}_{O_2}$ with the fiberoptic PA catheter is that it may allow earlier detection of an imbalance between D_{O_2} and $\dot{V}_{O_2}$. If Sa_{O_2} is being monitored simultaneously and is unchanged, then a reduction in $S\bar{v}_{O_2}$ should predict either a primary reduction in $\dot{Q}_T$ or a rise in $\dot{V}_{O_2}$ unmet by a compensatory increase in $\dot{Q}_T$, provided that conditions of flow-independent $\dot{V}_{O_2}$ are present. For example, acute myocardial dysfunction or gastrointestinal hemorrhage could result in a widening of the $Sa_{O_2} - S\bar{v}_{O_2}$ gradient before other indicators of reduced $\dot{Q}_T$ become apparent. Likewise, agitation or shivering that leads to an increased $Sa_{O_2} - S\bar{v}_{O_2}$ gradient could indicate limited cardiac reserve and the need to control excess skeletal muscle activity. Whether or not continuous monitoring of $S\bar{v}_{O_2}$ by reflectance oximetry actually leads to improved patient care is uncertain, but the limited evidence to date would suggest that this technology might not be as clinically useful as originally anticipated.[65–67] In particular, the septic patient who demonstrates flow-dependent O_2 uptake would seem to benefit little from continuous monitoring of $S\bar{v}_{O_2}$ because of the dissociation of $S\bar{v}_{O_2}$ and $\dot{Q}_T$ in this setting.[61,64] Perhaps the most rational use of the fiberoptic PA catheter is in the management of the nonseptic patient with primary cardiac dysfunction in whom rapid changes in $\dot{Q}_T$ might be expected to occur on the basis of the underlying disease process or in response to pharmacologic interventions. This would be particularly true when measurement of $\dot{Q}_{Ttd}$ is rendered unreliable by significant tricuspid regurgitation or by a markedly variable heart rhythm. In the latter two instances, the $Sa_{O_2} - S\bar{v}_{O_2}$ gradient assumes primary importance as an indicator of $\dot{Q}_T$, and continuous fiberoptic monitoring might be more convenient than frequent blood sampling from the catheter's distal lumen.

Besides assessing the balance of D_{O_2} and $\dot{V}_{O_2}$, measurement of the $S\bar{v}_{O_2}$ may be of value when the absolute level of $\dot{V}_{O_2}$ is of interest. It has been shown that the $\dot{V}_{O_2}$ is a predictor of outcome from critical illness, with survivors having higher levels of $\dot{V}_{O_2}$ than nonsurvivors.[68] It has even been shown in one study that aggressive upward manipulation of D_{O_2} and $\dot{V}_{O_2}$ in patients with flow-dependent $\dot{V}_{O_2}$ may reduce mortality;[69] however, this practice remains controversial. Perhaps a less controversial reason for measuring $\dot{V}_{O_2}$ is to help guide nutritional support. Caloric needs are a function of overall metabolic activity, which in turn can be assessed by measuring $\dot{V}_{O_2}$. Resting energy expenditure (REE) is the caloric intake required to meet ongoing metabolic demands. Prediction of REE by the Fick method using PA catheter-derived data and assuming a respiratory quotient of 0.85 has been shown to correlate well with measurement of REE by indirect calorimetry.[70] The Fick-derived formula is REE (kcal/d) = $\dot{V}_{O_2} \times 7.0$, or REE = $\dot{Q}_T \times$ hemoglobin $\times (Sa_{O_2} - S\bar{v}_{O_2}) \times 95$.[70]

A final use of the $S\bar{v}_{O_2}$ is to aid in the diagnosis of intracardiac left-to-right shunts, in which case a significant step-up in O_2 saturation from RA to PA is found (vide infra).

Miscellaneous Diagnostic Applications of the Pulmonary Artery Catheter

For the most part, the PA catheter is used in the ICU to help in the management of fluids and vasoactive drug therapy during critical illness. There are, however, additional diagnostic applications of the catheter that may on occasion prove useful in the ICU. These include bedside balloon occlusion pulmonary angiography,[71] microvascular cytology,[72] arrhythmia evaluation,[20] and detection of intracardiac shunts.[20]

Pulmonary angiography has been performed successfully at the bedside with aid of the PA catheter.[71] This technique has been used to investigate the pulmonary circulation for evidence of microvascular thrombi in ARDS complicated by significant pulmonary hypertension. The rationale behind this technique is that microvascular thrombosis that contributes to pulmonary hypertension should be diffuse, thus sampling only 5 to 10 percent of the pulmonary arterial bed should be adequate for its detection.[71] Angiograms are obtained with a bedside film that is exposed after 15 to 20 mL contrast medium has been injected through the distal port of a PA catheter whose balloon has been inflated to achieve a wedge position. Balloon occlusion angiography has demonstrated filling defects due to thrombi, in vessels 1 to 3 mm in diameter, in almost 50 percent of patients with ARDS.[71] It has not been demonstrated, however, that treatment of these microvascular thrombi alters prognosis, and for this reason this technique has not achieved widespread use.

Microvascular cytology of blood drawn through the distal port of the wedged PA catheter has been used successfully to diagnose lymphangitic carcinoma.[72] It is unlikely that this technique will replace bronchoscopy with transbronchial biopsy and bronchoalveolar lavage as the initial diagnostic approach for this condition. However, if a PA catheter is inserted to measure the Ppw in a patient with diffuse

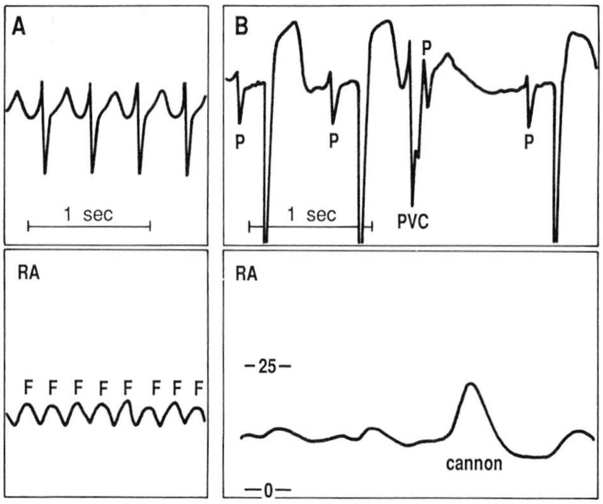

FIGURE 25-28 ***a*****. Surface ECG indicates a narrow complex tachycardia (*****top*****) of uncertain nature. Simultaneous RA pressure tracing (*****bottom*****) shows mechanical flutter waves (F) at a rate exactly twice that of the ventricular response, indicating atrial flutter with 2:1 block.** ***b*****. Premature wide complex (PVC) beat (*****top*****) is defined as ventricular in origin by the presence of a cannon "A" wave in a simultaneous RA pressure tracing. (From Reference 19 with permission.)**

lung disease of unknown etiology, a blood sample for microvascular cytology should be obtained if lymphangitic carcinoma is a diagnostic consideration. Also, very breathless patients with suspected lymphangitic carcinoma may find PA catheterization preferable to bronchoscopy. Microvascular cytology should prove to be a useful technique for diagnosing microscopic tumor embolism.

Narrow complex, regular tachyarrhythmias at a rate of 140 to 180 beats/min are common in the ICU. Differentiation of atrial flutter from sinus tachycardia and paroxysmal supraventricular tachycardia is sometimes difficult, even with the aid of a 12-lead ECG. It is sometimes possible to diagnose atrial flutter by observing the mechanical events in the RA via pressure recording from the proximal port of the PA catheter (Fig. 25-28*a*).[19] Also, an RA pressure recording may be of value in defining wide complex premature beats as ventricular in origin if clear-cut cannon "a" waves are seen (Fig. 25-28*b*).[19]

Ventricular septal perforation following myocardial infarction is not reliably diagnosed by bedside clinical examination. A VSD will result in a significantly higher Sa_{O_2} in blood obtained from the distal PA port than in blood obtained from the proximal RA port. (Also, the patient with an acute VSD may appear to be in shock clinically despite a normal, or even elevated, $\dot{Q}$Ttd.) In contrast, acute mitral regurgitation (another cause of a new postinfarction systolic murmur) is characterized by the appearance of a large V wave. A step-up in Sa_{O_2} from RA to PA can occasionally occur in acute mitral regurgitation, due to reflux of pulmonary venous blood into the PA,[19] and a VSD can occasionally produce a large V wave. Thus, differentiation of VSD and acute mitral regurgitation by pressure waveform and O_2 saturation criteria could prove to be difficult.[19] Doppler echocardiography should clarify confusing cases.

References

1. Goldenheim PD, Kazemi H: Current concepts: Cardiopulmonary monitoring of critically ill patients (Part 2). N Engl J Med: 770, 1984.
2. Robin ED: The cult of the Swan-Ganz catheter. Ann Intern Med 103:445, 1985.
3. Boyd KD: A prospective study of complication of pulmonary artery catheterizations in 500 consecutive patients. Chest 84:245, 1983.
4. Putterman CE: The Swan-Ganz catheter: A decade of hemodynamic monitoring. J Crit Care 4:127, 1989.
5. Sprung CL, Jacobs LJ, Caralis PV, et al: Ventricular arrhythmias during Swan-Ganz catheterization of the critically ill. Chest 79:413, 1981.
6. Shah KB, Rao TLK, Laughlin S, et al: A review of pulmonary artery catheterizations in 6,245 patients. Anesthesiology 61:271, 1984.
7. Morris D, Mulrihill D, Lew WYW: Risk of developing complete heart block during bedside pulmonary artery catheterization in patients with left bundle-branch block. Arch Intern Med 147:2005, 1987.
8. Chastre J, Corund F, Bouchoma A, et al: Thrombosis as a complication of pulmonary artery catheterization: Prospective evaluation by phlebography. N Engl J Med 306:278, 1982.
9. Foote GA, Schobel SI, Hodges M: Pulmonary complications of the flow directed balloon tipped catheter. N Engl J Med 290:927, 1974.
10. Hoar PF, Wilson RA, Mangarro DT, et al: Heparin bonding reduces thrombogenecity of pulmonary artery catheters. N Engl J Med 305:993, 1981.
11. Fletcher EC, Mihalick MJ, Siegel CO: Pulmonary artery rupture during introduction of the Swan-Ganz catheter: Mechanism and prevention of injury. J Crit Care 3:116, 1988.
12. O'Quinn R, Marini JJ: Pulmonary artery occlusion pressure: Clinical physiology, measurement and interpretation. Am Rev Respir Dis 128:319, 1983.
13. Civetta JM: Pulmonary artery catheter insertion, in Spring CL (ed): *The Pulmonary Artery Catheter. Methodology and Clinical Application*. Rockville, MD, 1979, Aspen, pp 22–33.
14. Gardner RM: Direct blood pressure measurement—dynamic response requirements. Anesthesiology 54:227, 1981.
15. Rapaport E, Dexter L: Pulmonary "capillary" pressure, in Warren JV (ed): *Methods in Medical Research*. Chicago, Year Book Medical Publishers, 1958, pp 85–93.
16. Morris AH, Chapman RH, Gardner RM: Frequency of technical problems encountered in the measurement of pulmonary artery wedge pressure. Crit Care Med 12:164, 1984.
17. Morris AH, Chapman RH: Wedge pressure confirmation by aspiration of pulmonary capillary blood. Crit Care Med 13:756, 1985.
18. Suter PM, Lindauer JM, Fairley HB, Schlobolym RM: Errors in data derived from pulmonary artery blood gas values. Crit Care Med 3:175, 1975.
19. Sharkey SW: Beyond the wedge: Clinical physiology and the Swan-Ganz catheter. Am J Med 83:111, 1987.
20. Pichard AD, Kay R, Smith H, et al: Larve V waves in the pulmonary wedge pressure tracing in the absence of mitral regurgitation. Am J Cardiol 50:1044, 1982.
21. Quinn K, Quebbeman EJ: Pulmonary artery pressure monitor-

ing in the surgical intensive care unit. Benefits vs. difficulties. Arch Surg 116:872, 1981.
22. Shuster DP, Seeman MD: Temporary muscle paralysis for accurate measurement of pulmonary artery occlusion pressure. Chest 84:593, 1983.
23. Sibhald WJ, Paterson NAM, Holliday RL, et al: Pulmonary hypertension in sepsis. Measurement by the pulmonary arterial diastolic-pulmonary wedge pressure gradient and the influence of passive and active factors. Chest 73:583, 1978.
24. Zapol WM, Snider MT, Rie MA, et al: Pulmonary circulation during adult respiratory distress syndrome, in Zapol WM, Falke KJ (eds): *Acute Respiratory Failure.* New York, Marcel Dekker, 1985, p 241.
25. Raper B, Sibhald WJ: Misled by the wedge. The Swan-Ganz catheter and left ventricular preload. Chest 89:427, 1986.
26. Cassidy SS, Schweip F: Cardiovascular effects of positive end-expiratory pressure, in Scharf SM, Cassidy SS (eds): *Heart-Lung Interaction in Health and Disease.* New York, Marcel-Dekker, 1989, p 463.
27. Jardin F, Genevisy B, Brun-Ney D, Bourdarais JP: Influence of lung and chest wall compliances on transmission of airway pressure to the pleural space in critically ill patients. Chest 86:653, 1985.
28. Cassidy SS, Robertson CH, Pierce AK, et al: Cardiovascular effects of positive end-expiratory pressure in dogs. J Appl Physiol 44:743, 1978.
29. Pharnant JF, Devaux JY, Monsallier JF, et al: Mechanisms of decreased left ventricular preload during continuous positive pressure ventilation in ARDS. Chest 90:74, 1986.
30. Maunder RJ, Shuman WP, McHugh JW, et al: Preservation of normal lung regions in the adult respiratory distress syndrome. Analysis by computed tomography. JAMA 255:2463, 1986.
31. Caster RS, Snyder JV, Pinsky MR: Left ventricular filling pressure during PEEP measured by wedge pressure after airway disconnection. Am J Physiol 249:770, 1985.
32. Pinsky M, Vincent J-L, DeSmet J-M: Estimating left-ventricular filling pressure during positive end-expiratory pressure in humans. Am Rev Respir Dis 143:25, 1991.
33. Shasby DM, Dauber JM, Pfister S, et al: Swan-Ganz location and left atrial pressure determine the accuracy of the wedge pressure when positive pressure, end-expiratory pressure is used. Chest 80:666, 1981.
34. Hassan FM, Weiss WB, Braman SS, Hoppin FG: Influence of lung injury on pulmonary wedge-left atrial pressure correlation during positive end-expiratory pressure ventilation. Am Rev Respir Dis 131:246, 1985.
35. Pepe PE, Marini JJ: Occult positive end-expiratory pressure in mechanically ventilated patients with airflow obstruction. Am Rev Respir Dis 126:166, 1982.
36. Benson MS, Pierson DJ: Auto-PEEP during mechanical ventilation of adults. Respir Care 33:557, 1988.
37. Rice DL, Chon KE, Gaasch WN, et al: Wedge pressure measurements in obstructive pulmonary disease. Chest 66:628, 1974.
38. Rao BS, Chon KE, Eldridge FL, et al: Left ventricular failure secondary to chronic pulmonary disease. Am J Med 45:229, 1968.
39. Harms BA, Kramer GC, Bodai BI, Demling RH: Effect of hypoproteinemia on pulmonary and soft tissue edema formation. Crit Care Med 9:503, 1981.
40. Gaar KA, Taylor AI, Owens LJ, Guyton AC: Pulmonary capillary pressure and filtration coefficient in the isolated perfused lung. Am J Physiol 213:910, 1967.
41. Palevsky HI, Pietra GG, Fishman AP: Pulmonary veno-occlusive disease and its response to vasodilator agents. Am Rev Respir Dis 142:426, 1990.
42. Cope DK, Allison RC, Parmentier JC, et al: Measurement of effective pulmonary capillary wedge pressure using the pressure profile after pulmonary artery occlusion. Crit Care Med 4:16, 1986.
43. Wood LDH, Prewitt RM: Cardiovascular management in acute hypoxemic respiratory failure. Am J Cardiol 47:963, 1981.
44. Holloway H, Perry M, Downey J, et al: Estimation of effective pulmonary capillary pressure in intact lungs. J Appl Physiol 54:846, 1983.
45. Collee GG, Lynch KE, Hill RD, Zapol WM: Bedside measurement of pulmonary capillary pressure in patients with acute respiratory failure. Anesthesiology 66:614, 1987.
46. Oppenheimer L, Goldberg HS. Pulmonary circulation and edema formation, in Scharf SM, Cassidy JS (eds): *Heart-Lung Intersection in Health and Disease.* New York, Marcel-Dekker, 1987, p 93.
47. Braunwald E, Ross J Jr: Control of cardiac performance, in Berne RM, Sperelakis N, Geiger SR (eds): *Handbook of Physiology.* Section 2, *The Cardiovascular System.* Vol I, *The Heart.* Bethesda, American Physiological Society, 1979, pp 533–573.
48. Sibbald WJ, Driedger AA, Myers ML, et al: Biventricular function in the adult respiratory distress syndrome: Hemodynamic and radionuclide assessment, with special emphasis on right ventricular function. Chest 84:126, 1983.
49. Parker J, Case R: Normal left ventricular function. Circulation 60:4, 1979.
50. Packman MI, Rackow EC. Optimum left heart filling pressure during fluid resuscitation of patients with hypovolemic and septic shock. Crit Care Med: 165, 1983.
51. Crexalls C, Chatterjee R, Forrester J, et al: Optimal level of filling pressure in the left side of the heart in acute myocardial infarction. N Engl J Med 289:1064, 1973.
52. Weisel RD, Berger RL, Hechtman HB: Measurement of cardiac output by thermodilution. N Engl J Med 292:682, 1975.
53. Elkayam U, Berkley R, Azen S, et al: Cardiac output by thermodilation technique. Effect of injectate's volume and temperature on accuracy and reproducibility in the critically ill patient. Chest 84:418, 1981.
54. Cigarroa RG, Lange RA, Williams RH: Underestimation of cardiac output by thermodilution in patients with tricuspid regurgitation. Am J Med 86:417, 1989.
55. Snyder JV, Powner DJ: Effects of mechanical ventilation on the measurement of cardiac output by thermodilation. Crit Care Med 10:677, 1987.
56. Stevens JH, Raffin TA, Milum FG, et al: Thermodilution cardiac output measurement. Effects of the respiratory cycle on its reproducibility. JAMA 253:2240, 1985.
57. Reves JG, Frazen RJ, Vinik HR, Greenblatt DJ: Midazolam: Pharmacology and uses. Anesthesiology 62:310, 1985.
58. Dorin RI, Kearns PJ: High output circulatory failure in acute adrenal insufficiency. Crit Care Med 16:296, 1988.
59. Dantzbe DR, Lynch JP, Weg JG: Depression of cardiac output is a mechanism of shunt reduction in the therapy of acute respiratory failure. Chest 77:636, 1980.
60. Hasinoff I, Ducas J, Prewitt RM: Increased cardiac output increases lung water in canine permeability pulmonary edema. J Crit Care 3:225, 1988.
61. Schumacher PT, Samsel RW: Oxygen delivery and uptake by peripheral tissues: Physiology and pathophysiology. Crit Care Clinics 5:255, 1989.

62. Lee J, Wright F, Barber R, Stanley L: Central venous oxygen saturation in shock. Anesthesiology 5:472, 1972.
63. Sperinte JM, Senelly KM: The oximetric opticath system: Theory and development, in Fahey PJ (ed): *Continuous Measurement of Blood Oxygen Saturation in the High Risk Patient.* Vol 2. San Diego, Beach International, 1985, pp 59–80.
64. Cain SM: Review: Supply dependency of oxygen uptake in ARDS: Myth or reality? Am J Med Sci 288:119, 1984.
65. Jastremski MS, Chelluri L, Beney KM, Bailly RT: Analysis of the effects of continuous on-line monitoring of mixed venous oxygen saturation on patient outcome and cost-effectiveness. Crit Care Med 17:148, 1989.
66. Vaugh S, Puri VK: Cardiac output changes and continuous mixed venous oxygen saturation measurement in the critically ill. Crit Care Med 16:495, 1988.
67. Rajput MA, Richey HM, Bush BA, et al: A comparison between a conventional and a fiberoptic flow-directed thermal dilution pulmonary artery catheter in critically ill patients. Arch Intern Med 149:83, 1989.
68. Russell JA, Ronco JJ, Lockhat D, et al: Oxygen delivery and consumption and ventricular preload are greater in survivors than in nonsurvivors of the adult respiratory distress syndrome. Am Rev Respir Dis 141:659, 1990.
69. Shoewisher WC, Appel PL, Krom HB, et al: Prospective trial of supranormal values of survivors as therapeutic goals in high-risk surgical patients. Chest 94:1176, 1988.
70. Liggett SB, St John RE, Lefrak SS: Determination of resting energy expenditure utilizing the thermodilution pulmonary artery catheter. Chest 91:562, 1987.
71. Greene R, Zapol WM, Snider MT, et al: Early bedside detection of pulmonary vascular occlusion during acute respiratory failure. Am Rev Respir Dis 124:591, 1981.
72. Masson RG, Krikorian J, Luke P, et al: Pulmonary vascular cytology in the diagnosis of lymphangiitic carcinomatosis. N Engl J Med 321:71, 1989.

Chapter 26

CARDIAC CATHETERIZATION, BALLOON ANGIOPLASTY, AND PERCUTANEOUS VALVULOPLASTY

TED FELDMAN
JOHN D. CARROLL

Diagnostic and therapeutic procedures in the cardiac catheterization laboratory are performed routinely on patients with life-threatening cardiovascular disease. This chapter, however, will focus on patients who have cardiovascular disease in addition to some other major illness or organ system failure. Patients with major organ system compromise requiring management in an ICU often have cardiovascular disease complicating their primary disease process. The management of these patients is highly complex and requires many special considerations.

To fully understand the role of cardiac catheterization-related procedures in these patients, some understanding of the basic elements of catheterization procedures is necessary (Table 26-1).

TABLE 26-1 Catheterization Procedures

RIGHT HEART CATHETERIZATION
Hemodynamic study
Temporary pacing
Pulmonary angiography
Endomyocardial biopsy
Electrophysiologic testing
Pulmonic valvuloplasty
Drug infusion
LEFT HEART CATHETERIZATION
(Brachial and Femoral Techniques)
Hemodynamic study
Coronary angiography
Left ventriculography
Peripheral arterial angiography
Balloon valvuloplasty
Balloon angioplasty

Diagnostic Cardiac Catheterization and Angiography

A patient may walk into the cardiac catheterization laboratory, undergo percutaneous femoral arterial catheterization with coronary arteriography and left ventriculography, and then be discharged from the hospital, ambulatory, a few hours after the procedure is completed.[1] At the other extreme, in the patient with multisystem organ failure (MSOF) and a prolonged hospital stay, transportation to the catheterization laboratory alone may involve movement of the patient, a respirator, and multiple infusion pumps. Transfer onto the angiography table may be an exercise in itself. The intraprocedure management of the patient may be complicated by difficulty with venous or arterial access, and hemodynamic instability may limit the extent of the procedure performed.

Among the more important steps in accomplishing a catheterization procedure is the preprocedure evaluation of the patient. A clear definition of both the indications and goals of the procedure must be established at the outset.

INDICATIONS

The indications for a cardiac catheterization in patients with MSOF or in highly complex and severely ill ICU patients are no different from those in the elective cardiac catheterization population.[2] The evaluation of ischemic heart disease, left or right ventricular heart failure, and the etiology of arrhythmias constitute the major categories of indications (Table 26-2). What is clearly different in the severely ill patient are the goals of therapy. Although coronary artery disease (CAD) may be present in a large proportion of older patients in ICU settings, its definition by coronary arteriography is warranted only when therapy for the CAD may affect the patient's overall course. In the simplest cases, definition of CAD may allow for more directed drug therapy. In some settings revascularization by angioplasty or coronary bypass surgery may be the desired goal, but this is often precluded or tempered by the patient's general condition. One common scenario involves ventilator-dependent

TABLE 26-2 Indications for Cardiac Catheterization

Clarification of chest pain or other findings suggestive of myocardial ischemia
Assessment of coronary anatomy when clinical condition suggests severe CAD (unstable angina, post MI angina, markedly positive ETT)
Assessment of nature and severity of valvular, myocardial, or pericardial disease
Assessment of cardiac transplant status
Sudden death evaluation
Preoperative assessment
Treatment of valvular stenosis
Treatment of CAD
Clarification of nature or treatment of rhythm disorder

patients who have paroxysmal elevations of the pulmonary capillary pressures suggesting that ischemic left ventricular dysfunction contributes to the ventilator dependence. These patients are very high risk for revascularization procedures. Nonetheless, specific elucidation of the extent of their myocardial ischemia may be necessary for their management. Similarly, patients with intractable arrhythmias complicating another illness such as acute respiratory failure may not be easily managed unless an ischemic etiology can be either demonstrated or excluded as the basis for the arrhythmia.

A third major group of patients who may benefit from diagnostic cardiac catheterization are those with significant left or right ventricular failure. The pathophysiology of a patient's heart failure syndrome must be defined precisely in terms of broad categories (i.e., cardiomyopathy, valvular, pericardial) and specific subtypes (diastolic versus systolic dysfunction, dilated versus restrictive cardiomyopathy, etc.). Simultaneous measurement of left and right heart pressures and cardiac output during a catheterization procedure with trials of drug therapy may be extremely helpful. Afterload reduction with nitroprusside, inotropic therapy with a catecholamine agent, or therapy with intravenous nitroglycerine during left and right heart catheterization may provide extremely useful guides to the ongoing management of these patients once pathophysiology is defined.

RISKS

The safety of catheterization procedures in unstable and acutely ill patients is highly variable (Table 26-3). There are no absolute contraindications to cardiac catheterization procedures. The relative risks have to be considered carefully in view of the potential benefits.[3–5] The risk of death during coronary arteriography is less than $\frac{1}{1000}$ (0.098 percent) and has fallen in the last decade. Age over 60, New York Heart Association Class IV, and left main coronary artery stenosis are factors which increase the risk to the 0.1 to 0.5 percent range.[4]

TABLE 26-3 Complications of Cardiac Catheterization—Results from 222,553 Patients

	Total (%)	Age > 60 (%)	NYHA Class IV (%)
Death	0.10	0.12^a	0.29^a
MI	0.06	0.06	0.12^a
Cerebrovascular accident	0.07	0.09^a	0.08
Arrhythmia	0.47	0.51^a	0.65^a
Vascular	0.46	0.49^a	0.46
Hemorrhage	0.07	0.10^a	0.09
Contrast	0.23	0.20	0.21
Other	0.28	0.35^a	0.43^a
Total	1.74	1.92^a	2.34^a

$^a p < 0.05$ vs total
SOURCE: *Cathet Cardiovasc Diag* 17:5, 1989.

Transportation of the patient to the cardiac catheterization laboratory is often a highly complex process. In addition to transporting a patient with a monitor and defibrillator, it is useful to have assistance from the ICU nurse and a respiratory therapist for ventilated patients (see Chap. 48). Allowing time for the transfer is also important, and procedures in these patients are ideally scheduled for early in the day.

CATHETERIZATION PROCEDURE CONSIDERATIONS

Arterial access is generally from the right femoral artery.[6] In patients with shock it is useful to prepare both femoral areas so that the left femoral artery may be used for intraaortic balloon counterpulsation if necessary during the catheterization. Either brachial artery may be used for retrograde catheterization if necessary.[7] Circumstances under which brachial arterial catheterization is important include severe peripheral vascular disease with diminished or absent femoral pulses, aortic dissection with absent femoral pulses, or patients with severe bleeding diatheses, in whom direct exposure and then repair of the brachial artery is preferable to an attempt at prolonged compression of percutaneous femoral arterial puncture. Patients with severe thrombocytopenia or prolonged prothrombin time (PT) caused by liver failure, malnutrition, or antibiotic therapy may have brachial cutdown performed by a vascular surgeon, with the aid of a cautery unit in the catheterization laboratory. When necessary for a right heart catheterization, venous access may be obtained by any central venous route. When the need for right heart catheterization is clearly short-term, femoral venous puncture is the simplest approach. If a longer term indwelling right heart catheter is desired, jugular, subclavian, or brachial venous approaches are preferable. Among patients at high risk for internal jugular cannulation, or those in whom it has been unsuccessful, a brachial venous cutdown is frequently used. If the line is to be left for longer than the catheterization procedure, it is introduced through a subcutaneous tunnel to eliminate the need for later suture removal and potentially diminish the possibility of infection (Fig. 26-1).

Patients with right bundle branch block who are to undergo left heart catheterization are at risk for complete heart block if a catheter is introduced into the left ventricle, impinging on the interventricular septum and the conducting system. With complete right bundle branch block, a temporary pacemaker is routinely used for left heart catheterization. A temporary pacemaker is also used for left bundle branch block with right heart catheterization. This necessitates venous access to accompany left heart catheterization in these cases. A "paceport" type pulmonary artery catheter is often useful for this purpose, but the pacing wire must be tested carefully.

The patient's volume status must be evaluated carefully by both the catheterization and ICU teams before and after the procedure. Since the catheterization will yield highly specific information regarding the patient's state of hydra-

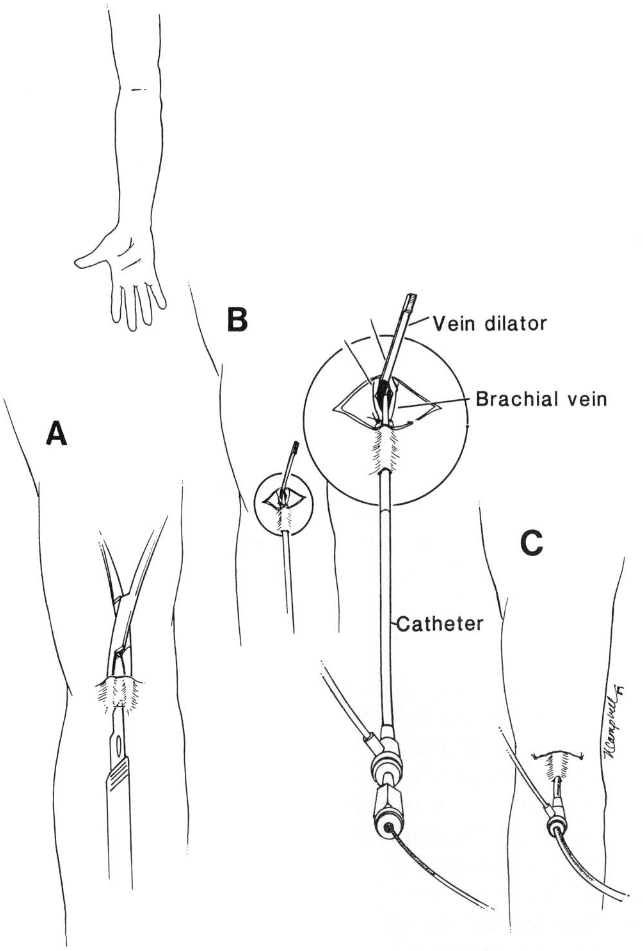

FIGURE 26-1 After a brachial venous cutdown, the catheter may be introduced through a subcutaneous tunnel and the incision closed with subcutaneous absorbable suture. After the vein is isolated, a small incision is made about 2 cm distal to the skin incision. *a.* Hemostat may be used to lift the skin and allow a small stab to be made safely. *b.* The introducer sheath is passed through the subcutaneous tunnel into the venotomy. *c.* The skin incision is closed with running subcutaneous absorbable suture.

tion, it is preferable to have a patient slightly hypovolemic rather than volume overloaded unless the patient is at high risk for dye-induced acute tubular necrosis, i.e., a diabetic with renal insufficiency. If a patient is volume overloaded at the beginning of a procedure, it is often impossible to give the necessary amount of contrast or volume during the procedure to complete a study. In this circumstance, low osmolarity contrast agents and digital processing of images can reduce the amount of dye needed and its hemodynamic effects.

Hemodynamically unstable patients often benefit from early therapy with inotropic or catecholamine agents.[8,9] Similarly, patients whose ventilation is marginal may be intubated prior to catheterization, under controlled circumstances, rather than in the midst of a complicated angiographic procedure.

If the patient has a history of allergy to radiographic contrast agents, premedication with steroids and antihistamines should be administered.[10,11] Hydrocortisone, 100 mg, and 25 mg Benadryl may be given orally or intravenously both 6 h before and 1 h before the procedure. In addition, patients allergic to conventional contrast media do not consistently cross-react to nonionic agents. Thus, nonionic agents should be used when contrast allergy is known or suspected.

Among patients with an elevated serum creatinine level, the relative risks of contrast administration must be weighed carefully. Low osmolarity contrast agents are of some use in this setting, not because they have been demonstrated to have less nephrotoxicity, but rather because a smaller osmolar load is given to the patient, thus diminishing the likelihood of left ventricular failure following the procedure.[12] In patients on chronic hemodialysis, plans for dialysis shortly after the procedure must be made. Among those with elevated creatinine levels, but no need for dialysis, hydration is useful. If the patient's volume status will not allow it prior to the procedure, then saline and furosemide may be given at the end of the catheterization procedure.

Other efforts to limit the contrast load are important. In most patients an examination of the left ventricle can be accomplished using gated blood pool studies, first-pass radionuclide studies, or echocardiography. Coronary arteriography may be performed afterward. This obviates the need for radiocontrast left ventriculography in these patients. When conventional noninvasive imaging does not adequately demonstrate the level of left ventricular function, injection of contrast echocardiographic agents directly into the ventricle during catheterization with simultaneous two-dimensional echocardiography provides excellent quality images.[13,14] This method is useful for the evaluation of valvular regurgitation without the use of radiocontrast. With careful attention to the amount of contrast material used, coronary arteriography can be accomplished in most patients with well under 50 mL of dye. Biplane coronary arteriography may be an important adjunct to the conservation of dye in these patients. However, a few good quality single-plane coronary views are preferable to poor quality or incomplete biplane pictures. Obese patients or those with large pleural effusions are poor candidates for biplane coronary arteriography.

When a high cardiac output is present and the patent has a dynamic precordium, concern regarding the administration of iodinated contrast agents to a hyperthyroid patient may be raised. If hyperthyroidism is present, then the short-term consequence of iodine administration will be suppression of thyroid function. Thus, the immediate concern regarding a catheterization procedure is unwarranted.

CATHETERIZATION PROCEDURE

After the patient arrives in the laboratory and is placed on the table, the arterial and venous access sites are prepared with iodine and then covered with sterile drapes. Superficial and then deep local anesthesia with lidocaine is given.

The dose of lidocaine may be relatively high for very old patients or those with compromised liver function, particularly if it is mistakenly given intravenously rather than subcutaneously. New onset lethargy, confusion, or loss of consciousness during the procedure may be due to lidocaine toxicity. Both a lidocaine level and careful neurologic examination must be done. A decision regarding completion of the procedure must be individualized.

For the awake patient, a sedative may be given. When hypotension or hypoventilation are problems, this need not be done. For the agitated patient or, for example, the patient with generalized seizures, the procedure may be accomplished under general anesthesia.

For the comatose patient it is unusual for cardiac catheterization to be needed. Yet, when it is necessary care must be taken to avoid complications which are usually prevented by the recognition of problems from patient's ability to voice complaints (i.e., vascular dissection from catheter advancement in the wall of an artery).

ANTICOAGULATION

Though cardiac catheterization is commonly done with the use of heparin anticoagulation, for simple diagnostic coronary arteriography this may be omitted. The use of anticoagulants is often highly problematic in critically ill patients who may have prolonged partial thromboplastin time (PTT), prolonged PT, or decreased platelet count. It must be remembered that for angioplasty or coronary bypass surgery high doses of heparin therapy are necessary. Right ventricular biopsy requires that no clotting disorder, including heparin, be present.

SELECTIVE CORONARY ARTERIOGRAPHY

When specific information regarding the distribution and severity of coronary stenoses is necessary, nonselective coronary arteriography is entirely inadequate. Likewise, the use of the surface electrocardiogram (ECG), echocardiogram, or nuclear scans to determine the anatomic distribution of coronary stenoses is extremely uncertain. Coronary arteriography provides information useful not only in directing invasive therapy, such as surgery or angioplasty, but also in the approach to medical management as well. For example, the patient suspected of having severe CAD, but found to have only mild or no CAD may be managed much more simply than the patient found to have unsuspected left main coronary stenosis.

The procedure is performed by local insertion of coronary catheters and injection of contrast material into the coronary ostia.[6,7] The risks of coronary arteriography are particularly high in patients with severe generalized vascular disease, where embolic stroke may result from dislodgement of fragments along the aortic arch or embolization of clots that form in catheters when the procedure time is prolonged due to difficult anatomy.

LEFT VENTRICULOGRAPHY

Imaging the left ventricle can be accomplished by a number of means. In severely ill patients, it is useful to characterize the level of left ventricular performance and the presence or absence of valvular regurgitation prior to a catheterization study. Echocardiography may be performed easily at the bedside in these patients. The utility of these studies is sometimes limited in mechanically ventilated patients because air between the chest wall and heart interferes with the imaging quality. Furthermore, echocardiography is least helpful when regional dysfunction is present. Portable gated blood pool studies and thallium scans may be obtained in many institutions. Since left ventricular ejection fraction is the single most powerful predictor of cardiovascular prognosis overall, its measurement will often help in defining the goals of a catheterization procedure. Conversely, when it is certain that both coronary arteriography and left ventriculography will be performed, preprocedure noninvasive testing may not be useful. After left ventriculography has been performed, other imaging modalities may be used to obtain complementary information. Because these additional tests require expense, time, and often transportation of the patient, they may have limited applicability. Newer modalities such as magnetic resonance imaging (MRI) and fast computed tomography (CT) scans are too cumbersome for many ICU patients.

Left ventriculography requires the introduction of a pigtail or other ventriculographic catheter into the ventricle retrograde across the aortic valve or antegrade across the mitral valve when transseptal left atrial catheterization has been performed. The presence of a foreign body (the catheter) in the ventricle may precipitate ventricular ectopy. This is usually limited to the period during which the catheter is present, but ventricular tachycardia or fibrillation may result. In patients with severe left ventricular dysfunction, left ventricular aneurysm, or recent myocardial infarction, (MI), left ventricular thrombus may be dislodged by the catheter with resultant embolic sequelae.

Left ventriculography provides an unequaled image quality for assessment of regional wall motion. The presence or absence of mitral regurgitation may be evaluated as well. The hemodynamic information recorded during a left ventricular radiographic examination is extremely important. The left ventricular end-diastolic pressure is measured and is the best single assessment of the patient's volume status and is often useful as a single index of chamber compliance. On a pullback of the catheter from the left ventricle to the aorta, the presence or absence of a transaortic valve pressure gradient is evaluated.

HEMODYNAMIC EVALUATION

The critically ill patient often needs a hemodynamic evaluation. The raw data of such an evaluation include the measurement of pressures in all major chambers and the arterial and venous systems, cardiac output, oxygen saturation in all cardiac chambers, and chamber size and geometry. From these values an analysis of pump, muscle, and valvular function is possible. Commonly derived indices include vascular resistance, valve area, ejection fraction, and shunt magnitude. Furthermore, more sophisticated approaches can be used to quantify left ventricular systolic and diastolic function, arterial mechanical properties, and the obstructive load imposed by stenotic valves.

The critically ill patient poses special problems for a hemodynamic study. Fast heart rates may produce artifacts in fluid-filled catheter assessment of pressures. Combined with a high cardiac output, the quality of angiographic studies is often compromised. Lung disease and ventilators may distort the true distending pressure of cardiac chambers.

STRUCTURAL ANALYSIS BY ENDOCARDIAL BIOPSY

Important diagnoses may be made by direct examination of cardiac tissue. Endomyocardial biopsy can be performed easily in virtually all patients. A bioptome is introduced by right internal jugular, femoral, or subclavian routes, and small tissue samples are obtained from the right ventricular septum. Because perforation of the right ventricular free wall is the most serious potential complication of the procedure, normal or near normal coagulation parameters are important. Perforation, air embolism, or bleeding from central venous puncture are extremely rare.

Biopsy is used most commonly to evaluate rejection after cardiac transplantation. It may be useful in the diagnosis of heart failure. Acute fulminant heart failure syndromes are more likely to represent acute myocarditis than cases with established dilated cardiomyopathy. Other causes of heart failure, such as amyloidosis, hemochromatosis, and sarcoidosis may be detected as well. Left ventricular biopsy is occasionally positive when right ventricular specimens are not.

POSTPROCEDURE MANAGEMENT

The major elements of concern immediately following a cardiac catheterization procedure are problems related to the disease process itself, volume overload from the large amount of contrast agent used, or problems related to hemostasis at the arterial and venous access sites or the arterial and venous sheath management. Close attention to the patient's status during the first hours after the cardiac catheterization almost always results in freedom from these complications.

The catheterization procedure may easily aggravate the underlying cardiac disease process. Coronary angiography in patients with left main stenosis is particularly dangerous. These patients may become very unstable after the lesion has been disturbed by a catheter and often require immediate coronary bypass surgery. Patients with valvular heart disease, particularly aortic valve stenosis, may have marked decompensation following the angiographic dye load. On occasion, the dehydration that accompanies preprocedure fasting may result in deficient preload with a fall in cardiac output or blood pressure or both. Failure to replace volume loss associated with postcatheterization osmotic diuresis may result in hypovolemia, hypotension, or an increased risk for dye-induced nephrotoxicity.

Management of the puncture site is also of critical importance. Following removal of catheters after an uncomplicated diagnostic procedure, pressure is applied to the puncture until hemostasis is achieved. This usually requires between 5 and 20 min. On occasion, particularly when the pulse pressure is wide as in patients with aortic insufficiency or hypertensive heart disease, prolonged pressure application for up to an hour may be necessary. Some available Velcro and plastic devices may aid with prolonged groin compressions. Clamp compression devices are dangerous when used by inexperienced personnel. A 5- to 10-lb sandbag may be left on the puncture site to aid in preserving hemostasis for the first few hours after catheterization. Among patients who are ambulatory or able to get out of bed and into a chair, 6 h of bed rest following the procedure is usual.

In the era of interventional cardiology and in those patients undergoing catheterization while anticoagulated with heparin, it is common to leave arterial and venous sheaths in place after the procedure. The management of these sheaths requires special attention. Heparin anticoagulation is important when indwelling arterial sheaths are left for prolonged periods lasting up to 48 h following catheterization. Endocarditis prophylaxis should be administered to patients with prosthetic valves or significant native valvular disease when prolonged sheath times are planned. Among anticoagulated patients, oozing around the sheaths is frequent. When the sheaths must be left in place and bleeding is more than a slow ooze, changing the sheath to a larger size may result in better hemostasis. The importance of careful nursing care cannot be overemphasized in the management of sheaths. Arterial sheaths should be connected to a pressure manometer so that the waveform may be used as an indication of cannula patency. Venous sheaths should at least have a "keep open" infusion. Complications that may result from long sheath times include arterial pseudoaneurysm, arteriovenous fistula, and hematoma. A vascular surgeon should be consulted early when any of these are suspected. Surgical repair is relatively simple when undertaken early.

When sheaths have been left in place for more than a few hours, the removal can be painful. Sheath removal after 24 h is complicated by severe vagal reactions in as many as 5 percent of patients. The resulting hypotension and bradycardia are particularly deleterious in patients with CAD or valvular heart disease. To avoid vagal reactions to the pain of sheath removal, infiltration with local anesthesia prior to sheath removal is useful. In addition, the intravenous administration of morphine or fentanyl before sheath removal is helpful.

Percutaneous Transluminal Coronary Angioplasty

Since first described by Andreas Gruentzig in 1978, percutaneous transluminal coronary angioplasty (PTCA) has come into common use.[15] When first introduced, the procedure was applied only to patients with proximal discrete, concentric, and noncalcified coronary artery stenoses (Fig. 26-2). With improvements in both technique and technol-

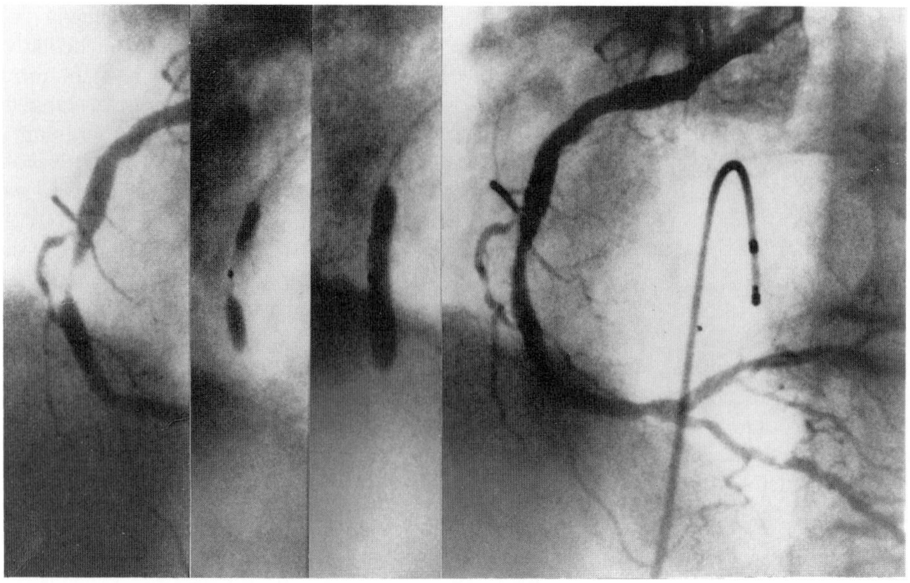

a b c d

FIGURE 26-2 *a.* **Subtotal mid right coronary artery stenosis. The lesion is concentric and fairly discrete.** *b.* **A radio-opaque dot marks the center of a coronary angioplasty balloon. The negative impression of the stenosis or "waist" demonstrates the location and severity of the stenosis.** *c.* **The fully expanded balloon relieves the stenosis, shown angiographically in** *d.*

ogy, the angioplasty procedure is now used in a wide spectrum of patients with single and multivessel CAD and with complex anatomy and lesion morphology.[16]

PATIENT SELECTION

It is useful to view patients as potential candidates for revascularization therapy, rather than considering them as candidates for angioplasty or coronary bypass surgery. The decision to pursue a mechanical revascularization should be made on the basis of the patient's clinical picture and the coronary artery anatomy. The specific technique used for revascularization depends on a variety of both technical and clinical factors. PTCA may be attempted in a wide spectrum of patients; the probability of success of the angioplasty procedure is highly variable and can be inferred before the procedure. It is the selection of patients in whom the risk benefit ratio is favorable that primarily determines patient selection. Clinical situations in which revascularization therapy may be useful include: patients with intractable chest pain despite medical therapy, unstable angina with reversible ECG changes associated with ischemia, objective evidence of severe ischemia in the asymptomatic patient, acute MI, and early post MI ischemic pain. In addition, revascularization therapy may be very important in the care of patients with ischemic syndromes following coronary artery bypass graft (CABG) surgery. This may be in both the very early postoperative phase and also in patients who are experiencing progression of either graft or native disease many years after bypass surgery.

RESULTS

The results of angioplasty for patients with one-, two-, and three-vessel disease have been summarized in a registry from the National Heart, Lung and Blood Institute (Table 26-4).[16] Single discrete lesions in patients with good left ventricular function can be treated with a greater than 90 percent success rate and a <0.5 percent procedure mortality rate. The rate of vessel closure with need for emergency CABG surgery is 3 percent and the periprocedure MI rate approximately 4 percent. As the complexity of the coronary anatomy and the number of vessels dilated increases, the risk of angioplasty increases as well. Among patients with multivessel CAD undergoing multivessel angioplasty procedure, mortality may exceed 2 percent.

EXPANDING ROLE OF PTCA

The settings in which angioplasty may be performed have been expanded considerably over the past decade. Angioplasty is now also feasible in patients with highly complex lesion morphology. Situations such as bifurcation lesions involving large side branches (Fig. 26-3) and patients with multilesion disease in a single vessel or multivessel disease may be dilated.

Chronic total occlusions remain one of the major limitations of balloon angioplasty. Total occlusions of more than 6 months' duration are often impossible to cross with a wire and recanalize. Those of even more than a few weeks' duration likewise have a lower success rate than elective angi-

TABLE 26-4 National Heart, Lung and Blood Institute PTCA Registry 1985–86[a]

	Single Vessel (%)	Double Vessel (%)	Triple Vessel (%)	Total (%)
Nonfatal MI	3.5	5.1	5.1	4.3
Emergency CABG	2.9	3.7	4.3	3.4
Death	0.2	0.9	2.8	1.0

[a]n = 1802

SOURCE: *N Engl J Med* 318:265, 1988.

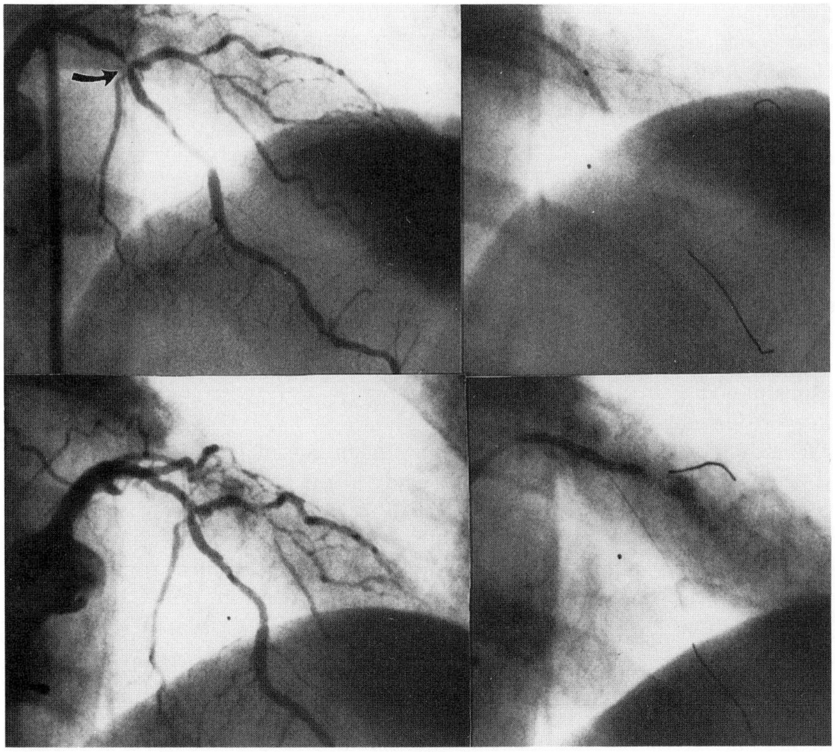

FIGURE 26-3 *Upper left.* **Bifurcation stenosis with subtotal occlusion of the left anterior descending artery and a multibranching diagonal vessel (arrow) are seen.** *Upper right.* **Balloon catheter is inflated in the left anterior descending stenosis and a small guidewire is in the diagonal artery.** *Lower right.* **Balloon catheter is inflated in the diagonal artery with a guidewire protecting the left anterior descending.** *Lower left.* **Widely patent bifurcation is apparent.**

oplasty for less than total occlusions and also have a higher restenosis rate in the first year after dilation. The likelihood of success in dilating total occlusions varies directly with their duration. In patients with acute MI and chest pain of less than 48 h duration, the likelihood of success in crossing a total occlusion and having a good angioplasty result approaches 90 percent.

Direct angioplasty for acute MI is a highly viable and useful modality (Fig. 26-4).[17,18] Those institutions capable of moving a patient into the catheterization laboratory and accomplishing an angioplasty within 1.5 h after symptom onset often favor direct angioplasty over thrombolytic therapy as a primary treatment for early evolving acute MI. PTCA may be used in conjunction with thrombolytic therapy. After intravenous thrombolytic therapy, successful recanalization of the infarcted artery may be expected in between 60 and 70 percent of patients. Among the remainder, urgent angioplasty as a "rescue" procedure has a great deal of efficiency.[19] A patent infarct vessel may be achieved in over 90 percent of patients with the combined approach of lysis and angioplasty. Some evidence suggests that the complications of urgent angioplasty are greater following thrombolysis than when angioplasty is performed without thrombolysis.[20] The mortality rate for patients with acute MI and mitral regurgitation or shock due to power failure is extremely high. Emergency angioplasty even beyond 24 h after onset of infarct symptoms has been shown to have benefit in these patients.[21] This group represents a difficult and challenging population of critically ill patients.

Revascularization therapy is sometimes attempted in the ventilator-dependent patient who has signs of high filling pressures, suggesting that this contributes significantly to

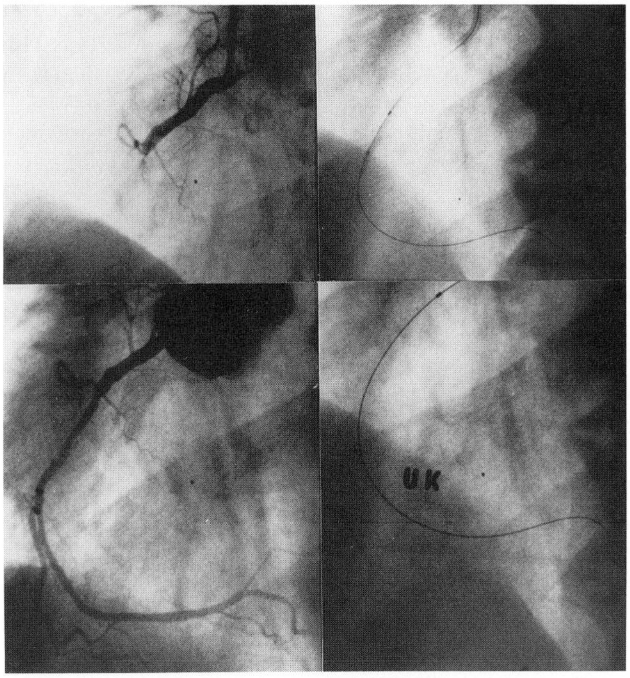

FIGURE 26-4 Coronary angioplasty for acute myocardial infarction. *Upper left.* **Stump of a totally occluded right coronary artery is seen.** *Upper right.* **An inflated balloon is seen across the stenosis.** *Lower right.* **Intracoronary urokinase is given to lyse residual thrombus.** *Lower left.* **Widely patent right coronary artery is seen with only irregularity at the site of the occlusion.**

the inability to wean from the ventilator.[22,23] It is important to realize that improvement in left ventricular function, when it is possible, occurs over a period of days or weeks following revascularization. Thus, the expectations for improvement in these patients must be tempered, and medical management for some number of days or weeks after the intervention should be accounted for.

Angioplasty has been of increasing benefit also in patients who have previously undergone CABG surgery.[24,25] Angioplasty is technically feasible in both saphenous vein bypass grafts and mammary artery grafts. Though the early success rate for angioplasty in saphenous vein grafts is high, the restenosis rate varies depending on the site within the graft. Aorto-ostial anastomotic lesions have an extremely high restenosis rate. Though they may be dilated with high initial success, the likelihood of restenosis within 6 months is high, and this must be considered when deciding on the goals of therapy. Midbody bypass graft lesions are also usually easy to dilate, but have a recurrence rate that approaches or possibly exceeds 50 percent. Distal anastomotic lesions have a restenosis rate similar to that of native coronary arteries and are most amenable to dilatation with long-term success. Mammary artery grafts may be dilated,[26] but are technically difficult due to their length and tortuosity. It is also imperative that the operator be experienced, because the ostium of the internal mammary artery is delicate and easy to dissect. The durability of results in internal mammary artery grafts is excellent, and the restenosis rate may be lower than that of native coronary arteries. Patients requiring angioplasty after coronary artery bypass may present early, after surgery with acute occlusion of one or more grafts, or very late, after operation with progression of both graft and native disease. The dilatation of native vessels in patients with some grafts open is feasible. These patients with severe multivessel disease may be revascularized adequately by careful selection of a few target lesions.

PTCA RISK ASSESSMENT

Among critically ill patients with other organ system dysfunction, case selection becomes exceedingly important. As a rule, patients who are poor candidates for CABG surgery are similarly poor candidates for angioplasty. The viability of a patient for surgical therapy in the event of immediate hemodynamic deterioration during an angioplasty procedure is a major consideration in assessing the patient risk. Risk may be divided into *lesion factors* and *patient factors*. Lesions likely to close acutely during the angioplasty procedure include those that are complicated by filling defects, reflecting thrombus in the vessel (Fig. 26-5), lesions that are long or extremely irregular or eccentric, stenoses on acute-angled bends in the artery, and subtotal stenoses.

The major patient factor associated with higher risk is significant left ventricular dysfunction. This includes patients who have, for example, an occluded right coronary artery and present for angioplasty of the left coronary artery, in whom a large area of myocardium would cease to contribute to pump function in the event of an acute vessel closure during the angioplasty procedure.

TABLE 26-5 Techniques for Supported Angioplasty

Mechanical
Intra-aortic balloon pump
Passive autoperfusion catheters
Roller pump perfusion catheters
Coronary sinus retroperfusion
Left atrial-aortic roller pump perfusion
Extracorporeal right atrium to aorta (femoral-femoral) bypass
Pharmacologic
Artificial hemoglobins
Fluosol
Intracoronary β-blockade

Renal insufficiency is another major consideration, since the contrast load given during an angioplasty procedure is often as much as 200 to 500 ml. Previous cardiac operation is also a significant factor. If these patients require emergency bypass surgery following a failed angioplasty attempt, dissection of previous adhesions is difficult and time consuming.

HIGH-RISK PTCA

Very high-risk patients may be supported using intra-aortic balloon counterpulsation[27–29] or percutaneous cardiopulmonary support.[30,31] A number of techniques are available for supported angioplasty (Table 26-5). These techniques are valuable when patients are very unstable, have severe left ventricular dysfunction, or a large territory of myocardium at risk. For example, a patient with prior anterior MI, left ventricular aneurysm, and aortic stenosis presented with new angina and left main coronary stenosis. Because of a left ventricular ejection fraction <20 percent and the risks of reoperation, he was deemed an inordinate risk for repeat bypass surgery. PTCA was performed with intra-aortic balloon pump support and a perfusion balloon catheter[32] (Fig. 26-6).

LASERS, MECHANICAL DEVICES, AND STENTS

New devices are being developed as alternatives and adjuncts to balloon angioplasty. Although all have great promise, significant technical problems exist as well. In addition, results to date have not been superior to conventional angioplasty with most of these devices. Among the more promising roles many of these technologies have are the salvage of abrupt vessel closure from balloon angioplasty and treatment of very diffuse CAD. Unfortunately, chronic total coronary occlusions have not yet given way to these new devices; restenosis has likewise been resistant to even mechanical stents and atherectomy shavers.

Catheter Balloon Valvuloplasty

Balloon dilation for intravascular obstruction has a relatively short history.[33] The technique was first used in 1962 by Rashkind for creating an atrial septal defect in patients

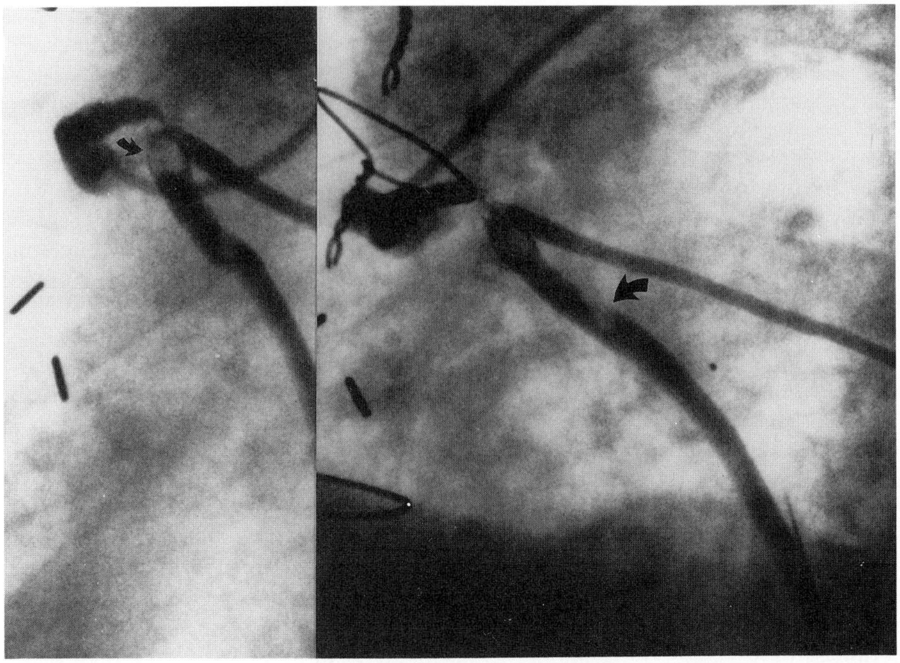

FIGURE 26-5 "Y" vein graft with a bifurcation stenosis. *Left.* Arrow points to a large filling defect that represents a thrombus in one limb of the graft. *Right.* An arrow pointing at a filling defect more distal in the vein graft demonstrates that the thrombus extends for some distance.

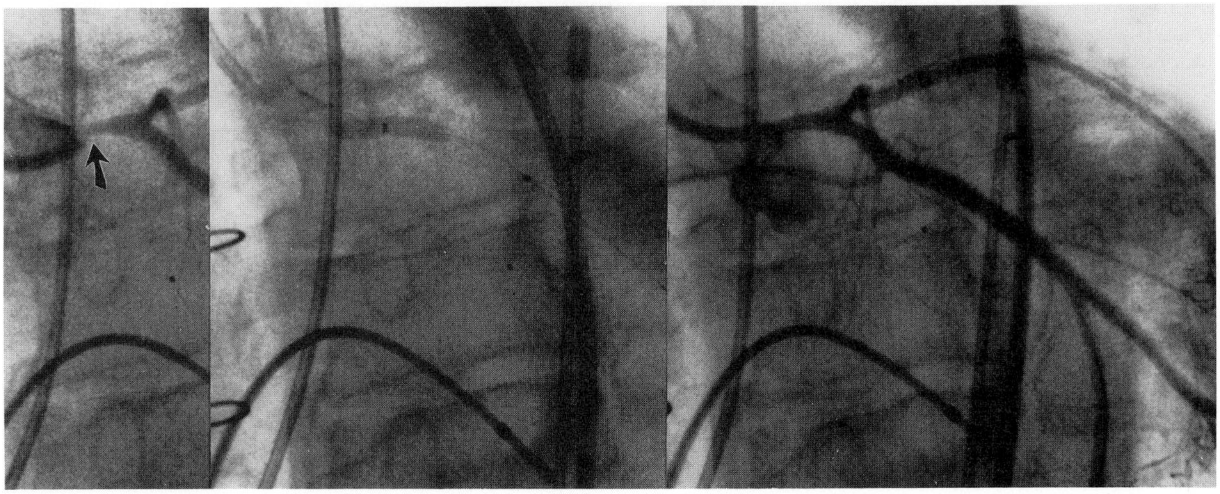

a *b* *c*

FIGURE 26-6 Coronary angioplasty of a left main coronary artery stenosis. *a.* Catheter is engaged in the left main coronary artery. The ostium is severely narrowed (arrow). *b.* Inflated balloon catheter is in the left main coronary artery. This is a perfusion balloon that allows flow of blood through the catheter shaft into the distal vessel. *c.* Widely patent left main coronary artery is seen. This patient had a negative 6-month follow-up stress test examination.

with transposition of the great arteries. Atrial septostomy was followed by application of balloon dilation for peripheral arterial stenoses and then for PTCA in 1978.[15] Balloon valvuloplasty was first reported by Kan in 1983 for use in children with pulmonic stenosis.[34] The technique was used initially in children, because the relatively pliable, noncalcified valves offered little concern regarding embolization and because pulmonic stenosis is a common congenital defect on the right side of the circulation. Thus, any deleterious hemodynamic consequences would not immediately and directly affect the left side of the circulation. The great success of this procedure led rapidly to its application to both children and adults with mitral and aortic valve stenosis.

AORTIC STENOSIS

Until recently, the only treatment available for significant aortic stenosis was valve replacement with a bioprosthetic or mechanical valve. The short-term results of these procedures are excellent for most patients, and the long-term durability of the prostheses has been established. Symptomatic patients with aortic stenosis usually have aortic valve area less than 1.0 cm^2. Prosthetic valves have an in vivo area of between 1.0 and 1.5 cm^2.[35] Though substantially less than the normal 2.5 to 4 cm^2 valve area, these valves provide adequate hemodynamics, and newer models such as the St. Jude's valve have better hemodynamics. Surgery for aortic valve stenosis has a number of limitations. The mortality rate for aortic valve replacement in patients over age eighty may be as high as 30 percent in the hospital and almost 50 percent by 6 months postoperatively.[36] Hospital mortality rates may range between 5 and 25 percent for patients with severe left ventricular dysfunction with ejection fraction under 30 percent and patients with other complicating illnesses such as severe lung disease or renal failure.

Balloon aortic valvuloplasty has emerged as an alternative to surgical therapy in these elderly or severely ill patients.[37,38] Balloon aortic valvuloplasty is performed during a regular catheterization procedure. The diagnosis of aortic valve stenosis is confirmed at the beginning of the procedure, and if Doppler echocardiographic assessment of the presence of aortic regurgitation has been inadequate or unclear, aortography is performed to ensure that aortic regurgitation is not the predominant hemodynamic lesion. After coronary arteriography, the transaortic valve gradient is measured and cardiac output is determined for calculation of the aortic valve area using the Gorlin formula for valve area. Using a long exchange wire, the diagnostic catheter is removed from the left ventricle, and a large caliber femoral arterial sheath is placed for passage of the balloon catheter. Although the first generation of aortic dilation devices required a No. 14 French femoral arterial sheath, newer balloons may be passed through a No. 12.5 French sheath. After the sheath is placed in the femoral artery, the balloon catheter is passed over the exchange wire retrograde across the aortic valve. Serial balloon inflations are performed (Fig. 26-7). The fully inflated balloon has a diameter ranging from 15 to 23 mm. The catheter shaft is No. 9 or 10 French. This large foreign body slides to and fro across the aortic valve as the ventricle attempts to eject it during each systole. Thus, the patient generally experiences a great deal of ventricular ectopy during balloon inflations (Fig. 26-8). Surprisingly, with balloon occlusion of the aortic outflow tract, there is usually some maintenance of aortic pressure. The irregular contour of the aortic orifice seems to be only partially obstructed by the round balloon. After a "waist" or indentation in the balloon is no longer seen with balloon inflation, the balloon is removed over an exchange wire, and a diagnostic catheter replaced in the ventricle for reassessment of the transaortic valve gradient[39] (Fig. 26-9). With an additional cardiac output determination, the valve area can be calculated, and if improved appreciably, the procedure is then terminated.

RESULTS OF AORTIC VALVULOPLASTY

The acute hemodynamic results of aortic valvuloplasty are often very dramatic. The mean predilation area seen in our own patient population is 0.6 cm^2 and following valvuloplasty increases to between 0.9 and 1.2 cm^2 with a mean of 1.1 cm^2.[40] Cardiac output usually increases slightly. Many patients have a dramatic fall in the pulmonary wedge pressure and left ventricular end-diastolic pressure. In the most dramatic examples, filling pressures may fall from the 30 to 40 range to the low 20s within a half hour after balloon dilation.[41] Unfortunately, in a substantial number of patients these results are not sustained. The restenosis rate of 1 year following balloon dilation is at least 50 percent and may be higher.[42] The mechanism of restenosis may be better understood if the mechanisms responsible for relief of stenosis in successful procedures are understood. The vast majority of elderly patients with aortic stenosis have calcific trileaflet aortic stenosis with calcification and thickening of the cusps and no commissural fusion. The calcium deposits are nodular when viewed grossly. Histologically, these nodules are densely encased in fibrous tissue, explaining in part the striking lack of embolization during this procedure. After balloon dilation, small fractures or cracks may be seen in the calcific nodules. This allows a great deal of leaflet mobility due to the presence of many small hinge points. The restenosis process involves regrowth of granulation tissue, fibrosis, and possibly true ossification of the fissures

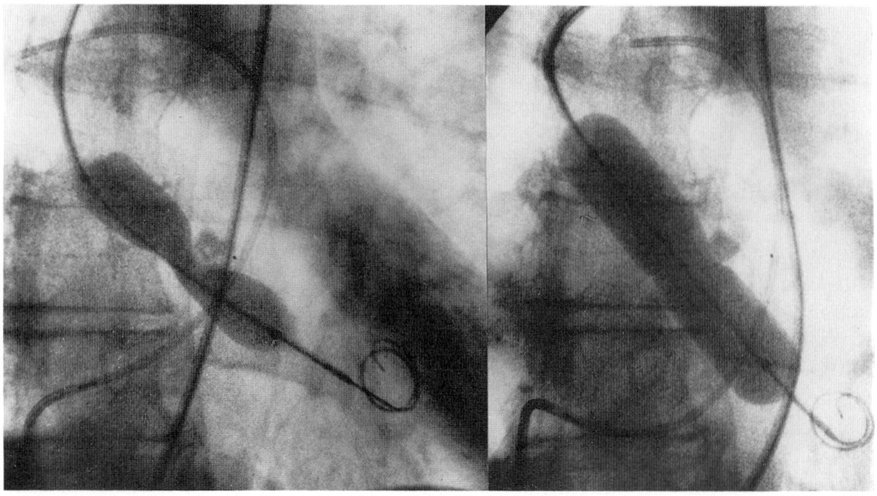

FIGURE 26-7 ***Left.*** **An aortic valvuloplasty balloon catheter is passed retrograde across the aortic valve. The stenotic valve indents the catheter. A large calcific density is seen in the indentation. A guidewire is curled in the left ventricular apex.** ***Right.*** **After full inflation of the balloon, the stenosis is substantially relieved.**

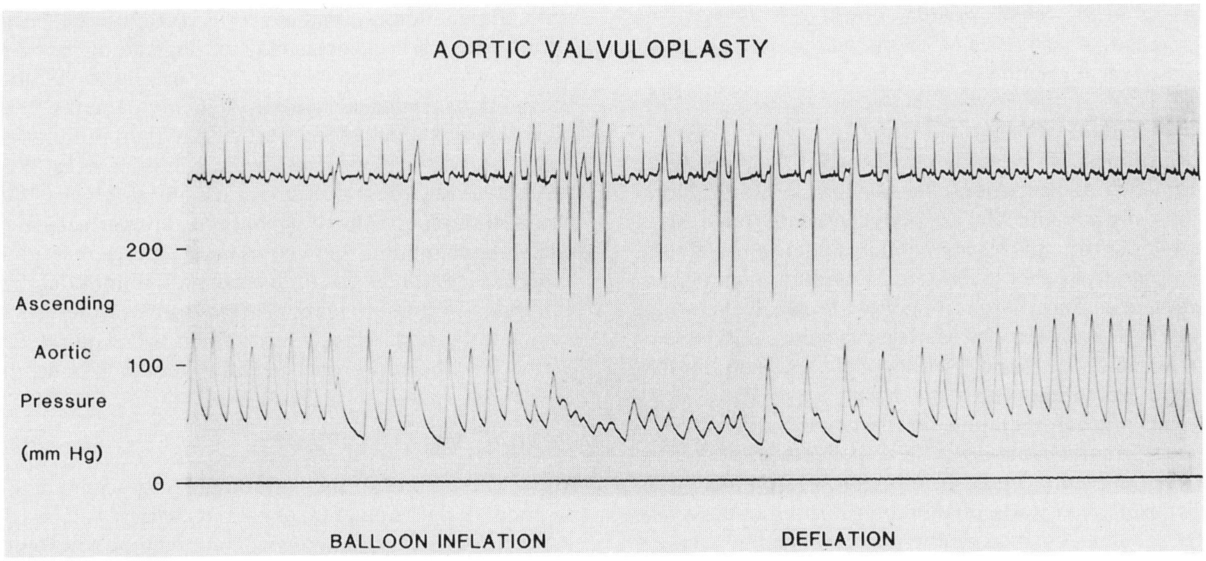

FIGURE 26-8 Aortic pressure and ECG during an aortic valvuloplasty balloon inflation. During balloon inflation marked hypotension and ventricular tachycardia are present. Normalization of the ECG and pressure recovery occur after balloon deflation.

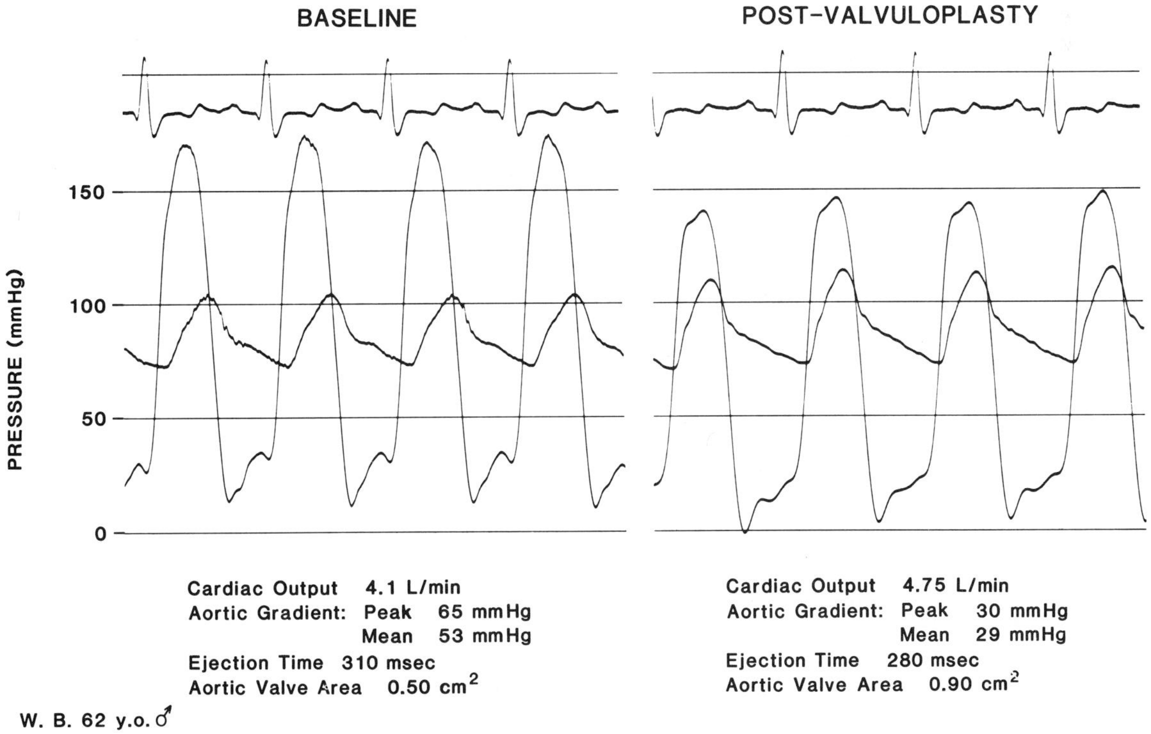

FIGURE 26-9 Simultaneous left ventricular and aortic pressure before and after balloon valvuloplasty. Base line recording shows a significant transaortic valve pressure gradient. Following valvuloplasty, the gradient is markedly reduced and the valve area is increased significantly.

and cracks in the calcific nodules on these leaflets.[42] This active process of restenosis follows a time course consistent with new scar formation.

PATIENT SELECTION

Since the long-term hemodynamic results of aortic valve replacement are so superior to those of balloon aortic valvuloplasty, only patients who are poor candidates for surgical therapy for aortic stenosis are good candidates for valvuloplasty. The ideal patients for aortic valvuloplasty are often identified in a critical care setting and are usually very old. Patients with end-stage left ventricular failure and pulmonary edema may be found after hospital admission, intubation, and stabilization to have aortic valve stenosis on screening echocardiographic examination. The physical diagnosis of aortic stenosis is these patients is, of course, often very difficult. The echocardiographic examination is usually prompted by auscultation of a murmur of uncertain origin. Occasionally, a screening echocardiogram discloses aortic stenosis as a previously unsuspected finding. Patients with severe left ventricular failure may be good candidates for initial valve dilation, followed by valve replacement surgery if some recovery of left ventricular performance occurs. In addition, patients with other serious illnesses and associated aortic stenosis in need of urgent noncardiac surgery are excellent candidates for valve dilation. For example, patients undergoing major thoracic or abdominal cancer surgery with associated aortic stenosis may be treated for the short-term with balloon valvuloplasty and, after further definition of their prognosis, may or may not undergo surgical valve replacement.

Relative contraindications for aortic valvuloplasty include significant aortic insufficiency, which may be made worse by valvuloplasty, or more importantly, not improved by relief of the associated aortic stenosis. Patients with significant bleeding diatheses are at high risk to need femoral arterial repair surgically following the dilation procedure. Percutaneous removal of No. 14 French sheaths has been accompanied by a 3 to 10 percent need for arterial repair even in patients with normal hemostasis. Severe CAD is not by itself a contraindication. Although certainly procedure risk is increased for these patients, the majority will tolerate valvuloplasty. Patients with left main or severe three-vessel CAD and symptomatic or severe aortic stenosis probably do not have any improvement in prognosis with valvuloplasty; thus, the procedure should be reserved for palliation of symptoms in that setting. Simultaneous PTCA and balloon valvuloplasty may be performed successfully.

COMPLICATIONS

The procedure mortality for balloon aortic valvuloplasty is usually reported in the 1 percent range. Embolization from the catheters or guidewires may result in transient ischemic attack or stroke in between 1 and 3 percent of patients. Between 5 and 15 percent of patients may require transfusion due to femoral arterial bleeding during and after the procedure. The aortic valve annulus is adjacent to the His bundle and atrioventricular node in the intraventricular septum. With the dilation, a calcified, rigid aortic valve in patients with calcific aortic stenosis may impinge on the conducting system and result in complete heart block. Temporary transvenous pacemakers are used in any patient with complete bundle branch block, particularly right bundle branch block, or bifascicular block. When complete heart block is precipitated by the procedure, it usually resolves within 24 hours, though occasional patients require permanent pacemaker implantation. Between 1 and 3 percent of patients experience catheter or guidewire perforations of the left ventricle. Though as many as two-thirds of these may be managed by pericardiocentesis, some will require surgical drainage of the pericardial space and repair of the ventricle.

MITRAL VALVULOPLASTY

Mitral valvuloplasty has proven to be efficacious in a large segment of the population of patients with rheumatic mitral valve disease. Percutaneous balloon commissurotomy has excellent results in patients who previously would have been considered good candidates for surgical mitral commissurotomy. In addition, patients for whom surgical therapy is not an option because of extremes of age or associated illnesses now have an option for mechanical therapy. Those patients with moderate valvular deformity who in the past would have received mitral valve replacement will often respond favorably to mitral valvuloplasty and have the potential now for deferring the need for a valve prosthesis and the associated lifetime anticoagulation therapy for a few years.

Most patients with symptomatic mitral stenosis have a mitral valve area between 0.5 and 1.5 cm^2. It is unusual for patients to have symptoms at rest until the valve area falls below 1.2 cm^2. The normal mitral valve area is 3.5 to 6.0 cm^2. Both mechanical and bioprosthetic mitral valves have areas in vivo that range between 1.5 and 2.5 cm^2.[35] As is the case with aortic valvuloplasty, very small increases in valve area result in marked clinical improvement in these patients. Thus, a patient with severe end-stage mitral stenosis and a valve area of 0.5 cm^2 may have a dramatic hemodynamic and symptomatic improvement if the valve area is increased to 0.9 or 1.0 cm^2.

Percutaneous Balloon Commissurotomy Procedure

Mitral valvuloplasty represents one of the most complex catheterization procedures performed today. After diagnostic catheterization and pressure measurement, which are usually performed prior to the valvuloplasty procedure, complete right and left heart catheterization is performed. In addition to placement of a left femoral arterial pigtail catheter, a Swan-Ganz catheter is placed in either the left femoral vein, a brachial vein, or a jugular vein. The right femoral vein is cannulated with a standard diagnostic catheter which is then exchanged for a transseptal catheter and needle. Transseptal puncture represents a necessary first step in the mitral valvuloplasty procedure.

Antegrade access to the mitral valve from the left atrium cannot be gained without first traversing the interatrial septum from the right atrium to the left atrium. To accomplish this, a transseptal needle inside a transseptal sheath is placed in the superior vena cava and withdrawn slowly under fluoroscopic guidance.[43] The tip of the sheath is felt to course over the bulge of the aortic root above the right atrium and then engage in the limbus of the fossa ovalis. The tip of the 21 gauge needle is directed posteriorly and then advanced into the left atrium through the interatrial septum (Fig. 26-10). Before advancing the No. 8 French sheath over the needle, arterial blood is aspirated from the left atrium, and if any question about the position of the needle exists, contrast is injected. Biplane fluoroscopy is very important to confirm the position of the transseptal catheter. When the left atrial position is clearly established, No. 8 French sheath is advanced over the transseptal needle as the needle is withdrawn. The left femoral arterial pigtail catheter can then be advanced retrograde across the aortic valve to measure the left ventricular pressure and simultaneous left atrial pressure for determination of the transmitral pressure gradient. In conjunction with the cardiac output, the Gorlin formula can be used to determine the mitral valve area prior to dilation.

Since transseptal puncture may be complicated by passage of the transseptal needle into the aorta or the pericardial space, heparin is not given until the transseptal portion of the procedure is completed successfully. We then administer 100 U/kg to ensure adequate anticoagulation for the long catheter and wire times necessary for this procedure.

Conventional Mitral Valvuloplasty

A balloon flotation catheter is passed through the left atrial transseptal sheath.[44] The balloon is inflated in the left atrium and floated across the mitral valve into the left ventricle and then out through the left ventricular outflow tract into the aortic root. A long exchange wire is passed through the balloon catheter into the aorta and around the aortic arch into the iliac artery (Fig. 26-11). The transseptal sheath and balloon catheter are removed, and a double-lumen catheter is passed over the wire into the aortic root. A second wire is then threaded through the inferior vena cava, right atrium, across the interatrial septum, through the left atrium and left ventricle, and into the descending aorta. This leaves two long exchange wires traversing the entire venous and arterial circulations. An 8- or 10-mm diameter peripheral arterial balloon is passed along one of the guidewires into the interatrial septum and inflated to dilate the septum (Fig. 26-11). This is necessary to allow passage of the very bulky dilation balloons. This smaller balloon is removed and an 18- or 20-mm diameter balloon is then advanced over the interatrial septum into the mitral valve and inflated one or two times. A second balloon is then advanced into the mitral valve and the two balloons inflated simultaneously until the "waist" or indentation in the balloon disappears (Fig. 26-11). The balloons severely impede flow across the mitral valve, with resultant hypotension. Some patients experience syncope at this point. There is often a great deal of ventricular ectopy. Left ventricular systole may eject the balloons; stability of the balloons is one of the difficulties in performing the procedure. In addition, careful attention must be paid to the proximal position of the balloons. If they are too close to the interatrial septum,

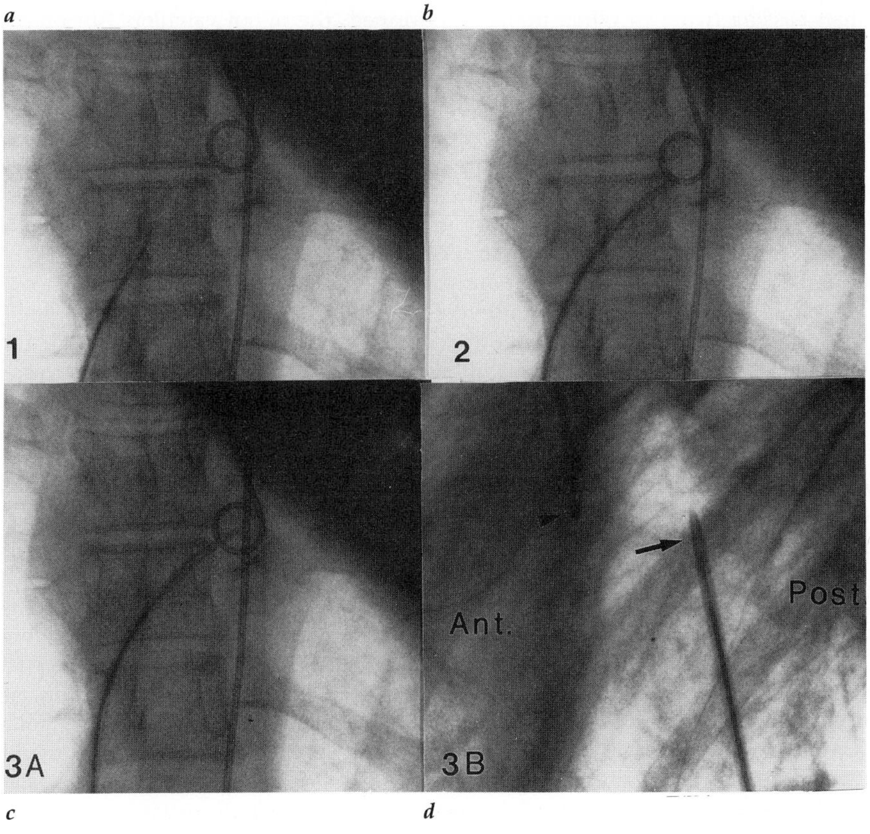

FIGURE 26-10 ***a.*** **The transseptal needle is below a pigtail catheter sitting on the aortic valve. In the anteroposterior projection as the needle is advanced *(b)* it appears as though it is about to puncture the aorta *(c)*. *d.* Simultaneous lateral view. The transseptal needle (arrow) can be seen pointing posteriorly toward the spine, a few centimeters away from the pigtail catheter sitting on the aortic valve (arrowhead).**

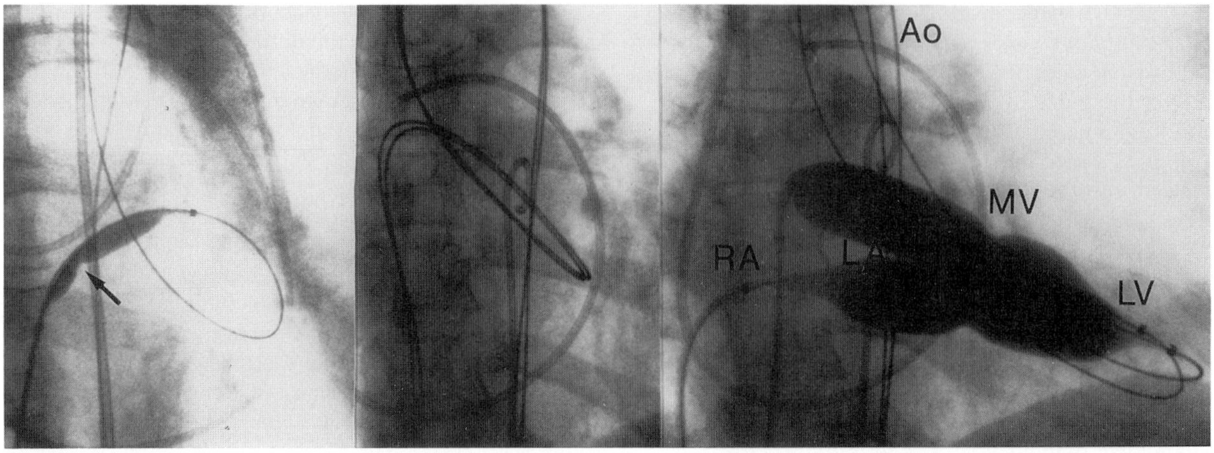

FIGURE 26-11 *Left.* **An 8-mm balloon is inflated in the interatrial septum. The arrow points at the indentation caused by the septum on the balloon.** *Center.* **Two guidewires are looped through the circulation.** *Right.* **Two 20-mm diameter balloons are inflated in the mitral valve. The balloons can be seen to span the valve from the left atrium, with their tips in the left ventricular apex. The double guidewires can be seen coiled from the right atrium (RA), through the left atrium (LA) and left ventricle (LV), and into the aorta (Ao).**

they will produce a large atrial septal defect. In addition, the distal tips of the balloons are long and relatively stiff and may perforate the ventricular apex.

An alternative method involves placing a catheter across the interatrial septum, the mitral valve, and into the left ventricular apex. Two wires can then be placed directly in the left ventricular apex and the transseptal sheath withdrawn. Double balloons are then passed over these wires. Though this procedure is much simpler than passing two wires through the left ventricle and into the aorta, there is less balloon stability when the guidewires are simply placed in the ventricular apex, and the procedure cannot be performed in this manner in some patients.

Inoue Mitral Commissurotomy

An alternative to conventional single or double balloon valvuloplasty has been developed recently.[45,46] The Inoue balloon device is entirely unique. After transseptal puncture a spring guidewire is introduced into the left atrium (Fig. 26-12). The Inoue balloon is advanced into the atrium where its distal portion is inflated with CO_2. The balloon is floated directly across the mitral valve into the left ventricle. The CO_2 is then purged, and a saline contrast mixture is used to inflate the balloon. The distal third inflates, and this is withdrawn until it engages the valve. Further inflation results in the proximal portion of the balloon inflating, leaving a "dog bone" appearance that firmly engages the mitral valve. Further expansion results in opening of the middle portion of the balloon with dilation of the valve. This firm engagement of the valve allows for use of a much shorter balloon with virtually no concern for dilation of the atrial septum or left ventricular apical puncture. Crossing from the left atrium into the left ventricle is made much simpler by this balloon flotation mechanism. The balloon is latex rather than polyethylene or polyvinyl chloride and thus, is very elastic. This allows the balloon to be stretched or "slenderized" for more easy passage across the interatrial septum, with less chance of resultant atrial septal defect. Furthermore, the same balloon can be inflated to a variety of diameters which makes for a much more controlled dilation that is individualized to the patient's anatomy.

RESULTS OF PERCUTANEOUS MITRAL COMMISSUROTOMY

When initially performed, the mitral valvuloplasty procedure was done with a single balloon, usually 25 mm in diameter. The resultant valve areas ranged between 1.0 and 1.5 cm^2 after dilation. In an effort to improve the results, the double balloon technique was used. This resulted in postdilation areas of between 1.8 and 2.2 cm^2. Single balloon dilation with the Inoue balloon yields results between 1.5 and 1.9 cm^2 in most patients. This is accomplished with fewer balloon inflations and a shorter procedure time, points that are particularly important when managing patients with severe end-stage disease. The patient in pulmonary edema who cannot lie flat will not tolerate the longer double balloon procedure. In addition, many elderly patients are not able to tolerate a conventional double balloon procedure and do very well with the significantly shorter Inoue balloon procedure.

PATIENT SELECTION

Patients with symptomatic mitral stenosis and pliable mitral valve leaflets with little evidence on echocardiography for leaflet thickening or rigidity or for subvalvular thickening or calcification are ideal candidates for percutaneous mitral commissurotomy (Fig. 26-13). These patients have excellent early hemodynamic results and, in addition, at follow-up studies between 6 and 12 months show no significant incidence of restenosis.[47,48] It is likely that they will have long-term results similar to those seen for surgical mitral valve commissurotomy. Elderly patients with end-

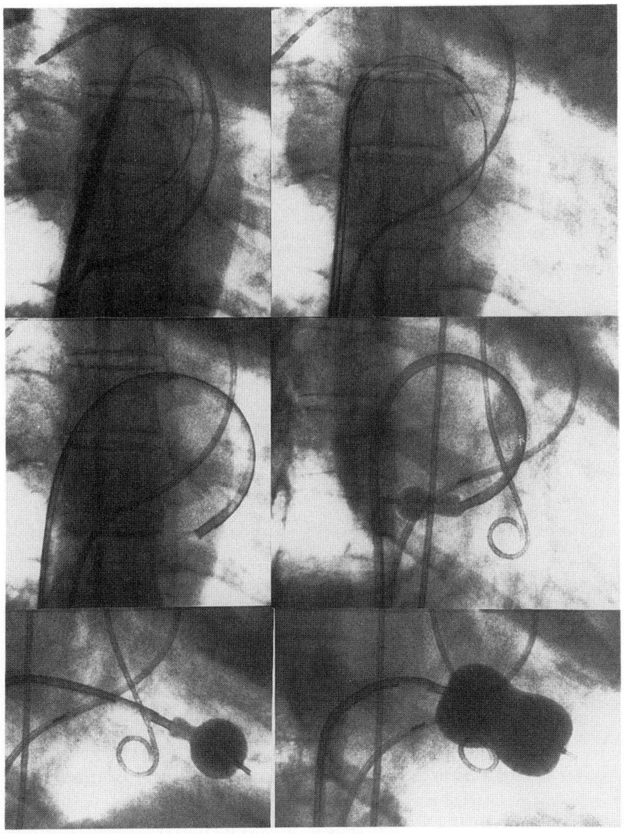

FIGURE 26-12 Balloon dilation using the Inoue rubber-nylon mesh single balloon technique. ***Upper left.*** **A No. 14 French dilator traverses the interatrial septum over a 0.025-in. spring guidewire.** ***Upper right.*** **A balloon tracks around the wire in the left atrium.** ***Center left.*** **The balloon catheter lies over the mitral valve.** ***Center right.*** **The tip of the balloon is inflated.** ***Lower left.*** **The inflated tip of the balloon is across the mitral valve. At that point, the balloon is withdrawn until it abuts on the mitral leaflets.** ***Lower right.*** **The fully inflated balloon is seen with some residual indentation from the valve commissures.**

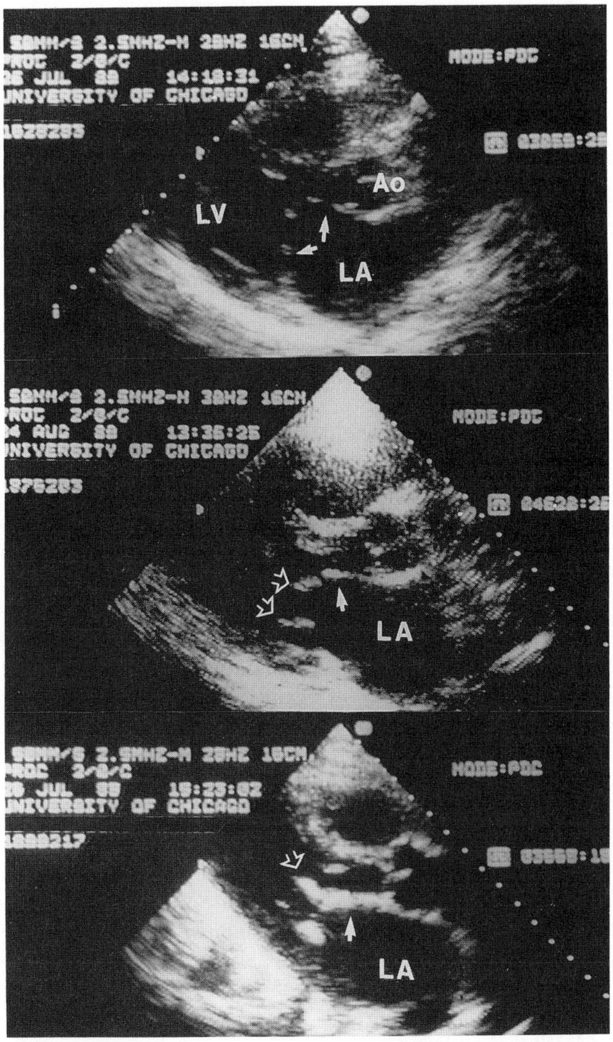

FIGURE 26-13 Two-dimensional echocardiographic long axis parasternal views of patients with mitral stenosis. ***Top.*** **Arrows point to the thin, domed, pliable mitral leaflets seen in patients who are excellent candidates for balloon commissurotomy.** ***Center.*** **The solid arrow points to a thickened valve leaflet and the open arrows point to thickened and probably calcified subvalvular apparatus. This is a moderately deformed valve and has somewhat higher risk for restenosis.** ***Bottom.*** **From patient aged eighty-seven. The solid arrow points to a dramatically thickened anterior mitral valve leaflet and the open arrow points to a densely calcified, ridged, and thickened subvalvular apparatus. This patient is far from an ideal candidate for valve dilation, but because of high surgical risk underwent balloon dilation with excellent clinical results.**

stage mitral stenosis and severely deformed valves are also patients for whom valvuloplasty is an excellent alternative (Table 26-6). In the past, many of these patients were considered not to be candidates for surgical valve replacement and subsequent long-term anticoagulation. Though the risks of valvuloplasty are increased in these patients, very good early hemodynamic results may be achieved. In our own experience, the oldest patient treated to date has been eighty-seven. Patients with moderate valvular thickening and deformity are traditionally considered candidates for mitral valve replacement with a prosthesis. These patients have a variable response to percutaneous commissurotomy. The vast majority have an excellent initial hemodynamic result. The restenosis rate in these patients may be increased, and it remains to be seen in our relatively early experience with valvuloplasty for what proportion of these it will be a useful therapy.

CONTRAINDICATIONS

Mitral regurgitation of more than moderate degree (2+ of 4) is the most important relative contraindication to catheter valvuloplasty. If mitral regurgitation rather than mitral stenosis is the predominant lesion, balloon dilation is unlikely to result in any benefit. In addition, it can certainly make the mitral regurgitation worse. Patients with contraindica-

TABLE 26-6 Percutaneous Mitral Commissurotomy

PATIENT SELECTION	
Inclusions	Exclusions
• Valve area <1.5 cm^2 • Mitral regurgitation $\leq 2+/4$ • Symptomatic	• MR $> 2+/4$ • Endocarditis • Left atrial thrombus • Severe subvalvular fibrosis[a] • Severe mitral calcification[a]

[a]May include if nonsurgical candidate.

tions to transseptal puncture must have mitral valvuloplasty deferred. These include severe thoracic spinal deformity that makes the landmarks necessary for safe transseptal puncture very obscure and left atrial thrombus. When possible, a patient should have Coumadin anticoagulation for 4 to 6 weeks prior to mitral valvuloplasty. This is especially true for patients with chronic atrial fibrillation. In addition, a two-dimensional echocardiogram, ideally a transesophageal study, is obtained prior to the valvuloplasty to exclude echocardiographically demonstrable thrombus in the left atrium. Coumadin is discontinued for 4 or 5 days prior to the valvuloplasty procedure. If the PT approaches normal more than 24 h prior to the procedure, heparin anticoagulation may be instituted and then discontinued 6 h prior to the procedure. Maintaining nearly continuous anticoagulation is especially important in patients with a history of thromboembolic complications from their mitral stenosis. Patients with significant bleeding diatheses are at high risk for transseptal puncture. Patients with normal coagulation parameters will tolerate a 21 gauge needle puncture of the aorta or right atrial free wall with relatively few complications.

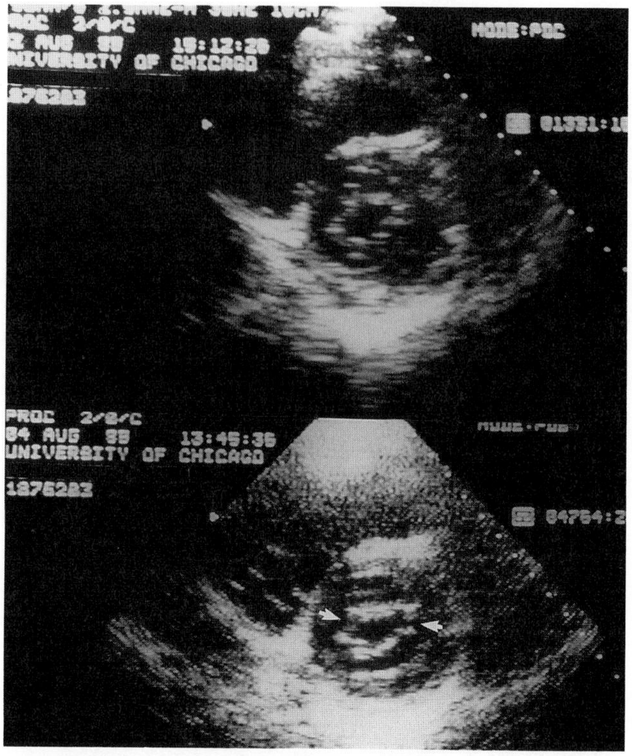

FIGURE 26-14 Short axis two-dimensional echocardiographic view of the mitral valve. *Top.* The fish mouth mitral valve orifice is noted in the center of the left ventricular cavity. The lateral and medial commissures are completely fused. *Bottom.* Following balloon valvuloplasty splitting of the commissures is shown by the solid white arrows. Commissural splitting is the mechanism of balloon mitral valvotomy.

COMPLICATIONS

Complications of the transseptal puncture represent a large proportion of the complications of mitral valvuloplasty. In addition, with conventional valvuloplasty the guidewires or balloon tips may perforate the left ventricular apex. Mitral regurgitation may be caused or increased by the valvuloplasty procedure. In the vast majority of patients there is no or only a slight increase in mitral regurgitation. Oversizing balloons must be avoided. In addition, with the Inoue balloon it is important to examine the patient with Doppler echocardiography for changes in mitral regurgitation after each balloon inflation, before proceeding to a larger inflated balloon diameter. Transient ischemic attack or stroke may result from dislodgement of thrombus in the left atrium or from embolization of clot fragments from catheters or wires. This occurs in 1 or 2 percent of patients undergoing mitral valvuloplasty. Remarkably, even though two No. 14 French profile balloons may be passed in the right femoral vein, bleeding following compression of this site after the procedure is rare.

MECHANISM OF MITRAL VALVULOPLASTY

Virtually all patients with mitral stenosis have rheumatic valvular disease. The leaflet edges are thickened and the commissures are fused. Balloon inflation results in splitting of the fused commissures (Fig. 26-14). Thus, balloon dilation results in a true commissurotomy. This is in contrast to aortic valvuloplasty in senile calcific aortic stenosis. Here no commissural fusion is present and balloon dilation results in fracture of the calcific nodules responsible for leaflet immobility.

References

1. Block PC, Ockene I, Goldberg RJ et al: A prospective randomized trial of outpatient versus inpatient cardiac catheterization. N Engl J Med 319:1251, 1988.
2. King SB III, Douglas JS Jr: *Coronary Arteriography and Angioplasty.* New York. McGraw-Hill, 1985.
3. Folland ED, Oprian C, Giacomini J et al and the participants in the VA Cooperative Study on Valvular Heart Disease: Complications of cardiac catheterization and angiography in patients with valvular heart disease. Cathet Cardiovasc Diagn 17:15, 1989.
4. Johnson LW, Lozner EC, Johnson S et al and the Registry Committee of the Society for Cardiac Angiography and Interventions: Coronary arteriography 1984–1987: A report of the registry of the society for cardiac angiography and interventions. I.

Results and Complications. Cathet Cardiovasc Diagn 17:5, 1989.
5. Lozner EC, Johnson LW, Johnson S et al and the Registry Committee of the Society for Cardiac Angiography and Interventions: Coronary Arteriography 1984–1987: A report of the registry of the society for cardiac angiography and interventions. II. An analysis of 218 deaths related to coronary arteriography. Cathet Cardiovasc Diagn 17:11, 1989.
6. Judkins MP: Selective coronary arteriography: A percutaneous transfemoral technic. Radiology 89:815, 1967.
7. Sones FM Jr: Cine coronary arteriography, in Abstracts of the 32nd Scientific Session of the American Heart Association. Circulation 20:773, 1959.
8. Carroll JD, Lang RM, Neumann A et al: Differential effects of positive inotropic and vasodilator therapy on diastolic properties in dilated cardiomyopathy. Circulation 74:815, 1986.
9. Rajfer SI, Carroll JD, Lang RM et al: Effects of dopamine on left ventricular afterload and contractile state: Relationship to the activation of beta-1 adrenoceptors and dopamine receptors. J Am Coll Cardiol 12:498, 1988.
10. Greenberger PA, Patterson R, Radin RC: Two pretreatment regimens for high-risk patients receiving radiographic contrast media. J Allergy Clin Immunol 74:540, 1984.
11. Greenberger PA, Patterson R: Adverse reactions to radiocontrast media. Review. Prog Cardiovasc Dis 31:239, 1988.
12. Schwab SJ, Hlatky MA, Pieper KS et al: Contrast nephrotoxicity: A randomized controlled trial of a nonionic and an ionic radiographic contrast agent. N Engl J Med 320:149, 1989.
13. Feinstein SB, Lang RM, Dick C et al: Contrast echocardiographic perfusion studies in humans. Am J Cardiac Imaging 1:29, 1986.
14. Lang RM, Feinstein SB, Feldman T et al: Contrast echocardiography for evaluation of myocardial perfusion: Effects of coronary angioplasty. J Am Coll Cardiol 8:232, 1986.
15. Gruentzig AR: Transluminal dilatation of coronary-artery stenoses. Letter to the Editor. Lancet 1:263, 1978.
16. Detre K, Holubkov R, Kelsey S et al: Percutaneous transluminal coronary angioplasty in 1985–1986 and 1977–1981. The National Heart, Lung and Blood Institute Registry. N Engl J Med 318:265, 1988.
17. Rothbaum DA, Linnemeier TJ, Landin RJ et al: Emergency percutaneous transluminal coronary angioplasty in acute myocardial infarction: A 3 year experience. J Am Coll Cardiol 10:264, 1987.
18. O'Keefe JH Jr, Rutherford BD, McConahay DR et al: Early and late results of coronary angioplasty without antecedent thrombolytic therapy for acute myocardial infarction. Am J Cardiol 64:1221, 1989.
19. Topol W: Coronary angioplasty for acute myocardial infarction. Review. Ann Intern Med 109:970, 1988.
20. Topol EJ, Califf RM, George BS et al: A randomized trial of immediate versus delayed elective angioplasty after intravenous tissue plasminogen activator in acute myocardial infarction. N Engl J Med 317:581, 1987.
21. Lee L, Bates ER, Pitt B et al: Percutaneous transluminal coronary angioplasty improves survival in acute myocardial infarction complicated by cardiogenic shock. Circulation 78:1345, 1988.
22. Carroll JD, Hess OM, Hirzel HO et al: Left ventricular systolic and diastolic function in coronary artery disease: Effects of revascularization on exercise-induced ischemia. Circulation 72:119, 1985.
23. Carroll JD, Hess OM, Hirzel HO et al: Effects of ischemia, bypass surgery and post infarction on myocardial contraction, relaxation and compliance during exercise. Am J Cardiol 63: 65E, 1989.
24. Ernst SM, Van der Feltz TA, Ascoop CA et al: Percutaneous transluminal coronary angioplasty in patients with prior coronary artery bypass grafting. Long-term results. J Thorac Cardiovasc Surg 93:268, 1987.
25. Corbelli J, Franco I, Hollman J et al: Percutaneous transluminal coronary angioplasty after previous coronary artery bypass surgery. Am J Cardiol 56:398, 1985.
26. Pinkerton CA, Slack JD, Orr CM et al: Percutaneous transluminal angioplasty involving internal mammary artery bypass grafts: A femoral approach. Cathet Cardiovasc Diagn 13:414, 1987.
27. Bolooki H: Current status of circulatory support with an intraaortic balloon pump. Cardiol Clin 3:123, 1985.
28. Weber KT, Janicki JS: Intraaortic balloon counterpulsation. A review of physiological principles, clinical results and device safety. Ann Thorac Surg 17:602, 1974.
29. Whitman G: Intra-aortic balloon pumping and cardiac mechanics: A programmed lesson. Heart Lung 7:1034, 1978.
30. Shawl FA: Percutaneous cardiopulmonary bypass support in high risk interventions. Review. J Invasive Cardiol 1:287, 1989.
31. Tommaso CL: Management of high-risk coronary angioplasty. Review. Am J Cardiol 64:33E, 1989.
32. Quigley PJ, Hinohara T, Phillips HR et al: Myocardial protection during coronary angioplasty with an autoperfusion balloon catheter in humans. Circulation 78:1128, 1988.
33. Lock JE, Keane JF, Fellows KE: The use of catheter intervention procedures for congenital heart disease. J Am Coll Cardiol 7:1420, 1986.
34. Kan JS, White RI, Mitchell SE et al: Percutaneous balloon valvuloplasty; a new method for treating congenital pulmonary valve stenosis. N Engl J Med 307:540, 1982.
35. Khuri SF, Folland ED, Sethi GK et al, and the participants in the VA Cooperative Study on Valvular Heart Disease: Six month postoperative hemodynamics of the Hancock heterograft and the Bjork-Shiley prosthesis: Results of a Veterans Administration cooperative prospective randomized trial. J Am Coll Cardiol 12:8, 1988.
36. Edmunds LH Jr, Stephenson LW, Edie RN et al: Open-heart surgery in octogenarians. N Engl J Med 319:131, 1988.
37. Letac B, Cribier A, Koning R et al: Results of percutaneous transluminal valvuloplasty in 218 adults with valvular aortic stenosis. Am J Cardiol 62:598, 1988.
38. Safian RD, Berman AD, Diver DJ et al: Balloon aortic valvuloplasty in 170 consecutive patients. N Engl J Med 319:125, 1988.
39. Feldman T, Carroll JD, Chiu YC: An improved catheter design for crossing stenosed aortic valves. Cathet Cardiovasc Diagn 16:279, 1989.
40. Feldman T, Chiu C, Carroll JD: Single balloon aortic valvuloplasty: Increase valve areas with improved technique. J Invasive Cardiol 1:295, 1989.
41. Ford LE, Feldman T, Chiu YC et al: Hemodynamic resistance as a measure of functional impairment in aortic valvular stenosis. Circulation Res 66:1, 1990.
42. Feldman T, Glagov S, Chiu YC et al: Second dilatation for restenosis following successful balloon aortic valvuloplasty: Results, pathology and mechanism. Abstract. J Am Coll Cardiol 13:17A, 1989.
43. Ross J Jr: Considerations regarding the technique for transseptal left heart catheterization. Circulation 34:391, 1966.
44. Feldman T, Brill DM, Chua KG et al: Balloon dilatation for mitral stenosis. Ill Med J 173:315, 1988.
45. Nobuyoshi M, Hamasaki N, Kimura T et al: Indications, com-

plications, and short-term clinical outcome of percutaneous transvenous mitral commissurotomy. Circulation 80:782, 1989.

46. Feldman T, Carroll JD, Chisholm RJ et al: Effect of valve deformity on results and mitral regurgitation after Inoue balloon commissurotomy. Circulation 82(III):546, 1990.
47. Palacios IF, Block PC, Wilkins GT et al: Follow-up of patients undergoing percutaneous mitral balloon valvotomy. Analysis of factors determining restenosis. Circulation 79:573, 1989.
48. Wilkins GT, Weyman AE, Abascal VM et al: Percutaneous balloon dilatation of the mitral valve: An analysis of echocardiographic variables related to outcome and the mechanism of dilatation. Br Heart J 60:299, 1988.

Chapter 27

PERICARDIAL WINDOW AND PERICARDIOCENTESIS

LARRY M. GENTILELLO
ALEX G. LITTLE

The number of patients with pericardial effusive disease is increasing due to such factors as the prolonged survival of patients with chronic renal failure or disseminated malignancy and the widespread availability of cardiac surgery. In addition, victims of penetrating mediastinal injuries may present with possible cardiac injury. The diagnosis of these pericardial disorders or associated effusions is challenging, and various diagnostic and therapeutic strategies exist.

In the clinical setting, when elevated central venous pressure is associated with hypotension, pericardial effusion with tamponade must be considered among the possible causes, which also include tension pneumothorax, pulmonary embolism, and right ventricular failure. Pulsus paradoxus (a systolic blood pressure difference >10 torr between expiration and inspiration) is almost always present in patients with tamponade, and its absence may help differentiate tamponade from other conditions. While pulsus paradoxus is highly sensitive, it is not very specific and may occur with airflow obstruction, obesity, ascites, pulmonary embolism, and cardiomyopathy. The amount of pulsus parodoxus does not correlate with the degree of tamponade since the actual value depends on the systolic blood pressure and pulse pressure. In patients who are hypotensive and who have a narrow pulse pressure, severe tamponade may be present with minimal paradoxus. Occasionally, patients with tamponade will not have pulsus paradoxus as defined above.

When the diagnosis or etiology of tamponade/effusion is uncertain or when the diagnosis is established and therapeutic decisions must be made, two realistic diagnostic and therapeutic interventional alternatives exist—pericardiocentesis and pericardial window. These are the subjects of this chapter.

Patient Management

MALIGNANCY

Mesothelioma is the most common primary pericardial malignancy; however, pericardial involvement by metastases is a far more common cause of pericardial effusions which occur in as many as 11 percent of patients with disseminated malignancies, most commonly lung or breast cancer, leukemia, or lymphoma.[1,2] Symptoms develop in 29 percent of patients, and 16 percent develop tamponade. The clinical importance of these effusions is considerable since they are either an immediate or contributory cause of death in 86 percent of patients who become symptomatic. Symptoms and signs can be dramatic (including hemodynamic collapse and shock) or subtle. It has been demonstrated, for example, that tamponade can increase interstitial lung water to an extent sufficient to decrease lung compliance significantly.[3] This could increase the work of breathing enough to produce dyspnea. Therefore, strict definition of the indications for therapeutic intervention is difficult. Certainly all patients in whom a hemodynamically or echocardiographically significant effusion is present should be treated if a reasonable, in terms of both quantity and quality, life expectancy can be predicted by controlling the effusion.

It is important to realize, however, that it has recently been demonstrated that nearly half of all pericardial effusions arising in cancer patients are not malignant.[4] These nonmalignant effusions in cancer patients are probably related to prior radiation or chemotherapy. A few are caused by infection induced by immunosuppression, and others are sympathetic in nature. Patients with a reasonable prognosis, assuming relief of tamponade, should therefore not be denied palliative relief of chest pain, dyspnea, and obstructive symptoms on the supposition that the effusion is a preterminal event signifying pericardial metastases. Not all effusions in a patient with a malignancy are "malignant effusions." In addition, approximately 40 percent of cancer patients with pericardial effusions will have a secondary cause for their elevated central venous pressure, such as constrictive disease, heart failure, or vena cava obstruction. Incomplete resolution of symptoms after treatment should lead to a search for one of these causes. Effusive constrictive pericarditis occurs when effusion and constriction are present simultaneously. Most patients present with dominant tamponade physiology. A constrictive component is suggested when elevated venous pressure without paradoxus occurs after drainage of the effusion.

Techniques available for treating malignant pericardial effusions include antineoplastic therapy, pericardiocentesis with or without injection of sclerosing agents, subxiphoid pericardial window, and pericardiectomy.

Radiation therapy can be effective in treating effusions secondary to leukemia or lymphoma through its effect on the malignancy. It is ineffective in treating epithelial tumors such as bronchogenic carcinoma, however, and may itself induce constrictive pericarditis. These factors limit the usefulness of radiation. In addition, due to the inability to be certain of the malignant status of pericardial effusions in cancer patients, the diagnosis must be confirmed prior to instituting radiation or other forms of cancer therapy.

Pericardiocentesis is often unsuccessful or ineffective and may not prevent recurrent effusions. Furthermore, 10 percent of all cases are complicated by pain, fever, and arrhythmias.[5] Although the reported success rate ranges from 81 to 91 percent, most patients require repeated instillation of sclerosing agents and, therefore, a relatively lengthy hospitalization. Accordingly, a pericardial catheter should be left in place to avoid the risks associated with repeated pericardial puncture.

A subxiphoid pericardial window provides both definitive diagnosis and treatment for malignant effusions with low morbidity and mortality.[4,6] It provides both diagnosis and effective treatment for patients with malignant effusions of all causes with little likelihood of recurrence. Further, it avoids side effects such as systemic toxicity, arrhythmia, and pain associated with pericardial instillation of chemotherapeutic agents.

Pericardiectomy is rarely appropriate in the absence of constriction. When the management of patients undergoing subxiphoid pericardial window includes an emphasis on postoperative drainage of the pericardial space (as discussed in the section on technique), results are as good as for pericardiectomy.[7] Therefore, exposing the patient to the increased morbidity and mortality of the larger procedure is not justified.

RENAL FAILURE

Uremic pericarditis can occur as a result of untreated severe uremia or in dialysis patients. Dialysis-associated pericarditis does not correlate with the degree of uremia and may be an autoimmune phenomenon. Hemodynamic compromise due to cardiac tamponade is common and may occur in as many as 89 percent of patients who develop this disease.[8] The diagnosis is suggested by the detection of a friction rub in patients with renal failure or by the onset of hemodynamic instability during dialysis. When fluid overload or cardiac failure lead to symptoms and signs which cannot be distinguished from tamponade, echocardiography is helpful.[9]

In uremic pericarditis, the pericardium is friable and layered with granulation tissue. Systemic heparinization is contraindicated, because it may precipitate hemorrhage and acute tamponade. Uremic pericarditis is, therefore, an urgent indication for dialysis using regional heparinization, and such patients should be managed in the ICU. Although pericarditis may improve with intensive dialysis, it remains unchanged in half the patients. There may be a role for nonsteroidal anti-inflammatory drugs in patients with mild effusions, but the risk of gastric complications is high. Because of the high incidence of hemodynamic compromise, effusions that do not readily resolve with dialysis should be treated with either pericardiocentesis or a subxiphoid pericardial window.

TRAUMA

Since tamponade due to cardiac injury is often occult, signs and symptoms may not become evident until the patient arrives in the ICU. Any patient with penetrating chest trauma, including cardiac catheterization, subclavian or jugular venipuncture, or transvenous pacemaker placement who develops shock must be suspected of having cardiac tamponade. Lack of acute pericardial elasticity allows tamponade with as little as 200 mL fluid, so that a normal cardiac silhouette may be present. Jugular venous distention and elevated venous pressure may be absent during hypovolemia. Conversely, patient agitation, shivering, hemothorax, pneumothorax, upper airway obstruction, or respiratory distress may cause jugular venous distention and even pulsus paradoxus in the absence of tamponade.

Although pericardiocentesis may provide dramatic relief, it may be either falsely positive or falsely negative. A false-negative result occurs when the needle is not placed accurately within the small pericardial sac. One may also falsely assume that a clotted aspirate signifies a ventricular rather than pericardial blood source. Thus, in the acute setting, defibrination may not be complete and clotting blood may be obtained. On the other hand, ventricular puncture is not uncommon in the emergency setting and may be falsely interpreted as a positive result.

The major role for pericardiocentesis in acute traumatic tamponade is as a temporizing measure and as a means of facilitating safe induction of anesthesia.[10] Decreased right heart filling caused by mechanical ventilation and anesthetically induced vasodilation may cause circulatory collapse. Prior to induction, pericardiocentesis may therefore be necessary. If cardiac injury is suspected, immediate thoracotomy is mandatory if there is impending or actual circulatory collapse. The role of prethoracotomy pericardiocentesis in these patients is controversial. Patients who are more stable should be transported to the operating room for performance of a subxiphoid pericardial window, which reliably yields the diagnosis and can be extended for treatment of an injury if one is encountered.[11]

Technique

The procedures which may be performed as treatment for effusion with or without tamponade include pericardiocentesis, pericardial window, and pericardiectomy. These procedures may be performed for diagnostic purposes, treatment of circulatory compromise, or for relief of symptoms.

PERICARDIOCENTESIS

There are two approaches to pericardiocentesis: subxiphoid and parasternal. In the absence of specific echocardiographic indications favoring the parasternal approach, the subxiphoid technique is preferable. Inadvertent coronary artery laceration is less likely to occur when approaching the heart inferiorly, and fluid is more likely to be obtained since it tends to pool in a dependent posteroinferior position. Since pericardiocentesis has inherent risks and a number of conditions may mimic tamponade, it should never be performed on an elective basis without confirming the diagnosis by echocardiography or cardiac catheterization.

Prior to its performance, patients should not eat or drink in the event of a complication requiring emergency operation. Atropine should be available at the bedside, because pericardial puncture sometimes causes a vagal response. The technique is shown in Fig. 27-1. The patient is placed in the Fowler's position to promote fluid collection inferiorly. Local anesthesia using lidocaine without epinephrine is

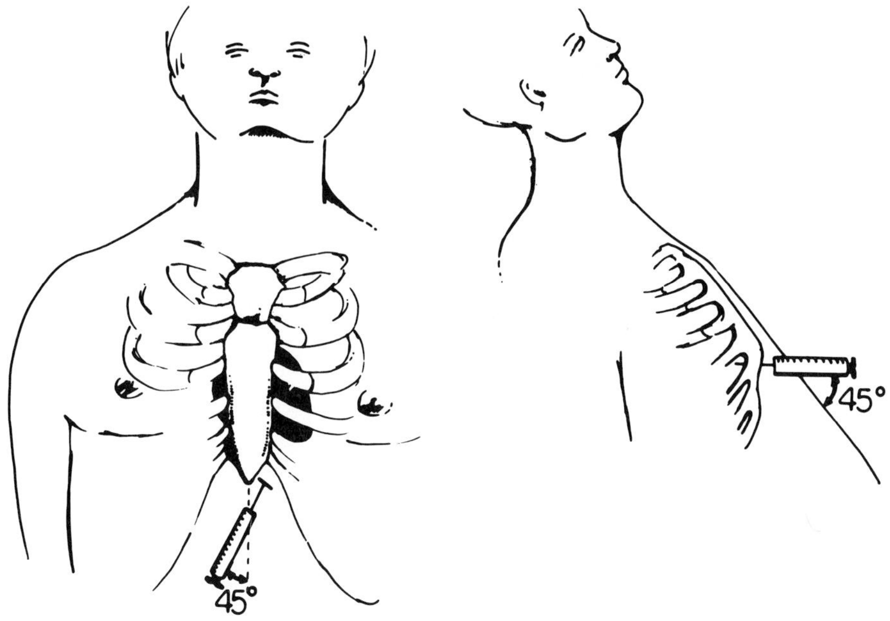

FIGURE 27-1 Technique for pericardiocentesis. The patient is positioned in the Fowler's position to cause inferior pooling of free flowing pericardial fluid. After local anesthesia, a 20 to 23 gauge spinal needle is inserted just below and to the left of the xiphoid process. The needle is inserted at a 45° angle from the midline and from the skin and directed toward the midclavicular point. The average distance from the xiphoid to the heart is 6 to 8 cm in the adult.

administered at a point just below and to the left of the xiphoid process. A 20 to 23 gauge spinal needle is inserted at a 45° angle to the skin and directed toward the midclavicular point. With thicker fluid or blood a larger needle, e.g., 18 gauge, is required. The average distance from the xiphoid to the heart is 6 to 8 cm in the adult, less in the child. Constant suction is maintained as the needle is advanced.

Any bloody fluid obtained should be tested for clotting. Blood in the pericardium for a period of time will defibrinate and, therefore, nonclotting blood confirms that aspiration from the pericardium has occurred. The presence of clot suggests inadvertent ventricular puncture. An unambiguous method for determining whether bloody fluid is being aspirated from the pericardium or the heart is to assess the patient's response. If removal of fluid improves the patient's clinical condition, then the needle is within the pericardial space. Conversely, if the patient deteriorates, then the needle is inside the heart. If access for continued drainage or injection of sclerosing or chemotherapeutic agents is needed, the needle can be removed over a guide wire and a catheter placed into the pericardium. A chest x-ray should be taken after the procedure to rule out the presence of pneumothorax.

When performed blindly, without the benefit of electrocardiographic (ECG) or echocardiographic guidance, serious complications leading to emergency surgery and even death have been reported in 7 to 20 percent of cases. Continuous cardiac movement relative to a needle fixed at the skin causes occasional ventricular or coronary artery laceration, pneumothorax, phrenic nerve injury, internal mammary artery laceration, or arrhythmia. The incidence of complications is related to the size of the effusion. Small, difficult to access effusions leave minimal space available for the exploring needle and are therefore prone to complications. Large chronic effusions increase the size of the pericardial space and are therefore less prone to complications.

When performing pericardiocentesis with ECG guidance, the limb leads should be in place for grounding, and the needle connected to V lead by means of an alligator clip. As the needle is advanced, contact with the epicardium is signalled by ST segment elevation or reversal of polarity of the QRS complex. Echocardiography usually allows visualization of the needle during pericardiocentesis, helps confirm intrapericardial placement, and may reduce the incidence of complications.

Although the use of ECG or echocardiographic guidance makes pericardiocentesis safer, when complications occur the effects on compromised patients can be life-threatening. The risks associated with pericardiocentesis are justified in an emergency situation when used as a potentially lifesaving measure. When used electively or semielectively to treat symptomatic effusions, the risk:benefit ratio is more equivocal. Furthermore, between 25 and 40 percent of patients with pericardial effusions treated with pericardiocentesis will ultimately require pericardial window or pericardiectomy for recurrent effusion, pericarditis, or constrictive pericardial disease. These considerations have led to the frequent use of alternative means of draining the pericardium, such as subxiphoid pericardial window.

SUBXIPHOID PERICARDIAL WINDOW

Subxiphoid pericardial window (Fig. 27-2) is carried out under local or general anesthesia through a small incision and provides access to the pericardial space under direct vision. The procedure requires a short incision over the xiphoid process, which is then excised. Vigorous upward traction on the sternum exposes the mediastinum, which is then dissected in the midline until the pericardium is clearly identified. The pericardium is then opened and a

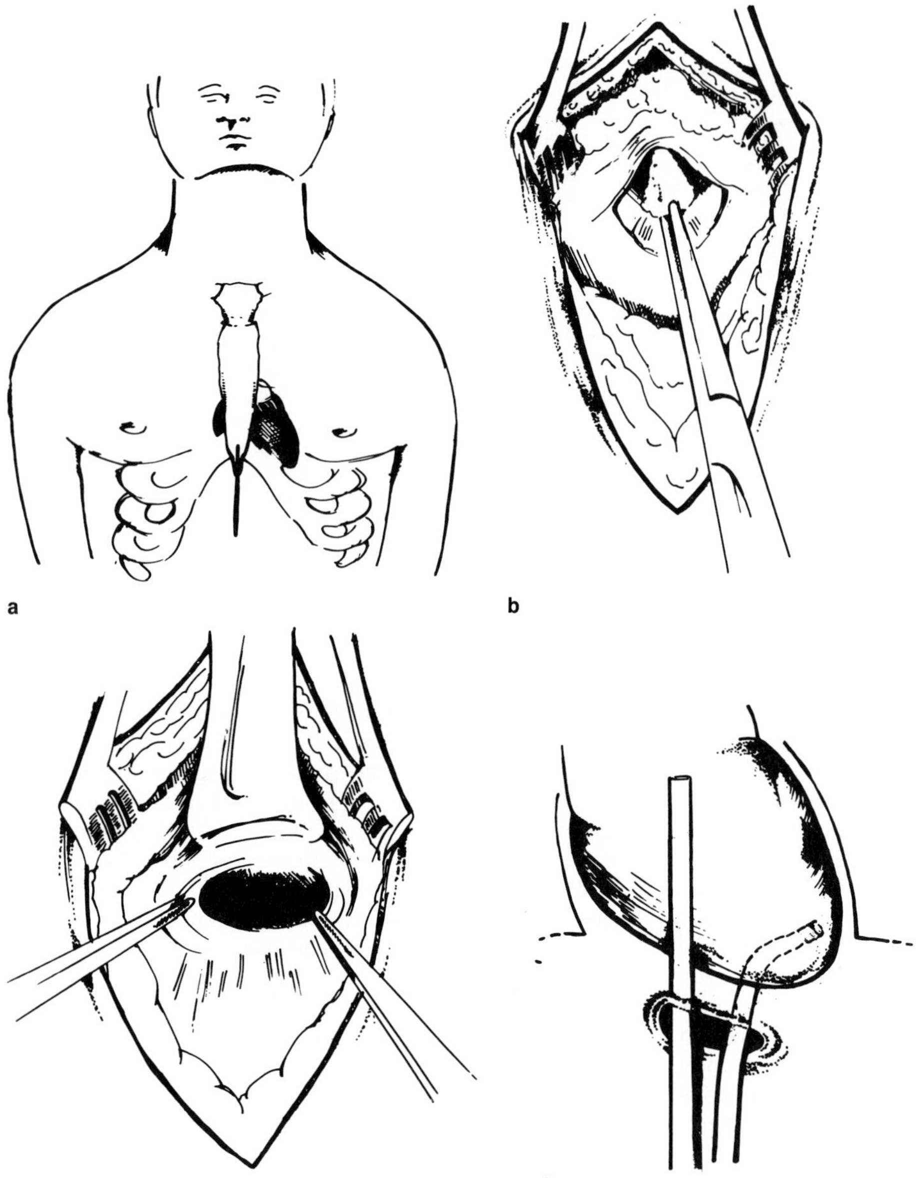

FIGURE 27-2 Technique for subxiphoid pericardial window. *A* shows the location of the 5- to 7-cm skin incision made for this procedure. *B* shows the xiphoid process being held by a clamp; resection provides access to the mediastinum. *C* shows that following resection of the xiphoid, a "window" of pericardium is resected to allow evacuation of fluid, disruption of loculations, and placement of drainage catheters. *D* shows two drainage catheters, routinely placed, both anterior and posterior to the heart.

generous "window" of pericardium is excised. The pericardial cavity is then explored visually and digitally to disrupt loculations and to detect tumor implants which are biopsied.

Contrary to the implications of the name, this window does not provide a permanent route for fluid drainage, since all mesothelial defects heal quickly. The reason this technique is successful is that fusion of the epicardium and pericardium occurs; the pericardial space is obliterated in analogous fashion to the use of pleurodesis to treat pleural effusions.[12] A critical aspect of performing this operation, therefore, is placement of pericardial drainage tubes. These remain in place to ensure continued removal of fluid until coaptation of these two surfaces occurs. These drainage tubes are removed when the volume of drainage is < 50 mL/day, which rarely takes more than 2 or 3 days.

A thoracotomy can be used for access to the pericardium for the purpose of creating a window for fluid drainage. However, this approach is both more painful and more morbid for the patient and should be abandoned except for patients requiring a thoracotomy for other purposes. Likewise, formal pericardiectomy is rarely necessary in treating effusive disease since subxiphoid window provides effective treatment. Pericardiectomy is too extensive a procedure for most debilitated patients, though it is still needed for treatment of constrictive pericarditis and as a form of pericardial debridement in cases of suppurative pericarditis.

Complications

Pulmonary edema is rare in tamponade, since impaired right heart filling decreases pulmonary blood flow. Typically, patients present with symptoms of myocardial failure and cardiomegaly, with clear lung fields on chest x-ray. Dyspnea, however, is a common symptom in patients with significant pericardial effusions. Sufficiently elevated left atrial pressure can increase interstitial lung water despite decreased pulmonary blood flow. Lung water may also be increased by elevated right heart pressure, which impairs drainage of lung lymph. Despite the confinement of pulmonary edema to the interstitium in most cases, compliance may decrease enough to cause the sensation of dyspnea. In contrast, however, the dramatic onset of pulmonary edema can follow the relief of tamponade.[13] In chronic tamponade, decreased cardiac output leads to compensatory fluid accumulation to sustain cardiac filling, and associated hypotension causes an increase in catecholamines and afterload. On relief of tamponade, the sudden increase in left ventricular end-diastolic volume due to an increased preload may lead to the onset of acute pulmonary edema. Patients with poor myocardial compliance, such as those with chronic hypertension, ventricular hypertrophy, and coronary artery disease with ventricular dysfunction, as well as patients with fixed cardiac output due to stenotic mitral or aortic valvular disease may be particularly prone to this phenomenon. Posttamponade pulmonary edema occurs after both pericardiocentesis and subxiphoid window. In the elective setting, patients should be screened for the above risk factors with preoperative echocardiography. If judged to be at risk, preoperative pulmonary artery catheter placement and postoperative ICU monitoring should be performed.

References

1. Skhvatsaja LV: Secondary malignant lesions of the heart and pericardium in neoplastic disease. Oncology 43:103, 1986.
2. Press OW, Livingston R: Management of malignant pericardial effusion and tamponade. JAMA 257:1088, 1987.
3. Sznajder JI, Evander E, Pollak ER, et al: Pericardial effusion causes interstitial pulmonary edema in dogs. Circulation 76:843, 1987.
4. Little AG, Kremser PC, Wade JL, et al: Operation for diagnosis and treatment of pericardial effusions. Surgery 96:738, 1984.
5. Sheperd FA, Morgan CD, Ginsberg JS: Control of malignant pericardial effusion by tetracycline sclerosis. Proc Am Soc Clin Oncol 5:246, 1986.
6. Palatianos GM, Thurer RJ, Pompeo MD, Kaiser GA: Clinical experience with subxiphoid drainage of pericardial effusions. Ann Thorac Surg 48:381, 1989.
7. Piehler JM, Pluth JR, Schaff HV, et al: Surgical management of effusive pericardial disease. J Thorac Cardiovasc Surg 90:506, 1985.
8. Conty CM, Cohen SL, Shapiro FL: Pericarditis in chronic uremia and its sequelae. Ann Intern Med 75:173, 1971.
9. Luft FC, Gilman JK, Weyman AE: Pericarditis in the patient with uremia: Clinical and echocardiographic evaluation. Nephron 25:160, 1980.
10. Trinkle JK, Marcos J, Grover FL, et al: Management of the wounded heart. Ann Thorac Surg 17:230, 1974.
11. Miller, FB, Bond SJ, Shumate CR, et al: Diagnostic pericardial window. A safe alternative to exploratory thoracotomy for suspected heart injuries. Arch Surg 122:605, 1987.
12. Sugimoto JT, Little AG, Ferguson MK, et al: Pericardial window: Mechanisms of efficacy. Ann Thorac Surg 50:442, 1990.
13. Naunheim KS, Wood LDH, Little AG: Pulmonary edema as a complication of pericardial drainage. Surg Gynecol Obstet 165:166, 1987.

Chapter 28

MECHANICAL ASSISTANCE OF THE FAILING HEART

STEPHANIE J. BRISTER
B. WILLIAM SHRAGGE

Ventricular assistance may salvage viable myocardium after a severe ischemic insult. The effects of myocardial ischemia have been studied extensively over the last 25 years. The concept of an "all or none" phenomenon of myocyte necrosis has been replaced by the concept of a gradation of injury. The resultant functional and structural changes depend on the duration of the coronary occlusion, the extent of collateral flow, the metabolic and hemodynamic conditions during which the myocardium is made ischemic, and the timing and nature of reperfusion.

Several modalities may be used to modify the conditions under which reperfusion occurs. Ventricular assist devices (VADs) have been developed to decrease the workload of the myocardium or replace the heart altogether. These devices may limit ischemic damage and facilitate the recovery of the injured myocardium. In canine models, left heart bypass decreased myocardial oxygen consumption,[1] and increasing left ventricular bypass flow rates further decreased myocardial oxygen consumption and decreased electrocardiographic (ECG) ST segment elevations.[2] Myocardial necrosis was reduced following 45 min of warm ischemia in dogs supported with a left ventricular assist device (LVAD) compared to dogs supported with an intraaortic balloon pump (IABP) and dopamine.[3] VADs may permit recovery in patients with reversible myocardial damage and hemodynamic compromise who cannot be supported with an IABP or inotropes.

Intraaortic Balloon Pumping

In 1967, Kantrowitz reported the first successful clinical use of the IABP in man.[4] Today, the balloon is usually inserted via the femoral artery and positioned in the descending thoracic aorta (Fig. 28-1). Phased inflations are synchronized to the ECG. Inflation of the balloon occurs with the closure of the atrioventricular (AV) valve and deflation occurs prior to the onset of systole. These mechanical events result in an increase in coronary perfusion pressure during diastole, a time during which coronary resistance is at its lowest. This results in an improvement in coronary blood flow. With deflation during systole, the left ventricle ejects against a low impedance and widely dilated vascular bed. In clinical studies, use of the IABP results in a 10 to 20 percent increase in cardiac output, a decrease in systolic pressure, an increase in diastolic pressure, a decrease in heart rate and usually, an increase in urine output.[4,5]

INDICATIONS AND CONTRAINDICATIONS

IABPs are most commonly used in postcardiotomy patients. The principal indication for insertion (Table 28-1) is inability to be weaned from bypass despite the use of moderate inotropes, development of low output syndrome in the ICU following cardiac surgery, and development of ischemic changes or electrical instability as a result of ischemia in postcardiotomy patients. Preoperative support with an IABP is indicated in patients with acute ventricular septal defects, acute mitral regurgitation secondary to ruptured papillary muscles, and failed angioplasties with subsequent hemodynamic instability or ischemia.[5] IABPs have also been used in patients in cardiogenic shock secondary to myocardial infarction (MI) who do not have specific mechanical defects. The results in these situations are mixed, depending on the reversibility of the underlying pathology. Patients who are appropriate for subsequent surgery or angioplasty have a better long-term prognosis than those who are inappropriate candidates for interventional procedures.[6,7] In addition, IABPs are often used to support critically ill patients who are waiting for transplantation.

Absolute contraindications for IABP insertion (Table 28-2) include aortic insufficiency and the presence of irreversible cardiac disease.[5] Relative contraindications are the presence of abdominal aortic aneurysm, severe peripheral vascular disease, and the presence of tachyarrhythmias. The latter present problems for the tracking of the ECG; therefore, the balloon counterpulsation cannot be appropriately timed for the arterial pressure.

TECHNIQUE FOR INSERTION AND REMOVAL

Initially, IABPs were inserted through an open incision in the groin. A vascular graft was sewn to the artery, and the IABP was passed through the graft and into the correct po-

TABLE 28-1 Indications for Intraaortic Balloon Pump

Absolute
- Inability to wean from cardiopulmonary bypass
- Low output syndrome postcardiotomy
- Acute ventricular septal defect secondary to MI
- Acute mitral regurgitation secondary to MI
- Failed angioplasty with hemodynamic compromise or evidence of ischemia

Relative
- Severe left ventricular dysfunction in a surgical candidate
- Development of ischemic changes on ECG in postcardiotomy patient
- Development of electrical instability in a postcardiotomy patient

Controversial
- Cardiogenic shock secondary to MI
- Unstable angina
- Major noncardiac operations in patients with known severe coronary artery disease

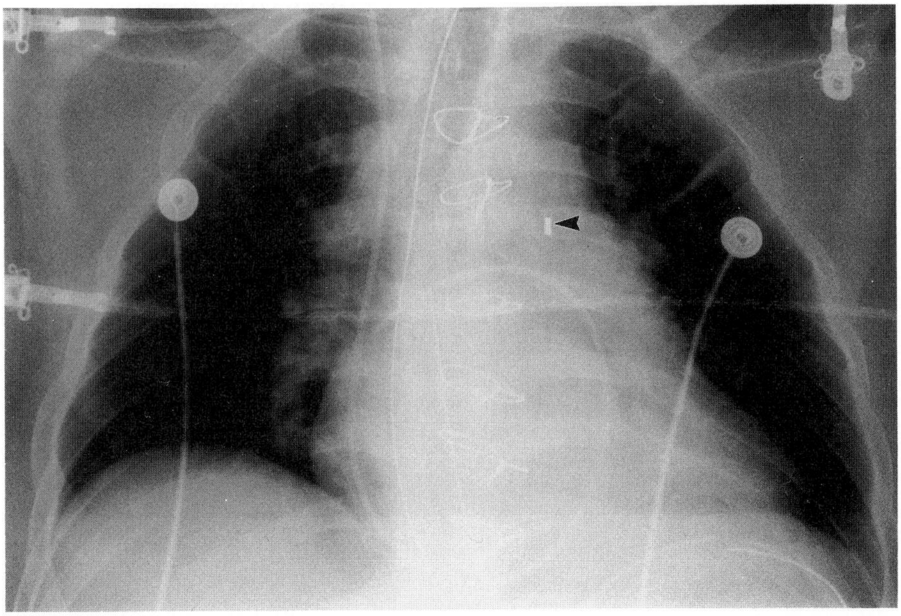

FIGURE 28-1 In this AP chest film the large arrow indicates the radiopaque marker demonstrating the tip of the IABP. It is in correct position, several centimeters below the aortic knob.

TABLE 28-2 Contraindications for Intraaortic Balloon Pump

Absolute
- Aortic insufficiency
- Irreversible cardiac disease
- Chronic end-stage disease

Relative
- Abdominal aortic aneurysm
- Severe peripheral vascular disease
- Tachyarrhythmias

sition in the thoracic aorta. Removal required a second trip to the operating room. This technique is now rarely used. Now, the majority of IABPs are inserted percutaneously through the femoral artery in the right or left groin. Occasionally in the operating room, the femoral artery will be exposed for insertion. The cannula, however, will still be inserted through a separate incision through the skin prior to entering the artery. Under these conditions, the balloon pumps can be removed in the ICU. When the IABP is removed, the balloon is deflated and some bleeding back from the artery is allowed. The groin should then be compressed for 45 to 60 min to achieve hemostasis. In rare instances, when peripheral vascular disease is extensive or an aortic aneurysm is present, the intraaortic balloon can be placed transthoracically. This is only appropriate for postcardiotomy patients. In this situation, a pursestring is placed in the ascending aorta and the insertion cannula and balloon are passed through the ascending aorta, through the arch, and positioned in the descending thoracic aorta. Removal after this approach is used requires a return to the operating room.

COMPLICATIONS

Complications of IABP arise from the insertion or from the device itself. Complications as a result of insertion include dissection of the aorta or the common femoral artery (which can result in vascular rupture or paraplegia), dislodgement of plaque or thrombus-forming emboli to major arteries, or perforation of the common femoral artery, iliac artery, or aorta. Complications arising from the device itself include obstruction of the common femoral artery with resultant peripheral ischemia, systemic infection, occlusion of a major artery, thrombocytopenia, hemorrhage, hemolysis, and rupture of the balloon with gas embolization.[5]

OUTCOME

Results of IABP insertion are difficult to assess. They depend primarily on the underlying pathology for which the balloon was inserted. Good results can be achieved in appropriate postcardiotomy patients. Mortality associated with acute ventricular septal defect or acute mitral regurgitation secondary to papillary muscle rupture is high because of the nature of the disease. Patients with cardiogenic shock secondary to MI can be supported hemodynamically with an IABP, but long-term success depends on the underlying nature of their disease and on whether or not it can be corrected by angioplasty or surgery.[5,7]

Ventricular Assist Devices

The development of VADs has occurred over the past 30 years. Three principal categories of devices are in clinical use at this time (Table 28-3). Centrifugal pumps, roller pumps, and hemopumps are nonpulsatile systems (type I) in which blood is removed from the heart by centrifugal force, gravity drainage, or a rotating shaft and pumped back into the patient. Roller pumps are simply an extension of the cardiopulmonary bypass apparatus. Centrifugal pumps are a newer adaptation which involves development of a centrifugal force by movement of a fluid through

TABLE 28-3 Categories of Ventricular Assist Devices

1. *Nonpulsatile Pump*
   - Centrifugal pump
   - Hemopump
   - Roller pump

II. *Heterotopic Ventricles*
   - Pneumatic pump
   - Hydraulic pump
   - Pusher plate pump

III. *Orthotopic Ventricles*
   - Jarvik heart
   - Penn State heart
   - Berlin heart
   - Unger heart

a constrained vortex.[8] Because of the nonocclusive nature of the pump, there should be less trauma to the blood elements than would occur with an occlusive roller pump. Arterial outflow obstruction or an increase in afterload decreases the output at the pump, even though the head continues to rotate. A decrease in preload will decrease output and an increase in preload will increase output. Pumping air is difficult because the pump's output stops when the inflow line cavitates. The centrifugal pump may also produce less gaseous microembolization, minimize hemoglobinemia and result in less postoperative blood loss than a roller pump.[9]

Heterotopic ventricles (type II) are pulsatile devices which augment the function of the intact ventricle. The native heart is not explanted, so the devices are connected to the existing heart and provide some hemodynamic support. These devices usually involve a sac which is compressed pneumatically, by plates or hydraulically. The original designs were cumbersome and not entirely implantable. Researchers are currently working on modifications such that these devices may be totally implantable and permanent.

Orthotopic ventricles (type III) have been developed for use as bridges to transplantation or to permanently replace a failing heart. They require explantation of the native heart with subsequent replacement by the device. The best known of these devices is the "Jarvik heart."

Over the last 10 years, the appropriate clinical use for VADs has been better defined. Currently, they are inserted for temporary support and as a bridge to transplantation in patients with reversible myocardial damage who are unable to support their circulation despite the use of inotropes and IABPs. Ultimately, these devices may serve as a permanent cardiac replacement.

Temporary Ventricular Support

The vast experience in temporary support of the patient with failing myocardium with VADs has occurred in postcardiotomy patients. Centrifugal pumps, impeller pumps, hemopumps and heterotopic ventricles that are pneumatically, hydraulically, or electrically driven have been used for this purpose.

INDICATIONS AND CONTRAINDICATIONS

Indications (Table 28-4) for placement of a VAD in a postcardiotomy patient include the inability to wean from bypass despite the use of IABPs or maximal inotropes, the development of shock in the ICU following cardiac surgery which is unresponsive to inotropes and IABP, age <65, the absence of other major medical illnesses, completion of a technically adequate operation, and the conduct of an expeditious bypass. The definition of shock may vary from institution to institution.

As outlined by Balakumaran and coworkers, cardiogenic shock can be divided into four classes (Table 28-5).[10] Although this classification is designed for cardiogenic shock developing prior to cardiac surgery, it does provide definitive parameters on which therapy can be based. Postcardiotomy patients in class I and II should be treated with inotropic agents. Class III patients should initially be given inotropes and if they fail to respond or deteriorate, an IABP should be placed. If further deterioration occurs, a VAD should be inserted. Class IV patients require prompt therapy with inotropes, followed by IABP and VAD if these agents fail.

Inotropic support can include combinations of epinephrine, dopamine, dobutamine, amrinone, or norepinephrine. If necessary, an IABP is inserted. When these measures fail, a VAD should be considered. The therapeutic alternatives must be instituted quickly and a prompt decision made as to their efficacy, since the early insertion of a VAD is paramount to its success.

Specific hemodynamic criteria which can be used for institution of LVAD support[11] include a cardiac index (CI) <2 L/min/m^2, systemic vascular resistance (SVR) >2100 dyne · s/cm^5, left atrial pressure >20 mmHg, and urine output <20 mL/hour. These criteria must exist in the presence of optimal preload, maximal drug therapy, corrected metabolism, and the presence of an IABP. Hemodynamic criteria for insertion of a right ventricular assist device (RVAD) include an elevated central venous pressure (>20 mmHg), a low left atrial pressure (<6 to 8 mmHg), systemic hypotension (systolic blood pressure <70 mmHg), a low CI (<1.5 L/min/m^2), and an elevated pulmonary vascular resistance.[11] A trial of atrial or AV sequential pacing, inotropic agents, pulmonary vasodilators, and IABP should be undertaken prior to insertion of an RVAD. A biventricular assist device should be considered when both ventricles are affected. Hemodynamic criteria for this are less specific but include a CI <2 L/min/m^2, high SVR, high pulmonary vascular resistance, and elevated central venous pressures.

TABLE 28-4 Indications for Insertion of Ventricular Assist Devices

- Inability to wean from bypass despite institution of IABP and maximal inotropes
- Development of cardiogenic shock postcardiotomy unresponsive to IABP and maximal inotropes
- Absence of other major medical illnesses
- Completion of a technically adequate operation
- Short cardiopulmonary bypass time

TABLE 28-5 Classification of Cardiogenic Shock

Hemodynamic Signs	Class I	Class II	Class III	Class IV
Heart rate (beats/min)	70–85	85–100	90–110	> 110
Blood pressure (mmHg)	> 90	80–90	60–80	< 60
Pulmonary capillary wedge pressure (mmHg)	< 12	12–14	14–18	> 18
Cardiac index (L/min/m^2)	> 3.0	2.5–3.0	2.0–2.5	< 2.0
Left ventricular work (L · mmHg/min/m^2)	> 270	200–270	120–200	< 120
Stroke work index (mL · mmHg/m^2)	> 3000	2000–3000	1200–2000	< 1200

Absolute contraindications to the procedure include irreversible cardiac damage, preoperative bleeding diathesis, and active infection (Table 28-6). Relative contraindications include cerebral vascular disease, hepatic failure, and multiple organ failure.

Predictive factors for survival of patients undergoing implantation of VADs include presence of a perioperative infarct, severe obstructive lung disease, and the "urgent" status of patients as they arrive in the operating room. Patients who arrive in the operating room in full cardiac arrest or in cardiogenic shock with IABP support tend to do poorly. In one series of 11 patients arriving in the operating room in this state, none survived 30 days after the operation.

TECHNIQUE

Most devices are now inserted in the operating room through an open chest. More recently, systems which can be inserted percutaneously or through open cutdown through the groin have been developed. The assist devices can be used for left ventricular assist, right ventricular assist, biventricular assist, or extracorporeal membrane oxygenation (ECMO). For left ventricular assistance, the outflow cannula is placed in the left atrium (Fig. 28-2). It can be inserted in the left atrial appendage, through the interatrial groove, through the superior pulmonary vein, and through the roof of the left atrium. The left ventricular apex can also be used for the outflow cannula, but proper placement in the left ventricle is important to allow appropriate percutaneous exit and to allow the heart to lie in its normal anatomic position. Care must be taken with insertion of this cannula because once in place, it is impossible to use additional sutures, and fatal hemorrhage can occur from the apex cannulation site.

TABLE 28-6 Contraindications for Insertion of Ventricular Assist Device

Absolute
- Irreversible cardiac damage
- Preoperative bleeding diathesis
- Active infection

Relative
- Cerebral vascular disease
- Hepatic failure
- Multiple organ failure

There are theoretical advantages to using the ventricular apex as the outflow site. Studies have shown that left ventricular bypass provides better decompression of the ventricle and decreases myocardial oxygen consumption to a greater extent than left atrial bypass. These theoretical advantages have not been translated into clinical benefit because of the technical difficulties of using the left ventricular apex; at this time most experienced surgeons use the left atrium.[12,13] The inflow cannulation occurs via a synthetic graft which is anastomosed to the ascending aorta.

For right ventricular support, the inflow cannula is placed first. The synthetic graft or cannula is placed in the pulmonary artery and appropriate de-airing is undertaken. The outflow cannulation is done through the right atrial free wall (Fig. 28-3). Biventricular support requires two devices. The LVAD is inserted initially in the manner previously described (see Fig. 28-2), and the RVAD is subsequently placed (see Fig. 28-3). For ECMO (Fig. 28-4), only a single device is necessary, but there must be a membrane oxygenator in line. Centrifugal pumps or roller pumps are the most frequently used devices for this type of support. The outflow cannulation is via the right atrium and the inflow cannulation is via the aorta.[9] The cannulas exit percutaneously for most heterotopic ventricles below the costal

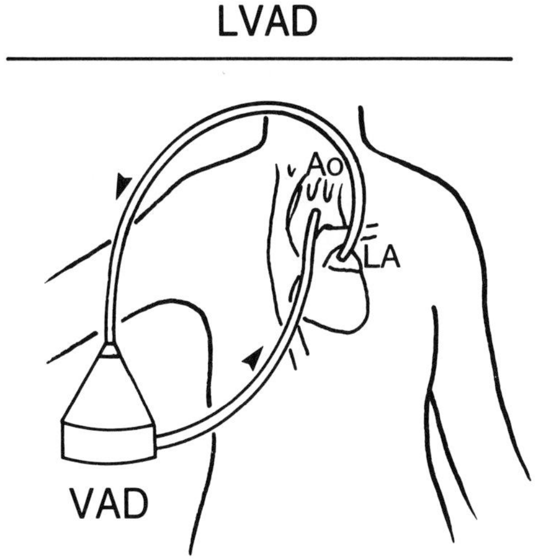

FIGURE 28-2 Depiction of correct cannulation sites for a left ventricular assist device (LVAD) with an outflow cannula in the left atrium (LA) and inflow cannula in the aorta (Ao).

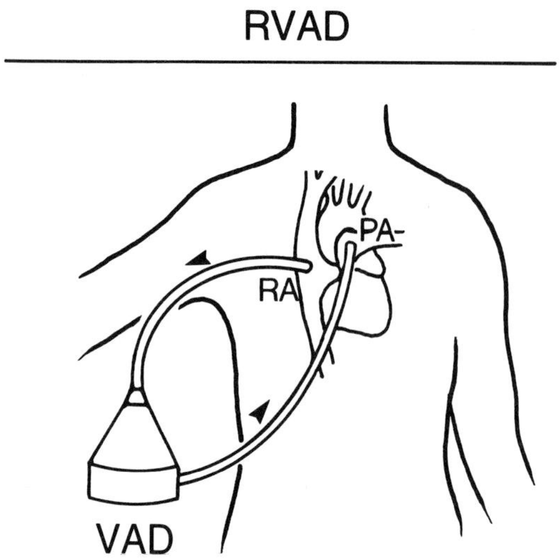

FIGURE 28-3 Depiction of proper cannulation sites for a right ventricular assist device (RVAD) with an outflow cannula in the right atrium (RA) and inflow cannula in the pulmonary artery (PA).

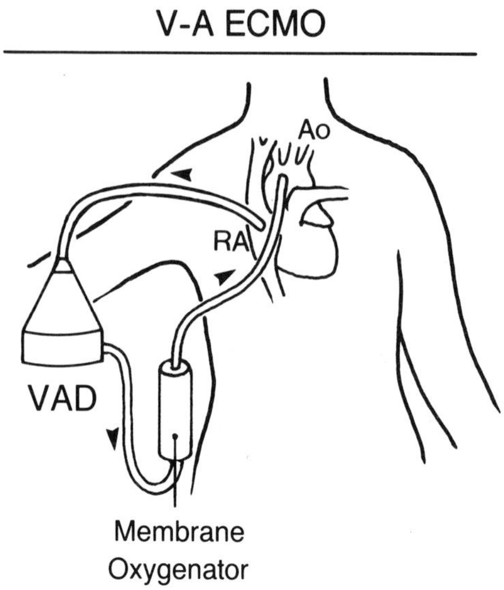

FIGURE 28-4 Depicts veno arterial extracorporeal membrane oxygenation (V-A ECMO) with an outflow cannula in the right atrium (RA) and an inflow cannula in the Aorta (Ao).

margin. For centrifugal pumps or roller pumps, cannulae can exit through the anterior portion of the chest. Most surgeons prefer to avoid having them exit directly through the sternum in case the patient requires subsequent transplantation.

DISCONTINUATION OF SUPPORT

Once in place, the device should be left alone for at least 24 hours. The myocardium must be given an opportunity to recover. The decision to wean is based on hemodynamic monitoring. In most situations, a left atrial line and Swan-Ganz catheter are present. During assistance a minimal flow of 4 L/min or CI of >2 L/min/m^2 is recommended. When weaning is attempted, pump flow is decreased and hemodynamic measurements are made. If there is a drop below the acceptable cardiac output or a rise in either pulmonary artery pressures or pulmonary wedge pressures, then a full flow must be reinstituted. Eventually the patients are weaned to the IABP and moderate inotropic agents.[14] Once successfully weaned, the patient must return to the operating room to have the device removed. Important predictors for the ability to be weaned are improvements in mixed venous oxygen saturation, CI, mean arterial pressure, ventricular ejection fraction, and atrial pressures.[14]

COMPLICATIONS

Bleeding is the principal complication related to use of VADs.[15] The bleeding diathesis associated with cardiopulmonary bypass is exacerbated with the use of VADs. Activation of platelets in the blood coagulation system is a result of the abnormal flow conditions introduced by the device and the biomaterial surfaces with which the blood interacts. It is very important that hemostasis be achieved prior to leaving the operating room. This is usually attainable by securing hemostasis at the suture lines and using platelet and plasma transfusions. Most surgeons do not institute heparin therapy in the operating room. Once the patient has arrived in the ICU and bleeding from the chest tubes is controlled, heparin therapy may be instituted. The optimal level achieved varies with the type of device inserted. For the centrifugal pump some investigators will institute full heparinization within several hours of discontinuing bypass. The goal is to achieve a partial thromboplastin time one and one-half times normal. Other investigators will not use anticoagulation as long as the centrifugal pump is running high flow rates.[15] When weaning is begun and the flow rates drop below 2 L/min/m^2, then full anticoagulation with heparin must be instituted again. Full anticoagulation is not essential with pulsatile assist devices. The difficulties with thromboembolism are greater, but this must be traded off against the risks of bleeding in any particular patient.

There is a significant number of other postoperative complications.[16] Inadequate cardiac output may develop in a patient who has a circulatory assist device in place. It may be related to hypovolemia, cannula obstruction, or right ventricular failure. Patent foramen ovale (PFO) in a patient with high right atrial pressures may result in shunting with desaturation of the arterial blood. When placing a VAD, the right atrium should be opened and checked for a PFO. Hemolysis is a problem which is worsened by prolonged cardiopulmonary bypass. It is unusual, but can occur. End-organ failure is a late complication of VAD and is often related to the length of time which the patient has been in cardiogenic shock prior to institution of the device. Device failure can also arise, though it is becoming less common. It is most often related to fractured valves, splitting of tubing in roller pumps, and drive unit failures. Infection is a problem arising in devices which are in place for a longer period of time. With the orthotopic devices, a mediastinal infection may develop from the percutaneously inserted driveline. With the centrifugal pumps, systemic sepsis can arise as a result of the percutaneous lines.

OUTCOME

In appropriately selected postcardiotomy patients, discharge from the hospital can be achieved in 30 to 40 percent of patients.[18] It is difficult to evaluate long-term results in these patients. At follow-up ranging from a few months to several years, the majority of patients are still alive. Sixty to 70 percent will be in New York Heart Association Class I or II. It appears that if a patient can walk out of the hospital, the chance of returning to a reasonable life-style is very good.[19]

Ventricular assistance has also been used for patients in cardiogenic shock secondary to acute MI. Extensive experimental evidence indicates that left ventricular assist reduces myocardial ischemia and the size of the infarct. It is also able to support the circulation during the period of infarction and circulatory instability.[20] However, outcomes reported in the literature are not encouraging. The circulation can certainly be supported by these devices in the acute period, but the difficulty comes with weaning the patient. If the underlying disease is not correctable by surgery, angioplasty, or transplantation, the prognosis of the patient is grim.[21] The centrifugal pump has been used via femoral cut down or an open chest insertion to support patients during high risk angioplasties, during cardiovascular collapse following percutaneous transluminal coronary angioplasty, for support during lung transplantation or liver transplantation, for support following pulmonary embolization, in thoracic aortic surgery to decrease spinal cord complications, and during surgery for renal cell carcinoma. The advantage of the centrifugal pump in the latter situations is the minimal heparinization which is needed.[22,23]

Bridging to Transplantation

As early as 1969, Denton Cooley used a VAD in a patient for 64 h until a donor heart became available.[24] IABPs have been used extensively as bridges to transplantation. The first successful use of a total artificial heart as a bridge to transplantation was reported by Copeland, and the first successful use of the Pierce Donachy VAD (a pneumatic sac pump), was reported in 1986.[25] Centrifugal pumps, impeller pumps, orthotopic prosthetic ventricles, and heterotopic prosthetic ventricles have all been used as bridges.[26–28] The indication for using an assist device as a bridge to transplantation[15] is the presence of a patient within minutes to hours of death, who is an appropriate transplant candidate and no donor heart is available.[28] The principal complications encountered in patients who are bridged include bleeding, infection, renal failure, hemolysis, respiratory failure, thrombosis, biventricular failure with inadequate cardiac output, perioperative infarction, emboli to the central nervous system, disseminated intravascular coagulation, and mechanical failure of the device. Results of bridging with a variety of devices are outlined in Table 28-7. Forty to 80 percent of patients who have devices implanted survive for transplantation. Thirty to 80 percent of patients who are transplanted survive to be discharged, and 25 to 70 percent of patients who initially have the device implanted as a bridge to transplantation survive to be discharged from the hospital. The results appear to be best with the Thoratec device, a heterotopic prosthetic ventricle.[29–31]

TABLE 28-7 Survival Results Following Use of Ventricular Assist Device as a Bridge to Transplantation[a]

Pump	No. Patients	Transplanted	Discharged	Survived
Centrifugal	25	16(64%)	10(62.5%)	10(40%)
Jarvik	81	58(72%)	31(53%)	31(38%)
Novacor	17	7(41%)	5(71%)	5(29%)
Thermedics	4	3(75%)	1(33%)	1(25%)
Thoratec	57	46(81%)	38(83%)	38(67%)

[a]See text for explanation of categories.

Permanent Total Artificial Heart

No device available at this time is a permanent artificial heart. The most widely known of the orthotopic ventricles, the Jarvik 7 or Jarvik 70,[32] have been used only as a bridge to transplantation. Mediastinitis following transplantation is a significant problem. Thromboembolism within the device has limited its use.[33] Totally implantable artificial hearts are being investigated by several centers. Davis and colleagues from the University of Pennsylvania are working on a pneumatically powered total artificial heart.[34] They have currently used it in six calves for an average survival time of 46 days. Other investigators have developed an electromechanically driven dual pusher plate blood pump.[33] It has been implanted in 20 patients. Total support of the systemic circulation and substantial left ventricular unloading were achieved with synchronous counterpulsation for periods of up to 90 days. Again, this device has not been left in place as "permanent." It has been used only as a bridge to transplantation. The ultimate cardiac replacement has not yet been designed. Further research must be done in terms of developing the implantable power systems and less thrombogenic surfaces.[32]

Biomechanical Ventricular Assistance

There are a large number of patients with diffuse cardiomyopathies. Cardiac transplantation, although a successful alternative, is limited because of the number of donors. At the present time, VADs are not able to support the ventricle on a permanent basis. Research interests have turned to utilization of the patient's own skeletal muscle as a source of ventricular assistance. Skeletal muscle is comprised of fast and slow muscle fibers. The former generate contractions of considerable force, but are easily fatiguable. The latter, slow muscle fibers, are more fatigue resistant. It is known that fast fibers can be transformed to slow fibers in any muscle by altering the neurostimulus.[35] Researchers have undertaken to transform skeletal muscle to slow fibers and then use that muscle in a variety of configurations for support of the left ventricle. The latissimus dorsi is the most commonly used muscle, and it has been used as a pedicle patch to the left ventricle,[36] to power an accessory ventricle,[37] as a wrap around the ventricle,[38] as a wrap around the aorta, or as a power source for an intrathoracic IABP.[39] Skeletal muscle has been used clinically by Carpentier in France[40] and McGovern in the United States.[41] It has been used as a pedicle muscle flap to the left ventricle following excision of a large portion of the ventricle. Muscle is then paced in synchrony with the left ventricle to augment ventricular output. No deaths have been reported. This is a new and innovative approach and may eventually replace cardiac transplantation as the treatment of choice for patients with end-stage cardiomyopathy.

References

1. Dennis C, Hull DP, Moreno JR, Senning A: Reduction of the oxygen utilization of the heart by left heart bypass. Circ Res 10:298, 1982.
2. Pennock JL, Pierce WS, Waldhauser JA: Quantitative evaluation of left ventricular bypass reducing myocardial ischemia. Surgery 79:523, 1976.
3. Mickleborough LL, Rebeyka I, Wilson GJ, et al: Comparison of left ventricular assist and intra-aortic balloon counterpulsation during early reperfusion after ischemic arrest of the heart. J Thorac Cardiovasc Surg 93:547, 1987.
4. Kantrowitz A, Krakauer JS, Rosenbaum A, et al: Phasic shift balloon pumping in medically refractory cardiogenic shock: Results in 27 patients. Arch Surg 99:739, 1969.
5. Scheidt S, Collins M, Goldstein J, Fisher J: Mechanical circulating assistance with the intra-aortic balloon pump and other counterpulsation devices. Prog Cardiovasc Dis 25(1):55, 1982.
6. Bardet J, Marquet C, Kahn C, et al: Clinical and hemodynamic results of intra-aortic balloon counterpulsation and surgery for cardiogenic shock. Am Heart J 93:280, 1977.
7. Scheidt S, Wilner G, Mueller H, et al: Intra-aortic balloon counterpulsation in cardiogenic shock: Report of a co-operative clinical trial. N Engl J Med 288:979, 1973.
8. Brister SJ, Weisel RD, Birnbaum P, Madonik M: Ventricular assistance with a centrifugal pump. Biomater Appl 4:391, 1990.
9. Frazier OH, Wampler RK, Duncan JM, et al: First human use of the hemopump, a catheter-mounted ventricular assist device. Ann Thorac Surg 49:292, 1990.
10. Balakumaran K, Hugenholtz PG: Cardiogenic shock; current concepts in management. Drugs 32:372, 1986.
11. Rose D, Connolly M, Cunningham JN, Spencer FC: Technique and results with a roller pump left and right heart assist device. Ann Thorac Surg 47:124, 1989.
12. Ganzel BL, Gray LA, Slater AD, Mavroudis C: Surgical techniques for the implantation of heterotopic prosthetic ventricles. Ann Thorac Surg 47:113, 1989.
13. Magovern GJ, Golding LAR, Oyer PE, Cabrol C: Weaning and bridging, Panel 5: Circulatory Support Symposium of the Society of Thoracic Surgeons, St. Louis, Feb 6–7, 1988. Ann Thorac Surg 47:102, 1989.
14. Termuhlen DF, Swartz MT, Pennington DG, et al: Predictors for weaning patients from ventricular assist devices. Trans Am Soc Artif Intern Organs Vol 34, 1988.
15. Copeland JG, Harken LA, Heinich J, Devries WC: Bleeding and anticoagulation, Panel 3: Circulatory Support Symposium of the Society of Thoracic Surgeons, St. Louis, Feb 6–7, 1988. Ann Thorac Surg 47:88, 1989.
16. Pierce WS, Gray LA, McBride LR, Frazier OH: Other postoperative complications, Panel 4: Circulatory Support Symposium of the Society of Thoracic Surgeons, St. Louis, Feb 6–7, 1988. Ann Thorac Surg 47:96, 1989.
17. Pennington PG, McBride LR, Swartz MT, et al: Use of the Pierce-Donachy ventricular assist device in patients with cardiogenic shock after cardiac operations. Ann Thorac Surg 47:103, 1989.
18. Pae WE, Pierce WS, Pennock JL, et al: Long term results of ventricular assist pumping in post cardiotomy cardiogenic shock. J Thorac Cardiovasc Surg 93:434, 1987.
19. Pennock JL, Pierce WS, Wisman CB, et al: Survival and complications following ventricular assist pumping for cardiogenic shock. Ann Surg 198:469, 1983.
20. Zumbio GL, Kitchens WR, Shearer G, et al: Mechanical assistance for cardiogenic shock following cardiac surgery, myocardial infarction and cardiac transplantation. Ann Thorac Surg 44:11, 1987.
21. Position Paper. The case of extra-corporeal circulation for circulatory support during PTCA. J Thorac Cardiovas Surg 99(3):385, 1990.
22. Reichman RT, Joyo CI, Dembitsky WP, et al: Improved patient survival after cardiac arrest using a cardiopulmonary support system. Ann Thorac Surg 49:101, 1990.
23. Hess PJ, Howe HR, Rohisek F, et al: Traumatic tears of the thoracic aorta: Improved results using the biomedicus pump. Ann Thorac Surg 48:6, 1990.
24. Cooley DA, Liotta D, Hallman GL, et al: Orthotopic cardiac prosthesis for two staged cardiac replacement. Am J Cardiol 24:723, 1969.
25. Hill JC, Farran DJ, Hushen JJ, et al: Use of a prosthetic ventricle as a bridge to cardiac transplantation for post infarction cardiogenic shock. N Engl J Med 314:626, 1986.
26. Levinson MM, Smith RG, Cork RC: Three recent cases of total artificial heart prior to transplantation. Heart Transplant 5:170, 1984.
27. Hill JP: Bridging to cardiac transplantation. Ann Thorac Surg 47:167, 1989.
28. Joyce LD, Emery RW, Cales F, et al: Mechanical circulatory support as a bridge to transplantation. J Thorac Cardiovas Surg 98:935, 1989.
29. Pennock JL, Pierce WS, Campbell DB, et al: Mechanical support of the circulation followed by cardiac transplantation. J Thorac Cardiovasc Surg 92:994, 1986.
30. Bolman RM, Cox JL, Marshall W, et al: Circulatory support with a centrifugal pump as a bridge to cardiac transplantation. Ann Thorac Surg 47:108, 1989.
31. Griffith BP: Interim use of the Jarvik-7 artificial heart: Lessons learned at Presbyterian-University Hospital of Pittsburgh. Ann Thorac Surg 47:158, 1989.
32. Muneretto C, Solis E, Pavic A, Leger PH: Total artificial heart: Survival and complications. Ann Thorac Surg 47:151, 1989.

33. Portner PM, Oyer PE, Pennington DG, et al: Implantable electrical left ventricular assist system: Bridge to transplantation and the future. Ann Thorac Surg 47:142, 1989.
34. Davis PK, Rosenberg G, Snyder AJ, Pierce WS: Current status of permanent total artificial hearts. Ann Thorac Surg 47:172, 1989.
35. Kochamba G, Chiu RC-J: The physiologic characteristics of transformed skeletal muscle for cardiac assist. Trans Am Soc Artif Intern Organs 33:404, 1987.
36. Walsh G, Chiu RC-J: Skeletal muscle for cardiac repair and assist: A historical review, in Chiu RC-J (ed): *Biomechanical Cardiac Assist: Cardiomyoplasty and Muscle Powered Devices*. Mount Kisco, NY, Futura, 1986, p 1.
37. Brister SJ, Fradet G, Dewar M, et al: Transforming skeletal muscle for myocardial assist: A feasibility study. Can J Surg 28(4):341, 1985.
38. Mannion JD, Hammond R, Stephenson LW: Hydraulic pouches of canine latissimus dorsi potential for left ventricular assistance. J Thorac Cardiovasc Surg 91:534, 1986.
39. Nielson IR, Brister SJ, Khalafalla AS, Chiu RC-J: Left ventricular assistance in dogs using a skeletal muscle powered device for diastolic augmentation. Heart Transplant 4:343, 1985.
40. Carpentier A, Chachques JC: The use of stimulated skeletal muscle to replace diseased human heart muscle, in Chiu RC-J(ed): *Biomechanical Cardiac Assist: Cardiomyopathy and Muscle Powered Devices*. Mount Kisco, NY, Futura, 1986, p 85.
41. Magovern GJ, Heckler FR, Park SB, et al: Paced skeletal muscle for dynamic cardiomyoplasty. Ann Thorac Surg 45:614, 1988.

Chapter 29

EXTRACORPOREAL MEMBRANE OXYGENATION AND CO_2 REMOVAL

JACOB IASHA SZNAJDER
ALAN H. MORRIS

Extracorporeal systems with access to the systemic circulation are used frequently in medicine. One very common application is hemodialysis, used to remove toxic waste products. Other extracorporeal systems that remove "unwanted" metabolites or other blood components include plasmapheresis, leukopheresis, hemofiltration, and extracorporeal carbon dioxide removal ($ECCO_2R$). Methods for delivering substances into the circulation are also used, such as insulin infusion pumps, extracorporeal membrane oxygenators, intravascular oxygenators, and again, $ECCO_2R$. This chapter will focus on the critical care uses of extracorporeal oxygenators, the intravenacaval hollow-fiber oxygenator, and CO_2 removers.

Extracorporeal bubble and membrane oxygenators are used in all open heart surgery procedures. Their use has increased significantly with the introduction of coronary artery bypass graft and heart and lung transplant surgery. These devices are also used to support gas exchange during bilateral lung lavage in the treatment of severe alveolar proteinosis, and more recently with operations to remove thrombi from the pulmonary circulation in the treatment of chronic pulmonary embolism. During surgery these systems provide total cardiopulmonary bypass with no blood flow to the natural heart and lungs for minutes to a few hours. During prolonged procedures extracorporeal membrane oxygenation (ECMO) is preferred over bubble oxygenators because the risk of air embolism and bleeding appears to be reduced. The tolerance of the natural lung to ischemia is a controversial subject. The risk of ischemia-reperfusion injury of the natural lung is real. The lung is somewhat protected against ischemia-reperfusion injury because of its double circulation, but in animal models there is evidence of significant lung injury and deterioration in gas exchange after 4 h of ischemia. Therefore, most forms of ECMO use partial heart-lung bypass.

Clinical Results of Extracorporeal Support

VENOARTERIAL ECMO STUDIES

Studies in Adults

In the mid 1950s it was first shown that gas exchange can be achieved for short periods of time with cardiopulmonary bypass.[1] In the 1960s, the feasibility of long-term cardiopulmonary support for open heart surgery and for treatment of hyaline membrane disease in neonates was established. Successful treatment of patients with acute hypoxemic respiratory failure (AHRF) with venoarterial extracorporeal membrane oxygenation (VA ECMO) was first reported in 1972.[2] Between 1974 and 1977, the National Heart Lung and Blood Institute supported a randomized, prospective, clinical trial of ECMO in 90 patients (12 to 65 years old) from nine medical centers who had the adult respiratory distress syndrome (ARDS) of less than 3 weeks' duration. The blood-gas entry criteria included "slow entry" patients (12 h of $Pa_{O_2} \leq 50$ mmHg, fraction inspired oxygen [FI_{O_2}] $\geq$ 0.6 and positive end-expiratory pressure [PEEP] $\geq$ 5 cmH_2O after 48 h of ICU care), and "rapid entry" patients (2 h of $Pa_{O_2} \leq 50$ mmHg, $FI_{O_2} = 1.0$ and PEEP $\geq$ 5 cmH_2O). Only 9 percent of patients with severe ARDS survived, and the survival rates were the same in VA ECMO and control patients.[3,4] These results halted widespread clinical application of VA ECMO in adults.

Neonatal Clinical Experience

VA ECMO has been used extensively in neonates with the neonatal respiratory distress syndrome (RDS) with significant success. It has been postulated that the higher survival rates in neonatal ECMO as compared to adults is due in part to the uniformity of technology and personnel training (modeled after the pioneering program at the University of Michigan). Further, RDS is different from the multietiologic ARDS and has a larger salvageable population (e.g., no terminal carcinomas or overwhelming postsurgical sepsis).[5–7] Finally, the neonatal lung heals after RDS, not only by scarring and repair, but also with maturation and growth. In several nonrandomized and uncontrolled clinical trials in patients with a predicted survival rate of 20 percent (by historical controls), treatment with VA ECMO resulted in a survival rate close to 80 percent.[6,7] However, nonrandomized studies using historical controls have limitations. Two studies have been conducted using randomization. In one, a "play-the-winner" approach was adopted, wherein the first patient had equal chances to be assigned to ECMO or conventional therapy.[7,8] Assignment of subsequent patients was determined by success or failure of the previous therapy. The first patient received conventional therapy and died, and the next 11 patients were treated with ECMO and survived. Another randomized controlled clinical trial of ECMO and conventional therapy addressed the ethical concerns regarding therapies which might prove to have very different survivals, and permitted only four deaths in either arm of the study.[9] During the randomized phase of the trial 6 of the 10 conventionally treated patients survived, whereas all 9 of the ECMO treated patients survived. During the subsequent, nonrandomized phase of the study 19 to 20 patients treated with ECMO survived the acute phase.

Simultaneously with the ECMO clinical trials in the pediatric population, changes were also introduced in the armamentarium of "conventional" therapy. In children with pulmonary hypertension, the combination of pharmacologic paralysis, hyperventilation, and the pulmonary vasodilator tolazoline resulted in survival rates of 50 to 65 percent.[10] Some centers that did not develop ECMO programs also compared their survival rates to ECMO-treated patients and reported survival rates of 60 to 90 percent in the late 1980s using entry criteria which predicted an 80 percent mortality.[9,11,12] The marked differences in reported survival rates have been attributed to improvements in conventional therapy, but they underscore the need for carefully controlled randomized clinical trials.

Although survival rates in both ECMO and conventional treatment groups are encouraging, attention should also be directed to long-term morbidity. In the ECMO-treated patients the carotid artery and jugular veins are ligated and several studies have reported subsequent motor abnormalities and cerebral atrophy. The ECMO registry reported up to a 25 percent incidence of neurologic sequelae in children after ECMO therapy,[13] and other investigators found that 45 percent of 145 ECMO survivors had intracranial abnormalities assessed by neurologic imaging studies.[14] These lesions were distributed on both sides without correlation to the arterial ligation site. In patients treated with conventional therapy, about 50 percent also had neurodevelopmental impairment.[15] Although there are no conclusive data on the incidence of chronic lung disease after ECMO or conventional therapy in neonates with respiratory failure, it is estimated to be as high as 10 percent.[13] A comparison of hospital charges revealed that ECMO was 43 percent less costly than conventional therapy, although the per diem charges for this latter group are 57 percent less than for the ECMO-treated babies.[16] The reduced total cost with ECMO was due to a reduction in the average length of stay.

Despite several unanswered questions, the American Academy of Pediatrics acknowledges that ECMO is an acceptable therapeutic alternative[17] and recommends that it be limited to centers with an established referral base, an adequate number of subspecialties, and an established record of research. As of 1988, 37 centers in the United States reported that 715 patients had been treated with ECMO and 81 percent survived the acute phase.[13]

VENOVENOUS ECMO AND $ECCO_2R$

Venovenous ECMO

Venovenous (VV) ECMO and VA ECMO are similar in the technical aspects and required support personnel. The major technical difference is that VV ECMO does not require arterial cannulation, which greatly reduces the risks of bleeding, systemic thromboembolism, and hemodynamic instability. It is also substantially less complicated surgically. In VV ECMO (Fig. 29-1), a large catheter with several side holes is inserted via the femoral vein into the inferior vena cava, and venous blood is drained by gravity. Blood is then pumped through the membrane oxygenator and returned through a cannula inserted into the other femoral vein. The return catheter is advanced near to the right atrium but far away from the "draining" catheter to avoid recirculation. Thus, there is no bypass of the pulmonary circulation which still receives all the cardiac output. One-quarter to one-half the cardiac output passes through one or two membrane oxygenators to remove CO_2 and add O_2.

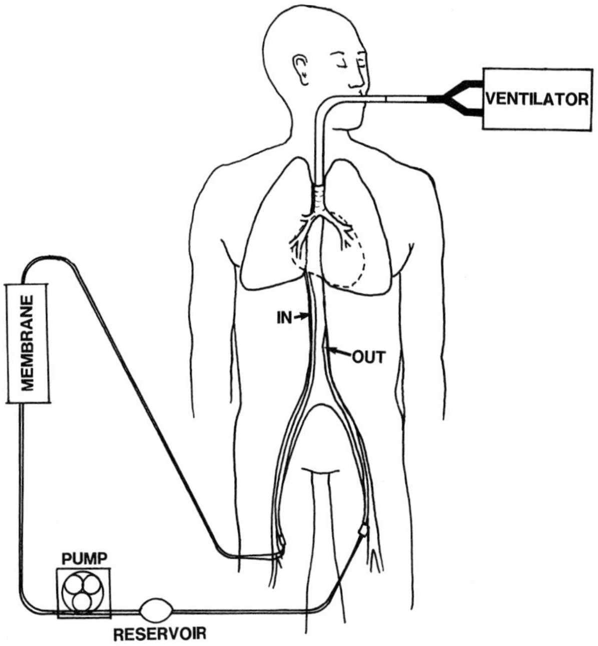

FIGURE 29-1 This diagram schematically depicts the ECMO circuit. During VV ECMO the outflow cannula is placed through the femoral vein into the inferior vena cava, whereas the inflow line is placed near the right atrium in such a way as to avoid recirculation.

Clinical Use of $ECCO_2R$

This technique was first described in the treatment of adults with ARDS. The investigators used VV ECMO primarily to remove CO_2, thus diminishing the need for alveolar ventilation. In this uncontrolled study the respiratory frequency was reduced from the usual 20 or more breaths/min to 4 breaths/min, and the peak airway pressure was limited to 45 cmH_2O, allowing the lungs to "rest." In these patients with severe ARDS, the survival rate was 49 percent, contrasting markedly with the historical survival rate of 9 percent.[18]

In Europe more than 200 patients have been supported with $ECCO_2R$, with a survival rate of approximately 50 percent, and 3 of 6 patients with ARDS and severe barotrauma have survived in the United States.[5,19]

THE LDS HOSPITAL TRIAL. A randomized, prospective, NIH-supported, single center clinical trial is currently being carried out at the Shock Trauma/Intermountain Respiratory ICU at the LDS Hospital, University of Utah.[20] Patients are randomly assigned to a traditional therapy group (continuous positive-pressure ventilation) or to a three-step therapeutic program.[18] This sequential three-step approach uses: **1.** pressure-controlled inverse ratio ventilation (PC-IRV), **2.** continuous positive airway pressure (CPAP) if the patient improves with PC-IRV, and **3.** low frequency positive-pressure ventilation with extracorporeal CO_2 removal (LFPPV-$ECCO_2R$) if the patient does not improve with PC-IRV. The goal is ventilation with respiratory rates of 2 to 4 breaths/min, peak airway pressures of up to 35 cmH_2O and an $F_{IO_2} < 0.6$.

Patients with ARDS meeting criteria for the $ECCO_2R$ trial and without $ECCO_2R$ exclusions are enrolled after signing informed consent. The $ECCO_2R$ exclusion criteria ensure that enrolled patients will not have underlying conditions, other than ARDS, which would preclude survival. This study plans to randomize 60 patients with stratification by age (≤ or >40 years) and history of trauma. At this early stage, the overall survival rate is 39 percent in both $ECCO_2R$ and conventional therapy groups.[20]

PROTOCOL CONTROL OF THERAPY. Patient care can vary not only between hospitals, but between ICUs within a hospital, between attending physicians within an ICU, and between patients cared for by the same resident-attending physician team. This lack of uniformity may confound the interpretation of much ARDS research. Application of clinical care protocols may alleviate some of these problems and document more precisely the standard of care. These protocols themselves may have an impact on outcome and are described in more detail in Chap. 41. The investigators at the LDS hospital established protocol-controlled uniformity of care, with equal intensity and frequency of monitoring, and consistent management decisions for ARDS patients randomized to the two different therapies of their clinical trial. Respiratory therapy for both traditional therapy and PC-IRV plus LFPPV-$ECCO_2R$ is guided by specific protocols. Paper-based flow diagrams (see Chap. 41), outline the directions for therapy, followed by a nurse, a respiratory therapist, or a physician. The flow diagram protocols meet four basic investigative needs of the clinical trial.

1. Use of uniform logic in decision-making
2. Examination of a uniform data base for decision-making
3. Equal frequency of monitoring
4. Equal intensity of care for all patients

The requirement to ensure uniformity of care for patients supported by the two therapeutic modalities is being achieved, and the flow diagram protocols have been applied for >27,000 h of care (representing approximately 25,000 bedside therapy decisions). The protocols successfully control therapy 94 percent of the time (there is an obligate fraction of time during which protocols must be suspended as a result of surgery, diagnostic procedures such as computed tomography scanning, or treatment procedures such as chest tube placement).

Rationale and Potential Pitfalls of Extracorporeal Support

BAROTRAUMA AND "RESTING" THE LUNGS

The rationale of all ECMO modalities is based on the fact that in ARDS the lungs become "stiffer" or "smaller" because part of their volume previously available for gas exchange is filled with proteinaceous-bloody fluid.[21] Ventilating with nominally "normal" tidal volumes of 10 to 12 mL/kg could overdistend areas of relatively normal and compliant lung, increasing the risk of barotrauma. The concept of barotrauma in this setting includes not only the traditional concepts of gas leakage from the parenchyma into adjacent spaces as seen in patients with pneumothorax or pneumomediastinum, but also parenchymal lung injury with capillary leak and high permeability pulmonary edema.[22,23] In ARDS lung injury is heterogeneous, with both flooded and normal alveoli coexisting within the same lobe.[21] Applying increased pressure to the whole lung (usually 50 to 70 cmH_2O in a patient with severe ARDS) may not reopen damaged, "unrecruitable" alveoli but rather may overdistend relatively normal and more compliant alveoli, worsening the overall lung damage. Studies in normal goats, sheep, and rats have shown that ventilation for up to 2 weeks with low peak pressures does not result in lung injury. However, ventilation with high tidal volumes and pressures results in pulmonary edema and severe hypoxemia after 24 h in sheep and after 20 min in rats.[22,23] One study in normal rats further demonstrated that tidal volume excursions rather than the peak pressures are probably responsible for the lung edema.[23] In the canine acid aspiration model of AHRF, it was shown that ventilation with high tidal volumes and low PEEP results in more edema formation than ventilating with small tidal volumes and high PEEP, although the plateau elastic airway pressure was similar in these two animal groups.[24]

ANIMAL STUDIES WITH VENOARTERIAL ECMO

In unanesthetized lambs and patients undergoing coronary surgery, the use of extracorporeal circulation does not influence lung fluid dynamics or result in increased extravascular lung water,[25] although VA ECMO has been reported to activate complement and promote neutrophil degranulation. In dogs undergoing cardiopulmonary bypass with the bubble oxygenator, other investigators have found increased lung neutrophil sequestration and increased tissue peroxidation. In a canine model of AHRF, early (1 h after induction of lung injury with intratracheal instillation of kerosene) VA ECMO reduced the pulmonary blood flow by 30 percent and the pulmonary capillary wedge pressure

(Ppw) from 10 to 5 mmHg.[26] After 4 h of ECMO treatment the animals had 50 percent less edema than a control group of dogs maintained at Ppw of 10 mmHg. However, in an oleic acid canine lung injury model where VA ECMO was started after edema was fully established, reduction of pulmonary blood flow and Ppw did not affect edema or gas exchange.

These animal studies suggest that VA ECMO probably does not injure normal lungs and if applied early in the exudative phase of lung injury may help in reducing edema and improving gas exchange. However, no definitive human data concerning these points are available.

INCREASED PULMONARY SHUNT DURING VENOVENOUS ECMO

A potential drawback in treating patients with AHRF with LFPPV-$ECCO_2R$ is suggested from studies in animal models of lung injury. In a canine hydrochloric acid aspiration model, increasing the oxygenation of the mixed venous blood with VV ECMO reduced pulmonary artery pressure, probably by blocking hypoxic vasoconstriction.[27] This was associated with a higher shunt than in control animals without VV ECMO. Conceivably, VV ECMO increases perfusion to nonventilated alveoli by raising mixed venous oxygen saturation, thereby relieving hypoxic vasoconstriction. Perfusion of more injured areas of the lung could also increase pulmonary capillary leak and enhance lung edema. Since these changes were observed during acute injury in an animal model, it could be argued that after several days in patients with ARDS, hypoxic vasoconstriction is less important. Therefore, the potentially detrimental effects of increased mixed venous oxygen saturation would be less important.

Methodologic Aspects

VA ECMO is the most frequently used extracorporeal system during open heart surgery. The heart is arrested and almost all of the cardiac output bypasses the natural heart and lungs. In patients with ARDS where the heart and lungs are only partly bypassed, the withdrawal cannula is usually inserted through the right internal jugular or femoral vein with the tip sitting close to the right atrium. The return-oxygenated blood is delivered at the aortic root by a cannula inserted in the carotid, axillary, or femoral artery. Care is taken to place the return cannula such that the carotid artery is not bypassed and blood supply to the brain is adequate. In adults No. 28 French drainage and No. 22 French reinfusion cannulae are normally used. The drainage cannula has multiple side holes and rounded tips. The connecting catheters are thin walled to minimize hydraulic resistance. The tubing bringing the blood to and from the membrane oxygenator is usually medical grade polyvinylchloride with polycarbonate connectors. Silicone rubber tubing is also used but it is significantly more expensive. Most centers using this technology outside the operating room employ the Sci-Med spiral membrane oxygenator although other membrane lungs manufactured by Sarns and Travenol are also being used. Some of the membrane oxygenators have incorporated a countercurrent heat exchanger within the oxygenator; others have the heat exchanger in series within the circuit. In VV ECMO or $ECCO_2R$, the circuit is similar but both inflow and outflow cannulae are placed through the femoral veins and advanced to the inferior vena cava, taking care to place the inflow line close to the right atrium to avoid recirculation. The membrane oxygenators have microporous polypropylene or nonporous silicone rubber membrane envelopes wound in tight spirals. The interior of the envelope has a gas compartment. Blood flows into a dispersal manifold and passes between the envelope layers. Oxygen from the gas compartment diffuses across the membrane into the bloodstream. Carbon dioxide diffuses across the membrane from the bloodstream into the gas compartment and is flushed from the oxygenator by the gas flow. Thus, the gas and bloodstreams flow in opposite directions (countercurrent flow) and the rate of O_2 and CO_2 exchange is highly dependent on their flow rates.

The gas exchange capacity of a membrane oxygenator is limited. The human lung has a surface area for gas exchange of approximately 70 m^2, whereas the membrane oxygenator surface area ranges from 1 to 5 m^2. The thin portions of human alveoli have a blood-alveolar barrier of around 0.6 μm, whereas the blood-gas barrier of membrane oxygenators is between 70 and 200 μm. The human lung can achieve a maximum transfer of O_2 and CO_2 of >2500 mL/min while the maximum transfer of O_2 and CO_2 of a typical membrane oxygenator is 200 to 400 mL/min.

The VA ECMO circuit utilizes roller or centrifugal pumps to propel the blood from the venous drainage site through the membrane oxygenator and into the aortic root. Roller pumps propel blood in a pulsatile manner by intermittent compression of the tubing. These pumps are less expensive than centrifugal pumps but induce significant cumulative wear on the tubing which lies beneath the rotating roller heads and represents the most frequent cause of breakdown. Some programs mount two roller pumps in parallel so that wear is distributed and the tubing under one rolling head or the complete roller pump can be replaced while the ECMO circuit is in operation. Other programs that use one pump rotate the tubing periodically to diminish wear.

The centrifugal circuit consists of a pump and disposable pump heads of variable capacity and generates flow by magnetic coupling of the pump head to the console. The resultant flow (measured by a calibrated flow probe placed on-line between the pump and the lung) is nonpulsatile and demand responsive. Thus, the pump automatically responds to both the resistance against which it is pumping and to venous return with appropriate changes in flow and pressure. These pumps were proposed to be more safe because they "stall" and do not generate suction or high outflow pressures when the circuit gets inadvertently occluded. However, hemolysis and damage to other blood cells can be greater with the centrifugal pump system. The cost of the centrifugal pumps is higher than the roller pumps and the disposable pump head ($250 cost) should be changed with each patient (for short procedures) or after 24 to 48 h of operation (for longer term use). During ECMO and other extracorporeal circulation techniques, frequent monitoring of activated clotting time (ACT) is necessary. The ACT should be maintained at 150 to 250 s by continuous infusion of heparin. Newer catheters coated with heparin are also being introduced as part of the circuit, but ACT should still be followed closely when administration of blood, platelet concentrates, fresh frozen plasma, or cryoprecipitate is necessary, because these may lower the ACT abruptly and cause thrombosis within the extracorporeal circuit. However, despite close monitoring of ACT and even with normal-low ACT values, bleeding continues to be a major problem in most ECMO operating centers.

It is difficult to accurately determine the cardiac output during VA ECMO because of the "steal" effect of the cannulae placed at the right atrium and the mixing of the left ventricular output with the returning, oxygenated, extracorporeal flow.

As Fig. 29-2 shows, "hosting" an ECMO facility requires a significant commitment of personnel, economic resources, and dedicated space. Also, it is very important to have access to a significant patient referral base. The centers that perform ECMO outside the operating room usually designate a spacious room at least 20 by 15 feet with extra AC, gas, and vacuum outlets, with dedicated telephone lines and quick access to the operating room. The room is ideally within the ICU structure, although away from main traffic so as to reduce infection risk and control access of visitors.

Operation of these complex circuits in the operating room, and especially in critically ill patients in the ICU, requires the assembly of technologic and human resources including nurses, perfusionists, technologists, social workers, and physicians. Table 29-1 depicts approximate charges of starting and operating ECMO, which may vary from $6,000 to as high as $20,000 daily in the presence of complications, with an average of around $80,000 to $100,000/patient. Also, it includes specialized personnel dedicated to the extracorporeal program. This is reflected by the fact that only a few centers can afford to establish these programs in the ICU setting.

Complications during ECMO (Table 29-2)

HEMORRHAGE

Bleeding due to disseminated intravascular coagulation (DIC), thrombocytopenia, or over-anticoagulation can occur in patients treated with ECMO. Infusion of heparin to maintain a high ACT can also result in bleeding. Bleeding usually occurs at the site of cannulation, or where trauma has been sustained, particularly in association with chest tubes. Bleeding is usually treated with fresh frozen plasma,

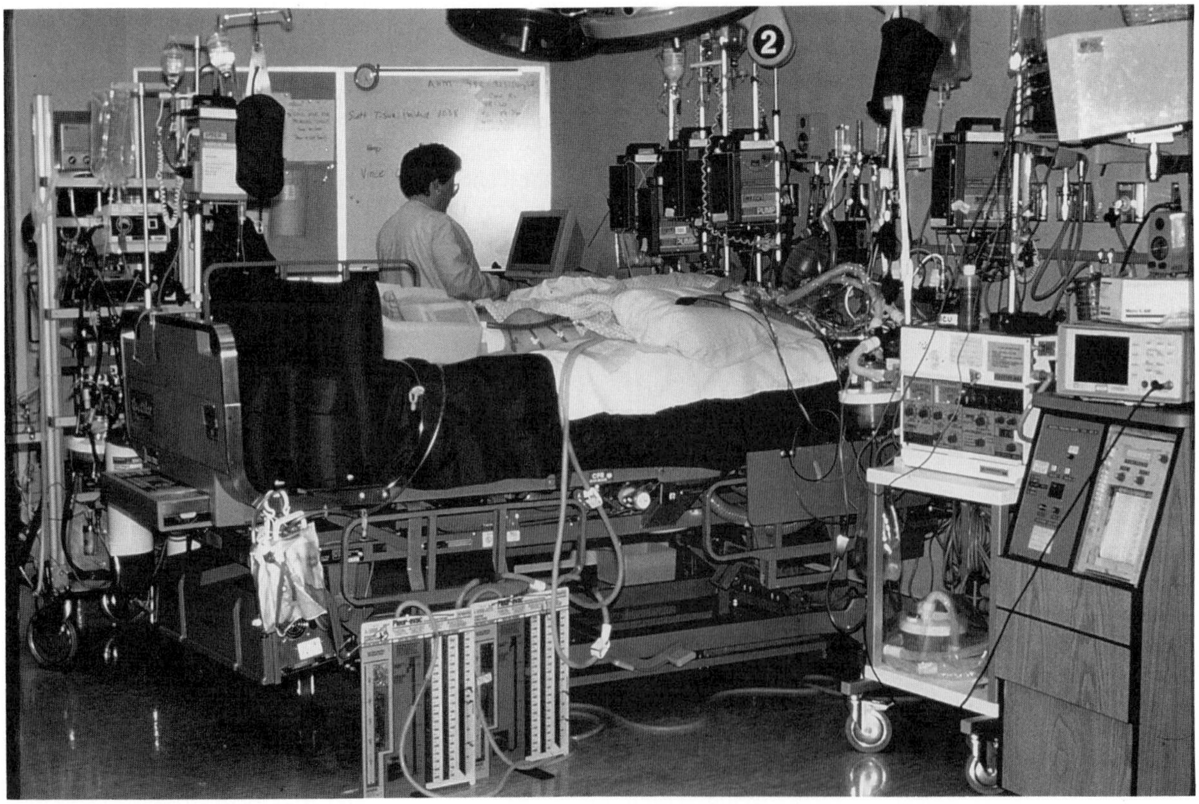

FIGURE 29-2 An ECMO facility.

TABLE 29-1 Approximate 1990 Charges of Operating ECMO

Personnel	
Anesthesia fee for cannulation	$ 950
Surgery for cannulation	$2,000
Circuit operation by perfusionist	$1,000
Nursing management	$1,000
Physician management	$1,400
Hospital Fees	
Operating room	$2,300
ICU fees	$1,250
Equipment	
Roller pump (two)	$8,000
or centrifugal pump	$7,000
Heater/cooler	$4,000
ACT tester	$1,800
Lab Products and Tests	
Blood	$140/500 mL
Fresh frozen plasma	$ 87/300 mL
Platelets	$430/10 unit
Antibiotics	$380/day
Drugs (miscellaneous)	$420/day
Blood-gas measurements (15/day $42/sample)	$630/day
Data base—chemistry and CBC	$182/day
Blood and other cultures	$175/day
Disposables	
Membrane oxygenators	$860 2/day
Hemofilter	$82 1/day
Tubing connectors, reservoir bags, gloves, cannulas	$380
Centrifugal pump head	$250/day

TABLE 29-2 Potential Complications during ECMO

Hemorrhage
Tubing obstruction
Tubing fracture leading to hemorrhage, air embolism
Air embolism from malfunctioning stopcocks
Pulmonary embolism
Thrombus formation
Bleeding caused by DIC or thrombocytopenia
Hemolysis caused by the pump
Neurologic damage due to bleeding or systemic embolism
Infection and sepsis

platelets, and red blood cells. When the fibrinogen levels fall to below 150 mg/dL, cryoprecipitate should be used.

TUBING OBSTRUCTION

Tubing obstruction is a potentially severe problem. If a roller pump is in use and the obstruction is not immediately corrected, the tubing or membrane may rupture, risking air embolization and blood loss with dangerous hemodynamic consequences. Also, discrete tubing fracture may be caused by overocclusion of the roller pump or prolonged use and wear. Usually, complications due to tubing fracture can be avoided by switching to the alternate circuitry and isolating and replacing the ruptured tubing.

AIR EMBOLIZATION

Air embolization can be a serious complication if the extracorporeal circuit is not primed correctly or if air bubbles arise from malfunctioning connections, stopcocks, tubing, or an incompletely flushed reservoir. Therefore, in most programs the stopcocks are positioned in areas within the circuit where blood pressure is significantly greater than the atmospheric pressure, thus reducing the risk of air entrainment.

THROMBUS FORMATION

Thrombus formation within the ECMO circuit can occur because of inadequate heparinization or when a malfunctioning membrane activates clotting factors. Clots usually form within the dispersal manifolds of the membrane, in the internal blood surfaces of the membrane lung envelope, and within large reservoir bags. Regions of stagnant blood are likely sites for blocking.

HEMOLYSIS

Hemolysis is seen with both roller and centrifugal pumps and is due to the exposure of erythrocytes to high shear forces at the cannulae tips and other regions of the circuit. An overocclusive roller pump will increase the rate of hemolysis. Levels of up to 10 mg/dL of plasma free hemoglobin are commonly observed due to erythrolysis during ECMO. Levels should not exceed 15 mg/dL.

STROKE

Severe neurologic damage may be caused by intracerebral bleeding and thromboembolic phenomena. Neurologic damage may be overlooked because patients are usually sedated and paralyzed. These complications are less frequently observed in the adult population (VV ECMO) compared to neonatal RDS patients (VA ECMO).

INFECTION

Infection and sepsis may also occur and may require stopping ECMO when uncontrollable. Sepsis is diagnosed when there is a raised white blood cell count, lactic acidosis, and hemodynamic deterioration with a fall in arterial blood pressure and systemic vascular resistance.

Other Less Common Gas Exchange Systems

$ECCO_2R$ WITHOUT OXYGENATION

Peritoneal or hemodialysis with CO_2 removal by alkali administration during apnea has been investigated in normal animals and used in newborns with respiratory failure.[28,29] This procedure is at an experimental stage; for adults, the potential overload of sodium during the infusion of alkali may limit its use.

ARTERIOVENOUS (AV) ECMO

With AV ECMO, blood flows from the arterial side and through the oxygenator before returning to the venous side. This method does not require a pump to drive blood flow, since the AV pressure gradient is sufficient. Nevertheless, the maximal oxygen transfer in the pumpless system is estimated to be only 30 mL/min. In the past this technique was tried unsuccessfully in children and it is not used currently for oxygenation or CO_2 removal in clinical practice. In adults the AV pumping system is commonly used for hemofiltration and hemodialysis.

VENOVENOUS INTRAVENACAVAL OXYGENATOR (IVOX)

An intravenous hollow-fiber oxygenator has recently been designed.[30] This device consists of a large number of small diameter, elongated hollow fibers mounted in parallel within an intravenous catheter. This intravenacaval oxygenator (IVOX) is inserted into the vena cava through a peripheral venotomy and simplifies the complex setup and instrumentation of other extracorporeal circulation techniques. After insertion, the device is twisted and the fibers become unfurled. Venous blood in the vena cava flows around the fibers, while O_2 is pumped through the fibers at subatmospheric pressure. The IVOX device allows up to 150 mL/min of O_2 to be transferred into the blood and up to 120 mL/min of CO_2 to be removed from the venous circulation. The safety and applicability of IVOX have been tested in more than 70 normal, awake sheep for periods of up to 19 days without apparent deleterious effects on hemodynamics, coagulation, or metabolic parameters. Gas exchange did not deteriorate during 7 days of continuous IVOX testing, and the device normalized gas exchange in animals made hypoxemic or hypercapnic. Currently, a phase I clinical trial in patients with respiratory failure is underway in four medical centers in the United States. The use of IVOX in the first patient with ARDS has been reported recently.[31]

Perspective

To introduce a new therapy that involves invasive technology can have enormous medicolegal, ethical, and economic ramifications. This is especially true for patients who are seriously ill and unable to consent to, question, or refuse therapy. In these cases it is medically and ethically obligatory to provide the standard or accepted therapy.[32] In the case of ECMO, clinicians started in an uncontrolled way treating desperately ill, almost moribund patients, with the hope that reducing the blood flow through the lungs would decrease their "work load" and allow them to recover. Use of VA ECMO was then expanded to many patients with ARDS, a common, yet poorly defined syndrome. ECMO seemed a reasonable attempt to salvage critically ill patients, since those who survive often go on to almost complete recovery of lung function.[33] However, VA ECMO in adults with ARDS proved ineffective, when submitted to a carefully controlled, multicenter, prospective clinical trial.[3] As of 1990, it appears that no medical centers in the United States routinely use VA ECMO in adults other than during open heart surgery. However, in the pediatric field VA ECMO is accepted by the American Academy of Pediatrics[17] as one of the therapeutic options in the treatment of neonates with respiratory failure, including pulmonary hypertension, sepsis, congenital diaphragmatic hernia, meconium aspiration, and RDS.

ECMO achieved its status in the therapy of neonates with respiratory failure without satisfying ideal, rigorous, randomized norms of research that many believe should govern the development of new medical therapy. The process by which this therapeutic modality is coming of age is not so unusual. ECMO emerged as part of standard pediatric medical care with some degree of uncertainty and with the limitations and the complexity of the clinical and ethical options that this therapy raised.[6] Now it provides access to invasive, potentially efficacious, and also potentially harmful treatment, allowing the physicians, patients, and their families to have choices in situations when no therapies are obviously preferable.

The utilization of historical controls is a serious limitation of most ECMO studies, although data from uncontrolled adult studies has made a randomized clinical trial possible by establishing a high probability that the new therapy is effective. The absence of standardized therapy for ARDS is another limitation in evaluating ECMO. For example, in pediatric pulmonary hypertension there was no conventional therapy established. "Conventional" therapy evolved simultaneously with the development of ECMO. It is therefore difficult to determine which alternative, ECMO or "conventional" should be considered experimental or standard therapy, which should require consent for research, and which should be obligatory. This was illustrated in an extreme case when investigators were accused in a newspaper of denying life-saving therapy to infants who were not treated with VA ECMO.[34]

Another limitation is the difficulty in comparing survivals of ECMO-treated neonates with other therapies where the "whole" outcome question is not easily comparable. As previously mentioned, ECMO may be "cheaper" and have better short-term survival than conventional therapy in neonates. However, the risk of long-term neurologic damage, stroke, and chronic lung disease may be worse in ECMO survivors. Therefore, it is unclear whether research will prove unequivocally that one therapy is better than another. Rather it can help to delineate the relative risks and benefits of the alternative approaches. This approach in neonates supports clinical judgments and helps clinicians as they work with patients and their families in evaluating the treatment recommendations. It is becoming more accepted that ECMO and conventional therapy in neonates with respiratory failure are not mutually exclusive. Rather, the focus is on how to maximize the available therapeutic resources to benefit neonates with specific clinical problems.

This "pragmatic" approach used in the clinical introduction of ECMO contrasts with what scientists would consider ideal for introducing new therapy. This ideal requires that careful controlled prospective trials establish the risk and benefit of the proposed therapy. A controlled clinical trial of a new therapy showing its benefit can establish whether this therapy can be considered standard, ethically and legally acceptable rather than experimental. Both in the adult and especially in the pediatric arena, ECMO therapy points out the weaknesses of this approach in clinical research, where the gold standard is prospective controlled clinical trials.[35,36] An alternative approach where medical sense can accept a reasonable degree of uncertainty will depend on how investigators, their patients, the medical community, insurance companies, and policy makers may view this issue.

In adult medicine more than a decade after the VA ECMO clinical trial, $ECCO_2R$ has also been introduced in an uncontrolled way. The drive to develop this modality was based on physiologic effects, clinical relevance, and feasibility. The early reports from Europe on survival when compared to historical controls and the survival of patients treated with VA ECMO were encouraging.[18] The struggle to scientifically define the role of this new modality in the treatment of ARDS stimulated the carefully designed, controlled, prospective clinical trial described above.[20] Now $ECCO_2R$ is undergoing an extensive evaluation in several centers in Europe and the United States. Although the final results of the uncontrolled clinical trials and the randomized trial are as yet inconclusive, it seems that $ECCO_2R$-treated patients have survival rates which are similar to those of conventionally (with the same "intensity" of care) treated patients. Therefore, it appears that $ECCO_2R$ might have a role in a very selected patient population in whom other therapies failed, as in the pediatric field.

References

1. Clowes GHA Jr, Hopkins AL, Neville WE: An artificial lung dependent upon diffusion of oxygen and carbon dioxide through plastic membranes. J Thorac Surg 32:630, 1956.
2. Hill JD, O'Brien TG, Murray JD, et al: Prolonged extracorporeal oxygenation for acute post-traumatic respiratory failure (shock-lung syndrome). N Engl J Med 286:629, 1972.
3. Zapol WM, Snider MT, Hill JD, et al: Extracorporeal membrane oxygenation in severe acute respiratory failure: A randomized prospective study. JAMA 242:2193, 1979.
4. Extracorporeal support for respiratory insufficiency: A collaborative study in response to RFP-NHLI 73-20. Bethesda, US Department of Health, Education and Welfare, National Institutes of Health, 1979.
5. Snider MT, Campbell DB, Kofke WA, et al: Venovenous perfusion of adults and children with severe acute respiratory distress syndrome—The Pennsylvania State University experience from 1982–1987. Trans Am Soc Artif Intern Organs 34:1014, 1988.
6. Lantos JD, Frader J: Extracorporeal membrane oxygenation and the ethics of clinical research in pediatrics. New Engl J Med 323:409, 1990.
7. Bartlett RH, Roloff DW, Cornell RG, et al: Extracorporeal circulation in neonatal respiratory failure: A prospective randomized study. Pediatrics 76:479, 1985.
8. Paneth N, Wallenstein S: Extracorporeal membrane oxygenation and the play-the winner rule. Editorial. Pediatrics 76:622, 1985.
9. O'Rourke PP, Crone RK, Vacanti JP, et al: Extracorporeal membrane oxygenation and conventional medical therapy in neonates with persistent pulmonary hypertension of the newborn: A prospective randomized study. Pediatrics 64:957, 1989.
10. Cohen RS, Stevenson DK, Malachowski N, et al: Late morbidity among survivors of respiratory failure treated with tolazoline. J Pediatr 97:644, 1980.
11. Dworetz AR, Moya FR, Sabo B, et al: Survival of infants with persistent pulmonary hypertension without extracorporeal membrane oxygenation. Pediatrics 84:1, 1989.
12. Nading JH: Historical controls for extracorporeal membrane oxygenation in neonates. Crit Care Med 17:423, 1989.
13. Toomasian JM, Snedecor SM, Cornell RG, et al: National experience with extracorporeal membrane oxygenation for newborn respiratory failure: Data from 715 cases. Trans Am Soc Artif Intern Organs 34:140, 1988.
14. Taylor GA, Fitz CR, Glass P, et al: CT of cerebrovascular injury after neonatal extracorporeal membrane oxygenation: Implications for neuro-developmental outcome. AJR 153:121, 1989.
15. Bifano EM, Pfannestiel A: Duration of hyperventilation and outcome in infants with persistent pulmonary hypertension. Pediatrics 81:657, 1988.
16. Pearson GD, Short BL: An economic analysis of extracorporeal membrane oxygenation. J Intensive Care Med 2:116, 1987.
17. Committee on Fetus and Newborn: Recommendations on extracorporeal membrane oxygenation. Pediatrics 85:618, 1990.
18. Gattinoni L, Pesenti A, Mascheroni D: Low-frequency positive-pressure ventilation with extracorporeal CO_2 removal in severe acute respiratory failure. JAMA 256:881, 1986.
19. Pesenti A, Gattinoni L, Kolobow T, et al: Extracorporeal circulation in adult respiratory failure. Trans Am Soc Artif Intern Organs 34:43, 1988.
20. Morris AH, Menlove RL, Rollins RJ, et al: A controlled clinical trial of a new 3-step therapy that includes extracorporeal CO_2 removal for ARDS. Trans Am Soc Artif Intern Organs 11:48, 1988.
21. Hall JB, Wood LDH: Pulmonary edema: in Cherniack R (ed): *Current Therapy in Respiratory Medicine.* Toronto, pp 222–227, 1986.
22. Kolobow T, Moretti MP, Fumagalli R, et al: Severe impairment in lung function induced by high peak airway pressure during mechanical ventilation. Am Rev Respir Dis 135:312, 1987.
23. Dreyfuss D, Soler P, Basset G, et al: High inflation pressure pulmonary edema. Respective effects of high airway pressure, high tidal volume, and positive end-expiratory pressure. Am Rev Respir Dis 137:1159, 1988.
24. Corbridge TC, Wood LDH, Crawford GP, et al: Adverse effects of large tidal volume and low PEEP in canine acid aspiration. Am Rev Respir Dis 142:311, 1990.
25. Delaney AG, Zapol WM, Erdmann AJ III: Lung transvascular fluid dynamics with extracorporeal membrane oxygenation in unanesthetized lambs. J Thorac Cardiovasc Surg 77:252, 1979.
26. Zucker AR, Wood LDH, Curet-Scott M, et al: Partial lung bypass reduces pulmonary edema induced by kerosene aspiration in dogs. J Crit Care (In press).
27. Yanos J, Presberg K, Crawford G, et al: The effect of hypoventi-

lation on low pressure pulmonary edema. Am Rev Respir Dis 142:316, 1990.

28. Chang BS, Garella S: Complete extracorporeal removal of metabolic carbon dioxide by alkali administration and dialysis in apnea. Int J Artif Organs 6:295, 1983.
29. Nolte SH, Jonitz WJ, Grau J, et al: Hemodialysis for extracorporeal bicarbonate/CO_2 removal (ECBicCO_2R) and apneic oxygenation for respiratory failure in the newborn. Trans Am Soc Artif Intern Organs 35:30, 1989.
30. Mortensen JD: An intravenacaval blood gas exchange (IVCBGE) device: A preliminary report. Trans Am Soc Artif Intern Organs 33:570, 1987.
31. York DP, Clemmer TP, Orme JF, et al: The first human use of an intracorporeal gas exchange device (IVOX). Chest 98:75S, 1990.
32. Levine RJ: *Ethics and Regulation of Clinical Research.* 2d ed. Baltimore, Urban & Schwarzengerg, 1986.
33. Elliot CG, Rasmusson BY, Crapo RO, et al: Prediction of pulmonary function abnormalities after adult respiratory distress syndrome. Am Rev Respir Dis 136:634, 1987.
34. Knox RA: A Harvard study on newborns draws fire: Doctors faulted for limiting life-saving therapy. Boston Globe, August 7, 1989, p 25.
35. Jonsen AR: Research involving children: Recommendations of the National Commission for the Protection of Human Subjects of Biomedical and Behavioral Research. Pediatrics 62:131, 1978.
36. Chalmers TC: A belated randomized control trial. Pediatrics 85:366, 1990.

Chapter 30

ELECTROCARDIOGRAPHY

RORY CHILDERS

Technological Considerations

In broad terms, the electrocardiograph (ECG) machine housed in an ICU (a mandatory item) is either "free-wheeling" or computer-linked. Nurses and house staff tend to prefer the former over the latter. The unlinked device is unconcerned with patient identity, will perform under the most adverse circumstances, and can tolerate all manner of physical abuse. But the price paid for this durability can be substantial. Tracings are often unlabelled as to time and date; not infrequently, they remain anonymous. Moreover, since they are recorded by residents or nurses, there is no routine for their processing, storage, billing, and above all, professional interpretation in light of previous tracings. Thus, tracings are often lost and seldom recovered. The adverse circumstances alluded to above are often simply poor or sloppy application of the ten electrodes, thereby ensuring a defective recording. On the other hand, a computer-linked ECG device will ensure permanent storage, unlimited copies, availability for comparison with other tracings, and billing and reportage. Moreover, the machine will insist on proper lead application and noise-free deflections. In emergencies it can be overriden and made to perform in the absence of identifying patient data (or data can be reduced to a bed number). The most essential stimulus for ensuring record identification is the demand for name and identification number by personnel from the ECG department (Heart Station) who know that the ECG has been recorded.

DIAGNOSTIC ADVANTAGES OF THE COMPUTER-LINKED ECG

The optimal data gathering system in computerized electrocardiography will deliver the usual three-channel tracing of four lead groups, each 2.5 s in duration. Most systems also provide a 10-s rhythm strip, optimally of three channels (I, II, V_1), or at a minimum, lead II alone. Systems which internally record and store 10 s of all the leads (as opposed to recording each lead group for only 2.5 s and confining the 10-s rhythm strip to lead II alone) are the most versatile. They allow one, on demand, to see what an ectopic complex in say, V_4, looks like in aVF. This provides the following diagnostic advantages: **1.** the lead-for-lead (LFL) comparison of a single premature ventricular contraction (PVC) (recorded during previous sinus rhythm) with the complexes of a wide QRS tachycardia, **2.** a similar LFL comparison in the case of the aberrant QRS generated by a single premature atrial beat, **3.** in intermittent left bundle branch block (LBBB), the "unblocked" QRS can be scrutinized LFL for Q waves, hypertrophy, ST elevation, and other features concealed or blunted by the BBB. Only one normalized beat (spontaneous or achieved by carotid massage) is needed for this purpose. In addition, these machines allow examination, in all 12 leads, of a single supraventricular beat in a tracing otherwise showing only artificially paced and diagnostically useless QRS complexes. Similarly, one can analyze the normalized QRS in intermittent preexcitation (note: delta waves both conceal and simulate infarction Q waves) or the supraventricular capture(s) in ventricular tachycardia or idioventricular rhythm (including its accelerated form). Finally, one also has the opportunity to display any complex rhythm at twice the recorded amplitude, selecting all 12 or any preferred leads, for analytical scrutiny (frequently, the solution to complex rhythm sequences is found in leads other than I, V_1, II, or V_5).

ECG NETWORKING

ECG interpretation in the ICU can be reinforced by electric, telephonic, or radio connections with the outside. Considered here are connections with the Heart Station mainframe computer via telephone or cable and connections with the ICU attending or other ECG expert via telephone or cellular phone.

OBTAINING ALTERNATIVE ECG DISPLAY FORMATS. The advantages of the computer-linked ECG outlined above depend on rescripting the 10-s ECG as simultaneous 12 leads on one page, 6 and 6 on two pages, or as a simple three-channel rhythm strip. These options can be fetched or summoned from the Heart Station, since none of these situations constitutes an emergency. If the ICU houses a retrieval terminal and writer, however, these options are immediately available and enable one to retrieve any tracing in any given format. Also available, though seldom used in ICUs, are operations performed on given tracings to elucidate the rhythm. Chief among these is the process of QRS subtraction[1] in wide QRS tachycardia. The QRS is computer averaged over the 10-s period and then subtracted from the actual tachycardic QRS/T complexes. If atrioventricular (AV) dissociation is present, the P waves formerly distorting the T and ST segments are shown in their naked isolated state (Fig. 30-1) and at a differing rate from that of the wide QRS tachycardia, which is probably thus ventricular in origin.

INTERACTIONS WITH PHYSICIANS REMOVED FROM THE ICU. Input from off-site attending staff is possible by means of a portable ECG writer (in car, office, or home). A 12-lead ECG can be transmitted in digital form via telephone or cellular telephone[2] immediately after it has been taken. Faxing the tracing is an increasingly attractive proposition, since it permits the transmission of rhythm strips from either an ECG machine or the monitor without special analog-to-digital conversion. These suggested improvements in communication should not be construed as advocating diagnosis and management of the ICU patient by

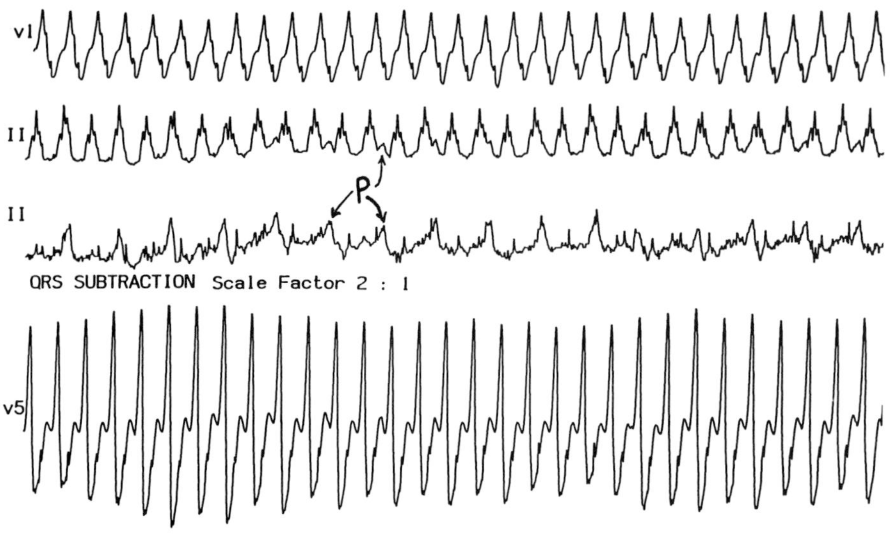

FIGURE 30-1 Wide QRS tachycardia; the QRST is computer-averaged. The mean is then subtracted from the actual lead II recording, revealing the slower sinus P waves, regular except for a single premature atrial contraction (PAC). The rhythm is ventricular tachycardia with complete AV dissociation.

remote control. They simply reflect the realities of modern practice.

MAXIMIZING DATA COLLECTION

It is important to record the 12-lead ECG during all forms of paroxysmal arrhythmia, be it tachycardia, bradycardia, or a new rhythm at approximately the same rate. A single strip from the monitoring write-out is simply not enough, though it is better than absolutely nothing. The ECG can be recorded while preparing for the conversion of the arrhythmia (lidocaine, adenosine, and others). The apotheosis of data gathering in this setting is to record the arrhythmic 12-lead ECG, and then to record selected leads (or another standard 12-lead) during the conversion. The rationale for the latter is as follows: **1.** many paroxysmal tachycardias only reveal their nature or mechanism at the moment of termination; **2.** the final beat of the tachycardia may be the only unencumbered beat that will be recorded (Fig. 30-2); **3.** the patient with paroxysmal supraventricular tachycardia (SVT) may show gross ST segment depression, especially if hypokalemia, digitalis, or both, are present. This ST depression is either rate related, ischemic (i.e., subendocardial injury, Fig. 30-3), or fixed. One selects for the rhythm strip those leads (often V_4 through V_6) which show the maximal ST deviation. Among the three cited causes, the deviation will disappear, respectively, in 1 to 3 beats of normal sinus rhythm, after 8 to 30 s, or not at all. In the case of the second, this recording sequence might be regarded as the equivalent of a stress test. Optimally, the mechanism of arrhythmia and the final unencumbered beat are best displayed in all 12 leads. Certain ECG machines can be programmed to start acquiring, in "loop mode," all ECG signals the moment the final ECG electrode is placed on the skin. Thus, the act of recording the 12-lead ECG simply secures the acquisition and graphic display of the previous rather than the prospective 10 s. This is very useful with any rhythm problem. The physician can watch the rhythm leads being recorded at the usual speed or at a slower, paper-conserving, speed. As soon as the beats of interest appear (e.g., the termination of tachycardia following lidocaine, verapamil, or carotid massage) one counts 3 or 4 s, and with the rhythm strip still running, presses "record ECG." The moment of conversion shows up in the middle of the 12-lead ECG. The tachycardia, final beat, and sinus rhythm morphologies are permanently stored.

ELECTRODES

ICUs require electrodes which can be rapidly applied. The strap electrodes used on limbs take longer than suction cups but do not fall off. The swiftest limb electrode is the clamp, though it has the disadvantage of being heavy and falling off the cart if not kept clamped to some sort of a bar when not is use. The chest electrode of choice is probably the temporary adhesive; it offers a free lip to which the ECG lead is attached by alligator clamp. Suction cups are satisfactory leads if one avoids an excess of electrode jelly, the major cause of disconnection. Esophageal electrodes are useful when flutter (Fig. 30-4), atrial tachycardia, or low voltage P waves are suspected, but not seen in the ECG. Of the two forms of esophageal electrode, catheter and "pill," the latter is easier to work with. If the patient is dyspneic, a good recording will be difficult to obtain because respiration causes dramatic wandering of the base line. In the cardiac surgical ICU a similar query about rhythm can often be answered by recording directly from the two atrial wires left in place. Commercial atrial electrogram "switchboxes" are available. The basic recording arrangment for both esophageal electrode and surgical wires is attachment to the two arm leads. Lead I of Einthoven then becomes essentially a bipolar atrial lead, with the atrial electrograms resembling mini QRS complexes and the actual QRS being either absent or small. If the wires are used for stimulation, in particular for the entrainment of atrial flutter, care must be taken to use atrial rather than ventricular wires.

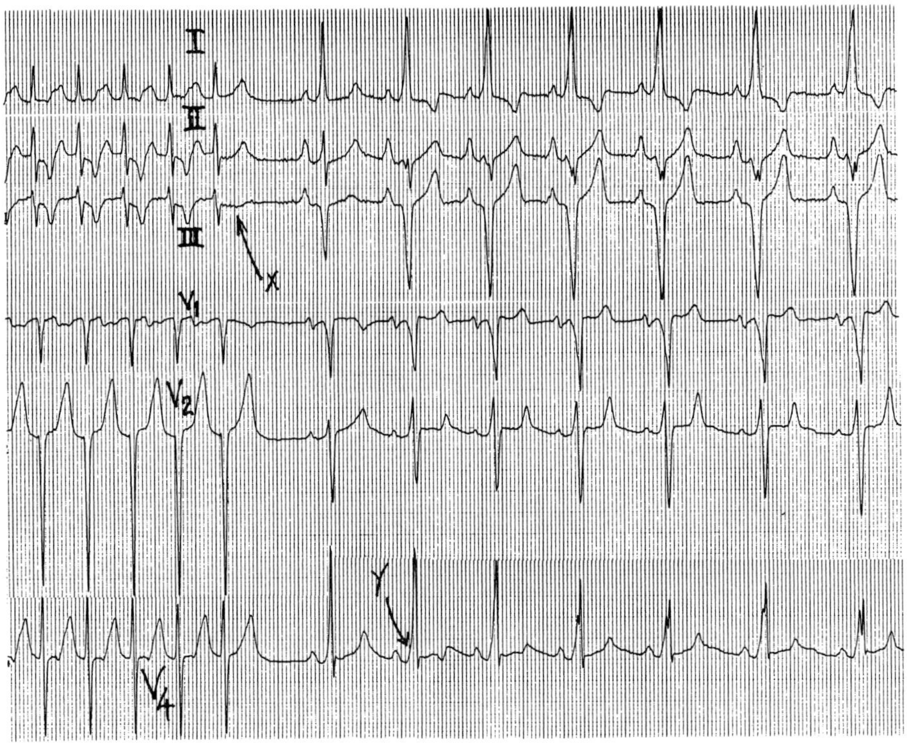

FIGURE 30-2 Termination of paroxysmal circus tachycardia in the Wolff-Parkinson-White (WPW) syndrome. Inferior ischemia is simulated by the retrograde P waves in II and III. Retrograde conduction fails in the final beat (X), the only truly unencumbered complex in the strip. The subsequent sinus beats show an increasing degree of preexcitation (Y), as sympathetic influence is withdrawn (or vagal effect returns).

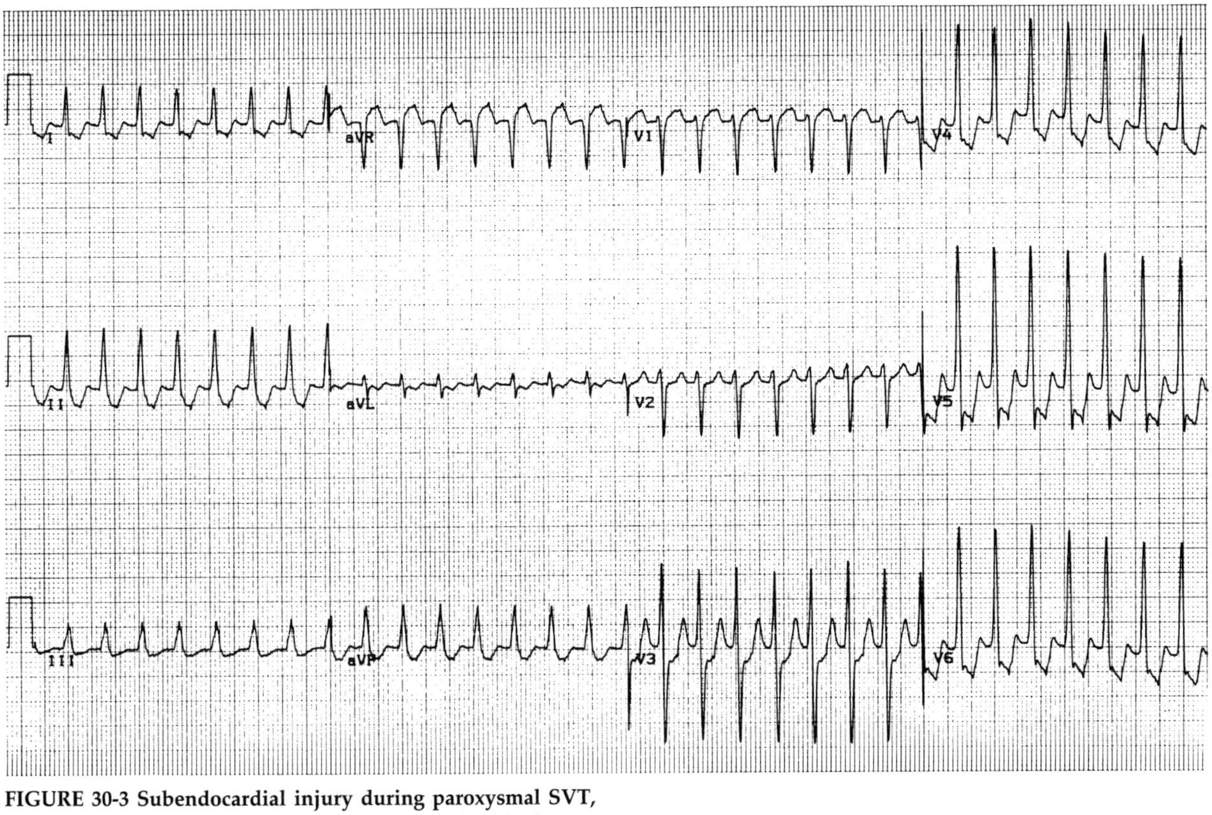

FIGURE 30-3 Subendocardial injury during paroxysmal SVT, rate 188 beats/min. The ST is grossly depressed with slope reversal; the deviation extends into V_3 and V_2.

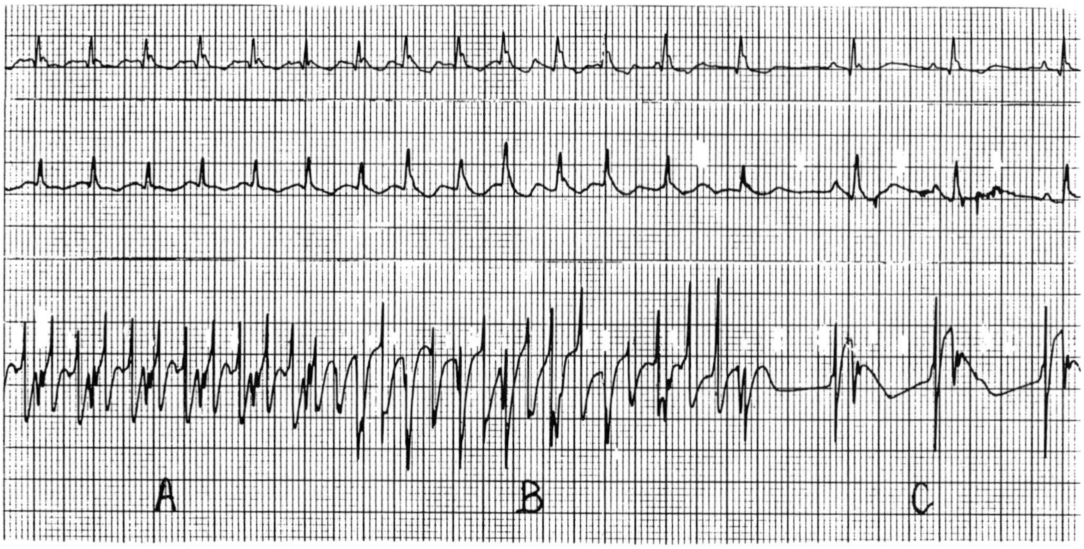

FIGURE 30-4 Esophageal electrograms recorded during spontaneous conversion of atrial flutter, to a brief fibrillation, thence to sinus rhythm. The atrial electrograms look like QRS complexes. The actual QRS is small.

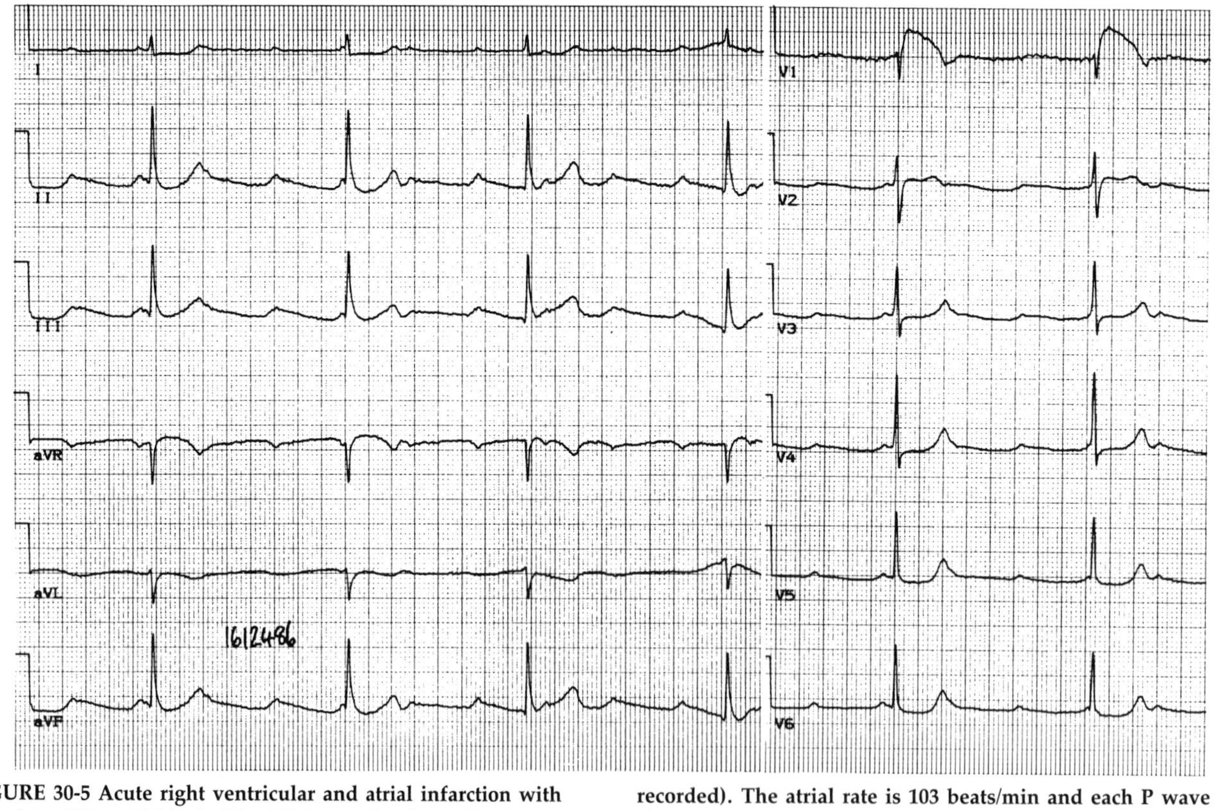

FIGURE 30-5 Acute right ventricular and atrial infarction with complete AV nodal block. The ST is grossly elevated only in V_1 (and presumably in V_{3R} and V_{4R}, though these were not recorded). The atrial rate is 103 beats/min and each P wave shows elevation of its T_a segment (atrial ST) which slopes down making it impossible to define P duration.

LEAD PLACEMENT

Serial ECGs taken in ICUs probably show greater day-to-day variation than in any other situation. For this reason, it is preferable to reduce to a minimum those variations which can be credited to a change in electrode placement. This is achieved by indelibly marking the V lead electrode sites at the time the first ECG is recorded. The limb leads do not enter this discussion since the same ECG deflections are recorded from the arm whether the electrode is on the shoulder or on the hand. When surgical wounds or burns overlie a V lead site on the chest, the electrode has to be displaced. The ECG technician should note this variation on the request form for the benefit of the physician interpreter. Right precordial lead positions (mirror-imaging the left) should be used when acute right ventricular infarction (Fig. 30-5) is suspected, when dextrocardia is present, and in pediatrics. These leads are designated V_{3R}, V_{4R}, etc.

Computer Diagnosis of ECG Abnormalities

ICUs with a computer-linked ECG system can choose to have the computer diagnosis announced or concealed by simply programming the ECG cart. The veracity of computer interpretations is not a subject for detailed discussion here, though some important points can be made. **1.** In rhythm disorders the physician is more reliable than the computer diagnosis. **2.** With few exceptions, the computer is better at measuring the standard ECG intervals than the physician. **3.** The existing computer programs are extremely cautious about the diagnosis of acute myocardial infarction (MI), with very few false-positive and numerous false-negative calls. Thus, as a purely theoretical consideration, if the program announces acute MI, and the physician bases the decision to give plasminogen activator solely on the ECG diagnosis, he will give it in the absence of acute MI in only 1 case in 50.[3] **4.** The computer is excellent at picking out the normal ECGs. **5.** The computer seldom calls "nonspecific" those T and ST disorders which signify something more serious.

Artifacts

Artifacts in the ECG are much more common in the ICU than elsewhere.[4] They are either intrinsic to the ECG-patient continuum (Epc) or extrinsic. The electromagnetic artifacts generated by other electrical devices in the room are of the latter kind (suction, ventilators, humidifiers). They may give regular signals totally out of phase with the rate and rhythm of the patient ECG. The most common of these are those that regularly register with a ventilator (Fig. 30-6). The only genuine competing rhythms which might be construed as artifacts are the native P waves of the original heart in cardiac transplantation and very rare cases of putative atrial dissociation (uniatrial fibrillation and others). In these instances, the "artifacts" do, in fact, resemble atrial deflections and are best seen in those leads (II and V_1) which show P waves to maximum advantage.

ARTIFACT IN MONITORING SYSTEMS

Although distortions in hemodynamic tracings are common, one can always repeat the measurements. One cannot ask the patient to repeat an arrhythmia. ECG monitoring systems in the very best of hands are still subject to a vast array of artifacts. For many patients, the greater the reliability of the electrode adhesive in the face of skin oil and perspiration, the greater the likelihood that it will cause pruritus. Scratching is a notorious cause of artifact, commonly mimicking ventricular tachycardia. Since electrodes seldom fall off entirely, there are gradations of electrode failure and loss of signal. In general, the high frequencies are subtracted first, with drastic reduction in QRS voltage.

Figure 30-7 is an interesting example of electrode failure which could have been the cause of a major error in management. The patient was an 84-year-old with bifascicular block, who had fallen and fractured his femoral neck 5 days previously. It was not clear whether the fall was accompanied by a disturbance of consciousness or not. The patient was being monitored in an ICU because of acute pulmonary embolism 8 h previously. The initial interpretation of the rhythm strip was Mobitz type II second degree AV block,

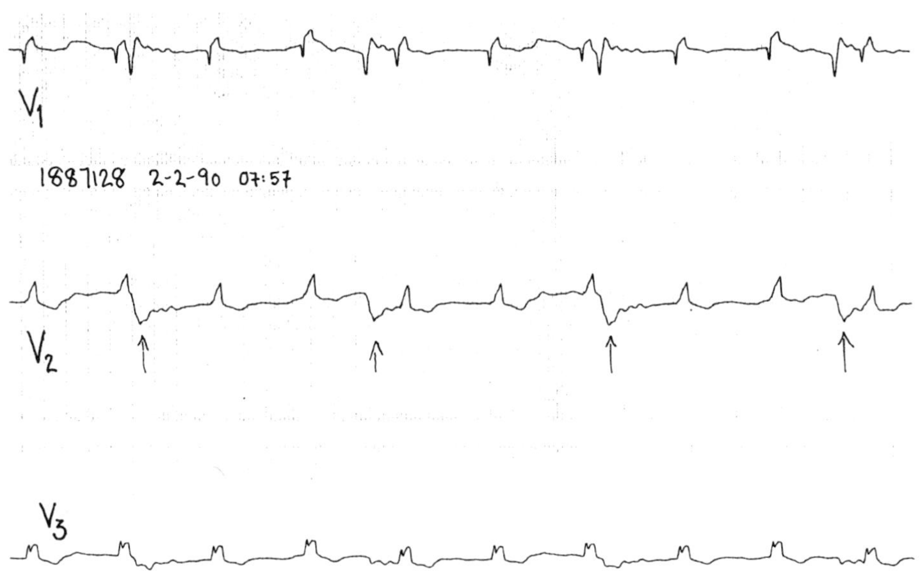

FIGURE 30-6 Regular ventilator artifacts (arrows) which mimic the QRS in V_1.

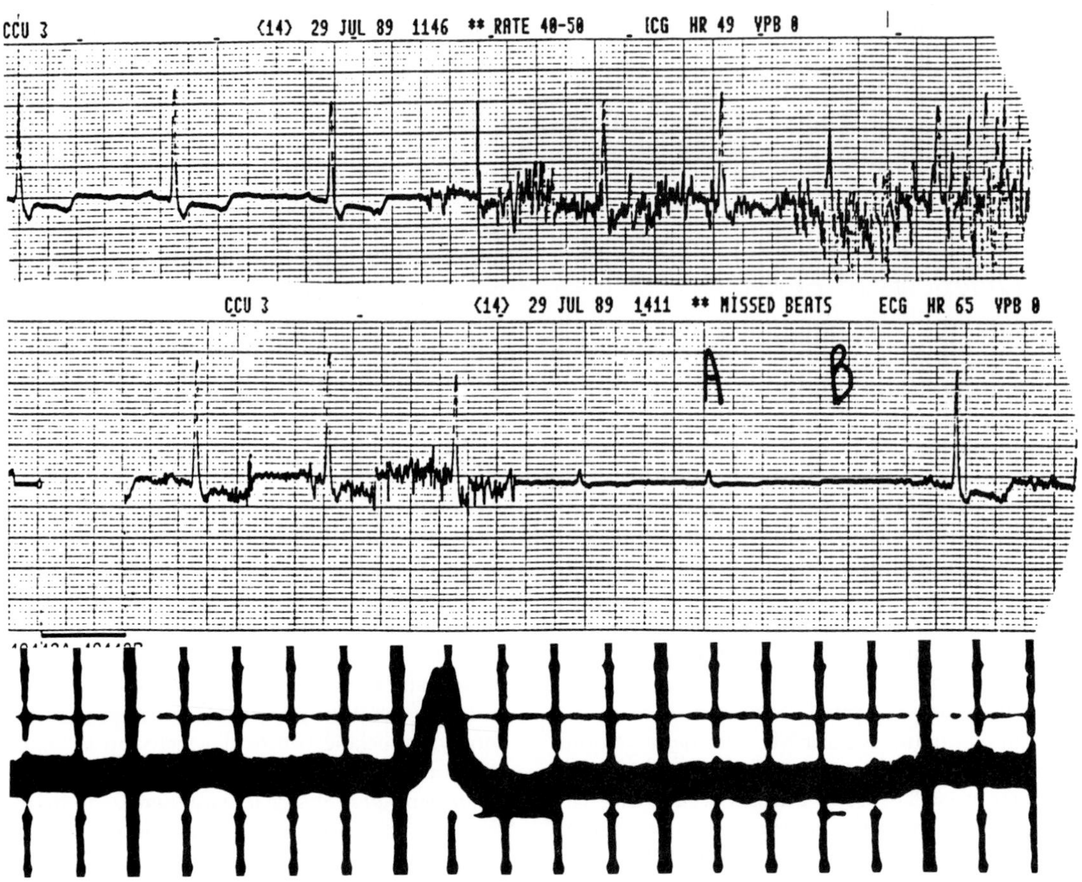

FIGURE 30-7 Monitor strip suggesting a dropped QRS (A) and then a dropped P (B). See text for description.

an expected event in such a patient. But close analysis with calipers raised disturbing questions. **1.** If the QRS was being acutely "dropped," why was there a subsequent "dropped P wave" (why should type II sinoatrial (SA) and AV block occur simultaneously here and only here)? **2.** Why did the P wave change its shape and amplitude just as it was about to drop a QRS? **3.** Why was the QT interval following the pause the same length as the earlier QT interval, not longer? **4.** Finally and decisively, why did the calipers show that the P wave under scrutiny was located where the next QRS, not P, was supposed to fall? The enlargement of the diminutive ECG signal shows the correct durations for both the QRS (120 msec) and the QT interval (400 msec). Thus, the putative P is the QRS of partial electrode failure, which thereafter became transiently total: the missing P wave.

RECOGNITION OF ECG MONITOR ARTIFACTS

Recognition of artifact depends on several simple precepts.

1. *Paper speed is rarely at fault.* It is important to realize that the rhythm strip, if poorly edited or trimmed, may sometimes include a stop and start. The printed time, minutes, and seconds, is helpful in this regard.

2. *Electrode failure simulates bradyarrhythmia (false pauses).* With these types of artifacts, the tracing is likely to show more than the usual amount of noise during and contiguous to the event. Also, the amplitudes of the QRS complexes on either or both sides of the putative pause will almost certainly show attenuation, from partial electrode failure. Bradyarrhythmias other than the true sudden pauses of type II second degree SA, AV, or idiorhythmic exit block will all show reinforcing diagnostic information in the clusters of beats adjacent to the longest pause. Thus, it would be hard to support a diagnosis of vagal bradycardia if the rates on either side of the pause were regular and similar elsewhere.

Although type II block can come without warning, it is more common for single beat dropping to be in evidence before an episode of sustained asystole (Fig. 30-8). Moreover, one has to consider whether the patient is a substrate for the problem; 90 percent of all type II AV block sequences occur in the presence of established bifascicular block (including LBBB, Fig. 30-9).

One type of genuine bradyarrhythmic crisis that may frequently be regarded as an artifact is the tachycardia-bradycardia pause. In this instance, a very "busy" tracing suddenly becomes flatline (Fig. 30-10). Atrial fibrillation arrests and is not replaced by a sinus, atrial, junctional, or ventricular escape for a prolonged period (3 to 6 s). The following

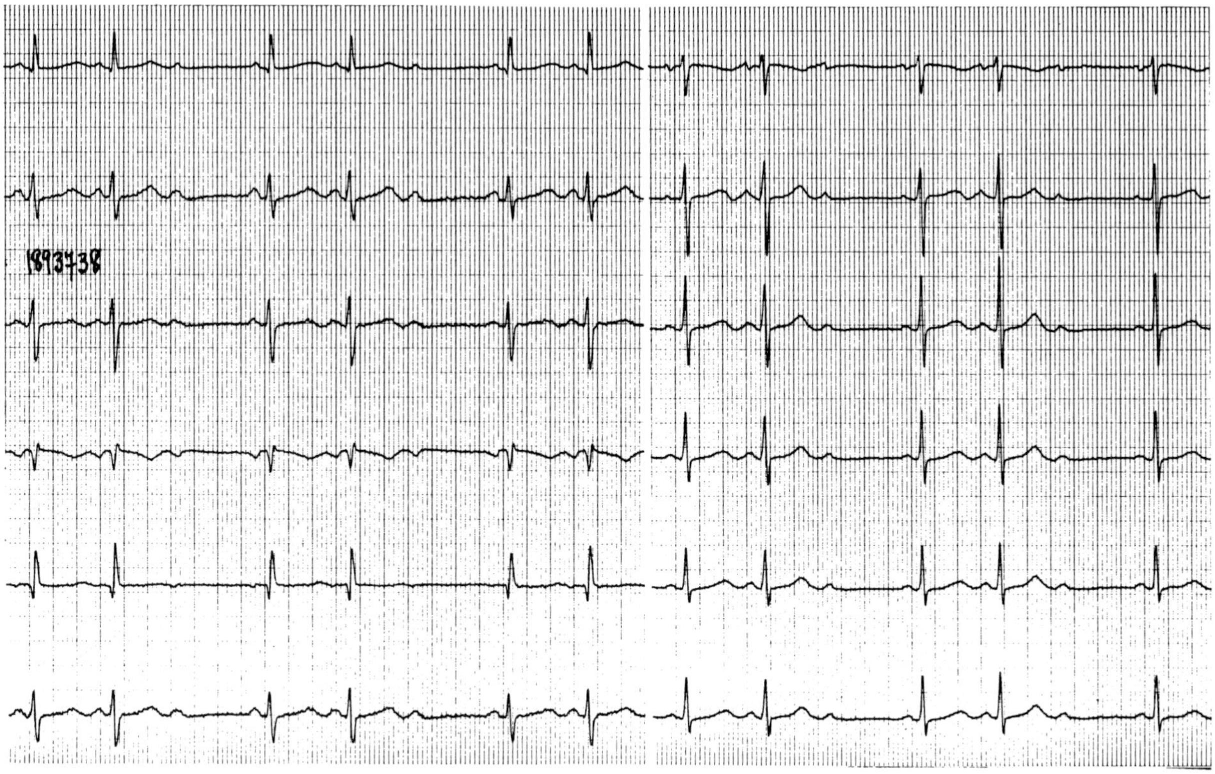

FIGURE 30-8 Mobitz type II second degree AV block at the level of the main His bundle. Every third QRS is dropped; the PR is constant. The patient had liver failure and hepatic encephalopathy, treatment of which restored normal AV conduction by 48-h Holter.

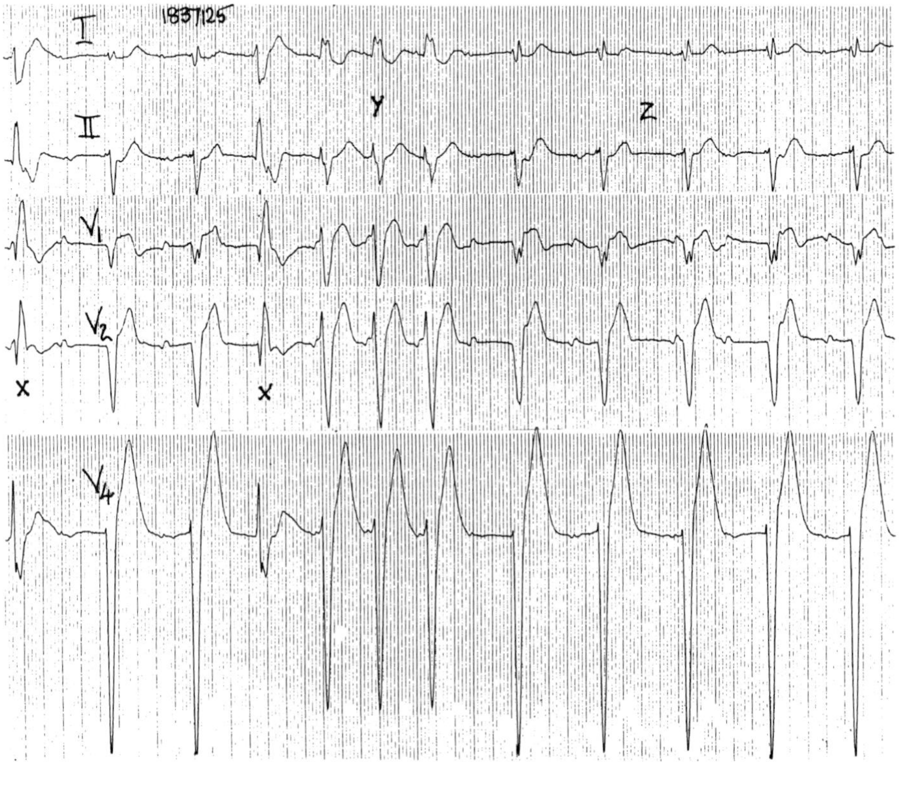

FIGURE 30-9 Renal and hepatic failure. The sinus is replaced by an accelerated ectopic atrial rhythm at 107 beats/min (see V_2). Except for the three beats (Y) consecutively conducted with complete LBBB, there is complete AV block due to bilateral bundle branch conduction failure. At Z can be seen the idioventricular QRS which is right ventricular in origin, simulating LBBB but clearly different from it (see Y). X marks left ventricular extrasystoles. In Mobitz II AV block, the resumption of atrioventricular capture (Y) is just as capricious as the initial conduction failures.

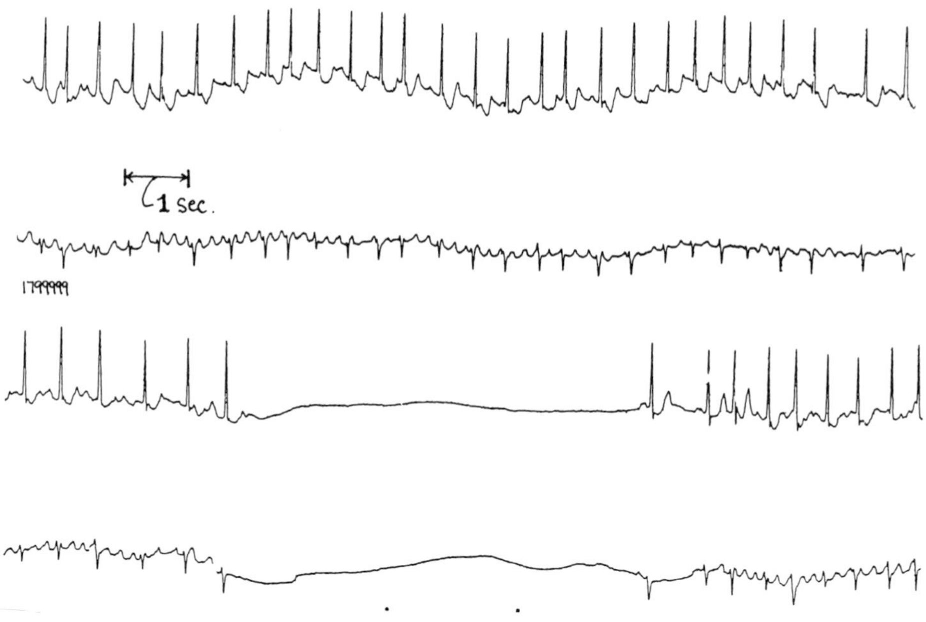

FIGURE 30-10 Monitor strip of the tachycardia-bradycardia syndrome. Immediately following the termination of paroxysmal atrial fibrillation there is a 6-s pause with a flatline tracing, due to absence or gross deficiency of the sinus, atrial, junctional, subjunctional, and idioventricular escape apparatus. Thereafter atrial fibrillation recommences.

features may simulate electrode failure: the "busyness" of the tracing may be accentuated just prior to the pause; the diastolic oscillations of fibrillation may increase in size as the atrial rate slows, prodromal to stopping; the faster the ventricular rate preceding the arrest, the longer the asystolic pause; finally, the eventual escape may be instantly followed by the resumption of fibrillation at a fast rate because of the baroreceptor recruitment of the sympathetic nervous system. Thus, one looks at a flatline pause at either end of which is atrial fibrillation and closely grouped RR intervals.

Artificial pacemakers notoriously interfere with the faithful registration of the paced QRS, a function of the defense mechanisms built into monitor systems against noise. The strip may show only stimulus artifacts. The quickest exclusion of true asystole is feeling the patient's pulse.

3. *Artifacts simulating ventricular tachycardia.* These artifacts are notorious in ICUs. All computer recognition programs can be fooled by them. It must be stressed, however, that those monitoring systems which use more than one pair of electrodes are less easily fooled; the arrhythmia will not be called if the second ECG channel fails to show the same perturbations (monitoring with two or more electrodes is endorsed in the most recent American Heart Association report on ICU monitoring).[5] When scrutinizing a strip which could be artifactual or true ventricular tachycardia, one should remember that a rate of 280 to 300/min, though not frequent with the latter does not in any way exclude it. Rates in excess of 345/min are either artifact, cardiac arrest (ventricular flutter), or atrial fibrillation down a Kent bundle. The latter should show delta waves in the previous tracing. The quickest way to "rule in" artifact is to caliper the QRS spikes to the left of the salvo and find that they continue to be inscribed throughout the putative tachycardia (Fig. 30-11), mixing in with the "QRS complexes" of the latter (if the adjacent ventricular rate is not regular, this maneuver is less useful). Keep in mind also that the earliest a ventricular tachycardia can start after the last supraventricular QRS is 300 msec, though this is exceptionally premature. Both true and artifactual ventricular tachycardia may show premonitory single or couplet deflections of the same shape before and after the actual salvo. Genuine complexes must obey the usual ECG decencies: their QRS cannot run into the QRS of the resumed dominant rhythm. Single PVCs most often generate a pause. If they are interpolated, the subsequent sinus P should show a prolonged PR interval. Finally, remember that artifacts generated by other electric devices in the patient's room are more likely to affect the 12-lead ECG than a monitored lead and are just as easily recognized (vide supra).

Impact of Extracardiac Thoracic Perturbations on the ECG

Many patients in ICUs have ECG changes due to altered volume conductor properties rather than intracardiac processes. Acute pneumothorax[6] can move the axis toward the vertical (regardless of which side is affected); it can also promote QS in V_1 to V_4, or poor R wave progression; it can decrease the voltage of both QRS and T in the chest leads; and it can prolong the QT interval. Bronchospasm and emphysema[7] can likewise provide a false pattern of completed anteroseptal MI. In asthma it will disappear after the acute attack. In these cases, V_1 (and occasionally other leads) shows gross swings in the depth of S. The respiratory rate can easily be measured from this. It should be emphasized that emphysema alone, in the complete absence of right ventricular hypertrophy or hypertension, can profoundly alter the ECG. Although flattening of the dia-

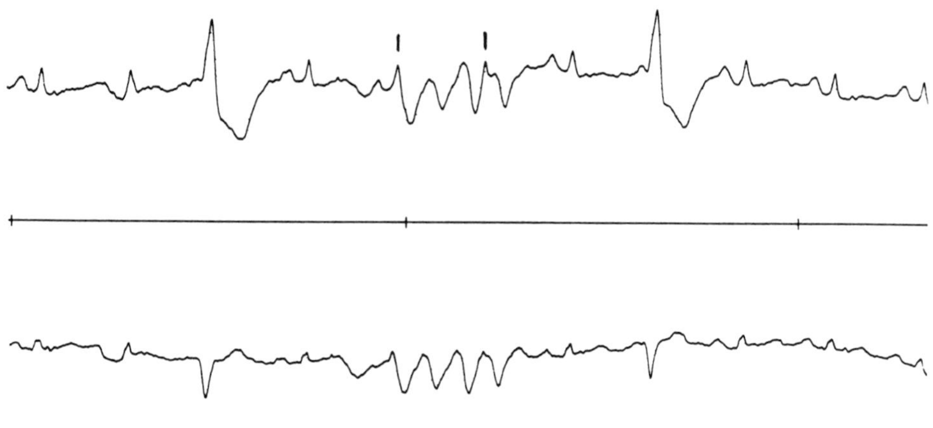

FIGURE 30-11 Typical artifactual 4-beat ventricular tachycardia which, on the bottom strip, resembles the true PVCs. The sinus QRS can be calipered through the disturbance (vertical bars).

phragm, with resulting verticalization of the heart is often invoked to explain these changes, they are more aptly related to the alteration in the volume conductor produced by lung hyperinflation. Typically, the P, QRS, and T wave axes all move toward the verticosagittal plane. Lead I will thus show almost no deflections. Less commonly, the QRS axis is $-90°$ (270°) or falls to either side of this midline axis. The inferior leads often show QS in the absence of MI. The chest leads show the already mentioned false pattern of anteroseptal MI, and the QRS in V_6 is a third or less the total amplitude of V_4.

Left pleural effusion and the atelectasis or effusion that follow sternotomy in cardiac surgery cause a local voltage reduction in the lateral chest leads. One factor powerfully affecting the amplitude of V_4 to V_6 in the ICU is the water content of the lungs. Both interstitial and alveolar edema (cardiac or noncardiac) will cause a reduction in voltage in these leads.[8] Hemodialysis reverses these changes,[9] as does diuresis. Apart from the specific artifact (see Fig. 30-6) already discussed, the impact of the ventilator on the ECG is almost entirely a question of how emphysematous or edematous the lungs are. Radical mastectomy causes an increase in QRS and T voltage (the latter disproportionately greater) over the precordium.[10] Although this effect is most pronounced on the left side following left-sided surgery, QRS voltage also increases on the contralateral side. These changes are a complex function of a major alteration of the thoracic volume conductor and cannot be explained by greater proximity of the electrodes to the heart.

Pneumonectomy on the left causes a leftward shift of the precordial transition, a poor R wave progression, or even a simulated anteroseptal MI.[11] Incomplete right bundle branch block (RBBB) is a common postoperative sequel. The axis moves to the right. Right-sided pneumonectomy shifts the transition to the right and causes leads I, II and V_5 and V_6 to show prominent Q waves, a function of cardiac rotation. It should be emphasized that pneumonectomy, esophagectomy, and even lobectomy will often show postoperatively the same patterns of surgical pericarditis observable after cardiac surgery, presumably as a result of incidental myocardial bruising. A similar ECG picture is sometimes seen following blunt chest trauma.

The ECG in Abnormal Metabolic States

THE HYPOENDOCRINE STATES

Generalized low voltage is found in Addison's disease, hypopituitarism, myxedema, anorexia nervosa, and untreated malabsorption diseases such as sprue. Addison's disease may show T waves suggestive of hyperkalemia; the PR interval may be prolonged. All the hypoendocrine states tend to show sinus bradycardia. The latter is partially counteracted when the anemia accompanying advanced precomatous myxedema conspires to produce a hyperkinetic circulation. The T wave of myxedema is flatter than the lowered voltage would dictate, a feature absent in anorexia nervosa. Nearly pathognomonic of the latter is the constellation of teenage female, low voltage with proportionate T waves, and sinus bradycardia. These conditions are all characterized by a low basal metabolic rate. Although pericardial effusion also produces low voltage, bradycardia is absent. Low voltage is also seen in hyperosmolar coma.

THE HYPERENDOCRINE STATES

Cushing's syndrome, like cortisone administration, shows a short PR interval. Hyperthyroidism commonly shows sinus tachycardia even during sleep. The P may increase more in magnitude than the tachycardia licenses. Thyrotoxic atrial fibrillation (rare in adolescents, common after age 40) is frequently coarse, with large fibrillatory (f) waves. It responds poorly to rate control with digoxin unless the latter is fortified by a β-blocking drug. Monofascicular conduction defects may occur. Left ventricular hypertrophy ultimately develops. Thyrotoxicosis is one of the few conditions where left ventricular "strain" disappears regularly when its cause is removed (i.e., with restoration of the euthyroid state).

CHRONIC RENAL FAILURE

Chronic hemodialysis patients often show a distinctive ECG constellation consisting of left ventricular hypertrophy (LVH) and strain (from hypertension), incomplete LBBB (the QS in V_5 and V_6 being replaced by an initial slurred upstroke), a short PR interval, and a sinus tachycardia of about 100 beats/min. The latter two features are related to the hyperkinesis generated by the combined effects of anemia and the arteriovenous fistula. The combination of a short PR and the slurred upstroke of the QRS in V_5 and V_6 often suggests the WPW pattern of preexcitation (and explains why the term pseudodelta wave is often used in describing the incomplete form of LBBB).

HYPOTHERMIA

In hypothermia the rate is slow and the PR and the QT intervals are long.[12] Osborne "J waves" may be in evidence. They are seemingly a terminal addition to the QRS complex, the polarity of which is positive in lead II and V_2 to V_6 (the elevated J wave of early repolarization occasionally simulates Osborne waves in V_4 to V_6, but of course, the QT is normal). The T waves lose their amplitude in hypothermia. The resulting appearance is vaguely reminiscent of an epicardial injury pattern, particularly in the inferolateral leads. But the putative ST elevation is of short duration, sinking below the base line after 180 to 200 msec, with two-thirds of the QT interval still to come. This negative portion does not resemble the terminally negative T waves seen in the midphase of acute MI. In V_2 the Osborne wave looks like a fat R′. Although these waves appear to widen the QRS, they should be regarded as expressions of rapidly changing voltage during the initial portion of repolarization. Atrial fibrillation, junctional rhythm, and PVCs are common. The colder the body temperature, the greater the danger of ventricular fibrillation. Obligatory shivering is likely to cause interference and wandering of the base line.

The ECG in Noncardiac Catastrophes

HYPOVOLEMIC SHOCK

Acute hemorrhage, substantial enough to induce weakness or syncope, is sometimes followed by symmetrical T wave inversion, even in the absence of coronary disease or chest pain.

PANCREATITIS

Acute pancreatitis has long been known to induce ECG changes suggestive of acute MI, even in patients with a normal coronary arteriogram.[13] These changes include reversible T wave inversion in one or more leads (I, II, V_2 through V_6). Less commonly, ST elevation and even transient Q waves have been noted. Attempts to attribute these changes to electrolyte depletion, shock per se, or myocardial digestion by circulating enzymes have failed to gain acceptance. The cause of the changes remains unknown.

CEREBROVASCULAR DISEASE

Acute cerebrovascular accidents commonly induce ECG changes, especially in the case of subarachnoid hemorrhage, cryohypophysectomy, and cerebral hemorrhage.[14] The changes involve expansion of the QTc, increased voltage (>0.5 mV) of the upright or inverted T wave, increased voltage of the U wave (especially with subarachnoid bleeds) (Fig. 30-12), and combinations of the preceding. The U wave may be inverted companion to an inverted T wave. These changes are being increasingly attributed to hypothalamic damage. A clinical error can arise with the following sequence of events: acute non-Q wave MI with typical T inversion and QT expansion—mural thrombus formation—cerebral embolism—ECG changes attributed entirely to the cerebrovascular accident.

PERICARDITIS

Pericarditis can directly influence the ECG by virtue of an associated ventricular and atrial epicarditis or by virtue of a resulting effusion around the heart.[15] Quite frequently the ECG is unaffected. The presence, absence, or loudness of the rub are not determinative in this regard. In the emergency room and in the doctor's office, the most common cause of acute electrocardiographically overt pericarditis is a viral infection. In the hospital ICU, the more common cause is the postoperative state: surgical pericarditis. Its incidence is virtually 100 percent following cardiac surgery and considerably less following esophagectomy, pneumonectomy, or lobectomy. In the latter three instances the pericardium does not have to be opened; the heart undergoes benign bruising during contiguous surgery. The same phenomenon can be seen following blunt injury to the chest, with cardiac contusion.

ECG CHANGES IN PERICARDITIS. The ventricular epicarditis typically causes a pattern of acute inferolateral injury. The ST becomes elevated in leads II, III, aVF, I, and V_4 to V_6 $\pm$ V_2 and V_3. ST is invariably depressed in aVR, and in 10 to 20 percent of cases, in V_1 alone among the chest leads. The second change that occurs, a function of atrial epicarditis, is the depression of PR segment in the same inferolateral leads (the PR segment is in effect the atrial ST segment), with elevation in aVR (Fig. 30-13). On rare occasions, the PR segment is elevated in V_1, an abnormality generally associated with ectopic atrial impulse formation and a short PR interval (inferior elevation suggests atrial infarction, see Fig. 30-5). It should be emphasized that the reference base line for judging ST elevation is the TP segment, not the PR segment. Not infrequently, the ST in the inferior leads is markedly elevated with respect to the depressed PR, though in fact only slightly above the TP segment. However, it will be elevated in the lateral leads. The diagnosis can be safely made if the PR segment depression is new (two tracings are thus needed), and the comparison is made at approximately the same resting heart rate (sinus tachycardia and primary AV block preclude discovering true PR depression if the P climbs the T descent). PR depression is also seen with gross atrial hypertrophy (the P wave being both wide and enormous), and in occasional cases of thyrotoxicosis before the tachycardia is prohibitive (hyperthyroidism directly impacts on atrial tissue).[16] The ST shape may be of the plateau variety, suggesting injury, but resem-

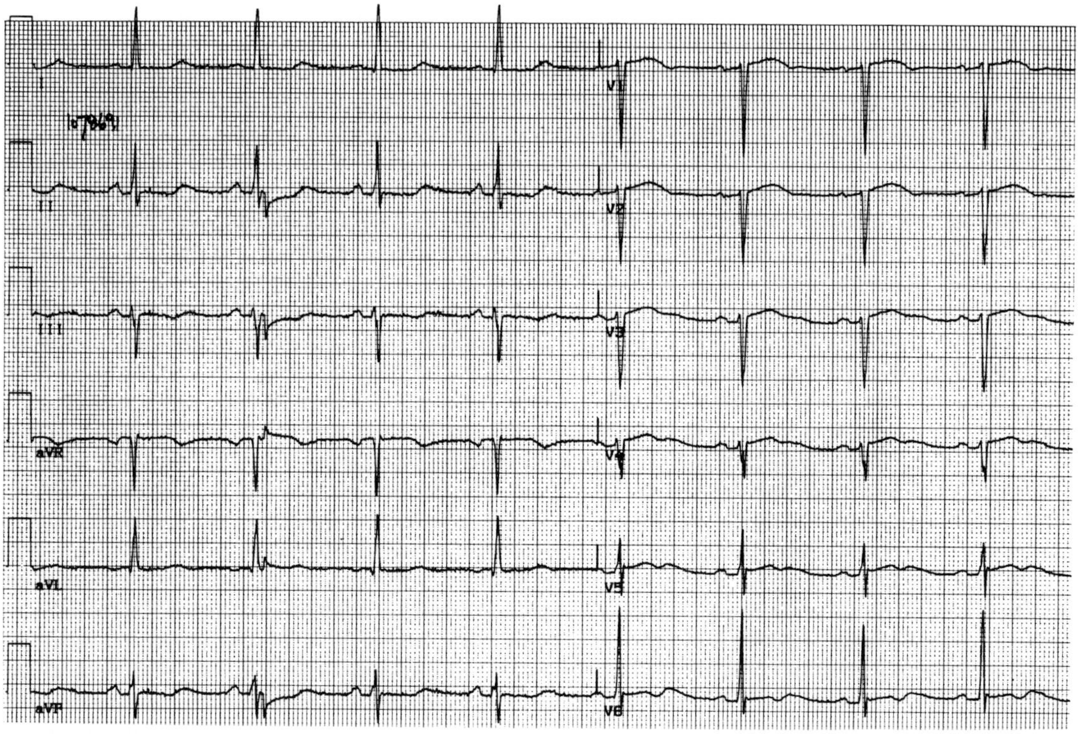

FIGURE 30-12 Subarachnoid hemorrhage. The QT is prolonged with exaggeration of the U wave which climbs on the descent of the T in V_3 to V_5. U is the only prominent repolarization wave in the inferior frontal leads.

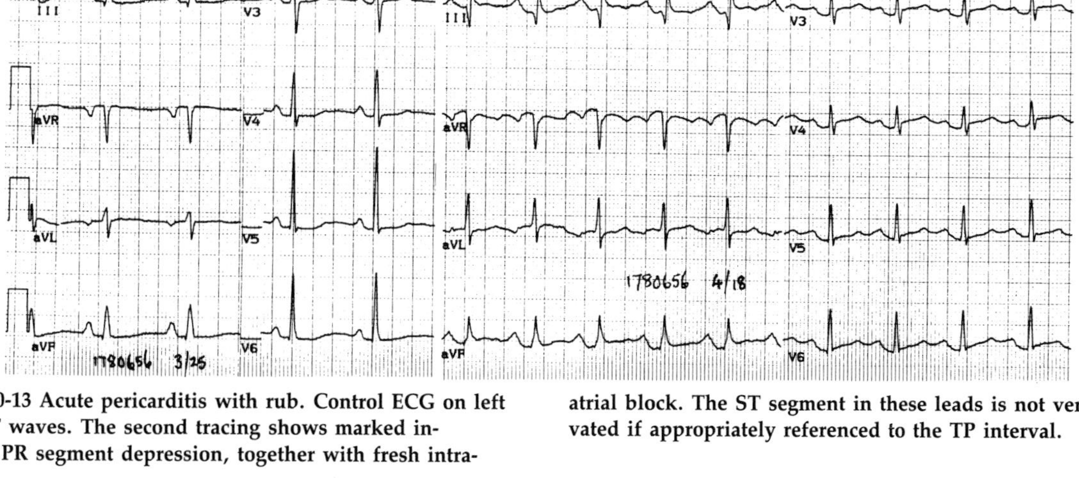

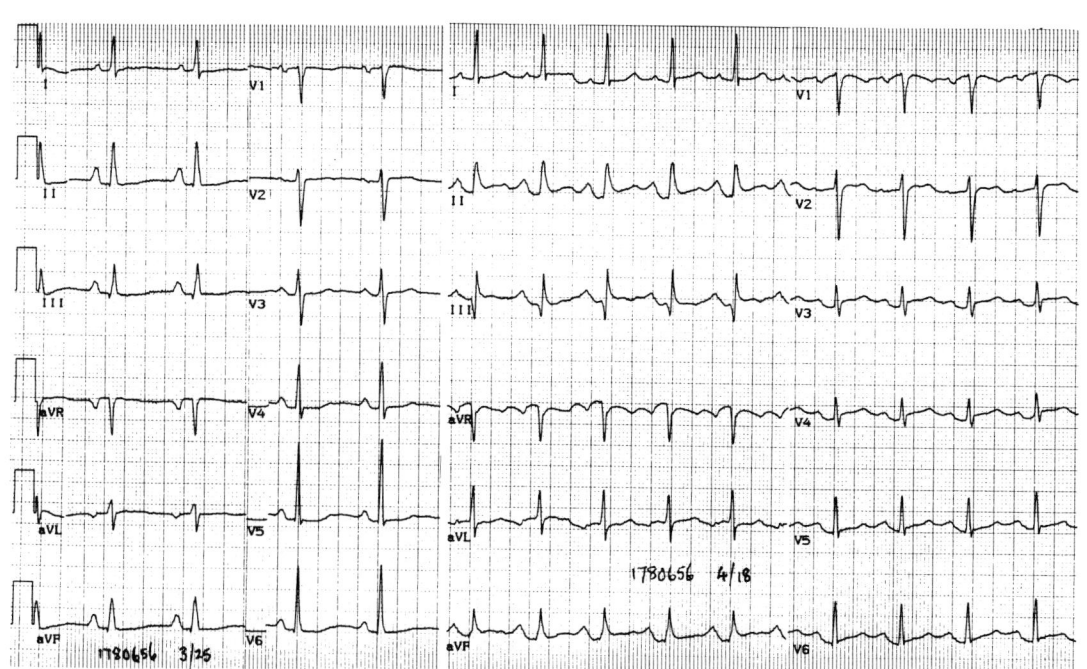

FIGURE 30-13 Acute pericarditis with rub. Control ECG on left with flat T waves. The second tracing shows marked inferolateral PR segment depression, together with fresh intra-atrial block. The ST segment in these leads is not very elevated if appropriately referenced to the TP interval.

bles early repolarization often enough to make the PR segment signs exceptionally valuable. The ST elevation can remain for hours or days. Not infrequently, it disappears only to return, a phenomenon not seen with early repolarization in the absence of interim exercise or hyperkalemia. The inferolateral ST elevation of acute pericarditis is distinguished from ischemic injury in the same locations by the absence of any change in the QRS even after prolonged ST elevation.

ELECTRICAL ALTERNANS.[17] A modest fall in ECG voltage is seen in many cases of pericarditis that do not require pericardiocentesis. The decision concerning pericardiocentesis should not depend on the ECG, but on the hemodynamic profile at the bedside. The one exception to this statement is the presence of total electrical alternans. In this infrequent but dramatic situation, neoplastic involvement of the serosa is usually the cause of effusion, often without inflammation. The sac may have thickened walls or may become paper thin; the absence of exudate precludes adhesions. The heart is suspended in a relatively huge bag of fluid, unrestrained by the lungs or diaphragm in its contractile motion. The latter involves not only the cyclic systolic flinch in heart volume, but also a native rocking or swinging motion of the organ, relative to its vascular anchoring (the great veins and arteries). At a critical heart rate, the mechanical impedance of the surrounding fluid may be such that it prevents the heart from returning, at the end of each cardiac cycle, to its precise original location in space. In electrical alternans, it only manages such a return after every other beat. At other heart rates a "cycle of motion" may require a different beat number or fraction thereof, making recognition of the above mechanism less overt.

The ECG in total electric alternans (Fig. 30-14) shows a regular sinus rhythm (the RR intervals do not alternate), an extreme of low voltage in the frontal, though frequently in both planes, an alternation of QRS morphology which in most leads registers in the R:S ratio, and a similar alternation in P and T amplitude or polarity. The presence of electrical alternans is an indication for pericardiocentesis. Rarely, the cause of the pericarditis in this syndrome is something other than neoplasia (e.g., tuberculosis). QRS alternans without low voltage is common in paroxysmal supraventricular tachycardia. Its registration is restricted to lead V_4 or V_5 or both.

ECG MONITORING DURING PERICARDIOCENTESIS. The V_1 lead is attached by alligator clamp to a short bevel aspirating needle. The latter is introduced either at the putative apex, 2 cm inside the border of percussible dullness and directed at the fourth vertebra, or directed at the right shoulder from the left paraxiphoid puncture site. It is advanced until ST elevation is visible in the V_1 lead. The needle is then withdrawn a few millimeters and aspiration is attempted. The ST elevation is a function of epicardial injury.

ACUTE PULMONARY EMBOLISM

Whether or not the ECG is altered by acute pulmonary embolism is a function of the magnitude of vascular obstruction and the timing of the subsequent ECG recording. Thus, the changes vary from none, or nonspecific ST-T abnormalities, to major deviations from the norm, or more importantly, from the ECG preceding the event.[18,19] The mechanisms by which this event has an impact on the ECG include sympathetic stimulation generated by acute arterial hypoxemia and hypotension, acute right ventricular hypertension and dilation, and occasional unmasking of latent ischemic heart disease as a result of systemic hypotension and hypoperfusion of the myocardium.

ECG CHANGES IN ACUTE PULMONARY EMBOLISM. Sympathetic stimulation often results in sinus tachycardia or a gross increase in ventricular rate in atrial fibrillation previously well controlled. Incomplete or complete RBBB may appear for the first time as a result of acute right ventricular hypertension (the RBB is extremely "exposed" on the right ventricular endocardial surface). The development of certain findings suggests right ventricular dilation. These include acute right axis shift of more than 30° and acute clockwise rotation. This leftward displacement of the transitional chest lead is the result of backward displacement of the left ventricle by the right ventricle, the dilation of which is limited anteriorly by the sternum. The development of the SI/QIII pattern (Fig. 30-15) is also suggestive of right ventricular dilation. This highly specific change is the result of the posterior displacement and reorientation in space of the interventricular septum. It should be noted that this pattern by itself is not in any way abnormal. Its fresh appearance, however, makes the diagnosis. Accompanying the SI/QIII pattern is a specific repolarization disorder in the same leads: ST depression in leads I, or II and elevation in III. This has to be distinguished from acute inferior MI, which does not, in its early phase, generate an S in lead I. Finally, the fresh appearance of acute right ventricular strain T inversion in V_1 through V_3 with or without ST depression, (the mechanism is not well understood) also suggests right ventricular dilation. Other less reliable changes such as fresh QS or QR in V_1, poor R wave progression, and fresh P pulmonale (these alterations may be related to those cases of pulmonary embolism that develop significant bronchospasm) have been noted.

The ECG may become complicated by the manifestations of ischemia. Subendocardial injury is common in this exigency, the ST segments being drastically depressed with slope reversal with or without inversion in the lateral and inferior leads, and to some extent, in V_3 and V_2.

SPECIFICITY OF THE ECG IN ACUTE PULMONARY EMBOLISM. It is important not to exaggerate the usefulness of these ECG changes. With the exception of sinus tachycardia, these changes are seen in only 20 to 30 percent of proven cases. An earlier ECG is essential for the changes outlined above to have diagnostic value. Frequently, the

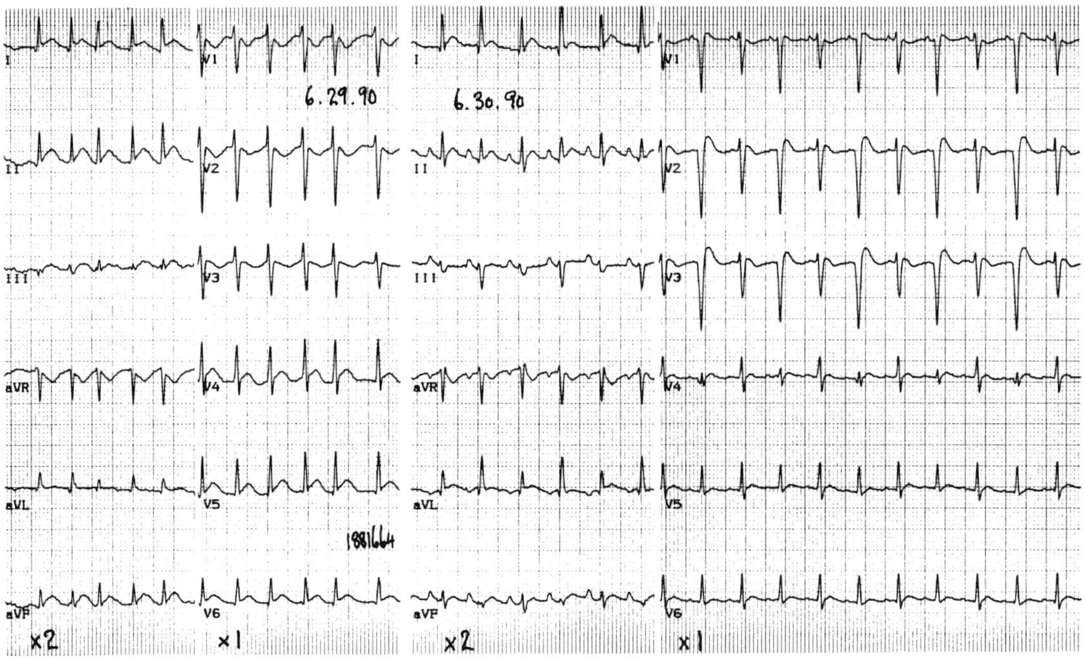

FIGURE 30-14 Acute pericarditis in a patient with inoperable lung cancer. At left, fresh onset atrial fibrillation with inferolateral ST elevation. At right total electrical alternans. The reduced frontal plane voltages are amplified two times in both ECGs.

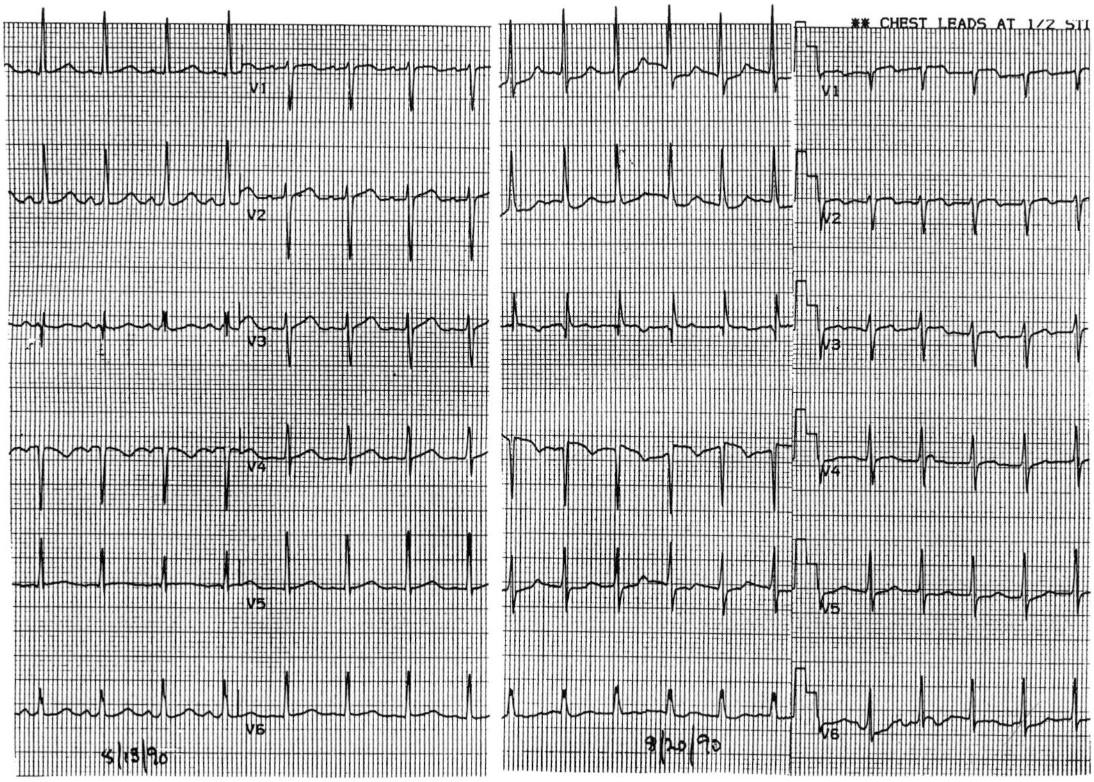

FIGURE 30-15 Acute pulmonary embolism, with control postoperative trace on left. Lead I and lead III, respectively, develop a fresh S and Q as a marker of acute right ventricular dilation.

diagnosis is retrospective: the ECG axis moves to the left, and the SI/QIII disappears. The fresh appearance of the latter pattern is highly specific because it does not occur with other forms of acute dyspnea (acute hyperventilation, acute bronchospasm, acute pulmonary edema). Moreover, it cannot be induced by any change in posture or by the Valsalva maneuver, and so on. It is important to state, however, that it is specific for acute right ventricular dilation, not for a clot in the lungs. We have seen it in the immediate postoperative period of coronary bypass surgery when a large retrosternal hematoma started to obstruct the right ventricular outflow tract. It can disappear quite suddenly if the pulmonary artery thrombus breaks up or lyses. Clockwise rotation is seen with many cases of new left axis deviation. Both RBBB and posterior fascicular block (with right axis deviation) can acutely develop in coronary heart disease, but an accompanying increase in rate would not be expected. Unusual presentations of acute pulmonary embolism include acute complete heart block, with patients showing a complete LBBB in the substrate ECG.

Electrolyte Disturbances

HYPOCALCEMIA

Hypocalcemia prolongs the QT interval, generally preserving both the shape, polarity, and even the amplitude of the T wave, which is simply "lifted and moved bodily" to the right (Fig. 30-16). Less typically, hypocalcemic expansion of the QT is attained by splaying out of the T wave, with the apex becoming rounded. When hypocalcemia is gross, the T wave may invert. Beat-to-beat alternation of T wave shape and QT interval may rarely be observed (Fig. 30-17). T wave alternation is also seen transiently following a PVC (an extension of postextrasystolic T inversion). Immediate QT prolongation due to hypocalcemia occurs if a coronary artery catheter is flushed with ordinary saline solution.

HYPOMAGNESEMIA

Hypomagnesemia, like hypocalcemia, affects repolarization, though less reliably. Since it is most commonly seen in alcoholics, there is almost always accompanying sinus tachycardia. Torsades de pointes or R-on-T events have been documented when these disorders occur in combination (low K^+, Ca^+, Mg^+) but are otherwise rare.

HYPERCALCEMIA

Hypercalcemia may shorten the QT with serum values above 15 mg/dL (Fig. 30-18).

HYPOKALEMIA

Hypokalemia (serum K content <3.5 meq/L) is extremely common. The specific ECG findings include the U-on-T phenomenon. In its classic form, the QT interval is prolonged and an enlarged U wave occupies its usual diastolic

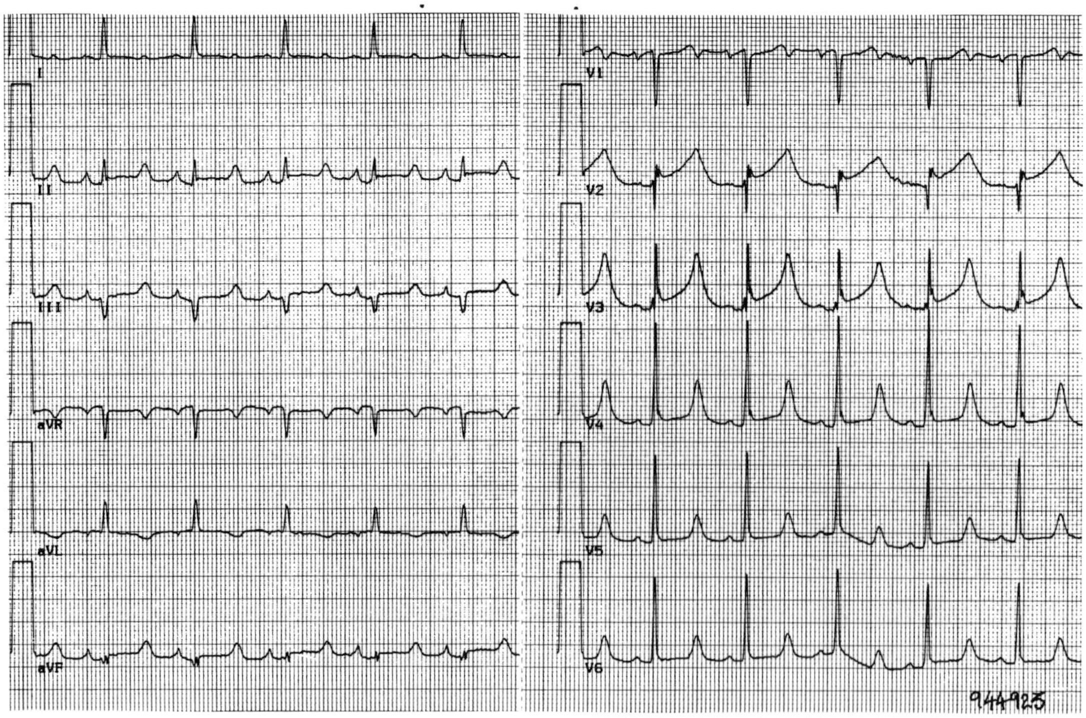

FIGURE 30-16 Chronic renal failure. Serum K level is 5.7 meq; serum calcium level is 6.5 mg. QT prolongation; the inferolateral leads show a T "lifted and moved bodily" to the right. The ST elevations may be pericarditic.

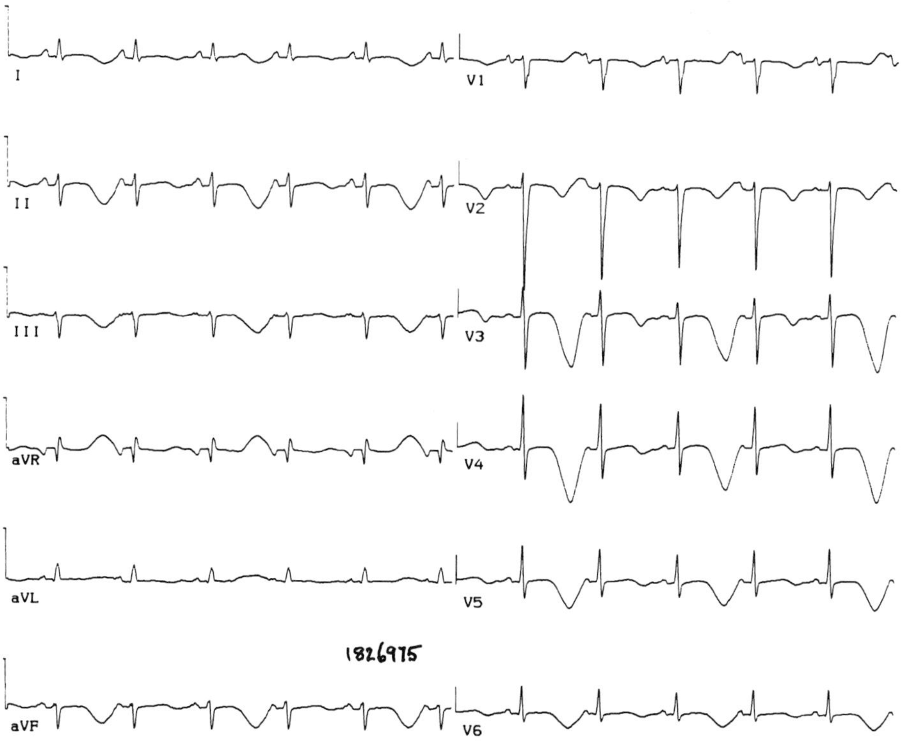

FIGURE 30-17 Severe hypocalcemia (4.7 mg/dL). Alternation of both the QT interval and the T wave are present. Note the instability of amplitude in the more prominent T, being deepest in the final beat of lead V_3.

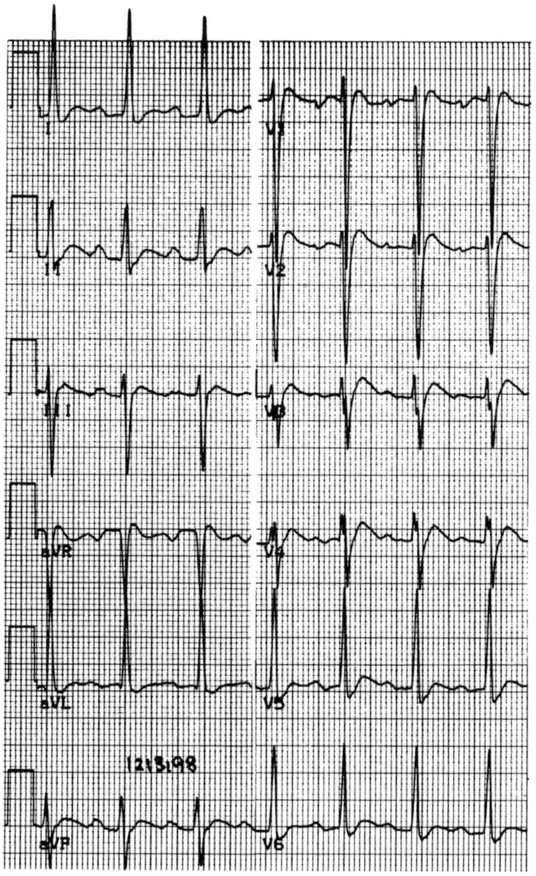

FIGURE 30-18 Severe hypercalcemia in terminal myelomatosis. Serum calcium level is 19.3 mg/dL. The QT seems excessively short in V_1; the ascent to the T apex is steeper than the descent in most leads.

position. It thus comes to sit on the descending limb of T. The actual QT can only be measured by extrapolation. The U-on-T phenomenon is best seen in V_2 and V_3, but the diagnosis requires the phenomenon to be seen in both frontal (lead II) and lateral leads (V_4 and V_5). In II and V_5, the U is not generally seen as a positive hump. Instead, it is seen as a sloping shelf starting from some point on the upper third of the T wave descent. It delays the return to the isoelectric line, often to the next sinus P wave (Fig. 30-19). Variants include ST depression in V_2 and V_3, with a terminally positive low voltage T and U wave (often of equal amplitude). Hypokalemia is sometimes represented by ST depression alone in V_1 through V_3 with no other abnormalities and T waves flattish in V_2 through V_4; the U wave is unduly large (especially in V_4) and is the most prominent repolarization feature in these leads.

T wave inversion is also seen in V_1 through V_3 with a positive U wave. Its ascending limb appears to be an overshoot of the returning limb of the T wave. T inversion is seldom seen with a serum K level >2.6 meq/L. Less specifically, hypokalemia is often associated with ectopic atrial or junctional rhythm and with premature ectopy from both chambers. Accelerated idioventricular rhythm is not a common complication of potassium depletion until extremely low serum values are obtained. Figure 30-20 was recorded with a K concentration of 1.0 meq/L. Digitalis effect, optimally seen in V_5 and V_6, often accompanies hypokalemia. The latter may be missed if the observer attributes ST depression in V_2 and V_3 to the glycoside.

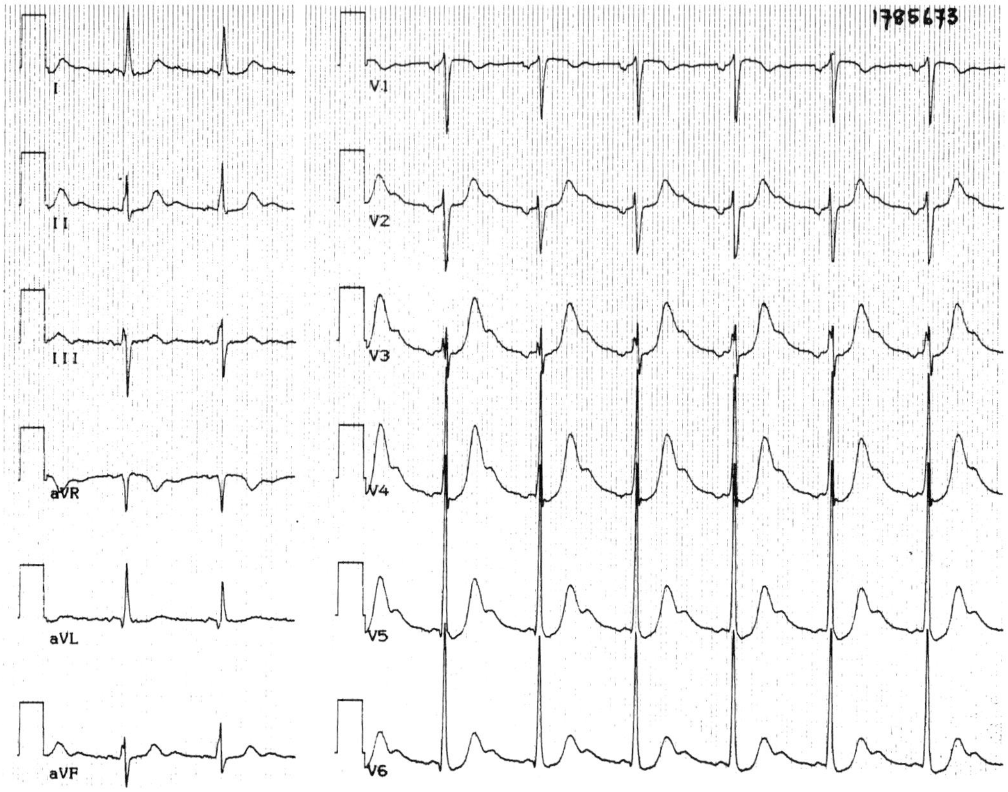

FIGURE 30-19 Severe hypokalemia (serum K level is 1 meq/L). The U-on-T phenomenon is marked everywhere. The T amplitude is atypically large in this case. P is ectopic.

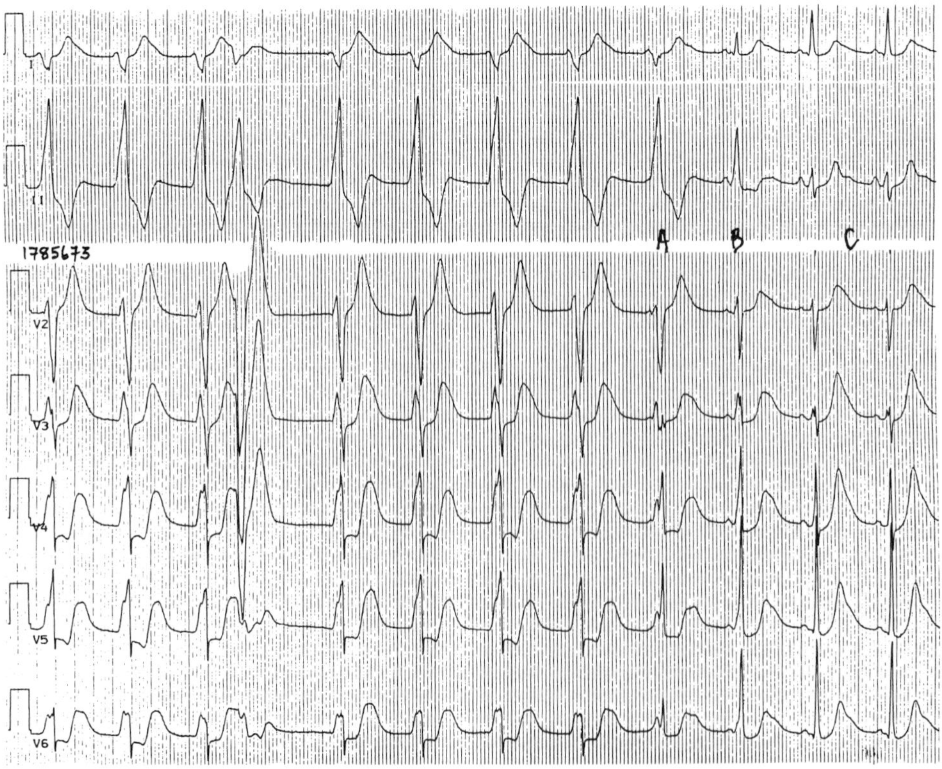

FIGURE 30-20 Same patient and time period as in Fig. 30-19. Accelerated idioventricular rhythm (rate 75 beats/min) with a single PVC. After two fusion beats (A, B) sinus rhythm appears with typical hypokalemic repolarization.

FALSE PATTERNS OF HYPOKALEMIA

A number of conditions may mimic hypokalemia on the ECG, including benign U waves, digitalis or amiodarone therapy, LVH, and subarachnoid hemorrhage.

BENIGN U WAVES. Benign U-on-T waves may be confined to V_2, though equally often to V_3 and V_4. The U takes off very low down on the returning limb of the T wave (lower half), slopes steeply, and rapidly attains the isoelectric line. The U is not a "second hump" in these leads. The frontal and lateral leads are normal.

DIGITALIS AND AMIODARONE. In prolonged digitalis therapy, the characteristic ST depression of digitalis effect is followed by a terminally positive T wave in V_5. The descent of the latter to the base line is for some reason delayed, simulating the shelf described above. The U-on-T pattern is absent in V_2 and V_3. Amiodarone's QT prolongation often simulates hypokalemia.

LEFT VENTRICULAR HYPERTROPHY. Prominent U waves may be seen in severe LVH, possibly due to hypertrophy of Purkinje fibers. Occasionally, the enlarged U wave sits on the descending limb of the T in a single lead, V_2 through V_4.

SUBARACHNOID HEMORRHAGE. In subarachnoid hemorrhage the U-on-T phenomenon is often greatly exaggerated. The T wave, of modest voltage in true hypokalemia, is often augmented, as is the U wave. When hypokalemia is extreme (e.g., 1.0 meq/L), both of these features may be present, making differentiation even more difficult (see Fig. 30-19).

HYPERKALEMIA

The first major manifestation of hyperkalemia is a change in the T wave, which becomes taller in amplitude, peaked or pointed at its apex, and narrowed at its base. This classic T wave of hyperkalemia is optimally displayed in V_4, especially if the latter is posttransitional with an R:S ratio of between 3 and 4:1. The T wave is tall but shows an isosceles triangulation in its entirety, or more frequently, in its upper two-thirds. The ascent during the latter is as steep as the descent. The T wave appears to have been squeezed at its base (Fig. 30-21). This basal abbreviation may start at the isoelectric line (if the ST remains "straightened" or isoelectric), but is more likely to start 1 to 2 mm above it, the ST being at first of gentle upward slope or horizontal but elevated. V_1 through V_3 show high amplitude but retain their asymmetry. In those leads with a shallow T wave (III, aVR, aVL, V_6, and in some instances, aVF), the ST may be isoelectric right up to the base of a generally perfect isosceles triangle 3 or 4 mm in height. The major variants of this characteristic T wave include instances where the isosceles triangulation is late in starting: it will then form sort of a narrow nipple on top of an otherwise nondescript T wave,

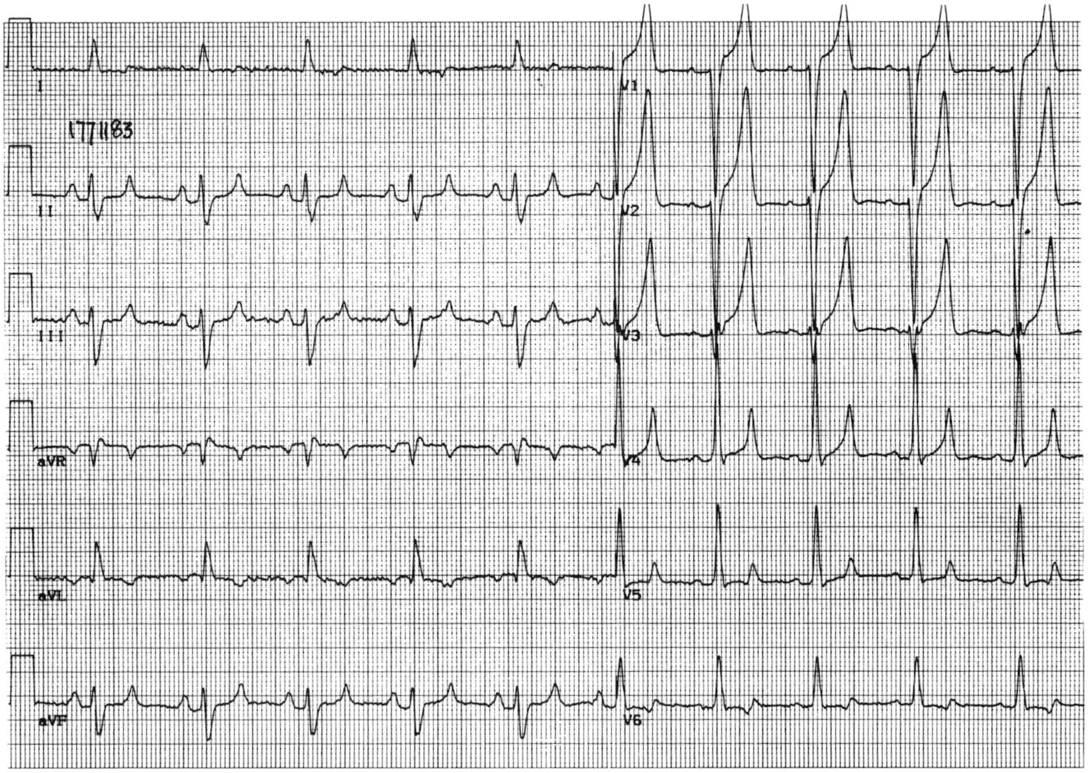

FIGURE 30-21 Hyperkalemia (6.9 meq). QRS is widened to 120 msec. The upper part of the T in V_4, and the T's of leads II and aVR, show perfect isosceles triangles.

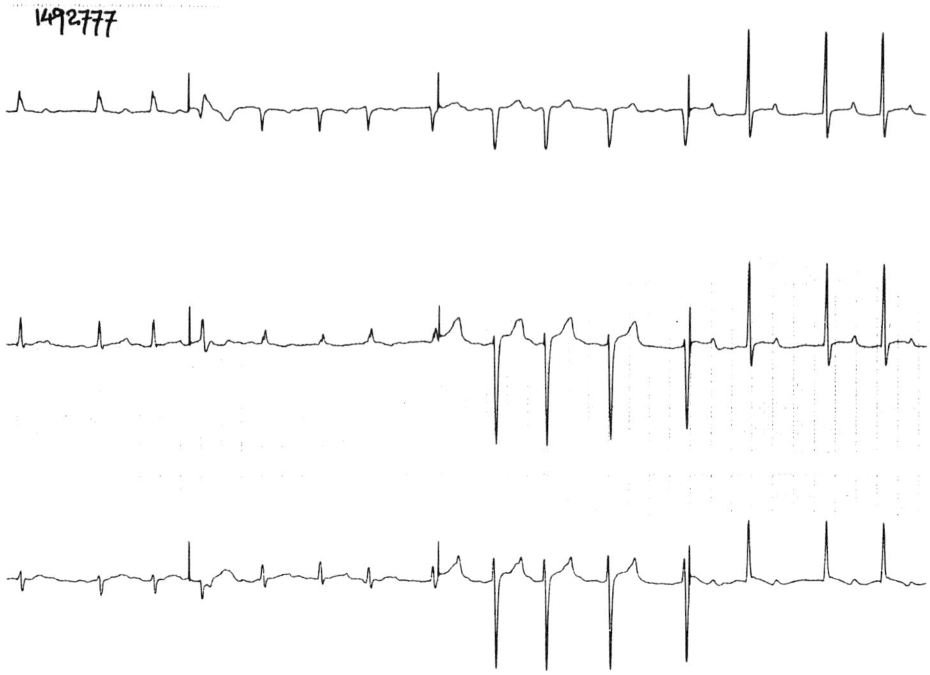

FIGURE 30-22 Hyperkalemia (5.9 meq/L). Atrial fibrillation. Hyperkalemia is suggested by the rapid ascent nipples on the top of T in V_3 and in V_4 and V_5.

instances where the T is of low amplitude and symmetrically steep only in V_4 (Fig. 30-22), and instances where the T is inverted but otherwise shows all the classic morphologic features described above.

THE THREE PHASES OF HYPERKALEMIA. In the earliest phase of hyperkalemia (approximately 5.5 to 6.3 meq/L) the QRS and P wave duration is unchanged. The classic T wave of hyperkalemia is either frankly present or strongly suggested. In the middle phase, the QRS and P wave durations are expanded (the lower voltage of the latter often making measurement problematic). About 15 percent of patients will alternatively have developed one of the classic intraventricular conduction defects,[20] not excluding the rare septal fascicular block;[21] bifascicular block and RBBB alone are the most common in this regard. For some reason, the latter combination often shows accompanying ST elevation in V_1 and V_2 (vide infra—ST elevation), creating case reports of pseudo MI. Diabetic ketoacidosis seems to encourage this simulation.[22] In the middle phase of hyperkalemia, the QRS widening seen in the majority of patients (85 percent) preserves lead for lead the same morphologic features of the control QRS, including individuated notchings and slurs. This fidelity in the splayed out hyperkalemic QRS is found in at least 11 of 12 leads (V_3, whether from lead placement differences or not, is the most likely to be divergent). The T wave remains "classic." It may be present in V_4 even in the minority of subjects who show a RBBB or bifascicular block. It is not often seen with hyperkalemic LBBB.

In late hyperkalemia (>8.2 meq/L), the QRS is grossly widened (still faithful to the past in its shape), and P waves are absent, since the atrium is paralyzed. Generally there is a tachycardia and often some irregularity in the dominant QRS rhythm. The T wave is no longer of the classic pointed variety, lacking both the voltage and the rapid ascent/descent typical of the earlier stages. The QT is only prolonged *pari passu* with the QRS, unless there is accompanying hypocalcemia. It is well known that the ECG can sometimes fail to show any of the above changes in the face of severe hyperkalemia.[23] In all such cases, the physician should be sure he is not dealing with spurious hyperkalemia, notoriously seen in massive leukocyte lysis in leukemia and thrombocythemia. In such instances, plasma potassium will be normal in the face of serum hyperkalemia (the serum K^+ normally exceeds that of plasma by <0.6 meq/L, and is due to platelet K^+, surrendered during the clotting of the sample).[24] When the ECG shows, in full, the signs of hyperkalemia, treatment with intravenous calcium or hypertonic saline solution can transiently normalize or almost normalize the tracing, even though the serum K value is as yet unchanged.[25]

Differential Diagnosis of Common ECG Abnormalities

THE SPLAYED OUT QRS

When QRS widening retains, LFL, the precise features of the complex in its normal narrow state, one should consider toxicity from quinidine, procainamide, or disopyramide (QT prolonged), drug effect with flecainide (QT not prolonged), global ischemia, typically seen with angina due to left main coronary stenosis (Fig. 30-23), or during cardio-

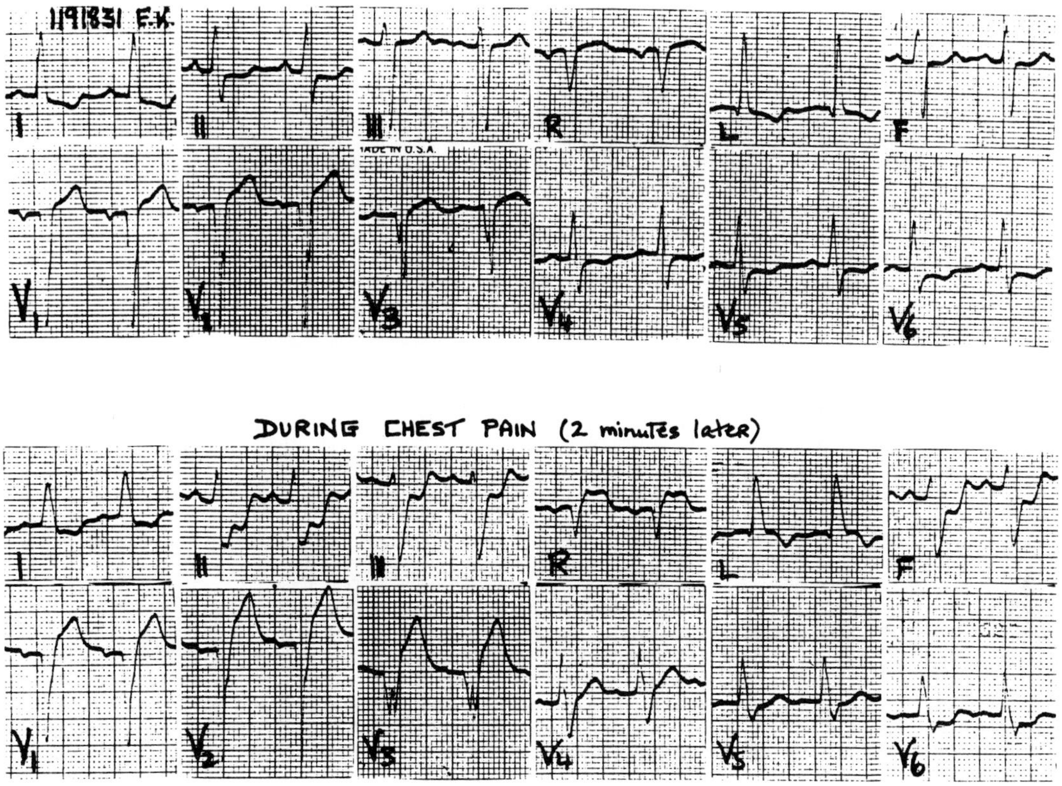

FIGURE 30-23 Global ventricular ischemia during anginal pain. Cicatricial left main coronary ostial stenosis is secondary to surgical cannulation 1 year previously. The widened QRS (bottom) preserves the individual slurs and notches of the baseline QRS.

pulmonary resuscitation (vide infra), and hyperkalemia. One should remember that the P wave may be absent in the late phase of hyperkalemia, requiring the physician to differentiate the tracing from idioventricular rhythm, or even from agonal rhythm, which severe hyperkalemia can sometimes resemble or deteriorate into.

ST ELEVATION

NORMAL. Normal J-point elevation is more often than not present in V_2, and to a lesser extent, in V_1 and V_3. In contrast to other epicardial leads (II, V_5, etc.), the J-point and the subsequent 80 msec of the ST segment are hardly ever isoelectric in these leads. All computer programs for ECG diagnosis make generous allowance for this deviation, lest acute anteroseptal infarction be incessantly overcalled. It should be emphasized that this ST elevation is not a variant like early repolarization, requiring actual mention in the ECG report.

INJURY. When ST elevation signals injury, most commonly it is the initial stigma of acute MI (or of balloon inflation in angioplasty). Depending on the affected leads, it is described as inferior, lateral, septal, anteroseptal, anterior, anterolateral, inferolateral, and occasionally, inferoseptal or high lateral (see Chap. 116).

ANEURYSM. ST elevation may be seen in ventricular aneurysm. Here the elevations are chronic, appearing in leads with pathologic Q waves. The ECG at all times resembles acute evolving MI in the middle phase. When the aneurysms are due to myocardial sarcoidosis there are seldom any Q waves. Only one-fourth of aneurysms announce themselves with a perpetual injury pattern.

TUMOR. When ST elevation is due to direct tumor invasion, echocardiography will generally reveal a focal myocardial fixation. The tumor anchors the heart at the site of local invasion. Under these circumstances each contraction generates mechanical stress at this site. The resulting ST elevation is the same as that which can be elicited by direct pressure on the myocardium by a catheter electrode, by a hook electrode in the dog heart, by epicardial pressure with an intraoperative mapping electrode, or by a needle during pericardiocentesis. The ECG shows ST elevations only. A mistaken diagnosis of pericarditis may be made (Fig. 30-24), but the pattern is quite fixed and nonevolving.

CORONARY SPASM. In coronary artery spasm (variant angina, Prinzmetal's angina), ST elevation will resolve with coronary dilators or antispasmodics. Additional to the injury pattern, the QRS may transiently show increased R amplitude in the injury leads; less often, Q waves appear

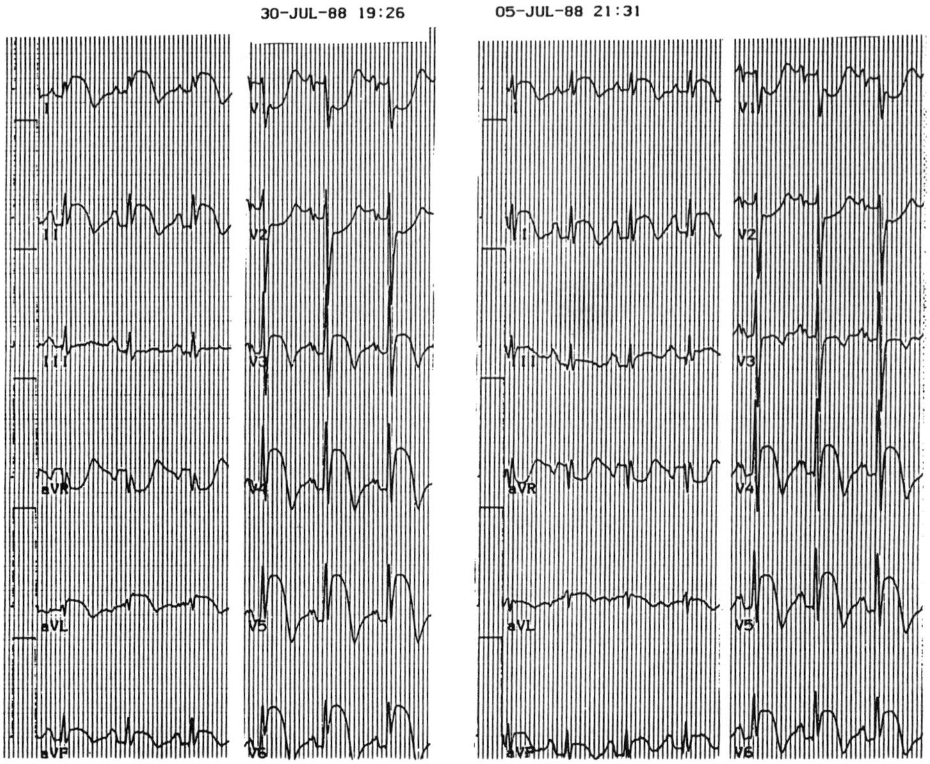

FIGURE 30-24 Chronic injury pattern secondary to invasion and fixation of the myocardial wall by tumor (confirmed by echocardiography). The two ECGs are identical. See text.

transiently, even with subsequent exclusion of necrosis by enzymes.

EARLY REPOLARIZATION. Early repolarization,[26] a variant of normal repolarization, is so named because repolarization appears to commence before depolarization is concluded, or in other words, before the descending limb of the R wave has reached the isoelectric line. QRS duration is not abbreviated, however. The ST segment is elevated in the inferolateral leads and is depressed in aVR. The T is invariably taller than the ST, with the normal curvature and concavity still present (Fig. 30-25). The ECG would be completely normal if the J-point were restored to the isoelectric line. The descending limb of R may smoothly horizontalize as a rounded J-point 1 to 6 mm above the base line, or even slope downward at first. Alternatively, the latter is seemingly preceded by an "attempt" at an S wave. The PR segment is normal and horizontal. The T wave is often inverted in V_1. The pattern is most marked in youth, the elevations becoming progressively less marked through the years. Early repolarization generally disappears with sinus tachycardia over 105/min, and with hyperkalemia. Digitalis also eliminates the elevation, restoring the J-point to the isoelectric line, frequently making the junction so smooth and rounded that the QRS duration may be difficult to measure. Early repolarization should not be invoked for those normals who have a "high takeoff" in V_2 and in V_1 and V_3. Conversely, in early repolarization, the ST in the inner precordial leads is generally unremarkable. Early repolarization should not be regarded as especially common in blacks; the particular variant of normal repolarization found in the inner precordial leads of some black males is neither early repolarization nor the juvenile pattern. If early repolarization is extreme in one plane and barely visible in the other, the diagnosis is probably wrong, and acute injury should be considered. Apart from ventricular aneurysm (and direct tumor invasion), early repolarization is the sole condition in which ST elevations in multiple leads fail to evolve (i.e., do not go on to develop terminal T inversion, Q waves, or timely normalization of the ST). The two diagnoses with which it may be confused are acute pericarditis and acute MI. In making this differentiation, two time-separated tracings are more useful than one. Comparisons are invalid if either tracing shows sinus tachycardia. The mechanism for early repolarization is unknown.

ACUTE PERICARDITIS (see Figs. 30-13, -14, and -16). As noted above, in pericarditis the ST segment elevations generally match in shape those of true ischemic injury. Unlike the latter, however, their distribution is more widespread. They are seen in the inferior and lateral leads: II, III, aVF, I, and V_4 through V_6. ST elevations may extend into V_3 and V_2, while ST in aVR is depressed. In 10 to 20 percent of patients, ST is also depressed in V_1 (but not in V_2, etc.). This finding is more specific if the T remains positive. The PR segment is depressed in leads II, aVF, and in V_4 and V_5. The record may resemble early repolarization in which the ST elevations are also inferolateral. But the latter does not produce PR segment depression or ST depression in V_1. Pericarditis evolves just like true ischemic injury, the T wave becoming first terminally, and then symmetrically, inverted, with the ST finally returning to the isoelectric line.

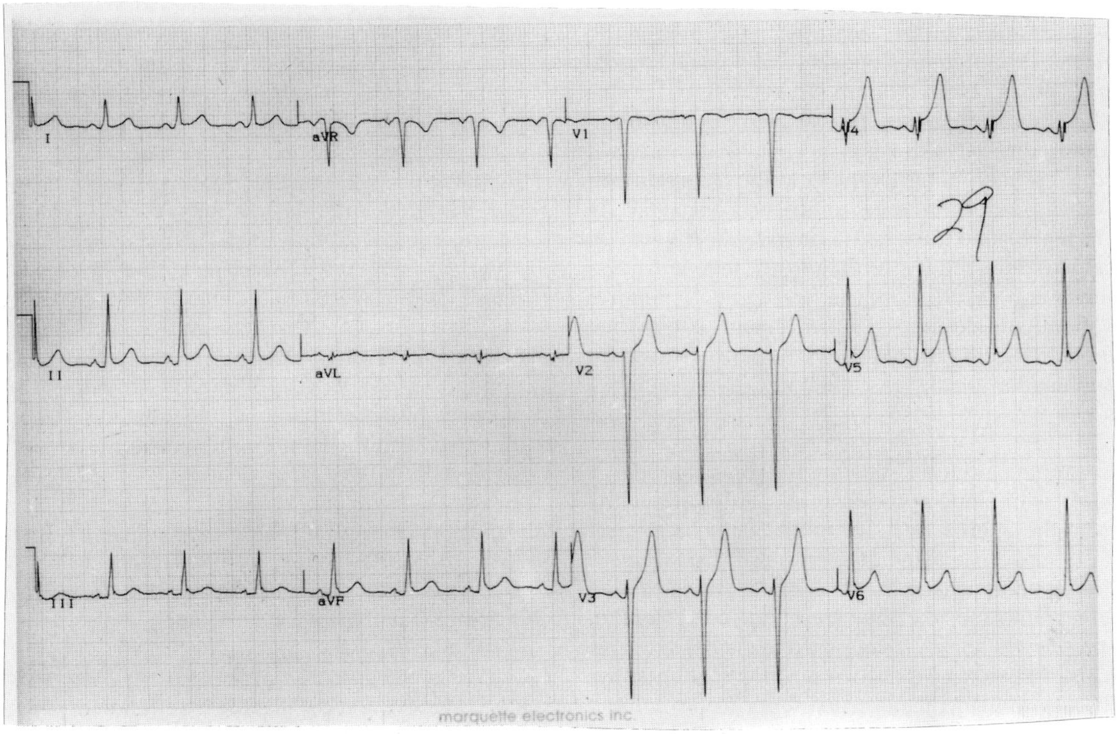

FIGURE 30-25 Early repolarization in a 24-year-old patient. See text.

Pathologic Q waves do not appear. Evolution of the process can vary in the following ways: **1.** it may be compressed into hours; **2.** the ST elevations may disappear only to reappear again after some hours; the T waves in between may invert completely, suggesting a conclusion of the process; and **3.** the PR segment depressions may be delayed or never appear.

BUNDLE BRANCH BLOCK. ST elevation is also seen in LBBB as a secondary ST-T change. There is marked J-point elevation and a tall T in V_1 through V_3. In incomplete RBBB an unusual ST elevation in V_2, or less frequently, in the complete form, in V_1, may be seen. In both instances the ST appears to be hoisted up by the R′.

ATRIAL ECTOPIC RHYTHM. In many cases of low atrial ectopic rhythm in which the P wave axis is $-90°$ and the T_a or atrial repolarization wave has an opposite polarity, some ST elevation will be apparent. The rhythm disturbance elevates both the QRS and ST segment in leads II, III, and aVF.[27]

PSEUDOINJURY. In pseudoinjury, acute MI is inexplicably simulated by diverse conditions such as acute pancreatitis, hyperkalemia, or wasp sting anaphylaxis. ST elevation of this kind has not been reported in the absence of at least one of the following: electrolyte imbalance, diabetic ketoacidosis, alcoholism, or severe allergic reaction.

ST DEPRESSION

RECIPROCAL DEPRESSION. The literature often uses the phrase "reciprocal" to describe certain kinds of ST depression, notably those seen in V_2 through V_4, in acute inferior MI. Such ST depression signifies in reciprocal, or mirror image fashion, an actual elevation of the ST segment on the posterior epicardial surface. But such reciprocal change may not be evident in other seemingly identical transmural inferior infarcts, since it is a question of transplanar infarct geometry. By way of contrast, in the frontal plane leads in acute inferior MI, if the ST is markedly and symmetrically elevated in II and III, it will always be depressed in aVR and aVL. This change should not be described as reciprocal, however. It is obligatory or mandatory, a function of lead structure in the Einthoven triangle (equally mandatory are the positive P waves in these two arm leads with "low atrial rhythm" when the P is retrograde and negative in the inferior leads).

DIGITALIS EFFECT. With digitalis effect, there is a rounded sagging of the ST, seen best in left ventricular leads (i.e., those with a qR configuration: V_4 through V_6, I, aVF, sometimes aVL). It is most often asymmetric, the concavity being maximal in the last third of the negative wave (southeast), and the ascent-return to the base line being relatively steep. The magnitude of ST depression may be greatly exaggerated, even suggesting subendocardial injury, at very rapid rates, particularly in paroxysmal supraventricular tachycardia.

LEFT VENTRICULAR STRAIN. To ascribe ST depression to left ventricular strain requires unequivocal voltage criteria: the R in aVL should exceed 13 mm. The QRS-T axial angle is wide, the T and companion ST axes being in the southwest quadrant or, if the QRS axis is more vertically inclined, in the northwest quadrant. Morphologically, the strain pattern is a triad: T inversion in left ventricular leads, ST depression in these same leads, and an upward convexity in the ST segment. Frequently overdiagnosed, left ventricular strain cannot appear or disappear overnight. It requires weeks or months to develop. It often remains even when the cause is successfully treated. It is notoriously simulated by the combination of digitalis effect and a symmetric T inversion.

ANGINA. Angina pectoris shows ST depression, either horizontal or with slope reversal. It is seen in either the lateral leads, the inferior leads, or both. Such changes reverse with nitrates. The magnitude of the ST displacement is 1 to 3 mm, and the change is generally confined to one, two, or three unipolar leads. The time-honored explanation for ST depression in angina (as opposed to elevation in coronary occlusion) invokes a selective sensitivity of endomyocardial tissues to inadequate coronary perfusion, a function of the relative sparseness of collaterals at this depth, of a metabolic fragility, or of both. The resulting ST segment vectors point toward the right shoulder. Not all of the endocardial lining is thus affected, otherwise the vectors would tend to cancel out. The most complete and severe expression of this process is called subendocardial injury.

SUBENDOCARDIAL INJURY. Subendocardial injury is invoked when there is gross depression of the ST segment, slope reversal, T wave inversion (or at best, inconsequential final positivity) affecting not only the lateral leads, but also "leaking" into the inner precordial leads as far as V_2. The ST depression, measured 80 msec after the J-point, may reach 7 mm in V_5. The inferior leads are seldom excluded. Other features attend this diagnosis. There is sinus tachycardia, and the patient is often apprehensive and in pain. This picture is very common in ICUs. It may develop in the postoperative patient or even at the moment anesthesia is being induced (particularly if coronary disease has gone unnoticed). It may also develop in a patient with coronary disease following substantial hemorrhage, with prolonged paroxysmal SVT (see Fig. 30-3), hypotension, or arterial hypoxemia, when an exercise test is performed on a patient with left main coronary artery stenosis or its three-vessel equivalent, or as the initial presentation of acute coronary occlusion, (the patient thereafter developing Q waves, completing a non-Q wave infarct, or retaining the pattern through cardiogenic shock and death). Autopsy in some cases has shown necrosis of the inner subendocardial lining of the left ventricle. Electrocardiographically, subendocardial injury must be distinguished from digitalis effect at very fast heart rates (if due to digitalis alone, the ST will normalize in the first 2 or 3 beats following conversion of the SVT, rather than in 12 to 30 beats or for minutes as in true subendocardial injury), from acute dorsal infarction where V_6 generally shows an isoelectric ST (the ST depression being maximal in V_2 and V_3), and from severe fixed left ventricular strain which gets worse with sinus tachycardia, but does not "leak" into inner pretransitional leads.

NONSPECIFIC CHANGES. Nonspecific ST changes (inferior, lateral, or anterolateral leads) are fairly common. The T waves are normal, and the ST depression is minor though often diffuse. If the ST were restored to the isoelectric line, repolarization would be normal.

LOCAL ST DEPRESSION. ST depression limited to V_2 through V_4 and V_5 is seen in acute true dorsal MI (the MI most likely to be missed), in some cases of hypokalemia (together with the U-on-T phenomenon), and in right ventricular strain (with T inversion).

SECONDARY ST CHANGES. Secondary ST depression is seen with LBBB (I, aVL, V_5 and V_6), and RBBB (V_1, V_2), in each case accompanied by T inversion. It is also seen with the WPW pattern of preexcitation and with ventricular rhythm/tachycardia.

MANDATORY ST DEPRESSION. Mandatory ST segment depression in frontal plane leads is seen with acute inferior injury, (ST down in aVR, sometimes aVL), acute lateral injury (ST down in aVR and III), acute pericarditis (ST down in aVR), early repolarization (ST down in aVR), and in acute pulmonary embolism (ST down in I). In all these instances the actual abnormality is conceptualized as a cause for ST elevation; ST depression is demanded in the opposing frontal leads.

PRIMARY T INVERSION

The causes of this common finding include: **1.** MI: Q wave, non-Q wave, recent or old; **2.** active ischemia or immediately following same (ST depression companion to the former); **3.** pericarditis, epicarditis, myocarditis, myocardial contusion; **4.** ventricular hypertrophy with strain; **5.** cardiomyopathy of all kinds; **6.** cerebrovascular accidents, brain surgery; **7.** the QT syndromes; **8.** drugs: digitalis, emetine, and others; **9.** systemic disease, e.g., lupus erythematosus; **10.** unexplained mild T inversion, correctible by intravenous Isuprel, by exercise, or by neither; **11.** mitral prolapse; and **12.** following ventricular pacing, sustained paroxysmal tachycardia, the remission of BBB, or the functional closure of a Kent bundle.

GIANT T WAVE INVERSION

Regardless of cause, giant (>1 mV, exceptionally as much as 2.7 mV)[28] T wave inversions are typically associated with QT prolongation, ST segment depression in lateral or inferior leads, and a discrete shelf somewhat suggestive of a "negative U-on-T" phenomenon in the final returning limb of T in the chest leads. Giant T inversion is seen with cerebrovascular accidents, evolving non-Q wave MI, apical hypertrophic cardiomyopathy (common among Japanese

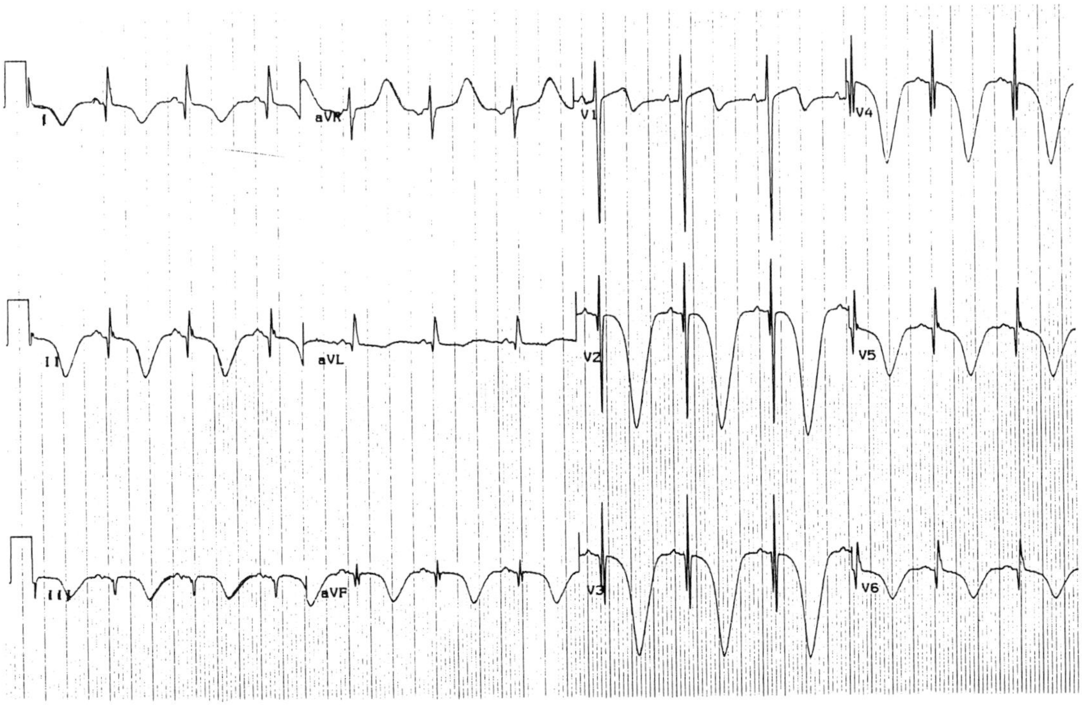

FIGURE 30-26 Giant T wave inversion and QT expansion following chest pain and negative enzymes in a patient with old inferolateral infarction. Note the Qs of the latter remain deep but narrow (seen also with IHSS).

and often missed in routine echocardiography since it must be actively sought). The giant T negativity is lateral, sometimes inferolateral (Fig. 30-26). Giant T inversion can also be seen with congenital long QT syndromes (where the T wave is bizarre in shape and undergoes extraordinary changes in the course of a 24-h Holter, including giant inversion), and with occasional cases of sustained severe electrolyte depletion, especially hypocalcemia. In both of these last two situations the T inversion may accompany T wave alternation. Inversion is also seen transiently following the inadvertent injection of calcium-free saline solution into a coronary artery, following the arrest of prolonged paroxysmal tachycardia, postpacing (in which the leads previously showing negativity of the paced QRS complex now show T inversion in the sinus beats, infrequently of giant proportions), and with complete AV block and prolonged QT syndrome. These cases tend to be in the older literature, predating artificial pacing, and are more likely to be seen when complete block and idioventricular rhythm have long been present. Furthermore, they show recurrent, often nonsustained, ventricular tachycardia (and sometimes torsades de pointes). Ventricular fibrillation, when it occurs in these cases, may spontaneously terminate. Some of these cases are variants of the congenital long QT syndrome. Finally, giant T inversion is seen with catechol injury of the myocardium, both in pheochromocytoma and following excessive use of adrenaline in asthma.

TALL T WAVES

Disproportionately tall T waves are seen in hyperkalemia (especially V_2 through V_4), in isolated "true" dorsal, or inferodorsal transmural MI, or ischemia (the tall T's in V_1 and V_2 mirror T wave inversion in the posterior left ventricular wall; Fig. 30-27), and with the combination of sinus tachycardia, PR prolongation, and P pulmonale: the latter sitting astride the T wave can cause leads II and III and aVF to resemble hyperkalemia. Tall T waves are also seen in the opening phase of some cases of acute MI: the "hyperacute" T wave is seen in one or some of chest leads, V_2 through V_5. The T is exceptionally tall, exceeding the height of the associated R wave (Fig. 30-28 *right*), and pointed if it follows a gross ST elevation (the latter may start near the top of the R and climb steeply to the T). Alternatively, the tall T is rounded rather than pointed and emerges from an ST only (as yet) modestly elevated (Fig. 30-28 *left*). The diagnosis of hyperacute T wave, perennially popular among housestaff, is less common than its familiarity would suggest. Finally, tall T waves are also seen in normal young males, with or without some degree of early repolarization (V_3 through V_5), and in a small minority of patients with subarachnoid hemorrhage where the T wave may be excessively large in V_3 or V_4, while showing an exaggerated U-on-T phenomenon and a long QT interval.

PROLONGED QT INTERVALS

Prolonged QT intervals[29] are found with some cases of BBB, hypocalcemia, hypokalemia (where the prolongation expands into a U wave), hypomagnesemia, hypothermia, liquid protein diets,[30] in drug-free depressed patients,[31] certain forms of complete AV block, infrequently with mitral prolapse,[32] in the occasional postoperative wake of a radical neck dissection, with evolving Q wave and non-Q wave

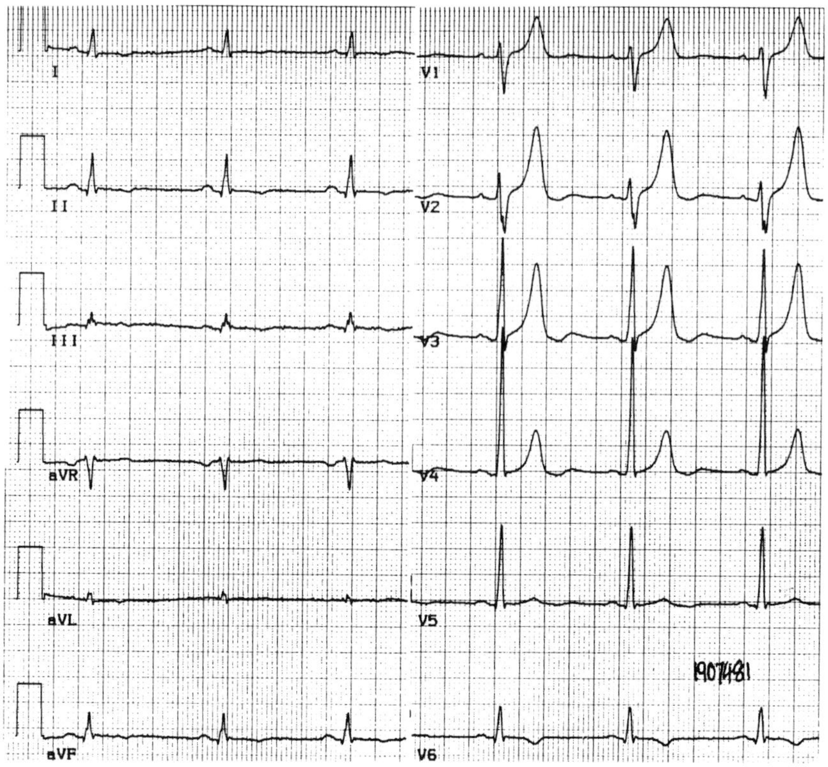

FIGURE 30-27 Angiographically confirmed true dorsal infarction of the non-Q wave type. The tall T in V_1 through V_3 mirrors posterior wall T inversion.

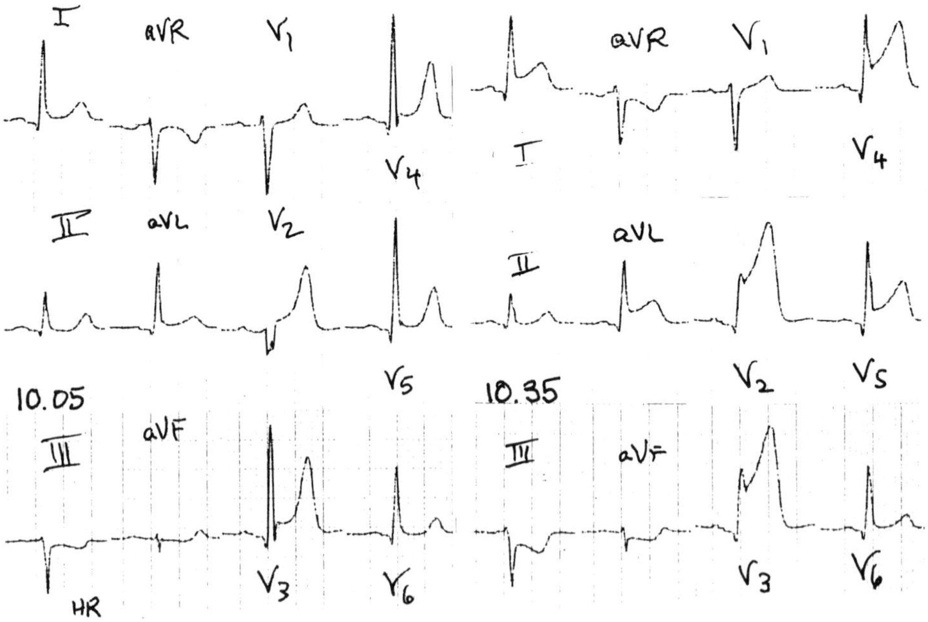

FIGURE 30-28 Types of hyperacute T wave (V_3) in the same patient, minutes apart: acute anterior MI.

MI,[33] in other cases of ischemia where MI fails to be documented (see Fig. 30-26), with many cerebrovascular accidents, and certain cases of intracranial surgery (notably hypophysectomy), in subarachnoid hemorrhage, following liver transplantation,[34] with the hereditary or familial QT syndromes, acquired or sporadic QT expansion, poisoning due to phenothiazines, cyclic antidepressants, or organophosphate insecticides, and finally, as a therapeutic or toxic drug effect of quinidine, procainamide, disopyramide, or amiodarone.

THE QT AND VULNERABILITY TO VENTRICULAR ARRHYTHMIA. Torsade de pointes has been documented in almost all of the above causes of QT expansion. It must be remembered however that ventricular tachycardia can also be of the traditional type: sustained, unifocal, and tidy looking.

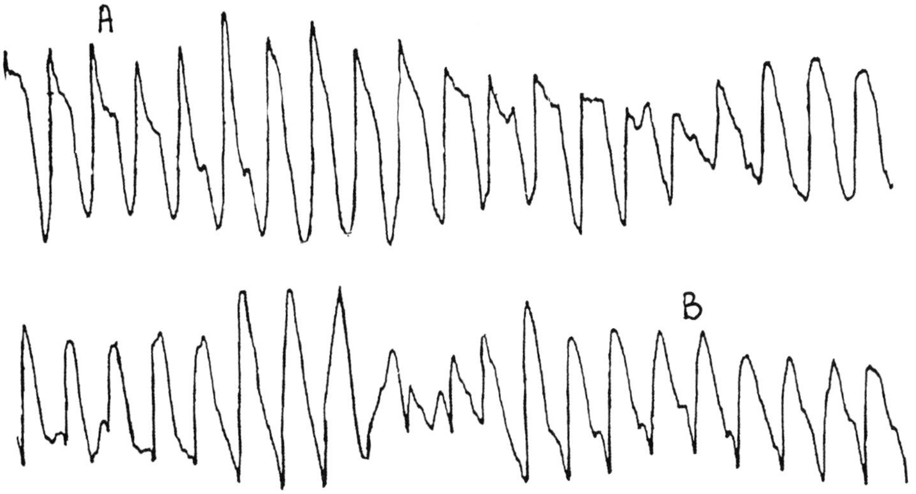

FIGURE 30-29 Torsades de pointes in a patient with the long QT syndrome. See text for the full description.

Equally, short salvos of nonsustained polymorphic tachycardia may follow an R-on-T phenomenon (also referred to as "multiple ventricular responses"). Finally, the R-on-T phenomenon may produce ventricular fibrillation too soon, making it impossible to decide if the initial venticular deflections constituted a torsade.

TORSADE DE POINTES. The visible impact of the QRS cadences in this particular form of ventricular tachycardia is, by the use of this descriptive term, likened to a specific choreographic sequence in ballet. Torsade (Fig. 30-29) is most often seen in the context of QT interval prolongation, most commonly as a proarrhythmic consequence of quinidine, procainamide, or disopyramide therapy. Generally, the R-on-T phenomenon is observed with the first ventricular ectopic beat and invariably with the subsequent beats, each of which seemingly climbs out of the apex of the preceding T wave. The rightward displacement of the T wave by the expanded QT facilitates this encroachment. The tachycardia is untidy looking and superficially reminiscent of the artifactual "V tacs" often recorded on monitor strips in ICUs. It is neither unifocal nor polymorphic. Each beat differs slightly from its neighbor in shape, size, and crudity. Additionally, many of the beats are frankly curvaceous and sinusoidal in shape, failing to look like real QRS deflections. Their duration is wide (>120 msec), but generally impossible to measure (either QRS initiation cannot be pinpointed or the J-point cannot be discerned).

The beats can be crudely grouped in repeating morphologic sequences, each constituting a single torsade of 5 to 10 beats. Most episodes consist of no more than two complete cycles after which the tachycardia spontaneously aborts or becomes fibrillation. The torsade shows, in consecutive beats, a gradual increase (Fig. 30-29*a*) and then decrease in overall amplitude. Accompanying these shifting voltages are changes in shape and polarity. Although the torsades can be said to "repeat," the morphology is never precisely the same. The overall visual impression at a distance suggests the graphic multibeat portrayal of a crescendo-decrescendo murmur or a taut vibrating guitar wire. As for the phasic change in polarity, if one were to extend the last visible sinus beat isoelectric line through the tachycardia, one would often bisect the QRS complexes, rather than find them grouped in turn, above and below, the isoelectric line (in practice, however, the tachycardia more often than not will generate patient movement and wandering of the base line). The postulate of change in polarity resides on the changing placement of QRS spikes.

In torsades, each large amplitude QRS most commonly shows but one spike and one rounded opposing extremity (see Fig. 30-29*a*). The seeming change in polarity coincides with the moment when consecutive beats showing positive R wave spikes yield to negative S wave spikes (Fig. 30-29*b*). In each prototype the opposite end of the complex is rounded. One infrequently sees a large amplitude wave with both R and S spikes. Distinct from each prototype are the sine wave complexes and those of low amplitude. The latter, in groups of two to six beats, serve as bridges between the high amplitude cadences. The low amplitude beats are invariably polyphasic with rapidly changing polarities.

The rate of torsade de pointe ranges from 185 to 240. It almost invariably fluctuates by as much as 15 beats/min, with the slower rates separating the sine wave beats, and the faster rates seen with spike-containing complexes. Variations from the foregoing description include a relatively abrupt change in amplitude (small to big rather than the converse), and instances where the ectopics are briefly "spiky" at both ends. Occasionally one will see a choreographically perfect torsade.

The triggering event in torsade is generally a pause which often follows an atrial premature beat. In some cases a type of U wave develops after the long QT, exclusively in the wake of such pauses. The first ventricular complex of the tachycardia arises from this U wave. It has been suggested that this U wave is an early afterpotential (the hallmark of one type of triggered automaticity), and that shifting QT intervals, common in all long QT syndromes, may be expressions of the presence or absence of such afterpotentials.[35] In torsades associated with the congenital, familial, or sporadic QT syndromes, the triggering factor is often some form of adrenergic stimulation: fright, anxiety, a loud noise, bad news, a phone call, etc.

The differential diagnosis of torsades de pointes includes only artifact. It resembles nothing else. In artifacts of this kind, the spikes discussed above are those of the bona fide generally sinus, QRS. By means of calipers, they can be demonstrated to traverse the putative wide complex tachycardia. The spikes will fail to be either the R or S waves of the latter, falling between or on the sides of the artifactual deflections.

QS, Q, POOR PROGRESSION OR REGRESSION OF R IN V_1 THROUGH V_3

In the absence of septal or anteroseptal MI, these changes are seen with emphysema, during an attack of bronchial asthma, with WPW preexcitation (the delta waves being negative in V_1 through V_3), in hypertrophic obstructive myocardopathy, with severe right ventricular hypertrophy (RVH) (qR in V_1 and V_2), with LBBB (where R is not, in fact, septal), with corrected transposition of great vessels (and bundle branches), primary myocardiopathy, severe LVH and strain (QS in V_1 and V_2), septal abscess in endocarditis, septal fibrosis, septal fascicular block, pneumothorax, left anterior fascicular block (tiny Qs in V_2 and V_3), acute pancreatitis, lead reversal (e.g., V_1 for V_3) or malplacement, transiently with wasp sting anaphylaxis, in occasional normals (minuscule Qs in V_2 and V_3, the R wave progressing normally), or with normals where QS in V_1 through V_3 or poor R wave progression, remain unexplained.

Abnormalities of Rhythm in the ICU

CLASSIFICATION BY CONTEXT

ICU patients who become subject to abnormalities of cardiac rhythm include those who are **1.** postcardiac surgery, in whom the rhythm problems are well defined (e.g., atrial flutter) and relatively easy to manage; **2.** those with coronary heart disease, the familiar arrhythmias of which are often temporary, but potentially disastrous—however, the management prerogatives are extensive, not infrequently involving invasive or surgical treatment; **3.** those with other heart diseases, where the rhythm disorder may or may not be part of the natural history, but where treatment is inexorably linked to the management of the cardiac disease itself; and **4.** those with all other critical illnesses.

Rhythm problems in this latter group are the most difficult to interpret and evaluate because most of the patients have no known cardiac disorder. Although the rhythm problem may be linked to cryptic heart disease, it is more likely a function of the severe illness that placed the patient in the ICU in the first place. Not uncommonly, multiple organ failures are present. A specific ECG diagnosis may be hampered by low voltage and other manifestations of grossly abnormal metabolism. The cause of a given arrhythmia is seldom obvious. Even when there is an obvious arrhythmogenic presence, such as electrolyte imbalance, its correction may not abolish the arrhythmia. Alternatively, the rhythm disorder may disappear well before the correction, and aggressive antiarrhythmic therapy may get the intensivist into additional and unneeded trouble. The management formulation is nearly always tactical rather than strategic. The presumption is that treatment for the problem will not be required in the long term.

Some of the diagnostic constellations associated with major dysrhythmia encountered by the author include acute respiratory failure, the adult respiratory distress syndrome, acute, drug-induced liver necrosis, subdiaphragmatic abscess, rupture of the esophagus, neglected bowel gangrene, septic pulmonary emboli, hypothermia plus brain abscess, myelogenous leukemia in blast crisis, drug purpura, sickle cell crisis, coumadin necrosis, disseminated lupus, and every kind of septicemia. None of these conditions is inexorably linked to a particular type of rhythm disturbance, but certain generalizations are possible.

SINUS DEPRESSION

Sinus depression (or even suppression) is common in situations where sinus tachycardia would otherwise be the expected rhythm (see Fig. 30-9). In its stead one often finds accelerated junctional rhythm with rates of 70 to 100 beats/min. Alternatively, P waves may only seem to be absent, because of a temporary low voltage, metabolic in origin.

SECOND DEGREE AV BLOCK

Second degree AV block is frequently seen in the absence of the usual causes. Wenckebach sequences occur without digitalis or diltiazem toxicity or acute inferior MI. Less commonly, Mobitz type II AV block may transiently appear and, with successful treatment or spontaneous resolution of the primary affliction, not return thereafter (see Fig. 30-8). In viral syndromes, fresh AV nodal block of any degree always suggests acute or subacute myocarditis. In such instances, myocardial biopsy is indicated.

PAROXYSMAL ATRIAL FIBRILLATION

Paroxysmal atrial fibrillation is common with any severe ICU illness. The ventricular rate is least likely to be controlled by digitalis in this setting. Such recalcitrance is seen with infection, (especially pneumonia with pyrexia), shock (hemorrhagic, cardiogenic, septic), acute pulmonary embolism, severe arterial hypoxemia, unrecognized hyperthyroidism, during the intravenous administration of adrenergic medications, pheochromocytoma, delirium tremens, WPW syndrome (the rapid transit and recovery time of Kent bundle conduction permits the ventricular rate to approach 400 beats/min), other conditions with a short PR interval (patients on hemodialysis, the Lown-Ganong-Levine syndrome, etc.), other clinical states in which sinus tachycardia would be present in the absence of atrial fibrillation, in some cases of acute asthma, and, finally, in a small subset of patients in whom rapid rate fibrillation is resistant to all AV nodal blocking agents (such patients may require His bundle ablation).[36]

The intensivist contemplating the use of AV nodal blocking drugs (digitalis, β blockers, and calcium antagonists) should never try to slow the ventricular response below the rate he would anticipate if the mechanism were sinus. In the case of pneumonia, the best management of the fibrillation is an antibiotic.

JUNCTIONAL RHYTHM AND ITS SIMULATORS

JUNCTIONAL RHYTHM. In junctional rhythm[37] the QRS resembles, LFL, the supraventricular QRS recorded during sinus rhythm. The rate is normally 45 to 64/min, but it is notoriously accelerated in the ICU setting (range 65 to 140/min). The tracing should be frisked for subtle or retrograde P waves by comparing, where possible, the ST-T's of II, III, aVF, V_1 and V_2 with the "unencumbered" deflections of a previous sinus rhythm tracing. A retrograde P may be visible in lead II as a fat S wave terminating (and perhaps "widening") the QRS, or as a negative indentation (axis $-90°$) in early to late in repolarization (Fig. 30-30*b*), sometimes simulating inferior T inversion. These P's form positive spikes in V_1, where they can mimic an r′ if early. The RP interval may be constant or progressively lengthen, culminating in an early "reciprocal" QRS, or echo. The sinus may then regain control, preempting the retrograde P. Uncommonly, RP intervals alternate long and short (Fig. 30-30*b*).

Sinus P waves may also be found on careful examination. If both QRS and P rhythms are regular, and PR is constantly changing, then complete AV dissociation is present. Early QRSs preceded by Ps are most probably captures (incomplete AV dissociation, Fig. 30-30*c*). Dissociation is seen when the sinus or atrial rate drops below that of the junction or other escape centers, when such centers become accelerated beyond the sinus rate, when the AV node is blocked, or most commonly, with mixtures of these three factors. In isorhythmic AV dissociation there is approximation of sinus and junctional rates. The sinus is seen to "run into" the QRS, and emerge to the right of it, remaining for several beats in the ST segment, and thereafter moving back, or advancing rightward to the point of capturing a QRS.

Finally, there may be no visible Ps of any kind (fluctuating ST-T morphology means P waves are present). The P may be retrograde and buried in the QRS, invisible to the closest scrutiny. It may slightly reduce the voltage of R in II compared with that of a previous sinus rhythm tracing. Alternatively there may be a junctional rhythm with no retrograde conduction and complete atrial standstill, with paralyzed sinus and ectopic atrial pacemakers.

SINUS WITH FIRST DEGREE AV BLOCK. In sinus rhythm with marked first degree AV block, the P may be submerged in the previous ST-T. If its shape is known from a previous ECG, it should be easy to recognize early in the inferior ST segments (Fig. 30-31). When superposed on a tall T, it may mimic hyperkalemia. In V_1, as a plus-minus deflection, it is relatively easy to see on the upsloping ST segment, but difficult if its positive phase is rounded and it

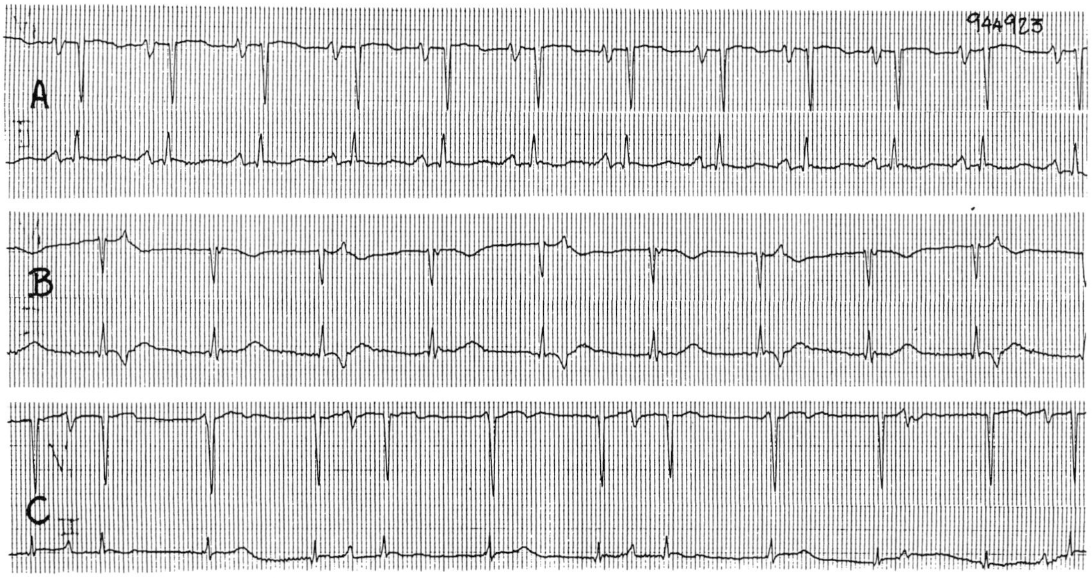

FIGURE 30-30 Twin channel recordings (V_1 and II) at different times in a subject with: *a*. Sinus rhythm. *b*. Junctional rhythm with alternating long and short RP intervals (dual AV nodal pathways). The long show P negative in II and positive in V_1. The short retrograde interval places the inverted P within the QRS of II, deepening its s wave. In V_1 it gives a tiny notch in the wake of an r′. *c*. Incomplete AV dissociation. The final two P waves show the bradycardic sinus rate (48/min). Many P's are buried in the junctional QRS beats (65/min). Others capture the ventricle with long PR's.

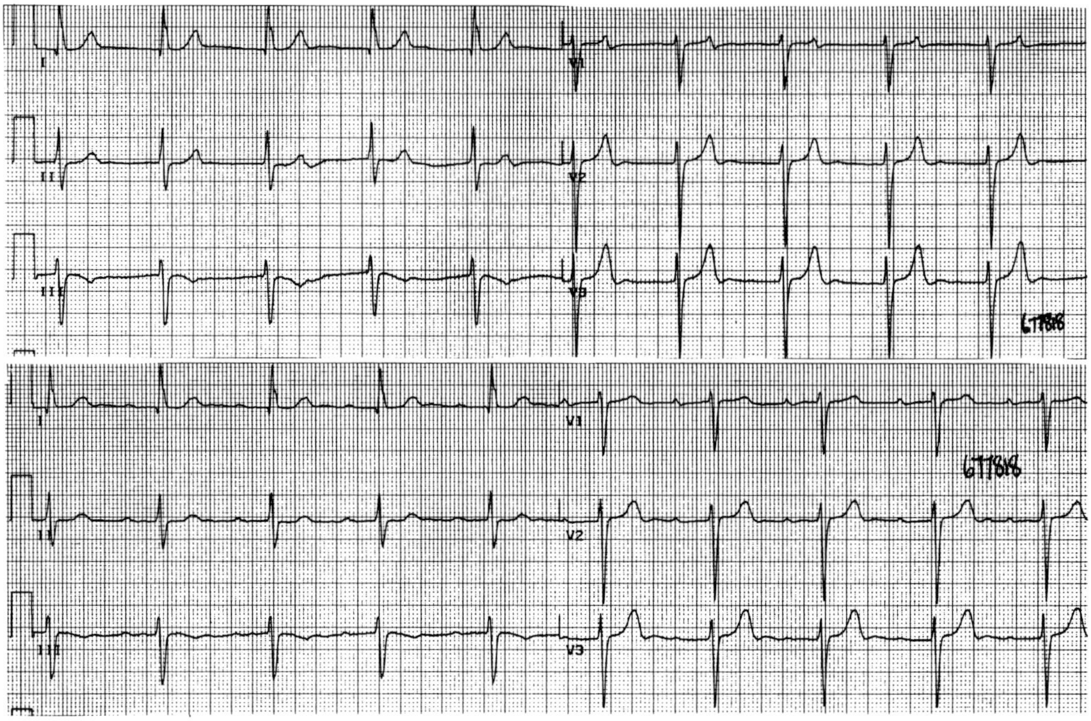

FIGURE 30-31 Junctional rhythm simulated by sinus rhythm and marked first degree AV block. The PR interval is 680 msec placing the sinus P wave invisibly in the T wave. The previous tracing shows that PR was already prolonged and displays the true shape of P and T in V_1.

sits precisely astride the apex of the T. If the P falls during the T descent, it will add a ripple to the slope. If it starts in mid descent, the final negative part of the P may be perceived as a terminal inversion of the T wave.

CONDUCTED ATRIAL RHYTHMS WITH LOW VOLTAGE P OR FLUTTER WAVES. Excessively low voltage P or flutter (F) waves may be regularly conducted, yet be hard to discern. Examples include ectopic atrial rhythm, atrial flutter with 4:1 block, atrial tachycardia with 2 or 3:1 block, and rarely, sinus rhythm.

OVERT ATRIAL RHYTHMS WITH COMPLETE AV BLOCK. Atrial fibrillation with complete AV dissociation and junctional rhythm yields a narrow QRS complex rhythm with fibrillatory (f) waves but no P. Overt flutter or atrial tachycardia with complete AV dissociation and junctional rhythm may only be recognizable by the failure of the RR intervals to be an arithmetic function of the flutter or atrial rate. They will not "fit" on the F waves or ectopic P waves, as in 4:1 or 5:1 block.

LOW ATRIAL VOLTAGE RHYTHMS WITH COMPLETE AV BLOCK. In cryptic atrial fibrillation with complete AV nodal block and junctional rhythm, the f waves are invisible or excessively reduced in voltage (often as a consequence of digitalis toxicity). Low voltage or absence of f waves is common in atrial fibrillation even outside ICUs, and, in the absence of complete AV block, generally ignored if the RR irregularity is gross enough to permit the fibrillation diagnosis (Fig. 30-32). Finally, low voltage atrial activity in flutter, atrial ectopic rhythm, atrial tachycardia, or even sinus rhythm will, with superimposed complete AV nodal block and junctional rhythm, resemble the garden variety of this arrhythmia described at the outset of this section.

EXAMINING FOR LOW VOLTAGE ATRIAL ACTIVITY. Not infrequently, junctional rhythm will be the computer diagnosis in the presence of low voltage, minuscule P waves, or atrial activity. The human eye is more discerning than the computer in this respect, and thus, not only every lead of the ECG, but every RR interval should be carefully scanned. A low voltage P may only be visible in V_1. It can be a tiny perturbation in the diastolic base line, recognizable because, unlike an artifact, it keeps cropping up in the same presystolic position. Having found such a P wave, one should immediately consider the possibility of 2:1 block. A second hidden P wave should be sought with the calipers at exactly double the apparent rate. The extra P may be seen only in the pause following a PVC or during carotid sinus massage. Low atrial voltage f, F, retrograde, ectopic, paroxysmal atrial, or sinus P waves is particularly difficult to visualize at fast rates, since tachycardia abbreviates diastole where atrial activity shows up best. It may be better seen by doubling ECG amplitude (now retrospectively possible with certain retrieval programs in the newer generations of ECG computer systems). In some instances atrial activity is only visible in intracavitary electrograms.

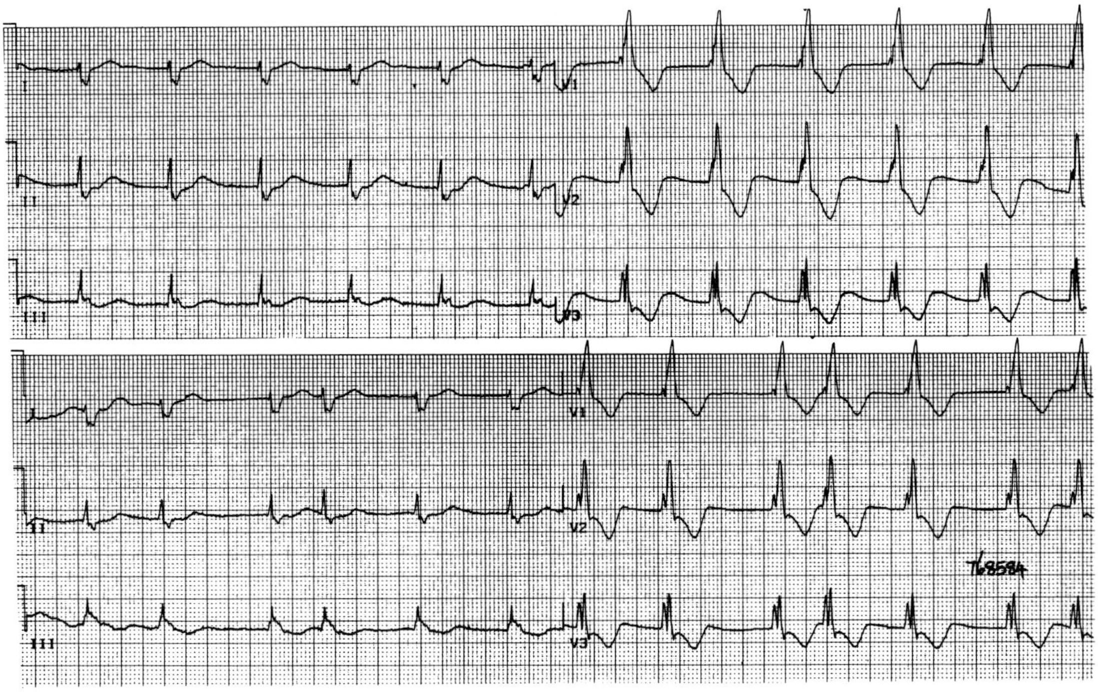

FIGURE 30-32 Concealment of complete heart block (at AV nodal level) by the total absence of atrial f waves. The tracing suggests either junctional rhythm with bifascicular block or accelerated idioventricular rhythm. Only the gross irregularity of the previously recorded RR intervals on the bottom trace revealed the presence of atrial fibrillation. The digoxin level was 4.9 mμg/mL, causing the complete AV nodal block.

When the low atrial voltage is permanent, there may be extensive atrial fibrosis (the atria may be inexcitable). In this context, an ectopic rather than sinus P wave is generally seen. In ICU patients, however, the atrial low voltage is often temporary and not easily explicable except with the catch-all phrase "metabolic disorder."

NARROW QRS TACHYCARDIA

PAROXYSMAL SUPRAVENTRICULAR TACHYCARDIAS. Narrow QRS tachycardia is either paroxysmal, nonparoxysmal, or unspecified. Paroxysmal SVTs are very common in the ICU, but in this setting, they differ from the generic profile offered in the literature. The latter is concerned with recurrent, sometimes lifelong, often therapeutically troublesome, paroxysmal SVT. The majority of such patients are subject to reentrant AV nodal tachycardia or circus tachycardia involving either a concealed bypass tract or the overt variety typical of the WPW syndrome. Paroxysmal tachycardia originating in the atrium is relatively uncommon (1 to 4 percent). In gross contrast, paroxysmal SVT in the typical ICU patient is most commonly unexpected and not destined to reappear after recovery and discharge. Atrial tachycardia is more common. The triggering factor for the paroxysm is least likely to be psychosocial. Because of the singularity of incidence and causation, treatment is often more a question of controlling ventricular rate than of total suppression and prevention. By the time the right prescription is found for achieving the latter, the arrhythmogenic morbid state may no longer be present. On the other hand, extreme rapidity of rate in paroxysmal SVT can cause organ failure when there is stenosing atherosclerosis of the relevent nutrient artery in a critically ill patient. This can produce myocardial, cerebral, or mesenteric infarction. In the kidney, it can result in acute tubular necrosis, and in the compromised distal limb, gangrene.

NONPAROXYSMAL TACHYCARDIA. The rate of sinus or nonparoxysmal junctional tachycardia[38] is related to the severity of the illness. It can accelerate or slow down only relatively gradually and only in accord with changing metabolism, tissue pathology, or both. By way of contrast, a paroxysmal tachycardia can terminate suddenly without change in the patient's morbid state. The ventricular rate is only decisively influenced by the latter in fibrillation, atrial tachycardia, and flutter.

IS IT SINUS TACHYCARDIA? The question arises when an increase in rate (up to 175/min) places the sinus P wave on top or within the T wave (tachycardia contracts diastole, the TP interval disappears). Such P waves do not stand out. In frontal leads they tend to have the same respective polarity as the T. If, from the same admission, a previous tracing in sinus rhythm is available, it will show what to expect with regard to P wave axis, PR interval base-line prolongation is likely to remain during a sinus tachycardia), and P wave shape, particularly in V_1. In the tachycardic tracing the sinus P wave(s) may be obvious following the pause generated by premature atrial or ventricular ectopics.

PAROXYSMAL CIRCUS TACHYCARDIA. Paroxysmal circus tachycardia may arise from a concealed AV bypass tract (CBT). The tract is said to be concealed because it is incapable of antegrade conduction. There is thus no delta wave during sinus rhythm; the tract is essentially a unidirectional Kent bundle. The tachycardia will show a P early in the ST segment (see Fig. 30-2). Although functionally "retrograde," the P morphology depends on the location of the tract. Since the latter is generally left-sided, the P is often frankly negative in Einthoven's lead I (the garden variety retrograde P hardly registers at all in this lead, having an axis of −90°). The rate is 180 to 230/min. Sustained aberration of the LBBB variety is common. Circus tachycardia arising in the WPW syndrome is similar except that on conversion to sinus rhythm the usual short PR, wide QRS, and delta wave can be seen. The "retrograde" P is less likely to be negative in lead I (because the Kent bundles are right- and left-sided). Aberration is not necessarily LBBB in type.

PAROXYSMAL AV NODAL REENTRY. Paroxysmal AV nodal reentry is a common tachycardia in which the retrograde P is either completely invisible, recognizable by the advent of an R′ in V_1, or overtly located in the ST segment (20 percent of such tachycardias, Fig. 30-33). In the case of the latter it may be difficult to distinguish from tachycardia with a CBT (see Fig. 30-2). The rate is 180 to 204. Sustained aberration of any kind is less common.

NONPAROXYSMAL JUNCTIONAL ACCELERATION. Nonparoxysmal junctional acceleration is seen with acute infarction and ischemia, with digitalis intoxication, during the first 48 h following cardiac surgery, in many cases of septicemia, multiorgan failure, systemic diseases such as lupus, in hypokalemia, in a variety of clinical situations characterized by high adrenergic drive, and with the administration of adrenergic drugs and theophylline. ECG recognition of the various interactions between junction and atrium has been described with junctional rhythm. They include AV dissociation (complete, incomplete, isorhythmic, etc.), retrograde conduction (1:1, Wenckebach, etc.).

ECTOPIC ATRIAL TACHYCARDIAS. Ectopic atrial tachycardias include simple accelerated ectopic atrial rhythm, paroxysmal reentrant atrial tachycardia, paroxysmal "automatic ectopic" atrial tachycardia, nonparoxysmal atrial tachycardia due to digitalis, nonsustained "benign" atrial tachycardia, chaotic multifocal atrial tachycardia, atrial flutter and atrial fibrillation.

Simple accelerated ectopic atrial rhythm has a rate of 100 to 165/min (see Fig. 30-9). In some patients the rate may be seen to accelerate over a number of tracings. Conceptually, an atrial escape focus has become accelerated. The sinus is either slower, transiently suppressed, or pathologically destroyed (in which case the patient is permanently depen-

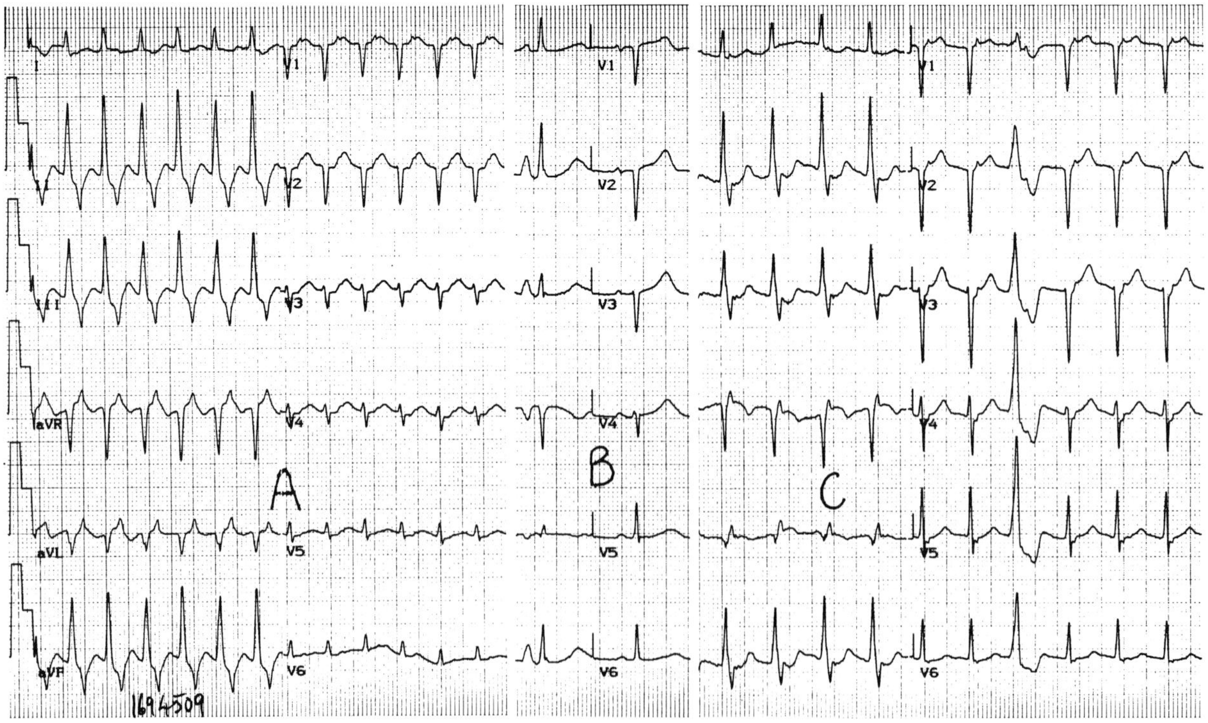

FIGURE 30-33 Paroxysmal SVT shows two different retrograde conduction times (probably AV nodal reentry). In A the inverted P is a negative spike in the ST segment of the inferior leads. The rate is 188 beats/min. The P shows as a positive deflection on the ST in V_1. B Sinus rhythm. C The retrograde P is buried in the QRS giving it a false inferior s wave and giving V_1 an early spike.

dent on the atrial and other downstream, ectopic pacemakers). In few instances the ectopic focus exists only in accelerated form and continuously usurps the sinus.

In *paroxysmal reentrant atrial tachycardia* the rate is 160 to 240/min, usually with 2:1 block (less commonly with 1:1 or variable AV conduction). Very often every other P wave is submerged in the QRS falsely suggesting accelerated ectopic atrial rhythm at half the actual atrial rate. Equally common is low voltage of the atrial deflection, falsely suggesting accelerated junctional rhythm. The presenting regular ventricular rate may be 170/min changing abruptly to 85. Only when the relationship of the rates is noted is the tracing more carefully scrutinized for low amplitude P waves. Incidentally, quinidine administered to such cases invariably restores 1:1 conduction with a gross increase in the ventricular rate.

Paroxysmal "automatic ectopic" atrial tachycardia is uncommon and differs from accelerated ectopic atrial rhythm in its sudden start and stop. It is attributed to automaticity rather than reentry because PACs frequently reset the atrial pacemaker, which often shows waxing and waning in its rate.

Nonparoxysmal atrial tachycardia is due to digitalis intoxication, with or without hypokalemia. Popularly known as "PAT with block," this rhythm is now thought to be an example of triggered automaticity due to late afterpotentials.[39] The 2:1, 3:1, or variable AV block is in no way specific for digitalis intoxication.

Nonsustained "benign" atrial tachycardia[40] appears as a recurrent 3 to 14 beat salvo of unifocal or multifocal atrial extrasystoles, seldom regularly spaced, sometimes showing accelerans or deccelerans structures. The salvos are separated by long periods of sinus rhythm. Variable AV block is seen with rapid rates. When the coupling of the first one or two ectopic Ps is very short the cause may be encroachment on a fragile atrial vulnerable period. The sequence cannot be distinguished from paroxysmal bursts of fibrillation; thyrotoxicosis should be excluded.

Chaotic multifocal atrial tachycardia is seen with acute or acute on chronic lung ailments and arterial hypoxemia. The atrial ectopics are early and late, blocked and conducted, of numerous morphologies, seldom permitting more than two consecutive sinus beats. The latter are invariably tachycardic.

Atrial flutter, paroxysmal or chronic, should always be considered with ventricular rates of 150 (140 to 165). The atrial rate of 300/min is remarkably common; rates in excess of 340 are probably coarse fibrillation. Slower rates (220 to 300) are seen with grossly diseased atria and with antiarrhythmic drugs. Atrial flutter most commonly shows negative P waves or saw teeth in the inferior leads, with positive spikes in V_1. The latter come 40 to 60 msec after the nadir of the lead II flutter wave. As with PAT, alternate F waves may be buried in the QRS. If this is so in V_1 the missing F wave may nevertheless be visible immediately to the left of the lead II QRS (because of the frontohorizontal time delay). A slow atrial rate of flutter is easily confused with the higher atrial rates of PAT, especially if the P of the latter is negative in the inferior leads, or if the rarer type of flutter with an upright inferior P wave is showing. Not uncommonly patients shift from paroxysmal flutter to PAT, the P waves of each being obviously different. Atrial flutter is a very common postoperative complication of coronary artery bypass graft surgery, probably related to atrial involvement in surgical pericarditis.[41] It can be abolished by stimulating the atrial wires left in place by the surgeons at a rate slightly in excess of the measured flutter rate. This technique will fail if the atrial rate exceeds 330/min. *Atrial fibrillation* has special features already noted above.

WIDE COMPLEXES IN SINUS RHYTHM

The QRS duration of the sinus beat is increased when the sinus impulse is delivered asynchronously to the two ventricles or segments thereof (as in bundle branch, fascicular block, or WPW), when there is a gross increase in the ventricular tissue mass (hypertrophy), or when there is diffuse conduction delay in the distal Purkinje system or ventricular muscle. The causes of such conduction delay include hyperkalemia, gross or global ventricular ischemia, and drugs and poisons (quinidine, procainamide, etc.). In hyperkalemia the QRS may simply be "splayed out" retaining, lead for lead, the former characteristics of the patient's QRS. Less commonly hyperkalemia (or procainamide) may induce a bundle branch or fascicular block which disappears when normal conditions are restored. The predictive value of this event for future pathologic conduction disturbance of the same type is unknown. Temporary QRS widening due to global ventricular ischemia is seen during cardiopulmonary resuscitation. As proof of this mechanism the sinus QRS will narrow down without essential change in its components following improved coronary perfusion (after optimal closed chest massage, ventilation, correction of acidemia, etc.). Gross ventricular ischemia is occasionally seen during angina pectoris with left main coronary ostial stenosis (see Fig. 30-23), or its three-vessel equivalent, especially following cardiac catheterization. In all these contexts the ST segment is drastically depressed, often qualifying as subendocardial injury. Patients who develop this pattern during an exercise test, with exercise hypotension or cardiac slowing, are invariably admitted to the ICU. Similar QRS widening is infrequently seen in the early phase of acute MI and is a dangerous sign.

References

1. Slocum J, Byrom E, McCarthy L, et al: Computer detection of atrioventricular dissociation from surface electrocardiograms during wide QRS complex tachycardias. Circulation 72:1028, 1985.
2. Grim P, Feldman T, Martin M, et al: Cellular telephone transmission of 12-lead electrocardiogram from ambulance to hospital. Am J Cardiol 60:715, 1987.
3. Kudenchuk PJ, Ho MT, Litwin PE, et al: Accuracy of cardiologist vs. computerized ECG analysis in selecting patients for out-of-hospital thrombolytic therapy. Circulation 80 (suppl II):354, 1989.

4. Zywietz C: Technical Aspects of Electrocardiogram Recording, in MacFarlane PW, Lawrie TDV (eds): *Comprehensive Electrocardiography 1.* New York, 19, pp 378–380.
5. Mirvis DM, Berson AS, Goldberger AL, et al: Instrumentation and practice standards for electrocardiographic monitoring in special care units. Circulation 79:464, 1989.
6. Feldman T, January C: ECG changes in pneumothorax. Chest 86:143, 1984.
7. Littmann D: *Textbook of Electrocardiography.* New York, Harper & Row, 19, pp 383–396.
8. Ishikawa K, Berson AS, Pipberger H: Electrocardiographic changes due to cardiac enlargement. Am Heart J 81:635, 1971.
9. Ishikawa K, Nagasawa T, Shimada H: Influence of hemodialysis on electrocardiographic wave forms. Am Heart J 97:5, 1979.
10. LaMonte CS, Freiman AH: The electrocardiogram after mastectomy. Circulation 32:746, 1965.
11. Calleja HB: Diagnostic value of electrocardiographic changes in pneumonectomies. Cardiologia 49:228, 1966.
12. Trevino A, Razi BM, Beller B, Antonio S: The characteristic electrocardiogram of accidental hypothermia. Arch Intern Med 127:470, 1971.
13. Mautner RK, Siegel LA, Giled TD, Kayser J: Electrocardiographic changes in acute pancreatitis. South Med J 75:317, 1982.
14. Harumi K, Chen CY: Miscellaneous electrocardiographic topics, in MacFarlane PW, Lawrie TDV (eds): *Comprehensive Electrocardiology 1.* New York, 19, pp 682–684.
15. Spodick DA. Electrocardiogram in acute pericarditis. Am J Cardiol 33:470, 1974.
16. Arnsdorf M, Childers RW: Atrial electrophysiology in experimental hyperthyroidism in rabbits. Circ Res 26:575, 1970.
17. Gabor GE, Winsberg F, Bloom HS: Electrical and mechanical alternation in pericardial effusion. Chest 59:341, 1971.
18. Chou TC. *Electrocardiography in Clinical Practice.* Orlando, Grune & Stratton, 1986, pp 309–319.
19. Stein PD, Dalen JE, McIntyre KM, et al: The electrocardiogram in acute pulmonary embolism. Prog Cardiovasc Dis 17:247, 1975.
20. Punja MM, Schneebaum R, Cohen J: Bifascicular block induced by hyperkalemia. J Electrocardiology 6:71, 1973.
21. Arnsdorf MF: Electrocardiogram in hyperkalemia. Arch Intern Med 136:1161, 1976.
22. Simon BC: Pseudomyocardial infarction and hyperkalemia: A case report and subject review. J Emerg Med 6:511, 1988.
23. Szerlip HM, Weiss J, Singer I: Profound hyperkalemia without electrocardiographic manifestations. Am J Kidney Dis 7:461, 1986.
24. Chumbley LC: Pseudohyperkalemia in acute myelocytic leukemia. JAMA 211:1007, 1970.
25. Ettinger PO, Regan TS, Oldewurtel HA: Hyperkalemia, cardiac conduction, and the electrocardiogram: Overview. Am Heart J 88:350, 1974.
26. Spodick DH: Differential characteristics of the electrocardiogram in early repolarization and acute pericarditis. N Engl J Med 295:526, 1976.
27. Puletti M, Curione M, Pozzar F, et al: Atrial repolarization: Its role in ST elevation. J Electrocardiol 12:321, 1979.
28. Jacobson D, Schrire V: Giant T wave inversion. Br Heart J 28:768, 1966.
29. Jackman WM, Clark M, Friday AJ, et al: Ventricular tachyarrythmias in the long QT syndrome. Med Clin North Am 68:1079, 1984.
30. Isner JM, Sours HA, Paris AL, et al: Sudden unexpected death in avid dieters using the liquid-protein-modified-fast diet. Circulation 60:1401, 1979.
31. Rainey JM, Pohl RB, Bilolikar SG: The QT interval in drug-free depressed patients. J Clin Psychiatry 43:39, 1982.
32. Bekheit SG, Ali AA, Deglin SM, Cain AC: Analysis of QT interval in patients with idiopathic mitral valve prolapse. Chest 81:620, 1981.
33. Doroghazi RM, Childers R: Time-related changes in the QT interval in acute myocardial infarction: Possible relationship to local hypocalcemia. Am J Cardiol 41:684, 1978.
34. O'Toole M, Mayer TA, Winters R, et al: Torsades de pointes and QT prolongation after orthotopic liver transplantation. J Am Coll Card 11:201A, 1988.
35. Zipes DP: Cardiac electrophysiology: Promises and contributions. J Am Coll Card 13:1329, 1989.
36. Gallagher JJ, Svenson RH, Kasell JH, et al: Catheter technique for closed-chest ablation of the atrioventricular conduction system. N Engl J Med 306:194, 1982.
37. Fisch C, Knoebel SB: Junctional rhythms. Prog Cardiovasc Dis 13:141, 1970.
38. Konecke LL, Knoebel SB: Nonparoxysmal junctional tachycardia complicating acute myocardial infarction. Circulation 45:367, 1972.
39. Wit AL, Rosen MR: Cellular electrophysiological mechanisms of cardiac arrhythmias, in MacFarlane PW, Lawrie TDV (eds): *Comprehensive Electrocardiology 2.* New York, 19, pp 810–818.
40. Stemple DR, Fitzgerald JW, Winkle RA: Benign slow paroxysmal atrial tachycardia. Ann Intern Med 87:44, 1977.
41. Waldo AL, MacLean WAH, Karp RB, et al: Entrainment and interruption of atrial flutter with atrial pacing. Studies in man following open heart surgery. Circulation 561:1309, 1977.

Chapter 31

ELECTRICAL CARDIOVERSION AND DEFIBRILLATION

JEFFREY S. SOBLE
THOMAS E. BUMP

Indications

Direct current cardioversion has the broadest spectrum of antiarrhythmic activity of any therapy (Table 31-1). Properly applied, it is nearly always effective against those arrhythmias which are thought to result from reentry, including atrioventricular (AV) nodal reentrant tachycardia, AV reentrant tachycardia using a bypass tract, atrial flutter, and most cases of paroxysmal atrial tachycardia and paroxysmal ventricular tachycardia (VT). In addition, high doses of electricity can defibrillate the heart, which is not surprising since atrial and ventricular fibrillation probably often arise from a reentrant mechanism. Finally, direct current can terminate one rhythm, *torsade de pointes,* which may result from a nonreentrant mechanism, namely triggered activity.

With the exception of *torsade de pointes,* electrical shock is ineffective against tachycardias which arise from enhanced automaticity. Arrhythmias in this category include sinus tachycardia, some forms of ectopic atrial tachycardia, multifocal atrial tachycardia, accelerated junctional rhythm, and even some cases of VT. Any rhythm that occurs in the setting of digitalis intoxication can be exacerbated by direct current shock, probably because shocks depolarize sympathetic nerve terminals in the heart, causing them to release their norepinephrine, which then accelerates the tachycardia or even causes a more malignant arrhythmia to appear. Finally, electrical shock can fail to terminate incessant VT which is caused by Class IC antiarrhythmic drugs (i.e., flecainide, encainide, and possibly propafenone) even though this rhythm is probably caused by reentry.[1]

TABLE 31-1 Effectiveness of Electrical Cardioversion

Usually effective
Paroxysmal supraventricular tachycardia: AV nodal reentrant tachycardia, AV reentrant tachycardia using a bypass tract, reentrant atrial tachycardia
Atrial flutter
Atrial fibrillation
Ventricular tachycardia (most cases): torsade de pointes, monomorphic ventricular tachycardia
Ventricular fibrillation
Usually ineffective
Sinus tachycardia
Multifocal atrial tachycardia
Nonparoxysmal atrial tachycardia (digitalis toxicity)
Accelerated junctional rhythm
Ventricular tachycardia (unusual cases): VT due to digitalis intoxication, incessant VT (including that due to proarrhythmia from Class IC antiarrhythmic drugs)

Mechanism of Action of Cardioversion

In order to terminate fibrillation, a shock must produce a sufficient voltage gradient throughout the fibrillating chamber to bring all myocardial cells to the same electrical state. When all the cells within a reentrant circuit are depolarized, a condition of electrical homogeneity is established which is inimical to reentry. This is because ongoing reentry requires that at all times some part of the chamber not be depolarized, so that this part can be next in line to be activated. In order to be successful, a shock must produce a period of electrical homogeneity which persists for a sufficient period of time. In an elegant series of animal experiments, fibrillation was demonstrated to reappear immediately if the period of homogeneity lasted for less than 130 ms.[2]

Reentrant arrhythmias that are more organized, like atrial flutter or VT, may require depolarization only of the excitable portion of the reentry circuit. This may explain the clinical observation that less energy and current are necessary to terminate these arrhythmias.

The minimum amount of energy required to defibrillate the heart is called the defibrillation threshold. Even in a single individual, the defibrillation threshold is not a single value but rather is a sigmoidal dose-response relationship: the greater the energy in a shock, the more likely it is to defibrillate a given heart.[3] Typical energy thresholds for transthoracic defibrillation of the atria or ventricles are between 50 and 100 J. There is marked variability from patient to patient in the energy threshold, mainly because of interpatient differences in transthoracic impedance. The latter has several determinants: interelectrode distance (chest size), electrode size, electrode–chest wall contact pressure and couplant ("electrode paste"), and respiratory phase. Increases in transthoracic impedance during lung expansion have implications for patients receiving mechanical ventilation and positive end-expiratory pressure. Impedance declines after repeated shocks, partly because of hyperemia and edema in the current pathway.[4] Since current, not energy, is the determinant of successful defibrillation, a defibrillator has been developed which automatically delivers more energy when the impedance has been found to be high.[5]

Other factors beside transthoracic impedance can influence the defibrillation threshold. Lidocaine reversibly increases the defibrillation threshold by as much as 50 percent.[6] Anecdotal reports suggest that amiodarone may as much as double the defibrillation threshold.[7] However, systematic experiments in animals have not shown this adverse effect of amiodarone.[8] Beta agonists and aminophylline, on the other hand, lower the defibrillation threshold.[9,10]

The duration of ventricular fibrillation prior to attempted defibrillation affects defibrillation threshold in a biphasic manner. The energy requirement may actually decrease after 2 min of ventricular fibrillation, perhaps because of favorable changes in extracellular potassium.[11] When ventricular fibrillation has persisted for more than 10 min, it becomes increasingly difficult and ultimately impossible to defibrillate the heart.

Equipment

A defibrillating system includes a bank of capacitors which can be charged from a voltage source (either line current or a battery) via a step-up transformer. Up to 7000 V may be needed to charge capacitors for delivery of 400 J. Inductance is usually added to the circuit in order to dampen the rise and fall of the current and voltage waveforms that are produced when the capacitors are discharged. Experimental evidence has suggested that dampened waveforms are safer and more effective than undampened capacitor discharges.[12] The optimal duration of a defibrillator shock has been found to be 4 to 12 ms.[13]

It is also possible to cardiovert the heart with alternating current. The first defibrillators used 200-ms pulses of alternating current (60 Hz), with a typical energy level of 500 J. A drawback of alternating current is that it faces a greater impedance than does direct current, and more energy must be delivered in order to pass the same amount of current across the heart. In addition, alternating current is a potent fibrillating agent and is more dangerous to use than direct current, both for the patient and the physician. Therefore, alternating current defibrillators were supplanted in clinical practice by direct current defibrillators.

SYNCHRONIZATION

All defibrillators have a feature which permits shock delivery to be synchronized to the QRS complex when patients are being cardioverted out of supraventricular tachycardia, atrial flutter, atrial fibrillation, or VT (but not ventricular fibrillation). This is to prevent delivery of shocks during the vulnerable period of the cardiac cycle, a brief period just before the apex of the T wave when part of the ventricle has repolarized and the rest is still depolarized. A shock which is delivered at this point will depolarize only the excitable (repolarized) part of the ventricle, with the remainder free to repolarize on schedule during the next few milliseconds. This results in inhomogeneously activated myocardium, which is a perfect substrate for ventricular fibrillation. Most, but not all, defibrillators can be synchronized by recording the electrocardiogram (EKG) through the paddles.

Unfortunately, the availability of synchronization can lead to a serious problem. A defibrillator in the synchronous mode will fail to deliver a shock to a patient in ventricular fibrillation, because there is no discrete QRS with which to synchronize. Inadvertently setting a defibrillator to the synchronous mode will lead to unacceptable and even lethal delays in therapy for a patient with ventricular fibrillation.

ELECTRODE PADDLES

Electrode paddles are a key component of a defibrillating system. The optimal electrode size for elective cardioversion has been shown to be in the range of 8 to 12 cm in diameter.[14] Smaller paddle electrodes (4.5 cm) are available for infants. There are no studies comparing the safety and efficacy of different-sized paddles in children, but it has been recommended that adult-sized (8-cm) paddles should be used for children over 10 kg in weight. Self-adhesive electrode pads represent a significant advance, in that these increase the likelihood of proper electrode placement and are safer and more convenient for the operator. However, they may slip out of position and make poor contact with the chest wall in the diaphoretic patient.

ADDED FEATURES

Several other recent advances have been made in the design of external defibrillators. Defibrillators have been developed that can both defibrillate and perform ventricular pacing through the same pair of self-adhesive pads. This has obvious advantages in the setting of cardiopulmonary resuscitation as well as elective cardioversion where occasional patients may develop asystole or bradyarrhythmias following cardioversion. Several new defibrillators automatically store information about each resuscitation effort on tape or floppy disk. This greatly assists documentation and should lead to better quality assurance. A new type of defibrillator presently undergoing clinical testing automatically measures the transthoracic impedance using a "test pulse" technique and then charges the capacitor to an energy sufficient to generate the desired peak current. This will ensure that enough current is delivered to patients with high transthoracic impedance and will protect against delivery of excessive current to patients with low transthoracic impedance. Finally, automated external defibrillating systems are now available which analyze the electrocardiographic signal which is recorded through the electrode pads. When these devices diagnose ventricular fibrillation, they flash and sound a warning and either deliver a shock or advise the operator to push a button which triggers the device to give a shock. This type of system is clearly more applicable to out-of-hospital cardiac arrests than it is to the situation in the intensive care unit.

ROUTINE MAINTENANCE OF DEFIBRILLATORS

Faulty maintenance is a leading cause of defibrillator failure. Table 31-2 presents a variety of maintenance problems which have occurred.[15] In a recent survey, 20 percent of defibrillators were found to lack scheduled periodic maintenance, and 14 percent failed to meet performance standards such as ability to deliver energy within 15 percent of the selected value, ability to charge to 360 J within 15 s, and

TABLE 31-2 Errors in Defibrillator Maintenance

Unit damaged by testing with paddles shorted together
Batteries depleted because alternating current main switch was turned off
Defibrillator incorrectly placed into its charger base
Fluids (coffee, D5W or normal saline) spilled onto the defibrillator
Dirty paddles (from dried electrode paste)
Connector cable from paddles to unit loosely connected
Inconsistent checking of equipment by clinical users
Operational problems not reported to clinical engineering personnel
Inadequate periodic maintenance

ability of the batteries to maintain the charged state over time.[15] Recommendations for defibrillator maintenance are listed in Tables 31-3 and 31-4.

Procedures for Defibrillation and Elective Cardioversion

EMERGENCY DEFIBRILLATION

Emergency defibrillation and elective cardioversion are handled with completely different techniques. *Emergency defibrillation* should be used to treat rhythms such as ventricular fibrillation or rapid VT which have caused the patient to be pulseless and unresponsive. In this situation speed should be given the highest priority, since the strongest determinant of survival is the interval between the onset of a cardiac arrest and the delivery of an effective electrical shock. If the defibrillating system has electrode paddles, these should be well coated with a gel, particularly around the edges. Although salt-containing electrode paste is usually used, ultrasound gel or surgical lubricant may also be used with equal success.[16] The electrodes must then be applied firmly to the chest wall (with about 25 lb of pressure). This compresses the thorax, leading to a shorter interelectrode distance and lower transthoracic impedance. Alternatively, flexible adhesive electrode pads might be applied to the chest wall.

With either type of electrode, the standard placement is with one just to the right of the upper sternum below the clavicle and the other with its center in the left midaxillary line at the level of the cardiac apex. The electrodes should not be placed over the sternum, vertebral column, or scapula because bone has a high impedance and will cause current to travel circumferentially around the chest wall rather than through the heart. Care must be taken that the electrodes do not touch each other and that there is no bridging between the electrodes by conductive gel. The respective polarity of each electrode is not an important determinant of either the safety or the efficacy of the procedure.

Once the electrodes are in place, the defibrillator capacitors should be charged to around 200 J and then discharged *asynchronously* (no shock will be delivered if the patient is in ventricular fibrillation and the unit is in the synchronous

TABLE 31-3 Periodic Care and Maintenance of Defibrillators

Nickel-cadmium batteries
- Battery dates: Label each battery for date manufactured and date placed in service. Useful life is generally 2 years, though periodic testing and reconditioning can extend this. Maintain traceable record for each battery.
- Exercise procedure: Perform a reconditioning or exercise procedure (deep discharge/charge three times) of the batteries every 3 months with battery support system available from the manufacturer.
- Battery capacity: Check the capacity of the batteries following the exercise procedure every 3 months. They should have greater than 70% of their rated capacity after being run through the exercise procedures. If not, remove battery from service.
- Self-discharge test: Perform a self-discharge test of the batteries every 6 months. They should self-discharge no more than 25% of measured capacity after 1 week. If they exceed this rate, remove battery from service.
- Charge time test: Measure the defibrillator charging time on battery power every 3 to 6 months. The defibrillator should charge to maximum rated energy level within 12 s with battery at room temperature (20 to 25°C). If not, remove battery from service.
- Energy accuracy test: Perform energy accuracy test every 3 to 6 months. Charge to 50 J, then to 360 J, and discharge each time into a 50-Ω load energy meter. To pass, the battery must deliver ±15% of selected energy; otherwise, remove from service.

Sealed lead-acid batteries
- Full charging: Sealed lead-acid batteries should be kept fully charged. Recharge fully as soon as possible after each use by plugging the defibrillator into a source of alternating current line power.
- Constant charging: Keep defibrillator (or battery if separate from the defibrillator) plugged into AC line power during standby periods to provide constant battery charging.
- No deep discharge cycling: Avoid periodic deep discharge cycling because this may damage lead-acid batteries (unlike nickel-cadmium batteries).
- Measure battery voltage: Certain defibrillators incorporate circuitry and displays for the management of battery voltage and recommended voltage ranges. If such is the case, a monthly check of battery voltage is recommended.
- Avoid uncharged batteries: A battery left uncharged for excessive periods (4 to 6 months) may be damaged and require replacement. Certain defibrillators are capable of testing for damage and required battery replacement.
- Battery age: Check the date code on battery. With proper maintenance and depending on use, battery life should exceed 2 years and may exceed 5 years.

NOTE: These are generic periodic maintenance recommendations that should be performed by the persons responsible for long-term periodic maintenance. While these checks usually will be performed by clinical engineers, they are within the capabilities of most clinical operators, without highly specialized testing equipment. They note the general areas that must be checked on a regular basis. Users should consult clinical engineering or manufacturer's service manuals for specific and complete details. Whenever replacement batteries are not immediately available, mark the defective unit and notify clinical engineering.
SOURCE: Cummins et al.[15]

TABLE 31-4 Shift Checklist for Defibrillators

Preparedness check before any clinical use
- Ensure that the unit is clean, with no fluid spills and nothing stored on unit.
- Check that paddles and electrode surfaces are clean and free of pitting.
- Verify presence and proper condition of all cables, cord, and connectors. Check for fraying, cuts, damaged insulation, and broken connector pins.
- Verify presence and proper condition of all disposable supplies (conductive medium, pads, monitor electrodes, recorder paper, recorder cassette, alcohol swabs, and razors).
- Check that spare charged batteries are available for units with user-serviceable batteries as a primary power source. Verify that operators know how to replace batteries.
- Check that defibrillator and monitor are pugged into a "live" outlet and that batteries are charging (where applicable). Ensure that battery contacts with charger and device are secure.
- Turn on power to defibrillator and to monitor (if separate) and inspect all indicators (charge light, energy display, power on, and monitor screen). This check may require attachment to brand-specific simulators.
- Check that electrocardiographic recorder advances paper, that paper is present in sufficient amount, and that spare paper is available.
- Verify that charge/discharge cycle functions correctly by charging device to a low energy level (50 to 100 J) and discharging into an appropriate test load. (See manufacturer's instructions for specific devices.)
- For those defibrillators that have capability for transcutaneous pacing: check that pacer output cable is connected, that pacer electrodes (set of two) are present, and that pacing indicators work.
- For automatic external defibrillators: verify that rhythm analysis is operable by attaching electrodes to appropriate simulator: check against normal sinus rhythm, ventricular fibrillation, asystole, and loose electrodes; for ventricular fibrillation, allow device to charge to lowest energy level and discharge into the test simulator; check that all indicators and messages are appropriate for each rhythm.
- Confirm presence of event documentation mechanism (i.e., tape cassette, solid-state memory module, or card), that it is properly inserted, and that a spare is available. Check that the tape recorder works.
- Correct, when possible, simple problems (e.g., unplugged charger cord) or supply shortages noted.
- Place out of service if problems cannot be corrected immediately and ensure that another defibrillator is readily available.
- Report problems with an out-of-service unit to the individual responsible for dealing with equipment problems.
- Sign that the unit is ready for clinical use.

Preparedness check after any clinical use
- Clean electrodes and equipment.
- Inspect unit, cables, and electrodes for visual damage.
- Recheck disposable supplies (pads); replace as needed.
- Restart battery-charging procedure, if appropriate.
- Place all items and unit in ready state for immediate use.

NOTE: These are the generic areas that the Defibrillator Working Group recommends for the shift checklist. Specific products may need more or fewer items on the shift checklist. Consult manufacturer's operating instructions and clinical engineering personnel for brand-specific details.
SOURCE: Cummins et al.[15]

TABLE 31-5 Confounding Variables in Defibrillation

Metabolic acidosis
Metabolic alkalosis
Hypoxia
Hyperkalemia
Hypokalemia
Hypomagnesemia
Digitalis intoxication
Proarrhythmia from encainide, flecainide, or other antiarrhythmics
Acute ischemia
Acute reperfusion injury

mode). If this first attempt fails to convert the rhythm to a hemodynamically stable one, a second shock with an intensity of 200 to 300 J should be delivered. If the first two shocks fail to defibrillate the patient, a third shock of 360 J should be delivered immediately.

If all these attempts fail, the physician should look for confounding factors such as inadequate electrode pressure, improper electrode position, and insufficient gel on the electrodes. Also, it should be determined if defibrillation has failed because of high transthoracic impedance due to a pneumothorax. An attempt should be made to correct any of the other conditions which can negate the effects of electrical defibrillation (Table 31-5). Epinephrine can be used to lower the energy requirement for defibrillation.[9]

Defibrillation of the patient who has an automatic implantable cardioverter-defibrillator (AICD) deserves special mention. In the presence of rapid VT or ventricular fibrillation, the AICD will deliver successive countershocks which are detectable by the patient's muscle contractions. When no further shocks are delivered, in the presence of persistant VT or ventricular fibrillation in an unconscious patient, the AICD has gone into the disabled mode, and external cardioversion should be undertaken. Discharge of the implantable defibrillator itself may cause a perceptible shock but does not pose a danger to persons in direct contact with the patient.

In summary, electrical defibrillation is a cornerstone of cardiopulmonary resuscitation, but of course it should be applied in the context of a complete resuscitative protocol such as that described in *Textbook of Advanced Cardiac Life Support*.[17]

ELECTIVE CARDIOVERSION

Elective cardioversion is used to treat rhythms such as supraventricular tachycardia, atrial flutter, atrial fibrillation, and hemodynamically stable sustained VT. The decision to use electrical countershock in the treatment of these rhythms should be based on the clinical setting and may be influenced by such factors as refractoriness to drug therapy (either for conversion or rate control) or the presence of angina, congestive heart failure, hypotension, or low output state which may be exacerbated by the arrhythmia. In general, it should not be done for stable patients scheduled

TABLE 31-6 Preparations for Elective Cardioversion

1. Prophylactic anticoagulation and/or temporary pacemaker if indicated (see text).
2. Administration of an antiarrhythmic agent to achieve chemical cardioversion and/or maintain sinus rhythm if indicated.
3. Laboratory studies including electrolytes and digoxin level.
4. No food by mouth (at least 6 h).
5. Informed consent.
6. Intravenous access.
7. Twelve-lead electrocardiogram prior to procedure.
8. Continuous recording of rhythm during procedure.
9. Proper equipment and personnel for airway management and resuscitation.
10. Administration of 100% O_2.
11. Anesthesia (see text).
12. Postcardioversion 12-lead electrocardiogram.

to undergo cardiac surgery in the near future. Elective cardioversion is most safely and effectively performed when the physician takes time for thorough preparation (Table 31-6).

ANTICOAGULATION

Particular attention must be paid to preventing thromboembolic complications. Left atrial thrombi are found during heart surgery in 40 to 50 percent of patients with atrial fibrillation, compared with 10 percent in patients with sinus rhythm.[18] These can be dislodged from the heart when atrial contractility is restored. Cardioversion of patients with atrial fibrillation has been reported to be associated with a risk of embolism of 1 to 7 percent if anticoagulation has not been administered.[19,20] The largest prospective study of anticoagulation in this setting found a 5.3 percent incidence of embolic episodes following cardioversion in patients who were not anticoagulated, compared to a 0.8 percent incidence in patients who had been anticoagulated.[21] The risk period for embolism may extend for as long as 4 weeks or more after the cardioversion, since it can take several weeks for an atrium to fully regain its contractility, especially if the patient had previously been in atrial fibrillation for many months.[22]

It is now generally accepted that selected patients should be anticoagulated before and after cardioversion for atrial fibrillation. On the other hand, it is not completely clear how long the duration of warfarin therapy need be; nor is it clear how long an episode of atrial fibrillation must have persisted before anticoagulation is indicated. The Second American College of Chest Physicians (ACCP) Conference on Antithrombotic Therapy strongly recommended that if atrial fibrillation has been present for at least two days, the patient should be anticoagulated with warfarin (INR of 2.0 to 3.0; prothrombin time 1.3 to 1.5 times control using North American thromboplastin) for at least 3 weeks before elective cardioversion and that anticoagulation be continued until normal sinus rhythm has been maintained for 2 to 4 weeks.[23] It is possible that anticoagulation should be administered when atrial fibrillation has persisted for less than 2 days in patients with mitral stenosis or prosthetic mitral valve, dilated cardiomyopathy, or myocarditis, or when there is a history of a stroke or transient ischemic attack which may have been embolic in origin. These guidelines also apply to patients in atrial fibrillation referred for cardiac surgery (e.g., bypass), as restoration of sinus rhythm when the heart is defibrillated may result in systemic embolization.

Of course, the decision of whether or not to anticoagulate must be guided not only by the presence of indications but also by the presence of relative and absolute contraindications to anticoagulation. Also, it is likely that these guidelines for anticoagulation will be revised in the future. A recent study in a small group of patients showed that transesophageal two-dimensional echocardiography was accurate in detecting clot in the left atrial appendage.[24] If these results are borne out by further experience, it may become common practice to use this method to identify patients who do not need anticoagulation prior to cardioversion.

There appears to be less risk of embolism when cardioversion is performed for arrhythmias other than atrial fibrillation. This may be due to the presence of effective atrial contractions during supraventricular tachycardia and atrial flutter. The second ACCP Conference on Antithrombotic Therapy recommended that anticoagulation not be given to patients with "pure" atrial flutter or supraventricular tachycardia. However, some physicians do anticoagulate patients with atrial flutter, arguing that the left atrium can fibrillate while the right atrium is fluttering. In these cases, fibrillation in the left atrium cannot be appreciated on the surface electrocardiogram because it is hidden by the right atrial flutter waves. In addition, patients can alternate between coarse atrial fibrillation and flutter, further strengthening the case for anticoagulation.

PROPHYLACTIC TEMPORARY PACING

Indications for temporary pacemaker placement prior to elective cardioversion of atrial fibrillation are based on anectdotal experience and are not well defined. Atrial fibrillation may occur in the setting of sick sinus syndrome (SSS) as a form of escape rhythm. A slow ventricular response to atrial fibrillation (40 to 60 BPM) in the absence of AV nodal blocking agents may be indicative of widespread conduction system disease and has been advocated as an indication for temporary pacing.[25] Of course, a known prior history of SSS mandates prophylactic pacing, and in both known and suspected SSS the patient must be evaluated as a candidate for permanent pacemaker placement prior to cardioversion. The presence of conduction block alone [right and left bundle branch block (RBBB, LBBB), bifascicular block, or intraventricular conduction delay] does not increase the risk of elective cardioversion.[26]

PREPARATION OF THE PATIENT

Prior to elective cardioversion the patient should be given nothing by mouth (other than medicines) for at least 6 h, or longer in patients with slow gastric emptying, because the electric shock can provoke vomiting and aspiration. Serum electrolytes should be measured and corrected if necessary. If the patient has received digoxin, a serum digoxin concentration should be measured because electrical shocks can cause refractory VT or ventricular fibrillation in patients with digitalis intoxication. However, it should be emphasized that it is safe to cardiovert patients with no symptoms of digitalis toxicity and with serum digoxin concentrations of up to 3 ng/mL.[27] It is common to pretreat patients with quinidine, procainamide, or another antiarrhythmic drug, both in the hope of achieving a pharmacologic conversion of the arrhythmia (which may occur in 10 or 15 percent of cases) and to prevent immediate recurrence of the arrhythmia following the cardioversion.

The procedure should be fully explained to the patient and informed consent obtained. Anxiety should be allayed. Pharmacologic sedation may be added as needed. A 12-lead EKG should be obtained, both to document the arrhythmia and to serve as a base line for comparison with EKGs obtained following the procedure.

Elective cardioversion should be performed only in a room which is equipped for electrocardiographic monitoring and resuscitation. A physician skilled in airway management (preferably an anesthesiologist) should be in attendance. There should be facilities for oxygen administration, suction, chest compression (i.e., a board), and emergency pacing. Intravenous access must be established. The patient should be given 100% oxygen prior to receiving anesthesia to increase the margin of safety should brief apnea occur. There should also be equipment for continuous recording of the EKG during the procedure on paper, tape, or some other recording medium.

The electrodes can be placed in the locations described above (anterolateral), or an anteroposterior configuration can be used in which one electrode is positioned to the right of the sternum under the clavicle and the other electrode is positioned at the angle of the left scapula. A prospective study discovered that both methods were equally successful at converting atrial fibrillation.[28] Once the patient has been connected to the electrocardiographic monitor, the physician should become satisfied that the defibrillator can be synchronized to the patient's QRS complexes. This is done by switching the defibrillator to its synchronous mode and then observing its oscilloscope screen or indicator light for properly timed flashes (superimposed on the QRS complexes). A sedative agent can then be administered, preferably one with potent amnestic effects such as one of several benzodiazepines (e.g., diazepam or midazolam). Alternatively, a short-acting barbiturate such as methohexital may be administered. Control over the airway should be established and maintained.

SYNCHRONIZED CARDIOVERSION

Once anesthesia has been administered, a synchronized shock can be given after the operator has ensured that no personnel are in direct or indirect contact with the patient. The intensity of the shock should be selected according to the rhythm which is being treated and according to the principle that the degree of myocardial injury, if any, is determined by the maximal single shock strength, not by cumulative energy.[29] In other words, for elective cardioversion it is better to start with low energies which might be ineffective than with high energies which might be excessive. Twenty-five joules is a good starting dose for treating atrial flutter, supraventricular tachycardia, and hemodynamically stable VT. Even 10 J can be sufficient to terminate tachycardia in some patients. If 25 J fails, it is then reasonable to try 50 and then 100 J. If 100 J fails to convert the tachycardia, then the physician should reassess the situation before deciding to go ahead with 200, 300, or 400 J; a tachycardia which does not respond to 100 J is likely also to be refractory to the higher energies.

In the case of atrial fibrillation, higher energies are required for conversion than is the case with paroxysmal supraventricular tachycardia, atrial flutter, and hemodynamically stable VT. A good starting dose is 50 J, to be followed if necessary by 100, 200, 300, and up to 360 or 400 J.

Complications

Potential complications of cardioversion include respiratory depression secondary to sedation, embolic phenomena, bradyarrhythmias or asystole, aspiration (during emergency cardioversion), and operator injury, all of which have been mentioned previously. Direct current cardioversion can rarely induce ventricular fibrillation, most often related to inaccurate synchronization and delivery of a low-energy shock. Synchronization is most difficult in the setting of wide complex tachycardias, where the machine may have difficulty distinguishing QRS from T wave, and initial defibrillation with 200 J should be considered in this situation. In any event, the operator should be prepared to deliver rapid defibrillation should the need arise. In addition, thermal chest wall injury may occur after repetitive, high-energy shocks or when inadequate paddle contact is maintained.

Direct current shock can also damage myocardium. At higher energies, myocardial necrosis and inflammation can be detected histologically.[30] Transient T wave abnormalities occur in approximately 2 to 3 percent of cases,[29] and transient ST elevation has been reported in the absence of evidence for myocardial damage.[31] Levels of creatine phosphokinase (CPK) are generally elevated after cardioversion, but are almost entirely secondary to elevation in MM isoenzyme. Two of 30 patients studied prospectively had modest elevations in CPK-MB isoenzymes (11 and 13 mIU/mL) after direct current cardioversion.[30]

Pacemaker malfunction has also been reported as a complication of defibrillation and cardioversion of patients with implanted unipolar pacing systems.[32] Most commonly encountered is a transient loss of pacemaker capture (seconds to minutes); chronic increases in stimulation threshold can also occur. Damage to the pulse generator has also been reported less commonly. Also, current may be shunted down the pacemaker lead, causing local injury at the endocardial surface. Defibrillator paddles should therefore ideally be placed 5 in. (12.7 cm) from the pulse generator of permanent pacemakers, and sequential measurements of stimulation threshold should be done immediately and then at intervals for up to 2 months following electrical countershock.

Efficacy

Success rates are high for electrical conversion of ventricular arrhythmias immediately after their onset. In the electrophysiologic laboratory, 80 percent of induced VT and ventricular fibrillation is converted after a single 200-J shock.[33] Cumulative effectiveness is 95 percent after a second 200-J shock, and 99 to 100 percent after a third 300-J shock. Defibrillation of spontaneous ventricular fibrillation is in large part related to the time delay to initiation of therapy. In a retrospective analysis of patients requiring defibrillation, 91 percent of patients treated within 10 min were successfully defibrillated, as opposed to only 50 percent of those treated after 10 min.[34] The amplitude of the ventricular fibrillation waveform has been shown to correlate with the time interval from initial cardiac arrest and to be a powerful predictor of outcome, with only 6 percent survival in patients with very low amplitude ("fine") fibrillation.[35]

Successful cardioversion is the rule for supraventricular tachycardias due to reentry at the AV node or using a bypass tract, and failure of electrical cardioversion should prompt a search for confounding variables such as misdiagnosis (e.g., of sinus tachycardia). However, as effective pharmacologic therapies are available for these rhythms, cardioversion should be reserved for instances of significant hemodynamic compromise. Successful cardioversion of atrial flutter occurs in over 95 percent of cases, although occasional patients will convert from atrial flutter to fibrillation, often with improvement in rate control or subsequent spontaneous conversion to sinus rhythm.

Overall immediate success rates for cardioversion of atrial fibrillation are in the range of 85 to 90 percent.[36] Best results can be expected in situations where the precipitant has been treated but atrial fibrillation remains, such as following thyrotoxicosis, pulmonary embolism, myocarditis, or pericarditis. Factors which mitigate against successful cardioversion include those which predispose to a lower likelihood of maintaining sinus rhythm over the ensuing 12 months: duration of atrial fibrillation of greater than 1 year, left atrial enlargement (45 mm or more), and the presence of mitral valve disease.[20] Although sinus rhythm may not be maintained over months, even short-term hemodynamic improvement may be important in the critically ill patient and should be considered in the decision to cardiovert in this setting. Additional consideration should be given to factors such as exogenous or endogenous catecholamine excess, aminophylline administration, and exacerbations of obstructive lung disease or congestive heart failure which may predispose to failure or recurrence of atrial arrhythmias after cardioversion.

References

1. Winkle RA, Mason J, Griffin JC, Ross D: Malignant ventricular tachyarrhythmias associated with the use of encainide. Am Heart J 102:857, 1981.
2. Chen PS, Shibata N, Dixon EG, Wolf PD, Danieley ND, Sweeney MB, Smith WM, Ideker RE: Activation during ventricular defibrillation in open-chest dogs. Evidence of complete cessation and regeneration of ventricular fibrillation after unsuccessful shocks. J Clin Invest 77:810, 1986.
3. Davy J-M, Fain ES, Dorian P, Winkle RA: The relationship between successful defibrillation and delivered energy in open-chest dogs: Reappraisal of the "defibrillation threshold" concept. Am Heart J 113:77, 1987.
4. Sirna SJ, Kieso RA, Fox-Eastham KJ, Seabold J, Charbonnier F, Kerber RE: Mechanisms responsible for the decline in thoracic impedance after direct current shock. Am J Physiol 257:H1180, 1989.
5. Kerber RE, Martins JB, Kienzle MG, Constantin L, Olshansky B, Hopson R, Charbonnier F: Energy, current, and success in defibrillation and cardioversion: Clinical studies using an automated impedance-based method of energy adjustment. Circulation 77:1038, 1988.
6. Dorian P, Fain ES, Davy J-M, Winkle RA: Lidocaine causes a reversible, concentration-dependent increase in defibrillation energy requirements. J Am Coll Cardiol 8:327, 1986.
7. Guarnieri T, Levine JH, Veltri EP, Griffith LSC, Watkins L, Jr, Juanteguy J, Mower MM, Mirowski M: Success of chronic defibrillation and the role of antiarrhythmic drugs with the automatic implantable cardioverter/defibrillator. Am J Cardiol 60:1061, 1987.
8. Fain ES, Lee JT, Winkle RA: Effects of acute intravenous and chronic oral amiodarone on defibrillation energy requirements. Am Heart J 114:8, 1987.
9. Ruffy R, Schechtman K, Monje E, Sandza J: Adrenergically mediated variations in the energy required to defibrillate the heart: Observations in closed-chest, nonanesthetized dogs. Circulation 73:374, 1986.
10. Ruffy R, Monje E, Schechtman K: Facilitation of cardiac defibrillation by aminophylline in the conscious, closed-chest dog. J Electrophysiol 2:450, 1988.
11. Babbs CF, Whistler SJ, Kim GKW, Tacker WA, Geddes LA: Dependence of defibrillation threshold upon extracellular/intracellular K^+ concentrations. J Electrocardiol 13:73, 1980.
12. Kouwenhoven WB, Milnor WR: Treatment of ventricular fibrillation using a capacitor discharge. J Appl Physiol 7:253, 1954.
13. Ewy GA: Cardiac arrest and resuscitation: Defibrillators and defibrillation. Curr Probl Cardiol 2:1, 1978.
14. Kerber RE, Grayzel J, Kennedy J, Jensen SR: Elective cardioversion; influence of paddle electrode location and size on success rates and energy requirements. N Engl J Med 305:658, 1981.
15. Cummins RO, Chesemore K, White RD, Defibrillator Working Group: Defibrillator failures. Causes of problems and recommendations for improvement. JAMA 264:1019, 1990.
16. Sirna SJ, Ferguson DW, Charbonnier F, Kerber RE: Electrical cardioversion in humans: Factors affecting transthoracic impedance. Am J Cardiol 62:1048, 1988.
17. American Heart Association: *Textbook of Advanced Cardiac Life Support.* Dallas, Texas, American Heart Association, 1987.
18. Hay WE, Levine SA: Age and auricular fibrillation as independent factors in auricular mural thrombus generation. Am Heart J 24:1, 1942.
19. Myers DG, Gonzalez ER, Nelson WP: The role of prophylactic

anticoagulation in cardioversion of atrial fibrillation. Cardiovasc Rev Rep 6:647, 1985.
20. Mancini GBJ, Weinberg DM: Cardioversion of atrial fibrillation: A retrospective analysis of the safety and value of anticoagulation. Cardiovas Rev Rep 11:18, 1990.
21. Bjerkelund CJ, Orning OM: The efficacy of anticoagulant therapy in preventing embolism related to D.C. electrical conversion of atrial fibrillation. Am J Cardiol 23:208, 1969.
22. Manning WJ, Leeman DE, Gotch PJ, Come PC. Pulsed doppler evaluation of atrial mechanical function after electrical cardioversion of atrial fibrillation. J Am Coll Cardiol 13:617, 1989.
23. Dunn M, Alexander J, de Silva R, Hildner F: Antithrombotic therapy in atrial fibrillation. Chest 95:118S, 1989.
24. Aschenberg W, Schluter M, Kremer P, Schroder E, Siglow V, Bleifeld W: Transesophageal two-dimensional echocardiography for the detection of left atrial appendage thrombus. J Am Coll Cardiol 7:163, 1986.
25. Mancini GB, Goldberg AL: Cardioversion of atrial fibrillation: Consideration of embolization, anticoagulation, prophylactic pacemaker, and long-term success. Am Heart J 104:617, 1982.
26. Cascio WE, Foster JR, Sheps DS: Elective cardioversion in the presence of conduction disturbances. J Electrocardiol 1:63, 1984.
27. Mann DL, Maisel AS, Atwood JE, Engler RL, LeWinter MM: Absence of cardioversion-induced ventricular arrhythmias in patients with therapeutic digoxin levels. J Am Coll Cardiol 5:882, 1985.
28. Kerber RE, Jensen SR, Grayzel J, Kennedy J, Hoyt R: Elective cardioversion: Influence of paddle-electrode location and size on success rates and energy requirements. N Engl J Med 305:658, 1981.
29. Resnekov L, McDonald L: Complications in 220 patients with cardiac dysrhythmias treated by phased direct current shock and indications for electroconversion. Br Heart J 29:926, 1967.
30. Eshani A, Ewy GA, Sobel BE: Effects of electrical countershock on serum creatine phosphokinase (CPK) isoenzyme activity. Am J Cardiol 37:12, 1976.
31. Chun PCK, Davia JE, Donohue DT: ST-segment elevation with elective DC cardioversion. Circulation 63:220, 1981.
32. Levine PA, Barold SS, Fletcher RD, Talbot P: Adverse acute and chronic effects of electrical defibrillation and cardioversion on implanted unipolar cardiac pacing systems. J Am Coll Cardiol 1:1413, 1983.
33. Waldecker B, Brugada P, Zehender M, Stevenson W, Wellens H: Dysrhythmias after direct-current cardioversion. Am J Cardiol 57:120, 1986.
34. Kerber RE, Sarnat W: Factors influencing the success of ventricular defibrillation in man. Circulation 60:226, 1979.
35. Weaver WD, Cobb LA, Dennis D, Ray R, Hallstrom AP, Copass MK, Ray R: Factors influencing survival after out-of-hospital cardiac arrest. J Am Coll Cardiol 7:752, 1986.
36. Morris JJ, Peter RH, McIntosh HD: Electrical conversion of atrial fibrillation. Immediate and long-term results and selection of patients. Ann Intern Med 65:216, 1966.

Chapter 32 CARDIAC PACING

THOMAS E. BUMP
JEFFREY S. SOBLE

Cardiac pacing is an invaluable technique for treating arrhythmias. In fact, for some patients it is the only effective therapeutic option. It can be administered by wholly implantable systems *(permanent pacing)* or by systems that can more easily be removed from the patient *(temporary pacing)*. The intensivist should be skilled in the application of temporary pacing systems and capable of determining which patients should be referred for implantation of permanent systems, and should be able to trouble-shoot pacemakers that are malfunctioning.

Principles of Pacing

In cardiac pacing, brief electric pulses are used to depolarize the heart. Each pulse directly depolarizes only a small volume of myocardium; but when sufficient myocardium has been depolarized, a self-propagating wave front of activation spreads from the site of stimulation. At this point, the stimulus is said to have *captured* the heart. In order to trigger a propagating depolarization, the stimulus must have at least a certain minimum intensity, the *threshold for capture,* which can be measured in terms of current (milliamperes, mA) or voltage (volts, V).

The threshold for capture is a function of the duration of the stimulus, being greater as the pulse width is shortened. The threshold is also highly dependent on the degree of contact between the pacing electrode and the heart. In the case of electrodes that are applied to the skin over the chest wall, the threshold for ventricular capture is generally between 35 and 70 mA at a pulse width of 40 ms. In the case of electrodes that are in direct contact with ventricular endocardium, the threshold is usually less than 0.5 mA at a pulse width of 0.5 ms.

The modern cardiac pacemaker not only stimulates the heart but also is capable of sensing the occurrence of spontaneous heartbeats. In order for sensing to occur, the spontaneous beat must produce a signal whose amplitude exceeds the preset sensing threshold of the pacemaker. For pacing electrodes in direct contact with ventricular endocardium, the R wave of a spontaneous beat usually exceeds 5 mV in amplitude. The amplitude of spontaneous atrial beats, as transmitted by intraatrial electrodes, is smaller—often around 1 mV in amplitude.

Pacemakers respond in different ways to sensed beats. Single-chamber pacemakers are usually *inhibited* from delivering stimuli whenever the native ventricular rate exceeds the preset rate of the pacemaker. Dual-chamber pacemakers can exhibit more complex behavior: spontaneous ventricular beats inhibit ventricular stimuli, and spontaneous atrial beats inhibit atrial stimuli and trigger the delivery of ventricular stimuli after a preset atrioventricular (AV) interval.

A code has been devised to identify the different types of pacemakers. The first letter indicates the chamber(s) that are paced: *A* for atrium, *V* for ventricle, *D* for dual-chamber pacing, or *S* for single-chamber pacing—which may be applied to either atrium or ventricle. The second letter indicates the chamber(s) that are sensed. An *O* is used if the pacemaker is incapable of sensing. The third letter indicates whether the pacemaker's stimuli are inhibited (*I*) or triggered (*T*), or both (*D*), by sensed spontaneous beats. Ventricular demand pacemakers are therefore labelled *VVI* or *SSI*. Dual-chamber pacemakers that pace and sense in both chambers are labelled *DDD* (the third *D* refers to the fact that spontaneous atrial beats both inhibit atrial output and trigger ventricular output). Temporary dual-chamber pacing systems usually are incapable of sensing atrial activity; these are therefore labelled *DVI.*

Dual-chamber pacemakers, though more complex than ventricular pacemakers, provide significant advantages because of atrioventricular synchrony. This enables atrial systole to contribute to ventricular filling, which is particularly important in several groups of patients. The first such group are those in whom left ventricular filling during atrial systole plays a major role in maintaining stroke volume. These might include patients with severe congestive cardiomyopathy; hypertrophied, noncompliant ventricles; mitral stenosis; and acute myocardial infarction. For example, in one study the average contribution of atrial contraction to left ventricular stroke volume was 20 percent in subjects without heart disease and 35 percent in patients with an acute myocardial infarction.[1] A second group of patients who benefit from atrioventricular synchrony are those who have intact ventriculoatrial conduction.[2] In these patients, single-chamber ventricular pacing results in a retrograde P wave after every QRS complex. With every paced beat the atria contract against closed mitral and tricuspid valves, producing cannon *a* waves. Dual-chamber pacing eliminates retrograde conduction by placing a P wave before every QRS complex. Finally, atrioventricular synchrony appears to be especially important in maintaining cardiac output and blood pressure in the setting of right ventricular infarction.[3]

In the intensive care unit (ICU) and elsewhere, pacing is used not only to treat bradycardias but also to terminate episodes of sustained reentrant tachycardia. Reentrant tachycardias are vulnerable to pace termination when the reentry circuit is anatomically defined and there is an excitable gap between a circulating wave front and its wake of refractoriness. Given these conditions, it should be possible for a stimulated impulse to invade the circuit and create bidirectional block. The latter will occur if the invading impulse proceeds in both directions in the circuit, clockwise and counterclockwise. In one direction the invading impulse will collide with and extinguish the reentering wavefront; in the other direction, it will itself be extinguished when it runs into the wake of refractoriness of the reentering impulse.

The usual technique of pace termination is to deliver a train of stimuli at a somewhat faster rate than that of the tachycardia. A train of stimuli is more likely than a single stimulus to produce an impulse that penetrates the reentrant circuit. With trains of stimuli, though, there is a risk that one stimulus will terminate a tachycardia and a subsequent one will restart the tachycardia. It may be necessary for the physician to deliver literally dozens of trains of stimuli of different rates and durations, until finally a train is delivered that fortuitously ends with a pulse that extinguishes the tachycardia rather than reinducing it.

Indications for Pacing

TEMPORARY PACING

Temporary pacing is the treatment of choice whenever sinus bradycardia or heart block contributes significantly to hypotension or a low-output state. It can provide immediate relief of symptoms due to hypoperfusion, provided bradycardia is the cause and provided it can be treated before irreversible organ damage has set in. Compared to pharmacologic options, such as repeated doses of atropine or continuous infusion of a β agonist, pacing produces fewer side effects and usually is better tolerated by patients—especially those with coronary artery disease, in whom drugs can cause angina.

Temporary pacing is also indicated for certain patients who are thought to be at high risk for developing lethal bradycardia. For example, patients who develop bundle branch block during acute myocardial infarction may suddenly have progression of their conduction disturbance, leading to asystole or complete heart block.[4] In a recent study of 698 patients, complete heart block developed in 36.4 percent of patients with three or more of the following characteristics: first degree atrioventricular block, Mobitz type I atrioventricular block, Mobitz type II atrioventricular block, left anterior hemiblock, left posterior hemiblock, right bundle branch block, and left bundle branch block.[5] It has been argued that patients who develop bundle branch block during myocardial infarction should receive a prophylactic temporary pacemaker to stay in place until it is clear that worse heart block will not occur.[6] This is a widely accepted practice, even though no study has ever shown that prophylactic temporary pacing reduces mortality in this group of patients. A recent American College of Cardiology/American Heart Association task force recommended the indications for temporary pacing in acute myocardial infarction that are found in Table 32-1.[7]

Traditionally, temporary pacing has also been indicated for patients with left bundle branch block who are about to undergo catheterization of the right side of the heart. In these patients, pacing is used as a prophylactic measure against catheter-induced mechanical injury to the one remaining fascicle in the conduction system. However, these precautions may not be necessary. A recent retrospective study found that flow-directed, balloon-tipped catheters caused complete heart block in 0 of 38 patients with left bundle branch that was old (more than 1 month in age) or of indeterminate age.[8]

TABLE 32-1 Indications for Temporary Pacing in Acute Myocardial Infarction

Class I: Usually indicated, always acceptable and considered useful/effective.
- Asystole.
- Complete heart block.
- Right bundle branch block with left anterior or left posterior hemiblock developing in acute myocardial infarction.
- Left bundle branch block developing in acute myocardial infarction.
- Type II second degree AV block.
- Symptomatic bradycardia not responsive to atropine.

Class IIa: Acceptable, of uncertain efficacy; may be controversial. Weight of evidence favors usefulness/efficacy.
- Type I second degree AV block with hypotension not responsive to atropine. During ventricular pacing, if ventriculoatrial conduction causes the atrial contraction to fall within ventricular contraction, atrial or AV sequential pacing may be necessary.
- Sinus bradycardia with hypotension not responsive to atropine.
- Recurrent sinus pauses not responsive to atropine.
- Atrial or ventricular overdrive pacing for incessant ventricular tachycardia.

Class IIb: Acceptable; of uncertain efficacy; may be controversial. Not well established by evidence; can be helpful; probably not harmful.
- Left bundle branch block with first degree heart block of uncertain duration.
- Bifascicular block of uncertain duration.

Class III: Not indicated; may be harmful.
- First degree heart block.
- Type I second degree AV block with normal hemodynamics.
- Accelerated idioventricular rhythm causing AV dissociation.
- Bundle branch block known to exist before the myocardial infarction.

Temporary pacing can also be used to prevent tachycardias, especially in the case of patients with a prolonged Q-T interval and recurrent *torsade de pointes* (rapid, polymorphic ventricular tachycardia that often arises after a pause or during bradycardia). In these patients, ventricular pacing is performed at rates of up to 100 beats per minute (bpm). When this fails to prevent recurrences of ventricular tachycardia, it usually is not helpful to pace the ventricles more quickly, though this is sometimes done as a last resort.

Temporary pacing can serve a diagnostic function in that direct recordings of atrial activity can be made via transvenous, epicardial, or transesophageal leads. These recordings can be invaluable during tachycardias when P waves are not clearly distinguishable on the surface electrocardiogram (ECG). For example, a normal-QRS tachycardia can be proved to be atrial flutter if the atria are found to be beating at 300 bpm while the ventricles are beating at 150 bpm. A wide-QRS tachycardia can be proved to be ventricular tachycardia if atrioventricular dissociation is found.

Or, temporary pacing of the atria or ventricles can be used to terminate reentrant tachycardias, including paroxysmal supraventricular tachycardia (including both AV nodal reentrant tachycardia and AV reciprocating tachycardia using an accessory pathway), atrial flutter, and some cases of ventricular tachycardia. There is seldom any call for pace-terminating the paroxysmal tachycardias, though, because verapamil and adenosine are so effective. However, atrial flutter and some cases of ventricular tachycardia can be highly refractory to drugs, and for patients with these arrhythmias pacing can be a very attractive alternative to electrical cardioversion.

PERMANENT PACING

The intensivist faces special problems in deciding which patients should be referred for permanent pacing. The acutely ill patient is more likely than the ambulatory patient to have a reversible cause for bradycardia. The patient with sepsis or with a bleeding diathesis is not a good candidate to undergo surgical implantation of a device. The terminally ill patient may be just as well served by temporary pacing as by a permanent pacemaker. These considerations must be weighed alongside the usual guidelines for implanting permanent pacemakers.

In 1984, a task force recommended the indications for permanent pacemaker implantation that are summarized in Table 32-2.[9] They separated indications for permanent pacemakers into three classes: class I, conditions for which there is general agreement that permanent pacemakers should be implanted; class II, conditions for which permanent pacemakers are frequently used but there is divergence of opinion with respect to the necessity of their insertion; and class III, conditions for which there is general agreement that pacemakers are unnecessary.

TABLE 32-2 Indications for Permanent Pacing in Adults

Class I: Conditions for which there is general agreement that permanent pacemakers should be implanted.

- Acquired complete heart block, permanent or intermittent, at any anatomic level, with any of the following complications: symptomatic bradycardia,* ventricular ectopy or other conditions that require treatment with drugs that suppress the automaticity of escape foci, documented pauses of 3.0 s or longer, or any escape rate of less than 40 bpm in symptom-free patients.
- Second degree AV block, permanent or intermittent, regardless of the type or the site of the block, with symptomatic bradycardia.*
- Atrial flutter or fibrillation or supraventricular tachycardia with complete or advanced AV block and any of the complications mentioned under "Acquired complete heart block" above.
- Persistent advanced second degree or complete heart block after acute myocardial infarction, regardless whether complications are present.

TABLE 32-2 Indications for Permanent Pacing in Adults (Continued)

- Bifascicular block with intermittent complete heart block or type II second degree AV block, with symptomatic bradycardia.*
- Sinus bradycardia, chronic or intermittent, with documented symptomatic bradycardia.*
- Recurrent syncope with spontaneous events clearly provoked by carotid sinus stimulation, when minimal carotid sinus pressure induces asystole longer than 3 s in the absence of any medication that depresses the sinus node or AV conduction.

Class II: Conditions for which permanent pacemakers are frequently used but for which there is disagreement about the need for their insertion.

- Asymptomatic complete heart block, permanent or intermittent, at any anatomic site, with ventricular rates of 40 or more bpm.
- Asymptomatic type II second degree AV block, permanent or intermittent.
- Asymptomatic type I second degree AV block at intra-His or infra-His levels.
- Persistent first degree AV block in the presence of bundle branch block not documented previously, following acute myocardial infarction.
- Transient advanced AV block and associated bundle branch block, following acute myocardial infarction.
- Bifascicular or trifascicular block with intermittent type II second degree AV block without symptoms.
- Bifascicular or trifascicular block with syncope that is not proven to be due to complete heart block, when no other possible causes for syncope are identifiable.
- Atrial pacing–induced infra-His block.
- Sinus node dysfunction, occurring spontaneously or as a result of necessary drug therapy, with heart rates below 40 bpm when no clear association between significant symptoms consistent with bradycardia and the actual presence of bradycardia has been established.
- Recurrent syncope without clear provocative events, when minimal carotid sinus pressure produces asystole longer than 3 s.

Class III: Conditions for which there is general agreement that pacemakers are unnecessary.

- First degree AV block.
- Asymptomatic type I AV block at the supra-His (AV nodal) level.
- Transient AV conduction disturbances in the absence of intraventricular conduction defects, in the setting of acute myocardial infarction.
- Transient AV block with isolated left anterior hemiblock, in the setting of acute myocardial infarction.
- Acquired left anterior hemiblock in the absence of AV block, in the setting of acute myocardial infarction.
- Fascicular block without AV block or symptoms.
- Fascicular block with first degree AV block without symptoms.
- Sinus node dysfunction, even if the rate is below 40 bpm, in asymptomatic patients or patients whose symptoms have clearly been shown not to be caused by bradycardia.

* *Symptomatic bradycardia* is used to refer to the following clinical manifestations, which are directly attributable to the slow heart rate: transient dizziness; light-headedness; near-syncope or frank syncope; exercise intolerance; and frank congestive heart failure.

In the 6 years since the appearance of these recommendations there have been only a few changes in attitudes toward the indications for permanent pacing. In 1985, Medicare began reimbursing for pacemaker implantation in patients with type I second degree heart block at any anatomic level, symptomatic or asymptomatic, with associated intraventricular conduction delay. In the same year, it was reported that permanent pacing appeared to prolong survival in patients with chronic type I second degree heart block, even in the absence of associated QRS widening.[10]

Temporary Pacing Systems

Temporary pacing systems incorporate a pulse generator, which is external to the patient, and pacing electrodes. External pulse generators all have the following characteristics: variable rate, variable stimulation amplitude, and variable sensing threshold (including the possibility of setting the threshold so high that spontaneous beats are not sensed and do not inhibit the pacemaker). There are also indicators (lights or needles) that show when a stimulus is delivered or when a spontaneous beat is sensed. In other respects, there are considerable differences between pulse generators that are intended for transvenous, transesophageal, or noninvasive (transcutaneous) pacing. Of course, temporary systems also differ from one another in the configuration of their pacing electrodes.

TRANSVENOUS PACING

Transvenous pacing systems incorporate at least a pair of electrodes which are mounted at the tip of a catheter or lead. The pulse generator for transvenous pacing is a small, portable unit powered by a 9-V battery. The pacing rate is adjustable from between 30 and 50 to between 180 and 200 pulses per min. The pulse width is generally fixed at 0.5 to 1.0 ms, but the pulse amplitude can be adjusted to up to 20 V or 20 mA. The sensing threshold is also adjustable from 1 mV to as much as 10 mV or more. Most external pulse generators accommodate only single pacing leads for single-chamber pacing; but dual-chamber units are also available. At present, the only type of external dual-chamber pacemaker approved by the Food and Drug Administration (FDA) is the DVI pacemaker, which permits sensing and pacing in the ventricle but only pacing (not sensing) in the atrium. External pulse generators that sense and pace in both the atrium and the ventricle (DDD) are presently undergoing clinical trials.

PLACEMENT

The transvenous pacing lead can be inserted into an antecubital vein, an internal or external jugular vein, a subclavian vein, or a femoral vein. Insertion via an antecubital vein has fewer initial complications than the other routes, but is associated with a higher frequency of dislodgement because of arm movement.[11] There is also a higher incidence of phlebitis with the antecubital route.[12] Insertion by a subclavian or jugular vein is associated with a small incidence of complications such as pneumothorax or inadvertent puncture of a subclavian or carotid artery; but the position of the pacing lead is more stable than with antecubital insertion. Femoral insertion seems to be relatively free of complications; some physicians permit patients with femoral pacing leads to sit and even to ambulate freely.

Usually, fluoroscopy is used to guide the catheter's advancement to the right atrium or the apex of the right ventricle. Once the catheter tip appears by fluoroscopy to be in good position, this can be verified by determining whether there is an appropriately low threshold for capture—for example, less than 1.0 mA in the ventricle. If the lead tip is in the right ventricular apex, the paced QRS complex should have a left bundle branch block morphology and a negative frontal axis (Fig. 32-1). The lead should be repositioned if either the pacing threshold is too high or the signal generated by spontaneous beats is too small to be sensed.

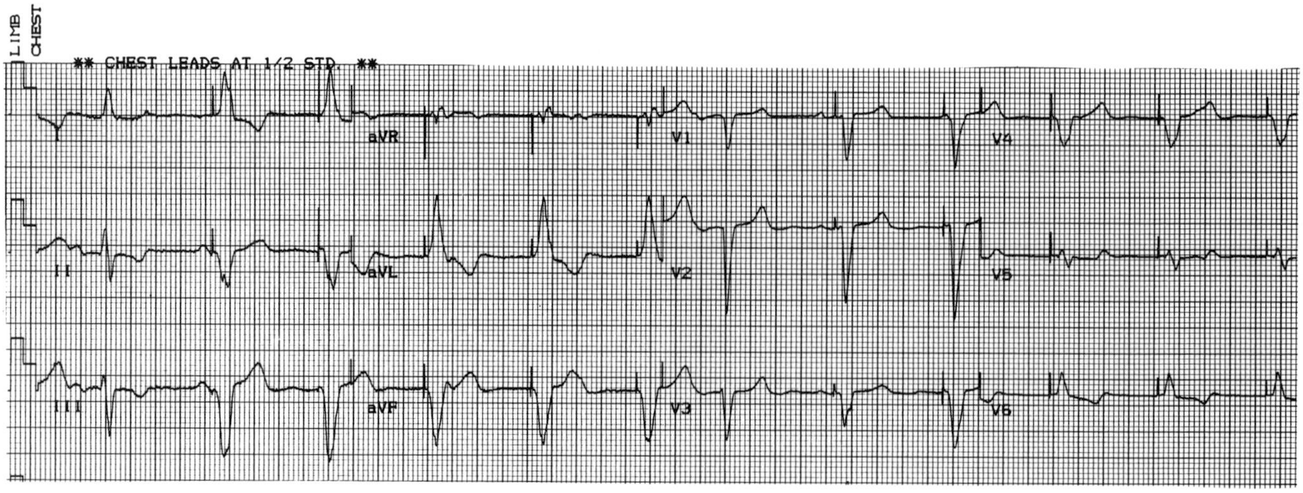

FIGURE 32-1 A 12-lead ECG of a patient being paced at the right ventricular apex.

There should be slack left in the lead so that it is less likely to be pulled out of the right ventricular apex, and care must be taken that the tip is not bearing on the endocardium with too much pressure.

If fluoroscopy is not available, there are alternative techniques. Balloon-tipped pacing catheters can be positioned using electrocardiographic guidance.[13] The distal electrode of the catheter is connected to the V lead of an ECG, while the four limb leads are attached in the usual way to the patient. The ECG machine must be well grounded (i.e., with a leakage current less than 10 μA) because higher levels of current can induce ventricular fibrillation. As the catheter floats into the right atrium, a large P wave is inscribed on the ECG (Fig. 32-2). If the catheter tip is in the high right atrium, a downgoing P wave will be recorded, because atrial activation will be spreading away from the sinus node, which lies at the junction of the superior vena cava and the right atrium. If the catheter tip is in the low right atrium, a positive P wave will be recorded during sinus rhythm, because atrial activation will be proceeding toward the electrode. With the catheter tip in the mid–right atrium, the large P wave will be biphasic, with first an upgoing and then a downgoing component.

A limitation of the balloon-tipped catheter is that it cannot be floated into the heart during a cardiac arrest, when there is minimal or no blood flow. Under these circumstances, blind insertion can sometimes be accomplished with No. 3 or 4 French pacing catheters.[14] Blind insertion is extremely difficult when there is not only no blood flow but also no electrocardiographic activity with which to guide the placement of the catheter.

Other types of transvenous pacing leads are also available. Some leads have four or more electrodes at their tip. This enables the physician to connect the distal pair of electrodes to a pulse generator, and the proximal pair to recording equipment. Other catheters have electrodes at their tip and electrodes farther back along the shaft. These are meant to enable pacing of both the atria and the ventricles through one catheter; in practice, reliable atrial stimulation through the shaft electrodes is virtually impossible. The problem of temporary atrial pacing has inspired numerous catheter designs, including a J-shaped lead designed to be seated in the right atrial appendage[15] and a dual-chamber pacing system that incorporates a No. 2 French "J" lead for the atrium and a No. 3.5 French balloon-tipped ventricular lead for the ventricle.[16] Combined pacing and hemodynamic monitoring systems are available, in which a balloon-tipped thermodilution catheter has an extra right ventricular port through which a flexible, thin bipolar pacing lead can be introduced into the ventricle.[17] This system can rapidly provide access to ventricular pacing if the catheter tip is in the pulmonary artery. If the catheter tip is not yet in the pulmonary artery, ventricular pacing may be difficult to establish. Thus this system does not provide sufficient protection for patients who are at risk of developing complete heart block during right heart catheterization. Once the catheter is in place, pacing will be interrupted if the balloon of the thermodilution catheter is inflated in order to measure the pulmonary capillary wedge pressure (because of migration of the catheter to the wedge position).

Once a transvenous pacing lead is positioned, one should determine that its function is not compromised by deep breaths or coughs. Then the lead can be secured with tape or suture. If the pacing threshold is less than 1.0 mA, the maintenance output can be left at 5.0 mA. A chest x-ray

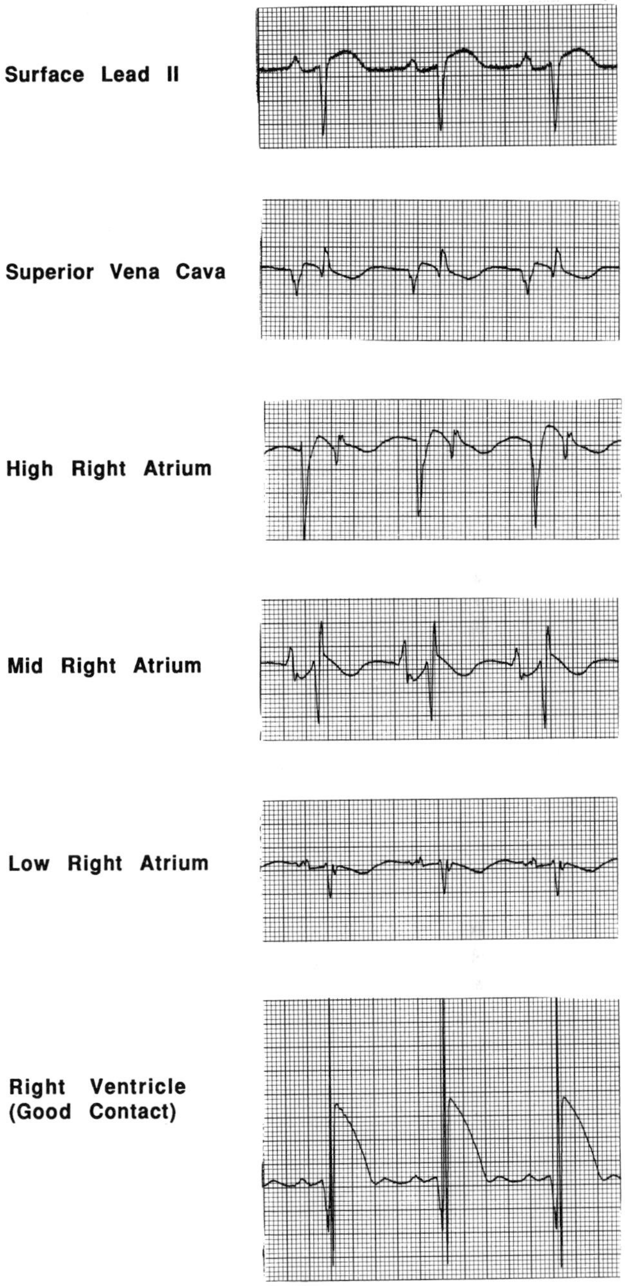

FIGURE 32-2 Recordings made during passage of a transvenous pacing lead. The distal electrode of the lead is connected to the *V* terminal of the ECG, and the limb leads are connected in the usual way to the patient. In the superior vena cava (SVC) tracing the first component of each pair of complexes represents atrial depolarization (P wave). The P wave is negative in the SVC and high right atrium since the depolarization wave front is moving away from the pacing lead tip.

should be obtained to verify the position of the lead and to rule out complications such as pneumothorax or hemothorax. The entry site should be observed frequently and kept clean and dry, and an antibiotic ointment should be applied.

One must remember that the lead is a direct route for environmental electricity to reach the heart; noninsulated components of the system, such as the lead terminals, should be protected in some way—for example, by flexible plastic tubing. The entire pulse generator should be placed in an insulating pouch or, for example, in a rubber glove. People who handle the connectors must avoid contact with any electrically operated devices, including lights, monitors, and other appliances. The battery should not be replaced while the lead is connected to the pulse generator, because there may be a low-impedance pathway between the battery terminals and the output terminals of the pulse generator.

Routine surveillance of a transvenous pacing system should include daily measurement of the pacing threshold and the ability of the pulse generator to sense spontaneous beats. Of course, one should ensure that the battery in the generator is fresh.

COMPLICATIONS

The complications of temporary transvenous pacing are varied but infrequent, at least in experienced hands. Placement of the lead can be complicated by inadvertent puncture of an artery, pneumothorax, air embolism, catheter embolism, hematoma, infection, or perforation of the heart or some other part of the vascular tree. Ventricular perforation is more common with stiffer pacing wires; when placement is done without fluoroscopic guidance; when the catheter tip is being manipulated in the thin-walled right atrium or coronary sinus; and when it is being manipulated in an infarcted right ventricle. The diagnosis of perforation is suggested when there is a rise in pacing threshold, chest or shoulder pain, a pericardial friction rub, or stimulation of the chest wall or diaphragm by pacing stimuli. Electrocardiographic signs of perforation include a change in the frontal plane axis of the pacing spike and a change in the QRS morphology of the paced beats from left bundle branch block to right bundle branch block, signifying that the left ventricle is now being paced. This nearly always responds immediately to repositioning of the lead, as the muscular ventricular wall reseals itself when the catheter is withdrawn. The physician should be aware that extra heart sounds can be caused by the contact between the endocardium and the pacing lead.[18] Thus a lead does not have to be removed or repositioned if a friction rub is heard on auscultation, when no other evidence of perforation is present.

The pacing lead may mechanically irritate the heart, leading to arrhythmias ranging from atrial premature beats to ventricular fibrillation. Serious arrhythmias are more likely to arise in the settings of digitalis intoxication, right ventricular infarction, hypoxia, and excess catecholamine levels.[19] Continued presence of the lead, especially beyond 3 days, exposes the patient to risks of phlebitis and sepsis.

The pacing system may also fail either to sense or to capture the heart successfully. These problems are discussed below.

EPICARDIAL PACING

Epicardial pacing is performed through electrodes that have temporarily been loosely left on the epicardial surface at the time of cardiac surgery. Often leads are left on both the atrium and the ventricle. The electrodes are attached to very thin insulated wires that are brought through the chest wall via small stab wounds. These wires can be connected to recording equipment so that atrial activity can be monitored during arrhythmias that arise in the postoperative period; in this way atrial flutter or atrial fibrillation can be diagnosed and distinguished from sinus tachycardia, and ventricular tachycardia can be differentiated from supraventricular tachycardia with aberrant ventricular conduction.

In addition, the epicardial leads can be connected to the same kind of pulse generator that is used for transvenous pacing. The pacing threshold is usually a little bit higher than is the case with endocardial electrodes, but should be less than 5 mA as long as the leads have not become dislodged. The heart can be paced if a bradycardia complicates the postoperative course, or if pace termination of a tachycardia is desired.[20] These leads are easily polarized by pacing, so it can be impossible to record signals from them for up to 30 s after they have been used for pacing.

Temporary epicardial leads are virtually free of infectious complications, and never lead to hematomas or perforation of vascular structures. Their chief limitations are that they are available only following cardiac surgery and that they may come free of the epicardial surface, leading to unacceptably high pacing thresholds and poor recordings of cardiac activity.

TRANSESOPHAGEAL PACING

Transesophageal pacing systems incorporate their electrodes into a lead that can be introduced through the nose or mouth to the esophagus; the lead passes immediately behind the heart along its course through the chest. At its closest point, the esophageal lumen is only 5 to 10 mm away from the posterior surface of the left atrium and 30 mm away from the posterior wall of the left ventricle. Electrodes can fairly easily be positioned in the esophagus for recording of an electrocardiographic signal with large, sharp P waves. Atrial pacing via esophageal electrodes is also possible.[21] Ventricular pacing from esophageal electrodes usually is not possible with stimuli that can be tolerated by the patient.

A variety of esophageal electrodes have been used for atrial recording and pacing. Early studies employed a single electrode in the esophagus with a reference electrode on the chest wall. This led to undesirable stimulation of the chest wall and diaphragm. More acceptable results have been obtained with bipolar pacing from the esophagus.[22] Electrode pairs can be mounted on catheters that are inserted through the nares like nasogastric tubes. Alternatively, bipolar pacing or recording can be performed through a pill electrode consisting of a pair of stainless steel electrodes attached to a twisted pair of very thin, Teflon-insulated stainless steel wires and enclosed in an ordinary pharmaceutical gelatin capsule.[23] The pill electrode is swallowed with a gulp of water while a nurse, technician, or physician gradually releases the wires. The capsule dissolves in a few minutes, and peristalsis advances the electrode toward the stomach.

The optimal pacing site in the esophageal lumen is usually that location where the largest atrial deflection can be recorded in the ECG. A P-to-QRS ratio of 2:1 or 3:1 in a bipolar recording is a reliable indicator of excellent left atrial approximation. This type of electrocardiographic signal is usually found at a distance of 35 to 45 cm from the lips of an adult, or 7 to 11 cm above the gastroesophageal junction. The signal can be recorded by connecting the esophageal leads to an electrophysiologic amplifier or to the right and left arm leads of a standard ECG, with the leg leads connected in the usual manner. A special-purpose preamplifier is available that can be inserted between the electrodes and the ECG and that eliminates low-frequency artifact from peristalsis, respiration, and cardiac contraction.

With the electrodes in their optimal location, one can expect to be able to capture the atrium with a current of 15 to 25 mA, if a pulse width of 10 ms is used. The threshold for capture is not any less for pulse widths greater than 10 ms. With pulse widths narrower than 10 ms, the threshold for capture is usually prohibitively high. Thus, transesophageal pacing mandates the use of a specialized stimulator that can deliver pulses with a width of 10 ms and an amplitude of up to 30 mA (i.e., 60 V, since bipolar esophageal electrodes typically have an impedance of 2000 Ω).

Transesophageal pacing has found its greatest utility in the management of paroxysmal atrial flutter. It has been reported to terminate flutter successfully in about 85 percent of cases.[24] Transesophageal pacing rarely plays a role in managing patients with sinus bradycardia and intact atrioventricular conduction, since it is less well tolerated than transvenous pacing. Because only the atrium is captured, transesophageal pacing plays no role in the management of patients with heart block.

Transesophageal pacing produces a sensation of pulsatile heartburn that disappears immediately upon cessation of pacing. Endoscopic studies have revealed minimal damage, if any, to the esophageal epithelium. Rarely, inadvertent ventricular pacing can occur, with the possibility of accidental induction of ventricular tachycardia or fibrillation. Also, when the electrodes are positioned proximal to the optimal pacing site, coughing can be provoked. A placement that is too distal may cause diaphragmatic stimulation and hiccuping.

TRANSTHORACIC PACING

In temporary transthoracic pacing the pacing electrode(s) are placed into a ventricle through a long hollow needle that is introduced through the skin and advanced until it has punctured the ventricular wall. Various approaches for inserting the needle have been advocated, with insertion in the subxiphoid space or at various spots in the left fifth intercostal space (next to the left edge of the sternum, or 4 cm to the left of the midsternal line, or 6 cm to the left of the midsternal line). From the subxiphoid position it has been recommended that the needle be directed at an angle of 30° to the skin toward either the left or right shoulder. From any of the positions in the fifth intercostal space, it has been recommended that the needle be directed at an angle of 30° to the skin toward the right second costochondral junction.

None of these approaches is certain to get the tip of the needle into either the right or the left ventricle. Autopsy studies have shown that these approaches successfully puncture the left or right ventricle in only 25 to 90 percent of attempts.[25] Even if blood can be freely withdrawn there is no guarantee that the tip of the needle is in a position that will permit pacing, since the above approaches can lead to puncture of the inferior vena cava, right atrium, or pulmonary artery, or laceration of a coronary artery, instead of puncture of a ventricle.

It is extremely rare for a patient to be successfully paced by transthoracic pacing; it is even rarer for a patient to survive the procedure. In one series of 139 patients who underwent temporary transthoracic pacing, none survived.[26] Undoubtedly the reasons for the high failure rate of this technique are many. Foremost is the fact that transthoracic pacing is almost always used as a last-ditch maneuver in patients who have not responded to any other efforts at resuscitation. With the availability of external pacing, the indications for transthoracic pacing will certainly shrink, and it is conceivable that the procedure will become extinct.

TRANSCUTANEOUS PACING

Temporary transcutaneous pacing (also called *noninvasive* or *external* pacing) involves the use of a pair of large electrodes that are placed on the chest wall.[27] Each electrode is incorporated into a flexible adhesive pad so that good contact is made with the skin over a large surface area. This permits large total currents to be delivered to the heart, with low current density at the skin or chest wall muscles. Transcutaneous pacing can be used only for ventricular pacing; it is not possible to selectively pace the atria by this technique. At least one system is available that can both pace and defibrillate through the same pair of electrode pads.

In order to capture the ventricles using these electrodes, a special stimulator must be used that can provide pulses with a 40-ms pulse width. Even with pulses this wide, the threshold for ventricular capture is generally 35 to 70 J. In our experience, stimuli of this intensity usually cause stimulation of skeletal muscles and the diaphragm. The resultant twitching of the chest wall is not well tolerated by most patients.[28]

The advantages of transcutaneous pacing lie in the speed and ease with which it can be employed. It does not require special skill or experience in the operator. It is particularly useful in the setting of a bradycardiac arrest. In most instances it should be considered a temporary measure, a "bridge" to a transvenous pacemaker. To a lesser extent it may be useful for pace-terminating supraventricular or ventricular tachycardia in certain patients.[29] It is often tempting to rely on transcutaneous pacing when patients need a standby pacemaker (i.e., when they do not yet have a bradycardia but are at high risk for developing one). This can eliminate the need for a prophylactic transvenous pacing system, but the trade-off is that the physician must check the pacing threshold of the patches in order to be certain that it will be possible to pace the heart transcutaneously if necessary.

Troubleshooting

The different types of pacemaker malfunction are listed in Table 32-3. With both temporary and permanent pacemakers, the worst malfunction is a failure of the pacemaker to produce a spike that captures the heart in a patient who is "pacemaker-dependent" (i.e., one who has a dangerously slow rhythm in the absence of pacing) (Fig. 32-3). This malfunction can often be corrected by increasing the stimulus amplitude or by increasing the pulse width, if possible. At the same time, the integrity of the lead system should be checked, including the positioning of the electrodes and the connection of the leads to the pulse generator. The power source of the pulse generator should be evaluated through a battery check or by making sure that the device is plugged in; and it should be determined that the device is set or programmed to pace.

If none of these measures results in effective stimulation, the possibility should be considered that the pacing system is being inappropriately inhibited, either by itself, by the patient, or by external electromagnetic interference. Dual-chamber pacemakers can inhibit themselves, in the sense that atrial stimuli can be sensed by the ventricular channel and can inhibit ventricular output through a process called *cross-talk inhibition*. Pacemakers can also be inappropriately inhibited by electric signals ("myopotentials") generated by skeletal muscle contraction (Fig. 32-4). In the ICU, microwave blood warmers, electrocautery, and diathermy units are notorious for inhibiting demand pacemakers. Inappropriate inhibition can be ruled out by setting the pulse generator to an asynchronous mode (i.e., to VOO pacing). With permanent pacemakers this can be accomplished by placing a magnet over the device. If pulses still fail to be produced, then the problem is *not* inappropriate inhibition.

In some cases, stimuli may fail to appear because of the way that the pacemaker has been programmed, and not

TABLE 32-3 Types of Pacemaker Malfunction

Failure to produce stimuli.
- Battery failure.
- Disconnected lead or lead fracture.
- Inappropriate inhibition.
  - P-wave sensing.
  - T-wave sensing.
  - Myopotential sensing (in implanted unipolar pacemakers).
  - Artifact sensing (e.g., lead fracture).
  - Cross-talk inhibition (in dual-chamber pacemakers).
  - Hysteresis (in which the escape interval between the last spontaneous beat and the first pacing stimulus can be programmed to a much longer value than the interval between consecutive pacing stimuli).

Failure of stimuli to capture the heart.
- Threshold higher than selected output.
  - Lead dislodgement or perforation.
  - Threshold elevated by infarction, fibrosis, antiarrhythmic drugs, hyperkalemia, hypoxia, etc.
  - Inappropriately low stimulus amplitude or pulse width.
- Partially disconnected lead or lead fracture.
- Battery failure.

Undesired stimulation.
- Failure to sense.
  - Lead dislodgement or perforation.
  - Cardiac signal reduced in amplitude by infarction, fibrosis, antiarrhythmic drugs, etc.
  - Inappropriately high selected sensing threshold.
  - Electromagnetic interference causing reversion to asynchronous pacing.
  - Spontaneous QRS occurring during the blanking period (in dual-chamber pacemakers).
- Triggered pacing.
  - Triggered mode (VVT) in which a stimulus is delivered whenever a spontaneous QRS is sensed.
  - Ventricular stimuli triggered by sensed atrial activity (in DDD pacemakers).
    - Sensing of atrial fibrillation or flutter.
    - Sensing of retrograde P waves (pacemaker-mediated tachycardia).
  - Runaway pacemaker (battery failure).

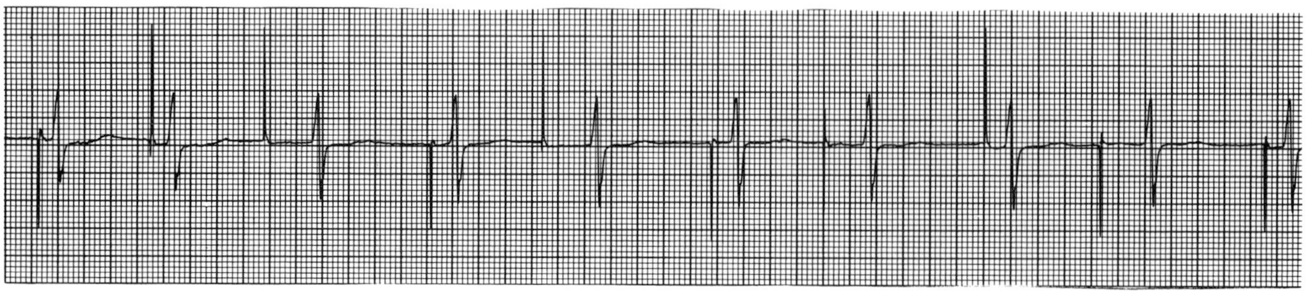

FIGURE 32-3 Failure to capture.

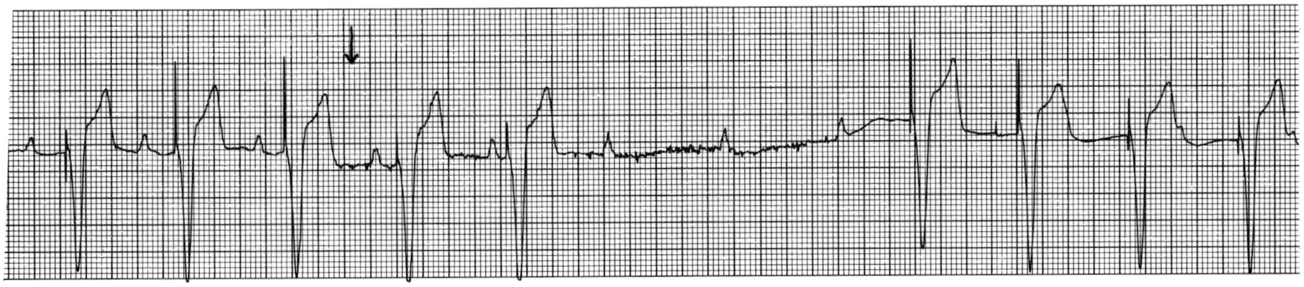

FIGURE 32-4 Myopotential inhibition of a unipolar permanent pacemaker. The pulse generator was placed next to the pectoral muscle, and inappropriate inhibition of the pacemaker occurred whenever the patient adducted her arm. Forcible arm adduction begins at the arrow where muscular artifact can be discerned in the tracing.

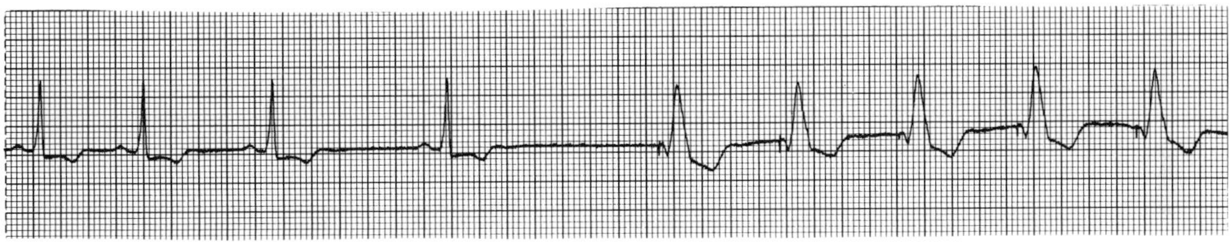

FIGURE 32-5 Pacemaker hysteresis. The pacemaker is programmed to pace at 70 pulses per min, but not to start pacing until the heart rate has fallen below 40 bpm.

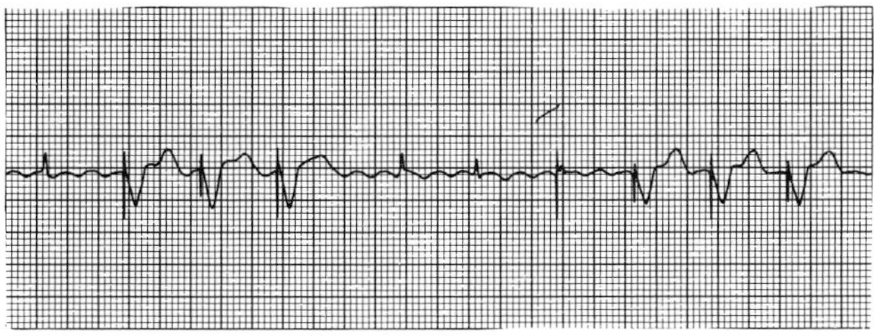

FIGURE 32-6 Rapid ventricular pacing delivered by a dual-chamber pacemaker (DDD) during atrial flutter. The atrial channel of the pacemaker senses every other atrial beat, and each sensed atrial beat triggers the ventricular channel to deliver a stimulus.

because of pacemaker malfunction. For example, pulses may fail to appear at a rate of 70 per min simply because the pacemaker has been set to pace at 40 pulses per min. In fact, some permanent pacemakers can be programmed to an OOO mode in which no pacing is delivered. A more common source of confusion is pacemaker hysteresis, which is a feature of some permanent pacemakers in which the pause that a pacemaker takes before pacing is independent of the pacing rate (Fig. 32-5). In other words, a pacemaker that is set to pace at 70 pulses per min can be programmed, using hysteresis, to wait up to 2 s after the last spontaneous beat before delivering the first stimulus.

A very serious type of pacemaker malfunction is the appearance of unwanted stimuli, either occurring at a faster rate than desired or delivered too soon after the previous beat. Uncurtailed rapid ventricular pacing can cause palpitations, angina, or heart failure. Rapid ventricular pacing can result from runaway pacing by a pulse generator with a dying battery, though recently manufactured devices are designed to protect themselves against this malfunction.[30] Patients with dual-chamber pacemakers can experience rapid ventricular pacing through two common mechanisms: (1) development of an atrial tachyarrhythmia, with rapid atrial activity triggering rapid ventricular pacing (Fig. 32-6); and (2) pacemaker-mediated tachycardia, in which each paced ventricular beat conducts retrogradely to the atria and the retrograde P waves are sensed by the pacemaker and trigger the delivery of ventricular stimuli (Fig. 32-7).[31] Both of these problems can be immediately controlled by placing a magnet over the pacemaker; this disables sensing by the pacemaker and prevents ventricular stimuli from being triggered by sensed atrial beats. In order to prevent the rapid pacing from recurring, the pacemaker must be reprogrammed.

Unwanted stimuli can also appear when spontaneous beats are not sensed. This can result from lead dislodgement, placement of the lead next to infarcted myocardium, a failing pulse generator battery, or an inappropriately high setting of the sensitivity threshold (Fig. 32-8). Patients with dual-chamber pacemakers can receive unwanted ventricular stimuli if spontaneous QRS complexes occur simultaneously with atrial pacing spikes, because in order to prevent cross-talk inhibition (discussed above) the ventricular channel is prevented from sensing during the atrial extrastimulus and for the next 20 ms or so (the "blanking period").

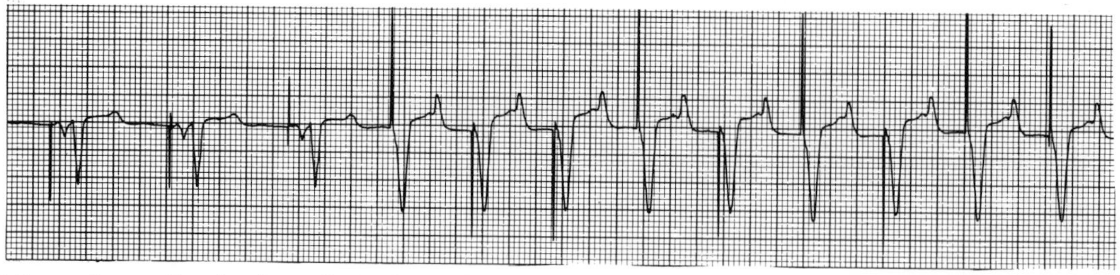

FIGURE 32-7 Pacemaker-mediated tachycardia. Each paced ventricular beat conducts retrogradely to the atria; the retrograde P waves are sensed, and each triggers another ventricular stimulus. Shifting of the axis of the pacing stimulus, as in this tracing, is a common phenomenon seen in normal circumstances.

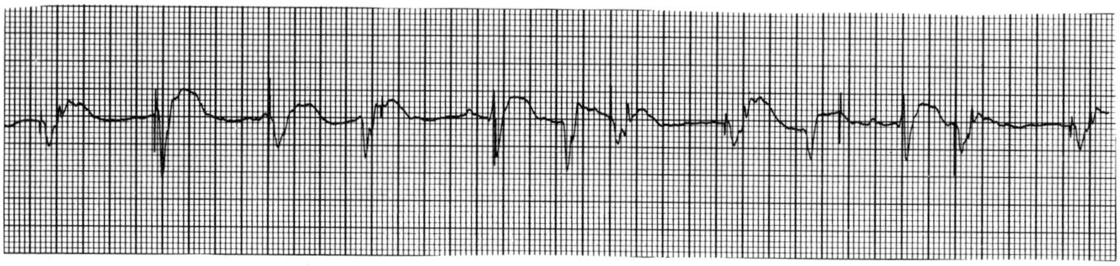

FIGURE 32-8 Failure to sense. Pacing stimuli occur at a rate of 70 pulses per min and are not inhibited by spontaneous beats. Stimuli fail to capture only when they fall during the refractory period of the patient's ventricle; otherwise, capture is intact.

References

1. Rahimtoola SH, Ehsani A, Sinno MZ, et al: Left atrial transport function in myocardial infarction. Importance of its booster pump function. Am J Med 59:686, 1975.
2. Johnson AD, Laiken SL, Engler RL: Hemodynamic compromise associated with ventriculoatrial conduction following transvenous pacemaker placement. Am J Med 65:75, 1978.
3. Love JC, Haffajee CI, Gore JM, Alpert JS: Reversibility of hypotension and shock by atrial or atrioventricular sequential pacing in patients with right ventricular infarction. Am Heart J 108:5, 1984.
4. Hindman MC, Wagner GS, JaRo M, et al: The clinical significance of bundle branch block complicating acute myocardial infarction. 1. Clinical characteristics, hospital mortality, and one-year follow-up. Circulation 58:679, 1978.
5. Lamas GA, Muller JE, Turi ZG, et al: A simplified method to predict occurrence of complete heart block during acute myocardial infarction. Am J Cardiol 57:1213, 1986.
6. Hindman MC, Wagner GS, JaRo M, et al: The clinical significance of bundle branch block complicating acute myocardial infarction. 2. Indications for temporary and permanent pacemaker insertion. Circulation 58:689, 1978.
7. Gunnar RM, Bourdillon PDV, Dixon DW, et al: Guidelines for the early management of patients with acute myocardial infarction: a report of the American College of Cardiology/American Heart Association Task Force on Assessment of Diagnostic and Therapeutic Cardiovascular Procedures (Subcommittee to Develop Guidelines for the Early Management of Patients With Acute Myocardial Infarction). J Am Coll Cardiol 16:249, 1990.
8. Morris D, Mulvihill D, Lew WYW: Risk of developing complete heart block during bedside pulmonary artery catheterization in patients with left bundle-branch block. Arch Intern Med 147:2005, 1987.
9. Frye RL, Collins JJ, DeSanctis RW, et al: Guidelines for permanent cardiac pacemaker implantation: a report of the Task Force on Assessment of Diagnostic and Therapeutic Cardiovascular Procedures (Subcommittee on Pacemaker Implantation). J Am Coll Cardiol 4:434, 1984.
10. Shaw DB, Kekwick CA, Veale D, et al: Survival in second degree atrioventricular block. Br Heart J 53:587, 1985.
11. Austin JL, Preis LK, Crampton RS, et al: Analysis of pacemaker malfunction and complications of temporary pacing in the coronary care unit. Am J Cardiol 49:301, 1982.
12. Hynes JK, Holmes DR Jr, Harrison CE: Five-year experience with temporary pacemaker therapy in the coronary care unit. Mayo Clin Proc 58:122, 1983.
13. Bing OHL, McDowell JW, Hantman J, Messer JV: Pacemaker placement by electrocardiographic monitoring. N Engl J Med 287:651, 1972.
14. Drozd P, Escher DJW, Furman S: Pacing by a bipolar transvenous "semifloating" elecath electrode. Circulation 40:III, 1969.
15. Littleford PO: Physiologic temporary pacing: techniques and indications, Barold SS (ed): *Modern cardiac pacing*. Futura Publishing, Mount Kisco, NY, 1985 p 239.
16. Breivik K, Oie S: Clinical performance of a new atrioventricular sequential temporary pacing electrode system, in Gomez FP (ed): Cardiac pacing. Futura Publishing, Mount Kisco, NY, 1985, p 390.
17. Gessler CJ Jr, Jaffe AS: Hemodynamic monitoring and pacing with one catheter. Cathet Cardiovasc Diag 13:141, 1987.
18. Glassman RD, Noble RJ, Tavel ME, et al: Pacemaker-induced endocardial friction rub. Am J Cardiol 40:811, 1977.
19. Resnekov L, Lipp H: Pacemaking and acute myocardial infarction. Prog Cardiovasc Dis 14:475, 1972.
20. Waldo AL, MacLean WAH, Karp RB, et al: Entrainment and interruption of atrial flutter with atrial pacing. Studies in man following open heart surgery. Circulation 56:737, 1977.

21. Santini M, Ansalone G, Cacciatore G, Turitto G: Transesophageal pacing. PACE 13:1298, 1990.
22. Gallagher JJ, Smith WM, Kerr CR, et al: Esophageal pacing: a diagnostic and therapeutic tool. Circulation 65:336, 1982.
23. Jenkins JM, Dick M Jr, Collins S, et al: Use of a pill electrode for transesophageal atrial pacing. PACE 8:512, 1985.
24. Crawford W, Plumb VJ, Epstein AE, Kay GN: Prospective evaluation of transesophageal pacing for the interruption of atrial flutter. Am J Med 86:663, 1989.
25. Brown CG, Hutchins GM, et al: Placement accuracy of percutaneous transthoracic pacemakers. Am J Emerg Med 3:193, 1985.
26. White JD: Transthoracic pacing in cardiac asystole. Am J Emerg Med 3:264, 1983.
27. Zoll PM, Zoll RH, Falk RH, et al: External noninvasive temporary cardiac pacing: clinical trials. Circulation 71:937, 1985.
28. Klein LS, Miles WM, Heger JJ, Zipes DP: Transcutaneous pacing: patient tolerance, strength-interval relations and feasibility for programmed electrical stimulation. Am J Cardiol 62:1126, 1988.
29. Estes NAM, Deering TF, Manolis AS, et al: External cardiac programmed stimulation for noninvasive termination of sustained supraventricular and ventricular tachycardia. Am J Cardiol 63:177, 1989.
30. Reddy CVR, Gould L, Singh BK, et al: Runaway temporary pacemaker. N Engl J Med 302:1030, 1980.
31. Furman S, Fisher JD: Endless loop tachycardia in an AV universal (DDD) pacemaker. PACE 5:486, 1982.

Chapter 33

ENDOSCOPY

IRA M. HANAN

Diagnosis and potential treatment of acute gastrointestinal bleeding is the most common indication for upper gastrointestinal endoscopy in the ICU patient. Upper gastrointestinal endoscopy allows complete examination of the esophagus, stomach, and duodenum—the most common sites of gastrointestinal tract bleeding—as well as examination of the duodenal papilla and proximal jejunum. Esophagogastroduodenoscopy (EGD) identifies the source of upper gastrointestinal tract bleeding in >85 percent of patients. However, despite the excellent sensitivity of EGD in the bleeding patient, the overall mortality rate for patients with upper gastrointestinal tract bleeding remains approximately 10 percent,[1] a figure noted in such patients prior to the standard use of EGD. Nevertheless, selected patients, such as those carrying a high risk for surgery or those with liver disease, may benefit from early diagnostic and therapeutic endoscopy. Colonoscopy is occasionally indicated to evaluate bleeding, diarrhea, or pseudo-obstruction in the critically ill patient (Table 33-1).

Less frequently, EGD or colonoscopy is necessary for nonbleeding indications in the ICU patient. These will generally be well-tolerated and carry less risk than when performed in the bleeding patient.

Esophagogastroduodenoscopy

INDICATIONS FOR EGD IN ICU PATIENTS

Suspected upper gastrointestinal tract bleeding is the most common indication for EGD in the ICU patient. Although bleeding usually is evident by a presentation of melena or hematemesis, brisk upper gastrointestinal tract bleeding, such as from a deep duodenal ulcer, may present with hematochezia and signs of hemodynamic instability. In such instances, EGD should be undertaken as the first diagnostic study prior to endoscopic evaluation of the rectum and colon. Patients presenting with hypotension or orthostasis of 20 mmHg or greater, in conjunction with bright red blood or maroon stool per rectum, should be evaluated by EGD first. The relative ease with which the procedure is performed and tolerated by the ICU patient warrants this approach. As many as 14 percent of patients presenting with significant acute gastrointestinal bleeding will have a "negative" nasogastric aspirate, despite an upper gastrointestinal cause of the bleed.[1] Enteral nutritional support of critically ill patients may necessitate the placement of nasoenteric or percutaneous feeding tubes. EGD may be required for proper positioning of these tubes.

Less frequently, the critically ill patient may require EGD to evaluate infectious esophagitis. The immunocompromised patient is susceptible to esophagitis from candidal, herpetic, or cytomegaloviral infection. Each form of esophagitis has a characteristic endoscopic appearance. Cytology brushings and biopsy may confirm the infectious etiology of esophagitis in the immunocompromised patient. Emergent endoscopy allows drainage of infected bile in biliary sepsis.

CONTRAINDICATIONS (Table 33-2)

Conscious patients undergoing EGD must be cooperative prior to undertaking the procedure. Although this is usually best achieved with conscious sedation, special circumstances may require the use of general anesthesia or no sedation. The failure to achieve cooperation from the patient is frequently a cause for aborting or postponing endoscopy. Uncooperative conscious patients place not only themselves at risk during the procedure, but the critical care personnel as well. Bite- and fingernail-induced skin wounds, as well as blunt trauma from flailing arms or legs, may put the medical personnel at substantial risk, particularly if the patient carries transmissible disease. The comatose and muscle-relaxed patients require no sedation as they are easily examined.

Suspicion of gastrointestinal perforation or impending perforation contraindicates performance of EGD. Perforation of the stomach or duodenum from trauma, tumor infiltration, or peptic ulcer disease will present with signs of pneumoperitoneum and peritonitis. Fever and a high white blood cell count, with a left shift initially, may be absent. Appropriate upright chest and lateral abdominal x-rays should be obtained before endoscopy in patients suspected of having a perforation. Carcinoma, trauma, or emetogenic injury (Boerhaave's syndrome) may cause perforation of the esophagus as well as bleeding. Subcutaneous emphysema and pneumomediastinum would suggest this diagnosis, which contraindicates endoscopy.

Gastrointestinal obstruction at any level heightens the potential risk of aspiration of gastrointestinal contents dur-

TABLE 33-1 Indications for Endoscopy in the ICU Patient

Diagnosis and treatment of gastrointestinal bleeding
Decompression of acute colonic pseudo-obstruction
Biliary decompression in biliary sepsis
Diagnosis of infectious esophagitis
Proper positioning of nasoenteric feeding tube; percutaneous placement of gastrostomy tube

TABLE 33-2 Contraindications to Endoscopy

Uncooperative patient
Suspected or documented gastrointestinal perforation
Suspected or documented gastrointestinal obstruction
Hemodynamic instability (systolic pressure <100 mmHg, pulse >120/min), signs of respiratory distress

ing EGD. Additionally, room air is used to insufflate the gastrointestinal tract during endoscopy. In the presence of an obstruction, perforation of the small intestine could ensue.

Hemodynamic instability is the most common contraindication to safely performing EGD in the critically ill patient. Hypotension, profound orthostasis, and tachycardia may be the direct result of acute blood loss in these patients. Inadequate volume replacement heightens the risk of complications (see below). Effort should be made to restore the blood pressure to systolic >100 and pulse <120.

SEDATION AND CHOICE OF ENDOSCOPE

The use of premedication to achieve conscious sedation prior to endoscopy is widespread, yet not essential. The National American Society for Gastrointestinal Endoscopy (ASGE) Survey on Upper Gastrointestinal Bleeding reports premedication given in 85 percent of examinations. The most commonly used agent was diazepam; 40 percent received meperidine. Some argue that premedication is not essential prior to endoscopy,[2] yet generally it is preferred by the patient. In one series, nearly half the patients examined without sedation considered the experience unpleasant. In selective, cooperative patients, the judicious use of a topical anesthetic, such as Xylocaine or lidocaine, may be sufficient. Most endoscopists agree that patient cooperation and comfort are improved by the use of sedatives. Yet, whether an endoscopic examination is completed may not be influenced by whether the patient received sedation.[1] Commonly used sedatives include diazepam or midazolam, with or without narcotics, such as meperidine. Midazolam, an imidazobenzodiazepine, has greater potency and a shorter half-life than diazepam. When compared to diazepam in patients undergoing EGD, midozolam decreases induction time, whereas recovery time is unaffected. Importantly, the amnestic effect of midazolam is superior to that of diazepam. The dose range of midazolam required to achieve conscious sedation is 0.01 to 0.07 mg/kg. Lower doses are required for the elderly patient or when narcotic agents are used concomitantly. Higher doses are often needed in alcoholic patients or those who chronically use benzodiazepines. The average dose requirement of diazepam is two to three times that required for midazolam.

Both diazepam and midazolam produce respiratory depression when administered parenterally as a premedication for endoscopy. Both agents cause respiratory depression by direct depression of central respiratory drive and perhaps by simultaneous depression of respiratory muscle efficiency. The degree to which diazepam and midazolam depress central respiratory drive appears similar.[3] The endoscopist must be aware of the potential hyperagitation resulting from the use of diazepam. This paradoxical response may initially result in additional administration of the sedative, with the eventual catastrophe of coma or respiratory arrest. Close monitoring must be advised after the endoscope is removed in patients receiving large doses of diazepam or midazolam, as the "noxious agent," i.e., the endoscope, which has driven the respiratory center, has been withdrawn. Profound hypoventilation is likely to occur at the completion of the examination.

Narcotic agents are frequently used in conjunction with benzodiazepines to achieve conscious sedation for endoscopy. Some prefer concomitant use of a narcotic agent, such as meperidine, because it augments the sedative effects. However, concomitant use of a narcotic with benzodiazepine also augments respiratory depression, especially in the elderly patient. The vasodilatory effects of some narcotic agents may limit their use in the hemodynamically compromised bleeding patient. In such instances, the sole use of a nonnarcotic agent is preferred.

Some endoscopists use parenteral atropine as a premedication agent. Its prime function is to decrease oral secretions and gastrointestinal motility during the examination. It does not improve the patient's tolerance for the examination nor the endoscopist's ability to adequately complete the examination. Although it does decrease oral secretions, it does not reduce the risk of aspiration.

A pediatric endoscope, with a small outer diameter, may be used in an elderly patient with pronounced cervical lordosis. This allows easier esophageal intubation through the pyriform sinus, as well as easier intubation of a potentially scarred pyloroduodenal channel, which is critical in the bleeding patient to exclude a bleeding duodenal ulcer. However, a pediatric endoscope has a small biopsy/suction port, limiting the suctioning capability, as well as limiting the use of various therapeutic devices. "Therapeutic" endoscopes, with a 13-mm outer diameter, may have one or two large suction ports, allowing greater suctioning and therapeutic capabilities; yet they may be difficult to use in elderly or uncooperative patients. Standard adult endoscopes generally suffice for adequate diagnostic and therapeutic endoscopy in the bleeding patient. Selective use of a large diameter endoscope in the actively bleeding younger patient may be warranted.

COMPLICATIONS OF EGD (Table 33-3)

Significant hypoxemia may occur during routine EGD. Although this may rarely occur in young patients with normal lungs, it is likely in elderly patients or those with obstructive pulmonary disease. As great as an 18 percent fall from base-line values of oxygen tension (Pa_{O_2}) has been noted during EGD in elderly patients.[4] Patients with moderate to severe obstructive pulmonary disease, identified as those with forced expiratory volume in 1 s/forced vital capacity (FEV_1/FVC) less than 60 percent, desaturate significantly as well.[5] The probable causes include hypoventilation due to sedative agents, the partial airway obstruction produced by the endoscope, and aspiration of gastric contents, resulting in bronchospasm and ventilation/perfusion ($\dot{V}/\dot{Q}$) mismatch[5]. Of these factors, sedative-induced hypoventilation probably plays the paramount role. Some question the effect of sedation on oxygen desaturation, having shown no greater fall in oxygen saturation in sedated than unsedated patients undergoing EGD.[6]

The diameter of the endoscope used may influence the

TABLE 33-3 Complications of Endoscopy

Respiratory depression, hypotension secondary to sedatives
Aspiration of gastric contents during EGD, especially in the bleeding patient
Perforation of esophagus, pylorus during EGD
Perforation during colonoscopy
Bleeding secondary to endoscope-induced Mallory-Weiss tear
Tissue necrosis, perforation, or bleeding secondary to therapeutic intervention

degree of desaturation. Thin endoscopes (8.5 mm diameter) cause less desaturation during endoscopy than do standard (11.5 mm diameter) or large therapeutic endoscopes (13 mm diameter). Thinner endoscopes may be better suited for use in the elderly patient or those with significant obstructive pulmonary disease. Cautious use of sedative drugs and the administration of low flow nasal oxygen during sedation and endoscopy are recommended in these patients at risk, particularly if concomitant anemia from gastrointestinal bleeding is present. The use of pulse oximeters during EGD in high-risk patients is becoming standard.

Although significant aspiration of gastric contents is rare in the nonbleeding patient, massive aspiration causing pneumonitis may occur in the patient with an exsanguinating upper gastrointestinal bleed, such as from varices. In such a patient, if the airway cannot be protected from refluxed blood or hematemesis, endotracheal intubation should be performed before undertaking endoscopy.

Serious cardiac arrhythmias may occur even during nonemergent EGD. Holter monitoring of patients before, during, and after EGD demonstrates an increased occurrence of sinus tachycardia and frequent premature ventricular beats, even if anticholinergic agents are not administered prior to the procedure.[7] Those patients with a prior history of cardiovascular disease carry a greater risk of developing arrhythmias. Though cardiac arrest has occurred and been attributed to EGD, its incidence is exceedingly rare. The role transient hypoxemia plays in induction of arrhythmia, as opposed to the effects of the augmented sympathetic drive which occurs during endoscopy, is not known.

Endoscopy-induced injury may cause bleeding or perforation. Perforation may occur at the cricopharyngeal region on intubation of the esophagus or less commonly at the pylorus/duodenal junction when intubation of the duodenum is blind.[8] Cervical esophageal perforation from endoscope intubation is more likely to occur in the elderly patient with cervical spine osteophytes. Esophageal intubation under direct visualization and the use of smaller, more flexible endoscopes are likely to reduce this potential complication. An endoscope-induced Mallory-Weiss tear may result from excessive retching or vomiting during endoscopy. Typically, a mucosal tear occurs at the cardioesophageal junction, usually along the posterior wall. Although only a few cases of such endoscope-induced injury are reported,[9] its occurrence approaches $\frac{1}{1000}$.[1] As with noninstrument-induced Mallory-Weiss tears, the bleeding is generally self-limited. However, it may cause confusion as to the etiology of bleeding in the patient undergoing endoscopy for upper gastrointestinal tract bleeding.

Bacteremia following endoscopy has been well-documented, with rates varying according to the procedure performed. Incidences of bacteremia as high as 27 percent following colonoscopy[10] and 8 percent following EGD are reported.[11] Despite its frequency, transient bacteremia following endoscopic procedures generally is of little clinical significance. However, concern and controversy exist regarding the risk of endocarditis in patients with valvular heart disease undergoing endoscopy. Although the American Heart Association (AHA) has recommended prophylactic antibiotic coverage for patients with valvular heart disease who undergo endoscopy,[12] some feel there is little basis for this recommendation[13] because only few poorly documented cases of endocarditis following EGD are known.[14] Patients with prosthetic valves are theoretically at greater risk of developing endocarditis should bacteremia occur; therefore, the AHA recommendation regarding antibiotic prophylaxis in such patients is widely accepted (see Chap. 122).

TIMING OF EGD IN THE BLEEDING PATIENT

Questions frequently arise concerning the timing of EGD in the bleeding patient. Although each case needs to be individually assessed, some general guidelines can be derived. These recommendations are based on consideration of potential benefits versus risks of performing EGD early in the assessment and management of the bleeding patient (Table 33-4). The primary assumption which some make is that prompt diagnosis will alter the outcome of the bleeding episode. This postulate rests on a second assumption that prompt diagnosis permits prompt institution of specific therapy to control hemorrhage. Athough these two basic assumptions may hold true for selected patients, they do not hold true for many bleeding patients. In fact, since the standard use of fiberoptic endoscopy for diagnosis of gastrointestinal bleeding, overall mortality from ongoing and recurrent bleeding has not been reduced.[1]

Early endoscopy does not affect mortality or prevent the need for surgical intervention in patients with upper gastrointestinal bleeding.[15] The primary reason lies in the fact that most bleeding is self-limited and not recurrent. When all forms of upper gastrointestinal bleeding are considered, nearly 75 percent will be self-limited, single episodes. Furthermore, management initiated prior to endoscopy is not often altered once the results of the endoscopy are known.[15] Therefore, many patients do not require early endoscopy and should not be subjected to the increased

TABLE 33-4 Indications for Early EGD

Over age 60
History of chronic liver disease
Bright red blood or maroon stool per rectum in association with hypotension or orthostasis
More than 4 U blood required in 6 h

complication rate associated with it. The risk of endoscopy in the bleeding patient rises the sooner the procedure is performed. The national ASGE survey reported a 0.9 percent endoscopy-related complication rate in patients undergoing EGD for acute hemorrhage compared with a rate of 0.13 percent in routine instances. Most complications occurred when the procedure was performed in the emergency setting. Poor fluid and blood volume replacement likely accentuate the hypotensive and respiratory depressive effects of sedatives. Limited time to properly evacuate blood from the stomach heightens the potential for aspiration during endoscopy.

Proponents of early endoscopy in the assessment of the bleeding patient argue that it may be helpful in altering the clinical course of selected patients. Early endoscopy identifies the patient with ongoing hemorrhage and the patient likely to have a recurrent bleed. Endoscopic findings of a clean, nonbloody ulcer crater are associated with only a 10 percent recurrent bleeding rate. On the other hand, an adherent clot or nonbleeding visible vessel in an ulcer base alerts one to a 50 percent likelihood of rebleeding. Furthermore, actively bleeding lesions, i.e., oozing or pumping vessels, which carry a high mortality, generally signify the need for surgical intervention. By identifying high-risk patients, it is possible that early endoscopy may affect management to limit mortality. This is particularly true in patients with peptic ulcer bleeds, where earlier operation results in lower blood transfusion requirements and lower operative mortality.[16]

Presence of liver disease raises the suspicion that esophageal varices may be the source of hemorrhage. However, up to 40 percent of alcoholic cirrhotic patients may bleed from nonvariceal sources. In such patients, early differentiation is vital because management strategies will be different (see Chap. 163).

Finally, proponents of early endoscopy can argue that early diagnostic endoscopy allows early therapeutic endoscopy intervention. Initial studies assessing the impact of early endoscopy on the outcome of bleeding could not assess the potential influence of therapeutic endoscopy, because it did not exist to any degree. The benefits of endoscopic means to control gastrointestinal bleeding are still forthcoming. Initial reports favor their use, suggesting impact on the need for surgical intervention and mortality.[17,18]

A selective approach to endoscopy in the bleeding patient considers: **1.** the questions to be answered by endoscopy, i.e., what is bleeding and will it continue or recur; **2.** the potential for endoscopic therapy; and **3.** the risk of early endoscopy. Following vigorous blood and fluid resuscitation in an attempt to adequately stabilize both heart rate and blood pressure, emergent endoscopy should be considered in selected groups of patients. Patients over age sixty with peptic ulcer disease carry a high mortality rate if bleeding continues and if surgery is delayed.[6] In this group, early endoscopy may assess the need for early surgical intervention before excessive transfusion is required.[6]

Patients with known or suspected liver disease should undergo early endoscopy. This particular group of patients may require various nonsurgical interventions to control variceal hemorrhage. Precise identification of the source of bleeding is essential in patients with liver disease, prior to the institution of specific therapeutic interventions such as tamponade tubes and sclerotherapy.

Patients with bleeding significant enough to cause hypotension or orthostasis or those in whom more than 4 U blood are required in the first 6 h should undergo early endoscopy, because this constitutes a group at risk of continued bleeding and higher surgical necessity.[6]

PREPARATION OF THE PATIENT FOR ENDOSCOPY

Informed consent, outlining the purpose and nature of the endoscopic procedure and the potential risks, is required prior to proceeding. Such consent should anticipate possible therapeutic procedures to control bleeding, i.e., endoscopic variceal sclerotherapy, thermal coagulation, and injection therapy. Because it may not be apparent which modality will be necessary, it is prudent to discuss briefly the potential risks and benefits of each therapy with the patient. By so doing, the endoscopist does not compromise management because adequate consent was not obtained.

Adequate preparation of the patient includes measures to limit potential complications. Therefore, attempts to correct coagulopathy or thrombocytopenia should be initiated prior to endoscopy, but need not be fully corrected before proceeding. Proper resuscitation includes replacement of blood volume as well as crystalline fluid replacement. Thus, patients in whom emergency endoscopy is warranted should have generally received at least 2 U packed red blood cells prior to beginning endosocpy. In the elderly, anemic patient or one with a history of pulmonary disease, oxygen via nasal cannula is prudent, especially if low oxygen saturation is documented by pulse oximetry.

Nasogastric lavage is usually preferred to "clear" the stomach prior to endoscopy. Yet frequently, the volume of fluid instilled exceeds the amount recovered. This can result in large volumes of blood and fluid remaining in the stomach, increasing the risk of aspiration. Therefore, the medical personnel must be watchful that "overlavaging" does not occur. If there is little nasogastric tube return, further instillation of fluid should not continue. The use of iced saline to control bleeding is commonly practiced, but poorly supported by current literature reports.

The risk of aspiration during endoscopy is greater in the bleeding patient. If hematemesis of large quantities of blood is occurring, endoscopy should be delayed until the airway is protected by endotracheal intubation. This frequently may be required in the setting of a massive variceal hemorrhage. Persistent hematemesis despite nasogastric suction warrants endotracheal intubation for airway protection.

An adequate intravenous access line for administration of sedatives is essential. This line should not be simultaneously used for other products such as blood or vasopressin infusion. The specific intravenous access used by the endoscopist should be easily recognizable and accessible during the procedure, such that it can promptly be used to administer additional sedation or narcotic antagonists as the situation may warrant.

The endoscopist must be adequately prepared before beginning any endoscopic procedure. The endoscopist must carefully select the appropriate endoscope, as previously discussed. A well-equipped endoscopy cart is essential. In anticipation of bleeding esophageal varices, an actively bleeding ulcer, or nonbleeding visible vessel within an ulcer, sclerotherapy needles, sclerosing agents, thermal coagulation devices, and solutions for injection therapy should be at hand. Preparation for either endoscopic variceal sclerotherapy or injection therapy of nonvariceal lesions requires solutions to be drawn into syringes and properly labeled prior to beginning endoscopy.

Ideally, an assistant trained in gastrointestinal endoscopy should assist the physician during the procedure. In some situations, e.g., after working hours, critical care nursing personnel will be asked to assist. The individual attention and experience of the assistant is essential. Responsibilities include proper positioning of the body and head during the procedure and monitoring of the patient's secretions during endoscopy to prevent aspiration. The assistant must ensure that the patient does not dislodge the bite-block protecting the endoscope. Additionally, a member of the critical care team should be present to monitor the cardiopulmonary status of the patient during endoscopy. Monitoring of the vital signs, oxygen saturation by means of pulse oximetry, and prevention of endotracheal tube dislodgement are best handled by this critical care member who is not immediately involved in the endoscopic procedure.

THERAPEUTIC INTERVENTION DURING EGD

Within the past decade, endoscopy has evolved from predominantly a diagnostic modality to one which includes a variety of therapeutic options. Therapeutic gastrointestinal endoscopy includes endoscopic control of bleeding, removal of obstructing foreign bodies, and provision of access for enteral feeding. Clearly, the endoscopist most frequently is called on to control bleeding in the critical care patient. Several therapeutic modalities are currently available to control gastrointestinal bleeding. Although many require "high tech" devices not generally available to most endoscopists, injection therapy and thermal coagulation are quickly becoming standard interventions.

ENDOSCOPIC VARICEAL SCLEROTHERAPY

The use of endoscopic variceal sclerotherapy (EVS) was first reported in 1939.[19] Over the ensuing four decades, EVS was used sparingly to control recurrent hemorrhage from esophageal varices. Reports that shunt operations for treatment of recurrent variceal hemorrhage fail to prolong survival[20] while precipitating further hepatic failure have led to a resurgence in the use of EVS to control acute variceal hemorrhage, as well as to prevent future bleeds. Formerly performed using rigid endoscopes, EVS has been adapted to use with flexible fiberoptic endoscopes at the time of the diagnostic endoscopy. Various techniques exist for injecting a variety of sclerosing agents. Although some advocate paravariceal injection,[21] i.e., into the esophageal mucosa next to the varix, most prefer the technique of intravariceal injection, as it may result in less mucosal ulceration. Since good results are reported despite the technique used, both are likely to be effective.[22] Depending on the technique used, from 1 to 5 mL of sclerosing agent per varix is used. The sclerosant is injected into each varix in the distal esophagus, within 3 cm of the gastroesophageal junction (see Plate 24). Most endoscopists inject sclerosant into only one site of each varix. Multiple injections along the course of each varix are not necessary.

Sodium tetradecyl sulfate, ethanolamine oleate, and sodium morrhuate are the most frequently used sclerosing agents in the United. States. Polidocanol, used for paravariceal injections, is available only in Europe. Sclerosing agents cause thrombosis of the submucosal esophageal vessels, with surrounding tissue necrosis. Several days after injection, mucosal ulceration develops. After several weeks, mucosal and submucosal fibrosis occurs, further obliterating the varices.

During the injection of the sclerosing agent, the patient may experience pain in the substernal region. This is generally short-lived, but if persistent may require narcotic analgesic for pain control. Dysphagia and odynophagia may develop because of mucosal edema and ulceration. Sucralfate, in suspension form, may provide symptomatic relief of these symptoms.

Complications related to EVS vary widely, being higher in prospective studies than in retrospective series. Significant complications occur in an estimated 10 to 15 percent of patients undergoing EVS.[23] Pneumonia, pleural effusions, mediastinitis, esophageal perforation,[23] pericarditis,[24] sepsis,[25] and acute respiratory failure[26] have been reported as acute complications related to EVS. Esophageal strictures may result after repeated EVS. These benign strictures, forming after successful obliteration of varices, are amenable to bougienage dilation with good results.

Ideally, EVS is performed after the acute bleeding episode has abated. The endoscopist may choose to proceed with EVS after other bleeding sources are excluded in the patient with large esophageal varices. EVS can be performed in the presence of thrombocytopenia or coagulopathy. The procedure should not be postponed to allow correction of these bleeding diatheses. Certain endoscopic stigmata, e.g., an adherent clot over a varix or "red spots" on varices, correlate well with recent hemorrhage. It is important that the endoscopist assess whether the presence of varices warrants EVS. Many cirrhotic patients have large esophageal varices which do not bleed. Such patients should not be treated, since prophylactic EVS in the patient without prior bleeding is of unproven benefit and carries risk.[27]

Gastric varices, generally found in the cardiofundic region of the stomach, originate from various channels deeper in the submucosa of the stomach wall. They may develop in conjunction with esophageal varices in the cirrhotic patient. However, the finding of large gastric varices in the absence of large esophageal varices should raise the suspicion of extrahepatic portal vein or splenic vein occlusion. Regardless of the etiology, gastric veins generally are not sclerosed. Results have been unfavorable.

A nasogastric tube need not be reinserted unless the patient continues to bleed actively. Insertion of a tamponade tube (e.g., Sengstaken-Blakemore tube) need not be inserted following EVS, unless variceal bleeding continues.

THERMAL COAGULATION

Thermal therapy is commonly used when an ulcer is actively bleeding at the time of endoscopy or when significant rebleeding is apt to occur. This generally occurs from a single artery within the base of the ulcer. Alternatively, oozing of blood from the perimeter of the ulcer crater may be encountered. Thermal therapy is indicated when acute bleeding, either from a visible vessel or margin of the ulcer, is noted or when a nonbleeding visible vessel is present. The latter circumstance carries approximately a 60 percent likelihood of rebleeding. Thermal therapy is designed to produce coagulation and dehydration in the ulcer base surrounding the bleeding vessel. Such efforts result in constriction and destruction of the submucosal feeding vessels supplying the actively bleeding surface artery.

Initially, monopolar electrocoagulation probes passed through the biopsy channel of the endoscope were used and proved effective in controlling active bleeding and limiting rebleeding.[28] Monopolar electrocoagulation generates a current which passes through the patient to a grounding pad. The depth of electrocoagulation extends into the submucosa, producing the desired necrosis of submucosal tissue. However, concern regarding potential perforation with this device has limited its use.

Bipolar (or multipolar) electrocoagulation is the most commonly used device for controlling acute bleeding. This device allows the endoscopist to produce the desired electrocoagulation of the submucosal tissue, while the probe also serves to rinse the ulcer base, allowing better visualization of the lesion. The depth of penetration of energy is less than that of the monopolar device but sufficient to provide the desired effect. The probe is brought in direct contact with the tissue surrounding the visible vessel or active bleeding site while pressure is applied. Such "coaptation" tamponades the tissue while current is applied. The bipolar electrocoagulation unit has the advantage that it is portable and affordable for most endoscopists.

Despite its availability, bipolar electrocoagulation has been critically evaluated only recently. Blinded, sham control studies in patients with active upper gastrointestinal tract bleeding have suggested that the rebleeding rate, transfusion requirements, and hospital length of stay are decreased when bipolar electrocoagulation is used.[17] However, it has not significantly improved mortality.

Endoscopic laser therapy provides deep tissue necrosis without probe contact. Both Nd:YAG and argon lasers have been used for control of gastrointestinal bleeding. Limited data from nontreatment control studies suggest that laser therapy does not influence the outcome of acute upper gastrointestinal tract bleeding.[29] Though laser therapy may be advantageous for treatment of multiple telangiectasias (as in Rendu-Osler-Weber syndrome), the immobility of the laser unit, high cost, and unproven effectiveness have limited its use.

INJECTION THERAPY

Injection of hemostatic agents, in a manner similar to sclerotherapy, has been widely used in Japan for several years with good results. This technique consists of local injection of hypertonic saline-epinephrine or pure ethanol into the ulcer crater surrounding a bleeding vessel (see Plate 25) or into an oozing lesion, such as a Mallory-Weiss tear. Hypertonic saline-epinephrine solutions provide the vasoconstrictive effect of epinephrine, while the hypertonic saline creates tissue swelling, fibrinoid degeneration of the arterial wall, and thrombosis of the vessel.[18] Pure ethanol causes tissue dehydration and contraction with necrosis of the vessel. Using a sclerotherapy needle, 0.1 to 0.2 mL of pure ethanol is injected in four quadrants, 1 to 2 mm from the bleeding vessel.[30] Pure ethanol must be injected slowly, and the total volume administered should not exceed 1 mL because extensive ulceration may occur.[30] When using hypertonic saline-epinephrine as the hemostatic agent, 3 mL of a solution consisting of 1:10,000 epinephrine and 2.7% saline is injected into four quadrants surrounding the vessel. Both agents provide excellent hemostasis (approaching 90 percent in cases of acute bleeding), even when pulsating bleeding vessels are observed.[30] Furthermore, injection therapy provides permanent hemostasis, thereby preventing rebleeding hours or days later. Uncontrolled studies suggest that it prevents rebleeding from nonbleeding visible vessels. Experience suggests that it can be effective regardless of the cause of nonvariceal bleeding.

The rate of emergency operation for patients with nonvariceal bleeding may be reduced by the use of injection therapy.[18] As with other hemostatic endoscopic modalities, injection therapy carries a small risk of perforation, particularly when pure ethanol is used.

THERAPEUTIC ENDOSCOPY IN THE NONBLEEDING PATIENT

Although the majority of therapeutic endoscopic procedures performed in the critically ill patient are done to control hemorrhage, various other procedures may be helpful in special instances. Overwhelming sepsis secondary to ascending cholangitis (generally caused by choledocholithiasis) may necessitate emergent biliary drainage. This can be performed percutaneously or endoscopically following initial stabilization and antibiotic administration. Following diagnostic endoscopic retrograde cholangiography, a nasobiliary stent can be inserted by an experienced endoscopist, using a side-viewing duodenoscope. The placement of a nasobiliary stent through the ampulla of Vater does not require a sphincterotomy, since the 6 to 7-mm diameter stent can be easily passed over a guidewire past the obstruction. Fluoroscopic guidance is required, necessitating the use of a C arm or transport of the patient to the radiology suite. The initial use of the nasobiliary stent, as opposed to an internal stent, allows assurance that proper positioning and functioning of the stent continues, ensuring adequate drainage. Several days following the placement of a nasobiliary stent, definitive endoscopic or surgical therapy to remove a calculus or relieve obstruction can be undertaken. Alternatively, in the high-risk patient, the nasobiliary stent may be used to perfuse a gallstone dissolution agent, such as monooctanoin, in an attempt to dissolve stones without surgical intervention. Emergent endoscopic retrograde cholangiography, followed by sphincterotomy, may be necessary in the setting of gallstone pancreatitis. This form of pancreatitis carries a higher mortality rate. If gallstone pancreatitis is fulminant, surgical or endoscopic intervention is often indicated. Endoscopic sphincterotomy facilitates the removal of small- and medium-sized gallstones, relieving obstruction of the common channel formed by the pancreatic and common bile ducts. Cholangitis, or worsening pancreatitis, may follow diagnostic endoscopic retrograde cholangiopancreatography, which should not be performed unless an endoscopist experienced in performing endoscopic sphincterotomy is available or emergent surgery is planned.

POSTPROCEDURAL CONSIDERATIONS

Following upper gastrointestinal endoscopy, attention must be given to the respiratory and circulatory status of the sedated patient. Removal of the endoscope reduces patient stimulation and may result in diminished respiratory drive. Gastric distention, resulting from air insufflation during endoscopy, may cause emesis after endoscopy. To prevent aspiration, the patient should be maintained in the lateral decubitus position for one-half hour following completion of the examination. After endoscopy in the nonbleeding patient, oral intake may be resumed once the effects of topical anesthesia have resolved.

In the setting of acute bleeding, a previously removed nasogastric tube may need to be reinserted. The nasogastric tube should be used for gastric aspiration when massive bleeding continues. Patients in whom bleeding has stopped generally can be managed without continued nasogastric suctioning.

Immediately on completion of the endoscopic procedure, the endoscopist must complete the endoscopic report. This report should include not only objective findings, but also the endoscopist's impressions of these findings. The endoscopist must interpret the significance and relevance of abnormal findings. The report must also include any complications and the completeness of the examination. Photodocumentation of abnormal findings is advisable when possible. The endoscopist should verbally report the results of the endoscopy to the management team, including the surgical consultant. Ideally, the managing physicians and surgical consultants should be present at the time of endoscopy. Decisions regarding surgical or endoscopic therapy of the bleeding patient can be made jointly when both the surgeon and endoscopist are present.

Colonoscopy

Common indications for colonoscopy in the critically ill patient include evaluation of acute gastrointestinal bleeding and diarrhea. Suspected perforation or obstruction of the colon contraindicates colonoscopy. Fulminant colitis, whether idiopathic or infectious in origin, may contraindicate colonoscopy since toxic megacolon may ensue.

Colonoscopy may be helpful in the evaluation of massive lower gastrointestinal bleeding, providing a diagnosis in 40 to 70 percent of cases.[31,32] However, in light of the difficulty encountered in performing colonoscopy in the actively bleeding patient, it generally is performed after an EGD has ruled out an upper gastrointestinal source of the rectal bleeding. Colonoscopy may localize the site of bleeding to a particular segment of the colon, limiting the extent of resection in instances in which surgical treatment is necessary. Ideally, colonoscopy should be performed after bleeding has stopped, allowing some preparation of the colon. This waiting period allows a more complete examination with a higher diagnostic yield, yet may raise questions as to the origin of the bleed. In the patient in whom extensive diverticular disease is noted throughout the colon, delayed colonoscopy may fail to identify the precise site of diverticular bleeding. Furthermore, the acute bleeding episode may be amenable to therapeutic colonoscopic interventions, such as electrocoagulation of a bleeding angiodysplastic lesion. Lavage of a bleeding diverticulum with epinephrine to control bleeding has been reported.[33]

Alternatively, massive bleeding resulting in hemodynamic instability may be evaluated by angiography. Angiography localized bleeding in 72 percent of patients presenting with lower gastrointestinal bleeding in one series. Furthermore, it allowed segmental resection with a lower mortality than in patients undergoing resection without angiography.[34] It has not been established whether colonoscopy or angiography should be performed as the first diagnostic procedure for massive lower gastrointestinal bleeding. Both procedures are useful in assessing the bleeding patient when used at the appropriate time.

Colonoscopy may be used to establish the diagnosis of ischemic injury to the colon. Bright red blood per rectum, with or without diarrhea, is commonly seen in patients with colonic ischemia. Patients in whom the diagnosis is suspected should undergo a "gentle" colonoscopic examination, since distention of the bowel with insufflating gas may result in perforation. If ischemic changes are noted in the left colon, complete examination of the entire colon is not necessary.

Colonoscopy is indicated for the treatment of acute pseudo-obstruction of the colon, which occurs in patients critically ill from noncolonic causes. Frequently, trauma or sepsis precedes the onset of massive colonic distention. If unattended, acute colonic pseudo-obstruction may result in colonic necrosis and perforation, generally in the thin-walled cecum, with a mortality rate of >40 percent.[35] The risk of cecal perforation is highest when the cecal diameter

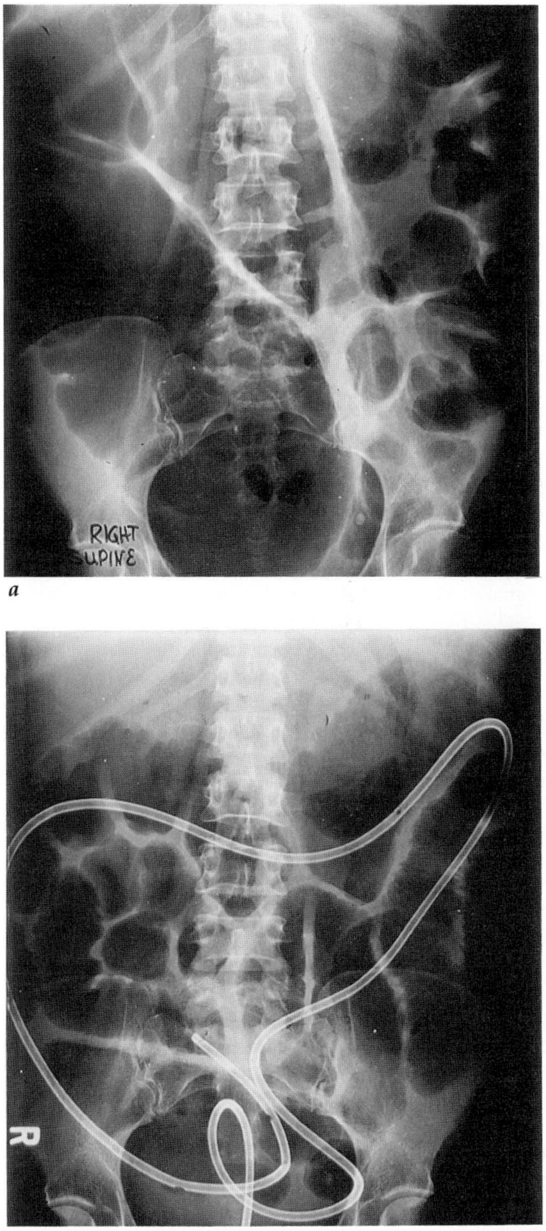

a

b

FIGURE 33-1 ***a.*** **Abdominal x-ray demonstrates massive colonic pseudo-obstruction.** ***b.*** **Significant improvement is accomplished after colonoscopic decompression and placement of enteroclysis tube.**

on a plain radiograph exceeds 12 cm. Colonoscopic decompression (Fig. 33-1) is a safe and effective means of preventing cecal perforation. Following a brief trial of intestinal decompression by nasogastric suction, correction of any electrolyte imbalances and discontinuation of narcotic agents which may precipitate pseudo-obstruction, decompressive colonoscopy should be undertaken. After a tap water enema is gently administered, the colonoscope is inserted into the rectum and advanced as far as possible. It is paramount that the endoscopist limit the air insufflation during colonoscopy, because failure to do so may result in progressive distention of the colon. When available, carbon dioxide is preferred for insufflation, since it is readily absorbed by the colonic epithelium, transported by the bloodstream to the lungs, and excreted in the breath. Once maximum insertion is achieved, the colonoscope is used to suction gas as it is withdrawn from the colon. In nearly half the cases, an experienced endoscopist can reach the cecum in the unprepared patient with pseudo-obstruction. Even in instances in which the cecum is not reached with the tip of the colonoscope, suctioning in the distal colon may achieve partial cecal decompression.

Following colonoscopic decompression, acute colonic distention may recur in 75 percent of patients. Several techniques have been designed to place a decompression tube into the cecum at the time of colonoscopy. Such tubes (usually a cantor tube or enteroclysis tube) can be "pulled" to the cecum using the colonoscope, or passed over a soft tip guidewire passed through the colonoscope's biopsy channel.[36] The placement of a decompression tube can significantly diminish the likelihood of recurrent pseudo-obstruction. An attempt to place a decompression tube should be made whenever possible.

Intraoperative Endoscopy

Intraoperative endoscopy may be indicated in selected circumstances in which gastrointestinal bleeding is believed to arise from the small bowel. Although intraoperative endoscopy is frequently used for assessment of chronic intermittent blood loss following a negative conventional evaluation in the elderly patient, it may occasionally be useful in the setting of acute gastrointestinal bleeding. Intraoperative endoscopy should be considered only after conventional colonoscopy and EGD have failed to identify a bleeding source. It may be particularly useful to identify suspected angiodysplasia of the ileum, which may coexist in patients with cecal angiodysplasia. By identifying the uppermost extent of small bowel angiodysplasia, the length of resected small bowel can be limited. Intraoperative endoscopy may aid in localizing small bowel polyps in patients with Peutz-Jeghers syndrome. In such instances, intraoperative endoscopy may facilitate endoscopic removal of hamartomatous lesions or direct the surgeon to the bowel segment to be resected.

Intraoperative endoscopy can be performed through oral, rectal, or enterotomy introduction of the endoscope. Following incision of the abdominal wall and exposure of small bowel, the endoscope can be introduced orally. The endoscope, generally a pediatric colonoscope, can be advanced easily to the ligament of Treitz. Thereafter, examination of the entire small bowel is facilitated by pleating the small bowel over the colonoscope. The endoscopist must take care to limit the amount of air insufflation, because excessive distention of the bowel will result in prolonged postoperative ileus. Following inspection of the small bowel to the ileocecal valve, a second inspection is performed as the colonoscope is slowly withdrawn. The surgeon assists the examination by carefully inspecting the serosal side of the bowel, looking for a transilluminated angiodysplastic lesion.

Alternatively, a sterilized colonoscope may be placed through an enterotomy site in the small bowel. It can then be passed proximally and distally into the small bowel to facilitate examination. This approach carries a risk of contamination of the exposed peritoneum.

Complications encountered during intraoperative endoscopy include serosal laceration and prolonged ileus. These can be minimized by teamwork between the surgeon and endoscopist during the procedure.

References

1. Silverstein FE, Gilbert DA, Tedesco FJ et al: The national ASGE survey on upper gastrointestinal bleeding: II. Clinical prognostic factors. Gastrointest Endosc 27:80, 1981.
2. Al-Atrakchi HA: Upper gastrointestinal endoscopy without sedation: A prospective study of 2000 examinations. Gastrointest Endosc 35:79, 1989.
3. Forster A, Gardaz J-P, Suter PM et al: Respiratory depression by midazolam and diazepam. Anesthesiology 53:494, 1980.
4. Rozen P, Oppenheim D, Ratan J et al: Arterial oxygen tension changes in elderly patients undergoing upper gastrointestinal endoscopy: I. Possible causes. Scand J Gastroenterol 14:577, 1979.
5. Rostykus PS, McDonald GB, Albert RK: Upper intestinal endoscopy induces hypoxemia in patients with obstructive pulmonary disease. Gastroenterology 78:488, 1980.
6. Lavies NG, Creasy T, Harris K et al: Arterial oxygen saturation during upper gastrointestinal endoscopy: Influence of sedation and operator experience. Am J Gastroenterol 83:618, 1988.
7. Segawa K, Nakazawa S, Yamao K et al: Cardiac response to upper gastrointestinal endoscopy. Am J Gastroenterol 84:13, 1989.
8. Blackstone MO: *Endoscopic Interpretation.* New York, Raven Press, 1984.
9. Baker RW, Spiro AH, Trnka YM: Mallory-Weiss tear complicating upper endoscopy: Case reports and review of the literature. Gastroenterology 82:140, 1982.
10. Pelican G, Hentges D, Butt J: Bacteremia during colonoscopy. Gastrointest Endosc 23:33, 1976.
11. Baltch AL, Buhac I, Agrawal A: Bacteremia after upper gastrointestinal endoscopy. Arch Intern Med 137:594, 1977.
12. American Heart Association Committee on Rheumatic Fever and the Committee on Congenital Cardiac Defects: Prevention of bacterial endocarditis. Circulation 46(suppl V):3, 1972.
13. Vennes JA: Infectious complications of gastrointestinal endoscopy. Dig Dis Sci 26 (July suppl):60, 1981.
14. Meyer GW: Prophylaxis of infective endocarditis during gastrointestinal procedures: Report of a survey. Gastrointest Endosc 25:1, 1979.
15. Peterson WL, Barnett CC, Smith HJ et al: Routine early endoscopy in upper-gastrointestinal-tract bleeding: A randomized, controlled trial. N Engl J Med 304:925, 1981.
16. Hunt PS, Hansky J, Hillman H et al: Reduction in mortality from upper gastrointestinal hemorrhage. Med J Aust 2:552, 1983.
17. Laine L: Multipolar electrocoagulation in the treatment of active upper gastrointestinal tract hemorrhage: A prospective controlled trial. N Engl J Med 316:1613, 1987.
18. Hirao M, Kobayashi T, Masuda K et al: Endoscopic local injection of hypertonic saline-epinephrine solution to arrest hemorrhage from the upper gastrointestinal tract. Gastrointest Endosc 31:313, 1985.
19. Crafoord C, Frenckner P: New surgical treatment of varicose veins of the oesophagus. Acta Otolaryngol Stockh 27:422, 1939.
20. Reynolds TB, Donovan AJ, Mikkelsen WP: Results of a 12-year randomized trial of portacaval shunt in patients with alcoholic liver disease and bleeding varices. Gastroenterology 80:1005, 1981.
21. Paquet KJ, Feussner H: Endoscopic sclerosis and esophageal balloon tamponade in acute hemorrhage from esophagogastric varices: A prospective controlled randomized trial. Hepatology 5:580, 1985.
22. Westaby D, MacDougall BRD, Williams R: Improved survival following injection sclerotherapy for esophageal varices: Final analysis of a controlled trial. Hepatology 5:827, 1985.
23. Marzuk PM, Schwartz JS: Endoscopic sclerotherapy for esophageal varices. Ann Intern Med 100:608, 1984.
24. Knauer CM, Fogel MR: Pericarditis: Complication of esophageal sclerotherapy: A report of three cases. Gastroenterology 93:287, 1987.
25. McGrew W, Goodin J, Stuck W: Fatal complication of endoscopic sclerotherapy: *Serratia marcescens* bacteremia with delayed esophageal perforation. Gastrointest Endosc 31:329, 1985.
26. Monroe P, Morrow C, Millen J et al: Acute respiratory failure and sclerotherapy. Gastroenterology 85:693, 1983.
27. Santangelo WC, Dueno MI, Estes BL et al: Prophylactic sclerotherapy of large esophageal varices. N Engl J Med 318:814, 1988.
28. Papp JP: Endoscopic electrocoagulation in the management of upper gastrointestinal tract bleeding. Surg Clin North Am 62:797, 1982.
29. Krejs GJ, Little KH, Westergaard H: Laser photocoagulation for the treatment of acute peptic-ulcer bleeding: A randomized controlled clinical trial. N Engl J Med 316:1618, 1987.
30. Chen P-C, Wu C-S, Liaw Y-F: Hemostatic effect of endoscopic local injection with hypertonic saline-epinephrine solution and pure ethanol for digestive tract bleeding. Gastrointest Endosc 32:319, 1986.
31. Forde KA: Colonoscopy in acute rectal bleeding. Gastrointest Endosc 27:219, 1981.
32. Jensen DM, Machicado GA: Abstract. Emergent colonoscopy in patients with severe lower gastrointestinal bleeding. Gastroenterol 80:1184, 1981.
33. Ballardini G, del Poggio P: Therapeutic use of colonoscopy in active diverticular bleeding. Letter. Gastrointest Endosc 31:290, 1985.
34. Browder W, Cerise EJ, Litwin MS: Impact of emergency angiography in massive lower gastrointestinal bleeding. Ann Surg 204:530, 1986.
35. Strodel WE, Nostrant TT, Eckhauser FE et al: Therapeutic and diagnostic colonoscopy in nonobstructive colonic dilatation. Ann Surg 197:416, 1983.
36. Harig JM, Fumo DE, Loo FD: Treatment of acute nontoxic megacolon during colonoscopy: Tube placement versus simple decompression. Gastrointest Endosc 34:23, 1988.

Chapter 34

INTRACRANIAL PRESSURE MONITORING AND TREATMENT OF INTRACRANIAL HYPERTENSION

LAWRENCE H. PITTS
BRIAN T. ANDREWS

Over the past 15 years, intracranial pressure (ICP) monitoring and control have been hallmarks of aggressive management of traumatic brain injury, and their use has been increasingly common in management of other cerebral disorders such as subarachnoid hemorrhage (SAH), intracerebral hematomas (ICH), brain tumors, and liver disease. ICP monitoring and control are routine features of intensive care in most major neurosurgical centers and are done commonly in community hospitals. Although definitive proof of their efficacy is lacking, substantial anecdotal or suggestive data support their use and growing application.[1–4]

ICP is the pressure measured from some intracranial site generally recorded as mmHg or torr. The measured site is within the cerebral ventricles, or in the subdural or epidural space, or rarely from within the brain parenchyma. While the brain is reasonably plastic and the ICP measured at a single place within the skull fairly well reflects the pressure at any other place, tissue pressure in or around very focal pathology such as a tumor or hematoma probably is higher than the "whole box" ICP. Cerebral perfusion pressure (CPP) is the difference between mean arterial pressure (MAP) and ICP (CPP = MAP − ICP).

In normal brain, cerebral blood flow (CBF) remains fairly constant around 50 mL/100 g brain tissue/min as long as cerebral autoregulation is intact, i.e., cerebral vessels change their diameter and resistance with pressure changes so that a constant CBF is maintained as long as CPP is about 50 to 150 mmHg. If MAP falls substantially or ICP rises substantially, then CPP becomes lower than autoregulation can correct for and CBF falls with resulting cerebral ischemia. With marginal CPP around 50 to 60 mmHg, one must remember that "focal" CPP can be lower than the "whole box" CPP if there are focal brain lesions, and a more generous CPP of 60 to 80 may be necessary to prevent focal ischemia. Intracranial hypertension is potentially injurious elevated ICP. While the precise level of abnormal ICP is not agreed on and undoubtedly varies among different pathologies, ICP levels above 20 or 25 mmHg for 10 to 15 min generally would be considered pathologic and require treatment.

ICP monitoring has taken its place as an important tool in the intensive management of patients with a diversity of acute neurologic disorders including congenital (aneurysm), traumatic, and metabolic abnormalities. Physiologic monitoring of ICP, MAP, central venous pressure (CVP), and metabolic parameters such as arteriovenous oxygen content difference $(a - v)_{O_2}$ all can supplement the neurologic examination in determining the progression of the initial injury or the development of a new problem and can help to guide their management. When intracranial hypertension threatens to add a new insult to the neurologic injury, a number of successful strategies can be used to reduce ICP to acceptable levels. However, several different treatments are possible and the problems to be treated are varied; thus therapy must be tailored to the specific patient to be optimally effective. This chapter reviews the indications for ICP monitoring and the various therapeutic alternatives which facilitate this optimal intensive care.

Indications for ICP Monitoring (Table 34-1)

HEAD INJURY

Since Lundberg[5] described ICP monitoring in 1960, its use in adults has been preponderantly in patients with severe head injury, both because of the large number of such patients treated each year and because intracranial hypertension is common when the injury is severe. We cannot tell in individual patients whether severe head injury produces a bad outcome and that brain swelling and increased ICP are epiphenomena, or the injury produces intracranial hypertension which in turn directly causes more brain injury and worsens outcome. The first of these two choices has no remedy—the injury is so severe from the outset that treatment will be ineffective. Most neurosurgeons assume and hope the second of these two possibilities to be true, i.e., that intracranial hypertension itself is adding to brain in-

TABLE 34-1 Conditions in Which Early Detection and Treatment of Intracranial Hypertension May Prevent Secondary Brain Ischemia

Head Injury
Postevacuation of large subdural or epidural hematoma
Delayed intracerebral hematoma
Coma-producing diffuse head injury
Subarachnoid Hemorrhage (SAH)
Pre- and postoperative hydrocephalus
Post SAH infarction
Brain Tumors
Posttumor removal
Postoperative tumor-induced hydrocephalus
Fulminant Hepatic Failure
Hepatic coma awaiting transplant
Reye's syndrome

jury, and also believe that ICP elevations should be detected and controlled. Each experienced neurosurgeon can relate specific anecdotal cases where detection and treatment of elevated ICP reversed neurologic deterioration and contributed to a good outcome. For example, detection of a delayed expanding intracranial hematoma by observing rising ICP can lead to more prompt, possibly life-saving clot removal.

CBF falls when ICP increases to 20 to 30 mmHg or CPP decreases to 40 to 50 mmHg. Multimodality evoked potentials (MEPs) also deteriorate with rise of ICP and reduction of CPP, presumably from cerebral ischemia. MEPs were moderately or severely abnormal over 75 percent of the time that ICP rose above 30 mmHg, confirming with this particular functional measure the likely direct role of intracranial hypertension in causing brain injury and worsening outcome in some patients.[6]

One particularly dangerous situation for patients with severe head injury is that of a large subdural or epidural hematoma with subsequent massive swelling of one hemisphere subjacent to the extracerebral hematoma following its removal. The severe unilateral ischemia undoubtedly arises from the mass effect of the overlying hematoma, but the effect is dramatically worsened by accompanying hypoxia or hypotension which is present in about half the patients who develop this particularly severe postoperative complication. Even if ICP is normal shortly after the initial operative procedure, intracranial hypertension occurs in virtually all of these patients and may be uncontrollable and fatal in a high percentage.[7]

Only a small percentage of patients with intracranial hematomas develop delayed traumatic ICHs not seen on the initial computed tomographic (CT) scan, some after previous surgery for extracerebral hematomas and sometimes more than a day after injury.[8] ICP monitoring and recognition of intracranial hypertension can lead to earlier repeat CT scanning, clot identification, and removal than relying only on the neurologic examination,[9] although earlier removal has an uncertain effect on outcome.[10]

Numerous reports suggest a beneficial effect of ICP monitoring and treatment of intracranial hypertension although there are no controlled trials of this technology. In a group of patients with Glasgow coma scores (GCS)[11] of 3, 4, or 5, the mortality rate was 39 percent when ICP was monitored and 67 percent when it was not; the patients were not randomly allocated into the two groups.[12] In another series using patients evaluated in sequential time periods with slightly different treatment protocols, the mortality rate fell from 46 percent to 33 percent when ICP was rigorously controlled below 15 mmHg.[2] There is pathologic evidence of intracranial hypertension as measured by medial temporal lobe necrosis, secondary brain stem damage, or cerebral ischemic changes in as many as 75 percent of patients who die after head injury.[13] These and other reports have convinced most neurosurgeons that ICP monitoring is appropriate in patients with traumatic coma.

Elevated ICP clearly correlates with a poor outcome in head injured patients. In one series of patients with severe head injury, 74 percent whose ICP remained below 20 mmHg had a satisfactory outcome, while only 55 percent of patients who required therapy to control ICP to this level had a similar outcome; if ICP could not be controlled, 92 percent of patients died and only 3 percent had satisfactory outcomes.[14] In another series, the number of patients who died or remained institutionalized more than doubled when ICP was higher than 15 mmHg (57 versus 23 percent) than when it remained below that level.[15] In addition to its effects on survival, intracranial hypertension affects brain function in survivors. Neuropsychologic assessment done 1 year after severe head injury revealed that hyperemia during the acute phase correlated better with poor intellectual and memory function than did low flow states, and that patients with intracranial hypertension had more memory deficits than did those patients with normal ICP.[16]

SUBARACHNOID HEMORRHAGE

Optimal intensive care of patients with SAH following rupture of an intracranial aneurysm or arteriovenous malformation is complex and involves a variety of issues including control of blood pressure, circulating blood volume, and ICP. Intracranial hypertension is common after SAH, particularly in poorer grade patients. ICP typically is higher in patients with poor clinical grade or thick subarachnoid clots than in better grade patients, and patients who had persistent elevation of ICP have significantly worse outcomes than those patients with normal ICP, probably reflecting some degree of ischemia or infarction with brain swelling in the poorer grade patient.[4] Even when good grade patients are included, elevated ICP is present during surgery in most patients independent of preoperative neurologic grade or the quantity of subarachnoid or intraventricular hemorrhage. Following surgery, intracranial hypertension is usually not a problem although brain swelling can occur in a few patients. Hydrocephalus, requiring either ventricular drainage transiently for 5 to 10 days or permanent cerebrospinal fluid (CSF) shunting, can occur following SAH; ICP monitoring by ventriculostomy can facilitate identifying these patients fairly early in their course and allow CSF drainage to control elevated ICP.[17]

Following SAH, high pressure or low pressure hydrocephalus may develop. Blood can obstruct outflow of CSF at the pacchionian granulations and cause communicating hydrocephalus; blood in the ventricular system can occlude the aqueduct of Sylvius and cause obstructive hydrocephalus. Both forms of obstruction can cause intracranial hypertension which may add to the cerebral ischemia often caused by vasospasm which can accompany SAH.

BRAIN TUMORS

Intracranial hypertension can cause the presenting complaints of patients with brain tumors, including headaches, nausea, vomiting, lethargy, and memory changes. Such symptoms lead to radiologic studies and the diagnosis of the tumor; ICP monitoring rarely finds a use at this stage of care. When CT scans show large amounts of peritumoral edema, ICP has a substantial risk of being elevated at the time of craniotomy. In such patients, ICP monitoring might be started before surgery to facilitate control of intracranial hypertension at the time of surgical anesthesia.[18] ICP monitoring can have an important role in following patients after surgery for tumor removal. In one large series in which ICP was monitored postoperatively in over 500 brain tumor patients, 18 percent of patients with supratentorial tumors and 13 percent of those with infratentorial tumors had intracranial hypertension following surgery. Factors associated with the highest risk of postoperative ICP elevation were glioblastoma resection, tumor reoperation, and prolonged operations. In some instances, ICP elevation preceded neurologic deterioration and allowed quicker realization of a complication; in others, deterioration and ICP elevation occurred simultaneously. In only a minority of patients did ICP not rise until after neurologic worsening. The elevated ICP was treated by medical means predominantly; a few patients required reoperation for tumor bed hemorrhage or brain necrosis when nonoperative management was not effective in restoring normal ICP.[19]

HEPATIC FAILURE

Brain swelling has been recognized as a major cause of death and disability with liver necrosis for several decades,[20] and ICP monitoring has been used in the care of patients with hepatic disease and neurologic dysfunction for longer than 10 years.[21] Hepatic failure can arise from a number of factors including drug intoxication, Reye's syndrome, and congenital or infectious abnormalities of the liver. Reye's syndrome is a reversible metabolic encephalopathy and hepatopathy which causes mitochondrial dysfunction although the actual metabolic aberration is unknown. Glial and neuronal function are disrupted, possibly by direct toxic effects or by altered transmitter metabolism and signal transduction. Increased vascular permeability from circulating toxins may contribute to the cerebral swelling seen.[22] Intracranial hypertension often accompanies severe liver failure; its cause is unclear, but its treatment has improved outcome in patients with liver disease. In some instances, liver function recovers or a liver transplantation is successful, but neurologic recovery is less than satisfactory, probably due in part to brain injury from cerebral ischemia during intracranial hypertension and reduced CPP.[3] Recognition of raised ICP as a treatable complication of liver disease, particularly fulminant hepatic failure, and management of intracranial hypertension has improved outcome from these previously poorly treated entities and is a critical tool in the care of patients with reversible failure or irreversible failure requiring liver transplantation.[3,23]

Monitoring Techniques

A variety of monitoring techniques have been used over the past 30 years. Lundberg first used a ventriculostomy coupled to a fluid-filled manometer.[5] This system was cumbersome and ran considerable risk of infection. As electronic transducers became available, closed monitoring systems came into use. Although a few implantable transducers have been used experimentally, they are not in regular clinical use today. The two most common ICP monitoring systems now are fluid-filled catheters or rigid "bolts"[24] attached to an electromechanical transducer or a fiberoptic system that detects deflection of a sensing mirror to measure ICP.[25] The former is generally less expensive but can be prone to blockage and may require more practice to keep functioning optimally; the latter may provide more accurate data for longer periods of time without the need for intervention by doctors or nurses. The fluid-filled systems may be best in hospitals where ICP monitoring is done often, frequently in a number of patients at one time; in such settings, medical personnel become familiar with the system and can recognize and correct problems as they arise. The fiberoptic systems may be better in facilities where fewer patients who require ICP monitoring are treated.

We currently use either subdural or intraventricular catheters for monitoring ICP which we either place in the operating room at the time of surgery or at the bedside in the ICU (Fig. 34-1). We prefer an intraventricular position so that CSF can be drained when necessary to lower ICP. This can be done through a craniotomy opening in the operating room or by twist-drill ventriculostomy in the operating room or ICU when we feel the ventricles are sufficiently large to be entered. When the ventricles are compressed by brain swelling, we prefer a subdural catheter which can only be placed in the operating room; a twist-drill hole is perpendicular to the skull and brain and precludes catheter insertion parallel to the inner table of the skull over the brain surface. Placement of an ICP device requires meticulous sterile technique; if any part of the system is contaminated during insertion or attachment, it must be discarded and replaced. Intracranial infection is a devastating complication when added to the brain dysfunction for which monitoring is required. We feel that ICP monitors should be

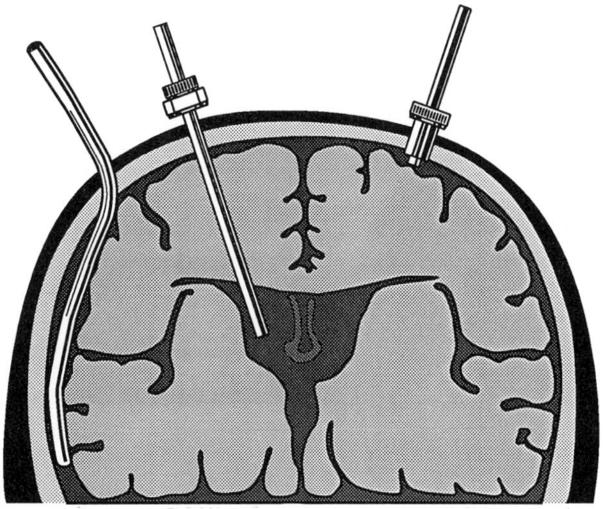

FIGURE 34-1 Schematic drawing of a sagittal section of the brain showing (left to right) the placement of a subdural flexible catheter, an intraventricular catheter, and a rigid subarachnoid "bolt."

placed by neurosurgeons since they are most familiar with manipulating brain tissue and are least likely to induce brain hemorrhage, a risk which is always present and which can be fatal. Epidural catheters must be placed through a burr hole in the operating room and are used less frequently than subdural or intraventricular monitors.

We attach the ICP catheter to pressure transducers connected to monitors which provide continuous digital and waveform displays of ICP as well as arterial, central venous, or pulmonary vascular pressures as needed either in the operating room or ICU. The data can be sampled by a central ICU computer so that these and other parameters can be analyzed over a few hours or days. Usually a good pressure tracing is easily recognized, having a regular pulse pressure of 3 to 7 mmHg which can be greater at elevated ICP. The ICP base line gently drifts up and down with respiratory or ventilatory excursions as intrathoracic pressure changes with breathing and slightly alters the intracranial venous pressure and ICP. A "flat" ICP tracing cannot be interpreted; a grave error in ICP monitoring is accepting a meaningless digital readout number as the actual ICP when the tracing clearly does not reflect a valid waveform. A flat tracing usually is due to blockage by blood or brain occluding the catheter tip or the catheter being kinked along its course. After the extracranial portion of the monitor is inspected for proper placement, it may be necessary to inject a small amount (use 0.25 mL initially) of an irrigating solution to clear the catheter tip; a larger amount, even only 1 mL, can markedly increase ICP when the brain is tight. It is helpful to turn the system stopcock from the injection position back to the monitoring position *while the irrigant is being injected;* if the stopcock is turned after the injection is completed, brain under pressure may immediately occlude the catheter tip when the injection pressure is stopped. Even if a catheter reoccludes and produces a flat waveform, a valid estimate of the ICP usually can be made. After a small amount of irrigant is injected, the ICP will be briefly elevated and have large pulse pressures but drift asymptotically toward the true ICP before becoming a flat line again.

The ICP catheter and transducer are filled with an antibiotic solution containing gentamicin, 1 mg/mL, which is stable in solution for 4 to 6 days and has wide antibacterial activity. It is important to maintain a closed system as much as possible; this requires tight connections throughout the monitoring system. It is imperative that no CSF leak around the catheter; any such leakage greatly increases the risk of infection. If leakage is noted, a new purse string suture must be placed around the catheter's exit from the scalp. If the monitoring device is sufficiently flexible, it should be brought out through a stab wound a short distance from the incision made to insert it to further reduce infection risk. Our intracranial infection rate among a variety of open or penetrating brain injuries is <2 percent so that the infection rate attributable to ICP monitoring is extremely low. Infection rates vary from 0.7 to 6.3 percent in other series using different devices.[26,27] In 378 patients, several different fluid-filled systems for monitoring ICP were compared regarding their propensity to become blocked or infected. The rigid Richmond bolt[24] became occluded 16 percent of the time; subdural or intraventricular catheters became blocked only 3 percent of the time, but the intraventricular catheters were associated with complications of infection or intracerebral hemorrhage and led the authors to recommend the subdural catheter as the best of the methods.[28] However, intraventricular catheters allow withdrawal of CSF as one sometimes critical method of ICP control. Some prefer to measure the change in ICP produced by withdrawal of a measured volume (ΔV) of CSF to determine the intracranial compliance ($\Delta V/\Delta ICP$); we have not found this additional measurement to provide a sufficient increment in useful data to warrant the time and risk.

Intracranial Hypertension in Specific Disorders

HEAD INJURY

When head injured patients are arousable and can obey commands, we follow them with serial neurologic examinations. However, deterioration is difficult to detect in comatose patients (GCS 8 or less), and we monitor ICP to warn us of a worsening brain status and allow us to take new diagnostic or therapeutic measures. In a few patients (<5 percent of patients in traumatic coma), the clinical examination suggests that the patient might emerge from coma in a few hours and ICP monitoring is not established at the outset of care. Such patients do not open their eyes or speak, but have an intact brain stem examination and localize a painful stimulus so that any deterioration usually can be determined from the examination. If such a patient does not regain consciousness as anticipated, we usually place an ICP catheter within a few hours of admission.

CT scanning may be normal in patients after severe head injury, possibly reflecting complicating events such as hypoxia or hypotension soon after injury. Although a normal CT scan does not necessarily confer a good outcome in such patients,[29] it does indicate that the risk of intracranial hypertension is exceedingly low and ICP monitoring may be omitted in such patients. In another series, a normal CT scan also correlated with a normal ICP except in patients who were hypotensive, older than 40 years or had a Glasgow motor score <4; these patients should have ICP monitors placed.[26] An initial CT scan excluding lesions requiring surgical evacuation does not preclude delayed development of an intracerebral[8] or extracerebral hematoma. Thus, if ICP is not being monitored, a new CT scan should be obtained when there is any deterioration in neurologic status. Even if ICP is monitored and remains normal, a current CT scan is mandatory whenever there is unexplained neurologic worsening.

Hyperemia with increased cerebral blood volume (CBV) is common, occurring in perhaps two-thirds of head injured patients with intracranial hypertension. Hyperventilation to cause vasoconstriction and lowered CBV is an appropriate therapy in such patients. However, other patients do not have particularly increased CBV, and lowered Pa_{CO_2}

may cause ischemia in this group. A distinction can be made between those patients in whom hyperventilation does not reduce CBF too severely, and those patients in whom hyperventilation may cause injurious ischemia, by measuring the cerebral metabolic rate for oxygen (CMR_{O_2}) or arteriovenous differences in oxygen content $(a - v)_{O_2}$ or lactate $(a - v)_L$[30] (vide infra).

Traumatic ICH may be small or may not cause a mass effect even when somewhat larger depending on the degree of brain atrophy or ventricular size which can compensate for the hematoma volume. Deciding whether or not to remove an ICH in a given patient can be one of the most difficult decisions in the management of head injured patients. When the ICH is causing relatively little mass effect, one may decide merely to observe the patient. In one series, about 30 percent of 244 patients, all of whom had remained neurologically stable since injury, were selected for ICP monitoring to assist in the decision regarding operative hematoma removal. Two-thirds of those patients with ICP monitoring had intracranial hypertension and underwent operative removal. However, ICP was normal in 30 patients and the hematomas were not evacuated; 5 of these patients suddenly deteriorated or died later than 1 week after injury, indicating that delayed brain injury or secondary insult, perhaps unrecognized, such as hypoxia or hypotension may worsen the patient's status in the setting of an ICH.[31] Somewhat more prolonged ICP monitoring or evaluating CT data, such as the amount of edema around a hematoma or compromise of the basal subarachnoid cisterns, might lead to a more liberal judgment regarding ICH evacuation before neurologic deterioration.

Medical management of intracranial hypertension after head injury is generally successful in the vast majority of patients with severe head injury (8 to 23 percent).[32–34] In one series when standard medical management was unsuccessful, pentobarbital coma was induced but only controlled intracranial hypertension in about 30 percent of such refractory intracranial hypertension. A subtemporal decompression was then performed with a significant further reduction in ICP and a 60 percent survival compared with $<$20 percent survival when subtemporal decompression was not done.[33] This surgical adjunct perhaps deserves consideration for a very small number of head injured patients who are failing all other avenues of ICP control.

SUBARACHNOID HEMORRHAGE

After SAH, high pressure hydrocephalus can occur early and is related to obstruction of the outflow from the cerebral ventricles or by obstruction of CSF drainage into the venous dural sinuses at the pacchionian granulations. The high pressure hydrocephalus is either diagnosed by elevated ICP when a ventriculostomy is in place or with patient deterioration, CT scanning, and the discovery of progressive hydrocephalus. The definitive treatment of high pressure hydrocephalus is drainage of CSF through an existing ventriculostomy or one that is established. If intracranial hypertension remains present when the ventriculostomy is periodically occluded and ICP monitored, CSF shunting may be required. The low pressure hydrocephalus that follows subarachnoid hemorrhage typically develops weeks or months thereafter and is diagnosed by progressive neurologic problems of headache, gait disturbance, and urinary incontinence, and generally requires shunting for its resolution.

LIVER FAILURE

It is not always easy to differentiate between hepatic encephalopathy and brain dysfunction due to raised ICP in patients with significant lethargy or coma who have acute liver disease. ICP monitoring may be required to differentiate between these two clinical states. Since liver failure usually is accompanied by coagulation disorders, it is imperative that a patient's clotting status be treated with appropriate factors such as fresh frozen plasma or platelets before an ICP monitor is placed. Fatal intracranial hemorrhage has occurred at our institution even when parameters were only mildly abnormal; one patient developed a fatal intracerebral hemorrhage after ventriculostomy placement with a platelet count of 49,000. Most of the treatments for intracranial hypertension listed below have been used in patients with liver failure or after liver transplantation, including hyperventilation, osmotherapy, ventricular drainage, diuretics, and barbiturates.[1,3,23]

Intensive Care Management of Intracranial Hypertension

Initial care of the patient with grave neurologic dysfunction involves appropriate diagnosis and management. In acute situations such as head injury or SAH, emergency resuscitation of ventilatory and circulatory disturbances is imperative and usually is done in the emergency department. Proper diagnostic tests will determine the need for urgent operative intervention for intracranial mass lesions or acute hydrocephalus, or more elective procedures such as brain tumor removal. When there is substantial risk of intracranial hypertension as defined above for the various disorders, ICP monitoring is established using careful sterile technique either in the operating room or at the bedside, usually in the ICU.

ICP monitoring is done in relationship to other clinical information, foremost of which is the neurologic examination. When done sequentially, neurologic assessment provides essential information regarding the patient's status. A patient's neurologic deterioration with or without ICP increases will be a critical factor in determining when management should be altered, such as obtaining new radiologic studies or adding new therapy. Sequential neurologic assessments are done by the ICU nursing staff and recorded on a standardized form (Fig. 34-2). Examination features include the GCS (eye opening, verbal and motor responses), pupillary responses to light and limb strength, and the ICP. Any worsening of these features should be discussed with the neurosurgeon and ICU physician.

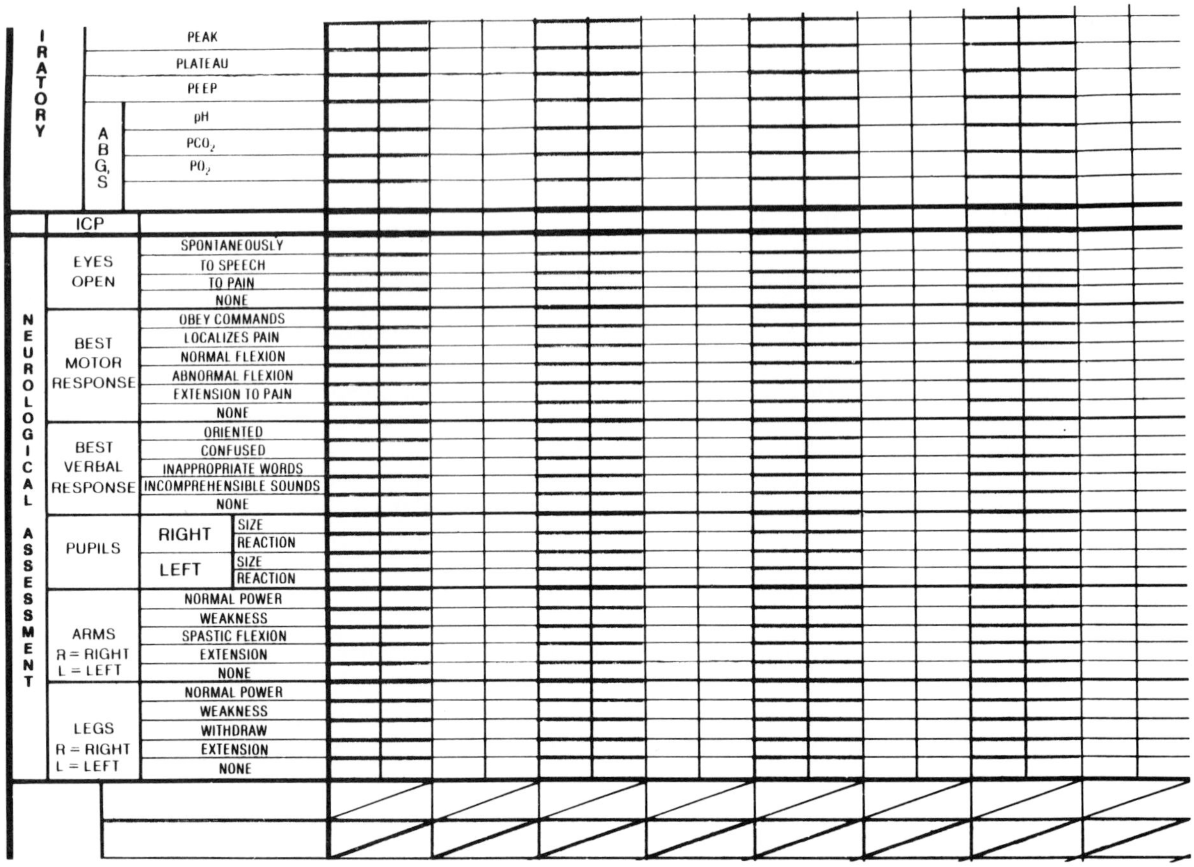

FIGURE 34-2 Portion of an ICU patient flow sheet showing the area for recording the neurologic examination including GCS, pupillary response, and upper and lower extremity motor function.

Drugs such as anticonvulsants, narcotics, sedatives, or paralyzing agents probably will affect the examination as will shock or hypoxia and must be considered. If no cause for patient worsening can be found and corrected, cranial CT scanning should be done to search for possible correctable lesions.

Surgical removal of intracranial masses is the most direct way to lower ICP. Delayed formation of intracranial hematomas (particularly epidural hematomas not seen on initial or "zero time" CT scans or ICHs which can arise in areas of cerebral contusion) can directly raise ICP and their removal immediately lower ICP. Surgical removal of infarcted or severely contused tissue can reduce intracranial volume and lower ICP. Hydrocephalus developing after head injury, SAH, or brain tumor surgery also can immediately increase ICP, but can be rapidly and effectively treated by CSF drainage by ventriculostomy. These measures generally should be tried before other treatment for intracranial hypertension is used.

If no lesions requiring surgical removal are present, medical management must be used to control ICP. While the exact level of injurious ICP has not clearly been determined and undoubtedly varies from patient to patient, aggressive treatment to prevent ICP elevations above 20 mmHg or CPP below 60 mmHg has generally been recommended.[2,32,34–36] Methods to accomplish this are described below, generally in order of safety and simplicity (Table 34-2).

BLOOD PRESSURE CONTROL

Continuous monitoring and management of arterial blood pressure is as important as control of elevated ICP in the severely head injured patient to prevent hypotension or excessive hypertension and maintain an adequate CPP. It is crucial that secondary ischemic brain injury due to systemic hypotension be prevented or rapidly corrected.

TABLE 34-2 Treatments for Intracranial Hypertension

Surgical removal of intracranial masses
Sedation
Paralysis
Ventricular drainage
Controlled hyperventilation
Hyperosmotic therapies
Diuretics
Barbiturate coma
Subtemporal decompression

In the trauma patient, hemorrhagic or hypovolemic shock is not uncommon although in the multiply injured patient there may be additional causes for hypotension, such as hemorrhage, a low cardiac output due to cardiac contusion or cardiac tamponade, or loss of peripheral vascular tone due to an injury of the cervical spinal cord. It is important to consider these additional causes of shock, especially when the blood pressure does not respond to initial volume resuscitation. Arterial pressure is a less accurate measure of shock than are pulse rate, skin perfusion, and urine output, because compensatory mechanisms may allow for the blood pressure to remain relatively stable during hemorrhage until there is an abrupt fall due to profound volume loss.[37]

Patients with clinical manifestations of hypoperfusion should be resuscitated to a systolic pressure of at least 100 mmHg or higher. Excessive volume expansion should be avoided because it may increase cerebral edema or produce pulmonary edema especially if there is an associated pulmonary contusion. When there is uncertainty about a patient's fluid status, a CVP catheter should be placed via the jugular or upper extremity veins for monitoring pressures to assist in fluid management. Fluid repletion with balanced salt (crystalloid) solutions significantly improves cellular and clinical response to shock. There is little difference in the hemodynamic or pulmonary effects of crystalloid solutions versus colloid solutions in the initial resuscitation of trauma victims, as long as each is given to the same hemodynamic end point.[37] A greater absolute volume of crystalloids will be required, given their greater distribution in the interstitial space. An elevated serum glucose level appears to be harmful to the injured and ischemic brain,[38] and we avoid crystalloid solutions containing glucose during resuscitation. During ICU care, we monitor and control serum glucose to levels of 100 to 200 mg/dL. An hematocrit of 32 to 35 percent should be maintained to provide optimal perfusion and oxygen-carrying capacity.[37] In one series where CPP was maintained about 70 to 80 mmHg with volume expansion and catecholamines to elevate mean arterial pressure to 100 to 110, escaped ICP only occurred in 8 percent of patients.[34]

Head injury can adversely alter cerebral autoregulation and systemic hypertension can produce excessive CBF and volume and raise ICP. Patients have increased catechol levels and sympathetic activity with hypertension, tachycardia, increased cardiac output, and low or normal systemic vascular resistance.[39] This hypertension can be managed with β-adrenergic blocking agents such as propranolol or esmolol.

SEDATION AND MUSCLE RELAXATION

A struggling patient will increase intrathoracic pressure and CVP and produce a subsequent rise in intracranial venous volume and ICP. Sedation with intravenous morphine sulfate will prevent or reduce this muscle activity and maintain a more stable ICP. Diazepam will add to the sedative effects of narcotics. Midazolam is a favorite sedating drug used by anesthesiologists during and following surgery, but its effect on the injured brain is uncertain and we prefer not to use it.

If patient struggling is not adequately controlled by sedation, chemoparalysis with vecuronium or pancuronium will further prevent venous pressure increases with their effects on intracranial hypertension. Obviously, this can be done only in mechanically ventilated patients. Temporary chemoparalysis with succinyl choline is more effective for controlling ICP rises during nursing maneuvers such as suctioning, bathing, or turning than is intravenous or intratracheal lidocaine or thiopental.[40]

VENTRICULAR DRAINAGE

When a ventriculostomy is in place, CSF drainage is the simplest method of lowering ICP. This may be the only technique needed for ICP control when excessive CSF is all or part of the cause of intracranial hypertension, such as with hydrocephalus due to aqueductal or ventricular obstruction from intraventricular hemorrhage, SAH, tumors, or cysts. When diffuse brain swelling is present such as with head injury, hepatic failure, or cerebral ischemia, the cerebral ventricles often are small and relatively little CSF can be removed. Even in these situations, if the neurosurgeon can place a ventricular catheter, small amounts of CSF drainage can be used along with other techniques to control or reduce ICP better than if the other techniques are used alone.

CONTROLLED HYPERVENTILATION

Hyperventilation lowers Pa_{CO_2}; the respiratory alkalosis that occurs raises the CSF pH. Decreased pH is a primary and potent cause for cerebral arteriolar vasodilation, so that respiratory alkalosis produces cerebral vasoconstriction[31,41] and a decrease in CBV which causes a decrease in the volume of the brain with an immediate effect of lowering the ICP. Hyperventilation causes progressive cerebral vasoconstriction down to a Pa_{CO_2} of about 22 to 25 mmHg[42] although lower levels are sometimes used. Extremely low levels resulting from excessive hyperventilation can cause cerebral ischemia, which is best determined by calculating the CMR_{O_2}. This calculation is somewhat complex since it requires a knowledge both of CBF and $(a - v)_{O_2}$ [$CMR_{O_2} = CBF \times (a - v)_{O_2}$]. Since CBF is not commonly available in most clinical situations, one nonetheless can rely in part on the $(a - v)_{O_2}$ and $(a - v)_L$.[30] A normal $(a - v)_{O_2}$ is about 3 to 6 mL O_2/100 mL blood; levels below this are consistent with hyperemia for which hyperventilation is appropriate. When the $(a - v)_{O_2}$ is above 6.5, there is greater than normal oxygen extraction by the brain and cerebral ischemia probably is present to some degree; hyperventilation might accentuate that ischemia. When the $(a - v)_{O_2}$ is abnormally high, other measures for controlling ICP should be used, such as hyperosmolar therapy and ventricular drainage.

The $(a - v)_{O_2}$ and $(a - v)_L$ are derived by sampling arterial blood (by a radial artery or other arterial monitoring line) and jugular venous blood, calculating their contents of oxygen or lactate, and deriving the $(a - v)_{O_2}$ or $(a - v)_L$. Jugular blood is obtained from a catheter inserted into the jugular vein (found just lateral to the carotid artery) and directed superiorly from the puncture site. A $3\frac{1}{2}$-inch 25 gauge spinal needle can be passed through the catheter insertion needle to initially find the jugular vein; even if the carotid artery is punctured with the small gauge needle, there is no likely harm and gentle finger pressure over the artery after the needle is removed will prevent a hematoma. After venous blood is obtained from the spinal needle, the larger insertion needle is passed over the spinal needle guide into the vein. The guide needle is removed and the catheter inserted, tilting the insertion needle superiorly toward the skull base. A second method is to place the catheter insertion needle immediately parallel to a smaller needle placed into the jugular vein. The catheter is gently inserted until a mechanical obstruction is palpated (the skull base at the jugular bulb) and the catheter pulled back 5 to 10 mm. A lateral or anterior-posterior cervical spine x-ray will confirm that the catheter tip is at the skull base and has not inadvertently been passed down the jugular vein toward the chest. Venous samples for determining the brain $(a - v)_{O_2}$ or $(a - v)_L$ must be taken from the jugular bulb only; other sample sites distal to the bulb will be contaminated by facial or other neck veins which typically have higher oxygen extraction values than does the proximal jugular vein. Although $(a - v)_{O_2}$ and $(a - v)_L$ determinations offer an excellent adjunct for optimizing control of ICP, they are not yet commonly used, but we believe are likely to become more so in the future.

Prolonged hyperventilation (Pa_{CO_2} maintained at 25 mmHg) experimentally becomes less effective with time so that by the twentieth hour vasoconstriction diminishes back to control vessel diameters; subsequent return to normocapnia results in actual vasodilation and an increase in CBV. During this prolonged period of hyperventilation, arterial and CSF pH also return to normal in animals[41] and human beings.[43] These results suggest that continuous hyperventilation may be ineffective after 20 to 24 h, and later normalization of Pa_{CO_2} may result in vasodilation and rises in ICP.[41] We, therefore, recommend that hyperventilation be used only for acute elevations in ICP while other methods to lower ICP are initiated. When ICP returns to acceptable levels, we return Pa_{CO_2} toward more normal values around 30 to 33 mmHg to maintain arteriolar responsiveness and allow us to use acute hyperventilation again should it be necessary.

Direct injuries to the chest can prevent adequate spontaneous ventilation and will require careful management. Penetrating chest trauma with pneumothorax or hemothorax may require thoracostomy. Blunt trauma such as rib fractures, a flail segment of the chest, or pulmonary contusions may cause pulmonary insufficiency and require positive-pressure ventilation. Even without obvious chest or pulmonary injury, many injured patients will be hypoxic on arrival at the hospital. While increasing the fraction of inspired oxygen (FI_{O_2}) will correct the hypoxemia in many patients, intubation and institution of controlled ventilation with or without positive end-expiratory pressures (PEEP) may be necessary for some patients to be well oxygenated. Mild increases in PEEP usually do not cause significant increases in ICP.

HYPEROSMOTIC THERAPY

We commonly administer mannitol (0.25 to 0.5 g/kg body weight intravenously) to treat intracranial hypertension. Mannitol infusion has several beneficial effects: it reduces brain water where the blood-brain barrier is intact; it increases circulating volume and arterial blood pressure; and it causes hemodilution and reduces blood viscosity.[44] Red blood cell deformability increases and improves blood viscosity independently of hemodilution. It has been reported that mannitol improves intracranial compliance even more than it lowers ICP.[45] Cerebral vasoconstriction follows blood viscosity lowering after mannitol infusion, possibly related to improved red cell oxygen transport, and, if there is intact autoregulation, resulting vasoconstriction.[44,46] Patients with a reduced CPP have a greater effect of mannitol lowering ICP than patients with a high CPP, possibly because mannitol increases arterial pressure and CPP which in turn causes cerebral vasoconstriction. Thus by multiple effects, mannitol infusions can produce cerebral vasoconstriction and a decrease in ICP in addition to osmotic effects on the brain.[47]

Repeated mannitol usage can dehydrate a patient and we do not use it when the serum osmolarity exceeds about 330 mM, as such a rise can cause neural , cardiopulmonary, and renal dysfunction. Excessive fluid loss should be replaced to prevent decreased cardiac output which can be measured with a pulmonary artery catheter. CVP probably should be maintained at 2 to 5 mmHg or pulmonary wedge pressure at about 5 to 10 mmHg in patients needing mannitol.

DIURETICS

Furosemide can be used to reduce intracranial hypertension and probably works by diuresis, increasing intravascular oncotic pressure, removing brain water, and possibly reducing CSF production.[48] The combination of mannitol and furosemide may be more effective in lowering ICP than either drug alone. This synergistic effect is not from an altered renal excretion of mannitol but may help sustain the elevated serum osmolarity induced by mannitol, or sustain the osmotic gradient across the blood-brain barrier induced by mannitol.[48] However, some caution is advised since the combined use of mannitol and furosemide can cause rapid dehydration, hypotension, and a reduced CPP with the risk of brain ischemia.

BARBITURATE COMA

Iatrogenic barbiturate coma has been induced to lower ICP when other measures have failed.[32,49–51] Barbiturates lower cerebral metabolism and blood flow in addition to lowering

ICP.[49] However, systemic hypotension is common when these agents are used so that arterial and pulmonary artery catheters are advised for monitoring circulating fluid status; pressor agents such as dopamine or norepinepherine may be required to support blood pressure and to maintain an adequate cardiac output.[50,51]

Although barbiturates are effective in lowering ICP, their effect in improving outcome is uncertain.[32,50,51] In one randomized and controlled prospective trial of barbiturate coma in severe head injury, there was no improvement in survival and no difference in the incidence or duration of elevated ICP.[51] In another large series of patients with severe head injury, only about 12 percent had intracranial hypertension uncontrolled by standard medical and surgical support. In a controlled series evaluating this subgroup of patients with refractory intracranial hypertension, half were given large doses of pentobarbital; the other half were managed similarly but without the use of barbiturates. ICP control was successful more than twice as often in patients receiving barbiturates, and this advantage was increased to a fourfold improvement in the ability to control intracranial hypertension when patients were excluded who had been hypotensive at some point during their earlier treatment. Patients who had been hypotensive and received barbiturates had worse outcomes than the other groups, suggesting that barbiturates should be avoided when hypotension has complicated the patient's early management. Because of the relatively small number of patients with "escaped ICP" available for study entry and crossover of patients between the various treatment groups, no definite conclusion could be reached regarding the possible benefit of barbiturates on outcome.[32] One other prospective controlled trial of barbiturates for "escaped ICP" reported that outcome was worse and that ICP was no better controlled with barbiturates than with mannitol.[50]

When ICP exceeds 25 mmHg for 15 min and cannot be lowered by the various methods described, we give pentobarbital, 10 mg/kg slowly, followed by 1.5 mg/kg/h to achieve encephalographic burst-suppression. Pentobarbital levels are determined periodically and the administered dose adjusted to give a serum level of about 3 mg/dL. This barbiturate level generally will prevent any response to pain and may suppress brain stem reflexes; thus, this therapy should only be given when ICP is being monitored. Therapy can be stopped when ICP has been controlled for 2 to 3 days or when ICP cannot be controlled and rises to the level of arterial pressure (CPP = 0, consistent with brain death). Brain death can be determined even when there are excessive barbiturates levels by determining CBF by bedside isotope studies of cerebral perfusion.

References

1. Brajtbord D, Parks RI, Ramsay MA, et al: Management of acute elevation of intracranial pressure during hepatic transplantation. Anesthesiology 70:139, 1989.
2. Saul TG, Ducker TB: Effect of intracranial pressure monitoring and aggressive treatment on mortality in severe head injury. J Neurosurg 56:498, 1982.
3. Potter D, Peachey T, Eason J, et al: Intracranial pressure monitoring during orthotopic liver transplantation for acute liver failure. Transplant Proc 21:3528, 1989.
4. Takeuchi S, Koike T, Sasaki O, et al: Intracranial extradural pressure monitoring after direct operation on ruptured cerebral aneurysms. Neurosurgery 24:878, 1989.
5. Lundberg N: Continuous recording and control of ventricular fluid pressure in neurosurgical practice. Acta Psychiatr Neurol Scand 36(suppl 149):1, 1960.
6. Shigemori M, Nakashima H, Moriyama T, et al: Noninvasive study of critical thresholds of intracranial pressure and cerebral perfusion pressure for cerebral circulation and brain function. Neurol Res 11:165, 1989.
7. Lobato RD, Sarabia R, Cordobes F, et al: Posttraumatic cerebral hemispheric swelling. Analysis of 55 cases studied with computerized tomography. J Neurosurg 68:417, 1988.
8. Soloniuk D, Pitts LH, Lovely M, Bartkowski H. Traumatic intracerebral hematomas. Timing of appearance and indications for operative removal. J Trauma 26:787, 1986.
9. Bullock R, Golek J, Blake G: Traumatic intracerebral hematoma—which patients should undergo surgical evacuation? CT scan features and ICP monitoring as a basis for decision making. Surg Neurol 32:181, 1989.
10. Gentleman D, Nath F, Macpherson P: Diagnosis and management of delayed traumatic intracerebral haematomas. Br J Neurosurg 3:367, 1989.
11. Teasdale G, Jennett B: Assessment of coma and impaired consciousness. Lancet 2:81, 1974.
12. Bowers SA, Marshall LF: Outcome in 200 consecutive cases of severe head injury treated in San Diego County: A prospective analysis. Neurosurgery 6:237, 1980.
13. Graham DI, Lawrence AE, Adams JH, et al: Brain damage in nonmissile head injury secondary to high intracranial pressure. Neuropathol Appl Neurobiol 13:209, 1987.
14. Miller JD, Butterworth JF, et al: Further experience in the management of severe head injury. J Neurosurg 54:289, 1981.
15. Marshall LF, Smith RW, Rauscher LA, Shapiro HM: The outcome with aggressive treatment in severe head injuries. Part II. J Neurosurg 50:20, 1979.
16. Uzzell BP, Obrist WD, Dolinskas CA, Langfitt TW: Relationship of acute CBF and ICP findings to neuropsychological outcome in severe head injury. Neurosurg 65:630, 1986.
17. Auer LM, Mokry M: Disturbed cerebrospinal fluid circulation after subarachnoid hemorrhage and acute aneurysm surgery. Neurosurgery 26:804, 1990.
18. Bedford RF, Morris L, Jane JA: Intracranial hypertension during surgery for supratentorial tumor: Correlation with preoperative computed tomography scans. Anesth Analg 61:430, 1982.
19. Constantini S, Cotev S, Rappaport ZH, et al: Intracranial pressure monitoring after elective intracranial surgery. A retrospective study of 514 consecutive patients. J Neurosurg 69:540, 1988.
20. Ware AJ, D'Agostino AN, Combes B: Cerebral edema: A major complication of massive hepatic necrosis. Gastroenterology 61:877, 1971.
21. Hanid MA, Davies M, Mellon PJ, et al: Clinical monitoring of intracranial pressure in fulminant hepatic necrosis. Gut 21:866, 1980.
22. Livingstone AS, Potvin M, Gorewsky CA, et al: Changes in the blood-brain barrier in hepatic coma after hepatectomy in the rat. Gastroenterology 73:697, 1977.
23. LeRoux PD, Elliott JP, Perkins JD, Will HR: Intracranial pres-

sure monitoring in fulminant hepatic failure and liver transplantation. Lancet 335:1291, 1990.
24. Vries JK, Becker DP, Young HF: A subarachnoid screw for monitoring intracranial pressure. Technical note. J Neurosurg 39:416, 1973.
25. Ostrup RC, Luerssen, TG, Marshall LF, Zornow MH: Continuous monitoring of intracranial pressure with a miniaturized fiberoptic device. J Neurosurg 67:206, 1987.
26. Narayan RK, Kishore PRS, Becker DP, et al: Intracranial pressure: To monitor or not to monitor? Review of our experience with severe head injury. J Neurosurg 56:650, 1982.
27. Rosner MJ, Becker DP: ICP monitoring: Complications and associated factors. Clin Neurosurg 23:494, 1976.
28. North B, Reilly P: Comparison among three methods of intracranial pressure recording. Neurosurgery 18:730, 1986.
29. Lobato RD, Sarabia R, Rivas JJ, et al: Normal computerized tomography scans in severe head injury. Prognostic and clinical management implications. J Neurosurg 65:784, 1986.
30. Robertson CS, Narayan RK, Gokaslan ZL, et al: Cerebral arteriovenous oxygen difference as an estimate of cerebral blood flow in comatose patients. J Neurosurg 70:222, 1989.
31. Lassen NA: Brain extracellular pH: The main factor controlling cerebral blood flow. Scan J Clin Lab Invest 22:247, 1968.
32. Eisenberg HM, Frankowski RF, Contant CF, et al: High-dose barbiturate control of elevated intracranial pressure in patients with severe head injury. J Neurosurg 69:15, 1988.
33. Gower DJ, Lee KS, McWhorter JM: Role of subtemporal decompression in severe closed head injury. Neurosurgery 23:417, 1988.
34. Rosner MJ, Daughton S: Cerebral perfusion pressure management in head injury. J Trauma 30:933, 1990.
35. Bruce DA, Alavi A, Bilanuik L, et al: Diffuse cerebral swelling following head injuries in children: The syndrome of "malignant brain edema." J Neurosurg 54:170, 1981.
36. Tsutsumi H, Ide K, Mizutani T, et al: The relationship between intracranial pressure, cerebral perfusion pressure and outcome in head-injured patient: The critical level of cerebral perfusion pressure, in Miller JD, Teasdale GM, Rowan JO, et al (eds): *ICP VI*. Berlin, Springer-Verlag, 1985, pp 661–666.
37. Lewis FR: Initial assessment and resuscitation. Emerg Med Clin North Am 2:733, 1984.
38. Rehncrona S, Rosen I, Siesjo B: Brain lactic acidosis and ischemic cell damage: 1: Biochemistry and neurophysiology. J Cereb Blood Flow Metab 1:297, 1981.
39. Robertson CS, Clifton JL, Taylor AA, Grossman RG: Treatment of hypertension associated with head injury. J Neurosurg 59:455, 1983.
40. White PF, Schlobohm RM, Pitts LH, Lindauer JM: A randomized study of drugs for preventing increases in intracranial pressure during endotracheal suctioning. Anesthesiology 57:242, 1982.
41. Muizelaar JP, van der Poel HG, Li Z, et al: Pial ateriolar vessel diameter and CO_2 reactivity during prolonged hyperventilation in the rabbit. J Neurosurg 69:923, 1988.
42. Paul RL, Polanco O, Turney SZ, et al: Intracranial pressure responses to alterations in arterial carbon dioxide pressure in patients with head injuries. J Neurosurg 36:714, 1972.
43. Christensen MS: Acid-base changes in cerebrospinal fluid and blood, and blood volume changes following prolonged hyperventilation in man. Br J Anaesth 46:348, 1974.
44. Muizelaar JP, Wei EP, Kontos HA, Becker DP: Mannitol causes compensatory cerebral vasoconstriction and vasodilatation in response to blood viscosity changes. J Neurosurg 59:822, 1983.
45. Leech PJ, Miller JD: Intracranial volume-pressure relationships during experimental brain compression in primates. Part 3: The effect of mannitol and hypocapnia. J Neurol Neurosurg Psychiatry 37:1105, 1974.
46. Muizelaar JP, Lutz HA, Becker DP: Effect of mannitol on ICP and CBF and correlation with pressure autoregulation in severely head-injured patients. J Neurosurg 61:700, 1984.
47. Rosner MJ, Coley I: Cerebral perfusion pressure: A hemodynamic mechanism of mannitol and the postmannitol hemogram. Neurosurgery 21:147, 1987.
48. Roberts PA, Pollay M, Engles C, et al: Effect on intracranial pressure of furosemide combined with varying doses and administration of mannitol. J Neurosurg 66:440, 1987.
49. Nordstrom CH, Messeter K, Sundbarg G, et al: Cerebral blood flow, vasoreactivity and oxygen consumption during barbiturate therapy in severe traumatic brain lesions. J Neurosurg 68:424, 1988.
50. Schwartz ML, Tator CH, Rowed DW, et al: The University of Toronto Head Injury Treatment Study: A prospective, randomized comparison of pentobarbital and mannitol. Can J Neurol Sci 11:434, 1984.
51. Ward JD, Becker DP, Miller JD, et al: Failure of prophylactic barbiturate coma in the treatment of severe head injury. J Neurosurg 62:383, 1985.

Chapter 35

BLOOD PRODUCTS AND PLASMAPHERESIS

BEVERLY W. BARON
JOSEPH M. BARON

General Indications for Transfusion

With increased awareness of infectious diseases that can be transmitted by blood transfusion—especially acquired immunodeficiency syndrome (AIDS) and hepatitis, but also malaria, Epstein-Barr virus (EBV), cytomegalovirus (CMV), Chagas' disease, and others—criteria for transfusion have become more stringent, and the indications are more strictly monitored by hospital accrediting agencies. Hospital transfusion committees, in conjunction with the medical staff, establish the criteria and evaluate the circumstances leading to apparent inappropriate transfusions. In general, there is no justification for transfusing anemic patients with adequate cardiovascular compensation whose anemia will respond to specific medical therapy (e.g., iron, folic acid, or vitamin B_{12}). On the other hand, many critically ill patients have severely limited oxygen delivery in the face of increased oxygen demand. Transfusion may improve oxygenation of critical organs or allow adequate oxygenation at lower cardiac outputs.

In recent years, use of whole blood largely has been replaced by component therapy. This practice advocates transfusion of only those blood components needed to fulfill specific needs.

WHOLE BLOOD

Hemorrhagic shock is the usual indication for requests for whole blood. However, in the absence of coagulation factor abnormalities, aggressive therapy with red blood cells and crystalloid solutions usually is sufficient to stabilize the patient.

RED BLOOD CELLS

Red blood cells are given to improve the oxygen-carrying capacity of blood. Standard indications for red blood cell transfusions include: major trauma with bleeding; shock secondary to acute blood loss [when coagulation factors are abnormal, fresh frozen plasma (FFP) may be added]; intraoperative blood loss >750 mL or 15 percent of total blood volume; and anemia. A "safe" level for hemoglobin depends on the clinical circumstances. This issue is discussed more fully in Chap. 145.

PLATELETS

Template bleeding time usually is normal if platelet count is at least 100,000/mm^3, but as the count approaches 50,000, bleeding time becomes twice normal. Below this level, an inverse relationship exists between bleeding time and platelet count. At platelet counts ≤20,000/mm^3, bleeding time is >25 to 30 min, and many patients will continue to bleed from the small incision made for the test.

Thrombocytopenia <20,000/mm^3 usually is the typical indication for prophylactic platelet transfusion, but some authorities believe a safe platelet threshold may be even lower in a stable patient who has no other significant risk factors for bleeding.[1,2] Platelet transfusions may be warranted to achieve higher platelet levels in patients who have significant active bleeding in the face of thrombocytopenia or thrombocytopathy (e.g., in uremia). Since adequate hemostasis generally can be achieved when the platelet count reaches 70,000 to 100,000/mm^3 1 h after transfusion, it is usually not necessary to raise the platelet count to normal levels for most surgical procedures. Patients who are on cardiopulmonary bypass tend to have a moderate fall in platelet count, and their platelets may show transient functional abnormalities; bleeding time may help assess the need for platelet transfusion better than the platelet count, although both parameters are needed in bypass patients who do not cease to bleed after protamine neutralization.[3]

Platelet transfusions usually are not effective in patients with rapid platelet destruction, e.g., idiopathic thrombocytopenic purpura (ITP), or in drug-related thrombocytopenia, and they are contraindicated in patients with thrombotic thrombocytopenic purpura (TTP) or hemolytic uremic syndrome (HUS), unless there is life-threatening bleeding. Drug-related thrombocytopenia is most often caused by cardiac drugs (e.g., quinidine), quinine, heparin, penicillins, cephalosporins, hydrochlorothiazide, and sedatives.[4–7] Platelet transfusions may not be effective in patients with hypersplenism, fever, sepsis, disseminated intravascular coagulation (DIC), platelet antibodies, or alloimmunization to major histocompatibility (HLA) antigens.

GRANULOCYTES

Granulocyte transfusions may be given to febrile neutropenic patients (<500 neutrophils/μL) with bacterial or fungal infections unresponsive to antibiotic therapy and a good chance of bone marrow recovery. Since bone marrow neutrophil reserve and granulocyte function in neonates may be decreased by severe stress or infection,[8–11] granulocyte transfusion should be considered for septic, granulocytopenic neonates with decreased bone marrow reserve.

PLASMA

Infusion of plasma is indicated for the bleeding or presurgical patient with coagulation factor deficiency, for the treatment of TTP and HUS, for rapid reversal of vitamin K deficiency or warfarin overdose, and for deficiencies of substances, such as antithrombin III, which are found in plasma. Factor concentrates may be indicated for certain factor deficiencies (e.g., factor VIII).

Blood Components

WHOLE BLOOD

Whole blood stored for more than 24 h contains few viable platelets or granulocytes; factors V and VIII are decreased, but stable clotting factors are maintained.

When a unit of whole blood is transfused to an average-sized adult, hemoglobin will increase by 1 g/dL and hematocrit by 3 percent in the absence of bleeding. Red blood cells and crystalloid should be used rather than whole blood for patients who do not need replacement of coagulation factors.

RED BLOOD CELLS

Removal of 200 to 250 mL of plasma from whole blood results in "packed" red cells. A unit of packed red cells will increase the hematocrit and hemoglobin of a normal-sized adult by the same amount as will one unit of whole blood.

Red cells may be stored frozen after addition of glycerol, thawed at 37°C, washed to remove the glycerol, maintained at 1 to 6°C, and transfused within 24 h. Freezing of red cells may be indicated for rare or autologous blood units. Because of the multiple washes involved in deglycerolization, such red cells contain minimal quantities of plasma, white cells, and platelets. However, the time and expense involved in the preparation precludes the routine use of this product.

PLATELETS

Single-donor platelet packs are obtained from whole blood units and contain at least 5.5×10^{10} platelets/mm^3 in approximately 50 mL plasma. Individual platelet packs may be pooled into a single bag to facilitate administration and then must be transfused within 6 h. For patients who cannot tolerate the plasma volume, who have adverse reactions to plasma, or who are to receive ABO-incompatible platelet products, it may be desirable to "concentrate" the platelets by removing the plasma; they then must be transfused within 6 h.

Although platelets stored at room temperature may require as much as 24 h following transfusion to acquire normal in vivo function,[12] they have an average normal life span of at least 8 days.[13,14] However, platelets stored at 4°C for up to 18 h are said to be more effective hemostatically, and have an average life span of only about 48 h.[15] These observations suggest that platelets stored at room temperature might be most effective for prophylactic transfusions in patients with hypoplastic bone marrows, whereas patients with active bleeding might benefit most from platelets stored at 4°C.[16] Recent data indicate that warming platelets to 37°C prior to transfusion has a beneficial effect on efficacy, resulting in more normal morphology and higher count increments.[17]

Platelet packs contain white and red blood cells, which may sensitize the recipient to leukocyte and red cell antigens. Since red cell contamination is usually <0.5 mL, hemolysis is not a problem even in a recipient with antibodies to antigens present on the donor red cells. If Rh-positive platelets must be given to an Rh-negative woman with childbearing potential, concurrent administration of Rh immune globulin should be considered (although care should be taken when intramuscular injections are given to thrombocytopenic patients). ABO-incompatible plasma in platelet packs may cause a positive direct antiglobulin test and, occasionally, hemolysis. ABO-incompatible platelets may not have optimum survival.

In a normal 70-kg adult, one platelet pack should increase platelet count by 5000 to 10,000/mm^3. Since one-third of the platelets administered are sequestered in the spleen, a useful formula for estimating the expected increase in platelet count (per mm^3) from a platelet pack containing 5.5×10^{10} platelets is:

$$\frac{5.5 \times 10^{10} \times 2/3 \times 10^{-3}}{\text{patient's blood volume (mL/kg)}} \qquad (35\text{-}1)$$

Single-donor plateletpheresis products, which are collected by an apheresis procedure, contain at least 3×10^{11} platelets (the equivalent of about 6 U random donor platelets) suspended in approximately 300 mL plasma and help reduce multiple donor exposure. For patients who are alloimmunized to HLA antigens and therefore often fail to have a significant rise in 10-min[18] or 1-h posttransfusion platelet counts, these products may be HLA-matched. If HLA-matched platelets are not available, alloimmunized patients may show a rise in platelet count if they receive platelets from family members, especially siblings.

Some alloimmunized patients do not respond even to HLA-matched products. If this is the case or if no histocompatible donors are available, management is problematic. Administration of several units of platelet concentrates at short intervals (e.g., 4 U every 4 to 6 h) may be tried; transfusions of multiple units from different donors increase the chance of selection of histocompatible units that may be beneficial. Antibodies against platelet-specific antigens may account for refractoriness in a small percentage of patients,[19] who might benefit from crossmatched platelets.

Another approach is transfusion of autologous platelets collected during clinical remission and stored frozen. Problems with this practice have included: uncertainty of the length of clinical remission, which may be too short to collect adequate numbers of platelets; inability to collect enough platelets because of low blood counts; and failure of frozen, thawed platelets to provide good in vivo recoveries. Yet another possible way to circumvent some of these difficulties is to freeze platelets from donors for future use for histocompatible, alloimmunized patients.

LEUKOCYTE-POOR AND WASHED BLOOD PRODUCTS

Patients who receive transfusions and pregnant women may become alloimmunized to antigens present on the cell membranes of leukocytes or platelets, or they may develop allergies to plasma substances. Such individuals then may experience febrile, allergic, or anaphylactic reactions or noncardiogenic pulmonary edema when transfused with blood products containing white cells or plasma.

Most of the white cells can be removed from blood products by centrifugation, saline washing, or use of microaggregate blood filters. Leukocyte-poor products are indicated for patients who have had severe or recurrent (two or more) nonhemolytic febrile reactions associated with transfusion. With the introduction of improved filters for removal of white blood cells, the possibility of routine use of leukocyte-poor blood products to reduce the incidence of alloimmunization in certain patient groups, e.g., those who will require long-term platelet transfusions, is under investigation.[20–22] For patients with severe or repeated allergic or anaphylactic reactions, plasma may be removed from blood products by washing.

The disadvantages of saline washing include use of an open system, thus subjecting the product to risk of bacterial contamination and shorter shelf life (24 h for red cells at refrigerator temperature, 6 h for platelets at room temperature), and partial loss of the product. These drawbacks may be circumvented with the use of microaggregate filters for removal of white blood cells (however, filters cannot be used to remove plasma).

GRANULOCYTES

Granulocyte concentrates prepared by leukapheresis should have at least 1×10^{10} granulocytes and usually also contain hydroxyethyl starch (HES, a sedimenting agent), platelets, lymphocytes, and red cells in 200 to 300 mL plasma. Granulocytes are stored at room temperature (20 to 24°C) and must be transfused within 24 h, but they are most beneficial if used as soon as possible.

Side effects during infusion are common and include chills, fever, and allergic reactions. It may be advisable to administer nonaspirin antipyretics, diphenhydramine, meperidine, and steroids before granulocytes are given. Severe pulmonary insufficiency has been reported, and some authors believe the risk of this complication increases when amphotericin B and granulocyte concentrates are given concurrently.[23] As much time as possible should elapse between these therapies, and amphotericin should be given more slowly than usual, with careful observation of the patient.

Granulocytapheresis products should be ABO compatible with the recipient because of the large numbers of red cells they contain. CMV-negative recipients should receive granulocytes from CMV-negative donors, if possible. Some authorities believe that alloimmunized patients should not receive granulocytes from random donors; alloimmunization can be suspected when reactions occur in association with platelet transfusions in a recipient who then has poor posttransfusion platelet increments. It has been recommended that platelet donors, preferably family members, who are closely HLA-matched with the recipient also serve as granulocyte donors.[24] However, patients who are to undergo bone marrow transplantation preferably should not receive granulocyte transfusions from the marrow donor or the donor's close relatives prior to transplantation because of the possibility of alloimmunization with subsequent rejection of the graft.

Granulocyte transfusions should be administered slowly to minimize the pulmonary side effects. They should not be transfused through microaggregate filters, which will remove the white cells. Since granulocytes leave the circulation rapidly, efficacy must be monitored by clinical improvement rather than by an increase in granulocyte count.

PLASMA PRODUCTS

Fresh frozen plasma (FFP, 200 to 250 mL) is separated from freshly drawn whole blood and then frozen. Once thawed, it should be stored at 1 to 6°C and used within 24 h to obtain maximal levels of labile coagulation factors (V and VIII). One milliliter supplies approximately one unit of coagulation factor activity.

It is not appropriate to administer FFP for volume expansion, because crystalloid or colloid solutions are safer and as effective. Patients with severe coagulopathies may not be able to tolerate the volume of FFP required for correction, and more concentrated factor preparations may be indicated (vide infra). Therapy should be monitored with prothrombin time (PT), activated partial thromboplastin time (PTT), or specific factor assays.

FFP should be ABO compatible, but crossmatching is not required. Rh type need not be considered.

Liquid plasma (200 to 250 mL), prepared by separating plasma from a whole blood unit up to 5 days after the expiration date, contains the stable coagulation factors, but levels of factors V and VIII are decreased. Plasma may be used to treat stable coagulation factor deficiencies. Compatibility considerations are the same as for FFP.

Cryoprecipitate is made by thawing a unit of FFP at 4°C. A white precipitate forms; most of the supernatant plasma is then removed. The cold precipitated protein and the approximately 10 ml of residual plasma in the bag are refrozen. A pack of cryoprecipitate contains von Willebrand factor, lesser amounts of factor VIII coagulant (minimum of 80 U), fibrinogen (at least 150 mg), factor XIII, and fibronectin.

Cryoprecipitate is used for therapy of von Willebrand's disease, mild to moderate hemophilia A, factor XIII deficiency, and fibrinogen deficiency. ABO-compatible cryoprecipitate is preferred because of the presence of anti-A and anti-B agglutinins. Infusion of large amounts of cryoprecipitate can cause hyperfibrinogenemia, which may be associated with hemorrhagic problems.

The *factor concentrates* make it possible to deliver large quantities of clotting factors in small volumes, thus reducing the risk of circulatory overload encountered with FFP.

Factor VIII concentrate is a lyophilized product made by fractionation of pooled plasma. Newer methods of preparation have decreased the risk of disease transmission. Factor VIII concentrate is used to treat patients with moderate to severe hemophilia A and with low titer factor VIII inhibitors; DDAVP (1-deamino-8-D-arginine vasopressin) should be used instead, if possible, in patients with mild to moderate hemophilia A or von Willebrand's disease. Since factor VIII concentrate lacks the von Willebrand factor, it should not be used alone for treatment of von Willebrand's disease. When large doses of factor VIII concentrate are administered, hyperfibrinogenemia may occur.

Factor IX concentrate (prothrombin complex), which is prepared by fractionation and lyophilization of pooled plasma, contains factors II, VII, IX, and X. Newer processing methods have decreased the risk of disease transmission with this product as well. Factor IX concentrate is used to treat patients with hemophilia B (Christmas disease), factor II, VII, or X deficiency, or factor VIII inhibitors (prothrombin complex contains activity which may bypass factor VIII). Immediate side effects of therapy can include chills, fever, headache, nausea, flushing, thrombosis, and DIC.

PLASMA SUBSTITUTES

Albumin and *plasma protein fraction* (PPF), which are derived from plasma, contain albumin, globulins, and other proteins. These products are heat treated to eliminate disease transmission. Testing for ABO compatibility is not a concern. Serum albumin is prepared as a 5% or 25% solution and PPF as a 5% solution; each contains about 145 meq/L sodium. The 5% solutions have osmotic and oncotic properties equivalent to plasma.

These products are indicated for patients who are both hypovolemic and hypoproteinemic; they should not be given to promote wound healing or for nutritional support. Since 25% albumin solutions may enhance interstitial dehydration by causing absorption of tissue fluids into the intravascular space, it is advisable to supplement administration with crystalloid infusions to offset this effect.[25]

Rapid administration of PPF has caused hypotension attributed to the vasodilatory effects of sodium acetate, which is present as a buffer.[26] PPF should not be given intra-arterially or during cardiopulmonary bypass; these contraindications do not apply to albumin.[25]

Volume expanders include *crystalloid* solutions (e.g., normal saline, Ringer's lactate) and *colloid* substitutes such as Dextran and HES. The possibility of fluid overload must be considered with the use of volume expanders, particularly in patients with cardiac or renal failure. HES can cause prolongation of PT and PTT, pruritus,[25] and anaphylactoid reactions.[27] Likewise, Dextran can cause anaphylactoid reactions, as well as fever, rash, tachycardia, hypotension, and increased bleeding due to interference with platelet function and to stimulation of fibrinolysis; infusion of low molecular weight products has been associated with renal failure.[25]

IRRADIATED BLOOD PRODUCTS

Graft-versus-host disease (GVHD) can occur 3 to 30 days after transfusion when an immunocompromised patient receives immunologically competent, allogeneic lymphocytes.[28] A radiation dose of 1500 to 5000 rad renders 85 to 95 percent of the lymphocytes in a unit of blood, granulocyte, or platelet concentrate incapable of replication,[29] apparently without significantly affecting function of red blood cells, granulocytes, or platelets.[28]

Irradiation of all cellular blood products as well as fresh plasma components is indicated for patients with congenital immune deficiencies and for recipients of allogeneic or autologous bone marrow transplants. Irradiation of blood is also recommended for patients with hematologic malignancies when transfusions are given during periods of severe therapy-induced immunosuppression.

There have been several recent reports of fatal GVHD following blood transfusion in patients who apparently were not immunocompromised.[30–32] One proposed explanation is that the donors were homozygous for HLA haplotypes for which the recipients were heterozygous,[30,32] and thus the immune system of the recipients did not "recognize" the transfused lymphocytes as foreign; however, the latter "recognized" the recipient as HLA incompatible. Since homozygosity for HLA haplotypes for which a family member is heterozygous would be most likely to occur among first-degree family members, it has been recommended that blood components from such donors be irradiated.[33]

BLOOD SALVAGED INTRAOPERATIVELY OR POSTOPERATIVELY

Intraoperative blood salvage, or intraoperative autotransfusion, is a process whereby blood collected during surgery subsequently is reinfused. With the use of modern technologic devices, blood is aspirated from the surgical field, anticoagulated with heparin, filtered, washed, centrifuged, and reinfused as red cells suspended in the wash solution with a hematocrit of about 60 percent. Plasma, platelets, and white blood cells are not salvaged. The procedure with the newest machines is quite safe, but air embolism, hemolysis,[34–36] hypofibrinogenemia[34,36] or other coagulopathies, and bacterial contamination of the blood have been reported occasionally. Most authorities believe this practice is contraindicated in patients with bacteremia or potential for bacteremia (e.g., nonsterile surgical fields) and in patients with malignancies until further studies prove the procedure is safe under these conditions.[37]

Patients with hemothorax are suited for autotransfusion after trauma, but reinfusion of abdominal hemorrhage without knowledge of extent of injury carries a greater risk of contamination (from the bowel, gallbladder, or urinary bladder).

Postoperatively or posttrauma, autologous blood may be reinfused within 6 h following collection from tube drainage.[38]

Transfusion Therapy

EMERGENCY TRANSFUSION

When the time needed for routine processing of blood may jeopardize the welfare of a patient, wise transfusion practices may necessitate different standards. Complete transfusion work-up, which includes antibody screen and crossmatch, requires at least 30 to 45 min (Table 35-1). The clinicians should inform the blood bank of the degree of urgency. Emergency situations in previously unhospitalized individuals are accompanied by special problems of patient identification and accurate labeling of blood specimens.

If the patient's identity is not known, the blood tube and request should display an identification number assigned in the Emergency Department. If the patient is in the hospital, the blood tube should be labeled at the bedside with the patient's first and last name, hospital identification number, and date. The request for the blood must include the phlebotomist's signature. Most hemolytic transfusion reactions result from ABO incompatibility secondary to clerical errors; mislabeling of the patient's blood sample is the most common.

Even in extremely urgent situations, a properly labeled patient sample must be delivered to the blood bank before blood is administered. If the patient must be transfused immediately, group O, Rh-negative packed red cells can be given and will avoid transfusion of significant quantities of anti-A and anti-B in group O plasma. Alternatively, group O whole blood with anti-A and anti-B titers predetermined to be <1:200 in saline may be used. Transfusion can be enhanced by placement of a pressure cuff around the unit. If time permits, determination of ABO and Rh type, which takes approximately 5 min, can be performed, and then type-specific blood can be issued. Reliance must not be placed on old records or typing results from other institutions.

TABLE 35-1 Compatibility Testing Times for Packed Red Cell Products

Packed Red Cell Product	Approximate Blood Bank Testing Time
O negative	None
Type-specific	5 min
Immediate-spin crossmatch	10 min for first 2 U (includes typing time)
Type and antibody screen	30–45 min
If negative	5 additional min for immediate-spin crossmatch
If positive	Antibody identification required (minimum 45 min), with procurement of compatible units; testing time depends on nature of antibodies and number of units needed

An abbreviated immediate-spin crossmatch procedure, which takes approximately 5 min, involves reaction of the recipient's serum and donor red cells after immediate centrifugation and detects IgM antibodies of the ABO blood groups. This practice is appropriate in emergency situations and for massively transfused patients. When blood is issued before full compatibility testing is completed, as in the situations mentioned above (O-negative, type-specific, and immediate-spin crossmatch prior to antibody screen), the records must contain a statement signed by the requesting physician that the clinical situation is sufficiently urgent to warrant the increased risk. The label attached to the blood must indicate that compatibility testing was incomplete. The antibody screen (and, if positive, also complete major crossmatch) must be performed promptly after the blood is issued; however, this is not necessary for patients whose entire blood volume has been replaced. If clinically significant unexpected antibodies or incompatibilities are discovered during subsequent complete compatibility work-up, the units issued must be retrieved. If the blood has been transfused, the patient's physician must be notified; appropriate monitoring of the patient and therapy should be discussed (see Complications and Hazards). If a patient has received more than 4 U group O packed cells, the decision to switch to group-specific blood depends on whether or not anti-A or anti-B antibodies are found in the recipient. The levels of these isoagglutinins in the recipient vary with the volume of plasma present in the red cell unit and the titers of anti-A and anti-B.

In a hospitalized patient who has had a "type and screen," the blood type has been identified, and the screen has enabled detection and then identification of significant antibodies. For such a patient, type-specific blood lacking antigens to which the patient has significant antibodies may be provided after an immediate-spin crossmatch is performed with a properly identified current blood sample.

MASSIVE TRANSFUSION

Massive transfusion means transfusion within a 24-h period that approximates a patient's blood volume. The clinical results of massive transfusion of red cells are influenced largely by two factors: the effects of shelf storage and the dilutional effects on platelets and coagulation factors (Table 35-2). The aging of banked packed red cells results in seepage of intracellular potassium into the plasma, fall in plasma bicarbonate level, rise in lactate concentration, fall in 2,3-diphosphoglycerate (DPG) level, rise in plasma hemoglobin, rise in plasma lactate dehydrogenase level, deterioration of some of the coagulation factors, and rise in ammonia content.[39]

Because plasma potassium concentration increases during storage, one might postulate that massive transfusion could cause hyperkalemia; however, in practice this is rarely the case. Hypokalemia actually is more common for two reasons: **1.** the transfused hypokalemic red cells may take up potassium,[40] and **2.** metabolism of citrate (the anticoagulant in blood) to bicarbonate causes metabolic alkalo-

TABLE 35-2 Potential Complications of Massive Transfusion

Dilutional Effects
Thrombocytopenia
Coagulopathy
Consequences of Prolonged Blood Storage
Hyperkalemia (in renal impairment)
Left shift of the oxyhemoglobin dissociation relationship (temporary)
Miscellaneous
Hypothermia
Volume overload
Metabolic alkalosis
Hypocalcemia

sis, resulting in a compensatory exchange of intracellular hydrogen ions for extracellular potassium ions. However, in patients with shock, acidosis, and compromised renal perfusion, the potential for development of hyperkalemia does exist, and monitoring of serum potassium is appropriate.

Lactic acid content increases during blood storage, with a fall in pH, leading to decreased glycolysis and a decrease in 2,3-DPG level. Since 2,3-DPG competes with hemoglobin for oxygen binding, massive transfusion may result in a temporary shift of the oxygen dissociation curve of hemoglobin, with tighter binding of oxygen to hemoglobin and impaired tissue oxygenation. However, 2,3-DPG ordinarily is regenerated rapidly by red cells in vivo,[41] returning to more than 50 percent of the final level within 24 h of transfusion and exhibiting normal affinity for oxygen at 24 h,[42] although this process may take longer in patients with metabolic derangements.[43] As long as anemia is corrected by transfusion, the temporary increase in the oxygen affinity of hemoglobin can be compensated for by an increase in cardiac output. Blood <14 days old and cryopreserved red cells contain enough 2,3-DPG for near-normal oxygen release immediately after transfusion.

Normally functioning platelets are virtually absent in stored blood. Thrombocytopenia correlates with the amount of blood transfused and may become clinically significant in an adult after administration of 15 to 20 U (equivalent to approximately one and a half to two times the blood volume).[44] Although the labile coagulation factors (V and VIII) deteriorate with storage, other coagulation factors, including fibrinogen, are retained. Coagulation abnormalities in massively transfused patients are associated closely with the extent of trauma and development of DIC rather than with the number of blood units transfused.[24,44,45] The plasma present in administered platelet packs may be sufficient to correct clotting factor deficiencies. The most useful tests for guiding management are platelet count and fibrinogen level; PT, PTT, and bleeding time are often moderately abnormal in patients who do not develop generalized bleeding, although they correlate with bleeding when markedly prolonged.[44]

In massive transfusion, hypocalcemia may result from the binding of calcium by the citrate anticoagulant in banked blood. However, with the possible exceptions of premature infants, patients with severe liver disease, patients in the anhepatic phase of liver transplantation, and those receiving infusions of citrated products at the rate of more than 100 mL/min,[46] citrate ordinarily is rapidly metabolized by the liver, and therefore clinically significant hypocalcemia usually does not develop during massive transfusion. The serum ionized calcium level and prolongation of the QT interval should be monitored to determine the need for supplemental calcium therapy.

Rapid transfusion of refrigerated blood can cause hypothermia with its attendant complications. An external blood warmer is recommended during massive transfusion.

TRANSFUSION IN PATIENTS WITH CHRONIC DISEASE

Patients with *chronic anemia,* such as those with chronic renal failure, tolerate hematocrits in the range of 20 percent. With the introduction of erythropoietin therapy, it may be possible to minimize red cell transfusion further in some patients with anemia secondary to chronic disease.

Patients with increased plasma volume or incipient *heart failure* may develop chest tightness, shortness of breath, cough, and pulmonary edema if blood is infused rapidly. Transfusion of packed red cells, if necessary, should be performed slowly with the patient sitting upright or should be guided with invasive hemodynamic monitoring. It may be desirable to remove an aliquot for transfusion from a blood unit in sterile fashion and to store the remainder of the unit in the blood bank for subsequent use by the same patient.

Patients who develop *autoimmune hemolytic anemia* are often elderly and have underlying cardiac abnormalities. Their autoantibodies usually react with the red cells of virtually all donors, which may make it difficult to detect the presence of significant alloantibodies. The best approach is to transfuse only if absolutely necessary with least incompatible blood and to treat the autoimmune process with medication (e.g., steroids, intravenous gamma globulin, immunosuppressive drugs), if possible. The transfused cells usually will have shortened survival, but they may be destroyed no more rapidly than the patient's own red cells.

Because transfusion of patients with *aplastic anemia* may induce sensitization to antigens that increase the risk of bone marrow graft rejection and that make platelet transfusion difficult,[47] administration of blood products is best avoided in such patients unless absolutely necessary. If transfusions are needed, usage of modern types of filters that deplete leukocytes to at least 5×10^6 per transfusion from red cell and platelet units may help prevent alloimmunization.[22,48] It has been advocated that transfusions of blood products from a potential marrow donor and the donor's close relatives are best avoided prior to transplantation. Although a study by Ho and colleagues[49] failed to show an increase in graft rejection in leukemic patients who had been transfused with blood products from their relatives, including the marrow donor, it has been argued that patients with acute leukemia, who are under the immunosuppressive effects of chemotherapy, are less likely to become sensitized to HLA antigens through transfusions than are patients with aplastic anemia, who are immunologically competent.[50]

ADMINISTRATION OF BLOOD PRODUCTS

Before transfusion, the blood product with the compatibility tag must be compared with the patient's wrist band; no discrepancies in name or identification number should exist. The patient should be observed for 5 to 10 min after the start of the transfusion and thereafter should be checked periodically throughout the transfusion period.

Because of the potential for bacterial growth in blood, if the time for infusion is to be more than 4 h, the unit should be divided into aliquots, and portions should remain refrigerated in the blood bank until needed.

Infusion sets must be sterile and pyrogen free, and all blood components (but not plasma substitutes) must be given through a filter. Standard filters (170 to 260 μm pore size) remove large clots and other debris. Microaggregate blood filters (20 to 40 μm pore size) remove the small aggregates that form in blood after 5 days of storage. They are not indicated for routine transfusion but should be used for patients transfused during cardiopulmonary bypass, when microaggregates enter the systemic circulation directly.[25] Such filters also may be used to prevent febrile transfusion reactions, but they should not be used with granulocyte transfusions. Blood less than 5 days old, washed red cells, and deglycerolized red cells have few microaggregates.

To decrease viscosity and increase infusion rate, red cells usually are diluted with normal saline (0.9% USP). ABO-compatible plasma can be used if indicated but increases the risk of transfusion-transmitted diseases. Dextrose, hypotonic sodium chloride, and lactated Ringer's solution are contraindicated. Medications should not be added to blood. Tubing should be flushed with normal saline when blood is administered through an existing intravenous line.

Mechanical infusion devices may induce hemolysis when used to administer packed red cells. The manufacturer should be consulted regarding the suitability of the instrument for this purpose. For maximum effect, large gauge needles and tubing are recommended.

Complications and Hazards

DISEASE TRANSMISSION

Individuals at risk for transmission of *AIDS* are prevented from donating blood products when a history for risk factors is elicited, when the donor describes symptoms suggestive of the syndrome, or when blood test results (usually, enzyme-linked immunosorbent assay [ELISA] screening test, Western blot confirmatory test) are positive. It has been estimated that the likelihood of the screening test missing a donor, who may be in the "window period" following exposure but before the human immunodeficiency virus (HIV) antibody screen becomes positive, is in the range of 1:40,000 to 1:200,000,[51] depending mainly on the prevalence of the disease in the area where the donor resides.

The precise incidence of *hepatitis* following blood transfusion is unknown, but estimates have ranged from 1 to 10 percent. Most of the patients are anicteric. Steps taken to decrease this risk include elimination of paid donors and testing for hepatitis B surface antigen, antibody to hepatitis B core antigen, and elevation of alanine aminotransferase. The vast majority of cases of posttransfusion hepatitis currently are due to the non-A, non-B virus(es). New methods of treating blood products and institution of testing for hepatitis C virus promise to decrease the risk further.

In the rare instances when *bacteria* are present in blood components, septic reactions may occur in the recipient. Most reactions are due to endotoxin produced by cold-growing, gram-negative bacteria, which have included *Pseudomonas* species, *Citrobacter freundii*, *Escherichia coli*, and *Yersinia enterocolitica*. Reactions are characterized by high fever, shock, hemoglobinuria, DIC, and renal failure. The skin is dry and flushed. Abdominal cramps, diarrhea, vomiting, and muscle pain may occur.[29]

If bacterial contamination is suspected, transfusion should be discontinued and the blood unit inspected for purple color, clots, or hemolysis; however, often the blood bag is not remarkable. Gram stain of the product if positive for organisms is confirmatory, but the absence of organisms does not rule out this possibility. The patient's blood, the blood product, and intravenous solutions should be cultured for aerobic and anaerobic organisms at refrigerator, room, and body temperatures. Treatment includes appropriate antibiotics and supportive measures.

Screening of blood donors for *human T lymphotropic virus type I (HTLV-1)* was instituted to minimize the spread by blood transfusion of acute T cell leukemia and tropical spastic paraparesis (also called HTLV-I-associated myelopathy).

CMV and *EBV* can be transmitted by leukocytes and can cause a *postperfusion syndrome* at 3 to 6 weeks, characterized by fever, splenomegaly, liver dysfunction, and lymphocytosis with atypical cells. Most prone to this syndrome are premature infants, transplant patients on immunosuppressive therapy, and patients who have had open heart surgery.

Treponema pallidum cannot survive at refrigerator temperatures for more than 2 to 3 days, but syphilis could be transmitted by fresh blood or by platelets which are stored at room temperature. Most of the serologic tests for syphilis are negative during the spirochetemic phase.

Blood transfusions are not a significant means of *malaria* spread. Donors are deferred for a period of time if they have traveled in areas where malaria is endemic or if they have had malaria.

Since *rickettsiae* are blood-borne, rare individuals who are asymptomatic carriers could transmit infection.

Because of increased immigration from areas in Central or South America where *Chagas' disease* is endemic, concern has been raised regarding increased spread of the disease from asymptomatic donors who carry the causative agent, *Trypanosoma cruzi*. Although most infected individuals are asymptomatic, serious complications such as cardiomyopathy and dilatation of the esophagus or colon can occur, particularly in immunosuppressed patients. Currently, no commercial screening test is available. Most authorities believe that national screening is not indicated, but local screening may be useful in areas where the incidence of positive donors is likely to be high.[52,53]

RED CELL RELATED

Acute hemolytic transfusion reaction usually is due to an antibody in the recipient's plasma that reacts with donor red cells. Depending on the nature of the antibody and its ability to bind complement, the reaction can result in intravascular or extravascular hemolysis.

Intravascular hemolysis with destruction of erythrocytes within the lumen of blood vessels can occur if the antibody is of an IgM or IgG type capable of activating complement through C9. Such antibodies include most anti-A and anti-B, some anti-Lewis, anti-Kidd, and others. Intravascular hemolysis is frequently rapid, occurring with only a few milliliters of blood, and can lead to shock, acute renal failure, or bleeding due to DIC and hypofibrinogenemia. Symptoms include chills and fever, a burning sensation along the course of the vein, headache, oppressive chest pain, back pain, fever, or facial flushing. If the patient is unconscious, as when under anesthesia, after trauma, or in shock, or if the patient is in the pediatric age group, hypotension, pink or red-tinged urine, shock, or a bleeding diathesis may be the only indication of a hemolytic transfusion reaction.

Even in the absence of symptoms, a patient transfused with a unit of blood that is incompatible because of an antibody associated with intravascular hemolysis should be treated as though an intravascular hemolytic reaction is occurring. The following steps should be taken:

1. Discontinue transfusion immediately. Leave intravenous line open with saline (use fresh tubing).
2. Perform rapid check of labels, forms, and patient identification.
3. Record and monitor urinary output.
4. Maintain urine output of at least 30 mL/h.
5. Measure blood pressure and institute therapy for shock, if present.
6. Notify the blood bank and initiate reaction work-up; send unused blood bag and freshly drawn blood samples to the blood bank with transfusion reaction work-up request forms.
7. Perform base line and follow-up laboratory studies, including:
   - **a.** Blood urea nitrogen (BUN), creatinine, electrolytes.
   - **b.** PT, PTT, fibrinogen, platelet count, fibrin degradation products (DIC screen), D dimer.
   - **c.** Hemoglobin or hematocrit.
   - **d.** Urinalysis for evaluation of hemoglobinuria.
   - **e.** Plasma or serum evaluation for hemoglobinemia (precipitous decrease in haptoglobin level occurs early but is not as reliable as hemoglobinemia; since visible hemoglobinemia develops only after haptoglobin depletion, little is gained by measuring haptoglobin if there is visible hemoglobinemia).
   - **f.** Base line serum bilirubin at the time of the suspected transfusion reaction and subsequent serum bilirubin 5 to 7 h later (rising unconjugated bilirubin may be detectable as early as 1 h postreaction; peak levels occur at 4 to 6 h and disappear in 24 h if bilirubin excretion is normal).
8. Since the renal failure which may accompany hemolytic transfusion reactions is thought to be secondary to damage caused by hypotension and vasoconstriction following destruction of red cells, with formation of red cell stroma-antibody complexes, the clinical service attending physician, in consultation with the attending physicians of the blood bank and hematology department, may wish to initiate prompt whole blood or plasma exchange, dialysis, or heparin therapy (for DIC), depending on the nature of the transfusion reaction, results of the transfusion work-up, and clinical condition of the patient.
9. Give compatible blood transfusions if clinically indicated after the blood bank evaluation is complete.

Extravascular hemolysis, with phagocytosis and destruction of erythrocytes by macrophages, occurs with IgG or IgM antibodies that do not bind complement or activate only a portion of the complement pathway. Most antibodies other than anti-A and anti-B react in this manner. The reaction usually is not clinically severe, but chills and fever, hyperbilirubinemia, and decreased survival of incompatible erythrocytes can occur. Specific therapy for a purely extravascular hemolytic reaction usually is not necessary, but it is wise to keep the patient well-hydrated and to monitor urinary output and hematocrit or hemoglobin level.

Often, hemolytic reactions are a combination of intravascular and extravascular hemolysis. The clinical manifestations and therapy depend on which predominates.

Occasionally a recipient develops detectable antibody levels several hours, days, or weeks after transfusion of erythrocytes containing the corresponding antigen *(delayed hemolytic transfusion reaction).* Usually extravascular hemolysis occurs, resulting in anemia, possibly associated with fever and hyperbilirubinemia. The detection of spherocytes on the peripheral blood smear may be the first indication of red cell destruction. Blood bank work-up reveals that a positive direct antiglobulin test has developed, and a "mixed-field" reaction usually is detected microscopically. Since fever and chills may not occur until several hours after transfusion, the patient's reaction may not be due to the blood being infused at the time of the reaction; thus, it is desirable to perform a serologic work-up on each blood unit in a multiple unit transfusion.

Delayed transfusion reactions rarely can be associated with intravascular hemolysis, with life-threatening consequences. Treatment recommendations are discussed in the previous sections on intra- and extravascular hemolysis.

WHITE CELL RELATED

Febrile nonhemolytic reaction is defined as a temperature rise of 1°C or more occurring in association with transfusion without any other explanation. It is thought to be caused by antibodies in recipient plasma reacting against antigens on the cell membranes of transfused leukocytes. Prior transfusions or pregnancies contribute to development of the antibodies. A febrile reaction may also occur if the recipient's antigens react with antibodies in donor plasma.

Once a febrile reaction occurs, it must be distinguished from the early manifestations of a hemolytic transfusion reaction by laboratory investigation. When the patient's temperature reaches high levels, it may be advisable to culture the blood product to rule out bacterial contamination.

If the reaction is severe, an antipyretic may be given to ameliorate the symptoms. Future reactions usually can be prevented by premedication with an antipyretic and use of leukocyte-poor blood products.

Since only about 15 percent of patients who have a febrile nonhemolytic reaction are likely to experience a similar subsequent reaction, it has been recommended that leukocyte-poor products not be administered unless a patient has had at least two febrile nonhemolytic reactions.[54] However, it may be desirable to modify this approach to be less stringent with regard to the availability of leukocyte-poor blood products for patients who are clinically unstable.

Some patients develop *transient dyspnea* (noncardiogenic pulmonary edema) in association with transfusion, which has been attributed to a reaction between leukoagglutinins and leukocytes, resulting in transient pulmonary infiltrates. The chest film is typical of pulmonary edema. Transfusion should be stopped; treatment is supportive and may include intravenous steroids. Washed blood products may prevent subsequent reactions.

Alloimmunization to HLA antigens is discussed in the section on platelets and GVHD in the section on irradiated blood products (see Blood Components).

PLASMA RELATED

Allergic reaction usually manifests as urticaria (hives), but other types of rashes may be noted. Allergy to a substance in the donor plasma is suspected. Treatment with an antihistamine usually is effective, and the transfusion then may be continued if the reaction was minor. Rarely, asthma or glottal edema may occur. Epinephrine, diphenhydramine, steroids, and fluid replacement should be administered intravenously, if needed. Allergic reactions can be ameliorated by administration of an antihistamine prior to transfusion. Washed blood products are indicated for patients with severe or repeated reactions.

About 1 individual in 500 to 1 in 1000 is IgA deficient. When initially transfused and exposed to IgA, these patients may produce anti-IgA. When subsequently transfused, the IgA and anti-IgA may react, causing an *anaphylactic reaction.* Features that distinguish anaphylactic from other immediate reactions are occurrence after infusion of only a few milliliters of blood or plasma and lack of fever. Symptoms include coughing, bronchospasm, respiratory distress, vascular instability, abdominal cramps, vomiting, diarrhea, shock, and loss of consciousness.[29] Anaphylactic reactions should be treated in the usual manner. Subsequently, patients should be transfused with red cells washed multiple times or with deglycerolized frozen red cells, which virtually lack plasma containing IgA. When time permits, elective predonation of autologous blood or selection of homologous donors who are IgA deficient are other approaches for prevention of this complication.

PLATELET RELATED

Posttransfusion purpura is a rare, life-threatening condition resulting from thrombocytopenia, which usually occurs about 7 to 10 days after blood transfusion to a rare patient who lacks the Pl^{A1} platelet antigen (present in about 98 percent of people). Individuals who develop this complication are most often women with a prior history of pregnancy. The induced alloantibody destroys transfused platelets as well as the recipient's Pl^{A1}-negative platelets by a mechanism that is not well understood. Favorable responses have been reported in patients who have received high dose intravenous gamma globulin.[55] Red cells should be washed prior to subsequent transfusions to such individuals to remove residual platelets and thereby minimize further antigenic exposure.

OTHER

Alloimmunization and reactions to other components in platelet packs are discussed in prior sections.

Therapeutic Apheresis

Therapeutic apheresis is performed when it is desirable to remove a portion of a patient's blood that contains a pathologic component. Although the processing can be done manually, several liters usually are processed more easily by a machine that separates the unwanted component and reinfuses the remainder of the patient's blood.

Machines used for apheresis may have continuous or discontinuous types of flow; the former variety is preferred because of less risk of hypotension. The machines separate blood components by centrifugation or membrane filtration (membrane filtration is for separation of plasma only). It may be preferable to use a blood warmer and cardiac monitor in association with subclavian access, particularly for elderly patients who may be prone to cardiac arrhythmias from infusion of cold or citrated solutions.

Anticoagulation can be with citrate or heparin. Since the effect of heparin lasts for at least 6 h, it should be used cautiously in patients with bleeding tendencies, abnormal coagulation tests, or who are immediately pre- or postoperative. If citrate is given too rapidly or to a patient whose liver cannot readily metabolize it, symptoms of hypocalcemia can occur. Treatment includes slowing the return of blood and administration of calcium after flushing the intravenous tubing to avoid clotting.

Other complications include those associated with venous lines, hypotension, volume overload, vasovagal reactions, protein depletion (during a series of plasmapheresis procedures, patients should be followed with total protein and immunoglobulin levels), sensation of coldness, cardiac arrhythmia or arrest, respiratory arrest, anaphylaxis, seizures, or death. Serious complications are rare.

Plasmapheresis usually involves the removal of one to one and a half plasma volumes, which ordinarily is replaced with an albumin-saline mixture to maintain oncotic properties. This is considered standard therapy for the acute symptomatology of hyperviscosity, myasthenia gravis, idiopathic rapidly progressive glomerulonephritis, Goodpasture's syndrome (without anuria or with pulmonary hemorrhage), rapidly progressive glomerulonephritis secondary to vasculitis, Refsum's disease, TTP, thyroid storm or thyroid hormone overdose, overdose with certain drugs, and severe acute polyradiculoneuropathy (Guillain-Barré syndrome).[56] FFP replacement (plasma exchange) has been effective for patients with TTP, HUS, or significant coagulation factor abnormalities (e.g., in liver disease).

Excessive numbers of platelets, granulocytes, or lymphocytes may be removed from symptomatic patients by plateletpheresis or leukapheresis. During red cell exchange, a patient's red cells are removed (e.g., for hemoglobinopathy such as sickle cell disease) and replaced with normal red cells.

With the use of immunoadsorption treatment columns, a patient's plasma is percolated through a column inserted in the extracorporeal circuit. Columns have been designed for selective removal of circulating immune complexes and IgG molecules. It is speculated that removal of these "immunomodulation molecules" may stimulate the immune system, effect a change in the composition of circulating immune complexes such that free antibody is released into the patient's circulation, or generate activated complement components, which stimulate further removal of circulating immune complexes by the patient's reticuloendothelial system.[57] To date, studies with the columns have shown some success in treatment of ITP, thrombocytopenia secondary to HIV infection, and in the HUS/TTP-like syndrome occasionally seen in patients with various types of cancer or related to antineoplastic drug therapy.[58]

References

1. Freireich EJ, Kliman A, Gaydos LA et al: Response to repeated platelet transfusions from the same donor. Ann Intern Med 59:277, 1963.
2. Tomasulo PA, Petz LD: Platelet transfusions, in Petz LD, Swisher SN (eds): Clinical Practice of Transfusion Medicine, 2d ed. New York: Churchill Livingstone, 1989, pp 432, 436.
3. Harker LA, Malpass TW, Branson HE et al: Mechanism of abnormal bleeding in patients undergoing cardiopulmonary bypass: Acquired transient platelet dysfunction associated with selective alpha-granule release. Blood 56:824, 1980.
4. Cimo PL, Pisciotta AV, Desai RG et al: Detection of drug-dependent antibodies by the ^{51}Cr platelet lysis test: Documentation of immune thrombocytopenia induced by diphenylhydantoin, diazepam, and sulfisoxazole. Am J Hematol 2:65, 1977.
5. Schiffer CA, Weinstein HJ, Wiernik PH: Methicillin-associated thrombocytopenia. Ann Intern Med 85:338, 1976.
6. Karpatkin S: Drug-induced thrombocytopenia. Am J Med Sci 262:69, 1971.
7. Hackett T, Kelton JG, Powers P: Drug-induced platelet destruction. Semin Thromb Hemost 8:116, 1982.
8. Hill HR: Phagocytic transfusion—ultimate therapy of neonatal disease? J Pediatr 98:59, 1981.
9. Wright WC Jr, Ank BJ, Herbert J et al: Decreased bactericidal activity of leukocytes of stressed newborn infants. Pediatrics 56:579, 1975.
10. Shigeoka AO, Santos JI, Hill HR: Functional analysis of neutrophil granulocytes from healthy, infected and stressed neonates. J Pediatr 95:454, 1979.
11. Christensen RD, Rothstein G: Exhaustion of mature marrow neutrophils in neonates with sepsis. J Pediatr 96:316, 1980.
12. Handin RI, Valeri CR: Hemostatic effectiveness of platelets stored at 22°C. N Engl J Med 285:538, 1971.
13. Murphy S, Gardner FH: Platelet preservation: Effect of storage temperature on maintenance of platelet viability—deleterious effect of refrigerated storage. N Engl J Med 280:1094, 1969.
14. Murphy S, Sayar SN, Gardner FH: Storage of platelet concentrates at 22°C. Blood 35:549, 1970.
15. Becker GA, Tuccelli M, Kunicki T et al: Studies of platelet concentrates stored at 22°C and 4°C. Transfusion 13:61, 1973.
16. Kattlove HE: Platelet preservation—what temperature? A rationale for strategy. Transfusion 14:328, 1974.
17. Hutchison RE, Kunkel KD, Schell MJ et al: Beneficial effect of brief pre-transfusion incubation of platelets at 37°C. Lancet I(8645):986, May 6, 1989.
18. O'Connell B, Lee EJ, Schiffer CA: The value of 10-minute post-transfusion platelet counts. Transfusion 28:66, 1988.
19. Brand A, van Leeuwen A, Eernisse JG et al: Platelet transfusion therapy: Optimal donor selection with a combination of lymphocytotoxicity and platelet fluorescence tests. Blood 51:781, 1978.
20. Murphy MF, Metcalfe P, Thomas H et al: Use of leukocyte-poor blood components and HLA-matched-platelet donors to prevent HLA alloimmunization. Br J Haematol 62:529, 1986.
21. Sniecinski I, O'Donnell MR, Nowicki B et al: Prevention of refractoriness and HLA-alloimmunization using filtered blood products. Blood 71(5):1402, 1988.
22. Meryman HT: Transfusion-induced alloimmunization and immunosuppression and the effects of leukocyte depletion. Trans Med Rev III(3):180, 1989.
23. Wright DG, Robichaud KJ, Pizzo PA et al: Lethal pulmonary reactions associated with the combined use of amphotericin B and leukocyte transfusions. N Engl J Med 304:1185, 1981.
24. Schiffer CA: Annotation: Some aspects of recent advances in the use of blood cell components. Br J Haematol 39:289, 1978.
25. Pisciotto, PT (ed): *Blood Transfusion Therapy: A Physician's Handbook,* 3d ed. Arlington, VA, American Association of Blood Banks, 1989.
26. Olinger GN, Werner PH, Boncheck LI et al: Vasodilator effects of the sodium acetate in pooled protein fraction. Ann Surg 190:305, 1979.
27. Ring J, Messmer K: Incidence and severity of anaphylactoid reactions to colloid-volume substitutes. Lancet 1:466, 1977.
28. Leitman SF, Holland PV: Irradiation of blood products: Indications and guidelines. Transfusion 25:293, 1985.

29. Walker RH (ed): *Technical Manual,* 10th ed. Arlington, VA, American Association of Blood Banks, 1990.
30. Thaler M, Shamiss A, Orgad S et al: The role of blood from HLA-homozygous donors in fatal transfusion-associated graft-versus-host disease after open-heart surgery. N Engl J Med 321:25, 1989.
31. Juji T, Takahashi K, Shibata Y et al: Host-transfusion graft-vs-host disease in immunocompetent patients after cardiac surgery in Japan. Letter. N Engl J Med 321:56, 1989.
32. Otsuka S, Kunieda K, Hirose M et al: Fatal erythroderma (suspected graft-versus-host disease) after cholecystectomy: Retrospective analysis. Transfusion 29:544, 1989.
33. American Association of Blood Banks: Blood Bank Week 6(42):4, Nov. 10, 1989.
34. Stillman RM, Wrezlewicz WW, Stanczewski B et al: The haematological hazards of autotransfusion. Br J Surg 63:651, 1976.
35. Smith RN, Yaw PB, Glover JL: Autotransfusion of contaminated intraperitoneal blood: An experimental study. J Trauma 18:341, 1978.
36. Bell W: The hematology of autotransfusion. Surgery 84:695, 1978.
37. Popovsky MA, Devine PA, Taswell HF: Intraoperative autologous transfusion. Mayo Clin Proc 60:125, 1985.
38. Holland PV (ed): *Standards for Blood Banks and Transfusion Services,* 13th ed. Arlington, VA, American Association of Blood Banks, 1989, p 43.
39. Bailey DN, Bove JR: Chemical and hematological changes in stored CPD blood. Transfusion 15:244, 1975.
40. Holland PV: The diagnosis and management of transfusion reactions and other adverse effects of transfusion, in Petz LD, Swisher SN (eds): Clinical Practice of Transfusion Medicine, 2d ed. New York, Churchill Livingstone, 1989, p 728.
41. Beutler E, Wood L: The in vivo regeneration of red cell 2,3-diphosphoglyceric acid (DPG) after transfusion of stored blood. J Lab Clin Med 74:300, 1969.
42. Valeri CR, Hirsch NM: Restoration in vivo of erythrocyte adenosine triphosphate, 2,3-diphosphoglycerate, potassium ion, and sodium ion concentrations following the transfusion of acid-citrate-dextrose-stored human red blood cells. J Lab Clin Med 73:722, 1969.
43. O'Brien TG, Watkins E Jr: Gas-exchange dynamics of glycerolized frozen blood. J Thoracic Cardiovasc Surg 40:611, 1960.
44. Counts RB, Haisch C, Simon TL et al: Hemostasis in massively transfused trauma patients. Ann Surg 190:91, 1979.
45. Hewson JR, Neame PB, Kumar N et al: Coagulopathy related to dilution and hypotension during massive transfusion. Crit Care Med 13:387, 1985.
46. Committee on Trauma, American College of Surgeons: Blood and fluid replacement in shock, in Walt AJ (ed): *Early Care of the Injured Patient,* 3d ed. Philadelphia, Saunders, 1982, p 22.
47. Storb R, Thomas ED, Buckner CD et al: Marrow transplantation in thirty "untransfused" patients with severe aplastic anemia. Ann Intern Med 92:30, 1980.
48. Fisher M, Chapman JR, Ting A et al: Alloimmunization to HLA antigens following transfusion with leukocyte-poor and purified platelet suspensions. Vox Sang 49:331, 1985.
49. Ho WG, Champlin RE, Winston DJ et al: Bone marrow transplantation in patients with leukaemia previously transfused with blood products from family members. Br J Haematol 67:67, 1987.
50. Storb R, Weiden PL: Transfusion problems associated with transplantation. Semin Hematol 18:163, 1981.
51. American Association of Blood Banks: Blood Bank Week 6(10):1, Mar. 10, 1989.
52. American Association of Blood Banks: Blood Bank Week 6(35):6, Sept. 15, 1989.
53. American Association of Blood Banks: Blood Bank Week 6(21):2, May 26, 1989.
54. Menitove JE, McElligott MC, Aster RH: Febrile transfusion reaction: What blood component should be given next? Vox Sang 42:318, 1982.
55. Berney SJ, Metcalfe P, Wathen NC et al: Post-transfusion purpura responding to high dose intravenous IgG: Further observations on pathogenesis. Br J Haematol 61:627, 1985.
56. Council on Scientific Affairs of the American Medical Association: Current status of therapeutic plasmapheresis and related techniques. JAMA 253(6):819, 1985.
57. Introducing the Prosorba Immunoadsorption Treatment Column. Seattle, Imré Corp, 1988.
58. Miescher PA, Jaffe ER, Pinsky CM (eds): Selective removal of plasma components to achieve immune modulation. Semin Hematol 26, No 2, suppl 1, 1989.

SECTION B

MANAGEMENT OF THE INTENSIVE CARE UNIT

Chapter 36

STAFFING AND MANAGEMENT OF THE INTENSIVE CARE UNIT

DAVID D. RALPH
DAYLE HOSEK GLEASON

Delivery of high-quality critical care to patients requires bringing together a variety of highly trained personnel and providing them with the physical facilities, equipment, and organizational structure that will enable them to operate effectively.

There are many different ways of organizing and staffing critical care units. Some hospitals have individual critical care units for specific services, e.g., cardiac, respiratory, surgery, or neurosurgery. Other hospitals have general intensive care units or intensive care units that combine two or more services, e.g., cardiology and cardiac surgery. The organization that works best for a hospital will depend on the individual needs of that hospital and its clients. In this chapter we will emphasize what factors need to be considered in managing intensive care units, rather than offering a specific plan of organization of the units. We will consider the purpose of the intensive care unit, the personnel who staff the intensive care units, optimizing interactions between nurses and physicians, policy development, the relationship of the intensive care unit with hospital administration and other services, and development of new programs. Other important aspects, including the physical plant, computer applications, and quality assurance are considered in detail in Chap. 40, 41, and 42 and will be only briefly mentioned here.

All critical care units are not created equal. The quality of an intensive care unit is not determined just by the age of the physical plant, the level of technology available, or the years of education or number of advanced certifications held by the staff. A critical care unit is first and foremost a team. It is the effectivensss of the teamwork which determines if a unit is mediocre even with superb assets or superb even though resources are limited.[1] In better critical care units leaders will seek to enhance the skill, communication, and coordination that engender greatness in any team regardless of the setting or industry. The responsibility of those who participate in the administration of critical care units is to create an environment in which personnel can properly apply their expertise, compassion, and enthusiasm to improve the clinical status of patients. Ineffective management can lead to poor organization, lack of essential facilities and supplies, poor planning of new programs, and lack of staff motivation and satisfaction. On the other hand, overmanagement or micromanagement can lead to demoralization and excessive inefficiencies and costs in patient care.[2]

Purpose of the Intensive Care Unit

The primary purpose of a critical care unit is to provide exemplary intensive medical and nursing care for critically ill patients who require life-supporting services. Certain hospitals will also have as additional important goals the teaching of nurses, physicians, or other personnel. Other hospitals will include clinical research as part of the purpose of the intensive care unit. In any case, it is important to first consider what kind of patients will be admitted to the intensive care unit and what kinds of patients will be routinely excluded (see Chap. 46). Patients should be specifically excluded when they have diagnoses for which physician or nursing expertise is not available in the hospital. They should also be excluded if special procedures such as extracorporeal membrane oxygenation (ECMO) are needed but are not available. It is important that reasons for exclusion be determined in advance so that patients are not inappropriately admitted to an intensive care unit that does not have the facilities and expertise to care for them. The unit must have predetermined procedures for referring or transferring such patients elsewhere.

Special functions must also be assumed by the intensive care unit when other hospital areas are understaffed or overwhelmed. Some intensive care units are used at times as surgical recovery areas. Others provide temporary holding areas for emergency department patients who are waiting for admission to the general wards of the hospital. Intensive care units are sometimes used as temporary placement areas for patients who require procedures such as cardioversion. Intensive care unit personnel may go to other areas of the hospital for purposes such as supporting the care of unstable patients in a cardiac catheterization laboratory or responding to cardiac arrests elsewhere in the hospital. Practice standards in these situations must be uniform for all critical care patients and all procedures. Patient admission criteria need to be defined in advance as do the circumstances in which intensive care personnel will leave the intensive care unit to support other hospital functions. The purpose of the unit, the admission criteria, the responsibilities of the personnel, and the standards of care adopted all help determine what staffing is needed.

Exceptions to general admitting and staffing policies are indicated occasionally but should be carefully monitored. For example, deploying highly trained critical care nurses to general nursing wards can be demotivating, while sharing between intensive care units with different orientations can be educational and exhilarating. Similarly, in times of bed shortage, admitting a patient with a critical medical illness to a surgical unit (or vice versa) can promote good interdepartmental critical care. On the other hand, abrupt early transfer of such a patient to the "correct" unit as soon as a bed becomes available is often inefficient and exasperating to the patient and nursing staff.[3]

Personnel

The fundamental patient care relationship in a critical care unit is the triangle of patient, physician, and nurse with the central focus on improving the health of the patient. Although there are many people contributing specialized functions to the critical care team, only the physician and the nurse have overall patient care responsibility across all functions. Another group of health care professionals, the respiratory therapists, plays a significant role on the critical care team in many units (see Chap. 38). The effectiveness of the unit is measured and evaluated in terms of the quality and cost effectiveness of patient care and the intangible feelings of satisfaction by the patient, family, and the primary care personnel. Too little or inappropriate care compromises the physical health of the patient; excess or unnecessary care compromises the fiscal health of the patient and the hospital. Active and personal communication, cooperation, teamwork, and organizational pride exhibited in the critical care unit are significant indicators of unit effectiveness.

The personnel who work in an intensive care unit must be well trained. Their level of training must be adequately documented for monitoring agencies. Managers of the intensive care unit are responsible for coordinating the activities of physicians, nurses, and a variety of therapists, technicians, and other support personnel. The success of this coordination will in large part determine the quality of the intensive care unit. Patients rate the quality of their care based upon assessment of the care delivered by physicians, nurses, and all other personnel, so attention to all participants in unit life by unit managers improves the patients' perceptions of the care.

PHYSICIANS

MEDICAL DIRECTOR

The physician medical director will often be the person ultimately responsible for management of the intensive care unit. In other hospitals a partnership model exists which includes an administrative or nursing manager who is at a management level equal with that of the medical director. The director needs to set general policies, principles, and decision criteria for the intensive care unit but must also be able to react quickly to the special situations which often arise in intensive care units. The medical director must be responsible 24 hours a day to respond to situations where there is a question about the quality of medical care being delivered. Although ensuring the quality of care delivered to individual patients is always the major task of the medical director, it is also extremely important to ensure that the hospital personnel who work in the intensive care unit are adequately supported and enthusiastic. It is clear that having an experienced staff leads to earlier identification of clinical complications, faster and more appropriate treatment of these complications, and greater job satisfaction.

The medical director, in conjunction with hospital administration, should determine the training and credentials required before physicians are allowed to admit patients to the intensive care unit. It is also the medical director's responsibility to ensure that physicians who perform procedures such as central line insertion in the intensive care unit have adequate training. The medical director should also define policies for required continuing medical education for physicians who practice in the intensive care unit.

ATTENDING PHYSICIANS

In some hospitals, all physicians with admitting privileges to the hospital will be able to admit to the intensive care unit. In other hospitals physicians who are able to admit to the intensive care unit are chosen based upon their training and expertise in delivering intensive care. In any case, the role and responsibilities of the primary attending physicians need to be described. The admitting physician should be expected to examine the patient and write an initial history and physical in the chart within a defined period after the patient's admission to the hospital. If initial orders are given verbally, they should be countersigned as soon as possible. Subsequent orders should be initially written whenever possible or, if given by telephone, signed the next time the physician sees the patient. Daily progress notes should be required and discharge summaries promptly dictated. Since many patients in the intensive care unit will have multisystem disease, general criteria should exist for determining when a consultant should be called. The medical director should have the authority to intervene if consultation appears necessary but has not been ordered by the attending physician. The attending physician should be expected to have regular meetings with patients' families. A cross-coverage physician must be clearly identified in advance to the nursing staff at times when the primary physician is not on call. Similarly, if an attending physician is outside the hospital and cannot respond immediately to an emergency situation, it is imperative that a mechanism has been established to determine which physician will respond and be in charge of the case until the regular attending physician can respond. Delays in responding to pages caused by confusion about which physician is responsible for the patient and difficulties in contacting the attending physician cannot be tolerated.

CONSULTANT PHYSICIANS

The complexities of modern intensive care mean that most patients will have one or more consultations while in an intensive care unit. Consultants should be expected to respond in a timely manner when requested by the attending physician. When patients are comanaged by the regular attending physician and a consultant, the division of responsibilities must be clear to the nursing staff. For example, it must be clear whether both the attending physician and the consultant will be writing orders. The consultant should be expected to write prompt initial consultation notes and regular follow-up notes. Consultants should document in the chart any procedures performed.

HOUSE STAFF AND STUDENTS

It is extremely important that intensive care units in teaching hospitals have a clear definition for the role of house staff physicians. If a clinical service has several patients in an intensive care unit, it is usually more efficient to have residents and fellows assigned to that service for the intensive care unit only. This allows the physicians to be more available to the patients and enables the nursing staff to interact with a smaller number of physicians, thus fostering teamwork and effective and timely communication. It also allows teaching to be more efficiently organized and directed toward intensive care problems. Because of the complexity and acuity of intensive care patients, medical students should participate in their care only when directly supervised by residents, fellows, or attending physicians. It is inappropriate for medical students to write the progress notes on these patients unless their notes are carefully and promptly reviewed.

NURSING

This section provides the job descriptions of critical care nursing personnel, emphasizing their roles as participating members of the critical care team. A more complete description of critical care nursing is presented in the next chapter (see Chap. 37).

STAFF NURSES

As the physician is the medical expert, responsible for the assessment and medical management of patient care, the nurse is the bedside provider who administers most of the care. A skilled nurse is a sensitive, caring person who quickly makes both clinically competent and cost-effective decisions daily for and with the patient. Most knowledgeable about the patient's current condition and recent changes, staff nurses have 24-hour responsibility for providing and coordinating care for the patient. They have the primary role for monitoring the changing clinical, physiologic and psychosocial status of the patient and communicating to the physician and other team members necessary information in a timely manner. Other responsibilities include identification of the need for psychosocial interventions for patients and families and initiation and evaluation of actions.

Nursing staff are integral members of the health care team and as such they function independently, interdependently, and dependently in providing care to patients and families. They are the interface between the physician team and the organization and the patient/family group and the organization. They plan, direct, provide, and evaluate interventions in an effort to maximize patient outcomes during an era in which the ever shortening length of hospital stay requires rapid assessment and decision making.

Unlike the physician who is usually an independent practitioner, the nurse is the agent of the hospital organization. The nurse has a responsibility to the patient and physician and to the organization. Although the task skills and patient care decisions of the individual staff nurse determine the quality of care for their patients on each shift, the quality of care also depends heavily on the effectiveness and efficiency of the nurse-physician team and the hospital organization. A well-managed nursing organization is essential to the effective operation of a critical care unit. There are different roles within the organization which are provided by nursing personnel. These nursing roles determine the availability and effectiveness of the individual nursing care. Decisions relating to any specific patient should be discussed with the patient's primary nurse.

CHARGE NURSES

Although the staff nurse is responsible for the clinical and cost decisions associated with an assigned patient or patients, individual patients have different needs and individual nurses have different skills and abilities. The charge nurse on each shift has the responsibility to allocate limited nursing resources to match patient needs with available nursing skills in a safe and cost-effective manner. When bed capacity becomes limited, it is the responsibility of the charge nurse to communicate with the appropriate nurses and physicians to determine if a current intensive care patient may be transferred to make a critical care bed available to a more critically ill patient. While the staff nurse makes decisions at the patient level, the charge nurse makes organizational decisions which have a significant impact on the availability, quality, and cost of nursing care. Since staff nurses and charge nurses make different types of decisions, charge nurses should receive additional training prior to holding this responsibility.

On any given shift, the number of nurses allocated to patient care by the charge nurse depends on actual patient census and acuity for the next shift as well as anticipated needs for the next 24-hour period. Excess nurses are often reassigned to another nursing unit in the hospital, thus utilizing scarce intensive care resources elsewhere, or are required to take a day off. Since nurses from other clinical areas seldom have the skills necessary to function safely in an intensive care unit, there are limited supplemental nurses to cover intensive care shift shortages. Overtime, additional shifts, and nurse registry staff may be utilized with varying effects upon the operational and cost effectiveness of the unit.

NURSE MANAGERS

The next level of decision making tends to be less tangible, occurs over a longer period of time, and addresses issues relating to organizational development and coordination. Nursing managers need to be skilled at selecting team members, creating individualized training, and fostering team building processes. Selection of nursing personnel should be based on how well their clinical and interpersonal skills will complement the existing team. By individualizing formal and informal training, nursing personnel effectiveness is improved. Ad hoc and ongoing communication and team building processes improve coordination, operational effectiveness, and levels of job satisfaction.

The nurse manager is responsible for the operational management of the critical care unit. This includes responsibility for the daily operation of the nursing unit on all three shifts and for coordination and collaboration with the medical staff as well as with other department managers and with the Division of Nursing Administration. The position carries the responsibility and authority to identify and resolve problems affecting the critical care unit both directly and indirectly in all clinical and managerial areas.

NURSING DIRECTOR FOR CRITICAL CARE

The hospital may have a director for critical care in addition to the nursing managers and the physician medical director. The director for critical care provides leadership for managers of all the critical care and related nursing care units in the hospital through the interpretation and implementation of the philosophy, objectives, and policies of the hospital as a whole. The director collaborates with the medical staff, including the medical director and administrative team, in the planning and coordination of patient care programs and facilitates the implementation and evaluation of these programs.

The director and nurse manager are responsible for the nurse-bed capacity, staff availability, unit economics, patient care skills, effective decision criteria, and culture which fosters teamwork and sensitivity. To provide quality patient care, it is necessary to have adequate bed and nursing capacity, availability of nursing resources, technical skills and decision making, and communication and caring sensitivity.

Adequate nurse availability depends on nursing capacity, scheduling, and staffing. Nursing capacity, in terms of having an adequate number of skilled nurses to support available beds, is essential for an effective intensive care unit. Maintaining adequate nursing capacity requires a long-term program based on up-to-date forecasts of patient census and acuity and planning for new programs. Appropriate recruiting, selection, and training by the nurse manager and director determines nursing capacity. If there is inadequate nursing capacity, no unit will be effective. If there is excess nursing capacity, no unit can be cost-effective. Effective allocation of nursing capacity is essential to match varying patient care demands for these skills. Without proper scheduling and staffing, adequate nursing capacity may be inappropriately allocated, thereby limiting nurse availability to match patient demand and cost effectiveness of care. Monitoring patient care and acuity is important for forecasting future demand. Scheduling practices which attempt to match nursing capacity with the variation in forecast demand over a four- to eight-week period are important for cost-effective utilization of nursing resources.

Effective scheduling and staffing requires data collection and interpretation to understand the demand for nursing services by identifying patterns, trends, and variability. Data collection is reduced to key leverage points. Activity and acuity by shift and days of week can be used in a basic analysis. Identification and modification of the controllable aspects of the process will minimize variability of patient care requirements. The allocation of staff must be adjusted to match the uncontrollable but partially predictable demand for patient care.

OTHER NURSING PERSONNEL

Depending on the size of the nursing unit and the number of nursing personnel, there may be other nursing leadership personnel who develop, influence, and support the staff nurse in providing quality cost-effective patient care. Assistant nurse managers are prospective unit managers in training. They have clinical and administrative responsibilities and may serve as resources and role models in dissemination of information and implementation of unit objectives, policy, standards, and staff development.

Clinical nurse specialists, advanced practitioners in an on-line position, are responsible for clinical role modeling for nursing staff. They assist with the clinical development of the staff and standards development and participate in problem identification and resolution on a consultative basis.

Administrative nursing supervisors function both as supervisors of staff and patient care and as the administrative support and resource person to staff throughout the hospital. They focus on the ongoing implementation of the division of nursing, hospital, and unit standards; identification of and communication of problems; and active participation in problem resolution.

OTHER HEALTH CARE PERSONNEL

Important nonnursing personnel include (but are not limited to) respiratory therapists and utilization management/discharge planners. The role of respiratory therapists varies between different hospitals, but generally it is to support the physician-nurse team. Their responsibilities include very active participation in the care of patients on mechanical ventilators, with special attention to the initial intubation and ventilator setup, to chest physiotherapy, to weaning and extubation, and to blood gas and oximetry monitoring. The respiratory therapist is also the expert in troubleshooting the ventilators when mechanical problems occur. It is important that the critical care unit policies make clear the division of patient care responsibilities between the nurses and the respiratory therapists (see Chap. 38).

Utilization management/discharge planners may be social workers or registered nurses who are instrumental in the placement of patients at the time of discharge from the critical care unit. Based on standards from the hospital and on diagnosis-related group data, they review the length of stay of patients, identify outliers, and develop discharge plans in consultation with the physicians and nurses. In many hospitals they also coordinate the care conferences in which the physicians, nurses, and family members participate in planning placement after patient discharge.

Impact of Nursing Shortage

When there is less nursing capacity or coverage than is required, there is a nursing shortage. At times, this condition exists with all intensive care units. In the best units, it is an uncomfortable but temporary condition based on planned risk and resources to provide cost-effective quality patient care. On poorly managed units, the nursing shortage is pronounced, protracted, and the result of dramatically changing conditions, poor planning, or weak organization or leadership. The national demand for intensive care nurses already exceeds the supply. As career options for women continue to expand, the competition to attract skilled nurses will further intensify. Nursing leaders who are most effective at building teams with a reputation for sensitive, high-quality, and cost-effective patient care and who foster a positive unit culture will ensure the nursing shortage is more likely to happen to another critical care unit. These leaders will be proactive in anticipating and preventing staffing and operational problems before they occur. They will continually strive for performance improvement which boosts team pride. They foster a work climate which is attractive to prospective employees and encourages current employees to stay.

In some situations and for a variety of reasons, an inadequate supply of competent, qualified registered nurses will exist. An organization may choose to reduce the financial resources available to a nursing unit as revenues become more and more limited. Other means of staffing an intensive care unit must be established to continue to meet the goals of the unit. At this time, the staffing configuration may be changed such that some of the tasks traditionally performed by registered nurses are now delegated to and performed by other personnel. In this environment, the registered nurse reduces the range of functions to those requiring registered nurse training and licensure. Other specialized skills and tasks may be performed by ancillary personnel such as cardiac monitoring technicians who are trained in arrhythmia analysis and are responsible for observing and identifying abnormal rhythms and notifying nursing personnel; hospital assistants or technicians who provide nursing personnel with equipment and supply support; and licensed practical nurses, graduates of a one-year nursing program, who perform delegated patient care tasks under the supervision of the registered nurse.

The quantity, quality, and timeliness of the individual nursing tasks determine the quality and cost of nursing care received and perceived by the patient. The morale and attitude of nursing personnel are influenced not only by the quality of their work but also by the ability to influence operational processes, the perceived value of the unit culture, and the personnel maintenance activities performed by the unit leadership.[4] Effective unit leaders work to ensure that the following are perceived as important functional goals in the unit: (i) three-way communication, (ii) support, (iii) humor, and (iv) making the unit an enjoyable place to work.

As with other professionals, nursing personnel seek significance and security in their work. Job satisfaction is most positively influenced by the following factors:

1. The nature of work itself must be seen as activity having purpose and value. The matching of personal responsibility and ability to influence the outcome improves individual job satisfaction.
2. Quality supervision maintains unit goal focus and minimizes the frequency and duration of emergent organization and personnel problems.
3. Peer association becomes a significant job satisfaction factor in the selection and retention of personnel. Leaders will select personnel with the necessary skills and values coherent with others in the intensive care unit.
4. Promotion opportunity must be real and visible via a clinical ladder, unit management, or educational pathway.
5. Compensation must be competitive (and be perceived as being competitive) with other health care organizations in the same market and with other professions requiring like academic preparation and experience to continue to maintain job satisfaction and attract adequate numbers of nursing personnel. In situations where compensation and promotion opportunities are less competitive, it is all that much more important for leaders to enhance the perceived value of the less tangible aspects of job satisfaction.

The Nurse-Physician Team

Patients receive optimal care only when their nurses and physicians are aware of the expertise that each other can provide. Informed awareness is often associated with mutual respect, providing an efficient, complementary division of labor. In contrast, lack of this awareness leads to less efficient exchange and utilization of essential diagnostic and management data and is associated with rancor and divisiveness.[5] As previously noted, the critical care nurse monitors the current clinical physiological state of the patient and is in a position to recognize early signs of clinical deterioration. Nurses also have valuable information and insights gained from their bedside presence into the psychological state of the patient and the needs and concerns of the family. The physician's expertise in disease states is the primary determinant of the therapeutic measures initiated. If the physician has had a long-term relationship with the patient, then valuable information will be available regarding the patient's psyche and the family's dynamics.

The simplest, yet most powerful method to assure that nurses and physicians share their expertise is for them to routinely meet before or at the time the physician makes rounds. If the clinical situation is not straightforward, they should review the care plan after examination of the patient and clarify any complex orders. Physicians should be especially alert to identify anything about the care plan that is unusual compared to the typical care given to patients with the same diagnosis. Nothing builds trust and respect between nurses and physicians and other intensive care personnel better than having them struggle together to devise the best way to care for a patient who is in a difficult situation.[6]

Nursing-physician communication is also strengthened by having both groups jointly participate in educational activities, case reviews, and the development of new protocols and new programs.

Development of Policies for the Intensive Care Unit

Intensive care units are required by the Joint Commission on Accreditation of Health Organization (JCAHO) and other federal, state, and local agencies to have a responsible administrative structure. This structure must include representation from the physician staff, nursing staff, and administration of the hospital. The management committee of the intensive care unit should have a clear relationship to the hospital medical staff, hospital nursing staff, and administrative structure of the hospital. It should be clear what the responsibilities and decision-making power of the management committee are. As a minimum the committee should be responsible for reviewing recurrent problems in the day-to-day operations of the unit, approving internal intensive care unit policies, and advising the hospital on policies which involve the relationship of the intensive care unit to other hospital departments. Committee members should be close enough to the daily operations of the clinical care in the intensive care unit to be aware of what is needed to improve patient care at the bedside.

Intensive care unit internal policies should address the following issues:

ADMISSION AND DISCHARGE CRITERIA

It is important to have criteria for which patients will require admission to the intensive care unit. These policies need to take into account the acuity of the patient's illness, the level of nursing expertise needed to care for the patient safely, and the need for ventilator management or other procedures that would automatically require intensive care unit management. A mechanism must also always exist where physicians and nurses from the intensive care unit can make on-the-spot decisions in borderline or controversial situations. For example, what will the intensive care unit do if all the beds are full but an additional patient needs admission? Will an existing intensive care unit patient be automatically discharged or transferred or will the admission be referred to another facility? Criteria for discharge also need to be established so that intensive care unit services will not be inappropriately extended too long to patients who no longer require or will benefit from them. A system for triage must be available for application when there is excessive demand for intensive care unit facilities. This should be the responsibility of both the medical director and the nursing director or their representatives.

STANDING ORDERS

It is essential that the intensive care unit have standing orders to cover matters such as drugs to be administered during cardiopulmonary resuscitation (CPR), vital signs, routine frequency of recording data from pulmonary artery catheters and other monitoring devices, routine protocols for care of intravascular catheters, ranges of abnormal laboratory values which must be immediately reported to the physician, etc. Formulating the standing orders for these situations will make patient care more uniform and will decrease the need for additional written orders.

STANDARDS FOR PHYSIOLOGICAL MONITORING

Standards need to be developed for calibration of equipment, e.g., pressure transducers, and for the frequency of quality checks and the frequency with which the data they provide will be recorded in the chart.

QUALITY ASSURANCE AND QUALITY IMPROVEMENT

Quality assurance is considered in detail in Chap. 42. The challenge to intensive care management is to develop a quality assurance program that will actually make a difference in the quality of care delivered yet be efficient and meet JCAHO standards.

IDENTIFICATION AND SOLVING OF PROBLEMS

One of the most important activities of the intensive care unit administrative team is to develop mechanisms which allow problems to be identified, either at the bedside in the day-to-day management of patients or by review of statistics on morbidity/mortality and patient outcome. Most of the inadequacies or inefficiencies in patient care are best identified by those who work at the bedside. For example, a delay in delivery of medications from the pharmacy is immediately obvious to the bedside nurse. The intensive care unit needs to have a system whereby nurses and physicians can note these problems for review by the management team. The task of the management team then is to prioritize the problems, suggest solutions, and communicate with other hospital departments as needed to solve them. Progress in addressing these problems can be monitored by the overall unit quality assurance plan.

ETHICS

Although ethical considerations have always been important in intensive care medicine, the evolution of intensive care over the past several years has seen more emphasis on an organized approach involving guidelines for ethical issues. This should be coordinated with the hospital's general policies on ethics, but many of the issues such as prolongation of mechanical support, do-not-resuscitate policies, and issues of patient competence are magnified in the intensive care unit setting. It is extremely important that the intensive care unit have policies regarding ethics and have mechanisms for resolution of the conflicts which inevitably arise in complicated situations among patients, their families, and hospital personnel as well as those between hospital personnel.

DISASTER PLANS

A major disaster will place great stress upon an intensive care unit. An intensive care unit disaster plan must be coordinated with the hospital and community disaster plan and consider the mechanism for triaging those patients who will be admitted to the intensive care unit, triaging those patients who no longer need intensive care, calling in additional hospital personnel to care for patients, and potentially changing the level of care given to patients. During a disaster situation the intensive care unit may temporarily admit patients it would not otherwise take. For example, burn patients may be admitted to intensive care units for stabilization before being transferred to a distant burn facility. These special situations should be anticipated, and adequate supplies available for responding to them should be provided. Any disaster will require on-the-spot decisions to be made by the medical and nursing directors to best utilize intensive care unit resources.

EDUCATION

Continuing education should be expected for physicians, nurses, and therapists who work in an intensive care unit. It is best if the hospital provides this as part of its ongoing activities. Educational forums can provide a major mechanism for increasing the morale as well as the knowledge and teamwork of intensive care unit personnel. A quality continuing education program should increase retention of personnel.

RESEARCH

In intensive care units where clinical research occurs, it is extremely important that the research not interfere with patient care. Quality research should be encouraged. In addition to being approved by the hospital's human subjects committee, research protocols should be reviewed by the intensive care committee so that the impact on patient care can be considered. Research protocols frequently involve extra observations and recording activities as well as interventions. If these are to be done by clinical nurses, the impact on the hours of care required for the patients should be considered in advance by the intensive care committee so that these activities will not detract from patient care (see Chap. 188).

Relationship of the Intensive Care Unit to Other Hospital Services and to Hospital Administration

Just as it is important that there be clear reporting lines and clear responsibilities within the intensive care unit, it is equally important that the relationship of the intensive care unit management be clearly delineated with respect to the hospital administration, the hospital medical administration, and the hospital nursing administration. Intensive care unit management should be proactive and anticipate future needs such as the need for additional beds, new services, or the expansion of current services. Excessive duplication of responsibilities between various hospital departments can easily create a situation in which nobody is really responsible for the efficiency or quality of services.

The relationship between the intensive care unit and the emergency department is especially important. Since the timing of admissions from the emergency department cannot be easily anticipated, the intensive care unit needs to have mechanisms for calling in additional staff for new admissions when needed. The ability of emergency departments to hold patients for periods of time varies widely depending on their abilities and staffing. Accordingly, the flexibility of the intensive care unit in taking admissions through the emergency department needs to be well coordinated with the emergency department's facilities and needs. Admissions from the operating rooms are generally easier to anticipate because these patients can be identified prior to going to surgery. However, the intensive care unit still needs to maintain some flexibility to accommodate unanticipated admissions from the operating areas.

Hospital diagnostic areas such as radiology and cardiac catheterization laboratories raise special problems. Some intensive care units send nurses to accompany unstable patients who need to have procedures done in these areas. Other hospitals are organized with nurses in the radiology and catheterization laboratories who will care for these patients while they are there. In the latter case it is important that intensive care nurses properly communicate with the nurses in the diagnostic areas about patient condition and needs. When intensive care nurses do travel out of the intensive care unit, the flexibility of the unit is decreased. Accordingly, the timing of diagnostic procedures should ideally be coordinated so as to have a minimum impact on the intensive care unit nursing while also facilitating the efficient functioning of these diagnostic areas. Protocols that identify which department will provide emergency drugs, monitoring equipment, and resuscitation equipment for patients during transportation between departments should be established as well. The status of a patient vis-à-vis cardiopulmonary resuscitation has to be clearly identified during transportation (see Chap. 48).

A system should be established whereby transportation of clinical specimens to the clinical laboratories is prompt and does not require highly trained personnel. In addition, reports from the laboratory need to be noted and received in a timely manner that minimizes delays and maximizes clarity. The intensive care unit and pharmacy need to work out protocols so it is clear which medicines are immediately available in the intensive care unit and which must be obtained from the pharmacy. As part of this, the intensive care unit personnel need to know how to obtain special medications only occasionally required, such as unusual antidotes or digitalis antibodies.

As the bed occupancy grows in hospitals, it becomes all the more important that coordination of discharges from the intensive care unit to the hospital wards be carefully monitored so that beds become available in a timely manner. One mechanism to assist in this coordination is to have a meeting shortly after the start of each nursing shift between the charge nurses for the intensive care unit and the nursing wards to which intensive care patients are discharged. This meeting also serves to identify patients on the ward who are deteriorating and may possibly need intensive care nursing later.

A dedicated telephone line for discussing transfer of patients into the unit can be used for accepting unscheduled admissions. Any physician desiring to transfer a patient can thus be immediately placed in contact with the charge nurse who best knows the availability of beds and nurses to care for the potential admission. If there is any question about the appropriateness of the admission or difficulty in accepting the patient for admission, the nurse will notify the medical director, who can then talk to the referring physician. This mechanism decreases the number of inappropriate transfers and the number of phone calls that must be made to ensure acceptance of appropriate transfer admissions.

Initiating New Programs

A new program can be regarded as something as simple as a variation on a type of surgery that has previously been performed in the hospital but where the variation will require different postoperative care. This requires advance education of the nursing staff, evaluation of the required intensity of nursing, and proper planning so that the appropriate resources and supplies are available. A major new program, such as organ transplantation, requires a much more extensive evaluation before it is started, but the principles for planning which are followed are the same as for small programs. Appropriate intensive care and hospital personnel need to evaluate the proposed program for its impact in several areas. These include the need for additional personnel, the need for additional or expanded educational programs, access to supplies, alterations in the physical plant, coordination with other hospital departments, and an assessment of any adverse impact on other ongoing hospital programs. Advice and input should be sought from any department or staff who would participate in or be affected by the program change. Resistance to change can always be expected, but the reasons for any resistance should be dissected to separate valid from invalid concerns. Frequently it is wise to review with other hospitals which have similar programs what resources are realistically required and what the impact has been on the intensive care unit.

As medical advances continue to be introduced at a rapid pace and as patterns of hospital care are constantly altered by nonclinical factors such as patterns of funding and the requirements of regulatory agencies, planning for new programs and changing current programs has to be thought of as an ongoing activity in the intensive care unit rather than as an intermittent activity. In this way the intensive care managers will better smooth the difficulties inherent in managing change.

References

1. Lynch BL: Team building: Will it work in health care? J Allied Health 10:240, 1981.
2. Herzberg F: One more time: How do you motivate employees? in Harvard Business Review on Management. New York, Harper & Row, 1975, p 372.
3. Allen M, Jackson D, Younger S: Closing the communication gap between physicians and nurses in the intensive care setting. Heart Lung 9:836, 1980.
4. Dear MR, Weisman CS, Alexander CC, et al: The effect of the intensive care nursing role on job satisfaction and turnover. Heart Lung 11:561, 1982.
5. Altschul A: With all due respect . . . Interprofessional relations. Nursing Mirror 157:20, 1983.
6. Mausch IG: Nurse-physician collaboration: A changing relationship. J Nurs Admin 11:35, 1981.

Chapter 37

CRITICAL CARE NURSING MANAGEMENT

PAMELA H. MITCHELL

"Formal training in medicine and nursing is concerned with the art and science of healing, not with its administration. Yet it is the latter that places the greatest demands on the clinician's time."*

The high degree of expertise and coordination required in modern critical care places some amount of nonclinical managerial responsibility on nearly every professional participant. Although formal responsibility for administrative management of the unit rests with the designated nursing and medical directors and managers, achievement of the highest degree of clinical coordination and skills increasingly rests on an understanding of principles of modern management by all critical care professionals. Further, there is increasing evidence that effective clinical practice requires a base of effective administrative practice.

Therefore, this chapter is written for critical care clinicians as well as administrators and managers. Management is presented as a practice intended to create organizational environments that foster optimal clinical care. Components of effectively managed units will be described, along with evidence linking these components to optimal patient care outcomes. Though the subject of this chapter is critical care nursing management, the principles are applicable and relevant to all professional disciplines that provide care to critically ill patients.

Management: Creation of Environments for Optimal Patient Care

In the not too distant past, the hospital, like industry, operated as a mechanical bureaucracy, with management considered a means to control the work and the workers. Although this management style was well suited for efficiently accomplishing routine work by relatively unskilled workers, patient care in acute hospitals did not remain either routine or unskilled. During the past 10 to 15 years, hospitals have been joining industry in instituting new forms of organization and management for complex and dynamic organizations, recognizing the crucial role of participation and joint management by staff and administrators. In this new environment, managers are not controllers and supervisors; rather they are facilitators and enablers. In the case of hospital care, the work of clinical staff is to manage the patient care, whereas the work of managers and administrators is to create an organizational environment that supports excellent clinical care.

This approach to management suggests there are at least two kinds of environments in critical care: clinical environments and organizational environments. The clinical environment is comprised of the physical environment and the interpersonal environment for patient care. Components of the physical environment are discussed in Chap. 40. The interpersonal environment is comprised of the clinicians providing direct care, other professionals who move in and out of the direct care-giving arena, and the patients' families and significant others. Management of the clinical environment is the direct responsibility of the various professionals involved in care of the critically ill patient. Most often the nursing staff coordinates this level of management, either by default or by design.

Organizational environments are both external and internal. The external environments are many and include such factors as economic conditions, competition in the larger hospital industry, human and financial resources available, governmental factors such as regulation, and the sociopolitical environment of local, regional, and national health care.

Internally, the hospital organization can be thought of as an environment for patient care units. There is evidence that the nature of that larger hospital organizational environment measurably influences the care delivered in the clinical environment. Managers directly involved with the delivery of patient care are crucial in mediating the impact of the hospital's internal environment on patient care.

MANAGEMENT OF CRITICAL CARE NURSING STAFF: THE CRUCIAL LINK BETWEEN ORGANIZATION AND PATIENT CARE OUTCOMES

The evidence that organization and management influence patient care comes from various sources—general hospital literature, popular management literature, and a smaller portion from investigations in critical care units.

For the most part, surveys of highly regarded hospitals and businesses have identified consistent beliefs regarding effective hospital environments. The Magnet Hospital study, National Commission on Implementation for Nursing, and variations of the "search for excellence" theme are key examples. However, there has been little rigorous testing of the relationship between these approaches and measures of hospital or critical care unit effectiveness.

Beliefs about what creates an effective nursing environment were explicated in the Magnet Hospital study, conducted by the American Academy of Nursing in 1982.[1] Forty-two hospitals were nominated on the basis of high nursing retention in the midst of an acute nursing shortage, and interviews were conducted with staff and administrative nurses about the characteristics of those hospitals. Several themes were evident, including a high proportion of

*Fein IA, Strosberg MA: *Managing the Critical Care Unit*. Rockville, MD, Aspen, 1987, p xxii.

registered nurses in the nursing staff, decentralized management, participatory management, and professional practice models for nursing. More recently, the National Commission on Nursing Implementation Project[2] conducted extensive hearings and interviews regarding the features of high quality and cost-effective nursing care delivery systems. Similar to the Magnet study, these included positive working relationships among nurses and physicians, systems that obtain and retain competent nurses, and sound financial management and planning.

Other management characteristics were identified in follow-up studies to the Magnet survey.[3,4] Sixteen of the original 42 hospitals were sampled randomly, with more extensive interviews conducted among staff nurses, nursing, and hospital administration. Both low turnover and high nurse satisfaction were again evident, coupled with many features described in America's best run businesses. These features included a bias for action, being close to the consumer, opportunities for autonomy, and entrepreneurship among the staff. Self-governance and participatory management were cited as examples of the principle of productivity through people. Excellence and becoming excellent were considered key values. Few studies have been designed to explicitly test the relationship of these beliefs to measures of clinical effectiveness. Two studies do so in general hospitals and four in critical care.

ORGANIZATION AND PATIENT CARE IN GENERAL HOSPITALS. Large studies of general hospitals in the late 1950s and mid 1970s attempted to determine how aspects of organization and management related to quality of patient care. Georgopoulos and Mann surveyed 12 community general hospitals in Michigan regarding quality of care, measured as the judgments of various professional groups.[5] Both nursing and overall hospital care were judged. These were implicit judgments as no specifications were given to participants regarding what the nature of outstanding to poor quality might be. The investigators concluded that better quality care was correlated with higher proportion of registered nurses, higher nurse:patient ratios, lower nursing absenteeism, better overall organizational coordination (particularly in the nursing department), less intraorganizational strain, and greater shared expectations about the nature of the work among various groups, particularly nurses and physicians. No relationships were found between quality of care and physical facilities or hospital affluence. Although the quality of medical and nursing care were strongly related to one another, only the quality of nursing care was significantly related to perception of overall hospital quality.

The Stanford Health Care Research Group used data from their survey of 1224 hospitals to examine the relationship of aspects of hospital management to outcome in surgical patients.[6] Data were obtained through the chart abstraction services of the Commission on Professional and Hospital Activities (CPHA) for the year 1972. Although numerous variables were analyzed (including the proportion of ICU beds to general beds to represent intensity of treatment), relatively few were significantly associated with the primary outcome measures of risk of death and surgical complications. A greater proportion of salaried (versus privately practicing) physicians was associated with poorer outcomes, whereas a higher nurse:patient ratio, higher proportion of part-time nurses and higher proportion of registered nurses to all nursing staff were all associated with better outcomes.

ORGANIZATIONAL FACTORS AND PATIENT OUTCOMES IN CRITICAL CARE. Several studies have addressed the relationships between clinical outcomes in critical care and organizational factors. One evaluated the impact on quality of care of cost-saving measures instituted in a surgical ICU.[7,8] The ten cost-cutting measures were administratively instituted and can be interpreted as representing a variety of structural and organizational process changes. For example, elimination of standing orders and institution of written guidelines (or protocols) provide for a more discretionary structure, while providing some degree of programmed coordination (organizational process). Formal feedback (process) was another explicit component of the cost-control measures. Laboratory charges and the number of blood-gas tests were significantly lower following the cost-control measures, yet mortality was not significantly different. Since patient severity of illness was equivalent for the two time periods, the authors concluded that quality of care was not adversely affected by measures shown to control costs.

Another study capitalized on the opening of an ICU and a subsequent change in the method of physician staffing from office-based private practitioners to full-time ICU physicians, to evaluate the impact of this structural arrangement on clinical processes and outcomes.[9] Patient data were compared retrospectively for all admissions for the year before and the year following the change in physician staffing. The authors statistically adjusted mortality outcomes to account for differences in severity of illness between the two groups of patients, and concluded that adjusted mortality was less for patients in the year staffed by ICU physicians, and that the decreased mortality was associated with an increased use of ICU-appropriate tests and interventions. They were careful not to suggest a direct causal relationship among the variables. However, they failed to note that the improved outcomes could be explained, or at least influenced, by the increased experience of the staff during year 2 just as much as it was by having full-time ICU physicians.

The landmark study suggesting an important relationship between organizational and management factors and critical care mortality was conducted by the George Washington University ICU Research Group.[10] A qualitative cross-tabulation approach was used to identify critical care unit structure and process factors associated with mortality outcomes in 13 tertiary care hospitals. Structural indicators were based on recommendations of the National Consensus Conference on Critical Care for administrative structure to differentiate levels of critical care units.[11,12] These included indicators of centralization or decentralization of medical decision-making (presence of full-time medical director, 24-h in-unit physician coverage, director versus attending physician control over admission/discharge), nursing expertise (senior nurses designated as charge nurses; nurse:patient ratios) and standardization (provisions for continuing education, formal orientation for nurses, research and training for physicians). Processes included amount and type of treatment and interaction/coordination of medical and nursing staff.

The standardized mortality ratios (SMR) (the ratio of actual to predicted deaths × 100 percent) ranged from 59 percent to 158 percent, with a median of 93 percent. Contrary to the authors' expectations, these ratios did not form a rank order based on the degree of full-time medical administration, teaching/nonteaching hospital status, or intensity of medical therapies. Rather, the only factor that discriminated the high ranking (low SMR) from the low ranking (high SMR) hospitals was the continuity of nursing care, adequacy of nurse staffing and interaction among nurses and physicians. The authors conclude that ". . . a high level of intensive care can be provided by hospitals lacking a full-time, dedicated intensive care physician team if adequate attention is given to unit coordination, especially coordination between nursing and physician staffs."

The American Association of Critical Care Nursing (AACN) Demonstration Project also shed light on the relationship between organization and clinical outcomes through an intensive prospective description of organizational and clinical structure, process, and outcome in a single critical care unit.[13] The authors described the characteristics of this unit to test a general proposition that desirable patient and organizational outcomes should be associated with structure and process attributes that have been proposed in the literature as determinants of those outcomes. Decentralized administration and participatory management (decentralization), high rate of nurse and physician specialty certification, all registered nurse staff (expertise), use of specialty based standards (standardization), and high nurse-physician collaboration (coordination) were all present. Further, organizational and clinical outcomes were as predicted: nurse satisfaction was high, job turnover was low, the SMR was 51 percent, the complication rate was low, and patient satisfaction was high.

Taken together, the critical care and general hospital studies are consistent in the finding that the organization and quality of nursing care, and the coordination of interdisciplinary care at the unit level, is an important factor in patient outcomes. There is also support for the notion that physician-nurse interactions influence patient outcomes. However, the specific organizational and clinical structures and processes that are most important for these desirable outcomes are not entirely clear. Nonetheless, the experiences of critical care clinicians and administrators do provide some guidelines for effective management and day-to-day provision of care.

Components of Effectively Managed Critical Care Units

Organizational contingency theory is a useful way to pull together the components of organizational environments and processes to predict effectiveness. This way of looking at organizations suggests there is no "one best way" to design an organization. Rather, the effectiveness of an organization depends on (or is contingent on) the complexity and stability of the external environment and the technology or type of work to be done.

Van de Ven and colleagues[14,15] have specified three general patterns of structure and process at the work unit level that best fit the nature of the work to be done: systematized, discretionary, and developmental. Routine work in a stable environment (e.g., an industrial assembly line) can be accomplished efficiently and effectively with a highly systematized pattern of work design, in contrast to discretionary and developmental patterns for nonroutine work in more unstable environments.

Hospital nursing, particularly critical care nursing, is characterized by a moderate to high degree of instability of the environment and of the patients cared for, moderate to high uncertainty about the outcomes and processes of care, with little routine care. In the Van de Ven formulation, this combination would call for a discretionary work design, characterized by decentralization of decision-making to the unit level, moderate degree of standardization of care processes (procedures, protocols), high degree of professionalism (standardization of skills), a variety of methods of coordination of work (standardization of skills and procedures, mutual adjustment, formal and informal meetings) and a moderate to low degree of specialization (people understand and can do some of the work of others). This mode of operating specifies formalization of process and procedure and training for those things that are familiar and well understood (e.g., the protocol for a cardiac arrest), but relies on professional judgment and discretion for those things that are not well understood (e.g., monitoring and managing a patient with complex arrhythmias).

The developmental work pattern is called for in situations in which little is known about the technology and the processes, for example, fourth generation computer design. Such situations require a loose structure that promotes considerable interchange and rapid shifts in procedures. The developmental work pattern might be seen in critical care units when pioneering new surgical techniques or mechanical technologies.

Guidelines for Creating Optimal Critical Care Unit Environments

The discretionary nature of critical care unit work design has been implicitly and sometimes explicitly evident in major textbooks and position papers attempting to define standards and guidelines for critical care unit administration. For example, the 1983 NIH Consensus Development Conference Statement on Critical Care Medicine[11] explicitly endorsed the contingent nature of critical care technology and organizational structure: "Any organizational structure must, therefore, match technology with the correct blend of personnel. . . ." With respect to nursing organization, the consensus conferees noted, "Nurses are the key element in critical care. They provide continuity while physicians and other health care professionals come and go. The organizational structure must support rather than detract from this role."

Adoption of discretionary work patterns does not mean everyone does anything they please. It means that those aspects of the work that are well understood are formalized into policies, procedures, and protocols. It means that professional training, staff development, continuing education, and in-service training are used to attain and maintain the high level of technical skill required. In organizational language, this is standardization of skills and replaces close supervision or other means to standardize work. It also means that those doing the work are involved in decision-making not only about the immediate aspects of patient care, but about the formalized policies, procedures, and the like.

The discretionary pattern of work design provides some categories into which we can group key questions that nursing administrators might ask about the functioning of a given critical care unit.

TECHNOLOGY

In organizational theory, technology refers to the means by which inputs are transformed to outputs.[16] In critical care, the inputs are actual or potentially unstable and critically ill patients. Outputs are the patient's state of health at discharge from the unit, hopefully more stable or in better health, while the means of transformation include not only the technologic monitoring and therapeutic instruments but also the judgments and skills of critical care personnel. Therefore, key questions about technology have to do with the nature of the patients as well as the nature of the work being done.[17]

- Why are patients admitted to this critical care unit? What is the mix of those who need active intervention and those admitted for close monitoring only?
- What proportion of patients have high nursing dependency requirements in addition to or in place of requirements for active medical intervention?
- Do the patient classification data used measure all dimensions: physiologic instability, nursing dependency, active medical interventions?
- Are there clear admission and discharge policies with joint medical and nursing input on individual admission/discharge decisions?
- Is there an adequate mechanism to adjust staffing based on patient acuity?
- What is the skill mix of personnel (education, certification, experience, specific critical care training)?

STRUCTURE OF NURSING MANAGEMENT SYSTEM

Similarly, a number of key questions guide nursing management to determine the level of expertise necessary, the degree of decentralization that is desirable, standardization of procedures, and means of feedback.

- What are the means for recruiting experienced staff, for maintaining skills, for training for new skills?
- To what extent are administrative and clinical decision-making delegated to the unit level?
- Are nursing and medical administrators allowed full authority and responsibility for decisions within their spheres of influence and competence?
- When participatory management by staff is present (e.g., self-staffing, shared governance), is appropriate skill training made available?
- Are there policies, procedures, and protocols for the well-understood aspects of critical care? Are these readily available to staff? Are they used when staff are in an unfamiliar situation?
- Are new technologies and procedures developed by those directly involved in their use?
- Are there general and individualized standards of nursing care?
- Are multiple means of work coordination used (formal and informal verbal and written communication, mutual adjustment, in-service training, professional development, for example)?
- Is collaboration evident among nurses, physicians, and other critical care professionals? Is there a mechanism to promote active collaboration?
- Are multiple means used for conflict resolution? Are direct, constructive methods preferred over indirect and destructive means?
- What formal mechanisms exist for feedback about organizational and clinical functioning?
- Do the professional staff judge the unit to be effective?
- Do all relevant critical care professionals sit on quality assurance committees?
- What quality assurance data are gathered? Are mortality, morbidity, untoward incidents, patient and family satisfaction routinely monitored?
- Are changes in administrative or clinical practice made based on the feedback?

These questions and their answers form a basis for critical care nursing management intended to create organizational environments that foster optimal clinical care. Growing evidence indicates that organization and management structures and processes directly influence patient care outcomes. The critical care and general hospital studies are consistent in their findings that the organization and quality of nursing care and the coordination of interdisciplinary care at the unit level are important factors in patient outcomes. There is also support for the importance of physician-nurse interactions in mediating the impact on patient outcomes.

References

1. Task Force on Nursing Practice in Hospitals: Magnet Hospitals: Attraction and Retention of Professional Nurses. Kansas City, MO, American Academy of Nursing, 1983.
2. National Commission on Nursing Implementation Project. Report of Work Group II: Management of practice. Milwaukee, NCNIP, 1987.
3. Peters TJ, Waterman RH: *In Search of Excellence.* New York, Warner Books, 1982.
4. Kramer M, Schmalenberg C: Magnet hospitals: Institutions of excellence. JONA 18(1):13 (Part 1); 18(2):11 (Part 2), 1988.
5. Georgopoulos BS, Mann FC: *The Community General Hospital.* New York, MacMillan, 1962.
6. Flood A, Scott WR, Ewy W: Hospital characteristics and hospital performance, in Flood AB, Scott WR (eds): *Hospital Structure and Performance.* Baltimore, Johns Hopkins University Press, 1987, pp 311–342.
7. Civetta JM, Hudson-Civetta JA: Maintaining quality of care while reducing charges in the ICU. Ann Surg 202:524, 1985.
8. Hudson-Civetta JA, Civetta JM, Weppler D, Dorotea M: Improved nursing efficiency and productivity. Crit Care Med 15:351, 1987.
9. Li TCM, Phillips MC, Shaw L, et al: On-site physician staffing in a community hospital intensive care unit. JAMA 252:2023, 1984.
10. Knaus WA, Draper EA, Wagner DP, Zimmerman JE: An evaluation of outcome from intensive care in major medical centers. Ann Intern Med 104:410, 1986.
11. National Institutes of Health Consensus Development Conference: Critical care medicine. JAMA 250:798, 1983.
12. Parillo JE, Ayres SM: *Major Issues in Critical Care Medicine.* Baltimore, Williams & Wilkins, 1984.
13. Mitchell PH, Armstrong S, Simpson TF, Lentz M: AACN demonstration project: Profile of excellence in critical care nursing. Heart Lung 18:217, 1989.
14. Van de Ven AH: A framework for organizational assessment. Acad Manag Rev 1(1):64, 1976.
15. Van de Ven AH, Drazin R: The concept of fit in contingency theory. Res Org Behav 7:333, 1983.
16. Perrow C: *Complex Organizations: A Critical Essay.* 3d ed. New York, Random House, 1986, pp 140–156.
17. Leatt P, Schneck R: Nursing subunit technology: A replication. Admin Sci Q 26:225, 1981.

Additional Reading

Adler DC, Shoemaker NJ: *AACN Organization and Management of Critical-Care Facilities.* St. Louis, Mosby, 1979.

American Association of Critical-Care Nurses and Society for Critical Care Medicine: Position Statement. Collaborative practice model: The organization of human resources in critical care units. Newport Beach, CA, AACN, 1983.

American Association of Critical-Care Nurses: Position Statement. Use of technical personnel in critical care settings. Newport Beach, CA, AACN, 1984.

American Association of Critical-Care Nurses: Position Statement. Role expectations for the critical care manager. Newport Beach, CA, AACN, 1986.

American Association of Critical-Care Nurses: Position Statement: Guidelines for admission/discharge criteria in critical care. Newport Beach, CA, AACN, 1987.

Committee on Trauma of the American College of Surgeons: Hospital and prehospital resources for optimal care of the injured patient. Appendix A: Qualifications of trauma-care personnel. ACS Bull 71(10):4, 1986.

Mintzberg H: *Structure in Fives: Designing Effective Organizations.* Englewood Cliffs, NJ, Prentice-Hall, 1983.

Mudd DL: Monitoring productivity and quality indicators in a critical care setting. Nurs Manag 19(10):96A, 1988.

Shortell SM, Kaluzny AD: *Health Care Management: A Text in Organizational Theory and Behavior.* 2d ed. New York, Wiley, 1988.

Spicer JG, Robinson M (eds): *Managing the Environment in Critical Care Nursing.* Baltimore, Williams & Wilkins, 1990.

Stahl LD: Demystifying critical care management. JONA 15(10):27 (Part 1), 15(11), 14 (Part 2), 1985.

Task Force on Guidelines, Society of Critical Care Medicine: Recommendations for services and personnel for delivery of care in a critical care setting. Crit Care Med 16(8):809, 1988.

Chapter 38

CRITICAL CARE MANAGEMENT: THE RESPIRATORY CARE COMPONENT

JOHN S. CAPPS

The critical care setting has become the primary site for management of respiratory care services in most large medical centers. The demand for skilled direction of this service is apparent in three areas of emphasis: quality management, resource management, and information management. Resource management is closest to the focus of classical management theory, but the contribution of respiratory care practitioners to the treatment of seriously ill patients depends on effective management of all three.

These charges for management will not be well-coordinated or administered unless management begins by working to build or join a cohesive critical care team. Respiratory care practitioners are legitimate members of the team comprised of medical staff, nursing staff, and specialty staff who provide threshold-to-threshold care for the critically ill. To effect this level of critical care, management must make a conscious effort to establish mutual respect among team members, assist and defer to each other appropriately, and plan patient care jointly through rounds, conferences, and day-to-day contact. Once the team concept is established, important associations which advance the management of quality, resources, and information are also facilitated.

Quality Management

In all direct patient care, quality delivered and quality perceived do not necessarily coincide. Delivery of quality respiratory care to the critically ill depends on technical quality—the effective, reliable completion of physician orders. Perception of quality—by the physician, the patient, the patient's family—depends on coordination, promptness, and satisfaction.[1] Not only is quality assurance of both aspects desirable, but continuous quality improvement is recommended.[2,3]

The quality delivered by respiratory care services in the critical care unit begins with the knowledge base, skills, and training of the practitioners. At point of entry, new employees or those newly entering critical care can be given practical or written tests to determine their preparedness. Testing, a management option, is not a substitute for careful observation by preceptors during the orientation period. Documentation of critical care orientation should be specific, detailed, dated, and initialed by orientor and orientee. Orientation of new employees assesses and augments the employees' knowledge in several areas: basic physiology, pathophysiology, respiratory equipment, techniques, and response to emergencies and unusual situations. Emphasis should be placed on knowledge of problems and responses most often encountered in the particular institution. For example, trauma centers typically encounter large numbers of head injured and cervical spine injured patients. As part of orientation, new therapists need to review levels of dysfunction associated with injuries to the spine at different levels and current respiratory management techniques used in the patient with recent closed head injury and with increased intracranial pressure. In this way, orientation is the time to correct deficient areas of knowledge, build skilled responses into personnel before they are required to operate independently, and to document this process.

Quality delivery problems can often be traced and corrected by referring to this documentation. Scoring to rate performance during orientation is used in some institutions.[4,5] To deliver quality respiratory care in critical care units where mistakes can literally be fatal, these or other methods must be used to exclude inadequate performers whenever standards are not met.

Standards for respiratory care have historically been developed by individual institutions. In 1990, the Society of Critical Care Medicine published specific recommendations for standards for the care of patients with acute respiratory failure on mechanical ventilatory support.[6] These recommendations detail the services, equipment, monitored variables, airway management techniques, ventilatory support techniques, and guidelines for removal of ventilatory support that should be considered part of the minimum knowledge base for respiratory care practitioners working in critical care settings.

Ongoing staff education is one means of maintaining the quality of the service delivered. New techniques, monitoring devices, research results, and therapeutic advances, as well as periodic reviews of the most demanding services, need ongoing attention. Staff input is the best method of pinpointing specific needs; top-down decisions about educational needs often miss the most important topics. Educational resource people within a department include the manager, medical director, a designated education coordinator (perhaps an assistant manager or supervisor), and motivated staff members who are expert in a particular aspect of care. Other medical staff participants depend on the size and type of institution. The medical director, by the Joint Commission on Accreditation of Healthcare Organizations (JCAHO) standards, always participates; attending physicians, fellows, and house staff, as they are available, are used.[7]

Quality assurance is a formalized process that requires establishment of indicators, thresholds for review, methods for collecting performance data, data analysis, and actions to correct any inadequate performance. Quality improvement is an evolving concept in health care that will require applying techniques already in use in other industries: process flow analysis, control charts, cause-and-effect diagrams, and others.[3,8]

Four aspects of quality in critical care must be researched: efficacy, appropriateness, execution, and purposes of care. The challenge to respiratory care management is to address these quality issues without exceeding budgetary constraints. Also, respect for the health care worker must be a primary consideration. Quality studies that focus on improved outcomes, engage staff in data collection, and do not emphasize "deficiency" in employees will be successful in achieving goals without adversely affecting cost per occupied bed.[2,3,9]

One model that focuses on patient outcome improvement is the multidisciplinary quality group. The quality group consists of one or two members each from medical staff, nursing, and respiratory care, along with a hospital quality assurance representative and meets regularly to discuss specific concise data that reflect critical care quality issues. For example, any documented self-extubation or readmission to an ICU could be reviewed by this group for performance of all concerned. If a problem is identified, either system changes can be implemented or individuals can be contacted by the group (physicians, nurses, respiratory therapists, as necessary) to reduce undesired outcomes in the future (fewer self-extubations or readmissions). Necessarily, the same items must be reviewed following any action to see if quality has been improved.

Medical staff, patients, and family members perceive quality in terms of promptness, coordination, and satisfaction. Respiratory care may be technically advanced and consistently meet all standards for delivery, but be poorly coordinated with other care—nursing, physical therapy, laboratory—or fail to build confidence and satisfaction with the patient/family component. Management must establish objective measures of quality as it is perceived outside the department. A mechanism for nondefensive, investigative response to complaints and well-written, summarized patient surveys (filled out by family if patients are unable) are two methods to assess perceived quality. In making improvements, it is vital to provide respiratory care staff with positive examples. Employees who are providing technically correct care under stressful circumstances, perhaps in the presence of inappropriate hostility from appropriately concerned family members, will not improve in the future if all they receive is censorship. The Japanese management concept of this process is called *kaizen*—the continuous search for opportunities for all processes to get better.[3] Accomplishing needed care of the critically ill with available resources is usually the greatest priority for respiratory care management, but perceived quality is assuming increasing importance.

Resource Management

Resources are an important focus for the management of respiratory care, especially in critical care units. The two categories of resources are human and equipment resources, both of which consume significant portions of the hospital's most carefully controlled resource, budgeted expense. Critical care services, in total, are responsible for as much as 15 to 20 percent of hospital costs,[10,11] of which respiratory care can represent a significant portion. The efficiency of human resources is typically controlled through productivity systems retrospectively and through acuity systems prospectively. Effectiveness of human resources in critical care operations must be addressed through more staff-oriented processes.

Productivity systems which address the efficiency of human resources management, in simplest terms, require measurement of activities or time (both measure volume) spent directly providing services relative to total hours worked or paid by the department.[1] Time worked or paid represents the labor component of the cost of care, expressed in hours or full-time equivalents (FTEs) equal to 40 h/week. Most often, it is assumed that staffing of critical care with respiratory therapists can be done with variable staffing, requiring a flexible labor budget. When volume increases, more FTEs are allowed by the budget; when volume decreases, fewer FTEs are allowed. Volume, or units of service, can be expressed in a variety of ways, most often procedure or time based. Charge or charting systems may be used to collect volume data as a secondary function, whether manual or computerized data base systems are used.

For example, if a department records all activities (ventilator checks, suctioning, intubations, extubations, blood-gas measurements, treatments) performed by therapists in 24 h, the number of hours spent providing the services is totalled, assuming standard times for charting and average length of the procedure. The number of staff per shift for first, second, and third shifts is totalled and multiplied by 8 to determine the total hours worked or productive hours. A typical productivity target will assume an acceptable percentage of time at work is nonproductive. For example, 15 percent of 8 h to allow for nonproductive activities such as breaks and interruptions, results in an 8:6.8 ratio of hours worked:hours of volume produced. This can be reduced to 1.18 as a productivity target. The following example is for a department which has multiple critical care units, which on day X staffs 12, 12, and 10 therapists for first, second, and third shifts, respectively.

$12 + 12 + 10 = 34$ therapists $\times$ 8 h worked = 272 therapist hours
Hours of volume produced from daily records = 240 h volume
$272/240 = 1.13$ productivity ratio Target ratio is 1.18
$1.18/1.13 \times 100 = 104$ percent productivity

If the budgeted acceptable range is 90 to 110 percent, then the manager responsible for respiratory care must decrease or increase staff if the percent productivity falls outside of the range and expected volume remains the same. Depending on the system used, productivity and management's response can be generated monthly, weekly, daily, or shift-by-shift but remains a retrospective technique.

Acuity systems, formal or informal, allow prospective adjustment of staff. Although guidelines more specific than

JCAHO are now suggested by the Society of Critical Care Medicine regarding respiratory care training and staffing for critical care, an acuity system or staffing method is needed to implement flexible staffing.[6] The numbers of ventilated patients and expected activities or procedures are estimated prior to each shift. Detailed acuity systems can assign greater weights to patients with greater severity of illness. An appropriate workload is then assigned to each therapist with allowances for expected excess activities made according to the acuity system. The total number of staff required is determined following appropriate advance assignment of patient care. Nonscheduled staff are cancelled or additional staff obtained if the required numbers indicated by the acuity system do not match those previously scheduled. An ideal combination of acuity system and productivity system takes minimum time to calculate and apply, and productivity consistently confirms that acuity-based staffing decisions were correct.

Although these methods work well for critical care units when the patient mix and census fall within particular ranges, the spectrum of circumstances extends to situations requiring other staffing methods. For instance, critical care units in large hospitals typically maintain, even at times of low census, enough activity to maintain one therapist in the unit 24 h a day, or at least, a therapist with a "split" assignment (between two units). However, the small community hospital may use a two-tiered system. An example would be maintaining 24-h coverage, levels determined by productivity and acuity, when ventilator patients are present, but when the critically ill patient census is lower and no ventilator patients are present, it may make sense to maintain a respiratory therapist in-house for day or day and evening hours only. Management can determine what the lowest level, considered "fixed" staffing, will be.

Another special circumstance that does not fall in the scope of most productivity or acuity systems is respiratory care participation in highly labor-intensive specialized care. For example, out-of-house transports may need staffing support from stand-by respiratory therapists, either to go out on transports or to replace the therapist who leaves the hospital abruptly for a transport. Extracorporeal membrane oxygenation (ECMO) uses therapists in busy, expanded roles in some medical centers, and at key times such as during cannulation/decannulation procedures, extra staff may need to be deployed rapidly for limited periods of time. Economic considerations put pressure on staffing decision-makers to preserve low labor expense when possible, but inappropriate understaffing can result in lower quality, more costly patient care that eliminates any expected savings.[12]

Operational effectiveness—how to get the best function out of existing human resources through best techniques, team-building, and attention to job satisfaction—increases the impact of respiratory care services in critical care units. Although mechanistic systems such as productivity and acuity systems address the most easily documented management responsibilities, human resource development and support require attention to staff needs.

Leadership by department managers begins with articulating a common departmental vision of the role of respiratory therapists in critical care and their relationship with other departments. By incorporating staff input and consistently reinforcing a vision which supports and develops the staff, effectiveness of the staff's provision of respiratory care can be addressed and improved.[8] If the vision, as accepted by the staff, includes "we are the resident experts on the technical aspects of ventilatory support, and our mission is to share knowledge with other team members, house staff and nurses," potential to improve effectiveness results. With such a departmental vision, staff are more likely to find techniques which result in the best outcomes for ventilator patients and will not hesitate to initiate changes which coordinate the respective roles of all care givers. Level of job satisfaction cannot be assumed, but can be improved by attention from department management. Respiratory therapists consider the quality of the work performed and the nature of supervision the most important factors which affect job satisfaction.[13] Greater satisfaction encourages improved performance and effectiveness of care.

Supply and equipment management requires maintaining adequate permanent (capital) equipment as well as consumable supplies. Capital equipment is generally expected to last longer than a year and requires a significant dollar amount of the hospital capital budget. For use in critical care, respiratory care is responsible for providing and maintaining capital equipment. Support, diagnostic, and monitoring equipment (e.g., ventilators, oxygen and analyzers, pulse oximeters, capnographs, blood-gas machines) are the highest priorities. Although financial decision-making techniques (break-even, internal rate of return, net present value, and others) are used to determine an institution's purchases, relevance to the hospital's mission is equally important. If adequate levels of items such as mechanical ventilators are not owned, they will frequently be leased or rented. Objective evaluation of new capital equipment is a managerial responsibility which has both financial and patient care implications.

Respiratory monitoring equipment has proliferated in usage in many hospitals, at times in excess of cost-conscious levels of utilization. Some institutions have sought to regulate usage of instruments such as pulse oximeters, apnea monitors, and capnographs. Methods such as developing appropriateness guidelines in conjunction with medical staff or setting an upper limit of available instrumentation have been used to successfully limit utilization. For the well-equipped critical care unit, availability may not be an issue, as every bed may be provided with pulse oximetry, capnography, waveform displays of respiratory indices such as airway pressure and volume versus time, in addition to cardiac and other standard monitoring. Department management, however, has an obligation to perform a gatekeeping function through technology assessment.

Respiratory care has evolved intertwined with the growth of new technology. When the new technology (device, method, or treatment) is properly assessed for clinical, economic, and ethical impact, unnecessary proliferation is less likely to occur. If technology is not fully assessed as it is introduced, in-depth reassessment for common techniques such as pulse oximetry could be required later to correct improper application or burgeoning costs. An example of reassessment of technology in another field is electronic fetal monitoring, which by 1979 cost $411 million in the United States. The same year, the National Institutes of Health declared auscultation an acceptable substitute, in most cases, and much less costly.[14]

Supplies and consumable equipment for respiratory critical care require a materials management perspective. These supplies (tubing, portable oxygen for transports, among others) must be readily available and retained at the minimum required inventory level to maintain low operating costs. Respiratory supplies can be delivered efficiently via a just-in-time or stockless inventory system the same as any basic medical or surgical supplies.

Information Management

Data collection and data management are of increasing importance to respiratory care. Although well-designed handwritten flow sheets are commonly used, greater capability with computerized bedside information systems is now possible. Some systems are designed to automatically record ventilator settings, alarm settings, and patient data such as respiratory rate, oxygen saturation, end-tidal carbon dioxide levels, lung compliance, and airway resistance. The capability of capturing extensive data is accompanied by the responsibility to utilize, screen, and review clinical data. The three primary uses for respiratory data collected in the critical care unit are direct patient care, quality assurance/risk management, and research.

Monitored patient care information includes complete ventilator settings and physiologic data. A partial list of settings includes mode, fraction inspired oxygen (F_{IO_2}), set/total respiratory rate, set/corrected tidal volume, positive end-expiratory pressure, pressure support or control level, inspiratory flow, inspiratory pause, airway temperature, and all alarm settings. Certain information, such as F_{IO_2} and airway temperature, are not only useful, but are required monitoring by the JCAHO guidelines.[7] Peak and plateau pressures, static lung compliance, total respiratory rate, spontaneous ventilatory parameters (maximum inspiratory force, vital capacity, rate, tidal volume, and minute ventilation) are, in part, required physiologic data for ventilator patients. Therapists also track assessment information such as breath sounds, arterial blood-gas values, hemodynamic values, and clinical signs of increased work of breathing. All of the information is only valuable in terms of patient care if acceptable and unacceptable ranges are known and if appropriate responses to unacceptable values are known to the therapists.

Current noninvasive patient data monitoring technology, such as respiratory inductance plethysmography, pulse oximetry, and capnography, has been used to reduce the load of patients in ICUs with higher staff:patient ratios and to place them in lower cost noninvasive respiratory care units.[15–17]

Analysis of key data is required to use them for quality assurance and risk management purposes. The statistical treatment of the data can be simple and yet effective. Yes or no answers to quality of care questions such as "F_{IO_2} analyzed and charted every 8 h?" or "endotracheal tube placement checked on x-ray within 1 h of admission?" are used to determine the percentage of successful completions of quality indicators in a random sample of critical care flow sheets. Risk management issues occur when patient safety is questionable due to an undesirable event, such as unplanned extubation. The patient data recorded by the therapist should capture the circumstances surrounding the event and help uncover any process problems such as absence of two-point restraints.[18]

Clinical research involving respiratory care most often occurs in university-associated teaching hospitals, but can be achieved in any facility. Department management determines the scope and depth of research done in critical care. The central function in research efforts involving respiratory critical care patients is data collection. Staff cooperation and understanding of randomization, consistency, and clarity of data collection are crucial to the success of a project. The challenge to management is to develop well-planned protocols, with attention to efficient use of human resources, and to communicate them to the staff. With a highly developed departmental vision, therapists will energetically screen patients regarding entry criteria and collect and analyze data.

References

1. Griffith JR: *The Well-Managed Community Hospital.* Ann Arbor, Health Administration Press, 1987.
2. McLaughlin CP, Kaluzny AD: Total quality management in health: Making it work. Health Care Manage Rev 15:7, 1990.
3. Berwick D: Continuous improvement as an ideal in health care. N Engl J Med 320:53, 1989.
4. Ritz R, Pierson DJ: Managing respiratory care at Harborview. Respir Care 31:1049, 1986.
5. Respiratory Care Services Policy, Emanuel Hospital & Health Center, Portland, OR, 1990.
6. Bekes C, Bayly RW, Branson RD, et al: Society of Critical Care Medicine guidelines. Concern (Summer):38, 1990.
7. Joint Commission for Accreditation of Healthcare Organizations: *Accreditation Manual for Hospitals, Respiratory Care Services.* Chicago, 1990.
8. Kaluzny AD: Revitalizing decision-making at the middle management level. Hosp Health Serv Admin 34:39, 1989.
9. Berwick D: Health services research and quality of care. Med Care 27:763, 1989.
10. Strauss MJ, LoGerfo JP, Yeltatzie JA, et al: Rationing of intensive care unit services: An everyday occurrence. JAMA 255:1143, 1986.

11. Wagner DP, Wineland TD, Knaus WA: The hidden costs of treating severely ill patients: Charges and resource consumption in an intensive care unit. Health Care Finance Rev 5:81, 1983.
12. Behner KG, Fogg LF, Fournier LC, et al: Nursing resource management: Analyzing the relationship between costs and quality in staffing decisions. Health Care Manage Rev 15:63, 1990.
13. Akroyd HD, Robertson R: Factors affecting the job satisfaction of respiratory therapists who work in adult general and critical care: A multivariate study. Respir Care 34:179, 1989.
14. Banta HD, Thacker SB: The case for reassessment of health care technology. JAMA 264:235, 1990.
15. Krieger BP, Ershowsky P, Spivack D, et al: Initial experience with a central respiratory monitoring unit as a cost-saving alternative to the intensive care unit for Medicare patients who require long-term ventilator support. Chest 93:395, 1988.
16. Bone RC, Balk RA: Noninvasive respiratory care unit: A cost effective solution for the future. Chest 93:390, 1988.
17. Souhrada L: Technology makes patient monitoring less costly. Hospitals 62:84, 1988.
18. Little LA, Koenig JC, Newth CJL: Factors affecting accidental extubations in neonatal and pediatric intensive care patients. Crit Care Med 18:163, 1990.

Chapter 39

ECONOMIC ISSUES IN CRITICAL CARE

T.W. NOSEWORTHY
P. JACOBS

The Critical Care Product

Critical care originated in the early 1950s in response to patient mortality associated with respiratory failure caused by poliomyelitis. From such focused innovation, intensive care units (ICUs) have evolved to specialized centers offering monitoring or support (or both) for patients with threatening or established organ dysfunction. Civilian violence, vehicular trauma, and the Vietnam, Korean, and World wars have expanded understanding of severe trauma, shock, sepsis, and multisystem organ failure (MSOF). As a result, ICUs are now used for a spectrum of problems and offer a variety of products. Neonatal, pediatric, medical and surgical, coronary, cardiovascular, burn, and some trauma units all fall within the designation of an ICU and are part of critical care. By definition, ICUs are distinguished by the presence of concentrated medical and nursing services and both technologic support and sophisticated monitoring, most saliently exemplified by the mechanical ventilator and 24-h electrocardiographic (ECG) and hemodynamic monitoring.

Within the ICU, the inputs to production include capital and human resources. The output is the critical care "product" delivered to patients. By far, nursing services represent the largest resource consumed by critical care. Thus, nursing represents the largest cost.

The organizational structure of the ICU varies by unit and institution, related to such factors as internal resources, hospital size, location, the operation of regional programs, and the case mix.

At a senior administrative level, the principal medical care provider is the ICU director who, with other critical care physicians, renders patient care with the help of consultants. This model is the *closed ICU*. As critical care progressively becomes a recognized discipline, with demonstrable knowledge and skills, and as tertiary care units and graduates from training programs increase in number, this organizational structure is likely to predominate. Conversely, a more common model of the past has been the *open ICU* in which patient care is conducted by individual attending physicians, often with critical care consultant input. There is a debate on the propriety and pitfalls of each approach. Surprisingly, there has not been rigorous assessment of the utilization and cost impacts of these models. Many ICUs have residents or interns who provide medical care in conjunction with attending staff. This additional input has significant implications for costs and utilization.

Not surprisingly, in some sizable hospitals, up to 15 to 20 percent of all medical patients receive some portion of care in an ICU.[1] In the average United States hospital of 200 beds or larger, approximately 6 percent of beds are devoted to ICUs. In France, ICUs are believed to account for approximately 5 percent of beds, whereas New Zealand devotes 1.5 percent of its hospital beds to ICUs.[2] The Canadian government recommends an allocation of 4 percent of hospital beds to intensive care.

By 1983, over 90 percent of all United States acute care hospitals had at least one ICU. In the preceding 7 years, the number of ICU beds increased at a rate of 29 percent, as compared to 5 percent for general acute care beds.[3]

Basic Economics and Definitions of Cost

ICUs have drawn an enormous amount of attention in recent years, in large part because of their economic characteristics. Despite this attention to the economics of ICUs, there remains a great deal that we don't know. The economic issue most broadly stated is; Do we get as much for our dollars spent on ICUs as we could from alternative uses of these resources?

The economic dimensions of ICUs can be summarized from two distinct vantage points—that of the individual institution and that of society (Table 39-1).

THE INSTITUTIONAL PERSPECTIVE

From the perspective of individual hospitals, a number of different measures of cost can be used to quantify ICU resource consumption. Which concept is used will depend on the purpose of the analysis. One reason for classifying costs is to identify the impact of various activities on resource use. From this standpoint, the fixed/variable distinction is important.

Fixed costs are those costs which do not change as output changes over the relevant time frame. Thus, in the ICU, certain costs are generated, irrespective of whether any patients are occupying beds.

Variable costs refer to the values of those resources which do increase with the level of care. For example, the variable cost of a patient-day in a unit not fully occupied is the cost of additional labor and materials consumed by the patient.

Fixed and variable costs can be either *direct* (costs incurred in the treatment of patients) or *indirect* (costs which cannot be directly traced to the patient). Direct variable costs include medical and nursing care, medical/surgical

TABLE 39-1 Alternative Measures of Institutional and Societal Benefits and Costs

Institutional Measures	
Charges	Fixed costs
Revenues	Variable costs
Societal Measures	
Benefits	Economic costs

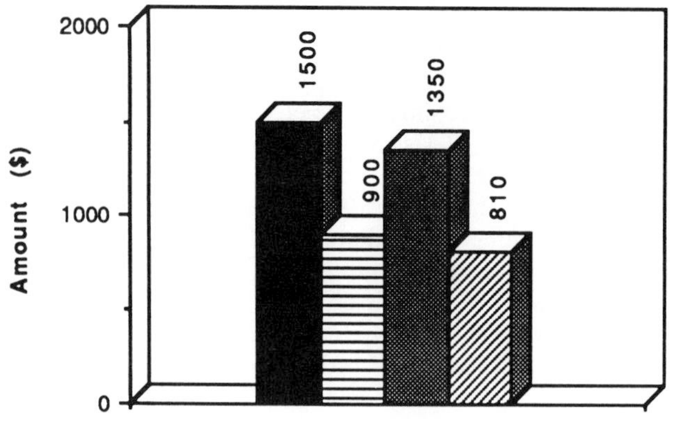

FIGURE 39-1 Revenue and cost measures. Categories (from left to right): charges, revenues, full cost, and marginal cost.

supplies, pharmacy, laboratory, and diagnostic imaging. Indirect variable costs included patient billing, housekeeping, and similar items.

Some accounting practices, such as those found in Medicare cost reports, allocate all hospital costs to revenue centers, of which an ICU is one. *Allocated costs* load a share of a hospital's nonrevenue-producing, or overhead, costs onto revenue-producing centers, such as the ICU. There are numerous accounting methods for doing this. This approach is particularly relevant when the revenue-producing departments are reimbursed on a cost recovery basis. Thus, all costs (direct and indirect) are related to a product.

The result of adding direct and indirect unit costs to allocated costs is the *full cost*.

From an institutional viewpoint, there are two separate revenue measures. The first of these is *charges* (or billings) which are the amount the hospital designates as a "sticker price" for these services. A number of reimbursement agencies, for example Blue Cross, and some Medicaid programs, pay less than full charges, thus charges are not representative of revenues. For example, if the hospital's charge for a patient day in the ICU is \$800, and Blue Cross pays at a discount of 10 percent, then the hospital receives \$720. This net amount actually received by the hospital is the true *revenue*. The difference between revenues and full costs are the hospital's surplus or *profit*. To the extent that different payers (e.g., Medicaid, Blue Cross) pay different revenues for similar patients, profits or losses will also differ among payers.

The following is an example to illustrate the above definitions (Fig. 39-1). Assume that the total charges for a typical day in the ICU are \$1500. These include the "hotel," or room and board charges, and the diagnostic and therapeutic services. Because some paying agencies pay less than charges, net revenues will be less than \$1500. Although there is no standard proportion paid, a number of studies show that some Medicaid reimbursements approximate 60 percent of the charges, or in this case, \$900. The ratio of full costs to charges might be 90 percent. Thus, in this case full cost would be \$1350/day. If the revenue is \$900 and the full cost is \$1350, for each patient there will be an accumulated deficit of \$450. However, assume that the hospital decides to assess the impact of a contract to add one extra patient per day to the ICU. The *marginal cost* of an extra patient is typically estimated at approximately 60 percent of full cost. Thus, in this case, the additional cost of adding another patient day will be 60 percent of \$1350 or \$810. The correct figure for estimating whether the hospital is losing or gaining money, by adding this additional patient, is the difference between revenues and marginal costs. In this case, the hospital is earning a *contribution margin* of \$900 minus \$810 or \$90.

It is important to illustrate a salient problem in identifying ICU-specific revenues. When hospitals are paid on the basis of diagnostic-related groups (DRGs), revenues are received on a case-by-case basis, for all services during the hospital stay. This incorporates the ICU portion. Distinguishing ICU from non-ICU revenues, when payment is made on a per case (DRG) basis, is arbitrary and imprecise. Thus, it is impossible to identify an ICU's contribution margin. A potential alternative is to measure the revenues generated by a case, which includes an ICU stay, and to compare this with the marginal cost of the entire stay (ICU and non-ICU). This allows one to measure the contribution margin generated by cases which include a portion of ICU care, but fails to provide a measure of the contribution margin from ICU operations per se.

THE SOCIETAL VIEWPOINT

The foregoing analysis is at the institutional level. For policy purposes, a broader societal vantage point is necessary. From this perspective, *benefit* rather than revenue is the relevant measure. Benefits refer to the physical impact of ICU treatment on the patient or to the dollar value of these benefits. The typical measure of benefits is years of life saved, attributable to the treatment. If the quality of these years varies significantly from productive, healthy years, they may be indexed in one fashion or another, into *quality-adjusted life-years* (QALYs).

While obtaining a figure for the net impact of ICU treatment may be heroic enough for most observers, intrepid souls may wish to carry the analysis one additional step by placing a dollar value on benefits, i.e., the value of human life. We shall return to this topic later in this chapter.

The concept of revenues is replaced by that of benefits when one moves from an institutional to a societal perspective; correspondingly, societal costs replace institutional costs. This measure is known as *economic or opportunity costs* or the value to society of the resources used in the ICU. In most cases, economic costs may be well approximated by institutional costs, but in some instances they may be much broader. For instance, the economist would count as a social cost the market value of any unpaid resources used for equipment operation, donated buildings, volunteer services, and so on. In general, then, social cost exceeds full cost, but we have no information on exactly how much this excess is.

What Do ICUs Cost?

The cost of caring for critically ill patients may be analyzed from a microeconomic or macroeconomic perspective. Microeconomic costs are examined on an individual sample, unit, or institutional basis, whereas macroeconomic estimates are on a population, aggregate, or national basis.

MICROECONOMIC STUDIES

Most of the information available on the cost of ICUs is derived from microeconomic analyses. The generalization of this information beyond the specific setting studied has understandable limitations. In addition, these studies do not use consistent methods. Although not conclusive, the following illustrations serve as useful indicators of the magnitude of resource consumption by ICUs.

The sickest group of patients (Class IV on the Therapeutic Intervention Scoring Scale) in the ICU have been estimated to generate an average of $22,000 in charges per patient for the entire stay.[4] Mean total ICU cost per patient (i.e., the ICU-generated costs) for all groups has been estimated at $3100, accounting for 50 percent of mean total hospital costs per patient, though accumulated in 20 percent of the hospitalization time.[5] In both Canada and the United States, a ratio of 3:1 for daily ICU bed cost to general acute care bed cost appears to be an accepted and commonly used estimate.[6]

The ICU cost of patients with specific disorders, such as gastrointestinal bleeding associated with cirrhosis, has been documented to generate costs up to $260,000/survivor. With adequate recognition that accurate costing of individual patients remains to be fully and accurately elucidated, recent attempts at assessing the cost in relation to the benefit of certain types of care have produced comparative information.[7] One estimate of ICU cost has suggested a figure of $460/year of extended life for patients suffering from respiratory failure secondary to asthma, versus $8026/year for patients experiencing cardiac failure. On average, it costs $1826/year of extended life for patients requiring greater than 48 h of mechanical ventilation. At the extreme, cardiovascular surgical patients cost $116,000/life-year saved. These figures do not include physician reimbursement or follow-up care.

Other data propose that the cost of saving a life in the neonatal ICU may be only one-tenth the cost per death averted during adult life.[8]

Although such figures are interesting, they require careful interpretation. Obviously, individual costs per patient and disease entity will be strikingly different. It has been suggested that resource consumption by patients in the ICU may vary by as much as 1000-fold.[9]

There is unquestionably a substantial basis for proposing that intensive care is expensive care. Not surprisingly, this raises the question: Is intensive care worth it, not merely in postponing death, but in terms of prolonging an acceptable quality of life?

MACROECONOMIC STUDIES

Despite interest in the macroeconomic characteristics of ICUs, data appear sparse. Most United States standards of ICU cost are based on annual surveys conducted by the American Hospital Association (AHA). These estimates encompass neonatal, pediatric, cardiac, and adult ICUs. In 1976, 5.2 percent of all beds in community hospitals were within ICUs or coronary care units (CCUs). Using this figure, together with an estimate of total per diem cost of an ICU bed (calculated as three times the cost of a general ward bed), it was concluded that ICUs add 10 percent to the total cost of each hospital patient-day. By 1979, it was estimated that the aggregate cost of ICUs in the United States was $12.8 billion or 15 percent of global hospital costs.[2]

AHA data from 1986 indicate that there were 85,000 ICU beds. Using the occupancy rate of 84 percent reported in a survey conducted by the American Association of Critical Care Nurses (AACCN), there were 26.1 million ICU patient days, or 108 ICU patient days per 1000 population. At an ICU to non-ICU bed cost ratio of 3:1, this resulted in an estimated national cost of $33.9 billion. This figure represented 20 percent of all inpatient costs, and 0.8 percent of the gross national product (GNP) in 1986.[10]

Comparative data from Canada suggest that ICUs represent less than 10 percent of inpatient costs and approximately 0.2 percent of GNP. While there has been unrelenting growth in cost and utilization of Canadian ICU services, such growth has been proportionately greater in the United States. This has resulted in 2.5-fold greater utilization of ICU services by the United States than by Canada.[10]

Available data have marked limitations, and calculations made from these may render misinformation. The direct and indirect cost of ICU beds is unknown and customarily calculated from the estimated cost of non-ICU beds and the 3:1 ratio. Setting aside the limitations of the 3:1 ratio, the calculated cost of non-ICU beds has inherent inaccuracies. This information can only be generated by detailed cost accounting and management information systems, as yet not widely used throughout North America.

Not surprisingly, we are a long way from being capable of accumulating data from patient-specific cost accounting systems, as a means of estimating aggregate cost of ICUs from a national, state, or provincial perspective.

Nonetheless, using conservative figures and estimates, the message remains unalterable: ICUs use a tremendously large and rapidly growing volume of resources. It remains to be determined if the utilization and costs are congruent with the benefits.

Who Generates ICU Costs?

SUPPLY AND DEMAND

The economist's categorization of supply and demand has proved to be a useful means of identifying pressure points in resource allocation decisions. Such an analysis helps to answer questions related to how costs are generated. Thus, it is a prerequisite to determining how costs can be controlled.

The complexity of applying the supply/demand framework to ICUs lies with the difficulty of identifying the suppliers and demanders in a complex hospital setting. A framework has been developed[11] in which doctors are identified as demanders and hospital administrators as suppliers, with the supply arrangements being regarded as passively responsive to physician demand though this may be changing. The application of this framework to ICUs requires some refinement, however. *Admission demand* and *demand for services* (intensity and length of stay) once the patient is admitted may come from different sources. Further, the organizational structure of the ICU, closed or open, has implications for ICU demand as well.

DEMAND

The traditional view of demand focuses on product price as the major influence of allocation. From this perspective, when consumers are faced with higher prices for a product, to the extent possible, they will shift their preferences and purchases to substitute products. For a number of reasons, such a framework is of limited use in understanding ICU operations. Firstly, the ICU product is frequently demanded under emergency circumstances and there are limited or no substitutes for this care. This is true for both the monitoring and supportive functions offered by the ICU. Secondly, because of the presence of health insurance, cross-subsidization from profit centers, and other forms of discretionary funding, price is not a significant issue in the admitting decision. Finally, clinical decisions are made by the physician, as an agent of the patient, and medical facts and practice patterns become the principal variables which determine demand. Added to this is the increasingly sophisticated technology offered by ICUs, making care within them more applicable to a growing population of patients. The demand spotlight, therefore, falls on the physician.

To analyze demand, the ICU product has to be dissociated into two components, admissions and services. The reason for this distinction is that the demand pressures of each component come from different directions. This particularly applies to the open and closed organizational structures, discussed in a previous section of this chapter.

With an open unit structure, demands for admissions and services will come from a wide spectrum of the hospital's attending physicians. With a closed structure, the demand for admissions will similarly come from the hospital's attending physicians, but the demand for services created by patients in the ICU will come from critical care physicians on behalf of their patients. Research on practice patterns has uncovered remarkable variation in resource consumption by ICU patients. Virtually no research has been reported, however, on the relationship between practice patterns, costs, and ICU organizational structure.

SUPPLY AND TECHNOLOGY

Ostensibly, ICU services are "supplied" by hospital administration and, in the past, supply appears to have been very responsive to demand.[11] This has potentially led to a blurred distinction between supply and demand. But, they should be kept separate, particularly because there is growing evidence that the relationship between these forces may be changing.

Supply is determined by *both* cost and reimbursement. Costs have been driven by more intensively trained personnel and technology, such as modern positive-pressure ventilators, dialysis equipment, and cardiac assist devices. Cost-based reimbursement, at least until the introduction of DRGs by Medicare in 1983, facilitated the hospital's ability to respond to physician-demanders. With DRGs and a fixed payment per case, there has been progressive pressure on hospital administrations to place limitations on the supply of ICU services. Indeed, a number of post-1983 studies have documented the shortfall between revenues and costs for patients admitted to ICUs with specific DRGs.

How To Control ICU Costs

UNDERSTANDING PHYSICIAN VARIATION

Doctors' decisions have a profound and direct impact on the cost of medical care.[12] Although physicians' fees represent only 20 percent of health care costs, as much as 80 percent of expenditures for services are prescribed by physicians. A rich literature, not directly related to critical care, describes marked variations in physicians' practice patterns. Intuitively, it is reasonable to suspect that a wide range of practice variation may also exist in the ICU.

Simplistic analyses of variation of physician practice have proposed simple explanations such as financial motivation and fear of litigation. This is naive and not surprisingly, cost control mechanisms arising from such presumptions attempt to arrive at simplistic or unrealistic proposals to control physician behavior. To effectively alter physicians' clinical practice and behavior patterns, one must attempt to understand the complex entanglement of factors that influence decision-making. Only then can interventions be designed to alter observed patterns and behaviors.

Physician-initiated demand may be either physician or patient induced. Both apply in the ICU. Furthermore, patients' families often act as surrogate decision-makers for their relatives and may augment patient-induced demands, particularly in situations where patients have lost competence and may not have expressed their personal views regarding the extent or nature of therapy they wish. Thus, clinical decision-making by ICU physicians is a complex interaction between attempts to satisfy the professional goals and desires of the physician and the personal health care goals of the patient, as expressed by themselves or their families.

The threshold that the ICU physician uses for initiating a diagnostic test or using specific monitoring or technologic supports ought to be based on the perception of the benefits and costs involved. Under ideal circumstances, care would be initiated or continued whenever benefits were seen to exceed costs. Problems exist with this paradigm. Firstly, costs are poorly understood. Costs of patient care

are not usually captured or known. Secondly, the costs do not fall directly on those who generate them, namely, physicians. Indeed, this reduces the incentive for physicians to measure these costs. Problems on the benefit side stem from the fact that outcomes for a given patient are not known with certainty. ICU physicians may have the best available information on the outcome of admissions to the ICU, but this is "aggregate" information and not case specific. Thus, it is often too general in nature to be useful. Furthermore, some outcome studies suffer from a short length of follow-up, insufficient to be an appropriate index of benefit. As longer follow-ups are examined, however, the influence of many other factors, besides the ICU intervention, may confound the validity of the outcome results. A central question is: What outcome indicator is the desirable target? Mortality, though easy to measure, may not be a sensitive or relevant end point. Yet, morbidity and quality of life assessments are only now being properly studied. The information derived has to be interpreted in light of health status prior to ICU admission.

In situations where the outcome measure is survival, the benefit of ICU appears to be substantial, with up to two-thirds of patients alive a year later.[5] The quality of life achieved, in those situations where it has been measured, appears to be directly proportional to the premorbid functional status.[13]

MECHANISMS FOR COST CENTER CONTROL

PREDICTION OF OUTCOME. The ability to control the cost of ICUs must be examined in relation to any adverse impact on the quality of health care delivered or the outcome. However, there is insufficient and, at times, conflicting information on the benefits derived from the ICU.

One might attempt to initiate cost control maneuvers in relation to predicted benefits and outcomes. However, even if there were a perfect prediction tool, problems would exist. Firstly, it is not clear to what extent intensive care would be used or rejected, related to the given outcome prediction. The problem here is achieving medical, if not societal consensus, on the predicted survival rate below which intensive care would be withdrawn or withheld. There is no evidence that explicit prediction levels, arguably with the exemption of 0 and 100 percent, would promote a consensus. Secondly, there is evidence that patients in intermediate prediction ranges may actually cost the most, dashing the hope that a predictive tool would necessarily lead to specific patterns of intensive care allocation.[14]

Alarm has been expressed that it is difficult to die in hospital, without doing so in the ICU.[15] The allegation is made that hopelessly ill patients are frequently admitted for aggressive terminal care deemed to be both costly and medically not beneficial. However, the absence of a perfect prediction tool raises a dilemma for the ICU physician. The ideologic basis of the physician/patient interaction is not grounded on allocation of care in relation to cost, but rather the premise that the physician shall provide whatever reasonable and beneficial care believed necessary. It is problematic to expect physicians, ICU or otherwise, to be resource allocators at the individual patient bedside.

How might ICU cost be controlled? The answer, at least in part, would appear to be eliminating unnecessary admissions and generating a greater efficiency in patient care and services provided following admission. In CCUs, it has been shown that during periods of reduced bed capacity, physicians' admitting thresholds may vary, and admissions may be controlled without apparent reductions in outcome or quality of care.[16] To an extent, this is likely to be true in other types of ICUs, though rigorously collected data are unavailable.

In terms of promoting increased efficiency, the management tools available to influence physicians' decision-making include education, with and without feedback, participation, incentives, sanctions, and administrative rules.[12] To a varying extent, in the non-ICU setting, each has been examined as a means of influencing physician performance. Unfortunately, virtually all research in this area is limited to the use of laboratory tests, diagnostic imaging procedures, or drug prescription. Although such information may be available for collection and analysis, it remains to be seen if it has general applicability to critical care services.

EDUCATION. Though it may be intuitively appropriate to implement educational programs as a means of reducing health care costs, the available evidence is conflicting, but tends to suggest that education alone either does not effect change in behavior or its effect is not prolonged. Cost awareness programs, as well, appear to provide mixed results in terms of altering test-ordering behavior. While one study has estimated that educational programs may reduce diagnostic tests by as much as 30 percent, the tests most reduced were in less acutely ill patients.[17]

The strategy of controlling cost by enunciating explicit guidelines for care, or standards, generally does not work, at least as it has been examined in relation to diagnostic tests, drugs, and blood transfusions.[18,19]

Educational programs appear to have their greatest potential when professional role models effect change in physicians' professional environments. It has been shown that when information from such sources is transmitted by mail, it is less effective than when communicated personally.[20]

The attributes necessary for successful personal communication appear to be: authenticity of source, the medium of presentation, the audience targeted, the nature of the message, and the setting in which it is delivered. Of course, equally important as these determinants for the success of education is the perceived need for change. Progressive economic pressures on critical care physicians may provide an incentive to develop or enhance procedures and programs aimed at maintaining quality of care within the limits of fiscal restraint. This would potentiate the value of concurrent educational programs.

FEEDBACK. Though education alone does not appear to effect lasting changes in decision-making, combining education with feedback appears to be complementary. When performance is compared to statistical standards, or peer groups, and the tenor of this performance information is constructive and not threatening, there is the potential for modifying decision-making.[18]

Performance feedback has been regarded as labor intensive. To be successful, it has to be used by clinical role models who may be professional leaders with diverse commitments. Thus, although feedback as an adjunct to education holds more promise than education alone in reducing utilization of services offered by physicians, feedback may be costly.

Earlier evidence from individual studies and professional review programs suggests that the cost of personalized feedback may not necessarily generate a net savings.[21] However, as management information systems (MIS) develop, the costs of feedback may fall significantly.

PARTICIPATION/INCENTIVES/PENALTIES/ADMINISTRATIVE RULES. Numerous studies show that physicians are resistant to changing their patterns of utilization, and so education and feedback may not be adequate. Participation, incentives, and penalties are additional management tools aimed at altering physicians' behavior for the purposes of controlling cost. Participation involves physicians in group decision-making; incentives appeal to physicians' personal or professional interests; and, penalties restrict their professional freedom or independence in decision-making. These measures have not been researched to the extent that education and feedback have, but nonetheless appear to be in common usage.

The theory of management accounting suggests that policies and procedures are more likely to achieve success, if the stakeholders actively *participate* in their formulation and implementation. Physicians are unlikely to respond favorably to "top-down" decision-making. By involving physicians in operational decisions, one is more likely to achieve an optimum and balanced result that is both administratively and medically acceptable.

Reimbursement methods, such as DRGs, potentiate greater mutual dependence between administrators and physicians. For administrators to accomplish the objective of controlling costs, they must invite physicians' participation.

Another management tool for cost control is an *incentive,* which may be of a financial, personal, or professional nature. Some health maintenance organizations are known for profit-sharing with physicians, provided that practice quotas, referral rates, or surgical activities fall within prearranged targets.

At an individual patient level, financial incentives appear to have failed in changing resident and medical staff behavior. This may be because insufficient rewards have been available or have been targeted at such specific points in physician practice that they were unlikely to effect significant alternations in practice patterns or behaviors.[22] Additionally, physicians' concerns for promoting suboptimal care, regardless of the quest for cost containment, balance and limit the ensuing success of incentive programs and may create an ethical conundrum.

The reverse of incentive is *penalty,* the success of which directly depends on the degree of dependence or autonomy the physician enjoys in relation to the paymaster or controller of resources. Models with few or single paymasters are more likely to effectively use penalties, either as a threat or reality.

Administrative rules are the final example of a management tool available for cost control. In general, a "top-down" source or edict has less chance for success than a participatory approach that involves physicians and administrators. Physician managers hold promise as important future contributors to developing administrative rules. The hope is that the input of management-trained physicians to the formulation and implementation of policies and procedures may lead to broader recognition of both administrative and clinical issues and the sensitivities of each.

An example of an administrative change directed at the ICU might be a rule to maintain an unoccupied bed for an absolute "emergency," such as a victim of a cardiac arrest. By doing so, the occupancy rate is potentially lessened and, to the extent that it is, the total cost of ICU care is lowered. Such a policy may also make good clinical sense.

It should be readily apparent that effective cost control is best achieved in a setting in which there is an understanding of what factors influence decision-making and the consumption of resources. Those who participate in decision-making must be provided proper information and feedback and be placed in a position of responsibility for cost control wherein they are rewarded for success or may be penalized for failure.

Examining the utility of these management tools within the context of ICU cost containment provides a bountiful opportunity for future research in the economics of ICUs.

MANAGEMENT CONTROL SYSTEMS

Cost control measures should always be examined in a cost-benefit framework. The foregone benefits resulting from reduced service must be recognized to properly assess the impact of cost reductions.

To analyze cost control in the ICU, it is necessary to distinguish controls at two levels of operation, hospital-wide and departmental (ICU). At the hospital level, a prime control is the reimbursement mechanism, as determined by the pay master. DRGs form one type of control, limiting the amount that Medicare will pay for a specific patient type or case mix. This rate is expected to encompass all hospital expenditures, including those incurred in the ICU. The incentives created by this form of payment are those which reward the hospital for reducing its costs. Doing so generates a larger contribution margin to apply to fixed costs.

Tighter control of reimbursement for hospitals does not automatically lead to lower operating costs. Management initiatives are needed to reduce these costs. Indeed, the fiscal goals of hospitals may be at variance with the care goals of ICUs. Such differences may lead to internal conflict. This may be particularly true for long-stay patients with MSOF.

To avoid excessive conflict, an internal mechanism may be set up to ensure that units within the hospital act in concert with institutional goals. Such a mechanism is called a *management control system* (MCS). An MCS is a series of policies and procedures designed to control the actions of the "manager" of an internal unit.

The prerequisite to establishing an MCS is to identify the responsibility centers within the hospital and to develop a *management information system* (MIS). An MCS can only be relationally applied if there is sufficient and accurate report information.

There are a number of different types of responsibility centers, including supportive or functional centers such as laboratory medicine and diagnostic imaging, and clinical centers such as emergency rooms and ICUs. A responsibility center can be organized as a *cost center* (which is judged by costs of operations), a *profit center* (judged by profits), or as a *program* (judged by how effectively it meets predetermined objectives). Which organizational design is chosen depends largely on the manner in which senior management and the ICU director want the ICU to contribute to the overall organizational goals and objectives. Designating the ICU as a cost or program center seems more realistic than viewing it as a profit center because of the difficulty in isolating ICU from non-ICU revenues in the overall hospital payment.

In targeting specific variables to be controlled and assigning responsibility for controlling these variables, the golden rule of responsibility accounting is: "Whoever can best control the targeted variable should be made responsible for controlling it." Viewing the ICU as a responsibility center, we posit that it be evaluated as a program set up to meet multiple objectives in a fiscally responsible manner. The principal objective is to contribute to the health of critically ill patients. The manager of the ICU responsibility center should be the ICU director, who is expected to "manage" the unit in accordance with the hospital's overall objectives. The unit manager participates in setting the unit's goals which should not be imposed by senior management. Indeed, current information suggests that a "top-down" MCS does not work in a highly technical setting.[23,24]

An effective MCS calls for objectives to be set by the manager, an MIS to measure actual performance, and a feedback system to inform the institution and the manager of performance and to reward successful efforts. Among the mechanisms used in an MCS are financial budgets, standard operating procedures, statistical reports, and performance appraisal.[24]

The application of an MCS to an ICU should concentrate on mechanisms for reducing cost without adversely affecting patients' health status. Costs are identified in three dimensions: intensity of services per day, number of days in the ICU, and admission (or not) to the ICU. Resource intensity per day includes the sum of all services used by the patient, including human resources, capital expenditures, and support and diagnostic services. More of these services lead to higher daily costs, but only a portion of the costs generated by these services can be best controlled by the ICU manager. ICU physicians cannot exert control over the cost of producing a laboratory test or an x-ray. Likewise, they cannot control the prices paid for nurses. What they can control, and thus, what they should be made responsible for, is the number of services per patient utilized on a daily basis. An MCS device should therefore focus on utilization variables.[25]

With regard to the number of days that the patient remains in the ICU, the longer the stay, the more the high daily costs multiply. Decisions about length of stay are highly subjective, the threshold varying as a result of such factors as bed availability, quantity and quality of nursing care on general wards, and the comfort level in decision-making by the ICU physician.

Another control variable is whether or not the patient is admitted to the ICU. Intensive care is much more costly than non-ICU care, and this variable clearly contributes to higher costs.

From a resource allocation viewpoint, the degree to which each of these variables is under the control of the ICU physician is of fundamental importance. If ICU physicians can best control these variables, they should be made responsible for them. Contrariwise, if admission, for instance, is the responsibility of some other (non-ICU) physician, then these other physicians should be assigned responsibility for these variables. Otherwise, cost control is not possible.

Unfortunately, current management practice falls short of the prescribed optimum. There exist few practice standards on which departmental objectives can be firmly grounded. Current MISs do not adequately allow for satisfactory performance appraisal. Furthermore, we have not developed sufficient reward systems to ensure congruence between hospital and physician objectives.[12]

One pioneering study has sought to identify and apply monitoring measures of service utilization in an ICU.[26] The methodology relied primarily on standard operating procedures, such as eliminating standing orders, repetitive orders, and verbal orders, and instituting specific guidelines for laboratory tests. Additionally, a mechanism was instituted whereby practitioners received feedback on the laboratory tests they performed. The authors reported dramatic reduction in laboratory charges per ICU patient—from $10,000/case in 1983 to $6300 in 1984, the year that the monitoring system was initiated. However, no specific motivating factor was identifiable as being responsible for this change. It has to be pointed out that experiments such as these often yield only temporary reductions in utilization and cost, the so-called Hawthorne effect. Furthermore, the impact on patient outcome has to be documented concurrently and has to be clearly shown not to be adversely affected.

How Much ICU Care—Economic Analysis?

COST EFFECTIVENESS AND COST BENEFIT

Under DRG payments, pressures have increased to reduce ICU costs. What guidance can economics give to helping ICU managers decide which cuts might produce the least harm? The approaches available in the economist's tool kit are referred to as *cost-benefit* and *cost-effectiveness analysis.* These methodologies have the virtue of providing the analyst with a framework with which to organize data used for optimizing resource allocation.

The prerequisite to any economic analysis is the clear identification of which intervention is being studied and the alternative which it is replacing. This can avoid a great deal of confusion. The next step is the definition and identification of the relevant health status indicators for the patients under study. Such a measure should enable one to assess the outcome, focusing on relevant aspects of patient health status subsequent to being discharged from the ICU. Postdischarge measures fall into three groups:

1. Basic, unadjusted health indicators
2. Health status weighted indicators
3. Dollar value of health status

The unadjusted indicator may be simply survival or nonsurvival, or it may be the number of years following ICU discharge until death. Recognizing that perceived quality of years can differ dramatically, the second set of measures attempts to assign weights indicating the level or QALY. Given the complexity of the subject, no single best measure of QALY has emerged. Analysts have worked with subjective, patient assessment indices,[27] and with indexed weights assigned by physicians.[28]

The third measure of outcome is the dollar value placed on the survivors' benefits. This is a highly controversial issue, and it is not surprising that a wide range of benefit measures have been developed. These range from the value of production lost,[29] to willingness to pay to avoid risks of injury, illness or death,[30] to the valuations on life designated by an elected or chosen body such as politicians or physicians.[31]

Let us demonstrate how the definition of intervention and the concept of health status can be used to define an economic measure of "outcome" in the ICU. First, look at the relationship between health status and resource use as measured by cost for three types of ICU patients, A, B, and C (Fig. 39-2). These hypothetical outcome curves illustrate how a patient progresses with additional resources (time or intensity or both) in relation to the discharge threshold. Case A responds quickly, reaching the threshold after only $200 worth of services, after which she is discharged. Case B also responds, but not as quickly, thus requiring $1000 worth of ICU services before she reaches the threshold. Case C does not respond, and despite the application of considerable resources, she dies after $3200 worth of services have been used.

The measures of probability of outcome, such as the mortality prediction model[32] are attempts to classify whether cases approximate the A, B, or C type. A high probability of survival is typified by patient A, a low probability is seen with patient C. Unfortunately, as we embark on the provision of care for many ICU patients, we are unable to tell with certainty whether a patient is one type or another. Nonetheless, these curves can be used to illustrate and ex-

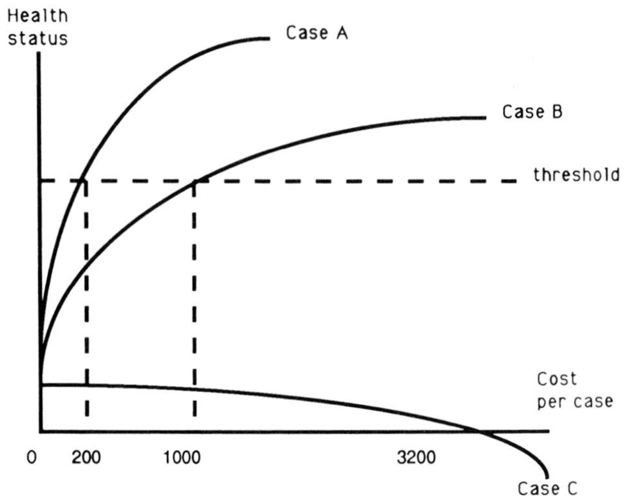

FIGURE 39-2 Health status in relation to cost per case—three scenarios.

plain the common observation that nonsurviving ICU patients cost more than survivors. An additional interpretation, common to all curves, is that there is a limit to the additional provision of ICU services, beyond which health status ceases to improve, and in fact may worsen. Avoiding so-called "flat of the curve" medicine is clinically and economically good sense.

A second observation worth making is that the TISS[33] and other severity scales can be used to measure progress in health status up to the discharge point. Beyond that point, health status is measured by life-years, QALYs, or perhaps some other scale.

Cost-effectiveness ratios measure the additional cost per additional outcome unit, *all else held constant.* Thus, holding the case type constant, cost effectiveness would measure the additional contribution to health status resulting from the use of additional ICU resources. If, for instance, an intervention of interest is an x-ray per day, and the alternative is none, then using an example of a patient whose x-rays cost $1000 for the entire stay and contributed 5 years of life, the cost-effectiveness ratio is $1000 divided by 5 years, or $200/life-year saved. If the 5 years were not of expected quality, but for whatever reason were valued by the patient as half of normal, then the cost effectiveness, or cost utility, would be $1000 for 2.5 life-years, or $400/QALY.

Great care should be exercised in interpreting existing data. For instance, much has been made of the difference in costs between survivors and nonsurvivors[14] yet, in no way can we draw clear inferences about the cost effectiveness of ICU service from this observation. Take cases B and C, for instance. Patient B was discharged with an acceptable health status and incurred $1000 in costs; C was discharged dead and incurred $3200 in cost. We cannot say from this data how effective the ICU resources were. Even though C died, there is no information about the effectiveness of the resources for B. B and C may represent different case types or severity of illness, and each will respond differently to therapies administered in the ICU. To judge the effectiveness of ICU resources consumed, all other relevant variables must be controlled for B and C.

This point can perhaps be best illustrated using case X and her twin, X′, both admitted to the hospital with identical conditions. X is admitted to the ICU and X′ is provided conventional care. With such care, the probability of survival is 20 percent, and the life span is 20 more years of complete health. With ICU care, the probability of survival increases to 60 percent, also for a life span of 20 more years. Expected life-years are 4 for conventional care and 12 for ICU care. Thus, the additional life-years expected from ICU care over the alternative is 8 additional life-years. The cost of ICU care is $12,000 and conventional care is $4000. The additional cost of ICU care is $8000. The cost-effectiveness ratio for ICU care over conventional care is 8 extra years for $8000 or $1000/life-year saved.

There have been only a few studies of the cost-effective or cost-benefit aspects of intensive care.[34] An evaluation of the effects of a regional neonatal intensive care program was undertaken in terms of cost per life-year, per QALY, and per dollar of benefits. The cost-benefit ratio was positive for birth weights between 1000 and 1499 g, but negative for weights from 500 to 999 g. However, the authors evaluated the *net* benefits of the program (comparing the net increase in life-years as compared to before the program was established) with the *total* program costs. Had they used the net change in cost above that of the old program, they would have had higher (and more appropriate) benefit-cost ratios, and perhaps even a positive one for the low-birth weight group. Other studies[35,36] of neonatal intensive care in Rhode Island have found a positive benefit-cost ratio for all neonatal size groups, although they did not seem to use the net change figure.

ECONOMICS, BIOMEDICAL ETHICS, AND PUBLIC POLICY

Regardless of how the economic characteristics of ICUs are assessed, the benefit in relation to the cost must be considered within the context of societal norms and values. Regardless of the fact that increasing dollars are being spent on ICUs, there is no consensus that it is appropriate to withdraw or withhold intensive care based solely on economic criteria. Rather, both economics and biomedical ethics have a place in discussions regarding ICU resource allocation.[37]

Policies and procedures that make good economic sense may not always be congruent with sound biomedical ethics. This should not connote that economics principles and practices are in direct conflict with biomedical ethics. Alternatively, the underpinnings of ethics and morality in medicine may result in decision rules or courses of action that exclude certain economic alternatives, while embracing others. Striking the balance between good economics and sound ethics should be implicit to all decisions from both a macroeconomic or microeconomic perspective.

From an ethics perspective, physicians are obligated to provide for the individual patient whatever additional resources may be seen to improve that patient's health status. The cost of these resources is of secondary importance. However, from an economics perspective, if resources are scarce, whether or not they are effective, someone has to reallocate these limited resources from elsewhere.

Although the role of physician/resource allocator has not been traditional for all physicians, the ICU physician has increasingly become both a prescriber/provider and one who is expected to allocate or ration the critical care product. In the absence of explicit public policies on utilization and cost of ICUs, not surprisingly this creates the dilemma of choosing between the best available economic and ethical courses of action.

References

1. Relman AS: Intensive care units: Who needs them? N Engl J Med 302:965, 1980.
2. Knaus WA, Thibault GE: Intensive care units today, in McNeil BJ, Cravalho EG (eds): *Critical Issues in Medical Technology.* Boston, Auburn House Publishing, 1982. p 193.
3. Berenson RA: Intensive care units, in *Health Technology Case Study 28:* Washington, Office of Technology Assessment.
4. Cullen DJ, Keene R, Waternoux C et al: Results, changes, and benefits of intensive care for critically ill patients: Update 1983. Crit Care Med 12:102, 1984.
5. Bams JL, Miranda DR: Outcome and costs of intensive care. Intensive Care Med 11:234, 1985.
6. Russell LB: *Technology in hospitals.* Washington DC, The Brookings Institute, 1979.
7. Schmidt CD, Elliott G, Carmelli D et al: Prolonged mechanical ventilation for respiratory failure: A cost benefit analysis. Crit Care Med 11:407, 1983.
8. Kaufman, SL, Shepard DS: Costs of neonatal intensive care by day of stay. Inquiry 19:167, 1982.
9. Bendixen JJ: The cost of intensive care, in Runker JP, Barnes BA, Mosteller F (eds): *Costs, Risks and Benefits of Surgery.* New York, Oxford University Press, 1984, p 372.
10. Jacobs P, Noseworthy TW: National estimates of intensive care costs in Canada and the United States. Crit Care Med 18:1282, 1990.
11. Harris J: The internal organization of hospitals: Some economic implications. Bell J Economics 8:467, 1977.
12. Eisenberg JM: Doctors' decisions and the cost of medical care. Ann Arbor, Health Administration Peers Perspectives, 1986.
13. Goldstein RL, Campion EW, Thibault GE et al: Functional outcomes following medical intensive care. Crit Care Med 14:783, 1986.
14. Detsky AS, Stricker SC, Mulley AG et al: Prognosis, survival, and the expenditure of hospital resources for patients in an intensive care unit. N Engl J Med 305:667, 1981.
15. Knaus WA: The use of intensive care: New research initiatives and their implications for national health policy. Milbank Memorial Fund Q, Health Soc 61:561, 1983.
16. Selker HP, Griggith JL, Dorey FJ et al: How do physicians adapt when the coronary care unit is full? JAMA 257:1181, 1987.
17. Cummings KM, Frisof KB, Long MJ et al: The effect of price information on physicians' test ordering behavior: Ordering of diagnostic tests. Med Care 20:293, 1982.
18. Soumerai SB, Avorn J: Efficacy and cost-containment in hospital pharmacotherapy: State of the art and future directions. Milbank Memorial Fund Q 62:447, 1984.

19. Gryskiewicz JM, Detner DE: Waste not, want not: Use of blood in elective operations—improved utilization of blood by use of blood-ordering protocols and the type of screen. Curr Surg 40:371, 1983.
20. Check WA: How to affect antibiotic prescribing practices, JAMA 244:2594, 1980.
21. Schroeder SA, Myers LP, McPhee SJ: The failure of physicians' education as a cost containment strategy: Report of a prospective controlled trial at a university hospital. JAMA 252:225, 1984.
22. Moore SH, Martin DP, Richarson WC: Does the primary care gate-keeper control the costs of health care? Lessons from the SAFECO experience. N Engl J Med 309:1400, 1983.
23. Eisenberg J: Physician utilization. Med Care 23:461, 1985.
24. Daft WL, MacIntosh NB: The nature and use of formal control systems for management control and strategy implementation. J Manag 10:43, 1984.
25. Young D, Saltman RB: Medical practice, case mix and cost containment. JAMA 247:801, 1982.
26. Civetta JM, Hudson-Civetta JA: Maintaining quality of care while undergoing changes in the ICU. Ann Surg 202:524, 1985.
27. Boyle MH, Torrance GW: Developing multiattribute health indexes. Med Care 22:1045, 1984.
28. Williams A: Economics of coronary by-pass grafting. Br Med J 291:325, 1985.
29. Rice D: Estimating the costs of illness. Am J Public Health 57:424, 1967.
30. Landefeld JG, Seskin EP: The economic value of life: Linking theory to practice. Am J Public Health 72:555, 1982.
31. Blades CA, Culyer AJ, Walker A: Health service efficiency: Appraising the appraisers. Soc Sci Ann Med 25:461, 1987.
32. Lemeshow S, Teres D, Pastides H et al: A method for predicting survival and mortality of ICU patients using objectively weighted scores. Crit Care Med 13:519, 1985.
33. Cullen RJ: Results and costs of intensive care. Anesthesiology 47:203, 1977.
34. Boyle MH, Torrence GW, Sinclair JC et al: Economic evaluation of neonatal intensive care of very-low-birth-weight infants. N Engl J Med 308:1330, 1983.
35. Walker DJ, Feldman A, Vohr BR et al: Cost benefit analyses of neonatal intensive care for infants weighing less than 1000 grams at birth. Pediatrics 74:20, 1984.
36. Walker DJ, Vohr BR, Oh W: Economic analysis of regionalized neonatal care for very low birth weight infants in the state of Rhode Island. Pediatrics 76:69, 1985.
37. Noseworthy TW: Resource allocation of adult intensive care. Ann R Coll Phys Surg Can 21:199, 1988.

Chapter 40

PHYSICAL PLANT AND TECHNOLOGY

TERRY P. CLEMMER
JAMES F. ORME, JR.

The physical plant of the intensive care unit (ICU) will vary depending upon the size of the hospital, the types of patients cared for in the unit, the desired level of care to be provided, local building codes, and space and economic restrictions. These considerations, along with a wide variety of personal styles of care, and the hospital politics, make it impossible to stipulate what an ideal unit should be like.

This chapter's goal is to bring the commonly encountered issues to the forefront for reflective consideration, and although the authors' bias may well come through, it is hoped that the spirit of suggestion and consideration will prevail. Most of the material will be taken from the literature and from experiences the authors have had in the planning and construction of two critical care units. In some instances, guidelines of the Society of Critical Care Medicine (SCCM),[1] The National Institute of Health (NIH) Consensus Conference on Critical Care Medicine,[2] and the Joint Commission on Accreditation of Healthcare Organizations (JCAHO)[3] are used. These represent attempts at providing guidelines that are representative of the thoughts of prominent workers in this area and the state of the art in the field.

Although the same principles apply whether one is building a new hospital or wing, or remodeling an existing area, the space constraints and geographical considerations with regard to the rest of the hospital are much more difficult during remodeling.

Initial Planning Process

COMPOSITION OF THE INITIAL PLANNING COMMITTEE

The initial planning should be done primarily by those persons who are expected to work in the unit. If more than one unit is being planned, each unit should be represented on the initial planning committee.[4] The initial planning committee should consist of at least the physician director of the unit(s), the head nurse(s), the administrator over the critical care unit(s), and an architect who is experienced in hospital projects, a good listener, and a willing communicator with medical personnel. In addition, where applicable, the biomedical, education, and research personnel should have input from the inception. Others may be invited according to the specific hospital needs and mission of the unit.

CHARGE OF THE INITIAL PLANNING COMMITTEE

This committee is to lay the philosophy and foundation for the construction of the critical care unit(s) (CCU). It should determine the total number of beds to be constructed, division of beds if more than one unit is required, outline the purpose of the unit(s) as to the type of patient population, the level of care to be delivered, the educational and research activities anticipated, relationship of the unit(s) with other departments, and the space and economic constraints of the construction. It should not become encumbered with the design details of the unit itself, but rather establish the broad guidelines and constraints within which the detailed design must fit.

TOTAL NUMBER OF BEDS

The number of beds to be constructed is an important issue in today's climate of medical economics. To have insufficient beds, which results in frequent closure of the unit to admissions, is a major political and economic headache. Conversely, to have empty beds is an economic disaster. Therefore, careful analysis and projection of needs is worth the effort early in the project. It is best to start with the current needs as projected from historical records. Examining current census needs and reviewing how many days all beds are full and how many requested admissions are denied, will help determine the needs. Formulas are available to predict from these the number of beds depending upon the percent of time the hospital is willing to be unable to accept admissions. One such formula[5] is as follows:

$$\text{Beds needed} = \text{Average census} + Z\sqrt{\text{Average census}}$$

The constant Z is a factor that is determined by the desired probability (P) of having a critical care bed available upon request as follows:

P (%)	Z
99	2.33
95	1.65
90	1.28
85	1.04
80	0.804

Other factors such as creative patient triage may help to keep the units open for admissions. Nurses and physicians skilled in this area can significantly change these formulas.

To the above calculated number, the projected community population and economic growth should be considered. This is more difficult, but past performance and national trends help with this projection, and fairly good estimates are usually available.

The more difficult projection is the impact of future hospital programs that are planned. This may alter the critical care census in different directions. For example, if a liver transplant program is planned, an increased demand will be created of not only the transplanted patient but also an influx of severe liver disease patients waiting for transplant. On the other hand, if the hospital has a large percentage of its patient population participating in prospective reimbursement plans, they may opt for more preventative medicine programs and outpatient services to avoid a large number of critically ill patients who frequently lose money under such reimbursement. Such a change in philosophy may reduce the needs for critical care beds.

STRUCTURING THE BEDS INTO UNITS

The NIH Consensus Conference on Critical Care Medicine,[2] the SCCM,[1] and our personal opinion is that units larger than 12 to 16 beds are difficult to manage from an administrative and quality care standpoint. Above 16 beds, it becomes a nightmare. On the other hand, small units with less than 6 beds are not economically efficient from a staffing and supply perspective. Therefore, it is recommended that the critical care beds should be clustered into units of 6 to 16 beds. Within this range, there may be reasons to choose the higher or lower number. Where there is a large number of one type of patient, such as postthoracic surgery patients, a 16-bed unit may be manageable. If the patient population is multidiscipline type patients, administration and control of quality care would be difficult in a 16-bed unit. This is an area where many administrators do not understand the care issues and for cost reasons want to create larger units with less supervisory, middle-management, and clerical personnel. The efforts required to keep on top of the quality of care delivered, handle the personnel's personal and psychosocial problems, deal with the supply problems, and resolve the political issues in the unit are not appreciated, and these issues increase with larger units.

The other constraints in determining the size of the units are architectural in nature. Most building codes now require that an outside window be provided for each bed, and that direct visualization of the patient be maintained from the central nursing station. Larger nursing units result in longer distances to be covered during the day by the personnel working in the unit and accentuate intraunit communication problems. The larger the staff, the more difficult it is to maintain an *esprit de corps,* which is so valuable to the unit's function.

The guidelines for deciding what type of units the hospital should have are variable depending upon defined needs. Small hospitals may need only one CCU to meet all their demands, one serving a multidisciplinary purpose for coronary, medical, and surgical care. Larger institutions that require more ICU beds will make divisions by either specialty or levels of care. Where there are large volumes of patients (enough to require at least six beds be available at all times) with one basic problem, such as myocardial infarction, postop thoracic surgery or neurosurgery, a separate unit that can establish specific patient care protocols is desirable. Another reason to create specialty units is political, because of dominant physicians and departments insisting on control. This need may be for support of a teaching program, for research reasons, or because they feel that patient care is better when they control the environment. Whatever the reason, political territories are frequently real and a driving force behind the division. Harmony within the unit is important, and these political issues can become very emotional. Where there are no overwhelming economic or administrative reasons preventing them, it may be best to permit the divisions to take place along these lines.

Where the political climate allows, units may be defined by level of care. More critically ill patients may be placed in a unit with physician coverage around the clock, increased space for high-tech procedures, and higher nurse staffing ratios.[7] Another unit would provide care for patients who require less direct physician care, lower nursing acuity, and less high-tech procedures. This second unit would be much less costly, allow for more economical delivery of care, and provide a less aggressive and more peaceful environment.

DEFINE THE PURPOSE OF EACH UNIT

What kind of patients will routinely be cared for in the unit, and what level of care is needed? This must take into consideration trends in patient acuity. Will the needs of the patients be primarily routine monitoring, or will the unit be an aggressive invasive monitoring and therapeutic life support ICU? Will new high-tech procedures be used routinely, such as right and left ventricular assist devices, balloon pumps, and extracorporeal support, or will these needs be met in another unit or even another hospital? Will the patients be confined to primarily one disease type, such as heart disease, or will there be frequent admissions from many departments with a large variety of diseases and failing organs? Will there be only a few physicians admitting to the unit, such as a thoracic surgery unit, or will it be most of the physicians on the hospital staff, such as with a combined medical–surgical unit? Will this unit be used in teaching programs for medical students and house officers? Will the unit be staffed by full-time, critical care physicians? Will teaching only be at the bedside, or in formal rounds and didactic sessions? Will the acuity of the patients require physician coverage 24 h per day? What role will the unit play in nursing education and what will be the nature of that education? Will research be conducted in the unit and what will be the nature of the research?[7] Will research be bedside data gathering of routine care, or will it include the evaluation of new technology and programs, and involve research teams and technicians? Will a special procedures room be required in the unit for special high-tech procedures and research purposes? All of these questions must be carefully considered and answered before one proceeds with the allotment of space and finalizing the unit design, for they will impact heavily on the requirements.

Careful consideration of future goals and programs is necessary to ensure that the units that will be finished several years in the future will still meet the needs then and not just now. This concern is obviously fraught with many pitfalls, but by applying the methods outlined for deciding the needed number of beds, reasonable estimates can be made of the mission of the unit in the future.

PHYSICAL RELATIONSHIP TO OTHER UNITS AND DEPARTMENTS[4,7,8]

This issue often generates an impossible "wish list," since those who work in the CCU would like to be near all other critical care units, the laboratory, computed tomography (CT) scanner, magnetic resonance imaging (MRI) scanner, angiography suite, nuclear medicine, respiratory therapy, the emergency room, the step-down unit or the nursing unit to which they most often transfer their patients, the operating suite, the helicopter landing site, and the cafeteria if at all possible! The task is to identify which of these needs is the most critical, and emotionally the most important to the nurses in the units, since all desires cannot be met. Where there are many units, many needs may be common, but some may be very different. They may therefore vie for priority locations. There are also budgetary and architectural constraints that may dictate differently from the requests. Some of these difficulties may be met by the use of satellite laboratory and x-ray facilities to support clustered ICUs. The use of dedicated elevators and stairwells may allow the stacking of units and help solve these problems. In the end this task will require a great deal of discussion, diplomacy, creative planning, and finally, compromise.

SPACE ALLOCATION

Once the number of beds has been determined and divided into units and the purpose of each unit identified, space requirements can be delineated. Once again, there will be a need for negotiations among the architect and administration members who are responsible for the final budget of the project and the requirements to stay within the legal codes and constraints, and the clinical team who want the best. Because the space requirements are different depending on whether the beds are in an open-bay configuration or in individual rooms, this decision must be made at this time. The SCCM recommends that each bed be allotted 150 to 200 $ft.^2$ if the unit is an open bay design, and 225 to 250 $ft.^2$ if in individual rooms.[1] This is based on the unit having an invasive high-tech mission. If its purpose is for lower acuity, and noninvasive monitoring, smaller rooms could be considered. These dimensions are only for patient care space. To this must be added about 100 $ft.^2$ per bed for patient support space that would include the nurses' station, physician dictating and work area, nutrition area, and dirty and clean utility and storage. In addition to these, family waiting area, nursing lounge, offices, laboratory, classroom(s), physician sleep areas, and research space are considered depending on unit needs.[1] In units where full-time critical specialists are employed, sufficient physician office space will be necessary.

A conflict between space and budget may well arise and create the need for the difficult decision of cutting beds or working in a smaller care area. This must be answered by careful analysis of how the total number of beds were determined, the accuracy of the predicted future community and new program needs, the accuracy of the projected future patient acuity, and how the demands for new technology will impact needs for additional space. It may be best to take a middle-of-the-road approach and eliminate a few beds and decrease space slightly. Where it is anticipated that patient acuity and higher-tech care delivery will increase, it is an error to limit working space significantly. It would be better to have fewer patients and adequate space to provide the level of care desired.

If an accredited program for teaching critical care physicians is a part of the hospital's mission, significant room for teaching, offices, and research is required. The Accreditation Council of Graduate Medical Education (ACGME) requires that sufficient space be provided for fellows to work and engage in scholarly activities.[10] Although this can be elsewhere in the hospital, space in or near the ICU is ideal.

Final Designing Process

COMPOSITION OF THE FINAL DESIGNING COMMITTEE

In addition to those on the initial planning committee for the detail design, input from the physicians, nurses, respiratory therapists, and technicians who work in the specific unit being designed should be solicited. Valuable insights are gained not only from the head nurse and/or the unit medical director, who are usually in more administrative positions, but also from those who work in the unit day to day.[4] In addition, others who interface in the unit frequently, such as radiology, pharmacy, respiratory and physical therapy, clinical and blood gas laboratory, housekeeping, central services, unit clerks, and those responsible for hospital epidemiology and infectious diseases, provide valuable insights and suggestions. It will not be necessary to have all of these persons attend all of the committee meetings on a regular basis, but their input will be needed when specific issues are discussed and before the plans are finalized.

OVERALL DESIGN CONSIDERATIONS

Unit access and traffic patterns: Control of unit access is desirable to reduce traffic and unwanted visitors.[11] Much control is accomplished by policy, but design is also very useful. Location of the unit away from the main corridors and hospital traffic is desirable. Having a family waiting area that is comfortable and designed to allow some privacy between families will help enforce unit policies with regard to visiting hours. It is helpful to the physician staff and the nurses if they do not have to pass by the waiting area each time they enter or exit the unit. On the other hand, physician communications with families can be encouraged by them passing the waiting area frequently. When they enter the unit, the visitors should be directed to or automatically encounter the clerk, who can greet them and prepare them and the nurses for the visit. The main doors used to move patients in and out of the unit should be as wide as the hallway and preferably automatic. The elevators that offer access to the ICU should also be generous in size to accommodate not only the bed but also equipment around the bed and four to five hospital personnel, since the movement of very ill patients with life support equipment is a frequent process performed many times per day. Traffic patterns within the unit should also be considered, since the reduction in steps within the unit can improve efficiency and reduce fatigue of the personnel. This is especially true with the very common 12-h shift staffing. The requirement that the patient be in constant view of the staff should be incorporated into the traffic pattern and nursing station design. Where units are large, multiple nursing stations and support areas are needed to meet this requirement and to allow efficiency of movement during patient care. Another solution is to install closed circuit video monitoring.

CONTROL OF NOSOCOMIAL INFECTIONS

Because hospital-acquired infections are so common, the unit design should facilitate practices that reduce this risk. The most important proven practice is frequent hand washing.[10] Having sinks conveniently located so that hand washing is done as personnel move between patients is desirable. Where possible, foot control of the water is best to discourage possible contamination while hand controls are turned off. In addition, locating facilities to dispose of body wastes within the patient room or near the bed saves having to carry bed pans and urinals across the unit to the dirty utility area. This also allows for any room to become an isolation room, if necessary. The control of air flow in individual rooms is of questionable value at present, and airborne hospital-acquired infections are extremely unusual except for some highly contagious viruses and perhaps tuberculosis. Walls and floors must be of materials that will allow cleaning and decontamination.

PATIENT COMFORT AND PSYCHOLOGIC SUPPORT

The comfort and psychologic support of the patient and staff should be maximized by ensuring control of the temperature between 65 to 85°F and humidity between 30 and 60 percent within the individual rooms, and by providing privacy and noise control.[1] This can be accomplished by using appropriate building materials, and curtains and carpets in appropriate areas. Carpets in the patient rooms, although not proved to be an infectious problem, usually retain odors with time and are best avoided. In addition, lighting control to allow dimming for rest periods, but brightness when basic procedures are performed, is necessary. Procedure lights are a must and can be portable or ceiling-mounted in the room, depending upon the frequency of use and budget. Windows and wall clocks that are easily seen by the patients help with orientation. Color patterns and decor will vary by preference and needs. In a neurosurgical unit, a more stimulating decor may be useful. In other circumstances, a restful, soothing color scheme might be preferable. The unit staff are more qualified to make this decision than a professional decorator.

In addition, designated rooms that are separate from the regular waiting room should be available near the intensive care unit for family and personnel counseling, and solitude. These areas can be used by the medical staff, clergy, and social services when dealing with specific family needs.

COMMUNICATIONS

The ability to call help is required.[3] This should include a mechanism for notifying the hospital cardiac arrest team and/or personnel within the unit immediately should a sudden life-threatening event occur. In addition, in larger units the ability to talk to the nurses' station or clerk's desk via intercom is frequently convenient and time-saving. Numerous telephones should be located throughout the unit, and a portable phone for rare patient use is occasionally useful, depending on the type of patient population. Where computers are used to interface with the laboratory, central services, and other departments, ample space for terminals and printers must be provided.

PATIENT ROOM CONFIGURATION

This is an area where once again there is a variety of individual difference in opinion. It is usually necessary that staff and equipment move freely around at least three sides of the bed. Many prefer 360 degree access to the patient. Special means to supply oxygen, suction, air, electrical power, and monitoring cables have been designed, such as the floor-to-ceiling power columns that are positioned at one corner of the bed or the ceiling, or floor-mounted columns commonly used in operating rooms.[12] As more and more high-tech equipment appears, the access around the patient becomes more limited. Any device that removes the equipment from the floor to the wall, bed, or ceiling is appreciated. Ceiling-mounted tracks for intravenous (IV) poles are a must. The number of poles needed on this track depends on the patient acuity and on the purpose of the unit. Most prefer circular tracks so that the poles can be moved from one side of the bed to the other for convenience, depending on the patient's IV access.

If at all possible, the sink should be located next to the door for convenience when one is entering and leaving the room. When possible, a square room design is best, but if rectangular, it is desirable to locate the head wall on the long side of the rectangle to maximize the space at the sides of the bed, since most equipment and care are provided from this position. A method to secure devices to the head wall in a reconfigurable and movable manner, such as a rail system, is preferred. It is extremely useful for the architect to provide a mock-up of a room with head wall and plumbing details so that the unit personnel are given an opportunity to recognize potential problems and give input prior to completion of the final plans. Windows in the head wall should be small as to not interfere with maximal utilization of this space. Ample oxygen, air, and suction outlets must be provided. The minimum would be two oxygen, two suction, and one air outlet. This would be for a unit with patients who primarily require monitoring. Active invasive units will minimally require four to six oxygen, four to six suction, and two to four air outlets. These should be located at waist-to-chin level and above floor-level equipment that might be placed in front of them. Where rail-type systems are used, they should be located between double horizontal rails or just above or below single rails. The minimal number of electrical outlets is 12–18, and in high-tech units as many as 30 may be necessary. One may be mounted low behind the bed, but all others are best located high. Those head wall outlets farthest away from the bed seem to be the most used. Having some mounted on other walls is also convenient. The room outlets should be 110-V connected to 20–30 A circuit breakers. A 220-V outlet may be necessary for every two beds when required for special equipment such as portable x-ray machines. Isolated electrical panels and grounds are not required in most states, and redundant grounding is seldom if ever used. In most newer hospitals, it is unnecessary. Still, where required by individual state building codes, they must be installed. The estimate of electrocutions by hospital equipment in the 1960s and early 1970s was exaggerated. With newer equipment standards, this problem has been almost eliminated. Good grounding and monitoring of the standard electrical outlets is necessary with frequent monitoring of the safety of the system, along with proper maintenance of equipment. Entry into the room should be wide enough so that the bed plus any life support equipment used during transport can easily pass through. The room should be arranged so that large equipment such as x-ray and fluoroscopy machines can be used at the bedside.

Rooms separated by movable partitions with the ability to create a single larger room for special procedures might be considered for those institutions planning procedures such as extracorporeal support, or other types of therapy requiring the long-term use of large or bulky equipment. If such needs are routine, a separate special procedures room may be better.

It is difficult to anticipate the problems as you plan the room design. When possible, a prototype construction or mock-up is very useful to help the planning by having the nurses and technicians function in the mock-up and make suggestions to improve the design.[8]

PATIENT SUPPORT AREAS

In addition to the patient room, support areas are needed. The nursing station(s) are to be located in such a manner that all beds can be viewed, or the use of video monitoring may be necessary. This usually affords a place for the nurse to chart, a bank of remote monitors where the patient's heart rate and other vital signs are displayed, a medication area with a locked narcotics cabinet, and a nutrition area for preparation of enteral diets. Separate refrigerators for medications and food are mandated by JCAHO.[3] An area for physicians to chart and to dictate is part of the nurses' station or immediately adjacent to it. The clerk's desk should also be located near the chart rack, where communication with the nurses and physicians can be easily accomplished. The location of computer terminals should be determined by those who use them most. If computers are used by nurses, physicians, and clerks, multiple terminals will be needed in the nurses' station area. The size and configuration of the nursing station will vary depending on the mission of the unit. Where there are major teaching commitments and several staff in the unit at all times, the physician area will need to be larger. If the nurses perform all the charting at the bedside and if bedside computer terminals are available, then the use of the nurses' station will be reduced. In units where the patients are more stable and the objective is to give them more uninterrupted rest, more nursing time will be spent at the nurses' station, where the patient can be monitored without being disturbed. Computers change the use of the central stations significantly and should be heavily considered in the design if their use is anticipated. Some hospitals have decentralized pharmacy programs, and some have clinical pharmacists in the critical care areas. If this is a major program, a separate pharmacy area may be required.

The clean utility area is used for storage of small, frequently used items that are stocked from central services and in turn may be used to stock patient rooms. The dirty utility area is for waste disposal, and cleaning equipment and instruments before they are sent for sterilization. The size and plan of these rooms will depend upon the type of activities of the unit. Sinks and hoppers are necessary in the dirty utility area, along with disposal mechanisms for contaminated materials. Whether or not a sink is needed in the clean utility area for hand washing will depend on the projected uses of the room.

In addition to the utility areas, most units have need for an adequate equipment storage area. Most such areas contain procedure lights, cooling blankets, portable oxygen and IV poles, scales, and other items requiring storage. Research-oriented units will have a variety of special monitors and carts that can significantly increase the size requirement of this room.

When the laboratory is not as responsive as needed, a satellite facility in the ICU may be a solution. The common procedures performed in this area are blood gases, complete blood count (CBC), electrolytes, lactates, gram stains, and some culture plating. Some units also develop x-rays in the unit to save time and technician steps. Other requirements include an area for housekeeping and a conference area for consulting with families. The family waiting area should be designed according to the style of use. If the unit has a strict policy forbidding family members from staying the night, the design should facilitate that policy. Where night vigilance is permitted or even encouraged, a design that allows resting and/or sleeping in the waiting area will be necessary. Some ICUs may even provide separate sleeping rooms for visitors.

SUPPORT AREA FOR NURSES

At a minimum, the staff should have their own restroom facilities; a locker area with a shower is preferred, and both male and female areas are needed. In addition, a nursing lounge area for breaks, meals, or study is highly recommended to reduce stress and promote congeniality among the nursing personnel. A nursing office and administrative area near the ICU is also recommended. With today's demands on quality assurance and credentialing of personnel, administration of units have become full-time jobs. Where education is a major activity in the unit, a classroom may be desirable or necessary.

PHYSICIAN SUPPORT AREA

This will vary from unit to unit depending upon its function. If the physicians only conduct their rounds for a short period of time each day on individual patients, a charting and dictation area is all that is needed. If there are full-time critical care physicians assigned to the unit, nearby physician offices are desirable. When there is a strong student and staff teaching program, larger areas near the nurses station and perhaps a nearby classroom will be required. Research activities place even more demands for special procedure rooms, equipment storage, and work stations. Computer usage consequently increases, and these space needs must be anticipated.

Equipping the Critical Care Area

BASIC MONITORING AND THERAPEUTIC EQUIPMENT REQUIRED BY ALL CCUs

There are basic equipment needs required for all units. This includes appropriately designed beds that are electrically safe. They should have removable head boards and be capable of being placed in Trendelenburg and reverse Trendelenburg positions. All the equipment necessary to carry out advanced cardiopulmonary resuscitation (CPR), including equipment for airway intubation, must be available in the unit. Hand ventilation devices, such as a bag-valve-mask with the capability of delivering 100% oxygen, other oxygen delivery devices, oxygen outlet connectors, suction, back board, IV catheters with tubing and fluids, monitor/defibrillator, and cardiac drugs must all be immediately available. All units should have noninvasive electrocardiogram (ECG) and blood pressure monitoring with audible and visual alarms, thermometers, oxygen and suction sources with quick connects, and sufficient electrical outlets. Some type of weighing device should be available in the unit. Medication refrigerator, proper hand-washing and waste disposal equipment, including contaminated materials, must be provided.

MONITORING EQUIPMENT DESIRABLE FOR MOST CCUs

In addition to basic equipment, it is desirable to have remote monitors at the nurses' station, unless the staff is able to stay at the bedside at all times. Most units have a need for multichannel monitors and the capability to perform invasive pressure monitoring. With these monitors come more sophisticated alarm systems for dysrhythmia detection and pressure alarms. This allows for arterial blood pressure, right and left heart filling pressures, and intracranial pressures to be continuously monitored. Cardiac output determination is desirable if care of a significant number of unstable patients is anticipated. In addition, noninvasive pulse oximetry and mixed venous oximetry are used in most larger units and have become almost standard. Data management systems are becoming more common and are now on the desirable list for most CCUs. Because of the enormous volume of information generated on ICU patients daily, the physicians and nurses need state of the art methods of data retrieval and organization.

THERAPEUTIC EQUIPMENT DESIRABLE FOR MOST CCUs

In addition to basic airway, ventilatory and cardiac support, most CCUs need ventilators that can provide safe, long-term support. Most volume ventilators today require compressed air to control the F_{IO_2}. Infusion pumps for titration of vasoactive, antiarrhythmic, and other continuous infusion drugs are standard equipment. Ceiling-mounted IV poles are desirable when multiple IV use is likely. Patient temperature control devices are frequently used in the ICU and should be available to the unit. Where a high number of cardiac patients are seen, pacemakers are necessary. This may also suggest the need for beds capable of permitting fluoroscopy to be used. Other commonly used devices include dialysis and hemofiltration equipment, and outlets for these devices should be provided. In addition, where a satellite clinical laboratory is included in the ICU, a blood gas machine, microscope, gram-staining materials, centrifuge, and basic chemistry analyzers should be available. In the nutrition area, a sink, refrigerator, and microwave are usually standard. Some units have small stoves or hot plates. Specialized beds that are thought to have therapeutic value are also commonly used and frequently require more space and consideration of how the tubes and cables will access the patient.

COMMONLY USED HIGH-TECH EQUIPMENT

There is some equipment that is used on a frequent basis in critical care today and may suggest a trend that hospitals may want to plan for, even though the effectiveness of the devices is still not clear. They include continuous electroencephalogram (EEG) monitors, metabolic measuring devices, and continuous cardiac output monitoring by ECHO or impedance techniques. Balloon cardiac assist devices are very popular and commonly used along with left and right ventricular assist devices. Ventilators are also becoming more sophisticated and provide a variety of ventilation modes including pressure-controlled inverse ratio ventilation (PC-IRV), pressure support ventilation (PSV), both volume and pressure ventilation along with synchronized intermittent mandatory ventilation (SIMV), controlled or assist/controlled ventilation, and continuous positive pressure breathing (CPPB) support. As the technology in this area expands, it brings with it new requirements for respiratory therapy education and standards. It is common to find that physicians and nurses in the ICU can no longer set up and troubleshoot the ventilators or readily access the various modes made available by the ventilator without consulting the therapist. Consequently, the therapist has become an integral part of the CCU and should be included in the space and equipment planning.

With the expansion of the new monitoring and therapeutic equipment, the routine ICU room may become crowded. Some critical care units that have a significant interest and desire to use high-tech equipment may consider building a special procedures room adjacent to the unit for such activities. This may be with or without built-in x-ray and fluoroscopic capabilities, depending on the type and frequency of procedures to be performed.

EXPERIMENTAL EQUIPMENT AND PROCEDURES

Some equipment being used in critical care medicine today should be considered experimental and should only be used in those facilities that are in the process of scientifically evaluating the efficacy of such therapy. This equipment includes artificial hearts, long-term extracorporeal support for respiratory failure, special experimental mode ventilation such as high-frequency jet ventilators for adults, and oscillatory ventilation. Although some justify the use of such equipment as being innovative and a last-ditch effort in a "sure to die otherwise" situation, (with very rare exception) it is difficult to justify such use outside of investigative protocols. When such equipment is introduced into practice by these methods, it is common not to know for years the efficacy and true hazards that might be associated with the therapy.

This abbreviated overview of ICU planning and design is to help direct and remind future planners of many of the considerations that must be made when designing a unit. It is obviously not all encompassing, nor does it answer all questions. Each planner will have to make decisions based on needs, budget, and local environmental factors. Hopefully this chapter has outlined the questions that should be asked and a method that may be useful in making decisions during the planning process.

References

1. Society of Critical Care Medicine, Committee on Guidelines: Guidelines for organization of critical care units. JAMA, 222:1532–1535, 1972.
2. *Critical Care Medicine. National Institute of Health Consensus Development Conference Summary,* Vol. 4, 1983. Washington, DC, U.S. Government Printing Office.
3. Joint Commission on Accreditation of Health Organizations: *Special Care Units: Accreditation Manual for Hospitals,* 1990, pp. 243–254.
4. Hudson LD: Design of the intensive care unit from a monitoring point of view. Respir Care, 30:549–559, 1985.
5. *Evaluation and Space Programming Methodology for Special Care Units: Medical, Surgical, Coronary and Respiratory Intensive Care.* Canada: Department of National Health and Welfare, Health Services Promotion Branch, 1979.
6. Design lines: Gradations of intensive care. Hospitals, 47:46–47, 1973.
7. Brackell CE: Administration, staffing and design of the intensive care unit. Clin Neurosurg, 22:389–410, 1975.
8. Thams J: Design and developing the critical care unit, in Adler D, Shoemaker N (ed): *AACN Organization of Management of Critical Care Facilities.* St. Louis, CV Mosby, 1979.
9. *Requirements for Accreditation of Programs: Section II of Graduate Medical Education Programs 1989–1990, by the Accreditation Council for Graduate Medical Education.* Chicago, AMA, 1989.
10. Sampson LK: Designing and equipping the critical care unit, in Adler D, Shoemaker N (eds): *AACN Organization and Management of Critical Care Facilities.* St. Louis, Mosby, 1979.
11. Stoddart JC: Design, staffing and equipment requirements for an intensive care unit. Int Anesthesiol Clin, 19:77–95, 1981.
12. Piergeonge AR, Cesarano FL, Casanova DM: Designing the critical care unit: A multi-disciplinary approach. Crit Care Med, 11:541–545, 1983.

Chapter 41
COMPUTER APPLICATIONS

ALAN H. MORRIS
REED M. GARDNER

Introduction

In the past 30 years there has been an explosion of information in medicine. This prodigious growth has resulted in a proliferation of medical journals and books and has found clear expression in the staggering amount of information produced by critical care patients. We recently counted 236 different variables being followed for one patient in the Shock Trauma/Intermountain Respiratory ICU at our institution, the LDS Hospital in Salt Lake City. This list did not include all the data and, though many variables changed as a function of time, did not include repeated (serial) measurements. It included variables in the following categories: hemodynamics (14), blood gases (15), ventilatory management (20), hemogram (20), urinalysis (20), ECG (11), blood chemistry (20), special blood chemistry (12), urine chemistry (4), bacteriology (10), bone marrow (17), nutritional balance (20), coagulation (7), temperature (1), weight (1), and medications (44). It did not include information from physical examination, x-ray, special studies (e.g., CT scans, ultrasound, angiography), physicians' consultation notes, nurses' notes, respiratory therapists' notes, physicians' progress notes, operating room notes, anesthesia notes, or pathologists' reports. We question whether any mere mortal could effectively assimilate all the variables and come to the "right clinical treatment decision" for this severely ill patient. Even acknowledging that not all variables are necessary for every treatment decision and that not all the data are independent, it still seems likely that most physicians would have difficulty dealing systematically with this large mass of clinical data. In fact, having to deal with as few as four variables has prevented experienced pulmonary and critical care physicians from systematically managing a mechanical ventilator in the inverse ratio ventilation mode (see Inverse Ratio Ventilation Protocol, below). The physician who attempts to integrate knowledge from the pertinent literature with all patient data, including results of the physical examination, frequently faces a nearly impossible task.

In critical care, computer applications have made multiple contributions, from coordinating data to assisting in medical decision-making. In most of these applications the digital computer system has been used as a tool to aid in the management and interpretation of large amounts of information. Computers can be expected to play an increasingly important role in medical practice,[1] although there is some controversy over the exact role computers should fill.[2] Although ICU computerization began at the LDS Hospital 20 years ago, only about one-fourth of the average LDS hospital medical chart is currently computerized.[3] It is noteworthy that attention paid to specific kinds of data by the medical staff seems unrelated to the fraction of the total medical record occupied by those specific data.[3,4] Computer applications in critical care take many forms. Computer systems vary in size from the isolated personal computer dedicated to a specific and constrained task (see Inverse Ratio Ventilation Protocol, below) to large, integrated hospital information systems. Three of the best-known hospital information systems are HELP, TMIS, and PROMIS.[5] We will illustrate some of the broad applications of computers in critical care by referring to our experience with the HELP (Health Evaluation through Logical Processing) computer system.[6,7]

Figure 41-1 illustrates the flow of information into and out of the HELP system. Information is entered and stored in coded format into the patient data base. Clinical staff members (physicians, registered nurses, and respiratory therapists—MDs, RNs, and RTs, respectively), laboratories, and others have access to all of the patient's information from bedside or other terminals and from printers. The HELP system knowledge base is then applied to the patient data. The knowledge base contains decision criteria from the published literature and from local, national, and international experts. The outputs of the HELP system can be reviewed from bedside and other computer terminals, or as printed reports. The reports include the derived variables, the interpretation of data sets, alerts (warnings) of potentially dangerous situations, and the instructions for therapy according to protocols, where applicable.

Acquisition and Integration (Coordination) of Data

Adding structure to the clinical data base, by itself, appears to have a favorable effect on physicians' performance.[8] Entry of data into a computerized data base can occur either manually (via a keyboard) or by automatic entry through an electronic connection such as the medical information bus (MIB), which is being developed as an industry standard.[9,10,11] Manual (keyboard) data entry is routinely used by nurses,[12,13] physicians,[6] respiratory therapists,[14] and others in the LDS Hospital. In some institutions the keyboard seems to be an obstacle to medical computer use. At the LDS Hospital the use of keyboards and simple screen menus has been readily accepted and is routinely used as a bedside tool. While automatic data entry through the MIB[10,11] simplifies data acquisition for clinical care team members, it raises questions about data quality, data representativeness, and data overload. It is easy to overload a computer, as well as a human being, with data. For example the storage of data collected from a modern mechanical ventilator for *one patient-day* in our ICU required more than 4 million bytes of space. (Our current typical ICU patient record amounts to fewer than 15,000 bytes per day.) Even if

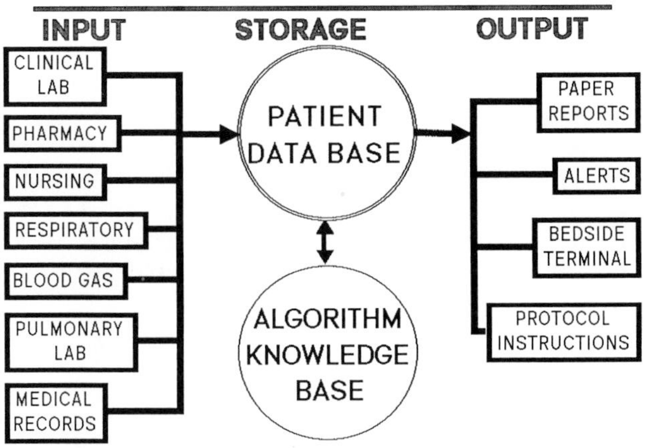

FIGURE 41-1 The HELP System. Data from many sources are stored in the computerized patient database. The data are then available for review or for use in reports or computerized decision-making. The HELP knowledge base consists of decision criteria developed from expert opinion, the literature, and experience.

high-quality data are assured, one must ask if they are "representative" if they are to be used for clinical decision-making. For example, an accurate measurement of blood pressure, or arterial or mixed venous oxygenation, during a period of endotracheal suctioning would not provide data representative of the patient's response to therapy. Such nonrepresentative data would not be pertinent to the planning of therapy.

The coordination of raw data and the generation of legible reports containing accurate information about medications, fluid intake and output, nutritional information, and basic monitoring are extremely important. They strike directly at the information overload problem facing the medical care delivery system. Derived data, such as arterial–mixed venous oxygen content difference, oxygen consumption, alveolar-arterial oxygen pressure difference, cardiac index, pulmonary vascular resistance, stroke work index, thoracic compliance, net fluid balance, caloric balance, etc., are easily obtained. Once algorithms, obtained both from published information and from consensus of experts both distant and local (MDs, RNs, RTs), are entered into the system's knowledge base (Fig. 41-1), they provide accurate derived data and avoid the large investments of time and energy required to do such work repetitively by hand.

Integration of data takes place in many areas. For example, blood gas analysis is performed in a blood gas laboratory and integrated with cardiac output measurements performed either at the bedside or in the cardiac catheterization laboratory. As a result of this integration, whenever a mixed venous and arterial blood sample pair is submitted for blood gas analysis (and an arterial–mixed venous oxygen content difference [$C(a-\bar{v})O_2$], calculated), the data base is automatically searched for a cardiac output measured within 15 min of the time at which the arterial and mixed venous blood samples were obtained. If a cardiac output is found, it is multiplied by the $C(a-\bar{v})O_2$ to compute the oxygen consumption ($\dot{V}O2$), which is included on the blood gas laboratory report (Fig. 41-2).

Figure 41-3 illustrates a 12-h ICU shift report containing vital signs, hemodynamic measurements, urine flow and analyses, weight, tube drainage, fluid intake and output, and drug administration with units and infusion rates every 15 min. Net fluid balance and complete hemodynamic and blood gas reports are included. The 7-day summary reports (Fig. 41-4) are derived from the two 12-h shift reports (Fig. 41-3) for each day. The identification of fluid balance, medication (with units and route of administration), and vital signs represents a major contribution to efficient management of large amounts of clinical information. Our clinicians consider this capability of collating and organizing data for reporting purposes to be a major and extremely valuable benefit associated with use of an integrated hospital information system.

Although it is not part of the official hospital record, a 24-h summary report has been used successfully as a brief précis for presentation at morning ICU rounds (Fig. 41-5). It has been useful as a means of quickly summarizing the most pertinent data, grouped by organ system. Transparencies of the report are projected on a screen at morning rounds, thus facilitating communication between clinical care team members (including trainees).

Computerized Medical Decision Making

Medical decision-making support is a major element of the HELP hospital information system. The concept of providing the practicing physician with decision-making aids capable of dealing with a large amount of information and of applying a well-defined set of decision-making rules is attractive. Interpretation of a patient's laboratory test results is one of the simplest applications of computerized medical decision-making. Measurements of blood gases (Fig. 41-2) and cardiac output (Fig. 41-6) measurements provide ready examples. The algorithms used to interpret these two sets of data are widely available in textbooks and other publications.[15] Computerized interpretations provide uniformity and prevent such common mistakes as errors in computation, transcription, and noncongruence of units. The rapid availability of the results and interpretations provides information that would not normally be obtained manually, because physicians and nurses are so busy.

The generation and presentation of alerts or warnings to physicians, nurses, therapists, and other members of the hospital staff represents another level of clinically valuable computerized decision-making. Alerts are generated as a result of automatic interpretations of data from the clinical laboratories,[16,17] the respiratory care department,[18] the pharmacy department,[19] and other sites, including the blood gas laboratory. Alerts include responses defined by recent and past medical history and current medication administration, as well as medications ordered but not yet administered. Table 41-1 includes examples of alerts for severe hypoxemia, sepsis, electrolyte abnormalities, and drug incompatibility. The respiratory therapy department

```
              L D S   H O S P I T A L   B L O O D   G A S   R E P O R T
                                                                                    SEX  AGE    ROOM
           R      K.                        NO.           DR. L    P                  F   48    DS

DEC 14 90    pH    PCO2    HCO3     BE   HB   CO/MT   PO2   SO2   O2CT   %O2  AVO2  VO2   C.O.   A-a  Qs/Qt  PK/ PL/PP  MR/SR
             --    ----                                ---
NORMAL HI   7.45   40.9    26.2    2.5  15.9   2/ 1                          5.5  300   7.30    22     5
NORMAL LOW  7.35   27.5    15.9    2.5  11.9   0/ 1    62    90   16.1       3.0  200   2.90           0

14 04:16 V  7.32   52.0    26.3         11.7   3/ 1    49    82   13.5   100                                54/ 47/30   3/
14 04:15 A  7.34   48.2    25.5     .2  12.0   3/ 1   162    95   16.4   100  2.55 212   8.30   383    35   54/ 47/30   3/
14 01:05 A  7.34   50.8    26.9     .9  12.3   2/ 1    59    89   15.3    40                     120        54/ 49/30   3/
            SAMPLE # 110, TEMP 36.1, BREATHING STATUS : IMV
            MODERATE MIXED CHRONIC AND ACUTE RESPIRATORY ACIDOSIS
            MODERATE HYPOXEMIA
            MILDLY REDUCED O2 CONTENT
            HYPOVENTILATION MARKEDLY IMPROVED
            PULSE OXIMETER SO2  93.0

13 17:35 A  7.36   57.9    32.2    5.8  12.1   2/ 0    70    92   15.7    60                     222        53/ 50/30   3/
            SAMPLE # 109, TEMP 36.3, BREATHING STATUS : IMV
            SEVERE CHRONIC RESPIRATORY ACIDOSIS
            MILDLY REDUCED O2 CONTENT
            HYPOVENTILATION NOT IMPROVED
            PULSE OXIMETER SO2  94.0

13 13:31 V  7.42   53.3    34.2    8.9  12.0   2/ 1    49    84   14.2    80                                55/ 50/30  20/
13 13:30 A  7.40   56.4    34.5    8.7  12.3   2/ 1    71    93   16.1    80  1.46 158  10.80   345    57   55/ 50/30  20/
            SAMPLE # 108, TEMP 36.5, BREATHING STATUS : IMV
            SEVERE CHRONIC RESPIRATORY ACIDOSIS
            MILDLY REDUCED O2 CONTENT
            NORMAL O2 SATURATION AND PO2
            HYPOVENTILATION WORSE
            PULSE OXIMETER SO2  93.0

13 12:10 A  7.42   52.6    33.8    8.5  12.3   2/ 0    67    93   16.0    90                     412        53/ 49/30   3/
            SAMPLE # 107, TEMP 36.3, BREATHING STATUS : IMV
            MODERATE CHRONIC RESPIRATORY ACIDOSIS
            MILDLY REDUCED O2 CONTENT
            HYPOVENTILATION NOT IMPROVED
            PULSE OXIMETER SO2  93.0

13 08:44 A  7.44   51.4    34.6    9.8  12.0   3/ 1    61    90   15.3   100                     481        54/ 48/30   3/
            SAMPLE # 106, TEMP 36.6, BREATHING STATUS : IMV
            MODERATE MIXED RESPIRATORY ACIDOSIS AND METABOLIC ALKALOSIS
            MILD HYPOXEMIA
            MILDLY REDUCED O2 CONTENT
            PULSE OXIMETER SO2  92.0

13 06:05 A  7.43   51.6    33.9    8.9  12.1   2/ 1    54    88   14.9   100                     487        56/ 51/30   3/
            SAMPLE # 105, TEMP 36.7, BREATHING STATUS : IMV
            MODERATE CHRONIC RESPIRATORY ACIDOSIS
            MODERATE HYPOXEMIA
            MILDLY REDUCED O2 CONTENT
            HYPOVENTILATION NOT IMPROVED
            PULSE OXIMETER SO2  87.0

13 04:59 O  7.53   35.0    29.3    7.5  12.3   1/ 1   412    98   18.1   100                                56/ 50/30   3/
13 04:57 I  7.41   55.0    34.5    8.9  12.3   1/ 1    34    72   12.4   100                                56/ 50/30   3/
13 04:56 V  7.43   50.3    33.1    8.2  12.2   2/ 0    38    78   13.4   100                                56/ 50/30   3/
13 04:55 A  7.42   51.3    32.9    7.9  11.9   1/ 0    47    86   14.3   100  1.28 156  12.20   495    74   56/ 50/30   3/
            SAMPLE # 104, TEMP 36.5, BREATHING STATUS : IMV
            MODERATE CHRONIC RESPIRATORY ACIDOSIS
            SEVERE HYPOXEMIA BREATHING OXYGEN **CONTACT MD OR RN!!!!
            MILDLY REDUCED O2 CONTENT
            HYPOVENTILATION NOT IMPROVED
            PULSE OXIMETER SO2  84.0

PRELIMINARY INTERPRETATION -- BASED ONLY ON BLOOD GAS DATA.  ***(FINAL DIAGNOSIS REQUIRES CLINICAL CORRELATION)***
KEY: CO=CARBOXY HB, MT=MET HB, O2CT=O2 CONTENT, AVO2=ART VENOUS CONTENT DIFFERENCE (CALCULATED WITH AVERAGE OF A &V HB VALUES),
 VO2=OXYGEN CONSUMPTION, C.O.=CARDIAC OUTPUT, A-a=ALVEOLAR arterial O2 DIFFERENCE, Qs/Qt=SHUNT, PK=PEAK, PL=PLATEAU, PP=PEEP
 MR=MACHINE RATE, SR=SPONTANEOUS RATE.       *** SPECIMEN IDENTIFICATION: BLOOD (A=ARTERIAL, V=VENOUS, C=CAPILLARY, W=WEDGE);
                                             FLUIDS (P=PLEURAL, J=JOINT, B=ABDOMINAL, S=ABSCESS); E=EXPIRED AIR;
                                             ECCO2R (I=INFLOW, M=MIDFLOW, O=OUTFLOW)
```

FIGURE 41-2 HELP System Blood Gas Report. The patient's arterial–mixed venous oxygen content difference (AVO2) and machine (ventilator) rate (MR) are reduced because this patient is supported with veno-venous extracorporeal oxygenation and carbon dioxide removal.[22,25] The diagnostic statements for oxygenation, acid-base balance, and ventilation are derived from a standardized interpretative scheme.[15]

```
AGE:  48    SEX: F    ADM WT:   70.50 KG    HT: 165 CM    BSA  1.97 SQM    DR: L     , P
          P HR TEMP
         SD *     C          DEC 13 90 18:01  -  DEC 14 90 06:00
                  18   19   20   21   22   23    0    1    2    3    4    5    6
         --------|+---+---+---+---+---+---+---+---+---+---+---+---+---+
          235 41|
                |
          220 40|
                |
          205 39|
                |
          190 38|
                |
          175 37|
                | CCCCCCCCCCCCCCC C
          160 36|                 C CCCCCCCCCCCCCCCCCCCCCCCCCCCCCCCCC
                |
          145 35|
                |
          130 34|                               S
                |-------------------S--SS-SSS-----------SS---------
          115   | *********S****S*S*S*  *****   S S    S S
                | SS S S           S    S*SS  S ****S****SS*S *****  ****
          100   |   S S SS SSS    S                S     *  S  S* S S
                |                                             SS SS S
           85   |
                |--------------------------------------------------
           70   |
                |
           55   |                                        D
                | D  D
           40   |  DD DDDDDDDDDDDDDDDDDDDDDDDDDDDDDDDDDD D D   DD  D
                |                                         D DDD  DD D
           25   |
                |
           10   |
                  18   19   20   21   22   23    0    1    2    3    4    5    6
         --------|+---+---+---+---+---+---+---+---+---+---+---+---+---+
```

```
     YESTERDAY'S WEIGHT:   90.00
     TODAY'S WEIGHT:       79.40
*                                  *
********** 06:00 TO 06:00 *********
*                                  *
   MAXIMUM TEMP: 36.9

  INPUT
     IV:          3232
     BLOOD:
     COLLOID:   1705
     TOTAL:      4977    NET: -10007
  OUTPUT
     URINE:     13750
     DRAIN:       661
     TOTAL:     14984
*                                  *
*********** LAB RESULTS ***********
*                                  *
  WBC     28.2    DEC 14 90 04:00
  HCT     36.7    DEC 14 90 04:00
  HGB     12.7    DEC 14 90 04:00
  PLATE   31      DEC 14 90 04:00

  NA     146      DEC 14 90 04:00
  K        5.5    DEC 14 90 04:00
  CL      96      DEC 14 90 04:00
  CO2     21      DEC 14 90 04:00
  BUN    118      DEC 14 90 04:00
  GLUC   126      DEC 14 90 04:00
  CREAT    3.1    DEC 14 90 04:00
```

```
WEIGHT (KG)                                                79.40
BED WEIGHT                                                    *
RAP (MMHG)                20   18   18   18   18   19   18   17   17   20   20   19
PA SP (MMHG)              38   38   38   38   42   36   36   36   40   44   44   44
PA DP (MMHG)              24   24   24   24   23   20   22   20   22   24   24   23
PA MEAN (MMHG)            29   29   29   29   29   25   26   26   27   31   31   30
PA WEDGE (MMHG)           20   20   20   17   19   18   17   17   18   22   22   20
CO (L/MIN)                                                       8.30
RESP RATE                  3    3    3    3    3    3    3    3    3    3    3    3
URINE SP G                 1.015
BLOOD GLU MG/DL              233            204            153
URINE PH                     5.0
URINE BLOOD                   3+
URINE PROTEIN                 3+
BILIRUBIN                     3+
KETONES                       5+
TUBE/DRAIN PH                7.0
OXIMETRY - SVO2           86   87        88   85   85   82   82   83   91   82   73
OXIMETRY - STO2 (F)       96   96        96   96   95   93   93   95   99   97   92
MEAN BP (MMHG)            60
FOLEY CATH URINE           0    5
ULTRAFILATION OUT        7001100 800  900  635  800  360                     400
ACT                      156       136       157       145       150  157

TIME              CO     CI   HR   SV   SI   MP   MSP   PA    RA   PW   PVR   SVR   RWI   LWI
NORMAL HI       7.30   3.50   89  101   48  105   123   19   5.0   12   1.0    18  11.0    85
NORMAL LOW      2.90   2.80   49   47   38   70    80    9   1.0    4   0.5    12   8.0    48

DEC 14 04:10    8.30   4.46  107   78   42   50    73   26  10.0E18    1.0     5   9.1    31
            DEC 14 03:56  DOPAMINE (INTROPIN) 8.00 MCG/KG/MIN
            DEC 13 09:00  DIGOXIN .125 MGM, INJ
            MILD LV DYSFUNCTION
```

```
                                                           DEC 13 90 18:01  -  DEC 14 90 06:00
                                                        18   19   20   21   22   23    0    1    2    3    4    5    6
                                           -------------|+---+---+---+---+---+---+---+---+---+---+---+---+---+
 IMIPENEM CILASTATIN (PRIMAXIN), INJ         500 MGM    IV            1                            1
 HUMULIN REGULAR, INJ                          3 UNITS  IV          1
 D5W, INJ                                    127 ML     IV      *****************************************
          INFUSION RATE                    5.000 CC/HOUR        111111111119999111111111111111111    11111
```

FIGURE 41-3 (See page 505 for legend.)

```
          INFUSION RATE                              65.00 CC/HOUR                                     111
  FAT EMULSION 10% (LIPOSYN), INJ                     350 ML     IV     *************
  DOPAMINE, INJ                                       332 MGM    IV     *****************************************
          INFUSION RATE                             1.000 MCG/KG/MIN     8888888888888888888888888888888888888888
          INFUSION RATE                             10.00 MCG/KG/MIN    1
    D5W, INJ                                           79 ML
  NORMAL SALINE, INJ                                  150 ML     IV     ********************
  VECURONIUN BROMIDE (NORCURON MG/HR), INJ              0 MGM    IV     *************************************************
    D5W, INJ                                            0 ML
  AMINOSYN RF, INJ                                     88 ML     IV     ******************
          INFUSION RATE                             55.00 CC/HOUR       11111111111111111
    DEXTROSE 70%, INJ                                 147 ML
    SODIUM                                            1.6 MEQ
    CALCIUM                                           1.3 MEQ
    ZINC                                              1.0 MGM
    COPPER                                            0.2 MGM
    MANGANESE                                         0.1 MGM
    CHROMIUM                                          2.1 MCG
    CHLORIDE                                          1.6 MEQ
    GLUCONATE                                         1.3 MEQ
    MVI-12, INJ                                       1.8 ML
    INSULIN REGULAR, INJ                                7 UNITS
    ELECTROLYTE VOLUME                                3.3 ML
    RANITIDINE HCL (ZANTAC), INJ                       29 MGM
  HEPARIN, INJ                                       4100 UNITS IV      *******************
          INFUSION RATE                              400. UNITS/HR      111111111111111111
    D5W, INJ                                           41 ML
  MIDAZOLAM (VERSED), INJ                            38.0 MGM    IV     *************************************************
          INFUSION RATE                             3.000 MGM/HR        1111111111111111111111111111111111111111111111111
    D5W, INJ                                           38 ML
  AMINOSYN 8.5%, INJ                                  208 ML     IV                      ********************************
          INFUSION RATE                             55.00 CC/HOUR                        11111111111111111111111111111111
    DEXTROSE 50%, INJ                                 208 ML
    SODIUM                                           14.5 MEQ
    POTASSIUM                                         8.3 MEQ
    CALCIUM                                           1.9 MEQ
    MAGNESIUM                                         2.1 MEQ
    ZINC                                              1.9 MGM
    COPPER                                            0.4 MGM
    MANGANESE                                         0.2 MGM
    CHROMIUM                                          3.7 MCG
    CHLORIDE                                         14.5 MEQ
    ACETATE                                          12.3 MEQ
    MVI-12, INJ                                       3.2 ML
    INSULIN REGULAR, INJ                               10 UNITS
    ELECTROLYTE VOLUME                                8.3 ML
  HEPARIN, INJ                                       3100 UNITS IV                        *******************************
          INFUSION RATE                              400. UNITS/HR                        1111111111111111111111111111111
    D5W, INJ                                           31 ML
  FRESH FROZEN PLASMA                                 205 ML     IV                       **
    O POSITIVE
    NO.                                           1326364
  FRESH FROZEN PLASMA                                 240 ML     IV                        *
    O POSITIVE
    NO.                                           1326390
  NORMAL SALINE, INJ                                  200 ML     IV                        ******************************
  DOPAMINE, INJ                                        76 MGM    IV                                              *********
          INFUSION RATE                             1.000 MCG/KG/MIN                                             888888999
    D5W, INJ                                           18 ML
  D5W, INJ                                             11 ML     IV                                              *********
          INFUSION RATE                             5.000 CC/HOUR                                                111111111
  FRESH FROZEN PLASMA                                 200 ML     IV                                                  *
    O POSITIVE
    NO.                                            110232
  FRESH FROZEN PLASMA                                 215 ML     IV                                                  *
    O POSITIVE
    NO.                                            110213
                                                                      18  19  20  21  22  23   0   1   2   3   4   5   6
                                                      --------------|+---+---+---+---+---+---+---+---+---+---+---+---+
   DEC 13 90 18:01 TO DEC 14 90 06:00   WA     , W     C, RN          ************************************************

  INTAKE (ML):  COLLOID          860   OUTPUT (ML):  INSENSIBLE LOSS            265
                NON-BLOOD IV    1712                 ULTRAFILTRATION OUT       5695
                                                     PHLEBOTOMY OUTPUT          101
                                                     NG TUBE DRG.               200
                                                     FOLEY CATH URINE             5
                  TOTAL         2572                   TOTAL                   6266       NET BALANCE     -3694

 DEC 14 90    pH   PCO2   HCO3   BE   HB   CO/MT   PO2   SO2   O2CT   %O2   AVO2   VO2   C.O.   A-a   Qs/Qt   PK/ PL/PP   MR/SR
              --   ----                            ---
```

FIGURE 41-3 (*continued*)

```
NORMAL HI    7.45    40.9    26.2   2.5  15.9   2/ 1                                  5.5  300   7.30   22    5
NORMAL LOW   7.35    27.5    15.9   2.5  11.9   0/ 1    62     90    16.1              3.0  200   2.90         0

14 04:19 O   7.45    33.2    22.9    .3  11.9   2/ 1   375     97    17.2   100                                      54/ 47/30   3/
14 04:17 I   7.31    54.9    27.1    .4  12.1   3/ 1    46     79    13.5   100                                      54/ 47/30   3/
14 04:16 V   7.32    52.0    26.3        11.7   3/ 1    49     82    13.5   100                                      54/ 47/30   3/
14 04:15 A   7.34    48.2    25.5    .2  12.0   3/ 1   162     95    16.4   100   2.55 212   8.30  383    35        54/ 47/30   3/
14 01:05 A   7.34    50.8    26.9    .9  12.3   2/ 1    59     89    15.3    40                      120              54/ 49/30   3/
             SAMPLE # 110, TEMP 36.1, BREATHING STATUS : IMV
             MODERATE MIXED CHRONIC AND ACUTE RESPIRATORY ACIDOSIS
             MODERATE HYPOXEMIA
             MILDLY REDUCED O2 CONTENT
             HYPOVENTILATION MARKEDLY IMPROVED
             PULSE OXIMETER SO2  93.0
```

FIGURE 41-3 Example of 12-h (6:00 PM, December 13, 1990, to 6:00 AM, December 14, 1990) shift report generated by computer. Top line shows patient's age, sex, admission weight, height, and body surface area (BSA). Moving down the sheet, physiologic data are plotted at 15-min intervals (systolic and diastolic pressures, heart rate, and temperature). To the right of the plot are weight comparison, daily maximum temperature, 24-h fluid input and output summary, and the most current laboratory results. Below the plot of the physiologic data is a summary of other measures, such as pulmonary artery pressures, oximeter readings [both arterial, from a finger (F) probe, and mixed venous], and cardiac output determinations. Note that full cardiac output reports follow this section; they have all appropriate values calculated, provide an interpretation (mild left ventricular dysfunction, in this case), and indicate what drugs and doses were present (and their starting times and dates) at the time of the cardiac output determination. Next is a list of all medications given and of IV solution infusion rates. Evidence of MIB IV pump infusion rate output data is indicated for several infusions (e.g., dopamine, first at 10 mcg (μg) per kg per min and then at 8 mcg/kg/min). After the list of medications, it can be seen that one nurse (WA, WC) cared for the patient for the full 12-h shift. An intake and output summary follows, and then blood gas study results with the interpretations are presented. Note particularly the arterial and mixed venous sample pair (samples labeled 04:15 A and 04:16 V). For this arterial and mixed venous blood sample pair, the computer system automatically calculates the arterial-venous oxygen content (AVO2) difference (2.55 mL per dL of blood), the oxygen consumption (383 mL/min) and right-to-left shunt (35 percent) from the data available in the HELP system. The report took only 24 s to generate. The report also illustrates how the computer integrates and organizes data for nursing and medical staff. A = arterial; A − a = alveolar-arterial O_2 pressure difference; ADM = admission; BE = base excess; BSA = body surface area; C = core temperature; CL = chloride; CO = cardiac output; CO/MT = carboxy- and methemoglobin saturation; CREAT = creatinine; D = diastolic arterial pressure (on graphic plot); D5W = 5% dextrose in water; DRG = drainage; GLUC = glucose level; HB or HGB = hemoglobin; HCO3 = bicarbonate; HCT = hematocrit; HR = heart rate; HT = height; K = potassium level; LAB = laboratory; LV = left ventricle; LVI = left ventricular stroke work index; MCG = micrograms; MP = mean systemic blood pressure; MR/SR = machine (ventilator) rate/spontaneous ventilatory rate; NA = sodium; NG = nasogastric; O2CT = oxygen content; PA = pulmonary artery mean pressure; PA DP = pulmonary artery diastolic pressure; PA SP = pulmonary artery systolic pressure; PA WEDGE or PW = pulmonary artery wedge pressure; PK/PL/PP = peak and plateau positive end-expiratory pressures from ventilators; PLATE = platelet count; PVR = pulmonary vascular resistance; Qs/Qt = right-to-left shunt (percent); RA or RAP = right atrial mean pressure; RESP = respiratory rate; RVI = right ventricular stroke work index; S = systolic arterial pressure (on graphic plot); SI = stroke volume index; SO2 = oxygen saturation; STO2 = pulse oximeter oxygen saturation (F = finger); SVO2 = mixed venous oxygen saturation; SVR = systemic vascular resistance; TEMP = temperature; V = venous; O2 = oxygen consumption; WT = weight; * = heart rate (on graphic plot).

alone generates and stores approximately 18,000 patient data elements in one day. Timely examination of this amount of information by hand is impossible. Not only is the task unmanageable by hand because of its large volume, but the percentage of data that deserve attention, and that should generate alerts (warnings), is low. Alerts are generated for only about 5 percent of LDS hospital patients[6] (Fig. 41-7).

A more comprehensive application of computers in medical decision-making is the use of computerized protocols to aid and guide physicians in the conduct of a patient's therapy. The total parenteral nutrition (TPN) protocol is an example of a broadly disseminated protocol applied throughout our hospital wards and on different clinical services. It provides recommendations and a standard set of default orders that ensure an adequate standard of care. The physician can, however, change the standard orders within constraints determined by patients' laboratory values. The options for tailoring an order to a particular patient's needs

TABLE 41-1 Representative HELP Alert (Warning) Statements for Hypoxemia, Sepsis, Electrolyte, and Pharmacy Problems

Hypoxemia
- Mixed venous P_{O_2} = 25 mmHg (critically low)
- Severely reduced O_2 content (12.7) due to anemia
- Severe hypoxemia breathing oxygen—Contact MD or RN!

Sepsis
- Nosocomial infection probability = .91, because of age (79), diagnosis (upper GI bleeding, metastatic colon Ca, bowel resection), and urinary catheter.

Electrolyte imbalance
- Suggest that patient's potassium chloride therapy be changed to another form of potassium, since patient's serum chloride level is elevated at 120 meq/L

Pharmacy
- Concurrent aminoglycoside and vancomycin therapy may result in increased risk of nephrotoxicity
- Antacids or Kaopectate, when given at the same time as digoxin, decrease absorption of digoxin; suggest these two drugs be given at least 2 h apart.
- Suggest that serum potassium level be monitored daily, since this patient is receiving a potassium-sparing diuretic and a potassium supplement

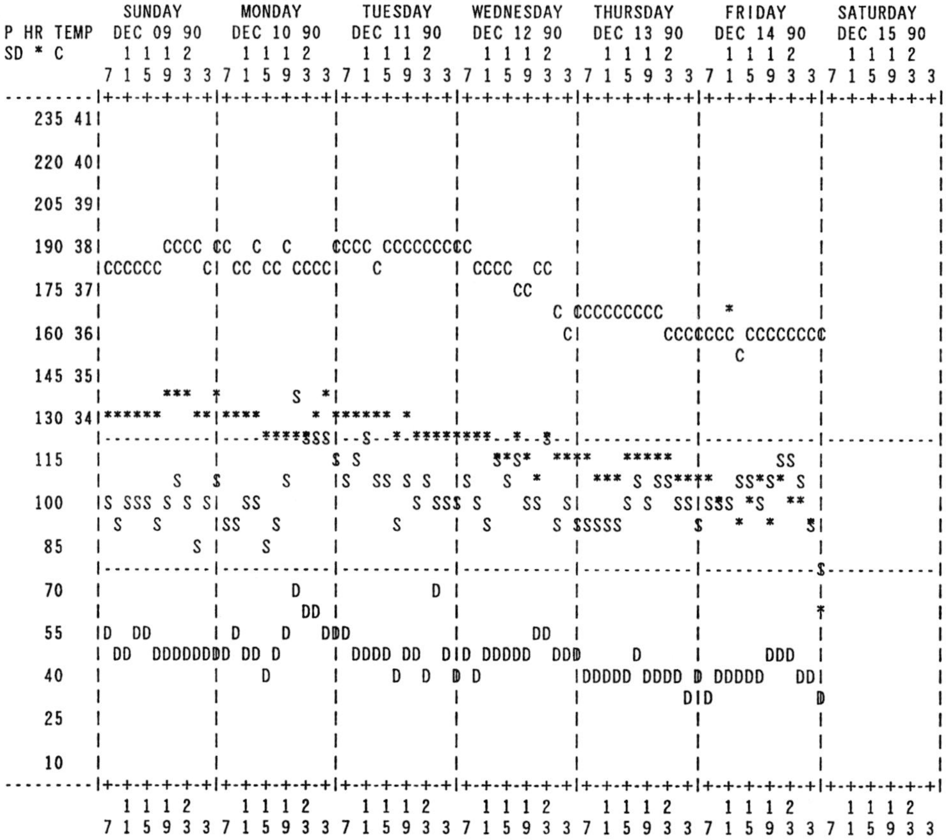

			DEC 09	DEC 10	DEC 11	DEC 12	DEC 13	DEC 14	DEC 15
MIDAZOLAM (VERSED), INJ	MGM	IV	105.0	70.0	87.0	68.0	73.0	11.0	
IMIPENEM CILASTATIN (PRIMAXIN), INJ	MGM	IV	2000	2000	2000	2000	2000	1000	
VANCOMYCIN (VANCOCIN), INJ	MGM	IV						1000	
NOREPINEPHRINE (LEVOPHED), INJ	MCG	IV						8080.0	
PHENYLEPHRINE (NEOSYNEPHRINE), INJ	MGM	IV	7.20	15.00	1.44			49.40	
DOPAMINE, INJ	MGM	IV	214	239	269	542	958	1940	
VECURONIUN BROMIDE (NORCURON MG/HR), INJ	MGM	IV	45	49			17	5	
VECURONIUM BROMIDE (NORCURON MCG/KG/MIN), INJ	MGM	IV		15	53	79	1		
ALBUTEROL (PROVENTIL), INHALATION SOLUTION	MGM	INHAL	10.00	10.00	15.00	2.50			
DIGOXIN, INJ	MGM	IV	0.250	0.250	0.250	0.125	0.125	0.125	
FUROSEMIDE, INJ	MGM	IV		40		3170	1660		
RANITIDINE HCL (ZANTAC), INJ	MGM	IV	192	103	116	100	109	102	
MAGNESIUM CITRATE, LIQUID	ML	NG			150				
MAALOX EXTRA STRENGTH, LIQUID	ML	NG			30				
HEPARIN, INJ	UNITS	IV				3800	12300	8200	
DURA-TEARS, OINT	APPLIC	OPTHN	12	12	12	10	6	12	
FRESH FROZEN PLASMA	ML	IV		1590		2815	1705	4615	
PACKED RBC	ML	IV				1500		1500	
PLATELETS (RANDOM DONOR)	ML	IV	400	400		800		1350	
ALBUMIN 25%, INJ	ML	IV				100			
D5W, INJ	ML	IV	435	960	515	725	846	2201	
NORMAL SALINE, INJ	ML	IV	191	444		650	400	8164	
FAT EMULSION 20% (LIPOSYN), INJ	ML	IV				200		200	
TAP WATER, LIQUID	ML	NG			40	20	40	20	
AMINOSYN RF, INJ	ML	IV				272	328	305	
DEXTROSE 70%, INJ	ML	IV				454	546	508	
SODIUM	MEQ	IV	43.8	13.7	12.9	5.9	20.5	33.3	
POTASSIUM	MEQ	IV	63.1	69.3	73.5	5.3	8.3	19.0	
CALCIUM	MEQ	IV	6.2	6.3	5.9	4.5	6.8	6.6	
ZINC	MGM	IV	6.0	6.2	5.8	3.6	5.7	5.6	
COPPER	MGM	IV	1.2	1.2	1.2	0.7	1.1	1.1	
MANGANESE	MGM	IV	0.5	0.5	0.5	0.4	0.6	0.6	
CHROMIUM	MCG	IV	12.1	12.3	11.6	7.2	11.4	11.1	
CHLORIDE	MEQ	IV	40.3	43.6	45.1	8.3	20.5	35.9	
ACETATE	MEQ	IV	39.8	9.6	9.0	0.7	12.3	20.7	

FIGURE 41-4

GLUCONATE	MEQ	IV	6.2	6.3	5.9	4.5	4.9	4.6
ELECTROLYTE VOLUME	ML	IV	62.5	50.0	50.2	13.8	20.5	30.2
SODIUM BICARBONATE, INJ	MEQ	IV						1200
AMINOSYN 8.5%, INJ	ML	IV	672	685	645	47	208	222
DEXTROSE 50%, INJ	ML	IV	672	685	645	97	208	247
MAGNESIUM	MEQ	IV	10.7	11.0	10.3	0.7	2.1	2.2
FAT EMULSION 10% (LIPOSYN), INJ	ML	IV	500	500	500		500	
IV FLUID, INJ	ML	IV				237	166	
NORMISOL-R, INJ	ML	IV				450		
NA POLYSTYRENE (KAYEXALATE) ENEMA	GM	RECT				100		
POTASSIUM CHLORIDE, INJ	MEQ	IV	49.0	65.9	5.5	0.6		
PHOSPHATE	MEQ	IV	38.4	42.5	45.7	3.3		
SULFATE	MEQ	IV	10.7	11.0	10.3	0.7		
D10W, INJ	ML	IV				479		
CALCIUM GLUCONATE, INJ	MEQ	IV				4.6		
POTASSIUM PHOSPHATE, INJ	MEQ	IV		20.0				
LACTATED RINGERS, INJ	ML	IV		300				
D5 IN 0.2 NACL, INJ	ML	IV	433					
HUMULIN REGULAR, INJ	UNITS	IV	14	6	3	16	24	3
INSULIN REGULAR, INJ	UNITS	IV	6	27	34	26	38	31
MVI-12, INJ	ML	IV	9.7	9.9	9.3	6.3	10.0	9.8
PHYTONADIONE (AQUA-MEPHYTON), INJ	MGM	IV				10.0	10.0	
PHYTONADIONE (AQUA-MEPHYTON), INJ	MGM	IM			10.0			
PHYTONADIONE (AQUA-MEPHYTON), INJ	MGM	SUBQ	10.0					
INTAKE (ML): BLOOD			400	400		2300		1350
COLLOID				1590		2915	1705	3745
NON-BLOOD IV			2961	3634	2364	3632	3232	5354
ENTERAL FEEDING					40	20	40	
NG DRUG					180			
OTHER DRUG						100		
TOTAL			3511	5624	3184	8997	4977	10449
OUTPUT (ML): INSENSIBLE LOSS			1124	1133	949	702	572	238
PHLEBOTOMY OUTPUT			41		35	100	161	116
ULTRAFILTRATION OUT							13345	10895
NG TUBE DRG.			525	100	112	400	500	225
STOOL			25			200		100
STOOL							1	4
FOLEY CATH URINE			1355	4055	1562	1870	405	8
TOTAL			3070	5288	2658	3412	14984	6693
NET BALANCE (ML):			441	336	526	5585	-10007	3756
WEIGHT (KG)			80.8	80.3	79.1		90.0	90.3
NUTRITIONAL: NP ENERGY	KCAL	(IV)	1837	1877	1734	1931	2346	914
TOTAL ENERGY	KCAL	(IV)	2066	2110	1953	2004	2485	1007
PROTEIN	GM		57	58	54	19	34	23
FAT	GM		50	50	50	40	50	0
CHO	GM		379	391	348	450	528	269
NP ENERGY/N2	KCAL/GM		204	208	216	643	391	228
N2 IN	GM		9	9	8	3	6	4

FIGURE 41-4 HELP system 7-day summary report. This report is a synthesis and summary of the information contained in the two 12-h shift reports (see Fig. 41-3) for each day. For explanation of abbreviations, see Fig. 41-3.

```
                         L D S   H O S P I T A L   I C U   R O U N D S   R E P O R T
                                           DATA WITHIN LAST 24 HOURS

NAME: K         R        K.                  NO.                    ROOM:                              DATE: DEC 12 06:00
DR. L     P                         SEX: F    AGE:  48   HEIGHT: 165   WEIGHT:   90.30    BSA: 1.97   BEE:  1577   MOF:   16
ADMT DIAGNOSIS:                                    ADMIT DATE: 04 DEC 90        APACHE II: 31   APS: 26
====================================================================================================================
CARDIOVASCULAR:   3                                                             EXAM: ____________________________
TIME                CO     CI    HR   SV   SI    VP  MSP   MP SVR LWI  PW   PA   PVR     RWI  ____________________________
DEC 12 04:30  10.00   5.35  122  82  44 18.0M  78   59  4  35  20   29    .9     6.6
         DEC 11 18:14  DOPAMINE (INTROPIN)  2.00 MCG/KG/MIN
         DEC 11 22:00  DIGOXIN .250 MGM, INJ
         MILD LV DYSFUNCTION
                    SP     DP     MP    HR  |  LACT          CPK          CPK-MB        LDH-1         LDH-2
  LAST VALUES      119     50     64   131  |
  MAXIMUM          136     74     98   148  |  4.3 (05:20)      (     )      (     )      (     )      (     )
  MINIMUM           34     20     53    24  |
====================================================================================================================
 RESPIRATORY:   3
              pH     PCO2     HCO3      BE     HB   CO/MT    PO2    SO2    O2CT    %O2  AVO2   VO2    C.O.   A-a  QS/QT   PK/ PL/PP  MR/SR
12 05:55 A  7.42    54.3     34.9      9.4  12.6    0/ 0     64     90    15.9     90                         414           0/  0/22  16/ 0
         SAMPLE # 83, TEMP 38.1, BREATHING STATUS : OTHER
         MODERATE CHRONIC RESPIRATORY ACIDOSIS
         MILD HYPOXEMIA
         MILDLY REDUCED O2 CONTENT
         HYPOVENTILATION IMPROVED
12 04:23 V  7.37    63.2     36.0      9.2  12.1    1/ 0     40     69    11.7    100                                       42/ 42/22  16/ 0
12 04:22 A  7.39    57.3     34.2      8.2  12.0    1/ 0     63     89    15.1    100   3.51                 473    47     42/ 42/22  16/ 0

         ------- machine settings ------- | -------------------------- patient values -----------------------------
         VENT  MODE  VR    VE    O2%    IT% PT%    MAP   PK    PL  PP  m-Vt   c-Vt  s-Vt  MR   SR   TR  m-VE  s-VE  t-VE  Cth   Pc
12 04:30  900c  V CL  16 75.6   90     67  10     37.7   45    45  21   467    419         16             6.7                17.5
12 04:30   5/04:32   INTERFACE: NASOTRACH;  BREATH SOUNDS: COARSE CRACKLES, THROUGHOUT INSPIRATION AND EXPIRATION, BOTH LUNGS,
        MODERATELY DECREASED, THROUGHOUT INSPIRATION AND EXPIRATION, BOTH LUNGS;  TEMP SETTING: 5.0; POSITION: SUPINE;
        PATIENT CONDITION: MEDICATED, PARALYZED;  THERAPIST: HEXEM, DAN,  RRT
                                                                                          EXAM: ____________________
  -- NO SPONTANEOUS PARAMETERS WITHIN THE LAST 24 HOURS --                                      ____________________
====================================================================================================================
NEURO AND PSYCH:   0
   GLASCOW   (      ) VERBAL ________    EYELIDS ________    MOTOR __________    PUPILS ________    SENSORY ________

   DTR __________    BABIN. ________    ICP __________    PSYCH __________
====================================================================================================================
COAGULATION:  3
   PT:    16.2   (05:20     ) PTT:      33 (05:20     ) PLATELETS:   36 (05:20     )  FIBRINOGEN:   0(00:00) EXAM:___________
   FSP-CON:   0 (00:00      ) FSP-PT:   0 (00:00      ) 3P:                (00:00     )                              ___________
====================================================================================================================
RENAL, FLUIDS, LYTES:  1
   IN   3184 CRYST    2364  COLLOID          BLOOD       NG/PO    220 | NA   147 (05:20) K   6.0   (05:20)  CL  101   (05:20)
   OUT  2658 URINE    1562  NGOUT        112 DRAINS    35 OTHER   949 | CO2 35.0 (05:20) BUN  101  (05:20)  CRE   1.9 (05:20)
   NET   526 WT     79.10   WT-CHG    -1.20  S.G.     1.022           | AGAP   17.0      UOSM               UNA     1OCRCL
====================================================================================================================
METABOLIC --- NUTRITION:  0
   KCAL     1953  GLU  153 (12 05:20)  ALB    2.2  (11 05:22) | CA   9.0 (11 05:22)  FE    .0 (00 00:00)  TIBC     0 (00 00:00)
   KCAL/N2  198   UUN   .0 (00 00:00)  N-BAL   .0              | PO4  6.1 (12 05:20)  MG   3.0 (12 05:20)  CHOL   101 (11 05:22)
====================================================================================================================
GI, LIVER, AND PANCREAS:  3                                                                                        EXAM:
   HCT    37.6 (12 05:20)  TOT BILI 14.9 (11 05:22)  SGOT  190 (11 05:22)  ALKPO4  140 (11 05:22) GGT  169 (11 05:22) __________
   GUAIAC NG 0+  (12 06:00) DIR BILI 12.4 (11 05:22)  SGPT   49 (11 05:22)  LDH  566 (11 05:22)  AMYL  356 (12 05:20) __________

====================================================================================================================
INFECTION:  3
   WBC 22.1(05:20 ) TEMP  38.2 (11/16:00) DIFF  38 B, 33P, 22L,  6M,  1E (05:20) GRAM STAIN: SPUTUM __________ OTHER __________

====================================================================================================================
SKIN AND EXTREMITIES:
   PULSES ________   RASH ________   DECUBITI ____________
====================================================================================================================
TUBES:
   VEN ________   ART ________   SG ________   NG ________   FOLEY ________   ET ________   TRACH ________   DRAIN______

   CHEST ____________  RECTAL ______   JEJUNAL ________   DIALYSIS ________   OTHER ______________________________
====================================================================================================================
MEDICATIONS:

MIDAZOLAM (VERSED), INJ                     MGM   IV        87    MAGNESIUM                          MEQ   IV       10.318
IMIPENEM CILASTATIN (PRIMAXIN), INJ         MGM   IV      2000    ZINC                               MGM   IV        5.804
ALBUTEROL (PROVENTIL), INHALATION SOLUTIMGM   INHAL       15    COPPER                             MGM   IV        1.161
VECURONIUM BROMIDE (NORCURON MCG/KG/MIN), MGM   IV        53    MANGANESE                          MGM   IV         .516
DOPAMINE, INJ                               MGM   IV    *8.800    CHROMIUM                           MCG   IV       11.607
                                                                                                              #960 - pg1
```

FIGURE 41-5

PHENYLEPHRINE (NEOSYNEPHRINE), INJ	MGM	IV	1.440	CHLORIDE	MEQ	IV	45.139
DIGOXIN, INJ	MGM	IV	.250	ACETATE	MEQ	IV	9.028
RANITIDINE HCL (ZANTAC), INJ	MGM	IV	*6.396	PHOSPHATE	MEQ	IV	45.655
MAGNESIUM CITRATE, LIQUID	ML	NG	150	SULFATE	MEQ	IV	10.318
MAALOX EXTRA STRENGTH, LIQUID	ML	NG	30	GLUCONATE	MEQ	IV	5.932
TAP WATER, LIQUID	ML	NG	40	ELECTROLYTE VOLUME	ML	IV	50.169
POTASSIUM CHLORIDE, INJ	MEQ	IV	5.500	INSULIN REGULAR, INJ	UNITS	IV	33.661
SODIUM	MEQ	IV	12.897	HUMULIN REGULAR, INJ	UNITS	IV	3
POTASSIUM	MEQ	IV	73.511	MVI-12 , INJ	ML	IV	9.286
CALCIUM	MEQ	IV	5.932	PHYTONADIONE (AQUA-MEPHYTON), INJ	MGM	IM	10

FIGURE 41-5 ICU rounds report. This is an organ system–oriented computer report designed to present important items of patient data concisely. Space has been left to allow the addition of pertinent information not contained in the computer record.

FIGURE 41-6 HELP system cardiac output report. CO = cardiac output; CI = cardiac index; HR = heart rate; SV = stroke volume; SI = stroke index; MV = mean systemic blood pressure; MSB = mean systolic blood pressure (systemic); PA = pulmonary artery mean pressure; RA = right atrial pressure; PW = pulmonary artery wedge pressure; PVR = pulmonary vascular resistance; SVR = systemic vascular resistance; RWI = right ventricular stroke work index; LWI = left ventricular stroke work index. The dates and starting times for the drugs indicated below the data sets indicate the times and dates at which particular drug therapies were begun.

```
                      C A R D I A C   O U T P U T   R E P O R T

K           R        K.          NO. 2         DR L    , P                  RM
HT        CM     WT 90.30   KG      BSA  1.97 SQM         AGE  48      SEX F
TIME                 CO       CI   HR   SV   SI   MP   MSP   PA    RA   PW   PVR   SVR   RWI   LWI
NORMAL HI          7.30     3.50   89  101   48  105   123   19    5.0  12   1.0   18   11.0    85
NORMAL LOW         2.90     2.80   49   47   38   70    80    9    1.0   4   0.5   12    8.0    48

DEC 15 04:09       8.70     4.42   95   92   46   51    77   36   30.0M32     .5    2    3.8    28
          DEC 15 02:00  DOPAMINE (INTROPIN)  20 MCG/KG/MIN
          DEC 14 21:54  LEVOPHED (LEVARTERENOL)   0.143MCG/KG/MIN
          DEC 15 02:56  NEOSYNEPHRINE   0.710MCG/KG/MIN
          DEC 14 09:00  DIGOXIN 0.125 MGM, INJ
          SEVERE LV DYSFUNCTION

DEC 14 13:00       9.30     5.00   96   97   52   58    88   30   22.0M22     .9    4    5.7    47
          DEC 14 11:10  DOPAMINE (INTROPIN)  30 MCG/KG/MIN
          DEC 14 12:51  LEVOPHED (LEVARTERENOL)   0.057MCG/KG/MIN
          DEC 14 12:39  NEOSYNEPHRINE   0.710MCG/KG/MIN
          DEC 14 09:00  DIGOXIN 0.125 MGM, INJ
          MILD LV DYSFUNCTION

DEC 14 12:00       9.20     4.95  167   55   30   56    81   31   20.0M22    1.0    4    4.4    24
          DEC 14 11:10  DOPAMINE (INTROPIN)  30 MCG/KG/MIN
          DEC 14 11:49  NEOSYNEPHRINE   0.190MCG/KG/MIN
          DEC 14 09:00  DIGOXIN 0.125 MGM, INJ
          MODERATE LV DYSFUNCTION

DEC 14 04:10       8.30     4.46  107   78   42   50    73   26   10.0E18    1.0    5    9.1    31
          DEC 14 03:56  DOPAMINE (INTROPIN)   8 MCG/KG/MIN
          DEC 13 09:00  DIGOXIN 0.125 MGM, INJ
          MILD LV DYSFUNCTION

DEC 13 13:33      10.80     5.48  109   99   50   57    73   33   20.0M28     .5    3    8.9    31
          DEC 13 09:50  DOPAMINE (INTROPIN)  12 MCG/KG/MIN
          DEC 13 09:00  DIGOXIN 0.125 MGM, INJ
          SEVERE LV DYSFUNCTION

DEC 13 04:48      12.20     6.56  113  108   58   67    83   39   26.0M30     .7    3   10.3    42
          DEC 13 00:58  DOPAMINE (INTROPIN)   8 MCG/KG/MIN
          DEC 13 00:00  DIGOXIN 0.125 MGM, INJ
          MILD LV DYSFUNCTION

DEC 13 04:00      12.20     6.56  113  108   58   65    81   38   26.0M34     .3    3    9.5    37
          DEC 13 00:58  DOPAMINE (INTROPIN)   8 MCG/KG/MIN
          DEC 13 00:00  DIGOXIN 0.125 MGM, INJ
          MODERATE LV DYSFUNCTION

DEC 13 00:00      12.90     6.94  124  104   56  104   102   36   26.0M26     .8    6    7.6    58
          DEC 12 23:57  DOPAMINE (INTROPIN)   4 MCG/KG/MIN
          DEC 13 00:00  DIGOXIN 0.125 MGM, INJ
          LV PARAMETERS ARE WITHIN NORMAL LIMITS
```

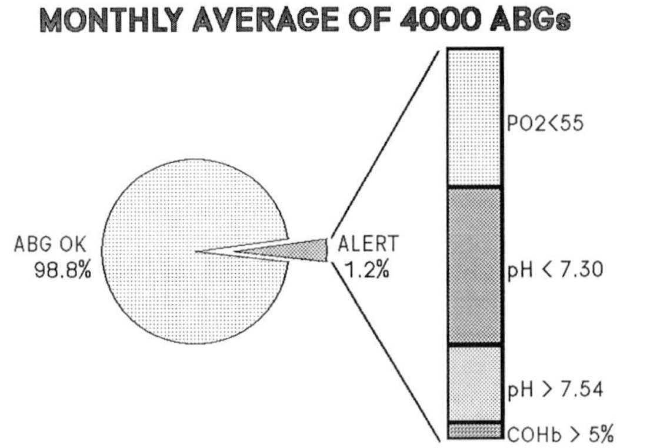

FIGURE 41-7 HELP blood gas alerts within the LDS Hospital's Respiratory Care Department quality assurance program.

are therefore limited by the patient's state and the patient's laboratory values; the physician is thus constrained to choose from among a set of options that appear to be appropriate for the patient. This prevents mistakes that might prove to be detrimental to the patient. Within the ordering program, guidance for therapy, as well as for education, is provided to the physician interacting with the computer terminal. These orders are intended to guide, but not rigidly constrain, the physician, and are available not only in the ICU but throughout the hospital.

The HELP protocol for management of arterial hypoxemia in patients with acute hypoxic pulmonary failure [adult respiratory distress syndrome (ARDS)][20,21,22,23] is an example of a detailed computerized protocol. This protocol application is limited to one of our hospital ICUs. It provides specific and detailed instruction and imposes greater limitations on a physician's options than the TPN protocol (see above). The physician is free to decline to follow a protocol instruction if he or she has a defensible reason, but the protocols provide a standard therapeutic response to the arterial hypoxemia in mechanically ventilated patients with severe ARDS. These hypoxemia-focused protocols have been generated using the best information available in the published literature, combined with input from local, national, and international experts. Physicians at our hospital have agreed to abandon personal style and adopt a "standard" protocol for the management of hypoxemia.

The protocol management of arterial hypoxemia is achieved primarily by manipulation of oxygen concentration and positive end-expiratory pressure (PEEP) during mechanical ventilator support of patients with severe pulmonary failure. This acceptance of protocol-controlled therapy has required a high level of collegiality and commitment from MDs, RNs, and RTs. The computerized versions of these protocols have been used for about 20,000 h in routine care around the clock and have proved to be much more easily applied than were manual paper-based flow diagram versions.[21,23] The computerized versions have proved to be more accurate than paper flow diagrams, as well. Computerized protocol instructions control therapy for arterial hypoxemia in severe ARDS patients for 94 percent of the day (23 of 24 h) in our ICU.[24,25] In addition, they provide an audit trail, which permits a detailed review of the performance of the protocols in the clinical environment. Figure 41-8 illustrates a simplified and selected portion of 1 of approximately 30 pages of protocols used for the control of arterial oxygenation in these patients. Three sets of representative instructions, generated during routine application to one patient, are also shown.

Inverse Ratio Ventilation Protocol

The result of application of an inverse ratio ventilation (IRV) protocol is particularly instructive, because of its implication regarding the limited number of variables that physicians are capable of managing.[26,27] The IRV protocol operates in a dedicated personal computer linked to a mechanical ventilator. Instructions from the HELP system protocols for arterial hypoxemia management (see above) display the patient's desired end-expiratory alveolar pressure on the HELP system bedside terminal. This desired end-

FIGURE 41-8 Selected elements of a protocol for direction of arterial hypoxemia. CORE = continuous respiratory evaluation (diagnostic protocol). Patient data and protocol instructions corresponding to numbers 1, 2, and 3 (at bottom) are those associated with the routes numbered 1, 2, and 3 in the flow diagram.

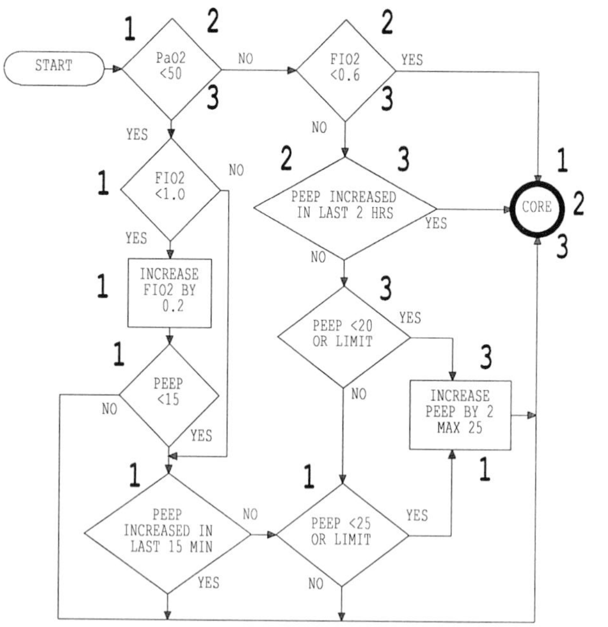

PATIENT DATA:

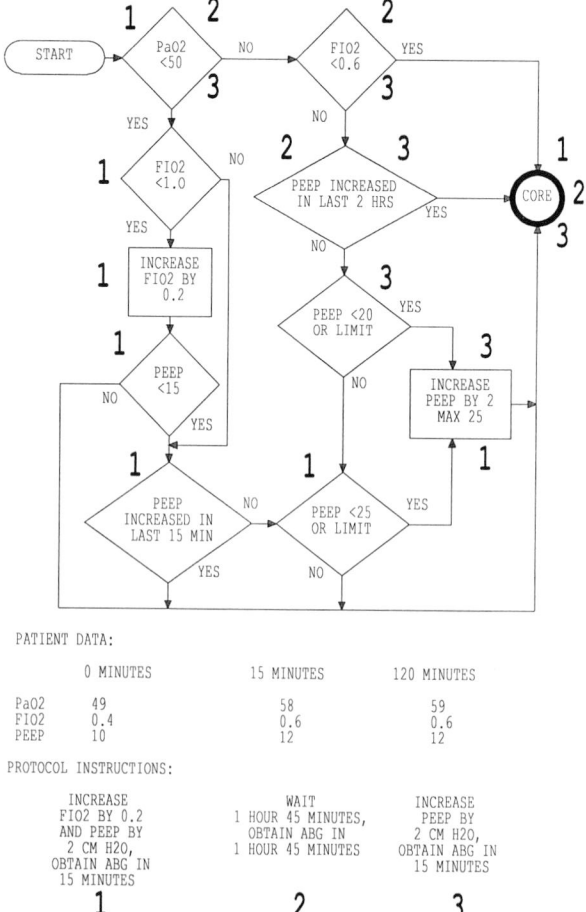

	0 MINUTES	15 MINUTES	120 MINUTES
PaO2	49	58	59
FIO2	0.4	0.6	0.6
PEEP	10	12	12

PROTOCOL INSTRUCTIONS:

INCREASE FIO2 BY 0.2 AND PEEP BY 2 CM H2O, OBTAIN ABG IN 15 MINUTES	WAIT 1 HOUR 45 MINUTES, OBTAIN ABG IN 1 HOUR 45 MINUTES	INCREASE PEEP BY 2 CM H2O, OBTAIN ABG IN 15 MINUTES
1	2	3

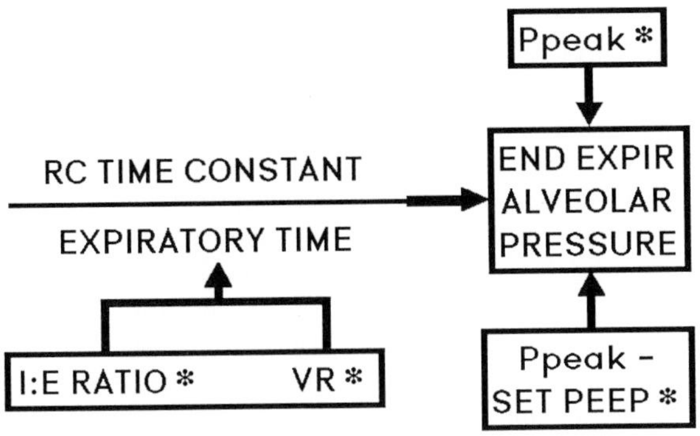

FIGURE 41-9 Conceptual diagram of inverse ratio ventilation "controlled air trapping" protocol. End-expiratory alveolar pressure is adjusted by regulating the four variables indicated by asterisks. I:E ratio = inspiratory:expiratory ratio; Ppeak = peak ventilator pressure; VR = ventilatory rate; SET PEEP = external PEEP setting, either with the ventilator knob or with a water column.

expiratory pressure is entered into the IRV personal computer as the new target value. Four variables (inspiratory/expiratory ratio, ventilatory rate, peak ventilator pressure, and PEEP setting—I/E, VR, Ppeak, and setPEEP, respectively) determine the end-expiratory alveolar pressure (Fig. 41-9). "Controlled air trapping" (end-expiratory alveolar pressure) is achieved as the clinical staff follows the protocol instructions displayed on the IRV personal computer screen. While many publications deal with IRV, there is no well-defined method, and published descriptions of the technique lack essential details.[28] Information gained from visits to domestic and international medical centers has confirmed our local experience that, though based on pathophysiologic principles, IRV is usually applied by trial and error. This implies that the application of IRV is not systematic and is, therefore, not reproducible in the clinical setting.

The computerized IRV protocol displays instructions for changing the four determining variables by small increments or decrements. Since its initial application in our ICU, IRV has been markedly simplified; IRV is now seen as a technique that can be used systematically, predictably, and reproducibly. This dramatic change in our perception of IRV performance has been noted by MDs, RNs, and RTs alike. We conclude that the four determining variables (I/E, VR, Ppeak, setPEEP) were not managed systematically before the computer protocol was applied, even though IRV was used by experienced pulmonary and critical care physicians within an academic training program. This suggests that experienced physicians, faced with the challenge of adjusting four variables, were not able to develop a systematic response to ventilatory support problems. We do not think we are unique in this inability; we suggest that other physicians likely face similar limitations in their ability to manage clinical problems that have at least four variable determinants. Within the more than 236 different variables noted in one ICU patient (see above) there are a number of clinically important problems involving at least four adjustable variables, including cardiac output (intracavitary pressures and pericardial or intrathoracic pressures on both the right and left sides of the heart, heart rate, ventricular septal position, electrical conduction and rhythm, arterial oxygenation, and medications); renal output (cardiac output, arterial oxygenation, venous pressure, abdominal pressure, intrathoracic pressure, and medications); and "tissue oxygenation" (cardiac output, arterial oxygen content, arterial oxygen pressure, oxygen consumption, bacteremia or infection, temperature, activity, and medications). These considerations led us to question our ability to come to the "right therapeutic decision" when dealing with multivariate problems in severely ill patients (see Introduction).

Quality Assurance

Quality assurance, measures of outcome, and documentation of performance are growing requirements in modern hospitals. Computer applications in critical care are an extremely valuable part of the response to the widespread demand for more cost-effective care and for better documentation to justify clinical decisions. The 18,000 data items recorded daily by our respiratory therapy department are a graphic expression of the enormous numbers of data that must be reviewed for quality assurance purposes. Quality assurance reviews in the respiratory care department utilize data from the blood gas laboratory, from the microbiology laboratory, and from the respiratory therapist's clinical chart. Manual surveys typically are limited to retrospective reviews and restricted to a small fraction of the patients—and to only a fraction of the hospital record data for these patients. Manual surveys are time-consuming and produce results that are frequently available months after the assignment is made. In contrast, off-line surveys of data by computerized review allow examination of all information and all patient records. Off-line computerized surveys are routinely carried out in our respiratory care,[19] infectious disease,[29,30] and blood bank[31] departments. Figures 41-10

FIGURE 41-10 HELP system alerts for the LDS Hospital's Respiratory Care Department off-line computerized quality assurance program.

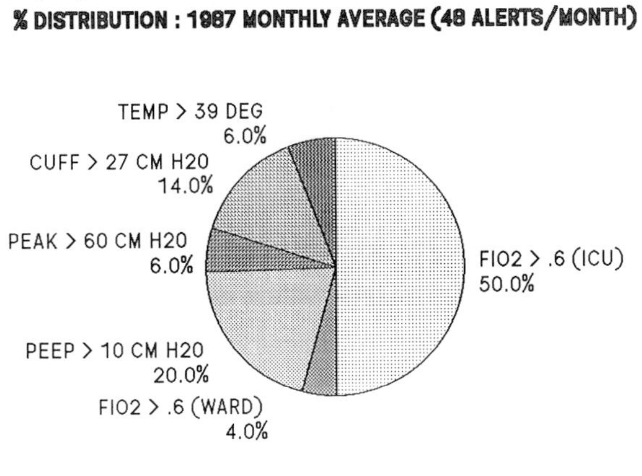

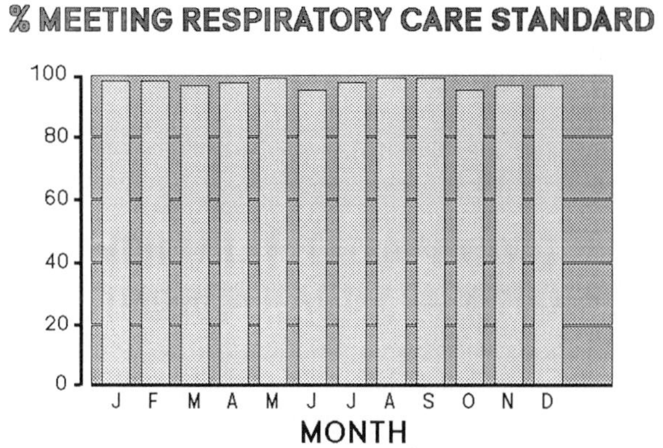

FIGURE 41-11 HELP system alerts for the LDS Hospital's Respiratory Care Department on-line computerized quality assurance program.

and 41-11 display representative outcome data from quality assurance activities in the Respiratory Care Department.

On-line computerized surveys provide an even more powerful tool for quality assurance in the clinical environment. The computerized data base can be surveyed completely with all information reviewed on a real-time, daily, weekly, monthly, or yearly basis. Such surveys not only increase the power of our departments but also provide opportunities for outcome research. An additional benefit is the ability to compare our hospital's performance with that of other centers, and with our own past performance, by referring to reference criteria such as the APACHE II score.[32] Figure 41-12 provides representative examples of results of such routine daily surveys from the respiratory care and infectious disease departments.

Clinical Trials and Research

Of the three major elements involved in clinical research—the content of clinical care, patient selection, and the process of clinical care (Fig. 41-13)—only the content is clearly defined in the Methods sections of most clinical research publications. The content represents the "what" that we do to patients. It is usually easy to assess whether the study in question involves penicillin, gentamicin, or other drugs; extracorporeal support; mechanical ventilation; or some other therapeutic modality. The patient selection—i.e., the "whom" to whom the "what" is delivered—is much more difficult to identify. For example, there is at present no uniformly accepted definition of adult respiratory distress syndrome (ARDS). Nevertheless, there is usually some useful information concerning patient selection in most medical publications. In contrast, the process of medical care—the "how" we deliver the "what" to "whom"—is almost never articulated. Therefore, the two most important goals of a Methods section in a scientific publication—the provision of enough detail to allow a reviewer to evaluate critically the results of the work and its conclusions, and the provision of enough detail to allow the interested investigator to duplicate the work—usually are not fulfilled. As a result, much "noise" is introduced into clinical settings from which medical publications are derived, making the interpretation of the outcomes of such work much more difficult for the medical community.

It is informative to examine the relationship of these three elements (content, patient selection, and the process of medical care) with the two major determinants of both the intensity of care to which a patient is subjected and the patient's ultimate outcome (Fig. 41-14). Our focus in medicine, both in clinical care and in clinical research, is patient outcome. The most desirable outcome is survival with resumption of a productive life. Unfortunately, the signal-to-noise ratio (S/N) associated with outcome differences in clinical trials is frequently very low. The noise in the clinical environment is both random and nonrandom (bias). Random noise can be dealt with by increasing the number of observations made (or the number of patients) in a clinical trial. Since the signal to noise ratio (S/N) for random noise is inversely proportional to the square root of the number of observations, increasing the number of observations (or patients) 100-fold would increase S/N by a factor of 10. This is a difficult challenge in critical care, since the acquisition of large numbers of patients in clinical trials is not easy and is very costly. Nonrandom noise (bias), quite common in clinical settings, is not influenced by increasing the number of observations (or patients) and therefore must be reduced by other means. Both of the major elements that determine the intensity of patient care and the patient outcome [the

FIGURE 41-12 HELP system alerts for the LDS Hospital's Respiratory Care Department on-line computerized quality assurance program.

W 820 PATIENT JJ
SPUTUM CULTURE 2/26/88 1045
PSEUDOMONAS AEROGINOSA

COMMON ORGANISM: WITH PATIENT AK E630
THERAPIST 23432 ALSO SAW PATIENT AK

FIGURE 41-13 Three major elements involved in the delivery of clinical care.

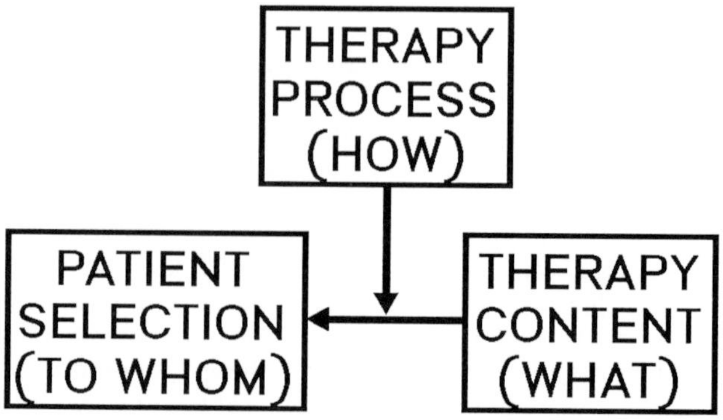

patient-disease complex and the response of the clinical care team (see Fig. 41-14)] are sources of both random and nonrandom noise. Noise is introduced in the patient-disease complex because of our inability to control host factors and the disease's etiology, extent, and duration. In addition, significant bias is introduced in patient selection, both in clinical care and—more pertinent to this discussion—in clinical trials. The patient identification and selection process is quite imperfect and incorporates much local bias because of the prejudices of individual clinical investigators and the specific characteristics of their local clinical environments, as well as the failure of the medical community to establish broadly accepted specific definitions of many diseases. Much work needs to be done, and much improvement can be achieved, in this regard. The other major element, the response of the clinical care team to the patient-disease complex, also introduces both random noise and bias. Strong bias is injected into the response of the clinical care team as a result of many factors that play upon their behavior, including general and local cultural factors, local technical abilities, and experience—all of which affect the process of therapy. This process is usually poorly articulated; frequently one cannot uncover the rules behind decisions relating to important stages in the delivery of care. For clinical trials, this deficiency means it is not possible to define "how" the investigation is actually conducted.

Few studies have dealt with the impact of controlling the process of medical care, although it is clear that interpretations of outcomes will be difficult as long as the process of care is poorly defined. There is some evidence that such control is beneficial.[33,34] This contrasts with the more common emphasis, in medical informatics, on understanding how human beings reason and matching medical expert system products to individual physicians' preferences.[35] In general it is believed that detailed protocols will not be able to replace the individual physician's judgment.[36] The minute-to-minute management demands of severely ill ICU patients, however, provide an unusually fertile field for application of detailed protocols. Our colleagues and we have attempted to reduce the noise associated with the clinical care team's response by defining, with computerized protocols, the process of medical care associated with the management of arterial hypoxemia in a clinical trial of two therapies for ARDS.[22,25] With more than 20,000 hours of application of computerized protocol control of clinical care, 24 hours a day, it is now clear that this approach is feasible and—with the appropriate computer infrastructure—practical.[21,23] Such computerized protocol control of the process of care does appear to control the intensity of care of severely ill patients.[25] Whether this approach will be generalizable is currently unknown. If it is generalizable, it may allow the performance of clinical trials that will have the potential of significantly decreasing the noise introduced by the response of the clinical care team and thus increasing S/N for outcome. This will very likely make a number of clinical studies more credible and more definitive.

FIGURE 41-14 Determinants of the intensity of care and of ultimate patient outcome. The two major elements are the patient-disease complex and the response to the patient-disease complex provided by the clinical care team. Both of these elements introduce noise, which reduces the signal-to-noise ratio (S/N) for outcome results.

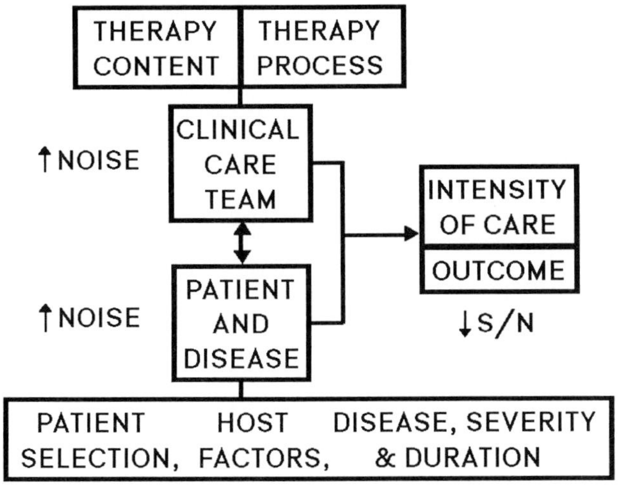

Summary

The availability of the computerized, fully integrated data base from a hospital information system allows the performance of a number of tasks that would, in the absence of such a system, be prohibitive because of the large investment of resources required for manual achievement of the same goals. Among these are the acquisition and integration of data and the generation of appropriate reports. The decision-making support that is now becoming more widely available in the HELP computer system extends the impact of computers on medical practice and provides the potential for much greater influence on ultimate patient outcome. The applications of computerized data bases to quality assurance questions address an extremely important and highly visible area of concern in the current medical climate in the United States.

Available evidence of the ultimate impact of such systems on costs and cost/benefit ratios in hospital practice suggests a favorable impact of computers in hospital pharmacy[19] and infectious disease[30] departments. Carefully controlled randomized clinical trials dealing with patient outcome, and especially with survival, are sorely needed. They will help provide the information base necessary for the establishment of appropriate medical policy relative to the future role of computerized data management systems in critical care medicine and in medicine at large. Nevertheless, the preliminary information currently available indicates the great potential for computer applications in critical care medicine and suggests a future with a much-expanded role for computers in medicine.

References

1. Rennels GD, Shortliffe EH: Advanced computing for medicine. Sci Am 257(4):154, 1987.
2. Gardner RM, Shabot MM: Computerized ICU data management: Pitfalls and promises. Intern J Clin Monitoring Computing 7:99, 1990.
3. Kuperman GJ, Gardner RM: The impact of the HELP computer system on the LDS Hospital paper medical record. Proceedings: 14th Annual Symposium on Computer Applications in Medical Care. Los Alamitos, CA, IEEE Computer Society Press, 1990, p 673.
4. Bradshaw KE, Gardner RM, Clemmer TP, et al: Physician decision-making: Evaluation of data used in a computerized ICU. Intern J Clin Monitoring Computing 1:81, 1984.
5. Shortliffe EH: Clinical decision-support systems, in Shortliffe EH, Perreault LE (eds): *Medical Informatics: Computer Applications in Health Care.* Reading, MA, Addison-Wesley, 1990, p 466.
6. Pryor TA, Gardner RM, Clayton PD, Warner HR: The HELP System. J Med Systems 7:87, 1983.
7. Pryor TA: Development of decision support systems. Intern J Clin Monitoring Computing 7:137, 1990.
8. Sutton GC: Computer-aided diagnosis: A review. Br J Surg 76:82, 1989.
9. Shabot MM: Standardized acquisition of bedside data: The IEEE P1073 medical information bus. Intern J Clin Monitoring Computing 6:197, 1989.
10. Hawley WL, Tariq H, Gardner RM: Clinical implementation of an automated medical information bus in an intensive care unit. Proceedings: 12th Annual Symposium on Computer Applications in Medical Care. Los Alamitos, CA, IEEE Computer Society Press, 1988, p 621.
11. Gardner RM, Tariq H, Hawley WL, East TD: Medical information bus: The key to future integrated monitoring (editorial). Intern J Clin Monitoring Computing 6:205, 1989.
12. Bradshaw KE, Sitig DF, Gardner RM, et al: Computer-based data entry for nurses in the ICU. MD Computing 6:274, 1989.
13. Gardner RM, Bradshaw KE, Holingsworth KW: Computerizing the intensive care unit: Current status and future directions. J Cardiovasc Nurs 4:68, 1989.
14. Andrews RD, Gardner RM, Metcalf SM, Simmons D: Computer charting: An evaluation of a respiratory care computer system. Respir Care 8:695, 1985.
15. Morris AH, Kanner RE, Crapo RO, Gardner RM: *Clinical Pulmonary Function Testing: A Manual of Uniform Laboratory Procedures,* 2d ed. Salt Lake City, UT, Intermountain Thoracic Society, 1984.
16. Bradshaw KE, Gardner RM, Pryor TA: Development of a computerized laboratory alerting system. Comput Biomed Res 22:575, 1989.
17. Tate KE, Gardner RM, Weaver LK: A computerized laboratory alerting system. MD Computing 7:296, 1990.
18. Elliott CG, Simmons D, Schmidt CD, et al: Computer-assisted medical direction of respiratory care. Resp Management 19:31, 1989.
19. Gardner RM, Hulse RK, Larsen KG: Assessing the effectiveness of a computerized pharmacy system. Proceedings: 14th Annual Symposium on Computer Applications in Medical Care. Los Alamitos, CA, IEEE Computer Society Press, 1990, p 668.
20. Sittig DF, Gardner RM, Pace NL, et al: Computerized management of patient care in a complex, controlled clinical trial in the intensive care unit. Comput Methods Programs in Biomed 30:77, 1989.
21. Henderson SE, Crapo RO, East TD, et al: Computerized clinical protocols in an intensive care unit: How well are they followed? Proceedings: 14th Annual Symposium on Computer Applications in Medical Care. Los Alamitos, CA, IEEE Computer Society Press, 1990, p 284.
22. Morris AH, Wallace CJ, Clemmer TP, et al: Extracorporeal CO_2 removal therapy for adult respiratory distress syndrome patients. Respir Care 35:224, 1990.
23. East TD, Morris AH, Clemmer T, et al: Development of computerized critical care protocols: A strategy that really works. Proceedings: 14th Annual Symposium on Computer Applications in Medical Care. Los Alamitos, CA, IEEE Computer Society Press, 1990, p 564.
24. Morris AH, Wallace CJ, Beck E, et al: Protocols control respiratory therapy of ARDS (abstract). Clin Res 38:138A, 1990.
25. Morris AH, Wallace CJ, Clemmer TP, et al: Extracorporeal CO_2 removal therapy for adult respiratory distress syndrome patients: A computerized protocol controlled trial. Réan Soins Intens Méd Urg 6:485, 1990.
26. Boehm SH, Peng L, East TD, et al: Computerized protocol management of pressure control inverse ratio ventilation (abstract). Chest 98:77S, 1990.
27. East TD, Böhm SH, Peng L, et al: Exquisite management of pressure control inverse ratio ventilation by a computerized protocol (abstract). Am Rev Respir Dis 141:A240, 1990.
28. Kaczmarek RM, Hess D: Pressure controlled inverse-ratio ventilation, panacea or auto-PEEP? Respir Care 35:945, 1990.
29. Evans RS, Burke JP, Pestotnik SL, et al: Prediction of hospital infections and selection of antibiotics using an automated hospital database. Proceedings: 14th Annual Symposium on Computer Applications in Medical Care. Los Alamitos, CA, IEEE Computer Society Press, 1990, p 663.
30. Evans RS, Pestotnik SL, Burke JP, et al: Reducing the duration of prophylactic antibiotic use through computer monitoring of surgical patients. DICP, Ann Pharmacother 24:351, 1990.
31. Gardner RM, Golubjatnikov OK, Laub RM, et al: Computer-critiqued blood ordering using the HELP system. Comput Biomed Res 23:514, 1990.
32. Knaus WA, Draper EA, Wagner DP, Zimmerman JE: APACHE II: A severity of disease classification system. Crit Care Med 13:818, 1985.
33. Wirtschafter DD, Scalise M, Henke C, Gams RA: Do information systems improve the quality of clinical research? Results of a randomized trial in a cooperative multi-institutional cancer group. Comput Biomed Res 14:78, 1981.
34. Dawes RM, Faust D, Meehl PE: Clinical versus actuarial judgment. Science 243:1668, 1990.
35. Rennels GD, Miller PL: Artificial intelligence research in anesthesia and intensive care. J Clin Monit 4:274, 1988.
36. Flanagin A, Lundberg GD: Clinical decision making: Promoting the jump from theory to practice (editorial). JAMA 263:279, 1990.

Chapter 42

QUALITY ASSURANCE IN CRITICAL CARE

JOHN P. CULVER
LEONARD D. HUDSON

The measurement and improvement of quality are topics of major interest and importance throughout health care. Unfortunately, quality can also be an elusive, problematic, and frustrating subject. As the social debate over the quality of health care has intensified, agencies charged with the regulation of quality have demanded increased efforts from providers to demonstrate their dedication to quality. The intent of this chapter is to lead the reader through the conceptual and regulatory maze of quality assurance toward an approach which should provide for monitoring and improving the quality of patient care, furnish enough flexibility to adapt to new approaches as research continues to define and elucidate better scientific models for evaluating quality, and meet regulatory and legal requirements for assessing quality of care.

History of Quality Assurance Regulation

It is probably safe to assume that as long as medicine has been considered worth doing, it has been considered worth doing well. It was not until the nineteenth century, however, that the average medical encounter came to have a probability of actually benefiting the patient. With the rapid advance of both basic biomedical science and new statistical tools, new interventions became possible. At the same time it also became possible to quantify the effectiveness of accepted practices as well as new interventions. A utilitarian epidemiologic approach to evaluating the effectiveness of old and new treatments was advocated by a number of workers. Early in the twentieth century, the "End Result System," essentially a method for tracking outcomes, was developed. It involved systematic evaluation of the final result in each case treated and attribution of responsibility for failure or success to the individual practitioner.[1] For a number of reasons, not the least of which was the abrasive personality of its creator, the system never achieved widespread acceptance. The regulation of hospital quality took a slightly different course, as the American College of Surgeons initiated its hospital standardization program and developed a "minimum standard" for hospitals. From 1919 until 1950, the standardization program gradually expanded until it involved half the hospitals in the United States. At that time, the College of Surgeons and four other associations joined to form the Joint Commission on Accreditation of Hospitals (JCAH) as an independent, voluntary, nonprofit organization. The JCAH continued the work which the College had begun, establishing standards and surveying hospitals.[2]

In the 1970s, the JCAH encouraged the medical audit as a tool to review the quality of care. This approach was not uniformly successful because hospitals tended to concentrate on the requirement itself rather than on how the audit could be used to measure quality. The Commission modified the standard in 1979 to encourage hospitals to focus on problems in patient care and on integration of all quality assurance activities. In the early 1980s, with the passage of national legislation aimed at curbing the cost of health care, quality came to the forefront of the professional and social debates on the status of health care delivery. The JCAH clarified its requirements by developing a fairly simple 10-step model for monitoring and evaluation.[3]

Along with the JCAH's evolving and gradualist approach to quality, researchers were developing models which were more scientifically sound and which reflected the rapidly developing information technology. The classic model was based on structure, process, and outcome perspectives.[4] Previous regulatory attempts to evaluate the quality of health care had emphasized chiefly the structure and process aspects of assessment. Outcome as an indicator of quality, however, has great social attractiveness in that patients are given a fairly precise idea of what the final result of their care might be. Unfortunately, a concomitant and often complex adjustment for case mix and severity of disease process is required to account for different patient populations and different stages of disease.[5] A number of methodologies have been developed for objectively weighting and scoring severity of disease. These have included the Physiologic Stability Index,[6,7] the APACHE,[8–13] the Therapeutic Intervention Scoring System,[9,14] the Simplified Acute Physiology Score, and the Mortality Prediction Model.[13,15–17] Some of these systems will be discussed below.

Independent of the tripartite model, but not necessarily in conflict with it, many other quality assessment strategies were developed to assist providers. These include generic and occurrence screening systems, tracer methods, criteria mapping, problem lists, and expansions of audit criteria.

In 1987, the JCAH embarked upon its "Agenda for Change" to develop specific outcome indicators allowing a more objective scientific approach to the quality of care both nationally and within any given hospital. Although a number of major problems remain to be worked out in the implementation of this program, it is clear that clinical indicators based on patient outcomes will be developed and promoted for use in all hospitals, and that this in turn will necessitate universal application of risk and severity adjustments in the near future.

Evaluating Quality of Care

The triad of structure, process, and outcome provides a convenient platform for conceptualizing and discussing quality and a reasonable approach to the subject. While Donabedian has provided a comprehensive discussion of the various interrelationships within the triad which will not be duplicated here,[4] it is probably important to understand how the three aspects fit together.

STRUCTURE

Structure can be defined as the relatively stable characteristics in the human, physical, technologic, and financial resources that must be present for patient care to occur. "Structure is relevant to quality in that it increases or decreases the probability of good performance."[4] The presence of quality structure does not necessarily assure that care will be provided in a quality manner, although conceptually it would seem to be a prerequisite for quality care to occur. Much of what can be considered structure is described in Chap. 40 on the physical plant characteristics and in Chap. 36 on staffing.

One additional but very important structural component to consider is the structure for reviewing quality of care. While each unit will need to carefully design the most appropriate structure, we have found that a multidisciplinary committee, perhaps an established critical care committee, is an effective and responsible body for looking at care. This multidisciplinary committee can establish policies and oversee and coordinate administration and patient care activities throughout a hospital's ICUs. Such a committee can also be very helpful in developing and carrying out a program of quality assurance. Development of such a committee is applicable whether there is one large general ICU or whether there are several specialized units. The membership of such a committee depends on which of these two situations exists in the local institution. If one large, general ICU exists, membership should include physician representatives of the medical disciplines most frequently admitting patients to the unit, nursing staff responsible for administering the critical care unit, as well as a representative of the respiratory care department. Nursing representatives may either include nurse managers of each unit or the membership of nurse managers may rotate among the various units, in addition to permanent membership of the nursing director of critical care, should such a position exist. If a director of quality assurance for the hospital exists, it is important to include this person as a committee member. Depending on the institutions and the issues dealt with, other representatives, such as social work or general hospital administration can be added as necessary. It is also useful to include a representative of the emergency department because of the need for coordination between the activities in these two areas of patient care. If the hospital has several specialized critical care units, the physician membership should include medical directors of each of the critical care units. The quality assurance activities can be carried out in the committee as a whole or can be assigned to a subcommittee with review by the entire committee. The committee is responsible for setting standards on quality assurance and for carrying out monitoring of compliance to these standards in the process described below. Such a multidisciplinary committee can identify unique circumstances or problems which require evaluation of quality, primarily limited to individual units, but with occasional use in other units—for example, use of intracranial pressure monitoring in the neurosurgical ICU, but also occasionally carried out in the surgical or trauma ICU or medical ICU. However, and perhaps more important, the committee can identify those issues which affect quality of care that are relevant to all of the critical care units. Examples include bed utilization between units when a given unit is full, infection control measures, patient transport procedures, hemodynamic monitoring measures, among others.

For the quality assurance process to receive meaningful participation by all of the necessary parties and, in our experience, particularly the involved physicians, the aspects of quality being monitored must be perceived as reflecting the important aspects of patient management or real problems in the management of the critically ill patient in the specific institution. The best way to ensure this perception is, in fact, to address these real concerns by having representatives of the actual caregivers, including the medical directors of the critical care units, the nurse managers, and respiratory care supervisors, involved in the identification of the areas to be monitored or the specific problems to be addressed by the quality assurance process. Assigning this responsibility to the multidisciplinary committee achieves this objective.

An important part of the structure for reviewing quality of care is a provision for resources to assist with or carry out data collection and analysis. In assessing measures of process and outcome as described below, it is obviously most economic to use data already being collected by existing hospital personnel. However, undoubtedly, some of the desired measurements of quality will entail collection of new data in addition to that already available. It is important to recognize that an effective program of quality assurance will require additional resources on the part of the hospital and this should be reflected in budgetary allocations. Whether this is reflected in the budgets of individual units or whether a centralized quality assurance data collection and analysis resource is established will depend both on those variables to be measured, whether an existing structure is in place in each unit to collect and analyze such data, and other decisions regarding the overall institutional quality assurance program.

PROCESS

After design or establishment of a structure for quality, the next aspect of quality which might be considered is the process of care. While licensing and regulatory agencies have historically looked at structure, the thrust over the last decade has increasingly been concerned with the process of care. The JCAH has developed a 10-step approach as part of the compliance monitoring of its standard on quality assurance. The following steps "are necessary for effective monitoring and evaluation in an organization, department, or service:[3]

1. Assign responsibility.
2. Delineate scope of care.
3. Identify important aspects of care.
4. Identify indicators related to these aspects of care.
5. Establish thresholds for evaluation related to the indicators.
6. Collect and organize data.
7. Evaluate care when thresholds are reached.
8. Take actions to improve care.
9. Assess the effectiveness of the actions and document improvement.
10. Communicate relevant information to the organization-wide quality assurance program."

Although this methodology is designed to apply to structure, process, and outcome, it is often applied to process since the process of care entails the various actions included under aspects of care.

Since procedures, policies, and guidelines are the expression of what the process of care generally involves and are intended to direct the process of care, these are often excellent sources for process types of indicators. The multidisciplinary critical care committee may be responsible for developing and improving ICU policies. This includes both nursing procedure policies as well as physician guidelines for management of particular medical problems. Such policies provide one means for allowing the committee to develop a rational basis for a quality assessment monitoring program, especially as it relates to process. The scope of care and the important aspects of care (steps 2 and 3 of the 10-step approach described above) should already be delineated in the policies or guidelines. The committee can assign responsibility for monitoring the care process defined by a given policy and for identifying the indicators to be monitored which relate to the aspects of care, as well as establishing thresholds for evaluation. After the data are collected and organized, they can be presented to the multidisciplinary critical care committee, which is then responsible for evaluating the care, taking actions to improve the care, and supervising assessment of the effectiveness of the actions taken and communication of relevant information to those parties involved. Thus the critical care policies and guidelines, together with the existing unit administrative oversight committee structure, can provide a means for carrying out clinically relevant quality assurance programs.

Unfortunately, a difficulty often encountered is that relatively simple compliance monitoring fails to take into account the real complexity of care and how it relates to a particular patient. In addition, the evaluation of compliance frequently takes on a punitive flavor which is not conducive to positive staff involvement. Indeed, one of the reasons why industrial models and theories of total quality improvement are becoming increasingly popular in the health care field is the negative aspect of focusing on compliance and correction of misbehavior.[18] This excessive emphasis on monitoring has been dubbed the "theory of bad apples," since identification and elimination of the practitioner has predominated in this model.

An additional resource issue which must be faced in using process-oriented indicators is the fact that often data are not available to answer the specific question being posed and therefore additional resources must be committed to retrieving the data. As an example, suppose that an ICU were concerned about communicable disease transmission. One way to look at the relevant process of care, which would presumably be that appropriate infection control policies were in place and followed, would be to evaluate compliance to a policy which stated that providers would wear gloves for all patient care interactions involving contact with patients' mucous membranes, open skin, or indwelling devices at the insertion site. It is unlikely that any data source currently extant would be able to give direct information on this topic, and so new data collection must be instituted. There are at least two possibilities for doing this: to have a closed circuit camera record all interactions, or a sample of interactions, between the practitioner and the patient and then evaluate whether for each interaction gloves were worn or not. The other possibility would be to have an on-site observer watching a sample of the interactions for compliance with the policy. In either example, the amount of personnel time devoted to obtaining enough data to indicate whether a problem exists will be considerable. Looking at the process of care may not always be the most efficient way to perform surveillance to discover problems, but it is often the best way to evaluate an issue once a problem or potential problem has been identified.

Using the same example, if an increase in nosocomial infections had been identified as a problem within the ICU (through monitoring of infections, essentially an outcome of care), then the expenditure of resources to evaluate compliance with the gloving policy might well be justified on the basis of the savings if compliance could be enforced and infections could be reduced.

In the JCAH 10-step model, a problem sometimes also arises when thresholds are to be assigned. Often little data exist to suggest what the threshold should be and the threshold is essential to the determination of quality in this model. Until historical and normative data are obtained, setting a threshold is often a matter of educated guessing with obvious concerns regarding lack of precision.

OUTCOME

The third leg of the Donabedian triad is outcome, an area of great current interest and research. An outcome is defined as "a change in patient's current and future health status that can be attributed to antecedent health care."[4] Outcomes measure the effectiveness of health care and can be used to target or prioritize process and structure for more intensive review.[19–24] Process and outcome are not always well correlated but, if forced to choose, most patients and practitioners would opt for a good outcome. Another advantage for studying outcomes is that often some raw data are already available, e.g., deaths, complications, hospital-acquired infections. It is important in terms of cost and availability to assess what types of information might be accessible on various data bases. Volume data is often a good place to begin: what are the numbers of discharges over successive months during preceding years, what are the most common admitting and discharge diagnoses, what are the most common procedures, how many deaths occur during a month, and how are they aggregated? Once these data have been retrieved and reviewed, further steps in data acquisition or use may become evident.

Clearly the need for precision and accuracy of data is great, and the role of risk (or severity) adjustment in data evaluation is a major one. It has been noted that "risk adjustment is a way to remove or reduce the effects of confounding factors in studies where the cases are not randomly assigned to different treatments."[5] This is certainly the case in trying to evaluate quality of patient care and has been quite extensively studied using mortality as an outcome of care. Individual case review has limitations in that patterns of problems may not be easily identifiable; it is also labor intensive, and so is best reserved for cases where there is a high suspicion of quality problems. However, if outcomes can be adjusted to correct for factors that affect the outcome but are not indicative of differences of quality, then differences in comparative rates or differences between observed and predicted rates may indeed be indicative of quality problems. Although many of the severity-indexing systems use subjective scores which are summed, it is preferable to attempt to use the categorical or continuous variable that went into the scores for each case.

Systems which predict outcomes of critical care can be used to establish predicted rates, to compare them with the observed rates, and to evaluate unfavorable differences for quality of care issues. These systems can also be used to stratify patients such that risk groups can be defined and evaluated separately. APACHE II is a well-known severity of disease classification system which uses a point score based on initial values of 12 routine physiologic measurements, age, and previous health status to provide a measure of severity of disease. The physiologic measurements include temperature, mean arterial pressure, heart rate, respiratory rate, oxygenation, arterial pH, serum sodium, serum potassium, serum creatinine, hematocrit, white blood count, and Glasgow coma score. The variables were initially selected and weighted based on a nominal group process, and the system was specifically designed for use in ICUs. It has been used to stratify groups of patients to examine whether differences in structure and process of intensive care influenced the effectiveness of care.

It may not be appropriate to apply APACHE II to diagnostic categories that do not include large numbers of patients or the high death rates seen in the original studies. For such categories, more clinically specific adjustments might be required (e.g., the Injury Severity Score in trauma patients). Another factor to keep in mind in using APACHE II is that it includes the worst physiologic derangements in the first 24 h of ICU admission and therefore is not totally independent of treatment that occurs in the emergency room or early in the ICU stay. This drawback may be corrected in future versions of the system.

Another classification system developed from the original APACHE system is the Simplified Acute Physiology Score (SAPS). This system uses 13 variables with the same weighting as the original APACHE system plus age. The 13 variables include heart rate, systolic blood pressure, body temperature, spontaneous respiratory rate, requirement for mechanical ventilation or continuous positive airway pressure, urinary output, blood urea nitrogen, hematocrit, white blood cell count, serum sodium, serum potassium, serum glucose, serum bicarbonate, and Glasgow coma scale. Some workers feel that the SAPS is comparable to APACHE II in sensitivity, specificity, and accuracy in patients with acute myocardial infarctions, and that both the nonspecialized systems work as well as the Coronary Prognostic Index, a clinically specialized system. Further testing will need to be done in other diagnostic categories to see if this is a consistent finding, but since different diagnostic categories have varying clinical classification systems one would suspect that it would not hold true in all diagnostic classifications. Because the SAPS was based on the original Acute Physiology Score, it too may be susceptible to the inclusion of treatment results in the index.

The mortality prediction model (MPM) is another severity indexing system. Multiple logistic regression was used to select from many variables those that were most predictive of mortality in a multivariate sense. After testing, the model was modified to consist of seven variables including level of consciousness, type of admission, cancer as part of present problem, infection, cardiopulmonary resuscitation before ICU admission, age, and systolic blood pressure. In a comparison study of MPM with APS and SAPS, each method was effective in analyzing the case mix in an ICU.

An advantage to the MPM is that it is entirely independent of ICU treatment factors, all scores being assigned at admission. The MPM also does not require assignment of a single precipitating factor or major organ system failure to convert the score to a probability. Thus, APACHE II may be more useful for specific disease categories while MPM may be more applicable to ICU patients in general.

Generally, the trend has been to make scoring systems as statistically and mathematically objective as possible. Increasing levels of precision are being obtained. However, it is still important to realize that variations between expected outcome rates and actual rates do not necessarily equate with differences in quality. These differences certainly point up areas where intensified review should occur, much the same as other outcome indicators would focus quality reviewers in certain areas.

Although the Outcome Index is not a severity index,[25] it is somewhat analogous to one in that it assigns a system outcome score to each patient, which allows ultimately a mortality rate prediction for an intensive care population. It approaches physiologic dysfunction from the standpoint of intervention and those categories of intervention that are simply and objectively assessed. The specifications for the system included brevity, simplicity, and objectivity. Thus, it is easy to apply and is intended to focus on variation in care which should lead to investigation. Part of the motivation for development of the system was a mysterious cluster of deaths and cardiopulmonary arrests within a special care unit; this was suspected to be due to "malicious inter-

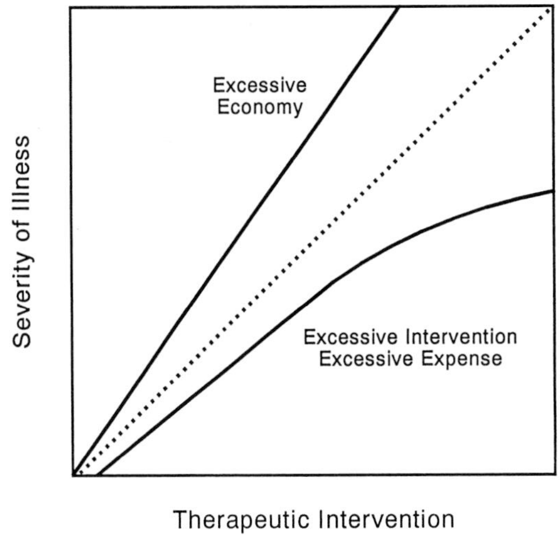

FIGURE 42-1 The dotted diagonal line represents a balance between severity of illness and the appropriate application of technology. The horizontal axis can be calibrated with a scale such as the Therapeutic Intervention Scoring System (TISS). The vertical axis representing severity of illness could be calibrated with a scoring system such as APACHE II. (From Sivak ED, Perez-Trepichio A: Cleve Clin J Med 57:273, 1990.)

ference'' by an unknown individual. While other systems for evaluating outcomes should make it possible to identify patterns suggestive of this source of poor quality, it is notable that this system was specifically designed to discover such trends.

The above discussion has focused on mortality as an obvious outcome variable. Other measures of outcome appropriate for evaluating quality of care include length of ICU stay, change in physiologic measurements, measures of functional recovery, and incidence and severity of complications. The outcome variables chosen for evaluation will depend in part on the patient population seen in a given institution or ICU. The above discussion on risk adjustment is equally applicable to evaluation of these other outcome variables as it is to assessment of mortality rates.

Another application of risk adjustment or severity of illness scales has been suggested by Sivak and Perez-Trepichio and is diagrammed in Figure 42-1.[26] They have suggested a model in which severity of illness is plotted against a measure of therapeutic intervention to evaluate whether the application of technology is appropriate to the severity of illness. Such a model allows consideration of the issues of over- or underintervention. Appropriate assessment of these issues involves comparison with other institutions. As these authors point out, excessive intervention with low or moderate severity of illness could be associated with excessive cost or with iatrogenic problems related to excessive intervention and thus a compromise in quality of care. On the other hand, high severity of illness with a low therapeutic intervention could result in high mortality, prolonged ICU stay, or compromised quality of life after discharge.

Summary

In summary, the issue of quality is clearly a permanent one. In developing a unit-appropriate method for evaluating quality, the accountability and communication structure should be carefully designed. Indicators may be developed based on structure, process, or outcome, but should always have clinical significance for the staff. The quality assessment structure should continually ask the question ''how do we know we are doing a good job?'' Outcome indicators, particularly, may be useful for both staff and regulators but will need to be adjusted for particular patient populations and disease severity.

References

1. Codman EA: *The Shoulder: Rupture of the Supraspinatus Tendon and Other Lesions in or about the Subacromial Bursa.* Boston, Thomas Todd Co Printers, 1934.
2. Roberts JS, Coale JG, Redman RR: A history of the Joint Commission on Accreditation of Hospitals. JAMA 258:936, 1987.
3. Joint Commission on Accreditation of Healthcare Organizations: *Examples of Monitoring and Evaluation in Special Care Units.* Chicago, 1988.
4. Donabedian A: *Explorations in Quality Assessment and Monitoring.* Vol. 1, *The Definition of Quality and Approaches to its Assessment.* Ann Arbor, Health Administration Press, 1980.
5. Blumberg MS: Risk adjusting health care outcomes: A methodologic review. Med Care Rev 43:351, 1986.
6. Yeh TS, Pollack MM, Ruttimann UE, et al: Validation of a physiologic stability index for use in critically ill infants and children. Pediatr Res 18:445, 1984.
7. Pollack MM, Ruttimann UE, Getson PR, and Members of the Multiinstitutional Study Group. Accurate prediction of the outcome of pediatric intensive care: A new quantitative method. N Engl J Med 316:134, 1987.
8. Dobkin JC, Cutler RE: Use of Apache II classification to evaluate outcome of patients receiving hemodialysis in an intensive care unit. West J Med 149:547, 1988.
9. Jensen NH, Dragsted L, Christensen JK, Jorgensen JC, Qvist J: Severity of illness and outcome of treatment in alcoholic patients in the intensive care unit. Intensive Care Med 15:19, 1988.
10. Knaus WA, Draper EA, Wagner DP, Zimmerman JE: An evaluation of outcome from intensive care in major medical centers. Ann Intern Med 104:410, 1986.
11. Knaus WA, Draper EA, Wagner DP, Zimmerman JE: APACHE II: A severity of disease classification system. Crit Care Med 13:818, 1985.
12. Kruse JA, Thill-Baharozian MC, Carlson RW: Comparison of clinical assessment with APACHE II for predicting mortality risk in patients admitted to a medical intensive care unit. JAMA 260:1739, 1988.
13. Moreau R, Soupison T, Vauquelin P, et al: Comparison of two simplified severity scores (SAPS and APACHE II) for patients with acute myocardial infarction. Crit Care Med 17:409, 1989.
14. Keene AR, Cullen DJ: Therapeutic intervention scoring system: Update 1983. Crit Care Med 11:1, 1983.
15. Lemeshow S, Teres D, Avrunin JS, Gage RW: Refining intensive care unit outcome prediction by using changing probabilities of mortality. Crit Care Med 16:470, 1988.

16. Lemeshow S, Teres D, Avrunin JS, Pastides H: A comparison of methods to predict mortality of intensive care unit patients. Crit Care Med 15:715, 1987.
17. Lemeshow S, Teres D, Pastides H, et al: A method for predicting survival and mortality of ICU patients using objectively derived weights. Crit Care Med 13:519, 1985.
18. Berwick DM: Continuous improvement as an ideal in health care. N Engl J Med 320:53, 1989.
19. Dragsted L, Jorgensen J, Jensen NH, et al: Interhospital comparisons of patient outcome from intensive care: Importance of lead-time bias. Crit Care Med 17:418, 1989.
20. Franklin C, Jackson D: Discharge decision-making in a medical ICU: Characteristics of unexpected readmissions. Crit Care Med 11:6166, 1983.
21. French Multicenter Group of ICU Research, INSERM Unit 169 of Statistical and Epidemiological Studies: Factors related to outcome in intensive care: French multicenter study. Crit Care Med 17:305, 1989.
22. Hannan EL, Bernard HR, O'Donnell JF, Kilburn H: A methodology for targeting hospital cases for quality of care record reviews. Am J Public Health 79:430, 1989.
23. Rubins HR, Moskowitz MA: Discharge decision-making in a medical intensive care unit: Identifying patients at high risk of unexpected death of unit readmission. Am J Med 84:863, 1988.
24. Schroeder SA: Outcome assessment 70 years later: Are we ready? N Engl J Med 316:160, 1987.
25. McFee AS, Gilbert J: The outcome index: A method of quality assurance in the special care area. Arch Surg 124:825, 1989.
26. Sivak ED, Perez-Trepichio A: Quality assessment in the medical intensive care unit: Evolution of a data model. Cleve Clin J Med 57:273, 1990.

Chapter 43

INFECTION SURVEILLANCE AND CONTROL IN THE ICU

JOHN P. FLAHERTY
TERESA CHOU
PAUL M. ARNOW

In United States hospitals, nosocomial infections cause increased morbidity and mortality and generate excess costs estimated at $5 to $10 billion per year.[1] ICU patients experience a disproportionate share of these infections. While about 5 percent of all hospitalized patients develop nosocomial infections, rates of nosocomial infection in ICU patients may exceed 30 percent.[2] Pneumonia and bacteremia, serious infections which contribute substantially to mortality and cost,[3,4] occur disproportionately in ICU patients.[2,5]

The increased risk of infection probably results both from the greater severity of underlying disease and from the resultant frequent use of medical devices that bypass normal barriers to infection. A patient's condition on admission to the ICU appears intuitively to be an important predictor of nosocomial infection risk, although few studies have examined this relationship. Britt and coworkers[6] demonstrated a progressive increase in nosocomial infection rate related to severity of illness in patients admitted to medicine services, and in an ICU-based study by Gross and colleagues, the number of comorbidities or active preexisting illnesses on admission was predictive of nosocomial infection risk.[7] The APACHE II score, a commonly used prognostic index, has been associated by univariate but not multivariate analysis with nosocomial infection risk.[2] Medical devices, which have become an integral part of ICU patient management, are significantly associated with nosocomial infection[2] and account for an estimated 50 percent of all nosocomial infections.[8] For example, endotracheal intubation has been shown to increase the risk of nosocomial pneumonia more than sixfold in ICU patients.[9]

Efforts to control infections in ICUs have evolved largely within the framework of hospital-wide infection control programs. These programs, which arose in response to the staphylococcal pandemic of the late 1950s and early 1960s, now are mandated by accrediting agencies and engage in a broad range of activities. Core activities include surveillance of nosocomial infections, establishment of isolation policies for patients with transmissible infections, development of infection control guidelines for patient care, education of hospital personnel, and investigation of nosocomial infection problems. The impact of well-directed infection control activities, when examined hospital-wide or on selected wards, has been to reduce nosocomial infection rates by about 30 to 50 percent.[6,10]

Surveillance

Infection surveillance involves the systematic collection, tabulation, and analysis of data on nosocomial infection occurrences. The usual goals of surveillance are to ascertain the incidence of nosocomial infections and to provide sufficient detail about these infections (site, pathogen, and host features), so that problems can be recognized and characterized. An extension of these goals has been proposed by Haley[9] who advocated that outcome objectives (i.e., targeted reductions in infection rates) be linked to traditional surveillance activities. Whether or not this approach is used, it introduces the critical point that surveillance data should be used in some productive manner to justify the substantial resources required for this activity.

Infection surveillance requires the cooperation of infection control and ICU personnel. To achieve unity of purpose, surveillance objectives should be set by infection control staff and the ICU medical and nursing directors. The individual then charged with conducting surveillance is usually an infection control nurse who works throughout the hospital. Alternatively, some hospitals have designated a staff nurse on each unit to perform surveillance and other infection control duties for that unit. In either system, surveillance personnel require special training in the diagnosis of infections and will need to consult periodically with ICU clinicians about cases where the presence of nosocomial infection is uncertain. Criteria for the diagnosis of nosocomial infections have been developed by the Centers for Disease Control (CDC)[11] and are widely accepted. Nonetheless, it is noteworthy that the demand for accuracy on the part of an infection control nurse who must decide the presence of nosocomial infection is greater than that on clinicians who may choose to treat patients for infection presumptively, even in situations where the likelihood of infection is low.

Surveillance in the ICU may take any of several forms, depending on the resources and objectives. Surveillance may be continuous or periodic; also, it may be directed at all infections or at targeted sites or devices. Examples of targeted surveillance activities are assessments of infection risk for specific types of intravascular catheters or of pneumonia risk in patients requiring tracheal intubation. Such surveillance can be used to gauge the effectiveness of measures intended to reduce infection risk or to assess adverse consequences of new devices or patient care procedures. Periodic or targeted surveillance can be supplemented by microbiology laboratory-based systems, which identify increased numbers of isolates of various organisms that then should be investigated to determine if they represent clusters of infections.

Several different techniques to detect nosocomial infections have been developed by workers seeking to maximize the efficiency of patient-based surveillance. Patients likely to have infection have been identified by review of pharmacy or ward records of antibiotic administration, nursing care plans, microbiology laboratory results, and patient charts. Whatever the starting point, it inevitably becomes necessary to review patient charts to confirm the presence of infection. Detection of ICU-acquired infections can be augmented by continuing to monitor for a few days patients transferred from an ICU to another unit and by review of autopsies performed on ICU patients.

Nosocomial infection rates commonly are expressed as incidence, that is, number of infections/number of patients at risk during a specific time period. The usual denominator is the number of patients discharged or admitted in a month. In burn units or other ICUs where patient stays are lengthy, alternative denominators such as number of patients hospitalized or number of patient-days may be used. Rates of nosocomial infection determined by standard methods can be compared to rates during earlier periods and from other hospitals. Higher than expected rates should prompt investigation by infection control and ICU staff.

Environmental Surveillance

The hospital environment contributes negligibly to the acquisition and spread of most endemic nosocomial infections. Consequently, in the absence of an epidemic problem, environmental culturing appears unwarranted and is discouraged by most authorities. Nonetheless, environmental culturing can be considered in selected situations. One such situation is when the care of substantial numbers of highly immunosuppressed patients, such as bone marrow or solid organ transplant recipients, is about to be undertaken. These patients have increased susceptibility to two life-threatening diseases, Legionnaires' disease and aspergillosis, caused by organisms whose reservoir is the inanimate hospital environment. Culturing of hot tap water for *Legionella* or air for *Aspergillus* may be worthwhile if it is anticipated that detection of these organisms will prompt measures to suppress them. Another use of environmental culturing is to assess aseptic practices or cleaning procedures. A culture survey to detect *Clostridium difficile* spores on floors or others surfaces could be one measure of the adequacy of housekeeping.

Control Measures

HANDWASHING

For more than a century handwashing has been widely recognized as an important measure for preventing nosocomial infections. The role of inadequate handwashing in sporadic cases of nosocomial infection has not been established, but in outbreak settings hand carriage of the epidemic organism by hospital personnel is commonly detected. Studies in ICUs have shown that, on average, hospital personnel wash their hands after contact with patients less than half the time.[12] Standard educational techniques have had limited success in improving compliance. Alternatively, use of less irritating, emollient handwashing agents and feedback to personnel regarding their handwashing practices have improved compliance.

ISOLATION PRECAUTIONS

Isolation precautions have traditionally involved separating patients with transmissible infections from other patients and health care workers and using barriers such as gloves, gowns, or masks to prevent direct exposure to transmissible organisms. The two major systems of isolation precautions are category-specific and disease-specific.[11] *Category-specific isolation* guidelines group transmissible diseases by their major route(s) of spread and provide techniques that prevent transmission of all diseases in a particular category (Table 43-1). Diseases grouped in any specific category may differ in their transmissibility by various routes, so certain category-specific precautions may be excessive for a particular infection. The disadvantage of "over isolation" for some infections is offset by having a small number of categories that are easily understood by most hospital personnel. *Disease-specific isolation* guidelines provide techniques specific to each infection. This system is very precise, but hospital medical and nursing staff who select precautions for each patient must be well trained in infectious disease epidemiology to use the system correctly.

Implementation of protective isolation precautions for uninfected patients has been of benefit in selected ICU populations. In a pediatric ICU, routine use of gowns and gloves by personnel caring for nonimmunocompromised mechanically ventilated children was associated with delayed colonization by nosocomial pathogens, a longer interval before the first infection, and a lower daily risk of infection.[13] Burn patients have also benefitted from strict environmental isolation in conjunction with topical and systemic antimicrobial prophylaxis. Barrier precautions (gowns and gloves) have limited the spread of multiresistant gram-negative bacilli[14] but have not benefitted granulocytopenic patients.[15] This is not surprising because most infections in these patients are caused by endogenous organisms colonizing the patient at the time of hospital admission. Increasing evidence indicates that presumed nosocomial gram-negative organisms, especially *Pseudomonas aeruginosa* or *Enterobacter cloacae,* frequently are present in patients on admission to ICUs. Barrier precautions would not prevent acquisition or infection with such organisms.

NURSE STAFFING

Nurse staffing has been reported to play a role in both epidemic and endemic infection transmission. Methicillin-resistant *Staphylococcus aureus* transmission in a burn unit increased during periods when nurse-to-patient staffing ratios were low and was controlled only when separate nurses were assigned to colonized patients.[16] A 50 percent increase in nurse staffing levels was credited as a major factor associated with a dramatic reduction in the nosocomial infection rate in a neonatal ICU.[17]

ICU Design

Suprisingly, the architectural design of general medical-surgical ICUs has had little impact on infections in the few

TABLE 43-1 Category-Specific Isolation

Category	Specifications	Diseases (examples)
Strict	Private room with door closed; masks, gown, gloves for all entering room	Varicella (chickenpox) Herpes zoster, localized in immunocompromised patients or disseminated
Contact	Private room; masks for close patient contact, gowns if soiling is likely, gloves for touching infective material	Methicillin-resistant *Staph. aureus* Aminoglycoside-resistant gram-negative bacilli Viral pneumonia in children Major skin, wound, and burn infection
Respiratory	Private room with door closed; masks	Pulmonary tuberculosis Meningococcal meningitis, pneumonia, or meningococcemia *Hemophilus influenzae* epiglottitis or pneumonia Measles
Enteric	Private room only if hygiene is poor; gloves if touching infected material; gown if soiling is likely	*C. difficile* colitis Encephalitis (unless known not to be caused by enteroviruses) Bacterial gastroenteritis Hepatitis A
Drainage/ Secretion	Gloves if touching infected material; gown if soiling is likely	Minor skin or wound infection Infected decubitus ulcer Conjunctivitis
Blood/ Body Fluid	Private room if hygiene is poor; gown if soiling by blood or body fluids is likely; gloves for touching blood or body fluids	HIV infection Hepatitis B or C

SOURCE: Adapted from Reference 11.

studies that have examined this issue.[17] Conversion of open ICUs to individual rooms and addition of handwashing sinks have not appreciably reduced nosocomial infection rates. Nonetheless, individual rooms appear desirable and are necessary for several types of isolation.

Infection Control Policies and Procedures

The Joint Commission on Accreditation of Healthcare Organizations requires that ICUs have written policies and procedures relating to infection control. Awareness of and adherence to these policies and procedures is important for all health care workers, especially those involved in direct patient care. Because of the considerable risk of nosocomial infection related to the use of invasive devices,[18] these devices should be addressed specifically in the infection control policies and procedures.

INTRAVASCULAR CATHETERS

Up to one-third of all endemic nosocomial bacteremias and the majority of candidemias result from intravascular catheter-related infection.[19] The incidence of catheter-related infection varies with the type of catheter, the site of placement, and the patient population studied. All intravascular catheters, whether used for infusion therapy or hemodynamic monitoring, must be recognized as potential portals for the entry of infection. Handwashing, the wearing of gloves, thorough disinfection of the site with a reliable germicide, and meticulous attention to aseptic technique throughout the insertion constitute the initial steps in the prevention of cannula-related infection. Thereafter, careful aseptic dressing technique, routine tubing changes, and maximal care when preparing and handling infusions are critical. The risk of infection is a function of time—the longer a catheter is in place, the greater the risk of infection. The risk of catheter-related infection in peripheral intravenous catheters increases substantially after 3 days in place; these should be changed to a new site every 48 to 72 h. There is disagreement, however, about the proper approach to other vascular catheters, including central venous, pulmonary artery, and arterial catheters. Arterial catheter infection has been associated with duration of placement >4 days in some studies but not others. As a result, CDC guidelines suggest but do not strongly recommend arterial catheter changes every 4 days. Some authorities have suggested a similar approach be used for central venous catheters (see Chap. 24). In some institutions, catheter changes to a new site are performed every 3 to 5 days to minimize infection risk. Others use guidewire exchange or infrequent catheter changes to new sites to minimize inconvenience and morbidity from mechanical complications. Available data from small prospective studies suggest that these methods of long-term maintenance have comparable infection risks.[20] Guidelines for the prevention of intravenous catheter-related infection are presented in Table 43-2.

PRESSURE TRANSDUCERS

Indwelling catheters connected to pressure transducers have become a routine part of intensive care patient management. The potential for these devices to serve as a source of bacterial and fungal bloodstream infection led to recommendations for preventing transducer-related bacteremia in the 1970s. Nonetheless, outbreaks of bacteremia related to contaminated transducers continue to occur. From 1977 to 1987, these devices were the most common source of epidemic bloodstream infection investigated by the CDC.[21]. These outbreaks were prolonged (mean 11

TABLE 43-2 Guidelines for Prevention of Intravenous Therapy-Related Infections

Insertion

- IV catheters should only be used for definite therapeutic or diagnostic indications.
- Wash hands vigorously before inserting a catheter. Wear gloves during insertion.
- The upper extremity should be used in preference to the lower extremity.
- Scrub the IV site in concentric circles starting from the site of insertion with an appropriate antiseptic (1–2% iodine, an iodophor,[a] chlorhexidine or 70% alcohol) for at least 2–4 min prior to insertion.
- Central catheters and catheters placed by cutdown should be inserted using sterile technique (sterile gloves, sterile gowns, mask, hair cover, and sterile drapes).
- Apply an antimicrobial ointment, preferably an iodophor (povidone-iodine), to the site immediately after insertion.
- Sterile gauze dressings secured with tape are preferable to occlusive, semipermeable transparent dressings.[b]

Maintenance

- Evaluate patients daily for evidence of catheter-related complications. This evaluation should include gentle palpation of the insertion site through the intact dressing. If the patient has unexplained fever or pain at the insertion site, the dressing should be removed and the site inspected.
- Inspect the insertion site, clean with an iodophor (or alcohol, if the patient is sensitive to iodine products), and redress with a new sterile dressing at least every 48–72 h or whenever dressings are moist or soiled.
- Change IV solutions and flush solutions every 24 h.
- Change IV tubing every 48–72 h and immediately after the administration of blood, blood products, or lipid emulsions.

Maintenance

- Carefully wipe all injection ports with an antiseptic (e.g., alcohol or an iodophor) prior to entry.
- Each port of a central venous catheter should be used for a single purpose, when possible.
- Keep ports covered with sterile caps.

Removal

- Catheters inserted without proper asepsis, such as those placed in an emergency, should be replaced at the earliest opportunity and always within 24 h.
- All peripheral IV catheters and peripherally placed central venous catheters (e.g., inserted through a peripheral vein, external jugular or femoral vein) should be removed 48–72 h after insertion and the insertion site changed, unless extenuating circumstances exist.
- Central catheters inserted aseptically through a subclavian or internal jugular approach need not be changed routinely.
- If a patient with a central venous catheter develops unexplained fever, bacteremia, or fungemia, the catheter insertion site should be inspected for purulence, cellulitis, or thrombophlebitis.
- If pus is present at the insertion site, remove the catheter immediately and culture the pus and the catheter tip.
- If pus is not present at the insertion site, but catheter-related infection is suspected, remove the catheter and culture the catheter tip; if the catheter tip culture is positive (>15 colonies by semiquantitative culture) and the catheter was exchanged over guidewire, the catheter should be removed and restarted at a new site.

[a]Since iodophors depend on the slow release of elemental iodine for their antibacterial properties, iodophors should not be wiped off with alcohol.
[b]Occlusive, semipermeable transparent dressings promote growth of bacteria and should be reserved for situations when skin integrity would be compromised by the routine removal of gauze and tape dressings, protection against contamination by secretions is needed, or the catheter cannot be adequately secured by a gauze and tape dressing.

SOURCE: Adapted from Simmons BP, Hooton TM, Wong, ES, et al: CDC Guidelines on Infection Control: Guidelines for prevention of intravascular infections. Infect Control 3:61, 1982.

months) and involved large numbers of patients (mean 24 patients). In each case, reusable transducers were either improperly disinfected or fitted with improperly sterilized domes. ICU personnel must be aware of the potential for bacteremia related to these devices and implement appropriate infection control strategies (Table 43-3).

UNINARY CATHETERS

The urinary tract is the most frequent site of infection in hospitalized patients. Approximately 80 percent of nosocomial urinary tract infections occur in patients with indwelling urinary catheters.[22] Most catheter-associated urinary tract infections appear benign; only 20 to 30 percent result in symptoms. The major complication is secondary bacteremia, and estimates of secondary bacteremia range from 0.5 to 2 percent of catheterized patients. Although the risk of urosepsis is small in any given patient, bacteremia arising from catheter-associated urinary tract infection still accounts for about 30 to 40 percent of all cases of gram-negative bacteremia. Prevention efforts should be focused primarily on aseptic care of the catheter and discontinuation at the earliest possible time (Table 43-4).

RESPIRATORY THERAPY EQUIPMENT

While pneumonia develops in 0.5 percent to 2 percent of all hospitalized patients,[9] the problem is particularly severe in mechanically ventilated ICU patients, whose rates of pneumonia are as high as 7 to 41 percent.[2,23] Nosocomial bacterial pneumonia is particularly common following acute lung injury such as adult respiratory distress syndrome, (see Chaps. 52 and 54). The risk of pneumonia correlates with the duration of mechanical ventilation and increases significantly with prolonged (>5 days) ventilator therapy.[24] Pneumonia is the most common fatal nosocomial infection, with mortality rates of 20 to 50 percent. Despite a substan-

TABLE 43-3 Guidelines for Prevention of Infections Related to Intravascular Pressure Monitoring Devices

Hospital personnel should wash their hands before manipulating a pressure monitoring system.
Glucose-containing solutions should not be used as flush solutions.
Maintain as closed flush systems. Stopcocks, if used, should be covered with sterile caps.
Keep manipulations to a minimum.
Obtain all specimens aseptically. Prior to entry, sample ports should be wiped with an antiseptic (e.g., alcohol or Betadine).
Flush solutions should be changed every 48 h.
Chamber dome, administration tubing and continuous flow devices (if used) should be replaced every 48–74 h.
Transducers should be changed every 4 days.
Arterial catheters should be replaced every 4 days, unless extenuating circumstances exist.
Nondisposable components, such as the transducer and dome, should either receive high level disinfection or be sterilized with ethylene oxide. Store in a manner that prevents recontamination prior to use.
Disposable components of the pressure-monitoring system should not be resterilized or reused.

SOURCE: Adapted from Simmons BP, Hooton TM, Wong ES, et al: CDC Guidelines on Infection Control: Guidelines for prevention of intravascular infections. Infect Control 3:61, 1982.

tial increase in the number of potent broad-spectrum antibiotics, there is little evidence that survival has improved in patients with hospital-acquired pneumonia, emphasizing the importance of prevention.

Although pneumonia may be caused by bacteria, viruses, fungi, or protozoa, the vast majority of nosocomial pneumonias are bacterial. Of these, most are caused by aerobic gram-negative bacilli and to a lesser extent, gram-positive cocci. Bacteria are believed to invade the lower respiratory tract by three routes—aspiration of oropharyngeal organisms, inhalation of contaminated aerosols, and hematogenous spread from a distant site of infection. Aspiration is believed to initiate most episodes of nosocomial pneumonia and is difficult to prevent. Efforts have focused on positioning patients to limit aspiration and the judicious use of devices that heighten aspiration risk (e.g., endotracheal tubes, nasogastric tubes). Unfortunately, current guidelines for pneumonia prevention appear to offer only limited benefit (Table 43-5).

Epidemics of gram-negative pneumonia have been associated with inhalation of aerosols from contaminated respiratory therapy equipment, specifically nebulizer reservoirs. When appropriate protocols for disinfection and maintenance of ventilator circuit tubing and nebulizers are followed, the rate of contamination of respiratory therapy equipments is low and contributes minimally to the endemic pneumonia rate. Neverthless, epidemics of pneumonia related to inadequate sterilization of respiratory therapy equipment continue to be reported.[25] ICU physicians should be particularly suspicious of pneumonia caused by bacteria having the potential to multiply in nebulizer solutions, for example, *Acinetobacter* and *Pseudomonas* species and *Serratia marcescens*.

TABLE 43-4 Guidelines for Prevention of Urinary Catheter-Related Infection

Catheterize only when necessary.
Emphasize handwashing before and after manipulation of the catheter.
Insert catheters using aseptic technique and sterile equipment.
Use a closed sterile drainage system.
Maintain gravity drainage.
Obtain urine samples aseptically.
Avoid irrigation unless needed to prevent or relieve obstruction.
Refrain from daily meatal care.
Do not change catheters at arbitrarily fixed intervals.
Avoid routine bacteriologic monitoring.

SOURCE: Adapted from Reference 22, with permission.

TABLE 43-5 Guidelines for Prevention of Nosocomial Pneumonia

- Use perioperative measures for prevention of postoperative pneumonia.[a]
- Emphasize handwashing before and after patient contact.
- Only sterile fluids should be nebulized or used in a humidifier.
- Position patients to decrease risk of aspiration.
- Promptly remove endotracheal tubes and nasogastric tubes whenever possible.
- Change ventilator circuit tubing every 48 h.
- Discard ventilator tubing condensate—do not allow it to drain back into the reservoir.
- Suctioning should not be done routinely but only when needed to reduce substantial secretions.
- Suction using a sterile catheter and "no touch" technique or gloved hands.
- Flush suction catheter with sterile fluid.
- Isolate patients with potentially transmissible respiratory infections.
- If an influenza epidemic is anticipated, institute a prevention program for all patient care personnel and high risk patients, including the use of influenza vaccine and amantidine chemoprophylaxis.

[a]Including: preoperative treatment and resolution of pulmonary infections; instruction on importance of frequent coughing, deep breathing, and early ambulation; incentive spirometer use; control of pain that interferes with coughing and deep breathing; avoidance of routine systemic antibiotic pneumonia prophylaxis.

SOURCE: Adapted from Simmons BP, Wong ES: CDC guidelines for the prevention and control of nosocomial infections: Guidelines for Prevention of Nosocomial Pneumonia. Am J Infect Control 11:230, 1983.

TABLE 43-6 Guidelines for Prevention of Ventriculostomy-Related Infections

Maintain a closed drainage system.
Limit irrigation.
If monitoring is required for more than 5 days, remove and reinsert at a different site.

TABLE 43-7 Infectious Diseases Encountered by ICU Employees

Infectious Agent	Incubation Period	Period of Communicability	General Precautions	Vaccines or Prophylaxis
HIV	Variable: 2 weeks to 6 months	Probably lifelong	Universal precautions are standard for all patients.	Possibly zidovudine after needlestick exposure (efficacy undocumented)
Hepatitis B	6-24 weeks	While HBsAg-positive	Blood precautions for patients HBsAg-positive personnel are informed, counseled to wear gloves, but not usually removed from work unless clinically ill.	Passive prophylaxis: HBIG 0.06 mL/kg body weight for HBsAg-positive needlesticks. Repeat at 1 month if not vaccinated. Active prophylaxis: hepatitis B vaccine, 20 μg doses at 0, 1, and 6 months.
Hepatitis C	3-18 weeks	Unknown	Same as for hepatitis B	No therapy or possibly IG (0.06 mL/kg body weight) for needlestick injuries.
Hepatitis A	2-7 weeks	2-3 weeks before jaundice; until 7 days after onset of jaundice	Stool precautions for patients Good handwashing by employees; remove from work for 7 days after onset of jaundice	IG, 0.02 mL/kg
Influenza	1-3 days	1 day before to 5 days after onset of symptoms	Respiratory precautions for patients Remove employees from work for period of communicability.	Influenza vaccine is given yearly. Amantidine, 100 mg orally twice a day, is effective prophylaxis against influenza A.
Varicella-zoster	Usually 10-21 days after exposure	2 days prior to onset of lesions until crusted (~7 days)	Patients with chickenpox require strict isolation in a room with negative pressure ventilation; patients with localized herpes zoster are placed on contact precautions. History of chickenpox is reliable. Exposed susceptible employees should not work from days 10–21 following exposure. Infectious employees are removed until lesions dry and crust. Employees with localized herpes zoster should cover lesions and not care for high-risk patients.	VZIG may attenuate or prevent disease and should be given to high-risk patients and considered for personnel.
Tuberculosis	Usual 3-5 weeks Range 2-8 weeks	Until three consecutive sputa are free of tubercle bacilli or the patient is on adequate therapy for 2 weeks	Evaluate contacts and monitor employees with PPD skin test. Respiratory precautions for patients Ventilation UV lights in high risk areas	Isoniazid prophylaxis if indicated BCG not recommended
Meningococcal disease	Variable 1-10 days	Variable	Close prolonged exposure required for transmission (mouth to mouth resuscitation or prolonged exposure to infected secretions) Respiratory precautions for 24 h after start of effective therapy	Rifampin, 600 mg orally twice a day for 2 days (sulfonamide, if sensitive); vaccine against meningococcal groups A,C,Y, and W135 is available.

TABLE 43-7 Infectious Diseases Encountered by ICU Employees (Continued)

Infectious Agent	Incubation Period	Period of Communicability	General Precautions	Vaccines or Prophylaxis
S. aureus	Variable; 4-10 days	During skin infection or as a nasal "disseminator"	Patients placed on contact precautions Infected personnel should be evaluated by employee health service and may be removed from work.	Topical or oral antibiotics sometimes used to treat carriers

Note: HIV, human immunodeficiency virus; HBsAg, hepatitis B surface antigen; HBIG, hepatitis B immune globulin; IG, immune serum globulin; HAV, hepatitis A virus; VZIG, varicella-zoster immune globulin; PPD, purified protein derivative; BCG, bacillus Calmette-Guérin; UV, ultraviolet.
SOURCE: Adapted from Reference 27, with permission.

INTRACRANIAL PRESSURE MONITORS

Intracranial pressure (ICP) monitoring via ventriculostomy catheter, subarachnoid catheter, or subarachnoid bolt has been of great value in neurosurgical patients. (see Chap. 34). However, the use of these devices is associated with a significant rate of complicating infection. Recent studies have demonstrated a 6 to 11 percent risk of ventriculitis or meningitis in patients undergoing ICP monitoring.[26] The risk of infection appears highest with ventriculostomy catheters and lowest with the subarachnoid bolt. Additional risk factors for infection include intracranial hemorrhage, elevated ICP (>20 mmHg), irrigation of the system, and duration of catheterization >4 to 5 days. While the risk of infection was 9 percent at day 5, it increased to 37 percent by day 10 in one study. Infection prevention efforts should focus on aseptic maintenance and early removal (Table 43-6). Prophylactic antibiotics do not appear to favorably influence infection risk. The use of fiberoptic devices as opposed to fluid-filled tubing connected to a pressure transducer may reduce the frequencies of manipulation, contamination, and infection.

Employee Health

ICU personnel are subject to various occupational hazards, among them the risk of infectious diseases.[27] Health care workers may acquire and transmit infection to other personnel, patients, or family members, and in the case of a pregnant employee, to the fetus. Certain viruses and bacteria may spread rapidly to other patients or hospital personnel. Many hospitals have an employee health service or infection control program to assist with decisions about when to remove employees from work and when prophylaxis is appropriate. Other institutions leave such decisions to supervising physicians. Therefore, it is important the ICU physicians be familiar with these issues (Table 43-7).

The concept of universal precautions was developed to protect health care workers from blood-borne infections. In essence, blood and body fluids containing blood should be presumed infectious, and health care workers should wear protective equipment when contact with these fluids is unavoidable. The protective equipment for a given situation depends on the risk of exposure to blood and blood-containing fluids. For example, because there is no likely risk of exposure when obtaining a pulse, blood pressure, or temperature, no protective equipment is needed. Gloves are recommended when placing an intravenous catheter or arterial line or when suctioning a patient. Gloves and a gown should be worn to change dressings, while gloves, a gown, mask, and goggles are necessary when intubating a patient. Training in the appropriate use of universal precautions may significantly decrease the risk of cutaneous exposures to blood and body fluids and thereby decrease the risk of transmission of human immunodeficiency virus (HIV), hepatitis B, and hepatitis C.[28] Gloves worn for the health care worker's protection during patient care should be removed when the activity is completed. Continued wearing of contaminated gloves in common areas where personnel handle telephones, charts, and so on may contaminate the ICU environment.

Antibiotic Use

Intensive antibiotic therapy, given to many ICU patients, suppresses the normal microbial flora and promotes colonization and ultimately infection with antibiotic-resistant organisms such as methicillin-resistant staphylococci, enterococci, multiresistant gram-negative bacilli, and yeasts. Most nosocomial outbreaks of resistant bacteria have occurred in ICUs, with antibiotic pressure implicated as important in many of these outbreaks.[29] Antibiotic control generally involves the restriction of broad-spectrum agents to selected circumstances.[30] Such controls may delay the emergence of resistance to specific antibiotics and reduce costs associated with antibiotic use, although evidence of reduction in infection risk has yet to be demonstrated.

Investigational Approaches to Infection Prevention

Conventional infection control approaches, such as dedicated surveillance and control programs and barrier isolation techniques, effectively interrupt acquisition of many pathogens and reduce infection rates in the ICU. However, a substantial number of infections result from endogenous rather than acquired organisms. Prevention of these infections will require novel strategies to halt the progression from colonization to infection.

Systemic antibiotic prophylaxis has consistently failed to prevent nosocomial pneumonia.[31] Topical endotracheal prophylaxis reduces the incidence of pneumonia but results in the emergence of intrinsically resistant gram-negative bacilli.[32] Selective decontamination of the oropharynx and gastrointestinal tract with nonabsorbable antibiotics directed against aerobic gram-negative bacilli has demonstrated promise for the prevention of infections, particularly pneumonia.[33–35] Almost all trials of selective decontamination have demonstrated reduced infection rates. Contrary to the experience with single-agent endotracheal or aerosol prophylaxis, prolonged (30 months) continuous use of selective decontamination regimens has not been associated with the emergence of resistant organisms. In fact, selective decontamination was used successfully to control nosocomial outbreak of colonization and infection with multiresistant gram-negative bacilli in a medical ICU.[36] Despite its apparent success in preventing infection, selective decontamination has not convincingly reduced mortality or length of stay. Further experience should define its role in selected patient populations and clarify the significance of the selection of resistance.

Because loss of gastric acidity is associated with bacterial overgrowth in the stomach and may lead to pneumonia, the need for routine stress ulcer prophylaxis with antacids or H_2 blockers in critically ill patients has been questioned. Prospective investigations have suggested a lower incidence of pneumonia in patients receiving sucralfate stress ulcer prophylaxis rather than antacids or H_2 blockers.[37] The avoidance of routine stress ulcer prophylaxis or the substitution of sucralfate for antacids or H_2 blockers may be an effective strategy to reduce the incidence of nosocomial pneumonia in the ICU (see Chap. 52).

Because so many nosocomial infections are device-related, there is a particular need to develop devices that resist rather than promote colonization and infection. Silver-impregnated indwelling urinary catheters and cuffs for central venous catheters are already available.[38] It is anticipated that other devices will be developed with colonization-resistant materials or features which limit damage to host defenses and the progression from colonization to infection.

Special Problems

HUMAN IMMUNODEFICIENCY VIRUS

As the HIV epidemic expands, the potential for occupational exposure among health care workers increases. Blood is the single most important source of HIV infection. ICU personnel are at particular risk because of the many invasive procedures they perform with the potential for exposure. Cumulative data from a number of prospective studies indicate that the risk of HIV transmission after accidental needlestick injury is approximately 0.3 percent.[39] The risks associated with occupational mucous membrane and cutaneous exposures to HIV-infected blood appear to be substantially smaller. HIV transmission does not occur during routine patient care. Accordingly, infection control efforts for HIV must then focus on preventing exposure to blood. Implementation of blood and body fluid precautions is useful in preventing exposure to HIV and of these, needlestick precautions are the most important (do not recap needles; discard needles and scalpels in puncture-resistant containers immediately after use). Universal precautions apply principally to blood and other body fluids containing visible blood but should also be applied to cerebrospinal fluid, synovial fluid, pleural fluid, peritoneal fluid, pericardial fluid, amniotic fluid, vaginal secretions, and semen. The risk of transmission of HIV from these fluids is unknown. Universal precautions do not apply to feces, nasal secretions, sputum, sweat, tears, urine, and vomitus unless they contain visible blood. The risk of transmission of HIV from these fluids and materials is extremely low or nonexistent.[40]

The management of the health care worker exposed to HIV is controversial. AZT chemoprophylaxis is frequently offered although only limited evidence supports its use.[41] If the decision is made to institute AZT chemoprophylaxis, treatment should be instituted as soon as possible after exposure.

TUBERCULOSIS

Tuberculosis is frequently unsuspected in hospitalized patients and this is also true for those admitted to ICUs.[42] This failure of diagnosis has emerged as an important contributor to mortality. Failed or delayed diagnosis may also increase risk of transmission to hospital personnel.[43,44] Delays in diagnosis may be particularly long in patients with tuberculosis and acute respiratory failure. ICU physicians who perform endotracheal intubation, fiberoptic bronchoscopy, and ventilator management (which are associated with respiratory aerosols) may be at particular risk for acquisition of tuberculosis. It should be noted that a negative acid-fast smear does not eliminate the possibility of transmission to medical personnel. The recent reversal of the downward trend in incidence of tuberculosis in the United States appears related to the HIV epidemic and warns of a potential for an increase in tuberculosis transmission to health care workers. ICU physicians must maintain a high level of suspicion for tuberculosis and initiate respiratory isolation precautions whenever the diagnosis is considered. In addition, all ICU personnel should undergo tuberculin skin testing annually. Patients with pulmonary tuberculosis are probably no longer contagious soon after starting effective treatment. By convention, patients are maintained on respiratory isolation precautions for 2 weeks following initiation of antituberculosis therapy.

METHICILLIN-RESISTANT *Staphylococcus aureus*

Methicillin-resistant *S. aureus* (MRSA) has been reported with increasing frequency in hospitals throughout the United States. The patients at highest risk for colonization and infection with this organism are the critically ill, the elderly, those with burns, and those with surgical wounds or intravascular catheters.[46] Once an outbreak occurs, colonized and infected patients act as reservoirs of MRSA, and health care personnel become transient carriers, transferring organisms to other patients. Surgical ICUs and burn units have been implicated as "epicenters" of hospital outbreaks so efforts to prevent spread of MRSA must be especially stringent in those units.[47]

Recommended control measures include isolation of colonized or infected patients, careful handwashing, and the use of barrier (gown and glove) isolation precautions for personnel having contact with the patient or the patient's immediate environment.[48] Attempts to eradicate the MRSA carrier state with topical antimicrobials (e.g., chlorhexidine, bacitracin, or mupirocin) or oral antibiotics (e.g., rifampin plus trimethoprim-sulfamethoxazole or ciprofloxacin) have had mixed results and cannot be recommended routinely.

RESPIRATORY SYNCYTIAL VIRUS

Respiratory syncytial virus (RSV) is the leading cause of lower respiratory tract infection among young children, and each year is responsible for outbreaks of nosocomial pneumonia and bronchiolitis on pediatric wards. Mortality and morbidity from RSV infection are highest among infants with congenital heart disease and immunosuppressed and critically ill children. Adults caring for these children appear to be important in the spread of the virus. Transmission occurs not only through staff becoming infected but also by the spread of contaminated secretions from infected children. Infected infants should be separated from other infants in the ICU. Furthermore, personnel with respiratory illness during RSV outbreaks should not care for children at risk for RSV infection. Careful handwashing is particularly important in controlling the spread of infection. In addition, the use of barrier (gloves and gown) isolation precautions may reduce nosocomial transmission.[49] The use of eye goggles and masks by personnel may further reduce the spread of nosocomial RSV infection, presumably by decreasing self-inoculation of the virus into the eyes and nose.[50]

References

1. Wenzel RP: Nosocomial infections, diagnosis-related groups, and study on the efficacy of nosocomial infection control: Economic implications for hospitals under the prospective payment system. Am J Med 78(suppl 6B):3, 1985.
2. Craven DE, Kunches LM, Lichtenberg DA, et al: Nosocomial infection and fatality in medical and surgical intensive care unit patients. Arch Intern Med 148:1161, 1988.
3. Leu HS, Kaiser DL, Mori M, et al: Hospital-acquired pneumonia: Attributable mortality and morbidity. Am J Epidemiol 129(6):1258, 1989.
4. Spengler RF, Greenough WB: Hospital costs and mortality attributed to nosocomial bacteremias. JAMA 240:2455, 1978.
5. Donowitz LG, Wenzel RP, Hoyt JW: High risk of hospital-acquired infection in the ICU patient. Crit Care Med 10:355, 1982.
6. Britt MR, Schleupner CJ, Matsumiya S: Severity of underlying disease as a predictor of nosocomial infection. JAMA 239:1047, 1978.
7. Gross PA, DeMauro PJ, Van Antwerpen C, et al: Number of comorbidities as a predictor of nosocomial infection acquisition. Infect Control Hosp Epidemiol 9:497, 1988.
8. Stamm WE: Prevention of infections: Infections related to medical devices. Ann Intern Med 89:764, 1978.
9. Celis R, Torres A, Gatell JM, et al: Nosocomial pneumonia: A multivariate analysis of risk and prognosis. Chest 93:318, 1988.
10. Haley RW, Culver DH, White JW, et al: The efficacy of infection surveillance and control programs in preventing nosocomial infections in US hospitals. Am J Epidemiol 121:182, 1985.
11. Garner JP, Simmons BP: Guideline for isolation precautions in hospitals. Infec Control 4(suppl):245, 1983.
12. Simmons B, Bryant J, Neiman K, et al: The role of handwashing in prevention of endemic intensive care unit infections. Infect Control Hosp Epidemiol 11:589, 1990.
13. Klein BS, Perloff WH, Maki DG: Reduction of nosocomial infection during pediatric intensive care by protective isolation. N Engl J Med 320:1714, 1989.
14. Weinstein RA, Kabins SA: Strategies for prevention and control of multiple drug-resistant nosocomial infection. Am J Med 70:449, 1981.
15. Nauseef WM, Maki DG: A study of the value of simple protective isolation in patients with granulocytopenia. N Engl J Med 304:448, 1981.
16. Arnow PM, Allyn PA, Nichols M, et al: Control of methicillin-resistant *Staphylococcus aureus* in a burn unit: Role of nurse staffing. J Trauma 22:954, 1982.
17. Goldmann DA, Durbin WA, Freeman J: Nosocomial infections in a neonatal intensive care unit. J Infect Dis 144:449, 1981.
18. Huebner J, Frank U, Kappstein I, et al: Influence of architectural design on nosocomial infections in intensive care units—a prospective 2-year analysis. Intensive Care Med 15:179, 1989.
19. Maki DG: Infections due to infusion therapy, in Bennett JV, Brachman PS (eds): *Hospital Infections.* Boston/Toronto, Little Brown, 1986.
20. Eyer S, Brummitt C, Crossley K, et al: Catheter-related sepsis: Prospective, randomized study of three methods of long-term catheter maintenance. Crit Care Med 18:1073, 1990.
21. Beck-Sague CM, Jarvis WR: Epidemic bloodstream infections associated with pressure transducers: A persistent problem. Infect Control Hosp Epidemiol 10:54, 1989.
22. Stamm WE: Nosocomial urinary tract infections, in Bennett JV, Brachman PS (eds): *Hospital Infections.* Boston/Toronto, Little Brown, 1986.
23. Ruiz-Santana S, Jimenez AG, Esteban A, et al: ICU pneumonias: A multi-institutional study. Crit Care Med 15:930, 1987.
24. Cross AS, Roup B: Role of respiratory assistance devices in endemic nosocomial pneumonia. Am J Med 70:681, 1981.
25. Hartstein AI, Rashad AL, Liebler JM, et al: Multiple intensive care unit outbreak of *Acinetobacter calcoaceticus* subspecies *anitratus* respiratory infection and colonization associated with contaminated, reusable ventilator circuits and resuscitation bags. Am J Med 85:624, 1988.
26. Mayhall CG, Archer NH, Lamb VA, et al: Ventriculostomy-related infections: A prospective epidemiologic study. N Engl J Med 310:553, 1984.
27. Patterson WB, Craven DE, Schwartz DA, et al: Occupational hazards to hospital personnel. Ann Intern Med 102:658, 1985.
28. Fahey BJ, Koziol DE, Banks SM, Henderson DK: Frequency of nonparenteral occupational exposures to blood and body fluids before and after universal precautions training. Am J Med 90:145, 1991.

29. Maki DG: Risk factors for nosocomial infection in intensive care: 'Devices vs nature' and goals for the next decade. Arch Intern Med 149:30, 1989.
30. Marr JJ, Moffet HL, Kunin CM: Guidelines for improving the use of antimicrobial agents in hospitals: A statement by the Infectious Diseases Society of America. J Infect Dis 157:869, 1988.
31. Mandelli M, Mosconi P, Langer M, et al: Prevention of pneumonia in an intensive care unit: A randomized multicenter clinical trial. Crit Care Med 17:501, 1989.
32. Feeley TW, du Moulin GC, Hedley-Whyte J, et al: Aerosol polymyxin and pneumonia in seriously ill patients. N Engl J Med 293:471, 1975.
33. Ledingham I McA, Alcock SR, Eastaway AT, et al: Triple regiment of selective decontamination of the digestive tract, systemic cefotaxime, and microbiological surveillance for prevention of acquired infection in intensive care. Lancet 1:785, 1988.
34. Unertl K, Ruckdeschel G, Selbmann HK, et al: Prevention of colonization and respiratory infections in long-term ventilated patients by local antimicrobial prophylaxis. Intensive Care Med 13:106, 1987.
35. Flaherty J, Nathan C, Kabins SA, Weinstein RA: Pilot trial of selective decontamination for prevention of bacterial infection in an intensive care unit. J Infect Dis 162:1393, 1990.
36. Brun-Buisson C, Legrand P, Rauss A, et al: Intestinal decontamination for control of nosocomial multiresistant gram-negative bacilli: Study of an outbreak in an intensive care unit. Ann Intern Med 110:873, 1989.
37. Driks MR, Craven DE, Celli BR, et al: Nosocomial pneumonia in intubated patients given sucralfate as compared with antacids or histamine type 2 blockers: The role of gastric colonization. N Engl J Med 317:1376, 1987.
38. Maki DG, Cobb L, Garman K, et al: An attachable silver-impregnated cuff for prevention of infection with central venous catheters: A prospective randomized multicenter trial. Am J Med 85:307, 1988.
39. Henderson DK, Fahey BJ, Willy M, et al: Risk for occupational transmission of human immunodeficiency virus type 1 (HIV-1) associated with clinical exposures: A prospective evaluation. Ann Intern Med 113:740, 1990.
40. Centers for Disease Control: Update: Universal precautions for prevention of transmission of human immunodeficiency virus, hepatitis B virus, and other bloodborne pathogens in health-care settings. MMWR 37:377, 1988.
41. Henderson DK, Gerberding JL: Prophylactic zidovudine after occupational exposure to the human immunodeficiency virus: An interim analysis. J Infect Dis 160:321, 1989.
42. Frame RN, Johnson MC, Eichenhorn MS, et al: Active tuberculosis in the medical intensive care unit: A 15 year retrospective analysis. Crit Care Med 15:1012, 1987.
43. Ehrenkranz NJ, Kicklighter JL: Tuberculosis outbreak in a general hospital: Evidence for airborne spread of infection. Ann Intern Med 77:377, 1972.
44. Catanzaro A: Nosocomial tuberculosis. Am Rev Respir Dis 125:559, 1982.
45. Malasky C, Jordan T, Potulski F, Reichman LB: Occupational tuberculous infections among pulmonary physicians in training. Am Rev Respir Dis 142:505, 1990.
46. Brumfitt W, Hamilton-Miller J: Methicillin-resistant *Staphylococcus aureus.* N Engl J Med 320:1188, 1989.
47. Boyce JM, White RL, Causey WA, Lockwood WR: Burn units as a source of methicillin-resistant *Staphylococcus aureus* infections. JAMA 249:2803, 1983.
48. Ayliffe GAJ, Duckworth GJ, Brumfitt W, et al: Guidelines for the control of epidemic methicillin-resistant *Staphylococcus aureus.* J Hosp Infect 7:193, 1986.
49. Leclair JM, Freeman J, Sullivan BF, et al: Prevention of nosocomial respiratory syncytial virus infections through compliance with glove and gown isolation precautions. N Engl J Med 317:329, 1987.
50. Gala CL, Hall CB, Schnabel KC, et al: The use of eye-nose goggles to control nosocomial respiratory syncytial virus infection. JAMA 256:2706, 1986.

Chapter 44

PSYCHOLOGIC SUPPORT IN CRITICAL CARE

CARROL ALVAREZ
SHELLEY MALAN

Critical care succeeds because of the speed with which aggressive procedures and continuous monitoring are carried out in patients who are at risk of death. The immediate and overriding focus is stabilization of the patients' physical condition. There is little time for emotional support to patients who may have already undergone severely traumatic events and who will certainly undergo others. Nevertheless, interventions that diminish emotional distress moderate its associated physiologic dysfunctions, thereby enhancing the likelihood of the success of the physiologic interventions. Moreover, pertinent items of emotional support can be given concurrently to physical assessment and treatment. Finally, during crises even brief interventions can precipitate permanent changes in emotional adjustment.

Stress: Emotional and Physiologic Connections

Stress in any form is a multidimensional phenomenon composed of autonomic, endocrine, cognitive, and behavioral components. The concept of the "fight-or-flight" response is heavily reliant upon an emotional reaction as the triggering mechanism for the physiologic response.

Typical psychologic reactions that trigger the physiologic stress response are anxiety, pain, grief, fear, sensory deprivation, and sleep deprivation.[1] These emotions and events are standard observed conditions of patients in a critical care environment. In fact, if patients do not display these reactions, they may be severely depressed, psychotically withdrawn, or in denial.

The psychologic stimulus involves an individual's response to a perceived threat that seems to take one of two routes based upon that person's interpretation of what is occurring, usual coping style, and experiences. If the experience is viewed as merely a threat to control, a fight-or-flight response appears to predominate with a preponderance of sympathetic nervous system-adrenal medullary activation. However, if the threat is interpreted as an actual loss of control, the pituitary-adrenal axis is activated and the individual displays helplessness and depression.[2] These two responses may occur sequentially, since prolonged periods of sympathetic nervous system stimulation become exhausting and the pituitary-adrenal system takes over.

Sources of Stress

Emotional stressors of the intensive care unit (ICU) fall into four categories. First is the event precipitating admission, the alien environment, its paradox of simultaneous sensory deprivation and sensory overload, and disrupted sleep. Second is friction that occurs at the boundary where the needs of the patients' personalities meet the requirements of the ICU environment. The third category includes dysfunctional behaviors and adversarial relationships that occur when patients who have had marginally adaptive coping skills attempt to use those same coping methods in the ICU. Finally, there are disrupted relationships with family members and supportive others.

ENVIRONMENTAL SOURCES OF STRESS

SENSORY DEPRIVATION AND SENSORY OVERLOAD

The ICU contains multiple stimuli that paradoxically create sensory deprivation yet bombard the patient with information that is difficult to interpret. Interpretation may be further confounded by a clouded sensorium. Nevertheless, the physiologic impact is a function of the patient's impression of his or her environment even if this impression is a distorted one. The cognitions regarding these stimuli are a primary focus of psychologic support. Recognition of the stressors themselves can also lend to moderation of their frequency and intensity.

The stress of sensory deprivation occurs when four conditions are met: reduction of stimulus input levels; reduction of stimulus variability; social isolation; and diminished kinesthetic input.[3] In the ICU, these conditions coexist with specific types of sensory overload. Stimulus heterogeneity in all spheres is limited, while the stimuli that are present are of the pathologic kind: of high intensity, meaningless, or open to negative interpretation. The available sights are monotonous, potentially frightening. Kinesthetic sense is diminished by patients' limited movement. Odors are diminished in variety and intensity; at times they are disagreeable. The same is true for taste. Affectional touch is diminished, while touch associated with pain, procedures, and invaded privacy is increased. Sound heterogeneity is decreased while intensity is increased, resulting in a variety of physiologic effects. An additional effect is disrupted sleep: frequent awakenings as well as changes in sleep stage.

When these environmental stressors cannot be modified, cognitive interventions can be powerful. For example, the number of natural killer cells in people undergoing a stressful life event has been shown to vary according to the interpretation of the stressor.[4] Patients who have had a presurgery interview addressing their concerns about their open heart surgery have shown as much as a 50 percent decrease in postoperative delirium, compared with a matched group of patients undergoing the same planned surgery but without the interview. Psychologic preparation can also affect the level of anxiety, the amount of pain medication used, and length of stay.[5]

Preparation before admission is not available for trauma patients or others with unexpected admissions to the ICU. However, an orientation of sorts can be provided as soon as the admission begins, via continuous, brief, and concrete explanations of each thing that is occurring. The most useful explanations include a description of the procedure, sensations the patient will be experiencing, and equipment that will be seen or felt. When multiple interventions are being made by several people, one member of the treatment team can take responsibility for keeping the patient informed; this provides the patient with an anchor of ongoing interpretation in a situation of potential sensory and emotional overload.

Such ongoing explanations are particularly important for patients who are delirious, therapeutically sedated, or comatose (a later ability to recall events that occurred during coma is not related to initial Glasgow Coma Score or lesion site).[6] Prevailing themes of the memories of these patients include being imprisoned, having committed a crime, being unable to flee, and having distorted perceptions of time passing. These perceptions are only briefly altered by reorientation and reexplanations, indicating the need for such orientation to occur frequently. In addition, the patients describe fear and startled responses when staff work near them without explanations or begin an intervention without warning.

Orientation to the ICU, whether occurring before or during the admission, can also acknowledge and normalize those aspects of noxious environmental stimuli, such as noise, which cannot be changed. A similar acknowledgment of delirium is particularly pertinent for patients who are experiencing it; they can be reassured that the delirium is not uncommon, is not permanent, and is not a sign of craziness.

Within formal preadmission and preprocedure teaching programs, those that include modeling and teaching of coping techniques decrease anxiety more than those that simply provide information. Modeling is visual information (e.g., video) by which patients see others who have gone or are going through the same procedure. During unplanned hospitalizations, an adaptation of modeling can occur; following acknowledgment of the patients' distress, a brief verbal description can be given of others who have successfully undergone the procedure being performed or who have recovered from similar injuries or illnesses.

Coping techniques, such as distraction, use of imagery, and relaxation strategies, can be taught by consultants in psychology, psychiatry, psychiatric nursing, social work, or recreation therapy. Use of relaxation and imagery in particular have been correlated with improved wound healing.[7]

Visual Stimuli

Few things can be done to alter the visual environment. Family members can be encouraged to bring in photographs and other personal items to be placed within the patients' view and to personalize the environment. However, patients are still left with a view of medical technology, their own bodies intruded upon by tubes and devices, and other patients around them. Therefore, visual stimuli are particularly apt for cognitive intervention.

Technology is reassuring for some patients, reminding them that they are monitored continuously and that a response would be immediate if their condition worsened. Other patients are frightened by the monitors, seeing them as evidence of dire future outcomes. For these patients, reinterpreting the technology and providing a more comforting meaning is helpful.

Touch

The ICU is home to the paradox of intimate human contact without corresponding emotional intimacy. Nevertheless, touch that is intended to be reassuring has been shown to decrease agitated behavior, decrease intracranial pressure, and be recalled as helpful by patients who were comatose.[8] Gentle touch has also been shown to increase nutritional intake in patients with dementia.[9] In contrast, touch that is procedure oriented has been shown to be stressful and potentially destabilizing of patients' cardiac conditions even when it is not painful.[10] Nevertheless, touch that produces pain or is procedure oriented occurs three times more frequently than does comforting touch. Differences in physiologic effect may be a function of caregiver intent and meanings ascribed to the touch by patients. It may be that the intent of the caregiver can change procedural touch to caregiver touch, with physiologic benefit. However, patients have different levels of tolerance for being touched and interpret it according to complex cultural and personal norms. Patients with a high need for privacy, for example, may find touch of any kind to be a further intrusion. Clearly the use of touch to comfort is of potential physiologic advantage and is a means of combating the sensory deprivation endemic to the ICU; however, it is best used in conjunction with observation of patients' responses.

Sound

Noise is the most universally distressing sensory aspect of the ICU. Noise is one of two major causes of sleep disruption and is a contributing factor in ICU psychosis. Other psychologic and physiologic consequences include peripheral vasoconstriction that leads to persistent hypertensive responses in patients with preexisting hypertension; changes in skeletal muscle tension; increased need for pain medication; startle responses, which increase catecholamine secretion and thereby increase heart rate, metabolism, and oxygen consumption; and decreased frustration tolerance.[11]

The impact of noise is pertinent, since noise levels in ICUs have consistently been found to exceed recommended levels. The two major sources of noise are equipment and conversation among staff. Noise levels from conversation can exceed those from equipment or treatments. In addition, patients have described person-generated noise as more annoying and even distressing than that from the machines. Conversation is also more disruptive when it is unwanted since it is open to erroneous interpretations by patients.

Interventions are readily available. Staff can moderate conversational noise; periodic monitoring of noise levels can cue staff who have become habituated to the sounds of what is, for them, a familiar environment. Conversations at the bedsides can be directed to patients, increasing the meaningful content of the sound environment. Phones can be muted, prompt attention given to alarms, overhead paging volumes decreased, and computer printers covered.

In addition, cognitive interventions can be added. These include preadmission description of noise levels that may occur as well as explanations of various machine-generated sounds. Potentially frightening noises, such as alarms, can be redescribed as signals for staff intervention, evidence that patients are in a safe, monitored environment. Finally, music can be used when patients' preferences are known. Soothing music within patient preferences has been shown to decrease situational anxiety, sympathetic nervous system activity, and pain.[12] Families can be asked to bring in audio equipment as well as favorite tapes.

SLEEP DEPRIVATION

Externally induced factors disrupting sleep include noise and interruption by care providers, while internally induced factors include pain, anxiety, and a decreased ability to change positions while asleep. The most frequent source of sleep disruption is treatment intervention and monitoring by nursing staff. Members of the health care team often view sleep deprivation as an expected and uncontrollable by-product of the critical care environment. Patients, however, identify disturbance of their sleep as a frequent and major stressor. Researchers corroborate these subjective reports by patients. One study of trauma patients using polysomnography as an objective measurement of sleep found that the average number of awakenings per night was 7 to 71, with a mean of 32.[13] Additional studies in a variety of critical care settings have shown similar findings. The longest uninterrupted time for sleep ranges from as little as 10 to no more than 60 min.[14] Given these factors, patients in critical care areas are clearly precluded from completing even one normal sleep cycle.

Patients are observed to be "asleep" almost all of the time (day or night) that noise, visitation, assessments, monitoring, or interventions are not being done. However, because of the short uninterrupted times for sleep, patients seldom progress any further than stage 1 or 2 non–rapid eye movement (NREM) sleep. Stages 3 and 4 NREM sleep are greatly diminished, and REM sleep is virtually nonexistent since this sleep stage occurs at the end of a typical 90-min cycle.

Consequences of Sleep Deprivation

Deprivation of stage 4 NREM sleep, the stage in which deep and restful sleep occurs, leaves patients fatigued and sleepy and without the benefit of physiologic restoration (e.g., decreased muscle tone, heart rate, blood pressure, temperature, metabolic rate, and increased release of growth hormone). Lack of REM sleep denies the patient the opportunity to process and integrate the harrowing experiences of critical illness; it fosters increased anxiety and irritability when mild and contributes to the development of psychosis when severe. Sleep deprivation is highly correlated with the development of ICU psychosis and in one study was found to precede the onset of delirium in 9 of 10 patients.[15] The response to sleep deprivation is highly individualized; the severity of symptoms is frequently, but not always, correlated with the duration of the deprivation. Patients most susceptible to sleep deprivation are the elderly, patients with a past psychiatric history, and those with severe illness.

When sleep deprivation occurs, the body tries to recover lost stage 4 NREM as well as REM sleep during subsequent sleep periods. These "rebound" sleep cycles entail entering the lost sleep cycle(s) more frequently and from stages in the sleep cycle normally not associated with the deprived stage. In the presence of both stage 4 NREM and REM sleep deficits, the body gives a higher priority to stage 4 rebounds over REM rebounds. As a result, REM sleep deficits are allowed to accumulate; when REM sleep rebound finally occurs, it can be intense and prolonged. Because of the sympathetic nervous system stimulation and changes in cerebral blood flow that occur with REM sleep, REM rebounds can produce significant physiologic risks to patients including increased oxygen demand by the myocardium leading to ischemia, infarct, dysrhythmias, or failure; increased tissue oxygen consumption; increased intracranial pressure; and increased sleep apneic episodes.[16]

Interventions

Many factors involved in producing sleep deprivation are controllable. First, it is imperative to recognize that sleep deprivation is undesirable and exposes patients to risk. It is crucial for all members of the health care team to value sleep as a significant therapy and to purposefully make and communicate to each other plans and goals for facilitation of sleep. The most helpful interventions address pain and anxiety, noise, and day-night orientation.

Pain and anxiety are most often treated with analgesics, sedatives, and hypnotic agents. Deliberation and care must be taken in prescribing these agents since many can interfere with sleep. Comfort measures (positioning for comfort, soothing touch, verbal reassurance, guided relaxation, music therapy) used in conjunction with medication can facilitate the drug effect and may help reduce dosage requirements. Noise can be normalized and diminished (vide supra).

Differentiation between day and night is not always possible in the ICU. Many units do not have windows, and bright lights are used 24 h a day. Desynchronization of normal circadian rhythms occurs and patients do not know when to sleep. Units with windows in the rooms are ideal, but even then, the bed must face the window and window coverings must be open. Unit lighting should be dimmed at night. Verbal orientation to time of day and clocks are useful.

Treatments should be clustered whenever possible to allow patients the maximum amount of sleep. The key to sleep facilitation is planning. Sleep charts (often a part of the documentation flowsheet) communicate the value of adequate sleep as part of the treatment regimen. All members of the health care team should frequently review the need for and timing of routine procedures, tests, and monitoring. For example, many critical care units have standing orders for vital sign monitoring every hour; however, this does not take into consideration the individual patient's actual needs as he or she stabilizes or improves. As a consequence, the patient may continue to be awakened every 60 min.

MALADAPTIVE BEHAVIORS

Maladaptive behaviors may represent patients' normal means of coping or they may simply indicate the breakdown of usual coping styles. In both instances, proactive plans that address early problem behaviors serve to maintain patients' dignity, avert negative staff-patient interactions, and support positive coping methods.

For patients whose coping behaviors have usually been adequate, ICU hospitalization may represent an overwhelming stressor leading to failure of normal coping. For other patients the requirements of the ICU may represent an intolerable abridgement of personality needs. In either situation, previously well-adjusted patients become angry, demanding, manipulative, sullen, uncooperative, sabotaging, withdrawn, dependent, or depressed. Problematic ICU requirements include immobility (particularly difficult for patients whose coping includes taking action in any crisis), invasion of privacy, loss of control, and reliance on others (difficult for patients who have a preexisting difficulty with trust).

Other patients may have marginal adaptive skills prior to hospitalization. These skills are often learned in settings that require extraordinary and unusual methods of coping. However, behavior that was adaptive in a dysfunctional family or on the streets is not likely to be adaptive in the hospital setting. For example, manipulation and intimidation (indirect ways of assuring that needs are met) may keep the individual safe and fed while living on the street but are more likely to lead to caregiver anger in the hospital.

Also frustrating to staff is the frequency with which the goals of such patients are in conflict with the goals of the treatment team. Drug-dependent patients may be more focused on receiving narcotics than on becoming weaned from the ventilator. Patients with a preexisting dependent personality may be more interested in continuing current levels of caretaking by others than in participating in and supporting recovery.

INTERVENTIONS

In all of these situations, the potential exists for control battles among patients and members of the treatment team. Setting of limits, alone, simply underscores the battle and often precipitates escalations in patients' maladaptive behaviors. Alternatively, consistent care plans that take into consideration the patients' previous abilities, coping methods, and current goals will usually lead to more cooperative behaviors.

In order to develop a meaningful plan of care, an accurate psychologic history is important. With patients who are using uncharacteristic responses to stress, lack of a history can, at the least, result in unfair labeling. With patients who have poorly developed coping skills, lack of a history delays the initiation of pertinent care plans. In both instances, cycles of negative staff-patient conflict can develop. Such histories can be obtained by the social worker on the treatment team, a psychologist, the liaison psychiatrist, or the psychiatric clinical nurse specialist. This person can also assist the team in setting up a care plan to minimize maladaptive behaviors.

Patients with a History of Adequate Coping

For patients who have functioned well prior to hospitalization, a history will indicate when current behaviors are atypical and thus potentially treatable, avert staff pessimism and labeling, provide information about possible points of friction between patient requirements and requirements of the hospital (since these may be negotiable), and inform staff of coping styles to support (i.e., those that patients have previously used with success).

A common example concerns control. For patients who do not want control, being given it leads to stress; for others an increased sense of control has been shown to decrease stress and autonomic activity while increasing the willingness to endure more of an unpleasant event.[17] For these straightforward control needs, cognitive strategies are helpful. Patients can be supported in focusing on attainable, interim goals; they can be supported also in seeing that their efforts make a difference. Treatment strategies and decisions can be discussed with patients. Even minor intervention decisions can be given as choices.

When the history suggests the evolution of a new problem in a formerly well-adjusted patient, treatment may include medication (e.g., for depression), increased emotional support, a behavioral care plan, or treatment of physiologic causes of psychosis.

Patients with a History of Marginal Coping

Other patients have never had other than marginal coping skills. An adequate history for these patients will allow for early identification of patients needing special care plans, identify early those needing referral for drug and alcohol treatment, and diminish the potential for staff frustration by altering expectations of patients' coping abilities.

Trauma patients in particular have been found to have preexisting psychiatric or behavioral problems: the frequency may be as high as 88 percent for patients with penetrating trauma and 50 percent for those with blunt trauma.[18] Yet documentation of these problems is uncommon. These patients are thus particularly at risk, facing unexpected and frightening events with limited coping skills that may have been further compromised by physiologic stressors.

Interventions often involve finding a therapeutic way to address patients' goals while in the hospital. For example, the drug-addicted patient's primary goals may include a constant supply of narcotic medication and complete relief of physical pain or emotional discomfort. The goal of recovery from illness is often secondary. In addition, these patients may appear to disbelieve or disregard the seriousness of their condition. To withdraw all narcotic drugs may leave such a patient with the same ego deficits that prompted drug abuse in the first place but in a setting where addressing these deficits is impossible, resulting in a likely outcome of increased drug-seeking behavior directed at a variety of sources. In addition, withdrawing the narcotics completely adds another stressor and another major task (i.e., drug rehabilitation) to recovery. In this instance methadone may be a useful interim measure while the patient is in the hospital, pending entry into a drug recovery program.

There will be patients for whom limit setting is a part of a care plan that includes negotiated and more functional ways to meet perceived needs. For example, a 17-year-old male admitted to the ICU with a C-4 injury following a gunshot wound to the neck was using his opportunities to have visitors to receive and sell illegal drugs. Limit setting was a necessary part of a care plan that included staff-generated ways to meet the patient's needs for challenge and control.

FAMILIES OF CRITICALLY ILL PATIENTS

Families can affect patient outcomes. Family members' responses to the crisis of their relatives' illnesses or injuries will be communicated, verbally and nonverbally, to patients. These responses can become destructive in several ways: family anxiety may precipitate increased anxiety in the patient, with physiologic consequences; families may support patients' maladaptive behaviors; and they may encourage noncompliance with treatments. Conversely, families who feel supported by the treatment team and believe that their needs are being addressed can become powerful adjuncts in promoting patient recovery. In addition, family members can serve as a buffer between the unfamiliar environment of the critical care area and the patient, more easily orient the patient, elicit more accurate descriptions of pain or other symptoms, and support patient compliance with treatments.

The previous sections of this chapter identify the stressors that patients in critical care environments experience. The stresses that their critical illnesses or injuries cause the family are not easily recognized. However, addressing these family responses is necessary in order to take advantage of family support for the patient. The focus of health care providers in critical care is primarily on the patient. Time spent with family members is often, of necessity, brief, and the problems discussed are those of prime concern to the practitioner rather than the family. In fact, families are often viewed as sources of stress for staff members. Health care providers are not always educationally prepared nor personally comfortable in addressing family concerns and needs.

A critical illness can severely disrupt even the most functional family unit. The family members' reactions to admission of a loved one to the ICU are likely to include a feeling of loss of control. Like patients, the families are plunged into a foreign environment consisting of strange sights, sounds, smells, and high technology upon which the patient's life depends. They are confronted with the frantic pace of a critical care unit and with people whose roles and jargon are unclear. Families are often not certain who is in charge and how decisions are made; they receive information from many different people and disciplines. Negative conclusions are often drawn about the way that important decisions are made.

TABLE 44-1 Needs of Families

1. To know the prognosis
2. To have questions answered honestly
3. To know specific facts concerning the patient's progress
4. To feel that hospital personnel care about the patient
5. To be called at home about changes in the condition of the patient
6. To feel there is hope
7. To have explanations given in terms that are understandable
8. To be assured that the best care possible is being given to the patient
9. To see the patient frequently
10. To know why things were done for the patient and exactly what is being done for the patient

FAMILY NEEDS

Recent research comparing health care providers' perceptions of families' needs with the families' perceptions of their own needs shows a significant discrepancy between these two points of view.[19,20] Clearly families must be asked what is needed. However, consistently self-identified needs of family members can be broken down into six major categories: the need for information, the need for hospital personnel to care about them and the patient, the need for hope, the need for emotional support, the need to be with the patient, and the need for physical comfort. A summary rank ordering from several studies of the average ratings by family members of critically ill patients is presented in Table 44-1.[19–25]

INTERVENTIONS

Families asked to identify the needs most often not met cited their desire to talk to the physician once a day, to be alone or have a place to be alone, to provide some physical care to the patient, and to have a bathroom near the waiting room.[23] While there is little that can be done to change the physical facilities of an institution, the other frequently unmet needs are amenable to intervention through awareness.

Need for Information

Communication among all members of the health care team is essential so that consistent messages can be given the family and team members are aware of information given by others. If possible, family members should be talked to in a quiet, private location. This helps them to focus on the information and provides privacy so they may express themselves freely. It may be useful to identify a family spokesperson or consistent family group to talk with; they can then accept responsibility to share the information with others. Whenever possible, the same physician should talk to the family each day at a consistent, specified time. Everything should be explained in layman's terms rather than medical jargon or terminology. It is an error to assume that because family members use medical terms, they understand them. Explanations should be specific, rather than general, and begin simply, building on previous information so as to not overload the family. When possible, the same references should be used each day (e.g., heart rhythm, pain, level of consciousness). It may be necessary to repeat information (possibly multiple times), since people experiencing anxiety are not always able to attend to communication. The communicator can obtain useful information by having the family members repeat their understanding of explanations. Covering physicians and other health team members should be notified regarding what families have been told. Questions should be encouraged and answered honestly. Advance warning about transfer or discharge from the ICU allows family members to adequately plan. Finally, a mechanism should be established to guarantee that families are called if the patient's condition changes.

Need That Personnel Care about Them and the Patient

A caring attitude toward patients and their families is manifested in the manner and attitude accompanying communication. Active listening as well as verbal and nonverbal behaviors communicate caring. When communicating with family members toward whom there are positive feelings, this is usually easy. When staff have negative feelings, self-monitoring is important.

It is important to direct attention to the person(s) being spoken to and stop other activities. If it is currently inconvenient to talk, establish a time with the family when it is convenient. Patients and their families should be treated as unique individuals. Acknowledging the patient and family members by name personalizes communication. Rather than anticipating what someone is going to say, it is preferable to listen actively to what is actually being said. Finally, the speaker should communicate concern and empathy for the family members' situation, encourage verbalization from family members of both positive and negative feelings, and use touch to communicate caring (remembering that some people feel uncomfortable when strangers touch them).

Need for Hope and Emotional Support

A family's perceptions of the situation should be identified. The family may request certainty in an uncertain situation or may express a degree of optimism that does not seem realistic. Although these situations can create conflict, acknowledgment of the family's wish for the patient to do well may be all that is required. Further approaches include acknowledgment of the family's difficulty with the "roller coaster" emotions often felt in unknown situations, allowing adequate time during family discussions for feelings to be expressed and questions answered, and helping family members identify others who are also able to support them: other family members, friends, other patient's families who are going through similar circumstances, and the clergy. Setting short-term goals may help the family see small steps toward progress.

Need to Be with the Patient

Caregivers must understand that the family has a long-term and intimate relationship with the patient and has a need to continue that relationship. Visiting hours in critical care units are restrictive at best and contribute to familys' feelings of loss of control. Visiting hours should be humane and flexible. The reason the family cannot have unlimited access should be explained. When patients have a poor prognosis, the patient and family may benefit from reduced sedation; a patient who is unresponsive to family members may negate the precious time that they have left together. Allowing family members to participate in the patient's care mobilizes them, decreases feelings of helplessness, and increases feelings of worth. Finally, family members should be reassured that it is all right for them to leave the hospital and, indeed, that it is crucial to their continued health and well being.

Need for Physical Comfort

There are not many changes that can be made to existing structures in order to make them more comfortable for family members. Every effort should be made, however, to provide minimum comforts. Families should be oriented to the location of the chapel (if available), cafeteria/coffee shop, and parking facilities. If they live a long distance away, efforts should be made to assist them in finding affordable accommodations and transportation to and from the hospital.

FAMILIES IN CRISIS

The sudden serious illness or injury of a loved one may precipitate a situational crisis within a family, throwing it into disequilibrium. A crisis situation exists when the family's usual problem-solving and coping mechanisms fail, leaving them feeling helpless and ineffective and escalating the underlying anxiety level.

A crisis may be precipitated when a family is exposed to stress with little or no preparation, exposed to a stressor for a prolonged period of time, exposed to multiple stressors at the same time, confronted with ambiguous or uncertain events, or exposed to an event that threatens an important aspect of life such as health or survival. When spouses were asked to identify stressors associated with a mate's sudden illness, the responses included[26,27,28] the following:

1. Possibility that husband or wife will die
2. Loss of healthy mate
3. New roles in the family unit
4. Total responsibility for child and household care
5. Worry about financial problems
6. Uncertain, unpredictable future
7. Change in self-esteem
8. Dealing with patient's reaction to illness
9. Fear that illness will reoccur

10. Separation from mate
11. Trying not to upset or worry patient
12. Thinking about difficulties when patient gets home
13. Not being able to sleep
14. Difficulty concentrating
15. Being lonely
16. Not being informed about changes in patient's condition
17. Problems with transportation to and from hospital
18. Recurrence of own illness

Whether or not a crisis will develop for individuals within the family is dependent upon several factors: the perception of the event, the functional support systems available to help resolve the problem(s), and the effectiveness of coping mechanisms used in the past to resolve other problems. Another factor that may have an influence is the patient's role in the family. If the role is central and significant, such as income provider or child care provider, the absence of this member materially affects family functioning and may require major role changes of other family members. The suddenness of the illness or injury as well as the predictability of the outcome can be major factors influencing the critical nature of the perceived event. If family members have had previous experiences or know others who have successfully problem-solved their way through a similar event, they have probably either learned or seen effective behaviors for coping with a similar crisis. This may make the difference between disequilibrium and equilibrium for the family.

Family members may display a wide range of behaviors when in a crisis situation. The reaction to and behavior displayed will depend on the individual's personality and past behaviors in similar situations as well as their cultural background. The range of behaviors extends from hysterical crying to anger and aggression to sitting quietly and acting as if nothing has happened.

Individuals also differ greatly in how they progress through the crisis state. Use of a model is helpful in determining appropriate interventions but serves only as a guide for the professional and is not intended to overly simplify the process or to pigeonhole individuals into types of behavior.

The following model identifies stages through which families progress during a crisis and is used to help order observations and suggest interventions. The stages are anxiety, denial, anger, remorse, grief, and reconciliation.[29] Individuals in crisis may experience several of these emotions simultaneously or go through them one at a time in no particular order. It is also not uncommon for people to reexperience an emotion once they have appeared to resolve it already.

Characteristic behaviors displayed during each stage are as follows:

- Anxiety—physical agitation, increased muscle tension, nausea, narrow focus, decreased ability to process information.
- Denial—refusal to acknowledge the reality of the situation, may be unrealistic about outcome (it is necessary to differentiate this from maintenance of hope).
- Anger or hostility—directing blame at the patient, other family members, and/or medical staff. This behavior provides relief from anxiety.
- Remorse—expression of guilt and sorrow, regret at not being able to have prevented the illness or injury.
- Grief—depression, sense of overwhelming loss, sleep disturbance, difficulty concentrating, loss of interest, anorexia, weight loss.
- Reconciliation—mobilization of self, increased ability to seek solutions to problems and find support, use of effective coping mechanisms.

While experiencing the crisis, the individual often becomes unable to hear or process information and may be unable to think clearly enough to problem-solve or make effective decisions. The crisis continues to heighten because of the inability to think of or use effective coping mechanisms and usually requires outside intervention for resolution.

INTERVENTIONS

As previously discussed, the key to successful intervention is the underlying communication of a caring, gentle, warm, kind, concerned, and human attitude.[30] Maintaining a nonjudgmental, nonreactive, calm approach without personalizing the family's expression of feelings combined with active and passive listening skills and appropriate use of touch can go far to help resolve the difficulties the family is experiencing.

Before beginning intervention it is important to assess the current state of the family:

1. Identify the family's perception of the situation: Is it realistic or distorted?
2. What coping mechanisms have they already tried? What coping skills have been successful/not successful in the past for other problems encountered?
3. What supports are currently available to the family?

This information is useful in determining approaches to the family as well as in mobilizing members' internal and external sources of support and problem solving. The following are suggestions for interventions for the six previously identified stages of crisis.

Anxiety

The manner in which information is given needs to be concise and concrete. Information should be repeated multiple times and reinforced with each encounter. Family members should be encouraged to repeat what they have heard, write down important information, and express their feelings. Allow the family as much control as possible within the hospital environment, as in allowing flexibility in visiting hours.

Denial

The family members' needs for psychologic protection against reality should be acknowledged, but their denial should not be actively facilitated. If the denial is becoming dysfunctional (family is not able to respond with necessary actions or treatment decisions), reality orientation should be provided without withdrawing hope but without giving false assurances. Since denial interferes with information processing, repetition of information is usually necessary.

Anger

It is useful to talk with the family in a quiet, private place, in a calm manner. Family members should be allowed to express anger, and it may be validated as understandable under the circumstances. Anger is frequently a mask for underlying, more primary emotions; naming what these might be can dissipate the anger (e.g., fear or feeling out of control, vulnerable, tired, or ignored). The real target of anger is sometimes the patient, but the family members feel guilty about feeling angry at an ill or injured person. Acknowledging that this is a normal reaction may help the person feel less guilty. It is crucial to avoid getting defensive or arguing with the family member. Reasonable demands can be met and explanations given when unreasonable ones cannot; in the latter instance, given the described constraints, families can then be asked to participate in resolving the dilemma. Limits may need to be set on behaviors if they are becoming violent, destructive, or harmful to others. On the other hand, it may be useful to allow the family as much control over the environment as is possible.

Remorse and Guilt

Feelings of guilt should be acknowledged and not rationalized away. It is useful to determine if guilt is real (the family member had a part to play in the illness) or is self-imposed. If guilt is self-imposed, the family member can be asked what he or she could have done to prevent the illness or injury (i.e., one cannot in reality control another person's behavior).

Grief

Quiet support should be provided. Feelings of grief must be acknowledged, since expressing them is necessary for future reconciliation. Verbally diminishing these feelings with reassurances only serves to communicate to individuals to remain silent about their sadness; they still feel sad but become reticent about sharing these feelings.

Reconciliation

The family member can be assisted in developing a plan of action by identifying support systems and resources available to help them (family, extended family, neighbors, church, community support services/groups). Adaptive and productive coping skills can be reinforced and alternate coping mechanisms explored. The goal of crisis intervention is to at least return the family to the precrisis level of functioning and to reestablish equilibrium. Sometimes following a crisis situation, the family may have gained new coping skills that can be used in the future to function at a higher level than before.

Resources

It may not always be feasible to personally intervene in all situations requiring psychologic support for patients or family members. This is especially true when the symptoms displayed indicate severe dysfunction that might require long-term intervention and follow-up or is beyond the expertise of the individual physician. Referral of patients or families to other resources for support in the assessment, planning, or intervention may be very helpful to all concerned. This, as with all other aspects of patient and family care responsibilities, is more effective if conducted and communicated as a team approach drawing on the strengths of each member of the team.

Each institution will differ in the type and availability of resources, but some individuals who may provide assistance include psychiatric liaison service personnel, psychiatric clinical nurse specialist, critical care clinical nurse specialist, social worker, chaplain, unit nurse manager or nursing supervisor, patient representatives, family life educators, institutional or community support groups, community crisis centers, financial aid personnel, and housing aid personnel. An important additional source of information and support is the primary nursing staff caring for the patient. Often, very comprehensive patient and family psychosocial assessments have already been completed as a part of the admission history.

Multidisciplinary patient/family conferences are highly effective in collecting information, developing a plan of action, and determining effective interventions. Involving primary nursing staff, clinical nurse specialists, the social worker, and others as appropriate helps to facilitate communication between the team members as well as provide a variety of perspectives in problem solving.

References

1. Selye H: *Stress in Health and Disease.* Boston, Butterworths, 1976, pp 728–784.
2. Mason JW, Maher JT, Hartler LH: Selectivity of corticosteroid and catecholamine responses to various natural stimuli, in Serban G (ed): *Psychopathology of Human Adaptation.* New York, Plenum Press, 1976, p 147.
3. Suedfeld P: Introduction and historical background, in Zubeck JP (ed): *Sensory Deprivation: 15 Years of Research.* New York, Appleton-Century-Crofts, 1969, p 4.
4. Irwin M, Daniels M, Weiner H: Immune and neuroendocrine changes during bereavement. Psychiatr Clin North Am 10:449, 1987.
5. Anderson KO, Masur FT: Psychological preparation for cardiac catheterization. Heart Lung 18:154, 1989.
6. Tosch P: Patients' recollections of their posttraumatic coma. J Neurosci Nurs 20:223, 1988.
7. Holden-Lund C: Effects of relaxation with guided imagery on surgical stress and wound healing. Res Nurs Health 11:235, 1988.
8. Walleck CA: Acute head injury, in Von Rueden K, Walleck CA (ed): *Critical Care Case Studies.* Rockville, MD, Aspen, 1990.
9. Eaton M, Mitchell-Bonair IL, Friedmann E: The effect of touch on nutritional intake of chronic organic brain syndrome patients. J Gerontol 41:611, 1986.

10. Mills ME, Thomas SA, Lynch JJ, Katcher AH: Effect of pulse palpation on cardiac arrhythmia in coronary care patients. Nurs Res 25:378, 1976.
11. Falk SA, Woods NF: Hospital noise-levels and potential health hazards. N Engl J Med 289:774, 1973.
12. Updike P: Music therapy results for ICU patients. Dim Crit Care Nurs 9:39, 1990.
13. Fontaine DK: Measurement of nocturnal sleep patterns in trauma patients. Heart Lung 18:402, 1989.
14. Walker BB: The postsurgery heart patient: Amount of uninterrupted time for sleep and rest during the first, second and third postoperative days in a teaching hospital. Nurs Res 21:164, 1972.
15. Helton MC, Gordon SH, Nunnery SL: The correlation between sleep deprivation and the intensive care unit syndrome. Heart Lung 9:464, 1980.
16. Orem J: Compendium of physiology of sleep, in Orem J, Barnes CD (eds): *Physiology of Sleep*. New York, Academic Press, Inc, 1980, p 315.
17. Thompson SC: Will it hurt less if I can control it? A complex answer to a simple question. Psychol Bull 90:89, 1981.
18. Whetsell LA, Patterson CM, Young DH: Pre-injury psychopathology in trauma patients. J Trauma 28:1099, 1988 (abstr).
19. Lynn-McHale DJ, Bellinger A: Need satisfaction levels of family members of critical care patients and accuracy of nurses' perceptions. Heart Lung 17:447, 1988.
20. Jocono J, Hicks G, Antonioni C, O'Brien K, Rasi M: Comparison of perceived needs of family members between registered nurses and family members of critically ill patients in intensive care and neonatal intensive care units. Heart Lung 19:72, 1990.
21. Bouman CC: Identifying priority concerns of families of ICU patients. Dim Crit Care Nurs 3:313, 1984.
22. Daley L: The perceived immediate needs of families with relatives in the intensive care setting. Heart Lung 13:231, 1984.
23. Rodgers CD: Needs of relatives of cardiac surgery patients during the critical care phase. Focus Crit Care 10:50, 1983.
24. Leske JS: Needs of relatives of critically ill patients: A follow-up. Heart Lung 15:189, 1986.
25. Norris LO, Grove SK: Investigation of selected psychosocial needs of family members of critically ill adult patients. Heart Lung 15:194, 1986.
26. Caplin MS, Sexton DL: Stresses experienced by spouses of patients in a coronary care unit with myocardial infarction. Focus Crit Care 15:31, 1988.
27. Bedsworth JA, Molen MT: Psychological stress in spouses of patients with myocardial infarction. Heart Lung 11:450, 1982.
28. Nyamathi AM: Perceptions of factors influencing the coping of wives of myocardial infarction patients. J Cardiovasc Nurs 2:65, 1988.
29. Epperson MN: Families in sudden crisis: Process and intervention in a critical care center. J Soc Work Health Care 2:265, 1977.
30. Kleeman KM: Families in crisis due to multiple trauma. Crit Care Nurs Clin North Am 1:23, 1989.

Chapter 45

LEGAL ISSUES IN CRITICAL CARE

MARSHALL B. KAPP

The making, implementation, and documentation of treatment decisions in the practice of critical care medicine raise a host of potential legal implications. This chapter briefly outlines some of the more salient issues and suggests avenues for their management and further exploration. Figure 45-1 depicts these issues as they arise within and impact upon the physician–patient relationship in intensive care units.

It must be noted that what is described here are the evolving legal ramifications particular to critical care practice in the United States. For comparison, international critical care presents a very different perspective where legal issues may impact much less on day-to-day decision making (see Chap. 189). It may be argued that the U.S. approach encourages greater sensitivity to and protection of the rights of patients. In contrast, the legal systems of many other countries have elevated the role of the critical care physician as advocate for the critically ill patient. A tangible outcome of this difference is that intensivists in the United States usually are more cautious in giving medical advice—especially advice with difficult ethical connotations—to their patients or surrogates compared to Australasian, European, or even Canadian intensivists, all of whom assume a more commanding presence at the physician–patient interface regarding critical care decision making. It is not uncommon to encounter U.S. critical care decision making suspended, awaiting the input of family or an institutional ethics committee that has yet to be apprised of the patient's condition or need for a decision; in contrast, quite similar situations are decided autocratically by the attending intensivist in other countries. Because critical care is evolving rapidly throughout the world, the contributions of the legal system—positive and negative—to health care and to society as a whole are not yet clear. It is clear, however, that legal issues become less dominating and intrusive, and ethical concerns become more central, when intensivists and their critical care teams initiate and continue sensitive, complete, consistent, and honest communication with their critically ill patients and "significant others."

Informed Consent[1]

The well-established legal doctrine of informed consent is based on the ethical principles of autonomy (personal self-determination) and beneficence (doing good for the patient).[2] Early lawsuits growing out of medical interventions conducted in the absence of informed consent were predicated on a battery, or unconsented-to touching of the person, theory. Most such cases today, though, are framed as negligence actions where the alleged unintentional wrong is the physician's violation of the fiduciary or trust duty to inform the patient adequately as part of the permission process.

In order to be considered legally effective, consent to medical treatment must meet three tests (in the absence of an exception such as an unforseeable emergency). First, consent must be voluntary—that is, not coerced—in nature. The patient (or surrogate decision maker) must retain the ultimate power to accept or reject the available interventions.

Second, consent must be adequately informed or knowing. The majority of U.S. jurisdictions still enforce a physician-oriented standard of information disclosure, inquiring whether the amount of information shared by the physician with the patient or surrogate was consistent with the usual practice of other prudent, competent physicians in similar circumstances. A large minority of states, however, have adopted a more patient-oriented standard, requiring physi-

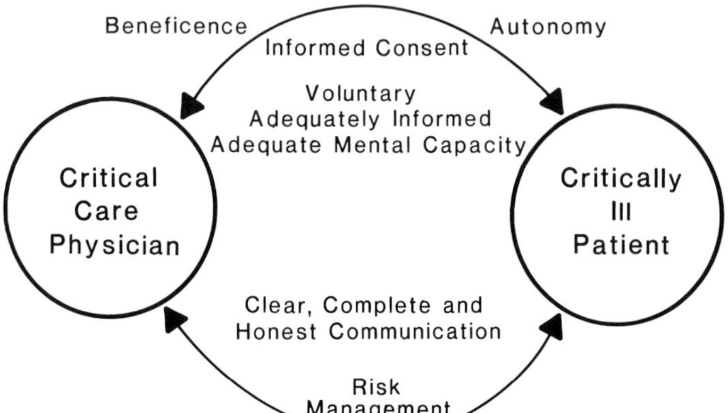

FIGURE 45-1 Outline of Legal Issues in Critical Care: The communication and interaction between critical care physician and critically ill patient involves areas (informed consent, risk management) with legal issues and precedents.

cians to disclose all the information that the patient would want to know under the circumstances. This latter approach is also termed the *materiality* standard, since it compels the disclosure of information that would be material—that is, which might affect the decision—for a patient.

Under either a physician- or patient-oriented approach, several particular kinds of information need to be disclosed in understandable lay language. These include: the nature of the patient's medical problem; prognosis with and without treatment; nature of the suggested intervention; likely benefits of treatment; reasonable alternatives; and foreseeable risks of the various alternatives. Additionally, many people today are interested in knowing the probable financial ramifications of their medical decisions.

Third, informed consent is sufficient only when it is given by an individual with adequate mental capacity and legal authority. This element of consent may be especially problematic in critical care and is discussed in the next section.

A note of caution regarding the legal value of written consent forms must be added here. Contrary to the usual mistake that health care providers make of treating the two things as synonymous, a written consent form is not the equivalent of legally effective informed consent. Informed consent is the process of mutual communication[3] and ultimate patient or surrogate choice as described earlier. The written form is only tangible documentation or evidence that the communication process occurred. This evidence may be very important to the physician in defending against a lawsuit claiming medical intervention in the absence of informed consent, by creating a legal presumption that consent was properly obtained. Where inadequate communication actually took place, however, the presumption created by the consent form may be successfully rebutted or overcome by the plaintiff. While broad, blanket consent forms used in many hospitals are sufficient to authorize routine, noninvasive medical treatments, more specifically tailored and informative forms are preferable for interventions that are nonroutine or invasive, and certainly for treatments that might be characterized as experimental or innovative.[4]

Application of these general principles is somewhat complicated in critical care by the fact that, in the intensive care unit (ICU) interventions can be nearly continuous for the most unstable patients. Informed consent is necessary any time the doctor proposes doing anything to a patient (i.e., any "intervention"). For quasi-continuous interventions, informed consent must certainly be obtained at the initiation of the intervention, and the patient or surrogate must be afforded the opportunity to withdraw that consent at any later point.

Most interventions in critical care may be categorized as "risky" or "invasive," that is, involving for the patient a higher degree of risk or intrusion than he or she would ordinarily face in normal, everyday life. However, this categorization is relevant only to the question of the extent of advisable documentation; the requirement of an informed consent process itself applies regardless of an intervention's level of risk or invasiveness.

Decisional Capacity and Surrogate Decision Making

Minor children (defined in almost every state for medical purposes as those younger than 18 years old) are presumed legally to be incapable of making their own medical decisions, and, in the absence of an exception based on the minor's "emanicipated" or "mature" status, the natural parent or court-appointed guardian is legally empowered as the medical decision maker. Adults, on the other hand, are presumed legally to be decisionally capable.[5] In critical care, many (although certainly not all) patients will be so ill and debilitated that they are not presently capable of making and expressing treatment choices resulting from a rational thought process of digesting and weighing information about the benefits and risks of different alternatives.[6]

Although in theory the same degree of mental capacity is necessary whether the patient is accepting or declining the recommended medical intervention, in practice a formal inquiry into patient capacity usually occurs only in the case of patient refusal. Ideally, a judgment about patient decisional capacity, which may fluctuate widely over time because of a variety of natural and iatrogenic factors, is being made at least implicitly by the attending physician each time the patient is seen. Such an inquiry ought to be inherently built into every physician–patient encounter. Where decisional capacity is seriously questioned, a more focused examination needs to be conducted. In especially ambiguous cases, documentation in the patient's medical record by consultants who have evaluated the patient's decisional capacity is good risk management for the physician proposing an intervention, who is the one ultimately responsible for assuring informed consent; the legal system affords psychiatrists a great deal (arguably an excessive amount) of deference as consultant capacity assessors.

For patients who in fact lack the ability to engage in a rational decision-making process, the presumption of capacity is rebutted or overcome. This does not, however, mean that the physician may dispense with informed consent prior to initiating particular interventions. Consent remains necessary for treatment of incapacitated patients, but the consent must be obtained from a surrogate or proxy acting on the patient's behalf. Several approaches to surrogate medical decision making have developed.

Approximately a dozen states in the past decade have enacted "family consent statutes," which specify relatives (ordinarily in a priority order) who may legally make medical decisions for an incapacitated family member. Advance directives (see next section), especially the durable power of attorney, may be used by currently capable persons to designate their own surrogates in the event of subsequent incapacity. A formal guardianship or conservatorship (precise terminology varies among jurisdictions) proceeding may be initiated, in which a probate court finds the patient (the ward) to be decisionally incapacitated (the legal term usually employed is *incompetent*) and appoints someone else (the guardian or conservator of the person) as the surrogate decision maker.

In most cases, however, the physician relies on family members as the surrogate decision makers for an incapacitated patient, even in the absence of a specific statute, advance directive, or court order empowering the family. This informal process of "bumbling through" using "next of kin," even without explicit legal authority, works well in the vast majority of situations where the family members agree on a course of conduct both among themselves and with the physician, and they appear to act consistently with the patient's values and preferences (the "substituted judgment" standard) or his best interests.

Decisions to Limit Treatment[7,8]

Some patients retain a sufficient degree of capacity to make and express their own medical decisions even after admission to a critical care unit (CCU). Legal precedent is very clear that, except where the welfare of a third party such as a minor dependent is jeopardized, a properly informed, capable patient has the right to make personal medical decisions, including a decision to refuse even life-prolonging treatment.

Where the patient is decisionally incapacitated, a more difficult scenario may confront the physician. A surrogate decision maker may be identified (see previous section) under a state family consent statute, the patient's prior execution of a durable power of attorney (See App. 1 for a model) naming a surrogate or health care agent, a court appointment of a guardian/conservator, or informally relying on available, willing family members.

The surrogate is legally expected in most states to make decisions consistent with what the patient would choose if he or she were presently able to make and express choices personally (substituted judgment standard, or "donning the mental mantle" of the incapacitated person). If there is no reliable indication (some states, e.g., New York,[9] require proof by "clear and convincing evidence") of the patient's preference under the circumstances, the surrogate must act in the patient's best interests, considering—from the patient's perspective—the proportionality of likely benefits and burdens associated with available medical alternatives.

An increasing percentage of patients, especially as the population ages, lack available, willing relatives or friends to act as surrogate decision makers. In such cases, there are several potential sources of guidance for the physician.

The patient may have executed a living will document while still decisionally capable. This type of advance directive, which is authorized by statute (frequently called a Natural Death Act) in 41 jurisdictions as of 1990, permits a capable adult to make a record of personal preferences regarding future medical treatment in the event of subsequent incapacity and critical illness. (see Appendix 2 for model). Although usually this directive is used to indicate a preference for the limitation of future medical intervention, it could be employed to request maximum medical intervention if there is any likelihood of benefit to the patient.[10] However, neither a patient nor his or her family have a legal right, nor does a physician have the obligation, to provide medical treatment that would be futile—that is, nonbeneficial—for that patient.[11]

Even in states that do not have living will statutes, documents purporting to be living wills can supply valuable guidance to the physician regarding the patient's values and wishes. In these states, as well as those with specific legislation, a physician who complies in good faith with the patient's expressed voluntary, informed wishes to limit life-prolonging treatment is on firm legal ground.[12] For the physician who, for ethical reasons or otherwise, chooses not to follow a living will's directive to limit treatment, there is at the least an ethical obligation to notify the patient or surrogate (if one is present) and to make a reasonable attempt to transfer the patient to another physician who is willing to comply with the living will. There have even been a few recent lawsuits placing civil liability on the physician for imposing medical treatment (e.g., a mechanical ventilator) against the previously stated wishes of the patient.[13]

In many states, a public guardianship system has been created to make surrogate decision makers available, either through a government agency or through a private agency under government contract, for incapacitated patients who lack available, willing relatives or friends. There are also some demonstration projects in progress exploring the use of privately funded private agencies acting as surrogate medical decision makers for incapacitated patients.[14] The physician should consult hospital legal counsel to determine possible sources of surrogate decision making for the incapacitated patient without relatives or friends.

The most controversial and complicated issue in the treatment limitation arena is the status of artificial feeding and hydration.[15] Throughout the 1980s, the courts exhibited a strong trend toward considering feeding tubes merely another form of medical intervention, which could be withheld or withdrawn under the same circumstances that would apply to the withholding or withdrawal of any other type of medical intervention.[7] The American Medical Association[16] (see Appendix 3) and other groups[17,18] endorse this analysis. However, some argue that feeding and hydration, even where accomplished through tubes surgically or forcibly inserted in the patient's body, are fundamentally different and more elemental than medical treatment and, therefore, ought to be continued as long as they can keep the patient alive.[19] A number of state legislatures have embodied this argument in living-will or durable power of attorney statutes that severely restrict the ability of surrogate decision makers to authorize the removal of feeding tubes.[20]

The case of Nancy Cruzan, decided by the United States Supreme Court on June 25, 1990, sheds light on the issue of limiting life-prolonging treatment. Cruzan is an automobile accident victim being kept alive in a persistent vegetative state within a state (Missouri)-operated, long-term care facility, through feeding and hydration tubes. Her parents asked that this intervention be discontinued, a request they claimed was consistent with the patient's previously expressed (although not documented) wishes. The physicians refused this request, and the Missouri Supreme Court upheld the lower-court decision and refused the parents' request to discontinue treatment.

The U.S. Supreme Court held that a mentally capable person does have a fundamental constitutional right, under the liberty provision of the Fourteenth Amendment's due process clause, to make personal medical decisions, even regarding life-prolonging treatments, including artificial feeding and hydration. For incompetent patients, though, the court ruled that a state's interest in preserving life was strong enough to permit a state, *if the state so chooses*, to require "clear and convincing" evidence of the treatment preference the patient would hold if currently able to make and express an autonomous choice before the state must allow the withdrawal of life-prolonging medical care. Presumably, a written declaration made while the patient was competent would suffice as evidence of treatment preference in the event of subsequent incapacity. Under the Cruzan decision, states are also free to set lower standards of proof than "clear and convincing" evidence for incapacitated patients, such as proof by a preponderance of the evidence (i.e., greater than 51 percent likelihood). In the Cruzan case itself, Missouri by statute imposed the "clear and convincing" evidentiary standard, and, since Cruzan had never clearly documented her treatment wishes while still competent, the proof was inconclusive, and the state was permitted to err on the side of continued treatment.

One form of treatment limitation around which there is a high degree of current consensus is the do-not-resuscitate (DNR) or no code order, which instructs caregivers to refrain from initiating cardiopulmonary resuscitation (CPR) for a patient who suffers an anticipated cardiac arrest. There have been very few legal cases in this arena,[21,22] but the well-accepted rule is that a decisionally capable patient has the right to refuse CPR and that surrogates may elect to forego CPR for a patient if the likely burdens of this intervention to the patient would be disproportionate to any benefits (e.g., continued existence until the next arrest) that might be derived.[23] As is true for all medical decisions, a DNR order should be made only after a thorough consultation with the patient or surrogates[24] and should be clearly documented in the medical record.

Where the patient or surrogate has declined aggressive, technologically oriented interventions, the physician still retains the legal obligation to continue basic palliative (comfort and pain control) and hygiene measures. Failure to do so could constitute the tort (civil wrong) of patient abandonment.[25]

The other side of the coin on treatment decision making is presented when the patient, or more usually the family, insists on initiation or continuation of medical treatment ("doing everything") that the clinician judges to be futile in terms of benefit to the patient. No court has ever ordered a physician to begin or perpetuate futile interventions for a critically ill patient, or has imposed liability for failure to do so, even in the face of family insistence on a "full-court press." In fact, judicial decisions have expressly upheld clinician nonintervention in the face of medical futility. Nonetheless, clinicians usually seem to take the path of least resistance in such circumstances and "treat the family," often out of misapprehension of potential liability exposure. In the vast majority of cases, better physician–family communication, in which the realistic implications of "doing everything" are spelled out clearly, can obviate serious disagreement over how to proceed.

Institutional Protocols and Institutional Ethics Committees

A growing number of hospitals have adopted or are in the process of adopting written policies and procedures concerning patient admission to, retention in, and discharge from CCUs. The ability of physicians to consult institutional guidelines generally leads to better, more consistent decisions that are easier to defend against later claims of impropriety.[26] Clear protocols facilitate communication and cooperation among members of the health care team, lessening both inadvertent mistakes and interpersonal tension. Institutional protocols are also essential as inevitable discussions of health care rationing take on increasing urgency.[27]

The development of institutional protocols regarding critical care, especially DNR orders, is now required by some states[28] and by the Joint Commission on Accreditation of Healthcare Organizations (JCAHO).[29] Formal mandating of such policies is likely to expand.[30]

Critical care physicians must be completely familiar, and must assure familiarity on the part of nurses and other staff working as members of their teams, with their own institutions' formal policies and procedures. Ideally, members of the medical staff should contribute to the drafting, continuing reevaluation, and revision of institutional protocols.[31] Questions regarding the meaning or implementation of these protocols should be addressed in timely fashion (i.e., before a crisis erupts) to hospital legal counsel.

Similarly, the physician must be knowledgeable about the operation of his or her hospital's institutional ethics committee (IEC), if any. In the past decade and a half, there has been a proliferation of entities within health care institutions designed to provide education, formulate policies and procedures, and offer advice regarding particular cases and issues with serious bioethical implications.[32] Although the emphasis of IECs is, and ought to be, on better ethical decision making, salutary legal by-products may also result from their activities. Effective use of an IEC may preclude resort to the judicial system, initiated either by the family or by a health care team member who feels his or her opinion has been inadequately taken into account, for definitive resolution of a case. Further, in the relatively unlikely event of the informal decision-making process breaking down and court involvement being invoked,[33] utilization of an IEC acts as powerful evidence of the provider's good faith and appropriate concern for patient autonomy and welfare.

Determinations of Death

One inescapable aspect of critical care medicine with important legal implications is the determination and declaration of when a patient has died. Traditional standards of death based on cessation of cardiorespiratory functioning are no longer sufficient by themselves in light of modern medical technology that frequently can maintain the human organism almost indefinitely. Questions relating to the discontinuation of medical intervention and the harvesting of organs for transplantation have demanded new approaches to the legal definition of death.

In response to these questions, almost all states have adopted, either by statute or court decision, a version of "brain death." This definition provides, either as an alternative to or a replacement for the traditional heart–lungs approach, that a person is legally dead when there is irreversible cessation of all (including stem) brain function.[34] Brain death should be confirmed clinically according to the Harvard criteria,[35] as updated by the President's Commission[36] (see Table 45-1). Once a patient has been declared dead, there are no longer any treatment decisions to be made (although autopsy and organ donation issues may remain). There is neither a legal duty nor a right to continue medical intervention on a patient who has become a corpse.[37]

TABLE 45-1 Brain Death Criteria

Either

A. An individual with irreversible cessation of circulatory and respiratory functions is dead.
   1. Cessation is recognized by an appropriate clinical examination.
   2. Irreversibility is recognized by persistent cessation of functions during an appropriate period of observation and/or trial or therapy.

Or

B. An individual with irreversible cessation of all functions of the entire brain, including the brainstem, is dead.
   1. Cessation is recognized when evaluation discloses findings of a and b:
      a. cerebral functions are absent, and
      b. brainstem functions are absent.
   2. Irreversibility is recognized when evaluation discloses findings of a and b and c:
      a. the cause of coma is established and is sufficient to account for the loss of brain functions, and
      b. the possibility of recovery of any brain functions is excluded, and
      c. the cessation of all brain functions persists for an appropriate period of observation and/or trial of therapy

SOURCE: Adapted from the Report of the Medical Consultants on the Diagnosis of Death to the President's Commission for the Study of Ethical Problems in Medicine and Biomedical and Behavioral Research. JAMA 246:2184, 1981.

Legal Responsibility and Vicarious Liability[7]

Critical care medicine is an interprofessional team enterprise, and the manner in which members of the team relate to each other and to the patient and family carries legal consequences. Under the longstanding doctrine of "captain of the ship," a physician in charge of a critical care unit automatically would be held legally answerable for any negligently caused patient injury happening in the unit, regardless of the physician's personal ignorance of or noninvolvement in the particular error or omission. The captain of the ship doctrine essentially has been abandoned by the courts over the past several years in recognition of the increasing complexity of health care delivery.

However, a physician may still be held responsible, under a vicarious liability rationale, for patient injuries proximately (directly) caused by negligent errors or omissions committed by nurses or other providers over whom the physician has supervisory duties. The key inquiry in potential vicarious liability situations is not whether the physician actually was exercising supervisory power at the time of the supervisee's negligence, but whether he or she had the authority and opportunity to supervise properly if he or she had chosen to exercise that power.[26]

Thus, the vicarious liability doctrine has significant legal ramifications for the interprofessional team's conduct in rendering critical care. The physician and other team members must understand their legal relationships to each other and their connotations for assignment of tasks, oversight, reporting, communication, and problem resolution. Physicians must take their obligations as legal leader of the team seriously without acting autocratically and thereby negating the benefits of broad interprofessional contributions to patient care.

Institutional protocols should delineate operational principles of the team and the individual physician's supervisory responsibilities. Where, as is the norm, there are multiple consultants on a particular case, medical staff bylaws must spell out the continuing coordination and monitoring obligations of an identified attending or primary care physician; failure to do so unambiguously will likely, in the event of a bad clinical outcome, increase the liability exposure of all involved physicians and the hospital. Consultants who are not hospital employees must be credentialed to practice within the hospital according to criteria contained in the bylaws. Hospital policies and procedures must designate their ICUs as either "closed" (where the patient is transferred to an intensivist who functions as the primary care physician) or "open" (where the original primary care physician retains ultimate authority and responsibility, but is permitted or required to consult with a critical care physician on the hospital's staff).

Similarly, methods of triaging patients into and out of the ICU should be delineated within the hospital's written policies and procedures. Included should be a specification of ultimate responsibility for a patient's admission or discharge.

As a general principle, where there is a question concerning allocation of responsibility for decisions or actions, development of an institutional policy may be advisable. Courts ordinarily grant hospitals broad leeway in the development and enforcement of the sort of institutional protocols discussed in this chapter, as long as policies and procedures appear to assure patient care within currently acceptable medical standards. As noted earlier, accreditation standards of the JCAHO also set permissible parameters for internal institutional protocols.

For physicians who function as clinical instructors in teaching programs, residents and medical students may expose the attending physician to vicarious liability for negligent acts or omissions done in the course of the educational activity. The exercise of due care in the monitoring, supervision, task assignment, and evaluation of residents and students who are supposed to be under the physician's supervision cannot be overlooked.[38]

Documentation

The courts have held that creating and maintaining accurate records of patient care is an integral part of the duty that a health care provider owes to a patient. Good documentation is imperative to providing competent patient care and, since avoiding unexpected bad outcomes is the best legal prophylaxis, is therefore wise legal practice. Furthermore, in the event of accusations of substandard care, the physician's best (and often only) defense will lie in the quality of documentation created to explain and justify decisions made and actions taken. In addition, institutional accreditation and third-party reimbursement turn heavily on information drawn from medical records.

The quality of medical records is especially important in critical care, where patient conditions are subject to rapid change, many different professionals may be involved in treating the patient, cost considerations are ever present,[39] and decisions (such as limiting the application of life-prolonging technology) may be controversial. The watchwords of documentation are the same from the legal and medical perspectives: completeness, legibility (dictation is preferable, but dictated entries should be read and corrected before being signed), accuracy or truthfulness, timeliness, corrections made in a clear and unambiguous fashion, and objectivity.

A corollary to the subject of medical record keeping is confidentiality. The physician must guard against unauthorized disclosures of personal information about the patient. The party who has authority to give or refuse consent for medical treatment (i.e., the patient or his surrogate) ordinarily controls the release of identifiable medical information to third parties, absent a court order or countervailing government regulation. Questions about the release of medical information to third parties in specific cases should be directed to the institution's medical records department or legal counsel.

The counterpart to the right of the patient or surrogate to control the release of information to others is their own right of access to the information contained in the medical record. This right of access is guaranteed, at least for in-hospital care, by the federal Privacy Act for federal facilities, and by state statute and JCAHO standards in most private and public institutions. Patients or their surrogates request access to records for a variety of reasons ranging from curiosity to serious questioning of quality of care. A physician who is informed of a patient's or surrogate's request for access to records should offer to go through the record with the patient or surrogate, explain matters to them, and answer their questions. In short, reacting to this circumstance as an opportunity to bolster, or correct existing but perhaps unnoticed deficiencies in, communication between the physician and patient or surrogate, rather than as a personal affront calling for defensive posturing, often can pay risk management dividends in obviating at an early stage potential misunderstandings that would otherwise eventually manifest themselves in the legal arena.

Risk Management Program

The hospital's overall program to identify, mitigate, and avoid potential problems that could result in legal and, therefore, financial loss to the institution, that is, the risk management program, should incorporate specific activities designed to address legal risks prevalent in the delivery of critical care.[32] Particular areas of attention in a critical care–sensitive risk management program should include the organization and administration of CCUs, the roles and responsibilities of the different professionals having contact with patients in those units, medical records, equipment maintenance, equipment modification, equipment records, analysis of equipment malfunctions, incident reporting, and trend analysis of unexpected incidents.

The physician should be knowledgeable about the institution's risk management program and cooperate with it to assure appropriate sensitivity to critical care practices and potential problems and their avoidance or mitigation. The physician should view the risk manager as a partner in pursuit of the common goal of providing, and if necessary proving after-the-fact, quality patient care.

Perhaps the single most influential aspect of effective risk management is the fostering of a positive relationship between the critical care team, led by the physician, and the patient and his or her family. There is a demonstrated correlation between patient (or family) psychologic satisfaction with the quality of the physician–patient (family) relationship and the propensity to file a lawsuit if a bad outcome happens.[40] Communicating openly and compassionately, especially acknowledging the vast uncertainty that pervades much of critical care medicine, is as important a tool in the malpractice prophylaxis arsenal as being proficient, up to date, and conscientious in knowing and applying technologic information and skills.[41]

References[1]

1. Annas GJ: *The Rights of Patients.* Carbondale, IL, Southern Illinois University Press, 1989, Chap. VI.
2. President's Commission for the Study of Ethical Problems in Medicine and Biomedical and Behavioral Research: *Making Health Care Decisions.* Washington, DC, Government Printing Office, 1982, pp 2–3.
3. Katz J: *The Silent World of Doctor and Patient.* New York, Free Press, 1984.
4. Curran WJ: The unwanted suitor: Law and the use of health care technology, in Reiser SJ, Anbar M (eds): *The Machine at the Bedside: Strategies for Using Technology in Patient Care.* New York, Cambridge University Press, 1984, p 122.
5. Annas GJ, Densberger J: Competence to refuse medical treatment: Autonomy v. paternalism. Toledo L Rev 15:561, 1984.
6. Applebaum P, Grisso T: Assessing patients' capacity to consent to treatment. N Engl J Med 319:1635, 1988.
7. Meisel A: *The Right to Die.* New York, John Wiley & Sons, 1989.
8. President's Commission for the Study of Ethical Problems in Medicine and Biomedical and Behavioral Research: *Deciding to Forego Life-Sustaining Treatment.* Washington, DC, Government Printing Office, 1983.
9. In re: Mary O'Connor, 534 N.Y.S. 2d 886, 531 N.E. 2d 607 (1988).
10. Kapp MB: Response to the living will furor: Directives for maximum care. Am J Med 72:855, 1982.
11. Annas GJ: *The Rights of Patients.* Carbondale, IL, Southern Illinois University Press, 1989, pp 217–218.
12. Taraska JM: *Legal Guide for Physicians.* New York, Matthew Bender & Company, 1988, sec. 11.05[2].
13. *Estate of Leach v. Shapiro,* 13 Ohio App. 3d 393, 469 N.E. 2d 1047 (1984).
14. Gibson J, Nathanson P: Temporary medical treatment guardians. In *Generations* San Francisco, American Society on Aging, 1991.
15. Congressional Office of Technology Assessment: *Life-Sustaining Technologies and the Elderly.* Washington, DC, Government Printing Office, 1987, chap 8.
16. American Medical Association: *Current Opinions of the Council of Ethical and Judicial Affairs.* Chicago, AMA, 1989, sec. 2.20, 2.21.
17. Hastings Center: *Guidelines for the Termination of Life-Sustaining Treatment and the Care of the Dying.* Bloomington, Indiana University Press, 1988, pp 57–62.
18. Wanzer SH, Federman DD, Adelstein SJ, Cassell CK, Cassem EH, Cranford RE, Hook EW, Lo B, Moertel CG, Safar P, Stone AA, van Eys J: The physician's responsibility toward hopelessly ill patients. N Engl J Med 310:955, 1984.
19. Siegler M, Weisbard AJ: Against the emerging stream: Should fluids and nutritional support be discontinued? Arch Intern Med 145:129, 1985.

[1]*Note:* For references to judicial decisions, usually (a) case name is listed first, followed by (b) state reporter citation, (c) regional reporter citation, and (d) date. References to state and regional reporters are in the form of volume number, name of reporter, and page number. Thus, one would find the reported 1983 opinion in *Kapp v. The World,* 25 Ohio 100, 400 A. 2d 150 (1983) at Vol. 25, p. 100 of the *Ohio Reports* or Vol. 400, p. 150 of the *Atlantic Reporter,* 2d ed.

20. Kapp MB: Ohio's new durable power of attorney. Vol. 14 p. 541, 1989. Univ Dayton L Rev
21. *Matter of Dinnerstein,* 6 Mass. App. 466, 380 N.E. 2d 134 (Mass. App. 1978).
22. *Hoyt v. St. Mary's Rehabilitation Center,* No. 774555, 4th Jud. Dist., Hennepin County, Minn. (Jan. 2, 1981).
23. Committee on Policy for DNR Decisions, Yale-New Haven Hospital: Report on Do-Not-Resuscitate Decisions. Conn Med 47:477, 1983.
24. Stephens RL: Do not resuscitate orders: Ensuring the patient's participation. JAMA 255:240, 1986.
25. Norton ML, Norton EV: Medicolegal issues in high-intensity care, in Norton ML, Finch JS, Finch EV (eds): *High-Intensity Care: Medical, Administrative, and Legal Issues.* Rockville, MD, Aspen Publishers, 1989, pp 147–152.
26. Miles SH, Gomez CF: *Protocols for Elective Use of Life-Sustaining Treatments.* New York, Springer Publishing Company, 1989.
27. Grument BR: Legal perspectives on the allocation of intensive care services, in Strosberg MA, Fein IA, Carroll JD (eds): *Rationing of Medical Care for the Critically Ill.* Washington, DC, Brookings Institution, 1989, p 79.
28. New York State Public Health Law Sections 2960–78 (1988).
29. Joint Commission on Accreditation of Healthcare Organizations: *Accreditation Manual for Hospitals.* Chicago, JCAHO, 1989, Standard M.A. 1.4.
30. Congressional Office of Technology Assessment: *Institutional Protocols for Decisions About Life-Sustaining Treatments.* Washington, DC, Government Printing Office, 1988, pp 26–29.
31. Meisel A, Grenvik A, Pinkus RL, Snyder JV: Deciding about life-sustaining treatment: The role of hospital guidelines, in Benesch K, Abramson NS, Grenvik A, Meisel A (eds): *Medicolegal aspects of critical care.* Rockville, MD, 1986, chap 9 and Appendix A.
32. Cranford R, Doudera AE (eds): *Institutional Ethics Committees and Health Care Decision Making.* Ann Arbor, MI, Health Administration Press, 1984.
33. Kapp MB, Lo B: Legal perceptions and medical decision making. *Milbank Quarterly* 64(suppl 2):163, 1986.
34. Capron AM: Determination of death, in Benesch K, Abramson NS, Grenvik A, Meisel A (eds): *Medicolegal Aspects of Critical Care.* Rockville, MD, Aspen Publishers, 1986, chap 6.
35. Ad Hoc Committee of the Harvard Medical School to Examine the Definition of Brain Death: A definition of irreversible coma. JAMA 206:337, 1968.
36. Guidelines for the determination of death: Report of the medical consultants on the diagnosis of death to the President's Commission for the Study of Ethical Problems in Medicine and Biomedical and Behavioral Research. JAMA 246:2184, 1981.
37. *Strachan v. John F. Kennedy Memorial Hospital,* 109 N.J. 523, 538 A. 2d 346 (1988).
38. Kapp MB: Legal implications of clinical supervision of medical students. J Med Educ 58:293, 1983.
39. Raffin TA, Shurkin JN, Sinkler W III: *Intensive Care: Facing the Critical Choices.* New York, WW Freeman and Company, 1989, chap 10.
40. Press I: The predisposition to file claims: The patient's perspective. *Law Med Health Care* 12:53, 1984.
41. Gutheil T, Bursztajn H, Brodsky A: Malpractice prevention through the sharing of uncertainty: informed consent and the therapeutic alliance. N Engl J Med 311:49, 1984.

APPENDIX 1

Durable Power of Attorney for Health Care

1) I, ______________________________, hereby appoint
Name of principal

______________________________, an adult,
Name of attorney in fact

of ______________________________ to be my attorney in
Address and telephone number

fact to make any and all health care decisions for me at any time at which I no longer have the capacity to make such decisions myself. Such decisions shall include, unless I indicate otherwise below, the decision to give, refuse or withdraw informed consent to any and all health care or treatment provided to me, including decisions to withhold or withdraw life-sustaining medical treatment.

2) In the event the person I appoint above is unable, unwilling or unavailable to act as my health care agent, I hereby appoint

______________________________ of ______________________________.
Name of alternate attorney in fact — Address and telephone number

3) My attorney in fact or alternate attorney in fact shall have the same right as I would have to receive information about proposed health care, to review health care records, and to consent to the disclosure of such records. My attorney in fact or alternate attorney in fact shall have full power and authority to do and perform all that he/she determines to be necessary or proper, as I might or could do if I had the capacity. THIS POWER OF ATTORNEY BECOMES EFFECTIVE WHEN I CAN NO LONGER MAKE MY OWN MEDICAL DECISIONS AND SHALL NOT BE EFFECTED BY MY DISABILITY.

4) I have discussed my wishes with my attorney in fact and alternate attorney in fact and authorize him/her to express and carry out my specific and general instructions and desires with respect to medical treatment, including my wishes on the subject of withholding or withdrawing all forms of life-sustaining medical treatment, including tubal feeding and medication.

A. I wish to limit the authority of my attorney in fact or my alternate attorney in fact as follows: (If you do not wish to limit the authority, write: "No limit").

____

____

B. My specific desires regarding health care and treatment are as follows: (If none, write: "NONE")

____

____

____

____
Principal's signature

____
Date

APPENDIX 1 *(Continued)*

ATTESTATION

We, the undersigned witnesses, hereby jointly and severally attest to the following:

1. We know the principal personally,
2. The principal signed or acknowledged his signature in the presence of ourselves as witnesses,
3. The principal appeared to be of sound mind and not under or subject to duress, fraud or undue influence,
4. We are not related to the principal by blood, marriage or adoption; not to the best of our knowledge entitled to benefit in any way from the death of the principal; not designated hereinabove as attorney in fact; not physicians; and not employees or agents of a physician or health care facility.

IN TESTIMONY WHEREOF, we hereunto set our hands as witnesses to the signature of the principal on the _______ day of _______________, 19_______.

______________________ Name	______________________ Name
______________________ (Printed)	______________________ (Printed)
______________________ Address	______________________ Address

STATE OF OHIO)
) SS:
COUNTY OF ______________________)

Before me, a Notary Public in and for said county and state, appear the aforesaid ______________________ who appears to
Name of Principal

be of sound mind and not under or subject to duress, fraud or undue influence, and who acknowledged the signing hereof to be his/her free act and voluntary deed.

IN WITNESS WHEREOF, I hereunto set my hand and official seal as a Notary Public, in and for the aforesaid county and state, on the _______ day of _______________, 19 _______.

____
Notary Public

SOURCE: Reprinted by permission of Society for the Right to Die, 250 West 57 Street, New York, NY 10107.
NOTE: Legal requirements of individual states may vary and should be consulted.

APPENDIX 2

LIVING WILL DECLARATION

To My Family, Doctors, and All Those Concerned With My Care:

I, ______________________, being of sound mind, make this statement as a directive to be followed if for any reason I become unable to participate in decisions regarding my medical care. I direct that life-sustaining procedures should be withheld or withdrawn if I have an illness, disease or injury, or experience extreme mental deterioration, such that there is no reasonable expectation of recovering or regaining a meaningful quality of life.

These life-sustaining procedures that may be withheld or withdrawn include, but are not limited to:

SURGERY ANTIBIOTICS CARDIAC RESUSCITATION
RESPIRATORY SUPPORT ARTIFICIALLY ADMINISTERED FEEDING AND FLUIDS

I further direct that treatment be limited to comfort measures only, even if they shorten my life.

You may delete any provision above by drawing a line through it and adding your initials.

Other personal instructions:

These directions express my legal right to refuse treatment. Therefore, I expect my family, doctors, and all those concerned with my care to regard themselves as legally and morally bound to act in accord with my wishes, and in so doing to be free from any liability for having followed my directions.

Signed ______________________ Date __________

Witness ______________________ Witness ______________________

PROXY DESIGNATION CLAUSE

If you wish, you may use this section to designate someone to make treatment decisions if you are unable to do so. Your Living Will Declaration will be in effect even if you have not designated a proxy:

I authorize the following person to implement my Living Will Declaration by accepting, refusing and/or making decisions about treatment and hospitalization:

NAME: ______________________

ADDRESS: ______________________

If the person I have named above is unable to act on my behalf, I authorize the following person to do so:

NAME: ______________________

ADDRESS: ______________________

I have discussed my wishes with these persons and trust their judgment on my behalf.

Signed ______________________ Date __________

Witness ______________________ Witness ______________________

SOURCE: Reprinted by permission of Society for the Right to Die, 250 West 57 Street, New York, NY 10107
NOTE: Legal requirements of individual states may vary and should be consulted.

APPENDIX 3

2.2 WITHHOLDING OR WITHDRAWING LIFE-PROLONGING TREATMENT.

The social commitment of the physician is to sustain life and relieve suffering. Where the performance of one duty conflicts with the other, the preferences of the patient should prevail. If the patient is incompetent to act in his own behalf and did not previously indicate his preferences, the family or other surrogate decisionmaker, in concert with the physician, must act in the best interest of the patient.

For humane reasons, with informed consent, a physician may do what is medically necessary to alleviate severe pain, or cease or omit treatment to permit a terminally ill patient to die when death is imminent. However, the physician should not intentionally cause death. In deciding whether the administration of potentially life-prolonging medical treatment is in the best interest of the patient who is incompetent to act in his own behalf, the surrogate decisionmaker and physician should consider several factors, including: the possibility for extending life under humane and comfortable conditions; the patient's values about life and the way it should be lived; and the patient's attitudes toward sickness, suffering, medical procedures, and death.

Even if death is not imminent but a patient is beyond doubt permanently unconscious, and there are adequate safeguards to confirm the accuracy of the diagnosis, it is not unethical to discontinue all means of life-prolonging medical treatment.

Life-prolonging medical treatment includes medication and artificially or technologically supplied respiration, nutrition or hydration. In treating a terminally ill or permanently unconscious patient, the dignity of the patient should be maintained at all times. (I,II,IV,V)

2.21 WITHHOLDING OR WITHDRAWING LIFE-PROLONGING MEDICAL TREATMENT-PATIENTS' PREFERENCES. A competent, adult patient may, in advance, formulate and provide a valid consent to the withholding or withdrawal of life-support systems in the event that injury or illness renders that individual incompetent to make such a decision. The preference of the individual should prevail when determining whether extraordinary life-prolonging measures should be undertaken in the event of terminal illness. Unless it is clearly established that the patient is terminally ill or permanently unconscious, a physician should not be deterred from appropriately aggressive treatment of a patient. (I,III,IV,V)

SOURCE: Reprinted by permission from 1989 *Current Opinions* of the Council on Ethical and Judicial Affairs of the American Medical Association.

Chapter 46

TRIAGE AND ASSESSMENT OF SEVERITY OF ILLNESS

CARL A. SIRIO
WILLIAM A. KNAUS

Our ability to extend and maintain life in the face of critical illness continues to improve as our diagnostic and therapeutic armamentarium becomes increasingly more sophisticated. At the same time physicians, patients and their families, and policy makers are more sensitive to the emotional and economic toll such care can exact. This awareness has encouraged the development of clinical tools critical care physicians can use to improve decisions regarding the scope and intensity of intensive care treatment. Most of these endeavors began with efforts to accurately assess and precisely measure the severity of patient illness. Several physiologically based severity of illness systems currently exist. These systems include the Acute Physiology and Chronic Health Evaluation (APACHE), the Simplified Acute Physiology Score (SAPS), and the Mortality Prediction Models (MPM). As these systems become more sophisticated, they will be used increasingly in the triage of patients, evaluation of outcome and quality of care, and the refinement of clinical trials.

Severity of Illness and Risk Assessment

Physicians admit patients with varied disease processes and degrees of physiologic impairment to ICUs. Admission is usually for intensive treatment of a severe illness, for expectant monitoring to detect and prevent complications, or for concentrated nursing care unavailable in other hospital settings. Thresholds for using ICUs vary greatly depending on practice styles and availability of resources.[1,2] Despite the presumed utility of critical care therapy, the clinical literature highlights conflicting evidence regarding this benefit in various disease states.[3,4] As a result, a consensus on the appropriate use of intensive care resources does not exist. Consequently, interest is growing in accurately assessing severity of illness and other pertinent patient risk factors to more exactly estimate probabilities for various outcomes. The most commonly studied outcome has been death. Other outcomes of clinical importance include the incidence of morbidity and the overall length and quality of survival (Table 46-1).

TABLE 46-1 Outcomes of Critical Care of Clinical Importance

Mortality
Morbidity
Nosocomial infection
Reintubation
Self-extubation
Readmission to the ICU within 24 h
Length of survival following hospital discharge
Quality of survival
Activities of daily living
Satisfaction with quality of life achieved
Return to work

The benefits of improved and accurate predictive models in critical care are fourfold. First, they allow physicians to focus aggressive intervention on those individuals most likely to benefit. As institutional resources become constrained, physicians are confronted with determining which clinical problems are most likely to benefit from ICU care. The Task Force on Guidelines of the Society of Critical Care Medicine has suggested that objective measures of illness should play a part in ICU admission and discharge decisions.[5]

Secondly, physicians caring for critically ill individuals are often faced with the decision to limit or withdraw therapy. These decisions are fraught with clinical uncertainty. Accurate prognostic information predicting outcome could serve as an adjunct for these difficult but unavoidable decisions. Work is currently in progress to determine the applicability of prognostic tools to individual patient care problems.[6]

Thirdly, precise prognostic assessment can facilitate the comparison of performance between ICUs. The demand for improved and formalized methods of monitoring quality and outcomes in health care has increased as the cost of medical and hospital care has soared. To date, governmental and institutional efforts to evaluate quality of care using a retrospective analysis of hospital mortality and morbidity have met with skepticism mainly due to the inability of this approach to adequately control for important patient risk factors, especially severity of illness.

Fourthly, prognostic scoring systems (PSS) will facilitate the assessment of new technologies and allow for comparative analysis with established modes of therapy.[7] Clinical trials using accurate and reliable pretreatment risk stratification controls will help us to better understand the value of critical care by reducing the amount of unexplained variation in patient risk. This enables investigators to use smaller sample sizes to reach statistically significant results.

Development of Prognostic Scoring Systems

Current efforts to assess severity of illness in critical care began with the development of disease-specific prognostic indices. Examples of such indices include the Glasgow Coma Score for patients with acute neurologic injury, the Killip classification system for patients with acute myocardial infarction, and the Ranson criteria in acute pancreatitis.[8–10]

Although accurate in providing relative risk stratification, these systems have been limited by their disease specificity. This prevents useful comparisons across diseases or for patients with complex disorders. Today, there is widespread recognition that general, not disease-specific, methods of assessing severity of illness are more useful because of their utility across a broad spectrum of diseases.

An important step forward in this regard was the development of the Therapeutic Intervention Scoring System (TISS).[11] TISS was designed to quantify the amount of skilled care a patient received. By measuring 78 distinct nursing, monitoring, and procedural responsibilities, TISS serves as an indirect measure of the severity of illness across differing diseases. This scoring system does not, however, promote understanding of the relationship between a patient's specific illness and the impact of ICU care. It is rather, an assessment of the level of care and monitoring.

Progress in the development of general severity of illness measures continued with the introduction of the APACHE, designed to capture those determinants of outcome felt to be significant prior to therapy.[12] The application and response to therapy were not included in the evaluation to avoid biasing the predictions with the impact of therapy. The important determinants of outcome are listed in Table 46-2.

Subsequently, other systems designed to assess illness severity have been created. These include the SAPS,[13] and the MPM.[14] Similar methods for assessing severity of illness in pediatric patients have also been developed. These include the pediatric Physiologic Stability Index (PSI)[15] and the Pediatric Risk of Mortality Score (PRISM).[16]

Severity of Illness Measures

APACHE

The first general system for assessing severity of illness in the critically ill, APACHE, was introduced in 1981. The original system consisted of two parts: the acute physiology score (APS), based on 34 physiologic measures designed to capture the severity of an acute illness, and a preadmission health evaluation describing a patient's prior health status. The APS consisted of variables available near the time of admission and felt to be clinically important by an expert panel of intensive care physicians in predicting mortality. Relative weights were assigned to each variable signifying the degree of abnormality from normal and the relative importance of that derangement when compared to the other variables. Studies evaluating the validity of APACHE in risk prediction demonstrated a direct relationship between the APS and the relative risk of death. The chronic health indicators were associated with an increased risk of death only for those patients with severe and failing health prior to admission.

The original APACHE model had several limitations. In addition to the lack of explanatory power using the bulk of the chronic health evaluation, many of the 34 data points in the APS were not routinely measured in all patients. This led to refinement and improvement of the methodology with the introduction of APACHE II in 1985,[17] which differed significantly from its predecessor. The number of physiologic variables incorporated in the initial assessment of severity was reduced to 12. In addition, several threshold values and weights for the physiologic measures were changed. For example, the importance of the Glasgow Coma Score and the importance attributed to acute renal failure were increased due to a better understanding of the impact of coma and renal failure on outcome. The impact of each of these changes was evaluated using multivariate comparisons to the original APACHE model.

The assessment of chronic health was changed as chronic health risk points were assigned for ongoing organ dysfunction. Chronological age was incorporated into the APACHE II model, with increasing age being given an increasing number of risk points. In addition, the impact of emergency surgery was integrated into the analysis of outcome since analysis revealed this to be independently associated with an increased risk of mortality.

The resultant APACHE II score was a sum of the acute physiology, age, and chronic health points. This point total, when combined with a patient's actual disease state in a multivariate logistic analysis, provided the basis for an assessment of severity of illness and risk of mortality. The APACHE II system was validated on 5815 patients from 13 United States medical centers and revealed a consistent relationship between APACHE II mortality predictions and observed hospital death rates. This relationship was found across the entire spectrum from a low to a high risk of death.

Currently, an updated and revised version of APACHE, APACHE III, is nearing completion. The APACHE III study is being undertaken with a nationally representative sample of 40 United States hospitals. This latest endeavor has several goals.

First, the APACHE III study is designed to improve the APACHE system. The physiologic variables measured are being reevaluated to determine the importance of additional physiologic measures such as bilirubin, albumin, glu-

TABLE 46-2 Determinants of Patient Outcome

Information Available	Patient and Treatment Factors
Before treatment	Type of disease (diagnosis)
	Severity of disease
	Physiologic reserve
	Age
	Chronic disease
After treatment	Therapy available
	Application of therapy
	Timing
	Process
	Response to therapy

cose, urine output, and blood urea nitrogen (BUN) on outcome. In addition, the weights assigned to each variable are being reexamined.

To date, APACHE II uses the most deviant measure within the first 24 h of a patient's ICU stay. The APACHE III study is designed to evaluate the importance of timing in capturing the physiologic measurements and their impact on outcome by measuring both the first ICU value, as well as the worst over 24 h. In addition, the impact of therapy prior to ICU admission will be assessed.

The importance of chronic health is being reevaluated. It appears likely that the comorbid conditions included in APACHE II will be further refined. In addition, the disease categories available for classification with APACHE II will be expanded.

APACHE III will improve the evaluation of the processes of clinical care as well as new therapeutic modalities. Physicians will be able to derive an accurate estimate of the number of excess deaths attributable to variations in quality of care, and, using the normative data base, identify areas in need of improvement and acknowledge areas of excellence. Further, physicians will have more reliable estimates of patient prognosis which can be incorporated into clinical decision-making.

SIMPLIFIED ACUTE PHYSIOLOGY SCORE

SAPS was developed in 1984 as an independent attempt to simplify APACHE.[13] Using multiple linear regression, 13 physiologic variables were chosen to stratify patients based on their pretreatment risk of mortality. The variables included age, heart rate, systolic blood pressure, respiratory rate, urine output, BUN, hematocrit, white blood cell count, serum glucose, sodium, potassium, bicarbonate, and Glasgow Coma Score. The physiologic weights assigned to each of these variables were nearly equivalent to those used in APACHE. The predictive results derived from an analysis using SAPS were comparable to the original APACHE system. However, comparisons using APACHE II with SAPS reveal measurable improvements in predictive accuracy for APACHE II using multidiagnostic data. These differences are negligible when comparing predictive ability within a diagnostic group because of the underlying similarities of the two systems.[18]

MORTALITY PREDICTION MODEL

The MPM differs from both APACHE and SAPS because the predictor variables were selected by a computer search technique.[19] The MPM was created using data from 755 consecutive admissions to the ICUs in a single hospital. On admission to the ICU, one hundred thirty seven background, disease-related, and treatment variables were monitored and 75 were further evaluated at 24 and 48 h after admission. Using stepwise linear discriminant function and multiple logistic regression techniques, 11 admission variables were identified as predictive of subsequent hospital mortality (Table 46-3). Variables such as cardiopulmonary resuscitation prior to ICU admission are not physiologic measurements. Some of the variables described, such as "infection part of the patient's major problem" are more prone to ascertainment or measurement bias than direct physiologic values.

TABLE 46-3 Components of the Admission Mortality Prediction Model

Level of consciousness
No coma/deep stupor
Coma or deep stupor
Type of admission
Elective
Emergency
CPR prior to ICU admission
No
Yes
Cancer part of present problem
No
Yes
History of chronic renal failure
No
Yes
Infection
No or not probable
Probable
Age
(10-year relative risk)
Previous ICU admission within 6 months
No
Yes
Heart rate at ICU admission
(10 beat/min relative risk)
Surgical service at ICU admission
No
Yes
Systolic blood pressure

SOURCE: Adapted from Reference 19, with permission.

The variables used in the MPM are influenced by the patients treated at the institution where the model was developed. This may explain in part why APACHE II performs better than the MPM in formal comparisons. The MPM is currently undergoing a multi-institutional validation designed to address this problem as well as refine the predictions made at 24, 48, and 72 h after admission to the ICU.

Potential Uses for Severity of Illness Measures

SEVERITY OF ILLNESS AND TRIAGE DECISIONS

Triage is the screening of patients to determine their relative priority for treatment. In the critical care setting it involves decisions that affect both the admission and discharge of patients from the unit. A central issue in the triage of patients is the allocation of resources to ensure appropriate and maximal potential outcomes for individuals, while using resources in the most effective overall manner.

The pressure to move patients into and out of the ICU can vary enormously between institutions, depending on a variety of factors. These include the size, location, and case mix of a hospital, as well as local practice styles. Bed availability and hospital protocols influence decisions to admit and discharge as well.[20] There is growing concern that patient outcome may be affected by the selection criteria used to admit or exclude patients from critical care services.

To fully evaluate these issues, an accurate assessment of patients' clinical characteristics prior to ICU admission is required. Using such an evaluation physicians will be able to better select those patients in greatest need of critical care services. Furthermore, it may allow for a more objective determination of those most likely to benefit from ICU admission. These determinations can help structure admission decisions for patients unlikely to receive active therapeutic intervention, as well as those destined to die regardless of treatment.

LOW RISK PATIENTS

Depending on the ICU examined, anywhere from 20 to 80 percent of admissions are for monitoring, not for acute life support, and are therefore potentially discretionary. Recent work indicates that acute physiologic abnormality is a powerful predictor of the potential risk for a patient admitted for monitoring subsequently requiring and receiving active ICU therapies.[21] For many patients designated as "low risk monitor," there are legitimate questions as to whether the patient is best treated in an ICU, in a less intensive step-down unit, or on the general hospital floor. In those instances when a patient is admitted, it would be helpful to know when discharge can be safely considered.

The utility of identifying patients who are admitted to medical and surgical ICUs with a low risk of receiving active therapy[22] was studied in 5790 patients in 13 United States tertiary care hospitals; 1941 patients required only monitoring during their critical care admission. Seventy percent of these patients were predicted to have a < 10 percent risk of needing active treatment by use of routine measures of severity of illness. Only 58 patients, or 4.3 percent, of these low risk patients actually received active therapeutic intervention. These results are summarized in Table 46-4.

Thus, a significant proportion of patients admitted to the ICUs studied were at low risk of requiring active critical care therapies. An objective appraisal of relative risks can complement physician judgment by providing a more precise evaluation of a patient's likelihood of requiring active therapy subsequent to admission.

PATIENTS UNLIKELY TO RECOVER

In addition to the patients who are not likely to receive active or distinctive ICU therapy, there are groups of patients for whom critical care is not successful in reversing the effects of a severe acute illness. Some individuals are at high risk of short-term mortality despite aggressive intervention. Some patients in these circumstances are candidates for setting therapeutic limits or for withdrawal of life-sustaining therapies (see Chap. 185). The decision to forego critical care treatment is complex and fraught with emotion. Nevertheless, such decisions are made with increasing frequency.

The systematic collection of fundamental patient characteristics such as disease and disease severity is leading to reliable and accurate estimates of the probability of mortality for many of these severely ill patients. The decision to withhold intensive care for these patients will hopefully be enhanced by better assessments of outcome. It is becoming increasingly evident that physicians will rely on these physiologic estimates of mortality risk as these appraisals of outcome become more accurate.[23] Although physicians may initially be uncomfortable with explicit probabilities, decisions incorporating such probability statements could improve the overall quality of patient care.[24,25] The crucial issue in the selection of patients for intensive care becomes ensuring access to those who will clearly benefit, while limiting admission of patients who will not. Strategies need to be developed to monitor outcomes of those denied ICU admission to ensure that they receive high quality care appropriate for their illness.

A recent study highlights how problematic these decisions may be.[26] This study was designed to ascertain pa-

TABLE 46-4 Characteristics of 5790 ICU Admissions Categorized by Initial Condition

	Low Risk Monitor (<10%)	High Risk Monitor (>10%)	Initially Actively Treated
No. of patients	1358	583	3849
Mean APS (first day)	4.67	11.34	12.35
Mean total TISS (entire ICU stay)	27.00	64.50	116.10
% actively treated	4.30	18.50	100.00[a]
ICU length of stay (days)	2.12	3.95	4.60
Death rates			
ICU	0.50	5.30	14.40
Hospital	420	16.30	22.00

[a] By definition.

SOURCE: Adapted from Reference 22, with permission.

tient and family preferences for life-sustaining care in a cohort of patients who had experienced ICU care. The results indicated that the vast majority of patients and immediate family members of those who died would be extremely willing to undergo ICU care even for a 1-month extension of life. This was irrespective of age, functional status, perceived quality of life, or the individual's actual ICU experience. Individual self-determination and societal needs to constrain utilization of health care resources may be difficult to reconcile.

ASSESSING QUALITY OF CARE

Within intensive care it is becoming apparent that hospital mortality rates, when properly risk adjusted, could be used to assess quality. In one review of outcome data for 13 United States hospitals (in which APACHE II scores and disease were used to control for variations in patient characteristics), 2 hospitals were identified with actual death rates significantly different from predicted.[27] One hospital had a standardized mortality ratio (observed death rate: predicted death rate) of 0.59 whereas another hospital had a ratio of 1.59. Substantial differences were noted retrospectively in the clinical and organizational process of care between the two institutions. The hospital with lower than expected mortality performance had 24-h in-unit physician coverage, a full-time ICU director, and comprehensive nursing continuing education. In addition, patients received, on average, larger amounts of skilled nursing as measured by TISS. Most importantly, the hospital with a better than predicted mortality performance had open and effective communication between the nursing and medical staffs. In contrast, the hospital with worse than expected outcome did not have such clinical or organizational characteristics and exhibited poor communication between physicians and nurses. This study supports the hypothesis that the process of care can have an impact on outcome in both positive and deleterious ways. These findings have led to a prospective multi-institutional study evaluating the potential links between the process of care and outcome in critical care.[6]

There are still serious obstacles to making this approach to quality assessment a valid and reproducible technique. Even if adequate control of all relevant patient attributes that influence outcome can be achieved, there are several other legitimate threats to the widespread use of mortality rates for review of the quality of care.

First, solely as a consequence of statistical selection and random variation, a hospital could become a statistical outlier. However, over time these aberrations are expected to be self-correcting.

Secondly, hospital discharge practices, patient and family preferences, and the selection of alternative sites for death, such as nursing home or hospice facilities, can also have an impact on hospital mortality statistics. As a consequence, in-hospital mortality should be assessed within a context of postdischarge deaths. Although deaths that occur after hospitalization may not entirely reflect hospital care because of intervening medical events, they may serve to uncover disparities in death rates because of the time selected for discharge.[28]

Until recently there has also not existed a national standard for comparison of outcomes in critical care. The completion of the APACHE III study may identify a tool for a national mortality-based performance assessment standard for all hospitals with more than 200 beds. This will be accomplished by including hospitals of varying size, location, and teaching status within the cohort of randomly selected participating study hospitals. The data base of approximately 17,500 patients will allow statistically powerful comparisons of outcome between individuals and hospitals. In time it is hoped that such a representative data base will continue to grow. This will allow for continued refinement in the accuracy of the outcome data and for incorporation of changes in clinical care over time as technology and knowledge evolve.

A final issue regarding the quality of ICU care and its link to mortality remains. If mortality rates are tied to the quality of clinical care and clinical decision-making, what are the normative standards that are most appropriately applied to an institution? Should hospital outcome be compared only to outcomes for hospitals with similar characteristics such as size, geographic location, and teaching status, or should universal standards apply for all institutions? To date no consensus on these questions has been achieved.

Hospital mortality data may prove to accurately distinguish those institutions providing better than expected care as well as those providing suboptimal care. The diagnostic and therapeutic decisions that make up the processes of care will remain open to scrutiny. Nevertheless, our current sophistication regarding the interpretation of these data does not allow us to make unqualified statements pertaining to the quality of care. It is apparent that many issues need to be addressed and understood when evaluating mortality data as a definitive marker for the quality of clinical care.

There is also a need to consider severity-adjusted outcomes other than mortality in an ongoing evaluation of quality in critical care. The occurrence of morbid events can have a profound impact on the length and quality of survival. To this end investigators are beginning to evaluate additional measures of outcome to study the process of care and the relationships to outcome and quality. These measures include an analysis of the association of length of stay to disease severity. In addition, evaluating events such as nosocomial infection, the use of invasive technology such as pulmonary artery flow directed catheters, and rates of reintubation after extubation or readmission to the ICU after recent discharge may help determine quality of care. Appropriate control for patient specific illness, physiologic abnormalities, age, and chronic health using well-validated severity of illness measures should facilitate these analyses.

CLINICAL INVESTIGATION

The most direct method of documenting the impact of new therapies or diagnostic strategies is by a randomized controlled clinical trial (RCT). RCTs are often difficult to perform because of their expense or the large numbers of pa-

TABLE 46-5 Base Line Characteristics of Two Randomly Selected Groups of Respiratory Failure Patients*

Characteristics	Group I	Group II	p-Value
No. of patients	26	24	
Age, year	64	61.6	0.62
Male, %	31	35	0.77
Poor chronic respiratory status, %†	21	26	0.52
FI_{O_2}	60.2	56.5	0.63
pH	7.38	7.35	0.44
P_{O_2}	74.8	85.3	0.36
P_{CO_2}	44.0	42.7	0.83
$(A - a)D_{O_2}$	326.6	297.4	0.54
Heart rate	122.2	129.0	0.35
Mean blood pressure	87.0	82.4	0.63
Unassisted respiratory rate	38.3	36.9	0.69
Temperature	36.9	38.4	0.30
Hematocrit, %	38.1	38.0	0.96
White blood cell count	17.5	12.6	0.02
Serum BUN	43.0	28.4	0.14
Serum creatinine	1.8	2.3	0.57

*All values reported are mean values except number of subjects, sex, and chronic health status.
†Defined as shortness of breath on mild exertion (<2 blocks) 6 months prior to hospitalization.
SOURCE: From: J Chron Dis 37(6):455–463, 1984, reprinted with permission.

tients required to demonstrate a statistically significant benefit of a new medical approach to diagnosis or treatment. For some scientific questions, performing a controlled trial is not ethically feasible. The alternative is to perform observational studies using historical or case control analysis.

In either type of study, the investigators need to know whether the study groups under consideration are comparable by virtue of having equivalent pretreatment risk for the outcome being assessed. Most commonly, researchers address susceptibility bias by randomizing patients and performing univariate comparisons of mean demographic and physiologic variables. Unfortunately, comparison of mean values is an imprecise measure of differences between groups because it does not accurately assess and account for the prior probability of an outcome for each patient. Additionally, in complex medical situations this comparison of means does not reflect the interaction between the variables studied nor does it account for threshold values of clinical importance. Consequently, univariate comparison of mean values does not identify the real distribution of individual patient risk across groups and is therefore an inadequate measure of severity of illness.

An example of a hypothetical research trial illustrates this more clearly. Using a data base of patients admitted to an ICU, 50 consecutive patients with respiratory failure secondary to infection were randomly assigned to group 1 or group 2. Severity of illness was compared using important mean values versus using APACHE II. As demonstrated in Table 46-5, with the exception of white blood cell count, there were no significant differences in mean values. Further, there was no difference in the need for ventilatory support. However, using the APACHE II risk stratification for each individual patient in the two groups, the two groups are not equivalent. Based on each patient's severity of illness and prior probability of risk, the patients in group 1 had a predicted death rate of 37 percent, whereas those in group 2 had a 27 percent predicted risk of death. Furthermore, there was a nonlinear relationship between the acute physiology score and outcome, demonstrating the interrelationship of other variables including age and chronic health status on outcome.

This example highlights that although a comparison of mean values appeared to ensure adequate randomization between two groups of patients, this was not actually true. Performing a multivariate risk assessment using APACHE in this hypothetical randomization revealed differences in the two groups that would not be otherwise apparent. Using these two groups of different patients in an actual trial might have led to erroneous conclusions regarding the efficacy of an intervention under investigation. It is therefore essential that accurate risk assessment of patients in clinical studies be performed to ensure the adequacy of randomization.

A recent clinical study comparing antibiotic therapy in intraabdominal infections demonstrates the use of severity of illness scores within an RCT.[29] The experimental design was intended to overcome deficiencies in previous studies limited by inadequate sample size and stratification of pretreatment patient severity of illness. Using strict entry criteria in this prospective, randomized trial and APACHE II as a single numerical descriptor of severity of illness to stratify patient risk, study participants were evaluated for outcome of the abdominal infection. Using APACHE II, the authors were able to ensure that the control arm was representative of the group of patients in the study arm. Furthermore, by using the APACHE score as a continuous variable, the authors were able to show a continuous relationship between treatment failure, mortality, and APACHE score, and succeeded in decreasing the size of the comparative groups while attaining sufficient statistical power.

Future Directions

Current research efforts are directed toward improving the accuracy and utility of prognostic scoring systems. The value of assessing severity of illness will become apparent to the clinician at the bedside when information is provided in real time to assist in individual patient decision-making. The capability of prognostic systems to provide this information will become a reality as current efforts to automate data collection are achieved. As data bases continue to expand, improvement and refinement in the predictive ability of these systems will be possible.

Serial predictions over time may prove to have clinical utility. Intuitively, patients who improve rapidly with ICU care are more likely to have successful outcomes. Investigators using the MPM have published models using that system at 48 and 72 h into ICU care. Others have used a modification of APACHE II to stratify the likelihood of ICU survival and eventual hospital discharge over time. These results indicate that proportional changes in scores between ICU admission and the fourth day of ICU stay were accurate in predicting outcome for 87 percent of survivors and 75 percent of nonsurvivors.[30]

The proliferation of new and expensive technologies will continue to expand our therapeutic capabilities. Our ability to determine which of these new modes of diagnosis and therapy are of actual benefit will improve with the continued refinement of prognostic scoring systems. Physicians will also continue to be called on to make difficult ethical decisions regarding the appropriateness of initiating, limiting, and withdrawing care. As prognostic scoring systems' data bases grow and are refined they should become useful for individual prognostication and provide assistance with these decisions.

References

1. Knaus WA, Wagner DP, Loirat P, et al: A comparison of intensive care in the USA and France. Lancet ii:642, 1982.
2. Zimmerman JE, Knaus WA, Judson JA, et al: Patient selection for intensive care: A comparison of New Zealand and U.S. hospitals. Crit Care Med 16:318, 1988.
3. Petty TL, Lakshminarayan S, Sahn SA, et al: Intensive respiratory care unit: Review of ten years experience. JAMA 34:322, 1975.
4. Hook EW, Horton CA, Schaberg DR: Failure of intensive care unit support to influence mortality from pneumococcal bacteremia. JAMA 249:1055, 1983.
5. Task Force on Guidelines—Society of Critical Care Medicine. Recommendations for intensive care unit admission and discharge criteria. Crit Care Med 16:807, 1988.
6. APACHE III Study Design: Analytic plan for evaluation of severity and outcome. Zimmerman, JE (ed): Crit Care Med 17:S169, 1989.
7. Kalb PE, Miler DH: Utilization strategies for intensive care units. JAMA 26:2389, 1989.
8. Jennett B: Resource allocation for the severely brain damaged. Arch Neurol 33:595, 1976.
9. Killip T III, Kimball JT: Treatment of myocardial infarction in a coronary care unit. A two year experience with 2150 patients. Am J Cardiol 20:457, 1967.
10. Ranson JHC, Rifkind KM, Roses DF, et al: Prognostic signs and the role of operative management in acute pancreatitis. Surg Gynecol Obstet 139:69, 1974.
11. Cullen DJ, Civetta JM, Briggs BA, et al: Therapeutic intervention scoring system: A method for quantitative comparison of patient care. Crit Care Med 2:57, 1974.
12. Knaus WA, Zimmerman JE, Wagner DP, et al: APACHE—Acute physiology and chronic health evaluation: A physiologically based classification system. Crit Care Med 9:591, 1981.
13. LeGall JR, Loirat P, Alperovitch A, et al: A simplified acute physiology score (SAPS). Crit Care Med 12:975, 1984.
14. Teres D, Lemeshow S, Avrunin JS, et al: Validation of the mortality prediction model for ICU patients. Crit Care Med 15:208, 1987.
15. Yeh TS, Pollack MM, Ruttimann UE, et al: Validation of a physiologic stability index for use in critically ill infants and children. Pediatr Res 18:445, 1984.
16. Pollack MM, Ruttimann UE, Getson PR: Pediatric risk of mortality (PRISM) score. Crit Care Med 16:1110, 1988.
17. Knaus WA, Draper EA, Wagner DP, et al: APACHE II: Severity of disease classification system. Crit Care Med 13:818, 1985.
18. Moreau R, Soupison T, Vauquelin P, et al: Comparison of two simplified severity scores (SAPS and APACHE II) for patients with acute myocardial infarction. Crit Care Med 17:409, 1989.
19. Lemeshow S, Teres D, Avrunin SJ, et al: Refining intensive care unit outcome prediction by using changing probabilities of mortality. Crit Care Med 16:470, 1989.
20. Sax FL, Charlson ME: Utilization of critical care units: A prospective study of physician triage and patient outcome. Arch Intern Med 147:929, 1987.
21. Wagner DP, Knaus WA, Draper EA, et al: Identification of low-risk monitor patients within a medical-surgical intensive care unit. Med Care 21:425, 1983.
22. Wagner DP, Knaus WA, Draper EA: Identification of low-risk monitor admissions to medical-surgical ICUs. Chest 92:423, 1987.
23. McClish DK, Powell S: How well can physicians estimate mortality in a medical intensive care unit? Med Decis Making 9:125, 1989.
24. Ruark JE, Raffin TA: The Stanford University Medical Center Committee on Ethics: Initiating and withdrawing life support: Principles and practice in adult medicine. N Engl J Med 318:25, 1988.
25. Griner PF: The relationship between managerial and clinical decision making in the hospital. Med Decis Making 8:151, 1988.
26. Danis M, Patrick DL, Southerland CJ, et al: Patients' and families' preferences for medical intensive care. JAMA 260:797, 1988.
27. Knaus WA, Draper EA, Wagner DP, et al: An evaluation of outcome from intensive care in major medical centers. Ann Intern Med 104:410, 1986.
28. Dubois RW, Rogers WH, Moxlet JH, et al: Hospital inpatient mortality: Is it a predictor of quality? N Engl J Med 317:1674, 1987.
29. Salomkin JS, Delline EP, Christou NV, et al: Results of a multicenter trial comparing imipenem/cilastatin to tobramycin/clindamycin for intra-abdominal infections. Ann Surg 212:581, 1990.
30. Bion JF, Aitchison TC, Edlin SA, et al: Sickness scoring and response to treatment as predictor of outcome from critical illness. Intensive Care Med 14:167, 1988.

SECTION C

STABILIZATION AND TRANSPORT OF THE CRITICALLY ILL

Chapter 47

PRINCIPLES OF CRITICAL CARE MEDICINE RESUSCITATION AND STABILIZATION

WILLIAM F. RUTHERFORD
EDWARD A. PANACEK

Resuscitation (from the Latin, *resuscitare:* to revive, to restore consciousness, to restore life) and stabilization may operationally be defined as the interventions designed to restore and maintain airway, breathing, and circulation in their broadest senses. Far from being separate processes designed to simply achieve and maintain normal values for pulse, blood pressure, and respiratory rate, when approached optimally, resuscitation and stabilization are integrated vertically and horizontally into a continuum of effort, the goal of which is to bring order out of physiologic chaos. Though the most extreme illustration, the patient in cardiopulmonary arrest is certainly not the only candidate in need of resuscitation. The concept of resuscitation applies equally well to the patient in septic shock for example, who is maintaining a "normal" systolic blood pressure, but yet is at risk for hypoperfusion-induced acute tubular necrosis; myocardial ischemia brought about by increased myocardial oxygen consumption; or respiratory failure secondary to adult respiratory distress syndrome (ARDS) or respiratory muscle fatigue.

The Tempo of Assessment and Treatment

Initially, achieving this goal often requires aggressive care ("resuscitation") based on a rapid but disciplined and methodical assessment of the situation, focused on the physical evidence of vitality. While there may be times when the classic internal medicine approach of a comprehensive history followed by the performance of a meticulous physical examination and the integration of laboratory data leading to the development of a hypothesis is appropriate, such times do not occur until after much of resuscitation and stabilization has been accomplished. Rather, during a resuscitation the intensivist must use an approach of simultaneous evaluation and treatment. By focusing initially on the *life-threatening* physiologic aberrations and immediately instituting measures to correct them, and then broadening the evaluation and therapy to include all organ systems in a progressively more detailed fashion, the intensivist will provide initial support for the patient, and ultimately identify the critical lesion or lesions in a timely fashion.

Simultaneously, the intensivist must develop a sense of direction of physiologic flow over some unspecified period of time (usually hours), as well as an estimate of where the patient is likely to equilibrate. This is most obvious in the case of a patient who may need to be transported either for diagnostic or therapeutic interventions. This can be accomplished by asking anticipatory questions such as "What is the worst that can happen if current physiologic trends continue?" and "What else is likely to or can possibly go wrong?" The answers to such questions are based on a sound knowledge of the disease processes, as well as deliberation on the facts of the case in a more systematic fashion than occurs during the stereotypical approach to resuscitation. As an example, a patient in septic shock from pneumonia may well respond with increased blood pressure when adequate intravascular volume is restored. However, experienced clinicians will be aware that the $(A - a)O_2$ is likely to increase over the next several hours, as the supplemental fluid is translocated into the alveoli. Anticipation of deterioration should lead to closer monitoring and earlier performance of ultimately necessary interventions such as intubation, when the patient is in relatively better shape to withstand the stresses imposed. This aspect of resuscitation and stabilization may be summarized as a "sooner rather than later" orientation.

It is useful to approach this objective by specifically considering the current status, physiologic reserve, and potential for deterioration of each organ system or problem rather than just the primary diagnosis, and to develop a plan of action. No disease or physiologic perturbation should be considered as an isolated entity. For example, the patient with urosepsis must have a detailed evaluation of cardiopulmonary sufficiency, renal function, hepatobiliary function, nutritional status, neurologic status, and immunocompetence including the integrity of the skin. The indicated interventions can be thought of as the formal "stabilization" phase, being mindful that such a separation of the resuscitation and stabilization components is largely artificial and best used for purposes of illustration.

Stabilization of the critically ill patient includes several specific points which must be addressed. First, it is imperative that pathophysiologic oscillations such as extreme swings in blood pressure be reduced. Second, the clinician must also provide for as much physiologic tolerance as possible to "buffer" the impact of new insults. For example, the patient with a gastrointestinal bleed may have a normal heart rate and blood pressure after resuscitation with crystalloid, but be far better able to tolerate a recurrence of the bleed if the hematocrit of 20 percent is elevated by transfusion. Third, the institution of appropriate prophylactic measures should occur promptly, such as restoring potassium and magnesium depleted by diuretic therapy in a chronically hypertensive patient with an acute myocardial infarction. Such efforts may result in the avoidance of ventricular arrhythmias altogether. Finally, the root cause of the deterioration, such as mucous plugging leading to hypoxemia, must be dealt with immediately during stabilization so that the cycle is not repeated.

The zeal to address each derangement must be tempered by an understanding of the consequences of each intervention. For example, while the patient in septic shock from pneumonia described above may well have an additional increase in cardiac output with further elevation of pulmonary artery wedge pressure above 6 to 10 cmH_2O, the resulting predictable increase in the $(A - a)O_2$ due to increased extravascular lung water may be prohibitive,[1] particularly in those patients with low plasma colloid oncotic pressure. Additionally, the desirable ideal range for measurable parameters may vary with the particular disease process. The individual suffering from an acute myocardial infarction may achieve an adequate cardiac output with little increase in myocardial oxygen consumption by elevating the pulmonary artery wedge pressure closer to 16 cmH_2O,[2] rather than by excessive use of β_2 agonist such as dobutamine. In reality, many patients require a combination of therapies, each used in a judicious fashion which maximizes the benefits and minimizes the cost of the particular intervention. Alternatively, different patients with the same acute problem may require substantially different approaches due to their underlying state of health. The 20-year-old with a subarachnoid hemorrhage can withstand greater cardiovascular stress imposed by attempts to overcome the cerebral vasospasm than the 68-year-old with the same diagnosis and complication.

Techniques of Resuscitation and Stabilization

As might be anticipated from the above comments, certain factors are common in all attempts at resuscitation and stabilization. It is not the intent of this section to regurgitate those fundamentals which are found in basic texts, but rather to emphasize their importance and to provide practical guidelines for their implementation in the care of the critically ill.

ASSESSMENT

As outlined above, the need to act must not replace the need to assess the patient in an organized and efficient fashion. Action and thought are not mutually exclusive in either time or space, and it is only when thought and action are combined that the patient receives the best possible care.

AIRWAY AND BREATHING

Control of the airway and provision of adequate ventilation are immediate objectives in all patients. The only circumstances which take precedence are the need to protect the patient from further injury (fire, electrocution, etc.), initial attempts at defibrillation, and compression of exsanguinating hemorrhage. This is not to say that every patient must be intubated, but rather that immediate assessment of airway and breathing coupled with measures to correct the deficiencies revealed are almost always the highest priorities.

Assessment of respiratory sufficiency must not be prolonged nor complicated. The agitated or confused patient should be presumed to be hypoxemic until proven otherwise, and supplemental oxygen should be administered. The patient breathing at the same rate as the examiner and speaking in full sentences does not require an arterial blood gas determination to know that intubation is not necessary immediately. Conversely, the hypotensive septic patient whose blood pressure continues to decline despite volume expansion and who is becoming irrational does not need an arterial blood-gas determination to indicate that intubation is necessary.

The classic indications for intubation include the need for control of the airway, excessive secretions, hypoxemia, and ventilatory failure, as well as the immediate likelihood of any of these. Those who care for the critically ill must be skilled in evaluating and responding to the above parameters clinically and be willing to act before laboratory confirmation is available.

A fifth, generic indication for intubation (and mechanical ventilation) exists when the cost of breathing contributes to the worsening of some pathophysiologic process or prevents resuscitation, stabilization, and/or recovery. For example, a patient in cardiogenic shock may maintain parameters such as respiratory rate, Pa_{O_2}, etc., which, narrowly interpreted, do not signal respiratory failure. However, intubation and mechanical ventilation may well reduce the work of breathing, and thus the overall burden on the failing myocardium, therefore benefiting the patient. Another common example is the therapeutic mechanical ventilation of a patient with a head injury to reduce intracranial pressure, even though the arterial blood-gas values are normal.

Almost any single measurement or value in the critically ill patient must be interpreted as it relates to other relevant values, and arterial blood-gas values are no exception. For example, a Pa_{O_2} of 70 mmHg has an entirely different significance depending on whether the accompanying Pa_{CO_2} is 15, 40, or 70 mmHg and on the value of the fraction inspired oxygen (FI_{O_2}). In the first example, the patient is *not* "oxygenating well" but rather is only "not hypoxemic" and is achieving adequate oxygenation only through extreme hyperventilation. In the last example, (assuming room air), the patient's lungs are indeed serving extremely well as an air-blood interface, but the patient may well die if attention is not turned to ventilation. Single parameter, noninvasive indicators such as pulse oximetry are extremely valuable, but must be interpreted in a fashion similar to arterial blood-gas determinations, where respiratory rate and tidal volume are considered. Additionally, presently available pulse oximeters often fail due to poor perfusion of the extremities in the patients most in need of rapid assessment. Capnometry depends on spontaneous circulation, so that its use during a cardiac resuscitation is primarily that of announcing the return of spontaneous circulation.[3] It may be extremely useful in detecting instability of a patient's respiratory drive. Increased end-tidal carbon dioxide values may indicate gradual loss of respiratory drive due to fatigue or altered mental status, whereas decreasing end-tidal carbon dioxide levels may herald hypoxemia.

CIRCULATION

Inadequate perfusion can certainly occur in the presence of an "adequate" blood pressure. Therefore, assessment of circulation should include not only blood pressure and heart rate, but indicators of end-organ perfusion such as the degree of pallor and the temperature of the extremities, the presence of mottling of the skin, nailbed return, the quality of mentation and level of consciousness, and urine output.

The three basic components of the circulatory system are the circulating volume and its composition, the adequacy of the heart as a pump, and the tone and integrity of the vascular pathway. Each component must be reviewed when inadequate perfusion is identified during a resuscitation. A pulmonary artery catheter facilitates such a review, but its absence does not preclude analyzing the problem in such a conceptual fashion.

VOLUME EXPANSION. The heart simply cannot pump what is not returned to it, and there is a maximum degree to which vessels can constrict. A variety of conditions produce either relative or absolute hypovolemia, as shown in Table 47-1. Therefore, provision of adequate circulating volume must be accomplished. Generally, this requires the administration of crystalloid or colloid solutions, or less often, cellular suspensions. While the choice of volume expanders[4] is beyond the scope of this chapter, hemoglobin must be adequate to provide adequate oxygen transport. However, evidence suggests that, at least in some organ beds, expansion of the red cell mass beyond a certain point does not increase tissue oxygen delivery due to the increase in viscosity and subsequent inefficiency in distribution of flow.

If it is decided that volume expansion is required, then such expansion should be achieved by bolus administration of the chosen fluid. The desired therapeutic goal is to elevate the ventricular filling pressure and assess the response. If low filling pressure is the only defect, then blood pressure, urine flow, mentation, etc. should respond rapidly. Simply increasing a normal saline drip to 200 mL/h (a common error) does not constitute a fluid bolus, and one may have to wait several hours to see the beneficial effect of such a maneuver. Rather, in such situations, volume expanders should be administered as rapidly as possible. If one is concerned about precipitating fluid overload, then the correct approach is to administer smaller volumes, for example, 250-mL aliquots.

TABLE 47-1 Examples of Hypovolemia

True Volume Loss
Bleeding (trauma, gastrointestinal ulceration, coagulopathy, etc.)
Interstitial translocation (third-spacing—burns, sepsis)
Excessive gastrointestinal loss (emesis, diarrhea)
Inappropriate diuresis (diabetes insipidus, diuretic abuse)
Inadequate intake
Excessive insensible loss
Expansion of Vascular Space
Medications
Loss of vasomotor tone ("spinal shock," hypoadrenalism)
Sepsis
Decrease in Venous Return
True volume loss, as above
Increased intrathoracic pressure (tension pneumothorax, PEEP, intrinsic PEEP)
Direct venous obstruction (superior vena cava syndrome, gravid uterus)
Decrease in Ventricular/Pericardial Compliance
Myocardial infarction
Constrictive pericarditis
Cardiac tamponade

The choice of catheters used for fluid bolus administration is not a mundane matter. It is worth understanding that the rate of flow is directly related to the fourth power of the diameter and inversely related to the length of the catheter (Pouiselle's law). Therefore, short, large bore catheters are preferable. A No. 8 to 8.5 French introducer connected directly to the solution administration set makes an ideal access, and it is our catheter of choice for rapid, massive volume resuscitation. An existing central venous pressure or pulmonary artery catheter may be the only route available, but one must understand that the rate of administration will be slow unless a pressure bag or infusion pump is applied, because of both the small diameter of such lines and their length.

VENTRICULAR FUNCTION. The components of cardiac output are well understood, and include heart rate, inotropic state, preload, and afterload. Any or all of these may need to be manipulated during resuscitation and stabilization. Even the most well-conditioned heart is unlikely to generate sufficient cardiac output to provide adequate cellular perfusion with a rate in the low 30s, and rarely will diastolic filling time be sufficiently preserved to achieve the same goal when the heart rate exceeds 160. Thus, the hypotensive, bradycardic patient should have either pharmacologic (atropine or a β_1 agonist) or electrical elevation of the heart rate, whereas the patient with supraventricular or ventricular tachycardia may require physiologic (Valsalva, carotid sinus massage), pharmacologic (adenosine, verapamil, digoxin, lidocaine), or electrical (overdrive pacing or synchronized cardioversion) therapy to restore cardiac output. Vasoconstrictive agents have no place in the therapy of tachycardic hypotensive patients, except in an indirect fashion to induce a vagal reflex in the tachycardic patient with a reentrant supraventricular tachycardia.

The inotropic state of the heart may be adversely affected by a variety of conditions, including electrolyte, acid-base, and metabolic disturbances; medications and toxins; extremes in body temperature; and chronic and acute disease states. Should the intensivist have reasonable suspicion of a depressed inotropic state, therapy directed at the above factors, including empiric use of inotropic catecholamines and vasodilating agents is warranted. Ideally, use of such agents is directed on a long-term basis by hemodynamic monitoring, but one must consider the additional physiologic stress and danger imposed by placing an unresuscitated patient with an unsecured airway under sterile drapes where he cannot be visually monitored to obtain central venous access. In some patients, resuscitation and stabilization may need to be well underway before it is safe to place a pulmonary artery catheter.

VASCULAR INTEGRITY AND TONE. At present no direct therapy is available to halt the diffuse capillary leak which can lead to impressive fluid loss in a large number of pathologic states. The extravascular fluid accumulation caused by such a leak is most problematic in the lungs, but direct effects on organs such as the brain and gastrointestinal tract, as well as the indirect burden imposed on the heart and other organs add significantly to morbidity and mortality.[1] The debate continues as to the contribution of various crystalloid versus colloid volume expanders to the rate and amount of leakage,[5–7] but by examining the Starling equation, it is clear that the oncotic pressure of the intravascular fluid is a major determinant of leakage, and should be addressed early in the patient's course, at least in terms of nutritional support.[8] The Starling equation also points to the role of intravascular hydrostatic pressure. In the quest to optimize ventricular output by providing adequate preload, the intensivist will need to refrain from volume overload which can worsen the effects of the capillary leak.

In contrast to vascular integrity, a number of agents, mostly catecholamines, can successfully alter vascular tone. For example, dopamine has vasodilating properties in low doses, positive inotropic properties in moderate doses, and vasoconstrictive properties in high doses, and exerts part of these effects indirectly through stimulation of release of endogenous norepinephrine.

The primary indication for the use of a vasoconstrictor is the absence of appropriate vasoconstriction in the setting of hypotension, such as the autonomic lability seen with high spinal injuries. Use of these agents in other situations should be considered a temporizing measure only, until the underlying problem can be adequately addressed. Extended use in the setting of hypovolemia is particularly fraught with complications such as ischemic damage to the extremities and organs such as the kidneys.

NEUROLOGIC FUNCTION

Neurologic status must be evaluated as part of the initial assessment, both because of the potentially devastating long-term impact of central nervous system lesions in their own right, as well as the obvious effect on airway and breathing. During the initial moments, neurologic status can be evaluated by the *AVPU* method;[9] that is, the patient is *alert*, or responds to *voice*, or responds only to *pain*, or is *unresponsive*. The second level of assessment includes evaluation of orientation and cognitive abilities, cranial and peripheral nervous function, cerebral motor and sensory function, cerebellar function, and elicitation of pathologic reflexes. It is imperative that hypoxia, hypercapnia, metabolic derangements such as acidemia and alkalemia, hypo- and hypercalcemia, and hyperammonemia, as well as drug effects always be prominently considered in the evaluation of a patient with altered mental status.

Special Situations

CARDIAC ARREST

Resuscitation, stabilization, and ultimate discharge of the patient who has suffered a cardiac arrest are only occasionally achieved. Successful resuscitation, defined as the presence of a pulse and blood pressure at the conclusion of the resuscitative effort, is accomplished in 0 to 50 percent,[10,11] depending on the setting and the diagnosis of the patient. Hospitalized patients who arrest tend to do poorly, since their deaths are often due to some progressive pathophysiologic process, as opposed to out-of-hospital patients who tend to suffer sudden death due to an arrhythmia. However, most studies indicate that 6 to 20 percent of patients who arrest in either setting are ultimately discharged.[12–14]

Though the percentage of successful resuscitations is quite low, the estimated 200,000 to 300,000 resuscitation attempts yearly result in a large number of patients who are returned to active lives. A major concern of those involved in resuscitation has been the impact of cerebral dysfunction both on survival and quality of life. The reported incidence of long-term neurologic dysfunction following resuscitation varies from 4 percent[15] to 59 percent.[16] Perhaps even more problematic is the finding in one study that more deaths in the immediate postresuscitation period of 1 week are associated with (and perhaps caused by) neurologic dysfunction than are associated with arrhythmias and cardiac pump failure.[17]

A concerted effort to develop a specific approach to cerebral resuscitation has been made over the past few decades.[18] This effort continues to explore both pharmacologic [e.g., barbiturates, calcium-entry blockers, free-radical scavengers, γ-aminobutyric acid (GABA)-inhibitors] and physical (e.g., hypothermia) methods for reducing the impact of ischemia and reperfusion injury, and methods such as hypertension-hemodilution-heparinization for promoting the return of cerebral circulation. Though brain-oriented intensive care seems to result in a modest improvement in outcome following resuscitation, none of the protocols investigated to date have resulted in a dramatic breakthrough. While the search for therapies to optimize cerebral resuscitation has by no means been abandoned,

TABLE 47-2 Treatment of Ventricular Fibrillation/Pulseless Ventricular Tachycardia

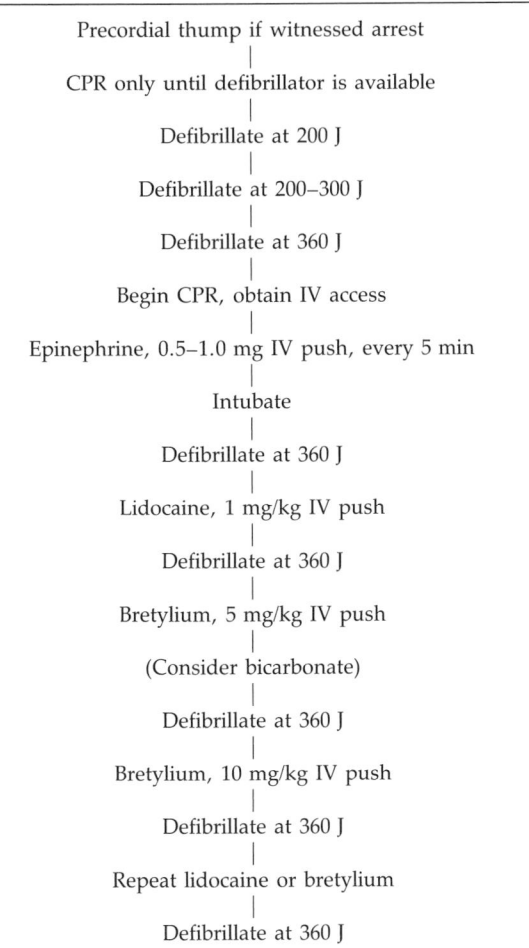

Precordial thump if witnessed arrest
|
CPR only until defibrillator is available
|
Defibrillate at 200 J
|
Defibrillate at 200–300 J
|
Defibrillate at 360 J
|
Begin CPR, obtain IV access
|
Epinephrine, 0.5–1.0 mg IV push, every 5 min
|
Intubate
|
Defibrillate at 360 J
|
Lidocaine, 1 mg/kg IV push
|
Defibrillate at 360 J
|
Bretylium, 5 mg/kg IV push
|
(Consider bicarbonate)
|
Defibrillate at 360 J
|
Bretylium, 10 mg/kg IV push
|
Defibrillate at 360 J
|
Repeat lidocaine or bretylium
|
Defibrillate at 360 J

there is a growing realization that the best thing for the brain is the rapid restoration of physiologically adequate circulation. As such, interest in methods of improving cardiac resuscitation, such as the use of higher doses of epinephrine or emergent cardiopulmonary bypass (both of which result in improved coronary and cerebral blood flow) are receiving increased attention.

Patients in cardiac arrest due to trauma have an even more dismal prognosis. There is some possibility of success with penetrating thoracic or abdominal trauma, provided the injury can be quickly located and adequate circulating volume restored. Beyond establishing control of the airway and ensuring adequate ventilation and initial volume resuscitation, continuation of efforts to resuscitate the victim of blunt trauma who is in cardiac arrest is without merit.

VENTRICULAR FIBRILLATION/PULSELESS VENTRICULAR TACHYCARDIA. Ventricular fibrillation is the most common cause of sudden death and the most amenable to treatment. Estimates of potential salvage from sudden death in this group of patients run as high as 80 percent, though large studies have generally reported a survival-to-discharge rate of approximately 30 to 40 percent.[19]

In an out-of-hospital population, one study documented that 84 percent of survivors of a cardiac arrest are defibrillated with one of the first two shocks. As such, the absolute priority in any attempt at resuscitation from ventricular fibrillation or pulseless ventricular tachycardia is defibrillation. All efforts should be directed at accomplishing this as rapidly as possible or facilitating its effectiveness. Patients in ICUs, cardiac catheterization laboratories, and special procedure areas should be defibrillated immediately, in accordance with current American Heart Association (AHA) recommendations (Table 47-2). Neither cardiopulmonary resuscitation (CPR) nor attempts at intubation should be instituted until after the failure of the first three defibrillation attempts, assuming a defibrillator is immediately available.

Once initial attempts at defibrillation have failed, attention should be turned to modifying the milieu of the heart so that it does respond to defibrillation. Major factors which are thought to influence cardiac responsiveness to defibrillation include oxygenation, acid-base status, and myocardial perfusion pressure.

Since oxygenation and ventilation are so critical, control of the airway is vital during a resuscitation. Though the guidelines set forth by the AHA indicate that intubation has a relatively low priority, many experienced clinicians perform intubation immediately after the initial defibrillation attempts, for the following reasons: **1.** Bag-valve-mask ventilation can result in gastric distention and embarrassment of diaphragmatic excursion, worsening the already poor ventilation which occurs with mask systems; **2.** In addition to poor ventilation, regurgitation and aspiration can occur unless the airway is protected; **3.** Since ventilation is ensured, the acid-base status can be more easily controlled (vide infra); **4.** Oxygenation is more easily achieved; and **5.** Epinephrine, atropine, and lidocaine can all be administered via the endotracheal tube, though their efficacy is not well established when given via this route.

Myocardial perfusion pressure (diastolic blood pressure minus right atrial pressure) of at least 15 mmHg appears to be critical for successful defibrillation.[11] The current recommendation for 0.5 to 1.0 mg epinephrine is based on work done in animals of approximately 10 kg in weight (0.1 mg/kg).[20] This suggests that the current dose of 0.01 to 0.02 mg/kg severely underdoses the adult patient. Recent work has established that myocardial perfusion pressure and myocardial blood flow in animal models is improved by using doses of epinephrine as high as 0.2 mg/kg.[21] Several case reports have appeared offering anecdotal evidence of superior efficacy of higher doses of epinephrine.[22] Numerous multicenter trials using higher doses of epinephrine during cardiac resuscitation are currently underway.

VENTRICULAR TACHYCARDIA WITH A PULSE. The appropriate measures in this condition depend on how well the patient is tolerating the arrhythmia, as shown in Table 47-3. Patients who have severe chest pain or who are hypotensive or otherwise evidencing poor tissue perfusion (pallor, diaphoresis, altered mental status) should be immediately cardioverted, whereas patients who are more tolerant of

TABLE 47-3 Ventricular Tachycardia with a Pulse

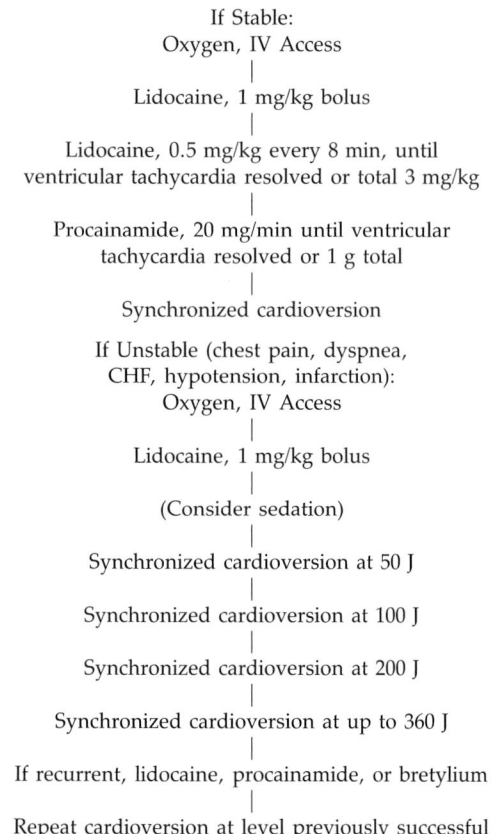

If Stable:
Oxygen, IV Access
|
Lidocaine, 1 mg/kg bolus
|
Lidocaine, 0.5 mg/kg every 8 min, until ventricular tachycardia resolved or total 3 mg/kg
|
Procainamide, 20 mg/min until ventricular tachycardia resolved or 1 g total
|
Synchronized cardioversion

If Unstable (chest pain, dyspnea, CHF, hypotension, infarction):
Oxygen, IV Access
|
Lidocaine, 1 mg/kg bolus
|
(Consider sedation)
|
Synchronized cardioversion at 50 J
|
Synchronized cardioversion at 100 J
|
Synchronized cardioversion at 200 J
|
Synchronized cardioversion at up to 360 J
|
If recurrent, lidocaine, procainamide, or bretylium
|
Repeat cardioversion at level previously successful

this rhythm may respond to antiarrhythmic medication or overdrive pacing. Should synchronized cardioversion become necessary in the "stable" patient, sedation with a short-acting barbiturate or benzodiazepine is imperative. It is likewise imperative to look for precipitating or aggravating conditions such as electrolyte disorders or drug toxicity.

ASYSTOLE/BRADYCARDIA. Resuscitation from asystole is quite rare, and it is the impression of many that successful resuscitations generally occur when the primary cause is hypoventilation. The patient who suddenly becomes asystolic in the ICU is probably quite different from the patient who progresses to asystole after passing through ventricular fibrillation or an idioventricular rhythm. There is some evidence that extreme vagal tone (as can be generated during intubation) can lead to asystole, and a very small trial resulted in the recommendation for the use of 1 mg atropine in this setting. Many intensivists instead recommend the initial use of a fully vagolytic dose of 2 mg, on the grounds that if the lack of cardiac activity is due to vagal tone, nothing is to be gained by stepwise elimination of such vagal tone, as recommended by the AHA (Table 47-4). Data in this area is sorely lacking.

Bradycardias should be treated when hemodynamically significant or when ventricular escape ectopy is apparent

TABLE 47-4 Asystole

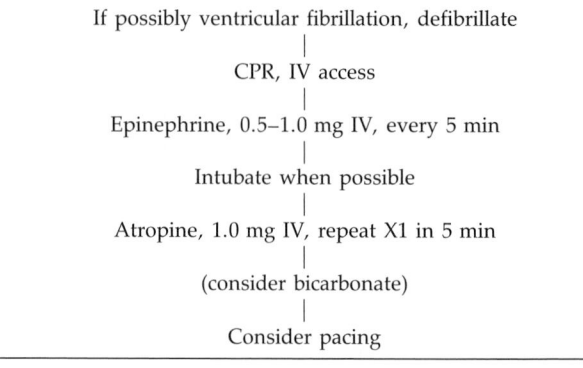

If possibly ventricular fibrillation, defibrillate
|
CPR, IV access
|
Epinephrine, 0.5–1.0 mg IV, every 5 min
|
Intubate when possible
|
Atropine, 1.0 mg IV, repeat X1 in 5 min
|
(consider bicarbonate)
|
Consider pacing

(Table 47-5). Atropine in progressive doses to a total of 2 mg can be followed by isoproterenol or a pacemaker. Because of the arrhythmogenic nature of isoproterenol as well as the increasing availability of transcutaneous pacemakers, many experienced clinicians might proceed to a pacemaker directly. Pacemakers are useful in the setting of disturbances in impulse conduction or formation, such as bradycardia with a pulse or 3° atrioventricular block without an adequate escape focus. Their efficacy in asystole has been generally disappointing.

ELECTROMECHANICAL DISSOCIATION (EMD). The presence of a complex with a very weak or absent pulse should immediately generate a search for the first six conditions in Table 47-6. Again, the heart simply cannot pump what it is not getting, and therefore hypovolemia should be considered whenever EMD is noted. Effective hypovolemia (absolute or relative) may occur because of exsanguination, vasodilating drugs, poor venous return due to high intrathoracic pressures, pericardial tamponade, or embolic obstruction of the pulmonary outflow tract.

Based on the above considerations, the presence of EMD should immediately lead to a rapid (<1 min) review of the

TABLE 47-5 Bradycardia

If sinus, junctional, 1° AVB, or type I 2° AVB, treat only if signs or symptoms present. If type II 2° AVB or 3° AVB, treat even if asymptomatic:

Atropine, 0.5 mg–1.0 mg IV
|
Repeat atropine every 5 min until total 2.0 mg
|
External pacemaker
or
Isoproterenol, 2–10 μg/min
|
Transvenous pacemaker

AVB = atrioventricular block.

TABLE 47-6 Electromechanical Dissociation—Causes and Therapy

Hypovolemia—Volume replacement
Tension pneumothorax—Needle thoracostomy, tube thoracostomy
Pericardial tamponade—Volume replacement, pericardiocentesis
Pulmonary embolus—Thrombolytic therapy
Acute valvular regurgitation—Afterload reduction, surgery
Myocardial wall rupture—Afterload reduction/pericardiocentesis, surgery
Idiopathic EMD—CPR, IV access, epinephrine, 0.5–1.0 mg, intubate, consider bicarbonate

patient's history and physical examination, focusing on predisposing conditions such as carcinoma of the lung or breast or suggestive physical findings such as unilateral decrease in breath sounds or a shift of the trachea. While the AHA guidelines recommend only epinephrine in standard dosages and supportive measures, many intensivists would recommend both a fluid challenge, as well as a high dose α agonist. In the adult patient who is easily ventilated and has no history of chest trauma or lung disease, empirical needle thoracostomy is probably not necessary. Pacemakers are of no value in EMD.

SUPRAVENTRICULAR TACHYCARDIA. The intensivist must differentiate situations such as hypoxemia, hypovolemia, pain, and fever, in which the resultant tachycardia is an appropriate physiologic response, from pathologic situations such as paroxysmal supraventricular tachycardia, accelerated junctional rhythm, and atrial fibrillation and flutter with rapid ventricular response. In the former, therapy is directed at removing the need for the increased heart rate by correcting whatever physiologic deficit exists. Therapy in the setting of pathologic rhythms is determined by the level of compromise. Patients who are hypotensive, experiencing chest pain, or are otherwise seriously threatened by the arrhythmia should be treated with synchronized cardioversion, using 50 to 360 J, whereas others less seriously threatened can be treated by vagotonic maneuvers and agents, overdrive pacing, and synchronized cardioversion if necessary. In this category, sedation and preparation for airway control must be achieved prior to cardioversion. It is imperative that precipitating and contributing factors such as hypoxemia, elevated right and left heart filling pressures, electrolyte disturbances, and drug toxicities be identified and corrected.

BICARBONATE. Recently some have pointed out the lack of efficacy of sodium bicarbonate in cardiac resuscitation.[23] It is clear that the best way to correct a metabolic acidosis produced by poor perfusion is to restore perfusion, independent of the controversy regarding the use of arterial or mixed venous blood-gas measurements as the standard by which acid-base balance is judged during a cardiac arrest. If bicarbonate administration is deemed necessary, it is imperative that the patient be adequately ventilated to handle the increased carbon dioxide which is rapidly generated. Because of the ease with which carbon dioxide crosses cell membranes compared to the more polar bicarbonate ion, some investigators are concerned about the generation of a paradoxical intracellular acidosis.[24] A few studies have used nonbicarbonate-based buffers, without clear results.

CALCIUM. Calcium is an excellent inotrope and may be effective in the patient with poor (but not absent) cardiac contractility secondary to decreased ionized calcium. Such situations may occur in the patient coming off a bypass pump or who has received massive transfusions such as in the setting of liver transplantation. Additionally, calcium is effective in reversing the vasodilation produced by calcium entry blockers such as verapamil. The use of calcium in the adult patient with asystole or EMD is without foundation or efficacy. Patients in asystole or EMD who receive calcium have the same survival rate as those who do not receive calcium.[25,26] Additionally, there is concern about the cytotoxic effects of calcium which could leak into ischemic cells.[27]

TRAUMA

Resuscitation and stabilization of trauma victims proceeds in the same methodical but efficient approach as outlined above, with certain specific practices which must be incorporated.[9] Since the subject is covered in more detail in other chapters, we will summarize the approach to the trauma patient and emphasize the differences from a primarily medical resuscitation.

During the *primary survey*, assessment and initial management of life-threatening conditions are addressed in the following order: **1.** airway maintenance with cervical spine control; **2.** breathing; **3.** circulation as measured by a capillary blanch test, with control of exsanguinating hemorrhage; **4.** assessment of neurologic deficit, using the AVPU method described above; and **5.** complete exposure of the patient. The crucial points which are commonly missed by those less familiar with resuscitation of the trauma victim are cervical immobilization until radiographic clearance to the C_7–T_1 interspace is obtained and exposure of the entire patient to identify all serious injuries.

Following the primary survey, the *resuscitation phase* is initiated with the provision of supplemental oxygen, institution of electrocardiographic (ECG) monitoring, and the placement of at least two short, large bore intravenous lines. Initial fluid resuscitation is begun with crystalloid solutions, with the use of type specific or low-titer O negative blood in patients unresponsive to 2 L crystalloid. The use of the pneumatic antishock garment is controversial, but may assist in placement of intravenous lines and initial resuscitation, as well as in stabilizing lower extremity and pelvic fractures. The garment does not produce an autotransfusion as had originally been thought, but rather, creates a high-resistance circuit in the lower extremities, leading to shunting of available blood into the relatively lower resistance torso. During this phase, a urinary catheter and naso- or orogastric catheter may be placed, provided they are not contraindicated by urethral transection or massive facial trauma, respectively.

At this point, the *secondary survey* is instituted, with reassessment of the vital signs, and rapid, thorough examination of the entire patient. The head and face must be closely examined for any signs of trauma and some gross estimation of vision attempted. Any sign of head or maxillofacial trauma leads to the presumption of cervical trauma until proven otherwise. In the absence of respiratory distress, protective helmets should be left in place until a lateral cervical radiograph is obtained. The chest, abdomen, pelvis, perineum, and extremities must be visually inspected, palpated, and auscultated where appropriate. Neurologic status is repeatedly assessed using the Glascow Coma Score as well as motor and sensory evaluation of the extremities. Appropriate laboratory studies are obtained during this phase, and usually include an arterial blood-gas determination, a complete blood count, a chemistry panel, blood for crossmatch, and a urinalysis. A toxicology screen is often appropriate. An ECG should be performed at this time, though the danger of an isolated myocardial contusion, as well as the sensitivity and specificity of the ECG for this condition, remain to be fully defined. Standard radiographic studies in the multiple trauma patient include cervical spine, chest, and pelvis, plus those dictated by clinical examination. At this point, the patient would generally proceed to indicated diagnostic testing or to definitive therapy for the identified injuries.

Philosophical and Ethical Considerations

One of the goals of resuscitation and stabilization (and indeed, of all of critical care) is the prevention of premature or unnecessary death, but not the prolongation of the act of dying. Those specializing in the care of the critically ill are often confronted with patients for whom the issues of appropriateness and desirability of resuscitation and stabilization have not been adequately addressed. The intensivist may be thrust into a role traditionally occupied by the primary care physician. In such settings the intensivist must usually presume that aggressive efforts are desired and appropriate and make the best effort to provide such care.

It is axiomatic that some patients become terminally ill, despite their own wishes and the wishes of family, as well as the heroic efforts and desires of the health care team. Should it be decided by an acceptable, ethical process that further care is inappropriate, futile, or simply not desired by the competent patient or legitimate surrogate decision-maker, the intensivist must be just as willing to shift the focus of care to issues of comfort and dignity. Such a decision may be appropriate in the early phases of resuscitation or after a lengthy and arduous course in the ICU. The change in focus must be accomplished without causing undue physical or emotional hardship on the patient or the patient's family. Perhaps all such decisions should be examined in the illumination provided by the late Jacob Javits, who stated, "It strikes me that in critical care the issues are three: realism, dignity, and love."

References

1. Rackow EC, Fein IA, Seigel J: The relationships of colloid osmotic-pulmonary artery wedge pressure gradient to pulmonary edema and mortality in critically ill patients. Chest 82:433, 1982.
2. Forrester JS, Diamond G, Chatterjee K, et al: Medical therapy of acute myocardial infarction by application of hemodynamic subsets. N Engl J Med 295:1356, 1976.
3. Garnett AR, Ornato JP, Gonzalez ER, et al: End-tidal carbon dioxide monitoring during cardiopulmonary resuscitation. JAMA 257:512, 1987.
4. Virgilio RW, Rice CL, Smith DE, et al: Crystalloid vs. colloid. Is one better? A randomized clinical study. Surgery 85:129, 1979.
5. Boutros AZ, Ruess R, Olson L, et al: Comparison of hemodynamic, pulmonary and renal effects of use of 3 types of fluid after major surgical procedures on the abdominal aorta. Crit Care Med 7:9, 1979.
6. Haupt MT, Rackow EC: Colloid osmotic pressure and fluid resuscitation with hetastarch, albumin and saline solutions. Crit Care Med 10:159, 1982.
7. Rackow EC, Falk JL, Fein IA, et al: Fluid resuscitation in shock: A comparison of cardiorespiratory effects of albumin, hetastarch, and saline solutions in patients with hypovolemic shock. Crit Care Med 11:839, 1989.
8. Blackburn GL, Thornton PA: Nutritional assessment of the hospitalized patient. Med Clin North Am 63:1103, 1979.
9. American College of Surgeons: *Advanced Trauma Life Support Student Manual,* Chap. 1. 1989.
10. Burns R, Graney MJ, Nichols LO: Prediction of in-hospital cardiopulmonary arrest outcome. Arch Intern Med 149:1318, 1989.
11. Paradis NA, Martin GB, Rivers EP, et al: Coronary perfusion pressure and the return of spontaneous circulation in human cardiopulmonary resuscitation. JAMA 263:1106, 1990.
12. Taffet GE, Teasdale TA, Luchi RJ: In-hospital cardiopulmonary resuscitation. JAMA 260:2069, 1988.
13. Bonnin MJ, Swor RA: Outcomes in unsuccessful field resuscitation attempts. Ann Emerg Med 18:507, 1989.
14. Eitel DR, Walton SL, Guerci AD, et al: Out-of-hospital cardiac arrest: A six-year experience in a suburban-rural system. Ann Emerg Med 17:808, 1988.
15. Bedell SE, Delbanco TL, Cook EF, et al: Survival after cardiopulmonary resuscitation in the hospital. N Engl J Med 309:569, 1983.
16. Longstreth WT, Inui TS, Cobb LA, et al: Neurologic recovery after out-of-hospital cardiac arrest. Ann Intern Med 98:588, 1983.
17. Myerburg RJ, Conde CA, Sung RJ, et al: Clinical, electrophysiologic, and hemodynamic profile of patients resuscitated from prehospital cardiac arrest. Am J Med 68:568, 1980.
18. Rogers MC, Kirsch JR: Current concepts in brain resuscitation. JAMA 261:3143, 1989.
19. American Heart Association. *Textbook of Advanced Cardiac Life Support, 2d ed.* Chap. 2, 1987.
20. Pearson JW, Redding JS: Epinephrine in cardiac resuscitation. Am Heart J 66:210, 1963.

21. Brown CG, Werman HA, Davis EA, et al: The effects of graded doses of epinephrine on regional myocardial blood flow during cardiopulmonary resuscitation in swine. Circulation 75:491, 1987.
22. Koscove EM, Paradis NA: Successful resuscitation from cardiac arrest using high-dose epinephrine therapy. JAMA 259:3031, 1988.
23. Guerci AD, Chandra N, Johnson E, et al: Failure of sodium bicarbonate to improve resuscitation from ventricular fibrillation in dogs. Circulation (suppl IV) IV:75, 1986.
24. Weisfeldt ML, Bishop RL, Greene HL: Effects of pH and P_{CO_2} on performance of ischemic myocardium, in Roy PE, Rona G (eds): *Recent Advances in Studies on Cardiac Structure and Metabolism*. Baltimore, University Park Press, 1975, 10:355.
25. Stueven HA, Thompson BM, Aprahamian C, et al: Calcium chloride: Reassessment of use in asystole. Ann Emerg Med 13:820, 1984.
26. Harrison EE, Amey BD: Use of calcium in electromechanical dissociation. Ann Emerg Med 13:844, 1984.
27. Fiskum G: Mitochondrial damage during cerebral ischemia. Ann Emerg Med 14:810, 1985.

Chapter 48

INTRAHOSPITAL TRANSPORT

WILLIAM F. RUTHERFORD
EDWARD A. PANACEK

It has been stated that when patients are transported from an ICU to a diagnostic area such as a radiology suite, they are not in a hospital, but only close to one. Such an indictment implies that patients do not receive the same level of care during the transport and in the diagnostic or procedure area as they receive in the ICU. Only a small amount of data support this position, yet it is likely that many ICU personnel would accept it as a truism.

Although this chapter deals with *intrahospital* transport, it is useful to briefly examine the evolution of *interhospital* transport. Twenty-five years ago the goal of the ambulance attendant was simply to transport the patient from point A to point B as rapidly as possible. This has been superseded for the most part by an emphasis on the controlled transport of critically ill patients in a supportive and protective environment that reproduces an ICU in many ways. Vast sums of money are now spent on interhospital transport systems, which include mobile ICUs and rotor- and fixed-wing air ambulances. These vehicles are staffed with physicians, nurses, medics, respiratory therapists, and perfusionists, who have in many cases received extra training specific to the problems associated with interhospital transport, such as altitude physiology. Further, the vehicles are equipped with support and monitoring devices including ventilators, invasive and noninvasive pressure monitors, pacing systems, pulse oximeters, and even blood-gas machines, as well as patient loading systems and sophisticated communications packages.

Judging from the relative volume of literature and the individual nature of some transport systems devised by some hospitals and units, little attention has been paid to the *intrahospital* transport of the same patient after arrival. It is imperative that the health care system address the issue of intrahospital transport in a systematic fashion so that no additional threat to survival is imposed.

Types of Patients

There are four types of patients to consider when designing a system to minimize the risks incurred and maximize the support provided during transport of the critically ill: **1.** patients from the emergency department or operating room; **2.** patients who are deteriorating in an area of less intense care such as a general ward; **3.** ICU patients being transferred to stepdown or intermediate care units; and **4.** ICU patients temporarily dislocated to some other area of the hospital, generally for a therapeutic intervention or diagnostic test.

Patients in the first and second groups must obviously be transported, but the degree to which the transport benefits the patient can be improved by reducing risk. Although critical interventions should have been initiated in these groups, this is by no means ensured. Those responsible for the care of the critically ill patient must be certain that the sense of urgency among care givers does not result in neglect of fundamental principles such as control of the airway *prior* to transport.

The number of patients being transported to intermediate and special care units is likely to increase in response to demands placed on critical care beds. By definition, these patients have not yet recovered their full physiologic stability. The increasing sophistication of such intermediate care units leads to the transport of patients still dependent on relatively high-risk devices such as endotracheal tubes and central lines. As such, their risk for the hazards associated with movement is increased over the general patient population.

The transport of the ICU patient to diagnostic or therapeutic procedures may be relatively elective, in the sense that there must be consideration of the patient's stability. Theoretically such a transport can be orchestrated to minimize patient risk. It must be appreciated that even though these patients may be considered "stable," their physiologic reserve is often minimal or nonexistent. Also, these patients may require diagnostic procedures [e.g., a head computed tomography (CT) scan] necessitating movement at the first recognition of new instability. The time frame for stabilization may well be compressed by the need to rapidly identify problems, such as a subarachnoid hemorrhage, which require immediate intervention. These patients are often the most logistically complex because of their accumulated support devices. They also undergo the greatest number of "moves" as the transport is a "round-trip." Therefore, they demand and deserve both the greatest number of personnel and the greatest amount of pretransport planning.

Risks and Benefits of Transport

The risk of anesthesia must be added to the risk of a particular surgical intervention to arrive at the overall assessment of danger to the patient. Likewise, the risk of transport must be added to the risk of any out-of-unit procedure or diagnostic test for a valid risk-benefit analysis to be performed by the physician or informed consent to be given by the patient or representative. As with anesthesia and surgery, the risk of transport may be less than, equal to, or exceed the risk of the procedure itself.

The risks and physiologic perturbations associated with transport are as yet sparingly documented, but there is evidence that in certain situations they can be considerable (Table 48-1). One study documented that 68 percent of 103 patients experienced a total of 113 serious physiologic

TABLE 48-1 Complications and Physiologic Changes Reported during Intrahospital Transport

Airway obstruction
Extubation
Deterioration in arterial blood gas
Respiratory arrest
Dysrhythmias
Hypotension
Hypertension
Cardiac arrest
Bleeding
Loss of vascular catheters
Pain/discomfort
Hypothermia
Gastric aspiration
Missed medications

changes of at least 5 min duration during intrahospital transport.[1] These included a 40 percent incidence of a change in systolic or diastolic blood pressure of at least 20 mmHg, a 21 percent incidence of a change in pulse by 20 beats/min or more, and a decrease in arterial hemoglobin oxygen saturation by 5 percent or more, in 17 percent of the patients. Thirty-one (30 percent) patients experienced a change in more than one of the measured parameters. In another study, 14 life-threatening events occurred in 31 critically ill ICU patients being transported for diagnostic imaging.[2] These included 5 episodes of systolic blood pressure <80 mmHg, 4 episodes of severe respiratory distress including 1 extubation, 3 disconnections of central lines, and 2 episodes of ventricular dysrhythmias which required pharmacotherapy or cardioversion. The fact that none of the patients in either study died may be more a comment on the efficacy of the response to the untoward event than the seriousness of the event or the wisdom of moving the patient. Such has not been the case in all studies, including one in which 3 deaths occurring in 86 transported patients were attributed to the transport itself.[3]

Acutely ill cardiac patients seem to be at particular risk during transport. Of 50 such patients moved within a hospital, 42 experienced dysrhythmias, over half requiring treatment.[4] These included 6 episodes of ventricular tachycardia and 3 occurrences of complete heart block.

Ventilator-dependent patients also appear to require special attention. Fifteen of 20 such patients ventilated manually by a bag-valve device demonstrated 14 episodes of significantly altered arterial blood-gas values (10 with hyperventilation and alkalosis, 4 with hypoventilation and acidosis), 5 episodes of hypotension (mean 40 mmHg), and 2 episodes of hemodynamically significant cardiac ectopy.[5] In a subsequent group of 16 patients, there was some improvement when the manual ventilation was replaced by a portable ventilator, though there were still 7 complications, including 6 clinically significant changes in arterial blood-gas values.

While the above data certainly support the association of complications and physiologic deterioration with transport, the causal relationship has yet to be firmly established. None of the studies cited has truly investigated the "background noise" of untoward events occurring in a population of critically ill patients. The independent contribution of transport to the risks accumulated during a several hour period must be determined by analyzing similar patients who do not leave the ICU. However, even if it is ultimately shown that there is no additional risk, the mere occurrence of the cited complications warrants the provision of care equivalent to that provided in the ICU.

Data are even more sparse regarding the value to patient management of studies performed which require patient transport. One series reports that only 24 percent of diagnostic studies performed on patients transported from an ICU resulted in a therapeutic change within 48 h.[1]

System Elements

The systematic approach to patient transport advocated in the introduction consists of 4 elements: the decision process, personnel, equipment, and planned responses.

TRANSPORT DECISION

The decision to transport a patient should be arrived at through the summation of the risks, benefits, and availability of alternatives. As with all procedures, the safest transport is one that does not take place at all. As such, optimum use must be made of tests which can be done at the bedside with acceptable results. Such optimum use may include "screening" tests (e.g., ultrasound or portable ventilation/perfusion scans), with reservation of the higher yield "gold standard" tests which require transport (e.g., CT or pulmonary angiography) for those situations in which the question remains unsettled. This may require consultation with the appropriate imaging specialists, enlightening them as to desirability of a test of perhaps lower diagnostic value. Also, critical care physicians must become vigorous advocates for the further refinement of portable imaging techniques capable of providing definitive answers.

The fact that 76 percent of diagnostic studies do not result in a change in therapy within 48 h[1] must be viewed with a great degree of circumspection. Changes in therapy may be individually invaluable to the remaining 24 percent, and thereby warrant the risks of transport. A test which "only" confirms that the current course of treatment is correct or rules out a new and potentially dangerous therapy may have similar value. However, these data do suggest that each potential transport be subjected to the following examination: **1.** What will be the response if there is a "positive" test? **2.** What will be the response if there is a "negative" test? **3.** If the response to **1** and **2** are the same, is there still *relative* value to the test?

PERSONNEL

Once the decision to transport the patient has been made, those accompanying the patient must understand that the degree to which the ICU environment can be reproduced during the transport determines to what extent the desire for pure speed of transport can be reduced. Quite simply, a smooth, controlled transport is far more important than one which exposes the patient to added risk due to inappropriate priorities.

Personnel accompanying the patient during transport must be capable of initiating a response to deterioration in the patient's condition in the same fashion and to the same degree as would be expected if the patient had remained in the ICU. Patient transporters or orderlies must at a minimum be trained in Basic Life Support. Professionals accompanying the critically ill should be proficient in Advanced Cardiac Life Support (ACLS) techniques, and there must be a sufficient number of care givers to address potential situations. For example, to isolate a single nurse in an elevator with a patient who is experiencing ventricular ectopy is not a reasonable approach, even if the nurse is ACLS certified. It makes even less sense to send a fourth year medical student as "the doctor," when he or she cannot legally even write a medication order, let alone resuscitate the patient.

Care givers at all levels should be impressed with the need for documentation of events occurring during transport. Most sophisticated interhospital transport systems routinely document all transports in a fashion similar to documentation which occurs in the ICU. Given the base line chance of a poor outcome in the critically ill patient and the need to objectively examine untoward events, the additional risk imposed by transport as well as the medicolegal climate today necessitate accurate and complete documentation. One approach is to document the indications, risks, benefits, and alternatives to the transport in a "procedure note" format.

Individual hospitals must develop their own policies regarding appropriate personnel for various categories of ICU patients. Most use some combination of the primary nurse, one or more patient transporters, a respiratory therapist, and perhaps a physician, typically a resident. It must be noted that several of the studies cited above used both the primary nurse and a physician during the transport, indicating that the presence of a physician is not necessarily protective. Though expensive, some institutions have advocated an organized critical care transport service whose chief responsibility is to provide the care necessary during transport of the critically ill. Such a system introduces at least the theoretical advantage of practical education and familiarity with the idiosyncrasies of a specific institution, as well as the general principles of transport.

To ensure that the patient is transported by sufficient numbers of adequately trained personnel, a systematic evaluation of each patient should be undertaken prior to transport. Though often done informally and on the basis of tradition, it is perhaps better to approach this aspect of critical care from a protocol-driven perspective, similar to a preoperative checklist. Predefined, objective criteria (Table 48-2) should be used to establish the risk level and individualize the support required for each patient. The more items identified on the checklist, the more support that will be required. Certain items or combinations (e.g., positive end-expiratory pressure [PEEP] >20 cm) or a total "point value" may be used to identify patients who should not be moved under any but the most emergent circumstances. Such an objective point system has yet to be developed.

Also included should be an assessment of the relative stability of the patient. The term "stable" should imply that the patient has not exhibited any recent changes in condition, nor is likely to do so: Its use to connote "wellness" of the patient should be discontinued, since critically ill patients are by definition physiologically compromised.

TABLE 48-2 Transport Checklist

Conditions	
—sedated/neuromuscular blockade	—combative
—seizures	—self-extubation risk
—excessive secretions/hemoptysis	
—acute ischemia/infarct	—dysrhythmia
—shock	
—fractures	—obesity
—positioning difficulty	—isolation required
—neutropenic precautions	—bleeding risk
Previous 24 h	
—cardiopulmonary arrest	—unstable
Resuscitation Status	
—limited resuscitation (specify in Comments section)	
—do not resuscitate	
Equipment/Medications	
—endotracheal/tracheostomy tube	—supplemental O_2
—ventilator-specify settings:	FI_{O_2}_____ Vt_____ RR_____ PEEP/CPAP/PS_____
—chest tube(s)	
—constant medication infusions	—temporary pacemaker
—CVP catheter	—PA catheter
—arterial line	—femoral line (any type)
—intra-aortic balloon pump	—dialysis catheters
—CAVH set-up	—urinary catheter
—NG/OG tube	—Minnesota/S-B tube
—splints/traction	—spinal immobilization
Comments: __________	

EQUIPMENT

The equipment must meet the needs of the patient and be compatible with the required movement in terms of transportability, shock resistance, power supply (preferably both battery and line power), and ability to function in the procedure area. All required and desirable support devices must fit within the elevator and still leave room for adequate numbers of personnel to function as needed. The patient should not be used as a "table," i.e., the equipment should not be placed on the patient's legs. In addition to the obvious impoliteness and discomfort of such an arrangement, to do so introduces the possibility of expensive equipment being thrown to the floor by a violent or seizing patient. Newer models of ICU beds often have footboards which double as equipment trays. Some institutions have designed trays or carts which mount on the patient bed or attach to it.[6] Monitoring and support devices should have a relatively broad base and a low center of gravity and should be secured to whatever surface that is in use. Various designs for self-contained adult "transport modules" are starting to appear, complete with ventilators, cardiac and hemodynamic monitors, and patient surfaces compatible with radiologic equipment. This feature may one day eliminate the need to move the patient onto another surface (with the attendant risks of extubation, line disconnection, and discomfort) on arrival at the particular scanner.

The care providers must be able to monitor the patient during the procedure. This may necessitate the installation of remote monitoring devices in the control areas of radiology suites where they are easily observed by the care providers. Not only should the electrocardiogram be displayed, but consideration should be given to automated blood pressure monitoring and respiratory monitoring. Ventilators must be equipped with alarms and placed so that alarms are audible and visible.

If equipment substitution occurs, it must be determined *prior to transport* that the transport equipment is capable of meeting the patient's physiologic demands. For example, current portable ventilators made of nonferrous parts may be compatible with a magnetic resonance imaging (MRI) scanner and provide adequate respiratory support in many patients. However, such ventilators may be incapable of providing the extremely high minute ventilation, airway pressures, and PEEP required by patients with acute respiratory distress syndrome.

The equipment accompanying the patient must function within the area of destination. For example, proper gas lines and fittings must be in place in the CT suite for patients on ventilators. The magnetic or electrical field generated by the scanner must not interfere with the electrical function of the support equipment. Monitoring and support devices must be compatible with the diagnostic device, such as the absence of ferrous metal components in infusion pumps and ventilators designed for use with an MRI scanner. Sufficient power outlets should be placed in easily accessible locations so that batteries may be reserved for transit.

In addition to the complement of monitoring and support devices, the patient must be accompanied by the standard resuscitation drugs as well as analgesics, sedative/hypnotic agents, and neuromuscular blocking agents. Airway adjuncts, including the equipment required for reintubation, must also accompany the patient. Rather than collect such medications and equipment each time a patient is to be transported, a portable "crash box" containing the essentials should be made up and checked periodically.

CONTINGENCY PLANNING

Responses to patient crises occurring during transport should be established before such an event occurs. Will the radiology technician perform cardiopulmonary resuscitation or call for help? Will an overhead page for help in the angiography suite result in a "thundering hoard" which prevents an efficient response to patient needs? Does the code team (which may have several junior houseofficers in a large academic center) even know where the nuclear medicine suite is located? Will a patient who arrests in the CT scanner be attended there or be expeditiously moved to the emergency department 50 feet away? Will the emergency physician be called to abandon patients in the emergency department, or will the patient's physician be called at home? Obviously not all such questions can be answered on a contingency basis, but those of most importance can be identified by reviewing previous experience through the quality assurance process. Hospitals may wish to formally analyze and codify their transport policies and procedures.

Summary

Deterioration in patient status is associated with transport of the critically ill. Portable studies and bedside procedures should be used to the extent allowed by good medical practice. When intrahospital transport of the critically ill is necessary, it should be accomplished with the same rigorous attention to detail that is applied to care of these patients within the ICU. Anything less results in a system which relies on speed and luck, and may add to the threat to life already present. Such an added threat should be deemed unacceptable by those responsible for the care of the critically ill.

References

1. Indeck M, Peterson S, Smith J et al: Risk, cost, and benefit of transporting ICU patients for special studies. J Trauma 28:1020, 1988.
2. Rutherford WF, Fisher CJ: Risks associated with in-house transportation of the critically ill. Clin Res 414A, 1986.
3. Waddell G: Movement of critically ill patients within hospital. Br Med J 2:417, 1975.
4. Taylor JO, Chulay JD, Landers CF et al: Monitoring high risk cardiac patients during transportation in hospital. Lancet 2:1205, 1970.
5. Braman SS, Dunn SM, Amico CA et al: Complications of intrahospital transport of critically ill patients. Ann Intern Med 107:469, 1987.
6. Nielsen MS, Bacon RJ: The transport of critically ill patients within the hospital. Intensive Care World 6:126, 1989.

Chapter 49

ORGANIZATION OF INTERHOSPITAL TRANSPORTS

CHARLES J. FISHER, JR.
DUDLEY G. SMITH

In the course of events it is inevitable that, for a variety of reasons, critically ill patients will require transport from one medical institution to another.[1] It is the responsibility of the physicians and hospital personnel involved to assure that the level of care and mode of transportation are adequate and appropriate for the patient's medical condition. The purpose of this chapter is to identify and discuss the cardinal features involved in organizing and accomplishing the safe transport of a critically ill patient from one health care facility to another.

Decision to Transfer

The first problem a physician faces is making the decision to transport a patient. This is true whether the physician is the referring physician or the receiving physician. The most common appropriate reasons for transferring a critically ill patient are the lack of currently available appropriate health care resources at the referring institution or a need to refer a patient for specialized care available only in a referral center. The most common inappropriate decision to transfer is lack of financial reimbursement for patient services. On August 1, 1986, the Consolidate Omnibus Budget Reconciliation Act (COBRA) became Public Law 99-272. The law affects every hospital that receives Medicare patients and places greater burden on transport services and referring and receiving physicians and hospitals.

Traditionally, transferring physicians have been held responsible for the safe transport of their patient through transportation and until the patient is received by a receiving physician. Under COBRA the transferring hospital assumes liability for the appropriateness of the transfer and the appropriateness and adequacy of the receiving institution. In some cases, the critical care physician may be exposed to increased liability if the patient is turned over to a "lesser" level of care during or after the transport. The impact of the COBRA legislation can be extensive, and every physician involved in transferring patients should be aware of the current laws affecting transfers.

Communication and Coordination of Patient Transfer

To ensure the smooth and safe transfer of a critically ill patient with an optimal outcome, it is imperative that the referring and receiving physician discuss the patient directly with each other. The failure to do this all too frequently leads to significant gaps in the transfer of significant patient information, resulting in missed or delayed diagnoses and therapy. This conversation further allows a dialogue that may prove educational to both parties as well as further enhance referral relationships. It is ideal if the receiving physician, or better, the referring and receiving physician, have a checklist to review while they discuss the patient. This checklist should include the referring physician's name and the call-back telephone number (particularly important if the call is cut off), the institution where the patient is located, the patient's name and diagnoses as well as the unit within the institution [emergency department or intensive care unit (ICU) including the floor and the bed number].

After the initial demographic information is shared, it is important to state a specific reason for the transfer of the patient. This should be followed by a pertinent but brief history and physical description of the patient and a working diagnosis or problem list. It is important to include the results of salient diagnostic tests that have been performed and a systematic list of the patient's current therapy. This list should include such items as number, site and gauge of intravenous lines, intravenous fluids infusing, current medications and intravenous drips, including rate and method of infusion. Additionally, the patient's vital signs, airway status and presence or absence of mechanical ventilation, specific FI_{O_2}, rate, volume, positive end-expiratory pressure, and blood gases should be stated. Further, there should be a specific statement regarding the patient's current rhythm and notation of any episodes of cardiac irritability.

After the above items are systematically reviewed, the receiving physician should state clearly whether he will or will not accept the patient. Once the patient has been accepted for transfer, a discussion regarding the most appropriate method of transport should ensue. In determining the most appropriate method of transport, discussion should include such issues as length of time out of hospital during transport, timeliness of response of the method of transport, the urgency and the timing of the referral, and the expectation of probable patient problems during transport such as management of ongoing arrhythmias, the need for intubation and ventilation, and other issues associated with patient stability during transport. It is very helpful if the referring physician speaks to both the patient and family to explain the reasons for transfer, to which facility and physician the patient will be transported, and the method of transport.

When the decision to transfer the patient has been made and the receiving physician has agreed to accept the patient and the method of transport has been agreed upon, a wide variety of logistical issues are brought to bear to affect the safe transport of the patient. It is imperative that the physician on each end clearly communicate to the nursing staff what has been discussed and agreed upon to allow a similar and effective communication between the nurses at the referring and receiving institutions. This nursing report is absolutely vital to assure that the proper preparations are made at both the referring and receiving institutions. The nursing report should include concentration of intravenous drips, need for invasive pressure monitoring, ventilator parameters, and need for specialized care such as intraaortic counterpulsation balloon or hemodialysis.

Once the referring institution has made arrangements for the patient to be accepted and transferred, all pertinent patient records including physician and nurses' notes as well as medication sheets, order sheet, flow sheets, electrocardiograms (ECGs), and x-rays should be copied and made available at the patient's bedside prior to the arrival of the transport team. Additionally, a legibly written or preferably typed discharge summary/transfer note summarizing all the major events diagnostically and therapeutically of the patient's course should be attached to the patient record and be made available for the transfer team. All of these records should then be clearly handed off directly to the receiving physician. It is important to emphasize that the absence of a clear hand-off of the information to designated people has led to loss of vital information and hours of frustration trying to track down missing records. The receiving physician must assure himself that the admissions office has been notified and appropriate preparations have been made for the patient to be admitted to the hospital so that there is no delay in doing laboratory tests or x-rays or getting blood products or other therapeutic agents as may be required when the patient arrives.

After discussion among themselves, either the referring or the receiving physician needs to designate one to function as the lead physician to organize the transport. This is typically done by contacting the transport service and stating clearly to the transport team the goals of the transport, the reason for the transport, and the problems anticipated with the patient during the time of the transport. Unfortunately it is all too common that this communication does not occur, leaving the transport team to arrive, assess an unknown critically ill patient, assimilate a great deal of information, make decisions on limited data, and then transport a critically ill patient. By taking the time to appropriately communicate with the transport team the above issues, significant improvement in patient transport will occur.

Similarly, on the receiving team, it is most appropriate that the leader of the transport team and the receiving physician have a clear hand-off of all patient information, including any issues or problems that developed during the course of the transport. This assures that the patient is not "dropped in the cracks" during the time of the transfer of services. Again, it is helpful to have a preprinted and regularly used checklist to review at the time of the patient hand-over.

Decision on Mode and Medical Configuration of Transport

Once a patient has been accepted for transfer, the mode of transport and medical configuration must be decided. In broad terms, there are two modes of transport: air medical and ground.[2] Air medical can be further divided into fixed winged aircraft with or without cabin pressurization and rotor wing aircraft (helicopter), which are unpressurized. Ground transport can range from basic ambulances with basic emergency medical technicians to mobile ICUs with physician staffing and full ICU capability. Therefore, the decision-making process includes distance to travel in terms of miles, time out of hospital, the stability of the patient, the ability to accept the problems or hazards in one mode of transportation versus another, and medical crew configuration. Typically ground ambulances are used within a 30-to-50-mile radius. Helicopters are used typically within a 30-to-150-mile radius but extending out to approximately 250 miles, and fixed winged aircrafts are typically used for 150 miles and beyond.

Transportation Modes

Removing a patient from the hospital exposes the patient to a far less stable environment. The floor of the ambulance moves, the number of medical personnel are limited, resources are limited by small operating spaces, and environmental control of lights, temperature, water, and electrical power are more susceptible to failure. The risk of the transport vehicle hitting or being hit by another vehicle or object is real. Yet despite the risk of transport, the patient may be better off than remaining in an environment that is understaffed, overoccupied, underequipped, or otherwise unable to handle the medical needs of the critically ill or injured patient. Unfortunately, the local services available may not always match the needs of the patient. In these cases, additional services may need to be explored, the service supplemented with hospital personnel or equipment, or transport must be done by the best of the inadequate services, realizing the liability.

BASIC GROUND TRANSPORT

By far the most common transport mode is the ground ambulance. Built on a truck chassis, the ground ambulance can take on a variety of shapes, sizes, and levels of sophistication. Federal guidelines exist for basic ambulance design. The guidelines define the minimum vehicle limits, patient access, structural design, emergency lighting, and other physical specifications. It is important to remember these are guidelines only. While some states have adopted these guidelines as state standards, some ambulances do not comply with even the basics for patient care equipment and space or patient and crew safety. Transport of a critically ill patient requires adequate space and ceiling height in the event of a cardiac arrest or other medical emergency. Effective care cannot be given in the back of a converted hearse or stationwagon. It is essential, therefore, that the critical care physician understand the type of equipment being used in the transportation of his or her patients.

The equipment and supplies carried in the basic ground ambulance are determined by state regulations, the medical crew training, and the financial situation of the ambulance service. A common basic transport unit contains portable and vehicle-mounted oxygen and suction, oral airway and basic respiratory management equipment, bandages and splints, backboards and other spinal immobilization equipment, kits for emergency childbirth, and some basic rescue equipment. In private or tax-supported public service with adequate financial resources and a commitment for optimum patient care, additional, more sophisticated supplies such as medical antishock trousers (MAST), the "Jaws of Life" rescue and extrication tool, automatic blood pressure monitors, and pulse oximeters may be carried.

ADVANCED GROUND TRANSPORT

Intermediate and paramedic ground units supplement this basic equipment with supplies and medications authorized by local protocol. Typically, drugs authorized for paramedic use center around emergency treatment of cardiac dysrhythmias, convulsions, respiratory distress, and shock. Depending on local protocol, supplies and equipment may include cardiac monitors and defibrillation, and supplies necessary to reduce a tension pneumothorax or perform a cricothyrotomy.

MOBILE INTENSIVE CARE UNIT (MICU) SPECIALTY TRANSPORTS

While the basic ground unit equipment and supplies set the foundation for the intermediate or paramedic unit, the MICU medical specialty vehicle may be significantly different. The medical team is organized and trained for a specific type of patient, and the equipment and supplies are focused for that patient population. For example, a pediatric transport vehicle would stock medications and supplies directed to pediatric dosages and pediatric spine immobilization. A vehicle established primarily for neonatal transports would accommodate one or two transport isolettes, additional staff, redundant electrical systems, and perhaps an air-oxygen blender. The adult cardiac care transport unit typically accommodates an intraaortic counterpulsation balloon pump, multiple infusion pumps, and monitoring equipment for invasive and noninvasive pressure and cardiac monitoring.[3] MICUs carry instrumentation to analyze arterial blood gases and blood chemistries such as electrolytes and glucose.

AIR MEDICAL TRANSPORT

Air medical transport can be divided into rotor wing or fixed wing.[4–6] By far the most common mode of air medical transport is a helicopter. Typically both rotor wing and fixed wing aircraft are equipped with the same basic medical capabilities similar to an advanced ground transport unit. The staffing may vary from program to program but ranges from a nurse-paramedic team to a physician-nurse team in addition to the pilot(s). The major advantage of the helicopter transport is that it can typically go from institution to institution and land directly on the hospital building, or just outside, and the patient can be transferred directly from the hospital bed onto the transport gurney from the helicopter. This is particularly effective where travel is affected by hazardous roads, terrain, or busy traffic.

Fixed wing capabilities are most useful for traveling long distances particularly when a patient is being transported back to the home environment or to a very specialized tertiary care center. The fixed wing transport typically requires an ambulance transfer from the ICU out to the airport at both ends of the trip. The problems associated with this additional transfer as well as time associated with it should be entered into the planning and decision to use fixed wing transport.[7] Issues of in-flight medical care in both unpressurized and pressurized aircraft are discussed in Chap. 50.

Medical Care Levels

Medical care during transportation can be divided into four categories: (1) basic; (2) intermediate; (3) paramedic; and (4) specialty care.[8,9]

BASIC CARE

Basic units usually contain basic life support equipment such as oxygen, airway control devices, first aid supplies, and a stretcher. The level of training of the medical attendants is usually mandated by the state and will vary from less than 100 h to more than 300 h of classroom and practical training. Typical training includes oral airway management, basic cardiopulmonary resuscitation (CPR), hemorrhage control, emergency childbirth, fracture stabilization, noninvasive shock treatment, and victim rescue.

The majority of the basic emergency medical services are staffed and operated by volunteer public service agencies such as the local fire department. While these services are less expensive than private services, they tend to avoid interhospital transfer because it temporarily takes them out of service, thus diverting them from their primary mission of providing rapid prehospital care to their community. Volunteer services are also facing a new challenge of decreased volunteerism and increased liability and can ill afford the increased risks resulting from interhospital transports.

Private basic ambulance services are best used for interhospital/facility transports or discharge transport of stabilized patients. The crew usually consists of two emergency medical technicians (EMTs), one of which is usually the driver. The additional crew member(s) ride with the patient and provide whatever care and intervention the patient requires. In general, basic services do not transport patients with intravenous life lines, monitors, or requirements for medications en route.

INTERMEDIATE CARE

Intermediate medical transport care builds upon the basic level with additional training that may include intravenous life lines, defibrillation, and the administration of specific medications. Certifications such as EMT-A (Emergency Medical Technician—Ambulance), EMT-A Advanced (EMT-A with additional training), EMT-D (EMT-A with training in automatic or manual defibrillation), and EMT-E (EMT with training in administration of epinephrine) or EMT-Advanced (with advanced airway skills) are distinctly different and even vary from state to state. Care should be taken to select a transport unit that is staffed to meet your patient's needs.

PARAMEDIC CARE

A paramedic transport vehicle is typically staffed by at least one certified paramedic and a driver. Often the driver is certified at the basic, intermediate, or paramedic level. Like the other EMT training, the extent of education is mandated by the state and may vary greatly from state to state. In addition to the skills learned by the basic and intermediate EMT, the paramedic studies such skills as intravenous access, defibrillation, drug administration, needle decompression of a tension pneumothorax, and needle cricothyrotomy for a blocked or crushed trachea. Continuing education requirements are higher for the paramedic level as are the quality assurance reviews. Each paramedic unit operates under the medical direction of a physician medical director. While some medical services require direct contact with the physician medical control, either by radio or telephone, before providing other than basic care, many operate under written standing orders that allow the medical crew to assess and actively intervene in patient care without direct physician contact.

SPECIALTY CARE

Specialty transport teams are organized around a patient's special needs. Most common of these are cardiac care patients, neonates, and burn victims. Specialty teams usually are hospital based and center around the specific types of patients seen by that hospital.

The crew member configuration and training vary and may include physicians, nurses, respiratory therapists, paramedics, and/or EMTs with additional training in the required specialty. In addition to direct patient care, training usually includes operation of specialty equipment designed for transport use.

Summary

The cardinal features to ensure the safe, efficient transfer of a critically ill patient from one medical institution to another include the following: clear decision making regarding the reason for the transfer; open communication between referring and receiving physician, nursing staff, and transfer team; and the selection of the appropriate medical team and mode of transport.

References

1. Cummins R: Interhospital transfer of acutely ill cardiac patients. JAMA 259:1988.
2. Burney R, Fischer R: Ground versus air transport of trauma victims: Medical and logistical considerations. Ann Emerg Med 15:1491, 1986.
3. Rubenstein D, Treister N, Kapoor A, Mahren P: Transfer of acutely ill cardiac patients for definitive care. JAMA 259:1695, 1988.
4. Schneider S, Borok Z, Heller M, Paris P, Stewart R: Critical cardiac transport: Air versus ground? Am Emerg Med 6:449, 1988.
5. Topol E, Fung A, Kline E, Kaplan L, Landis D, Strozeski M, Burney R, Pitt B, O'Neill W: Safety of helicopter transport and out-of-hospital intravenous fibrinolytic therapy in patients with evolving myocardial infarction. Catheter Cardiovasc Diag 12:151, 1986.
6. American College of Emergency Physicians Government Affairs Committee: Guidelines for transfer of patients. Ann Emerg Med 14:1221, 1985.
7. Association of Air Medical Services: Position paper on the appropriate use of emergency air medical services. J Air Med Transp 9:29, 1990.
8. General Services Administration: KKK-A-1822C, Federal Specifications for Ambulances. General Services Administration, Federal Supply Service, Washington, DC, January 1990.
9. Public Law 99-272, U.S. Government Printing Office, 42 U.S. Code Service, 1935 dd. Washington, DC, Lawyer Cooperative Publishing Company, 1986.

Chapter 50

CARE OF THE PATIENT DURING TRANSPORT

GARRETT E. FOULKE

With currently available technology, it is possible to replicate the critical care environment required for transportation of virtually any patient. However, features of the transport environment can aggravate a patient's condition as well as alter or interrupt ongoing therapy. These represent some of the major risks during patient transportation. The goal of care during transport is to minimize these risks and provide care as necessary. Transportation critical care, therefore, differs from in-hospital care largely in the degree that pragmatics, logistics, and anticipation of needs play a role. It is unlikely a controlled study will ever prove that transportation of the critically ill patient can be accomplished without alteration in outcome. However, large series of transport patients have been reported without evidence of major "untoward" events.[1,2] Such data support undertaking the transport of critically ill patients for the purpose of significantly improving care.

The composition of the transport team should vary based on the specialty needs of the patient and the skill of team members. Organization to allow obstetric, pediatric, and intensive care physicians, nurses, and respiratory therapists to accompany the patient should be available. While some reports have suggested that patients can be transported safely by staff possessing only basic health care skills,[3] it is the impression of the author that the skill level and resources of the transport team determine safety rather than the absolute speed of transport in most instances.

The precise role of physicians on medical transport teams remains controversial. Physicians accompany patients on transports throughout Europe. Several studies in the United States have shown that physician attendance improves patient outcome. The arguments against routine physician attendance on all transports are usually based on economic issues. The author feels it is in the best interest of the patient to provide (within the time frame allowed by patient condition and location) a physician skilled in transport medicine to accompany any critically ill patient during transport. In sending or accepting a patient in transfer, the intensivist shares responsibility for patient care during transport. Clearly there is a need to increase the (usually limited) involvement of critical care physicians in planning and supervising transportation.

The Transport Environment

GROUND TRANSPORTATION

Transport of patients in ground vehicles entails multiple movement risks. Extubation, dislodgement of intravascular lines or other equipment, and disconnection of drug infusions may occur. Scrupulous supervision to prevent such occurrences must be undertaken, particularly during transfers to and from gurney and vehicle. Ambulances used for ground transport may or may not arrive with adequate oxygen, suction equipment, or other supplies. These should be checked prior to departing. Ambulances dispatched for transport of a critically ill patient often provide only this basic life support equipment. It is best to maintain a preassembled collection of all transport equipment and supplies as part of the transport system. Suggested equipment lists are available.[4,5] Transport personnel should never assume that short distances equal short time. Ambulances are subject to the same mechanical breakdowns and traffic blockades that other vehicles are. Even for a five-block trip one should be prepared for the amount of time (minimum of 30 to 60 min in an urban setting) it would take to obtain and move to a secondary vehicle.

In moving a patient to and from an ambulance there will be short periods of Trendelenburg and reverse Trendelenburg position. The "one-man loading" ambulance gurney may accentuate this. These episodes are usually not long enough to exacerbate pathophysiologic states (e.g., shock, congestive heart failure, intracranial hypertension), but the patient on a transport stretcher may shift on the ambulance gurney even if the gurney is secured. In addition, axial load changes are applied to the patient in traction or in head or spine fixation devices. The team must be the "patient stabilizer" in these situations.

AIR TRANSPORT

Air transport of critically ill patients is usually carried out in unpressurized helicopters or small pressurized fixed-wing aircraft. The flying altitude of helicopters is generally maintained at <5000 ft (routinely <3500 ft). This must be exceeded in numerous parts of the country, however, by geographic constraints. In pressurized aircraft, the cabin pressure is maintained to provide an "effective altitude." This will vary with aircraft and flight altitude but should not exceed 8000 ft (except with emergency depressurization). To avoid hypoxia, one should identify the maximum effective altitude at which the patient may be safely transported. Table 50-1 indicates the barometric pressures at varying altitudes. This pressure can be substituted into the alveolar air equation for estimating the patient's physiology at altitude. Assuming A-aDO_2 and ventilation remain the same, one can solve for the maximum altitude (on 100% O_2) which allows adequate oxygenation (Table 50-1). Alternatively, at any given altitude, the fraction of inspired oxygen (F_{IO_2}) required to maintain oxygenation can be roughly calculated. The maximum altitude likely to be tolerated should

TABLE 50-1 Atmospheric Pressure and Oxygen Requirements at Altitude

Altitude (ft)	Pressure (mmHg)	Pa_{O_2} (mmHg)[a]
0	760	98
2000	707	86
4000	656	80
6000	609	64
8000	565	55

$(FI_{O_2}\ SL) \times (760\ mmHg) = (FI_{O_2}\ ALT) \times (Patm\ ALT)$

FI_{O_2} SL is fraction of inspired oxygen at sea level.
Patm ALT is atmospheric pressure at altitude.
FI_{O_2} ALT is fraction of inspired oxygen required at altitude.
[a] Arterial oxygen tension of healthy person breathing ambient air.

be communicated to the pilot and the feasibility of performing the transport assessed.

Barometric pressure changes during transport can affect many body cavities. A trip from sea level to 8000 ft will cause approximately a 30 percent increase in gas volume. The simple application of Boyle's law ($P_1V_1 = P_2V_2$) allows approximation of the volume effects at intermediate altitudes. This rough guideline is used to estimate the effect that expanding gases may have on patient care. Features that must be considered include preexisting middle ear or sinus congestion and gastrointestinal air (from obstruction, ileus, diverticulitis, hernia, volvulus, etc.). Expansion of gas within a cavity can cause pain and may restrict ventilation. Placement of nasogastric and rectal tubes may be necessary. It is important to not clamp such devices, which could prevent escape of gas during ascent. Any pneumothorax needs to be addressed prior to transport. Other abnormal gas collections may result from surgery or trauma, such as pneumocranium, intra-abdominal free air, gas gangrene, orbital air, or air trapped in tissues inside an orthopedic cast.

The supine patient is placed in Trendelenburg and reverse Trendelenburg positions on takeoff and landing of aircraft and is also subjected to significant acceleration and deceleration forces. These may be prolonged enough to exacerbate hypoperfusion or respiratory failure. The patient position (head fore or aft) should be carefully considered with regard to the effect of these forces. In addition, the pilot should be informed if such forces are considered a potential patient care problem. Landing conditions can generally be modified (to a much greater extent than takeoff forces) to reduce this effect.

Patient Care Issues

PATIENT ASSESSMENT AND STABILIZATION

Patients are usually transported because their condition has deteriorated and become less stable. Relative stabilization prior to transport will vary with the setting of transport origin (field, emergency department, transfer from one ICU to another). A reasonable attempt should be made to stabilize the patient prior to interfacility transport. This may include invasive procedures and monitoring. Decisions regarding the extent of intervention are complex, however. Many procedures carry particular risks during transport (e.g., air embolus if central catheters disconnect), and abundant time is often not available. If the patient is in need of definitive surgery, stabilization procedures, or other therapy that is only available at the receiving facility, one should delay only for items essential to a safe transport.

The transport team should accept medical responsibility for ongoing care of the patient. Specific subspecialty needs (e.g., pediatric, neonatal, obstetric) must be identified and met. Preflight consultation with the receiving physician is in order. Because family members are rarely transported, it is helpful to obtain consent from parents of underage patients for the transport and for any procedures that may become necessary in flight or on arrival.

Prior to transport, cervical spine stability (including adequate x-rays), potential intrathoracic injury, pelvic fracture, intestinal obstruction, and head or eye injury must always be considered. In air transport, the eye is particularly important since it is highly sensitive to hypoxia. In addition, depressurization can lead to extrusion of globe contents. Adequate assessment of the airway cannot be overemphasized. Noise confounds auscultation once transport has begun. The vehicle or aircraft configuration may make intubation extremely difficult. The decision to intubate the patient at the transferring facility is an individual one based on likelihood of need and the transport configuration. A lower threshold for intubation is appropriate compared to the in-hospital setting.

CARDIAC DISEASE

Transport of the patient with cardiopulmonary compromise is commonly undertaken. In cardiac ischemia, the anxiety and hypoxic stress of transport must be considered. Supplemental oxygen and pulse oximetry should be used liberally. Assessment for fluid overload and pulmonary edema by physical examination should precede transport. Central venous lines and right heart catheterization can be undertaken if necessary. It is important to remember that the Trendelenburg position is not possible in most transport settings. Adequate intravenous access and flow rates for resuscitation must be established. Although sometimes difficult, cardiopulmonary resuscitation can be accomplished in most transport settings. Cardiac countershock can be performed safely, but it is important to notify the pilot in an air transport (radio transmission may be affected) and check for clearance from the multiple metal parts of the environment. Several series have shown successful transport of patients with acute ischemia or infarct.[6,7] A large percentage of these patients received thrombolysis prior to transport without complications en route.

PULMONARY DISEASE

The patient with acute pulmonary disease will need oxygen for air transport. Assessment of the patient's F_{IO_2} need at altitude is essential. This can be accomplished by the formula previously discussed or by available tables.[8] Auscultation and chest x-ray to confirm endotracheal tube placement is essential. Patients can be transported with standard chest tube drainage systems (combination suction/water seal/drainage chamber units). Because they are cumbersome and difficult to keep upright, they should be used only when ongoing drainage of large amounts of blood or fluid is necessary. In other instances, a one-way valve (Heimlich valve) should be placed on the chest tube and suction applied if necessary.

Bronchospasm should receive maximal therapy before transportation. Although nebulized aerosol therapy is possible, it is rarely undertaken during transport. The simple methods now used to administer handheld metered-dose inhalers to intubated patients in the ICU can be applied during transport. Establishing an appropriate tidal volume, respiratory rate, and F_{IO_2} with current blood-gas levels is essential. These will serve to guide ventilation throughout transport. Ventilation is generally accomplished by bag-valve endotracheal tube with assessment of adequacy by observation and feel of the chest wall. Studies have confirmed that routine transport with this type of ventilation results in changes in blood-gas values. Fourteen of 20 patients had a rise in P_{CO_2} of 10 mmHg during transport.[9] This variability is reduced by the use of a transport ventilator. Even so, abnormalities occur in some patients. One group of authors suggested that the most optimal system is bag ventilation with careful monitoring of ventilation via a spirometric device attached to the system.[10] Other monitoring systems can be used (e.g., end-tidal and transcutaneous CO_2 monitors) but are more cumbersome. Regardless of whether a ventilator is used or bag ventilation is maintained, considerable work and time are involved in providing ventilation for a patient during transport. A respiratory therapist trained in transport techniques can be a valuable addition to the transport team for such patients.

CENTRAL NERVOUS SYSTEM DISEASE

The head injured patient may be disoriented, combative, or have elevated intracranial pressure. It is best to place the patient's head forward in air transports because the deceleration force (increasing intracranial pressure) at landing can be more controlled by the pilot than acceleration forces during takeoff. The combative patient presents a particular problem, especially in air transports. It is important to adequately restrain the patient and provide sedation. The ability of the patient to become agitated and overcome restraints should never be underestimated. If adequate sedation, restraint, or neuromuscular blockade cannot be provided, then the transport should not be undertaken. Failure to adequately restrain the patient (chemically and physically) can result in the death of all on board. Stabilization of cervical spine injuries is a distinct problem in transport. Collar and sandbag immobilization are generally used. For the patient who is already in cervical traction, the problem is more difficult. Most transport systems are not equipped to provide traction during transportation, although such systems have been described.[11] One air medical service has had success with the use of a specially built compact cervical traction and transport board system.[12]

PREGNANCY

Transport of the critically ill pregnant patient can be undertaken with appropriate planning. The patient must be positioned so that she can lie on the left side if hemodynamic instability is expected. The majority of high-risk obstetric transfers are undertaken because of preterm or complicated labor. All precautions should be taken to avoid delivery while in transport. The transport environment is difficult enough without having to provide care for two patients. Tocolytic agents (e.g., subcutaneous terbutaline, intravenous $MgSO_4$) are widely used in this setting. Careful examination for pelvic station and cervical dilation, as well as consultation with the receiving obstetrician prior to transport, are necessary. A key decision is whether to transport the patient or to allow delivery at the referring facility. With careful attention to this question, it is possible to avoid delivery during transportation in most cases. In one series, there was a single delivery during 445 air transports of pregnant patients.[13]

Despite taking all possible steps to avoid delivery during transport, the team must be prepared with umbilical catheters and neonatal resuscitation equipment should the need arise. Patient positioning for possible delivery must also be considered.

Equipment and Technology Issues

Many factors affect the use of critical care equipment in transportation. These include size, portability, ability to function on batteries, battery life, variation with altitude, and compatibility with avionics (both ability to function properly in the aviation environment and lack of electromagnetic interference). Any transport vehicle places some limits on the size and weight of equipment. One must also consider the loss of electrical power when aircraft are shut down. For both ground and air vehicles, one must confirm that there is an AC converter in the system and an adequate number of receptacles. Batteries must be fully charged with a known half-life. An extra battery should be carried for all equipment with removable batteries. Organizations such as the United States Air Force School of Aerospace Medicine have tested medical equipment for acceptability in air transport. A more detailed discussion of this issue with equipment specifications is available.[14] It is important to note that some equipment judged as "unacceptable" by strict guidelines has been used with success in aeromedical transport (such as a volume ventilator which delivers unreliable volume during rapid changes in altitude). This simply requires foreknowledge and careful monitoring.

Since blood pressure cannot be reliably auscultated, one must use palpation, a Doppler device, a noninvasive oscillometric device, or an arterial line. Oscillometric devices are in wide use in the transport setting and function well. Data suggest that there is mild to moderate inaccuracy with most oscillometric devices. Patients who are on vasoactive agents or in severe shock will not be monitored accurately. Arterial, central venous, and pulmonary artery pressure monitoring can be undertaken in most transport settings. Pulmonary artery catheter balloon inflation should not be performed during any altitude change due to the risk of balloon rupture. Truly transportable monitoring devices which allow cardiac, pressure transducer, and noninvasive blood pressure monitoring are now available. The Propaq series monitor (Protocol Systems, Inc., Beaverton, Oregon) is such a device and functions well in the transport environment.

Oxygen is supplied from compressed gas cylinders. One can make supply estimates based on cylinder pressure and maximum usable capacity (Table 50-2). It is important to recognize that in the unintubated patient a precise FI_{O_2} is never achievable, and requirements for oxygen are likely to vary with altitude. Accordingly, an approach to give enough oxygen titrated against some simple end point, such as saturation by pulse oximetry, is advised. Standard volume ventilators can be used on transports but are cumbersome and require large transport craft. Smaller "home" or transport ventilators are available, but their availability and characteristics may vary widely from equipment used in the ICU or emergency room. Prominent differences include maximal positive end-expiratory pressure (PEEP) level, maximal airway pressure, resistance of the inspiratory circuit, and maximal minute ventilation. When a patient must be switched from one type of ventilator to an alternative transport model, it is ideal to make this change within the hospital to demonstrate stability and respond to difficulties. Alternatively, if the patient can be adequately ventilated and oxygenated with hand-bag ventilation and tank oxygen, it is likely the same result can be achieved with most transport devices.

Both transcutaneous, temporary transvenous, and permanent transvenous pacemakers have been used in air transport. The transport environment presents two problems. Failure of pacemaker capture due to movement mandates stabilizing the patient as well as possible. Oversensing or other malfunction of a pacemaker may also occur as a result of avionic interference. At least one instance of dysfunction of a programmable pacemaker and inability to utilize a programming machine during flight has been noted.[15] Reduction in radio transmission (chief source of interference) to a minimum is the key modification that can be made to improve this situation.

TABLE 50-2 Approximate Oxygen Cylinder Capacity

Tank Size	Capacity (L)*
D	350
E	650
M	3000
H	5500

*Approximate usable volume at recommended 1800 lbs/in^2 maximum filling pressure.

Intravenous lines are a major problem when moving the patient. Glass containers should be avoided. Since there is limited hanging height during transport, gravitational pressure head is reduced and a pressure bag is used to increase flow. Multiple adjustments during changes in altitude are necessary. One must monitor fluid level in all reservoirs and drip chambers to prevent air embolism. Standard hospital intravenous infusion pumps are quite cumbersome when many are needed. Small portable intravenous infusion pumps are available. These should be used whenever necessary, but it is important to remember that all infusion and monitoring equipment must be moved as a unit with the patient during each transfer. In addition, all such equipment will require an electric receptacle during very long transports (limited battery life).

References

1. Harless K, Morris A, Cengiz M et al: Civilian ground and air transport of adults with acute respiratory failure. JAMA 240:361, 1978.
2. Ehrenwerth J, Sorbo S, Hackel A: Transport of critically ill adults. Crit Care Med 14:543, 1986.
3. Rubenstein D, Treister N, Kapoor A et al: Transfer of acutely ill cardiac patients for definitive care. JAMA 259:1695, 1988.
4. McNeil E: *Airborne Care of the Ill and Injured.* New York, Springer-Verlag, 1983, p 39.
5. Pearl R, Mihn F, Rosenthal M: Care of the adult patient during transport, in Hackel A (Ed): *Critical Care Transport.* Int Anesthesiol Clin 25:73, 1987.
6. Bellinger R, Califf R, Mark D et al: Helicopter transport of patients during acute myocardial infarction. Am J Cardiol 61:718, 1988.
7. Kaplan L, Walsh D, Burney R: Emergency aeromedical transport of patients with acute myocardial infarction. Ann Emerg Med 16:55, 1987.
8. McNeil E: *Airborne Care of the Ill and Injured.* New York, Springer-Verlag, 1983, p 121.
9. Braman S, Dunn S, Amico C et al: Complications of intrahospital transport in critically ill patients. Ann Intern Med 107:469, 1987.
10. Gervais H, Eberle B, Konietzke D et al: Comparison of gases of ventilated patients during transport. Crit Care Med 15:761, 1987.
11. McNeil E: *Airborne Care of the Ill and Injured.* New York, Springer-Verlag, 1983, p 144.
12. Rutledge G, Sumchai A, Stewart L et al: A safe method for transportation of patients with cervical spine injuries. Aeromed J 2:32, 1987.
13. Low R, Martin D, Brown C: Emergency air transport of pregnant patients: The national experience. J Emerg Med 6:41, 1988.
14. McNeil E: *Airborne Care of the Ill and Injured.* New York, Springer-Verlag, 1983, p 43.
15. Sumchai A, Sternbach G, Eliastam M et al: Pacing hazards in helicopter aeromedical transport. Am J Emerg Med 6:236, 1988.

Chapter 51

DISASTER MANAGEMENT

KEVIN L. FERGUSON
CONNIE WALLECK
MICHAEL JASTREMSKI

As with other areas of medicine, and for that matter life, the ability to cope, manage, and survive a disaster is improved by foresight and planning. It has been said that luck results when planning meets opportunity. To this end, a prearranged disaster plan and regularly scheduled drills are the keys to successfully dealing with a disaster. While some aspects of the plans must be fairly detailed, the plans must also be flexible enough to allow for the particular needs of the disaster at hand. A disaster plan that incorporates as much of the usual daily routine and standard operating procedures as possible will be the least confusing to the staff and the most likely to succeed. Table 51-1 summarizes the major considerations that must be addressed by a disaster plan and drilled in subsequent practice exercises.

Since by the very nature of most disasters there is little to no warning of the impending mass casualties, details of the demands to be placed on the intensive care services will not be known and cannot be anticipated. There are, however, enough predictable stresses that are likely to be involved in a mass casualty event that plans and drills have been shown to facilitate coping with disaster. Traumatic disaster situations such as air disasters, tornadoes, and terrorist bombings usually deliver few intensive care unit patients, since only a small percentage of these patients have delayed death. This is a reflection of the mechanism of injury. The majority of patients from these situations will have either injuries producing immediate death, obviously mortal injuries, or minor to mild injuries.[1,2] Medical mass-casualty incidents, such as toxic fume exposure, smoke inhalations from high-rise structure fires, and radiation exposures, are less frequent but more likely to deliver many patients to the intensive care unit.[3]

TABLE 51-1 Disaster Preparedness Plan: Key Elements*

Consideration of nature of likely disasters
Communications
Within and out of hospital
Central control center
Resource utilization (people, supplies, facilities)
What will be needed?
What is available?
What can be readily obtained?
How will resources be allocated?
Transportation
Staff to hospital
Patients within hospital
Supplies within hospital
Triage
Arriving patients
Existing inpatients
Practice
Blackboard
Drills

*Disaster management plans should address these general areas. The details are dependent on the specific situation and will be refined based on feedback from drills.

External Disasters

DISASTER PLANNING AND PREPARATION

Studies from military and civilian disasters emphasize preparation and rehearsal for mass-casualty situations as the single most beneficial factor in patient salvage. While on-the-scene, prehospital, and field triage and treatment of these patients is more appropriately the purview of the emergency department, it is important for a disaster planning committee to have the intensivist's input. Since disasters may involve entire communities and not simply one hospital, disaster planning must be coordinated broadly, including police, fire, and rescue units in the area. Plans must include the possibility that some of the health care institutions will be involved in the disaster and may not only be unable to accommodate disaster victims but may need to be relieved of their critical patients. These interinstitutional plans are perhaps best coordinated by the local Department of Public Health or other governmental agency.

Contingency plans must account for the expected natural disasters of the geographic region (earthquake, tornado, hurricane, or flood), as well as for those situations that are human-caused (accidents at amusement parks, resorts, and airports), where an otherwise simple incident can produce mass casualties.[4] The intensivist's responsibility should focus less on prehospital management and concentrate on preparing the hospital to receive and distribute the patient load so that the most seriously ill or injured are sent to the locations capable of handling each patient's specific needs as quickly as possible, as well as ensuring that no single unit is overwhelmed.

COMMUNICATION AND TRANSPORTATION

A central control center should be established immediately upon the declaration of a disaster. Those at the control center will coordinate the disaster response based on input from the various divisions concerned with their assignments. The hierarchy is established so that the information from the several divisions, such as nursing, police and emergency medical services (EMS), flows to the control center, and responses and decisions flow smoothly back to the appropriate departments (see Fig. 51-1). This limits those that have access to the control center and keeps the

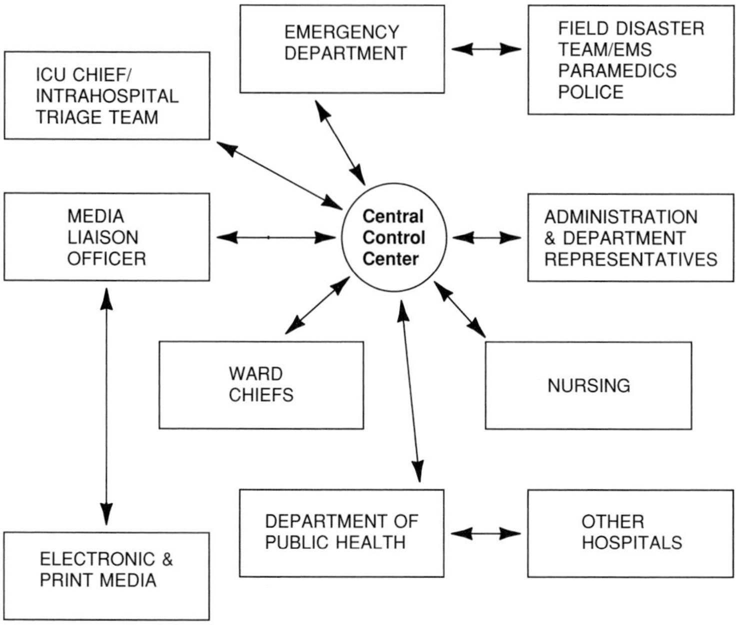

FIGURE 51-1 One possible organizational plan for delegation of responsibilities in a disaster response, including a mechanism for coordinating the overall effort and responding to the dynamics of the situation. In this plan, the field response and prehospital phase is controlled by the emergency department and EMS. Similarly, the central control center is buffered from other hospitals' situations and the media to avoid overburdening them with these problems. Individual plans may have other departments interface with the control center or may consolidate several departments' input via a single liaison officer.

sources to a manageable number. The situation where one or several departments make independent decisions without the knowledge and direction of the control center can at best result in wasted efforts and disorder. Information and decisions regarding interhospital transfers and allocation of personnel and resources to other facilities should be arranged through the Department of Public Health.

Plans for contacting additional personnel and providing for their transportation to the hospitals need to account for the possibility that the disaster will destroy or limit the usual means of communication and transportation.[5] Even if telephone service in the hospital area is not directly disrupted, there will be an increase in volume of use as friends and relative from outside the area attempt to contact loved ones. Dedicated phone lines and radio backup communications systems between vital services such as police, fire, other hospitals, and the disaster scene are vital. Systems have been devised where a cascade enables contact with as many people as possible. In such a system, each person contacted is given a list of others to contact, thus enabling exponential growth in the number of people contacted over time and minimizing the time needed to accomplish this phase of the disaster response.[5]

A preprinted disaster schedule for staff to work 8- to 12-h shifts over 5 to 7 days should be printed and known to the staff. Key supervisory personnel should know their department's role in a disaster by rote.

If the nature of the disaster inhibits regular transportation modes, the initial response to maintaining adequate staffing is to retain all personnel currently at the hospital until the magnitude of the disaster and both the number of casualties and availability of off-duty staff are estimated. Remember that the hospital staff needs food, clothing, and shelter. Provisions for these basic needs of the staff must be included in the disaster plan, especially if personnel will not be able to leave the hospital for long periods. Every member of the hospital staff should have adequate, scheduled, and enforced rest periods so that their own health and effectiveness can be preserved.

Since available helicopters may need to be reserved for transportation of the patients, alternate land transportation for vital hospital employees to the hospital should be arranged. However, it should be remembered that key personnel may be more important to the success of the disaster response than any given patient. If air transport becomes the only realistic means of transporting key staff to the hospital quickly, a helicopter should be diverted for this purpose. The disaster plan should incorporate this possibility, and a helicopter landing zone should be predetermined near the residence of such key personnel. If the area hospitals do not already receive air ambulances routinely, an appropriate landing area near each hospital should be designated. If the landing area is not immediately adjacent to or on the hospital grounds, land transport from the landing area to the hospital will be necessary and ground ambulances should be reserved and dispatched for this purpose. This site should be examined by the flight crew well in advance and any concerns about it addressed.[4]

For land transport of staff to the hospital, several alternate routes to gathering places should be laid out and personnel advised of the pickup site when they are contacted. Van pools and buses can be used to transport large numbers of personnel from the gathering sites for efficient use of time and vehicles. The addresses of personnel and their proximity to other hospital personnel should be available to facilitate transportation as efficiently as possible. This process may be more efficient if staff from multiple hospitals that are fairly contiguous are transported together (i.e., from the suburbs to inner city hospitals). The police or national guard may be needed to help transport employees to the hospital if normal land transportation is disrupted by the disaster.

The benefit of routine disaster drills is gained in the review process. Immediately after the disaster drill, the staff and its performance must be critiqued. Contingency plans have to be devised for all unanticipated problems. The difficulties experienced by the staff as well as any proposed solutions should be actively sought from all employees. Contingency plans for child care, food and laundry services, and other usual daily activities require creative planning.[6]

HOSPITAL TRIAGE AND RESOURCE ALLOCATION

All disaster patients should be reevaluated or triaged on arrival at the hospital or immediately postoperatively. The triage of critical care patients is similar to the emergency room triage; the intent is to identify those most likely to require and benefit from ongoing intensive care. The difference is that in addition to identifying those new patients who would benefit from intensive care, the critical care unit must also identify those existing patients who are to be discharged from the unit. These patients are also triaged into four groups, just as the disaster victims, corresponding to the military categories of minimal, delayed, immediate, and expectant. These can be redesignated as ill, severely ill, critically ill, and hopelessly ill, or simply category I, II, III, and IV, respectively. The category I group would be those stable patients requiring observation only, for instance, patients admitted to rule out myocardial infarction, those recently extubated or recently removed from cardiac drug infusions, or the patient with a now resolved gastrointestinal tract bleed who has stopped bleeding and has been transfused. Category II includes stable patients who require some active interventions that are usually administered in the intensive care unit (ICU) but which could probably be safely undertaken in a ward or intermediate care setting. An example would be the nonintubated patient with chronic obstructive pulmonary disease (COPD) receiving an aminophylline drip and frequent respiratory treatments. Category III, or critically ill patients, are those essentially as ill as those expected from the disaster. The hopelessly ill are those who will not benefit from intensive care but for policy or staffing reasons are in the ICU. An example is the patient who is intubated but now carries a "do not resuscitate" order and is receiving comfort care, or the patient with metastatic cancer, bone marrow suppression, and sepsis. The criteria for defining these patients need to be established in advance to avoid unpleasant arguments during the disaster's management. However these categories are defined, category I and IV patients are the first in line to be removed from the unit. Next to be discharged would be the patients in category II. Category III patients are not "bumped" out to accommodate new patients because they are, by definition, as ill and as salvageable as those arriving.

When only category III patients are left in the ICU, consideration should be shifted to either rerouting patients to other institutions or to expanding ICU capacity. The latter can be accomplished by upgrading ward and/or intermediate care beds and utilizing recovery unit space, placing pediatric patients in adult units and vice versa. Patients who need monitoring because of medications differ in the level of care compared to ventilator-dependent patients or those with invasive hemodynamic monitoring and multiple drips. Intermediate and intensive care beds can be created by temporarily suspending restrictive policies. Suspending policies, such as the conditions under which continuous drips or push medications are administered to permit their use under less stringently monitored conditions, or increasing the number of patients each nurse can care for, increases the capacity to care for category I, II, and IV patients in areas other than the ICU. If the patient-to-nurse ratio is increased, but the level of care needed is the same or greater, more ancillary staff will be needed to assist in patient care. Both patient care and paperwork should be reduced to the essentials to maximize the number of patients that can be treated, realizing that the niceties (e.g., back rubs and long care plans) may need to be sacrificed for a few days. Phlebotomy teams, intravenous teams, physician assistants, and respiratory therapists can be employed to relieve nursing staff of these duties and allow them to provide services requiring their skills. This increase in staff requirements highlights the importance of being able to communicate and transport hospital personnel rapidly and efficiently.

Consideration ought to be given to creating an expanded intermediate care unit to care for category II patients and those in the similar category coming from the disaster. The goal is to maximize the overall utility given the circumstances that exist during a disaster. Since the critically ill or injured will be the first to arrive, priority is given to opening up ICU and intermediate care beds.

Although the most immediate needs will be for the emergency department, operating room, and intensive care resources, eventually there will be a need for routine ward beds. In addition, if disaster strikes when a hospital has a high occupancy rate, it may be necessary to discharge patients to provide space for those patients triaged out of intensive care. Thus, there should also be a triage of all current inpatients performed early in the disaster response to identify those patients to be discharged. For expediency, this function is best carried out by a nurse-physician team or teams different from the ICU triage team. Since the disaster may disrupt transportation and communication, a comfortable holding area for the discharged patients should be available for them to wait in until they are able to leave.

The ICU triage is best performed by a team consisting of a critical care nurse and intensivist. Consideration of severity of illness and injury scales, degree of the patient's response to intensive care treatment already provided, and short- and long-term prognosis may be useful parameters and may provide an objective basis on which to make decisions. This removes some of the pressure on the triage team who will be called on to make crucial and even painful choices. Just as the field triage officer's authority to expedite or deny care to those at the scene is absolute, so too must the critical care triage team's authority be. Mortality and morbidity will increase if debates are allowed to impede the allocation of resources.

MEDIA MANAGEMENT

In this era of satellite communications, large disasters bring with them intense media attention. The presence of this mass communications can be used to the advantage of those coping with the disaster but is at best a double-edged sword. The difficulties can be minimized if the needs of the media are recognized and approached in a cooperative manner. Indeed, the media with its self-contained and mobile communications ability may be the only immediately available way to reach the outside world and communicate pressing needs. Disaster planning should include appropriate facilities to accommodate the press, and appointment of a press liaison officer. Early on, the media should be contacted by the press liaison officer and notified of the incident. The media should be told that reporters will be provided with regular bulletins, should be told where and when to meet, and should be introduced to the press liaison officer.[7] This approach establishes good rapport and an atmosphere of trust which will pay dividends later. By the end of the first hour, after notification of the media, the first press release should be issued even if it contains little detailed information. If the press gather at the scene and are ignored, it will only be a matter of time before they attempt to gain the information themselves. As long as they perceive that the best way to obtain the information they need is by staying at the designated press area, they are likely to remain there. The media area should be as close to the center of clinical activity as possible, since this reduces the area security officers need to contain the area and decreases the likelihood of reporters wandering around the hospital. It also avoids taking the medical staff far away from the areas where they are needed when they speak to the media. Senior members of the medical and nursing staff can also be encouraged to provide short interviews without being removed from the immediate areas where they are needed.

The press room should have several phone lines that bypass the hospital switchboard, several power outlets, blackboard or large display wall chart, and tables and chairs. Coffee, spare typewriters, paper, and other provisions are also appreciated and, again, a happy press corps that does not feel shut out is less likely to become mischievous in their pursuit of the story. Press releases should be provided at regular and announced intervals even if they are repetitious and do not include truly new information. This will dampen the spread of rumor. The scheduling of conferences and press releases should be timed to be convenient for the press deadlines for morning and evening papers.[7] Of course, the release of information must balance the need to inform the community and the right of the patient to privacy. The content of the press releases may include information helpful to the handling of the disaster as well, for instance, to request that friends and relatives refrain from calling the hospital to get information on patients, and to keep phone lines available for important communications needed to maintain contact with the scene and other agencies. The media can also be used to inform employees that a disaster has been declared, when and where to report, and to communicate what personnel and supplies are needed. The release of information on specific patients and deceased must be made after informing the nearest relatives. If the disaster is or possibly could be related to criminal or terrorist activity, press statements should be cleared by the responsible police agency. Requests to speak to patients are inevitable, but practical considerations preclude each press member from interviewing each disaster victim. Therefore, it would be advisable to arrange for group press conferences for any patient who was willing and medically fit to participate. No reporter should be granted an exclusive interview in the hospital since this will bring charges of bias and demands for equal treatment. Patients should be informed that if they wish to provide private and exclusive interviews, they should wait until they are released and are off hospital grounds.[7]

Internal Disasters

Disaster planning tends to focus on an institution's response to an external event. However, it is perhaps more probable that any ICU or hospital would have to cope with a unit-specific crisis such as a power failure, loss of medical gases, a flood (all which have occurred in our unit in the last few years), or a fire. Thus, it is equally important that each ICU have a unit-specific disaster plan.

The elements of an internal disaster plan are very similar to those of an external disaster plan. A planning committee representing a cross section of all hospital departments potentially involved in an ICU disaster should be put together and charged with the design of a plan. The committee would also be responsible for overseeing the implementation of the plan, should it become necessary. Mock evacuation exercises should be scheduled to review the comprehensiveness of the plan, to test needed procedures, and to determine the training needs of the staff.

Identification of areas within the hospital where the ICU could move should be done early in the planning process. These areas should be able to be accessed easily and must have enough space to contain the necessary equipment needed by critically ill patients, as well as the supplies necessary to deliver care. It is important to identify more than one such area for possible transfer of the ICU, depending on the type of disaster that occurs and the potential for more than one of the hospital's ICUs to be involved.

COMMUNICATIONS

The most important aspect of communication in an internal disaster is to be sure that the appropriate personnel are aware of the disaster. Most institutions use some type of special page to alert the in-house personnel of a disaster, including the name of the unit involved. Specific personnel should be assigned specific tasks during a disaster and should proceed to their tasks as soon as they are notified of the disaster. An example of this may be that all housekeeping personnel report to the unit to assist in moving equipment to the alternate location for the unit. Depending on the time of day the disaster occurs, there may be more support personnel than are actually needed. If this is the case, someone will be needed to exert crowd control and assure a calm, efficient movement of patients.

TRIAGE AND RESOURCES

The medical director or the person he or she designates will be responsible for triaging the patients in the ICU. He or she will need to be present in the unit during the evacuation to assess the patients and determine what level of care is actually needed by each patient. Decisions may also need to be made for transferring other patients to the ICU depending on the injuries suffered in the disaster. Triage must be done quickly so as not to endanger patients or staff caring for them in an unsafe area of the hospital.

The ability to mobilize staff and support personnel quickly is important. The staff may have to be split up so that a part of the staff can go to the receiving area to prepare it and receive the patients as they are brought to it. Again, it is important that all roles be specified in the plan so that long delays are not encountered in making assignments. Everyone involved should know clearly what is expected of them during this stressful time.

Depending on the extent of the disaster, additional personnel may be needed. The disaster list mentioned earlier in this article can be used to call in additional personnel that may be needed. It should be an expectation that staff already in the hospital will stay until relief is provided. This may affect staffing for the next shift or even the next day. Policies should be developed to meet staffing needs and to provide adequate time off for the staff involved.

It should be mentioned that the staff involved in the disaster area may also be experiencing some panic and disorientation. This is why it is important that the internal disaster plan be specific and become rote to those who may have to put it to the test. The ability to remain calm and make appropriate judgments will reduce the number of casualties among the patients and staff members. Hospitals need to provide education to the staff regarding the internal disaster plan and not just assume the staff will read the plan. In addition to education, mock evacuations should be done routinely to practice the plan under different types of disasters and assure that roles are clear. Evaluations of the mock evacuations should be done to reassure staff of the plan and to determine any necessary changes needed in the plan.

An internal disaster can place as much stress on the hospital system as any external disaster. The ability to respond appropriately to internal disasters is critical in preventing injury to staff and patients. A solid plan known to all, practice evacuations, and stringent evaluation can make the difference between successfully dealing with an internal disaster or having a panic situation.

References

1. Frykberg ER, Tepas JJ: Terrorist bombings lessons learned from Belfast to Beirut. Ann Surg 208:569, November 1988.
2. Frykberg ER, Tepas JJ: The 1983 Beirut airport terrorist bombing, injury pattern and implication for disaster management. Am Surgeon 55:134, March 1989.
3. Plante DM, Walker JS: EMS response at a hazardous material incident: some basic guidelines. Emerg Med 7:55, 1989.
4. Mahoney, LE, et al.: Disaster medical assistance teams. Ann Emerg Med 16(3):157, March 1987.
5. de Boer J, van der Slikke W: Disaster management: an alarm procedure. Emerg Med 2:195, 1985.
6. Orient JM: Disaster preparedness: an international perspective. Ann Intern Med 103:937, 1985.
7. Partington, AJ, Savage, PE: Disaster planning: managing the media. Br Med 291:590, August 1985.

PART III

DIAGNOSIS AND MANAGEMENT OF CRITICAL ILLNESS

EDITORS' INTRODUCTION

Even experienced critical care specialists are surprised to find 133 disease states, each requiring a chapter devoted to differential diagnosis and management. That these chapters are useful was affirmed by how much our students and fellows valued reading the preliminary drafts to obtain an updated understanding of and direction in approaching new patients. To meet this need for a reference book and yet avoid reproducing books of internal medicine and surgery, we invited our contributing authors to focus the discussion on the critical care of each disease; special emphasis on the subtleties of diagnostic techniques and clinical judgment was encouraged, and we invited them to highlight the controversies or their skepticism concerning established practices in critical care.

To facilitate a clear presentation of the clinical reality of each critical illness, we invited a case presentation and discussion to conclude each chapter. We believe this enables our contributors to address the real problems of diagnosis and management while minimizing esoteric discussion; each chapter will assist the reader in approaching a new patient with some practical, helpful guidance. In many instances, these are real cases; others were modified or fabricated to eliminate distractions and clarify important didactic issues. We also encouraged the citation of sufficient references to point out evidence bearing on areas of uncertainty or incomplete understanding, as well as to include the key citations in support of diagnosis and management. In this way, we hope to provide the interested reader with a bibliography with which to test the veracity of the approaches proposed. To make space within each chapter for this clinical scholarship, we invited our contributors to assume that the pathophysiology of each condition was discussed in Part I and the organization of critical care was available in Part II. Because readers in critical care often must extract the key points from each chapter for immediate application, we highlighted these at the beginning of each chapter for easy reference.

We found it convenient to arrange these chapters in 15 sections. So much of the origin and outcome of critical illness is related to the complications of critical care that we begin Part III with a review of the principles of their prevention: early detection and management. Because this evaluation of complications is so much a part of making rounds in an intensive care unit, we present that discussion with an organ system orientation not unlike the critical care rounding process observed in many units. Later in Part III, we return to the organ system approach to critical illness with successive sections addressing cardiovascular, pulmonary, neuropsychiatric, hematologic and oncologic, renal and metabolic, and gastrointestinal disorders in the critically ill. But before approaching these critical illnesses focusing on a single organ system, the early chapters address the evolution in understanding of multiple systems organ failure via six chapters written from differing perspectives.

We then proceed to important aspects of surgical critical care, from the perspective of the surgical intensivist, whose techniques and surgical judgment are essential to the management of critical illness associated with trauma, burns, and transplantation. Also included here are anesthesiologic and surgical management in the perioperative and peripartum periods. Of course, trauma is a topic to which separate books have been devoted. Yet much trauma care overlaps with critical care, especially in the period following emergency resuscitation and operative stabilization, when effective critical care requires on-going communication between the trauma surgeon and the intensivist. Transplantation surgery has been so facilitated by advances in immunotherapy that many surgical intensive care units are experiencing a rapid change in census toward posttransplant patients and their special problems, including infection and procurement of donor organs.

In the watershed between surgical and medical critical care, 24 chapters are devoted to the important topics of nutrition and infection in the critically ill. We conclude Part III with a section addressing overdose and poisoning in which each chapter attempts to address detoxification, where available, while emphasizing the supportive care required to sustain the patient during recovery. Because entire books have been written about each of these topics, our focus has been on their manifestations as critical illnesses.

We hope each chapter in Part III will present exemplary critical care through a questioning approach. Accordingly, our goals in this section are to provide both a manual for specific critical care of all conditions encountered, and a scholarly discussion through which a less hurried reading might reveal the reasons for controversies and skepticism concerning established practices. Further, we hope these chapters provide direction for investigations aimed to improve the diagnosis and management of critical illness in the future.

SECTION A

COMPLICATIONS OF CRITICAL CARE

Chapter 52

PREVENTION AND EARLY DETECTION OF COMPLICATIONS OF CRITICAL CARE

SUSAN K. PINGLETON
JESSE B. HALL

KEY POINTS

- *Assessment of patients for actual or potential complications of critical illness is a necessary aspect of daily rounds.*
- *Abnormal behavior or perceptions should only be ascribed to "ICU psychosis" when all other causes have been excluded.*
- *Hepatic failure, subclinical status epilepticus, and drugs are relatively inapparent causes of abnormal mental status, stupor, or coma.*
- *Endotracheal tube complications can be minimized by preventing overinflation, excessive tube movement, and obstruction due to prolonged use.*
- *Atelectasis can be minimized by three-point turning, chest physiotherapy, early mobilization from bed and the supine position, and ventilator maneuvers including sighs, positive end-expiratory pressure (PEEP), and early reexpansion.*
- *Pulmonary barotrauma during mechanical ventilation is best prevented by measures which reduce airway pressures (low tidal volume [V_T] least PEEP, relief of intrinsic PEEP, controlled hypoventilation).*
- *Pulmonary interstitial emphysema often precedes more gross forms of barotrauma.*
- *Pneumothorax in the critically ill patient is usually not apicolateral, and atypical presentations are common.*
- *Ventilated patients with high alveolar pressures have increases in dead space which may be lessened by reducing excessive ventilation or increasing cardiac output.*
- *In assessing worsened oxygenation in patients with lung disease, reductions in cardiac output, hematocrit, and arterial saturation resulting in diminished mixed venous oxygen saturation must be considered.*
- *Pulmonary artery catheter complications are best minimized by careful justification and implementation of the insertion procedures and by early discontinuation.*
- *Myocardial ischemia often presents without typical chest pain in critically ill patients, with agitation, abnormal vital signs, and pulmonary edema as early signs.*
- *Prophylaxis against thromboembolic disease should be considered in all critically ill adults; the vast majority of patients are candidates for heparin therapy.*
- *Complicating major gastrointestinal hemorrhage is most common in patients with coagulopathy requiring mechanical ventilation; hypoperfusion and renal failure may be additional risk factors.*
- *Neutralization of gastric pH reduces gastrointestinal hemorrhage in selected patients, but also carries a risk of gut colonization and nosocomial pneumonia.*
- *The diagnosis of nosocomial pneumonia is difficult to make by clinical criteria and may be assisted by quantitative cultures obtained by protected specimen brush or bronchoalveolar lavage (BAL).*
- *Heparin associated thrombocytopenia causes hemorrhage or thrombosis, is IgG mediated, and occurs in approximately 5 percent of patients treated with this drug.*
- *Drug side effects are extraordinarily common given the polypharmacy of critical care, and daily rounds should include medication review, with unit policies directed at minimizing systematic sources of error.*
- *Obscure sources of infection in critically ill patients are often identified as sinusitis; endocarditis; phlebitis; intravascular line sepsis; empyema; abdominal, pelvic, or rectal abscess; peritonitis; and decubitus ulceration. This differential diagnosis requires early aggressive escalation of diagnostic approaches when blood, urine, and sputum cultures are not revealing.*

In the course of critical illness, many complications of care are observed. Indeed, once specific disease processes are identified and management begun, survival from critical illness is often determined by the number and severity of complications related to life support and monitoring interventions. We contend that this "race" between cumulative risk and gradually returning organ function determines outcome. Accordingly, daily rounds of patients in the ICU attempt to anticipate and prevent these adverse effects.

Most of these problems are discussed elsewhere in Part III of this book, and the clinician must be prepared to exercise the full range of diagnostic and therapeutic considerations known to intensive care in the approach to the critically ill. Nonetheless, it seems helpful to collate the common complications in one chapter for orientation of the student of critical care to these problems. Of many possible organizational plans, this chapter follows an organ system review not unlike the systematic reviews of critically ill patients on daily rounds.

The reader will note that some complications emanate directly from a particular intervention (e.g., tracheal stenosis following intubation), some from the global ICU experience (e.g., "ICU psychosis"), and others from underlying and precipitating diseases (e.g., lung fibrosis following acute lung injury). Thus, our goal is to provide the reader with the information base which, when coupled to knowledge of the specific interventions and underlying diseases in a given patient, will heighten awareness and hasten identification and treatment of complications.

Neurologic Complications

ICU PSYCHOSIS

INCIDENCE AND PATHOGENESIS. The incidence of abnormal behavior, perception, or cognition in adult patients admitted to an ICU is somewhat disputed, but every observational study has reported some incidence of such abnormalities with the highest estimates placed at 70 percent.[1,2] These aberrations typically occur after 5 to 7 days of ICU stay, and risk of their development increases with duration of stay.

It is perhaps intuitively clear that life in the ICU is sufficiently stressful to result in overt psychiatric consequences for the patient. Physically, the patient often experiences substantial pain. Sleep is unlikely to even approximate the normal architecture, and sleep deprivation is common.[3] Perception is grossly distorted with loss of day-night cycles, immobilization, technology's noise, and overwhelming monotony. Emotionally, the patient must contend with the fear of death, the loss of self-control, the total invasion of privacy, and the dependence on staff and machines to perform even basic bodily functions. This physical and emotional crisis occurs most commonly in conjunction with polypharmacy and neurologic consequences of underlying disease.

DIAGNOSIS. Some authors[4] have objected to the use of the term "ICU psychosis," largely because it is a convenient catchall obscuring the identification of specific disorders. Nonetheless, it is our observation that when all organic causes of abnormal mentation described above have been excluded, many patients are encountered with persisting difficulties that do respond to modification of the ICU experience. *We emphasize, however, that this is a diagnosis of exclusion and that other possibilities must be rigorously considered and sought.*

Information which characterizes the patient's perceptions, mood, and cognitive function should be obtained daily. Because communication is often impaired or impeded by our interventions and many abnormal behaviors are intermittent and most often expressed at night, collateral history obtained from family and nursing and respiratory therapy staff is invaluable. Nurses may relate abnormal behavior from the prior night, with visual hallucinations, attempts or desires to leave the cubicle, and pulling at catheters, tubes, and dressings common. Subtle changes are often appreciated only by family members.

Once abnormal behavior or perception has been observed or related to the physician, evaluation should be directed to a wide range of diagnostic possibilities (Table 52-1). A thorough neurologic examination is necessary, and focal findings mandate appropriate laboratory investigations to identify a structural lesion. Evidence of infection (photophobia, meningismus, fever, and leukocytosis) should prompt consideration of meningoencephalitis and requires lumbar puncture. Metabolic disturbances to be sought include hypoxia, electrolyte abnormalities, hepatic failure, hypoglycemia, and, rarely, thyroid dysfunction. Intermittent hypoglycemia can be particularly difficult to identify but should be considered in patients with liver disease, and those receiving insulin, or undergoing major changes in parenteral or enteral nutrition. Withdrawal from several drugs of abuse (alcohol, cocaine) or prescription drugs (benzodiazepines, barbiturates) can manifest as abnormal behavior and hallucinosis. Withdrawal from street drugs most often manifests early in the hospitalization. Careful review of medication history is necessary, because critically ill patients receive numerous agents and toxicity is very common.[5] It is useful to determine if periods of abnormal behavior relate to the dosing schedule of a particular drug. Agents often associated with mental status changes are listed in Table 52-2. For some drugs (e.g., lidocaine), determination of serum levels can help in assessing the likelihood of toxicity; for other agents (e.g., cimetidine) dosing guidelines require adjustment for age, renal function, and so on, and the appropriateness of the given dose should be confirmed. Finally, one must consider whether the patient has experienced prior psychiatric illness that is recurring or worsening in the ICU environment.

The clinician should strongly consider a diagnosis of "ICU psychosis" only when the diagnostic exercise outlined above has been performed. As noted, some findings may lead to diagnostic tests (e.g., lumbar puncture, determination of serum electrolytes or arterial blood ammonia level). It is also frequently necessary to adjust, discontinue, or substitute for various medications which may contribute to abnormalities of mental status. The diagnosis of ICU psychosis is

TABLE 52-1 Evaluation of the Critically Ill Patient with Abnormal Behavior

Perform neurologic examination to exclude a focal abnormality suggesting structural injury
Seek evidence of CNS infection
Exclude metabolic disturbances
Consider withdrawal state
Consider prior psychiatric disorder
Review medication history to exclude drug side effects
Consider "ICU psychosis"

TABLE 52-2 Common Medications Used in the ICU Associated with Abnormal Mental Status

Lidocaine
H_2 blockers
Opiates
Benzodiazepines
Theophylline
Corticosteroids
Sodium nitroprusside

strengthened if the features are typical—emergence 5 to 7 days after admission to the unit, manifestations most florid in the evening, abnormal behavior or hallucination usually terminated by quiet assurance and constant attention to the patient, and periods of confusion followed by return to near normal function, particularly during the busy ICU morning rounds.

TREATMENT AND PREVENTION. It has been emphasized that a major risk associated with the tentative diagnosis of ICU psychosis is that it may be misapplied and delay the identification of life-threatening problems. In itself, this abnormal behavior (self-extubation, thrashing with an unstable orthopedic injury, yanking enteral feedings tubes or pulmonary artery catheters, etc.) can be lethal or at the least impede treatment and monitoring. When behavior is extremely inappropriate, the patient may require restraints and sedation until other measures have restored more normal function.

In all but the most severe forms of abnormal behavior, major tranquilizers (haloperidol, thorazine, etc.) have little place since they do not facilitate communication with the patient and usually complicate already existing polypharmacy. It is usually preferable to institute a number of measures directed at the presumed causes of ICU psychosis. Determination of the duration and quality of sleep should be made, and if possible, the procedures and physician visits rescheduled for the daytime. Sleeping medications (short-acting benzodiazepine, barbiturate, or opioid) can be considered for single-time use in the evenings. Lighting in the ICU should be adjusted to facilitate sleep. Family should be instructed as to the importance of this aspect of care. Communication with staff and family should be augmented, with constant attempts to orient the confused or hallucinating patient. Often hospital volunteers can be recruited for this activity when family members are not available. Staff and family should respond to inaccurate perceptions expressed by the patient with quiet assurance that they are not true, with attempts at reorientation to the immediate environment. During the patient's more lucid intervals, attempts to interrupt the monotony of the ICU routine are often helpful; we find television, reading to the patient, radios, and Walkman cassettes particularly useful. Finally, it is important to recognize underlying fears concerning death, desertion of family, and loss of control. Physicians, nurses, and clergy involved in patient care can begin the extended process of patient and family discussions to identify concerns, express feelings, and facilitate ongoing communication.

STUPOR AND COMA

Though many patients are admitted to the ICU with coma or stupor, it is equally common for a reduction in the level of consciousness to occur during their stay. Typical scenarios include the patient requiring sedation and paralysis during acute respiratory failure who "fails to wake up," the patient with status epilepticus controlled with various medications who does not regain full consciousness, and the patient with sepsis and multisystem organ failure (MSOF) with apparent profound central nervous system (CNS) depression. In many regards the situation is analogous to that of ICU psychosis; the daily task of the intensivist is the consideration and exclusion of specific diagnoses, pending which one must contend with the generic diagnosis of "metabolic encephalopathy of unknown cause."

DIAGNOSTIC CONSIDERATIONS. As for the patient with abnormal behavior or hallucinations, assessment begins with a thorough neurologic examination. Focal abnormalities mandate brain imaging with computed tomography (CT) or nuclear magnetic resonance (NMR) scanning; the latter is preferred if brain stem pathology is strongly suspected. Even for patients without focal findings, the threshold for imaging the brain should be low, unless another readily identifiable cause is present.

Similarly, lumbar puncture should be considered early in this setting, once significant elevations of intracranial pressure have been excluded by brain imaging or careful fundoscopic examination. This procedure will identify infectious meningoencephalitis, carcinomatous meningitis, and subarachnoid hemorrhage (SAH). SAH may be missed in as many as 10 percent of cases by routine brain imaging, and lumbar puncture may be indicated to make this diagnosis despite a negative CT or NMR.[6] Many patients with critical illness have profound coagulopathies and for them SAH is a prominent consideration. Of course, the same coagulopathy which raises concern for SAH constitutes a relative contraindication to lumbar puncture. This procedure should not be performed in the face of clinical evidence of disseminated bleeding or if platelet counts are below 20,000/mm^3. In addition, the procedure should not be performed in a critically ill patient if management will not be altered by possible findings.

Status epilepticus should be considered in all patients with profound reduction in level of consciousness. It is possible for intermittent seizure activity to produce coma without tonic-clonic motor activity.[7] Clues to this etiology of coma include a prior history of seizures and an examination that varies significantly over short periods of time or between observers. We find this diagnostic possibility to be one of the strongest indications for electroencephalography in the ICU, since identification of seizure activity and control with antiepileptics can result in improvement in level of consciousness.[7]

Certain encephalopathies are common in critically ill patients and must be excluded. Drug accumulations that are relatively common (Table 52-3) and must be considered include: **1.** long-acting benzodiazepines given intermittently for sedation, particularly in the elderly; **2.** lidocaine in the

TABLE 52-3 Drug Accumulations to Consider in Stupor and Coma

Benzodiazepines
Lidocaine
Sodium nitroprusside
Muscle relaxants

elderly, in patients with hypoperfusion, or in patients with liver disease; **3.** prolonged (beyond 72 h) infusions or large doses (>8 μg/kg/min) of sodium nitroprusside, with consequent cyanide or thiocyanate accumulation; and **4.** the muscle relaxant pancuronium if given on a regular schedule in patients with renal dysfunction; the ensuing prolonged paralysis may mimic coma, although the patient may actually be conscious.

Hypoxic and ischemic insult to the CNS must be considered, though in our experience it is invoked more frequently than is supported by available data. Patients with hypoxemia in combination with anemia and hypoperfusion are most likely to sustain injury. Following hypoxic insult to the brain, consciousness may be delayed or return after a period of initial improvement.[7] Electrolyte disturbances capable in and of themselves of producing stupor or coma are limited to marked hyponatremia, hypernatremia, and hypercalcemia. Milder perturbations may act synergistically with other CNS insults. Sepsis frequently causes mild obtundation and on occasion coma, without direct involvement of the CNS.[8] This effect may be mediated by alterations in amino acid metabolism that influence neurotransmitter levels in the CNS and by alterations in cerebral blood flow.[9,10] Hepatic failure may first manifest as coma or stupor. Most often routine liver function tests (total bilirubin, transaminases, albumin, prothrombin time) are markedly abnormal, but we have encountered patients with normal or near normal values, particularly those patients with endstage liver disease under evaluation for liver transplantation. In this setting, determination of the arterial blood ammonia level is useful, as described above. Hypoglycemia must be excluded in all cases of coma and stupor.

METABOLIC ENCEPHALOPATHY OF UNKNOWN ETIOLOGY
Frequently, vascular, infectious, drug-related, and known metabolic disturbances are all considered, with no specific cause of stupor or coma in a given patient identified. Speculation often focuses on a "missed" earlier insult but this is difficult to prove. This circumstance is frustrating for the physician for a number of reasons. Prognosis is difficult, and it is not advisable to apply information from large series of patients *presenting* with coma to this patient group. Since specific disorders have been excluded, therapy is supportive. Future observations in these patients may identify multiple etiologies of CNS failure. For example, Marini has raised the possibility that some patients with acute respiratory failure undergoing mechanical ventilation may have precipitous CNS injury resulting from ventilator-induced air embolization. The cases he has reported strongly suggest this mechanism of injury and suggest that patients should be monitored for this possibility.[11]

Pulmonary Complications

BAROTRAUMA

DEFINITION. Barotrauma is defined as the presence of extraalveolar air in locations where it is not normally found in patients receiving mechanical ventilation. Clinical manifestations of barotrauma include pulmonary interstitial emphysema (PIE), pneumothorax, subcutaneous emphysema, pneumoperitoneum, tension lung cysts, hyperinflated left lower lobe, subpleural air cysts, and air embolization.[11–14] All forms of ventilator-induced barotrauma develop after rupture of an overdistended alveolus (Fig. 52-1). When the alveolus ruptures, air is introduced into the perivascular adventitia, which results in interstitial emphysema. Gas may then dissect along perivascular sheaths into the mediastinum to produce a pneumomediastinum (Fig. 52-2). Accumulated mediastinal gas may decompress along cervical fascial planes into the subcutaneous tissue to produce subcutaneous emphysema. Gas may also escape retroperitoneally into the abdomen and eventually burst into the peritoneal cavity to cause pneumoperitoneum. If mediastinal pressures rise abruptly or decompression via other routes is not sufficient to relieve the tension, the mediastinal parietal pleura may rupture, resulting in pneumothorax. Ventilator-associated pneumothorax also occurs with rupture of subpleural air cysts, which are localized collections of interstitial gas beneath the visceral pleura.

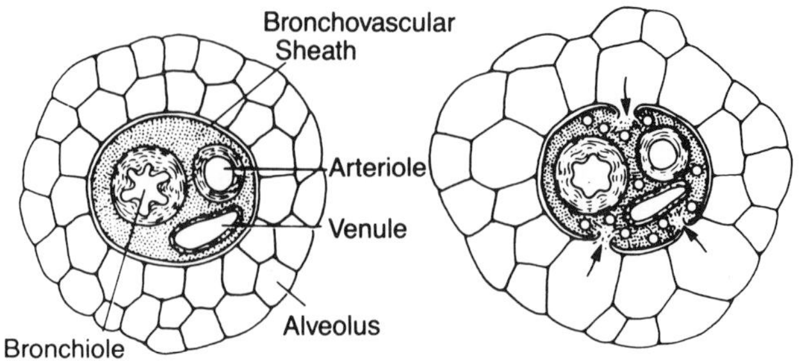

FIGURE 52-1 Cross-sectional diagram of bronchovascular bundle surrounded by alveoli in the normal state (left) and after alveolar rupture (arrows, right) resulting from over distention. Reproduced with permission from Reference 12.

PATHOPHYSIOLOGY. Risk factors thought to predispose to ventilator-associated barotrauma by producing alveolar distention include the use of volume ventilators, high tidal volumes, high inflation and inspiratory airway pressures secondary to low lung or chest wall compliance, and PEEP.[15,16] Barotrauma can also occur in patients with preexisting alveolar distention, i.e., in patients with primary diseases of high lung compliance (emphysema) and in patients with status asthmaticus. Of all the risk factors evaluated, the degree of lung distention (i.e., lung volume) and the integrity of lung tissue appear to be of greatest importance. Unfortunately, these parameters are difficult to quantitate and measure in the course of critical illness. Instead, the clinician relies largely on the proximal airway pressure, displayed on most ventilators breath to breath.

The precise magnitude of peak inflation pressures associated with pulmonary barotrauma is not well defined. In part this relates to the underlying lung compliance. Patients with normal or high compliance develop barotrauma at lower peak pressures, reflecting the higher lung volumes achieved with even modest airway pressures. Most pa-

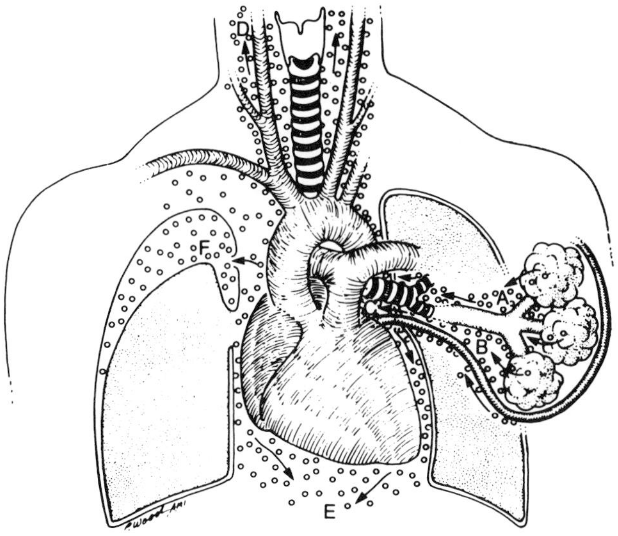

FIGURE 52-2 Following rupture of alveoli surrounding the bronchovascular sheath air may accumulate in the lung interstitium (areas A and B) resulting in pulmonary interstitial emphysema (PIE); may dissect back to the mediastinum and result in pneumomediastinum (area C); and from the mediastinum may further dissect to cause subcutaneous emphysema (area D), pneumoperitoneum (area E), or pneumothorax (area F). Reproduced with permission from Reference 12.

tients with acute hypoxemic respiratory failure (see Chap. 128) have stiff, noncompliant lungs. In general, the higher the peak airway pressure in patients with any given lung compliance, the greater the probability that barotrauma will occur. Inspiratory pressures of >70 cmH_2O were associated with a 43 percent chance of barotrauma, whereas inspiratory pressures between 50 and 70 cmH_2O had an 8 percent risk in patients with acute respiratory failure. No barotrauma was found with inspiratory pressures <50 cmH_2O.[16]

Dynamic pulmonary hyperinflation (intrinsic PEEP [PEEPi]) is common in ventilated patients with chronic obstructive pulmonary disease (COPD). Low levels (6 to 13 cmH_2O) are usually found, but PEEPi levels to 22 cmH_2O in acute exacerbations of airflow obstruction have been noted.[17] The severity of airflow obstruction is one of the prime determinants of pulmonary hyperinflation.[18] When extreme, dynamic hyperinflation could result in a significant incidence of barotrauma. On the other hand, the same severe airflow obstruction which results in dynamic hyperinflation limits large pressure excursions with ventilator breaths to the relatively robust proximal bronchi provided that low V_T, low respiratory rate, and high flow rate are used to minimize intrinsic PEEP and so alveolar rupture (see Chap. 130).[19] Another mechanism of pulmonary hyperinflation with potential for alveolar rupture is mechanical obstruction caused by inadvertent intubation of the right mainstem bronchus or by a foreign body.

DIAGNOSIS. Symptoms of barotrauma are unlikely to be specific in critically ill, ventilated patients unable to speak. Agitation, progressive hypoxemia, hypotension, or cardiovascular collapse may herald the appearance of pneumothorax, especially tension pneumothorax. Crepitation in the neck, face, chest, axillae, or abdomen by auscultation or palpation signifies subcutaneous emphysema. A "mediastinal crunch" is reported in 50 to 80 percent of patients with pneumomediastinum. The presence of subcutaneous or mediastinal air is rarely associated with hemodynamic compromise, but should alert the clinician to the possibility of subsequent pneumothorax and the potential for tension pneumothorax associated with increased mortality. Air embolization during mechanical ventilation may present with hypoxemia, CNS dysfunction, and livedo reticularis.[11]

Radiographic evaluation is the usual method used to diagnose pulmonary barotrauma. Theoretically, the earliest radiographic finding associated with barotrauma should be PIE. It has been described to be frequent in infants with the respiratory distress syndrome but is less well recognized in adults with respiratory failure. Recently, PIE was identified in 88 percent of 15 adult patients with adult respiratory distress syndrome (ARDS) evaluated retrospectively.[20] Pneumothorax never preceded the radiographic development of PIE. Radiographic findings of PIE included small parenchymal cysts, linear streaks of air radiating toward the hilus, perivascular halos, intraseptal air collection, pneumatoceles, and large subpleural air collections. The presence of PIE should be sought, as it can be the harbinger of potentially fatal barotrauma such as tension pneumothorax. Additionally, subpleural air collections may become secondarily infected.

The usual radiographic diagnosis of pneumothorax is made by identification of the apicolateral visceral pleural line separated from the chest wall by a radiolucent zone void of vascular markings. These findings are easily seen on upright posteroanterior and lateral chest films. Unfortunately, most critically ill patients are supine or semirecumbent at the time of radiologic examination. It is now clear that the radiographic appearance of pneumothorax is influenced by the patient's position as well as by the underlying pleuropulmonary disorder.[21,22] Alterations in lung recoil caused by consolidation or adhesions allow air to surround an incompletely inflated lung or exclude air from an area of obliterated pleural space. Locations of pneumothoraces in critically ill supine patients include, in addition to the usual apicolateral location, anteromedial, subpulmonic, and posteromedial pleural recesses. In 88 respiratory ICU patients, the most commonly involved pleural recesses included the anteromedial (38 percent) and subpulmonic (26 percent).[21] The classic location, apicolateral, was found in only 22 percent of patients. Anteromedial pneumothorax presents as a linear air density adjacent to the mediastinum or increased sharpness of the mediastinal border outlined by intrapleural air. Subpulmonic pneumothorax can be recognized by hyperlucency of the upper abdominal quadrants and visualization of the anterior costophrenic sulcus. Findings can be mimicked by pneumoperitoneum, bullous lung disease, or subcutaneous air. The radiographic determination of localized pneumothorax and ventilator-induced subpleural air cysts can be extremely difficult (Fig. 52-3). Diagnoses of

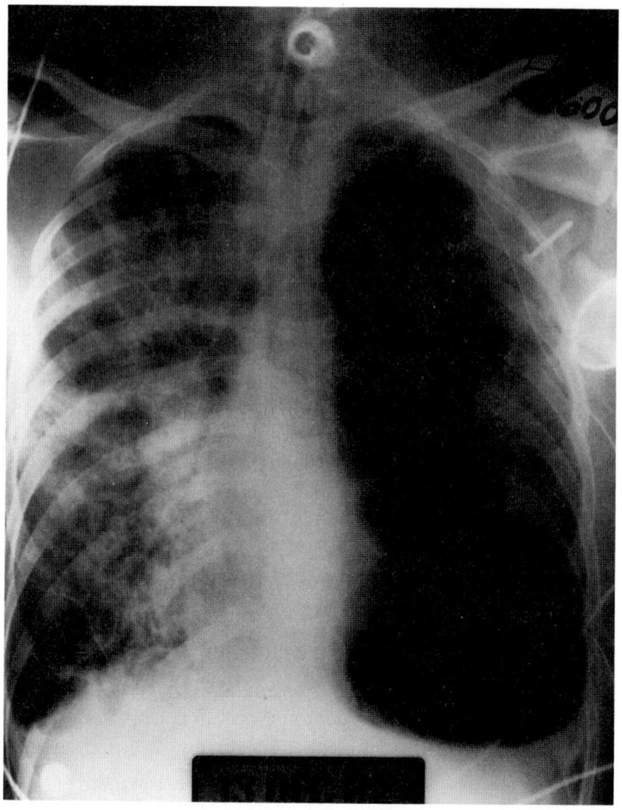

FIGURE 52-3 Radiograph of ventilated patient with ARDS. Note the large subpleural lung cyst in the lower left lung field. A localized pneumothorax is also present on the left, but determining anterior or posterior location is impossible from the film alone. This radiograph demonstrates the unusual presentation of barotrauma in the critically ill patient undergoing mechanical ventilation. (Reproduced with permission from Pingleton SK: Complications of acute respiratory failure. Am Rev Respir Dis 137:1463, 1988.)

pneumothoraces in unusual locations are frequently missed with important consequences. As many as one-third of pneumothoraces in supine, critically ill patients are missed by the clinician or radiologist.[22] Anteromedial and subpulmonary pneumothoraces are the types most frequently missed. More than one-half the missed pneumothoraces progress to tension pneumothorax. Tension pneumothorax can produce life-threatening pulmonary and cardiovascular deterioration. Usual radiographic signs of tension include striking collapse of the lung, contralateral shift of the heart and mediastinum, and inversion of the hemidiaphragm. Tension pneumothorax can also occur without the usual signs. Subtle signs of tension include slight flattening of the cardiac border and ipsilateral contour changes or depression of the diaphragm. It is to be emphasized that unusual locations of pneumothorax are common in ventilated patients. Exceptional care in the diagnosis of pneumothorax in high risk patients should be undertaken, since the risk of a missed pneumothorax is considerable. Special attention should be directed to the medial and basilar aspects of the lung. Decubitus and cross-table laterals can aid in the diagnosis. Although not inherently practical, CT examination can be very helpful in detecting pneumothoraces in this patient population.

THERAPY AND PROPHYLAXIS. Standard methods to reduce the frequency of barotrauma include measures to decrease alveolar inflation and pressures, V_T, PEEP, and PEEPi. Beyond a regular attempt to seek the least values of these variables while still achieving an acceptable end point of gas exchange and venous return, these measures include patient sedation and coordination with the ventilator, reduction in peak flow if it does not increase intrinsic PEEP, and perhaps adjustment of ventilator modes. Controlled hypoventilation to minimize peak airway pressures can reduce barotrauma in status asthmaticus[23] and perhaps in other forms of respiratory failure as well. Pressure-assisted ventilation may also help reduce barotrauma compared to inverse ratio ventilation,[24] since the latter may cause unduly large intrinsic PEEP.

Specific treatment modalities vary with the type of pulmonary barotrauma. Tube thoracostomy is appropriate therapy for pneumothorax or tension pneumothorax. Pulmonary interstitial emphysema is generally treated with nothing but the aforementioned methods to decrease lung distention. Pneumomediastinum and subcutaneous emphysema are generally thought to be benign but should heighten vigilance for further manifestations of barotrauma. The issue of "prophylactic chest tubes" in patients with pulmonary barotrauma but not pneumothorax is not resolved. We do not advocate routine tube thoracostomy unless pneumothorax has been identified or must be excluded. Nonetheless, individual patients with extremely high PEEP requirements and high airway pressures may be encountered in whom bilateral chest tube placement may be warranted.

PULMONARY FIBROSIS

PATHOPHYSIOLOGY. Diffuse interstitial fibrosis may follow lung injury of diverse causes, including ARDS. Pathologic patterns of structural change following ARDS can be divided into three phases: the acute or exudative phase (6 days), the subacute proliferative phase (4 to 10 days), and the chronic fibrotic phase (from 8 days on)[25] (Fig. 52-4). The initial exudative phase is characterized by alveolar and septal edema and hyaline membranes. Mononuclear infiltrates and alveolar epithelial hyperplasia appear between 7 and 10 days. Proliferation of alveolar type II cells, interstitial cells, macrophages and fibroblasts occurs, and mild interstitial fibrosis begins. Later, beyond 2 weeks, the chronic fibrotic phase begins.

DIAGNOSIS. The diagnostic criteria for pulmonary fibrosis following ARDS are not different from other causes of fibrosis. When proliferative phase ARDS evolves rapidly in the patient still on the ventilator, a rather characteristic clinical pattern is often noted. The chest radiograph exhibits a "honeycomb" appearance, distinct from the typical pulmo-

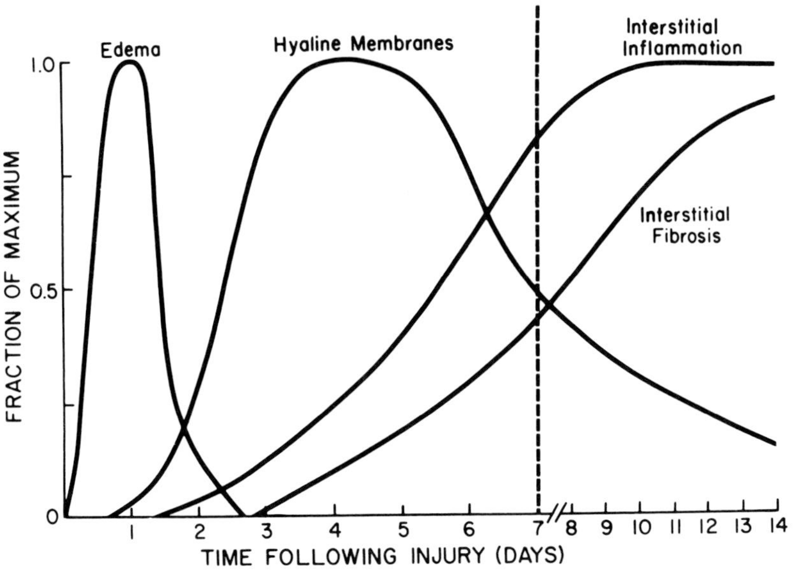

FIGURE 52-4 Schematized view of the time course of acute lung injury with diffuse alveolar damage. In the early exudative phase alveolar flooding is prominent, with histologic findings of edema and hyaline membranes. If the patient does not recover, disordered healing during the proliferative phase can appear as early as 1 to 2 weeks, with histology characterized by interstitial inflammation and interstitial fibrosis. Reproduced with permission from Katzenstein AA, Askin FB: *Surgical pathology of Nonneoplastic Lung Disease.* Philadelphia, Saunders, 1982, p. 10.

nary edema findings of the exudative phase. Lung compliance remains remarkably low, and the patient exhibits tachypnea and dyspnea. Shunt fraction often decreases relative to the acute phase of the illness, with lower PEEP and fraction inspired oxygen (F_{IO_2}) requirements necessary to maintain arterial hemoglobin saturation. In contrast, dead space fraction rises dramatically in these patients, with minute ventilations of 20 to 30 L/min typical. Often, even these high levels of ventilation are inadequate to maintain eucapnea. The destruction of lung parenchyma resulting in nonperfused air spaces no doubt causes much of this wasted ventilation, but patients with late ARDS pulmonary fibrosis are also at risk for development of physiologic dead space (zone I lung conditions, see Chap. 1). Alveolar pressure in the stiff, noncompliant lung rises parallel to the observed proximal airway pressure and can reach levels that are higher than the contiguous pulmonary vascular pressures (particularly in nondependent portions of the lung). Perfusion of these ventilated units is thus precluded, adding to total dead space. High V_T, PEEP, and breathing frequency will contribute to higher mean alveolar pressure, while hypovolemia will tend to make pulmonary artery pressures low. Accordingly, strategies used to maintain low pulmonary vascular pressures during earlier stages of edemagenesis may require modification in later stages of pulmonary fibrosis.

This pathophysiology may also be encountered during the postextubation, posthospital recovery phase of ARDS. During this time, continued pulmonary symptoms, restrictive lung dysfunction, and radiographic infiltrates suggest the diagnosis. Previously, survival of ARDS was thought to correlate well with complete recovery of pulmonary impairment. Recent data suggest persistence of pulmonary function abnormalities is more frequent than previously believed. One year after ARDS, spirometric abnormalities may be found in as many as 60 percent of survivors.[26] Impairment is mild in over three-fourths of those patients, but may be moderate or severe in one-fourth. Long-term pulmonary function abnormalities in ARDS survivors relate to the degree of ARDS severity as well as to the persistence of impaired lung function.[27] Evaluation of ARDS survivors should include assessment of physiologic status until stabilization or return to normal.

THERAPY AND PROPHYLAXIS. Specific therapies to prevent or reverse disordered healing and lung fibrosis have been entertained, but none demonstrated to be effective. Anecdotally, many clinicians advocate high dose corticosteroid treatment for patients with proliferative phase ARDS, but we cannot advocate this approach in the absence of supportive data.

Prevention of this entity centers on limiting exposure to toxic concentrations of oxygen and positive-pressure ventilation, the influences presumed to interact with the underlying lung injury to culminate in fibrosis.[28,29] A reasonable goal for the clinician in the early phases of ARDS is the use of PEEP to achieve 90% saturation of arterial hemoglobin on a nontoxic F_{IO_2}. We advocate the prompt titration of PEEP to a level which permits a reduction in F_{IO_2} to ≤ 0.6, which can be achieved in the majority of patients with acute hypoxemic respiratory failure. PEEP is usually well tolerated if used in conjunction with low V_T (6 to 7 mL/kg) to prevent barotrauma (vide supra). Adjunctive therapies to maintain high oxygen delivery (maintain hematocrit ≥ 35, use of vasoactive drugs to augment cardiac output) and lower oxygen consumption (sedation and muscle relaxation, treatment of hyperthermia, modification of nutrition) may also be used to support the patient at the brink of gas exchange failure (see Chap. 128). Duration of mechanical ventilation may be shortened by hemodynamic interventions during the early phase of acute lung injury which reduce pulmonary vascular pressures and limit edemagenesis.[30] Intricacies of these approaches are described elsewhere in this text, but as a generalization the clinician must assess the patient with acute hypoxemic respiratory failure daily, with an eye to diminishing the potentially dangerous therapies of oxygen and mechanical ventilation. Finally, for those patients with established pulmonary fibrosis in the wake of acute lung injury, particular attention must be paid to the possibility that even minor degrees of hypovolemia can result in large increases in dead space fraction, presumably by lowering pulmonary blood flow and thus pulmonary artery pressure below alveolar pressure. Observations supporting this include the typical setting of late ARDS and the fact that Pa_{CO_2} changes little (or even increases) with increases in PEEP, VT, or frequency. By contrast, significant reductions in PEEP, VT, and minute ventilation can *reduce* Pa_{CO_2} in this setting.

COMPLICATIONS RELATED TO AIRWAY MANAGEMENT

COMPLICATIONS DURING THE INTUBATION PROCEDURE. Complications are common during intubations performed in critically ill patients.[31] A prolonged intubation (>2 to 3 min) occurs in as many as 30 percent of attempts at the procedure in training centers. Sequelae of these prolonged attempts include cardiac arrest, generalized seizures, and gastric distention. Right mainstem intubation occurs in 7 to 9 percent of all intubations but is twice as frequent after prolonged attempts. Mainstem intubation places the patient at risk for alveolar hypoventilation, pneumothorax, and atelectasis. Right mainstem intubation often results in collapse of the right upper lobe, since the endotracheal tube tip or cuff is likely to obstruct this orifice at its origin. Self-extubation is a serious complication that increases mortality and requires reintubation in almost half the patients.

COMPLICATIONS AFTER TRANSLARYNGEAL INTUBATION. Complications of endotracheal intubation result from injury to the hypopharynx, larynx and trachea, and are related to both the tube and cuff (Fig. 52-5). Virtually all patients intubated for 2 to 6 days demonstrate laryngeal edema, ulceration, and hemorrhage.[31] Pathologic findings can translate to clinical findings of stridor or upper airway obstruction, but these symptoms are infrequent, occurring in <5 percent of translaryngeally intubated patients. Other postextubation symptoms are more common. Hoarseness occurs in three-fourths of patients but resolves within a month in the majority of patients. Paranasal sinusitis is found in as many as 25 percent of patients and can be the source of unexplained fever and sepsis. Aspiration can occur postextubation due to incomplete closure of the vocal cords resulting from laryngeal damage.[32]

Tracheal injury can also result from translaryngeal intubation. Tracheal stenosis is diagnosed in almost 20 percent of endotracheal intubations.[31] Stenosis occurs most often at the cuff site but may also be found in the subglottic area. Stenosis is not usually severe and most patients have <50 percent narrowing.

COMPLICATIONS ASSOCIATED WITH TRACHEOSTOMY. Potentially life-threatening complications of tracheostomy

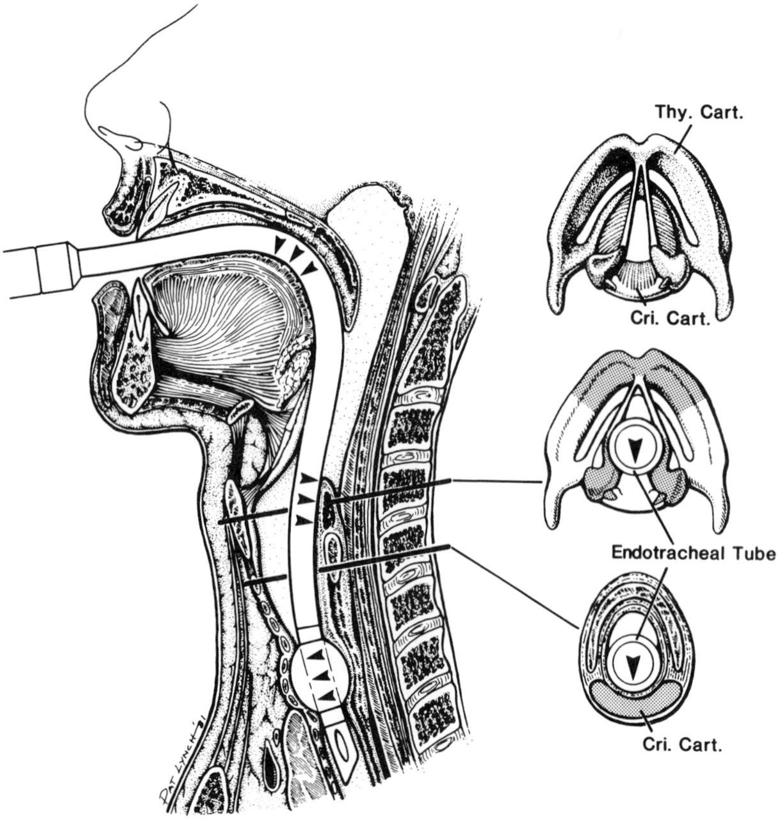

FIGURE 52-5 Sagittal section demonstrates endotracheal tube position. The arrows indicate areas susceptible to trauma and pressure necrosis and the cross-sectional views indicate the likely areas of laryngeal injury. Reproduced with permission from Colice G, Matthay R: Guidelines for doing tracheal intubation. J Respir Dis 3:43, 1982.

include tracheoinnominate fistula, tracheoesophageal fistula, and tracheal stenosis.[33] Tracheoinnominate fistula, although occurring in only 2 percent of patients, is a feared complication. Erosion into this vessel can produce sudden massive hemorrhage. Resultant airway bleeding occurs anytime from days to months after tracheostomy placement. With massive hemorrhage, tamponade should be attempted with hyperinflation of the tracheostomy cuff or with a newly placed endotracheal tube. Anterior compression of the innominate artery is a last resort. Surgery with ligation and resection of the affected artery must be performed later. The survival rate is only 25 percent. Tracheoesophageal fistula is also infrequent (<1 percent) and results from poor surgical techniques or a poorly fitting tracheostomy tube with excessive cuff pressure.

Tracheal stenosis is a major complication occurring after tracheostomy in as many as 65 percent of patients.[31] It occurs in three main regions of the airway. If the tracheostomy is placed too high with damage to the cricoid cartilage, subglottic stenosis occurs. Stenosis can also occur at the level of the cuff and stomal site. The stomal site is prevalent because of the indenting or caving in of the permanent defect of the anterior tracheal cartilage. After extubation, the cartilage and lateral margin fall in at the margins and are united by a fibrous scar. Of all potential stenotic sites, tracheal stenosis occurs most frequently at the stomal site.

Diagnosis of tracheal stenosis requires a high index of suspicion in patients developing respiratory symptoms after tracheostomy. Symptoms are rare unless there is a 75 percent reduction in tracheal lumen. History, physical examination, and flow-volume loops are sensitive indicators of stenosis. Inspiratory and expiratory lateral soft tissue views of the neck together with fluoroscopy or tomography are usually adequate to diagnose tracheal stenosis.

MANAGEMENT TO PREVENT AIRWAY COMPLICATIONS. Various factors have been implicated in laryngeal and tracheal injury, and daily management of the intubated patient is directed at minimizing the likelihood of complications (Table 52-4). Cuff pressure is clearly an important determinant. Cuff-related injuries result from ischemic damage to the tracheal mucosa when cuff pressure exceeds capillary perfusion pressure of 20 to 30 mmHg. Friction between the cuff surface and tracheal mucosa by patient movement, swallowing, or coughing may further accentuate the problem. The potential for cuff-related tracheal injury is less with the advent of high volume, low pressure cuffs. However, even the pressure-volume relationships of these cuffs can be altered by confinement within the tracheal walls, converting their behavior to a low volume high pressure cuff. Management strategies include careful cuff inflation with minimal inflation volume and measurement of intracuff pressure with a four-way stopcock.[33] Avoiding small endotracheal tubes helps prevent excessive cuff inflation. The cuff can also be deflated to allow a "minimal leak" (as assessed by auscultation or measurement of inspired and expired V_T). Finally, the patient should be managed to avoid kinking and torsion on the airway, which can increase its resistance, induce pain and coughing, and "fulcrum" the device on the larynx, thereby resulting in greater trauma.

TABLE 52-4 Daily Management of the Airway

Ensure adequately sized tube with normal patency
Minimize cuff pressure by minimal leak or measured pressure <25 mmHg
Minimize cuff movement and tube flexion or torsion
Confirm position by inspection, auscultation, palpation, and radiologic imaging
Assess duration of intubation

Airway position must be ensured at all times. Once position is confirmed after intubation, it is advisable to note the centimeter marking of the tube correlating to lip or "tip of the nose" position and inform nursing and respiratory therapy of the position to be maintained during the frequent retapings of the airway. Cuff position can be confirmed in some patients by palpating the cuff during inflation and deflation immediately above the sternal notch. Routine daily inspection of airway position with chest radiograph is advisable during the first week of critical illness. Appropriate endotracheal tube position is confirmed by chest radiograph when the tip is 3 to 5 cm above the carina. It is important to note that the tip will follow the direction of the patient's chin during neck flexion or extension and will move 2 to 4 cm from full extension to full flexion. Fiberoptic confirmation of tube position and patency can be useful in certain emergent circumstances.

The duration of "safe" endotracheal intubation before reversion to tracheostomy is not known. The common practice is 7 to 14 days of endotracheal intubation prior to tracheostomy. Some patients tolerate endotracheal intubation for as long as 22 days. Isolated cases of truly prolonged intubation (55 to 155 days) are reported. However, late complications can occur after only 3 days of endotracheal intubation. Thus, the safe period cannot be predicted for each patient. Goals should include appropriate therapy for the primary disease that results in prompt extubation. We assess all patients carefully approximately 7 to 10 days after intubation with a judgment as to whether extubation is likely within the next week; if it appears possible, we continue the translaryngeal intubation. If underlying disease has not been reversed and the course is likely to continue over a prolonged period of time, tracheostomy is recommended.

Since patient movement, particularly in the agitated or confused individual, can result in airway trauma and self-extubation, constant attention to the causes and treatment of patient discomfort, delirium, and inappropriate behavior is required. Also, all endotracheal tubes must be followed carefully on a daily basis for the development of obstruction, signalled by inability or difficulty in passing a catheter or by rising peak airway pressures. Evaluation of endotracheal tubes in mechanically ventilated patients has indicated significant increases above in vitro measurements of tube resistance,[34] contributing significantly to work of breathing.

On occasion the clinician will be required to evaluate the possibility of tube occlusion emergently. The usual setting is a distressed patient with ventilator alarms firing because of high airway pressure and failure to deliver an adequate VT. A concise and swift management plan is required. The patient should immediately be removed from the ventilator and hand-bagged with 100% oxygen. This eliminates ventilator malfunctions from consideration, and the clinician will be able to assess the resistance to inflation directly. If bagging is difficult and ventilation of the patient minimal, a catheter should be passed down the endotracheal tube. Failure to pass the catheter the full 25 to 35 cm to the trachea indicates tube obstruction. If immediately available, a fiberoptic bronchoscope is useful to determine tube patency and position. Preparation should be made for emergent reintubation. If the source of obstruction is clearly at the level of the teeth, as occurs on occasion in the thrashing patient undergoing alcohol withdrawal, a bite block may be applied or a paralyzing dose of succinylcholine may be given (see Chap. 83). If muscle relaxation does not immediately restore tube patency and ability to ventilate, the endotracheal tube should be removed, mask ventilation undertaken, and reintubation performed. In patients with obstruction below the level of the teeth, inability to pass a catheter, and complete inability to ventilate, cuff deflation should be performed. With older endotracheal tubes this was recommended because cuff herniation over the endotracheal tube tip was possible, with consequent obstruction. We rarely if ever encounter this difficulty, but cuff deflation will allow patients with continued respiratory efforts to partially ventilate "around" the tube. Since most tube obstructions result from concretized secretions and mucous plugs, it is unlikely they can be removed once complete obstruction has occurred; reintubation should be performed quickly, with special attention to measures to prevent aspiration (see Chap. 6). Patients who have completely obstructed their endotracheal tube are often those with small tubes, airway bleeding, excessive secretions, and high minute ventilations making humidification of inspired gas difficult. Following the emergent securing of the airway, the patient should be examined to determine if a larger endotracheal tube can be accommodated, if the frequency of suctioning should be increased, and if humidification is optimal. Patients with inability to ventilate but a patent endotracheal tube should be immediately assessed for tension pneumothorax, suggested by subcutaneous emphysema, tracheal deviation, and asymmetry of breath sounds, often in conjunction with indications of diminished venous return such as tachycardia, narrow pulse pressure, and hypotension (vide supra).

APPROACH TO ARTERIAL HEMOGLOBIN DESATURATION OR HYPOVENTILATION

Critically ill patients frequently require oxygen therapy and mechanical ventilation, and ongoing monitoring of arterial hemoglobin saturation by pulse oximetry or blood-gas analysis is routine. Of course, progression of primary causes of respiratory failure (ARDS, pneumonia, lung hemorrhage) or new lung insults (nosocomial pneumonia) may result in deterioration of gas exchange. These processes are usually readily identified by physical examination and chest radiograph.[35] It is also common for desaturation to signal one of the less apparent complications of critical illness, and we therefore offer an approach to this observation.

First and foremost, the clinician must seek an explanation for all unanticipated instances of worsened gas exchange, although initial response to severe desaturation should include administration of sufficient amounts of oxygen to restore adequate arterial hemoglobin saturation. The information base that is useful for evaluation of observed desaturation is the arterial blood-gas, true $F_{I_{O_2}}$, and mixed venous blood-gas values, coupled with bedside examination and assessment of the airway and ventilator.

A recommended approach is given in Table 52-5. Artifact in arterial blood-gas analysis (see Chap. 13) certainly occurs, but is an unlikely explanation when multiple determinations yield similar results, the clinical picture suggests hypoxemia, or pulse oximetry confirms the blood-gas determination. Much more confounding is the assumption of an $F_{I_{O_2}}$ that is higher than that actually achieved in the patient. *Patients with respiratory distress receiving nasal cannula or*

TABLE 52-5 Causes of Worsening Hypoxemia in the Critically Ill Patient

1. Artifact
2. Alterations in $F_{I_{O_2}}$
3. Hypoventilation ($[A - a]_{O_2}$ unchanged)
   a. Diminished patient effort (fatigue, depressed drive)
   b. Ventilator malfunction or inadvertent change in settings
   c. Gas leak
   d. Alterations in physiologic dead space
      Hypovolemia
      PEEPi
      Increased alveolar pressures in restrictive lung disease
4. $\dot{V}/\dot{Q}$ mismatch
   a. Airway
      Bronchospasm
      Secretions
      Mucous plugging
      Endotracheal tube suctioning
   b. Vasculature
      Use of vasoactive drugs (inhaled or intravenous)
5. Shunt
   a. Atelectasis
   b. Pulmonary edema
   c. Pulmonary hemorrhage
   d. Positional change in nonhomogeneous disease
   e. Lobar collapse (acutely)
   f. Pneumonia
   g. Cardiac shunt
6. Mixed venous hypoxemia
   Low O_2 delivery due to reduced flow, hematocrit, or saturation or to increased $\dot{V}_{O_2} \rightarrow$ low mixed venous saturation $\rightarrow$ arterial hypoxemia in shunt or lung disease with large numbers of low $\dot{V}/\dot{Q}$ units.
7. Miscellaneous
   a. Dialysis
   b. Pulmonary embolus

mask oxygen must be considered to have an unknown F_{IO_2}, although in most circumstances significant supplementation occurs.[36] This imprecision in the effective F_{IO_2} is attributable to entrainment of room air in these circumstances. F_{IO_2} is only fixed (known) when breathing room air or when intubated with a tight-fitting endotracheal tube. Even in this latter circumstance we have encountered ventilator malfunctions with specious readings of F_{IO_2}; if this is suspected, a gas analyzer must be connected to the ventilator circuit and F_{IO_2} directly measured. Indeed, some units send a sample of mixed expired gas with each blood-gas sample drawn from ventilated patients to calculate dead space (Vd/Vt) and P_{IO_2} ($= P_{EO_2} + P_{ECO_2}$).

Hypoventilation will be signaled by the fall in Pa_{O_2} correlating to a rise in P_{CO_2} as dictated by the alveolar gas equation (see Chap. 1). Again, use of the alveolar gas equation is contingent on the patient having a known F_{IO_2}. In hypoventilation, $(A - a)_{O_2}$ will be unchanged. Numerous complications resulting in hypoventilation are given in Table 52-5. Of particular note is the development of large regions of physiologic dead space (vide supra). This is likely to occur when alveolar pressure is high and pulmonary vascular pressure is low. Thus, it should be anticipated in hypovolemic patients with ARDS (particularly late, proliferative disease) or those with severe airflow obstruction with the development of dynamic gas trapping (PEEPi or occult PEEP).[37]

Ventilation/perfusion ($\dot{V}/\dot{Q}$) mismatching occurs with many processes complicating critical illness. Bronchospasm, increased airway secretions, and airway plugging are common in intubated patients and are likely contributors to nocturnal desaturation as the frequency of airway suctioning and inhalation therapy diminishes to facilitate sleep. Inhalational agents may acutely worsen ventilation/perfusion relationships[38] as do vasodilating drugs which increase blood flow to lung units with low ventilation. The combination of worsened $\dot{V}/\dot{Q}$ matching and an increase in dead space should prompt consideration of pulmonary embolus, which can be extremely difficult to diagnose in the critically ill patient (see Chap. 118). Increased $\dot{V}/\dot{Q}$ variance is suggested by increased $(A-a)_{O_2}$ in the absence of increased shunt ($\dot{Q}s/\dot{Q}t$) or worsened hypoxemia on an $F_{IO_2} < 0.6$ (above this F_{IO_2}, $\dot{V}/\dot{Q}$ mismatch rarely contributes to hypoxemia).

Development or worsening of intrapulmonary shunt is suggested by severe hypoxemia refractory to oxygen therapy. Shunt fraction can be calculated from simultaneously sampled arterial and mixed venous blood-gas samples collected on a known and high F_{IO_2}. A number of processes will increase intrapulmonary shunt, the common feature of which is filling or collapse of alveolar spaces. Thus, the chest radiograph will identify most such processes, with the exception of diffuse microatelectasis. As with $\dot{V}/\dot{Q}$ mismatch, vasoactive drugs like nitroprusside, dopamine, dobutamine, and other pulmonary vasodilators increase shunt and can worsen hypoxemia.[39] On occasion right-to-left shunting will occur within the heart; this is suggested when $\dot{Q}s/\dot{Q}t$ is out of proportion to the air space filling on the chest radiograph and can be confirmed with echocardiographic detection of infused bubbles or with early recirculation on a green dye dilution curve. This is rare but described to occur in acute pulmonary embolus, when increased pulmonary vascular resistance leads to increased right heart pressures and the opening of a patent foramen ovale with right-to-left flow at the atrial level.[40] Other causes of pulmonary hypertension combine with ischemia or congenital ventricular or atrial septal defects as remote causes.

Finally, it is important to determine if circulatory disturbances are resulting in arterial desaturation. In patients with substantial intrapulmonary shunts or $\dot{V}/\dot{Q}$ mismatch, mixed venous saturation will in part determine arterial desaturation. In hypoperfused states, anemia, and arterial desaturation, mixed venous desaturation may worsen, with arterial hypoxemia out of keeping with change in lung function. Thus, it is useful to follow the mixed venous oxygen saturation as well as parameters of perfusion (heart rate, blood pressure, cardiac output, urine output) when evaluating hypoxemia in patients with lung disease.

ATELECTASIS AND LOBAR COLLAPSE

Increasing age, obesity, volume overload, supine positioning, and smoking history are risk factors for diminished functional residual capacity and increased lung closing volumes, a confluence of lung abnormalities which can result in substantial atelectasis (see Chap. 1). In addition, patients undergoing intubation and mechanical ventilation are at risk for lobar collapse, particularly if airway secretions are tenacious, the artificial airway is malpositioned, or there is underlying neuromuscular weakness.

DIAGNOSIS. Atelectasis or lobar collapse is usually identified by abnormalities in gas exchange, physical examination, or chest radiograph. Diffuse atelectasis can occur with marked hypoxemia and minimal findings at the bedside or by chest radiography.

THERAPY AND PROPHYLAXIS. All critically ill patients should be considered at risk for this complication, and measures should be instituted to prevent its development. Three-point turning, early mobilization to a chair, incentive spirometry, and the upright position should be applied to patients at the earliest possible time. Mechanically ventilated patients often require ventilator adjustments to prevent atelectasis, and it is our clinical impression that sighs and low levels of PEEP (3 to 7 cmH_2O) are helpful in this regard. Large V_T should not be used to prevent atelectasis since they risk barotrauma (vide supra). Observation of collapse of the right upper lobe should prompt consideration of a right mainstem intubation; collapse of the left lower lobe is common in patients with neuromuscular disease undergoing mechanical ventilation. Once lobar collapse has occurred, reexpansion can often be accomplished by gradually increasing the V_T at the bedside. When recruitment of the lobe is accomplished, the airway pressure will be seen to no longer rise with the increased V_T and may actually fall, corresponding to the recruitment of collapsed lung providing a greater number of alveolar units to receive the fixed volume. If a collapsed lobe cannot be recruited before airway pressures of 50 to 55 cmH_2O are reached, chest physiotherapy, vigorous airway suctioning, and PEEP should be used for 12 to 24 h to achieve lobe expansion. If this is unsuccessful in reexpanding the lobe, or if initial concern for airway obstruction is high, fiberoptic bronchoscopy should be performed to confirm or establish airway patency. Most often inflammation and secretions are noted, without clear evidence of discrete, correctable obstruction. Nonetheless, fiberoptic bronchoscopy will often achieve partial or complete reexpansion.

Cardiovascular Complications

Common cardiovascular complications of critical illness that must be sought on a daily basis include pulmonary embolus, pulmonary artery catheter-associated problems, myocardial ischemia, and arrhythmias.

PULMONARY EMBOLI

INCIDENCE AND PATHOGENESIS. The frequency of pulmonary emboli complicating the course of patients with critical illness is difficult to ascertain. Conventional autopsy studies report an incidence from 8 to 27 percent[41,42] in patients with acute respiratory failure. On the other hand, pulmonary vascular lesions, thought to represent in situ pulmonary thrombi, not emboli, have been found in 90 percent of patients with ARDS.[43] Prospective clinical studies of pulmonary emboli in acute respiratory failure patients are largely unavailable. The source of pulmonary emboli in critically ill patients has been thought to be due primarily to deep venous thrombosis (DVT), especially of the lower extremity. Critically ill patients often possess many of the known risk factors for DVT, including prolonged venous stasis caused by bed rest, right and left ventricular failure, dehydration, obesity, and advanced age. Vessel injury and coagulation changes are likely important factors in patients with multiple trauma or undergoing surgical procedures. DVT has been found to occur in 13 to 29 percent of patients in an ICU.[44,45] Another source of pulmonary emboli in critically ill patients can be thrombus associated with intravenous catheters (vide infra).

DIAGNOSIS. The diagnosis of pulmonary emboli must be considered whenever acute unexplained dyspnea, hypoxemia, pulmonary hypertension, or hypotension develops in the critically ill patient. Accordingly, this diagnosis is considered very often in the ICU. The diagnosis, however, cannot be made on physical examination, laboratory, electrocardiographic (ECG), or hemodynamic abnormalities alone, since these tests are neither sensitive or specific. Definite diagnosis can be made with lung scanning in the appropriate setting, but this test loses value and can actually confound diagnosis in patients with radiographic infiltrates or clinical evidence of airway disease (see Chap. 118). Thus, in many instances, pulmonary angiography is necessary, although difficult to arrange due to the many impediments to transporting and investigating critically ill patients.[46]

PROPHYLAXIS AND TREATMENT. Prevention of pulmonary emboli in populations at risk is centered on prophylaxis of DVT or in the use of devices which prevent the migration of intravenous clot to the pulmonary circulation. As the precise frequency, cause, and impact of pulmonary emboli in patients with critical illness is unknown, the need for prophylaxis of DVT is controversial. Nonetheless, we feel the majority of critically ill patients are at risk for DVT and pulmonary embolus and will benefit from prophylactic therapy.[41,46] For most patients, we prefer the use of subcutaneous heparin at a dose of 5000 U every 8 to 12 h. If the patient does not have contraindications to anticoagulants but cannot tolerate heparin (i.e., heparin-induced thrombocytopenia), warfarin is an acceptable alternative.

Patients with absolute contraindications to low dose heparin therapy should have intermittent venous compression pneumatic devices applied to the lower extremities. Patients unable to receive anticoagulants should constitute only a small fraction of the critically ill and would include those individuals with active bleeding or recent brain or spinal cord injury.

Multiple trauma patients present a particular challenge for DVT prophylaxis. The incidence of this complication is high in this group, but lower extremity injury may preclude compression device use, and active bleeding may make anticoagulation unwise. Some authors have suggested placement of a Greenfield filter in the inferior vena cava to prevent pulmonary embolization in this group, but this approach has not been widely and prospectively evaluated.[46] As experience with these intravascular filters widens and as modifications are made to make them removable, their role in prophylaxis of pulmonary emboli during periods of critical illness may be expanded.

COMPLICATIONS ASSOCIATED WITH PULMONARY ARTERY CATHETERS

INSERTION COMPLICATIONS. Major complications of pulmonary artery catheter insertion include pneumothorax, air embolism, arrhythmias, phrenic or brachial nerve injury, carotid or subclavian injury, hemothorax, cardiac perforation with tamponade, and intrapleural or intramediastinal infusion of fluid. With experienced personnel, pneumothorax and venous air embolism are rare complications, although there exists a wide range of experience and training among housestaff performing this procedure among different academic centers. In patients requiring mechanical ventilation, any pneumothorax mandates tube thoracostomy. In spontaneously breathing patients with stable cardiopulmonary function, a small ($<$25 percent) pneumothorax may be observed with sequential examinations and radiographs, but the majority of patients will require tube drainage. Arterial punctures will usually respond to direct compression, which is difficult to achieve with subclavian puncture. On occasion bleeding from a carotid artery puncture will result in a large hematoma that compromises the airway; this is more likely in patients with an underlying coagulopathy.

Arrhythmias, especially ventricular arrhythmias, are frequent. Over 50 percent of patients whose severity of illness is described by a 51 percent mortality have advanced ventricular arrhythmias with placement of pulmonary artery catheters.[47] In general, premature ventricular contractions are self-limited and resolve with forward movement of the catheter. Risk factors for sustained ventricular tachycardia include myocardial infarction (MI) or ischemia, hypoxemia ($P_{O_2} < 60$ mmHg), and acidosis (pH < 7.20). Prolonged catheterization is another risk factor. Bundle branch block occurs much less frequently (estimated to occur in 3 to 5 percent of patients). Right bundle branch block is usually transient with resolution in 10 to 24 h.[47] Complete heart block is very infrequent. Treatment of ventricular tachyarrhythmia is standard. Prophylaxis is more controversial. Prophylactic lidocaine may be helpful in high risk patients with prolonged (>20 min) catheterization time. Transvenous pacemakers are not suggested in patients with chronic left bundle branch block but are recommended in patients with acute MI and right bundle branch block.[48] Pulmonary artery catheters with a pacemaker channel may be useful in this setting, as may external cardiac pacemakers.

COMPLICATIONS FOLLOWING INSERTION. Major complications seen after placement include pulmonary artery rupture, infection, and thrombosis. Pulmonary artery rupture is an infrequent complication occurring in <1/1000 insertions. Nevertheless, it is important because of its outcome. Mortality can be as high as 46 percent and increase to 75 percent in anticoagulated patients. Risk factors for the development of this complication include pulmonary hypertension, age >60 years, and improper location and inflation of the balloon.[49] Arterial trauma can also result in dissection of the pulmonary artery.[50] False pulmonary artery aneurysms secondary to the catheter present with hemoptysis. A well-developed mass or nodule adjacent to the pulmonary artery catheter position is seen radiographically. The mass persists 2 to 5 weeks. Diagnosis requires pulmonary angiography. Ablation of the aneurysm can be accomplished with steel coil transcatheter embolization. Guidelines for safe catheter use include anticipation and recognition of distal catheter migration, avoidance of permanent catheter wedging, and balloon hyperinflation. Infectious complications may either be local or systemic. Systemic infections include catheter-related sepsis (vide infra).

Thrombosis as a complication of the pulmonary artery catheter occurs in several ways. Persistent wedging in small pulmonary arteries causes thrombosis at the catheter tip with resultant infarction. However, this is an infrequent complication. Two other types of catheter-associated thrombus occur, fibrin sheath thrombus and mural thrombus. A *fibrous sheath or sleeve clot* is the most common form of catheter-associated clot.[51] It originates at the point of intimal injury where the catheter enters the vein. The clot then propagates downward toward the tip. Fibrin sheaths are visible only when contrast material is injected during catheter removal, but they do occur with most central catheter placements. The clinical significance of fibrin sheath formation is uncertain. Shearing of the fibrin sheath during catheter removal may cause pulmonary emboli. The second type of catheter-associated thrombus is *mural thrombus,* which begins where the catheter is in contact with the venous, endocardial, or pulmonary arterial wall and may be attached to the wall.[52] Clinical symptoms can result from occlusion of the vessel by the mural thrombus or embolization of thrombus into the pulmonary arteries. Although the potential for subclinical or clinically unrecognized or unrecorded problems seems high, the frequency of documented sequelae is low.

Effective measures to prevent catheter-associated thrombus have not been determined, although three areas of intervention are possible: catheter composition, anticoagulation, and duration of catheterization. Heparin-bonded catheters reduce thrombus with short-term use (1 to 2 days); however, thrombus can be identified in almost all catheters used for longer periods (6 days). Prophylaxis of catheter-associated thrombus with anticoagulation has not been evaluated and can only be inferred. Thrombosis is less frequent in patients with a history of coagulation disorders. Duration of catheterization affects the frequency of thrombosis. Catheterization for longer than 2 days increases the incidence and extent of thrombosis. Therefore, every effort should be made to use the pulmonary artery catheter for only the minimum time necessary.

In our view, the most commonly overlooked complication is misinterpretation of the hemodynamic data obtained and the consequent erroneous titration of patient care. In critical care training where fellows and housestaff occasionally regard completion of pulmonary artery catheter in numbers of procedures, emphasis must be refocused on integrating the hemodynamic interpretation with patient care as the end point of pulmonary artery catheterization. This obvious approach facilitates a questioning and skeptical approach to the indications for pulmonary artery catheterization and is the best way to encourage shorter use. When daily rounds encounter a patient with a pulmonary artery catheter, its continued use should be justified by answering the question: *What information am I obtaining to influence diagnosis and treatment which I would not have without the pulmonary artery catheter?*

ISCHEMIA

Myocardial ischemia is likely common during critical illness, although it is difficult to detect because of impaired patient perception and communication and atypical presentation. Although ischemia may be signalled by typical chest pain, other presentations are common and are listed in Table 52-6.

When phenomena listed in Table 52-6 are noted, further evaluation with ECG and serum enzyme analysis is recommended. Often the ECG is abnormal but not diagnostic for ischemic heart disease, i.e., the observed changes are consistent with electrolyte disturbances, the effects of mechanical ventilation, etc. In this circumstance, serial studies may

TABLE 52-6 Presentations of Myocardial Ischemia in the Critically Ill

Typical chest pain
Agitation with heart rate abnormalities
Sudden pulmonary edema
Sudden elevation of pulmonary capillary wedge pressure
ECG or echocardiographic abnormalities noted during "routine" monitoring

elicit subtle changes. Echocardiography may be useful here, with transient segmental wall motion abnormalities suggesting regional ischemia. All patients over the age of 40 or with known history of ischemic heart disease should have daily ECGs as a screening measure.

ARRHYTHMIAS

Continuous ECG monitoring is routine in virtually all critical care units. Heart rate or rhythm detection alarms and algorithms result in automatic recording of abnormal rhythms, and many units now have computerized storage of all recordings for 24 to 48 h for recall as needed.

Both bradyarrhythmias and tachyarrhythmias are extremely common in the course of critical illness, and the clinician must be familiar with the principles of specific diagnosis outlined elsewhere in the text (see Chap. 30). Although these rhythm disturbances may signal underlying cardiac disease, many are complications of therapy and should be recognized as such, obviating unnecessary diagnostics. Accordingly, it is helpful for the intensivist to have a list of anticipated arrhythmias complicating the disease and therapy of each critically ill patient so that early detection, prevention, and treatment plans are in place before they occur.

As noted above, atrial and ventricular tachyarrhythmias as well as heart block are common during right heart catheterization. Most often seen when the catheter is first passed through the right ventricle, they may occur with the catheter in place. These rhythm disturbances can also be noted when routine central venous catheters are placed, particularly during guidewire placement or if the catheter itself is advanced beyond the superior vena cava. The clinician should always be aware of the existence of intravascular devices when attempting to determine the cause of an arrhythmia, and should confirm appropriate catheter position.

Metabolic disturbances associated with arrhythmias include electrolyte disturbances (particularly hypokalemia and hyperkalemia, hypocalcemia, and hypomagnesemia) and hypoxia (see Chap. 120). Determination of serum electrolytes is advised in most patients with sustained or complex atrial or ventricular tachyarrhythmias, particularly if underlying metabolic abnormalities are suggested (e.g., prolonged QT interval, prominent U waves, T wave peaking, etc.). It can also be helpful to determine interventions and patient condition at the time the arrhythmia occurs. For example, bradyarrhythmia during airway suctioning or patient movement may suggest the effects of either hypoxia or excessive vagal tone. Ventricular tachycardia with QT interval prolongation during plasmapheresis may indicate a fall in ionized serum calcium resulting from the citrate load associated with this procedure.

Drug effects must be considered as a cause of observed atrial and ventricular arrhythmias in the critically ill. Catecholamine infusions frequently result in (worsened) sinus tachycardia and ventricular extrasystoles or ventricular tachycardia. Inhaled catecholamines rarely cause symptomatic arrhythmias in ambulatory patients. In critically ill asthmatic patients, however, these drugs are often titrated to an end point of undesirable side effects, often a heart rate or abnormal rhythm limit. Theophylline is a common cause of both atrial and ventricular tachyarrhythmias, and this side effect is a major reason for the need for frequent determination of serum methylxanthine levels. It is advisable to infuse theophylline through peripheral catheters to avoid high local concentrations in cardiac conduction tissue. All cardiac antiarrhythmic drugs are capable of adverse rhythm effects, and management of newly observed arrhythmias must include a careful review of these agents and their dosing, serum levels, and pharmacokinetics.

Severe lung disease and pulmonary hypertension are associated with atrial arrhythmias such as multifocal atrial tachycardia (MAT) and paroxysmal atrial tachycardia (PAT). These often respond to verapamil, but unfortunately this agent can result in significant hypotension in these patients due to arteriolar dilation with a fixed low cardiac output. More recently, adenosine infusion has been suggested in this setting, because its MAT-terminating effect is comparable and associated hypotension less.[53]

Gastrointestinal Complications

PNEUMOPERITONEUM

Pneumoperitoneum is often a diagnostic dilemma. Causes of free air in the peritoneal cavity detected by abdominal radiographic evaluation include ruptured viscus and barotrauma associated with mechanical ventilation (vide supra). When pneumoperitoneum is caused by barotrauma, other forms of barotrauma are also usually present, most commonly pneumothorax or pneumomediastinum. Thus, when mechanically ventilated patients are discovered to have pneumoperitoneum, the presence of thoracic manifestations of barotrauma and the absence of abdominal signs and symptoms of perforation suggest that barotrauma is the likely cause. If this association cannot be firmly established, the patient should undergo surgical evaluation for possible intraabdominal catastrophe.

Treatment of pneumoperitoneum caused by mechanical ventilation is guided by the amount of air present. Most often no specific therapy is required, but evacuation with a tube may be necessary if a large amount of air results in abdominal distention and difficulty in ventilation.

ALTERATIONS IN GASTROINTESTINAL MOTILITY

Alterations in gastrointestinal motility occur in patients with acute respiratory failure, especially those who are mechanically ventilated. Clinical manifestations include ileus and diarrhea. Decreased bowel sounds and abdominal distention may occur in as many as 50 percent of patients with respiratory failure.[54] Early aggressive correction of electrolyte abnormalities, reduction of morphine and other drugs which reduce motility, discontinuation of enteral feedings, and suction from above and below will decrease the morbidity from progressive bowel dilation. After digital disimpaction, a low threshold for colonscopic drainage and decompression may avoid late complications of megacolon or colonic rupture.

Likewise, the incidence of diarrhea in critical patients may also approach 50 percent. Multifactorial causes of diarrhea in the ICU include enteral alimentation, medications such as antacids or cimetidine, infection, hypoalbuminemia, and dietary lipids.[55] Definitive treatment of diarrhea requires modifying known causes of diarrhea.

COMPLICATIONS OF RECTAL TUBE USE

Rectal catheters have long been used for brief periods of time to achieve bowel decompression before or during surgery or to remove contrast material following radiologic investigations. Increasingly they are finding application for continuous colonic decompression in critically ill patients and are on occasion used for the patient with uncontrollable massive diarrhea. It should be signaled that complications with these devices are frequent and include discomfort, local ulceration and necrosis, secondary infection, and perforation with extraperitoneal migration and contamination.[56] It is recommended that rectal tubes be used only for clear indications and that these indications be reviewed on a daily basis so that the device does not become a nursing and physician "convenience." In addition, it is advisable to deflate the tube at least twice daily to inspect for related injuries.

GASTROINTESTINAL HEMORRHAGE

Much is discussed below and in Chap. 163 about this common complication. It is surprising how often the answer to the following relevant questions asked on daily rounds allow adjustments of therapy associated with demonstrated reduction in morbidity: *Is the patient receiving antacids, H2 blockers or sucralfate? What is the pH of gastric suckings? Is there blood or guaiac-positive reaction of the gastric secretions, stool, or ostomy liquid? Does intercurrent coagulopathy, shock, respiratory-renal-hepatic dysfunction invite increased prophylaxis for gastrointestinal hemorrhage?*

PATHOGENESIS. In general, two different types of upper gastrointestinal hemorrhage occur in the ICU. First are those patients who initially present with hemorrhage caused by a variety of diverse gastrointestinal disorders such as esophageal varices or acid-peptic disease. Second are those critically ill patients, often with multisystem disease, who present with nongastroenterologic disease such as acute respiratory failure but develop gastrointestinal hemorrhage later in their ICU course as a complication of critical illness. In these instances, hemorrhage is most commonly caused by, but not limited to, "stress" or acute gastric ulceration.

Pathologically stress ulcerations are erosions superficial to the muscularis mucosa. These multiple, shallow erosions predominately involve the stomach and are usually found in the fundus with sparing of the antrum. Stress ulcers develop from a temporary failure of one or more of the gastric defense mechanisms. Normally the intraluminal hydrogen ion concentration is enormous compared to the intramural hydrogen concentration. Even under these conditions, the gastric mucosa maintains this gradient and protects itself. This defense or self-protection can be defined as the gastric mucosal barrier. Originally the barrier was envisioned as a tangible physical impediment such as the mucus lining layer, but no anatomic barrier has been identified. Instead preservation of gastric mucosal integrity is a dynamic process dependent on systemic tissue and humoral factors. Normal gastric blood flow, systemic acid-base balance, and normal mucosal secretory state are essential to prevent mucosal breakdown and resultant ulceration.[56] Mucosal ischemia secondary to decreased gastric blood flow is one of the most important factors in stress ulceration. Ischemia reduces mucosal capacity to neutralize acid entering the tissue. Hydrogen ion accumulates with resultant mucosal acidification and ulceration. Ischemia may also affect gastric energy metabolism. Luminal acid and pepsin are important in the pathogenesis of stress ulceration, but not because of increased hydrogen ion concentration. Other than stress ulceration associated with diseases of the CNS (Cushing's ulcer), increased concentration of acid and pepsin are not found in critically ill patients. Acid and pepsin are generally thought to be required for the development of stress ulceration, but the primary mechanisms of ulceration are tissue acidosis or ischemia which result in impaired mucosal handling of hydrogen ion already present.

DIAGNOSIS. The clinical diagnosis of gastrointestinal hemorrhage is made by the appearance of hematemesis, melena, bright red blood per nasogastric tube, or signs of hypovolemic shock. Hematest-positive nasogastric aspirate in the absence of other signs of acute blood loss is a less reliable sign of significant gastrointestinal hemorrhage. It should be emphasized that nasogastric suction itself frequently causes multiple small mucosal erosions. Stress ulceration can be found in a majority of critically ill patients; however, not all ulcerations result in gastrointestinal hemorrhage. The frequency with which such bleeding occurs varies depending on the diagnostic method used and the patient population studied. Severe or massive gastrointestinal bleeding occurs in about 5 percent of medical ICU patients.[57] Risk factors for the development of gastrointestinal hemorrhage include major trauma, shock from any cause, sepsis, renal failure, jaundice, and acute respiratory failure.[57] Bleeding occurs more frequently in ARDS than in other causes of acute respiratory failure. Also, patients who are ventilated have a higher incidence of bleeding than nonventilated patients with lung disease. Bleeding occurs in 30 percent of ventilated patients compared to only 3 percent of nonventilated patients.[58] Prolonged mechanical ventilation (>5 days) is also associated with an increased risk of bleeding. Coagulopathy increases bleeding. Thrombocytopenia or prolonged prothrombin time (PT) or partial thromboplastin time (PTT) was found in over 75 percent of mechanically ventilated patients who bled.[59] Most studies show increasing risk of gastrointestinal hemorrhage with increasing number of risk factors or other evidence of MSOF, especially renal failure and jaundice. Patients with gastrointestinal hemorrhage are sicker as evidenced by longer ventilator and ICU days as well as increased mortality.

THERAPY. Therapy of stress ulceration should correct conditions favoring its development. Correction of hypoperfusion and acidosis are prime considerations. Indeed the frequency of stress ulceration may be decreased since its early description is due in large part to better control of hypotension and acidosis. At times, however, it may not be possible to control these conditions. Therefore, prophylaxis of stress ulceration and resultant hemorrhage has assumed great importance. Prophylactic measures have centered on neutralizing gastric acidity with antacids or decreasing gastric acid secretion with histamine-receptor blockade such as cimetidine or ranitidine. Sucralfate appears to provide stress ulcer protection without reducing levels of gastric acid. Although early individual studies indicated antacids to be superior to H_2 blockers, recent combined analysis suggest both are equal in efficacy.[60] In addition, complications associated with their use have limited initial enthusiasm for aggressive prophylaxis. In addition to other complications, antacids require large nursing time commitment to administer these agents every 1 to 2 h with intragastric pH measurement. Both antacids and H_2 blockers are associated with gastric colonization caused by alkalinization of gastric pH.[61] Resultant transmission of gastric organisms into the airways with the development of nosocomial pneumonia is a possibility. Sucralfate may lessen this complication.[61]

Nutrition may be a useful prophylaxis against stress ulceration. Enteral nutrition is associated with decreased gastrointestinal hemorrhage in burn patients and mechanically ventilated respiratory ICU patients.[62,63] The mechanism for this protective effect of enteral nutrition is not known. Enteral administration of metabolic substrate may achieve gastric cytoprotection without an effect on gastric acidity. The gastric mucosa has extremely low glycogen stores and therefore, may depend on a continuous supply of substrate for metabolism. Focal gastric necrosis results from any energy deficit, particularly severe in the fundus because energy metabolism is primarily aerobic. Gastric colonization with resultant nosocomial pneumonia can also occur with enteral feeding.[64]

A summary recommendation for prophylactic therapy of stress ulceration is difficult. It is important to know that mortality has not been shown to decrease with prophylaxis. Also, severe massive overt gastrointestinal hemorrhage is infrequent, but appears to occur in those patients with risk factors of prolonged mechanical ventilation and coagulopathy. The worrisome gastrointestinal hemorrhage occurs in a very critically ill patient population where bleeding may be yet another marker of multiorgan involvement and thus, not responsive to prophylaxis. Certainly not all ICU patients require prophylaxis. Mechanically ventilated patients with coagulopathy or other risk factors such as sepsis, hypotension, or renal failure should receive prophylaxis. Further information is needed to determine if prophylaxis will significantly alter long-term outcome.

NUTRITIONAL COMPLICATIONS

Nutritional complications in critical illness include the adverse effects of malnutrition on the cardiopulmonary system as well as complications associated with the administration of either parenteral or enteral nutrition. Helpful questions incorporated into daily rounds to ensure adequate early nutrition in each patient are: *What are this patient's protein and calorie requirements? What is this patient receiving? By what route? Why not enterally?*

ADVERSE EFFECTS OF MALNUTRITION. Malnutrition is virtually a universal problem in critically ill patients. Furthermore, nutritional status may deteriorate during hospitalization. Inadequate nutritional support on an iatrogenic basis occurs frequently in ventilated patients.[65] Poor nutritional status can adversely affect pulmonary function by impairment of respiratory muscle power generation and pulmonary defense mechanisms. These adverse effects are independent of the presence or absence of primary lung disease, but clearly can be additive in some patients with respiratory failure, especially those with COPD.

In critical illness, protein catabolism occurs to provide energy. In simple starvation without the stress of critical illness, energy sources are primarily fat. With inadequate caloric intake in critically ill patients, energy sources are derived from protein breakdown and gluconeogenesis. Of various protein "pools," the muscle protein pool is susceptible to catabolism to provide fuel. Respiratory muscles are skeletal muscles and, therefore, susceptible to this catabolic effect. Malnutrition reduces diaphragmatic muscle mass and diaphragmatic strength with an impairment in respiratory muscle function.[66,67] Nutritional repletion can improve or alter respiratory muscle strength in some patients.

Ventilatory drive is also affected by nutritional status and nutritional intake. Clinical semistarvation reduces ventilatory response to hypoxemia by almost half.[68] Refeeding returns the hypoxic drive to base line. It is not clear that these changes in ventilatory drive are clinically significant. Malnutrition also influences the immune system with the most profound effects found in cell-mediated immunity. Although serum levels of immunoglobulins are normal, turnover may be impaired. Clinical sequelae of altered respiratory muscle strength, ventilatory drive, and immune mechanisms could include precipitation of hypercapnic respiratory failure, difficulty in weaning from mechanical ventilation, and infection, particularly nosocomial lung infection.

COMPLICATIONS OF NUTRITIONAL SUPPORT. Complications associated with enteral nutrition can be classified into mechanical, gastrointestinal, and metabolic categories.[69] Mechanical complications relate to the size and position of the feeding tube and include inadvertent nasotracheal passage, clogging, obstruction of the tube, and aspiration of enteral feeding. Pleuropulmonary complications include pneumothorax, pneumomediastinum, subcutaneous emphysema, and death. A common finding in these cases is the use of a wire stylet to assist passage of the flexible feeding tube. Neurologically impaired or pharmacologically sedated patients are at high risk. Radiologic confirmation of placement is essential.

The incidence and sequelae of aspiration from enteral feeding is difficult to determine. Studies vary in the patient population, size of feeding tubes, methods of enteral feeding, and criteria for aspiration. Clinically significant aspiration appears infrequent when enteral feeding is administered continuously via a small bore feeding tube in intubated patients. Prevention of gastric content aspiration should be directed at minimizing the mechanical factors contributing to regurgitation such as patient elevation and improper tube placement. Gastric residual should be checked frequently, especially in patients at risk for slowed gastric emptying.

Gastrointestinal complications of enteral feeding include vomiting, abdominal distention, and diarrhea (vide supra). Metabolic complications of enteral nutrition include electrolyte abnormalities. Hyperglycemia and hypophosphatemia are common. Periodic evaluation of electrolyte levels should be undertaken in all patients fed enterally.

Complications related to total parenteral nutrition (TPN) are also multiple and can be the source of increased morbidity and mortality. They are classified into mechanical, infectious, or metabolic categories.[70] Mechanical complications include those of catheter placement. Pneumothorax and arterial injury occur in 1 to 8 percent of TPN catheters. Tension pneumothorax can develop and lead to death. Material for tube thoracostomy should be immediately available. Catheter-related sepsis is an important complication of TPN that appears to be more frequent with the use of multilumen catheters. The most common organisms isolated include staphylococci and fungi, particularly *Candida* species. Appropriate antimicrobial therapy is required in addition to removal of the catheter. Although many authors advocate a course of antibiotics in an attempt to sterilize an infected catheter in stable patients receiving home or long-term hyperalimentation, this is generally not an advisable course in the critically ill individual. Major metabolic complications include hyperchloremic acidosis, hyperglycemia, and hypophosphatemia. Hepatic abnormalities are frequent in patients receiving TPN.[71] Histologic findings of fatty liver, cholestasis, and triaditis develop after short-term TPN. Clinically these findings are heralded by abnormalities in serum hepatic function studies. The frequency of reported hepatic abnormalities varies widely. The cause of liver function abnormalities remains obscure. Current recommendations to diminish hepatic injury include avoidance of excessive quantities of carbohydrates and protein with 10 to 30 percent of nonprotein calorie supplied as lipid.[71] Serum enzyme studies should be performed weekly.

Worsening hypercapnia can occur in patients receiving either enteral or parenteral nutrition and is often associated with excess carbohydrate calorie administration. Carbon dioxide production increases because calories in excess of energy needs result in lipogenesis and a markedly increased respiratory quotient (RQ). The RQ is the ratio of carbon dioxide production to oxygen consumption during substrate utilization. The RQ of glucose is 1.0 and the RQ of fat is 0.7; however, the RQ of lipogenesis is approximately 8.8, reflecting the much greater production of carbon dioxide relative to oxygen consumed. Hypercapnia from increased CO_2 production is avoided in normal persons by a compensatory increase in ventilation. Patients with compromised ventilatory status such as COPD or weak respiratory muscles may be unable to increase ventilation appropriately. Hypercapnia may result. Clinical sequelae of excess carbohydrate calories in critically ill patients include precipitation of acute respiratory failure or difficulty in weaning from mechanical ventilation.[72,73] Quantitation of carbon dioxide production is accomplished by indirect calorimetry or by analyzing a timed collection of expired air. This problem can be avoided by identifying patients at risk (COPD, the "difficult to wean" patient), avoiding excessive calorie administration (follow nutritional formulae and nitrogen excretion), and providing of a high percentage (40 to 50 percent) of calories as lipids in the appropriate patient population.

Infectious Complications

It is quite common to encounter patients on daily ICU rounds with new onset leukocytosis or leukopenia with a shift to immature forms, with new onset fever or hypothermia, and with other suggestions of new infection such as high cardiac output hypotension, thrombocytopenia, tachycardia, increased bilirubin level, oliguria, or decreased level of consciousness. Of course, the discerning intensivist has a broad differential for each of these, but a low threshold for an early search for infection is indicated. Beyond the initial surveillance cultures of blood, sputum, or endotracheal secretions and urine, most such critically ill patients benefit from an aggressive systematic top-to-bottom search for additional sites of infection: meningitis, sinusitis, septic thrombophlebitis, line sepsis, endocarditis, nosocomial pneumonia, empyema, pericarditis/pleuritis, abdominal or pelvic abscess, rectal abscess, peritonitis, acalculous cholecystitis, decubitus ulceration, and arthritis. As always, the search begins with review of the history and course of each patient's critical illness followed by a focused physical examination to elicit evidence for the specific disorders listed above. Special diagnostic procedures can then be prioritized to initiate the search immediately with the highest yield probes: CT scan of head and sinuses, lumbar puncture, echocardiography, thoracentesis, ultrasound of right upper quadrant or kidney, CT of the abdomen or pelvis, etc.

NOSOCOMIAL PNEUMONIA

PATHOGENESIS. Nosocomial pneumonia is a frequent complication of critical illness with multiple adverse sequelae. It occurs in 20 percent of mechanically ventilated patients in a medical ICU and as many as 68 percent of patients with ARDS.[74] Morbidity is increased in terms of worsening lung function and lengthened duration of hospitalization. Nosocomial pneumonia is also associated with increased mortality. Only 12 percent of ARDS patients with nosocomial pneumonia survived in a recent analysis of 129 patients with ARDS.[74] The mortality rate was related directly to the infection and development of other complications.

Gram-negative bacilli represent over half the organisms responsible for infection. Sources for potential nosocomial pathogens are multiple and include invasive monitoring devices, respiratory therapy equipment, medical personnel, and sites in the ICU such as food or sinks. Despite these exogenous sources for nosocomial pathogens, however, most infections appear to result from endogenous sources. The incidence of nosocomial infection was not different in an old versus a new hospital even though major differences in environmental contamination were present.[75] Therefore, although many potential and, at times, real sources of nosocomial infection are present in the patient's environment, it is the host's response to serious underlying disease necessitating these support devices and not the environment itself that is usually most important.

The primary pathogenetic mechanism of nosocomial lung infection relates to oropharyngeal colonization with subsequent tracheobronchial colonization by gram-negative organisms. Colonization or the growth of potential pathogenic organisms in the absence of clinical infection is well recognized in critically ill patients. In early work colonization was found in 73 percent of moribund patients compared to only 6 percent in healthy hospital workers.[76] Later data indicated 37 percent of ICU patients developed colonization; nosocomial pneumonia developed in almost 23 percent of these patients.[77] Gram-negative colonization occurs rapidly in critically ill patients; more than three-fourths of the patients become colonized in the first 3 days. Rapid colonization, in the absence of subdetectible colonization in patients transferred into the ICU from another part of the hospital, suggests a "susceptible" patient pool. Susceptibility is largely due to changes in oropharyngeal and tracheobronchial cell adherence. Increased gram-negative colonization results from increased buccal and airway adhesion due to increased availability of bacterial receptor sites. The mechanism for this is not entirely known. Epithelial cell surface glycoproteins such as fibronectin may be depleted by high salivary protease activity and thus may expose receptors for gram-negative organisms.[78] Other possible mechanisms include loss of interbactericidal inhibition and alteration of pH.[79]

Although microorganisms can reach the airway by inhalation, inoculation from contiguous sites of infection, and hematogenous spread, aspiration of colonized oropharyngeal contents is generally thought to be responsible for most cases of tracheobronchial colonization and pneumonia. Recently, another mechanism of tracheobronchial colonization independent of oropharyngeal colonization has been described. Gastric colonization with subsequent tracheal appearance of gastric organisms has been found in patients undergoing gastric pH manipulation with antacids or cimetidine. Sterile acid gastric contents have been found on ICU admission, but within 24 to 48 h after alkalinization, multiple organisms including gram-negatives have been cultured from tracheal aspirate.[80] Enteral nutrition, in the absence of antacids or H_2 blockers may also result in gastric colonization. In a recent study of simultaneous gastric, tracheal, and oropharyngeal cultures, enteral feeding was associated with increased gastric colonization. Tracheal colonization occurred not only after oropharyngeal colonization but also after gastric colonization.[81] Thus, sources of tracheal colonization include not only aspiration of colonized oropharyngeal contents, but aspiration of colonized gastric contents as well. Tracheal colonization can also occur without prior appearance of the organism(s) in the oropharynx or stomach.[81] The source of these organisms is not entirely known.

DIAGNOSIS. The diagnosis of nosocomial pneumonia is very difficult, particularly in patients with radiographic infiltrates already present. These patients may also have other causes of fever, leukocytosis, and positive sputum cultures, the traditional diagnostic guidelines of pneumonia. Thus, the distinction between tracheobronchial colonization and pneumonia is difficult if not impossible. Andrews and associates compared the clinical predictors of bacterial pneumonia with postmortem histologic findings in patients with ARDS.[82] At autopsy, 58 percent of 30 consecutive patients had histologic pneumonia. Of these patients, 36 percent thought to have only ARDS had pneumonia, and 20 percent thought to have pneumonia had ARDS. The clinical predictors of pneumonia were not helpful in the diagnosis; in the nonpneumonia group 80 percent had fever and leukocytosis, 70 percent had sputum pathogens, and 30 percent had asymmetry on the chest x-ray. Also, the response to antibiotics was not helpful in correctly assessing the presence of pneumonia. More recent data confirm and extend these observations. In almost 150 mechanically ventilated patients clinically suspected of nosocomial pneumonia, stepwise logistic regression analysis of 16 clinical variables failed to find any combination which was useful in distinguishing patients with bacterial pneumonia.[83] Thus, it appears the diagnosis of nosocomial pneumonia cannot be reliably made by clinical criteria.

In the setting of clinically suspected nosocomial pneumonia in mechanically ventilated patients, empirical antibiotics are often administered either before or in lieu of culture data. Studies indicate even adequate or appropriate antibiotic therapy is not beneficial. In vitro microorganism susceptibility and antibiotics administered were studied in 108 infections in 129 ARDS patients.[74] Patients receiving adequate antibiotic therapy did not have a higher survival rate (29 percent) than those who received inadequate antibiotics (23 percent). Antibiotic therapy prior to the development of nosocomial pneumonia influences the frequency of various types of pneumonia. Prior antibiotic therapy was assessed in mechanically ventilated patients with nosocomial pneumonia.[84] The incidence of *Pseudomonas* and *Acinetobacter* pneumonia was 61 percent in those patients with prior antibiotic therapy compared to an incidence of only 19 percent in patients without prior antibiotics. The frequency of methicillin resistance in staphylococcal infection was increased from 33 percent to 100 percent in patients with prior antibiotics. These data suggest antibiotics may not only be ineffective but may also increase the rates of serious gram-negative or difficult to treat gram-positive pneumonia.

Because diagnosis is difficult, new techniques and technologies have been introduced to improve diagnostic sensitivity and specificity of nosocomial pneumonia. Most interest has centered around the use of the protected specimen brush (PSB) or BAL with bronchoscopy. The PSB attempts to bypass upper airway contamination by using a telescoping cannula brush to obtain lower airway secretions. Quantitative PSB cultures ($>10^3$ cfu/mL) have been shown to be highly accurate in diagnosis of nosocomial pneumonia. In early work, quantitative PSB culture was 100 percent sensitive and 60 percent specific in 26 ventilated patients where immediate postmortem PSB cultures were compared to corresponding histopathology.[85] In more recent work, the clinical utility of PSB culture was studied in a large group of ventilated patients.[82] The PSB diagnosis was rigorously confirmed or excluded. No patient with $<10^3$ cfu/ml was subsequently found to have pneumonia and only four or five patients diagnosed with pneumonia were subsequently found to have false-positive cultures. Quantitative BAL cultures may also have utility in the diagnosis of nosocomial pneumonia. Animal data suggest quantitative BAL culture correlated well with bacterial counts in the lung provided culture results are expressed as a "bactericidal index" defined as the sum of logarithmic concentrations of individual species.[86] The superiority of PSB or BAL in the diagnosis of nosocomial pneumonia is not known with certainty. Some data suggest PSB is more accurate,[87] other data suggest BAL is.[86] Excellent agreement between PSB and BAL cultures regarding the type of recovered organism has been demonstrated in mechanically ventilated patients.[88] BAL, however, may be associated with a higher degree of contamination by oropharyngeal bacterial flora.[89]

PREVENTION. General strategies aimed at the prevention of nosocomial pneumonia include efforts to improve host defense mechanisms as well as measures directed at decreasing airway colonization and bacterial inoculation into the lower airway. Although no generally accepted methods to decrease airway colonization exist, recent preliminary information suggests that specific antibiotic prophylaxis in high risk patients decreases not only airway gram-negative colonization but also gram-negative nosocomial pneumonia.[90–92] However, more controlled studies in patients with acute respiratory failure should be prospectively obtained, and routine antibiotic prophylaxis cannot be recommended at this time.

BACTEREMIA AND SEPSIS

Bacteremia is defined classically as the presence of bacteria in the bloodstream as determined by blood cultures. Clinical sepsis or the sepsis syndrome occurs when fever, hypotension, tachycardia, alterations in mental status, or leukocytosis occur with or without positive blood cultures. Sepsis, as a complication of critical illness, is associated with increased morbidity and mortality. Sepsis is a primary cause of death in ARDS.[93] It is also associated with nonpulmonary organ failure such as renal failure, hepatic failure, and coagulopathy.

Bacteremia can be primary or secondary.[94] Sources of secondary bacteremia are those secondary to a known infection. Primary bacteremia originates most frequently from intravascular devices. Pulmonary artery catheter-related sepsis is infrequent (1 to 4 percent), but colonized catheters may be the source of sepsis.[95] Bacteremia secondary to arterial catheters is likewise infrequent.[96] Other components of the system besides the catheter itself can cause bacteremia. Stopcocks, pressure transducers, and flush solutions can become colonized and release organisms into the circulation. Bacteremia may signal endocarditis as well as the sepsis syndrome. Pulmonary artery catheter-induced endothelial damage can result in damaged valvular leaflets with risk for subsequent endocardial infection.[97]

Line sepsis is best prevented by meticulous attention to detail in line maintenance and early discontinuation, generally within 48 to 72 h, for catheters placed in the ICU. When assessing the patient for possible line sepsis, culturing through the suspect catheter and from peripheral sites is helpful. Persistently positive cultures obtained through the catheter, with negative cultures at other sites, strongly suggests at least colonization of the catheter.

Renal Complications

ACUTE RENAL FAILURE

The development of renal failure in patients with critical illness, particularly acute respiratory failure, is an ominous prognostic sign. Mortality approaches 80 percent in patients with ARDS who develop renal failure.[98] An early response to oliguria or new increases in blood urea nitrogen (BUN) and creatinine levels should occur immediately. This approach excludes or treats prerenal and postrenal causes and reviews the list of potential nephrotoxins many patients are receiving.

TABLE 52-7 Common Nephrotoxic Drugs Used in Critical Illness

Antibiotics
Aminoglycosides
Amphotericin
Nonsteroidal Anti-inflammatories
Immunosuppressives
Cyclosporine
Anesthetics
Enflurane
Methoxyflurane
Contrast Media
Chemotherapy Agents
Cisplatin
Methyl-CCNU
Mitomycin-C
Adriamycin
Methotrexate

Common causes of acute renal failure in the ICU include hypoperfusion with prerenal azotemia, acute tubular necrosis (ATN) caused by decreased renal perfusion, and tubular dysfunction following nephrotoxic drug administration. Despite its relative rarity, *the index of suspicion for obstructive uropathy must be high,* since therapeutic approach will be different from other etiologies of renal dysfunction. Renal ultrasound is an excellent screening test for this possibility. Every patient with renal dysfunction in the ICU should have a careful review of medication history, with particular attention to the drugs listed in Table 52-7.

Therapy of acute renal failure should be directed at its apparent cause. Expansion of volume deficit or relief of urinary tract obstruction are obvious modalities in prerenal or postrenal azotemia. No specific therapy for ATN exists. Goals for ATN include preventing ATN, shortening its course, or increasing urine output. General management of the patient with acute failure includes preventing infection and bleeding, maintaining fluid and electrolyte balance, and providing adequate nutrition.

ASSESSMENT OF FLUID BALANCE

Alterations in renal hemodynamics and tubular function are common in critically ill patients as a result of hypoxemia, acidosis, mechanical ventilation, PEEP, and postoperative changes in water balance.[99] Adverse consequences include positive water balance, edema, hyponatremia, and possible increased mortality. Hormonal and nonhormonal mechanisms are responsible. Elevated antidiuretic hormone levels are found in almost half the hypoxemic and hypercapnic respiratory failure patients.[100] Patients with acute respiratory failure often have maximally compromised gas exchange. Further deterioration from fluid retention is neither desirable nor necessary. Close observation of renal status and fluid balance is important.[101] A daily answer to these questions allows early detection and treatment of abnormal trends in total body water, its distribution, and its effects on electrolyte balance: *What is the change in weight, serum sodium concentration, and fluid intake and output compared to yesterday and again compared to 3 days ago?*

Hematologic Complications

Perturbations in red, white, and megakaryocytic cell lines are common in critical illness. Hematocrit drops of more than 2 to 3 percent in 24 h should prompt consideration of excessive blood loss, underproduction, or both. In addition to obvious sites of blood loss (gastrointestinal tract, surgical drains, etc.), traumatized, anticoagulated, or instrumented patients may have loss at relatively occult sites. Retroperitoneal hemorrhage in the heparinized patient or thigh hematoma following intraaortic balloon pump removal are examples of sites that are somewhat difficult to evaluate. CT scanning can be of help in these settings. Not uncommonly, evidence of hemolysis is sought or reported late in the critically ill patient. A high index of suspicion in acute anemia can be tested by taping a blood sample to the cubicle wall and checking shortly thereafter for pink supernatant after the cells settle. Such evidence should prompt immediate evaluation for disseminated intravascular coagulation (DIC, vide infra) or drug-induced hemolysis. Dilutional contributions to anemia are frequently seen following massive fluid resuscitation. Finally, critically ill patients often have very significant volumes of blood removed for laboratory testing in combination with the frequent flushing and clearing of right heart and arterial catheters. While this is a "diagnosis by exclusion," it is a frequent contributor to the anemia observed in the course of critical illness.

Thrombocytopenia can be caused by both increased consumption and decreased thrombopoiesis in acute respiratory failure.[102] Other causes of increased platelet consumption include DIC and intravascular pressure monitoring devices. Platelet counts have been reported to drop (maximal decrease 50,000/mm^3) following the placement of right heart catheters.

Observation of significant thrombocytopenia should prompt careful medication review. Most drug-related thrombocytopenia results from diminished production. By contrast, heparin can induce antiplatelet antibody formation in approximately 5 percent of patients receiving this drug.[103] These antibodies cause platelet aggregation with resulting thrombotic and hemorrhagic complications. Thrombocytopenia via this mechanism most commonly occurs 7 to 8 days after initiation of treatment, although patients receiving a second course of heparin may manifest thrombocytopenia within 2 days. Since the causes of thrombocytopenia may be multiple in a given patient and anticoagulation may be a crucial component of management, it is often useful to assay for these IgG immunoglobulins.[104] Heparin-associated thrombocytopenia usually responds promptly to discontinuation of the drug, but patients with severe thrombotic and hemorrhagic complications have been treated with intravenous immunoglobulin.[105] Antiplatelet antibodies may result from even prophylactic doses of heparin and conceivably from exposure to heparin-coated catheters.[106]

Relatively acute depression of thrombopoiesis can also occur during critical illness. Acute folic acid deficiency can cause thrombocytopenia sometimes in the absence of leukopenia and anemia.[107] Clinical risk factors include postoperative status, renal failure, sepsis, and TPN. Folic acid replacement results in prompt improvement.

Endocrinologic Complications

Thyroid function tests are frequently abnormal in acutely ill patients with nonthyroidal disease. The term "euthyroid sick syndrome" is used to describe these patients. Thyroxin (T_4) levels are low, while free T_4 and thyrotrophin (TSH) values are within normal limits. Although a normal TSH value rules out primary hypothyroidism, pituitary abnormalities in critical illness occur which make interpretation of a normal TSH value difficult.[108] Thyroid function studies should not be routinely ordered in critically ill patients unless a clinical suspicion of hypothyroidism or hyperthyroidism exists.

Glucose intolerance is extremely common as well, particularly during sepsis or the hypermetabolic phase of MSOF. Euglycemia may be achieved only with great effort, and it is unclear what benefit is conferred on the previously nondiabetic patient to have blood sugar levels dropped from the 150 to 200 mg/dL range to normal by insulin infusion.

De novo adrenal insufficiency is uncommon in critical illness, but can result from shock (hemorrhagic and septic) and has been associated with certain drug use, in particular ketoconazole and rifampin. More common is the circumstance of iatrogenic adrenal insufficiency preceding or accompanying acute illness. When adrenal insufficiency is suspected and the patient is hemodynamically unstable, stress doses of dexamethasone should be administered while a cortisol level is obtained before and after an ACTH stimulation test is performed. (See Chap. 160.)

Pharmacologic Complications

Drug toxicity may manifest as dysfunction of any organ system (vide supra), but a few comments should be made about the generic problem of minimizing drug side effects. Daily rounds on critically ill patients should include a thorough review of all medications. Changes in agents, dose, or route of administration; reasons for drug administration; and possible toxicities should all be noted. Most of this information will be forthcoming by review of the medication sheet on rounds and discussion with the bedside nurse. Many critical care units regularly include pharmacy staff on rounds. Minimizing drug errors can be achieved by this review as well as by simple measures such as automatic discontinuation of orders at 48 to 72 h, thus mandating review and reordering. The clinician must be aware of and check drug delivery systems, which are increasingly varied and complex in the ICU (e.g., continuous infusion pumps, intrapleural or epidural administration of anesthetic, chemotherapy reservoirs, etc.). A number of complications arise from inappropriate administration site (e.g., aminophylline through a central line), inappropriate rate of administration (incorrectly set or functioning pump or flowguard giving vasoactive drugs at high rates), or from incorrectly placed devices (e.g., infiltration of vasoactive drugs around intravenous catheter sites).

CASE PRESENTATION

T.G., a 14-year-old white male was transferred to the University of Kansas Medical Center from a community hospital on May 12, 1989 complaining of fever and dyspnea. He had been in good health until 1 week prior to admission when an infected right great toenail was noted and removed with grossly black discharge present. He then developed right knee and leg pain and fever. Fever continued after admission to the local hospital, followed by the development of signs of coagulopathy (increased PT, PTT, and thrombocytopenia). One day prior to transfer he developed acute respiratory distress.

On admission to the ICU, he was dyspneic but alert and cooperative. The temperature was 37.8°C (100.3°F), pulse 120, blood pressure 100/50 mmHg, and respiratory rate 45. Cardiac examination was unremarkable. Chest examination showed decreased breath sounds in the right basilar area. His right lower extremity was tender, erythematous, and swollen. The chest x-ray revealed diffuse alveolar infiltrates consistent with pulmonary edema, a large right pleural effusion, and cavitary pulmonary nodules in all lung fields. Ventilation perfusion lung scan was consistent with pulmonary emboli. Arterial blood-gas values with oxygen by nasal cannula showed pH of 7.46, P_{O_2} of 60 mmHg, and P_{CO_2} of 32 mmHg. Hemoglobin and hematocrit were normal and the WBC count was 11,100 with left shift. The PT was 13.2, PTT 35.9, and platelets 76,000/mm^3. FDP was >40, BUN 38 mg/dL, and creatine 0.9 mg/dL. The remainder of his laboratory examinations were within normal limits.

On the second day, blood cultures were reported positive for *Staphylococcus aureus*. A venogram showed right femoral vein thrombosis. Gas exchange deteriorated and the patient was intubated. At that time diagnoses included staphylococcal sepsis, acute respiratory failure due to ARDS and pulmonary emboli, and DVT. Endotracheal intubation was accomplished orally with a 7.0-mm tube. Position was confirmed at 24 cm at the mouth, and nursing and respiratory therapy staff were informed of the appropriate position. Initial mechanical ventilation was F_{IO_2}, 1.0; VT, 6 mL/kg; and rate 24 in an assist-control mode, resulting in the patient triggering at rates of 24 to 28. PEEP was titrated to 12 cmH_2O, which permitted reduction of F_{IO_2} to 0.5 with 90% saturation of arterial hemoglobin and peak airway pressures of 40 to 45 cmH_2O. Vancomycin and gentamicin were started. Cimetidine was begun for prevention of gastrointestinal hemorrhage.

On the second hospital day, the patient was alternately agitated and lethargic. Morphine sulfate was used for sedation to prevent excessive airway pressures. A brain CT scan and lumbar puncture were performed and excluded CNS infection. Intermittent opiate use was necessary for continued agitation. Enteral feedings were deemed necessary and a nasoenteral tube was placed. Prior to instillation of feedings, a chest radiograph revealed that the tube had been misplaced in the lung, with wire-guide placement past the endotracheal tube cuff. The tube was replaced in the jejunem, but when feedings were started an ileus developed. TPN was started.

By the third hospital day airway secretions were copious with intermittent blood streaking and blood clot. On the evening of the fourth hospital day the patient became acutely agitated and ventilator alarms fired as airway pressures acutely rose to 75 cmH_2O. Set VT could not be delivered. The covering houseofficer quickly arrived and disconnected the patient from the ventilator and noted the patient could not be bagged. A bite-block was quickly passed between his clenched teeth, but a catheter could not be passed through the endotracheal tube. The cuff was immediately released and the tube removed and emergent reintubation performed, during which time the patient became briefly cyanotic and marked arterial desaturation was noted by pulse oximetry. His circulation remained stable throughout this emergent procedure and his neurologic status returned to its base line. The endotracheal tube removed was noted to be obstructed by encrusted blood and secretions. On the sixth hospital day the patient was judged to require long-term ventilatory support, and a tracheostomy was performed.

Over the first several days of intubation and mechanical ventilation the patient had been cautiously diuresed with the pulmonary capillary wedge pressure maintained at the lowest level consistent with an adequate cardiac output. By the seventh hospital day, intrapulmonary shunt had improved and PEEP could be decreased to 5 cmH_2O. On the evening of the eighth hospital day the patient became acutely hypoxemic on these unchanged ventilator settings and a chest radiograph revealed collapse of the left lower lobe. FI_{O_2} was increased to 1.0, achieving adequate arterial hemoglobin saturation, and VT was then gradually increased at the bedside. As the VT was increased from 900 to 1100 mL, the airway pressure did not increase, as it had with each incremental VT increase. It was actually noted to fall. Chest auscultation and radiograph confirmed recruitment of the collapsed lobe and the patient was placed on a VT of 9 mL/kg, with sighs and a PEEP level of 7.5 cmH_2O. No further lobar collapse was noted.

By hospital day 12, the diffuse alveolar infiltrates on presentation had resolved, though multiple bilateral lung abscesses persisted. Low grade temperatures persisted. On day 13, subcutaneous emphysema was present on physical examination and the morning chest radiograph revealed a small pneumomediastinum. On hospital day 14, despite peak airway pressures maintained at approximately 50 cmH_2O, the patient developed a tension pneumothorax, heralded by hypotension and a sudden rise in airway pressures with inability to ventilate. A right-sided chest tube was placed which evacuated 100 mL of bloody fluid which subsequently grew *S. aureus.*

By day 14 fevers had resolved and mental status had greatly improved. However, during the second and third weeks in the ICU progressive renal and hepatic failure developed. Bedside ultrasound excluded biliary or ureteral obstruction. Hemodialysis was required by day 21. Liver function abnormalities stabilized at this time, with a peak bilirubin concentration of 18 mg/dL.

By day 15, mild thrombocytopenia, which progressed to platelet counts of approximately 50,000/mm^3, was noted. Heparin was discontinued, coumadin begun, and heparin antibodies assayed but not found to be present. Review of medications and DIC panel failed to identify a specific etiology for the thrombocytopenia, which gradually resolved over the next 3 weeks.

During the course of thrombocytopenia the patient was noted to have gastrointestinal hemorrhage as manifested by guaiac-positive drainage of nasogastric suckings and blood loss requiring approximately 3 U RBC transfusion each week for 3 weeks. Coumadin was stopped and an inferior vena caval filter placed. Review of gastric pH indicated intermittent drops to <5.0, which resolved when the histamine blocker was given by continuous infusion. Endoscopic gastroduodenoscopy revealed multiple small erosions attributed to the nasogastric tube as well as a single larger gastric ulcer in the fundus. Bleeding slowed gradually and surgical repair was not undertaken.

By the sixth week fevers and an elevated WBC count recurred. Some sinus tenderness was present on examination and a head CT scan revealed a large fluid collection in the right maxillary sinus. Purulent fluid was drained at the bedside, and fevers diminished only to return in the seventh and eighth weeks. Chest CT scan revealed well-circumscribed lung cavities as well as an unexpected large right pleural air and fluid collection. Despite multiple attempts at chest tube placement, the pleural space could not be sufficiently evacuated and a decortication procedure was performed.

Again, there was a resolution of markers of infection as antibiotics were continued postdecortication. The patient again became febrile, however, and a purulent central venous catheter used for hyperalimentation was removed. Blood cultures were then positive for *Candida* species, and a course of amphotericin B was initiated.

By the ninth and tenth weeks in ICU the patient was eventually placed on enteral nutrition and gradually assumed full spontaneous ventilation. All evidence of infection resolved and antibiotic courses were discontinued. By week 11, renal and hepatic function had improved markedly and hemodialysis was no longer required. In week 12 the tracheostomy tube was removed and the patient began a rehabilitation program after transfer from the ICU. After 16 weeks of hospitalization he was discharged, to continue a gradual but continued rehabilitation as an outpatient in his own community.

CASE DISCUSSION

This patient's extremely complicated course is unfortunately typical of many critically ill individuals, although admittedly more protracted than most. The life-threatening processes of sepsis and acute respiratory failure requiring mechanical ventilatory support set the stage for myriad subsequent complications of therapy.

Early on, the patient's acute hypoxemic respiratory failure was managed with strategies to minimize the risks of oxygen toxicity and barotrauma—low VT, the least amount of PEEP titrated to an adequate circulation and nontoxic FI_{O_2}, and careful attention to maintain hematocrit and diminish oxygen consumption by sedating the patient and performing all the work of breathing. Also, nutrition was initiated early, with the first attempt to use an enteral route. A misadventure with the feeding tube was avoided by confirming position prior to use. Unfortunately, gut feedings were not tolerated. One might argue that opiate administration contributed to the ileus preventing use of the gut. One might continue this line of speculation and wonder whether the risks for subsequent gastrointestinal hemorrhage and line-related sepsis might have been favorably influenced by achieving earlier enteral nutrition.

The near-catastrophic airway problem on the third hospital day was likely due to the purulent and bloody secretions coupled to the use of a small airway. One certainly could argue that earlier tracheostomy would be appropriate, since this patient could have been anticipated to have a prolonged course under the best of conditions.

The cause of acute hypoxemia noted on hospital day 8, of course, had a long differential diagnosis but was quickly identified as lobar collapse. Atelectasis is common in bedridden mechanically ventilated patients and should have been anticipated in this patient as acute lung flooding resolved and PEEP requirements diminished. This introduces the notion of "tailoring" mechanical ventilation to the changing needs of the patient—early use of higher PEEP levels and smaller VT to reduce lung shunt with acceptable airway pressures, followed by increasing VT and sighs as PEEP is decreased during the resolution of lung edema.

Despite concerted efforts to avoid excessive lung inflation, barotrauma developed in this patient. The underlying pneumonia-associated lung necrosis likely resulted in greater susceptibility to this complication. The life-threatening pneumothorax was heralded by subcutaneous emphysema and pneumomediastinum, usually well-tolerated forms of ventilator-induced barotrauma.

Gastrointestinal hemorrhage was likely in this patient, given the risk factors of mechanical ventilation and coagulopathy, and occurred despite the use of prophylaxis. Diagnostic endoscopy indicated both nasogastric tube trauma and the typical form of "stress" ulceration.

The patient's late course was dominated by multiple organ dysfunctions and multiple infectious complications. Sinusitis likely resulted from early endotracheal intubation and subsequent nasogastric tube placement and required drainage. Pleural space infection occurred despite adequate antibiotics and earlier chest tube drainage, a not uncommon phenomenon in critically ill patients. Chest CT scan was particularly useful to identify this problem. Finally, line sepsis and fungemia were late complications. Continued vigilance for multiple new infectious sources was necessary, with constant modification and redirection of diagnostic strategies. With this constant attention to the reduction of risk for and early identification of complications, this patient survived and recovered from catastrophic illness.

References

1. Kleck R: Means to forestall ICU syndrome explored. Anesth News 10:10, 1984.
2. Eisendrath SJ: ICU syndromes: Their detection, prevention and treatment. Crit Care Update 7:5, 1980.
3. Cassem N: Critical care psychiatry; Shoemaker WC, Thompson L, Holbrook P (eds): *Textbook of Critical Care*. Philadelphia, Saunders, 1984, pp 981–988.
4. Smith J, Seidl L, Cluff L: Studies on the epidemiology of adverse drug reactions. Ann Intern Med 65:629, 1986.
5. Adams HP, Jergenson DD, Kassell NF, Sahs AL: Pitfalls in the recognition of subarachnoid hemorrhage. JAMA 244:794, 1980.
6. White SR, Hall JB, Dietrich M, Spire JP: Clinically inapparent status epilepticus as a cause of coma in the critically ill. J Crit Care 2(2):112, 1987.
7. Devereaux MW, Partnow MJ: Delayed hypoxic encephalopathy without cognitive dysfunction. Arch Neurol 32(10):704, 1975.
8. Jackson AC, Gilbert JJ, Young GB, Bolton CF: The encephalopathy of sepsis. Can J Neurol Sci 12(4):303, 1985.
9. Bowton DL, Bertels NH, Prough DS, Stump DA: Cerebral blood flow is reduced in patients with sepsis syndrome. Crit Care Med 17(5):399, 1989.
10. Mizock BA, Sabelli HC, Dubin A, et al: Septic encephalopathy: Evidence for altered phenylalanine metabolism and comparison with hepatic encephalopathy. Arch Intern Med 150:443, 1990.
11. Marini JJ, Culver BH: Systemic gas embolism complicating mechanical ventilation in the adult respiratory distress syndrome. Ann Intern Med 110(9):699, 1989.
12. Maunder RJ, Pierson DJ, Hudson LD: Subcutaneous and mediastinal emphysema. Arch Intern Med 144:1447, 1984.
13. Haake R, Schlichrig R, Ulstad DR, Henschen RR: Barotrauma-pathophysiology, risk factors and prevention. Chest 91:608, 1987.
14. Albelda SM, Gefter VB, Kelley MA, et al: Ventilator-induced subpleural air cysts: Clinical, radiographic, and pathologic significance. Am Rev Respir Dis 127:360, 1983.
15. Cullen DJ, Caldera DL: Pulmonary barotrauma in critically ill patients. Anesthesiology 50:187, 1979.
16. Petersen GW, Baier H: Incidence of pulmonary barotrauma in a medical ICU. Crit Care Med 11:67, 1983.
17. Broseghini C, Brandolese R, Poggi G, et al: Respiratory mechanics during the first day of mechanical ventilation in patients with pulmonary edema and chronic airway obstruction. Am Rev Respir Dis 138:355, 1988.
18. Tuxen DV: Detrimental effects of positive end-expiratory pressure during controlled mechanical ventilation of patients with severe airflow obstruction. Am Rev Respir Dis 140:5, 1989.
19. Hall JB, Wood LDH: Management of the critically ill asthmatic patient, in Dosman JA, Cockcroft DW, (eds): *Obstructive Lung Disease*. Med Clin North Am 74(3):1, 1990.

20. Woodring JH: Pulmonary interstitial emphysema in the adult respiratory distress syndrome. Crit Care Med 13:786, 1985.
21. Tocino IM, Miller MH, Fairfax WR: Distribution of pneumothorax in the supine and semirecumbent critically ill adult. AJR 144:901, 1985.
22. Ziter FMH, Westcott JL: Supine subpulmonic pneumothorax. AJR 137:699, 1981.
23. Darioli E, Perret C: Mechanical controlled hypoventilation in status asthmaticus. Am Rev Respir Dis 129:385, 1984.
24. Lain DC, DiBenedetto R, Morris SL, et al: Pressure control inverse ratio ventilation as a method to reduce peak inspiratory pressure and provide adequate ventilation and oxygenation. Chest 95:1081, 1989.
25. Meyrick B: Pathology of the adult respiratory distress syndrome. Clin Chest Med 2:405, 1986.
26. Ghio AJ, Elliot CG, Crapo RO, et al: Impairment after adult respiratory distress syndrome. Am Rev Respir Dis 139:1158, 1989.
27. Peters JI, Bell RC, Prihoda TJ, et al: Clinical determinants of abnormalities in pulmonary functions in survivors of the adult respiratory distress syndrome. Am Rev Respir Dis 139:1163, 1989.
28. Borelli M, Kolobow T, Spatola R, et al: Severe acute respiratory failure managed with continuous positive airway pressure and partial extra corporeal carbon dioxide removed by an artificial membrane lung. Am Rev Respir Dis 138:1480, 1988.
29. Rinaldo JE, Rogers RM: Adult respiratory distress syndrome: Changing concepts of lung injury and repair. N Engl J Med 306:900, 1982.
30. Humphrey H, Hall JB, Sznajder JI, et al: Improved survival in ARDS patients is associated with a reduction in pulmonary capillary wedge pressure. Chest 97:1176, 1990.
31. Stauffer JL, Olson DE, Petty TL: Complications and consequences of endotracheal intubation and tracheotomy. Am J Med 70:65, 1981.
32. Colice GL, Stukel TA, Dain B: Laryngeal complications of prolonged intubation. Chest 96:877, 1989.
33. Heffner JE, Miller KS, Sahn SA: Tracheostomy in the intensive care unit. Chest 90:430, 1986.
34. Wright PE, Marini JJ, Bernard GR: In vitro versus in vivo comparison of endotracheal tube airflow resistance. Am Rev Respir Dis 140:10, 1989.
35. Glauser FL, Polatty RC, Sessler CN: Worsening oxygenation in the mechanically ventilated patient. Am Rev Respir Dis 138:458, 1988.
36. Hall JB, Wood LDH: Oxygen therapy, in West JB, Crystal RG (eds): *The Lung:* Scientific Foundations. New York, Raven, 1990. (In press).
37. Pepe PE, Marini JJ: Occult positive end-expiratory pressure in mechanically ventilated patients with airflow obstruction. Am Rev Respir Dis 126:166, 1982.
38. Douglas JG, Rafferty P, Fergusson RJ: Nebulized salbutamol without oxygen in severe acute asthma: How effective and how safe? Thorax 40:180, 1985.
39. Prewitt RM, Wood LDH: Effect of sodium nitroprusside on cardiovascular function and pulmonary shunt in canine oleic acid pulmonary edema. Anesthesiology 55:537, 1981.
40. Huet Y, Lemaire F, Brun-Buisson C, et al: Hypoxemia in acute pulmonary embolism. Chest 88(6):829, 1985.
41. Harris (Pingleton) SK, Pingleton WW, Ruth WE: Prevention of pulmonary emboli in a respiratory intensive care unit. Chest 79:647, 1981.
42. Neuhaus A, Bentz RR, Weg JG: Pulmonary embolism in respiratory failure. Chest 73:460, 1978.
43. Tomashefski JF, Davies P, Boggis C, et al: The pulmonary vascular lesions of the adult respiratory distress syndrome. Am J Pathol 112:112, 1983.
44. Moser KM, LeMoine JR, Nachtwey FJ, Spragg RG: Deep venous thrombosis and pulmonary embolism. JAMA 246:1422, 1981.
45. Cade JF: High risk of the critically ill for venous thromboembolism. Crit Care Med 10:448, 1982.
46. Moser KM: Venous thromboembolism. Am Rev Respir Dis 141:235, 1990.
47. Sprung CL, Pozen RG, Rozanski JJ, et al: Advanced ventricular arrhythmias during bedside pulmonary artery catheterization. Am J Med 72:203, 1982.
48. Sprung CL, Elser B, Schein RMH, et al: Risk of right bundle branch block and complete heart block during pulmonary artery catheterization. Crit Care Med 17:1, 1989.
49. Hannan AT, Brown M, Bigman O: Pulmonary artery catheter-induced hemorrhage. Chest 85:128, 1984.
50. Dieden JD, Friloux LA, Renner JW: Pulmonary artery false aneurysms secondary to Swan-Ganz pulmonary artery catheters. AJR 149:901, 1987.
51. Hoshal V, Ause R, Hoskins P: Fibrin sleeve formation on indwelling subclavian central venous catheter. Arch Surg 102:353, 1971.
52. Bel-Kahn JVD, Fowler NO, Doerger P: Right heart catheter lesions: Any significance? Am J Clin Pathol 82:137, 1984.
53. Garratt C, Linker N, Griffith M, et al: Comparison of adenosine and verapamil for termination of paroxysmal junctional tachycardia. Am J Cardiol 64:1310, 1989.
54. Dark DS, Pingleton SK: Nonhemorrhagic gastrointestinal complications in acute respiratory failure. Crit Care Med 17:755, 1989.
55. Gottschlich MM, Warden GD, Micha M, et al: Diarrhea in tube-fed burn patients: Incidence, etiology, nutritional impact, and prevention. JPEN 12:338, 1988.
56. Channick R, Curley FJ, Irwin RS: Indications for and complications of rectal tube use in critically ill patients. J Intensive Care Med 3(6):321, 1988.
57. Silen W: Pathogenetic factors in erosive gastritis: Am J Med 79:45, 1985.
58. Schuster DP, Rowley H, Feinstein S, et al: Prospective evaluation of the risk of upper gastrointestinal bleeding after admission to a medical intensive care unit. Am J Med 76:623, 1984.
59. Harris (Pingleton) SK, Bone RC, Ruth WE: Gastrointestinal hemorrhage in patients in a respiratory intensive care unit. Chest 72:301, 1977.
60. Shuman RB, Schuster DP, Zuckerman GR: Prophylactic therapy for stress ulcer bleeding: A reappraisal. Ann Intern Med 106:562, 1987.
61. Driks MR, Craven DE, Celli BR, et al: Nosocomial pneumonia in intubated patients given sucralfate as compared with antacids or histamine type 2 blockers. N Engl J Med 317:1376, 1987.
62. Choctaw WT, Fujita C, Zawacki BE: Prevention of upper gastrointestinal bleeding in burn patients. Arch Surg 115:1073, 1980.
63. Pingleton SK, Hadizma S: Enteral alimentation and gastrointestinal bleeding in mechanically ventilated patients. Crit Care Med 11:13, 1983.
64. Pingleton SK, Hinthorn D, Liu C: Enteral nutrition in patients receiving mechanical ventilation. Multiple sources of tracheal colonization include the stomach. Am J Med 80:827, 1986.
65. Driver FAG, LeBrun M: Iatrogenic malnutrition in patients receiving ventilatory support. JAMA 244:2195, 1980.
66. Arora NS, Rochester DF: Effect of body weight and muscularity on human diaphragm muscle mass, thickness and area. J Appl Physiol 52:64, 1982.

67. Kelly SM, Rosa A, Field S, et al: Inspiratory muscle strength and body composition in patients receiving total parenteral nutrition therapy. Am Rev Respir Dis 130:33, 1984.
68. Doekel RC Jr, Zwillich CW, Scoggin CH, et al: Clinical semistarvation: Depression hypoxic ventilatory response. N Engl J Med 295:358, 1976.
69. Heymsfield SB, Erbland M, Casper K, et al: Enteral nutritional support: Metabolic, cardiovascular, and pulmonary interrelations. Clin Chest Med 7:41, 1986.
70. Wolfe BM, Ryder MA, Nichikawa RA, et al: Complications of parenteral nutrition. Am J Surg 152:93, 1986.
71. Baker AL, Rosenberg IH: Hepatic complications of total parenteral nutrition. Am J Med 82:489, 1987.
72. Covelli HD, Black JW, Olsen MS, Beckman JF: Respiratory failure precipitated by high carbohydrate loads. Ann Intern Med 95:579, 1981.
73. Dark DS, Pingleton SK, Kerby GR: Hypercapnea during weaning: A complication of nutritional support. Chest 88:141, 1985.
74. Seidenfeld JJ, Pohl DF, Bell RC, et al: Incidence, site, and outcome of infections in patients with the adult respiratory distress syndrome. Am Rev Respir Dis 134:12, 1986.
75. Maki DG, Alvarado CJ, Hassemer CA, Zila MS: Relation of the inanimate hospital environment to endemic nosocomial infection. N Engl J Med 307:1562, 1982.
76. Johanson WG, Pierce AKK, Sanford JP: Changing pharyngeal bacterial flora of hospitalized patients. N Engl J Med 281:1137, 1969.
77. Higuchi JH, Johanson WG Jr: Colonization and bronchopulmonary infection. Clin Chest Med 3:133, 1982.
78. Dal Nogare AR, Toews GB, Pierce AK: Increased salivary elastase precedes gram-negative bacillary colonization in postoperative patient. Am Rev Respir Dis 135:671, 1987.
79. Niederman MS, Rafferty TD, Sasaki CT, et al: Comparison of bacterial adherence to ciliated and squamous epithelial cells obtained from the human respiratory tract. Am Rev Respir Dis 127:85, 1983.
80. Hillman KM, Riordan T, O'Farrell SM, Tabaqchali S: Colonization of the gastric contents in critically ill patients. Crit Care Med 109:444, 1982.
81. Niederman MS, Mantovani R, Schoch P, et al: Patterns and routes of tracheobronchial colonization in mechanically ventilated patients. Chest 95:155, 1989.
82. Andrews CP, Coalson JJ, Smith JD, Johanson WG: Diagnosis of nosocomial bacterial pneumonia in acute, diffuse lung injury. Chest 80:254, 1981.
83. Fagon JY, Hance AJ, Guigueit M, et al: Detection of nosocomial pneumonia lung infection in ventilated patients. Am Rev Respir Dis 138:110, 1988.
84. Fagon JY, Chester J, Domart Y, et al: Nosocomial pneumonia in patients receiving continuous mechanical ventilation. Am Rev Respir Dis 139:877, 1989.
85. Chastre J, Viau F, Brun P, et al: Prospective evaluation of the protected specimen brush for the diagnosis of pulmonary infections in ventilated patients. Am Rev Respir Dis 130:924, 1984.
86. Johanson WG, Seidenfeld JJ, Gomez P, et al: Bacteriologic diagnosis of nosocomial pneumonia following prolonged mechanical ventilation. Am Rev Respir Dis 137:259, 1988.
87. Chastie J, Fagon JY, Golen P, et al: Diagnosis of nosocomial bacterial pneumonia in intubated patients undergoing ventilation: Comparison of the usefulness of bronchoalveolar lavage and the protected specimen brush. Am J Med 85:499, 1988.
88. Torres A, DeLa Bellacasa J, Xaubet A, et al: Diagnostic value of quantitative cultures of bronchoalveolar lavage and telescoping plugged catheters in mechanically ventilated patients with bacterial pneumonia. Am Rev Respir Dis 140:306, 1989.
89. Kirkpatrick MB, Bass JB Jr: Quantitative bacterial cultures of bronchoalveolar lavage fluids and protected specimen brush catheter specimens for normal subjects. Am Rev Respir Dis 139:546, 1989.
90. Crouch TW, Higuchi JH, Coalson JJ, Johanson WG Jr: Pathogenesis and prevention of nosocomial pneumonia in a nonhuman primate model of acute respiratory failure. Am Rev Respir Dis 130:502, 1984.
91. Stoutenbeek CP, Van Saene HKF, Miranda DR, Zandstra DF: The effect of selective decontamination of the digestive tract on colonization and infection rate in multiple trauma patients. Intensive Care Med 10:185, 1984.
92. Van Uffelen R, Rommes JH, Van Saene HKF: Preventing lower airway colonization and infection in mechanically ventilated patients. Crit Care Med 15:99, 1987.
93. Montgomery BA, Stager MA, Carrico CJ, Hudson LD: Causes of mortality in patients with the adult respiratory distress syndrome. Am Rev Respir Dis 132:485, 1985.
94. Maki DG: Nosocomial bacteremia: An epidemiologic overview. Am J Med 70:719, 1981.
95. Singh S, Nelson N, Acosta I, et al: Catheter colonization and bacteremia with pulmonary and arterial catheters. Crit Care Med 10:736, 1982.
96. Gardner RM, Schwartz R, Wong HC, Burke JP: Percutaneous indwelling radial-artery catheters for monitoring cardiovascular function. N Engl J Med 290:1277, 1974.
97. Rowley KM, Clubb KS, Smith FJW, Cabin HS: Right-sided infective endocarditis as a consequence of flow-directed pulmonary-artery catheterization. N Engl J Med 311:1152, 1984.
98. Ellison DH, Bia MJ: Acute renal failure in critically ill patients. J Intensive Care Med 2:8, 1987.
99. Sladen A, Lauer MP, Pontoppidan H: Pulmonary complications and free water retention in prolonged mechanical ventilation. N Engl J Med 279:448, 1968.
100. Szatalowicz UL, Goldberg JP, Anderson RJ: Plasma antidiuretic hormone in acute respiratory failure. Am J Med 72:583, 1982.
101. Simmons RS, Berdine GG, Seidenfeld JJ, et al: Fluid balance and the adult respiratory distress syndrome. Am Rev Respir Dis 135:924, 1987.
102. Schneider RC, Zapol WM, Carualho AC: Platelet consumption and sequestration in severe acute respiratory failure. Am Rev Respir Dis 122:445, 1980.
103. King DJ, Kelton JG: Heparin-associated thrombocytopenia. Ann Intern Med 100:535, 1984.
104. Kelton JG, Sheridan D, Santos A, et al: Heparin-induced thrombocytopenia: Laboratory studies. Blood 72:925, 1988.
105. Frame JN, Mulvey KP, Phares JC, Anderson MJ: Correction of severe heparin-associated thrombocytopenia with intravenous immunoglobulin. Ann Intern Med 111:946, 1989.
106. Laster JL, Nichols WK, Silver D: Thrombocytopenia associated with heparin-coated catheters in patients with heparin-associated antiplatelet antibodies. Arch Intern Med 149:2285, 1989.
107. Amos RJ, Hinds CJ, Amess AL, et al: Incidence and pathogenesis of acute megaloblastic bone-marrow changes in patients receiving intensive care. Lancet 2:835, 1982.
108. Wehmann RE, Gregerman RI, Burns WH, et al: Suppression of thyrotropin in the low thyroxine state of severe non-thyroidal illness. N Engl J Med 312:546, 1985.

SECTION B

MULTIPLE SYSTEMS ORGAN FAILURE (MSOF)

Chapter 53

MULTIPLE SYSTEMS ORGAN FAILURE: CLINICAL EXPRESSION, PATHOGENESIS, AND THERAPY

GEORGE M. MATUSCHAK

KEY POINTS

- *Multiple systems organ failure (MSOF) develops in up to 15 percent of patients requiring ICU admission.*
- *Failure of systemic host defense homeostasis in MSOF is linked to inappropriate regulation of acute immune and inflammatory responses.*
- *Organ systems differ in their host defense functions, sensitivity to damage, time course of expression of injury, metabolic requirements, and response to vasoactive agents.*
- *Occult dysfunction in immunoregulatory aspects of liver and gastrointestinal function both predispose to MSOF and impair its resolution.*
- *The liver is pivotal in host defense by mononuclear phagocytic defense, production and "export" of endogenous inflammatory mediators including cytokines and eicosanoids, hepatobiliary clearance of such mediators, and synthesis of acute-phase reactants.*
- *The physiologic definition of MSOF is severe acquired dysfunction in at least two organ systems lasting at least 24–48 h.*
- *Sepsis is the most common cause of MSOF.*
- *Infection as a microbiologic phenomenon should be differentiated from sepsis as the sum of host immune and inflammatory responses over time producing tissue injury, cardiovascular derangements, and hypermetabolism.*
- *Noninfectious stimuli such as ischemia and trauma also culminate in stereotypic pathophysiologic changes mediating tissue injury and host defense impairment.*
- *MSOF evolves through several stages, each of which has characteristic clinical features.*
- *Unresolved issues in MSOF are whether dysfunction of specific organs influences pathogenesis and outcome, and whether dysfunction in particular systems occurs more frequently than in others.*
- *Dysregulation of the acute response to sepsis can evolve initially by loss of host control of systemic endotoxemia and bacteremia.*
- *Derangement of organ system interactions in the gut–liver axis can result in endogenous endotoxemia and bacterial translocation.*
- *Enhanced and/or prolonged cytokine responses to bacteria and their products by tumor necrosis factor-α/cachectin (TNF-α) and interleukin (IL)-1, IL-2, and IL-6 can induce tissue injury, partly by platelet-activating factor (PAF) and eicosanoids together with local second-messenger systems.*
- *Synergistic interactions between immunologic responses and physiologic mechanisms amplify tissue injury by the complement, kinin, and coagulation cascades, O_2 radical-mediated oxidant injury, and local release of proteases, elastases, and collagenases by activated phagocytic cells.*
- *TNF-α is a pivotal early mediator in the host response to infection and has multiple pathophysiologic effects relevant to MSOF.*
- *The actions of TNF-α at the tissue level appear to be mediated by eicosanoid metabolites of arachidonic acid and/or PAF.*
- Progression *of initial infection or injury to MSOF does not depend on persistently elevated plasma TNF-α levels.*
- *Therapy for MSOF requires maintenance of global and local O_2 delivery, meticulous organ-specific support, prevention/eradication of primary and secondary septic foci (source control), and antimicrobial therapy to prevent bacteriologic complications.*
- *Management of time-varying derangements in immunologic and biochemical pathways characterizing MSOF will require combinations of mechanism-specific agents.*
- *Immunization against gram-negative organisms or endotoxin, monoclonal antibodies directed against cytokines, antagonists of PAF, and synthesis inhibition or receptor blockade of cyclooxygenase and lipoxygenase eicosanoids have all been established to reduce organ damage and MSOF in experimental models.*

Overview

The clinical syndrome of multiple systems organ failure (MSOF), also termed the *multiple organ failure syndrome,* has emerged over the past 15 years as the major therapeutic challenge facing intensive care physicians treating critically ill and injured patients, regardless of the specialty training or unit affiliation of the intensivist. Despite general agreement regarding its pathogenetic complexity, profoundly negative impact on the survival of patients otherwise expected to live, and enormous socioeconomic importance, there are both pragmatic and conceptual divergences of view with respect to its exact definition. As a basis for discussion of the current understanding of MSOF regarding its multifaceted clinical expression, pathogensis, and therapy, it is necessary to consider its origins.

MSOF has correctly been termed a disease of medical progress.[1–3] Initially recognized in 1973,[4] its acceptance as a distinct nosologic entity[1,2] was slower. Ironically, the causes of MSOF are linked to the success of the fundamental paradigm underlying evolution of intensive care units (ICUs) over the past three decades: monitoring and single organ-directed interventions to support failing organ systems during acute illness or after traumatic injury. Immediate goals of ICU care typically include preservation of organ-specific homeostasis to avoid life-threatening derangements in gas exchange, acid-base balance, and cardiovascular adequacy. This often necessitates pharmacologic or mechanical support of failing organ function until recovery occurs or death supervenes. Success or failure of such crisis-oriented therapy in the ICU has characteristically been evaluated over the short term and validated by stabilization and recovery of individual organ function. Thus, identification of single organ-related problems such as upper airway obstruction, acute ventilatory failure, acute renal failure, or circulatory shock from a variety of etiologies has led to a resuscitative approach appropriately focused on the specific failing system. This rationale is supported by clinical results. In the absence of promptly initiated, titrated management at the bedside, irreversible organ failure leading to death develops within hours or days. From a historical perspective, improvements in organ-specific resuscitation in the ICU have evolved through stages, deriving from recognition of major organ-specific problems, definition of the abnormal underlying physiology, and institution of single-organ-directed therapy, such as mechanical ventilation and dialytic techniques.

Vigorous application of this approach and advances in antimicrobial therapy, imaging procedures, and monitoring of the critically ill has largely succeeded in averting early mortality from life-threatening single organ physiologic derangements. However, global physiologic homeostasis requires moment-to-moment adaptive responses mediated by the sum total of differentiated functions of multiple individual organs. These act in concert to prevent progressively widening oscillations in the internal milieu after initial derangements in host defense homeostasis. Yet with regard to MSOF, the question posed in the first description of "sequential system failure" after rupture of abdominal aortic aneurysms remains as germane now as in 1973: ". . . how do a number of physiological liabilities, each in itself potentially reversible, combine to make survival exceptional. . . ?"[4] There is compelling evidence, which we will review, that development of MSOF has been unmasked by the combination of (1) the broad availability and increased utilization of ICU resources, and, more important, (2) activation of immune and inflammatory responses during the initial illness or injury that are not adequately addressed, or are exacerbated, by current organ-specific treatment protocols. These factors now permit an extended ICU course during which basic pathogenetic mechanisms produce a "malignant" form of intravascular inflammation, enabling tissue injury and organ damage to proceed unchecked.

DEFINITION OF MSOF

It is essential to clearly define what MSOF is and is not. There is no unequivocal answer to the simple but important question of what type and severity of organ system dysfunction in fact constitutes MSOF. The conventional definition of MSOF, derived from the perspective at the bedside, is pragmatic. Phenomenologically, MSOF is a clinical constellation of severe physiologic dysfunction occurring sequentially or concomitantly in multiple organs, usually in the setting of sepsis or widespread perfusion deficits after severe infection or trauma.[2,3,5] Initial studies of this problem focused indirectly on MSOF, since they were concerned primarily with single organ dysfunction, and MSOF was implicitly viewed as a collection of unrelated single-organ failures. For example, mortality and the relation of MSOF to outcome during supposed single-organ dysfunction, such as sepsis-related adult respiratory distress syndrome (ARDS), were evaluated using definitions independently developed by each investigator.[7–9] This resulted in two problems.

First, both lack of reproducibility of objective physiologic measurements of single organ dysfunction across studies, and the ensuing variability among indices of organ failure made it difficult to compare the effects of treatment among differing ICU patient populations.[7–11] We still lack a universally agreed-upon classification system of organ-specific failure. However, a significant advance in this direction was made with the development and validation of the Acute Physiologic and Chronic Health Evaluation Score II (APACHE II).[12–14] This established reproducibility in measurements of organ-specific failure in five systems (cardiovascular, respiratory, renal, hematologic, and neurologic). APACHE II represents a pragmatic tool to study the epidemiology and prognosis of MSOF, since it is based on objective data readily obtainable at the bedside or from routine laboratory tests. Since the initial description of APACHE II, there has been an appreciation of the role of liver function in MSOF.[15,16,17] Therefore, it has recently been suggested that APACHE II incorporate objective definitions for severe hepatic dysfunction as well.[14] The resulting amended definitions of organ system failure for six systems are shown in Table 53-1.

Although very useful prognostically, the narrow definition of MSOF in such tabulations implies that all organs are of equal pathogenetic significance (i.e., all organs are created equal). However, this concept, in terms of pathogenetic mechanisms, appears untenable. The following points demonstrate that organ systems (1) subserve different physiologic and immunologic functions, (2) show differential sensitivity to external and host-derived cellular damage, (3) manifest clinical manifestations of dysfunction at different times following global cellular injury, (4) have disparate substrate requirements for energy production and roles in intermediary metabolism after sepsis or trauma, and (5) respond by different regional circulatory changes after sys-

TABLE 53-1 Modified Apache II Criteria for Organ System Failure*

Cardiovascular failure (presence of one or more of the following):
- Heart rate ≤54/min
- Mean arterial blood pressure ≤49 mmHg (systolic blood pressure ≤60 mmHg)
- Occurrence of ventricular tachycardia and/or ventricular fibrillation
- Serum pH ≤7.24 with a Pa_{CO_2} of ≤40 mmHg

Respiratory failure (presence of one or more of the following):
- Respiratory rate ≤5/min or >49/min
- $Pa_{CO_2} \geq 50$ mmHg
- $(A - a)_{O_2}$ ≥350 mmHg $(A - a)_{O_2} = 713\ Fi_{O_2} - Pa_{CO_2} - Pa_{O_2}$
- Dependent on ventilator or CPAP on the 2nd day of OSF (i.e., not applicable for the initial 24 h of OSF)

Renal failure (presence of one or more of the following)†:
- Urine output ≤479 mL/24 h or ≤159 mL/8 h
- Serum BUN ≥100 μg/100 mL (>36 μmol/L)
- Serum creatinine ≥3.5 μg/100 mL (>310 μmol/L)

Hematologic failure (presence of one or more of the following):
- WBC ≤ 1000 μL
- Platelets ≤ 20,000 μL
- Hematocrit ≤ 20%

Neurologic failure
- Glasgow Coma Score ≤6 (in absence of sedation)
- Glasgow Coma Score: Sum of best eye opening, best verbal, and best motor responses
- Scoring of responses as follows (points):

Eye Open: spontaneously (4); to verbal command (3); to pain (2); no response (1)

Motor Obeys verbal command (6); response to painful stimuli–localized pain (5); flexion-withdrawal (4); decorticate rigidity (3); decerebrate rigidity (2); no response (1); movement without any control (4)

Verbal Oriented and converses (5); disoriented and converses (4); inappropriate words (3); incomprehensible sounds (2); no response (1)
If intubated, use clinical judgment for verbal responses as follows: patient generally unresponsive (1); patient's ability to converse in question (3), patient appears able to converse (5)

Hepatic failure (presence of both of the following):
- Serum bilirubin >6 mg %
- Prothrombin time >4 s over control (in the absence of systemic anticoagulation)

Abbreviations: WBC, white blood count; BUN, blood urea nitrogen; Pa_{CO_2}, partial arterial pressure of carbon dioxide; $(A - a)_{O_2}$, arterial-alveolar difference in oxygen tension; Fi_{O_2}, fraction of inspired oxygen; Pa_{O_2}, partial arterial pressure of oxygen; CPAP, continuous positive airway pressure.
*If the patient had one or more of the following during a 24-h period (regardless of other values), organ system failure (OSF) existed on that day.
†Excluding patients on chronic dialysis prior to hospital admission.
SOURCE: Modified from Knaus WA, Wagner D,[14] with permission.

temic administration of vasoactive agents. In addition, the critical care physician must understand that two further problems exist with the notion of "organ equivalence" in MSOF.

First, accurate and uniform definitions of organ "failure" remain problematic for certain organ systems having multiple immunoregulatory functions critical in host defense but that are inaccessible for direct clinical study. Few would argue that "true" renal failure corresponds with oliguria and azotemia, or that neurologic failure is present when the Glasgow Coma Score (GCS) is less than 6. The situation becomes more complex for the gastrointestinal (GI) system and the liver. Ideally, criteria of organ failure in MSOF should reflect pathogenetic mechanisms causing generalized cellular dysfunction within individual organs. The question may be posed: What constitutes "true" GI failure? Changes in mucosal barrier function permitting intraluminal bacteria or their products access to the systemic circulation is a final common pathway in circulatory shock.[18,19] However, these changes can be neither directly assessed nor accurately predicted from nonspecific indicators of other parameters of GI function such as motility or upper GI stress ulceration. With respect to the liver, hepatobiliary dysfunction or altered protein synthetic function may be dissociated from mononuclear phagocytic (Kupffer cell) performance or production of endogenous inflammatory peptide and lipid mediators that transduce pathophysiologic effects.[16]

Second, data suggest that a "summative" model of organ interactions in MSOF (based on the concept of organ equivalence) is inadequate to explain fundamental changes in host defense and regulation of acute immune and inflammatory responses that predispose to MSOF and amplify its expression (Fig. 53-1). On the other hand, the summative model has proven useful for prognosticating outcome in MSOF based on objective measurements of organ dysfunction.[13] However, by the time multiple organ dysfunction is clinically apparent, measurements such as serum bilirubin or creatinine may reflect epiphenomenal organ-specific cellular alterations caused by secondary events, which may not correspond to more proximal mechanisms of tissue injury. Consequently, reorientation to a "relational" model of organ interactions may offer greater insight (Fig. 53-2).

FIGURE 53-1 Summative model of organ system interactions in MSOF. Organs are assumed to have equivalent pathogenetic importance in the clinical expression of MSOF, the outcome of which depends on the numerical sum of organ-specific failures. Abbreviations: MSOF, multiple systems organ failure; ARDS, adult respiratory distress syndrome; DIC, disseminated intravascular coagulation; ATN, acute tubular necrosis.

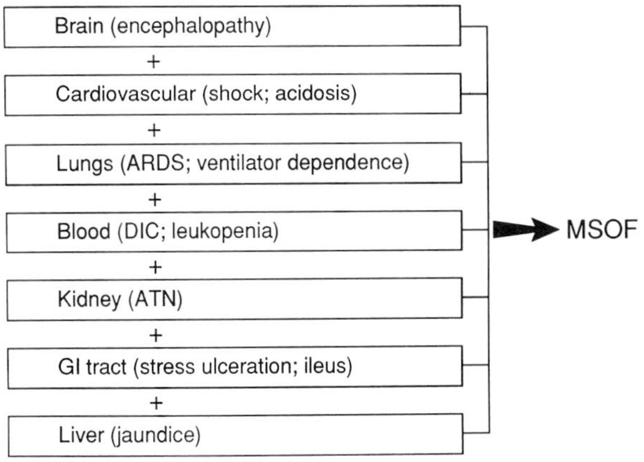

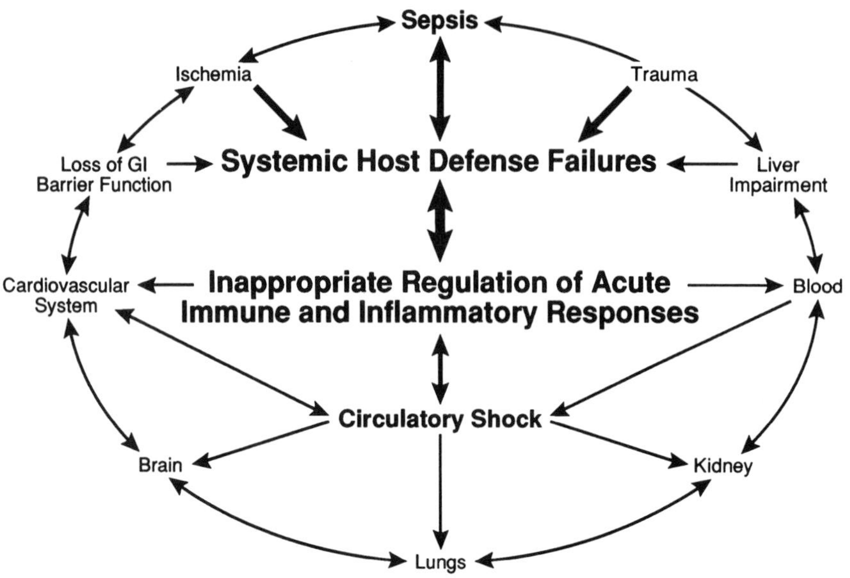

FIGURE 53-2 Relational model of organ system interactions in MSOF. Impairment of organs with immunoregulatory functions (e.g., liver, GI tract) amplify fundamental alterations in systemic host defense induced by severe sepsis, ischemia, or trauma. Subsequent inappropriate host regulation of acute immune and inflammatory responses caused by genetic factors or acquired derangements in organ function such as the liver involved in cytokine pathways produce circulatory shock and pan-systemic endothelial injury. Bi-directional arrows depict interdependent effects.

Epidemiology and Clinical Features

Information concerning the incidence, outcome, clinical predispositions, and bedside manifestations of MSOF derives from two sources: **1.** general surveys of organ-specific failures in medical and surgical ICU patients; and **2.** studies analyzing the outcome of a single-organ system dysfunction, such as ARDS, after development of MSOF. Incidence figures vary with the differing definitions of MSOF. Furthermore, both the number of dysfunctional organs *and* the duration of dysfunction are critical elements in establishing a rigorous definition of MSOF. Unfortunately, these have not been consistently taken into account. If MSOF is physiologically defined as severe acquired dysfunction in at least *two* organ systems after critical illness, injury, or major operation that lasts at least 24–48 h, then available prospective data indicate that MSOF complicates from 7 to 15 percent of all ICU admissions (Table 53-2). As can be inferred from Table 53-2, interpretation of incidence figures is limited by the following: **1.** different ICU patient populations and methods of study (e.g., prosepctive vs. retrospective analysis); **2.** lack of uniform, standardized criteria for organ-specific failures; and **3.** systematic exclusion of patients with preexisting chronic diseases of the liver, kidneys, or heart.[7] Although MSOF is a dynamic process, documentation of the time period over which organ failure is sustained has not been consistent. Because transient organ dysfunction is relatively common in the ICU, it is essential that both a minimum *time requirement* of organ failure be met and that the dysfunction meet established criteria as outlined in Table 53-1 before the organ system should be considered to have "failed."

TABLE 53-2 Incidence and Mortality of Multiple Systems Organ Failure*

				MORTALITY RATE PER # ORGAN SYSTEMS FAILED		
Study	Patients	ICU population*	Incidence *n* (%)	1	2	≥3
Knaus et al.[14]	5815	M,S†	891 (15)	40	60	100
ECMO[7]	490	M,S‡	74 (15.1)	40*	55	80–100
Fry et al.[10]	553	S§	38 (6.9)	30*	60	85–100
Montgomery et al.[9]	207	M,S‡	22 (10.6)	NE	NE	NE
Pine et al.[11]	106	S¶	21 (19.8)	10	50	100
Goris et al.[5]	92	S‖	92 (100)	0	0	19–100
Bell et al.[8]	84	M,S‡	40 (47.6)	40	54	80–100

*Multiple systems organ failure-(MSOF) defined as severe acquired dysfunction in ≥2 organ systems during critical illness or after trauma/major operation.
†Random ICU admissions prospectively followed.
‡Patients at risk for ARDS or with established ARDS prospectively identified.
§Emergency surgical patients retrospectively reviewed.
‖Patients with preexisting intraabdominal sepsis prospectively followed.
Abbreviations: M, medical patients; S, surgical patients; NE, not evaluable.
¶Patients with trauma or intraabdominal sepsis retrospectively reviewed.

The most extensive data base from which to evaluate incidence and mortality data in MSOF is a group of 5815 randomly selected ICU admissions from 13 U.S. medical centers studied using the APACHE II scoring system.[13,14] Of this number, 2843 patients (49 percent) met at least *one* of the definitions for organ failure lasting more than 1 day, and 891 (15 percent) met criteria for greater than two systems. There were three major risk factors for development of MSOF: (1) severity of disease (APACHE II score), (2) diagnosis of sepsis or infection at ICU admission, and (3) patient age greater than 65 years. This investigation and most others (Table 53-2) demonstrate that the greater the number of organ failures and the longer their duration, the more likely the patient will die. Nonetheless, it must be borne in mind that application of scoring system results to measure and predict ICU outcome in individual patients with MSOF is problematic, since both APACHE II and the Mortality Prediction Model (MPM) developed by Teres et al.[20] have a misclassification rate of 10 to 15 percent. Despite these caveats, the similarity of outcome data across the diverse studies of MSOF show remarkable agreement in relation to the close correspondence between mortality risk and the number of organs failing (Table 53-2). Any single-organ system failure lasting more than 1 day in the study cited above[13] resulted in an in-hospital risk of approximately 40 percent; persistent failure in two organs over the same interval led to 60 percent mortality, while failure of any three systems for >72 h led to mortality risks approaching 100 percent. In patients <65 years of age at risk for ARDS because of a variety of recognized predispositions in the Extracorporeal Membrane Oxygenation (ECMO) trial, failures in five nonpulmonary systems were evaluated: cardiovascular, renal, liver, central nervous system (CNS), coagulation, and the "host defense" system (where failure was defined by the presence of severe sepsis).[7] Despite the lack of standardized criteria for nonpulmonary organ dysfunction, single-organ system dysfunction (e.g., the lungs) also resulted in a mortality rate of nearly 40 percent. The incremental mortality risk paralleled the number of organ failures in addition to the lungs, so that the presence of three severely impaired organs plus ARDS caused mortality to exceed 75 percent (Table 53-2). This study also supported the concept that both MSOF predisposition and mortality are augmented by advanced age (>65 years), since age and development of MSOF were the only two predictive variables for nonsurvival in ARDS.[7] Advanced age thus increases both the probability of developing MSOF after a physiologic insult and the probability of dying with MSOF.

Multiple reports confirm that sepsis is the main predisposing factor in MSOF during critical medical and surgical illness.[8–10,21–23] Furthermore, acute inflammatory changes accompanying sepsis amplify cellular injury and promote hypermetabolism in acute conditions not of infectious origin, such as trauma. However, several recent observations suggest that *sepsis,* as the term is commonly understood, may be neither necessary nor sufficient to explain clinical features of MSOF under all circumstances. In trauma patients dying of MSOF, bacterial sepsis may be present in <50 percent despite the appearance of a clinically "septic" state.[5] Patients with trivial infections or no infections documentable by microbiologic, radiologic, operative, or pathologic methods may have severe MSOF.[21,23] Treatment of infection in patients with MSOF by appropriate antibiotics and drainage of purulent collections often fails to reverse organ failures.[24,25] Finally, bacteria-independent models of MSOF demonstrate similar physiologic and histopathologic abnormalities when compared to those caused by infection.[26] It is thus critically important that infection, sepsis, and the sepsis syndrome be distinguished to promote an understanding that the clinical expression of MSOF reflects generalized activation of humoral and cellular elements of the immune system and circulatory changes that escape normal host regulation. *Infection,* defined as a state of tissue invasion accompanying local growth of microorganisms in a normally sterile anatomic site, may or may not be the "trigger" of this process. Just as microbial colonization is not synonymous with infection, microbial infection is not equivalent to sepsis. It has been stressed that infection is a microbial phenomenon, while *sepsis* represents the sum total of host-derived immune and inflammatory responses over time, producing tissue injury, cardiovascular derangements, hypermetabolism, and the clinical syndrome of MSOF.[23] The *sepsis syndrome* is presently defined by microbiologic and physiologic data. These include the presence of a clinically significant bacterial infection accompanied by a concomitant, deleterious systemic response independent of the presence of bacteremia.[8,9,21,22] This can be summarized by the following features: temperature >39° or <36°C; white blood cell count >12,000 or <3000 cells/mm^3, or with >10 percent band granulocytes; positive blood culture of a commonly accepted pathogen; known or strongly suspected source for nonbacteremic infection such as pus in an enclosed space; plus unexplained systolic hypotension <90 mmHg or >30 percent decline in a previously hypertensive patient for >2 h, and at least one end-organ demonstrating inadequate perfusion or dysfunction, such as altered mentation, ongoing anion-gap metabolic acidosis caused by increased lactate production with a base deficit >5 mEq/L, oliguria, and systemic vascular resistance <800 dynes/s/cm^{-5}.

Although the clinical expression of MSOF cannot automatically be equated with uncontrolled infection even if the syndrome was initiated by sepsis, infection has been most closely associated with its development.[2,21,23,27] When infecting organisms trigger host responses leading to tissue injury, their microbiologic identity does not seem to matter, since gram-positive organisms, fungi, and viruses, as well as gram-negative bacteria, have been implicated.[22] As stated earlier, the magnitude of the underlying infection may correlate poorly with the observed septic response in individual patients. This suggests that once initiated, host inflammatory processes operative in sepsis-induced MSOF can be self-perpetuating by leading to a state of malignant intravascular inflammation.[3] While one recognizes these facts, vigorous monitoring of the patient to prevent, detect, and control local infection remains essential in preventing microbiologic complications, such as metastatic abscesses and the septic response. Clinical risk factors initiating

TABLE 53-3 Clinical Risk Factors for the Development and/or Lethal Progression of MSOF

Severity of disease (APACHE II score)
Sepsis or infection at ICU admission
Age >65 years
Systemic sepsis
Bacteremic
Nonbacteremic
Nonbacterial
Persistent deficit in O_2 delivery after resuscitation from circulatory shock
Focus of devitalized/injured tissue
Severe trauma/major operations
Preexisting end-stage liver failure

MSOF independent of infection or synergistic in its development and lethal progression are shown in Table 53-3.

Studies analyzing determinants of the continuing high mortality during two frequent organ-specific manifestations of MSOF, ARDS, and acute renal failure (ARF) demonstrate that complex interactions exist among sepsis and noninfectious factors in shaping the expression of MSOF. These investigations highlight the conceptual difficulties involved in determining systemic mechanisms underlying MSOF from a focus based on organ-specific clinical features. Two lessons have been learned. The first is that an initial single-organ system dysfunction such as nosocomial pneumonia can trigger systemic inflammatory responses that extend the organ-specific problem to a generalized process of host immune dysregulation affecting cardiovascular homeostasis and multiple secondary-organ function.[28,29] Alternatively, manifestations of individual organ dysfunction apparently limited to a single organ early in the course of a catastrophic illness or injury may instead be occurring as part of a generalized injury to the endothelium of multiple organs.[16]

ARDS WITH MSOF

Mortality in ARDS has not appreciably decreased over the past two decades despite improvements in supportive ICU management, including ventilatory techniques.[8,9,15,28] Bias in the selection of patients with more severe degrees of lung damage to meet eligibility criteria for ARDS may be a partial explanation. Conceivably, therepeutic advances such as invasive hemodynamic monitoring and more aggressive resuscitation of deficits in 0_2 transport have minimized the development of ARDS in many patients. This might allow those with comparably severe lung dysfunction who otherwise would have died early to survive longer, allowing factors that amplify lung injury and/or impede its resolution to come into play. Most studies of ARDS with nonpulmonary organ failures have implicitly analyzed organ interactions in MSOF by a summative model (Fig. 53-1), where separate dysfunctions in nonpulmonary organs were seen to complicate a primary pulmonary problem, e.g., acute lung injury. This clearly occurs after direct lung parenchymal insults (e.g., aspiration of gastric contents or toxic gas inhalation). However, blood-borne mediated injury to the lungs during nonpulmonary sepsis can result in ARDS being the pulmonary manifestation of a systemic disorder of host defense.[15,16]

In support of this, data from the ECMO trial have been confirmed showing that approximately 85 percent of patients with ARDS die of MSOF and not irreversible pulmonary failure. In one report, 141 patients with ARDS were prospectively studied to determine the impact of infection and MSOF on outcome.[8] Patients who died had a higher incidence of nonpulmonary failures in conjunction with nonbacteremic sepsis. Failure in eight organ systems was diagnosed when it was considered life-threatening on the basis of specific abnormalities. These stringent but arbitrary criteria for organ dysfunction, with resultant increased severity of organ failure at initial diagnosis, may partly account for the observed increased incidence of MSOF in this study compared with other investigations of MSOF (Table 53-2). Initial pulmonary variables reflecting gas exchange, the mechanical properties of the lung, or responses to ventilatory management with positive end-expiratory pressure (PEEP) did not predict survival. On the other hand, failures in the CNS, renal, GI, endocrine, and coagulation systems were strongly correlated with nonsurvival.[8] Relations among the anatomic focus of sepsis, likelihood of positive blood cultures, and mortality from MSOF were also established. Patients with a nonbacteremic clinical sepsis syndrome and lethal MSOF usually have occult intrapulmonary sepsis, whereas in patients with positive blood cultures, an abdominal source is usually responsible.[9] Others have confirmed a close association of ARDS with sepsis[25] but have not specifically evaluated the role of individual organ systems on nonresolution and mortality. Collectively, these findings support the concept of source control in MSOF—that nonresolving ARDS with MSOF mandates a vigorous search for surgically remediable foci of infection.[2] Although valid, a negative result of this search does not exclude the possibility of an occult focus, as indicated above. Furthermore, depending on the timing of positive findings and drainage of purulent collections relative to the duration of MSOF, such treatment does not guarantee clinical improvement.[24]

ACUTE RENAL FAILURE (ARF)

Severe renal dysfunction developing in critically ill patients appears to represent another example of failure of individual organ support to alter the natural history of MSOF. Similar to the situation with ARDS, the mortality rate in ARF has not been significantly lowered over the past two decades in spite of improvements in dialytic therapy. The clinical context in which the renal failure is occurring is a major determining variable of survival, and there is some evidence to confirm the intuition that the ICU patients of today are, as a group, sicker than they were previously. In one study, two groups of patients requiring hemodialysis were compared, one treated over the period 1962–1969 and the other from 1972 to 1982.[30] Acute reductions in the glomerular filtration rate caused by isolated episodes of hypovolemia-associated hypotension were the most common etiology in the first group. Because of increasing utilization of invasive hemodynamic monitoring to guide fluid management, ARF in the later cohort did not appear to be secondary to well-defined episodes of hypovolemia. Instead, ARF developed in the setting of complex hemodynamic derangements associated with critical medical and surgical illnesses. ARF, like ARDS, seems to have been in evolution over this time. Moreover, the epidemiologic factors governing such evolution are likely to continue, since it is expected that the progressively aging population will have a higher prevalence of chronic disease, limiting organ reserve prior to the onset of critical illness or injury. It is also desirable that continuing technical advances in single-organ support occur. Finally, it is proper that the drive for excellence in provision of care to ICU patients remains the goal of critical care medicine. Because of this, a synthesis is required to incorporate present standards of single-organ-directed support with newer knowledge of basic mechanisms of impaired immunoregulation and cellular injury if the incidence and clinical expression of MSOF are to be altered.

A major unresolved issue in MSOF concerns the relative importance of *specific* organ systems in modulating outcome. There are three considerations: **1.** Does intrinsic dysfunction in particular systems occur more frequently than in other organs during MSOF? **2.** Can such dysfunction in specific organs be directly implicated in impeding resolution of established MSOF? **3.** Does preexisting or acquired organ-specific dysfunction disproportionately influence the pathogenesis of MSOF?

In a retrospective series of emergency surgical patients having an overall mortality rate of 74 percent, the incidence of lung, liver, and kidney failures were comparable.[10] A 68 percent mortality was present in 47 patients with ARDS developing MSOF.[9] In this report, a third of ARDS-related deaths occurred <72 h after presentation and were attributable to the underlying illness or injury, whereas deaths >3 days after were primarily related to a sepsis syndrome inducing MSOF. Thus, sepsis preceding ARDS usually originates from an abdominal focus, but sepsis complicating ARDS most often derives from infection within the damaged lung.[28] In such patients with ongoing respiratory failure, the most direct causes of late death were the sepsis syndrome, cardiovascular dysfunction, and CNS failures.[9] To determine the incidence of organ-specific dysfunction and death in MSOF, a prospective study was performed in 106 patients found at operation to have intraabdominal sepsis.[11] An increased risk of death was present in patients with shock, age >65 years, history of alcoholism, bowel infarction, or malnutrition. Lung dysfunction occurred most frequently (30/106 patients or 28 percent) and all patients who died of MSOF had respiratory failure. Cardiovascular, liver, and CNS dysfunction were never observed in isolation; when present, they were uniformly fatal (Table 53-4). Data regarding the influence of specific organ system failure on mortality were also analyzed in a series of surgical patients divided into two groups: 55 patients with trauma and 37 with intraabdominal sepsis.[5] In both groups, pulmonary and cardiovascular failures were present in the 33 patients who died, with hepatic failure existing in 32/33 (97 percent). The high incidence and low mortality related to the number of organ failures in this investigation are atypical compared with other studies of MSOF (Table 53-2) and are possibly accounted for by lack of time-dependent criteria for organ dysfunction. In contrast with these findings, CNS failure conferred the highest mortality risk in the large multicenter APACHE II study alluded to above,[13] with an approximate 10 percent incremental risk (overall risk, 40 percent) of hospital death compared with other single-organ system dysfunctions.

TABLE 53-4 Incidence of Organ Dysfunction and Related Mortality in 106 Patients with Intraabdominal Sepsis

Dysfunction	No. of Patients (%)	No. of Deaths	Mortality (%)
Lungs	30 (28)	19	63
Kidneys	16 (15)	12	75
Heart	11 (10)	11	100
Liver	9 (8)	9	100
CNS	10 (9)	10	100
Any organ	31 (29)	19	61

SOURCE: Data from Pine et al.[11]

It is difficult to conclude at present that intrinsic dysfunction in a particular system occurs more frequently than in other organs during MSOF following sepsis or trauma. In terms of organ-specific failures impeding resolution from MSOF, cardiovascular failure poorly responsive to vasoactive agents will limit survival in MSOF, presumably because of the overriding effect on tissue 0_2 delivery. Similarly, persistent respiratory failure can amplify mortality in MSOF independent of correction of gas exchange abnormalities caused by the frequent development of nosocomial pneumonia and resultant nonbacteremic sepsis syndrome.[8,31] However, dysfunction in the liver and GI tract during MSOF have likely been underestimated. Further, these organ systems, along with the cardiovascular system, may have a major influence on the pathogenesis of MSOF. These organs have not been previously recognized as pivotal to clinical outcome in ARDS and MSOF for several reasons. Both hepatic and GI dysfunction have been nonspecifically defined. For example, there are significant shortcomings inherent in defining global liver dysfunction by standard liver function tests that are sensitive but not specific.[15] Transaminase levels reflect parenchymal injury, not clearance or synthetic function, and do not correlate with the severity of histologic damage or outcome from a variety of types of hepatic injury. Similarly, serum bilirubin levels can be elevated nonspecifically during a variety of critical illnesses and their therapy because of sepsis-induced depression of hepatobiliary secretion, hypoxemia, drug-induced cholestasis, red cell transfusions, or the effects of increased back pressure to hepatic venous outflow created by increases in intrathoracic pressure during positive-pressure ventilation.[32,33] Neither organ system is as accessible for study as the cardiovascular system, lung, or kidney; and acute dysfunction is not as immediately evident as is circulatory shock, acute lung injury, or renal failure. Very few data exist to evaluate whether preexisting or acquired organ-specific dysfunction has a proportionately greater influence on pathogenetic mechanisms in MSOF. The incidence and clinical characteristics of ARDS were analyzed in patients with end-stage liver failure (ESLF) who required intensive care while awaiting liver transplantation.[15] ARDS occurred in 23 of 29 patients with ESLF; sepsis was the most common predisposing factor (18/29 patients, 62 percent). In contrast, ARDS developed in 3 of 44 (6.8 percent) control ICU patients without ESLF. Once initiated, regardless of etiology, ventilatory support, and aggressive management of hemodynamic abnormalities, ARDS was irreversible in all ESLF patients. These limited data and others[17] suggest that compromise of systemic and pulmonary host defense by impaired hepatic mononuclear phagocytic (Kupffer cell) performance and parenchymal cell function may both predispose to ARDS with MSOF and critically modulate its resolution. Other reports have also found a poor ICU outcome in patients with severe liver disease, but the impact of preexisting organ dysfunction on the incidence, clinical features, and mortality associated with MSOF has not been clearly established.

As a clinical syndrome, MSOF typically evolves through several identifiable stages with rather characteristic clinical features at each stage, albeit at a highly variable tempo in individual patients. It has been suggested that the common 21 to 28-day course of MSOF leading to either recovery or death in the setting of modern ICU therapy passes through four phases: shock, resuscitation, hypermetabolism, and transition to MSOF by multiple convergent and divergent pathways of cellular injury and tissue damage.[6] As in any clinical syndrome, clinical features differ at each phase. A clinical picture of the sequential changes in a typical patient during and after the transition to the MSOF has been provided.[2] The evolving changes in general appearance and single-organ function, while none in themselves diagnostic, are highly characteristic when observed together at the bedside (Table 53-5A–D). Such descriptions imply that there is a typical sequence of sequential organ system failure in MSOF.[1]

Overall, the combined experience in medical and surgical studies suggests that this is probably not the case.[5,8–11,13] The apparent sequential nature of organ dysfunction may instead reflect time-dependent variability in the organ-specific expression of pathogenetic events simultaneously affecting endothelial cell integrity and inflammatory cell activation in all organs at an earlier point along the temporal spectrum of host immune responses.[16] Therefore, the absence of a "typical" constellation of progressive organ failures or the tempo of their development should not be a deterrent in diagnosing MSOF in its earliest clinical phases. Likewise, it is important to bear in mind that certain treatable multisystem diseases, particularly when of fulminating onset, may mimic the clinical picture presented by sepsis or trauma-related MSOF (Table 53-6).

TABLE 53-5A Stage 1 of MSOF

General appearance	Normal or mildly restless
Cardiovascular function	Increased volume requirements
Respiratory function	Mild respiratory alkalosis
Renal function	Oliguria, limited diuretic responsiveness
GI function	Distension
Hepatic function	Normal or mild cholestasis
Metabolism	Hyperglycemia, ↑ insulin requirements
CNS	Confusion
Hematology	Variable

SOURCE: Modified from Carrico et al.[2]

TABLE 53-5B Stage 2 of MSOF

General appearance	Ill appearing, restless
Cardiovascular function	Hyperdynamic, volume-dependent
Respiratory function	Tachypnea, hypocapnia, hypoxemia
Renal function	Fixed output, minimal azotemia
GI function	Intolerance to enteral feeding
Hepatic function	Hyperbilirubinemia, prolonged PT
Metabolism	Severe catabolism
CNS	Lethargy
Hematology	Thrombocytopenia, leukopenia, or leukocytosis

SOURCE: Modified from Carrico et al.[2]

TABLE 53-5C Stage 3 of MSOF

General appearance	Obviously unstable
Cardiovascular function	Shock, decreased cardiac output, edema
Respiratory function	Severe hypoxemia, ARDS
Renal function	Azotemia, indication for dialysis
GI function	Ileus, stress ulceration
Hepatic function	Clinical jaundice
Metabolism	Metabolic acidosis, hyperglycemia
CNS	Stuporous
Hematology	Coagulopathy

SOURCE: Modified from Carrico et al.[2]

TABLE 53-5D Stage 4 of MSOF

General appearance	Moribund
Cardiovascular function	Vasopressor dependent, edema, rising S_vO_2
Respiratory function	Hypercapnia, barotrauma
Renal function	Oligo-anuria, instability on dialysis
GI function	Diarrhea, ischemic colitis
Hepatic function	Transaminase elevations, deepening jaundice
Metabolism	Muscular wasting, lactic acidosis
CNS	Coma
Hematology	Uncorrectable coagulopathy

SOURCE: Modified from Carrico et al.[2]

Pathogenesis/Pathogenetic Mechanisms

MSOF can be viewed broadly as the cumulative effect of impaired host defenses and inappropriate host regulation of acute immune and inflammatory responses (Fig. 53-2).

TABLE 53-6 Conditions Producing Multisystem Disease that Simulate Sepsis-Induced MSOF

Common
- Severe acute pancreatitis
- Systemic vasculitides
  1. Polyarteritis nodosa
  2. Granulomatous vasculitis
     a. Wegener's granulomatosis
     b. Lymphomatoid granulomatosis
- Active connective tissue diseases
  1. Systemic lupus erythematosus
  2. Rheumatoid arthritis
- Infective endocarditis
- Thrombotic thrombocytopenic purpura

Uncommon
- Atrial myxoma
- Cholesterol emboli syndrome
- Acute poisoning
  1. Arsenic
  2. Mercury
  3. Methanol
  4. Ethylene glycol
  5. *Amanita*
- Nonbacterial infections
  1. Rocky Mountain Spotted Fever
  2. *Falciparum* malaria

After infectious stimuli and noninfectious processes, such as ischemia and tissue trauma, stereotypic pathophysiologic pathways mediating tissue injury culminate in organ-specific damage and perpetuation of host defense impairment. Although essentially a disorder of immunoregulation, multiple pathogenetic mechanisms have been postulated in MSOF that are not mutually exclusive (Table 53-7). Each likely plays an important role at differing times, although it is not yet clear which are fundamental and which are epiphenomena. Mechanisms differ with respect to their temporal activation after initiation of host responses, place within the hierarchy of host defenses, and operation at specific anatomic loci. In this regard, the influence of the organ-specific anatomic locus of tissue injury likely has a similar determinative role in shaping the clinical expression of MSOF as it does on the outcome of local bacterial infection. For example, leukostasis caused by abnormal polymorphonuclear neutrophil (PMN) adherence to endothelium with resultant increases in microvascular permeability is a generalized process after trauma,[5] but the structure–function relations within the gas-exchanging apparatus lead to early clinical pulmonary impairment. Despite the systemic nature of mechanisms of MSOF, the interplay between host-mediated local tissue damage and salvage is therefore modulated by the microenvironment. Furthermore, established mechanisms of tissue injury, such as circulatory shock, microthrombosis, activation of the complement, kinin, and coagulation cascades, and intravascular release of proteases, now appear to be preceded by immunologic events resulting in the release of peptide and lipid inflammatory mediators. Therefore, to follow the unfolding events leading to MSOF through multiple stages,

TABLE 53-7 Pathogenetic Mechanisms Implicated in Tissue Injury During Sepsis-Related MSOF

Microbiologic
- Overwhelming sepsis from primary infecting microorganisms
- ICU-acquired infection with multiply-resistant microflora (e.g., *S. epidermidis, Pseudomonas* sp., *Candida* sp.)
- Undrained purulent collections (abscesses) or persistent localized infection (e.g., pneumonia)
- Endogenous (gut-derived) endotoxemia
- Bacterial translocation

Immunoregulatory
- Inappropriate regulation via excessive synthesis/decreased clearance of
  - Cytokines
    - TNF-α
    - IL-1α and IL-1β
    - IL-2
    - IL-6
  - Platelet-activating factor (PAF)
  - Cyclooxygenase and lipoxygenase metabolites of arachidonic acid
- Loss of regulatory control of complement, kallikrein-kinin, coagulation, and ACTH/endorphin systems after intravascular activation
  - Acquired systemic immunosuppression

Hemodynamic
- Flow-dependent tissue VO_2
- Distributive shock (e.g., altered regional blood flow distribution)
- Myocardial depression
- Microcirculatory derangements caused by
  - PMN adherence to capillary endothelium
  - Increased microvascular permeability

Biochemical
- PMN-induced O_2 free radical-mediated oxidant injury (including reperfusion injury)
- Lipid peroxidation of cell membranes
- Lysosomal enzyme release

Metabolic
- Altered intermediary metabolism and substrate utilization (hypermetabolic response)
  - $\uparrow$ Energy expenditure
  - Proteolytic catabolism
  - IL-6 directed reprioritization of hepatic protein synthesis to acute-phase reactants
  - Hyperglycemia caused by $\uparrow$ counter-regulatory hormones

we will identify the general characteristics of the early phases of the integrated host response to sepsis. The early phases of this response encompass convergent and divergent cascades leading to dynamic changes at the genetic level, which in MSOF escape host control, resulting in augmented inflammatory mediator production and immune cell activation. Subsequent changes in cytokine kinetics, interorgan traffic of immune effector cells, and intraorgan recruitment and accumulation of these cells amplify intravascular inflammation that exacerbates generalized endothelial damage and critical organ injury. Preexisting impairment in parenchymal organ function important in MSOF predisposition may then synergize with acquired organ injury in altering organ interactions that modulate the kinetics of secondary inflammatory mediators. By poorly understood mechanisms, a state of systemic cellular immunosuppression can follow that further impairs host defense homeostasis. It must be understood that at each stage, physiologic derangements such as cardiovascular impairment may interact with immunologic changes, inextricably linking the two phenomena in a complex model of global cybernetic failure.

HOST CONTROL OF SYSTEMIC ENDOTOXEMIA AND BACTEREMIA

Circulating gram-negative endotoxin has been extensively implicated in the mediation of early pathogenetic events relevant to sepsis-induced MSOF.[34–37] Teichoic acid from the cell walls of gram-positive bacteria and mannan from fungal microorganisms induce similar pathophysiologic effects by interaction with host effector mechanisms.[38] However, much more information is available for endotoxin. Endotoxemia is associated with the characteristic features of sepsis such as fever, hypotension, and leukopenia. Endotoxin also has direct cytotoxic effects. Endothelial cells are damaged in vitro; other changes include activation of circulating and tissue-based phagocytic cells, "priming" of phagocytes to become fully activated in response to other stimuli, and triggering of the complement, kinin, and coagulation cascades that synergistically impair endothelial cell structural integrity and metabolic function.[27,39] It follows that impairment in systemic host defenses permitting sustained endotoxemia or bacteremia results in three main complications: **1.** generalized endothelial damage; **2.** augmented generation of host-derived inflammatory mediators; and **3.** bacteriologic complications, such as metastatic abscess formation. Endothelial damage and multiple-organ injury can be amplified by both increases in the rate of generation of circulating endotoxin during infection, or reductions in its detoxification and clearance. The time course of endotoxin-induced tumor necrosis factor-α/cachectin (TNF-α) appearance in blood after endotoxemia in experimental models is similar regardless of whether endotoxin is infused as a bolus, a bolus followed by a slow infusion, or a slow infusion alone.[40] However, in this study the magnitude of the TNF response was higher after slow infusions, suggesting that the "shape" of the plasma endotoxin time-activity curve may modulate production of endogenous inflammatory mediators. Since the characteristics of plasma endotoxin concentrations can influence host responses, concern has been raised that "too rapid" bacteriolysis after antibiotic therapy for severe infection might liberate large amounts of endotoxin that exceed intravascular clearance mechanisms.[41] In this respect, "appropriate" antimicrobial treatment of sepsis associated with ARDS and MSOF has not improved survival.[25] Recent study of this question has not confirmed that antibiotic therapy increases plasma endotoxin levels in critically ill patients with meningococcal infection.[35] On the other hand, plasma endotoxin levels >700 ng/mL in that study correlated with development of septic shock, ARDS, increased serum creatinine levels, and death from MSOF. Moreover, circulating endotoxin, acting in concert with other vasotoxic substances, such as activated complement fragments, may increase the risk of developing ARDS in infected patients.[39,42]

The major mechanism controlling the magnitude and duration of systemic endotoxemia and bacteremia is mononuclear phagocytic uptake and detoxification by the liver. This is mediated primarily by Kupffer cells lining the extensive sinusoidal network.[16,43,44] Under certain circumstances, hepatocytes also participate in the intravascular clearance of endotoxin. Several factors are responsible for the pivotal role of the liver in this aspect of host defense. Nearly 90 percent of the fixed tissues macrophages of the body are contained within the liver.[45] In addition, Kupffer cells are more efficient in clearing bacteria and their products than other tissue-based phagocytes, such as alveolar macrophages, probably reflecting differential characteristics of cellular activation and the blood:cell interface among organ systems. Endotoxemia leads to additional recruitment and activation of phagocytic cells in the liver.[46] Finally, the liver occupies a strategic position immediately downstream from the GI tract, where the large bowel constitutes a large reservoir of intraluminal endotoxin and bacteria. The entire splanchnic venous outflow (25 percent of the cardiac output) passes through the sinusoidal microvasculature. This affords a first-pass defense system by which vasoactive substances that escape the GI lumen can be taken up prior to their entry into the systemic circulation and clearance by the lungs, the next downstream organ system.[47]

Impairment of hepatic mononuclear phagocytic (reticuloendothelial system) performance by several mechanisms can exacerbate circulatory shock, multiple-organ damage, and mortality after sepsis or trauma[15–17,48] (Table 53-8). Results from experimental and clinical studies demonstrate three primary determinants of the efficiency of this host defense system: (1) The metabolic state of the cells, in terms of their phagocytic "history," is critically important. Prior/concomitant phagocytic burdens induce either depression or stimulation with respect to subsequent nonbacterial particulate challenges, such as tissue debris or fibrin degradation products as a complex function of time. Increased systemic generation of endotoxin, augmented intravascular entry from gut reservoirs, or overwhelming bacteremia can thus exceed Kupffer cell uptake capacity, leading to "spillover."[16,45] (2) The availability of essential nonimmune opsonic cofactors, such as the glycoprotein, plasma fibronec-

TABLE 53-8 Mechanisms that Compromise Hepatic Phagocytic Host Defense During MSOF

Preexistent significant parenchymal liver disease
Excessive intravascular endotoxin/bacteria with resultant systemic spillover
Alterations in gut–liver axis
Augmented systemic generation (e.g., abscesses)
Hypo-opsonemia (depletion of opsonic cofactors such as plasma fibronectin)
Mesenteric/hepatic ischemia

tin (440,000 to 450,000 kDa), also modulates tissue injury and organ failure.[48] Domains within fibronectin bind denatured collagen, fibrin, and *Staphylococcus aureus.* Increased consumption of plasma fibronectin synthesized by endothelial cells, hepatocytes, and fibroblasts results in a "hypoopsonemic state" in which microthrombotic organ injury is exacerbated in animal models and patients with septic or posttraumatic MSOF.[49] (3) The characteristics of global hepatic blood flow determine the rate of delivery of substances to be cleared by the liver. The partitioning between portal venous blood flow (70 to 80 percent of total hepatic flow) and the hepatic arterial circuit (25 to 30 percent of total flow) influence host defense vis à vis endotoxin clearance.[50] The intrahepatic distribution of microcirculatory perfusion at the blood:sinusoidal cell interface may further modulate mononuclear phagocytic performance. Thus, preexisting conditions associated with liver damage or treatments, such as vasopressor infusions inducing hepatic or mesenteric ischemia (which reduces portal venous inflow), can be regarded as having immunomodulatory effects. Failure of the hepatic mononuclear phagocytes to control high-grade systemic endotoxemia, bacteremia, and blood levels of vasoactive byproducts of sepsis, including activated coagulation factors, damaged red cells and platelets, and particulate tissue debris during their initial appearance, can therefore predispose to MSOF by several mechanisms (Table 53-9). Significant underlying liver disease can itself be viewed as a clinical predisposition to MSOF.[15] Support for this derives from models of hepatic mononuclear phagocytic system blockade, hepatocytic injury, or obstructive jaundice, which independently increase mortality and extrahepatic organ injury during bacteremia or endotoxemia.[47,48,51] Even in the absence of liver disease, alterations in organ interactions within the gut–liver axis represent key factors in the pathogenesis and perpetuation of MSOF. Two principal mechanisms have been identified.

Endogenous endotoxemia was initially described over 30 years ago in studies designed to clarify the nature of determinants of "irreversibility" in hemorrhagic and traumatic shock.[18,52] These studies remain highly relevant to an understanding of MSOF. The concept of endogenous endotoxemia must be integrated with newer immunologic information deriving from cellular and molecular biology to arrive at a comprehensive picture of homeostatic derangements in MSOF. In this regard, the GI tract can be viewed as a "motor" in processes eventuating in MSOF[2] by sequential changes schematically depicted in Fig. 53-3. Evidence confirming that endotoxemia of host origin represents a final common pathway to multiple-organ damage and death under conditions of mesenteric ischemia can be summarized as follows: **1.** animals dying of irreversible hemorrhagic shock despite restoration of blood volume or traumatic shock have elevated plasma endotoxin levels; **2.** animals made tolerant to endotoxemia by prior exposure to low doses are made tolerant to otherwise lethal shock; **3.** sublethal hemorrhagic shock associated with smaller increases in plasma endotoxin levels induces cross-tolerance with respect to mortality and endotoxin concentrations in subsequent traumatic shock; and **4.** prior sterilization of the gut by nonabsorbable antibiotics increases the threshold for circulatory shock by reducing endogenous endotoxemia.[19]

Bacterial translocation is defined as the passage of viable indigenous bacteria from within the GI tract through the epithelial mucosa and lamina propria to the mesenteric lymph nodes and other organs.[53] Key events in this process

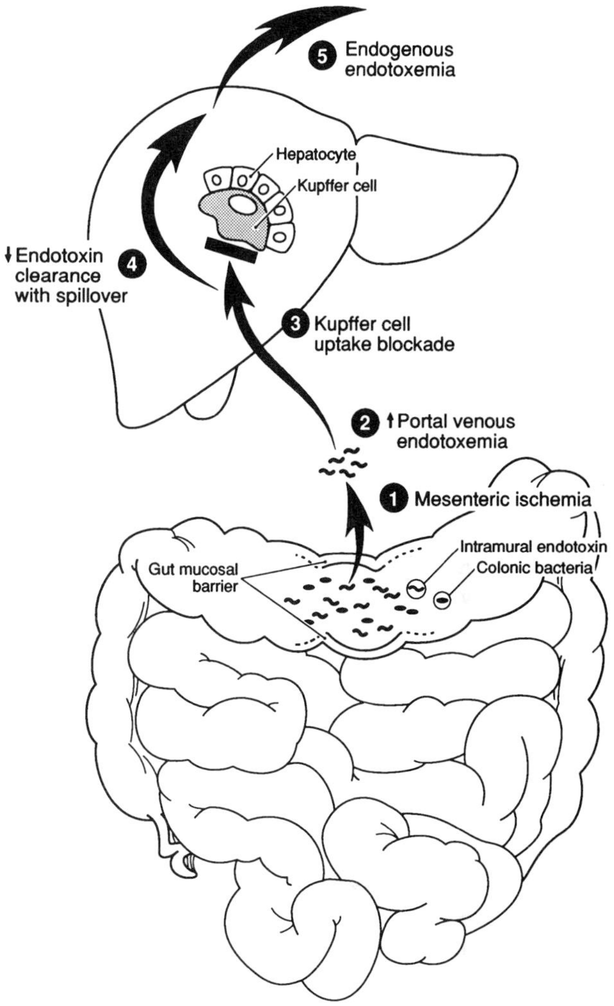

FIGURE 53-3 Sequence of events in the gut–liver axis involved in endogenous endotoxemia.

TABLE 53-9 Factors Promoting Bacterial Translocation in Animal Models and Man

Disruption of ecologic balance of normal indigenous microflora leading to overgrowth
Deficient T-cell mediated immunity
Systemic trauma
Endotoxemia
Endotoxin challenge in protein-calorie malnutrition
Total parenteral nutrition
Hemorrhagic shock
Intraabdominal abscess
Thermal injury
Intestinal obstruction

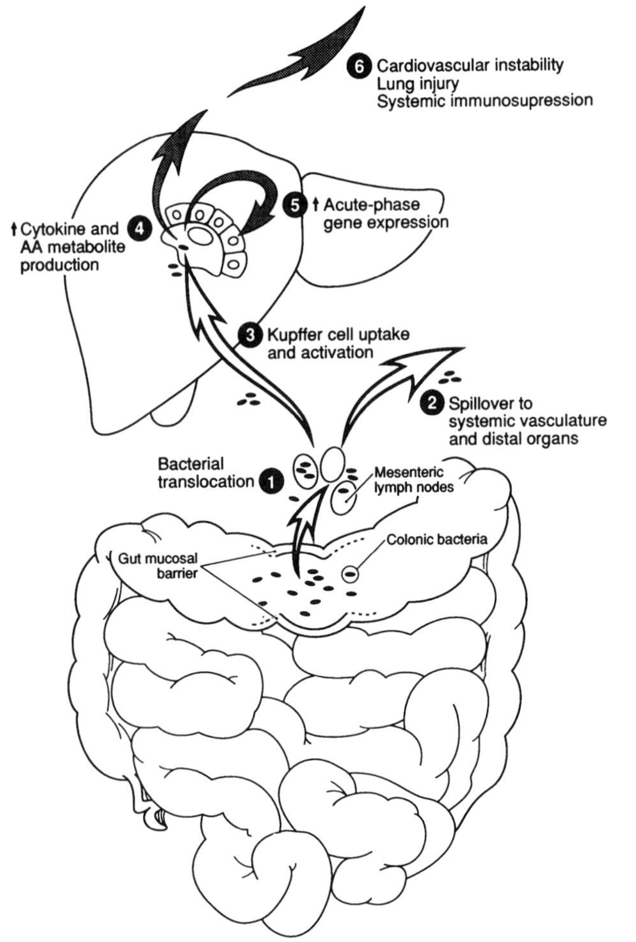

FIGURE 53-4 Sequence of events in the gut–liver axis involved in bacterial translocation.

and resultant organ system interactions among the gut, liver, and extrasplanchnic organs are schematically shown in Fig. 53-4. Several conditions and events common in the critically ill favor the development of translocation, particularly mesenteric ischemia and systemic endotoxemia (Table 53-9). Bacterial overgrowth, intestinal mucosa damage, or altered host immune functions underlie these conditions that lead to failure of gut antibacterial defenses.[54,56] Translocation has also been observed after acute intestinal obstruction in man,[57] presumably because of reductions in nutritive mucosal blood flow from gut distention accompanying high intraluminal pressures. A potential amplification loop in the pathogenesis of MSOF centering on the gut–liver axis, therefore, can be inadvertently produced by hemodynamic derangements accompanying a wide variety of acute diseases in the ICU, which have as a common denominator decreases in intestinal perfusion. After resuscitation from hypovolemic shock, pathologic changes in intestinal villus structure include an edematous lamina propria, separation of the epithelium from the basal lamina, and PMN infiltration, although the surface mucosal barrier superficially appears intact. These effects appear to be due partly to a reperfusion injury mediated by xanthine oxidase-derived oxidants.[58] Since α-adrenergic vasopressors support systemic perfusion pressure at the cost of mesenteric blood flow,[16] prolonged infusions or high doses may potentially exacerbate mesenteric ischemia and enhance endogenous endotoxemia and bacterial translocation. Like endogenous endotoxemia, bacterial translocation conceivably results in a large proportion of cases of severe or recurrent systemic sepsis in patients with nonresolving MSOF, in whom no localized anatomic focus of bacterial infection is ever detected radiologically, at operation, or by pathologic methods.

Early evidence supporting the importance of this process in systemic infection derived from experience with neutropenic patients, in whom the incidence of "autoinfection" with enteric flora is significantly increased. In these patients, prophylactic selective decontamination of the gut with antimicrobial drugs in turn decreases the incidence of sepsis. More recent reports in ICU patients without neutropenia have shown the efficacy of selective decontamination of the upper and lower digestive tracts in reducing colonization by pathogenic microorganisms and the overall infection rate. In trauma patients receiving mechanical ventilation for >5 days, topical oropharyngeal application and enteral administration of a combination of polymyxin E, tobramycin, and amphotericin B reduced gram-negative colonization without significant secondary overgrowth by resistant organisms.[59] When combined with systemic cefotaxime, the infection rate was reduced from 81 to 16 percent. A similar triple regimen was used in a prospective study of 324 ICU patients divided into control and treatment groups.[60] Consistent reductions in colonization of the digestive tract with aerobic gram-negative bacilli was demonstrated in treated patients, and the incidence of acquired infection decreased from 24 to 10 percent with reduction in mortality in certain groups. Other investigations have reported similar results.[61] However, it must be remembered that under normal circumstances, bacterial antagonism of GI levels of certain indigenous bacteria, such as *Escherichia coli*, by other members of the normal bacterial flora represents an important defense mechanism confining bacteria to the GI tract. Use of broad-spectrum antibiotics in the ICU to treat infections appropriately or prophylactically in other anatomic sites may upset this balance, favoring the development of pathogenic gram-negative bacterial colonization and translocation.

CYTOKINE RESPONSES IN SEPSIS

Along with the above mechanisms, circulatory shock, inflammation, and organ damage during gram-negative infection have been shown to be dependent on endogenous pro-inflammatory mediators after induction from host cells by the lipopolysaccharide component of endotoxin (LPS). Ischemia and trauma may activate cytokine responses in the absence of ongoing infection. It has been suggested that a cytokine cascade initiated by TNF-α, amplified by interleukin-1 (IL-1), IL-2, and IL-6, and modulated by the lipid mediators platelet-activating factor (PAF) and eicosanoid metabolites of arachidonic acid (AA) play major pathogenetic roles in sepsis-related MSOF.[3,62] The pathways by which cytokine kinetics and metabolism affect organ interactions during MSOF and how, in turn, they are influenced by them are just beginning to be clarified. Host regulatory control of TNF-α, IL-1, IL-6, PAF, and cyclooxygenase and lipoxygenase-derived eicosanoids have been analyzed individually. However, interactions among mediators parallel the complexity of interaction among organ systems in MSOF. Understanding such interactions offers both challenges and therapeutic opportunities. In the following discussion, we will review the pathophysiologic effects of each of these mediator classes, offering information concerning the parallel and convergent nature of their biologic effects.

TNF-α/CACHECTIN

TNF-α is a 157-residue polypeptide encoded by one of two linked genes on chromosome 6 within the major histocompatibility complex. The other closely related product, TNF-β or lymphotoxin, is secreted by activated lymphocytes and binds to the same cell receptor. TNF-β is likely of greater importance in such lymphocyte-mediated phenomena as chronic organ rejection. On the other hand, TNF-α is secreted primarily by endotoxin-activated monocytes/macrophages as a monomer that aggregates into biologically active trimers. TNF-α has been proposed as the principal cytokine mediating gram-negative shock and sepsis-related organ damage, the proximal mediator in a chain of mediators (Fig. 53-5; Table 53-10).[63] Cells do not contain preformed TNF-α. Instead, LPS-stimulated cells release TNF-α after a latency period of approximately 30 to 60 min that is requisite for gene transcription and translation of TNF-α-specific mRNA regardless of whether LPS is given in vitro or in vivo. Peak serum levels occur after 1 to 2 h.[63,64] TNF-α mediates cardiovascular and inflammatory phenomena previously attributed to LPS, including hypotension, fever, diarrhea, lung injury, leukopenia, platelet aggregation, and intravascular coagulation.[65] Generalized vascular endothelial injury and a cellular shift to a procoagulant state occurs after TNF-α. Further, the gut appears to be an early target organ with respect to increases in vascular permeability.[66] The vasculotoxic effects of TNF-α, thus, may enhance endogenous endotoxemia and bacterial translocation. Strong evidence for its central role in the events described earlier and the early phases of MSOF is provided by the following data: **1.** lethal endotoxemia or bacteremia is regularly accompanied by high circulating TNF-α lev-

TABLE 53-10 Biologic Actions of TNF-α/Cachectin

Microbiologic
- PMN activation, degranulation, enhanced O_2 radical release, phagocytic function, and Ab-dependent cytotoxicity
- Increased nonspecific host resistance
- Increased vascular permeability in the gut
- Neutrophilia, lymphopenia

Immunologic
- Promotion of IL-1, IL-2, IL-6, PAF, and eicosanoid production
- Expression of MHC antigens on tissue cells
- Hemorrhagic necrosis
- Induction of hepatic acute-phase reactant synthesis
- Diminished endothelial thrombomodulin activity
- Expression of adhesion molecules on vascular endothelium for PMNs and lymphocytes
- Release of plasminogen activator inhibitor
- Expression of tissue factorlike procoagulant activity
- Fever
- Growth-promoting and inhibiting effects on normal fibroblasts
- Stimulation of B- and T-lymphocyte proliferation

Hemodynamic
- Hyperdynamic circulatory shock
- Capillary leak syndrome
- Microvascular thrombosis
- Inhibition of cardiac myocyte β-adrenergic responsiveness

Biochemical
- Induction of stress hormone release
- Lactic acidosis
- Reduction in transmembrane resting potential in skeletal muscle
- Inhibition of hepatic drug metabolism

Metabolic
- Hyperglycemia → hypoglycemia
- Hypertriglyceridemia caused by inhibition of lipogenic gene transcription
- Hyperaminoacidemia and proteolysis
- Anorexia, cachexia

FIGURE 53-5 Schematic summary of the effects of lipopolysaccharide (LPS) and dexamethasone (Dex) on the stepwise expression of the TNF-α/cachectin gene product, demonstrating posttranscriptional amplification of LPS-induced biosynthesis of TNF-α. The defect imparted by the C3H/HeJ mutation is also shown. The upper × signifies a partial transcriptional blockade, and the lower × represents complete translational blockade. (From Beutler B et al: Science 232:997–980, 1986. Copyright 1986 by the American Association for the Advancement of Science.)

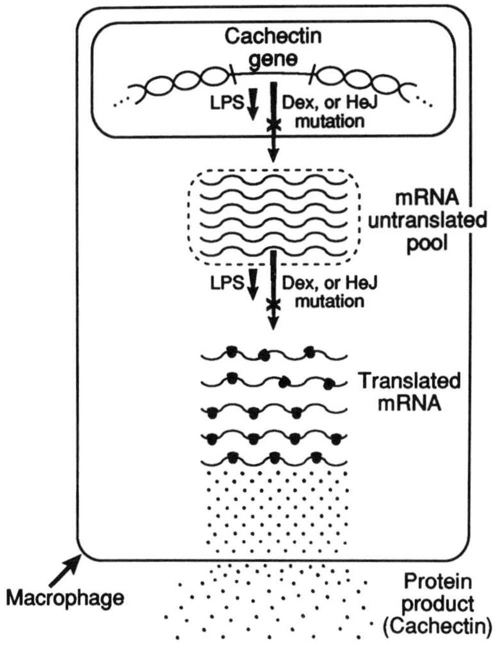

els.[63,67] In a study of 79 patients with meningococcemia, initial serum levels were highly predictive of survival, since 10 of 11 patients having values >0.1 ng/mL died of irreversible shock and MSOF.[68] **2.** Passive immunization of animals with monoclonal antibodies directed against TNF-α are protective against mortality and critical organ injury arising from lethal bacteremia.[69] **3.** Injection of LPS-free recombinant TNF-α leads to pathophysiologic changes similar to those seen after bacteremia or endotoxemia in MSOF. **4.** The biologic actions of TNF-α include effects on each pathogenetic mechanism implicated in the induction of tissue injury during MSOF (Table 53-7).

Once produced, the intravascular half-life of TNF-α is very brief, approximately 6.5 to 10.5 min. TNF-α binds to specific cell surface receptors similar to classic peptide hormones. Because of its wide-ranging cellular effects, several forms of host regulatory mechanisms have evolved, presumably in order for the organism to protect itself from progressive auto-injury after infection and trauma. Ligand–receptor interactions are influenced by prior exposure to endotoxin (or TNF-α) and other cytokines such as gamma-interferon, which increases TNF-α receptor number.[70] Intracellular signal transduction is modulated by changes in cytosolic concentrations of cyclic AMP induced by lipid mediators, particularly cyclooxygenase pathway metabolites (Fig. 53-6).[71] Finally, gene transcription and protein synthesis of TNF-α are regulated by mechanisms determining cytokine mRNA stability to RNases to permit subsequent message amplification by protein synthesis (Fig. 53-5).

Cells within multiple organs are capable of producing TNF-α. Since monocytes/macrophages are the principal cells in this regard, the lung and particularly the liver are key organs of TNF-α synthesis in quantitative terms.[72] For unclear reasons, monocytes from patients with alcoholic liver disease have an enhanced production rate for TNF-α.[73] Likewise, because many cell types have TNF-α receptors, many organs participate in its intravascular clearance. However, similar to its role in TNF-α production, the liver is one of the principal organs mediating TNF-α disposition.[51,73]

In spite of its importance, it is unlikely that TNF-α alone mediates all phases of the evolution of MSOF. Because it is released into the vasculature as a burst after endotoxemia, mechanisms determining TNF-α release seem to be activated within a narrow interval. Plasma TNF levels on the day that sepsis was diagnosed in 43 critically ill patients was accompanied by detectable circulating TNF in only 25 percent of cases,[74] although this group had a twofold increase in mortality. However, there was no significant difference in the incidence of MSOF between TNF-positive and -negative groups. Results may be explained by a functional block of TNF-α synthesis occurring despite continuing high LPS levels, compatible with a bidirectional tolerance phenomenon.[70] Furthermore, structural modifications of LPS that elminate in vivo toxicity continue to induce high plasma levels of TNF-α. Small amounts of endotoxin coinjected with recombinant TNF-α augment mortality in experimental models, suggesting that other mediators besides TNF-α that are induced by LPS modulate the clinical expression of shock and multiple organ injury. Finally, several lines of evidence show that many of the effects of TNF-α at the tissue level are mediated by cyclooxygenase pathway metabolites of arachidonic acid. In healthy humans receiving *E. coli* LPS, ibuprofen pretreatment attenuates fever and stress hormone responses, although circulating TNF-α levels are not affected.[64] Other data indicate that TNF-α normally plays a critical but nonspecific role in the early phase of the host response to a variety of acute conditions, such as acute myocardial infarction.[71,75] Nor should the effects of TNF-α be viewed in an entirely negative light. TNF-α mediated host responses to a septic challenge in most cases are probably beneficial,[76] associated with uneventful recovery of the patient. Humoral and cellular defenses are broadened and amplified at local and systemic levels, while increased substrate is made available for energy production. For example, the mutation in CH_3/HeJ mice that renders them resistant to lethal endotoxemia by the inability to produce TNF-α also results in an increased susceptibility to lethal bacterial infections. However, mechanisms integrating local synthesis and metabolism via autocrine and paracrine processes that assist in normal tissue repair after minor injury can escape host regulatory

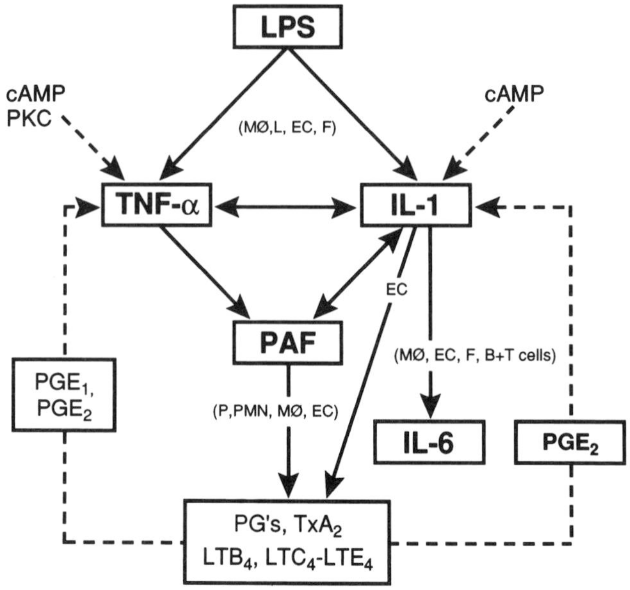

FIGURE 53-6 Endogenous peptide and lipid mediator interactions during gram-negative endotoxemia relevant to impaired regulation of acute immune and inflammatory responses and consequent cellular damage in MSOF. Directional arrows represent stimulatory pathways of interaction, except in the case of PGE_2, which is inhibitory to induction of TNF-α and I1-1. Increases in intracellular cAMP levels or protein kinase C activation (PCA) are also inhibitory to TNF-α and IL-1 gene transcription. Abbreviations of mediators: TNF, tumor necrosis factor-α/cachectin; IL-1, interleukin-1; PAF, platelet-activating factor; PG, prostaglandin; TxA_2, thromboxane A_2; LT, leukotriene. Abbreviations of cells: MO, monocyte/macrophage; L, lymphocyte; EC, endothelial cell; F, fibroblast; PMN, polymorphonuclear leukocyte; P, platelet.

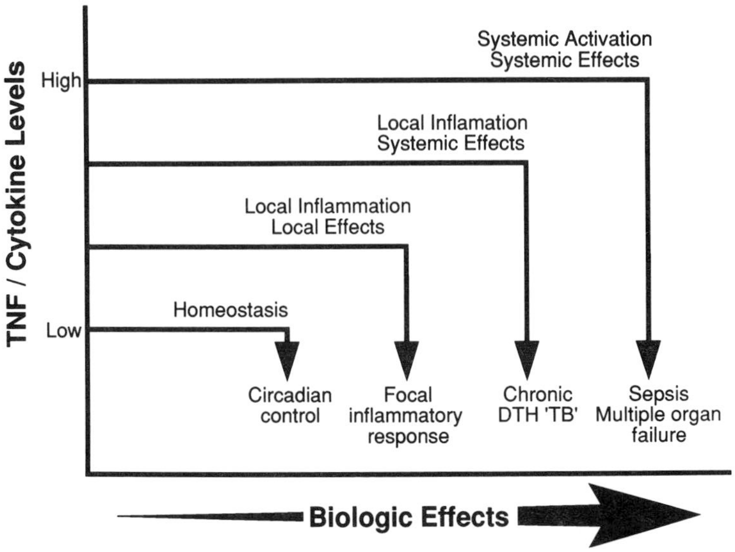

FIGURE 53-7 Schematic view of concentration-dependent and site-specific effects of TNF-α, showing a spectrum of effects ranging from paracrine to systemic actions. (Reprinted with permission from Kunkel SL et al: Crit Rev Immunol 9:93, 1989. Copyright CRC Press, Inc., Boca Raton, FL.)

control (Fig. 53-7). In addition to physiologic events mediated by the soluble form of cytokines such as TNF-α, membrane-bound forms may play an important local role in organ-specific immune responses and homeostasis. In contrast, high circulating levels that are rapidly released intravascularly characterize septic states accompanied by shock and MSOF. This exaggerated production and release may synergize with impaired clearance caused by preexisting or acquired critical organ system dysfunction as in the liver to produce a malignant form of intravascular inflammation involving secondary mediators (Fig. 53-6).

INTERLEUKINS

The interleukins are a group of peptide hormones involved in cell-to-cell communication during the evolution of immune and inflammatory responses. Ten different types have been described.[77] Of these, IL-1 and IL-6 are especially relevant to the early phases of MSOF, while IL-2 is an important mediator in subacute/chronic phases (Table 53-11). IL-1 exists in two molecular forms, IL-1α and IL-1β, which are 26% homologous yet bind to the same receptor that is distinct from the TNF-α receptor. IL-1α and IL-1β (IL-1) share many of the biologic actions described for TNF-α despite lack of structural homology and origin from a much larger array of cell types. For example, cyclic AMP is also an intracellular second messenger for IL-1. Like recombinant (r) TNF-α, rIL-1 injected into rabbits induces circulatory shock indistinguishable from that seen after endotoxemia.[78] Thus, TNF-α and IL-1 have overlapping activities with respect to both tissue injury and repair. Understanding interactions between these proximal mediators during endotoxemia and their individual roles in the clinical expression of MSOF is limited by this, their mutual induction by LPS, and potential for modulation by co-varying changes in eicosanoids (Fig. 53-6).

These considerations suggest four important concepts for understanding mediator involvement in MSOF: **1.** *Signal redundancy and convergency* characterize immunologic and physiologic responses. Multiple paths to similar immunologic, cardiovascular, and metabolic phenomena complicate assessment of the hierarchy of in vivo host responses to LPS in terms of the kinetics and metabolism of cytokines and other mediators such as PAF (Fig. 53-6). For example, induction of IL-1 from monocytes/macrophages or endothelial cells can proceed after TNF-α ligand-receptor interactions, or directly after stimulation by LPS and the complement fragment C5a. As with TNF-α, most effects of IL-1 at the cellular level are transduced by a variety of secondary mediators. The adverse circulatory effects in particular appear to be mediated by cyclooxygenase pathway metabolites.[78] **2.** *Bidirectional pathways* are frequent; mediator inter-

TABLE 53-11 Comparative Biologic Actions of IL-1, IL-2, and IL-6

Cytokine	Cellular Sources	Biologic Actions
IL-1α IL-1β	Monocytes/macrophages Endothelial cells Fibroblasts B and T cells Mesangial cells of kidney	Virtually identical to TNF except for limited effects on PMN chemotaxis and oxidative metabolism
IL-2	T cells	Proliferative signal for T and natural killer cells
IL-6	Fibroblasts Monocytes/macrophages Endothelial cells B and T cells Epidermal cells	Acute-phase gene expression Activation of thymocytes and T cells Induction of B cell differentiation Stimulation of hematopoietic precursors Inhibition of TNF-α gene expression ?Shock

actions are not necessarily unidirectional. For example, PAF can elicit production of IL-1, and IL-1 can induce TNF-α. **3.** *Synergism of physiologic with immunologic changes* at each stage of the host response influences the expression and outcome of MSOF. Dynamic physiologic changes affecting global blood flow and regional organ perfusion are interwoven with macrophage, lymphocyte, endothelial cell, and fibroblast activation signals that induce tissue injury. This is due in part to derangements in tissue-specific vascular integrity and partly by changes in the kinetics of mediator disposition. **4.** *Distinguishing beneficial from adverse effects* of physiologic and immunologic changes is difficult. As the other side of the biologic coin, IL-1 and other mediators, like TNF-α, have beneficial effects in host defense. In fact, the continuing ability of the host to synthesize IL-1 may be a determinant of survival during conditions of severe stress associated with sepsis, since decreased serum IL-1 activity and monocyte IL-1 production have been demonstrated in patients with a fatal outcome in sepsis-induced MSOF.[79]

Generation of IL-2 by T cells plays a pivotal role in amplifying subacute immune responses to sepsis and trauma by recruitment and activation of other T lymphocytes. Secondary mediators released by these cells subsequently transduce wide-ranging changes in the immune and hematopoietic systems.[77] Its relevance to MSOF is most likely if continuous antigenic stimulation persists. On the other hand, IL-6 (formerly β_2-interferon) has emerged as a major pleiotropic cytokine that functions as an intermediary to TNF-α, IL-1, and IL-2 to direct multiple immune and inflammatory changes (Table 53-11).[80,81] It appears to be the principal cytokine amplifying gene expression of acute-phase reactants such as C-reactive protein by reprioritizing protein synthesis in hepatocytes while diminishing production of "negative" acute-phase reactants such as albumin and transferrin. Acute-phase reactants in turn play diverse roles in up-regulating, down-regulating, or modulating immune and inflammatory responses. For example, C-reactive protein and complement components enhance bacterial phagocytosis, α_1-protease inhibitor modulates protease and elastase-induced acute lung injury, and ceruloplasmin and fibrinogen influence O_2 radical scavenging and coagulation, respectively.[16]

PLATELET-ACTIVATING FACTOR

PAF, also referred to as PAF-acether or AGEPC (acetyl glycerol ether phosphorylcholine) is a potent inflammatory lipid mediator with diverse effects on the homeostasis of multiple organs during ischemia and trauma (Table 53-12).[62] Pathways of synthesis and degradation after ischemia or trauma are depicted in Fig. 53-8. Although stimuli activating calcium-dependent phospholipase $A_2(PLA_2)$ activity also result in formation of arachidonic acid metabolites, synthetic pathways for PAF are distinct from those involved in cyclooxygenase and lipoxygenase eicosanoid production. PAF is not stored but formed de novo from alkylacyl-GPC within membrane lipids, with degradation occurring both intracellularly and in plasma.

TABLE 53-12 Biologic Actions of PAF

Bronchoconstriction; ↑ airway resistance
Dose-dependent arterial hypotension
Increases in total peripheral and pulmonary vascular resistance
Cardiodepression caused by
Induction of arrhythmias
Reduced contractility
Decreased coronary blood flow
Release of lysosomal hydrolases
Induction of platelet aggregation
Leukocyte margination
Bowel necrosis during endotoxemia
Enhanced microvascular permeability
Release of endogenous vasodilator substances (PGI_2, ADP, adenosine)

PAF has a variety of pathophysiologic effects capable of exacerbating ischemia and shock by functioning as a mediator of TNF-α and IL-1 (Fig. 53-6).[82] Intravenous injections cause cardiovascular collapse in animals,[62] similar to its effects when released endogenously in IgE-mediated anaphylactic shock. Consideration of the role of PAF on organ dysfunction during endotoxemia reemphasizes the principles alluded to earlier of signal redundancy, and synergism of physiologic with immunologic mechanisms of tissue injury. Like TNF-α and IL-1, PAF can mediate autocrine and paracrine tissue-specific pathologic changes with or without accompanying changes in circulating levels. The actions of PAF on target tissue also demonstrate mediator class interdependency with respect to transduction of cellular changes. The actions of PAF on the bowel during endotoxemia are illustrative (Table 53-13). PAF induces the synthesis of leukotrienes, which in turn transduce the effects of PAF.[83] Bowel necrosis after local PAF production during

FIGURE 53-8 Biosynthetic pathway for PAF.

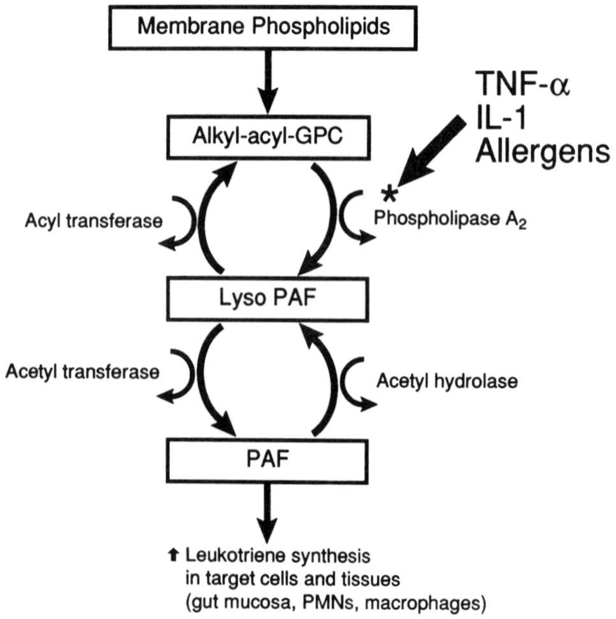

TABLE 53-13 Evidence for PAF Mediation of Bowel Necrosis in Endotoxemia

Normal gut contains PAF
Necrotic intestinal lesions are induced by LPS
Production of PAF increases in bowel after LPS
Isolated perfused intestine releases PAF after LPS
Pretreatment with PAF antagonists prevent LPS-related necrosis

SOURCE: From Hsueh et al.[83]

endotoxemia may set the stage to amplify generalized septic organ dysfunction by enhancing endogenous endotoxemia and bacterial translocation.

EICOSANOIDS

Individual eicosanoid products of the cyclooxygenase pathway (Fig. 53-9) and lipoxygenase pathway (Fig. 53-10) have been clearly implicated in the pathogenesis of tissue injury in individual organs during endotoxemia and septic MSOF (Tables 53-14, 53-15).[84–86] However, recent work has focused on interactions within a network of cell activation signals in which eicosanoids are broadly viewed as a heterogeneous second-messenger system for cytokines and PAF. Of these interactions, production of the immunodepressant eicosanoid, PGE_2, is of significant interest. PGE_2 is released along with cytokines, lipid mediators, proteases, and O_2 radicals during macrophage activation. A negative feedback loop has been defined with respect to TNF-α. Dose-dependent stimulation or suppression of TNF-α gene transcription and translation by PGE_2 and PGI_2 have been characterized in a series of studies (Fig. 53-6).[71] In turn, these effects are mediated by increases in intracellular concentrations of cyclic AMP. In this regard, cyclooxygenase pathway inhibition with ibuprofen, reducing PGE_2 levels, attenuates toxicity associated with TNF-α. PGE_2-induced suppression of IL-1 synthesis has also been described.[87] In

TABLE 53-14 Biologic Actions of Cyclooxygenase Metabolites of Arachidonic Acid

Prostaglandins
Vasodilation (PGI_2, PGE_1) or vasoconstriction ($PGF_{2\alpha}$)
Anti-aggregatory effects on platelets
Arterial hypotension
Enhanced capillary permeability
Arterial hypoxemia via changes in hypoxic pulmonary vasoconstriction
Thromboxanes
Platelet and PMN aggregation
Increased PMN adhesiveness
Vasoconstriction of regional vascular beds (especially pulmonary, coronary, splanchnic, and renal circuits)
Enhanced capillary permeability
Capillary leak syndrome
Increased airway resistance and reduction in dynamic compliance

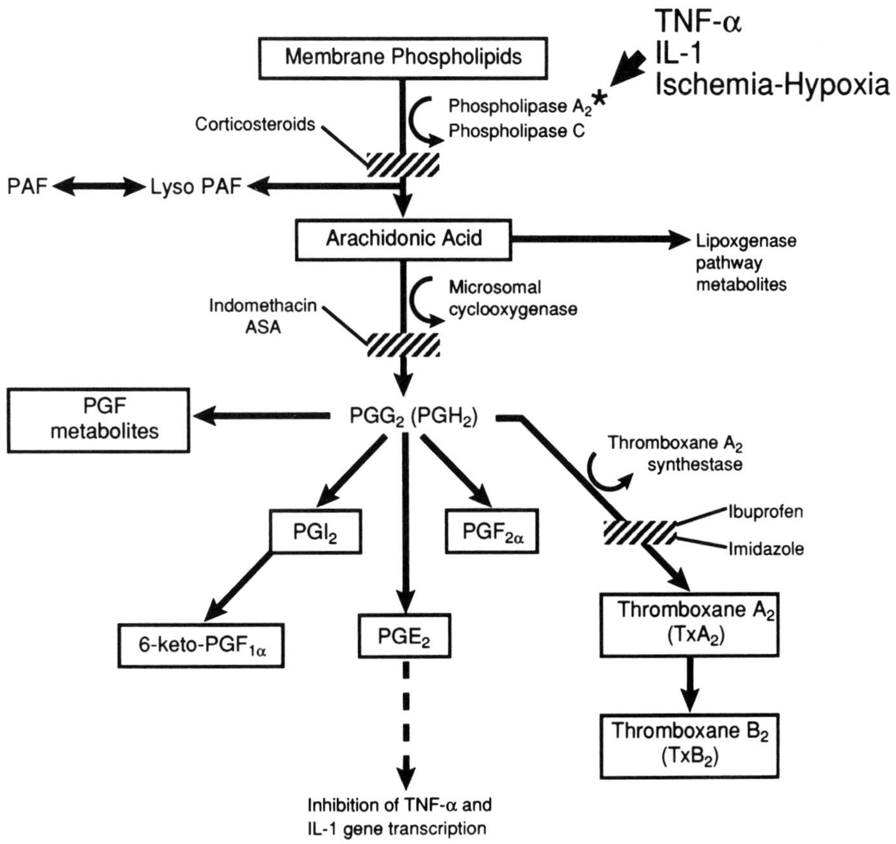

FIGURE 53-9 Biosynthetic pathway for cyclooxygenase eicosanoids.

TABLE 53-15 Biologic Actions of Leukotrienes

LTB_4	
	Chemoattractant + chemotactic for PMNs
	Enhanced capillary leakage
LTC_4, LTD_4, and LTE_4	
	Bronchoconstriction
	Vasoconstriction in vitro and in vivo
	Depression of cardiac contractility
	Enhanced capillary leakage

contrast, lipoxygenase products may enhance IL-1 production.

The liver and the lung play key roles in the production and disposition of arachidonic acid metabolites in the intact organism. However, it has been difficult to study the selective influence of preexisting or acquired organ system dysfunction on the metabolic fate of these substances in vivo after endotoxemia. Hepatobiliary elimination of systemically generated leukotrienes after endotoxemia or rTNF-α represents an example of the complex interplay among variables involving systemic host defense, organ interactions, and mediator-dependent tissue injury operative in MSOF (Fig. 53-11). Concentrations of LTB_4, LTC_4, and LTD_4 are elevated in the bronchoalveolar lavage fluid (BALF) of patients with ARDS and those at risk for ARDS.[85,86] Although endotoxemia causes the generation of leukotrienes in blood and BALF, LPS dose-dependently impairs the clearance of endogenously generated or exogenously administered peptide leukotrienes, even during normal liver function.[88] These interactions reemphasize the importance of source control during sepsis to reduce circulating endotoxin levels. Preexisting hepatocytic injury can therefore be seen to significantly impair host defense by sensitizing to the inflammatory and vascular effects of leukotrienes produced after endotoxemia.[89]

Therapy

The epidemiologic data described earlier confirm that outcome from established MSOF after sepsis or trauma remains poor. Accordingly, there has been great interest in the development and clinical testing of alternative approaches based on mechanisms identified, for the most part, in experimental models (Table 53-16). This is desirable, but such advances must complement, not supersede, meticulous bedside care of the critically ill using well-defined physiologic principles.

CASE PRESENTATION

B.R., a 58-year-old white man with biopsy-documented chronic liver disease attributable to long-standing ethanol abuse, was brought to the emergency room (ER) after two episodes of massive hematemesis. Prior to this, the patient had complained of mild upper gastrointestinal discomfort for several days. On initial examination, the

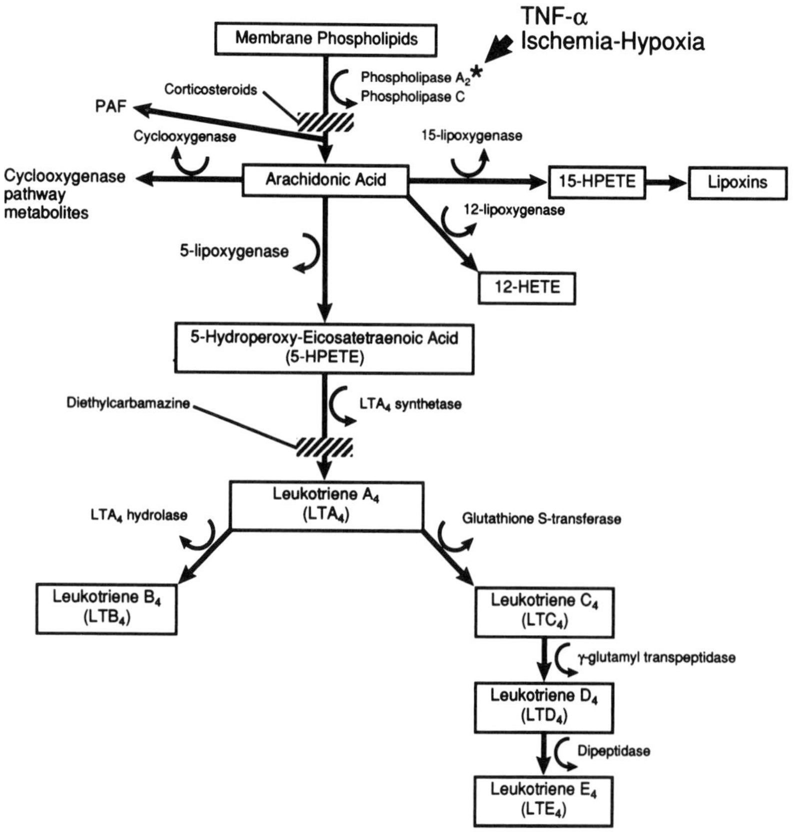

FIGURE 53-10 Biosynthetic pathway for lipoxygenase eicosanoids.

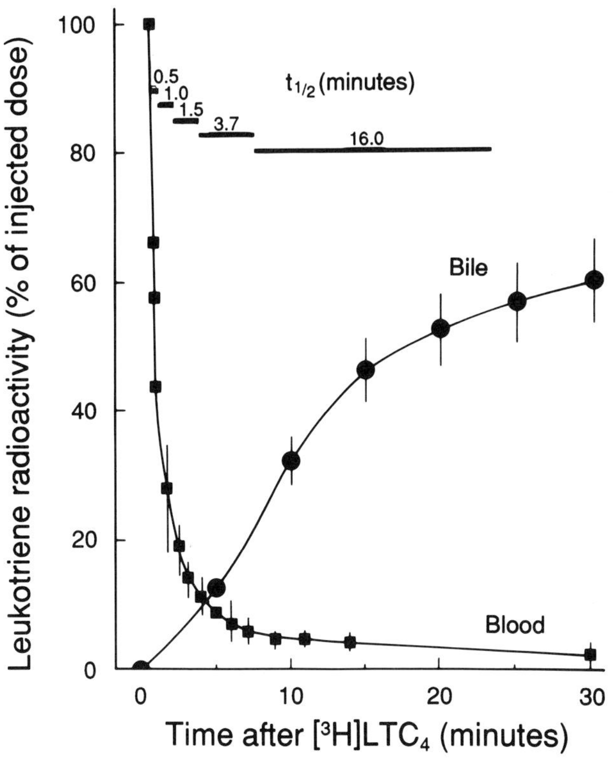

FIGURE 53-11 Role of the liver in the intravascular clearance of peptide leukotrienes. The dynamics of the hepatobiliary clearance of systemically administered radiolabeled LTD_4 are shown relative to concomitant blood concentrations. (From Denzlinger C et al: Science 230:330, 1985. Copyright 1985 by the American Association for the Advancement of Science.)

patient was restless but oriented. The skin was warm and flushed and revealed palmar erythema with several spider nevi over the trunk. The systolic pressure was palpable at 70 mmHg with a pulse rate of 130/min, respirations 34/min, and temperature of 38.1°C. The chest was clear. Bowel sounds were hypoactive, and the stool was melanotic. The liver was hard, irregular, and 16 cm in span; a spleen tip was felt. No ascites were detected. No focal sensory or motor deficits were present. Two liters of crystalloid solution were infused intravenously along with thiamine and vitamin K. Another episode of hematemesis of over 100 ml of dark blood led to endotracheal intubation. Bloody secretions were present in the endotracheal tube. A nasogastric tube was inserted without difficulty, and the aspirate was frankly bloody, clearing moderately with saline lavage.

Laboratory Findings

The hemoglobin was 8.1 g/dL with a hematocrit of 24%. The white blood cell (WBC) count was 14,500/mm^3 with 75 PMNs, 8 bands, 10 lymphs, and 7 mononuclear cells. Arterial blood gases were as follow: pH 7.2; Pa_{O_2} 88 mmHg; Pa_{CO_2} 25 mmHg during ventilation with a $FI_{O_2} = 0.5$. The serum sodium was 128 meq/L, chloride 98 meq/L, potassium 3.1 meq/L, and bicarbonate 9 meq/L. Blood urea nitrogen (BUN) was 10 mg/dL, creatinine 2.1 mg/dL, and aspartate aminotransferase was elevated >three times the upper limit of normal. Serum bilirubin was 5.5 mg/dL. A coagulation profile included a platelet count of 85,000 mm^3, a prothrombin time that was 4.5 s longer than control, and a borderline elevated partial thromboplastin time. Urinalysis disclosed 1 + proteinuria without red or white cells.

TABLE 53-16 Mechanism-Oriented Prophylactic and Therapeutic Options for Sepsis-Induced MSOF

Active immunization, passive protection by antisera/purified immunoglobulins against *Enterobacteriaceae, Pseudomonas sp.*, endotoxin
Reduction in frequency/duration of deficits in global O_2 delivery by maintenance of intravascular blood volume
Therapeutic goals for O_2 delivery based on values from survivors
Source control of infection
Antibiotics
Drainage of purulent collections
Prevention of mesenteric/hepatic ischemia during vasoactive drug infusions
Selective mesenteric dopaminergic receptor stimulation (e.g., dopamine 1–3 μg/kg/min)
Inhibition of xanthine oxidase-mediated generation of O_2 free radicals during resuscitation for circulatory shock
Allopurinol, other agents
Administration of opsonic plasma fibronectin during states of consumptive hypo-opsonemia
Extracorporeal filtration to dampen malignant intravascular inflammation
Plasma exchange
Specific absorption (e.g., polymyxin B for endotoxin)
Administration of monoclonal Abs directed against TNF-α
Pharmacologic modulation of intracellular cyclic AMP in inflammatory cells by therapy
Pentoxifylline
PGE_2
Dibutyryl cAMP
Pharmacologic modulation of cytokine gene expression or tissue effects
Corticosteroids
PAF synthesis inhibitors or PAF receptor blockade
Cyclooxygenase pathway inhibition (e.g., ibuprofen)
Lipoxygenase pathway inhibition or leukotriene receptor blockade, especially with preexisting liver damage
Preservation of gastric acidity to decrease incidence of nosocomial pneumonia
Meticulous management of intravascular lines

Clinical Course

On ICU admission, the patient's mental status and temperature were unchanged. Systolic blood pressure was 88 mmHg, pulse rate 120 min, and respirations 30/min during intermittent positive pressure ventilation (IPPV) in the assist-control mode at an $FI_{O_2} = 0.5$, V_T = 10 mL/kg, and positive-end expiratory pressure (PEEP) = 5 cmH_2O. The nasogastric aspirate was dark pink. The urine output was less than 30 mL/h. Femoral arterial and pulmonary artery catheters were inserted. The right atrial pressure was 5 mmHg, pulmonary artery pressure 48/10 mmHg, and the wedge pressure 8 mmHg. The cardiac index was 3.1 L/min/m^2, with an arteriovenous AV_{O_2} content difference of 2.8 vol %. The systemic vascular resistance index was 1677 dyne/s/cm^{-5}. The lactate level was 5 m*M*/L, and repeat arterial blood gases revealed pH 7.28; Pa_{O_2} 98 mmHg; and P_{CO_2} 28 mmHg. Three units of packed red cells, 10 U of platelets, and 4 U of fresh frozen plasma and lactulose were given. The arterial pressure was 110/60 mmHg. Flexible upper esophagogastroduodenoscopy confirmed the presence of large (>5 mm) esophageal varices, one of which was partially obscured by a large adherent clot, but minimal active bleeding. A diagnosis of variceal hemorrhage was made and an intravenous infusion of vasopressin was started at 0.4 U/min in combination with topical (2%) nitroglycerin. Repeat prothrombin time was 2 s over control values. After 24 h, the vasopressin infusion was discontinued without complication.

On the fourth hospital day, the patient was febrile to 38.7°C and exhibited a decreased mental status together with oliguria. Purulent secretions were present in the endotracheal tube and right lower lobe air-space consolidation was present. The white blood count (WBC) was 18,000/mm^3 with 90 PMNs, 15 bands, and 5 lymphs. Intravenous nafcillin and cefotaxime were begun. However, within 12 h the patient became hypotensive with an arterial pressure of 80/mmHg. The nasogastric (NG) aspirate was clear and hemoglobin and hematocrit values not significantly different. The wedge pressure was 8 mmHg. Several liters of crystalloid solution were administered without effect. A dopamine infusion was begun at 5 μg/kg/min and incrementally increased to 15 μg/kg/min. Arterial pressure increased to 92/48 mmHg. Two blood cultures grew *Enterobacter aerogenes,* and gentamicin was added to the antibiotic regimen. At this point, the arterial oxygenation began dropping, such that it required 15 cmH_2O PEEP to enable an $FI_{O_2} = 0.5$ to achieve a $Pa_{O_2} > 60$ mmHg. Bilateral pulmonary filtrates were present on a repeat chest radiograph. By 36 h later, the patient was stuporous and had deepening jaundice. Oliguria (output ≤20 mL/h) developed with limited responsiveness to large doses of metolazone and furosemide. Serum bilirubin was 8.1 mg/dL. The dopamine infusion could not be reduced below 10 μg/kg/min because of hemodynamic instability. Repeat blood cultures revealed *Staphylococcus epidermidis;* nafcillin was discontinued and vancomycin administered. The cardiac index was now 3.6 L/min/m^2 with an AV_{O_2} content difference of 2.5 vol %. The platelet count, which had increased earlier, now decreased to 65,000/mm^3. Enteral nutrition was started with branched-chain amino acids but was discontinued after ileus and diarrhea. Parenteral nutrition was initiated but resulted in hyperglycemia with blood sugar values ranging from 250 to 400 mg/dL that required exogenous insulin. Generalized edema and ascites developed over the next 48 h (7th day of hospitalization) in association with a decreasing albumin level (1.9 gm/dL). A repeat coagulation profile demonstrated progressive increases in the prothrombin time (5 s greater than control) and partial thromboplastin times; fibrin split products were present in a titer of 1:128. A paracentesis revealed sterile fluid. A computed tomography (CT) scan of the abdomen and pelvis with contrast confirmed ascites but showed no extraluminal masses or pockets of gas. The patient became responsive only to deep pain. A CT scan of the head excluded hemorrhage or mass lesion and a lumbar puncture after transfusion of fresh frozen plasma revealed no evidence for infection. Because of a rising BUN to 80 mg/dL and creatinine of 4.8 mg/dL together with hyperkalemia (potassium level 6.1 meq/L) and volume overload (wedge pressure 24 mmHg), an attempt was made at hemodialysis. Significant hemodynamic instability resulted, necessitating an infusion of norepinephrine titrated to maintain the systolic blood pressure ≥90 mmHg. On the 10th hospital day, the patient remained febrile and vasopressor-dependent with numerous hypotensive episodes. Blood cultures remained sterile. There was little change in neurologic function. A metabolic acidosis (pH 7.28) was present with an anion gap of 24 mEq. The arterial lactate concentration was 7 m*M*/L despite progressive increases in the mixed venous O_2 saturation to 70%. The bilateral pulmonary infiltrates persisted. While remaining on 18 cmH_2O PEEP, a tension pneumothorax developed resulting in a cardiopulmonary arrest from which the patient could not be resuscitated. Postmortem examination revealed bilaterally edematous lungs with numerous foci of bronchopneumonia and microabscesses, from which were cultured *E. aerogenes, E. coli,* and *Candida albicans.* The liver showed micronodular cirrhosis. Several renal parenchymal abscesses were detected that on staining disclosed hyphae consistent with *C. albicans.*

DISCUSSION

The presentation and course of this patient's illness are illustrative of MSOF in several respects. Following hypovolemic shock and resuscitation, the patient's condition was initially stabilized for a brief interval. Transition to MSOF subsequently occurred after sepsis supervened, resulting in the stepwise progression of severe physiologic dysfunction in multiple organ systems. During this transition, there was the evolution, in stages, of a rather stereotypic "gestalt" of clinical features (Table 53-5A–D). Treatment of the infectious process with appropriate antibiotics prevented death from overwhelming sepsis but was incapable of resolving the bacterial infections within the damaged lung partly because of the nonsterile conditions of the lower respiratory tract during ventilatory management of ARDS. The antibiotics may have further predisposed to gram-positive bacterial superinfection and subsequent opportunistic infections with fungal pathogens. Despite vigorous organ-specific support, including treatment of ARDS and ARF, secondary complications developed eventuating in death. After the onset of the initial organ system dysfunctions that were sustained over time, it was clear that this patient was at very high risk for dying from MSOF (Table 53-2).

Within the context of pathogenic interactions among immune effector cells, their products, and physiologic control mechanisms, iatrogenic organ system interactions may have altered the initial conditions sufficiently to create large differences in outcome. For example, although acute lung injury is treated by PEEP, PEEP may have adverse extrapulmonary consequences on the CNS, kidney, and liver. If PEEP-induced reductions in hepatic blood flow (QL) compromise flow-dependent mechanisms for hepatic clearance of blood-borne inflammatory mediators, the PEEP might modulate resolution of ARDS (Table 53-8). To further this analogy, PEEP can affect the liver by three mechanisms: **1.** reduction in cardiac output; **2.** increase the back pressure of hepatic venous outflow; and **3.** influence partitioning of flow between the portal venous and hepatic arterial circuits. Although sustained hepatic compression by the descending diaphragm has been postulated to alter the pressure gradient for sinusoidal perfusion or intrahepatic vascular resistance, the effect appears to be minimal at PEEP levels $\leq$ 10 cmH_2O.[32] Because of the multiple hemodynamic and intrinsic cellular variables regulating Kupffer cell and hepatocytic uptake mechanisms, the effects of positive-pressure ventilation on the liver remain unclear. Some clearance processes may be facilitated (Fig. 53-12), while others such as biliary flow may be reduced. Phasic increases in intrathoracic pressure (ITP) during IPPV also phasically elevate the effective hepatic backpressure. At ventilatory

Figure 53-12 Schematic representation of proposed mechanisms by which PEEP may alter clearance of diffusible substances during elevations in the back pressure to hepatic outflow. A: sinusoidal transit of indocyanine green (ICG molecules) (filled circles) in absence of PEEP-induced hepatic venous pressure (Phv) elevations. Dashed lines, sinusoidal microvascular fenestrae. Proportionally shaded arrows depict balance of sinusoidal vascular inflow and outflow forces (inflow pressure Pi) as a function of sinusoidal blood volume and flow. Thin arrows, transsinusoidal plasma movement containing ICG. Large open rectangles, hepatocytes. Diagonal-lined area, space of Disse. B: augmentation of plasma movement by PEEP-induced increases in hepatic back pressure, resulting in increased transsinusoidal ICG passage into extracellular space of liver and enhanced uptake. Not graphically depicted are potential co-varying changes in sinusoidal transit time and increases in hepatic vascular capacitance during PEEP-induced Phv elevations. (From Matuschak GM et al: J Appl Physiol 62(4):1377–1383, 1987, with permission.)

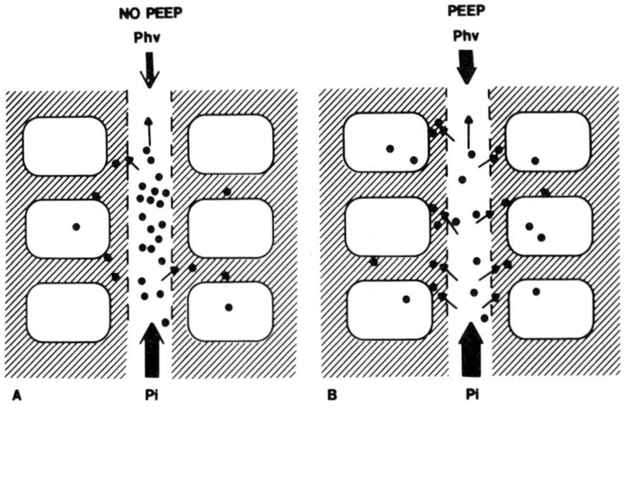

frequencies (f) $\leq$ 150 breaths/min during fixed levels of mean ITP, the hepatic outflow pressure is modulated in a postsinusoidal, flow-limiting segment caused by diaphragmatic compression that increases resistance to portal flow in a f-dependent manner.[90] However, the pharmacokinetics of substances whose extraction is dependent on QL primarily vary with determinants of inflow (e.g., cardiac output).

The management of individual problems in this patient, while correct in terms of their *specific* anticipated effects, nonetheless may have inadvertently promoted development of MSOF by several mechanisms (Table 53-7). Aggressive volume resuscitation to counteract initial hypovolemia was performed but was not guided by therapeutic goals based on hemodynamic and O_2 transport variables associated with improved survival. However, it is arguable whether targeted goals in O_2 delivery/uptake variables are achievable in patients with severe liver disease caused by derangements in vasomotor tone and peripheral arteriovenous shunting.[91] Similarly, the mesenteric ischemia therapeutically induced by vasopressin to reduce portal pressure may have led to occult but significant changes in the gut–liver axis (Figs. 53-3 and 53-4). Portal venous pressure–flow relations are characterized by lack of autoregulation; the vasopressin-induced reduction in portal pressure is achieved at the cost of reduced mesenteric inflow. While nitrate therapy combined with vasopressin ameliorates untoward systemic vasoconstrictive effects, the GI hemodynamic changes persist, potentially favoring endogenous endotoxemia and/or bacterial translocation. Support of systemic blood pressure to ensure a critical perfusion pressure with α-adrenergic agonists can have a similar effect on GI host defense.[18] It is presently unclear whether in the latter circumstance, selective stimulation of mesenteric dopaminergic receptors may ameliorate reductions in QL, although it has been suggested that such therapy improves postischemic liver function.[92]

Recently, the microbiology of ICU-acquired infections has been more fully defined.[23] Infections with *Pseudomonas sp., S. epidermidis,* and *Candida* are characteristic and associated with a poor outcome despite appropriate treatment. Infection with these organisms thus reflects the combined effects of antibiotic-induced suppression of other flora and systemic immunosuppression caused by endogenous substances released from inflammatory cells, particularly Kupffer cells.[38] The presence of severe chronic liver disease itself can be considered a risk factor that interacts with other clinical predispositions for MSOF (Table 53-3). In this patient, the hepatic host defense mechanisms described earlier were impaired. Functionally, the patient can be considered to have been an immunocompromised host. Kupffer cell phagocytic efficiency was likely reduced due to intrahepatic shunting of sinusoidal uptake sites and reduced synthesis of opsonic plasma fibronectin. Abnormal liver–lung interactions occur during gram-negative bacteremia in obstructive jaundice, in which spillover of microorganisms escaping normal hepatic uptake leads to their lodgement in the lungs.[47] Such a mechanism may have contributed to the pathogenesis of sepsis-induced ARDS and to its failure to resolve in this patient.

CT scans are frequently performed in patients with nonresolving organ failure in the setting of sepsis, particularly when MSOF follows a prior operation. There are very limited data to determine whether drainage of purulent collections discovered by CT scanning improves the outcome of established MSOF.[93] The timing of exploratory relaparotomy when CT scans are unrevealing and the patient is deteriorating is similarly unclear.[94]

Even in the absence of ongoing infection, the preexisting liver disease in this patient may have predisposed to malignant intravascular inflammation after endotoxemia. The signal redundancy and mediation of cytokine responses by eicosanoids during the inflammatory response to infection with liver damage may result in impaired clearance of mediators such as the leukotrienes.[95,96] Figure 53-11 demonstrates the importance of hepatobiliary metabolism in reducing circulating levels of peptide leukotrienes. In a model of *E. coli* endotoxemia in which preexisting liver injury was induced pharmacologically, mortality, albumin leak in the lungs, and PMNs in BALF were increased.[89] These changes were accompanied by increased blood and BALF levels of LTB_4 and LTC_4; lipoxygenase pathway inhibition with diethylcarbamazine (Fig. 53-10) decreased pathophysiologic effects and mediator levels, suggesting that impaired metabolism of endogenously synthesized leukotrienes underlies these phenomena. This mechanism may have enhanced septic lung injury during the liver dysfunction in this patient.

Until alternative therapeutic approaches listed in Table 53-16 are clinically validated, we are left with our clinical judgment and an extensive knowledge of organ-specific pathophysiologic mechanisms that are eminently treatable with current methods of ICU support. These physiologic principles evolved in response to acute organ failures during the resuscitation phase. The challenge for the critical care physician caring for septic or traumatized patients at the point of transition to MSOF is to integrate this data with newer information concerning immunoregulatory pathways of host defense homeostasis which transcend an organ-specific focus. As the whole is greater than the sum of its parts, so may this perspective optimize treatment for MSOF.

Acknowledgments

The author wishes to acknowledge the excellent secretarial assistance of Susan Lee during the preparation of this manuscript, which was supported in part by grants #GM-43513 and #HL-30572 from the National Institutes of Health.

References

1. Baue AE: Multiple, progressive, or sequential systems failure. Arch Surg 110:779, 1975.
2. Carrico CJ, Meakins JL, Marshall JC, et al: Multiple-organ-failure syndrome. Arch Surg 121:196, 1986.
3. Pinsky MR, Matuschak GM: Multiple systems organ failure: Failure of host defense homeostasis. Crit Care Clin 5:199, 1989.
4. Tilney NL, Bailey, Morgan AP: Sequential system failure after rupture of abdominal aortic aneurysms: An unsolved problem in postoperative care. Ann Surg 178:117, 1973.
5. Goris RJA, te Boekhorst TPA, Nuytinck JKS, Gimbrere JSF: Multiple-organ failure: Generalized autodestructive inflammation? Arch Surg 120:1109, 1985.
6. Cerra FB: Multiple organ failure syndrome, in Bihari DJ, Cerra FB (eds): *Multiple Organ Failure*. Fullerton, CA, Society of Critical Care Medicine, 1989.
7. National Heart, Lung, and Blood Institute, Division of Lung Diseases: *Extracorporeal Support for Respiratory Insufficiency: A Collaborative Study*. Bethesda, MD, NIH, 1979.
8. Bell RC, Coalson JL, Smith JD, Johanson WG Jr: Multiple organ system failure and infection in adult respiratory distress syndrome. Ann Intern Med 99:293, 1983.
9. Montgomery AB, Stager MA, Carrico CJ, Hudson LD: Causes of mortality in patients with the adult respiratory distress syndrome. Am Rev Respir Dis 132:485, 1985.
10. Fry, DE, Pearlstein L, Fulton RL, Polk HC: Multiple system organ failure: The role of uncontrolled infection. Arch Surg 115:136, 1980.
11. Pine RW, Wertz MJ, Lennard ES, et al: Determinants of organ malfunction or death in patients with intra-abdominal sepsis. Arch Surg 118:242, 1983.
12. Knaus WA, Draper EA, Wagner DP, Zimmerman JE: APACHE II: A severity of disease classification system. Crit Care Med 13:818, 1985.
13. Knaus WA, Draper EA, Wagner DP, Zimmerman JE: Prognosis in acute organ-system failure. Ann Surg 202:685, 1985.
14. Knaus WA, Wagner DP: Multiple systems organ failure: Epidemiology and prognosis. Crit Care Clin 5:221, 1989.
15. Matuschak GM, Rinaldo JE, Pinsky MR, et al: Effect of end-stage liver failure on the incidence and resolution of the adult respiratory distress syndrome. J Crit Care 2:162, 1987.
16. Matuschak GM, Rinaldo JE: Organ interactions in the adult respiratory distress syndrome during sepsis: Role of the liver in host defense. Chest 94:400, 1988.
17. Schwartz DB, Bone RC, Balf RA, Szidon JP: Hepatic dysfunction in the adult respiratory distress syndrome. Chest 95:871, 1989.
18. Ravin HA, Fine J: Biological implications of intestinal endotoxins. Fed Proc 21:65, 1962.
19. Gathiram P, Wells MT, Brock-Utne JG, et al: Oral administered nonabsorbable antibiotics prevent endotoxemia in primates following intestinal ischemia. J Surg Res 45:187, 1988.
20. Teres D, Lemeshow S, Harris D, Klar J: Mortality prediction models (MPM) for ICU patients, in Farmer JC (ed): *Prognostic Scoring Systems in the ICU. Problems in Critical Care*. Philadelphia, Lippincott, 1989, p 585.
21. Meakins JL, Wicklund B, Forse RA, McLean PH: The surgical intensive care unit: current concepts in infection. Surg Clin North Am 60:117, 1980.
22. Wiles JB, Cerra FB, Siegal JH, Border JR: The systemic septic response: Does the organism matter? Crit Care Med 8:55, 1980.
23. Marshall J, Sweeney D: Microbial infection and the septic response in critical surgical illness: sepsis, not infection, determines outcome. Arch Surg 125:17, 1990.
24. Norton LW: Does drainage of intraabdominal pus reverse multiple organ failure? Am J Surg 149:347, 1985.
25. Seidenfeld JJ, Pohl DF, Bell RC, et al: Incidence, site, and outcome of infections in patients with the adult respiratory dis-

tress syndrome. Am Rev Respir Dis 134:12, 1986.
26. Steinburg S, Flynn W, Kelley K, et al: Development of a bacteria-independent model of the multiple organ failure syndrome. Arch Surg 124:1390, 1989.
27. Sheagren JN: Mechanism-oriented therapy for multiple systems organ failure. Crit Care Clin 5:393, 1989.
28. Hudson LD: Multiple systems organ failure (MSOF): Lessons learned from the adult respiratory distress syndrome. Crit Care Clin 5:697, 1989.
29. Keenan RJ, Todd TRJ, Girotti, MJ: Experimental gram-negative pneumonia produces a hyperdynamic septic profile. Circ Shock 22:303, 1987.
30. Abreo K, Moorthy V, Osborne M: Changing patterns and outcome of acute renal failure requiring hemodialysis. Arch Intern Med 146:1338, 1986.
31. Craven DE, Kunches LM, Kilinsky V: Risk factors for pneumonia and fatality in patients receiving continuous mechanical ventilation. Am Rev Respir Dis 133:792, 1986.
32. Matuschak GM, Pinsky MR, Rogers RM: Effects of positive end-expiratory pressure on hepatic blood flow and performance. J Appl Physiol 62:1377, 1987.
33. Johnson EE, Hedley-Whyte J: Continuous positive-pressure ventilation and portal flow in dogs with pulmonary edema. J Apply Physiol 33:385, 1972.
34. Suffredini AF, Harpel PC, Parillo JE: Promotion and subsequent inhibition of plasminogen activation after administration of intravenous endotoxin to normal subjects. N Engl J Med 320:1165, 1989.
35. Brandtzaeg P, Kierulf P, Gaustad P, et al: Plasma endotoxin as a predictor of multiple organ failure and death in systemic meningococcal disease. J Infect Dis 159:195, 1989.
36. Natanson C, Danner RL, Elin RJ, et al: Role of endotoxemia in cardiovascular dysfunction and mortality: *Escherichia coli* and *Staphylococcus aureus* challenges in a canine model of human septic shock. J Clin Invest 83:243, 1989.
37. Pinsky MR, Matuschak GM: Cardiovascular determinants of the hemodynamic response to acute endotoxemia in the dog. J Crit Care 1:18, 1986.
38. Marshall JC, Christou NV, Meakins JL: Immunomodulation by altered gastrointestinal tract flora: The effects of orally administered, killed *Staphylococcus epidermidis, Candida,* and *Pseudomonas* on systemic immune responses. Arch Surg 123:1465, 1988.
39. Brigham KL, Meyrick BO: Endotoxin and lung injury. Am Rev Respir Dis 133:913, 1986.
40. Waage A: Production and clearance of tumor necrosis factor in rats exposed to endotoxin and dexamethasone. Clin Immunol Immunopathol 45:348, 1987.
41. Shenep JL, Flynn PM, Barrett FF, et al: Serial Quantitation of endotoxin and bacteremia during therapy for gram-negative bacterial sepsis. J Infect Dis 157:565, 1988.
42. Parsons PE, Worthen GS, Moore EE, et al: The association of circulating endotoxin with the development of the adult respiratory distress syndrome. Am Rev Respir Dis 140:294, 1989.
43. Rogers DE: Host mechanisms which act to remove bacteria from the blood stream. Bacteriol Rev 24:50, 1960.
44. Freudenberg MA, Freudenberg N, Galanos C: Time course of cellular distribution of endotoxin in liver, lungs, and kidneys of rats. Br J Exp Pathol 63:56, 1982.
45. Wardle EN: Kupffer cells and their function. Liver 7:63, 1987.
46. Pilaro AM, Laskin DL: Accumulation of activated mononuclear phagocytes in the liver following lipopolysaccharide treatment of rats. J Leukocyte Biol 40:29, 1986.
47. Katz S, Grosfeld JL, Gross K, et al: Impaired bacterial clearance and trapping in obstructive jaundice. Am Surg 199:14, 1984.
48. Saba TM: Fibronectin: Relevance to phagocytic host defense to injury. Circ Shock 29:257, 1989.
49. Saba TM, Blumenstock FA, Shah DM, et al: Reversal of opsonic deficiency in surgical, trauma, and burn patients by infusion of purified human plasma fibronectin. Am J Med 80:224, 1986.
50. Wolter J, Liehr M, Grun M: Hepatic clearance of endotoxins: Differences in arterial and portal venous infusions. J Reticuloendothel Soc 23:145, 1978.
51. Lehmann V, Freudenberg MA, Galanos C: Lethal toxicity of lipopolysaccharide and tumor necrosis factor in normal and D-galactosamine-treated mice. J Exp Med 165:657, 1987.
52. Cuevas P, Fine J: Demonstration of a lethal endotoxemia in experimental occlusion of the superior mesenteric artery. Surg Gynecol Obstet 133:81, 1971.
53. Steffen EK, Berg RD, Deitch EA: Comparison of translocation rates of various indigenous bacteria from the gastrointestinal tract to the mesenteric lymph nodes. J Infect Dis 157:1032, 1988.
54. Deitch EA, Berg R, Specian R: Endotoxin promotes the translocation of bacteria from the gut. Arch Surg 122:185, 1987.
55. Alverdy JC, Aoys E, Moss GS: Total parenteral nutrition promotes bacterial translocation from the gut. Surgery 104:185, 1988.
56. Burke DJ, Alverdy JC, Aoys E, Moss GS: Glutamine-supplemented total parenteral nutrition improves gut immune function. Arch Surg 124:1396, 1989.
57. Deitch EA: Simple intestinal obstruction causes bacterial translocation in man. Arch Surg 124:699, 1989.
58. Deitch EA, Bridges W, Baker J, et al: Hemorrhagic shock-induced bacterial translocation is reduced by xanthine oxidase inhibition or inactivation. Surgery 104:191, 1988.
59. Stoutenbeek CP, van Saene HKF, Miranda DR, Zandstra DF: The effect of selective decontamination of the digestive tract on colonization and infection rate in multiple trauma patients. Intensive Care Med 10:185, 1984.
60. Ledingham IMcA, Eastaway AT, Mckay IC, et al: Triple regimen of selective decontamination of the digestive tract, systemic cefotaxime, and microbiological surveillance for prevention of acquired infection in intensive care. Lancet 1:785, 1988.
61. Kerver AJH, Rommes JH, Mevissen-Verhage AE, et al: Prevention of colonization and infection in critically ill patients: a prospective randomized study. Crit Care Med 16:1087, 1988.
62. Lefer AM: Induction of tissue injury and altered cardiovascular performance by platelet-activating factor: Relevance to multiple systems organ failure. Crit Care Clin 5:331, 1989.
63. Hesse DG, Tracey KJ, Fong Y, et al: Cytokine appearance in human endotoxemia and primate bacteremia. Surg Gynecol Obstet 166:147, 1988.
64. Michie HR, Manogue KR, Spriggs DR, et al: Detection of circulating tumor necrosis factor after endotoxin administration. N Engl J Med 318:1481, 1988.
65. Millar AB, Singer M, Meager A, et al: Tumour necrosis factor in bronchopulmonary secretions of patients with adult respiratory distress syndrome. Lancet 1:712, 1989.
66. Remick DG, Kunkel RG, Larrick JW, Kunkel SL: Acute *in vivo* effects of human recombinant tumor necrosis factor. Lab Invest 56:583, 1987.
67. Damas P, Reuter A, Gysen P, et al: Tumor necrosis factor and interleukin-1 serum levels during severe sepsis in humans. Crit Care Med 17:975, 1989.
68. Waage A, Halstensen A, Espenik T: Association between tumor necrosis factor in serum and fatal outcome in patients with meningococcal disease. Lancet 1:355, 1987.
69. Tracey KJ, Fong Y, Hesse DG, et al: Anti-cachectin/TNF monoclonal antibodies prevent septic shock during lethal bacte-

remia. Nature 330:662, 1987.
70. Fraker DL, Stovroff MC, Merino MJ, Norton JA: Tolerance to tumor necrosis factor in rats and the relationship to endotoxin tolerance and toxicity. J Exp Med 168:95, 1988.
71. Kunkel SL, Remick DG, Strieter RM, Larrick JW: Mechanisms that regulate the production and effects of tumor necrosis factor-α. Crit Rev Immunol 9:93, 1989.
72. Matthews N: Tumour-necrosis factor from the rabbit. V. Synthesis *in vitro* by mononuclear phagocytes from various tissues of normal and BCG-injected rabbits. Br J Cancer 44:418, 1981.
73. Beutler BA, Milsark IW, Cerami A: Cachectin/tumor necrosis factor: production, distribution, and metabolic rate in vivo. J Immunol 135:3972, 1985.
74. Debets JMH, Kampmeifer R, van der Linden MPMH: Plasma tumor necrosis factor and mortality in critically ill septic patients. Crit Care Med 17:49, 1989.
75. Maury CPJ, Teppo A-M: Circulating tumour necrosis factor-α (cachectin) in myocardial infarction. J Intern Med 225:333, 1989.
76. Urbaschek R, Urbaschek B: Tumor necrosis factor and interleukin 1 as mediators of endotoxin-induced beneficial effects. Rev Infect Dis 9(suppl 5):S607, 1988.
77. Mizel SB: The interleukins. FASEB J 3:2379, 1989.
78. Okusawa S, Gelfand JA, Ikejima T, et al: Interleukin 1 induces a shock-like state in rabbits: synergism with tumor necrosis factor and the effect of cyclooxygenase inhibition. J Clin Invest 81:1162, 1988.
79. Luger A, Graf H, Schwarz H-P, et al: Decreased serum interleukin 1 activity and monocyte interleukin 1 production in patients with fatal sepsis. Crit Care Med 14:458, 1986.
80. Ramadori G, Van Damme J, Rieder H, et al: Interleukin 6, the third mediator of acute-phase reaction, modulates hepatic protein synthesis in human and mouse: comparison with interleukin 1β and tumor necrosis factor-α. Eur J Immunol 18:1259, 1988.
81. Le J, Vilcek J: Interleukin 6: A multifunctional cytokineregulating immune reactions and the acute phase protein response. Lab Invest 61:588, 1989.
82. Wang J, Dunn MJ: Platelet-activating factor mediates endotoxin-induced acute renal insufficiency in rats. Am J Physiol 253:F1283, 1987.
83. Hsueh W, Gonzalez-Crussi F, Arroyave JL: Platelet-activating factor: an endogenous mediator for bowel necrosis in endotoxemia. FASEB J 1:403, 1987.
84. Petrak RA, Balk RA, Bone RC: Prostaglandins, cyclo-oxygenase inhibitors, and thromboxane synthease inhibitors in the pathogensis of multiple systems organ failure. Crit Care Clin 5:303, 1989.
85. Sprague RS, Stephenson AH, Dahms TE, Lonigro AJ: Proposed role for leukotrienes in the pathophysiology of multiple systems organ failure. Crit Care Clin 5:315, 1989.
86. Antonelli M, Bufi M, De Blasi RA, et al: Detection of leukotrienes B_4, C_4 and of their isomers in arterial, mixed venous blood and bronchoalveolar lavage fluid from ARDS patients. Intensive Care Med 15:296, 1989.
87. Dinarello CA: Biology of interleukin 1. FASEB J 2:108, 1988.
88. Hagmann W, Denzlinger C, Keppler D: Role of peptide leukotrienes and their hepatobiliary elimination in endotoxin action. Circ Shock 14:223, 1984.
89. Matuschak GM, Pinsky MR, Klein EC, et al: Effects of D-galactosamine-induced acute liver injury on mortality and pulmonary responses to E. coli lipopolysaccharide: Modulation by arachidonic acid metabolites. Am Rev Respir Dis in press.
90. Matuschak GM, Pinsky MR: Effects of positive-pressure ventilatory frequency on hepatic blood flow and performance. J Crit Care 4:153, 1989.
91. Moreau R, Lee SS, Hadengue A, et al: Relationship between oxygen transport and oxygen uptake in patients with cirrhosis: effects of vasocative drugs. Hepatology 9:427, 1989.
92. Townsend MC, Schirmer WJ, Schirmer JM, Fry DE: Low-dose dopamine improves effective hepatic blood flow in murine peritonitis. Circ Shock 21:149, 1987.
93. Hoogewoud H-M, Rubli E, Terrier F, Hassler H: The role of computerized tomography in fever, septicemia and multiple system organ failure after laparotomy. Surg Gynecol Obstet 162:539, 1986.
94. Ferraris VA: Exploratory laparotomy for potential abdominal sepsis in patients with multiple-organ failure. Arch Surg 118:1130, 1983.
95. Huber M, Beutler B, Keppler D: Tumor necrosis factor α stimulates leukotriene production *in vivo*. Eur J Immunol 18:2085, 1988.
96. Waage A, Brandtzaeg P, Halstensen A, et al: The complex pattern of cytokines in serum from patients with meningococcal septic shock. Association between interleukin 6, interleukin 1, and fatal outcome. J Exp Med 169:333, 1989.

Chapter 54

ADULT RESPIRATORY DISTRESS SYNDROME

JEAN E. RINALDO

KEY POINTS

- *Adult respiratory distress syndrome (ARDS) is a physiologic syndrome characterized acutely by lung edema resulting from increased alveolar-capillary permeability, sometimes followed by a prolonged or aberrant process of pulmonary "wound healing."*
- *The mortality of ARDS is usually associated with pulmonary superinfection and multiple system organ failure.*
- *A major supportive goal is treatment of hypoxemia while avoiding hypovolemia and oxygen toxicity.*
- *Effective therapy requires reversal of the underlying predisposition, treatment of intercurrent infections, aggressive nutritional support, and vigilance for iatrogenic complications.*

The *adult respiratory distress syndrome* (ARDS) is a generic term denoting a constellation of symptoms and findings resulting from hypoxemia and noncardiogenic pulmonary edema. Although termed the "adult" respiratory distress syndrome, an identical presentation occurs in pediatric patients who have sustained similar insults. Patients usually have had no previous history of lung disease.

ARDS is precipitated by a spectrum of processes that injure the lung. These include aspiration of gastric contents, ingestion of lung toxins such as paraquat, smoke inhalation, blunt thoracic trauma, crush injuries, long bone fractures, burns, near drowning, pancreatitis, obstetric catastrophes, systemic infections, abacteremic sepsis syndrome, and primary pneumonia. The generic term *ARDS* disguises a covert nonuniformity of mechanism in these diverse clinical settings. Nonetheless, the term has retained its currency for over 20 years because a common strategy of supportive care can be followed in these patients.

Although the complexity of each case may seem enormous because of the plethora of detail involved, the basic principles of supportive care are simple:

1. Maintenance of arterial P_{O_2} at a level which provides adequate hemoglobin saturation, using a nontoxic inspired concentration of oxygen.
2. Maintenance of intravascular volume and cardiac output to minimize lung edema while maintaining renal perfusion.
3. Diagnosis and definitive treatment of underlying conditions.
4. Prevention, recognition, and therapy of superinfection, especially superimposed pneumonia.
5. Avoidance of, vigilance for, and when necessary, rapid treatment of the common life-threatening iatrogenic complications of cardiopulmonary support: barotrauma, oxygen toxicity, complications of vascular access, and complications of endotracheal intubation.
6. Avoidance of protein-calorie malnutrition.
7. Recognition and treatment of intercurrent medical problems such as electrolyte disorders, cardiac dysrhythmia, pulmonary embolism, and gastrointestinal hemorrhage.

Compulsive attention to these basic principles and constant review of the details they entail is the key to successful therapy of ARDS patients. The details of supportive therapy will be covered elsewhere in the text (see Chap. 128).

Definition and Incidence of ARDS

There are no sensitive and specific markers of pulmonary endothelial and/or epithelial injury. Therefore, ARDS is presently defined by physiologic criteria that are themselves controversial.[1] The "incidence" of the disease depends upon diagnostic criteria used. Commonly used criteria include a widened $(\text{A} - \text{a})_{O_2}$ (alveolar to arterial) oxygen tension difference, bilateral pulmonary infiltrates, reduced compliance and exclusion of congestive heart failure by clinical criteria or by measurement of pulmonary artery occlusion pressure (Table 54-1).

It was estimated in 1972 that the syndrome affected 150,000 patients per year, or 75 cases per 100,000 population.[2] However, the criteria used were not clearly defined, and the validity of this estimate is in question. Recent information suggests that the true incidence may be as low as 1.5 cases per 100,000 population.[3] The reason for this discrepancy is unclear. It is possible that the decreased "incidence" may be based on improvements in supportive care: Fewer patients may now deteriorate to the point where they meet the stringent diagnostic criteria commonly used for ARDS.[4] Those who do meet all of the standard criteria continue to have a mortality rate in excess of 50 percent in published series.

The use of a generic physiologic definition for ARDS obscures important epidemiologic factors. Patients with hematologic malignancies undergoing marrow ablative chemotherapy and/or bone marrow transplantation, patients awaiting organ transplantation, or patients with acquired immunodeficiency syndrome may manifest a much higher incidence and mortality rate from ARDS than young, previously healthy patients seen in level 1 trauma centers or ob-

TABLE 54-1 Common Physiologic Criteria for ARDS

1. Bilateral pulmonary infiltrates
2. PCWP* <18 mmHg
3. Pa_{O_2}/PA_{O_2} ratio† <0.2
4. Static compliance‡ <40 mL/cmH₂0

*PCWP, pulmonary capillary wedge pressure.
†Arterial P_{O_2}/alveolar P_{O_2} calculated from alveolar gas equation.
‡Tidal volume/(inspiratory plateau pressure − PEEP).

stetrical services. Several of these clinical subgroups have appeared within the past 10 years. Epidemiologic studies have not assessed their impact on ARDS incidence and outcome.

In general, the highest incidence of ARDS appears to occur in patients with the "sepsis syndrome." The sepsis syndrome is defined as the concurrence of leukocytosis or leukopenia, fever or hypothermia, and hypotension with or without documented bacteremia. It is reported that one-third of such patients develop ARDS. The incidence of ARDS is reported to approach 30 percent in patients witnessed to aspirate gastric contents. Other common predispositions have a lower incidence of inciting ARDS. The likelihood of developing ARDS increases if more than one predisposing feature is present.[5,6]

Pathophysiology and Clinical Sequelae of Pulmonary Microvascular Injury in ARDS Patients

CELLULAR CHANGES IN ARDS

The primary physiologic abnormality in ARDS is a derangement of lung microvascular permeability. The earliest morphologic abnormality in animal models of ARDS is injury to lung microvascular endothelial cells. Capillary endothelial cells detach from their basement membrane, and the connective tissue matrix between and beneath cells is probably disrupted as well. It has also been suggested that the endothelial cytoskeleton contracts, creating spaces between cells. Although the cause of these changes is uncertain, it is likely that they are caused at least in part by the activation of circulating blood granulocytes and/or alveolar and interstitial macrophages. The soluble products of activated inflammatory cells include substances that promote alterations in adhesive glycoproteins, proteolytic degradation of proteoglycans and collagen, and contraction of the actin filaments in endothelial cells. Also, cytokines released during inflammation, including interleukin-1, gamma interferon, and tumor necrosis factor signal direct changes in endothelial cell function that increase the adhesiveness of these cells, cause them to initiate blood clotting, and cause them to release chemotactic factors for neutrophils that further amplify damage.

Epithelial cells are probably injured as well. Severe ARDS is characterized by airspace flooding, evident from the suctioning of edema fluid from the endotracheal tube. The alveolar epithelium is normally much less permeable than the capillary endothelial cells. Thus, some major disruption in alveolar epithelial or small airway permeability must also occur for airspaces to be filled with fluid. Furthermore, it has recently been demonstrated that normal alveolar epithelial cells actively transport fluid out of airspaces and that this important protective mechanism is impaired in ARDS.

These cellular events characterize the acute phase of ARDS. After several days, a second phase is observed morphologically, termed the *proliferative* phase of ARDS. To replace the injured cells and restore the integrity of the breached alveolar barrier, progenitor cells begin to replicate rapidly. The cellularity of the lung parenchyma increases, and its functional efficiency as a gas exchange organ is diminished until the healing process is complete. Like other wound healing, complete architectural healing of the lung takes at least 2 weeks. In some cases, healing is deranged because of oxygen toxicity, malnutrition, or other unknown factors. Alternatively, ongoing injury resulting from superinfection may prevent normal sequential evolution of the healing process. In such cases, healing may be abnormal, and an exuberant fibrotic response is observed. It is intuitively obvious that manipulations of the circulation are more likely to be effective early, while late disordered healing is more likely to be associated with prolonged ventilator dependance, pulmonary superinfection, and multisystem organ failure.

ALTERED LUNG MICROVASCULAR PERMEABILITY IN ARDS PATIENTS

During the acute phase, increased lung microvascular permeability to fluid and solutes is thought to be the physiologic hallmark of ARDS. Although numerous experimental models support this notion, confirmatory data in human beings are difficult to obtain. In patients, altered permeability is generally inferred from indirect measurements indicating increased lung water (usually radiographic) in the absence of a sustained elevation in pulmonary artery occlusion pressure. A few studies have directly measured lung microvascular permeability in ARDS patients[7–9] and found it to be increased. A common problem with most measurements of permeability in the whole lung is that an increase in solute exchanging surface area (by microvascular recruitment) cannot be differentiated from an increase in permeability itself; rather, a "permeability-surface area product" is measured. Recently, it has been possible to measure lung microvascular permeability independent of surface area in a group of 39 ARDS patients.[9] It was shown that permeability abnormalities were present and were worse in patients who never reversed physiologic criteria for ARDS compared to patients who later reversed criteria for ARDS. This represents the first demonstration that the severity of abnormalities in lung microvascular permeability is correlated with severity of clinical illness.

RELATIONSHIPS AMONG HYPOXEMIA, ALTERED PERMEABILITY, AND PULMONARY VASCULAR RESISTANCE

When ARDS was first described, it was assumed that the severe hypoxemia observed in ARDS patients resulted from alveolar flooding and thus resembled the hypoxemia of congestive heart failure. However, later studies demonstrated that this concept was oversimplified.[7] As is shown in Fig. 54-1, neither extravascular lung water (Fig. 54-1*a*) nor increased lung microvascular permeability (Fig. 54-1*b*) area is well correlated with the degree of hypoxemia in groups of ARDS patients. It is likely that the hypoxemia is

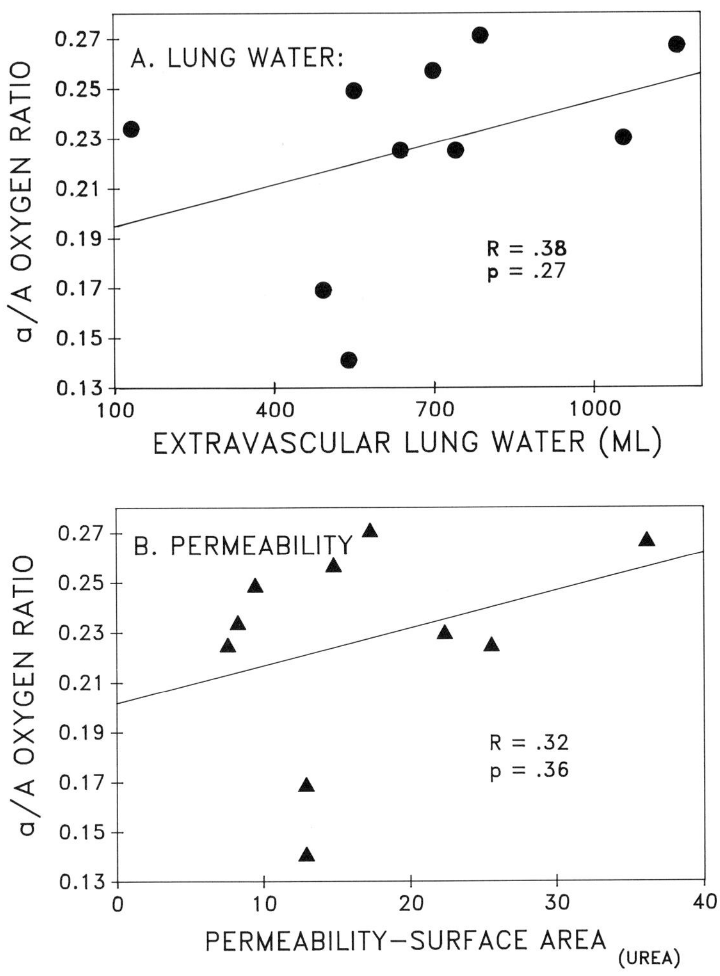

FIGURE 54-1 Failure of hypoxemia to correlate with degree of pulmonary edema or abnormal permeability in 10 ARDS patients. (*a*) (filled circles) Shows relationship between extravascular lung water and arterial/alveolar P_{O_2} ratio (defined in Table 54-1). (*b*) Shows relationship between permeability-surface area for urea (filled triangles) and arterial/alveolar P_{O_2} ratio. *(From data in ref. 8.)*

due at least in part to edema-independent alterations in ventilation-perfusion matching. Derangements in ventilation-perfusion matching probably arise from changes in both regional ventilation and regional perfusion. On the one hand, ARDS patients manifest significant abnormalities in airflow resistance.[10] On the other hand, it has been proposed that shunting of blood from injured vascular beds toward more normal ones is a critical defense mechanism against hypoxemia.[7] This defense mechanism can be subverted by both exogenous and endogenous vasodilators (such as prostacyclin) released by lung cells.[11] It is proposed that this protective vasoconstrictive mechanism results in increased vasomotor tone over a substantial fraction of the pulmonary vascular bed due to diffuse injury, resulting in a measurable increase in pulmonary vascular resistance during ARDS. Vascular occlusion with thrombi and vascular obliteration may also contribute to pulmonary hypertension in ARDS.

CLINICAL IMPLICATION: THERAPY OF HYPOXEMIA

The mechanism of hypoxic vasoconstriction (the presumed basis of ventilation-perfusion matching in the injured lung) remains uncertain. Because hypoxemia results from abnormal matching of ventilation and perfusion rather than from lung edema per se, it is difficult to treat definitively, i.e., at the level of the underlying mechanism. Hypoxemia is treated by manipulations of inspired oxygen concentration, intravascular volume and cardiac output, and positive end expiratory pressure.

Because refractory hypoxemia arises from ventilation-perfusion mismatching rather than simple interstitial edema and alveolar filling, vigorous diuresis may or may not reverse it. As noted earlier, in groups of patients the correlation of lung water to hypoxemia is poor. The benefit for individual patients to lessening lung water remains controversial and is under investigation by several groups at present. Diuresis poses potential problems. Covert intravascular hypovolemia is often present, especially at the onset of ARDS induced by sepsis. There are several reasons why intravascular hypovolemia is common in the early phase of ARDS. First, initiation of positive pressure ventilation or continuous positive airway pressure (CPAP) has often occurred recently. During respiratory distress, hyperpneic negative-pressure spontaneous breathing is characterized by an elevated respiratory drive and profoundly negative pleural pressure, which augments venous return.

Replacing it is markedly positive intrathoracic pressure [positive-pressure ventilation (PPV) and positive end-expiratory pressure (PEEP), or CPAP], often with concomitant use of sedative drugs, which both dilate venous capacitance vessels and reduce sympathetic tone. Furthermore, if a septic event has initiated the episode of respiratory failure, panendothelial injury has likely reduced intravascular volume caused by alterations in systemic capillary permeability. Adding to these factors is the likelihood that there has been recent empiric use of diuretics prior to intubation to forestall intubation or to increase urine output. All of these factors act in concert to promote intravascular volume depletion and to reduce venous return. Because the likelihood of inducing sepsis-related acute renal failure is enhanced by hypovolemia,[12] diuresis should be used with extreme caution as therapy for hypoxemia early in ARDS, despite evidence of pulmonary edema.

The most fruitful approach to hypoxemia is the application of increments of positive end-expiratory pressure (PEEP), in order to reverse microatelectasis, to increase resting lung volume, and accordingly, to improve the ventilation-perfusion ratio of poorly ventilated areas of the lung.[13,14] The goal of PEEP is to permit reduction of F_{IO_2} to nontoxic levels as rapidly as possible. The normal human lung appears relatively resistant to oxygen toxicity, but recent experimental insights suggest that the *injured* lung may be quite susceptible. Deoxyribonucleic acid (DNA) is a sensitive target of injury by oxygen-derived free radicals. An early manifestation of oxygen toxicity to human lung endothelial cells is an inability to replicate. Replication of endothelial cells is the critical process by which abnormalities in pulmonary microvascular permeability are reversed. There is provocative clinical evidence that in ARDS patients, oxygen toxicity promotes an abnormal healing response in the lung,[15] possibly by impairing endothelial replication. An F_{IO_2} of 0.5 appears to be the threshold at which replication is impaired.[16] Therefore, reduction of F_{IO_2} to 50 percent within a few hours is an important therapeutic goal.

During application of PEEP, it is important to recognize the possibility that PEEP may in fact decrease oxygen delivery to tissue while improving arterial P_{O_2}, because PEEP's effect on cardiac output is unpredictable. As noted, hypovolemic patients are likely to respond with a fall in cardiac output caused by decreased venous return. Euvolemic patients with left ventricular dysfunction are more likely to experience a rise in cardiac output because PEEP reduces left ventricular afterload. Patients with acute right ventricular failure may experience a fall in cardiac output because PEEP increases pulmonary vascular resistance. In such cases, septal bulging may compromise the left ventricle as well due to ventricular interdependence. PEEP as a therapeutic modality and the hemodynamic effects of PEEP will be covered elsewhere in the text in detail (see Chaps. 1 and 128).

It would be desirable to develop other therapies for hypoxemia arising from microatelectasis, as an adjunct to or even a replacement for PEEP. Surfactant abnormalities are not the primary defect causing ARDS. However, surfactant may be inactivated in the inflammatory milieu. Instillation of pulmonary surfactant as specific therapy for hypoxemia in ARDS is currently undergoing study in clinical trials.[17]

Pathophysiology and Clinical Sequelae of Extrapulmonary Microvascular Injury in ARDS Patients

ARDS AS A PANENDOTHELIAL PROCESS

In the preceding sections, ARDS is treated as an organ-specific abnormality of pulmonary capillary endothelial permeability. However, at least in the setting of trauma and sepsis, ARDS affects capillary beds throughout the body concurrently. The lung is a clinically conspicuous target because increased microvascular permeability results in alveolar flooding causing dyspnea, abnormal opacities on the chest X-ray, and death from hypoxemia. Other organs are not dependent upon intact microvascular permeability for physiologic function, and provide no radiographic clues since they are fluid density at baseline. Nonetheless, ARDS is a multisystem disorder from the outset. Sensitive techniques in humans and in animal models reveal evidence of injury at many vascular target sites.[18,19]

Complex inflammatory cascades involving granulocytes, macrophages, cytokines, lipid mediators, and other components interdigitate to cause microvascular damage. The complexity of the entire system is such as to elude complete understanding currently and will not be discussed here. Recent monographs have reviewed in detail what is presently known about the mechanisms and mediators of microvascular injury in ARDS.[20,21]

ONGOING INFECTION LINKS ARDS TO MULTIPLE SYSTEMS ORGAN FAILURE (MSOF)

Although panendothelial injury is probably always present in trauma and sepsis severe enough to cause respiratory compromise, dysfunction is often silent, and, if ARDS resolves, this silent transient injury may never present clinical manifestations. Why do some ARDS patients progress to fatal MSOF? It appears likely that ongoing infection is an essential link between early self-limited ARDS and progressive ARDS that terminates in multiple system organ failure.[22] Several studies support the hypothesis that unresolved inflammation is the "missing link" between ARDS and MSOF. In an early study, Bell and coworkers[23] observed that bacterial infection was present in 98 percent of autopsied patients who died with ARDS. These were the same patients who commonly had renal failure, hepatic failure, coagulopathies, and other extrapulmonary problems. Later, Montgomery and associates[24] found that patients who died of ARDS after 72 h of therapy usually had MSOF. More than 80 percent of the patients with MSOF had ongoing clinical evidence of the "sepsis syndrome," although a bacterial pathogen was usually never isolated.

THE GASTROINTESTINAL BARRIER

Where does the sepsis syndrome come from in abacteremic patients? The gastrointestinal tract appears to harbor the bacterial organisms that often sustain the inflammatory processes that permit ARDS to progress. As a result of panendothelial injury, ischemic lesions in the gastric and intestinal mucosa compromise the integrity of the body's barrier against enteric flora, allowing translocation of bacterial products into the portal circulation. Translocation of enteric organisms causes recurrent bacteremia if the organisms are incompletely cleared by the liver.[25] Even if effectively cleared by the liver, the abnormal load of enteric organisms stimulates hepatic macrophages to release sepsis syndrome-inducing peptide mediators, such as tumor necrosis factor.[26] Bacterial translocation may be enhanced by ileus and by alterations of the microbiologic flora by administration of antibiotics, antacids, and histamine blockers. By neutralizing gastric pH, the latter agents allow overgrowth of the normally aseptic stomach contents with enteric aerobic gram-negative organisms.[27]

It has been proposed that one reason why gastrointestinal tract lesions arise is impaired availability of nutritional substrate. The gastric mucosa has been observed to have low glycogen stores and to depend upon a continuous supply of food substrate in the lumen for normal metabolism.[28] Enteral feeding may be important for the integrity of the gut mucosal barrier. Despite parenteral hyperalimentation, absence of oral nutrient flow may result in atrophy of intestinal villi and ulcerations.

PULMONARY SUPERINFECTION

An occupational hazard for intensivists is to become so interested in the cardiopulmonary physiologic manifestations of a case of ARDS that they overlook the subtle transmogrification of ARDS into a severe nosocomial bacterial pneumonia, an extremely common event. The lung is infected in up to 80 percent of patients who die after several days of therapy for ARDS.[24] Lung infection is difficult to recognize and to diagnose[29] when superimposed upon ARDS. Usually the pneumonia is caused by gram-negative aerobes.[30–32] The lung with underlying injury (ARDS) is characterized by impaired antibacterial defenses and, like the injured gastrointestinal barrier, permits the systemic translocation of organisms from the airspaces.[33] Unfortunately, parenteral administration of appropriate antibiosis does not appear to improve statistically the outcome of nosocomial pneumonia superimposed upon ARDS.[23]

In addition to permitting transmucosal passage of enteric organisms, the stomach and duodenum may serve as a reservoir for pathogenic organisms to colonize the nasopharynx, then to infect the lung when aspirated. Administration of antacids, antibiotics, and histamine antagonists creates conditions that favor the colonization of the normally sterile upper gastrointestinal tract with bacteria. A recent study[27] suggests that the use of sucralfate instead of H_2-blockers may result in a lessening of the rate of gastric colonization by potential enteric pathogens that may then colonize the pharynx and be aspirated.

THERAPEUTIC IMPLICATIONS: PREVENTION OF INFECTION AND MSOF

The recognition that ARDS patients die of MSOF and infection, not of ARDS per se, has prompted a quiet therapeutic revolution. If this concept is accepted, many former therapeutic strategies for ARDS will be modified.

TREND TOWARD LIMITATIONS OF INVASIVENESS

What may have been an excessive emphasis on invasive cardiopulmonary monitoring and respiratory support is now tempered by the overriding fact that each invasive device is a nidus of infection. The indication for each invasive device should be carefully examined initially and if utilized, reviewed daily. Those not needed should be promptly eliminated.

MAINTENANCE OF ENTERAL NUTRITION

To maintain gastrointestinal mucosal barrier functional integrity, there is a growing emphasis on maintenance of enteral nutrition independent of the additional need for avoidance of protein-calorie malnutrition. Ileus-promoting approaches, such as heavy sedation and muscle paralysis, are avoided if possible. If caloric needs cannot be met by enteral nutrition, parenteral hyperalimentation should be added, although attempts to maintain enteral nutrition should continue.

MEASURES TO LIMIT NOSOCOMIAL PNEUMONIA

Intubation and mechanical ventilation are a major breach in pulmonary host defense mechanisms. Avoidance of intubation (as by use of mask CPAP in select patients) is desirable. More commonly, patients require intubation, but it is a major responsibility of clinicians to maximize weaning conditions and to proceed with weaning as soon as the patient's condition permits. Inexperienced physicians commonly have difficulty moving decisively to wean weanable patients. Weaning conditions are maximized throughout the patient's course by avoidance of protein-calorie malnutrition, by diuresis of patients with lung edema who are in positive fluid balance and not actively septic, and by vigilance for and treatment of secondary infections.

There is evidence from animal models that nasopharyngeal and gastric decontamination with topic antibiotics is efficacious in reducing colonization of the upper respiratory tract by pathogenic bacteria, which precedes pneumonia.[34] Clinical trials are in progress to evaluate this approach for ARDS patients.

BALANCING THE KIDNEYS AND THE LUNG

During sepsis, the same pathophysiologic events that are manifested in the lung as ARDS are occurring in the kidney, placing patients at high risk for acute renal failure.[12,18,19,35–37] An approach to ARDS based entirely on Starling forces with a single-organ orientation dictates enthusiasm for diuretics and adrenergic vasopressors, the "dry-lung" approach to ARDS. However, the addition of renal failure markedly diminishes the survival rate from ARDS. In a study to evaluate the utility of corticosteroids in ARDS, an incidental finding was that serum creatinine greater than 2.0 in the presence of ARDS (as defined in Table 54-1) resulted in a 90 percent mortality rate. Other studies confirm that addition of renal failure doubles the mortality rate of ARDS.[2]

This poses a difficult dilemma, and the means to achieve the proper balance is unclear. It is not clear under which conditions volume infusions preserve renal function; on the other hand, it is clear that the edematous lung is more easily infected and that persistently positive fluid balance in ARDS patients is associated with higher mortality.

We favor a three-phase approach to fluid therapy, based on the notion that hydration is probably most important during the acute septic episode when hypovolemia is likely, as discussed previously, and when renal hypoperfusion is likely because of sepsis-induced alterations in renal prostaglandin metabolism and renal endothelial injury.[35–37] In the early hours of therapy if oliguria is present and definitive hemodynamic data is not yet available, we generally favor liberal volume infusion during the initiation of positive-pressure ventilation and PEEP, assuming a likelihood of intravascular volume depletion because of the factors enumerated earlier. We risk erring, occasionally, on the side of overhydration in order to avoid renal compromise. In phase two, a pulmonary artery catheter is placed if needed to guide fluid therapy. In phase three, when sepsis has been controlled and intravascular euvolemia ensured, it is important to initiate diuresis to prevent lung infection and to facilitate weaning.

ANTI-INFLAMMATORY AGENTS

A decade ago, as the role of granulocytes in the pathogenesis of ARDS was emerging, there was enthusiasm that anti-inflammatory drugs would be of clinical benefit. This has not been borne out. To date, no controlled randomized double blind studies have shown benefit from corticosteroids or other inflammatory agents.[38,39] Therapies presently being evaluated in such studies are largely supportive, such as instillation of surfactant and nasogastric decontamination.

CASE PRESENTATIONS

Case 1

A 26-year-old male student was in good health until he sustained bilateral fractures of the femur in a motorcycle accident. On arrival at the emergency room, he was confused and dyspneic. Chest x-ray revealed bilateral infiltrates. Arterial blood gas revealed a P_{O_2} of 37. He was intubated and taken to the operating room (OR) for fixation of the fractures. Postoperatively, vital signs were stable, and urine output 100 mL/h.

After initial stabilization in the ICU, the arterial blood gases were pH 7.4, P_{CO_2} 40, P_{O_2} 70 on 70% oxygen and 15 cmH$_2$O PEEP. A central venous catheter, pulmonary artery catheter, and femoral arterial catheter were inserted. These remained in place.

By the second day, the P_{O_2} was 104. The F_{IO_2} was reduced to 50%; the P_{O_2} was 82. Blood gases were checked twice daily thereafter and remained essentially unchanged for 4 days. To achieve ventilator synchrony, morphine and pancuronium were begun on the first day and continued around the clock. The next day, bowel sounds were decreased. Intravenous hyperalimentation and continuous nasogastric suctioning were begun.

After 7 days of therapy, fever, leukocytosis, and mild hypotension occurred. There was abdominal distention with absent bowel sounds. The next day, positive blood cultures for *Enterobacter cloacae* were obtained. An exploratory laparotomy revealed no pathology.

Despite appropriate antibiotic therapy, fever, leukocytosis, and mild hypotension continued. Thrombocytopenia, a mild coagulopathy, and an elevated bilirubin were observed on the 12th day. On the 18th day, the patient became anuric. Hemodialysis was begun.

From the seventh day onward, small increments in F_{IO_2} and PEEP were needed daily to maintain a P_{O_2} of 80–85. There was progressive pulmonary hypertension and reduction in dynamic compliance. On the 23rd day, bilateral pneumothoraces occurred and were treated with chest tubes. Respiratory deterioration continued. The patient expired on the 27th day. At autopsy, multiple gastrointestinal ulcerations were found. Evidence of bacterial pneumonitis with gram negative organisms was found on histologic examination of the lungs.

Case 2

A 26-year-old male student was in good health until sustaining bilateral femoral fractures in a motorcycle accident. On arrival at the emergency room, he was confused and dyspneic. Chest x-ray revealed bilateral infiltrates. Arterial blood gas revealed a P_{O_2} of 37. He was intubated and taken to the OR for fixation of the fractures. Postoperatively, vital signs were stable, and urine output 100 mL/h.

After stabilization in the ICU, arterial blood gases were pH 7.4, P_{CO_2} 40, P_{O_2} 70 on 70% oxygen, and 15 cmH$_2$O PEEP. Vital signs were stable. As there was no history of heart disease and urine output remained at 100 mL/h, it was decided that an arterial catheter, pulmonary artery catheter, and central venous catheter were not needed. A 16-gauge peripheral IV was inserted and a pulse oximeter employed.

The vital signs remained stable, and the abdominal examination remained normal. On the second day, the patient awakened and appeared alert. A small nasogastric feeding tube was placed and full-strength oral alimentation begun. The pulse oximeter revealed an arterial saturation of 95%; accordingly, the F_IO_2 was promptly reduced with continuous monitoring of the pulse oximeter. Within 4 h, it had been determined that hemoglobin saturation of 90% could be maintained using 40% oxygen and 10 cmH_2O of PEEP. An arterial blood gas was obtained for confirmation; the P_{O_2} was 63.

By the third day, saturation had risen to 94% on these settings. PEEP was reduced in two increments to 5 cmH_2O with saturation remaining at 92%. An arterial blood gas confirmed a P_{O_2} of 74. It was believed that this degree of support of oxygenation could be delivered by face mask. The patient was alert. A 4-h trial of spontaneous breathing through the endotracheal tube on CPAP system was performed. Respiratory rate initially was 36 and did not increase; no respiratory muscle dysynchrony was observed, and after 4 h the patient wrote that he felt comfortable. Arterial saturation remained at 92%. He was extubated that day.

The patient was maintained on 50% face mask oxygen for several additional days, with monitoring of arterial saturation by pulse oximeter. Full enteral alimentation was maintained, with an oral diet replacing nasogastric feeding. He was discharged from the intensive care unit on the eighth day.

CASE DISCUSSION

These cases contrast a highly invasive approach to ARDS, as was popular in the 1970s, with a less invasive approach more common today. The first approach is aimed primarily at monitoring and manipulating physiologic variables. The second approach is aimed at preventing infectious complications.

Both cases had a good initial response to PEEP, portending a favorable outcome.[12] But in case 1, the "golden window" of improvement on day 2 was overlooked, perhaps because of the high degree of unnecessary "intensification" and the fact that the patient was rendered vegetative by morphine and pancuronium. The indicated reduction in respiratory support was never completely pursued. We might speculate that the physicians were distracted by the wealth of physiologic data made available to them by modern technology; it possibly never occurred to them that this patient was not really ventilator dependent. In time, the plethora of invasive devices and the iatrogenic ileus made him a candidate for the sepsis syndrome due to breaches in the gastrointestinal mucosal barrier and a secondary gram-negative pneumonia. Ultimately, these resulted in MSOF, progressive ARDS, and death.

By contrast, in case 2, there was thoughtful restraint in invasive monitoring, so that no unnecessary sources of infection were introduced. There was then a well-controlled decisive and expeditious withdrawal of ventilatory support and of the endotracheal tube as soon as was appropriate, removing a major breach in pulmonary antibacterial host defense. Enteral nutrition was maintained to minimize the chance for gastrointestinal atrophy and mucosal breakdown.

Obviously, ARDS cannot always be managed as easily as in case 2; these patients were young and previously healthy, with a single predisposition to ARDS. Nonetheless, the principles of management illustrated by case 2 are always appropriate, even if not always so easy to apply.

Acknowledgment

This work was supported by the Department of Veterans Affairs, Nashville, Tennessee.

References

1. Murray JF, Matthay MA, Luce JM, et al: An expanded definition of the adult respiratory distress syndrome. Am Rev Respir Dis 138:720, 1988.
2. National Heart and Lung Institutes. *Respiratory Diseases: Task Force Report on Problems, Research, Approaches, Needs.* DHEW publication NIH 74-432. Washington DC: U.S. Government Printing Office, 1972, 167.
3. Villar J, Slutsky AS: The incidence of the adult respiratory distress syndrome. Am Rev Respir Dis, 140:814, 1989.
4. Rinaldo JE: Prognosis of the adult respiratory distress syndrome: Inappropriate pessimism? Chest 90:470, 1986.
5. Pepe PE, Potkin RT, Holtman RD, et al: Clinical predictors of the adult respiratory distress syndrome. Am J Surg 144:124, 1982.
6. Fowler AA, Hamman RF, Zerbe GO, et al: Adult respiratory distress syndrome: prognosis after onset. Am Rev Respir Dis 132:472, 1985.
7. Brigham KL, Kariman K, Harris TR, et al: Correlation of oxygenation with vascular permeability-surface area but not with lung water in humans with acute respiratory failure and pulmonary edema. J Clin Invest 72:339, 1983.
8. Rinaldo JE, Borovetz HS, Mancini MC, et al: Assessment of lung injury in the adult respiratory distress syndrome using multiple indicator dilution curves. Am Rev Respir Dis 133:1006, 1986.
9. Harris TR, Bernard GR, Brigham KL, et al: Lung microvascular transport properties measured by multiple indicator dilutin methods in patients with adult respiratory distress syndrome. Am Rev Respir Dis 141:272, 1990.
10. Wright PE, Bernard GR: The role of airflow resistance in patients with the adult respiratory distress syndrome. Am Rev Respir Dis 139:1169, 1989.
11. Melot C, Naeije R, Mols P, et al: Pulmonary vascular tone improves pulmonary gas exchange in the adult respiratory distress syndrome. Am Rev Respir Dis 136:1232, 1237, 1987.
12. Ellison DH, Bia MJ: Acute renal failure in critically ill patients. J Intensive Care Med 2:8, 1987.
13. Bone RC, Maunder R, Slotman G, et al: An early test of survival in patients with the adult respiratory distress syndrome: the Pa_{O_2}/FI_{O_2} ratio and its differential response to conventional therapy. Chest 96:849, 1989.
14. Weisman IM, Rinaldo JE, Rogers RM: Positive end expiratory pressure in adult respiratory failure. N Engl J Med 307:1381, 1982.
15. Elliot CG, Rasmussen BY, Crapo RO, et al: Prediction of pulmonary function abnormalities after adult respiratory distress syndrome. Am Rev Respir Dis 135:634, 1987.
16. Martin WJ, Kuchel DL: Oxygen-mediated impairment of human pulmonary endothelial cell growth: evidence for a specific threshold of toxicity. J Lab Clin Med 113:412,4, 1989.

17. Enhorning G: Surfactant replacement in adult respiratory distress syndrome. Am Rev Respir Dis 140:281, 1989.
18. Kreuzfelder E, Joka T, Hein-Otto Keinecke, et al: Adult respiratory distress syndrome as a specific manifestation of a general permeability defect in trauma patients. Am Rev Respir Dis 137:95, 1988.
19. Mizer LA, Weisbrode SE, Dorinsky PM: Neutrophil accumulation and structural changes in nonpulmonary organs after acute lung injury induced by phorbol myristate acetate. Am Rev Respir Dis 139:1017, 1989.
20. Hyers TM, Gee M, Andreadis NA: Cellular interactions in the multiple organ injury syndrome. Am Rev Respir Dis 135:952, 1987.
21. Rinaldo JE, Christman JW: Mechanisms and mediators of the adult respiratory distress syndrome. Clin Chest Med, 11:621, 1990.
22. Heyman SJ, Rinaldo JE: Multiple System organ failure in the adult respiratory distress syndrome. J Intensive Care Med 4:192, 1989.
23. Bell RC, Coalson KK, Smith JD, et al: Multiple organ system failure and infection in adult respiratory distress syndrome. Ann Intern Med 99:293, 1983.
24. Montgomery BR, Stager MA, Carrico CJ, Hudson LD: Causes of mortality in patients with the adult respiratory distress syndrome. Am Rev Respir Dis 132:484, 1985.
25. Matuschak GM, Rinaldo JE: Organ interactions in the adult respiratory distress syndrome during sepsis: Role of the liver in host defense. Chest 94:400, 1988.
26. Colletti LM, Remick DG, Burch GD, et al: The role of TNF in pathophysiologic alterations following hepatic ischemia reperfusion. Cytokine 1:150, 1989.
27. Driks MR, Craven DE, Celli BA, et al: Nosocomial pneumonia in intubated patients randomized to sucralfate versus antacids and/or histamine type 2 blockers: The role of gastric colonization. N Engl J Med 317:1376, 1987.
28. Levine GM, Deren JJ, Steiger E, et al: Role of oral intake in maintenance of gut mass and disaccharidase activity. Gastroenterology 67:975, 1974.
29. Andrews CP, Coalson JJ, Smith JD, et al: Diagnosis of nosocomial bacterial pneumonia in acute, diffuse lung injury. Chest 80:254, 1981.
30. Fagon JY, Chastre J, Domart, et al: Nosocomial pneumonia in patients receiving continuous mechanical ventilation: prospective analysis of 52 episodes with use of a protected specimen brush and quantitative culture techniques. Am Rev Respir Dis 139:877, 1989.
31. Seidenfeld JJ, Pohl DF, Bell RC, et al: Incidence, site, and outcome of infections in patients with the adult respiratory distress syndrome. Am Rev Respir Dis 134:12, 1986.
32. Craven DE, Kunches LM, Kilinsky V, et al: Risk factor for pneumonia and fatality in patients receiving continuous mechanical ventilation. Am Rev Respir Dis 133:792, 1986.
33. Johanson WG, Higuchi J, Woods D, et al: Dissemination of *Pseudomonas aeruginosa* during lung infection in hamsters: Role of oxygen-induced lung injury. Am Rev Respir Dis 132:358, 1985.
34. Johanson WG, Seidenfeld JM, DeLos Sanots R, et al: Prevention of nosocomial pneumonia using topical and parenteral antimicrobial agents. Am Rev Respir Dis 137:265, 1988.
35. Zager RA: *Escherichia coli* endotoxin injections potentiate experimental ischemic renal injury. J Appl Physiol F988, 1986.
36. Oates JA, Fitzgerald GA, Branch RA, et al: Clinical implications of prostaglandin and thromboxane A2 formation. N Engl J Med 319:761, 1988.
37. Badr KF, Kelly VE, Rennke HG, et al: Roles for thromboxane A2 and leukotrienes in endotoxin-induced acute renal failure. Kidney Int 30:474, 1986.
38. Bernard GR, Luce JM, Sprung CL, et al: High dose corticosteroids in patients with the adult respiratory distress syndrome. New Engl J Med 317:1565, 1987.
39. Bone RC, Slotman G, Maunder R, et al: Randomized double-blind multicenter study of prostaglandin E-1 in patients with the adult respiratory distress syndrome. Chest 96:114, 1989.

Chapter 55
SEPSIS SYNDROME

R. BRUCE LIGHT

KEY POINTS

- *Sepsis syndrome is a constellation of clinical and laboratory findings present to varying degrees in patients with infection. Major findings include fever or hypothermia, tachypnea, mental obtundation or confusion, hypotension and tachycardia, oliguria, elevated or left-shifted white blood cell count, thrombocytopenia, and hyperglycemia or increase in insulin requirement.*
- *Detection of features of the syndrome in the absence of evident infection should prompt a systematic search for a source of sepsis.*
- *Patients with sepsis-associated cardiorespiratory instability require immediate resuscitation as the first priority. This always involves fluid resuscitation and may require endotracheal intubation and administration of vasoactive drugs in patients who do not respond promptly to plasma volume expansion.*
- *Empiric antimicrobial therapy directed at all likely sources of infection is indicated when bacteremia is suspected, with respiratory or hemodynamic instability, and whenever life or major organ system function is threatened.*
- *Definitive surgical therapy to drain or debride infectious processes producing serious hemodynamic instability should proceed as soon as is practical.*

The term *sepsis syndrome* refers to a complex of clinical and laboratory findings associated with serious infection of any body site. The concept is useful mainly because features of the syndrome may suggest the possibility of infection in the absence of obvious local symptoms at an infected site and because repeated assessment of these features forms the basis of the clinical determination of response to therapy. In addition, many of the major issues in the intensive care treatment of serious infection involve management of the physiologic consequences of infection in order to minimize their impact until the infection is successfully controlled by antimicrobials, surgery, and the host response.

Some of the Key Points listed above deserve comment. First, recognition of the sepsis syndrome is not always straightforward. Errors such as mistakenly attributing sepsis-induced hyperventilation and hypotension to pulmonary embolism or sepsis-associated mental obtundation to sedative drug administration are not always avoidable but can be minimized by considering infection in every critically ill patient every day. Second, in many critically ill patients empiric antimicrobial treatment must precede definitive diagnosis. The standard precept that antimicrobial therapy should be prescribed only after a diagnosis is made cannot be applied to patients with life-threatening cardiorespiratory instability, and empiric therapy in this situation necessarily involves wide-spectrum antimicrobial coverage for all potential sources of infection of more than trivial probability. A final point is that definitive management generally will precede the ability to reduce or withdraw intensive care supportive measures. This mainly applies to surgical treatment of inadequately drained or debrided infected tissue; delaying surgical treatment in such cases in the hope that continued antimicrobial and supportive therapy will allow the surgery to be done under more stable conditions is often tempting but usually mistaken.

General Pathogenesis

Pathogenic microbes infecting human beings produce disease in several different ways, among them production of compounds which are directly toxic to cells (e.g., diphtheria toxin), production of compounds which act on cellular receptors and disrupt normal function (e.g., tetanus), and intracellular parasitism exploiting cellular machinery to produce microbial proteins rather than functional cell proteins (e.g., most viral infections). However, the most common mechanism of disease is simply the proliferation of organisms within normally sterile body tissues after normal surface defenses against such invasion have been breached. Many of the clinical features that follow, including most manifestations of the "sepsis syndrome," are the result of the recognition of the presence of foreign microbe–associated macromolecules in tissues and in the blood stream by the host immune system leading to a local and systemic inflammatory response (Fig. 55-1).

The best studied and probably most potent of the microbial macromolecules capable of provoking the host inflammatory response is gram-negative endotoxin, or lipopolysaccharide (LPS).[1] However, it is clear that other microbial cell constituents are capable of inciting the host response and that compounds from other highly pathogenic organisms approach the potency of LPS in inciting an inflammatory response in the human host, for example, the peptidoglycans present in the cell wall of *Staphylococcus aureus* and other bacteria.[2]

The key recognition cell in the human host is the tissue macrophage, the first phagocytic cell to come in contact with the pathogen. Phagocytic activation by exposure to microbial cell constituents leads to production and release of a number of *cytokines*.[3] These are polypeptide molecules which modify the actions of other host cells by binding to and stimulating receptors on their surfaces. Local effects include chemotaxis, leading to an influx of phagocytic cells into the infection region and activation of these cells to promote phagocytosis and microbial killing efficiency. Phospholipases produced and released by phagocytes cleave phospholipids from cell membranes and increase the local availability of arachidonic acid and similar lipids, which in turn can be metabolized by leukocytes and other cells to produce prostaglandins and leukotrienes, potent mediators of local vasomotor changes. Microbial cell products may

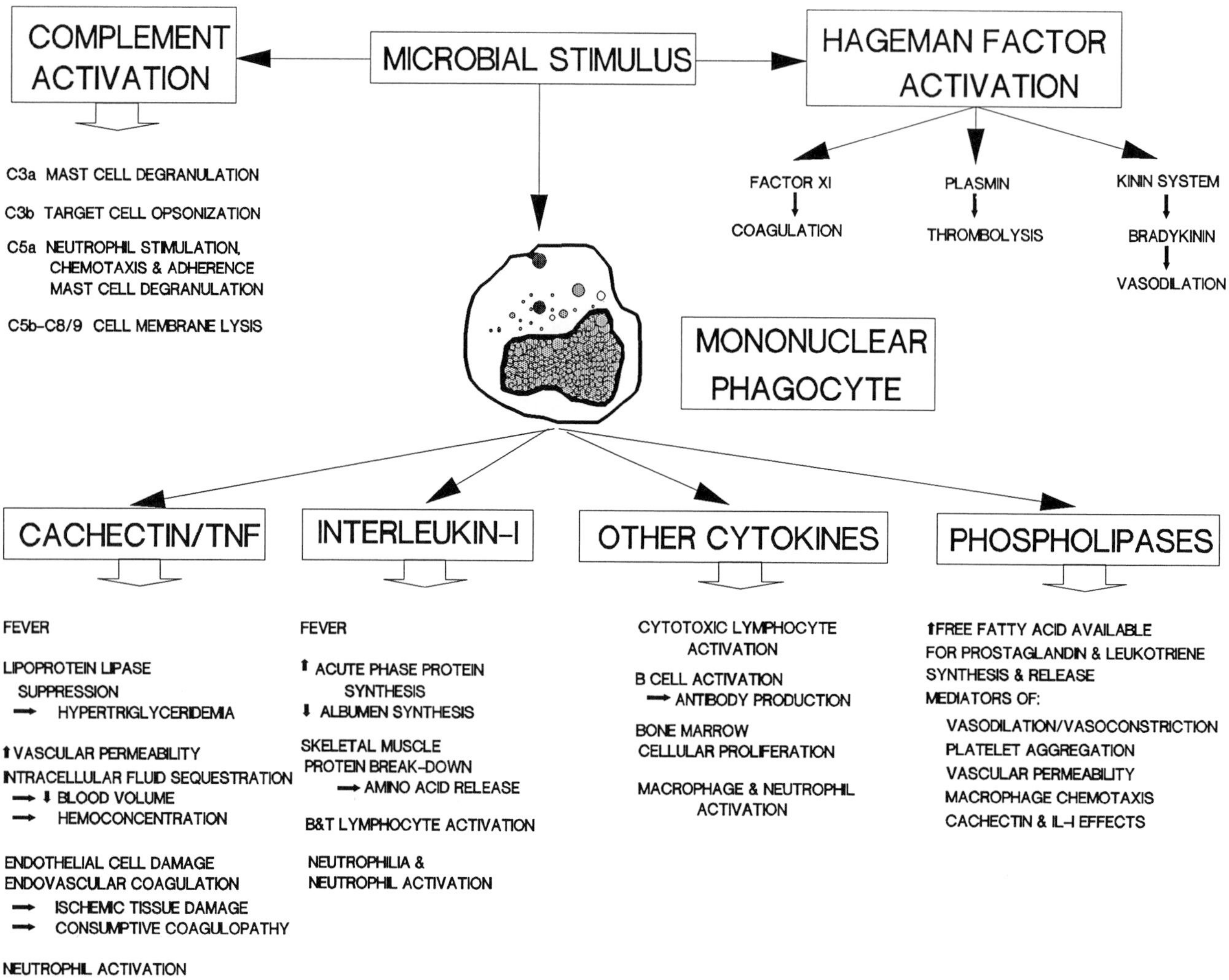

FIGURE 55-1 In the sepsis syndrome, gram-negative bacterial endotoxin and other microbial macromolecules do not act primarily as direct "toxins" but rather as stimuli to host phagocytic cells and to contact systems which then mediate the diverse manifestations of the sepsis. Among the cytokines produced and released by mononuclear phagocytes in response to this stimulus *cachectin,* also called *tumor necrosis factor (TNF),* is probably the most important, mediating directly or indirectly many of the major features of sepsis. Other cytokines, prostaglandins, and compounds derived from activation of direct contact systems such as the complement system and Hageman factor amplify the immunologic response to infection and mediate or contribute to many of the metabolic, hematologic, and cardiorespiratory features of sepsis.

also interact directly with other constituents of the host immune response, most notably the complement system.[4] This chain reaction cascade may begin with an antibody-mediated reaction between a complement-fixing preformed antibody and a microbial antigen, or with a nonspecific interaction between the alternate complement pathway and microbial antigen, and leads to the production of a number of biologically active molecules mediating chemotaxis, phagocytic cell activation, vasoactive effects, and even microbial cell lysis.

This local inflammatory process can be manifest systemically as the sepsis syndrome in one of two ways. First, bacteremia or systemic antigenemia may produce a systemic inflammatory response. Second, many of the mediators produced locally at the site of an infection act as hormones, producing changes in the function of cells in tissues remote from the site of the infection.

Interleukin-1 (IL-1) is the most completely described phagocytic cell cytokine with important systemic effects.[5] Previously named *leukocyte endogenous pyrogen,* it is known to induce prostaglandin E_2 synthesis in the anterior hypothalamus, resetting the thermoregulatory center to a higher set-point resulting in the symptom of "chills" and the clinical signs of shivering, rigors, and fever. It also mediates, at least in part, the marked reduction in liver albumen production and coincident increase in production of the acute-phase proteins such as haptoglobin, fibrinogen, C-reactive protein and proteins of the complement system. Skeletal muscle protein catabolism is also a result of IL-1 action. Effects on blood cells include release of neutrophils from bone marrow, neutrophil activation, T- and B-lymphocyte activation, and release of lactoferrin from neutrophils causing reduced bioavailability of iron, contributing to the anemia associated with inflammatory diseases.

More recently described and less completely understood, *cachectin* [also called *tumor necrosis factor* (TNF)] is another macrophage peptide hormone with important systemic effects.[6,7] In low concentrations in tissues it is known to have local proinflammatory effects and contributes to healing of local injury by stimulating angiogenesis. Given systemically in low concentrations to experimental animals, it produces progressive cachexia, leukocytosis, anemia, and low-grade inflammatory changes in many tissues. Acute injection of larger amounts of cachectin can reproduce many of the systemic effects of septic shock. Major effects so far described include an increase in procoagulant activity of vascular endothelium leading to microvascular thrombosis and tissue necrosis, damage to endothelial cells themselves causing microvascular fluid leakage, and shift of extracellular fluid into cells, particularly skeletal muscle, with consequent reduction in plasma volume. It is an endogenous pyrogen in its own right and also a stimulant to further release of IL-1. Many of its effects appear to be secondarily mediated by prostaglandins while others can be related to cachectin-induced release of other cytokines. However, the full extent of its actions and the mechanisms underlying its contribution to the sepsis syndrome in man remain to be worked out.

Additional cytokines of importance to sepsis and host defense continue to be described, and new roles for previously discovered cytokines continue to be defined. Interleukin-2 (IL-2) activates cytotoxic lymphocytes, induces synthesis of other lymphokines, and is a T cell growth factor; other interleukins promote proliferation and activation of lymphocyte populations and mast cells and amplify IL-1 effects. Colony-stimulating factors (CSFs) from activated lymphocytes promote growth of various bone marrow phagocytic cell lines. Gamma-interferon from activated T-lymphocytes activates macrophages, increases antibody production, and modulates TNF synthesis. The interactions between all of these mediators and the pathogenetic function of each in the sepsis syndrome are still far from being completely understood.

The role of the metabolites of *arachidonic acid* and related lipids in the pathogenesis of sepsis also remains to be defined, although many individual actions of these compounds are well described. It is known that phospholipases originating from phagocytic cells and other sources contribute to the increased availability of these lipids in sepsis.[8,9] Local tissue concentrations of leukotrienes, the products of the lipoxygenase pathway for arachidonic acid metabolism, are increased at inflamed sites and produce local vasoconstriction and increased microvascular permeability. Products of the main alternative metabolic pathway, mediated by cyclooxygenase, include the potent vasodilator prostacyclin as well as the vasoconstrictor and platelet aggregation stimulant thromboxane A_2. Prostacyclin has been found in increased amounts in the blood of septic humans and probably contributes to vasodilation and hypotension; the role of thromboxane A_2, if any, remains to be established. As noted above, it is also known that other prostaglandins mediate some of the cellular effects of cytokines. In the current state of knowledge we can conclude only that compounds of these classes are almost certainly important mediators of parts of the sepsis syndrome, but which particular compounds, in which tissues, and under what circumstances are for the most part obscure.

Platelet activating factor is another lipid mediator synthesized and released in increased amounts by a wide variety of cells during sepsis. A potent pulmonary and systemic vasoconstrictor, it also induces platelet aggregation and polymorphonuclear leukocyte adherence and increases microvascular permeability. Like some of the prostaglandins, it acts as a secondary mediator of some of the functions of the major cytokines.

Direct interactions between microbial macromolecules and host humoral defense mechanisms also account for some of the features of sepsis.[10] Endotoxins and other microbial cell constituents are known to directly activate Hageman factor (factor XII of the coagulation cascade). Activated Hageman factor is a fairly widely active protease which can initiate the activation of the plasma kinin system leading to the production of the potent vasodilator bradykinin. Factor XII activation of factor XI can lead to intravascular coagulation, while at the same time activated XII can initiate the protease cascade leading to fibrinolysis mediated by plasmin. Activated systemically, it therefore contributes to the consumptive coagulopathy and also to the systemic vasodilation of sepsis.

As noted earlier, activation of the complement cascade can also occur by either the usual or alternate pathways and, when activated systemically, contributes to increased vascular permeability, endothelial cell damage, and release of secondary mediators.[4] These secondary mediators include leukotrienes, prostaglandins, histamine and other compounds released by degranulating mast cells, and platelet activating factor.

The systemic inflammatory response with its associated reduction in functional blood volume, hypotension, and tissue damage also leads to the familiar neuroendocrine response to stress. Plasma levels of endogenous catecholamines, corticosteroids, endorphins, and insulin and glucagon are all increased and contribute to the cardiorespiratory and metabolic changes associated with sepsis detailed below.

Pathogenesis of the Major Clinical Manifestations of Sepsis

The sepsis syndrome features changes in the function of almost every organ system in the body, some on the basis of direct humoral effects of mediators involved in the systemic inflammatory response, others secondary to more general changes in circulatory control, metabolism, or in-

TABLE 55-1 Clinical Manifestations of the Sepsis Syndrome

	STAGE OR SEVERITY OF SEPSIS	
System	Early or Mild/Moderate	Advanced or Severe
Central nervous system	Fever (38–40°C), chills, confusion, obtundation	Fever >40°C, hypothermia, stupor, coma
Respiratory	Tachypnea, hypocapnia, mild arterial hypoxemia	Hypercapnic respiratory failure, hypoxemic respiratory failure
Cardiovascular	Tachycardia Hypotension Wide pulse pressure Warm skin Good response to volume expansion and vasoactive drugs	Tachycardia Hypotension Narrow pulse pressure Poor tissue perfusion Poor response to volume expansion and vasoactive drugs
Hematologic	Leukocytosis, left-shifted thrombocytosis, or mild thrombocytopenia; normal prothrombin time and partial thromboplastin time	Leukopenia, thrombocytopenia, disseminated intravascular coagulation
Renal	Prerenal oliguria	Acute Renal Failure
Hepatic/metabolic	Hyperglycemia, hypertriglyceridemia, mild hyperbilirubinemia and liver enzyme elevation, hypoalbuminemia	Hyperglycemia or hypoglycemia, lactic acidosis, hepatic failure

ternal milieu. The more usual and clinically most evident features of the syndrome are listed in Table 55-1.

CENTRAL NERVOUS SYSTEM EFFECTS OF SEPSIS

The common central nervous system (CNS) findings in sepsis include *fever* or *hypothermia* and disturbed level of consciousness, ranging from confusion through obtundation or coma. Fever is clearly attributable to the effects of IL-1 and cachectin release from macrophages involved in the inflammatory process.[11] The cause of hypothermia in some patients is less well understood but is probably related to respiratory and cutaneous heat loss due to hyperventilation and peripheral vasodilation, particularly in the elderly and in patients who have impaired muscular heat production due to low muscle mass, neuromuscular disease, or drugs which inhibit shivering.[12] Mental changes may be attributable to hypotension or hypoxia but often are not and, in the absence of other cause, are referred to as sepsis-associated encephalopathy. Global disturbances in the content or level of consciousness are usual while focal neurologic findings and significant brain stem dysfunction are absent. The pathogenesis is obscure. Reduced cerebral blood flow has been demonstrated in some septic patients,[13] while others have suggested that elevated plasma amino acid levels associated with protein catabolism penetrate the CNS and disturb neurotransmitter function.[14] Another possibility is a contribution by IL-1, which has been shown to possess sleep-inducing properties.[5] The encephalopathy is fully reversible in most cases.

RESPIRATORY SYSTEM CHANGES IN SEPSIS

One of the most characteristic early signs of sepsis, particularly gram-negative sepsis, is *tachypnea* with alveolar hyperventilation. This often occurs without demonstrable pulmonary disease and is of unknown cause, although direct stimulation of the respiratory center or of lung receptors has been suggested. Temperature elevation and the increase in metabolic rate associated with sepsis also increase body CO_2 production. In most cases primary hyperventilation results in hypocapnia despite this,[15] but in patients with limited respiratory reserve hypercapnic respiratory failure may be precipitated.

A degree of arterial hypoxemia may accompany the hyperventilation, but in the absence of a pulmonary infiltrate it is seldom severe. Fully developed hypoxemic respiratory failure associated with sepsis is usually due to pneumonia. However, subsequent to the onset of sepsis, generally after 24 to 72 h and particularly in patients with more severe sepsis complicated by shock, hypoxemic respiratory failure due to the adult respiratory distress syndrome may supervene (Chap. 54).

CARDIOVASCULAR EFFECTS OF SEPSIS

Vasodilation of both arterial and venous blood vessels is the predominant primary cardiovascular effect of sepsis.[16] Important mediators include bradykinin and other elements of the kinin system, vasodilator prostaglandins, and probably platelet activating factor, endogenous opioids, and β-adrenergic stimulation. *Hypotension* may result from the combination of reduced venous return and low systemic vascular resistance (SVR), but in patients who have been given intravenous fluid resuscitation or who have themselves compensated for the reduced SVR by increasing cardiac output (with *tachycardia* and endogenous *sympathetic stimulation*), the result is warm, flushed skin with a hyperdynamic circulation manifest as increased pulse volume and wide pulse pressure on clinical examination. If central vascular monitoring is done, there is an increased cardiac output with low systemic vascular resistance.

In addition to vasodilation, effective circulating blood volume is reduced by loss of intravascular volume into the extravascular portion of the extracellular fluid compartment. This is due to increased vascular permeability to fluids and protein, particularly albumen.[17] Consequences of this include an increase in the ongoing intravenous (IV) fluid infusion requirement to maintain a circulating blood volume and a tendency toward fluid retention with edema formation.

Once controversial, there is now reasonably compelling evidence in human beings that sepsis results in reduced myocardial contractility by an as yet incompletely defined mechanism.[18] In less severe sepsis this is usually not evident at the bedside since the other obvious cardiovascular effects of sepsis dominate the picture. In late sepsis complicated by shock, however, myocardial failure is increasingly important and becomes a factor limiting short-term survival (Chaps. 98 and 115).

RENAL EFFECTS OF SEPSIS

Oliguria (urine output <0.5 mL/kg/H) is common in sepsis but generally reflects inadequate renal perfusion related to reduced functional blood volume and corrects with intravascular volume expansion. In the absence of prior diuretic administration or underlying renal disease, prerenal oliguria is associated with low urine sodium concentration (<20 meq/L) and high urine osmolality (>450 mO/kg). With protracted oliguria or more severe sepsis acute renal failure may supervene and is signaled by oliguria despite demonstrably acceptable blood pressure and cardiac output with isosmotic urine containing a high concentration of sodium. In septic patients it is common to observe a deterioration in renal function that is intermediate between these extremes in which oliguria is not profound and does respond to treatment (volume repletion, diuretics, dopamine), urine sodium concentration is high and osmolality isosmotic, and serum creatinine rises two- or threefold.

GASTROINTESTINAL EFFECTS OF SEPSIS

Abnormal gastrointestinal motility is the most common sepsis-associated gastrointestinal problem. Impairment of gastric emptying, termed *gastric atony*, and more generalized small bowel *adynamic ileus* occur after abdominal surgery or trauma and in the presence of peritonitis but can also complicate systemic sepsis of any source, particularly when shock results in intestinal ischemia. Opiates given for pain relief and bowel wall edema due to vascular leak and low serum albumen concentration also contribute to this problem. Clinically significant upper gastrointestinal bleeding due to "stress ulceration," once extremely common in septic patients, is now unusual. This change may relate to the widespread use of agents for gastrointestinal bleeding prophylaxis but is more likely due to more aggressive and prompt resuscitation from shock leading to reduced gastric mucosal ischemia; in patients in whom shock is not reversed quickly, bleeding occurs much more commonly.

Abnormalities of liver function are also frequent in sepsis. Acute anoxic liver injury may occur associated with an episode of severe hypoxia or shock from which the patient is quickly resuscitated. This produces marked but transient elevations in blood transaminase levels which are not associated with significant functional impairment. Lower grade increases in liver enzymes, often with mild to moderate hyperbilirubinemia, regularly occur with systemic sepsis of any cause.[19–21] This seems to be related to focal hepatic necrosis and to cholestasis of unknown mechanism. In most cases the jaundice is associated with relatively preserved hepatic function in other respects, but in more severe and protracted sepsis this process can progress to frank hepatic insufficiency with hypoprothrombinemia, jaundice, lactic acidosis, and hypoglycemia; when this occurs, survival is unusual.

HEMATOLOGIC EFFECTS OF SEPSIS

The *leukocytosis* of sepsis is due in part to endogenous catecholamine-induced demargination of polymorphonuclear leukocytes and in part to cytokine-induced release of young and immature polymorphs from bone marrow. In patients who do not have a preceding underlying cause, *granulocytopenia* with sepsis implies utilization of neutrophils at a rate which exceeds bone marrow capacity to replace them and is a marker for uncontrolled sepsis with a poor prognosis unless it occurs only transiently early in the course. In these instances the white blood cell differential count reveals a predominance of immature polymorphonuclear neutrophils (PMNs).

Although *anemia* is not a feature of acute sepsis in the absence of an underlying cause, hemoglobin concentration may fall quite abruptly due to hemodilution after fluid resuscitation from hypotension, and few patients who are critically ill with sepsis for periods longer than a few days are capable of maintaining a stable hemoglobin concentration without transfusion. The gradually progressive anemia is due to a combination of shortened red cell survival due to sepsis, blood letting for laboratory testing, and the impaired hematopoeiesis accompanying any systemic inflammatory process.

Thrombocythemia may accompany infection of milder degree, but more severe sepsis is characterized by *thrombocytopenia*, which is usually moderate but may be severe. Frank *disseminated intravascular coagulation (DIC)* is defined as thrombocytopenia associated with clinical evidence of thrombosis with tissue ischemia, abnormal bleeding from puncture sites and wounds, and low blood levels of fibrinogen and factors II, V, and VIII with elevated fibrin degradation products.[22] It is fortunately rare, generally occurring in association with intractable septic shock and probably attributable to uncontained systemic Hageman factor activation. The more usual isolated thrombocytopenia of sepsis is likely related to adherence of platelets to damaged microvascular endothelium and to microaggragates lodging in tissue capillary beds. It reverses promptly when sepsis is controlled, and in this respect is a useful monitoring parameter. Mild to moderate elevations of the prothrombin time and partial thromboplastin time are also common in sepsis but do not usually imply DIC.

METABOLIC AND ELECTROLYTE CHANGES IN SEPSIS

Among the best established genuinely metabolic changes which occur are those attributable to the effects of the cytokines IL-1 and cachectin. The rapid development of *hypoalbumenemia* in septic patients, in part due to redistribution of albumen into the extravascular space, is contributed to by the IL-1-mediated shift in hepatic protein synthesis away from albumen toward production of acute-phase reactant proteins. Interleukin-1 also mediates protein catabolism in skeletal muscle. Presumably this has the function of providing a continuing source of amino acids for wound healing and acute-phase protein production during a period of reduced nutrition. In addition, amino acids from protein breakdown become a major energy source in sepsis. The result is negative nitrogen balance and rapid loss of body muscle mass.

Glucose utilization in sepsis is impaired, as in other stress situations, by increased levels of endogenous catecholamines, glucocorticoids, and glucagon.[23] *Hyperglycemia* is common, particularly with administration of glucose-containing intravenous solutions. *Hypoglycemia* is much less common and can usually be related to hepatic insufficiency when it occurs. Use of fat as a caloric source is also impaired in sepsis. The failure of tissues to effectively use free fatty acids for energy is described but not well explained. On the other hand, hypertriglyceridemia in sepsis is best explained by a cachectin-mediated reduction in plasma and tissue lipoprotein lipase activity. This can result in a degree of hyperlipidemia and even frank lipemia in patients receiving total parenteral nutrition with a substantial lipid component. The metabolic changes associated with sepsis are discussed in more detail in Chaps. 56 and 90.

A wide variety of electrolyte disturbances can accompany sepsis. Probably the most common is *hyponatremia* related to limited water excretion capability due to inappropriate secretion of antidiuretic hormone. This is particularly common in the presence of CNS infections[24] and in bacterial pneumonia.[25] *Hypocalcemia* is seen in as many as 20 percent of patients with bacterial sepsis. It is associated with increased mortality and with hypotension, which may improve with calcium administration.[26] *Hypomagnesemia* and *hypophosphatemia* are also often seen in septic patients but are common in critically ill patients in general and probably not directly attributable to sepsis.

Diagnosis

The full definition of the sepsis syndrome which has been used in a number of clinical trials of management of sepsis has included a definable serious infection, body temperature abnormality, tachypnea and tachycardia, and evidence of inadequate perfusion or function of one or more organ systems (altered mental status, oliguria, lactic acidosis, unexplained arterial hypoxemia).[27–29] However, infections in critically ill patients have a wide range of severity, progress to established sepsis syndrome or shock at varying rates, and manifestations vary considerably. Therefore strict application of the criteria listed above before the patient is considered potentially septic is inadvisable. The most useful approach is to be constantly alert for manifestations of sepsis (Table 55-1) and to consider the diagnosis when any of these findings are present and are otherwise unexplained. In critically ill patients there is usually no shortage of potential sources of sepsis. These are usually evident from the physical examination and the basic laboratory investigation. For a fuller discussion of an approach to etiology of sepsis or unclear origin, see Chap. 97.

PHYSICAL EXAMINATION

Clinicians often refer to patients with severe infections as looking "toxic" or "septic," an impression often based on unspecified features of the physical examination. Since these features are mainly nonspecific, it is best to carefully search for and document the basis for this impression, considering alternative explanations for each. Confusion, apprehension, or mental obtundation with hyperventilation may be the earliest or even only signs of sepsis, particularly in the elderly or debilitated. Detection of fever or hypothermia is best accomplished with a rectal thermometer or other core temperature measurement device, since oral temperature can be misleading in a hyperventilating patient.[30] Tachycardia is usual. In early sepsis or in adequately volume resuscitated patients blood pressure is usually only moderately depressed from base line, the pulse pressure widened, and the skin warm and well perfused or flushed. In relatively volume depleted patients, those with significant preexisting cardiac disease, and in advanced septic shock the blood pressure is markedly reduced, pulse pressure is narrow, and the skin is cold, pale, and mottled. In these patients assessment of the jugular venous pressure (JVP) is helpful in distinguishing relative hypovolemia (low JVP or empty neck veins while recumbent) from cardiac dysfunction (elevated JVP, full neck veins). Oliguria is almost always present. A careful search of the skin, nail beds, mucosal surfaces, conjunctiva, and eye grounds will occasionally be rewarding. Petechiae and ecchymoses, pustular or vesicular lesions, *ecthyma gangrenosum*, or areas of cellulitis may suggest bacteremia (perhaps even its cause), while prominent erythroderma, conjunctivitis, and other red mucosal surfaces suggest toxin-mediated staphylococcal or streptococcal disease (see Plates 35 and 40). Most patients with these nonspecific physical findings suggesting sepsis will also have evidence of a specific local infection on careful general clinical examination.

LABORATORY FINDINGS

Arterial blood gases often demonstrate an acute respiratory alkalosis. Mild arterial hypoxemia, easily corrected with oxygen, is also often present in the absence of lung disease. The polymorphonuclear leukocyte count is usually elevated and "left shifted" but may be depressed in fulminant sepsis or in patients with depressed bone marrow function. In patients already hospitalized with other illness, it is often an unexplained elevation of the white blood cell count that first prompts a search for occult infection. Similarly, unexplained thrombocytopenia is an early feature of sepsis. Hyperglycemia is prominent in patients with diabetes mellitus; a degree of glucose intolerance is a feature in nondiabetics as well. Serum creatinine may rise even in the absence of significant oliguria. Proteinuria is usual, and some patients will have an active urinary sediment suggesting nephritis. Hypoalbuminemia can develop quite quickly for reasons described above. The most common acute electrolyte abnormality is hypokalemia, probably due to endogenous catecholamine release, but hyponatremia, hypocalcemia, hypophosphatemia, and hypomagnesemia are also frequent if looked for. Mild elevation of transaminases and mild hyperbilirubinemia occur. In more severe sepsis with shock there is metabolic acidosis due to lactate accumulation, the coagulopathy of DIC may become prominent, and laboratory evidence of renal and hepatic failure become more florid.

DIFFERENTIAL DIAGNOSIS

Blood cultures demonstrate an organism in something less than half of cases with apparent sepsis, defined as abnormal body temperature together with hypotension, clinical findings suggesting sepsis (mental changes, unexplained hyperventilation) and hematologic changes consistent with sepsis.[27,28] There are really no reliable general clinical or laboratory features to act as a guide to the microbial etiology of sepsis, and in the absence of specific findings suggesting a particular organism (e.g., petechiae in meningococcemia, soft tissue gas with *Clostridium perfringens*) or findings in a particular organ system, the approach to diagnosis and to empiric therapy is necessarily broad (see Chap. 97).

Sepsis syndrome may be produced by a variety of nonbacterial infections including viral infections (severe acute influenza, viral hepatitis, unusually severe enteroviral or adenoviral infections), parasitic infections (particularly malaria due to *Plasmodium falciparum*), fungal infections, rickettsiae (especially Rocky Mountain spotted fever), and pathogens in the atypical pneumonia group (*Mycoplasma pneumoniae*, Q-fever, *Chlamydia psittaci*). Diseases which are not necessarily invasive infections but which are mediated by bacterial toxins must also be considered. These include hemolytic-uremic syndrome, usually following a diarrheal illness caused by a toxin-forming *Escherichia coli*, toxic shock syndrome (see Chap. 113), and a similar illness caused by toxin-producing group A β-hemolytic Streptococcus.

Most patients with apparent sepsis syndrome and negative blood cultures nevertheless prove to have infections, but the initial presentation of some noninfectious syndromes may be confused with sepsis. These include hypotension and hyperventilation after pulmonary embolism, which is distinguished from sepsis by the clinical context, absence of pyrexia, clinical evidence of pulmonary hypertension and right ventricular overload in association with reduced peripheral perfusion, and absence of immature neutrophils in the blood smear. On occasion a patient will come to lung scan, pulmonary angiography, or demonstration of high pulmonary artery pressure with low cardiac output by flow-directed pulmonary artery catheterization to make the distinction.

Drug-related pyrexial illnesses such as malignant hyperthermia, neuroleptic malignant syndrome, anticholinergic or sympathomimetic drug exposures, and allergic reactions must be distinguished from sepsis. Accidental hypothermia can be distinguished from sepsis-associated hypothermia by the absence of hematologic evidence of sepsis, lack of evidence of a primary source of sepsis, and demonstration of a low cardiac output and high systemic vascular resistance if a thermal dilution pulmonary artery catheter is placed.[31]

Tissue necrosis due to ischemic injury, trauma, or acute pancreatitis can also produce most of the features of the sepsis syndrome; these are usually fairly obvious because of the clinical context. Systemic lupus erythematosus and several of the systemic vasculitis syndromes can also be difficult to distinguish from sepsis when first seen. Indeed, since sepsis is a frequent complication in all of these entities, empiric antimicrobial therapy until sepsis is excluded is often warranted in critically ill patients.

In addition to making the determination that the sepsis syndrome is present, it is important to make an assessment of its relative severity to serve as a guide to the pace of investigation and to the need for empiric antimicrobial treatment. This assessment must include not only indices of the apparent severity of the infection but also host factors relating to the risk of rapid progression of the infection and the physiologic stability of the patient. In general terms, infectious syndromes associated with moderate pyrexia and elevated white blood cell count occurring in a patient who is immunologically intact and physiologically stable are not emergent situations, and delay of empiric therapy until a presumptive diagnosis is made is reasonable. On the other hand, marked pyrexia with more severe hematologic changes (neutropenia, thrombocytopenia) and hypotension even in an immunologically competent individual mandates urgent empiric therapy and an aggressive diagnostic approach; in patients who are seriously immunocompromised, as in granulocytopenia, unexplained pyrexia alone is sufficient to warrant this approach.

Management

TREATMENT OF INFECTION

The decision regarding whether to employ empiric antimicrobial therapy hinges on the assessment mentioned above. In general, new pyrexia of mild to moderate severity in a physiologically stable patient should not be treated with antibiotics in the absence of a supported presumptive diagnosis; examples of a supported presumptive diagnosis would include a pulmonary infiltrate consistent with pneumonia, a red, purulent intravenous cannula site or erythema, and tender swelling surrounding a surgical wound.

Antimicrobial choice depends on the site of the suspected or proven infection and on host factors associated with increased risk of infection with relatively antimicrobial resistant organisms. In general, antimicrobial coverage for seriously ill patients with infection of unclear origin should always include *S. aureus* and enteric gram-negative bacilli such as *E. coli* and *Klebsiella* spp. This can be achieved with a regimen such as cefazolin 1 to 2 grams IV every 8 h and an aminoglycoside such as gentamicin 1.5 mg/kg every 8 h, with adjustment of dose in patients with impaired renal function. Alternatives include cefotaxime 2 g every 8 h or ceftriaxone 2 g every 24 h. For granulocytopenic patients or others at increased risk for infection with relatively resistant aerobic gram-negatives such as *Pseudomonas aeruginosa,* a regimen such as piperacillin 3 g every 6 h with an aminoglycoside is preferable. A number of guidelines for modification of antimicrobial coverage can be stated: **1.** If CNS infection is suspected, cefazolin should not be used. Ampicillin 2 g every 4 h is preferred for suspected community-acquired meningitis in adults, while a third generation cephalosporin such as ceftazadime 2 g every 8 h with nafcillin 2 g every 4 h is indicated for possible gram-negative or staphylococcal meningitis following surgery or associated with bacteremia from another source. **2.** Respiratory infection in patients with chronic respiratory disease often involves *Hemophilus influenzae* or *Branhamella catarrhalis,* and in hospitalized or chronically institutionalized patients enteric gram-negatives are more common; for all of these Cefuroxime 0.75 to 1.5 g IV every 8 h or a third generation cephalosporin is preferable to cefazolin. **3.** Involvement of anaerobic bacteria is usual in intraabdominal infections, including those involving the female genital tract and in many necrotizing soft tissue infections. When this is suspected, add an effective antimicrobial for *Bacteroides fragilis* group, such as metronidazole 500 to 750 mg every 8 h, substitute cefoxitin 1 to 2 g every 6 h for cefazolin, or use clindamycin 450 to 900 mg every 8 h (which is also effective therapy for most gram-positive infections outside the CNS) together with an aminoglycoside, third-generation cephalosporin, or cotrimoxazole. **4.** Nosocomial infections in hospitals or intensive care units with locally endemic antimicrobial-resistant organisms require modification of these regimens. Examples include methicillin-resistant *S. aureus* (MRSA), usually requiring addition of vancomycin 500 mg every 6 h (with adjustment for renal failure), or enteric gram-negatives resistant to the first-line agents noted above necessitating use of alternative agents such as third generation cephalosporins, cotrimoxazole, imipenem, or fluoroquinolones. Recommendations for therapy of specific infectious syndromes can be found in the chapters dealing with them.

Surgical or percutaneous catheter drainage in the case of undrained infected fluid collections and surgical resection or debridement in the case of infected devitalized tissue is at least as important as appropriate antimicrobial therapy in critically ill patients with sepsis. Such treatment should proceed as soon as the diagnosis has been made, delaying only to correct immediately remediable electrolyte disturbances, severe anemia, and cardiorespiratory instability. Many such patients are necessarily at high operative risk because of their critical condition. However, if the infective process is a major cause of their unstable condition and surgical therapy is needed to correct it, delaying intervention in the hope that medical treatment will lead to the surgery being done under more favorable conditions is usually an error.

IMMUNOTHERAPY

At the time of this writing there are no widely available immunotherapeutic agents available which can yet be considered standard therapy in sepsis. However, clinical trials employing polyclonal human antiserum preparations against gram-negative endotoxin or whole gram-negative organisms have unequivocally demonstrated that this approach to adjunctive treatment can reduce mortality.[29] Encouraging preliminary results from clinical trials of monoclonal antibodies against endotoxin are now available, and an improvement in survival in patients with gram-negative sepsis appears to be achievable. It is extremely likely that use of monoclonal antibodies against gram-negative endotoxin will soon become a widely used adjunctive therapy in patients with presumed gram-negative sepsis syndrome. Monoclonal antibodies against components of the host response to endotoxin, notably cachectin,[32] have also been developed recently, and some are reaching the clinical trial stage; whether this approach will prove useful in patients with sepsis syndrome remains to be seen.

SUPPORTIVE THERAPY

Hypotension and oliguria due to sepsis are initially treated with rapid administration of intravenous fluids. Normal saline or lactated Ringer's solution are the best fluids to begin with because they are usually immediately at hand and can be infused rapidly. Repeated infusion of 0.5-L boluses of fluid, each over 5 to 15 min, is given until the blood pressure and urine output increase to an acceptable level or until signs of pulmonary congestion and elevated jugular venous pressure supervene. Patients poorly responsive to acute volume expansion will usually require central hemodynamic monitoring and vasopressor therapy, discussed in more detail in Chaps. 98 and 114. However, even in the majority of patients who do respond satisfactorily to volume expansion, it must be remembered that crystalloid solutions will rapidly redistribute from the intravascular to the extravascular extracellular fluid volume to an even greater extent in septic than in nonseptic patients. A high rate of continuing intravenous fluid administration (usually 150 to 200 mL/H or more of 0.5 N saline with or without 5% dextrose) will therefore be required to maintain an adequate circulating blood volume. Persistent positive fluid balance will eventually lead to accumulation of edema fluid in tissues. While it is probably reasonable to regard this as only a "cosmetic" problem if it is of mild degree, more severe edema can cause problems with vascular access and impair wound healing and gut function. In the presence of relatively "leaky" membranes and low colloid osmotic pressure, continuing positive fluid balance probably also contributes to the development of pulmonary edema. If the hemoglobin is less than 100 g/L, it is reasonable to transfuse packed red blood cells both to reduce fluid requirements and to ensure adequate blood oxygen carrying capacity. If hypoalbumenemia is significant, administration of albumen will usually permit maintenance of the blood volume with less crystalloid administration, as will use of 6% hetastarch in normal saline or dextran volume expansion solutions.

The importance of prompt resuscitation and reestablishment of a reasonable urine output is difficult to overstate, since oliguric renal failure greatly complicates the management of critically ill patients in many ways. If oliguria does not correct with initial plasma volume expansion, the first possibility to consider is inadequate renal perfusion due to low blood presssure or cardiac output. Inadequate resuscitation can usually be detected on clinical assessment of the mental state, heart rate, blood pressure (taking into consideration the patients' usual blood pressure, since chronically hypertensive individuals may require a higher than normal pressure for adequate organ perfusion), and perfusion of the skin of the extremities. If there is doubt about circulatory adequacy and there is no evidence of pulmonary or venous congestion, further fluid challenges are warranted. If doubt persists or if there is evidence of fluid overload, central hemodynamic monitoring is indicated. Oliguria in the presence of clinically adequate hemodynamics should prompt examination of the urinary electrolytes to help distinguish acute renal failure from prerenal oliguria and consideration of other possible causes of renal insufficiency (obstruction, primary renal disease). Management of oliguria complicating shock or hypotension is discussed in detail in Chap. 153.

Arterial blood gases should be measured in all cases of sepsis and oxygen administered to maintain arterial oxyhemoglobin saturation above 95%. Endotracheal intubation is indicated when oxygen saturation cannot be maintained at this level by oxygen enrichment of inspired gas alone or when a depressed level of consciousness threatens airway integrity. In addition, patients with persistent hypotension who cannot be promptly resuscitated with volume infusion alone should be intubated and given mechanical ventilatory support; without this intervention many will rapidly develop acute respiratory failure or even acute respiratory arrest with potentially catastrophic results.

Hemoglobin concentrations as low as 60 to 70 g/L are usually well tolerated by individuals with normal cardiorespiratory reserve; but since systemic oxygen delivery is often problematic in sepsis, transfusion of packed red blood cells should be considered when the hemoglobin concentration is below 100 g/L. The thrombocytopenia of sepsis is not often a cause of bleeding in the absence of frank disseminated intravascular coagulation. Platelet transfusion is not indicated unless there is uncontrollable nonsurgical bleeding associated with platelet counts below 40×10^9/L, since platelet survival is markedly reduced in sepsis. Significant elevations of the prothrombin time or partial thromboplastin time are most often related to depletion of liver-derived coagulation factors and can be treated with intravenous vitamin K once or twice a week and, if necessary, infusion of stored plasma. Neutrophil transfusions are of no proven value for either neutropenia caused by sepsis or sepsis complicating iatrogenic neutropenia.

Nutritional support should be established as early in the course of a septic illness as is practical (see Chap. 92). Sepsis is frequently associated with multiple blood electrolyte disturbances, notably, hypokalemia, hyponatremia, ionized hypocalcemia, hypomagnesemia, and hypophosphatemia. All of these should be looked for and corrected by intravenous administration of the electrolyte (in the case of low magnesium, ionized calcium, phosphate, or potassium) or by reduction of the water content and total volume of intravenous fluids in the case of hyponatremia (see Chap. 156).

Prognosis

Bacteremia with a sepsis syndrome not complicated by shock or by failure of one or more major organs systems is associated with a mortality of about 10 to 15 percent, lower for sepsis of milder degree without bacteremia. More severe sepsis carries a mortality of 30 to 70 percent and is heavily influenced by the presence of shock, the severity and nature of underlying disease, and the organism causing sepsis. Major negative prognostic host factors include severe immune dysfunction (granulocytopenia or hypogammaglobulinemia) and reduced cardiorespiratory reserve from preexisting lung or heart disease. Development of major organ system failure as a result of sepsis is also strongly associated with a fatal outcome, particularly acute respiratory failure from either pneumonia or acute respiratory disease syndrome (ARDS), renal failure, or hepatic failure. Bacteremia with particularly virulent organisms (e.g., fulminant disease due to *Cl. perfringens*, which produces a highly toxic lecithinase) or organisms which are often highly resistant to antimicrobials (e.g., *Pseudomonas* spp.) also carries a worse prognosis.

CASE PRESENTATION

Mr. ST, a 40-year-old, unemployed steroid-dependent chronic asthmatic, came to the hospital emergency room with complaints of nausea, vomiting, and abdominal pain for 5 days associated with increasing dyspnea over the preceding 2 days. Initial examination revealed a respiratory rate of 32 BPM, heart rate 100 BPM, blood pressure 130/95 mmHg, and temperature 38.5°C. He was moderately confused and diaphoretic, with labored respirations, an obvious wheeze, and pale, dusky skin. The rest of the examination was unremarkable. His initial arterial blood gas showed mild hypoxemia and a respiratory alkalosis. The $FEV_{1.0}$ was unmeasurably low. The white blood cell count was 16.3×10^9/L with >90% polymorphonuclear leukocytes, 20% young forms. The hemoglobin was 156 g/L and the platelets 120×10^9/L. Serum electrolytes and basic blood chemistry were normal.

The patient was kept in the emergency room and treated for severe asthma with intravenous theophylline, inhaled salbutamol, intravenous methylprednisolone, and oxygen by face mask. Vascular access was initially a problem because of sclerosed veins but was eventually achieved (during attempted venous cannulation the patient told the intern "if you can't do this, let me show you how it's done"). Over the ensuing 48 h the patient's $FEV_{1.0}$ steadily improved, reaching 1.8 L by the second day. However, he continued to complain of severe dyspnea and was visibly tachypneic. He remained diaphoretic and became increasingly confused and belligerent, despite acceptable arterial oxygenation. By this time he had also become more febrile to 39°C, and the blood pressure had fallen to 90/40 mmHg and remained there despite infusion of 1.5 L of normal saline. Repeat blood work showed a white blood cell count of 19.6×10^9/L, mostly PMNs with a "left shift," and the platelets were 89×10^9/L.

A consult to the intensive care unit staff was written. However, before they could be contacted, the patient suffered an acute respiratory arrest which was immediately complicated by extreme bradycardia and an unobtainable blood pressure. The arrest team intubated the patient and gave assisted ventilation with oxygen. Intravenous epinephrine was given and restored the heart rate and blood pressure, which were then maintained by infusion of Ringer's lactate at 400 mL/H and dopamine at 5 μg/kg/min. Physical examination at this time revealed a stuporous patient responsive to deep pain only. The chest was wheezy but otherwise clear. The neck was supple. The abdomen was distended, tympanitic, and quiet but not obviously tender. Scattered pustules were seen on all extremities and on the abdominal wall.

With a diagnosis of presumed sepsis and bacteremia of unclear origin, cefotaxime and clindamycin were given intravenously. Investigations included blood cultures, gram stain and culture of tracheal secretions, examination of cerebrospinal fluid (normal), an echocardiogram (normal), and a computerized tomography (CT) scan of the abdomen (also normal). The cutaneous pustules were opened, cultured, and gram stained, revealing clumps of gram-positive cocci. The following day, blood cultures obtained earlier in the hospital course and the skin pustule cultures demonstrated *S. aureus.* Cloxacillin was given intravenously; the clindamycin and cefotaxime were stopped. Over the next 5 days the patient gradually became afebrile and stable from a cardiorespiratory perspective. No primary source for the bacteremia was detected. He was extubated and transferred to a medical ward service to complete a 6-week course of intravenous cloxacillin for his bacteremia with possible infective endocarditis.

CASE DISCUSSION

The correct diagnosis of staphylococcal sepsis was missed for the first 48 h in this patient despite the presence of major risk factors for sepsis (chronic steroid therapy and reason to suspect IV drug abuse) and presence of a number of features of the *sepsis syndrome*: hyperventilation (admittedly confounded by the asthma also present), fever, confusion, thrombocytopenia, and an elevated left-shifted white blood cell count. Forty-eight hours later these findings became much more florid, and he developed hypotension which responded poorly to volume resuscitation. The correct diagnosis was entertained at this time. However, the response proved less than adequate, since the combination of increased respiratory work load (from sepsis and asthma) combined with hypotension resulted in a cardiorespiratory arrest which could have been avoided. Sepsis-associated hypotension of this degree, especially in a patient with labored respirations, is almost always an indication for immediate endotracheal intubation as part of the resuscitative effort.

Initial treatment for sepsis was fairly appropriate in that antimicrobial agents were given to cover *S. aureus,* most aerobic gram-negative bacilli and other organisms which might be implicated in primary bacteremia or pneumonia, and also *B. fragilis* in view of the equivocal abdominal findings at this time. This is in keeping with the principle that in life-threatening sepsis treatment should be conservative, covering all major diagnostic possibilities entertained until a diagnosis is established. However, the regimen chosen can be criticized for not including an agent effective against *P. aeruginosa,* a prominent pathogen in IV drug abusers; addition of an aminoglycoside or substitution of ceftazadime for cefotaxime would have been appropriate here.

The investigations ordered excluded many of the initially considered diagnoses, and the subsequent blood culture result eventually yielded the diagnosis. It should be pointed out that although no source could be demonstrated for the bacteremia, as occurs in about 50 percent of *S. aureus* bacteremias, the negative physical examination and echocardiogram cannot exclude the diagnosis of infective endocarditis; a full course of therapy for this potential diagnosis is therefore mandatory, and the patient should be followed closely for subsequent development of valvular insufficiency or other complications of this disease.

References

1. Wolff SM: Biological effects of bacterial endotoxins in man. J Infect Dis 128(Suppl):S259, 1973.

2. Kaplan MH, Tenenbaum MJ: *Staphylococcus aureus:* Cellular biology and clinical application. Am J Med 72:248, 1982.
3. Dinarello CA, Meir JW: Lymphokines. N Engl J Med 317:940, 1987.
4. Frank MM: Complement in the pathophysiology of human disease. N Engl J Med 316:1525, 1987.
5. Dinarello CA: Interleukin-I and the pathogenesis of the acute-phase response. N Engl J Med 311:1413, 1984.
6. Tracey KJ, Lowry SF, Cerami A: Cachectin: A hormone that triggers acute shock and chronic cachexia. J Inf Dis 157:413, 1988.
7. Beutler B, Cerami A: Cachectin: More than a tumor necrosis factor. N Eng J Med 316:379, 1987.
8. Vadas P, Pruzanski W, Stefanski E et al: Pathogenesis of hypotension in septic shock: Correlation of circulating phospholipase A_2 levels with circulatory collapse. Crit Care Med 16:1, 1988.
9. Ball HA, Cook JA, Wise WC et al: Role of thromboxane, prostaglandins and leukotrienes in endotoxic septic shock. Int Care Med 12:116, 1986.
10. Colman RW: Contact systems in infectious diseases. Rev Infect Dis 11:S689, 1989.
11. Dinarello CA, Cannon JG, Wolff SM: New concepts on the pathogenesis of fever. Rev Infect Dis 10:168, 1988.
12. Hudson LD, Conn RD: Accidental hypothermia: Associated diagnoses and prognosis in a common problem. JAMA 227:37, 1974.
13. Bowton DL, Bertels NH, Prough DS et al: Cerebral blood flow is reduced in patients with sepsis syndrome. Crit Care Med 17:399, 1989.
14. Jeppson B, Freund HR, Gimmon Z et al: Blood-brain barrier derangement in sepsis: Cause of septic encephalopathy? Am J Surg 141:136, 1981.
15. Simmons DH, Nicoloff J, Guze LB: Hyperventilation and respiratory alkalosis as signs of gram-negative bacteremic shock. JAMA 174:2196, 1960.
16. Hess ML, Hastillo A, Greenfield LJ: Spectrum of cardiovascular function during gram-negative sepsis. Prog Cardiovasc Dis 23:279, 1981.
17. Fleck A, Raines G, Hawker F et al: Increased vascular permeability: A major cause of hypoalbuminaemia in disease and injury. Lancet, April 6, 781, 1985.
18. Parillo JE, Burch C, Shelhamer JH et al: A circulating myocardial depressant substance in humans with septic shock: Septic shock patients with a reduced ejection fraction have a circulating factor that depresses *in vitro* myocardial cell performance. J Clin Invest 76:1539, 1985.
19. Pirovino M, Meister F, Rubli E et al: Preserved cytosolic and synthetic liver function in jaundice of severe extrahepatic infection. Gastroenterology 96:1589, 1989.
20. Franson TR, Hierholzer WJ, LaBreque DR: Frequency and characteristics of hyperbilirubinemia associated with bacteremia. Rev Infect Dir 7:1, 1985.
21. Zimmerman HJ, Fang M, Utili R et al: Jaundice due to bacterial infection. Gastroenterology 77:362, 1979.
22. Colman RW, Robboy SJ, Minna JD: Disseminated intravascular coagulation: A reappraisal. Ann Rev Med 30:359, 1979.
23. Mizock B: Septic shock: A metabolic perspective. Arch Intern Med 144:579, 1984.
24. Anderson RJ, Chung H-M, Kluge R et al: Hyponatremia. A prospective analysis of its epidemiology and the pathogenetic role of vasopressin. Ann Intern Med 102:164, 1985.
25. Dreyfuss D, Leviel F, Paillard M et al: Acute infectious pneumonia is accompanied by a latent vasopressin-dependent impairment of renal water excretion. Am Rev Respir Dis 138:583, 1988.
26. Zaloga GP, Chernow B: The multifactorial basis for hypocalcemia during sepsis. Ann Intern Med 107:36, 1987.
27. Veterans Administration Systemic Sepsis Cooperative Study Group: Effect of high-dose glucocorticoid therapy on mortality in patients with clinical signs of systemic sepsis. N Engl J Med 317:659, 1987.
28. Bone RC, Fisher CJ, Clemmer TP et al: A controlled trial of high-dose methylprednisolone in the treatment of severe sepsis and septic shock. N Engl J Med 317:653, 1987.
29. Ziegler EJ, McCutchan JA, Fierer J et al: Treatment of gram-negative bacteremia and shock with human antiserum to a mutant *Escherichia coli*. N Engl J Med 307:1225, 1982.
30. Tandberg D, Sklar D: Effect of tachypnea on the estimation of body temperature by an oral thermometer. N Engl J Med 308:945, 1983.
31. Morris DL, Chambers HF, Morris MG et al: Hemodynamic characteristics of patients with hypothermia due to occult infection and other causes. Ann Intern Med 102:153, 1985.
32. Tracey KJ, Fong Y, Hesse DG et al: Anti-cachectin/TNF monoclonal antibodies prevent septic shock during lethal bacteremia. Nature 330:662, 1987.

Chapter 56

THE SYNDROME OF HYPERMETABOLISM AND MULTIPLE SYSTEM ORGAN FAILURE

FRANK B. CERRA

KEY POINTS

- *Multisystem organ failure (MSOF) is a clinical syndrome that is manifest primarily as lung, liver, and renal failure.*
- *A patient with MSOF usually has a history of shock and resuscitation followed by a period of stable hypermetabolism.*
- *The risk factors for developing MSOF appear to be persistent shock, infection, inflammation, and dead or injured tissue.*
- *The irreversible form of the process is characterized by adult respiratory distress syndrome (ARDS) and progressively rising serum bilirubin and creatinine levels.*
- *Nosocomial infections usually occur during the clinical course of the disease, irrespective of the etiologic event.*
- *Once resuscitation has occurred, the presence of the cellular injury takes 7 to 10 days to appear clinically, and is poorly reflected in injury severity scores performed at or within several days of ICU admission.*
- *The postresuscitation phase of the MSOF process is characterized by a hyperdynamic physiology, hypermetabolic metabolism, and adequate availability of energy produced by the process of aerobic glycolysis.*
- *The pathogenesis of MSOF appears to reside in dysregulation of metabolism and microcirculatory physiology.*
- *Current therapy consists of source control, restoration and maintenance of oxygen transport, and nutritional and metabolic support.*
- *Future therapies might be designed to prevent the process from being initiated and to modulate the cellular components of inflammation and repair.*

Single organ failure has long been recognized as a cause of morbidity and mortality in surgical patients. In trauma centers in the late 1960s a new form of organ failure was recognized, that of sequential failure of lung, liver, and kidney, usually followed by death. By the mid 1970s, the syndrome of MSOF postinjury was well described[1–4] and had been observed following other etiologies such as ruptured abdominal aortic aneurysm[5] and infection.[6,7]

This distinction between isolated organ failure postinjury and the syndrome of MSOF is a relatively new clinical differential. It was recognized that although MSOF occurred in only a small fraction of polytrauma patients, it was a major cause of late mortality after trauma. In the setting of surgical sepsis, progressive MSOF continues to carry a high mortality risk, approaching 75 to 90 percent after septic shock. ARDS also occurs after a variety of etiologies and carries a mortality risk of 40 to 80 percent. It is increasingly recognized that death in this setting is frequently from the systemic process of MSOF.[8,9]

MSOF occurs in several time-dependent phases and patterns. The biology of MSOF also changes with time. In the initial shock and resuscitation phases, perfusion and oxygen transport appear central to injury development, with the endothelial cell the target cell. In the hypermetabolism-organ failure phase, the biology seems to involve mechanisms of metabolic regulation with the macrophage a key target cell. Current management consists of source control, resuscitation, and nutrition/metabolic support. Newer therapies are being developed based on the biology of the syndrome. In the clinical setting, each of the therapies necessitates trade-offs in its application. In turn, these trade-offs necessitate a clear understanding by critical care practitioners of the interaction of various disease states and our treatment of them.

This chapter will review the syndrome of MSOF including natural history, pathophysiology, metabolic dysregulation, microbiology, pathogenesis, and treatment modalities.

Natural History

In the surgical ICU, typical clinical patterns of MSOF have emerged.[6,7] The events initiating hypermetabolism include severe hemorrhage, sepsis, tissue injury or ischemia, and severe inflammation such as in pancreatitis. Common to all of these events is a relative or absolute perfusion deficit that may or may not be associated with the usual clinical signs of circulatory insufficiency such as hypotension and oliguria. The rapidity and adequacy of the resuscitation appears to be a major determinant of whether or not the patient will proceed to hypermetabolism and MSOF. A period of relative hemodynamic stability is then entered that is characterized by persistent hypermetabolism and is usually associated with some form of lung injury. If the process is not reversed, it progresses over a period of 14 to 21 days to MSOF and eventually death (Fig. 56-1, Table 56-1).

The clinical features of hypermetabolism include fever, leukocytosis, tachycardia, oliguria, and tachypnea. Lung infiltrates on chest x-ray and progressive arterial hypoxemia characterize the respiratory failure that is an integral feature of the syndrome. Mechanical ventilation with a high fraction inspired oxygen ($F_{I_{O_2}}$) and positive end-expiratory pressure (PEEP) are usually required. The patients are hyperdynamic with a cardiac index (CI) often exceeding 4.5 L/min/m^2, a decreased systemic vascular resistance (SVR) (often below 600 dyne/sec/cm^5), hyperglycemia, hyperlactatemia, elevated oxygen consumption index often exceeding 180 mL/min/m^2, and an elevated urinary urea nitrogen excretion often exceeding 15 g/day. This array of clinical and hemodynamic findings is identical to that seen

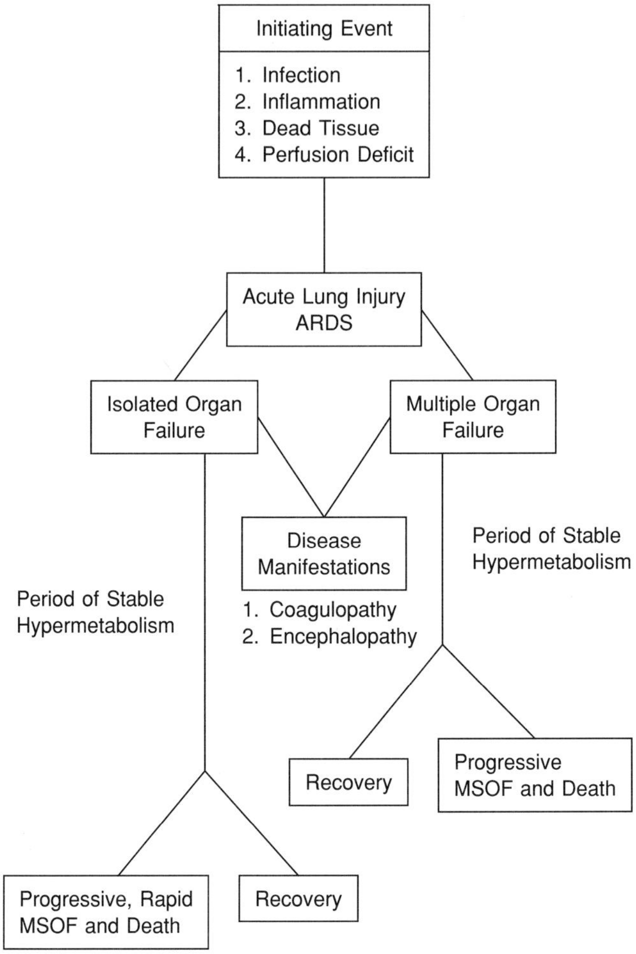

FIGURE 56-1 Following an initiating event, ARDS occurs as an isolated organ failure or as part of multiple organ injury. In both cases, after appropriate resuscitation, a period of stability is entered in which the patient is both hyperdynamic and hypermetabolic. In the ARDS-dominant pathway, MSOF is telescoped into the few days preceding death. In the multiple organ pathway, liver and renal dysfunction are present with the ARDS. After a period of stability, progressive organ failure ensues over several days and death occurs.

in surgical sepsis. Sepsis is distinct from hypermetabolism or "sepsis syndrome" only in that sepsis is associated with a documented bacterial, fungal, or viral etiology.

Following shock and resuscitation, control of the inciting source and supportive measures are associated with recovery of most patients. In a smaller group of patients, a phase of persistent hypermetabolism is entered. Once activated, even in the presence of control of the inciting source, this hypermetabolic phase can persist for 14 to 21 days. In those patients who recover, the hypermetabolism spontaneously abates. The mortality rate for this phase of persistent hypermetabolism is in the 25 to 40 percent range.

Most MSOF occurs in two forms relative to the initiating event (see Fig. 56-1). In the first form, frequently seen after a primary pulmonary event such as aspiration, the MSOF is a terminal event, becoming manifest only within a few days of death. In the second form, as in the case of septic shock with ARDS, the MSOF is present nearly from the time of injury, but does not become progressive for 7 to 14 days after injury. The onset of progressive MSOF is heralded by the onset of progressive jaundice and hyperbilirubinemia, usually by 6 to 10 days postinjury, and the onset of progressive renal failure with a rising serum creatinine value, usually 10 to 14 days postinjury (Table 56-2).

TABLE 56-2 Epidemiologic Characteristics of MSOF

	SURVIVED		EXPIRED	
Demographic	Mean	SE	Mean	SE
Age, years	49.2	4.4	60.3	2.6
ICU stay, days	11.0	4.4	17.1	1.2
Ventilator days	7.5	2.2	15.2	1.3
Hospital stay, days	23.3	2.9	27.8	2.0

	NUMBER OF INFECTIONS/PATIENT			
Nosocomial Infections	Total	Gram +	Gram −	Fungus
Survived	.54	.13	.33	.04
Died				
MSOF	1.4	.4	.44	.50
Non-MSOF	.43	.19	.25	0

	SURVIVED		EXPIRED	
Discriminator of Survival	Mean	SE	Mean	SE
$Pa_{O_2}:FI_{O_2}$	311	25	233	14
Lactate mg/dL	1.1	.2	3.4	.7
Bilirubin mg/dL	2.2	.6	8.5	2.2
Creatinine mg/dL	1.9	.6	2.9	.3

	OUTCOME
Persistent hypermetabolism	65% mortality
Progressive MSOF	95% mortality

TABLE 56-1 Overview of Clinical Stages of MSOF

Clinical Stage	Physiology	Therapy
Shock and resuscitation	Oxygen transport	Source control Resuscitation Nutrition
Hypermetabolism MSOF	Altered metabolic regulation	Modulation of inflammation, repair, and immune function

Several clinical settings are associated with the transition from hypermetabolism to organ failure. These include a persistent perfusion deficit (often unrecognized), a persistent focus of infection, the combination of a perfusion deficit and a persistent or new septic focus (e.g., recurrent episodes of septic shock), and a persistent inflammatory focus in the absence of infection, such as acute fulminant pancreatitis.

The terminal phase of MSOF is felt to represent clinical hepatic failure.[1,2,9–12] The data consistent with this hypothesis include the progressive jaundice, biliary stasis, reduced hepatic amino acid extraction, and reduced hepatic and total body protein synthesis, increased hepatic triglyceride production with reduced peripheral triglyceride clearance, increased ureagenesis in the absence of protein loading, reduced hepatic redox potential as reflected in the β-hydroxybutyrate:acetoacetate ratio, and, terminally, a failure of glucose release and hypoglycemia, seen in the terminal phase of MSOF.

The transition to clinical MSOF is a significant prognostic event. It heralds a change in mortality from the 25 to 40 percent range to the 40 to 60 percent range in the early stage and to the 90 to 100 percent range in the late stage of MSOF. Patients who survive hypermetabolism and MSOF are in a markedly debilitated state, even with the use of aggressive nutrition support throughout the entire course. A hallmark of this debilitation is the reduced skeletal muscle mass, which disappears so rapidly as to cause the phenomenon to be termed autocannibalism.[13] All muscle groups are affected. Consequently, weight-bearing and exercise are major rehabilitation problems. Frequently muscle power is insufficient to support ventilation even at low minute ventilation requirements, necessitating prolonged periods of ventilatory support. Rehabilitation becomes a long, slow process of rebuilding skeletal muscle mass, joint stability, and bone strength.

A form of peripheral neuropathy has been identified as a sequelum of hypermetabolism and MSOF.[14] The problem is characterized by a motor and sensory peripheral neuropathy together with evidence of skeletal muscle denervation. The clinical presentation is frequently one of failure to wean from the ventilator even after resolution of the hypermetabolism, together with inordinate muscle weakness. The cause is unknown, although some have speculated on the relationship to use of neuromuscular blocking agents. The treatment is supportive.

Admission severity indexing poorly predicts which patients will subsequently develop MSOF.[15] There are several reasons for this observation. **1.** Most surgical patients are postresuscitative when they enter the ICU. **2.** The injury in MSOF is at the cellular level where current severity indexes are not sensitive. **3.** The cellular injury takes time to develop. Over time various metabolic predictive variables may be useful and include the $Pa_{O_2}:FI_{O_2}$ ratio (early, day 1); the plasma lactate level (early, day 2), the serum bilirubin value (later, day 6), and the serum creatinine concentration (late, day 12 postinjury) (Table 56-2).

Pathophysiology

The systemic response is heralded by an increase in oxygen consumption.[11,16–18] This demand must be met by an increase in supply, with a consequent increase in cardiac output and minute ventilation. The high flow state is accompanied by a fall in SVR, a phenomenon referred to as the vascular tone abnormality of sepsis or sepsis syndrome. The absence of this hyperdynamic response is associated with an increased mortality risk and usually occurs for one of three reasons: inadequate preload, preexisting cardiac disease, or an acquired cardiac dysfunction. This latter phenomenon has only recently been described and consists of dilation of the ventricles, reduced diastolic compliance, and reduced systolic contractile function.[19,20] This cardiovascular response is also associated with an increase in vascular capacitance, further necessitating an expansion of blood volume to maintain adequate preload.

The decrease in SVR is independent of flow and may be a response to the primary increase in oxygen consumption demand.[21,22] This reduction in vascular resistance, however, is not homogeneous in all vascular beds. In the acute, unresuscitated shock state, flow is markedly reduced in the visceral compartment and increased in the muscle compartments. In the adequately resuscitated state, large fractions of flow go to the skeletal muscle and visceral compartments. This increase in visceral compartment blood flow and oxygen consumption may predict for survival.[23] The putative need for this increased visceral perfusion may relate to the synthetic activity present in this compartment, particularly hepatic amino acid clearance and protein synthesis. Failures of central amino acid clearance and hepatic protein synthesis both seem to be major determinants of mortality.[4,24]

As the patient proceeds toward organ failure, an oxygen extraction failure appears in the peripheral microcirculation. This is signaled by a rise in mixed venous hemoglobin saturation and a narrowing of the arteriovenous oxygen content difference $(a - v)_{O_2}$. It is not known how often this phenomenon occurs, nor whether it is secondary to a maldistribution of the high cardiac output or to a defect in the ability of tissues to extract oxygen. Many consider that the elevated lactate of MSOF confirms the extraction defect, but this increased lactate is not associated with the other metabolic characteristics of anaerobic metabolism. This problem increases in severity as the organ failure process worsens. Eventually, perfusion failure again becomes a dominant problem, tissue ischemia occurs, and death usually ensues.

Metabolic Dysregulation

Patients who develop MSOF generally proceed through the phases of shock, resuscitation, stable hypermetabolism, and then progressive MSOF. In the phase of stable postresuscitative hypermetabolism in which the plasma lactate level is usually elevated, the metabolic data indicate that energy production and availability are adequate. This energy, however, does not appear to be supplied in the usual form by Krebs cycle oxidation, and the carbon sources include substrates other than glucose alone. This form of energy production is referred to as *aerobic glycolysis*. This section will present the human data supporting these interpretations.

Energy expenditure is increased and is reflected in increased oxygen consumption and carbon dioxide production. The endogenous respiratory quotient (RQ) ranges from 0.78 to 0.82, reflecting a mixed fuel source, i.e., the carbon source for oxidative production of adenosine triphosphate (ATP) is not glucose alone, but rather a mixture of carbohydrate, fat, and amino acids. Because of the increase in total energy expenditure to 1.5 to 2.0 times basal energy expenditure, there is an absolute increase in the amount of glucose and fat oxidized relative to a comparable period of starvation. The fats oxidized are long-, medium-, and short-chain fatty acids. The carbohydrate carbon sources include glucose, glycerol, and lactate. The amino acids oxidized for energy production are predominantly the branched-chain amino acids, leucine, isoleucine, and valine. Amino acid oxidation appears to occur primarily in skeletal muscle. The production of ATP is efficiently maintained as long as appropriate resuscitation has occurred. A true failure of energy production seems to only occur during perfusion shock phase (see Fig. 56-1) and as a terminal event in MSOF.[1,2]

The increased energy expenditure in the phase of postresuscitative hypermetabolism may result from aerobic glycolysis (Fig. 56-2, Table 56-3). There are significant increases in plasma lactate and pyruvate with a normal lactate:pyruvate (L:P) ratio. There is a marked increase in the release of lactate and pyruvate from muscle, peripheral tissue, and the mononuclear cell mass. Thus, the cytosol redox potential may be normal. An index of the mitochondrial redox potential is the ratio of β-hydroxybutyrate:acetoacetate. When this ratio is evaluated in this phase, it is likewise within normal limits. The oxidation of pyruvate appears to be reduced, with a reduced activity of pyruvate dehydrogenase associated with it. There is increased oxidation of tricarboxylic acid (TCA) cycle fuels, primarily two carbon fat fragments and amino acids. There is a marked increase in the formation of alanine and glutamine from the alpha amino group that is released when the amino acids enter the TCA cycle. This amino-

TABLE 56-3 Characteristics of Aerobic Glycolysis during Postresuscitative Hypermetabolism

1. Adequate energy availability as evaluated from high energy phosphate levels and measurements of substrate oxidation rates and the rates of release of alanine and glutamine
2. Normal cytosol redox potential as evaluated by the L:P ratio
3. Functional mitochondrial redox potential as evaluated by the β-hydroxybutyrate:acetoacetate ratio
4. Reduction in the activity of pyruvate dehydrogenase and an associated reduction in the fractional oxidation of glucose
5. Increased fractional oxidation of amino acids and fatty acids

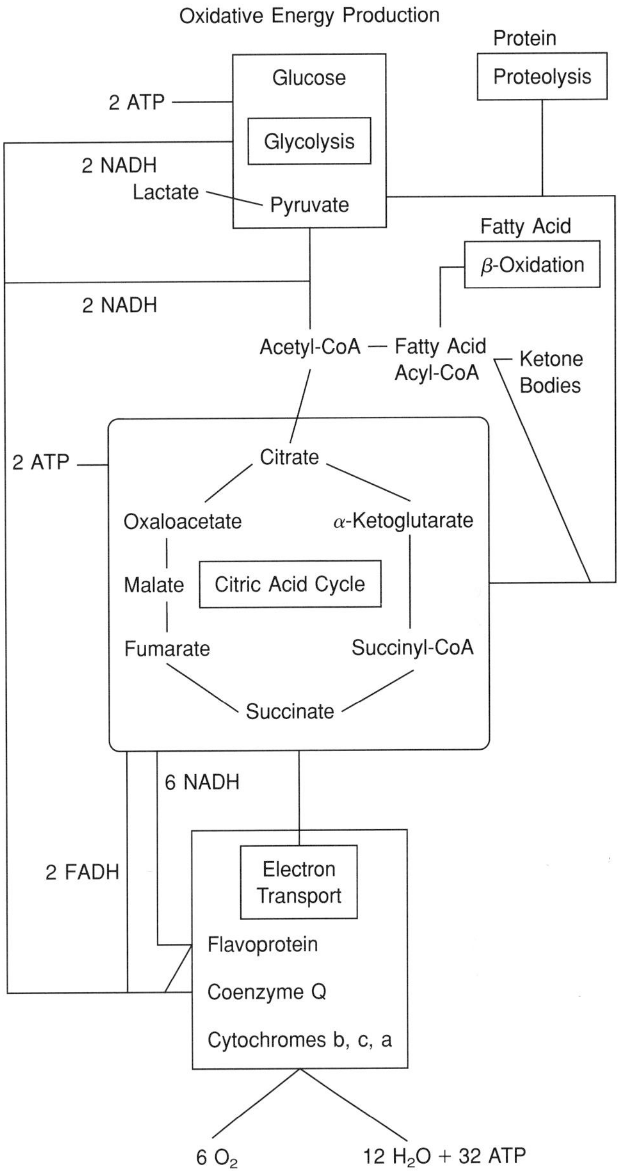

FIGURE 56-2 The majority of energy production occurs in the Krebs cycle. The production of energy is a function of relative redox states, i.e., the ability to transfer electrons and protons with the ultimate formation of carbon dioxide and water. Glycolysis occurs in the cytosol, Krebs cycle, and electron transport in the mitochondria. In anaerobic glycolysis, pyruvate and alternate carbon sources (protein and fat) do not enter the Krebs cycle, and excess lactate is formed relative to pyruvate. In the aerobic states, the major differences occur in the carbon sources that enter the Krebs cycle for energy production. In starvation, the early source is glucose and the adapted source is fat. In aerobic glycolysis, there is a reduction in the amount of pyruvate entering the Krebs cycle. The amino acid and two carbon fat fragments provide the carbon sources for the Krebs cycle and energy production is normal. The result is increased lactate, pyruvate, and alanine release with normal redox states in the cytosolic and mitochondrial compartments. CoA, coenzyme A; NADH, reduced nicotinamide-adenine dinucleotide; FADH, reduced flavin adenine dinucleotide.

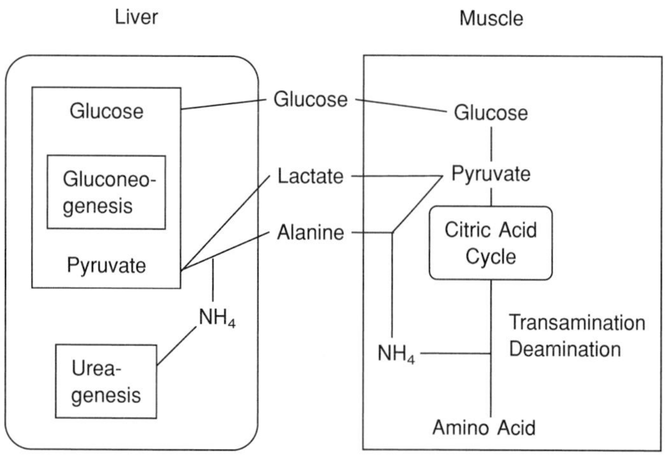

FIGURE 56-3 The Cori and alanine cycles are presented. The functions of these cycles are to transfer nitrogen from the periphery to the liver, to provide 3-carbon fragments for gluconeogenesis in the liver, and to produce heat. Both cycles are poor sources of net energy production. The amount of urea excreted becomes a marker for the amount of peripheral catabolism in the lean body mass.

nitrogen combines with lactate to form alanine and is transaminated with glutamate to form glutamine. There is a marked increase in the release of these two nitrogen carriers from peripheral tissue (Fig. 56-3). At least in the case of alanine, this release is stoichiometric with the release of lactate and pyruvate. Thus, this constellation of metabolic parameters is not consistent with persistent microcirculatory hypoxia or with persistent vascular shunting of significant magnitude to affect energy metabolism.[10,11,13]

The Cori cycle is likewise very active[8] (see Fig. 56-3). The lactate and alanine that are released are converted by the liver back into glucose that is recycled back to the periphery. This cycle produces no net energy, generates heat, and is biochemically futile. Thus, the available data are consistent with and are best explained by not an uncoupling of oxidation from phosphorylation but rather by the efficient energy production process of aerobic glycolysis in the presence of an active Cori cycle.

Hepatic glucose release is increased. This derives in part from increased gluconeogenesis and in part from increased glycogenolysis. The gluconeogenic substrates include lactate, alanine, glutamine, glycine, serine, and glycerol. A major source of this nitrogen reflected in the alanine and glutamine carriers is from amino acids whose carbon skeletons are entering the Krebs cycle for ATP production. This nitrogen and that from the other gluconeogenic amino acids entering into glucose production result in increased urea production. Gluconeogenesis appears to be driven by a number of mechanisms including the amount of substrate presented, the hormonal milieu (particularly a high glucagon : insulin ratio), and inflammatory mediators.[1,25–27]

An excess of total calories or an excess of glucose calories has a number of detrimental effects on metabolism and organ structure and function. These effects include fatty liver syndrome, hyperosmolar states, excess carbon dioxide production and oxygen consumption, stimulation of catecholamine release, increased lactate formation, a failure to suppress gluconeogenesis, a failure to alter catabolic or synthetic rates, and increased gas production and bowel distention when used enterally. Not exceeding the total caloric requirement and the substitution of fat calories for glucose calories can alleviate the adverse effects of excess glucose administration.

Use of exogenous insulin in this inherently hyperinsulinemic state increases peripheral uptake of glucose but does not appear to significantly alter its oxidative pathways. As the progression into MSOF occurs, lactate and pyruvate production progressively increase but without excess lactate production until the cardiac output falls. Ultimately, glucose release fails and hypoglycemia can occur as a terminal event.[10]

After resuscitation, lipolysis is increased, presumably reflecting a marked increase in beta stimulation. Plasma ketone levels are very low even in the absence of any glucose administration. The peripheral tissue and the peripheral mitochondria appear to have an increased capacity to oxidize two carbon fragments.

The turnover of medium- and long-chain fatty acids is also increased. A picture of long-chain fatty acid deficiency develops in the plasma immediately following injury.[28–30] The increase in oleic acid can be suppressed by the administration of fat emulsions, but the reductions in linoleic and arachidonic acid are not. Exogenous lipid can increase the metabolism of arachidonic acid with an increased production of its metabolites. Long-chain fatty acid triglyceride emulsions in doses exceeding 1.5 g/kg/day have been associated with increased bacteremia rates, acute hypoxemia, and suppression of in vitro tests of lymphocyte function.[30,31]

As MSOF progresses, the endogenous RQ exceeds 1.0, indicating net lipogenesis. The site of this increased lipogenesis appears to be primarily hepatic. The peripheral clearance of triglyceride is reduced, in part reflecting a reduced lipoprotein lipase activity in skeletal muscle and adipose tissue. The plasma polyunsaturated fatty acid profile comes to resemble that reported for hepatic failure.

Total body protein catabolism is markedly increased. Total body protein synthesis is increased relative to starvation but is significantly less than the increased rate of catabolism. Thus the rate of net catabolism is high.[1,2,13] The lean body mass can become significantly depleted in 7 to 10 days. The clinical correlates of this are rapid loss of skeletal muscle mass and high urine nitrogen excretions, frequently exceeding 20 g/day. The primary sites of amino acid mobilization are from skeletal muscle, connective tissue, and unstimulated gut. The uptake of amino acids by skeletal muscle is suppressed, further potentiating the net catabolism.

The hepatic uptake of amino acids is increased and is reflected in increased hepatic protein synthesis. Certain proteins such as albumin and transferrin have selectively decreased synthesis, while others such as the acute phase reactant proteins are increased. Other locations of increased amino acid use are active sites of inflammation, wounds, and in mononuclear cells producing cytokines. One of the manifestations of this increased flux and turnover of amino acids is an increase in urea production and the clinical manifestation of prerenal azotemia that becomes aggravated as the glomerular filtration falls, even in the absence of exogenous amino acids.

The catabolic rate is not very responsive to exogenous amino acids; the total body synthetic rate, however, is. As the load of exogenous amino acids is increased, the synthetic rate can increase until it equals the catabolic rate. At that point, nitrogen equilibrium is achieved and the rate of net catabolism is minimized by increasing the rate of synthesis and not so much by decreasing the rate of catabolism. In patients who are going to survive, this stimulation of protein synthesis rates in response to exogenous amino acids is characteristic. Patients in whom this phenomenon does not occur have a much higher mortality rate.

The dominant form of nitrogen in the urine is urea. The amount of urea excreted in the urine reflects the rate of net catabolism. It also reflects the disuse of muscle in patients who are at bed rest and the loss of muscle tone in such settings as quadriplegia, muscle paralysis, and heavy sedation. In addition, as the catabolism increases, other forms of nitrogen appear in the urine, including uric acid, ammonia, and metabolic acids. Thus, the total urine nitrogen excretion is poorly predicted from the urinary urea, an important nutritional assessment consideration.[32,33]

As MSOF progresses, total body and hepatic protein synthesis rates fall and the rates of absolute and relative catabolism increase. A reflection of this is in the increased rate of ureagenesis and the increased prerenal azotemia. In these latter phases, exogenous amino acid support is of little therapeutic benefit.

Microbiology

A number of etiologic events can initiate the hypermetabolism-organ failure response. One of these is infection. Irrespective of the etiologic event, however, nosocomial infections eventually present during the course of the disease. The origin of most of these nosocomial infections seems to be the patient's own flora, particularly that residing within the gastrointestinal tract. This section will discuss infection as an etiologic process and nosocomial infection as an event in the organ failure process. Although different infecting agents can produce variations in local inflammatory reactions, when the systemic response occurs, there seems to be little or no difference in the patterns of physiologic and metabolic response among the types of infecting organisms. Patients with gram-negative, gram-positive, aerobic, and polymicrobial bacterial sepsis all have similar clinical, physiologic, and metabolic characteristics. Viral sepsis as seen with cytomegalo-virus and fungal sepsis as seen with *Candida* species are also indistinguishable in their physiology from bacterial sepsis.[34,35]

The physiologic and metabolic responses observed following severe perfusion deficits (e.g., ruptured aneurysms) or following inflammation (e.g., pancreatitis or the tissue injury of polytrauma) are indistinguishable from those of microbial-induced hypermetabolism. These observations have led to the classification of a systemic inflammatory response called *sepsis* in the presence of an identified infecting source with an identified bacterial agent and called *sepsis syndrome or hypermetabolism* when a bacterial or other infectious source cannot be identified.

Once initiated, the bacterial process during the hypermetabolism phase is somewhat stereotypical. Colonic flora begin to overgrow the upper gut and pharynx and soon colonize the lower respiratory tract. Some of the principal organisms are *Pseudomonas, Enterobacter,* and *Candida* species. *Staphylococcus epidermidis* is also frequently seen in gastric aspirate culture. Gram-negative pneumonias tend to occur during this phase, as do episodes of line sepsis.

Some evidence relates nosocomial pneumonias to this respiratory tract colonization and relates the latter to stress ulcer prophylaxis with antacids or H_2-receptor antagonists.[36] Not all studies confirm the association between gastric pH control and nosocomial pneumonias, and some have also questioned the correlation between the bacteria causing pneumonias and those cultured from the gastric aspirates.[37]

Nosocomial infections are common in MSOF patients. However, gram-negative infections do not appear to discriminate survivors from nonsurvivors. Rather, nonsurvivors have an increased incidence of gram-positive and fungus infections[9] (see Table 56-2).

Anergy and alterations in nearly all in vitro tests of immune function are usually present. In hypermetabolism and in MSOF considerable controversy exists as to whether the episodes of nosocomial infection are symptoms of MSOF or the causes of it. The clinical impression is that one can usually cure the immediate infection with antimicrobial agents but that the MSOF metabolic processes will continue. Clinical studies on gut and oral cavity bacterial decontamination and antifungal prophylaxis as a means of reducing the incidence of enteric organism-induced pneumonias and septic episodes indicate that the incidence of nosocomial infections can be significantly reduced but that there is not an associated reduction in MSOF or mortality.[38,39] More data must be generated before a consensus can be reached.

Pathogenesis

A number of factors can initiate hypermetabolism. Dead or injured tissue, infection, and shock are currently recognized etiologic events. At least three mediator systems can translate the injury into a recognizable response: the central nervous system, the classic endocrine system, and the cell-cell system.[1,39–42] It is apparent that these systems interact with each other, that a maximum response requires all three systems, that deficiencies in one system can be compensated for, and that different pathways may predominate in response to different initiating events.

Most inciting events may be classified as trauma, infection, or lack of perfusion. A local inflammatory response occurs, presumably from the products of platelet activation, endothelial injury, and tissue factor release with subsequent activation of complement, coagulation, and the kallikreine systems. The local "soup" that develops can then initiate a systemic response. Local and systemic responses can also be induced by direct action of microbial toxins or components of the microorganism. The result is the systemic inflammatory response called hypermetabolism or sepsis syndrome.

Under these conditions, metabolism is controlled largely by these mediators (Table 56-4) and becomes less responsive to other regulatory mechanisms usually operative in starvation. The consequences of metabolic changes so mediated include:

1. an obligatory rise in energy demand manifested by an increase in oxygen consumption and in an increase in carbon dioxide and metabolic acid production;
2. gluconeogenesis and lipolysis that is much less responsive to downregulation by exogenous glucose;
3. energy production by the process of aerobic glycolysis; and
4. a change in body composition characterized by an unrelenting reduction in lean body mass that is poorly responsive to exogenous amino acids and anabolic hormone modulation; and by a redistribution of the body nitrogen to areas of active protein synthesis such as the viscera, wounds, and white blood cell mass.

TABLE 56-4 Potential Mediators of Hypermetabolism and MSOF

Cytokines
Interleukin 1–8
Interferon g
Platelet activating factor
Tumor necrosis factor
Eicosanoids
Prostaglandins (PGE_1, PGE_2, PGI_2)
Thromboxanes (TXA_2)
Leukotrienes (LTC_4, LTD_4)
Mediator Amines
Histamine
Serotonin
Epinephrine
Norepinephrine
Octopamine
Opioids/Other Neurotransmitters
Hormonal Amines/Peptides
Thyroxine
Growth hormone
Insulin
Glucagon
Catecholamine
Cortisol
Cortical releasing factors
Complement
Kinin
Fibronectin
Growth Factors
Enzymes
Proteases (acid and neutral)
Other Lysosomal enzymes
Nitric Oxide (derived from L-arginine)
Oxygen-Derived Intermediates

The transition from hypermetabolism to MSOF is a significant clinical and prognostic event and probably signals overt cell injury. The mechanisms of cell injury are multiple and include microcirculatory hypoxia, injury from inflammation, and microbial toxin-induced injury. When systemic resuscitation is inadequate, hypoxia may exist in the microcirculation. The available data would support the position that following resuscitation by current criteria, muscle perfusion is adequately restored, but visceral perfusion may not have been adequately achieved.[11,16–18,23]

Mediator-induced injury also seems to occur. White blood cell-mediated endothelial damage is a well-described phenomenon in acute lung injury. Oxygen radical generation with injury is a potential mechanism for reperfusion injury to intracellular organelles and membrane signal transduction mechanisms.[43] Excessive PGE_2 production is immunosuppressive and may potentiate infectious complications.[44] Leukotriene can cause profound cardiac contractility depression. Microbial toxins or components can cause cell injury. Endotoxin can directly inhibit intracellular glycolytic enzymes and can directly alter hepatocyte protein synthesis.[45] It can also produce indirect effects by stimulating the macrophage which then can alter target cell function.[46]

Another mechanism of injury is best categorized as metabolic dysregulation. In this model, products of metabolism in one area adversely alter metabolism in another area. As an example, plasma proteases may hydrolyse peptide mediators into smaller peptides that are also metabolically active. A major proteolytic inducing factor may be a peptide derived from interleukin-1 (IL-1).[47] Octopamine is a vasoactive amine derived from the nonoxidative metabolism of phenylalanine that can induce the low SVR and high cardiac output state.

Current Therapy and Future Directions

Current therapy of MSOF is aimed at prevention and at supportive care. Three general areas are emphasized—source control, restoration and maintenance of oxygen transport, and metabolic support.[2] Source control is a major emphasis because persistence of a source guarantees a high mortality risk from MSOF. Whenever possible, excision or removal of the inciting cause is desirable, as in early fracture fixation, abscess drainage, removal of an infected uterus, and full-thickness burn excision and skin grafting. In many cases, however, this is not possible (e.g., primary pneumonias, pancreatitis, soft tissue injury, and hematoma). Appropriate antimicrobial agents are particularly important where the septic focus cannot be removed. These agents are usually effective in eradicating these foci.

With the possibility of subclinical flow-dependent oxygen consumption in settings of pancreatitis, ARDS, sepsis, and hypovolemic shock, increased emphasis is being placed on invasive techniques of resuscitation using oxygen consumption criteria.[16–18,21,22] The usual clinical criteria of resuscitation, (i.e., pulse, blood pressure, urine output, skin perfusion) do not appear adequate to judge when oxygen delivery is adequate, at least from the total body perspective. Invasive monitoring during the shock-resuscitation phase with flow measurements and manipulations to increase oxygen delivery may improve outcome following resuscitation. Flow-dependent oxygen consumption is treated with a comprehensive approach. Oxygen content is increased by maintaining an arterial oxygen tension that will maintain over 90% saturation of the hemoglobin and maintaining a hemoglobin in the 13 g/dL range. Oxygen consumption is then measured and flow increased consecutively until there is no significant increase in oxygen consumption and the L:P ratio returns to a normal range. Flow is increased with a combination of preload, afterload reduction, and inotropic support modalities. Pre- and postoperative studies continue to indicate a decrease in mortality, infectious complications, and MSOF when these principles are used.[21,22,48]

Malnutrition is one of the primary manifestations of MSOF. It seems increasingly clear that nutrition support per se does not alter the course of underlying disease but can effectively control single nutrient and generalized nutrient deficiency. With such support, reductions in morbidity and mortality have been observed.[1,2,10] To effectively achieve these ends, several principles have evolved.

1. Avoid excess total calories and excess glucose by providing 25 to 30 kcal/kg/day with 3 to 5 g/kg/day as glucose, maintaining an RQ under 0.9.
2. Restrict fat emulsion (n-6 polyunsaturated fatty acids) to 0.5 to 1.0 g/kg/day to avoid fat overload syndromes and iatrogenic immunosuppression.
3. Achieve nitrogen equilibrium by adjusting the dose of amino acids. Current clinical studies indicate that the modified amino acids are a more efficient protein source and can facilitate nitrogen retention with a higher rate of protein synthesis and less ureagenesis than the standard amino acid formulas.
4. Achieve a rising or normal range of hepatic protein synthesis as reflected in the plasma transferrin or prealbumin.
5. Provide the necessary vitamins, minerals, trace elements, and micronutrients.

TABLE 56-5 Summary of Therapies in Clinical Testing

Rationale	Therapy
1. *Treatment of Infection*	1. Monoclonal antibodies against endotoxin 2. Passive antibody protection 3. Gut decontamination regimens to prevent nosocomial infections
2. *Support of Gut Function*	1. Mucosal stimulating agents: glutamine, bombesin, ketone bodies, epidermal growth factor 2. Early enteral feeding
3. *Improved Resuscitation*	1. Hypertonic saline 2. In-line sensors 3. Tissue-specific sensors 4. Noninvasive monitoring
4. *Endothelial Cell Protection*	1. Platelet activating factor inhibitors 2. WBC adherence inhibition 3. Antioxidant therapy 4. Eicosanoid modulation 5. Monoclonal antibodies directed against cytokines and cell surface receptors
5. *Modulation of Macrophage Function*	1. n-3 polyunsaturated fatty acids 2. Signal transduction modulation
6. *Stimulation of Lymphocyte Function*	1. Arginine 2. n-3 polyunsaturated fatty acids

The newer experimental approaches to therapy are based on modulation of inflammation and repair or more efficient and effective control of the initiating cause of MSOF. Based on experimental data bases, a number of new support and therapeutic regimens are in clinical testing (Table 56-5). Clinical trials of single-agent chemotherapy such as insulin, steroids, PGE_1, and the enteral route of nutrition have shown no significant improvement in survival or the occurrence of MSOF. Experimental studies with other single-agent chemotherapies are continuing to produce conflicting results. It appears as if there is no "magic bullet." Some encouraging results with experimental combination chemotherapy are beginning to be reported. Hopefully some of these newer approaches will provide improved therapeutic or support regimens.

CASE PRESENTATION

The patient was a 65-year-old, well-nourished man who entered the hospital with left lower quadrant pain, localized peritonitis, fever, and hemodynamic stability. He was treated with fluids and a third generation cephalosporin. One day later, his peritonitis was worse, his blood pressure fell to 90/60 mmHg, with a pulse of 120 beats/min, and he became oliguric. He was taken to the operating room, was found to have a ruptured sigmoid diverticulitis with peritonitis, and underwent a sigmoid resection with end-colostomy and Hartmann pouch. He was given more fluids and an aminoglycoside was added to the antibiotic regimen. On day 2, his hemodynamic status had not improved and he was transferred to a tertiary care center.

On ICU admission, the patient was responsive with blood pressure of 110/40 mmHg, pulse of 125 beats/min, and respiratory rate of 25. The extremities were warm with bounding pulses. The abdomen was slightly distended and tender as expected for his postoperative state. Bilateral interstitial infiltrates were noted on chest x-ray. The $Pa_{O_2}:FI_{O_2}$ ratio was 180 on mask oxygen of 60%. Pertinent laboratory data included a serum bilirubin of 2 mg/dL, an L:P ratio of 75, and an arterial pH of 7.29, with a Pa_{CO_2} of 30 mmHg. The hemoglobin was 12 g/dL, WBC count 15,500/mm^3, and the admission APACHE score was 13. He produced 30 mL urine for the first hour after ICU admission.

He was intubated and started on positive-pressure ventilation when gas exchange deteriorated. The endotracheal tube suckings and chest radiograph were consistent with ARDS. A pulmonary artery catheter was placed. The pulmonary capillary wedge pressure (PCWP) was 9 mmHg, CI 3.5 L/min/m^2, SVR 750 dyne/sec/cm^5, and oxygen consumption 140 mL/min/m^2. He was volume loaded and repeat measurements included PCWP 18 mmHg, CI 4.3 mL/m^2, SVR 700 dyne/sec/m^5, and oxygen consumption 175 mL/min/m^2. At this time the arterial lactate was 3.0 mg/dL and L:P ratio 50, with pH 7.35 and Pa_{CO_2} 35 mmHg. Dobutamine was begun and more fluids administered. Repeat studies revealed CI 6.0 L/min/m^2, SVR 600 dyne/sec/cm^5, oxygen consumption 198 mL/min/m^2 with a PCWP of 18 mmHg and arterial lactate 2.5 mg/dL and L:P ratio of 20 with pH 7.4 and Pa_{CO_2} 36 mmHg. Urine output was 1.2 mL/kg/h. Enteral nutrition was begun with a feeding tube passed beyond the pylorus. Initial feedings consisted of 2.0 g/kg/day of modified amino acids, 30 kcal/kg/day with 1.0 g/kg/day fat, and 4 g/kg/day glucose with multivitamins, magnesium, zinc, and trace elements.

Three days later microbiologic cultures were reported as growing no pathogens, and the patient was stable with mechanical ventilatory support. The serum bilirubin level was 2.5 mg/dL, glucose 195 mg/dL, and creatinine 2.0 mg/dL. The oxygen consumption was 210 mL/min/m^2, with a CI of 6.5 mL/min/m^2, $(a - v)_{O_2}$ of 3.2 vol %, and an arterial lactate of 1.8 mg/dL and L:P ratio of 15. Evidence of infection persisted with a temperature of 101°F (38.3°C) and WBC of 13,000/mm^3 with left shift. A computed tomography scan of the abdomen revealed a pelvic fluid collection. A percutaneous tap removed clear, yellow fluid with a negative Gram stain and no growth on culture. Antibiotics were continued.

On day 7 after ICU admission, the serum bilirubin was 8 mg/dL, the creatinine 2.8 mg/dL, temperature 101°F (38.3°C), WBC 10,000/mm^3, and gram-positive cocci were cultured from the blood. The lines were changed and gram-positive antibiotic coverage was begun. A *Pseudomonas* species was recovered from a tracheal aspirate, a more dense area was observed on chest x-ray, and WBCs were abundant in the tracheal secretions. The antibiotics were adjusted to reflect the in vitro antibiotic sensitivities of this organism.

The patient became encephalopathic and developed disseminated intravascular coagulopathy with thrombocytopenia. He continued to require mechanical ventilation. His nitrogen balance was negative 1.0 g/day, serum albumin 2.5 g/dL and BUN 100 mg/dL. A PCWP of 17 mmHg and inotropic support were titrated to maintain an arterial lactate value under 2.0 mg/dL with an oxygen consumption that ranged from 175 to 195 mL/min/m^2. The RQ was 0.9. The remainder of the clinical course was one of progressive MSOF and death. Dialysis was not instituted.

CASE DISCUSSION

In many respects, this case is typical of the patient with a hypermetabolic state and MSOF. The initial insult was sepsis from an abdominal source. To the extent that source control is important in limiting progression of hypermetabolism and related organ failure, even the modest delay in definitive surgical drainage may have set the stage for subsequent progression.

As has been noted, persistence of a hypoperfused state, as suggested by this patient's hemodynamics determined at the time of right heart catheterization, may be a risk factor for subsequent evolution of MSOF. As is often seen, acute hypoxemic respiratory failure followed closely on the heels of sepsis, and the patient exhibited a flow dependent oxygen consumption that has been suggested by some clinical studies to typify the response to volume loading and vasoactive drug use.

Nutritional support was started early with total calorie and specific composition guidelines directed at minimizing catabolism. The patient then entered a "stable hypermetabolism" that has been described in many postoperative and trauma patients. By the seventh hospital day evidence of lung colonization and conceivably lung infection appeared. Despite appropriate adjustment of antibiotics and continued supportive therapy, the patient made a transition to MSOF. Consistent with the general observation in these patients of an extremely poor prognosis, he died.

References

1. Cerra F: Hypermetabolism, organ failure, and metabolic support. Surgery 101(1):1, 1987.
2. Cerra FB: The syndrome of multiple organ failure, in Cerra FB, Bihari D (eds): *New Horizon III: Cell Injury and Organ Failure.* Fullerton, CA, Society of Critical Care Medicine, 1988, pp 1–14.
3. McMenany RC, Birkhahn R, Oswald G, et al: Multiple systems organ failure I: The basal state. J Trauma 21(2):99, 1981.

4. Moyer ED, Border JR, Cerra FB, et al: Multiple systems organ failure V: Alterations in the plasma proteins as a function of amino acid infusion in the trauma septic patient: Contrasts between survival and death. J Trauma 21:645, 1981.
5. Tilney N, Bailey G, Morgan A: Sequential systems failure after rupture of abdominal aortic aneurysms. Ann Surgery 118:117, 1973.
6. Pine RW, Wertz MJ, Lennard ES, et al: Determinants of organ malfunction or death in patients with intraabdominal sepsis. Arch Surgery 118:242, 1983.
7. Baue AE: Multiple, progressive or sequential systems failure: A syndrome of the 1970's. Arch Surgery 110:779, 1975.
8. Petty PE: ARDS: Definition and historical perspective. Clin Chest Med 3:3, 1982.
9. Pepe PE, Porkin RT: Clinical predictors of ARDS. Am J Surgery 144:124, 1982.
10. Cerra FB, Siegel JH, Border JR, et al: The hepatic failure of sepsis: Cellular vs. substrate. Surgery 86:409, 1979.
11. Siegel JH, Cerra FB, Border JR, et al: Physiological and metabolic correlation in human sepsis. Surgery 806:409, 1979.
12. Walvatne C, Cerra FB: Hepatic dysfunction in multiple organ failure, in Deitch EA (ed): *Multiple Organ Failure: Pathophysiology and Basic Concepts of Therapy.* New York, Thieme, 1990, pp 241–260.
13. Cerra FB, Siegel JH, Colman B, et al: Autocannibalism, a failure of exogenous nutritional support. Ann Surgery 192:570, 1980.
14. Bolton C, Young G: Sepsis and septic shock. Central and peripheral nervous systems, in Sibbald W, Sprung C (eds): *New Horizons: Perspectives in Sepsis and Septic Shock.* Fullerton, CA, Society of Critical Care Medicine, 1985, pp 157–171.
15. Cerra FB, Abrams J, Negro F: APACHE II score does not predict MOFS or mortality in postoperative patients. Arch Surgery 125:519, 1990.
16. Bihari D, Smithies M, Gimson A, et al: The effects of vasodilation with prostacyclin on oxygen delivery and uptake in critically ill patients. New Engl J Med 317:397, 1987.
17. Gutierrez G, Pohil R: Oxygen consumption is linearly related to the oxygen supply in critically ill patients. J Crit Care Med 1:45, 1986.
18. Danek S, Lynch J, Weg J, et al: The dependence of oxygen uptake on oxygen delivery in the adult respiratory distress syndrome. Am Rev Respir Dis 122:387, 1980.
19. Danner RL, Natanson C, Suffredini AE, et al: Microbial toxins: Role in pathogenesis of septic shock and MOF, in Bihari DJ, Cerra FB (eds): *New Horizons: Multiple Organ Failure Syndrome.* Fullerton, CA, Society of Critical Care Medicine, 1989, pp 351–193.
20. Stahl TJ, Alden PB, Ring WS, et al: Sepsis induced diastolic dysfunction in chronic canine peritonitis. Am J Physiol 27(3):H625, 1990.
21. Shoemaker WC: Hemodynamic and oxygen transport patterns in septic shock: Physiologic mechanisms and therapeutic implications, in Sibbald W, Sprung C (eds): *New Horizons: Perspectives in Sepsis and Septic Shock.* Fullerton, CA, Society of Critical Care Medicine, 1985, pp. 203–234.
22. Shoemaker W, Appel PL, Kram HB: Tissue oxygen debt as a determinant of lethal and nonlethal postoperative organ failure. J Crit Care Med 16:1117, 1989.
23. Dahn MS, Lange P, Lobdell, et al: Splanchnic and total body oxygen consumption in septic and injury patients. Surgery 101:69, 1987.
24. Pearl RH, Clowes GHA, Hirsch EF, et al: Prognosis and survival as determined by visceral amino acid clearance in severe trauma. J Trauma 25:777, 1985.
25. Giovannini I, Boldrini G, Castagnato M, et al: Respiratory quotient and patterns of substrate utilization in human sepsis and trauma. JPEN 7:226, 1983.
26. Shaw JHF, Wolfe RR: Glucose and urea kinetics in patients with early and advanced gastrointestinal cancer: The response to glucose infusion, parenteral feeding, and surgical resection. Surgery 101:181, 1987.
27. White RH, Frayn KN, Little RA, et al: Hormonal and metabolic responses to glucose infusion in sepsis studies by the hyperglycemic glucose clamp technique. JPEN 11:345, 1987.
28. Alden PB, Svingen BA, Deutschman CS, et al: Essential fatty acid status in isolated closed head injury. J Trauma 27:1039, 1987.
29. Alden PB, Svingen BA, Johnson SB, et al: Partial correction by exogenous lipids of abnormal patterns of polyunsaturated fatty acids in plasma phospholipids of stressed and septic surgical patients. Surgery 100:671, 1986.
30. Cerra FB, Alden PA, Negro F, et al: Sepsis, endogenous and exogenous lipid modulation. JPEN 12(6):63s, 1988.
31. Frases I, Neoptolemos J, Darby H, et al: Effects of intralipid and heparin on human monocyte and lymphocyte function. JPEN 10:381, 1986.
32. Konstantinides FN, Cerra FB: Can urinary urea nitrogen be substituted for total urinary nitrogen when calculating nitrogen balance in clinical nutrition. JPEN (suppl) 12(1):1, 1988.
33. Konstantinides F, Boehm KA, Radmer WJ, et al: Pyrochemiluminescence: Real-time cost-effective method for determining total urinary nitrogen in clinical nitrogen-balance studies. Clin Chem 34(12):2518, 1988.
34. Deutschman CS, Konstantinides FN, Tsai M, et al: Physiology and metabolism in isolated viral septicemia: Further evidence for an organism-independent, host response. Arch Surgery 122:21, 1987.
35. Wiles JB, Cerra FB, Calleri G, et al: The systemic septic response: Does the organism matter? J Crit Care Med 8(2):55, 1980.
36. Driks M, Craven DE, Bartolome R, et al: Nosocomial pneumonia in intubated patients given sucralfate as compared with antacids or histamine type 2 blockers. New Engl J Med 317:1376, 1987.
37. Ryan P, Dawson J, Teres D, et al: Continuous infusion of cimetidine vs sucralfate: Incidence of pneumonia and bleeding compared. J Crit Care Med 18(4):S253, 1990.
38. Guiot HF, Van der Meer JM, Van Furth R: Selective antimicrobial modulation of human microbial flora: Infection prevention in patients with decreased host defense mechanisms by selective elimination of potentially pathogenic bacteria. J Infect Dis 143:644, 1981.
39. Ramsey G, Lendingham I: Management of multiple organ failure: Control of the microbial environment, in Bihari DJ, Cerra FB (eds): *New Horizons: Multiple Organ Failure Syndrome.* Fullerton, CA, Society of Critical Care Medicine, 1989, pp 327–337.
40. Vilcek LEJ: Biology of disease TNF and IL-1: Cytokines with multiple overlapping biological activities. Lab Invest 56:234, 1987.
41. Chang S, Feddersen CO, Henson PM, et al: Platelet-activating factor mediates hemodynamic changes and lung injury in endotoxin-treated rats. J Clin Invest 79:1498, 1987.
42. Dinarello: Interleukin-1 and the pathogenesis of the acute-phase response. N Engl J Med 311:341, 1984.
43. Ward PA, Warren JS, Remick DG, et al: Cytokines and oxygen-radical-mediated tissue injury, in Bihari DJ, Cerra FB (eds): *New Horizons: Multiple Organ Failure.* Fullerton, CA, Society of Critical Care Medicine, 1989, pp 93–100.

44. Cook JA, Halushka PV: Arachidonic acid metabolism in septic shock, in Bihari DJ, Cerra FB (eds): *New Horizons: Multiple Organ Failure.* Fullerton, CA, Society of Critical Care Medicine, 1989, pp 101–124.
45. Mazuski JE, Platt JL, West MA, et al: Direct effects of endotoxin on hepatocytes. Arch Surgery 123:340, 1988.
46. West MA, Keller G, Hyland B, et al: Hepatocyte function in sepsis: Kupffer cells mediate a biphasic protein synthesis response in hepatocytes after endotoxin and killed *E. coli.* Surgery 98:388, 1985.
47. Clowes GHA, Georg BC, Villu CA: Muscle proteolysis induced by a circulating peptide in patients with trauma and sepsis. N Engl J Med 303:545, 1983.
48. Eyer SD, Cerra FB: Cost-effective use of the surgical intensive care unit. World J Surg 11:241, 1987.

Chapter 57

PATHOLOGIC SUPPLY DEPENDENCE OF OXYGEN UTILIZATION

RICHARD W. SAMSEL
PAUL T. SCHUMACKER

KEY POINTS

- *Oxygen uptake is normally set by metabolic need, rather than by oxygen delivery.*
- *When normal tissues are stressed by progressively lowering oxygen delivery, they maintain a normal oxygen uptake until oxygen delivery falls below a critical point, independent of whether anemia, hypoxemia, or falling blood flow was responsible for the drop in oxygen delivery.*
- *The oxygen extraction ratio (the fraction of oxygen extracted on a single pass through the circulation) is the best single indicator of the threshold of tissue hypoxia. In normal tissues, the threshold of hypoxia (the critical O_2 delivery) generally occurs when the oxygen extraction ratio is about 70 percent.*
- *Several clinical syndromes [notably adult respiratory distress syndrome (ARDS) and sepsis] have been reported to impair tissues' ability to extract oxygen from blood, resulting in delivery-dependent oxygen uptake even when the extraction ratio is 50 percent or less. This impaired oxygen extraction may represent occult tissue hypoxia and may contribute to the high incidence of multiple systems organ failure.*
- *Possible mechanisms for impairment of tissue oxygen extraction include anatomic or functional arteriovenous shunting, microembolization, and impairment of the autoregulatory systems that normally match tissue oxygen delivery to tissue oxygen demand. A better understanding of alterations in microcirculatory control in sepsis may permit a better understanding of oxygen extraction defects.*
- *Methodologic questions preclude definitive interpretation of human studies reporting oxygen extraction defects in humans. Nevertheless, a common clinical consensus holds that patients at risk for tissue hypoxia may benefit from therapies aimed at improving tissue oxygenation: increasing oxygen delivery and decreasing oxygen demand.*

Cardiopulmonary supportive care is the art of preventing tissue hypoxia. Knowing when tissue hypoxia is imminent or present can be challenging, particularly if tissue oxygen utilization is impaired. Tissue hypoxia can supervene whenever blood flow, hematocrit, or arterial oxygen saturation fall below minimum adequate levels. These three components of tissue oxygen transport can be summarized in a single factor, the oxygen delivery ($\dot{Q}_{O_2}$, the product of arterial oxygen content and blood flow). In normal animals, a single critical value of oxygen delivery can predict the threshold of tissue hypoxia regardless of how oxygen delivery was lowered.

Interpreting the oxygen delivery in the critical care setting is often more difficult. Evidence from human studies has suggested that ARDS and sepsis may alter the normal relationship between tissue oxygen uptake and delivery, impairing tissues' ability to extract oxygen from blood. Tissue oxygen availability can thus be impaired, even when total oxygen delivery is in its normal range. In this chapter, we will explore the physiology of tissue oxygen uptake, the evidence for impaired O_2 extraction in patients, possible mechanisms for this phenomenon, and its therapeutic implications.

The Normal Determinants of O_2 Uptake

Under normal, resting conditions, tissue oxygen demand rather than tissue oxygen supply determines the rate of oxygen uptake. However, in critical illness oxygen delivery is often reduced to the point where tissue hypoxia occurs. Understanding how normal and diseased tissues respond to falling oxygen delivery is critical to preventing tissue hypoxia.

SYSTEMIC OXYGEN TRANSPORT, CONSUMPTION, AND EXTRACTION LIMITS

The hallmarks of tissue hypoxia are falling oxygen consumption ($\dot{V}_{O_2}$), elaboration of reduced substrate forms such as lactate, and a decline in tissue function. Experimentally, the point where $\dot{V}_{O_2}$ begins to fall and arterial blood excess lactate begins to rise correlates with a critical level of tissue oxygen delivery ($\dot{Q}_{O_2}$ = blood flow times arterial O_2 content). Hence, the three ways to lower O_2 delivery are to lower blood flow (stagnant hypoxia), arterial hemoglobin saturation (hypoxic hypoxia), or blood hemoglobin concentration (anemic hypoxia). Oxygen delivery is the product of cardiac output ($\dot{Q}_T$, dL/min) and arterial O_2 content, and can be calculated as

$$\dot{Q}_{O_2} = \dot{Q}_T(\alpha \times Sa_{O_2} \times Hgb + \beta \times Pa_{O_2}),$$

where α represents the binding capacity for hemoglobin (1.39 mL O_2/g Hgb), Sa_{O_2} is the fractional arterial hemoglobin saturation, Hgb is the hemoglobin concentration (g/dL), β is the solubility of O_2 in plasma (0.003 mL O_2/torr/dL plasma), and Pa_{O_2} is the arterial partial pressure of oxygen (torr). The small value of β in physical terms reflects the low solubility of oxygen in plasma and renders the dissolved oxygen negligible except in cases of hyperbaric therapy, where Pa_{O_2} can reach the thousands. The relative insolubility of oxygen in water necessitates the presence of hemoglobin as an oxygen carrier. Despite hemoglobin, the high molar demand for oxygen compared to other metabolic substrates means that tissues deplete blood of oxygen

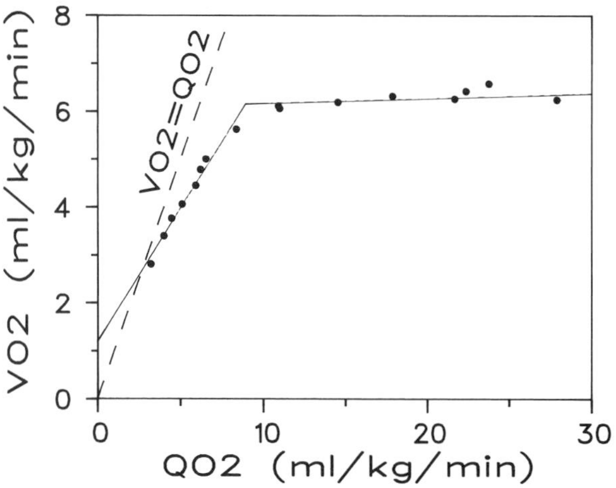

FIGURE 57-1 The normal relationship between oxygen delivery and uptake in tissues. Points reflect data taken from an anesthetized dog subjected to progressive hemorrhage leading to stagnant hypoxia. Best fit lines are drawn on the plot. Below a critical O_2 delivery, O_2 uptake is limited by supply. Above it, oxygen uptake is relatively constant. Even above the critical point, a slight positive slope is seen. This feature is reproducible in larger series and probably reflects flow dependent metabolic activity in tissues such as heart, kidney, and liver.

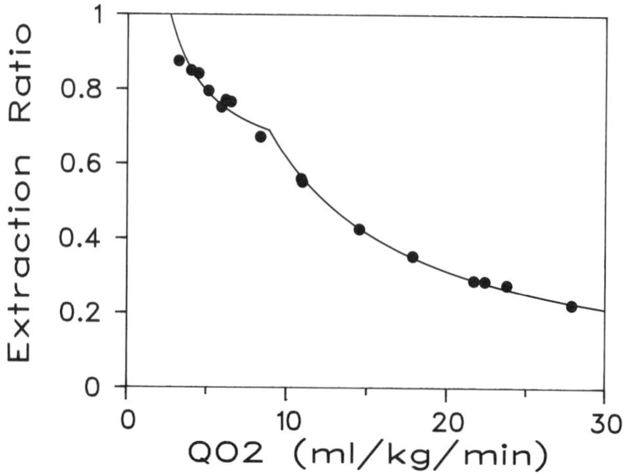

FIGURE 57-2 Oxygen extraction ratio as a function of oxygen delivery. Decreases in oxygen delivery require proportional increases in the extraction ratio to maintain $\dot{V}_{O_2}$. Below the critical O_2 delivery, increases in extraction are inadequate to maintain $\dot{V}_{O_2}$. Data points were taken from an anesthetized dog subjected to hemorrhage, resulting in stagnant hypoxia. Curves reflect the hyperbolic transformation of the best-fit oxygen supply–uptake relationship (see Fig. 57-1).

much sooner than of these other substrates. Thus, when oxygen delivery supply falls, tissues shift toward a chemically reduced state.

Oxygen uptake is fixed by metabolic need, and is essentially independent of O_2 delivery above a critical threshold (Fig. 57-1). As oxygen delivery falls along the "plateau phase," the oxygen extraction ratio (ER = $(Ca_{O_2} - Cv_{O_2})/Ca_{O_2}$, where Ca_{O_2} and Cv_{O_2} are the arterial and venous blood oxygen contents) must rise to compensate for the falling oxygen availability (Fig. 57-2).

Both active processes (such as compensatory redistribution of blood flow) and passive processes (the physics of convection and diffusion) contribute to the increase in the extraction ratio as oxygen delivery falls. However, these processes permit healthy tissues to extract only about 70% of the delivered oxygen before oxygen uptake begins to fall, and tissue hypoxia supervenes.

The critical oxygen delivery reflects the minimum delivery necessary to meet metabolic demands and thus will increase or decrease as metabolic demand changes. By contrast, the O_2 extraction ratio at the critical point is a dimensionless value, and thus reflects tissue O_2 extraction efficacy independent of metabolic demands. Thus, it is more useful in comparing individuals or tissues with very different demands for oxygen.

At deliveries below the critical point, a variety of physiologic changes accompany the decline in oxygen uptake. Lactic acid production increases[1] and its metabolic clearance falls.[2] As lactic acid concentrations increase, blood bicarbonate falls, and CO_2 is elaborated. The respiratory exchange quotient ($R = \dot{V}_{CO_2}/\dot{V}_{O_2}$) increases measurably, as long as the lactic acid level continues to increase. Most importantly, tissue function itself begins to fail.

Above the critical point, most animals subjected to stagnant hypoxia exhibit a slight dependence of O_2 uptake on O_2 supply, as indicated by a small slope seen in the supply-independent "plateau" (Fig. 57-1). This probably reflects the contributions of organs with a known positive relationship between flow and O_2 demand, such as liver and myocardium (vide infra).

CELLULAR OXYGEN AVAILABILITY AND UPTAKE

At the cellular level, the cardiopulmonary oxygen transport system functions to service mitochondria, so that they in turn can supply adenosine triphosphate (ATP) for cell synthetic, transport, and motile functions. Normally functioning mitochondria can ordinarily supply ATP as fast as it is required, so that substrates are not limiting. An exception to this is maximal exercise, where lactic acid production supplements aerobic activity even when local tissue hypoxia is not present.[3] While maximal exercise in athletes is interesting from the standpoint of learning about the limits of tissue oxygen transport, its relevance to patients in intensive care units is less certain. At rest, failure of cellular oxygen supply manifests itself as a shift of cellular metabolites toward reduced forms, with falling cellular pH, falling stores of phosphorylated adenosine species, buildup of hypoxanthine, inosine and xanthine, lactate elaboration, and a decline in cellular function.

With respect to oxygen use, the cytochrome aa_3 system is thought to be rate limiting and has an extraordinarily high oxygen affinity ($K_M = 0.05$ torr). Provided that intramitochondrial P_{O_2} is at least five times this K_M value, oxygen turnover should be normal. A diffusion gradient between extracellular fluid and intramitochondrial cytochrome oxidase increases the critical level of P_{O_2} by another order of magnitude, to 1–2 torr. Thus, single cells continue to use oxygen normally if pericellular P_{O_2} is greater than this level.[4] Moreover, there is little evidence that this critical threshold changes in any common clinical disease. In cellular terms, therefore, the cardiopulmonary system must generally maintain extracellular P_{O_2} above this minimal level.

Regional Contributions to Oxygen Demand

Overall oxygen supply–demand relationships, as described earlier, ultimately represent the contributions of each of the individual organ systems. Each organ has its own delivery–uptake relationship and has its own specific workload that generates oxygen demand. Full data are unavailable for many organ systems; below, we review available information for several systems.

MUSCULAR OXYGEN CONSUMPTION AND EXTRACTION

The large mass of skeletal muscle in the body accounts for a large share of resting oxygen use on the basis of its bulk alone. However, when normalized to its weight, resting muscle oxygen utilization is slightly lower than that of the body as a whole. The oxygen uptake–delivery relationship for skeletal muscle has been heavily debated. While some investigators studying smaller animals have argued that skeletal muscle $\dot{V}_{O_2}$ is normally supply dependent at rest, most investigators using larger animals have found a relationship between oxygen delivery and uptake similar to that reported for the body as a whole.[5] In either case, resting skeletal muscle produces lactic acid and is probably responsible for much of the lactic acid seen in blood under normal resting conditions.

Normal skeletal muscle appears able to extract as much as about 70% of oxygen under resting conditions; exercising skeletal muscle can extract more than 80%. This improvement in oxygen extraction with exercise may be explained by an increase in perfused capillary density, coupled with a partial desaturation of muscle myoglobin, which facilitates the diffusion of oxygen within the sarcomere.

ALIMENTARY OXYGEN CONSUMPTION

Like skeletal muscle, intestinal O_2 demand varies with its metabolic workload; the presence of foodstuffs in the lumen stimulates both intestinal hyperemia and an increase in oxygen uptake. The blood supply to the mucosa is regulated differently from the blood supply to the bowel wall; the former exhibits a reactive hyperemia following brief occlusion, while the latter does not. Adenosine receptor blockade appears to prevent this regulatory vasodilation, suggesting a central role for adenosine release and washout in intestinal autoregulatory control.[6]

The resting canine intestine displays an O_2 uptake of 25 mL O_2/min/kg gut weight, about five times larger than the mean systemic O_2 uptake. Much of the oxygen demand in the intestine is absorptive; the mucosa accounts for a large share of oxidative work. The alimentary canal is a highly metabolic system and accounts for a substantial share of systemic O_2 demand. In states of limited oxygen delivery, isolated intestine can extract as much as 70 percent of the delivered oxygen prior to the onset of supply dependence, a figure in line with that of the whole body.[7,8]

The splanchnic circulation is susceptible to profound vasoconstriction in the presence of arginine vasopressin, as well as sympathetic stimulation, consistent with the traditional view that splanchnic beds are sacrificed early in states of reduced O_2 delivery. Yet in dogs subjected to progressively falling blood flow, isolated, innervated intestine reached its critical point only a short time before the body as a whole became obviously supply dependent.[7] This suggests that the proclivity of the alimentary tract to fail in hypoperfusion states, manifested initially by sloughing of the mucosa, may reflect intrinsic sensitivity to hypoxia caused by a high metabolic rate, as much as to a preferential shutdown of splanchnic flow.

HEPATIC OXYGEN CONSUMPTION AND EXTRACTION

Metabolically, the liver is a relatively active organ, with estimates of its resting oxygen demand ranging from 25 to 50 mL O_2/min/kg liver mass. The work of the liver is absorptive, metabolic, and synthetic. Hepatic oxygen uptake is heavily influenced by the presence or absence of absorbed foodstuffs in the blood feeding it. The availability of these substrates likely limits both the synthetic ability of the liver and the transport-work of conditioning the perfusing blood. In many respects, the concentration of such substrates in portal blood, and the portal flow is a central determinant of hepatic oxygen demand.

Blood flow through the portal system is determined primarily by the arterioles in the intestinal mucosa. The portal circuit is a passive one, with little intrinsic contractility and little ability to control flow. In isolated livers, the sites of flow resistance appear to be largely venous, and portal pressure is very close to sinusoidal pressure. Portal blood typically carries three quarters of the oxygen of arterial blood; portal oxygen transport should be able to provide for the liver's needs alone. Yet a separate circulation exists. In the cat, the hepatic artery vasodilates in response to a drop in portal flow, and this effect is blocked by adenosine receptor antagonists.[9] Splanchnic vasoconstriction will not only decrease portal flow, it will also drop portal oxygen content. Thus, it seems plausible that a separate (and complementarily controlled) vascular system is required to allow the liver to adjust its oxygen delivery if splanchnic supply decreases. If this is the case, then simultaneous mesenteric artery constriction with hepatic artery dilation may be able to drop hepatic O_2 demand and may be a means for animals to readjust their O_2 requirements in response to falling O_2 availability.

In response to falling blood flow in both circuits, the oxygen uptake of the liver falls. The fall is gradual above a

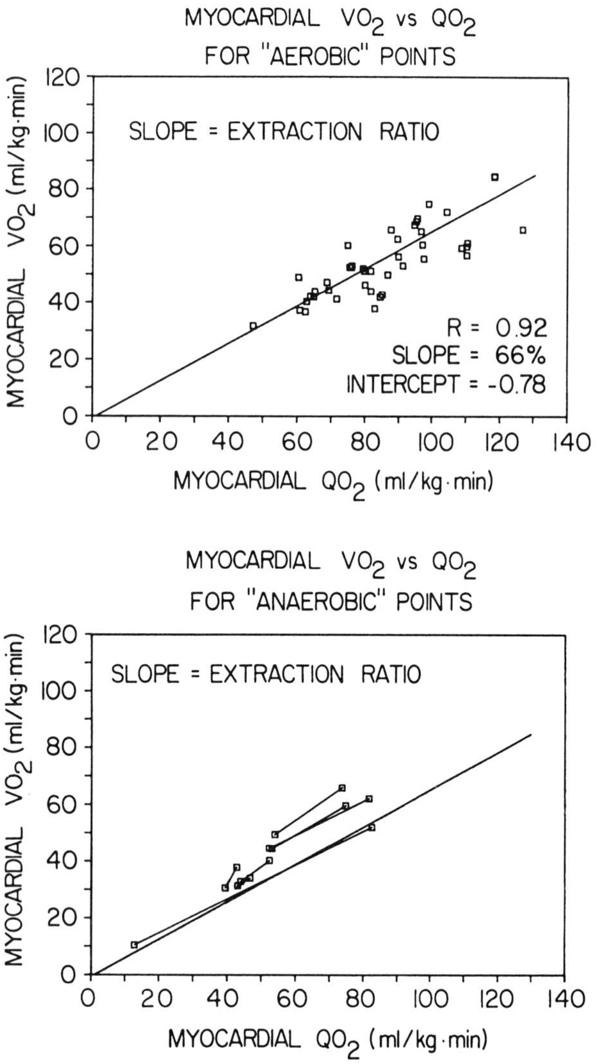

FIGURE 57-3 Myocardial oxygen consumption is related to myocardial oxygen delivery by a constant extraction ratio, as long as coronary autoregulation can maintain aerobic metabolism. (*From Walley et al,* **Circ Res** *62:849, 1988, with permission.*)

critical threshold and much steeper below it. The mild supply-dependency of hepatic oxygen uptake on the "plateau" phase may contribute to the gradual slope seen at the systemic level. The liver extracts about 10 percent of the delivered lactate at a variety of flows above the critical point but becomes a lactate producer below its critical point. Like the rest of the body, the liver extracts about 70 percent of the delivered oxygen at this critical level.

CARDIAC OXYGEN CONSUMPTION AND EXTRACTION

Cardiac oxygen demand is high; estimates are from 30 to 80 mL O_2/min/kg cardiac tissue. When left ventricular pressure is plotted against volume over the cardiac cycle, it has been shown that cardiac oxygen uptake varies directly with the pressure volume loop area, plus the area under the end-systolic pressure volume relationship, extrapolated back to the *x* intercept.[10] This means simply that increases in cardiac workload (either afterload expressed as pressure, or end-diastolic volume, or both) translate directly into increases in cardiac oxygen demand.

The relationship between O_2 uptake and delivery in the heart is difficult to define, because the heart ordinarily operates at an oxygen extraction ratio of about 60 percent. Unlike other tissues where a limitation in oxygen delivery is accompanied by an increase in O_2 extraction, the heart has little ability to increase its O_2 extraction before it encounters its critical O_2 extraction ratio, so it must rely on coronary vasodilation to augment myocardial O_2 delivery. Accordingly, the relationship between myocardial O_2 delivery and uptake normally has a positive slope for both aerobic and anaerobic states (Fig. 57-3). Limitations in myocardial oxygen delivery caused by limitations in coronary blood flow are associated with impaired pumping function. This in turn lowers coronary oxygen demand and V_{O_2}, leading to the apparent positive relationship between O_2 supply and uptake in the normal heart. This relationship is a natural consequence of the limited ability of the normal heart to increase its O_2 extraction ratio in response to changes in coronary O_2 supply.[11]

RENAL OXYGEN DELIVERY AND UPTAKE

Renal oxygen extraction remains essentially constant over widely varying blood flow rates; oxygen consumption varies almost linearly with blood flow over a wide range.[12] This contrasts sharply with behavior of the whole body, intestine, muscle, or even liver, where a relatively supply-independent plateau is seen at high levels of delivery.

Renal oxygen uptake fuels the metabolic work of the kidney. In energetic terms, most of this work is sodium reabsorption, and filtered sodium is proportional to the renal blood flow. It stands to reason that oxygen delivery is a less important determinant of renal O_2 uptake than the glomerular filtration rate itself. In a kidney with urinary outflow obstruction, where both filtration and reabsorption have come to a standstill, renal O_2 consumption falls to a much lower baseline and becomes essentially independent of flow.

Determining the limits of oxygen extraction in the kidney will require studies either of obstructed kidneys, or of kidneys subject to hypoxic or anemic forms of hypoxia, where flow remains high but O_2 delivery falls. Under such circumstances, kidneys appear to have O_2 extraction limits similar to those in the body as a whole[13]; a thorough characterization of renal O_2 extraction has not yet been made.

Mechanisms of Local O_2 Supply–Demand Matching

Organisms respond to limitations in oxygen delivery at many levels. At the behavioral level, injured animals become lethargic, thermally insulate themselves, and conserve energy to the best of their ability. As these somatic changes proceed, their tissues exhibit a variety of changes aimed at preventing or minimizing tissue hypoxia. We will consider, in turn, the interregional matching of supply to demand, the microcirculatory adjustments that permit autoregulation, and the cellular responses to impaired oxygen supply.

INTERREGIONAL MATCHING OF O_2 SUPPLY TO TISSUE O_2 DEMAND

As peripheral tissues are challenged by limitations in oxygen delivery, optimal vasoconstriction must gradually reduce each tissue's blood flow to its minimum requirement, so that one tissue will not be overperfused while others are starving for oxygen.[14] Mechanisms for this vasoconstriction include sympathetically mediated vasoconstriction and probably also humoral systems such as the renin–angiotensin and the arginine–vasopressin system.

Impairment of normal vasoconstriction (as, e.g., by α blockade) slows tissue compensation for falling O_2 delivery, lowering the systemic extraction ratio at the critical point.[14] Interestingly, α blockade does not impair regional oxygen extraction.[15] Since α blockade primarily affects regional perfusion, this suggests an important role for progressive systemic vasoconstriction in mediating optimal interregional distribution of blood flow with respect to oxygen demand. This view is further supported by the observation that intestine reaches its local hypoxic threshold at about the same level as the whole body.[7] Thus, even while individual organs must each compete for a limited supply of blood, the systemic response to hypoxia facilitates the coordinated response among many regional circulations.

Activation of each physiologic regulatory system causes a shift in blood flow among organs. Sympathetic nervous activity provokes both venoconstriction, to augment venous return and thus improve cardiac output, and arterial constriction, to maintain enough driving force that autoregulation can function effectively. Since the coronary and cerebral vascular resistances increase less with elevated sympathetic tone than other beds, there is thought to be a relative redistribution of blood flow toward these vital tissues. Moreover, release of arginine vasopressin causes splanchnic vasoconstriction, mild coronary vasodilation, and cerebral vasodilation. A relative shift in blood flow toward coronary cerebral vascular beds is thought to be advantageous for maintaining cardiac function and improving brain survival in states of circulatory crisis. Renin, whose release is triggered by sympathetic beta receptor stimulation, maintains overall arteriolar tone through the activation of angiotensin. Without these active processes, local metabolic control of blood flow would fail, from the loss of perfusion pressure.

LOCAL METABOLIC CONTROL

Autoregulatory processes are largely vasodilatory in nature. The peripheral circulation ordinarily maintains a high degree of active tone; from this baseline, local vasodilatory stimuli can substantially increase flow when necessary. Granger and colleagues[16] have identified a useful dichotomy in vessels controlling peripheral microcirculatory flow: flow controlling vessels and distribution vessels. Total regional flow is determined by large vessels (medium-sized arterioles) where the majority of the arteriovenous pressure gradient is dissipated. By contrast, local distribution of flow is determined downstream, by precapillary sphincters in tissues that have them, or by similarly sized precapillary arterioles in all tissues. It has been argued that these vascular regions are separately controlled. The distribution vessels are primarily under local control, responding to buildup of vasodilator metabolites, and largely refractory to sympathetic control. Upstream flow controlling vessels are mainly controlled by sympathetic and other regional control systems, although ultimately they are also subject to metabolic feedback.

Hypoxic stimuli affect both systems but appear to have a greater role in the distribution vessels. Dilation of precapillary sphincters will increase the number of conduits carrying the same flow; this enables the mean capillary transit time to increase and the average intercapillary distance to fall. As a result, diffusion distances are more advantageous and the necessary O_2 driving pressures are smaller. This is most important in organs with high O_2 demands, where the oxygen gradients between capillary and cell must be highest.

Endothelial cells appear to play a central role in the regulation of vascular tone, by the release of both vasodilator and vasoconstrictor substances. A variety of endogenous vasodilators (e.g., bradykinin, ADP) exert their action on smooth muscle through stimulating release of endothelium-derived relaxing factor (EDRF), an arginine-derived paracrine factor similar or identical with the free radical nitric oxide. These endothelial mechanisms seem ideally suited to mediate local autoregulatory vasodilation that is essential to normal distribution of blood flow, although other factors also participate.

CELLULAR ADAPTIVE RESPONSES TO A LIMITED OXYGEN SUPPLY

As tissue oxygen supply falls, cells may exhibit protective reductions in their own oxidative demands. On a physiologic scale, several mechanisms might contribute to a reduction in O_2 demand. Some known examples of this are somatic changes, such as muscle rest, thermal insulation, and omission of food intake—all of which can reduce tissue oxygen demands during states of impaired supply. Second, a fall in blood flow is expected to drop oxygen demand by organs whose workload is flow dependent: the kidney, heart, and liver. Cells have many avenues of energy loss that could conceivably be suppressed in times of threatened oxygen supply. Reductions in cell ionic permeability, synthesis of structural materials, and in futile cycling in actively regulated biochemical processes would be likely candidates for facultative control. Hochachka and Guppy[17] have argued that such adaptations are likely to accompany hibernation and similar states. However, there is little evidence to date that such processes can exist within humans, especially in states of acute illness.

Pathologic Supply Dependence in Critical Illness

Studies have reported that several patient populations exhibit a pathologic dependence of oxygen delivery on oxygen supply, even when the oxygen extraction ratio is within normal limits. This finding is closely associated with lactic acidosis in several patient groups. Most of these reports fit in three broad groups: adult respiratory distress syndrome (ARDS), sepsis, and chronic states of low oxygen delivery.

ARDS

As described in several recent reviews,[18-20] at least 10 studies since the first in 1973 have reported that patients with acute respiratory failure exhibited a dependence of oxygen uptake on oxygen delivery, despite normal or high levels of oxygen delivery. The implication is profound: that oxygen uptake is supply dependent in critically ill patients suggests that tissue hypoxia persists despite high levels of oxygen delivery.

ARDS appears to induce changes in the normal relationship of O_2 uptake and delivery, and one possible description of these changes is summarized in Fig. 57-4. These curves are an idealization drawn in part from data collected in animal experiments, and partly from analysis of grouped data in clinical studies. The relationship thought to exist in ARDS is characterized by an increase in O_2 demand, an increase in the critical O_2 delivery, and a decline in the O_2 extraction ability of the tissue. However, it should be noted that no clinical study of ARDS has generated such a relationship in a single patient, because of the technical and ethical problems that would be encountered. Nevertheless, the human studies of pathologic supply dependence suggest the presence of a defect in oxygen extraction ability, characterized by supply-dependent O_2 uptake even when extraction ratios are as low as 30 to 40 percent.

It is now widely recognized that patients with ARDS who die are frequently septic, and die more often of multisystem organ failure (MSOF) than of refractory hypoxemia. If widespread tissue hypoxia is a common accompaniment of ARDS, then it seems plausible that it may play a central role in the pathogenesis of MSOF. ARDS appears increasingly to be the pulmonary manifestation of a systemic disease. It seems likely that the common inciting feature is diffuse vascular damage, leading to increased permeability in the lung and impaired autoregulation in the periphery. Tissue hypoxia resulting from either hypoxemia or impaired regulation of blood flow distribution leads to diffuse tissue dysfunction and eventually tissue death. Although increasing tissue oxygen supply by increasing flow seems a logical treatment for pathologic supply dependence, ultimately only correction of the underlying defects will bring about the reversal of this problem.

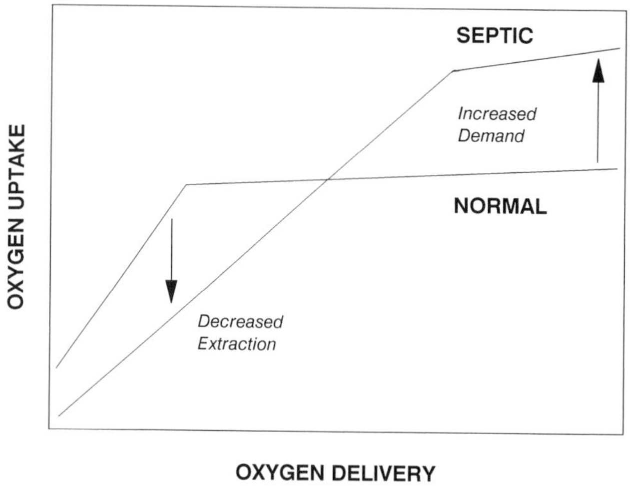

FIGURE 57-4 Idealization of the relationship between oxygen delivery and uptake in patients with pathological O_2 supply dependency associated with critical illness. Baseline O_2 demand is increased, while the extraction ratio at the point where O_2 uptake becomes supply limited is significantly reduced.

Although the existence of pathologic supply dependence in critically ill patients is widely accepted, two different lines of thinking have argued against this conventional interpretation. One line of argument suggests that "pathologic supply dependence of O_2 uptake" is not pathologic at all but instead represents the normal relationship in humans. The other suggests that the observation of pathologic supply dependence is a consequence of experimental error and coupled variables. We will consider these in turn.

The first line of thinking observes that supply dependence of O_2 uptake exists in most patient populations that have been studied and suggests that this may reflect a difference between human and animal physiology, arguing that humans cannot achieve the high extraction ratios seen in anesthetized animals. Against this argument is the observation that some patients with severe and acute reductions in O_2 delivery have been shown to exhibit high levels of O_2 extraction.[21] Moreover, it seems unlikely that human tissues differ so dramatically from the other species studied: dogs, pigs, sheep, and rats. Finally, many of the human studies have included control groups showing little or no supply dependence of O_2 uptake. An important point is illustrated by this debate: It is difficult to determine if parallel changes in oxygen delivery and uptake seen in a patient with critical illness reflect pathologic dependency of V_{O_2} on delivery, or just the normal cardiovascular response to acute changes in O_2 demand in patients with varying O_2 demand.

The second line of argument concerns a statistical problem with most of the studies of O_2 uptake in patients.[22] Because the measurement of oxygen uptake from the inspired and expired gas measurements is difficult, most studies have calculated O_2 uptake as the product of arteriovenous O_2 content difference and the measured cardiac output. Since delivery is also calculated as the product of arterial O_2 content and cardiac output, the two variables ($\dot{V}_{O_2}$ and $\dot{Q}_{O_2}$) share a dependence on both arterial content and cardiac output. Thus, measurement error in either of these variables will cause a related shift in both variables. Such related shifts will appear as supply-dependent O_2 uptake.

To rectify this experimental problem, two studies have measured oxygen uptake and delivery independently, calculating $\dot{V}_{O_2}$ from expired gas measurements, and delivery from cardiac output.[23,24] Neither of these studies found a correlation between oxygen uptake and oxygen delivery. The first study was limited to patients breathing inspired O_2 concentrations of 50% or less. Presumably, these patients were less severely afflicted than patients in the prior studies. Although the second study involved sicker patients, the changes in cardiac output were not large. It is difficult to reconcile these findings with those of the prior studies. It is important to note that the use of independent measurements on two axes predisposes to a failure to disclose pathologic supply dependence (a type II error) just as use of dependent measurements predisposes to spurious discovery of supply dependence (a type I error). The only way to avoid these difficulties is to ensure that imposed changes in oxygen delivery are large compared to the error in determining the oxygen delivery. It follows that improving technology to provide better clinically usable measurements of O_2 uptake is needed to resolve the debate. In the interim, it remains possible that the phenomenon of pathologic O_2 supply dependency exists only under specific clinical circumstances. It is also possible that sufficiently large increases in O_2 delivery are necessary to elicit an increase in $\dot{V}_{O_2}$, perhaps through recruitment of additional capillaries in tissues.

SEPSIS

Because of the reported prevalence of both sepsis and peripheral oxygen extraction defects in patients with ARDS, it is possible that sepsis, rather than simple ARDS, accounts for the peripheral changes. Several groups have reported pathologic supply dependence in patients with sepsis, but without ARDS. Pathologic supply dependence accompanied sepsis in patients with lactic acidosis but not in patients without lactic acidosis.[25,26] These results further suggest that pathologic supply dependence is really an indicator of tissue hypoxia. Yet lactic acidosis alone must be interpreted with caution, since elevations in lactate are elicited as a consequence of increased metabolic rate of glycolysis, even in the absence of anaerobic metabolism. In this regard, the measurement of excess lactate (or lactate:pyruvate ratio) is required to differentiate between the contributions of anaerobic metabolism on the one hand and increased aerobic glycolysis on the other.[27] The absence of lactate:pyruvate ratio measurements in many studies relates to the technical difficulty of measuring pyruvate accurately in a clinical setting.

Several lines of animal experimentation further support the notion that pathologic supply dependence may be related more directly to sepsis than to lung injury itself. Oleic acid-induced lung injury does not impair tissue's ability to extract oxygen.[28,29] By contrast, experimental bacteremia[30] and endotoxin infusion[8] in animals confer a defect in oxygen extraction by tissues. These models for sepsis provide further support for the notion that a peripheral circulatory change caused by sepsis, rather than lung injury per se, may be responsible for oxygen extraction defects seen in ARDS.

Further clinical studies involving subgroup analysis of patients with ARDS will be required to sort out whether different etiologies for ARDS (e.g., sepsis versus acid aspiration versus traumatic lung injury) differ in their ability to confer a defect in peripheral O_2 extraction.

CHRONIC STATES OF LOW O_2 DELIVERY

Several studies have now investigated the relationship between O_2 uptake and delivery in diseases where oxygen uptake is chronically limited, including obstructive pulmonary disease, congestive heart failure, pulmonary hypertension, and obstructive sleep apnea.[31–34] These studies have, with one exception, reported that oxygen uptake increased when oxygen delivery was increased. While the changes were somewhat less dramatic than in the patients with ARDS or sepsis, several were made with independent measurements of O_2 delivery and uptake, and so avoided the criticisms arising from the use of shared variables.

Patients with chronic hypoxic states differ from patients with sepsis and ARDS—it seems unlikely that pathologic supply dependence in such patients stems from occult tissue hypoxia. Patients with these diseases may demonstrate a qualitatively different pattern, and, if real, this phenomenon may reflect an exaggeration of the normal mild physiologic supply dependence seen in normals above the critical point. Such an exaggeration is consistent with active facultative control of oxidative demand. As previously noted, there is little precedent for this in human tissues. Further studies should aid in exploring mechanisms for facultative control of tissue oxygen demand.

Mechanisms of Pathologic Supply Dependence

Patients with ARDS appear to change their $\dot{V}_{O_2}$ when their normal or high levels of O_2 delivery are adjusted, but questions about the interpretation of these findings persist, as described earlier. Patients with sepsis show a similar relationship at high levels of O_2 delivery and exhibit increased levels of arterial lactic acid, but the lactic acid may not arise from anaerobic metabolism. Patients without ARDS or sepsis increase their $\dot{V}_{O_2}$ when delivery is increased during resuscitation, but this is seen when the starting O_2 delivery is at such low levels that even normal subjects might be expected to be O_2 supply dependent. Finally, patients with chronically low levels of systemic O_2 delivery appear to increase $\dot{V}_{O_2}$ when delivery is increased, although less so than patients with acute respiratory failure or sepsis. To the extent that pathologic O_2 supply dependence is real in some or all of these patient groups, several mechanisms that might contribute to the phenomenon are now discussed.

IMPAIRED VASCULAR CONTROL

Efficient peripheral oxygen transport requires tight regulation of blood flow distribution. Impairment of normal autoregulatory control may be manifest in tissues exhibiting pathologic supply dependence of oxygen transport. For example, α receptor blockade was associated with a decline in the ability of the body as a whole to extract oxygen from a limited supply.[15] Also, *Proteus aeruginosa* bacteria or *Escherichia coli* endotoxin reproduced a state of pathologic supply dependence in laboratory animals, qualitatively similar although less severe than that reported in human studies. Moreover, the regional distribution of oxygen extraction impairment varied, with relative sparing of skeletal muscle but substantial effects on intestine.[5,8] This tissue-dependent response paralleled a loss of the reactive hyperemia following transient arterial occlusion, occurring in intestine but not muscle. These findings are consistent with impairment of tissue autoregulation of blood flow distribution.

Sepsis itself is known to produce substantial effects on vascular reactivity. Vascular catechol responsiveness is abnormal in experimental sepsis,[35,36] and vessels fail to relax normally to topically applied vasodilators.[37,38] Impaired reactive hyperemia was reported in patients with sepsis, and it correlated with lethality of the syndrome.[39] Endothelial cells are known to exhibit structural changes during sepsis and septic insults.[40] Since endothelial cells play a central role in regulation of vascular tone, it is possible that changes in endothelial biology may underlie altered vascular responsiveness in sepsis.

One hypothesis holds that sepsis induces an activated endothelium, resulting in elaboration of a variety of endothelium-derived mediators, including EDRF, endothelin, and possibly others. According to this hypothesis, direct action of EDRF on vascular smooth muscle results in the profound vasodilation associated with sepsis. Moreover, *basal* activation of vasodilating systems may undermine the ability of metabolic stimuli to *induce* vasodilation necessary for autoregulatory control. Thus, mismatch of oxygen delivery to oxygen demand might result from inability for further compensatory vasodilation in response to the stimuli that ordinarily couple vasodilation to increases in oxygen demand. While extremely speculative, these hypotheses offer a new approach to understanding the genesis of extraction defects in peripheral tissues.

EMBOLIZATION

A second contributor to peripheral oxygen extraction deficits is microembolization. An increase in neutrophil margination in sepsis is well known, as is an increase in platelet aggregation. Either of these may act as microemboli. In the peripheral circulation, two possible effects may be expected. First, by plugging distribution vessels in the microcirculation, the average distance between perfused capillaries will increase. A widening of the spacing between capillaries increases the diffusion gradients that are needed to drive oxygen from erythrocyte to mitochondrion. This would be manifest as an increase in the minimum level of O_2 delivery required to prevent cellular hypoxia.[41] Second, neutrophils may also act by release of toxic metabolites, notably active oxygen radicals and elastase. Free radical damage to tissues might directly affect endothelial or smooth muscle function, thus contributing to or even causing the previously hypothesized blood flow distribution defects.

Arguments against microembolization as the sole mechanism are that many tissues have a reserve of recruitable capillaries and that geometric factors alone suggest that a large number of peripheral capillaries must be plugged to substantially increase intercapillary distance. For example, assuming hexagonally arrayed capillaries, occluding 75 percent of the perfused capillaries will roughly double the distance between perfused capillaries. In the presence of normal regulation of distribution vessels, substantial degrees of embolization might be well tolerated. It is plausible that a combination of microembolization with impaired autoregulatory response may be needed to account for peripheral extraction impairments reported in sepsis and ARDS.

DISORDERED CELLULAR UTILIZATION

Yet another possible mechanism for oxygen extraction changes is an impairment of cellular mechanisms for usage of oxygen. As noted earlier, mitochondria normally use oxygen at a rate determined by ATP turnover, provided that local P_{O_2} is above 0.25 torr. A variety of mitochondrial metabolic poisons have been explored, primarily as tools to gain greater understanding of mitochondrial function. Two major classes, "uncouplers" (e.g., 2,4-dinitrophenol) and electron transport inhibitors (e.g., cyanide) are useful as paradigms for what might happen to mitochondrial function. Uncouplers work by enabling the electron transport chain to function in a "short circuit mode," without ADP phosphorylation. They markedly increase oxygen demand, but have little effect on oxygen extraction capacity in vivo.[42] Cyanide inhibits electron transport by inhibiting oxidation; it is associated with a marked decline in O_2 uptake independent of O_2 delivery. Thus, its effects are global, and not delivery dependent. It seems unlikely that either of these paradigms might explain delivery dependent oxygen uptake.

A variety of studies have explored direct effects of sepsis on mitochondria. The reports are mixed; some suggest the presence of moderate uncoupling, while others suggest enhanced function. In vitro effects of endotoxin on mitochondria are seen but only at concentrations of endotoxin orders of magnitude greater than might be seen in tissues. Even if little evidence supports direct mitochondrial changes in pathologic supply dependence, one cannot rule out the possibility. The very observation of delivery-dependent oxygen uptake suggests that if the problem is intrinsically mitochondrial, then it must reflect a change in the critical threshold P_{O_2}. We are not aware of any reports that bear directly on this measurement.

Toward Physiologic Therapies

Three central approaches may contribute to an improvement in supply–demand matching. They are decreasing oxygen demand, increasing oxygen delivery, and improving oxygen distribution. The first two form the mainstay of cardiopulmonary supportive therapy; by minimizing demand and increasing supply, one can often support patients through acute disease. Improving oxygen distribution is more difficult and must remain a goal for the future.

DECREASING OXYGEN DEMAND

Critically ill patients increase their O_2 consumption because of fever, work of breathing, and the associated metabolic responses to sepsis and trauma. Decreasing oxygen demand represents one approach to patients who exhibit delivery-dependent O_2 uptake, because of either a low oxygen delivery or to peripheral O_2 extraction impairment. The accepted approaches to this are anxiolytic therapy, rest, muscular paralysis with sedation to allow mechanical ventilation, and correction of hyperthermia. Correcting hyperthermia is particularly challenging in some patients; despite conventional antipyretic therapy with acetaminophen, patients often remain febrile. In nonsedated and nonparalyzed patients, cooling blankets are very uncomfortable and may do more harm than good by stimulating shivering. Moreover, on thermodynamic grounds it can be argued that patients at a given temperature will be consuming more oxygen if they are artificially cooled. However, increases in temperature increase metabolic rate, and $\dot{V}_{O_2}$ usually decreases when febrile patients are cooled to 37°C. Canine studies suggest that minimal impairment of O_2 extraction ability should occur with such a procedure.[43] Antipyretic agents that inhibit prostaglandin synthesis may be no more effective, and carry the risk of precipitating renal failure in patients whose renal blood flow may be prostaglandin dependent. With studies of ibuprofen in septic shock underway, the safety of its use in sepsis should become clear.

Other approaches to this are enforced hypothermia and gas anesthesia. While both can lower oxygen demand, both also impair peripheral oxygen extraction.[43,44] Moreover, it is not clear what effect they may have on the underlying cause of the illness. Although they suggest interesting possibilities, their use seems inadvisable at this point.

INCREASING OXYGEN DELIVERY

Increasing oxygen delivery is another therapy when oxygen uptake is limited by excessively low deliveries. Although some have argued that it is appropriate therapy in all critically ill patients because they may have delivery-dependent O_2 uptake, implementation of increased O_2 delivery carries its own problems.

Increasing the hematocrit is sensible, if the hematocrit is below normal limits. However, blood viscosity increases monotonically over the entire range of hematocrit. Studies of optimal hematocrit done in other conditions may not apply in sepsis, and, in the absence of better data, it seems wise to limit therapy to a return of hematocrit to the normal range. Note that most critically ill patients have a low hematocrit which is not cause for blood replacement in other circumstances, yet raising the hematocrit from 30 to 40 percent may have a substantial effect on O_2 delivery.

One should likewise increase the arterial P_{O_2} to the normal range by administration of supplementary oxygen. Short of full hyperbaric therapy, further increases in O_2 content with supplemental oxygen tend to be small. Because of the nonlinearity in the oxyhemoglobin dissociation curve, increases in Pa_{O_2} from 40 to 60 torr produce large increases in O_2 delivery, whereas increases in Pa_{O_2} above 70 torr have relatively less influence on O_2 transport. When Pa_{O_2} is low, interventions designed to increase hemoglobin affinity for oxygen (decrease hemoglobin P_{50}) such as hyperventilation (to lower Pa_{CO_2}) or bicarbonate administration (to increase pH) would increase systemic oxygen delivery by increasing the arterial saturation, but this may necessitate a lower P_{O_2} in the tissues to effect unloading of oxygen from the hemoglobin. The effects of lowering P_{50} on the oxygen extraction ability of the tissues is controversial, with some animal studies suggesting that low P_{50} reduces O_2 extraction ability[45] while others suggest that tissue extraction ability is unaffected.[46]

Positive end-expiratory pressure (PEEP) is another effective way to increase oxygen transport in acute respiratory failure, through its improvement in arterial oxyhemoglobin saturation. PEEP can also increase, decrease, or not change cardiac output, depending upon its relative effects on venous return, ventricular afterload, lung volume, ventricular interdependence, and other cardiopulmonary interactions. Judicial titration of the level of PEEP can optimize O_2 transport by maximizing the increase in saturation while minimizing the depression in cardiac output.

Another effective way to increase oxygen delivery is to increase cardiac output. This can usually be achieved by increasing preload or contractility, or by decreasing afterload. Intravascular volume expansion is often necessary early in resuscitation of septic patients, yet administered fluid leaks from both pulmonary and peripheral beds. Increases in extravascular lung water may necessitate increases in ventilatory pressures and aggravate hypoxemia. Reducing afterload should be undertaken carefully if at all, since most patients with suspected pathologic O_2 supply dependence exhibit low blood pressures. Of course, if contractility is normal and afterload is low, end-systolic volumes tend to be low, and little is to be gained. Yet ventricular function is often depressed in ARDS or other forms of acute hypoxic respiratory failure, and vasodilator therapy has been reported to increase cardiac output and reduce wedge pressures.

Augmenting contractility remains a possibility; use of sympathetic amines (dobutamine in particular) has become a popular means to increase oxygen delivery in this patient population. Dobutamine therapy does not substantially increase oxygen demand in normal animals, so benefits of increased oxygen delivery are unlikely to be negated by calorigenic effects. Dobutamine therapy has its own difficulties: Tachycardia can occasionally be limiting. Often, cardiac output in patients with ARDS or sepsis is limited by right ventricular performance rather than by left ventricular performance. Accordingly, management of circulatory function requires careful attention to both ventricles.

As with any situation in critical care medicine, the optimal combination of therapies used is best determined by individual patient evaluation based on physiologic principles. Without a clear way to test for pathologic O_2 supply dependency, therapy aimed at increasing oxygen delivery must include an appropriate endpoint. There is currently no physiologic rationale for identifying an adequate O_2 delivery, so decisions must be made on reasonable clinical grounds. One approach is to increase oxygen delivery until it is in the normal range—but identifying a fixed "normal value" is difficult. A second is to increase oxygen delivery until further attempts to increase it fail, or complications of the attempts limit further increases. Neither of these approaches is fully satisfying. At present, we undertake to restore hematocrit to 30–40, to ensure a normal arterial saturation, and to maximize cardiac output, often using sympathomimetics as inotropes.

Ultimately, the reason for difficulty in defining endpoints for increasing oxygen delivery is the failure of any study to demonstrate a "plateau" of oxygen uptake in supply-dependent patients, a difficulty that may stem from coupled measurement errors and the growing inaccuracy of cardiac output measurements at high flow rates. Thus, further studies are critically needed to establish meaningful recommendations.

IMPROVING OXYGEN DISTRIBUTION

At the present time, questions regarding the prevalence, significance, and mechanisms underlying pathologic O_2 supply dependency remain. The potential significance of occult tissue hypoxia to the morbidity and mortality of critical illness is significant, yet the lack of understanding of mechanisms involved complicates the development of rational therapeutic approaches. As information on the pathogenesis of extraction defects improves, specific therapies directed at the physiologic, cellular, and molecular derangements may become possible. Specific approaches to come from this line include using drugs to redistribute blood flow at the organ or microvascular level, manipulations of blood rheology to improve distribution of erythrocytes among microcirculatory channels, and attempting to directly treat the vascular changes underlying the septic state. Until more specific therapies become possible, the mainstay of supportive therapy must rely on efforts to improve oxygen delivery and decrease oxygen demand. Even here, controlled trials to answer central questions have not been done, and so a reasoned approach, based on known physiology and pathophysiology, is the basis of our therapeutic approach.

CASE PRESENTATION

A 61-year-old woman came to the emergency room complaining of severe dyspnea. She had a prior history of hypertension and congestive heart failure, and had suffered a 3-month course of dyspnea and weight loss. Initial physical examination revealed a cachectic woman, sitting bolt upright and breathing 40 times per minute, with a heart rate of 140/min, a blood pressure of 130/80, and a temperature of 38.7°. There was no jugular venous distension, and the cardiac exam revealed only tachycardia. The chest exam revealed dullness to percussion at the bases and coarse low-pitched wheezes throughout. A large liver was palpated, but the abdomen was otherwise normal. There was no cyanosis or clubbing; there was moderate pitting pretibial edema. A chest radiograph revealed bibasilar infiltrates, and moderate four-chamber dilation, with a normal azygos shadow, without pulmonary vascular redistribution and without signs of pulmonary edema. Her initial hematocrit was 36, and her leukocyte count was 12,600 with 81 percent neutrophils and 13 percent bands. Presumptive clinical diagnoses of pulmonary embolus and pneumonia were made, and she was placed on heparin and appropriate antibiotics. She was transferred to the coronary care unit; she was initially felt to be too unstable to undergo further diagnostic procedures.

On the second hospital day, a screening thyroid stimulating hormone test sent at the time of admission returned as undetectable. At this point, doses of propylthiouracil, potassium iodide, and propranolol were given for a presumed diagnosis of thyroid storm. Several hours later, the patient abruptly coughed up 300 mL of bright red blood. Coagulation parameters were retested, and she was found to have a partial thromboplastin time above 100 s, and heparin was stopped. The hemoptysis gradually subsided.

A second dose of propranolol was given, and the patient became more bradycardic and lethargic. A room-air blood gas drawn at this point revealed a pH of 7.39, a P_{CO_2} of 28, and a P_{O_2} of 83. Shortly after this blood gas returned, the patient had a combined respiratory and asystolic cardiac arrest. Her trachea was rapidly intubated, and mechanical ventilation was begun; shortly after receiving epinephrine, her cardiac rhythm returned to a sinus tachycardia. Her initial blood pressure was 103/51, but over the next few minutes it fell to 66 systolic. The pulses were weak and thready, the nailbeds were dusky, and capillary refill was completely absent. A blood gas revealed a pH of 7.21, a P_{CO_2} of 22, and a P_{O_2} of 100. Rapid bolus infusion of intravenous saline was begun, and the blood pressure returned to 106 systolic, and peripheral perfusion improved by clinical examination.

At this point, further diagnostic studies were undertaken. A lactate level was 11 m*M*. A pulmonary artery catheter was placed, showing a right atrial pressure of 26 torr, a right ventricular pressure of 60/30, a pulmonary artery pressure of 58/30, pulmonary wedge pressure of 30, and a systemic arterial pressure of 110/32. Her cardiac output was measured to be 1.56 liters, and a mixed venous blood sample displayed a saturation of 48%. A simultaneous arterial sample had a saturation of 98 percent, giving an extraction ratio of 51 percent. An echocardiograph revealed severe diffuse hypokinesis and four-chamber enlargement, with no pericardial effusion.

With this information, the patient was felt to be in cardiogenic shock, precipitated in part by beta blockade used in treatment of her hyperthyroidism. Treatment consisted of lowering her oxygen demand and further increasing her oxygen delivery. To reduce her oxygen demand, her fever was reduced with antipyretics, she was sedated to prevent respiratory efforts, and treatment with potassium iodide and propylthiouracil was continued to suppress thyroid hormone release. To improve her oxygen delivery, propranolol therapy was discontinued, and infusions of dopamine (at 2 μg/kg/min) and dobutamine (at 2 μg/kg/min increasing to 10 μg/kg/min) were begun. With these manipulations, her cardiac output rose to 4.25 L/min, and remained stable there. Her oxygen extraction ratio fell to 26 percent. Assuming no change in her hematocrit between these measurements, her $\dot{V}_{O_2}$ rose by 39 percent. Similar delivery-dependent oxygen uptake is often seen in patients with resolving lactic acidosis.

By the third hospital day, her lactic acid level had fallen to 2 m*M*, and her metabolic acidosis resolved. Therapy to maintain a stable cardiac output was continued, and the patient remained physiologically stable. On the fourth hospital day, sedation was withdrawn, the patient began to breathe, and mechanical ventilatory support was discontinued. Her dobutamine and dopamine were tapered and discontinued. By the fifth hospital day, all intensive therapies had been discontinued, and the patient was alert and comfortable. She completed her course of antibiotics, with resolution of her cough, fever, and leukocytosis. The remainder of her hospital course was uneventful.

CASE DISCUSSION

This patient developed abrupt circulatory failure under the watchful eye of a hospital coronary care unit. In retrospect, the diagnosis of thyroid storm was clear and the early use of beta blockers contraindicated, as discussed elsewhere in this text. Once hypotension developed, appropriate therapy was undertaken (initially intravascular volume expansion), even as diagnostic procedures began. Pulmonary artery catheter data and echocardiographic demonstration of severe left ventricular hypokinesis identified her shock as primarily cardiogenic; in patients like this one, the drop in blood volume (as might result from 300 mL acute hemoptysis), and the additional cardiac compromise associated with positive pressure ventilation results in dramatic hypotension. As often happens, cardiac output, oxygen extraction, and filling pressures were not measured before an empiric resuscitation had restored systemic arterial pressures to her baseline state. In this patient, a modest volume infusion (under 1 L of saline) restored high filling pressures. Even after the filling pressures were raised, cardiac output remained very low and oxygen extraction very high, and inotropic agents were used to restore an acceptable cardiac output. Because invasive measurements are available only after, not before, her acute decompensation, one can only speculate on the magnitude of the changes in each of her hemodynamic parameters. As volume infusion occurred, cardiac output increased along with systemic arterial pressure; at the same time, the dilutional effect reduced oxygen-carrying capacity. Since it took only a little volume to restore this patient's filling pressure to the high values necessary for her to have an acceptable cardiac output, we conclude that her vasculature was relatively stiff, and the dilutional effect was more than offset by the difference in cardiac output.

Even after volume resuscitation had restored clinically apparent perfusion and a normal blood pressure, this patient exhibited a markedly elevated extraction ratio of 51 percent. Note that the extraction ratio was calculated from direct (optical) measurements of hemoglobin saturation in the arterial and mixed venous blood. Using saturations rather than contents eliminates errors from spurious hemoglobin measurements that accrue from red cell settling. When extraction ratios are calculated in this fashion, they offer a valuable measurement of adequacy of oxygen delivery, entirely independent of the thermodilution cardiac output measurement.

The very high extraction ratio (50 percent) this patient displayed even after resuscitation restored an acceptable arterial pressure suggests that the extraction ratio may have been much higher earlier, when the patient was still hypotensive and making lactic acid. Treatment measures appropriately focused on lowering oxygen demand and increasing oxygen delivery. With improvement in oxygen delivery, lactic acidosis eventually resolved, and the patient recovered uneventfully. While similar strategies (reduction of demand and increase in delivery) are also often considered in high flow states such as sepsis, the end points of therapy are often much more difficult to define.

References

1. Cain SM: Relative rates of arterial lactate and oxygen-deficit accumulation in hypoxic dogs. Am J Physiol 224:1190, 1973.
2. Arieff AI, Graf H: Pathophysiology of type A hypoxic lactic acidosis in dogs. Am J Physiol 253:E271, 1987.
3. Connett RJ, Gayeski TEJ, Honig CR: Lactate accumulation in fully aerobic, working dog gracilis muscle. Am J Physiol 246 (Heart Circ Physiol 15):H120, 1984.
4. Longmuir IS: Respiration rate of rat liver cells at low oxygen concentration. Biochem J 65:378, 1957.

5. Samsel RW, Nelson DP, Sanders WM, Wood LDH, Schumacker PT: The effect of endotoxin on systemic and skeletal muscle oxygen extraction. J Appl Physiol 65:1377, 1988.
6. Lautt WW: Effect of raised portal venous pressure and postocclusive hyperemia on superior mesenteric arterial resistance in control and adenosine receptor blocked state in cats. Can J Physiol Pharmacol 64:1296, 1986.
7. Nelson DP, King CE, Dodd SL, Schumacker PT, Cain SM: Systemic and intestinal limits of O_2 extraction in the dog. J Appl Physiol 63:387, 1987.
8. Nelson DP, Samsel RW, Wood LDH, Schumacker PT: Pathologic supply dependence of systemic and intestinal O_2 uptake during endotoxemia in dogs. J Appl Physiol 64:2410, 1988.
9. Ezzat WR, Lautt WW: Hepatic arterial pressure flow autoregulation is adenosine mediated. Am J Physiol 252:H836, 1987.
10. Suga H, Hayashi T, Sirahata M, Ninomiya I: Critical evaluation of left ventricular systolic pressure volume area as predictor of oxygen consumption rate. Am J Physiol 240:H39, 1981.
11. Walley KR, Becker CJ, Hogan RA, Wood LDH: Progressive hypoxemia limits left ventricular oxygen consumption and contractility. Circ Res 63:849, 1988.
12. Lassen NA, Munck O, Thaysen JH: Oxygen consumption and sodium reabsorption in the kidney. Acta Physiol Scand 51:371, 1961.
13. Gotshall RW, Miles DW, Sexson WR: Renal oxygen delivery and consumption during progressive hypoxemia in the anesthetized dog. Proc Soc Expt Biol Med 174:363, 1983.
14. Cain SM: Gas Exchange in hypoxia, apnea, and hyperoxia, in *Handbook of Physiology—The Respiratory System IV*. American Physiological Society. Baltimore, Williams & Wilkins, pp 403–420, 1964.
15. Cain SM, Chapler CK: O_2 extraction by canine hindlimb during α adrenergic blockade and hypoxic hypoxia. J Appl Physiol 48:630, 1980.
16. Granger HJ, Goodman AH, Cook BK: Metabolic models of microcirculatory regulation. Fed Proc 34:2025, 1975.
17. Hochachka PW, Guppy M: *Metabolic Arrest and the Control of Biologic Time*. Cambridge, MA, Harvard, 1987.
18. Schumacker PT, Samsel RW: Oxygen delivery and uptake by peripheral tissues: Physiology and pathophysiology. Crit Care Clin 5:255, 1989.
19. Cain SM: Supply dependence of oxygen uptake: Myth or reality? Am J Med Sci 288:119, 1984.
20. Schumacker PT, Cain SM: The concept of a critical oxygen delivery. Intensive Care Med 13:223, 1987.
21. Schlichtig R, Cowden WL, Chaitman BR: Tolerance of unusually low mixed venous oxygen saturation. Am J Med 80:813, 1986.
22. Archie JP: Mathematical coupling of data. A common source of error. Ann Surg 193:296, 1981.
23. Annat G, Viale J-P, Percival C, Froment M, Motin J: Oxygen delivery and uptake in the adult respiratory distress syndrome. Am Rev Respir Dis 133:999, 1986.
24. Carlile PV, Gray BA: Effect of opposite changes in cardiac output and arterial P_{O_2} on the relationship between mixed venous P_{O_2} and oxygen transport. Am Rev Respir Dis 140:891, 1989.
25. Gilbert EM, Haupt MT, Mandanas RY, Huaringa AJ, Carlson RW: The effect of fluid loading, blood transfusion, and catecholamine infusion on oxygen delivery and consumption in patients with sepsis. Am Rev Respir Dis 134:873, 1986.
26. Haupt MT, Gilbert EM, Carlson RW: Fluid loading increases oxygen consumption in septic patients with lactic acidosis. Am Rev Respir Dis 131:912, 1985.
27. Cerra FB: Hypermetabolism-organ failure syndrome: A metabolic response to injury. Crit Care Clin 5:289, 1989.
28. Pepe PE, Culver BH: Independently measured oxygen consumption during reduction of oxygen delivery by positive end-expiratory pressure. Am Rev Respir Dis 132:788, 1985.
29. Long GR, Nelson DP, Sznajder JI, Wood LDH, Schumacker PT: Systemic oxygen delivery and consumption during acute lung injury in dogs. J Crit Care 3:249, 1988.
30. Nelson DP, Beyer C, Samsel RW, Wood LDH, Schumacker PT: Pathological supply dependence of O_2 uptake during bacteremia in dogs. J Appl Physiol 63:1487, 1987.
31. Albert RK, Schrijen F, Poincelot F: Oxygen consumption and transport in stable patients with chronic obstructive pulmonary disease. Am Rev Respir Dis 134:678, 1986.
32. Mohsenifar Z, Amin D, Jasper AC, Shah PK, Koerner SK: Dependence of oxygen consumption on oxygen delivery in patients with chronic congestive heart failure. Chest 93:447, 1987.
33. Williams AJ, Mohsenifar Z: Oxygen supply dependency in patients with obstructive sleep apnea and its reversal after therapy with nasal continuous positive airway pressure. Am Rev Respir Dis 140:1308, 1989.
34. Mohsenifar Z, Jasper AC, Koerner SK: Relationship between oxygen uptake and oxygen delivery in patients with pulmonary hypertension. Am Rev Respir Dis 138:69, 1988.
35. Zweifach BW, Thomas L: The role of epinephrine in the reactions produced by the endotoxins of gram negative bacteria. The changes produced by endotoxin in the vascular reactivity of epinephrine of the rat mesoappendix and the isolated perfused rabbit ear. J Exp Med 104:881, 1956.
36. Baker CH, Wilmoth FH: Microvascular responses to *E. coli* endotoxin with altered adrenergic activity. Circ Shock 12:165, 1984.
37. Altura BM, Gebrewold A, Burton RW: Reactive hyperemic responses of single arterioles are attenuated markedly after intestinal ischemia, endotoxemia and traumatic shock: Possible role of endothelial cells. Microcirc Endothelium Lymphatics 2:3, 1985.
38. Altura BM, Gebrewold A, Burton RW: Failure of microscopic metarterioles to elicit vasodilator responses to acetylcholine, bradykinin, histamine and substance P after ischemic shock, endotoxemia and trauma: possible role of endothelial cells. Microcirc Endothelium Lymphatics 2:121, 1985.
39. Hartl WH, Gunther B, Inthorn D, Heberer G: Reactive hyperemia in patients with septic conditions. Surgery 103:440, 1988.
40. Lee MM, Scheussler GB, Chien S: Time-dependent effects of endotoxin on the ultrastructure of aortic endothelium. Artery 15:71, 1988.
41. Schumacker PT, Samsel RW: Analysis of oxygen delivery and uptake relationships in the Krogh tissue model. J Appl Physiol 67:1234, 1989.
42. Cain SM, Chapler CK: Circulatory responses to 2,4-dinitrophenol in dog limb during normoxia and hypoxia. J Appl Physiol 59:698, 1985.
43. Schumacker PT, Rowland J, Saltz S, Nelson DP, Wood LDH: Effects of hyperthermia and hypothermia on oxygen extraction by tissues during hypovolemia. J Appl Physiol 63:1246, 1987.
44. Hershenson MB, O'Rourke PP, Schena JA, Crone RK: Effect of halothane on critical levels of oxygen transport in the anesthetized newborn lamb. Anesthesiology 64:174, 1988.
45. Gutierrez G, Andry JM: Increased hemoglobin O_2 affinity does not improve O_2 consumption in hypoxemia. J Appl Physiol 66:837, 1989.
46. Schumacker PT, Long GR, Wood LDH: Tissue oxygen extraction during hypovolemia: role of hemoglobin P_{50}. J Appl Physiol 62:1801, 1987.

Chapter 58

ROLE OF FREE RADICALS IN CRITICAL ILLNESS

A. NAHUM
J. I. SZNAJDER

KEY POINTS

- *Toxic oxygen metabolites, O_2^-, H_2O_2, and $OH\cdot$, are produced during sequential single electron reduction of O_2 to H_2O.*
- *O_2^- and H_2O_2 in the presence of metal ions (Fe^{2+}, Cu^+) can form the extremely reactive and toxic hydroxyl radical $OH\cdot$.*
- *Toxic O_2 metabolites can lead to cell injury via protein degradation, lipid peroxidation, deoxyribonucleic acid (DNA) and membrane damage, and activation of inflammatory mediators.*
- *Major antioxidant defenses either neutralize O_2^- or H_2O_2 or sequester metal ions to prevent $OH\cdot$ formation.*
- *High concentrations of inspired O_2 (F_{IO_2}) are toxic; oxygenation should be maintained with the lowest tolerable F_{IO_2}.*
- *Ischemia reperfusion in various organs induces injury mediated by toxic O_2 metabolites.*

The sequential single electron reduction of oxygen (O_2) with subsequent production of toxic O_2 metabolites was described by chemists in the early 1930s. The biologic importance of these reactions was appreciated after the discovery of superoxide dismutase (SOD) in 1969 and by the discovery that neutrophils (PMNs) can generate superoxide radicals.[1] Since then, many investigators have sought to elucidate the role of toxic O_2 metabolites in a variety of disease states.

It is clear that toxic O_2 metabolites can be produced intracellularly in a variety of cell types.[1–3] Cell injury occurs when production of toxic O_2 metabolites overwhelms the antioxidant defense mechanisms of the cell. When a sufficient number of cells is affected, end organ dysfunction is evident. The tissue injury produced by toxic O_2 metabolites can be limited or amplified by both intra- and extracellular inflammatory mechanisms. For instance, production of arachidonic acid products, activation of complement or coagulation cascades, and activation and recruitment of platelets or neutrophils can all affect the degree and character of the tissue injury.

Studies examining involvement of toxic O_2 metabolites in disease are often indirect, since these metabolites are very short-lived, are produced at very low concentrations and are difficult to assay.[1] In order to prove an association between the disease process and the production of toxic O_2 metabolites, three criteria should be met: production of toxic O_2 metabolites during the disease process, protection against the injury by agents that remove the toxic O_2 metabolites, and reproduction of the disease process by application of toxic O_2 metabolites at the organ of interest. Many animal models of tissue injury satisfy these criteria. However, extrapolation of these studies to humans is difficult, and unequivocal evidence for involvement of toxic O_2 metabolites in human disease requires clinical studies that demonstrate that these criteria are satisfied.

Chemistry

Molecular oxygen in its ground state contains two unpaired electrons with parallel spins, whereas most organic compounds contain a single outermost electron. For O_2 to react with such organic compounds, the spin of one of its outermost electrons must be reversed. This energy requirement for spin reversal makes O_2 a relatively nonreactive substance in the absence of a catalyst. Nevertheless, under certain conditions, O_2 forms reactive metabolites that can lead to tissue injury.

Singlet O_2 is produced when absorption of sufficient energy shifts one of oxygen's unpaired electrons to a higher orbit with inversion of spin. Singlet O_2 can dissipate its excess energy by light emission, chemical reaction, or thermal decay. These processes can lead to local thermal and chemical injury.

As shown schematically in Fig. 58-1, toxic O_2 metabolites are produced during sequential single-electron reduction of O_2 to water. Univalent reduction of O_2 leads to the formation of superoxide anion radical (O_2^-), which is unstable, with a lifetime of milliseconds at neutral pH.[1,3] Superoxide anion protonates to the weak acid perhydroxyl radical ($OH_2\cdot$) with a pK_a of 4.8, therefore, at physiologic pH, O_2^- predominates. $OH_2\cdot$ is a stronger oxidant than O_2^- and can react with polyunsaturated fatty acids. In acidic cellular microenvironments, $OH_2\cdot$ can be the major form and can increase the toxicity of O_2^-.[1,3,4] Superoxide anion dismutates spontaneously to hydrogen peroxide (H_2O_2) and O_2 with a rate constant of 2×10^5 L/mol/s at pH 7.4.[5] Consequently, production of O_2^- in physiologic systems invariably leads to formation of H_2O_2. Because of its negative charge, O_2^- is not very lipid soluble. However, it is transported across membranes through anion channels.[1,6] Superoxide anion is a weak oxidant but a potent reductant. The low reactivity of O_2^- suggests that O_2^- by itself is not the major mediator of cytotoxicity but rather a precursor to more reactive O_2^- derived metabolites.[1,6]

Two electron reduction of O_2 or single electron reduction of O_2^- leads to the formation of hydrogen peroxide (H_2O_2), which is a relatively stable oxidant.[7] H_2O_2 has approximately the same lipid solubility as O_2 and can readily traverse membranes.[1,7] H_2O_2 has a vapor pressure of about 5 mmHg at 37°C and, because of its volatility and high lipid solubility, can be excreted by the lungs.

Three electron reduction of O_2 to form the hydroxyl free radical ($HO\cdot$), a powerful oxidizing agent, cannot occur.

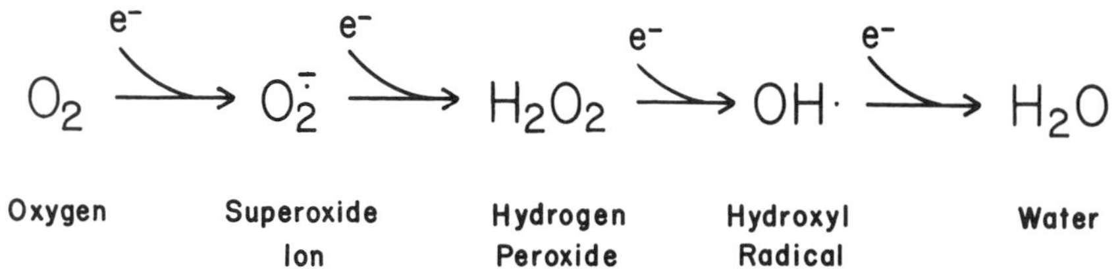

FIGURE 58-1 Sequential single electron (e^-) reduction of oxygen (O_2) to water (H_2O).

However, in the presence of certain transition metals (Fe^{2+}, Mn^{2+}, Cu^{+}), metal chelates, or hemoproteins, O_2^- and H_2O_2 can undergo the following reactions to form the hydroxyl radical ($HO\cdot$):[1,3,4]

$$\begin{array}{rl} O_2^- + Fe^{3+} & \longrightarrow O_2 + Fe^{2+} \\ H_2O_2 + Fe^{2+} & \longrightarrow HO\cdot + OH^- + Fe^{3+} \\ \hline O_2^- + H_2O_2 & \longrightarrow HO\cdot + OH^- + O_2 \end{array}$$

This reaction is known as the iron-catalyzed Haber-Weiss reaction, or O_2^- driven Fenton reaction. Since O_2^- production is always associated with the production of H_2O_2, during formation of O_2^- the presence of trace quantities of metal ions can lead to the formation of $HO\cdot$. Organic peroxides, as well as H_2O_2, can yield $HO\cdot$.[8] Hydroxyl radical can react with virtually any organic molecule, with reaction rates that approach diffusion limited rates of 10^7 to 10^{10} L/mol/s.[1,3,4] Because $HO\cdot$ is extremely reactive, it survives for only a few collisions after it is formed. This implies that $OH\cdot$ reacts at the sites of production. Hence, the quantity of $OH\cdot$ produced may be less critical than the specific location. For instance, even small quantities of $OH\cdot$ formed on the surface of DNA or membrane proteins could lead to cellular dysfunction.

The hydroxyl radical can initiate lipid peroxidation by hydrogen abstraction from lipids (LH). The resulting lipid radical ($L\cdot$) reacts rapidly with O_2 to form a lipid peroxy radical ($LOO\cdot$), which itself can abstract a hydrogen atom from an unsaturated lipid molecule and form a lipid hydroperoxide (LOOH) and a lipid radical.[1,8]

$$\begin{array}{lrl} \text{Initiation} & LH + HO\cdot & \longrightarrow L\cdot + H_2O \\ \text{Propagation} & L\cdot + O_2 & \longrightarrow LOO\cdot \\ & LOO\cdot + LH & \longrightarrow LOOH + L\cdot \\ \text{Termination} & L\cdot + L\cdot & \longrightarrow LL \\ & LO_2\cdot + LO_2\cdot & \longrightarrow LOOL + O_2 \\ & LO_2\cdot + L\cdot & \longrightarrow LOOL \end{array}$$

In this manner, lipid peroxidation is propagated until two lipid radical species react with each other and terminate lipid peroxidation. In physiologic systems iron leads to partial reduction of O_2 and can initiate lipid peroxidation. Iron can also enhance the rate of lipid oxidation by converting lipid hydroperoxides (LOOH) to reactive alkoxyl ($LO\cdot$) or peroxyl ($LOO\cdot$) radicals.[8]

Iron absorbed from the gut is transported in plasma bound to transferrin. One transferrin molecule binds two ferric iron molecules.[1,3] Iron bound to transferrin cannot catalyze $OH\cdot$ formation or induce lipid peroxidation at physiologic pH. However, at pH < 6, iron easily detaches from transferrin. Therefore, iron can be made available to catalyze radical reactions if the microenvironment is made acidic, as occurs during phagocytosis. Intercellular iron is stored in the ferric state bound to ferritin. Superoxide anion can release ferrous iron from ferritin.[3] Consequently, despite the tight control of iron in physiologic systems, under the proper conditions, iron, as well as other metal ions, can be available to catalyze free radical reactions. Cellular injury appears to enhance the availability of free iron.[3] Therefore, cellular injury can potentially amplify the formation of radical species and contribute to the deterioration of tissue injury. For instance, cerebrospinal fluid lacks any appreciable iron-binding capacity despite the fact that certain areas of the brain are rich in iron.[9,10] Injury of the brain leads to release of iron, which initiates lipid peroxidation and may extend post injury tissue degradation.

Certain hemoprotein peroxidases, like myeloperoxidase (MPO) and eosinophilic peroxidase (EPO), have the ability to combine with H_2O_2 and a halide anion (Cl^-, I^-, Br^-), or a pseudohalide (like thiocyanate, SCN^-) to form potent oxidizing agents.[1,11,12] Oxidation of Cl^-, I^-, and Br^- anions by an oxidase and H_2O_2 leads to the formation of hypochlorous (HOCl), hypoiodous (HOI), and hypobromous (HOBr) acids, respectively. All these hypohalous acids are potent oxidizing and halogenating agents. On a molar basis, the ability of halides to promote MPO- and H_2O_2-induced cytotoxicity follows the order $I^- > Br^- > Cl^-$. Since the physiologic concentration of Cl^- is much greater than other halides, with few exceptions, the most commonly formed hypohalous acid is HOCl. Of physiologic interest is the rapid reaction of HOCl with primary-amines to form *N*-chloramine derivatives (RNHCl).[12] Since physiologic concentrations of primary-amines are high and some forms of RNHCl are very lipophilic, RNHCl is the likely final mediator of cell toxicity of the MPO–H_2O_2–Cl^- system.[12]

Peroxidases can also catalyze the oxidation of SCN^- by H_2O_2 to form the hypothiocyanate anion ($OSCN^-$). The $OSCN^-$ anion can oxidize sulfhydryl compounds (RSH) to sulfinic acid (RSOH), while regenerating SCN^-.[5] Lactoperoxidase, H_2O_2, and SCN^- are present in relatively high concentrations in human saliva, tears, and milk. This reaction system is thought to control oral and gastrointestinal bacterial growth and maintain the sterility of human tears and milk.[1]

A number of compounds can enhance production of toxic oxygen metabolites by redox cycling.[1,4,13] In this process the compound is first reduced, then reacts with O_2 to regenerate the parent compound and produce O_2^-. Paraquat, adriamycin, and nitrofurantoin are such compounds and contribute to toxic O_2 metabolite generation. Some xenobiotics produce free radicals during their metabolism. For instance, carbon tetrachloride is reduced in the liver by nicotinamide adenine dinucleotide phosphate (NADPH)-cytochrome P_{450} reductase to form trichloromethyl radical, which can then react with O_2 to form the more reactive $CCl_3OO\cdot$ radical. Other compounds, such as nitrogen dioxide, are free radicals themselves and can initiate lipid peroxidation.

Defense Mechanisms Against Toxic Oxygen Metabolites

ANTIOXIDANT ENZYMES

Superoxide dismutase (SOD) catalyzes the dismutation of O_2^- to H_2O_2 and O_2, increasing the rate of spontaneous dismutation 10,000-fold.[1,6] SOD exists as a Mn-containing protein in the mitochondria and as a Cu–Zn containing protein in the cytoplasm. Hydrogen peroxide formed during spontaneous dismutation or SOD catalyzed reaction is decomposed to water by the enzyme catalase.[1] SOD and catalase act in concert to remove both O_2^- and H_2O_2 and, thus, prevent formation of the most potent radical, $HO\cdot$. Catalase is specific for H_2O_2 and does not decompose organic hydroperoxides. Organic peroxides, as well as H_2O_2, are decomposed by a Se-containing enzyme, glutathione peroxidase (GPO). GPO uses glutathione (GSH) as the reducing agent to catalyze the decomposition of organic hydroperoxides (ROOH) to water and an organic alcohol (ROH)

$$2GSH + ROOH \xrightarrow{GPO} GSSG + ROH + H_2O$$

As shown earlier, during this reaction GSH is oxidized to GSSG, which is recycled by the glutathione reductase catalyzed reaction. GPO is specific for GSH as the reductant, but can reduce a variety of other hydroperoxides, including H_2O_2, cumene hydroperoxide, and lipid hydroperoxides.[1] Enhanced production of O_2^- can initiate lipid peroxidation or lead to increased cellular H_2O_2 concentrations. Removal of H_2O_2 by glutathione peroxidase (GPO) will deplete the cell of glutathione (GSH) and leave it susceptible to peroxidative damage.[7]

CuZn–SOD is found in relatively high concentrations in the liver and brain, in moderate concentrations in the kidneys and heart, and in low concentrations in the lungs and red blood cells. Catalase is found in high concentrations in the liver and red blood cells; in moderate concentrations in the kidney, lung, and adipose tissue; and in low concentrations in the brain and muscle. GPO activity is high in the liver; moderate in the heart, lung, and brain; and low in the muscle.

ANTIOXIDANTS AND CHELATORS OF METAL IONS

Several biologic compounds have the ability to inhibit free-radical generated reactions or directly scavenge free radicals. α-Tocopherol (vitamin E) has been shown to prevent lipid peroxidation and prevent oxidant injury in some models. β-Carotene, a precursor of vitamin A, can scavenge $HO\cdot$ and HOCl. Sulfhydryl compounds and other oxidizable compounds, such as GSH, methionine, and ascorbate, reduce reactive O_2 metabolites and decrease their oxidizing potential. However, ascorbate can also reduce Fe^{3+} to Fe^{2+}, which in the presence of H_2O_2 can stimulate $HO\cdot$ formation. The role of GSH as a substrate for GPO was discussed earlier. In addition, GSH can scavenge $HO\cdot$. Uric acid is also a powerful scavenger of hydroxyl radicals and can inhibit peroxidation. Glucose in physiologic concentrations has the ability to scavenge $HO\cdot$. Albumin can act as a radical scavenger. It binds copper tightly, and iron weakly. Iron bound to albumin can still participate in radical producing reactions, but radicals formed in this manner on the surface of albumin react with albumin and are effectively removed from the solution.

Antioxidant defense systems and their interaction with toxic O_2 metabolites are schematically illustrated in Fig. 58-2. Antioxidant defense systems are located in specific locations within the cell, where they can neutralize the effects of toxic O_2 metabolites most effectively.[14] Intracellularly the defenses consist of enzymatic neutralization of toxic oxygen metabolites and containment of lipid peroxidation.[1,2,9] Intracellular antioxidant defenses consist largely of specific enzymes, such as SOD, catalase, GPO, and small molecules such as vitamin C (see Fig. 58-2). SOD, GPO, and vitamin C form the main cytoplasmic defenses. Catalase is mainly found in peroxisomes, whereas mitochondria contains SOD and GPO.[7] Vitamin E and β-carotene are part of the antioxidant defenses of cellular membranes. Extracellular defenses are tailored for scavenging free radicals and chelation of transition metals to limit the formation of $OH\cdot$.[1,3,9] Most extracellular fluids contain very low SOD, catalase, and GPO activity.[1,3,9] For instance, plasma catalase activity is about 4000-fold less than that of red blood cells. In extracellular fluids, antioxidant defenses are performed by low molecular weight compounds that act as scavengers and/or chelate metal ions and prevent them from participating in reactions that form radicals.[3,9] In plasma the major metal ion chelators are transferrin and ceruloplasmin. Transferrin can effectively chelate iron and prevent the generation of $HO\cdot$. Ceruloplasmin can react with O_2^- and also possesses ferroxidase activity, i.e., it can oxidize Fe^{2+} to Fe^{3+} and prevent the iron-catalyzed Haber-Weiss reaction. The iron-binding protein lactoferrin released by activated neutrophils also binds iron and limits radical production. Many antioxidant defense systems require micronutrients. For instance, Se is essential for GPO. Therefore, the nutritional state of the cell also affects the level and characteristics of antioxidant defenses.[14]

Generation of Toxic O_2 Metabolites and Subsequent Tissue Damage

Toxic oxygen metabolites can be produced intracellularly or extracellularly by inflammatory cells or through redox cycling of xenobiotics. The bulk of oxygen reduction in the

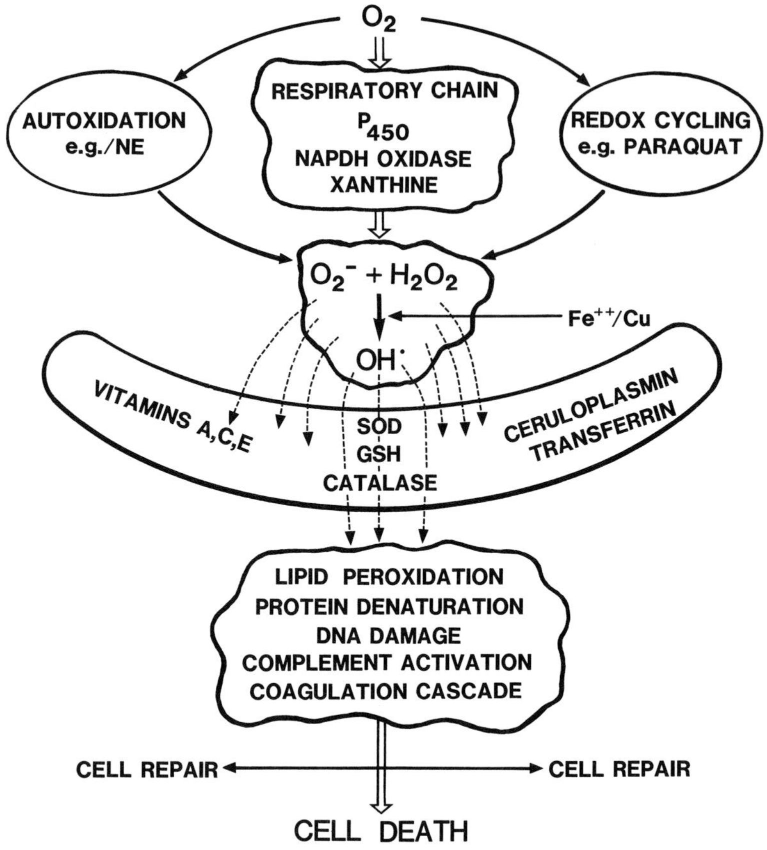

FIGURE 58-2 Schematic representation of the sequence events that lead to cell toxicity from production of toxic oxygen metabolites.

cell occurs in the mitochondrial cytochrome oxidase pathway. During this reaction, four electrons are transferred to O_2 to form H_2O.[2,13] The flow of electrons in the respiratory chain of the mitochondria leads to sequential reduction of flavoproteins, ubiquinone, and mitochondrial cytochromes. Single-electron transfer occurs during the reduction of ubiquinone and possibly flavins, where leakage of the electrons to O_2 could result in generation of O_2^-. Inhibition of the respiratory chain distal to the site of ubiquinone reduction results in increased production of O_2^-. Similarly, ubiquinone-repleted mitochondria demonstrate an enhanced ability to produce toxic oxygen metabolites relative to ubiquinone-depleted mitochondria.[13] These results suggest that the reduced form of ubiquinone, ubisemiquinone,

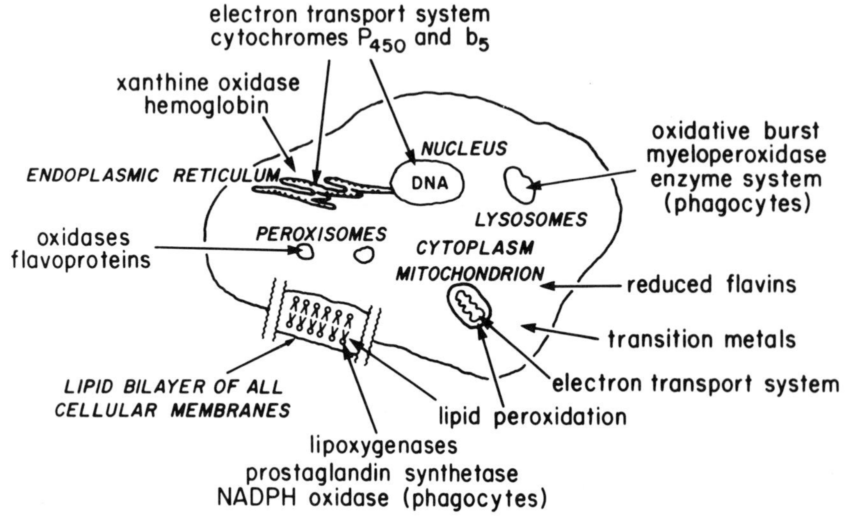

FIGURE 58-3 Cellular sources of toxic oxygen metabolites. (Adapted with permission from Machlin LJ, Bendich A: Free radical tissue damage: Protective role of antioxidant nutrients. FASEB Monogr 1:441–445, 1987.)

reacts with O_2 to form O_2^- during reoxidation by the cytochrome *b* complex. The major source of intracellular O_2^- production appears to be leakage of electrons from the electron transport chain in the mitochondria and the cytochrome P_{450} system.[2,13] Under normal conditions, up to 5 percent of O_2 that is consumed by the respiratory chain is converted to toxic O_2 metabolites that are neutralized by intracellular antioxidant defense mechanisms.[1,2,13] In inflammatory cells like neutrophils and eosinophils, specific enzymes, such as NADPH oxidase, produce toxic oxygen metabolites.[11,12] In all systems, the increased availability of O_2 during hyperoxia leads to increased generation of toxic oxygen metabolites. The O_2^- generated in the mitochondria is mainly dismutated to H_2O_2 by SOD.

Several other reactions in the cell result in univalent or divalent reduction of O_2 leading to the formation of O_2^- and H_2O_2.[1,5,13,14] The electron transport system of the endoplasmic reticulum that utilizes cytochrome P_{450} transfers one electron from reduced flavin to cytochrome P_{450}-substrate complex. Auto-oxidation of the partially reduced flavin can then transfer the electron to O_2 forming O_2^-. Superoxide anion and H_2O_2 are also produced in specific peroxisomal enzymatic reactions. NADPH oxidase that resides in the plasma membrane of the neutrophil produces O_2^-. Urate oxidase generates H_2O_2 during the conversion of urate to allantoin, xanthine oxidase and aldehyde oxidase produce H_2O_2 or O_2^- during conversion of hypoxanthine to uric acid, and D-amino oxidase and monooxidase can generate H_2O_2. Cellular sources of toxic O_2 metabolites are schematically illustrated in Fig. 58-3.

Auto-oxidation of physiologic or pharmacologic compounds can also generate O_2^-.[1] Quinones and catechols are two classes of biologic compounds that are susceptible to auto-oxidation. Radical production from thiols, hydropterins, flavins, and hemoglobin has also been demonstrated.

Toxic oxygen metabolites can lead to tissue injury in a variety of ways. They can initiate lipid peroxidation with subsequent cell membrane dysfunction. They can also activate a variety of biologic cascades, including complement and coagulation components. They can cause depletion of cellular adenosine triphosphate (ATP) levels, denature enzymes and proteins, activate proteinases, deactivate antiproteinases, damage DNA, and act as substrates for the formation of other toxic substances. The cell copes with oxidative stress through antioxidant defenses, as outlined earlier.

Neutrophils have the ability to generate large quantities of toxic oxygen species and convert H_2O_2 that they produce to hypohalous acid through MPO.[11,12] Similarly, eosinophils can generate hypohalous acid utilizing H_2O_2 and eosinophil peroxidase. Toxic O_2 metabolites and proteinases can interact to augment tissue injury.[12] Oxidants can inactivate plasma-derived proteinase inhibitors, allowing cellularly secreted proteinases to function freely.[12] For instance, neutrophils use chlorinated oxidants to inactivate the antiproteinases, like alpha$_1$-proteinase inhibitor, while activating latent metallo-proteinases collagenase and gelatinase. At the same time, secretion of elastase and other metalloproteinases by the neutrophils inactivates the proteinase inhibitors. Thus, neutrophils can create a microenvironment where neutrophil elastase and other plasma-derived proteinases as well as neutrophil-derived oxidants can damage host tissues free of inhibitors.[12]

Markers of Oxidative Injury

EXPIRED BREATH H_2O_2

Hydrogen peroxide can be excreted by the lungs because of its volatility, high lipid permeability, and stability.[15] The H_2O_2 measured in the expired breath arises either from toxic oxygen metabolite production by inflammatory cells or by an oxidative process involving the lungs. The fraction of H_2O_2 that escapes the body's defense mechanisms is available for excretion by the lungs. Hence, not all oxidative or inflammatory processes lead to increased concentrations of H_2O_2 in the expired breath. Also, contamination by mouth flora and saliva may erroneously elevate expired breath H_2O_2 ($EB_{H_2O_2}$) levels.[15] For this reason, only intubated patients can be examined for the amount of H_2O_2 present in their expired breath. Elevated $EB_{H_2O_2}$ levels have been reported in patients with adult respiratory distress syndrome (ARDS).[16] In a more extensive study, $EB_{H_2O_2}$ was measured in four groups of patients.[15] In otherwise healthy patients undergoing elective nonthoracic surgery, $EB_{H_2O_2}$ levels were undetectable. However, all patients studied in the intensive care unit demonstrated elevated levels of $EB_{H_2O_2}$. Specifically, patients with hypoxemic respiratory failure who had either adult respiratory distress syndrome (ARDS) or focal lung infiltrates demonstrated the highest levels of $EB_{H_2O_2}$, as shown in Fig. 58-4. The importance of these observations, for patient management, as early markers of oxidative load that may contribute to lung injury requires further study.

MARKERS OF LIPID PEROXIDATION

There are a number of techniques for measuring lipid peroxidation,[1,3,17,18] but no single method accurately reflects overall lipid peroxidation. Two techniques, expired breath hydrocarbon gases and thiobarbituric acid test for malondialdehyde, have been used most extensively in humans.

EXPIRED BREATH ETHANE AND PENTANE

The volatile gases ethane and pentane are produced as minor side products during transition metal-catalyzed oxidation of lipid hydroperoxides. These volatile gases are excreted by the lungs and are easily measured by the technique of gas-liquid chromatography. However, the methodology suffers from the fact that the gases are minor end products of peroxidation, and measurements can be confounded by elevations in the availability of metal ions catalyzing lipid peroxidation.[3]

In experimental animal models, the amount of pentane or ethane detected in the expired breath depends on the nutritional status of the animal.[8] Animals that are fed diets

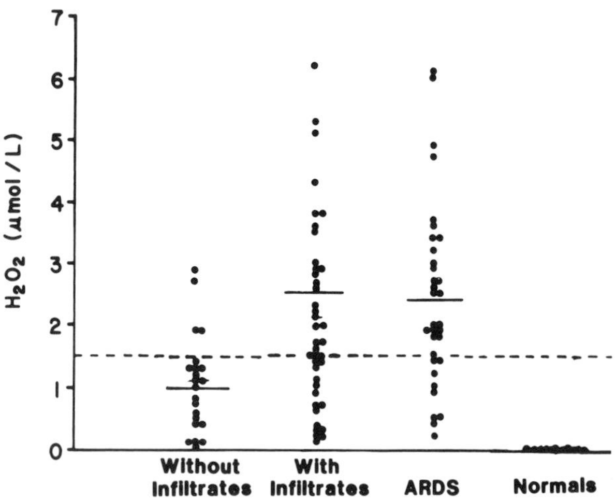

FIGURE 58-4 Hydrogen peroxide levels in the expired breath condensate of patients with adult respiratory distress syndrome (ARDS) versus acute hypoxic respiratory failure (AHRF) patients with focal pulmonary infiltrates, mechanically ventilated patients without pulmonary infiltrates, and patients undergoing elective nonthoracic surgery (normals). (Adapted with permission from Sznajder JI, Fraiman A, Hall JB et al: Increased hydrogen peroxide in the expired breath of patients with acute hypoxemic respiratory failure. Chest 96:606–612, 1989.)

poor in vitamin E and Se demonstrate increased expired pentane. Animals fed polyunsaturated fats to increase the available substrate for lipid peroxidation also have increased pentane excretion. These results suggest that expired breath pentane and ethane measurements could be used as in vivo markers of lipid peroxidation. However, certain precautions must be applied to interpretation. Pentane is also metabolized by the liver, introducing a further source of error. Drugs or conditions that affect the metabolism of pentane would lead to misleading conclusions regarding lipid peroxidation. Moreover, control experiments measuring gas production by gut bacteria and purification of inhaled air for volatile hydrocarbon contamination are necessary to interpret the results.[8] In humans expired breath pentane or ethane measurements require a 60- to 90-min equilibration period prior to the measurement to wash out the tissue stores absorbed from the atmosphere. Expired breath pentane levels increased 60 to 400 percent in six healthy volunteers within 30 min of exposure to 100 percent oxygen. This suggested rapid onset of lipid peroxidation in hyperoxia.[19]

THIOBARBITURIC ACID TEST

The thiobarbituric acid (TBA) test is one of the oldest and most frequently used methods to evaluate lipid oxygenation.[1,3,17–20] The test relies on formation of malondialdehyde (MDA), which is a byproduct of lipid peroxide decomposition in the presence of trace quantities of iron salts.[20] The sensitivity of the test is high, but other physiologic compounds, such as prostaglandin endoperoxides, also react with TBA. Usually the TBA test is calibrated with MDA, and the results are expressed as amount of MDA produced per unit time. In human studies the amount of TBA reactive material changes with sex and age.[17]

Serum lipid peroxide levels were found to be elevated in active hepatitis, fulminant hepatitis, and fatty liver.[21] Similarly, in heavy drinkers, liver lipoperoxide levels measured from liver biopsy samples were higher than in nondrinkers.[21] These results suggest that certain liver diseases lead to lipid peroxidation. Whether lipid peroxidation causes liver injury or occurs as a result of liver dysfunction still remains to be determined. It has also been demonstrated that the erythrocytes of patients with circulatory shock contain a larger amount of lipid peroxidation-derived aldehydes than those of normal adults.[22] This suggests that plasma levels of lipid peroxidation could be a marker of increased oxidative stress in critically ill patients. However, it is difficult to interpret the significance of increased levels of lipid peroxides measured in the plasma or tissues because tissue injury and hypoxia accelerate lipid peroxidation.[1,8]

Toxic O_2 Metabolites in Critical Illness

NORMOBARIC HYPEROXIA

Oxygen is one of the most common therapies used in patients with respiratory illnesses in the intensive care unit (ICU). Room air oxygen is not sufficiently reactive to cause tissue injury, yet prolonged exposures to high concentrations of oxygen can result in lung damage.[23] Hyperoxia increases the rate of production of intracellular toxic O_2 metabolites.[2,13,23,24] When production of toxic O_2 metabolites exceeds their consumption by antioxidant defense systems, tissue damage ensues.

The organs that are most susceptible to O_2 toxicity include the lungs, the eyes, and the central nervous system (CNS).[23,24] The lung is the organ most severely affected by normobaric hyperoxia in adults. Clinically, oxygen toxicity manifests itself as three often related entities: acute tracheobronchitis; acute lung injury resulting in ARDS; and chronic lung injury, such as bronchopulmonary dysplasia.[23] Characteristic symptoms of tracheobronchitis are substernal chest pain and nonproductive cough.[23] In healthy volunteers, tracheal mucus velocity is depressed within 3 h after breathing 100 percent O_2.[25] After 6 h of 100 percent O_2 exposure, the trachea contains focal areas of redness, edema, and injection of small vessels.[25] Chest pain develops between 12 to 16 h and resolves by 24 to 48 h if exposure is continued. Prolonged exposure to hyperoxia causes damage to capillary endothelial cells and alveolar epithelial cells with exudation of plasma caused by increased permeability.[26] Patients develop progressive arterial hypoxemia with alveolar infiltrates on chest roentgenograms. In healthy volunteers, 17 h of hyperoxia causes alveolar-capillary leak as detected by the presence of increased concentrations of albumin and transferrin in the bronchoalveolar lavage fluid.[27] In the chronic stages of O_2 toxicity, proliferation of lung fibroblasts with increased collagen synthesis leads to severe pulmonary fibrosis and bronchopulmonary dysplasia.[23,26] The lung fibrosis observed at this stage is not specific for O_2 toxicity but follows a number of lung injuries.

Oxygen toxicity of the lung parenchyma proceeds in three phases.[23] During the first phase of exposure to 100 percent O_2, there is a latent period where no pathologic change can be detected in the lungs. In animals, this period usually ranges between 24 to 72 h. Tissue injury occurs during the second and third phases. The second phase is characterized by acute inflammation with atelectasis, edema, and alveolar hemorrhage. In the third phase, there is chronic proliferation of Type II pneumocytes, hyaline membrane formation, and, eventually, fibrosis.[26] During the latent period, cellular defense mechanisms appear to cope with the increased flux of toxic oxygen metabolites. Over time the antioxidant defense mechanisms are overwhelmed, and the formation of oxygen radicals exceeds consumption. At this point a number of side reactions, such as lipid peroxidation and loss of membrane integrity, DNA damage, and oxidation and denaturation of cellular enzymes and proteins, lead to tissue injury. When this occurs, the second inflammatory phase of O_2 toxicity starts.

The earliest pathologic changes are swelling of endothelial cells followed by damage to alveolar pneumocytes and interstitial edema.[26] With continued O_2 exposure, these cells slough by 2–6 days with denuding of the basement membrane. Type I pneumocytes are much more sensitive to hyperoxia than type II pneumocytes because of their increased surface area to volume ratio and their relative deficiency of antioxidant defenses. When prominent injury is observed in type I pneumocytes, only minor changes are observed in type II pneumocytes. However, hyperoxia significantly decreases the ability of type II pneumocytes to synthesize surfactant. Septal edema develops due to loss of endothelial cell integrity, and fibrin deposition occurs in denuded areas. Type II pneumocyte hyperplasia becomes prominent after 6 days. After that time, septal fibrosis progresses with continued O_2 exposure.

Large numbers of neutrophils infiltrate the lung during the late stages of cellular injury. There is some controversy regarding the contribution of neutrophils to lung injury during hyperoxia. It is clear that neutrophils have the capacity to cause damage if they are recruited into the tissues.[11] However, there is also ample evidence that during hyperoxia, intracellular generation of toxic oxygen metabolites is sufficient to cause cellular injury.[2,13,23,24] The pathogenesis of hyperoxic lung injury is currently thought to occur via intracellular production of toxic oxygen metabolites that cause endothelial and epithelial damage. During the inflammatory phase and after the initiation of cellular injury, recruitment of polymorphonuclear leukocytes (PMNs) into the tissues may then contribute to or modify the tissue injury.

The exact nature and amount of O_2-induced damage in human studies is difficult to separate from the underlying pulmonary disease which necessitates therapy with O_2.[23] Nevertheless, there are a few prospective studies examining the toxic effects of O_2 in patients. In a now classic study, 10 patients with irreversible brain damage were exposed to either room air ($n = 5$) or 100 percent O_2 ($n = 5$) for periods of 30 to 72 h.[28] After 40 h, the Pa_{O_2} on 100% O_2 was around 200 mmHg in the hyperoxia group as opposed to 360 mmHg in the room air group. The hyperoxia group developed an intrapulmonary shunt ($\dot{Q}s/\dot{Q}_T$) of 35 percent versus 20 percent in the group exposed to room air. Examination of four of the five chest roentgenograms in the hyperoxic group demonstrated diffuse alveolar infiltrates. After 40 h, there were no significant gross or histologic differences between the two groups, but ultrastructural changes were not examined. In another report, five patients with neuromuscular disease were described who were ventilated unintentionally with $F_{I_{O_2}} > 0.85$ for 10 to 32 days.[29] After 4 to 10 days, all patients developed patchy pulmonary infiltrates, fevers as high as 102°F, and leukocytosis ranging from 14 to 36×10^3 cells/mm^3. No infectious etiology was found, and a presumptive diagnosis of pulmonary O_2 toxicity was made. Inspired O_2 concentrations were decreased to less than 50 percent, and within 2 to 5 days pulmonary infiltrates improved, and all but one patient was extubated. These cases underscore the importance of suspecting pulmonary O_2 toxicity in critically ill patients requiring high concentrations of O_2. The arterial hypoxemia resulting from oxygen toxicity otherwise is treated with ever-increasing concentrations of O_2, only worsening the lung injury. Our therapeutic solution to this problem is to employ the lowest concentration of O_2 to maintain hemoglobin saturation of 90% and to prevent development of pulmonary edema and atelectasis by judicious fluid management, application of positive end-expiratory pressure (PEEP), and meticulous pulmonary toilet. The exact threshold for O_2 toxicity in patients is unknown. The effect of underlying lung injury on the risk of O_2 toxicity is also not clear. We advocate reducing oxygen concentrations below 60% as early as possible. Most patients who require $F_{I_{O_2}} > 0.6$ manifest large amounts of intrapulmonary shunt and only marginally benefit from higher inspired concentrations of O_2. The guiding principle in oxygen therapy is to deliver the lowest possible O_2 concentration necessary to correct tissue hypoxia.

HYPERBARIC HYPEROXIA

Hyperbaric oxygen (HBO) therapy is used therapeutically in decompression sickness, carbon monoxide poisoning, arterial air embolism, burns, and necrotic tissue infections.[30] These conditions are discussed in detail elsewhere in this book. In this section, we will briefly discuss the pathophysiology of HBO toxicity.

One hundred percent oxygen is lethal to animals within days when given at 1 atm, whereas at 5 atm of 100% O_2, animals survive for only 1 h.[24] The first manifestation of HBO toxicity in man is seizures and is related to the inhibition of γ-aminobutyrate. As the pressure of O_2 is increased, the time to onset of seizures is shortened. During HBO therapy, the lungs are exposed to much higher O_2 tensions than the brain.[24] For instance, in normobaric hyperoxia O_2 tensions in the lung and brain are approximately 670 and <80 torr, respectively. At 4 to 5 atm of O_2 the corresponding O_2 tensions become 3000 versus <600 mmHg. At equivalent O_2 tensions of around 600 mmHg, the toxic symptoms in the brain manifest within hours, whereas lung toxicity takes days to develop. Current evidence indicates that this difference is due to differences in the amount of antioxidants present in the brain versus the lung. Moreover, the brain contains modest quantities of unchelated iron that can initiate $OH\cdot$ radical production and lipid peroxidation.[9,31] The areas of the brain most susceptible to O_2 toxicity are also areas rich in iron, and brain tissue forms lipid peroxides very readily under hyperoxic conditions.[24,31] Presumably generation of O_2^- with dismutation to H_2O_2 can form $OH\cdot$ in the presence of iron, which leads to lipid peroxidation, DNA damage, and protein oxidation and denaturation.

Despite the vulnerability of the CNS to HBO, the current protocols of HBO therapy are quite safe.[30] The cumulative rate of seizures estimated from the published literature is about 1 in 10,000. In 15 burn patients, after 90 min of HBO therapy at 2 atm, we could not detect any increase in their $EB_{H_2O_2}$ or plasma MDA levels. These results are consistent with the notion that patients can tolerate the oxidative stress induced by current HBO protocols.

PARAQUAT TOXICITY

Paraquat (1,1″-dimethyl-4,4″-bipyridium dichloride) is a commercially available herbicide that can be fatal if accidentally or deliberately ingested. Toxicity is seen with accidental or intentional drinking, or after percutaneous absorption in field workers. The time course of toxicity varies from a couple of days to several weeks. The organs most affected are the kidneys, liver, and lungs. During the phase of lung injury, paraquat toxicity is augmented if the patient is exposed to high concentrations of O_2. This can be a clinical dilemma because hypoxemia is a frequent result of lung toxicity. Mortality in paraquat poisoning is very high, and therapeutic success requires aggressive supportive therapy, including hemodialysis with a Fuller's earth column, charcoal hemoperfusion, and mechanical ventilation with low F_{IO_2}.[32] Treatment of paraquat toxicity is discussed elsewhere in this book. Here we will focus on the role of O_2 radicals in the pathogenesis of paraquat-induced injury.

Paraquat lung toxicity is thought to occur via intracellular production of O_2 metabolites via cyclic reduction and oxidation, especially in epithelial cells.[33] Autoradiographic studies show active paraquat uptake by alveolar epithelium, supporting the notion that selective pulmonary toxicity of paraquat is due to the ability of alveolar epithelium to concentrate paraquat via the basal (bloodstream) and apical (airways) cell membranes.[33] Paraquat is directly cytotoxic to lung parenchymal cells. Light and electron microscopic examination shows: **1.** signs of alveolar wall disruption; **2.** type II epithelial cell hyperplasia; **3.** mobilization of macrophages and neutrophils; and **4.** migration and accumulation of fibroblasts.[34] Further studies suggest that lung injury is mediated by the cyclic reduction and oxidation of paraquat by NADPH–NADP, resulting in the ongoing generation of O_2^-.[1] Paraquat cation (PQ^{2+}) in tissues is enzymatically reduced to the paraquat cation radical ($PQ^+\cdot$) possibly by the flavin at the active site of NADPH-cytochrome P_{450} reductase. The $PQ^+\cdot$ reacts with O_2 to form O_2^-. Superoxide anion causes lipid peroxidation within cell membranes that may be the dominant mechanism of epithelial and endothelial cell death in paraquat poisoning. SOD inhibits paraquat toxicity in one model, whereas catalase, dimethyl sulfoxide (DMSO), and deferoxamine fail to protect against injury.[35] This and other subsequent studies support the concept that superoxide anion is a major mediator of paraquat poisoning, and H_2O_2 or $HO\cdot$ have minor roles in paraquat lung toxicity. Plasma MDA levels were found to be elevated 6 to 10 days after ingestion of paraquat in three out of four patients who eventually died.[32] Plasma MDA levels of these patients ($n = 4$) were 2.7-fold greater than the plasma MDA levels of three patients who survived paraquat poisoning. This observation suggests that paraquat may lead to lipid peroxidation. However, plasma MDA levels are usually elevated in critically ill patients, hence the specificity of plasma MDA elevations in paraquat toxicity is unclear.

Paraquat-induced lung injury may in part be mediated by neutrophils that accumulate in the lung parenchyma during the acute alveolitis.[34] After the neutrophil component of the alveolitis resolves, the bronchoalveolar lavage (BAL) fluid contains increased amounts of the fibroblast chemoattractant glycoprotein fibronectin and a growth factor for fibroblasts. The "early" neutrophil alveolitis may contribute independently to the lung injury preceding paraquat-induced fibrosis. The neutrophils are by themselves a source of toxic oxygen metabolites and proteinases and may compound the lung injury.

ARDS

ARDS is characterized by increased pulmonary capillary permeability that leads to pulmonary edema. ARDS is associated with many clinical settings but primarily occurs with sepsis, aspiration, and trauma. Although ARDS carries a high mortality, not many patients die from respiratory failure. Many investigators have hypothesized unifying mechanisms of lung injury to explain how diverse clinical entities can lead to ARDS. A central theme implicates toxic O_2 metabolites generated by neutrophils sequestered in the lung.[10,36] Lung sequestration of neutrophils is known to occur in hemorrhagic shock, burn, trauma, sepsis, hyperoxia, after microembolization, and during extracorporeal circulation. Similarly, neutrophils and their products, such as elastase, are increased in the BAL fluid of ARDS patients during the course of their illness.[36,37] In one study, the number of neutrophils recovered in the BAL correlated with the alveolar-to-arterial P_{O_2} gradient, suggesting a causality between neutrophil sequestration and gas exchange impairment.[37] ARDS patients also demonstrate an increased oxidative stress in their lungs, demonstrated by elevated levels of H_2O_2 in their expired breath.[15,16]

Both in vivo and in vitro animal models of increased permeability pulmonary edema using endotoxin, microemboli, zymosan-activated plasma, and toxic O_2 metabolite generating systems have been shown to be neutrophil-dependent.[36] In these models, permeability changes are prevented or attenuated by the use of antioxidants, suggesting the participation of toxic O_2 metabolites in lung injury.[36] It could be postulated that clinical settings that predispose the patient to the development of ARDS, such as sepsis and aspiration, result in retention of neutrophils in the pulmonary circulation. Subsequent insults that lead to neutrophil chemotaxis, sequestration, and activation can then lead to generation of toxic O_2 metabolites and can overwhelm the lung defenses and contribute to tissue injury and amplification of the inflammatory responses. Neutrophils can also modulate tissue response to toxic O_2 metabolites directly via coproduction of proteinases and leukotrienes. Nevertheless, the exact pathophysiologic role of neutrophils in ARDS remains to be elucidated.

Neutrophil-mediated lung injury may not be central to all forms of acute lung injury. It is well known that neutropenic patients can develop ARDS.[10,38] Nonetheless, neutrophil functions are known to be up-regulated in ARDS,[39] and neutrophils are retained in the lungs of ARDS patients.[40] We believe that the conflicting evidence regarding the role of neutrophils in acute lung injury simply reflects the diverse etiologies that can lead to the clinical syndrome of ARDS. Moreover, there is growing evidence that intracellular toxic O_2 metabolite production, apart from the neutrophil, can lead to endothelial injury and potentially yield ARDS.

ISCHEMIA REPERFUSION INJURY

The participation of toxic oxygen metabolites in ischemia reperfusion was first demonstrated in the small intestine.[41] Since then, O_2 radicals have been implicated in the ischemia-reperfusion damage of multiple tissues, including small intestine, brain, heart, kidney, liver, lungs, muscles, skin, and stomach.

Reperfusion injury is thought to hinge on two events occurring during ischemia. During ischemia, ATP stores are depleted, and increased ADP and AMP lead to formation of hypoxanthine. At the same time, ischemia converts xanthine dehydrogenase to oxidase. Consequently, ischemia primes the xanthine oxidase for the formation of O_2^-. The only factor that prevents the formation of O_2^- is the lack of O_2. With reperfusion, oxygen availability shuttles the purine substrate accumulated during ischemia to uric acid via a xanthine oxidase-catalyzed reaction. The byproducts of this reaction are O_2^- and H_2O_2. These toxic oxygen metabolites, in the presence of iron, participate in the Fenton reaction and produce $HO\cdot$. Hydroxyl radical is very toxic and initiates lipid peroxidation and protein denaturation. Inhibition of xanthine oxidase can limit the formation of O_2^- and H_2O_2 during reperfusion. Also, chelating iron impairs the ability of O_2^- and H_2O_2 to form $HO\cdot$.

Conversion of xanthine dehydrogenase to xanthine oxidase proceeds at different rates in various tissues. Recently it was shown that xanthine dehydrogenase conversion to xanthine oxidase at 25°C in the intestine of the rat is extremely rapid and occurs within only 1 min. The heart requires around 15 min to convert xanthine dehydrogenase completely to oxidase, whereas other organs, such as kidney, lung, spleen, and liver, might require more than 1 h of ischemia for complete conversion.[42]

SMALL INTESTINE

Figure 58-5 depicts one model proposed to explain the formation of oxygen radical in the ischemic bowel. During ischemia, ATP is metabolized to hypoxanthine, which then accumulates in the tissue. During the low-energy state, Ca^{2+} moves into the cells and triggers the conversion of NAD^+-reducing xanthine dehydrogenase to the oxygen radical, producing xanthine oxidase via a Ca^{2+}-regulated proteinase. During reperfusion, molecular oxygen reacts together with hypoxanthine and xanthine oxidase to form the superoxide radical. Therefore, the damage in the small bowel occcurs not so much during the ischemic period but rather during reperfusion (reoxygenation). The rate-limiting factor in the formation of O_2^- appears to be oxygen, which falls to low values during ischemia. Upon reperfusion, oxygen is no longer a rate-limiting substrate and toxic oxygen metabolites are produced.

BRAIN

Toxic oxygen metabolites have been implicated in central nervous system damage following trauma or ischemia.[43] During middle cerebral artery occlusion in cats, there is a significant reduction of ATP with accumulation of ADP. During reperfusion, there is a progressive reduction in forebrain ascorbate, α-tocopherol, ubiquinone, and glutathione levels suggestive of O_2 radical generation. The levels of these antioxidants do not decrease during ischemia but rather after reperfusion. Also, generation of O_2^- by infusion of xanthine oxidase and hypoxanthine into the brain increases the permeability of the blood-brain barrier, producing cellular injury and edema. Recently, we found increased levels of H_2O_2 in the expired breath of patients with brain injury.[15]

HEART

Reoxygenation of hypoxic myocardium can result in tissue injury rather than improvement, a phenomenon called the oxygen paradox.[44] Studies in hearts subjected to ischemia reperfusion showed that pretreatment with SOD, SOD plus catalase, and allopurinol reduced the infarct size and reduced damage to mitochondrial membranes. Pretreatment with allopurinol reduced the S-T segment elevation in dogs with coronary artery occlusion.[41] The combination of SOD and mannitol also protects left ventricular function following ischemia–reperfusion, as does the combination of SOD and catalase or DMSO.[41] In other models, SOD alone, but not catalase, is protective against ischemia reperfusion of the heart, suggesting that O_2^- but not H_2O_2, is mediating the injury. Further evidence supporting the toxic oxygen

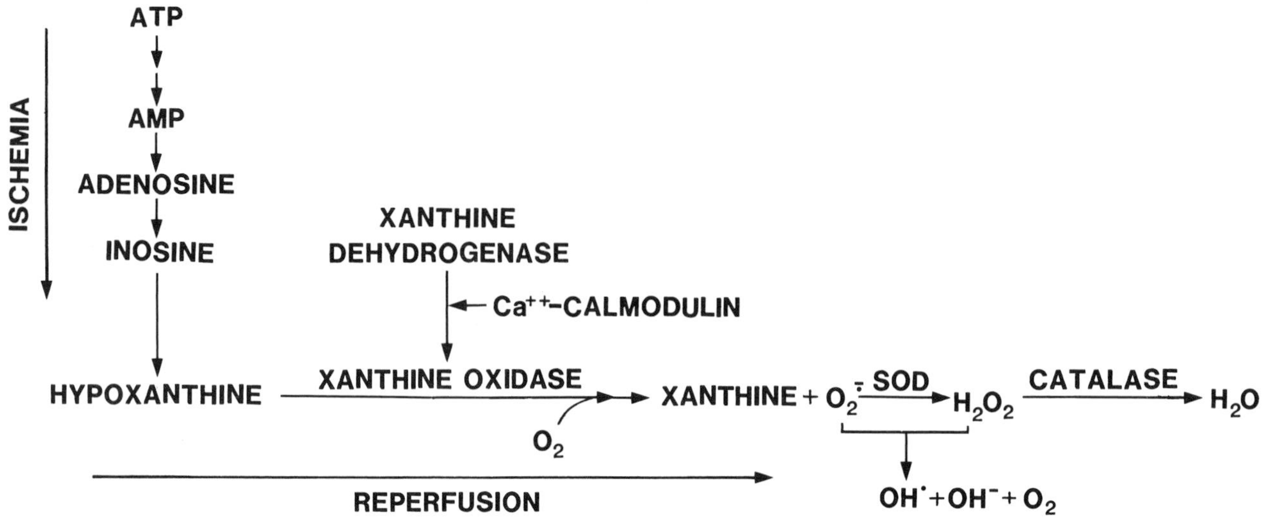

FIGURE 58-5 Mechanism of toxic oxygen metabolite production during ischemia reperfusion.

radical involvement in myocardial ischemia reperfusion was shown by increased lipid peroxidation and decreased glutathione peroxidase, catalase, and SOD activities during hypoxia reoxygenation.

Clinically, situations such as percutaneous transluminal coronary angioplasty, open-heart surgery, heart transplantation, and even coronary reperfusion after thrombolytic therapy could contribute to myocardial injury. Several clinical trials are being conducted to test the usefulness of O_2 radical scavengers in attenuating myocardial damage after coronary reperfusion.[45]

KIDNEY

Acute tubular necrosis is a frequent occurrence after renal hypoperfusion. During ischemia, there is a 10 to 300-fold increase in renal tissue hypoxanthine levels, suggesting generation of O_2 radicals.[46] Pretreatment with allopurinol or SOD 1 h prior to renal artery occlusion significantly reduces plasma creatinine and improves inulin clearance following reperfusion. Pretreatment with SOD also reduces lipid peroxidation products in renal cortex. Mannitol and DMTU, both OH · scavengers, protect against elevations in postischemic creatinine, thereby suggesting that OH · is the main offender in renal ischemia-reperfusion injury.[47] While mannitol is usually used as an osmotic diuretic, it may also have protective effects caused by its OH · scavenging properties. Other studies show that in norepinephrine-induced renal failure, the Ca^{2+} channel blockers verapamil and nifedipine offer protection by decreasing mitochondrial Ca^{2+} accumulation that inhibits the conversion of xanthine dehydrogenase to oxidase.

LIVER

Liver transplantation has drawn much attention to the mechanisms of injury during the period of ischemia and to ways of preserving organ function. Human liver can be preserved successfully with hypothermia for up to 10 h. Nevertheless, organ preservation remains a major challenge for successful transplantation. The combination of SOD and catalase pretreatment significantly protects against ischemia-reperfusion liver injury in rats and dogs. Formate, which prevents the accumulation of H_2O_2 and acts as an OH · scavenger, penetrates cell membranes, reduces lipid peroxidation, and prevents depletion of GSH.[41]

Oxidative stress leads to the oxidation of GSH to GSSG, causing an increased cellular GSSG:GSH ratio. Ischemia-reperfusion injury increases the GSSG:GSH ratio of hepatocytes. Pretreatment with allopurinol reduces this elevation in GSSG:GSH and implicates xanthine oxidase as a major source of free radical generation.[48] The liver is very well equipped against oxidizing agents. It contains significantly more CuZn SOD (2000 U/g) and glutathione (4 to 10 m*M*) than other tissues. It is also rich in α-tocopherol, catalase, and coenzyme Q. Therefore, oxidative stress in the liver is thought to lead to cellular injury after the depletion of antioxidants and inhibition of endogenous scavengers during ischemia.

LUNGS

Recently a model of reperfusion injury was developed in rabbit lungs.[49] During reperfusion there was a threefold increase in lung O_2^- production. Injury was prevented by the xanthine oxidase inhibitor allopurinol and SOD. The iron chelator deferoxamine, DMTU, and *N*-acetylcysteine also protected against the reperfusion injury. The protective effect of SOD could be abolished by the anion channel blocker, 4,4′-diisothiocyano-2,2′-stilbene disulfonic acid, which indicates that SOD consumes O_2^- in the extracellular medium, thereby creating a concentration gradient favorable for diffusion of superoxide anion out of the cells.

Reperfusion pulmonary edema has also been reported in patients after pulmonary artery thromboendarterectomy.[50] Clinically, reperfusion injury might play a role in acute pulmonary embolism as well, and after re-expansion of a collapsed lung. Reperfusion injury might also be important during pulmonary inflammation and the adult respiratory distress syndrome where parts of the pulmonary vasculature can be occluded by microemboli or in situ thrombosis.

SKELETAL MUSCLE

Skeletal muscle is relatively resistant to ischemia. However, edema occurs after 30 min of ischemia followed by reperfusion. The amount of edema is dependent on the duration of the ischemic period. This sequence of events likely contributes to the development of compartment syndromes after trauma. Pretreatment with SOD, catalase, and DMSO reduces the injury to skeletal muscle, suggesting that HO· is mainly responsible for this injury. The skeletal muscle resistance to ischemic injury is due to the fact that only small amounts of xanthine dehydrogenase are converted to oxidase after 1 h of ischemia.[41] In addition, ATP does not decrease significantly in the first 3 h of ischemia.

During prolonged periods of ischemia in skeletal muscle, there is a no-reflow phenomenon after reperfusion. This is manifested by an increase of muscular vascular resistance. The role of toxic O_2 metabolites in increased vascular resistance is questionable as allopurinol, SOD, and DMSO only slightly attenuate the rise in vascular resistance associated with ischemia.

STOMACH

Critically ill patients have a high incidence of life-threatening gastric and bowel "stress" ulcers, and studies in animal models suggest a role for O_2 radicals in their pathogenesis. It has been shown that "stress" ulcers in rats can be induced by cold or hemorrhagic shock. In hemorrhagic shock, reducing the celiac perfusion pressure to 30 mmHg for 1 h followed by reperfusion causes significant loss of radiolabeled albumin and red blood cells across the gastric mucosa. Pretreatment with allopurinol, SOD, and DMSO reduces the loss of red blood cells, suggesting that HO· has a major role in inducing the injury.[41]

Therapeutic Approaches

Understanding the role of toxic O_2 metabolites in the development of tissue injury opens up completely new avenues of therapy. The ultimate goal of this therapy is the preservation of tissue function. The treatment strategy of toxic O_2 metabolite-induced injury includes augmenting antioxidant defenses, eliminating reactions that produce radicals, and minimizing initiation of destructive inflammatory responses through activation of alternative pathways, such as neutrophil recruitment, eicosanoid production, and complement activation.

Exogenous Antioxidant Delivery

Historically, three problems have hindered the therapeutic potential of SOD and catalase. First, enzymes derived from other species produce an immunogenic response in humans. Second, these enzymes have very short half-lives. SOD's half-life is less than 5 min, which necessitates massive continuous infusions to maintain plasma or tissue levels.[51] Finally, they penetrate the cells very poorly. Recombinant DNA technology has already solved the first problem, as human SOD is now commercially available.[51] Modification of the enzymes by polyethylene glycol (PEG) eliminates the second and third problems. PEG-SOD and PEG-catalase have markedly prolonged half-lives and have been shown to penetrate endothelial cells.[52] Delivery of antioxidant enzymes can also be achieved by packaging them into liposomes and by either aerosolizing them into the lungs or by intravenous infusion. We expect rapid application of this technology to a variety of disease states in the next few years.

Chelation Therapy

In physiologic systems, the most reactive radical, OH·, is produced mainly in the presence of metal ions, especially iron. Appropriate chelation of Fe^{2+} eliminates its participation in redox reactions such that it can no longer catalyze formation of OH·.[3] This concept has been proven experimentally by the protective use of deferoxamine in animal models. However, toxicity of deferoxamine limits its use in patients. Chelation therapy is most promising in CNS injury because, unlike other organs, the brain contains free iron, with production of O_2^- resulting in the formation of OH·.[9,10,31] Another limitation of chelation therapy is that it carries the risk of mobilizing iron from body stores and increasing local iron concentrations.[3] Clinical application of chelation therapy awaits development of new drugs with minimal toxicity and a wide margin of therapeutic safety.

Enzyme Induction

It is well known that rats exposed to 85 percent O_2 atmosphere or given endotoxin develop tolerance to subsequent exposure to 100 percent O_2 through induction of lung SOD, catalase, and GPO activities.[1] However, not all species, including humans, demonstrate such activity. As such, induction of antioxidant enzymes currently remains a research tool. Another recently explored approach is transvection of human cells with a genetically engineered plasmid that can express human SOD, catalase, and GPO. Such genetic modification of the cells during the time they are exposed to oxidant stress can theoretically protect them from toxic O_2 metabolite-induced injury.

Scavengers

Scavengers are a group of compounds that can react rapidly with toxic O_2 metabolites providing an alternative target. The main problem with most known scavengers is their toxicity and inability to gain access to intracellular sites.

Modulation of Inflammatory Response

Production of free radicals can initiate a cascade of events that can amplify the inflammatory response. Lymphocytes, monocytes, neutrophils, alveolar macrophages, platelets, and endothelial cells all can release soluble mediators and influence each others' cellular function. Further characterization of cellular communication and interactions can allow for pharmacologic modification of the cellular responses that will lead to better tissue preservation. For instance, use of pentoxifylline that down-regulates neutrophil function can decrease neutrophil-induced tissue injury. Similarly, monoclonal antibodies aimed specifically to neutralize neutrophil adherence molecules can prevent neutrophil sequestration and modify neutrophil-induced tissue injury.

Augmentation of Cofactors

One of the main cofactors involved in antioxidant defense is GSH. GSH provides reducing equivalents to GPO and also protects disulfide bonds of proteins from oxidation. Supplementation of alternate —SH groups is already applied in clinical therapy. *N*-Acetylcysteine, which contains an —SH group and is a precursor of GSH, is used as an antidote in acetaminophen toxicity where depletion of intracellular GSH stores makes cells more susceptible to free radical attack.

Modulation of Lipid Peroxidation

Another potential set of compounds that can find application in toxic O_2 metabolite-induced injury are lipid peroxidation inhibitors. Inhibition of lipid peroxidation can protect membrane integrity and may preserve cell function despite toxic O_2 metabolite production.

Most antioxidant therapeutic modalities discussed earlier are in their infancy. However, the rapid expansion of free radical biology since the discovery of SOD 20 years ago suggests that the field will create multiple therapeutic modalities with potential applications in a variety of disease states. Without a doubt, these approaches will be explored more extensively in the future in the form of controlled clinical trials in human disease states and will expand the therapeutic armamentarium of the critical care physician.

CASE PRESENTATION

A 26-year-old male developed symptoms of shortness of breath and nonproductive cough 1 day after a routine appendectomy. The patient was diagnosed with testicular carcinoma 1.5 years earlier and was successfully treated with orchiectomy and chemotherapy with cisplatin, VP-16, and bleomycin. His total bleomycin dose was 300 mg. Three days earlier, he had presented to the emergency room with fevers, leukocytosis, and right lower quadrant pain and underwent appendectomy the same day. His chest x-ray prior to surgery was normal. One day after surgery, he developed a nonproductive cough, nausea and vomiting, followed by shortness of breath. He was afebrile, his respiratory rate was 26/min; his supine heart rate and blood pressure were 100 beats/min and 120/80 mmHg, respectively; and, upon his standing, they became 110 beats/min and 104/67 mmHg, respectively. His physical exam was remarkable for dry mucous membranes and bi-basilar crackles at the lung bases. His room air blood gas revealed a pH of 7.48, P_{CO_2} of 30 mmHg, P_{O_2} of 62 mmHg, and O_2 saturation of 88 percent. His white blood cell count was 12×10^3 cells/mm^3 with a normal differential. His chest x-ray demonstrated patchy infiltrates most prominent in the lower lobes. He was admitted to the medical intensive care unit and hydrated with normal saline, while his oxygenation was monitored by pulse oximetry. He received 3 L of saline over 4 h, and his O_2 saturation fell to 79 percent. Pulmonary artery catheterization revealed a wedge pressure of 16 mmHg, cardiac output of 7.0 L/min, and an arterial-mixed venous O_2 content difference of 3.5 mL O_2/dL of blood. The patient was initially placed on nasal cannula O_2, and his O_2 therapy was titrated to an arterial saturation of 85–90 percent using the pulse oximeter. He was treated with diuretics while his oxygenation, wedge pressure, and cardiac output were monitored. He responded well to diuresis and within a few hours, his room air blood gas improved to P_{O_2} of 75 mmHg with O_2 saturation of 92 percent. He continued to maintain O_2 saturation above 90 percent at room air and was discharged from the intensive care unit after 36 h.

CASE DISCUSSION

This patient's clinical course highlights one of the dilemmas critical care physicians face in applying O_2 therapy. The differential diagnosis of this patient's condition included pneumonia, aspiration, cardiogenic pulmonary edema, and O_2-enhanced bleomycin toxicity. The first three etiologies are unlikely given the lack of signs of infection and rather low wedge pressure despite fluid resuscitation. A review of the anesthesia report revealed that during the appendectomy, the patient was ventilated with F_{IO_2} of 0.40. Development of noncardiogenic pulmonary edema after bleomycin therapy upon exposure to inspired O_2 fractions greater than 0.30 has been described. This is thought to occur because of synergy between O_2 and bleomycin toxicity with increased production of toxic O_2 metabolites during exposure to increased F_{IO_2}. Hence, therapy should be directed at minimizing inspired O_2 concentrations while maintaining an adequate cardiac output and O_2 delivery to the tissues.

References

1. Halliwell B, Gutteridge MC: *Free Radicals in Biology and Medicine.* Oxford, England, Clarendon Press, 1985.
2. Fisher AB: Intracellular production of oxygen-derived free radicals, in Halliwell B (ed): *Oxygen Radicals and Tissue Injury.* Bethesda, MD, American Societies for Experimental Biology, 1988, pp 34–42.
3. Halliwell B, Gutteridge JMC: The importance of free radicals and catalytic metal ions in human diseases. Mol Aspects Med 8:89–193, 1985.
4. Southorn PA, Powis G: Free radicals in medicine. I. Chemical nature and biologic reactions. Mayo Clin Proc 63:381–389, 1988.

5. Grisham MB, McCord JM: Chemistry and cytotoxicity of reactive oxygen metabolites, in Taylor AE, Matalon S, Ward P (eds): *Physiology of Oxygen Radicals*. Baltimore, MD, Waverly Press, 1986, pp 1–18.
6. DiGuiseppi J, Fridovich I: The toxicology of molecular oxygen. CRC Crit Rev Toxicol 12:315–342, 1983.
7. Chance BH, Sies A, Boveris A: Hydroperoxide metabolism in mammalian organs. Physiol Rev 59:527–605, 1979.
8. Horton AA, Fairhurst S: Lipid peroxidation and mechanisms of toxicity. CRC Crit Rev Toxicol 18:27–79, 1987.
9. Cross CE, Halliwell B, Borish ET et al: Oxygen radicals and human disease. Ann Intern Med 107:526–545, 1987.
10. Hammond B, Kontos HA, Hess ML: Oxygen radicals in the adult respiratory distress syndrome, in myocardial ischemia and reperfusion injury, and in cerebral vascular damage. Can J Physiol Pharmacol 63:273–287, 1985.
11. Lehrer RI, Ganz T, Selsted ME, et al: Neutrophils and host defense. Ann Intern Med 109:127–42, 1988.
12. Weiss SJ: Tissue destruction by neutrophils. N Engl J Med 320:365–372, 1990.
13. Fisher AB, Forman HJ: Oxygen utilization and toxicity in the lungs, in Fishman AP, Fisher AB (eds): *Handbook of Physiology*. Baltimore, Waverly Press, 1985, pp 231–254.
14. Machlin LJ, Bendich A: Free radical tissue damage: Protective role of antioxidant nutrients. FASEB Monogr 1:441–445, 1987.
15. Sznajder JI, Fraiman A, Hall JB et al: Increased hydrogen peroxide in the expired breath of patients with acute hypoxemic respiratory failure. Chest 96:606–612, 1989.
16. Baldwin SR, Simon RH, Grum CM et al: Oxidant activity in expired breath of patients with adult respiratory distress syndrome. Lancet 1:11–14, 1986.
17. Yagi K: Assay for serum lipid peroxide level and its clinical significance, in Yagi K (ed): *Lipid Peroxides in Biology and Medicine*. New York, Academic Press, 1982, pp 223–242.
18. Tappel AL: Measurement of and protection from in vivo lipid peroxidation, in Williams AP (ed): *Free Radicals in Biology*, Vol. 4, 1981, pp 123–144.
19. Morita S, Snider MT, Inada Y: Increased N-pentane excretion in humans: A consequence of pulmonary oxygen exposure. Anesthesiology 64:730–733, 1986.
20. Gutteridge JMC: Lipid peroxidation: Some problems and concepts, in Halliwell B (ed): *Oxygen Radicals and Tissue Injury*. Bethesda, MD, American Societies for Experimental Biology, 1988, pp 9–19.
21. Suematsu T, Abe H: Liver and serum lipid peroxide levels in patients with liver disease, in Yagi K (ed): *Lipid Peroxides in Biology and Medicine*. New York, Academic Press, 1982, pp 285–294.
22. Poli G, Biasi F, Chiarpotto E et al: Lipid peroxidation in human diseases: Evidence of red cell oxidative stress after circulatory shock. Free Rad Biol Med 6:167–170, 1989.
23. Jenkinson SG: Oxygen toxicity. J Intensive Care Med 3:137–152, 1988.
24. Jamieson D: Oxygen toxicity and reactive oxygen metabolites in mammals. Free Rad Biol Med 7:87–109, 1989.
25. Sackner MA, Landa J, Hirsch J et al: Pulmonary effects of oxygen breathing; a 6 hour study in normal men. Ann Intern Med 82:40–43, 1975.
26. Katzenstein ALA, Bloor CM, Leibow AA: Diffuse alveolar damage: the role of oxygen, shock and related factors. Am J Pathol 85:210–228, 1976.
27. Davis WB, Rennard SI, Bitterman PB et al: Pulmonary oxygen toxicity: early reversible changes in human alveolar structures induced by hyperoxia. N Engl J Med 309:878–883, 1983.
28. Barber RE, Lee J, Hamilton WK: Oxygen toxicity in man. A prospective study in patients with irreversible brain damage. N Engl J Med 283:1478–1489, 1970.
29. Hyde RW, Rawson AJ: Unintentional iatrogenic oxygen pneumonitis: Response to therapy. Ann Intern Med 71:517–524, 1969.
30. Thom SR: Hyperbaric oxygen therapy. J Intensive Care Med 4:58–74, 1989.
31. Braughler JM, Hall ED: Central nervous system trauma and stroke: Biochemical considerations for oxygen radical formation and lipid peroxidation. Free Rad Biol Med 6:289–301, 1989.
32. Yasaka T, Okudaira K, Fujito H et al: Further studies of lipid peroxidation in human paraquat poisoning. Arch Intern Med 146:681–685, 1986.
33. Bus JS, Aust SK, Gibson JE: Lipid peroxidation: A possible mechanism for paraquat toxicity. Res Commun Chem Pathol Pharmacol 11:31–38, 1975.
34. Schoenberger CI, Rennard SI, Bitterman PB et al: Paraquat induced pulmonary fibrosis. Role of the alveolitis in modulating the development of fibrosis. Am Rev Respir Dis 129:168–173, 1984.
35. Bagley AC, Krall J, Lynch RE: Superoxide mediates the toxicity of paraquat for Chinese hamster ovary cells. Proc Natl Acad Sci 83:3189–3193, 1986.
36. Ward PA, Johnson KJ, Till GO: Oxygen radicals, neutrophils, and acute tissue injury, in Taylor AE, Matalon S, Ward P (eds): *Physiology of Oxygen Radicals*. Baltimore, Waverly Press, 1986, pp 145–150.
37. Weiland JE, Davis WB, Holter JF et al: Lung neutrophils in the adult respiratory distress syndrome. Clinical and pathophysiologic significance. Am Rev Respir Dis 133:218–225, 1986.
38. Ognibene FP, Martin SE, Parker MM et al: Adult respiratory distress syndrome in patients with severe neutropenia. N Engl J Med 315:547–551, 1986.
39. Zimmerman GA, Renzetti AD, Hill HR: Functional and metabolic activity of granulocytes from patients with adult respiratory distress syndrome. Evidence for activated neutrophils in the pulmonary circulation. Am Rev Respir Dis 127:290–300, 1983.
40. Warshawski FJ, Sibbald WJ, Driedger AA et al: Abnormal neutrophil-pulmonary interaction in the adult respiratory distress syndrome. Qualitative and quantitative assessment of pulmonary neutrophil kinetics in human with in vivo ^{111}indium neutrophil scintigraphy. Am Rev Respir Dis 133:797–804, 1986.
41. Korthius RJ, Granger DN: Ischemia reperfusion injury: role of oxygen derived free radicals, in Taylor AE, Matalon S, Ward P (eds): *Physiology of Oxygen Radicals*. Baltimore, Waverly Press, 1986, pp 217–249.
42. Roy RS, McCord JM: Superoxide and ischemia: Conversion of xanthine dehydrogenase to xanthine oxidase, in Cohen G, Greenwald MD (eds): *Oxy-Radicals and Their Scavenger Systems*. Vol. 2, New York, Elsevier, 1983, pp 143–153.
43. Kontos HA: Oxygen radicals in cerebral vascular injury. Circ Res 57:508–516, 1985.
44. Hearse DJ, Humphrey SM, Chain EB: Abrupt reoxygenation of the anoxic potassium-arrested perfused rat heart: a study of myocardial enzyme release. J Mol Cell Cardiol 5:395–407, 1973.
45. Cohen MV: Free radicals in ischemic and reperfusion myocardial injury: Is this the time for clinical trials? Ann Intern Med 111:918–931, 1989.
46. Paller MS, Hoidal JR, Ferris TF: Oxygen free radicals in ischemic acute renal failure in the rat. J Clin Invest 74:1156–1164, 1984.

47. Ouriel K, Smedira NG, Ricotta JJ: Protection of the kidney after temporary ischemia: free radical scavengers. J Vasc Surg 2:49–53, 1985.
48. Nordstrom G, Seeman T, Hasselgren PO: Beneficial effect of allopurinol in liver ischemia. Surgery 97:679–684, 1985.
49. Kennedy TP, Rao NV, Hopkins C et al: Role of reactive oxygen species in reperfusion injury of the rabbit lung. J Clin Invest 83:1326–1335, 1989.
50. Levinson RM, Shure D, Moser K: Reperfusion pulmonary edema after pulmonary artery thromboarterectomy. Am Rev Respir Dis 134:1241–1245, 1986.
51. Greenwald RA: Superoxide dismutase and catalase as therapeutic agents for human diseases: A critical review. Free Rad Biol Med 8:201–210, 1990.
52. Beckman JS, Minor RL Jr, White CW et al: Superoxide dismutase and catalase conjugated to polyethylene glycol increases endothelial enzyme activity and oxidant resistance. J Biol Chem 263:6884–6892, 1988.

SECTION C
TRAUMA

Chapter 59
PRIORITIES IN MULTISYSTEM TRAUMA

J. ALI

KEY POINTS

- *Management of the multiply injured patient must be conducted on a priority basis in order to improve chances of survival.*
- *Order of priority among injuries is related to the degree to which survival is threatened by each injury.*
- *Airway control, maintenance of ventilation, and adequacy of perfusion take first priority in management.*
- *Cervical spine precautions are crucial during airway intubation.*
- *Concept of a trauma team leader is important in coordinating management in the multiply injured patient.*
- *Complete familiarity with techniques for airway control, chest decompression and establishing intravenous (IV) access is essential in multiple trauma management.*
- *Treatment of fractures and complete in-depth assessment of the multiply injured patient are required only after the respiratory and hemodynamic status has been stabilized.*
- *Repeated assessment is necessary to diagnose and treat injuries that are not immediately obvious on initial presentation.*

Mortality from multiple injuries follows a trimodal distribution.[1] The first peak represents death occurring at the scene of the accident and arises as a result of such injuries as cardiac rupture or disruption of the major intrathoracic vessels and severe brain injury that is incompatible with life. Death from such injuries occurs within minutes of the traumatic event, and there is very little that can be done to improve the possibility of survival. The second peak in mortality following multiple injuries occurs from minutes to approximately 1 h. Mortality during this phase is related to injuries that are immediately life-threatening, such as tension pneumothorax and cardiac tamponade. This is also a period during which appropriate resuscitative measures could affect the outcome significantly. The third peak occurs as a result of complications of the injury, such as sepsis or multiple systems organ failure. However, this third phase can be significantly affected by the type of intervention during the second phase. The intensivist dealing with the multiple trauma patient is very likely to be involved in the institution of resuscitative measures during the second phase as well as the management of the complications of the injury or complications arising from inadequate treatment of the trauma patient during the third phase. Many of the chapters in this text deal with the complications of trauma, such as sepsis and multiple organ failure. This chapter will deal with the priorities that must be adhered to during the second peak of the trimodal distribution of trauma-related mortality.

Blunt trauma from motor vehicle accidents is the most frequent cause of injuries in general. This type of impact usually results in injuries to many different parts of the body simultaneously. Over a 2-year period at the Sunnybrook Health Science Centre Trauma Unit, 338 motor vehicle drivers were admitted with multiple injuries. There were 2566 injuries in theses 338 patients; Fig. 59-1 shows the distribution of these injuries. Head and neck injuries were the most frequent, occurring at a frequency of 1.88 per patient, with the overall frequency of 7.6 injuries per patient.

When faced with multisystem injury, the intensivist must prioritize his or her treatment according to the threats to the patient's survival. Prioritization of assessment and intervention requires a coordinated team approach. Where personnel are available from different specialities, it is of paramount importance that the entire resuscitative effort be coordinated through an identified team leader. This very simple decision should be made prior to institution of therapy and can be critical in determining the outcome in the patient with multisystem trauma. The leader of the resuscitation, who may be an intensivist, must be completely familiar with a wide variety of injuries and their relative threat to life in order to prioritize his or her intervention and direct personnel appropriately.

Certain fundamental concepts underly the approach to resuscitation of the multiply injured patient. The most im-

FIGURE 59-1 Injuries in 338 motor vehicle drivers (total: 2566 injuries). As indicated in the text, most of these patients had injuries to the head and neck area, and the average number of injuries per patient was 7.6.

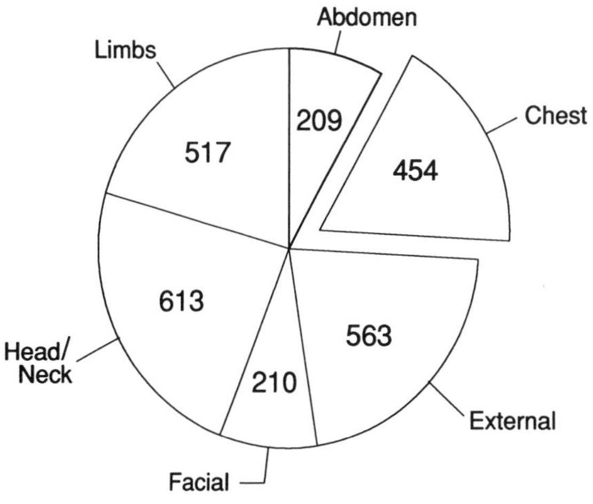

portant of these is that immediately life-threatening injuries should be treated as they are identified. Therefore, assessment and resuscitation must proceed simultaneously. The initial goal in managing the trauma patient is to provide adequate oxygenation and perfusion. This goal is achieved by approaching our assessment and treatment so that abnormalities in the injured patient that affect oxygenation and perfusion would take top priority. It is also of prime importance to recognize the findings that suggest a need for emergent surgical intervention.

Priorities

As indicated earlier, the order of priorities is a key feature for successful management of the multiply injured patient and should follow the following sequence:

1. Establishment of the airway and ventilation with cervical spine control
2. Maintaining adequacy of perfusion
3. Providing hemorrhage control
4. Assessment and correction of neurologic abnormalities
5. Stabilization of fractures
6. Detailed systematic assessment and provision of definitive care

The basis for this order of priorities is related to the degree to which abnormalities in the different systems threaten the life of the patient. Although the patient with multiple fractures requires treatment of these fractures, such treatment should take lower priority compared to injuries affecting the airway or respiratory status.

AIRWAY AND VENTILATION AND C SPINE CONTROL

The most frequent cause of airway obstruction in the multiply injured patient is loss of tone of the muscles supporting the tongue because of hypoperfusion of the brain from hypovolemic shock or because of central nervous system (CNS) injury. As outlined in Chap. 6, the simple maneuvers of chin lift and jaw thrust move the mandible forward, and, since all the muscles of the tongue are attached to the mandible, this action brings the tongue forward and allows patency of the upper airway. It is essential in the trauma victim that one inspects the oropharynx to ensure that there is no foreign material (including vomitus) in the pharynx that will occlude the airway. Quick observation of the patient's nares and mouth and listening for unobstructed passage of air through the upper airway, together with inspection for the presence of foreign objects in the oropharynx, are all very simple maneuvers that should be undertaken in the initial care of the multiply injured patient. The patient who is fully conscious, vocalizing and breathing adequately, and who is not in shock does not require any artificial airway. The underlying principle of establishing an airway in the trauma victim is to institute the simplest measure that allows effective ventilation. Over 90 percent of patients will not require endotracheal intubation. Measures short of endotracheal intubation include the insertion of oropharyngeal or nasopharyngeal airways. However, when endotracheal intubation is necessary, this should be performed promptly and expeditiously. Prolonged unsuccessful attempts at endotracheal intubation without ventilation should be avoided. Mask ventilation with oxygen and an oropharyngeal airway should be performed intermittently to avoid hypoxia during prolonged attempts at endotracheal intubation. In very rare circumstances, the patient's airway may not be patent, but it is impossible to establish an airway through the nose or mouth, and in those situations one should be prepared to proceed to cricothyroidotomy. This procedure should only be done when there is inability to establish an airway by other means. The landmarks for the cricothyroid membrane are indicated in Fig. 59-2. A cricothyroidotomy may be done using a large-bore needle or scalpel, the former being preferable in children because the cricoid cartilage is essential to the stability of the upper airway of infants and young children. A 14-gauge needle and cannula may be inserted through the cricothyroid membrane for temporary oxygenation, but this is not a very efficient means of ventilation. In order to maximize oxygenation and avoid hypercapnea, the needle cricothyroidotomy should be followed by tracheostomy in an operating room under ideal circumstances if a surgical airway is still required. The placement of the cricothyroidotomy needle allows approximately 30 to 45 min of adequate oxygenation without severe hypercapnea. The surgical cricothyroidotomy is preferable and more effective in adults. A transverse skin incision is made directly over the cricothyroid membrane, and, after reflecting the subcutaneous structures, the cricothyroid membrane is identified and incised transversely. A forcep is then inserted to spread the opening, and an appropriate caliber tube, usually a #6 or a

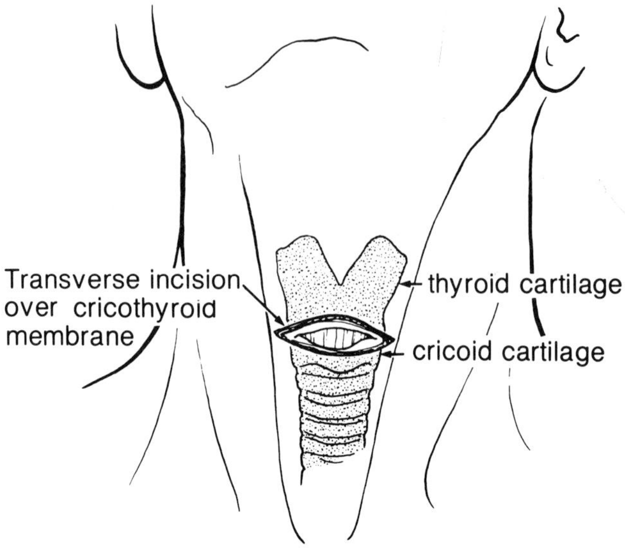

FIGURE 59-2 Landmarks for cricothyroidotomy.

#7 French tracheostomy or endotracheal tube, is inserted through the opening and secured.[2]

The types of oxygen delivery systems for both oropharyngeal airways and through endotracheal tubes are discussed in earlier chapters (see Chaps. 6 and 11).

Many techniques of establishing an artificial airway potentially put the cervical spine at risk of injury. Awareness of this potential for C-spine injury during airway intubation is crucial in preventing spinal cord injury in the multiply injured patient. Inappropriate manipulation of the C-spine during airway intubation could convert an unstable cervical spine injury without neurologic deficit into one with permanent neurologic deficits, including paraplegia and even death. The patient who is unconscious or who is suspected of having a cervical spine injury should not have the neck flexed, extended, or rotated. In-line immobilization should be maintained with the neck in the neutral position while the airway is being intubated. If the patient is conscious and breathing, then a blind nasotracheal intubation may be attempted with cricoid pressure anteriorly. If the patient is apneic, then orotracheal intubation with in-line cervical immobilization will need to be attempted. Failure to secure the airway by either of these means will necessitate cricothyroidotomy. Although it is controversial, there may be a role for proceeding directly to cricothyroidotomy for establishing an airway in patients with cervical spine injury who cannot be intubated by the blind nasotracheal technique, since adequate visualization of the vocal cords for facilitating oral intubation may not be achieved while in-line cervical immobilization is maintained. The opposing view is that most patients could be intubated by the endotracheal route while in-line cervical immobilization is maintained. Where fiberoptic bronchoscopy is immediately available, it may be used to facilitate endotracheal intubation. All unconscious patients or patients suspected of cervical spine injury should have a lateral cervical spine x-ray done as a minimum, and all seven cervical vertebrae should be clearly visualized. Failure to visualize all seven vertebrae should necessitate other views of the spine, including a swimmer's view. If there is doubt, the patient should be treated with a semirigid cervical collar until tomograms or computed tomography (CT) scans are performed to assess the integrity of the cervical spine. In the presence of clinical signs of spinal cord injury, the C-spine is considered to be abnormal in spite of a normal appearing lateral x-ray.[3]

Adequacy of ventilation is quickly assessed by observation of the chest for asymmetrical movement or paradoxical movement followed by quick auscultation and percussion to determine whether there is any hyperresonance or dullness to suggest pneumothorax or hemothorax. Deviation of the trachea suggests the diagnosis of a pneumothorax or hemothorax, but this finding is not always evident. Although one may confirm the diagnosis of a simple traumatic pneumothorax with upright chest x-ray, suspicion of a tension pneumothorax requires immediate decompression, without prior x-ray confirmation. Further examination of the chest should be conducted to determine the presence of other life-threatening thoracic injuries, such as cardiac tamponade, open pneumothorax, flail chest, ruptured thoracic aorta and massive hemothorax (see Chap. 63).

ADEQUACY OF PERFUSION

Once control of the airway and ventilation have been established, the next priority is maintenance of adequate perfusion. The most common source of hypoperfusion in the multiply injured patient is major hemorrhage. Its clinical presentation will depend on such factors as the patient's age as well as the duration and magnitude of the hemorrhage. In this regard, it is important to remember that the presence of a normal or even elevated blood pressure, particularly in the young patient, does not rule out hypoperfusion. The physiologic response to hypovolemia includes sympathetic discharge with vasoconstriction and tachycardia, all of which will tend to maintain the blood pressure for long periods of time. Older patients tend to manifest hypotension much earlier in the course of hypovolemia. Other signs of hypoperfusion, therefore, should be sought in assessing the trauma patient. The location and character of the pulse, the skin color, and capillary refill time are all signs that are immediately accessible to the examining physician and should be used in determining adequacy of perfusion. Failure to palpate a radial pulse may signify hypotension of the order of 70 to 80 mmHg. Tachycardia with cool extremities suggests hypoperfusion until proven otherwise. This is usually as a result of hemorrhage, although other causes of hypoperfusion must be considered. Hemorrhage may be classified into classes I to IV,[1] each class having an associated clinical response as indicated in Table 59-1. The patient who has a normal heart rate with a strong bounding radial pulse, warm skin, and a capillary refill time of less than 2 s would be considered not to have lost any significant blood, whereas the degree of deviation from these clinical parameters would correlate with the magnitude of blood loss.

Though the most common cause of hypoperfusion in trauma patients is hemorrhage, other causes such as tension pneumothorax, cardiac tamponade, myocardial contusion, open pneumothorax, and flail chest must be considered.

Once the trauma patient is considered to be hypoperfusing, then the source of hemorrhage should be identified and controlled. Any external source of hemorrhage should be controlled by direct pressure without resorting to blind application of clamps or tourniquets. This is followed by attempts to stabilize the hemodynamic status. This should be accomplished by aggressive fluid replacement through large bore (minimum 14 to 16 gauge) intravenous catheters. It is very helpful to establish multiple IV catheters not only because this facilitates rapid volume infusion but it also ensures an IV site should one of these sites become disconnected, plugged, or otherwise nonfunctional. Failure to establish intravenous access by venipuncture should prompt establishment of intravenous access by the venous cutdown technique. The usual site is the saphenous vein at the ankle. Once this vessel is identified, IV extension tubing may be advanced into the vein and used as a route for rapid fluid infusion. A temporary venous access may also be es-

TABLE 59-1 Clinical Classification of Shock in a 70-kg Male

	Class I	Class II	Class III	Class IV
Blood loss (ml)	Up to 750	750–1500	1500–2000	2000 or more
Blood loss (% BV)	Up to 15%	15–30%	30–40%	40% or more
Pulse rate	<100	>100	>120	140 or higher
Blood pressure	Normal	Normal	Decreased	Decreased
Pulse pressure (mmHg)	Normal or increased	Decreased	Decreased	Decreased
Capillary refill test	Normal	Positive	Positive	Positive
Respiratory rate	14–20	20–30	30–40	>35
Urine output (mL/h)	30 or more	20–30	5–15	Negligible
CNS-Mental status	Slightly anxious	Mildly anxious	Anxious and confused	Confused—lethargic
Fluid replacement (3:1 Rule)	Crystalloid	Crystalloid	Crystalloid + blood	Crystalloid + blood

The clinical signs of shock are very subtle at the levels of classes I and II, but it is crucial to make the diagnosis at this stage before deeper levels of shock ensue. This is ensured by prompt fluid resuscitation. In replacing crystalloid for estimated blood loss, a very rough guide is the 3:1 rule, in which the amount of estimated blood loss should be replaced by three times the volume of crystalloid in order to have a similar effect on vascular volume. This, however, is to be used only as a guideline, and the adequacy of perfusion of the patient should be the end point for determining adequacy of fluid resuscitation.

SOURCE: Reproduced from the *Advanced Trauma Life Support Manual,* Committee on Trauma, American College of Surgeons, 1989, with permission.

tablished by femoral vein puncture in the groin. In situations where the intensivist is confident and experienced in establishing percutaneous central venous access, the internal jugular or subclavian veins may be used for inserting large bore catheters for intravenous fluid administration in trauma resuscitation. As a general rule, it is best to avoid placing IV catheters in limbs that have major soft tissue or bony injuries. Occasionally, the application of the pneumatic antishock garment may increase venous pressure and allow catheterization of veins in the upper limbs that would otherwise be not easily cannulated. Therefore, the intensivist must be completely familiar with the usual sites for venous access and also be prepared to proceed to venous cutdown promptly, since cannulation of the veins becomes more difficult as shock persists due to venoconstriction and venous spasm.

Once temporary control of external hemorrhage and IV access have been established, the patient should be taken to the operating room (OR), where adequate lighting would allow better visualization and definitive control of the bleeding points. In establishing the intravenous access, blood is simultaneously drawn for complete blood count, cross matching of blood, coagulation, and toxicology screens. Prior to the availability of blood products, it is essential to maintain adequate perfusion as judged by clinical assessment, including blood pressure, pulse, status of the neck veins, and urinary output. In most circumstances, there is sufficient time to obtain the patient's blood type. However, if after approximately 2 to 3 L of crystaloid, the patient's vital signs do not stabilize or stabilize only temporarily, and typed blood is not available, then emergency blood (Group O) will be required for resuscitating the patient. Packed cells in the amount of anywhere from 4 to 10 U should be ordered for resuscitating the patient with major hemorrhage.

If there is no obvious external source of hemorrhage, one should observe for the presence of pelvic or extremity fractures that would account for the blood loss. Failure to demonstrate blood loss in these areas means that the blood loss is either in the thorax or the abdomen. Most sources of thoracic hemorrhage can be identified by a combination of physical examination and chest x-ray. By a process of elimination, therefore, it is usually possible to determine the source of the hemorrhage. If the areas identified earlier do not represent the source of hemorrhage, the most likely source is intraabdominal. These patients will therefore require laparotomy for identification and control of hemorrhage. In certain instances, there may be an easily identifiable source of blood loss, such as an extremity fracture, but one is uncertain about whether or not there is concomitant intraabdominal hemorrhage, and in these situations the use of peritoneal lavage or CT scan (see Chap. 63) is helpful in detecting whether or not there is an intraabdominal source of hemorrhage as well.[4]

As indicated earlier, other causes of hypoperfusion should be sought in the trauma patient by assessing for the signs of cardiac tamponade, myocardial contusion, tension pneumothorax, etc. with prompt institution of corrective measures. These intrathoracic causes of hypoperfusion will be discussed in Chap. 63.

When the pneumatic antishock garment has been applied in the field in order to maintain blood pressure,[5,6] it should not be removed until volume resuscitation has been initiated. Once adequate IV access has been achieved, the pneumatic antishock garment should be slowly deflated starting with the abdominal compartment. Deflation should continue as long as blood pressure is maintained. If there is a drop in blood pressure of greater than 5 mmHg with deflation, further volume infusion is required prior to further deflation. If volume infusion is not adequate to maintain blood pressure with the pneumatic antishock garment deflated, the patient should be taken to the operating room, where the garment could be deflated and the search for the source of hemorrhage instituted immediately. If it is impossible to deflate the garment because of persistent hypotension, thoracotomy and temporary clamping of the aorta above the diaphragm may be required before deflating the garment and proceeding to laparotomy. The pneumatic antishock garment should not be considered a substitute for adequate volume resuscitation and is a device that should be only used on a temporary basis until adequate volume is given and control of hemorrhage is established.

In any event, application of this garment should not be prolonged because of the recognized complications, such as compartment syndrome and ischemia necessitating amputation which can result when the garment is left inflated for periods approaching 4 h duration.[8,9]

In an evaluation of the patient's response to volume infusion, it is important to recognize that massive blood loss may trigger a vagal mediated bradycardia and that in these circumstances the absence of tachycardia does not represent adequate volume resuscitation. When one is judging the amount of fluid required and the requirement for blood, a useful guideline is that if stabilization of blood pressure is not accomplished after 50 mL/kg of crystalloid infusion, then blood should be administered.[10] As indicated earlier, if type specific blood is not available, then emergency type O packed red blood cells may be used. Whenever large volumes of blood are administered, facilities for warming the patient and warming the infused blood should be made available. One of the most common causes of hypothermia and its complications is the rapid infusion of cold solutions in the resuscitation of trauma patients. In addition to electrocardiographic monitoring, and continued assessment of vital signs, core temperature monitoring is therefore important, utilizing a device that is capable of reading at hypothermic levels.[11]

In situations where the patient fails to respond to massive fluid infusion emergency thoracotomy allows **1.** identification and treatment of pericardial tamponade, **2.** internal cardiac massage, **3.** identification and control of intrathoracic hemorrhage, and **4.** cross clamping of the thoracic aorta in order to maintain cerebral perfusion and coronary blood flow while decreasing bleeding from a subdiaphragmatic source.[12] Emergency thoracotomy also allows the diagnosis and treatment of air embolism, which is discussed in Chap. 63.

Although volume deficit is the major cause of hypoperfusion in the trauma patient, failure to respond to adequate volume infusion may represent cardiovascular decompensation. If such causes as cardiac tamponade or tension pneumothorax have been ruled out as the cause of this cardiovascular decompensation, consideration should be given to the use of inotropes and vasoactive agents to support the circulation in these circumstances. Such intervention is accomplished with close hemodynamic monitoring as outlined in earlier chapters.

NEUROLOGIC STATUS

Following control of the respiratory and circulatory status, attention is next directed to assessment and management of the neurologic status. The hallmark of CNS injury is a change in the level of consciousness. Therefore, it is essential that the level of consciousness be defined in such a manner that repeated assessment of the level of consciousness would allow one to determine whether there has been change from examination at one point in time to a subsequent examination. Although detailed assessment of the neurologic status including assessment of the Glasgow Coma Score (GCS) (see Chap. 60) is of importance in the definitive management and assessment of the head-injured patient, initial examination does not need to be as detailed in order to detect a change in the level of consciousness. A simple method of initial assessment of the level of consciousness is to determine whether the patient responds appropriately to all commands and is completely oriented in all spheres (the A level). A second level is whether the patient responds to voice alone (the V level). A third level is indicated by responsiveness to pain (the P level), and a fourth level is unresponsiveness (the U level) to stimuli.[1] This simple grading of the level of consciousness, in conjunction with the status of the pupils and any lateralizing signs, should be noted in the initial evaluation of the patient. Any change of these parameters reflects a change in the level of consciousness and necessitates further investigation or surgical intervention if there is deterioration.

The brain is very susceptible to hypoxia and hypoperfusion, and one of the commonest causes of a depressed level of consciousness in the multiply injured patient is uncorrected hypovolemia resulting in hypoperfusion and cerebral hypoxia. Overall resuscitative measures aimed at maintaining vascular volume and arterial oxygenation, therefore, are of prime importance in treating the patient with a possible head injury. Volume restriction in order to decrease intracranial pressure and decrease cerebral edema is inappropriate in treating the hypovolemic patient who has a head injury. This approach, in fact, is more likely to further aggravate the head injury and increase cerebral edema and intracranial pressure. These are the key features of initial assessment and resuscitation of the brain-injured patient. Further discussion of the detailed assessment and need for intervention as well as sophisticated monitoring, including intracranial pressure monitoring are discussed in Chaps. 60 and 34.

FRACTURE STABILIZATION

Although the most dramatic injury in the multiply injured patient is the mangled limb resulting from major fractures, the fractures do not pose an immediate threat to life and, therefore, are of much lower priority. However, the secondary effect of fractures may require a higher level of prioritization. For instance, massive hemorrhage associated with a fracture will require reduction of the fracture and the institution of such techniques as external fixation in the case of massive hemorrhage from pelvic fractures. Time is also of the essence in managing fractures when there is interference with the blood supply to the limb that may result from spasm of the blood vessels or direct injury to the blood vessels adjacent to the fracture. Early assessment of neurovascular integrity and the correction of any abnormality are essential features of management of fractures in order to ensure limb salvage and to prevent rhabdomyolysis and compartment syndrome. Limb ischemia associated with the fracture should be initially treated by reduction of the fracture and immobilization. If this manipulation fails to restore perfusion, early angiographic assessment should be undertaken. In order to improve limb salvage, the period of limb ischemia should be less than 4 to 6 h. All efforts, therefore, should be made to obtain early angiography and definitive repair of the vascular injury associated with fracture. The possibility of compartment syndrome should be kept in mind particularly after perfusion has been reestablished to a previously ischemic limb. Definitive management of the fracture itself will be discussed in Chap. 65.

DETAILED SYSTEMATIC ASSESSMENT AND DEFINITIVE CARE

Once the initial rapid assessment of the patient has been completed, then a more in-depth assessment of the patient is conducted in a systematic fashion beginning with the head and ending with the lower extremities. The multiply injured patient must be completely undressed so that a complete physical examination is undertaken. This includes assessment of the back and requires careful "log rolling" of the patient in order to visualize the back while protecting the spinal column. X-rays of the thoracolumbar spine should be considered in unconscious patients or those with major torso trauma with or without neurologic deficit and those in whom the mechanism of injury suggests the possibility of spinal column injury. Until adequate radiologic assessment is complete, these patients should be moved with caution by "log rolling" and avoidance of any rotatory, flexion, or extension movement of the thoracolumbar spine.

All multiply injured patients should have (a) large-bore intravenous access, (b) a nasogastric tube inserted in order to decompress the stomach and monitor for evidence of upper gastrointestinal (GI) hemorrhage unless contraindicated as discussed below and (c) a transurethral Foley catheter for monitoring urine output unless contraindicated by the presence of a urethral injury. The patient with a possible urethral injury may present with a major pelvic fracture, perineal and scrotal ecchymosis or bleeding through the urethral meatus or the presence of a high-riding boggy prostate on rectal examination. If these signs are present, a urethrogram should be performed; only if this is normal should the Foley catheter be inserted per urethra. The presence of a cribriform plate fracture is a relative contraindication to insertion of a nasogastric tube.[13,14] Gastric decompression in these situations should be achieved by orogastric intubation.

If a rectal examination has not been conducted until this point to rule out a urethral injury prior to inserting a urethral catheter, it should be done as part of the complete assessment. The rectal examination not only assesses the integrity of the rectum but provides information on the presence of blood in the GI tract, the possibility of extrarectal pelvic injury (bony as well as soft tissue, e.g., prostatic urethra) and the presence of rectal sphincter tone, which may be abnormal in spinal cord injury. During this phase of the assessment of the multiply injured patient, potentially life-threatening injuries or injuries that are likely to produce morbidity and require correction on a nonurgent basis are detected. If one utilizes the techniques of inspection, percussion, palpation, and auscultation where appropriate, injuries such as simple pneumothoraces, uncomplicated fractures, and soft tissue wounds are detected and plans for management instituted.

Reduction and stabilization of uncomplicated fractures are conducted once the life-threatening injuries have been treated. The tetanus immunization status of the patient should be determined and appropriate prophylactic measures instituted. The trauma flow sheet should be completed, and the use of agents such as tetanus toxoid should be clearly documented and must be available for continued reference during the patient's stay in the intensive care unit (ICU).

It is at this point in the assessment and management of the multiply injured patient that subspecialities such as plastic surgery and otolaryngology may be consulted.

Repeated examination of the trauma patient is important so that injuries that are not immediately obvious at initial presentation may be diagnosed and treated appropriately. The history of the mechanism of the injury should be carefully noted, and a high index of suspicion is required so that occult injuries may not be missed. Patients who are relatively stable who were involved in accidents in which there is an associated fatality must be monitored very carefully in an ICU setting, since it must be assumed that such patients have been exposed to the same force and energy transfer as the dead patient. Such patients may have temporarily contained hematomas of the spleen, liver, retroperitoneum, or around major vascular structures. These patients could decompensate abruptly with sudden spontaneous hemorrhage. Slowly progressive tachycardia, hypotension or fall in hemoglobin, or any worsening of abdominal findings, such as increasing pain or signs of peritoneal irritation, should warrant aggressive investigation and consideration of intervention, including surgical exploration. These high-risk patients should have available at all times in the early phase of treatment approximately 4 to 6 U of blood available. Unexplainable fall in hemoglobin must be considered a sign of continued hemorrhage, and any sudden increase in heart rate or decrease in blood pressure must be considered signs of major hemorrhage. The source of this hemorrhage should be promptly identified and treated appropriately. A more subtle sign of impending hemodynamic instability is a progressive decrease in urine output with what appears to be adequate volume replacement based on the recognized injury. Deterioration in the respiratory status should prompt assessment for the presence of a pneumothorax, lung contusion, or other subtle injuries, such as a ruptured esophagus with pleural effusion that may present later in the patient's course. Delayed cardiac decompensation without obvious blood loss should warrant investigation for myocardial contusion, cardiac tamponade, or tension pneumothorax. The latter may occur on institution of positive pressure ventilation in a patient who sustained an unrecognized simple pneumothorax. Respiratory deterioration may also occur in spontaneously breathing patients who have sustained ruptures of the diaphragm with early containment of the abdominal viscera within the abdominal cavity but later displacement above the diaphragm with respiratory compromise. For these reasons, continuous close monitoring in an ICU setting is crucial to improving survival of the multiply injured patient.

X-ray examinations are conducted as indicated. In most multiply injured patients, these x-rays would include lateral cervical spine if there is any suggestion of cervical spinal injury, chest x-ray, and an x-ray of the pelvis. Other radiologic investigations will be undertaken based on the assessment, such as the presence of deformity in an extremity warranting x-ray to confirm fracture of that extremity.

Deciding on Surgical Intervention

One of the most important decisions to be made in the emergency management of the trauma patient is whether or not surgical intervention is necessary. If the decision based on the initial assessment is that surgery is not warranted, then continued observation in an intensive care setting is usually required in most multiply injured patients. This approach combined with a high index of suspicion will avoid missing occult injuries, such as the presence of subcapsular hepatic hematoma in a patient who is initially stable but has the potential of major sudden hemorrhage and hypovolemic shock.

In considering the need for surgical intervention, the common emergency indications are for thoracic and abdominal injuries. For thoracic injuries, this includes an uncontrollable pneumothorax representing a major airway laceration, a massive hemothorax usually representing a laceration of a systemic blood vessel or central pulmonary vessel, a widened mediastinum or other sign of aortic disruption, or signs of a ruptured esophagus, cardiac tamponade, or air embolism. The hypovolemic patient who suddenly becomes asystolic or suffers electromechanical dissociation is also a candidate for emergency thoracotomy. The details of assessment and management of these indications for thoracic surgery will be considered in Chap. 63. Likewise, the indications for laparotomy in the multiply injured patient are signs of penetration, perforation, or hemorrhage in general; these will be discussed in further detail in Chap. 63.

Summary

Patients frequently present to the intensivist in a trauma center with injuries affecting several systems simultaneously. The approach to such multiply injured patients requires prioritization of assessment and intervention. This should begin with a rapid overall assessment of the patient, during which life-threatening injuries are identified and resuscitative measures instituted. The identification of these life-threatening injuries is done in a sequence that allows attention to the airway first of all, followed by assessment of the breathing mechanism, the circulatory status, and then the neurologic status of the patient. Optimum assessment in this manner requires that the patient be completely exposed.

Following this rapid period of assessment, a more in-depth examination of the patient is conducted in an organized manner beginning with the head and ending with the toes, in order to diagnose conditions that may not be immediately life-threatening but if left unattended for a period of time could eventually threaten the patient's life as well.

CASE PRESENTATION

The following case history serves to demonstrate the process of prioritization in the multiply injured patient.

A 27-year-old intoxicated driver was brought into the emergency room approximately 15 min after having struck his car against a telephone pole. The ambulance personnel could not detect a radial pulse, but they were able to feel a femoral pulse, and the patient had a heart rate of 130. There was minimal bleeding from his nostrils, but he was vocalizing and complaining of right-shoulder pain and chest pain as well as shortness of breath. He did not remember the details of the accident. He also had an obvious deformity of his left thigh with marked swelling in this area. Because of the femoral fracture and his obvious state of hypoperfusion, the pneumatic antishock garment was applied, and the lower-limb and abdominal compartments were inflated until his radial pulse was palpable. He arrived in the emergency room within 15 min of being picked up at the scene of the accident.

Within minutes of arriving in the emergency room, he began to bleed massively through his mouth, and there was obvious ecchymosis around the eyes and evidence of a massive facial injury. Attempts were made to suction out the oropharynx and gain access for endotracheal intubation while maintaining C-spine control by in-line cervical immobilization, but repeated attempts to visualize the upper airway through the mouth were unsuccessful, and suction was continued and the patient underwent a surgical cricothyroidotomy with insertion of a No. 6 French endotracheal tube; the cuff was inflated. Suction of the oropharynx was then continued, and the bleeding subsequently ceased. The patient still appeared to be in severe respiratory distress, and assessment of the chest revealed that there was decreased air entry on the right side with hyperresonance. A large-bore needle was inserted in the second intercostal space on the right side, immediately relieving respiratory symptoms. This was followed by the insertion of a No. 32 French chest tube on the right side. The patient's respiratory status improved considerably, and his color improved with the administration of oxygen through the cricothyroidotomy tube.

Large-bore intravenous lines were established in both antecubital fossae and 3 L of normal saline were administered over $\frac{1}{2}$ h. The pneumatic antishock garment was slowly deflated, allowing maintenance of a blood pressure of 100 systolic and a pulse rate of 120. In order to maintain the blood pressure at this level, however, the patient required infusion of 3 U of type specific blood, which stabilized his blood pressure to 110 systolic. With this blood pressure, it was noted that the dorsalis pedis pulse on the left side was not as strong as on the right side. Application of a splint and realignment of the femur on the right side resulted in return of the pulse to the right dorsalis pedis artery.

A lateral cervical spine x-ray and supine chest x-ray were considered normal. An orogastric tube was inserted, and, after assessment of his abdomen and pelvis, which did not indicate any evidence of fracture of the pelvis, a Foley catheter was inserted per urethra. This revealed grossly bloody urine.

Because of the transient loss of consciousness, the patient was taken to the computed tomography (CT) scanner, where a scan of the head failed to reveal any evidence of a space-occupying lesion. CT scan of the abdomen failed to reveal any evidence of intraabdominal solid visceral injury or intraabdominal blood. Both kidneys also appeared intact, and there was no evidence of retroperitoneal hematoma on the CT scan. Over the next 2 h, he stabilized hemodynamically and was taken to the operating room, where his fractures were treated surgically. He was then transferred to the ICU with his cricothyroidotomy tube in place. Forty-eight hours later, the patient was taken back to the operating room for formal treatment of his facial fractures, at which time the cricothyroidotomy was converted to a formal tracheotomy. Over the next 10 days, the patient was successfully extubated and discharged from the ICU to the ward.

CASE DISCUSSION

It was quite evident on initial examination of this patient that he had a major problem with oxygenation and maintaining patency of his airway. Therefore, the first priority was to establish an airway. Attempts to intubate the airway through the mouth and nose were unsuccessful because of massive hemorrhage and failure to visualize the upper airway. The indication for cricothyroidotomy was failure to establish an airway by nonsurgical method. In addition, the patient had obviously sustained the following injuries: a tension pneumothorax, facial fracture, fractured femur and humerus on the right side, concussion, and hematuria. Of these injuries, according to our prioritization as outlined in this chapter, the tension pneumothorax would appear to be the lesion that would require our immediate attention. However, even though the facial fracture per se does not require immediate treatment, the effect of the facial fracture, i.e., major upper airway hemorrhage, necessitated an intervention prior to the insertion of the chest tube.

In situations where more than one member of the medical team is available, it should be possible to perform the cricothyroidotomy while at the same time decompressing a tension pneumothorax by needle insertion. However, the diagnosis of tension pneumothorax was not immediately made, and the order of priority was appropriate in attending to the airway before examining the chest for evidence of tension pneumothorax. Once the tension pneumothorax was diagnosed, this received immediate attention in the form of needle decompression, which was followed by formal decompression with the insertion of a large-bore chest tube. It is entirely inappropriate to wait for a chest x-ray in these circumstances, when one considers the possibility of a tension pneumothorax.

Although it is quite clear that this patient was in hypovolemic shock, one could not be certain whether there may have been concomitant intraabdominal hemorrhage to account for the hypovolemic shock. It was quite possible that the hemorrhage from the fractured femur and humerus could account for significant blood loss and hypotension. In these circumstances, concomitant blood loss in the abdomen and chest could not be ruled out. The insertion of a chest tube and failure to demonstrate massive amounts of blood from the pleural space and a chest x-ray that did not show any blood in the opposite chest suggested that the only other possible source of hemorrhage other than the fractures would be intraabdominal. Ordinarily under these circumstances, a diagnostic peritoneal lavage would have been undertaken, particularly as one could not rely entirely on the patient's assessment of the abdomen because of his concussion. However, because the patient had stabilized hemodynamically and required a CT scan for assessment of his head injury, it was decided to forego diagnostic peritoneal lavage and to assess the abdomen by performing a CT scan of the abdomen. In situations where a CT scan is not immediately available, it is reasonable to assess the abdomen by a diagnostic peritoneal lavage. Similarly, an intravenous pyelogram would have been considered if the patient had gross hematuria and a CT scan was not being considered. However, with the CT scan being available and being conducted, it was possible to assess the integrity of both kidneys by this technique. It should be pointed out, however, that the CT scan does not assess the excretory function of the kidneys as well as intravenous pyelography would. If the hematuria had not cleared within 48 to 72 h, then consideration would still need to be given for the performance of an intravenous pyelogram to assess the excretory function of both kidneys. The indication for the CT scan of the head in this patient is the transient loss of consciousness that he must have suffered because of his inability to remember the details of the accident.

Gastric decompression was accomplished through the oral route rather than the nasal route because the presence of a cribriform plate fracture was not ruled out previously.

In the order of priorities, the definitive treatment of the extremity fractures was conducted only after the airway and hemodynamic status of the patient had been stabilized and temporary early reduction and splinting of the fracture was required to maintain perfusion of the limb. Similarly, formal definitive treatment for the facial fractures was not conducted until the other life-threatening injuries had been attended to.

This case demonstrates the principle that the multiply injured patient sustains injuries that all require treatment at some time. However, it is crucial that the intensivist managing such a patient has a clear rationale for the order of intervention. This order is based on the degree to which the individual injuries threaten the patient's life and begins with an assessment of the airway, the adequacy of breathing, and correcting of any deficiencies in these areas before going on to correction of identifiable causes of hypoperfusion. Once these areas of oxygenation and hypoperfusion have been corrected, attention is directed to the neurologic status, which is followed by a detailed assessment of the entire patient for identification and treatment of other injuries that do not pose an immediate threat to life.

Acknowledgment

The author acknowledges the assistance of Sunnybrook Studios of the Sunnybrook Health Science Centre, Toronto, for preparation of the illustrations.

References

1. Committee on Trauma, American College of Surgeons: *Advanced Trauma Life Support Manual.* Chicago, American College of Surgeons, 1989.
2. Narrod JA, Moore EE, Rosen P: Emergency cricothyrostomy, technique and anatomical considerations. J Emerg Med 2:443, 1985.
3. Shaffer MA, Doris PE: Limitation of the cross table lateral view in detecting cervical spine injuries: A retrospective analysis. Ann Emerg Med 10:508, 1981.
4. Moore JB, Moore EE, Markovchick VJ, Rosen P: Diagnostic peritoneal lavage for abdominal trauma: Superiority of the open technique at the infra-umbilical ring. J Trauma 21:570, 1981.
5. Gaffney FA, Thal ER, Taylor WF: Hemodynamic effects of medical anti-shock trousers (MAST Garment). J Trauma 21:931, 1981.
6. Johnson G III, Bond RF, Stack LB, Class CA: Efficacy of Military antishock trousers in compensatory and decompensatory hemorrhagic hypotension. Circ Shock 21:233, 1987.
7. Bickell WH, Geer MR, Rubal BJ: Hemodynamic response to rapid pneumatic antishock garment deflation. Ann Emerg Med 15:886, 1986.
8. Brotman S, Browner BD, Cox EF: MAS trousers improperly applied causing a compartment syndrome lower extremity trauma. J Trauma 22:598, 1982.
9. Templeman D, Lange R, Harms B: Lower extremity compartment syndromes associated with use of pneumatic antishock garment. J Trauma 27:79, 1987.
10. Rush BF Jr, Richardson JD, Bosomworth P, Eiseman B: Limitations of blood replacement with electrolyte solution: A control clinical study. Arch Surg 98:49, 1969.
11. Reuler JB. Hypothermia: Pathophysiology, clinical settings and management. Ann Intern Med 89:519, 1978.
12. Baxter BT, Moore EE, Moore JB, et al: Emergency department thoracotomy following injury: Critical determinants for patient salvage. World J Surg 12:671, 1988.
13. Bouzarth WF: Intracranial nasogastric tube insertion, editorial. J Trauma 18:319, 1978.
14. Fremstad JD, Martin GH: Lethal complication from insertion of nasogastric tube after severe basilar skull fracture. J Trauma 18:820, 1978.

Chapter 60

CLOSED AND OPEN HEAD INJURY

RICHARD J. MOULTON

KEY POINTS

- *Early diagnosis and surgical evacuation of operable intracranial hematomas is essential.*
- *Monitoring and aggressive treatment of intracranial pressure should be undertaken in appropriately selected patients.*
- *Hypoxia and ischemia must be prevented by appropriate airway and respiratory management, including mechanical ventilation for all comatose patients, and maintenance of appropriate extracellular fluid volume and blood pressure.*
- *Prophylaxis and aggressive treatment of seizures following head injury must be instituted.*
- *Maintenance of normal fluid and electrolyte balance and early provision of enteral or parenteral nutrition is necessary.*
- *Risk of central nervous system (CNS) infection is reduced by surgical debridement and restoration of dural integrity in cases of open cranial injury.*
- *Systemic sepsis often complicates recovery and should be diagnosed and treated aggressively.*

Epidemiology and Etiology of Head Injury

The incidence of head injury in the United States is approximately 200 to 400 per 100,000 population per year. Similar incidence rates have been documented for other countries. Male to female incidence ratios vary between 2:1 and 3:1, and the peak age incidence occurs in the second and third decades.[1] Severe injuries [i.e., those admitted in coma, Glasgow Coma Score (GCS) $\leq$8; see Table 60-1][2,3] comprise a minority of patients admitted to hospital but account for most morbidity and mortality (Fig. 60-1). Those hospitals with a large primary care population will see a relatively smaller proportion of severely injured patients than will those functioning primarily as a tertiary referral center.

The most common cause of closed head injury is road traffic accidents. These include injuries to vehicle occupants, pedestrians, motorcyclists, and bicyclists. Falls are the next most common cause of injury. Gunshot injuries are a major cause of penetrating head injury in the United States and comprise up to 44 percent of head injuries in some series.[1] Etiology varies considerably with local patient demographics, proximity to major highways, etc., and the resulting case mix will vary from center to center in terms of intracranial hematoma incidence, mean patient age, and, consequently, outcome from injury. Younger adults are more often involved in vehicular trauma, and there is a lower incidence of intracranial mass lesions in this patient population. Older patients are more often injured as a result of falls and have a higher incidence of mass lesions. At an equivalent depth of coma, both increasing age and presence of intracranial hematomas predispose patients to a poorer outcome.

Intoxication with alcohol or other agents is a significant factor in all causes of injury and across virtually all age groups except the very young and very old. Depending on etiology, 10 to 50 percent of our patients were obviously intoxicated at admission (Fig. 60-2).

The social and economic costs of head injury are enormous. Severe injury carries a high mortality, and patients who survive severe and moderate injuries may remain substantially disabled for years after the injury. The persistent effects of head injury on personality and mentation may be devastating for both patients and their families.

Pathophysiology of Craniocerebral Trauma

ACCELERATION–DECELERATION INJURY

Injury to the brain is produced by energy transfer to the cranium and its contained structures. In blunt injury, angular acceleration–deceleration forces cause shear strains within the cerebral parenchyma, which in turn are responsible for the characteristic diffuse axonal injury. The force may be applied directly to the head (i.e., impact injury) or indirectly via the body (i.e., impulse injury). The physiologic hallmark of diffuse injury to the brain is loss of con-

TABLE 60-1 The Glasgow Coma Score[2,3]

Eye opening	
Spontaneous	4
To voice	3
To pain	2
None	1
Verbal response	
Oriented	5
Confused speech	4
Inappropriate words	3
Incomprehensible sounds	2
None	1
Motor response	
Obeys commands	6
Localizes pain	5
Withdraws	4
Abnormal flexion	3
Extension	2
None	1

Although the score in the three categories is frequently summed for convenience, the most information is conveyed by reporting the three response categories separately. The motor score from the patient's "best" side is used if there is a discrepancy in response between sides. Intubation may be designated by a "T" in the verbal response.

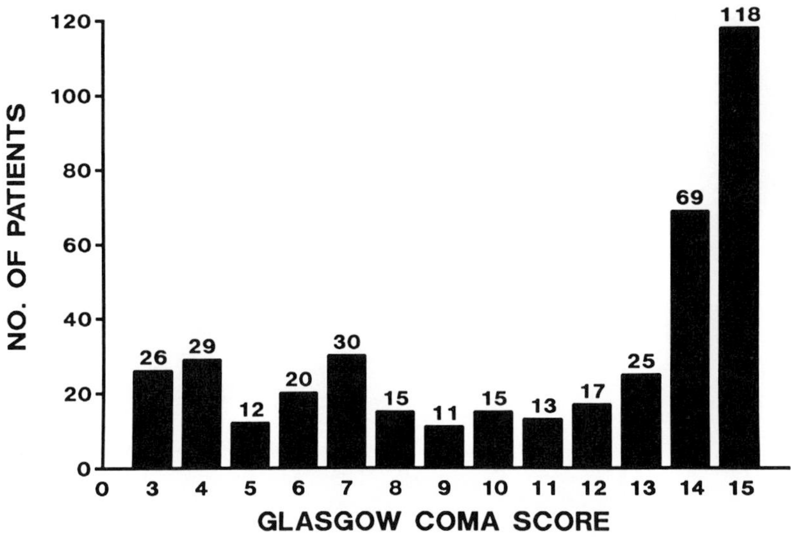

FIGURE 60-1 Distribution of head injury severity (measured by Glasgow Coma Score at admission) in 400 consecutive admissions to a tertiary care hospital neurosurgical unit.

sciousness. Concussion is a brief loss of consciousness without obvious sequelae. Coma is defined as a state of unconsciousness wherein the patient neither opens his or her eyes, follows commands, nor utters any recognizable words. The severity of brain injury may be gauged by the depth and duration of coma or the duration of posttraumatic amnesia. Both the duration of coma and posttraumatic amnesia can be judged only in retrospect, so that the depth of coma as quantified by the GCS has been widely adopted as the most convenient measure of injury severity. With severe and prolonged coma, the patient may reach a state characterized by observable periods of eye opening and sleep without appreciation of the environment or of people or objects in it. This has been called the persistent vegetative state.

Acceleration–deceleration injury occurring as a result of impact or impulse mechanisms may produce gross disruption of brain tissue (laceration and/or contusion), diffuse axonal injury, or both. The characteristic histologic findings of diffuse injury consist of axon retraction balls and microglial stars. Hemorrhagic lesions of the anterior corpus callosum may be seen on careful post mortem examination

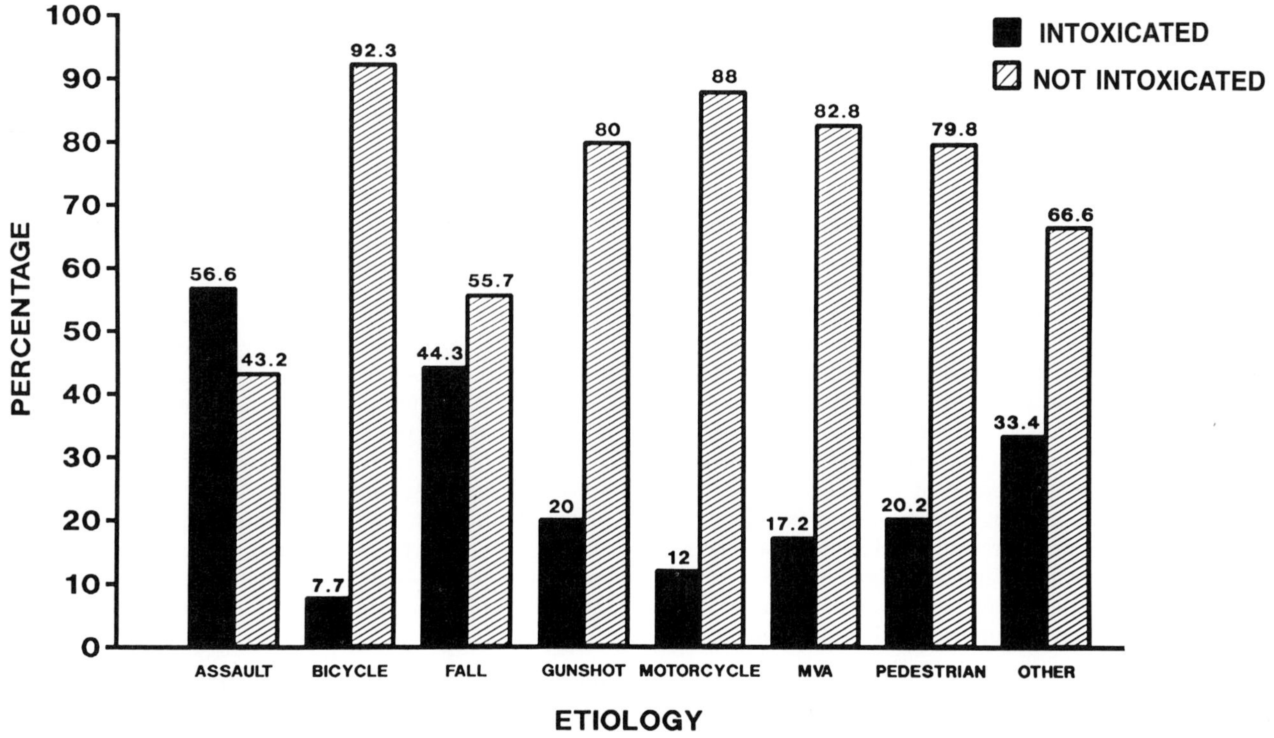

FIGURE 60-2 Proportional incidence of alcohol intoxication by injury etiology in 400 consecutive head injury patients. MVA refers to injuries to motor vehicle occupants.

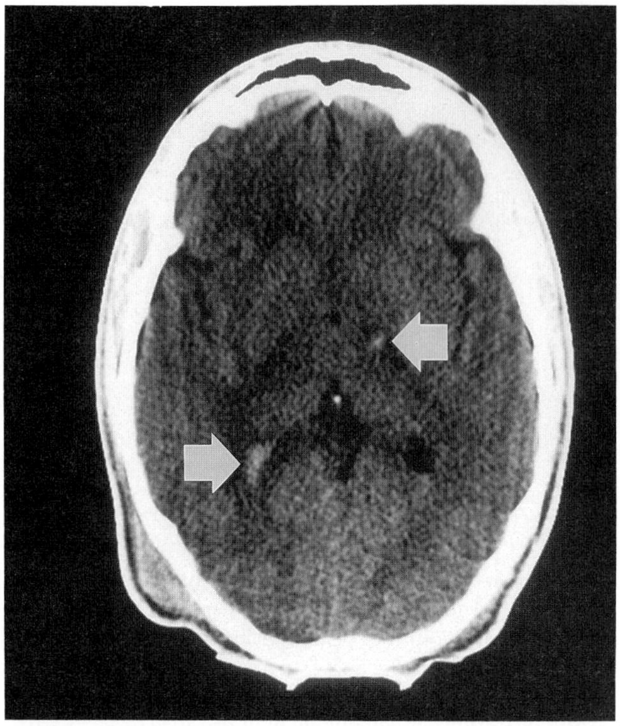

FIGURE 60-3 CT scan of a 16-year-old patient with a typical diffuse head injury. The patient's GCS at admission to hospital was four. There is a small amount of blood in the trigone and occipital horn of the right lateral ventricle *(lower arrow)*. There is a small punctate hemorrhage in the left internal capsule *(upper arrow)*.

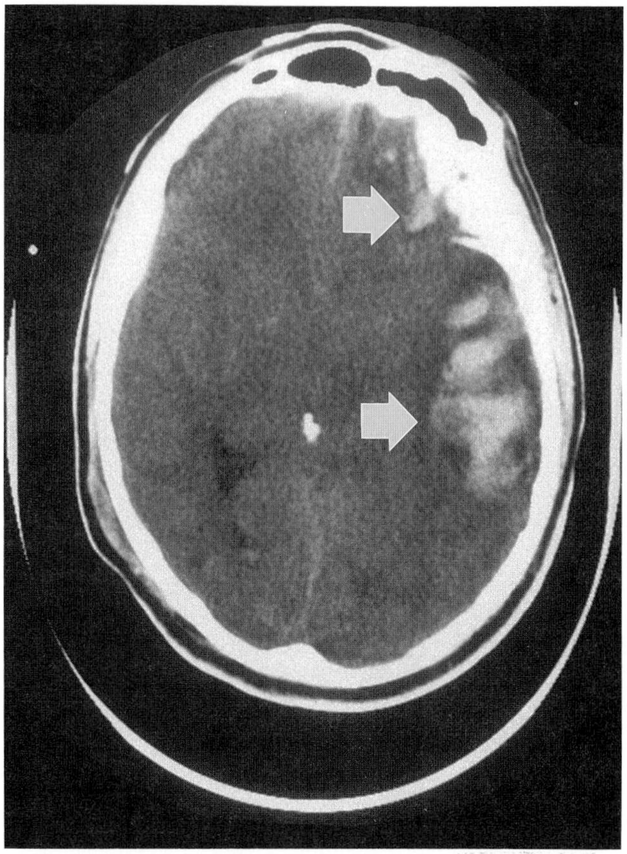

FIGURE 60-4 CT scan of a 50-year-old man injured in a fall. There is a large mixed-density lesion in the left temporal lobe *(lower arrow)* and a similar, smaller lesion in the left orbito-frontal cortex *(upper arrow)*. The appearance is typical of cerebral contusions.

or may be apparent on computed tomography (CT) scan, as may small punctate hemorrhages deep within the hemispheres, or small amounts of blood within the ventricular system (Fig. 60-3). For a given force, the greatest degree of injury occurs in the white matter of the hemispheres with relatively less injury to the brainstem.

Laceration/contusion of the brain surface may underlie the site of a blow (coup contusion) or more typically is found on the orbito-frontal surface of the frontal lobes and/or the anterior portion of the temporal lobes remote from the site of the blow (contre-coup injury) (Figs. 60-4, 60-5). To and fro motion of the brain over the uneven surfaces of the anterior and middle fossae has been postulated as the underlying mechanism of contre-coup contusion. Cavitation of the brain produced by the rapid acceleration of the skull away from the brain at contusion sites is an alternate hypothesis. Both cerebral parenchyma and blood vessels are disrupted at the sites of contusion, and the bleeding may be sufficient to produce a subdural hematoma, a large confluent intracerebral hematoma, or both.

In addition to the disruption of cerebral parenchyma, direct impact injury may disrupt the skull and meninges, or their blood vessels. Skull fractures are of importance primarily because they may trigger epidural bleeding, provide a portal of entry for infective organisms if compound (either directly or indirectly via the middle ear or paranasal sinuses), or lacerate the meninges and underlying brain if depressed fragments are present. Cranial nerves may be injured as they exit the skull base, and fractures involving the petrous temporal bone may injure the auditory and/or vestibular end-organs, or disrupt the ossicles of the middle ear.

PENETRATING INJURY

Penetrating injury produces direct disruption and laceration of brain tissue. In low-velocity injuries (stab wounds, impalement), damage is confined to the directly disrupted tissue. There is often no loss of consciousness. In missile injuries, cavitation occurs along the tract of the missile, and depending on the size and velocity of the missile, disruption of surrounding cerebral tissue is often widespread and severe. Both high- and low-velocity-penetrating injuries disrupt the overlying skin, skull, and meninges of the brain, thereby allowing contamination of cerebrospinal fluid (CSF) or brain with infective microorganisms.

SECONDARY INJURY TO THE BRAIN

Direct and immediate disruption of the brain tissue consequent to blunt or penetrating trauma constitutes primary injury. Secondary processes may be initiated at the time of injury or at any subsequent time, and these may aggravate

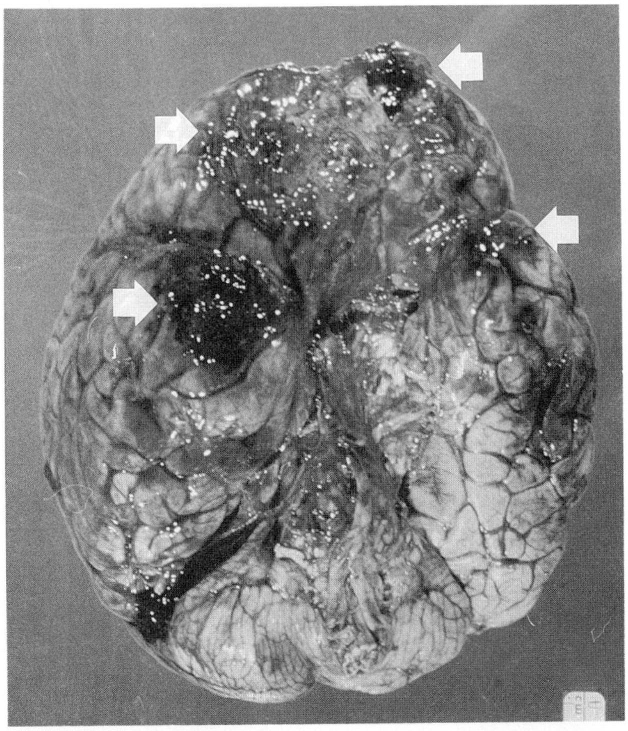

FIGURE 60-5 Pathologic specimen showing asymmetric hemorrhagic contusions of both temporal lobes *(lower arrows)* and both frontal poles *(upper arrows)*. These are the usual locations of cerebral contusions.

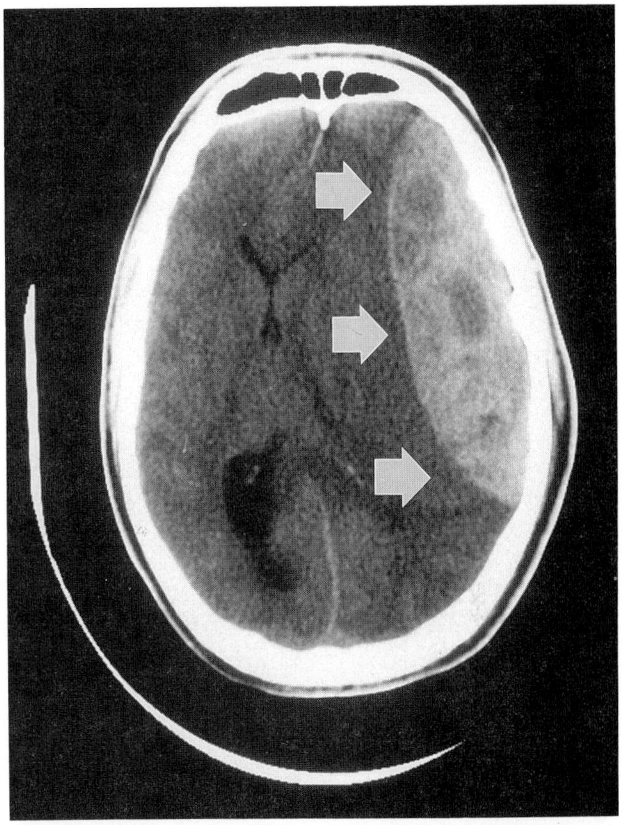

FIGURE 60-6 CT scan of a large acute extradural hematoma *(arrows)*. Extradural hematomas have a convex medial border producing the "lens" shape, which distinguishes epidural from subdural hematomas.

existing injury to the brain. Secondary injuries include intracranial bleeding, hypoxia, ischemia, raised intracranial pressure (ICP), infection, and electrolyte and metabolic disturbances.[4] The incidence of secondary injury generally increases with the severity of the primary injury, although the relationship is not completely congruent. Patients with devastating primary injuries may initially have very little secondary injury. Conversely, patients with little primary injury may die or be crippled as a result of an enlarging intracranial hematoma or uncontrolled ICP. Clinically, the neurologic disturbance produced by primary injury is maximal at onset and then lessens or remains stable. In contradistinction, secondary injuries produce worsening of the patient's clinical neurologic status as their effects are added to those of the primary injury. Of considerable importance is the fact that secondary injuries are treatable and/or preventable.

Intracranial hematomas occur between the skull and dura mater (epidural; Fig. 60-6), between the dura mater and brain (subdural; Fig. 60-7), or within the substance of the brain (intracerebral; Fig. 60-8). As intracranial hematomas enlarge, they produce compression and shift of the adjacent brain. This enlargement produces rapid and large increases in ICP as the volume-buffering capacity of the cranial contents is exhausted (see Chap. 34). ICP may also increase from edema adjacent to a contusion or present diffusely throughout the white matter of one or both hemispheres, or from engorgement of the cerebral vasculature. Often all three mechanisms are operative to some extent. The combination of brain shift, high intracranial pressure, and pressure gradients across dural and bony partitions (i.e., falx cerebri, tentorium, and foramen magnum) cause herniation of brain tissue from higher to lower pressure compartments. The most important of these is transtentorial herniation, signalled by the presence of an ipsilateral dilated and fixed or sluggishly reactive pupil (see Chap. 34). Increased ICP also reduces cerebral perfusion pressure [CPP = mean arterial blood pressure (MABP) − ICP]. In cases of uncontrolled ICP, the terminal event is usually an increase of the ICP to a level at or slightly above MABP.

Hypoxia may occur as the result of central depression of respiration consequent to loss of consciousness, injury to the thorax, aspiration of gastric contents, or any combination of the above.

Evidence of ischemia is frequently found at autopsy following blunt head injury.[5] Focal ischemia may occur at the site of contusions or may be the result of vasospasm induced by traumatic subarachnoid hemorrhage. Global ischemia may be induced by systemic hypotension or reduction in CPP secondary to increased ICP.

Infection may be local (e.g., meningitis, brain abscess) or systemic. The former occurs when the integrity of the meninges is compromised as a result of penetrating injuries or compound fracture of the vault or skull base. Meningitis or ventriculitis may be iatrogenic as a result of insertion of

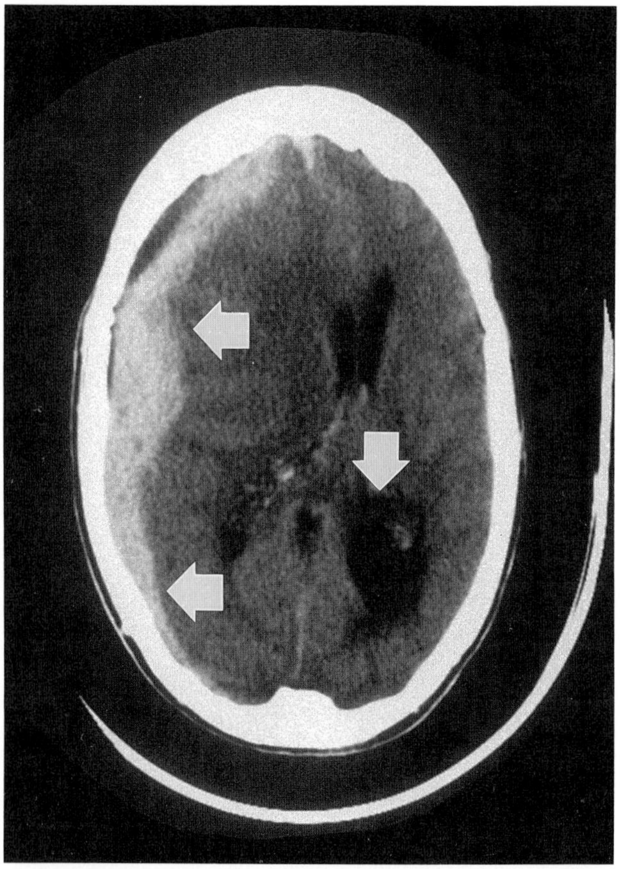

FIGURE 60-7 CT scan of a large acute subdural hematoma ***(horizontal arrows).*** **The hematoma spreads over the entire convexity of the hemisphere so that the medial border of the hematoma is concave. Note also the large amount of midline shift. The occipital horn of the left lateral ventricle is acutely enlarged as a result of "trapping" of CSF by ventricular distortion and obstruction of CSF flow** ***(vertical arrow).***

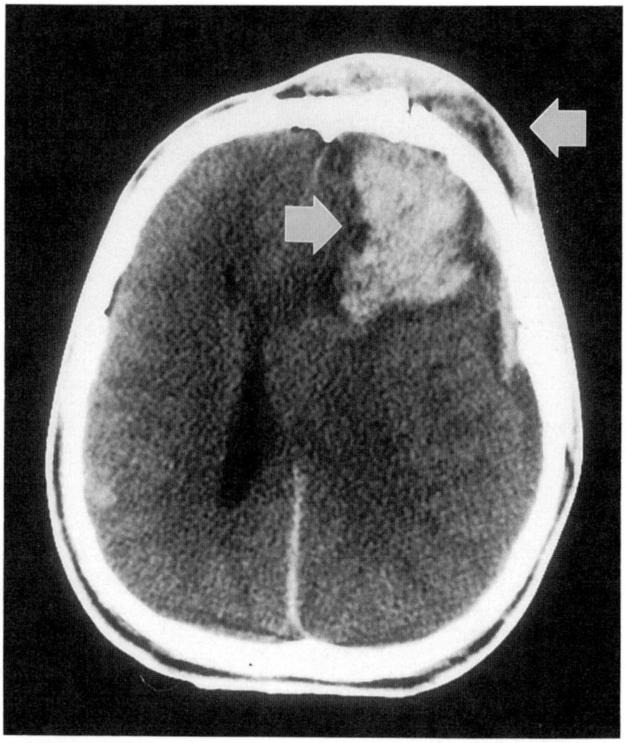

FIGURE 60-8 CT scan of a confluent traumatic intracerebral hematoma in the left frontal lobe of a patient struck by a motor vehicle ***(lower arrow).*** **There is overlying scalp swelling and contusion at the site of the blow to the head** ***(upper arrow).***

ICP-monitoring apparatus. Systemic infection typically involves the lungs or genitourinary tract. Systemic sepsis often causes neurologic deterioration that may improve with resolution of the infection. The accompanying hyperthermia often aggravates existing ICP problems.

Electrolyte disorders are common in moderate and severe head injuries. The most frequent is the syndrome of inappropriate ADH secretion (SIADH). Serum sodium may fall significantly, and deterioration in patients' neurologic status usually occurs at levels below 120 to 125 meq/L. Diabetes insipidus usually occurs in more severe injuries, often as a preterminal event in patients with progressive rostral–caudal neurologic deterioration caused by uncontrollable ICP. In a much smaller number of patients, diabetes insipidus may be the result of focal injury to the hypothalamic–pituitary axis.

Severe head injury induces a state of catabolism with net excretion of nitrogen similar to that seen in other injuries. Catecholamine-induced tachycardia, increased blood pressure, and increased cardiac output are common. Myocardial ischemia may occur as a result of closed head injury.[6]

Abnormalities of blood coagulation are known to occur as a result of brain injury and are predictive of a poor outcome.[7] The reported incidence of coagulopathy depends to a certain extent on the diligence with which it is sought and is often confounded by other potential causes of coagulation disturbance, such as massive transfusion in the multiple-injured patient. Delayed and recurrent hematomas, including those related to placement of ventricular catheters, have been described in patients with disseminated intravascular coagulation.[8] In patients in whom a bleeding diathesis is known or suspected, it is preferable to use a subarachnoid bolt or epidural transducer rather than a ventricular catheter for ICP monitoring when there is a high likelihood of increased ICP (e.g., in the presence of a mass lesion). In those patients who are known to have a low incidence of raised ICP (i.e., normal CT scans), monitoring can be deferred until the coagulation abnormality is reversed.

Management of Acute Head Injury

As may be inferred from the discussion of pathology and pathophysiology presented earlier, the management of head injury during the acute period is based primarily on the timely diagnosis and treatment of secondary insults to the injured brain. Management of the primary injury consists of providing the best possible physiologic milieu in order that the recovery of sublethally injured neurons may proceed unimpeded. At the present time, there is no medical or surgical therapy directed at the primary injury, and the cellular pathophysiology of primary brain injury has not been fully elucidated.

DIAGNOSIS

Diagnosis in closed head injury is based on history, physical examination, and radiologic investigation. The relevant elements to be ascertained from the history are the mechanism of injury, whether there was any initial loss of consciousness, and whether the level of consciousness has improved or deteriorated since the injury. This last item is of paramount importance, since worsening of the patient's neurologic state subsequent to injury always implies the presence of secondary injury to the brain. Patients who have talked at some point after injury and who subsequently lapse into unconsciousness almost invariably are harboring an intracranial hematoma. One should determine whether or not there has been any witnessed seizure activity, since this may produce transient profound deterioration in level of consciousness that may mimic that induced by an expanding intracranial hematoma.

Neurologic examination consists of two components: determination of the level of consciousness, and establishing the presence of focal deficits to aid in lesion localization and measurement of severity. The former is the single-most-important measure following traumatic brain injury and is best accomplished by use of the GCS. In patients with a disturbed level of consciousness, the scope of the traditional neurologic examination is severely limited because of its considerable dependence on patient cooperation. In unconscious patients, crude localization may be achieved by observing discrepancies between sides in the patient's motor response to pain. Evidence of brainstem dysfunction should be sought, and the common measures are pupillary reaction to light, oculocephalic (Doll's eye maneuvers) or oculocaloric responses, and corneal reflexes. Doll's eye testing should be deferred until it is known that the cervical spine is intact, and oculocaloric testing should not be carried out in the presence of a ruptured tympanic membrane. Unless there has been local ocular trauma, the presence of unilateral pupillary dilatation and unreactivity implies the presence of a mass lesion, and urgent diagnosis and evacuation of the mass are essential. This is particularly important in cases of unwitnessed unconsciousness, and investigation of metabolic causes of coma should be deferred until a CT scan has been obtained.

Other relevant physical examination consists of an examination of the head for signs of trauma. These include bruising or laceration of the face and scalp, open skull fractures, hemotympanum and bruising over the mastoid process (Battle's sign) indicating fracture of the petrous temporal bone, and periorbital hematoma (raccoon eye) indicating fracture of the floor of the anterior fossa. One should also look for signs of CSF leakage from the nose or ears. CSF may be admixed with blood, and "targeting" of the drainage on a piece of filter paper indicates the presence of CSF. Biochemical determination of the presence of CSF by means of glucose or chloride measurement is usually not possible because of the difficulty in collecting a sufficient amount of drainage. Ordinarily the CSF glucose level is approximately half that in serum. The CSF chloride level is 116–122 meq/L.

CT scanning is essential to the proper management of unconscious head injury patients. It allows the precise diagnosis of all types of intracranial hematoma, their location, and the extent of the mass effect produced by the hematoma, measured by the displacement of the septum pellucidum from the midline. The scan should be obtained as soon as the patient is stable and any more urgent management priorities have been attended to. It is occasionally necessary to forgo CT scanning to deal with life-threatening injuries to other systems or because of an unacceptable delay in obtaining a scan in a patient with a high likelihood of having an intracranial surface clot. Unconscious patients should have lateral and anterior–posterior (AP) x-rays of the cervical spine to the level of T_1 in order to rule out cervical fracture. In the absence of x-ray evidence of an intact cervical spine, one must presume there is a fracture and continue to immobilize the head and spine until appropriate x-rays are obtained and the necessary treatment instituted.

Magnetic resonance imaging (MRI) has been used on a limited basis with head injury patients. There is a greater ability to detect some types of small extra-axial fluid collections and parenchymal injuries. However, there is no advantage in detecting hematomas requiring surgical treatment, and the difficulties inherent in having to exclude metallic objects from the scan environment render the technique somewhat impractical in the acute posttrauma setting. A potential application is the improved identification of parenchymal changes following mild and moderate head injury that have been shown to correlate with the neuropsychologic sequelae of head injury.[9,10]

PREOPERATIVE MANAGEMENT

In the initial phase of head injury management, the usual diagnostic and treatment priorities for treatment of trauma patients are followed. Establishment of an adequate airway is of paramount importance in unconscious patients. All patients with a GCS ≤ 8 should have endotracheal or nasotracheal intubation and mechanical ventilation regardless of whether other indications for intubation are present or not. Nasotracheal intubation should be avoided in patients with signs of basal skull fracture. Patients should be hyperventilated to a modest degree (P_{CO_2} 30–35 mmHg) in order to reduce raised ICP. In patients who are comatose, or in whom there has been clearcut deterioration in neurologic status, a bolus of 20% solution of mannitol should be given in a dose of approximately 1 g/kg patient weight. Contraindications to the use of mannitol are hypotension, anuria, or severe congestive heart failure. Corticosteroids are of no benefit in reducing ICP in head injury, and their use has

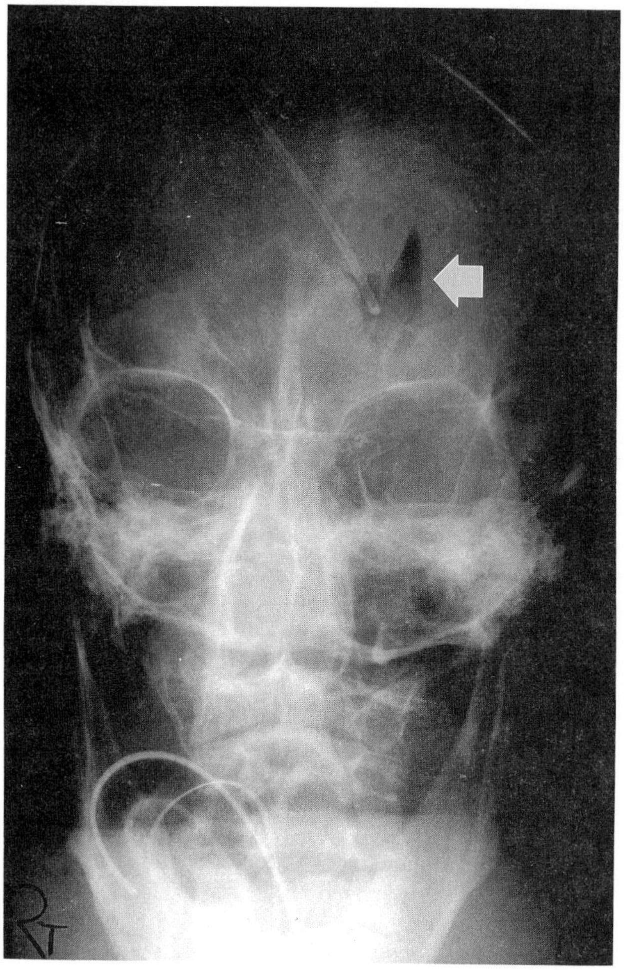

FIGURE 60-9 Air ventriculogram done in the operating room in a multiple-injured patient. Air (4 mL) was injected into the ventricular catheter and an AP skull film obtained. The displacement of the frontal horns of the ventricles *(arrow)* away from the midline toward the left side indicates a mass lesion on the right side. Subsequent craniotomy revealed a large right frontal intracerebral hematoma.

been abandoned in most centers. As soon as other management priorities have been dealt with, the patient should undergo CT scanning.

OPERATIVE MANAGEMENT

INTRACRANIAL HEMATOMA

The cornerstone of acute head injury management is the rapid diagnosis and prompt surgical evacuation of intracranial hematomas. Twenty-five to fifty percent of patients rendered comatose as a result of acute head injury will have an operable intracranial hematoma.[3,4,11–13] Approximately 20 percent of patients with intracranial hematomas have an extradural hematoma, and the rest will have hemispheric acute subdural hematomas, significant brain contusions, or both.[4,11,13] Traumatic hematomas in the posterior fossa are unusual. The diagnosis is ordinarily made with a CT scan. Surgical evacuation is then accomplished via craniotomy with wide exposure and evacuation of the hematoma and coagulation of sources of hemorrhage. Occasionally, when there is clearcut evidence of neurologic deterioration with progression to signs of uncal herniation (i.e., pupillary dilatation) it is necessary to proceed directly to operation, bypassing CT scan. The other circumstance in which exploratory burr holes may be necessary is in comatose patients with signs of brainstem compromise who must be taken to the operating room for life-threatening systemic injuries without benefit of a CT scan. An alternate strategy in these patients is twist-drill air ventriculography in the operating room. The standard landmarks are used for cannulation of the frontal horn of the lateral ventricle. Once the ventricle is cannulated, 3 to 4 mL of air are introduced into the ventricles, and a brow-up AP skull film is obtained. The presence of a mass lesion is inferred from shift of the ventricular system (Fig. 60-9).

The frequent coexistence of acute subdural hematomas and temporal and/or frontal cortical laceration/contusion dictates the necessity of a wide operative exposure, allowing access to both the frontal and temporal lobes, as well as the medial convexity adjacent to the sagittal sinus, where there may be torn bridging veins (Fig. 60-10). The operative approach to an isolated extradural hematoma may be more circumscribed. Contusions of the frontal and temporal lobes, or confluent blood clots producing greater than 5 mm midline shift should be evacuated operatively through the standard large flap. Often removal of the contused brain must be accompanied by formal frontal or temporal lobectomy in order to provide adequate internal decompression in the face of a traumatized swollen brain. In this circumstance, the question of whether or not to leave out the craniotomy bone flap (or remove it later), in order to provide more room for the swollen brain, has engendered some controversy. The prevalent view holds that this does not improve functional outcome. It is probable, however, that poor outcome is more likely the result of performance of the procedure in someone with overwhelming primary injury, and that decompressive craniectomy may be useful in patients in whom the degree of primary injury is compatible with a reasonable neurologic outcome.

At the conclusion of the evacuation of a hematoma, an ICP monitoring device is placed in almost all cases. The exceptions are patients whose level of consciousness was only mildly depressed preoperatively (GCS > 10) and in whom the brain is not significantly contused or swollen at the time of operative exposure. The techniques and indications for ICP monitoring are discussed in Chap. 34.

PENETRATING INJURY

The same principles of prompt evacuation of intracranial hematomas and debridement of contused brain apply to penetrating injuries. The other indication for operating on compound lesions is the restoration of the integrity of the dura and overlying tissues in order to prevent bacterial infection of CSF (i.e., meningitis) or cerebral parenchyma (brain abscess). Indriven bone fragments should all be removed as well as underlying hematoma and devitalized brain. It is not necessary to attempt to remove inaccessible

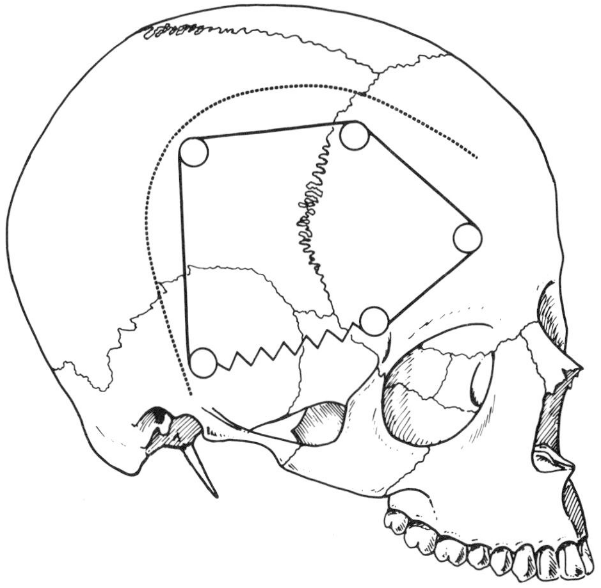

FIGURE 60-10 Diagram of the operative exposure for the removal of a traumatic intracranial hematoma. The skin incision is shown with the dotted line. The skull flap is outlined with a solid line. The exposure permits access to the major portion of the hemisphere convexity as well as sufficient access for debridement/lobectomy of the frontal or temporal lobes.

missile fragments from the depths of the brain. Prophylactic antibiotics are used to reduce the incidence of delayed infection in cases of penetrating injury. Broad spectrum coverage with antibiotics capable of crossing the blood-brain barrier should be used (e.g., cloxacillin 4 to 6 g/day and chloramphenicol 4 g/day given intravenously).

BASAL SKULL FRACTURE

A special case of compound injury is the basal skull fracture with CSF leakage through the paranasal sinuses or into the mastoid air cells, middle ear, and external ear or pharynx. CSF otorrhea almost always stops spontaneously, and surgical repair of the leak is rarely necessary. Rhinorrhea is more prone to continue, and the continued presence of a CSF fistula will eventually lead to delayed meningitis. Surgical repair of an anterior fossa fistula may be undertaken early when there is an obvious bony disruption of the anterior fossa floor, often coincident with complex facial fractures. In this case, repair of the CSF leak is undertaken at the time of facial reconstructive surgery. In cases of persistent CSF leak without obvious bony disruption, the site of the fistula may sometimes be localized with coronal CT cuts through the anterior fossa following the instillation of water soluble radiographic contrast material into the CSF. Investigation of persistent CSF leakage should be deferred until the patient is stable with respect to both ICP and coexisting systemic injuries. Occasionally bilateral anterior fossa exploration is necessary in the face of persistent CSF rhinorrhea, the site of which cannot be identified radiologically.

There is considerable debate about the merits of prophylactic antibiotics for CSF rhinorrhea and otorrhea. Unfortunately there are no good clinical studies to support either their use or abandonment, and this remains largely a matter of personal preference. We do not use prophylactic antibiotics for CSF leak in our unit for fear of selecting multiply-resistant organisms. When there is established infection, the diagnosis and treatment is the same as for meningitis of any cause. Operative repair of the dural fistula should not be undertaken until the infection has been cleared with appropriate antibiotic therapy.

CRITICAL CARE MONITORING

Monitoring of the head-injured patient is designed to detect and treat secondary injuries before they further compromise the injured brain. Ideally one would like to monitor neurologic function, cerebral blood flow (CBF) and metabolism, the intracranial pressure, and those systemic parameters required for the maintenance of adequate perfusion and oxygenation of the brain. Measurement of all these parameters is possible although difficult in the case of cerebral blood flow and metabolism measurements, and the ideal situation described here is infrequently practiced.

CLINICAL EXAM

Monitoring of neurologic function is most commonly and simply carried out by means of hourly repetition of the abbreviated version of the neurologic examination described earlier under diagnosis. Any deterioration in the patient's neurologic status should trigger an investigation for treatable causes. Neuromuscular blocking agents used to treat raised ICP or respiratory problems prevent the conduct of a meaningful neurologic examination. In this circumstance, only the pupillary responses are available for assessment, and significant deterioration in the patient's neurologic function may occur before pupillary changes are evident.

ICP monitoring is then essential in order to have some information about the status of the patient. Although ICP is not a measure of neurologic function per se, many of the pathologic processes that endanger the head-injured patient in the early phase after injury manifest themselves with raised ICP in addition to neurologic deterioration. In a patient who is pharmacologically paralyzed for ICP control, paralysis should be allowed to wear off at intervals of 12 to 24 h so that a neurologic assessment may be carried out. Occasionally the effects of reversal on ICP are intolerable, and reversal is not possible. A potential alternative to clinical neurologic monitoring is electrophysiologic measurement of neurologic function. The common techniques are EEG and evoked potentials (EPs).

EEG

EEG recordings in comatose patients typically show slowing of the background frequencies with correlation between the degree of slowing and the depth of coma in most cases. Conventional strip chart EEG is impractical because of the amount of data generated. Various methods of data compression have evolved, the most common being Fast Fourier Transformation of the EEG. Fourier transformation yields quantitative frequency and amplitude data from the

EEG and is well suited to long-term trending of the background frequencies and to quantitative analysis thereof. Specific pattern recognition (e.g., seizure spikes) is sacrificed. Survival from head injury has been correlated with a return of higher frequency activity in the first week after injury.[14]

EPs

EPs have been demonstrated to be particularly useful in predicting outcome from head injury. The single most useful measure is the somatosensory evoked response,[15] although combinations of EPs (somatosensory, auditory, and visual) yield the highest prognostic accuracy.[16] Deterioration in serially measured EPs, occurring as a result of secondary injury to the brain, have been shown to correlate with poor patient outcome.[17] In the past, EPs have been used primarily in an intermittent manner for determination of prognosis. With further technologic improvements and increased automation of data collection, these techniques may see more widespread use for continuous monitoring in an ICU setting.

ICP MONITORING

The use of ICP monitoring has become widespread in the treatment of head injuries since the 1970s, when a number of reports indicated a reduction in mortality in severe head injury (i.e., GCS $\leq$ 8) with aggressive management, including routine ICP monitoring.[4,11,18] The data from these series are confounded somewhat by the presence of a number of management innovations in addition to ICP monitoring, including CT scanning and routine mechanical ventilation of comatose patients. Nonetheless, there is an established association between raised ICP and poor outcome, although causation has not been proven. Two large nonrandomized studies have shown beneficial effect on mortality with ICP monitoring and aggressive treatment.[12,13] We feel that ICP monitoring should be used initially in all comatose patients, patients who have had mass lesions evacuated and who are not sufficiently conscious to follow commands, selected patients in whom nonoperative treatment of significant cerebral contusions has been elected (see Case Discussion), and patients with head injuries and a disturbed level of consciousness in whom pharmacologic paralysis is necessary for respiratory management.

BLOOD FLOW AND METABOLIC RATE

CBF and metabolism have been measured in a number of units engaged in clinical research. The common techniques rely on measurement of washout curves from the brain of nitrous oxide or radioactive xenon. The equipment and techniques for conducting CBF measurements are complicated and expensive, and this has discouraged widespread adoption of these measures. Furthermore, in the case of xenon CBF measurement, the number of studies that can be carried out in a given patient is limited by radiation safety concerns. Although the incidence of ischemic levels of blood flow is very low in published series, knowledge of CBF may be useful in determining patients in whom hyperemia is contributing substantially to increased ICP. In addition, these studies may aid management in cases where vigorous hyperventilation is necessary to control raised ICP and reduction of CBF is a possibility. CBF, the cerebral metabolic rate for oxygen ($CMRO_2$), and the arterial–jugular oxygen content difference (AVD_{O_2}) are related by the following equation:

$$CMR_{O_2} = (AVD_{O_2} \times CBF)/100.$$

When CMR_{O_2} is relatively constant, AVD_{O_2} varies inversely with CBF; therefore, the use of AVD_{O_2} measurements has been suggested as an index of the adequacy of cerebral blood flow.[19] The jugular oxygen content may be measured by advancing a central venous catheter rostrally in the internal jugular vein upward to the base of the skull. The normal arterial–jugular oxygen content difference is 4 to 9 volume percent. Higher values indicate increased oxygen extraction and potential ischemia. While the idea of a relatively straightforward blood test to determine the adequacy of CBF is appealing, the utility of this test has not been unequivocally shown, and there is some evidence that it may be misleading in the presence of ischemic levels of blood flow.[20]

HEMODYNAMICS

Hemodynamic monitoring in the acute phase of head injury management should include arterial pressure monitoring and detailed measurement of fluid input and output. In those cases where repeated large doses of mannitol are used, pulmonary artery pressure measurement may be required to maintain an accurate assessment of intravascular volume status in the face of massive diuresis and consequent fluid replacement (vide infra).

MEDICAL MANAGEMENT

MANIPULATING ICP

The medical management of acute head injury focuses primarily on the detection and treatment of raised intracranial pressure. Although the ICP is less than 10 torr in normal individuals, 20 to 25 mmHg is generally accepted as the point at which ICP requires treatment in head injury patients. Transient elevations above this level are common when patients are restless or coughing; therefore, persistence of the ICP elevation for 5 to 10 min in a nonagitated patient should be observed prior to initiating treatment. In all cases, a cause for the elevation should be sought. There may be a problem with ventilation or obstruction of jugular venous return. Unless contraindicated by other injuries, patients should be positioned head-up 30 degrees with the neck neutral between flexion and extension. If the ICP elevation persists after having assured adequacy of ventilation and unimpeded jugular venous return, it is incumbent on the physician to rule out a surgically treatable cause of the ICP elevation with a CT scan. In cases of unoperated cerebral contusion, an increase in ICP may signify the need for surgical evacuation of the contused brain.[21]

Once it has been determined that there is no surgically treatable cause of the ICP increase, management depends on pharmacologic reduction of ICP and manipulation of the patient's P_{CO_2}. If the patient is not ventilated, intubation and mechanical ventilation should be instituted with moderate hyperventilation (i.e., P_{CO_2} 30–34 mmHg). If the patient is already ventilated, sedation with morphine or an analogue should be given. If this is insufficient to reduce the ICP, then pharmacologic paralysis with pancuronium bromide should be carried out. In patients who are febrile, reduction of the core temperature to 37°C by means of a cooling blanket frequently results in reduction of raised ICP. Often these measures alone are sufficient.

If the ICP elevation persists, and there is a ventricular drain in place, intermittent drainage of CSF may be instituted. It may be necessary to repeat drainage several times an hour. Continuous drainage should not be used because drainage will often cease as the ventricles undergo progressive compression, and during ventricular drainage the ICP is not being measured. One is then in the unfortunate situation of not reducing the ICP and not being aware of the true ICP. If ventricular drainage is not feasible or effective, then mannitol must be used.

Mannitol, an osmotic diuretic, is the single-most-useful pharmacologic agent in the management of raised ICP following head injury. The dosage is .5 to 1.0 g/kg of a 20% solution infused as a bolus. Typically the effects of mannitol on ICP will last from 2 to 6 h depending on the severity of the underlying pathologic process. Mannitol may be administered repeatedly as long as the serum osmolarity does not exceed 320 mosm/L. At osmolarities greater than this, the effectiveness of the drug is reduced, and there is an increasing risk of renal toxicity.[22] With frequent repeated doses of mannitol and the consequent diuresis, the patient may become systemically dehydrated, resulting in hypotension and increased serum osmolarity. Systemic dehydration is not necessary to achieve reduction in ICP. Therefore, the excess urine loss caused by mannitol should be replaced. The amount and type of replacement fluid should be calibrated to maintain a high normal pulmonary wedge pressure, serum osmolarity <300 mosm/L, and normal serum electrolytes. With this regimen, it may be possible to give mannitol at intervals of 2 h for several days at a time using aggregate volumes of 2 to 3 L of mannitol per day. Aggressive hyperventilation to a P_{CO_2} of 25 mmHg or less combined with mannitol therapy is often necessary with increased ICP secondary to hyperemia, a condition most often found in children and young adults.[23]

In situations where the combination of measures listed above is insufficient to control ICP, or where mannitol can no longer be used because of extant or incipient renal failure, pentobarbital may be a useful adjunct in the management of ICP.[24] It is not a first-choice agent, since it is clearly less effective than mannitol in lowering raised ICP,[25] may cause harmful cardiovascular side effects, and has no demonstrated protective effects on the brain when administered prophylactically to head-injured patients with or without raised ICP.[26] The dosage regimen varies in the published literature, and pentobarbital may be given by bolus infusion or by drip. The end point of administration is reduction of ICP or an unacceptable decrease in arterial blood pressure. Adequate hemodynamic monitoring (i.e., arterial line and pulmonary artery catheter) must be in place prior to giving pentobarbital, and the pulmonary wedge pressure should be in the high-normal range prior to administration. Infusion of dopamine or other vasoactive agents is often necessary to maintain an adequate arterial pressure. Administration of high doses of pentobarbital will result in pupillary dilatation and unreactivity so that no clinical neurologic examination is possible. Brainstem auditory evoked responses (BAEPs) are preserved, and their recording may be a useful adjunct to the management of patients in barbiturate coma.[27]

The surgical options available for the treatment of refractory ICP include frontal or temporal decompressive craniectomy, removal of an existing bone flap, or internal decompression by removal of a swollen or damaged frontal or temporal lobe. The controversy surrounding decompressive craniectomy has been alluded to above. We have used the procedure in young patients with refractory ICP who have a reasonable potential for neurologic recovery (i.e., GCS ≥ 7).

SEIZURES

Seizures may aggravate an existing brain injury; therefore, their prompt treatment is essential. Factors increasing the risk of late epilepsy include severe injuries, intracranial hematomas, and the presence of seizures early after injury. Ordinarily, patients in these risk categories are given prophylactic phenytoin at the time of admission, and the medication is continued for 6–12 months, depending on the injury type and whether or not any seizures have occurred. The value of prophylactic anticonvulsants has been neither convincingly demonstrated nor disproved, and they are routinely used in most neurosurgical units. A discussion of acute seizure management is given in Chap. 142.

NUTRITION

The caloric requirements of head injury patients are comparable to those present in a 20 to 40 percent body surface area burn. The requirements are increased by motor posturing and reduced by barbiturate coma or muscle relaxants. Enteral feeding via nasogastric tube is usually possible and is certainly desirable early after injury, unless there has been major abdominal trauma, in which case parenteral alimentation may be used. Although the nitrogen loss resulting from a severe head injury may be mitigated by early feeding, it may not be possible to reverse it consistently.[28]

FLUID AND ELECTROLYTES

SIADH is usually successfully managed by restricting fluid intake to 1 L/24 h or less. Demeclocycline may be a useful adjunct with persistence of the syndrome beyond a few days. Hypertonic saline (3%) is occasionally necessary to correct profound hyponatremia in the presence of serious neurologic symptoms (e.g., seizures). Diabetes insipidus may be managed with desmopressin acetate (DDAVP). The dosage is 1 to 2 μg (0.25–0.5 mL) intravenously two to four times daily as necessary to control urine output. Serum and urine osmolarity and electrolyte measurements are necessary to distinguish true diabetes insipidus from excessive diuresis caused by mobilization of fluids used during resuscitation or as a result of the use of mannitol for control of ICP (see Chap. 157).

REHABILITATION

Attention to the rehabilitation needs of the patient should begin on or shortly after admission to the critical care unit. In the early days after admission, this consists of proper positioning, regular turning, skin care, and movement of patients' limbs through a full range of movement to minimize or prevent the incidence of late joint contractures and skin decubiti, either of which may significantly retard recovery, and more active rehabilitation once consciousness has been regained. Sensory stimulation programs to facilitate the return of normal consciousness are theoretically attractive but unproven by randomized clinical trials. As the patients' level of consciousness improves, the goals of rehabilitation therapy change from maintenance of normal limb posture and movement to the retraining of simple and then progressively more complex physical and mental activities. Although at this time, the patient will normally be out of the intensive care unit, it is important that these measures be initiated in the ICU.

OUTCOME FROM TRAUMATIC BRAIN INJURY

The mortality from severe head injury varies from 30 to just over 50 percent in most published series.[3,4,11–13,18] Factors associated with a decreased likelihood of survival are low GCS, advanced age, presence of significant intracranial hematomas, and the presence of significant systemic injuries in addition to the head injury. Approximately 50 percent of patients dying from head injury do so from uncontrollable ICP, and this occurs early in the patients' course. The portion of patients with a good outcome or moderate disability varies from 30 to 60 percent. In contrast, the number of patients with good outcome or moderate disability following hypoxic–ischemic coma was 13 percent in one large series.[29] In addition to those patients who die, small numbers will be left in a persistent vegetative state or alert but totally dependent. The numbers of such patients have not been increased in those series of patients with reduced mortality from early aggressive management of head injury.[4] Recovery may continue for up to 18–24 months after head injury, although the most significant gains are made during the first 6 months.[3]

CASE PRESENTATION

R.L., a 35-year-old male, was referred to the trauma unit of St. Michael's hospital on September 24, 1988, following a motor vehicle accident. He was a passenger in a van that was struck by another vehicle. The patient was thrown from the van.

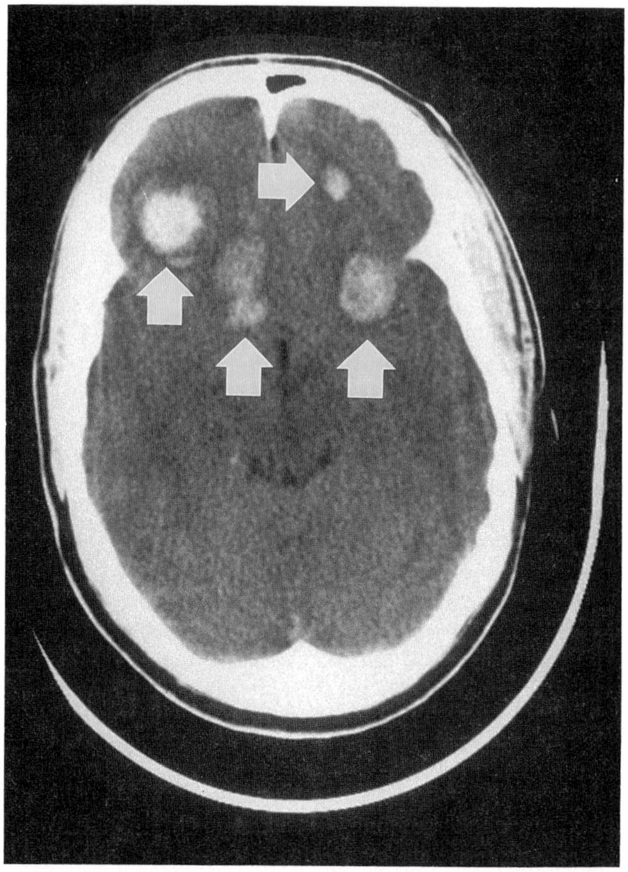

FIGURE 60-11 Bilateral frontal intracerebral hematomas *(arrows)* in a patient injured in a motor vehicle accident. (See text for history.)

On examination at the time of admission, the blood pressure was 120/80, pulse 76 and regular, respiratory rate 18. The patient was localizing pain bilaterally, opening his eyes to pain, and muttering some recognizable words (GCS: motor, 5; eye, 2; verbal, 3). There were no other significant injuries. Blood gases on room air were P_{O_2}, 76; P_{CO_2}, 31; pH, 7.46. A CT scan showed deep bilateral frontal intracerebral hematomas (Fig. 60-11). It was felt that operative evacuation of the hematomas carried substantial risk of incurring permanent neurologic deficit. Therefore, operation was not undertaken, and the patient was admitted to the intensive care unit for observation.

Approximately 30 h after admission, the patient stopped speaking and opening his eyes (GCS motor, 5; eye, 1; verbal, 2). A repeat CT scan was carried out and was unchanged from the admission scan. The patient was taken to the operating room for insertion of a ventricular catheter for ICP monitoring. Postoperatively the patient remained intubated, mechanically hyperventilated, and pharmacologically paralyzed for ICP control. In addition to the above measures, mannitol was used at approximate intervals of 2 to 3 h in doses from 1.5 to 3.2 L/day, over the next 10 days, in order to maintain ICP at less than 25–30 mmHg. Between doses of mannitol, the ICP intermittently exceeded 50 mmHg. Serial somatosensory and brainstem auditory evoked response measurements were carried out, and, in spite of the very difficult problems with ICP, no deterioration in evoked responses was observed. (The patient was continuously paralyzed for ICP control, so no clinical examination was possible.) On the 10th day postinjury, the serum osmolarity reached 320 mosm/L, limiting usage of mannitol in the face of an as-yet uncontrolled ICP. Intravenous pentobarbital was given without effect. Bifrontal decompressive craniectomy was undertaken on the same day in order to achieve ICP control. The patient's mannitol requirement was initially halved and progressively fell thereafter. By the 21st day postinjury, the ICP was under control, pharmacologic paralysis was reversed, and the ICP monitor was removed. The patient opened his eyes spontaneously, was following commands, and was able to say a few simple words (GCS = 13). The frontal bone flaps were replaced at 2 months postinjury, and the patient was transferred to a rehabilitation hospital. At 1 year postinjury, the patient is living independently at home.

CASE DISCUSSION

The case of R.L. illustrates a number of principles described in this chapter that are integral to the management of patients with acute head injury. Most important is careful monitoring of the patient to detect evolving secondary injury (in this case, increasing ICP) and begin treatment before further irreversible neurologic damage occurs. In this case, mechanical ventilation and monitoring and treatment of ICP were begun before the onset of motor posturing or signs of brainstem dysfunction. Continuous evoked potential monitoring while the patient was pharmacologically paralyzed did not show any worsening of the patient's neurologic condition and aided in the decision to undertake decompressive craniectomy when the ICP became medically uncontrollable. In the future, routine use of electrophysiologic monitoring may have a role to play in determining levels of ICP at which treatment is necessary, and in selecting patients in whom very aggressive treatment is likely to be helpful. In those patients who do not have clinical evidence of an overwhelming primary injury immediately following injury (i.e., motor posturing and bilateral pupillary and oculomotor dysfunction), there is often considerable potential for recovery if further insult to the injured brain can be avoided.

References

1. Frankowski RF, Annegers JF, Whitman S: Epidemiological and descriptive studies part 1: The descriptive epidemiology of head trauma in the United States, in Becker DP, Povlishock JT (eds): *Central Nervous System Trauma Status Report*. Bethesda, MD, NINCDS, National Institutes of Health, 1985, p 33.
2. Teasdale G, Jennett B: Assessment of coma and impaired consciousness: A practical scale. Lancet 2:81, 1974.
3. Jennett B, Teasdale G, Galbraith S, et al: Severe head injury in three countries. J Neurol Neurosurg Psychiatry 40:291, 1977.
4. Becker DP, Miller JD, Ward JD, et al: The outcome from severe head injury with early diagnosis and intensive management. J Neurosurg 47:491, 1977.
5. Graham DI, Adams JH, Doyle D: Ischaemic brain damage in fatal non-missile head injuries. J Neurol Sci 39:213, 1978.
6. Robertson CS, Clifton GL, Taylor AA, Grossman RG: Treatment of hypertension associated with head injury. J Neurosurg 59:455, 1983.
7. Olson JD, Kaufman HH, Moake J, et al: Incidence and significance of hemostatic abnormalities in patients with head injuries. Neurosurgery 24:825, 1989.
8. Kaufman HH, Moake JL, Olson JD, et al: Delayed and recurrent intracranial hematomas related to disseminated intravascular clotting and fibrinolysis in head injury. Neurosurgery 7:445, 1980.
9. Snow RB, Zimmerman RD, Gandy SE, Deck MDF: Comparison of magnetic resonance imaging and computed tomography in the evaluation of head injury. Neurosurgery 18:45, 1986.
10. Levin HS, Amparo E, Eisenberg HM, et al: Magnetic resonance imaging and computerized tomography in relation to the neurobehavioral sequelae of mild and moderate head injuries. J Neurosurg 66:706, 1987.
11. Miller JD, Butterworth JF, Gudeman SK, et al: Further experience in the management of severe head injury. J Neurosurg 54:289, 1981.
12. Saul TG, Ducker TB: Effect of intracranial pressure monitoring and aggressive treatment on mortality in severe head injury. J Neurosurg 56:498, 1982.
13. Marshall LF, Smith RW, Shapiro HM: The outcome with aggressive treatment in severe head injuries. Part 1: The significance of intracranial pressure monitoring. J Neurosurg 50:20, 1979.
14. Steudel WI, Kruger J: Using the spectral analysis of the EEG for prognosis of severe brain injuries in the first post-traumatic week. Acta Neurochir *[Suppl]*. 28:40, 1979.
15. Lindsay KW, Carlin J, Kennedy I, et al: Evoked potentials in severe head injury—analysis and relation to outcome. J Neurol Neurosurg Psychiatry 44:796, 1981.
16. Narayan RK, Greenberg RP, Miller JD, et al: Improved confidence of outcome prediction in severe head injury. J Neurosurg 54:751, 1981.
17. Newlon PG, Greenberg RP, Hyatt MS, et al: The dynamics of neuronal dysfunction and recovery following severe head injury assessed with serial multimodality evoked potentials. J Neurosurg 57:168, 1982.
18. Bowers SA, Marshall LF: Outcome in 200 consecutive cases of severe head injury treated in San Diego County: A prospective analysis. Neurosurgery 6:237, 1980.
19. Obrist WD, Langfitt TW, Jaggi JL, et al: Cerebral blood flow and metabolism in comatose patients with acute head injury. J Neurosurg 61:241, 1984.
20. Robertson CS, Narayan RK, Gokaslan ZL, et al: Cerebral arteriovenous oxygen difference as an estimate of cerebral blood flow in comatose patients. J Neurosurg 70:222, 1989.
21. Galbraith S, Teasdale G: Predicting the need for operation in the patient with an occult traumatic intracranial hematoma. J Neurosurg 55:75, 1981.
22. Becker DP, Vries JK: The alleviation of increased intracranial pressure by the chronic administration of osmotic agents, in Brock M, Dietz H (eds): *Intracranial Pressure: Experimental and Clinical Aspects*. New York, Springer-Verlag, 1972, p 309.
23. Bruce DA, Alavi A, Bilaniuk L, et al: Diffuse cerebral swelling

following head injuries in children: The syndrome of "malignant brain edema." J Neurosurg 54:170, 1981.
24. Eisenberg HM, Frankowski RF, Contant CF, Marshall LF, Walker MD, Comprehensive Central Nervous System Trauma Centers: High-dose barbiturate control of elevated intracranial pressure in patients with severe head injury. J Neurosurg 69:15, 1988.
25. Schwartz ML, Tator CH, Rowed DW, et al: The University of Toronto head injury treatment study: A prospective, randomized comparison of pentobarbital and mannitol. Can J Neurol Sci 11:434, 1984.
26. Ward JD, Becker DP, Miller JD, et al: Failure of prophylactic barbiturate coma in the treatment of severe head injury. J Neurosurg 62:383, 1985.
27. Newlon PG, Greenberg RP, Enas GG, Becker DP: Effects of therapeutic pentobarbital coma on multimodality evoked potentials recorded from severely head-injured patients. Neurosurgery 12:613, 1983.
28. Clifton GL, Robertson CS, Grossman RG, et al: The metabolic response to severe head injury. J Neurosurg 60:687, 1984.
29. Levy DE, Coronna JJ, Singer BH, et al: Predicting outcome from hypoxic-ischemic coma. JAMA 253:1420–1426, 1985.

Chapter 61
SPINE INJURIES

G.E. JOHNSON

KEY POINTS

- *Spinal injuries must be considered unstable until they are thoroughly evaluated.*
- *Life-threatening injuries must be managed first.*
- *Vertebral injuries must be assessed in terms of the potential to create early neurologic injury or late deformity.*
- *Spinal cord injury is minimized by limiting the secondary ischemic phase.*
- *Complete spinal cord injuries have no potential for functional recovery. Incomplete injuries have recovery potential which must be maximized.*
- *Considerations in rehabilitation must be initiated at the outset.*

It is estimated that approximately 20 percent of patients suffering from multiple trauma also have injuries to the spinal column. The severity of the spinal injury is variable and may constitute a major component of multiple-system injury, or, if the spinal injury is less severe, it may impact greatly on overall management considerations. The purpose of this chapter is to review **1.** the mechanism, classification, and clinical picture of spinal injuries, and **2.** the principles of management of each of the vertebral and neurologic injuries.

It is extremely important in management of the multiply injured patient that longer-term rehabilitation considerations not be forgotten, as this may result in serious long-term disability. The possibility of cervical spine injury must be considered in anyone who has suffered significant injuries to the face or head, especially those unconscious from trauma. However, patients predisposed on the basis of preexisting abnormalities of the cervical spine (e.g., ankylosing spondylitis and congenital anomalies) may suffer serious neck injury as a result of what otherwise may appear to be trivial trauma. Knowledge of the mechanism of injury is helpful in considering the possibility of spinal injury (e.g., fractures at the thoracolumbar junction associated with falls from a height).

Anatomy

The vertebral column may be considered to consist of three components:[1]

1. The anterior column consisting of the anterior two-thirds of the vertebral body, the disc, annulus, and anterior longitudinal ligament.
2. The middle column consisting of the posterior one-third of the vertebral body, disc, annulus, and posterior longitudinal ligament.
3. The posterior column consisting of the pedicles, lamina, facets, capsule, interspinous and supraspinous ligament (Fig. 61-1).

An injury is considered to be stable if only one of the columns is involved and does not pose a risk of damage to neural structures. Any injury resulting in damage to two or more columns or risking neurologic injury (i.e., damage to the middle column) is considered to be unstable. There is a great variety of forces or combination of forces which may be applied to the vertebral column (e.g., flexion, extension, flexion rotation, shear, axial load). The resultant effect of the application of these forces to the vertebral column depends upon

1. The magnitude and direction of the force
2. The underlying anatomy

A flexion force applied to the cervical spine may result in a pure soft-tissue ligamentous injury and dislocation, because of the relatively horizontal alignment of the facets. A similar force applied to the lumbar spine would most commonly result in fracturing due to the vertical orientation of the facets. An exception to this is ankylosing spondylitis where the force is dissipated across the vertebral column much as it would be in a long bone.[2]

FIGURE 61-1 The anterior, middle, and posterior columns are illustrated. SSL—supraspinous ligament, ISL—interspinous ligament, LF—ligamentum flavum, C—capsule, PLL—posterior longitudinal ligament, AF—annulus fibrosis, ALL—anterior longitudinal ligament. (Courtesy F. Denis.[1])

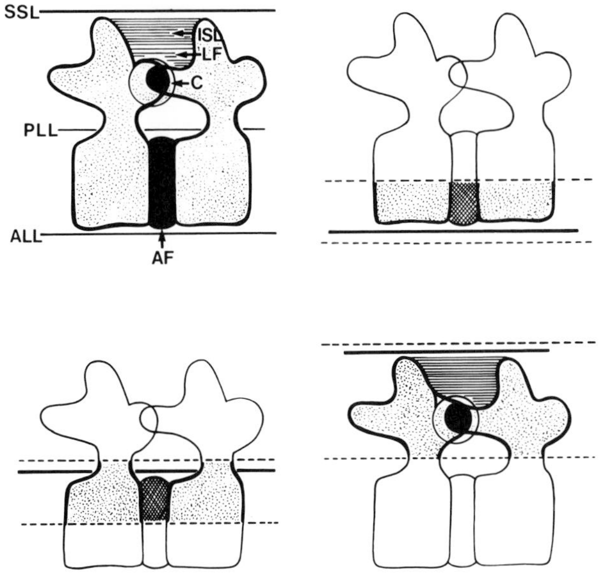

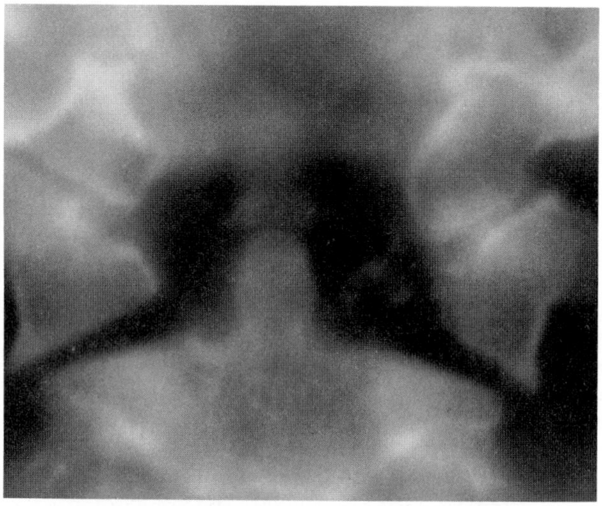

a

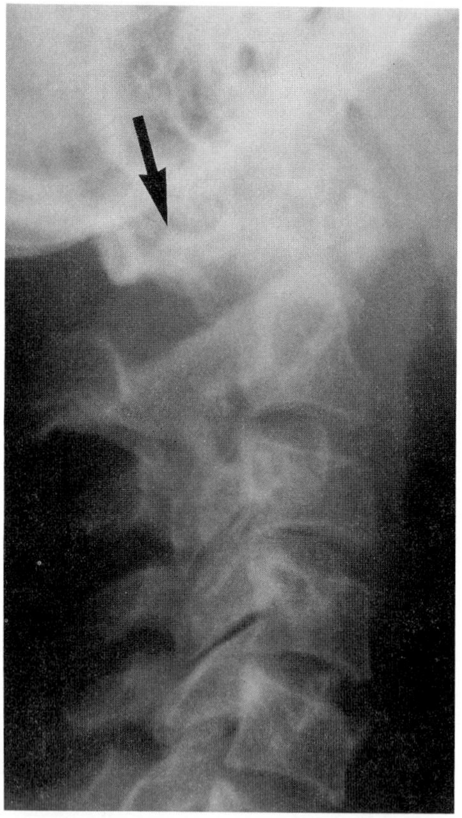

b

FIGURE 61-2 ***(a)*** **A–P tomogram. Confirming an unstable Jefferson's fracture, with avulsion of the transverse ligament from the lateral mass of C1.** ***(b)*** **Lateral view. Fracture of posterior arch of C1 (arrow).**

Classification of Vertebral Injuries

CERVICAL

UPPER CERVICAL SPINE

Because of the unique anatomy of the occipito-atlanto axial complex, applied forces result in characteristic injury patterns.

Jefferson's Fracture

This is a four-part fracture of the ring of the atlas (C1) caused by axial loading (e.g., a fall on the vertex of the skull). If the combined lateral displacement of the lateral masses exceeds 7 mm, disruption of the transverse ligament has occurred indicating a greater degree of instability (Fig. 61-2*a*).[3] This must be differentiated on a lateral x-ray view from a stable fracture involving only the posterior arch of C1 caused by extension (Fig. 61-2*b*).

Atlantoaxial Instability (C1 and C2)

SAGITTAL A gap greater than 4 mm between the anterior arch of the atlas and the odontoid is due to insufficiency of the transverse ligament. This may be from trauma or inflammatory erosion (e.g., rheumatoid arthritis).

ROTATIONAL This is a subluxation of variable degree, recognized by asymmetry of the gap between the lateral side of the odontoid and the lateral mass of C1 on each side and also a decreased joint space between the lateral masses of C1 and C2.

Fractures of the Odontoid

These are caused by shear forces in the sagittal plane. The level of the fracture is variable and has been classified by Anderson and D'Alonzo into three types (Fig. 61-3).[4]

Hangman's Fracture

This is a traumatic spondylolisthesis of C2–C3. It is a bipedicle fracture of C2 usually from an extension force, with anterior displacement of the body of C2 on C3. There is a low incidence of neurologic injury.

LOWER CERVICAL SPINE

These injuries are classified on the basis of the force applied to the neck.[5]

Flexion

The applied force may be either compressive or distractive.

COMPRESSIVE The force acting through the anterior column results in fracturing of the vertebral body. The extent

FIGURE 61-3 Fractured odontoid. (Courtesy Anderson and D'Alonzo.[4])

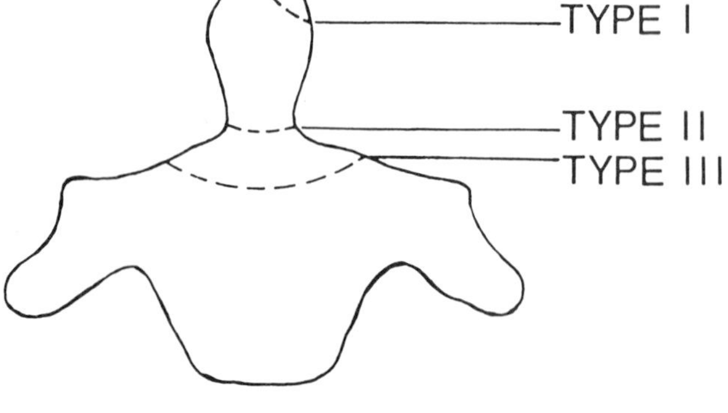

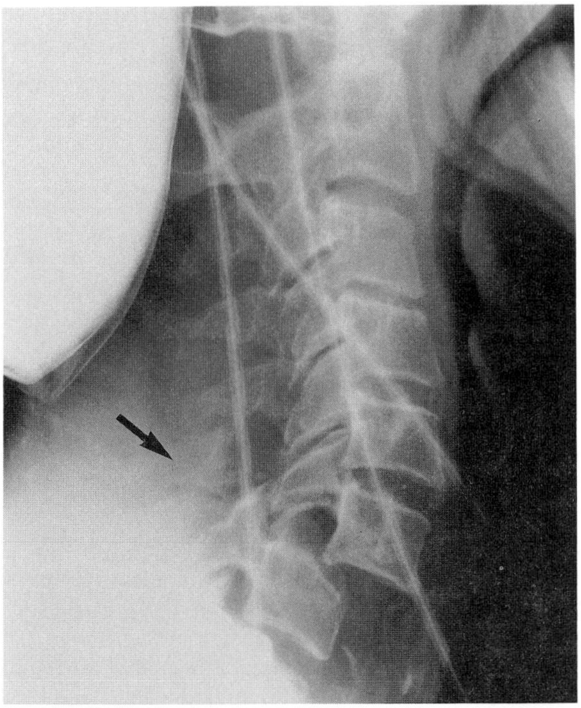

FIGURE 61-4 Compressive extension fracture dislocation of C6–C7. There is dislocation of the facets, but, as the spinous process and lamina were sheared off (arrow), there was minimal neural canal encroachment and the patient suffered only bilateral C7 root injury.

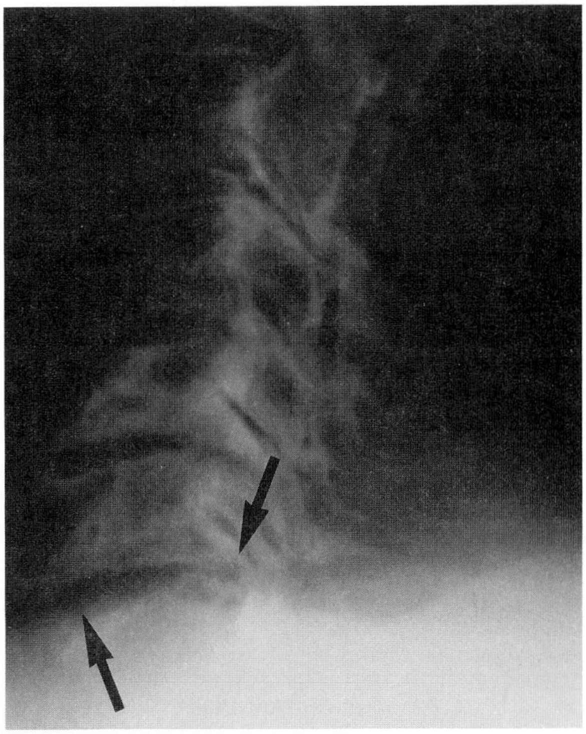

FIGURE 61-5 Distractive extension injury with severe preexisting osteoarthritis of the cervical spine. The disc space is opened anteriorly (arrow). Posterior osteophytes encroach on neural canal with myelographic block (arrow).

of the injury varies from stable minor wedging of the anterior vertebral body only, and no neurlogic loss, to marked intrusion into the neural canal, and frequent severe neurologic loss. There is usually associated facet subluxation and instability (e.g., teardrop and quadrangular fracture).

DISTRACTIVE The applied force begins posteriorly, involving the posterior ligamentous complex and, if severe, may involve all three vertebral columns. The extent of the injury varies from relatively stable subluxation, through unilateral and bilateral facet dislocations to a complete vertebral body dislocation. The extent and frequency of neurologic injury usually is in proportion to the vertebral injury, but the initial displacement of the vertebrae may have been much more severe than that seen on x-ray.

Extension

The applied force may also be compressive or distractive.

COMPRESSIVE This type of force results in fractures through the laminae which may be sheared off. These fractures can be unilateral or bilateral, and at the extreme there may be displacement of the vertebral body anteriorly and severe instability. However, as the laminae are sheared off, there may be little intrusion into the neural canal, so the extent of neurologic injury may be less severe than the vertebral injury (Fig. 61-4).

DISTRACTIVE There is failure of the anterior column (anterior longitudinal ligament and disc) in tension, and therefore the anterior column is usually stable in flexion. In young individuals, this may be easily missed clinically and radiologically and is associated with a low incidence of neurologic involvement. However, in the elderly with associated preexisting degenerative changes, there may be avulsion of bony spurs from the anterior vertebral body. The cervical spinal cord may be pinched between osteophytes on the posterior vertebral body and infolded ligamentum flavum posteriorly, typically resulting in incomplete injury (usually central cord syndrome, Fig. 61-5).

Vertical Compression

Axial load causes centrifugal displacement and intrusion into the neural canal and subsequent serious neurologic injury.

Lateral Flexion

Results in compression and fracturing of the lateral mass and also frequent contralateral ligament disruption. This is usually associated with nerve root injury on the compression side.

THORACOLUMBAR

As the underlying anatomy in the thoracic and lumbar spine is similar, the mechanistic classification proposed by Denis is helpful.[1]

COMPRESSION
This is usually stable and only involves the anterior column, so there is a low incidence of neurologic injury.

BURST
This results from axial load force, causing major injury to the centrum of the vertebral body, intrusion of bone into the neural canal, often associated with lateral displacement of the pedicles and a vertical fracture of the laminae. There frequently is associated neurologic injury.

SEAT BELT TYPE (CHANCE FLEXION-DISTRACTION)
This is caused by a severe flexion force with the axis of rotation anterior to the vertebral body, resulting in failure of all three columns in tension. The pattern may vary between combinations of bony and ligamentous injury. There is minimal encroachment into the neural canal, and the most common neurologic injury involves the nerve root unilaterally or bilaterally exiting beneath the involved pedicle.

FRACTURE DISLOCATIONS
These are usually caused by a combination of forces (flexion, rotation, shear) and result in translation of the vertebrae and severe neurologic loss.

The Neurologic Injury

Nerve tissues can be injured by stretching, compression, or laceration. Physical disruption of the spinal cord would result in complete irreversible loss of function. However, autopsy examination of the spinal cord in patients who clinically had a complete injury showed the spinal cord frequently to be structurally intact but suffering fibrous and cystic degeneration resembling end-stage ischemic changes.[6] Experimentally, in drop-weight tests, the initial finding is hemorrhage into the gray matter of the central cord which may coalesce and form a central hematomyelia, surrounding edema, and increased interstitial pressure and local ischemia as evidenced by a severe decrease in oxygen tension and increased lactic acid.

A second ischemic phase begins shortly afterward and may persist for more than 24 h, involving both gray and white matter and spreading both proximally and distally from the site of injury.[7,8] The mechanism for this secondary vascular injury may be caused by local high concentrations of norepinephrine[9–11] or other vasoactive amines. In addition to vascular injury, direct axonal injury would result in permanent functional loss due to the limited ability of central axons to recover.

It has been clearly shown that the effect of injury is directly related to the magnitude of the force and the duration of application of the force.[12,13] Since the initial force cannot be changed, we can only prevent further force application initially by immobilizing the unstable area and then relieving the continued compression by early reduction of displaced bony fragments and discs.

SPINAL SHOCK AND SPINAL CORD INJURIES

The direct force applied to the spinal cord results in a physiologic block to conduction recognized clinically as complete cessation of all neurologic function—motor, sensory, and autonomic below the level of the injury. In slight injuries this lasts only minutes, but in more severe injuries it may last weeks. During this phase of spinal shock, predictions of neurologic recovery should be avoided.

The *pattern of spinal cord* injury is determined when the patient is out of spinal shock.

COMPLETE
Clinically there is no voluntary movement, no sensation, but spinal reflexes are present or exaggerated.

INCOMPLETE

Anterior Cord Syndrome
This syndrome is characterized by complete motor loss below the level of injury, loss of light touch, with preservation of position, vibration, and deep touch sensation. This is caused by anterior compression of the spinal cord, injuring the lateral corticospinal and spinothalamic tracts. The posterior tracts are preserved.

Central Cord Syndrome
Clinically there is disproportionate loss of motor power in the upper extremities with less severe loss seen in the lower extremities. Sensation is variably altered. This is caused by central hemorrhage in the cord affecting the lower motor neurons and decussating tracts with preservation of the lateral corticospinal tracts.

Brown-Séquard
Rarely, this is seen as a pure injury, with blunt trauma but may be seen in penetrating injuries. Motor power is lost on the ipsilateral side, and pain and temperature are lost on the contralateral side up to one or two segments below the level of the injury.

POSTERIOR CORD SYNDROME
This is rare but results in loss of position sense.

CAUDA EQUINA SYNDROME
The degree of neurologic loss may vary greatly depending upon the extent of nerve root damage. The motor and sensory loss is symmetrical, and there may be loss of bladder and bowel control.

ROOT LOSS
There are a few specific vertebral injuries associated with loss of function of individual nerve roots. For example, a C5–C6 unilateral facet dislocation may cause ipsilateral C6 root injury. In a seat belt injury it is not uncommon that the nerve root exiting below the affected pedicle either unilaterally or bilaterally may be injured.

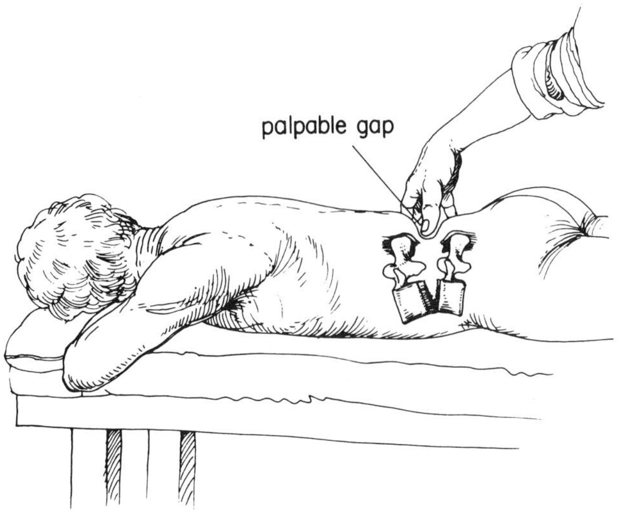

FIGURE 61-6 A palpable gap between the spinous processes indicates complete disruption of the supraspinous and infraspinous ligament and severe posterior column injury. (Courtesy Hoppenfield, Orthopedic Neurology, Saunders.)

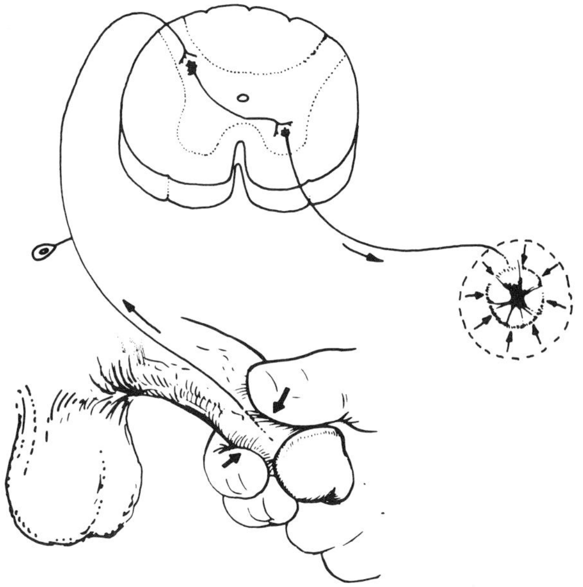

FIGURE 61-7 Bulbocavernosus reflex produced by stimulation of the dorsum of the glans penis resulting in anal sphincter contraction. (Courtesy Hoppenfield, Orthopedic Neurology, Saunders.)

CLINICAL ASSESSMENT

Assessment of patients specifically for possible spinal injury requires that the initial general assessment and resuscitative measures have been instituted. The patient must have an intact airway, adequate ventilation and circulation, and control of hemorrhage.

A history of the mechanism of injury is helpful in anticipating the type of injury which has occurred. Other important information includes a history of previous neurologic abnormalities. Observations by the patient, witnesses, or primary care giver of the occurrence of transient or persistent weakness or sensory changes or loss of bladder function related to the injury are very helpful.

On examination, any evidence of head or facial trauma such as bruises, laceration, or abrasion would suggest the direction of an applied force. Especially important is any asymmetry of head position and tenderness along the sternomastoids. In a patient with an injured cervical cord, the arms may be held in the typical position of shoulder abduction and elbow flexion of a C5 quadriplegic. An ominous sign of neurologic loss would be the presence of a paradoxical pattern of respiration. Priapism in a male patient with an injured cervical cord indicates loss of thoracolumbar sympathetic outflow. Examination of the trunk may show bruises or abrasions of the shoulders, the periscapular area, or buttocks suggesting a rotatory or flexion force to the spine.

A detailed neurologic examination should then be performed and recorded on a flow sheet to allow for serial examinations. The patient in a cervical collar and with gentle manual traction may be carefully log-rolled to allow examination of the back for tenderness, malalignment of the spinous processes, or a boggy gap in the supraspinous ligament, suggesting disruption of the posterior column (Fig. 61-6). While the patient is turned, sensation in the perianal area and rectal examination to include resting tone and voluntary contraction should be performed, along with a bulbocavernosus reflex (Fig. 61-7).

RADIOLOGIC EXAMINATION

In multiple trauma, the initial films are the scout lateral cervical spine film and an anteroposterior (AP) view of the chest and pelvis. Other more detailed films would be based upon the clinical findings. In addition to the configuration and alignment of the vertebral bodies, general alignment of the facets, posterior vertebral bodies, and interspinous distances, the specific points to observe on each film are listed in Table 61-1.

Following these x-rays, further detail may be required and the following techniques are helpful, but since they require movement or turning of the patient, they should only be done when no instability has been demonstrated on plain films.

CERVICAL SPINE

Swimmer's View
This technique helps to visualize the cervicothoracic junction but is difficult to interpret and may show only gross malalignment.

Oblique and Pillar Views
This method is used to show the facets and lateral masses, respectively, and can be done with minimal movement of the patient. Occasionally when routine films are negative and a ligamentous injury to the cervical spine is suspected, flexion and extension films are indicated. They must be

TABLE 61-1 Radiologic Evaluation of Spine Injuries

Location of Injury	Lateral	Anteroposterior
Cervical spine	Adequacy of the film, to see the top of T1 Retropharyngeal swelling at C3 (>3 mm) and C6 (>15 mm)	
Upper	Odontoid Gap anterior arch to odontoid <4 mm	(Through-mouth) Odontoid Interval odontoid to C1 lateral mass General alignment occipital condyle to lateral mass C1, and C1–C2 Joint space C1–C2
Lower (C3–C7)	Disc space height Compression or avulsion of the anterior vertebral body Widening or asymmetry of interspinous distance	Fracture of lateral mass Abrupt change in alignment of the spinous processes
Thoracic and lumbar spine	Vertebral body configuration especially the posterior wall Pedicles	Vertebral body height H-shape of the lamina Interpedicular distance Interspinous distance

done only actively, and therefore in an awake patient, with medical supervision.

LUMBAR SPINE

Oblique Views
This shows the lamina, pars interarticularis, and facets.

Tomography
This considerably improves detail and helps to show difficult areas (e.g., cervicothoracic junction). It should always be done in two planes (AP and lateral), and therefore requires turning of the patient.

Computed Tomography
This is a very valuable assessment and requires only a single transfer of the patient which can be done on the spine board or patient mobilizer. Routine, coronal, and sagittal reconstructions should be obtained. It is important that this examination be coordinated with other disciplines so that the patient with known or suspected spinal injury can have the appropriate areas examined at the same time as examination for other injuries (e.g., head, intrathoracic, intraabdominal).

Myelography
This technique is indicated only under the following conditions:

1. The extent of the neural injury cannot be explained on the basis of plane films or computed tomography (CT) scan.
2. Progressive neurologic loss occurs in the absence of severe encroachment on the neural canal suggesting that the loss is ischemic in nature.
3. It is necessary to demonstrate possible dural defects or avulsed nerve roots.

Pitfalls in Assessment of Spinal Injuries

ANKYLOSING SPONDYLITIS

The fracture may not be seen initially. The patient should be managed as an unstable injury until further investigations (tomograms, bone scan) are performed.[2]

MULTIPLE NONCONTIGUOUS INJURIES

The occurrence of fractures in the spine occurring at two nonadjacent levels simultaneously is becoming more common, especially in high-velocity injuries. The primary injury is considered to be that injury associated with neurologic deficit. This is most often in the upper thoracic level. When a fracture in the spine is diagnosed, the entire spine should be x-rayed.[14]

UNCONSCIOUS OR HEAD-INJURED PATIENTS

The absence of symptoms and/or compromised neurologic exam make assessment very difficult.

Management of Spinal Injuries

IMMEDIATE

PREHOSPITAL
Multiple-trauma victims and patients with spinal injuries, especially involving neurologic loss, should be taken directly to a level-1 tertiary care center, if physiologically sta-

ble, and if the transport time is reasonable. It is incumbent on any major trauma receiving center that a formal team be identified for the management of spinal injuries.[15]

PRIORITIES
The presence of a spinal injury, although serious and possibly associated with severe late disability, does not alter the priorities of a clear airway, adequate ventilation, and adequate circulation.

SPINAL INJURY
Trauma patients with suspected or proven spinal injuries must continue to be immobilized with a cervical collar and/or spine board as indicated until definitive care can be instituted. It is important that this initial assessment and resuscitation be expedited to avoid prolonged pressure on insensitive areas such as the sacrum and heels.

It is imperative to maintain adequate perfusion of well-oxygenated blood to the injured spinal cord, and therefore supplemental oxygen is given by face mask to maintain an arterial P_{O_2} of greater than 100 mmHg. Other measures as outlined below are used to maintain a blood pressure of at least 100 mmHg systolic.

Other general measures that should be instituted in the emergency department include insertion of intravenous lines, a nasogastric tube, and a Foley catheter.

LOCATION
Immediately upon arrival of the patient in the emergency room, the spine injury team should be notified. They then may supervise the spinal aspects of overall patient management and participate in decision making. Patients requiring manipulation for reduction of the spine should be managed where they can be carefully monitored and have easy access to x-ray facilities for serial films. Spine injury patients with other multiple trauma, all high spinal cord injured patients (above C5), and patients with low cervical or thoracic cord injury, with significant preexisting disease, are best treated initially in the intensive care setting, until stabilized.

DRUGS
The use of drugs to minimize secondary injury to the spinal cord is controversial, and the rationale for each is outlined below.

NEUROLOGIC SHOCK
Patients with neurologic loss, especially those in spinal shock from injuries above the level of T6, will be hypotensive and bradycardiac due to the combination of

1. Loss of thoracic sympathetic outflow, vasodilation, and pooling of blood
2. Relative preponderance of vagal stimulation to the heart

In the absence of associated hypovolemia, the patient should be given maintenance crystalloid infusion. If tissue perfusion is inadequate and/or the response to infusion is unsatisfactory, the patient should be investigated for concealed bleeding. Central lines are indicated and monitoring of pulmonary artery pressure used to gauge further fluid resuscitation. Extremes of crystalloid administration to maintain a normal pressure should be avoided and colloids given as a volume expander, as repeated challenges. A persistently low perfusion pressure in spite of adequate fluid resuscitation warrants consideration of small doses of vasopressors.

Management of Complications of Spinal Injuries

Respiratory complications are greatest in cervical cord injuries where the patient has lost intercostal function and abdominal muscles needed to support a vigorous cough. The phrenic nerve is involved in lesions above C5. In lesions below C5, with a functioning diaphragm, and accessory muscles and in the absence of lung injury or preexisting disease, most patients can support satisfactory ventilation. There is a tendency even with good general care for deterioration of ventilatory function by the third or fourth day, because of fatigue and retained secretions, and intubation and ventilation may be required early. While the patient is being ventilated, the position of the cervical vertebrae can be maintained by traction, giving access to the chest for therapy. Once the respiratory compromise has stabilized and weaning can begin, it is advantageous to mobilize the patient in a halo vest. (Fig. 61-8). The vest restricts access to the chest and increases chest wall stiffness. However, the upright, or semiupright position facilitates diaphragmatic

FIGURE 61-8 Halo vest.

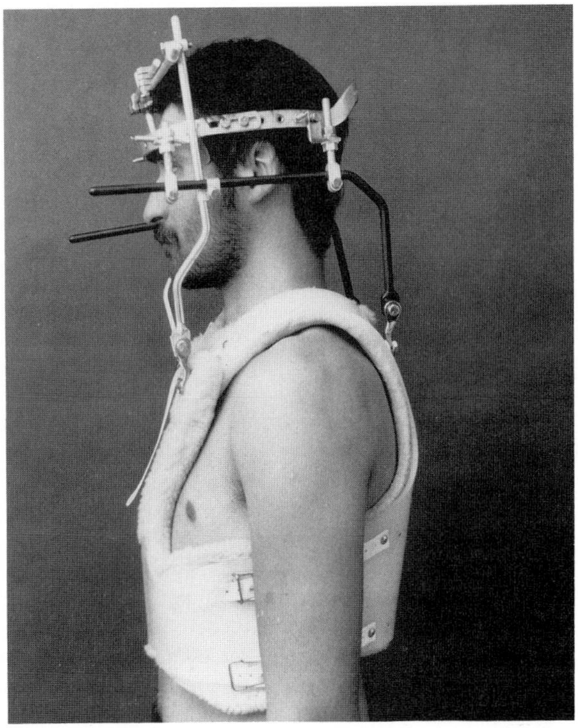

excursion improving pulmonary function especially in patients lacking intercostal function. While the patient is in spinal shock, postural hypotension will not allow maintenance of the upright position.

CARDIAC

Acute spinal cord injury may be associated with pulmonary edema. This usually occurs early, possibly secondary to a massive sympathetic outflow increased after load and a predisposition to arrhythmia.[16,17] A more persistent feature following acute spinal cord injury above the T6 level is hypotension and bradycardia, even after sufficient administration of fluid and colloid to fill the venous capacitance vessels. This may respond to atropine (0.2 to 0.4 mg), or if hypotension persists, vasopressors may be required.

GASTROINTESTINAL

Almost every patient with spinal cord injury and most patients with significant fractures of the thoracic or lumbar spine in the absence of neurologic injury will have a transient ileus, and a nasogastric tube should be inserted.

THROMBOEMBOLIC PREVENTION

Approximately 15 percent of patients with spinal cord injuries develop deep venous thrombosis, and one-half of these lead to pulmonary embolism.[18] The use of compression stockings and low-dose[19] or adjusted-dose heparin is recommended.

SKIN CARE

Avoidance of decubitus ulceration depends upon meticulous attention to frequent turning and protection of pressure points. This is made easier by the use of special mechanized beds for turning (e.g., Stoke-Mandville bed).

NUTRITION

Following acute spinal cord injury, the patient becomes catabolic. In order to minimize this and encourage early rehabilitation, early alimentation is encouraged as soon as the ileus resolves.

MANAGEMENT OF THE NEUROLOGIC INJURY

Decision making is based upon accurate neurologic assessment initially, serial examinations, and accurate documentation.

In the presence of neurologic injury the two fundamental principles of management are

1. Provision of an adequate perfusion pressure with well-oxygenated blood: The patient must not be allowed to become hypotensive or hypoxic.
2. Decompression: The degree of injury, and conversely the ability of the spinal cord to recover, vary according to the magnitude of the applied force and the duration of compression. Decompression of the injured cord must be achieved as quickly as possible usually by reducing displaced fracture fragments, either by closed (e.g., halo traction, postural reduction on bolsters) or open means. The adequacy of decompression must be proven radiologically.

Principles of Surgical Management

1. Decompression should be performed from the direction of encroachment on the neural canal (anterior or posterior).
2. Adequacy of decompression should be proven intraoperatively by direct visualization or myelography or postoperatively by CT scan.
3. Following decompression, a stable construct must be achieved by internal stabilization.[20]

Indications for surgical decompression of spinal cord and cauda equina or root injuries are

1. Progressive neurologic loss: This is seen clinically as either an ascending level or progression from incomplete to complete injury. Not infrequently in the very early stages following injury the neurologic level may rise by one segment. This is due to ischemia and subsequently usually recedes to the original level.
2. Failed or anticipated inability of nonoperative decompression (retained bone or disc fragments). Generally the reduction seen on plain x-rays represents the residual encroachment on the neural canal. Only in 3 percent of cases is there residual soft-tissue compression.
3. Incomplete cord and/or cauda equina lesions with residual compression.

Under the following situations, surgical decompression will be of no benefit or may even be harmful.

1. Complete spinal cord lesion in a patient out of spinal shock
2. Progressive neurologic loss due to ischemia, with no block or significant residual compression as seen on myelography

TECHNIQUES OF SPINAL CORD DECOMPRESSION

Anterior decompression of the cervical spinal cord[21] is the technique of choice in the following injuries:

1. Axial load (burst) fractures
2. Cervical disc
3. Distractive extension injuries with residual neural canal encroachment by posterior vertebral body osteophytes

Excision of one or more vertebral bodies is usually required. Stabilization may then be achieved by a tricortical iliac crest graft and small plate.

Residual encroachment on the cervical neural canal and posterior spinal cord compression is usually caused by failed reduction of distractive flexion injuries (i.e., unilateral or bilateral facet dislocations). These should be reduced and stabilized posteriorly. A variety of internal fixation devices is available for this.

Extremely complex patterns of fractures and fracture dislocations (e.g., quadrangular,[22] teardrop,[23] compressive extension) may be approached by a combination of anterior and posterior approaches.

The most common type of injury to the upper thoracic spine which may require decompression is a fracture dislocation which is extremely unstable and difficult to reduce nonoperatively. When decompression is indicated, the reduction can best be performed posteriorly, followed by stabilization using either segmental spinal instrumentation technique[24] or Harrington rod fixation supplemented with sublaminar wires for stabilization.

Harrington rod instrumentation has been the most frequently used technique. Recently there has been increasing recognition of the limitation of this.[25]

A new, versatile technique has recently been developed.[26] Variations of this technique (e.g., fixateur interne),[27] successfully achieves reduction of burst fractures by axial distraction (ligamentotaxis) if used within a few days of injury and has the benefit of limiting the extent of fusion. It can also be used in compression for seat belt injuries and gives excellent stability for fracture dislocations. Anterior decompression of burst fractures[28] is indicated for severe residual canal encroachment.

ADJUNCTIVE TECHNIQUES TO REDUCE SPINAL INJURY

Other adjunctive methods of management of spinal cord injury are intended to alter the secondary ischemic effects which follow the initial injury. To be effective, these must be instituted almost immediately as the secondary effects are established by 4 h posttrauma.[29]

COOLING

Cooling of the cord to decrease metabolic requirements and alter the effect of locally released norepinephrine has not given improved results clinically[30] and experimentally[31] has been inconsistent.

STEROIDS

The glucocorticoids (e.g., dexamethasone) are presumed to act by decreasing the effect of norepinephrine, stabilizing cell membranes, preventing lysosomal enzyme release, inhibiting complement activation, and reversing the sodium and potassium electrolyte imbalance resulting from tissue edema and necrosis.[32] Considerable controversy exists regarding the effectiveness of steroids experimentally. Clinically, in a Second National Acute Spinal Cord Injury study, Bracken et al.[33] have shown that the administration of methylprednisolone 30 mg/kg within 8 h of injury, followed by infusion of 5.4 mg/(kg · h) for 23 h resulted in significant improvement in neurologic function. Further studies are required to give guidance regarding optimal dosage and duration of administration. As there may be complications associated with the use of steroids, their administration on an ad hoc basis is to be discouraged. The use of steroids should be a policy decision of the spine injury team, standardizing dosage, time of administration, and duration.

OPIOID ANTAGONISTS

Locally released endogenous opioids also have a vasospastic effect. Clinical trials are currently in place to determine the effectiveness of the narcotic antagonist naloxone. Faden et al.[34] have demonstrated that both naloxone and thyrotropin-releasing hormone (TRH) improve neurologic recovery following impact injury to the spinal cord.

Methods designed to improve the microcirculation, such as mannitol and dimethyl sulfoxide (DMSO), have experimentally shown some improvement in spinal cord injury. Hyperbaric oxygen has been used to advantage in primates but may aggravate lipid peroxidation, increasing injury to neuronal tissue.

Perhaps one of the more promising experimental treatment modalities is the use of the calcium channel blocking agent, Nimodipine, in combination with adrenalin. The use of vasopressors alone has not been shown to improve spinal cord blood flow and may even result in an increase in medullary hemorrhage. However, this combination of drugs has been shown to increase spinal cord blood flow experimentally by 60 percent.[35] Further clinical and laboratory data are required to determine the optimal vasopressor effect.

Management of the Vertebral Injury

When considering the bony injury, the principles of fracture management (reduction, maintenance, and mobilization) apply. This may be accomplished nonoperatively. With failed closed reduction, inability to maintain position, or the desire for early mobilization, an open reduction and internal stabilization is indicated. Stable fractures of the cervical or thoracolumbar spine can be mobilized early with limited use of an orthosis for pain relief.

In the cervical spine, unstable fractures, not requiring reduction, may be managed in an orthosis only (e.g., undisplaced type III fracture of the odontoid), but careful monitoring is necessary to demonstrate that the position is maintained. When a reduction is necessary, halo traction should be used so that once reduced, the patient can be mobilized in a halo vest (Fig. 61-8). The initial enthusiasm regarding the ability of the halo vest to control unstable cervical injuries has been challenged.[36] Patient selection criteria for halo vest management are outlined in Table 61-2.

When open reduction and internal stabilization is indicated, the fracture pattern must be carefully analyzed in preoperative planning to assure that the force causing the injury is neutralized in order to achieve sufficient stability so that minimal if any external support is required. Using modern implant techniques this result is for the most part achievable.[37,38]

In fractures of the thoracic and lumbar spine, similar principles may be applied. Unstable fractures not requiring

TABLE 61-2 Halo Vest Management of Cervical Injuries

Suitable	Unsuitable
Fracture odontoid types II and III	Axially unstable fractures (e.g., Jefferson's)
Hangman's fracture	Primarily ligamentous injuries (e.g., distractive flexion causing unilateral and bilateral facet dislocations)
Minimal compressive flexion injuries	Obesity
Lateral mass fracture	Noncompliance
	Multiple-level injuries

reduction may be treated with bed rest and log-rolling for 2 to 3 weeks followed by a well-fitted, rigid polypropylene brace. Closed postural reduction of some displaced thoracolumbar fractures can be achieved by positioning of the patient on corrective bolsters[39] and careful log-rolling until sufficient bony healing has occurred to allow mobilization in an orthosis. However, this requires skilled personnel in specialty units. With the advent of improved stabilization, there is an increasing trend toward surgery, but careful attention must be given to achieving sufficient stability to allow early mobilization.[40,41]

Pitfalls in the Management of Spinal Cord Injury

HYPOTHERMIA

This is particularly important in patients with cervical or high thoracic cord injury during the stage of spinal shock. The patient is unable to vasoconstrict because of loss of the thoracic sympathetic outflow and is also unable to shiver to maintain core temperature. This results in hypotension and bradycardia. The temperature must be carefully monitored, with the patient kept covered or warmed by radiant heaters.

AUTONOMIC DYSREFLEXIA

This potentially dangerous complication occurs in patients with spinal cord injuries above the T6 level, at any time after the stage of spinal shock. The presenting symptoms may be quite variable, the most consistent of which are hyperhydrosis, headache, and vasodilatation above the level of the neurologic loss and nasal stuffiness. Paroxysmal hypertension is the cardinal sign, bradycardia is inconsistent. The usual precipitating events are bladder or rectal distention or manipulation or intraabdominal pathology. These stimuli result in reflex massive sympathetic outflow causing hypertension and reflex bradycardia and vasodilatation in that part of the body above the level of the spinal cord lesion. Immediate management should consist of placing the patient in an upright position and removal of the stimulus, e.g., bladder decompression. Vasodilator therapy may be required for severe hypertension.[42]

THE SWOLLEN LIMB

The neurologically impaired patient may at any time following the neurologic injury present with a painless swollen limb. The differential diagnosis includes fracture, venous thrombosis, and myositis ossificans. Myositis ossificans is a frequent occurrence in association with spinal cord injury. In total joint arthroplasty the use of indomethacin may decrease its occurrence and severity, but its use is unproven in spinal injuries. Physiotherapy to maintain range of motion should be reduced but probably not discontinued.

Considerations in Rehabilitation

The restoration of the patient with a spinal injury to the highest possible level of function begins with initial management. As function is directly related to the level of neurologic injury, preservation of even a single nerve root or segment, especially in the cervical cord, may make the difference between independence or the need for attendant care. For example, a C6 quadriplegic with good shoulder muscles and some active wrist extension is capable of independent feeding and grooming because of fairly strong tenodesis grip. The patient can turn independently in bed, assist with transfers, operate a regular wheelchair, and even operate a car with hand controls, whereas at a C5 level the patient is capable of very limited self-care, cannot turn in bed, and can only use an electric wheelchair.

Maintaining range of movement of joints which can be actively moved is essential to obtain maximum function. This is also important in joints which have lost active movement as flexion contractures of hips and knees severely interfere with independent transfers.

In some instances it may be advantageous to leave an imbalance of certain muscle groups in order to facilitate function. For example, some tightness of the long finger flexors will assist in improved grip in those patients dependent upon tenodesis effect for grasping objects.

Active therapy must begin during the phase of spinal shock and continue as the patient passes into the stages of spasticity.

CASE PRESENTATION

Mr. A.B., a 40-year-old obese truck driver, suffered a burst fracture of the lumbar spine in a motor vehicle accident. On arrival at a tertiary care hospital 36 h postinjury, he was disoriented, hypoxic, and hypercarbic. His abdomen was grossly distended. Neurologic examination showed him to be areflexic in the lower extremities. He had a mixed cauda equina injury, with marked weakness in both legs, asymmetrically; diffuse loss of sensation including the perianal area; and marked weakness of voluntary anal sphincter contraction.

X-ray of the lumbar spine showed a burst fracture of L2 with loss of vertebral body height and widening of the

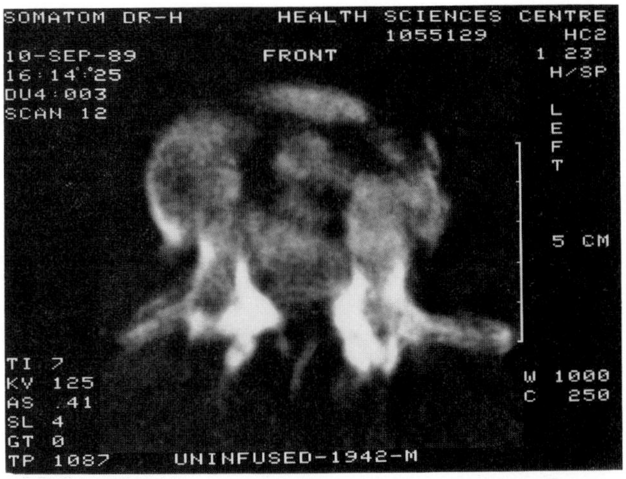

FIGURE 61-9 CT scan showing nearly total encroachment on the neural canal.

intrapedicular distance. A CT scan (Fig. 61-9) showed nearly total encroachment on the neural canal.

In addition to intravenous fluids, nasogastric intubation, log-rolling, chest physiotherapy, and analgesia, the recommended treatment was decompression of the neural canal and stabilization of the unstable lumbar fracture to facilitate mobilization and chest care. He underwent open reduction with decompression of the neural canal using the fixateur interne to provide distraction of the fracture, and reduction of the fracture fragment by ligamentotaxis of the posterior longitudinal ligament. An intraoperative myelogram confirmed relief of the block and minimal residual canal compromise. Postoperatively he was extubated within 48 h and immobilized in a semireclining position with frequent turning. He was transferred from the intensive care unit to the regular ward in 72 h. He was discharged from the hospital 26 days later, ambulant with assistance, and subsequently regained normal bowel and bladder function. A follow-up CT scan showed residual canal encroachment of 20 percent. X-rays showed healing of the fracture.

CASE DISCUSSION

This man's impending respiratory failure was contributed to by the following factors:

1. Prolonged recumbency without turning
2. Obesity
3. 20 pack years of smoking
4. Ileus, abdominal distention
5. Splinting, secondary to pain

The severity of the fracture of L2 was underestimated on the initial x-rays, with failure to recognize the disproportionately severe neurologic loss. Under these circumstances further investigations such as myelogram or CT scan are indicated. The initial CT scan demonstrated the severe extrusion of bone into the neural canal and residual cauda equina compression.

His clinical picture neurologically was that of a mixed cauda equina injury which has a good prospect for functional recovery. There were two indications for surgery:

1. Decompression of the cauda equina
2. Stabilization of the spine to allow early mobilization of the patient with minimal external support

An anterior retroperitoneal vertebral body excision offers excellent canal clearance. However, in this obese man it would be technically difficult and is more painful postoperatively causing further splinting and prolongation of the ileus. Anterior stabilization also requires external support.

Posterior pedicle screw decompression by distraction in this patient gave good decompression, proven intraoperatively, and sufficient stability for mobilization without external support.

References

1. Denis F: The three column spine and its significance in the classification of acute thoracolumbar spine injuries. Spine 8(8):817, 1983.
2. Hunter T, Dubo H: Spinal fractures complicating anklyosing spondylitis. Arthritis Rheum 26:751, 1983.
3. Spence KF, Decker S, Sell KW: Bursting atlantal fracture associated with rupture of the transverse ligament. J Bone Joint Surg 52A(3):543, April 1970.
4. Anderson LD, D'Alonzo RT: Fractures of the odontoid process of the axis. J Bone Joint Surg 56A:1663, 1974.
5. Allen RL, Ferguson RL, Lehman TR, et al.: A mechanistic classification of closed, indirect fractures and dislocations of the lower cervical spine. Spine 7(1):1, 1982.
6. Tator CH: Acute spinal cord injury: A review of recent studies of treatment and pathophysiology. Can Med Assoc J 107:143, 1972.
7. De la Torre JC: Spinal cord injury: Review of basic and applied research. Spine 6(4): 315, 1981.
8. Tator CH, Rivlin AS, Lewis AJ, et al.: The effect of acute spinal cord injury on axonal counts in the pyramidal tract of rats. J Neurosurg 61:118, 1984.
9. Osterholm JL, Mathews GJ: Altered norepinephrine metabolism following experimental spinal cord injury. Part 1: Relationship to hemorrhagic necrosis and post-wounding neurological defects. J Neurosurg 36:386, 1972. Part 2: Protection against traumatic spinal cord hemorrhagic necrosis by norepinephrine synthesis blockade with alpha methyl tyrosine. J Neurosurg 36:395, 1972.
10. De la Torre JC, Johnson CM, Harris LH, et al.: Monoamine changes in experimental head and spinal cord trauma: Failure to confirm previous observations. Surg Neurol 2:5, 1974.
11. Naftchi NE, Demeny M, DeCrescito V, et al.: Biogenic amine concentrations in traumatized spinal cords of cats. J Neurosurg 40:52, 1974.
12. Rivlin AS, Tator CH: Effect of duration of acute spinal cord compression in a new acute cord injury model in the rat. Surg Neurol 10:38, 1978.
13. Tator CH, Rowed DW: Current concepts in the immediate management of acute spinal cord injuries. Can Med Assoc J 121:1453, 1979.

14. Powell JN, Waddell JP, Tucker WS, et al.: Multiple level noncontiguous spinal fractures. J Trauma 29(8):1146, 1989.
15. Donovan WH, Carter RE, Bedbrook GM, et al.: Incidence of medical complications in spinal cord injury: Patients in specialized compared with non-specialized centres. Paraplegia 22:282, 1984.
16. Albin MS, Buregin L, Wolf S: Brain and lungs at risk after cervical spinal cord transection. Surg Neurol 24:191, 1985.
17. Evans DF, Kobrine AL, Rizzoli HV: Cardiac arrhythmias accompanying acute compression of the spinal cord. J Neurosurg 52:52, 1980.
18. Casas ER, Sanchez MP, Arias CR, et al.: Prophylaxis of venous thrombosis and pulmonary embolism in patients with acute traumatic spinal cord lesions. Paraplegia 14:178, 1976.
19. Watson N: Anticoagulant therapy in the prevention of venous thrombosis and pulmonary embolism in spinal cord injury. Paraplegia 16:265, 1978–1979.
20. White AA, Manohan M, Panjabi D: The role of stabilization in the treatment of cervical spine injuries. Spine 9(5):512, 1984.
21. Aebi M, Hohler J, Zach GA, et al.: Indication, surgical technique, and results of 100 surgically treated fractures and fracture dislocations of the cervical spine. Clin Orthop 203:244, 1986.
22. Favero KJ, Van Peteghem PK: The quadrangular fragment fracture: Roentgenographic fractures and treatment protocol. Clin Orthop 239:40, 1989.
23. Schneider RC, Kahn EA: Chronic neurologic sequelae of acute trauma to the spine and spinal cord. Part 1: The significance of the acute flexion or "tear-drop" fracture dislocation of the cervical spine. J Bone Joint Surg 38A:985, 1956.
24. Luque ER, Cassis N, Ramirez-Wiella G: Segmental spinal instrumentation in the treatment of fractures of the thoracolumbar spine. Spine 7(3):312, 1982.
25. Gertzbein SD, MacMichael D, Tile M: Harrington instrumentation as a method of fixation in fractures of the spine: A critical analysis of deficiencies. J Bone Joint Surg 64B:526, 1982.
26. Roy-Camille R, Saillant G, Berteaux D, et al.: Osteosynthesis of thoracolumbar spine fractures with metal plates screwed through the vertebral pedicles. Reconstr Surg Traumatol 15:2, 1976.
27. Dick W, Kluger P, Magerl F, et al.: A new device for internal fixation of thoracolumbar and lumbar spine fractures. The "fixateur interne." Paraplegia 23:225, 1985.
28. Kostuik J: Anterior spinal cord decompression for lesions of the thoracic and lumbar spine, techniques, new methods of internal fixation, results. Spine 8(5): 512, 1983.
29. White RJ, Albin MS, Harris LS, et al.: Spinal cord injury: Sequential morphology and hypothermic stabilization. Surg Forum 20:432, 1969.
30. Tator CH, Deecke L: Value of normothermic perfusion, hypothermic perfusion, and durotomy in the treatment of acute spinal cord trauma. Neurosurg 39:52, 1973.
31. Albin MS, White MS, Acosta-Rua G: Study of functional recovery produced by delayed localized cooling after spinal cord injury in primates. J Neurosurg 29:113, 1968.
32. Lewin MG, Hansebout RR, Pappius HM: Chemical characteristics of spinal cord edema in cats: Effects of steroids on potassium depletion. J Neurosurg 40:65, 1974.
33. Bracken MB, Shepard MJ, Collins WF, et al.: A randomized, controlled trial of methylprednisolone or naloxone in the treatment of acute spinal-cord injury. N Engl J Med 322:1405, 1990.
34. Faden AI, Jacobs TP, Smith MT, et al.: Comparison of thyrotropin releasing hormone (TRH), naloxone and dexamethasone treatments in experimental spinal cord injury. Neurology 33:673, 1983.
35. Guha A, Tator CH, Smith CR, et al.: Improvement in posttraumatic spinal cord blood flow with a combination of a calcium channel blocker and a vasopressor. J Trauma 29(10):1440, 1989.
36. Whitehill R, Richman JA, Glaser JA: Failure of immobilization of the cervical spine by the halo vest. J Bone Joint Surg 68A(3):326, 1986.
37. Bohler J, Gaudernak T: Anterior plate stabilization for fracture dislocations of the lower cervical spine. J Trauma 20:203, 1980.
38. Holness RO, Huestis WS, Howes WJ, et al.: Posterior stabilization with an interlaminar clamp in cervical injuries: Technical note and review of the long-term experience with the method. Neurosurg 14:318, 1989.
39. Frankel HL, Hancock DO, Hyslop G, et al.: The value of postural reduction in the initial management of closed injuries of the spine with paraplegia and tetraplegia. Paraplegia 7:179, 1969.
40. Luque ER, Cassis N, Ramirez-Wiella C: Segmental spinal instrumentation in the treatment of fractures of the thoracolumbar spine. Spine 7(3):312, 1982.
41. Dick W: The "fixateur interne" as a versatile implant for spine surgery. Spine 12(9):882, 1987.
42. Jant MJ, Freehafer AA, Hazel C, et al.: Autonomic dysreflexia: A cause of morbidity and mortality in orthopedic patients with spinal cord injury. Clin Orthop 169:151, 1982.

Chapter 62

OTHER NECK INJURIES

D. IAN SOUTTER

KEY POINTS

- *For the purposes of trauma management, the neck is divided into three anatomic zones.*
- *Penetrating neck wounds may harbor significant visceral or vascular injury with little or no clinical findings.*
- *Wounds should never be explored in the emergency department.*
- *Airway compromise and bleeding are the common modes of death.*
- *Indications for immediate neck exploration include airway compromise, shock, uncontrolled bleeding, or rapidly expanding hematoma.*
- *Without signs of vital structure injury, one may expect equivalent mortality and morbidity from policies of mandatory or selective exploration if appropriate resources are available.*

Injuries to the neck are potentially fatal and associated with significant morbidity. Most injuries result from acts of violence and are penetrating in nature (e.g., stab wounds, gunshot wounds, or wounds from other sharp instruments). Blunt injury to the neck is more likely to cause spinal or spinal cord damage, but it may result in airway, visceral, or vascular injury. Prior to World War II, the treatment of penetrating neck wounds was primarily nonoperative, with mortality rates in the range of 10 to 15 percent. Most urban centers now record mortality rates in the range of 2 to 6 percent, a reduction attributed to the principle of mandatory exploration of all neck wounds that penetrate the platysma.[1–6] This policy has now been effectively challenged by numerous centers reporting equivalent low mortality with a policy of selective exploration based upon clinical examination supplemented with radiologic and endoscopic investigations.[7–14] The intensivist needs to be familiar with the principles of management if he or she is to take over care or give effective consultative advice.

Anatomy

The neck is a small and relatively unprotected area that contains vital structures from four systems (airway, vascular, digestive, neurologic). For purposes of clinical assessment and surgical management, the neck is divided into three zones (Fig. 62-1). Zone I extends from the cricoid cartilage down to the level of the clavicle and represents the thoracic outlet or the root of the neck. Included in this area are the proximal carotid and subclavian vessels, trachea, esophagus, thoracic duct, and apex of the lung. Zone II includes the area from cricoid to the angle of the mandible and represents the midneck. Penetrating injuries are most frequent in this area and are easiest to evaluate; however, it is this area that has generated the management controversy between mandatory and selective exploration. Zone III is the area located between the angle of the mandible and the base of the skull.

The neck is divided into anterior and posterior regions by the palpable transverse processes of the midcervical vertebrae. The superficial fascia is a thin layer that encloses the platysma muscle in the anterior neck. Penetration of this muscle (easily determined clinically) is used by many clinicians as a guideline for mandatory exploration. The deep cervical fascia supports and separates the viscera, vessels, and neck muscles. The neck is "packaged" into an anterior visceral unit containing the laryngotracheal and pharyngoesophageal passageways by the pretracheal fascia, and a posterior vertebral unit, including the spine, spinal cord, and the bulk of the neck musculature by the prevertebral fascia (Fig. 62-2). Both units are enclosed by an outer investing fascia, which incorporates the sternomastoid and trapezius muscles. The pretracheal layer extends into the chest, blending with the pericardium. The carotid sheath, containing the common and internal carotid arteries, the internal jugular vein, and the vagus, blends with the pretracheal fascia anteriorly, the prevertebral fascia posteriorly, and the investing fascia laterally. The posterior half of the neck contains no major vessels or nerves, except those nerves to individual muscles.

Iatrogenic Neck Injury in the Intensive Care Unit (ICU) Patient

Significant complications may occur as a result of intubation, endoscopy, or attempted vascular access. Perforation of the cervical esophagus has occurred after attempted translaryngeal intubation, diagnostic flexible endoscopy, or

FIGURE 62-1 Zones of the neck.

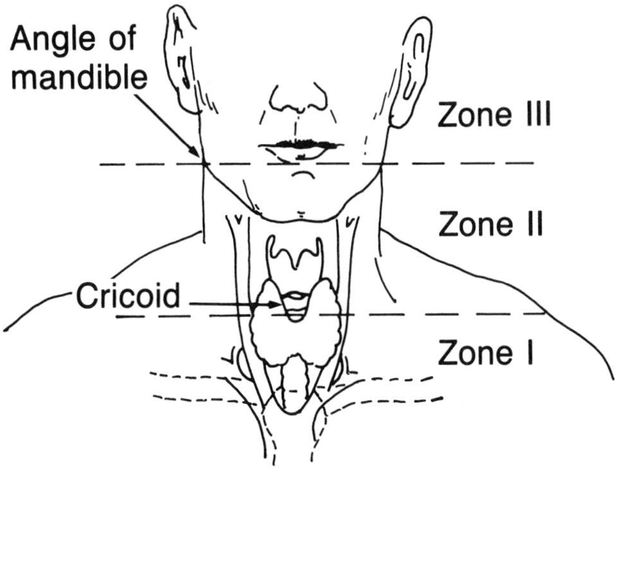

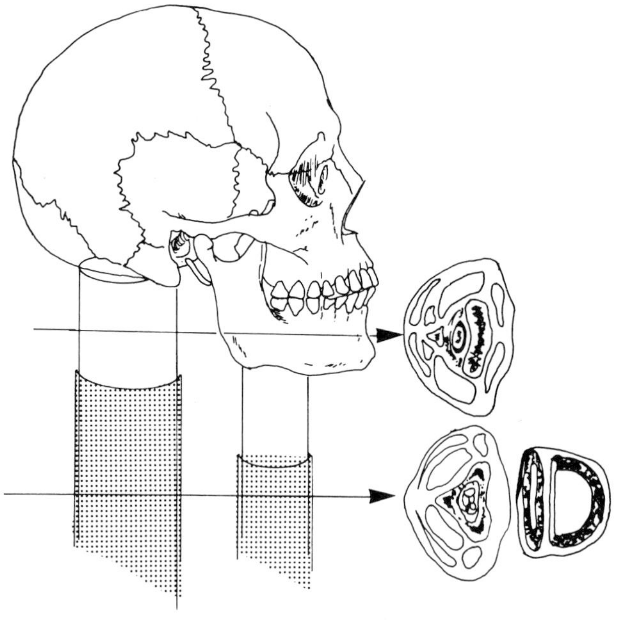

FIGURE 62-2 "Packaging" of the neck by investing fascia illustrating an anterior visceral (laryngotracheal and pharyngoesophageal) unit and a posterior vertebral unit.

even passage of a nasogastric tube. Although rare, it should be kept in mind in a patient who develops fever, leukocytosis, or subcutaneous emphysema in the neck after these procedures. Soft-tissue x-rays of the chest and neck may demonstrate air within deep tissue planes that may not be clinically palpable. If a perforation is suspected, the diagnosis should be confirmed with a Gastrografin swallow, followed by barium if no leak is seen. Demonstration of a leak demands prompt intervention to control the soilage, restore continuity, and deal with the surrounding soft tissue infection. This usually requires surgical drainage, repair, and appropriate antibiotics. Oral feeding should be resumed only after one obtains clinical and radiologic evidence that the leak has ceased, usually 1 week later.

Attempted central venous access may result in arterial puncture or pneumothorax. Penetration of the trachea or esophagus, although reported, should not occur when attention is paid to proper technique. Inadvertent arterial puncture is usually easily identified by the color of the blood and its pulsatile flow, although in a hypotensive or hypoxemic patient, this may be difficult. Direct pressure for 10 min after withdrawal of the needle should prevent significant neck hematoma. Pneumothorax is more frequent in patients receiving positive pressure ventilation and positive end-expiratory pressure (PEEP). Mandatory chest x-ray (CXR) immediately after central line insertion will detect many but not necessarily all pneumothoraces, as they may become clinically apparent hours later. Whenever possible, the CXR should be done in the upright position, since pneumothoraces may be missed on supine film. An acute increase in airway pressure or hemodynamic deterioration after the procedure in a ventilated patient should prompt immediate clinical evaluation for the presence of a tension pneumothorax. If present, it requires immediate decompression by needle, followed by a tube thoracostomy.

Penetrating Neck Injury

Penetrating wounds are more likely than blunt trauma to require operative intervention. Penetrating wounds may harbor significant injury with little or no initial clinical findings.[1,12,16] Exsanguination and airway compromise caused by major vessel injury are the most common causes of death following a penetrating neck wound. Vascular injuries may also result in air embolism, false aneurysms, arterial venous fistulae, or stroke. Unrecognized pharyngeosophageal penetration, although not a cause of early mortality, may result in significant delayed morbidity from mediastinitis.

Injuries from stab wounds are somewhat more predictable because of the linear nature of the trauma. Injuries from gunshot wounds are unpredictable because of the possibility of deflection, tumbling, shattering, and venous or arterial embolization. The amount of soft-tissue damage is primarily related to the velocity of the missile, as expressed by the formula $K = MV^2/2$, where K is the kinetic energy, M is the mass, and V is the velocity. Significant tissue damage out of the direct path of the missile may result from tissue compression and cavitation, depending on the missile mass and velocity. Hematomas in the neck usually predict underlying visceral or vascular injury. They may be associated with profuse external bleeding, bleeding into the oral pharynx, or no obvious external blood loss. A hematoma deep in the neck may cause airway obstruction as it enlarges, by direct tracheal compression and by secondary glottic edema from ongoing blood loss.

Airway compromise may result from **1.** direct laryngotracheal injury, **2.** compression and edema secondary to unrecognized expanding deep hematoma, or **3.** massive intraoral bleeding, resulting in drowning. Venous air embolism may result from the consequences of a lacerated major vein in a patient who is spontaneously breathing in the upright position. Although rare, it may be the result of ill-advised wound exploration in the emergency room without preliminary intubation and positive pressure ventilation.

Clinical Evaluation

Patients with penetrating neck injuries should be rapidly and thoroughly evaluated, after airway patency is ensured and after assessment and management of life-threatening breathing or circulatory disturbances. It is helpful to approach the evaluation looking for clinical evidence of underlying vital structure injury in any of the four systems (airway, vascular, digestive, and neurologic). Information from prehospital personnel, such as blood loss at the scene, nature of the weapon, and time from injury is valuable in making an accurate assessment. Historical details, such as pain, dyspnea, dysphagia, odynophagia, and past neurologic history, should be sought. A detailed physical exam is important. Features suggestive of underlying vital structure injury of the laryngotracheal apparatus include pain and marked tenderness, hoarseness, and subcutaneous emphysema. Dysphonia depends upon the magnitude of vocal cord injury or edema. Cough may be secondary to aspiration or endotracheal bleeding. Specific signs indicative of injury to the laryngeal framework include a tender flat thyroid prominence and crepitus. These clinical features are usually readily evident, and the diagnosis of injury to the laryngotracheal apparatus is usually not difficult. Vascular injury may be manifested by bruit, expanding hematoma, decreased pulses, significant bleeding, or hemispheric signs. Serious vascular injury, however, may occur in the absence of clinical signs.[15,16] Absent clinical findings are more likely to occur with injuries to zones I and III of the neck. Detection of neurologic injury requires a careful sensory and motor examination of the ipsilateral arm and of cranial nerves 10 to 12. The patient may also present with Horner's syndrome. Injury to the digestive tract may be suggested by tenderness, dysphagia, crepitus, or x-ray evidence of subcutaneous air in the prevertebral tissue planes. Clinical signs are often absent with esophageal injuries.

FIGURE 62-3 Soft-tissue swelling of the prevertebral space from C_2 to C_6 indicative of deep cervical hematoma (see Case Presentation).

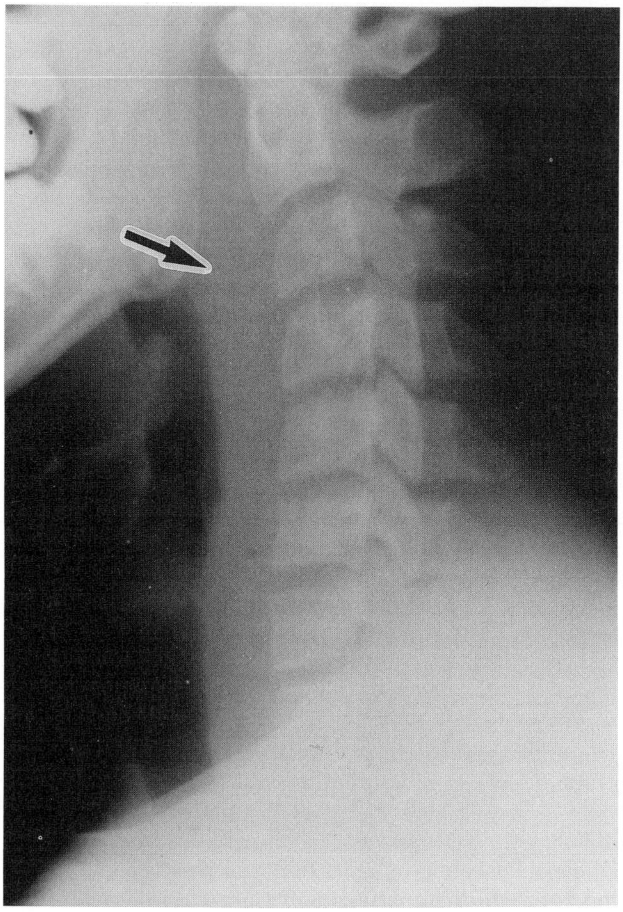

The following interventions should never be done in the emergency room:

1. Do not probe or explore wounds. At best this will result in a false negative evaluation and at worst may result in resumption of bleeding with possible airway compromise, exsanguination, or air embolism.
2. Do not clamp bleeders deep in the wound. Ongoing hemorrhage is best controlled with direct pressure. Further hemostasis need not be obtained until the airway has been secured. The blind clamping of vessels deep in the wound is often unsuccessful and may lead to irreversible neurologic injury.
3. Do not pass a nasogastric tube. The associated retching and vomiting usually seen with the passage of a nasogastric tube may result in the resumption of hemorrhage with its attendant complications. It is best to pass a nasogastric tube after endotracheal intubation. This will often take place in the operating room, with rapid sequence induction and cricoid pressure.
4. Do not remove the weapon until after the airway has been secured.

Soft tissue x-rays of the neck may be useful in detecting subcutaneous air that is not palpable clinically. In addition, the x-ray is helpful in determining the location of a missile but does not ordinarily delineate its path. One may also see evidence of deep cervical hematoma or deviation of the tracheal air column, suggestive of underlying vascular injury (Fig. 62-3).

EMERGENCY AIRWAY MANAGEMENT

Endotracheal intubation can almost always be secured via the orotracheal route. With penetrating injury, the cervical spine will usually be stable. Even in the face of massive intraoral hemorrhage, orotracheal intubation is usually possible with the aid of tonsil suction. In the presence of major structural deformity from hematoma and edema, or inability to secure orotracheal intubation, a cricothyroidotomy is the procedure of choice. Formal tracheostomy should be reserved for those few patients with direct injury to the larynx. In patients with direct laryngeal trauma (usually blunt), attempted orotracheal intubation may further damage the delicate laryngeal apparatus or may convert a partial to a complete obstruction. Cricothyroidotomy may result in the airway being placed in the retrolaryngeal space.

It is important to realize the possibility of ipsilateral chest injury, particularly when the penetrating wound is located in zone I. Clinical and radiologic assessment for the presence of pneumothorax or hemothorax is mandatory.

INDICATIONS FOR SURGERY

Indications for immediate neck exploration after penetrating trauma include **1.** airway obstruction, **2.** shock, **3.** uncontrolled bleeding, and **4.** rapidly expanding hematoma. These patients should have orotracheal intubation secured

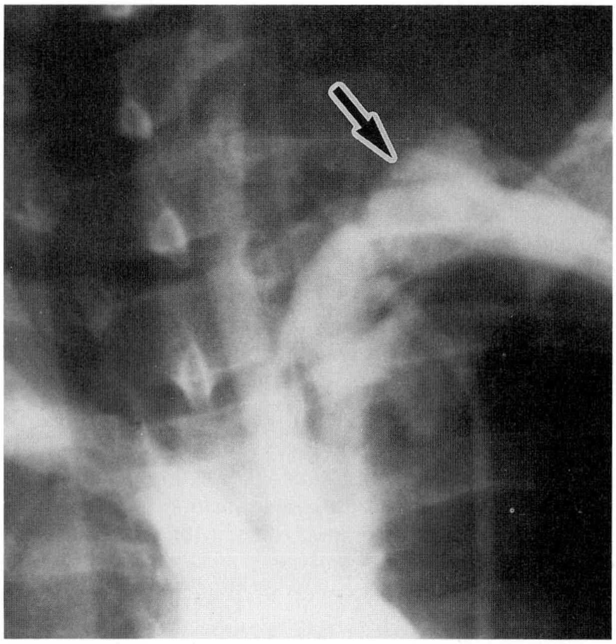

FIGURE 62-4 Arteriography in a zone I injury illustrating injury to the left subclavian artery.

in the resuscitation area, followed by rapid transfer to the operating suite. A supine chest x-ray should be obtained that should not significantly delay neck exploration.

Patients without these obvious indications for surgery should be clinically evaluated for signs suggestive of vital structure injury. With evidence of platysma muscle penetration in zone I, routine operative exploration is ill-advised. Since injuries may involve structures of the superior mediastinum, thoracotomy is often required for control or repair. Arteriography is essential in all stable patients with zone I injuries to define the presence of vascular injury and allow for planning of the operative procedure (Fig. 62-4).

Similarly, angiography is recommended for stable patients with penetrating wounds in zone III. These injuries are located high in the neck, above the angle of the mandible, and exploration of this area requires difficult exposure techniques. Routine exploration is therefore not advised.

Controversy exists regarding policies of mandatory exploration versus selective management (based upon ancillary studies), for penetrating trauma in zone II (midneck). Proponents of mandatory exploration justify their position claiming the possibility of mortality or morbidity with missed injuries in patients who do not undergo routine exploration.[1–6] It should be pointed out that both vascular and esophageal injuries are occasionally missed at surgical exploration, resulting in delayed morbidity.[11,12,17] This underscores the need for thorough surgical evaluation of the carotid sheath, hypopharynx, and esophagus. Those authors who advocate selective management claim a much lower incidence of negative neck exploration with equivalent results.[7–14]

Although a few authors base the policy of selective operation on clinical evaluation primarily, most utilize ancillary studies in the routine evaluation of the stable patient without obvious clinical signs of vital structure injury. With the exception of an occasional report,[1] angiography will reliably exclude arterial injury.[2,8,11,14,18,19] Angiography may also be of value in documenting vertebral artery injuries that may be missed at neck exploration and require difficult surgical exposure. Four-vessel angiography is required (a) to evaluate the cerebral circulation, (b) to determine if the injury noted may possibly require ligation, and (c) to exclude vertebral injury. Multiple views and the use of digital subtraction may be required to identify subtle arterial injuries.

Nonoperative evaluation of the cervical esophagus and hypopharynx requires contrast radiography or endoscopy. Hypopharyngeal and esophageal injuries, however, may be overlooked with contrast studies or esophagoscopy.[1,8,14] False-negative rates from contrast studies are typically in the range of 10 to 20 percent but have been reported as high as 52 percent.[15] The results of endoscopic evaluation depend upon the type of instrument (rigid vs. flexible) and the skill of the examiner. The hypopharyngeal and cricopharyngeal regions are notoriously difficult to evaluate endoscopically. Missed esophageal injuries have occurred in 11 percent of patients evaluated by rigid endoscopy and up to 62 percent of patients evaluated by flexible endoscopy.[8] No single test is as reliable as angiography in ruling out injury. The combination of barium esophagography and rigid endoscopy, however, is accurate in ruling out pharyngoesophageal injury.[8]

It appears that a policy of selective exploration based upon clinical evaluation, arteriography, barium esophagography, and endoscopy yields equivalent results with fewer negative neck explorations.[7–14] Stable patients without obvious indications for surgery should undergo four-vessel angiography. If positive, exploration is indicated, and a thorough search should be made for esophageal or hypopharyngeal injury. This may be supplemented by direct laryngoscopy and rigid endoscopy if deemed necessary. Patients with negative angiography should proceed to barium esophagography. If results are positive or equivocal, rigid endoscopy under general anesthesia is indicated, followed by neck exploration. If the barium examination is negative, the patient may be observed. The subsequent clinical development of findings would warrant exploration. A policy of selective management can only be recommended, however, if there is immediate availability of these procedures and expertise in their evaluation. Although associated with a high negative exploration rate, the time-honored policy of mandatory surgical exploration is associated with extremely low morbidity and mortality.

SURGICAL APPROACH

The surgical approach to penetrating neck injury is dictated primarily by the zone of injury.

ZONE I

Of major concern is injury to the great vessels at the base of the neck. Many of these patients present in shock. A left tube thoracostomy is indicated in these patients to determine if there is active bleeding into the chest cavity and to reexpand a pneumothorax. Occasionally patients will present with exsanguinating hemorrhage into a hemithorax and require emergency thoracotomy for resuscitation. A gauze sponge should be placed at the apex of the pleural cavity and the suspected subclavian or innominate artery injury compressed between the gloved fist within the chest and the open hand in the supraclavicular fossa. The patient is then moved to the operating room (OR) for definitive repair.

The key to successful repair of zone I injuries involves proximal vascular control in the upper mediastinum prior to neck exploration (Fig. 62-5). This can be done through a median sternotomy or a left third interspace anterior thoracotomy for control of the innominate or left subclavian arteries, respectively. With injuries to the carotid arteries, it is best to extend the median sternotomy along the anterior border of the sternomastoid muscle on the appropriate side. With proximal subclavian artery injuries, exposure is gained by extension along the superior aspect of the clavicle with or without resection of its medial half. Proximal control of the left subclavian artery is best obtained through a left third or fourth interspace thoracotomy, which provides greater access to the posterior aspect of the chest than a median sternotomy. This incision can be extended through the sternum and manubrium and joined with the supraclavicular incision to form a trapdoor, allowing for greater exposure on the left side.

ZONE II

Exposure for all injuries of the anterior neck within zone II can be obtained though anterior sternocleidomastoid incisions from the angle of the jaw to the suprasternal notch on the appropriate side. Proximal and distal vascular control should be obtained prior to entering the periarterial hematoma. Active arterial hemorrhage can usually be controlled with digital pressure. After proximal control is obtained, the hematoma may be entered and the artery dissected. Debridement, followed by direct suture repair, is usually possible.

Exposure of the pharyngoesophageal region involves division of the omohyoid muscle, middle thyroid vein, and occasionally the common facial vein.

ZONE III

Surgical exposure of zone III injuries is gained by extending the anterior sternomastoid incision superiorly, anterior to the pinna, and by subluxation of the ipsilateral temporomandibular joint. The jaw may be wired in this subluxed state prior to surgical incision (Fig. 62-6). Further access to the area is gained by division of the posterior digastric, stylohyoid, and styloglossus muscles. Mandibular osteotomy is occasionally necessary.

Management of Specific Neck Injuries

VASCULAR INJURIES

Arteriography in the stable patient, as indicated, is useful in

1. defining the presence and nature of the injury;
2. determining the persistence or absence of prograde flow;
3. planning operative approach; and
4. allowing for embolization of expendable (branches of external carotid) or poorly accessible (vertebral) vessels.

Injuries to the external carotid may be ligated. Management of common and internal carotid injuries is more controversial. Ligation of these injured structures was initially performed because of the fear of inducing a hemorrhagic infarction with reperfusion of ischemic tissue after vascular repair. Ligation, however, was associated with very high morbidity and mortality rates. Most authorities recommend revascularization in all cases (including patients with preoperative neurologic signs) except those with **1.** profound coma, **2.** no prograde flow angiographically and the absence of significant neurologic findings, or **3.** injuries to the internal carotid at the base of the skull.[20–22] Neurologic deficits have been significantly improved in more than 50 per-

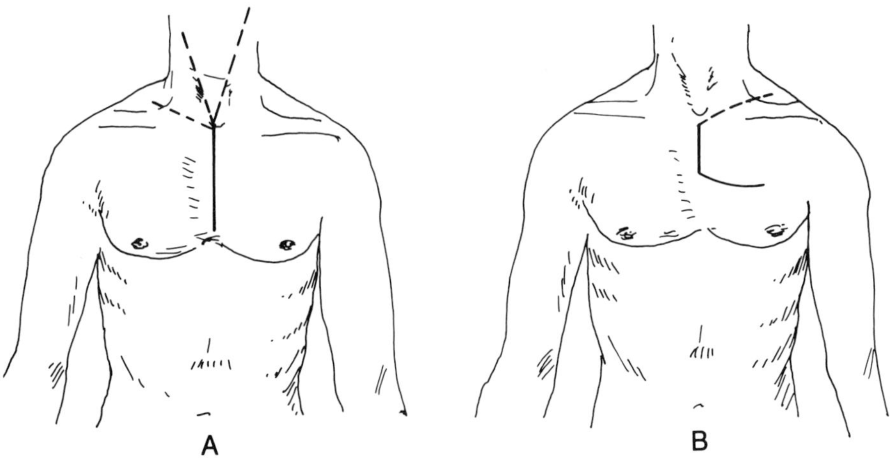

FIGURE 62-5 The surgical approach to proximal vascular control for zone I injuries of the (*a*) innominate, proximal right subclavian or right carotid, proximal left carotid; and (*b*) proximal left subclavian.

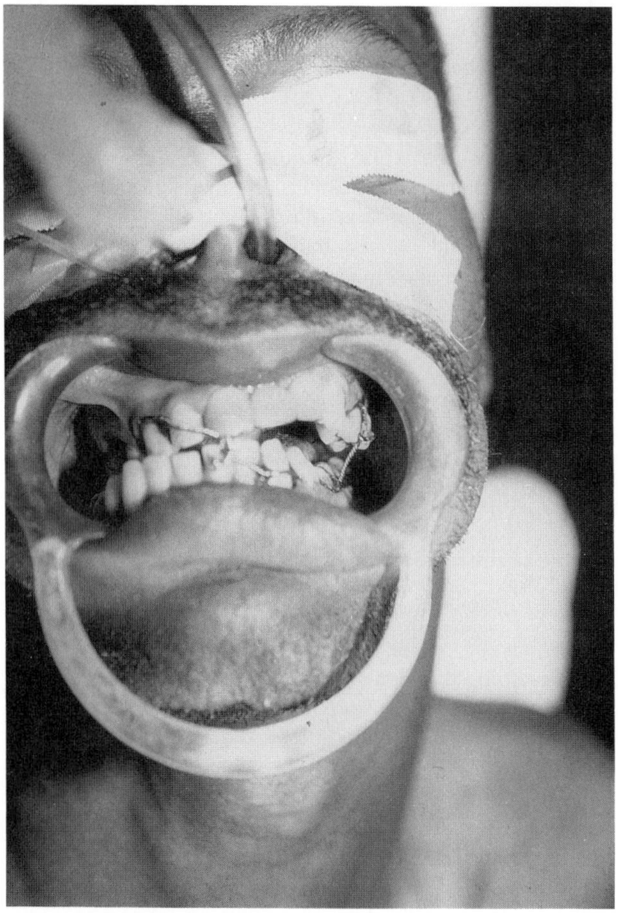

FIGURE 62-6 Dislocation of temporomandibular joint held by temporary interdental wiring. Note malocclusion.

cent of patients with revascularization.[20] Techniques of repair may involve lateral arteriorrhaphy, segmental resection with reanastomosis, saphenous vein or gortex grafts, patch angioplasty, and occasionally transposition of the proximal external carotid. The repair of complex injuries may require intraluminal shunting. Systemic anticoagulation is rarely necessary for patients who require uncomplicated revascularization.

Injuries to the vertebral artery are infrequent and are usually symptom free at presentation. These injuries require repair since pseudoaneurysms, A-V fistula, or occlusion may present as late complications. The vertebral artery may be angiographically occluded if good flow is documented in the contralateral vertebral artery such that the basilar and posterior inferior cerebellar arteries fill. Balloon occlusion may be used distal to A-V fistulae for control.

Injuries of the internal jugular vein should be repaired if the repair is easily performed. Unilateral ligation, however, is well tolerated and should be done if repair is difficult.

PHARYNGOESOPHAGEAL INJURIES

Lacerations to the oropharynx can be sutured transorally with associated antibiotic coverage. Wounds of the hypopharynx and cervical esophagus require neck exploration, direct two-layer suture repair, and drainage. Extensive wounds may require exteriorization. Missed injuries result in mediastinitis with serious consequences and have strengthened the case for mandatory exploration. Esophageal injuries, however, may be overlooked at surgery without deliberate attention to the area. Intraoperative esophageal air insufflation via nasogastric (NG) tube or rigid esophagoscopy may aid in documenting injury.

LARYNGOTRACHEAL INJURIES

Laryngeal injury, in particular, should be dealt with early and by experienced laryngeal surgeons in order to obtain best functional results. The initial therapeutic decision involves establishment of an airway. Endotracheal intubation is not indicated with laryngeal trauma, as it may compound the injury or be unsuccessful with intubation of the extralaryngeal tissues. Direct laryngeal trauma is an indication for formal tracheotomy. Techniques of laryngeal repair are beyond the scope of this chapter.

Tracheal injury most commonly involves the proximal rings. Endotracheal intubation, with insertion of the tube distal to the laceration, will ensure airway patency. Following blunt injury, the trachea may be completely divided. Intubation over a flexible bronchoscope may be of value. One should be prepared for tracheal exploration on an immediate basis in this setting. Direct suture repair is usually possible with minor lacerations. One must ensure a tension-free anastomosis to reduce wound dehiscence and tracheal stenosis. This may involve the use of tracheal retention sutures, neck flexion, and laryngeal release maneuvers.

BLUNT NECK INJURY

Forces impacting upon the head or chest, such as seen in motor vehicle trauma, are more likely to cause musculoskeletal injury resulting in spine and spinal cord damage, rather than visceral or vascular damage. Direct neck trauma may occur, such as seen with "clotheslining" from snowmobile accidents or striking the dashboard with a hyperextended neck.

Laryngotracheal injuries are most common because of their anterior position. Blunt esophageal perforation is exceedingly rare but has been reported. Blunt vascular injury is often not diagnosed. Patients with blunt vascular injury will have few, if any, local neck findings, and associated neurologic findings are usually presumed to be secondary to commonly associated head injury.

In the initial assessment of patients with blunt neck trauma, it is of primary importance to protect the cervical spine until injury can be excluded. Patients with blunt laryngotracheal injury often present with dysphonia, stridor, cough, hemoptysis, and neck pain. On examination, one may find flat thyroid prominence, extreme tenderness, crepitation on movement of the larynx, or subcutaneous emphysema.

Evaluation of suspected laryngotracheal injuries must be done promptly, since airway compromise is a potential delayed problem. Methods of evaluation include indirect mirror examination, flexible fiberoptic direct laryngoscopy, soft tissue x-rays, and computed tomography (CT) scanning.

Follow-up in the Intensive Care Unit

Patients may be admitted to the ICU after neck injury for observation or for postoperative care. Significant injuries may be clinically occult initially and present hours or days later. Vascular injuries could result in hematoma formation and progressive airway problems within 6 h. At the early signs of enlarging hematoma or airway compromise, translaryngeal intubation should be accomplished, followed by surgical reevaluation. Ongoing deep hemorrhage in the neck may make translaryngeal intubation difficult and at times impossible. Cricothyroidotomy may then be indicated.

Delayed manifestations of a hypopharyngeal or esophageal injury are usually those of systemic sepsis. Because of the continuity of the mediastinal and deep cervical planes, these patients will frequently develop mediastinitis with signs of hypovolemia and sepsis or mediastinal abscess. Delayed diagnosis of this complication may result in significant mortality. One must keep in mind that injuries may be missed during neck exploration if all of the vital structures have not been closely inspected.

Most patients who have prompt surgical therapy have little or no postoperative complications. Hemorrhage is possible after vascular repair, and hypertension should be controlled to minimize this possibility. Bulky neck dressings should be avoided to facilitate early detection of an enlarging hematoma or airway compromise. A leak from a missed or repaired esophageal injury will usually present with excessive wound drainage or local wound infection. If the leak is well drained, then systemic sepsis is unlikely to result.

Extubation of the patients after neck exploration is usually uneventful; however, one must be certain that significant upper airway edema is not present. A large air leak around a deflated cuff suggests extubation should be successful. If there is any concern, then extubation over a flexible bronchoscope will allow evaluation and immediate reintubation.

CASE PRESENTATION

A 25-year-old man arrived in the emergency room (ER) 30 min after sustaining gunshot wounds from a small-caliber handgun to the left side of the neck and to the right side of the back, lateral to the midscapula. The entrance wound on the neck was immediately adjacent to the angle of the mandible. There was no exit wound. The patient was sitting upright and had hemoptysis but was able to speak with a normal voice. There was no stridor, respiratory distress, or odynophagia. Vital signs were: pulse, 88; BP, 130/85; and respiratory rate, 24/min. There was no obvious hematoma, crepitus, or bruit in the neck.

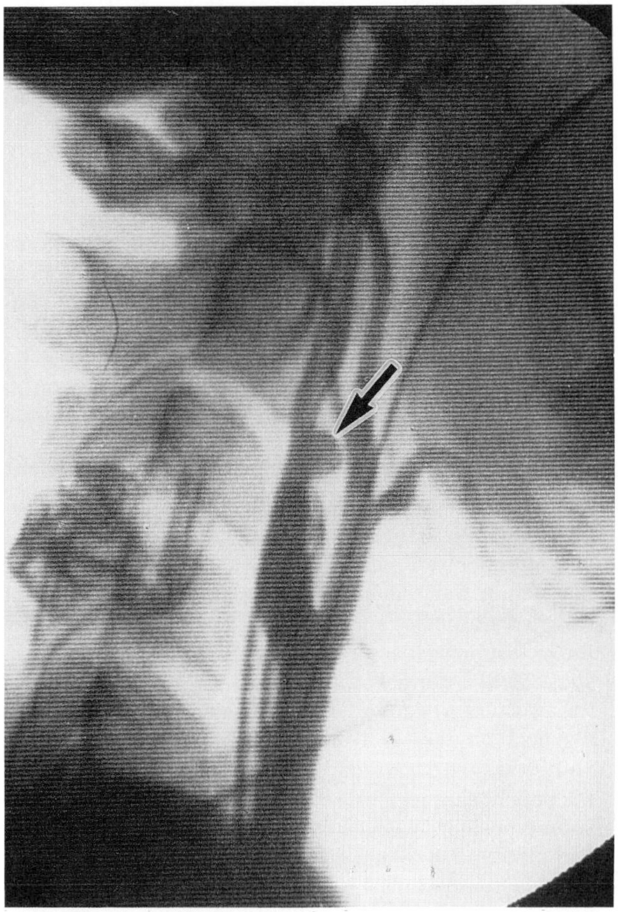

FIGURE 62-7 Angiogram demonstrating injury to the left internal carotid artery above the bifurcation at the junction of zones II and III. Good distal flow is preserved.

Examination of the oropharynx revealed a small amount of fresh blood in the posterior pharynx with no obvious swelling and no obvious laceration. Neurologic evaluation was unremarkable. Air entry over the chest was equal bilaterally, and the trachea was midline.

Blood was drawn for crossmatching and baseline hematologic and biochemical studies. Large-bore venous access was established in the left antecubital vein, and infusion of crystalloid was begun. Supplemental oxygen and electrocardiographic monitoring were begun. A nasogastric tube was not passed. Portable x-rays of the chest and neck were obtained. The CXR revealed a bullet in the lateral soft tissues with a small, right-sided pneumothorax.

Soft tissue x-rays of the neck revealed marked prevertebral swelling (Fig. 62-3). No bullet was seen in the neck films. A subsequent abdominal film revealed a bullet in the left upper quadrant, presumably in the stomach.

A right-sided No. 36 French chest tube was inserted. The patient's airway was secured in the ER. Orotracheal intubation was performed utilizing neuromuscular blockade and cricoid compression. Four-vessel angiography was performed. This revealed a laceration of the internal carotid artery just above the bifurcation (Fig. 62-7). Flow was preserved distally, and the vertebral arteries were normal.

Direct laryngoscopy in the operating room (OR) revealed a small laceration on the left side of the oropharynx posteriorly. The left temporomandibular joint was subluxed anteriorly and held open with temporary arch bars and wires.

The neck was explored, with proximal control gained before the periarterial hematoma was entered. Attempted distal control resulted in brisk back bleeding, easily controlled with finger pressure, followed by temporary distal arterial occlusion with a Fogarty catheter. Arterial repair was performed uneventfully with debridement and primary end to end anastomosis. The postoperative recovery was uneventful.

CASE DISCUSSION

This relatively uncomplicated case illustrates the principles of management of a penetrating neck wound. Particular attention was paid to airway and breathing difficulties within the primary survey. The initial assessment revealed no obvious airway difficulty, as evidenced by the lack of hoarseness, stridor, and the patient's ability to speak with a normal voice. Nevertheless, concern about the airway is well founded in any patient with a penetrating neck wound, and more particularly in this patient with evidence of intraoral bleeding. The presentation of the patient sitting in an upright position suggests that the supine position may result in some difficulty with intraoral blood pooling and airway compromise. Despite the absence of any clinical indication of airway compromise, penetrating neck wounds should always raise the concern of delayed bleeding and airway compromise from glottic edema or tracheal compression. Further evidence of hemorrhage should be sought with soft tissue x-rays of the neck, such as a lateral C-spine film.

With no clinical evidence of respiratory distress, and stable vital signs, a tube thoracostomy may be deferred until after a CXR has been obtained. With evidence of penetrating injury to the chest in a patient with either respiratory distress or unstable vital signs, tube thoracostomy should precede CXR.

Although there is no evidence of circulatory instability at presentation, large-bore venous access remains necessary. Patients may have compensated well for significant blood loss prior to admission, or may bleed substantially after admission, because of coughing, retching, or attempted instrumentation of their oro- or nasopharynx. Central lines should be avoided, as this may interfere with subsequent evaluation or surgical management. Large-bore venous access is preferable in the upper extremity on the uninjured side. Passage of a nasogastric tube is contraindicated, as it may precipitate significant bleeding and airway compromise. Detailed neurologic examination in a cooperative and reliable patient should exclude injury to the cranial nerves or brachial plexus.

The soft tissue x-rays of the neck revealed significant prevertebral swelling, suggestive of hemorrhage from an underlying vascular injury. No bullet was seen in the neck, suggesting that it was either swallowed or expectorated. Pharyngeal penetration must be assumed from the clinical presentation and x-rays. This was confirmed by the presence of the bullet in the left upper quadrant on abdominal x-ray. Aside from direct inspection of the oropharynx with appropriate lighting, one should avoid further attempts at direct or indirect laryngoscopy for the same reason that passage of a nasogastric tube is contraindicated.

Because the wound was located relatively high in the neck, at the junction of zones II and III, and the patient remained stable, angiography was useful to document the exact location and extent of the vascular injury, the presence or absence of distal flow, and collateral circulation. This helped plan the operative approach and management. If the patient had presented unstable from hemorrhage, immediate neck exploration after intubation would have been preferred.

Because angiography usually involves moving the patient to a poorly equipped and attended area within the hospital, and takes time to perform, the airway should be secured first if there is clinical suspicion of future compromise. Significant prevertebral swelling and ongoing intraoral bleeding requiring the patient to maintain a semi-upright position, necessitated orotracheal intubation prior to angiography. Orotracheal intubation should be performed in a well-lighted and -equipped area. This may involve a crash induction technique or topical pharyngeal anesthesia and minimal sedation with a semi-awake patient. Regardless of the method used, good suction is necessary, and a surgeon should be in attendance to gain access if a surgical airway is required.

Angiography revealed injury to the internal carotid artery above the bifurcation. The operative strategy involved good exposure and proximal plus distal control. Exposure was aided by subluxation of the left temporomandibular joint, in order to improve control to the distal internal carotid artery behind the ramus of the mandible. Wide exposure was obtained with an anterior sternomastoid incision, extending anterior to the pinna. Proximal vascular control was relatively straightforward; however, the periarterial hematoma often extends up the carotid sheath behind the angle of the mandible, making distal arterial control difficult at times. Attempt at distal control prior to entering the periarterial hematoma was unsuccessful and, therefore, digital pressure over the lacerated carotid artery temporarily stopped bleeding, until a Fogarty catheter could be inserted distally. Following this, vascular loops and clamps were placed distally as required. With minimal tissue loss, primary anastomosis is usually possible. Vascular repair to the common or internal carotid arteries should always be performed unless the patient has profound coma or lack of prograde flow in the absence of a neurologic deficit. Systemic anticoagulation was deemed unnecessary.

Postoperatively, one must be sure that the airway remains patent after extubation. In patients who have significant arterial hemorrhage in the neck, prolonged intubation may be required until glottic and subglottic edema resolves. The patient should not be extubated until fully awake. This should be performed with an anesthetist or surgeon in attendance. Listening for a large air leak with the endotracheal balloon let down prior to extubation suggests a patent airway will be present. If there is concern, extubation over a flexible bronchoscope will allow for better evaluation and for immediate reintubation, using the bronchoscope as a guide.

References

1. Meyer JP, Barrett JA, Schuler JJ, Flanigan DP: Mandatory vs selective exploration for penetrating neck trauma. Arch Surg 122:592, 1987.
2. Roon AJ, Christensen N: Evaluation and treatment of penetrating cervical injuries. J Trauma 16:391, 1979.
3. Saletta JD, Lowe RJ, Lim LT, et al: Penetrating trauma of the neck. J Trauma 16:579, 1976.
4. Williams JW, Sherman RT: Penetrating wounds of the neck—surgical management. J Trauma 13:435, 1973.
5. McInnis WD, Cruz AB, Aust JB: Penetrating injuries to the neck: Pitfalls in management. Am J Surg 130:416, 1975.
6. Ashworth C, Williams LF, Byrne JT: Penetrating wounds of the neck: Re-emphasis of the need for prompt exploration. Am J Surg 121:387, 1971.
7. Rao PM, Bhatti FK, Gaudino J, et al: Penetrating injuries of the neck: Criteria for exploration. J Trauma 23:47, 1983.
8. Weigelt JA, Thal ER, Snyder WH, et al: Diagnosis of penetrating cervical esophageal injuries. Am J Surg 154:619, 1987.
9. Campbell FC, Robbs JV: Penetrating injuries of the neck: A prospective study of 108 patients. Br J Surg 67:582, 1980.
10. Ordog GJ, Albin D, Wasserberger J, et al: 110 bullet wounds to the neck. J Trauma 25:238, 1985.
11. Wood J, Fabian TC, Mangiante EC: Penetrating neck injuries: Recommendations for selective management. J Trauma 29:602, 1989.
12. Jurkovich GJ, Zingarelli W, Wallace J, Curreri PW: Penetrating neck trauma: Diagnostic studies in the asymptomatic patient. J Trauma 25:819, 1985.
13. Metzdorff MT, Lowe DK: Operation or observation for penetrating neck wounds? Am J Surg 147:646, 1983.
14. Noyes LD, McSwain NE, Markowitz IP: Panendoscopy with arteriography versus mandatory exploration of penetrating wounds of the neck. Ann Surg 204:21, 1986.
15. Sheely CH, Mattox KL, Beal AC, DeBakey ME: Penetrating wounds of the cervical esophagus. Am J Surg 130:707, 1975.
16. McCormick TM, Burch BH: Routine angiographic evaluation of neck and extremity injuries. J Trauma 19:384, 1979.
17. Massac E, Siram SM, Leffall LD: Penetrating neck wounds. Am J Surg 145:263, 1983.
18. Merion RM, Harness JK, Ramsburgh SR, Thompson NW: Selective management of penetrating neck trauma. Arch Surg 116:691, 1981.
19. O'Donnell VA, Atik M, Pick RA: Evaluation and management of penetrating wounds of the neck: The role of emergency angiography. Am J Surg 138:309, 1979.
20. Brown MF, Graham JM, Feliciano DV, et al: Carotid artery injuries. Am J Surg 144:748, 1982.
21. Liekweg WG, Greenfield LJ: Management of penetrating carotid arterial injury. Ann Surg 188:587, 1978.
22. Unger SW, Tucker WS, Mrdeza MA, et al: JG: Carotid arterial trauma. Surgery 87:477, 1980.

Chapter 63

TORSO TRAUMA

J. ALI

KEY POINTS

- *Because of the close anatomic relations, abdominal and thoracic injuries should be considered as one complex, torso trauma.*
- *Treatment of patients with torso trauma requires prioritizing interventions based on the threat to life.*
- *In managing torso trauma, the surgeon must be prepared to explore the chest and abdomen when the source of instability is uncertain.*
- *Indications for surgical intervention in abdominal trauma are perforation, penetration, and hemorrhage.*
- *Peritoneal lavage and other ancillary investigations are important tools in assessing the traumatized abdomen when physical examination alone is not possible or is unreliable.*
- *Emergency thoracotomy should be considered in the unstable patient who has a potentially correctable source of the instability in the thorax.*

Consideration of thoracoabdominal injuries as a single, complex, torso trauma is a useful concept for several reasons. Configuration of the diaphragm and attachment to the rib cage result in marked variability in position and, hence, demarcation of the thoracic and abdominal cavities. It is not unusual for the diaphragm to traverse distances of over 15 cm between the inspiratory and expiratory phase of respiration. The diaphragm may be at the level of the nipple line during full expiration and well below the costal margin during full inspiration, with corresponding shift of the abdominal and thoracic contents (Fig. 63-1). This, together with the variable trajectory of penetrating missiles and objects, makes it virtually impossible in many instances to determine whether intrathoracic or intraabdominal injury has been sustained based on the external point of impact or penetration. The concept of torso trauma ensures that injuries in one cavity will not be overlooked while one is managing injuries in the other.

As outlined elsewhere (see Chap. 59), the initial approach in trauma management is to secure the airway, maintain respiration, and identify and control hemorrhage as well as institute immediate fluid resuscitation. During this resuscitative phase, definitive management of intraabdominal or thoracic injury may be required as part of this process, particularly if the source of instability is major hemorrhage within the thoracic or abdominal cavity. Although it may be possible to specify a thoracic or abdominal source of instability in the trauma patient, it is frequently impossible to be absolutely certain. Therefore, a decision has to be made to approach the unstable patient through either a laparotomy or thoracotomy if a source outside the thorax or abdomen has been ruled out as the cause of the instability. With this approach, one must be prepared to stop exploration of one cavity when it becomes obvious that the source of the instability is in the other cavity.

Classification of Torso Trauma

Generally, torso trauma may be classified into two broad groups: penetrating and blunt. As indicated above, any penetrating missile inferior to the nipple line can produce diaphragmatic, intrathoracic, or abdominal injuries. Similarly, blunt injuries may disrupt intrathoracic contents as well as intraabdominal contents either directly or indirectly through fractures of the lower ribs, which then puncture intraabdominal organs such as the spleen, liver, stomach, etc.

A more clinically applicable method of classifying torso trauma involves two categories. The first category consists of injuries requiring immediate intervention because of cardiorespiratory or hemodynamic instability. The other category includes injuries in a stable patient. These latter injuries are considered to be potentially life-threatening, since, if left unattended, they may result in a threat to the patient's survival.

FIGURE 63-1 Principle of torso trauma. Note that at the same level of impact on the chest wall, intraabdominal or intrathoracic injury may occur depending on missile trajectory or location of the diaphragm.

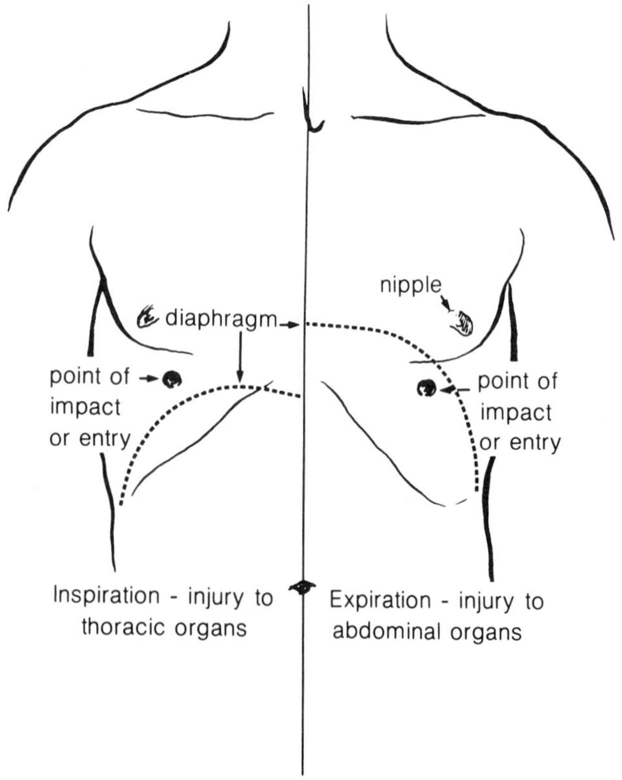

Apart from major intraabdominal hemorrhage, most injuries to the torso requiring immediate intervention involve the thoracic organs. Rapidity of intervention in these injuries is related to the immediate threat to life that the injuries present. The injuries therefore, will be dealt with as two separate groups, namely, those requiring immediate intervention and others with a potential for threatening survival.

Thoracic Injuries Requiring Immediate Intervention

Although 25 percent of trauma related deaths have an associated thoracic injury, 85 percent of these injuries do not require formal open surgical intervention.[1] The life-saving skills in most cases are quite simple and within the scope of any practicing intensivist. Of the 15 percent that require open surgical intervention, the majority do not require the expertise of a trained thoracic surgeon. From the intensivist's standpoint, resuscitative measures are aimed at correcting hypoxemia and maintaining hemodynamic stability. These two aims are achieved by techniques for establishing patency of the airway (see Chap. 59), chest decompression for evacuating fluid or air, pericardiocentesis, and vascular access for fluid administration.

Apart from upper airway obstruction, which has been discussed (see Chaps. 6 and 59) and which poses an immediate threat to life, following is a list of thoracic injuries requiring immediate intervention:

1. tension pneumothorax
2. open pneumothorax
3. cardiac tamponade
4. massive hemothorax
5. massive pneumothorax
6. traumatic air embolism
7. flail chest

Since all of these conditions require immediate intervention, the intensivist who sees such patients must be prepared to institute therapy before any other physician is available. To guide appropriate intervention, a brief description of the pathophysiology, diagnosis, and treatment principles for each of the above conditions follows. In all cases, the airway must be secured and adequate intravenous (IV) access established (see Chap. 59).

TENSION PNEUMOTHORAX

This lesion arises whenever there is a one-way valve mechanism on the chest wall or lung side of an injury. Gas enters the pleural space but has no escape, and with each subsequent respiratory cycle, there is increased intrapleural pressure and gas accumulation. This increased tension causes the ipsilateral lung to be compressed as well as to be displaced to the opposite side. With this shift of the mediastinum, there is not only compromise of ventilation and gas exchange but also kinking of the major veins at the thoracic inlet of the neck and at the diaphragmatic entrance of the inferior vena cava, with compromise of venous return. This combination of hypoperfusion and hypoxemia can be lethal, and immediate treatment is required. The diagnosis is suspected in a patient who presents with chest trauma, tachypnea, severe dyspnea, ipsilateral decreased air entry, and hyperresonance, tracheal shift to the opposite side, and hypotension.

The treatment is immediate decompression of the pleural space, which is accomplished initially by inserting a large-bore needle or incising with a scalpel down through the chest wall into the pleural space at the second intercostal space in the midclavicular line. If a plunger syringe is used with the needle, an immediate spontaneous rise of the plunger in the barrel will be seen. Similarly, when the scalpel enters the pleural space, there is a massive loud decompression of the pleural space followed by immediate respiratory improvement. Either procedure should be followed by formal insertion of a chest tube (see Chap. 16). Briefly, the technique of chest tube insertion requires an incision into the pleural space in the fourth to fifth intercostal space in the anterior axillary line. The large-bore chest tube is inserted directly with a clamp after verification with finger palpation that the pleural space has been entered. Prior to insertion of the chest tube, a needle may be inserted through the finger portion of a glove so that air may exit but not enter the pleural space from the atmosphere (Fig. 63-2). Once the chest tube is inserted, it is connected to an underwater seal system with the option of applying suction.

OPEN PNEUMOTHORAX

In open pneumothorax, there is free communication through a chest wall wound between the pleural space and the atmosphere. Entry of air with each respiratory cycle results in progressive collapse of the ipsilateral lung. The

FIGURE 63-2 Needle decompression of pleural space. Finger portion of glove prevents air entry into pleural space.

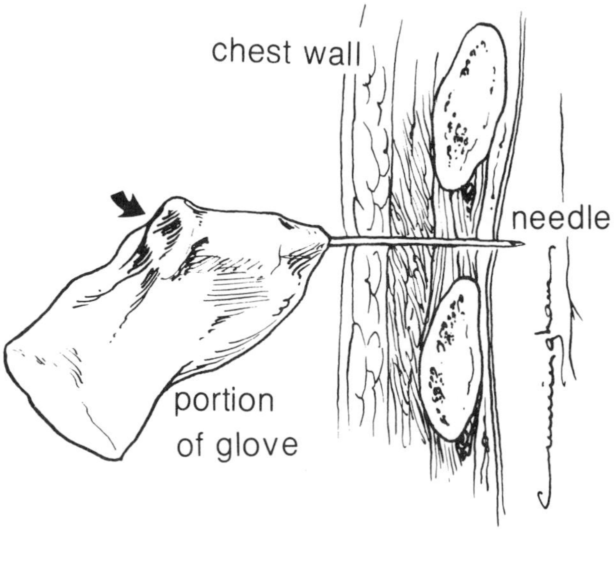

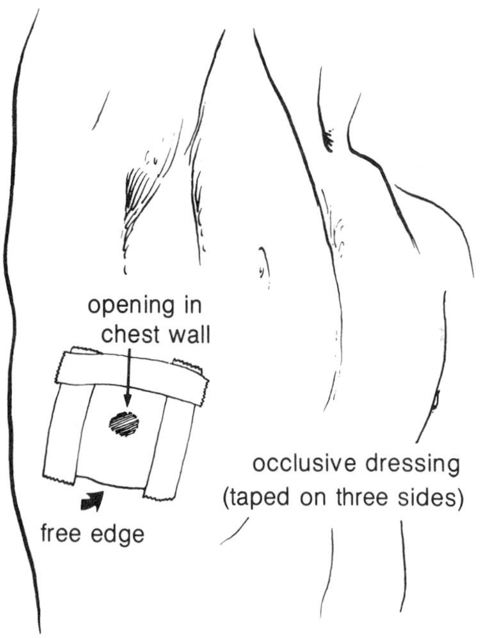

FIGURE 63-3 Temporary occlusive dressing for open pneumothorax. This allows egress of air but prevents air entry into pleural space.

larger the defect in the chest wall, the greater is the rate at which pleural air accumulates, and the more rapid the collapse of the ipsilateral lung. This pathophysiology is similar to that in tension pneumothorax, since collapse of the lung and shift of the mediastinum to the opposite side will cause hypoxemia and decreased venous return. The diagnosis is usually obvious with a visible open wound in the chest wall and a characteristic loud noise created from air entry into the pleural space.

The basic principle in treating this injury is occlusion of the open wound. This can usually be accomplished with an occlusive gauze dressing (Fig. 63-3). Larger defects will require much larger dressings, and major defects that cannot be readily occluded by dressing technique will require support of the patient with endotracheal intubation and positive pressure ventilation until formal repair of the chest wall defect can be performed. Once the opening in the chest wall is occluded, a chest tube should be inserted through a separate opening. Figure 63-3 shows a technique whereby an occlusive dressing can be applied that allows decompression of the pleural space as well as occlusion of the opening. The nonpermeable dressing is applied over the opening and secured on all but one side. This allows egress of air from the pleural space but prevents air entering the pleural space from the atmosphere.

CARDIAC TAMPONADE

Cardiac tamponade occurs when fluid accumulation in the pericardial sac interferes with cardiac filling and emptying. Elevated pericardial pressure decreases transmural filling pressures of the cardiac chambers, resulting in diminished filling and stroke volume of the right and the left side of the heart. Cardiac output falls with an attendant decrease in systolic blood pressure and pulse pressure.

The diagnosis of cardiac tamponade is one that requires a high index of suspicion and should be considered in any patient who has blunt or penetrating trauma to the chest and is hypotensive without any obvious signs of blood loss. The classic triad described by Beck of hypotension, elevated venous pressure, and muffled heart tones is not always present or easily discernible.[2] The status of the neck veins is particularly important in distinguishing hypotension caused by hypovolemia as opposed to hypotension caused by cardiac tamponade. In the former, the neck veins are flat, whereas in the latter, the neck veins are distended. However, a struggling or straining patient may produce misleading bulging of the neck veins, which must be taken into consideration. An increase in pulsus paradoxus (the difference in systolic blood pressure between inspiration and expiration) above 10 mmHg suggests the diagnosis of cardiac tamponade. However, in the emergency setting it can be difficult to quantitate the degree of paradox. During arterial pressure transduction in the intensive care unit (ICU), it is possible to measure pulsus paradoxus accurately. The physician should note the difference between systolic blood pressure during inspiration and expiration. The pressure waveform will exhibit a lower peak level in inspiration, with higher peak levels in expiration. The difference between the two peaks is the pulsus paradoxus. The degree of pulsus paradoxus may be determined at the bedside by listening for the first set of sounds with the sphygmomanometer slowly deflating. The first set of sounds represents the systolic blood pressure on expiration. As the pressure in the cuff is slowly released, the gaps in systolic blood pressure sounds between inspiration and expiration disappear, and there is a more constant frequency of sounds heard with the stethoscope. The difference between the initial pressure and the pressure when the gaps in sounds have disappeared is the degree of pulsus paradoxus. Since distended neck veins and hypotension are present in both tension pneumothorax and cardiac tamponade, differentiation between these two conditions is important but at times difficult. The physician must rely on evidence of hyperresonance and decreased breath sounds that will suggest tension pneumothorax, and if, in spite of this, there is still doubt, the patient should be first treated as having a tension pneumothorax by inserting a needle in the pleural space. This can be quickly done and will give the diagnosis as well as be therapeutic for a tension pneumothorax. Having ruled out a tension pneumothorax, one should proceed to treatment of the patient for cardiac tamponade if signs of circulatory compromise persist.

Although performance of a subxiphoid pericardial window (see Chap. 27) in the relatively stable patient is acceptable, the initial treatment of cardiac tamponade consists of prompt pericardiocentesis.[3] This is usually performed with a 16 to 18 gauge needle that is at least 6 in. in length, incorporates a catheter, and is attached to a 50-mm empty syringe with a three-way stopcock. If time permits, the skin below the xiphoid process is anesthetized, and an electrocardiographic lead is attached to the hub of the needle as the needle is inserted below the skin at roughly a 45° angle and advanced cephalad toward the tip of the left scapula.[1,3] Gentle aspiration is maintained as the needle is advanced. A sense of "give" may be noted as the needle enters the pericardial sac. Nonclotting blood aspirated at this time confirms a pericardial position of the needle. If the needle is advanced into the myocardium, an injury pattern is seen on the electrocardiogram (ECG) monitor. If this is noted, the needle should be withdrawn slightly and then aspirated coincident with the return to the previous baseline electrocardiogram tracing. Other ECG patterns, including premature ventricular contractions, may occur when the needle contacts the myocardium.

Although the pericardial sac can accommodate large volumes of fluid that accumulate chronically, in acute pericardial tamponade as small a volume as 100 cm^3 is capable of compromising cardiac function significantly. Similarly, withdrawal of as little as 50 mL of blood from the pericardial sac results in significant improvement in hemodynamic status.[4] Apart from the signs noted earlier that suggest successful aspiration of the pericardial sac, recovery of blood that immediately clots in the syringe, particularly if the patient's hemodynamic status does not improve, should raise the concern that the needle has penetrated the ventricular wall and ventricular blood rather than pericardial blood is being aspirated. As pericardiocentesis is being conducted, the operating room (OR) should be prepared, and if there is failure of pericardiocentesis or successful pericardiocentesis with stabilization of the hemodynamic status, the pericardiocentesis should be followed by formal thoracotomy and repair of the lacerated heart.[5] This is usually conducted through an anterolateral thoracotomy incision in the fifth intercostal space. However, a median sternotomy is an alternate route for this procedure. On entering the thoracic cavity, the pericardium is identified, and an incision is made in the pericardium with care taken to avoid transection of the phrenic nerve. Blood is aspirated and the laceration in the heart is quickly identified and controlled by digital pressure. With finger control of the bleeding point, interrupted sutures are placed and secured with Teflon pledgets to repair the laceration, and the pericardium is then resutured with a small opening (approximately 1 cm) left to prevent reaccumulation of blood in the pericardial sac. In very rare circumstances, the laceration may involve the coronary arteries. Formal repair of the artery will require heart-lung bypass and should not be done in the emergency setting. If the patient's condition stabilizes and the bleeding and laceration have been controlled with primary sutures, then definitive therapy for the coronary artery laceration may be subsequently pursued on an elective basis.

Massive Hemothorax

Although most patients with traumatic hemothorax are relatively stable and do not require immediate surgical intervention, there is a small group of patients who present with massive intrathoracic hemorrhage, which requires prompt diagnosis and immediate treatment to ensure survival. The mechanism of injury may be blunt or penetrating and generally involves disruption of a major central vascular structure or lacerated intercostal artery. Intrathoracic hemorrhage usually arises from parenchymal lesions of the lung and stops spontaneously, particularly with re-expansion of the lung. The patient with massive intrathoracic hemorrhage presents initially with severe hypotension from blood loss and later with hypoxemia from collapse of the lung caused by the mass effect of the blood in the involved thoracic cavity. Apart from severe hypotension and tachycardia, these patients demonstrate dullness to percussion and decreased air entry on the involved side and a shift of the mediastinum to the opposite side. The central venous pressure or jugular venous pressure is usually low but may be elevated in the unusual circumstance of mass effect from the blood contained within the thorax producing a mechanical obstruction to venous inflow into the chest.

The diagnosis is confirmed and treatment instituted by insertion of a large-bore chest tube from which usually at least 2000 mL of blood drains immediately, followed by a continuous drainage of blood at the rate of at least 100 mL/h. If either of these conditions is present, the patient is considered to have a massive hemothorax requiring surgical intervention. These should not be considered absolute indications for thoracotomy but merely guidelines. The most important criterion for surgical intervention is whether or not the patient remains stable after chest decompression and with fluid resuscitation. If bleeding continues at a rapid rate or if the patient's hemodynamic status cannot be stabilized with rapid infusions of blood and crystalloid, surgical intervention is warranted. Therefore, the patient is taken to the OR, and the involved chest is opened through a posterolateral incision. Once the blood has been evacuated from the pleural space, a search is made for the bleeding point. It is frequently necessary to temporarily clamp the hilum of the lung and intermittently release it in order to identify the area of bleeding that is repaired by direct suture. Occasionally massive hemorrhage requires resection of the involved lung, which should be accomplished quickly using staple devices. Very occasionally, the bleeding point may be from a ruptured thoracic aorta. Usually patients with free bleeding into the thoracic cavity from a ruptured aorta exsanguinate at the scene of the accident or immediately thereafter. However, in certain instances, it is possible to salvage some of these cases by clamping the aorta proximal and distal to the laceration and expeditiously repairing the laceration or inserting an aortic graft prosthesis. If available, a preheparinized shunt may be of use in these circumstances to bypass the lacerated area of the aorta and maintain perfusion of the distal aorta and spinal cord while the repair is undertaken.[6]

Massive Pneumothorax and Airway Injury

Most patients with traumatic pneumothoraces will present with the signs characteristic of a pneumothorax but without any major degree of instability, and the pneumothorax responds very promptly to chest tube insertion. Occasionally, however, the pneumothorax will persist in spite of adequately functioning large-bore chest tubes with attendant massive subcutaneous emphysema and continued hypoxemia and respiratory instability. The patient usually also has some degree of hemoptysis, and this may be evident by blood draining through the endotracheal tube if the patient has been intubated, as is often the case. This scenario suggests the presence of a large airway laceration and requires immediate surgical intervention.

The patient is immediately placed on 100% oxygen. If time allows, a bronchoscopy should be performed in order to identify the level of the lacerated airway. However, thoracotomy is warranted even if the lesion is not identified or there is insufficient time to perform bronchoscopy. It is essential that one is certain that the chest tubes are functioning adequately in these circumstances, and, if mechanical problems are ruled out, the patient should be taken to the operating room promptly. Occasionally, for a right-sided bronchial leak, insertion of a balloon-tipped catheter down the right-main-stem bronchus may allow ventilation of the normal lung after occluding the bronchus by inflation of the balloon. This temporarily stabilizes the patient by decreasing the air leak on the involved side. This, however, is technically very difficult to accomplish and should not take priority over getting the patient to the operating room as quickly as possible. For a left-sided bronchial tear, the endotracheal tube may be directed into the right-main-stem bronchus and the cuff of the endotracheal tube inflated. This would allow ventilation of the right lung until the left lung lesion has been repaired.[7] At surgery, the lesion is identified and repaired directly. If there is massive destruction of the airway with failure to achieve an anastomosis or high risk of subsequent stenosis of the airway, lung resection should be considered.

Massive Bleeding and the Unstable Patient

As indicated previously, it is not always possible to determine precisely whether massive bleeding arises from a thoracic or abdominal source. Therefore, it is crucial that the entire abdomen and chest be prepared and draped for exposure in the OR. In these circumstances, if the bleeding is into the right chest with the apparent impact or penetrating injury in the lower right chest below the nipple line, laparotomy through an upper midline incision should be conducted, since the source of the hemorrhage is usually from a liver injury with penetration of the right hemidiaphragm. Failure to reveal an abdominal source of hemorrhage will necessitate an anterolateral thoracotomy on the right side, which would usually reveal lacerated intercostal arteries that should be identified and ligated. As indicated earlier, injuries to the low-pressure pulmonary vasculature are not usually associated with massive hemorrhage, and the bleeding stops spontaneously, particularly with re-expansion of the lung and decompression of the pleural space. If the impact is to the right upper chest or any portion of the left chest, then massive hemorrhage should be treated by anterolateral thoracotomy on the bleeding side and the incision extended as necessary in order to obtain control of the bleeding site. Occasionally, bleeding into the chest may arise from a penetrating injury to the base of the neck (see Chap. 62). In these circumstances, the chest should be opened through a median sternotomy with the option of extending laterally into the chest as well as above the clavicle, in order to convert the incision to a trap door type of exposure. The median sternotomy under these circumstances allows better exposure of the vascular structures of the base of the neck than would otherwise be available through an anterolateral thoracotomy.

TRAUMATIC AIR EMBOLISM

The exact incidence of this entity in patients with multiple injuries is not determined. However, in order to make the diagnosis, a very high index of suspicion must be maintained, and this diagnosis should be suspected in any patient with sudden cardiovascular collapse who demonstrates a neurologic deficit after chest injury, especially if these signs occur with the initiation of positive pressure ventilation.[8] In most cases, the diagnosis of traumatic air embolism is made at thoracotomy that is conducted on the basis of sudden collapse of a patient who has sustained major chest trauma. Occasionally these patients may be quite stable initially, only to suddenly develop a focal neurologic deficit with cardiovascular collapse immediately after being placed on positive pressure ventilation. Other signs suggestive of the diagnosis are the presence of bubbles within arterial blood drawn by arterial puncture, usually for blood gas analysis. It must be recognized, however, that the most common cause of air bubbles in the syringe is a loosely fitting syringe connector; this must be ruled out prior to making the diagnosis. Occasionally air may be seen in the retinal arteries on fundoscopic examination as well.

An anterolateral thoracotomy should be performed on the side of the penetrating injury, or on the left side if no penetration is apparent. On entry into the thoracic cavity, prevention of further embolization is attempted by cross-clamping the pulmonary hilum. A #18 needle should be used for venting the most anterior surfaces of the left atrium, left ventricle, and ascending aorta. This maneuver is followed by compressing the root of the aorta between the thumb and index finger, which are placed in the transverse sinus. Massaging the heart should drive air bubbles out of the coronary microvasculature. Maintenance of a high systemic blood pressure, with alpha agonists if necessary, should help force trapped air from the heart and brain through the microvasculature into the venous circulation. With the reestablishment of cardiac activity, the left-sided chambers and the aorta should be vented once more. Attention is then directed to the pulmonary lesion that will require repair by direct suture, lobectomy, or pneumonectomy as necessitated by the nature of the injury.

FLAIL CHEST

This condition arises whenever a portion of the chest wall becomes completely discontinuous from the rest of the rib cage. It usually results from blunt chest trauma in which several adjacent ribs are fractured on both sides of the sternum or at least at two locations on each of the ribs involved. This leads to a free-floating segment of the chest wall that positions itself in response to changes in intrapleural pressure rather than to the mechanical positions of the rest of the chest wall. The result is paradoxical movement of this portion of the chest wall. During spontaneous breathing, the flail segment moves inward with the negative intrapleural pressure of inspiration and moves outward with expiration. The diagnosis is frequently missed initially if one relies entirely on the detection of paradoxical movement of the chest wall, since muscle spasm and pain restrict movement of the chest wall and make it very difficult to detect the paradoxical movement. This is particularly so in injuries involving the posterior thorax where the muscle mass makes it even more difficult to detect paradoxical movement. Also, if the patient has been intubated and positive pressure ventilation is instituted, paradoxical movement of the chest wall will not be seen. The presence of multiple adjacent rib fractures involving the same rib in different segments on chest x-ray (CXR) would suggest the entity of flail chest, even though it is not clinically apparent under these circumstances. The degree of pulmonary and hemodynamic disability that arise are related to the extent of the flail, the degree of underlying lung contusion, and the restrictive effect of chest wall pain from the multiple fractures. There is, therefore, a wide spectrum of presentation of patients with flail chest.

In the severely hypoxemic patient with a large flail and/or hemodynamic instability, immediate endotracheal intubation and positive pressure ventilation are indicated with prompt chest tube insertion on the involved side in order to prevent a tension pneumothorax with institution of positive pressure ventilation. Patients who are able to maintain adequate oxygenation and ventilation with supplemental oxygen may be maintained without mechanical ventilation and endotracheal intubation, particularly if adequate pain control can be achieved. This may require frequent or continuous intravenous analgesia in the form of titrated fentanyl, morphine, or other agents. In other circumstances, epidural or less preferable intercostal blockade with long acting local anesthetic agents may be used for controlling the pain. With adequate analgesia, it is possible to avoid endotracheal intubation and mechanical ventilation in most patients with flail chest.[9]

Emergency thoracotomy is not required for treating the flail chest. Also, mechanical fixation of the rib fractures is not usually necessary. It is still controversial as to whether formal thoracotomy and mechanical fixation of the fractured ribs should be considered at all in these patients.[10] However, in situations where thoracotomy may be required for other reasons, it may be appropriate to reduce and plate the fractures involved.

If a decision is made to ventilate the patient with a flail chest, the timing of weaning will not necessarily depend on the disappearance of the paradoxical movement of the chest wall. Rather, weaning from the respirator may be initiated when the gas exchange abnormality associated with underlying lung contusion is resolved. In fact, frequently these patients are completely weaned off respiratory support with adequate pain control and clearing of the lung contusion with residual paradoxical movement apparent for several weeks. A potential disadvantage of the nonsurgical and conservative nonventilating approach to flail chest is the acceptance of a high degree of ultimate chest wall deformity. These chest wall abnormalities are of questionable significance in terms of producing a long-term restrictive defect in these patients.

Other Chest Injuries

Although the following injuries do not produce an immediate threat to life, early diagnosis and treatment are essential, since these conditions will result in mortality if not appropriately treated. These chest injuries are

1. lung contusion
2. myocardial contusion
3. aortic rupture
4. esophageal disruption
5. diaphragmatic hernia
6. rib fractures
7. simple hemopneumothorax

A very brief discussion of the pathophysiology, diagnosis, and treatment of these entities will follow.

LUNG CONTUSION

This lesion results from direct trauma to the lung parenchyma usually by a blunt mechanism, although it can occur from penetrating injuries as well. There is a wide spectrum of pulmonary contusion, ranging from very minor localized hemorrhage into the lung parenchyma to complete obliteration of an entire lung or even bilateral involvement. This injury is often missed because the respiratory failure that develops is not immediately evident, and, indeed, CXR examination may be completely normal initially. It is essential, therefore, that one considers the diagnosis whenever there is significant direct injury to the chest wall. Initially, there may be chest pain and minimal dyspnea or hypoxia. However, within hours there may be slow deterioration in gas exchange and a progressive development of radiologic densities on CXR. As pointed out earlier, there may or may not be an associated flail chest component to this lesion.

The treatment is selective and is based on the degree of respiratory impairment.[11] Minimal gas exchange abnormality in which oxygenation and ventilation can be maintained without endotracheal intubation requires close attention to fluid balance. However, fluid should not be restricted in a patient with lung contusion if fluid resuscitation is required in an otherwise hemodynamically unstable patient. It is essential that close continuous monitoring of the hemodynamic and respiratory status be maintained; if stable, the patient will not require mechanical ventilation. The criteria for initiation of mechanical ventilation are outlined in earlier chapters of this volume, but certain associated disorders will make the likelihood of mechanical ventilation greater. These include preexisting chronic respiratory failure and associated abdominal, thoracic, or central nervous system (CNS) injuries.

MYOCARDIAL CONTUSION

This lesion probably occurs much more commonly than was previously suspected because of the subtle nature of its presentation among other associated injuries.[12] It usually results from the blunt trauma to the sternum, most commonly caused by steering wheel impact. In fact, whenever a fractured sternum is diagnosed in chest trauma, one must assume underlying myocardial contusion. The patient's symptoms frequently are clouded by associated chest wall contusion and other causes for chest wall discomfort and cardiorespiratory dysfunction. The diagnosis is suggested by the presence of ECG abnormalities, serial CPKMB enzyme elevations or abnormal two-dimensional echocardiography, and MUGA scans. ECG abnormalities may vary from few to multiple premature ventricular contractions, persistent tachycardia, dysrhythmias such as atrial fibrillation, bundle branch block, ST segment changes, or even changes indistinguishable from acute myocardial infarction. None of these tests is specific for myocardial contusion.

Because of the nature of this entity and the propensity for developing certain life-threatening dysrhythmias, consideration should be given to monitoring these patients in an ICU environment. Oxygen should be administered. Pain should be treated with parenteral analgesics and the patient treated as outlined in other chapters of this book, as one would treat a patient with myocardial ischemia. The indications for inotropic agents, vasoactive drugs, and other forms of cardiac support are comparable to any patient with myocardial ischemia. Most patients with minor degrees of contusion do not require ICU admission.

AORTIC RUPTURE

Traumatic disruption of the thoracic aorta is frequently lethal. Of those patients who reach the hospital alive, the rupture tends to occur at the point of fixation of the aorta just distal to the take off of the left subclavian artery at the ligamentum arteriosum that coincides with the junction between relatively fixed and mobile portions of the vessel. Therefore, the mechanism is a shear force commonly seen with acceleration–deceleration injuries. Other locations of aortic rupture at the root of the aorta usually result in death at the scene of the accident. Patients who survive the initial injury have their hematoma contained within an intact adventitial layer. Because of the possibility of free rupture and exsanguination whenever this diagnosis is suspected, investigations and treatment should be prompt. Although several radiologic signs are described (such as widened mediastinum, fractures of the first and second ribs, obliteration of the aortic knob, deviation of the trachea to the right, presence of a pleural cap, elevation and rightward shift of the right main stem bronchus, depression of the left main stem bronchus, and obliteration of the space between the pulmonary artery and the aorta), frequently the only suggestive sign is a widening of the mediastinum on plain CXR (Fig. 63-4). Other suggestive signs are the presence of a thoracic bruit or a discrepancy in blood pressure between the upper limb and lower limb or between the right and left upper limbs. Placement of a nasogastric tube may highlight

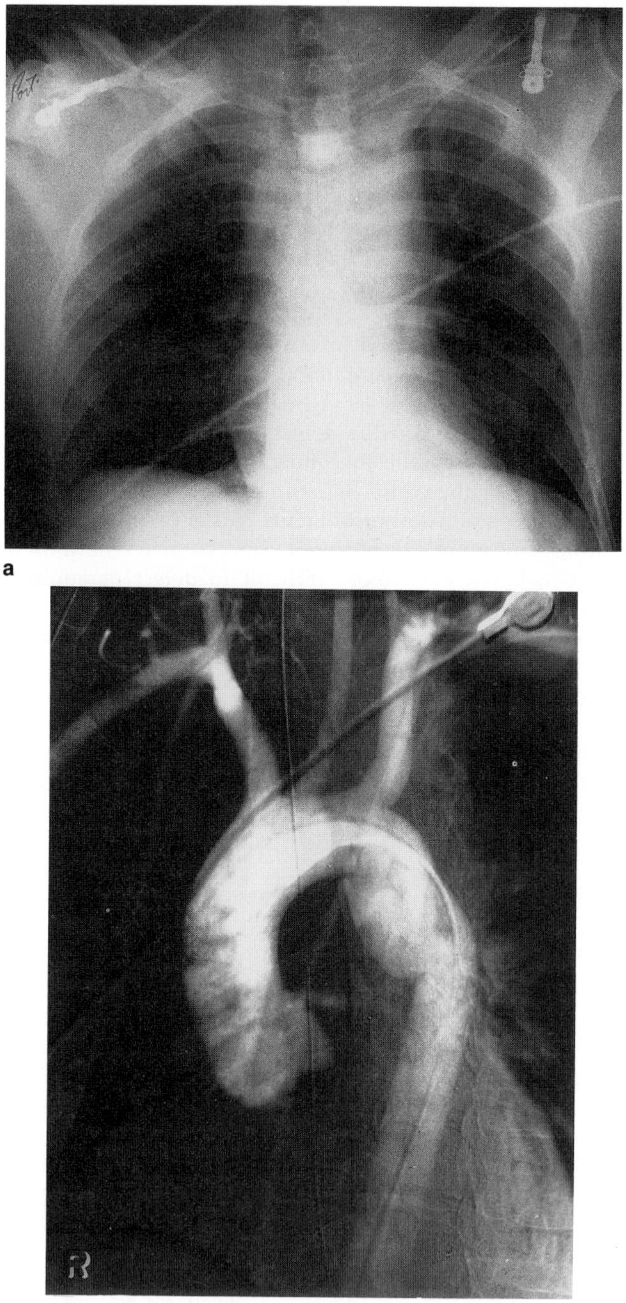

FIGURE 63-4 Ruptured thoracic aorta: *(a)* CXR showing widened mediastinum. *(b)* Aortogram on same patient showing lacerated aorta.

the degree of esophageal deviation and hematoma size on the CXR. Since most CXRs in traumatized patients are done in the supine position, mediastinal size is exaggerated, and this diagnosis is considered in a large percentage of patients who do not indeed have a traumatic aortic rupture. However, because of the lethal nature of this disease, it seems justified that aortography should be performed whenever it is seriously suspected. With this approach, approximately 10 percent of aortograms will be positive for aortic rupture.[13]

Although there is some controversy regarding the use of computed tomography (CT) scan in diagnosing aortic rupture, most authorities recommend that definitive diagnosis requires angiography.[14] The CT scan may be used if the diagnosis is seriously considered. If the CT scan is questionable, then an aortogram should be conducted. In any event, prior to surgery most surgeons will insist on angiography.

The approach to the management of the patient with aortic rupture is surgical repair that frequently requires a resection with placement of a prosthetic graft, although direct repair without the use of a prosthetic graft is sometimes possible. As soon as immediate life-threatening injuries are addressed, the aortic lesion should be surgically treated.

ESOPHAGEAL DISRUPTION

The most common cause of esophageal rupture is iatrogenic during endoscopic maneuvers. However, this injury may result from both penetrating as well as blunt injury. A severe blow to the upper abdomen in the presence of a closed glottis can result in sudden increase in intraesophageal pressure with rupture. The resulting tear allows leakage of gastric contents into the mediastinum with severe mediastinitis.

The patient presents with severe retrosternal chest pain and very soon develops profound hypotension and tachycardia. Frequently, pneumothorax or hemothorax is evident without a rib fracture, and, if a chest tube is inserted, particulate matter may appear in the drainage. The drainage of pleural fluid with a very low pH and high amylase should also suggest the diagnosis. Other radiologic signs include the presence of mediastinal air. The diagnosis may be confirmed by gastrograffin swallow or esophagoscopy.

Treatment consists of massive infusion of crystalloid to maintain hemodynamic stability, antibiotic coverage, and early thoracotomy with repair of the lesion. If the diagnosis is made late in the onset of the disease, direct repair of the laceration may not be possible, and esophageal diversion techniques may become necessary as part of the surgical therapy. This may require the formation of an esophagostomy in the neck as well as a gastrostomy and pleural drainage through chest tubes and parenteral nutrition.[15]

DIAPHRAGMATIC RUPTURE

Lacerations of the diaphragm may occur from blunt and penetrating injuries, and the injury may originate either from the thorax or abdomen. The injury is most frequently diagnosed on the left side, but this does not necessarily mean that left-sided diaphragmatic laceration is more common. Penetrating injuries tend to be small and sharply demarcated, whereas blunt injuries often result in large irregular lacerations with herniation of intraabdominal contents into the chest.

The diagnosis is often missed because of misinterpretation of the CXR, which is often thought to represent an elevated left hemidiaphragm, gastric dilatation, or loculated hemopneumothorax or hematoma. The placement of a nasogastric tube and its location above the diaphragm after entry into the stomach is frequently noted and confirms the diagnosis.

Depending on the degree of herniation of abdominal contents into the thoracic cavity, the symptoms may be very minimal or very significant. A patient with blunt chest or abdominal trauma exhibiting sudden deterioration in respiratory status with inflation of the pneumatic antishock garment should be considered as having a ruptured diaphragm, and the pneumatic antishock garment should be deflated as promptly as possible. If a chest tube has been placed, and during peritoneal lavage the lavage fluid drains through the chest tube, diaphragmatic rupture is likely.

The urgency of treatment of this lesion depends on the degree to which the patient's hemodynamic and respiratory status is compromised. In most instances, an isolated diaphragmatic hernia can be repaired within several hours of admission after the patient is stabilized. Repair is through a midline upper abdominal incision. This allows the complete examination of the abdominal cavity, and the abdominal contents can be reduced quite easily and the repair conducted from within the abdomen. Associated injuries, such as splenic rupture, may then be attended to during the laparotomy. If the diagnosis is made several weeks after the incident, then it is preferable to approach the lesion through a thoracotomy, since any intraabdominal injury would have already declared itself prior to this; also it will be much easier to reduce the abdominal contents from within the thoracic cavity.

RIB FRACTURES

Rib fractures occur very commonly following injuries to the chest. Frequently they are missed on x-ray examination unless special rib views are ordered. However, the diagnosis is suspected when there is localized chest wall pain. The diagnosis is also suggested when one is able to elicit crepitus over the fracture site or auscultate a "click" with inspiration over the fracture site. Tenderness on compression of the chest wall is also suggestive of rib fractures.

The treatment of rib fractures consists of analgesics that may be administered orally, parenterally, or epidurally, depending on the degree of discomfort and the number of ribs involved. In the ICU setting, parenteral analgesics or regional blocks are preferable. Generally the fractured ribs do not require any treatment. However, in the setting of a patient with preexisting pulmonary dysfunction, the restriction produced by fractured ribs can make the difference between normal gas exchange and severe respiratory failure. Maintenance of adequate respiratory function is therefore the mainstay of treatment in these patients.

SIMPLE HEMOPNEUMOTHORAX

In contrast to a tension pneumothorax, the simple hemopneumothorax is usually diagnosed by a combination of physical examination and CXR. Generally if a hemo or pneumothorax is noted following trauma, a chest tube should be inserted regardless of the size of the air or blood collection. This allows decompression of the pleural space as well as monitoring of the drainage from the pleural space. It is particularly important that chest tube decompression of the pleural space is secured before institution of mechanical ventilation or the administration of a general anesthetic.

Abdominal Injuries

GENERAL PRINCIPLES

Apart from pericardial tamponade and traumatic air embolism, any unstable patient with torso trauma with adequately functioning chest tubes demonstrating no free blood or continued major air leak must be considered to have an intraabdominal source of persistent cardiovascular instability. Hence, when the decision is unclear in an unstable patient with torso trauma, the combination of chest x-ray and chest tube insertion will frequently allow one to determine whether or not the lesion is located in the chest. With a negative CXR and no chest tube drainage, in the absence of cardiac tamponade or air embolism, laparotomy is urgently required in the unstable patient with torso trauma.

All such patients should have the entire abdomen and chest prepared and draped for surgical exposure. They should also receive preoperative antibiotics with aerobic gram-negative and anaerobic coverage. It is crucial that the antibiotics be administered prior to the incision in order to minimize septic complications.[16] If there is no fecal contamination within the peritoneal cavity, the antibiotics may be stopped within 24 h. However, in the presence of contamination, antibiotics should be maintained until the temperature is normal and there is no leukocytosis. If the temperature and white blood cell (WBC) count increase after cessation of antibiotics, one must consider that there is residual sepsis that often is in the form of an undrained intraabdominal abscess.

A generous upper midline incision extending from the xiphoid process to just below the umbilicus is the exposure of choice, since most of the lesions producing instability arise from injuries to the upper abdominal contents. This incision can be easily extended up into the chest through lateral thoracotomy or a median sternotomy, or extended into the lower abdomen for lower abdominal injuries. Occasionally the history may suggest an isolated lower abdominal injury, and in these circumstances a lower midline incision beginning at the umbilicus may be undertaken.

Prior to laparotomy, the surgeon needs only to decide that surgical intervention is necessary without having a specific diagnosis. In deciding on laparotomy, one looks for the signs of penetration, perforation, or hemorrhage. Penetration of the peritoneum in stab wounds is diagnosed by exploration of the abdominal wound under local anesthesia with good lighting; once one determines that the peritoneum has been violated, in most instances this will lead to laparotomy. This approach has recently been questioned, and peritoneal lavage has been conducted in conjunction with exploration of the wound (see later for interpretation of peritoneal lavage) in order to determine need for laparotomy on a more selective basis.[17] In these circumstances, demonstration of violation of the peritoneum plus positive peritoneal lavage will be used as indications for laparotomy. All bullet wounds to the abdomen are treated by laparotomy.[18] The signs of perforation are abdominal pain, tenderness, guarding, or rigidity. Signs of hemorrhage may also present with signs of peritoneal irritation, shoulder tip pain, or variable degrees of hemodynamic instability.

On entry into the peritoneal cavity, the presence of dark blood usually suggests a liver injury, whereas bright red blood suggests an arterial source of the bleeding. Rapid evisceration of the small intestine and liberal use of packs wherever blood is accumulating allows identification of the source of the blood loss. One must avoid concentrating on the first site of bleeding and approach the lesions in the order of severity, i.e., the areas that are bleeding most briskly should receive one's attention first.

In deciding on surgical intervention, one relies frequently on the presence of abdominal findings. There are certain situations, however, where the signs may be equivocal or impossible to elicit. In these circumstances, peritoneal lavage is a very helpful technique in determining the need for laparotomy.

As pointed out earlier, massive intraabdominal hemorrhage may require thoracotomy in order to clamp the supradiaphragmatic aorta for controlling intraabdominal hemorrhage and maintaining perfusion to the brain and myocardium. Such a situation may arise when the pneumatic antishock garment is used to tamponade intraabdominal bleeding, and one is unable to deflate the garment without severe hypotension. In these circumstances, thoracotomy should be conducted with clamping of the supradiaphragmatic aorta before deflation of the pneumatic antishock garment and formal laparotomy.

ROLE OF PERITONEAL LAVAGE IN ASSESSING ABDOMINAL TRAUMA

As with any other investigative tool, peritoneal lavage should only be conducted if the results of the procedure will affect the decision to perform a laparotomy. If there is an obvious need for laparotomy, then peritoneal lavage is not indicated.

INDICATIONS

1. Equivocal abdominal findings: Certain conditions such as fractured lower ribs, pelvis, or lumbar spine may pro-

duce abdominal signs that are difficult to separate from injury to intraabdominal structures.
2. Abdominal findings may be impossible to elicit when pain perception is abnormal, such as following severe head injury, drug intoxication, or spinal cord injuries.
3. In certain circumstances, the patient may be unavailable for long periods of time to allow continued repeated physical examination and observation, such as occurs during lengthy surgical or radiologic investigation. Peritoneal lavage may be warranted in these circumstances.
4. When there is an obvious source of hemorrhage, such as a pelvic or extremity fracture that may account for hypotension, it is not always possible to rule out simultaneous intraabdominal blood loss. In these circumstances, peritoneal lavage allows the detection of intraabdominal hemorrhage.

Contraindications

As stated, an absolute contraindication is an existing indication for laparotomy. Relative contraindications include previous abdominal operations with scars in the abdomen, morbid obesity, a preexisting coagulopathy, and advanced pregnancy. An incision can be made above the umbilicus in advanced pregnancy or distant from prior surgical wounds and the open technique performed if necessary.

Technique

The urinary bladder and stomach should be decompressed by urinary catheter and nasogastric tube, respectively. The abdomen should be surgically prepared with an antiseptic solution and local anesthetic infiltrated below the umbilicus in the midline if the patient perceives pain. The skin is incised in the midline, and an opening is made that permits visualization of the subcutaneous tissue and fascia. After one ensures hemostasis in the skin and subcutaneous tissue, the fascia is incised and the peritoneum grasped with clamps. A purse string suture is then inserted in the peritoneum and an opening made for insertion of the peritoneal dialysis catheter into the peritoneal cavity. The catheter is directed toward the pelvis, connected to a syringe, and aspirated. If there is no gross blood or obvious enteric contents aspirated, 10 mL/kg of Ringer's lactate or normal saline is allowed to drain by gravity into the peritoneal cavity. The abdomen is gently palpated and agitated to allow distribution of the fluid throughout the peritoneal cavity. After approximately 5 to 10 min, the fluid is siphoned off and examined. In a controlled environment with appropriately trained personnel an alternative approach involves introduction of the catheter through the Seldinger technique.

INTERPRETATION

1. Aspiration of >5 mL of gross blood or obvious enteric contents signifies a positive peritoneal lavage.
2. A positive result is also suggested by the inability to read newsprint through the IV tubing containing the drained fluid.
3. The fluid is sent for microscopic analysis, and the following criteria are used for positivity: $>10^5$ red blood cells (RBC)/mm^3 or >500 WBC/mm^3 or the presence of bacteria, vegetable fibers, etc. on Gram stain.

With the use of these criteria, the peritoneal lavage findings are false negative in approximately 2 percent of cases, and these are usually in isolated injuries of the pancreas, duodenum, diaphragm, small bowel, or bladder.[19] In general, retroperitoneal injuries are frequently missed by peritoneal lavage.

Recently, CT of the abdomen and, to a lesser extent, ultrasonography of the abdomen have been suggested as substitutes for diagnostic peritoneal lavage in evaluating patients with abdominal trauma. This has arisen chiefly because of the high incidence of false positivity of diagnostic peritoneal lavage. In situations where the patient could be observed very closely in an ICU setting and CT scan is being conducted for other reasons, then the CT scan of the abdomen may be undertaken and conducted instead of diagnostic peritoneal lavage. It must be borne in mind, however, that CT scanning of the abdomen may miss life-threatening intraabdominal injuries.[20]

SPECIFIC ABDOMINAL INJURIES—DIAGNOSIS AND MANAGEMENT PRINCIPLES

Although the nonsurgeon intensivist does not require detailed knowledge of the surgical management of specific intraabdominal injuries, some familiarity with diagnostic and management principles to be applied in the surgical treatment of specific intraabdominal organ injuries is likely to improve the confidence with which these patients are managed in the ICU setting.

Penetrating abdominal injury differs significantly from nonpenetrating injury. Penetrating injury may result from stab wounds or other sharp objects, or from bullet or shotgun wounds. Stab wounds tend to be the least serious in that they involve organs only within the short trajectory of the weapon, and unless the stab wound impales major vessels directly, major hemorrhage is not as likely as in other forms of penetrating or blunt abdominal injury. Patients with stab wounds require exploration of the wound to determine whether or not the peritoneum has been violated. Once the peritoneum has been violated, a decision has to be made to proceed with formal laparotomy unless one is prepared to use peritoneal lavage as an adjunctive test in determining whether laparotomy should be conducted.[17] All bullet and shotgun wounds to the abdomen require laparotomy.[18] These missile injuries usually result in damage to more than one organ. Since kinetic energy transfer is most significantly affected by missile velocity ($K = \frac{1}{2}MV^2$), low-velocity missiles tend to produce limited surrounding injury, whereas high-velocity missiles produce greater damage. Organ involvement, therefore, is very unpredictable because of the variable trajectory and the fact that a straight line joining the point of entry and exit does not usually represent the pathway of the missile. In shotgun injuries, much less damage is inflicted when the injury occurs from far range rather than close range.

The crushing force produced by blunt injuries results in very irregular lacerations. Multiple injuries are also common. Diagnosis and therapy are more challenging and should be more aggressive with blunt injury. Hemorrhage, devitalization of tissue, morbidity, and mortality are all increased in blunt injury as compared to penetrating injuries of the abdomen.

The frequency of organ involvement in penetrating trauma is also different from blunt trauma to the abdomen. In penetrating trauma, the organ involvement in order of frequency is liver, small bowel, stomach, colon, major vessels, and the retroperitoneum. In blunt injuries, the solid organs, namely, the spleen, kidney, and liver, are highest in frequency, followed by the intestines.[21]

STOMACH INJURIES

The diagnosis of stomach injury is suggested by epigastric pain and pain at the shoulder tip if there is free perforation. Usually there is very minimal hemorrhage, and the patient's hemodynamic status is not particularly affected. Upright CXR reveals free air under the diaphragm. The diagnosis may also be suggested by bloody aspirate from the nasogastric tube.

The surgical treatment of stomach injuries is straightforward and involves debridement of devitalized tissue and usually primary suture or anastomosis if resection is required for wide areas of devitalization. It is essential that complete mobilization of the stomach is accomplished so that the entire organ is visualized.

DUODENAL INJURIES

These injuries are often seen in association with other injuries, and the second portion of the duodenum is most commonly involved. Because the duodenum is a retroperitoneal structure, frank peritonitis is a very late sign, and the diagnosis is made only with a very high index of suspicion based on the mechanism of injury. A useful sign is the identification of retroperitoneal air on plain film of the abdomen (Fig. 63-5). Occasionally a free perforation of the first portion of the duodenum will produce pneumoperitoneum and be identified on an upright CXR.

In the surgical treatment of injuries to the duodenum complete mobilization and visualization of the entire duodenum are crucial. Patients with intramural hematoma of the duodenum may present with vomiting and gastric outlet obstructive symptoms; radiologic examination of the stomach and duodenum with contrast agents reveals the presence of an intramural hematoma. If this is the only injury, treatment can be conservative with nasogastric suction and intravenous fluids until the hematoma resolves. If the lesion is found at laparotomy, an incision in the wall of the duodenum with evacuation of the hematoma is easily accomplished.[22] The principle of treatment is to debride the area of injury, removing all devitalized tissue. If, after this is accomplished, the edges of the duodenum can be approximated without undue tension, primary anastomosis is appropriate. The defect may also be closed by a serosal patch from adjacent small bowel or a resection and end-to-end anastomosis. When these techniques are not possible, then Roux-en-Y anastomosis between the duodenal ends

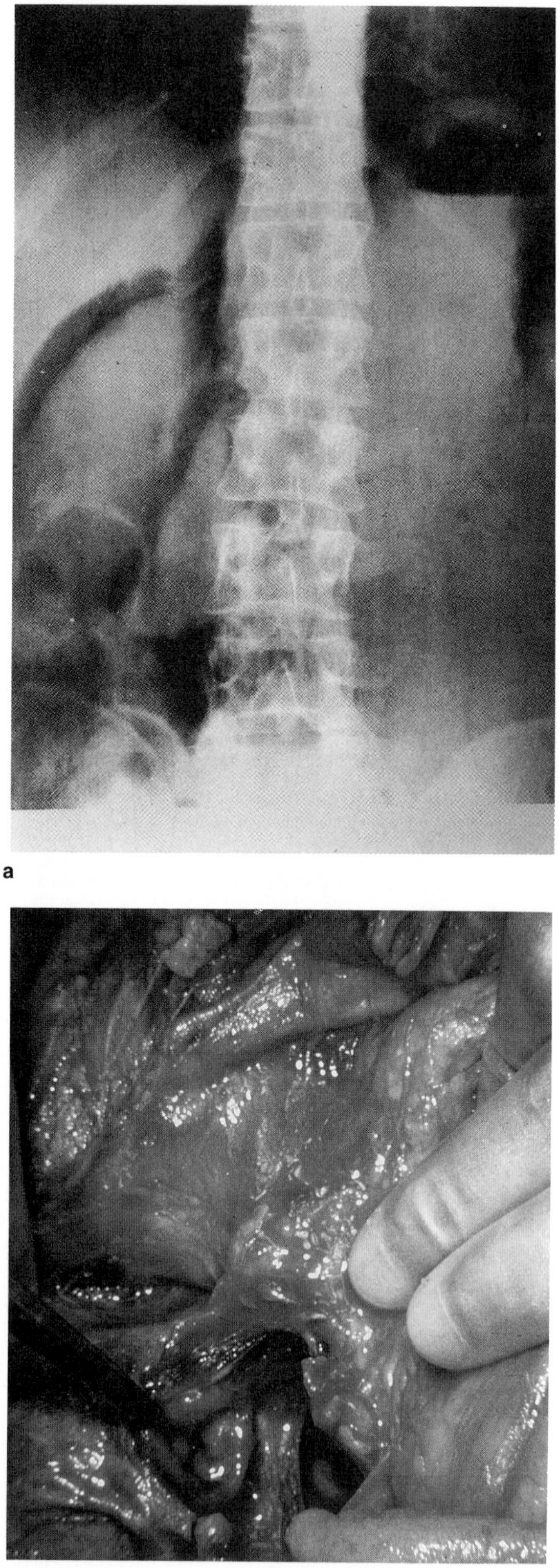

a

b

FIGURE 63-5 Ruptured duodenum: *(a)* Plain radiograph showing retroperitoneal air around right kidney. *(b)* Transected duodenum found at laparotomy on the same patient.

and the small bowel needs to be conducted. When there is concern about the duodenal closure, it is wise to place a duodenal catheter brought out as a duodenostomy. If the anastomosis is not secure, the resulting duodenal fistula will be controlled and can be treated by observation and parenteral nutrition.

PANCREATIC INJURIES

Injuries to the pancreas usually result from blunt trauma when the pancreas impacts against the vertebral column. Diagnosis is often difficult because the retroperitoneal position of this organ prevents early physical signs of peritoneal irritation. Frequently, the diagnosis is made at laparotomy for other associated conditions. However, the diagnosis is suggested by an increase in serum amylase. If the diagnosis is suspected and physical examination is minimal, upper gastrointestinal (GI) radiographic studies with gastrograffin may demonstrate a widening of the duodenal loop. CT scan of the abdomen allows assessment of the retroperitoneum and pancreatic area for evidence of retroperitoneal hematomas or even ductal injury. Peritoneal lavage is frequently negative in the presence of severe retroperitoneal pancreatic injuries.

Treatment of these injuries depends largely on whether or not the pancreatic duct has been violated. In simple contusions of the pancreas, drainage of the area is all that is required after mobilization of the pancreas and full inspection to rule out any associated ductal injury. Any devitalized area should be debrided and bleeding points controlled by direct suture ligations combined with cautery.

When the duct has been injured, there is often a mixture of pancreatic fluid and blood over the surface of the pancreas that should be exposed for complete inspection. Although ductal injury involving the body and tail of the pancreas may be treated by transection and anastomosis of the ends of the duct to the small bowel, this injury is more appropriately treated by distal pancreatic resection without an enteroanastomosis. When the head of the pancreas is involved, a Roux-en-Y anastomosis of the distal pancreatic segment is advisable.[23] This type of injury usually is a combined pancreaticoduodenal injury and may require a Whipple procedure (pancreaticoduodenectomy). This procedure carries a high mortality and should be conducted only when more conservative measures are unsuccessful. An alternative approach to combined pancreaticoduodenal injury is the diverticulization procedure,[24] in which the pylorus is closed internally, and a gastrojejunostomy is constructed with an added option of drainage of the duodenum through a tube duodenostomy after repairing the duodenal injury by primary sutures. The entire area is drained with drains placed around the peripancreatic and duodenal area and exiting posteriorly. It should be emphasized that pancreaticoduodenal resection should be a last resort because of the high associated mortality. Less aggressive treatment should be instituted initially if possible.[25] Even though this approach is more likely to result in complications such as pancreatic abscess, the overall mortality is still less with drainage rather than resection.

Postoperatively, patients with pancreatic injury are at risk for development of complications such as pancreatic abscess and pseudocyst. The former is suggested by a continued septic course with the development of a peripancreatic mass with the consistency on CT scan that is characteristic of liver necrosis and abscess. The presence of this lesion requires drainage and antibiotic coverage.

The complication of pseudocyst of the pancreas results from localization of pancreatic secretions and debris in the lesser sac. Symptoms may be those of a mass effect and may include gastric outlet obstruction with vomiting. The presence of a symptomatic mass in these patients requires decompression of the pseudocyst. However, if the pseudocyst is not symptomatic, it may be observed for up to 6 weeks, at which time, if there are no signs of spontaneous decrease in size, it should be drained. There is much controversy as to whether drainage should be conducted internally or externally. If the external route is chosen, percutaneous drainage may be done under ultrasound or CT scan control. In any event, if this technique is attempted, and the catheter is incapable of handling the secretions because of their consistency, internal drainage should be performed via pseudocystgastrostomy or cystenterostomy.[26] Apart from the mass effect of the pseudocyst, these patients require frequent monitoring of the serum amylase, which frequently remains elevated during the active process of increasing size of the pseudocyst.

INTESTINAL INJURIES

Acceleration-deceleration injuries are most likely to occur at points of fixation of the bowel, e.g., the ligament of Treitz, ileocecal junction, rectosigmoid area. Blow-out perforations of the small bowel, however, can occur at any point in the small bowel. Another mechanism for bowel perforation and injury is related to the lap seat belt. The presence of contusion on the abdominal wall from a lap seat belt often makes it difficult to assess the abdomen for signs of peritoneal irritation. In these circumstances, diagnostic peritoneal lavage with the possible addition of CT scan examination of the abdomen is quite helpful in determining whether or not there is a seat-belt-related intestinal injury. The presence of peritoneal signs will necessitate laparotomy.

Treatment of injuries to the small bowel involves debridement of devitalized tissue and control of any associated bleeding points with primary suture. Devitalized areas may require formal resection of segments of bowel; this is usually followed by primary anastomosis with excellent results. The treatment of injuries to the colon depends on the time elapsed between injury and surgery, the degree of contamination, the stability of the patient, and the presence of associated injuries. If there is minimal gross contamination, and the patient has been operated upon within 3 to 4 h and is not in shock, primary anastomosis may be conducted safely. Devitalization of a large portion of the right colon often requires resection of the ileum and ascending colon with an ileocolic anastomosis. Left colonic lesions are more likely to be associated with frank fecal spillage. However, if there is very minimal spillage and no evidence of continued hemorrhage or associated injury, even these injuries may be treated by primary closure.[27] Whenever there is doubt, however, the safest technique for treating left-sided colonic injuries is the fashioning of a colostomy together with repair of the laceration and irrigation of the peritoneal cavity. In situations where the lacerated bowel can be exteriorized, the resection may be performed and the ends of the bowel brought out as a proximal defunctioning colostomy and a mucous fistula. This technique is preferable to a defunctioning colostomy and Hartman's procedure (oversewing of the rectal stump in the pelvis), because of the greater difficulty in subsequent reconstruction of the large bowel with Hartman's procedure.

Injuries to the rectum should be assessed in the operating room and frequently require general anesthesia with a proctosigmoidoscopic assessment to determine whether or not the anorectum has been violated. Because of the propensity for major septic complications, particularly in the multiply injured patient, patients with rectal injuries should be treated by a proximal defunctioning colostomy and the fashioning of a mucous fistula through which a catheter may be inserted for performing complete rectal washout.[28] The irrigation of the rectum is conducted with the anus being held dilated. The perirectal space is then drained with appropriately placed drainage tubes. Once the gross fecal contents have been irrigated, the rectal mucosa and major lacerations should be approximated and the sphincter muscles reapproximated with interrupted sutures. This approach in the acute phase prevents retraction of the transected sphincter muscles, which makes later repair and maintenance of continence very difficult. Failure to adhere to the system of drainage, irrigation, and proximal defunctioning colostomy can lead to a protracted septic course with multiorgan failure and death from rectal injuries. A patient with a rectal injury with gross fecal contamination in the perineal area may require reexploration if the patient continues to run a septic course in the ICU.

As indicated on the chapter on intraabdominal sepsis, the abdomen remains a frequent source of sepsis in surgical patients in the ICU setting. These complications arise primarily from operations on the bowel, so that any traumatized patient who has had bowel lesions treated surgically and who remains septic should be considered as having an intraabdominal source for that sepsis. This requires intensive investigation that uses modalities such as CT scan and ultrasound technique and drainable lesions may be treated by percutaneous techniques under CT scan or ultrasound control. When such techniques are contraindicated or when the source is not obvious in spite of investigations, laparotomy may be the last resort to identify and treat septic complications. With the availability of sophisticated technology in the form of CT scan and ultrasound investigations, it is usually possible to make a diagnosis prior to laparotomy, and only under very unusual circumstances is the lesion not identified prior to laparotomy. One of the areas of sepsis in patients with perforated bowel is wound infection. Although the incisions in these patients are frequently left packed open rather than closed primarily, in some instances the wound is closed primarily. One has to be aware of the possibility of suppuration in the wound; at the first sign of sepsis, the wound should be opened to determine whether or not there is infection in the wound. Although there is not very good experimental evidence to substantiate it, most abdominal wounds are left packed open when there is gross intraabdominal contamination in order to prevent wound infections.

LIVER INJURIES

Although liver injuries may occur from both blunt and penetrating trauma, patients with blunt injury to the liver tend to carry a higher morbidity and mortality because of the irregular type of laceration and its involvement of an entire lobe or frequently both lobes of the liver. The signs of liver injuries are very nonspecific, and the diagnosis is frequently made only at laparotomy, the patient presenting with signs of intraabdominal hemorrhage. Liver hemorrhage may be the chief cause of a patient presenting in hemorrhagic shock. In the patient who has minimal signs and in whom peritoneal lavage is indicated, liver injuries may be suggested by a positive diagnostic peritoneal lavage.[19] These injuries are very clearly outlined by CT scan or ultrasound of the abdomen, and in an otherwise stable patient, these investigative techniques may replace diagnostic peritoneal lavage. Other signs that suggest the possibility of liver injuries include bruising of the lower chest, particularly on the left side; contusions over the upper abdomen; fractured lower ribs, particularly on the left side; an elevated hemidiaphragm, and increased size of the liver shadow on plain films of the abdomen. The usual indication for surgery in a patient with liver injury is intraabdominal hemorrhage.[29]

Although the reported mortality rate from major liver trauma varies from 20 to 60 percent, most of the deaths are due to severe associated injuries, particularly of the head and thorax. When death is attributed to the liver injury itself, it is usually secondary to uncontrollable hemorrhage and later in the course is due to sepsis and multiorgan failure. Careful surgical technique and postoperative management of these patients will decrease the morbidity and mortality. The objectives of surgical management of liver injuries are **1.** control hemorrhage, **2.** remove nonviable tissue, and **3.** provide adequate drainage.

Exposure must be adequate and requires midline upper abdominal incision with the ability to extend into the chest. The liver itself should be completely mobilized by transection of the triangular ligaments as well as the falciform ligament, with care taken to secure the inferior phrenic artery.

CONTROL OF HEMORRHAGE

In most instances, once the peritoneal blood has been aspirated, a nonbleeding hepatic laceration is identified. Such lacerations require drainage and no further surgical exploration. If hepatic bleeding is still active at the time of laparotomy, then the initial maneuver is to pack the liver area very tightly with dry gauze and continue with the remainder of the laparotomy for approximately 15 min. This allows time for stabilization of the patient's hemodynamic status as well as time for replacement of fluid deficits. If, on removal of the pack, the bleeding has stopped, as is frequently the case, then the treatment is drainage of the perihepatic space. Failure to control bleeding by this technique requires clamping the portal triad with examination of the wounds to determine the source of hemorrhage and direct suture ligation of the bleeding points. Intermittent release of the clamp will allow examination for hemostasis. Hepatic artery ligation may be of benefit in some patients, although its effectiveness has been questioned.[30] When bleeding arises from the retrohepatic vena cava as evidenced by failure to control the bleeding by clamping of the portal triad, it is necessary to rotate the liver medially and visualize the retrohepatic vena cava. In such instances, the use of an intracaval shunt would assist in preserving a dry field so that the injured hepatic veins and retrohepatic vena cava may be identified and sutured.[31] In extreme circumstances complete vascular isolation of the liver by also clamping the suprahepatic and infrahepatic vena cava may be successfully applied, although this maneuver frequently results in cardiac arrest of the already hypovolemic patient. In some instances, formal resection of liver tissue is required to control hemorrhage, particularly when there is major devitalization of liver tissue. This usually does not require formal anatomic lobectomy but instead consists of resectional debridement of the bleeding devitalized liver tissue as demarcated by the edges of the laceration itself. The bare area of the liver is then treated with suture ligature, cautery, and the application of microfibrillar collagen or other types of topical hemostatic agents. In some instances, the patient may lose several units of blood and also have other injuries that require attention. In addition, with the massive blood transfusions, the patient may show signs of coagulopathy. In those instances, it is advisable to pack the liver temporarily, close the abdominal wound, and correct the coagulopathy in the ICU with the hope of stabilizing the patient. The patient may then be taken back to the operating room in 48 h for removal of the pack, after which the bleeding will have either ceased or decreased considerably, allowing formal treatment of the bleeding points.[32]

RESECTION OF DEVITALIZED TISSUE

As pointed out earlier, formal hepatic lobectomy is seldom necessary for trauma. Resection is usually confined to removal of frankly nonviable tissue. The area for resectional debridement is usually well demarcated by the nature of the liver laceration itself. Manual compression is maintained on the liver, while the resection is conducted in order to control hemorrhage. Intermittent packing and compression of the liver may be required to allow hemodynamic stabilization of the patient during the procedure.

DRAINAGE

The lacerated liver continues to drain bile, blood, and tissue fluid for a considerable length of time postoperatively. Accumulation of this fluid in the peritoneal cavity is prevented by appropriately functioning peritoneal drains. T-tube drainage of the common bile duct is not required unless there is a central ductal injury requiring surgical repair or unless the common bile duct is enlarged because of previous pathology.

During the postoperative period, these patients frequently run a febrile course, which makes it difficult to determine whether or not there is underlying sepsis. Therefore, antibiotics are continued in the immediate perioperative period. With major hepatic resection, glucose infusions are required to treat hypoglycemia, and hypoalbuminemia needs to be treated temporarily with plasma and albumin infusion until the nutritional status of the patient is improved. Coagulation defects are treated with fresh frozen plasma, vitamin K supplement, and platelets when indicated. Most of these patients also develop some degree of jaundice that is usually transient and may last from several days to several weeks. Because many of the signs indicated earlier are common in uncomplicated liver injuries, the presence of septic complications may go unnoticed unless one is quite vigilant. Frequent radiologic investigation and monitoring of the WBC are necessary, and baseline estimate of these parameters would allow one to determine whether the patient is progressing satisfactorily or not. A patient whose bilirubin and WBC are decreasing, who suddenly increases his serum bilirubin or has a spike in his temperature, should be investigated carefully for a source of sepsis in the abdomen. Another complication that may arise in hepatic injury is hemobilia which may present with upper GI hemorrhage, as evidenced by hematemesis or blood-stained nasogastric drainage. This lesion requires immediate investigation in the form of hepatic angiography and CT scan or ultrasound. Once the source of the intrahepatic hemorrhage is identified, hepatic artery embolization or balloon tamponade is a viable option for controlling the hemobilia.[33] Failure of this may require formal hepatic resection in order to treat this complication.

SPLEEN INJURIES

Injuries to the spleen should be suspected in patients who present with left upper quadrant pain, especially in the presence of left lower rib fractures. There may be associated shoulder tip pain on the left side. A frequent mode of presentation, however, is a patient with signs of massive intraperitoneal hemorrhage requiring immediate laparotomy for hemorrhagic shock. In situations where the signs are equivocal, peritoneal lavage may be necessary. CT scan or ultrasound examination of the abdomen in the otherwise stable patient can help diagnose splenic injury. Although there is some argument for treating splenic injuries in children conservatively without laparotomy,[34] whenever there is suggestion of associated injury or whenever there is an acute splenic injury in the adult, laparotomy is advised.

At laparotomy, the aim should be to control hemorrhage with splenic salvage if possible. In order to assess the splenic injury adequately, complete mobilization and delivery of the spleen into the wound is necessary. Superficial supcapsular tears of the spleen may be treated by initial packing for approximately 15 min. Failure to control the hemorrhage by this means will require such techniques as the application of microfibrillar collagen or fine sutures. Identifiable bleeding points are coagulated as well as suture ligated, particularly when bleeding points occur near the hilum of the spleen. Ligation of the short gastric vessels in certain instances will also arrest splenic hemorrhage. In some instances, a lacerated portion of the spleen may be excised with suturing of the remainder of the spleen with large chromic sutures with Teflon pledgets for securing the sutures. When multiple lacerations are evident, it is possible to control the hemorrhage by placing the spleen in a net of Dexon mesh, which can be tightened to produce compression and control of hemorrhage.[35] If control of hemorrhage by a combination of these techniques is impossible, then splenectomy should be conducted. Also, if the patient remains unstable from other major injuries and bleeding from the spleen is a major problem, splenectomy should be conducted most expeditiously in order to decrease the operating time and improve the patient's chances at survival.

Postsplenectomy patients are particularly prone to septic complications; prior to discharge from the unit, these patients should be given Pneumovax. Patients should also be warned that any infective process is cause for seeking medical attention because of the potential risk for overwhelming sepsis in postsplenectomized patients.[36] One of the areas of concern in monitoring patients postsplenectomy in the ICU is the frequent occurrence of leukocytosis and thrombocytosis. This makes monitoring for intraabdominal sepsis difficult, and one has to follow WBC until it plateaus. A deviation or a sudden increase from a plateau high WBC could be considered as evidence of occult sepsis. In patients who are in the ICU for prolonged periods of time with platelet counts above 1 million, consideration should be given to prophylactic anticoagulation to prevent thrombotic complications.

INJURIES TO THE EXTRAHEPATIC BILIARY TRACT

These injuries are relatively infrequent but when present are usually diagnosed at laparotomy because there are no specific signs on physical examination for this type of injury.

Although it may be possible to repair an injury to the gall bladder, in most circumstances cholecystectomy is performed because no data are available to determine whether primary suture of the gall bladder results in further episodes of gall bladder symptomatology. Certainly in the presence of other intraabdominal injuries cholecystectomy should be performed if the gall bladder is injured.

Injury to the extrahepatic bile ducts will be evidenced by bile drainage into the peritoneal cavity, and the type of repair necessary will depend on the nature of the injury itself. Usually debridement of the wound and primary anastomosis are possible, and a proximal T-tube is used for stenting the anastomosis. In situations where the ends of the bile duct cannot be approximated, resection and enteroanastomosis with T-tube drainage will be necessary. An alternative approach utilizes the gall bladder for the anastomosis between the biliary tract and the bowel.

Patients with injury to the biliary tract are also prone to septic complications, and the most common cause of septic complications in this setting is failure to decompress and drain the biliary tract, resulting in continued drainage of infected bile into the peritoneal cavity. The aim of postoperative management, therefore, is to maintain patency of the biliary tract and decompression of the biliary tract until adequate healing is accomplished. In observing patients with biliary drainage, assessment of the nature of the drainage is important. Clear, thin liquid drainage that suddenly becomes thick or purulent, especially in the presence of fever or leukocytosis, should be cause for immediate Gram stain and culture of the bile and the initiation of appropriate antibiotics. Similarly, change in the volume of drainage (either an increase or sudden decrease or cessation of drainage) should be cause for investigating adequate function of the drainage tube by instilling contrast material through the tube and visualizing the biliary tract.

RETROPERITONEAL HEMORRHAGE

Frequently at laparotomy one is faced with hemorrhage in the retroperitoneal space. This can be very difficult to deal with, and wherever possible preoperative investigation of the genitourinary tract in the form of intravenous pyelogram and CT scan as well as x-ray of the pelvis will allow one to consider specific diagnostic possibilities. When the patient is taken to the OR prior to any of these investigations because of instability, however, a decision needs to be made regarding the proper handling of the retroperitoneal hemorrhage.

In general, hemorrhage that is associated with a major pelvic fracture and confined to the pelvis or originating in the pelvis should be treated without exploration unless there is a penetrating injury that is likely to involve the iliac vessels. Exploration of the retroperitoneal hematoma usually results in massive uncontrollable hemorrhage when the source is arising from the pelvic fracture. This type of hemorrhage is often best treated by external fixation of the fractured pelvis and blood transfusions (see Chap. 64). Angiography may be done in circumstances where hemorrhage is continuing with a view to embolizing any identifiable bleeding artery. The mainstay of controlling hemorrhage from pelvic fractures, however, is immediate stabilization of the pelvis to prevent undue motion of the fracture fragments, and this is most expeditiously accomplished by external fixator application.

Apart from hematomas arising from the pelvis, those hematomas that are not pulsatile or expanding and located in the lateral retroperitoneal spaces should also be left unexplored and further investigation done postoperatively in the form of CT scan and IV pyelography if indicated. If the lesion is expanding or pulsatile, the retroperitoneal space has to be explored to identify the bleeding point and control it, as indicated by the nature of the lesion. As pointed out earlier, temporary control of an infradiaphragmatic source of hemorrhage can be achieved by thoracotomy and clamping of the supradiaphragmatic aorta. However, when the hematoma or bleeding does not extend to the aortic hiatus, temporary control may be achieved by compressing the aorta at the diaphragmatic crura after dividing the gastrohepatic ligament. This compression can be achieved by an assistant's hand, an aortic compressor, or a sponge stick. By incising the peritoneum and mobilizing the esophagus to the left, a clamp may also be applied directly to the aorta in order to gain temporary control of intraabdominal hemorrhage.

When the retroperitoneal hematoma is centrally located in the midabdomen, this represents possible injury to the pancreas and peripancreatic area. These hematomas require exploration with a view to determining the extent of the injury to the pancreas and particularly to determine whether or not the pancreatic duct has been violated. The lesion is then treated as outlined earlier for pancreatic trauma.

Occasionally, retroperitoneal hemorrhage, particularly in the pelvis, cannot be controlled by surgical means, and one has to resort to packing of the retroperitoneal space and closure of the abdomen with a view to exploring the patient within 48 h, hopefully after cessation of the bleeding. These patients require very close observation in the ICU with correction of any coagulopathy and should be covered with appropriate antibiotics to prevent sepsis from complicating their massive blood loss.

GENITOURINARY INJURIES

Although hematuria is absent in 5 to 10 percent of patients with genitourinary trauma,[37] this still is a most important sign of injury. The patient frequently has sustained injury to the flank or diffuse transfer of force to the abdomen. Occasionally there may be direct penetrating injury into the bladder or kidney. Penetrating injury resulting in ureteric lacerations is very rare. Although in the past 15 years, traumatic hematuria of any degree has been investigated with IV pyelography, a more selective approach has been adopted recently. This change in approach has resulted from the low yield of IV pyelography in all patients with trauma; also in the presence of hematuria, the yield in terms of positive lesions identified varies from 15 to 60 percent.[38] Most of the injuries discovered (65 to 70 percent) are considered minor, involving a parenchymal laceration or contusion that does not require surgical intervention. Major parenchymal laceration through the corticomedullary junction and often into the collecting system usually causes gross hematuria and represents 10–15 percent of renal injuries.[39] The remainder of renal injuries are associated with a shattered kidney or renal pedicle injury. These facts, together with the cost of the procedure as well as the incidence of allergic reaction (5.7 percent) including anaphylaxis, renal failure, and death 0.0074 percent), have led to a change in the approach to hematuria in assessing genitourinary trauma. In most instances, the major cause of death from genitourinary trauma is due to the associated injuries, and the investigation using intravenous pyelography has had very little effect on management or outcome in general. Microhematuria without shock has not been shown to be associated with lesions requiring surgical intervention, while gross hematuria or microhematuria with shock or a major abdominal injury has been associated with lesions requiring surgery in up to 10 percent of cases.[38,39] Penetrating renal injuries are associated with lesions requiring surgery both with and without hematuria.[39] Based on these observations, the recommendation at present is that IV pyelography should not be routine in abdominal trauma as it has been in the past. Also, if the patient is having a CT scan of the abdomen for another reason or if there is only microhematuria without shock or any evidence of severe injury, IV pyelography is not recommended. The IV pyelogram, however, is indicated in the following circumstances: (a) if a CT scan is not being done and there is gross hematuria or microhematuria with shock, (b) hematuria in the presence of a major abdominal injury, or (c) if there is a penetrating injury and one suspects from the trajectory the possibility of renal injury even without hematuria. One other relative indication for IV pyelography is if the patient is unstable but hematuria is present, a one-shot IV pyelography, if time allows, may be conducted in order to assess the functioning of both kidneys in the event that nephrectomy may be required during laparotomy.

The main indication for surgical intervention in renal trauma is an injury with major hemorrhage such that the patient's hemodynamic stability could not be maintained with rapid crystalloid and blood transfusions. Otherwise, most patients with renal trauma are treated initially nonoperatively (Fig. 63-6). They should be observed very closely in an ICU setting for any deterioration in hemodynamic status suggesting continued major hemorrhage that requires surgical intervention. If there is failure to visualize both kidneys on IV pyelography, then CT scan or angiography should be conducted to determine the extent of the injury producing a nonfunctioning kidney.

Hematuria may also result from injury to the bladder, and the suspicion of bladder injury should be investigated by cystography with at least three views being taken with the bladder filled as well as emptied to determine whether or not there is any extravasation of bladder contents that is an indication for surgical intervention.

Although in most multiply injured patients, urinary catheterization per urethra is routine for monitoring the urine volume and consistency as a reflection of the hemodynamic status, there are certain contraindications, as indicated in Chap. 59, to catheterization per urethra. Blood at the urethral meatus or the presence of scrotal or perineal hematomas with a large high-riding boggy prostate may signal injury to the urethra; these findings require a urethrogram to exclude urethral laceration prior to Foley catheter placement. Urethral rupture requires urologic consultation and treatment.

Postoperative care of these patients requires maintenance of renal perfusion; thus, careful attention to maintenance of hemodynamic stability is important. In addition, maintenance of good urinary output and close monitoring of the degree of hematuria as well as the volume of urine is also required in the ICU setting. An occult injury to the genitourinary tract with extravasation of urine that is left undiagnosed is another means whereby the ICU patient following multiple trauma may develop septic complications. This type of complication should be investigated by ultrasonog-

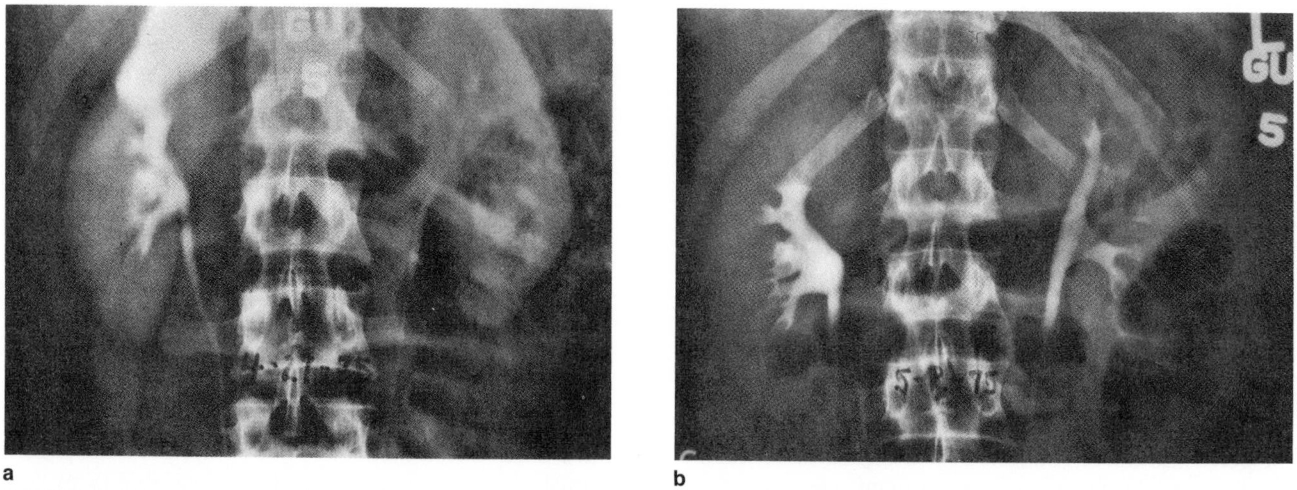

FIGURE 63-6 Spontaneous resolution of renal injury: *(a)* IVP showing extravasation of contrast immediately after blunt trauma with hematuria. *(b)* Repeat IVP after 5 days of observation with no extravasation.

raphy or CT scan, although IV pyelography may also allow visualization of the extravasation. Drainage of the urinoma may be necessary if it results in sepsis.

CASE ILLUSTRATION

The following case history demonstrates some of the principles outlined earlier in the management of patients with torso trauma.

Mrs. S.M. is a 47-year-old female who was transferred to the Toronto General Hospital following a fight with her husband in which she was shot in the right upper quadrant of the abdomen with a small-caliber handgun at close range. There was no loss of consciousness at the scene and when brought in to the emergency room (ER) she had a Glasgow coma score of 15, a heart rate of 110, and a blood pressure of 100 systolic. She had been previously well, and on examination, she was in moderate distress, alert, and oriented. Head and neck examination was negative. Examination of the chest revealed an exit wound at the left lower chest in the posterior axillary line (Fig. 63-7). However, she had good air entry and was breathing spontaneously. The entrance wound was in the right subcostal area as indicated. She had a left chest tube inserted, and this revealed very minimal blood and no air; oxygen was applied by mask. The remainder of her physical examination apart from diffuse tenderness in the upper abdomen was negative, including a rectal examination. She had a Foley catheter inserted, and this failed to reveal any gross hematuria. The remainder of her examination showed an entry and exit wound of the left elbow. Her hemoglobin on admission was 109 g/L with a WBC of 8.4 × 10^9/L; her electrolytes, PT, and PTT were within normal limits. Arterial blood gases on 60% O_2 by face mask were: pH of 7.34 with a P_{CO_2} of 24, P_{O_2} of 219, and bicarbonate of 13. CXR after insertion of the left chest tube showed no abnormalities.

She was taken to the operating room (OR) for laparotomy within $\frac{1}{2}$ h of admission to the ER, and surgery was commenced 55 min after arrival at the Toronto General Hospital. Thirty-five minutes into surgery, she was started on IV antibiotics.

At surgery she was found to have approximately 1.5 L of fresh blood in the peritoneal cavity, and there was a through and through injury of the right lobe of the liver involving the inferior surface. This required minimal debridement of devitalized liver tissue and suture ligation of a small artery on the inferior surface of the liver.

Anterior examination of the stomach was normal. The lesser sac was entered, and a hole was demonstrated in the posterior wall of the stomach that was not evident on initial examination of the stomach. The entry site was also identified on the lesser curvature at the incisura. Both these lesions were closed by two layers of sutures. A hematoma was noted in the omentum of the splenic flexure, and dissection revealed a 7 × 1.5 cm tangential wound in the colon with a small amount of fecal contamination. A loop colostomy was constructed at the site of

FIGURE 63-7 Entrance and exit wounds traversing abdomen and chest.

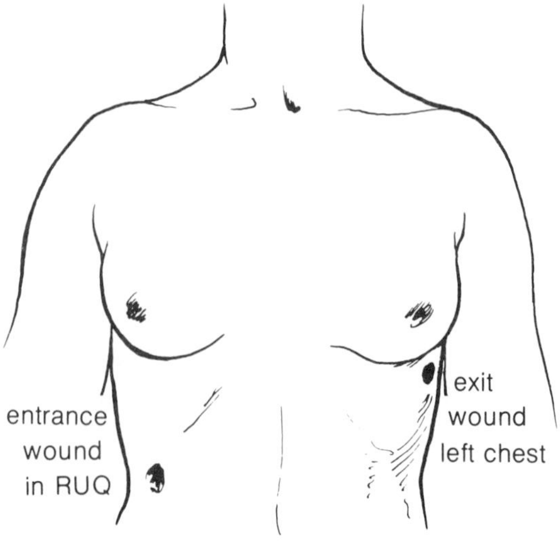

colonic perforation. The abdomen was irrigated with normal saline profusely, and a right upper quadrant drain was placed. The skin was closed with skin clips after closing the fascia. She was taken to the surgical ICU immediately postoperatively, and, after 48 h in the ICU, she was transferred to the ward. By 1 week postop, she was on a regular diet, and she was afebrile with a WBC cell count of 7000 at the time. The antibiotics were then stopped. Three days later, her temperature increased to 38.3°C but she was asymptomatic and physical examination was not abnormal. Reassessment on the 13th postoperative day revealed an obvious redness to the wound with marked tenderness. The staples were removed and pus drained from the wound. The day after, the wound was packed open with Hygeol solution packs. She still remained febrile and at 16 days postoperative, under CT scan control, one of two identified collections of fluid was aspirated and yielded thick, foul-smelling pus (Fig. 63-8). This was considered to be an infected hematoma, and the patient was taken to the OR on the next day, when a subhepatic infected hematoma was drained and further debridement conducted. The peritoneal cavity was lavaged again with saline, and the patient was started on Ancef. She did well and was discharged on the 22nd postoperative day. Her colostomy was then closed 2½ months later.

CASE DISCUSSION

The points illustrated in this case history regarding management of the patient with torso trauma are as follows:

1. The patient was taken to the OR without any peritoneal lavage or CT scan of the abdomen, since the results of these tests would not alter the decision for laparotomy.

FIGURE 63-8 CT scan of abdomen showing anterior right subhepatic abscess.

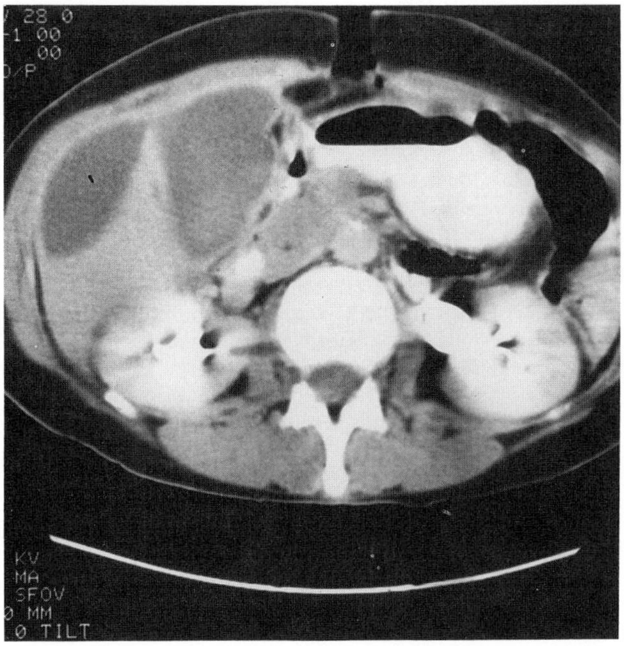

The two indications for laparotomy in this patient were (a) the patient had a penetrating injury with a handgun. Had this been a penetrating injury inflicted by a knife wound, it would have been necessary to explore the wound to demonstrate penetration of the peritoneal cavity. (b) The patient also had physical signs on abdominal examination suggesting the possibility of peritonitis.

2. Although the bullet entered from the right and extended to the left, there was concern about injury to the chest as well as the abdomen, and the chest tube was inserted first on the left side to ensure that there was no continued intrathoracic bleeding. The chest tube was also inserted even though there was no evidence of a pneumothorax because the patient was going to undergo a laparotomy under general anesthesia, and under those circumstances whether pneumothorax is present or not, a prophylactic chest tube should be inserted. The rationale is that the development of a pneumothorax under anesthesia could well be a tension pneumothorax leading to sudden instability of the patient, and it is far safer to have the left chest decompressed by a chest tube to avoid this complication. Once significant injury in the chest was excluded, laparotomy was required. However, the entire chest and abdomen were prepared in the event that there was some instability that could not be accounted for during laparotomy that would then require thoracotomy. Esophageal injury was not completely excluded prior to laparotomy.

3. In previous years, this patient would likely have had an intravenous pyelogram (IVP). However, the absence of hematuria and the stability of the patient as well as the trajectory of the bullet outside the path of the kidneys suggested that an IVP would not have given useful information.

4. The patient's hemoglobin was 109 g/L and for an otherwise healthy 47-year-old female, this indicates a substantial drop in hemoglobin. With no demonstrated blood loss in the pleural space or extremity trauma, the source of the blood loss had to be within the abdomen. Indeed, at laparotomy, 1.5 L of fresh blood was found in the peritoneal cavity.

5. IV antibiotics were commenced on this patient. However, whether the delay in use of antibiotics (approximately 35 min after the beginning of the operation) contributed to the septic complication is uncertain. However, it has been previously shown that perioperative antibiotics are most effective in decreasing septic complication if the antibiotics are administered prior to the beginning of the laparotomy as opposed to after surgery.

6. Although the laceration of the right lobe of the liver was through and through, there was no active bleeding at the time of laparotomy, and only local control of the hemorrhage was required with minimal debridement and drainage. Therefore, it was not necessary to probe the entire depth of the liver wound because this might induce further bleeding. The postoperative intraabdominal abscess probably resulted from a combination of inadequate drainage of the liver wound and contamination from the colon contents. In this setting, patients must be

observed very closely for signs of postoperative sepsis, and the abdomen should be a prime suspect as the source.

7. Because of the trajectory of this missile, it is imperative that all portions of the stomach be examined completely; hence, the decision to enter the lesser sac and the discovery of a hole in the posterior wall of the stomach. Once one hole in the stomach is identified, then one should look for a second hole, which was discovered on the lesser curvature at the incisura. A common principle is that perforating missiles should always result in an even number of holes and one should look for the second hole when a first one is identified.

8. Injuries of the stomach as opposed to injuries to the large bowel can be sutured primarily, as indicated in this case.

9. A hematoma in the omentum at the splenic flexure without any obvious injury to the colon should be followed by freeing of the splenic flexure so that all surfaces of this part of the bowel can be inspected. As seen in this case, without mobilization of the splenic flexure, a potentially lethal injury in the splenic flexure of the colon could have been missed.

10. Because of the multiplicity of injuries, including a bleeding liver laceration and because of the presence of gross fecal contamination, it was decided to exteriorize this bowel rather than do a primary closure of the colon laceration.

11. The skin was closed with skin clips in spite of the fact that there was gross contamination, and this may or may not have resulted in the wound abscess that developed 10 days later.

12. Antibiotics in the perioperative period are usually administered for approximately 24 h if there is no spillage or contamination. However, in the presence of contamination, the criteria for stopping antibiotics are the following: The patient should be afebrile and there should be a normal white blood cell count. All of these were present, and the antibiotics were therefore stopped. However, within 3 days, fever recurred, demonstrating that antibiotics may mask infection.

13. Persistence of a fever after draining a source of infection should raise concern about another source or incomplete drainage of the previous abscess. Thus, CT scan examination of the abdomen was conducted, since this is often the source of the sepsis. In this case, as is done generally, other sources, such as the chest and extremities, were investigated. When other sites are excluded, the source of infection is very likely within the abdomen, as pointed out on the percutaneous aspiration. This type of abscess does not respond generally to ultrasonic aspiration because of its consistency, having arisen within an infected hematoma. Thin bile or a cavity containing very thin pus can be treated successfully by the percutaneous route, but an infected hematoma with thick purulent material that is difficult to aspirate through a large bore tube is better treated by formal surgical drainage of the abscess.

Acknowledgment

We acknowledge the assistance of Sunnybrook Studios of the Sunnybrook Health Science Centre, Toronto, for preparation of the illustrations.

References

1. Committee on Trauma, American College of Surgeons: *Advanced Trauma Life Support Manual.* Chicago, American College of Surgeons, 1989.
2. Fowler NO: Physiology of cardiac tamponade and pulsus paradoxus in cardiac tamponade. Mod Concepts Cardiovasc Dis 47:109, 1978.
3. Spodick DH: Acute cardiac tamponade pathologic physiology, diagnosis and management. Prog Cardiovasc Dis 10:64, 1967.
4. Kilpatrick ZM, Chapman CB: On pericardiocentesis. Am J Cardiol 16:722, 1965.
5. Pories WJ, Guadiani VA: Cardiac tamponade. Surg Clin North Am 55:573, 1975.
6. Watkins L Jr, Gott VL: Blunt and penetrating trauma to the great vessels. *Thoracic and Cardiovascular Surgery,* 4th ed. Norwalk, CT, Appleton-Century-Crofts, 1983, pp 1489–1497.
7. Barone JE, Pizzi WF, Nealon TF: Indications for intubation in blunt chest trauma. J Trauma 26:334, 1986.
8. King MW, Aitchison JM, Nel JP: Fatal air embolism following penetrating lung trauma: An autopsy study. J Trauma 24:753, 1984.
9. Shackford SR, Virgilio RW, Peters RM: Selective use of ventilator therapy in flail chest injury. J Thorac Cardiovasc Surg 81:194, 1981.
10. Trinkle JF, Richardson RD, Franz JL, et al: Management of flail chest without mechanical ventilator. Ann Thorac Surg 19:355, 1975.
11. Richardson JD, Adams L, Flint LM: Selective management of flail chest and pulmonary contusion. Ann Surg 196:481, 1982.
12. Tenzer ML: The spectrum of myocardial contusion: A review. J Trauma 25:620, 1985.
13. Marnocha KE, Maglinte DDT, Woods J: Blunt chest trauma and suspected aortic rupture: Reliability of chest radiograph findings. Ann Emerg Med 14:644, 1985.
14. Miller FB, Richardson JD, Thomas HA, et al: Role of CT in diagnosis of major arterial injury after blunt thoracic trauma. Surgery 106:596, 1989.
15. Ajalal GM, Mulder DG: Esophageal perforations—the need for an individualized approach. Arch Surg 119:1318, 1984.
16. Oreskovich MR, Dellinger EP, Lennard ES, et al: Duration of preventive antibiotics administration for penetrating abdominal trauma. Arch Surg 117:200, 1982.
17. McAlvanak MJ, Shaftan GW: Selective conservatism in penetrating abdominal wounds: A continuing re-appraisal. J Trauma 18:206, 1978.
18. Moore EE, Moore JB, VanDuzer-Moore S: Mandatory laparotomy for gunshot wounds penetrating the abdomen. Am J Surg 140:847, 1980.
19. Fischer RP, Beverlin BC, Engrav LH: Diagnostic peritoneal lavage: Fourteen years and 2586 patients later. Am J Surg 136:701, 1978.
20. Federle MP, Cross RA, Jeffrey RB, Trunkey DD: Computed tomography in blunt abdominal trauma. Arch Surg 117:645, 1982.

21. Blaisdell FW, Trunkey DD: *Abdominal Trauma*. New York, Thieme-Stratton, 1982, p 11.
22. Fullen WD, Selle JG, Whitely DH, et al: Intramural duodenal hematoma. Ann Surg 179:549, 1974.
23. Cogbill TH, Moore EE, Kashuk JL: Changing trends in the management of pancreatic trauma. Ann Surg 187:555, 1978.
24. Vaughan GD III, Frazier OH, Graham DY, et al: The use of pyloric exclusion in the management of severe duodenal injuries. Am J Surg 134:785, 1977.
25. Sims EH, Mandal AK, Schlater T, et al: Factors affecting outcome in pancreatic trauma. J Trauma 24:125, 1984.
26. Bradley EL III, Clements JL Jr, Gonzalez AC: The natural history of pancreatic pseudocysts: A unified concept of management. Am J Surg 137:135, 1979.
27. Stone HH, Fabian TC: Management of perforating colon trauma: Randomisation between primary closure and exteriorization. Ann Surg 190:430, 1979.
28. Trunkey DD, Haves RJ, Shires FT: Management of rectal trauma. J Trauma 13:411, 1973.
29. Ali J: Abdominal trauma with special reference to hepatic trauma. Can J Surg 21:512, 1978.
30. Moore FA, Moore EE, Seagraves A: Non resectional management of major hepatic trauma. Am J Surg 150:725, 1985.
31. Schrock TR, Blaisdell FW, Mathewson C Jr: Management of blunt trauma to the liver and hepatic veins. Arch Surg 96:698, 1968.
32. Feliciano DV, Mattox KL, Jordan GL Jr: Intra-abdominal packing for control of hepatic hemorrhage: A reappraisal. J Trauma 21:285, 1981.
33. Neilson ML, Mygind T: Selective arterial embolization in trauma hemobilia. World J Surg 4:357, 1980.
34. Wesson DE, Filler RM, Ein SH, et al: Ruptured spleen—when to operate? J Pediatr Surg 16:324, 1981.
35. Delany HM, Porreca F, Mitscido S, et al: Splenic capping: An experimental study of new techniques for splenorrhapy using polyglycolic acid mesh. Ann Surg 196:187, 1982.
36. Francke EL, Neu HC: Postsplenectomy infection. Surg Clin North Am 61:135, 1981.
37. Bright TC, White K, Peters PC: Significance of hematuria after trauma. J Urol 120:445, 1978.
38. Thomason RB, Julian JS, Mortellar HC, et al: Microscopic hematuria after blunt trauma—is pyelography necessary? Am Surg 55:145, 1989.
39. Mee SL, McAninch JW, Robinson AL, et al: Radiographic assessment of renal trauma: A 10 year prospective study of patient selection. J Urol 141:1095, 1989.

Chapter 64

PELVIC TRAUMA

MARVIN TILE

KEY POINTS

- *Stabilization of those pelvic fractures which increase pelvic volume (type B1, C) is an essential part of hemodynamic stabilization in the acute resuscitative phase.*
- *Treatment of the musculoskeletal injury depends on the type of pelvic disruption and the presence or absence of shock.*
- *Stable pelvic ring fractures (type A) require no specific orthopedic treatment.*
- *In unstable fractures, operative stabilization may be required to control hemorrhage, facilitate critical care management, and prevent long-term disability.*
- *Early orthopedic management consists of a simple anterior external fixator with femoral skeletal traction.*
- *If laparotomy is performed, internal fixation of the symphysis pubis is desirable.*
- *Posterior internal fixation should be reserved for the difficult unstable pelvis.*
- *Avoid undertreatment of unstable fractures and overtreatment of stable fractures.*

Traumatic disruption of the pelvic ring is a major focus of interest for intensivists as well as orthopedic surgeons especially with respect to the approach to stabilization of this injury. Whether stabilization of the pelvis reduces the high mortality rate associated with pelvic trauma and whether it improves the long-term functional results of such injuries is still unanswered. Despite improvements in management, the mortality rate from major pelvic fractures continues to be high, at approximately 10 percent,[1,2] especially in high energy injury. High energy injury is associated with a higher Injury Severity Score (ISS) and major associated injuries to the head, chest, and gastrointestinal and urologic systems. The management of hemorrhage associated with pelvic trauma is a major problem which may be facilitated by early stabilization of the pelvic fracture.[3]

The natural history of the musculoskeletal injury suggests that stable injuries to the pelvis have minimal long-term effects, whereas vertically unstable pelvic fractures are associated with long-term unsatisfactory results more than 50 percent of the time.[4] Therefore, to reduce the mortality and improve outcome, knowledge of pelvic anatomy, biomechanics, survival studies, and natural history is necessary. From such knowledge a classification and management protocol can be developed to aid in decision-making.[5]

Survival Studies

The mortality rate of patients with fractures of the pelvis continues to be high. Despite more aggressive early resuscitation, including early application of external fixators, the mortality rate has remained constant at 10 percent in our center in the last 494 cases managed over the past 5 years.[6] The associated injuries, especially head injuries, as well as massive pelvic bleeding may account for this. There is a direct correlation between mortality and the ISS.

Early open reduction and stable internal fixation of long bone fractures is safe and improves survival.[3] Similarly, open reduction and internal fixation of unstable pelvic fractures has repeatedly reduced the mortality rate from such fractures.[7] Of 111 patients with unstable pelvic ring fractures, the overall mortality rate was 19 percent, with mortality in those patients undergoing operation being 8.3 percent, with ISS similar between the groups. Although open reduction and internal fixation (ORIF) appears to be safe and may reduce mortality, this course of action should only be undertaken in well staffed and equipped trauma centers because the complication rate is potentially high.

Natural History

It is generally thought that patients surviving a disruption of the pelvic ring have few late musculoskeletal problems, regardless of initial management. A review of the natural history of pelvic disruption may clarify whether stabilization of pelvic fractures, especially by ORIF, is justified. Holdsworth reported that 15 of 27 patients with a sacroiliac dislocation were unable to return to their regular work because of continuing disability, whereas the 23 with a sacral or iliac fracture had more satisfactory results.[8] In a study of 359 cases, Pennal suggested that patients with unstable vertical shear injuries had many late complications, including nonunions which had not previously been reported.[9] In other series, 33 to 52 percent of patients with pelvic fractures have been reported to suffer long-term discomfort.[10]

In reviewing the literature, it is difficult to determine whether fractures of a similar type and prognosis are being compared. In an attempt to further clarify the natural history of this injury, we reported on 248 patients with pelvic

TABLE 64-1 Classification of Pelvic Fractures

Type A—Stable	
A1	Avulsion fractures
A2	Isolated fractures of the iliac wing, undisplaced ring fractures
A3	Transverse fractures of the sacrum and coccyx
Type B—Vertically Stable, Rotationally Unstable	
B1	Open book injury
B2	Lateral compression
B3	Bilateral partially stable injuries
Type C—Vertical and Rotational Instability	
C1	Fracture of the ilium
C2	Fracture or fracture-dislocation of the sacroiliac joint
C3	Fracture of the sacrum

ring disruptions.[11] In this study each patient was recalled, personally interviewed and examined by the authors, and radiographed using inlet, outlet, and anteroposterior views. The fractures were classified according to their degree of instability and severity (Table 64-1). Of the 248 patients available for follow-up at a mean of 5.6 years (range 2 to 18 years), 30 patients were eliminated because of major acetabular involvement, leaving 218 patients for evaluation. Of these 218 patients, 118 were treated in community hospitals with traditional methods of traction and bed rest; 100 were the first consecutive group in the Sunnybrook Trauma Unit. Twenty-one were treated with external fixation. The conclusions from the study were as follows:

1. Stable pelvic injuries gave few major long-term problems. If present, pain was usually mild or moderate.
2. Patients with unstable pelvic disruptions behaved differently.

Sixty percent of this group had continuing pain. The pain was usually in the posterior sacroiliac area or the lower lumbar spine and was most often associated with an unreduced sacroiliac dislocation or a nonunion. Nonunion occurred in 3.5 percent of patients and malunion, defined as having a >2.5 cm leg length discrepancy, in 4 percent. Also, 12 patients (5.5 percent) had permanent nerve injury and 6 (2.5 percent) permanent urethral damage.

It appears, therefore, that the outcome from a pelvic fracture depends on the degree of initial force, the type of injury, (stable or unstable), the method of treatment, and the presence of associated disorders such as permanent nerve damage, urethral tear, malunion, malreduction of the sacroiliac joint, or nonunion. Of these factors, the stability of the fracture is paramount in determining the prognosis. Therefore, pelvic fractures must be classified according to their degree of instability. Simple treatment of stable fractures produces good results, whereas vertically unstable injuries, especially with a sacroiliac dislocation, often result in a significant disability. Therefore, surgical stabilization should be limited to this group. Even in major trauma centers, more than 60 percent of all injuries to the pelvis are vertically stable and therefore rarely require operative stabilization.[12] At Sunnybrook Hospital in the past 5 years, we have managed 494 cases of pelvic disruption, of which only 68 required external fixation and 24 internal fixation.[6]

Anatomic and Biomechanical Considerations

The bony pelvis, lacking inherent stability, is held together by the ligamentous structures, anteriorly by the symphysis, posteriorly by the anterior and posterior sacroiliac ligaments (Fig. 64-1*a*). The pelvic floor, which includes the sacrotuberous and sacrospinous ligaments, as well as the muscles of the pelvic floor and their investing fascia, also play a major role in the stability of the pelvic ring (Fig. 64-1*b*). To

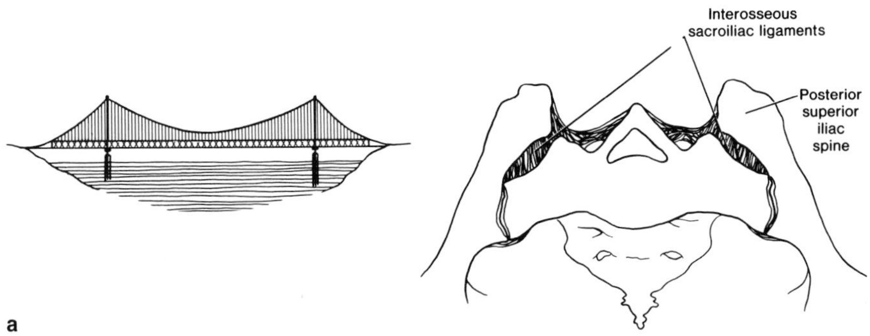

a

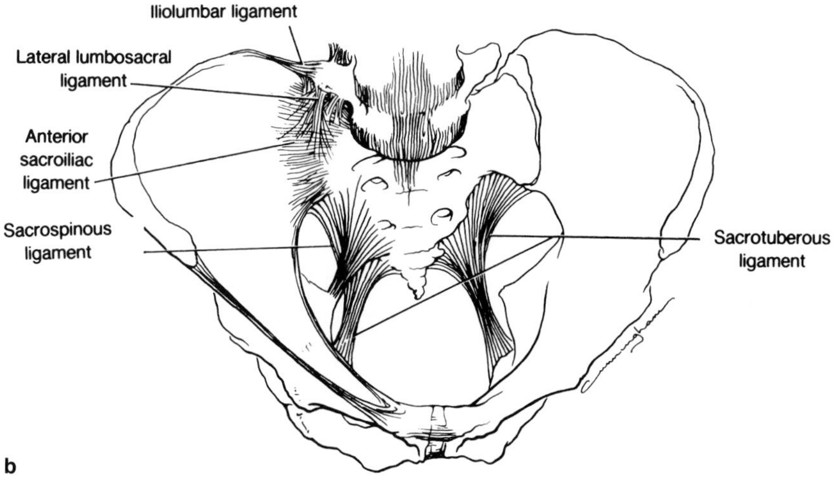

b

FIGURE 64-1 *a*. **Drawing depicting the suspension bridge-like appearance of the ligaments binding the posterior sacroiliac complex. Note the vertical direction of the interosseous posterior sacroiliac ligaments, noted by Grant to be the strongest in the body.** *b*. **The ligamentous structures of the pelvis from the anterior view. Note the flat sacroiliac ligaments, the triangular sacrospinous ligament lying anterior to the sacrotuberous ligament; a strong band outcropping from the pelvic floor extending from the lateral portion of the sacrum to the ischial tuberosity. (Reproduced from Reference 5, with permission.)**

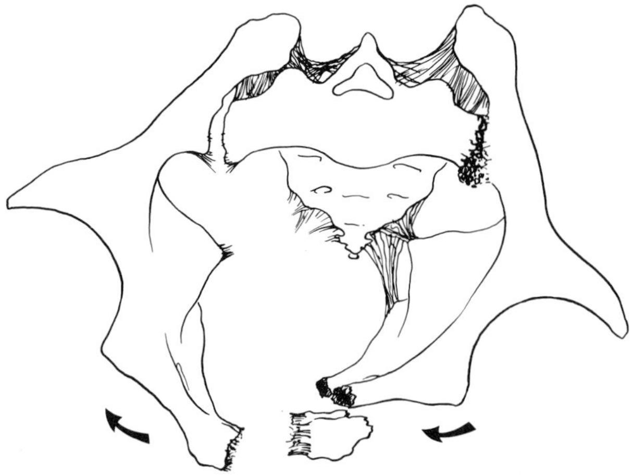

FIGURE 64-2 Diagram to show rotational instability of the pelvis, with no vertical instability. On the right hemipelvis an external rotation force has disrupted the symphysis pubis as well as the sacrospinous and anterior sacroiliac ligaments, but the posterior ligaments remain intact. The posterior iliac spine abuts against the sacrum. On the left hemipelvis an internal rotation force has fractured the rami and crushed the posterior sacroiliac complex, but the posterior ligaments and the pelvic floor are intact. (From Tile M: Pelvic ring fractures: Should they be fixed? J Bone Joint Surg [Br] 70-B:1, 1988.)

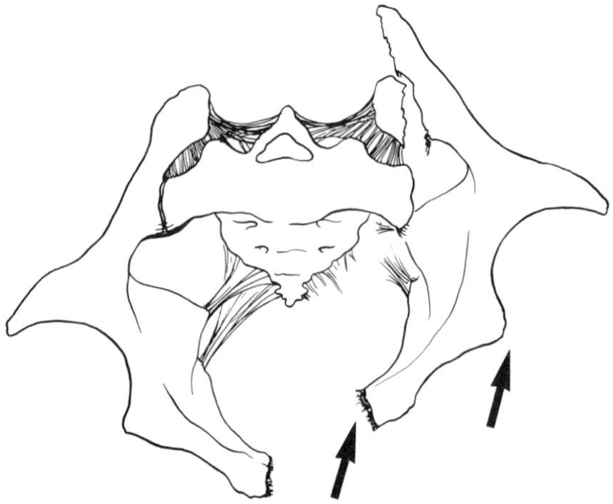

FIGURE 64-3 Diagram depicting vertical instability of the pelvis. A vertical shearing force has disrupted the symphysis and the sacrospinous ligament and caused a fracture-dislocation of the sacroiliac joint. The posterior sacroiliac complex has been disrupted. (From Tile M: Pelvic ring fractures: Should they be fixed? Bone Joint Surg [Br] 70-B:1, 1988.)

understand the injury patterns and the subsequent classification it is important to consider the pelvis as a true ring structure. If the ring is broken in one area and the fragments displaced, then there must be a fracture or dislocation in another portion of the ring.

PELVIC STABILITY

The stability of the pelvic ring depends on the integrity of the posterior weight-bearing sacroiliac complex as well as the muscles and ligaments of the pelvic floor. The major posterior ligamentous structures are the sacroiliac ligaments including the strong interosseous ligaments, which maintain the normal position of the sacrum in the pelvic ring. The major ligamentous structures of the pelvic floor are the sacrospinous ligament which limits external rotation and the sacrotuberous ligament which limits superior or inferior migration in the sagittal plane. The entire complex has the appearance of a suspension bridge (see Fig. 64-1*a*).

FORCES ACTING ON THE PELVIS

The major forces acting on the pelvis are external rotation, internal rotation (lateral compression), or vertical shear. In some complex high energy injuries, the actual forces operating may defy precise description, but generally these three are identified as largely responsible for injury.

External rotation is caused by a direct blow on the posterior iliac spines or more commonly by forced external rotation of the femur and produces an open book type of injury (Fig. 64-2). This is characterized by a disruption of the symphysis pubis and as the force continues, by a rupture of the anterior sacroiliac and sacrospinous ligaments. The end point is reached when the posterior ilium abuts against the sacrum. If the force continues, the hemipelvis may be sheared off, resulting in gross instability.

Internal rotation (*lateral compression*) is caused by a direct blow on the lateral aspect of the iliac crest or by an indirect force through the femoral head and is characterized by compression fractures of the posterior complex and rami fractures anteriorly (Fig. 64-2). These injuries may be of two types, those in which the anterior and posterior lesions are on the same side (ipsilateral type) or those where the anterior and posterior lesions are on opposite sides (bucket handle type). This latter type may cause major rotational deformities and result in malunion. In some instances, the lateral compression force stops short of rupture of the posterior structures; in others, this end point is exceeded and the posterior structures may rupture. However, in all lateral compression types, the pelvic floor remains intact; therefore, vertical displacement *cannot* occur.

Vertical shearing forces cross the main trabecular pattern of the pelvis and cause marked displacement of bone, gross disruption of soft tissues, and complete instability (Fig. 64-3). There is generally no end point to this force; therefore, in the extreme, even a traumatic hemipelvectomy may result.[13,14]

FORCE TRANSMISSION TO THE VISCERA, VESSELS, AND NERVES

External rotation and shearing forces cause tearing of the pelvic viscera and the pelvic blood vessels. Traction on the lumbosacral nerve plexus may also result from this force (see Fig. 64-4). In contrast, lateral compression forces cause visceral and blood vessel injury by direct penetration of bone. Lumbosacral plexus nerve injury is usually caused by compression of the sacral nerve roots in the foramina.

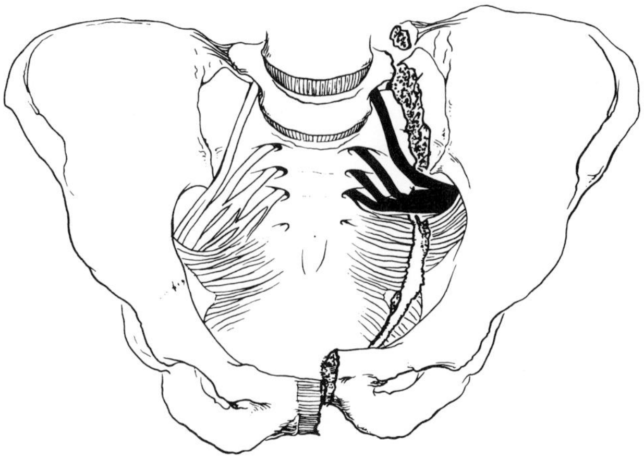

FIGURE 64-4 The drawing demonstrates that external rotation and shearing forces cause major visceral injuries including traction on the lumbosacral nerve plexus and disruption of pelvic blood vessels. (Reproduced from Reference 5, with permission.)

Classification

Fractures of the pelvis may be divided into three types (Table 64-1):

Type A—Stable
Type B—Vertically stable, rotationally unstable
Type C—Unstable (rotationally + vertically)

Also, any injury to the pelvis may be either unilateral or bilateral. Completely unstable (type C) fractures make up no more than 30 to 35 percent of the total number of cases. To understand this classification a knowledge of the concept of pelvic stability is essential. The bony pelvis with its intact ligamentous structures may be considered a stable anatomic structure; that is, *it is able to withstand physiologic forces without abnormal deformation.* This concept must be understood in "relative" rather than "absolute" terms. All pelvic injuries may be placed on a *scale of stability,* depending on the precise pathologic anatomy. In this classification, by definition, an unstable vertical shear injury means instability in the *vertical plane.* Displacement in the vertical plane allowing posterior and cephalad migration of the hemipelvis is only possible if the posterior sacroiliac complex and the pelvic floor are disrupted. An injury which is vertically stable cannot, by definition, be vertically displaced, but there may be rotational instability which can be caused by external (open book) or internal rotatory forces (lateral compression).

With type A stable fractures (see Table 64-1), the pelvic ring is stable and the amount of displacement insignificant. Included in this type are:

A1—Avulsion fractures seen mainly in adolescents
A2—Isolated fractures of the iliac wing not involving the pelvic ring, undisplaced fractures of the ring, or the four rami fracture with no posterior injury
A3—Transverse fractures of the sacrum and coccyx distal to the pelvic ring

In type B injuries, there is vertical stability, but rotational instability (see Table 64-1). In type B1, the open book injury (Fig. 64-5) is caused by external rotatory forces resulting in a disruption of the symphysis pubis. The injury may be unilateral or bilateral. If the symphyseal disruption is <2.5 cm, no lesions of the pelvic floor or sacroiliac ligaments are present, whereas if >2.5 cm, the sacrospinous and anterior sacroiliac ligaments are disrupted. The hemipelvis is unstable in external rotation, but if the force does not continue beyond the yield strength of the posterior sacroiliac ligaments, vertical stability is maintained. Stability may be returned to the pelvic ring by internal rotation, easily accomplished by placing the patient in the lateral position.

Type B2 injuries result from lateral compression. In this injury pattern the rami may rotate inwardly until they impact on the opposite hemipelvis, allowing internal rotatory instability or impaction of the sacrum. However, the pelvic floor remains intact so that vertical displacement is not possible. The subgroups of lateral compression depend on the sites of the anterior and posterior lesion.

In the *ipsilateral* type (B2-1) (Fig. 64-6), the rami are commonly fractured anteriorly and the posterior complex crushed on the same side. Other varieties include those with an overlapped locked symphysis or a so-called tilt fracture in which the superior ramus is rotated into the perineum.

In the *contralateral* (bucket handle) types (B2-2) (Fig. 64-7), the major anterior displacement is on the side opposite to the posterior lesion, even if all four rami may have fractured anteriorly. The affected hemipelvis rotates anteriorly and superiorly like the handle of a bucket so that even if the posterior structures are relatively intact, the patient may have a major leg length discrepancy. Reduction requires derotation of the hemipelvis rather than traction in the vertical plane. Bilateral partially stable injuries (type B3) may occur but are rare.

Therefore, external rotatory forces may cause external rotatory instability—an open book injury—and internal rotatory forces—a lateral compression or closed book injury, but both remain vertically stable unless the posterior ligaments and the pelvic floor rupture. In those cases, the injury must be considered *unstable* because vertical migration is possible.

The vertically unstable pelvic disruption (type C, see Table 64-1) implies a rupture of the pelvic floor including the sacrospinous and sacrotuberous ligaments, as well as the posterior sacroiliac complex (Fig. 64-8). The anterior injury may be a disruption of the symphysis, a fracture of two or all four pubic rami, or a combination of the above. The posterior injury may be a fracture of the ilium (C1), a dislocation or fracture-dislocation of the sacroiliac joint (C2), or a fracture of the sacrum (C3). Combinations of bilateral injuries may occur. Bilateral C type injuries represent the most unstable pelvic injuries.

Some pelvic fractures defy precise classification because of the complex forces resulting in a bizarre pelvic ring injury. Those pelvic ring disruptions associated with *acetabular fractures* should be considered separately, since the

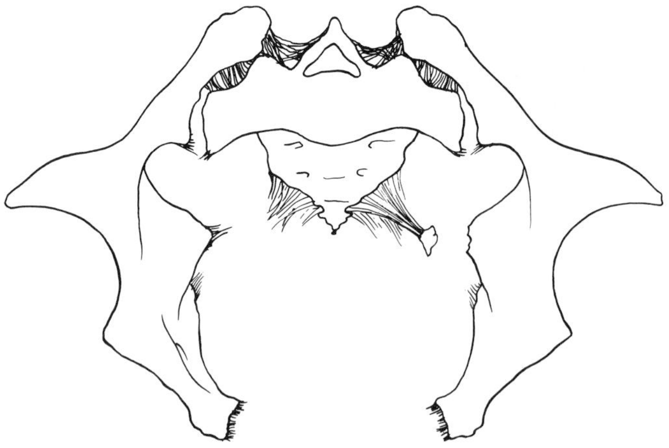

a

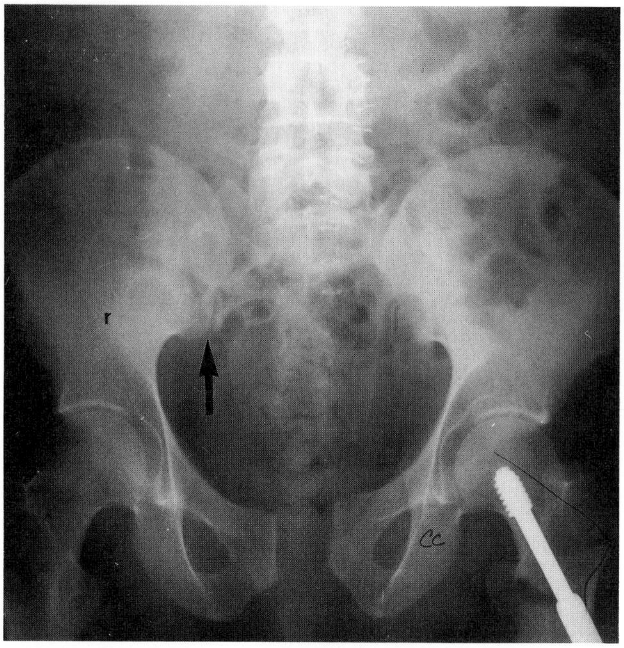

b

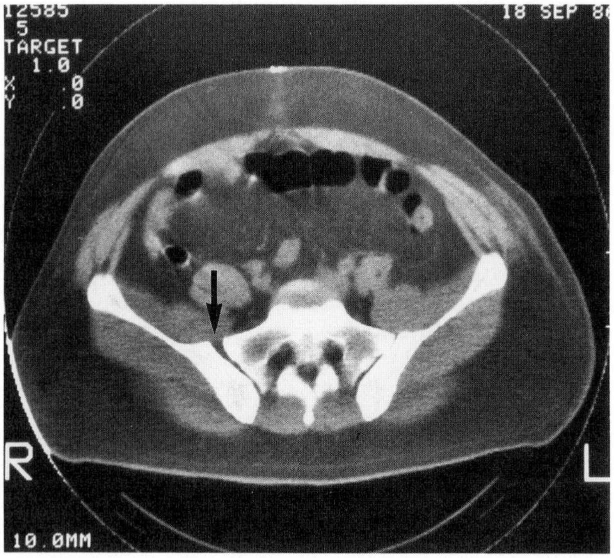

c

FIGURE 64-5 Type B1 open book injury. The drawing (*a*) demonstrates a typical open book injury. Note the intact posterior sacroiliac ligaments preventing posterior or vertical migration of the hemipelvis despite the wide disruption of the symphysis and anterior sacroiliac ligaments. A typical unilateral injury is noted in the radiograph (*b*) and the computed tomography (CT) scan (*c*). Note the symphysis disruption and the anterior opening at the sacroiliac joint with no posterior displacement.

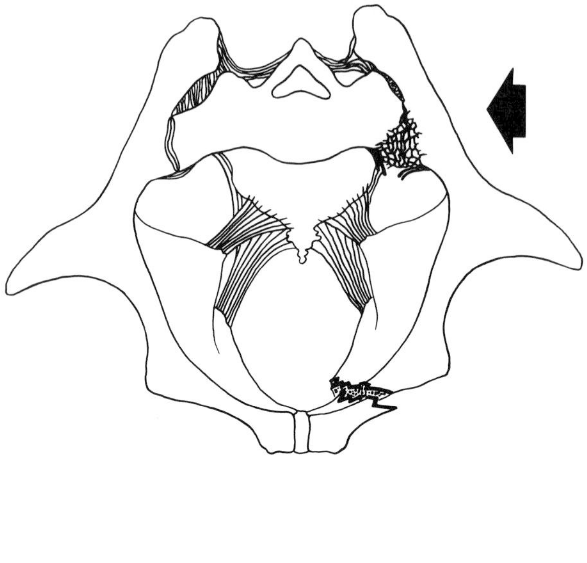

FIGURE 64-6 A lateral compression injury depicting a posterior sacral crush and an ipsilateral anterior fracture of both pubic rami. Note the intact posterior sacroiliac ligamentous complex. With internal rotation, even if that complex is disrupted, only minimal vertical displacement will be possible because of the intact pelvic floor. (Reproduced from Reference 5, with permission.)

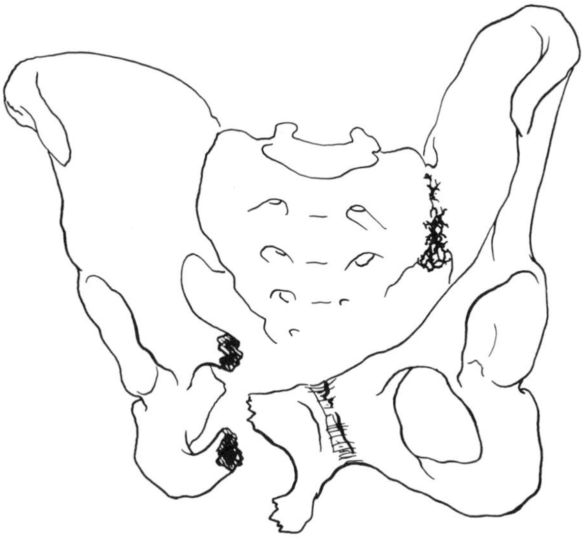

a

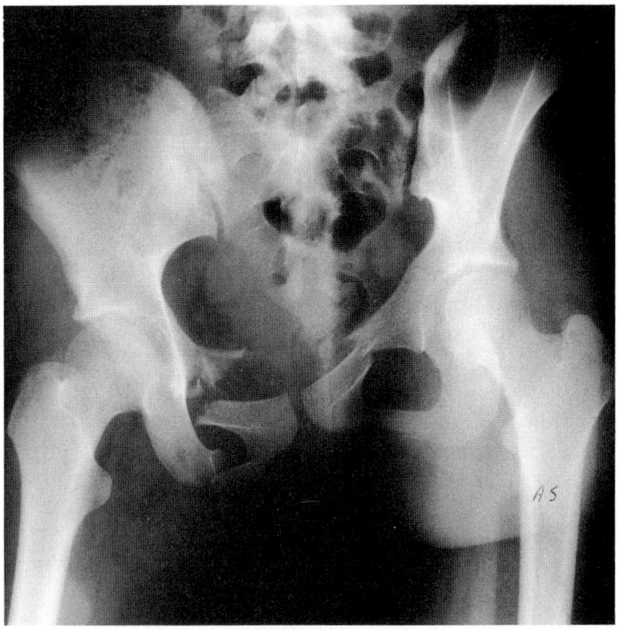

b

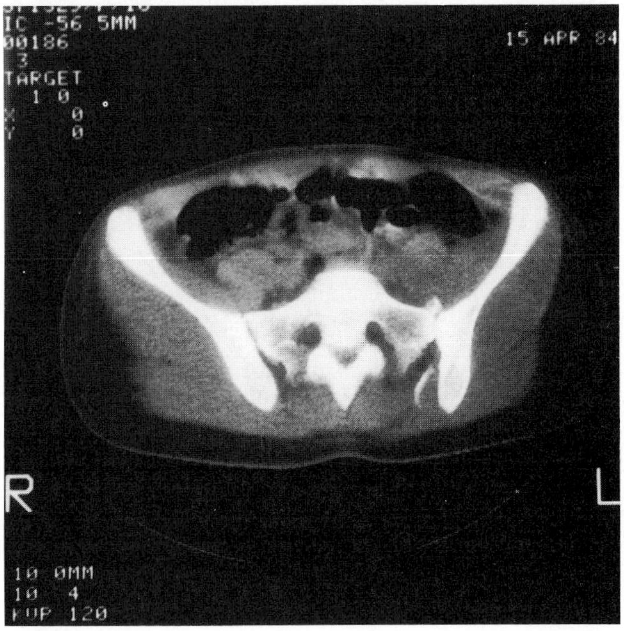

c

FIGURE 64-7 Bucket handle lateral compression injury—type B3. The diagram (*a*) shows the typical appearance of a bucket handle injury, with the left hemipelvis internally and superiorly rotated by 40°. The radiograph (*b*) shows internal rotation of the left hemipelvis with fracture of all four pubic rami. The CT scan (*c*) confirms the internal rotation of the hemipelvis and the crush injury of the anterior sacrum. It shows avulsion of the posterior iliac apophysis. (From Tile M: Pelvic ring fractures: Should they be fixed? J Bone Joint Surg [Br] 70-B:1, 1988.)

prognosis will clearly depend more on the results of treatment of the acetabular fracture than on the pelvic ring.

Management

ASSESSMENT

Other portions of this book have dealt with the assessment and resuscitation of the polytraumatized patient (see Chap. 59). These extremely ill patients with pelvic fractures require rapid general assessment and resuscitation.

RESUSCITATION

The key elements of resuscitation of the patient with pelvic fractures are massive fluid replacement and hemorrhage control. The latter may be accomplished by pneumatic antishock garment, stabilization of the unstable pelvic disruption, embolization of the pelvic vessels, or surgical intervention.[3,15,16] In the presence of adequate fluid replacement, the early application of an external skeletal frame may reduce pelvic venous and bony bleeding to the extent that other intervention is rarely required.[16] Embolization of small arterial vessels should not be attempted prior to stabilization of the pelvis by an external fixator.[2] In many cases, packing of the pelvis is the only means of controlling the hemorrhage. Direct surgical intervention is rarely successful in hemorrhage control.

Determining the stability of the pelvic ring by clinical and radiographic means is an important step in decision-making. Palpation and manipulation of the pelvis and application of traction will readily determine whether vertical instability is present. Other clinical signs of instability include severe displacement of the pelvis noted on examination, marked bruising posteriorly, severe associated injuries to nerves or vessels, and the presence of an open wound. Instability is confirmed by radiographic examination. Of greater importance than the routine anteroposterior view is the inlet view, which clearly illustrates posterior displacement, and the outlet view showing superior migration or rotation.[17] CT scanning is the best single investigative tool for determining instability, because the sacroiliac complex is best visualized by this technique (Fig. 64-9a). The recent added refinement of three-dimensional CT scanning allows clear visualization of the injury pattern (Fig. 64-9*b*).

Radiographic evidence of pelvic instability is implied by posterior or superior displacement of the posterior complex by >1 cm through either a fracture, a dislocation, or a combination of both. As well, the presence of a large gap posteriorly rather than impaction is evidence of vertical instability (see Fig. 64-9).

Fractures with complete instability (type C) are at much greater general risk (mortality 10 percent) than those with a stable pelvis and require immediate resuscitation.

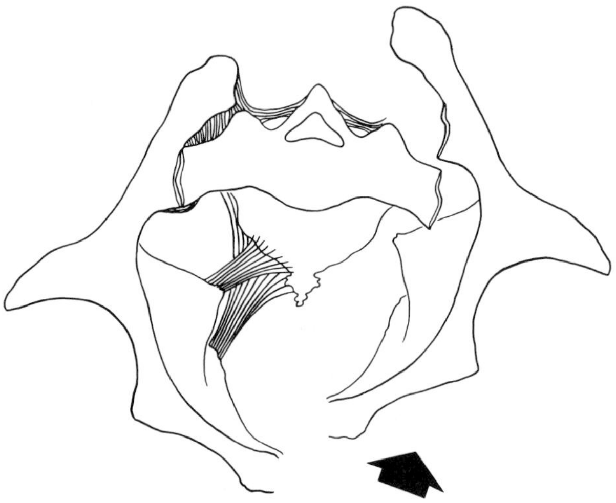

a

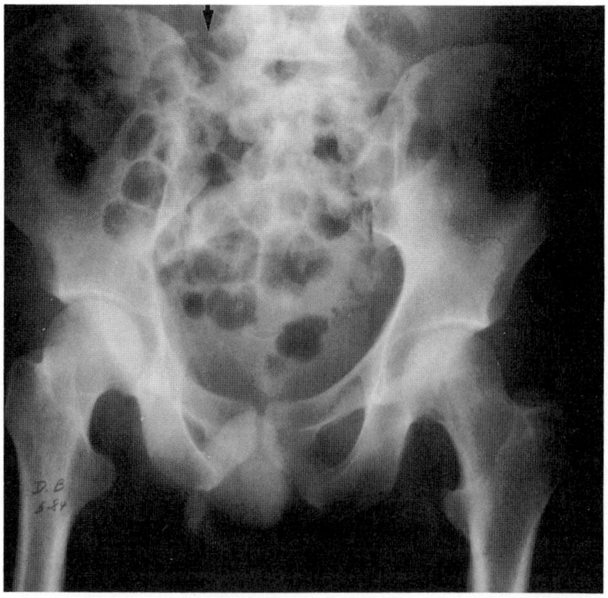

b

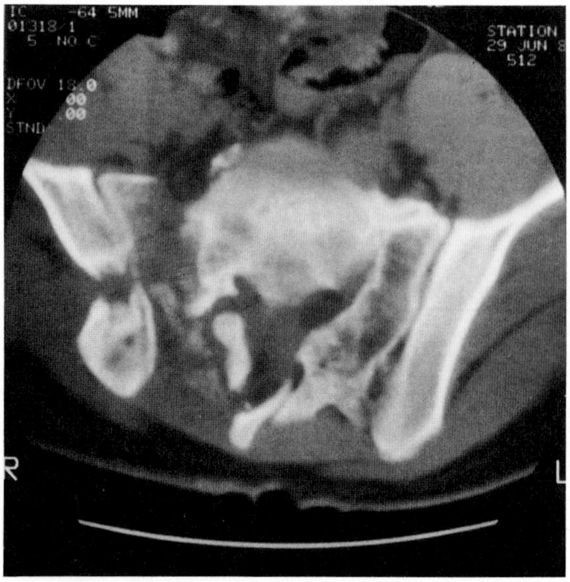

c

FIGURE 64-8 *a*. An unstable vertical shear injury (type C) causing gross disruption of both the anterior and posterior portions of the pelvis, including disruption of the pelvic floor resulting in major pelvic instability allowing posterior and vertical migration. *b*. The radiograph shows the fracture line through the sacrum and avulsion of the tip of the transverse process of L5 (arrow). Displacement appears to be minimal, but the unstable nature of this injury is best shown on the CT scan (*c*) by the wide displacement of the sacral fragments. (Reproduced from Reference 5, with permission.)

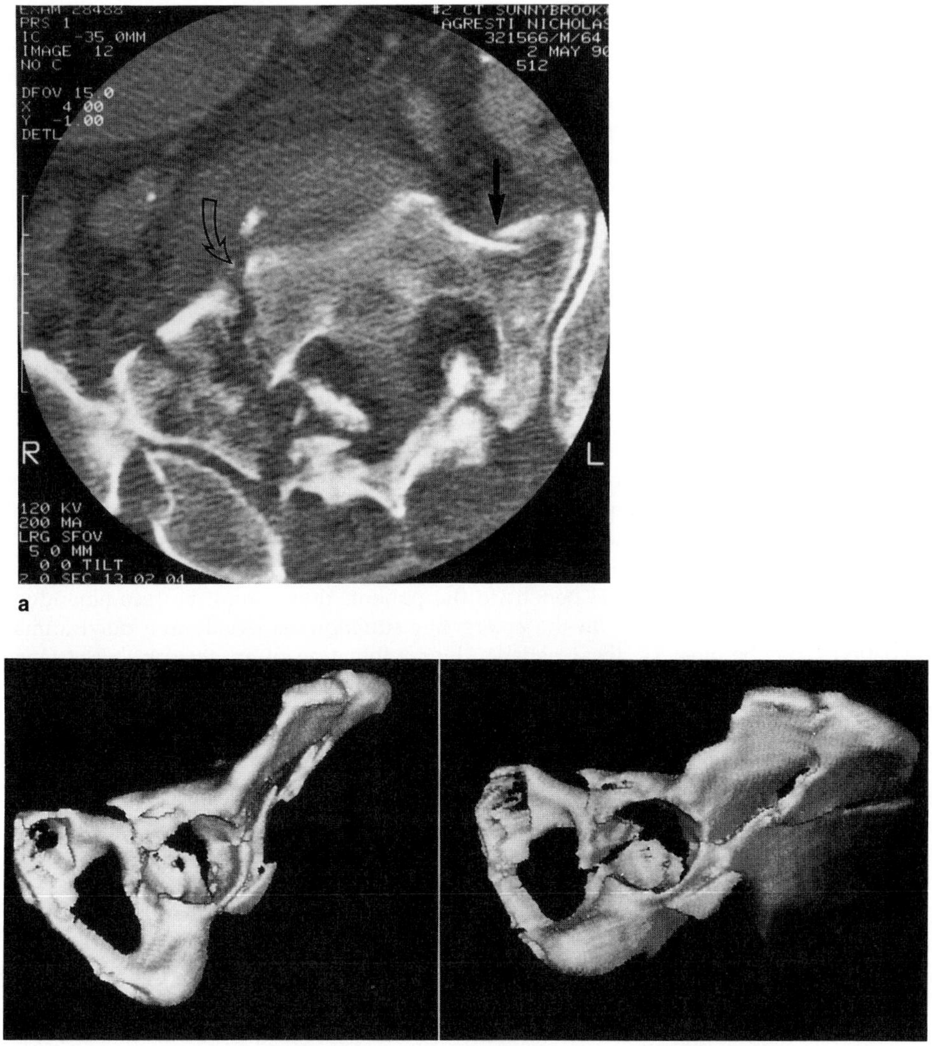

FIGURE 64-9 ***a*****. This CT demonstrates a type C unstable sacral fracture on the right (curved arrow) and a Type B2 compression fracture of the sacrum on the left (straight arrow).** ***b*****. Three-dimensional CT; note the anatomic detail in this acetabular fracture.**

PROVISIONAL STABILIZATION

For those pelvic fractures which result in an increased pelvic volume, namely the open book injury (B1), and the unstable injury (C), stabilization of the pelvic ring should be performed early. Provisional fracture stabilization belongs in the resuscitative phase of management. It is most safely and quickly achieved with an external frame applied percutaneously or with a pelvic clamp which may be applied in the emergency room. Biomechanically, in the vertically unstable injury, the external skeletal frames of any commonly used configuration cannot restore full pelvic stability allowing ambulation of the patient. However, they will reduce the volume of the pelvis, thereby restoring the tamponade effect of the bony pelvis resulting in a reduction of hemorrhage.[15,16]

Because these patients are usually extremely ill, a simple frame configuration is preferable. Two pins are placed percutaneously in the ilium, one in the anterior superior spine and one at the iliac tubercle approximately 45° to each other. The frame is completed in the form of an anterior rectangular configuration (Fig. 64-10). The more sophisticated external frames requiring dissection to the anterior inferior spine are not indicated in the acute resuscitative period.[18] They have a slight biomechanical advantage but cannot stabilize an unstable pelvic fracture to allow ambulation. Therefore, the added risk of the operative procedure is not worthwhile. Also, skeletal traction (30 lb) through a supracondylar femoral pin should be applied to prevent cephalad migration of the hemipelvis. Although these various simple frames and traction commonly used cannot fully stabilize the unstable pelvic ring biomechanically, the patient can be placed in the upright position for proper ventilation even in the traction. Some redisplacement usually occurs, but this may be dealt with when the general state of the patient improves.

DEFINITIVE STABILIZATION

The definitive management of displaced fractures of the pelvic ring depends on the stability of the fracture. In treating these displaced fractures, the risks and benefits of pel-

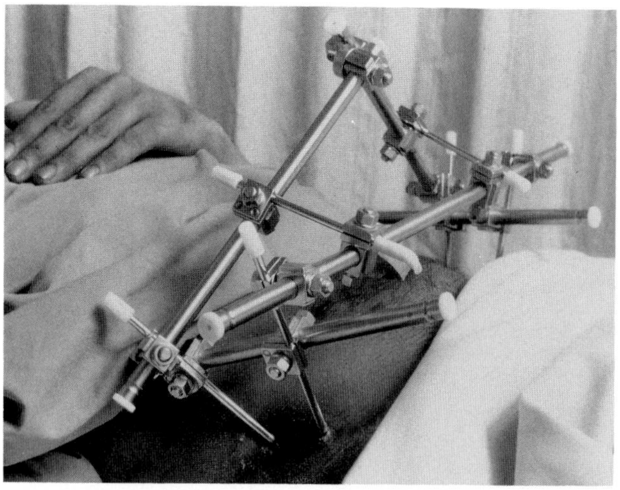

FIGURE 64-10 Anterior external fixation of the pelvis.

vic stabilization must be considered. If the pelvic ring is *stable* with insignificant displacement (type A), only symptomatic treatment is necessary. These patients may be mobilized quickly and the pelvic fracture largely ignored.

With type B1 (open book) injuries, no specific stabilization is required if the symphysis is open <2.5 cm. A good result may be expected in most cases although rarely, some pain may persist at the symphysis for months or even permanently. If the symphysis is open more than 2.5 cm, external rotatory instability is present. The pelvic ring may be closed by placing the patient in the lateral position, thereby closing the open book. The position is maintained by a simple external skeletal fixator or by a plate on the symphysis pubis. Both are biomechanically sound and will allow the patient to ambulate. If the patient requires a laparotomy and there has been no fecal contamination, we favor plating of the symphysis at that time. In other cases, external fixation is used.

Type B2 (lateral compression) injuries are the most common type of pelvic ring fracture, and are by definition, vertically stable, because of the intact pelvic floor. In most cases of ipsilateral injuries (B2-1), the elastic recoil of the pelvis usually restores the anatomy to near normal; therefore, no form of stabilization is required.

In the bucket handle type injury (B2-2), the sacrum is usually compressed; therefore, the pelvic ring may not move even with a closed manipulation under general anesthesia. For this particular injury, assessment of degree of stability is subtle. Stabilization will depend on the state of the patient and the degree of displacement. It is usually preferable to accept a leg length discrepancy of up to 1.5 cm with some internal rotation of the hemipelvis in preference to destabilizing the pelvis with the subsequent need for an external frame or internal fixation. If the leg length discrepancy is >1.5 cm or if the pelvic deformity is excessive, more aggressive management may be indicated, but only with the patient informed of the inherent risks and benefits. In that circumstance reduction may be obtained by externally rotating the hemipelvis through pins in the iliac crest (Fig. 64-11). After reduction has been achieved, the anterior frame is completed and held in external fixation. In rare instances of the tilt fracture, where bone is protruding into the female perineum, open reduction and internal fixation may be required.

In polytrauma patients with a lateral compression type B2 injury, an external skeletal frame is desirable. The frame should be applied early and the fracture reduced by external rotation. With the restoration of pelvic stability, pain will be reduced even with movement, which in turn will greatly facilitate the critical care management of the patient.

The options for definitive fixation of the vertically *unstable* pelvis (type C) include complex external fixation with or without skeletal traction, or open reduction and internal fixation. Complex frames have a biomechanical advantage over the simple frames. However, none can restore adequate stability to the pelvis, which would allow the patient to ambulate without loss of reduction. Therefore, since the added risks of the procedure do not substantially increase the benefit to the patient, they cannot be recommended.

In the emergency situation, especially in a polytraumatized patient, the combination of an *anterior skeletal frame with skeletal traction* provides the surgeon with a safe method of treatment. A supracondylar traction pin in the femur is favored. Often, up to 40 lb of traction is necessary to maintain the posterior sacroiliac complex in the reduced position. In polytrauma, the patient's course is unpredictable. The patient may become septic so that further surgical intervention to the pelvis would be contraindicated. The anterior frame plus traction might then become definitive treatment. This is especially true in those patients in whom an adequate reduction of the posterior sacroiliac complex is obtained and those in whom the posterior injury is a fracture.

For traction to be successful, it must be maintained for a minimum of 8 to 12 weeks, depending on the rate of healing as monitored by radiographs. Therefore, especially with posterior fracture rather than dislocation of the sacroiliac joint, where surgery is contraindicated, patients treated with provisional external fixation and femoral traction may be adequately managed with the expectation of a good result. The major disadvantage is the long period of enforced bed rest with its inherent risks in the polytraumatized patient. For this reason, open reduction and internal fixation of the vertically unstable pelvic ring may be the preferred option in selected patients.

For the unstable pelvic disruption with the potential for relatively poor long-term results, open reduction and internal fixation of the pelvis offers many advantages. Biomechanically, stable internal fixation can restore excellent stability to the pelvic ring, thereby allowing early ambulation of the patient, a distinct advantage to the polytraumatized patient. As well, the large cancellous surfaces of the pelvis are amenable to interfragmental compression to prevent both malunion and nonunion. However, the many risks include increased bleeding, wound problems, and nerve injury. Complication rates approaching 25 to 50 percent

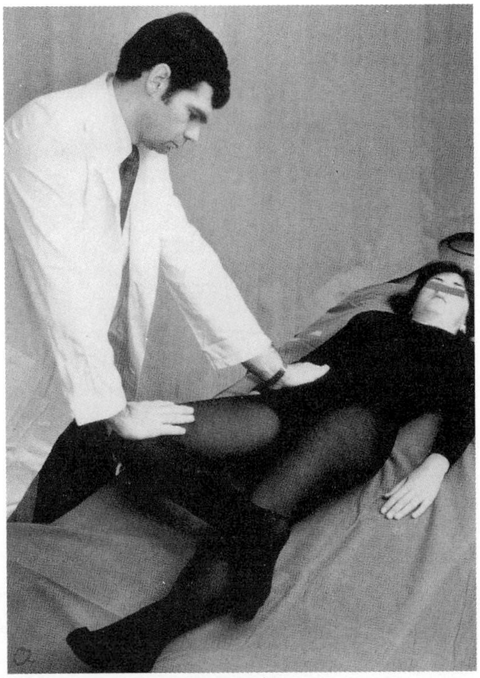

a

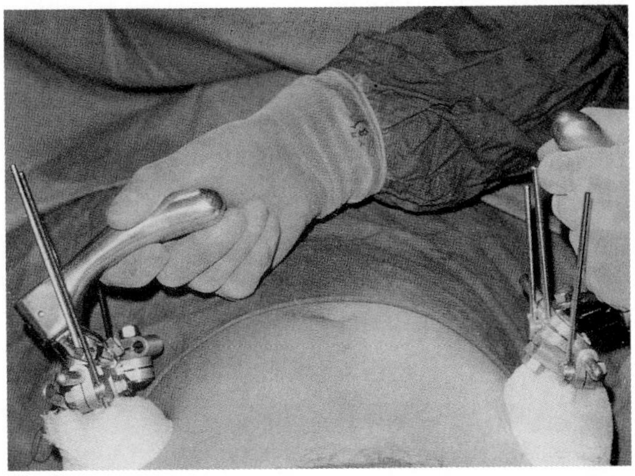

b

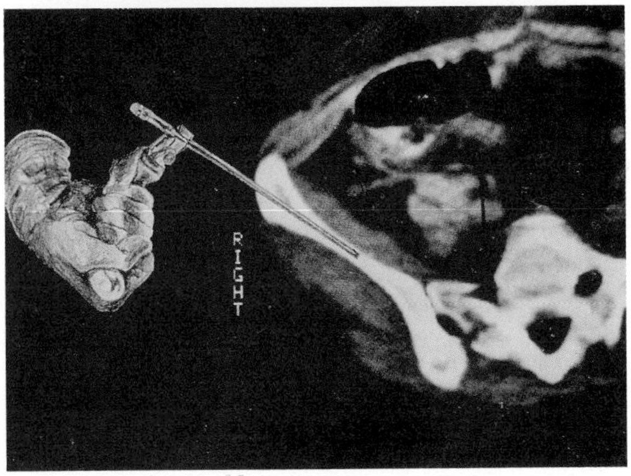

c

FIGURE 64-11 Lateral compression injuries may be reduced closed by external rotation of the hemipelvis (*a*). Insertion of pins for an external fixator as noted in the photograph (*b*) and the CT (*c*) allow direct external rotation forces to be applied to the hemipelvis, thereby simplifying the reduction. (From Schatzker J, Tile M: *The Rationale of Operative Fracture Care.* Heidelberg, Springer-Verlag, 1987.)

have been reported.[12] Theoretically, opening the pelvis may cause a loss of tamponade which may increase hemorrhage. Also, if massive transfusion becomes necessary, the patient's clotting mechanism may be deficient, thereby increasing the risk of further hemorrhage during a surgical procedure. These risks are so potentially devastating that some centers have recommended preoperative angiography and embolization, when necessary, for all patients in whom internal fixation is planned.[3,19] Posterior pelvic wounds are especially prone to skin necrosis.

Probable causes of this high rate of posterior wound breakdown include a crush injury to the skin at the time of injury and avulsion of the gluteus maximus fascia from its origin leaving the skin with an inadequate blood supply. Neurologic damage is another major risk of internal fixation. In posterior approaches, a misplaced screw may enter the first sacral foramen or the spinal canal, damaging the cauda equina with the sacral nerve roots. In anterior approaches to the sacroiliac joint the fifth lumbar nerve root is at risk.

Anterior internal fixation of a disrupted symphysis pubis will greatly simplify the management of the patient especially one undergoing abdominal or pelvic surgery for associated injuries, unless the wound is grossly contaminated by feces or a long-standing suprapubic drain is contemplated. If possible, suprapubic drains should be avoided in areas of fracture fixation. In that situation, external fixation is safer. The technique is quick and relatively safe since the dissection is usually completed by the trauma. In the open book (type B1) lesion, with no posterior instability, biomechanical tests have shown that good stability to the pelvic ring can be achieved with either anterior plating or anterior external fixation. However, if the symphysis disruption is associated with an unstable (type C) pelvic disruption, an-

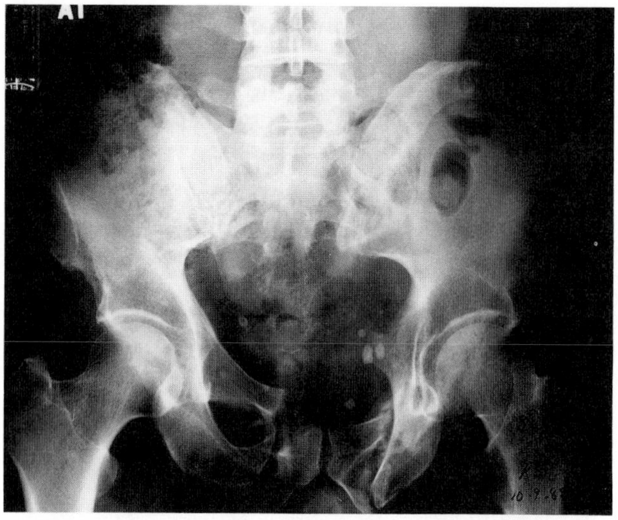

a

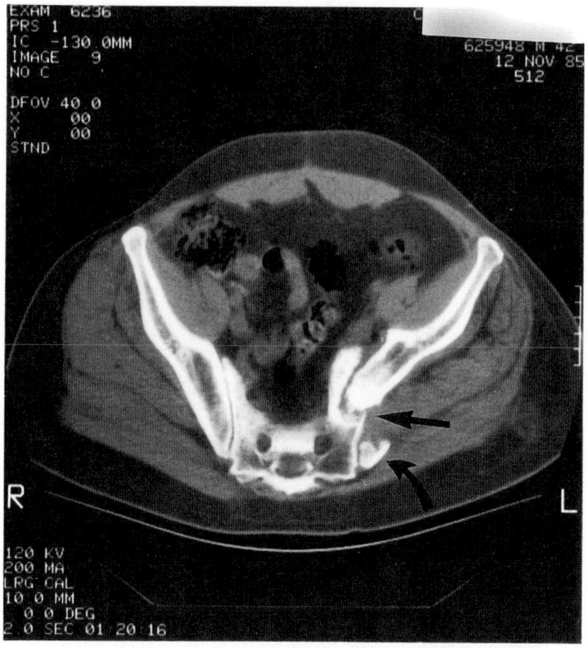

b

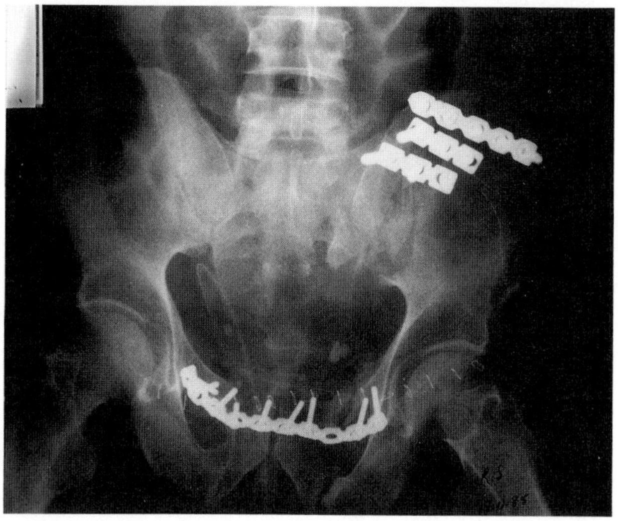

c

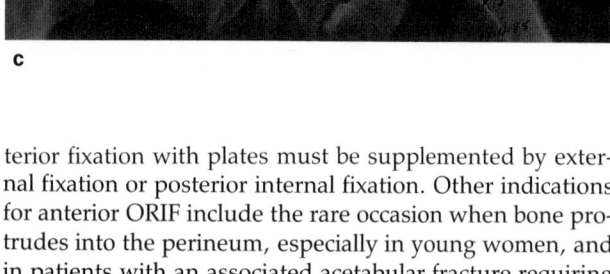

FIGURE 64-12 Reduction of the posterior sacroiliac complex. ***a.*** **The radiograph shows marked external rotation of the left hemipelvis with fractures of all four pubic rami.** ***b.*** **The degree of displacement is best seen on the CT scan, which shows that the left hemipelvis has been externally rotated and driven to the anterior surface of the sacrum (straight arrow), where it had caused a complete lumbosacral trunk injury. The remaining portion of the ilium is indicated by the curved arrow.** ***c.*** **The radiograph shows the result after ORIF with plates across the sacroiliac joint, the iliac fracture, and the rami. (From Tile M: Pelvic ring fractures: Should they be fixed? J Bone Joint Surg [Br] 70-B:1, 1988.)**

terior fixation with plates must be supplemented by external fixation or posterior internal fixation. Other indications for anterior ORIF include the rare occasion when bone protrudes into the perineum, especially in young women, and in patients with an associated acetabular fracture requiring ORIF.

Fixation of laterally placed pubic rami fractures is much more difficult, requiring an ilioinguinal approach. In most cases, the risks are greater than the benefits; therefore, this procedure is rarely indicated in pelvic ring trauma unless associated with an anterior acetabular fracture. In those particular unstable patterns, it is more advantageous to fix the posterior lesions and control the rami fractures with an anterior external frame.

The major indication for posterior internal fixation is an unstable, unreduced posterior sacroiliac complex, especially an unreduced sacroiliac dislocation with a gap of >1 cm (Fig. 64-12). If fractures are present posteriorly, especially through the ilium, and a minimal gap is noted, other methods such as external frames plus skeletal traction will suffice, but if the sacroiliac joint is dislocated, open reduction is the preferred option. Other indications for posterior fixation include those rare instances where the posterior sacroiliac complex is disrupted and the posterior skin has been lacerated. Since the wound is already open, posterior fixation is indicated. However, if the wound is in the perineum, then all forms of internal fixation are contraindicated. Treatment should include cleansing and careful debridement of the wound followed by stabilization with an external skeletal frame and skeletal traction. Both bowel and bladder diversion are essential to prevent sepsis. Posterior ORIF may also be indicated in those pelvic disruptions associated with an acetabular fracture requiring ORIF.

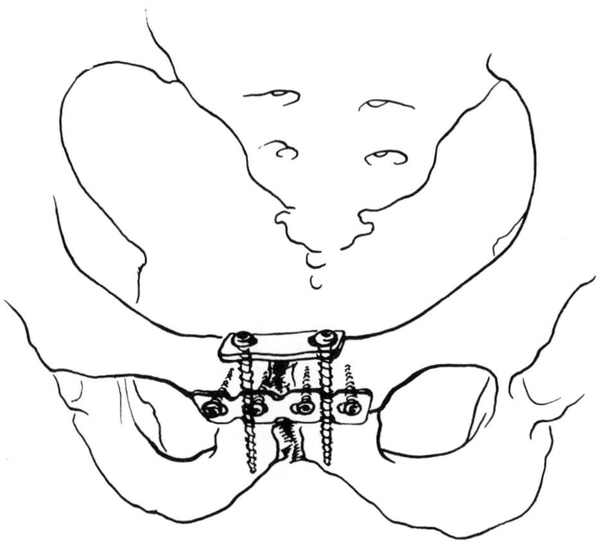

FIGURE 64-13 Plating the symphysis pubis. For stable injuries, a superiorly placed two-hole plate may be used. For vertically unstable injuries where posterior fixation will not be used, two plates at right angles to each other are recommended. (From Tile M: Pelvic ring fractures: Should they be fixed? J Bone Joint Surg [Br] 70B:1, 1988.)

SURGICAL METHOD

TIMING. It is preferable to wait until the patient's general state is improved, usually between the fifth and seventh post-operative day, to perform posterior ORIF of the pelvis. The use of percutaneous techniques, however, may allow immediate internal fixation with fewer complications. This would be contraindicated in the hemodynamically unstable patient, but in the hemodynamically stable patient it may be desirable.

ANTIBIOTICS. Prophylactic antibiotics are routinely given for these major operative procedures. Intravenous cefazolin (2 g daily) supplemented by tobramycin (160 mg daily) in cases of potential gram-negative contamination should be given for a minimum of 48 h.

POSITIONING AND REDUCTION. For disruption of the symphysis pubis in vertically stable (type B1) open book injuries, a two- to four-hole reconstruction plate should be placed on the superior surface and fixed with fully threaded cancellous screws. For unstable (type C) injuries where no posterior fixation is planned, two plates at 90° to each other, anteriorly and superiorly (Fig. 64-13), should be used to prevent movement in two planes.

The posterior sacroiliac complex may be approached either anteriorly or posteriorly. The anterior approach has the advantage of good soft tissue cover and is indicated if the posterior skin is crushed. The precise method used will depend on the pattern of fracture or fracture dislocation.

METHODS OF FIXATION. For *sacral fractures,* two transiliac bars from one posterior iliac spine to the other will provide good stability and compression of the sacral fracture with little risk to the neural elements[5] (Fig. 64-14). Care must be taken to avoid overcompression. Posterior screw fixation under image intensification, either open or closed, is another option but it increases the risk of damage to the neural elements.[5,10,12]

For *sacroiliac dislocations* with or without an iliac fracture, anterior plating of the sacroiliac joint is preferred.[5] Care must be taken to avoid the L_5 nerve root as it crosses the

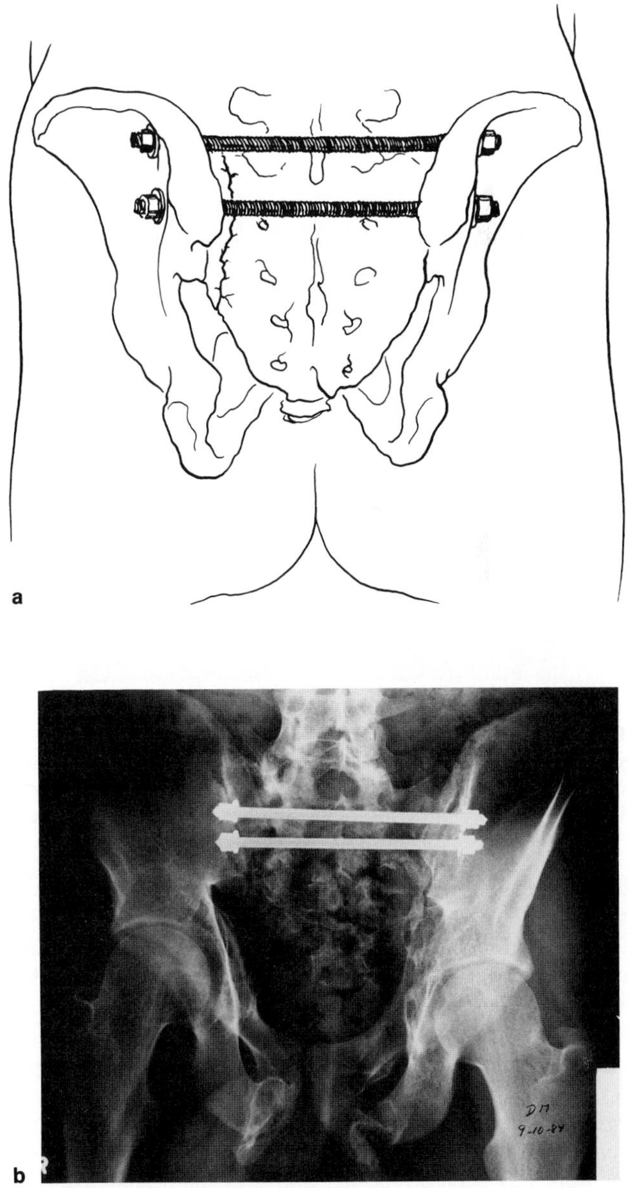

FIGURE 64-14 Transiliac bars. For sacral fractures, two transiliac bars provide good stability and compression of the fracture as noted on the diagram (*a*) and radiograph (*b*). (From Tile M: Pelvic ring fractures: Should they be fixed? J Bone Joint Surg [Br] 70B:1, 1988.)

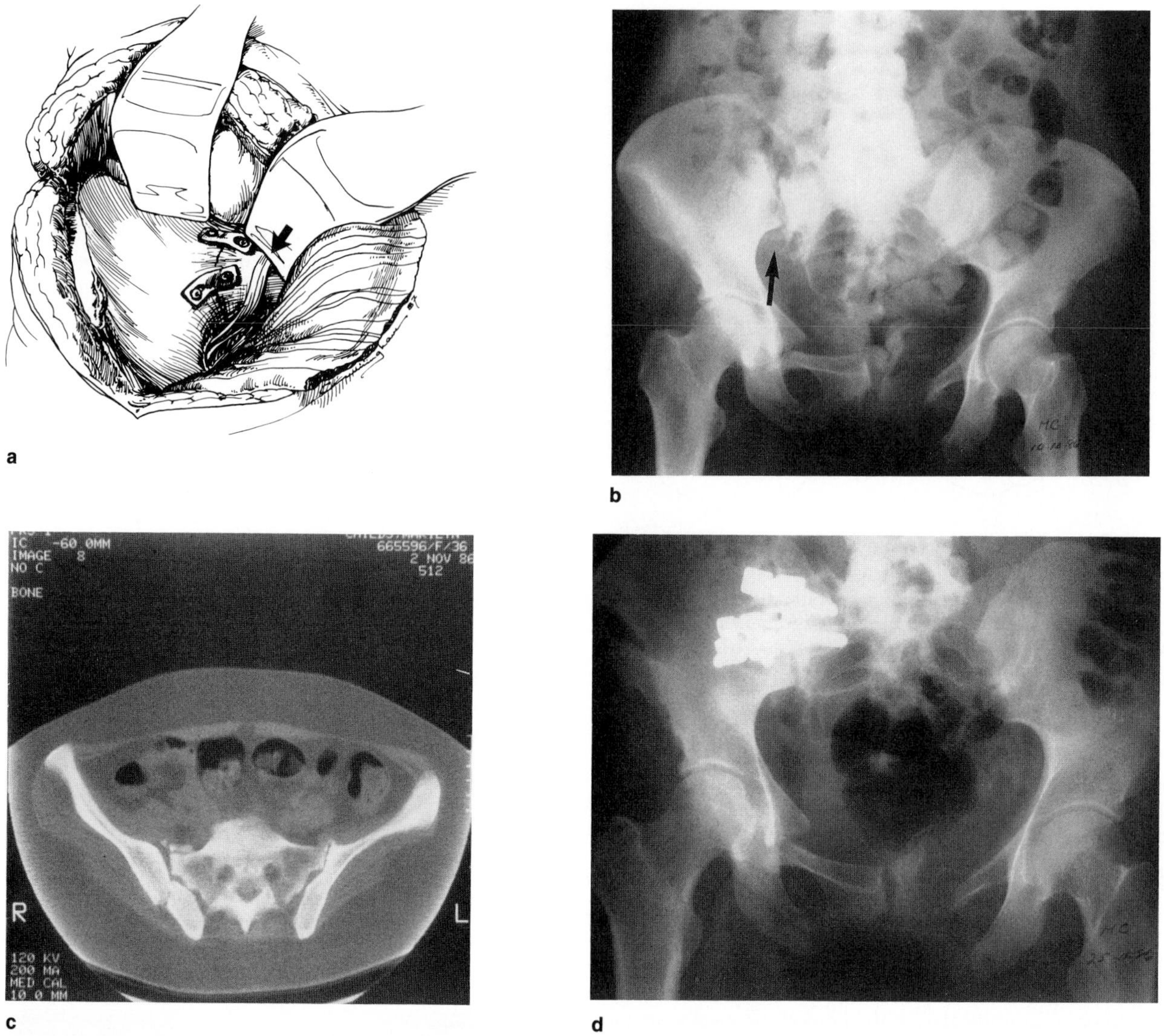

FIGURE 64-15 Anterior plating of the sacroiliac joint. *a*. The sacroiliac joint is exposed anteriorly by subperiosteal dissection of the iliacus muscle. Note the proximity of the L_5 nerve root (arrow). *b*. Anteroposterior radiograph shows a posteriorly displaced ununited sacroiliac fracture-dislocation (arrow). *c*. CT of the same patient. *d*. Fixation of the right sacroiliac joint using three pelvic reconstruction plates.

lateral mass of the sacrum (Fig. 64-15). Posterior screw fixation may provide equally good stability and is especially useful if an iliac fracture is also present, but there is the added risk of skin breakdown after a posterior approach. This method is safe when the screws penetrate only the lateral mass of the sacrum, but if the technique is used in patients with a sacral fracture the screws must enter the body of the sacrum, resulting in an increased risk of damage to the cauda equina or sacral nerves (Fig. 64-16). Recently, percutaneous posterior screw fixation of the sacroiliac joint has been advocated under image intensification, the major advantage being a decrease in the incidence of skin necrosis.[20]

Iliac fractures may be fixed by interfragmental screws or plates using standard techniques of internal fixation. The most common plates used are 3.5-mm reconstruction plates, which are more malleable and allow easier contouring.

MANAGEMENT OF PELVIC FRACTURES IN THE ICU

The foregoing discussion is intended to inform the critical care physician as to fundamental aspects of orthopedic decision-making and surgical intervention in the management of pelvic fractures. A number of general points should also be made in regard to the pre- and postoperative management of these patients.

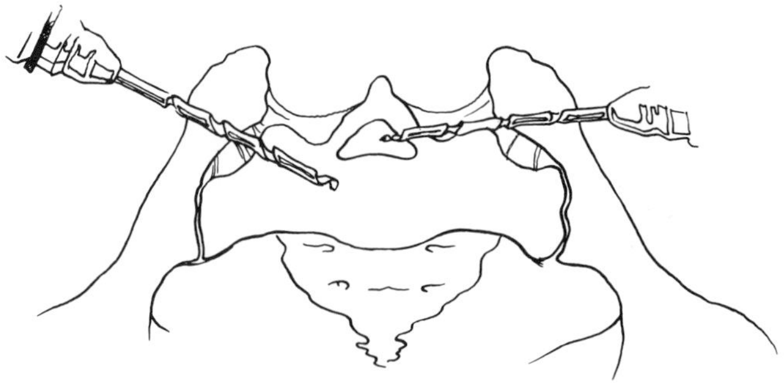

FIGURE 64-16 Posterior screw fixation of the sacroiliac joint for sacral fractures is a difficult technique which must be controlled by image intensification. Note the direction of the drill into the body of the sacrum (right). Even slight changes in the direction of the drill may produce major complications, such as penetration of the spinal canal and cauda equina or penetration of the anterior surface of the sacrum into the great blood vessels (left).

As noted, the trauma resulting in pelvic fracture often causes neurologic, torso, or other injuries. Most often, triage requires that assessment of injury at these other sites take precedence over extensive evaluation for pelvic bone and soft tissue injuries. It must be appreciated, however, that blood loss into the pelvis can be massive and life-threatening and may require extremely aggressive fluid resuscitation and during early management, use of pneumatic antishock garments. When life-threatening hypovolemia has occurred in the trauma patient, it can be difficult to partition blood loss between the abdomen, pelvis, and thighs by physical examination alone. CT scanning is remarkably helpful in this regard and should be used early in the stabilized patient when the potential for blood loss in multiple sites below the diaphragm exists.

In addition to possible occult blood loss, another early risk for these patients is thromboembolic disease, a risk that likely arises almost immediately after injury and remains high over a prolonged period of time until tissue repair and mobilization are achieved. Precise determination of the incidence of thromboembolism in pelvic trauma has not been made, but judging from patients with similar but even more limited injury (e.g., following hip surgery), virtually all of these patients likely develop venous thrombosis. Accordingly, measures to prevent pulmonary embolization should be routine (see Chap. 118). Full anticoagulation is unacceptable early in the course because of the risk of major hemorrhage in an occult site. If not contraindicated because of central nervous system injury or active ongoing bleeding, prophylactic doses of heparin should be considered. Intermittent pneumatic compression cuffs can be used in addition to or in place of heparin, but often are not feasible for technical reasons in patients with pelvic and extremity injuries. Noninvasive serial examination of the patient for venous thrombosis (see Chap. 23) is also often difficult technically. Recent experimental work with removable devices that interrupt the inferior vena cava may lay the groundwork for a useful intervention in these traumatized patients in the near future.

Another early complication of patients with pelvic trauma is fat embolization (see Chap. 118); it may also occur later in the course in association with intentional or unintentional movement of unstable bone fragments. In and of itself, fat embolism produces a syndrome characterized by acute hypoxemic respiratory failure (AHRF), thrombocytopenia, petechiae, mental status abnormalities, and fat microemboli recoverable from a number of different sites. The respiratory failure from uncomplicated fat embolization is generally well tolerated and self-limited, with resolution over 2 to 3 days, even if mechanical ventilatory support is required. During the early phase, AHRF in these patients may also result from lung contusion, adult respiratory distress syndrome (ARDS) following hypovolemic shock with blood product resuscitation, or other pulmonary manifestations of trauma; late in the course, AHRF often arises from nosocomial pneumonia or sepsis.

Late complications of pelvic trauma arise largely from infection and multisystem organ failure (see Chaps. 67 and 97). Immobilization from pelvic trauma and other contingencies of multisystem injury place these patients at high risk for nosocomial pneumonia. Within the limitations of their injuries, aggressive early mobilization and chest physiotherapy for selected patients with underlying lung disease is appropriate (see Chap. 84). For those patients requiring near immobilization for extended periods of time because of their orthopaedic and other injuries, devices such as rotating beds may find increasing application. Infection may also arise later in the course directly from pelvic or associated intraabdominal injuries. This can be particularly difficult diagnostically, since the physical examination is often nonspecific, the manifestations of infection such as fever and leukocytosis often have multiple noninfectious explanations, and the prior antimicrobial history is complex. When other obvious sites of infection cannot be identified and the pelvis remains a possible source, liberal use of imaging techniques such as CT scanning and ultrasound, with percutaneous tapping or draining of fluid collections, is advisable.

Thus, the range of complications in these patients during their management in the ICU is wide, and diagnostic and therapeutic strategies require frequent reformulation. This is best accomplished by an integrated approach to care, with careful consultation between orthopedist, other trauma surgeons, and the critical care team to optimize outcome.

CASE PRESENTATION

A 19-year-old man was the driver of a car which was hit from the side. He required extrication from the car and was taken to a local hospital where he was noted to have amnesia for the event, but was conscious on arrival at the primary hospital. Following initial resuscitation he was sent to Sunnybrook Medical Centre Trauma Unit by helicopter. On route the patient received 6 U packed cells and 4 L crystalloid. On arrival at Sunnybrook Medical

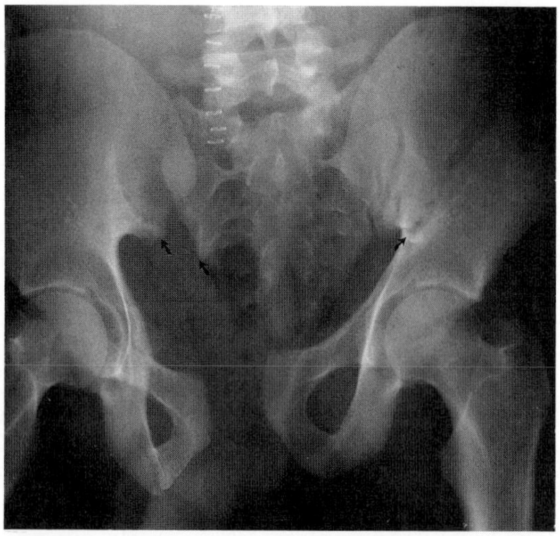

a

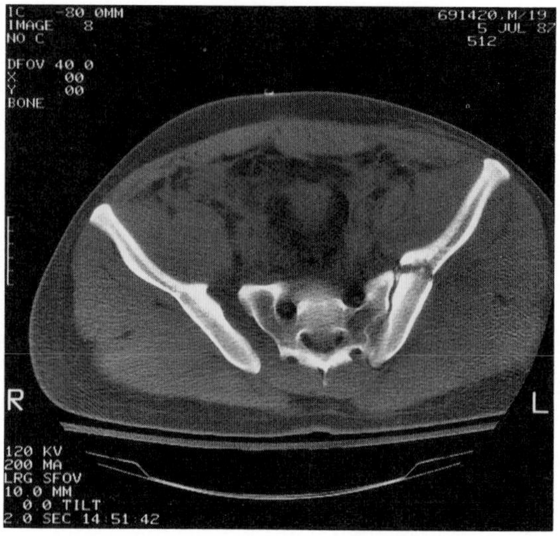

b

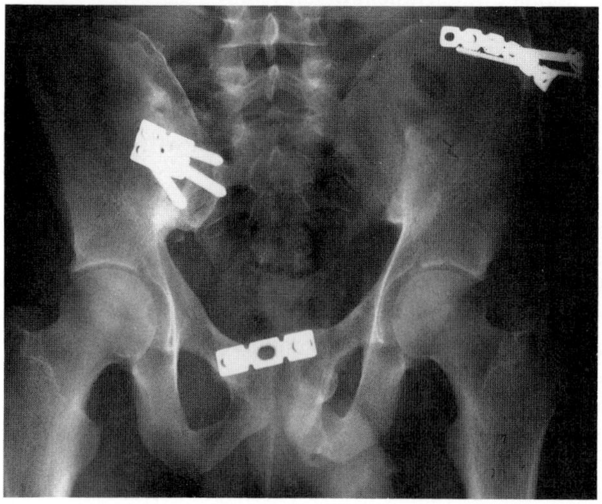

c

FIGURE 64-17 ***a*****. Anteroposterior pelvic radiograph shows a diastasis of the symphysis pubis, an unstable, displaced, right sacroiliac joint, and a fracture of the left ilium.** ***b*****. CT of the same patient demonstrates the markedly widened right sacroiliac joint. On the left side, the sacroiliac joint is stable. Note the fractured ilium.** ***c*****. The pelvis was stabilized with 3.5-mm reconstruction plates on the symphysis, the right sacroiliac joint anteriorly, and the left iliac fracture; also supplemented with lag screws.**

Centre his blood pressure was 130/80 and heart rate 110 beats/min. There was blood in his nasogastric tube. His abdomen was distended with generalized tenderness. Other findings were: a decrease in rectal tone, absent bulbocavernosus reflex, clinically unstable pelvis, weakness of the left extensor hallucis longus, peroneus longus and brevis, right tibialis anterior, peroneae and extensor hallucis longus muscles.

X-rays of the chest and cervical and thoracic spine were normal. A pelvic x-ray showed a disruption of the right sacroiliac joint with displacement (Fig. 64-17*a*), a fracture in the left iliac wing, and a diastasis of his symphysis pubis. A peritoneal lavage revealed gross blood.

He was taken directly to the operating room where a formal laparotomy revealed colonic serosal tears which were repaired and a retroperitoneal hematoma which was not opened. He was hemodynamically stable and a traction pin was placed in his right femur to temporarily maintain the right hemipelvis in good position. This was followed later by a CT scan which demonstrated a fracture of the left acetabulum (Fig. 64-17*b*).

The patient did well in the early posttrauma period. The neurologic abnormalities in his lower extremities resolved quickly. Four days posttrauma the patient was returned to the operating room where ORIF of all fractures of the pelvis were carried out using plates (Fig. 64-17*c*). All the procedures were done in the supine position through anterior approaches. He had an uncomplicated postoperative course, and at discharge, his neurologic deficit had completely resolved.

Three years following his fractures, the patient was doing extremely well. He was working full-time at a heavy job, and he considered himself completely normal. His neurologic picture had completely resolved as previously noted. He had mild low back pain on occasion. At that time both sacroiliac joints had fused. His metal was still in place.

CASE DISCUSSION

This patient had a massive pelvic disruption including a symphysis pubis disruption, an unstable right sacroiliac dislocation, and a left iliac fracture. He had a grossly positive peritoneal lavage, but was at all times hemodynamically stable. The decision to perform the laparotomy was made in consultation with the orthopedic surgeons, demonstrating the importance of a team approach to the management of such patients.

Because of the left iliac fracture and because he was hemodynamically stable, external fixation was not required. This allowed further investigation and pelvic stabilization was not performed at the time of laparotomy. However, a skeletal traction pin was inserted on the right side to temporarily maintain the reduction of the right sacroiliac joint and CT scan later allowed more precise definition of the injury so that formal surgical treatment could be planned. Early ORIF of the left iliac fracture, the symphysis pubis, and the right sacroiliac joint were all performed in the supine position using anterior approaches. The patient did extremely well and demonstrates that with a planned team approach through management and adherence to the principles outlined in this chapter a good outcome can be achieved from seemingly devastating fractures of the pelvis.

References

1. McCowan S, Kellam JF, Tile M: Unstable pelvic ring disruptions—Results of open reduction and internal fixation. Orthop Trans 11(3):478, 1987.
2. McMurtry R, Walton D, Dickinson D et al: Pelvic disruption in the polytraumatized patient: A management protocol. Clin Orthop 151:22, 1980.
3. Goldstein A, Phillips T, Sclafani SJA et al: Early open reduction and internal fixation of the disrupted pelvic ring. J Trauma 26(4):325, 1986.
4. Huittinen VM, Slatis P: Fractures of the pelvis, trauma mechanism, types of injury and principles of treatment. Acta Chir Scand 138:563, 1972.
5. Tile M: *Fractures of the Pelvis and Acetabulum*. Baltimore, Williams & Wilkins, 1984, pp 10–35.
6. Personal communication.
7. Hesp WL, van der Werken C, Keunen RW et al: Unstable fractures and dislocations of the pelvic ring: Results of treatment in relation to the severity of injury. Neth J Surg 37:148, 1985.
8. Holdsworth FW: Dislocations and fracture-dislocation of the pelvis. J Bone Joint Surg [Br] 30B:461, 1948.
9. Pennal GF, Tile M, Waddell JP et al: Pelvic disruption: Assessment and classification. Clin Orthop 151:12, 1980.
10. Raf L: Double vertical fractures of the pelvis. Acta Chir Scand 131:298, 1966.
11. Dickinson D, Lifeso R, McBroom R et al: Disruptions of the pelvic ring. J Bone Joint Surg *64B*(5):635, 1982.
12. Kellam JF, McMurtry RY, Paley D: The unstable pelvic fracture: Operative treatment. Orthop Clin North Am 8:25, 1987.
13. Raffe J, Christensen NM: Compound fractures of the pelvis. Am J Surg 132:282, 1976.
14. Morales GR, Phillips T, Conn AK et al: Traumatic hemipelvectomy: Report of 2 survivors and review. J Trauma 23:615, 1983.
15. Gylling SF, Ward ME, Holcroft JW et al: Immediate external fixation of unstable pelvic fractures. Am J Surg 150:721, 1985.
16. Mears DC, Rubash HE: Acute resuscitation, in Mears DC, Rubash HE: *Pelvic and Acetabular Fractures.* Slack, Thorofare, NJ, 1986, p 163.
17. Pennal GF, Sutherland GO: Fractures of the pelvis. (Motion Picture) American Academy of Orthopedic Surgeons Film Library, 1961.
18. Mears DC, Fu FH: Modern concepts of external skeletal fixation of the pelvis. Clin Orthop 151:665, 1980.
19. Delal S, Burgess A, Young J et al: Pelvic fractures: Classification by force vector in relationship to associated injuries. Presented at The Orthopedic Trauma Association Meeting, Oct. 27–28, 1988, Dallas, TX.
20. Tompkins RG, McCabe CJ, Burke JF et al: Rectal necrosis after pelvic crush injury. J Trauma 28(5):697, 1988.

Chapter 65

EXTREMITY INJURIES

G.E. JOHNSON
A.R. DOWNS

KEY POINTS

- *Knowledge of the mechanism of injury helps in anticipating the type and severity of extremity injury.*
- *Compartment syndrome must be recognized and treated early to avoid serious late morbidity.*
- *Peripheral nerve injuries may be difficult to recognize clinically in multiple trauma and must be specifically looked for.*
- *Vascular injuries must be anticipated, and any patient with questionable or proven vascular injury must be assessed by a vascular surgeon.*
- *Complications of extremity vascular injuries are best avoided by prompt treatment of surgically correctable lesions.*
- *Fractures, although not life threatening, are important considerations in general patient management. Management must facilitate early control of hemorrhage and ischemia and general patient care and must also result in the best possible functional outcome.*
- *Postfracture hypoxemia from fat embolism, although not common, may be life threatening and require ventilatory support.*

Injuries to the extremities frequently accompany multisystem trauma and require important consideration in the overall management of critically ill patients. Exsanguinating hemorrhage must be controlled as part of the initial resuscitation. In addition, the method of management of extremity injuries can seriously impact on a patient's overall management. Complications associated with extremity injuries, such as sepsis, hemorrhage, shock, and crush syndrome, can, of themselves, also be life threatening. It is also extremely important that long-term function remain a consideration, even in the critically ill, as all too often extremity injuries receiving less than optimal care in the early stages result in serious long-term morbidity.

Mechanism of Injury

Knowledge of the mechanism of injury is helpful in **1.** anticipating the combination of trunk and extremity injuries, **2.** determining the degree of soft-tissue injury, **3.** prioritizing management, and **4.** identifying late complications as early as possible.

Following a fall from a height, the victim may, in addition to injuring solid viscera, sustain fractures of the calcaneus, a vertical shear fracture of the pelvis, and fractures of the spine, usually at the thoracolumbar junction. The unrestrained driver of a car in a head-on motor vehicle accident may suffer chest and abdominal injuries from impacting with the steering wheel, but additionally the knee striking the dash may cause a fractured patella or posterior cruciate ligament tear. With the force transmitted along the shaft of the femur, a fracture of the neck of the femur or posterior fracture/dislocation of the hip may result.

A car-pedestrian accident frequently results in a predictable pattern of musculoskeletal injuries if close attention is focused on an accurate history. The point of initial impact may cause a valgus force to the knee on the side of contact and a varus force on the contralateral knee, resulting in tearing of the medial collateral and lateral collateral ligaments, respectively. The victim may then be thrown over the hood of the car, strike the windshield with the head and shoulder, and subsequently land on the ground, fracturing his pelvis.

In anticipating the degree of soft-tissue injury, it is obvious that a direct crushing injury increases the likelihood of skin and subcutaneous tissue necrosis as well as the possibility of compartment syndrome and deep vein thrombosis. The effect of a rolling mechanism, as when a vehicle wheel passes over a limb, can be particularly misleading. On initial inspection, there may be only minor abrasions or skin lacerations. However, the shearing forces that develop between the subcutaneous tissue and fascia tear the perforating vessels, resulting in a large area of necrotic soft tissue and devitalized skin flap.

Compartment Syndrome

The intensivist dealing with multisystem trauma must maintain a high index of suspicion for development of a compartment syndrome. This is defined as an elevation of the interstitial pressure in a closed osseofascial compartment, resulting in microvascular compromise.[1] Compartment syndrome may result from prolonged external pressure, direct trauma, with or without an underlying fracture, and vascular injury, especially following revascularization of an ischemic limb. Other risk factors, especially associated with multiple trauma, may include a history of hypotension, the use of pneumatic antishock trousers, and coagulopathy. Compartment syndromes are particularly common in multiple-system trauma related to high-speed motor vehicle accidents; when the patient has sustained a crushing injury, the likelihood of development of compartment syndrome in a second anatomic site is high.[2]

Compartment syndrome is precipitated by increased fluid within a rigid fibro-osseous compartment, resulting in pressure elevation, venous stasis, decreased capillary flow, tissue hypoperfusion, and eventually, anaerobic metabolism. Tissue hypoperfusion may lead to muscle and nerve necrosis while distal pulses are still maintained. Although most frequently seen in the forearm or leg, compartment syndromes are now being recognized with much greater frequency in other areas, such as the hand, foot, and thigh.[3,4]

DIAGNOSIS

In the conscious patient with no local nerve or spinal cord injury, the cardinal symptom is pain disproportionate to the known cause of pain (e.g., fracture). Other helpful clinical findings are swelling and tenderness over the involved compartment. In the patient able to cooperate with physical examination, the most important signs of an impending compartment syndrome are severe pain on passive stretch of the muscles within the compartment, hypoesthesia in the area of cutaneous innervation from nerves lying within the compartment, and severe weakness of the involved muscles.

A greater diagnostic problem occurs in the unconscious patient with the above risk factors and a swollen tense extremity. In this situation, intracompartmental pressure measurement, which should not be elevated above 30 to 40 mmHg, is helpful in making the diagnosis. However, because of considerable individual variation, there is no single intracompartmental pressure which indicates irreversible muscle or nerve ischemia, and injury appears related to both absolute pressure and its duration.

In one investigation utilizing ^{31}P magnetic resonance spectroscopy to quantitatively study intracellular high-energy phosphate compounds, it was found that the perfusion pressure (the difference between the mean arterial pressure and compartment pressure) is the key determinant of the degree of injury and ischemia postfasciotomy,[5] emphasizing the importance of avoiding hypotension. In some studies nerve conduction velocity was shown to better predict the degree of ischemic injury and potential for recovery than blood flow measurements or muscle enzyme determinations.[6] Most authors agree that the decision to proceed to fasciotomy is a clinical one and that a complete fasciotomy performed early (less than 8 h following onset) will result in good functional recovery.

MANAGEMENT

Nonoperative management is possible only in the earliest stages and consists of removing all sources of external pressure (including cutting the cast and padding to expose skin throughout the length of the case). It is also important to maintain the limb at the same level as the heart to maintain perfusion and minimize further fluid collection. Success of nonoperative management is indicated by complete resolution of symptoms and signs within 1 h.

Surgical management consists of a thorough open release of the entire compartment involved, and in some areas (large multipennate muscles, e.g., glutei and deltoid) epimysiotomy.[7] Associated underlying fractures should be stabilized and the fasciotomy incisions packed open to await secondary suturing or skin grafting within 4 to 7 days.[8] Complications of compartment syndrome include myoglobinuria and acute renal failure, infection of the fasciotomy site, loss of range of movement of the affected joints, and muscular weakness.

Peripheral Nerve Injury

Injuries to a peripheral nerve may be easily overlooked in multisystem injury, especially in the unconscious patient. Some nerve injuries occur in common association with fractures and dislocations; for example, radial nerve palsy caused by oblique fracture of the distal third of the humerus, median nerve injury in Colles' fracture, anterior interosseous nerve injury with supracondylar fractures of the humerus, and sciatic or common peroneal nerve injury with posterior dislocations of the hip.

DIAGNOSIS

A detailed neurologic examination should be conducted with special attention to those extremities with a known injury. A screening examination may be performed quickly by identifying the specific nerve to be tested, examining for sensation in the isolated zone of cutaneous innervation of that nerve, and choosing a single muscle which best satisfies the three following criteria: **1.** most distal, **2.** least cross innervation, **3.** not inhibited by pain. For example, examination of the radial nerve in association with a fracture of the shaft of the distal third of the humerus should include determination of sensation in the first dorsal web space and motor function of the extensor pollicis longus. In the unconscious or impaired patient, one may observe for altered or asymmetric spontaneous movements in the extremities.

MANAGEMENT

Once the peripheral nerve injury has been identified, the next decision is whether the injury is a lesion in continuity or a physical disruption of the nerve (neurotmesis). Any nerve injury which is felt to be in continuity and does not recover within 3 to 6 weeks is likely an axonotmesis. With this injury the first muscle to be innervated upon regeneration of the axons is identified and an approximate schedule is set, based upon axonal regeneration at the rate of approximately 1 mm/day plus 1 month delay at the site of the injury. During this waiting period, following the patient with a Tinel's sign is helpful. A positive Tinel's sign (pain or paresthesia in the distribution of the nerve upon tapping over the course of the nerve distal to the level of the injury) which is progressive indicates that nerve regeneration is taking place. If this does not occur according to the above schedule, then a neurotmesis is likely and the nerve should be explored. The nerve repair may either be primary (within 7 days) or secondary. Under optimal circumstances (a clean incision with a healthy, well-vascularized bed of soft tissue), primary repair is recommended.[9] In the multiply traumatized patient, primary nerve repair is rarely indicated as this may unduly prolong the surgical procedure. Further, the soft-tissue injury is often extensive and requires multiple debridements, increasing the risk of ischemia and infection. If in the course of extremity surgery for other purposes the nerve ends are identified and require more than simple suturing, they should be apposed and tagged to maintain length and facilitate identification at a later time.

Vascular Injuries

Most patients with isolated vascular injuries of the extremities do not qualify for admission to an intensive care unit unless there is massive blood loss and shock. If a patient has an open injury due to penetrating or blunt trauma with continuing bleeding, direct transfer to the operating room from the emergency room is usually indicated. The patient may require intensive care postoperatively for shock management or the effects of reperfusion injury.

The multiple-trauma patient with head, torso, and extremity injuries is more likely to be admitted directly to the intensive care unit for assessment and management. It is this type of patient who will require appropriate assessment for vascular injuries associated with extremity soft-tissue injury or fractures. The mechanism of trauma will lead one to suspect particular injuries.

BLUNT VASCULAR INJURIES

UPPER EXTREMITY

Traction injuries of the shoulder girdle may be associated with brachial plexus palsy and innominate, subclavian, or axillary artery injury. Fracture or dislocation about the shoulder or elbow is potentially associated with arterial injuries, especially supracondylar humeral fractures in children.

LOWER EXTREMITY

The most common and most serious site of lower extremity vascular injury associated with skeletal injury is the popliteal artery.[10] Fractures about the knee (dislocation of the joint, upper tibia and fibula fractures, or supracondylar fractures of the femur) are the skeletal injuries most commonly associated with popliteal artery occlusion and account for the majority of amputations required for these injuries. Femoral shaft fractures due to blunt trauma are less commonly associated with femoral artery occlusion. Since the collateral circulation about the midsuperficial femoral artery is much better than it is about the popliteal artery, limb-threatening ischemia is less frequent with isolated femoral shaft fractures, even with involvement of the femoral artery. Dislocation of the hip is rarely associated with an arterial injury.

When arterial occlusion has occurred in the presence of shock, ischemic injury to the muscle and nerves will be more severe because of the poor collateral circulation. Time is of the essence in managing the acutely ischemic limb, and it is important to recognize that muscle cell death occurs after 6 h of ischemia. Revascularization must be accomplished within this time frame to preserve the function of the limb.[11] Recognition of the presence of an ischemic extremity is of paramount importance if normal function is to be preserved and amputation avoided.

CLINICAL ASSESSMENT

The clinical diagnosis of an ischemic extremity is usually not difficult. The type of injury should raise the suspicion of vascular insult; then the five p's—pain, pallor, paresthesias, paralysis, and pulselessness—will usually confirm the diagnosis. When local pain is out of proportion to the apparent injury, vascular injury (or compartment syndrome) should be suspected. Unfortunately the patient with multiple injuries may be in shock or have an associated head injury, so one must rely upon assessment of the peripheral pulses. These may be misleading, however, in the hypotensive patient.

NONINVASIVE ASSESSMENT

The continuous wave Doppler may be used to assess peripheral flow. However, in the patient in shock, this may not be reliable. If a flow signal is present at the ankle or wrist, at least the safe time frame for assessment is longer.[12]

If pulses are still absent after the patient is hemodynamically stabilized, one has to presume occlusion is present: An arteriogram should be performed either in the angiography suite or in the operating room (see Fig. 65-1).

If there are multiple fractures in the extremity, it is most helpful to have multiple film angiography to determine the site of occlusion. However, in the unstable or hypotensive patient angiography may be unreliable in determining the site of occlusion because of slow flow. Arterial spasm may be present and is characterized angiographically by thread-like arteries in continuity which fill distal to the level of the suspected injury (see Fig. 65-2). Angiographic documentation of a patent circulation allows one to safely observe the patient with the expectation that normal flow will resume when the patient's general condition has improved. Ischemia must not be attributed to spasm with the expectation of spontaneous resolution unless there is angiographic proof or the continuous wave Doppler demonstrates adequate distal flow.

MANAGEMENT

The ischemic limb should be protected from additional external trauma. Wounds should have occlusive dressings and fractures should be stabilized. The dislocated knee has often been reduced at the scene of the accident or before transport of the patient. Prophylactic antibiotics are given depending on the nature of the injury.

The objective of treatment is restoration of blood flow within 6 h of the onset of the ischemia. As soon as the patient's general condition permits, arterial reconstruction should begin. All critical artery injuries should be repaired (e.g., common femoral, superficial femoral, popliteal, subclavian, axillary, brachial). The radial, ulnar, profunda femoral, or profunda brachial arteries may be sacrificed in isolation if collateral flow is adequate. The principles of arterial repair require adequate exposure at the site of the injured artery to allow appropriate assessment and debridement of the injured artery.

An end-to-end anastomosis is the best type of repair; this can be done in the superficial femoral, popliteal, and axillary arteries with excision of up to 1.5 cm of artery with

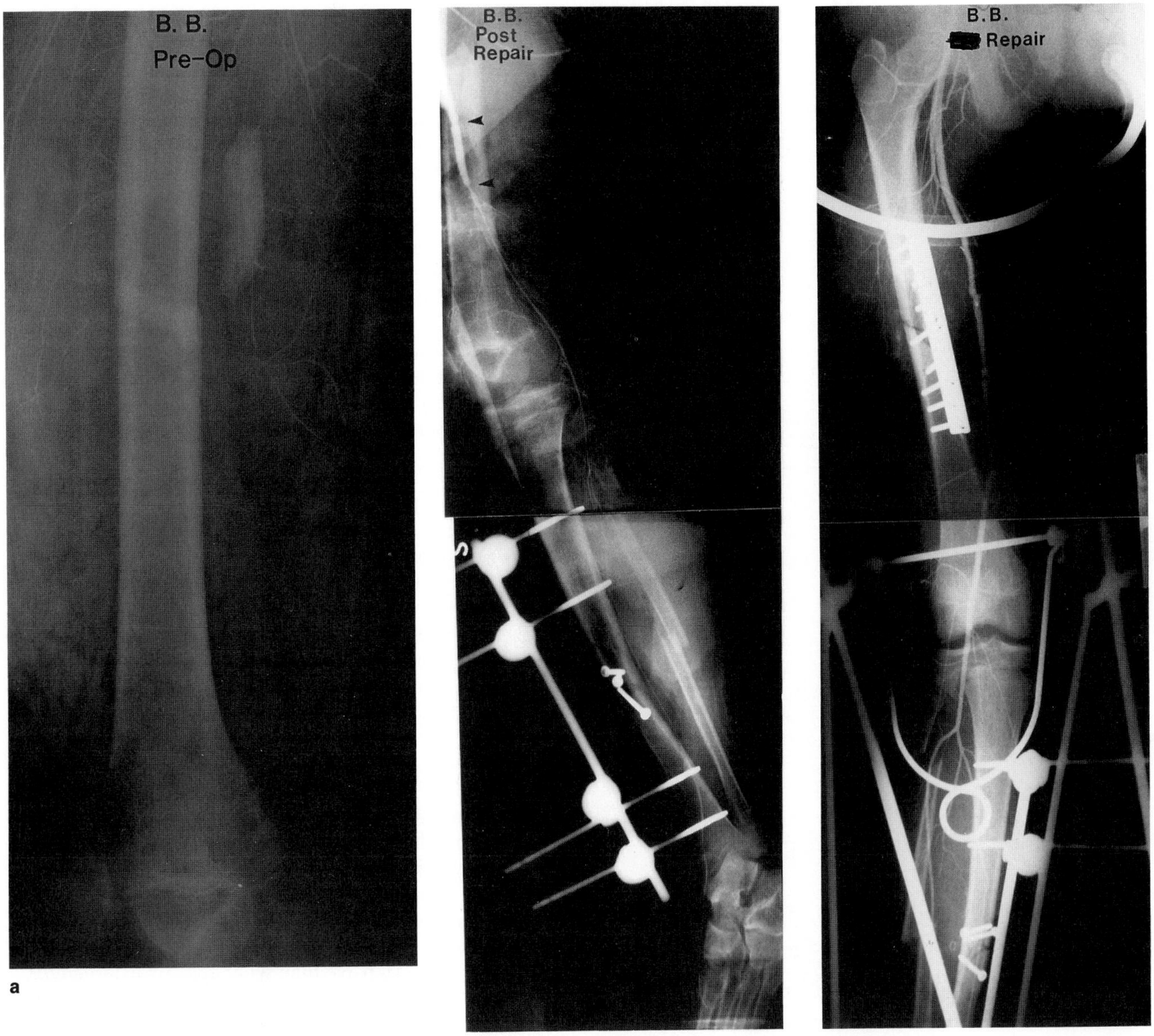

a b c

FIGURE 65-1 *(a)* **A 16-year-old male presented 2 h after a car–pedestrian accident, with a blood pressure of 90/48, pulse of 108, a compound fracture of the right femur, degloving of the thigh, and an open fracture of the tibia and fibula. The lower leg was cold, anesthetic, pulseless, and without movement. The patient was stabilized with crystalloid, but there was no improvement in the distal circulation. An angiogram demonstrated a superficial femoral artery occlusion and little distal flow through collaterals.** *(b)* **Operative repair with a vein graft restored flow, but the distal arteries were in severe spasm. The postoperative arteriogram demonstrates vein graft at arrows, with distal spasm.** *(c)* **Angiogram 10 days postoperatively shows excellent distal arteries.**

adequate mobilization.[10] If this cannot be accomplished without tension, then a graft segment replacement will be necessary. Usually an autogenous saphenous vein from the opposite limb is used, and, therefore, its use for resuscitation should be avoided when possible. An autogenous artery such as the hypogastric artery may also be used, but this is rarely immediately accessible. If the saphenous vein is not adequate, then a prosthetic graft such as PTFE or dacron may be used, but this is very much a second choice because of higher early and late occlusion.[13] Upon completion of the repair, angiography is essential.

When there is an associated fracture, stabilization is achieved by external or internal fixation depending on the site of injury and the degree of contamination. It is usually preferable to perform the arterial repair before the fracture fixation to reduce the ischemia time. Rarely is the limb so unstable that fixation is necessary to facilitate the vascular repair. If it is deemed advisable to stabilize the limb prior to

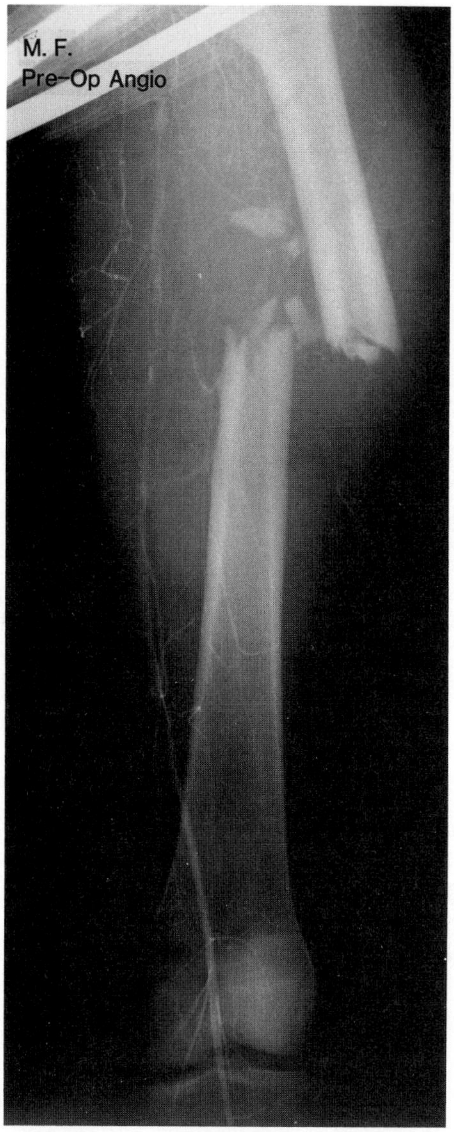

FIGURE 65-2 Preoperative angiogram shows spasm in superficial femoral artery and good distal filling. The foot was cool and pulseless, but Doppler signals were present over the pedal arteries. Following internal fixation, normal circulation and pulses returned.

the arterial repair, it may be helpful to use a temporary shunt to restore flow while awaiting the definitive repair. It is necessary to appropriately reassess the vascular repair following fracture stabilization. Soft-tissue coverage should be attained over the site of arterial repair.

Concomitant venous repair is usually performed, especially at the popliteal level. This may be accomplished by lateral suture, end-to-end anastomosis, or vein graft.

Local heparin is generally used, and, in the absence of bleeding problems, systemic heparin may be used during the vascular repair and then reversed with protamine sulfate. Postoperative anticoagulation is not recommended.

Concomitant fasciotomy should be performed if the ischemia is over 6 h or if there is evidence of compartment swelling before or after revascularization. If there is no definite indication for fasciotomy at the time of the vascular repair, subsequent observation for increasing compartment pressure is essential. Postoperative assessment of motor or sensory function as an index of increasing intracompartmental pressure is frequently inaccurate because of associated neurologic injury. Compartment pressure measurement may be helpful postoperatively with an acceptable maximum pressure of 40 mmHg. However, the need for fasciotomy is usually determined clinically and is best made by the experienced vascular or orthopedic surgeon.

Close monitoring of the adequacy of circulation postoperatively is essential. Palpation of pulses and assessment with continuous wave Doppler are the best techniques. Frequently after peripheral arterial repair, the distal pulses do not return immediately because of arterial spasm, and Doppler assessment may be necessary to determine adequacy of flow and continued patency of the arterial reconstruction.

The revascularized limb should be in a neutral position in relation to the level of the heart and protected from external pressure, since it is often insensate because of associated nerve injury or ischemic neuropraxia. It is essential to avoid pressure sites which may cause tissue necrosis. The sites most vulnerable in the lower extremity are the heel and the Achilles tendon area. These sites must be protected by frequent position changes. Fasciotomy wounds should be closed within 4 to 7 days to avoid infection.

PENETRATING VASCULAR INJURIES

Most penetrating civilian vascular injuries are due to low-velocity missiles such as handguns or stab wounds. Shotgun injury may cause multiple vascular lesions.

A high-velocity missile may cause extensive internal tissue damage because of the concussive force, particularly if it has caused a fracture. The internal soft-tissue injury may be much more extensive than what appears externally.[14] A penetrating injury may present with massive blood loss and shock, pulsating hematoma, arteriovenous fistula, or ischemia.

When the site of the penetrating injury is in the vicinity of the neurovascular bundle, there is always the possibility of a vascular injury. The presence of peripheral pulses does not exclude an arterial injury since it may be a noncritical artery such as the deep femoral. Alternatively, a major artery may have a partial laceration without occlusion, or an arteriovenous fistula may be present. It is important to identify these nonlimb-threatening injuries early, since they are more easily repaired in the acute setting, and late sequelae such as false aneurysm and arteriovenous fistulae can be avoided.[15]

DIAGNOSIS

An arterial injury is suspected in any penetrating injury in proximity to the neurovascular bundle. There may be evidence of ischemia with the five p's present, but a significant number of arterial injuries will not cause ischemia. Venous injuries do not cause ischemia. Evidence of massive blood

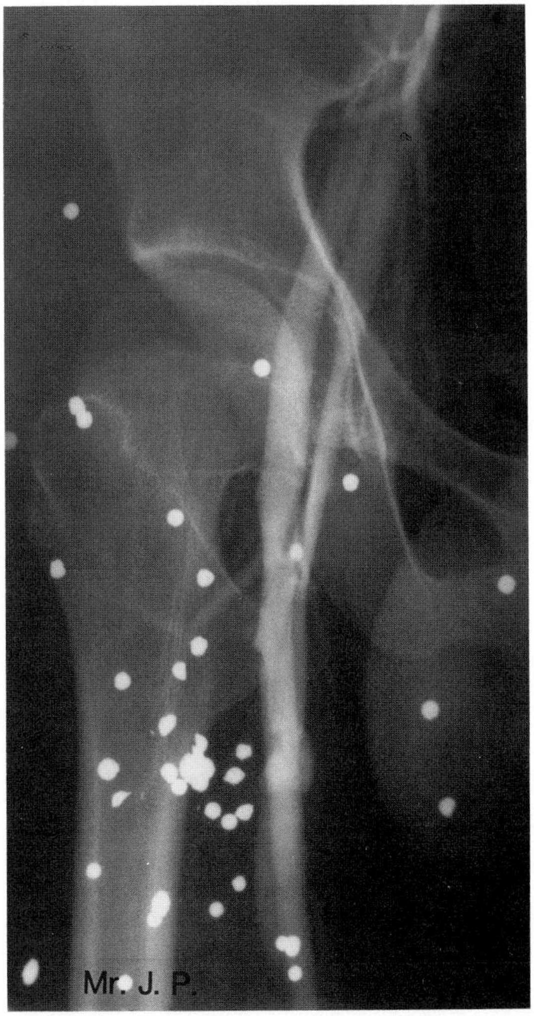

FIGURE 65-3 Preoperative angiogram shows filling of superficial femoral artery and vein due to arteriovenous fistula. Vein graft repair of the artery and vein restored normal circulation.

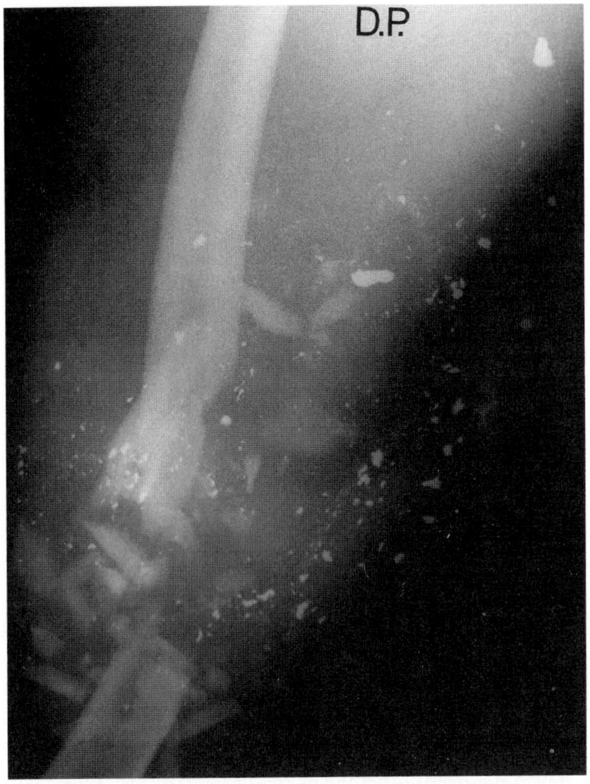

FIGURE 65-4 Plain x-ray of the femur shows shattered femur and metallic fragments due to high-velocity missile. Massive hemorrhage necessitated immediate surgical exploration which revealed frank muscle necrosis requiring amputation.

loss, which has often stopped by the time the patient arrives in the hospital, is sufficient evidence to warrant either exploration or angiography. The presence of a pulsating or expanding hematoma is indicative of an arterial injury. A systolic bruit or continuous bruit may be present with stenosis, pseudoaneurysm, or arteriovenous fistula. In the stable patient, an angiogram should be performed to identify the site and nature of the lesion (see Fig. 65-3).

In the unstable patient direct transfer to the operating room for control of the bleeding and vessel repair is indicated. Wounds should not be explored except in the operating room. Bleeding can usually be controlled by pressure dressings or direct compression. Dressings or penetrating foreign bodies should not be removed until the patient is in the operating room and anesthetized.

MANAGEMENT

The patient should receive antibiotic and tetanus prophylaxis (see Table 65-1). The injured site is explored under general anesthesia. A donor site for a saphenous vein graft should also be prepared. Usually proximal and distal control is obtained; however, it may be simpler to proceed directly through the site of the injury. Finger control of the severed artery and compression of the accompanying veins can usually be readily accomplished. When bleeding is under control, complete assessment of the associated soft-tissue injury is performed. With high-velocity missile injury the internal explosion may have caused so much damage that primary amputation is indicated (see Fig. 65-4).

When there is extensive muscle destruction with bone and major nerve disruption, it may be safer to proceed with amputation. In any case all dead muscle must be debrided. Appropriate arterial and venous repair is accomplished with direct anastomosis or vein graft. In severely contaminated wounds an extra-anatomic placement of the graft may be preferable. If a vein is not readily available, a prosthetic graft may be used, although with potentially inferior results.

Grafts should be covered with soft tissue, and fractures stabilized with internal or external fixation. It is usually preferable to repair the vessels first, although if ischemia is absent or of short duration, fracture stabilization may be performed first. Angiography upon completion is usually desirable in the lower extremity but may not be necessary in the upper extremity since the pulses are usually more easily palpated at the wrist.

TABLE 65-1 Tetanus Immunization Schedule

History of Absorbed Tetanus Toxoid, Number of Doses	NONTETANUS-PRONE WOUNDS		TETANUS-PRONE WOUNDS	
	Td[a]	TIG[b]	Td	TIG
Unknown or less than three	Yes	No	Yes	Yes
Three or more[c]	No[d]	No	No[e]	No

[a]Td: Tetanus and diphtheria toxoids absorbed—for adult use. For children under 7 years old diptheria and pertussis (dPT) (Td, if pertussis vaccine is contraindicated) is preferred to tetanus toxoid alone. For persons 7 years old and older, Td is preferred to tetanus toxoid alone.
[b]TIG: Tetanus immune globulin—human.
[c]If only three doses of fluid toxoid have been received, a fourth dose of toxoid, preferably an absorbed toxoid, should be given.
[d]Yes, if more than 10 years since last dose.
[e]Yes, if more than 5 years since last dose. (More frequent boosters are not needed and can accentuate side effects.)

Close postoperative observation for evidence of compartment syndrome or reperfusion injury is essential. Monitoring of the pulse or continuous wave Doppler assessment is necessary to determine the continued patency of the arterial reconstruction.

Penetrating injuries of noncritical arteries (profunda brachial, profunda femoral, radial, ulnar, or tibial) are less likely to cause serious sequelae. Angiographic demonstration of a laceration or arteriovenous fistula of noncritical vessels may allow indirect treatment by embolization. Loss of either the radial or ulnar artery, or one of the tibial arteries, will not lead to dysfunction;[16] however, disruption of both arteries makes repair mandatory to preserve limb function.

Fractures and Joint Injuries

The importance of fractures and joint injuries in the extremities is that they may occasionally pose a life-threatening problem (hemorrhage, fat embolism, or sepsis); they may be easily overlooked; they may interfere with the optimal care of life-threatening conditions; and late recognition or inadequate care may result in serious long-term morbidity. The extremity injuries seen in the intensive care unit are usually a result of high-velocity forces and, therefore, are often multiple, associated with more extensive soft-tissue injury, greater comminution, and a higher incidence of complications. The blood loss for isolated long-bone fractures may range from 500 to 2000 mL[17] and, especially if multiple, may account for considerable concealed blood loss, hypovolemia, and shock.

The extremity injury may be obvious, such as an unstable deformity in the midshaft of a long bone, or a joint held in a fixed deformed position, but subtle injuries may be masked—swelling, bruising, or loss of voluntary use of an extremity may be recognized late upon serial examination.

Initial clinical assessment of the local area should be followed by evaluation of the associated joints and other areas of transmission of the force, as well as by examination of the soft tissues and the neurovascular status. Immediate management of fractures requires gentle realignment in an anatomical position and splinting to include the joints above and below the fracture. In dislocations where a fixed position is present, the limb should be splinted in situ. Open wounds should be cleaned of gross contamination and a sterile dressing applied, and the tetanus immune status checked (see Table 65-1).

MANAGEMENT

The principles of definitive management of fractures are reduction, maintenance, and rehabilitation. Frequently this can be accomplished by closed techniques, through manipulation, application of external splints, or traction, emphasizing the need to mobilize both the injured extremity and the patient as quickly as possible in order to minimize the complications of recumbency, as well as joint stiffness and muscle wasting. Operative fracture management is indicated for failed closed reduction, inability to maintain the fractures in an external splint, mobilization of the patient, or facilitation of early rehabilitation of the injured extremity. Internal fixation of the following fractures is necessary for fracture management and early mobilization, ipsilateral femur and tibia (floating knee), bilateral lower extremity, combined upper and lower extremity, intraarticular fracture, and association with ligamentous injury. Recent advances in techniques of internal fixation have further expanded the indications for surgery (e.g., locked intramedullary nail).[18]

FRACTURE MANAGEMENT IN MULTISYSTEM TRAUMA

Until recently it was considered that a victim of multiple trauma was too sick to undergo definitive management of extremity injuries. Several authors have clearly shown that immediate operative stabilization of fractures and early mobilization of the patient result in a significantly decreased incidence of pulmonary complications.[19,20] It has been suggested that extended traction in patients with severe trauma results in evolution of multiple-system dysfunction ("the pulmonary failure septic state"),[21] and that complications accrue during conservative fracture management. Immediate operation also reduces immediate perioperative complications such as the fat embolism syndrome.[19]

Additional benefits are attributed to early initiation of oral alimentation. Multisystem trauma patients have been shown to experience protein malnutrition affecting the integrity of the gut mucosa allowing translocation of endotoxins[22] and bacteria from the gut into the circulation (see Chaps. 5, 53, and 67). Measures to avoid this potential septic state include ensuring at least 2 to 4 g of protein, plus 30 to 40 calories of energy per kilogram per day (preferably enterally), and debridement of necrotic material from the wound at the time of the internal stabilization.

COMPOUND FRACTURES

The open wound adds the risks of infection, soft-tissue necrosis, and late complications. The factors determining outcome are the magnitude of the force and, therefore, the degree of soft-tissue injury; the circumstances under which the fracture occurred (e.g., farmyard); and delay in management.

The classification of open fractures by Gustilo et al.[23,24] focuses attention on those factors associated with an increased incidence of complications.

TYPE I. This type is a low-velocity injury less than 1 cm long, usually compound from within, with minimal soft-tissue injury or comminution of the fracture.

TYPE II. This type is a laceration more than 1 cm long, with minimal to moderate soft-tissue crushing.

TYPE III. This type is a high-velocity injury with severe crushing and the presence of skin flaps.

A. No soft-tissue loss. Infection rate of 4 percent; amputation rate of 0 percent.
B. Soft-tissue loss with periosteal stripping. Infection rate of 52 percent; amputation rate of 16 percent.
C. Associated vascular injury. Infection rate of 42 percent, amputation rate of 42 percent.

Management of Compound Fractures

The most common organism contaminating these wounds in the past has been *Staphylococcus aureus,* although recently an increased frequency of gram-negative organisms has been noted.[25] Specific bacterial contamination may occur depending upon the circumstances of the injury (e.g., clostridium in a farmyard). The initial antibiotic of choice is cefazolin (Ancef) with a loading dose of 2 g and then 1 g intravenous (IV) every 8 h.

When gram-negative contamination is more likely, or with Type III wounds, an aminoglycoside should be added. Penicillin G should be added for those wounds possibly contaminated by clostridium. Antibiotics should be used for 3 days, then discontinued, cultures taken, and, if necessary, restarted based on the culture results.

The initial cleaning and debridement of the wound is a surgical emergency, and failure to achieve this within 8 h postinjury will convert a contaminated wound to an infected wound. The debridement must be meticulous, and specimens must be taken for culture. Type I wounds may be closed if treated within 8 h. Other compound fractures must be packed open, and the patient must be returned to the operating room for dressing change and possible further debridement or delayed primary closure in 48 h. Definitive closure of the wound may require extensive soft-tissue reconstruction.[26]

Generally, the simplest form of fracture fixation which allows access to the soft tissues is the most appropriate.[27] The presence of internal fixation devices does not increase the risk of infection, but care must be taken not to further devitalize bone or soft tissue during the fixation. Accordingly, Type I and II compound fractures can be managed by either external splinting or internal fixation as required by the configuration of the fracture itself.

Type III fractures require special attention. The most important factor in management is achieving stability in order to allow access to the soft tissues. This can most often be provided by some form of external fixator which accomplishes excellent fracture stability, does not require placing foreign material in the wound, yet allows easy access for dressing changes, further debridement, or even reconstructive procedures such as flaps (see Fig. 65-5*a* and *b*). Generally, other methods of internal fixation such as plates or intramedullary rods can be avoided, but occasionally these are necessary.[28]

DISLOCATIONS

Complete disruption of a joint results in severe ligamentous tearing, is frequently associated with intraarticular fractures, and has a high incidence of neurologic and vascular injury. Reduction of the dislocation should be performed as quickly as possible in order to avoid prolonged pressure on articular cartilage, soft tissues, nerves, vessels, and skin, and the limb should then be splinted.

Posterior dislocation of the hip deserves special mention. The main blood supply to the head of the femur is provided by two retinacular vessels, branches of the extraarticular circumflex femoral artery, which pass through the posterior capsule to enter the neck of the femur. These vessels become kinked by the displaced proximal femur, making reduction of the dislocation in less than 8 h mandatory to avoid late avascular necrosis.[29,30] Definitive soft-tissue repair and internal fixation of associated fractures may be performed electively (see Fig. 65-6).

Fat Embolism

The association of hypoxemia with long-bone or pelvic fracture, even in the absence of chest injury, is well known.[31] Criteria for a positive diagnosis of fat embolism syndrome (FES) include respiratory insufficiency, cerebral involvement, and petechial rash (fat embolism is discussed more fully in Chap. 118).[32] Minor features are pyrexia, tachycardia, retinal changes, anemia, thrombocytopenia, and lipiduria. Most authors have emphasized that the critical consideration is the diagnosis of potentially severe respiratory impairment and not fat embolism per se.[33,34]

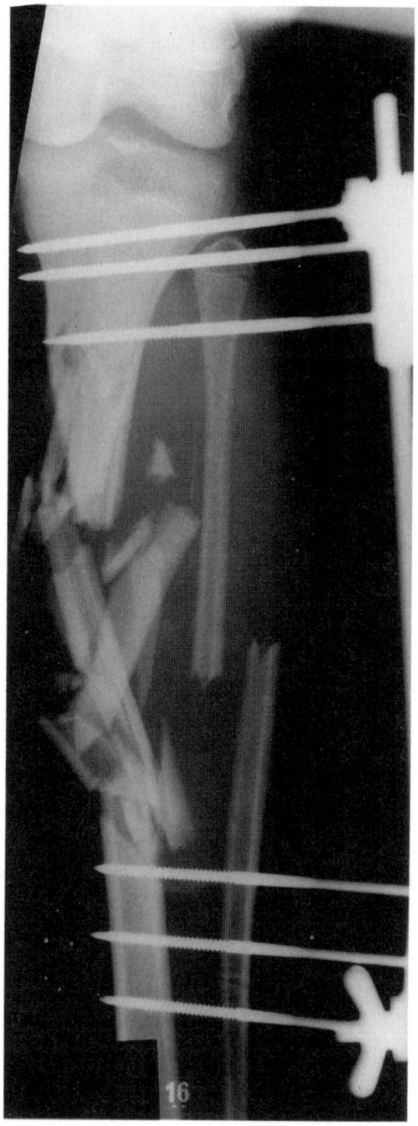

a

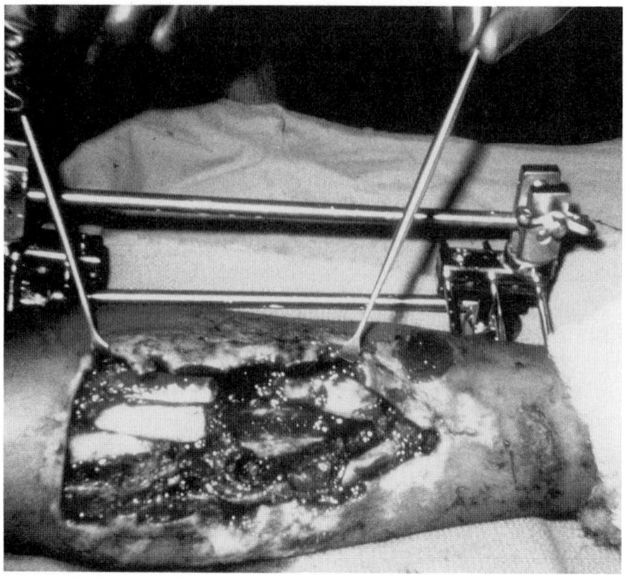

b

FIGURE 65-5 (*a*) This Type IIIB compound fracture occurred in an 18-year-old man whose leg was run over by the track of a snowmobile. Following debridement (*b*), an external fixator was used to provide fracture stabilization and allow access for further debridement, dressing changes, and subsequently a free vascularized latissimus dorsi flap. Subsequently cancellous bone grafting resulted in fracture healing.

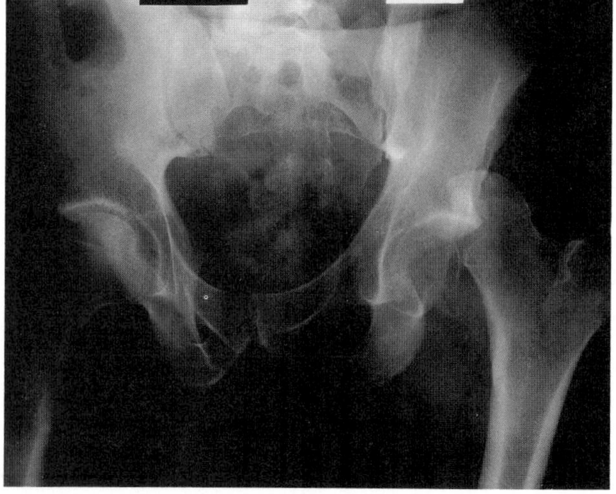

FIGURE 65-6 Posterior dislocation of the hip with associated fracture of the head of femur. The hip is flexed, adducted, and internally rotated. This patient had been involved in a head-on motor vehicle accident striking the knee against the dash.

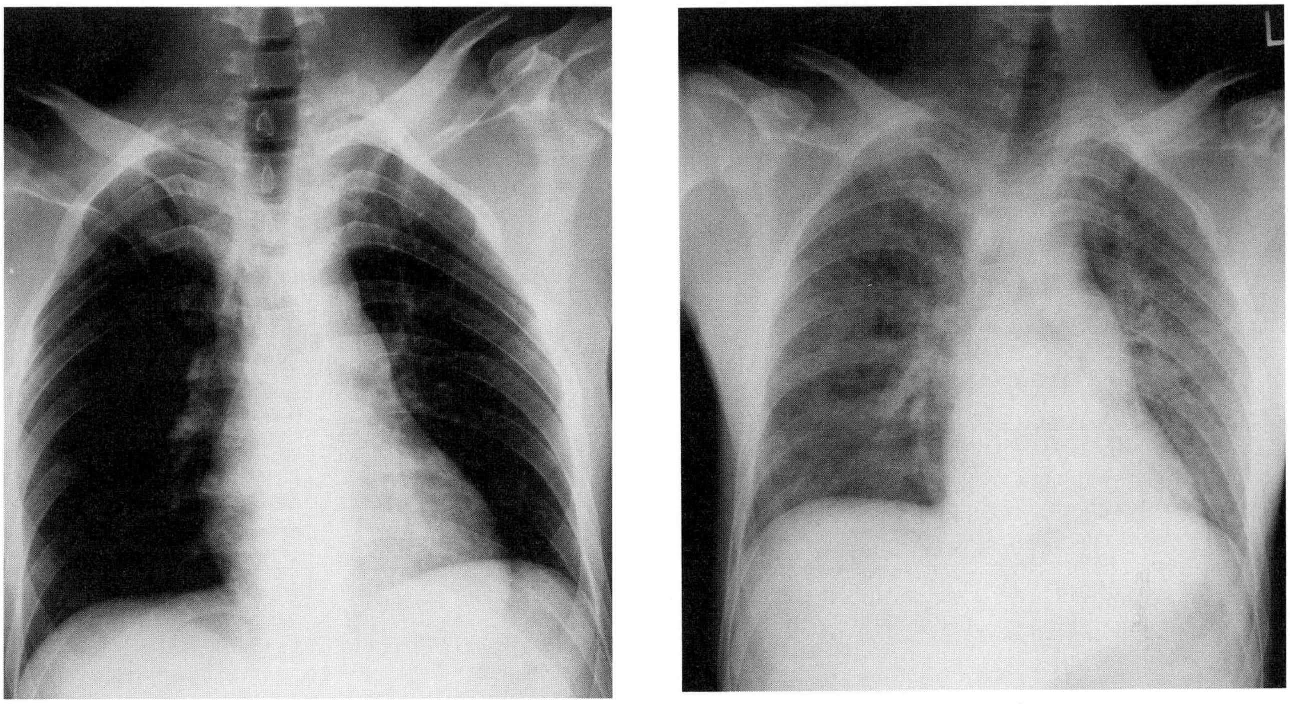

a

b

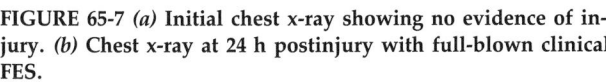

FIGURE 65-7 ***(a)*** **Initial chest x-ray showing no evidence of injury.** ***(b)*** **Chest x-ray at 24 h postinjury with full-blown clinical FES.**

Clinically apparent FES occurs in approximately 0.5 to 2 percent of patients with long-bone fractures.[35] This frequency rises to 5 to 10 percent in the face of multiple fractures and especially multisystem trauma and is therefore one of the more frequent and life-threatening complications which the intensivist is likely to deal with.

The full-blown FES usually occurs within 48 to 72 h following injury. The patient may be disoriented, lethargic, irritable, and appear to have a head injury, withdrawal symptoms, or severe sepsis. The patient is usually febrile and may be anemic. Petechiae are present in 50 to 60 percent of patients, usually in the upper trunk, axillary folds, conjunctiva, or fundi. Lipiduria is an inconsistent finding. Most commonly there is an additional 3- to 4-g drop in hemoglobin, superimposed on the previous blood loss secondary to trauma. Depending on the timing, there is also usually thrombocytopenia and increased fibrin breakdown products, although a clinical bleeding disorder is rare. Chest x-ray may show a diffuse alveolar infiltrate (see Fig. 65-7*a* and *b*). Electrocardiographic findings may show ST segment changes and other abnormalities indicative of right ventricular strain. The degree of hypoxemia is variable but may be extreme.

Early, adequate fracture splinting is probably the most effective method of avoiding this syndrome. Concern has been expressed that early, operative fracture management may increase the risk of fat embolism; however, this has not been substantiated. On the contrary, there is a decreased incidence of FES in association with early operative stabilization of long-bone fractures.[19] In addition, avoidance of hypotension may also decrease the severity of FES. Early recognition, however, remains the most important factor in initiating treatment and ultimately a satisfactory outcome. When hypoxemia is severe, mechanical ventilatory support is required. Drug therapy of FES is controversial and is more fully discussed in Chap. 118. The most commonly used agents are corticosteriods, although controversy still exists regarding optimal dosage and whether steroids should be used prophylactically or are of benefit if initiated upon the diagnosis of established FES.

Early recognition of hypoxemia and its treatment including mechanical ventilation, aggressive correction of hypoperfusion, and early stabilization of long-bone fractures remain the most reliable treatment modalities in FES.

CASE PRESENTATION

A 70-year-old obese female with long-standing, severe rheumatoid arthritis requiring the use of steroids was an unrestrained rear-seat passenger in a car involved in a head-on motor vehicle accident. She suffered bilateral fractures of both femurs and tibias (floating knees). Three of the fractures were compound (Types I and II). She had no other significant injuries. The night of the accident, with two operating teams, she was taken to the operating room where the compound wounds were debrided and both femurs were internally stabilized simultaneously. The wounds were packed open. She was immobilized in bed in bilateral long-leg casts. Careful serial assessments for hypoxemia, respiratory distress, cardiac ischemia, and skin petechiae were performed. Two days later the dressings were changed and cultures were taken. Four days after injury her cultures were negative and she was returned to the operating room where she underwent bilateral closed intramedullary rodding of the tibias and bone grafting of the femoral fractures. Postoperatively, she was mobilized as a bed-and-chair patient, but while in bed, continuous passive movement devices were used. Her subsequent course was uneventful, and she was discharged from the intensive care unit 6 days postinjury. All four fractures eventually healed, she regained 0 to 90° range of movement in both knees, and was able to resume independent walking using a walker 4 months postinjury.

CASE DISCUSSION

This patient was at high risk for morbidity related to her fractures because of age, obesity, and corticosteroid use. Several complications were appropriately anticipated and possibly prevented by meticulous attention to detail. Had these complications occurred, the careful ongoing assessment of cardiorespiratory function might have led to early recognition, allowing institution of therapy. In particular, the following complications were anticipated:

1. Fat embolism related to four long-bone fractures
2. Pneumonia, pulmonary embolism, or respiratory failure related to obesity and prolonged recumbency if treated in traction
3. Deep venous thrombosis, caused by direct soft-tissue injury and recumbency
4. Increased risk of nonunion or malunion of fractures (related to "floating knee")
5. Increased risk of sepsis with three compound fractures in a patient on steroids
6. Poor fixation of the devices because of severe osteoporosis
7. Severe knee stiffness related to supracondylar fractures of the femur in a patient with preexisting severe rheumatoid arthritis of the knees

The following measures were taken to avoid these anticipated complications:

1. The patient was given an increased dosage of steroid to avoid adrenal cortical insufficiency from chronic suppression.
2. Since the femoral fractures were both internally stabilized the night of injury, the patient could be mobilized in a sitting position in long-leg casts, easily turned, and given maximal chest care.
3. Prophylactic anticoagulants were not used because of the risk of bleeding. Efforts were concentrated on early mobilization, and the patient resumed her usual salicylates once an oral diet could be resumed in about 72 h.
4. The ipsilateral fractures of the femurs and tibias were internally stabilized.
5. The patient was given cefazolin prophylactically. Her tissue was generally thin and friable from steroid use. Although the soft-tissue wounds were not severe, and the initial debridement was performed within 8 h, the wounds were packed open and recultured in 48 h.
6. There was risk of the screws not holding in the femur, but, since the fractures were near the joint, no other fixation device was available. The fractures were grafted early anticipating delayed healing. The choice of closed, minimally seamed, locked, intramedullary nails for the tibias was to avoid further injury to skin overlying the fractures, and to interfere as little as possible with the intramedullary blood supply while giving sufficient stability to avoid external splints.
7. The use of continuous passive movement devices facilitates early joint range of movement but confines the patient to bed. Therefore, this was used only intermittently when the patient was in bed and was discontinued to allow mobilization.

References

1. Mubarak SJ, Hargens AR, Owen CA, et al.: The wick catheter technique for measurement of intramuscular pressure. J Bone Joint Surg 58:1016, 1976.
2. Schwartz JT, Brumback RJ, Lakatos R, et al.: Acute compartment syndrome of the thigh. J Bone Joint Surg 71:392, 1989.
3. Halpern AA, Green R, Nichols T, et al.: Compartment syndrome of the interosseous muscles. Clin Orthop 140:23, 1979.
4. Bonutti PM, Bell GR: Compartment syndrome of the foot. J Bone Joint Surg 68:1449, 1986.
5. Heppenstall RB, Sapega AA, Izant T, et al.: Compartment syndrome: a quantitative study of high-energy phosphorus compounds using ^{31}P-magnetic resonance spectroscopy. J Trauma 29:1113, 1989.
6. Bourne RB, Rorabeck CH: Compartment syndromes of the lower leg. Clin Orthop 240:97, 1989.
7. Mubarak SJ, Owen CA, Hargens AR, et al.: Acute compartment syndromes: diagnosis and treatment with the aid of the wick catheter. J Bone Joint Surg 60:1091, 1978.
8. Matsen FA, Winquist RA, Krugmire RB: Diagnosis and management of compartmental syndromes. J Bone Joint Surg 62:286, 1980.
9. Tupper JW, Crick JC, Matteck LR: Fascicular nerve repairs: A comparative study of epineurial and fascicular (perineurial) techniques. Orthop Clin North Am 19:57, 1988.
10. Downs AR, MacDonald P: Popliteal artery injuries: Civilian experience with sixty-three patients during a twenty-four year period (1960 through 1984). J Vasc Surg 4:55, 1986.
11. Miller HH, Welch CS: Quantitative studies on time factor in arterial injuries. Ann Surg 130:428, 1949.
12. Strandness DE, Jr: Non-invasive tests in vascular emergencies, in Bergan JJ, Yao JST (eds): *Vascular Surgical Emergencies*. Orlando, Grune & Stratton, Inc., 1987, p 104.
13. Feliciano DV, Mattox KL, Graham JM, et al.: Five year experience with PTFE grafts in vascular wounds. J Trauma 25:71, 1985.
14. Perry MO: Penetrating trauma to the extremities, in Bergan JJ, Yao JST (eds): *Vascular Surgical Emergencies*. Orlando, Grune & Stratton, Inc., 1987, p 166.
15. Rich NM, Hobson RW, II, Collins GJ, Jr: Traumatic arteriovenous fistulas and false aneurysms: A review of 558 lesions. Surgery 78:817, 1975.

16. McNutt R, Seabrook GR, Schmitt DD, et al.: Blunt tibial artery trauma: Predicting the irretrievable extremity. J Trauma 29:1624, 1989.
17. O'Donnell TF, Belkin SC: The pathophysiology, monitoring and treatment of shock. Orthop Clin North Am 9:1478, 1978.
18. Wiss DA, Flemming CH, Matta JM, et al.: Comminuted and rotationally unstable fractures of the femur treated with an interlocking nail. Clin Orthop 212:35, 1986.
19. Riska EB, Vonbonsdorff H, Hakkinen S, et al.: Primary operative fixation of long bone fractures in patients with multiple injuries. J Trauma 17:111, 1977.
20. Meek R, Vivoda E, Crichton A, et al.: Comparison of mortality of patients with multiple injuries according to method of fracture treatment. J Bone Joint Surg 63:456, 1981.
21. Seibel R, LaDuca J, Hassett JM, et al.: Blunt multiple trauma (ISS 36), femur traction, and the pulmonary failure—septic state. Ann Surg 202:283, 1985.
22. Border JR, Chenier R, McManamy RH, et al.: Multiple systems organ failure: Muscle fuel deficit with visceral protein malnutrition. Surg Clin North Am 56:1147, 1976.
23. Gustilo RB, Anderson JT: Prevention of infection in the treatment of one thousand and twenty-five open fractures of long bone. J Bone Joint Surg 58:453, 1976.
24. Gustilo RB, Mendoza RM, Williams DN: Problems in the management of type III (severe) open fractures: A new classification of type III open fractures. J Trauma 24:742, 1984.
25. Patzakis MJ: Management of open fractures and complications—Part 1, in Frankel VA (ed): *Aaos Instructional Course Lectures*, vol. 32. St. Louis, CV Mosby, 1983, pp 62–64.
26. Burgess AR, Poka A, Brumback RJ, et al.: Management of open grade III tibial fractures. Orthop Clin North Am 18:85, 1987.
27. Chapman MW: Role of bone stability in open fractures, in Frankel VA (ed): *Aaos Instructional Course Lectures*, vol. 32. St. Louis, CV Mosby, 1983, pp 75–87.
28. Chapman MW: The role of intramedullary fixation in open fractures. Clin Orthop 212:26, 1986.
29. Stewart WJ: Aseptic necrosis of the head of the femur following traumatic dislocation of the hip joint. Case Study and Experimental Studies. J Bone Joint Surg 15:413, 1933.
30. Morton KS: Traumatic dislocation of the hip: A follow-up study. Can J Surg 3:67, 1959.
31. Fabian C, Hoots AV, Stanford DS, et al.: Fat embolism syndrome: A prospective evaluation in 92 fracture patients. J Trauma 27:820, 1987.
32. Gurd AR: Fat embolism: An aid to diagnosis. J Bone Joint Surg 52:732, 1970.
33. Chan KM, Tham Kt, Chiu HS, et al.: Post-traumatic fat embolism—its clinical and subclinical presentations. J Trauma 24:45, 1984.
34. McCarthy B, Mammen E, Leblanc LP, et al.: Subclinical fat embolism: A prospective study of 50 patients with extremity fractures. J Trauma 13:9, 1973.
35. Blumenstock TA, Weber P, Saba TM, et al.: Electro immuno assay of alpha-2-opsonic protein during reticulo-endothelial blockade. Am J Physiol 232:80, 1977.

Chapter 66
ELECTRICAL TRAUMA

LAWRENCE J. GOTTLIEB
JONATHAN SAUNDERS
RAPHAEL LEE

KEY POINTS

- *Aggressive and prolonged life support maneuvers should be performed on all electrical injury patients.*
- *All patients are to be regarded as multisystem blunt trauma patients and appropriate prophylactic measures and diagnostic tests should be utilized.*
- *Volume resuscitation should not be underestimated.*
- *Selected patients should be monitored for cardiac arrhythmias for 24 to 48 h after injury.*
- *Renal function prophylaxis is largely directed toward adequate volume resuscitation.*
- *The neurologic exam should be carefully followed and documented.*
- *Early recognition and decompression of compartment syndromes is critical for maximizing extremity salvage and long-term function.*
- *Adequate wound care necessitates complete debridement of nonviable tissue followed by wound closure as expeditiously as possible.*

The typical victim of high-voltage electrical injury is a young industrial worker or lineman. Immediate death can result from cardiac arrhythmia, central respiratory arrest, or asphyxia due to tetanic contraction of the muscles of respiration. If the victim survives the initial cardiopulmonary or central nervous system (CNS) insult, he then may face potential limb and life-threatening sequelae from cutaneous injury, occult soft tissue destruction, and multiple organ damage. The distribution of the tissues and organs damaged is dependent upon the path of the current. Frequently the injury is complicated by associated blunt trauma when the patient falls from a height or is thrown by the force of the electric current.

The duration of contact with the high-voltage power source is an important factor in the magnitude of the injury. If the contact is brief, cell damage is theoretically related to the nonthermal component of electrical injury, called electroporation.[1] If the contact is longer, both heating caused by electrical conduction (Joule heating) and electroporation play important roles. Prolonged contact can lead to complete thermal destruction of tissues in the current path.

Many cells, such as muscle and nerve, utilize electrical signals to control their function. The application of weak electric fields from a nonphysiologic source can interfere with cell function and, if the field is strong enough, cause direct cell damage.

At the commercial frequency of 60 Hz the threshold for human perception of a current passed hand to hand is approximately 1.0 mA. If the current is raised to 16 mA, the muscle in the arm develops involuntary spasm. Within 10 to 100 ms (the excitation-contraction response time of human skeletal muscles), muscles located in the current path will contract. If the hand is grasping the conductor at the time of current passage, the strong forearm flexor muscles will contract, causing the victim to be unable to let go. This is called the no-let-go phenomenon. Alternately, if the victim is close to but not yet in contact with the conductor at the time of current passage, the strong muscle contractions will propel him away from the contact. Judging from eyewitness reports, the latter may be more common. When a current of 60 mA traverses the adult thorax, the heart will fibrillate in 30 s in most victims. When the current ampli-

TABLE 66-1 Criteria for Admission of Electrically Injured Victims

Any one of the following qualifies a patient for admission to an intensive care unit:

1. Thermal injury (arc or flash) to greater than 20% body surface area (BSA)
2. Thermal injury (arc or flash) to hands, feet, face, or perineum
3. Suspicion of inhalation injury or upper airway swelling
4. Evidence or suspicion of direct electrical contact with more than 100 V across the body (or at least one limb) and more than 200 mA
5. History of loss of consciousness
6. Abnormal neurologic examination (central or peripheral)
7. Cardiac arrythmia (at scene or in emergency room)
8. Abnormal electrocardiogram (ECG)
9. History of cardiopulmonary arrest (at scene or in emergency room)
10. Evidence of (or suspicion of developing) increased muscle compartment pressure
11. Creatine phosphokinase (CPK) greater than 400 I.U.
12. Pigments (hemochromogens) in urine
13. History of a fall or being thrown from a power source (r/o blunt trauma)
14. Abdominal signs

TABLE 66-2 Criteria for Transfer Out of Intensive Care Unit

All of the following criteria need to be met for safe transfer at 48 h

1. Less than 20% BSA thermal injury
2. No evidence of inhalation injury or upper airway edema
3. Neurologically stable
4. No cardiac arrythmia for 24–48 h
5. Hemodynamically stable for 24–48 h
6. Normal acid-base balance
7. Compartment syndrome has been ruled out or treated appropriately
8. Peak CPK less than 400 I.U. in first 48 h[a]
9. Urine has cleared of pigments

[a] See Ahrenholz et al.[2]

tude reaches 1500 mA through the upper extremity, skeletal muscle and peripheral nerve cells are damaged by electrical forces independent of heat. Smaller current in the range of 200 to 500 mA can generate enough Joule heating to cause tissue damage if the duration of current passage is sufficient.

While the spectrum of electrical injury ranges from minor cutaneous trauma to severe multisystem injury, the victims of high-voltage electrical injury are usually the patients who are admitted to a critical care unit (see Tables 66-1 and 66-2).

Initial Evaluation

Upon arrival to the critical care facility, the *ABCs* of airway, breathing, and circulation are assessed and appropriate therapeutic maneuvers enacted. Cardiopulmonary resuscitation should be started or continued, if needed, and routine Advanced Trauma Life Support (ATLS) procedures and protocols should be performed. Life support activities should be continued for prolonged periods of time as complete functional recovery has been well documented despite lengthy resuscitatory efforts.[3] Precise time limits for the continuation of life support have not been well elucidated.

After stabilization of the patient, a complete history should be obtained if possible and a careful physical examination should be performed. Witnesses and family members often give pertinent information regarding the accident as well as significant medical history. On physical exam, particular attention should be paid to the sites of electrical contact. The terms of entry and exit sites are actually incorrect because when the electrical source is 60 Hz alternating current, all contact points carry current either in or out of the body 120 times per second. Contact points, which are usually full-thickness burns, enable one to establish the likely pathway of the current and the regions where tissue damage may have occurred. Typically, obvious cutaneous injury is only the tip of the soft tissue iceberg. Victims of electrical trauma frequently require large volumes of isotonic intravenous fluids during resuscitation. These large fluid requirements are due to considerable third-space losses secondary to deep or occult tissue damage. Unlike purely thermal burn injuries, resuscitation formulas such as the Parkland formula are not helpful guides to fluid management. Isotonic fluids should be given liberally with the initial goal of resuscitation being a urine output of between 0.5 and 1 mL/kg/h. Any electrolyte abnormalities should be corrected immediately. If myoglobin or free hemoglobin is found in the urine, the fluid rate is increased to obtain a urine output of twice this amount. Obtaining the appropriate urine output may require mannitol. The urine may also be alkalinized (to pH >7.0) with bicarbonate to prevent precipitation of urine myoglobin in the renal collecting system. The recommended dosage is 12.5 g, administered as an intravenous bolus, then 12.5 g/h continuously until myoglobin clears. Loop diuretics should rarely, if ever, be used to improve urine output.

Reliable, large-bore intravenous access is essential, as is an arterial line and a urinary catheter. A pulmonary artery catheter is not necessary in most patients, but may be necessary if the volume status cannot be ascertained on other grounds. It may be helpful to view all victims of electrical trauma as having the potential of suffering from blunt trauma. These patients should be evaluated as one would multisystem blunt trauma victims (see Chap. 59). A large percentage of high-voltage electrical trauma patients have either fallen from a height or been thrown secondary to the force of the electric current. Cervical spine as well as other orthopedic injuries should be suspected, appropriately investigated, and treated with conventional splinting devices. A falling hematocrit or hemodynamic instability should be thoroughly investigated with the appropriate diagnostic tests. Unexplained changes in level of consciousness are not to be assumed to be due to *changes secondary to electricity* until surgically correctable head trauma has been eliminated. The initial physical exam should also include a careful evaluation and documentation of both the central and peripheral nervous systems. As neurologic deficits may manifest in a delayed fashion, these evaluations should be repeated daily.

Appropriate tetanus prophylaxis is provided as delineated by the ATLS Committee on Trauma Guidelines. Antistreptococcal and anticlostridial antibiotics should be administered prophylactically.

CARDIAC

A major cause of immediate mortality secondary to electrical injury is malignant ventricular arrhythmia. If the initial arrhythmia is able to be corrected and the patient stabilized, then the recurrence of potentially fatal arrhythmias secondary to cardiac pathology is unusual. It is important to reemphasize that when faced with a patient who is requiring cardiopulmonary resuscitation (CPR) due to an arrhythmia, long-term ATLS should continue, as reports of complete functional survival after significant periods of CPR do exist.[3]

Close to 50 percent of patients exhibit ECG changes or rhythm disturbances after injury. The most common ECG alterations are nonspecific ST-T wave changes, which usually revert with time, and sinus tachycardia. Most arrhythmias are transient, and therapeutic pharmacologic intervention is rarely needed. The difficulty lies in attempting to identify the existence of new myocardial damage as well as determining its physiologic significance.

The usual criteria for the diagnosis of myocardial infarction include ECG changes and elevation of cardiac isoenzymes in a setting compatible with myocardial ischemia. These pieces of evidence are not reliable, however, in the circumstance of electrical injury. Electrocardiographic abnormalities after electrical trauma are common, temporary, and usually physiologically insignificant. The CPK-MB isoenzymes may be falsely positive as elevation may occur with large-scale skeletal muscle damage.[4] Clinical symptomatology of cardiac ischemia, which is subjective in the best of times, is usually unhelpful in the face of multisystem electrical trauma. The technetium 99m pyrophosphate scan has also been used to try to identify myocardial damage. However, transmural myocardial damage is rare, and this test is not able to accurately assess nontransmural injury. Since diagnostic tests are not helpful and significant myocardial injury is historically known to be unlikely, aggressive volume resuscitation and surgical intervention should proceed as required. The exception to this principle is the patient who has been hemodynamically unstable as a result of congestive heart failure, malignant arrhythmia, or clinically obvious myocardial ischemia.

The evaluation of these patients includes daily ECGs for 3 days following injury as well as serial cardiac isoenzymes. The results of these tests are interpreted in light of the clinical situation. It has been suggested that not all patients need to have continuous cardiac monitoring after injury unless they have a history of (1) loss of consciousness or cardiac arrhythmia at the scene, (2) recurrent arrhythmia in the field or emergency room, (3) abnormal ECG on admission, or (4) other injuries which would themselves require monitoring.[5]

RENAL

Renal dysfunction occurs in approximately 10 percent of patients who suffer high-voltage electrical trauma. The most frequent cause of renal toxicity and the most simply remediable is hypovolemia. It is a common mistake to grossly underestimate volume requirements in electrically injured patients. The quantity of soft tissue damage and the resultant third-space losses are not always immediately apparent and inadequate fluid resuscitation occurs. Intravascular depletion can lead to a decrease in glomerular filtration rate, renal cortical ischemia, and acute tubular necrosis. Aggressive volume replacement is therapeutic with 0.5 to 1 mL/kg/h of urine output being the goal.

The precipitation of intravascular hemochromogens in the renal tubules is another cause of renal dysfunction. Hemochromogens can be visualized in the urine in approximately 25 percent of patients with electrical injuries. Myoglobin, secondary to myonecrosis, and free hemoglobin, from lysed red blood cells, are the responsible pigments. The detrimental effect of pigments deposited in the tubules is thought to increase with hypovolemia, which further underscores the need for adequate fluid resuscitation.

The best prophylactic and therapeutic regimen to prevent renal toxicity secondary to hemochromogen deposition is to maintain a high urine output. This is done with lactated Ringer's solution and mannitol, infused hourly in 12.5-g increments. The resulting solute diuresis must be followed carefully in order to prevent inadvertent intravascular depletion. In the presence of urine pigments, the goal is to create a flow of urine of at least 1 to 2 mL/kg/h.

It is established that myoglobin is much more soluble and less likely to be retained by the kidney when the urine is alkaline. Some feel that by providing adequate resuscitation and a solute diuresis, a urine pH which is clinically therapeutic will have been created. However, others recommend that sodium bicarbonate be utilized to help maintain urinary alkalinity.[6] An ampule of $NaHCO_3$ is given in every liter of lactated Ringer's with the goal being a urinary pH greater than 6.5 This is continued until urinary myoglobin has cleared, which may take from 48 to 60 h. Systemic alkalemia may need to be corrected with acetazolamide. Incidentally, there is evidence that bicarbonate also participates in the solute diuresis; hence its value may be twofold.[7] If the urine does not clear of hemochromogens within 24 h and the serum CPK isoenzymes continue to rise, then a source of undetected muscle ischemia or myonecrosis should be actively investigated. Careful, repeated physical examination, specifically looking for areas of swelling and tenderness should be performed. Technetium 99 nuclear medicine scanning may be helpful in localizing areas of ischemic muscle, although its lack of specificity may lead to false-positive results. Xenon 131 scan and arteriography have both been shown to be generally unhelpful in localizing areas of muscle ischemia or myonecrosis. On the horizon, magnetic resonance imaging (MRI) will likely provide a reliable method of evaluating injured muscle. When occult muscle ischemia is discovered, decompression or debridement may not lead to functional recovery of that muscle group but may alleviate the systemic problems related to toxic effects of dying or dead muscle.

PULMONARY

There are relatively few pulmonary abnormalities which are characteristic of electrical injury. Acute ventilatory failure secondary to electrical injury is usually related to CNS injury or to chest wall impairment. Depressed respiratory drive due to CNS damage may lead to respiratory failure, necessitating mechanical ventilation. The chest wall and the muscles of respiration may be directly injured, compromising neuromuscular efficiency and also leading to the need for ventilatory support.

Long-term pulmonary sequelae such as pneumonia or effusion are treated as in any traumatic injury. There are isolated reports of current-induced bronchopleural fistula, but in the majority of cases the need for ventilatory support is not due to current injury to the pulmonary parenchyma.

When the transient path of the current passes through the pharynx, significant upper airway swelling may develop. All patients at risk should undergo serial fiber-optic, endoscopic examination of their upper airway and should be prophylactically intubated if hypopharyngeal edema is found.

GASTROINTESTINAL

Abdominal complications following electrical trauma are relatively infrequent. Most often, gastric atony and adynamic ileus are seen. These usually resolve with nasogastric suction, intravenous fluids, nutrition, and time. More serious complications such as gastrointestinal bleeding and acalculous cholecystitis have been reported. It is difficult to know whether these processes are due to electricity or the stresses of severe shock and systemic illness. If a contact point on the abdomen has caused a full-thickness burn, the wound should be surgically excised. If this wound includes the posterior fascia of the abdominal wall, then formal exploratory celiotomy should follow. Intraabdominal pathology may be present even without abdominal wall injuries, however. Systemic signs of sepsis or changes on serial physical examination of the abdomen should alert the clinician to intraabdominal pathology. White blood cell counts, liver function tests, amylase and lipase levels, as well as abdominal ultrasound, computed tomography (CT) scans, MRI scans, and peritoneal lavage may come into play in making the correct diagnosis and directing therapy. Virtually any abdominal catastrophe can be caused by electrical current, and thus the physician must be alert and react to subtle changes in abdominal signs and symptoms.[8]

NEUROLOGIC

It is possible for any aspect of the human nervous system to be affected by high-voltage trauma. Neurologic deficits may appear in either the central or peripheral nervous system. Evidence of injury may be immediate or delayed in appearance. Finally, the duration of neurologic deficit ranges from transient to permanent.

Neurologic changes are often poorly described and documented when they do occur, and hence assimilation of retrospective data is difficult. Immediate neurologic deficits occur in more than 40 percent of all patients. The most common symptom is loss of consciousness. This occurs in up to 65 percent of symptomatic patients and usually resolves without permanent sequelae. However, long-term complaints include headache, dizziness, vertigo, and seizure activity as well as psychosocial behavioral disorders such as impotence and personality changes.

Spinal cord injuries can have acute or delayed presentations. Acute neurologic deficiencies can demonstrate a frighteningly complete motor and sensory loss. Yet acute deficits have a tendency to resolve over hours or days. Delayed spinal cord symptomatology is much more ominous and less likely to resolve. The pathophysiology of these delayed findings is not well understood.[9]

Peripheral nerve injuries account for 5 to 23 percent of all posttraumatic neurologic sequelae. The most common injury is to the median nerve, followed by the ulnar, radial, and peroneal nerves. In the acutely damaged edematous arm and hand, immediate operative decompression of the carpal tunnel, cubital tunnel, and Guyon's canal is urgent if peripheral neuropathy develops. Following appropriate release, signs of acute peripheral nerve compression should dissipate if thermal injury to the nerve has not occurred.

EXTREMITY AND WOUND

The care of the extremity as well as the wound caused by electrical trauma will be discussed concurrently. The rationale behind this is that the attempted salvage of the extremity, particularly the arm and hand, best demonstrates the principles of maximal tissue preservation with optimal residual function.

After life-threatening emergencies are addressed, attention should be turned toward documenting the soft tissue injury. The injury should always be suspected of being more extensive than it initially appears, as visible cutaneous injury is only a portion of the total tissue destruction.

Compartment syndromes are a common manifestation of the electrically traumatized extremity. Within minutes after injury, tissue edema begins to increase due to increased vascular permeability and release of intracellular contents into the extracellular space. Pain with passive movement is an early finding. Tense compartments may be recognized by palpation, but compartment pressure should be documented.

Compartment fluid pressures in excess of 30 mmHg are abnormal and indicate the need for fasciotomy. Measurement of pressure in smaller compartments such as the intrinsic muscles of the hand is notoriously unreliable. Exploration of the fascial compartments of the acutely swollen hand should be performed empirically whenever high-voltage trauma involves the hand and there is a high index of suspicion of compartment syndrome. Fasciotomy of any fascially bound muscle group may salvage an otherwise moribund muscle. Complete release may be facilitated by incising the epimysium of each muscle.

All nonviable skin is debrided. Deciding which tissue is irretrievably injured and requires debridement is often a difficult problem. We define healthy muscle as that which is of normal color and contracts with electrocautery stimulation. All noncharred nerves and tendons are preserved, as is marginal muscle when intermixed with healthy muscle.

It is at this point in management where controversy exists. The most widely practiced surgical approach is to reinspect the wound and debride obviously necrotic tissue every 48 h.[10] Between debridements allograft is applied to decompressed, exposed, viable muscle, and Sulfamylon is applied to marginal tissue every 8 h. Closure usually awaits a wound which is in bacteriologic balance and is free of all dead or marginal tissue. Whether the recognition of additional nonviable tissue at each of the serial debridements represents *progressive necrosis* or *progressive recognition* of fatally damaged tissue remains an unresolved question.

Based on the hypothesis that marginally viable tissue is potentially salvageable if covered acutely with well-vascularized tissue, another more aggressive therapeutic regimen exists for selected patients with extremity injuries. After decompression of tense compartments, debridement of obviously nonviable muscle and skin is performed. Exposed, devascularized tendons and nerves, as well as marginal muscle, are acutely covered with well-vascularized tissue. Due to the limited availability of suitable local tissue, distant flaps or microvascular free tissue transfers are usually utilized for coverage.[11]

The decision to salvage an injured extremity must involve careful weighing of the potential morbidity and mortality. A cold insensate stiff extremity will be of less service to the patient than a functional prosthesis. This decision should be made soon as possible in order to minimize the risks as well as the physical and psychological effort invested in salvaging an extremity that will eventually be amputated.

Lightning Injury

Injuries due to lightning are often fatal, and the pathophysiology is relatively complex. Lightning occurs when the electric field strength in the air exceeds the electrical breakdown strength of 3×10^6 V/m. The lightning arc temperature is roughly 3000°C. The current flows transiently, probably for less than 1 μs. Therefore, there is a high transient electrical field and resultant magnetic field. Because of its high-frequency characteristics, the electric field only penetrates the outer surface of the body. However, the huge magnetic field can penetrate throughout. Because of this complexity, little work has been accomplished in describing the mechanisms of cardiac and CNS injury. However, hundreds of fatalities occur in the United States alone each year as a result of lightning injury.[12] Treatment of lightning injury should follow the guidelines stated for major electrical trauma. In addition to the electrical effects, one may expect tissue injury from the electrothermal-acoustic shock waves that also occur.

Survivors of lightning injury are not likely to be the victims of a direct hit. Rather, they are likely to be in the vicinity and experience surface burns and arc effects.

Late Sequelae of Electrical Injury

The late sequelae of electrical injury are generally consequent to acute tissue loss or damage. The extent of tissue damage may not be recognized acutely. Neuromuscular problems are usually due to muscle fibrosis and peripheral neuropathies coupled with loss of tissue from debridements and joint stiffness. Sensorimotor neuropathies, paresthesias, dysesthesias, and reflex sympathetic dystrophy may manifest long after the wounds have healed. Cold intolerance may persist for up to 2 to 3 years, and growth disturbances producing skeletal deformities in children are frequent long-term sequelae.

There are also late sequelae of electrical trauma in which the etiology is unknown. Cataracts occur in 1 to 2 percent of victims even though the current path did not necessarily involve the head and neck. A full spectrum of central neurologic disorders has been described as late sequelae of electric shock. Paraplegia and quadriplegia have become manifest 5 years after the injury. In addition, subtle mental status and personality changes may severely affect the patient's motivation and participation in the rehabilitation program that is crucial to optimum function.[13]

CASE PRESENTATION

A 54-year-old gentleman was helicoptered into the medical center after having sustained a severe electrical injury. The patient was working on a fire hydrant when a high-voltage power line fell and landed on his neck. He was witnessed to fall to the ground, but a history of loss of consciousness could not be confirmed. After initial volume resuscitation was started, he was transported.

On arrival the patient was alert and oriented but had no recollection of the incident. The past medical history obtained was generally unremarkable. On physical exam, contact sites were noted to be his posterior neck, right hand, left hand, and left thigh. Chest and abdomen exams were normal. The right wrist was acutely flexed as were the fingers. Peripheral pulses were intact. He had absent sensation in both the median and ulnar nerve distributions of his right hand, but the left hand was neurologically normal. Both forearms were swollen and tense. Compartment pressures in each forearm were greater than 30 mmHg. A urinary catheter was placed and tea-colored urine returned. However, this cleared rapidly over the next hour with crystalloid and mannitol. The ECG, chest radiograph, and admission labs were all normal except for an admission CPK, which was 7500. An arterial line and a central venous pressure line were inserted.

After hemodynamic stabilization he was taken to the operating room within 3 h of admission. He underwent bilateral fasciotomies of each of the muscle compartments below the elbow. His right forearm demonstrated a significant amount of nonviable muscle and a firm, constricted median nerve for a distance of 16 cm. After decompression fasciotomies, debridement of all clearly nonviable muscle, and neurolysis of the right median nerve, the exposed tendons, nerves, and remaining injured muscle were covered with a free rectus abdominus muscle flap, which was itself covered with a split-thickness skin graft. The inferior epigastric artery and vein of the rectus abdominus muscle were anatomosed to the proximal radial artery and the brachial vein using microvascular techniques. The left forearm musculature rapidly regained normal color and contractibility following decompressive fasciotomy and was temporarily covered with fresh allograft skin graft.

Postoperatively he did well, although he did suffer from persistent hypopharyngeal edema which did not allow him to be extubated for approximately 3 weeks. His serum CPK isoenzymes gradually returned toward normal. During his hospital course, he underwent two additional major operative procedures. His posterior neck soft tissue injury was debrided and closed with a trapezius myocutaneous flap. Then, after demonstrating good adherence of the previously applied allograft, his left arm wound was closed with autologous split-thickness skin graft. Six weeks after injury the patient was discharged from the hospital. During the past 9 months he has undergone comprehensive physical therapy and at present has a fully functional left hand. His right hand has regained some ulnar nerve sensation and function with an advancing Tinnel's sign. The median nerve deficit remains profound. Future care will involve tendon transfers and nerve grafting.

CASE DISCUSSION

This case was managed expeditiously with the ultimate goal being maximal tissue salvage. It is crucial that hemodynamic stability is assured prior to proceeding with a lengthy limb salvage procedure. This patient was operated upon prior to the clearance of his cervical spine due to difficulties in radiographically visualizing C_7 in the presence of bilateral upper extremity compartment syndromes. Because the accident was witnessed and with the capability of flexible fiber-optic intubation techniques, operative intervention proceeded with his neck extensively splinted. If his cervical spine had been able to be cleared, his posterior neck might also have been surgically addressed at the initial operation.

Also of note is the persistent hypopharyngeal edema which did not permit extubation for approximately 3 weeks. This edema was felt to be secondary to current injury in the peripharyngeal region and was monitored by serial fiber-optic endoscopic evaluation of his hypopharynx every 2 to 3 days.

The expeditious decompression of his compartment syndrome, coupled with immediate debridement and closure of his wounds, enabled this patient to start rehabilitation rapidly, permitting an early attainment of maximal function. It must be stressed that this approach should not be utilized on all patients. In patients with more severe extremity injuries or those with multisystem injuries, the classic multiple debridement regimen and delayed closure or amputation may indeed be the treatment of choice.

Fortunately, this patient's serum CPK isoenzymes progressively dropped following his initial operation and returned to normal after the injury on his neck was addressed. If indeed it had remained elevated, then a careful systematic appraisal of all the major muscle groups within the current path would have begun. A persistent elevation may have led to surgical re-exploration of his upper extremities seeking unrecognized myonecrosis.

References

1. Lee RC, Kolodney MS: Electrical injury mechanism: Electrical breakdown of all membranes. Plastic Reconstruc Surg 80(5):672, 1987.
2. Ahrenholz DH, Schubert W, Solem LD: Creatine kinase as a prognostic indicator in electrical injury. Surgery 741, 1988.
3. Taussig HB: Death from lightning and the possibility of living again. Ann Intern Med 68(6):1345, 1968.
4. McBride JW, Labrosse KR, McCoy HG: Is serum creatine kinase-MB in electrically injured patients predictive of myocardial injury. JAMA 255(6):764, 1986.
5. Purdue GF, Hunt JL: Electrographic monitoring after electrical injury: Necessity or luxury. J Trauma 26:2, 1986.
6. Better OS, Stein JH: Early management of shock and prophylaxis of acute renal failure in traumatic rhabdomyolysis. N Engl J Med 322(12):825, 1990.
7. Zagaer RA: Studies of mechanism and protective maneuvers in myoglobinuric acute renal injury. Lab Invest 60(5):619, 1989.
8. Miller FE, Peterson D, Miller J: Abdominal visceral perforation secondary to electrical injury: Case report and review of the literature. Burns 12(7):505, 1986.
9. Lee RC, Cravalho EG, Burke JF (eds): *Electrical Trauma: The Pathophysiology, Manifestations, and Clinical Management.* Cambridge Press Publishers, Cambridge, Engl, 1991.
10. Artz CP: Electrical injury simulating crush injury. Surg Gyn Obstet 125:1316, 1967.
11. Gottlieb LJ, Saunders J, Krizek TJ: Surgical technique for salvage of electrically damaged tissue, in Electrical Trauma: Pathophysiology. Cambridge Press Publishers, 1990.
12. Monafo WW, Freedman BM: Electrical and lightning injury, in Boswick JA, Jr (ed): The Art and Science of Burn Care. Aspen Publishers 1987.
13. Rosenberg DB, Nelson M: Rehabilitation concern in electrical burn patients: A review of the literature. J Trauma 28(6):808, 1988.

Chapter 67

PREVENTION AND MANAGEMENT OF MULTIPLE SYSTEMS ORGAN FAILURE FOLLOWING TRAUMA

JAMES R. MACHO

KEY POINTS

- *Tissue oxygenation should be maintained during trauma resuscitation.*
- *Avoidance of and surveillance for infection are essential.*
- *Antibiotics should be used appropriately.*
- *Gastrointestinal function and microflora should be preserved.*
- *Early support of nutritional and metabolic status should be provided.*
- *Support of individual organ systems is essential.*

Multiple system organ failure (MSOF) is a syndrome of progressive and cumulative organ system dysfunction that can occur following severe trauma, major surgery, intraabdominal sepsis, and other forms of critical illness.[1] Patient mortality ranges between 90 and 95 percent when three or more organ systems become severely impaired.[2,3] MSOF is often associated with uncontrolled infection and invariably involves the respiratory and cardiovascular systems early, followed by involvement of the kidneys, gastrointestinal (GI) tract, and liver.[4] The central nervous system (CNS), coagulation system, and the immune system often become involved.[5] Despite the focus on individual organ systems, the overall degree of cellular dysfunction is likely the important determinant in patient survival. The similar presentations of MSOF despite the different etiologies has led to the consideration of a common mechanism involving the normal host response to infection, such as the activation of inflammatory mediators including the complement system, the products of arachidonic acid metabolism, and tumor necrosis factor.[6,7] MSOF may therefore be considered as a failure of host defense homeostasis. The tissue destruction in MSOF appears to be due to an inappropriate inflammatory response rather than to a direct effect of invading organisms.[8,9]

Although most frequently associated with sepsis, MSOF can occur without an identifiable source of infection. MSOF may be perpetuated by certain factors, including the overgrowth of bacteria in the GI tract and the passage of organisms and their toxins across the gut mucosal barrier through a process known as translocation.[10]

Traumatized patients are at particular risk for developing MSOF because of such factors as prolonged shock, direct tissue injury, intestinal ischemia, and effects on cell-mediated immunity.[11] While trauma patients may be at increased risk, the otherwise healthy patient who develops the syndrome after a severe injury may have the greatest chance for recovery, even from the advanced stages of MSOF.[12] By careful management of tissue oxygenation and avoidance or control of infection, the syndrome may, to some extent, be preventible. This chapter focuses on strategies of prevention and treatment. Therapy specifically directed at attenuation or reversal of the inflammatory response is desirable but is not available. In established MSOF, treatment is aimed at support of individual failing organ systems.[13] The advantages of a treatment for a particular organ system must be weighed against the potential detrimental effects of this treatment on other organ systems. These considerations represent the major challenge to the physician managing the patient with MSOF.

Prevention of MSOF

Prevention of MSOF begins with the initial resuscitation. The major goals are maintenance of tissue oxygenation, prevention of infection, support of the integrity and function of the gut, and maintenance of an adequate nutritional and metabolic status.[14]

A common event preceding MSOF is the development of circulatory shock. Circulatory shock represents an imbalance between oxygen supply and demand at the tissue level. Oxygen transport is the product of cardiac output and arterial oxygen content. It is frequently reduced in patients with trauma and other risk factors for MSOF, particularly those in hypovolemic shock. Prolonged tissue hypoxia may result in irreversible damage to susceptible organs and serve as a stimulator for the inflammatory response. Injury to the gut may result in translocation of bacteria and endotoxin, which may initiate the inflammatory response that culminates in organ failure. In addition, reperfusion injury may occur due to the generation of oxygen radicals with toxic effects on the tissues.[9]

Hopefully, MSOF can be prevented or attenuated in such patients by improving tissue oxygenation through support of the cardiovascular, pulmonary, and hematologic systems. Once adequate arterial oxygenation has been achieved, tissue oxygen delivery is optimized by insuring an adequate volume status and cardiac output with judicious use of fluids, blood, vasoactive agents, and close hemodynamic monitoring. During the initial resuscitation of trauma patients, it is preferable to err on the side of increased fluid administration to avoid the possibility of hypoperfusion of organs such as the kidneys. Nevertheless, conservative fluid management aided by dopamine and perhaps dobutamine, if cardiac output is depressed, may be appropriate in patients during the postresuscitative phase.[15]

Prevention of sepsis is a major goal in the initial resuscitation of trauma patients. These patients must be thoroughly reexamined in the intensive care unit (ICU) to identify injuries that may predispose to infection. Surgical intervention may be required for soft tissue debridement or fracture stabilization to avoid further tissue injury and to facilitate patient mobilization.[16] Prophylactic antibiotics should be used for those injuries in which they have been shown to be effective, such as open fractures and bowel perforation.[17] In most cases, a second- or third-generation cephalosporin is used.[11] When prophylactic antibiotics are used, a short course of 24–48 h of therapy is efficacious while it reduces the selection of resistant organisms.[18]

Patients must be followed closely for signs of infection in the postresuscitative period. Wounds and incisions should be carefully inspected on a regular basis. All intravascular lines placed with suboptimal technique during the initial resuscitation must be removed within 12 to 24 h and replaced if necessary, using sterile technique. Infection at a catheter site or persistent fever without an obvious source, especially in the presence of positive blood cultures, should prompt removal of the catheter and local wound care. Generally, the devices are removed whenever they have served their monitoring purpose. The same is true of intracranial pressure monitors and indwelling catheters of the urinary tract. Catheter-related bacteremia and fungemia will occur in 5 to 20 percent of patients with central venous catheters used for parenteral hyperalimentation.[19] The complication is frequently heralded by unexplained fever and leukocytosis. An obviously infected catheter should be removed and replaced at an alternate site if necessary. However, in most cases, catheter sepsis will not be present, and removal of the catheter for each case of suspected infection would subject the patient to the increased risk of replacement. Suspected catheters should be changed with a Seldinger guidewire technique. If catheter sepsis is present, this usually results in a resolution of the signs of sepsis. The finding of positive blood and catheter tip cultures for the same organism confirms the diagnosis.[20]

Endotracheal tubes can predispose to the development of pneumonias as well as to colonization of the respiratory tract; sputum cultures are frequently positive, despite the absence of true infection. Radiographic infiltrates can be misleading in the presence of pulmonary contusion or pleural effusion. Therefore, patients should be treated for presumed pneumonia only if they demonstrate fever, leukocytosis, and discrete radiographic changes in the presence of white blood cells, abundant organisms, and a lack of epithelial cells on Gram stains of tracheal secretions.[21] Initial antibiotic choice is best made on Gram-stained results and then tailored to sputum cultures if large growth of a single organism is present, recognizing that such cultures may reflect oropharyngeal colonization.[22]

In addition to the skin and the respiratory tract, the gut represents a major interface of the patient with the external environment. Many studies have shown that the gut is adversely affected in critically ill patients.[10,23,24] Circulatory shock can result in loss of the barrier function of the intestine with the development of increased permeability to organisms and their toxins, particularly endotoxin. Critically ill patients frequently are treated with antacids or histamine-2 receptor blocker therapy to prevent the development of stress ulceration of the stomach. The use of these agents with or without broad spectrum systemic antibiotics may alter the flora of the gastrointestinal (GI) tract and lead to the overgrowth of some organisms, such as gram-negative rods and fungi.[23,25] This overgrowth may increase the likelihood of translocation of these organisms. In addition, patients with colonization of the proximal GI tract frequently will develop pneumonias caused by the same organisms.[23] This is thought to be due to retrograde colonization of the pharynx and tracheal aspiration facilitated by the presence of a nasogastric tube. The use of sucralfate, a cytoprotective agent, for stress ulcer prophylaxis has been associated with less perturbation of the GI flora and a decreased incidence of pneumonia and infectious complications in critically ill patients.[25]

Despite preventive measures, infections frequently develop in traumatized patients. Intraabdominal infections and lower respiratory infections are the most difficult to diagnose and treat. Bacteremia with multiple organisms is particularly suggestive of intraabdominal infection. Earlier studies suggested that the sudden development of MSOF was an indication for exploratory laparotomy.[26,27] Presently, computed tomography (CT) is the standard for detection of abscesses and other intraabdominal infections.[12] CT is particularly advantageous because high-resolution images of the entire abdomen are obtained without interference from overlying bone or bowel gas. In addition, CT may provide information about other noninfectious processes and allow therapeutic as well as diagnostic percutaneous approaches to intraabdominal pathology. It has prevented unnecessary laparotomies, which rarely reveal infectious sites if the CT is normal.[12] In the case of a patient who is too unstable for transport, bedside sonography may provide diagnostic information. Sonography and/or nuclear scanning may offer some advantage over CT in the evaluation of the biliary tract.

Chest CT is generally less useful, but it may provide valuable information about intrathoracic abscesses, empyema, and other conditions that may benefit from surgical or percutaneous drainage. Nevertheless, CT rarely resolves the issue of colonization versus infection in patients with suspected pneumonia. Because of this problem and the limitations of sputum Gram stains and cultures alluded to earlier, clinicians have employed a variety of techniques to obtain lower airway secretions for analysis. Such techniques have included transtracheal aspiration, transthoracic needle aspiration, transbronchial biopsy via the bronchoscope, and open lung biopsy. Transtracheal aspiration is rarely useful, since its results may be affected by oropharyngeal colonization. It is contraindicated in intubated and mechanically ventilated patients. Transthoracic needle aspiration cannot be used safely in severely tachypneic patients or in those receiving mechanical ventilation because of risk of pneumothorax.[21] This is also true of transbronchial biopsy. Open-lung biopsy allows both culture and histologic confirmation of infection; this procedure is the "gold standard" in determining the presence of bacterial pneumonia.[21] However, the value of the information obtained has to be weighed against the relatively high risks of the biopsy.

A double-sheath-protected specimen brush catheter introduced by the bronchoscope can be used to obtain secretions from the lower airways and can be used with fluoroscopic guidance.[28,29] This technique is relatively safe in intubated and ventilated patients and may well provide appropriate samples for analysis. However, although the protected catheter technique has been shown to be sensitive, it lacks specificity, particularly in ventilated patients receiving antibiotics. Techniques to detect antibody-coated bacteria in bronchoalveolar lavage in an attempt to differentiate between lung infection and colonization have been used, but these techniques probably have limited specificity as well.[30]

The lower urinary tract is the most common site of nosocomial infection but rarely causes manifestations of sepsis. In patients with sepsis without an identifiable source, some unusual causes should be considered. Chronic sinusitis is frequently encountered in intubated patients, especially those with nasotracheal tubes. Acute acalculous cholecystitis may be a cause of occult sepsis in trauma patients receiving hyperalimentation. Perianal abscess should be considered, particularly in patients who have required placement of a rectal tube.

The organisms recovered from MSOF patients who are bacteremic or have intraabdominal or pulmonary infections vary, but *Staphylococcus epidermidis* and *aureus*, gram-negative organisms such as *Escherichia coli* and *Pseudomonas aeruginosa*, and anaerobic organisms predominate. When a decision is made to treat with empiric therapy, broad spectrum coverage consisting of nafcillin or vancomycin, an aminoglycoside, and metronidazole should be given to most trauma patients who are thought to be septic until specific culture results are available. When the culture and sensitivity results are available, the antibiotic therapy should be adjusted to provide the most specific and least toxic therapy possible. When *Pseudomonas* infection is documented, it generally should be treated with an aminoglycoside and a third-generation cephalosporin. When aminoglycosides are used, the dosage should be determined relative to the level of renal function. Serum levels should be checked at frequent intervals to insure that the levels are therapeutic and to prevent toxicity. Even with appropriate levels, nephrotoxicity may develop, and, in that setting, the drug should be discontinued if possible. Critically ill patients with altered cellular immune function who are treated with broad spectrum antibiotics for extended periods frequently become superinfected with *Candida albicans* and other opportunistic organisms. Ideally, parenchymal involvement by *Candida* or other fungi should be demonstrated before amphotericin B is given. Nevertheless, the presence of *Candida* in three or more surveillance cultures of sputum, urine, or peritoneal fluid in patients who manifest persistent fever or leukocytosis should prompt therapy.

As noted earlier, MSOF cannot be controlled in some patients despite appropriate antibiotics. In these patients, the gut may serve as an occult reservoir for bacterial overgrowth and systemic translocation of organisms and their toxins. This has led to the suggestion that the GI tract be selectively decontaminated by the administration of enteral, nonabsorbable antibiotics. Oral ketoconazole has been shown to be effective in preventing *Candida* sepsis in certain susceptible patients.[31] However, antibiotic therapy aimed at GI tract organisms has not improved survival in critically ill patients.[32,33] Such broad spectrum therapy may contribute to colonization and infection with more resistant organisms. In the absence of proven efficacy, this technique cannot be recommended.

The concept of blunting the inflammatory processes that lead to MSOF with antiinflammatory agents may seem attractive. However, the use of corticosteroids in septic patients or those at risk of developing the adult respiratory distress syndrome (ARDS) has not improved outcome in several large trials.[34,35] Other antiinflammatory or vasoactive agents such as ibuprofen, prostacyclin, prostaglandin E_1, anticomplement antibodies, and anticachectin antibodies are currently being studied.[36] Their use cannot be recommended in the absence of positive clinical trials.

Nutritional and Metabolic Support

Nutritional and metabolic support is essential to the support of all organ systems, particularly in patients with MSOF. A hypercatabolic, hypermetabolic state develops early in the syndrome, and severe malnutrition can become a prominent feature within days of the onset of illness.[37] The alterations observed with the hypermetabolic state include increases in resting energy expenditure and oxygen consumption; increased use of carbohydrate, fat, and amino acids as energy substrates; and increased loss of nitrogen in the urine. If the hypermetabolic state is not supported by exogenous substrate, profound protein catabolism results, which can have deleterious effects on organ function and the immune response. The hypermetabolic state observed in patients with MSOF appears to be caused by the inflammatory mediators and the hormonal response to injury and is not readily altered by therapy.[38] However, when adequate nutritional support has not been provided, organ dysfunction will likely be accelerated. Malnutrition has also been associated with an alteration of intestinal flora and an increase in bacterial translocation from the GI tract in experimental studies.[10] Glucose intolerance is observed frequently in patients with MSOF, and excess administration may lead to hepatic steatosis and hyperosmolar coma.[37]

The goal of nutritional support in patients with or at risk for MSOF is to prevent substrate limited metabolism and to support, rather than attempt to alter, the hypermetabolism. Recent studies strongly suggest that nutritional support started within the first 12 to 72 h after injury may attenuate the hypermetabolic response and facilitate the attainment of positive nitrogen balance.[39] The preferred route of nutritional support is enteral because the potential septic complications of intravenous hyperalimentation are avoided, and cholestasis and the development of biliary sludge may be eliminated, thereby reducing the risk of acalculous cholecystitis. Furthermore, immunologic function and the integrity of the mucosal barrier appear to be dependent on this route of administration.[40] Early enteral feedings have been associated with improved animal survival in burn models.[41] Recent clinical studies demonstrate that enteral nutrition is well tolerated in critically ill trauma patients when administered by jejunostomy and that septic complications, particularly pneumonias, are significantly reduced.[39] As an alternative to a surgical jejunostomy, nasojejunal tubes may be placed. An elemental formula may be started at a low rate and concentration and increased at intervals until adequate nutritional support is attained.

Standard regimens of hyperalimentation may not meet metabolic needs and actually may be harmful because of the effects of excessive glucose administration. Improved metabolic support is achieved by decreasing the caloric and glucose loads and increasing the protein load.[37] A regimen of 35 to 40 nonprotein calories/kg/day with 2 to 3 gm/kg/day of amino acids has been described as a starting point, with the regimen adjusted by determination of resting energy expenditure and the respiratory quotient. Intravenous (IV) fat emulsions should be included to reduce the problems of excess glucose administration and to prevent essential fatty acid deficiency.[41] The fat emulsions may be used to provide 30 to 40 percent of the nonprotein calories; excessive administration can lead to hepatic steatosis and interference with macrophage function. The use of solutions of branched chain amino acids and the use of formulations with supplemental glutamine may offer some benefit in supplying amino acids for which there is an increased demand.[42]

Support of Failing Organ Systems in MSOF

The multisystem effects of any treatment modality must be considered in the patient with MSOF, since treatment that supports one organ system may be detrimental to another. The discussion in this section will emphasize these interactions.

Most patients with MSOF develop early respiratory failure, with hypoxemia caused primarily by intrapulmonary shunt. The clinical presentation is characterized by severe hypoxemia, dyspnea, and diffuse chest radiographic infiltrates in the presence of a normal pulmonary artery wedge pressure. As in ARDS, treatment consists of supplemental oxygen, positive pressure ventilation, and the use of positive end-expiratory pressure (PEEP) to decrease shunt and allow for a lower, less toxic fraction of inspired oxygen (F_{IO_2}).

High frequency jet ventilation has not been shown to reduce mortality in patients with MSOF. Similarly, other modes of ventilatory support such as pressure support ventilation, inverse ratio ventilation, and extracorporeal CO_2 removal by veno-venous circuit have not been subjected to randomized trials and cannot be recommended.[43]

The goal of support of the cardiovascular system is to optimize oxygen delivery and oxygen consumption. However, the extent to which oxygen delivery should be improved in a patient with MSOF is a matter of speculation.[15] Lactic acidosis caused by tissue hypoxia has been shown to be a poor prognostic factor in critically ill patients.[44] Many patients will manifest oxygen transport or delivery dependence in that their tissue oxygen consumption is determined by oxygen transport. At normal levels of oxygen delivery, such patients frequently manifest lactic acidosis and a high mixed venous oxygen content, reflecting a failure of tissue oxygen extraction. The outcome for such patients, including the generation and perpetuation of their MSOF, might improve with enhanced oxygen delivery. Whenever possible, an attempt should be made to increase oxygen delivery to the point of correcting lactic acidosis. This may require fluid loading, blood transfusion, or the use of vasoactive drugs.[15] However, the efficacy of such therapy in improving survival has not been established. This therapy will require invasive hemodynamic monitoring with its attendant risks. Catheters with capability for continuous monitoring of mixed venous oxygen saturation have not proven to be useful in patients with MSOF because of the high values related to the decreased extraction of oxygen by the tissues.

In many patients with MSOF, volume repletion is not always successful in restoring tissue oxygenation. Inotropic support may be required. Dopamine, which has inotropic properties and preferentially increases renal and mesenteric blood flow, would appear to be an ideal vasoactive agent in patients with MSOF. However, dopamine may also increase the intrapulmonary shunt. Dobutamine has been shown to be useful in hypervolemic patients because it lowers the wedge pressure and may have less effect on gas exchange.[15] Vasodilators such as nitroprusside would seem to have a theoretic advantage in patients with MSOF because they increase cardiac output and because they may improve regional perfusion. Recent experimental studies with prostacycline have demonstrated an improvement in oxygen transport and uptake.[36] Nevertheless, vasodilator therapy did not improve the outcome of the patients in this study, and vasodilators are contraindicated in the face of hypotension. The effects on respiratory function must be considered, since drugs such as nitroprusside may increase intrapulmonary shunt by their effects on hypoxic pulmonary vasoconstriction. For these reasons, vasodilator therapy cannot be recommended for patients with MSOF.

Although the liver is involved early in MSOF,[38] and bacterial overgrowth in the gastrointestinal tract may fuel the process, little specific therapy for the hepatic and GI systems exists for patients with MSOF beyond the general objectives of limiting infection and improving tissue oxygen delivery. However, therapy is available to prevent or treat stress ulceration, which otherwise occurs commonly in the setting of MSOF, and which is associated with a high morbidity and mortality.[25] The most common approach in recent years has been to use antacids or histamine blockers to titrate the gastric pH to a level of 4.0 or greater. One potential problem with this approach is that it may allow the overgrowth of gram-negative bacteria in the stomach. These organisms may then cause pneumonia through retrograde oropharyngeal colonization, facilitated by the presence of a nasogastric tube.[23] Several studies have now demonstrated that nosocomial pneumonia occurs more frequently in patients treated with antacids and/or histamine blockers than it does in patients who receive sucralfate, which does not alter the gastric pH and thereby tends to preserve normal gastric flora.[25] The use of sucralfate has not been associated with an increase in the incidence of stress ulceration and should be used preferentially in this group of patients.

Renal insufficiency and failure commonly occur in patients with MSOF and predisposes to fluid overload as well as intensifying nutritional and metabolic derangements. Furthermore, renal disease may either cause or potentiate acid-base disturbances in critically ill patients. The altered renal clearance must be considered in drug therapy such as antibiotic administration. In the patient with MSOF, every attempt should therefore be made to preserve renal function, including the avoidance of nephrotoxic drugs such as aminoglycosides whenever possible. Patients receiving radiographic contrast dye should be well hydrated prior to the procedure, and fluid administration should be maintained at a high level until the dye load is cleared.[12]

The nutritional and metabolic support with high levels of protein administration required in patients with MSOF may worsen renal failure. A more conservative approach to nutritional support may be necessary to control the blood urea nitrogen level. However, provision of metabolic substrates should be maintained and innovative techniques such as hemofiltration utilized to augment hemodialysis.[45]

Although mild degrees of metabolic acidosis may be disregarded in patients with MSOF, a new agent, dichloroacetate, may be effective in treating more severe metabolic acidosis.[46]

Red blood cell transfusions may be required to maintain adequate oxygen delivery when hematocrit is low in MSOF. Coagulation disorders, including DIC, may also occur in such patients and require treatment with platelets and factor replacement, particularly in the presence of clinical bleeding. In the absence of clinical bleeding, this therapy can often be cautiously withheld.

Despite a high mortality rate, patients do recover from MSOF and return to a fully functional state. The approach to a patient at risk for MSOF must be aggressive, with meticulous attention given to the smallest details of care. Constant surveillance is necessary to avoid potential sources of infection and to identify and treat infections early and appropriately. In patients with established MSOF, infection control continues to be of major importance, and careful monitoring is required to avoid adverse interactions between the various therapies for the support of failing organ systems.

CASE PRESENTATION

Ms. L.N. is a 42-year-old female pedestrian who was struck by a motor vehicle. She was conscious but in profound shock on admission to the emergency room (ER). She was resuscitated with crystalloid that was administered via saphenous vein cutdowns. Chest x-ray (CXR) revealed a right hemothorax with multiple rib fractures. A right chest tube was placed. There was an obvious left femur fracture, which was splinted and placed in traction. The patient continued to manifest hemodynamic instability and was noted to have a decreasing hematocrit. She was taken to the operating room (OR) for laparotomy. Massive intraperitoneal (IP) hemorrhage resulted from a liver laceration that was controlled and repaired. Peritoneal soilage from jejunal laceration was identified and repaired. A feeding jejunostomy tube was placed distal to the injury. Since the patient was then stable, open reduction and internal fixation of the femur fracture was performed. Ten units of blood were administered during surgery. The patient received a single dose of cefazolin preoperatively and two additional postoperative doses.

After transfer to the intensive care unit (ICU), a thorough physical examination was performed, and this did not reveal any other injuries. A CXR demonstrated right-sided infiltrates consistent with pulmonary contusion. Arterial blood gases revealed a P_{O_2} of 60 on an F_{IO_2} of 0.6. The patient was continued on mechanical ventilation with increased PEEP.

All lines placed during the resuscitation were removed and replaced during the first 24 h in the ICU. Jejunostomy feedings were begun 18 h after surgery and increased in volume and concentration until calculated caloric needs were attained. Sucralfate was administered for prophylaxis against the development of stress ulceration.

The patient improved over the subsequent 72 h and attempts were initiated to wean her from mechanical ventilation. On postoperative day 5, the patient was noted to have worsening gas exchange. Hypotension and low urine output developed and required increased administration of fluid. The WBC count was elevated to 22,000/mm^3, and the blood glucose was elevated to 410 mg/dL. CXR revealed bilateral infiltrates, but sputum Gram stain failed to reveal the presence of white cells and predominant organisms. Broad spectrum antibiotics were administered, and an abdominal computed tomography scan was obtained. This revealed a left subphrenic abscess, which was drained by percutaneous technique. Antibiotics were changed when culture and sensitivity results were available.

The patient's condition improved, and she was extubated on postoperative day 10. She was discharged from the hospital on postoperative day 20.

CASE DISCUSSION

The multiple, severe injuries, the period of shock and resuscitation, the need for multiple blood transfusions, and the peritoneal contamination all increase the risk of the development of MSOF in this patient. Initial concern should always be directed to rapid resuscitation from the shock state and identification and early appropriate management of all injuries. In this case, resuscitation required emergency operation to control hemorrhage. Early stabilization of the fracture was performed to avoid further tissue inflammation and to improve postoperative mobilization of the patient. After transfer to the ICU, a thorough reevaluation was performed to avoid the possibility of an overlooked and untreated injury.

Control of sepsis is the next consideration in the management of this patient. This often requires continued resuscitation to maintain adequate tissue oxygenation. Suspect lines placed during the emergency resuscitation are removed early to eliminate a possible source of sepsis. Prophylactic antibiotics are administered for a short course.

Nutritional support is provided early by an enteral route whenever possible. Gut function is maintained, and the complications of intravenous hyperalimentation are avoided. Stress ulcer prophylaxis with sucralfate avoids bacterial colonization of the stomach and decreases the likelihood of the development of pneumonia.

The failure of the patient to wean from mechanical ventilation, the increasing fluid requirement, the leukocytosis, and the elevated blood glucose all suggest the development of sepsis. Identification of these signs necessitates an urgent and thorough evaluation for the source of the sepsis. In this case, the pulmonary infiltrates prompted concern regarding the development of a pneumonia but this was not supported by the findings on sputum Gram stain. An abdominal CT scan was obtained because of the risk of intraabdominal sepsis in this patient, and an intraabdominal abscess was identified and treated early.

This case demonstrates the importance of (a) rapid resuscitation and early identification and treatment of all injuries, (b) avoidance of and surveillance for infection, (c) early support of nutritional and metabolic status with support of gut function and flora, and (d) early identification and treatment of sepsis. Prevention of MSOF is a primary consideration, since available treatment options are limited to support of failing organ systems.

References

1. Baue AE: Multiple, progressive or sequential systems failure: a syndrome of the 1970s. Arch Surg 110:779, 1975.
2. Carrico CJ, Meakins JL, Marshall JC, et al: Multiple-organ failure syndrome. Arch Surg 121:196, 1986.
3. Knaus WA, Draper EA, Wagner DP, et al: Prognosis in acute organ-system failure. Ann Surg 202:685, 1985.
4. Fry DE, Pearlstein L, Fulton RL, et al: Multiple system organ failure: the role of uncontrolled infection. Arch Surg 115:136, 1980.
5. Nishijima MK, Takezawa J, Hosotsubo KK, et al: Serial changes in cellular immunity of septic patients with multiple organ failure. Crit Care Med 14:87, 1986.
6. Stephens KE, Ishizaka A, Larrick JW, et al: Tumor necrosis factor causes increased pulmonary permeability and edema. Comparison to septic acute lung injury. Am Rev Respir Dis 137: 1364, 1988.
7. Weinberg PF, Matthay MA, Webster RO, et al: Biologically active products of complement and acute lung injury in patients with the sepsis syndrome. Am Rev Respir Dis 130:791, 1984.
8. Goris RJ, te Boekhorst TP, Nuytinck JK, et al: Multiple organ failure: generalized autodestructive inflammation? Arch Surg 120:1109, 1985.
9. Pinsky MR, Matuschak GM: Multiple Systems Organ Failure: failure of host defense homeostasis. Crit Care Clin 5:199, 1989.
10. Deitch EA, Winterton BS, Li M, et al: The gut as a portal of entry for bacteremia. Rolé of protein malnutrition. Ann Surg 205:681, 1987.
11. Nichols RL, Smith JW, Klein DB, et al: Risk of infection after penetrating abdominal trauma. N Engl J Med 311:1065, 1984.
12. Macho JR, Luce JM: Rational approach to the management of multiple systems organ failure. Crit Care Clin 5:379, 1989.
13. Matuschak GM, Rinaldo JE: Organ interactions in the adult respiratory distress syndrome during sepsis. Chest 94:400, 1988.
14. Macho JR, Meyer AA: The management of sepsis following injury. Crit Care Clin 2:869, 1986.
15. Gilbert EM, Haupt MT, Mandanas RY, et al: The effect of fluid loading, blood transfusion, and catecholamine infusion on oxygen delivery and consumption in patients with sepsis. Am Rev Respir Dis 134:873, 1986.
16. Lozman J, Deno DC, Feustel PJ, et al: Pulmonary and cardiovascular consequences of immediate fixation or conservative management of long bone fractures. Arch Surg 121:992, 1986.
17. Jones RC, Thal ER, Johnson NA, et al: Evaluation of antibiotic therapy following penetrating abdominal trauma. Ann Surg 201:576, 1985.
18. Dellinger EP, Oreskovich MR, Wertz MJ, et al: Efficacy of short course antibiotic prophylaxis after penetrating intestinal injury. A prospective, randomized trial. Arch Surg 121:23, 1986.
19. Sitzmann JV, Townsend TR, Siler MC: Septic and technical complications of central venous catheterization: A prospective study of 200 consecutive patients. Ann Surg 202:766, 1985.
20. Bozzetti F, Terno G, Bonfanti G: Prevention and treatment of central venous catheter sepsis by exchange via a guidewire. A prospective controlled trial. Ann Surg 198:48, 1983.
21. Davidson M, Tempest B, Palmer DL: Bacteriologic diagnosis of acute pneumonia. Comparison of sputum, transtracheal aspirates and lung aspirates. JAMA 235:158, 1976.
22. Montgomery AB, Luce JM: Infection monitoring. Respir Care 30:489, 1985.
23. Marshall JC, Christou NV, Horn R, et al: The microbiology of multiple organ failure. The proximal gastrointestinal tract as an occult reservoir of pathogens. Arch Surg 123:309, 1988.
24. Wilmore DW, Goodwin CW, Aulick LH, et al: Effects of injury and infection on visceral metabolism and circulation. Ann Surg 192:491, 1980.
25. Driks MR, Craven DE, Celli BR, et al: Nosocomial pneumonia in intubated patients given sucralfate as compared with antacids or histamine type 2 blockers: the role of gastric colonization. N Engl J Med 317:1376, 1987.
26. Ing AF, McLean PH, Meakins JL: Multiple-organism bacteremia in the surgical intensive care unit: a sign of intraperitoneal sepsis. Surgery 90:779, 1981.
27. Polk HC, Shields CL: Remote organ failure: A valid sign of occult intra-abdominal infection. Surgery 81:310, 1977.
28. Chastre J, Viau F, Brun P, et al: Prospective evaluation of the protected specimen brush for the diagnosis of pulmonary infections in ventilated patients. Am Rev Respir Dis 130:924, 1984.
29. Wimberley NW, Bass JB, Boyd BW, et al: Use of a bronchoscopic protected brush for the diagnosis of pulmonary infections. Chest 81:556, 1982.
30. Winterbauer RH, Hutchinson JF, Reinhart GN, et al: The use of quantitative cultures and antibody coating of bacteria to diagnose pneumonia by fiberoptic bronchoscopy. Am Rev Respir Dis 128:98, 1983.
31. Slotman GJ, Burchard KW: Ketoconazole prevents candida sepsis in critically ill surgical patients. Arch Surg 122:147, 1987.

32. Ledingham IM, Alcock SR, Eastway AT, et al: Triple regimen of selective decontamination of the digestive tract, systemic cefotaxime, and microbiological surveillance for prevention of acquired infection in intesive care. Lancet 1:785, 1988.
33. Stoutenbeek CP, van Saene HK, Miranda DR, et al: The effect of selective decontamination of the digestive tract on colonisation and infection rate in multiple trauma patients. Intens Care Med 10:185, 1984.
34. Bernard GR, Luce JM, Sprung CL, et al: High-dose corticosteroids in patients with the adult respiratory distress syndrome. N Engl J Med 317:1565, 1987.
35. Bone RC, Fisher CJ, Clemmer TP, et al: A controlled clinical trial of high-dose methylprednisolone in the treatment of severe sepsis and septic shock. N Engl J Med 317:653, 1987.
36. Bihari D, Smithies M, Gimson A, et al: The effects of vasodilation with prostacyclin on oxygen delivery and uptake in critically ill patients. N Engl J Med 317:1565, 1987.
37. Cerra FB: Hypermetabolism organ failure syndrome: a metabolic response to injury. Crit Care Clin 5:289, 1989.
38. Cerra FB, Siegel JH, Borden JR, et al: The hepatic failure of sepsis: Cellular vs. substrate. Surgery 86:409, 1979.
39. Moore FA, Moore EE, Jones TN, et al: TEN versus TPN following major abdominal trauma—reduced septic morbidity. J Trauma 29:916, 1989.
40. Alverdy JC, Chi HS, Sheldon GS: The effect of parenteral nutrition on gastrointestinal immunity. Ann Surg 202:681, 1985.
41. Cerra FB: Hypermetabolism, organ failure, and metabolic support. Surgery 191:1, 1987.
42. Bower RH, Muggin-Sullam M, Vallgren S, et al: Branched chain amino acid enriched solutions in the septic patient: a randomized, prospective trial. Ann Surg 203:13, 1986.
43. Gattinoni L, Pesenti A, Mascheroni D, et al: Low-frequency positive-pressure ventilation with extracorporeal CO_2 removal in severe acute respiratory failure. JAMA 256:881, 1986.
44. Broder G, Weil MH: Excess lactate: an index of reversibility of shock in human patients. Science 143:1457, 1964.
45. Kaplan AA, Longnecker RE, Folkert VW: Continuous arteriovenous hemofiltration: A report of six months' experience. Ann Int Med 100:358, 1984.
46. Stacpoole PW, Harman EM, Curry SH, et al: Treatment of lactic acidosis with dichloroacetate. N Engl J Med 309:390, 1983.

SECTION D

BURNS AND ENVIRONMENTAL INJURY

The burn patient changes dramatically over the course of the injury. The initial postburn period is characterized by cardiopulmonary instability caused by fluid shifts and direct smoke injury to the airways. With the onset of intense wound inflammation, immunosuppression, and infection, physiologic and metabolic parameters change substantially from those seen initially. Treatment must therefore be based on a clear understanding of these changes over time.[1,2] This discussion will therefore be divided into three time periods—the initial resuscitation period (0 to 36 h) (Chap. 68), the early postresuscitation period (2 to 6 days) (Chap. 69), and the inflammation-infection period, which is usually most evident after the first week (Chap. 70).

To say that the major burn patient is complex and difficult to manage is truly an understatement. Many of the problems are predictable and must be prevented rather than treated as they develop. The burn patient is a very fragile, compromised host who tolerates complications poorly. The optimal environment is a burn center with a team approach to care, all members being highly experienced. If this is not available, an ICU environment is adequate if it is modified for the special needs of the burn patient. Increased room temperature is essential as are standard isolation techniques. Infection control principles, however, are the same as for any other critically ill patient. The major cause of cross-contamination remains personnel in the unit.

Monitoring requirements are also no different from those for any other ICU patient. However, vascular access is much more of a problem, and noninvasive measures are often all that are available. A typical burn unit has a procedure room for wound care and often an operating room, but wound care in the ICU is very feasible and actually essential in the unstable patient. Hyperbaric oxygen chambers are not a necessary component and are really only indicated in patients with such severe carbon monoxide exposure that the cytochrome system is saturated with carbon monoxide, not readily displaced with 100% oxygen alone. It is safe to say that 99 percent of major burns with some degree of carbon monoxide inhalation do not require hyperbaria.

The secret to a successful patient outcome, however, remains in the knowledge base, judgment, and decision-making skills of the personnel, not in the external environment.[1,2]

Chapter 68

BURNS: RESUSCITATION PHASE (0 to 36 h)

ROBERT H. DEMLING

KEY POINTS

- *A burn patient is a trauma patient; therefore, look for other traumatic injuries.*
- *Obtaining an adequate airway means an adequately sized tube for both ventilation needs and pulmonary toilet. Changing the tube can be extremely dangerous.*
- *Hypothermia is a major concern, and early aggressive attempts at prevention are required.*
- *Modification of the standard lactated Ringer's resuscitation is often necessary in the massive burn or inhalation injury patient or in the very young and old. Additions of colloid, blood, low dose dopamine, and inotropes are often very useful in restoring hemodynamic stability. Do not get locked into a formula.*
- *Watch for local perfusion problems and chest wall constriction caused by the burn.*
- *Once the fire is out, the burn itself is a low priority for care.*

Cardiopulmonary instability characterizes this period. Life-threatening airway and breathing problems are major concerns at this time with carbon monoxide poisoning, upper airway edema, and the immediate effect of smoke inhalation injury being the most common. The initial phase is also characterized by hypovolemia as plasma volume is lost into the burn tissue. The burn itself is of less immediate concern, but the adequacy of initial treatment of pulmonary and circulatory abnormalities sets the stage for subsequent management. Any early management error will lead to a dramatic increase in morbidity and mortality during the subsequent injury phases. It is of critical importance to remember that the burn patient is a trauma patient with the potential for many other traumatic injuries in addition to the obvious skin burn. The standard approach to trauma resuscitation must therefore be followed, including assessment for cervical-spine and head injuries, pulmonary and abdominal trauma, fractures, etc. Management of these problems is the same as that in the nonburn patient.

Airway and Pulmonary Abnormalities

Abnormalities of ventilation and oxygenation are common in the immediate postburn period. Several fairly distinct critical disease processes must be recognized and managed aggressively.[3] The first three are associated with the inhalation injury complex and are presented in the approximate order in which symptoms will develop (carbon monoxide toxicity, upper airway obstruction, chemical burn to the lung). Following this is a discussion of lung changes due to the skin burn, and last, the effects of impaired chest wall compliance.

SMOKE INHALATION INJURY COMPLEX

Pulmonary insufficiency caused by the inhalation of heat and smoke is the major cause of mortality in the fire victim, accounting for over 50 percent of fire-related deaths.[4,5] The magnitude of the problem has been much better appreciated in recent years. The use of many new synthetics in home furnishings and clothing has resulted in a much more complex form of injury due to extremely toxic combustion products. The exposure time, concentration of fumes, elements released, and degree of concomitant body burn are critical variables in determining ultimate morbidity and mortality. In addition to lung injury, a closed-space fire can cause a severe hypoxic insult. Improved knowledge of the pathophysiology combined with an aggressive treatment plan has made it possible to improve the outcome.

CARBON MONOXIDE (AND CYANIDE) TOXICITY

Carbon monoxide, a by-product of incomplete combustion, is one of the leading causes of death in fires. Hydrogen cyanide is also a well-recognized cause of morbidity and mortality, especially with burning of synthetics such as polyurethane (see Chap. 176).

Symptoms of carbon monoxide toxicity are usually not present until the carboxyhemoglobin concentration exceeds 15 percent. Symptoms are those of decreased tissue oxygenation with initial manifestations being neurologic. Cyanide toxicity presents in a very similar fashion with severe metabolic acidosis and obtundation. Diagnosis, however, is more difficult since cyanide levels are not always readily available or very reliable. Normal levels are <0.1 mg/L (even in smokers). A level near 1 mg/L is lethal. Neurologic dysfunction can also be caused by noncarbon monoxide-induced processes such as alcohol, drugs, or blunt head trauma. A toxicology screen is therefore warranted. A head computed tomography (CT) scan is warranted based on the same criteria used in the trauma patient.

The persistence of a metabolic acidosis in the patient with adequate volume resuscitation and cardiac output suggests impairment of oxygen transport and utilization by carbon monoxide or cyanide. Arterial P_{O_2} can remain relatively normal since the chemical alteration of hemoglobin by carbon monoxide will not affect the amount of oxygen dissolved in arterial plasma. However, the measured oxygen saturation of hemoglobin (S_{O_2}) will be markedly decreased relative to the P_{O_2}.

A high carboxyhemoglobin level also indicates a significant smoke exposure, and therefore, a chemical burn to the airways. A low carboxyhemoglobin does not always indicate a minimal smoke exposure because administration of oxygen at the scene can displace some of the carbon monoxide prior to arrival at the emergency room.

Treatment of carbon monoxide toxicity is more fully covered in Chap. 175, but briefly consists of the early displacement of carbon monoxide from hemoglobin by administration of 90 to 100% oxygen. Treatment of cyanide toxicity involves restoration of hepatic blood flow to clear the cyanide (see Chap. 176). Hyperbaric oxygen is best used in cases when the patient has severe neurologic compromise with a high carboxyhemoglobin level (>50 percent) but no major burns or severe pulmonary injury, and is not responding to high flow oxygen with clearance of symptoms. However, the vast majority of cases can be successfully managed using simply 90 to 100% oxygen. Endotracheal intubation and use of 100% oxygen is indicated for those patients with impaired neurologic function and a high carboxyhemoglobin level.

UPPER AIRWAY OBSTRUCTION FROM AIRWAY EDEMA

Direct heat injury caused by the inhalation of air heated to a temperature of 150°C (318°F) or higher ordinarily results in burns to the face, oropharynx, and upper airway (above the vocal cords). Even superheated air is rapidly cooled before it reaches the lower respiratory tract because of the tremendous heat-exchanging efficiency of the oropharynx and nasopharynx.

Heat produces an immediate injury to the airway mucosa, resulting in edema, erythema, and ulceration. Although these mucosal changes may be anatomically present shortly after the burn, physiologic alterations will not be present until the edema is sufficient to produce clinical evidence of impaired upper airway patency. This may not occur for 12 to 18 h. The presence of a body burn magnifies the injury to airways in direct proportion to the size and depth of the skin burn. The massive fluid requirements necessary to treat the skin burn are in part responsible.

A face or neck burn will accentuate these problems by producing marked anatomic distortion and in the case of the deep neck burn, external compression of the larynx. A particularly dangerous injury is the third-degree facial burn with minimal external edema. The lack of external edema is due to the nonelastic third-degree burn, which does not allow expansion. Intraoral edema in this case is usually massive but may go unrecognized unless specifically investigated.

Symptoms of obstruction, such as stridor, dyspnea, and eventually cyanosis, do not develop until a critical narrowing of the airway is present. The airway edema and the external burn edema have a parallel time course such that by the time symptoms of airway edema develop, external and internal anatomic distortion will be extensive. The local edema usually resolves in 4 to 5 days.

Inspection of the oropharynx for soot or evidence of a heat injury should be routine in every burn victim. Numerous techniques have been used to further assess the degree of injury and to determine the need for endotracheal intubation. Spirometry and flow-volume curves detect early airway changes but require a cooperative patient without severe facial burns. Fiberoptic bronchoscopy or laryngoscopy will determine whether physical evidence of pharyngeal or laryngeal mucosal injury is present. Laryngoscopy will demonstrate the presence of mucosal irritation at and above the cords and provide information about the need for endotracheal intubation.[4,5] Unfortunately, unless serial studies are performed, none of these tests can accurately predict the severity of subsequent airway compromise since the edema is progressive during the first 18 to 24 h. Repeated examination for airway compromise is feasible using laryngoscopy or fiberoptic bronchoscopy in the patient without a facial burn or without other reasons for immediate intubation. However in the presence of a large burn, it is best to proceed with intubation if there is concern about the potential development of airway problems rather than performing serial examinations. Absence of upper airway changes almost always means absence of lower airway injury.

Maintaining an adequate airway is essential for successful early management. Intubation of the trachea impairs cough and increases the risk of nosocomial infection. A judgment must be made in the initial assessment as to whether the airway can be managed safely without an endotracheal tube. When in doubt, it is safer to intubate. There are many other indications in the burn patient besides airway edema for the need for intubation, such as hemodynamic instability and impaired consciousness. A large oral endotracheal tube (at least 7 mm internal diameter) should be used in adults because very thick secretions develop as a result of lung injury. If the initial tube is too small, it will be dangerous to change once massive facial and airway edema develops. Although the nasotracheal route may be more comfortable for the patient, the tube may need to be smaller and lead to later problems for secretion clearance.

A patient with a significant inhalation injury and deep facial burns should usually be managed by early endotracheal intubation. Management without intubation is allowed only when close monitoring for obstruction is available and *only* if intubation can be safely and rapidly performed when needed. Progressive anatomic distortion caused by face and neck burns usually makes delayed intubation very difficult. Patients not intubated need to be placed with the head elevated and with experienced ICU personnel ready to intervene if necessary. Patients with small second-degree facial burns from flashes of flame or hot liquids, but no smoke exposure or intraoral burns, are at less risk for airway compromise. Elevation of the head of the bed and controlled fluid resuscitation usually allow conservative management. An algorithm for this approach is presented in Fig. 68-1.

CHEMICAL BURN TO UPPER AND LOWER AIRWAYS

This aspect of inhalation injury is often an extension of the upper airway injury just described but is generally much more serious than that produced by heat alone. Toxic gases contained in smoke as well as carbon particles coated with irritating aldehydes and organic acids can injure both upper and lower airways (Table 68-1). The location of injury will depend on the duration of exposure, the size of the particles, and the solubility of the gases.

Water-soluble gases found in smoke from burning plastics or rubber such as ammonia, sulfur dioxide, and chlorine react with water in mucous membranes to produce strong acids and alkalies that lead to irritation, broncho-

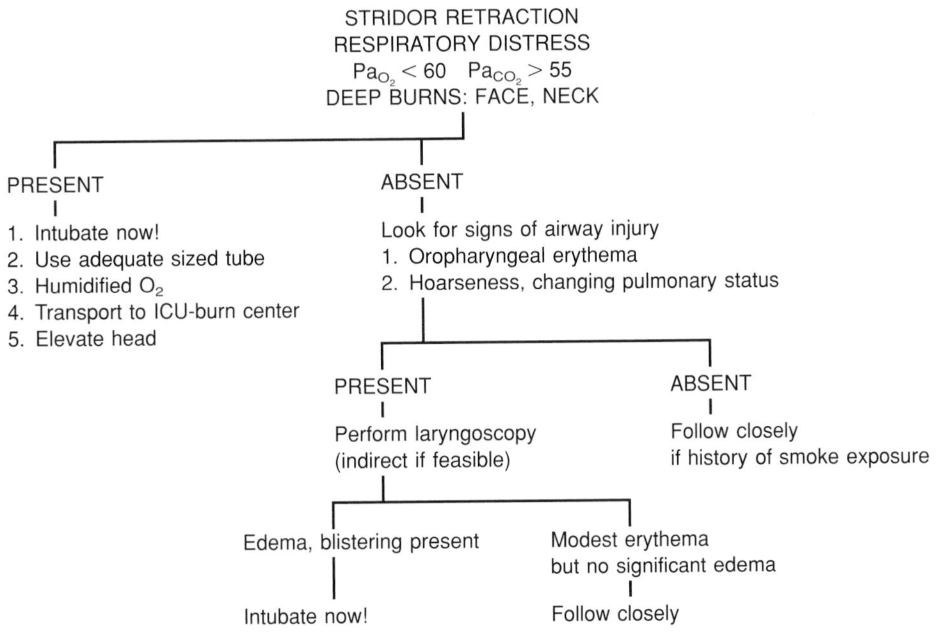

FIGURE 68-1 Initial assessment of airway (to intubate or not to intubate).

TABLE 68-1 Toxic Elements in Housefire Smoke

Gas	Source	Effect
Carbon monoxide	Any organic matter	Tissue hypoxia
Nitrogen dioxide	Wallpaper, wood	Bronchial irritation Dizziness Pulmonary edema
Hydrogen chloride (from phosgene)	Plastics (Polyvinyl chloride)	Severe mucosal irritation
Hydrogen cyanide	Wool, silk, nylons (Polyurethane)	Headache Respiratory failure Coma
Benzene	Petroleum plastics	Mucosal irritation Coma
Aldehydes	Wood, cotton, paper	Severe mucosal damage Extensive lung damage
Ammonia	Nylon	Mucosal irritation

spasm, mucous membrane ulceration, and edema. Severe damage to the ciliary mechanism of the mucosa leads to impairment of the removal of particles and mucus. Lipid-soluble compounds such as nitrous oxide, phosgene, hydrogen chloride, and toxic aldehydes are transported to the lower airways on carbon particles which, in turn, adhere to the mucosa. All these agents produce cell membrane damage.

Breath-holding and laryngospasm are protective mechanisms against excessive exposure in the conscious patient. The unconscious patient, however, loses this protection and sustains more severe injury to the lower airways. Information regarding loss of consciousness at the scene should be sought in the history.

A history of confinement in a closed space during the burning process is a good indicator of potential lung damage. However, single breath exposures to toxic chemicals are sufficient to produce major airway damage. An absence of a history, especially by transferring medical personnel, often means a lack of detailed information about the circumstances of injury. The true story often takes hours or days to determine.

Symptoms may well be absent on admission with the true magnitude of injury only becoming evident after 24 to 48 h. Early symptoms usually consist of wheezing and bronchorrhea. This intense initial bronchorrhea caused by the irritation of the airway mucosa in combination with increased oral and nasal secretions can give the false appearance of fulminant pulmonary edema. Soot in the lung secretion is certainly evidence of smoke exposure but is not a necessary finding.

Physical findings on admission which suggest smoke exposure include a facial burn, soot in the sputum, dyspnea, coughing, wheezing, and bronchorrhea. If present, these findings are helpful. However, many patients demonstrate minimal symptoms early after injury and only when airway edema develops do symptoms become evident.

Early bronchospasm and bronchiolar edema initiated by the irritant gases cause a marked decrease in dynamic lung compliance and increased work of breathing. Impaired clearance of secretions will accentuate this problem.

Impairment of gas exchange is due to ventilation/perfusion ($\dot{V}/\dot{Q}$) mismatching related to airway injury rather than to alveolar edema.[6] Several clinical studies have verified that alveolar edema is present in the first 24 h only after massive inhalation injuries where damage has extended beyond the small airways.[7,8] Alveolar flooding in these severe cases may well be due to retrograde flow of bronchorrhea. A body burn markedly potentiates the inhalation-induced lung dysfunction caused by chemical injury. The mortality rate for patients with severe inhalation injury alone is 5 to 8 percent. The combination of a major burn and smoke inhalation is more lethal than either injury alone.

Initial treatment of this component consists of an aggressive approach to upper airway maintenance and pulmonary support, which includes maintenance of small airway patency and removal of soot and the mucopurulent secretions. A careful well-monitored fluid resuscitation is necessary to avoid accentuation of the process. The addition of positive end-expiratory pressure (PEEP) is frequently necessary to maintain small airway patency and an adequate functional residual capacity (FRC), assisting in holding the edematous airway open until edema resolves. Endotracheal intubation and PEEP have been reported to decrease early pulmonary deaths after severe burns and smoke inhalation.[9] The use of humidified oxygen to maintain adequate oxygen delivery as well as to assist in the clearance of secretions is indicated. Elevation of the patient's head and chest 20 to 30° is also helpful. Bronchospasm can be treated with parenteral or inhaled bronchodilators.

Beginning about 18 to 24 h after a burn, increasing airway resistance is often due to bronchiolar edema and airway plugging rather than to bronchospasm. The associated impairment of gas exchange often responds to further increases in PEEP in addition to bronchodilators. The injured airway mucosa will frequently become colonized with bacteria, especially if an endotracheal tube is present. Prophylactic antibiotics will only select for resistant organisms and are, therefore, not indicated. Corticosteroids increase morbidity and mortality in the presence of a body burn and are, therefore, contraindicated. Even in the absence of a burn, steroid treatment of inhalation injury has shown no benefit.[10,11]

Close monitoring of the adequacy of gas exchange is necessary particularly during the early evolution of the inhalation injury. An indwelling arterial line or a pulse oximeter is required.

LUNG CHANGES FROM SKIN BURN

Pulmonary complications seen after burns, even in the absence of inhalation injury, have previously been attributed to increased lung protein permeability. Recent evidence indicates that this is not the case.[12,13] Although biochemical changes occur in lung tissue, particularly increased lipid peroxidation (reflecting oxygen radical injury), there is no measurable lung microvascular protein leak, at least not in man, until later when sepsis evolves. A number of human studies have verified no increase in lung water during the resuscitation phase despite massive burn soft tissue edema. Also nonburn tissue edema does not appear to be due to increased permeability but rather to the profound hypoproteinemia that occurs with protein loss into the burn itself.[12]

Lung changes as a result of the body burn, however, do include a transient increase in pulmonary artery pressure and a modest, but significant, decrease in P_{O_2}. An increase in closing volume and increased airway resistance indicate small airway pathology. A number of bronchoconstrictor and vasoactive mediators are released from burn tissue. The effects of these mediators are relatively modest in degree, however, in the absence of concomitant inhalation injury. Nevertheless, the two injuries together may dramatically compound the injury produced by either alone.

IMPAIRED CHEST WALL COMPLIANCE

Respiratory excursion can be markedly impaired by a burn to the chest wall, especially with a circumferential third-degree burn. The loss of elasticity of the chest wall will markedly increase the work of breathing. Developing subeschar edema compresses the chest wall, reducing FRC. The loose areolar tissue in the axilla and lateral chest wall sequesters huge amounts of edema fluid which leads to a very heavy, tense chest wall. Full-thickness burns produce more severe limitation since tissue expansion is markedly impaired. The reduced FRC, in conjunction with the elevated closing volume, causes airway closure with ($\dot{V}/\dot{Q}$) mismatching and atelectasis. In addition, the increased work of breathing can lead to hypoventilation and respiratory failure. Any process which compromises the necessary increase in inspiratory force and muscle activity, such as hypoxia, hypovolemia, pain, or sedation, will accentuate lung dysfunction.

Symptoms may not be clearly evident until edema formation peaks. The first clinical evidence of chest wall restriction is often labored breathing, followed by rapid respiratory deterioration, particularly in the patient who is not receiving ventilatory support. Clearance of secretions can be impaired due to the inability to generate a hyperinflation. The increased intrathoracic pressure required to expand the stiff chest wall leads to impaired venous return in the mechanically ventilated patient. The hemodynamic instability is difficult to treat simply by volume loading since any increase in central venous pressure (CVP) will dramatically increase the rate of fluid and protein loss into the burn tissue, accentuating the chest wall edema.

Treatment involves edema reduction, possibly with surgical decompression of the chest wall. As soon as the patient is hemodynamically stable, the head and chest should be elevated 30° to decrease anterolateral chest wall edema. Fluid resuscitation should be well controlled, especially in the immediate postburn period to avoid both under and overhydration. If symptoms compatible with chest wall restriction develop in a third-degree burn, escharotomy is required. Longitudinal incisions placed in the midaxillary lines should be connected across the lower chest wall. Bleeding is usually easily controlled if the incisions stay within the margins of the third-degree burn, since the dermal vessels are thrombosed. The incision must extend into the subeschar area to allow adequate chest wall expansion. If a charred chest wall is present on admission, reflecting extension of the burn into fat and possibly fascia (i.e., fourth-degree burn), escharotomy should be performed on admission. An extremely deep burn results in tissue contraction due to dessication, making the chest wall tight even before edema develops. Use of microcrystalline collagen to pack the incision sites can help control punctate bleeding. Larger vessels usually require suture ligatures or cautery. Even with an escharotomy, the restrictive process can be of such magnitude that hypoventilation is clearly evident. In these patients, endotracheal intubation and positive-pressure ventilation should be initiated prior to obvious pulmonary deterioration. Escharotomies are usually not required in a second-degree burn unless the burn is very deep or the edema is so massive that the burned skin is tight. (This approach is diagramed in Fig. 68-2.)

Restoration and Maintenance of Hemodynamic Stability

Massive fluid shifts occur during this period, which can lead to severe impairment in oxygen delivery to tissues. An understanding of these early fluid shifts is necessary to avoid hemodynamic instability and to initiate appropriate treatment.

PATHOPHYSIOLOGY OF BURN SHOCK

With a major burn, intravascular volume is lost into burned tissue as well as nonburned tissue. Increased vascular per-

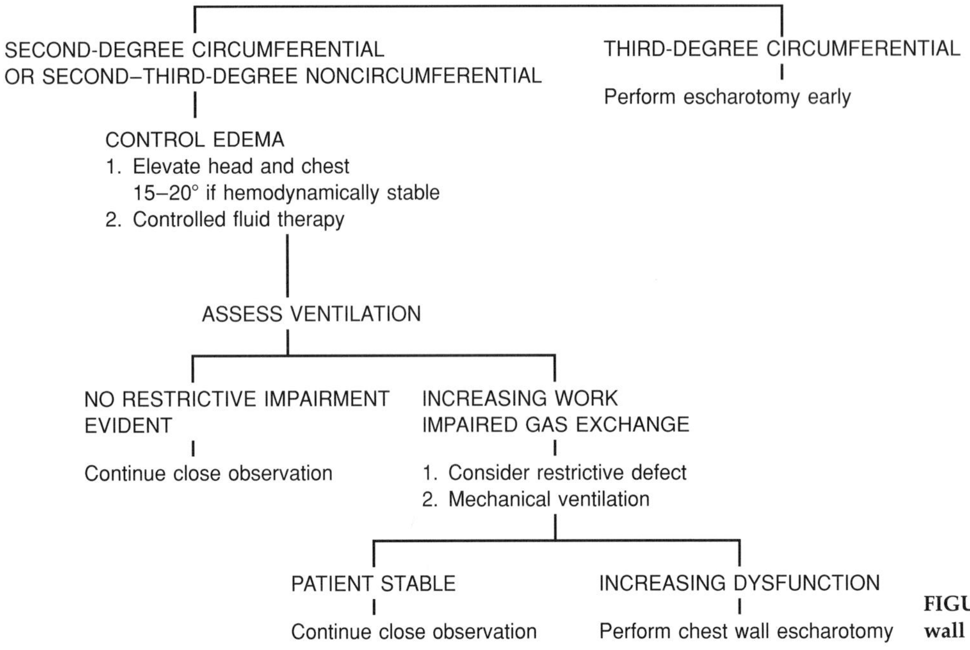
SECOND-DEGREE CIRCUMFERENTIAL
OR SECOND–THIRD-DEGREE NONCIRCUMFERENTIAL
THIRD-DEGREE CIRCUMFERENTIAL
Perform escharotomy early
CONTROL EDEMA
1. Elevate head and chest
15–20° if hemodynamically stable
2. Controlled fluid therapy
ASSESS VENTILATION
NO RESTRICTIVE IMPAIRMENT
EVIDENT
Continue close observation
INCREASING WORK
IMPAIRED GAS EXCHANGE
1. Consider restrictive defect
2. Mechanical ventilation
PATIENT STABLE
Continue close observation
INCREASING DYSFUNCTION
Perform chest wall escharotomy

FIGURE 68-2 Treatment of chest wall burn.

meability, raised burn tissue osmotic forces, and cellular swelling contribute.[14]

BURN EDEMA

Massive fluid and protein shifts occur in the burn tissue itself as a result of alterations in vascular permeability. The most pronounced shift occurs in the first several hours as a result of the increased protein permeability and the apparent increase in burn tissue osmotic pressure.

The concept of a mediator-induced injury is of considerable importance since it allows the possibility of modulating burn edema by mediator inhibition.[15] Vasoactive mediators such as vasodilator prostaglandins, histamine, bradykinin, and oxygen radicals can produce edema by a direct increase in vascular permeability or indirectly by increasing microvascular hydrostatic pressure. The markedly abnormal vascular permeability in burn tissue leads to a loss of the gradient between plasma and interstitial protein contents, even for very large macromolecules. This fact means that the rate rather than the type of resuscitation fluid controls the burn edema process.

The rate of the initial fluid loss from the microcirculation into the interstitium of the burn tissue exceeds that due simply to an increase in vascular permeability. An increase in burn tissue osmotic pressure estimated at 200 to 300 mmHg has been hypothesized to explain the rapid water shift. This increase in osmotic forces is felt to be due to sodium binding to injured collagen.[16]

The fluid and protein shifts are the greatest in the first several hours because of the combined effect of increased permeability and an imbalance of osmotic forces. After the first several hours, the rate of edema formation depends on the adequacy of wound perfusion and on capillary pressure. Edema formation in a small wound is maximum at about 6 h after injury, since blood volume and vascular pressures to the wound are maintained. The degree of systemic hypovolemia caused by fluid loss into a large burn surface will retard the rate of edema formation. Subsequently, the quantity of edema depends on the adequacy of the fluid resuscitation.

Severe hypoproteinemia also occurs as a result of the protein loss into the wound. The major protein losses occur in the first 6 to 8 h during the peak of the fluid loss. Plasma proteins can decrease to <50 percent of normal. The protein-rich edema in burn tissue is present primarily in the now expanded interstitial space. This interstitial edema fluid appears to form a gel after about 12 h, leading to obstruction of local lymphatics. The gel is probably due to leakage of clotting proteins and to fibrin deposition. Edema clearance is therefore markedly impaired. Tissue oxygen tension also decreases with edema as the distance between viable cells and the closest capillary increases. This process will have the most deleterious impact on the marginally viable cells. Resolution of edema depends on restoration of lymphatic patency which may take a number of days to weeks. Edema in deeper burns resolves more slowly than in superficial burns.

CHANGES IN NONBURN TISSUE (NONBURN EDEMA)

Generalized tissue edema in nonburned tissues is clearly evident in patients with burns exceeding 30 percent of the total body surface area (TBS). The process is not due simply to an increase in vascular permeability since permeability is only transiently altered in nonburned tissues. The edema appears to be due, at least in part, to an alteration in the microvascular interstitium itself related to the low protein content.[12]

There is also a generalized alteration in the cell membranes of nonburned tissue, especially in muscle. A decrease in cell membrane potential occurs, as is seen in other forms of shock, leading to a shift of sodium and water from the extracellular space into the cell. The significance of this process depends on the degree of shock and can be minimized by early restoration of tissue perfusion.

SYSTEMIC HEMODYNAMIC CHANGES

Cardiac output is initially depressed, related primarily to hypovolemia. Afterload is also increased due to a marked increase in systemic vascular resistance (SVR) from vasoactive mediators such as catecholamines. Systemic hypertension is seen in about 10 percent of burn patients due to this mediator response. A decrease in cardiac contractility from a circulating myocardial depressant factor has been reported, but the factor has yet to be identified. A decrease in cardiac contractility is most evident in third-degree burns in excess of 40 percent of TBS and is probably due to myocardial edema rather than to a circulating factor. Positive-pressure ventilation frequently required in the early postburn period may further decrease perfusion. As a result of the increased heart rate typically present, cardiac output is usually restored toward normal well before a normal plasma volume is restored. The CVP and pulmonary artery wedge pressure (PAWP) usually remain low even when cardiac output and perfusion are adequate. All of these contributors to impaired perfusion are summarized in Fig. 68-3.

TREATMENT

INTRAVENOUS ACCESS

A peripheral vein catheter through nonburn tissue is the route preferred for fluid administration. A central line or pulmonary artery line, preferably through nonburned tissue, is only occasionally needed to monitor the patient during the initial resuscitation period and is removed as soon as it is no longer needed.

Monitoring lines are required primarily for the elderly patient or the patient with severe heart disease. An extremely high complication rate has been reported with central catheters in burn patients as a result of infection and embolic episodes related to the hypercoagulable state. Because of the high infection rate, an intravenous catheter should not be placed through burn tissue unless no other possible route exists. Central line sites (when not dedicated to total parenteral nutrition) should be rotated every 3 days to minimize the risks of catheter sepsis.

WHAT TO MONITOR

No one parameter of perfusion in the burn patient can be considered to be a completely reliable indicator of tissue oxygenation (perfusion) and, therefore, several standard hemodynamic monitors and laboratory tests should be used.

Base-line body weight is used to help estimate the initial fluid infusion rate (via various formulas). The preburn weight (if available) should be used for assessing nutrition needs and drug dosage.

The increased sympathetic tone characteristic of this early period makes arterial pressure an insensitive measure of volume status. However, a minimum perfusion pressure, for example, a mean arterial pressure of >85 mmHg must be maintained.

Tachycardia is inevitable due to hypovolemia and catechol release. The degree of tachycardia can be useful for determining adequacy of volume replacement. Exceptions are elderly patients or those with preexisting heart disease in whom the heart rate cannot increase in proportion to the stimulus. In most patients, a pulse <120 usually indicates adequate volume, while a pulse >130 usually indicates that more fluid is needed. Arrhythmias are uncommon in the young patient as long as oxygenation is adequate, but become a major concern in the older patient.

Renal blood flow is another reflection of the adequacy of systemic perfusion during this early phase of injury. A urine output of 0.5 to 1 mL/kg/h normally reflects adequate renal blood flow assuming there are no factors such as hyperglycemia, mannitol, or alcohol to alter the relationship between renal perfusion and urine output. A value <0.5 mL/kg/h indicates renal hypoperfusion, unless an acute renal insult has also occurred or there is inappropriate renal sodium and water retention (as for example with the syndrome of inappropriate antidiuretic hormone [SIADH]). A value >1.0 mL/kg/h usually means that too much fluid is being given and therefore, that excess edema is being produced. Because of the need for continuous assessment of urine output, an indwelling urinary catheter is necessary for burns in excess of 30 percent TBS or in smaller burns with other complicating factors.

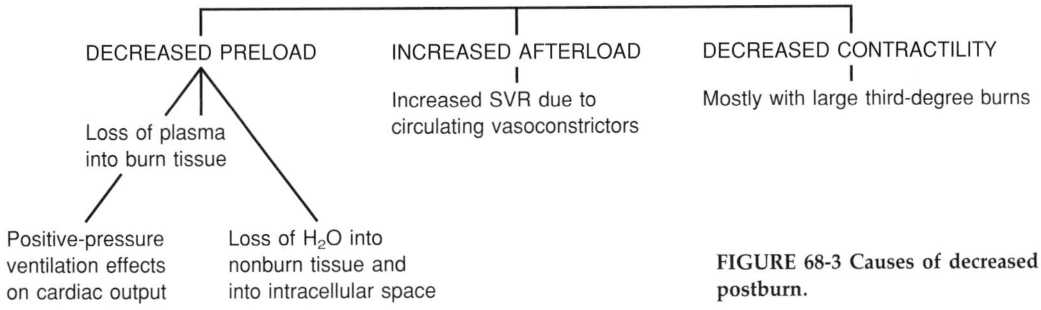

FIGURE 68-3 Causes of decreased oxygen delivery to tissues postburn.

The measurement of pH is extremely useful for the assessment of tissue oxygenation. A base deficit during this phase usually reflects impaired tissue oxygenation due to hypovolemia or carbon monoxide (or cyanide) toxicity. If an arterial line cannot be placed safely, a pulse oximeter can be used for assessment of arterial saturation, complemented by measurement of venous pH and P_{CO_2}.

The burn patient is very prone to hypothermia during this early period, especially with infusion of cool fluids. A decrease in temperature will lead to further hemodynamic instability and impaired perfusion. The external environment must be altered to allow for maintenance of a normal temperature for this period (which is 37 to 37.5°C, 98.6 to 99.9°F). At a later phase, a higher core temperature will be required.

The CVP in the large burn at his stage is usually low (0 to 5 cm H_2O), even with adequate fluid resuscitation. This fact is understandable if one remembers that the burn-injured circulation is acting like a sieve. The rate of fluid loss is markedly accentuated by any increase in capillary pressure. Therefore, it can be very dangerous to use an arbitrary value of CVP as an end point of resuscitation.

Most young patients, even with massive burns, do not require pulmonary artery catheterization for initial resuscitation. Hypoperfusion is almost always due to hypovolemia. In this population, the risks of a pulmonary artery line may well exceed its benefits in assessing adequacy of perfusion. As with the CVP, PAWP is usually 6 to 10 mmHg even when adequate perfusion is present. Some patients can benefit from invasive measurement of hemodynamics. These include elderly patients and patients with burn and smoke inhalation not responding to what appears to be adequate fluids.

A cardiac index of about 2.5 L/min/m^2 is normal for a noninjured person. However, injured tissue requires greater oxygen delivery. In this setting, even a normal measured cardiac index does not guarantee that tissue oxygen needs are met. The mixed venous P_{O_2}, however, can greatly assist in this determination (described in Chap. 114).

CHOICE OF RESUSCITATION FLUID

In general, fluids which contain at least as much salt as is contained in plasma are appropriate for use in resuscitation. Restoration of sodium lost into the burn is essential. Fluids should be free of glucose (except in small children), since glucose intolerance is characteristically present. The oral route can be used for small burns, but intestinal ileus occurs after deep burns in excess of 20 percent TBS. A number of salt-containing intravenous fluids are used, including colloids, to minimize edema in nonburned tissues and maintain a better blood volume.

Blood volume in severe burns can remain decreased for days in view of the ongoing fluid and protein losses. Even with massive fluid replacement, blood hematocrit of over 50 is not uncommon in the early postburn period. Blood volume can be more effectively restored once the leak begins to slow up at about 24 to 36 h. An overzealous attempt at restoring blood volume over and above that necessary for adequate perfusion can markedly accentuate edema-related complications.

CRYSTALLOID (ISOTONIC, HYPERTONIC) Crystalloid, in particular lactated Ringer's solution, is the most popular resuscitation fluid in the United States. Isotonic crystalloid, if given in large enough amounts, can restore cardiac output toward normal in most patients, the exceptions being at the extremes of age and in massive burns. Lactated Ringer's is preferred to normal saline because it more closely matches extracellular fluid. The amount of isotonic crystalloid required in the first 24 h is adjusted based on the parameters used to monitor the adequacy of resuscitation (vide infra).

Since sodium appears to be the key element in crystalloid infusion, solutions with increased sodium concentration have a theoretical advantage in that less water is infused. The hypertonic salt solutions used clinically have a milliosmolar content of 400 to 600 (280 to 300 mO is isotonic), thereby transiently generating potential osmotic pressures of several thousand mmHg in excess of normal until an isosmolar state is produced. This equilibrium occurs as the extracellular space is expanded by a shift of intracellular water. The current practice is to use a solution with a sodium content of approximately 240 meq/L by adding 2 ampules sodium lactate to each liter normal saline. The serum sodium level should not be allowed to exceed 160 meq/L.[17] A more isotonic solution should be instituted once a hyperosmolar state develops. Complications of the use of this solution relate primarily to those of the hyperosmolar state which occurs if too much salt is given.

COLLOIDS (PROTEIN, NONPROTEIN). Since nonburned tissue appears to regain normal permeability very shortly after injury and since hypoproteinemia may accentuate the nonburn edema, protein restoration beginning at about 8 to 12 h seems appropriate if edema in noninjured tissue and total fluid requirements are to be minimized. The use of fresh frozen plasma should be reserved for correction of documented clotting abnormalities. A 6% albumin solution replaces only the albumin losses. The amount of 6% albumin to be infused remains undefined. Many investigators have arbitrarily used between 0.5 and 1 mL/kg/% burn during the first 24 h. The amount depends on the magnitude of injury and the degree of hemodynamic instability. The protein should be infused at a constant rate over time rather than pulsed since the pulsed approach will transiently increase pressure and increase the rate of edema formation.

Nonprotein colloids are advantageous if colloids are required early to maintain hemodynamic stability since the more expensive protein is lost into the burn. Hetastarch, a 6% starch solution, has colloid properties similar to those of a 6% protein solution and generates an oncotic pressure comparable to that of protein. The molecules are much larger than those of most dextrans and vascular clearance is, therefore, much slower. As with dextran, volumes exceeding several liters can lead to clotting abnormalities and to the potential for immune dysfunction from reticuloendothelial blockade.

BLOOD. Because there is no early red blood cell deficit with a burn alone (unless severe hemolysis occurs), blood replacement is usually not needed. Occasionally however, blood can be a useful volume expander to restore cardiac output if perfusion is not adequately maintained by other fluids, especially if the patient has lost red blood cells, for example, from escharotomies or from hemolysis, in the early postburn period.

RATE OF INFUSION

Rate of fluid administration depends on the rate of loss, which is assessed by the perfusion monitors. An initial rate can be estimated using the size of the burn (combined second-degree and third-degree) relative to TBS and body weight.

$$\text{24 h volume} = 4\ \text{mL} \times \%\ \text{burn} \times \text{weight (kg)}(\tfrac{1}{2}\ \text{in first 8 h}) \quad (68\text{-}1)$$

However, the amount of fluid required is that necessary to maintain perfusion. Any formula is only an initial guide. If shock is present on admission, a bolus of fluid should be given (colloid is more effective than crystalloid). After perfusion is restored, fluid, usually isotonic crystalloid, should be infused at a relatively constant rate over a several hour period, making small changes to maintain perfusion. Once shock is corrected, boluses are disadvantageous since these transiently increase pressure and increase the rate of loss into the burn. Approximately half of the first 24 h requirements will need to be given in the first 8 h. Once a fluid infusion rate is reached which produces adequate perfusion, only modest hourly changes should be made so as to avoid large fluctuation in hemodynamic stability. Beginning at 8 to 10 h, an attempt should be made to gradually decrease the rate to that which is the least amount necessary to maintain adequate perfusion.

INDICATIONS FOR INOTROPIC SUPPORT

Inotropic support to supplement fluids is indicated if adequate perfusion cannot be maintained without excessive fluid administration. In contrast to the nonburned patient, it is very difficult to increase preload to values above normal levels in order to increase cardiac output. This maneuver may simply lead to a marked accentuation in tissue edema which, in turn, can further impair perfusion. Poor cardiac output is most commonly seen in the elderly burn patient or the patient with smoke inhalation who requires increasing positive pressure. Since improved renal blood flow is a major goal, low dose dopamine (1 to 3 μg/kg/min) is often useful. If an inotrope is needed, dopamine or dobutamine, depending on the hemodynamic status, is the agent of choice. Digoxin is not recommended in the immediate postburn period since the rapid fluid shifts can lead to digitalis toxicity. Hemodynamic management is summarized in Fig. 68-4.

Hematologic Changes

A number of hematologic disorders are seen after major burns.[18,19] Hemolysis commonly occurs after deep third-degree burns or any prolonged exposure to a heat source, as evidenced by free plasma hemoglobin and hemoglobinuria. In addition, red blood cell fragility is markedly in-

Large bore peripheral IVs
Begin lactated Ringer's; estimate initial rate according to % TBS and weight
Monitor: pulse, blood pressure, urine, ECG, temperature, electrolytes, CBC, I + O
Maintain: BP > 90 systolic, urine 0.5–1 mL/kg/h, pulse < 130, temperature 36–38°C (96.8–100.4°F)

MODIFY PROTOCOL WITH

MASSIVE BURNS, INHALATION INJURY, ELDERLY, SHOCK

MONITORING
1. Add arterial line if BP cannot be adequately monitored, if unstable or for access of blood gases
2. Pulse oximeter (ideal for O_2 saturation)
3. Pulmonary artery catheter:
   if preexistent heart disease is severe
   if hemodynamic instability persists and
   if inotrope is needed
4. Monitor cardiac output, PCWP, mixed venous P_{O_2}
5. Add BUN, creatinine, coagulation panel, plasma proteins

FLUID INFUSION TO INCLUDE:
1. Colloid or
2. Hypertonic lactated saline (for first 8–10 h)

CONSIDER
1. Inotrope if fluid alone not adequate (low dose dopamine first choice)
2. Vasodilator if severe systemic hypertension present (Nipride is best initial choice)

FIGURE 68-4 Treatment summary (0 to 24 h) for maintaining hemodynamic stability. All patients had burns > 20 percent TBS.

creased. Increased cell wall lipid peroxidation is evident, and fragmented cells are often seen on smear. The injured red cells will have a markedly shortened life span, leading to an anemia beginning in the first week. Red cell hemopoiesis is also markedly impaired and remains so until the burn is closed, resulting in a persistent anemia. A leukocytosis is also characteristic during this early phase. A marked consumption of platelets, fribrinogen, and plasminogen is seen in the burn wound as well as a marked depletion of hemostatic components. A hypercoagulable state can be seen in the initial period in moderate burn injuries. A hypocoagulable state, resulting from a depletion of clotting factors, is frequently seen with massive burns. Thrombocytopenia will be evident in this latter group as well. This is most likely the result of the tremendous stimulus to clotting from the large area of injured collagen.

Management of the Burn Wound

The recognition of the magnitude of burn injury, which is dictated by its depth and size as well as the prior health of the host, is of crucial importance in the overall care plan. Decisions regarding wound management are based on this assessment. In addition, it is important to understand that the wound itself in this early period can rapidly evolve toward a deeper injury. The type of early care provided will have a major impact on the prognosis for healing and on morbidity and mortality.[20]

PATHOPHYSIOLOGY OF THE EARLY BURN WOUND CHANGES

ANATOMY AND FUNCTION OF THE SKIN

The skin is the largest organ of the body, ranging from 0.25 m^2 in the newborn to over 2 m^2 in the adult. It consists of two layers, epidermis and dermis (or corium). The outermost cells of the epidermis are dead cornified cells that act as a tough protective barrier against the environment. The second, thicker layer, the corium (0.06 to 0.12 mm) is composed chiefly of fibrous connective tissue. The dermis contains the blood vessels to the skin and the epithelial appendages of specialized function. The nerve endings that mediate pain are also found in the dermis. Partial-thickness injuries are extremely painful, because the nerve endings are exposed. Full-thickness burns are usually anesthetic due to heat destruction of the nerves.

The skin is also the barrier that prevents loss of body fluids through evaporation and limits the loss of body heat. Sweat glands help maintain body temperature by controlling the amount of heat lost by evaporation. Increased loss of water and heat through burned skin are the major pathophysiologic changes seen early postburn. In addition, the skin is the primary protective barrier against penetration of microorganisms into the subdermal tissues. Loss of this function results in increased risk of invasive infection. Another protection the skin provides is adaptation to changes in the physical environment initiated by the sensory nerve endings in the dermis which detect the sensation of touch, pressure, pain, cold, and heat. Loss of this function will lead to long-term impairment.

DEPTH OF BURN INJURY

Traditionally, burn depth has been classified in degrees of injury based on the amount of epidermis and dermis injured. At present, depth is estimated by physical appearance, pain, and skin texture or pliability. A number of noninvasive diagnostic techniques are being evaluated; however, none has replaced the accuracy of experienced clinical assessment. A *first-degree burn* involves only the thin outer epidermis and is characterized by erythema and mild discomfort. Tissue damage is minimal and protective functions of the skin are intact. Pain, the chief symptom, usually resolves in 48 to 72 h, and healing takes place uneventfully.

Second-degree burns are defined as those in which the entire epidermis and variable portions of the dermis are destroyed. A *superficial second-degree burn* involves heat injury to the upper third of the dermis. The microvessels perfusing this area are injured, and permeability is increased, resulting in the leakage of large amounts of plasma into the interstitium. This fluid lifts off the thin heat-destroyed epidermis, causing blister formation. Despite loss of the entire basal layer of the epidermis, a burn of this depth will heal in 7 to 14 days due to repopulation by the epithelial cells present in hair follicles, sweat glands, and other skin appendages anchored deeply in the dermis. Minimal scarring is expected to occur, if the burn does not increase in depth, because the wound inflammation which stimulates excessive collagen deposition is short-lived due to the rapid wound closure.

A *deep dermal (or deep second-degree) burn* extends well into the dermal layer, and fewer viable epidermal cells remain. Therefore, reepithelialization is extremely slow, sometimes requiring months. In these patients, blister formation does not characteristically occur since the dead tissue layer is sufficiently thick and adherent to underlying viable dermis that it is not readily lifted off the surface by the edema. The exceptions are very young or old patients with a thin dermis. The wound surface is usually red, with white areas in deeper parts. Only modest plasma surface leakage occurs because of the severe impairment in blood supply. Because the remaining blood supply is marginal, there is a high probability of deepening of the tissue damage with time. Dense scarring is usually seen if the wound is allowed to heal primarily rather than if it is excised and skin grafted.

A *full-thickness* or *third-degree burn* occurs with destruction of the entire epidermis and dermis, leaving no residual epidermal cells to repopulate. Therefore, this wound will not reepithelialize. The area of the wound not closed by wound contraction will require skin grafting. A characteristic appearance of the burn tissue is a waxy white color typical of any avascular tissue. If the burn extends into the fat or there is prolonged contact with a flame source, a leathery brown or black appearance can be seen along with coagulated veins, characterizing charred tissue. Full-thickness flame burns usually lead to immediate occlusion of the in-

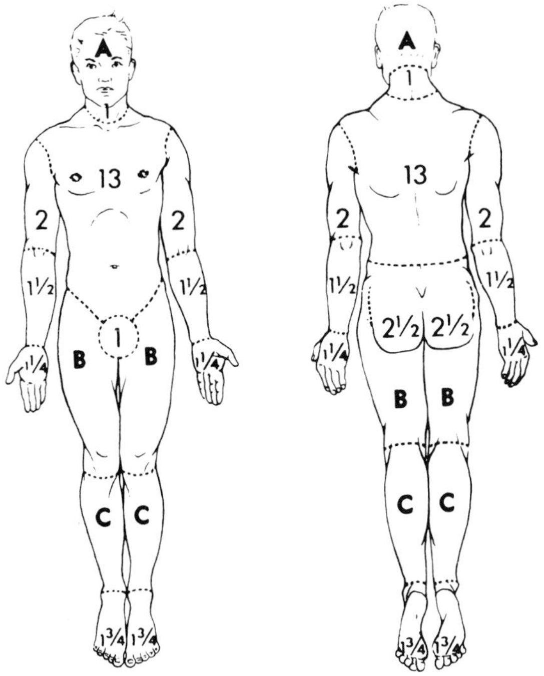

Relative Percentages of Areas Affected by Growth

Area	Age 10	Age 15	Age Adult
A = half of head	5½	4½	3½
B = half of one thigh	4¼	4½	4¾
C = half of one leg	3	3¼	3½

FIGURE 68-5 Lund and Brower method of calculating percent body burn.

TABLE 68-2 Data Obtained from Specialized Burn Facilities Mean Survival Rate (%) According to Age and Burn Size

% TBS BURN*	AGE (YRS) 0–1	2–4	5–34	35–49	50–59	60–74	>75
0–10	>95	>95	>95	>95	>95	95	90
10–20	95	>90	>95	>90	>85	80	50
20–30	90	90	95	90	75	50	25
30–40	75	80	90	80	60	30	<10
40–50	50	65	80	60	40	10	<5
50–60	40	50	60	45	30	<10	<5
60–70	20	30	40	20	15	<5	0
70–80	5	20	25	10	5	0	0
80–90	0	<10	10	<10	<5	0	0
90–100	0	<5	<5	<5	0	0	0

*Combined second-, third-degree

jured capillaries by thrombosis, as with electrocautery. The lack of any painful sensation is due to the heat destruction of the nerve endings. This characteristic can be used to distinguish a third-degree burn from a second-degree injury. The exact depth of many deep burns cannot be clearly defined on first appearance. A zone of ischemia is present beneath the dead superficial tissue and above the deeper living tissue. Whereas some vessels to this area are thrombosed, others are patent but have endothelial damage. This marginally viable tissue can be readily converted to nonviable tissue by a further decrease in blood flow caused by local mediator release or infection. A deep second-degree or healable burn can therefore progress to a third-degree burn.

SEVERITY OF INJURY

The size of the burn is defined in terms of percent of TBS. A useful initial guide is the use of the *rule of nines* where the body is divided into areas each with 9 percent of TBS. The head and each arm are considered 9 percent of the total while the chest and abdomen, the back and each lower extremity are considered to be 18 percent of TBS. However, the Lund and Browder chart (Fig. 68-5) is more accurate and should be used for more precise calculation. The surface area of the body involved, the depth and location of injury, the patient's age, and the presence of associated injuries determine morbidity and mortality.[20] Age and presence of associated injury appear to be the most significant parameters dictating survival (Table 68-2).

Survival statistics are best for patients 10 to 30 years old whose burns are not complicated by smoke inhalation injury, since the latter markedly increases mortality. Age is a major factor in survival, with increased mortality seen in children under 2 and adults over 50.

TREATMENT

The initial management of the burn wound is based on a knowledge of the skin anatomy and of functional losses with injury. The major objectives are to decrease the potential for further local damage and to decrease the systemic abnormalities which can be produced by the loss of the barrier function. The early treatment, therefore, focuses on neutralizing the source of burn injury, avoiding excess heat loss, determining the extent of injury, cleaning and debriding the wound, controlling infection, and maintaining tissue perfusion.

NEUTRALIZING THE SOURCE OF BURN INJURY

With a flame or scald burn, the clothing can retain heat for considerable periods of time. Rapid removal of burned clothing is, therefore, essential. Cooling the burn wound has a number of advantages. First, immediate cooling will help neutralize retained heat, decreasing injury. Cooling also appears to stabilize skin mast cells, which decreases histamine release and resulting edema. Cooling must be applied within seconds to minutes of the burn to obtain these gains. Cooling also decreases pain from the irritated nerve endings of a partial-thickness burn. This improvement can be seen anytime in the first several hours after injury. Deeper burns are relatively anesthetic and therefore do not need cooling.

However, cooling has a number of major disadvantages as well. First, cooling will increase body heat loss through the burn wound. A decrease in body temperature is deleterious in that the initial shivering, which invariably occurs, produces a marked increase in oxygen consumption and calorie demands at a time when oxygen delivery is compromised.[21] Hypothermia can result from severe heat loss and lead to shock. Rewarming is extremely difficult after a burn not only because of hypovolemia but also because of the inability of burned skin to vasoconstrict and minimize continued losses. Also, available glycogen stores can be exhausted during shivering. The rate of loss of body heat in water (wet dressings or hydrotherapy) is 25 times greater than in air. Wet burn dressings accentuate bacterial migration from environment to wound. Finally, local cooling will decrease skin blood flow. Ice directly applied to the wound will produce further tissue injury similar to that seen with frostbite. Cooling is therefore only used for initial heat neutralization and to control pain in superficial second-degree burns <15 percent of TBS.

TABLE 68-3 Standard Burn Categorization

CRITICAL BURNS
1. Second-degree burns involving >30% TBS
2. Third-degree burns involving >10% TBS
3. Burns complicated by respiratory tract injury or fractures or involving critical areas such as face, hands, feet, perineum
4. High voltage electrical burns
5. Lesser burns in patients with significant preexisting disease
MODERATE BURNS
1. Second-degree burns involving 15–30% TBS
2. Third-degree burns involving 2–10% TBS
3. Areas above not involving face, hands, feet, perineum
MINOR BURNS
1. Second degree burn <15% TBS
2. Third-degree burns <2% TBS

AVOIDING EXCESS HEAT LOSS

With a deep burn the barrier to evaporative water loss is markedly impaired. This also means impairment of the barrier to heat loss, a fact extremely important to recognize in the resuscitation period. Heat loss can be decreased by closing the wound under dressings, thereby limiting the air movement and decreasing the air-to-wound temperature gradient.

The major burn patient must be placed in a warmed external environment to minimize heat loss. Wound debridement and washing should not be initiated on a large burn until the external temperature is controlled. Once the heat source has been neutralized and the depth and extent of injury determined, wounds should be covered with dry dressings until the problem of external heat loss can be controlled. Burns of a magnitude which will lead to this problem should be transferred to a burn facility where more definitive wound care in a controlled environment can be provided.

DETERMINING THE EXTENT OF INJURY

The depth and extent of injury can be determined using the characteristics previously described. However, exact determination will require cleaning of the wound and some debridement of nonviable epidermis. The wound can be categorized based on size, depth, age, and other complicating factors. Table 68-3 presents the standard categorization used by the American Burn Association.

CLEANING AND DEBRIDING THE WOUND

The management of the burn wound itself depends on the status of initial cardiopulmonary function. Adequate control of the airway, gas exchange, and restoration of fluid loss must precede attempts at wound cleaning and debridement. The optimum environment for cleaning of the major burn is not the emergency room where temperature control and aseptic technique are difficult to maintain. The superficial second-degree burn is the most painful and will require analgesics before any cleaning can be performed. The burn-induced sympathetic discharge, as well as hypovolemia with large burns, will produce a relative decrease in skin and muscle blood flow. Intramuscular narcotics are contraindicated because of erratic absorption, except in minor burns. Intravenous narcotics are indicated because of greater safety and better pain control.

The solution used to clean the burn should be nontoxic yet effective against the organisms present. Chlorhexidine diluted in sterile saline or water is the most commonly used agent. Loose tissue, broken blisters, and dirt should be gently removed since they all add to subsequent infection risk. It is important to wash and gently mechanically debride the wound not only to remove loose devitalized tissue but also to determine the true depth of the burn. Initial assessment prior to cleaning may be very inaccurate.

CONTROLLING INFECTION

Once the wound is initially debrided, control of potential infection in the injured tissue is the next priority. Tetanus prophylaxis is necessary.

SYSTEMIC ANTIBIOTICS. Numerous studies have demonstrated that prophylactic systemic antibiotics in either the minor or major burn are of no benefit in decreasing the rate of wound infection.[22] The relatively avascular deep burn will not receive a sufficient blood supply to provide adequate tissue antibiotic levels. In addition, any open wound will become colonized with bacteria. The only exception is the use of low dose penicillin for protection against β-hemolytic streptococcus, particularly if the patient is at high risk for this organism (a known carrier or has had recent exposure).

TOPICAL ANTIBIOTICS. The recommendation for the use of topical antibiotics is based on the fact that nonviable tissue is present and will act as a nidus for infection and on the lack of effectiveness of systemic antibiotics. The specific types and use of topical antibiotics is discussed more fully in Chap. 70.

1. Assure adequate ventilation and perfusion
2. Remove heat source and any constricting items
3. Cool water for small second degree burns only
4. Assess depth and size—"rule of nines"
5. Tetanus prophylaxis

PATIENT NOT STABLE

1. Remove clothing
2. Cover with warm dry dressing
3. Wait until ABC's controlled to initiate aggressive wound care
4. Do not put in hydrotherapy tank or move away from adequate monitoring

PATIENT REASONABLY STABLE

1. Maintain warm external temperature during wound cleaning
2. Use adequate pain control (small doses IV narcotics for major burn)
3. Chlorhexidine wash: dilute contents of one packet in 1–2 quarts warm (85–90°F, 29.4–32.2°C) H_2O
4. Remove dirt, loose skin
   May leave large blisters intact

SUPERFICIAL SECOND-DEGREE BURN

WOUND RELATIVELY CLEAN

1. Can use petrolatum gauze with dressing
2. Consider temporary skin substitutes: biobrane
3. Elevate burned extremity: bacitracin
4. Perineum, feet: use Silvadene

WOUND DIRTY

1. Use topical antibiotic: Silvadene 1st choice
2. Elevate burned extremity

DEEP BURN

1. Use topical antibiotic cream: Silvadene 1st choice
2. Closed dressing technique exception: face, perineum
3. Monitor perfusion to distal extremity

THIRD-DEGREE BURN

1. Use topical antibiotic cream Silvadene: if wound not grossly infected; Sulfamylon for small to moderate size infected burn
2. Parenteral antibiotics if infected, not for prophylaxis
3. Closed dressing technique except: face, perineum
4. Monitor perfusion: may need escharotomy

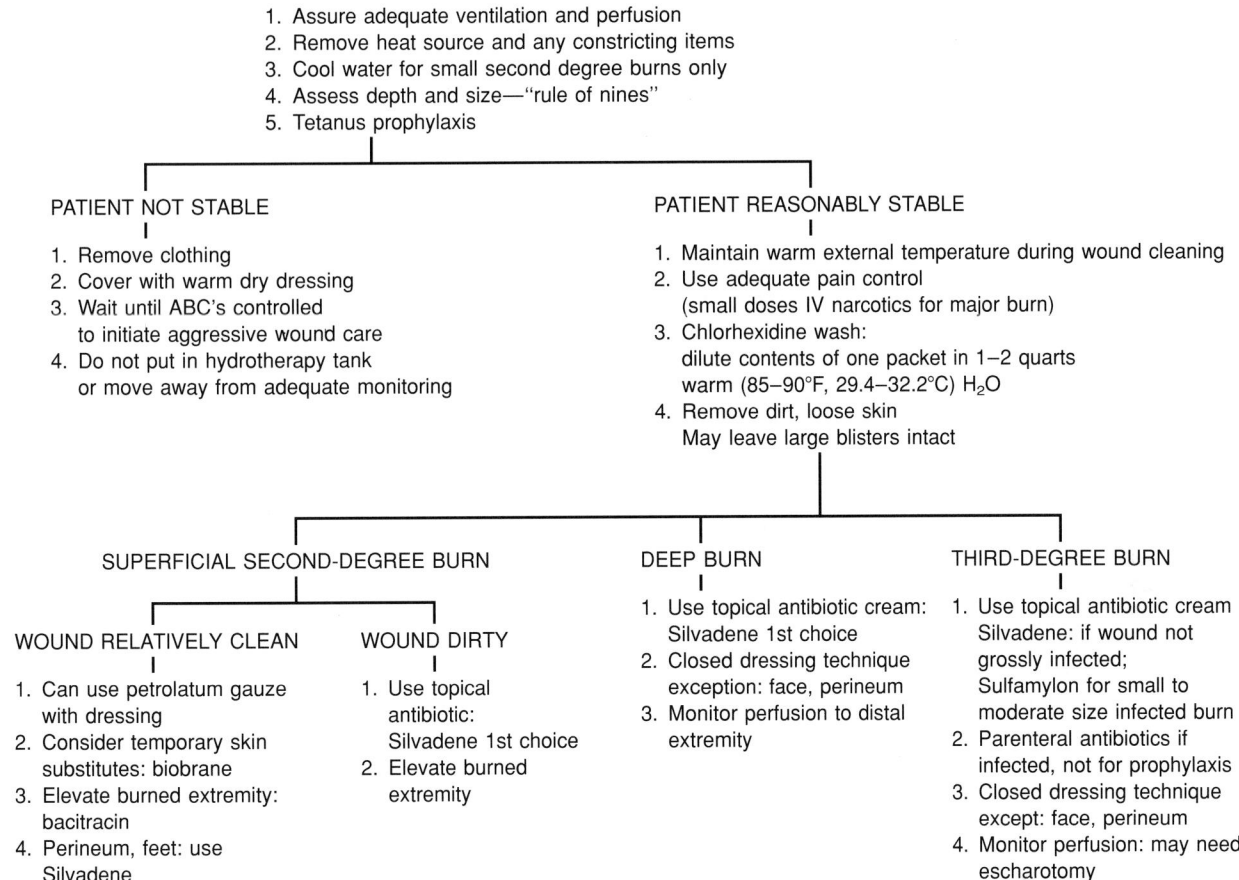

FIGURE 68-6 Treatment summary (0 to 24 h). Wound management.

IMPAIRED DISTAL PERFUSION AND NEED FOR ESCHAROTOMY

As subeschar edema develops under the burn tissue, pressure increases. This is of particular concern in extremities with a circumferential burn where the increasing pressure cannot be dissipated by expansion of neighboring tissue. The pressure initially impedes venous return which produces an increase in capillary hydrostatic pressure. Increased capillary pressure markedly accentuates further edema production, raising tissue pressure to a level which then impedes arterial blood flow. Injury to local lymphatics and veins impairs clearance of the edema fluid once it is formed.

Perfusion to the distal extremity must be closely monitored. Pain and color are unreliable indicators of perfusion in the presence of a burn. A warm extremity invariably indicates good flow during this period but cool skin does not always indicate that the problem is due to proximal burn constriction. Hypovolemia may well be the problem. The monitoring of distal pulsatile flow initially by palpation and then by the use of a Doppler flowmeter is the most practical manner of assessment. Tissue pressure measurements using a small needle, similar to the method of measuring subfascial compartment pressure, can be obtained. This approach, however, carries the risk of infecting the subeschar space with surface bacteria and is not used routinely. A tissue pressure exceeding 25 to 30 mmHg indicates the need for escharotomy since this pressure exceeds capillary hydrostatic pressure. Decreasing distal flow with a proximal deep burn is also an indication for an escharotomy. The incision is usually placed both medially and laterally on the involved extremity and must extend completely through the nonviable tissue to subcutaneous tissue in order to relieve the underlying tissue pressure. Wound management is summarized in Fig. 68-6.

CASE PRESENTATION

W.O., a 28-year-old male, was involved in a chemical plant explosion and fire in January 1989. He crawled from the building, where he was found by firefighters. He was transferred to a local emergency room, intubated, then quickly evacuated by helicopter to a referral center. Upon admission to the burn center, he was noted to be obtunded and in respiratory distress, being very difficult to bag ventilate with a peak inspiratory pressure (PIP) of 60 cmH_2O on a 10 mL/kg tidal volume when placed on a ventilator. A #6 endotracheal tube was in place. Vital signs included a blood pressure of 80/50, pulse of 140, body temperature <31.6°C (89°F), and weight was 70 kg. Initial blood gases, corrected for temperature on a fraction inspired oxygen ($F_{I_{O_2}}$) of 1.0, revealed a Pa_{O_2} of 65 mmHg, Pa_{CO_2} of 35, pH of 7.18, and carboxyhemoglobin <5 percent. The burn was estimated to involve 60 percent TBS.

The primary initial concerns were airway maintenance and ventilation. A suction catheter could not be passed down the small tube, and visualization of the cords via direct laryngoscopy was not possible due to massive oral edema. Thus, changing the tube, even over a bronchoscope, was not considered safe. In addition, no breath sounds were heard on the right side. Percussion to demonstrate hyperresonance was not conclusive. A chest film was taken immediately and a bedside cricothyroidotomy performed for placement of a #8 tracheal tube. The foreshortening of the neck from thick eschar and edema made a standard tracheostomy not feasible. Airway resistance decreased with PIP decreasing to 45 cmH_2O. However, breath sounds on the right remained diminished, and a right chest tube was therefore placed immediately with return of breath sounds. Initial chest x-ray, now available, revealed a tension pneumothorax and metallic fragments in the lung. Because of circumferential burns, a standard chest wall escharotomy was also performed. The PIP on 10 mL/kg TV now decreased to 30 cmH_2O, and 5 cmH_2O of PEEP was added. Blood-gas values improved.

A femoral artery line was placed since radial pulses were absent. It revealed a BP of 90/60 and pulse of 140. A urinary catheter was placed with an initial removal of 100 mL clear urine, followed by red-colored urine, at a rate projected to be 15 mL for the first hour. Because of the severe hypothermia, the adequacy of volume resuscitation was more difficult to determine. Therefore, a pulmonary artery catheter was placed via the internal jugular vein on the side of the chest tube. Initial PCWP was 16 mmHg, and cardiac index was 2 L/min/m^2. Fluids were warmed and initially set at a liter of lactated Ringer's per hour (4 mL × 70 kg × 60% TBS × $\frac{1}{2}$ per first 8 h ÷ 8 h = 1000 mL/h) with as much additional 6% albumin as needed to maintain a wedge of 14 to 16 mmHg. Low dose dopamine was also begun. Overhead and additional radiant heaters were used and the patient's burns were kept covered with dry dressings until temperature and hemodynamic stability were restored. No wound care was initiated except for bilateral arm escharotomies, after which radial pulses returned.

Over the next 8 h, body temperature was restored, the metabolic acidosis resolved and urine output was maintained at 0.5 to 1 mL/kg/h. Urine and plasma pigment, which was hemoglobin rather than myoglobin, cleared. Lung function was improved compared to admission but remained severely impaired with Pa_{O_2} of 90 mmHg on an $F_{I_{O_2}}$ of 0.7. Increasing PEEP to 7.5 resulted in improvement. Pa_{CO_2} remained at 40 mmHg with a minute ventilation of 10 L. C_{DYN} remained at 30 mL/cmH_2O and C_{STAT} at 40 mL/cmH_2O. An airway injury from smoke inhalation was evident, and an aerosolized bronchodilator was added. Heart rate was too rapid to initiate aminophylline.

As the patient stabilized, extreme agitation was evident, especially with wound management, which impaired ventilation. The patient was placed on a midazolam and fentanyl continuous infusion of 1 mg and 50 μg/h, respectively. After temperature was restored from muscle heat generation, a nondepolarizing paralytic agent was used as needed. A strong history of alcoholism was obtained with initial alcohol levels also being elevated. Thiamine and tetanus toxoid were given. Wounds were covered with silver sulfadiazine and Cefazolin (1 g every 6 h) was started not for the burns but because of the vascular and chest tube catheters placed through burn tissue. Coagulation tests at 12 h revealed a prothrombin time of 18 s (control 14), partial thromboplastin time of 60 (normal < 30 s), and a platelet count of 60,000. Fibrin split products were not increased.

CASE DISCUSSION

The burn patient is a trauma patient first since traumatic injuries are usually more immediately life-threatening than the burn itself. In this case, a shrapnel-induced tension pneumothorax was present, which was missed on initial assessment since there were many other reasons for respiratory problems. Airway maintenance is of critical concern. Since massive edema will soon develop with deep facial burns, the first tube has to be big enough to ventilate and clear secretions because changing the tube even within 4 to 6 h is often impossible. Decreased compliance caused by lung injury or by a noncompliant chest wall cannot be easily distinguished. Chest wall escharotomy is indicated under these circumstances. Hypothermia is a major and often unappreciated problem to emergency room and transport personnel and rewarming is difficult in the absence of a skin barrier. The hypothermia accentuates the problem of perfusion restoration. Normally monitoring of filling pressures and cardiac index is not necessary in a young healthy male no matter how big the burn. However, hypothermia, inhalation injury, and a large burn together often necessitate more invasive monitoring until adequate perfusion is restored. Fluid formulas are not particularly helpful in this type of patient except as a beginning point. Colloid is used early if crystalloid alone and in large quantities (4 mL/kg/percent burn) is not adequate to maintain perfusion. Low dose dopamine will assist renal perfusion as in any other critically ill patient. Urine output can also be better maintained, especially in the presences of high antidiuretic hormone and aldosterone levels seen postburn. The wound is the least important component, except for the need for escharotomies and wound cleaning, and debridement should not be initiated until the ABCs (airway, breathing, circulation) and body temperature are under control. Finally, a consumptive coagulopathy is a typical finding in a burn of this size.

References

1. Demling RH: Medical progress: Burns. N Engl J Med 313:1389, 1985.
2. Demling RH: Improved survival after massive burns. J Trauma 23:179, 1983.
3. Cahalan M, Demling RH: Early respiratory abnormalities from smoke inhalation. JAMA 251:771, 1984.
4. Moylan J, Alexander G: Diagnosis and treatment of inhalation injury. World J Surg 2:185, 1978.
5. Head J: Inhalation injury in burns. Am J Surg 139:508, 1980.
6. Robinson W, Hudson L, Robertson H: Ventilation and perfusion alterations after smoke inhalation injury. Surgery 90:352, 1982.
7. Peitzman A, Shires T, Corben W, et al: Measurement of lung water in inhalation injury. Surgery 90:305, 1981.
8. Tranbaugh R, Elings V, Lewis F: Effect of inhalation injury on lung water accumulation. J Trauma 23:597, 1983.
9. Venus B, Matsuda T, Copiozo J: Prophylactic intubation and continuous positive airway pressure in the management of inhalation injury in burn victims. Crit Care Med 9:519, 1981.
10. Robinson W, Hudson L, Riem M, et al: Steroid therapy following isolated smoke injury. J Trauma 22:876, 1982.
11. Levine B, Petroff P, Slade L: Prospective trials of dexamethasone and aerosolized gentamycin in the treatment of inhalation injury in the burned patient. J Trauma 18:188, 1978.
12. Harms B, Bodai B, Demling RH: Microvascular fluid and protein flux in pulmonary and systemic circulations after thermal injury. Microvasc Res 23:77, 1982.
13. Jin L, LaLonde C, Demling RH: Lung dysfunction after thermal injury: Relationship to prostanoid and oxygen radical release. J Appl Physiol 61:103, 1986.
14. Demling RH: Fluid resuscitation after major burns. JAMA 250:1438, 1983.
15. Demling RH, LaLonde C: Early post burn lipid peroxidation: Effect of ibuprofen and allopurinol. Surgery 1990.
16. Arturson G: Microvascular permeability to macromolecules in thermal injury. Acta Physiol Scan 463:111, 1979.
17. Monafo W, Halverson J, Schechtman K: The role of concentrated salt solutions in the resuscitation of patients with severe burns. Surgery 95:129, 1984.
18. Peterson V, Robinson W: Hematologic changes in burn patients, in Boswick J (ed): *The Art and Science of Burn Care.* Rockville, MD, Aspen Publications, 1987.
19. Sasaki J, Cottam G, Baxter C: Lipid peroxidation following thermal injury. JBCR 4:251, 1983.
20. Feller I, Tholen D, Cornell RG: Improvements in burn care, 1965–1979. JAMA 244:2074, 1980.
21. Wilmore D, Mason A, Johnson D: Effect of ambient temperatures on heat production and heat loss in burn patients. J Appl Physiol 38:593, 1975.
22. Boxx W, Brand D, Acampara D: Effectiveness of prophylactic antibiotics in the treatment of burns. J Trauma 25:224, 1985.

Chapter 69

BURNS: POSTRESUSCITATION PHASE (DAY 2 TO DAY 6)

ROBERT DEMLING

KEY POINTS

- *Pulmonary problems must be controlled during this period to allow for an aggressive surgical excisional approach. Pulmonary toilet is of primary concern.*
- *Fluid management changes dramatically, to a strategy of replacing evaporative water losses.*
- *Postburn anemia will develop and necessitate increased blood transfusions.*
- *Monitoring must be primarily noninvasive, to avoid line sepsis.*
- *Nutritional support should begin now, using the parenteral route until full enteral alimentation is possible.*
- *Controlled surgical excisions should begin as soon as the patient is hemodynamically stable, to avoid having extensive burns still in place when entering the infection-inflammation phase.*

The early postresuscitation phase is a period of transition from the ebb, or shock, phase to the flow, or hypermetabolic, phase. Major cardiopulmonary and wound changes occur that substantially alter patient care from that given during resuscitation. In general, cardiopulmonary stability is optimal during this period, since wound inflammation and infection have not yet developed. However, cardiovascular changes will only get worse with the evolving hypermetabolism and sepsis, unless the wound is aggressively managed. The early wound excision and grafting approach is initiated during this period, because increased wound blood flow and infection have not yet peaked. Operative risks, especially blood loss and septicemia, are substantially less than after inflammation and infection develop. The exceptions to this rule are patients with severe smoke inhalation in whom major lung dysfunction is present, and patients who are hemodynamically unstable.

Pulmonary Abnormalities

There are five major abnormalities that impair pulmonary function during this period. These are **1.** continued upper airway obstruction; **2.** decreased chest wall compliance; **3.** tracheobronchitis; **4.** pulmonary edema; and **5.** surgery- (and anesthesia-) induced lung dysfunction. Recognition of these potential problems will allow preventive measures to be initiated before severe dysfunction results, avoiding what would otherwise be a major impediment to an aggressive surgical approach to the burn wound.

CONTINUED UPPER AIRWAY OBSTRUCTION

Upper airway and facial edema caused by the heat-induced tissue and mucosal damage begins to resolve between days 2 and 4 with superficial injuries. With full-thickness burns, however, this edema will resolve more slowly. Continued airway maintenance with an endotracheal tube may be required. Placement of the patient in the head-elevated position (30 to 45°) will allow faster resolution of edema.

The decision to extubate (see Fig. 69-1) is a difficult one, since there is no good test for determining the adequacy of airway patency. Laryngoscopy to determine the presence of cord edema is helpful, as is deflation of the cuff to determine if air moves around the tube. If air can pass around the tube, laryngeal edema has sufficiently resolved. However, the lack of an air leak may simply reflect the use of a large tube in a small trachea. Edema of the false cords and oropharynx, as well as external compression from a neck burn, can also impair the airway, even if minimal cord edema is present. Therefore, one must be prepared to reintubate, since no test of airway patency is foolproof. Even extubation over a bronchoscope is not totally reliable, since the supraglottic edematous tissue can be stented out of the way by the bronchoscope. Major airway problems can then develop when the tube is removed, usually over the ensuing hours rather than minutes, as the patient begins to fatigue from the added work of breathing.[1]

DECREASED CHEST WALL COMPLIANCE

The impaired compliance of the chest wall caused by deep burns is improved, but certainly not eliminated, by escharotomy. A significant impairment in compliance will persist as a result of the loss of elasticity in burn tissue. In addition, tissue edema itself remains for many days and impairs expansion and, in turn, decreases functional residual capacity (FRC) and vital capacity. Work of breathing and energy requirements will remain increased. This process is particularly relevant for operative procedures requiring general anesthesia. The effect of impaired chest wall compliance on hemodynamic function will be accentuated with the use of a general anesthetic.

Maintenance of a semi-erect position will assist in movement of edema away from the chest wall to more dependent tissues. Continued careful volume replacement will minimize further edema formation. Mechanical ventilation with positive pressure may be needed to help maintain FRC and minimize atelectasis, as well as to diminish oxygen demands during this period of impaired energy stores. Early excision of the full-thickness wound can improve chest wall motion by removing both edema and noncompliant tissue.

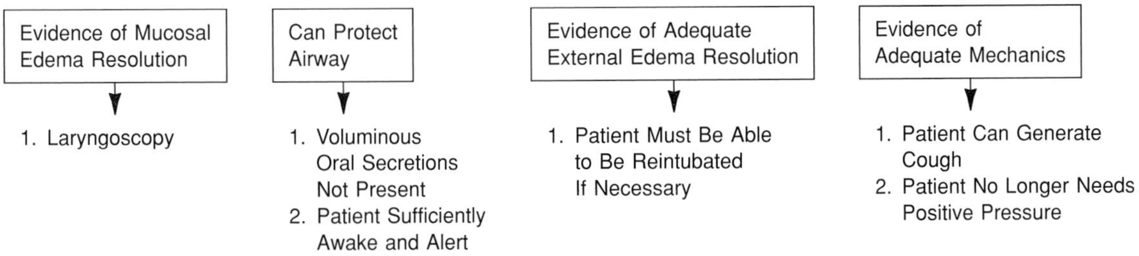
Evidence of Mucosal Edema Resolution
1. Laryngoscopy
Can Protect Airway
1. Voluminous Oral Secretions Not Present
2. Patient Sufficiently Awake and Alert
Evidence of Adequate External Edema Resolution
1. Patient Must Be Able to Be Reintubated If Necessary
Evidence of Adequate Mechanics
1. Patient Can Generate Cough
2. Patient No Longer Needs Positive Pressure

FIGURE 69-1 Criteria for deciding when to extubate a patient: all criteria should be met to ensure safe extubation.

TRACHEOBRONCHITIS FROM INHALATION INJURY

The chemical burn to the airways results in a spectrum of clinical manifestations during this period. At the very least, mucosal irritation will persist for several days and cause bronchorrhea, increased cough, and increased mucus production. The damaged ciliary function of the airways leads to a high risk for infection, manifested first (in the next 3 to 4 days) by a bacterial tracheobronchitis, which is often followed by bronchopneumonia. Bacterial colonization is inevitable. Characteristically with a severe injury, the damaged mucosa becomes necrotic 3 to 4 days after injury and begins to slough. Increased viscous secretions can lead to distal airway obstruction, atelectasis, and a high risk of a rapidly developing bronchopneumonia. If infection can be controlled and secretions cleared, the acute process will resolve over the next 7 to 10 days. However, the risk of infection persists for several weeks, extending well into the inflammation period. Clinical evidence of continued respiratory compromise, such as dyspnea, tachypnea, diffuse wheezing, and rhonchi, precedes x-ray changes. The more common radiologic abnormalities are diffuse atelectasis, pulmonary edema, or bronchopneumonia.[2] Repeated blood gas analysis and assessment of changes in sputum characteristics are the most useful parameters to monitor.

The clearance of soot, mucopurulent exudate, and sloughing mucosa is essential to avoid progression of the lung injury. An endotracheal tube may be necessary if clearance of secretions is inadequate. Mechanical ventilation may also be necessary if the patient fatigues or if gas exchange worsens. Bronchodilators, particularly those provided by aerosols, are also very helpful, along with frequent changes in position and chest physiotherapy. A continuously rotating bed is ideal for the patient with an inhalation injury and a large body burn in whom movement for pulmonary toilet is limited by pain and stiffness. The constant postural drainage assists in removing airway plugs.

Infection surveillance is crucial during this early period in order to detect bacterial bronchitis prior to development of pneumonia. Unlike typical bronchopneumonia presenting with a localized infiltrate, the entire tracheobroncheal tree becomes colonized with pathogens, and the resulting infection is often a diffuse bronchopneumonia. Sputum smears and monitoring of the character of the sputum are useful as early guides. However, as with any other form of nosocomial lung infection, the reliability of the sputum in reflecting infection and the organisms involved is fair at best. The issue of when to initiate antimicrobial therapy remains unresolved; waiting too long may lead to severe bilateral disease, while treating too soon can result in colonization with more virulent organisms. Systemic antibiotics are not given prophylactically, but are initiated when a bacterial tracheobronchitis becomes evident. It is not necessary to wait until there is obvious x-ray evidence of bronchopneumonia, since the process, once well established, will be difficult to reverse. Broad-spectrum antibiotics can be used until the specific sensitivities return and a more tailored antibiotic regimen can be instituted. This approach is summarized in Fig. 69-2.

PULMONARY EDEMA

The most common causes of pulmonary edema during this period are volume overload and progression of the chemi-

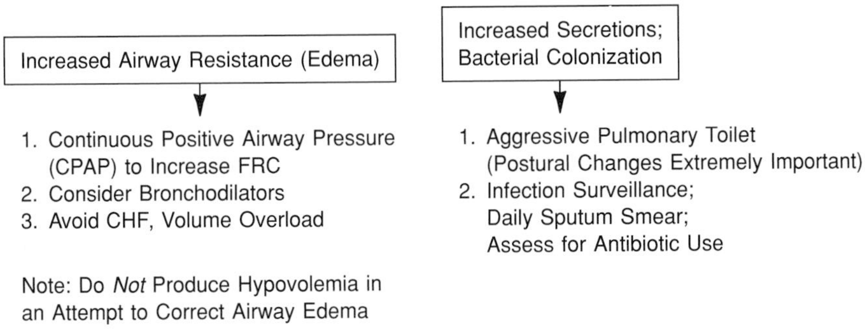
Increased Airway Resistance (Edema)
1. Continuous Positive Airway Pressure (CPAP) to Increase FRC
2. Consider Bronchodilators
3. Avoid CHF, Volume Overload
Note: Do Not Produce Hypovolemia in an Attempt to Correct Airway Edema
Increased Secretions; Bacterial Colonization
1. Aggressive Pulmonary Toilet (Postural Changes Extremely Important)
2. Infection Surveillance; Daily Sputum Smear; Assess for Antibiotic Use

FIGURE 69-2 Treatment of tracheobronchial injuries.

cal tracheobronchitis of a smoke inhalation injury. Volume overload is frequently due to a combination of systemic resorption of tissue edema at a rate faster than that which can be cleared by the kidney, and to a continued excess infusion of salt-containing fluid on the basis of an assumption that oliguria and tachycardia together indicate hypovolemia, when in fact heart failure may be the cause.

The usual clinical findings one expects to see with pulmonary edema may be relatively unreliable diagnostic clues. If an inhalation injury has occurred, increased secretions, rhonchi, and wheezing are already present, making the determination of added cardiogenic pulmonary edema difficult. Additional information, gained by way of using a pulmonary artery catheter for determination of pulmonary capillary wedge pressure, may be necessary.

If the patient is intubated, it is usually best to make appropriate adjustments in fluid infusion rate and protein replacement aimed at reducing the severity of the pulmonary edema while the patient is still being supported with positive pressure. Low-dose dopamine will assist in the diuresis by increasing renal blood flow and by its antialdosterone effects. The continued losses from the burn wound can result in a gradual decrease in blood volume. Therefore, vigorous diuresis is normally not needed to correct hypervolemia.

SURGERY– AND ANESTHESIA–INDUCED LUNG DYSFUNCTION

Repeated excision and grafting procedures, especially on large body burns, usually result in a situation in which the patient either is recovering from an inhalation anesthetic or is awaiting surgery. These patients often remain intubated between excision procedures if there is a concomitant inhalation injury and the burn is large. Most general anesthetics cause deterioration in an already marginal respiratory status and put the patient at further increased risk for pneumonia and respiratory failure during the subsequent phase of injury. Muscle relaxants further compound this problem. Ketamine anesthesia helps by decreasing the anesthesia-induced respiratory depression. Early recognition of hypoventilation in the early postanesthesia period is essential, and mechanical ventilation should be added early, to avoid the development of frank respiratory failure.[3] The treatment of lung dysfunction during this phase is summarized in Fig. 69-3.

Maintaining Hemodynamic Stability

PATHOPHYSIOLOGIC CHANGES IN THE POSTRESUSCITATION PERIOD

FLUID AND PROTEIN LOSSES

Edema in burned tissue is maximal between 24 and 30 h after injury in well-controlled fluid resuscitation. However, loss of skin integrity leads to continued losses of fluid, protein, and red cells. Evaporation from the surface of the burn becomes a major source of water loss that persists until the wound is closed. This loss is related to the water vapor pressure at the surface.[4,5] In normal skin the vapor pressure is 2 to 3 mmHg, while on a full-thickness burn where the eschar is soft and hydrated the pressure is about 32 mmHg. In addition, the rate of loss increases with sur-

Airway Maintenance

1. Maintain Artificial Airway Until Face and Neck Edema and Intraoral Have Adequately Resolved
2. Laryngoscopy or Bronchoscopy Prior to Tube Removal

Maintain Pulmonary Toilet

1. Do Not Underestimate Inhalation Injury
2. Avoid Airway Plugging from Inhalation Injury; Vigorous Cough, Suctioning, Broncho-
3. Aggressive Chest Physiotherapy
4. Avoid Nosocomial Pneumonia

Maintain Adequate Gas Exchange

1. Avoid Pulmonary Edema from Volume Overload
2. Aggressively Treat CHF (May Need Inotropes)
3. Avoid Hypoventilation (Especially Prevalent in Perioperative Period)
4. Consider Partial Mechanical Ventilation, Especially with Frequent Operative Interventions

Maintain Infection Control

1. Primary Therapy is Pulmonary Toilet
2. Initiate Antibiotics with Early Evidence of Bacterial Tracheobronchitis

FIGURE 69-3 Summary of treatment of pulmonary abnormalities from 36 h to 6 days after burn.

face blood flow. A reasonable estimate of loss can be obtained from the following formula:

$$\text{Evaporative water loss (mL/h)} = (25 + \%\ \text{burn}) \times (\text{m}^2\ \text{body surface area}) \quad (69\text{-}1)$$

Although edema usually peaks during the resuscitation period, the increase in vascular permeability persists for days after injury, until the basement membrane and endothelial integrity are restored. Increasing vascular hydrostatic pressure with hypervolemia, positive end-expiratory pressure (PEEP), or impaired venous return will accentuate the edema. Careful volume replacement, especially during operative procedures, is necessary to avoid magnifying the edema.

RED BLOOD CELL LOSSES

Red blood cell mass can decrease markedly during this period because of red blood cell breakdown and decreased production.[6] A large portion of the red blood cell mass is exposed to heat with a large flame burn, a long exposure to scald, or an electrical burn. In addition, many absorbed chemicals increase red cell fragility. Lipid peroxidation of the red cell membrane is well described after burn injury. The hematocrit characteristically falls to between 30 and 35, or lower, several days postburn. If there are additional external losses, or hemolysis is evident, the hematocrit will decrease more rapidly and to a greater degree. In addition, losses from escharotomies and blood drawing become more evident. Also, as plasma volume is restored over the next several days, the red cell distribution space increases and the hematocrit decreases. Besides increased red cell breakdown, there is decreased red cell production by the bone marrow—characteristic of any chronic injury state. Red cell production does not return to normal until after the wound is closed. Therefore, unlike transient blood loss in an otherwise healthy host, the decreased red cell mass will not correct itself.

FLUID GAINS

Intravascular fluid is gained during the postresuscitation period, from the absorption of edema. The rate of absorption is variable and depends on burn depth and subsequent lymphatic damage. While water can cross the endothelial barrier from interstitium to plasma, protein must be cleared by lymphatics. Edema resorption is much more rapid in superficial burns where lymphatics are intact, and begins at about day 2 or 3. Edema resorption is much slower after full-thickness injury, because of the lack of local lymphatics and venules. In addition, fibrin deposition in burn edema produces a gel that requires some fibrinolysis prior to resorption. Edema resorption can also be impaired by high central venous pressures, retarding venous and lymphatic return. However, a hypovolemic state will not accentuate fluid resorption from sequestered burn edema fluid. Increased muscle activity improves edema resorption by increasing venous return and lymphatic function. For all of these reasons, the magnitude of tissue edema is not a valid reflection of the circulating volume and should never be used to judge the rate of fluid replacement.

Real mechanisms are also important in the genesis of expanded intravascular fluid volume. Any impairment in renal perfusion impairs clearance of intravascular fluid. Heart failure, which is not uncommon in elderly patients, leads to further fluid gains. In addition, stress-induced antidiuretic hormone (ADH) and aldosterone release accentuate water and sodium resorption and potassium loss. Hyponatremia caused by infusion of hypotonic solutions increases sodium resorption. Hypernatremia, caused by infusion of isotonic solutions to replace hypotonic losses, will stimulate ADH release. Urinary potassium losses are usually very high.

SYSTEMIC METABOLIC AND HEMODYNAMIC CHANGES

The "ebb" phase, or hypometabolic phase, characteristic of the initial burn shock period begins to be transformed to the "flow" phase, or hypermetabolic state, over the next 3 to 5 days.[7,8] Patients are usually hemodynamically stable in the immediate postresuscitation period if adequate fluid has been infused during resuscitation. However, cardiac output usually begins to increase and to exceed normal values as a hyperdynamic state evolves. A modest-to-significant tachycardia (100 to 120 beats per minute) is usually seen, in part because of persistently elevated catecholamines from hypothermia, hypoxia, or pain. Systemic vascular resistance (SVR) begins to decrease. The vasodilation results in an increase in the capacity of the vascular space and, therefore, an increased need for colloid and red cells.

Surgical procedures are often performed during this period, since morbidity from early wound excision and closure is much less during the first week.[9,10] The repeated anesthetics, volume loss, and replacement make it very difficult to determine blood volume and hemodynamic stability.

Oxygen consumption usually peaks 5 to 7 days postburn.[7] The transition to the "flow" state also initiates an increase in body temperature, which increases further with burn wound pyrogen release. The characteristic increase in body temperature of 1 to 2°F makes it more difficult to diagnose infection. Patients with subclinical glucose intolerance (typically obese or elderly) may develop hyperglycemia, especially with a large burn. Increased catabolism leads to increased urea production, especially if inadequate glucose calories are being provided. This leads to difficulty in distinguishing a rise in blood urea nitrogen (BUN) due to renal dysfunction or hypovolemia from that due to catabolism.

The restoration of blood flow to the burn tissue results in the resorption of a large load of osmotically active solutes from disrupted cells and fragments of denatured proteins. This results in an obligate solute diuresis manifested by the increased output of high–specific gravity urine. This osmotic effect is very evident in second degree burn blisters, which increase in size and pressure over a period of days. An increase in urine output may be mistaken for fluid resorption and hypervolemia unless the specific gravity is followed carefully.

HEMODYNAMIC MANAGEMENT

Understanding the physiologic and metabolic changes during this period is the key to successful management. The major decisions relate to fluid therapy and the ongoing assessment of adequacy of perfusion.

TYPE OF FLUID

A common error is continued infusion of isotonic crystalloid during a period when major losses of sodium do not occur. A 5% glucose-containing solution with a low sodium content is the primary replacement fluid for evaporative and urinary losses during this period. Glycogen stores have been depleted and exogenous glucose is required, especially for the brain and red blood cells. The addition of 20 to 30 meq of potassium per L is usually necessary to match urinary potassium loss and intracellular shift of potassium (due to carbohydrate infusion). The high fluid requirements of large burns make it easier to give the needed calories and nitrogen. Sufficient volume to maintain adequate tissue oxygen transport to tissues is necessary. The rate of infusion requires frequent readjustment to compensate for fluid shifts. Even though evaporative losses are fairly constant, the rate of edema mobilization varies considerably. In addition, frequent surgical procedures with creation of new wounds (donor sites) and blood loss require frequent readjustment in volume replacement.

Hepatic albumin synthesis is markedly diminished in favor of acute-phase protein synthesis.[11] In order to restore blood volume and maintain the protein binding required for predictable pharmacokinetics, protein losses should be replaced. A serum albumin level of 2.5 g/dL is a reasonable goal. Infusion of albumin should be avoided while the patient is volume-overloaded.

It is also frequently necessary to replace red cells. The hematocrit should be kept at least in the low 30s to optimize delivery of oxygen to tissues. Preoperative maintenance of a reasonable hematocrit is essential for minimizing operative morbidity, since blood loss can occur very rapidly early in the procedure.

WHAT TO MONITOR

Assessment of the adequacy of perfusion, tissue oxygenation, and fluid and electrolyte balance can be difficult during this period of evolving hemodynamics. Oxygen consumption gradually increases with the transition from the "ebb" state to the "flow" state. The same parameters are monitored as before. However, interpretation of some of the specific physiologic values differs from that during initial resuscitation.

Urine output usually exceeds 0.5 mL/kg per h as edema fluid and solute load are mobilized, but may not reflect adequacy of perfusion due to the obligatory solute diuresis. Intake continues to exceed urine output for several days at least. However, the major output, constituted by wound surface and evaporative losses, cannot be accurately quantitated. As edema is mobilized, a gradual decrease toward, but not to, preburn body weight should be anticipated. Therefore, the absolute value of body weight cannot be used to reflect blood volume during this transition period. However, if weight is increasing, excess fluid (and salt) is probably being given. Arterial blood pressure becomes dependent on the effects of pain, elevated temperature, narcotics, and increasing metabolic rate. The heart rate initially decreases, as compared to that seen in the resuscitation phase. It then begins to increase again, as the "flow" phase evolves. One must also consider the effects of temperature, pain, etc. A rising hematocrit usually implies hemoconcentration and indicates hypovolemia. One should anticipate a gradual increase of 1 to 2°F over normal; this is due to hypermetabolism. Further increases are common with wound manipulation.

A central venous pressure greater than 15 mmHg indicates hypervolemia or impaired venous return—for example, from PEEP. A pulmonary capillary wedge pressure greater than 15 mmHg suggests the possibility of heart failure, hypervolemia, or PEEP. An increase in $\dot{V}O_2$ of between 50 and 100 percent of normal is expected by the end of this period. Since oxygen demands increase, a cardiac output that was adequate during resuscitation will now be insufficient. In a burn greater than 30 percent of total body surface (TBS), the cardiac output usually doubles.

PHARMACOLOGIC SUPPORT

Congestive heart failure is commonly seen in the fluid resorption period in elderly patients. Salt load and excessive release of ADH and aldosterone can impair water clearance as edema is resorbed. Low-dose dopamine (1 to 3 μg/kg per min) is a very effective agent to maintain renal perfusion and increase both sodium and water loss. It is very safe, with few complications at this dosage. In the setting of increased filling pressures and a catechol-induced tachycardia ("flow" phase), the inotrope of choice is usually dobutamine.

Diuretics may be helpful during this period if there is fluid retention and hypervolemia, but it is important to remember that the amount of tissue edema does not accurately reflect blood volume. Small quantities of a loop diuretic (e.g., 10 to 20 mg furosemide) will often initiate a controlled diuresis. Hemodynamic management is summarized in Fig. 69-4.

Care of the Burn Wound

The wound undergoes dramatic changes during this period as inflammation develops. In addition, wound colonization and the potential for wound infection increase. Of particular importance is the potential for change in the zone of ischemia—that tissue that is injured, but still viable, on admission. Changes in local wound microcirculatory blood flow, as a result of vasoactive inflammatory agents or local infection, can convert the zone of ischemia to a zone of necrosis. This process (called *wound conversion*) is most commonly seen in deep second degree burns and can occur even with optimum management. Processes such as wound dessication, hypovolemia, increased tissue pres-

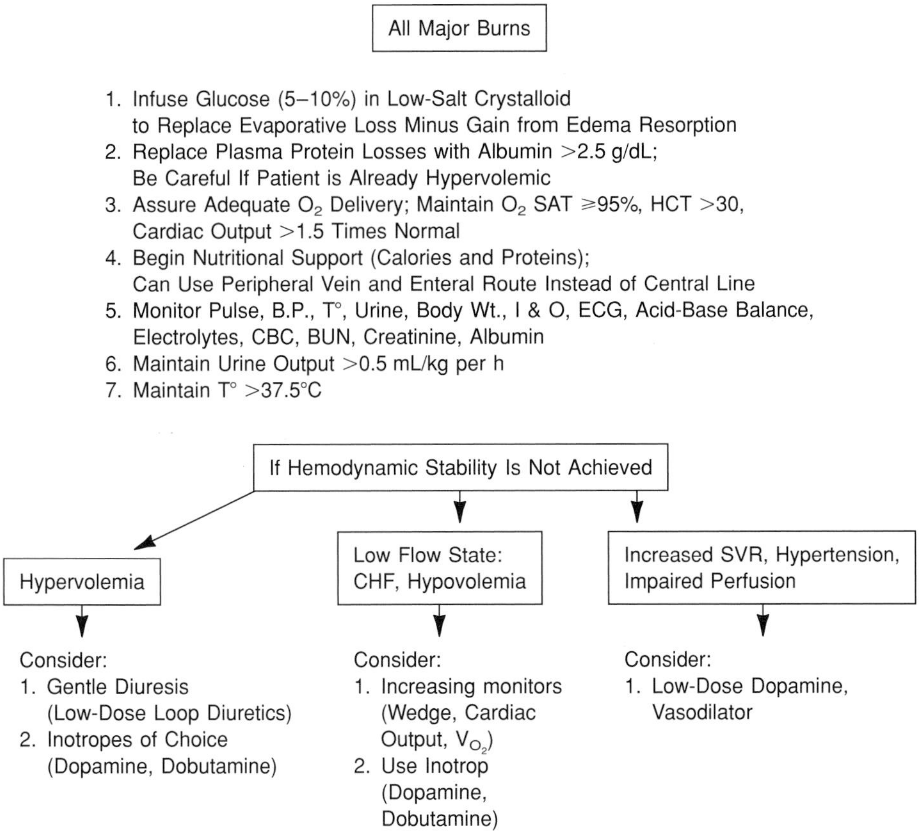

FIGURE 69-4 Maintenance of hemodynamic stability from 36 h to 6 days after burn.

sure, and hypothermia can all accentuate the potential for conversion. The most common cause, however, is local infection.

PATHOPHYSIOLOGIC CHANGES IN THE BURN WOUND

The relatively inert burn wound, as seen at 24 h, changes to a focus of intense inflammation at about 7 to 10 days in full-thickness burns and several days sooner in partial-thickness burns. The rate of onset of inflammation is dependent on the blood flow to the wound, with inflammation occurring more rapidly in more superficial burns. A marked increase in wound vascularity is seen beginning at about day 3 to day 5 in partial-thickness burns and at day 7 to day 10 in full-thickness burns. This neovascularization is initiated by, and essentially parallels, the degree of acute inflammation. Increased vascularity leads to an increasing release of inflammatory mediators. In addition, blood loss with wound debridement will be in direct proportion to the vascularity of the wound.

A deep burn develops a more prominent eschar during this period. The eschar is made up of nonviable upper dermis, initially adherent to the lower dermis; surface coagulated protein; and residue from topical antibiotics. The yellow-to-white adherent eschar can give the wound an appearance indistinguishable from that initially seen with a full-thickness injury.

The subeschar tissue changes dramatically as neutrophil infiltration (at 2 to 3 days) is followed by an intense macrophage infiltration. This turns the relatively inert tissues into an inflammatory focus, with peak inflammation usually occurring at about 7 to 10 days. White cell proteases begin to liquefy and macerate the eschar. Some bacterial colonization is usually evident in 2 to 3 days, but invasive wound infection is not common during the first week unless the initial wound was grossly contaminated and initial wound debridement and topical antibiotics were delayed. Conversion characteristically occurs during this period, as injured ischemic dermis becomes nonviable on account of local vasoconstriction or occlusion of dermal vessels.

In general, the inflammatory response is delayed in deep burns as compared to shallower ones, since the impaired blood flow limits inflammatory cell migration and hyperemia. Impaired oxygen delivery to the eschar impairs local immune defenses, since bacterial killing by neutrophils is impaired. Increased vascularity begins in the subeschar space toward the end of the first week. Spontaneous surface sloughing, due to loss of integrity of the thick eschar, begins toward the end of this period.

The rate of eschar sloughing is accentuated by wound bacteria, which create an additional stimulus to inflammation and local protease release. Progressive invasion by bacteria is difficult to prevent since there is penetration of topically applied antimicrobials into the subeschar space through the thicker eschar of deep burns. Nevertheless, as with second degree burns, invasive infection is not common in the first several days unless initial gross contamination was present.

As wound blood flow increases, so do water loss and heat loss.[11–13] This is particularly true for deep second degree burns. Superficial second degree burns still have some remaining skin barrier, and third degree burns, until eschar separation, have limited perfusion. Heat and water losses are further accentuated by the increase in core temperature that develops with the onset of hypermetabolism. Pain and anxiety increase during this period, as more aggressive wound care is initiated, blood flow to the wound increases and furthers eschar separation, and the patient becomes more aware of the threatening ICU environment. The pain and anxiety further increase metabolic demands.

MANAGEMENT OF BURN WOUND INFECTION

PATHOGENESIS OF BURN WOUND INFECTION

The burn wound is a major site of infection for three reasons: **1.** loss of the skin barrier, **2.** presence of dead tissue, and **3.** systemic immunosuppression.[14–16] The stratum corneum is a relatively impermeable barrier to bacterial invasion through the skin. With the loss of the outer skin barrier, bacteria can populate the burn wound. Most of these early colonizing bacteria are endogenous, originating from the heat-injured skin (especially in hair follicles, glands, etc.), the nares and oropharynx, or the perineal and stool microflora. The bacteria find their way to the wound by way of migration in wet dressings; water immersion; hand contact; and, to a lesser extent, via aerosolized particles. The impaired blood flow to the surface of the burn results in decreased local immune defenses, since oxygen is required for white cell–mediated bacterial killing. In addition, the phagocytes and opsonins must reach the wound by way of the circulation. The wound itself releases immunosuppressive substances that impair phagocytic and cell-mediated immunity. Finally, systemic host defenses are significantly impaired after a major burn[17] (see Table 69-1).

TABLE 69-1 Effects of a Major Burn on the Immune System

Impaired Cell-Mediated Immunity
Altered skin test reactivity (anergy)
Increased allograft survival
Decreased T cell response to mitogen
Decreased T cell numbers and response to antigen
Increase in suppressor relative to helper T cells
Impaired Neutrophil Function
Decreased chemotaxis
Decreased phagocytosis
Decreased bacterial killing
Alterations in Humoral Defenses
Decreased immunoglobulins
Decreased fibronectin
Decreased 1^0 antibody response

Movement of organisms via hand contact, by patient and personnel, from area to area on the patient—or between patients—is the major factor leading to bacterial contamination of the wound. This process is particularly prevalent with nonnursing personnel, who, in general, are less compulsive about standard infection control techniques. The problem can be markedly attenuated by the enforcement of hand washing between encounters with patients and the avoidance of breaks in standard aseptic techniques. Aerosolized bacteria from drying wound crusts, airborne by turbulent airflow, represent another known method of cross contamination. Common sources are vents and airflow systems not regularly dusted and disinfected. Hydrotherapy equipment is a further source of contamination. A warm, moist environment and the repeated use of the same equipment for multiple patients with little time for decontamination have been implicated. The addition of hypochlorite to the water does *not* sterilize the water.

DIAGNOSIS OF WOUND INFECTION

In order to assess the wound for infection, a definition of *infection* must be well understood. Burn wounds are never sterile, even in the presence of topical agents or systemic antibiotics. The presence of bacteria on the wound surface or in the nonviable tissue is called *colonization*. Colonization may occur with a single type of organism or with multiple organisms. Although endotoxin may be released locally and absorbed, the bacteria are not invading underlying viable tissue. *Infection* of the wound (or *local wound sepsis*), in contrast, indicates invasion of the underlying viable tissue. As infection progresses the viable tissue and its blood vessels are invaded, and sepsis develops. The risk of infection overcoming local defenses is high when the blood flow in the subeschar space is marginal, as is the case prior to neovascularization and granulation tissue formation. After several weeks, when the highly vascularized granulation tissue develops at the interface, local resistance to invasive infection increases.

The clinical diagnosis of wound infection can be quite difficult. Fever, leukocytosis, tachycardia, and intermittent temperature spikes are characteristically seen in the burn patient with or without infection. However, sudden accentuation of these abnormalities indicates an infection someplace. Wound purulence is a reliable indicator of infection only if the purulence is in the subeschar space. What looks like purulence on the surface when the dressing is initially removed is often surface exudate mixed with residue of the topical antibiotic.[14] This appearance is especially prominent with silver sulfadiazine. Wound inspection is more valid after the previously applied topical agent and surface exudate have been wiped off.

Surface cultures of the wound invariably grow bacteria. It is impossible to distinguish bacterial colonization from wound infection by the results of surface cultures. However, identification of the type of bacteria on the surface is useful in assessment of the effectiveness of the topical agents being used. Cultures are taken after the wound exudate has been removed. The most common organism involved in wound infection, particularly in the first week, is

Staphylococcus aureus. Infection with *β-hemolytic streptococci* can also be seen early, but these organisms are recovered in fewer than 5 percent of burn patients.[14,18] Infection with gram-negative organisms is more evident after the first week. *Pseudomonas aeruginosa* is present on the wounds of approximately 25 percent of burn patients. Enterococci and *Candida albicans* are now seen with increasing frequency, each found in the wounds of about 50 percent of burn patients.

The most reliable method of diagnosing a burn wound infection is bacterial analysis of a wound biopsy.[19] A small, full-thickness portion of eschar is removed using a punch biopsy instrument or scalpel. The biopsy must include some underlying viable subcutaneous tissue. It has been established that 10^5 organisms per of tissue is the bacterial load that is preinvasive. The pitfall of this method is the possible overestimation of infection when only superficial eschar is obtained for analysis. A reproducible technique of obtaining an accurate sample of eschar is essential for the validity of this method. The second and more reliable technique is that of histologic inspection of the biopsy, sectioning the sample so that the interface between viable and nonviable tissues is seen. Bacterial invasion of viable tissue indicates true infection rather than colonization, and the need for systemic antibiotics. Routine monitoring of the wound, with biopsies every 3 to 4 days, provides continuing information on microbiologic changes in the wound.

INFECTION CONTROL

Infection control is a major component of burn management. Virulent antibiotic-resistant organisms on the healing or freshly grafted wound can lead to a marked delay in healing and to loss of graft. Movement of organisms from dirty to clean areas, or to other, previously noninfected, patients, will lead to a significant increase in morbidity and mortality. A vigorous infection control policy is necessary for any burn unit or ICU managing burn patients. Antibiotic management is discussed more specifically in Chap. 70.

EARLY WOUND EXCISION AND GRAFTING

Early excision and grafting should be considered for all burns that will not heal by primary intention within 3 weeks. Full-thickness burns require grafting unless they are smaller than 3 to 4 cm in diameter. The more rapidly the wound is closed, the better.[9,20] Burns covering less than 30 percent of TBS can, at least theoretically, be rapidly closed, because adequate donor sites are available. Larger burns are more difficult, if not impossible, to completely graft early. Deep partial-thickness burns are also difficult to assess clearly as regards time to healing. Considerable judgment and assessment skills, therefore, are essential.

The key issue is to balance the risks of a surgical procedure against the benefits gained by early wound closure. Risk assessment requires accurate assessment of cardiopulmonary stability. It must also take into account the skill of the operating team, the anesthesiologist, and the postoperative team. Complications in a severely compromised host can lead to severe morbidity or even death.

Assessing the benefits of early wound closure is similarly difficult. The surgeon must project 7 to 10 days ahead to predict the ability of the patient to tolerate intense inflammation, hypermetabolism, and infection if the wound is not closed. Accurate prediction of the delayed effects of a burn (i.e., what will heal and what will not) requires careful determination of wound depth (see Fig. 69-5).

PAIN AND STRESS CONTROL

Management of pain and anxiety is of extreme importance, beginning early postburn, to avoid loss of control of the patient. Since pain and stress are present at all times and are amplified with wound management, a continuous background use of narcotics—often patient-regulated or continuously infused—is used. Low doses of benzodiazepines are also used. Drug dosages are then increased during the period of stress response to wound management. Antipsychotic agents are also often necessary. It must be remembered, however, that burn patients are very prone to the extrapyramidal side effects of these drugs.[21] In many cases all drug dosages must be increased because of rapid clearance of drugs when the patient is in the hypermetabolic state.[22]

CASE PRESENTATION (continued from Chap. 68)

Beginning on day 2, the patient's respiratory status stabilized but remained compromised, necessitating vigorous pulmonary toilet and positive-pressure ventilation. Minute ventilatory needs began to increase as CO_2 production increased. Vital signs were: BP, 100/70; P, 120; temperature, 100.5°F. Blood gases on an $F_{I_{O_2}}$ of 0.5 with a TV of 12 mL/kg, PEEP of 7.5 cmH_2O, and rate of 16 were: Pa_{O_2}, 98 mmHg; Pa_{CO_2}, 42 mmHg; pH 7.38. The VD/VT was 0.6 and $\dot{V}_{O_2}$ 180 mL/min. Urine output was 50 mL/h, with a specific gravity of 1.022. Fluids were changed to 10% dextrose with 3% amino acids and electrolytes, at a rate of 4 L per day, plus 1000 lipid calories. In addition, 6% albumin was given as needed. Minimal sodium was added, since the serum Na^+ level was 145 meq/L, but 200 meq K^+ was given per day, along with increased doses of magnesium and phosphate (which are characteristically decreased postburn). Tube feedings at 30 mL/h were initiated. Surgical excision was begun on day 2 with excision to fascia of the neck, entire chest, and abdomen, limiting the operating time to less than 2 h. All transportation was done with a portable ventilator. Only the neck around the tracheostomy was skin grafted; the rest was covered with artificial skin substitutes (e.g., Biobrane). The preoperative platelet count was 60,000; platelets were given along with fresh frozen plasma to correct the abnormal PTT of 60 s and decrease surgical bleeding sites. The hematocrit was maintained at 30 with a reticulocyte count of 1 percent. A similar excisional procedure involving both arms and legs with full-thickness burn was performed on days 4 and 6. All available donor sites except those in the groin, where the venous vascular catheters were placed, were removed and widely

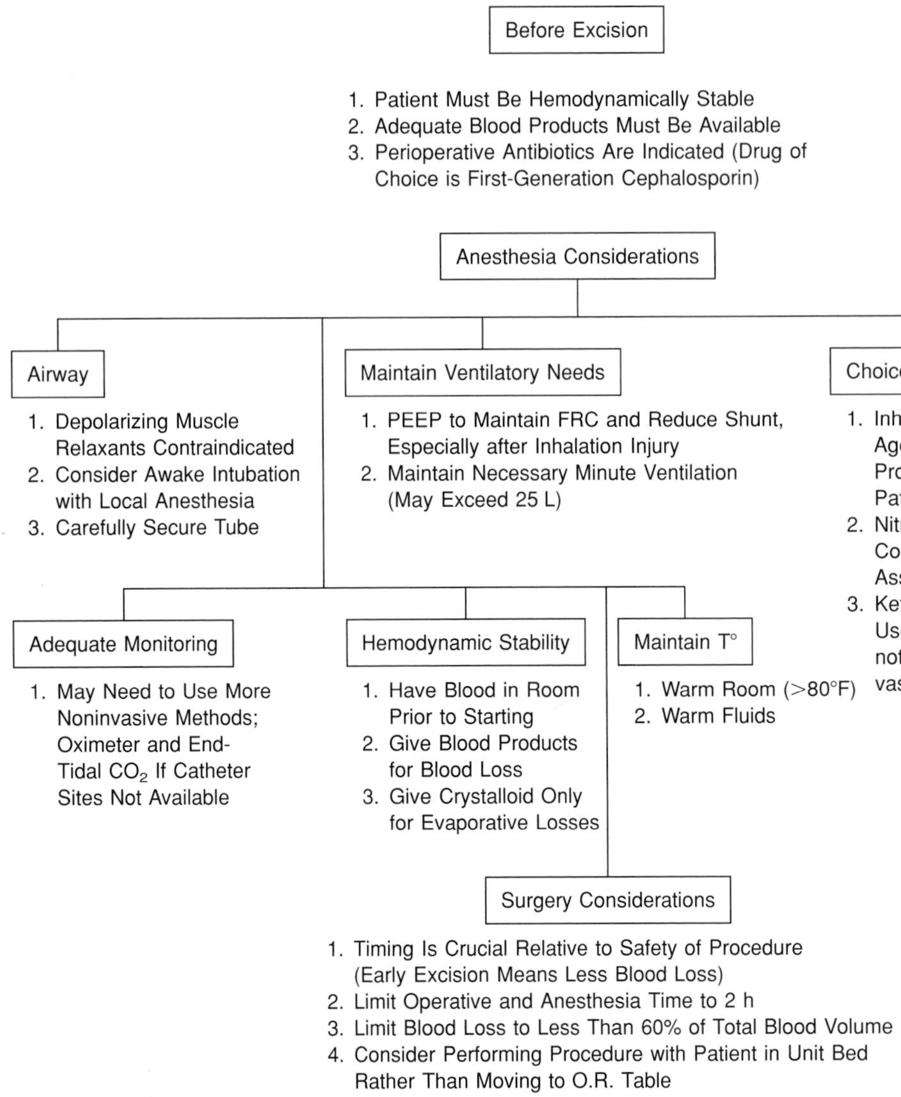

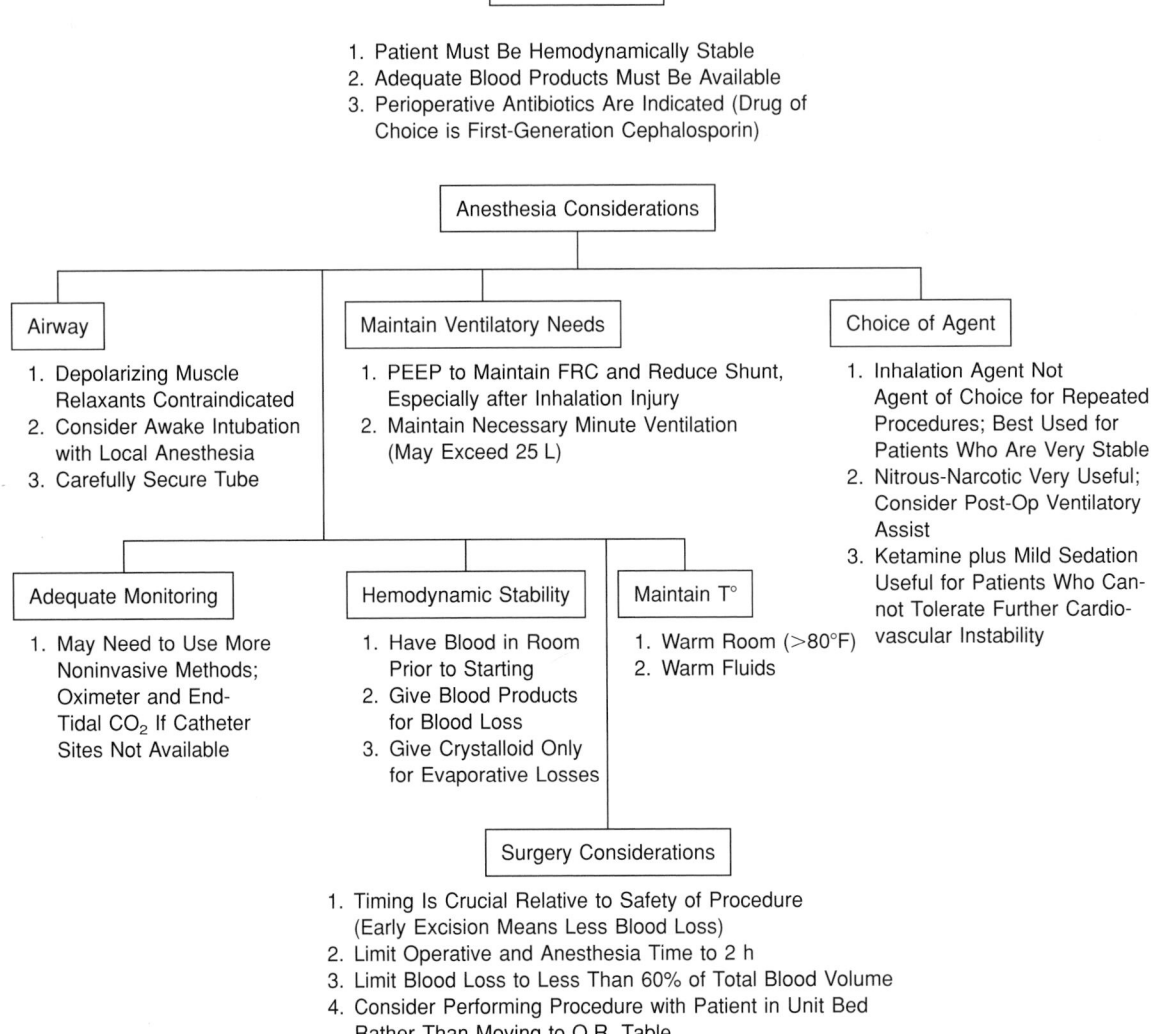

FIGURE 69-5 General principles of burn excision.

meshed. Coverage of the excised areas was begun. Blood loss averaged 4 U per procedure. The patient was kept heavily sedated, on continuous narcotics and benzodiazepines, between procedures. Room temperature in the ICU and in the operating room was maintained in excess of 85°F in order to avoid hypothermia. All wound care was performed at the bedside, since the presence of a central venous catheter precluded any other approach. The pulmonary artery catheter initially placed through the burn was removed at 36 h. Venous groin lines were rotated every 72 h. No other lines were used. O_2 SAT was monitored using pulse oximetry, and P_{CO_2} was followed by noting changes in central venous gases. Nonexcised areas were managed with twice-a-day applications of silver sulfadiazine.

A picture of hypermetabolism evolved over the first 6 days which was difficult to distinguish from infection, although hemodynamic stability was not a problem. Wound surface and sputum cultures grew *Staphylococcus aureus,* and the patient was treated perioperatively with cefazolin. No thick eschar remained after 6 days.

CASE DISCUSSION

This patient illustrates the relative physiologic stability characteristic of this period, when initial resuscitation has been accomplished but infection and severe hypermetabolism have yet to develop. Ventilatory function usually remains compromised if inhalation injury has occurred, though the inevitable nosocomial infection usually has not yet developed. Major fluid shifts do continue to occur during this period, but the major losses are now water lost through evaporation and blood products lost with surgical procedures. Red cell longevity is also decreased, and by this time at least one exchange of blood has already occurred. The maintenance fluid, therefore, is water plus electrolytes (to replace wound losses). Nutrition is begun early, and the need for increased free water allows the use of peripheral lines. In a case such as this only the fewest catheters possible are used. Aggressive surgical removal of burn is performed during this period, limiting operative time and blood loss. Surgeons need to work quickly, but must cautiously control blood loss. Two or more teams work simultaneously. Once the dead tissue is removed and the clean wound temporarily covered, further grafting can be performed as donor sites become available. The period of transportation out of the ICU is one of high risk; cardiopulmonary complications must be minimized. Optimal monitoring and the use of the portable ventilator reduce complications. Since the patient is either pre- or postsurgery almost continuously during this period, sedatives and analgesics are used literally to allay pain and anxiety. Very little weaning from ventilatory support is possible in any case. Continuous infusion of narcotics, however, does compromise the potential for oral feeding.

References

1. Demling R, Read T, Lind L et al: Incidence and morbidity of extubation failure in surgical intensive care patients. Crit Care Med 16:573, 1988.
2. Petroff P, Pruitt B: Pulmonary disease in the burn patient, in Artz C, Moncrief W, Pruitt B (eds): *Burns: A Team Approach.* Philadelphia, WB Saunders, 1979, p. 95.
3. Demling R, Crawford G, Lind L et al: Restrictive pulmonary dysfunction caused by the grafted chest and abdominal burn. Crit Care Med 16:743, 1988.
4. Wilson J, Moncrief J: Vapor pressure of normal and burned skin. Ann Surg 162:130, 1965.
5. Lamke L: Evaporative water loss from normal and burnt skin. Scand J Plas Reconst Surg 5:17, 1971.
6. Wallner S, Vantrin R: The anemia of thermal injury: mechanism of inhibition of erythropoesis. Proc Soc Exp Biol Med 181:144, 1988.
7. Wilmore D, Long J, Mason A: Catecholamines: mediators of the hypermetabolic response to thermal injury. Ann Surg 180:653, 1974.
8. Wilmore D, Aulick L, Mason A: Influence of the burn wound on local and systemic responses to injury. Ann Surg 156:444, 1977.
9. Demling RH: Effect of early burn excision and grafting on pulmonary function. J Trauma 24:410, 1984.
10. Demling R, Katz A, LaLonde C: The effect of immediate versus delayed burn care wound excision on pulmonary function. J Crit Care 1:154, 1986.
11. Wilmore D, Goodwin C, Aulick L: Effect of injury and infection on visceral metabolism and circulation. Ann Surg 192:491, 1980.
12. Gump F, Price J, Kinney J: Blood flow and oxygen consumption in patients with severe burns. Surg Gynecol Obstet 130:23, 1970.
13. Aulick L, Hander E, Wilmore D: The relative significance of thermal and metabolic demands on burn hypermetabolism. J Trauma 19:559, 1979.
14. Alexander JW: The role of infection in the burn patient, in Boswick J (ed): *The Art and Science of Burn Care.* Rockville, MD, Aspen Publications, 1987, p. 108.
15. Shuck J: Infection control in burns: topical and systemic. Surg Clin North Am 52:1425, 1972.
16. Boyce J, White R, Causey W et al: Burn units as a source of methicillin resistant *Staphylococcus aureus* infections. JAMA 249:2803, 1983.
17. Miller C: Burns and the immune network. J Trauma 19:880, 1979.
18. Demling RH: Infection following burns, in Hoeprich P (ed): *Infectious Diseases,* 4th ed. Philadelphia, JP Lippincott, 1989, p. 1424.
19. Pruitt B, Foley F: The use of biopsies in burn patient care. Surgery 73:887, 1973.
20. Gray D, Pine R, Harnon T et al: Early surgical excision versus conventional therapy in patients with 20 to 40% burns. Am J Surg 144:76, 1982.
21. Huang V, Figge H, Demling R: Haloperidol complications in burn patients. J Burn Care Rehabil 8:269, 1987.
22. Sawchuk R, Rector T: Drug kinetics in burn patients. Clin Pharm 5:548, 1980.

Chapter 70

BURNS: INFLAMMATION–INFECTION PHASE (DAY 7 TO WOUND CLOSURE)

ROBERT DEMLING

KEY POINTS

- *This period is characterized by hypermetabolism and sepsis syndrome due to wound inflammation.*
- *Sepsis from infected vascular catheters is common, because of colonization of even normal skin with pathogens.*
- *Inappropriate use of systemic antibiotics in common during this period, since the assumption is often made that infection must be the cause of the sepsis syndrome.*
- *During this period wound manipulation and operative procedures must be limited, because of wound colonization and hypervascularity.*
- *Pulmonary complications are the most common cause of mortality during this period; general anesthesia and transport are high-risk periods.*
- *Anemia is characteristic of this period, because of decreased red cell production and continued red cell losses.*
- *Pain and stress management are major problems often necessitating extensive use of narcotics, sedatives, and antipsychotic drugs. These agents often impair the effective use of enteral nutrition as the sole route of nutrient administration.*

The interval from day 7 postburn to wound closure is the most complicated phase of management of a large burn. The systemic effects of burn wound inflammation alter the function of all organ systems and magnify any preexisting organ dysfunction—especially cardiopulmonary dysfunction. The changes in metabolism resulting from the inflammatory response are very complex, requiring of the physician or surgeon a working knowledge of metabolism and nutrition in order to provide adequate care. The remaining wound is now colonized with bacteria, and wound sepsis is a prominent concern. The use of topical and systemic antibiotics leads to emergence of resistant organisms, further complicating the control of infection. The hyperdynamic hypermetabolic state makes it increasingly difficult to diagnose wound and lung infection. Multisystem organ failure (MSOF) may develop. Prevention is the only real mode of management, since mortality approaches 100 percent for MSOF in burn patients.

Pulmonary Abnormalities

Pulmonary problems remain a major cause of morbidity and mortality during this phase.[1,2] Respiratory failure and pneumonia surpass burn wound sepsis as causes of mortality. The burn patient is especially prone to infection after smoke inhalation. In addition, the hypermetabolic state produces a marked increase in oxygen consumption and CO_2 production at a time when respiratory function may be seriously impaired by pneumonia, pulmonary edema, or muscle weakness. Particularly ominous is the adult respiratory distress syndrome (ARDS), a severe complication of sepsis, which may be very difficult to reverse in burn patients[1] (see Chap. 54).

NOSOCOMIAL TRACHEOBRONCHITIS AND PNEUMONIA

PATHOGENESIS

Burn patients with the combination of inhalation injury and a major body burn have the greatest risk of pneumonia, with a rate approaching 50 percent. The high incidence is due to the presence of virulent organisms in the ICU environment and the immunosuppressed state of burn patients. In nearly 100 percent of major-burn patients with respiratory burns the oropharynx has been colonized with pathogens. There are a number of routes and events by which colonization occurs. Up to 50 percent of burn unit personnel have been shown to carry either gram-negative bacilli or *Staphylococcus aureus* on their hands; compulsive hand washing has been shown to markedly reduce such transmission. The burn wound is another major source of bacteria that can be transmitted to the oropharynx. The patient's gastrointestinal tract also contributes. Aerosol nebulizers and ventilator tubing are also potential sources, because of the moist environment. The recent introduction of more disposable equipment and unit-dose packaging of aerosols has decreased the incidence of contamination via this route. Broad-spectrum antibiotics reduce the normal oral flora, allowing overgrowth of pathogens.

Aspiration of infected secretions is the next step following colonization. Aspiration is potentiated by sedation, or any apparatus or process that impairs the normal clearance of oral secretions (such as a nasogastric tube). Adequate cough will be impaired by a chest burn and also by muscle weakness from catabolism. The endotracheal tube, while necessary for maintaining an airway, decreases the ability to generate a cough. Under these conditions microorganisms contained in aspirated infected oral secretions will have the opportunity to proliferate.

The airways are lined with a ciliated, mucus-coated epithelium that clears particles and microorganisms. This is particularly important in the smaller airways, which are less effectively cleared by coughing. Ciliary action is directly injured by heat and by chemicals in inhaled smoke and often does not adequately regenerate, contributing further to the risk of retention of contaminated secretions and development of pneumonia.

The usual criteria for diagnosing pneumonia are fever, leukocytosis, purulent sputum, new or increasing infiltrates on x-ray, and pathogens growing from the sputum. These criteria are of much less value in burn patients, where wound inflammation and other sources of infection can mimic pneumonia. Examination of expectorated sputum remains the most common method of detecting a respiratory tract infection. Although sputum is reliable in about half of patients, cultures obtained by invasive means are discordant with sputum cultures in the rest. The major reason is contamination of sputum by organisms colonizing the upper airways. As with the diagnosis of pneumonia in other critically ill patients, there are numerous problems yet unsolved in defining the presence of infection and the organisms involved.

PREVENTION AND TREATMENT

Since eradication of an established pneumonia in a burn patient is very difficult, prevention is of primary importance.[3] When using antibiotics, it is important to remember that the doses of most antimicrobials required to obtain adequate levels are much higher in hypermetabolic burn patients.[4] An approach to antimicrobial selection for pneumonia in critically ill patients can be found in Chap. 102.

Improving Host Defense

Systemic host defenses are best maintained by assuring adequate oxygenation and perfusion of all tissues while providing proper nutrition.

Local defenses are similarly important. Maintaining an adequate cough is of utmost importance in the patient at risk for pneumonia, particularly in the absence of positive-pressure support (where there is a greater risk of atelectasis). Analgesics and sedation must be used carefully. It is necessary to provide adequate pain relief, especially if chest wall splinting is present. In addition, adequate sleep is required to maintain muscle activity. On the other hand, oversedation is counterproductive unless mechanical ventilatory support is being provided.

If continued intubation is expected for many weeks, conversion to a tracheostomy in the first 7 to 10 days will greatly assist the clearance of secretions. The tracheostomy should not be placed through burned tissue. If the neck is burned, early excision and grafting is indicated. The tracheostomy can be performed through the skin graft 24 to 48 h later.

Postural drainage is necessary to move the small airway secretions to the proximal airways, so that cough clearance can occur. Ambulation is the ideal approach. An intubated, ventilated patient with a lung injury who cannot ambulate is best managed using side-to-side position changes.

Minimizing Colonization

Decreasing the potential for cross contamination of bacteria from personnel or equipment to the patient's airway will certainly decrease the risk of colonization with a virulent, resistant hospital organism. Avoiding unnecessary use of broad-spectrum antibiotics will also decrease risks.

HYPERMETABOLISM-INDUCED RESPIRATORY FATIGUE (POWER FAILURE)

The increase in oxygen consumption and CO_2 production during this period imposes increased demand on the respiratory system relative to that seen in the previous periods.[5,6] A 50 to 100 percent increase in CO_2 production will be seen with burns in excess of 50 percent of total body surface (TBS). In addition, the severe catabolism initiated by the inflammatory response can lead to weakness of the chest wall. Chronic pain and anxiety cause sleep deprivation and fatigue. While impaired oxygenation is common (because of cardiogenic and noncardiogenic edema, as well as atelectasis), hypercapnic respiratory failure is usually the major problem. A doubling of CO_2 production requires a doubling of alveolar ventilation. Increased ventilation entails increased work of breathing, especially if a decrease in compliance or an increase in dead space is also present. These multiple causes of increased ventilatory load and decreased neuromuscular competence commonly lead to respiratory failure (see Chap. 84).

This syndrome is relatively common in the perioperative period. The immediate postoperative period is the time of greatest vulnerability, since oxygen consumption and CO_2 production return to preoperative values almost immediately after the anesthetic is withdrawn.

TREATMENT

Protection of the lungs against processes that would impair their function is the best form of support. Controlling edema and infection, maintaining nutrition, and provision of adequate rest, as well as chest wall exercise, are key components. CO_2 production should be limited by avoiding excess carbohydrate calories and controlling hyperthermia. Partial ventilatory support via a tracheostomy may be useful, especially if recovery is not anticipated for several weeks. A narcotic infusion is advantageous, if the patient is already on partial mechanical ventilatory support, to decrease the stress response.

Hemodynamic and Metabolic Support

The onset of the hypermetabolic state and infection, along with continued fluid and protein losses, makes this a challenging period in which to maintain hemodynamic stability. A good understanding of the metabolic and physiologic changes is necessary in order to determine fluid, electrolyte, and nutrient requirements.

FLUID, PROTEIN, AND RED BLOOD CELL LOSSES

Fluid, protein, and red blood cell losses during this period occur primarily through evaporation and wound debridement. Evaporative water losses remain increased until the wound is closed. Even after closure, evaporative losses through the grafted wound are much higher than through normal skin. Water losses from the now-soft eschar or granulation tissue may be considerably greater than from the earlier thick, dry eschar, since surface blood flow is much higher. Donor sites for skin grafts are an added source of loss. Losses are further increased by the inevitable increase in body temperature.

The friable vascularized wound tends to be a source of constant blood loss even with very gentle daily care. Frequent blood sampling also contributes. Decreased red cell production (until the wound is closed) and continued daily losses cause a constant need for blood replacement. Losses from the wound excisions can be massive during this phase, because of wound hypervascularity.

Protein losses from wound exudation and from bleeding persist until wound closure. Albumin production by the liver is markedly decreased during the hypermetabolic state, in favor of acute-phase protein synthesis. Therefore, albumin losses are not compensated by albumin synthesis, despite adequate nutritional support.

Administration of excess salt in the face of large evaporative water losses can lead to hypernatremia. Potassium abnormalities are common, particularly with the onset of nutritional support. Calcium, magnesium, and phosphate abnormalities are also common; these levels must be monitored.

THE HYPERMETABOLIC STATE

Beginning at day 5 or 6 there is a gradual increase in the metabolic rate, from a normal level of 35 to 40 cal/m^2 per h (25 cal/kg per day) to levels ranging from 2 to 2.5 times normal at about day 10.[5,9,12] The increase in metabolic rate after burns far exceeds those seen after other severe injuries, including sepsis. The magnitude of the increase is directly related to burn size. Young patients appear to generate higher postburn metabolic rates than elderly patients.

The hypermetabolic state is characterized by increased oxygen consumption, increased heat production, increased body temperature, hyperglycemia, and increased protein catabolism. Body temperature increases from a normal of 98°F (37°C) to between 100 and 101°F (38 to 38.5°C). This is thought to be due to a resetting of the hypothalamic temperature center caused by the altered hormonal environment. The decrease in tissue responsiveness to insulin may result in the necessity for exogenous insulin supplementation (see Chap. 90 and 92).

Much of the glucose generated by the liver is used anaerobically by the burn wound in generating lactate, which is then transported back to the liver for gluconeogenesis. Lactate is rapidly cleared, so plasma levels are usually not increased unless sepsis or hypovolemia is also present. There is clear evidence of a CNS modulation in this hypermetabolic response. High-dose narcotic infusions or general anesthesia can substantially attenuate the response.

The hypermetabolic state leads to major physiologic changes. Cardiac output increases two- to threefold. O_2 consumption increases from a normal value of about 125 mL/m^2 per min to values approaching 300 mL/m^2 per min. CO_2 production can also reach values over two times normal. Urine output remains 1 to 2 mL/kg per h as long as an increased solute load is present. The pulse rate again increases, as was seen in the initial hypovolemic phase; but now systemic vascular resistance is decreased. Systemic hypertension is relatively common, particularly in patients with a relatively noncompliant vascular tree. Heart failure may occur during this period in patients with an impaired myocardium.

TREATMENT

FLUID REPLACEMENT

The extra free-water losses allow the use of more dilute solutions of nutrients and, often, the use of peripheral veins instead of central veins to supplement enteral feeding. It is preferable to maintain a serum albumin level above 2.5 g/dL to avoid hypoproteinemia-induced tissue edema. Although a hematocrit of less than 30 may be sufficient for a young patient after nonburn trauma, the tissue oxygen needs of a major burn are considerably greater; therefore severe anemia is less well tolerated. The hematocrit should be maintained between 30 and 35.

NUTRITION

It is expected that nutritional support has been started in the early post-resuscitation period; however, this support will require adjustment during this period of increasing metabolic activity. The first requirement is an estimation of energy requirements; this is followed by an organized approach to nutrient delivery, tailoring the proportions of carbohydrate, protein, and fat to the individual patient's needs.

The objective of nutritional support is to provide the necessary calories for the required energy needs. The energy required depends on *energy expenditure.* This quantity represents the basal metabolic rate (BMR), muscle activity, and stress-induced energy needs. The BMR is the energy required to maintain cell integrity in the resting state and to maintain body temperature. Body size is a principal factor, so BMR is normalized to body surface area. Other variables include age and, to a lesser extent, sex. A general discussion of evaluation of metabolic requirements is found in Chap. 91; factors specific to burn patients are detailed below.

In the burn patient in ICU, muscle activity is usually quite limited and considered to be no more than an additional 25 percent of the BMR. Excessive muscle activity from "fighting the ventilator," from excessive work of breathing, or as a result of a combative, disoriented state will markedly increase the energy expenditure. Sedation or, if necessary, muscle paralysis may be needed to control this component of the total energy expenditure.

The third component, stress-induced energy needs, includes the "stress factor," which defines the hypermetabolism induced by the burn. The stress factor is a multiple of the BMR. The value takes into consideration the type and size of burn and the average metabolic response seen with this degree of injury (see Table 70-1).

TABLE 70-1 Stress Factors for Use in Calculating Nutritional Energy Requirements of Burn Patients

Burn Size (%TBS)	Stress Factor
10	1.25
20	1.5
30	1.7
40	1.85
50	2.0
60–100	2.1

An estimation of caloric needs is based on the following simple formula:

$$\text{Energy requirement} = \text{BMR} \times 1.25\ (\text{Activity}) \times \text{stress factor} \quad (70\text{-}1)$$

Since over 95 percent of energy generated requires oxygen, there is a direct relationship between oxygen consumption and metabolic rate. The increase in V_{O_2} can be used to calculate the increase in metabolic rate.

Approximately 60 percent of estimated nonprotein calorie requirements should be given as glucose in order to effectively spare nitrogen. Fat can be used for the remaining 40 percent of nonprotein calories. Monitoring of triglyceride levels is necessary to avoid exceeding a value of 250 mg/dL 4 h after cessation of the lipid infusion. Lipid clearance is not impaired in the majority of burn patients; in fact, lipid utilization may be increased.

Protein (nitrogen) requirements can be calculated in a number of ways. A standard estimate of 1.5 to 2 g of protein per kg body weight can be used for all major burns. A more specific quantitative estimate is based on the calorie/nitrogen ratio. A calorie/nitrogen ratio of 150:1 has been the standard used for a number of years. Recent data in burn patients indicate that a 100:1 ratio may be preferable. This is based on the finding that a protein-rich diet is more effective in reversing the immune deficiencies seen in the postburn period. Noninjured man normally consumes a diet with a calorie/nitrogen ratio of about 250:1 (see Chap. 91).

A number of vitamins are lost in burn patients both because of loss in wound secretions and because of increased metabolism. Vitamins A and C are of particular concern, since they are essential for healing. Vitamin A should be given in a daily dose of 10,000 to 50,000 units, and vitamin C in a daily dose of about 1 g. Zinc, a trace element required for healing, is also lost in increased amounts.[11] Replacement is usually 220 mg $ZnSO_4$ twice daily, given orally, or 45 mg daily, given parenterally. The vitamin B complex is also essential, doses for burned patients being 5 to 10 times the RDA. The specific added needs for other trace minerals are not well defined.

Nutritional support is best managed during this period by the enteral route, usually through a combination of a balanced tube feeding and voluntary intake. Parenteral hyperalimentation through a central vein is occasionally required if the gastrointestinal tract is not functioning adequately.

Infection and Sepsis

PATHOPHYSIOLOGY

Sepsis is the leading cause of morbidity and mortality during this period. The sepsis syndrome often looks very much like the postburn hypermetabolic state; it can be characterized initially by fever, leukocytosis, tachycardia, and a hyperdynamic state reflected by increased cardiac output, decreased vascular resistance, and increased oxygen consumption. Evidence of impaired tissue oxygenation is, however, also present. This includes lactic acidosis and hypotension, which are not seen with hypermetabolism alone. There is considerable variability in the initial sepsis symptom complex.

The most common sites of infection in the burn patient are the lungs, the burn wound, and vascular catheters. Intraabdominal processes, in particular acalculous cholecystitis, are uncommon, but are well recognized as sources of sepsis in critically ill patients. Pancreatitis, with superimposed infection, is another potential cause of intraabdominal sepsis.

The high risk of intravascular lines cannot be overemphasized.[13] Although a positive blood culture is evidence of septicemia, lack of a positive blood culture does not rule out an infected line. A strict infection policy on vascular catheters is required. Diagnosis demands a high index of suspicion. Sometimes the only proof is defervescence and resolution of the septic episode after removal of the catheter.

TREATMENT

FLUID TREATMENT

The primary treatment for the inadequate tissue oxygenation in sepsis syndrome is restoration of an adequate blood volume by infusion of fluids intravenously. With successful volume restoration, the degree of lactic acidosis should decrease. Only a minority of patients will require infusion of vasoactive drugs for maintenance of adequate blood pressure and cardiac output; this problem is discussed more fully in Chaps. 98 and 114.

ANTIBIOTIC THERAPY

Empiric antibiotics should be started if the presumed infection is a greater immediate threat to the patient than the antibiotic therapy. The antibiotic regimen can be altered when culture data and diagnostic studies become available. Combined antibiotic therapy, usually using a first-generation cephalosporin and an aminoglycoside, is the most effective initial management of the septic patient.

Appropriate antibiotic dosing is a crucial aspect of management. Because of the hypermetabolic state, as well as the loss of antibiotics from the wound, the burn patient generally requires a larger total antibiotic dose and increased frequency of doses to maintain adequate levels. This increased requirement is well documented for the aminoglycosides. Renal impairment may mandate lower doses. Monitoring antibiotic levels is the only valid approach to the use of systemic antibiotics in major-burn patients.

Because of the immunocompromised nature of the burn patient, as well as the use of topical and systemic antibiotics, fungal sepsis—especially due to *Candida albicans*—relatively common. The prodrome is often more subtle than with other microorganisms, with patients appearing more chronically ill and just "not doing well."

SURGICAL MANAGEMENT

As with any form of sepsis, the removal or control of the septic focus is of primary importance. Mafenide cream is the agent of choice for topical management of wound infection, if the wound is not massive in size and the carbonic anhydrase inhibitor effect caused by absorption of this drug can be tolerated. Debridement should be gently performed to unroof pockets of infection and allow for better local wound and topical antibiotic care. Large excisions are often poorly tolerated during this period, because of dissemination of infection and blood loss.[14] Septic thrombophlebitis should always be considered, especially in the presence of repeatedly positive blood cultures. A tender peripheral vein, or a vein with overlying induration, should be inspected via a cutdown. If there is any question of purulence the vein should be surgically removed. Central veins cannot be readily removed, but usually do not become directly involved in a closed-space abscess. However, a soft-tissue abscess in proximity to central veins is not uncommon in the subclavicular area or in the neck. Any small local induration should lead to a limited local exploration (at least) looking for a deeper abscess. The approach to infection is summarized in Fig. 70-1.

CASE DISCUSSION (continued from Chap. 69)

Beginning after day 7, the patient developed a persistently febrile state with a steady-state temperature of 100.5°F and intermittent spiking to 104°F, usually 1 to 2 h after burn care. Infections were not evident to explain the majority of temperature spikes. Over the ensuing weeks, the remaining excised but nongrafted wounds were grafted as donor sites became available. The feet were used eight times for donor sites. Several bacteremias were documented, and were thought to be due to contaminated vascular catheters, even though lines were alternated between the left and right groin every 3 days (these areas were spared from the burn). Eventually, vascular lines were moved to the subclavian areas, after these areas were covered with skin graft. An episode of candidemia, with candida also in lungs and wound, was treated with a course of amphotericin B. The patient received partial mechanical ventilatory support for the next 3 months, gradually being weaned to a continuous posi-

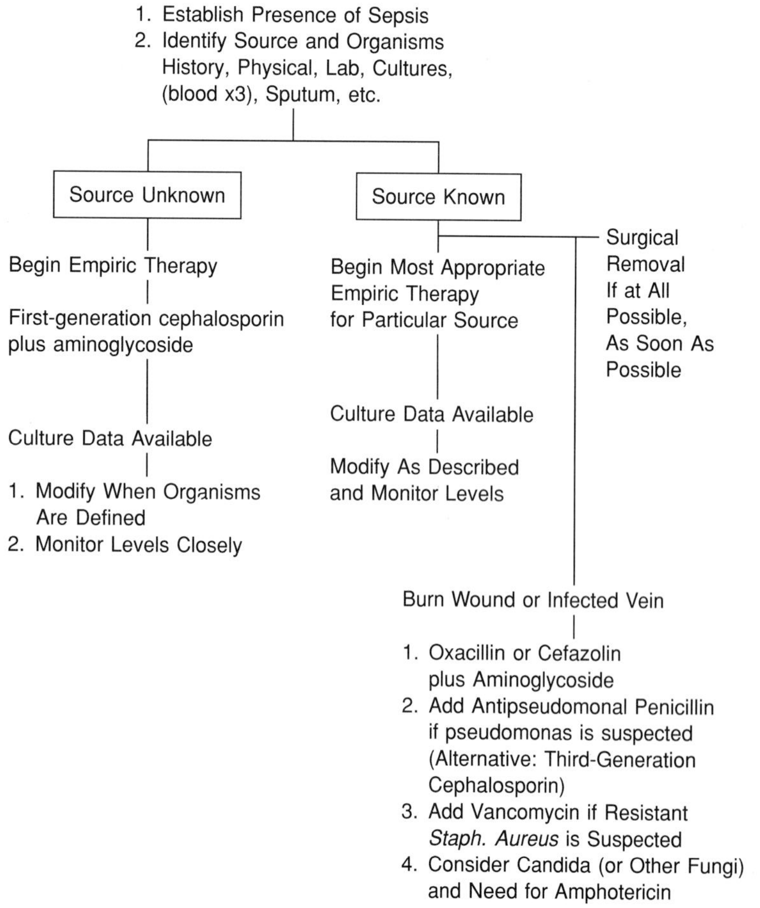
1. Establish Presence of Sepsis
2. Identify Source and Organisms
History, Physical, Lab, Cultures, (blood x3), Sputum, etc.
Source Unknown
Source Known
Begin Empiric Therapy
First-generation cephalosporin plus aminoglycoside
Culture Data Available
1. Modify When Organisms Are Defined
2. Monitor Levels Closely
Begin Most Appropriate Empiric Therapy for Particular Source
Culture Data Available
Modify As Described and Monitor Levels
Surgical Removal If at All Possible, As Soon As Possible
Burn Wound or Infected Vein
1. Oxacillin or Cefazolin plus Aminoglycoside
2. Add Antipseudomonal Penicillin if pseudomonas is suspected (Alternative: Third-Generation Cephalosporin)
3. Add Vancomycin if Resistant *Staph. Aureus* is Suspected
4. Consider Candida (or Other Fungi) and Need for Amphotericin

FIGURE 70-1 Treatment of infection during inflammation-infection phase in burn patients.

tive airway pressure (CPAP) mode with 7.5 cmH_2O. Eventually spontaneous ventilation without CPAP was achieved and the tracheostomy was removed. During this time the rigid chest and abdominal wall had been replaced with a thin layer of epidermis over a fibrous tissue bed. This process made the patient very prone to atelectasis, especially in the early postoperative period, as vital capacity remained low at 10 to 12 mL/kg. Several episodes of nosocomial pneumonia, diagnosed by purulent sputum and new lung infiltrates, were treated. Each new infection involved increasingly resistant gram-negative organisms.

Enteral nutrition was initiated early, but, because the frequent small operative procedures and the need for continuous fentanyl infusion to control pain impaired GI motility, supplementary parenteral nutrition was required. In addition, low-dose dopamine was used over a 3-month period. Initial attempts at discontinuation led to oliguria. Modest volume loading, used on several occasions to treat the oliguria, led to pulmonary edema. Neither a pulmonary artery catheter nor an arterial line was used, because of lack of clean sites and fear of infection. Daily fluid requirements were considered to be 4 to 5 L of low-salt-content fluid to replace evaporative losses. Between 1 and 2 U of packed red blood cells was given on a weekly basis to keep the hematocrit at 30, especially before surgery. Nutritional requirements were estimated at 40 cal/kg with protein needs of 2 g/kg, since O_2 consumption was measured at nearly double the normal value during this period. Agitation and intermittent psychosis also developed, necessitating thorazine up to 1.2 g/day. Systemic hypertension also developed, but was well controlled with the thorazine. Aggressive physical therapy was continued throughout the patient's hospital course. Despite this fact, significant muscle wasting and extremity rigidity developed, which gradually resolved as the amount of physical therapy increased and the dosage of thorazine decreased. Benadryl was used routinely to attenuate any extrapyramidal side effects of the antipsychotic agents. The patient gradually recovered and was transferred to a local rehabilitation facility.

CASE DISCUSSION

During this period, following burn wound inflammation and bacterial colonization, the patient developed a sepsis syndrome that persisted until the wound was closed. In addition, this period was characterized by recurrent infections arising from the combination of an immunosuppressed host, invasive catheters, and an external environment where resistant organisms were to be found. The profound pyrogen release from any wound manipulation, with or without bacteria, made the diagnosis of infection versus inflammation alone difficult to determine. Pulmonary function was of major concern, since patients are very prone to nosocomial pneumonia, especially from an impaired cough. Narcotics (used to control pain), impaired chest wall compliance from a burn, and the presence of an endotracheal tube all impaired effective clearance of secretions in this patient. The increased CO_2 production and O_2 consumption led to accentuation of any lung dysfunction. Because of these pulmonary changes and intense burn inflammation and colonization, the patient was very prone to operative complications, especially sepsis and atelectasis. Procedures by necessity must be small, lasting less than 90 min, with much less wound manipulation than in the post-resusitation period. The lack of red cell formation and the losses during operative procedures and daily care necessitated the frequent use of blood products. But perseverance and attention to detail, along with an experienced team, produced a successful outcome even in this massively burned young man.

References

1. Marshall W, Dimick A: The natural history of major burns with multiple subsystem failure. J Trauma 23:102, 1983.
2. Fein A, Leff A, Hopewell P: Pathophysiology and management of the complications resulting from fire and the inhaled products of combustion: Review of the literature. Crit Care Med 8:94, 1980.
3. Demling RH: Nosocomial pneumonia, Wilmore D (ed): *American College of Surgeons, Pre and Post Operative Care Manual.* New York, Scientific American Publishers, 1989.
4. Zaske D, Sawchuk R, Strate R: The necessity of increasing doses of amikacin in burn patients. Surgery 84:603, 1978.
5. Wilmore D, Aulick L, Becker R: Hormones and the control of metabolism, in Fischer J (ed): *Surgical Nutritions.* Boston, Little, Brown and Company, 1983, p. 65.
6. Goodwin C: Metabolism and nutrition in the thermally injured patient. Crit Care Clin 1:97, 1985.
7. Wolfe R, Durkot M, Allsop J: Glucose metabolism in severely burned patients. Metabolism 28:1031, 1979.
8. Watters J, Bessey P, Dinarello C: Both inflammatory and endocrine mediators are necessary to stimulate host responses to sepsis. Arch Surg 121:179, 1986.
9. Aulick L, Wilmore D: Increased peripheral amino acid release following burn injury. Surgery 85:560, 1979.
10. Matsuda T, Kagan R, Hanumadass M et al: The importance of burn wound size in determining the optimal caloric nitrogen ratio. Surgery 94:562, 1983.
11. Larson D, Maxwell R, Aboton S: Zinc deficiency in burn children. Plast Reconst Surg 46:13, 1970.
12. Curreri P, Luterman A: Nutritional support of the burned patient. Surg Clin North Am 58:1151, 1978.
13. Pruitt B, McManus W, Kim S: Diagnosis and treatment of cannula related intravenous sepsis in burned patients. Ann Surg 191:546, 1980.
14. Peterson S, Umpherd E, Warden G: The incidence of bacteremia following wound excision. J Trauma 22:274, 1982.

Chapter 71

DERMATOLOGIC CONDITIONS IN THE CRITICALLY ILL

KAREN TIMPE SCHMIDT
GREGORY A. SCHMIDT

KEY POINTS

- *It is essential to establish the appearance and evolution of any skin condition in order to effectively communicate with the dermatology consultant.*
- *All surfaces must be examined, including mucous membranes (oral, ocular, nasal, genital, and perianal), hair, nails, and skin*
- *Since dermatologic conditions often evolve, yielding additional information over time, patients must be reassessed, retested, and rebiopsied until the diagnosis is made.*
- *Painful, red skin may be the first sign of toxic epidermal necrolysis (TEN).*
- *Palpable purpura is an important marker of vasculitis.*
- *Pressure sores are often more extensive than suggested by the surface lesion; they can be an overlooked source of sepsis in the critically ill patient.*
- *Extensive skin involvement can cause significant fluid, protein, and electrolyte losses and, ultimately, sepsis.*

This chapter will be divided into four general sections to illustrate the range and character of different dermatologic conditions that the intensivist may encounter during the routine care of critically ill patients. In the first section, a general approach to dermatologic disease is given. In the second section, five classic life-threatening dermatoses are described, including toxic epidermal necrolysis (TEN), pemphigus vulgaris, pustular psoriasis, exfoliative dermatitis, and erythema multiforme (EM). The third section addresses several common dermatologic complications of critically ill patients, including cutaneous reactions to drugs, contact dermatitis, decubitus ulcer, dopamine infusion-induced ischemia, steroid acne, asteatotic eczema, and milia. Finally, the fourth section will cover selected conditions with distinctive cutaneous findings, including acquired immunodeficiency syndrome (AIDS), subacute bacterial endocarditis, sepsis, purpura, leukemic and lymphomatous infiltrates, herpes simplex and herpes zoster, necrotizing vasculitis, bullous pemphigoid, disseminated candidiasis, systemic lupus erythematosus, Osler-Weber-Rendu syndrome, porphyria cutanea tarda, carbon monoxide poisoning, necrolytic migratory erythema, loxoscelism, and erythema chronicum migrans.

An Approach to Skin Disease in the Intensive Care Unit (ICU)

CRITICAL FUNCTIONS OF THE SKIN

There are many important functions of the skin that may be deranged when large areas of skin are involved in the life-threatening dermatoses. The pathophysiologic pathways for many of these complications are similar for many of the life-threatening dermatoses, and these general principles will be discussed as a group.

The skin acts as a crucial barrier between the internal milieu and the outside environment. A selective filtration barrier exists at the basement membrane zone, reducing water and electrolyte permeability. Additionally, the skin provides mechanical protection to underlying structures and performs wound repair and vital immune functions.

Loss of the barrier function leads to massive fluid and electrolyte imbalances, dehydration, shock, deep venous thrombosis, pulmonary embolism, and acute tubular necrosis with renal failure. Profound caloric losses from the surface lead to negative nitrogen balance and subsequently a catabolic state with hypoalbuminemia and its sequelae. An example is exfoliative dermatitis; up to 30 g of cells are lost daily from the skin surface in rapid turnover. Increased capillary permeability and excess cell turnover lead to hypoalbuminemia and occasionally to iron and folic acid deficiencies, contributing to anemia. The catabolic state leads to an inability to protect against mechanical trauma and to heal even minor wounds; this leads to pressure sores and extensive denudation of affected skin. One of the most crucial consequences of loss of the barrier function is invasion by microorganisms leading to local infection and subsequently to sepsis. This is compounded by the inability of affected skin to process foreign antigens and to mount an inflammatory response.

Maintenance of body temperature through insulating fat deposits, arteriovenous shunts, countercurrent vascular mechanisms, and eccrine sweating are also compromised in life-threatening dermatoses. When this capacity is lost, hypothermia occurs, leading to dysfunction of multiple cellular mechanisms. For instance, in exfoliative dermatitis, despite a doubling of metabolic heat production, impaired cutaneous vasoconstriction leads to hypothermia. Due to this impaired local vasoconstriction, the skin often feels warm. No shivering occurs until a profound drop in core temperature has occurred. In some conditions, such as pustular psoriasis and exfoliative dermatitis, increased cutaneous blood flow leads to high-output congestive heart failure with secondary compromise of crucial organ blood flow.

APPROACH TO THE PATIENT

The intensivist must process the visual data presented by dermatologic disorders in order to arrive at a differential diagnosis and plan the diagnostic workup. Although substantial information is "right in front of the eyes," the task is complicated by the fact that the skin reacts to multiple stimuli through a relatively limited number of reaction patterns. Therefore, the physician must employ a careful, methodical approach to diagnosis.

A careful history should be obtained from the patient or family, including the site of the initial abnormality, appearance and pattern of individual lesions, overall grouping, manner of evolution of lesions, relationship of eruption to drugs and other provocative factors (including proximity to tubes and catheters that disrupt the mucocutaneous barrier function), and response to therapy. Also, inquiry into the patient's general health, previous allergies and skin disorders, and past medical, family, social, and occupational history may yield important clues for diagnosis.

Physical examination should include a description of the lesions themselves, including the type (macule, papule, etc.), configuration, arrangement of multiple lesions, and overall distribution, including extent, pattern, and relationship to instrumented sites and external devices; color, consistency, and depth of involvement should also be noted. Certain clinical signs, such as Nikolsky's sign (ability to dislodge affected and adjacent epidermis with lateral finger pressure on the skin), give essential clues to diagnosis and should be sought and described. A good assessment should include a description of the patient's overall condition along with the appearance of the entire integument including hair, nails, and all mucous membranes (oral, ocular, nasal, genital, and perianal).

Workup is aided by several laboratory tests, including a gram stain, culture and dark-field examination of tissue or exudates, Tzank smear of vesicles and bullae, and KOH preparation of scrapings. The accessibility of the skin makes a skin biopsy a very useful tool. Either a Keyes punch or full-thickness excisional biopsy is done followed by formalin fixation and histopathologic analysis. Immunofluorescence and electron microscopy of skin also give additional information. Factors such as age and location of skin lesions influence the success of biopsy. Since many skin conditions evolve over time, retesting is important until the etiology is established.

GENERAL PRINCIPLES OF TREATMENT

Principles of treatment that apply to most serious dermatologic conditions include elimination of suspicious precipitating factors, withdrawal of nonessential drugs, aggressive volume status monitoring and nutritional support, prevention of anemia, surveillance culturing of denuded and affected skin, bed rest with frequent turning on fluidized beds, physical and respiratory therapy, administration of mild sedation and antihistamines, and meticulous mucous membrane and eye care. Frequent debridement may also be necessary. Specifics of topical therapy vary, from wet dressings, whirlpool and topical antibiotics for EM, and topical antibiotics such as 1% silver sulfadiazine cream, silver nitrate 0.5% cream, or bacitracin dressings (among others) for toxic epidermal necrolysis to frequent wet dressings with normal saline for pemphigus or frequent applications of bland emollients or low-potency steroids for pustular psoriasis and exfoliative erythroderma. Further details of therapy are included in the discussion of the specific life-threatening dermatoses.

Life-threatening Dermatologic Conditions

TOXIC EPIDERMAL NECROLYSIS (TEN)

Toxic epidermal necrolysis consists of widespread erythema and epidermal sloughing that resembles scalding. Adults are affected more often than children, there is no racial or sex preponderance, and the syndrome carries a high morbidity and mortality. Many etiologic factors have been identified, and multiple inciting factors may coexist in a given patient. Drug reactions from multiple drug classes can cause TEN; sulfonamides, butazones, and hydantoins are identified most frequently. An immune mechanism may be responsible for TEN, but the exact mechanism is unknown.[1]

Early TEN (before confluence of erythema and vesiculation) cannot be distinguished clinically from EM or drug reactions. At its peak it resembles EM, scalding kerosene or paraffin burns, staphylococcal scalded skin syndrome, generalized bullous fixed drug eruption, chemical burns (e.g., boric acid, ethylene oxide, nitrogen mustard), the blistering phase of psoriasis, and pressure/anoxia blisters.[2] Histologically, vacuolization of epidermal basal cells occurs in affected skin, followed by eosinophilic necrosis and subepidermal bullae formation above the epidermal basement membrane. There is endothelial swelling of dermal vessels but no necrosis or vasculitis.

Prodromal symptoms are frequent and include skin tenderness, conjunctival burning, fever, malaise, and arthralgias. These are followed hours to days later by a morbilliform rash that begins on the face and extremities and then becomes confluent and diffusely erythematous. Vesicles appear, followed by bullae, which rupture resulting in large denuded areas on the back, shoulders, and face. The hallmark of TEN is necrolysis, large areas of erythema in which Nikolsky's sign is positive (dislodging of the epidermis with lateral finger pressure, uncovering underlying dermis). Up to 50 percent or more of the body surface can be denuded. Mucous membranes are often severely involved, with diffuse erythema, vesiculation, and widespread erosions on oral, conjunctival, genital, and anal mucosa. In addition, eyebrows, cilia, fingernails, and toenails can be shed. Occasionally, targetlike lesions can be seen on the palms and soles, and some cases of TEN clinically resemble EM major (vide infra). In fact, many believe that EM major (also called Stevens-Johnson syndrome) and TEN are manifestations of a spectrum of related diseases.

Typical complications include hypovolemic or septic shock, pulmonary edema, and renal failure. Involvement of the gastrointestinal and respiratory tracts leads to tracheitis, bronchopneumonia, esophageal and gastrointestinal bleeding, acute tubular necrosis (ATN), and membranous glomerulitis. The mortality rate is 25 to 50 percent. Recovery is related to adequacy of supportive care. Scarring is common, leading to symblepharon, entropion, ectropion, corneal opacities, and alopecia.

When TEN is diagnosed, high-dose corticosteroids (e.g., prednisone, 250 mg per day) have traditionally been given, continued until the progression of skin lesions ceases (up to 3 weeks), then tapered. However, efficacy is unproven and this approach has fallen out of favor. In addition to the basic supportive measures discussed (e.g., use of topical antimicrobials such as 1% silver sulfadiazine cream, silver nitrate 0.5% cream, and bacitracin dressings), the use of tissue grafts to aid in reepithelialization of the skin is under investigation. The specialized nursing care required to manage TEN is often facilitated by transferring the patient to a burn ICU.

PEMPHIGUS VULGARIS

Pemphigus is an autoimmune blistering disease with several forms, differentiated by both clinical findings and level of blister formation. Only pemphigus vulgaris will be treated in this section.

Pemphigus vulgaris occurs in all age groups but is usually seen in the fourth and fifth decades. It has been described in all races and ethnic groups but predominates in people of Jewish or Mediterranean descent. A genetic link has been suggested by the increased incidence of leukocyte antigens HLA-A10, HLA-A13, and Dw4. The disease is mediated by serum IgG autoantibodies, which bind to antigenic sites on the surface of the keratinocytes, localize in the intercellular spaces, and do not require complement to cause acantholysis. When exposed to pemphigus antibody, epidermal cells release plasminogen activator, which dissolves intracellular cement and leads to edema and blistering.[3] Antibody levels can fluctuate with disease activity. Direct immunofluorescent staining of skin or mucous membranes is positive for both IgG and C3 early in the disease in virtually all cases.

Clinically, flaccid weeping bullae appear on either erythematous or normal-appearing skin. They rupture easily, leaving large denuded areas of skin. Often, crusting is the only evidence of the blistering process. Nikolsky's sign is frequently present. Scalp, mucous membrane, umbilical, and intertriginous areas are commonly involved. Lesions involving the pharyngeal, laryngeal, conjunctival, nasal, vaginal, or anal mucosa are tender and painful. They heal slowly with hyperpigmentation but seldom scar. After a few weeks the disease extends beyond its initial localization. Typically, the lesions can appear fleetingly on the oral mucosa for weeks before presenting more extensively on the torso and extremities.

A Tzank preparation made by scraping a freshly unroofed early blister often reveals acantholytic cells. This finding should prompt further histologic as well as immunofluorescent studies. Skin biopsy reveals acantholysis of the epidermis, with loss of cohesion of epidermal cells, and suprabasal intraepidermal bullae formation. There is little inflammation, but a distinctive finding of eosinophilic spongiosis (accumulations of eosinophils in the epidermis) is often present. Direct immunofluorescence of lesions demonstrates intercellular IgG and complement (C3). Indirect immunofluorescence measuring IgG levels in the blood can be used in a qualitative fashion to follow disease progress.

Until the advent of the steroid era, this disease had a high mortality rate, often greater than 70 percent. Even now, the course is variable depending on the timing of the diagnosis and institution of therapy, making prompt diagnosis essential. Topical therapy includes frequent wet dressings with normal saline. There is no substitute for high-dose corticosteroids in the acute phase of the illness. Typically, 240 mg or greater of prednisone is administered daily until new blister formation is suppressed. Weekly serum pemphigus antibody titers should be followed. Using titers and clinical activity, steroids can be tapered to maintenance levels that keep the patient blister free. Alternate day therapy can be considered once the prednisone has been tapered to 40 to 60 mg per day. At this time, immunosuppressive agents can be added for their steroid-sparing effect. Azathioprine (50 to 150 mg by mouth daily), methotrexate (25 to 35 mg weekly by mouth or intramuscular), and cyclophosphamide (100 to 200 mg daily tapered to 100 mg daily after 3 weeks) have been used. Often, after roughly 1 month of adjuvant therapy, steroids can be reduced or switched to an alternate-day regimen.[4]

Adjuvant treatment with immunosuppressive drugs or gold has been proposed for the following indications: (1) in the initial treatment of patients with relative contraindications to steroid use—peptic ulcer, diabetes, cataracts, osteoporosis—or patients with known side effects from corticosteroids; (2) in patients unresponsive to high doses (240 mg per day) of corticosteroids given for adequate periods of time; and (3) in patients in whom repeated attempts to taper corticosteroid doses are associated with recurrence of disease.[5] Intramuscular gold is typically given as 10 mg intramuscular with weekly doses adjusted according to the clinical response. Although still considered experimental, plasmapheresis may be useful for initial control in patients with high levels of circulating intercellular pemphigus antibodies and rapidly progressive disease unresponsive to high-dose corticosteroids.[5]

PUSTULAR PSORIASIS

Pustular psoriasis is a potentially lethal variant of psoriasis characterized by extensive generalized erythroderma and pustule formation along with systemic symptoms. There is an association of pustular psoriasis with HLA-B27. Provocative factors include infection, pregnancy, sunlight, and drugs such as salicylate, iodide, lithium, phenylbutazone, and oxyphenbutazone. Topical and systemic corticosteroids can destabilize psoriasis vulgaris to generalized pustular psoriasis, particularly after abrupt discontinuation.[6]

Apprehension, nausea, and shivering begin hours before existing psoriatic plaques become bright red and tender and new areas of inflammation appear. The affected areas develop pinhead-sized pustules, which rapidly enlarge and coalesce to form lakes of pus. Within a day, the stratum corneum exfoliates, leaving a denuded surface on which new pustules appear. After a few waves of pustule formation the process may subside or it may persist for weeks. This process can appear anywhere, but marked involvement of the face is unusual. Up to one-third of these patients have concomitant exacerbation of inflammatory polyarthritis.

Biopsy of affected skin reveals intense inflammation. An early dermal lymphocytic infiltrate is followed by intracellular and intercellular edema in the epidermis. Neutrophils invade the epidermis, forming spongiform pustules and micro- and macroabscesses. The stratum corneum becomes parakeratotic. Laboratory findings include leukemoid reactions, hypoalbuminemia, elevated erythrocyte sedimentation rate, and hyperlactatemia.[7]

Initial topical therapy includes frequent application of low-potency steroids or bland emollients. Occasionally, more aggressive therapy may be necessary. Photochemotherapy with psoralen (8-MOP) and ultraviolet A light (PUVA) is an option.[8] The results of a double-blind, controlled study of etretinate (initial dose, 0.75 mg/kg daily) suggest that it is a drug of choice.[9] Pustules disappear in an average of 1 week, but a maintenance dose has to be administered for 3 months or longer to maintain clearance.[10] Another alternative is methotrexate in doses of 5 to 10 mg intramuscular weekly.[11] In general, oral steroids should be avoided.

EXFOLIATIVE DERMATITIS

Exfoliative dermatitis, or erythroderma, is an inflammatory disorder in which generalized erythema and scaling occur, either as a specific phase of processes such as drug eruptions and T cell lymphomas or in the absence of preexisting disease. In a review of 101 cases, 75 percent of patients were male with a mean age of 50 years. The mean duration of illness was 5 years.[12] A clinicopathologic study of 135 cases[13] revealed that 54 patients had erythroderma attributable to drugs (primarily sulfonamides, penicillins, barbiturates, and antimalarials), 36 had preexisting dermatosis (including eczema, atopic dermatitis, stasis dermatitis, and psoriasis), and 23 had associated malignancy that usually antedated the skin eruption (such as mycosis fungoides, Hodgkins disease, leukemia, or lymphoma) (Table 71-1). Eighty-seven of these died from a disease related to the exfoliative dermatitis (pneumonia, septicemia, cardiac failure), and in the remainder no other cause of death other than exfoliative dermatitis could be found.[13]

In idiopathic cases, erythema begins over the head, trunk, or genitals and usually extends to cover the whole cutaneous surface over the next several days to weeks. Palms and soles are involved but mucous membranes are usually spared. Although the skin initially seems thinned, with time it becomes thickened and dry. Scaling and hair loss occur. Dermatopathic lymphadenopathy occurs in 60 percent (in the absence of myeloproliferative syndromes). Hepatomegaly occurs in 35 percent, often associated with drug reactions or preexisting dermatoses. If splenomegaly occurs, it is usually in association with an underlying lymphoproliferative disorder. The histologic findings on biopsy of affected skin are nonspecific, and laboratory workup is usually nondiagnostic.

TABLE 71-1 Factors Associated with Exfoliative Erythroderma

Cutaneous disorders	Drugs
Atopic dermatitis	Allopurinol
Contact dermatitis	Arsenic
Nummular dermatitis	Aspirin
Dermatophytosis	Barbiturates
Congenital icthyosiform erythroderma	Captopril
Mycosis fungoides	Cephalosporins
Lichen planus	Chlorpromazine
Pemphigus foliaceus	Codeine
Pityriasis rubra pilaris	Dimercaprol (BAL)
Psoriasis	Diphenylhydantoin
Reiter's syndrome	Ethylenediamine
Stasis dermatitis	Gold
Systemic diseases	Iodine
Carcinoma of lung and rectum	Isoniazid
Hodgkins disease	Mercurials
Leukemia	Mercury
Lymphoma	Penicillin
Multiple myeloma	Phenindione
Reticulum cell sarcoma	Practolol
	Quinidine
	Sulfonamides
	Trimethoprim

Systemic corticosteroids (100 to 300 mg per day cortisone acetate initially, tapered to 50 mg daily) should only be used with great caution but may be useful in the idiopathic form when conservative therapy (frequent application of low-potency steroids and emollients) fails. Antimetabolites have been used in the treatment of psoriatics with exfoliative dermatitis but they prevent overall healing. Photochemotherapy with PUVA can benefit patients with exfoliation due to mycosis fungoides. Exfoliative dermatitis resistant to therapy should arouse suspicion of an underlying malignancy.

ERYTHEMA MULTIFORME

Erythema multiforme (Fig. 71-1, Plate 28) is an acute episodic cutaneous or mucocutaneous syndrome defined primarily by the characteristic "target" skin lesions, which are the sine qua non for diagnosis. Although the term *multiforme* was initially meant to highlight the changing nature of the individual lesions in this syndrome, EM is now regarded as a spectrum of manifestations and is divided into two relatively distinct patterns (Table 71-2). The mild cutaneous form of the disease with a tendency for recurrences is referred to as EM minor. The more severe form, with significant morbidity and occasional mortality due to the systemic and mucocutaneous involvement, is called EM major (also known as Stevens-Johnson syndrome) (Fig. 71-2, Plate 29). In some patients, extensive epidermolysis develops that is indistinguishable from that seen in TEN, suggesting a relationship between these two conditions.

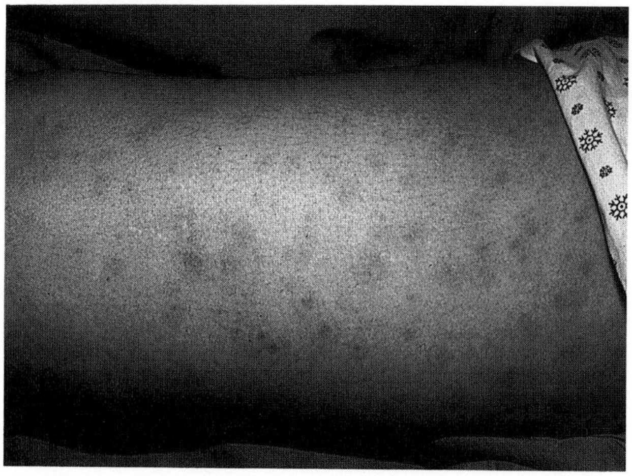

FIGURE 71-1 EM: typical "target" lesions on legs with central necrosis and peripheral erythema. See Plate 28.

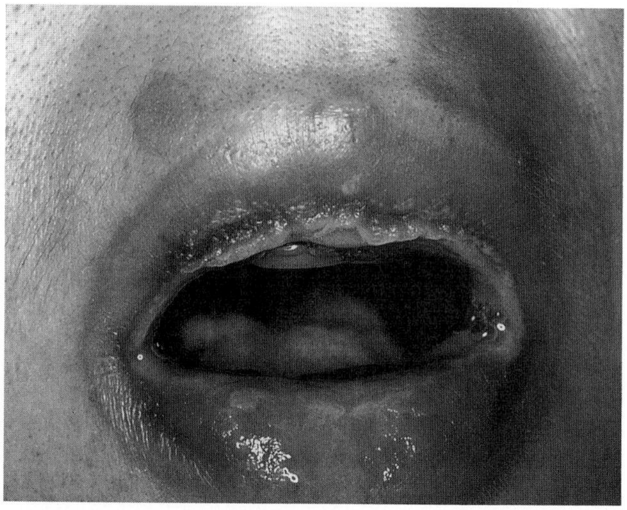

FIGURE 71-2 Stevens-Johnson syndrome: erosive involvement of lips and oral mucosa. See Plate 29.

Erythema multiforme occurs primarily in young healthy individuals.[14] There is no firm seasonal pattern of occurrence, and recurrences are common. It may be a delayed hypersensitivity reaction. Although vasculitic changes are not seen, the initial event is local vascular damage leading to marked edema, subepidermal vesiculation, and necrosis of the overlying epidermis. Foreign antigens, sequestered within the epithelium, may act as immune stimuli provoking the specific cytologic mechanism that produces the epidermal cell damage.[15]

Numerous etiologic factors have been identified (Table 71-3). Three associations have been well described: herpes (EM minor), mycoplasma (EM major), and drugs (EM major). Primarily the sulfonamides, but also the sulfonamide derivatives, phenylbutazone, diphenylhydantoin, and penicillin derivatives, have been implicated in drug-induced EM. Typically, EM major follows drug exposure by 1 to 3 weeks but may occur hours to days after drug administration when there has been prior exposure, as typifies a hypersensitivity reaction.[16]

Prodromal symptoms such as malaise, fever, headache, pharyngitis, rhinorrhea, cough, chest pain, nausea, vomiting, diarrhea, and arthralgias may occur a week or more prior to the onset of symptoms of EM. Prodromal symptoms are more common in EM major and may in reality be manifestations of the precipitating illness. The earliest lesions of EM are often red, edematous papules surrounded by blanching that enlarge to small plaques with concentric alterations in color and morphology. The characteristic target lesion is a central area of epidermal necrosis with or without blister formation (Fig. 71-1, Plate 28). These lesions

TABLE 71-2 Preliminary Diagnostic Criteria for EM

Parameter	EM Minor	EM Major
Course	Acute, self-limited, or episodic	Acute, self-limited, or episodic
Duration	Attack or episode 1–4 weeks	Attack or episode 1–6 weeks
Skin lesions	Symmetrically distributed, fixed (lasting >7 days) discrete, round erythematous skin lesions	Symmetrically distributed, fixed (lasting >7 days) discrete, round erythematous skin lesions
Evolution of skin lesions	Concentric color changes in at least some lesions	Concentric color changes in at least some lesions
Mucous involvement	Absent or limited to one surface (usually mouth)	Severe, involving at least two surfaces
Histopathology	"Compatible" (primarily mononuclear cell infiltrate, no leukocytoclastic vasculitis)	"Compatible" (primarily mononuclear cell infiltrate, no leukocytoclastic vasculitis)

SOURCE: Huff JC, Weston WW, Tonnesen MG: Erythema multiforme: A critical review of characteristics, diagnostic criteria, and causes. J Am Acad Dermatol 8:763, 1983.

TABLE 71-3 Etiolotic Associations of EM Mentioned in Medical Literature

A. Infections
  1. Viral
    a. Herpes simplex*
    b. Infectious mononucleosis*
    c. Vaccinia*
    d. Orf
    e. Milker's nodules
    f. Mumps
    g. Measles
    h. Influenza
    i. Psittacosis
    j. Varicella/herpes zoster
    k. Lymphogranuloma venereum
    l. Enterovirus infections
    m. Adenovirus infections
    n. Hepatitis B
  2. Bacterial
    a. Streptococcus
    b. Typhoid fever
    c. Pseudomonas
    d. Proteus
    e. Tularemia
    f. *Vibrio parahemolyticus*
    g. Dental infections
    h. Vincent's angina
    i. Pneumococcus
    j. Yersinia infections*
    k. Legionnaire's disease
  3. Mycobacterial
    a. Tuberculosis*
    b. Bacille Calmette Guérin
  4. Spirochetal—syphilis
  5. Mycoplasmal—*Mycoplasma pneumonia**
  6. Protozoan—*Trichomonas*
  7. Fungal
    a. Histoplasmosis*
    b. Coccidioidomycosis
    c. Dermatophyte infections

B. Immunizations or hyposensitization
  1. Horse serum
  2. Diphtheria-pertussis
  3. Polio vaccine
  4. Typhoid vaccine
  5. Pollen hyposensitization
  6. Poison ivy hyposensitization
  7. Measles vaccine

C. Systemic drugs*
  1. Sulfonamides
  2. Penicillins
  3. Diphenylhydantoin
  4. Phenylbutazone
  5. Chlorpropamide
  6. Barbiturates
  7. Phenolphthalein
  8. Tetracycline
  9. Acetylsalicylic acid
  10. Alkylating agents
  11. Estrogens
  12. Arsenic
  13. Ethanol
  14. Carbamazepine
  15. Thiouracil
  16. Codeine
  17. Trimethadione
  18. Chloramphenicol
  19. Thiacetazone
  20. Meprobamate
  21. Glutethimide
  22. Quinine
  23. Isoniazid
  24. Furosemide
  25. Rifampin
  26. Glucocorticoids
  27. Zomepirac
  28. Cimetidine
  29. Clindamycin
  30. Methotrexate
  31. Thiabendazole
  32. Ibuprofen
  33. Ethosuximide
  34. Benoxaprofen
  35. Fenoprofen
  36. Minoxidil
  37. Sulindac
  38. Methaqualone
  39. Dapsone
  40. Glucagon

D. Topical agents (chemical and drugs)
  1. 9-Bromofluorene
  2. Sulfonamides
  3. Anticholinergic eye drops
  4. Primula antigen
  5. Tropical woods
  6. Fire sponge

E. Neoplasms
  1. Leukemia
  2. Lymphoma
  3. Pelvic tumors
  4. Leiomyoma

F. Connective tissue disease—lupus erythematosus

G. Physical agents
  1. Sunlight
  2. X-irradiation of tumors*

H. Food—margarine (emulsifying agent)

I. Inhalant—methylparathion

J. Other diseases or conditions
  1. Inflammatory bowel disease
  2. Sarcoidosis
  3. Pregnancy
  4. Menstruation

*Well-documented precipitating factor.

SOURCE: Huff JC, Weston WW, Tonnesen MG: Erythema multiforme: A critical review of characteristics, diagnostic criteria, and causes. J Am Acad Dermatol 8:763, 1983.

vary considerably. Centrally there is a red, whitish, or greyish area of epidermal necrosis with a darker grey or bluish rim surrounded by shades of red and pink. These lesions can evolve by coalescing, developing central erosions, crusting, or clearing. Acral areas are usually involved initially followed by centripetal spread of the eruption. Up to 60 percent of cases have mucous membrane lesions in some form, involving primarily the vermillion border of the lips, buccal mucosa, and palate. Mucosal involvement and cutaneous manifestations usually occur simultaneously.

Erythema multiforme minor appears symmetrically on the extensor aspects of the extremities and then involves the flexor surfaces and trunk. The dorsal hands and extremities are often involved; palms, soles, flexor aspects of extremities, neck, perineum, ears, and face are involved less frequently. Ultraviolet light[12] and trauma may affect the distribution of lesions. In EM minor lesions occur in successive crops for 3 to 5 days; however, this can continue for as long as 2 weeks. Healing usually begins within 2 weeks; recurrent attacks can occur before healing is complete.

Erythema multiforme major typically begins with sudden onset of inflammatory bullous lesions that rapidly evolve into confluent erosions of the oral mucosa, lips, and bulbar conjunctiva, coated by greyish white pseudomembranes and hemorrhagic crusts. The pain from these lesions is severe, making eating and breathing difficult. Erythema multiforme major can be atypical, with variably distributed maculopapular eruptions, large areas of erythema, bullae and plaques, and extensive denudation of the epidermis. The course of EM major is prolonged, usually with resolution within 6 weeks. The most severe complications are due to ocular disease and include corneal opacities, synechiae, and blindness[16]; permanent visual impairment is seen in up to 10 percent of patients. An ominous cutaneous complication of EM major is evolution to TEN in which the mortality rises to at least 50 percent. Disease can also involve the nasopharynx, esophagus, larynx, trachea, and urogenital tract with significant morbidity. When the genital mucosa is involved, balanitis and vulvovaginitis may lead to urinary retention, phimosis, and intravaginal scarring bands. Gastrointestinal complications include esophagitis and stricture. Pneumonia (which can occur as a precipitant or complication of EM) leads to death in 18 percent of severely affected patients.[14] In severely afflicted patients, fibrinoid necrosis is seen at autopsy in many organs such as the stomach, spleen, trachea, and bronchi.[17]

Laboratory findings are not diagnostic. The initial pathologic changes on skin biopsy are a perivascular lymphohistiocytic infiltrate in the upper dermis, endothelial cell swelling, hydropic degeneration of basal cells with a bandlike infiltrate at the dermal-epidermal junction, necrosis of individual keratinocytes, and subepidermal blister formation. Direct immunofluorescence of skin is nonspecific and is usually done primarily to rule out other diseases. Mucosal lesions have similar histologic changes; but blisters are transient and usually erosions are seen.

Atypical cutaneous presentations of EM must be differentiated from chronic urticaria, necrotizing vasculitis, toxic erythemas (secondary to infection or drugs), septic infarcts (such as gonococcemia or meningococcemia), serum sickness, secondary syphilis, viral exanthems (such as variola, echo 9, and hand-foot-mouth disease), TEN, Rocky Mountain spotted fever, collagen-vascular diseases, and mucocutaneous lymph node syndrome. Oral lesions must be differentiated from mucosal pemphigoid, pemphigus vulgaris, erosive lichen planus, Bechet's syndrome, recurrent aphthous ulcers, and primary herpetic gingivostomatitis. Prompt mucous membrane biopsy can often differentiate between these.

In an ICU, the typical patient is one with extensive tissue necrosis due to EM major. The usefulness of systemic steroids in this setting is not proven, but in the absence of controlled studies, they are often administered. An initial adult dose of 50 to 80 mg prednisone is given as a short tapering course, and the condition usually resolves in 4 to 6 weeks. Since EM minor is a mild self-limited disorder, conservative management is appropriate; local or systemic corticosteroids are not indicated. Classic treatment of recurrent EM consists of conservative topical or systemic corticosteroids. Although many reports suggest that systemic corticosteroids may shorten the course and reduce disease severity, this has not been substantiated.[18]

Dermatologic Complications of Critically Ill Patients

CUTANEOUS REACTIONS TO DRUGS

The skin responds to a wide variety of insults through a limited number of morphologic patterns. Although some drug reactions are associated with specific morphologic patterns (Table 71-4), the mechanism of most drug reactions is unknown and cannot be identified clinically. Cutaneous reactions to drugs occur by both immunologic and nonimmunologic mechanisms (e.g., cumulative toxicity or interaction of multiply administered drugs and exacerbation of underlying skin diseases). Postmarketing drug surveillance is not rigorous, and unfortunately most information on cutaneous drug reactions comes from voluntary reporting and epidemiologic reviews. In a study of 22,227 medical inpatients,[19] an overall rate of 3 skin reactions per 1000 courses of drug therapy was found. Over two-thirds of these were caused by sulfonamides, penicillins, and blood products. Risk of reaction could not be associated with age, diagnosis, or admission blood urea nitrogen. Using algorithms for multiple drug use, quantitative reaction rates for many different drugs were obtained (Tables 71-5 to 71-8).

Typical cutaneous reactions to drugs include urticaria and angioedema as well as morbilliform eruptions that often begin over the trunk and spread peripherally in a symmetric fashion. These reactions recur on rechallenge, persist until the offending drug is withdrawn, and are pruritic. Urticarial eruptions occur within 36 h of onset of the offending drug while most other reactions typically occur within a week of onset (some can begin as late as 2 weeks after cessation of the offending drug).

Less common reactions include cutaneous vasculitis and fixed drug eruptions. Cutaneous vasculitis typically presents with palpable purpura that can urticate, become hemorrhagic, or ulcerate. Fixed drug eruptions consist of one or a few well-demarcated erythematous burning lesions typically occurring on the face or genitals. They recur in the same location on rechallenge and display postinflammatory hyperpigmentation. The key to treatment is identification and discontinuation of the responsible drug(s). Symptomatic relief can be obtained with bland emollients and oral antihistamines.

CONTACT DERMATITIS

This eczematous dermatitis is caused by exposure to substances that act as irritants or sensitizers. Both primary irritant and allergic contact forms can be seen in an ICU setting. In irritant dermatitis, the barrier function created by the water-protein-lipid matrix of the outer epidermis is damaged, often by substances such as strong alkalis, which destroy the lipid barrier, or acids, which cause dehydration. Repeated use compromises the skin and allows weak irritants to sustain the inflammation. The intensity is related to the concentration of the irritant and the exposure time. The mode of onset is gradual, with dryness, fissuring, and erythema evolving into an eczematous reaction. Individual patients vary in their ability to withstand exposure to irritants. Colostomy sites and the perineum and adjacent skin of incontinent or catheterized patients are areas that are often moist and are frequently washed. Frequent "surgical scrubbing" done by conscientious medical personnel can be a cause of irritant dermatitis seen in the ICU.

Allergic contact dermatitis is a form of delayed hypersensitivity reaction affecting some individuals after a few expo-

TABLE 71-4 Selected Drugs Associated with Cutaneous Eruptions with Distinctive Morphologies

- Acneform
  - Hormones (adrenocorticotropic hormone, corticosteroids, oral contraceptives, androgens)
  - Halogens
  - Dilantin
  - Isoniazid
  - Amoxapine
  - Trazodone
  - Lithium
  - Haloperidol
- Alopecia
  - Chemotherapeutic agents
  - Anticoagulants
  - Hormones (oral contraceptives, androgens)
  - Dilantin
  - Retinoids
  - Nonsteroidal anti-inflammatory agents
  - Imipramine
  - Valproate-sodium
  - Bromocriptine
  - Piroxicam
- Erythema multiforme
  - Penicillin
  - Barbiturates
  - Dilantin
  - Sulfonamides
  - Phenothiazines
  - Griseofulvin
  - Phenolphthalein
  - Nitrogen mustard
  - Nonsteroidal anti-inflammatory agents
  - Codeine
  - Tetracycline
  - Minocycline
  - Trimethoprim-sulfa
  - Glutethimide
  - Cimetidine
  - Methotrexate
  - Prazosin
  - Ethinyl estradiol
  - Ketoconazole
  - Sulfasalazine
  - Cefaclor
  - Allopurinol
  - Methaqualone
  - Furosemide
  - Streptomycin
- Erythema nodosum
  - Oral contraceptives
  - Sulfonamides
  - Halogens
  - Tetracycline
  - Penicillin
  - 13-*cis*-Retinoic acid
- Fixed drug eruptions
  - Oral contraceptives
  - Barbiturates
  - Phenolphthalein
  - Phenacetin
  - Salicylates
  - Glutethimide
  - Naproxen
  - Tolmetin
  - Nystatin
  - Methaqualone
  - Fiorinal
  - Butazolidin-alka
  - Sulindac
  - Tetracycline
  - Minocycline
  - Sulfonamides
  - Chlorphenesin carbamate
  - Metronidazole
- Lichenoid
  - Gold
  - Antimalarials
  - Thiazides
  - Levamisol
  - Molindone hydrochloride
  - Tetracycline
  - Phenothiazines
  - Furosemide
  - Chlorpropamide
  - Orphenadrine citrate
  - Diflunisal
  - Penicillamine
  - Propranolol
  - Captopril
- Photosensitivity
  - Griseofulvin
  - Phenothiazines
  - Thiazides
  - Sulfonamides
  - Nonsteroidal anti-inflammatory agents (benoxaprofen, piroxicam)
  - Tetracyclines (including minocycline and doxycycline)
  - DTIC (Dacarbazine)
  - Chloroquine
  - Methotrexate
  - Sulfonylureas
  - Fluorouracil
  - Vinblastine
- Toxic epidermal necrolysis
  - Dilantin
  - Nonsteroidal anti-inflammatory agents
  - Allopurinol
  - Trimethoprim-sulfa
  - Prazosin
  - Thiabendazole
  - Penicillin
  - Dilantin
  - Mithramycin
  - Sulfasalazine
  - L-Asparaginase
  - Streptomycin
  - Nitrofurantoin
  - Amoxapine
- Vasculitis
  - Allopurinol
  - Thiazides
  - Gold
  - Sulfonamides
  - Levamisole
  - Hydralazine
  - Nonsteroidal anti-inflammatory agents
  - Propylthiouracil
  - Dilantin
  - Ketoconazole
  - Quinidine
  - Tetracycline
  - Penicillin
  - Cimetidine
- Vesiculobullous
  - Nonsteroidal anti-inflammatory agents
  - Griseofulvin
  - Thiazides
  - Barbiturates
  - Furosemide
  - Mellaril
  - Dipyridamole
  - Chemotherapeutic agents
  - Amoxapine
  - Nalidixic acid

SOURCE: Wintroub BU, Stern RS, Arndt KA: Cutaneous reactions to drugs, in Fitzpatrick TB (ed): *Dermatology in General Medicine*, 3rd ed. New York, McGraw-Hill, 1987.

sures to an antigenic substance. On reexposure to the antigen, sensitized T cells bring about an eczematous pruritic inflammatory response in the area of exposure within 12 to 48 h. *Para*-aminobenzoic acid derivative local anesthetics (such as procaine) are potent sensitizers. Topical antibiotics such as neomycin, nitrofurazone, and penicillin can cause severe dermatitis. Most topical antihistamines are sensitizers and can cause photosensitivity dermatitis upon subsequent use of oral antihistamines. Patients allergic to balsam of Peru can develop allergic contact dermatitis on subsequent use of tincture of benzoin. Benzoyl peroxide, used as topical treatment in ulcer care and for acne patients, rubber

TABLE 71-5 Allergic Skin Reactions to Drugs Received by at Least 1000 Patients

Drug	Number of Reactions	Number of Recipients	Reaction Rate*
Ampicillin	156	2988	52
Penicillin G	51	3286	16
Cephalosporins†	17	1308	13
Packed red blood cells	11	1366	8.1
Heparin	12	1553	7.7
Nitrazepam	7	1118	6.3
Barbiturates‡	22	4658	4.7
Chlordiazepoxide	9	2161	4.2
Diazepam	18	4692	3.8
Propoxyphene	10	2976	3.4
Guaifenesin§	7	2440	2.9
Furosemide	9	3497	2.6
Phytonadione	1	1111	0.9
Flurazepam hydrochloride	1	1862	0.5
Chloral hydrate	1	4809	0.2

*Reactions per 1000 recipients.
†Cephalexin monohydrate, cephaloglycin dihydrate, cephaloridine, cephalothin sodium.
‡Amobarbital, barbital, butabarbital, butethal, mephobarbital, pentobarbital, phenobarbital, secobarbital.
§Guaifenesin and theophylline.
SOURCE: Arndt KA, Jick H: Rates of cutaneous reactions to drugs: A report from the Boston Collaborative Drug Surveillance Program. JAMA 235:918, 1976.

TABLE 71-6 Allergic Skin Reactions to Drugs Received by 500–999 Patients

Drug	Number of Reactions	Number of Recipients	Reaction Rate*
Semisynthetic penicillins†	27	760	36
Blood, whole human	32	908	35
Gentamicin sulfate	10	607	16
Quinidine	8	652	12
Dipyrone	10	876	11
Mercurial diuretics‡	6	630	9.5
Trimethobenzamide hydrochloride	5	752	6.6
Isoniazid	2	675	3.0
Chlorothiazide	2	707	2.8
Isophane insulin suspension	1	777	1.3
Phenytoin	1	905	1.1

*Reactions per 1000 recipients.
†Carbenicillin, cloxacillin sodium monohydrate, dicloxacillin, methicillin, nafcillin, oxacillin.
‡Meralluride, mercaptomerin sodium.
SOURCE: Arndt KA, Jick H: Rates of cutaneous reactions to drugs: A report from the Boston Collaborative Drug Surveillance Program. JAMA 235:918, 1976.

TABLE 71-7 Allergic Skin Reactions to Drugs Received by 100–499 Patients

Drug	Number of Reactions	Number of Recipients	Reaction Rate*
Trimethoprim-sulfamethoxazole	10	169	59
Corticotropin	3	106	28
Blood platelets	4	145	28
Erythromycin	11	481	23
Sulfisoxazole	8	462	17
Practolol	2	128	16
Plasma protein fraction	3	245	12
Nitrofurantoin	2	219	9.1
Chloramphenicol	2	292	6.8
Phenazopyridine hydrochloride	1	153	6.5
Methenamine	1	157	6.4
Cyanocobalamin	3	486	6.2
Glutethimide	1	221	4.5
Indomethacin	1	229	4.4
Metoclopramide hydrochloride	1	247	4.0
Nystatin	1	342	2.9

*Reactions per 1000 recipients.
SOURCE: Arndt KA, Jick H: Rates of cutaneous reactions to drugs: A report from the Boston Collaborative Drug Surveillance Program. JAMA 235:918, 1976.

TABLE 71-8 Allergic Skin Reactions to Drugs Received by Less Than 100 Patients

Drug	Number of Reactions	Number of Recipients
Colistimethate sodium	1	97
Salicylazosulfapyridine	2	95
Perphenazine	1	90
Desipramine hydrochloride	1	60
Levodopa	1	46
Methimazole	1	34
Glyburide	1	28
Gold sodium thiomalate	1	21
Primaquine phosphate	1	20
Antihemophilic factor, human	2	12
Anileridine	1	12
Dehydrocholate sodium	1	10
Vancomycin hydrochloride	1	10
Phenoxybenzamine hydrochloride	1	9
Diethylcarbamazine citrate	1	4

SOURCE: Arndt KA, Jick H: Rates of cutaneous reactions to drugs: A report from the Boston Collaborative Drug Surveillance Program. JAMA 235:918, 1976.

gloves, glutaraldehyde, and the acrylic monomers used as cement for orthopedic procedures can all lead to similar reactions. Nickel, present in orthopedic implants and surgical instruments, is a potent sensitizer and a common source of allergic contact dermatitis.

Both of these forms of contact dermatitis can be treated similarly. The most important task is identification and elimination of the offending agent. For the moist exudative eruptions of acute eczematous dermatitis, soaks or wet dressings with cool tap water, saline, or Domeboro (aluminum sulfate and calcium acetate at 1:40 dilution) compresses applied 2 to 4 times daily for 20 min followed by application of a potent topical corticosteroid such as 0.05% fluocinonide in an ointment or cream base applied two to three times daily are used. For subacute eczematous dermatitis, a moderate-potency topical steroid such as 0.025 to 0.1% triamcinolone in a cream base should be applied two to three times per day. Severe eruptions may require oral corticosteroids (prednisone 20 to 40 mg daily for 3 to 5 days, then tapered over 10 to 14 days). As long as a sensitizing topical antihistamine is not suspected, oral antihistamines are useful for the associated pruritis. If the skin is secondarily infected with skin flora, erythromycin (250 mg by mouth four times daily for 7 to 10 days) is given. Topical antibiotics can also be compounded into corticosteroids for topical application to impetiginized areas.

DECUBITUS ULCER

Up to 5 percent of newly admitted patients develop pressure sores during hospitalization. They occur over bony prominences: 65 percent in the pelvic area and 30 percent on the lower extremities. Risk factors include pressure, fecal incontinence, diarrhea, fractures, urinary catheter use, weight loss, dementia, and hypoalbuminemia.[20]

Of these, the most important effect is pressure. Prolonged direct pressure above 32 mmHg produces tissue anoxia followed by epidermal and superficial dermal necrosis (Fig. 71-3, Plate 30). The average supine patient generates 70 mmHg at the sacrum and 45 mmHg at the heels. With these conditions, pressure sores can arise from less than 1 h of total immobility. Shearing forces (e.g., when an immobile patient is placed in the Trendelenburg position) and friction (e.g., pulling instead of lifting the patient's body) as well as moisture all contribute to the formation of pressure sores. Loss of subcutaneous fat (as in aging) as well as drugs and conditions decreasing baseline cutaneous blood flow contribute to an unfavorable tissue milieu.

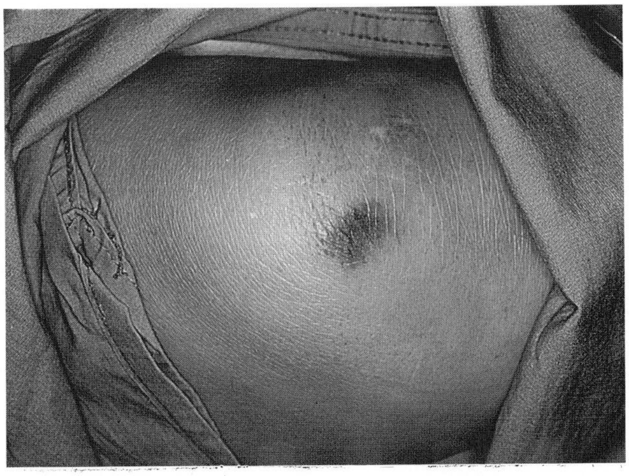

FIGURE 71-3 Decubitus ulceration: superficial necrosis and erythema in a lesion of unknown depth. See Plate 30.

Physical examination is critical for early detection of pressure sores. Developing ulcers are usually irregularly shaped. The ulcer base must be palpated; due to the pressure gradients, very small surface openings often overlie much larger defects. Classification of pressure sores is as follows:[21] stage 1—reversible epidermal involvement (irregular, ill-defined area of soft tissue swelling, induration, and warmth); stage 2—reversible inflammatory and fibroblastic response (extending through the dermis to the subcutaneous fat); stage 3—full-thickness skin defect (extension into the subcutaneous fat with undermining); and stage 4—penetration into deep fascia (muscle and bone involvement). Once pressure ulcers become established, there is a high complication rate. Polymicrobial sepsis (with anaerobes such as *Bacteroides fragilis*) and osteomyelitis occur frequently and carry a 50 percent mortality.

Up to 90 percent of pressure sores are superficial and can be managed with conservative therapy. General principles of wound care apply. The first principle of treatment is relief of pressure; therefore, high-quality nursing care is essential. Pressure must be redistributed away from bony prominences with frequent turning of bedridden patients (every 2 h) and use of fluidized beds. Friction should be minimized and moisture avoided. Sheepskin bed pads absorb water vapor and help minimize stress to the dependent skin.

Stages 1 and 2 lesions can be managed with local therapy and wound debridement. Initial debridement can be done with wet to dry dressings using fine mesh gauze soaked in normal saline and loosely packed in the wound and changed every 3 to 4 h. Routine systemic antibiotic use should be avoided unless systemic infection or local cellulitis are present; ideally therapy should then be influenced by cultures of tissue taken from the ulcer crater. Early surgical consultation should be obtained when more advanced pressure sores are found. Surgical objectives include excision of ulcerated areas, resection of bony prominences, resurfacing defects, and formation of flaps (for filling in defects and padding).

CUTANEOUS COMPLICATIONS OF DOPAMINE INFUSION

It is no surprise that complications of dopamine (and other vasoconstrictor) therapy including digital ischemic necrosis and gangrene are seen in the ICU. Elderly patients who have Raynaud's disease, diabetes, atherosclerosis, or other vascular diseases are at particular risk.[22] Depending on the nature of the indication for dopamine, topical nitroglycerine can be administered. If discoloration, sloughing, or skin necrosis occur after local extravasation of dopamine, the infusion should be stopped immediately. Affected areas should be infiltrated as soon as possible with phentolamine (an α-adrenergic blocker), by liberally infiltrating the ischemic area with 5 to 10 mg phentolamine dissolved in 15 mL normal saline. This should yield immediate obvious local hyperemia if given within 12 h of extravasation.

STEROID ACNE

This symmetric eruption of small, uniform, follicular pustules and papules can follow the initiation of oral corticosteroid therapy and is usually distributed over the neck, chest, and back. This eruption is not a contraindication to continued or future use of oral steroids. Good general skin care (avoiding excess heat and sweating, especially for the back), along with topical tretinoin (0.025% cream) and benzoyl peroxide (2.5 to 5% aqueous) once daily is effective therapy.[23]

ASTEATOTIC ECZEMA

A primary irritant, asteatotic eczema occurs frequently in elderly patients with xerotic skin. Patients with a tendency toward atopy are more susceptible. Although it can occur anywhere on the skin surface, it is most commonly seen on the anterolateral aspects of the legs. The skin becomes dry, cracked, and scaly with accentuation of the skin lines followed by the appearance of red plaques with thin, horizontal, superficial fissures. Short vertical fissures connect with the horizontal fissures, giving the skin the appearance of cracked porcelain. Scratching or application of drying lotions often leads to impetiginization and crusting with painful, deep, oozing fissures.

Treatment of the initial phases involves compresses with Domeboro solution (1:20 to 1:40 dilution of aluminum sulfate and calcium acetate) or saline applied four times daily to remove crusts followed by application of an equal mixture of topical antibiotic (such as polymyxin B sulfate and zinc bacitracin) and a midstrength steroid ointment or cream three or four times daily. In mild cases, the steroid ointment or cream can be applied alone. In all instances, frequent lubrication with water-in-oil or fatty hydrophobic medications (such as lanolin or petrolatum) should be undertaken in order to rehydrate the skin. Oral steroids are contraindicated.

MILIARIA

Miliaria, or "heat rash," is a common sequela of excess heat exposure in the ICU. The eccrine sweat ducts become occluded, then rupture and leak sweat, which induces an inflammatory response. While these papules and vesicles resemble folliculitis, on close inspection it can be seen that they are not follicle based.

The two common forms of milia will be described. Miliaria crystallina represents occlusion of the eccrine duct at the skin surface and accumulation of sweat under the stratum corneum. The clear-fluid-filled vesicle is close to the skin surface and appears as a clear "dew drop." The lesions appear frequently in bedridden patients either singly on in clusters, are usually asymptomatic, and do not appear erythematous. Rupture produces clear fluid. This self-limited process responds to improved air circulation and saline compresses.

Miliaria rubra, known as "prickly heat," is the most common sweat retention phenomenon. It arises from occlusion of the intraepidermal portion of the eccrine sweat duct in areas prone to sweating with overheating. Tiny papules and vesicles, which are often surrounded by a red halo or diffuse erythema, erupt diffusely, accompanied by a stinging or prickling sensation. Treatment consists of establishing good skin ventilation with frequent turning, changing of bed linens, and use of air conditioning. Use of a topical steroid such as 0.1% betamethasone valerate lotion three to four times daily relieves symptoms and shortens the duration of inflammation.

Selected Conditions with Distinctive Cutaneous Findings

ACQUIRED IMMUNODEFICIENCY SYNDROME

Initial human immunodeficiency virus (HIV) infection can produce a transient macular roseolalike eruption. Persistent seborrheic dermatitis is also seen in increased frequency in asymptomatic HIV-positive patients, although its prognostic significance is unknown.[24]

Most dermatologic manifestations of AIDS arise from severe T cell immunodeficiency complicated by opportunistic infections. Many commonplace infections can present in florid, aggressive, or complicated forms. These include dermatophyte infections [which can coexist with viruses such as herpes or cytomegalovirus (CMV)], molluscum contagiosum, candidiasis (aggressive mucocutaneous disease), warts (widespread persistent lesions, often with foci of atypia), and huge condyloma acuminata. Large, painful, plantar warts can be resistant to local destructive measures. Scabies and tinea versicolor can present in aggressive forms. Herpes infections are prevalent and may alter HIV expression; as the immune response decreases, herpes simplex lesions become chronic and fail to heal. Persistent herpes zoster may be a reliable indicator of HIV infection; both simplex and zoster lesions can appear as nondescript localized or disseminated lesions. AIDS patients can contract unusual primary and disseminated cutaneous fungal infections such as cryptococcosus, histoplasmosis, and sporotrichosis as well as mycobacterial infections with *Mycobacterium tuberculosis, M. avium-intracellulare,* and other atypical mycobacteria. Reiter's disease, disseminated amebiasis, strongyloides, alternariosis, and phaeohyphomycosis are less common cutaneous infections that have also appeared in AIDS patients.

Several types of cutaneous malignancies are seen in patients with AIDS. Lesions of Kaposi's sarcoma appear as solitary or disseminated light tan to dark blue or purplish brown macules, papules, or nodules. In the skin they can appear anywhere in linear, follicular, or zosteriform patterns and are often found on the palatal or buccal mucosa. Characteristic biopsy features include a profusion of capillarylike spaces, atypical spindle cells, and extravasated red blood cells. In AIDS patients there is an increased frequency of oral squamous cell carcinoma, cloacogenic rectal carcinoma, and lymphoma.

Several mucous membrane lesions appear in AIDS pa-

TABLE 71-9 Frequencies of Cutaneous Diseases in HIV-Infected Patients

Skin Condition	Frequency (%)*
Oral hairy leukoplakia	21
Seborrheic dermatitis	19
Tinea unguium	12
Tinea pedis, inguinalis	8
Oral candidiasis	7
Acne vulgaris	6
Folliculitis (truncal)	5
Psoriasis	3
Herpes zoster	3
Cheilitis angularis	3
Pityriasis versicolor	3
Herpes simplex	3
Condylomata acuminata	3
Aphthous ulceration	3
Asteatotic eczema	2
Dry skin	2
Hair disease	1
Molluscum contagiosum	1
Rashes (unknown)	1
Syphilis	1
Other	4

*Percentage of a cohort of 150 known HIV-infected patients serially followed by dermatologists and dentists.

SOURCE: Sindrup JH, Weisman K, Petersen CS, et al: Skin and oral mucous changes in patients infected with human immunodeficiency virus. Acta Derm Venereol 68:440, 1988.

tients. The white adherent plaques of oral candidiasis are a marker of disease progression; papilloma virus and herpes virus can also produce oral lesions. "Oral hairy leukoplakia" is a mixed infection with Epstein-Barr, herpes, and other viruses that appears as "hairy" plaques on the sides of the tongue. Disseminated infections such as histoplasmosis also produce mucosal lesions in AIDS patients.[25] Complex cutaneous infections can arise from the coexistence of more than one pathogen in the mucous membranes as well as in the skin.

Drug reactions are seen with increased frequency in AIDS patients. Diffuse maculopapular erythematous eruptions to trimethoprim-sulfamethoxazole are seen in patients infected with *Pneumocytis carinii.* Other common skin conditions associated with AIDS include worsening of preexisting psoriasis and atopic dermatitis, granuloma annularelike eruptions, vasculitis, eosinophilic folliculitis, telangiectasias, yellow nail syndrome, alopecia areata, vitiligo, persistent urticarial eruptions, and hypertrichosis of the cilia (Table 71-9.)[26]

The combination of KOH and Tzank preparations of skin scrapings along with skin biopsy with special stains for light microscopy and culture can give a preliminary diagnosis in many of these conditions.

SUBACUTE BACTERIAL ENDOCARDITIS

Frequent cutaneous manifestations of subacute bacterial endocarditis include petechiae, splinter hemorrhages, Osler nodes, and Janeway lesions. Petechiae occur as crops of small, reddish brown macular nonblanching lesions, often on the extremities and upper chest. They usually darken and fade within a few days. Histologic evidence of small-vessel inflammation (endothelial proliferation, hemorrhage, and lymphocytic inflammation) is present. Splinter hemorrhages are dark red streaks usually occurring near the middle third of finger and toenails. As the nail grows out, they move distally. Osler nodes (Fig. 71-4, Plate 31) are small, erythematous, painful, nodular lesions with whitish centers often located on the finger and toe pads, on the thenar and hypothenar eminences, and over the arms. They occur in crops lasting only hours to a few days, and they do not ulcerate. Histologic examination reveals evidence of immunologic phenomena with small-vessel arteritis of the skin. Janeway lesions (Fig. 71-5, Plate 32) are small

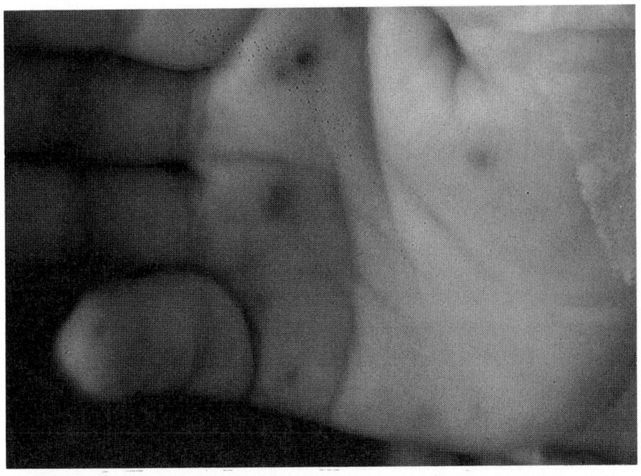

FIGURE 71-4 Osler's nodes: randomly distributed tender nodules on the palm of the hand in a patient with *Staphylococcus aureus* endocarditis. See Plate 31.

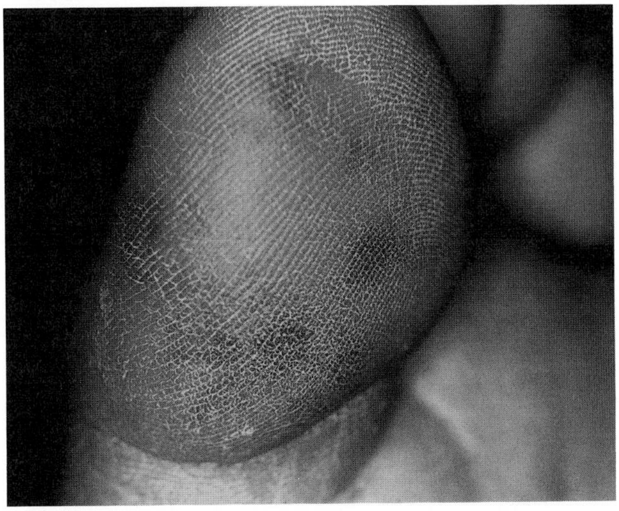

FIGURE 71-5 Subacute bacterial endocarditis: nontender, purpuric macules with irregular borders scattered on the toes (Janeway lesions). See Plate 32.

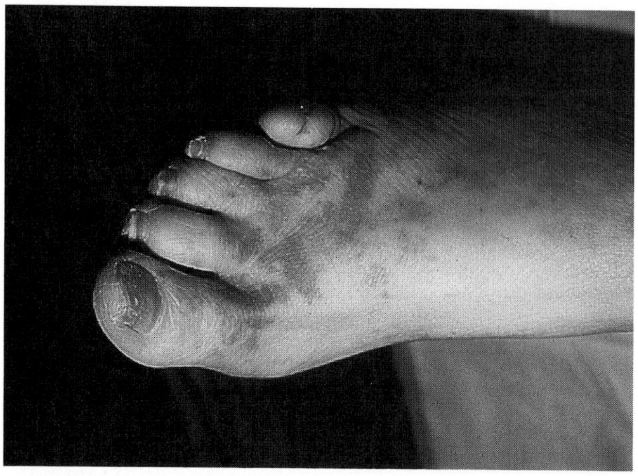

FIGURE 71-6 Meningococcemia: purpuric lesions with irregularly angulated borders. See Plate 33.

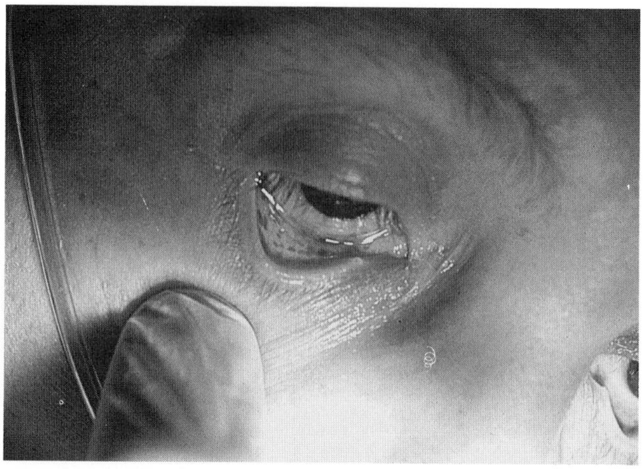

FIGURE 71-7 Meningococcemia: petechiae of the bulbar and palpebral conjunctivae. See Plate 34.

erythematous macules or nodular hemorrhages in the palms and soles. They are usually numerous and painless. On biopsy, polymorphonuclear infiltration of capillary walls, extravasated red blood cells, and dermal microabscesses are present.

SEPSIS

Patients with certain forms of sepsis, notably with *Neisseria gonorrhoeae, N. meningitidis,* and *Pseudomonas aeruginosa,* present distinctive cutaneous findings. The characteristic skin lesions of gonococcemia appear in crops of usually less than 10 lesions. They are distributed distally, especially near the joints. The primary macule rapidly evolves into a small, tender, hemorrhagic papule or umbilicated pustule with a red halo. Rarely, a hemorrhagic subepidermal bulla may become necrotic and heal with scarring. The skin lesions rarely yield organisms on conventional smears or cultures. Immunofluorescence studies demonstrate antigenic material both intra- and extracellularly around dermal blood vessels.

Although meningococcemia can be preceded by a prodrome (headache, nausea, vomiting, and fever), fulminant meningococcemia can present with rapidly progressing symptoms including hemorrhagic rash (Fig. 71-6, Plate 33), stupor, and hypotension within a few hours of the start of the disease. Petechiae are a prominent cutaneous sign, but urticarial or maculopapular eruptions are also seen initially. The petechiae are often palpable, with a smudgy appearance and pale, grey, vesicular centers. They are usually seen on the torso and extremities but can also appear on the palms, soles, head, and mucous membranes (Fig. 71-7, Plate 34). Bullous and hemorrhagic lesions with central necrosis and purpura fulminans (vide infra) occur when disseminated intravascular coagulation supervenes.

Several skin lesions can be seen with *Pseudomonas* septicemia, including vesicles and bullae, scattered either singly or in groups. They frequently become hemorrhagic. Ecthyma gangrenosum (Fig. 71-8, Plate 35) often evolves from these hemorrhagic vesicles as a round, indurated, painless lesion with surrounding erythema and a central necrotic grey-black eschar. It often presents in the axillae or anogenital region. Gangrenous cellulitis, a superficial, painless, sharply demarcated, necrotic ulcerlike lesion, arises in nonpressure-bearing areas. Multiple small painless maculopapular lesions can appear scattered over the torso. Nodular cellulitis appears after days or weeks as red, warm, fluctuant plaques that suppurate. Other lesions include scattered petechiae, ecchymoses, purpura fulminans, and erythema multiforme.

Similar cutaneous manifestations can complicate sepsis from many other sources seen in critically ill patients, including disseminated fungal infections such as candidiasis (Fig. 71-9, Plate 36) and aspergillosis.

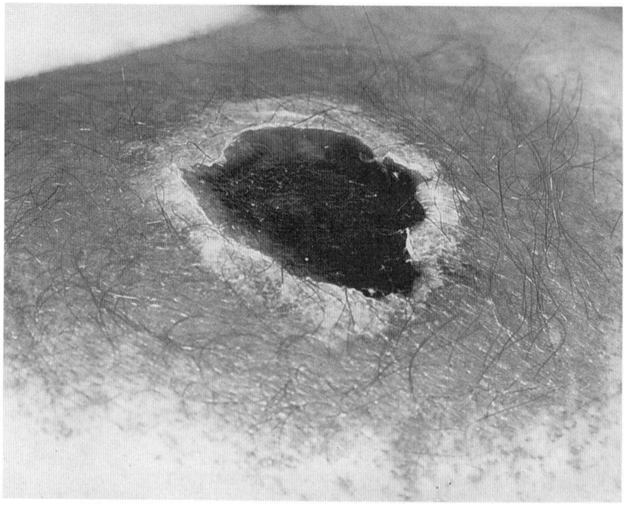

FIGURE 71-8 Ecthyma gangrenosum: necrosis and eschar formation on an erythematous base. See Plate 35.

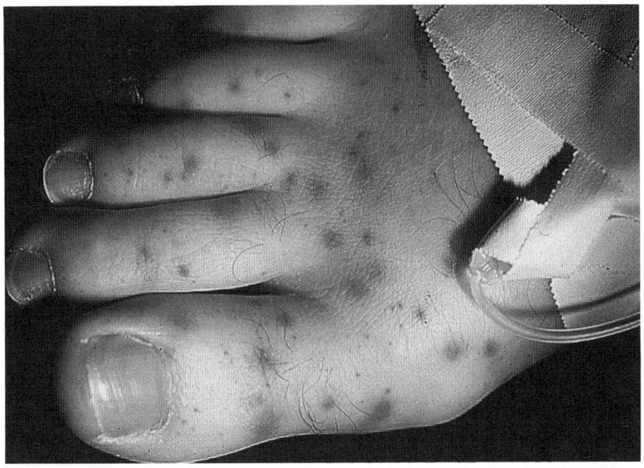

FIGURE 71-9 Candida sepsis: scattered papules, many of which progressed to pustules. See Plate 36.

PURPURA

Senile purpura is a noninflammatory purpura that arises from an age-related deficiency of the collagen surrounding cutaneous capillaries. On the dorsa of the hands and forearms of the elderly, these present as well-defined ecchymoses.

Drug purpura can be caused by numerous drugs; ampicillin, chlorothiazide, phenylbutazone, and sulfonamides are common culprits. The usual histologic picture is that of lymphocytic vasculitis. An infiltrate of mononuclear cells and eosinophils is clustered in and around small vessels of the skin. All areas of skin are involved and palpable purpura is the typical clinical picture. The vasculitis can involve multiple organ systems such as heart, lung, and kidneys, and death can occur.

Purpura fulminans is an uncommon, acute, often fatal nonspecific hemorrhagic infarction and necrosis of the skin secondary to disseminated intravascular coagulation occurring as a sequela of a variety of infections (mainly group A streptococcal infections, scarlet fever, staphylocccal and pneumococcal bacteremias, meningococcemia and varicella). The clinical manifestations appear during or after infection, with fever and rigors followed by the appearance of localized, massive ecchymoses with sharp, irregular borders. These lesions typically appear symmetrically over pressure points of the extremities but can also present on the lips, ears, nose, and trunk. They may be surrounded by a zone of erythema. They become edematous, develop hemorrhagic bullae, and can rapidly progress to gangrene over 48 to 72 h. Biopsy of involved skin shows fibrin thrombi occluding arterioles in the dermis. In the patients who survive, extensive skin grafting and amputation of affected areas are often necessary.

MALIGNANT INFILTRATES OF THE SKIN

Adenocarcinomas metastatic to the skin arise from all internal organs, including the prostate, kidney, colon, stomach, breast, and pancreas. A classic cutaneous finding is metastatic adenocarcinoma from the stomach or colon to the umbilicus, the "Sister Mary Joseph's nodule."

Several lymphoproliferative diseases can involve the skin. Cutaneous lesions of B cell lymphoma occur as a late event. Clinically these occur as indurated plaques or nodules, red to plum colored, smooth surfaced, solitary or multiple, either widespread or localized. They are usually palpable as firm, nontender, asymmetic, subcutaneous masses. Histologically the lymphocytes appear as dense nodular and diffuse monomorphic infiltrates with frequent central and adnexal necrosis. A zone of normal dermal collagen is usually present between the thin epidermis and the lymphomatous infiltrate that extends from the reticular dermis into the subcutis where it is most dense.

Cutaneous lesions of Hodgkins disease appear as small, reddish papules or nodules that often are adjacent to involved lymph nodes and tend to ulcerate. Histologically a lymphocytic infiltrate containing Reed-Sternberg cells is usually present.

Lymphocytoma cutis is a reactive cutaneous process that resembles a B cell lymphoma clinically and histologically but has a benign course. It often arises secondary to the trauma of an insect bite, scabies, tatoos, or ruptured cysts and presents as single to multiple red to plum-colored smooth papules or nodules that tend to spontaneously regress. Histologic examination permits differentiation from lymphoma. The infiltrate of lymphocytoma cutis is symmetric, well circumscribed, polymorphous, and more dense in the upper portion of the skin. Germinal centers and adnexal structures are unaffected, and there are no increased mitotic figures or necrosis present.

Leukemia cutis (Fig. 71-10, Plate 37) presents with localized or widespread erythroderma, nodules, plaques, or ulcers. Hemorrhage may be present in the lesions, which appear as purpura, petechiae, or ecchymoses. Erythema multiforme, erythema nodosum, and pyoderma gangrenosum can appear in these patients. Patients with myeloblastic leukemia can present with a particular greenish cutaneous nodule called a *chloroma,* which consists of myeloblasts containing myeloperoxidase. Histologic exam

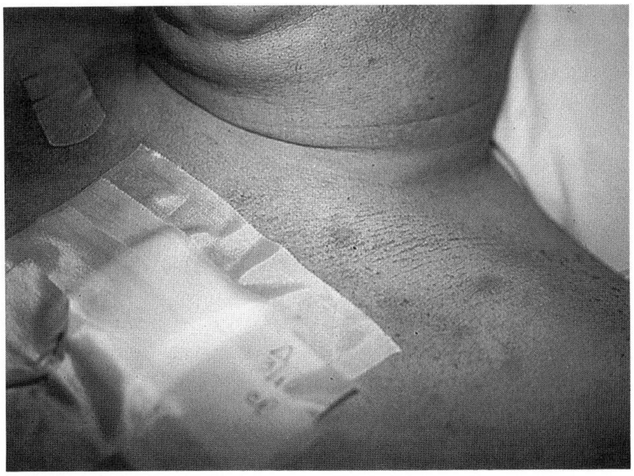

FIGURE 71-10 Leukemia cutis: soft, plum-colored nodules. See Plate 37.

of leukemic infiltrates reveals a zone of normal dermal collagen adjacent to the epidermis. Infiltrates of leukemic cells can be superficial or deep, perivascular, interstitial, or diffuse. There is often invasion of blood vessels by leukemic cells with abundant nuclear debris and extravasation of red cells.

HERPES SIMPLEX AND ZOSTER

Orofacial herpes simplex, caused by herpes simplex virus (HSV) type 1, produces an acute gingivostomatitis that occurs primarily in childhood or early adult life. Recurrences occur most commonly as herpes labialis, but any part of the skin or mucous membranes can be affected with grouped vesicles appearing on an erythematous base. Primary infection with HSV-2 usually occurs on the genitalia after genital contact with an infected individual. It also presents with grouped vesicles on an erythematous base, often with associated localized burning pain. With time, the cutaneous lesions of both of these become pustular and then crust over. Mucosal lesions quickly become eroded and appear as shallow ulcers.

Herpes zoster usually appears as grouped vesicles on an erythematous base along the dermatomal distribution of a sensory nerve. The erythematous base can appear hemorrhagic, and lesions can become necrotic and ulcerate. Occasionally satellite lesions appear beyond the dermatome, even on mucosal surfaces.

Immunosuppressed patients often have much more extensive involvement with herpes simplex and zoster. Herpes simplex lesions can develop into progressive deep facial, oral, and anogenital ulcerations. They can coalesce into large lesions leading to painful stomatitis from which the virus can be isolated for months and occasionally result in herpes esophagitis and pneumonitis. Immunocompromised patients develop disseminated herpes viremia and hepatitis; both the incidence and severity of herpes zoster infections are increased. The typical eruption can be either localized (often necrotic) or disseminated, and more than one episode may occur. Fatal systemic manifestations including pneumonia, gastroenteritis, and encephalitis can occur as complications. The incidence of zoster is notably increased in patients with advanced Hodgkin's disease.

Diagnosis can be made by Tzanck smear of material scraped from the base of a freshly unroofed vesicle found on the skin or mucous membrane; this shows multinucleated giant cells. Skin biopsy reveals intraepidermal vesicles with ballooning and reticular degeneration of epidermal cells as well as characteristic epithelial giant cells with intranuclear inclusion bodies. Immunomorphologic tests such as peroxidase-antiperoxidase and avidin-biotin tests on fixed tissue or smears can distinguish between HSV-1, HSV-2, and varicella, as can immunofluorescence using monoclonal antibodies. Virus isolation in tissue culture is still considered the gold standard for diagnosis.[27]

Therapy in these conditions has traditionally been with acyclovir. In immunocompromised patients with mucocutaneous herpes simplex, acyclovir seems to shorten the period of viral shedding, the time interval to healing, and the duration of pain. Since a single lesion can be a nidus for dissemination of disease, some suggest that topical acyclovir is useful in immunosuppressed patients; however it cannot suppress recurrence of disease. Oral acyclovir is more effective than topical acyclovir, but for severe or life-threatening infections, the intravenous route should be used. Oral doses of acyclovir are 400 mg by mouth five times daily for 10 days; intravenous doses are 5 mg/kg every 8 h for 7 days.

Resistance to acyclovir, associated with loss of viral thymidine kinase activity, has occurred infrequently in states of severe immunodeficiency. Severe persistent ulcerating mucocutaneous infections with acyclovir-resistant HSV-1 and HSV-2 are being seen with increasing frequency in patients with AIDS. Alternate therapies include foscarnet (trisodium phosphoformate), a pyrophosphate analog that inhibits HSV deoxyribonucleic acid (DNA) polymerase without requiring prior activation by viral thymidine kinase, and vidarabine, which is activated by cellular enzymes and inhibits HSV DNA polymerase.[28]

Acyclovir is also the mainstay of treatment of herpes zoster in immunocompromised patients. Topical acyclovir may benefit immunosuppressed patients by accelerating cutaneous healing. Oral acyclovir appears to be effective in zoster, not only when initiated in early stages but also in later stages. Intravenous acyclovir decreases new lesion formation, decreases pain, halts viral dissemination, and lessens visceral complications. Doses are slightly higher than for herpes simplex since the varicella virus is less sensitive to acyclovir: oral doses of 800 mg by mouth five times a day and intravenous doses of 500 mg/m^2 or 10 mg/kg every 8 h are recommended.[29]

Topical therapy for both herpes simplex and zoster is with saline compresses or Burow's solution (1:20 to 1:40) for 20 min every 8 h followed by the application of a topical antibiotic ointment (unless topical acyclovir is being applied).

CUTANEOUS NECROTIZING VASCULITIS

Necrotizing vasculitis refers to a group of disorders caused by immunologic or inflammatory mechanisms resulting in segmental inflammation and fibrinoid necrosis of blood vessels. The usual manifestation of hypersensitivity vasculitis in the skin, leukocytoclastic vasculitis, has distinctive histologic features: neutrophilic infiltration of vessels with karyorrhexis of nuclei. The most frequently postulated mechanism for this condition is local deposition of circulating immune complexes in venules with subsequent activation of the complement system.

Palpable purpura (Fig. 71-11, Plate 38) appears on dependent portions of the body (such as the lower extremities) or in areas subjected to pressure. Individual lesions can appear anywhere (usually sparing the palms, soles, face, and mucous membranes) and last up to 1 month before resolving, leaving hyperpigmentation or atrophic scars. Recurrent episodes can continue for weeks to years. Lesions are pruritic or produce a sensation of burning and can be preceded by fever, myalgias, arthralgias, and malaise. Other

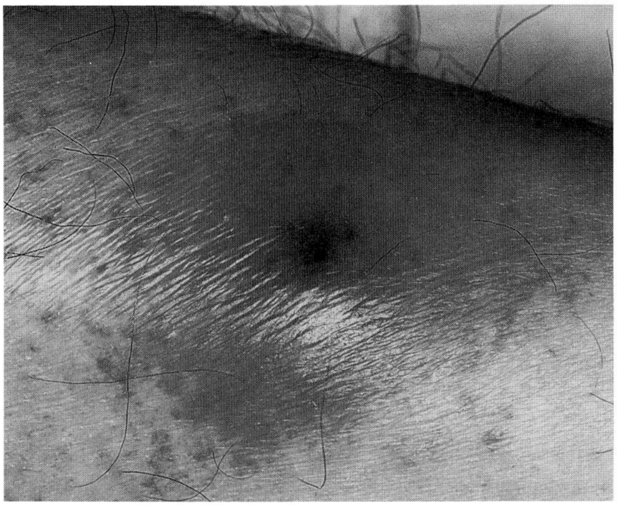

FIGURE 71-11 Vasculitis: erythema with nodular, grey, necrotic center. See Plate 38.

clinical manifestations such as urticaria, angioedema, nodules, pustules, vesicles, ulcers, livedo reticularis, and gangrene can accompany palpable purpura.

Clinical conditions signaled by cutaneous necrotizing vasculitis can be divided into three categories—coexistent chronic disorders, recent precipitating events, and idiopathic disorders. Coexistent chronic disorders include rheumatoid arthritis, Sjögren's syndrome, systemic lupus erythematosus, hypergammaglobulinemic purpura, lymphoproliferative disorders, cryoglobulinemia, ulcerative colitis, and cystic fibrosis. Recent precipitating events include infections with agents such as hepatitis B, group A β-hemolytic streptococci, *S. aureus,* and *Mycobacterium leprae.* Offending drugs precipitating a serum-sickness-like reaction mediated by immune complexes include sulfonamides, thiazides, penicillins, and radiocontrast media. Idiopathic disorders include Henoch-Schonlein purpura, chronic urticaria/angioedema syndromes, erythema elevatum diutinum, nodular vasculitis, livedoid vasculitis, and inherited C2 deficiency.[30]

BULLOUS PEMPHIGOID

Bullous pemphigoid is produced by the interaction of an IgG autoantibody with antigen(s) in the lamina lucida portion of the basement membrane zone of the skin. This is followed by activation of complement, neutrophil and eosinophil chemotaxis, enzyme activation, destruction of the basement membrane, and blister formation. This disease typically affects ages 50 to 70 with no racial or sex predominance.

Clinically, bullous pemphigoid is characterized by large, tense bullae appearing on normal or erythematous skin. These bullae often rupture, leaving denuded areas that usually heal without scarring. Urticarial, erythematous areas may be present and form round or serpiginous configurations. Usual sites for bullae are inner thighs, axillae, groin, flexor aspects of the forearms, lower abdomen, palms, and soles. Oral lesions, usually intact blisters, occur in one-third of patients. Other mucous membranes can be affected also. Pruritis may or may not be present.

Histologically, subepidermal microvesicles appear and evolve into subepidermal blisters containing neutrophils, eosinophils, lymphocytes, and fibrin. Direct immunofluorescence staining of individual blisters primarily reveals deposits of IgG and C3.

The patient's health is generally good, but those with widespread disease may appear quite ill. Treatment has traditionally been with corticosteroids (such as 50 to 100 mg prednisone daily), which are tapered to the lowest possible doses that suppress new blister formation. Immunosuppressive agents such as azathioprine can be used in combination with steroids to achieve a steroid-sparing effect. During therapy, monitoring for hyperglycemia, infections, and other side effects is essential. For elderly patients at excess risk of steroid side effects, high-dose erythromycin, sulfapyridine, and sulfones have been used.[31] If left untreated, this disease persists for months to years with periodic remissions and exacerbations, which are often less severe than the initial episodes.

DISSEMINATED CANDIDIASIS

This typically occurs against a background of hematologic malignancy, neutropenia, AIDS, thermal burns, major surgical procedures, intravenous alimentation, drug abuse, or extensive antibiotic therapy. Clinically, fever and myalgias precede the eruption of red to violaceous papules and nodules that appear predominantly over the trunk (Fig. 71-9, Plate 36).

Diagnosis is based on clinical background, skin biopsy specimens stained with PAS and Gomori silver stains for fungal elements, aspiration and culture of skin lesions, blood cultures, and frozen section muscle biopsy in certain cases.

The mainstay of therapy remains intravenous amphotericin B. Ketoconazole is useful for localized infections but not disseminated disease. Mortality remains high despite therapy. Attention has understandably focused on prophylaxis. Clotrimazole is useful for prevention of local oral disease. Ketoconazole is probably more effective than nystatin for oral prophylaxis but is not better for candida at other sites. Fluconazole, a newly developed imidazole agent, has a similar mechanism of action as other antifungals but does not inhibit mammalian sterol synthesis, and therefore has a higher safety profile. It is useful for localized disease.

SYSTEMIC LUPUS ERYTHEMATOSUS (SLE)

Approximately 20 percent of patients with SLE present with cutaneous signs. These usually consist of poorly demarcated, erythematous, slightly edematous patches primarily seen in the malar region. Any area of skin can be involved, particularly the palms and fingers. These lesions can be petechial, ulcerative, or vesicular (Fig. 71-12, Plate 39). In approximately 15 percent, well-defined discoid lesions [similar to discoid lupus erythematosus (DLE)] ap-

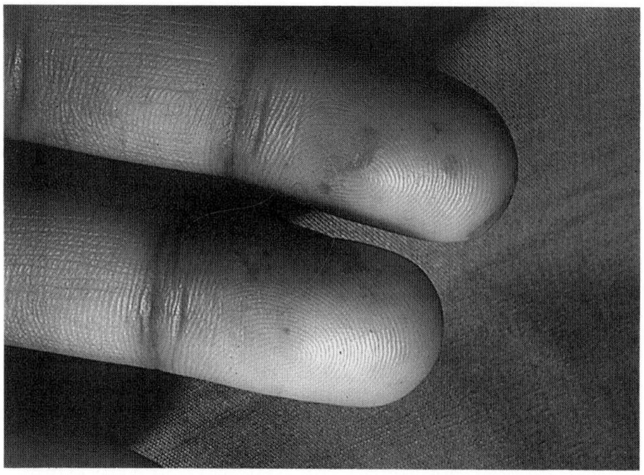

FIGURE 71-12 SLE: irregularly distributed and shaped erythematous, macular, digital infarcts. See Plate 39.

pear with atrophic scarring. These lesions precede other clinical signs of SLE and are associated with a more benign course. Occasionally overlap syndromes with features of scleroderma or dermatomyositis are seen. The other clinical findings and laboratory abnormalities will be discussed in Chap. 126 and will not be repeated here, except for the characteristic skin biopsy findings. In well-developed lesions there is hydropic degeneration of the basal layer, edema of the upper dermis, and extravasation of erythrocytes. Thickened dermal collagen bundles occur as a result of the deposition of fibrinoid material. A mild perivascular lymphohistiocytic infiltrate is often present. The subcutaneous fat often shows mucoid degeneration with a reactive lymphocytic infiltrate. Occasionally, nonpurpuric, pruritic urticaria-like lesions are present that show signs of leukocytoclastic vasculitis on biopsy.

Several drugs, notably procainamide, hydralazine, and diphenylhydantoin, can induce a syndrome identical to SLE. Drug-induced SLE is clinically, pathologically, and serologically similar to spontaneous SLE, but cutaneous manifestations are less common. Clinical and laboratory manifestations of this syndrome subside when the drug is discontinued.

OSLER-WEBER-RENDU SYNDROME

This familial disease is characterized by ectatic vessels in the skin, mucous membranes, and viscera. Epistaxis, the first manifestation of the disease, begins around puberty. The skin lesions appear after puberty and increase in number with advancing age. Telangiectases appear over the face, lips, nares, tongue, ears, hands, chest, and feet. Histologically they consist of dilated, thin-walled vessels often no larger than a single endothelial cell in thickness. Three morphologic types of superficial telangiectases occur in this disease. Puncta are most common and occur on skin and mucous membranes. They are discreet, red, and tiny (typically a few millimeters in diameter). They may be flat or slightly raised and are typically located on fingers, face, lips, and oral and nasal mucous membranes. These are prone to ulceration and hemorrhage. Spider and linear or branched telangiectases also occur. Because of intrapulmonary vascular lesions, brain abscess occasionally occurs. Treatment is symptomatic and directed toward prevention of hemorrhage. There is no spontaneous resolution of the lesions and prognosis must be guarded.

PORPHYRIA CUTANEA TARDA (PCT)

The symptoms of this disorder of heme biosynthesis usually present in the third or fourth decade. The biochemical defect, a deficiency in uroporphyrinogen decarboxylase, leads to an accumulation of uroporphyrinogens I and III as well as coproporphyrin and isocoproporphyrinogen. Patients develop moderate to severe photosensitivity leading to vesicular bullous and ulcerative lesions primarily on light exposed skin. Their skin has increased fragility to mechanical trauma. They develop hypertrichosis, periorbital violaceous coloration, scarring alopecia, hyperpigmentation, and sclerodermatous plaques along with milia on the fingers and hands.

Certain drugs (furosemide, tetracycline, nalidixic acid, and sulfonamides) and other conditions (hemodialysis, variegate porphyria, and epidermolysis bullosa acquisita) can mimic the skin lesions of PCT and must be excluded. In addition to a detailed history, skin biopsy of an intact blister with PAS staining gives a characteristic picture of hyaline deposition in upper dermal capillary walls and subepidermal bullae. Patients with PCT excrete increased amounts of porphyrins in the urine, which, when exposed to Wood's light, often shows pink-red fluorescence. Twenty-four-hour urine collections reveal increased uroporphyrin, coproporphyrin, and isocoproporphyrin. Isocoproporphyrin and coproporphyrin are elevated in the feces and uroporphyrin is elevated in the blood. The treatment of choice is phlebotomy; chloroquine in varying dose schedules is an alternative.[32]

CARBON MONOXIDE

The most characteristic sign of carbon monoxide poisoning is the cherry red color of the patient's skin and mucous membranes caused by the bright red compound carboxyhemoglobin. However, this sign is very insensitive, being seen in a small minority of cases. The pathophysiology, manifestations, and treatment of carbon monoxide poisoning are described in Chap. 175.

NECROLYTIC MIGRATORY ERYTHEMA

This condition consists of superficial, migratory, circinate and gyrate areas of erosive erythema accompanied by blistering. Intertrigo and stomatitis are also frequently present. The erythema occurs on dependent areas of the body, particularly over the extremities, trunk, and perioral and genital regions. These annular and arcuate lesions develop peripheral blisters that then desquamate and become necrotic. The oral and intertriginous erosions resemble mucocutaneous candidasis. Although classically seen in patients with glucagonomas, virtually identical skin lesions are also observed in patients with zinc, fatty acid, and amino acid deficiencies. Biopsies of skin lesions reveal characteristic epidermal destruction with dyskeratotic cells. Ultrastructural analysis shows vacuolar degeneration and lysis of organelles in the upper epidermis.

LOXOSCELISM

Five of the 13 species of *Loxosceles* have been associated with cutaneous loxoscelism. The brown recluse spider (*L. reclusa*) is widely distributed in the Midwest and Southwest and can be identified by the characteristic "violin" shape on its thorax. It usually bites humans during March and October when its habitat (closets, outbuildings) is disturbed. Among other proteins, its venom contains sphingomyelinase D, which produces skin necrosis (see Chap. 182).

The initially painless bite begins as a central papule followed by an irregular erythematous reaction within 6 to 12 h. This is followed by blister formation and often necrosis. The wound is usually nontender and nonpruritic. The necrotic areas heal slowly and may need skin grafting to promote healing. They are usually nontender and nonpruritic. The actual bite is hard to detect, and this syndrome is often confused with allergic reactions, abscesses, tick bites, and wasp stings. On biopsy, involved skin demonstrates platelet thrombi and acute vasculitis with leukocytic infiltrates.

Treatment includes application of ice and elevation to reduce local erythema and swelling, antihistamines for pruritis, and administration of oral dapsone (50 to 100 mg per day) to inhibit leukocytic infiltration. For patients with large lesions, antibiotics are indicated to reduce the incidence of secondary infection. Patients with marked systemic symptoms may benefit from corticosteroids, but they are not considered routine therapy. Primary excision is also not indicated for routine management of these bites.

ERYTHEMA CHRONICUM MIGRANS

In addition to fever, headache and myalgias, an early cutaneous marker of Lyme disease is erythema chronicum migrans. A large erythematous ring develops around the site of the tick bite (*Ixodes dammini* in the northeast and midwest United States and *I. pacificus* in California and Oregon) and gradually expands peripherally. The border is one or more centimeters wide, firm, smooth, and bluish red. In untreated patients, secondary annular lesions develop. Nearly all patients with erythema chronicum migrans have elevated Clq binding activity, and many are found to have circulating cryoglobulins.

Skin biopsy reveals epidermal spongiosis and parakeratosis at the bite site along with dermal edema and perivascular accumulation of mononuclear cells both at the bite site and elsewhere in the lesion.

CASE PRESENTATION

A 46-year-old white woman was an unrestrained driver in a motor vehicle accident, sustaining left-sided rib fractures, pulmonary contusion, a deep scalp laceration, and a small intracerebral hemorrhage. She was begun on dilantin, her mentation improved to near baseline, and she was promptly transferred from the ICU to the ward. Despite a therapeutic dilantin level a seizure on the fourth hospital day prompted the addition of phenobarbital. She thereafter remained seizure free, and her recovery was uneventful.

Discharge was planned for the eleventh day, but the patient complained of burning eyes, skin tenderness over the extremities, and malaise. Later that day the temperature rose to 38.0°C. The blood pressure was 110/70 mmHg, respirations 22/min, and heart rate 104/min. An erythematous, morbilliform rash with a pale, livid hue developed over the face and extremities. In the next 12 h, erythema deepened and became confluent and generalized. Vesicles appeared within the rash and expanded into large, irregularly shaped, flaccid bullae. Nikolsky's sign was positive and a tentative diagnosis of TEN was made. The patient was transferred to the burn ICU.

On examination the patient was ill-appearing, lethargic, and in mild respiratory distress. The blood pressure was 90/65 but improved with 3 L of saline. The respirations were 34 and shallow, the heart rate 122, and the temperature 38.8°C. The skin was diffusely erythematous, with widespread necrolysis affecting 70 percent of the body. The oral mucosa, lips, and conjunctivae were also erythematous, displaying few vesicles but widespread erosions. Abnormal laboratory findings included transaminases that were elevated three times above the upper limit of normal, bilirubin 2.3 mg/dL, albumin 2.4 g/dL, glucose 295 mg/dL, hemoglobin 8.6 g/dL, white blood cell count 19,000/mm^3 with 23 percent band forms. Arterial blood gas results were P_{O_2} 86 mmHg on 2 L/min nasal cannula, P_{CO_2} mmHg 30, ph 7.32. The lactate concentration was 3.5 mmol/L. The chest x-ray revealed scattered patchy infiltrates and recent rib fractures.

Blood, urine, and skin cultures were drawn, and empiric antimicrobial therapy was begun. Methylprednisolone, 50 mg every 6 h, was given intravenously and dilantin was discontinued. A soft feeding tube was placed to begin enteral feeding, and antacids and subcutaneous heparin, 5000 U twice daily, were initiated for prophylaxis. Necrotic skin was widely debrided and silver sulfadiazine cream, 1%, was applied. The patient was placed on a fluidized bed.

The next day oliguria developed and persisted despite fluid challenge. A pulmonary artery catheter was placed to exclude hypovolemia and revealed a pulmonary capillary wedge pressure of 16 mmHg and a cardiac output of 8.8 L/min. Dopamine, 2 μg/kg/min, was infused to improve renal perfusion. Fluid requirements reached 6 L per day, and a warming blanket was needed to maintain normal body temperature. Insulin was given to control hyperglycemia. On skin biopsy there was widespread eosinophilic necrosis of the epidermis with a plane of cleavage above the basement membrane, diagnostic of TEN.

Over the next 3 days, eyebrows and nails were shed. Progressive obtundation and respiratory distress mandated endotracheal intubation. Guaiac positive nasogastric aspirate and a fall in hemoglobin led to esophagogastroduodenoscopy, which showed diffuse, erosive esophagitis. Blood transfusions were required. Surveillance cultures of skin grew methicillin-resistant *Staphylococcus aureus* (MRSA). On the sixth ICU day, refractory hypotension led to cardiac arrest. Postmortem blood cultures grew MRSA.

CASE DISCUSSION

This case is, unfortunately, typical of the course in patients with severe destruction of the skin. The resulting fluid losses, temperature disregulation, and infectious complications are typical of TEN but can also be seen in EM major, severe pemphigus, exfoliative erythroderma, pustular psoriasis, and burns. In fact, the differential diagnosis in this patient initially should have included EM major, staphylococcal scalded skin syndrome, and generalized bullous fixed drug eruption. Early skin biopsy is often useful to provide a firm foundation for therapy, and here confirmed the clinical suspicion of TEN. Dilantin was considered the most likely precipitant, but barbiturates are also well-known causes.

The initial subjective complaints of the patient were harbingers of the subsequent devastating necrolysis. Repeated examinations of the skin were crucial for early diagnosis and showed a rapidly evolving eruption. Mucous membranes were involved and likely contributed to respiratory failure (aspiration) and possibly to infection. Had the patient survived, mucous membrane disease (especially conjunctival) might have created the greatest long-term morbidity.

Therapy for many severe skin disorders, including TEN, is largely supportive and has the potential to harm as well as aid the patient. For example, invasive monitoring devices may facilitate fluid management but also contribute to risk of infection. In order to maximize the benefit from these devices, they should always be placed to answer a well-formulated question (e.g., "Is oliguria due to a prerenal state?") and should be withdrawn when no questions remain. Similarly, antibiotics were prudently given in response to the sepsis syndrome but may have contributed to superinfection with the resistant *S. aureus* that led to death. The most controversial aspect of care is the use of high doses of corticosteroids. Lacking data from clinical investigations, the clinician faces a hopeless task of weighing incalculable risks and unproven benefits. In our patient, despite care that was meticulous, prompt, and well informed, the outcome was death. It is unclear whether this septic death was encouraged by our therapies or was merely the unavoidable consequence of catastrophic dermatologic illness.

References

1. Reinhoff HY. Toxic epidermal necrosis. John Hopkins Med J 51:326, 1982.
2. Lyell A. Toxic epidermal necrolysis: A reappraisal. Br J Derm 100:69, 1979.
3. Hashimoto K, Shafran KM, Webber PS, et al: Anti-cell surface pemphigus autoantibody stimulates plasminogen activator of human epidermal cells. A mechanism for the loss of epidermal cohesion and blister formation. J Exp Med 57:259, 1983.
4. Lever WF, Lever, GS: Treatment of pemphigus vulgaris: Results obtained in 84 patients between 1961 and 1982. Arch Dermatol 20:44, 1984.
5. Bystryn JC: Adjuvant therapy of pemphigus. Arch Derm 20:941, 1984.
6. Ryan TJ, Baker H: The prognosis of generalized pustular psoriasis. Br J Derm 85:407, 1971.
7. Yung CW, Ell SR, Soltani K, et al: Hyperlactatemia associated with pustular psoriasis and leukocytosis. Arch Dermatol 18:432, 1982.
8. Konrad K, Wolff K: Photochemotherapy for pustular psoriasis (von Zumbusch). Br J Derm 77:119, 1977.
9. Wolska H, Jablonska S, Bounameaux Y: Etretinate in severe psoriasis: Results of double blind study and maintenance therapy in pustular psoriasis. J Am Acad Dermatol 9:883, 1983.
10. Orfanos CE. Oral retinoids-present status. Br J Derm 103:473, 1989.
11. Baker H: Pustular psoriasis. Derm Clin 2:455, 1984.
12. Abrams I, McCarthy JT, Saunders SL: 101 cases of exfoliative dermatitis. Arch Dermatol 87:136, 1963.
13. Nicolis GD, Helwig EB: Exfoliative dermatitis: A clinicopathologic study of 135 cases. Arch Dermatol 108:788, 1973.
14. Huff, JC, Weston WL, Tonnesen MG: Erythema multiforme: A critical review of characteristics, diagnostic criteria, and causes. J Am Acad Dermatol 8:763, 1983.
15. Howland WW, Golitz LE, Weston WL, et al: Erythema multiforme: Clinical, histopathologic and immunologic study. J Am Acad Dermatol 10:438, 1984.
16. Edmond BJ, Huff JC, Weston WL: Erythema multiforme. Ped Clin N Am 30:631, 1983.
17. Elias PM, Fritsch PO: Erythema multiforme, in Fitzpatrick TB (ed): *Dermatology in General Medicine,* 3rd ed. New York, McGraw-Hill, 1987, pp 555–562.
18. Fitzpatrick JE, Thompson PB, Aelig JL, et al: Photosensitive recurrent erythema multiforme. J Am Acad Dermatol 9:419, 1983.
19. Arndt KA, Jick H: Rates of cutaneous reactions to drugs. JAMA 235:918, 1976.
20. Minaker RL, Rowe JW, Besdine RW. The geriatric patient, in Noble J (ed): *Textbook of General Medicine and Primary Care,* 1st ed. Boston, Little Brown and Company, 1987, pp 2239–2250.
21. Reuler JB, Cooney TG: The pressure sore: Pathophysiology and principles of management. Ann Intern Med 94:661, 1981.
22. Alexander CS, Sako Y, Mikulic E: Pedal gangrene associated with the use of dopamine. JAMA 12:591, 1975.
23. Hitch JM: Acneiform eruptions induced by drugs and chemicals. JAMA 200:879, 1976.
24. Berger RS, Stoner MF, Hobbs ER, et al: Cutaneous manifestations of early human immunodeficiency virus exposure. J Am Acad Dermatol 19:298, 1988.
25. Penneys NS: Cutaneous signs of AIDS. Derm Clin 7:571, 1989.
26. Sindrup JH, Weismann K, Petersen CS, et al: Skin and oral

mucous changes in patients infected with human immunodeficiency virus. Acta Derm Venereol 68:440, 1988.
27. Solomon AR: New diagnostic tests for herpes simplex and varicella zoster infections. J Am Acad Dermatol 18:218, 1988.
28. Chatis PA, Miller CH, Schrager LE, et al: Successful treatment with foscarnet of an acyclovir-resistant mucocutaneous infection with herpes simplex virus in a patient with acquired immunodeficiency syndrome. N Engl J Med 320:297, 1989.
29. Huff JC: Antiviral treatment of chickenpox and herpes zoster. J Am Acad Dermatol 18:204, 1988.
30. Soler NA, Wolff SM: Necrotizing vasculitis, in Fitzpatrick TB (ed): *Dermatology in General Medicine,* 3rd ed. New York: McGraw-Hill, 1987, pp 1300–1311.
31. Jordan RE: Bullous pemphigoid, cicatricial pemphigoid and chronic bullous dermatosis of childhood, in Fitzpatrick TB (ed): *Dermatology in General Medicine,* 3rd ed. New York: McGraw-Hill, 1987, pp 580–582.
32. Bickens DR, Pathak MA: The porphyrias, in Fitzpatrick TB (ed): *Dermatology in General Medicine,* 3rd ed. New York: McGraw-Hill, 1987, pp 1666–1715.

Chapter 72

HYPOTHERMIA

MITCHELL F. KEAMY III
JESSE HALL

KEY POINTS

- *Hypothermia is often obvious, as in victims of outdoor winter exposure or cold water immersion; however, a high index of suspicion of hypothermia is appropriate in the evaluation of the elderly or drug-intoxicated patient presenting with depressed mental status in winter months and in patients returning to the ICU following prolonged operative procedures.*
- *The goals of therapy are to institute methods of rewarming appropriate for the severity of body cooling and to anticipate cardiovascular instability during the rewarming phase which is not predictably responsive to usual vasoactive drug therapy.*
- *Abnormalities are noted in many organ systems in the hypothermic patient; in most cases these are best corrected by rewarming and do not need correction primarily.*
- *Below 30° to 32°C (86° to 89.6°F) shivering ceases, level of consciousness progressively declines and cardiac arrhythmias become more common; ventricular fibrillation and asystole are common below 28°C (82.4°F).*
- *Regulation of body pH is likely altered during cooling, with alkalemia relative to normothermia appropriate for the physicochemical changes that occur; when adjusting Pa_{CO_2} via controlled ventilation in the hypothermic patient, blood-gas values uncorrected for temperature may be used.*
- *The J or Osborne wave is a typical electrocardiographic (ECG) finding below a temperature of 33°C (91.4°F).*
- *The airway should be secured in any hypothermic patient who is not readily responsive and able to follow simple commands.*
- *During rewarming, massive volume infusion is often necessary as arterial and venous dilation occur.*
- *For patients with a core body temperature above 32°C (89.6°F), passive rewarming and supportive therapy are usually preferred; for lower temperatures with hemodynamic stability, peritoneal, gastric, bladder, and pleural lavage may be considered.*
- *If available, cardiopulmonary bypass should be considered for profoundly hypothermic patients or those with hemodynamic instability.*

Unlike ectotherms or hibernators, man does not respond to heat loss by orderly physiologic slowdown. Minimal or subclinical hypothermia (below 36.5°C, 97.7°F), results in shivering, peripheral vasoconstriction, and increased sympathetic activity, mechanisms which are directed at preventing further heat loss and restoring body temperature.[1] When core temperature falls below 30° to 32°C (86° to 89.6°F), shivering ceases and obtundation appears which progresses to coma with further cooling (Fig. 72-1). Hypothermia causes heart block and disorganization of cardiac rhythm, with ventricular fibrillation or asystole common below 28°C (82.4°F). This is the typical mechanism of hypothermia-induced death. Mortality from profound hypothermia is high, in some studies reaching 70 percent, reflecting the difficulties in resuscitating cold patients, the typical severity of intercurrent disease processes, and, in older literature, a lack of understanding of hypothermia physiology.

On the cellular level, hypothermia does result in an orderly attenuation of cellular metabolic and enzymatic processes. The loss of cellular membrane integrity and protein disorganization which characterizes cell death does not usually occur until freezing. Typically, mammalian cell injury from hypothermia is not manifested until rewarming provokes a reactivation of normal cellular respiration. Subsequent cell viability depends on adequate nutrient blood flow during the rewarming period and the degree and duration of ischemia experienced during hypothermia. From the standpoint of single cell processes and organ physiology, function is generally well preserved when normothermia is reestablished.

The goals of therapy in the management of severely hypothermic patients are to **1.** identify and treat the metabolic derangements which predispose to or complicate hypothermia; **2.** institute a definitive method of rewarming appropriate to the degree of hypothermia; and **3.** anticipate and treat the cardiac rhythm and cardiovascular instability that frequently arise during rewarming. This chapter will review approaches to each of these problems.

Heat Loss and Thermoregulation

Body temperature is not homogeneous. From a thermoregulatory perspective, the body is separated into two compartments, the core and the shell. The shell is those tissues, mainly the limbs, in which temperature varies under control from the hypothalamus to preserve or shed thermal energy. The core is that group of tissues which requires stable temperature and constant, high blood flow to maintain normal function.

Heat is transferred from the body by radiation, convection, conduction, and evaporation. The relative importance of the latter three is intuitive to anybody who has climbed from a bath or pool into a breeze (evaporation and convection) or who has lain on a concrete floor (conduction). Radiation is also a significant route for thermal loss, accounting for >50 percent of heat loss in the exposed individual at room temperature. In certain circumstances, environmental conditions may dramatically increase the rate of heat loss. Immersion in cold (<24°C [75.2°F]) water causes enormous and rapid heat loss by conduction. Wind may cause convective heat loss to increase fivefold, as reflected by the meteorologist's declaration of "wind-chill factors."

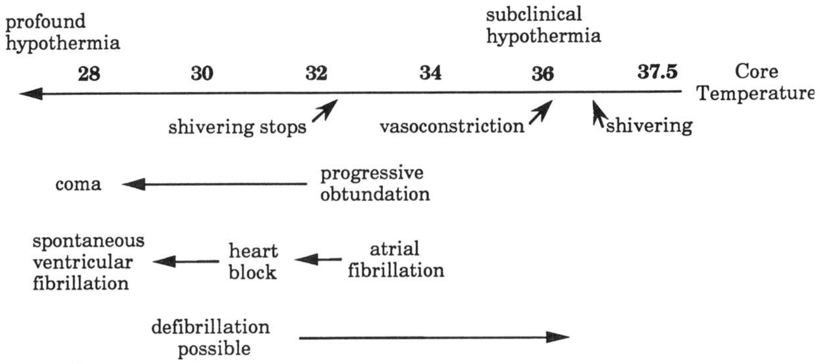

FIGURE 72-1 Major clinical events in relation to core temperature during hypothermia.

Heat is generated in the body by inherently inefficient metabolic processes. Under normal circumstances this inefficiency provides the heat energy required to maintain body temperature. In situations where losses exceed production, additional heat can be liberated by muscular shivering. Shivering can increase the normal muscle heat production fourfold, and the actual muscular work is expended moving internal elastic muscular elements, which likewise ends up as thermal energy. In infants, temperature can also be maintained by nonshivering thermogenesis through the metabolism of brown fat. Over periods of days to weeks, the normal thyroid axis can also adjust for increased heat loss by stimulating metabolism to foster greater heat generation as a by-product.

An additional important hypothermia defense is shell isolation. This is accomplished by progressive peripheral vasoconstriction, which begins at 36°C (96.8°F), and can become sufficiently intense to occlude limb blood flow. This can be accompanied by anaerobic metabolism in the extremities, which proceeds at an attenuated rate due to the decreased metabolism engendered by tissue hypothermia.

TABLE 72-1 Organ System Effects of Hypothermia

CNS
Reversible coma
Metabolism and Endocrine Disturbances
Increased metabolic rate with shivering
Oxygen consumption falls to 50% of normal at 26°C (78.8°F)
Hyperglycemia
Respiration and Acid-Base Disturbances
Diminished minute ventilation
Altered pH regulation
Increased aspiration risk
Cardiovascular and Renal Disorders
Dysrhythmias
Peripheral vasoconstriction
Typical ECG changes
Diuresis
Hematologic and Coagulation Disorders
Granulocytopenia
Platelet dysfunction
DIC?
Gastrointestinal Disturbances
Ileus
Pancreatitis

Hypothermic Effects on Organ System Function

Much of the previously documented mortality in hypothermia resuscitation has derived from lack of knowledge regarding intravascular volume shifts during resuscitation, lack of understanding of cardiac physiology during hypothermia, and lack of appreciation of other organ system effects of hypothermia. A thorough historical review of research in this field is available to the interested clinician.[2] Three decades of cardiac surgery, usually performed with hypothermic protection, have enhanced this understanding, and have placed the acute resuscitation of accidental hypothermia on more rational and less empirical grounds (Table 72-1). One key lesson acquired from induced hypothermia is that the intensivist should display a slow hand in dealing with the many secondary organ system derangements of accidental hypothermia because they are corrected by rewarming.

CENTRAL NERVOUS SYSTEM

The brain is largely impervious to permanent cold-induced injury in the range of body temperatures of 15° to 35°C (59° to 95°F). Indeed, cold is therapeutic to brain in the context of ischemia and hypoxia. Temperatures below 20°C (68°F) are well tolerated and allow total circulatory arrest for periods in excess of an hour with no deficits on rewarming. Acutely, intellectual function begins to be impaired at approximately 34°C (93.2°F), with progressive somnolence leading to unconsciousness below 28°C (82.4°F).[3] This is accompanied by an orderly decrease in electroencephalographic (EEG) activity with electrocerebral silence occurring below 26° to 28°C (78.8° to 82.4°F). These changes are fully reversible on rewarming.

METABOLISM AND ENDOCRINE DISTURBANCES

Initially, shivering provokes an increase in metabolic rate, which can increase oxygen consumption 400 to 600 percent above basal rate.[4] Once shivering abates, metabolic rate diminishes rapidly; at 26°C (78.8°F), the oxygen consumption will be <50 percent of basal. As a result of this decreased metabolic rate, a lesser cardiac output and lower perfusion pressure are well tolerated. Such circulation "abnormalities" need not be corrected until metabolism is increased by rewarming (vide infra).

Hypothermia provokes moderate elevations in glucose in a minority of patients. Other endocrine physiology remains essentially normal. Although cold does not induce endocrinopathy, the converse is not true. Hypoglycemia, diabetic ketoacidosis, and hyperosmolar coma may all cause hypothermia by suppressing hypothalamic temperature regulation or through the inhibition of shivering. Hypothyroidism is an uncommon finding in hypothermia but should always be considered in the differential diagnosis.

RESPIRATION AND ACID-BASE DISTURBANCES

Respiration slows and becomes shallow with hypothermia, once the added metabolic stimulus of shivering has abated. Pulmonary mechanics and gas exchange properties are preserved as hypothermia progresses. The observed hypopnea, which may be quite profound (respiratory rate <5/min at 25°C [77°F]) primarily reflects decreased respiratory requirements rather than pathologically depressed drive, although with temperatures below 24°C(75.2°F) apnea has been observed.

As body temperature falls, vertebrate blood pH regulation can follow two courses. Hibernators maintain pH constant at 7.4. This necessitates a relative respiratory acidosis to overcome temperature-induced shifts in the neutral pH of water. This is termed *pH-stat control.* Alternately, cold blooded animals (and probably man) allow an alkaline shift by relative hyperventilation. This shift is 0.015 pH units/°C and is termed *alpha-stat,* referring to the dissociation of the imidazole moiety of histidine. Alpha-stat regulation better preserves protein and enzyme function during hypothermia, preserves and stabilizes myocardial function, and facilitates normal cerebral autoregulation.[5] Thus, during hypothermia man is likely best allowed to be alkalemic, an appropriate adaptation to the chemical changes induced by the temperature drop. In cases in which Pa_{CO_2} is controlled by the physician (e.g., mechanical ventilatory support), this can be achieved by *not temperature correcting* pH and Pa_{CO_2} (measured at 37°C [98.6°F]) and taking the uncorrected values of $Pa_{CO_2} = 40$ mmHg and pH = 7.40 as desirable end points (vide infra).

The depressed consciousness that accompanies hypothermia causes a blunting of protective airway reflexes. The high incidence of pneumonia that accompanies successful hypothermia resuscitation likely results from pulmonary aspiration of gastric contents, combined with the progressive atelectasis that accompanies hypothermia-induced hypopnea.

CARDIOVASCULAR AND RENAL DISORDERS

From a cardiac standpoint, hypothermia is primarily an electrophysiologic disorder. Myocardial mechanics in the otherwise normal heart, while depressed with decreasing temperature, are sufficient to maintain adequate blood flow provided venous return is maintained and a perfusing rhythm is present. The cardiac ouput progressively decreases as the temperature drops below 30°C (86°F), partially as a result of decreased heart rate and partially as a response to decreased oxygen demand. Blood pressure and systemic vascular resistance are preserved until temperatures below 25°C (77°F) are attained. Most patients with accidental hypothermia are hypotensive due to reduced cardiac ouput and impaired sympathetic reflex increase in the systemic vascular resistance. This is less evident in induced hypothermia in the operating room, suggesting that accidental hypothermia is often complicated by relative hypovolemia (vide infra).

Arrhythmias are preceded by the appearance of characteristic J-junction elevation on the ECG (Fig. 72-2) which occurs below 33°C (91.4°F) and becomes more pronounced as temperature decreases. Atrial fibrillation is common below 33°C (91.4°F). Prolongation of the PR and QT intervals may be noted, and higher degrees of atrioventricular (AV) block or sinus bradycardia will accompany lower temperatures, until the heart becomes asystolic below 20°C (68°F). At 28°C (82.4°F) the heart becomes extremely irritable, and ventricular fibrillation may occur spontaneously or with mechanical, thermal, or biochemical irritation as might occur with line placement, pleural rewarming, or ischemic limb rewarming. This instability is evident during rewarming when ventricular arrhythmias have a higher incidence as the patient is warmed from 28° to 32°C (82.4° to 89.6°F). Once ventricular fibrillation occurs, it is difficult to convert until the temperature is increased above 30°C (86°F);[6] yet it is also difficult to prevent, so lidocaine or other antiarrhythmics are less effective than immediate detection and electrical conversion during rewarming.

Hypothermia results in a central redistribution of intravascular volume and causes an increase in peripheral vascular resistance as a result of shell vasoconstriction. Conversely, limb rewarming results in peripheral veno- and arteriodilation, likely potentiated by local ischemic metabolic influences. This has the effect of placing an increased demand on the heart for blood flow at the same time that venous blood is being pooled in the venous capacitance beds with impaired venous return. Thus, it is logical that immersion rewarming of profound hypothermia victims, if not accompanied by aggressive volume resuscitation, could result in abrupt cardiovascular collapse, as the cold heart is confronted with the burden of a reviving shell. The available evidence suggests that inotropic agents have little effect on the hypothermic heart, so therapy is directed at restoring circulating volume and rewarming. Meanwhile, the myocardium is subject to transient depression of contractility due to the effects of limb wash-out of ischemic products such as lactic acid and potassium.

Renal blood flow and glomerular filtration rate (GFR) decrease with hypothermia. Despite this decreased flow and GFR, urine output increases. The "cold diuresis" observed during hypothermia represents a response to the increase in core intravascular volume as blood distributes back to the trunk. Cold also blunts the renal tubular response to antidiuretic hormone.[7] Accordingly, oliguria is a later sign of hypoperfusion states in the hypothermic pa-

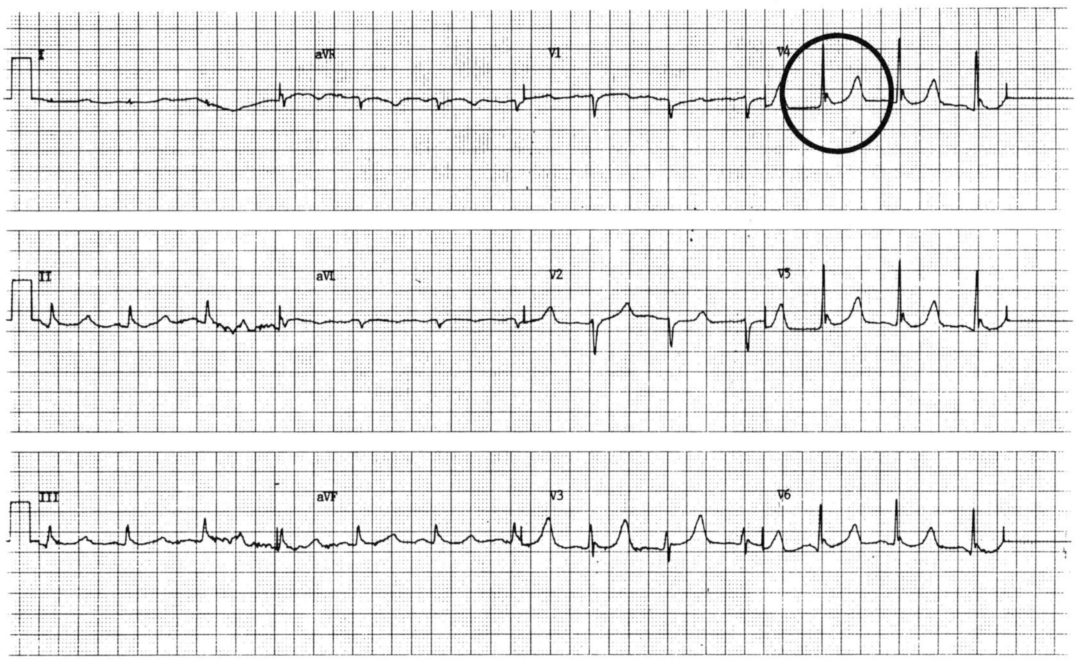

FIGURE 72-2 Typical ECG changes in hypothermia. Typically the rate is slow and the PR and QT intervals are long. Osborne or 'J waves' may be in evidence. They appear as a terminal addition to the QRS, with positive polarity in leads II and V_2 through V_6. Note circled complex in V_4. This tracing is atypical in that bradycardia is absent.

tient. On the plus side, bladder perfusion is maintained, so warmed lavage is a convenient method of core rewarming.

HEMATOLOGIC AND COAGULATION DISORDERS

Profound hypothermia (below 28°C, [82.4°F]), provokes granulocytopenia and may increase hematocrit by hemoconcentration.[8] Platelet count is diminished and function is impaired. Surgical hemostasis is consistently impaired by hypothermia; this coagulopathy is reversible if temperature can be elevated, but is not responsive to component therapy in the hypothermic patient.[9] Bleeding time is prolonged as temperature decreases, and this almost certainly represents cold-induced impairment of platelet function and enzymatic protein activity on which effective clotting depends. Tests such as the activated clotting time, prothrombin time, or partial thromboplastin time may yield normal results in the face of clinical coagulopathy, because these tests are performed in heated chambers which warm the blood to normal physiologic temperatures. Provided adequate factor levels are maintained (so that dilutional coagulopathy is avoided), coagulation should return to normal on rewarming. Disseminated intravascular coagulopathy (DIC) has been reported as a sequel to profound hypothermia, although convincing evidence of a specific etiologic link is lacking.

GASTROINTESTINAL DISTURBANCES

Ileus is a common gastrointestinal response to many systemic stresses; hypothermia is not an exception. Ileus typically resolves rapidly following rewarming. Asymptomatic pancreatitis is a common complication of hypothermia; more than half of recovered hypothermics have marked elevation in serum amylase, and autopsy evidence of pancreatitis is common.[10] These disturbances not withstanding, the upper gastrointestinal tract remains well perfused, so it is an ideal site for core rewarming with gastric or peritoneal lavage.

Clinical Presentation (Table 72-2)

Hypothermia is an obvious consideration in cold water immersion or winter outdoor exposure. In the modern urban hospital, hypothermia is likely to present in an obtunded elderly patient, often transported after being discovered indoors, with a host of apparent or potential organ system dysfunctions. A high index of suspicion is necessary, and a reliable measurement of body temperature should be made immediately on presentation. It should be suspected and excluded in all patients whose presentation or disease process suggests a long period of immobility, whether in a cold environment or not.

Hypothermia is frequently present in the elderly, either as a result of the prolonged muscular inactivity that can accompany the interlude between collapse (i.e., from stroke or hip fracture) and discovery or from chronic exposure to a mildly stressful thermal environment, such as a cool apartment. The elderly rely on the heat by-product of muscular activity to supplement waning metabolic processes. The decreased muscular activity and diminished cognitive compensatory capacity in the elderly render them particularly susceptible to hypothermia.

TABLE 72-2 Clinical Presentation of Hypothermia

Clear Instances of Exposure
Immersion
Winter outdoor exposure
Postoperative state
Extensive burns
Hypothermia Complicating Other Disorders
Elderly patients with diverse injuries
Prolonged immobility, even indoors
Drug use
Alcohol
Psychotropics
Barbiturates
Endocrinopathies
Hypoglycemia
Hyperosmolar coma and diabetic ketoacidosis
Myxedema coma
Spinal cord injuries
Sepsis

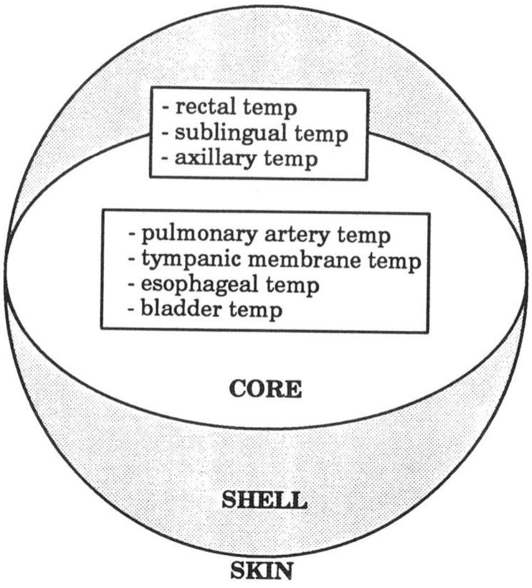

FIGURE 72-3 Temperature monitoring sites during hypothermia.

Alcohol and other sedating drugs simultaneously provoke lethargy, which diminishes muscular heat generation, and cause peripheral vasodilation, which enhances heat loss. Drugs such as alcohol and barbiturates may also act to directly suppress hypothalamic function. Hyperosmolar coma and diabetic ketoacidosis are associated with hypothermia; the mechanism has not been elucidated, but may relate to impaired hypothalamic functioning or decreased cellular metabolic activity. Hypoglycemia impairs hypothalamic temperature regulation, inhibits shivering, and provokes perspiration and vasodilation. Myxedema coma is a rare endocrinopathy, but the majority of patients present in winter and with subnormal temperatures. Spinal cord injury results in both decreased activity and impairs vasoconstriction in the affected limbs. Skin disruption from burns, bullous disease, or erythroderma greatly increases evaporative heat loss, which can rapidly provoke hypothermia. Finally, sepsis may produce mild hypothermia and remains a constant threat to the patient during the recovery from hypothermia with multisystem dysfunction.

Management

INSTRUMENTATION AND MONITORING

Diagnosis of hypothermia depends on measuring an accurate temperature (Fig. 72-3). The decline in use of the glass/mercury thermometer, with a lower limit of measured temperature of 32° to 33°C (89.6° to 91.4°F), in favor of electronic devices has dramatically aided the diagnosis of hypothermia. Virtually all electronic thermometers currently in clinical use will measure temperatures in the severe hypothermia range. Continuous electronic temperature systems are an integral part of all anesthesia monitoring locations and are easily transportable to the ICU.

No single site measurement can be expected to give an accurate picture of the patient's thermal status; better perspective can be obtained by measuring multiple sites sequentially, or optimally, continuously. Traditionally, sublingual, rectal, or axillary sites have been used. Site selection should reflect physiologic awareness of anatomic core and shell boundaries, tempered by the knowledge of local influences on individual sites (see Fig. 72-3). Axillary temperatures are obviously situated on a core-shell boundary and are probably poorly suited to assessing temperature in profound hypothermia. The rectal temperature should reflect visceral core temperature, provided the probe is not insulated by stool. Pulmonary artery blood temperature (by pulmonary artery catheter) and esophageal temperature are good measures of core temperature. Like sublingual temperature, these can be influenced somewhat by respiratory gas temperature and flow. Bladder temperature, which is commonly measured using special Foley catheter systems, is a good measure of visceral core, especially if urine output is brisk. Small probes which fit the external auditory canal allow measurement of tympanic membrane temperature. Tympanic membrane temperature is an excellent measure of core temperature since this region is warmed by cerebral blood flow.

In cases of profound hypothermia, it is generally preferable to monitor two sites simultaneously, and if possible, continuously. Logical site selection suggests at least one core temperature, and preferably, one that is not influenced excessively by the chosen rewarming technique. For instance, pulmonary artery monitoring may not reflect true core temperature during rewarming by cardiopulmonary bypass. Likewise, bladder temperature may be artificially elevated during warming by peritoneal irrigation.

Right heart catheterization may be difficult in profound hypothermia due to the low cardiac output. Literature which suggests excessive irritability of the hypothermic heart is anecdotal, and there are many equally anecdotal reports of successful instrumentation.[11] In patients with known or suspected intercurrent cardiomyopathy or other indications for the procedure, a pulmonary artery catheter is certainly worth the potential arrhythmia risk, but the intensivist needs to interpret the hypothermic hemodynamic data in such patients cautiously.

For example, a patient at a temperature of 28°C (82.4°F) with an arterial blood pressure of 90/70 with a cardiac index of 2 L/min/m^2 and a pulmonary artery wedge pressure of 15 mmHg probably needs no cardiovascular intervention except rewarming. In otherwise healthy, hemodynamically stable patients, management may not require invasive monitoring, provided the practitioner is willing to rapidly and empirically infuse the massive volume which is frequently required (2 to 8 L of warmed crystalloid) during rewarming.

An arterial line is mandatory for serial blood-gas and laboratory assays and to provide a measure of central blood pressure. Just as automated oscillometric blood pressure monitors may be foiled by peripheral vasoconstriction, peripheral percutaneous arterial catheter placement may be problematic. If peripheral pulses are not palpable or locatable by Doppler probe, a femoral cutdown should be performed. Pulse oximetry on the digits or ear lobes is ineffective due to hypothermia-induced vasoconstriction. A disposable finger probe arched over the bridge of the nose will often provide an adequate signal, but initial readings should be confirmed by arterial blood-gas analysis. Alternately, a pulmonary artery oximetry catheter will allow continuous mixed venous oxygen saturation, but interpretation to guide judgments concerning adequacy of tissue oxygen delivery is confounded by changing regional redistribution of cardiac output between core and shell.

Endotracheal intubation should be performed for airway protection unless the patient is reasonably alert and able to follow commands. Nasal intubation should be avoided because of the risk of epistaxis from hypothermia-induced coagulopathy. An orogastric tube should be inserted to aspirate gastric contents. This reinforces the imperfect protection against pulmonary aspiration offered by the cuffed endotracheal tube, and begins early treatment of hypothermia-induced ileus. This may be changed to a nasogastric tube for patient comfort if it is still required once the patient is rewarmed. A Foley catheter and a continuous ECG should be used for obvious reasons.

REWARMING

Rewarming is the single most effective therapy for the hypothermic patient. It should be initiated immediately in all hypothermic patients admitted to the ICU. Current rewarming strategies segregate into three categories based on invasiveness, ranging from minimally invasive surface rewarming to cardiopulmonary bypass (Fig. 72-4). No matter which techniques are selected, care should be taken to minimize further thermal loss by keeping the patient dry and covered, by humidifying inspired gases, and by using warm intravenous fluids. A convenient way to effect adequate warming of intravenous solutions is to use a blood warming coil. Alternately crystalloid solutions can be heated in a microwave unit, but extreme care must be taken to avoid overheating, since this can result in hemolysis on infusion. Fluid should be warmed to 36° to 39°C (96.8° to 102.2°F). As such, it does not result in significant warming of the patient, but does avoid further hypothermic insult.

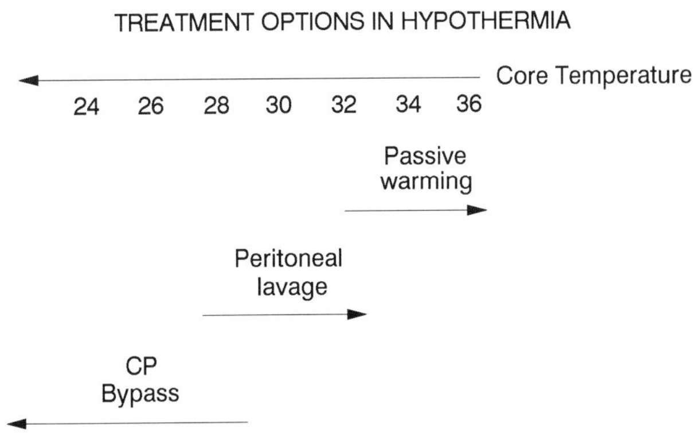

FIGURE 72-4 Treatment options in hypothermia. Treatment should not be determined only by core temperature, but should also take into consideration age, cardiovascular stability, and associated disorders (see text).

The decision as to whether to actively rewarm, and by what technique, depends on judgments concerning the patient's physiologic ability to participate in rewarming and the severity of the hypothermia. Above 32°C (89.6°F), virtually all patients will rewarm themselves, provided external hypothermic stresses are removed. With proper insulation, patients will rewarm at 1 to 3°C/h, depending on their metabolic state and intensity of shivering. Blankets, humidified inspired gas, and warm fluids are typically sufficient. Exceptions include patients for whom the cardiovascular stress of shivering needs to be avoided (such as patients with myocardial ischemia). Minimally invasive active rewarming is probably indicated in these individuals. Shivering, in particular, can induce fivefold increases in oxygen consumption and consequently, increases in myocardial work load. Shivering is regulated centrally by the hypothalamus and peripherally by skin temperature.[12] Shivering can be suppressed somewhat by radiant skin warming or warm blankets. Demerol in moderate doses (25 mg intravenously) is also effective in suppressing shivering. In patients who are intubated, ventilated, and sedated, neuromuscular blockade will dramatically decrease oxygen consumption due to shivering, allowing exogenous rewarming.

Below 32°C (89.6°F), warming should be more aggressive, especially in the elderly or in patients with intercurrent disease processes. Somewhere below 32°C (89.6°F) shivering will stop, heralding the onset of metabolic slowdown to a hibernation-like state. An otherwise fit young person will likely self-warm from this temperature with simple heat-preserving measures and with no systemic sequelae expected.

Heat-preserving measures rely on limiting loss through the mechanisms of radiation, evaporation, conduction, and convection. The scalp has particularly high blood flow, and especially in bald patients, dramatic radiative and convective losses can occur through the head. In the operating suite, where patients are unconscious and intubated, plastic trash bags placed over the head provide a convenient barrier to evaporation and convection, although radiation is only slightly impeded. Evaporation is a potent source of heat loss because the heat of vaporization of water is high. Well-humidified inspiratory gas eliminates the loss of heat required to otherwise humidify respiratory gas in the tracheobronchial tree. Skin surfaces should be kept dry. Convection can be countered simply by keeping the patient covered and by ensuring that the circulating air from flotation beds is properly warmed.

A wide variety of techniques have been used for minimally invasive active rewarming of mild or moderate hypothermia (>30°C [86°F] and <36°C [96.8°F]). Warm water immersion is slow and is intuitively impractical because it limits care giver access to the patient. It can be dangerous for the reasons cited earlier, but may be acceptable for patients with mild hypothermia. In general, efforts at conductive surface warming (i.e., warming blankets) will be unsuccessful due to the low body surface area: mass ratio of adults. In patients with mild hypothermia, surface rewarming will probably be adequate if augmented by convection, as in some of the newer warm air circulating systems (BAIR Hugger). Radiative warmers are likewise likely to be ineffective in adults, both because of low body surface area, and because the exposed integument which is required for heat lamps to work allows evaporative, conductive, and radiative losses to the surroundings.

Administration of warm respiratory gases is largely ineffective, because of the low specific heat (and thus, low heat transport capacity) of nitrogen and oxygen.[13] The use of extremely hot (60°C [140°F]), inspired gas, although advocated by some, should be avoided because of the risk of airway mucosal injury. Although never formally investigated, helium, with its much higher specific heat, might have a role in airway warming. On the other hand, the heat of vaporization of water is high. The administration of dry inspired gases at any temperature forces humidification by the respiratory system at a high thermal cost to vaporize airway water. This is to be assiduously avoided in hypothermics, lest other efforts at rewarming be foiled.

Warm gastric or bladder irrigation is probably insufficient in profound hypothermia and unnecessary in mild hypothermia. Yet these sites are usually immediately accessible and many more effective measures are rendered unnecessary when a member of the care-giving team is assigned to these irrigations while the patient awaits access sites for the more effective measures. If undertaken, isotonic solutions should be used, exchange volume should be measured to ensure appropriate volume return, and solution temperature should be <41°C (105.8°F) to avoid mucosal injury.

Pleural lavage has been studied with intercurrent open-chest cardiac massage and has been found to be effective in heat transfer to hypothermic patients. A more practical technique is peritoneal lavage with warmed (up to 43°C [109.4°F]), isotonic peritoneal dialysate. This transfer process can be hastened with the insertion of two catheters to allow flow-through irrigation and is the current technique of choice for profoundly hypothermic patients with intact cardiac function.[14] Rewarming can be expected to occur at 1.5° to 3°C/h.

If available, mechanical bypass of blood flow should be instituted in patients with unstable hemodynamics.[15] In those patients in frank arrest, the femoral vessels should be cannulated to institute venoarterial bypass. In these patients, even with membrane oxygenation on bypass, if external cardiac massage is elected, it should be accompanied by ventilation, lest deoxygenated blood from the external massage flow up the carotids and provoke cerebral hypoxia. In patients with intact cardiac function, venovenous bypass can theoretically be instituted; while inherently safer, it does not allow for artificial circulatory support in the case of ensuing arrest. Warming can proceed in excess of 10°C/h with extracorporeal warming, although the rate of warming is limited somewhat by the need to avoid extreme transmyocardial thermal gradients; a gradient of >2°C can provoke ventricular fibrillation.

Cardiopulmonary bypass requires pharmacologic anticoagulation. Prolonged extracorporeal membrane oxygenation can be accomplished with a partial thromboplastin time of 80 s or less, or an activated clotting time of 180 s, if careful attention is paid to maintaining low turbulence connections and a membrane oxygenator is used.[16] Even minimal anticoagulation may provoke lethal hemorrhage in the traumatized hypothermic patient, however. Recent clinical trials of a passive arteriovenous fistula heat exchanging device which does not require anticoagulation have been undertaken. A commercial device is not available as yet and, of course, it requires intact hemodynamics.

A protocol should be established in advance with the cardiothoracic surgical team which includes entrance criteria, notification procedure, and whether cannulation must be performed in the operating suite. Indications include core temperature below 25°C (77°F) or core temperature below 30°C (86°F) with cardiac arrest without other intercurrent processes that preclude anticoagulation. The recent interest in emergency cardiopulmonary bypass for cardiovascular support of the arresting patient should facilitate the future availability of perfusion support for the resuscitation of hypothermia victims.

SUPPORTIVE THERAPY

RESPIRATORY. Blood-gas levels should be managed using an alpha-stat protocol. Evidence has mounted over the past decade to suggest that myocardial electrophysiologic stability and mechanical performance is enhanced with alpha-stat regulation, and cerebral blood flow autoregulation is better maintained.[9] This coincides with theoretical formulations which encourage alpha-stat pH management based on enzyme performance and isolated blood behavior.[17]

Blood pH shifts alkalotic with decreasing temperature just as the whole body does. This makes alpha-stat management simple and straightforward. Arterial blood is, of course, drawn at patient temperature. The blood-gas analyzer then warms the blood to a standard 37°C (98.6°F) prior to analysis. In warming, the isolated blood sample rapidly temperature equilibrates the pH down, becoming more acidotic by 0.015 pH units/°C. Thus, if arterial pH and Pa_{CO_2} are reported to the practitioner at 37°C (98.6°F) (*not* corrected to the patient's body temperature), the practitioner may adjust ventilation to set the pH to 7.4 at 37°C (98.6°F), knowing that the patients' actual pH is appropriately more alkalotic at 0.015 pH units per degree below 37°C (98.6°F). Thus, the clinician is advised not to use nomogram temperature correction for pH and Pa_{CO_2}. Temperature correction is important, however, for Pa_{O_2} and hemoglobin saturation (Sa_{O_2}) determination. Thus, in our blood-gas laboratory both 37°C (98.6°F) and patient temperature corrected blood-gas values are reported. The corrected Pa_{O_2} and Sa_{O_2} are used in assessing cardiopulmonary function and oxygen delivery. The uncorrected pH and Pa_{CO_2} are used to regulate ventilation in those hypothermic patients requiring mechanical support.

CARDIOVASCULAR. Patients with a perfusing rhythm require early repletion of their circulating volume; all intravenous solutions should be warmed as described above. When hypotension persists after a volume challenge, care to ensure adequate volume repletion includes central venous pressure or pulmonary artery pressure monitoring. Persistent hypotension with adequate circulating volume focuses therapy on rewarming, for otherwise indicated inotropic and vasoactive drugs (dobutamine, dopamine) are ineffective and arrhythmogenic.

The majority of patients who are cold and asystolic on initial presentation are, in fact, dead. The adage "nobody is dead unless they are warm and dead" begs the necessity for triage based on scarce resource allocation in the modern intensive care and emergency departments. Once instituted, resuscitation of the hypothermic patient must proceed until a core temperature of 30°C (86°F) or better is obtained, at which time spontaneous cardioversion becomes likely in survivors. Separating the potential survivors from the nonsalvageable requires consideration of history and current patient condition.

Any sign of viability should prompt aggressive resuscitative efforts. Such signs may be subtle, given the tendency for profound bradycardia, hypopnea, and the vasoconstrictive obliteration of peripheral pulses. No single prognostic indicator precludes successful resuscitation in the apparently lifeless hypothermic patient. Patients have been resuscitated from well below 20°C (68°F), as have patients who have been in apparent arrest for over 2 h. Severe hyperkalemia (>10 mM/L) is a probable marker of death preceding hypothermia, provided specific nonlethal etiologies (such as hemolysis, chronic renal failure, crush injury) are excluded.[18,19] Gradual hypothermia promotes mild hypokalemia through "cold diuresis," and rapid hypothermia does not affect serum potassium.

External cardiac massage is as effective as open-chest massage in these patients. Intubation is, of course, mandatory. There is no evidence to suggest that intrapleural warm irrigation is more effective than peritoneal lavage, and peritoneal lavage is safer and more easily instituted. In general, antiarrhythmics are ineffective in profound hypothermia. The notable exception may be bretylium, which decreases the occurrence of ventricular fibrillation in a hypothermic dog model, and facilitates defibrillation.[20] Transvenous pacing cannot be relied on to capture the cold myocardium and may stimulate ventricular fibrillation. A trial of electrical defibrillation is probably indicated, although results should not be expected until the core temperature is >30°C (86°F). Lifelessness persisting as the temperature approaches 31°C (87.8°F) may be reasonably considered to indicate death.

Postrewarming and postresuscitation therapy consists of routine supportive cardiorespiratory care, along with diagnostic efforts to exclude common causative or related pathologic processes, such as drug or alcohol toxicity, renal failure, frostbite, or rhabdomyolysis. Glucose metabolism must be monitored closely, and many patients will require laboratory testing for hypothyroidism. The threshold for using empirical antibiotics or investigating for sources of sepsis should be low.

Areas of frostbite should be initially treated with rapid rewarming at 40° to 44°C (104° to 111.2°F). Regional vasodilator therapy with reserpine or by sympathectomy has been successful in reversing the intense local vasospasm that accompanies this injury, whereas anticoagulation is controversial. In the absence of secondary infection, demarcation of necrotic areas is typically allowed to proceed to salvage as much viable tissue as possible.[21]

CASE PRESENTATION

A 65-year-old woman was brought unresponsive to the emergency room in the month of March. She was said by her neighbors to have a history of heavy alcohol use. When she was not seen for 2 days, her landlord entered her apartment and found her unresponsive on the floor. Paramedics were called and obtained a Dexi-stick of <100 mg/dL. An ampule of 50% dextrose was given with minimal response and she was transported to the hospital.

On arrival the patient grimaced to deep pain but was unresponsive to voice. Distal pulses were absent, but a carotid pulse was readily palpable and a brachial blood pressure by Doppler probe appeared to be 80 systolic. The heart rate was 76 and respirations 8. A glass rectal thermometer was inserted and a temperature of 33°C (91.4°F) recorded. The patient's neurologic examination was nonfocal and no meningeal signs were present. The cardiac and lung examinations were unremarkable, as was the abdomen. Examination of the extremities revealed a shortened and outwardly rotated right leg.

The patient was promptly intubated via an oral approach and placed on a ventilator with F_{IO_2} of 1.0, tidal volume 500 mL, and respiratory rate of 10; 50% glucose, naloxone, and thiamine were given intravenously without obvious clinical response. Venous blood was sent for routine chemistries, CBC, thyroid functions, alcohol level, and toxic screen. A chest radiograph revealed good endotracheal tube position and right and left midlung field infiltrates suggesting aspiration. An ECG revealed prominent J waves (see Fig. 72-2). Multiple attempts at arterial puncture were unsuccessful and an adequate pulse oximetry signal could not be obtained. The patient was covered with a warming blanket and transferred to the ICU.

On arrival in the ICU a thermocouple rectal temperature of 27°C (80.6°F) was recorded. An inspired gas humidification system set at 41°C (105.8°F) was put in place and the rectal temperature probe left in place for continuous readings. Intravenous saline solution was run through a warming coil set at 40°C (104°F). A large bore catheter was placed in the stomach and a Foley catheter placed; lavage with 42°C (107.6°F) saline solution was conducted at both sites with recording of lavage volumes. A peritoneal catheter was placed at the bedside under direct vision and peritoneal lavage begun. A right femoral cutdown was performed and an arterial catheter placed; the initial blood pressure measured at this site was 100/75. The initial blood-gas determination was:

	37°C (98.6°F)	Corrected to 27°C (80.6°F)
pH	7.38	7.54
Pa_{CO_2}	37	23
Pa_{O_2}	108	53
Sa_{O_2}	98%	98%

The minute ventilation was not altered but positive end-expiratory pressure (PEEP) at 10 cmH_2O was added and the FI_{O_2} decreased to 0.6. Antibiosis with a third generation cephalosporin and aminoglycoside was begun.

A repeat blood-gas study revealed:

	37°C (98.6°F)	Corrected to 28.5°C (83.9°F)
pH	7.32	7.45
Pa_{CO_2}	39	26
Pa_{O_2}	80	44
Sa_{O_2}	95%	95%

The patient's body temperature rose approximately 1 to 1.5° each hour. At a temperature of 30.5°C (87°F) the patient manifested atrial fibrillation with a slow ventricular response. The systolic blood pressure fell to 70 mmHg, with an increase to 90 mmHg after 2 L normal saline solution was given by rapid infusion. A repeat ECG suggested lateral ischemic changes. Right heart catheterization was performed but was difficult and fluoroscopy was necessary for placement. This revealed a right atrial pressure of 6 mmHg, right ventricular pressure of 28/4 mmHg, pulmonary artery pressure of 26/15 mmHg, and pulmonary capillary wedge pressure of 4 mmHg. The cardiac output was 2.1 L/min with an $(a - v)_{O_2}$ of 6 vol%. With further volume infusion of 2 L crystalloid the wedge pressure rose to 8 mm Hg, the cardiac output to 3 L/min, and the $(a - v)_{O_2}$ decreased to 4 vol%.

At a temperature of 32°C (89.6°F) the patient had spontaneous ventricular fibrillation which responded to defibrillation. The right heart catheter was discontinued and bretylium infusion started.

The patient's hypothermia fully corrected over the next 6 h. Increasing amounts of minute ventilation were necessary to maintain an uncorrected Pa_{CO_2} of 40 mmHg. Her toxic screen was unremarkable, as was a lumbar puncture. Her mental status steadily improved with warming, and her thyroid studies were normal. She required mechanical ventilatory support for a presumed aspiration pneumonia for 3 days. Enteral feedings were delayed because of biochemical evidence of pancreatitis and parenteral nutrition was started instead. One week following admission she underwent surgical repair of her fractured hip.

CASE DISCUSSION

This is a typical case of hypothermia as encountered in the modern urban hospital—the elderly patient discovered indoors but incapacitated for a sufficiently long time for even mild environmental stress to cause moderate to severe hypothermia. The initial use of a glass thermometer was inappropriate and resulted in a delay of appreciation of the severity of her environmental injury. The inability to detect peripheral pulses, the need to perform a cutdown for arterial access, and the need for immediate protection of the airway are also typical features of early management.

When the severity of the hypothermia was appreciated, active rewarming was undertaken. In most instances, this can be accomplished without establishing extracorporeal circulation. The initial ventilatory management of the patient was accomplished by using uncorrected blood-gas values for adjustment of Pa_{CO_2} and pH, and corrected Sa_{O_2}. Remarkably little minute ventilation was necessary initially since oxygen consumption and carbon dioxide production are markedly reduced during hypothermia.

Cardiovascular instability is common during rewarming and usually relates to either vasodilation and a requirement for massive volume infusion or cardiac arrhythmias. Both occurred in this patient. When clinical data became confusing, pulmonary artery catheterization was conducted which confirmed ongoing hypovolemia. Interestingly, this invasive data also demonstrated the low oxygen consumption typical of these patients until hypothermia is corrected.

Longer term complications of her illness included aspiration pneumonia and pancreatitis, common problems in the hypothermic patient. Appropriately, complicating disorders such as drug overdose and hypothyroidism were sought and excluded.

References

1. Hardy JD: Body temperature regulation, in Mountcastle VB: *Medical Physiology*. Mosby, St. Louis, 1980, pp 1417–1456.

2. Moss JM: Accidental severe hypothermia. Surg Gynecol Obstet 162:501, 1986.
3. Michenfelder JD: The hypothermic brain, in Michenfelder JD: *Anesthesia and the Brain.* Churchill Livingstone, New York, 1988, pp 23–34.
4. Bay J, Nunn JF, Prys-Roberts C: Factors influencing arterial P_{O_2} during recovery from anaesthesia. Br J Anaesth 40:398, 1968.
5. Ream AK, Reitz BA, Silverberg GS: Temperature correction of Pc_{O_2} and pH in estimating acid-base status. Anesthesiology 56:41, 1982.
6. Mouritzen C, Andersen N: Myocardial temperature gradients and ventricular fibrillation during hypothermia. J Thorac Cardiovas Surg 49:937, 1965.
7. Rosenfeld JB: Acid-base and electrolyte disturbances in hypothermia. Am J Cardiol 12:673, 1963.
8. Kanter GS: Hypothermic hemoconcentration. Am J Physiol 214:856, 1968.
9. Curley FJ, Irwin RS: Disorders of temperature control: Hypothermia, part III, J Intensive Care Med 1:270, 1986.
10. Maclean D. Murison J, Griffiths PD: Acute pancreatitis and diabetic ketoacidosis in accidental hypothermia and hypothermic myxoedema. Br Med J; 4:757, 1973.
11. Harari A, Regnier B, Rapin M, et al: Hemodynamic study of prolonged deep accidental hypothermia. Eur J Intensive Care Med 1:65, 1975.
12. Simon E, Pierau-FK, Taylor DC: Central and peripheral thermal control of effectors in homeothermic temperature regulation. Physiol Rev 66(2):235, 1986.
13. Hendrickx HH, Trahey GE, Argentieri MP: Paradoxical inhibition of decreases in body temperature by use of heated and humidified gases. Anesth Analg 61(4):393, 1982.
14. Pickering BG, Bristow GK, Craig DB: Core rewarming by peritoneal irrigation in accidental hypothermia with cardiac arrest. Anesth Analg 56:574, 1977.
15. Wickstrom E, Ruiz E, Lilja GP, et al: Accidental hypothermia: Core rewarming with partial bypass. Am J Surg 131:622, 1976.
16. Snider MT, Campbell DB, Kofke WA, et al: Venovenous perfusion of adults and children with severe acute respiratory distress syndrome. The Pennsylvania State University experience from 1982–1987. ASAIO Trans 34(4):1014, 1988.
17. Swain JA: Hypothermia and blood pH, a review. Arch Intern Med 148:1643, 1988.
18. Schaller MD, Fischer AP, Perret CH: Hyperkalemia: A prognostic factor during acute severe hypothermia. JAMA 264:1842, 1990.
19. Auerbach PS: Some people are dead when they're cold and dead. JAMA; 264:1856, 1990.
20. Buckley JJ, Bosch OK, Bacaner MB: Prevention of ventricular fibrillation during hypothermia with bretylium tosylate. Anesth Analg 50:587, 1971.
21. Imparato AM, Riles TS: Peripheral arterial disease, in Schwartz SI (ed): *Principles of Surgery.* 4th ed. McGraw-Hill, New York, pp 964–966.

Chapter 73

HYPERTHERMIA

G. BRISTOW
L. PATEL

KEY POINTS

- *Malignant hyperthermia (MH) and neuroleptic malignant syndrome (NMS) are life-threatening pharmacologic syndromes, classically induced by inhalation anesthetics or depolarizing muscle relaxants in the case of MH and certain neuroleptic agents in the case of NMS.*
- *The manifestations of these syndromes result to a variable extent from massive heat production in the skeletal muscles.*
- *In contrast, heat stroke results from the inability of the body to dissipate normal or moderately increased heat production, usually in the face of a heat gain from the environment.*
- *MH, NMS, and heat stroke share clinical and laboratory features such as tachycardia, tachypnea, muscular rigidity, hyperthermia, hypercapnia, hypoxemia, acidosis, hyperkalemia, and rhabdomyolysis.*
- *If not recognized early and treated expediently, all of these entities are associated with a high mortality rate or irreversible sequelae.*
- *Management includes discontinuation of triggering agents in the case of MH and NMS and removal from the environmental stress in the case of heat stroke, specific drug therapy, hyperventilation with 100% oxygen, correction of acidosis, and systemic cooling.*
- *Early administration of dantrolene has significantly reduced the mortality and morbidity in the case of MH and NMS.*
- *Patients must be monitored for 24 to 48 h in the ICU for recrudescence and management of late events.*

Human beings, as homeotherms, maintain their core body temperature within the relatively narrow range of 36.2°C (96.5°F) to 38.2°C (101.8°F). The anterior hypothalamus orchestrates this control by balancing heat production and external heat gain with heat loss. The anterior hypothalamus thermostat functions at a set point, which is maintained. Elevation of the core body temperature above 38.2°C (101.8°F) is known as *hyperthermia*. The differential diagnosis of extremely elevated body temperature includes meningitis, sepsis, hypothalamic injury (trauma or hemorrhage), thyroid storm, pheochromocytoma, cholinergic (and other drug) overdose, heat stroke, malignant hyperthermia (MH), and the neuroleptic malignant syndrome (NMS).

Most causes of hyperthermia in human beings reset the anterior hypothalamic set point, a phenomenon called fever. This is usually the result of pyrogens reacting with the anterior hypothalamus. Fever will not be dealt with in this chapter. The several important causes of hyperthermia that occur in the presence of a normal anterior hypothalamic set point will be the subject of discussion in this chapter.

Because MH and NMS are two important disease entities with many similarities, they are discussed together. Heat stroke is discussed separately.

Malignant Hyperthermia and Neuroleptic Malignant Syndrome

BACKGROUND

MALIGNANT HYPERTHERMIA. MH is a true pharmacogenetic disease in that both an inherited predisposition and a triggering drug are necessary to induce the acute clinical manifestations of a reaction.[1] In North America, the incidence of fulminant MH in association with general anesthesia is reported to be 1:15,000 in children and 1:50,000 in adults.[2] In contrast, the incidence is reported as 1:250,000 in Denmark, 1:200,000 in the United Kingdom, and variously reported as from 1:7,000 to 1:110,000 in Japan. The true incidence of MH in the general population is difficult to ascertain.

Malignant hyperthermia susceptibility (MHS) is inherited, probably through one or more genes or alleles.[3] The autosomal dominant inheritance is the only form of unequivocally established inheritance, comprising 50 percent or more of the cases.[4] In other families, the pattern of inheritance includes multifactorial recessive, multigenic, and even fresh mutations.[4]

Anesthetic drugs that can trigger MH include the inhalation agents halothane, enflurane, isoflurane, sevoflurane, methoxyflurane, cyclopropane, and ether, as well as the depolarizing muscle relaxants succinylcholine and decamethonium.[1,2,21] The most fulminant form of the disease is usually associated with administration of halothane with succinylcholine.[5] Physical and emotional stress have been reported to trigger the syndrome in awake patients.[6] It is believed that MH and the human stress syndrome are variants of the same disease.[7,8] The use of depressant drugs, such as barbiturates or tranquilizers, and the use of nondepolarizing muscle relaxants delay the onset of MH in susceptible swine, sometimes for hours.[9,10] In addition, many affected individuals have previously tolerated potent anesthetic triggers without any obvious problems.[11]

Several musculoskeletal disorders have an inconsistent association with MH. These include central core disease (almost certainly related), Duchenne muscular dystrophy, and King-Denborough syndrome. Other myopathies may also be related. The association with sudden death syndrome, heat stroke, osteogenesis imperfecta, club feet, squints, and hernias appears quite coincidental.

The mortality rate from the fulminant syndrome was approximately 70 percent before the use of dantrolene.[12] With early recognition and optimal therapy it is now reported as 7 to 10 percent.[12] The use of prophylactic dantrolene prevents MH in the majority of susceptible persons.

An excellent model of human MH was discovered in stress-susceptible pigs (the Landrace, Pietrain, Poland, and

China breeds of pigs).[13] Human and porcine MH syndromes are nearly identical with respect to changes in vital signs, muscular activity, and metabolism. Thus, our knowledge of the biochemical changes and the efficacy of treating this syndrome is derived by liberal extrapolation of data from numerous controlled experiments on MH-susceptible pigs and only to a lesser extent from case reports of acute episodes in human beings.

The only currently reliable test for diagnosis of susceptibility to MH is the in vitro contracture test with halothane and (separately) caffeine. Skeletal muscle from MHS patients undergoes a hypercontracture in response to caffeine and halothane. This forms the basis for the test. Most North American and European centers performing these tests have agreed on a standardized protocol describing in detail how this test should be performed.[14,15]

NEUROLEPTIC MALIGNANT SYNDROME. NMS is likewise caused by trigger agents in susceptible individuals. These agents, as the name implies, are the major antipsychotic neuroleptic medication groups such as the phenothiazines, the thioxanthenes, and the butyrophenones. Neuropleptic drugs are also used as antiemetics and for dissociative anesthesia ("neurolept anesthesia"). Other agents such as the tricyclic antidepressants, lithium, and metoclopramide have also been suggested as possible trigger agents, although the evidence is poor.

NMS was first described in 1959,[16,17] and although considerable knowledge has been gained regarding this entity, it is not nearly as well understood as MH. The incidence of this entity has been variously described from rare to 1 percent of the population receiving the neuroleptic agents. Part of the reason for this wide discrepancy may be that NMS, unlike MH, may often present in a relatively mild form and escape detection. The syndrome appears to affect males more than females and the young more than the old. A genetic predisposition has not been discovered. Furthermore, some individuals who in one instance have received a neuroleptic agent that triggered the disorder fail to react on subsequent reexposure, and vice versa.

Although weak, some evidence indicates a possible association between MH and NMS such that the conduct of anesthesia for individuals with a history of NMS should be undertaken as if they were MH susceptible.[18]

PATHOPHYSIOLOGY

MALIGNANT HYPERTHERMIA. MH is now recognized as a metabolic disorder of skeletal muscle rather than as an essential loss of temperature control.[19,20] The systemic consequences are marked because skeletal muscle comprises about 40 percent of the adult body mass.[21] The muscle is normal in structure, function, and appearance until exposed to triggering agents. It appears to be a subclinical primary myopathy with an exaggeration of normal rather than different physiologic responses.

The precipitating cause of an MH reaction seems to be a loss of calcium control, with a sudden rise in the myoplasmic concentration of ionized calcium in the presence of triggering anesthetics.[22] This increase in myoplasmic ionized calcium in affected individuals has been confirmed recently by microelectrode studies.[23]

The sarcoplasmic reticulum (SR) with its calcium storage sites, the terminal cisternae, is the focus of the current theories of malfunction during MH episodes.[24] Enhanced calcium-induced calcium release, by increasing the permeability of the SR, may be a part of the abnormal response in MH.[25–27] On the other hand, SR function in MH may be adversely affected by abnormal mitochondrial release of fatty acids.[28]

The primary structure of the skeletal muscle ryanodine receptor (the calcium release channel of the SR) that is probably responsible for excitation-contraction coupling has been expressed from complementary DNA and sequenced.[29,30] Since then the ryanodine receptor gene that codes this calcium release channel of the SR has been cloned.[31] Preliminary genetic linkage studies with MH families strongly suggest that a mutation in this gene on region 13.1 of chromosome 19 may be a candidate for predisposition to MH.[32]

Calcium is central to the cells' metabolic and contractile processes. The presence of triggering anesthetics distorts the role of calcium in cellular metabolism in MHS individuals. The cellular defect is believed to rest in the excitation-contraction coupling mechanism. The level of calcium rises to the point of observable muscle rigidity in 75 percent of patients. This rise also sets off a cascade of compensatory events. Mitochondria actively sequester calcium ions. If this is marked, adenosine triphosphate (ATP) production by mitochondria is decreased, leading to insufficient energy stores for cellular functions. Initially, aerobic and then anaerobic metabolism increases dramatically to provide more ATP required to drive the calcium pumps that maintain calcium homeostasis across the SR and mitochondria as well as the sarcolemma.[24,33] These responses produce large amounts of lactate (as much as 30 μm/mL, a 15 to 20-fold increase), increase oxygen consumption (approximately three-fold), and significantly increase carbon dioxide production.[21] The acids from the cell diffuse into the extracellular fluid and into the effluent venous blood from the skeletal muscles and result in systemic acidosis. Lactate production is therefore the main cause of metabolic acidosis in MH. These changes occur before any detectable increase in temperature, heart rate, or circulating catecholamines is noted.[34,35]

With massive depletion of creatine phosphate and ATP, the sarcolemma of the muscle fiber becomes permeable to the movement of smaller molecules such as potassium, calcium, inorganic phosphate, creatine kinase (CK), and later, to larger molecules such as myoglobin. These molecules move from the cell into the extracellular space and plasma. The concomitant acidotic conditions and high temperature aggravate membrane damage and denaturation of enzymes and other functional proteins.

Sources of heat during active MH include aerobic and anaerobic metabolism, neutralization of hydrogen ions, and hydrolysis of the high-energy phosphates involved in ion transport and contraction-relaxation.

During the acute episode the products of this extreme metabolic activity initiate responses in several other tissues, resulting in multisystem organ failure. Secondary central nervous system (CNS), myocardial, renal, pulmonary, and coagulation derangements result from acidosis, hypoxia, high temperature, hyperkalemia, myoglobinemia, and increased catecholamines.[21,36] A considerable controversy exists regarding the time scale of sympathetic nervous system involvement. Levels of serum catecholamines are increased 30-fold during MH, as a result of increased skeletal muscle metabolism. However, indirect parameters support the view that catecholamines exacerbate but do not initiate the MH reaction.

NEUROLEPTIC MALIGNANT SYNDROME. For several reasons, including the absence of an animal model, the pathophysiology of NMS has been much less studied and is much less understood than that of MH. Virtually all agents that trigger NMS in susceptible individuals antagonize the brain effects of dopamine.[37] In fact, it appears that the likelihood of a neuroleptic agent being able to trigger NMS is directly related to the strength of its central dopamine antagonism properties.[38] It is likely that the central sites of dopamine antagonism are the hypothalamus and basal ganglia.[37] Antagonism of dopamine at these sites is in turn believed to be responsible for the CNS and cardiovascular effects to be described later, as well as for the muscle rigidity and hyperthermia. Hyperthermia, then, is felt to result from muscle contracture. Unlike MH, however, the muscle contracture is caused by a central rather than muscular abnormality. As will be seen later, this has important implications in the choice of treatment modalities.

As in MH, secondary myocardial, renal, pulmonary, and coagulation derangements result from acidosis, hypoxia, high temperature, hyperkalemia, myoglobinemia, and increased catecholamine levels.

CLINICAL PRESENTATION

MALIGNANT HYPERTHERMIA. Clinical presentation of MH is not uniform. The onset may occur suddenly or insidiously, intraoperatively, or occasionally, postoperatively. It is often abrupt when halothane and succinylcholine are used together. It varies in the severity of the acute episodes and all clinical features may not be present in every case. It ranges from the "classic" case to those with unusual presentations and mild symptomatology.

The classic clinical features are those of a malignant hypermetabolic state and include muscle rigidity, tachypnea, tachycardia, arrhythmias, hyperthermia, cyanosis, mottling of the skin, metabolic acidosis, rhabdomyolysis, increased end-tidal CO_2, central venous hypercapnia, and oxygen desaturation (Table 73-1).

Muscle rigidity may be the first indication of MH after administration of succinylcholine. It may be limited to the masseter muscles only, or it may be generalized. Tracheal intubation in these circumstances may be readily accomplished, difficult, or impossible. The incidence of isolated masseter muscle spasm is reported to be 1:100 when halothane and succinylcholine are used.[39] On the other hand, general muscular rigidity (80 percent) may develop insidiously if succinylcholine is not used.[1]

TABLE 73-1 Identification of Malignant Hyperthermia

Early Indicators
Muscle rigidity
Sinus tachycardia
Skin cyanosis with mottling
Increased end-tidal CO_2
Increased mixed venous CO_2
Late Indicators
Marked hyperthermia
Hypotension
Complex arrhythmias
Metabolic acidosis
Electrolyte disturbances
Rhabdomyolysis

Sudden unexplained sinus tachycardia is another early consistent sign (96 percent).[1] Other causes of tachycardia, such as anticholinergic drugs, hypovolemia, hypoventilation, hypoxemia, light general anesthesia, thyroid storm, unrecognized pheochromocytoma, and porphyria, must be ruled out.

As the hypermetabolic state progresses, other commonly seen arrhythmias include bigeminy, premature ventricular contractions, and ventricular tachycardia. These occur secondary to the direct action of hyperkalemia, acidosis, hypoxemia, hyperpyrexia, and increased catecholamines on the myocardium. Ventricular fibrillation is a terminal event.

Blood pressure is frequently unstable (85 percent).[1] At first, increased catecholamine levels result in hypertension. Later arrhythmias and decreased myocardial contractility result in hypotension.

Although hyperthermia is the hallmark of MH, the sustained increase in temperature is a late sign.[1] Although temperature may increase as fast as 1°C every 5 min, and may rise as high as 43 to 44°C (109.4 to 111.2°F), a rate of 1 to 2°C every hour is significant. The rate of change of temperature is more important than the actual temperature alone. The objective of the physician is to diagnose the condition and commence treatment before the temperature begins to rise!

The skin may be flushed and there may be profuse diaphoresis. These signs may rapidly progress to cyanosis (70 percent)[1] and mottling secondary to increased catecholamines. Unexplained cyanosis and mottling plus tachycardia in a well-oxygenated, previously healthy patient is almost pathognomonic of MH.

An increase in end-tidal CO_2 is the earliest consistent sign (85 percent), despite compensatory hyperventilation. Tachypnea (85 percent) occurs secondary to increased carbon dioxide production and oxygen consumption. The patient may breathe against a ventilator if insufficiently paralyzed. If a carbon dioxide absorber is used, it will overheat secondary to a greatly accelerated chemical reaction in the soda lime.

In the very early stages, mixed venous carbon dioxide is increased while Pa_{CO_2} may be normal, and mixed venous oxygen decreased more than Pa_{O_2}.[21] Therefore, a mixed venous blood-gas sample (from a central line if possible) would be more helpful in assessing the onset of MH than an arterial blood-gas determination. With extreme venous desaturation and intrapulmonary shunting, hypoxemia develops. Suggested limits for venous blood-gas values include a Pa_{CO_2} of 55 mmHg, and P_{O_2} of 35 mmHg. A base deficit of −5 mM/L is significant.[34]

Electrolyte disturbances are severe, with acute hyperkalemia and hypercalcemia developing from altered muscle membrane permeability to these ions. During the postcrisis diuresis or too zealous treatment, the reverse may occur with hypokalemia and hypocalcemia ensuing.

Rhabdomyolysis is a function of the severity of the acute MH episode and occurs later in the course of the syndrome. Serum myoglobin concentration increases above the threshold for renal damage. Myoglobinemia and myoglobinuria are more immediate and can be transient, anywhere from several hours to days. The CK value rises into the thousands. Levels of serum CK peak at 18 to 24 h after the acute episode and can take a few days to several weeks to become normal.

Erythrocyte lysis, likely caused by the acidosis, can also occur. Disseminated intravascular coagulation (DIC), which is one of the leading causes of death in MH, may develop in the more severe forms of MH.

Patients die of ventricular fibrillation, DIC, acute pulmonary edema, renal failure, or most frequently, brain death induced by cerebral edema.

NEUROLEPTIC MALIGNANT SYNDROME. NMS is usually triggered in patients with psychiatric disorders being treated with one of the major tranquilizer-neuroleptic agents. Both oral and parenteral neuroleptic agents cause this disorder. The dose of medication at the time of onset is usually in the therapeutic range and the syndrome often begins within several days of establishing treatment, though it may occasionally be within hours and rarely may take weeks.[38] As in MH, the presentation of NMS is not uniform and the rapidity of onset is variable. On the whole, it tends to be much slower and more insidious than in MH, and may easily go undetected.

There are four cardinal clinical manifestations of NMS (Table 73-2): fluctuating level of consciousness, cardiovascular lability, muscle stiffness, and increased temperature.[40] Typically, the signs manifest in this order and often develop over days, though they may progress from onset to the full blown syndrome within hours. Level of consciousness may range from random nonpurposeful movements, mutism, and confusion to coma. Autonomic instability is manifest by wide fluctuations in blood pressure and pulse rate, from hyper- to hypotension and tachy- to bradycardia associated with flushing and profuse diaphoresis. Muscle stiffness, which is pronounced, is of the "lead pipe" variety. To a large extent, because of the increased metabolism due to muscular stiffness, the core body temperature finally begins to rise and, although usually not as rapid as in MH, may reach levels in excess of 42°C (107.6°F).

TABLE 73-2 Cardinal Manifestations of Neuroleptic Malignant Syndrome

- Fluctuating level of consciousness
- Cardiovascular lability
- Muscle stiffness
- Increased temperature

Increased muscle tone (which reduces chest wall compliance), rising temperature, and impaired consciousness (frequently compounded by upper airway obstruction or gastric aspiration) lead to hypoxemia, hypercapnia, and a mixed respiratory and lactic acidosis. Although electrolyte disturbances, rhabdomyolysis, erythrocyte lysis, DIC, and cardiac arrhythmias may occur, the most common serious abnormality is acute respiratory failure. The usual cause of death, which has been cited at 20 to 30 percent in untreated cases, is therefore usually due to hypoxia and acidosis.

TREATMENT

MALIGNANT HYPERTHERMIA. Management of the acute MH crisis must be immediate and aggressive, whether the onset is slow or fulminant. It includes treatment with the only known specific therapeutic drug, dantrolene, and supportive care (Table 73-3).

Dantrolene. Dantrolene is a muscle relaxant that acts specifically on skeletal muscles. In isolated muscle preparations, dantrolene uncouples the excitation and contraction of skeletal muscles. It prevents the release of calcium from

TABLE 73-3 Treatment of Malignant Hyperthermia

1. Stop procedure, change anesthesia machine to a vapor-free machine, increase minute ventilation to three times normal using 100% oxygen.
2. Give sodium bicarbonate, 1–2 meq/kg.
3. Give dantrolene as soon as possible, 2.5 mg/kg, IV. If no response is evident within minutes, give further doses of 1–2 mg/kg at 10-min intervals. The maximum recommended dose is 10 mg/kg.
4. Cool the patient (surface cooling; intravenous cold saline; irrigation of wound, rectum, or stomach; cardiopulmonary bypass, if needed).
5. Maintain intravascular access. Monitor vital signs and rhythm. Consider invasive hemodynamic monitoring or esophageal echocardiography.
6. Initiate volume loading and osmotic diuretics.
7. Remain alert for coagulation disturbances and hyperkalemia (ECG signs may necessitate therapy before blood tests are available). Calcium should not be given.
8. Observe for 24–48 h, continue dantrolene 2.5 mg/kg IV every 5–8 h for three doses, followed by oral therapy 4 mg/kg/day for 2–3 days. Monitor for renal failure, DIC, and temperature instability.

the SR but does not affect its reuptake.[41] Thus, it prevents the increase in myoplasmic calcium and subsequent acute catabolism within the muscle cell, if given before calcium is released from storage sites.

It is packaged in vials containing a sterile lyophilized mixture of 20 mg dantrolene sodium, 3000 mg mannitol (which improved the solubility and makes the solution isotonic), and sufficient sodium hydroxide to yield a pH of approximately 9.5 (to make it soluble when reconstituted). Each 20 mg dantrolene must be dissolved with 60 mL sterile water (dextrose solutions lead to greater difficulty in dissolving dantrolene). If it does not dissolve immediately to produce a clear yellow-orange solution, it should be heated under tap water. In a dire emergency it should be administered through a filter without worrying about crystals. In a 70-kg adult, as many as nine to ten vials may be required to provide a 2.5-mg/kg dose. This will require several assistants.

The Malignant Hyperthermia Association of the United States (MHAUS) has developed a protocol to be put into effect at the first sign of MH. It recommends that operating room personnel stop the surgery, discontinue the inhalation anesthetic, and increase minute ventilation to at least three times normal using 100% oxygen. This is followed by the intravenous administration of 1 to 2 meq/kg of sodium bicarbonate ($NaHCO_3$), (in the absence of blood-gases). Intravenous dantrolene, 2.5 mg/kg, is given as soon as possible.[42] Response usually occurs within minutes. If no response occurs, the dose may be increased to the recommended upper limit of 10 mg/kg in increments of 1 to 2 mg/kg at 10-min intervals.[42] However, this dose may be exceeded if necessary.[42] The need for repeat doses of dantrolene should be guided by clinical or laboratory signs, especially changes in heart rate, rigidity, temperature, and metabolic acidosis. If dantrolene is given early enough while skeletal muscle perfusion is adequate, it rapidly halts the hypermetabolic process. Catecholamines and potassium return to normal levels, the vital signs soon become normal, and the patient regains consciousness.

In human beings, dantrolene metabolism is rapid via hepatic enzymes. The mean half-life of dantrolene after intravenous administration is about 5 to 8 h. Calcium antagonists interact with dantrolene and cause profound myocardial depression. Prophylactic intravenous dantrolene, 2 mg/kg, 15 min prior to induction of anesthesia is given to MHS patients to avoid a reaction.[12]

Supportive Care. Simultaneous cooling in almost any way to lower the patient's temperature should be commenced—surface cooling, intravenous cold saline, wound, rectal, or nasogastric irrigation with sterile cold solutions, and even bypass cooling may be required. A temperature of 41 to 42°C (105.8 to 107.6°F) is compatible with survival and normal brain function. Cooling should be halted at about 38°C (100.4°F) to avoid inadvertent hypothermia.

The anesthetic machine should be changed to a vapor-free machine or at the very least, the rubber tubing and carbon dioxide absorbers should be changed to unused ones.

Volume loading and osmotic diuretics are given to induce a brisk diuresis to avoid renal myoglobin deposition and failure. Hyperkalemia, common in the acute phase, may require treatment based on the level of potassium, presence of arrhythmias, or electrocardiographic (ECG) changes. Treatment may include hyperventilation, intravenous $NaHCO_3$, and intravenous glucose and insulin (1 ml/kg of a mixture of 5 units regular insulin in 50 mL of 50% glucose). The use of calcium to treat hyperkalemia is inappropriate in this condition.

Arrhythmias usually respond to treatment of acidosis and hyperkalemia. If they persist, a starting dose of procainamide, 1 mg/kg, may be tried, up to a total of 15 mg/kg. Procainamide must be administered no faster than a rate of 50 mg/min to avoid hypotension. ECG control is recommended.

Vital signs and temperature must be closely monitored. ECG monitoring for arrhythmias is imperative. Intravascular monitoring of cardiac filling and arterial pressures is desirable. Vascular access is necessary for serial blood-gas and biochemical analysis. The bladder should be catheterized to monitor urine output and the presence of myoglobinuria or hemoglobinuria. Clotting function should be assessed.

If the patient is stabilized, the surgery may be completed with no anesthetic, regional anesthetic, or a "safe" general anesthetic using nitrous oxide, narcotics, and nondepolarizing muscle relaxants.

The patient recovering from an episode of MH will need to be monitored closely in the ICU for 24 to 48 h. Recrudescence of MH (even after the triggering agents are removed) can occur 4 to 6 h and up to 36 h after the first episode.[43,44] Intravenous dantrolene therapy (2.5 mg/kg) should be continued every 5 to 8 h for approximately three doses, followed by oral dantrolene (4 mg/kg/24 h) for 2 to 3 days. These patients also need to be monitored for the late complications of the syndrome; temperature instability may continue for several days and DIC and renal failure are frequent findings.

NEUROLEPTIC MALIGNANT SYNDROME. Appropriate treatment of NMS, like MH, depends in the first instance on a high index of suspicion and early recognition. As with MH, the principles of treatment of NMS are to discontinue the triggering agents, provide supportive care, institute specific measures to control heat production, and finally to begin cooling. The treatment of victims of NMS, by and large, should be undertaken in an ICU with similar monitoring and general treatment as described for MH.

Any suspect medication should be discontinued immediately. The duration of the adverse action, however, will depend on the rate of elimination from the body, quite variable for the psychotropic medications. The effect may therefore last for several hours to days and in the case of the long-acting depot phenothiazines, weeks.

Because the most likely immediate life-threatening event is related to hypoxemia and a combination of respiratory and metabolic acidosis, the control of the airway with tracheal intubation should be accomplished and hyperventilation with 100% oxygen instituted. Tracheal intubation may be facilitated by the use of one of the nondepolarizing muscle relaxants. Vigilance for and the treatment of myoglobinuria, cardiac arrhythmias, and acid-base disturbances should proceed along the lines described for MH.

Although the etiology of NMS is incompletely understood and there have been no controlled studies of drug treatment efficacies, several modalities have been found useful in reducing an otherwise high mortality rate. Because the increase in muscle tone in NMS is essentially muscle mediated, nondepolarizing muscle relaxants are useful (unlike in MH) in terminating increased muscle tone, fever, and lactic acidosis.[45] Tracheal intubation and artificial ventilation are mandated by such therapy. This treatment is likely the single most useful intervention in the case of severe NMS because it not only protects the airway and ensures adequate alveolar ventilation but also stops the production of heat. Dantrolene, as used in MH, has also been shown to be effective in the treatment of NMS.[46] More specifically, drugs with dopamine agonist activity have been reported successful in the treatment of less severe NMS reactions.[38] Bromocriptine in oral doses of 2.5 to 10 mg three times daily has been effective, as has amantidine in oral doses of 100 mg twice daily. It is probably reasonable to treat a severe NMS reaction initially with a nondepolarizing muscle relaxant and dantrolene for 12 to 24 h, followed by one of the oral dopamine agonist agents for several days or more depending on the triggering drug half-life and the patient's clinical state.

Although core body temperature usually begins to fall with the institution of the treatment noted above, it may be necessary to expedite this by using one of the cooling methods discussed for MH.

Heat Stroke

Heat stroke is the most serious manifestation of the heat stress illnesses. Although it is not triggered by drugs, it may be facilitated by certain medications. More common than MH or NMS, heat stroke occurs predominantly in hot climates, in both sexes, and in all age ranges. Like NMS and MH, it is usually fatal if untreated.

PATHOPHYSIOLOGY

Heat production in man under resting conditions is approximately 70 kcal/m^2/h. The majority of this heat arises from metabolism. Fever, certain medications such as the salicylates, thyroid hormone, and the amphetamines, and most especially increased muscle activity as found in tremor, shivering, and exertion may increase heat production in excess of tenfold. To maintain the core body temperature this potentially massive heat production must be balanced by a commensurate increase in heat loss. Heat loss, under normal circumstances, occurs mainly from the skin through radiation, convection, and usually to a minimal extent, from conduction. Evaporative heat loss occurs from both the airway and skin. With the exception of sweating, skin heat loss is mediated through the cardiovascular system via skin blood flow, which may increase dramatically to subserve thermal regulation. As ambient temperature rises toward body temperature, heat loss through radiation, convection, and conduction diminishes. At temperatures above body temperature, heat will be gained from the environment. Sweating, with its attendant loss of 540 kcal for each liter evaporated, becomes increasingly important in maintaining normal body temperature as the ambient temperature rises. However, unacclimatized man's ability to sweat is limited to approximately 1 L/h and rises to approximately 2 to 3 L/h in the acclimatized person. Increasing humidity reduces the effectiveness of sweating to control body temperature. Although very important in maintaining normal body temperature, sweating is not without adverse effects because fluid, sodium and, to a lesser extent, potassium are lost in large quantities (particularly in the unacclimatized individual). Certain drugs, notably those with anticholinergic effects, may predispose to heat stroke by diminishing sweating.

Heat stroke in the elderly is often seen following several days of the lesser heat syndromes including heat cramps and heat exhaustion.[47] The onset is usually slow and related to a high ambient temperature and humidity in unacclimatized, chronically ill individuals with cardiovascular disease and often suffering an intercurrent febrile illness. Furthermore, the use of antihypertensive agents including diuretics may increase the risk of heat stroke in these individuals. In the young individual, however, the onset of heat stroke is usually more rapid, often over hours, and is associated with exercise and exertion in a hot environment.[48] Alcohol is often involved. Heat stroke resulting from alcohol use while in hot tubs has become much more common during the last decade.

The clinical manifestations are related to two abnormalities. First are those abnormalities produced by the body's attempt to dissipate the heat load during the incipient stages. Fluid loss may be on the order of 30 percent of the body fluid and associated with total body sodium and potassium depletion of considerable magnitude. The second abnormality is related to the rise of core body temperature.[49] Once the compensatory mechanisms have failed, evolution of the hyperthermic state is usually rapid; temperatures in excess of 42°C (107°6.F) are not uncommon. Core body temperatures of 45°C (113°F) have been reported. Above 41 to 42°C (105.8 to 107.6°F), enzyme and other protein denaturation begins, and cellular lipid membrane dissolution occurs. Therefore, if the hemodynamic effects of dehydration and its attendant morbidity have not resulted in death by the time the core temperature reaches 42°C (107.6°F), the direct thermal effects cause extensive morbidity and mortality. Many, if not all, organ systems are affected by this combination of hypovolemia and hyperthermia. Notable effects occur in the CNS, cardiovascular system, liver, kidneys, and coagulation mechanism.

CLINICAL PRESENTATION

A victim of heat stroke characteristically presents with a core body temperature >40°C (104°F). Characteristically the skin is flushed and dry, but there may be evidence of sweating. At one time it was believed that the absence of sweating was a characteristic if not a cause of heat stroke. It is now recognized, however, that in most instances sweating occurs profusely during the development of heat stroke. It is only in the later stages that this mechanism of compensation fails, likely due to severe dehydration. Usually severe hypovolemia with hypotension and tachycardia are evident. Although the central venous pressure (CVP) is usually low, consistent with the severe hypovolemia, evidence of cardiogenic shock with a high CVP may be present in the case of myocardial infarction or decreased myocardial contractility due to acidosis. Although the temperature and cardiovascular findings are the most obvious in the case of heat stroke, the CNS abnormalities are usually outstanding as well. These include cerebral disorders ranging from confusion to stupor and coma, as well as psychosis and seizure disorders. Muscle stiffness if often present. Although not necessarily evident immediately, coagulation disorders due to thermal effects on platelets and hepatic coagulation factors may develop quickly. DIC is not uncommon. If the patient survives, rhabdomyolysis with hyperkalemia, myoglobinemia, and myoglobinuria occur within 24 h. This is likewise caused by the thermal effect on the skeletal muscle. Rhabdomyolysis, in conjunction with the direct thermal effect on the kidneys, leads to renal failure. Typial laboratory findings include hemoconcentration with an increased hematocrit and hemoglobin, prolonged prothrombin (PT) and partial thromboplastin times (PTT), hyperkalemia, and a variable serum sodium, increased blood urea nitrogen (BUN) and creatinine, increased CK and myoglobinemia, decreased pH (due to a lactic acidosis), and variable values for Pa_{CO_2} and Pa_{O_2}. Many of the abnormalities related to hepatic, coagulation, and renal function do not appear for 24 h or more.

TREATMENT

Treatment in the first instance should be directed toward life support and temperature-lowering efforts. If the victim is unconscious, the airway should be secured by tracheal intubation facilitated by a muscle relaxant if necessary. Ventilation should then be provided to ensure a Pa_{O_2} >100 mmHg and Pa_{CO_2} <40 mmHg. $NaHCO_3$ should be administered for a pH <7.2. Severe hypovolemia should be treated by the administration of cold normal saline intravenously. Six to 10 L may be required, several in the first hour. Volume replacement should be undertaken with CVP monitoring and direct arterial measurements. In older patients, especially those with myocardial compromise, right heart catheterization is advisable. Once the victim is removed from the thermal stress, temperature lowering is usually not difficult.[50] Surface cooling is usually successful but often stimulates shivering. This can be controlled with paralysis with nondepolarizing muscle relaxants or with small doses of a phenothiazine, such as chlorpromazine given intravenously. Once the core temperature reaches 38°C (100.4°F) cooling should be discontinued to prevent an overshoot and hypothermia. The initial treatment of less severe episodes of heat stroke may require little more than the removal from the stressful environment, fluid replacement, and surface cooling.

All individuals suffering from heat stroke whose temperature has been >40°C (104°F) should be followed in the ICU for at least 48 h to ensure cardiovascular stability and to monitor CNS, hepatic, renal, and coagulation function. Much of the heat-related tissue dysfunction does not occur for 24 h or more and may last weeks.

CASE PRESENTATIONS

Case 1.

A 12-year-old boy, weighing 65.5 kg, with a diagnosis of spina bifida occulta and bilateral equinovarus deformities, was scheduled for bilateral Achilles tendon lengthening. Medical history and physical examination were otherwise negative. The patient had had no previous general anesthetic and no family history of any adverse reaction to general anesthetics was reported.

Intramuscular atropine, 0.6 mg, was given as premedication. Anesthesia was induced by inhalation with a mixture of halothane, nitrous oxide, and oxygen, using a circle system with a CO_2 absorber. Generalized fasciculations followed the intravenous administration of 100 mg succinylcholine. During laryngoscopy it was noticed that the patient had developed moderate trismus. However, it was possible to intubate the patient without difficulty. Vital signs on induction were a heart rate of 112 beats/min, respiratory rate of 23/min, and blood pressure of 128/70 mmHg. Soon after induction and intubation, the patient developed ventricular bigeminy which resolved to sinus rhythm after hyperventilation with 100% oxygen. At this time the heart rate was 120/min, respiratory rate was 26/min, axillary temperature was 36°C (96.8°F), and blood pressure was 120/65 mmHg. Although the possibility of masseter muscle spasm, as an early sign of MH was considered, it was not thought to be significant, and surgery was commenced. Of interest, the surgeons commented that the muscle tone in the lower limbs seemed to be increased compared to the preoperative examination.

During the next 30 min the patient developed significant sinus tachycardia (140/min) and tachypnea (38/min), and the axillary temperature increased to 39°C (102.2°F). The skin was flushed and hot to touch, and the patient was profusely diaphoretic. Muscle tone was increased in all four limbs. At the same time, the soda lime carbon dioxide absorber was warm to touch. An arterial blood-gas determination (with spontaneous ventilation and an FI_{O_2} of 0.35) revealed a Pa_{O_2} of 150 mmHg, Pa_{CO_2} of 31 mmHg, pH of 7.23, HCO_3^- of 13.2 meq/L, and base deficit of −13 meq/L. A presumptive diagnosis of MH was made based on the tachycardia, tachypnea, a rapid rise in temperature (an increase of 3°C in 30 min), muscular rigidity, and the moderate metabolic acidosis.

Treatment was begun immediately. Halothane and nitrous oxide were discontinued. Concomitantly, the anesthetic machine was exchanged for an inhalation vapor-free machine (reserved especially for this purpose on the operating room floor) and the patient was hyperventilated with 100% oxygen. Dantrolene, 2.5 mg/kg, was given intravenously (as soon as it was mixed by assistants). Cold intravenous saline (stored routinely in the operating area) was infused at a rate of 15 ml/kg/h. The ambient temperature of the operating room was lowered and a cooling blanket was placed under the patient. Treatment of the metabolic acidosis was initiated using 1 meq/kg of $NaHCO_3$. Intravenous furosemide, 40 mg, was given to ensure diuresis. The patient was given 5 mg intravenous morphine twice and the surgery was completed promptly.

A radial arterial line for direct blood pressure monitoring and repeated blood sampling, an internal jugular venous line to assess fluid replacement, and a urinary catheter to monitor urine color and output were established.

Over the next half hour the temperature returned to 37°C (98.6°F), at which time active cooling measures were stopped. Heart rate decreased to 80 to 90/min (sinus rhythm), the blood pressure stabilized at 130/76 mmHg, and the muscular rigidity of the limbs was noted to be markedly decreased. The patient began diuresing dark pink-colored urine. The blood serum potassium level, drawn with the first blood-gas sample, was 5.8 meq/L. Since there were no life-threatening arrhythmias, hyperkalemia was not treated but revolved with diuresis. A repeat arterial blood-gas determination revealed a Pa_{O_2} of 535 mmHg, Pa_{CO_2} of 23 mmHg, pH of 7.42, HCO_3 of 14.8 meq/L, and base deficit of −10 meq/L. Further $NaHCO_3$ was not given.

Forty minutes after instituting treatment, the vital signs including temperature were within normal limits. The muscle tone was normal and the patient was awake. Arterial blood-gas sampling with an $F_{I_{O_2}}$ of 1 and spontaneous ventilation showed a Pa_{O_2} of 405 mmHg, Pa_{CO_2} of 33 mmHg, pH of 7.35, HCO_3 of 19 meq/L, and a base deficit of −6.4 meq/L. It was felt that further treatment with dantrolene, $NaHCO_3$, and controlled ventilation was not required at this time. The trachea was extubated and the patient transferred to the ICU, breathing oxygen via a rebreathing mask, for further monitoring and treatment.

The patient remained in the ICU for 48 h, during which time he was treated with a single repeat dose of intravenous dantrolene 2.5 mg/kg, 6 h postcrisis. Oral dantrolene 4 mg/kg/24 h was continued at 6 hourly doses for 2 days. Brisk diuresis was maintained with intravenous fluids only. Vital signs remained stable. Arterial blood-gas determinations showed normocapnia and a base deficit ranging from −5 to −2.6 meq/L. No evidence of DIC was seen. Significant serum myoglobinemia and myoglobinuria persisted for 2 days, but renal function remained normal. The initial CK value at the time of the crisis was 21,800 IU and peaked at 184,000 IU 20 h later. The patient developed swollen muscles and complained of severe soreness, especially with movement the next day. He was discharged to the ward on the third ICU day.

Follow-up neurologic assessment 3 months later did not reveal an underlying myopathy nor any residual neurologic deficit. The resting CK value was 235 IU. A diagnostic muscle contracture test was felt to be unnecessary because the MH crisis confirmed the diagnosis.

Case 2.

A healthy 23-year-old man (weight 100 kg) suffering from dislocations of his right shoulder was admitted to the hospital on the day before surgery for an elective Putti-Platt repair and capsulotomy of his right shoulder. He was seen by the attending anesthetist on the day prior to surgery and judged to be fit for surgery. He had had a prior general anesthetic complicated by postoperative nausea and vomiting. He denied a family history of problems with anesthesia.

Morphine, 10 mg, was administered intramuscularly 1 h preoperatively. Anesthesia was introduced intravenously with 100 μg fentanyl, 350 mg thiopentone, and 120 mg succinylcholine and was maintained with oxygen, nitrous oxide, and halothane. Fentanyl (total dose of 150 μg) was administered as required. Pancuronium, 3 mg, was administered for muscle relaxation. Intravenous metoclopramide, 10 mg, and 5 mg droperidol were administered intraoperatively, because of the history of postoperative nausea and vomiting. Following completion of the surgical procedure, the muscle relaxation was reversed with 1.2 mg atropine and 2.5 mg neostigmine, given intravenously. The patient was extubated while in the lateral decubitus position and transported to the post-anesthesia recovery room (PARR).

On arrival in the PARR, the patient's vital signs were normal. Nasal oxygen was administered. He was somnolent and unresponsive to verbal commands. He demonstrated nonpurposeful and random movements of his extremities. Muscle tone was moderately increased. His skin was flushed and he was diaphoretic. Respirations were normal. The blood pressure and pulse were labile and fluctuated from 120/80 mmHg to 180/120 mmHg and 100 to 180 beats/min, respectively. Serum electrolytes, blood glucose, and arterial blood-gas determinations were normal. Three hours following admission to PARR the patient's status was unchanged. Intravenous naloxone, 0.4 mg, was given without effect. Because some of the signs suggested idiosyncratic anticholinergic effects, the patient was given 1 mg physostigmine intravenously, which was also ineffective. With the possibility that the patient was suffering from the extrapyrimidal side effects of droperidol or metoclopramide, intravenous benztropine, 1 mg, was given, without effect.

Seven hours postoperatively the patient had not improved. The rectal temperature was 38.4°C (101.5°F). A neurological consultation was sought, but a diagnosis was not made. The patient was subsequently admitted to the ICU for further observation and monitoring.

In the ICU the patient's status deteriorated. He became hypertensive (pressure 222/86 mmHg) and tachycardia (pulse 160 to 180 beats/min). He was flushed and profusely diaphoretic. His skin was mottled over the trunk. The respiratory rate was 30 to 40 breaths/min. The rectal temperature rose to more than 40°C (104°F) over 1 h. He remained obtunded and unresponsive to painful stimuli. The extremities, trunk, and neck were rigid, and the eyes were deviated to the left. No overt seizure activity was noted.

A presumptive diagnosis of NMS related to droperidol or metoclopramide was made. Oxygen was administered by a facemask. An arterial line was established, and normal saline infused intravenously. An initial arterial blood-gas sample revealed a Pa_{O_2} of 84 mmHg, Pa_{CO_2} of 25 mmHg, pH of 7.22, HCO_3 of 10 meq/L, and a base deficit of −14.9 meq/L. Fifty meq sodium bicarbonate was administered. Dantrolene, 2 mg/kg (total dose 200 mg), and 12.5 g mannitol were given intravenously. After the first dose of dantrolene (20 mg), a priming dose of atracurium (10 mg) was given, followed by 30 mg intravenously, which rapidly resulted in profound muscle relaxation. The patient was intubated and mechanically ventilated. The remaining dantrolene was subsequently given. Paralysis was maintained with pancuronium as needed, and the patient was sedated with morphine and diazepam.

He was placed on a cooling blanket and covered with a water-soaked blanket on which ice was placed. With these measures, the temperature rapidly decreased to 38°C (100.4°F) (esophageal). Repeat arterial blood-gas samplings with controlled ventilation demonstrated a small alveolar-arterial oxygen difference $(A-a)_{O_2}$, mild hypocapnia, and a pH and HCO_3 returning to normal over 8 h.

A computed tomographic scan of the brain and lumbar puncture performed shortly after admission to the ICU gave normal results. On the following day, an EEG showed diffuse slow wave activity, most likely secondary to a metabolic dysfunction. Cultures of the blood, urine, endotracheal tube aspirate, and cerebrospinal fluid were negative. Laboratory results showed a leukocytosis with a left shift. CK, drawn 18 h following admission to the ICU, was elevated to 2168 units, urea 2.4 mM/L, creatine 0.08 mM/L. There was no gross evidence of myoglobinurea.

On the second postoperative day, the patient's status had improved considerably. He was oriented and responded appropriately. No focal neurologic signs were seen. His temperature had decreased to 37.5°C (99.9°F). He was then extubated and discharged to the ward where his recovery continued uneventually. He displayed generalized muscle pain and tenderness for several days. He was provided with a Medic Alert bracelet warning of his sensitivity to neuroleptic agents. He was discharged from the hospital on the tenth postoperative day without obvious sequelae.

CASE DISCUSSION (*Cases 1* and *2*)

These cases illustrate the dramatic speed with which MH and NMS can appear. Although in each case there was some delay in appreciating the signs of an ongoing hypermetabolic state, early treatment with appropriate medications and supportive care was instituted, with rapid resolution of hyperthermia, muscle rigidity, tachycardia, tachypnea, and metabolic acidosis. The outcome was fortunate in these cases and serious complications were averted.

These cases emphasize the need for the high index of clinical suspicion, under appropriate conditions for both MH and NMS by the attending physicians, appropriate monitoring for anesthetized patients, early diagnosis, and timely therapy. With appropriate therapy, there is generally rapid normalization of clinical and biochemical signs and recovery without complications. Due to greater awareness of these symdromes, definitive therapy would normally be instituted as soon as there is any indication of the disease. Although fatalities are still being reported, as well as recurrence of symptoms with a prolonged recovery, appropriate therapy has made a significant contribution to the treatment of these very severe conditions.

CASE PRESENTATION

Case 3.

An 88-year-old woman, in good health apart from hypertension (controlled with 40 mg furosemide daily), was admitted to the emergency department with a rectal temperature of 42.5°C (108.9°F). The patient lived alone in a small non–air-conditioned apartment and had been feeling ill for several days with nausea and loss of appetite. On the day of admission, the patient had been noted by her family to be confused. Later, she was found in her apartment unconscious. The daytime high temperature on the day of admission and for the preceding week had been in excess of 30°C (86°F) with high humidity, and on the day of admission the temperature had reached 36.8°C (99°F).

On examination the patient was unconscious, responding to deep pain only, areflexic, flaccid, with no lateralizing signs or evidence of neck stiffness. Her skin was hot and dry to the touch, her chest was clear, and there was no evidence of trauma or heart failure. Vital signs disclosed a rectal temperature of 42.5°C (108.9°F) blood pressure of 90/48 mmHg, and pulse rate of 104 with ventricular ectopy.

Initial investigation disclosed cardiomegaly and sinus tachycardia with ventricular ectopy and nonspecific ST and T wave changes. A temperature-corrected arterial blood-gas determination while ventilated with an FI_{O_2} of 1 disclosed: Pa_{O_2} 216 mmHg, Pa_{CO_2} of 31 mmHg, pH 7.33, HCO_3 12 meq/L, and a base deficit of −13 meq/L. Serum sodium content was 130 meq/L, serum potassium 2.5 meq/L, BUN 9.9 meq/L, creatinine 226 meq/L, hemoglobin 13.5 g/dL, platelets 100,000, PT 16.1 s, and PTT normal. The CK was 686 units/L with a normal CP-MB band.

Initial treatment included tracheal intubation and ventilation with 100% oxygen, rapid administration of lactated Ringer's solution, Foley catheter insertion, and institution of a cooling blanket.

Within 2 h the patient had received 3 L fluid, her esophageal temperature had dropped to 38°C (100.4°F), and she was moving spontaneously and opening her eyes. Lorazepam 1 mg intravenously was given for restlessness, and the patient was transferred to the ICU.

In the ICU, ventilation was maintained and arterial and pulmonary artery catheters were established for blood sampling and pressure measurements. Cardiovascular parameters disclosed ongoing hypotension, tachycardia, a cardiac index of approximately 2 L/m^2, and a pulmonary capillary wedge pressure (PPW) of 28 mmHg. Physical examination disclosed bilateral rales, and a chest x-ray indicated evidence of pulmonary edema. Treatment consisted of dopamine 7.5 μg/kg/min, nitroglycerine 0.5 μg/kg/min, furosemide 80 mg intravenously and, sometime later, mannitol 20 g every 6 h intravenously. Within 16 h of admission to the ICU the patient was afebrile, responsive, and cooperative. She was extubated and the dopamine and the nitroglycerine discontinued. Her vital signs at that time included a blood pressure of 120/64 mmHg, with a mean of 83 mmHg, pulse rate of 83, sinus rhythm, and a cardiac index of 3.1 L/m^2. Her extubated blood-gas values disclosed a small $(A-a)O_2$ with a normal acid-base status. Within 16 h of admission to the ICU her serum sodium and potassium levels were normal and remained that way throughout the remainder of her hospital stay. The BUN and serum creatinine values rose slightly from admission values to return to normal on the third hospital day. Her hemoglobin stabilized at 11.5 g/dL over 24 h, her platelet count rose to normal within 2 days, and her PT returned to normal within 48 h. There was never any evidence of bleeding. The CK value rose to 13,650 units/L within 48 h, and after several days returned to normal. The CK-MB band remained normal. Myoglobin estimations were between 3200 and 6400 μg/L on admission. Within 24 h of admission the myoglobin reached a peak of between 12,800 and 25,600 μg/L. Over the subsequent 4 days, with ongoing fluid, mannitol, and furosemide diuresis, the myoglobin level fell to less than 400 μg/L.

The patient was discharged from the ICU to the ward in 72 h and from the ward to home 10 days later. At the time of discharge she was feeling well, and all of her laboratory values had returned to normal.

CASE DISCUSSION (*Case 3*)

This case graphically demonstrates the magnitude of heat stress that can be encountered under conditions of high ambient temperature and humidity by the elderly, particularly. The presentation with severe mental aberration, cardiovascular collapse, hot dry skin, and high core temperature was a classic presentation of heat stroke. The ease with which the core temperature could be reduced was also expected, as was the ease with which pulmonary edema was caused in this elderly, cardiovascularly compromised victim, This points out the need for aggressive monitoring during fluid replacement and cooling in such individuals.

The greatest threat to this woman's life after initial airway and cardiovascular control were established was the threat to her renal function with dehydration and myoglobinemia. Aggressive treatment with diuresis and monitoring prevented this complication.

References

1. Britt BA, Kwong FHF, Endreny L: The clinical and laboratory features of malignant hyperthermia management—a review, in Henschel EO (ed): *Malignant Hyperthermia: Current Concepts*. New York, Appleton-Century-Crofts, 1977, pp 9–46.
2. Britt BA, Kalow W: Malignant hyperthermia: A statistical review. Can Anaesth Soc J 17:293, 1970.
3. Kalow W, Britt BA, Chan FY: Epidemiology and inheritance of malignant hyperthermia. Int Anesth Clin 17:119, 1979.
4. McPherson E, Taylor CA, Jr: The genetics of malignant hyperthermia: Evidence for heterogenicity. Am J Med Genet 11:273, 1982.
5. Fletcher JE, Rosenberg H: In vitro interaction between halothane and succinylcholine in human skeletal muscle: Implications for malignant hyperthermia and masseter muscle rigidity. Anesthesiology 63:190, 1985.
6. Gronert GA, Thompson GL, Onfrio BM: Human malignant hyperthermia: Awake episodes and correction by dantrolene. Anesth Analg (Paris) 59:377, 1980.
7. Wingarg DW: Malignant hyperthermia—acute stress syndrome of man, in Henschel EO (ed): *Malignant Hyperthermia: Current Concepts*. New York, Appleton-Century-Crofts, 1977, pp 79–95.
8. Wingard DW: Malignant hyperthermia: A human stress syndrome? Letter. Lancet 2:1450, 1974.
9. Gronert GA, Milde JH: Variations in onset of porcine malignant hyperthermia. Anesth Analg 60:499, 1981.
10. Hall GM, Lucke JN, Lister D: Porcine malignant hyperthermia: IV neuromuscular blockade. Br J Anaesth 48:1135, 1976.
11. Halsall PJ, Cain PA, Ellis FR: Retrospective analysis of anesthetics received by patients before susceptibility to malignant hyperpyrexia was recognized. Br J Anaesth 51:949, 1979.
12. Gronert GA: Malignant hyperthermia. Semin Anesth 2:197, 1983.
13. Hall LW, Woolf N, Bradley JWP, Jolly DW: Unusual reaction to suxamethonium chloride. Br Med J 2:1305, 1966.
14. North American Malignant Hyperthermia Group: Standardization of the caffeine-halothane muscle contracture test. Anesth Analg 69:511, 1989.
15. European Malignant Hyperpyrexia Group: A protocol for the investigation of malignant hyperpyrexia (MH) susceptibility. Br J Anaesth 56:1267, 1984.
16. Preston J: Central nervous system reactions to small doses of tranquilizers. Am Pract Digest Treatment 10:627, 1959.
17. Delay J, Pichot P, Lemperier MT, et al: Un neuroleptique majeur non phenothiazinque et non reserpine, l'haloperidol, dans le traitment des psychoses. Ann Med Psychol 118:145, 1960.
18. Carroll SN, Rosenberg H, Fletcher JE, et al: Malignant hyperthermia susceptibility in neuroleptic malignant syndrome. Anesthesiology 67:20, 1987.
19. Kalow W, Britt BA, Terrau ME, et al: Metabolic error of muscle

metabolism after recovery from malignant hyperthermia. Lancet 2:89, 1970.
20. Britt BA: Malignant hyperthermia: A pharmacogenetic disease of skeletal and cardiac muscle. N Engl J Med 290:1140, 1974.
21. Gronert GA: Malignant hyperthermia. Anesthesiology 53:395, 1980.
22. Endo M: Calcium release from the sarcoplasmic reticulum. Physiol Rev 57:71, 1977.
23. Lopez JR, Alamo L, Caputo C, et al: Intracellular ionized calcium concentration in muscles from humans with malignant hyperthermia. Muscle Nerve 8:355, 1985.
24. Britt BA: Etiology and pathophysiology of malignant hyperthermia. Fed Proc 38:448, 1979.
25. Nelson TE: Abnormality in calcium release from skeletal sarcoplasmic reticulum of pigs susceptible to malignant hyperthermia. J Clin Invest 72:862, 1983.
26. Mickelson JR, Ross JA, Reed BK, Louis CF: Enhanced calcium-induced calcium release by isolated sarcoplasmic reticulum vesicles from malignant hyperthermia susceptible pig muscle. Bichem Biophys Acta 862:318, 1986.
27. Ohta T, Endo M: Inhibition of calcium-induced release by dantrolene at mammalian body temperature. Proc Jap Acad 62:Ser B:329, 1986.
28. Cheah KS, Cheah AM: Skeletal muscle mitochondrial phospholipase A_2 and the interaction of mitochondria and sarcoplasma reticulum in porcine malignant hyperplexia. Biochem Biophys Acta 638:40, 1981.
29. Takeshima H, Nishimura S, Matsumoto T, et al: Primary structure and expression from complementary DNA of skeletal muscle ryanodine receptor. Nature 339:439, 1989.
30. Gronert GA: Cloning of the SR foot. Literature Scan: Anesthesiology 3(5):6, 1989.
31. Zorzato F, Fujii F, Otsu K, et al: Molecular cloning of DNA encoding human and rabbit forms of the Ca++ release channel (ryanodine receptor) of the skeletal muscle sarcoplasmic reticulum. J Biol Chem 265:2244, 1990.
32. MacLennan DH, Duff C, Zorzato F, et al: Ryanodine receptor gene is a candidate for predisposition to malignant hyperthermia. Nature 343:559, 1990.
33. Berman MC, Conradie PJ, Keach JE: The mechanism of accelerated skeletal muscle glycogenolysis during malignant hyperthermia in swine. S Afr Med J 46:1810, 1972.
34. Gronert GA, Theye RA: Halothane induced porcine malignant hyperthermia: Metabolic and hemodynamic changes. Anesthesiology 44:36, 1976.
35. Lister D, Hall GM, Lacke JN: Catecholamines in suxamethonium induced hyperthermia in Pietrain pigs. Br J Anaesth 46:803, 1974.
36. Heffron JJA: Malignant hyperthermia: Biochemical aspects of the acute episode. Br J Anaesth 60:274, 1988.
37. Gibb WRG, Lees AJ: The neuroleptic syndrome—a review. Q J Med, New Series 56:421, 1985.
38. Guze BH, Baxter LR: Current concepts—neuroleptic malignant syndrome. N Engl J Med 313:163, 1985.
39. Schwartz L, Rockoff MA, Koka BV: Masseter spasm with anesthesia; incidence and implication. Anesthesiology 61:772, 1984.
40. Delay J, Deniker P: Drug-induced extrapyramidal syndromes, in Vinken PJ, Bruyn GW (eds): *Handbook of Clinical Neurology 6: Diseases of the Basal Ganglia*. Amsterdam, North Holland Publishing, 1968, pp 248–266.
41. Morgan KG, Bryant SH: The mechanism of action of dantrolene sodium J Pharmacol Exp Ther 201:138, 1977.
42. Rosenberg H: International workshop on MH. Anesthesiology 54:530, 1981.
43. Mathieu A, Bogosian AJ, Ryan JF, et al: Recrudescence after survival of an initial episode of malignant hyperthermia. Anesthesiology 51:454, 1979.
44. Murphy AL, Conlay L, Ryan JF, Roberts JT: Malignant hyperthermia during a prolonged anesthetic for reattachment of a limb. Anesthesiology 66:680, 1987.
45. Sangal R, Dimitrijevic R: Neuroleptic malignant syndrome—successful treatment with pancuronium. JAMA 245:2795, 1985.
46. Patel P, Bristow G: Postoperative neuroleptic malignant syndrome. Can J Anaesth 34:515, 1987.
47. Stine RJ: Heat illness—Collective review. JACEP 8:154, 1979.
48. Shapiro Y, Seidman DS: Field and clinical observation of exertional heatstroke patients. Med Sci Sports Exerc 22:6, 1990.
49. Hubbard RW, Matthew CB, Durkot MJ, Francesconi RP: Novel approaches to the pathophysiology of heatstroke: The energy depletion model. Ann Emerg Med 16:1066, 1987.
50. Costrini A: Emergency treatment of exertional heatstroke and comparison of whole body cooling techniques. Med Sci Sports Exerc 22:15, 1990.

Chapter 74

DIVING MEDICINE AND NEAR DROWNING

STEVEN D. BROWN
CLAUDE A. PIANTADOSI

KEY POINTS

- *The physiologic effects of immersion and diving are a direct consequence of the physical behavior of gases and the mechanical effects of hydrostatic pressure.*
- *Decompression sickness (DCS) is the result of inert gas coming out of solution in body tissues after diving with compressed gas, thereby producing ischemia by obstructing the vasculature and triggering inflammatory biochemical events.*
- *Therapy of DCS and gas embolism includes immediate administration of O_2 and rehydration. Recompression, even if it is delayed 1 or 2 days, is the therapy of choice.*
- *Gas embolism is second to near drowning (ND) as a cause of sports diving-related fatalities. It is usually the result of pulmonary barotrauma during ascent from shallow depths.*
- *The pathophysiology of ND is caused by asphyxia. The major target organs are the lung, brain, heart, and kidneys.*
- *In adults ND is associated often with drug or alcohol ingestion and may be associated with other injuries.*
- *Hyperventilation prior to breath-hold diving may result in shallow water blackout which is a common predisposition to ND.*
- *Adult respiratory distress syndrome (ARDS) complicates 40 percent of NDs, may be delayed, and can be aggravated by aspiration of stomach contents and other foreign debris.*
- *Pneumonia or sepsis induced by unusual organisms from contaminated water may complicate the ND victim's course. Prophylactic antibiotics, however, are not indicated.*

Millions of people enjoy the beauty and salutary effects of aquatic environments each year. Swimmers, boaters, and divers of all ages, with various degrees of physical skill and judgment, participate regularly in recreational activities involving water. The physical environment of the recreational swimmer and underwater diver, however, is deceptively hazardous. Any individual can be placed in imminent danger of drowning from even a relatively minor incident. Too often, swimmers or divers impair their faculties with alcohol or ignore their physical limitations and venture into unsafe conditions with tragic results. In some situations, such as with young children, the encounter with the aquatic environment is inadvertent or unsupervised. The number of drownings, diving accidents, and other aquatic misadventures each year is difficult to estimate. There are at least two million underwater divers and many more recreational swimmers in the United States. This activity translates to hundreds of diving accidents and thousands of drownings and near drownings each year. Many victims survive the actual event only to die hours or days later in the hospital. Thus, it is incumbent on the intensivist to be knowledgeable about the potentially life-threatening clinical consequences of diving accidents and ND.

The Biophysics of Underwater Environments

The physiologic responses to underwater environments are a direct consequence of the physical behavior of gases and the mechanical effects of hydrostatic pressure. Pressure measurements, force per unit area, can be expressed in a variety of ways (Table 74-1). Normal atmospheric pressure is approximately 760 mmHg or 14.7 pounds per square inch (psi). The pressure of a column of water varies linearly with its height and must be added to the normal atmospheric pressure to obtain absolute pressure. As shown in Table 74-1, a column of sea water 33.1 ft deep (fsw) exerts the same pressure as the normal atmosphere at sea level. Thus, a diver immersed in seawater at 33.1 ft is exposed to a total pressure of 2 atm (ATA). In diving with compressed gas, the pressure of the diver's breathing gas must be increased in proportion to the absolute pressure in order for the diver to inhale against the pressure of the water column above him. As a result, more gas molecules must occupy the lungs and other gas containing cavities of the body to maintain constant volume at a given temperature. The relationship between pressure (P), volume (V), temperature (T) and the number of moles of gas (n) can be described by the *ideal gas law:*

$$PV = nRT \quad (74\text{-}1)$$

where R is the universal gas constant. The special gas laws relevant to diving can be derived easily from the ideal gas law. Three special cases of the ideal gas law, where one of the three variables is held constant, are also shown in Table 74-1.

TABLE 74-1 Pressure Equivalents and Gas Laws

Condition	Depth	Pressure mmHg	psig[a]	(ATA)[b]
Sea level	0	760	0	1.0
Sea water	33 fsw[c]	1,520	14.7	2.0
Sea water	66 fsw	2,280	29.4	3.0
Sea water	330 fsw	8,360	147.0	11.0

Boyle's law $P_1V_1 = P_2V_2$
Charles' law $V_1/T_1 = V_2/T_2$
Gay Lussaac's law $P_1/T_1 = P_2/T_2$

[a]psig = pounds per square inch gauge. Note that a pressure gauge at sea level reads zero.

[b]ATA = atmosphere absolute. Note that depth in ATA = $\frac{\text{fsw} + 33}{33}$

[c]fsw = feet sea water

Air and other respirable gases are mixtures of oxygen and other molecules. In a mixture of gases, the total pressure is equal to the sum of the partial pressures of each of the gases (Dalton's law). This means that each gas in the mixture behaves as though it alone occupies the available space. The uptake of gas by body tissues is determined primarily by the diffusion of gas into or out of blood from the alveolar spaces. The amount of a gas dissolved in liquid at any temperature, e.g., blood or tissues of the body at 37°C (98.6°F), is also proportional to its partial pressure (Henry's law). The gas concentration is related to the partial pressure times its solubility coefficient. In general, the physiologic effects of diving gases, such as inert gas narcosis, correlate directly with the partial pressure of the gas in the tissues of the body.

Immersion and Breath-Hold Diving

Immersion in water produces physiologic adjustments by the respiratory, cardiovascular, renal, and endocrine systems.[1] Three prompt physiologic consequences of immersion are a decrease in thoracic gas volume, a sustained increase in cardiac output, and an increased urine output leading to dehydration. These responses are related to the effects of hydrostatic pressure and to the high density of water relative to air. During upright immersion, the extrathoracic blood vessels are supported by the water, and the body is exposed to a hydrostatic pressure gradient proportional to its vertical height. The hydrostatic pressure surrounding the body compresses the abdomen relative to the thorax, causing negative pressure breathing of approximately −20 cmH_2O. By displacing the diaphragm upward, these hydrostatic effects decrease the thoracic gas volume and expiratory reserve volume. The pressure gradient across the diaphragm created by immersion, together with hydrostatically decreased venous capacitance in the legs, increases the volume of blood in the intrathoracic vasculature including the heart. The increase in intrathoracic blood volume during immersion also is facilitated by the high density of water. Central blood volume may be augmented by peripheral arterial vasoconstriction if the water temperature is below thermoneutrality (34°C, 93.2°F).

Cardiovascular distention during immersion activates cardiac mechanoreceptors which normally respond to hypervolemia. Although there is no immediate change in circulating blood volume, the apparent hypervolemia is detected at the hypothalamus via vagal afferents. The ensuing immersion response has two components: diuresis and natriuresis. Diuresis and natriuresis after immersion have time profiles which suggest that they operate by different mechanisms. Peak diuresis occurs in the first 1 to 2 h of immersion, whereas peak natriuresis occurs after 4 to 5 h. Fluid restriction and administration of vasopressin before immersion prevent diuresis but do not affect natriuresis. There is a correlation between the amount of distention of the central circulatory organs and excretion of urinary sodium. The mechanism of the response to increased water loss during immersion is suppression of antidiuretic hormone (ADH) release. This is also known as the Gauer-Henry response. The mechanism of the natriuresis is related to decreased tubular reabsorption of sodium and not to an increase in filtered sodium. The most important factors in the natriuresis appear to be **1.** aldosterone suppression via decreased renin-angiotensin activity, **2.** increased release of atrial natriuretic factor, **3.** increased release of renal prostaglandins, and **4.** decreased sympathetic activity.

The increase in central blood volume during immersion distends the cardiac chambers and enhances ventricular diastolic filling, which increases cardiac output.[2] The increase in cardiac output is attributable almost entirely to an increase in stroke volume which may increase twofold. The increase in cardiac output persists and occurs with no measurable increase in systemic oxygen uptake. The mechanism of the increase in stroke volume appears to be primarily an increase in cardiac preload.

During immersion, the physiologic responses to breath-holding have special significance.[3] With apnea, the lungs act as a reservoir for exchange of O_2 for CO_2 in pulmonary capillary blood. During breath-hold in air, the mean alveolar P_{O_2} decreases linearly with time and its rate of change is a function of the decline in the mixed venous P_{O_2}. As alveolar P_{O_2} declines, whole body O_2 uptake eventually falls and anaerobic metabolism increases. Carbon dioxide enters the lungs during apnea in proportion to both the pulmonary blood flow and the diffusion gradient for CO_2 between mixed venous P_{CO_2} and alveolar P_{CO_2}. The rate of CO_2 transfer is initially high, but decreases rapidly because its diffusion gradient decreases as alveolar P_{CO_2} approaches the mixed venous value. Further CO_2 production increases mixed venous P_{CO_2} which again causes alveolar P_{CO_2} to rise. The point at which high P_{CO_2} causes breathing to resume is the break point. The time to the break point can be extended by maneuvers that lower P_{CO_2} or raise P_{O_2} such as hyperventilation or oxygen breathing. Notably, the body's O_2 store is not increased appreciably by hyperventilation because the increase in alveolar P_{O_2} resulting from a fall in alveolar P_{CO_2} increases blood O_2 content only slightly. Therefore, hyperventilation greatly extends breath-hold time though it can produce profound hypoxia before the CO_2 rises to the break point. Alveolar gas exchange during breath-holding is altered by underwater descent when lung volume decreases from thoracic compression and the partial pressures of O_2, CO_2, and N_2 increase in the lungs (Fig. 74-1). On descent, alveolar O_2 and CO_2 concentrations decrease due to a greater transfer of those gases to pulmonary capillary blood compared to inert gas (N_2). Alveolar P_{O_2} also is higher during breath-hold diving than during simple breath-holding, and the transfer of CO_2 during early descent is opposite normal, i.e., CO_2 moves from alveoli to pulmonary capillary blood. During ascent, the lung reexpands and alveolar P_{O_2} and P_{CO_2} decline. Near the surface, the alveolar P_{O_2} may be almost as low as the mixed venous P_{O_2}. In strenuous dives, expansion of hypoxic alveoli during ascent may result in reverse O_2 transfer from mixed venous blood to alveoli (see Fig. 74-1). Carbon dioxide retained in the blood during the dive also leaves the blood on

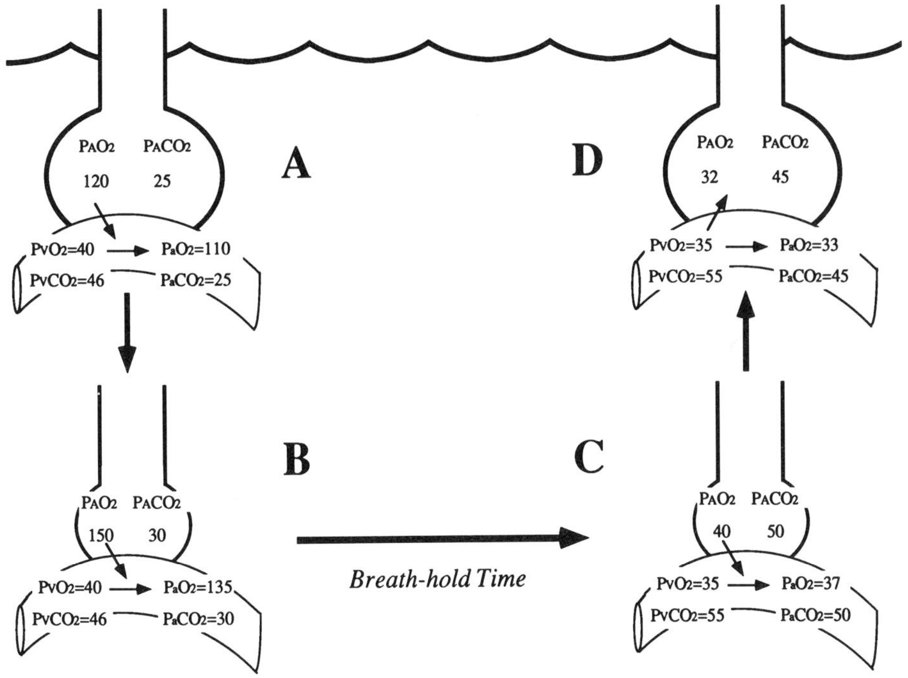

FIGURE 74-1 Proposed mechanism of shallow water blackout. All values are expressed in mmHg. *a.* The breath-hold diver begins by hyperventilating before the dive. *b.* At depth, Pa_{CO_2} and Pa_{O_2} increase as the alveoli are compressed by hydrostatic pressure. *c.* At the end of the breath-hold dive, CO_2 increases toward the break point, and the diver begins to ascend. Note the decreased PA_{O_2} and Pa_{O_2} at this point. *d.* On approaching the surface, PA_{CO_2} and PA_{O_2} decrease as the alveoli reexpand. O_2 leaves the pulmonary capillaries and enters the alveoli. This may result in profound hypoxemia and produce unconsciousness.

ascent as the alveolar P_{CO_2} decreases. Carbon dioxide elimination usually continues postdive as does exchange of the small amount of N_2 that entered the blood during the dive.

Hyperventilation before breath-hold diving is a dangerous way to extend the dive. During the dive, compression of the lungs causes the alveolar P_{O_2} to increase. Thus, the primary signal to return to the surface is the P_{CO_2}. When the diver hyperventilates before the dive, the arterial P_{CO_2} begins at a lower level, and the time to the breath-hold break point is extended. Alveolar O_2 concentration, however, is depleted more severely during longer dives and life-threatening hypoxia may occur when the diver approaches the surface. Loss of consciousness by this mechanism is called *shallow water blackout*. It undoubtedly causes a large number of drownings.

The body's response to breath-hold diving can be modified by a diving response induced by apnea and facial immersion, particularly in cold water. This diving response, manifested primarily as bradycardia, is most pronounced in young children. The diving response has been interpreted as an O_2-conserving response that redistributes blood flow from organs resistant to hypoxia to organs with continuous requirements of oxygen such as heart and brain. This interpretation in man is controversial, although a diving response may contribute to survival of children resuscitated up to an hour after submersion in cold water.

Diving with Compressed Breathing Gases

The limitations of breath-hold diving have been circumvented by diving systems which provide the diver access to a continuous supply of breathable gas at any depth. Diving in shallow water, e.g., 0 to 150 fsw, is usually carried out with compressed air as the breathing gas because air is inexpensive and can be obtained readily, even at remote dive sites. Air divers may be free swimming, e.g., self-contained underwater breathing apparatus (SCUBA), or tethered by an umbilical line to the surface. For SCUBA, the maximum safe depth is about 140 fsw and for tethered air diving, approximately 200 fsw.[4] These safety considerations are brought about by three factors including nitrogen narcosis, decompression time, and oxygen toxicity. To dive beyond the practical range of compressed air, special gas mixtures must be supplied. Usually helium is substituted for nitrogen as the diluent gas. In current helium-oxygen operations, the oxygen pressure is usually maintained at a constant 0.4 to 1.0 ATA, with the diver often operating out of a diving bell. The helium may be recycled by gas reconditioning equipment located on the bell. Surface supplied heliox diving is expensive but effective and relatively safe to depths of 400 fsw. Most dives deeper than 400 fsw require saturation of the diver with inert gas at the approximate working depth of the dive. Divers can live and work for many weeks under saturation conditions and then undergo a single slow ascent to the surface.

PRINCIPLES OF DECOMPRESSION

The use of compressed air in diving can cause physiologic problems on ascent due to release of excess gas from tissues. The process of inert gas elimination from the body after a decrease in pressure during ascent from diving or to altitude is known as *decompression*.

The rate of uptake or elimination of nitrogen and other

inert gases from the body after a change in pressure is exponential with respect to time. Inert gas exchange is determined primarily by gas solubility in blood and tissue, blood flow, and the volume of tissue. This assumes that the diffusion resistance between blood and tissue is inconsequential for nitrogen and other inert gases. Tissues that behave this way are perfusion limited, with the characteristics of their inert gas exchange defined by a half-time. Because the tissues of the body are perfused differently and nitrogen is more soluble in fat than other tissues, the half-times for different tissues may vary considerably. This principle was used to calculate the original tables for safe decompression, assuming that gas bubbles would form and DCS would occur only if the tissues were supersaturated, i.e., the nitrogen partial pressure were about twice the absolute pressure. Most current decompression tables are still based on multiple parallel exponential models, although other concepts also have been used successfully.[5] Even though decompression models are useful, two great unknowns still remain in decompression research, namely the extent and the duration of supersaturation with inert gas in living tissue. Although perfusion is the primary variable affecting uptake and elimination of inert gas, diffusion may limit the rate of inert gas exchange under some conditions. Diffusion limitation may occur if the rate of exchange of inert gas by perfusion is extremely rapid, if the tissue perfusion is very low or if part of the tissue such as the capillary endothelium has a high diffusion resistance. Diffusion may be important when two adjacent tissues have very different rates of perfusion. In such a situation, the elimination of inert gas from the faster tissue may allow additional inert gas to enter by diffusion from the slower tissue. Thus, the faster tissue may maintain supersaturation for a longer time. Diffusion is also important after gas bubbles have formed in a tissue during decompression. Gas bubbles contain large amounts of inert (N_2) gas which can be removed by tissue perfusion only after the N_2 diffuses back into the tissue. The rate at which N_2 diffuses away from a gas bubble is determined by the bubble surface area, the intrabubble pressure, and the partial pressure difference between bubble and tissue.

During decompression, bubble formation presumably occurs at specific nucleation sites in the body. The number and location of these nucleation sites varies according to physiologic condition. For example, exercise may increase the number of bubbles formed by tribonucleation, a mechanism that creates bubbles in areas such as joints, where large negative pressures can be generated by traction between surfaces lubricated by a liquid. Bubbles created by this vacuum mechanism may arise from either preexisting gas nuclei or by de novo formation. Tiny unstable bubbles, or gas nuclei, may exist for a long time in the body if they stabilize at hydrophobic sites. Such gas nuclei may grow into bubbles during decompression. There is little doubt experimentally that gas bubbles cause DCS, although clinically silent bubbles can be detected ultrasonically in the circulation during normal decompression. There is still uncertainty, however, about the mechanisms of bubble formation in the body and precisely how bubbles are related to the diverse manifestations of DCS.

DECOMPRESSION SICKNESS

The factors that govern the formation of bubbles during decompression have been used to develop tables for safe decompression. The computation of depth-time profiles for decompression usually assumes that DCS is related to some critical supersaturation threshold. This assumption conflicts with data indicating that DCS occurs as a statistical rather than a threshold event.[6] Therefore, even proper use of well-tested decompression tables is associated with a small but definite risk of DCS for dives of approximately 27 fsw or deeper. Most serious DCS, however, is the result of omitted decompression.

The clinical manifestations of DCS are attributed to growth of bubbles in body tissues. Primary sites of bubble growth are the joint spaces, tendon sheaths, and periarticular tissues, including peripheral nerve endings. Bubbles in these locations produce pain that is known as type I DCS, or bends. Bubble formation also occurs in the spinal cord and other areas of the central nervous system (CNS). This is called type II or serious DCS. DCS involving the audiovestibular system also occurs though it is relatively rare. The common clinical manifestations of DCS are summarized in Table 74-2. DCS in military and commercial divers occurs with a 4:1 predominance of type I symptoms. Altitude bends, or dysbarism, is generally accompanied by mild to moderate type I DCS. Tunnel workers have a reported incidence of DCS of 0.7 to 1.5 percent, primarily consisting of type I symptoms of the knee and lower leg.[7] In contrast, recent statistics suggest a 3:1 predominance of type II symptoms in recreational divers.[8] The reasons for this difference in DCS after sports diving are uncertain, although underreporting of type I DCS is likely, and in some cases, prolonged delays in the diagnosis and treatment of type I DCS may allow it to evolve into more severe disease. Also, recreational divers are more likely to omit a decompression

TABLE 74-2 Clinical Manifestations of DCS

Type I (mild DCS)

Limbs

- Pain (bends), niggles, lymphatic obstruction, numbness, and paresthesias usually involving the large joints, e.g., shoulders, elbows and knees

Skin

- Mottling, itching, rash, pallor, urticaria, edema

Type II (serious DCS)

CNS

Brain

- Headache, seizures, loss of consciousness, visual disturbances, hemiparesis, aphasia, tremor, ataxia (staggers)

Spinal cord

- Low back or pelvic girdle pain, paraparesis, urinary retention, incontinence

Audiovestibular DCS

- Tinnitus, vertigo, nystagmus, decreased hearing, nausea and vomiting

Cardiopulmonary DCS (chokes)

- Dyspnea, cough, wheezing, hemodynamic collapse

obligation than are professional divers, thus increasing the probability of serious DCS.

One of the most troublesome forms of serious DCS is spinal cord injury.[9] The precise mechanisms of spinal cord DCS are not yet fully understood. In experimental animals this injury may be precipitated by intravascular bubbles that form in the low pressure, epidural venous plexus of the spinal cord.[10] This venous lake is susceptible to bubble formation because of its low, bidirectional blood flow. Bubble-induced thrombi can easily obstruct venous outflow from the plexus, leading to ischemic injury of the spinal cord. Despite evidence for bubble formation in the spinal venous plexus, intravascular formation of bubbles appears to be otherwise uncommon. Most intravascular bubbles probably originate at the tissue-blood interface and stream into the circulation to be absorbed by the lungs. In the circulation, the surface active effects of bubbles at the blood-to-bubble interface produce hematologic changes. These include complement activation, platelet aggregation and destruction, mediator release, and procoagulant activity. Precise roles for these factors in the pathogenesis of decompression sickness are undetermined.

When many bubbles are released into the venous circulation, they may interact with and overwhelm the pulmonary circulation and cause chest pain, shortness of breath, pharyngeal irritation, and cough. This syndrome, known as *the chokes,* may lead to cardiovascular collapse and death if untreated. Some of these bubbles also may cross the pulmonary capillary bed as micro air emboli. Intravenous bubbles may pass into the arterial circulation in divers with type II DCS by a right-to-left intracardiac shunt, e.g., patent foramen ovale (PFO).[11] This cardiac anomaly, however, is present in about 20 percent of the normal population, and its precise role as a risk factor for decompression sickness is uncertain.

Divers with "the chokes" may develop symptoms minutes to hours after decompression. The symptoms may be progressive and if arterialization of venous bubbles occurs, severe type II symptoms may occur. Physical examination reveals tachypnea, tachycardia, cyanosis, crackles, wheezing and gasping in advanced cases. Arterial blood-gas determinations often reveal hypoxemia and hypo- to normocapnia. The chest radiograph may show diffuse pulmonary infiltrates similar to ARDS.[12]

PULMONARY BAROTRAUMA

Pulmonary barotrauma is a potentially serious consequence of the failure of expanding gases in the lung to escape from alveoli during ascent. Overinflation of the lung may lead to alveolar rupture and pulmonary interstitial emphysema. Alveolar rupture may cause pneumothorax, mediastinal or soft tissue emphysema, pneumopericardium, or arterial gas embolization (AGE). Pulmonary overinflation during ascent while diving on compressed gas is most likely to occur with breath-holding, loss of consciousness, or local obstruction of airways with trapping of gas. It also may occur after explosive decompression of aircraft at altitude. Lung rupture during a high-risk ascent also depends on several physiologic factors including pulmonary compliance, transpulmonary pressure and lung volume. Airway closure and air trapping induced by immersion in the upright position may increase the risk of lung rupture in free ascent.[13] When the pressure within the lung exceeds that at the body surface by about 100 cmH_2O, the lung will rupture. During breath-holding at total lung capacity (TLC), the difference between the alveolar and ambient pressure is approximately 50 cmH_2O. Thus, ambient hydrostatic pressure outside the body during ascent must fall another 50 cmH_2O for the lung to rupture. If the compliance of the lung and chest wall at TLC is 15 mL/cmH_2O, then the lung volume during ascent must increase by 15 mL × 50 cmH_2O or 750 mL before the lung will rupture. Using Boyle's law (see Table 74-1), the approximate ambient pressure from which a diver must ascend for pulmonary rupture during a breath-hold at TLC can be determined. At the surface, P_1 = 1.0 ATA, and suppose V_1 = 7000 mL. Then, V_2 = 7000 − 750 or 6250 mL. Therefore,

$$(1.0)(7000 \text{ mL}) = P_2(6250 \text{ mL}) \qquad (74\text{-}2)$$

and

$$P_2 = 1.0(7000/6250) = 1.12 \text{ ATA or } 4.0 \text{ ft.} \qquad (74\text{-}3)$$

This calculation illustrates how pulmonary overinflation and arterial air embolization may occur in shallow water when a compressed gas diver ascends too rapidly. The calculation also points out that fractional volume changes are greatest at low hydrostatic pressures. This principle accounts for the fact that the amount of gas released into the pulmonary venous system after overpressurization of the lungs during ascent can be quite great.

Venous and Arterial Gas Embolism

Intravascular gas emboli occur fairly often in compressed gas diving, as well as in diverse clinical settings. As previously mentioned, asymptomatic venous gas bubbles occur often in divers during and after decompression. In clinical settings, even careful intravenous infusion of solutions or contrast materials may be accompanied by venous gas emboli (VGE). Such emboli are usually clinically silent if the total volume of the gas is small and does not cross to the arterial side of the circulation. VGE create pathophysiologic consequences in four situations: **1.** arterialization of bubbles across the pulmonary vasculature, **2.** arterialization of bubbles across a PFO, **3.** obstruction of the heart or major vessels by VGE, and **4.** biophysical interaction between air and blood. When venous gas bubbles become arterialized, even a small amount of gas can produce substantial morbidity or death.[14,15]

The pulmonary vasculature is an effective filter for VGE larger than about 20 μm in diameter.[16] This barrier is not absolute since 500-μm bubbles have been demonstrated to cross the lung in some situations. Spillover of VGE through the pulmonary vasculature has been demonstrated in a number of animals. In dogs, spillover to the pulmonary veins occurs with an intravenous air bubbling rate of 0.3 mL/kg/min.[14] The rate of crossover and minimum filtering size of VGE increases in the setting of an increased pulmonary arterial minus pulmonary venous (Pa − Pv) pressure gradient. The pulmonary arterioles vasoconstrict in response to VGE and pulmonary artery pressures rises.[17] As more VGE mechanically obstruct the vasculature, the Pa − Pv gradient increases, thereby decreasing the filtering effectiveness of the pulmonary vasculature and allowing passage of VGE.[18] Intrapulmonary shunts further decrease the filtering efficiency of the pulmonary vasculature.

Paradoxical air embolism may occur when VGE are arterialized via a PFO, either in divers or in patients.[11] Detection of PFOs by echocardiography relies on microcavitated VGE for ultrasonic contrast. Right-to-left atrial crossover of bubbles is variable and may require special maneuvers to elevate right atrial pressure. Bubble crossover also may occur spontaneously during some phases of the cardiac cycle in asymptomatic individuals.[19] The probability of paradoxical gas embolism increases in patients who develop pulmonary hypertension due to regional pulmonary vasoconstriction and vascular obstruction from VGE.

VGE also become physiologically significant when a large quantity of gas overtly obstructs major vessels. Significant obstruction may occur at the level of the pulmonary vasculature or the heart. In the heart, gas is churned to a foam which obstructs inflow and outflow, thus diminishing cardiac output. In addition to obstructing the pulmonary vasculature, venous gas or foam triggers pulmonary arterial vasoconstriction, pulmonary hypertension, bronchospasm, and dyspnea.[20]

Biophysical interactions at the blood-bubble interface complicate simple mechanical obstruction of the circulation and amplify the physiologic effects of small volumes of intravenous gas. The blood-bubble interface stimulates numerous biochemical events including initiation of the coagulation cascade via activation of Hageman factor, complement activation and neutrophil and platelet aggregation. These events are associated with release of several inflammatory mediators with subsequent damage to the vascular endothelium. Noncardiogenic pulmonary edema may develop quickly as extravasated fluids flood the alveoli and interstitium and may advance to frank ARDS.[21] Compressed gas divers have long recognized a similar sequence of events as the postdecompression syndrome of the chokes.[22]

AGE may occur in the diver who breathes compressed gas either by VGE arterialization or by direct arterial embolization. AGE is second to drowning as the leading cause of fatal accidents during sports SCUBA diving. The most common source of AGE in the diving population is pulmonary barotrauma with rupture of the pulmonary vasculature and entry of gas under pressure into the pulmonary veins as discussed above. Similar pathophysiology occurs in mechanically ventilated patients who require high airway pressures for ventilation or have areas of poor pulmonary gas exchange. Pulmonary barotrauma which produces AGE either in the diver or the mechanically ventilated patient may not produce other evidence of barotrauma such as pneumothorax, pneumomediastinum, or pneumopericardium. As gas in the vasculature is detected unreliably by radiography, the diagnosis is suggested by clinical evidence of end-organ embolization, primarily manifest as ischemia of the heart or brain.[23] Therefore, prolonged procedures to visualize the air may compromise recovery of a critically ill patient and proper management of air embolism needs to start with a heightened suspicion of the diagnosis in the appropriate setting.

Like VGE, AGE are obstructive, induce vasoconstriction, activate the clotting cascade and complement, and stimulate neutrophil and platelet aggregation, which leads to release of various mediators of inflammation, with subsequent damage to vascular endothelium. Even small AGE carry the potential for permanent injury and should never be regarded as benign. Although small AGE, e.g., 0.5 mL, may produce death in animals if the gas obstructs portions of a critical vascular bed, the magnitude of the injury in general appears to be related to the dose of intravascular gas. In the heart, the myocardial response to AGE is similar to coronary insufficiency of any etiology. Ventricular arrhythmias and ST segment elevation or depression are common and may progress to infarction.[24] Cerebral manifestations of AGE are similar to those of thromboembolism and include focal neurologic deficits, loss of consciousness, seizures, and death. The distinction between AGE and VGE may become blurred clinically because the possibility of arterial spillover is difficult to exclude and either event may be heralded by cardiovascular collapse.

Compressed gas divers who suffer AGE are most often inexperienced and frequently appear suddenly at the surface after diving. Typically, they cry out upon surfacing, indicating a rapid ascent with a closed glottis, or they may surface unconscious. The embolism occasionally is complicated by pneumothorax or pneumomediastinum and is accompanied by clinical signs of pulmonary barotrauma, including mediastinal crunch (Hamman's sign), subcutaneous air, and tension pneumothorax. The clinical onset of AGE is quite sudden and generally present with ischemic symptoms involving the brain. Neurologic symptoms and signs usually appear within a few seconds to a few minutes after the ascent. Otherwise, the signs and symptoms are those of type II DCS and tend to be progressive. Initial symptoms of AGE rarely appear more than 2 h after ascent and delayed onset of symptoms suggests DCS. Common clinical findings of acute AGE include headache, pleuritic chest pain, confusion, nausea, vomiting, loss of vision, hemiparesis, seizures, and unconsciousness.

Therapy for Gas Bubble Disease

ADJUVANT THERAPY

The immediate management of VGE or AGE begins with identification of the problem and prevention of further embolization. In significant VGE of any etiology, a "mill-wheel" murmur produced by air in the right ventricle may be audible precordially with a stethoscope.[25] Positioning the patient in the left lateral decubitus and Trendelenburg position in an effort to avoid PFO crossover and brain embolization is a time-honored and standard clinical practice, both for gas embolism and type II DCS.[25,26] Also, the Trendelenburg position has been proposed to reduce cerebral bubble diameter by increasing hydrostatic pressure in the cranium. Recent animal studies suggest, however, that these positioning efforts are not efficacious since blood flow rather than buoyancy of the bubble determines the course of air emboli.[26] Furthermore, prolonged Trendelenburg positioning has been associated with increased cerebral edema in animals and may be counterproductive. Immediate ventilation with 100% O_2 will help correct hypoxemia, increase the diffusion gradient for nitrogen out of the bubbles, and cause them to shrink.[27] Vasopressors and antiarrhythmics may be required to combat hypotension and ventricular arrhythmias associated with significant air embolism. Lidocaine at 2 to 4 mg/min intravenously after a 1 mg/kg loading dose has ameliorated cerebral injury after experimental cerebral AGE.[28,29]

Adjuvant therapy, i.e., other than oxygen, for gas embolism and DCS is limited and consists of correction of hemoconcentration and supportive management of the complications of air embolism. Parenteral corticosteroids such as dexamethasone, 4 mg every 6 h, have been recommended in an effort to reduce cerebral or spinal cord edema following AGE and serious DCS. Experimental evidence demonstrating the efficacy of corticosteroids in either setting is lacking. Stress ulceration may occur after cerebral AGE, and prophylaxis for this complication should be used routinely. Because of the blood-bubble biophysical interactions discussed earlier, treatment of cerebral AGE with heparin was once recommended. Heparin therapy, however, has not proven efficacious and is associated with hemorrhage into areas of cerebral infarction induced by the air embolus.[28]

RECOMPRESSION THERAPY

Gas bubbles in tissues or the circulation will resolve spontaneously, but the rate at which they are removed can be enhanced greatly by oxygen breathing and recompression. Recompression and hyperbaric oxygen (HBO) administration are primary therapy for both DCS and AGE.[29] The resolution of bubbles is related to their size and the partial pressure difference that exists between the gas cavity and respiring tissue. This partial pressure difference is due to the inherent unsaturation of venous blood, which in turn is a result of the difference in solubility of O_2 and CO_2 in tissue. CO_2 is 20 times more soluble in body tissues than is O_2. As O_2 is consumed, it is replaced by CO_2 from substrate oxidation at a ratio of about 0.8 moles of CO_2 for each mole of O_2 reduced. Thus, oxygen entering a tissue at an arterial P_{O_2} of 100 mmHg leaves the venous capillary at a P_{O_2} of 40 mmHg. In contrast, CO_2 enters at 40 mmHg and leaves at only 46 mmHg. The remainder of the gas pressure in the tissues is primarily N_2, which at equilibrium has the same partial pressure, 573 mmHg, on both sides of the circulation. Therefore, the sum of the partial pressures in the venous system is 54 mmHg less than in the arterial system. This "oxygen window" provides a potential pressure gradient for elimination of N_2. As a gas pocket or bubble collapses from removal of O_2 by metabolism, the internal P_{N_2} must rise above tissue P_{N_2} because the total pressure in the bubble remains in equilibrium with ambient pressure. In this way, the N_2 is resorbed gradually. The oxygen window can be expanded during and after decompression and during recompression by administration of high partial pressures of O_2. Oxygen decreases the tissue P_{N_2} and increases the partial pressure gradient for N_2 between the bubble and tissue. Immediate O_2 administration at the scene of a diving accident before recompression therapy is clearly beneficial in the management of DCS and AGE.

A variety of available recompression schedules are effective for DCS if the treatment is begun promptly. Recompression tables which use minimal recompression and HBO have become the treatment of choice. US Navy Treatment Table 6, which uses intermittent HBO at a maximum depth of 2.8 ATA (60 fsw), has become a therapeutic standard for primary DCS as well as for recurrent symptoms.[4] Recurrent or persisting symptoms should be retreated with Table 6 once a day or with Table 5 twice a day. Persistent bladder and bowel dysfunction or neuromuscular weakness also may respond to saturation therapy, e.g., US Navy Table 7, if resources and expertise are available in conducting prolonged treatments.[4] In some instances of DCS, oxygen recompression is not available, and air recompression tables must be used. Air treatment tables are longer and less effective than oxygen tables and are more likely to produce DCS in the attendants inside the chamber.

The rationale for treatment of both AGE and clinically significant VGE with HBO is threefold. First, the increase in ambient pressure mechanically compresses the gas embolus and increases the surface area:volume ratio of the bubble, thus improving nitrogen diffusion from the bubble. Second, the higher the oxygen tension in the blood, the greater the nitrogen gradient across the blood-bubble interface. Third, the amount of O_2 physically dissolved in plasma (approximately 6 mL O_2/dL plasma at 2.8 ATA) during HBO may be sufficient to avert or reverse ischemia if plasma streaming occurs around small emboli which obstruct erythrocyte flow.

The optimal depth and duration for HBO treatment of air embolism are still uncertain. Experience by the US Navy with air embolism after military diving accidents led to the development of Table 6A.[4] Table 6A uses initial recompression of the patient breathing air to an equivalent pressure of 165 fsw (6 ATA) followed by prompt decompression to 60 fsw (2.8 ATA) where the patient breathes 100% O_2. The chamber is then decompressed slowly to the surface while the patient breathes O_2 in cycles alternating with air. The intent of the initial, deep compression in Table 6A is mechanical reduction of the emboli to 55 percent of their original diameter (assuming spherical geometry). This approach may be appropriate for very recent AGE or when the quantity of intravascular gas is very large. Deep compression on air, however, may actually allow influx of nitrogen into the emboli so that they are larger after decompression than before compression. This disadvantage can be circumvented in part by having the patient breathe a mixture of 50% O_2 and 50% N_2 during compression to decrease the driving force of N_2 into the emboli. Of note, recent experience using US Navy Table 6 to treat air embolism suggests that equally efficacious results are obtained when initial compression to 6 ATA is eliminated and the patient breathes 100% O_2 during compression to 2.8 ATA. This compresses the emboli to about 70 percent of the original diameter and expedites release of nitrogen. Table 6, originally designed for the treatment of type II DCS, is more amenable to hospital-based chambers and is particularly well suited to critically ill patients who suffer air embolism at normal barometric pressure. Like DCS, recurrent or persisting symptoms from gas embolism may respond to repetitive daily Table 6 treatments until no further improvement is noted.

Many hospitals may not have the experience or equipment to manage a critically ill patient in a hyperbaric chamber. In that case, the patient may require transfer to a suitably equipped facility. This can be accomplished by ground or air transportation as long as the aircraft can be pressurized to 1 ATA or safely fly below 1000 ft of altitude to avoid any further increase in the size of the gas emboli. Advice from a diving medicine physician concerning the management or referral of diving-related injuries is available 24-h a day by calling the Divers Alert Network (DAN) at (919) 684-8111. DAN is a nonprofit organization which collects and disseminates information about diving safety and related injuries and is associated with the FG Hall Hypo-Hyperbaric Center at Duke University Medical Center.

Near Drowning

PATHOPHYSIOLOGY

The immediate consequences of ND are attributable to asphyxia. Effective pulmonary gas exchange ceases, and the victim suffers the physiologic consequences of hypoxia and hypercapnia. Excellent reviews of the on-site management of ND and its demographics have been published and will not be repeated here.[30,31] This section will summarize the pathophysiology of the systems most frequently injured during ND and supported in the ICU: the lungs, brain, heart, and kidneys.

LUNG

The pathophysiology of lung injury in ND is complex. Airway obstruction is initiated when either fresh water (FW) or sea water (SW) contacts the mucosa of the lower respiratory tract and stimulates intense laryngospasm. Laryngospasm may be protective in some cases if the duration of hypoxemia is limited by a brief immersion time. Approximately 10 to 15 percent of ND victims aspirate trivial volumes of water, yet some of these individuals develop O_2 deprivation of sufficient magnitude and duration to produce hypoxic encephalopathy or ventricular arrythmia as a direct result of laryngospasm.[32] Aspiration of both SW and FW also induces mechanical airway obstruction with a small airway component. Small airway obstruction is aggravated by bronchoconstriction, mucosal edema, and plugging by water and suspended debris such as algae, diatoms, sand, mud, teeth, and stomach contents.[33]

Aspiration of even small quantities of either SW or FW produces a prompt and profound decrease in lung compliance and results in persistent areas of low ventilation/perfusion ratio ($\dot{V}_A/\dot{Q}$) and shunt.[33,34] Therefore, aspiration of water may produce a longer lasting hypoxemia than laryngospasm alone. Some of the mechanisms of the early changes in pulmonary gas exchange have been elucidated in animal models and are attributable, in general, to loss of surfactant or its activity, damage to the alveolar epithelium and capillary endothelium, and alveolar flooding. In human beings, vomiting and aspiration of stomach contents during ND is common and also aggravates mucosal and alveolar epithelial injury.

The combination of alveolar flooding, loss of surfactant, or its function with atelectasis and alveolar damage may give rise to progressive hypoxemia due to intrapulmonary shunting, which may reach 70 percent of the cardiac output in severe cases.[33,35] The pathophysiologic injury culminates in ARDS several hours to days after the ND event in about 40 percent of ND victims.[36,37] Hypoxemia usually necessitates treatment with supplemental oxygen at high inspired oxygen fraction (F_{IO_2}) which may superimpose pulmonary oxygen toxicity on ARDS. Fortunately, ARDS which develops after ND is more likely to be reversible relative to ARDS of other etiologies.[37]

BRAIN

The pathophysiology of brain injury in ND is that of global anoxia or severe hypoxia and differs little from other etiologies. Prolonged anoxia or hypoxia produces diffuse neuronal damage which, if severe, compromises the function of the blood-brain barrier with resultant cerebral edema. Intracranial pressure (ICP) may rise as edema develops, further decreasing brain perfusion, exacerbating intracellular hypoxia and, in severe cases, leading to herniation. Profound increases in ICP are infrequent after ND, but tend to appear more than 24 h after initial resuscitation in patients who already have some evidence of neurologic dysfunction.[37] Some authors consider a spiraling increase in ICP an indicator of the severity of initial and ongoing neuronal injury rather than a major source of the insult.[37,38]

The major potential differences between ND and anoxic brain insults of other etiologies are the diving reflex and body cooling (hypothermia).[39] In human beings, the diving reflex is vestigial and most demonstrable in young children during exposure to cold water.[39,40] ND in cold water with prompt hypothermia slows cerebral metabolism and thereby postpones the deleterious effects of anoxia.[41] These factors may be important as they are associated with a better prognosis after apparently severe ND in some patients.[40–42]

HEART

Atrial and ventricular arrhythmias, particularly ventricular fibrillation, occur in severe ND although some authors only report "cardiac arrest."[43] Older studies of drowning in animals demonstrated hemolysis and large rapid shifts in the concentrations of blood electrolytes after instillation of FW and SW into the lungs. These responses were correlated with the occurrence of ventricular arrhythmias. Human studies have failed to confirm significant electrolyte changes even in patients with ventricular fibrillation.[44] A notable exception is drowning in the waters of the Dead Sea which has a much higher mineral content than other SW. Dead Sea drowning victims developed hypernatremia, hyperchloremia, hypermagnesemia, and hypercalcemia slowly over 24 h following exposure because of absorption of electrolytes from the gastrointestinal tract after swallowing large volumes of water during the episode. These electrolyte changes were associated with fatal ventricular fibrillation in one of eight patients reported.[42]

ND in human beings differs in a major way from animal studies in the volume of fluid aspirated; human victims rarely aspirate enough water to produce significant electrolyte changes.[44] In addition, pathologic studies in humans after SW or FW drowning demonstrate myocyte hypercontraction and hypereosinophilic sarcomeres in the heart. These pathologic changes are characteristic of catecholamine excess and suggest that intense adrenergic stimulation contributes to the arrhythmias after ND.[45] Thus, the etiology of ventricular fibrillation in human beings is most likely related to hypoxia, respiratory and metabolic acidosis, and catecholamine excess.

KIDNEY

The incidence of renal insufficiency following ND is unknown but far less frequently reported than lung, brain, or cardiac injury. The renal complication cited most often is oliguria, attributable to acute tubular necrosis (ATN).[46] The etiology of ATN in this setting is likely hypoxemia and hypotension. Infrequently, ND may be complicated by rhabdomyolysis and hemolysis with disseminated intravascular coagulation (DIC).[47] Hemolysis and DIC also may contribute to ATN. Although patients with acute renal failure after ND may require transient dialysis, recovery of adequate renal function can be expected in the majority of patients.

MANAGEMENT

GENERAL MEASURES

ND in adults and adolescents is associated with a number of predisposing factors and complicating injuries. These factors are easily overlooked in the unconscious, critically ill ND patient. They must be suspected in every case because they may affect the treatment and prognosis of the patient.

Alcohol and other CNS-altering drugs are commonly implicated in adult ND.[48] Sedatives and alcohol in particular may complicate the patient's initial ICU course by exacerbating hypothermia and hypotension, impairing mental status, and depressing respiratory drive. Toxic drug and blood alcohol levels should be measured in complicated patients admitted to the ICU.

Other predispositions to ND include untoward pathophysiologic events in the otherwise unimpaired adult swimmer. Myocardial infarction, cardiac arrhythmias, seizures, subarachnoid hemorrhage, and AGE in the SCUBA diver have been implicated in many episodes of ND.[48] These events may require extraordinary diagnostic efforts in the immediate postresuscitation environment of the ICU. Electrocardiography (ECG) should be obtained routinely because the heart is a target organ for hypoxemia in ND victims. Serial measurements of cardiac enzymes in ND are useful in confirming the diagnosis of myocardial infarction when ECG changes are nondiagnostic. Acute intracranial hemorrhage or status epilepticus may need to be excluded in patients whose course in the ICU is complicated by neurologic dysfunction. Recompression and HBO therapy should be considered in the near drowned SCUBA diver with obtundation, coma, or other neurologic deficit (see section on VGE and AGE).

Injuries to the spine and skull are common in ND victims. These most often occur when a swimmer dives into shallow water and strikes the head on the bottom or on a submerged object.[48] Another common scenario involves a motor vehicle accident which leaves the passenger submerged in a body of water. Burst fractures of the cervical vertebrae resulting in tetraplegia have been reported in these settings. Additionally, skin, middle ear, or sinus trauma sustained during ND may serve as portals of entry for infection.[49] Such injuries must be considered in the unconscious ND victim in the ICU.

MANAGEMENT IN THE ICU

The major indications for admitting the ND patient to the ICU are respiratory failure, cardiac arrest or arrythmia, and obtundation or coma. The patient is often intubated prior to arrival in the ICU. Clinically, the patient may exhibit cyanosis, tachycardia, hypo- or hypertension, hypothermia (which may require a low temperature thermometer to measure), respiratory distress with frothy, blood-tinged sputum, diffuse crackles, and wheezing on examination. Initial laboratory evaluation often reveals a metabolic acidosis (due to lactic acid) and hypoxemia on arterial blood-gas analysis. Serum electrolytes, with the exception of a decreased bicarbonate concentration, rarely are perturbed significantly.[50] Hypoglycemia is common.[51] Hemolysis and rhabdomyolysis, if seen, tend to occur early in the clinical course unless they are the result of late sepsis. ECG abnormalities include evidence of ischemia or injury and ventricular and atrial arrhythmias. Initial chest radiographic findings range from patchy infiltrates to diffuse air space disease (Fig. 74-2). Progressive increase in parenchymal infiltrates over hours to days is not unusual.

RESPIRATORY CARE

Mechanical ventilation can be a major challenge in the severely injured ND victim. As discussed previously, atelectasis and pulmonary edema from the lack of functional surfactant and epithelial damage with intrapulmonary

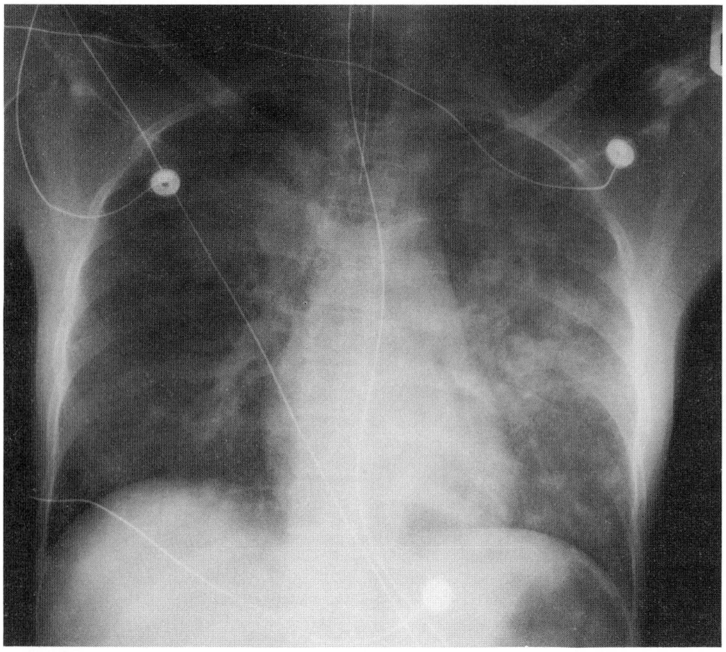

FIGURE 74-2 Chest radiograph 2 h after an ND episode shows typical patchy infiltrates.

shunting are encountered in all types of ND. ARDS can develop with accompanying elevated airway pressures which predispose to pulmonary barotrauma and air embolism. These conditions can be further complicated by the presence of foreign bodies in the airways. Sedation or paralysis with drugs such as pancuronium are best avoided in ND patients because they impair the clinician's ability to follow the neurologic examination. Careful use of these agents, however, may improve mechanical ventilation by synchronizing the patient with the ventilator and decreasing peak airway pressures and the risk of barotrauma. The advantages of positive end-expiratory pressure (PEEP) in decreasing intrapulmonary shunt can be dramatic in severe hypoxemia after ND.

Respiratory insufficiency in ND may be complicated by factors other than atelectasis and intrapulmonary shunt. Airway obstruction may occur either as bronchospasm or from a foreign body. Bronchodilator therapy with inhaled β-agonist agents and theophylline may benefit the patient with diffuse wheezing. Patients with localized atelectasis that fails to improve with effective ventilation or those who exhibit localized wheezing should undergo fiberoptic bronchoscopy to exclude or remove a foreign body.

Many ND accidents occur in water which is contaminated with human or animal waste or naturally contains pathogenic bacteria or fungi. The lung is the most common portal of entry for a wide variety of these organisms. Infection is heralded by fever 2 to 7 days after the ND event and should prompt sputum and blood cultures prior to initiation of antibiotic therapy.[52] Prophylactic antibiotic coverage has not improved outcome after ND, and routine use of antibiotics is not indicated. Reported infections have been summarized in Table 74-3. Awareness of infection by more unusual organisms is crucial, because they may have specific culture requirements not offered routinely in many hospital microbiology laboratories.[49]

BRAIN RESUSCITATION

Therapeutic measures for brain resuscitation after ND are controversial. The debate is complicated by the diverse parameters which influence brain injury and recovery, including the age of the victim, the water temperature and submersion time (or period of asphyxia), coexisting injuries, and preexisting disease.[57] The matter is complicated further by anecdotal reports of complete or near complete neurologic recovery in association with specific therapeutic measures after prolonged immersion. The initial prognostic uncertainties about brain recovery after ND mandate a full effort at cardiopulmonary resuscitation including correction of hypothermia.[58]

Classification of the victims' neurologic status 1 to 2 h after resuscitation allows systematic assessment of prognosis. A system with reasonable discrimination for outcome in human beings subclassifies patients after resuscitation into three categories as shown in Table 74-4.[40,41]

The best discrimination for outcome using this system has been found in children where all category A and B victims (n = 57) recovered completely. Level C victims (n = 39) suffered 33.3 percent and 23.9 percent cerebral morbidity (mortality + morbidity = 56.2 percent) with the lowest survival in the C.3 group.[41] In another series of patients which included 52 adults, the category A patients recovered completely while 2 adults and 1 child in category B eventually succumbed to barotrauma or other complications.[40] Eight of 11 (73 percent) adult and 8 of 18 (44 percent) child category C patients recovered completely in that series.

Early reports of a brain resuscitation regimen known as

TABLE 74-3 Microbial Isolates Associated with Infection in ND Victims[a]

Bacteria	Type of Water	Reference
Klebsiella oxytoca	FW	53, 49
Herellea spp	FW	47
Neiserria meningitidis	FW	47
Pseudomonas aeruginosa	FW	53
Listeria monocytogenes	FW	53
Plesiomonas shigelloides	FW	53
Edwardsiella tarda	FW	53
Chromobacterium violaceum	FW	67
Aeromonas hydrophila	SW, FW	53, 49
Escherichia coli	SW, FW	53, 49
Proteus mirabilis	SW, FW	49, 53
Staphylococcus aureus	SW, FW	53, 54
Neiserria mucosus	Brackish	55
Pseudomonas putrefaciens	SW	49, 54
Francisella philomiragia	SW	52
Vibrio parahemolyticus	SW	49
Fungus		
Pseudoallescheria boydii	FW	53
Aspergillus fumigatus	FW	56, 53

[a]Organisms isolated from sputum or blood of clinically infected ND victims soon after admission. This list does not include organisms recovered from infected wounds.
FW = fresh water; SW = sea water

TABLE 74-4 Classification of ND Victims Following Initial Resuscitation

Category A	Awake, fully conscious
Category B	Blunted consciousness, stuporous but arousable
Category C	Comatose

Category C is further subclassified into:

C.1	Decorticate posturing
C.2	Decerebrate posturing
C.3	Flaccid

HYPER (hyperhydration, hyperpyrexia, hyperexcitability, and hyperrigidity) suggested that the fraction of category C child ND victims with subsequent complete recovery could be increased.[41] The acronym addressed the overhydration, fever, excitability, and muscular rigidity noted in some category C patients. These findings were thought to affect outcome adversely, and aggressive therapy was recommended to minimize them.

HYPER therapy consists of systemic corticosteroids, osmotic diuretics, hyperventilation, barbiturate coma, and muscle relaxants administered to minimize cerebral edema and reduce ICP. Controlled hypothermia (32°C, 89.6°F) to decrease neuronal metabolism also was advocated.[42] Monitoring of ICP is necessary to guide such aggressive therapy. The basic rationale for this therapy assumed that control of ICP would minimize neuronal damage after diffuse anoxia. The pathophysiology of brain injury following ND suggests, however, that the increase in ICP which develops 24 to 48 h after ND may be a result of severe neuronal injury rather than its cause.

Critical reviews and subsequent experience with HYPER therapy have failed to confirm its efficacy and highlighted its potentially detrimental effects.[32,37,58] A retrospective review of 40 ND patients from the same institution that reported the original experience with HYPER found an increased incidence of sepsis and multiple organ failure in patients treated with hypothermia.[57] This may be due to cold-induced immune suppression (including neutropenia) complicated by cold-induced bronchorrhea and decreased mucociliary clearance.[57]

Corticosteroids are efficacious in reducing edema surrounding brain tumors but are of no proven benefit in reducing brain edema associated with trauma, intracerebral hemorrhage, or stroke. In the absence of convincing evidence that corticosteroids reduce edema and hence ICP, and that reduction of ICP improves neurologic outcome after ND, these agents should be avoided as they are immunosuppressive and predispose to infection and gastric ulceration.[59]

Although hypothermia and barbiturates can reduce ICP in some circumstances, their use has not been demonstrated to improve neurologic outcome. Attempts to decrease ICP by osmotic diuresis also have not been shown to improve neurologic outcome after ND and may induce hyperosmolarity and renal insufficiency. Thus, routine use of corticosteroids, hypothermia, and osmotic diuresis cannot be advocated in category C ND patients. Mild hyperventilation is a comparably benign intervention to reduce ICP temporarily, and ICP monitoring may help direct therapy in the subset of ND patients with elevated ICP and poor prognosis.

PROGNOSIS

Overall, about 80 percent of child and adult ND victims recover without sequelae while 2 to 9 percent survive with brain damage. Approximately 12 percent of all ND victims die. About 90 percent of category A and B and approximately 50 percent of category C patients survive with full recovery while 10 to 23 percent of the later group survive but have permanent neurologic sequelae.[36,37,40,44] Thus, respiratory insufficiency in the absence of sepsis or infection is seldom the cause of death in ND victims in hospitals with modern intensive care capabilities.

A number of indicators such as serum electrolytes, arterial blood-gas and pH values, electroencephalographic findings or clinical features (body temperature, absence of pupillary responses, cardiac arrest, duration of submersion, and initial resuscitative efforts) have been examined for use as early markers of prognosis. None is sufficiently discriminating to guide early therapy. The absence of spontaneous respirations after resuscitation, however, is a particularly ominous sign and uniformly associated with severe neurologic impairment or death.[58]

Therapeutic Whole Lung Lavage

Therapeutic flooding of the whole lung is a form of controlled ND used for many years to treat alveolar filling diseases including lipoid pneumonia, cystic fibrosis, and pulmonary alveolar proteinosis (PAP). Whole lung lavage is currently used primarily for PAP, a rare diffuse lung disease of unknown etiology.[60] In PAP, a combination of lipoproteins and noninflammatory cellular debris accumulates in the alveoli and creates a physiologic picture of low ventilation/perfusion ratio which may progress to severe shunting and refractory hypoxemia. The disease affects men twice as often as women and begins commonly in the fourth to sixth decade of life. Occasional onset in childhood is also well documented. Approximately one-third of patients with PAP spontaneously remit, one-third do not progress and one-third die of progressive respiratory or right ventricular failure or infection.

Indications for whole lung lavage include resting hypoxemia, e.g., <90% hemoglobin oxygen saturation or hemoglobin oxygen desaturation with routine activities. The frequency of lavage is variable; some patients require only one lavage and others require lavage every 8 weeks for extended periods of time. Therapeutic whole lung lavage with saline is more effective for physical removal of the debris than segmental lavage via a bronchoscope in patients with PAP. The efficiency of protein clearance is increased by manual percussion of the chest during the emptying phases of the lavage but not by additives such as proteolytic enzymes or heparin in the lavage fluid.[61] Complications of the procedure include hydropneumothorax, inadvertent flooding of the contralateral lung, hypoxemia, infection, and arrhythmias.[62,63]

LAVAGE TECHNIQUE

Lung lavage usually is performed under general anesthesia with muscle relaxation. Standard clinical monitoring during the procedure includes pulse oximetry, ECG, blood pressure by indwelling radial artery catheter, core temperature, and volume of exchange in and out of the lung.[61,64] The trachea and left main bronchus are intubated with a dual-lumen endotracheal tube (Fig. 74-3). Although intubation of the left main bronchus is technically more difficult than the right main bronchus, the greater length of the left mainstem before the first bifurcation provides better mechanical stability of the endotracheal tube and less chance of obstruction of a bronchial orifice. Proper placement of the endotracheal tube is crucial for success in separating the lungs for independent lavage and ventilation. Tube placement is verified anatomically by fiberoptic bronchoscopy and functionally by auscultation and inflation of one lung to 50 cm H_2O pressure to ensure that the contralateral main bronchus has been isolated. This is accomplished by connecting the appropriate bronchial tube via a connecting tube to a beaker of sterile saline and observing for bubbles. Although a few bubbles are seen initially from compression by the pressurized lung, persisting bubbles indicate a leak and incomplete separation of the lungs.

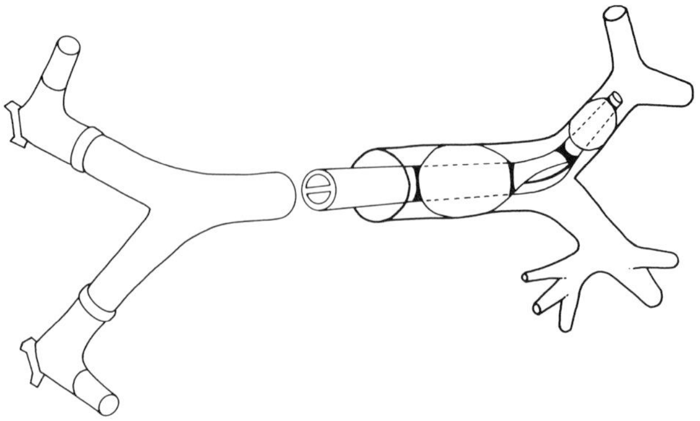

FIGURE 74-3 Schematic drawing of left main bronchus intubation with a dual-lumen endotracheal tube (Broncho-Cath, Mallinckrodt).

In our center, a number of patients with PAP are referred with advanced lung disease and severe hypoxemia despite supplemental O_2. All therapeutic lung lavages are performed by a team composed of the anesthesiologist, pulmonologist, and a physical therapist in a large hyperbaric chamber. This permits HBO to be used to maintain adequate oxygenation of arterial blood during the procedure if necessary.[65] Many patients with severe hypoxemia worsen during unilateral lavage, particularly during the emptying phases of the lavage. Worsening hypoxemia during the emptying phase occurs because pulmonary blood flow increases to the lavaged lung when the hydrostatic compression of the pulmonary capillaries is alleviated by the lung emptying. Therefore, we simulate the emptying phase of the lavage before the procedure by ventilating the lung to be lavaged with 6% O_2 (to approximate mixed venous P_{O_2}) and the other lung with 100% O_2 for 5 min.[66] Hemoglobin saturation is monitored by pulse oximetry, while an arterial blood-gas value at the nadir of the response is used to confirm the level of hypoxemia. Hemoglobin saturations below 85% ($P_{O_2} < 55$ mmHg) during this maneuver dictate that the lavage be performed under hyperbaric conditions (1.2 to 2.8 ATA). This test serves as a "worst case scenario" for arterial oxygenation and is useful to determine which patients will need HBO. If HBO will be required, bilateral myringotomies are performed to avoid middle or inner ear barotrauma during compression and decompression of the anesthetized patient.

The first phase of the lavage procedure is to wash N_2 out of the lungs by ventilating the patient with 100% O_2. This prevents relatively insoluble and nonmetabolizable N_2 from creating an "air lock" in the lavaged lung. The lung is then flooded with normal saline at 37°C (98.6°F) at a rate based on one-half the patient's O_2 uptake (1 to 2 mL O_2/kg body weight/min). This is accomplished via a tube connected to a reservoir of saline 45 to 50 cm above the patient's midaxil-

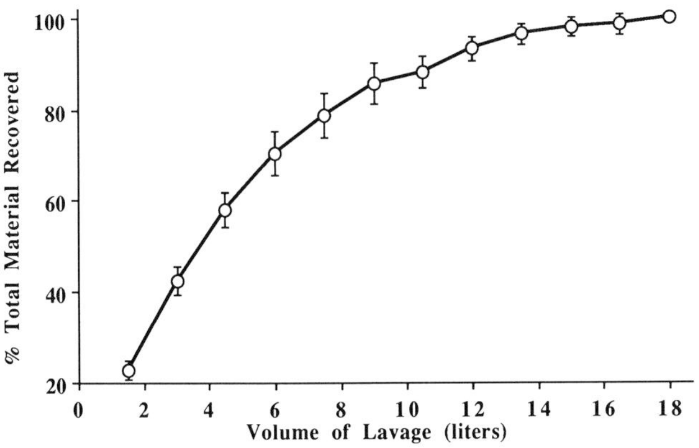

FIGURE 74-4 Cumulative recovery of wet debris in lavage fluid compared to lavage volume in six patients with alveolar proteinosis. Approximately 95 percent of the debris is recovered within 12 to 15 L lavage. (Data courtesy Dr. Alexander Spock, Division of Pulmonary Disease and Gastroenterology, Department of Pediatrics, Duke University Medical Center.)

lary line. Recent lung volume measurements are used to estimate the total volume of fluid that the lung will hold. If HBO is required, compression begins during flooding as the hemoglobin saturation declines. Compression of the chamber continues until a saturation of at least 90% can be maintained.

After filling the lung, that hemithorax is percussed vigorously as 400 to 500 mL fluid is drained by gravity to a graduated receiver 40 to 45 cm below the patient. Some authors advocate nearly complete emptying of the lung with each lavage aliquot. We use smaller tidal aliquots of lavage to minimize the hypoxemia associated with the emptying phases of the lavage.[64,65] After emptying, another tidal aliquot of saline is instilled, and the process is repeated until the effluent is nearly clear to inspection. This requires 10 to 20 L lavage fluid per lung. The efficiency of this method with respect to yield of wet debris is comparable to that achieved with near complete emptying of the lung and is shown in Fig. 74-4. After lavage, the lung is drained completely and suctioned before reinflating with large tidal volumes of 100% O_2 and PEEP. The availability of HBO allows the patient with a freshly lavaged lung to be oxygenated during the contralateral procedure. Using this procedure, both lungs can be lavaged sequentially on the same day. This allows the patient to undergo a single period of general anesthesia and a shorter hospitalization. Some institutions require a 2- to 7-day recovery period after the first lavage before lavaging the second lung. After lavage and anesthetic recovery, the patients are weaned rapidly from 10 to 15 cmH_2O PEEP and a high F_{IO_2} in the ICU and usually can be extubated 4 to 12 h after the procedure.

CASE PRESENTATION

A 21-year-old white male was completing his first open water dive in his SCUBA course when he found a fishing reel in 20 ft of water. In his excitement, he retrieved the tackle and quickly ascended to the surface where he shouted and sank underwater. He was unconscious and cyanotic but breathing spontaneously when retrieved from the water. Oxygen was applied by mask, and he regained consciousness within a few minutes. He was confused, but reported generalized weakness, tingling in the extremities, headache, chest pain, and shortness of breath. Nausea, vomiting, and worsening headache ensued before he again lost consciousness and developed decerebrate posturing. Oxygen by mask was continued, and he was taken to the emergency room of a local hospital where a physician suspected air embolism and ND. After bilateral chest tubes were inserted to relieve pneumothoraces, and tracheal intubation, he was transferred to a hospital with a hyperbaric chamber.

On arrival at the second hospital, the patient was comatose with decerebrate posturing and had crackles and wheezing on chest examination. He had persistent air leaks from the chest tubes. Arterial blood-gas determinations revealed a widened alveolar-arterial gradient; chest radiograph revealed patchy infiltrates and no pleural air. Computed tomography (CT) of the head obtained prior to consultation with a diving physician did not reveal intravascular gas or other abnormalites. Mechanical ventilation was complicated by high airway pressures and a requirement for a high F_{IO_2} and PEEP. The patient was first treated in the hyperbaric chamber nearly 24 h after the accident for presumed cerebral air embolism using US Navy Table 6A, with some improvement in his neurologic status. He was treated again 12 h later using US Navy Table 6 and recovered consciousness. His pulmonary status quickly improved, he was extubated, and the chest tubes were removed. Three days after the accident, he developed cough, fever to 39°C (102.2°F), dyspnea, leukocytosis of 16,700, and pulmonary infiltrates in the right lower lobe on chest radiograph. Sputum Gram stain revealed gram negative rods and culture grew *K. oxytoca* sensitive to cefazolin. He was treated initially with penicillin and subsequently was changed to cefazolin. His response to the therapy was excellent, and he was transferred out of the ICU on the fifth hospital day where he made an uneventful recovery.

CASE DISCUSSION

This case is typical of sports diving accidents in several respects. The diver was a novice making a shallow dive. The most common serious injury in the sports diver is ND, followed by AGE caused by rapid ascent either with a closed glottis, as in this case, or underlying lung disease, e.g., asthma, bleb, or other potentially obstructive airway defect. Injury often occurs in ascent from a shallow depth. This diver had clinical features of both ND and AGE. He also developed ARDS consistent with ND. Later, in the course of his hospitalization, he contracted pneumonia with an unusual organism, given his previous state of good health. Of note, SCUBA diving is typically practiced far from competent medical care. Delays in therapy are common even in catastrophic accidents. Recompression therapy, however, can be effective 1 to 2 days after the accident and must be offered.

One unnecessary delay in this case was the head CT scan on arrival at the second hospital. The clinical setting which suggested AGE and the rare detection of AGE by radiographic study made the CT unwarranted prior to recompression. Finally, physicians with experience in diving medicine do not all agree about the choice of a recompression treatment table for AGE. Evidence to suggest that the longer and deeper US Navy Table 6A is superior to Table 6 is lacking in treating the patient with AGE. Lidocaine, 2 to 4 mg/min after an appropriate loading dose, and intravenous fluids could have been administered in an attempt to reduce cerebral injury, prevent cardiac arrhythmias, and provide rehydration when the patient presented to the first hospital.

References

1. Epstein M, De Nunzio A, Ramachandran M: Characterization of the renal response to prolonged immersion in normal man: Implication for an understanding of the circulatory adaptation to manned space flight. J Appl Physiol: Resp Environ Exercise Physiol 49:184, 1980.
2. Lin YC: Circulatory functions during immersion and breath-hold dives in humans. Undersea Biomed Res 11:123, 1984.
3. Mithoefer JC: Breath holding, in Fenn W, Rahn H (eds): *Handbook of Physiology, Respiration.* Washington, American Physiology Society, 1965, p 1011.
4. US Navy Diving Manual, Washington, DC, US Department of the Navy, Vol 1, Air Diving, Revision 1, 1985 (NAVSEA 0994-LP-001-9021).
5. Vann RD: Decompression theory and application, in Bennett PB, Elliott DH (eds): *The Physiology and Medicine of Diving.* San Pedro, Best Publishing, 1982, p 352.
6. Weathersby PK, Homer LD, Flynn ET: On the likelihood of decompression sickness. J Appl Physiol 57:815, 1984.
7. Lam TH, Yau KP: Manifestations and treatment of 793 cases of decompression sickness in a compressed air tunneling project in Hong Kong. Undersea Biomed Res 15:377, 1988.
8. Divers Alert Network. *Report on 1987 Diving Accidents.* Duke University Medical Center, Durham, NC.
9. Hallenbeck JM, Bove AA, Elliott DH: Mechanism underlying spinal cord damage in decompression sickness. Neurology 25:308, 1975.
10. Leitch DR, Hallenback JM: Neurological forms of decompression sickness, in Shilling CW, Carlston CB, Mathias RA (eds): *The Physician's Guide to Diving Medicine.* New York, Plenum Press, 1984, p 326.
11. Moon RE, Camporesi EM, Kisslo JA: Patent foramen ovale and decompression sickness in divers. Lancet 1:513, 1989.
12. Clark MC, Flick MR: Permeability pulmonary edema caused by venous air embolism. Am Rev Respir Dis 129:633, 1984.
13. Dahlback GO, Lundgren CEG: Pulmonary air-trapping induced by immersion. Aerospace Med 43:768, 1972.
14. Katz J, Leiman BC, Butler BD: Effects of inhalation anaesthetics on filtration of venous gas emboli by the pulmonary vasculature. Br J Anaesth 61:200, 1988.
15. Pearson RR: Diagnosis and treatment of gas embolism, in Schilling CW, Carlston CB, Mathias RA (eds): *The Physician's Guide to Diving Medicine.* New York, Plenum Press, 1984, p 333.
16. Butler BD, Hills BA: The lung as a filter for microbubbles. Am J Physiol: Respir Environ Exercise Physiol 47:537, 1979.
17. Neuman TS, Spragg RG, Wagner PD, et al: Cardiopulmonary consequences of decompression stress. Respir Physiol 41:143, 1980.
18. Butler BD, Katz J: Vascular pressures and passage of gas emboli through the pulmonary circulation. Undersea Biomed Res 15:203, 1988.
19. Black S, Cucchiara RF, Nishimur RA, et al: Parameters affecting occurrence of paradoxical air embolism. Anesthesiology 71:235, 1989.
20. Ence TJ, Gong H Jr: Adult respiratory distress syndrome after venous air embolism. Am Rev Respir Dis 119:1033, 1979.
21. Lamm WJE, Luchtel D, Albert RK: Sites of leakage in three models of acute lung injury. J Appl Physiol 64:1079, 1988.
22. Zwirewich CV, Muller NL, Abboud RT, et al: Noncardiogenic pulmonary edema caused by decompression sickness: Rapid resolution following hyperbaric therapy. Radiology 163:81, 1987.
23. Marini JJ, Culver BH: Systemic gas embolism complicating mechanical ventilation in the adult respiratory distress syndrome. Ann Intern Med 110:699, 1989.
24. Hadjimiltiades S, Goldbaum TS, Mostel E, et al: Coronary air embolism during coronary angioplasty. Cathet Cardiovasc Diagn 16:164, 1989.
25. Gottlieb JD, Ericsson JA, Sweet RB: Venous air embolism: A review. Anesth Analg 44:773, 1965.
26. Butler BD, Laine GA, Leiman BC, et al: Effect of the Trendelenburg position on the distribution of arterial air emboli in dogs. Ann Thorac Surg 45:198, 1988.
27. Bulter BD, Luehr S, Katz J: Venous gas embolism: Time course of residual pulmonary intravascular bubbles. Undersea Biomed Res 16:21, 1989.
28. Dutka AJ: A review of pathophysiology and potential application of experimental therapies for cerebral ischemia to the treatment of cerebral arterial gas embolism. Undersea Biomed Res 12:403, 1985.
29. Committee Report. Hyperbaric Oxygen Therapy. Undersea and Hyperbaric Medical Society, Inc. UMS Publication #30, Bethesda, 1986.
30. Shepherd S: Immersion injury: Drowning and near drowning. Postgrad Med 85:183, 1989.
31. Shaw KN, Briede CA: Submersion injuries: Drowning and near-drowning. Emerg Med Clin North Am 7:355, 1989.
32. Modell JH: Near drowning. Circulation 74(suppl IV):27, 1986.
33. Colebatch HJH, Halmagyi DFJ: Lung mechanics and resuscitation after fluid aspiration. J Appl Physiol 16:684, 1961.
34. Modell JH, Moya F: Effects of volume of aspirated fluid during chlorinated fresh water drowning. Anesthesiology 27:662, 1966.
35. Lheureux P, Vincent JL, Brimioulle S: Fulminant pulmonary edema after near-drowning: Remarkably high colloid osmotic pressure in tracheal fluid. Intensive Care Med 10:205, 1984.
36. Kaukinen L: Clinical course and prognostic signs in near-drowning patients. Ann Chir Gynaecol 73:34, 1984.
37. Oakes DD, Sherck JP, Maloney JR, et al: Prognosis and management of victims of near-drowning. J Trauma 22:544, 1982.
38. Sarnaik AP, Preston G, Lieh-Lai M, et al: Intracranial pressure and cerebral perfusion pressure in near-drowning. Crit Care Med 13:224, 1985.
39. Siebke H, Breivik H, Rod T, et al: Survival after 40 minutes' submersion without cerebral sequelae. Lancet 1:1275, 1975.
40. Modell JH, Graves SA, Kuck EJ: Near-drowning: Correlation of level of consciousness and survival. Can Anaesth Soc J 27:211, 1980.
41. Conn AW, Montes JE, Barker GA, et al: Cerebral salvage in near-drowning following neurological classification by triage. Can Anaesth Soc J 27:201, 1980.

42. Yagil Y, Stalnikowicz R, Michaeli J, et al: Near drowning in the Dead Sea. Arch Intern Med 145:50, 1985.
43. Sarnaik AP, Vohra MP: Near-drowning: Fresh, salt, and cold water immersion. Clin Sports Med 5:33, 1986.
44. Modell JH, Graves SA, Ketover A: Clinical course of 91 consecutive near-drowning victims. Chest 70:231, 1976.
45. Karch SB: Pathology of the heart in drowning. Arch Pathol Lab Med 109:176, 1985.
46. Neale TJ, Dewar JM, Parr R, et al: Acute renal failure following near drowning in salt water. NZ Med J 97:319, 1984.
47. Ports TA, Deuel TF: Intravascular coagulation in fresh-water submersion. Ann Intern Med 87:60, 1977.
48. Manolios N, Mackie I: Drowning and near-drowning on Australian beaches patrolled by life-savers: A 10-year study, 1973–1983. Med J Aust 148:165, 1988.
49. Sims JK, Enomoto PI, Frankel RI, et al: Marine bacteria complicating seawater near-drowning and marine wounds: A hypothesis. Ann Emerg Med 12:212, 1983.
50. Modell JH, Davis JH, Giammona ST, et al: Blood gas and electrolyte changes in human near-drowning victims. JAMA 203:99, 1968.
51. Boles JM, Mabille S, Scheydecker JL, et al: Hypoglycemia in salt water near-drowning victims. Correspondence. Intensive Care Med 14:30, 1988.
52. Wenger JD, Hollis DG, Weaver RE, et al: Infection caused by Francisella philomiragia (formerly *Yersinia philomiragia*). Ann Intern Med 110:888, 1989.
53. Dworzack DL, Clark RB, Borkowski WJ, Jr et al: *Pseudallescheria boydii* brain abscess: Association with near-drowning and efficacy of high-dose, prolonged miconazole therapy in patients with multiple abscesses. Medicine 68:218, 1989.
54. Rosenthal SL, Zuger JH, Apollo E: Respiratory colonization with *Pseudomonas putrefaciens* after near-drowning in salt water. J Clin Pathol 64:382, 1975.
55. Manser TJ, Warner JF: *Neisseria mucosus:* Septicemia after near-drowning. South Med J 80:1323, 1987.
56. Vieira DF, Van Saene HKF, Miranda DR: Case reports: Invasive pulmonary aspergillosis after near-drowning. Intensive Care Med 10:203, 1984.
57. Bohn DJ, Biggar WD, Smith CR, Conn AW, Barker GA: Influence of hypothermia, barbiturate therapy, and intracranial pressure monitoring on morbidity and mortality after near-drowning. Crit Care Med 14:529, 1986.
58. Jacobsen WK, Mason LJ, Briggs BA, et al: Correlation of spontaneous respiration and neurologic damage in near-drowning. Crit Care Med 11:487, 1983.
59. Modell JH: Treatment of near-drowning: Is there a role for H.Y.P.E.R. therapy? Crit Care Med 14:593, 1986.
60. Claypool WD, Rogers RM, Matuschak GM: Update on the clinical diagnosis, management, and pathogenesis of pulmonary alveolar proteinosis (phospholipidosis). Chest 85:551, 1984.
61. Selecky PA, Wasserman K, Benfield JR, et al: The clinical and physiological effect of whole-lung lavage in pulmonary alveolar proteinosis: A ten-year experience. Ann Thorac Surg 24:451, 1977.
62. Hudes ET, Bradley JW, Brebner J: Hydropneumothorax—An unusual complication of lung lavage. Can Anaesth Soc J 33:662, 1986.
63. Ramirez-R J: Alveolar proteinosis: Importance of pulmonary lavage. Am Rev Respir Dis 103:666, 1971.
64. Smith LJ, Ankin MG, Katzenstein AL, et al: Management of pulmonary alveolar proteinosis: Clinical conference in pulmonary disease from Northwestern University McGaw Medical Center, Chicago. Chest 78:765, 1980.
65. Jansen HM, Zuurmond WA, Roos CM, et al: Whole-lung lavage under hyperbaric oxygen conditions for alveolar proteinosis with respiratory failure. Chest 91:829, 1987.
66. Brown SD, Camporesi EM, Moon RE, et al: Therapeutic lung lavage for pulmonary alveolar proteinosis in hyperbaric conditions. Am Rev Respir Dis 141:A53, 1989.
67. Macher AM, Casale TB, Fauci AS: Chronic granulomatous disease of childhood and *Chromobacterium violaceum* infections in the southeastern United States. Ann Intern Med 97:51, 1982.

Chapter 75

SEVERE ILLNESSES OF HIGH ALTITUDE

ROBERT B. SCHOENE

KEY POINTS

- *Severe high altitude illnesses have a number of similarities to commonly encountered critical illnesses at sea level.*
- *Impaired oxygen delivery is the primary similarity.*
- *A review of normal adaptation to high altitude is important to understanding the maladaptive processes that lead to severe illness.*
- *An awareness of the settings of high altitude illnesses is essential to recognizing and treating them effectively.*
- *The severe forms of altitude illness include high altitude cerebral edema (HACE) and high altitude pulmonary edema (HAPE).*
- *Other severe illnesses may occur concomitantly with altitude illness.*

Adaptation to Hypobaric Hypoxia

At high altitude hypoxia is global. Although the fraction of oxygen in our atmosphere is constant at 0.2093, the barometric pressure decreases with increasing altitude, thus decreasing the availability of oxygen (Table 75-1). The drop of P_{O_2} from the air to the blood to the tissues that occurs at sea level also occurs at high altitude. The main difference is that, at high altitude, the inspired partial pressure (PI_{O_2}) is lower, resulting in a proportional lowering of the P_{O_2} at each step in the oxygen cascade (Fig. 75-1).

If given enough time, the human body normally adapts quite well to moderate altitudes, e.g., below 16,000 ft, even though it may never completely adapt to these altitudes. Anecdotal evidence suggests that human populations have never been able to adapt in a way that ensures long-term survival at altitudes higher than 16,000 ft. Of course, individuals with preexisting medical problems may never adapt well to even lower altitudes; their underlying maladies may worsen in the environment of low oxygen. An overall review of altitude adaptation is available.[1]

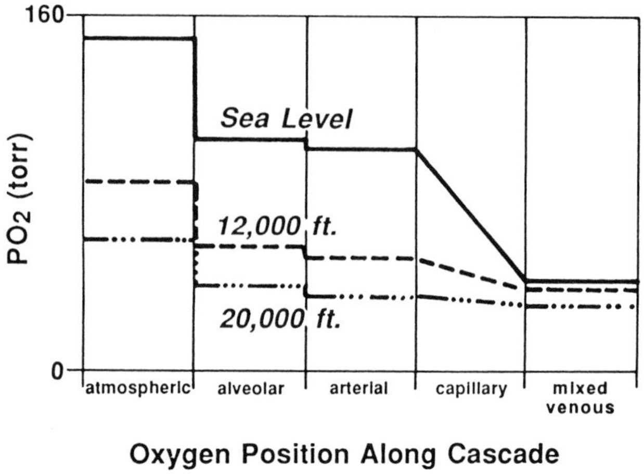

FIGURE 75-1 The oxygen cascade.

On acute ascent to high altitude, the first notable response is an increase in ventilation.[2] Although this response is immediate and is mediated primarily by the peripheral chemoreceptor, the carotid body,[3] ventilation may continue to increase for a number of weeks at any given altitude.[2] The increase in ventilation is a result of complex physiologic interactions that are not yet fully understood. An acute respiratory alkalosis develops and is followed by a much slower renal excretion of bicarbonate, such that the ensuing metabolic acidosis may eventually play a role in ventilatory stimulation. Despite the compensatory metabolic acidosis, persistent, mild alkalemia occurs because the respiratory alkalosis predominates. The increase in alveolar ventilation results in a higher PA_{O_2}.

A mild increase in cardiac output[4] and an improved ventilation/perfusion ($\dot{V}/\dot{Q}$) matching optimize gas exchange.[5,6] Hypoxic pulmonary vasoconstriction causes the more homogeneous distribution of perfusion throughout the lung which matches the increased ventilation.[7] At rest with this improved $\dot{V}/\dot{Q}$ match, there is adequate time for equilibration of the oxygen between air and blood. On the other

TABLE 75-1 Resting Ventilation and Arterial Blood-Gas Values[a]

Altitude (f)	Barometric Pressure (mmHg)	PI_{O_2} (mmHg)	Minute Ventilation (L/min)	pH	P_{CO_2} (mmHg)	P_{O_2} (mmHg)	Oxygen Saturation (%)
0	760	150	11.0 ± 1.0	7.43 ± 0.04	33.9 ± 3.5	99.3 ± 9.3	97.6 ± 0.1
15,000	429	80	14.6 ± 2.7	7.46 ± 0.02	25.0 ± 2.2	52.4 ± 4.0	84.8 ± 4.0
20,000	347	63	20.9 ± 6.3	7.50 ± 0.04	20.0 ± 2.8	41.1 ± 3.3	75.2 ± 6.0
26,500	282	49	36.6 ± 7.9	7.53 ± 0.03	12.5 ± 1.1	36.6 ± 2.2	67.8 ± 5.0
29,029	240	43	42.3 ± 7.7	7.56 ± 0.03	11.2 ± 1.7	30.3 ± 2.1	58.0 ± 4.5

[a] Measured during a simulated 40-day ascent of Mount Everest, in a chamber in 7 subjects ("Operation Everest II"). Values are mean ± standard deviation. Modified from Reference 16.

hand, exercise increases the already augmented cardiac output which subsequently decreases transit time across the pulmonary capillary. This rapid transit may not allow adequate time for oxygen transfer and may result in diffusion limitation.[5,8–10]

The next link in the chain of oxygen transport from the air to the tissues is the blood. Hypoxia stimulates an increased production of red blood cells, resulting in an increased oxygen-carrying capacity.[11] This erythropoiesis is mediated by an increase in erythropoietin which, in most individuals, is a beneficial adaptation. However, this response may be exaggerated, particularly in some high altitude natives, such that polycythemia with its inherent hyperviscosity ensues.[12] Hematocrit values of approximately 58 percent or more result in an impaired perfusion of the microvasculature and a decrease in oxygen delivery to the cells.[13] Isovolemic hemodilution improves the clinical status of polycythemic subjects.[14] At moderate altitudes, due to increased production of 2,3-diphosphoglycerate, the relationship of oxygen to hemoglobin is affected by a rightward shift of the oxygen-hemoglobin dissociation curve. This shift presumably improves the unloading of oxygen to the tissues. On the other hand, at extreme altitude, the marked respiratory alkalosis predominates and results in a leftward shift of the curve. Increased affinity of hemoglobin for oxygen is probably beneficial to the loading of oxygen in the lungs where the driving pressure for this process is very low.[15]

Other adaptations occur at the tissue level and presumably result in facilitation of oxygen transfer from the blood to the mitochondria.[16] The capillary: cell ratio increases and is probably secondary to an increase in capillary number and recruitment, as well as to a mild decrease in skeletal muscle size. The distance for diffusion of oxygen from the blood to the mitochondria is therefore decreased. The number of mitochondria also increases and the functioning of oxidative enzymes improves.

Spectrum of Altitude Illnesses

An important point to emphasize is that individuals undergo these adaptations at different rates. Some individuals acclimatize relatively quickly and well. Others may acclimatize just as well though more slowly. Still others may never adapt in a way that allows them to thrive or survive. This knowledge allows one to understand individual variation in susceptibility to illness.

All the altitude illnesses are probably on a spectrum of the same process mediated by hypoxia.[17,18] Although the mechanism is not well understood, fluid retention and a leak of fluid from the vascular to extravascular space takes place. All the symptoms and signs and subsequent pathophysiologic events are attributable to extravascular fluid in the brain, lungs, and peripheral tissues (Fig. 75-2).

The urgency with which one approaches altitude illness depends entirely on the severity and extent of tissue dysoxia, while the incidence and severity of altitude illness is directly proportional to the rapidity of ascent. Quick ascent does not allow time for adequate adaptation.

Acute Mountain Sickness

Acute mountain sickness (AMS) is primarily a common, self-limited form of mild altitude illness. The classic signs of AMS—headache, nausea, lethargy, loss of appetite, and insomnia—may be present in as many as two-thirds of the individuals who make a rapid ascent to 3000 to 4000 m (9842 to 13,123 ft). Mild peripheral edema and a decrease in urine output are also associated with AMS. These symptoms are very common in lowlanders who ascend rapidly to modest altitudes of 2500 to 3000 m (8202 to 9842 ft) for recreational activities such as skiing and hiking. Compared to healthy individuals who respond normally with diuresis, individuals with AMS have been shown to have a retention of fluid.[19,20] Also, individuals with a relatively blunted ventilatory response on ascent to altitude appear to be predisposed to developing AMS.[21,22] AMS usually resolves with 1 to 2 days of rest at the same altitude. However, the symptoms may worsen and evolve into severe altitude illness. If symptoms worsen, then the subject should descend immediately. It should also be emphasized that AMS symptoms usually precede severe, potentially fatal mountain sickness.

Severe Altitude Illnesses

The severe forms of altitude illness include HACE and HAPE. Both of these entities usually occur at higher altitudes (above 12,000 ft) and may take several days or even weeks to appear. The hallmark symptom of HACE is severe headache which is not relieved with mild analgesics. Additionally, there are further neurologic manifestations which may include ataxia, focal motor dysfunction, vomiting, visual impairment, confusion, stupor, and even coma. The onset of these symptoms may be rapid, and death may follow alarmingly quickly.[23]

HIGH ALTITUDE CEREBRAL EDEMA

The role of brain blood flow in the evolution of HACE is not fully understood. On ascent to altitude, hypoxia results in cerebral vasodilation. This is in part offset by the vasoconstriction caused by hypocapnia from the increase in alveolar ventilation. There is an increase in intracranial pressure in HACE which may be secondary to vasogenic or cytotoxic mechanisms of edema formation. Proponents of the vasogenic theory contend that hypoxic cerebral vasodilation overrides hypocapnic vasoconstriction which results in an increase in cerebral blood flow. A redistribution of blood volume caused by an increase in cardiac output from exercise and peripheral vasoconstriction from cold may increase the hydrostatic pressures in the microcirculation of the brain. This can in turn lead to leak of fluid from the intravascular to extravascular space. Hypoxia-induced cytotoxicity may also play a role in the fluid leak. Hypoxia may

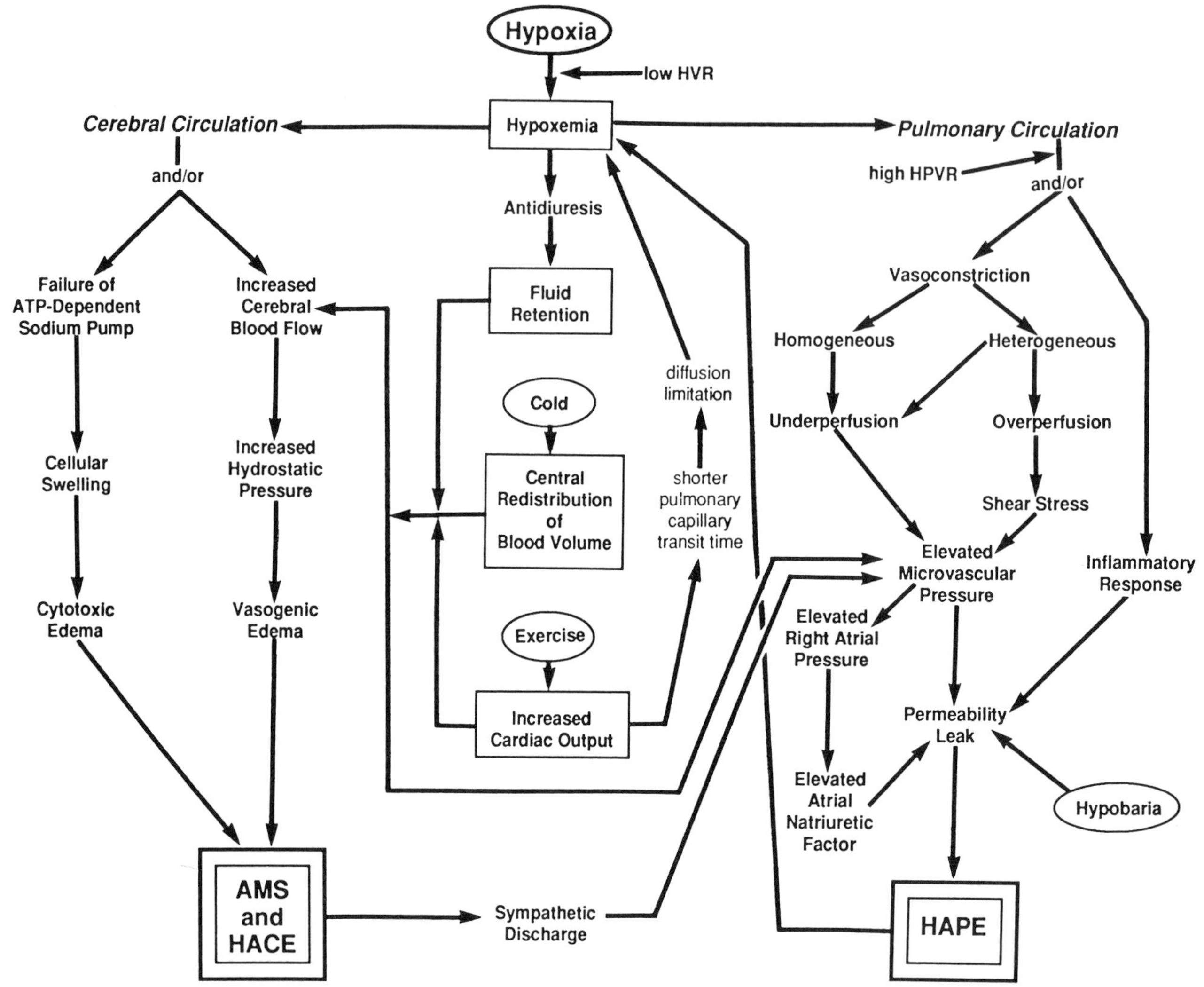

FIGURE 75-2 Schema of possible pathophysiology of acute mountain sickness (AMS), high altitude cerebral edema (HACE), and high altitude pulmonary edema (HAPE). HVR, hypoxic ventilatory response; HPVR, hypoxic pulmonary vascular response. (Reprinted with permission from Reference 44.)

cause a failure in the cellular adenosine triphosphate (ATP)-dependent sodium pump, resulting in sodium and water accumulation within the cells. Whatever the mechanism, brain swelling and petechial hemorrhages occur. It is also conceivable that people who are relative hypoventilators on ascent to altitude have not only a decreased oxygenation of the blood but also relative cerebral vasodilation which may predispose to fluid leak.

HIGH ALTITUDE PULMONARY EDEMA

Most commonly, symptoms of HAPE and HACE coexist in unpredictable proportions. Some of the same concepts of microvascular leak that pertain to HACE may pertain to HAPE. HAPE was not clearly described as a distinct clinical entity until the early 1960s.[24] Previously it had been thought to be pneumonia or congestive heart failure. Although the chest x-ray shows diffuse bilateral infiltrates, the cardiac silhouette is not enlarged and the pulmonary capillary wedge pressures are low or normal. The symptoms of HAPE are inordinate shortness of breath at rest, which worsens with exercise; a dry cough, which may evolve into a severe cough productive of frothy yellow or pink fluid; tachycardia; and cyanosis. Physiologic markers which may predispose individuals to developing HAPE are an accentuated hypoxic pulmonary vasoconstrictive response (HPVR)[25] and relative hypoventilation in response to hypoxia.[26] Although the normal response of the pulmonary vasculature to hypoxia is that of vasoconstriction, individuals with or who have had HAPE have a much more accentuated response. Additionally, they may have patchy as opposed to homogeneous vasoconstriction.[27] This response may result in overperfusion of some areas of lung which may lead to distention of the microvasculature endothelium and increased microvascular pressures in other areas. This may lead to leak directly into the interstitial space or into the alveolar space. As in AMS, individuals with blunted hypoxic ventilatory responses may be more predisposed to HAPE. Their relatively lower alveolar hypoxia may lead to a more profound HPVR which, if inherently more brisk or patchy may then lead to more stress on the microvasculature as mentioned above.

Alveolar fluid in patients with HAPE, obtained by bronchoalveolar lavage on Mt. McKinley, has been characterized[28,29] and shows a remarkably high protein content which is even higher than that demonstrated in patients with the adult respiratory distress syndrome (ARDS), another form of noncardiogenic pulmonary edema. Additionally, there is a marked cellular response which is primarily composed of alveolar macrophages. Evidence of the presence of vasoactive (thromboxane B_2) and chemotactic (leukotriene B_4) mediators is also present. The mechanism which leads to this profound protein leak is probably different from that in ARDS.

Approach to the Patient

Although the clinical setting may strongly suggest severe altitude illness, the clinician must concomitantly treat for HAPE or HACE while searching for other etiologic or confounding disease entities. High altitude hypoxia may precipitate other disease entities which may complicate the diagnostic and therapeutic course.

Furthermore, though many patients with high altitude edema have a low-grade temperature, a persistent fever should merit work-up for some infectious source, especially concomitant pneumonia. If the victim is hemodynamically unstable and if gas exchange does not improve with oxygen therapy, pulmonary embolism must also be considered. A number of anecdotal cases have been reported of individuals who have become intravascular volume depleted with accentuated polycythemia and hyperviscosity, who have developed pulmonary embolism at high altitude. Therefore, the entire status of the patient in the setting must be considered. Indeed, initial evaluation of the patient with HAPE or HACE should include examination for hypothermia, hypoglycemia, dehydration, infection, thromboemboli, and exhaustion.

In terms of cerebral dysfunction, the presence of lateralizing signs or a delay in improvement should also merit a search for other potential causes. The hyperviscosity of volume depletion and accentuated polycythemia at high altitude may also predispose individuals to intravascular cerebral events. Anecdotal cases have also been reported. A computed tomography (CT) scan and other appropriate neurologic work-up would be indicated.

Whether in an emergency setting in the field or in a hospital's ICU, the primary goal of the health care team is to improve oxygen delivery. Given that the cardiac function in most subjects with severe altitude illness is maintained, the improvement of oxygen delivery relies primarily on improving oxygenation of arterial blood by directing attention to the lung. First, alveolar ventilation must be maintained since central ventilatory depression may play a role in the profound hypoxemia. Therefore, it is mandatory that ventilation be ensured either with a self-inflating bag and facemask or intubation at the scene or in the hospital. Aim for a P_{CO_2} in the high 20 mmHg range until the patient can regulate his own ventilation adequately. Second, gas exchange must be improved. Assuming an adequate cardiac output and tidal volumes from the assisted ventilation, the clinician should be able to decrease shunt with modest levels of positive end-expiratory pressure (PEEP). Field studies have shown that use of an expiratory positive airway pressure mask can improve arterial oxygen saturation without increasing ventilation.[30] This lightweight mask may provide an easily administered measure which may temporize until more definitive therapy can be instituted. If the patient is still sick enough on admission to the hospital, the hypoxia should also respond to modest levels of PEEP. It is important to note that most individuals, even those with severe altitude illness, recover remarkably quickly merely by descending a few thousand feet. It would therefore be an unusual situation, but not unheard of, to have the victim sick enough to merit admission to the ICU.

Pharmacologic Intervention

Very few data support the benefit of pharmacologic intervention in severe altitude illness. Acetazolamide, a carbonic anhydrase inhibitor, has been shown in a number of studies to be an effective preventive measure for AMS.[31] However, no data are available to support its efficacy in treatment of either AMS or severe altitude illness. Therefore, there may be no benefit for its use in this setting. On the other hand, several studies have shown that dexamethasone is an effective drug in preventing AMS[32] and in treating more severe forms of cerebral AMS.[33] Its efficacy is presumably based on its ability to maintain the integrity of the capillary or arteriolar endothelium and thereby prevent leak of fluid from the intravascular to extravascular space. Neither acetazolamide nor dexamethasone is fully effective in preventing altitude-related illness, however, so that these diseases are possible even when prophylaxis has been taken. Nevertheless, one should be especially vigilant for an alternative underlying illness in the patient who has been taking these preventive medications.

Dexamethasone may also be effective in HAPE as well as in HACE. It is therefore an important medication to have in the field setting in case of emergency to improve one's cerebral and physical function, particularly if ambulation can be achieved. If the patient still has neurologic signs on arrival at the hospital, it would seem prudent to use parenteral dexamethasone as well. An initial dose of 8 mg dexamethasone intravenously should be followed by 4 mg every 6 h.

Diuretics, such as furosemide, may or may not be effective and may be dangerous in the field where victims usually have intravascular volume depletion despite increased total body fluid. Careful use of a low dose diuretic in the hospital may be helpful, but again, the clinician must be careful not to treat a patient who may be hypovolemic with a potent diuretic. Recent data suggest that the calcium channel blocker, nifedipine, when given intravenously improves gas exchange for a short period of time (Hackett, Oelz, personal communication). The mechanism of this salutory effect may be related to nifedipine's effect on decreasing pulmonary vascular resistance, though this possibility is only speculative. Also, there should be no reason to use cardiac glycosides, aminophylline, or morphine sulfate, all of which are used for left ventricular dysfunction.

CASE PRESENTATION

A previously healthy and physically very active 35-year-old man who lived in San Francisco took a backpacking trip into the High Sierras. On the first day he and his companions drove from San Francisco to the trailhead in the mountains (at 4000 ft altitude). They then ascended to a site at 9000 ft where they made camp. Throughout the night the man periodically awakened short of breath but easily fell back to sleep. In the morning he awoke with a severe headache which was not relieved with aspirin. He felt well otherwise and broke camp. He spent the day on a vigorous hike to their next camp site at 13000 ft altitude. His headache improved throughout the day, and he was able to keep up with his friends. His headache worsened while making camp that night, and he seemed more short of breath at rest than the others. He slept poorly that night because of a persistent cough, shortness of breath, and restlessness. The next morning his symptoms were even worse. Because he was able to walk and because his friends wanted to continue the high traverse, they broke camp and proceeded. His pace was markedly slower than that of his friends, and he had to take frequent rest stops. Their route did not entail any descent. They were only able to achieve a few miles that day, and camp was made earlier than hoped for. His symptoms persisted; his friends had to take over all of his camp chores. That night his headache was worse, he had trouble walking, and his thinking became cloudy. To improve his sleep his friends gave him a couple of sleeping pills and bedded down for the night. His cough persisted although he was quite drowsy. His compatriots slept soundly through the night. On waking the next morning they found him unresponsive. Finally recognizing the gravity of the situation, one decided to stay with him, and the other left without a load to make as rapid a descent as possible and initiate a rescue. Fortunately, he was in excellent condition, the weather remained good, and he was able to make a rapid descent by midafternoon to a ranger station. Access to their camp site was possible by air; by dinnertime a helicopter was at their camp site.

On examination the medics found him still unresponsive, with a blood pressure of 90/60, pulse 130 beats/min, respirations 18 beats/min with overt gurgling in his throat and temperature 38.0°C (100.4°F). He was cyanotic but had no lateralizing signs neurologically. His pupils were dilated but reactive. Cardiac examination revealed tachycardia with a prominent P_2 of his second heart sound but no murmur, rub, or gallop. Chest examination revealed shallow respirations with bilateral diffuse crackles from the midlung fields to the bases. The rest of his examination was unremarkable.

The medics placed him on a litter and gave him high flow oxygen which was delivered with a continuous positive airway pressure (CPAP) mask that effectively gave 10 cmH_2O pressure at end-expiration. An intravenous line was placed, hypertonic glucose was given in a bolus, and a drip of D_5W in 0.5 *N* saline solution at 100 mL/h was given. His clinical status did not change during the hour-and-a-half flight of evacuation. On arrival at the hospital he was immediately admitted to the ICU. A chest x-ray showed diffuse bilateral pulmonary infiltrates with a normal cardiac silhouette. His ECG showed a right bundle branch block and tachycardia. He had a slightly elevated white blood cell count. His electrolytes and metabolic parameters were all normal. Arterial blood-gas determinations showed a pH of 7.48, a Pa_{O_2} of 48 mmHg, and a Pa_{CO_2} of 32 mmHg. He was intubated with an endotracheal tube and placed on positive-pressure ventilation with 10 cmH_2O PEEP. He was given 8 mg dexamethasone intravenously and 40 mg furosemide. A CT scan of his brain showed diffuse cerebral edema but no focal lesions. His vital signs improved and over the next 12 to 24 h his gas exchange improved such that the PEEP and supplemental oxygen could be decreased. Within the first 12 h his mental status gradually improved so that he was stuporous but responsive to pain and voice. At 24 h he was extubated and put on face mask breathing with supplemental oxygen maintaining adequate oxygenation. By 36 h he was slightly lethargic but oriented and responsive. A day later his examination was normal and his chest x-ray had cleared except for a residual infiltrate in his right middle lobe. On day 3, he was discharged.

CASE DISCUSSION

This case illustrates both the proper and improper things to do when approaching altitude illness. First and foremost, the individuals involved in this trek foolishly did not recognize or heed the signs of worsening altitude illness. If signs of AMS do not abate, 1 to 2 days of rest are essential. If the signs worsen, descent is mandatory. If the signs and symptoms of oncoming severe altitude illness are recognized and unless there is severe trauma or weather conditions, descent should occur immediately. No one should die of HAPE or HACE. In that regard, these backpackers to the High Sierra made a nearly fatal error. Fortunately, once the severity of the illness was recognized all the right things were done by his colleagues, the medics, and the medical team at the hospital.

He was certainly in a moribund state at the time of the helicopter rescue. He was probably suffering tissue dysoxia as profound as that seen in an ICU. As his pulmonary edema progressed, his gas exchange and subsequent arterial blood oxygenation progressively worsened, largely due to various degrees of intrapulmonary shunting and development of low $\dot{V}/\dot{Q}$ areas. Additionally, as his cerebral hypoxia worsened, his alveolar ventilation may have been suppressed by central depression.

Endotracheal intubation allowed protection of the airway in this obtunded patient, while facilitating the use of PEEP to reduce shunt. Since dexamethasone is likely to be beneficial in severe altitude illness, it was given here. Once hypovolemia was excluded, furosemide was given to speed resolution of edema; however, it is not clear that this is helpful and in many cases these patients have intravascular depletion in which furosemide might be detrimental. The prompt recovery demonstrated by this case is typical of that of severe altitude illness.

References

1. Schoene RB, Hornbein TF: Respiratory adaptation at high altitude, in Murray JF, Nadel JA (eds): *Textbook of Respiratory Medicine*. Philadelphia, Saunders, 1988, pp 196–220.
2. Weil JV: Ventilatory control at high altitude, in *Handbook of Physiology: The Respiratory System, Vol 2: Control of Breathing, part 2*. Bethesda, American Physiological Society, 1986, chap 21.
3. Arias-Stella J: Human carotid body at high altitude. Am J Pathol 55:82a, 1969.
4. Reeves JT, Groves BM, Sutton JR, et al: Operation Everest II: preservation of cardiac function at extreme altitude. J Appl Physiol 63:531, 1987.
5. Gale GE, Torre-Bueno JR, Moon RE, et al: Ventilation-perfusion inequality in normal humans during exercise at sea level and simulated altitude. J Appl Physiol 58:978, 1985.
6. Wagner PD, Sutton JR, Reeves JT, et al: Operation Everest II: Pulmonary gas exchange during a simulated ascent of Mt. Everest. J Appl Physiol 63:2348, 1987.
7. Groves BM, Reeves JT, Sutton JR, et al: Operation Everest II: Elevated high-altitude pulmonary resistance unresponsive to oxygen. J Appl Physiol 63:521, 1987.
8. West JB, Wagner PD: Predicted gas exchange on the summit of Mt. Everest. Respir Physiol 42:1, 1980.
9. West JB, Boyer SJ, Graber DJ, et al: Maximal exercise at extreme altitudes on Mount Everest. J Appl Physiol 55:688, 1983.
10. Sutton JR, Reeves JT, Wagner PD, et al: Operation Everest II: Oxygen transport during exercise at extreme simulated altitude. J Appl Physiol 64:1309, 1988.
11. Winslow RM, Monge CC: Red cells, red cell and plasma volumes, and their regulation, in *Hypoxia, Polycythermia and Chronic Mountain Sickness*, Baltimore, Johns Hopkins, 1987, pp 31–54.
12. Winslow RM, Monge CC: High altitude natives and chronic mountain sickness. Ibid., pp 19–30.
13. Fan FC, Chen RYZ, Schuessler GB, Chien S: Effect of hematocrit variations on regional hemodynamics and oxygen transport in the dog. Am J Physiol 238:H545, 1980.
14. Sarnquist FH, Schoene RB, Hackett PH: Exercise tolerance and cerebral function after acute hemodilution of polycythemic mountain climbers. Aviat Space Environ Med 57:313, 1986.
15. Winslow RM, Monge CC: The structure and function of hemoglobin at high altitudes, in *Hypoxemia, Polycythemia and Chronic Mountain Sickness*. Baltimore, Johns Hopkins, 1987, pp. 55–74.
16. Green HJ, Sutton JR, Cymerman A, et al: Operation Everest II: Adaptations in human skeletal muscle. J Appl Physiol 66:2454, 1989.
17. Hackett PH, Hornbein TF: Disorders of high altitude, in Murray JF, Nadel JA (eds): *Textbook of Respiratory Medicine*. Philadelphia, Saunders, 1988, pp. 1646–1663.
18. Schoene RB: Adaptation and maladaptation to high altitude, in Baum GL, Wolinsky E (eds): *Textbook of Pulmonary Diseases*. 4th ed. Boston, Little, Brown, 1989, pp 1035–1054.
19. Hackett PH, Rennie D, Grover RE, Reeves JT: Acute mountain sickness and the edemas of high altitude: A common pathogenesis? Respir Physiol 46:383, 1981.
20. Hackett PH, Rennie D, Hofmeister SE, et al: Fluid retention and relative hypoventilation in acute mountain sickness. Respiration 43:321, 1982.
21. King AB, Robinson SM: Ventilation response to hypoxia and acute mountain sickness. Aerospace Med 43(4):419, 1972.
22. Larson EB, Roach RC, Schoene RB, Hornbein TF: Acute mountain sickness and acetazolamide: Clinical efficacy and effect on ventilation. JAMA 248:328, 1982.
23. Hamilton AJ, Cymmerman A, Black PM: High altitude cerebral edema. Neurosurgery. 19(5): 841, 1986.
24. Houston CS: Acute pulmonary edema of high altitude. N Engl J Med 263:478, 1960.
25. Hultgren HN, Grover RF, Hartley LH: Abnormal circulatory responses to high altitude in subjects with a previous history of high altitude pulmonary edema. Circulation 44:759, 1971.
26. Hackett PH, Roach RC, Schoene RB, et al: Abnormal control of ventilation in high-altitude pulmonary edema. J Appl Physiol 64:1268, 1988.
27. Viswanathan R, Subramanian S, Radha TG: Effect of hypoxia on regional lung perfusion by scanning. Respiration 37:142, 1979.
28. Schoene RB, Hackett PH, Henderson WR, et al: High-altitude pulmonary edema: Characteristics of lung lavage fluid. JAMA 256(1):63, 1986.
29. Schoene RB, Swenson ER, Pizzo CJ, et al: The lung at high altitude: Broncho-alveolar lavage in acute mountain sickness and pulmonary edema. J Appl Physiol 64:2605, 1988.
30. Schoene RB, Roach RC, Hackett PH, et al: High-altitude pulmonary edema and exercise at 4,400 meters on Mount McKinley: Effect of expiratory positive airway pressure. Chest 87(3):330, 1985.
31. Larson EB, Roach RC, Schoene RB, Hornbein TF: Acute mountain sickness and acetazolamide: Clinical efficacy and effect on ventilation. JAMA 248:328, 1982.
32. Ellsworth AJ, Larson EB: A randomized trial of dexamethasone and acetazolamide for acute mountain sickness prophylaxis. Am J Med 83:1024, 1987.
33. Hackett PH, Roach RC, Wood RA, et al: Dexamethasone for prevention and treatment of acute mountain sickness. Aviat Space Environ Med 59:950, 1988.

SECTION E

TRANSPLANTATION

Chapter 76

ORGAN PROCUREMENT AND MANAGEMENT OF THE MULTIORGAN DONOR

THOMAS G. HEFFRON

KEY POINTS

- *Although transplantation has developed into an important treatment for both acute and chronic organ failure, donor organ shortage is the rate-limiting factor in most types of transplantation.*
- *Exclusionary criteria for organ donation vary with recipient's needs and from transplant center to transplant center. The regional transplant team should be contacted before a possible organ donor is rejected.*
- *The diagnosis of brain death should be clearly documented in the chart by a physician not directly associated with organ procurement or transplantation and should be in compliance with state law.*
- *Acceptance of death is an absolute prerequisite to approaching a donor family for consent. The professional who is knowledgeable about organ transplantation and brain death is the person best able to interact with the donor family in an objective, yet compassionate, manner.*
- *The goal of management is to maximize organ function until these organs can be removed; volume resuscitation, maintenance of adequate cardiac output, and management of pulmonary edema are necessary to maintain organ perfusion and tissue oxygenation.*
- *Prompt recognition and treatment of common complications associated with the organ donor are essential to continued organ viability prior to transplantation. These include hypotension, arrhythmia, pulmonary edema, massive diuresis, coagulopathy, hypothermia, and infection.*

In the past 10 years, transplantation has developed into an important treatment for both chronic and acute organ failure. This has come about through recent advances in immunosuppression, surgical technique, critical care medicine, and organ preservation. From 1984 to 1989, the number of liver transplants performed annually in the United States increased from 308 to 2188; heart transplants, from 346 to 1687; and pancreas transplants, from 87 to 416 (Table 76-1). In 1989 there were 13,388 organ transplants performed in the United States.[1] Despite the rapidly increasing numbers of transplants, the numbers of people waiting for organs continue to increase. As of July 1, 1990, there were more than 20,000 people waiting for organ transplants. It has been estimated that up to 27,000 potential donors die each year in the United States.[2] However, only a small percentage of these potential donors become organ donors.[3] In 1989 there were only 3993 donors in the United States. This was an actual decrease in total number from 1988, in which there were 4090 total donors in the United States. Through early recognition of potential organ donors, accurate and efficient declaration of brain death, appropriate involvement of organ procurement agencies and skillful donor management prior to procurement, it will be possible to better utilize the donor organ pool in the United States.

Recognition of a Potential Organ Donor

Delayed recognition of a potential organ donor can result in significant loss of transplantable organs. One in five poten-

TABLE 76-1 Numbers of Transplants Performed in the United States, pre-1982–1989

Organ Type	1989	1988	1987	1986	1985	1984	1983	1982	Before 1982
Kidney	8935	9004	9094	8976	7695	6968	6112	5358	33,799
CAD*	7071	7229	7190	7082	5819	5264	4328		
LRD†	1864	1775	1904	1878	1876	1704	1784		
Liver	2188	1709	1199	924	602	308	164	62	119
Heart	1687	1662	1438	1368	719	346	172	103	403
Heart-lung	66	74	49	45	30	17	13	8	5
Lung	92	33	—	—	—	—	—	—	—
Pancreas	416	250	142	140	130	87	35	38	113

*CAD = Cadaveric Donor
†LRD = Living Related Donor
United Network for Organ Sharing (UNOS) began collecting data on October 1, 1987. Prior data were compiled from individual transplant registries and the Department of Health and Human Services.
SOURCE: UNOS.[1] Reprinted with permission.

TABLE 76-2 General Exclusionary Criteria for Organ Donation

Age greater than 70 years
Malignancy (primary cerebral, skin, and lip malignancies not regarded as exclusions)
Hepatitis
AIDS
Active tuberculosis
Systemic infection
Current IV drug abuse

tial donors dies within 6 h of hospital admission, and over half will die within 24 h if not managed appropriately.[4,5] It has been estimated that approximately 80 percent of all multiorgan donors are trauma victims. Cerebrovascular accidents account for an additional 10 percent.[6] A small percentage result from drug overdose, cerebral anoxia (e.g., drowning, smoke inhalation), brain tumor, and cardiopulmonary arrest.

INDICATORS OF ADEQUATE FUNCTION OF DONOR ORGANS

There are both general and organ-specific exclusion criteria (see Table 76-2). However, these require individual assessment depending on the urgency of recipients' need for life-sustaining organs (e.g., heart, liver) and the current organ shortage. Arbitrary age limits have been used in the past; however, in recent years these have been extended without the compromise of recipient transplantation results, and they are routinely extended when a recipient is deteriorating rapidly.[7,8] Accordingly, we encourage an approach to the evaluation of potential organ donors that is based on flexible criteria of adequate function of the donor organs, as opposed to use of a list of exclusion criteria for reasons to reject a donor candidate.

General absolute exclusion criteria of a donor include age greater than 70; malignancy (primary cerebral malignancy, skin cancer, and lip cancer are usually not regarded as exclusions); documentation of hepatitis [although donors who are hepatitis B surface antigen (HBsAg)–positive but e antigen–negative have been accepted], human immunodeficiency virus (HIV) infection or active tuberculosis; systemic infection; and current intravenous drug abuse. It must be stressed that other than these absolute organ exclusion criteria, all other indications are relative and may be disregarded, depending on a recipient's need.

KIDNEY AND PANCREAS DONORS

In addition to general exclusion criteria, there are organ-specific issues. Kidneys usually are not procured if there is evidence of long-standing severe hypertension or diabetes, or evidence of chronic renal disease. Specific exclusionary criteria for the pancreas include a history of diabetes and compelling evidence of pancreatitis. An increased serum amylase level is seen in large numbers of pancreas donors and, by itself, does not exclude transplantation. When a recipient is to receive both a kidney and a pancreas, both organs should come from the same donor, for immunologic reasons (see Chap. 77).

LIVER DONORS

Livers are not obtained from donors who have histories of chronic alcoholism or show other evidence of liver disease. We usually like to see the total bilirubin concentration less than 2.0 mg/dL and the serum glutamic-pyruvic transaminase (SGPT) concentration less than 300 U/L. However, total bilirubin can be elevated for other reasons (such as hemolysis). We accept donor livers with the SGPT level greater than 300 or the bilirubin level greater than 2.0 only if the trend is downward on serial testing. Isolated liver function tests have been notably inaccurate in predicting subsequent liver allograft function.[9] Dopamine is sometimes used for blood pressure support in organ donors. It interferes with portal venous flow and should be kept at as low a dose as possible. However, we have used liver donors receiving dopamine dosages as high as 20 μg/kg per min without adverse results.

LUNG DONORS

Potential lung donors are usually less than 45 years of age (although donors over 45 years of age may be considered, depending on a recipient's need). There must be no history of preexisting cardiac or pulmonary disease. The chest radiograph must be clear, with no evidence of major pulmonary injury or contusion. ABO blood group compatability is required. A direct crossmatch is not performed unless testing against a random pool of lymphocytes shows cytolytic antibodies. The recipient's total lung capacity (TLC) has already been measured; by knowing the donor's height, weight, and sex, it is possible to predict his or her TLC and thus obtain a suitable donor-recipient size match. Sputum cultures must confirm no evidence of ongoing infection. Bronchoscopy is indicated to exclude anatomic lesions, to rule out aspiration and aspirated foreign body (more than 80 percent of donors have died of massive head trauma), and to acquire sputum for Gram stain and culture. The Pa_{O_2}:FI_{O_2} ratio should be at least 250 to 300 mmHg. Peak airway pressures should be less than 30 cmH_2O when ventilated with a tidal volume of 15 mL/kg and a positive end-expiratory pressure (PEEP) of 5 cmH_2O. A pulmonary consultation should be obtained at the time of brain death if the donor is being considered for lung donation.

HEART AND HEART-LUNG DONORS

Heart donors usually are not accepted over the age of 45 years. However, donors older than this can be considered, depending on the acute need of the recpient and actual physiologic, versus chronological, age of the donor. A history of previous coronary or valvular heart disease excludes heart donation, as do pathologic Q waves.[4] A chest x-ray is also obtained to evaluate heart size and the lungs. If the physical examination and above mentioned tests are normal and the donor can maintain a systolic blood pressure of 90 mmHg or above on moderate doses of dopamine, the cardiac function is considered to be adequate for donation. Echocardiography should be performed, if available. The potential heart-lung donor should meet the respective criteria for both lung and heart donation. In addition, long-distance procurement poses an additional problem, because of the short period of tolerable heart-lung preservation. In summary, the workup consists of electrocardiogram (ECG), chest radiograph, echocardiogram, and cardiology consultation. A decision about the need for coronary angiography is left to the discretion of the cardiac team.

OBTAINING PERMISSION FOR ORGAN DONATION

At the time of brain death in a patient who meets the criteria for organ or tissue donation, the designated hospital representative, or the local organ procurement coordinator, should approach the legal next of kin to offer the family of the deceased the option of organ or tissue donation. The Uniform Anatomical Gift Act is in force throughout the United States and generally allows any individual over the age of 18 to donate all or part of his or her body after death for research, education, or transplantation, and permits the legal next of kin to consent for donation.

The order of priority, for granting consent, of next of kin for donors 18 years or older is: (1) the spouse, (2) an adult son or daughter, (3) either parent, (4) an adult brother or sister, (5) a legal guardian. The order of priority for donors under 18 years is: (1) both parents, (2) one parent (if both parents are not available and no contrary indications of the absent parent are known), (3) the custodial parent (if the parents are divorced or legally separated), (4) the legal guardian (if there are no parents).

The decision as to who will approach the donor family is made by the attending physician, in line with hospital policy. In most cases, the attending physician introduces the concept of organ donation to the next of kin. The informed consent is then usually obtained by the transplant coordinator. A professional who is knowledgeable and comfortable with brain death and organ transplantation is best able to interact with the next of kin in an objective, yet compassionate, way.

Acceptance of death is an absolute prerequisite to approaching the donor family. The family must be able to make an informed decision. To facilitate this, brain death must be explained thoroughly and succinctly. Until the family accept the reality of death, they should not be approached about organ donation. When they are approached, the family are given the opportunity to grant or deny permission for organ and tissue donation; they are not pressed. They should be reassured that their relative will be treated with respect, whether they give consent for donation or not.

Brain Death

Brain death is a medically and legally definable state synonymous with death of a human being. Brain death is defined as the total lack of function of the whole brain, including the brain stem. More than 20 years have passed since the Ad Hoc Committee of the Harvard Medical School attempted to define brain death on the basis of clinical characteristics.[10] Although all potential donors that meet the Harvard criteria are dead, many suffer cessation of cardiac and respiratory function before the mandatory 24-h observation period has passed. It was thought by many practitioners that the Harvard criteria were too exclusionary. Other groups developed different criteria, the major differences being a shorter observation period and less emphasis on the electroencephalogram (EEG). Finally, because of the different criteria used by different groups, 56 neurologic consultants compiled "Guidelines for the Determination of Death" for a presidential commission.[11] These guidelines are accepted as the standard for determining brain death in the United States today.

Neurologic death is defined as the irreversible cessation of all functions of the entire brain, including the brain stem. Neurologic death is equivalent to death of a human being. Cessation of brain function is recognized when (1) cerebral functions are absent, and (2) brain stem functions are absent. Irreversibility is recognized when (1) the cause of coma is established and is sufficient to account for the loss of brain functions, (2) the possibility of recovery of any brain functions is excluded, and (3) the cessation of cerebral and brain stem function persists for an appropriate period. The full neurologic examination of patients with suspected brain death is detailed in Chap. 144.

The determination of brain death can be complicated in several circumstances. Drug intoxication, especially with sedative and anesthetic drugs, can cause clinical cessation of brain function and electrocerebral silence. Where there is any likelihood of drug overdose, toxicologic screening for all likely drugs is necessary. Neuromuscular blockers can lead to prolonged paralysis, mimicking the clinical findings of death. This can be excluded by EEG, peripheral nerve stimulation, or extended observation. Hepatic, uremic, and hyperosmolar encephalopathies can produce deep coma. Such metabolic abnormalities should be corrected when possible, or confirmatory tests of brain death employed (EEG, cerebral angiogram). Hypothermia may mimic brain death in all respects; therefore a core temperature above 32.2°C is necessary in order for the clinical determination of brain death to be reliable. Infants and children under 5 years of age are much more resistant to neurologic damage than adults are. They may recover substantial function even after extended unresponsiveness. For this reason, extra caution is necessary when making a diagnosis of brain death in young children, and a more prolonged observation period may be in order. A special task force has outlined a useful set of criteria for the determination of brain death in children.[12] For term newborns, however, these criteria are useful only 7 days after the neurologic insult. The recommendations differ from those for adults in the length of the observation period and the ancillary tests required, depending on the age of the donor. As a final complicating situation, hypotension may contribute to coma, especially when associated with an elevated intracranial pressure

(ICP). The diagnosis of brain death in the presence of shock may not be reliable.

Once the criteria for brain death have been satisfied, an apnea test should be performed. This test should always be done last, on account of the possible complications of hypoxia, hypotension, and arrhythmia. To minimize these, the patient should be ventilated with 100% O_2 for at least 10 min prior to testing. The minute volume should be adjusted to allow the arterial P_{CO_2} to rise above 40 mmHg, thereby shortening the required duration of the apnea trial. The ventilator is disconnected and O_2 is delivered through a cannula in the trachea at a rate of 10 L/min. Pulse oximetry is a useful adjunct; severe O_2 desaturation is a reason to discontinue the trial. If there are no adverse events, the trial should continue for 10 min in order to allow the P_{CO_2} to rise adequately. The presidential commission advocated an arterial P_{CO_2} of 60 mmHg as reflecting a sufficient stimulus to breathe. This is supported by studies showing that some comatose patients may begin spontaneous breathing with P_{CO_2} measurements in the high 50s.[13,14] If there are no respiratory efforts in the face of a P_{CO_2} of 60 mmHg, apnea is confirmed.

The diagnosis of brain death should be clearly documented in the chart by a physician not directly associated with organ procurement or transplantation, prior to the organ procurement procedure, and in accordance with state law.

Management of Multiorgan Donors

The only purpose of continuing care of brain-dead multiorgan donors is to maximize donor organ function until these organs can be removed. This entails a multisystem approach and should begin as soon as brain death has been declared and the family has consented to organ donation. The primary goals of routine donor care are to maintain organ perfusion and tissue oxygenation, reduce the risk of infection, and monitor for complications.[4]

ROUTINE MANAGEMENT

Regular nursing care must continue after the declaration of death. Skin care, three-point turning, catheter and dressing changes, and charting of vital signs are essential for maintaining organ function and minimizing infection. Urine, blood, wound, and tracheal aspirates should be cultured routinely, and these results provided to the transplant team.

CARDIOVASCULAR MONITORING

As discussed below, cardiovascular instability is very common in brain-dead patients. A central venous catheter, arterial line, and Foley catheter are necessary to monitor the adequacy of perfusion and tissue oxygenation. These and all other invasive monitoring devices must be placed under sterile conditions. Maintenance fluids may need to include compensation for prior therapies, such as mannitol and diuretics, and should contain some glucose to preserve stores of hepatic glycogen. Minimal monitoring includes frequent determination of core temperature, heart rate, blood pressure, urine output, and arterial blood gas values, with continuous ECG surveillance. The use of a right heart catheter should be avoided unless it will provide information necessary to manage a hypoperfusion state (vide infra).

The best signs of an acceptable cardiac output are adequate systolic blood pressure and good urine output (at least 0.5 to 1 mL/kg per h). The most crucial aspect of maintaining organ viability is obtaining adequate systemic perfusion. There is an increased incidence of acute tubular necrosis (ATN) and allograft failure in renal transplantation when the donor's systolic blood pressure has been less than 80 mmHg for an extended period. In addition, liver grafts have a high primary nonfunction rate if the donor has been persistently hypotensive. A systolic pressure of 100 mmHg is the goal to ensure adequate perfusion. While the primary aim is to maintain organ perfusion, fluid overload should be avoided as well, because of the deleterious effects on lung function.

VENTILATORY MANAGEMENT

Routine respiratory care should not be neglected in the potential donor. Frequent suctioning, turning, and manual lung expansion help to prevent atelectasis and pneumonia. Up to 5 cmH_2O of PEEP may also be helpful in this regard, although higher levels may impair venous return or selectively reduce hepatic perfusion. High concentrations of O_2 must be avoided in patients who are potential lung donors to avoid O_2 toxicity. In patients who are not suitable for heart-lung donation, it is preferable to use a high F_{IO_2}, rather than a high level of PEEP, to maintain oxygenation when necessary. In a lung donor, the endotracheal tube should be placed high in the trachea to avoid injury at potential suture lines.

COMPLICATIONS ENCOUNTERED AFTER BRAIN DEATH

HYPOTENSION

The most common cause of hypotension is inadequate volume resuscitation. Organ donors are often in a state of massive diuresis due to diabetes insipidus, hyperglycemia, or the administration of mannitol or diuretic drugs. Fluid restriction instituted earlier for management of increased ICP may also contribute. In addition, the loss of autonomic tone following brain death blunts the vasomotor reflexes generally counted on to maintain cardiac output. Cardiac function may also be impaired, on account of the original trauma or underlying disease that led to brain death.

Half or more of organ donors require treatment for hypotension. The central venous pressure should first be increased to 8 to 10 cmH_2O by boluses of colloid, crystalloid, or blood, and the hematocrit should be kept in the range of 25 to 35 percent. If the blood pressure is still low after adequate hydration, vasoactive drugs may be necessary. Dopamine is added first in low doses (2 to 3 μg/kg per min).

When an inotrope is needed in addition, dobutamine or a higher dosage of dopamine is used. Doses of dopamine higher than 10 μg/kg per min can adversely affect the kidney and liver and should be avoided if possible. Epinephrine and norepinephrine, which cause vasoconstriction and organ hypoperfusion, should be avoided as well. If adequate systemic perfusion cannot be maintained without resorting to high doses of vasoactive drugs, right heart catheterization is essential to exclude continued hypovolemia and to guide further therapy. Because of the risk of infection, right heart catheters should be removed once the hemodynamic status stabilizes.

ARRHYTHMIAS

Bradyarrhythmia and systemic hypertension (Cushing's reflex) may be seen at the time of brain herniation. Unless these are associated with instability, treatment is unnecessary. Bradyarrhythmias are not responsive to atropine, since the vagal nuclei are nonfunctional after brain death. Treatment entails a catecholamine, such as isoproterenol, or electrical pacing. There may also arise tachyarrhythmias related to the release of catecholamines; these often respond to beta blockers.

CARDIAC ARREST

Cardiac arrest by itself does not exclude the use of an organ donor. Treatment should be undertaken in the same manner as for patients who are not brain-dead, with two exceptions: (1) atropine is ineffective; and (2) organ viability is the most important limiting factor, so the tolerances acceptable to the transplant teams should be known.

PULMONARY EDEMA

Pulmonary edema may be due to aspiration, fluid overload, myocardial decompensation, or neurogenic causes. Hypoxemia may be severe and rapid in onset. Treatment involves reducing filling pressures to the lowest level consistent with an adequate cardiac output and using PEEP to recruit alveoli (see Chap. 128). A right heart catheter is a necessity under these circumstances.

DIABETES INSIPIDUS (see Chap. 157)

Diabetes insipidus (neurogenic or hypothalamic) has been reported in 38 to 87 percent of brain-dead organ donors.[6] With massive fluid loss, urine electrolyte levels should be measured so that the appropriate electrolyte solutions can be given to replace urine output unit for unit.[15] Alternate explanations for diuresis should be sought, such as mannitol, hyperglycemia, and hypothermia. Vasopressin is often given to avoid electrolyte disturbances, hypovolemia, and hypotension; but it has the deleterious side effects of vasoconstriction, which can be especially harmful to donor organs. A synthetic analogue of AVP, desmopressin (DDAVP), is now the agent of choice. It lacks the side effects of AVP, with the added advantage of enhanced antidiuretic activity and a longer duration of action.[16] The dose of DDAVP should be titrated to keep urine output greater than 100 mL/h and less than 250 mL/h. Excessive loss of free water can result in hypernatremia and hypokalemia, which can be corrected by hypotonic saline solution with potassium. Hypophosphatemia may result from the massive diuresis, and should be promptly treated.

COAGULOPATHY

Coagulopathy and disseminated intravascular coagulation (DIC) are seen in a high percentage of head-injured patients. Manifestations include a low platelet count, a low fibrinogen level, and a prolonged prothrombin time. Hypothermia, dilutional thrombocytopenia from massive volume resuscitation, and acidosis can also contribute to coagulopathy. ϵ-Aminocaproic acid should not be used, because of the risk of inducing microvascular thrombosis with resultant ischemic organ damage. Appropriate therapy may include warming of the patient (for hypothermia), platelet transfusion, or component therapy (See Chap. 146).

HYPOTHERMIA

Hypothermia is a common finding in brain-dead donors. Contributing factors include massive cold-blood and crystalloid resuscitation, loss of sympathetic tone with consequent vasodilation, and loss of hypothalamic temperature regulation. Hypothermia may cause coagulation defects, cardiovascular arrhythmias, decreased cardiac output, and other adverse effects. It can usually be prevented or managed by heating blankets, warmers for blood and fluid infusions, and warming (to 40°C) of the humidified gas supplied through the mechanical ventilator. All possible donors should have core temperatures measured through the rectum or esophagus, with early, aggressive rewarming when a reduction is first noted.

INFECTION

At the first sign of infection, cultures of urine, blood, and wound and endotracheal secretions should again be collected. Since the recipient of the donor organ will be immunosuppressed, transplantation of infected organs can have disastrous consequences.[17] Communication of the findings on any microbiologic specimens from the primary team to the transplant service must be assured.

CASE PRESENTATION

A 63-year-old male was transferred to the ICU from the emergency room after being involved in a motor vehicle accident. He was intubated and had large-bore intravenous catheters and a Foley catheter in place. He was deeply comatose, with pupils fixed and dilated. A CT scan of the head revealed a large intracerebral bleed. His social history revealed him to be a divorced businessman with no history of drug or alcohol abuse. His vital signs were stable; his temperature was 36°C.

After 24 h of aggressive supportive management, he remained unresponsive to deep pain and had no spontaneous respirations. A neurologist found that the patient had no spontaneous motor activity, nor oculocephalic, pupillary, corneal, or pharyngeal reflexes. By adjustment of the minute ventilation, the P_{CO_2} was allowed to rise to high-normal levels prior to an apnea test. After the patient was ventilated with 100% O_2 for 10 min he was disconnected from the ventilator. He had no respirations for 10 min, despite an arterial P_{CO_2} of 62 mmHg. The pulse oximeter read more than 90 bpm, and no arrhythmias were noted. The neurologist noted in the chart that the patient had met the qualifications for brain death.

The organ procurement agency was notified, and the family gave consent for heart, liver, and kidney donation. It had been 48 h since the patient's admission. Liver enzymes on admission included an SGPT of 385 and a total bilirubin of 2.2. The prothrombin time was normal, the BUN 30, and the serum creatinine 1.1. Repeat measurements at the time of brain death were unchanged, except that the SGPT was 200 and the total bilirubin was 0.9. Serologic tests for HIV, syphilis, and hepatitis were all negative. The organ procurement team arranged for donation of liver and kidneys. The pancreas and heart were not donated, on account of the age of the patient.

The patient's urine output rose to more than 800 mL/h, his central venous pressure fell to less than 1, and he became hypotensive. A bolus of 1 L of Ringer's lactate was given, the central venous pressure rose to 3, and the systolic blood pressure rose to more than 100. A bolus injection of 2 μg of DDAVP was administered, after which the urine output dropped to 100 mL/h; it remained at that level with DDAVP, 1 μg subcutaneously q 12 h. The patient began to bleed from around his intravenous access sites and from abrasions on his arms that previously had been dry. The prothrombin time was found to be 25, the platelet count 15,000, and the fibrinogen level low. In addition, the core temperature was 32°C. Through a blood warmer were given 2 U of fresh frozen plasma, 2 U of packed red blood cells, and platelets. Warming blankets were placed above and below the patient, and warmed humidified air was given via the ventilator. His temperature rose to 36°C, the platelet count increased to 74,000, and the hematocrit remained stable at 32. The P_{O_2} dropped to 55 (saturation 88%) on F_{IO_2} of 40%, PEEP 5 cmH_2O, and tidal volume 700. The F_{IO_2} was increased to 60% and the P_{O_2} rose to 75 (saturation 93%).

The donor procurement proceeded without incident. The liver was transplanted into a 45-year-old female with sclerosing cholangitis. She was discharged from the hospital 15 days after her transplant. Both kidney recipients had immediate function and were discharged home 6 days after transplant.

CASE DISCUSSION

This case illustrates some of the major points necessary for successful management of the multiorgan donor. Several common, but preventable, errors in care could have led to the loss of life-saving organs. For example, this patient became hypotensive because of the lack of adequate volume resuscitation in the setting of diabetes insipidus (DI). Since DI is seen in up to 90 percent of brain-dead donors, it could have been better anticipated here, allowing earlier volume replacement and DDAVP therapy. Hypothermia, which contributed to coagulopathy, could have been prevented or minimized as well; for example, passive means, such as the use of extra blankets, can limit heat loss. When temperature first begins to fall, aggressive rewarming with warmed fluids and warming blankets should be initiated.

The physician has many incentives, after the declaration of a patient's brain death, to turn his or her attention to the family or to other patients. While the grieving family and living patients certainly deserve the physician's greatest efforts, *the brain-dead patient must be considered a potential source of life for others.* It is therefore appropriate and essential to continue "life-sustaining" measures aggressively, even in the face of death, until issues of organ donation can be addressed. In this case, the heart and lungs were rejected because of the age of the donor, but the liver and kidneys were passed on to waiting recipients, whose lives thereby were bettered.

References

1. UNOS (United Network for Organ Sharing). Am J Public Health July 1990, p 3.
2. Stuart FP: Need, supply and legal issues related to organ transplantation in the United States. Transplant Proc 16:87, 1984.
3. Merz B: The organ procurement problem: many causes, no easy solutions. JAMA 254:3285, 1985.
4. Darby JM, Stein K, Grenvik A, et al: Approach to management of the heartbeating "brain dead" organ donor. JAMA 261:2222, 1989.
5. Bark KJ, Macon EJ, Humphries AL: A response to the shortage of cadaveric kidneys in transplantation. Transplant Proc 11:455, 1979.
6. Evans RW, Manninen DL, Garrison LP, et al: Donor availability as the primary determinant of the future of heart transplantation. JAMA 255:1892, 1986.
7. Wall WJ, Mimeault R, Grant DR, et al: The use of older liver donors for hepatic transplantation. Transplantation 49:377, 1990.
8. Rao KV, Ney AL: Donor age does not affect the outcome of cadaver renal transplantation. Transplant Proc 20:773, 1988.
9. Makowka L, Gordon RD, Todo S, et al: Analysis of donor criteria for the prediction of outcome in clinical liver transplantation. Transplant Proc 19:2378, 1987.
10. Beechin HK: A definition of irreversible coma. Report of the Ad Hoc Committee of the Harvard Medical School to examine the definition of Brain Death. JAMA 205:337, 1968.
11. Guidelines for the determination of death: Report of the medical consultants on the diagnosis of death to the President's Commission for the Study of Ethical Problems in Medicine. JAMA 246:2184, 1981.
12. Annar GJ, Bray PF, Bennett DR, et al: Report of special task force: Guidelines for the determination of brain death in children. Pediatrics 80:298, 1987.
13. Schafter JA, Caronna JJ: Duration of apnea needed to confirm brain death. J Neurosurg 55:942, 1981.
14. Belsch JM, Blatt R, Schiffman PL: Apnea in brain death. Arch Intern Med 146:2385, 1986.
15. Mackersie RC: Organ procurement and brain death in trauma patients. J Intensive Care Med 4:137, 1989.
16. Debelak L, Pollack R, Rechkard R: Arginine vasopressin versus desmopressin for the treatment of diabetes insipidus in the brain dead organ donor. Transplant Proc 22:351, 1990.
17. Vandervliet JA, Tidwo G, Koostra G, et al: Transplantation of contaminated organs: Br J Surg 67:596, 1989.

Chapter 77

IMMUNOTHERAPY IN THE TRANSPLANT PATIENT

DAVID S. BRUCE
J. RICHARD THISTLETHWAITE

KEY POINTS

- *Improvements in immunosuppression have led to dramatic expansion in organ transplantation and hence in the number of transplant recipients in the general population.*
- *Immunosuppressive drugs have many side effects and predispose patients to infection.*
- *Immunosuppressive regimens can be modified to avoid toxicities of particular agents.*
- *Rejection should be suspected in any transplant patient with fever or evidence of graft dysfunction; liberal use should be made of relevant biopsy techniques to aid in the diagnosis.*
- *Immunosuppression may mask the signs and symptoms of infections such as peritonitis or meningitis.*
- *Pneumonia may progress rapidly in transplant patients and must be aggressively evaluated and treated; bronchoscopy and open lung biopsy are often required.*
- *Immunosuppression must often be reduced or withheld in the presence of severe infection.*

The transplantation of vascularized organ grafts represents a remarkable interface between surgical innovation, critical care, and immunology. Although experimental organ transplantation was described 80 years ago by Alexis Carrel, practical application was not achieved until immunosuppression using a combination of azathioprine and corticosteroids for renal transplantation was introduced in the early 1960s. Cyclosporine revolutionized transplant immunosuppression in the early 1980s and has stimulated dramatic growth in transplantation of the liver, heart, lung, and pancreas. Monoclonal antibody therapy and other recent advances may further improve outcome. However, acute rejection remains common, and modern immunosuppression imposes the hazards of a range of complications, both infectious and noninfectious. End-stage organ failure necessitating transplantation also predisposes patients to problems requiring astute management following the complex transplant surgical procedures. As shown in Table 77-1, outcomes following transplantation have dramatically improved in the last 15 years. In turn, improved outcome has stimulated a large increase in the number of institutions performing transplantation. The transplant patient thus offers an increasingly common challenge to the critical care physician.

TABLE 77-1 One-year Graft Survival Rates in Organ Transplant Recipients, in Percent

	1975	1990
Kidney	60	85
Heart	45	80
Liver	30	75
Pancreas	25	80

Mechanisms of Allograft Rejection

A transplant to an individual from another of the same species is called an *allograft*. Allograft rejection can occur in three histopathologically distinct forms. *Hyperacute rejection* is apparent soon after revascularization of the grafted organ. It is the result of preformed alloantibodies which cause complement activation, thrombosis, and irreversible graft destruction. There is no treatment for this devastating complication, which is now rare due to appropriate screening of donor/recipient pairs for most organ allografts. Interestingly, preformed alloantibodies do not usually result in hyperacute rejection in liver transplantation. This may be due to the sinusoidal nature of the venous bed of the liver.[1]

Chronic rejection is characterized by progressive vasculitis leading to graft ischemia, fibrosis, and loss of function. The pathogenetic mechanisms are unknown at the cellular and molecular levels, although the absence of cellular infiltration and the presence of alloantibodies within the graft implicate a humoral mechanism.[2] Chronic rejection tends to be refractory to immunologic therapy and is slowly progressive. It is the most frequent cause of late graft failure and is often an indication for retransplantation.

Clinical transplant immunosuppression represents an attempt to prevent or reverse the process of *acute rejection*. Although a variety of effector mechanisms may be involved, this is clearly a T cell-initiated process. The cellular and molecular basis of T cell alloreactivity is now reasonably clear.[3] Thymic selection creates a repertoire of T cells that recognize foreign antigenic peptides bound to one's own major histocompatibility complex (MHC) molecules, in humans called HLA (human leukocyte antigens).[4] T cell specificity is determined by an antigen-specific T cell receptor (TCR) which is associated with a group of proteins called CD3. Because HLA molecules are highly polymorphic, the HLA molecules on the graft nearly always will be different from those of the recipient. The T cell receptors of the recipient interpret foreign HLA as self-HLA plus foreign peptide and become activated.

TCR engagement, whether by antigen plus self-HLA, by foreign HLA, or by anti-CD3 monoclonal antibodies, initiates a complex chain of intracellular events leading to T cell activation.[5,6] Figure 77-1 illustrates some of these events, which include protein phosphorylation, calcium flux, turnover of phosphatidylinositol phosphates, and transcription of at least 50 different genes.[7] Two key events are the pro-

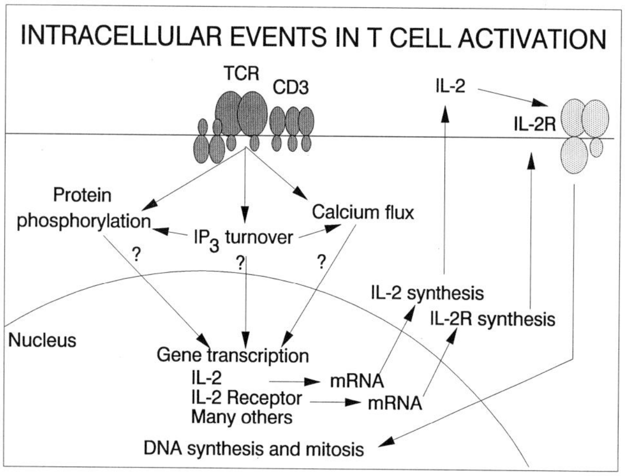

FIGURE 77-1 Schematic depiction of some of the intracellular events which occur after engagement of the T cell receptor/CD3 complex. Emphasis is placed on the production of IL-2 and the expression of IL-2 receptors on the cell surface, both of which are needed for T cell proliferation. Note that IL-2 can act either on the cell which produced it (autocrine effect) or on an adjacent cells (paracrine effect).

duction of interleukin-2 (IL-2) and the expression of IL-2 receptors on the cell surface. IL-2 acts in an autocrine fashion to drive T cell proliferation, creating clones of activated T cells specific for donor HLA.

$CD8^+$ cells and $CD4^+$ cells are distinct T cell subsets which respond to class I and class II MHC, respectively. Although both subsets can directly kill target cells, $CD8^+$ cells appear to be specialized for this function. $CD4^+$ cells function mainly by producing lymphokines which provide help to other cell types, including $CD8^+$ cells. Lymphokine production by alloreactive lymphocytes also recruits antigen-nonspecific effector cells, such as macrophages, which augment the tissue destruction. By providing help to B cells, T cell activation generates alloantibodies that bind vascular endothelium and promote fibrin deposition. Figure 77-2 illustrates some of the intercellular interactions involved in allograft rejection. This complex process offers many potential targets for intervention by immunosuppressive agents.

Mechanisms of Action and Toxicities of Immunosuppressive Agents

CYCLOSPORINE

Perhaps no single drug has advanced transplantation as greatly as has cyclosporine, an 11 amino acid cyclic peptide derived from the fungus *Tolypocladium inflatum*. First used clinically in 1978, cyclosporine is now an integral part of nearly all immunosuppressive regimens. Cyclosporine has significantly improved graft survival rates in renal transplant recipients.[8,9] Additionally, cyclosporine has been a major factor in the development of clinical heart, liver, pancreas, and lung transplantation, procedures which were justifiably considered experimental in the precyclosporine era.

The mechanisms of action of cyclosporine remain an area of intense investigation.[10,11] A major site of action of cyclosporine is the T lymphocyte (see Fig. 77-1). Cyclosporine prevents the production of IL-2 by T cells by interfering with production of its mRNA.[12] This prevents the development of the expanded clones of alloreactive effector cells which would normally initiate graft rejection. Most studies have found IL-2 receptor expression to be unaffected by cyclosporine. At the molecular level, evidence suggests that cyclosporine interferes with the correct folding of DNA-binding proteins required for IL-2 gene transcription. Peptidyl-prolyl isomerases are enzymes that allow newly synthesized proteins to fold into their correct conformations. The putative cyclosporine receptor is a peptidylprolyl isomerase termed cyclophilin. Cyclosporine binds to this protein and inhibits its enzymatic function. Although it has not been conclusively shown that this enzymatic inhibition is the means by which cyclosporine exerts it immunosuppressive effect, it is notable that FK506, an experimental immunosuppressive agent with actions similar to those of cyclosporine, also binds to a protein with peptidyl-prolyl isomerase activity. FK506 will be discussed later in this chapter.

Cyclosporine is currently used in combination with prednisone (and often azathioprine) as the mainstay of maintenance immunosuppression. Its administration is generally begun near the time of transplantation at approximately 8 to 10 mg/kg/day divided into two daily oral doses. When oral administration is not possible, cyclosporine is given intravenously in one-third the oral dose to correct for better bioavailability via the intravenous route. Of particular relevance to liver transplantation is the enterohepatic circulation of cyclosporine. This predictably results in significant loss via T tube drainage. Higher doses of cyclosporine are frequently required with T tube drainage of bile than after the T tube is clamped or removed. Children also generally require higher doses of oral cyclosporine than adults because of their shorter intestinal length and the low bioavailability of cyclosporine through gastrointestinal absorption.

Cyclosporine levels may be measured by either high pressure liquid chromatography (HPLC) or radioimmunoassay (RIA) methods. HPLC is more time-consuming and operator dependent but has the advantage of being able to distinguish between cyclosporine and its metabolites. A recently introduced anticyclosporine monoclonal antibody may provide similar metabolite specificity to cyclosporine RIA measurements. Cyclosporine levels must be interpreted with caution, because they do not reliably indicate either the presence of toxicity or the adequacy of immunosuppression.

Cyclosporine toxicity is significant (Table 77-2). The most important adverse effect is nephrotoxicity, which occurs to varying degrees in all recipients of this drug. The pathogenetic mechanisms involve vasoconstriction of preglomerular arterioles and resultant glomerular hypoperfusion. Ultimately, myonecrosis can occur in the arteriolar wall and

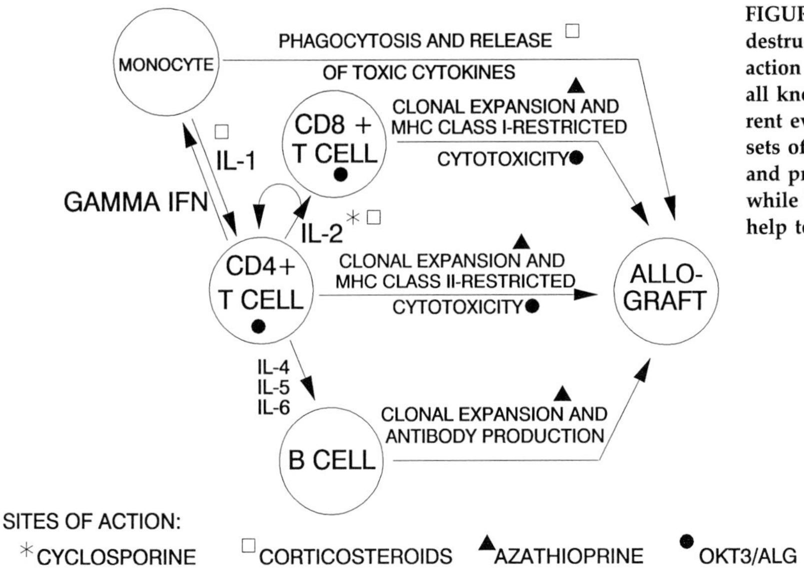

FIGURE 77-2 Cellular interactions leading to allograft destruction with depiction of the probable major sites of action of currently used immunosuppressive drugs. Not all known interactions are depicted. In particular, current evidence suggests the existence of two distinct subsets of CD4$^+$ T cells. T_{H1} cells produce IL-2 and γ-IFN and provide help to macrophages and cytotoxic T cells, while T_{H2} cells produce IL-4, IL-5, and IL-6 and provide help to B cells.

lead to a fixed lesion. Cyclosporine delays recovery from ischemic acute tubular necrosis (ATN) in recipients of cadaveric kidney transplants. Hypertension is encountered in most transplant recipients on cyclosporine, most likely as a result of decreased renal perfusion. To avoid these complications, immunosuppressive strategies have been devised in which cyclosporine is switched to azathioprine after several months of successful engraftment. Although this may improve renal function, the risk of acute rejection and graft loss is also increased. Alternatively, cyclosporine doses may be reduced to a minimal level (3 to 4 mg/kg/day) after stable graft function is achieved. Another strategy is to use anti-T cell agents such as antilymphocyte globulin (ALG) or OKT3 for induction immunosuppression and to delay cyclosporine until graft function is well-established. This may facilitate recovery from ATN in kidney transplantation. A more direct approach to the prevention of cyclosporine nephrotoxicity is to use calcium antagonists to reverse cyclosporine-induced vasoconstriction.[13] Although the efficacy of this approach in preventing the fixed vascular lesions is not known, the use of a calcium channel blocking agent as a first drug in control of hypertension seems warranted. Certain calcium antagonists, however, appear to increase blood cyclosporine levels by interfering with its metabolism in the liver. A marked increase in cyclosporine levels is seen with the initiation of diltiazem therapy. Ver-

TABLE 77-2 Non-infectious Complications of Immunosuppressive Drugs

Side Effects of Cyclosporine	Nephrotoxicity Hypertension Tremor Psychosis	Seizures Hypertrichosis Hyperkalemia Hepatotoxicity
Side Effects of Corticosteroids	Hyperglycemia Muscle wasting Impaired wound healing Gastritis Cataracts	Masking of infections Adrenal suppression Bone demineralization Cushingoid facies
Side Effects of Azathioprine	Neutropenia Hepatotoxicity	Squamous and basal cell skin cancer
Side Effects of ALG	Fever Chills Thrombocytopenia	Hypertension Pruritis Serum sickness
Side Effects of OKT3	Fever Bronchospasm Seizures Tachycardia Hypertension Headache	Pulmonary edema Rigors Formation of anti-OKT3 antibodies Nausea and vomiting Diarrhea

TABLE 77-3 Cyclosporine Drug Interactions

Drugs Causing Increased Cyclosporine Levels	Drugs Causing Decreased Cyclosporine Levels
Erythromycin	Corticosteroids
Ketoconazole	Phenytoin
Calcium channel blockers	Phenobarbital
Androgens	Carbamazepine
Oral contraceptives	Rifampin
Metoclopramide	
Drugs Causing Synergistic Nephrotoxicity	
Amphotericin B	
Aminoglycosides	

SOURCE: Modified from reference 14.

apamil results in a moderate increase in cyclosporine levels, whereas nifedipine appears to cause no increase. Many other commonly used drugs have significant interactions with cyclosporine and may cause either increased cyclosporine levels, decreased cyclosporine levels, or synergistic nephrotoxicity (Table 77-3).[14]

The other major complication of cyclosporine is neurotoxicity. Presentations range from mild nervousness and tremors to psychosis and convulsions. Headache, somnolence, and paresthesias are also observed. An increased incidence of severe neurotoxicity has been reported in patients with low cholesterol levels, suggesting a reduction in a plasma lipid carrier and an increase in free cyclosporine. Discontinuation or reduction of cyclosporine doses generally leads to improvement. Distinguishing cyclosporine neurotoxicity from the many other potential causes of abnormal neurologic status in the ICU patient may be difficult. Other adverse effects of cyclosporine include hyperkalemia, hypertrichosis, and hepatotoxicity. Hepatotoxicity usually presents as cholestasis and mild transaminase elevation and should be considered in the differential diagnosis of liver dysfunction in a transplant patient. Hypersensitivity to the intravenous carrier cremaphor infrequently causes anaphylactoid responses in patients receiving intravenous cyclosporine.

CORTICOSTEROIDS

Corticosteroids have been an integral part of immunosuppressive regimens since the early 1960s.[15] Although their clinical anti-inflammatory effects are well-known, the molecular basis of their immunosuppressive action is complex and incompletely understood. Administration of glucocorticoids results in circulating lymphopenia and redistribution of lymphocytes into lymphoid tissues, presumably by disrupting lymphocyte homing mechanisms. Corticosteroids block T cell proliferation and IL-2 synthesis in response to stimulation by anti-CD3 antibodies or by allogeneic cells (see Fig. 77-1 and 77-2). This inhibitory action may in part be due to direct effects on T cells, but the T cell regulatory effect of corticosteroids is probably a result of the inhibition of cytokine (especially IL-1) release by the monocytes participating in antigen presentation. Corticosteroids also inhibit the phagocytic functions of macrophages and in high doses prevent neutrophil degranulation. Corticosteroids are used in large doses for the induction of immunosuppression and for treatment of acute rejection episodes. Much smaller doses are used in multiple-drug regimens for maintenance immunosuppression, as will be discussed in a later section. Because administration of even small amounts of corticosteroids suppresses endogenous adrenal glucocorticoid production, care must be taken to administer adequate corticosteroids to prevent acute adrenal insufficiency in times of stress.

Corticosteroids have many potential adverse effects. Several of these are of particular relevance to the critical care physician. All immunosuppressive drugs render patients more susceptible to infections, but because of their effect on nonspecific host defense mechanisms, corticosteroids are most problematic. Corticosteroids cause insulin resistance. This may result in marked hyperglycemia in the immediate postoperative period or other times of stress, even in patients with no previous history of diabetes. These agents also predispose to gastrointestinal hemorrhage. Transplant patients should receive routine prophylaxis for stress gastritis with antacids or inhibitors of hydrogen ion secretion. Corticosteroids significantly impair wound healing and contribute to the risk of anastomotic leaks and other surgical complications. Perhaps most importantly, corticosteroids can greatly mask the signs and symptoms of infections. For example, frank peritonitis may present as mild abdominal discomfort. This can delay the diagnosis of a perforated viscus, leaking anastomosis, or other condition requiring surgical intervention. Because outcome is strongly influenced by such delays, a high index of suspicion must be maintained in any transplant patient with abdominal complaints. In a similar fashion, the most common presentation of meningitis is the complaint of a headache with no other signs or symptoms. Any headache which does not promptly resolve demands full investigation, including lumbar puncture.

AZATHIOPRINE

Azathioprine is a purine analogue that is converted in the liver to its active metabolite, 6-mercaptopurine (6-MP). 6-MP interferes with DNA and RNA synthesis by competitively inhibiting purine metabolism. Azathioprine acts predominantly on rapidly proliferating cells such as those of the bone marrow. Its antiproliferative action blocks the clonal expansion of antigen-specific T and B cells and their concomitant differentiation into effector cells (see Fig. 77-2). Azathioprine revolutionized transplantation in the early 1960s by providing, in combination with corticosteroids, the first immunosuppressive regimen of significant practical value.[16] With the introduction of cyclosporine, its role has been reduced to an adjunct in maintenance immunosuppression in combination with cyclosporine and corticosteroids, arguably allowing lower doses of the latter two agents and reducing their toxicity.

The principal side effects of azathioprine are bone marrow depression and hepatotoxicity. The bone marrow toxicity is predictable and dose dependent and is monitored by daily leukocyte counts in the early postoperative period. Leukopenia generally responds to temporary reduction or withholding of azathioprine. Hepatotoxicity is rare and manifests itself in clinical syndromes ranging from mild elevations of serum transaminases to fulminant acute hepatitis. Hepatotoxicity may occur at any time in the first several weeks after transplantation. A similar antimetabolite, cyclophosphamide, can be used as a substitute for azathioprine in the event of hepatotoxicity. The increased incidence of nonmelanoma skin cancers in transplant recipients also appears to be attributable to azathioprine.

POLYCLONAL ANTILYMPHOCYTE GLOBULIN

Polyclonal antilymphocyte antibodies have been widely used in transplant immunosuppression since the introduction of ALG in 1968. However, their efficacy is limited to immediate posttransplant induction and to the treatment of acute rejection episodes. The use of ALG for induction clearly prolongs the initial rejection-free interval after transplantation, although the overall incidence of rejection may not be decreased.[17] The immunosuppressive effects of ALG most likely result from both lymphocyte depletion and interference with a variety of T cell surface molecules, such as TCR/CD3, CD4, CD8, CD2, and LFA-1. Although administration may cause fevers, chills, hypertension, and pruritus, the chief adverse effect is an increased risk of viral infections, especially cytomegalovirus (CMV), as a result of T cell dysfunction. Serum sickness may occur with repeated use. A major drawback of polyclonal antibody therapy is the difficulty in obtaining preparations of uniform immunosuppressive activity. In addition, most ALG preparations contain antibodies cross-reactive with platelets which may lead to thrombocytopenia. ALG doses vary widely, depending on the weight of the patient and the potency of the ALG preparation.

OKT3

OKT3 is a murine monoclonal antibody which binds to the human CD3 ϵ chain. It was first used clinically in 1981 and is the most effective agent known for reversal of acute rejection. Success rates for OKT3 are 90 to 95 percent as compared to 65 to 75 percent for high dose corticosteroids.[18,19] OKT3 is administered intravenously and results in extremely rapid disappearance of T cells from the peripheral circulation. However, T cell depletion from lymph nodes is much less complete. OKT3 initially causes extensive T cell activation and release of several lymphokines, including IL-2, IL-6, γ-interferon, and tumor necrosis factor.[20] These lymphokines appear to mediate the acute toxicity seen with OKT3, particularly after the first dose. Despite this widespread T cell activation, OKT3 prevents the immune system from mounting a coordinated, antigen-specific response. The net result is usually the prompt reversal of an acute rejection episode. OKT3 has also been used for induction of immunosuppression for kidney, liver, pancreas, and heart transplantation.[21] Like ALG, OKT3 is given daily for a 7- to 14-day course. The usual dose of OKT3 for adults is 5 mg/day, as compared to 1000 to 1500 mg/day for many ALG preparations. These doses reflect the much greater purity of the monoclonal preparation.

Side effects of OKT3 are frequent and can be very severe. The lymphokine-mediated acute toxicity can be significantly attenuated by pretreatment with corticosteroids, antihistamines, and acetaminophen. Pulmonary edema appears to occur only in patients who are volume overloaded at the time of treatment. Uremia and hypocalcemia appear to predispose to seizures following OKT3 administration; these abnormalities should be corrected before the initiation of OKT3 therapy. Although pyrexia is almost uniform following OKT3, fevers during OKT3 therapy should be evaluated carefully, because intercurrent infection is common.

A troublesome complication of OKT3 therapy is the formation of anti-OKT3 antibodies.[22] These may be directed against either the constant portion of the antibody molecule (antimurine antibodies) or the hypervariable regions (anti-idiotypic antibodies). These anti-OKT3 antibodies can interfere with retreatment should another course of OKT3 become necessary. This problem has been cited as an argument against the prophylactic use of OKT3 for induction immunosuppression. However, retreatment with OKT3 in the presence of anti-OKT3 antibodies often can be successfully accomplished using larger doses of OKT3. Nevertheless, effective suppression of the humoral response to OKT3 would be a significant advance and is an area of active investigation.

IMMUNOSUPPRESSION-RELATED NEOPLASMS

Immunosuppressed transplant recipients experience an increased incidence of malignancies.[23] Prior to the introduction of cyclosporine, central nervous system (CNS) lymphomas and skin cancers predominated. Cyclosporine appears to be more closely associated with B cell lymphomas which usually occur outside the CNS. Immunosuppression appears to allow reactivation of Epstein-Barr virus with subsequent polyclonal B cell proliferation.[24] If immunosuppression is not reduced or withdrawn, this premalignant condition may lead to a frankly malignant, monoclonal B cell lymphoma which will no longer respond to mere reduction of immunosuppression. The risk of malignancy appears to be greater in patients receiving triple-agent (cyclosporine, azathioprine, and corticosteroid) maintenance immunosuppression.

General Strategies of Immunosuppression

Although the details of immunosuppression vary according to the preferences of the transplant team, the overall approach is reasonably constant. Intense immunosuppression

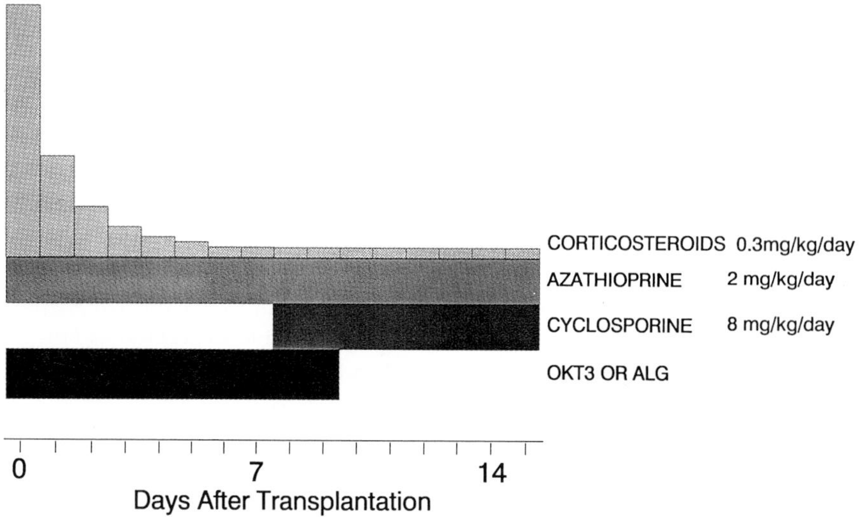

FIGURE 77-3 Sample regimen for perioperative immunosuppression, illustrating the use of induction OKT3.

is used perioperatively with subsequent tapering to lower dose maintenance regimens. The long-term goal of current immunosuppression is to balance prevention of rejection against avoidance of toxicity. The variety of immunosuppressive agents now available allows the basic strategy to be modified in certain situations without significantly increasing the risk of rejection.

INDUCTION OF IMMUNOSUPPRESSION

The perioperative induction of immunosuppression generally involves several components (Fig. 77-3). Corticosteroids are given in large doses intraoperatively (typically methylprednisolone, 500 to 2000 mg intravenously) and tapered rapidly to oral prednisone in doses of approximately 0.3 to 0.5 mg/kg/day. Azathioprine is begun with an intraoperative dose of 3 to 5 mg/kg and continued at doses of 1 to 2 mg/kg/day. Cyclosporine is begun at or shortly after transplantation with oral doses of 8 to 12 mg/kg/day for renal transplant recipients, and intravenous doses of one-third this amount for liver transplant recipients and others incapable of taking cyclosporine by mouth. All these doses vary significantly from one transplant center to another.

There is a progressive trend toward use of OKT3 or polyclonal antilymphocyte antibodies for 7 to 14 days postoperatively as induction immunosuppression. Both agents clearly prolong the initial rejection-free interval, allowing the patient greater time to recover from surgery and any posttransplant organ dysfunction. Diagnostic confusion between early rejection and graft dysfunction from other reasons in the postoperative period can thus be avoided. Induction immunosuppression with OKT3 also appears to reduce the overall incidence of acute rejection.

Certain clinical situations may call for modifications of this general strategy. The nephrotoxicity associated with cyclosporine has prompted withholding of cyclosporine from renal transplant recipients until graft function is established. The use of OKT3 for induction immunosuppression allows this to be done without increasing the incidence of acute rejection episodes. Severe infection is a common posttransplant complication of liver transplantation; thus, many liver transplant centers choose not to use the potent anti-T cell antibody induction except for special circumstances. In lung and heart-lung transplantation, healing of the critical bronchial or tracheal anastomosis can be significantly impaired by postoperative corticosteroids. The use of induction OKT3 or ALG allows steroids to be omitted until anastomotic healing is ensured.

MAINTENANCE IMMUNOSUPPRESSION

Current maintenance immunosuppression is most commonly a triple-drug regimen consisting of prednisone (approximately 0.2 to 0.3 mg/kg/day), cyclosporine (approximately 4 to 6 mg/kg/day), and azathioprine (1 to 2 mg/kg/day). The inclusion of azathioprine allows lower doses of cyclosporine and corticosteroids and thus helps to minimize toxicity.

Diagnosis and Therapy of Acute Rejection

Acute rejection remains a common problem despite the best immunosuppression currently available. Most rejection episodes occur within the first year after transplantation. The clinical presentation is highly variable and depends on the severity of the episode, the immunosuppressive agents being used, and on the organ transplanted. Although it is difficult to describe an approach to the diagnosis of acute rejection without reference to a particular organ graft, certain parallels can be drawn. First, rejection must be considered in any transplant patient with fever or symptoms or laboratory results suggestive of graft dysfunction or inflammation (vide infra Case Discussion). Second, the suspicion of rejection should initiate a thorough clinical evaluation and an immediate determination of simple parameters of graft function. These would include serum creatinine for a renal transplant, transaminases and bilirubin for a liver transplant, and so on. Third, liberal use should be made of relevant biopsy techniques should any suspicion of rejection remain following the initial evaluation. Because the morbidity of a single bolus dose of corticosteroids is limited, it may frequently be advisable to initiate this therapy on semiempirical grounds pending histologic confirmation of the diagnosis. Fourth, OKT3 represents the current "gold standard" for highly effective reversal of acute rejection, although its use is often restricted to rejection resistant to other therapeutic modalities because of the toxicity of this agent. Finally, it should be emphasized that the distinction between rejection and other causes of graft dysfunction can be extremely difficult and that even histologic analysis can be equivocal. Because the diagnosis of heart, lung, and liver rejection is addressed elsewhere in this text, this discussion will focus on kidney and pancreas rejection.

DIAGNOSIS OF RENAL ALLOGRAFT REJECTION

In patients not receiving cyclosporine, acute renal allograft rejection classically presents with fever, graft tenderness, decreased urine output, and a rise in the serum creatinine level. In patients receiving cyclosporine, however, the onset of rejection can be much more insidious, with a small elevation in serum creatinine content being the only clinical sign. An elevation in serum creatinine level can also be caused by cyclosporine nephrotoxicity, making rejection doubly difficult to diagnose. Transplant pyelonephritis can also mimic allograft rejection but can be more easily distinguished by the presence of neutrophils and casts in the urine. Rejection is rarely the cause of immediate posttransplant graft dysfunction. Because acute rejection requires several days to develop, lack of graft function in the first few days can reliably be attributed to ATN once technical problems with the vascular and ureteral anastomoses have been excluded. Obstruction of the urinary catheter by clots must be ruled out by gentle irrigation. It is also important to correct hypovolemia, but care must be exercised because excessive fluids may precipitate pulmonary edema. A posttransplant radionuclide renal scan is of great importance in patients with oliguria. A pattern of slightly delayed renal perfusion but absent excretion of isotope is characteristic of ATN. Absent perfusion suggests vascular occlusion, and appearance of isotope outside the collecting system indicates a ureteral anastomotic leak.

Once correctable technical problems have been excluded, the diagnosis of ATN is confirmed and the patient is maintained on hemodialysis with care taken to avoid hypovolemia. If oliguria does not quickly resolve, repeat renal scans and percutaneous renal biopsies can be obtained to rule out concomitant rejection, because it is particularly difficult to diagnose rejection occurring during graft dysfunction. Although severe rejection can cause decreased renal perfusion, a radionuclide scan showing normal perfusion does not rule out rejection and should not deter biopsy if otherwise indicated. Injury to a major renal vessel is a rare sequela of percutaneous core biopsy. Fine-needle aspiration cytology of the renal transplant has been proposed as a less invasive alternative, but this procedure is not yet widely used.

DIAGNOSIS OF PANCREATIC ALLOGRAFT REJECTION

A major obstacle to the development of clinical pancreatic transplantation has been the inability to diagnose acute rejection episodes in time for successful antirejection therapy. Hyperglycemia does not occur until 80 to 90 percent of the graft has been destroyed. For uremic diabetics, pancreatic transplantation is often performed concomitantly with a renal transplant from the same donor. Since both grafts bear the same foreign HLA molecules and kidney graft rejection is more easily detectable, the diagnosis of rejection is usually made based on renal rather than pancreatic graft dysfunction. For this reason, synchronous renal and pancreatic transplantation has achieved the greatest pancreatic graft survival of any technique yet developed.[25] Combined kidney/pancreas transplantation obviously applies only to diabetics who have progressed to end-stage renal failure. The application of pancreatic transplantation to diabetic patients prior to the development of irreversible target organ complications is potentially of much greater benefit, but a reliable means of detecting rejection in the isolated pancreatic graft is needed. Since current methods of pancreatic transplantation drain the exocrine secretions into the bladder, one possibility is to monitor urinary levels of pancreatic products. In particular, urinary amylase concentration has been reported to drop abruptly at the onset of rejection.[26] Unfortunately, exceptions occur frequently. Determinations of serum anodal trypsinogen or of pancreas-specific protein have also been advocated as screening tests for pancreatic rejection.[27,28]

DIAGNOSIS OF HEPATIC, CARDIAC, AND PULMONARY ALLOGRAFT REJECTION

Because the diagnosis of rejection of these organs is addressed elsewhere in this text, only brief mention will be made here. Hepatic allograft rejection should be suspected in the liver transplant recipient with elevated bilirubin and transaminase levels. The differential diagnosis includes viral hepatitis (including CMV), drug-induced hepatitis (including azathioprine), hepatic artery or portal vein thrombosis, cholangitis, cholestasis due to sepsis or biliary tree concretions, and technical problems with the biliary reconstruction. Percutaneous needle biopsy is the diagnostic procedure of choice; care should be taken to correct any platelet or coagulation deficits to minimize bleeding complications. Cardiac allograft rejection may present with decreased cardiac function (often as amelioration of cyclosporine-induced hypertension) but usually is clinically silent. Transvenous endomycardial biopsy is relatively simple and is performed frequently during the early postoperative period when the incidence of rejection is greatest.

Pulmonary allografts may similarly be surveyed by bronchoscopy with transbronchial biopsy. Interestingly, some histologic evidence of rejection is often seen in heart and liver biopsies without clinical evidence of rejection.

TREATMENT OF ACUTE REJECTION

On diagnosis of acute rejection, therapy is immediately initiated with either high dose corticosteroids, ALG, or OKT3. Prior to the introduction of OKT3, approximately 65 to 75 percent of acute rejection episodes eventually responded to high dose steroids, typically 500 mg methylprednisolone daily for 1 week with a subsequent slow taper.[15] The prolonged use of high dose corticosteroids greatly increased the risk of major bacterial and fungal infections. ALG and OKT3 are more effective in reversing acute rejection, with a success rate of 80 to 90 percent for ALG and $>$ 90 percent for OKT3. However, the toxicity of these agents is substantial. A short series of steroid pulses (e.g., 500 mg/day for 3 days) can identify the subset of patients whose rejection is easily reversed. If no improvement is seen within 3 or 4 days, a biopsy for histologic confirmation of the diagnosis should be considered, and ALG or OKT3 therapy should be initiated. This strategy allows easily reversible rejections to be treated without the toxicity of ALG or OKT3, while preventing patients with more refractory rejection from being subjected to the morbidity of prolonged high dose steroids before initiation of other therapy.[16,17]

Infectious Complications of Immunosuppression

The primary complication of immunosuppression is increased susceptibility to infection. Because current immunosuppression is not antigen specific, there is a balance between more effective suppression of rejection on the one hand and decreased ability to combat infection on the other. Successful management of these infectious complications demands prompt diagnosis and appropriate pharmacologic or surgical treatment of the infection. Modification of the immunosuppressive regimen is often required. The complexity of the management of transplant-related infection requires a vigilant and systematic approach on the part of the transplant physician. Although antigen-specific immunosuppression may ultimately be achieved and allow transplantation without immunodeficiency, expertise in the care of immunocompromised patients will remain essential for transplant physicians for the foreseeable future. The reader is referred to Chap. 99 for further discussion of this topic.

BACTERIAL INFECTIONS

Bacterial infections are normally cleared by the actions of neutrophils, macrophages, and the humoral immune system, with less involvement of T cells. Cyclosporine and OKT3 thus cause much less impairment of resistance to usual bacterial pathogens than do azathioprine and high dose corticosteroids. Bacterial infections are most frequent in the first month after transplantation. The organisms involved reflect the flora of the transplant site. For example, gram-negative aerobes and enterococci are the most common bacterial pathogens in liver transplant recipients. Many of these infections are more properly considered complications of surgery than of immunosuppression per se, although the adverse effects of corticosteroids on wound healing are certainly a contributing factor. Corticosteroids may also mask the symptoms of intraabdominal sepsis and contribute to dangerous delay in recognition of anastomotic leaks, abscesses, and other conditions requiring surgical intervention. A high index of suspicion of intraabdominal infection must be maintained in any transplant patient with ileus, abdominal pain, or unexplained sepsis, even if the abdominal findings are equivocal. A negative laparotomy, though undesirable, poses a much smaller risk than unrecognized peritonitis. Broad-spectrum antibiotic coverage is indicated but is only adjunctive therapy in the setting of an intraabdominal abscess, a perforated viscus, or a biliary or enteric anastomotic leak. Other common sites of bacterial infection in transplant patients are the urinary tract, the respiratory tree, and indwelling devices such as central venous catheters. The early removal of urinary, endotracheal, and intravascular catheters is advisable for all patients but is even more advisable in the setting of immunosuppression. An unexplained fever demands a diligent search for a site of infection. For example, long-term nasogastric intubation can cause sinusitis, and unattended dental caries can lead to mandibular osteomyelitis.

FUNGAL INFECTIONS

Fungal infections also usually occur within the first 1 to 2 months after transplantation. The risk of fungal infection is markedly increased by excessive corticosteroid use. Repeated courses of broad-spectrum antibiotics, multiple reoperations, and a prolonged ICU stay also predispose to fungal infections. *Candida* is the most common organism, although many other fungal pathogens are occasionally seen. Common sites of relatively minor infection are the oral cavity, the urinary bladder, and the upper respiratory tract. Oral candidiasis can be minimized by routine prophylaxis with nystatin. Colonization of the sputum or urine with *Candida* does not in itself warrant systemic amphotericin, although amphotericin bladder irrigation may be performed with little morbidity. Again, the importance of timely removal of indwelling catheters is stressed.

Major *Candida* infections include invasive pneumonitis, candidemia (often due to infection of central venous lines), and intraabdominal infection, usually in the reoperated patient. Although candidal sepsis can often be reversed with appropriate therapy, systemic infections with other fungi, such as *Aspergillus* or *Cryptococcus* organisms, carry a very high mortality rate in the transplant patient. *Aspergillus* organisms are particularly hazardous to immunocompromised patients exposed to dust from construction work. Any hospital renovation project involving replacement of walls or ceilings should be accompanied by specific measures to protect transplant recipients and other immunocompromised individuals. Treatment of major fungal infection includes both systemic amphotericin and elimination of any localized fluid collections or infected catheters. The nephrotoxicity of amphotericin is well-known and is synergistic with that of cyclosporine. Newer antifungal agents, such as fluconazole, may provide a less toxic alternative for the treatment of *Candida* and *Cryptococcus* infections.[29] However, fluconazole is fungistatic rather than fungicidal.

VIRAL INFECTIONS

The immune response to viral infection resembles the acute cellular response to a transplanted organ in that both are highly dependent on cytotoxic T cells. As clinical immunosuppression becomes increasingly targeted at T cells, it is no surprise that viral infections have become a major problem. CMV is the most common and important viral pathogen in transplant patients, particularly in those who have been treated extensively with OKT3 or ALG.[30] Infections range in severity from mild to lethal. CMV infections may be caused by reactivation of latent virus in a CMV-seropositive recipient. These reactivation infections occur 1 to 4 months after transplantation and are frequently less severe than primary infection, although their course may be more virulent in patients receiving ALG or OKT3. Primary CMV infection occurs in patients who are CMV-seronegative at the time of transplantation and receive an organ from a CMV-seropositive donor. CMV-positive blood products are a much less frequent cause of infection in solid organ recipients.

CMV causes several different clinical syndromes, including pneumonitis, hepatitis, nephritis, and gastrointestinal ulceration. The latter may result in perforation or hemorrhage and should be suspected in any transplant patient with gastrointestinal bleeding. However, the most common presentation of CMV is one of fever and leukopenia, occasionally with thrombocytopenia or atypical lymphocytes. Tissue invasion on liver or bronchoscopic biopsy serves to confirm the diagnosis.

The therapy of CMV infections depends on the severity of the disease. Many minor infections resolve without specific treatment. For more severe infections, immunosuppression should be reduced (vide infra) and antiviral therapy begun with ganciclovir. The use of ganciclovir, CMV immune globulin, or high dose oral acyclovir for CMV prophylaxis is currently under investigation.

Many other herpes viruses are commonly seen in transplant recipients. These include herpes simplex virus (HSV) reactivation and dermatomal varicella zoster virus (shingles). These infections are troublesome to the patient but are generally not life-threatening. Low dose oral acyclovir is effective for mucocutaneous HSV lesions.

PARASITIC INFECTIONS

Pneumocystis carinii pneumonia is the most common parasitic infection in the transplant recipient. This typically occurs several months after transplantation and should be suspected in any transplant patient presenting with a pulmonary infiltrate. The frequency of this complication can be reduced by prophylaxis with low dose oral trimethoprim/sulfamethoxazole (TMP/SMX). Intravenous TMP/SMX is the agent of first choice for documented infection. Pentamidine is an alternative agent which may be used when TMP/SMX is contraindicated due to allergy or adverse reaction. Although sputum specimens are usually nondiagnostic, the diagnosis can often be made by bronchoscopy with bronchoalveolar lavage and transbronchial biopsy.

APPROACH TO PULMONARY INFILTRATES IN TRANSPLANT RECIPIENTS

The most common serious infection occurring more than 1 month after transplantation is pneumonia. Pulmonary infections may be caused by a wide variety of organisms, including gram-negative aerobes, fungi, legionella, *P. carinii,* and viruses, especially CMV. As these infections may progress rapidly in the immunocompromised host, an expeditious evaluation is essential (Fig. 77-4).

Although invasive diagnostic procedures are often necessary, much information can be obtained from a chest radiogram and sputum examination. Bacterial pneumonias are more likely to present with lobar or unilateral infiltrates, whereas viruses and *P. carinii* usually cause diffuse, bilateral infiltrates. For example, a community-acquired lobar infiltrate associated with a sputum Gram stain dominated by gram-negative rods and neutrophils may be treated with an aminogylcoside and an antipseudomonal penicillin until culture results are obtained. Frequently, however, the chest film reveals diffuse, bilateral infiltrates. In this setting, expectorated sputum is usually nondiagnostic. Presumptive coverage should be broadened by adding erythromycin and TMP/SMX to cover *Legionella* and *Pneumocystis* species, respectively. Bronchoscopy should be performed promptly in transplant patients with diffuse infiltrates and should include bronchoalveolar lavage to optimize culture yield. Transbronchial biopsy may demonstrate CMV inclusions or may reveal *Pneumocystis* on silver stain. A nondiagnostic bronchoscopy should immediately lead to open lung biopsy. The empirical antibiotic regimen is modified as indicated once a specific diagnosis is made. In addition, the transplant patient with pneumonia must be closely monitored for evidence of incipient respiratory failure. Early intubation may be indicated, because deterioration can be rapid.

MODIFICATION OF IMMUNOSUPPRESSION IN TRANSPLANT PATIENTS WITH INFECTIONS

Although minor infections in transplant recipients may be managed without altering immunosuppression, severe or persistent infections often require that immunosuppression be reduced or withheld (vide infra Case Discussion). A life-threatening infection in a renal transplant recipient requires discontinuation of all immunosuppression except for hydrocortisone in sufficient doses to prevent adrenal crisis.

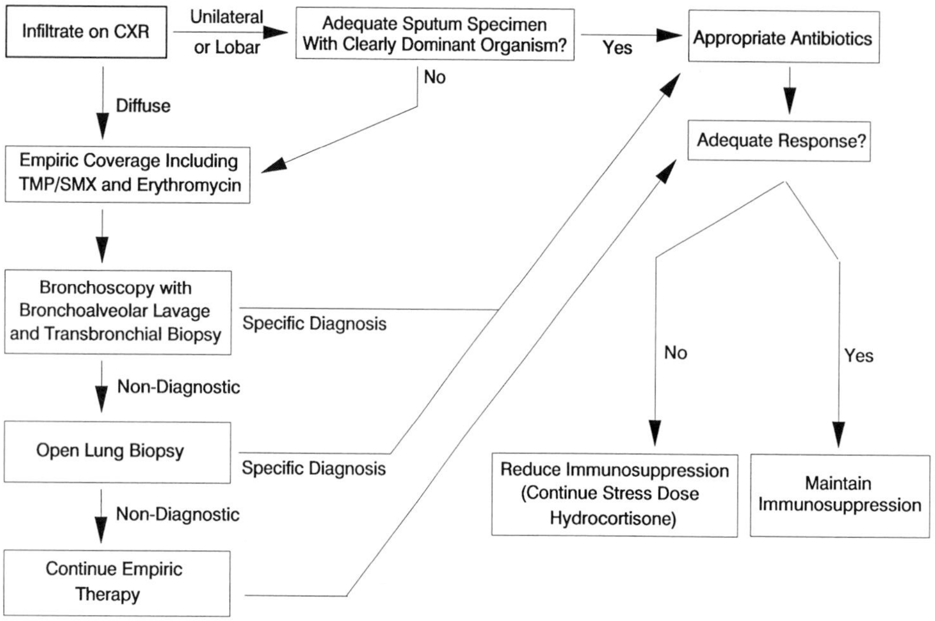

FIGURE 77-4 Approach to evaluation of pneumonia in transplant patients. Evaluation must be expeditious and should generally be completed within 48 h of presentation.

Severe infection in the heart or liver transplant recipient presents a dilemma, as life depends on continuing function of these grafts. However, it should be noted that the discontinuation of immunosuppression does not always lead to rejection in critically ill patients, particularly those with viral infections.

Future Directions in Immunotherapy for Transplantation

The ultimate goal of transplant immunotherapy is to produce permanent graft tolerance without otherwise compromising the immune response. Neither objective has been achieved by any available immunosuppressive regimen. Although graft-specific tolerance in human beings is not expected in the near future, it is likely that significant improvement in outcome will result from some of the immunotherapeutic modalities presently under investigation. Current research may be broadly grouped into three categories. The first of these is the preclinical and investigational use of a variety of new immunosuppressive drugs, including FK506, RS61143, and rapamycin.[31,32] A second major area of investigation is the refinement of monoclonal antibody therapy. Finally, much progress has been made in understanding the mechanisms by which self-tolerance is maintained, namely clonal deletion and clonal anergy.[33] Manipulation of these physiologic processes offers the best hope of eventually achieving the goal of graft acceptance without general immunoincompetence.

FK506 is a macrolide antibiotic with immunosuppressive properties similar to those of cyclosporine. Like cyclosporine, FK506 binds to a peptidyl-prolyl isomerase, although the two proteins are distinct from one another. FK506 is nephrotoxic but its therapeutic index appears to be much more favorable than that of cyclosporine. Rapamycin, another macrolide, also inhibits T cell proliferation. RS61143 is a lymphocyte-specific inhibitor of purine metabolism which acts by interfering with clonal expansion of activated lymphocytes.[34] Because RS61143 appears to inhibit antibody responses better than immunosuppressive agents presently in use, it is hoped that it will be more effective at preventing chronic rejection.

CASE PRESENTATION

A 17-year-old girl with end-stage renal disease received a living related kidney transplant from her father. Induction immunosuppression consisted of intraoperative administration of 2 g methylprednisolone and 200 mg azathioprine, with subsequent taper to daily doses of 15 mg prednisone and 75 mg azathioprine. Cyclosporine was begun the day of surgery at a total daily dose of 7.5 mg/kg and continued at this level. Induction OKT3 was not used because ATN is rare in living related transplants. Graft function was immediate, and she was discharged 6 days after surgery with a creatinine level of 1.1.

Four weeks after transplantation, the patient presented with a temperature of 39°C (102.2°F) and a rise in creatinine level to 1.9. Acute rejection was suspected, and treatment was initiated with 500 mg methylprednisolone on each of 3 consecutive days. After a transient improvement, she again became febrile, and her creatinine level rose to 2.1. Percutaneous renal biopsy confirmed acute cellular rejection, and the patient was admitted for OKT3 therapy. Although she experienced typical fever, chills, and rigors following the first dose of OKT3, no seizures, pulmonary edema, or other serious toxicity occurred. Her creatinine level began to fall after 4 days, and she was discharged the following day. OKT3 was continued as an outpatient via daily clinic visits. Total leukocyte counts fell progressively despite withholding azathioprine, and she was readmitted after 7 days of OKT3 with the presumptive diagnosis of CMV. Therapy consisted of neutropenia precautions and ganciclovir, 100 mg (2 mg/kg) every 12 h. OKT3 was discontinued after nine doses, and cyclosporine was reduced to 2.5 mg/kg/day.

The patient subsequently developed dyspnea and bilateral pulmonary infiltrates and was transferred to the ICU and electively intubated. Bronchoscopy was performed and broad-spectrum antibiotic coverage was initiated with vancomycin, erythromycin, and tobramycin. Bronchoscopic washings grew *Klebsiella pneumoniae*. Her respiratory function gradually improved, and she was extubated 4 days later. She was transferred out of the ICU shortly thereafter, and her general status was much improved.

Three weeks after admission, the patient developed hematemesis. Upper gastrointestinal endoscopy was performed, but the extent of bleeding within the stomach did not allow visualization of a specific source. An emergency laparotomy was performed with oversewing of a bleeding gastric ulcer. Although another episode of respiratory failure required a third ICU admission, she improved thereafter and was discharged after a 9-week hospitalization. She has since been maintained on only 10 mg prednisone daily and 2 mg/kg/day of cyclosporine with no evidence of rejection. Her creatinine level was 1.3 7 months after transplantation. The patient is now fully rehabilitated and is in her first year of college.

CASE DISCUSSION

Living related donor renal transplantation is associated with a short duration of graft ischemia and hence a low incidence of postoperative ATN. Therefore, it was possible to begin cyclosporine immediately and avoid the use of OKT3 for induction immunotherapy. Corticosteroids and azathioprine were tapered promptly, and the patient was maintained on a typical triple-drug regimen.

The occurrence of both fever and a rise in creatinine content strongly suggested the diagnosis of acute rejection. As is common in patients receiving cyclosporine, graft tenderness was not present. Antirejection therapy was begun immediately with a steroid pulse, but only transient improvement resulted. In view of the toxicity associated with OKT3, a biopsy was performed to confirm the diagnosis before beginning monoclonal therapy. OKT3 promptly reversed the rejection episode.

CMV infection is a well-recognized complication of immunosuppression and particularly of anti-T cell antibody treatment, because T cell responses are essential for immunity to this virus. CMV infection should be suspected in any transplant patient with falling leukocyte counts. Although CMV was not obtained from either the patient's lung or stomach, it is a notoriously difficult infection to document. It was suspected as the primary cause of the patient's pneumonitis and her gastric ulcer, as these are two of the most common complications of CMV infection. This case also illustrates the frequent occurrence of secondary bacterial infections in patients who have become neutropenic from CMV, as well as the early use of invasive diagnostic procedures.

The reduction in immunosuppression played a key role in the patient's recovery from life-threatening infection. The decision to decrease or withhold immunosuppression is complex and must take into account the severity of the infection and the specific infectious agent involved. In this case, the use of azathioprine was clearly contraindicated once the patient became neutropenic.

Finally, it should be noted that it was possible in this patient to taper immunosuppression to very low levels without evidence of recurrent rejection. This is common not only in recipients of living related donor renal transplants, but also in recipients more poorly matched with their donor who experience overwhelming sepsis. Of final note, the acute rejection episode, once reversed, characteristically had no late effect on graft function.

References

1. Kakizoe S, Yanaga K, Starzl T, et al: Evaluation of protocol before liver transplantation and after reperfusion biopsies from human orthotopic liver allografts: Considerations of preservation and early immunological injury. Hepatology 11(6):932, 1990.
2. Fellstrom B, Dimeny E, Larsson E, et al: Importance of PDGF receptor in accelerated atherosclerosis-chronic rejection. Transplant Proc 21(4):3689, 1989.
3. Halloran PF, Cockfield SM, Madrenas J: The molecular immunology of transplantation and graft rejection. Immunol Allergy Clin North Am 9:1, 1989.
4. Blackman M, Kappler J, Marrack P: The role of the T cell receptor in positive and negative selection of developing T cells. Science 248:1335, 1990.
5. Altman A, Coggeshall KM, Mustelin T: Molecular events mediating T cell activation. Adv Immunol 48:227, 1990.
6. Clevers H, Alarcon B, Wileman T, Terhorst C: The T cell receptor-CD3 complex: A dynamic protein ensemble. Annu Rev Immunol 6:629, 1988.
7. Crabtree GR: Contingent genetic regulatory events in T lymphocyte activation. Science 243:355, 1989.
8. Calne RY, White DJ, Thiru S, et al: Cyclosporin A in patients receiving renal allografts from cadaver donors. Lancet 2:1323, 1978.
9. Kramer NC, Peters TG, Rohr MS, et al: Beneficial effect of cyclosporine on renal transplantation. Transplantation 49:343, 1990.
10. Kahan BD: Cyclosporine. N Engl J Med 321:1725, 1989.
11. Foxwell BMJ, Ryffel B: The mechanisms of action of cyclosporine. Immuno Allergy Clin North Am 9:79, 1989.
12. Elliot JF, Lin Y, Mizel SB, et al: Induction of interleukin-2 messenger RNA inhibited by cyclosporin A. Science 226:1439, 1978.
13. Dawidson I, Rooth P, Fry WR, et al: Prevention of acute cyclosporine-induced renal blood flow inhibition and improved immunosuppression with verapamil. Transplantation 48:575, 1989.
14. Riotte B, Hull D: Cyclosporine drug interactions. Infect Surg July 1990, 5.
15. Dupont E, Wybran J, Toussaint C: Glucocorticoids and organ transplantation. Transplantation 37:331, 1985.

16. Murray JE, Merrill JP, Harrison JH, et al: Prolonged survival of human kidney homografts by immunosuppressive drug therapy. N Engl J Med 268:1315, 1963.
17. Cosimi AB, Wortis HH, Delmonico FL, et al: Randomized clinical trial of antilymphocyte globulin in cadaver renal allograft recipients: Importance of T-cell monitoring. Surgery 80:155, 1976.
18. Ortho Multicenter Transplant Study Group. A randomized clinical trial of OKT3 monoclonal antibody for acute rejection of cadaveric renal transplants. N Engl J Med 313:337, 1985.
19. Thistlethwaite JR, Haag BW, Gaber AO, et al: The use of OKT3 to treat steroid-resistant renal allograft rejection in patients receiving cyclosporine. Transplant Proc 19:1901, 1987.
20. Chatenoud L, Ferran C, Legendre C, et al: In vivo cell activation following OKT3 administration. Transplantation 49:697, 1990.
21. Benvenisty AI, Cohen D, Stegall MD, Hardy MA: Improved results using OKT3 as induction immunosuppression in renal allograft recipients with delayed graft function. Transplantation 49:321, 1990.
22. Schroeder TJ, First RM, Mansour ME, et al: Antimurine antibody formation following OKT3 therapy. Transplantation 49:48, 1990.
23. Penn I: Collective review—Cancer is a complication of severe immunosuppression. Surg Gynecol Obstet 162:603, 1986.
24. Hanto DW, Gajl-Peczalska KJ, Frizzera G, et al: Epstein-Barr virus (EBV) induced polyclonal B-cell lymphoproliferative disease occurring after renal transplantation. Clinical, pathologic, and virologic findings and implications for therapy. Ann Surg 193:356, 1983.
25. Sutherland DER, Moudry KC, Fryd DS: Results of pancreas transplant registry. Diabetes 38(suppl 1):46, 1989.
26. Prieto M, Sutherland DER, Fernandez-Cruz L, et al: Urinary amylase monitoring for early diagnosis of pancreas allograft rejection in dogs. J Surg Res 40:597, 1986.
27. Marks WH, Borgstrom A, Sollinger H, et al: Serum anodal trypsinogen is a predictive biochemical marker for pancreatic allograft rejection. Transplant Proc 22(2):673, 1990.
28. Fernstad R, Tyden G, Brattstrom C, et al: Pancreas-specific protein. New serum marker for graft rejection in pancreas transplant recipients. Diabetes 38(suppl 1):55, 1989.
29. Conti DJ, Tolkoff-Rubin NE, Baker GP, et al: Successful treatment of invasive fungal infection with fluconazole in organ transplant recipients. Transplantation 48:692, 1989.
30. Preiksaitis JK: Cytomegalovirus infection in transplant recipients. Immunol Allergy Clin North Am 9:137, 1989.
31. Metcalfe SM, Richards FM: Cyclosporine, FK506, and rapamycin: Some effects on early activation events in serum-free, mitogen-stimulated mouse spleen cells. Transplantation 49:798, 1990.
32. Thomas J. Matthews C, Carroll R, et al: The immunosuppressive action of FK506. Transplantation 49:390, 1990.
33. Ramsdell F, Fowlkes BJ: Clonal deletion versus clonal anergy: The role of the thymus in inducing self tolerance. Science 248:1342, 1990.
34. Morris RE, Hoyt EG, Murphy MP, et al: Mycophenolic acid morpholinoethyl ester (RS-61443) is a new immunosuppressant that prevents and halts heart allograft rejection by selective inhibition of T- and B-cell purine synthesis. Transplant Proc 22(4):1659, 1990.

Chapter 78
LUNG TRANSPLANTATION

E. VALLIERES
T. R. TODD

KEY POINTS

- *End-stage pulmonary fibrosis is best treated by single-lung transplantation; end-stage bilateral septic lung disease by double-lung transplantation.*
- *The donor lungs must be normal by chest x-ray and must be capable of maintaining the donor's* Pa_{O_2} *above 300 mmHg while being ventilated at a* F_{IO_2} *of 1.0 with a PEEP of 5 cm of* H_2O *for 5 min.*
- *During single-lung implantation, cardiopulmonary bypass is required in about 20 percent of cases.*
- *Cardiovascular instability is the rule in the first 24 h following double-lung transplantation.*
- *Two episodes of acute rejection are seen on average during the first 3 weeks after lung transplantation.*
- *Infections represent the greatest threat to long-term lung transplant recipient survival.*
- *Late airway stenosis can usually be successfully managed by repeated dilations and the use of endoluminal silicone stents.*
- *Bronchiolitis obliterans, which complicates a large proportion of heart-lung recipients, occurs in a few recipients of both single- and double-lung transplants.*

The lung is the only solid organ wherein the systemic arterial blood supply is not routinely reestablished at the time of transplantation. It is also the only transplanted organ which remains in direct and constant contact with the outside environment. These two peculiarities account in part for two of the main problems encountered with isolated pulmonary transplantation, namely airway ischemia with its related consequences and the constant threat of pulmonary sepsis.

Experimental lung transplantation began in the 1940s, and the first human lung transplantation was attempted by Hardy in Mississippi in 1963.[1] This was followed by over 40 unsuccessful attempts over the next 20 years. Airway ischemia and dehiscence, pulmonary sepsis, poor recipient selection, poor donor lung preservation, allograft rejection, and respiratory failure were the main reasons for these universally fatal attempts.

The arrival of cyclosporine led to a major improvement in immunosuppression, and two laboratory observations helped overcome the problem of airway healing, leading to the first successful single-lung transplantation in humans in 1983.[2] First, it was discovered that corticosteroid use contributed to impaired bronchial anastomotic healing,[3] a finding not seen with cyclosporine.[4] Second, bronchial omentopexy was shown to promote healing and augment blood supply to the bronchial anastomosis.[5] The first successful double-lung transplantation was performed in 1986.[6] As of October 1990, 302 single- and 130 double-lung transplantations have been performed worldwide in various centers.[7] These procedures have been accepted as therapeutic options in the management of end-stage pulmonary disease. A third option, heart-lung transplantation (see Chap. 79), was successfully reported in human beings in 1981.[8] Initially used exclusively in patients with primary or secondary pulmonary vascular disease, only recently has it been extended to patients with intrinsic lung disease.[9]

These recent advances and the reported successes of the three procedures are the result of a multidisciplinary approach to lung transplantation. Even today, each individual lung transplant remains a major clinical challenge and involves the combined efforts of many individuals; beginning with the assessment of potential recipients, their preoperative preparation, the proper donor selection, adequate intraoperative and postoperative care, and long-term surveillance. This chapter will review these various aspects of pulmonary transplantation with emphasis on donor preparation and maintenance as well as on early postoperative critical care.

Preoperative Preparation

SELECTION AND EVALUATION OF THE LUNG TRANSPLANT RECIPIENT

The main indication for single-lung transplant (SLTX) is end-stage fibrotic lung disease. Other indications are listed in Table 78-1. Though initially thought to be contraindicated in the treatment of chronic obstructive pulmonary disease, SLTX has now been utilized with success in its management in well-selected cases.[10] Double-lung transplant (DLTX) is almost exclusively used for end-stage bilateral septic disease, particularly cystic fibrosis and bronchiectasis, both of which constitute contraindications to SLTX (Table 78-1). Pulmonary hypertension, either primary or due to congenital heart disease or chronic thromboembolic disease, remains the classical indication for heart-lung transplant (HLTX) (Table 78-1). Nonetheless in situations where right ventricular function is considered reversible by preoperative assessment or where the congenital heart defect is correctable, SLTX is an option.[11] Because of technical difficulties due to cardiomegaly, DLTX in its initial version, using a single tracheal anastomosis, is considered a contraindication in such patients.[12] The new approach to DLTX by bilateral sequential SLTX is an option, however. Obviously, patients with end-stage parenchymal lung disease and separate cardiac dysfunction are best served by HLTX.

Stringent recipient selection criteria are probably the most important factors in predicting the success of lung transplant programs (Table 78-2). Patients should be oxygen dependent at rest. Age limits have been set at 60 years or younger for SLTX and 50 years or younger for DLTX and

TABLE 78-1 Indications for Lung Transplantation

Single-lung transplantation
- A. Treatment of choice for end-stage fibrotic lung disease: idiopathic, hypersensitivity, occupational, toxin sarcoidosis, others
- B. As a therapeutic option
  1. Chronic obstructive lung disease: emphysema, alpha-1 antitrypsin deficiency
  2. Pulmonary hypertension: primary, Eisenmenger's (if congenital heart defect is reversible)
  3. Lymphangioleiomyomatosis

Double-lung transplantation
- A. Treatment of choice for end-stage bilateral septic lung disease: cystic fibrosis, bronchiectasis
- B. As a therapeutic option
  1. Chronic obstructive lung disease: emphysema, alpha-1 antitrypsin deficiency, bronchiolitis obliterans
  2. Eosinophilic granulomatosis, lymphangioleiomyomatosis
  3. Pulmonary hypertension (bilateral sequential single-lung technique)

Heart-lung transplantation
- A. Treatment of choice for
  1. Pulmonary vascular disease: right ventricular ejection fraction less than 20%, primary pulmonary hypertension, chronic thromboembolic disease, Eisenmenger's with cardiac anomaly not correctable
  2. Pulmonary parenchymal disease: with separate heart disease; cardiac function not reversible
- B. As a therapeutic option for pulmonary vascular disease: right ventricular ejection fraction at or better than 20%; Eisenmenger's physiology with cardiac anomaly surgically correctable

HLTX. Patients over 50 should have coronary angiography as part of their assessment. Patients must be ambulatory to participate in preoperative rehabilitation programs, and ventilator dependency is a definite contraindication. Steroid dependency is considered a contraindication to lung transplantation by the Toronto Lung Transplant Group due to the impact of steroids on bronchial healing.[2,3,6] Other groups have reported using steroids as early as day 1 after transplant with good results,[13] but the risk of preoperative steroid administration remains a concern.

TABLE 78-2 Medical Criteria for Potential Recipients of Lung Transplantation

Life expectancy <18 months
Age <60 years for SLTX, <50 years for DLTX and HLTX
Ambulatory, but oxygen dependent at rest
Adequate nutrition, nonobese

Contraindications
- Steroid dependency
- Ventilator dependency
- Bilateral pulmonary sepsis (SLTX)
- Right heart failure (RVEF <20%)
- Malignancy
- Other end organ damage
- Coronary heart disease
- Psychiatric/drug abuse

Patients must be well nourished but nonobese. Previous major abdominal surgery was at one time considered a contraindication for fear of not finding sufficient residual omentum to use intrathoracically. The capability of using the pericardial fat pad, thymic fat, or even an intercostal muscle bundle to protect the anastomosis has led to the elimination of this exclusion criterion. In the same vein, prior major violations of the pleural space, initially considered a contraindication to DLTX and HLTX because of bleeding secondary to pleural adhesions and intraoperative anticoagulation, no longer contraindicate these procedures.

Candidates on the active transplant list have a life expectancy estimated at 18 months or less. Such evaluation is very difficult and often inaccurate. The fact that in Toronto 16 candidates out of 66 died while on the waiting list reflects the end-stage nature of the disease process.[11] Prediction remains difficult particularly in patients with chronic obstructive lung disease. However, the prognostic determination will become less important as continued success is realized.

Arbitrarily, the minimal preoperative right ventricular ejection fraction acceptable for SLTX has been set at 20 percent. Major improvements in right ventricular output have been observed following single-lung procedures.[14] This fact suggested that SLTX might be employed in the treatment of pulmonary hypertension.[15]

Candidates and family undergo full psychosocial evaluation. Patients must be well motivated and have adequate social and financial support. Major psychological disturbances or history of drug abuse are contraindications to transplantation.

In SLTX, the left side has traditionally been preferred because of technical ease in accessing the left atrium and pulmonary artery. The left side also allows better reexpansion of excessively large grafts by pushing down the diaphragm. Other factors that may influence the choice of the surgical side are avoidance of a previous thoracotomy site, disproportionate V/Q abnormalities, or asymmetry in the quality of the donor lungs. A preoperative quantitative perfusion scan will determine the side receiving the major proportion of pulmonary perfusion. Obviously, the contralateral side should be selected for transplantation in order to minimize acute changes in pulmonary vascular resistance during the procedure.

SELECTION AND MANAGEMENT OF THE LUNG DONOR

Head injury victims represent the main source of donors for solid organ transplantation (Pittsburgh; 45 percent closed head injury from motor vehicle accident (MVA); 40 percent gun shot wound to the head).[16] Scarcity of donors remains the major obstacle to the expansion of transplant programs despite an increase in demands (see Chap. 76). Intensivists play a major role in the initial selection of potential donors and more importantly in their preparation and maintenance. The paucity of donors is a particular problem in pulmonary transplantation because there is a high association between traumatic brain and lung injuries, neurogenic pulmonary edema is commonly associated with brain death, and many MVA victims suffer from aspiration pneumonitis. It is estimated that only 10 to 15 percent of heart donors had suitable lungs for transplantation.[17]

The successful care of the potential multiorgan donor requires maintaining adequate tissue perfusion and oxygenation. The management of hypotension may require aggressive fluid resuscitation. One should however aim to achieve the lowest central venous pressure or pulmonary capillary wedge pressure achieving adequate blood pressure and perfusion, in an effort to keep the lungs as dry as possible. The addition of inotropic support is often needed to achieve adequate perfusion at these low filling pressures (see Chap. 76).

The ventilator should be set at the lowest fraction of inspired oxygen ($F_{I_{O_2}}$) required to maintain oxygen saturations above 90%. Positive end-expiratory pressure (PEEP) is kept at 5 cm of water to minimize the risk of barotrauma. Similarly, in order to avoid peak inspiratory pressures greater than 30 cmH_2O, tidal volumes of 10 to 15 mL/kg are recommended. Although the risk of pulmonary sepsis is increased, prolonged mechanical ventilation does not preclude lung donation.

Hypothermia may complicate central nervous system injury with loss of central thermoregulating control. In addition, infusions of large amounts of fluids necessary to maintain adequate filling pressures may lower temperature. Measures applicable to preserve heat are important, including heating of the intravenous (IV) fluid tubing, adding a heated humidifier to the ventilator circuit, lavaging through the nasogastric tube with warm saline, and using heated blankets.

Donor selection criteria are listed in Table 78-3. The age limit has been set at 55. Abstinence from tobacco use would be ideal, but most centers accept a moderate history of smoking. It is important to evaluate potential donors over time. Serial chest radiographs are essential, and a chest x-ray done within 2 h of procurement must be normal (at least on one side) to permit unilateral transplantation. Serial blood gas measurements should be performed at regular intervals (6 to 8 hours) with the patient briefly on 100% $F_{I_{O_2}}$ and a PEEP of 5 cmH_2O. The Pa_{O_2} must be above 300 to be acceptable. Bronchoscopy is also part of the donor evaluation to determine the presence or absence of aspiration, intraluminal hemorrhage, or intraluminal foreign body aspirated at the time of initial injury. Sputum samples are obtained for gram stain. Specimens are also obtained for culture, sensitivities, and fungal studies.

The donor-recipient match involves group ABO matching. The donor's weight and height are also obtained in order to estimate thoracic volume. A standard chest anteroposterior (AP) film is used to determine horizontal dimensions taken from one costophrenic angle to the other. Vertical measurements are from the peak of the diaphragm to the highest point of the apex. One should attempt to match predicted lung volumes between donor and recipient, although discrepancies have been tolerated. For example, in SLTX for chronic obstructive pulmonary disease one generally accepts oversizes of 20 to 30 percent to minimize the risk of residual pleural spaces and to minimize ipsilateral mediastinal shift. However, oversizing in patients with fibrotic lung disease could lead to serious complications of cardiac compression and contralateral mediastinal shift with its consequent hemodynamic compromise. Details of lung donor extraction are well described elsewhere,[18] and methods of preservation are constantly being modified in an effort to minimize reimplantation injury[19] and improve ischemic times (which are usually less than 6 h).

TABLE 78-3 Selection Criteria for Pulmonary Donors

A.	Absolute
	Age <55 years
	Normal chest x-ray
	No previous chest surgery
	Pa_{O_2} >300 ($F_{I_{O_2}}$ 1.0, PEEP 5, ×5 min)
	Major ABO compatibility
	Similar projected lung volumes
	HBsAg and human immunodeficiency virus negative
B.	Desirable
	No infected sputum
	Normal bronchoscopy
	No history of smoking

Intraoperative Management

Single-lung transplantation offers specific challenges, particularly in the maintenance of adequate oxygenation, ventilation, and cardiac function during the period of one-lung ventilation.

Details of the induction and maintenance of anaesthesia have been published.[20] Continuous monitoring of systemic and pulmonary arterial pressures, pulse oximetry, end tidal CO_2, and cardiac output is helpful. Attempts are made to position the distal end of the pulmonary artery catheter in the lung which is not to be removed; keeping the patient turned on that side while placing the catheter may help. To eliminate the risk of air embolism during the insertion of the various venous lines, it is recommended that these be inserted after the patient has been anesthetized and ventilated. The exaggerated negative pleural pressure, particularly in pulmonary fibrosis, has resulted in air embolism. A left-sided bronchial blocker (14 French Fogerty venous catheter) is employed to allow single-lung ventilation during left lung transplant; for the right-sided procedure, a left-sided double-lumen endotracheal tube is used (see Chap. 10).

A fully primed bypass machine with oxygenator is always on standby in the room (see Chap. 29) even though the majority of SLTXs can be done without arterial venous bypass. It is difficult to predict in whom bypass will be required. Despite all the preoperative evaluation and assessments, the final decision to go on bypass can only be made once the pulmonary artery has been clamped. Thus, the ipsilateral groin should always be prepared and accessible whenever there is a concern that bypass will be required.

Early in the operation, the lung to be removed is collapsed for 15 min, and pulmonary artery pressure, cardiac index, and Pa_{O_2} are measured and compared to the initial values. In the first 15 Toronto patients, 11 patients had their femoral vessels exposed based on the following criteria: (1) preoperative mean pulmonary artery pressure over 35 mmHg which rose to 40 mmHg or more on one-lung ventilation; (2) preoperative (or a single-lung ventilation) cardiac index measured at less than or equal to 2.0 L/min/m^2 without concomitant use of inotropes or pulmonary vasodilators; and (3) O_2 saturations less than 85 at an FI_{O_2} of 1 on single-lung ventilation. Once the pulmonary artery is clamped (5 min), many of the patients may require pharmacological support (dopamine ± nitroglycerin). Only if this fails to bring the cardiac index over 2, the saturation over 90 or the mixed venous O_2 saturation over 60 does the patient go on bypass. Of the 11 patients identified by the above criteria, only 3 required cannulation and bypass. Retrospective analysis of these patients determined that preoperative room air P_{O_2}, systolic, diastolic, and mean pulmonary artery pressure, and pulmonary vascular resistance were significantly different from the other 8 patients. Right ventricular function as assessed by radionuclide angiography was of no predictive value in that respect.[20]

Traditionally, the sequence of events in implantation has involved anastomoses of the left atrium, then the pulmonary artery, and finally the bronchus. The lung is inflated, while the pulmonary artery is deaired. Omentum is wrapped over the bronchial anastomosis. To minimize trauma to the graft from excessive handling, a more recent technique has emphasized that the bronchus undergo anastomosis first followed by the left atrium and finally the pulmonary artery.

Initially DLTX was performed via sternotomy on full cardiopulmonary bypass. Recently, a bilateral thoractomy with transverse sternotomy and sequential bilateral single-lung implantation has been adopted.[12,21] This facilitates exposure of the pleural spaces and the division of vascular pleural adhesions. In addition, cardiopulmonary bypass may be avoided.

The First 24 H

Immediate postoperative care of lung recipients requires continuous monitoring and adjustment of hemodynamic function. This is particularly the case with DLTX recipients who universally have experienced a very rocky initial postoperative period. The latter require a tremendous amount of intravascular fluid administration as well as the judicious use of inotropic support. Beta-adrenergic doses of dopamine are standard. Double-lung transplant recipients have all sustained, in this early phase, a hyperdynamic state with high cardiac output and low peripheral vascular resistance. Alpha-adrenergic agents (norepinephrine, phenylephrine) have usually been required.[22]

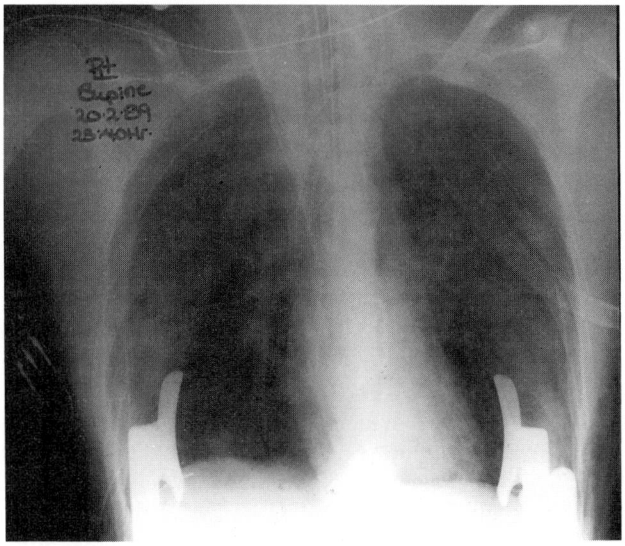

FIGURE 78-1 AP supine chest radiograph demonstrating sternal retractor in place to maintain relief of intrathoracic tamponade.

Double-lung transplant recipients potentially present with specific complications related to the use of cardiopulmonary bypass and systemic anticoagulation during surgery. Hemorrhage is of major concern, particularly with the chronic infected chest cavities of patients with cystic fibrosis and bronchiectasis, in whom dense adhesions are the rule. Bleeding may also result in intrathoracic tamponade from blood or fibrin clots which may render mediastinal drainage tubes nonfunctional. Tamponade has also resulted from an increase in intrathoracic pressures from oversized lungs. Pulmonary edema from poor preservation, cardiopulmonary bypass, or both leads to parenchymal swelling and noncompliance of the lungs. Treatment requires immediate reopening of the chest to release the intrathoracic tension. In three patients, the chest had to be kept open for 2 to 3 days with a sternal retractor while awaiting resorption of the edema (see Fig. 78-1). The incidence of this complication is high enough to suggest that double-lung recipients in shock not responding to fluid and inotropes have their chest immediately reopened. Sternal infection did complicate one of these three patients. Finally, left ventricular failure may be seen, either as a result of poor myocardial preservation while on extracorporeal circulation or possibly from coronary air embolism which may complicate inadequate deairing of the transplanted lung or lungs. The utility of pulmonary artery catheter monitoring in these patients cannot be overemphasized, and even the presence of a fresh vascular anastomosis is not considered a contraindication to its insertion. With the technique of bilateral SLTX via bilateral thoractomy and transverse sternotomy, bypass may not be required, thus decreasing the risk of these complications.

Capillary damage is still a major drawback of suboptimal organ preservation, and even though various techniques of preservation have been developed, the problem has not been eliminated. This, combined with the large amount of intravenous fluids required during and immediately after surgery, leads to some degree of edema in the transplanted lung postoperatively. In addition, as 80 percent of SLTXs are done without cardiopulmonary bypass,[20] there is a period during implantation when the native lung must accommodate the entire cardiac output. This results in a further increase of the often already elevated pulmonary artery pressure which leads to edema of the native lung as well. These pulmonary changes dictate postoperative management wherein an effort is made to give as little intravenous fluids as possible, followed by a forced diuresis once cardiovascular stability is achieved.

Ventilatory management in the first 24 h aims at maintaining adequate oxygenation and ventilation in the face of cardiovascular instability. The F_{IO_2} and peak inspiratory airway pressure should be as low as possible to avoid further injuries to the already damaged lungs. Peak inspiratory airway pressures over 50 cmH_2O should be avoided, as they tend to be associated with increased mean airway pressures which may produce hemodynamic impairment and may risk barotrauma to the bronchial anastomosis and pulmonary parenchyma. A PEEP of 5 cmH_2O is usual and may need to be increased to higher levels to maintain adequate oxygenation. When oxygen requirements are excessive or PEEP levels high, there are specific measures that may reduce the alveolar arterial oxygen difference. With SLTX, regional disparities in pulmonary artery flow distribution produced by postural changes may lead to significant changes in oxygenation. Laying the patient on the side with the best lung may thus improve ventilation perfusion matching. Selective reduction of the pulmonary artery flow to areas that are poorly ventilated can be achieved by PA balloon catheter occlusion.[22] Jet ventilation and extracorporeal membrane oxygenation (ECMO) have been utilized as last resorts on four occasions in the Toronto experience. The former has been useful, but the latter has universally been associated with a fatal outcome.

The airway should be endoscopically assessed either in the operating room or soon after arrival in the intensive care unit. Evaluation of the vascularity of the pulmonary artery anastomosis is important. Pallor this early after surgery is of major concern. Pulmonary toilet with a soft endotracheal suction catheter may be insufficient and bronchoscopy may have to be repeated.

Initial immunosuppression differs from center to center. In Toronto the patients receive a 500-mg bolus of intravenous methylprednisolone intraoperatively once the vascular anastomoses are completed. A skin test to verify reactivity to anti-lymphocyte globulin (ALG) is done preoperatively. If nonreactive, ALG at a dose of 10 to 20 mL/kg/day by continuous infusion is started immediately postoperatively. Azathioprine at a dose of 2 mg/kg is also started. Cardiovascular stability and adequate urinary output are assured prior to initiating cyclosporine administration.

If reactivity of the skin test to horse ALG is documented, goat ALG may be used. Assuming normal renal function, 100 to 150 mg cyclosporine is infused intravenously over the first 24 h postoperatively. In the face of severe hemodynamic instability, it is probably best to delay initiating the cyclosporine infusion for fear of nephrotoxicity.

During the first 7 years of the Toronto lung transplant program, corticosteroids were avoided as maintenance immunosuppression for the first 3 weeks postoperatively. More recently, however, following an intraoperative 500-mg bolus of methylprednisolone, daily doses of 100 to 125 per day have been utilized for 3 days and then decreased to the equivalent of 0.5 mg/kg of prednisone per day for the following 3 to 4 weeks (personal communication, G.A. Patterson).

Prophylactic antibiotics are employed routinely. The Pittsburgh group has recently adopted the routine use of ceftazidime, clindamycin, and amphotericin.[23] These are continued until the results from the tracheal cultures taken from the donor's airway prior to harvesting are available. If the cultures are negative, antibiotics are stopped. If positive, therapy is adjusted accordingly. The Toronto group uses a first generation cephalosporin to which gram-negative coverage may be added, depending on the gram stain of the initial donor tracheal aspirate. When culture results are available, therapy is modified accordingly.

Finally, systemic anticoagulation by continuous infusion of heparin 25,000 U, with dipyridamole, 150 mg in 250 mL normal saline at 10 mL/h is begun on day 1. The need for such anticoagulation measures is theoretical only, and its efficacy is unproven. There have been no hemorrhagic complications from such a practice.[22]

Day 2 and Then

Once cardiovascular stability has been achieved (24 to 36 h), emphasis is placed on eliminating the expanded third-spaced volume the patient has accumulated during and immediately after surgery. Forced diuresis with beta-adrenergic doses (less or equal to 5 μg/kg/min) of dopamine and regular intravenous doses of furosemide are the rule for the first week. Eliminating this extra fluid will improve gas exchange and facilitate weaning. The goal is a return to the patient's preoperative body weight without damaging renal function. Daily weights and careful monitoring of serum creatinine and blood urea nitrogen (BUN) are important. If the BUN rises before the baseline weight is attained, cyclosporine toxicity should be considered and intravascular hypovolemia excluded.

The use of cyclosporine very often results in refractory oliguria despite normal levels of serum creatinine.[22] This usually responds to increasing doses of furosemide. As long as the preoperative body weight has not been reached, hypovolemia is a less likely cause of oliguria.

A sudden rise in creatinine may signify hypovolemia, sepsis, cyclosporine toxicity, or nephrotoxicity from other drugs. Cyclosporine toxicity may occur even if serum levels are within the normal therapeutic range. Again, determination of the patient's weight may be helpful in differentiating the cause of such changes. When renal function is impaired for whatever reason, ultrafiltration will help decrease the extra volume load in a steady fashion without sudden drops in systemic perfusion pressures that could impair anastomotic healing.

Preoperative rehabilitation and preparation facilitate liberation from the ventilator. Extubation is usually achieved around days 3 to 7, but difficulties may be experienced if hemodynamic instability, poor graft preservation, or preoperative malnutrition is present. Mild to moderate hypercapnia is not unusual for the first 24 to 48 h and probably relates to the diuretic-induced metabolic alkalosis. Single-lung recipients may experience a sensation of dyspnea and anxiety as a reflex from the still innervated diseased native lung despite adequate gas exchange. All these patients need is reassurance. Specific problems may impede progress in weaning. Diaphragmatic paralysis secondary to phrenic nerve injury may be present. Airway ischemia and/or stenosis may increase the work of breathing.

Surveillance bronchoscopy before extubation is recommended. At this stage, the anastomosis should appear fully patent, but there may be white slough about the suture line. This should be of no concern. Isolated islands of dark mucosa distal to the anastomosis may also be seen under normal circumstances. However, the presence of grey slough or blackened mucosa at the level of the suture line predicts future dehiscence or stricture formation. Should the mucosa appear devascularized in a uniform fashion from the anastomosis to the segmental bronchial bifurcation, dehiscence is likely and consideration should be given for retransplantation.

Nutrition is also very important at this stage as most of these chronically debilitated patients come to surgery in a less than optimal nutritional state and are in negative nitrogen balance as a result of surgery. Theoretically, the oral route should be usable early postoperatively. However, we have observed prolonged gastrointestinal ileus as a result of the omentopexy. When this precludes enteral feeding, total parenteral nutrition should be started immediately. All DLTX recipients are placed on domperidone, 10 mg four times a day postoperatively, in view of the frequently observed gastric atony, which is probably secondary to inadvertent vagotomy at the time of the recipient's native lung extraction.[24]

Prophylactic antibiotics should be stopped at this stage. Beyond 3 weeks, *Pneumocystis carinii* infections become a potential problem and prophylactic cotrimoxazole should be initiated.

IMMUNOSUPPRESSION

ALG infusion is maintained until oral cyclosporine levels are adequate and not fluctuating. To monitor ALG therapy, daily lymphocyte counts are necessary, the aim being a count of 0.075 to 0.110×10^3 lymphocytes per milliliter. ALG therapy is maintained for 7 to 8 days.

Azathioprine is given intravenously at a dose of 2 mg/kg for the first week and then tapered to a dose of 1 mg/kg at which time the oral route is usually available. If the white blood cell count dips under 4000, the dose is either decreased or the medication temporarily stopped. Serum levels to monitor the therapeutic range are not available.

Cyclosporine is given intravenously until the oral route becomes feasible, the dose determined by daily serum levels. The oral dose necessary to maintain the therapeutic range approximates three times the intravenous dose, divided into two doses given every 12 h. With the initial oral intake of cyclosporine, the intravenous dose is reduced by half. Trough levels are obtained 1 h prior to the next oral dose. Difficulties in obtaining adequate serum levels of cyclosporine may be decreased by administering erythromycin, 125 mg three times a day, either orally or intravenously to inhibit cyclosporine metabolism.[25] The optimal long-term maintenance dose of cyclosporine has yet to be determined.

Steroids given as maintenance immunosuppression were until recently initiated around the third week, after bronchial healing has been judged adequate by bronchoscopic assessment, at an initial dose of 30 to 40 mg prednisone per day, gradually tapering over the next 6 months to a dose of 10 to 15 mg/day. Episodes of rejection will be discussed separately but are usually treated with boluses of methylprednisolone, 1 g intravenously followed by 500-mg boluses on day 2 and 3. Episodes refractory to this regimen may benefit from an additional 7- to 14-day course of ALG, or OKT-3 (see Chap. 77).

In most North American and European centers, the maintenance immunosuppression regimen consists of cyclosporine, azathioprine, and steroids. In Great Britain a two-drug regimen is used which includes cyclosporine and azathioprine.

ANTICOAGULATION

In centers where routine systemic anticoagulation is employed, sodium warfarin is initiated once the gastrointestinal tract is usable, aiming at a prothrombin time of 16 to 19 s (INR 2.0 to 3.0).

PSYCHIATRIC DISTURBANCES

Problems of insomnia, agitation, delirium, confusion, and noncompliance are common in the first weeks after lung transplant and affected half of the first 30 recipients in Toronto.[26] Use of cardiopulmonary bypass and cyclosporine are the most common etiologic factors mentioned to explain these behavioral abnormalities. The routine use of prophylactic haloperidol at a dose of 1 mg IV every 4 to 6 h titrated to the patient's mental state is effective in controlling these symptoms. It does not however replace the constant physical contact and support these patients need from the medical/paramedical staff and family members.[27]

REJECTION

In the first 3 weeks after transplant, two episodes of acute rejections are seen on average. The first occurs around days 5 to 8, the second by the end of the second week. The symptoms may resemble those of sepsis: fever, tachycardia, increased Aa gradient, decreased O_2 saturation, and leucocytosis. The classic radiological findings of rejection are a perihilar flare, homogenous diffuse infiltrate, or appearance or an increase in pleural effusion. However, air bronchograms and localized infiltrates, more typical of pneumonia, have been described with acute rejection.

A histological diagnosis of lung allograft rejection remains difficult and is not always practical. As a result, the presence of a clinical picture compatible with acute rejection without overt pulmonary infection (purulent sputum with localized infiltrate or air bronchogram) should be treated as an acute episode of rejection with intravenous steroids. If the diagnosis is correct, one should expect a clinical amelioration within the first 12 hours after the initial dose of corticosteroids. If the picture is less characteristic or the response poor (particularly if this occurs after the second week posttransplant), a bronchoscopy with transbronchial biopsies, bronchoalveolar lavage, and protected brushings is performed to exclude bacterial or other types of infection. Once the specimens are taken, one may initiate broad spectrum antibiotic therapy while waiting for the results.

Transbronchial biopsies are being used routinely by the Cambridge group to diagnose acute rejection.[28] A peribronchial or perivascular lymphocytic infiltration is characteristic but a nonspecific acute lung injury may be all that is found. Twenty or more biopsies are taken from the same lung during a single procedure. The Cambridge data are interesting in that in a significant proportion of patients, microscopic features of rejection have been noted in association with specific bacterial or viral infection. Other centers have not had the same success with transbronchial biopsies and thus continue to rely on clinical presentation and response to the bolus of steroids to confirm the diagnosis of an acute rejection episode. Rarely, despite steroid boluses and endoscopic sampling to rule out infection, does one have to go to open lung biopsy to establish a firm diagnosis.

Technetium 99 macro aggregated perfusion scans have been used with SLTX to diagnose rejection.[2] Anecdotally, it has been found that a decrease in quantitative perfusion to the transplanted lung antedates the onset of radiographic abnormality. Hence, to be useful, specific scans must be ordered routinely. Pulmonary function tests are useful in detecting chronic rejection and bronchiolitis obliterans, and small airway flow changes [forced expiratory flow (FEF) 25 to 75] have been shown in acute rejection episodes, similar to those seen in bronchiolitis obliterans.[29] Finally, bronchoalveolar lavage (BAL) may show a neutrophilic alveolitis pattern with rejection but is not very specific. The possibility of utilizing serial immunologic markers such as serum interleukin-2 receptors may prove to be useful in the future.[30]

BRONCHIOLITIS OBLITERANS

Bronchiolitis obliterans following transplantation was first reported in five HLTX recipients, and subsequently it was reported in 10 to 50 percent of heart-lung recipients, although a decreased incidence has been reported in later series.[29] A few cases have now been reported following SLTX and DLTX, but the incidence remains low.[31,32] It is an inflammatory disorder of the small airways which leads to destruction of the respiratory bronchioles. The clinical picture is one of chronic obstructive disease, but its course is much more rapid. There are no spontaneous remissions reported. However, early diagnosis followed by augmented immunosuppression using mainly steroids and azathioprine has been shown to reverse the clinical process.[29] If diagnosed at a later stage, increasing immunosuppression may stabilize but will not allow regression. The pathogenesis of bronchiolitis obliterans is unknown. It probably represents a chronic ongoing rejection triggered by small airway injury initiated by previous infection or repeated episodes of acute rejection. An association with cytomegalovirus (CMV) infection has been suggested. The most sensitive test for its early detection is pulmonary function testing with measurements of forced expiratory flow (FEF 25 to 75). The Standford Group recommends repeating pulmonary function tests every 2 weeks for the first 3 months after transplant and then every month.[29] As this process is not distributed uniformly throughout the lungs, a transbronchial biopsy may not be diagnostic.

INFECTIONS

BACTERIAL INFECTIONS

Pulmonary septic complications represent the greatest threat to long-term pulmonary transplant recipient survival and in most series are the leading cause of death. Many factors including systemic immunosuppression and the possibility of a preharvest donor infection have been incriminated. The absence of surgical reestablishment of lymphatics and innervation interfering with normal defense mechanisms as well as a major decrease in mucociliary clearance in the transplanted lung or lungs may also account for this susceptibility.

Bacterial infections account for almost all of the early infectious episodes (before 3 weeks) and 66 percent of all pneumonias seen.[24] Gram-negative rods are the major culprits (70 percent overall) and in one series accounted for all posttransplant pneumonias seen in the first 2 weeks.[23] In Pittsburgh, a change in the prophylactic antimicrobial approach has been followed by a dramatic decrease in the incidence of early pneumonia.[23]

CYTOMEGALOVIRUS

Cytomegalovirus is the most common cause of pneumonia in weeks 4 to 8, either as a reactivation or a primary infection. Though rare before week 4, it has been seen as early as the second week. Matching CMV seronegative donors and seronegative recipients and avoiding the transfusion of seropositive blood products to seronegative recipients has led to a dramatic decrease in the incidence of primary CMV infections (as high as a 50 percent drop in the Pittsburgh experience).[23] CMV pneumonia accounts for most of the symptomatic CMV infections seen. Unfortunately, the symptoms, radiological and BAL cellular profiles of CMV pneumonia, and rejection may be very similar. Diagnosis can be made by identification of viral inclusion bodies in cells obtained by BAL or transbronchial biopsies with a specificity of around 90 percent but unfortunately with a lack of sensitivity (around 20 percent). Immunostaining for viral antigens in BAL material is less specific (84 percent) but sensitive at 86 percent. The negative predictive value of this test is over 95 percent. Viral cultures are 100 percent sensitive but take weeks to complete. Shell-vial culture systems are faster and may be more applicable to the day-to-day practice.[33] Their sensitivities and specificities need to be evaluated.

CMV pneumonia was fatal in 22 percent of the Pittsburgh series.[29] The recent introduction of ganciclovir to the therapeutic armamentarium will hopefully improve these figures. Ganciclovir has been shown to increase survival and quality of life in patients with disseminated CMV disease.[34] Unfortunately its role in lung recipients is still unknown, but it appears that ganciclovir has no effect in the prognosis of severe CMV pneumonia.[23] It is possible that earlier use of the drug in the course of the disease may be of some help.

Prophylaxis for CMV with oral acyclovir has shown a decrease in prevalence of both primary infection and reactivation of disease in renal allograft recipients.[35] Its role in the pulmonary transplant population is being evaluated. Hyperimmune globulin prophylaxis should be given to sero-mismatched recipients.[36] Several regimens exist, but 5 g administered daily for 3 days is a common practice.

PNEUMOCYSTIS CARINII

Pneumocystis carinii pneumonia (PCP) is not seen in the first 3 weeks. The prophylactic use of cotrimoxazole in various regimens has in fact almost eliminated this complication in lung recipients. In Pittsburgh's most recent series, the only cases of PCP were in patients poorly compliant with their prophylactic regimen of cotrimoxazole double strength, one tablet twice a day for 1 week every month.[23] The Toronto program uses double-strength cotrimoxazole twice a day every Monday, Wednesday, and Friday. Aerosolized pentamidine can be used in patients allergic to sulfa medication. *Pneumocystis carinii* can be identified in BAL or transbronchial biopsy samples with proper stains. Treatment of established PCP is with intravenous cotrimoxazole, which is usually effective. Severe PCP is frequently complicated by combined bacterial infection as well.

Pneumocystis carinii, CMV, and Epstein-Barr virus infections often precede the development of bronchiolitis obliterans and may in fact be one of the triggering factors to this long-term complication.[29]

AIRWAY COMPLICATIONS

Airway anastomotic ischemia may lead to segmental stenosis or, in more severe situations, bronchial dehiscence. Omentopexy designed to prevent ischemia has also been shown to prevent a free communication to the pleural space. Early dehiscence was a particular problem with DLTX when a single low tracheal anastomosis was used. The recent adoption of bilateral main bronchial anastomoses may solve this problem. Late stenosis can usually be managed by repeated dilations or the endoluminal placement of silastic stents with good success rates.[37]

LONG-TERM RESULTS

The experience with SLTX is just over 7 years and that of DLTX 4 years. Long-term survival figures with these procedures are still unknown. However, the 2-year actuarial survival rates for SLTX and DLTX are 62 and 72 percent, respectively.

Physiological evaluation of the recipients shows progressive improvement up to the first year in both pulmonary function testing and exercise tolerance. Double-lung transplants show normal spirometry with slightly decreased gas transfer measurements. Single-lung transplant recipients have a mild restrictive pattern (72 percent predicted) with a moderate decrease in gas transfer measurements. Room air blood gases at 3 months document Pa_{O_2} at 79 to 80 in SLTXs and around 100 in DLTXs. The 6-min walk test, stage I exercise test, and modified BRUCE protocol have also shown an improvement with time up to the 1-year period at which a plateau is seen.[31]

Bronchiolitis obliterans which affects a large proportion of heart-lung recipients seems to be emerging in isolated lung recipients as well. It could very well be that longer follow-up may reveal an incidence as high as that of the HLTX population.

CASE PRESENTATION

A 21-year-old man with cystic fibrosis underwent a DLTX via a sternotomy. A bibronchial anastomosis was performed. Cardiopulmonary bypass was prolonged and blood loss was excessive secondary to vascular pleural adhesions. Perfusion pressures during bypass were low and the patient was oliguric throughout. At the completion of the procedure the sternum could not be closed due to aggravated hypotension. The patient arrived in the intensive care unit with a systolic blood pressure of 75 mmHg and an oxygen saturation of 83% on a fraction of inspired oxygen of 100% and 10 cm of water PEEP.

Table 78-4 details the changes of ventilatory parameters over several hours. Success was achieved in the end with high-frequency jet ventilation (HFJV) although the time frame was such that the improvement in gas exchange could be attributed to changes in lung compliance, pulmonary edema, and hemodynamics.

Hemodynamic interventions are noted in Table 78-5. Throughout this period his preload remained in the high normal range with pulmonary wedge and central venous pressures measured between 18 and 25 mmHg. At

TABLE 78-4 Changes of Ventilatory Parameters over Time

Time	Ventilator	Settings	Pa_{O_2}
1145	Bagging	100%, PEEP 10 cm	47
1300	Servo	100%, PEEP 15 cm	35
1330	Servo	100%, PEEP 17.5 cm	31
1520	HFJV	100%, rate 80, PEEP 10 cm	42
1830	HFJV	100%, rate 80, PEEP 10 cm	75

TABLE 78-5 Hemodynamic Interventions over Time

Time	Blood Pressure	Drugs
1120	60/40	Norepinephrine, calcium, dopamine
1128	80/40	Phenylephrine added
1134	60/40	Volume infusion
1140	120/60	Volume and dobutamine
1210	80/50	Epinephrine added
1250	90/50	Sternum reopened
1300	70/40	Phenylephrine bolus every $\frac{1}{2}$ h

1230 h the skin was reopened and the sternal spreader inserted (see Fig. 78-1). This did provide some transient improvement in hemodynamic parameters. However, blood pressure quickly fell again and further polypharmacy was required to regain a satisfactory perfusion pressure. By 1400 h the patient required a phenylephrine bolus (200 μg) each half hour in addition to norepinephrine, dopamine, and epinephrine to maintain a systolic pressure of 100 mmHg.

By 2300 h hemodynamic function and gas exchange had stabilized. Inotrope requirements decreased over the next several hours, and the sternal retractor was removed 36 h following the procedure. The sternum and skin were closed. The patient developed oliguric renal failure, and hemodialysis was initiated. By 48 to 60 h inotropes were required in only small amounts (dopamine 4 to 5 μg/kg/min) and volume cycled ventilatory support on a fraction of inspired oxygen 50% was all that was required to maintain saturation.

The patient survived the initial postoperative course. Two weeks later the donor bronchial tree was noted to be necrotic from the anastomoses to the segmental orifices. Subsequent sepsis developed before another donor could be found, and he succumbed to septic shock.

CASE DISCUSSION

The above case illustrates several points. First, ventilatory and hemodynamic management is often challenging and may require innovative interventions and polypharmacy. Second, DLTXs do experience several unique problems not seen in the single-lung population. At present, median sternotomy should not be undertaken for patients with cystic fibrosis and bronchiectasis. Rather a transverse-sternotomy has become a more efficient means of exposing the pleural spaces and controlling the ubiquitous vascular adhesions.

References

1. Hardy JD, Webb WR, Dalton ML, et al: Lung homo-transplantation in man. JAMA 186:1065, 1963.
2. Toronto Lung Transplant Group: Unilateral Lung Transplantation for Pulmonary Fibrosis. N Engl J Med 314:1140, 1986.
3. Lima O, Cooper JD, Peters WJ, et al: Effects of methylprednisolone and azathioprine on bronchial healing following lung autotransplantation. J Thorac Cardiovasc Surg 82:211, 1981.
4. Goldberg M, Lima O, Morgan E, et al: A comparison between cyclosporin A and methylprednisolone plus azathioprine on bronchial healing following canine lung autotransplantation. J Thorac Cardiovasc Surg 85:821, 1983.
5. Dubois P, Choiniere L, Cooper JD: Bronchial omentopexy in canine lung allotransplantation. Ann Thorac Surg 38:211, 1984.
6. Patterson GA, Cooper JD, Dark JH, et al: Experimental and clinical double-lung transplantation. J Thorac Cardiovasc Surg 95:70, 1988.
7. Cooper JD: International Lung Transplant Registry, October 1990 (personal communication).
8. Reitz BA, Wallwork JL, Hunt SA, et al: Heart-lung transplantation. Successful therapy for patients with pulmonary vascular disease. N Engl J Med 306:557, 1982.
9. Penketh A, Higenbottam T, Hakin M, et al: Heart and lung transplantation in patients with end-stage lung disease. Br Med J 295:311, 1987.
10. Mal H, Andreassian B, Fabrice P, et al: Unilateral lung transplantation in end-stage pulmonary emphysema. Am Rev Respir Dis 140:797, 1989.
11. Morrison DL, Maurer JR, Grossman RF: Preoperative assessment for lung transplantation. Clin Chest Med 11(2):207, 1990.
12. Patterson GA: Double lung transplantation. Clin Chest Med 11(2):227, 1990.
13. Novick RJ, Menkis AH, McKenzie FN, et al: Prednisone is not deleterious to airway healing following lung and heart-lung transplantation (abstract). Chest 98(2):7S, 1990.
14. The Toronto Lung Transplant Group: Experience with single lung transplantation for pulmonary fibrosis. JAMA 259:2258, 1988.
15. Fremes SE, Patterson GA, Williams WG, et al: Single lung transplant enclosure of patent ductus arteriosus for Eisenmenger's syndrome. J Thorac Cardiovasc Surg 100:1, 1990.
16. Griffith BP, Zenati M: The pulmonary donor. Clin Chest Med 11(2):217, 1990.
17. Harjula A, Baldwin JC, Starnes VA, et al: Proper donor selection for heart-lung transplantation. J Thorac Cardiovasc Surg 94:874, 1987.
18. Todd TR, Goldberg M, Koshal A, et al: Separate extraction of cardiac and pulmonary grafts from a single organ donor. Ann Thorac Surg 46:356, 1988.
19. Hachida M, Morton DL: The protection of ischaemic lung with verapamil and hydralazine. J Thorac Cardiovasc Surg 95:178, 1988.
20. Demajo WAP: Anesthesia for single lung transplantation, in Cooper DKC, Novitzky D (eds), *The Transplantation and Replacement of Thoracic Organs.* Kluwer Academic Publishers, Boston/London, 1990, pp 375–379.
21. Pasque MK, Cooper JD, Kaiser LR, et al: Improved technique for bilateral lung transplantation: Rationale and initial clinical experience. Ann Thorac Surg 49:785, 1990.
22. Todd TR: Early postoperative management following lung transplantation. Clin Chest Med 11(2):259, 1990.
23. Dauber JH, Paradis IL, Dummer JS: Infectious complications in pulmonary allograft recipients. Clin Chest Med 11(2):291, 1990.
24. Maurer JR: Therapeutic challenges following lung transplantation. Clin Chest Med 11(2):279, 1990.
25. Freeman DJ, Martell R, Carruthers SG, et al: Cyclosporin-erythromycin interactions in normal subjects. Br J Clin Pharmacol 23:776, 1987.
26. Craven JL, The Toronto Lung Transplant Group: Post-operative organic mental syndromes in lung transplant recipients. J Heart Transplant 9:129, 1990.

27. Craven JL, Bright J, Lougheed Dear C: Psychiatric, psychosocial, and rehabilitative aspects of lung transplantation. Clin Chest Med 11(2):247, 1990.
28. Higenbottam T, Stewart S, Wallwork J: Transbronchial lung biopsy to diagnose lung rejection and infection of heart/lung transplants. Transplant Proc 20(suppl 1):767, 1988.
29. Theodore J, Starnes VA, Lewiston NJ: Obliterative bronchiolitis. Clin Chest Med 11(2):309, 1990.
30. Waldmann TA: The multichain interleukin-2 receptor: A target for immunotherapy in lymphoma, autoimmune disorders, and organ allografts. JAMA 263:272, 1990.
31. Williams TJ, Grossman RF, Maurer JR: Long-term functional follow-up of lung transplant recipients. Clin Chest Med 11(2):347, 1990.
32. LoCicero J, Robinson PG, Fisher M: Chronic rejection in single lung transplantation manifested by obliterative bronchiolitis. J Thorac Cardiovasc Surg 99:1059, 1990.
33. Jespersen DJ, Drew WL, Gleaves CA, et al: Multisite evaluation of a monoclonoal antibody reagent (Syva) for rapid diagnosis of cytomegalovirus in the shell-vial assay. J Clin Microbiol 27:1502, 1989.
34. Keay S, Bissett J, Merigan T: Ganciclovir treatment of cytomegalovirus infections in iatrogenically immunocompromised patients. J Infect Dis 156:1016, 1987.
35. Balfour HH Jr, Chace BA, Stapleton JT, et al: Randomized placebo controlled trial of oral acyclovir for the prevention of cytomegalovirus disease in recipients of renal allografts. N Engl J Med 320:1381, 1989.
36. Snydman DR, Werner NG, Heinze-Lacey B, et al: Use of cytomegalovirus immune globulin to prevent cytomegalovirus disease in renal transplant recipients. N Engl J Med 317:1049, 1987.
37. Patterson GA, Todd TR, Cooper JD, et al: Airway complications following double lung transplantation. J Thorac Cardiovasc Surg 99:14, 1990.

Chapter 79

CRITICAL CARE OF THE RECIPIENTS OF HEART AND HEART-LUNG TRANSPLANTS

CHRIS DENNIS
JOHN WALLWORK
TIM HIGENBOTTAM

KEY POINTS

- *Heart-lung transplantation (HLT) is now an effective therapy for patients with end-stage pulmonary and cardiopulmonary disease.*
- *Refinements in methods of procuring and preserving donor organs and in matching donor and recipient for cytomegalovirus (CMV) status have improved survival and reduced the morbidity of the operation.*
- *Early, accurate diagnosis of rejection or opportunistic infection by transbronchial lung biopsy (TBB) in the ICU enables definitive treatment of pulmonary complications after HLT.*
- *Ambulatory patients can detect pulmonary complications after HLT by daily recording of spirometry using a pocket turbine spirometer.*
- *The occurrence of opportunistic infection is associated with recent augmented immunosuppression using high dose intravenous methylprednisolone.*
- *Obliterative bronchiolitis, a major long-term problem following HLT, may be prevented by early detection and treatment of acute lung rejection.*

Following early discouraging experience during the 1950s and 1960s, clinical heart transplantation was continued as part of an investigational program at Stanford University during the 1970s. Early results from this center[1] together with the development of endomyocardial biopsy to monitor rejection[2] encouraged others to enter the field. Success was facilitated by the effective use of cyclosporine as an immunosuppressive treatment in the early 1980s.[3] Similarly, both clinical and experimental HLT and lung transplantation had been unsuccessful until the 1980s. High mortality had been attributed to poor early graft function, infection, or dehiscence of the tracheal or bronchial anastomoses. Cyclosporine,[4] effective donor organ preservation,[5] and transbronchial biopsy to obtain lung tissue for histology to monitor for rejection[6] have enabled HLT and lung[7] transplantation to become effective clinical treatments, comparable to cardiac transplantation.

This chapter discusses early postoperative care of HLT patients; for comparison heart transplant patients are included. However, because of the importance to long-term survival of careful recipient selection, donor procurement, and long-term management, these activities are also described in detail. The most vital consideration in clinical practice is to optimally use a limited resource, i.e., limited availability of donor organs.

Selection of Patients

EVALUATION OF HEART AND HEART-LUNG RECIPIENTS

HEART TRANSPLANTATION

Selection is based on the development of class IV grade of disability using the New York Heart Association classification. In most centers, including our own, idiopathic cardiomyopathy is the most common cardiac disease requiring cardiac transplantation (Table 79-1). Pretransplant assessment involves careful clinical and laboratory investigation. Prior cardiac catheterization is usually required to provide the diagnosis and to indicate whether medical or surgical therapy will be effective. However, demonstration of reduced ejection fraction <15 percent and elevated pulmonary artery wedge pressure >25 mmHg with echocardiographic evidence of normal valve function may avoid full left cardiac catheterization with coronary angiography. Choice of recipients depends on clinical judgment that life expectancy is curtailed, supplemented by guidelines derived empirically.[8] Indications and contraindications are listed in Table 79-2.

Details of the contraindications to heart transplantation

TABLE 79-1 Types of Disease Treated by Cardiac Transplantation

Idiopathic cardiomyopathy	50%
Ischemic heart disease	45%
Miscellaneous, including end-stage valvular heart disease	5%

TABLE 79-2 Heart Transplant Patient Selection Criteria

Indications	Contraindications
Refractory heart failure with class IV disability (NYHA)	Elevated pulmonary vascular resistance >8 Wood units
	Significant systemic or cerebral vascular disease
Age <55	Continued alcohol or drug abuse
Normal or reversible renal or hepatic function	Malignancy
	Severe pulmonary dysfunction
No active systemic infection	
No pulmonary embolus in last 3 months	
Good psychosocial setting	

are not necessary here, but certain observations are important for postoperative care. An elevated pulmonary vascular resistance in excess of 8 Wood units remains an absolute contraindication to cardiac transplantation. In the immediate postoperative period these patients often have a catastrophic decrease in cardiac output despite inotropic support and pulmonary vasodilators. Pulmonary disease associated with a reduction of forced expiratory volume in 1 s (FEV_1) <40 percent predicted or DLCO (diffusing coefficient for carbon monoxide) <40 percent contributes to persisting long-term disability after cardiac transplantation alone, as well as being associated with a more hazardous postoperative period.

HEART-LUNG TRANSPLANTATION

Patients are selected for HLT because of end-stage cardiopulmonary disease. A clinical assessment of survival chance without transplantation is made, the criteria for which depend on the underlying disease process. A wider range of diseases are considered for HLT in our institution than for cardiac transplantation (Table 79-3). Pretransplant assessment follows the same pattern as for cardiac transplantation. Pulmonary function measurement and exercise testing using a 12-min walk assess survival chance without transplant surgery.[9] Although effective for chronic lung disease, such tests offer little in the assessment for pulmonary vascular disease. For example, in primary pulmonary hypertension (PPH) right-sided cardiac catheterization is necessary to measure mixed venous oxygen saturation ($S\bar{v}_{O_2}$) and cardiac index (CI), both of which offer valuable guides to prognosis.[10] An $S\bar{v}_{O_2}$ below 60% indicates <20 percent survival chance at 3 years. Unfortunately, with Eisenmenger's syndrome there is no measurement which evaluates prognosis. Most clinicians consider a worsening in exercise tolerance and the development of right ventricular failure as indications in these patients for transplant surgery.

Indications and contraindications for HLT are shown in Table 79-4. Other contraindications have been eliminated, but previous pleural surgery and high dose steroids remain. Previous pleurectomy or chemical pleurodesis are still associated with severe postoperative chest wall bleeding even where new measures such as preoperative use of aprotinin have been introduced (vide infra). Traditionally, a daily maximum dose of 10 mg prednisolone remains a limitation. It is important to beware of Addison's syndrome after surgery unless steroids are given postoperatively. As a result of an inability to completely remove *Aspergillus fumigatus* from the pleura, mycetoma remains a contraindication to HLT. As in heart transplant recipients, a good social and family background is essential to a good long-term result. For patients who are not severely ill, in our institution we also have a provisional waiting list where patients are regularly reviewed for deterioration. When deterioration occurs, patients are moved to the active waiting list. Patients with PPH have been treated with long-term continuous infusions of prostacyclin (PGI_2).[11] This appears to prolong survival and provides a reasonable quality of life, but in most patients HLT becomes necessary eventually.

TABLE 79-3 Diseases Treated by Heart-Lung Transplantation

	Percentage
Cystic fibrosis	27
Eisenmenger's syndrome	26
Primary pulmonary hypertension	15
Cryptogenic fibrosing alveolitis	4
Emphysema	5
Sarcoidosis	5
Miscellaneous, including eosinophilic granuloma	10

TABLE 79-4 Heart-Lung Transplant Patient Selection Criteria

Indications	Contraindications
Age <55	Other nonreversible organ dysfunction or disease
FEV_1 <25% of predicted value	Mycetoma
12-min walking distance <300 m	Pleurectomy or previous chemical pleurodesis
A minimal Sa_{O_2} during a 12-min walk of <60%	High dose steroid therapy; daily dose >10 mg prednisolone
For primary pulmonary hypertension an $S\bar{v}_{O_2}$ <60%	

In addition to careful clinical examination and detailed history-taking to exclude patients with evidence of irreversible changes of the central nervous system and poor renal and hepatic function, a number of investigations are undertaken. The ABO blood group is determined. Serologic tests for Epstein-Barr virus (EBV), toxoplasmosis, CMV, and herpes simplex virus (HSV) are made. Certain infections can be transmitted by the donor organs;[12,13] in other instances augmented immunosuppressive treatment after surgery can lead to reactivation of latent infections.[14] Preventive therapy on such occasions after surgery may avoid a fatal illness. Radiologic and bacteriologic evidence of pulmonary tuberculosis is sought. In the presence of disease, a full course of antituberculosis therapy is given before the patient proceeds to transplant surgery.

The only immunologic studies carried out to identify a suitable match between donor and recipient are based on ABO blood type. The limited time available between donor identification and the surgery as well as limited donors, makes routine use of HLA typing impractical. In any case, few studies show much advantage because of the introduction of cyclosporine as the immunosuppressive therapy.[15] Potential recipients are screened, however, for preformed antibodies using a broad panel of HLA antigens. An increase in preformed antibodies in a potential recipient makes finding a compatible donor more difficult. In practice, such patients are seldom given transplants.[16]

SELECTION AND CARE OF THE DONOR

A state of irreversible brain stem injury is now recognized with the use of the guidelines published in a report of the medical consultants to the President's Commission for the

Study of Ethical Problems in Medicine, Biomedical and Behavioral Research (1981) in the United States. In the United Kingdom, the Department of Health and Social Security provided a code of practice in 1983. Various means of obtaining consent for organ donation are used and are discussed in Chap. 76. In many countries, national and international schemes are available for organizing the distribution of referred organ donations.

The management and physiologic monitoring of heart and heart-lung donors up to the time of surgery remain crucial elements to ensure a satisfactory outcome to surgery but also to maintain adequate numbers of donors. Many potential organs are lost through poor donor care. The brain dead patient has usually been fluid-restricted and treated with diuretics in an attempt to lower intracranial pressures. With pronouncement of death, this is no longer a concern. Vasomotor instability associated with brain death, diabetes insipidus, and previous fluid restriction requires resuscitation with colloid or plasma substitutes and crystalloids. Care needs to be taken in heart-lung donors to avoid excessive replacement of fluid with resulting pulmonary edema. The central venous pressure and urine output should be monitored; diabetes insipidus is managed with intravenous aqueous vasopressin. Arterial pressure is monitored by an arterial line; if hypotension persists after adequate fluid replacement, inotropic support is often necessary. We use intravenous dopamine or dobutamine. Low hemoglobin concentration should be corrected by transfusion. Hypothermia is treated by warming blankets. Mechanical ventilation is established using a pattern of breathing to maintain eucapnia and provide a normal value of Pa_{O_2}. Excessive values of positive end-expiratory pressure ought not to be used to mask poor lung oxygen exchange.

The selection criteria for heart-lung donors are necessarily more strict than for cardiac donors (Table 79-5). Medical history is taken to exclude postpulmonary disease or cardiac disease. An asthma history is a contraindication but light cigarette smoking is not. A long period of assisted (mechanical) ventilation raises concern about pulmonary infection; at Papworth, HLT donors had an average of 34 h of ventilation, ranging from 10 to 95 h.[17] The chest radiograph must be clear of abnormal shadows for heart-lung donation. Pulmonary function can be assessed from the adequacy of lung oxygen exchange without excessively high fractional inspired oxygen (FI_{O_2}) and ventilation settings. Cardiac function can be assessed from the electrocardiogram (ECG) and requirements for inotropic support after adequate fluid replacement. Great importance is attached to bacterial and fungal culture of tracheal aspirate. Donor-transmitted infections are not uncommon and postoperative selection of antibiotic is aided by specific antimicrobial sensitivity results. For heart-lung donation, the upper age range is 45; for heart donors the age is 55. Causes of death include intracranial hemorrhage, traffic accidents, and gunshot wounds (in the United States).

TABLE 79-5 Criteria for Selection of Heart-Lung Donors

Age <45
No major thoracic trauma
No past history of pulmonary disease, including asthma
A short period of mechanical ventilation
No systemic or pulmonary infection
Normal chest radiograph
Normal lung compliance (this can be crudely judged from peak inspiratory airway pressure below 30 cmH_2O when tidal volume <15 mL/kg and respiratory rate is 10–14/min)
Normal gas exchange (Pa_{O_2} >13 kPa (100 mmHg) with FI_{O_2} of 30%)
Small degree of inotropic support, e.g., <10 μg/kg/min dopamine or dobutamine
Normal ECG
No history of neoplastic disease and negative serology for HIV

SPECIAL DETAILS OF COMPATIBILITY BETWEEN DONOR AND RECIPIENT

For HLT surgery, only CMV serologically negative donors are used for serologically negative recipients.[13] This avoids serious early CMV pneumonia with associated morbidity and mortality. Toxoplasmosis is another donor-transmitted infection. When seropositive toxoplasmosis donors are used in seronegative recipients, preventive pyrimethamine is used during the postoperative period.[12]

Size matching is important for heart-lung transplants.[18] Presently we predict the donor's total lung capacity (TLC) from age, height, and sex. The recipient's TLC is measured preoperatively so that approximate matching on size can be made.

The Operative Procedures

The surgery is described in detail elsewhere for heart transplantation[19] and HLT.[5] After HLT, reexploration for chest wall bleeding is common, up to 20 percent in some series of patients. It is seen more often in patients who have an earlier history of thoracotomy or Eisenmenger's complex. Recently, the use of the antiproteinase aprotinin (Trasylol) during surgery has reduced the reoperation rate for bleeding.[20] With multiple organ donation becoming more common, careful planning and administration of the donor teams is necessary.

PRESERVATION TECHNIQUES FOR DONOR ORGANS

CARDIAC TRANSPLANTATION

Adequate preservation of myocardium enables return of cardiac function at the end of the cross-clamp time while allowing distant transportation of the heart. A combination of topical hypothemia and cold hyperkalemic cardioplegia is used by most centers. The total ischemic time accepted by most centers is approximately 4 h beginning with the interruption of the blood supply of the donor organ and ending with revascularization in the recipient.[21]

HEART-LUNG TRANSPLANTATION

A number of different methods are used to preserve heart-lungs for transplantation.

AUTOPERFUSION. For this, both coronary and pulmonary arterial blood flows are maintained to preserve the heart and lungs in a modified Starling preparation. Although results from this technique are encouraging,[22] its complexity has limited widespread use.

CORE COOLING BY EXTRACORPOREAL CIRCULATION. This method requires the institution of cardiopulmonary bypass with cooling until the donor core temperature is 10°C (50°F). Depending on the donor's size, this takes between 15 and 45 min.[23] The major concerns with this method are the complications of cardiopulmonary bypass, which include acute lung injury.

ORGAN HYPOTHERMIA BY PULMONARY ARTERY FLUSH. As with established methods for preservation of liver, kidneys, and heart, this technique involves a single perfusion into the donor lungs after cardioplegia using a solution at 4°C (39.2°F).[5] The lungs are maintained inflated after excision in the cold storage box for transportation. Many different solutions have been used to "flush" the lung.[24] At Papworth we introduced the technique of infusing PGI_2 into the donor's pulmonary artery, before cardioplegia is instituted.[5] This was to vasodilate the pulmonary vascular bed before the cold perfusate was introduced to enable even cooling of the lung. Certainly excellent postoperative results have been achieved with alveolar-arterial oxygen gradient values similar to those seen after coronary artery bypass surgery.[5] Many centers have adopted this simple technique. In the United States, where PGI_2 is not available, the alternative PGE_1 is used as the precooling vasodilator. Similar total ischemic times to cardiac transplantation have been obtained by these techniques, increasing the available numbers of heart-lung donor organs.

IMMUNOSUPPRESSION

Immunosuppressive treatments are administered to the recipients before surgery, when the patient arrives in hospital (see Table 79-6). This includes intravenous azathioprine and methylprednisolone, which is given on induction of anesthesia and then when the donor organs are reperfused. Antithymocyte globulin (ATG) is administered when the recipient is put on cardiopulmonary bypass.

Cyclosporine is usually given orally by the second postoperative day, by which time the patients are usually taking oral food and fluids. Maintenance of sufficient immunosuppression is usually achieved using azathioprine and cyclosporine (see Table 79-6). Augmentation of immunosuppression for the control of diagnosed acute rejection is daily 0.5 to 1.0 g intravenous methylprednisolone for 3 days followed by daily oral prednisolone 1 mg/kg in decreasing doses for 10 days.

TABLE 79-6 Immunosuppression

Perioperative
Azathioprine, 2–3 mg/kg IV (on arrival in hospital)
Methylprednisolone, 1 g IV (500 mg on induction of anesthesia/500 mg on reperfusion of donor organs)
Equine ATG, 10 mg/kg (on cardiopulmonary bypass)
Day 1
Azathioprine, 2 mg/kg
Methylprednisolone, 125 mg IV × 3 doses at 2 h, 16 h, 24 h
ATG, 10 mg/kg
Day 2
Azathioprine, 2 mg/kg
ATG, 10 mg/kg
Cyclosporine, 4–6 mg/kg
Maintenance
Azathioprine, 2 mg/kg—adjusted to keep WBC 5000/mm^3
Cyclosporine, 6–10 mg/kg/day—adjusted according to trough levels and renal function

Postoperative Care of Heart and Heart-Lung Transplant Patients

CARDIOPULMONARY MANAGEMENT AND COMPLICATIONS IN THE IMMEDIATE POSTOPERATIVE PERIOD

The preoperative clinical condition of both heart and heart-lung patients is often poor with multiorgan dysfunction. Despite this, it is remarkable how rapidly function returns to normal following successful transplant surgery.

Liver dysfunction and expanded blood volumes are likely to lead to problems of reversal of heparinization. For those patients who preoperatively had disturbed coagulation, fresh frozen plasma should be available at the end of bypass.

Currently patients are transferred to a cubicle where they remain during the 3 days of ATG treatment. However, the rationale for this has been questioned. In the past, up to 2 weeks of isolation was thought necessary. Assisted mechanical ventilation of the lung is required only until the patient is hemodynamically stable, is awake, and has no neuromuscular disturbance. For HLT patients, over 60 percent are breathing spontaneously by 24 h.[17] This reflects the careful selection of donor organs as well as the efficacy of the preservation system. Most cardiac transplant patients are extubated by 12 h after return to the ICU.

Monitoring is simple; arterial and central venous pressures are displayed, together with ECG and oxygen saturation with a pulse oximeter. The response of the denervated heart is abnormal, both in heart and HLT patients; in particular hypovolemia and hypotension do not cause a reflex tachycardia. While hypovolemia is to be avoided, it is vital in HLT patients to prevent excessive fluid administration, so aggressive diuresis is helpful in these patients. The aim is to return the patient to the preoperative weight by 24 h after surgery. Hypotension and bradycardia are managed by direct-acting drugs—isoprenaline for its chronotropic action, dopamine or dobutamine for inotropic effects, and a direct-acting vasoconstrictor.

Following lung transplantation the cough reflex is lost.[25] As soon as patients are spontaneously breathing, mobilization and active physiotherapy are started; patients usually use exercise pedals during the second and third postoperative days. If continued assisted ventilation is required in HLT patients, then a minimum length of endotracheal tube is inserted with care to avoid the tracheal anastomosis. A bacterial filter is used over the endotracheal tube to lessen the risk of infection. Routine antibiotics are not used postoperatively in patients without cystic fibrosis but antibiotics are given to all patients with bacteria observed in the donor tracheal aspirate.

It should be stressed that while pulmonary complications are commonly reported in the immediate postoperative period in HLT recipients,[26] careful donor and recipient selection and improved organ preservation appear to have simplified postoperative ICU care. Early restoration of spontaneous ventilation and mobilization not only reflect this but also act to lessen potential problems.

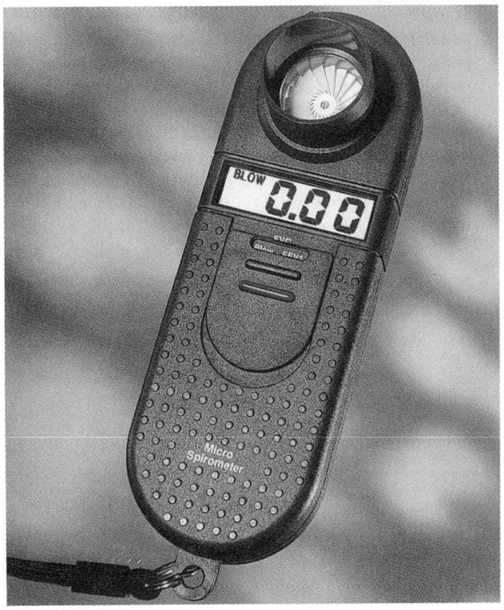

FIGURE 79-1 Pocket battery-operated spirometer.

REJECTION VERSUS OPPORTUNISTIC INFECTION

The principal problem in the management of HLT patients is that clinically it is impossible to separate opportunistic infection of the lungs from lung rejection.[27] Both complications can be present with respiratory symptoms of dyspnea and chest tightness, together with cough. The physical signs are comparable on auscultation of the chest. Both crackles and wheezes may be evident.[27]

The chest radiograph is not helpful in this situation; bilateral pulmonary shadows are often seen in both infection and rejection. Additionally, the chest radiograph may be entirely normal in patients experiencing acute rejection. This is particularly true after the first month following transplantation. After this time up to 70 percent of patients may have a normal chest radiograph.[28]

EARLY DETECTION OF PULMONARY COMPLICATIONS WITH HOME SPIROMETRY

During most episodes of acute rejection and infection the dynamic lung volumes diminish significantly. This change in function recovers with treatment. Dynamic lung volumes, such as FEV_1 and vital capacity (VC), can be measured daily by giving the patient a pocket battery-operated spirometer (see Figs. 79-1 and 79-2). Changes as small as 5 percent reduction on 2 consecutive days are sufficient to require patients to refer themselves to hospital for assessment and possible biopsy.[29]

Hence, unlike other solid organ transplants, the HLT patient can be monitored very closely and easily in terms of the physiologic function of the graft. These patients can also undergo repeated biopsies of the lung if necessary.

DIAGNOSIS OF REJECTION BY TRANSBRONCHIAL LUNG BIOPSY

The diagnosis of rejection is considered when a combination of clinical signs and symptoms is supported by chest radiograph changes and results of pulmonary function tests. A TBB is performed when patients complain of breathlessness in association with fever, crackles, or wheezes on auscultation. Further indications for biopsy are the findings of pulmonary shadows on chest radiograph or a reduction in FEV_1 and forced vital capacity (FVC).[30]

Additionally, biopsy specimens are routinely obtained when the patient is well at 3 months and then annually. The use of alligator forceps[31] enables specimens to be taken with sufficient tissue for histologic assessment of vascular, parenchymal, and mucosal change. Up to four biopsies are taken from the region of maximal radiographic abnormality or, when the radiograph is normal, three biopsies from each lobe.

We began using TBBs at Papworth in 1984. Use of the alligator forceps has enabled us to obtain biopsies up to 5 mm in size. It is customary to look for three elements in the biopsy: the bronchiolar mucosa, alveolar structures, and blood vessels, principally venules. It is essential that all three elements are present within the biopsy to accurately diagnose infection and rejection.[6]

The principal morphologic changes found in acute rejection are those of a circumscribed perivascular infiltrate. The infiltrate may extend into alveolar septa at later stages of rejection and, indeed, may cause alveolar infiltration. The presence of perivascular lymphocytic infiltrates is clearly distinguishable from the changes seen in opportunistic infection of the lung. With infection, perivascular edema

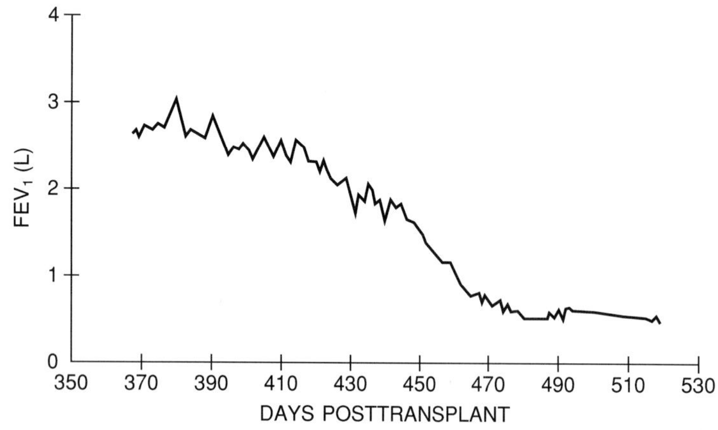

FIGURE 79-2 Graph shows FEV_1 in obliterative bronchiolitis.

without densely cellular circumscribed adventitial infiltration occurs. Intraalveolar exudates are common, together with pathognomonic features of infection.

In our prospective study of 95 occasions when TBB was performed, in just under half was rejection found alone, some 17 percent were entirely normal, and 8 percent showed infection alone. In just under one-quarter of the biopsy occasions, both infection and rejection were found. Indeed, on three occasions two infections in addition to rejection were found. This illustrates the importance of systematically sampling each of the lobes as infection was found in one lobe with rejection found in another.[32]

DIAGNOSIS OF INFECTION

Sputum bacteriology and viral serologic studies are performed regularly. Bronchial lavage is combined with TBB when indicated. CMV infection is diagnosed serologically, by viral culture or by histologic demonstration of viral inclusion bodies. *Pneumocystis carinii* pneumonia is diagnosed by the demonstration of foamy exudate containing trophozoite on silver staining of tissue obtained by TBB. HSV pneumonia may also occur and is usually diagnosed histologically. Both previous CMV infection and augmented immunosuppression are associated with the development of HSV pneumonia. Likewise, *Aspergillus* pneumonia has developed in patients who have had preexisting CMV infection.

With close monitoring and repeated biopsy sampling, it has become possible to reduce the number of fatalities due to infection. In our 80 patients only 13 deaths were attributable to fatal infections. Three of these were due to bacterial pneumonia associated with donor lung infection and only one to aspergillus. CMV pneumonia caused the death of four patients. Three of these were among our original 17 patients where donor and recipients were not matched for CMV. By this we mean that organs from a donor who is CMV positive serologically are not used in a recipient who is CMV negative. In the first 17 patients this occurred in seven patients and six of these developed primary CMV infection. Five infections occurred in the lung and one in the gastrointestinal tract. Three of the patients died.[13]

Although effective treatment for CMV pneumonia is now available with intravenous ganciclovir,[33] it is our current policy to match all donors and recipients for CMV so that no recipient who is CMV negative will receive organs from a donor who is serologically positive for CMV. Following the institution of this policy there have been only two instances of primary CMV pneumonia, one of which was related to the use of infected blood. There have been 11 cases of reactivation of CMV. All of these patients had sustained one episode of rejection requiring augmentation of immunosuppression prior to the development of the infection. We infer from this that augmentation of immunosuppression is probably the major contributing cause to the reactivation of CMV.[33]

Herpes simplex virus pneumonia has occurred in seven of our patients. All had positive serology for HSV prior to transplantation or had developed mucocutaneous lesions prior to the development of the pneumonia. As a result of these observations, patients who are HSV positive prior to transplantation now receive acyclovir for a period of at least 3 months following surgery. Furthermore, patients receiving augmentation of immunosuppression for episodes of rejection with corticosteroids are given prophylactic treatment with trimethoprim/sulfamethoxazole for *P. carinii*. Selected patients who have sustained an episode of CMV infection are considered for prophylactic therapy for *A. fumigatus* with econazole.

REJECTION VERSUS OPPORTUNISTIC INFECTION AS A CAUSE OF BRONCHIOLITIS OBLITERANS

Bronchiolitis obliterans can be defined as irreversible severe airflow obstruction as measured with physiologic lung function tests (FEV_1) where decline in lung function has not been prevented by recurrent use of augmented immunosuppression.[34] This process accounted for the deaths of four of our patients as a late complication of transplantation.

The pathology of the condition is one of obliteration of the bronchioli that are left as fibrous bands extending out to the pleura with associated dilatation and bronchiectasis of the proximal airways.[35] This unusual pattern of distribution of fibrosis and dilatation indicates that the major impact of the disease process falls on the airways. The transplanted

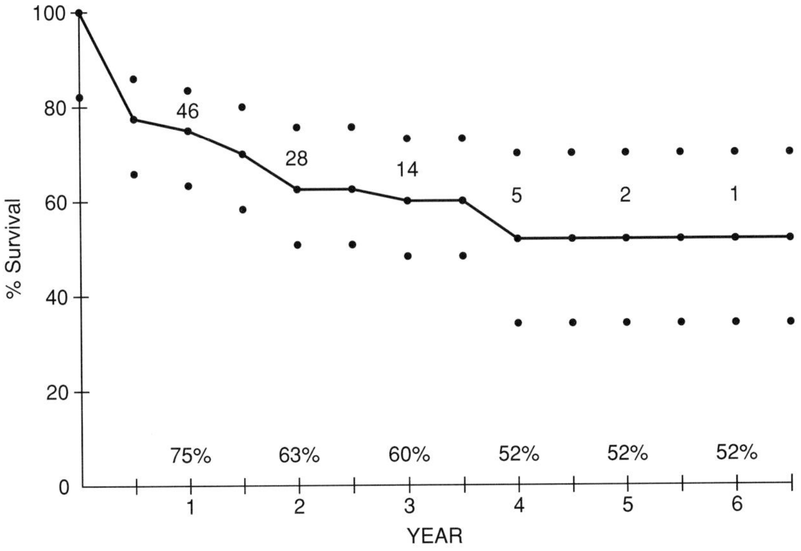

FIGURE 79-3 Graph showing actuarial heart-lung transplant patient survival (n = 80) for the patient population at Papworth up to 1990.

lung relies on the pulmonary artery for intrapulmonary airway blood flow, which follows a retrograde course up the bronchial arteries.[36] This is likely to be compromised during acute rejection because the rejection process principally affects blood vessels (venules and arteries) not only of the lung but also of the airways. For this reason a vascular etiology for bronchiolitis obliterans has been suggested.

Transbronchial biopsy specimens have revealed obliteration of the airways, but in addition submucosal fibrosis is seen in association with vascular sclerosis.[34] Although these changes are found in obliterative bronchiolitis they are by no means diagnostic of the condition which requires, as we have defined, irreversible airflow obstruction to be present clinically. Our observations clearly suggest that the development of obliterative bronchiolitis is closely related to the incidence and severity of rejection that occurs within the first 6 to 12 months following transplantation.

Our strategy to overcome this problem has involved close monitoring of the patients with lung function measurements via the home spirometer and repeated TBB to establish the presence and severity of rejection and to monitor the response to augmented immunosuppression. As a result, the incidence of obliterative bronchiolitis in our long-term survivors is currently 18 percent. This represents a considerable reduction from the initial figures of early experience in which between 20 and 50 percent of patients developed this complication (Fig. 79-3).

Outcome for Heart-Lung Transplant Recipients

Survival has progressively improved after HLT surgery. This reflects a reduction in the numbers of perioperative and immediate postoperative deaths.[26] The early diagnosis of opportunistic infection and accurate diagnosis of pulmonary rejection has also contributed to improved survival.[6] Considering our institute's results up to 1990, of 80 patients treated by HLT surgery, 51 are alive. The calculated actuarial survival rate is 76.3 percent at 1 year and 63.1 percent at 2 years (see Fig. 79-3). The causes of death are shown in Fig. 79-4. Over 50 percent of patients have values of FEV_1 in excess of 100 percent predicted. For the remainder only 20 percent have reduced FEV_1 values below 40 percent.

Early good function of the donor lung is not only important in lessening complications in the immediate postoperative period but also appears associated with better long-term outcome. Careful donor and recipient selection with improved donor organ preservation have greatly lessened the intensity of postoperative care.

CASE PRESENTATION

A 26-year-old man suffering from cystic fibrosis was referred for assessment for HLT. Cystic fibrosis had been diagnosed at the age of 6 months when he presented with failure to thrive. He remained well throughout childhood and had no further admissions until age 11 years. He sustained occasional chest infections throughout adolescence but generally remained well and active.

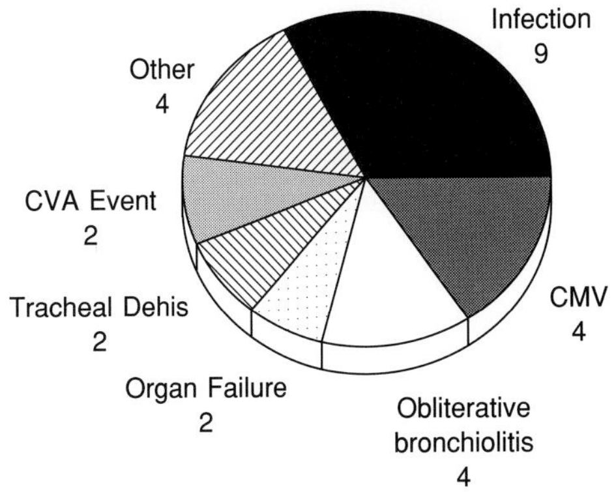

FIGURE 79-4 Pie chart shows major causes of death as a percentage of total number of deaths (n = 27).

He was able to undertake full-time work up until 18 months prior to assessment. During this period he developed progressive dyspnea on exertion and increasing cough productive of large amounts of purulent sputum. His respiratory tract was colonized with *Pseudomonas aeruginosa,* and he required repeated admissions to hospital for intravenous antibiotics during this period. Immediately prior to assessment he had required admission to hospital for an episode of right ventricular failure. Following this he remained on continuous oxygen therapy and was housebound because of his dyspnea. In addition his weight had fallen by about 6 kg in the 6 months prior to assessment. He suffered from no other medical problems. Specifically, he was not diabetic and had no history of liver disease. The family history was unremarkable. He suffered from no allergies and his regular medications consisted of nebulized salbutamol, vitamins A, D, and E, 10 mg prednisolone daily, ciprofloxacin, and pancreatic enzyme supplements.

On examination he appeared thin but not cachectic. He was centrally cyanosed on room air and tachypneic at rest with a respiratory rate of 22 breaths/min. There was clubbing of the fingers and his chest was hyperinflated with widespread crackles present. No signs of cardiac failure or chronic liver disease were seen.

Laboratory investigation revealed normal full blood count and clotting screen. Biochemical profile was normal apart from mild elevations in the globulin fraction and serum alkaline phosphatase. Arterial blood-gas values on room air revealed a P_{O_2} of 42 mmHg and saturation of 84%. The chest radiograph showed widespread tramline and ring shadows consistent with cystic bronchiectasis. Lung function tests revealed FEV_1 0.7 L, FVC 2.3 L, ratio 31 percent, and TLC 7.8 L. He was able to walk 500 m on the 12 min walking test with a reduction in Sa_{O_2} during this to 72%. Sputum culture revealed a heavy growth of *P. aeruginosa.* Echocardiogram and abdominal ultrasound results were normal.

The patient was admitted to hospital for a period of 4 days for this assessment. During this time he became acquainted with the details of transplantation and was assessed from the psychosocial point of view in addition to the medical considerations. After discussions with the transplant surgeon on the final day of his visit, he was placed on the definite waiting list for HLT.

One month following the assessment he underwent HLT. The surgical procedure was uncomplicated and he returned to the ICU after an operation of 3.5 h duration. He received immunosuppression with azathioprine and methylprednisolone and antithymocyte globulin and cyclosporine was introduced on day 1.

The only immediate postoperative problem was hyperglycemia, which was controlled by an insulin infusion. The patient was given a third generation cephalosporin and floxacillin to cover the organisms cultured from his bronchial tree prior to transplantation. He was extubated 6 h after return to the ICU and discharged from the unit on day 3.

Good progress was made until postoperative day 7 when dyspnea occurred and bilateral shadowing developed on chest radiograph. The patient was empirically given three daily doses of methylprednisolone (1 g) for a clinically diagnosed episode of rejection. Satisfactory progress was then made until day 16 with FEV_1 reaching 2.8 L. On day 16 the patient developed fever to 38°C (100.4°F), crackles in both lower zones, and a fall in FEV_1 to 1.7 L. TBB on this occasion confirmed the presence of features consistent with grade III rejection of the lung. Following this finding the patient again received three daily doses of methylprednisolone (1 g). This resulted in rapid clinical improvement with FEV_1 reaching 3.0 L over the subsequent 7 days. Repeat TBB on day 23 showed no evidence of rejection.

The patient was discharged home on day 30 with a clear chest radiograph and FEV_1 of 3.5 L. He remains well now some 3 months postoperatively with FEV_1 of 4.0 L. He is fully active and hopes to return to work soon.

CASE DISCUSSION

This patient is a typical example of many young adults with end-stage respiratory disease who are referred for assessment for HLT. Clearly this patient had deteriorated rapidly and was severely restricted and disabled by his lung disease. There were no contraindications to transplantation and laboratory investigations confirmed the severity of his condition. The reduction in FEV_1 and degree of oxygen desaturation during the walking test help us predict more accurately candidates for transplantation who are likely to deteriorate rapidly following assessment.

There were no significant problems in the perioperative period, which is the rule now since the operative technique for HLT has become highly refined.

Postoperatively no significant problems appeared until day 7 when clinical signs suggesting rejection were found. This is a typical time frame for such a problem to occur and is usually successfully treated with augmentation of immunosuppression. TBB allowed differentiation of the second episode of clinical deterioration from infection and also provided quantitation of the intensity of the rejection process.

It has been our policy to ensure that patients are clear of rejection on TBB prior to discharge after transplantation.

References

1. Baumgartner WA, Reitz BA, Bieber CP, et al: Current expectations in cardiac transplantation. J Thorac Cardiovasc Surg 75:525, 1978.
2. Caves PK, Billingham ME, Stinson EB, Shumway NE: Serial transvenous biopsy of the transplanted heart. Improved management of acute rejection episodes. Lancet 1:821, 1974.
3. Oyer PE, Stimson EB, Jamieson SW, et al: Cyclosporin in cardiac transplantation: A 2 and a half year follow up. Transplant Proc 15:2546, 1983.
4. Reitz BA, Wallwork J, Hunt SA, et al: Heart-lung transplanta-

tion: A successful therapy for patients with pulmonary vascular disease. N Engl J Med 306:557, 1982.
5. Hakim M, Higenbottam TW, Bethune D, et al: Selection and procurement of combined heart and lung grafts for transplantation. J Thorac Cardiovasc Surg 98:474, 1988.
6. Higenbottam TW, Stewart S, Penketh ARL, Wallwork J: Transbronchial lung biopsy for the diagnosis of rejection in heart-lung transplant patients. Transplantation 46:532, 1988.
7. Cooper JD, Pearson FG, Patterson GA, et al: Technique of successful lung transplantation in humans. J Thorac Cardiovasc Surg 93:173, 1987.
8. Permock JL, Oyer PE, Reitz BA, Jamieson SW, et al: Cardiac transplantation in perspective for the future. Survival, complications, rehabilitation and costs. J Thorac Cardiovasc Surg 83:168, 1982.
9. McGavin CR, Gupta SP, McHardy GJR: Twelve minute walking test for assessing disability in chronic bronchitis. Br Med J 1:822, 1976.
10. Fuster V, Steele PM, Edwards WD, et al: Primary pulmonary hypertension: Natural history and importance of thrombosis. Circulation 70:580, 1984.
11. Jones DK, Higenbottam TW, Wallwork J: Long-term treatment of primary pulmonary hypertension with prostacyclin. Br Heart J 57:270, 1987.
12. Hakim M, Wreghitt TG, English TAH, et al: Significance of donor-transmitted disease in cardiac transplantation. Heart Transplant 4:302, 1985.
13. Hutter JA, Scott JP, Wreghitt T, et al: The importance of cytomegalovirus in heart-lung transplantation recipients. Chest 95:627, 1989.
14. Smyth RL, Higenbottam TW, Scott JP, et al: Herpes simplex virus infection in heart-lung transplant recipients. Transplantation 49:735, 1990.
15. Stinson EB, Griepp RB, Payne R, Dony E: Correlation of histocompatibility matching with graft rejection and survival after cardiac transplantation in man. Lancet 2:459, 1981.
16. Rabin S: Immunological aspects of human cardiac transplantation. Heart Transplant 2:188, 1983.
17. Hutter J, Despins P, Higenbottam TW, Stewart S, Wallwork J: Heart-lung transplantation: Better use of resources. Am J Med 85:4, 1988.
18. Otulana BA, Mist BA, Scott JP, Wallwork J, Higenbottam TW: The effect of donor lung size on lung physiology after heart-lung transplantation. Transplantation 48:625, 1989.
19. Copeland JG: Heart transplantation. Med Tech Surg Cardiothorac Surg 66:1, 1984.
20. Bisstrup BP, Royston D, Sapsford RN, Taylor KM: Reduction in blood loss and blood use after cardiopulmonary bypass with high dose aprotinin (Trasylol). J Thoracic Cardiovasc Surg 97:364, 1984.
21. Watson DC, Reitz BA, Baumgartner WB, et al: Distant heart procurement for transplantation. Surgery 86:56, 1979.
22. Hardesty RL, Griffith BP: Autoperfusion of the heart and lungs for preservation during distant procurement. J Thorac Cardiovasc Surg 93:11, 1987.
23. Wahlers T, Haverich A, Fiegath HG, et al: Flush perfusion using Eurocollins solution vs cooling by means of extracorporeal circulation in heart-lung preservation. J Heart Transplant 5:89, 1986.
24. Haverich A, Scott WC, Jamieson SW: Twenty years of lung preservation—A review. Heart Transplant 4:234, 1985.
25. Higenbottam TW, Jackson M, Woolman P, et al: The cough response to ultrasonically nebulized distilled water in heart-lung transplantation patients. Am Rev Respir Dis 140:58, 1989.
26. Griffith BP, Hardesty RL, Trento A, et al: Heart-lung transplantation: Lessons learned and future hopes. Am Thorac Surg 43:6, 1987.
27. Penketh ARL, Higenbottam TW, Hutter J, et al: Clinical experience in the management of pulmonary opportunistic infection and rejection in heart-lung recipients. Thorax 43:762, 1988.
28. Millet B, Higenbottam TW, Flower CDR, et al: The radiographic appearances of infection and acute rejection of the lung after heart-lung transplantation. Am Rev Respir Dis 140:62, 1989.
29. Otulana BA, Higenbottam TW, Ferrari L, et al: The use of home spirometry in detecting acute lung rejection and infection following heart-lung transplantation. Chest 97:353, 1990.
30. Otulana BA, Higenbottam TW, Scott J, et al: Lung function associated with histologically diagnosed acute lung rejection and pulmonary infection in heart-lung transplant patients. Am Rev Respir Dis 141:329, 1990.
31. Clelland C, Higenbottam TW, Scott JP, Wallwork J: The histological changes in transbronchial biopsy after treatment of acute lung rejection in heart-lung transplants. J Pathol 161:105, 1990.
32. Igboaka G, Higenbottam TW, Scott JA, et al: A rationale for systematic transbronchial lung biopsy of all lobes of one lung in heart-lung transplant patients. Thorax 1991. (In press).
33. Collaborative DHPG treatment study group. Treatment of serious cytomegalovirus infections with 9 - (1,3 dihydroxy - 2 propoxymethyl) guanine in patients with AIDS and other immunodeficiences. N Engl J Med 314:801, 1986.
34. Scott JP, Higenbottam TW, Clelland C, et al: Natural history of chronic rejection in heart-lung transplant recipients. J Heart Transplant 9:510, 1990.
35. Burke CM, Theodore J, Baldwin JC, et al: 28 cases of human heart-lung transplantation. Lancet 1:517, 1986.
36. Sadeglu AM, Guthoner DF, Wexler L, et al: Healing and revascularization of the tracheal anastomosis following heart-lung transplantation. Surg Forum 33:236, 1982.

Chapter 80

CRITICAL CARE OF LIVER TRANSPLANT PATIENTS

JEAN C. EMOND

KEY POINTS

- *Liver transplantation is a standard therapy for end-stage liver disease.*
- *Critical care of liver transplant patients is required in three settings: the management of complications of liver disease prior to transplantation, the perioperative and immediate postoperative period, and the management of acute complications in the chronically immunosuppressed liver transplant recipient.*
- *Operative blood loss can quantify the magnitude of the surgical injury and is correlated with preoperative risk factors as well as postoperative prognosis.*
- *The overall strategy of postoperative care attempts to achieve rapid withdrawal of invasive therapy to minimize iatrogenic complications.*
- *Postoperative recovery results in gradual restoration of multisystem physiology deranged by liver failure and cirrhosis and can require days to months depending on the duration and severity of preoperative liver disease.*
- *Following discharge from the ICU the patient remains at risk for catastrophic events due to vascular complications or cardiopulmonary decompensation. The risk of life-threatening infections persists despite apparent full recovery following liver transplantation.*

Orthotopic liver transplantation (OLT) has become a widely accepted treatment for patients with end-stage liver disease. Between 1963, the year of the first procedure in man, and 1980, immediately prior to the introduction of cyclosporine (CY) to control rejection, the role of OLT was in serious question.[1,2] In the decade of the 80s, due in large part to the introduction of CY, OLT has been performed with increasing frequency and steadily improving results. In 1989, over 2200 liver transplants were performed in the United States with a 1 year patient survival rate of over 70 percent.[3] The increased utilization of OLT makes it likely that intensivists will increasingly be called on to manage patients with liver disease who are either candidates for or who have already received the procedure. OLT is resource intensive and the management of critically ill patients is intrinsic to its success. Intensive care is required both preoperatively in the process of selection and preparation of the recipient as well as postoperatively for the restoration of normal physiology and the management of complications. Because hepatic replacement is an operation of enormous magnitude with unique implications for physiologic derangement, successful management is an interface between hepatology, transplantation surgery, and critical care.

This chapter reviews the process of selection, preparation, and treatment of a patient with liver disease requiring transplantation. Attention will be given to physiologic derangements, commonly practiced approaches to critical care, and innovative strategies. Although this presentation is based on concepts applied in our institution, variations in practice exist between successful programs and efforts will be made to focus on generic issues.

Preoperative Considerations

PATIENT SELECTION

Patient selection has implications for resource requirements both in the treatment of the individual patient and in the results of the overall program. Evidence indicates that selection of patients based on preoperative variables is a key determinant of prognosis after hepatic replacement.[4,5] In our experience this difference has been more prominent in the adult population than in the pediatric patients (unpublished observations). The overall strategy of selection differs markedly in adults and children; whereas in adults only one-third of patients referred specifically for transplantation are suitable candidates, nearly all children with chronic irreversible liver disease are candidates. Indications for transplantation in a representative series are given in Table 80-1. These cover the range of diagnoses in clinical hepatology and represent a variety of stages in cirrhosis. Survival after OLT varies by diagnosis; in general, patients with cholestatic liver disease have had a better prognosis than those with parenchymal cirrhosis.[6] Although nearly all forms of liver disease have been treated by OLT, two conditions are of particular interest to the intensivist in terms of patient selection and determination of prognosis. These are fulminant hepatic failure and alcoholic liver disease.

Fulminant hepatic failure (FHF) is defined as severe liver injury in the absence of underlying liver disease progressing to hepatic encephalopathy within 8 weeks of onset.[7] Although a survival rate of 50 percent has been observed in patients with acetaminophen toxicity,[8] the prognosis with medical therapy for a patient with FHF due to most other etiologies is <5 percent.[8] In contrast, hepatic transplantation for FHF has resulted in survival between 50 and 80 percent.[9–11] Patients with FHF require intensive care in both the initial assessment and perioperative management. Multisystem derangements are the rule, and evaluation and treatment require a comprehensive approach which we have described elsewhere.[10] Although the use of OLT for FHF has been criticized by some for lack of controlled clinical trials, the efficacy of OLT and the absence of medical therapy have led to its widespread adoption. Therefore, the intensivist will be frequently confronted with these challenging patients.

TABLE 80-1 Indications for OLT in a Representative Series (University of Chicago 1985–1990)[a]

Indications and Results Adults N = 118	Diagnosis	N	Alive (%)
	Biliary cirrhosis	4	2 (50)
	Budd Chiari	2	1 (50)
	Cancer	13	4 (31)
	Chronic hepatitis with cirrhosis	42	33 (79)
	Cirrhosis (B Ag+)	12	7 (58)
	Cirrhosis (cryptogenic)	7	2 (29)
	Alcoholic cirrhosis	6	4 (67)
	Fulminant hepatic failure	13	9 (70)
	Primary biliary cirrhosis	7	4 (57)
	Sclerosing cholangitis	7	6 (86)
	Other	5	3 (60)
	TOTAL	118	75 (64)
Indications and Results Children N = 112	**Diagnosis**	**N**	**Alive (%)**
	α 1 Antitrypsin deficiency	5	3 (60)
	Biliary atresia	69	48 (70)
	Cholestasis	11	10 (91)
	Cirrhosis	8	6 (75)
	Fulminant hepatic failure	10	6 (60)
	Hepatoblastoma	1	0
	Tyrosinemia	3	3 (100)
	Other	5	4 (80)
	TOTAL	112	80 (72)

[a] Actual survival as of 7/1/90 is given. Follow up is from 1 to 5 years.

Alcohol is the most frequent cause of death due to liver disease in western countries. However, alcoholics have accounted for a small proportion of patients receiving OLT due to concerns about patient compliance and allocation of a limited resource. In addition, poor results in early series and the frequency of systemic disease in alcoholics have posed medical contraindications to OLT. However, recent reports have demonstrated that OLT can be successful in alcoholic cirrhosis,[12,13] and there has been an increasing trend to individualize patient selection and consider OLT more frequently in these patients. Those most likely to become eligible are patients with chronic cirrhosis who are experiencing deterioration despite abstinence from alcohol. In general, complications of alcoholic liver disease which require intensive care management pose prohibitive risks for OLT and must be resolved before the patient can be considered for the procedure. Occasionally, the young patient with acute alcoholic hepatitis and severe decompensation may be considered; in our experience, the prognosis is poor and the costs are high.

The contraindications to OLT have undergone reevaluation with increasing application of the procedure. A representative list of contraindications is presented in Table 80-2. Disseminated malignancy, systemic sepsis, or cardiovascular instability renders hepatic replacement futile. Patients with disabling extrahepatic conditions such as severe neurologic deficits excluding hepatic coma will probably not benefit from the procedure. Since the maintenance of a transplant requires a responsible, compliant patient or caretaker, uncontrolled substance abuse is also a contraindication.

In contrast to these clear contraindications, other criteria have been modified with increased experience. Age limits have been relaxed at both ends of the spectrum, and newborn infants as well as patients up to the age of 70 have been successfully transplanted. Extrahepatic organ failure in previously healthy patients with FHF does not preclude successful OLT, whereas it is rarely overcome in the cirrhotic. The technical difficulties of previous abdominal surgery such as portosystemic shunts and the Kasai operation for biliary atresia have been a source of increased morbidity but no longer represent contraindications in most centers. Increased awareness of the availability of OLT has resulted

TABLE 80-2 Contraindications to Orthotopic Liver Transplantation

Absolute
Disseminated malignancy
Systemic sepsis
Uncontrolled substance abuse
Life-threatening extrahepatic organ failure
Cardiovascular instability
Relative
Age >60
Disabling extrahepatic condition
Inability of patient or care giver to comply with a complicated medical regimen

in reevaluation of the role of palliative operations in patients with cirrhosis.[14,15]

The timing of liver transplantation depends on the form of liver disease. In acute conditions the patient is transplanted as soon as it is clear that spontaneous recovery will not occur. In patients with chronic liver disease, optimal transplantation should be performed after the onset of disability or the presence of complications and yet prior to deterioration of the patient which would result in unacceptable risk. Selection is more readily accomplished in cholestatic liver diseases (both in children and adults) such as primary biliary cirrhosis or biliary atresia in which the relationship between the rate of decompensation and the extent of cholestasis is well understood.[16] In contrast, timing is extremely difficult in adult patients with postnecrotic cirrhosis who can decompensate rapidly despite surprisingly good liver function.

ASSESSMENT OF THE TRANSPLANT CANDIDATE

Patients are most frequently referred to liver transplant centers after they have sustained a complication of liver disease. In these cases, the initial evaluation for transplantation coincides with treatment of the acute complication. Life-threatening events such as acute hemorrhage from esophageal varices, ascitic decompensation, hepatic encephalopathy, or acute bacterial infections herald the end stage of liver disease.

The modalities used for the evaluation of the liver are summarized in Table 80-3. These can be divided in three groups: morphologic studies, functional tests, and parameters of injury. Morphologic tests are used to determine the anatomy and structural abnormalities which may be present. These include information supplied by clinical examination as well as radiographic studies. Measures of injury are supplied by biochemical tests for the detection of enzymes which are normally present in low levels in the circulation. The presence of elevated levels of alanine aminotransferase (ALT or SGPT), aspartate aminotransferase (AST or SGOT), or glutamate dehydrogenase (GLDH) is consistent with direct injury to the hepatocyte, either due to ischemic, toxic, or viral injury. Alkaline phosphatase (AP) is present in biliary canaliculi and reflects biliary tract pathology or portal tract inflammation or infiltration. γ-Glutamyl transpeptidase (GGTP) is also present in the hepatocyte on the canalicular side and reflects injury similar to AP. GGTP can also reflect activation of microsomal enzyme systems and is elevated with chronic use of alcohol or drugs metabolized by that route. Liver function tests, strictly defined, include those studies which provide information

TABLE 80-3 Clinical and Laboratory Modalities for Assessment of the Liver

Type of Information	Test	Utility
Morphology	Physical examination findings	
	Hepatic size	Estimate parenchymal reserve
	Collateral veins	Severity of portal hypertension
	Ascites	
	Splenomegaly	
	Sonography	Parenchymal texture, masses
		Identify ductal dilation
		Vascular patency and flow
	Tomographic scans	Liver size, shape, masses
	(CT, MRI)	Relations to other organs
	Angiography	Precise vascular anatomy
Parameters of injury	Serum tests	
	ALT, AST, GLDH[a]	Hepatocyte death or compromise
	AP, GGTP	Biliary tract injury or intrahepatic cholestasis
Parameters of function	Clinical examination	
	Hepatic encephalopathy	Detoxification
	Laboratory tests	
	PT	
	Factor II, V	Synthetic function
	Albumin	
	Ammonia	Detoxification
	Bilirubin	Excretory function
	Nuclear scans	Hepatic uptake and excretion
		Function of focal lesions
	Quantitative liver function tests	Precise measures of hepatic function
	Galactose elimination	
	Indocyanin green clearance	
	Caffeine clearance	
	Aminopyrine breath test	
	Lidocaine elimination	

[a]See text for abbreviations.

about the functional capabilities of the liver. Most common functional tests remain in the normal range until critical depletion of hepatic reserve, so abnormalities of mentation, coagulation, or synthetic failure indicate advanced liver disease. Excretory failure reflected by elevation of the serum bilirubin is more sensitive to injury and therefore, cholestasis can occur with lesser degrees of hepatic injury. The quantitative liver function tests listed in Table 80-3 have been used in numerous investigations and provide valuable information about gradations in hepatic reserve. Although they have primarily been used as research tools, quantitative function tests are occasionally helpful in selecting patients for OLT.

In the evaluation of the patient for OLT, clinical examination can determine the extent of hepatic encephalopathy, the state of nutrition, and the severity of portal hypertension. Clinical experience suggests that liver size is an important prognostic variable, and a small nonpalpable liver is particularly ominous in both chronic and fulminant liver disease. Routine blood testing, including hepatic enzymes, serum bilirubin, albumin, prothrombin time (PT), and serum ammonia level, permits estimation of the level of hepatic function as well as the presence of acute hepatocyte injury. The presence of pancytopenia provides an estimate of the severity of portal hypertension and hypersplenism. Radiographic assessment of the liver is carried out to determine hepatic size and document the patency of the portal vein. Though it has become possible to successfully perform hepatic transplantation in the absence of a patent portal vein, this information is essential in preoperative planning. Imaging of the parenchyma is important to identify the development of primary liver cancer as the cause of clinical deterioration. Malignant transformation of the cirrhotic liver parenchyma can occur and pose a contraindication to OLT. Additional investigations are carried out to identify contraindications. Cardiopulmonary reserve is estimated with echocardiography and routine pulmonary function testing. In patients at risk for coronary artery atherosclerosis, radionuclide stress testing and occasionally angiography are performed. Although it has been difficult to determine the extent to which abnormalities of cardiac or pulmonary function should be regarded as contraindications, patients with limited cardiopulmonary reserve are clearly at higher risk. While these patients may withstand the initial procedure, complications are poorly tolerated, particularly if reoperation is required. We have observed acute cardiac decompensation in our patients including sudden death from myocardial infarction.

Routine bacterial cultures of the throat, skin, urine, and stool have been obtained to provide a general screening program and assess the presence of colonization by pathogens. There has been some evidence that preoperative alteration of the intestinal flora, using orally administered antibiotics, is of benefit.[17] Serologic studies are performed to test for present and prior exposure to the following viruses: hepatitis A, B, and C; Epstein-Barr virus (EBV), which has been associated with lymphoproliferative disorders after transplantation; cytomegalovirus (CMV), a common postoperative pathogen; and herpes simplex virus (HSV). Base-line assessment of renal function with calculation of creatinine clearance is performed and may be of assistance in evaluating the multiplicity of renal insults which may arise during the process of OLT. Most complicated postoperative courses are associated with renal insufficiency rendering base-line assessment useful.

MANAGEMENT OF SPECIFIC COMPLICATIONS IN THE TRANSPLANT CANDIDATE (Table 80-4)

CENTRAL NERVOUS SYSTEM (CNS). Neurologic derangements are common in patients with liver disease. Symptoms are most frequently due to portosystemic encephalopathy (PSE). The mechanisms for this syndrome have been the subject of extensive investigation and are only partially clarified.[18] In general, PSE is caused by presence in the intracerebral circulation of substances which are the breakdown products of protein metabolism and interfere with normal function. Clinical assessment of PSE is based on a reliable grading system. Derangements range from mild disorientation and deficits of memory and calculation ability (stage I) to frank coma (stage IV). Measurement of the arterial ammonia level correlates roughly with PSE stage.

The presence and severity of PSE is of particular prognostic value in the assessment of patients with FHF. In general, patients who reach stage IV hepatic coma have an extremely poor prognosis and are likely to require liver transplantation. Management of encephalopathy includes airway protection, withdrawal of neurodepressant medications, induction of intestinal catharsis to remove blood products and other protein material from the gastrointestinal tract, as well as the use of nonabsorbable oral antibiotics to reduce the activity of intestinal flora and the catabolism of proteins in the gut.

In cirrhotics, the onset of PSE is often precipitated by gastrointestinal bleeding or the presence of an infection such as spontaneous bacterial peritonitis. Therefore, the initial management of the cirrhotic with PSE must include evaluation of the gastrointestinal tract for bleeding and a search for a source of infection including culture of peritoneal fluid. In the absence of these complications, an unusual protein load, dehydration due to poor intake or excessive diuresis, or the use of sedatives can usually be causally implicated.

Several other intracranial events can complicate CNS function in the transplant candidate. Patients with acute liver disease can develop intracerebral hemorrhage due to poor coagulation and present with focal deficits. Liver failure can also result in alterations of intracranial capillary permeability and the development of cerebral edema.[19] Therefore, patients in whom transplantation is contemplated, who have significant neurologic defects, should have radiologic assessment of the CNS such as a computed tomography (CT) scan. Cerebral edema can be controlled by the usual measures of mannitol, diuresis, and hyperventilation. Steroids are not clearly of benefit in this situation. Intracranial pressure monitoring has been used,[20] but questions persist about its morbidity in patients with abnormal coagulation. Herniation as a consequence of intracranial

TABLE 80-4 Complications of Liver Disease in Candidates for Transplantation

Organ System	Complication	Causes
Neurologic	Encephalopathy	Abnormal nitrogen metabolism Gastrointestinal hemorrhage Infection Volume depletion Drugs
	Stroke	Coagulopathy Underlying cerebrovascular disease
	Brain edema	Liver failure, permeability
Cardiovascular	High output state	Peripheral shunting Metabolic
	Shock	Gastrointestinal hemorrhage Bacterial sepsis
Pulmonary	Edema	Volume overload Increased capillary permeability (Liver failure) Sepsis
	Pneumonia	Aspiration from coma or gastrointestinal hemorrhage
Renal	Hepatorenal syndrome	Liver failure
	Acute tubular necrosis	Drugs Hypovolemia Shock
Gastrointestinal	Bleeding	Varices Peptic ulcer Gastritis
	Ileus	Liver failure Bacterial peritonitis
	Ascites	Portal hypertension Hypoalbuminemia
Infections	All types	Bacterial common Cirrhotics are often immunosuppressed and can develop opportunistic infection

edema is a cause of death in approximately 30 percent of patients with FHF and can occur during OLT.

RESPIRATORY SYSTEM. Pulmonary complications are seen in both acute and chronic liver disease. Fluid overload due to volume resuscitation or hepatorenal dysfunction is a common cause of pulmonary edema. In chronic cirrhosis, pulmonary edema is frequently a lethal event and can be a consequence of unsuspected infection. Evidence suggests that patients in liver failure are particularly susceptible to pulmonary failure, possibly because of structural alterations of the microcirculation.[21] Cirrhotics with pulmonary decompensation should probably not be transplanted unless their condition improves. Patients with cirrhosis who require intubation for any cause have a mortality rate exceeding 90 percent,[22] and the prognosis of these decompensated patients has not been appreciably improved with OLT. Pulmonary shunting causing chronic hypoxemia has been observed in chronic liver disease[23,24] characterized by hypoxemia which is poorly responsive to exogenously administered oxygen. Until recently, this was believed to be an absolute contraindication to OLT; however, a recent report suggests that this syndrome can be reversible after OLT[25] suggesting that the large pulmonary shunt may be due to the circulating blockers of hypoxic pulmonary vasoconstriction.[26]

Patients with FHF can experience low pressure pulmonary edema which appears to be part of a systemic syndrome which results in structural alterations of the pulmonary microcirculation.[21] These changes may be part of systemic alterations in capillary permeability which are also manifested in the CNS by the formation of brain edema. Pulmonary edema in patients with FHF tends to respond rapidly to supportive therapy and reverses after hepatic transplantation. Management is aided by pulmonary arterial catheterization and hemodynamic measurements adjusted to maintain the least pulmonary vascular pressures compatible with adequate cardiac output. The goal of ventilator management is to provide the least positive end-expiratory pressure (PEEP) compatible with 90% saturation of an adequate circulating hemoglobin on a nontoxic fraction of inspired oxygen ($F_{I_{O_2}}$), as well as the least tidal volume maintaining eucapnia.

CARDIOVASCULAR AND RENAL SYSTEMS. The base-line circulatory state in cirrhosis is characterized by systemic hypotension with low systemic vascular resistance and high cardiac output.[27] We have measured resting cardiac outputs of 10 to 20 L/min in cirrhotics undergoing transplantation. This hemodynamic state is clinically similar to sepsis and yet can occur in cirrhotics without documentable bacterial infection and may be due to presence in the circulation of vasoactive substances which interfere with normal circulatory homeostasis.[28] The high output state is potentiated by the extensive portosystemic shunting occurring in the intraabdominal and retroperitoneal circulation; propranolol reduces the cardiac output and the portal pressure in these patients.[29]

Cardiovascular instability is often a consequence of hemorrhagic shock due to gastrointestinal bleeding from esophageal varices. Patients with FHF can also develop massive gastrointestinal hemorrhage due to gastritis and poor coagulation. Adult transplant candidates occasionally have underlying heart disease that is difficult to detect due to the great disability caused by liver disease which would mask additional cardiac symptoms. In our experience, echocardiography, while useful, has not been successful in detecting cardiac compromise prior to transplantation. Conceivably, the low systemic afterload allows even a damaged left ventricle to eject well. In the acute setting, circulatory instability is incompatible with successful OLT and must be corrected prior to attempting the procedure. Our approach to severe hypotension in the transplant candidate is to ensure adequate preload (up to a pulmonary wedge pressure of 20 mmHg), add dobutamine (10 μg/kg/min) and dopamine (5 μg/kg/min), and as a last resort, phenylephrine. While these measures may produce improved circulation, control of the cause of hypotension, whether bleeding or infection, must be obtained prior to attempting OLT.

Renal insufficiency frequently develops in patients with hepatic failure. Acute tubular necrosis is often associated with infected ascites and is due to a combination of decreased perfusion due to sepsis potentiated by the use of nephrotoxic antibiotics. Hepatorenal syndrome is frequently an end-stage complication in patients with both acute and chronic liver disease, although it is completely reversible if hepatic function can be restored.[30] Although the mechanisms are incompletely understood, there is redistribution of renal cortical blood flow with resulting fluid retention and oliguria despite adequate intravascular volumes. The diagnosis of this condition can be made in patients with very low urinary sodium content (<10 meq/L), low urine volume, and normal to elevated intravascular volumes as measured by hemodynamic monitoring. This should be contrasted to prerenal azotemia which is more common in liver disease and is a consequence of hypoalbuminemia and volume depletion, frequently caused by the use of diuretics.

LIVER AND GASTROINTESTINAL SYSTEM. Functional hepatic failure is manifested as synthetic failure in both acute and chronic disease. Coagulopathy is best measured by the PT and factor V levels and, along with PSE, provides an acute measure of hepatic function. PTs do not need to be normalized prior to OLT since the rapid volume shifts which occur during the operation provide the opportunity for intraoperative resuscitation. The benefit of controlling coagulopathy in the prevention of intracranial hemorrhage is controversial. Malnutrition is frequently present in chronic liver disease and nutritional support, either enteral or parenteral, should be part of the regimen as soon as hemodynamic stability is achieved. When nutritional depletion is due to hepatocyte failure, exogenous support is of little benefit. In many cases, however, it is appropriate as empirical therapy since poor intake is a contributing factor. Hypoalbuminemia is common in cirrhosis and can result in reduced circulating blood volumes despite the presence of ascites and peripheral edema. As a temporary measure in efforts to manage fluid overload, albumin infusion with diuretic therapy can be used to maintain the albumin in the normal range.

Hepatocellular failure also causes insufficiency of detoxification function. This is commonly manifested as PSE (vide supra) as well as delayed elimination of drugs which require hepatic metabolism. The complex of hepatic failure and portosystemic shunting results in failure of the reticuloendothelial system, leaving the patients more susceptible to sepsis and effects of enterically absorbed endotoxins.

The most dramatic complication of cirrhosis is hemorrhage due to esophageal varices. In addition, both gastritis and peptic ulceration are frequent in patients with liver disease. Esophageal varices account for at least 50 percent of bleeding episodes in patients with known cirrhosis. Management of this catastrophic circumstance requires aggressive volume repletion and invasive monitoring. In massive bleeding, stabilization of the airway is essential and early diagnosis with endoscopy is of benefit. Sclerotherapy should be part of the initial management and can be performed at the time of diagnosis. Experienced centers have reported up to 90 percent success in acute control of hemorrhage.[31] Subsequent hospital mortality, however, is dictated by the stage of the liver function, in some series approaching 50 percent. We use both vasopressin and balloon tamponade as adjunctive therapy. Although some have argued that shunt surgery is obsolete, it is occasionally required in the stabilization of potential transplant candidates and as definitive therapy in patients with contraindications to OLT.[32]

Paralytic ileus can complicate acute liver failure and may be the consequence of metabolic abnormalities including hypokalemia induced by excessive diuresis. Ileus also occurs in patients with ascites and can be a sign of bacterial infection of the ascitic fluid. Portal hypertension is also associated with edema of the bowel wall and decreased absorptive function. Ileus can pose significant problems for performance of OLT due to the massive enlargement of the gut. During OLT, with clamping of the portal vein, additional congestion occurs worsening the edema. These changes complicate the operation by making exposure difficult and can interfere with abdominal closure.

DONOR SELECTION AND MANAGEMENT

This is an important subject which is addressed in detail in Chap. 76. In general, the quality of the donor organ is a crucial element in successful OLT. Though it is obvious that

TABLE 80-5 Selection Criteria for Liver Donors[a]

Heart beating donor with declaration of brain death
Systolic blood pressure at least 80 mmHg (60 mmHg for infants)
Moderate doses of vasopressors are acceptable
Age between 3 months and 70 years
No evidence of active alcohol or intravenous drug use
No risk factors for HIV infection
No history of liver disease
Normal renal function
No previous biliary tract operation
Hepatitis, HIV serology negative
Bilirubin <3 mg/dL
AST, ALT <200 U/L
AP <200 U/L

[a]These criteria are representative and vary substantially among individual centers. In addition, modifications in practice often occur depending on the severity of the recipient's disease.

a young, physiologically stable individual is more likely to supply a liver with good initial function, the parameters for donor assessment remain empirical. A recent study of a large number of liver donors was unable to identify donor risk factors for poor graft function.[33] In most transplant programs, arbitrary selection criteria have been applied to the selection of donors based on intuitive relationships between risk factors and hepatic ischemia. Selection criteria used in our program are presented in Table 80-5.

Donors over 60 years of age have been used successfully for OLT. Although there is evidence that hepatocytes do not undergo senescence, atherosclerosis of the arterial system is usually the limiting factor to the health of the older liver. Livers from newborn donors appear to have a high incidence of vascular complications and nonfunction. Young victims of trauma are usually excellent liver donors despite having experienced initial circulatory instability. Victims of violent crime, most common in urban hospitals, must be assessed carefully for a history of alcohol or drug abuse and the risk of transmission of human immunodeficiency virus (HIV) or hepatitis virus. Brain death caused by asphyxia from drownings, burn inhalation injury, or strangulation is often associated with hepatic ischemia or hypoxia and requires careful evaluation. Spontaneous intracranial catastrophes generally result in a donor with stable circulation, but there is an increased likelihood of atherosclerotic disease.

Circulatory stability and acceptable serum liver chemistries are required for the selection of a suitable liver donor. Other general criteria such as the absence of systemic disease, malignancy, and infections are required for optimal liver procurement. The operative procedure for multiorgan retrieval has been described elsewhere[34] and is a complex procedure in a critically ill patient requiring aggressive anesthetic management including hemodynamic monitoring, pulse oximetry, and volume resuscitation.

At present, livers are obtained from just over 50 percent of cadaver renal donors in the United States.[3] Conceivably, up to 80 percent of kidney donors could supply livers with optimal management and distribution. The continued linear growth of OLT will require further use of this potential donor pool, beyond which absolute shortages of livers for transplantation will occur. Although every liver recipient requires an optimal donor, selection criteria are occasionally relaxed in emergent situations. For example, although immunologic matching is not performed prior to OLT, blood group compatibility is required, but mismatched livers are used in emergent situations.

Surgical reduction of the liver graft to overcome differences in size between donor and recipient has been one of the major surgical innovations in OLT. This procedure has been developed and promoted in the United States in our institution[35] and also in Europe and Australia.[36,37] We have demonstrated that the use of graft reduction to overcome size disparities has increased the likelihood of finding suitable donors, particularly in children, and has reduced pretransplant mortality.[38] While making livers smaller can improve the distribution of livers, it does not increase the overall supply of organs. We have demonstrated in a recent series that it is possible to transplant two patients with one liver,[39] thereby increasing the number of organs which can be obtained from a fixed donor supply. The final step in overcoming the crisis produced by the limited supply of liver donors is the use of living related donors for liver transplantation. Until recently, this was thought to be technically impossible; however, we have demonstrated the feasibility of this operation in a series of children receiving partial livers obtained from parent donors.[40]

Perioperative Management

SURGICAL PROCEDURE

Three distinct operative phases occur during OLT. The first period is that of the recipient hepatectomy, the difficulty of which varies depending on the severity of the portal hypertension and local conditions such as surgical adhesions or anatomic alterations which can be congenital or due to previous surgery. The initial step is the exposure and control of the porta hepatis. Ligation of the common bile duct and the hepatic artery is performed. Subsequently the portal vein is skeletonized and prepared for clamping. The final step is division of the ligamentous attachments and control of the inferior vena cava above and below the liver. Excessive hemorrhage during this period can produce circulatory instability and dilutional coagulopathy leading to complications during implantation.

The second phase is the anhepatic phase during which the liver is removed and vascular anastomoses are performed. This phase usually lasts 1 to 2 h depending on the technical difficulties encountered. The suprahepatic vena cava is anastomosed first, followed by the infrahepatic anastomosis. The arterial and portal anastomoses are then completed and the liver is reperfused. Occasionally, due to technical difficulties, completion of the arterial anastomosis prior to reperfusion will unduly extend the anhepatic period and expose the graft to warm ischemia. In these cases the arterial anastomosis is completed after reperfusion since there is no evidence that the initial period of portal perfusion causes any harm to the liver. Circulatory instability can occur during the anhepatic period, requiring volume resuscitation and the use of the venous bypass pump to return blood from the lower body and the mesenteric circulation to the heart while the portal vein and vena cava are clamped. The progressive effects of the anhepatic state can affect coagulation and other metabolic functions.

The final stage is reperfusion which can be associated with circulatory instability due to metabolic causes. Subsequently, hemostasis and biliary reconstruction are accomplished, usually during a period of remarkable stability, associated with the rapid onset of function of the graft. In fact, persistent metabolic and coagulation problems can be the initial signs of a poorly functioning liver. The biliary anastomosis is accomplished last. When possible, primary approximation of donor and recipient bile ducts is performed; otherwise, Roux en Y cholangiojejunostomy is required.

ANESTHETIC MANAGEMENT

Operative blood loss has been a useful index of technical difficulties and varies markedly between recipients. Several studies have demonstrated a relationship between preoperative variables and operative blood loss as well as hospital survival.[4,41] In general, significant correlations have been identified between variables which measure the degree of deterioration in liver function and the severity of complications and the course and outcome of OLT. Our study of 187 patients undergoing OLT (unpublished) identified ascites, previous operations, and inverse of the transplant number as the strongest predictors of blood loss and hospital survival. These variables roughly estimate liver function, technical complications, and the experience of the team. Others have noted the more favorable prognosis of patients with cholestatic disease. Such analyses may eventually be useful in refining indications and cost projections in the application of OLT.

The circulatory consequences of OLT are due in large part to the interruption of both systemic and portal venous flow which occurs during the anhepatic period which can last up to 2 h. Although infants generally experience little circulatory change, most adults experience decreased venous return with resultant hypotension and intestinal congestion and an increased risk of postoperative renal insufficiency. The use of external venous bypass which returns blood from the lower body and the visceral circulation to the central circulation has been adopted by most adult transplant centers.[42] Despite clear advantages in intraoperative stability, the use of bypass has not been demonstrated to improve survival and some groups use it selectively or not at all.[43] Volume losses are replaced with fresh frozen plasma and red blood cells. Excess plasma is usually required due to preexisting hypoproteinemia, as well as to maintain optimal coagulation.

The dramatic physiologic alterations of the reperfusion phase are multifactorial in etiology. Reperfusion of the ischemic organ introduces acid and potassium into the circulation. Products of oxidative injury and other substances with hemodynamic effects immediately enter the pulmonary circulation, a potent endocrine organ. The body temperature falls and air emboli also enter the pulmonary circuit.[44] Although intraoperative cardiac arrest occurs in <1 percent of cases, the period immediately after reperfusion is the most common time for intraoperative death. This period combines acute myocardial dysfunction from metabolic causes with acute blood loss as the liver fills with blood and new anastomoses are challenged. Despite the complexity of these events, circulatory instability is generally short-lived and is managed by simple measures to counteract hyperkalemia and acidosis and by warming the patient. Intraoperative deficits in coagulation are common due to hypothermia, hemorrhage, and replacement leading to dilution of platelets and coagulation factors, the absence of hepatic synthetic function, and the development of fibrinolysis. Thromboelastography has been advocated for the diagnosis and management of coagulopathy; however, with the exception of aminocaproic acid therapy used in some centers for control of fibrinolysis,[45] the mainstay of therapy has been empirical blood component replacement.

POSTOPERATIVE CARE

The recovery period can be divided into three phases corresponding to gradually reduced intensity of support. The initial phase begins when the patient arrives from the operating room and extends through the first 6 to 12 h, during which circulatory instability may be present. Complete hemodynamic monitoring, including arterial and pulmonary arterial catheterization, and hourly attention to abdominal drain and urinary output is routine. The patient is maintained on controlled ventilation during this early period. Volume resuscitation with packed red blood cells (PRBC) and fresh frozen plasma (FFP) is indicated for replacement of losses which can be estimated by vital signs, output of abdominal drainage catheters, and serial measurement of hematocrit. The patient who continues to require PRBC must be constantly evaluated for return to the operating room for hemostasis. The management of postoperative bleeding varies depending on the circumstances of the transplant procedure. Bleeding occurring after an uneventful procedure with good hemostasis mandates immediate reoperation, since the cause of bleeding is usually surgical and readily controlled. In contrast, patients with difficult operations and severe coagulopathy should be stabilized prior to attempting hemostasis. Reoperation is usually required if postoperative PRBC replacement exceeds the equivalent of one blood volume. The reoperation is usually performed at least 12 h posttransplant, to allow rewarming, correction of dilutional coagulopathy, and onset of synthetic function by the transplant. In our series, approximately 20 percent of patients have required laparotomy for hemostasis or clot evacuation.

Following establishment of good oxygenation, adequate renal function and a stable circulation, the patient enters the second phase. Maintenance intravenous therapy can be initiated using intravenous hyperalimentation as soon as initial fluid shifts are under control. Determination of the adequacy of the graft follows the parameters described in Table 80-3. Evaluation of the liver after OLT follows the same principles described for the transplant candidate. Ischemic injury is quantified by ALT and AST, while GGTP and AP are indicators of cholestatic injury. Functional measures are provided by the clinical evaluation of PSE, the PT, and the serum bilirubin.

Mechanical ventilation is usually required for 24 to 48 h, but early extubation is performed whenever possible. In our series, about 20 percent of patients can be extubated within the first 6 h. Five cm of H_2O of positive end-expiratory pressure (PEEP) is routinely used to prevent atelectasis, but higher pressures are used as needed to maintain oxygenation when pulmonary edema develops. While higher PEEP may increase pressure in the hepatic veins, in practical terms, adequate oxygenation takes precedence and PEEP should be instituted when necessary. Extubation criteria include the usual indices of respiratory function and ventilatory parameters. Other criteria to be considered in the liver transplant patient include the adequacy of graft function, mental status, and the absence of expected early surgical complications requiring reoperation. Volume sequestration of up to 20 L can occur with OLT, requiring diuretic therapy and the onset of mobilization of excess fluid prior to safe extubation. In our experience, patients with severe preoperative ascites are most likely to experience postoperative pulmonary edema and require ventilatory support.

Hypertension is an additional consequence of excess volume accumulation after OLT which is potentiated by the effects of CY. The first-line therapy for hypertension should be diuresis to be started once hemodynamic stability is achieved. This often requires supplementation with calcium channel blockers which can be continued as chronic therapy. Despite the initial prevalence of hypertension <25 percent of our patients have required long-term therapy.

Hemodynamic monitoring is discontinued as soon as possible to reduce the risk of infection. Central venous catheters are retained for administration of nutritional support which is generally required prior to the onset of satisfactory intestinal function. Since adult patients generally have a primary bile duct anastomosis without intestinal suture, nasogastric decompression is usually discontinued within 24 h. In patients with Roux en Y anastomosis, nasogastric decompression (gravity drainage only) is continued until restoration of peristalsis.

The strategy used for immunosuppression in our program is summarized in Table 80-6. In general, triple therapy including CY, azathioprine, and steroids is used in the initial period with the aim of achieving therapeutic serum levels of CY before the end of the first week after OLT. In the patient with severe renal impairment after surgery, CY is given at a lower dose. Other medications routinely administered postoperatively are summarized in Table 80-7. A brief period of antibacterial prophylaxis is routine, while trimethoprim-sulfa is added for protection against pneumocystis. Acyclovir has activity against herpesvirus which is commonly reactivated following the stress of transplantation and may also have activity against CMV. Antacids or H_2 blockers are used to diminish the risk of peptic ulceration or gastritis. The medical regimen which poses unique challenges for the management of the transplant patient is the group of agents used to prevent allograft rejection. Immunosuppression is a dynamic field which is reviewed in Chap. 77 reflecting the substantial variation in the agents and protocols existing between transplant centers. Although CY has been the mainstay of immunotherapy for OLT in the 1980s recent promising results obtained with FK506 may lead to changes in our approach in OLT.[46] Dis-

TABLE 80-6 Immunosuppression for Orthotopic Liver Transplantation at the University of Chicago

BASELINE REGIMEN

Timing	Methylprednisolone (Prednisone, when able to take PO)	Azathioprine	Cyclosporine
In OR	40 mg/kg (max 2 g)	5 mg/kg (max 500 mg)	none
Day 1–2	1 mg/kg twice daily	1 mg/kg/day	1 mg/kg twice daily
Day 3–4	0.75 mg/kg twice daily	1 mg/kg/day	3 mg/kg twice daily[a]
Day 5–6	0.5 mg/kg twice daily	1 mg/kg/day	3 mg/kg twice daily
Day 7–14	0.5 mg/kg/day	1 mg/kg/day	3 mg/kg twice daily
Day 15–28	0.4 mg/kg/day	1 mg/kg/day	3 mg/kg twice daily
Day >28	0.3 mg/kg/day	1 mg/kg/day	3 mg/kg twice daily

REJECTION THERAPY

Primary therapy (initiated on diagnosis of rejection): Bolus therapy of methylprednisolone (10 mg/kg × 3 days).
Rescue therapy (begun on laboratory and biopsy confirmation of continuing rejection): OKT3 5 mg/day × 14 days.
FK506 (begun on laboratory and biopsy confirmation of continuing rejection): 0.3 mg/kg daily.

[a]CY doses are adjusted based on serum levels as measured by HPLC in our center (see Chap. 77).

TABLE 80-7 Summary of Routine Postoperative Medications

Ranitidine 50 mg IV every 8 h (adjust for renal function)
Mycostatin 500,000 U swish and swallow 4 times daily
Cefotaxime 2 g IV every 8 h × 6 doses only
Ampicillin 500 mg every 6 h × 8 doses only
Morphine sulfate 2–4 mg IV every 10 min for pain, not to exceed 10 mg/2 h
Acetaminophen with codeine 1 or 2 PO every 4 h for pain when diet is tolerated
Diphenhydramine 50 mg IV ½ h before each IV dose of CY (discontinue when oral CY is initiated)
Bactrim DS 1 tab PO or per NG (to be started within 1 week of OLT, adjust to renal function)
Acyclovir 200 mg PO every 8 h (to be started within 1 week of OLT, adjust to renal function)

charge from the ICU and entry into the third phase occurs by the third postoperative day in approximately one-third of patients. Early cardiopulmonary, hepatic, and renal complications usually respond to therapy, and over 80 percent of patients in our series are able to be moved from the ICU within 10 days; however, the remainder enter into a difficult cycle of sequential complications requiring many weeks of ICU care. Such patients have an extremely poor prognosis and are extraordinarily resource intensive.

Management of Specific Complications in the Postoperative Period

HEPATIC COMPLICATIONS

The fate of the graft is ultimately the most important variable determining the course of the patient after OLT. With good graft function patients have a remarkable ability to overcome serious complications. Graft complications are summarized in Table 80-8 which, along with the patterns of liver test abnormalities summarized in Fig. 80-1, provide an outline of the range of events which can disturb the function of the transplanted liver.

NONFUNCTION OR NONVIABLE GRAFT. The early function of the graft is of paramount importance immediately following OLT. Despite the current selection criteria for identification of the optimal donor, discussed briefly above and in Chap. 76, 5 to 10 percent of livers fail to function and require replacement. Early functional assessment of the liver is based on the clinical evaluation and the PT. Levels of hepatocellular enzymes in the circulation are correlated with the severity of ischemic injury but do not necessarily have functional implications. Though levels of ALT and AST > 5000 U/L signal major ischemic damage, recovery can occur. Peak aminotransferase levels under 1000 U/L usually signal a graft with little injury. A PT < 15 s within 12 h after OLT is consistent with excellent initial function, although approximately one-half of grafts will have some delay in functional recovery with PTs between 15 and 25 s in the first 24 h.

Clinical evaluation of mental status is the most important indicator of early function; the patient should be awake and alert within 12 h after OLT. An organ search should begin immediately after OLT in the somnolent patient with poor coagulation or high aminotransferase levels (or both). In other patients, although the grafts meet criteria for initial function as described above, progressive cholestasis develops over 5 to 7 days, with serum bilirubin levels exceeding 25 mg/dL within 7 days. In these cases, if rejection and biliary or vascular obstruction are excluded, graft replacement will be required due to the severe defect in excretory function. Although the liver has the capacity to regenerate, the risk of complications is unacceptable during the period of marginal function.

Occasionally, the implanted liver is nonviable, manifested by immediate circulatory instability of the recipient due to circulating products of cell death. Immediate removal of the graft with creation of a portocaval shunt may be the only way to stabilize the recipient.[47] In these cases, it is usually not possible to maintain the anhepatic patient for more than 24 h during the urgent search for a replacement organ. Death occurs due to progressive brain edema or multiorgan failure.

VASCULAR THROMBOSIS. Arterial thrombosis occurs in <5 percent of adult recipients and up to 20 percent of infants receiving OLT.[48] Although it can present clinically as massive hepatic necrosis, arterial thrombosis is most commonly identified by sudden elevations of aminotransferase levels or the development of biliary complications. Although arterial thrombosis occasionally occurs intraoperatively, requiring immediate reconstruction, the diagnosis is most commonly made after 7 days. Doppler ultrasound is practical and reliable for identifying vascular complications and can be used for early screening.[49] Although it is possible to perform early reconstruction of the hepatic artery, most patients require graft replacement. Since the blood supply of the bile duct is predominantly arterial, thrombosis usually leads to anastomotic leakage. Late stricture formation or hepatic abscesses can also be caused by loss of the artery. Arterial thrombosis can also occur late after OLT, usually in the setting of poorly controlled acute or chronic rejection.

Portal vein thrombosis is less common (<2 percent) and can be asymptomatic. The clinical presentation is usually the formation of ascites and the development of bleeding varices. Reoperation with direct reconstruction is usually successful. Since liver function usually remains normal with portal thrombosis, retransplantation is rarely required. Obstruction of the hepatic vein does not occur with standard OLT but has been observed following implantation of partial liver transplants leading to a syndrome of graft enlargement with dysfunction with fluid retention.[50] Obstruction of the vena cava is uncommon and is usually due to excessive length with kinking. This complication rarely causes clinical problems but is occasionally detected in postoperative ultrasonography.

EPISODES OF REJECTION. Rejection is the most common cause of hepatic dysfunction after OLT; approximately two-

TABLE 80-8 Summary of Graft Complications in Recipients of OLT

Complication	Etiology	Time of Diagnosis	Incidence (%)
Graft nonfunction	Donor injury	Within 48 h	5–10
	Recipient hypotension		
Nonviable graft	Multifactorial	Immediate	1
Vascular thrombosis			
Arterial	Technical	Immediate	5–10
	Parenchymal resistance	Within 14 days	
	Chronic rejection	Months to years	
Portal vein	Technical	Immediate	<5
	Parenchymal resistance	Within 30 days	
Hepatic vein	Technical	Within 30 days	1
	Recurrent Budd Chiari	Months to years	<1
Rejection	Acute	5 days to 3 months	70
	Chronic	Months to years	10
Biliary			
Leakage	T tube complications	Within 30 days	5–10
	Anastomotic dehiscence	Within 14 days	
Obstruction	Sludge syndrome	Within 3 months	5–10
	Stricture	Months to years	
Infections			
Bacterial	Cholangitis	Days to weeks	5
	Hepatic abscess	Within 3 months	5
Hepatitis	CMV	After 3 weeks	5
	Hepatitis viruses	After 6 weeks	5–10
	Drugs	Acute or chronic	5?

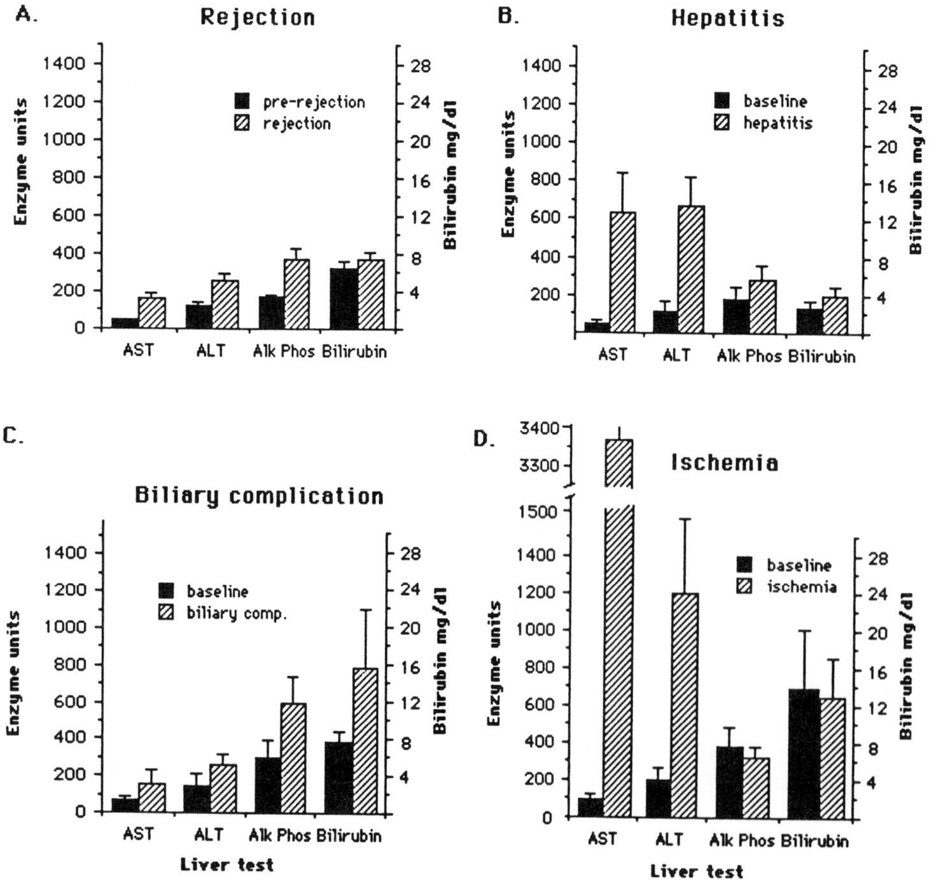

FIGURE 80-1 Biochemical patterns of graft dysfunction after liver transplantation. *a.* Rejection; *b.* Hepatitis; *c.* Biliary complication; *d.* Ischemia. Mean liver test values for base line (defined as the test value on the day prior to the onset of liver dysfunction) and on the day of diagnosis ± standard error (SE) are displayed except in *d* in which the SE of AST is 1419 U. (Reprinted with permission from Reference 53.)

thirds of patients experience at least one episode of acute rejection.[51–53] Clinical signs of rejection are nonspecific and include fever, malaise, fluid retention, and graft enlargement. Biochemically, both parenchymal and cholestatic markers of injury are usually present. Although rejection can occasionally cause massive hepatic injury, systemic decompensation due to hepatic failure is uncommon, and rejection episodes are usually managed outside the ICU. It is uncommon for rejection to occur prior to the fifth postoperative day although acute episodes can occur late after OLT. Typical patterns of liver biochemical changes occurring with various forms of injury are presented in Fig. 80-1. Although strongly suggestive, none of the clinical or biochemical findings associated with rejection is pathognomonic, so most centers perform liver biopsy prior to initiating therapy.[51] Typical histologic findings of hepatic rejection have been well characterized and include portal infiltration, vein endothelialitis, and bile duct injury.[52] In addition, exclusion of vascular or biliary complications by ultrasonography and cholangiography is often required. We have described our approach in the diagnosis and management of rejection after OLT.[53] The diagnosis and treatment of rejection is made most difficult by the possibility of infection, both as a diagnostic possibility as well as a side effect of therapy. Treatment of rejection episodes is summarized in Table 80-7; we used bolus high dose steroid therapy followed by OKT3 in the 15 percent of episodes which did not respond to steroids. In addition, FK506 has shown promise as a second-line agent for rescue therapy. Side effects of steroid therapy include peptic ulceration and potentiation of the risk of bacterial infection. OKT3, a monoclonal antibody directed against T cells, has been highly effective in reversing resistant rejection after OLT, but also promotes the development of viral illness, particularly CMV. Administration can cause seizures as well as acute pulmonary edema.

In most cases, complications of therapy, rather than rejection itself are the cause of return to the ICU. Chronic rejection is characterized by progressive destruction of biliary and arterial elements in the liver, which, in its end stage leads to biliary cirrhosis. In chronic rejection, cholestasis is the main feature, while functional failure is uncommon. Approximately 90 percent of rejection episodes are reversed by medical therapy, while 10 percent of grafts are replaced due to rejection.[53]

BILIARY TRACT COMPLICATIONS. Biliary tract complications have become less common since the early experience, but the exclusion of leakage or obstruction is mandatory in evaluating episodes of graft dysfunction. The diagnosis is suggested and distinguished from hepatitis and ischemia by the biochemical profile showing elevated AP and bilirubin levels without the extreme abnormalities of AST and ALT (see Fig. 80-1). Several options exist for reconstruction after OLT, each with risks and benefits. In most adults, the recipient bile duct is healthy and can be anastomosed to the donor duct, thereby reconstituting normal anatomy and avoiding intestinal surgery. Biliary drainage with a T tube is usually added to improve drainage and provide ready access for cholangiography. In patients in whom the recipient duct is not suitable, Roux en Y cholangiojejunostomy is performed. While it is a more reliable biliary anastomosis, it involves opening the gastrointestinal tract and creating two intestinal suture lines.

Complications occur with each technique. Primary duct anastomoses are prone to T tube dislodgement and local biliary leaks and seem to be more susceptible to obstruction by sludge and late strictures.[54] In contrast, leakage from breakdown of a Roux en Y repair, while uncommon (<5 percent) can result in catastrophic problems. Biliary complications can occur at any time following OLT, so the investigation of episodes of liver dysfunction should include cholangiography which is readily performed while the T tube is still in place (T tubes are usually removed between 6 and 12 weeks after OLT). In patients without T tubes, sonography is the initial screening measure for biliary problems, although false-negative studies are common. Cholangiography can be performed either by percutaneous puncture or via the endoscopic route. Surgical repair is usually performed for biliary problems and is well tolerated if graft function is good. As discussed earlier, determination of the patency of the artery should be performed prior to attempted biliary repair since graft replacement is nearly always required if the biliary problem is due to arterial thrombosis.

HEPATIC INFECTIONS. Infectious complications unique to the liver graft include septic cholangitis, hepatic abscess, and viral hepatitis. Both cholangitis and abscess can be caused by arterial thrombosis, which must be excluded in patients with bacterial sepsis. In the absence of obstruction, cholangitis is managed by systemic antibiotics. Extensive destruction of the biliary epithelium can occur and lead to graft loss. Gram-negative bacteria are most often responsible, including *Enterobacter* and *Pseudomonas*. Hepatic abscesses are also due to similar organisms and are often the result of poor graft perfusion or biliary tract sepsis. Localized lesions can be managed by percutaneous drainage while more extensive lesions which contain solid material or loculated collections require surgical drainage. Multiple abscesses can occasionally be treated with antibiotics; however, prolonged therapy is required and graft replacement must be considered unless convincing control of the infection is obtained.

Viral hepatitis occurs in about 10 percent of patients following OLT. Hepatitis A exposure occurs occasionally, usually leading to a self-limited syndrome similar to that observed in nontransplant patients. Hepatitis B most often represents recurrence of disease in patients infected prior to transplantation. There is at present no effective therapy for hepatitis B and most patients develop recurrence in their transplanted livers. In most cases this is a subclinical chronic disease; however, fulminant hepatitis can develop in about 10 percent requiring retransplantation, and is usually fatal. Hepatitis B DNA can be detected in the serum of patients with liver disease whose serologic tests are negative for hepatitis B suggesting that its incidence is higher than that detected by routine serologic tests.[55] Non-A non-B hepatitis was diagnosed clinically in about 5 percent of OLT patients due to their exposure to large numbers of blood products and our inability to diagnose hepatitis C infection until recently. With the development of hepatitis C serologic assays, it is now possible to ensure the safety of the blood supply and correctly diagnose the majority of patients with either non-A non-B hepatitis or cryptogenic liver disease. For both hepatitis B and C the management is expectant since effective antiviral therapy has not been available. While recent information suggests that interferon may have activity against both viruses,[56] response rates are low and the immune activation caused by interferon has led to caution in adopting this therapy in liver transplant patients. CMV is a common infection in patients receiving OLT. This virus can cause hepatitis, either mimicking or coexisting with rejection. Diagnosis can be made by liver biopsy and effective therapy with ganciclovir is available.[57]

DRUG HEPATOTOXICITY. If all other causes of liver dysfunction can be excluded, drug hepatotoxicity may be implicated as the cause of liver dysfunction. Azathioprine, CY, dilantin, and H_2 blockers have all been associated with hepatic injury and are usually administered in OLT patients. Most medications have at least theoretical possibility of hepatotoxicity and therefore any new medication may be implicated. Management of suspected hepatotoxicity requires empirical alteration of drug regimens to test the hypothesis and evaluate the response. In our experience it has rarely been possible to convincingly establish a diagnosis of drug hepatotoxicity, in part, because other causes of graft injury are so common and may coexist.

RETRANSPLANTATION FOR SEVERE GRAFT COMPLICATIONS. Retransplantation of the liver has been used liberally in most centers for the management of severe graft complications. It became clear several years ago that, despite the apparent prohibitive risks of performing OLT in the face of complications, an aggressive approach to graft replacement ultimately reduced patient mortality.[58] The indications for graft replacement in our series is presented in Table 80-9. Although rejection, both acute and chronic, accounted for one-third of cases, retransplantation was most often performed for the management of technical problems or nonfunction. Most large centers report overall retransplant rates between 10 and 20 percent.

TABLE 80-9 Summary of Indications for Retransplantation in 59 Cases[a]

Indication	Number (%)
Rejection	21 (36)
Arterial thrombosis	9 (15)
Portal thrombosis	1 (2)
Bile duct complications	4 (7)
Nonfunction	
Immediate	12 (20)
Delayed	10 (17)
Recurrent hepatitis	2 (3)

[a]From a representative series (University of Chicago 1985–1990). Overall incidence of retransplantation was 21%.

EXTRAHEPATIC COMPLICATIONS

Complications can develop in every organ system following OLT and are summarized in Table 80-10. In addition to surveillance of the graft, diagnosis and management of extrahepatic complications and the avoidance of iatrogenic injury are essential in obtaining a successful outcome after OLT.

CARDIOPULMONARY COMPLICATIONS. Cardiovascular complications are more common in the older patient after OLT, presumably due to the coexistence of underlying atherosclerosis or pulmonary disease. Sudden cardiac decompensation either due to infarction or congestive failure has occurred in several older patients in our series. These complications are inevitable, because despite optimal intraoperative management including pulmonary artery catheterization and cardiac sonography, OLT necessarily entails substantial blood loss and periods of hemodynamic change during mobilization of the native liver and on reperfusion of the graft. At the present time preoperative screening is the only method for reducing the incidence of these complications (vide supra), but attentive monitoring and early management of new ischemic or hypotensive events limits their progression. The management of hypertension has been described earlier.

Pulmonary edema is common after OLT and is due to several etiologies. Volume overload causes cardiogenic edema, in part aggravated by hypoalbuminemia, or aggravates edema due to increased pulmonary capillary permeability associated with liver failure (either FHF or acute transplant failure) or with perioperative sepsis or aspiration. Increased circulating volume is common in cirrhotics with severe ascites who may have delayed restoration of the hepatorenal fluid axis after chronic diuretic therapy and adaptation of renal function to the cirrhotic state. These early fluid-related problems can be managed with measurement and titration of the pulmonary vascular pressures. If edema develops, O_2 and PEEP therapy support oxygen delivery until diuresis or other reduction of circulating volume allows edema to clear. Early hemofiltration should be instituted if renal function is not adequate because increases of total body water of 5 to 20 L can occur during a difficult transplant procedure.

These large increases of body water can also increase the work of breathing and may compromise ventilation in the malnourished patient. Impaired ventilation can also be due to diaphragm paralysis caused by injury to the right phrenic nerve during cross-clamping. Although usually asymptomatic in adults, this problem can require surgical plication of the diaphragm in infants, occurring in about 5 percent of patients. Nutritional depletion is a more common cause of failure to wean from the ventilator, so early institution of protein-calorie supplementation and correction of electrolyte abnormalities (especially Mg^{2+}, PO_4^{3-}

TABLE 80-10 Summary of Extrahepatic Complications after OLT

Organ system	Complication	Etiology	Incidence (%)
Cardiovascular	Myocardial infarction	Undiagnosed coronary artery disease	2
	Congestive heart failure	Underlying cardiac or pulmonary disease	2
	Hypertension	Fluid overload, medications	50
	Shock	Hemorrhagic, septic, cardiogenic	10
Pulmonary	Edema		
	cardiogenic	Fluid overload, heart failure	20
	ARDS	Drugs (CY, OKT3), sepsis, aspiration	5
	Pneumonia	Bacterial, other	20
	Atelectasis	Reduced functional residual capacity; airways closure	20
	Pneumothorax	Iatrogenic	5
	Hemothorax		
	Prolonged pulmonary failure (tracheostomy)	Respiratory muscle weakness Increased respiratory load	8
CNS	Seizures	Medications, mass lesion	10
	Cerebral edema	Fulminant liver or graft failure	5
	Stroke with deficit	Cerebrovascular, air embolus?	7
Gastrointestinal	Bleeding	Varices	5
		Ulcer, gastritis	5
		CMV gastroenteritis or colitis	3
	Ileus	Multifactorial	10
	Perforation	Anastomotic	10
	Intraabdominal abscess	Perforation, infected hematoma, loculated ascites	10
Renal	Acute failure	Hemorrhage Residual hepatorenal syndrome Drugs: CY, antibiotics Infection	15
	Chronic failure	CY toxicity	2
Infections		Bacterial	30
		Viral	20
		Fungal	10

and K^+) help avoid prolonged intubation. Many OLT patients develop a postoperative metabolic alkalosis which causes them to hypoventilate. We find that correction of the multiple factors producing alkalemia can proceed while the patient is weaned from the ventilator usually with a P_{CO_2} closer to 50 mmHg than to 40 mmHg. Despite these measures approximately 10 percent of adults in our series have required tracheostomy with prolonged respiratory and nutritional support.

Acute respiratory insufficiency can develop after discharge from the ICU and is usually associated with systemic sepsis or the development of opportunistic pneumonia. Aggressive respiratory support and diagnostic measures including bronchoscopy are required to establish an early diagnosis. Empirical use of broad-spectrum antibiotics is appropriate and should include agents with activity against opportunistic pathogens including fungal, viral, and pneumocystis infections. This is essential if the pulmonary decompensation occurs more than 2 weeks after the initiation of immunosuppression or following aggressive rejection therapy. Further discussion of the management of infection in the transplant patient is presented in Chap. 99. Episodes of respiratory insufficiency can also be due to acute cardiac decompensation. Empirical heparinization should not be used in liver transplant patients due to the risk of hemorrhage and the low incidence of clinically significant pulmonary embolization in the postoperative period. Both CY (intravenously) and OKT3 have been associated with acute pulmonary insufficiency after OLT. Finally, a sudden respiratory decompensation may signal a surgical complication, such as a bile leak or intestinal perforation leading to intraabdominal sepsis. The investigation of any sudden change in the cardiopulmonary status of the patient after OLT must include a surgical evaluation.

CENTRAL NERVOUS SYSTEM. Neurologic complications are the most devastating events to occur in the perioperative period because of the implications for chronic disability and the lack of therapy if significant brain injury occurs. Fortunately, these events occur in only 5 to 7 percent of patients. Strokes are attributed to poor coagulation, increased intracranial pressure, or underlying cerebrovascular disease although it is rarely possible to precisely identify the etiology. Brain injury occurring after OLT has been most common in FHF, in which brain edema, already present due to the underlying disease, is worsened due to the volume resuscitation required during OLT. Pre- and intraoperative hemofiltration may be of benefit in preventing increased ICP and is essential if the patient is anuric preoperatively. Some groups have advocated the use of ICP monitoring which, although not beneficial in earlier studies of FHF, may permit earlier treatment of brain edema.[20] Brain edema can also occur during the anhepatic time with a nonfunctioning or nonviable liver and can lead to brain death from herniation. Intracranial hemorrhage can occur during OLT and is presumably related to coagulopathy although the presence of underlying pathology may also be required. Air embolization caused major complications in the early experience[59] and may continue to account for small deficits in speech or coordination which are occasionally observed. Management is based on accurate clinical and CT diagnosis. Where the intracranial injury is massive, early consideration of the decision to withdraw or withhold further life-sustaining therapy is indicated.

Seizures occur commonly after OLT and are usually due to side effects of immunosuppressive medication, including CY, and OKT3. Management includes standard measures for control of seizures and morphologic investigations to exclude mass lesions, hemorrhage, or abscess. Drug levels are of assistance in determining the role of CY.

DIGESTIVE SYSTEM. Gastrointestinal complications generally occur after the first postoperative week. Bleeding can occur from either varices or ulceration and requires endoscopic diagnosis. Persistence of dilated varices after OLT can be due to portal vein thrombosis or graft enlargement due to rejection. Sclerotherapy should be performed to control the varices acutely followed by sonography to assess the portal vein.[31] When possible, surgical ligation of a large coronary vein at the time of OLT may be useful in preventing postoperative bleeding from varices. Ulceration can occur due to an underlying peptic ulcer diathesis, postsurgical stress, or infection due to CMV disease. Operation is rarely required for peptic or stress ulceration, which is best managed by medical therapy aimed at prevention of acid secretion and protection of the mucosal barrier. CMV infection of the gastrointestinal tract causing ulceration and hemorrhage generally occurs later after OLT. Diagnosis is made by identification of viral infection in the serum or urine in a patient with a consistent clinical picture. Biopsy of the mucosa of the gastrointestinal tract by endoscopy with demonstration of CMV by histology or specific staining techniques can provide a specific diagnosis. In any case, therapy with ganciclovir is usually effective at controlling gastrointestinal infection.[57] Before the availability of antiviral medical therapy, surgery to control bleeding was occasionally performed, usually with disastrous results due to the high rate of dehiscence in intestinal anastomoses in bowel infected with the virus. Lower gastrointestinal hemorrhage occurring after the first postoperative week can also be the sign of an anastomotic dehiscence in patients with intestinal anastomosis such as a Roux en Y hepaticojejunostomy.

Ileus is common after OLT and usually is associated with an underlying complication such as residual hematoma, peritonitis, or the onset of rejection. Nasogastric intubation and intravenous hyperalimentation are appropriate as the initial approach to this problem, but aggressive efforts to exclude or treat an underlying etiology must be made. These include examination of the liver biochemical tests for evidence of rejection and abdominal scan or sonography to identify fluid collections. Occasionally laparotomy is required for the exclusion of a more serious complication such as peritonitis. In the absence of these findings ileus can be attributed to liver failure or metabolic derangements which are generally self-limited.

Intestinal perforations occur in as many as 10 percent of children after OLT,[60] usually in patients with extensive prior surgery and intestinal adhesions. These are usually the consequence of pinpoint perforations which occur during mobilization of the liver at the time of OLT. Intraabdominal abscesses are often due to contamination of residual hematoma causing infectious complications between 1 and 3 weeks after OLT. Management of these potentially life-threatening complications requires aggressive radiologic diagnosis and liberal use of surgical exploration whenever clinical suspicion exists. Peritonitis can also occur in the absence of a specific lesion in patients with severe immune decompensation several weeks after OLT. While mechanical lavage and surgical drainage is of some benefit, successful treatment requires broad-spectrum antibiotic therapy, which includes antifungal therapy, as well as reduction of immunosuppression.

RENAL COMPLICATIONS. Renal complications have become less frequent in the recent experience with OLT with the overall incidence of acute failure requiring dialysis of 10 percent in our series. Renal injury is most often associated with a difficult transplant requiring large volumes of blood replacement. Hemorrhage is poorly tolerated in cirrhotics with ascites who often have preexisting renal compromise due to hepatorenal syndrome and chronic diuretic therapy. Other causes of renal injury after OLT include medications, most commonly CY or antibiotics. Since renal failure can occur due to intraabdominal sepsis or bile leakage, a search for a surgical complication should be undertaken in the evaluation of unexplained deterioration of renal function. We have used continuous hemofiltration liberally in the management of volume excess associated with renal impairment in adult patients. This is best accomplished using an external Silastic arteriovenous shunt. In patients who require dialysis for metabolic indications, azotemia, hyperkalemia, or acidemia, continuous dialysis is advantageous since the circulatory instability associated with intermittent machine hemodialysis is avoided. In addition the flow rate is regulated by the patient's perfusion pressure rather than an arbitrary rate required for machine dialysis. In our experience, OLT patients who require dialysis due to ATN nearly always recover within 4 to 6 weeks. Chronic renal failure in survivors of OLT is infrequent and has occurred once in our series in a patient who failed to recover from ATN; an incidence of 0.5 percent. Overall, despite causing a reduction of renal function in most patients, chronic renal failure due to CY has been uncommon and chronic dialysis or renal transplantation has been required in <1 percent of patients.

EXTRAHEPATIC INFECTION. Infections are common after OLT and occur in close to 50 percent of patients. Although specific infections have been discussed earlier, liver transplant patients are vulnerable to the wide spectrum of infections which occur in immunocompromised patients. The risk of opportunistic infection is thus superimposed on the surgical complications inherent in patients undergoing major abdominal surgery. While bacterial infections are most common in the early postoperative period, viral infections tend to occur following 1 to 3 weeks of immunosuppressive therapy. Cirrhotics are immunocompromised hosts and are therefore susceptible to a wide range of infections which may be subclinical at the time of OLT. The most dramatic complication related to the underlying compromised state of the cirrhotic is the occurrence of fungal sepsis which can occur within 72 h following OLT. Fungal infection of the peritoneal cavity occurs relatively frequently due to opening of the gastrointestinal tract in the creation of biliary anastomoses. Further discussion of individual infections and management approaches occurring in immunocompromised patients is presented in Chaps. 77 and 99. Apart from meticulous surgical technique and rational use of prophylactic agents for control of likely pathogens, the management of infection is based on early aggressive diagnosis and treatment.

CASE PRESENTATION

A 31-year-old previously healthy woman was transferred to our institution with rapidly worsening liver function. She was well until 1 month previously, when she underwent tubal ligation under halothane anesthesia. Subsequently, she began to feel malaise and approximately 1 week prior to transfer she noted onset of jaundice. Liver chemistry tests were performed by her physician, which revealed an ALT of 5540 IU, AST of 3750 IU, AP of 215 IU, and a serum bilirubin of 12 mg/dL. At that time, the PT was 13 s. Her mental status was completely unremarkable. In the ensuing 7 days, she developed increasing confusion and insomnia and was transferred to our institution.

Initial evaluation revealed a well nourished woman who was lethargic but arousable, able to respond to questions and was oriented to self and place. Her weight was 63 kg. She was deeply jaundiced and her vital signs were normal. No skin lesions were identified and her cardiovascular examination was unremarkable. Abdominal examination revealed a slightly distended but soft abdomen, which was tympanitic. The liver was not palpable nor was it identified by percussion. Neurologic examination revealed normal deep tendon reflexes and intact cranial nerve function.

Past history was unremarkable; there were no previous operations and no medications. The patient's blood count was essentially unremarkable although the platelet count was slightly decreased at 147,000. Serum chemistries were remarkable for a creatinine level of 1.8 mg/dL. Liver tests were as follows: ALT 2523 IU, AST 2175 IU, AP 195 IU, bilirubin 28.7 mg/dL; PT was 36 s.

Intravenous fluids were started using 10% dextrose and water with a small amount of potassium for repletion. FFP was begun at 50 mL/h to attempt to correct coagulopathy. Nasogastric intubation was performed and lactulose, 30 mL every 2 h, was administered by nasogastric tube. Urinary catheterization was performed, which revealed diminished urine output. The urinary sodium value was 12 meq/L. Right heart catheterization was performed revealing a cardiac output of 8.2 L/min, with a pulmonary wedge pressure of 9 cmH_2O. Central venous pressure was 6 cmH_2O.

Because of encephalopathy and severe coagulopathy, the patient was listed as an urgent candidate for liver replacement. In the ensuing 12 h, her mental status deteriorated and she was no longer responsive. Her urine output diminished despite volume repletion to achieve a pulmonary wedge pressure of 16 cmH_2O and the creatinine level increased to 2.5 mg/dL. Because of deteriorating mental status, endotracheal intubation and ventilatory support were instituted providing F_{IO_2} 40% with 5 cmH_2O PEEP. Broad-spectrum antibiotics were administered for coverage of gastrointestinal flora. Under local anesthesia an arteriovenous shunt was inserted in the left ankle with the initiation of continuous hemofiltration to achieve a net loss of filtrate of 200 mL/h. Since the PT was still prolonged despite FFP, the rate of the replacement was increased to 100 mL/h. Thirty-six hours following admission, the patient had a stable circulation with an unchanged neurologic status. She was unresponsive except to deep pain, but cranial nerve reflexes were intact and there were no focal neurologic deficits. An ABO compatible donor was identified and, following successful procurement, she was transferred to the operating room. A CT scan performed after identification of the donor revealed no evidence of cerebral edema or intracranial focal lesions.

At surgery, a shrunken liver was removed. There was mild visceral congestion, consistent with ileus. Intraoperative blood replacement was 4 U PRBC and 16 U FFP and 16 U platelets. The pulmonary artery catheter was utilized intraoperatively to ensure accurate volume replacement. Intraoperative transesophageal echocardiographic monitoring demonstrated normal cardiac function. A small amount of urine output persisted during the transplant procedure and between 200 and 500 mL/h of ultrafiltrate was removed. There were no episodes of circulatory instability during a total anesthetic time of 7.5 h. The graft was of good quality and biliary reconstruction using a primary anastomosis was possible.

Postoperatively, the patient had a stable circulation with relatively clear outputs from the abdominal drains. The abdomen was soft, and within 6 h she was responsive to light touch and exhibited some spontaneous movement but was not awake. Initial laboratory evaluation revealed a PT of 15 s, ALT 721 IU, AST 915 IU, bilirubin 12 mg/dL. Due to mild hypoxemia occurring during the operation, $F_{I_{O_2}}$ was set at 50% with a PEEP of 8 cmH_2O. Within 12 h the patient was increasingly awake with eye opening and purposeful movement. Abdominal examination remained unremarkable. On the second postoperative day, the patient was fully awake and cooperative with simple commands. Abdominal examination was benign, abdominal drainage was clear with production of clear bile from the T tube. Liver tests showed ALT of 350 IU, AST 280 IU, AP 250 IU, and bilirubin 8.5 mg/dL. Because of renal impairment, CY was not initiated until day 2 when increased urine output signaled return of renal function. CY was begun at an IV dose of 2 mg/kg/day. The patient was fully alert and oriented with normal ventilation by day 5, at which time the endotracheal tube was removed. Ultrafiltration, which had been maintained at a net fluid loss of 100 mL/h was discontinued at this time. By day 6, ALT was 110 IU, AST 90 IU, serum bilirubin was 4.1 mg/dL, and PT 12 s, at which time she was transferred out of ICU.

On day 8, there was an increase of the ALT to 275 IU with an increase in serum bilirubin to 6.5 mg/dL. A T tube cholangiogram revealed a patent biliary anastomosis with good drainage. A percutaneous liver biopsy was performed which was consistent with acute rejection. Methylprednisolone, 10 mg/kg, was administered daily for the following 3 days. The CY level was 120 ng/mL and therefore the daily dose was increased to 4 mg/kg IV. The liver chemistry tests responded to steroid bolus therapy with gradual return of liver function to normal. The subsequent hospital course was marked by a gradual recovery of complete neurologic function. At the time of discharge, the patient had an ALT of 65 IU, AST of 48 IU, and serum bilirubin of 1.3 mg/dL with a normal PT. Renal function was excellent with a serum creatinine of 1.4 mg/dL. At the time of discharge, the patient was taking 250 mg CY orally twice daily, 100 mg azathioprine once daily and 30 mg prednisone once daily for immunosuppression. The patient returned to work 3 months following the procedure and has remained well 24 months after OLT.

CASE DISCUSSION

This case illustrates several features of the management of FHF requiring emergency OLT. In contrast to acetaminophen, FHF following halothane exposure is nearly always lethal and early consideration of OLT is mandatory. The rapid deterioration in neurologic status is not unexpected due to the small liver and the highly abnormal liver function. Medical management during this time is aimed at controlling coagulopathy, preventing infection, and supporting pulmonary and renal function during the organ search. The presence of normal cardiac function with a slightly hyperdynamic circulation was consistent with acute liver failure in a healthy patient. Although initially volume depleted, the progressive renal impairment with sodium retention despite volume repletion is consistent with hepatorenal syndrome which reversed promptly following OLT. While hemofiltration does not remove toxins, it permits the administration of large volumes of plasma even while renal function is compromised, thereby decreasing the risk of pulmonary or cerebral edema. We have used clinical evaluation of neurologic status and CT scanning to rule out the presence of brain edema, although some groups have recommended routine monitoring of intracranial pressure. The only absolute contraindication to OLT, in our opinion, is the loss of brain stem reflexes since we have observed recovery in the face of signs of early brain edema such as seizures or focal deficits. Ideally, however, the operation should be performed prior to the development of stage IV coma.

The continuation of hemofiltration during OLT in patients with renal failure gives much greater flexibility to the anesthesiologist in managing volume replacement. In general, patients with FHF are healthy and experience few circulatory problems during OLT, and, since the liver anatomy is normal, the operation poses few technical problems. Operative blood loss was below the mean for our group, equivalent to less than one-half the patient's blood volume, and is consistent with the absence of chronic liver disease or previous surgery.

Postoperatively, deficits are corrected by the new liver in proportion to their chronicity. For example, in this patient, renal failure was not fully developed and of short duration. In contrast, patients who are fully anuric require over a month to recover despite normal liver function. In this patient, PSE cleared within 48 h, whereas if cerebral edema is present preoperatively, up to a week may be required for recovery of neurologic function. The tragic outcome of brain death due to progressive edema and herniation during OLT with a normal liver after surgery occurs in about 5 percent of cases of FHF. Pulmonary derangements usually resolve prior to resolution of PSE; therefore, extubation is delayed until the patient is alert and able to protect the airway.

We delay the first dose of CY in patients with marginal renal function for 48 to 72 h to minimize renal injury. If anuric renal failure requiring dialysis is present, CY is given at usual doses since rejection is likely before renal function recovers and therefore immunosuppression takes priority. OKT3 can also be used in such cases to prevent rejection while the patient is off CY.

In this case, no graft complications requiring reoperation occurred, making it possible to discharge her from the ICU within the first week. Up to 50 percent of patients require at least one reoperation, so attention to each step of recovery is mandatory. The rejection episode described is typical; over 75 percent of rejection episodes can be managed without resort to rescue therapy.

The length of stay in the ICU of 6 days is below average in our center but is slightly above the median stay of 5 days. The period of hospitalization of 23 days is slightly above the mean for our patients; however, the distribution of durations is not symmetric. While over 50 percent of patients can be discharged between 10 and 20 days following OLT, outliers can require many months in the hospital and account for much of the excess in patient days, and obviously account for correspondingly high hospital charges. The problem of escalating costs in the face of complications will be one of the major challenges to the liver transplant community in the coming decade.

Since many points addressed in this review and the case discussion arise from the perspective of our own experience, the reader is referred to several reviews of the intensive care of OLT patients from other major centers.[61–63]

References

1. Starzl TE, Marchioro TL, BonKaulla KN, et al: Homotransplantation of the liver in humans. Surg Gynecol Obstet 117:659, 1963.
2. Starzl TE, Iwatsuki S, Shaw BW, et al: Evolution of liver transplantation. Hepatology 4:475, 1984.
3. United network for organ sharing, Richmond VA. Communication 1990.
4. Shaw BW, Wood RP, Gordon RD, et al: Influence of selected patient variables and operative blood loss on six month survival following liver transplantation. Semin Liver Dis 5:385, 1985.
5. Motschmal TL: Intraoperative blood loss and patient and graft survival in orthotopic liver transplantation: Their relationship to clinical and laboratory data. Mayo Clin Proc 64:346, 1989.
6. Cuervas-Mons V, Millan I, Gavaler JS, et al: Prognostic value of preoperatively obtained clinical and laboratory data in predicting survival following orthotopic liver transplantation. Hepatology 6:922, 1986.
7. Trey C, Davidson CS: The management of fulminant hepatic failure, in Schaffner F, Popper H (eds): *Progress in liver diseases*. Vol 3. New York, Grune & Stratton, 1970, pp 282–298.
8. O'Grady JG, Gimson AES, O'Brien CJ, et al: Controlled trials of charcoal hemoperfusion and prognostic factors in fulminant hepatic failure. Gastroenterology 94:1186, 1988.
9. Peleman RR, Gavaler JS, Van Thiel DH, et al: Orthotopic liver transplantation for acute and subacute hepatic failure in adults. Hepatology 7:484, 1987.
10. Emond JC, Aran PP, Whitington PF, et al: Liver transplantation in the management of fulminant hepatic failure. Gastroenterology 96:1583, 1989.
11. Bismuth H, Samuel D, Gugenheim J, et al: Emergency liver transplantation for fulminant hepatitis. Ann Intern Med 107:337, 1987.
12. Starzl TE, Van Thiel D, Tzakis AG, et al: Orthotopic liver transplantation for alcoholic cirrhosis. JAMA 260:2542, 1988.
13. Schenker S, Perkins HS, Sorrell MF: Should patients with end-stage alcoholic liver disease have a new liver? Hepatology 11:314, 1990.
14. Iwatsuki S, Starzl TE, Todo S, et al: Liver transplantation in the treatment of bleeding esophageal varices. Surgery 104:697, 1988.
15. Wood RP, Langnas AN, Stratta RJ, et al: Optimal therapy for patients with biliary atresia: Portoenterostomy ("Kasai procedure") versus primary liver transplantation. J Ped Surg 25:153, 1990.
16. Markus BH, Dickson ER, Grambsch PM, et al: Efficacy of liver transplantation in patients with primary biliary cirrhosis. N Engl J Med 320:1709, 1989.
17. Wiesner RH, Hermans PE, Rakela J, et al: Selective bowel decontamination to decrease gram-negative bacterial and *candida* colonization and prevent infection after orthotopic liver transplantation. Transplantation 45:570, 1988.
18. Zieve L: Hepatic encephalopathy, in Schiff L, Schiff ER (eds): *Diseases of the Liver*. Lippincott 1982, pp 433–460.
19. Hanid MA, Davies M, Mellon PJ, et al: Clinical monitoring of intracranial pressure in fulminant hepatic failure. Gut 21:866, 1980.
20. Potter D, Peachey T, Eason J, et al: Intracranial pressure monitoring during orthotopic liver transplantation for acute liver failure. Transplant Proc 21:3528, 1989.
21. Williams A, Trewby P, Williams R, et al: Structural alterations to the pulmonary circulation in fulminant hepatic failure. Thorax 34:447, 1979.
22. Shellman RG, Fulkerson WJ, Delong E, et al: Prognosis of patients with cirrhosis and chronic liver disease admitted to the medical intensive care unit. Crit Care Med 16:671, 1988.
23. Krowka MJ, Cortese DA: Pulmonary aspects of chronic liver disease and liver transplantation. Mayo Clin Proc 60:407, 1985.
24. Agusti A, Roca J, Bosch J, et al: The lung in patients with cirrhosis. J Hepatol 10:251, 1990.
25. Stoller JK, Moodie D, Schiavone WA, et al: Reduction of intrapulmonary shunt and resolution of digital clubbing associated with primary biliary cirrhosis after liver transplantation. Hepatology 11:54, 1990.
26. Rodriguez-Roisin R, Roca J, Agusti A, et al: Gas exchange and pulmonary vascular reactivity in patients with liver cirrhosis. Am Rev Respir Dis 135:1085, 1987.
27. Kowalsky HJ, Abelman WH: The cardiac output at rest in Laennec's cirrhosis. J Clin Invest 32:1025, 1953.
28. Fischer JE, Baldessarini RJ: False neurotransmitters and hepatic failure. Lancet 2:1038, 1971.
29. Agusti AG, Roca J, Bosch J, et al: Effects of propranolol on arterial oxygenation and oxygen transport to tissues in patients with cirrhosis. Am Rev Respir Dis 142:306, 1990.
30. Ellis D, Avner ED, Starzl TE: Renal failure in children with hepatic failure undergoing liver transplantation. J Pediatr 108:393, 1986.
31. Terblanche J, Burroughs AK, Hobbs KE: Medical progress: Controversies in the management of bleeding varices. N Engl J Med 320:1393, 1469, 1989.
32. Emond JC, Broelsch CE: Should portosystemic shunt be avoided in potential liver transplant candidates? HPB Surgery 1990.
33. Makowka L, Gordon RD, Iwatsuki S, et al: Analysis of donor criteria for the prediction of outcome in clinical liver transplantation. Transplant Proc 19:2378, 1987.
34. March CL, Perkins JD, Sutherland DE, et al: Combined hepatic and pancreaticoduodenal procurement for transplantation. Surg Gynecol Obstet 168:346, 1989.
35. Broelsch CE, Emond JC, Thistlethwaite JR, et al: Liver transplantation with reduced-size donor organs. Transplantation 45:519, 1988.
36. Otte JB, Yandza T, de Ville J, et al: Pediatric liver transplantation: Report on 52 patients with a 2-year survival of 86%. J Pediatr Surg 23:250, 1988.
37. Lynch SV, Balderson G, Armstrong G, et al: Mortality in pa-

tients on liver transplant waiting lists; an avoidable tragedy. Transplant Proc 21:1, 1989.
38. Emond JC, Whitington PF, Thistlethwaite JR, et al: Reduced-size orthotopic liver transplantation: Use in the management of children with chronic liver disease. Hepatology 10:867, 1989.
39. Emond JC, Whitington PF, Thistlethwaite JR, et al: Transplantation of two patients with one liver: Analysis of a preliminary experience with "Split liver" grafting. Ann Surg 212:14, 1990.
40. Broelsch CE, Emond JC, Whitington PF, et al: Application of reduced size liver transplants as split grafts, auxiliary orthotopic grafts, and living related segmental transplants. Ann Surg 212:368, 1990.
41. Lichtor JL, Emond JC, Chung MR, et al: Pediatric orthotopic liver transplantation: Multifactorial predictions of blood loss. Anesthesia 68:607, 1988.
42. Griffith BP, Shaw BW, Hardesty RL, et al: Veno-venous bypass without systemic anticoagulation for transplantation of the human liver. Surg Gynecol Obstet 160:270, 1985.
43. Wall WJ, Grant DR, Duff JH, et al: Blood transfusion requirements and renal function in patients undergoing liver transplantation without venous bypass. Transplant Proc 19:17, 1987.
44. Ellis J, Lichtor JL, Feinstein S, et al: Right heart dysfunction, pulmonary embolism, and paradoxical embolization during liver transplantation: A transesophageal two-dimensional echocardiographic study. Anesth Analg 68:777, 1989.
45. Kang YG, Martin DJ, Marquez J, et al: Intraoperative changes in blood coagulation and thromboelastographic monitoring in liver transplantation. Anesth Analg 64:888, 1985.
46. Starzl TE, Todo S, Fung J, et al: FK506 for liver, kidney, and pancreas transplantation. Lancet 2:1000, 1989.
47. Ringe B, Pichlmayr R, Lubbe N, et al: Total hepatectomy as a temporary approach to acute hepatic or primary graft failure. Transplant Proc 20(supp 1):552, 1988.
48. Mazzaferro V, Esquivel CO, Makowka L, et al: Hepatic artery thrombosis after pediatric liver transplantation—A medical or surgical event? Transplantation 47:971, 1989.
49. Segal MC, Zajko AB, Bowen A, et al: Doppler ultrasound as a screen for hepatic artery thrombosis after liver transplantation. Transplantation 41:539, 1986.
50. Emond JC, Whitington PF, Heffron T, et al: Hepatic vein obstruction: A unique complication of reduced size liver grafting. Hepatology 12:860, 1990.
51. Aran PP, Bostwick DA, Bissell M, et al: The clinical utility of liver biopsy in the diagnosis of post liver transplantation graft rejection. (Unpublished paper)
52. Snover DC, Sibley RK, Freese DK, et al: Orthotopic liver transplantation: A pathological study of 63 serial liver biopsies from 17 patients with special reference to the diagnostic features and natural history of rejection. Hepatology 4:1212, 1984.
53. Emond JC, Thistlethwaite JR, Baker A, et al: Rejection in liver allograft recipients: clinical characterization and management. Clin Transplant 1:143, 1987.
54. Rouch DA, Emond JC, Thistlethwaite JR, et al: Choledochocholedochostomy without a T-tube or internal stent in liver transplantation. Surg Gynecol Obstet 170:239, 1990.
55. Brechot C, Degos F, Lugassy C, et al: Hepatitis B virus DNA in patients with chronic liver disease and negative tests for hepatitis B surface antigen. N Engl J Med 312:270, 1985.
56. Davis GL, Hoofnagle JH: Interferon in viral hepatitis: Role in pathogenesis and therapy. Hepatology 6:1038, 1986.
57. Erice A, Jordan MC, Chace BA, et al: Gancyclovir treatment of cytomegalovirus disease in transplant recipients and other immunocompromised hosts. JAMA 257:3082, 1987.
58. Shaw BW, Gordon RD, Iwatsuki S, et al: Retransplantation of the liver. Semin Liver Dis 7:476, 1985.
59. Starzl TE, Schneck SA, Mazzoni G, et al: Acute neurological complications after liver transplantation with particular reference to intraoperative cerebral air embolus. Ann Surg 187:236, 1978.
60. Kelly DA, Kaufman SS, Shaw B, et al: Risk factors in gastrointestinal complications in children following orthotopic liver transplantation. Hepatology 8:215, 1988.
61. Pinsky MR, Grenvik A, Gordon RD, Starzl TE: Intensive care of liver transplant patients, in Civetta JM, Taylor RW, Kirby RR (eds): *Critical Care.* Philadelphia, Lippincott, 1988, pp 1605–1620.
62. Plevak DJ, Southorn PA, Narr BJ, et al: Intensive care unit experience in the Mayo liver transplantation program: the first 100 cases. Mayo Clin Proc 64:433, 1989.
63. Thompson AE: Aspects of pediatric intensive care after liver transplantation. Transplant Proc 19(suppl 3):34, 1987.

SECTION F

SPECIAL ANESTHESIOLOGIC AND SURGICAL MANAGEMENT

Chapter 81

PREOPERATIVE ASSESSMENT OF THE HIGH-RISK SURGICAL PATIENT

JOHN D. HAIGH

KEY POINTS

- *Positive and negative predictive values are the most useful test parameters to assess risk.*
- *At present there is no good method of screening the general surgical population to stratify patients for cardiac or pulmonary risk.*
- *Congestive heart failure, especially in the presence of ischemic heart disease, is by far the most significant risk factor for perioperative cardiac complications.*
- *Perioperative cardiac morbidity appears to have improved with aggressive medical management but which component of therapy is responsible is unclear.*
- *Postoperative pulmonary complications can be reduced by aggressive pre- and postoperative care, but improvements in outcome of clinical significance are achieved in a small subgroup of patients.*
- *Patients with worsening multisystem organ failure (MSOF) and an unidentified source of sepsis should be considered for diagnostic laparotomy even if noninvasive radiologic evaluation of the abdomen is unrevealing.*
- *Intra- and perioperative care of the critically ill requires close communication between medical disciplines, monitored transport with skilled personnel, and cautious titration of therapy to physiologic end points.*

Frequently the intensivist is consulted for the management of patients felt to be at high risk for perioperative morbidity and mortality. Two assumptions underlie such a consultation. The first is that the risk for a given category of patient can be determined in some way so as to aid in clinical decision-making. The second is the assumption that risk may be modified by pre-, intra-, or postoperative medical intervention. This section will examine the evidence available to support these assumptions. It will focus on cardiac and pulmonary risk because these are the most common reasons for requesting preoperative assessment by the intensive care physician. The management of the critically ill ICU patient requiring surgery will also be discussed.

Assessment of Surgical Risk

RISK PREDICTION

Four important properties of a symptom, sign, or test relate to its ability to identify those patients at risk. These are the sensitivity, specificity, positive predictive value (PPV) and negative predictive value (NPV) of the test.[1,2] They are summarized and defined in Table 81-1. The sensitivity and specificity are the more stable properties of a test, that is, their values tend not to change if a test is applied to a population with a low or high prevalence of the condition being sought. A test with high sensitivity detects most of the people who are truly at risk, i.e., it has a low false-negative rate. A test with high specificity identifies most of the people who are truly not at risk, i.e., it has a low false-positive rate. What is clinically relevant, however, is not the sensitivity and specificity of a test but its ability to predict the probability of a specific patient being at risk based on the results of the test in that patient. This is the PPV. To exclude risk the NPV is the pertinent property. These properties are not constant but are dependent on the prevalence (pretest likelihood) of the condition being sought. As the prevalence of a condition increases, the PPV of a test will increase and the NPV will decrease. When prevalence decreases, the converse occurs. Decision-making is facilitated most when the prevalence of the condition placing the patient at risk is 40 to 60 percent. A test provides little additional predictive information if the pretest likelihood is very high or very low.

TABLE 81-1 The Statistical Properties of a Test

	OUTCOME	
Test	Event Occurs	Does Not Occur
Test positive	True positive a	False positive b
Test negative	False negative c	True Negative d
Stable properties		
Sensitivity	a/(a + c)	
Specificity	d/(b + d)	
Prevalence	(a + c)/(a + b + c + d)	
Prevalence-dependent properties		
PPV	a/(a + b)	
NPV	d/(c + d)	

RISK MODIFICATION

Studies dealing with risk modification and improved outcome should meet the following criteria.[3]

1. To avoid bias it should be prospective and randomized. Information should be provided to demonstrate that randomization has led to comparable groups.
2. It should have all patients entered into the study accounted for at the conclusion of the study and have all clinically relevant outcomes reported.
3. The change in outcome must be not only statistically significant (a low probability that the difference occurred by chance, or alpha error $p < .05$) but also be of clinical significance (a difference in outcome of sufficient magnitude to warrant a change in clinical practice). A study reporting no change in outcome should also have a reasonable probability of detecting a change (low beta error, $p < .2$) Confidence intervals should be used to give a better understanding of the strength of the conclusions reached.
4. The report should be applicable to physicians' institutions of practice and patient population.

Cardiac Risk

ASSESSMENT OF CARDIAC RISK FOR NONCARDIAC SURGERY

A patient undergoing major abdominal or thoracic surgery has approximately a 10 percent chance of experiencing a perioperative cardiac complication such as myocardial infarction (MI), arrhythmia, cardiac failure, or cardiac death.[4] For patients undergoing surgery of the abdominal aorta or who are elderly, over half the perioperative mortality is cardiac in nature.[5] Understandably, attempts to predict cardiac risk and reduce it have been prominent in the literature.

MULTIFACTORIAL PREDICTORS OF RISK. Presently the two most commonly used multifactorial systems for risk assessment are the American Society of Anesthesiologists (ASA) classification of physical status[6] and the cardiac risk index (CRI).[4] The ASA physical status is listed in Table 81-2. Although not originally designed for this purpose, the ASA classification is used as an index of surgical risk because of its close correlation with surgical mortality.

The components of the CRI are listed in Table 81-3. The strongest predictors relate to the severity of coronary artery disease or poor myocardial function. Although stable angina is not listed as a risk factor, unstable angina may be closer to recent MI in terms of risk. Arrhythmias per se, in the absence of cardiac disease, are associated with a low risk of perioperative cardiac mortality.[7]

The retrospective analysis of 1001 patients from whom the CRI was derived is shown in Table 81-4. Those patients in class IV had a 22 percent incidence of a major cardiac event and a 56 percent mortality rate. Table 81-5 compares the predictive values of the CRI with the ASA system and with other tests used to assess cardiac risk. The CRI has since been examined prospectively. Class IV patients were still a high-risk group but the PPV was lower at 0.3.[8] The ASA has a low PPV because of the high number of false-positive results, i.e., although it is sensitive, it is not very specific. Although a patient falling into the CRI class IV is at high risk, the utility of the test is reduced by its low sensitivity. Only 55 percent of patients at risk were class III or IV. The sensitivity may be even less when dealing with patients undergoing abdominal aortic surgery in the CRI class I risk group.[9] Both the ASA and CRI have the advantage that they do not incur additional costs above those usually associated with surgery.

TABLE 81-2 ASA Preoperative Patient Classification

Class	Definition
I	Healthy patient
II	Mild systemic disease
III	Severe systemic disease, limits activity but is not incapacitating
IV	Incapacitating systemic disease which is a constant threat to life
V	Moribund, not expected to survive 24 h with or without operation
E	Added to class if an emergency

TABLE 81-3 Computation of the CRI

Criteria	Points
1. *History*	
a. Age >70 year	5
b. MI within previous 6 months	10
2. *Physical examination*	
a. S_3 gallop or JVD	11
b. Important valvular aortic stenosis	3
3. *ECG*	
a. Rhythm other than sinus or PACs on last preop ECG	7
b. >5 PVCs/min documented at any time before operation	7
4. *General status*	3
$P_{O_2} < 60$ or $P_{CO_2} > 50$ mmHg, $K < 3.0$ or $HCO_3 < 20$ meq/L, BUN > 50 or Cr > 3.0 mg/dL, abnormal SGOT, chronic liver disease, or bedridden from noncardiac causes	
5. *Operation*	
a. Intraperitoneal, intrathoracic, or aortic operation	3
b. Emergency operation	4
Total possible	53

JVD, jugular vein distention; PAC, premature atrial contraction; PVC, premature ventricular contraction

SOURCE: From ref. 4. Reprinted by permission of the New England Journal of Medicine (297:848, 1977.)

TABLE 81-4 CRI

Class	Point Total	No or Only Minor Complication ($N = 943$)	Life-Threatening Complication[a] ($N = 39$)	Cardiac Deaths ($N = 19$)
I($N = 537$)	0–5	532 (99)[b]	4 (0.7)	1 (0.2)
II($N = 316$)	6–12	295 (93)	16 (5)	5 (2)
III($N = 130$)	13–25	112 (86)	15 (11)	3 (2)
IV($N = 18$)	≥26	4 (22)	4 (22)	10 (56)

[a]Documented intraoperative or postoperative MI, pulmonary edema, or ventricular tachycardia without progression to cardiac death.
[b]Figures in parentheses denote percentage.
SOURCE: From ref. 4 with permission.

TABLE 81-5 Comparison of Predictors of Cardiac Risk

Risk Index	Reference	PPV	NPV
I. *Multifactorial Risk Indices*			
ASA ≥ III	4	0.11	0.98
ASA IV		0.23	0.96
CRI ≥ III		0.21	0.97
CRI IV		0.77	0.96
CRI IV	8	0.30	0.98
II. *Detecting Ischemic Heart Disease*			
A. Exercise stress testing			
ECG positive	10	0.32	0.93
ECG positive	11	0.81	0.91
Unable to attain HR > 100 for >2-min duration	13	0.28	0.92
B. 24-h Holter monitor—documented ischemia	13	0.38	0.99
C. DTS	15	0.50	1.00
III. *RF + DTS*			
CRF	17	0.32	0.96
CRF + DTS		0.42	0.95
1–2 CRF		0.16	0.97
1–2 CRF + DTS		0.30	0.97
≥3 CRF		0.50	0.89
≥3 CRF + DTS		0.64	0.67
MI within 6 months of operation	22		
1973–76		0.29	0.95
1977–82		0.04	0.98

CRF, clinical risk factors (see text); DTS, dipyridamole-thallium scanning; HR, heart rate.

ISCHEMIC HEART DISEASE. Exercise stress testing before vascular surgery has been shown to be quite sensitive, with variable specificity depending on the end points chosen and the investigator. The patients at highest risk were those with abnormal electrocardiograms (ECGs) at heart rates <75 percent of maximum predicted.[10] A better PPV was obtained by applying the ECG stress testing to a group pre-selected by history to have a higher incidence of cardiac disease.[11] These are retrospective studies and have not been confirmed by prospective testing.

The inability of a patient to exercise may be a more important factor.[12] Prospective assessment of patients over age 65 undergoing major abdominal and thoracic surgery revealed only the inability to exercise as a significant predictor of perioperative cardiac morbidity. Neither the CRI and other clinical indices nor radionucleotide ventriculography provided any additional predictive information. What is not clear is why the inability to exercise was predictive. Impaired joint mobility, dementia, and muscle weakness were felt to be more limiting than claudication or angina. However, the PPV of such prospective assessment when applied as a screening test is poor.

The detection of myocardial ischemia by preoperative Holter monitoring has recently been shown to be predictive of postoperative unstable angina, pulmonary edema, and MI.[13] This is a relatively inexpensive investigation which gave good PPV when applied to an unselected population scheduled for vascular surgery.

Coronary artery angiography has not been of value in predicting outcome although the ventriculogram may be more useful.[14] The lack of correlation of angiography is not surprising as the coronary anatomy itself does not give any idea of the physiologic reserve of the vascular supply to the heart.

To quantify such reserve in patients who could not exercise, dipyridamole-thallium scanning (DTS) has been used.[15] When patients with known stable ischemic heart disease scheduled for aortic or peripheral vascular surgery were studied, the test was very sensitive and quite specific and had a good PPV. If the patients whose repeat DTS was normal after coronary artery bypass grafting are included, the specificity increases to 90 percent. None were high risk by CRI criteria. Clinical data did not correlate with outcome. Angina or ST segment depression during the test also were not predictive. The usefulness of DTS has been confirmed prospectively by others and appears to be superior to exercise stress testing.[16]

Unfortunately DTS is less useful as a screening procedure for the general population.[17] In a retrospective analysis of 200 patients undergoing vascular surgery, multivariate analysis revealed five factors which were independently correlated with postoperative unstable angina, pulmonary edema, MI, or death. These were a history of ventricular arrhythmias requiring treatment, age over 70, Q waves on the ECG, a history of angina, and diabetes mellitus. Only Q waves on the ECG, a history of angina, and diabetes were significant risk factors when the end points of MI and death were chosen. Although DTS retained a high sensitivity, its specificity and predictive value fell when applied generally. It was only of value in aiding clinical decision-making in those of moderate risk (one to two clinical risk factors). The clinically low-risk group (no risk factors) had only a 3 percent incidence of cardiac events. The high-risk group (more than two risk factors) had a 50 percent risk of a cardiac event. While the PPV was high (0.64) in the high-risk group (more than two risk factors), DTS did little to improve risk prediction from that of clinical data (PPV = 0.50). Furthermore, the NPV fell, such that a negative DTS in this high-risk group was less predictive of an uncomplicated perioperative course. The greatest improvement in prediction came in the moderate-risk group where the PPV doubled from 0.16 to 0.30. DTS differentiated a group with a 3 percent risk from that of a 30 percent risk. This analysis shows how the clinical usefulness of a test depends on the selection of the population to which it is applied. Prospective evaluation and comparison with Holter monitoring is now required. Further improvements in risk stratification may be possible by quantifying the extent and severity of thallium redistribution.[18]

RECENT MI. For MI, early studies reported a perioperative reinfarction rate around 6 percent with a mortality rate of 50 to 70 percent.[19] The risk increased substantially if the infarct occurred within 6 months of surgery, being 15 percent between 3 and 6 months and increasing to 30 percent if within 3 months. A more recent retrospective study reported a reinfarction rate of 1.9 percent in a series of 733 patients operated on from 1977 to 1982.[20] Perioperative reinfarction rates for surgery performed within 3 and 6 months of infarction were 5.7 percent and 2.3 percent, respectively. Patients operated on in an earlier period (1973 to 1976) had rates similar to studies published from the same time period. Mortality from reinfarction was still 36 percent in the more recent series of patients. If these data are confirmed prospectively, recent MI (<6 months) may not necessarily be a predictor of bad outcome (see Table 81-5).

CONGESTIVE HEART FAILURE. In the above report, reinfarction was associated with congestive heart failure whether angina was present or not.[20] Congestive heart failure is also the greatest risk factor in the CRI. Others have found that it is the degree of myocardial dysfunction after MI rather than the time from infarction which determines perioperative mortality.[21] Also, nonsurgical patients after an MI who have no left ventricular dysfunction have a 7 percent 1-year mortality rate, whereas those with ejection fractions <30 percent or who cannot complete an exercise test have a 44 percent 1-year mortality rate.[22] This latter group also has a higher incidence of reinfarction, ischemia during exercise, and ischemic events at the time of death. It would not be surprising if their perioperative morbidity and mortality rates were higher.

AGE. Although multivariate analysis has shown age to be a risk factor in some studies, recent reports suggest that age itself may not be a major risk factor independent from the overall health of the patient.[13,17,20,23] In two studies of patients over the age of 90, long-term survival was comparable to the age-matched general population. Morbidity and mortality were closely associated with concurrent systemic disease.

DIABETES. Diabetes, like age, may not be a risk factor per se.[13,24] A retrospective multivariate analysis of 282 diabetics who underwent operation found that the risk of a major cardiac event was related to preexisting congestive heart failure, valvular heart disease, and age over 75.[24] The age relation may reflect the duration of diabetes. Although risk increased with increasing CRI class, the risk index was not an independent predictor of risk. Congestive heart failure or valvular heart disease was the only predictor of perioperative congestive heart failure, MI, and death (PPV = 0.55).

RISK MODIFICATION

CANCELLATION OR MODIFICATION OF SURGERY. Cancellation of surgery is frequently either not practical or the risks of surgical versus nonsurgical management are too ill defined to make this a viable option. While it seems intuitively correct that substituting a "less stressful" procedure should reduce the risk, there are no confirming prospective randomized trials. Major abdominal and thoracic procedures are in themselves risk factors.[4,20] Furthermore, patients with prior MI undergoing a "minor procedure" such as cataract operation have a very low incidence of reinfarction. Whether this is the nature of the surgery or the anesthesia is not clear. For patients with peripheral vascular disease, however, the available data suggest the cardiac risk is the same for aortic or peripheral vascular repair.[15,25]

PROPHYLACTIC CORONARY ARTERY BYPASS GRAFTING (CABG). Prophylactic CABG has been recommended to reduce cardiac risk.[5,14,25] Patients who survive cardiac surgery and subsequently undergo noncardiac surgery are at no greater risk than those without known cardiac disease.[26] However, the recommendations for prophylactic CABG are based on retrospective data and either do not include the mortality associated with CABG[25] or utilize historical controls for comparison of outcome.[5] The Collaborative Study in Coronary Artery Surgery (CASS) group did find a difference in the noncardiac surgical mortality (0.9 versus 2.4 percent) of post-CABG versus medically managed patients with ischemic heart disease, but the time from angiogram to noncardiac surgery was significantly longer for the medically treated group.[14] Furthermore, the mortality rate associated with CABG reported by the same group was 2.3 percent (range 0.3 to 6.4 percent, increasing with increasing age).[27] It would appear that prior bypass grafting offers no improvement in overall survival and may simply select lower risk patients.

DTS now allows the identification of a group of patients scheduled for noncardiac surgery who have a predicted cardiac mortality rate of 10 to 20 percent and a high incidence of surgically correctable coronary disease.[15,17] If confirmed, the risk reduction by prophylactic CABG could be considerable. With the advent of coronary angioplasty, which carries a reported 6 percent infarction rate and a mortality rate of <1 percent, the preoperative management of the patient at risk for a myocardial event needs to be reexamined. Randomized prospective studies in this area are badly needed.

INTENSIVE PERIOPERATIVE MANAGEMENT. The rationale for using aggressive medical intervention to reduce cardiac risk is compelling. Many of the major cardiac risk factors such as congestive heart failure, myocardial ischemia, and arrhythmias are detectable and amenable to therapy. By the use of a pulmonary artery catheter, hemodynamic assessment and manipulation are greatly facilitated. Intuitively, early intervention should reduce morbidity and mortality.

Preoperative ICU admission for investigation and physiologic "fine tuning" has been done in some centers. Data obtained from pulmonary artery catheterization and arterial blood-gas analysis have been used to stratify patients based on the degree of abnormal cardiopulmonary function.[28] Although a high-risk group could be determined clinically, the use of the pulmonary artery catheter and arterial blood-gas values allowed determination of the specific cardiopulmonary abnormality and guided its correction. These measures also detected a subgroup whose cardiopulmonary profile could not be restored to normal values by medical intervention. For those patients in the latter group who went to surgery, the perioperative mortality rate was 100 percent. Lack of randomization, the small percentage of high-risk patients who went to operation, the lack of information on outcome of those whose surgery was cancelled, and the absence of morbidity figures for line placement make it impossible to determine if this approach improved outcome. Similarly, it is not possible to determine if improvement of the cardiopulmonary profile changed mortality or selected for a less sick group.

The use of invasive monitoring along with aggressive perioperative control of hemodynamics (i.e., admission to the ICU for 72 to 96 h postoperatively) has been credited for the five to sevenfold reduction in the reinfarction rate of patients undergoing surgery within 6 months of MI.[20] The factors responsible for this reduction are difficult to determine. The same study demonstrated a significant reduction in reinfarction in the more recent patient group when the length of stay in the ICU was extended from 24 to 72–96 h. Others have also reported low perioperative infarction rates in high-risk groups when a similar preoperative and postoperative strategy was used.[13,17] However, the better outcomes could be due to factors such as better general medical management of the postinfarct patient prior to surgery or an inequality of the severity of myocardial dysfunction between the two groups.

If monitoring and ICU management are responsible for improved survival, the financial implications are staggering. More than 1300 ICU days of care were required to bring about a 2.4 percent reduction in the reinfarction rate.[20] If, however, only those patients with congestive heart failure, angina plus congestive heart failure, or angina and hypertension were admitted to the ICU, this would account for almost 80 percent of the perioperative infarctions but reduce the ICU days to <300. Interestingly, although the absolute numbers of reinfarctions were reduced in the more intensely monitored group, the above subgroups account for a similar percentage of reinfarctions in both cohorts. A more recent study found that 77 percent of postoperative ischemic events occurred within 26 h of surgery and 100 percent within 48 h suggesting a shorter period of monitoring may be sufficient.[13]

ANESTHETIC TECHNIQUE. Though not randomized prospectively, most studies have not shown a difference in outcome with the various forms of general anesthetic.[29] The controversy over regional versus general anesthesia is not settled. Only for ophthalmologic procedures and transurethral prostatectomy does regional anesthesia appear to offer significant advantages in terms of morbidity and mortality. A recent prospective randomized controlled study found that the combination of general anesthesia with intraoperative epidural anesthesia and postoperative epidural analgesia resulted in less cardiac morbidity and overall mortality when compared to general anesthesia with prn intramuscular narcotic analgesia.[30] It is not possible to say how much of the reduction in morbidity and mortality was due to intraoperative versus postoperative management or whether the level of analgesia was equivalent between the two groups. Other studies have failed to show any difference in total complications postoperatively.

In summary, DTS and preoperative Holter monitoring for the detection of myocardial ischemia are the best tests for separating high- and low-risk patients. DTS appears to offer advantages over clinical data but only in a specific subgroup of patients at intermediate risk. Preoperative Holter monitoring may be a less expensive way of identifying high-risk patients. The characteristics of the population which will maximize its predictive value are not yet defined. At the present time little evidence suggests sophisticated investigation offers any advantage over clinical impression of risk when dealing with the general population. No screening test or management algorithm is available for mass screening of preoperative patients. Of the clinical variables used to assess risk, congestive heart failure, especially in the presence of ischemic heart disease, is the most powerful. There is suggestive evidence, but no proof, that aggressive monitoring and tight physiologic control in the perioperative period may improve outcome in high-risk patients.

Risks of Pulmonary Morbidity and Mortality Associated with Nonpulmonary Surgery

RISK PREDICTION

The reported incidence of pulmonary complications following abdominal procedures is 25 to 56 percent. This large range results from varying definitions of what constitutes a pulmonary complication and whether any attempt was made to prevent such complications. In a recent prospective randomized study, respiratory failure necessitating mechanical ventilation ranged from 0 to 21 percent. Respiratory complications (cough, sputum production, dyspnea, chest pain, fever, tachycardia, radiographic changes) ranged from 30 to 88 percent depending on perioperative management.[31]

Spirometry has been used to identify high-risk patients, but these studies suffer from a number of design flaws such as retrospective or unblinded assessment of outcome, lack of randomization, and selection bias, which invalidate their conclusions.[32] Also, end points of morbidity are used which are of questionable clinical importance, such as radiographic changes or minor differences in Pa_{O_2}. The value of spirometry as a screening procedure for high-risk patients is at present unproven. Bedside spirometry is, however, a noninvasive, relatively inexpensive way of communicating to others an objective assessment of the severity of the patient's lung disease.

The inability to improve abnormal spirometry preoperatively may be a better indicator of risk.[33] In a prospective study those at risk for developing respiratory failure (ventilation for > 48 h) were best identified by the inability of 48 to 72 h of preoperative preparation to improve vital capacity (VC), forced expiratory flow over 25 to 75 percent of forced vital capacity ($FEF_{25-75\%}$) and maximal voluntary ventilation (MVV). The preoperative preparation consisted of chest physiotherapy, bronchodilators, intermittent positive-pressure breathing (IPPB), and cessation of smoking. The data do not allow calculation of PPV but 5 percent of the study group developed respiratory failure. All these patients had an $FEF_{25-75\%} < 50$ percent of predicted and an MVV < 50 percent of predicted, which had not improved with therapy. The mortality rate in this group was 60 percent.

Patients who are malnourished have significantly increased risk of pneumonia and prolonged hospital stay postoperatively.[34] Malnutrition is known to be associated with respiratory muscle impairment and pulmonary infection.[35] Postoperative complications have also been associated with obesity, duration of anesthesia >3.5 h and upper abdominal surgery.[31,36] Age and smoking have also been identified as risk factors, but not consistently.

Thus, in the general surgical population, respiratory complications and respiratory failure are as much markers of the severity of systemic disease as they are for pulmonary disease. As lung disease becomes more marked, the utility of pulmonary function as a predictor of poor outcome will increase. To date, there is no good multifactorial risk index for this patient population, but the severity of lung disease, smoking history, obesity, duration of anesthesia, nutritional status, and type of surgery are all factors which must be considered in assessing risk. Risk should be evaluated in terms of clinically relevant morbidity and survival. The prognosis and quality of life resulting from withholding surgery must also be considered. Furthermore, indices of risk must be tested prospectively. When 16 patients assessed to be at prohibitive risk actually underwent major surgery, only 1 died. Three had complications requiring ventilation > 24 h but all eventually survived.[37]

RISK REDUCTION

PREOPERATIVE PREPARATION. Prospective randomized trials have shown that pulmonary complications can be modified by preoperative and postoperative medical care.[31,38] High-risk patients who received intensive pre- and postoperative chest therapy consisting of cessation of smoking, bronchodilator drugs, inhalation of nebulized air, chest physiotherapy, delay of surgery if necessary, and antibiotics "when indicated," had a 22 percent incidence of complications compared to a 60 percent incidence in high-risk patients whose preoperative management was at the discretion of the attending physician.[38] Aggressive pulmonary therapy resulted in less severe pulmonary complications and a shorter hospital stay (24 versus 12 days). This occurred even though the treatment group had surgery delayed to improve pulmonary function.

CESSATION OF SMOKING. Cessation of smoking has been shown to result in the improvement of lung function over a period of 1 to 12 months. Since most of the postoperative pulmonary problems are felt to be due to a reduction in functional residual capacity (FRC) in relation to closing capacity, the improvements in closing volume and closing capacity should reduce the incidence of postoperative complications.[39] A retrospective analysis of pulmonary complications in CABG patients suggested that at least 8 weeks or greater abstinence from smoking is needed to cause a statistically significant reduction in complications.[40] Smoking history was significantly related to morbidity when the amount smoked reached 20 pack years. However, pulmonary function tests were not different between those who quit smoking and those who did not; these data have not been confirmed in a prospective study or in other types of surgical patients.

CHEST PHYSIOTHERAPY. While the deep breathing components of chest physiotherapy are effective as prophylaxis for postoperative pulmonary problems, chest physiotherapy per se is of value only in the treatment of established atelectasis or in those patients with copious sputum production.[31,41] In a prospective randomized study, deep breathing exercises, IPPB (intermittent positive-pressure breathing) and incentive spirometry all reduced postoperative pulmonary complications to approximately 30 percent of nontreated controls.[31] The reduction in hospital stay reached statistical significance only in the incentive spirometry group and only when high-risk patients were analyzed. IPPB was more expensive and not well tolerated by patients. Deep breathing exercises were the least expensive form of therapy. Others have also found that deep breathing exercises are as effective as incentive spirometry.

TYPE OF SURGICAL INCISION. Lung volumes are little affected postoperatively by peripheral surgical intervention. Lower abdominal operation results in a 25 to 30 percent decrease in VC and a mild decrease in oxygenation. Reduction in lung volumes and function is poorest with upper abdominal procedures. Upper abdominal surgical intervention results in an immediate 50 to 60 percent reduction in VC and 20 percent reduction in tidal volume. FRC deteriorates steadily to about 70 percent of preoperative values at 16 to 24 h postoperatively. This is accompanied by a deterioration in gas exchange and postoperative hypoxemia. The reduction in VC and FRC are thought to be a major factor in the development of pulmonary complications.[36,39] A two-incision thoracotomy-laparotomy affects pulmonary function less than a single thoracoabdominal incision. Similarly, a subcostal incision for cholycystectomy results in less reduction in VC and pulmonary complications than a midline incision. Laparotomies performed via a horizontal incision as compared to a vertical incision are associated with less atelectasis and hypoxemia.[36]

IMPROVING NUTRITIONAL STATUS. Evidence suggests that improvements in nutritional status will improve pulmonary function, but the hypothesis that preoperative nutrition will prevent respiratory complications and infections is unproven.[35]

TYPE OF ANESTHESIA. For hip surgery, epidural anesthesia results in higher Pa_{O_2} postoperatively than general anesthesia.[42] For abdominal surgery, anesthetic technique does not seem to be of importance.[31,43] Combined general and epidural anesthesia with postoperative epidural analgesia reduces the incidence of respiratory failure postoperatively when compared with general anesthesia and prn systemic narcotic analgesia.[30] The improvement in oxygenation observed with such a technique is likely due to the use of postoperative epidural analgesia.

POSTOPERATIVE ANALGESIA. All forms of regional analgesia such as epidural narcotics, epidural local anesthetics, intercostal nerve blocks, and intrapleural local anesthetics, improve postoperative variables such as forced expiratory volume in 1s (FEV_1), FVC, and Pa_{O_2}.[44,45] Transcutaneous nerve stimulation appears to improve FRC.[46] These techniques are attractive in terms of the degree of analgesia obtained for the amount of sedation. They may also improve mobilization. However, the beneficial changes in pulmonary function by any of these techniques have not been proven to influence outcome in terms of respiratory failure, pneumonia, or death or to be superior to standard narcotic analgesia.[47] This may be because although good postoperative analgesia will partially restore VC and flow rates, there is little influence on the delayed reduction in FRC postoperatively. It is this reduction in FRC which is felt to be the major factor in causing atelectasis and hypoxemia.[39] Furthermore, the immediate changes in pulmonary function may be due to reflex-induced diaphragm dysfunction rather than pain-induced changes in phrenic nerve activity.[48] Aminophylline may improve diaphragmatic dysfunction after cholecystectomy.[49]

In summary, the majority of studies use end points which have not been shown to affect long-term morbidity, mortality, or hospital costs. Therefore, the whole question of prevention of clinically significant pulmonary complications remains unanswered. From the available data a few conclusions may be tentatively drawn. Likely to benefit the patient preoperatively are cessation of smoking (at least 4 weeks and more than likely 8 weeks of abstinence to be beneficial), weight loss if morbidly obese, and optimization of pulmonary function. Intraoperative management which may benefit the patient are choosing an incision with less pulmonary compromise and limiting the duration of surgery. Postoperatively good analgesia combined with deep breathing exercises appear to reduce morbidity. The type of analgesia should be individualized to the patient's needs. Regional techniques may offer advantages in situations where early mobilization and limited sedation are advantageous. Chest physiotherapy is of proven value only for atelectasis but is useful as part of a program to stimulate deep breathing. Other methods of obtaining frequent deep inspirations appear to be as effective and may be less costly.

Surgical Risk in the ICU Patient

RISK ASSESSMENT

The risks of surgery for the critically ill patient in the ICU are much harder to quantitate. Perhaps the most difficult of this group are those patients with multisystem organ failure (MSOF) requiring laparotomy because of suspected intraabdominal sepsis (IAS). Few data are available to guide decision-making. The available literature is retrospective and the patient populations are diverse in terms of the primary disease process.

DIRECTED VERSUS UNDIRECTED LAPAROTOMY. Whether a laparotomy should be directed or undirected is controversial. A *directed laparotomy* is one in which clear clinical signs or radiologic/isotopic/ultrasonic evidence for IAS are present. An *undirected laparotomy* is one performed when extraabdominal sources are not considered adequate to explain the severity of the sepsis and an occult focus is sought. In a retrospective study of patients in an ICU who had a laparotomy prior to the development of septic shock, there was a higher percentage of positive laparotomies when laparotomy was directed versus nondirected (89 versus 58 percent).[50] However, the eventual mortality was similar for both groups whether the laparotomy was positive (48 versus 57 percent) or negative (75 versus 80 percent). In the presence of septic shock the mortality was uniformly high and was not different whether the laparotomy was directed or undirected, positive or negative.

Although computed tomography (CT) scanning has been shown to be the most accurate imaging technique for predicting the need for reexploration, a retrospective analysis of patients in the ICU found that 70 percent of CT scans were either of no help or not used in the decision to perform a laparotomy.[51,52] For CT scanning in patients with MSOF and sepsis, the PPV was 71 percent and the NPV 33 percent. Only 20 percent of the CT results were actually used in clinical decision-making for this subgroup of patients. No CT scan was positive within 8 days of the original operation. They also found that the financial and human resources expended in getting the patients to and from the scanner were considerable. The fact that CT scanning is generally only supplementary in clinical decision-making has been documented by others.[50–52]

The unexplained development of MSOF has been shown to be predictive of IAS. One study found 60 percent of undirected laparotomies and 73 percent of directed laparotomies located an intraabdominal source when unexplained organ failure was used as the indication for laparotomy.[53] In another retrospective study, 55 percent of patients who had laparotomy based on MSOF were positive and 33 percent survived. Two-thirds of those with drainable collections of pus had had negative radiologic imaging. Those with a negative laparotomy had a mortality rate of 100 percent.[52] In an analysis of ICU patients with MSOF, 80 percent of patients were found to have died of sepsis. Whereas only 25 percent of the nonsurvivors had IAS documented at surgery, 40 percent of the survivors had surgical drainage of an intraabdominal focus of infection.[51]

It is not possible to assess the negative impact of an unnecessary laparotomy on morbidity or mortality from the available literature. The high mortality associated with a negative laparotomy is probably an indicator of overwhelming sepsis. Untreated IAS with MSOF has a mortality rate approaching 100 percent as does MSOF of three or more organ systems lasting for >72 h.[50–54] It is difficult, therefore, to withhold surgery in this critically ill group of people. It must be considered, however, that in the elderly, survival will be approximately 10 percent or less even if a treatable focus is found. In the young, 75 percent will survive.[53]

In summary, unguided laparotomy is reasonable in the face of progressive unexplained organ failure, although with established MSOF the chances of finding a treatable source of sepsis or changing outcome are not good. In the elderly, the poor overall survival should be considered before proceeding to laparotomy. The available literature suggests that radiologic investigation of the abdomen is useful for confirming a clinical suspicion but is not useful for searching for an occult focus of infection or for ruling out IAS. This is especially so in patients with MSOF.

General Management of the ICU Patient Requiring Surgery

Although there is a paucity of literature to guide the perioperative management of these critically ill patients, several aspects need to be addressed to optimize patient outcome. The first is the need for good communication between all physicians involved. Since there are few hard data, the strength of the indication for operation and the risk of the procedure should be decided by the collective opinion of the surgeon, anesthesiologist, and intensivist. The local experience and skill of the individuals involved should decide the course of management.

The transportation of the patient to and from the operating room is frequently complicated. All the support systems of the ICU environment must be transported with the patient. Ideally the patient should never leave the technologic cocoon established in the ICU. This implies good quality transport monitors (ECG and pressure monitoring, preferably with defibrillation capability), a small portable ventilator or bag ventilator capable of administering positive end-expiratory pressure (PEEP) and 100 percent O_2, and portable infusion pumps. Skilled personnel should accompany the patient. This will usually involve an ICU nurse, a respiratory technologist, and either the ICU physician or the anesthesiologist. The continuity of care should likewise be uninterrupted for the return trip. It is surprising that while most intensivists, anesthesiologists, and surgeons would be concerned about a 15-min failure of monitors in the ICU or operating room, many elect to make a quick dash to and from the operating room without monitoring the patient. Frequently the failure to monitor occurs during periods of hemodynamic instability associated with the transfer of critically ill patients from bed to stretcher or operating table or when the patient is emerging from anesthesia.

The ICU and intraoperative management of these patients requires clinical judgment and common sense based on data extrapolated from other patient populations with isolated organ failure. Therapeutic goals require evaluation of all organ systems to identify which organ system is most likely to be responsible for mortality. Therapy can then be directed primarily at this organ system. Often therapy directed at one organ system may be at the expense of another. Therapy may have to be modified if there is impending failure of another organ system. For example, the low left atrial pressure and application of PEEP for management for adult respiratory distress syndrome (ARDS) may compromise renal perfusion. In a young individual with severe ARDS, it may be elected to allow a certain degree of physiologic insult to the kidneys. In the elderly, even transient renal dysfunction is much more serious, and therapy will have to be modified accordingly.

A discussion of anesthesia for the critically ill is beyond the scope of this chapter. However, no evidence suggests that one anesthetic technique is superior to another for this patient population, but derangements of physiology should be considered in managing such patients.[54] All of these patients either already have ARDS or are at risk for developing it. The present way of managing these patients is to keep the left atrial pressure as low as possible to lower transcapillary fluid flux. Cardiac output and oxygen delivery to the tissues are maintained with inotropes if necessary. Frequently the patient will be on PEEP. Both the hypovolemia and the PEEP will predispose the patient to marked hemodynamic instability if drugs with myocardial depressant or vasodilating properties are administered. Any drug should be given cautiously and titrated to both therapeutic and deleterious effects. Drug clearance may be markedly altered due to concomitant renal and hepatic dysfunction, and the volume of distribution of many drugs may be different because of extensive tissue edema and protein depletion.

The ventilator found on the anesthetic machine may be inappropriate for ventilating a patient with severe ARDS and high levels of PEEP. A more sophisticated ventilator may need to be brought to the operating theater. Inhalation anesthetics cannot be administered with the majority of these ventilators. The time required to obtain and set up such a ventilator and the necessary modifications in anesthetic technique necessitate anticipation of such problems and good communication between physicians.

Intraoperative fluid management should be conservative for reasons stated earlier. The goal should be to achieve adequate organ perfusion and oxygen delivery. This may be relatively simple such as maintaining a minimal urine output or more complicated such as assessing oxygen delivery and utilization with a pulmonary artery catheter. In general, when septic, this population is hyperdynamic with a high cardiac output and low systemic vascular resistance. The interpretation of mixed venous oxygen saturation is difficult in this situation as it is usually high and may not reflect peripheral oxygen supply-demand matching. Blood pressure may be maintained by increasing the cardiac output further with inotropes or by the judicious addition of vasoconstrictors. If ischemic heart disease is present, vasoconstrictors may be preferable.

When the patient is returned to the ICU, it is important that the patient again be transported with the same level of care given intraoperatively. The surgeon and anesthesiologist should inform the intensivist of the patient's intraoperative management and any problems encountered. This ensures that continuity of care is unbroken, allowing potential perioperative problems to be anticipated and prevented.

CASE PRESENTATION

A 71-year-old man presented for elective resection of an abdominal aortic aneurysm. The ICU was consulted for preoperative assessment, possible preoperative admission for hemodynamic assessment, and consideration for postoperative management. His past history was significant for coronary artery and pulmonary disease. He had sustained an anterior MI 2 years earlier, complicated by congestive heart failure. Since that time he had been pain free but complained of shortness of breath with exertion. He could walk up a flight of stairs at his home if he did not rush. He had had no episodes of overt congestive failure but was taking 40 mg furosemide and 0.125 mg digoxin daily. He was also using nitroglycerin sublingually prn which seemed to help the shortness of breath. He denied orthopnea, paroxysmal nocturnal dyspnea, or anginal type chest pain. He also had a history of claudication and was scheduled for vascular surgery prior to his MI. Because of the infarct, his surgery was not performed.

He continued to smoke one-half pack a day, having reduced his consumption from one and a half packs a day prior to the MI. He had some sputum production and cough in the morning but denied any major pulmonary problems other than as mentioned above. The rest of his history was unremarkable. Physical examination revealed an elderly man who looked his chronologic age. Relevant findings were a blood pressure of 150/85 mmHg and a regular pulse of 80 beats/min. Jugular venous pressure was not elevated. The carotid upstroke was normal, and no bruits were heard. All peripheral pulses were diminished and were absent in his feet. There was no peripheral edema. His apical impulse was somewhat diffuse. Heart sounds were normal apart from an S_4, and a III/IV systolic ejection murmur, which was aortic in nature. His color was good. He had a respiratory rate of 12 without use of accessory muscles or pursed lip breathing. Auscultation of the chest revealed scattered coarse rhonchi with wheezing throughout all lung fields. Apart from the abdominal aortic aneurysm, the rest of the examination was unremarkable.

Laboratory investigations were hemoglobin of 14 g/dL with a normal white cell count, platelet count, prothrombin, and partial thromboplastin times. Results of serum electrolyte and liver function tests were normal. His creatinine was mildly elevated at 140 μmol/L ($N < 124$). The BUN and urinalysis were normal. Chest x-ray showed mild cardiomegaly with no sign of pulmonary congestion or edema. The ECG revealed Q waves in leads V_{1-3} with T wave inversion V_{1-6}.

It was recommended that a cardiologist be consulted to obtain an echocardiogram to assess the degree of valvular stenosis and ventricular function. A stress thallium test was also recommended. The echocardiogram showed a thickened aortic valve with a mild degree of stenosis and a slightly dilated left ventricle with dyskenesis of the anterior wall. The DTS showed a fixed defect compatible with his old infarction placing him at low risk for perioperative MI. Further investigation of his coronary anatomy was thought to be unnecessary. A MUGA scan was also obtained, which showed an ejection fraction of 46 percent.

Bedside spirometry was requested and showed an FEV_1 50 percent of predicted and an FVC 80 percent of predicted. The ratio of FEV_1:FVC was 60 percent. There was no improvement with bronchodilator therapy. The chest physiotherapist began preoperative education on deep breathing exercises.

In light of his left ventricular function, it was considered desirable to have a pulmonary artery catheter intraoperatively to manage the hemodynamic consequences of aortic cross-clamping. After discussions with the anesthesiologist, it was decided to optimize the cardiopulmonary profile gradually overnight. The patient was admitted to the ICU for placement of an arterial line and pulmonary artery catheter. Cardiac index was 1.9 L/min/m^2 with a pulmonary artery occlusion pressure (PAOP) of 4 mmHg. The mixed venous oxygen saturation (MV_{O_2}) was 58 percent. Our opinion was that he had been aggressively diuresed and that he would be improved with a higher preload, especially since he would be without oral intake for over 13 h. Ringer's lactate (2L) administered over 8 h brought the PAOP to 14 mmHg and the cardiac index to 2.9 L/min/m^2. The MV_{O_2} increased to 70 percent. Combined general and epidural anesthesia were used. During aortic cross-clamping his blood pressure rose to 189/90 mmHg, the wedge pressure rose to 24 mmHg and the cardiac index fell to 1.3 L/min/m^2. This responded well to an infusion of nitroprusside. With unclamping of the aorta, blood pressure fell slightly to

95/40 mmHg with a PAOP of 12 mmHg and cardiac index of 2.5 L/min/m^2. This was treated with a volume infusion and a brief period of neo-Synephrine infusion. Urine volume was adequate throughout. The patient was admitted to the ICU for monitoring and epidural analgesia. Analgesia was obtained using a continuous fentanyl-0.125 percent bupivacaine infusion. He was extubated shortly after arrival. He developed some left lower lobe atelectasis but his oxygenation was good on 40 percent O_2 by mask. In anticipation of his return to the floor, the bupivacaine component of the epidural analgesia was discontinued. As the sympathetic tone and venous capacitance returned to normal, the PAOP increased to 20 mmHg and the gas exchange deteriorated requiring 70 percent O_2. This was treated with 20 mg furosemide intravenously. He was observed for a further 12 h and discharged to the surgical floor. The atelectasis resolved with mobilization and chest physiotherapy. The rest of his hospital stay was without incident.

References

1. Department of Clinical Epidemiology and Biostatistics, McMaster University Health Sciences Centre: How to read clinical journals: II. To learn about a diagnostic test. Can Med Assoc J 124:703, 1981.
2. Department of Clinical Epidemiology and Biostatistics, McMaster University: Interpretation of diagnostic data: 3. How to do it with a simple table (part B). Can Med Assoc J 129:705, 1983.
3. Department of Clinical Epidemiology and Biostatistics, McMaster University Health Sciences Centre: How to read clinical journals: V. To distinguish useful from useless or even harmful therapy. Can Med Assoc J 124:1156, 1981.
4. Goldman L, Caldera DL, Nussbaum SR, et al: Multifactorial index of cardiac risk in noncardiac surgical procedures. N Engl J Med 297:845, 1977.
5. Hertzer NR, Beven EG, Young JR, et al: Coronary artery disease in peripheral vascular patients. Ann Surg 199:223, 1984.
6. Keats AS: The ASA classification of physical status—A recapitulation. (Editorial). Anesthesiology 49:233, 1978.
7. Goldman L: Cardiac risks and complications of noncardiac surgery. Ann Intern Med 98:504, 1983.
8. Zeldin RA: Assessing cardiac risk in patients who undergo noncardiac surgical procedures. Can J Surg 27:402, 1984.
9. Jeffrey CC, Kunsman J, Cullen DJ, et al: A prospective evaluation of cardiac risk index. Anesthesiology 58:462, 1983.
10. Cutler BS, Wheeler HB, Paraskos JA, et al: Applicability and interpretation of electrocardiographic stress testing in patients with peripheral vascular disease. Am J Surg 141:501, 1981.
11. McCabe CJ, Reidy NC, Abbott WM, et al: The value of electrocardiogram monitoring during treadmill testing for peripheral vascular disease. Surgery 89:183, 1981.
12. Gerson MC, Hurst JM, Hertzberg VS, et al: Cardiac prognosis in noncardiac geriatric surgery. Ann Intern Med 103:832, 1985.
13. Raby KE, Goldman L, Creager MA, et al: Correlation between preoperative ischemia and major cardiac events after peripheral vascular surgery. N Engl J Med 321:1296, 1989.
14. Foster ED, Davis KB, Carpenter JA, et al: Principal investigators of CASS, and their associates: Risk of noncardiac operation in patients with defined coronary disease: The coronary artery surgery study (CASS) registry experience. Ann Thorac Surg 41:42, 1986.
15. Boucher CA, Brewster DC, Darling RC, et al: Determination of cardiac risk by dipyridamole-thallium imaging before peripheral vascular surgery. N Engl J Med 312:389, 1985.
16. Leppo J, Plaja J, Gionet M, et al: Noninvasive evaluation of cardiac risk before elective vascular surgery. J Am Coll Cardiol 9:269, 1987.
17. Eagle KA, Coley CM, Newell JB, et al: Combining clinical and thallium data optimizes preoperative assessment of cardiac risk before major vascular surgery. Ann Intern Med 110:859, 1989.
18. Eagle KA, Boucher CA: Cardiac risk of noncardiac surgery. Editorial. N Engl J Med 321:1330, 1989.
19. Steen PA, Tinker JH, Tarhan S: Myocardial reinfarction after anesthesia and surgery. JAMA 239:2566, 1978.
20. Rao TLK, Jacobs KH, El-Etr AA: Reinfarction following anesthesia in patients with myocardial infarction. Anesthesiology 59:499, 1983.
21. Dirksen A, Kjøller E: Cardiac predictors of death after noncardiac surgery evaluated by intention to treat. Br Med J 297:1011, 1988.
22. Dwyer EM Jr, Greenberg HM, Steinberg G: Clinical characteristics and natural history of survivors of pulmonary congestion during acute myocardial infarction. The Multicenter Postinfarction Research Group. Am J Cardiol 63:1423, 1989.
23. Hosking MP, Warner MA, Lobdell CM, et al: Outcomes of surgery in patients 90 years of age and older. JAMA 261:1909, 1989.
24. MacKenzie CR, Charlson ME: Assessment of perioperative risk in the patient with diabetes mellitus. Surg Gynecol Obstet 167:293, 1988.
25. Arous EJ, Baum PL, Cutler BS: The ischemic exercise test in patients with peripheral vascular disease. Arch Surg 119:780, 1984.
26. Crawford ES, Morris GC, Howell JF, et al: Operative risk in patients with previous coronary artery bypass. Ann Thorac Surg 26:215, 1978.
27. Kennedy JW, Kaiser GC, Fisher LD, et al: Clinical and angiographic predictors of operative mortality from the collaborative study in coronary artery surgery (CASS). Circulation 63:793, 1981.
28. Del Guercio LRM, Cohn JD: Monitoring operative risk in the elderly. JAMA 243:1350, 1980.
29. Mangano DT: Anesthetics, coronary artery disease, and outcome: Unresolved controversies. Editorial. Anesthesiology 70:175, 1989.
30. Yeager MP, Glass DD, Neff RK, et al: Epidural anesthesia and analgesia in high-risk surgical patients. Anesthesiology 66:729, 1987.
31. Celli BR, Rodriguez KS, Snider GL: A controlled trial of intermittent positive pressure breathing, incentive spirometry, and deep breathing exercises in preventing pulmonary complications after abdominal surgery. Am Rev Respir Dis 130:12, 1984.
32. Lawrence VA, Page CP, Harris GD: Preoperative spirometry before abdominal operations, a critical appraisal of its predictive value. Arch Intern Med 149:280, 1989.
33. Gracey DR, Divertie MB, Didier EP: Preoperative pulmonary preparation of patients with chronic obstructive pulmonary disease. Chest 76:123, 1979.
34. Windsor JA, Hill GL: Risk factors for postoperative pneumonia, the importance of protein depletion. Ann Surg 208:209, 1988.
35. Lewis MI, Belman MJ: Nutrition and respiratory muscles. Clin Chest Med 9:337, 1988.

36. Jackson CV: Preoperative pulmonary evaluation. Arch Intern Med 148:2120, 1988.
37. Williams CD, Brenowitz JB: "Prohibitive" lung function and major surgical procedures. Am J Surg 132:763, 1976.
38. Stein M, Cassara EL: Preoperative pulmonary evaluation and therapy for surgery patients. JAMA 211:787, 1970.
39. Craig DB: Postoperative recovery of pulmonary function. Anesth Analg 60:46 1981.
40. Warner MA, Divertie MV, Tinker JH: Preoperative cessation of smoking and pulmonary complications in coronary artery bypass patients. Anesthesiology 60:380, 1984.
41. Kirilloff HL, Owens GR, Rogers RM, et al: Does chest physical therapy work? Chest 88:436, 1985.
42. Hole A, Terjesen T, Breivik H: Epidural versus general anaesthesia for total hip arthroplasty in elderly patients. Anaesth Scand 24:279, 1980.
43. Tisi GM: Preoperative identification and evaluation of the patient with lung disease. Med Clin North Am 71:399, 1987.
44. Bromage PR, Camporesi E, Chestnut D: Epidural narcotics for postoperative analgesia. Anesth Analg 59:473, 1980.
45. Symreng T, Gomez MN, Rossi N: Intrapleural bupivacaine v saline after thoracotomy—Effects on pain and lung function—A double-blind study. J Cardiothorac Anesth 3:144, 1989.
46. Ali J, Yaffe CS, Serrette C: The effect of transcutaneous electric nerve stimulation on postoperative pain and pulmonary function. Surgery 89:507, 1981.
47. Rosenberg PH, Heino A, Scheinin B: Comparison of intramuscular analgesia, intercostal block, epidural morphine and on demand-iv-fentanyl in the control of pain after upper abdominal surgery. Acta Anaesth Scand 28:603, 1984.
48. Ford GT, Whitelaw WA, Rosenal TW, et al: Diaphragm function after upper abdominal surgery in humans. Am Rev Respir Dis 127:431, 1983.
49. Dureuil B, Desmonts JM, Mankikian B, et al: Effects of aminophylline on diaphragmatic dysfunction after upper abdominal surgery. Anesthesiology 62:242, 1985.
50. Sinanan M, Maier RV, Carrico CJ: Laparotomy for intra-abdominal sepsis in patients in an intensive care unit. Arch Surg 119:652, 1984.
51. Norwood SH, Civetta JM: Abdominal CT scanning in critically ill surgical patients. Ann Surg 202:166, 1985.
52. Hinsdale JG, Jaffe BM: Re-operation for intra-abdominal sepsis. Ann Surg 199:31, 1984.
53. Ferraris VA: Exploratory laparotomy for potential abdominal sepsis in patients with multiple-organ failure. Arch Surg 118:1130, 1983.
54. Pinsky MR, Matuschak GM (eds): Multiple systems organ failure. Crit Care Clin 5:2, 1989.

Chapter 82

CONTROL OF PAIN AND ANXIETY

KENNETH DRASNER
JEFFREY A. KATZ
ANTHONY SCHAPERA

During the last decade, there has been a fundamental change in our perception of the role of pain and anxiety in the outcome of critically ill patients. These patients have been perceived as at risk primarily from side effects of treatment; now, the contribution of pain and anxiety to morbidity, and possibly even mortality, is appreciated. Simultaneously, we have made significant advances in our ability to treat pain and anxiety due to the availability of better analgesic and sedative agents, greater use of regional anesthetic techniques, and, most significantly, the development of better methods of drug delivery.

Deleterious Effects of Pain and Anxiety

Acute pain and anxiety in the postoperative period or following traumatic injury may have harmful physiologic and psychologic effects. That is, pain and anxiety may adversely affect respiratory function, contribute to the development of a stress response, and increase cardiac morbidity.

RESPIRATORY DYSFUNCTION

Abnormalities of mechanical pulmonary function and gas exchange consistently occur following major abdominal and thoracic surgery.[1] Most often, a restrictive pattern develops, characterized by marked decreases in vital and inspiratory capacities and a smaller, but clinically important, decrease in functional residual capacity (FRC). Patients breathe with smaller tidal volumes and have a decreased ability to take deep breaths and cough effectively. The magnitude of these changes is a function of the proximity of surgery to the diaphragm. Similar changes in pulmonary function occur following blunt thoracic trauma complicated by multiple rib fractures.[2] The actual mechanisms of reduced lung volumes and hypoxemia following abdominal and thoracic surgery and thoracic trauma are not completely known, but spasm and splinting of the abdominal and intercostal muscles,[3] limited diaphragmatic movement,[4] and pain[5] appear to be the primary factors.

Changes in pulmonary function are most severe immediately after upper abdominal surgery. The patient's forced vital capacity (FVC) and forced expiratory volume in 1 s (FEV_1) decrease 60 percent below their preoperative levels, and FRC declines by 30 percent.[1] Gradually, these deficits improve, returning to preoperative levels within 2 weeks. After lower abdominal surgery, FVC and FEV decrease to a lesser extent, i.e., by only 30 and 10 percent, respectively. (Lung volumes remain normal following minor or peripheral surgery.)

Gas exchange abnormalities, primarily defective pulmonary oxygen exchange, are common after all types of surgery and occur in two phases. The first phase occurs in the immediate postoperative period and is a consequence of general anesthesia and its known effects on respiratory function, including residual central or peripheral ventilatory depression, increased venous admixture, and shivering after anesthesia. Administration of supplementary oxygen generally prevents serious hypoxemia secondary to most conditions causing hypoventilation postoperatively, but persistent hypoventilation may result in atelectasis, particularly after upper abdominal surgery. In the absence of preexisting abnormalities in pulmonary function, gas exchange returns to normal within 2 h following an uncomplicated general anesthetic for a peripheral procedure.

The second phase of abnormal gas exchange is attributable to the changes in lung mechanics following operations on the abdomen and thorax. Hypoxemia correlates with decreased FRC and is most severe in the elderly, the obese, and those with preoperative cardiopulmonary disease (conditions that increase the tendency for airway closure). When closing capacity exceeds FRC, regions in the lung with low ventilation perfusion ($\dot{V}/\dot{Q}$) matching and right-to-left shunting develop and cause hypoxemia.

THE STRESS RESPONSE

The pattern of biochemical changes following traumatic injury, sepsis, and surgery is known as the stress response. Stimulation of the peripheral, central (CNS), and autonomic nervous systems, and release of humoral factors, such as kinins, leukotrienes, and prostaglandins from tissue injury, produce these changes. Catecholamine, cortisol, and glucagon levels increase, as do vasopressin, growth hormone and β-endorphin levels. The magnitude of the hormonal changes is roughly proportional to the extent of trauma.

Hypercoagulability may occur because coagulation is activated (e.g., increased levels of factor VIII and increased fibrinogen-platelet activity), and fibrinolysis is inhibited (for up to 5 days).[6,7] Because the patient is immobile, changes in coagulation may result in arterial and venous thrombosis.

The elevated stress hormones also produce an altered endocrine/metabolic state characterized by hyperglycemia, insulin resistance, increased gluconeogenesis, increased metabolic rate, sodium and water retention, and protein catabolism. An impaired immune response also may be observed, characterized by a reduction in the number and function of lymphocytes and by granulocytosis.[8]

CARDIAC MORBIDITY

The stress response activation of the sympathetic nervous system increases heart rate, blood pressure, and myocardial contractility, thereby increasing myocardial oxygen consumption. Myocardial oxygen supply may decrease in response to systemic factors such as hypotension, tachycardia, anemia and hypoxemia, or to local factors, e.g., coronary artery thrombosis and spasm. Combined, these changes can precipitate myocardial ischemia or infarction (MI). Interestingly, the highest levels of plasma catecholamines have been observed immediately after surgery and have a positive correlation with changes in blood pressure and heart rate.[9]

Patients with cardiac risk factors who undergo abdominal or thoracic surgery have a high incidence of perioperative cardiac morbidity (e.g., MI, unstable angina, congestive heart failure, serious arrhythmia and cardiac death).[10] The incidence of MI after noncardiac surgery in the general population is 0.0 to 0.7 percent, but increases to 1.1 to 1.8 percent in patients with coronary artery disease. Reinfarction rates range from 1.9 to 8 percent for patients with previous infarction (i.e., >6 months), up to 37 percent for those with recent infarction (i.e., <3 months), and from 1 to 15 percent in patients undergoing vascular surgery. Mortality associated with perioperative MI ranges from 36 to 70 percent.

The peak incidence of perioperative MI occurs postoperatively. Similarly, myocardial ischemia is more common postoperatively (38 percent) than in the intraoperative (21 percent) or preoperative (24 percent) period.[11] However, both postoperative myocardial ischemia and MI often are clinically "silent," but are frequently associated with a chronically elevated heart rate.[10] Invasive intraoperative monitoring and extended postoperative care in an ICU appear to help reduce morbidity, e.g., overall infarction rate decreased to 1.9 percent in one study of high-risk patients and increased to 5.7 percent when MI was recent.[12]

DELETERIOUS EFFECTS OF ANXIETY

The ICU environment is frightening and stress-evoking. A survey of critically ill patients conducted after discharge from the ICU revealed that many recall having pain (40 percent) and anxiety (55 percent) during their treatment in the ICU.[13] Nearly 50 percent described mechanical ventilatory support as unpleasant and stressful and reported feelings of helplessness, fear, agony, and panic.[14] Particularly stressful were difficulties with synchronization, suctioning episodes, the inability to communicate, and fear of equipment failures. The period of resuming spontaneous breathing was especially stressful. Anxiety was increased by disorientation, desperation regarding the seriousness of their illness, and loss of control. Emotional suffering is heightened if therapeutic paralysis is induced without adequate analgesia and sedation. Some patients may develop a postoperative/traumatic neurosis characterized by anxiety, irritability, repetitive nightmares, preoccupation with death, and a reluctance to discuss their experience.[15]

Assessment of Pain and Sedation

In 1986, the Subcommittee on Taxonomy of the International Association for the Study of Pain adopted the following definition: "Pain is an unpleasant sensory and emotional experience associated with actual or potential tissue damage, or described in terms of such damage."[16] By definition, pain is always subjective and cannot be measured directly. This intrinsic subjectivity imposes obvious limitations to any analysis of pain management in the critically ill.

A wide variety of methods are available for assessing pain. However, rating scales are most commonly used. A major strength of this technique, particularly in the critical care setting, is its simplicity: patients simply rate their level of pain relative to a visual, verbal, or numerical scale. The most widely accepted of these instruments, the visual analog scale (VAS), requires patients to rate their pain by locating a point along a line whose poles represent extremes such as "no pain" and "the worst pain I've ever had." (A horizontal line appears to provide the most reliable results.) The degree of pain is identified by the distance from the poles. Despite its obvious simplicity, the VAS has been shown to have a high degree of reliability and validity.[17] Nevertheless, even this simple pain scale can often be too difficult to administer to critically ill patients.

A major weakness of rating scales is their unidimensionality (i.e., they ignore the qualitative aspects of the pain experience). More sophisticated instruments, such as the McGill Pain Questionnaire, designed to assess the qualitative aspects of the pain experience generally are too complex to administer to critically ill patients. However, these tools can provide useful retrospective data.

Methods have been developed to codify behavioral parameters, such as facial expressions, when pain must be assessed indirectly. Hemodynamic parameters also can be used to assess pain state, but the type of illness and drugs administered can significantly alter hemodynamic variables and thereby influence pain assessment.

ASSESSING SEDATION

Monitoring the degree of sedation in the ICU is inexact. The parameters most commonly used are the qualitative state of consciousness and assessment of the patient's hemodynamic and intracranial pressure responses to invasive procedures (e.g., endotracheal suctioning and chest physiotherapy). Scoring scales available for assessing the level of consciousness include the Glascow Coma Scale, which, although widely used, has established validity only in patients with neurologic deficits. Additionally, full scoring is often difficult in tracheally intubated patients. We prefer a six-point sedation scale which incorporates identifiable clinical end points (Table 82-1).[18] This scoring system has

TABLE 82-1 Sedation Scoring for Critically Ill Patients

Level	Response
1	Anxious and agitated or restless or both
2	Cooperative, oriented, and tranquil
3	Responding to commands
4	Brisk response to stimulus[a]
5	Sluggish response to stimulus[a]
6	No response to stimulus[a]

[a]Light glabellar tap or loud auditory stimulus

been widely used in clinical studies assessing sedation in critically ill patients.

Routine sampling of plasma concentrations of sedative agents has limited usefulness because of the time required to obtain blood assay results and marked interindividual variability in response to drugs. However, periodic determination of plasma concentrations may prevent overdosage and help to determine the cause of unexplained comatose states during sedation.

Other monitoring techniques include intermittent or continuous electroencephalography (EEG) and recording the frequency and amplitude of lower esophageal contractions. However, EEG recording is complicated, expensive, and indicated only in selected cases (e.g., monitoring the depth of barbiturate-induced coma). Lower esophageal contractions increase and intensify during stress and surgery and decrease with anesthesia, but do not appear to be useful in determining the depth of sedation in the ICU because of large interindividual variability and the differential effects of analgesic and sedative agents.[19]

Methods of Pain Control

The two major modes of pain control for critically ill patients are systemic administration of analgesic agents and regional analgesic and anesthetic techniques.

PARENTERAL NARCOTICS

Low plasma concentrations of narcotics do not significantly alter pain perception. As plasma narcotic concentration increases, an analgesic threshold is achieved.[20] Above this threshold, analgesia will be adequate; below this minimum effective analgesic concentration (MEAC), analgesia will be inadequate. At concentrations near MEAC, small changes in serum levels result in relatively large changes in analgesia, i.e., the dose-response curve for analgesia is relatively steep. However, a significant ceiling effect occurs at higher concentrations, where little additional analgesia is obtained while the risk of deleterious side effects is increased. Therefore, the goal of parenteral narcotic therapy is to maintain plasma levels within a range that will provide adequate pain relief with minimal side effects.

INTRAMUSCULAR ROUTE OF ADMINISTRATION

Intramuscular administration of narcotics results in highly variable absorption of drug. For example, standard intramuscular injections of meperidine can produce peak serum levels that vary by a factor of five, with a sevenfold difference in the time at which peak serum levels are achieved.[21] Additionally, there is considerable delay between the assessment of pain, administration of narcotic, and its absorption, resulting in wide swings in plasma levels. Consequently, the intramuscular route is inappropriate for treatment of severe pain in most critically ill patients.

INTRAVENOUS ROUTE OF ADMINISTRATION

Intravenous administration results in more rapid and predictable plasma drug levels than the intramuscular route. Although significant fluctuations still occur, intermittent intravenous regimens can be selected that will produce trough levels above MEAC. However, intermittent bolus regimens that will maintain plasma drug concentrations above MEAC will produce relatively high peak concentrations and thereby increase the likelihood of significant side effects. Although some side effects may be relatively unimportant or even desirable (e.g., respiratory depression may be a desirable feature for the patient whose trachea is intubated and who is receiving mechanical ventilation), increased narcotic consumption will contribute to the development of tolerance. Increased narcotic consumption can be minimized by administering a continuous infusion, which may produce stable serum concentrations and improve analgesia.

PATIENT CONTROLLED ANALGESIA (PCA)

Few critically ill patients are capable of using PCA, but the sense of control provided by this technique may be of tremendous psychologic benefit. The concept of using small intravenous doses of narcotics determined by the patient was initially described in 1968.[22]

Although MEAC for a given patient tends to be relatively stable, there is wide interpatient variability. Consequently, the conventional practice of administering fixed dosages based on weight will result in a significant degree of oversedation or inadequate analgesia for many patients. PCA devices permit the patient to self-administer analgesics at doses and intervals preset by the physician. When in pain, the patient depresses a button, causing delivery of a fixed intravenous dose from an infusion pump. The purpose of the "lock-out" interval is to permit sufficient time for a dose to achieve near-peak effect before a subsequent dose can be obtained, thereby safeguarding the patient against overdosage due to cumulative effects. In fact, oversedation and respiratory depression appear to be rare and, when present, are associated with other contributing factors[23,24] or with programming errors.[25] Studies have shown that patients using PCA tend to maintain serum drug concentrations around a particular "set point." As expected, this "set point" varies extensively among patients but tends to be relatively constant for the individual. Some studies document improved control of pain with PCA, whereas others do not. However, patient acceptance is very high. In one controlled study, the use of PCA resulted in a greater patient satisfaction than epidural morphine, despite the fact

TABLE 82-2 Pharmacology of Intravenous Narcotics

	Distribution Half-Life (min)	Elimination Half-Life (h)	Peak Effect (min)	Approximate Equinalagesic Dose	SUGGESTED INITIAL DOSE		
					Bolus	Continuous Infusion	PCA Bolus
Morphine	20	2–4	30	10	2–5 mg	2–10 mg/h	0.5–1.0
Meperidine	10	3–5	4	100	25–50 mg	Not recommended	5–10
Fentanyl	3	2–5	4	0.1	25–100 μg	25–100 μg/h	10–50
Sufentanil	1	2–3	8	0.01	2–10 μg	2.5–10 μg/h	2–5
Alfentanil	3	1–3	1	0.5	2–3 mg	0.5–3 mg/h	Not recommended

that patients given epidural morphine had more complete analgesia.[26]

CHOICE OF PARENTERAL NARCOTIC

Severe pain in the critically ill is best treated with a pure opiate agonist. Because the commonly used opiate agonists have similar receptor profiles, they are pharmacodynamically alike and differ little in their opiate-related effects. Choice of agent is therefore primarily based on pharmacokinetic characteristics (Table 82-2) and nonopiate-mediated effects. The clinical significance of these characteristics depends on the method of drug delivery and the patient's illness.

MORPHINE. Morphine remains the most commonly used narcotic in the ICU setting because most clinicians are familiar with its pharmacokinetic and pharmacodynamic properties and it is inexpensive. Disadvantages include a relatively slow onset of action and release of histamine. In addition, morphine-6-glucuronide, a metabolite with a potency four times greater than morphine, accumulates in critically ill patients with impaired renal function.[27]

MEPERIDINE. Meperidine is relatively lipid soluble and thus has a rapid onset of action. Compared with the other compounds, it is slowly eliminated (half-life 3 to 5 h). Meperidine is a fairly potent suppressor of shivering,[28] which may be of particular benefit in the immediate postoperative period. An important limitation of this drug is that a major metabolite, normeperidine, is a convulsant and may accumulate, particularly in patients with impaired renal function.[29]

FENTANYL. Fentanyl is a lipid-soluble compound having a more rapid onset of action than morphine. When small doses are administered, the duration of action is short because the drug is rapidly redistributed from the brain to other tissues. When large doses are administered, termination of effect requires elimination. Because fentanyl's elimination half-life is 2 to 5 h, duration of action following large doses is similar to that of morphine. The pharmacokinetics of fentanyl are not significantly altered in the presence of hepatic cirrhosis, and clearance appears to remain normal in renal failure.[29] Unlike morphine, fentanyl does not release histamine and therefore may be a better choice for patients who are hemodynamically unstable or have significant reactive airway disease.

ALFENTANIL. Of the available narcotics, alfentanil has the fastest onset and shortest duration of action. Its relatively short duration of action is a result of both rapid redistribution from brain to blood and a short elimination half-life of 90 min. Alfentanil is eliminated rapidly from the body because it has a relatively small steady-state volume of distribution.[30] Following a bolus of 2 to 3 mg, an infusion is started at an initial rate of 0.5 to 3.0 mg/h, and adjusted according to patient requirements. Interindividual variablity is great: 30 percent for initial distribution and 50 percent for clearance.[31] Hepatic disease prolongs elimination, but renal failure has little effect. Because alfentanil does not accumulate, rapid recovery follows discontinuation of therapy. In one study, patients treated with a combination of alfentanil and midazolam awakened sooner at the end of the infusion than those treated with fentanyl and midazolam.[32]

SUFENTANIL. Sufentanil is a highly potent lipid-soluble narcotic. Recent animal data suggest that receptor occupancy may be an important factor in the development of tolerance.[33] Thus, from a theoretical standpoint, the use of highly potent narcotics such as sufentanil which can produce a full effect with less receptor occupancy may be of benefit if patients require long-term administration of narcotic.

REGIONAL TECHNIQUES

EPIDURAL LOCAL ANESTHESIA

Epidural local anesthesia offers the easiest method to provide complete abdominal, thoracic, and lower extremity analgesia. In contrast to narcotic analgesia, the complete afferent blockade produced by local anesthetics results in profound analgesia, while avoiding the risk of respiratory depression. However, despite the excellent pain relief and potential benefits, its use remains limited because its side effects include hypotension, urinary retention, motor blockade, and the requirement for intensive monitoring. Sepsis, coagulation defects, and local skin inflammation generally contraindicate the use of epidural anesthesia.

TABLE 82-3 Continuous Epidural Bupivacaine for Pain Relief

		BOLUS INJECTION		CONTINUOUS INFUSION	
Location of Pain	Preferred Interspace	Conc (%)	Vol (mL)	Conc (%)	Vol (mL/h)
Thoracic	T_4–T_6	0.25	5–10	0.125	8–10
Upper abdomen	T_7–T_9	0.25–0.5	5–10	0.125–0.25	8–10
Lower abdomen	T_{12}–L_1	0.25	8–10	0.125	10–20
Extremity	L_2–L_4	0.25	8–10	0.125	10–15

Epidural local anesthetics inhibit neural transmission of spinal nerves by reducing the permeability of the cell membrane to sodium ions. Neural blockade of sympathetic, sensory, and motor fibers depends on the concentration of local anesthetic. Sympathetic blockade generally occurs with more dilute solutions and sensory and motor blockade at progressively increasing concentrations. Similarly, sympathetic blockade is present at a higher level than sensory blockade, which, in turn, is several dermatomes higher than the level of motor blockade. For postoperative pain control, segmental neural blockade of the wound is desirable, leaving autonomic and motor function as unaffected as possible.

Anesthesia is best achieved using a catheter technique which permits intermittent or continuous infusions. Following insertion of an epidural catheter, it is important to check for correct placement. Accidental intrathecal injection can result in profound spinal blockade, while intravascular injection can result in CNS toxicity or cardiovascular collapse. After checking for the presence of cerebrospinal fluid or blood, a "test dose" (generally 3 mL of a 1.5% lidocaine solution containing 10 to 15 μg epinephrine) is administered. A significant increase in heart rate occurring within 3 min indicates intravascular placement of the catheter, while significant sensory and motor blockade of the lower extremities suggests subarachnoid placement.

Ideally, the catheter should be placed at a spinal level that is approximately at the center of the desired analgesic band: T_4 to T_6 following thoracotomy, T_7 to T_9 for upper abdominal surgery, T_{12} to L_1 for lower abdominal surgery, and L_2 to L_4 to provide analgesia to the lower extremities and the perineum (Table 82-3).[34] The distribution of analgesia depends on the concentration and volume of local anesthetic used. High volume, low concentration regimens are preferred because higher volumes provide greater spread and lower concentrations produce less profound motor blockade. Bupivacaine is widely used because of its long duration of action and its relative sparing of motor nerve fibers.[35]

An initial bolus of 5 to 10 mL 0.25 to 0.5% bupivacaine is required to ensure effective neural blockade. The higher concentration is preferred following upper abdominal and thoracic procedures. Following the bolus injection a continuous infusion of a more dilute solution should be started (see Table 82-3). Dose requirements and infusion rates may vary and should be assessed periodically. If pain recurs, it may also be necessary to administer an additional bolus. Duration of treatment is commonly 1 to 3 days.

SIDE EFFECTS. The main side effects of epidural anesthesia result from autonomic and motor blockade. Autonomic blockade will affect cardiovascular, gastrointestinal, and genitourinary function. Hypotension results from sympathetic blockade, with magnitude generally dependent on the extent of sympathectomy (e.g., hypotension is more common following thoracic than lumbar blockade). Hypotension can be profound and potentially life-threatening, particularly in the presence of even minor degrees of hypovolemia. Therefore, hypovolemia must be corrected before administering an epidural local anesthetic. In addition, postural hypotension is relatively common in patients who have a sympathectomy. Thus, patients must be monitored closely if they are permitted to sit or stand; and clinically-significant alterations in blood pressure should be treated quickly and aggressively. Initial treatment includes Trendelenburg positioning, restoring or increasing intravascular volume by rapid infusion of fluids, and 5 to 10 mg intravenous ephedrine. Glycopyrrolate (0.2 mg) or atropine (0.4 mg) may be useful during periods of unopposed vagal activity.

Urinary retention will occur following parasympathetic blockade of nerve roots S_2 to S_4. In those patients in whom a urinary catheter has not been inserted, the urinary volume must be monitored and evidence of a full bladder checked. This is particularly important when neural blockade advances to low thoracic levels, because the patient may not experience the discomfort of a full bladder.

Motor blockade rarely results in respiratory depression. In patients with normal pulmonary function, epidural anesthesia to high thoracic levels does not decrease ventilation or the ventilatory response to added CO_2 because blockade of phrenic nerves rarely occurs.[36] FRC and gas exchange are well maintained.[37] However, depending on the level of motor blockade, ventilatory reserve is decreased, principally the expiratory reserve volume (ERV), i.e., the ability to cough.[38] For example, motor blockade to T_5 decreases ERV by 48 percent and inspiratory capacity by only 8 percent. Total thoracic motor blockade nearly eliminates ERV, while inspiratory capacity is decreased by only 20 percent. In contrast, a T_1 to T_5 segmental thoracic block resulted in minimal decrease in inspiratory capacity and no change in ERV or maximal expiratory flow at 75 percent of vital capacity.[39]

Cerebral and cardiovascular toxicity from excessive drug accumulation are seldom encountered, provided the drug is infused into the epidural space and care is taken to avoid excessive administration. An epidural bupivacaine infusion

TABLE 82-4 Epidural Narcotic/Local Anesthetic Standing Orders

1. The patient has received the following:
   Narcotic: (circle)
   (Preservative-free) Morphine: ________ dose ________ time
   Fentanyl: ________ dose ________ time
   Local anesthetic: ________ mL of ________% ____________ drug ________ time
   Route: Epidural Intrathecal (circle)
   Catheter insertion: Site: ____________ Time: ____________

2. Drug for continued analgesia—complete those that apply:
   Narcotics: Preservative-free morphine ____________ mg/mL
   Fentanyl ________ μg/mL
   Local anesthetics: ________ % ____________ drug
   Infuse at ____________ mL/h

3. Monitor vital signs:
   Following epidural narcotics:
   Respiratory rate, pattern and sedation scale q 30 min × ________ h, then q 1 h until ________ h after the last dose of narcotic.
   Following epidural local anesthetics:
   a. Arterial blood pressure via direct or automatic BP monitor:
      Following a bolus injection: q 1–2 min × 10 min
      While infusion is in progress: q 15 min
      Prior to and immediately following sitting or standing
   b. Sensory level and motor function q 1h

4. Ephedrine ampule at bedside

5. No narcotics are to be given for 24 h, except by order of intensivist.

6. Notify intensivist if:
   Following epidural narcotics:
   a. Respiratory rate $<$10/min
   b. Evidence of airway obstruction
   c. Decreased respiratory effort
   d. Pinpoint pupils
   e. Sedation scale level 3 or greater
   f. Severe itching, urinary retention, nausea, or vomiting not improved by treatment with naloxone
   g. Incomplete pain relief
   Following epidural local anesthetics:
   a. Systolic blood pressure $<$90 mmHg and/or pulse $<$60/min
   b. Patient is unable to move legs or feels tingling in fingertips
   c. Sensory level above the nipple line
   d. Patient complains of numbness around the mouth, ringing in the ears or light-headedness
   e. Muscle twitching, new arrhythmias or an increase in the frequency of arrhythmias
   f. Incomplete pain relief
   g. Postural decrease in systolic blood pressure of $>$15 mmHg or heart rate increase of $>$20/min

7. Management and treatment of side effects:
   Respiratory depression:
   a. Naloxone 0.4 mg IV *stat* for respiratory rate $<$8/min or sedation scale $\geq$3
   b. Repeat naloxone 0.4 mg IV q 5 min × 3 prn
   Nausea, vomiting and pruritus:
   a. Naloxone 0.08 mg q 15 min IV prn × 3. If symptoms relieved by IV bolus may repeat q 1 h prn
   b. Metoclopramide 10 mg IV q 8 h × 3 for nausea/vomiting not relieved by naloxone and then q 8 h prn
   c. Droperidol 0.625 mg IV repeat × 1 prn for nausea/vomiting not relieved by metoclopramide
   Urinary retention:
   a. Naloxone 0.08 mg q 15 min IV prn × 3
   b. Notify intensivist if not relieved by 45 min

8. Catheter dressings:
   Examine site daily

rate of >25 mg/h is seldom required, and 30 mg/h should be considered the upper limit.

Catheter-related infections are rare, but the catheter and site should be inspected periodically and a dressing similar to that used with central venous catheters should be applied.

Accidental dural puncture can result in a postdural puncture headache. The resulting postdural headache may be incapacitating. An epidural blood patch is 90 percent effective and is indicated if headache is limiting ambulation.

Every institution should devise standard orders for the care of critically ill patients. An example of standing orders for the management of patients who have received epidural local anesthesia or intraspinal narcotics is given in Table 82-4.

SPINAL NARCOTICS

Spinal opiate receptors were first identified in 1976,[40] and intrathecal administration of morphine was shown to produce profound analgesia in the rat.[41] By 1984, the effectiveness of spinal opiates was demonstrated in human beings[42] and the Food and Drug Administration approved the use of preservative-free morphine sufate for epidural or intrathecal administration. The prolonged and profound analgesia produced by a single spinal injection of morphine led to rapid widespread acceptance of the technique, which is now a routine component of pain management.

Selective spinal analgesia can be achieved using either epidural or intrathecal opioid injection. Analgesia following intrathecal injection tends to be more profound, but is associated with a higher incidence of side effects.[43] For the critically ill, we prefer to use an epidural catheter technique. This permits repeated injections to achieve a desired effect, administration of smaller incremental doses or a continuous infusion, maintenance of analgesia for prolonged periods, and substitution or addition of local anesthetics.

Analgesia produced by spinal narcotics is mediated primarily through activation of both pre-synaptic and postsynaptic opiate receptors within the dorsal horn of the spinal cord.[44] The effect produced, unlike that following application of local anesthetic, is selective for pain transmission. Thus, spinal opiates offer a distinct advantage over local anesthesia because they leave autonomic and motor function intact. Unlike systemic narcotics, spinal opiates do not produce a significant depression of sensorium. The magnitude of analgesia produced by spinal administration of morphine cannot be achieved by systemic administration without producing significant CNS depression.

Analgesia following spinal opiate administration tends to be segmentally distributed, with the extent of rostral spread related to lipid solubility of the drug.[43] The more lipid-soluble narcotics, such as fentanyl and meperidine, are rapidly absorbed into the CNS and other tissues, and the distribution of their effect is limited. In contrast, significant rostral spread occurs with morphine, a relatively lipid-insoluble compound. Thus, the analgesia associated with spinal morphine is minimally affected by the site of injection relative to the location of pain. For example, the pain following thoracotomy is reported to be equally well controlled when epidural morphine is injected at either a lumbar or thoracic level.[45]

TABLE 82-5 Starting Dose of Epidural Morphine (mg) for Incisional Pain[a]

Patient Age (years)	Nonthoracic Surgery (Lumbar or Caudal Catheter)	THORACIC SURGERY: Thoracic Catheter	THORACIC SURGERY: Lumbar Catheter
15–44	5	4	6
45–65	4	3	5
66–75	3	2	4
76+	2	1	2

[a]Reprinted with permission from Reference 46.

The relatively slow absorption of the more lipid-insoluble narcotics also confers a long duration of action. Of those commonly administered, morphine has the longest duration of action: analgesia following a single spinal dose can last 16 to 24 h. Thus, morphine can be administered either by single injection (1 to 6 mg epidural or 0.1 to 1.0 mg intrathecal) or by a continuous infusion of 0.2 to 1.5 mg/h. When administered as a single injection, the dose should be modified based on factors such as operative site and patient age (Table 82-5).[46] Epidural administration of fentanyl (50 to 100 μg) provides analgesia lasting only 2 to 4 h, and is therefore suitable only for administration by repeated bolus or continuous infusion (25 to 100 μg/h).

Sufentanil has been used effectively as an epidural agent, but the dose required is close to that used intravenously. This implies that the removal of the drug from the epidural space limits its dural penetration. Thus, when administered epidurally, sufentanil is less selective for activation of spinal cord opiate receptors, and there is greater risk of respiratory depression if it is accidentally injected intravenously. Consequently, we do not recommend the use of this drug epidurally.

Spinal narcotics may be particularly useful for the management of patients who have developed tolerance to opioids. There is evidence that the production of systemic opiate analgesia results from a synergistic or multiplicative interaction between spinal and supraspinal (brain stem) sites.[47] The development of tolerance to this multiplicative interaction appears to occur before the development of tolerance at individual sites (brain stem or spinal cord).[48] Because spinal opiates function primarily at the spinal level and therefore act independently of this synergistic mechanism, previous exposure to opiates should have less impact on the analgesia produced.

SIDE EFFECTS. The slow uptake of the more lipid-insoluble drugs can result in significant cephalad migration leading to activation of brain stem opiate receptors. This can result in life-threatening respiratory depression. Onset of this depression is delayed because the drug must migrate from the site of injection to the brain stem; the peak vulnerable period is 6 to 10 h after a lumbar injection of morphine. The incidence of significant respiratory depression after epidural narcotic administered in general surgical patients ranges from 0.25 to 0.9 percent; in a retrospective study of approximately 9000 patients, the incidence of ventilatory depression requiring naloxone reversal was 0.25 to 0.40 percent.[49]

The incidence of nausea, vomiting, and urinary retention appears to be similar for patients treated with epidural or intramuscular morphine. The incidence of pruritus requiring therapy is approximately 10 percent, which is significantly higher than that due to systemic narcotics. However, pruritus is almost invariably reversed with very small doses of naloxone (1 to 2 μg/kg/h) which have minimal effect on analgesia.

The use of continuous infusions or more lipid-soluble narcotics minimizes the cephalad migration of drug and reduces the risk of respiratory depression and other side effects.[50]

COMBINED EPIDURAL ANESTHETIC AND OPIOID

Local anesthetics have been combined with opioids epidurally to increase analgesia, delay tachyphylaxis, and reduce the side effects associated with each technique. Compared to either technique alone, this combination provides better analgesia.[51] The improved analgesic effect and prevention of tachyphylaxis due to this combination may result from their different modes of action. Drugs typically combined are bupivacaine (0.1 to 0.125%) and morphine (0.3 to 0.4 mg/h).[52] In one study, sensory blockade was better maintained when epidural morphine was added to a continuous bupivacaine infusion.[53]

INTERCOSTAL BLOCKADE

Intercostal nerve blockade can provide analgesia for somatic pain arising from thoracic and abdominal dermatomes, including the Kocher type incision for cholecystectomy, flank (e.g., nephrectomy) incisions, fractured ribs, and for placement of a tube thoracostomy. Because of overlap of cutaneous innervation, one segment above and one segment below the involved dermatome must be blocked. For example, relief of pain from the Kocher incision, which passes through the T_7 to T_9 dermatomes, requires a unilateral blockade of the sixth to tenth intercostal nerves.

It is recommended that the intercostal nerves be blocked as close as possible to the angle of the rib. This requires that the patient's back be accessible, which is not always the case for critically ill patients. However, recent data indicate that satisfactory blockade can be achieved from a midaxillary injection because the anesthetic spreads several centimeters along the subcostal groove to block the lateral cutaneous branch of the intercostal nerve.[54] Thus, the supine position can be used in patients in whom positioning is difficult.

Three to 5 mL 0.5% bupivacaine (with epinephrine 5 μg/mL) injected into each intercostal space provides pain relief lasting from 6 to 12 h.

SIDE EFFECTS. Clinically significant pneumothorax rarely occurs following intercostal blockade. One study reported an incidence of only 0.073 percent in more than 10,000 blocks performed by physicians in all stages of training.[55] Total spinal blockade is a rare complication that may be more likely with paravertebral approaches. It occurs when local anesthetic tracks along the peridural tissue.

Toxicity may occur because systemic absorption of local anesthetic is more rapid, and blood levels are higher after this than after any other regional nerve blockade. Adding epinephrine 5 μg/mL delays systemic absorption and decreases peak blood levels. However, toxicity is rare provided maximum dose guidelines are followed (e.g., <225 mg with epinephrine). To detect signs of spinal blockade or systemic toxicity, patients should be closely observed for 15 to 20 min.

INTERPLEURAL ANESTHESIA

Injection of local anesthetic directly into the pleural cavity via a catheter provides widespread analgesia in the dermatomes supplied by the intercostal nerves. The pleural space is entered over the superior aspect of the rib and a catheter is threaded 5 to 6 cm into the space. Analgesia results from absorption of local anesthetic through the posterior intercostal membrane and blockade of the intercostal nerves. This technique provides pain control for conditions similar to those successfully treated by intercostal nerve blockade.

Intermittent injections (every 4 to 6 h) of 20 mL 0.5% bupivacaine with epinephrine 5 μg/mL usually provide excellent analgesia, often with cutaneous anesthesia to pinprick over dermatomes T_2 to T_{10}. The onset of analgesia occurs within 15 min and the duration of action of a single injection varies from 3 to 6 h.[56] Arterial and venous concentrations of bupivacaine following interpleural injection of 100 mg bupivacaine with epinephrine are below toxic levels[56] and remain so, even with repeated injections every 4 h for several days.[57] Continuous infusions of bupivacaine (0.25 to 0.5%, 5 to 10 mL/h) have been administered, but the data describing duration of adequate analgesia and the risk of systemic toxicity are limited.[58,59]

Following cholecystectomy, interpleural injection provides nearly complete pain relief and improves pulmonary function.[60] However, pain relief following thoracotomy is inconsistent and may relate to residual fluid and drainage of bupivacaine via the tube thoracostomy under suction.[59,61] To improve pain relief when tube thoracostomy drainage is required, pleural suction should be discontinued during and for 10 min after each injection of local anesthetic.[57]

An obvious concern is the possible production of a pneumothorax. Although data are limited, minor signs of pneumothorax have been observed and, to date, do not appear to be a clinically significant problem.

Anxiety and Sedation

In most patients, a balanced combination of analgesic and sedative drugs is administered to provide pain relief, control anxiety, and permit sleep.

DESIRED LEVEL OF SEDATION

The desired level of sedation for critically ill patients depends on the patient's illness and the type and extent of ventilatory support. It is important to remember that agitation and confusion can signify respiratory distress and hypoxemia, and that inappropriate sedation can mask these clinical signs and delay appropriate corrective action.

Traditionally, heavy sedation was combined with neuromuscular blockade. A 1981 report of sedative techniques used in ICUs indicated that 68 percent of physicians felt that the ideal level of sedation was achieved when the patient was completely detached from the environment and awakened only occasionally.[62] More recently, 69 percent of physicians surveyed preferred that patients be sedated only to the point of no distress and only 21 percent preferred deep sedation (10 percent had no general strategy).[63]

Several factors have contributed to this change in sedation strategy in the ICU. First, the current trend in ventilatory support is to use techniques that maintain some degree of spontaneous breathing. Second, excessive sedation may prolong recovery time. Third, prolonged immobility may contribute to venous thrombosis, pressure damage to nerves and skin, and general muscle wasting. Finally, immunologic competence may be compromised by long and continued use of sedative drugs and may increase the patient's risk of infection.[64]

ADMINISTRATION OF SEDATION

As with analgesic agents, intravenous administration of sedatives is the preferred route and continuous intravenous infusion optimal. Initially, a bolus should be given to provide a therapeutic plasma level, followed by infusion; it may be necessary to supplement the infusion with repeated boluses before performing any painful procedure.

For most critically ill patients, adjusting the dosage of sedative drugs to maintain a level of sedation between levels 2 and 3 (see Table 82-1) will ensure that the patient is comfortable, yet minimize the risk of prolonged sedation and respiratory depression when administration is discontinued.

BENZODIAZEPINES

The anxiolysis, hypnosis, amnesia, and anticonvulsant effects of the benzodiazepines make them useful for sedation of the critically ill patient. Until recently, the use of diazepam was common. However, its long elimination half-life (24 to 40 h) and that of its active metabolite, *N*-desmethyl diazepam (elimination half-life up to 96 h), may prolong recovery of consciousness, particularly in the elderly, and in patients with impaired hepatic and renal function.[29] Diazepam also causes pain on injection and may induce thrombophlebitis when administered into a peripheral vein.

Midazolam has a rapid onset of action and relatively short elimination half-life (1 to 4 h). In critically ill patients, particularly those with impaired hepatic metabolism, its elimination half-life may be prolonged (4 to 12 h).[65] Additionally, midazolam may cause hypotension, particularly in the presence of hypovolemia.[66] Respiratory depression is an expected side effect, but infusions of midazolam need not be withdrawn to wean patients successfully from mechanical ventilation. Clinical and animal studies indicate that adrenal steroidogenesis is not suppressed by a 24-h infusion of midazolam.[67]

In critically ill patients, sedation is initiated by administering 0.5 to 1.0 mg increments of midazolam every 1 to 3 min until the desired level of sedation is achieved. There is wide interindividual variability in requirement; loading doses may vary between 0.1 to 0.5 mg/kg.[68] Maintenance infusion rates typically range from 0.01 to 0.20 mg/kg/h. In one study, the mean patient requirement was 0.1 mg/kg/h for 24 h, providing adequate sedation in 93 percent of patients; 74 percent were able to respond to commands at hourly assessments.[69] When infusion was discontinued, 61 percent were immediately able to respond to commands, and the longest time to response was 405 min. In 24 percent of patients, use of the drug was limited by cardiovascular depression.

Benzodiazepine-related sedation and respiratory depression are reversible using flumazenil, an imidazobenzodiazepine currently under investigation. Because flumazenil's half-life is short (50 min), reversal of benzodiazepine effects may require a prolonged infusion.[70] Although its properties in critically ill patients have not been fully investigated, preliminary reports are encouraging. Within 2 min, full reversal of midazolam-induced sedation was achieved in 13 critically ill patients without untoward hemodynamic or respiratory effects.[71] Titrating the dose of flumazenil to the point at which reversal of sedation occurs, rather than injecting large boluses, is important and probably avoids precipitating anxiety reactions and other hemodynamic and CNS effects. Flumazenil, when approved, may allow periodic assessment of neurologic status in patients who require prolonged deep levels of sedation and increase the flexibility and safety of sedation with the benzodiazepines.

MAJOR TRANQUILIZERS

Both the phenothiazines (e.g., chlorpromazine) and the butyrophenones (e.g., droperidol and haloperidol) can be used to control acute confusional states in critically ill patients. Generally, they are used to supplement other sedative and analgesic agents. However, chlopromazine is infrequently used because of its anticholinergic and relatively potent α-adrenergic blocking properties; the latter may precipitate significant hypotension. The α-adrenergic blockade produced by the butyrophenones is milder, and these agents generally have limited effect on cardiovascular dynamics. The use of halperidol, however, has resulted in sudden death and torsades de pointes.[72]

Both droperidol and haloperidol induce a state of apathy and general detachment and, when combined with a narcotic, may produce neuroleptic analgesia. This is characterized by a trancelike state of analgesia and clinical immobility. Patients sedated with these agents may appear calm and detached, but when later interviewed, report having been apprehensive. Combining these agents with narcotics appears to reduce this complication. The butyrophenones also may precipitate extrapyramidal reactions (dyskinesia) and laryngeal dystonia, probably due to their inhibition of central dopaminergic synapses.

The dose of haloperidol required to control agitation in critically ill patients varies markedly. One recommended approach is to administer an intravenous injection of 2.5 to 5.0 mg every 30 min until agitation ceases.[73] Peak plasma levels are reached in 11 min after intravenous injection, and the half-life of the drug is 10 to 24 h. Total doses of 100 to 300 mg/day have been used by some clinicians, but lower doses generally suffice.

Droperidol is commonly prescribed (0.625 to 1.25 mg) for its antiemetic effect but is equally useful in controlling agitation and confusion when administered in the dose range described for haloperidol. The onset of action after an initial intravenous dose ranges from 3 to 10 min, although the peak effect may not be achieved for 30 min. The duration of droperidol's tranquilizing effect may last only 2 to 4 h, but patients may not be alert for 6 to 12 h.

PROPOFOL

Propofol is a new intravenous anesthetic of the alkylphenol group. It is insoluble in water and formulated in a lipid emulsion. At low doses, it produces sedation. Recovery from a single injection or a short infusion is very rapid (5 to 10 min), due to rapid redistribution and extensive metabolism (elimination half-life 1 to 3 h). It has minimal cumulative properties, even with repeated administration. Clinical studies indicate that adrenal steroidogenesis is not suppressed by a 24-h infusion of propofol.[74]

There are only a few controlled trials of propofol administration at subanesthetic doses for sedation in critically ill patients requiring mechanical ventilation.[69,74,75] These studies have shown that doses of 1 to 3 mg/kg/h of propofol effectively sedate most critically ill patients, including those with head injury. Generally, rapid and predictable levels of sedation have been achieved, and recovery has occurred within 30 min when infusion was terminated. Additionally, prolonged administration does not appear to extend recovery time. When administered at an average infusion rate of 2.85 mg/kg/h for 4 days, recovery times were not delayed, and plasma concentrations were similar each day, indicating a lack of cumulative effects.[76]

Typically, propofol sedation for facilitating mechanical ventilation is initiated by bolus injection of 1 mg/kg, followed by a continuous infusion. Critically ill patients may become hypotensive after the bolus injection; therefore, some clinicians omit the bolus and begin with a higher infusion (e.g., 3 mg/kg/h). In one study comparing propofol to midazolam, cardiovascular depression limited the use of propofol in 23 percent of patients and of midazolam in 24 percent.[69] In both groups, hypotension responded to increases in intravenous fluid.

OTHER SEDATIVES AND ANESTHETICS

BARBITURATES

Barbiturates have several disadvantages that severely limit their usefulness as sedatives for critically ill patients. These include cardiovascular and respiratory depression, loss of thermoregulation, induction of hepatic microsomal enzymes, accumulation of drug with repeated doses or infusions, tolerance and subsequent withdrawal syndrome, and possible immune suppression. In addition, at subanesthetic doses, barbiturates result in hyperalgesia (i.e., decreased pain threshold).

KETAMINE

Ketamine, a phencyclidine compound, is the only intravenous anesthetic that produces analgesia at subanesthetic doses. It produces a dissociative or cataleptic state, in which occasional movement may occur unrelated to pain. Given as a bolus dose, ketamine has a very rapid onset and short duration (8 to 10 min). Its elimination half-life ranges from 1 to 3 h.[77] The drug may accumulate with continued administration.

Ketamine's undesirable effects include pulmonary and systemic hypertension, tachycardia, increased intracranial pressure, excessive upper airway secretions, and emergence reactions (e.g., vivid dreams and hallucinations). Ketamine may also produce myocardial depression. Administering drying agents, such as atropine and glycopyrrolate, or benzodiazepines immediately before ketamine may, respectively, attenuate secretions and emergence reactions.

Ketamine has been primarily used in the ICU during short painful procedures, such as dressing changes and minor debridement of wounds in burned patients. Low intravenous doses (0.5 to 1.0 mg/kg) provide 5 to 20 min of intense analgesia. An additional dose of 0.25 to 0.5 mg/kg is used for procedures lasting longer than 10 to 15 min. Alternatively, an intramuscular dose of 2 to 3 mg/kg will provide a similar effect and is less likely to cause respiratory depression. Tolerance develops with repeated use. Nonintubated burn patients should be kept NPO for 4 h prior to administration.

Ketamine is particularly useful as a sedative for patients with asthma requiring mechanical ventilation because hyperinflation and hemodynamic compromise may occur secondary to intrinsic positive end-expiratory pressure (PEEPi), limiting the administration of other sedative agents without pharmacologic support of the circulation.[78] In these cases, ketamine's sympathomimetic effects may be beneficial for maintaining circulatory stability and providing a bronchodilatory effect.

Ketamine has also been used to provide analgesia during postoperative mechanical ventilation.[79] It is given in relatively low (subhypnotic) doses (10 to 30 μg/kg/min), often in conjunction with diazepam. Although it provides profound analgesia, in one study, 20 percent of such patients complained of unpleasant hallucinations.[79]

INHALATION ANESTHETIC AGENTS

Inhalation anesthetics, such as nitrous oxide, halothane and isoflurane, are used in the ICU to provide analgesia and sedation and to treat refractory status asthmaticus and status epilepticus.[80–82] Because of the hazards associated with the use of the inhaled agents, most reports suggest that experienced anesthesia personnel administer them to critically ill patients. Adequate scavenging of exhaust gases is mandatory to prevent contamination with waste gases that can cause sedation of medical personnel and occupational risks related to long-term anesthetic exposure. Commonly used operating room ventilators have limited pressure and flow capabilities limiting their usefulness for patients with acute respiratory failure requiring high peak airway pressures (e.g., >50 cmH_2O) and high minute ventilation (e.g., >15 L/min).[83] Of the commonly used critical care ventilators, only the Siemens Servo 900C or D models have the capability of delivering anesthetic gases.

Nitrous oxide has analgesic activity at subanesthetic doses and has been used both intermittently and continuously in concentrations ranging from 30 to 70 percent. High concentrations limit the available inspired oxygen fraction, which limits the use of nitrous oxide in patients with acute hypoxemic respiratory failure. Its use is contraindicated if there is the potential to expand closed air spaces (e.g., pneumothorax, lung cysts, ileus). It will exacerbate increased pulmonary vascular resistance and should not be used in patients with adult respiratory distress syndrome (ARDS). Prolonged (greater than few days) or repeated administration of nitrous oxide disturbs DNA metabolism and may produce megaloblastic changes in the bone marrow. Because these disturbances may be particularly detrimental to critically ill patients, the use of nitrous oxide for analgesia and sedation in the ICU remains controversial.[84]

Recently, subanesthetic concentrations of isoflurane (0.1 to 0.4%) were evaluated and compared to midazolam for sedation in critically ill patients requiring postoperative mechanical ventilation.[85] The average concentration of isoflurane used for sedation was 0.21% (range 0.1 to 0.4%); the mean infusion rate of midazolam 0.05 mg/kg/h (range 0.014 to 0.14 mg/kg/h). In both groups, analgesia was provided with incremental doses of morphine, as needed; the median total doses of morphine were similar. Patients receiving isoflurane recovered more rapidly from sedation. Cardiovascular responses with both techniques were similar, and in the absence of hypovolemia, neither technique was associated with deleterious hemodynamic effects. This report suggests that isoflurane can be a useful alternative to intravenous sedation for patients receiving mechanical ventilation. However, further studies are needed to assess other, infrequent side effects and possible complications of prolonged administration.

Beneficial Effects of Analgesia and Sedation

The effects of pain therapy are a function of the quality of analgesia and the technique used for pain control. Except in very high doses, systemically administered narcotics do not provide analgesia comparable to that obtained using regional techniques. (And, as a result, patients treated with regional analgesia ambulate sooner, and may have a shorter hospital stay.[86]) Furthermore, independent of the analgesia, techniques for pain control have local or systemic effects. These, in turn, may alter outcome.

Treatment of anxiety relies on the appropriate use of sedation, adequate pain control, and frequent communication and reassurance from critical care staff. Effective therapy may reduce not only the acute emotional suffering but also decrease the incidence of postoperative/traumatic neurosis.

RESPIRATORY FUNCTION

There is always a respiratory deficit following upper abdominal and thoracic surgery or blunt thoracic trauma. Systemic administration of narcotics may exacerbate this deficit by inducing significant respiratory depression,[87] a particularly undesirable effect in critically ill patients. Regional techniques generally do not induce depression, but may fail to restore respiratory function to preoperative levels.[5] Regional analgesia has been reported to improve lung volumes and oxygenation and decrease pulmonary complications following abdominal[86,88,89] and thoracic surgery[90] or blunt thoracic trauma.[2,91–93] These findings, however, are not uniform; several studies have failed to document improved pulmonary function and reduced pulmonary complications with either epidural local anesthesia or epidural opioids.[93–96] Even with complete relief of pain, the epidural methods only partially restore FVC and FEV_1, minimally improve FRC and modestly increase oxygenation.[1] Thus, pain is only one of several factors leading to a restrictive pulmonary pattern postoperatively.

Diaphragm dysfunction has been suggested as a major determinant of the decreased lung volumes observed after upper abdominal[4,97] and thoracic surgery[98] and, to some extent, blunt thoracic trauma. This diaphragmatic dysfunction has been attributed to a visceral or somatic reflex decreasing phrenic nerve activity. Spasm and splinting of the abdominal and intercostal muscles also may be involved. This is supported by the observation in cats that stimulation of the intercostal muscle proprioceptive afferents reflexively causes a decrease in phrenic motor activity.[99] Thoracic epidural local anesthesia decreases diaphragmatic dysfunction, increases tidal volume, and decreases respiratory frequency,[100] while spinal opiates do not.[101,102] These effects of epidural local anesthesia may be direct or indirect. Visceral or somatic inhibitory afferents may be directly blocked at the level of spinal roots. Alternatively, or additionally, relaxation of abdominal muscle tone due to motor blockade or deafferentation of abdominal proprioceptors may indirectly benefit diaphragmatic mechanics. The decreased abdominal muscle tone might lessen the tension imposed on the diaphragm and reduce phrenophrenic inhibitory afferents and improve diaphragmatic excursion.

In summary, pain is a significant problem after major surgery and trauma, and its relief necessary not only for patient comfort but also for efficient respiratory therapy. However, pain does not appear to be the sole mechanism underlying respiratory muscle dysfunction. Inhibitory reflexes of the phrenic nerve are involved and do not appear to be blocked by spinal opiates but are partially blocked by thoracic epidural local anesthetics. Nevertheless, the analgesia provided by spinally administered opiates or local anesthetic solutions improves respiratory function more than systemically delivered narcotics and can be expected to reduce morbidity in some situations.

STRESS RESPONSE AND CARDIAC MORBIDITY

Traditionally, the stress response has been considered a homeostatic mechanism that helps to heal tissue and adapt to injury. However, recent data suggest that, at least in part, the response may be detrimental. The type and adequacy of pain relief may affect the magnitude of the pathophysiologic changes that occur following surgery or trauma.

Parenteral opioids decrease heart rate and myocardial wall tension and suppress the surgical stress response in a dose-dependent manner. In critically ill patients, intravenous doses of morphine ranging from 0.05 to 0.3 mg/kg/h decrease total body oxygen consumption by about 20 percent and energy expenditure by 10 to 30 percent.[103] Complete suppression of most endocrine and metabolic stress responses requires higher doses (e.g., 2 to 4 mg/kg of morphine or 100 μg/kg fentanyl).[104] Intravenous administration of high dose sufentanil (1 μg/kg/h) after coronary artery surgery resulted in a greater decrease in double product and in severity of ischemic episodes than the more conventional technique of intermittent intravenous administration of morphine (1 to 10 mg prn).[105]

The use of epidural local anesthetic solutions to induce a neural blockade from T_4 to S_5 markedly attenuates the stress response of lower abdominal or peripheral surgery.[104] Hormone levels are decreased, nitrogen balance and immunocompetence enhanced, and the incidence of thromboembolism reduced. However, epidural local anesthetic attenuation of the stress response is incomplete following upper abdominal and thoracic surgery; some hormonal responses are attenuated, but others are not (e.g., some studies have found a significant blunting of the hyperglycemic and catecholamine responses).[106] This incomplete suppression could be the result of unblocked vagal afferents, insufficient sympathetic blockade, or incomplete somatic afferent blockade.

Epidural local anesthetics also confer benefits derived from the associated sympathectomy. For example, they improve blood flow to the lower extremities. Additionally, they have both a fibrinolytic and an antithrombotic effect,[107] and reduce leukocyte locomotion, thereby preventing these cells from adhering to and invading venous endothelium.[108] A decreased incidence of thromboembolism has been documented following the intraoperative and postoperative use of epidural local anesthetics in patients requiring hip surgery[109] and retropubic prostatectomy.[110]

Spinally administered opioids provide a modest reduction in the stress hormone response. In one study of patients undergoing aortic reconstruction, postoperative epidural morphine decreased myocardial demand (heart rate and double-product) when compared to conventional parenteral morphine.[111] Following upper abdominal surgery, the suppressive effect of epidural morphine was found to be less than that of epidural bupivacaine but again greater than that of parenteral narcotics.[112] Thus, nonopiate-receptor mechanisms are also involved in activation of the stress response.

A major limitation in extending postoperative data to trauma-induced injury is that perioperative intervention is most often instituted prior to the stressful event. Although less effective, attenuation of the stress response has been shown to occur when epidural blockade is instituted following surgery or trauma.[113]

Postoperative cardiac complications appear to be fewer in high-risk patients whose anesthetic management combines intraoperative epidural and general anesthetic techniques with postoperative epidural analgesia. In one study, improved outcome was associated with attenuation of the cortisol response,[114] and in another, decreased cardiac complications (e.g., MI and arterial graft occlusion) were correlated with normalizing intraoperative and postoperative hypercoagulability.[115]

CASE PRESENTATION

A 38-year-old man was admitted to the hospital with progressive pleuritic chest pain and dyspnea. A chest x-ray and computed tomogram of the thorax showed bilateral bullous disease and an air fluid level in the left apex consistent with a lung abscess. His past medical history included a 20 pack-year history of smoking, substance abuse including intravenous heroin and inhalation of crack cocaine, and a previous admission for thoracic stab wounds requiring bilateral tube thoracostomies. On hospital day 5, the patient underwent a left posteriolateral thoracotomy for resection of the abscessed bulla. Preoperative pulmonary function revealed an FEV_1 of 2.9 L, a FVC of 4.4 L, and a diffusing capacity which was 70 percent of predicted. An arterial blood-gas sample taken while he breathed room air showed a pH of 7.39, a Pa_{CO_2} of 49 mmHg and a Pa_{O_2} of 64 mmHg. Medications included antibiotics and methadone, 40 mg/day.

After induction, anesthesia was maintained with isoflurane, supplemented by 23 mg intravenous morphine. Intraoperative pulmonary gas exchange was satisfactory. Before closing the thoracotomy, the surgeons directly infiltrated the intercostal nerves at three levels above the surgical site and two levels below using 5 mL 0.5% bupivacaine for each segment.

Soon after arrival in the postanesthesia care unit, an arterial blood-gas sample taken while the patient breathed 6 L/min of oxygen via nasal cannula revealed a pH of 7.29, a Pa_{CO_2} of 58 mmHg and a Pa_{O_2} of 63 mmHg. Postoperatively, he complained repeatedly of shortness of breath and persistent pain, despite treatment with 9 mg intravenous morphine. His respiratory rate varied between 20 and 24 breaths/min, and there was splinting of the left hemithorax. An arterial blood-gas sample taken while he breathed supplemental oxygen (15 L/min via face mask with a reservoir bag) indicated a pH of 7.33, a Pa_{CO_2} of 51 mmHg, and Pa_{O_2} of 113 mmHg. The patient remained tachypneic and required an additional 35 mg intravenous morphine for pain relief over the next 9 h. Respiratory therapy measures included placing the patient in the sitting position, encouraging deep breathing exercises via the incentive spirometer, and using inhaled bronchodilators. However, despite these measures, respiratory function deteriorated, the patient becoming progressively diaphoretic, lethargic, and more tachypneic. An arterial blood-gas sample obtained while breathing nearly 100% oxygen via a high flow nebulizer revealed a pH 7.25, Pa_{CO_2} of 73 mmHg, Pa_{O_2} of 70 mmHg. Chest x-ray examination revealed bilateral low lung volumes, elevated hemidiaphragms, and basilar atelectasis. Because of the worsening hypercapnia, the patient was treated with 0.2 mg intravenous naloxone. This action increased pain and caused a rapid decline in oxygen saturation. Arterial blood-gas values were pH 7.32, Pa_{CO_2} 67 mmHg, and Pa_{O_2} 68 mmHg. Respiratory rate had increased to 35 to 40 breaths/min and tidal excursion appeared limited, with obvious splinting. Respiratory failure appeared imminent. Tracheal intubation and mechanical ventilation were considered, pending trial of epidural analgesia and assessment of respiratory function.

After informing the patient of impending respiratory failure, he approved the placement of a thoracic (T_4 to T_5) epidural catheter. (Preoperatively, he had declined this method for postoperative analgesia.) Segmental epidural analgesia was provided by a bolus of 8 mL 0.5% bupivacaine preceded by an injection of 3 mL 1.0% lidocaine with 1:200,000 epinephrine. Onset of epidural analgesia occurred within 8 min and was associated with a rapid and dramatic improvement in respiratory function. Coincident with the subjective relief of pain and clear reduction in anxiety, respiratory rate decreased to 20 breaths/min and tidal volume significantly improved. Improvement in pulmonary gas exchange was reflected in arterial blood-gas values of pH 7.33, Pa_{CO_2} 55 mmHg, and Pa_{O_2} 189 mmHg. A continuous epidural infusion of 0.25% bupivacaine was combined with fentanyl 5 μg/mL at 8 mL/h to maintain excellent segmental analgesia from T_2 to T_8. There were no significant changes in hemodynamic function. Epidural infusion was continued for approximately 48 h, at which time the patient's pulmonary oxygen exchange was satisfactory while breathing room air. He was transferred to the ward and discharged from the hospital 48 h later.

CASE DISCUSSION

The patient's previous history of narcotic and cocaine abuse and daily methadone therapy complicated postoperative pain management by conventional parenteral narcotic techniques. This is dramatically illustrated by his obtaining only poor relief of pain with relatively large doses of morphine.

Postoperative analgesia was initiated with intraoperative intercostal blockade performed by the surgeon. Although this technique will block the thoracic dermatomes for 6 to 12 h, the thoracotomy wound involves not only the several intercostal spaces above and below the space through which the incision is made, but also the muscles of the shoulder girdle. In addition, the presence of tube thoracostomy drains irritates the parietal pleura, which usually involves a wider distribution than the several segments of intercostal blockade. Interpleural instillation of local anesthesia might be expected to improve the analgesia following thoracotomy better than an intercostal blockade, but was not chosen in this case because of the expected postoperative air leak and the requirement for continuous thoracostomy tube suction. Consequently, epidural blockade appeared to be the regional anesthetic technique most likely to succeed for this patient.

Respiratory dysfunction after thoracotomy manifested as tachypnea and hypopnea with splinting progressed to imminent respiratory failure with hypoxemia and hypercapnia nearly requiring tracheal intubation. Hypoxemia was most likely a consequence of hypoventilation-induced lung collapse, as suggested by the chest x-ray findings. Hypercapnia probably was due to respiratory depression from the large doses of narcotics or diaphragmatic dysfunction following thoracotomy. The basilar atelectasis and elevated hemidiaphragms visible on the chest x-ray may have reflected decreased contribution of the diaphragm to quiet tidal breathing. (Diaphragmatic dysfunction has been correlated with development of postthoracotomy respiratory failure.)

Following thoracic epidural blockade and complete pain relief, the patient showed steady improvement in lung mechanical function and gas exchange. Because local anesthetic agents were used, a thoracic epidural technique was chosen to permit segmental analgesia without inducing widespread blockade and increasing the potential for hypotension and motor blockade. Fentanyl was combined with bupivacaine to enhance the analgesia and prevent tachyphylaxis.

Epidural local anesthetics can provide complete pain relief and improve postoperative respiratory function. Specifically, FVC and tidal volume are increased and respiratory frequency decreased. Additionally, inhibitory reflexes of the phrenic nerve are partially blocked, improving diaphragm function. Whether the reversal of respiratory failure following thoracic epidural blockade was related to complete pain relief or to improved diaphragmatic function cannot be determined.

References

1. Craig DB: Postoperative recovery of pulmonary function. Anesth Analg 60:46, 1981.
2. Dittmann M, Wolff GA: A rationale for epidural analgesia in the treatment of multiple rib fractures. Intensive Care Med 4:192, 1978.
3. Duggan J, Drummond GB: Activity of lower intercostal and abdominal muscle after upper abdominal surgery. Anesth Analg 66:852, 1987.
4. Dureuil B, Cantineau JP, Desmonts JM: Effects of upper or lower abdominal surgery on diaphragmatic function. Br J Anaesth 59:1230, 1987.

5. Bromage PR, Camporesi E, Chestnut D: Epidural narcotics for postoperative analgesia. Anesth Analg 59:473, 1980.
6. Britton B, Hawkey C, Wood W, Peele M: Stress—A significant factor in venous thrombosis? Br J Surg 61:814, 1974.
7. Mansfield A: Alteration in fibrinolysis associated with surgery and venous thrombosis. Br J Surg 59:754, 1972.
8. Slade MS, Simmons CJ, Yunnis E, Greenberg LF: Immunodepression after major surgery in normal patients. Surgery 78:363, 1974.
9. Halter J, Pflug A, Porte D: Mechanisms of plasma catecholamine increase during surgical stress in man. J Clin Endocrinol Metab 45:936, 1977.
10. Mangano DT: Perioperative cardiac morbidity. Anesthesiology 72:153, 1990.
11. Mangano DT, SPI Group: Characteristics of electrocardiographic ischemia in high-risk patients undergoing surgery. J Electrocardiol 23:20, 1991.
12. Rao TK, Jacobs KH, El-Etr AA: Reinfarction following anesthesia in patients with myocardial infarction. Anesthesiology 59:499, 1983.
13. Bion JF: Sedation and analgesia in the intensive care unit. Hosp Update 14:1272, 1988.
14. Bergbom-Engberg I, Haljamae H: Assessment of patient's experience of discomforts during respiratory therapy. Crit Care Med 17:1068, 1989.
15. Blacher RA: Awareness during surgery. Anesthesiology 61:1, 1984.
16. Merskey H: Pain terms: A list with definitions and notes on usage. Recommended by the International Association for the Study of Pain Subcommittee on Taxonomy. Pain 6:249, 1979.
17. Chapman CR, Casey KL, Dubner R, et al: Pain measurement: An overview. Pain 22:1, 1985.
18. Ramsay MAE, Savege TM, Simpson BRJ, Goodwin R: Controlled sedation with alphaxalone-alphadolone. Br Med J 2:656, 1974.
19. Sessler DI, Stoen R, Olofsson CI, Chow F: Lower esophageal contractility predicts movement during skin incision in patients anesthetized with halothane, but not with nitrous oxide and alfentanil. Anesthesiology 70:42, 1989.
20. Austin KL, Stapleton JV, Mather LE: Relationship between blood meperidine concentrations and analgesic response. Anesthesiology 53:460, 1980.
21. Austin KL, Stapleton JV, Mather LE: Multiple intramuscular injections. A major source of variability in analgesic response to meperidine. Pain 8:46, 1980.
22. Sechzer PH: Objective measurement of pain. Anesthesiology 29:209, 1968.
23. Tamsen A, Hartvig P, Fagerlund B, et al: Patient-controlled analgesic therapy. Acta Anaesth Scand 74:157, 1982.
24. Gibbs JM, Johnson HD, Davis FM: Patient administration of i.v. buprenorphine for postoperative pain relief using the Cardiff demand analgesic apparatus. Br Anaesth 54:279, 1982.
25. White PF: Mishaps with patient-controlled analgesia. Anesthesiology 66:81, 1987.
26. Eisenach JC, Grice SC, Dewan DM: Patient-controlled analgesia following cesarean section: A comparison with epidural and intramuscular narcotics. Anesthesiology 68:444, 1988.
27. Osbourne RJ, Joel SP, Slevin ML: Morphine intoxication in renal failure: The role of morphine 6 glucuronide. Br Med J 292:1548, 1986.
28. Guffin A, Girard D, Kaplan JA: Shivering following cardiac surgery: Hemodynamic changes and reversal. Anesthesia 1:24, 1987.
29. Bodenham A, Shelly MP, Park GR: The altered pharmacokinetics and pharmacodynamics of drugs commonly used in critically ill patients. Clin Pharmacokinet 14:347, 1988.
30. Stanski DR, Hugg CC Jr: Alfentanil—A kinetically predictable narcotic analgesic. Anesthesiology 57:435, 1982.
31. Maitre PO, Vozeh S, Heykants J: Population pharmacokinetics of alfentanil: The average dose-plasma concentration relationship and interindividual variablity in patients. Anesthesiology 62:3, 1987.
32. Hoffmann P: Continuous infusions of fentanyl and alfentanil in intensive care. Eur J Anesth 1(suppl):71, 1987.
33. Sosnowski M, Yaksh TL: Symmetric tolerance after continuous spinal infusion of mu agonists in rats. Anesthesiology 71:A621, 1989.
34. Scott DB: Acute pain management, in Cousins MJ, Bridenbaugh PO (eds): *Neural Blockade in Clinical Anesthesia and Management of Pain*. Philadelphia, Lippincott, 1988, p 861.
35. Bromage PR: Mechanism of action of extradural analgesia. Br J Anaesth 47:199, 1975.
36. Moir DD: Ventilatory function during epidural analgesia. Br J Anaesth 35:3, 1963.
37. McCarthy GS: The effect of thoracic extradural analgesia on pulmonary gas distribution, functional residual capacity and airway closure. Br J Anaesth 48:243, 1976.
38. Freund FG, Bonica JJ, Ward RJ, Kennedy TJAF: Ventilatory reserve and level of motor block during high spinal and epidural anesthesia. Anesthesiology 28:834, 1967.
39. Sundberg A, Wattwil M, Arvill A: Respiratory effects of high thoracic epidural anaesthesia. Acta Anaesthesiol Scand 30:215, 1986.
40. Pert CB, Kuhar MJ, Snyder SH: Opiate receptor: Autoradiographic localization in rat brain. Proc Natl Acad Sci USA 73:3729, 1976.
41. Yaksh TL, Rudy TA: Analgesia mediated by a direct spinal action of narcotics. Science 192:1357, 1976.
42. Wang JK, Nauss LA, Thomas JE: Pain relief by intrathecally applied morphine in man. Anesthesiology 50:149, 1979.
43. Cousins MJ, Mather LE: Intrathecal and epidural administration of opioids. Anesthesiology 61:276, 1984.
44. Yaksh TL: Spinal opiate analgesia: Characteristics and principles of action. Pain 11:293, 1981.
45. Fromme GA, Steidl LJ, Danielson DR: Comparison of lumbar and thoracic epidural morphine for relief of postthoracotomy pain. Anesth Analg 64:454, 1985.
46. Ready LB, Oden R, Chadwick HS, et al: Development of an anesthesiology-based postoperative pain management service. Anesthesiology 68:100, 1988.
47. Yeung JC, Rudy TA: Multiple interaction between narcotic agonisms expressed at spinal and supraspinal sites of antinociceptive action as revealed by concurrent intrathecal and intracerebroventricular injections of morphine. J Pharmacol Exp Ther 215:633, 1980.
48. Roerig SC, O'Brien SM, Fujimoto JM, Wilcox GL: Tolerance to morphine analgesia-decreased multiplicative interaction between spinal and supraspinal sites. Brain Res 308:360, 1984.
49. Gustafsson LL, Schildt B, Jacobsen KJ: Adverse effects of extradural and intrathecal opiates: Report of a nationwide survey in Sweden. Br J Anaesth 54:479, 1982.
50. El-Baz NM, Faber LP, Jensik RJ: Continuous epidural infusion of morphine for treatment of pain after thoracic surgery: A new technique. Anesth Analg 63:757, 1984.
51. Cullen ML, Staren ED, El-Ganzouri A, et al: Continuous epidural infusion for analgesia after major abdominal operations: A randomized, prospective, double-blind study. Surgery 98:718, 1985.

52. Logas WG, El-Baz N, El-Ganzouri A, et al: Continuous thoracic epidural analgesia for postoperative pain relief following thoracotomy: A randomized prospective study. Anesthesiology 67:787, 1987.
53. Hjortso NC, Lund C, Mogensen T, et al: Epidural morphine improves pain relief and maintains sensory analgesia during continuous epidural bupivacaine after abdominal surgery. Anesth Analg 65:1033, 1986.
54. Thompson GE, Moore DC: Celiac plexus, intercostal, and minor peripheral blockade, in Cousins MJ, Bridenbaugh PO (eds): *Neural Blockade in Clinical Anesthesia and Management of Pain.* Philadelphia, Lippincott, 1988, pp 503–530.
55. Moore DC, Bridenbaugh LD: Pneumothorax: Its incidence following intercostal nerve block. JAMA 182:1005, 1962.
56. Stromskag KE, Reiestad F, Holmqvist ELO, Ogenstad S: Intrapleural administration of 0.25%, 0.375%, and 0.5% bupivacaine with epinephrine after cholecystectomy. Anesth Analg 67:430, 1988.
57. Scheinin B, Lindgren L, Rosenberg PH: Treatment of post-thoracotomy pain with intermittent instillations of intrapleural bupivacaine. Acta Anaesthesiol Scand 33:156, 1989.
58. Rocco A, Reiestad F, Gudman J, McKay W: Intrapleural administration of local anesthetics for pain relief in patients with multiple rib fractures. Reg Anesth 12:10, 1987.
59. Rosenberg PH, Scheinin BMA, Lepantalo MJA, Lindfors O: Continuous intrapleural infusion of bupivacaine for analgesia after thoracotomy. Anesthesiology 67:811, 1987.
60. VandeBoncouer TR, Riegler FX, Gautt RS, Weinberg GL: A randomized, double-blind comparison of the effects of interpleural bupivacaine and saline on morphine requirements and pulmonary function after cholecystectomy. Anesthesiology 71:339, 1989.
61. Kambam JR, Hammon J, Parris WC, Lupineti FM: Intrapleural analgesia for post-thoracotomy pain and blood levels of bupivacaine following intrapleural injection. Can J Anaesth 36:106, 1989.
62. Merriman HM: The techniques used to sedate ventilated patients. Intensive Care Med 7:217, 1981.
63. Ritz R, Spoendin M, Haefeli W: Long-term sedation in the critically ill. Update Intensive Care Emerg Med 10:723, 1990.
64. Watt I, Ledingham IM: Mortality amongst multiple trauma patients admitted to an intensive therapy unit. Anaesthesia 39:973, 1984.
65. Dirksen MSC, Vree TB, Driessen JJ: Clinical pharmacokinetics of long-term infusion of midazolam in critically ill patients—Preliminary results. Anaesth Intensive Care 15:440, 1987.
66. Adams P, Gelman S, Reeves JG, et al: Midazolam pharmacodynamics and pharmacokinetics during acute hypovolemia. Anesthesiology 63:140, 1985.
67. Shapiro JM, Westphal LM, White PF, et al: Midazolam infusion for sedation in the intensive care unit: Effect on adrenal function. Anesthesiology 64:394, 1986.
68. Michalk S, Moncorge C, Fichelle A, et al: Midazolam infusion for basal sedation in intensive care: Absence of accumulation. Intensive Care Med 15:37, 1988.
69. Aitkenhead AR, Willatts SM, Parks GR, et al: Comparison of propofol and midazolam for sedation in critically ill patients. Lancet 2:704, 1989.
70. Bodenham A, Park GR: Reversal of prolonged sedation using flumazenil in critically ill patients. Anaesthesia 44:603, 1989.
71. Geller E, Halpern P, Barzelai E, et al: Midazolam infusion and the benzodiazepine antagonist flumazenil for sedation of intensive care patients. Resuscitation 16:S31, 1988.
72. Zee-Cheng CS, Mueller CE, Seifert CF, Gibbi HR: Haloperidol and torsades de pointes. Ann Intern Med 102:418, 1985.
73. Bouckoms AJ: Pain relief in the intensive care unit. J Intensive Care Med 3:32, 1988.
74. Newman LH, McDonald JC, Wallace PM, Ledingham IM: Propofol infusion for sedation in intensive care. Anaesthesia 42:929, 1987.
75. Farling PA, Johnston JR, Coppel DL: Propofol infusion for sedation of patients with head injury in intensive care. Anaesthesia 44:222, 1989.
76. Beller JP, Pottecher T, Lugnier A, et al: Prolonged sedation with propofol in ICU patients: Recovery and blood concentration changes during periodic interruptions in infusion. Br J Anaesth 61:583, 1988.
77. White PF, Way WL, Trevor AJ: Ketamine—Its pharmacology and therapeutic uses. Anesthesiology 56:119, 1982.
78. Park GR, Manara AR, Mendel L, Bateman PE: Ketamine infusion: Its use as a sedative, inotrope and bronchodilator in a critically ill patient. Anaesthesia 42:980, 1987.
79. Joachimsson PO, Hedstrand U, Eklund A: Low-dose ketamine infusion for analgesia during postoperative ventilator treatment. Acta Anaesthesiol Scand 30:697, 1986.
80. Kofke WA, Snider MT, Young RSK, Ramer JC: Prolonged low flow isoflurane anesthesia for status epilepticus. Anesthesiology 62:653, 1985.
81. Bierman MI, Brown M, Muren O, et al: Prolonged isoflurane anesthesia in status asthmaticus. Crit Care Med 14:832, 1986.
82. Johnston RG, Noseworthy TW, Friesen EG, et al: Isoflurane therapy for status asthmaticus in children and adults. Chest 97:698, 1990.
83. Marks JD, Schapera A, Kraemer RW, Katz JA: Pressure and flow limitations of anesthesia ventilators. Anesthesiology 71:403, 1989.
84. Amos RJ, Amess JAL, Hinds CL, Mollin DL: Incidence and pathogenesis of acute megaloblastic bone-marrow change in patients receiving intensive care. Lancet 2:835, 1982.
85. Kong KL, Willatts SM, Prys-Roberts C: Isoflurane compared with midazolam for sedation in the intensive care unit. Br Med J 298:1277, 1989.
86. Rawal N, Sjostrand U, Christoffersson E, et al: Comparison of intramuscular and epidural morphine for postoperative analgesia in the grossly obese: Influence on postoperative ambulation and pulmonary function. Anesth Analg 63:583, 1984.
87. Catley DM, Thornton C, Jordan C, et al: Pronounced episodic oxygen desaturation in the postoperative period: Its association with ventilatory pattern and analgesic regimen. Anesthesiology 63:20, 1985.
88. Spence AA, Smith G: Postoperative analgesia and lung function: A comparison of morphine with extradural block. Br J Anaesth 43:144, 1971.
89. Cushieri RJ, Morran CG, Howie CJ, McArdle CS: Postoperative pain and pulmonary complications: Comparison of three analgesic regimens. Br J Surg 72:495, 1985.
90. Hasenbos M, Van Edmond J, Gielen M, Crul JF: Postoperative analgesia by high thoracic epidural versus intramuscular nicomorphine after thoracotomy. Acta Anaesthesiol Scand 31:608, 1987.
91. Bolliger CT, VanEeden SF: Treatment of multiple rib fractures: Randomized controlled trial comparing ventilatory with nonventilatory management. Chest 97:943, 1990.
92. MacKersie RC, Shackford SR, Hoyt DB, Karagianes VG: Continuous epidural fentanyl analgesia: Ventilatory function improvement with routine use in treatment of blunt chest. Trauma 27:1207, 1987.
93. Cicala RS, Voeller GR, Fox T, et al: Epidural analgesia in thoracic trauma: Effects of lumbar morphine and thoracic

bupivacaine on pulmonary function. Crit Care Med 18:229, 1990.
94. Hjortso NC, Andersen T, Frosig F, et al: A controlled study of the effect of epidural analgesia with local anesthetics and morphine on morbidity after abdominal surgery. Acta Anaesthesiol Scand 29:790, 1985.
95. Hendolin H, Lahtinen J, Lansimies E, Tuppurainen T: The effect of thoracic epidural analgesia on postoperative stress and morbidity. Ann Chir Gynaecol 76:234, 1987.
96. Jayr C, Mollie A, Bourgain JL, et al: Postoperative pulmonary complications: General anesthesia with postoperative parenteral morphine compared with epidural analgesia. Surgery 104:57, 1988.
97. Ford GT, Whitelaw WA, Rosenal WT, et al: Diaphragm function after upper abdominal surgery in humans. Am Rev Respir Dis 127:431, 1983.
98. Maeda J, Nakahara K, Ohno K, et al: Diaphragm function after pulmonary resection: Relationship to postoperative respiratory failure. Am Rev Respir Dis 137:678, 1988.
99. Shannon R: Intercostal and abdominal muscle afferent influence on medullary dorsal respiratory group neuron. Respir Physiol 39:73, 1980.
100. Mankikian B, Cantineau JP, Bertrand M, et al: Improvement of diaphragmatic function by a thoracic extradural block after upper abdominal surgery. Anesthesiology 68:379, 1988.
101. Clergue F, Montembault C, Despierre O, et al: Respiratory effects of intrathecal morphine after upper abdominal surgery. Anesthesiology 61:677, 1984.
102. Simonneau G, Vivien A, Sartene R, et al: Diaphragm dysfunction induced by upper abdominal surgery. Am Rev Respir Dis 128:899, 1983.
103. Swinamer DL, Phang PT, Jones RL, et al: Effect of routine administration of analgesia on energy expenditure in critically ill patients. Chest 92:4, 1988.
104. Kehlet H: Modification of responses to surgery by neural blockade: Clinical implications, in Cousins MJ, Bridenbaugh PO (eds): *Neural Blockade in Clinical Anesthesia and Management of Pain.* Philadelphia, Lippincott, 1988, p 145.
105. Siliciano D, Hollenberg M, Goehner P, Mangano D: Use of continuous vs intermittent narcotics after CABG surgery: Effects on myocardial ischemia. Anesth Analg 70:S371, 1990.
106. Hakanson E, Rutberg H, Jorfeldt L, Martensson J: Effects of the extradural administration of morphine or bupivacaine, on the metabolic response to upper abdominal surgery. Br J Anaesth 57:394, 1985.
107. Modig J, Borg T, Bagge L, Saldeen T: Role of extradural and of general anesthesia in fibrinolysis and coagulation after total hip replacement. Br J Anaesth 55:625, 1983.
108. Stewart G: Antithrombotic activity of local anesthetics in several canine models. Reg Anesth 7:S89, 1982.
109. Modig J, Borg T, Karlstrom G, et al: Thromboembolism after total hip replacement: Role of epidural and general anesthesia. Anesth Analg 62:174, 1983.
110. Hendolin H, Mattila M, Poikolainen E: The effect of lumbar epidural analgesia on the development of deep venous thrombosis of the legs after open prostatectomy. Acta Chir Scand 147:425, 1981.
111. Diebel LN, Lange MP, Schneider F, et al: Cardiopulmonary complications after major surgery: A role for epidural analgesia? Surgery 102:660, 1987.
112. Rutberg H, Hakanson E, Anderberg B, et al: Effects of the extradural administration of morphine, or bupivacaine, on the endocrine response to upper abdominal surgery. Br J Anaesth 56:233, 1984.
113. Moller IW, Rem J, Brandt MR, Kehlet H: Effect of posttraumatic epidural analgesia on the cortisol and hyperglycemic response to surgery. Acta Anaesthesiol Scand 26:56, 1982.
114. Yeager MP, Glass DD, Neff RK, Brinck-Johnsen T: Epidural anesthesia and analgesia in high-risk surgical patients. Anesthesiology 66:729, 1987.
115. Tuman KJ, McCarthy RJ, Spiess BD, Ivankovich AD: Epidural anesthesia and analgesia decreases postoperative hypercoagulability in high-risk vascular patients. Anesth Analg 90:S414, 1990.

Chapter 83

MUSCLE RELAXANTS

MITCHELL F. KEAMY III

KEY POINTS

- *Paralytics act at the neuromuscular junction by inhibiting acetylcholine-triggered depolarization.*
- *Smooth-muscle function is not directly influenced by these agents.*
- *Succinylcholine (Sch) is the only depolarizing agent used clinically.*
- *Sch has the advantage of brief duration of action but can cause hyperkalemia and elevation of intracranial pressure.*
- *Several nondepolarizing agents are available for use in the critically ill patient and offer longer duration of action and few side effects.*
- *Most depolarizing agents undergo hepatic and/or renal metabolism.*
- *Atracurium is a nondepolarizing agent which is autolytic and thus is preferred in severe renal and hepatic failure.*
- *Constant attention must be directed to the maintenance of adequate sedation in the paralyzed patient.*

The origin of curare is not known. When first encountered by western explorers at the beginning of the nineteenth century, it was being used by Caribbean tribal leaders in hunting and in ritual legal proceedings.[1] Following a century of quaint and sporadic experimentation, curare paralysis became a serious tool for anesthesiologists, who sought a way to facilitate abdominal and thoracic surgical procedures by decreasing skeletal muscle tone without the severe hemodynamic depressant effects provoked by high concentrations of inhalation anesthetics. The family of nondepolarizing neuromuscular junction blockers (NMBs), of which curare is the paradigm, is an example of the success of structure-activity relationship analysis in drug design; over the past 30 years, new NMBs have been developed which minimize the side effects associated with curare and which provide differing durations and mechanisms of elimination.

Pharmacology

All paralytics act primarily at the postsynaptic acetylcholine receptors (cholinoceptors) in the neuromuscular junction.[2] These receptors, when occupied by acetylcholine, cause myocyte membrane depolarization, which in turn activates cytoplasmic Ca^{2+} influx from the sarcoplasmic reticulum (SR) to trigger contraction. The nondepolarizing paralytics competitively inhibit these postsynaptic receptors, resulting in progressive weakness leading to a flaccid paralysis.[3] Succinylcholine (Sch) is the only clinically relevant member of the depolarizing class of paralytics. As its name suggests, its mechanism differs from the nondepolarizing muscle relaxants in that the molecule causes depolarization at the postsynaptic acetylcholine receptor. Unlike acetylcholine, which is rapidly metabolized at the receptor site by acetylcholinesterase, Sch must first diffuse from the receptor to the circulation, where it is deactivated by the less specific and slower enzyme pseudocholinesterase. The prolonged depolarization results in an initial tetanic twitch, followed by flaccidity because Ca^{2+} is not resequestered in the SR, and the actomyosin complex is not rearmed for further contraction.

Certain of the NMBs also act presynaptically at cholinoceptors on the nerve axon. Blocking these receptors inhibits the storage of acetylcholine at the nerve axon and decreases acetylcholine release from the axon. Considering the multitude of different cholinoceptors (central nervous system, preganglionic sympathetic, postganglionic parasympathetic, neuromuscular junction) it is remarkable that the paralytics are so specific for the skeletal muscle receptor. In fact, certain paralytic side effects are related to their effects at other cholinoceptors. Tachycardia is provoked by gallamine and pancuronium as a parasympatholytic effect, and curare is a weak preganglionic sympathetic blocker which causes hypotension at higher doses. Succinylcholine can provoke a profound bradycardia, occasionally resulting in transient sinus arrest. The paralytics have no effect on smooth-muscle function, and, provided ventilation is maintained, an individual can theoretically be subjected to complete and continuing paralysis with no ill effects. True anaphylactic reactions to the paralytics are extremely rare. There is no known organ toxicity associated with these drugs, and aside from some enhancement of their side effects, the only untoward consequences of overdosing will be a prolonged duration of action.

The placenta presents a variable barrier to pharmacologic paralytics. In anesthesia practice, this barrier is sufficient to allow maternal paralysis during general anesthesia for cesarean section, because of the short time from anesthesia induction to delivery.[4,5] During prolonged maternal paralysis, the fetus can be expected to develop clinically significant drug levels, which will depend on the specific placental transfer properties of the drug administered and on the fetal capacity to metabolize and excrete the drug. The teratogenic effects of these drugs and the influence of fetal paralysis on subsequent neuromuscular development have not been investigated.

Individual patient NMB dose response relationships are not linear, and interindividual relationships are quite variable, making predictable dosing problematic. For intubation, NMB drugs are usually dosed at 1.5 times their minimum effective dose to facilitate rapid onset and ensure complete neuromuscular junction blockade. At lesser doses, the degree of blockade may be unpredictable because of the abundance of receptors present at the neuromuscular junction and the interindividual variations in drug volume of distribution. Individual muscle group response is also variable. For instance, the extraocular muscles are quite sensitive to paralysis, while the diaphragm retains motor power until high drug concentrations are attained. Patients who are partially paralyzed present with a clinical pattern familiar to any clinician who has examined a symptomatic myasthenic patient. Frank weakness is preceded by easy fatigability; patients are able to initiate, but not sustain, muscular effort, leading to jerking or flopping activity. Peripheral nerve stimulation reveals a consistent pattern of fade of muscular contraction on continuing tetanic stimulation and of fade of twitch force with repetitive twitch stimulation.

None of these drugs is known to alter the kinetics or dynamics of other drugs. In general, the effects of other drugs on paralytic potency and duration are clinically insignificant. The nondepolarizing blockers will have their duration mildly prolonged by certain antibiotics, most notably the aminoglycosides, tetracycline, and clindamycin.[6,7] Antiarrhythmic agents, especially quinidine, may also potentiate paralysis. High magnesium levels, like those therapeutically generated by magnesium sulfate infusion for preeclampsia, profoundly increase sensitivity to pharmacologic paralysis. Acute hypokalemia will enhance NMB potency by the associated increase in cellular transmembrane potential. Chronic electrolyte abnormalities do not alter NMB kinetics or dynamics, presumably because transmembrane potentials are compensated.

Individual physiologic factors play a large role in determining paralytic potency and duration. As one might expect, factors that impair neuromuscular junction transmission (e.g., myasthenia gravis, Eaton-Lambert syndrome, hypothermia) potentiate the effect of the paralytics and may prolong their action.[8] Individual dose response relationships with these drugs vary so much that precise dosing requires careful empirical titration based on peripheral nerve stimulator assessment of block intensity. This issue is more germane to the use of paralytics as part of an anesthetic, where the drugs are dosed in a manner to facilitate the termination of paralysis at the completion of the procedure. In the ventilated patient in the intensive care unit (ICU), precise control of duration is less important.

NMBs are pharmacologically reversible. The receptor affinity of the drugs is quite high, resulting in continuing receptor occupancy and an effective duration of action that persists after serum concentrations have fallen. Drug action can therefore be terminated (once serum concentrations have decreased) by competitively dislodging the drugs from the receptor binding sites. This is accomplished by the administration of cholinesterase inhibitors such as edrophonium or neostigmine, which greatly increases acetylcholine concentrations and accelerates NMB displacement from receptors. In practice, the anticholinesterase is administered simultaneously with a parasympatholytic agent such as atropine to avoid the bradycardia and bronchospasm that would otherwise ensue.

Specific Drugs

SUCCINYLCHOLINE

Succinylcholine is the only clinically available member of the depolarizing class of muscle relaxants. Its unique advantage is its evanescence; the usual duration of Sch-induced paralysis is 2 to 4 min providing the patient has adequately functioning pseudocholinesterase. The intubating dose of Sch is 1.0 to 1.5 mg/kg (see Table 83-1). Rarely, a patient will present with genetically altered pseudocholinesterase which does not metabolize Sch; approximately 1:3200 patients will be homozygous for a defective pseudocholinesterase and demonstrate markedly prolonged block with Sch (3 to 8 h).[9] Patients who are heterozygous, pregnant, using echothiophate eyedrops for glaucoma, or have severe hepatic or renal dysfunction (the organs where pseudocholinesterase is elaborated) may have decreased levels of functional pseudocholinesterase, which may modestly prolong block (5 to 15 min).

Succinylcholine has notable side effects. It can raise intracranial pressure (ICP) dramatically. This may be partly due to increased venous pressure and carbon dioxide produced by the brief tetanic twitching, although when a subparalytic dose of a nondepolarizing NMB is administered prior to Sch to suppress the tetanic twitching, ICP still rises. It can induce a severe bradycardia by parasympathetic stimulation. In crush injuries, peritonitis, burns, and spinal cord injury, widespread membrane depolarization may result in massive potassium transfer from the intracellular to extracellular space, with consequent hyperkalemic arrest. The hyperkalemia is typically short lived, but if it is not immediately recognized and treated, or if the patient is fragile, fatal cardiac arrest can ensue. Finally, Sch is a potent trigger for malignant hyperthermia, which manifests as uncontrolled muscle contraction and hypermetabolism with fever, metabolic acidosis, ventricular tachycardia, and, potentially, death. Treatment with surface cooling and dantrolene should be promptly started. Despite these effects, Sch is still widely employed in the operating room, emergency room, and ICU by anesthesiologists, primarily because of its brief duration. In the operating room, a 3-min duration means that a properly preoxygenated patient will likely survive a dose of Sch even if intubation or mask ventilation are confounded by anatomic irregularities. In this setting, its brevity allows the anesthesiologist to revive the patient and try a different approach. In the ICU, where functional residual capacity is decreased, metabolic rate is increased, and patients have diminished cardiorespiratory reserve, 3 min may be too long to safely sustain apnea. In such a setting, the use of Sch may confer no advantage but may pose instead a considerable risk from its side effects.

NONDEPOLARIZING AGENTS

Tubocurarine is so named because when initially described by Waterston in 1812, it was produced in bamboo tubes

TABLE 83-1 Neuromuscular Junction Blockers

Paralytic	Initial Paralyzing Dose, mg/kg	Duration of Action of Bolus, min	Initial Drip Rate, mg/(kg · h)	Side Effects	Normal Elimination	Costs (average wholesale price), $/mg	Average daily cost of therapy (70-kg person), $
Vecuronium (Norcuron)	0.08	30–45	0.07	None	20% renal 80% biliary	1.71	201
Atracurium (Tracrium)	0.5	30–45	0.7	Slight histamine release on rapid bolus administration	Autolysis	0.37	621
Pancuronium (Pavulon)	0.08	60–80	0.025	Tachycardia	30% renal 70% biliary	1.34	56
Curare	0.6	60–80	0.15	Histamine release, hypotension by ganglionic blockade	60% renal 40% biliary	0.40	100
Metocurine	0.4	60–80	0.1	Slight histamine release	100% renal	0.45	76
Succinylcholine	1	2–5		Hyperkalemia, raised ICP trigger, malignant hyperthermia, increased intraocular pressure	Pseudo cholinesterase	0.06	

(tube wurali), as opposed to pot wurali, which was made in clay pots. Its use has decreased because of its ganglionic blocking properties and potent histaminergic effects. Nevertheless, it is inexpensive, widely available, and when slowly administered, it exhibits none of the dramatic hypotensive effects seen with bolus administration. The duration of the effect of curare following a bolus administration of 0.6 mg/kg is approximately 80 min.

Pancuronium (0.1 mg/kg) exhibits a duration of action similar to curare. It does not cause histamine release, but it does provoke a consistent tachycardia (10 to 30 beats per minute) presumably by parasympathetic blockade. This tachycardia is difficult to distinguish from other causes unless careful note is taken of the change in heart rate following the initial bolus administration. Both curare and pancuronium undergo renal and biliary excretion. Pancuronium is more dependent on renal excretion than curare and will have its duration prolonged in renal failure. Both drugs exhibit a decreased rate of excretion with biliary obstruction or cholestasis. Metubine (0.4 mg/kg) is a monoiodinated curare, originally marketed because of its lesser histaminergic tendencies; it is exclusively renally excreted, making it a poor choice in patients with impaired renal failure, in whom the drug will circulate indefinitely.

The current generation of NMBs (see Table 83-1) include atracurium (0.6 mg/kg) and vecuronium (0.08 mg/kg). Each has a duration of approximately 25 to 45 min. Vecuronium is eliminated primarily by biliary excretion, and its duration is prolonged in biliary obstruction, cholestasis, and cirrhosis. It has no side effects. Atracurium is mildly histaminergic and is autolytic; it does not depend on renal or hepatic elimination. At physiologic temperatures, it degrades by Hoffmann elimination making it an ideal brief-duration paralytic in patients with renal and hepatic insufficiency. The only pharmacologically significant metabolite of atracurium is laudanosine, which at high concentrations may cause hypotension, dysrhythmias, and seizures. Laudanosine is hepatically metabolized. For this reason, long-term drip infusion of atracurium should probably be avoided in patients with frank hepatic failure pending the results of further investigation. In patients with intact hepatic function laudanosine does not accumulate.[10]

Clinical Applications

Table 83-2 lists the indications for paralysis in the ICU. Most typically, paralysis is used to facilitate intubation by eliminating biting, gagging, combativeness, and laryngospasm. The use of paralytics in this role necessitates a clinician ac-

TABLE 83-2 Indications for Paralysis in the ICU

Facilitating intubation
Increased oxygen consumption associated with muscular activity
Abolishing ventilator-patient discoordination and "bucking"
Pharmacologic restraint
Septic shock—acute hypoxic respiratory failure
Resting fatigued respiratory muscle

complished in airway management, since the inability to intubate or mask ventilate following paralysis will at least require emergency cricothyrotomy, and, at worst, will result in an iatrogenic patient death.

In patients with hypoxia refractory to positive end-expiratory pressure (PEEP) and high inspired oxygen concentrations, paralysis can be employed to eliminate the aerobic costs associated with muscular activity. If effective, this decrease in oxygen consumption should increase mixed venous hemoglobin saturation, diverting oxygen supply from counterproductive muscular activity to vital organs. In patients who are quiescent prior to paralysis, no benefit is seen with neuromuscular blockade.[11] By contrast, shivering or respiratory muscle effort imposes a metabolic stress with increased oxygen consumption.[12] In such patients, paralysis may dramatically improve oxygen balance.

Certain patients demonstrate "discoordination" with the mechanical ventilator. The resulting bucking and straining may provoke pulmonary barotrauma and bronchospasm, as well as tracheal or laryngeal injury. On occasion, the pressure generated by the muscles of respiration is sufficient to overcome the ventilator driving pressure, which can give the impression of a patient struggling with an occluded endotracheal tube. The judicious use of a bolus of Sch accompanied by hand-bag ventilation facilitates the rapid diagnosis of such a life-threatening response. In addition, paralysis affords the ICU team an opportunity to optimize ventilation and modify the patient's sedation regimen. *It should be noted that discoordination most often signals ventilator settings that are not suited to the patient's requirements.* Hypoventilation, low inspiratory flow rates, and prolonged inspiratory hold can provoke bucking, which then self-perpetuates as the endotracheal tube movement provokes paroxysmal coughing. The clinician must always consider ventilator adjustment first before resorting to sedation and paralysis. In contrast, asthmatics typically respond to intubation with an exacerbation of their bronchospasm and with the tendency to increasing tachypnea which affords insufficient time for exhalation. In this population, early sedation and paralysis may be appropriate to facilitate the elective mechanical hypoventilation which characterizes the early stabilization of mechanically ventilated asthmatics.

A certain minority of patients, the paradigm of whom is the traumatized chronic alcoholic, may exhibit agitation which is refractory to sedation. Such patients are frequently combative; may flail actively, displacing invasive catheters and tubes; or may bite, obstructing endotracheal tube gas flow. Such behavior, when not responsive to intravenous sedation, necessitates paralysis as a form of pharmacologic restraint. These cases are rare, and aggressive attempts should be made to control the agitation with sedation prior to resorting to paralysis. In severe cases of tetanus, paralysis is indicated for relief of the muscle spasms; therapy is usually required for 1 to 3 weeks.

Paralysis is sometimes employed in patients with septic shock and acute hypoxic respiratory failure, the latter usually from noncardiogenic pulmonary edema. Paralysis in these patients is employed both to favorably influence oxygen balance and reduce lactic acid production by respiratory and other muscles. Sedation may be problematic in these patients. Narcotics, benzodiazepines, and major tranquilizers all tend to exacerbate the profound hypotension which is a common feature of septic shock, either directly by vasodilation and myocardial depression, or indirectly by decreasing catecholamine release. Clinical experience suggests that patients in septic shock are typically obtunded and survivors are usually amnestic, making concurrent sedation less urgent during paralysis.

Some practitioners advocate the use of pharmacologic paralysis to provide a period of rest for fatigued respiratory muscles. This interlude allows the muscles to recuperate, theoretically facilitating attempts to transfer the ventilatory power load from the ventilator to the patient's muscles. Such rest is most safely accomplished by increasing the ventilator minute volume in conjunction with narcotic sedation to depress central respiratory drive. However, when this is not feasible, the administration of a paralytic may be beneficial.

Complications

The side effects of paralysis are listed in Table 83-3. Most obviously, any respiratory reserve a patient may have had to overcome (i.e., ventilator failure, tube dislodgement, or tubing disconnect) is eliminated by paralysis. This shortens the available recognition and response time by the ICU team to minutes in order to avoid catastrophe. Thus, it is essential that all paralyzed and ventilated patients have functioning disconnect alarms and that the care team be conditioned to respond promptly to ventilation alarms in any patient room. The evolving standard of care also recommends that a secondary monitor of ventilation, such as an end-tidal CO_2 monitor or pulse oximeter, be employed on all ventilated patients. Anesthesia experience suggests that cerebral injury closely follows the hypoxia-induced bradycardia of hypoventilation; such episodes are sufficiently frequent in the ICU to sober the observant intensivist.

Physical examination of the central nervous system is impossible in a paralyzed patient; reflexes, gaze, meningismus, and limb movement all rely on skeletal muscle action. The iris is a smooth muscle; its tone, and consequently pupillary diameter, are autonomically mediated. While nondepolarizing relaxants do not paralyze the iris, pupillary size will be altered by the autonomic influences of pancuronium (anticholinergic) and Sch (cholinergic). In the setting where frequent neurologic examination is necessary, intermittent bolus administration of vecuronium or atracu-

TABLE 83-3 Risks of Paralysis

Loss of respiratory reserve
Loss of neurologic examination
Awake paralysis
Accelerated muscle wasting

rium will allow hourly examination. A clinical requirement for continuous neurologic assessment precludes the use of paralysis.

Pharmacologic paralysis raises the gruesome specter of conscious paralysis in the critically ill. It is clear from ICU survivor accounts that instances of iatrogenic "locking in" do occur and are terrifying. Inexperienced or careless clinicians are prone to equate patient immobility with insensibility, and senior members of the clinical team must be constantly vigilant for such transgressions as line insertions, tube changes, and minor surgical procedures performed without local anesthesia; all must strive to ensure an adequate level of sedation in these patients. To this end, it is inappropriate to refer to the paralyzed patient as being "relaxed" or (even worse) "pavulonized." Such euphemisms are typically employed to avoid upsetting the family of the critically ill patient. It is much more important to keep the family and health care team focused on the therapeutic situation, no matter how dire, and to avoid turning what could potentially be the last days of the critically ill patient's life into a conscious nightmare.

One might predict an acceleration of muscle wasting in patients who are paralyzed. It is clear that immobility results in muscle atrophy, especially in catabolic patients. Data to incriminate pharmacologic paralysis as a potentiating factor are unavailable. There are data to indicate that passive muscle stretching will delay muscle atrophy, although not indefinitely. Over the typical course of paralysis (which only occasionally lasts more than a week in survivors) this is probably not an issue, especially if an effort is made to institute passive range of motion exercise by physical therapy and nursing as part of patient care.

Long-term paralysis is most conveniently administered as an intravenous drip. Initial bolus doses and drip rates are listed in Table 83-1, with the proviso that interindividual dose response makes such information valuable only as an initial guide. Although current practice favors atracurium or vecuronium for their hemodynamic and kinetic advantages,[13,14] they are quite expensive, and in many instances, tubocurarine or pancuronium will offer satisfactory alternatives at a fraction of the cost.[15] Daily cost comparisons in Table 83-1 presume average wholesale price and a 70-kg adult requiring average dosing. Dosing should be empirically determined by patient observation as well as through the use of a nerve stimulator. Underdosing results in a typical flopping response; the patient will attempt an arm or head lift, which will stop as the neuromuscular junction fatigues. The appearance is of feeble jerking of the head or hand, which should alert the practitioner to the need for a higher relaxant dose, as well as a need to reassess the adequacy of sedation. Overdose has no consequence except for a long duration of paralysis following drip discontinuation. Once a day, the drip should be stopped, and the time to recovery noted. In many patients, the drip will be seen to have become unnecessary as, over the course of 6 to 8 h, the patient will remain immobile. In others, there will be a gradual return of the muscular activity which initially provoked paralysis; if feasible, the patient should be allowed to reverse sufficiently to assess the degree of sedation. In any case, the time to return of motor function should be noted, and bolus and drip reinstituted as required.

In patients who demonstrate no muscular activity for 8 h following drug discontinuation, an examination with a peripheral nerve stimulator is indicated. Such instruments are portable and readily available from the operating room. A brief demonstration from a cooperative anesthesiologist will provide the intensivist with the necessary skill to assess the intensity of blockade. The persistence of paralysis 8 h after the discontinuation of paralytic infusion should provoke a reassessment of the patient's hepatic and renal function; rising bilirubin or creatinine levels should alert the clinician to the possibility of impaired drug excretion; and a drug should be chosen from Table 83-1 that matches the patient's organ function. Alternate physiologic explanations should be sought (e.g., Eaton-Lambert syndrome, electrolyte imbalance), and the infusion concentration and drip rate should be recalculated to preclude overdosage. An anesthesiologist can be consulted and reversal attempted if the clinical situation so warrants, and when bolus and infusion is reinstituted, doses of 25 to 50 percent of the previous dose should be employed.

CASE PRESENTATION

A 32-year-old, 70-kg male was admitted to the emergency unit following blunt trauma. Admission hematocrit was 28 percent, ethanol level was 320 U, and peritoneal lavage was grossly positive. Chest radiograph was normal. The patient underwent laparotomy. Splenectomy was performed; the liver was noted to be cirrhotic. On admission to the ICU, a chest radiograph was performed to confirm central line position. A left lower lobe infiltrate was identified, and the differential diagnosis of pulmonary contusion versus aspiration pneumonia was entertained. Arterial blood gases demonstrated marked hypoxemia (P_{O_2} of 67 mmHg, P_{CO_2} 41 mmHg, pH 7.38) on 80 percent FI_{O_2}, assist-control of 14 breaths per minute, tidal volume of 750 mL, and PEEP 5 cmH_2O. PEEP was increased to 10 cmH_2O, with a rise in P_{O_2} to 87 mmHg. Six hours postoperatively, the patient was noted to be "straining" on the ventilator. Arterial blood gases and chest radiograph were obtained; the chest radiograph was unchanged, and the arterial blood gas had deteriorated (P_{O_2} 57 mmHg, P_{CO_2} 48 mmHg, pH 7.30). Peak airway pressures had risen from 38 cmH_2O to 55 cmH_2O. Morphine 10 mg in divided doses and midazolam 5 mg were administered, but the patient's agitation and apparent air hunger increased. Examination of the patient on brief continuous positive airway pressure revealed a respiratory rate of 28 shallow breaths. When coupled to the ventilator, the patient was noted to overdraw the triggered inspiratory flow, generating manometer readings of −5 cmH_2O on early inspiration, and exhaling at end inspiration, driving pressures to 55 to 60 cmH_2O. Inspiratory flow rate was increased until the triggered inspiration held positive pressure to at least 10 cmH_2O in early inspiration, and inspiratory: expiratory ratio was set so that there was no inspiratory plateau. With this change, the patient settled to a triggered rate of 20 breaths per minute, with peak airway pressures of 44 cmH_2O.

Forty-eight hours postoperatively, the patient became increasingly agitated and was refractory to massive doses of benzodiazepines and narcotics. He became combative, requiring four-point restraints, and an oral airway was required to keep him from biting his endotracheal tube. Constant thrashing made nursing care difficult, and the decision was made to paralyze the patient. The patient was given 6 mg of vecuronium, and an infusion was commenced at 5 mg/h. Narcotics and benzodiazepines were continued.

On the third day, the patient's oxygenation deteriorated, requiring 100 percent $F_{I_{O_2}}$ and PEEP of 12.5 cmH_2O to maintain a P_{O_2} of 65 mmHg. On the fourth day, the vecuronium infusion was discontinued at noon. By 8 p.m., no movement was noted. An anesthesiologist examined the patient with a nerve stimulator, and found the patient to be still paralyzed. It was felt that the prolonged duration of the vecuronium represented impaired biliary excretion, and after discussion with the primary team, the paralysis was reversed with 3 mg of neostigmine and 0.6 mg of the anticholinergic glycopyrrolate. Over 5 min, tonic-clonic contractions were noted; these persisted. The tonic-clonic activity interrupted pulse oximetry readings, but the mixed venous hemoglobin saturation measured by Swan-Ganz oximeter dropped from 64 to 42%. The patient was immediately reparalyzed with vecuronium, 10 mg, and an infusion was instituted with curare at 6 mg/h. Electroencephalogram monitoring was instituted and revealed continuous diffuse seizure activity. Control was achieved over 24 h using phenobarbital and phenytoin (Dilantin). A computed tomography scan of the head revealed moderate cerebral edema, in addition to a contusion noted on admission.

On the sixth day, with seizures suppressed and oxygenation improving, paralysis was again discontinued. Twelve hours after discontinuation, the patient remained immobile. Nerve stimulator examination demonstrated resolution of the block with intact neuromuscular response. The patient never regained consciousness and progressed to tracheostomy, weaning of mechanical ventilation, and subsequent nursing home placement.

CASE DISCUSSION

Initial ventilator adjustment avoided early paralysis, which was nevertheless later required for agitation due to ICU psychosis and delirium tremens. Vecuronium, which is eliminated primarily by biliary excretion, presumably accumulated because of the patient's cirrhosis, resulting in prolonged duration of blockade following discontinuation of the drip. Additionally, the paralysis prevented neurologic examination and obscured status epilepticus. Reestablishment of blockade was accomplished with curare, which relies less on hepatic excretion. In the event of combined renal and hepatic dysfunction, small doses of curare or Pavulon would be appropriate, titrated to nerve stimulator response. Atracurium might also be employed for brief duration (1 or 2 days).

References

1. Sykes WS: Curare, in Sykes WS (ed): *Essays on the First Hundred Years of Anaesthesia,* Churchill-Livingstone, Edinburgh, 1982.
2. Standaert FG: Basic physiology and pharmacology of the neuromuscular junction, in Miller RD (ed): *Anesthesia,* 2d ed, New York, Churchill Livingstone, 1986, pp 835–870.
3. Miller RD, Savarese JJ: Pharmacology of muscle relaxants and their antagonists, in Miller RD (ed): *Anesthesia,* 2d ed, New York, Churchill Livingstone, 1986, pp 889–943.
4. Shnider SM, Levinson, G: Anesthesia for cesarean section, in Shnider SM and Levinson G (eds): *Anesthesia for Obstetrics,* 2d ed, Baltimore, Williams and Wilkins, 1987, pp 169–171.
5. Dailey PA, Fisher DM, Shnider SM, et al.: Pharmacokinetics, placental transfer, and neonatal effects of vecuronium and pancuronium administered during cesarean section. Anesthesiology 60:569, 1984.
6. Sokoll MD, Gergis SD: Antibiotics and neuromuscular function. Anesthesiology 55:148, 1981.
7. Argov Z, Mastaglia FL: Disorders of neuromuscular transmission caused by drugs. N Engl J Med 301:409, 1979.
8. Feldman SA: Muscle relaxants in pathologic states, in, Feldman SA (ed): *Muscle Relaxants,* Philadelphia, WB Saunders, 1979, pp 108–116.
9. Whittaker M: Plasma cholinesterase variants and the anesthetist. Anaesthesia 35:174, 1980.
10. Yate PM, Flynn PJ, Arnold RW, et al.: Clinical experience and plasma laudanosine concentrations during the infusion of atracurium in the intensive therapy unit. Br J Anaesth 59(2):211, February 1987.
11. Palmisano BW, Fisher DM, Willis M, et al.: The effect of paralysis on oxygen consumption in normoxic children after cardiac surgery. Anesthesiology 61(5):518, November 1984.
12. Coggeshall JW, Marini JJ, Newman JH: Improved oxygenation after muscle relaxation in adult respiratory distress syndrome. Arch Intern Med 145(9):1718, September 1985.
13. Williams SG: Review of atracurium by continuous i.v. infusion. Br J Anaesth 58(suppl 1):51S, 1986.
14. Noeldge G, Hinsken H, Buzello W: Comparison between the continuous infusion of vecuronium and the intermittent administration of pancuronium and vecuronium. Br J Anaesth 56(5):473, May 1984.
15. Haraldsted VY, Nielsen JW, Madsen JV et al.: Maintenance of constant 95% neuromuscular blockade by adjustable infusion rates of pancuronium and atracurium. Br J Anaesth 60(5):491, April 1988.

Chapter 84

PERIOPERATIVE RESPIRATORY FAILURE

J. ALI

KEY POINTS

- *Pulmonary edema and atelectasis characterize perioperative respiratory failure; hypoventilation and aspiration contribute.*
- *A major therapeutic measure in decreasing lung water is the reduction of pulmonary capillary hydrostatic pressure.*
- *The concept of closing volume and its relationship to functional residual capacity (FRC) is important in understanding perioperative atelectasis.*
- *Risk factors for perioperative atelectasis include obesity, smoking, age, anesthesia, recumbency, and incisional pain.*
- *Diaphragmatic dysfunction is a major component of perioperative respiratory failure.*
- *Preoperative assessment of respiratory function predicts risk and allows the correction of abnormalities, particularly in the patient undergoing lung resection.*
- *Early ambulation, physiotherapy, treatment of sepsis and shock, adequate analgesia, and early operative stabilization of fractures are key elements in treating and preventing perioperative respiratory failure.*

In the period before, during, and after surgical treatment, patients are unusually vulnerable to respiratory failure through special manifestations of pulmonary edema, atelectasis, hypoventilation, and aspiration. Awareness of the factors promoting each of these interrelated processes allows an effective prevention program or early diagnosis and treatment regime for perioperative respiratory failure.

Pulmonary Edema

Of the forces in Starling's equation governing transcapillary fluid flux, the ones of particular relevance to surgical patients are microvascular hydrostatic pressure and pulmonary capillary permeability.

MICROVASCULAR PRESSURE

Secretion of antidiuretic hormone (ADH) and aldosterone is a major component of the metabolic response to operation and trauma.[1] Both tend to conserve water and decrease urine output in the postsurgical patient. However, the focus on increasing urine output by increasing fluid administration in the surgical patient without regard to this metabolic response could easily result in fluid overload and pulmonary edema leading to hypoxemia. Guidelines for fluid resuscitation in the perioperative period that focus on urine output and fluid replacements based on empirical values[2] could increase extravascular lung water and predispose the surgical patient to perioperative respiratory failure. Although the young healthy patient with significant cardiopulmonary reserve will undoubtedly tolerate these insults, the elderly surgical patient with a brittle cardiorespiratory status is more likely to develop respiratory failure unless extreme caution is taken in fluid resuscitation, with close constant monitoring of central hydrostatic pressures.

Pulmonary edema occurring in the head injured patient or *neurogenic edema* may be associated with a transient increase in hydrostatic pressure because of intense sympathetic discharge, although some workers have suggested that there may be a component of increased capillary permeability as well in this lesion.[3] Monitoring of pulmonary capillary hydrostatic pressure is important in determining therapeutic approaches to the head injured patient with pulmonary edema.

After normalization of vascular pressures, high pressure pulmonary edema does not immediately resolve.[4] The implication of this phenomenon is that the timing of the measurement of pulmonary artery wedge pressure (PAWP), which is used as a reflection of capillary hydrostatic pressure, is crucial in determining whether pulmonary edema is due to high vascular pressures or an increase in capillary permeability. Ordinarily, the presence of normal or low PAWP in the presence of pulmonary edema would be regarded as evidence of capillary leak pulmonary edema. However, if this measurement of a low PAWP is made during the lag phase of resolution of high pressure pulmonary edema, then therapy may be inappropriately directed by focusing on capillary leak as opposed to the already resolving, albeit slowly, cardiogenic edema.

Diuretics such as furosemide produce their effect of clearing edema by decreasing the central blood volume and pulmonary capillary hydrostatic pressure.[5] However, these agents may produce effects on gas exchange prior to the clearing of pulmonary edema.[6] Accordingly, diuretic therapy and fluid management of the oliguric hypoxemic perioperative patient may confuse the student of critical care at several levels. First, oliguria in the immediate postoperative period is not necessarily due to reduced blood flow to the renal cortex (prerenal oliguria), so fluid challenges aimed at increasing renal blood flow will not treat this metabolic response to surgery or other trauma. The consequent increase in pulmonary blood volume and pressure predictably increases pulmonary edema. On the other hand, diuretic therapy in such a patient will increase urine output even when the oliguria is due to reduced renal blood flow, thereby aggravating the prerenal failure. The best approach to this common perioperative conundrum recognizes that urine output could be a poor signal of adequate perfusion, so other indices of perfusion must be gained from careful history, physical examination and first-hand knowledge of the patient's perioperative course. For example, prior history of congestive heart failure predicts susceptibility to fluid overload to slow the physician's hand in administering fluid, while familiarity with the patient's preoperative blood pressure, heart rate, heart sounds, pulse volume, and digital perfusion allow the discerning physician to detect early signs of hypoperfusion requiring volume replacement. Often, the critical distinction between fluid overload and hypovolemia is not clear even to the astute clinician, when a low threshold for central hemodynamic measurements is indicated.[7] Then the combination of low pulmonary artery occlusion pressure, low cardiac output, and oliguria allows a volume challenge to return blood flow toward normal without risking edema; untoward increases in PAWP without much increase in blood flow warrants immediate reevaluation of the patient's cardiac function including an electrocardiogram (ECG) and cardiac enzymes and vasoactive drug therapy (low dose dopamine, 1 to 3 μg/kg/min to redistribute the flow toward the renal cortex; dobutamine, 2 to 10 μg/kg/min to increase ventricular contractility and output at reduced PAWP).

PULMONARY CAPILLARY PERMEABILITY

A frequent cause of increased capillary permeability and respiratory failure in the surgical patient is unrecognized sepsis which frequently is in the abdomen; this source often requires a surgical approach. Therefore, a major component of prevention and treatment of respiratory failure in the surgical patient is the early identification of occult sources of sepsis, aggressive investigation for abdominal causes of sepsis, and the provision of adequate drainage and treatment of septic foci, particularly within the abdomen.

Although increased microvascular hydrostatic pressure and pulmonary capillary permeability are important factors in the elaboration of extravascular lung water, manipulation of the microvascular pressure (by the use of vasoactive agents and regulation of the state of hydration) is the most direct means of altering pulmonary edema in the surgical patient. Search for a septic focus in the surgical patient is crucial whenever there is evidence of increased capillary permeability. Control of capillary permeability can then be achieved, although only indirectly, by treating the source of sepsis which may be surgically approachable. The link between sepsis and capillary permeability is thus broken, and the capillary permeability lesion is allowed to resolve with time with coincident improvement in perioperative respiratory failure. Until the permeability corrects itself, reduction of PAWP to the lowest level associated with adequate peripheral perfusion seems to reduce the edema.[5]

Atelectasis

In the normal lung, ventilation and perfusion are not equally matched because the shape of the thoracic cavity and the descent of the diaphragm result in greater expansion and ventilation of the lower lobes. Also, blood flow is greater in the dependent areas of the lung during spontaneous ventilation and changes with body position. The normal lung, therefore, has an average ventilation/perfusion ratio ($\dot{V}/\dot{Q}$) of approximately 0.8. Many factors in the surgical patient reduce this ratio to very low values causing hypoxemia, and similar factors lead to resorption of alveolar gas behind closed airways or to compression atelectasis.[8,9] This phenomenon of compression atelectasis in the dependent lung is thought to occur within 5 min after general anesthesia.

Shunt results from continued perfusion of nonventilated lung units, and the major cause for this in the surgical patient is perioperative atelectasis, although alveolar edema from fluid overload or capillary leak could also result in an increase in shunt.

AGE, POSITION AND AIRWAYS CLOSURE

Most surgical patients undergo procedures in the supine position, and we are increasingly operating on more elderly patients. Also, one of the major effects of surgery is the pain resulting from surgical incisions. Body position, incisional pain, and age all affect the relationship between the FRC and the closing volume. The FRC has been considered the most important index of mechanical abnormality in the lung because it represents the balance of opposing forces on the rib cage at resting lung volume. The closing volume is the measure of gas in the lung at the time when airway closure begins. When FRC exceeds closing volume, lower airway patency is maintained while airway closure begins when the FRC falls below the closing volume.[10] Age results in a fall in FRC, and all patients have the FRC at a lower volume in the supine position than in the upright position (Fig. 84-1). The commonly used lithotomy position results in a further decrease in FRC relative to closing volume.

When the difference between FRC and closing volume is plotted against alveolar-arterial (A − a) oxygen tension gradient,[11] it is evident that the A − a oxygen tension gradient increases as FRC falls below closing volume.

Areas of airway closure tend to occur in the most dependent areas of the lung, and in the supine position more areas of the lung are dependent, thus predisposing the patient to further areas of airway closure and hypoxemia. As indicated above,[8,9] general anesthesia itself may predispose to compression atelectasis in dependent areas of the lung. Also, in both normals and smokers increasing age is associated with an increase in closing volumes, predisposing the patient to airway closure at higher lung volumes.[12] As a group, smokers tend to have higher closing volumes so that the combination of age and smoking increases the likelihood of significant postoperative hypoxemia. It has generally been accepted that chronic cigarette smoking increases postoperative respiratory complications which may result not only from an alteration in the respiratory defense mechanisms but also an increase in airway resistance and the work of breathing. In fact, it has been demonstrated that cessation of smoking for over 8 weeks is an effective means of decreasing postoperative respiratory complications.[13]

Because small airways in the periphery of the lung are not supported by cartilage, they tend to be influenced significantly by changes in pleural pressures. The maintenance of a positive transpulmonary pressure resulting from the negative intrapleural pressure maintains patency of the

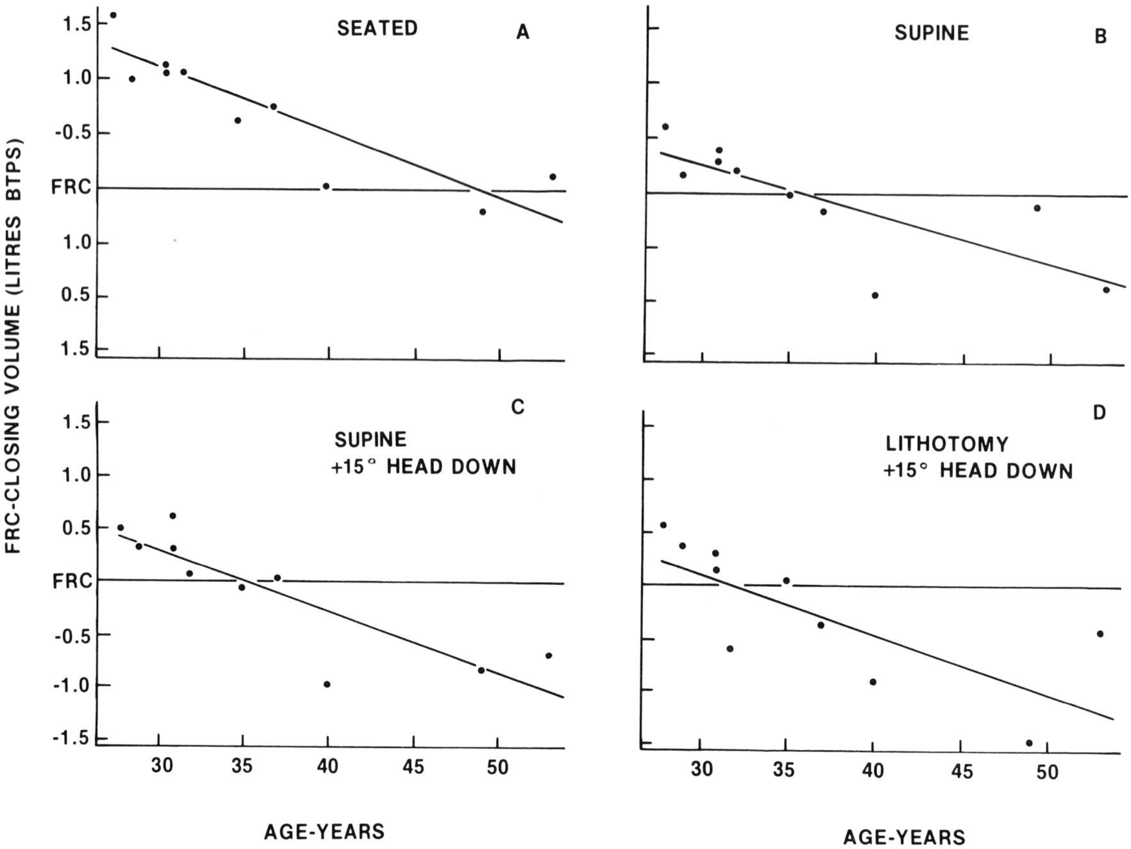

FIGURE 84-1 The difference between FRC and closing volume plotted against age in different surgical positions. Both age and position affect airway closure. (Reproduced with permission from Craig DB, et al: Can Anaesth Soc J 18(1):95, 1971.)

small airways. Breathing at a reduced FRC, such as occurs with abdominal pain, tends to lead to positive pleural pressures in the dependent areas of the lung and therefore predisposes to alveolar collapse. Complete collapse results in continued perfusion of nonventilated areas or shunt; when the airways are merely narrowed, low ventilation perfusion relationships occur, which also impair gas exchange and lead to hypoxemia.

The patient with multiple fractures is at increased risk for developing pulmonary complications not only from thromboembolic complications including fat embolism but also from atelectasis and pneumonia. A major predisposing factor in these patients is the prolonged period of imposed bed rest, particularly in the supine position, with its resultant effect on lung mechanics and lung volumes. Early operative stabilization of fractures in these patients has been shown to decrease pulmonary morbidity[14] because it allows more effective respiratory physiotherapy and early ambulation.

UPPER ABDOMINAL SURGERY AND DIAPHRAGM DYSFUNCTION

Although many of the factors indicated above are operative in patients undergoing most surgical procedures, the most serious sequelae are found in patients undergoing upper abdominal procedures. In these patients there is a significant fall in vital capacity (VC) almost immediately postoperatively within the first 4 h.[15] There is a slower but definite fall in FRC which is maximum at about 24 h, and this is associated with significant hypoxemia. In most patients who have no preexisting lung disease this effect of upper abdominal intervention on VC and FRC does not result in clinically significant respiratory complications. However, in patients who already have abnormalities of gas exchange, this superimposed effect due to operation can lead to severe respiratory failure. The decrease in VC seen in the postoperative period is a primarily restrictive rather than an obstructive phenomenon as evidenced by the maintenance of a normal forced expiratory volume at 1 s:forced vital capacity (FEV_1:FVC) ratio.[16] This restriction may be related to incisional pain which decreases the patient's ability to cough and clear secretions and eventually leads to an increase in closing volume and a decrease in FRC. A fall in VC is therefore the indication that the patient may progress to atelectasis and hypoxemia and a decrease in FRC if this is not corrected. To correct this abnormality, transcutaneous elective nerve stimulation has been used as an analgesic modality in the postoperative patient undergoing abdominal surgery.[17] Other workers have used epidural analgesia and intercostal blockade for the same purpose. Although all of these techniques have been successful in improving the VC and increasing the FRC compared to the nontreated

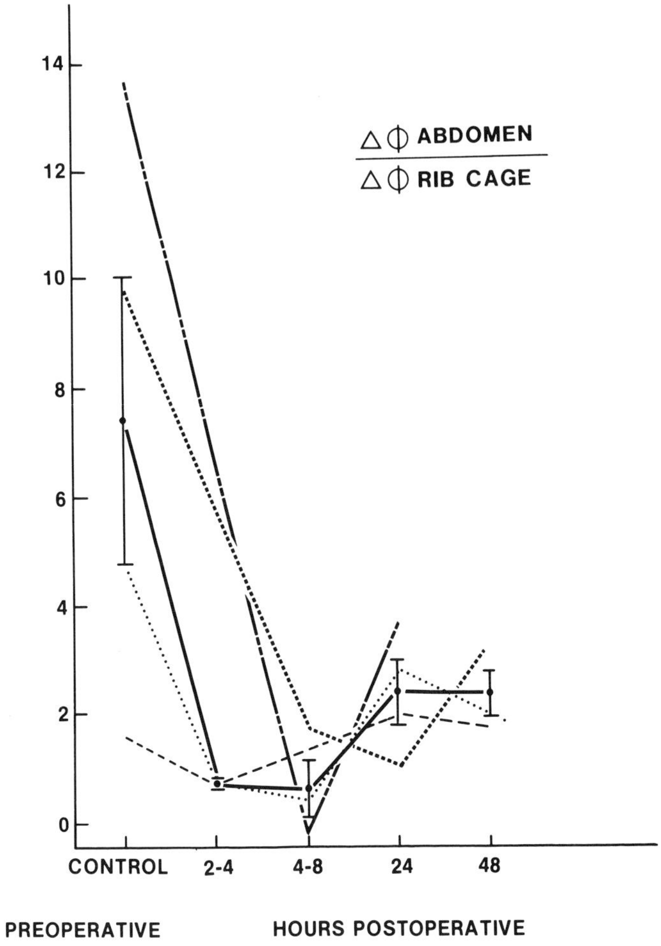

FIGURE 84-2 Relationship between the ratio of abdominal to rib cage diameter and time after abdominal surgery. Interrupted lines represent individual patients and the solid line represents the mean values for these four patients. Note the switch from predominantly abdominal breathing preoperatively to rib cage breathing postoperatively. (Reproduced with permission from Ford GT, et al: Am Rev Respir Dis 127:434, 1983.)

patients, none of these maneuvers is associated with complete recovery to the preoperative VC or FRC values. Either we are not controlling pain adequately by these techniques or else the restriction produced by pain is not the complete explanation for the postoperative respiratory dysfunction in upper abdominal interventions.

In patients undergoing upper abdominal operation, there is a significant decrease in the transdiaphragmatic pressure at FRC, and this is not altered by the institution of epidural analgesia.[18] These data suggest that there may be a primary effect of upper abdominal procedures on diaphragmatic function resulting in the respiratory dysfunction characteristic of upper abdominal surgery. Ford and coworkers showed that there is a switch from predominantly abdominal breathing to rib cage breathing in the postoperative period in patients undergoing upper abdominal surgery (Fig. 84-2).[19] Diaphragmatic function was similarly studied in an animal model undergoing cholecystectomy where the diaphragmatic dysfunction was again identified.[20] These studies established that general anesthesia was not responsible for the reduced diaphragm activities seen postoperatively and that the diaphragmatic dysfunction was not associated with lower abdominal surgery in dogs. Indeed, mere traction on the gallbladder is capable of producing similar effects on diaphragmatic function.[21]

Until the precise mechanism for diaphragmatic dysfunction has been identified other factors which contribute to respiratory failure must also receive attention to prevent this dire complication. Apart from the factors identified above, aging has been associated with loss of elastic lung recoil, decrease in respiratory flow rate, and diminished airway protective reflexes.[12] Obesity also poses a major risk for postoperative pulmonary complications, because these patients tend to breathe at reduced lung volumes so that closing volume frequently exceeds FRC, leading to hypoxemia and atelectasis. The increased work of breathing produced by the increased mass also contributes to respiratory dysfunction. Not only the type of operation but the particular location of the incision tends to affect the degree of respiratory impairment in the postoperative period.[22] In cholecystectomy the subcostal incision as opposed to the midline incision tends to produce less impairment, and lung impairment occurs with decreasing severity in the following surgical procedures: thoracic surgery, upper abdominal surgery, lower abdominal surgery, superficial surgery (Fig. 84-3).

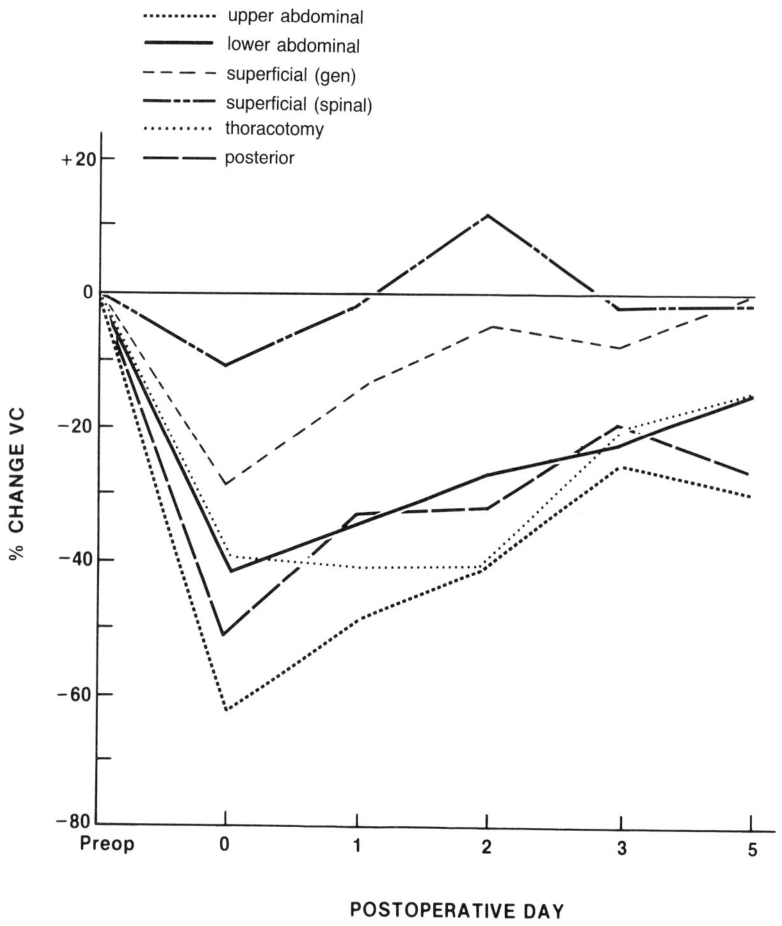

FIGURE 84-3 Postoperative changes in VC for different surgical incisions. Note that the upper abdominal surgery patients have the greatest postoperative depression in VC. (Reproduced with permission from Ali J, et al: Am J Surg 128:379, 1974.)

TABLE 84-1 Perioperative Atelectasis

Promoting	Preventing
Reduced FRC	
Supine position	45° upright
Obesity	Alternating postures
Ascites	Positive end-expiratory pressure (PEEP)
Peritonitis	Sighs
Upper abdominal incision	Analgesia
Increased Closing Volume	
Age	Preoperative physiotherapy
Smoking history	Cessation
Bronchospasm	Bronchodilation
Airway secretions	Cough, suction, deep breathing
Pulmonary edema	Avoid overhydration

As pointed out in earlier chapters in the text, shock and pulmonary edema in the form of cardiac failure also affect diaphragmatic function as indicated by changes in diaphragmatic force as well as glycogen depletion in diaphragmatic muscle.[23] Table 84-1 summarizes some of the factors which reduce the FRC and increase closing volume in the postoperative patient, with methods of prevention as identified.

Alveolar Hypoventilation

Hypoventilation characteristically is caused by impairment of ventilation resulting from the restrictive effect of painful incisions or peritonitis in surgical patients. Also, central nervous system (CNS) depression resulting from anesthesia, analgesia, or CNS injury could result in alveolar hypoventilation in the surgical patient.

The increased metabolic requirement after injury places a significant demand on the respiratory system. When calories, particularly in the form of carbohydrates, are provided to match this increased energy expenditure the increased CO_2 production requires significant increase in ventilation to maintain normocapnia. In surgical patients with significant pulmonary reserve, this added demand may be met without untoward effects. However, depleted surgical patients with borderline respiratory reserve may develop respiratory failure or show other signs such as failure to wean off the respirator in response to this demand.[24]

The respiratory system is protected from sepsis and atelectasis by a respiratory control mechanism that responds to hypoxemia, hypercapnia, acidosis, and the presence of irritative or noxious stimuli in the airway. These mechanisms can be significantly depressed in the postoperative patient as a result of the anesthetic agent or excessive narcotic analgesia. Inhalation anesthetics are known for their respiratory depressive effect, resulting in alveolar hypoventilation and a reduced response to carbon dioxide as well as blunting the response to hypoxemia and acidosis.[25] In the postoperative period, narcotic analgesics may have undesirable effects. Whereas in optimal doses they decrease abdominal pain and increase the ability to cough and clear secretions, in larger doses these agents may also depress the respiratory center producing alveolar hypoventilation as manifested by hypercapnia and secondary hypoxemia.

The clearance mechanism for particles in the upper airway is primarily the cough mechanism which is altered not only by anesthesia but also by narcotic agents. However, clearance of particles in the lower airways depends primarily on the mucociliary system, and several factors in the postoperative period may alter this function. Known effects of anesthetics on ciliary activity and mucous production lead to the production of mucous plugs which block the lower airways. In addition, the respiratory cellular defense mechanisms may also be altered by anesthetic agents.[26]

Aspiration

The supine position and depression of normal protective reflexes during general anesthesia predispose the surgical patient to gastric acid aspiration, which is one of the major causes of morbidity and mortality in the perioperative period.[27] This leads to early airway obstruction (from aspirated debris) to be followed by a chemical burn of the airway (with fluid loss into the injured area), then an intense inflammatory response, and finally an infective pneumonic process. The clinical presentation of these patients varies widely, with the very mild cases presenting with transient short-lived coughing and minimal bronchospasm. The most severe cases present with a progressive downhill course characterized by hypovolemia, hypoxemia, and finally fulminant bacterial pneumonia.

The treatment of acid aspiration consists of **1.** rapid removal of debris by immediate suction; endotracheal intubation and fiberoptic bronchoscopy may be necessary at this stage; **2.** placement of a nasogastric tube to evacuate the stomach and prevent further episodes; **3.** oxygen administration and mechanical ventilation if indicated by the degree of respiratory failure; **4.** bronchodilator therapy if bronchospasm is significant; **5.** maintenance of normovolemia and normal perfusion by monitoring and replacing fluid loss as well as instituting vasoactive and ionotropic support where necessary; and **6.** treatment of pneumonia by appropriate antimicrobial agents based on Gram stain and culture. Steroids have not been of any benefit in treating these patients.

Based on the recognized injurious effect of low pH gastric contents of the lung, preventive measures in high-risk patients include gastric decompression and the use of H_2 antagonists such as ranitidine.

Predicting and Preventing Perioperative Lung Dysfunction

Recognition of these postoperative abnormalities in lung function has resulted in many attempts at correction, including incentive spirometry, intermittent positive-pressure breathing (IPPB), and nasal continuous positive airway pressure, among others.[28,29] IPPB, incentive spirometry, and physiotherapy all improve postoperative respiratory function. However, when physiotherapy is maximized in the postoperative period, IPPB offers no advantage over physiotherapy.[29] Although nonyielding abdominal binders have a further restrictive effect on lung volumes postoperatively, the elastic binders may produce some benefit.[30] It must be recognized, however, that none of these interventions completely eradicates the postoperative respiratory dysfunction.

To decrease postoperative morbidity in surgical patients, apart from identifying the factors such as age, obesity, smoking, and location of incisions, attempts have been made to predict postoperative pulmonary morbidity by assessing respiratory mechanics preoperatively. No precise respiratory parameters will predict respiratory morbidity or mortality in an individual patient. In general, however, the more depressed the preoperative respiratory function, the more likely the patient is to have severe postoperative respiratory complications or even suffer postoperative mortality. Based on cumulative experience, spirometric criteria for predicting morbidity and mortality in postoperative adult patients have been proposed.[31,32] If the FEV_1 is <1 L, the FVC <1.5 L, the FEV_1/FVC <30 percent, or the forced expiratory flow [$FEF_{(25-75\%)}$] <0.6 L/s, and maximum minute ventilation <50 percent of predicted, then such patients are considered very high risk for postoperative pulmonary complications. The approach is to improve the preoperative pulmonary status to levels above these spirometric criteria by the treatment modalities indicated by the respiratory function. This may take the form of cessation of smoking, diaphragm muscle conditioning, weight loss, the treatment of heart failure and fluid overload, and the treatment of any identifiable reactive airway disease by removal from the stimulating agent or the administration of bronchodilator therapy (or both).

The patient who is at even greater risk of postoperative pulmonary complication is the one who undergoes lung resection, particularly if the lung removed is functioning lung tissue.[31,32] In these patients one has to consider not only the general effects of position, anesthesia and incisional pain, but also the effect of the lost lung volume. To predict the postoperative pulmonary spirometric performance of these patients, a quantitative perfusion lung scan would allow the determination of the fraction of the lung that will be remaining after the planned procedure. The postoperative FEV_1 is then the product of the preoperative FEV_1 and the fractional perfusion of the remaining lung. In applying this technique, it is generally regarded that if the adult patient is unable to maintain a predicted $FEV_1 > 0.8$ L in the postoperative period, the operative risk is prohibitive. The predictive value of these spirometric criteria is increased by measurement of the diffusing capacity which is an independent predictor of morbidity and mortality after major lung resection.[32] A useful guideline is to exclude from major lung resection all patients with diffusing capacity <60 percent of predicted even if spirometric values are considered satisfactory.[32] Arterial blood-gas criteria may also be used to exclude patients from major lung resection because of the prohibitive risk of postoperative morbidity and mortality. Patients with room air Pa_{O_2} of <50 mmHg or $P_{CO_2} > 45$ mmHg at rest are considered prohibitive operative risks and should not undergo major pulmonary resection. Other forms of surgical intervention are justifiable only if considered mandatory and lifesaving in the presence of these blood-gas criteria.

Treatment Principles

At present no specific therapy exists that can be directed at the underlying diaphragmatic dysfunction. The principles of respiratory care in the surgical patient, therefore, involve the following:

1. Maximization of the preoperative respiratory status. This includes cessation of smoking, diaphragmatic conditioning exercises, decreasing obesity, and treating any identified cardiorespiratory disease including congestive heart failure, bronchopneumonia, or bronchospasm.
2. Aggressive physiotherapy and early ambulation to overcome the effects of the supine position on changes in lung volumes, particularly their relationship between closing volume and FRC. In patients with multiple fractures early operative stabilization will decrease the period of recumbency.
3. Adequate treatment of sepsis and shock, recognizing the important role of surgery in identifying and draining areas of sepsis such as intraabdominal abscesses.
4. The judicious use of intravenous fluids to maintain adequate perfusion but yet not produce overhydration and pulmonary edema.
5. The optimum use of analgesics so that pain is controlled without producing respiratory depression.
6. The hypoxemic patient should receive supplemental oxygen to improve arterial oxygenation.
7. When a cause of hypoxemia can be identified, then this cause should be treated as specifically as possible, e.g., bronchodilator therapy for a patient with bronchospasm or antibiotic against a specific organism isolated in a patient with a pneumonic process.
8. Preoperative pulmonary assessment especially in patients with poor pulmonary reserve and particularly in those undergoing lung resection. This will allow an assessment of the relative risk of postoperative morbidity.
9. Institution of mechanical ventilation when the above measures fail.

Frequently mechanical ventilation can be avoided if strict attention is paid to the other measures pointed out above. Also, vigorous application of these principles immediately after stabilizing the patient can shorten the duration of mechanical ventilation considerably.[33] In particular, patients obviously susceptible to atelectasis are ventilated in the 45° upright position with a small amount of PEEP to maintain FRC and with sighs (one and a half to two times the tidal volume) to reexpand collapsing air spaces intermittently.[33]

CASE PRESENTATION

Mrs. A.H. is a 72-year-old woman who presented to a surgeon with a 3-month history of epigastric pain. She claimed to have smoked cigarettes in the amount of three packages a week for approximately 20 years. Otherwise her past history was unremarkable. Gastroscopy revealed a large antral ulcer, and biopsy was negative for malignancy. She was placed on the medical regime of frequent small meals, antacids, and cimetidine and 6 weeks later repeat gastroscopy failed to show any evidence of ulcer healing. Surgery was planned and the patient was seen by the anesthesia department preoperatively. A preoperative chest x-ray was regarded as normal; the arterial blood-gas values on room air were: P_{O_2}, 64; P_{CO_2}, 38; and pH, 7.40. Spirometry showed mild obstructive pattern with an FEV_1/FVC ratio of 65 percent and this was improved to a level of 78 percent on bronchodilator.

She was advised to stop smoking, put on a graded exercise program, and started on bronchodilator therapy with the plan to admit her for surgery in approximately 4 weeks. However, she presented to the emergency department 2 weeks later with melena and feeling "faint." A nasogastric tube was inserted, and bright red blood was aspirated from the stomach.

She was admitted to the ward; her blood pressure dropped to 90 systolic, and this promptly responded to saline infusion. It was decided to take her to the operating room on the day after admission. She had been placed on cimetidine, and the nasogastric tube was kept in place. At laparotomy she was still bleeding and a vagotomy and antrectomy were conducted. During the procedure she remained normotensive but received 8 U blood, 2 L crystalloid, and 4 U plasma. The operation lasted approximately 3 h during which time she had a urine output of 10 mL/h. Her central venous pressure (CVP) varied between 8 and 14 cmH_2O.

Toward the end of the procedure the anesthetist noted that it was very difficult to ventilate her, and her airway pressure rose to 50 to 60 cmH_2O. Attempts to ventilate her by bag produced significant resistance, and frothy

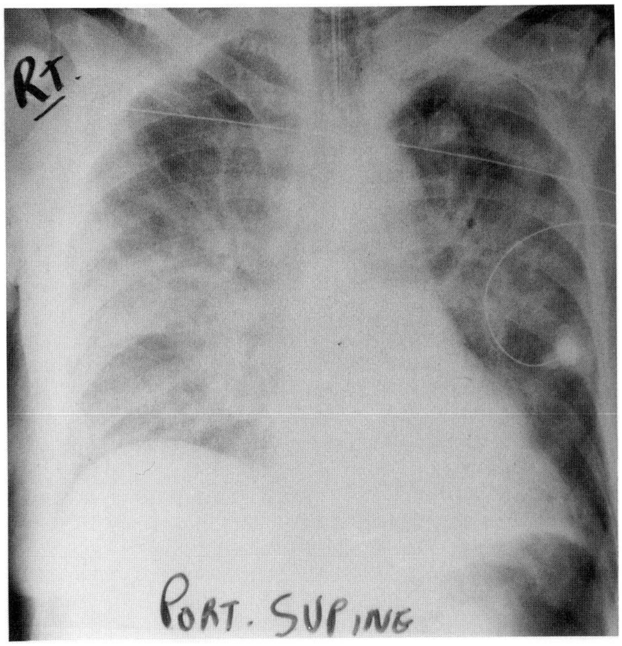

FIGURE 84-4 Postoperative chest x-ray of patient in the surgical ICU shows florid pulmonary edema.

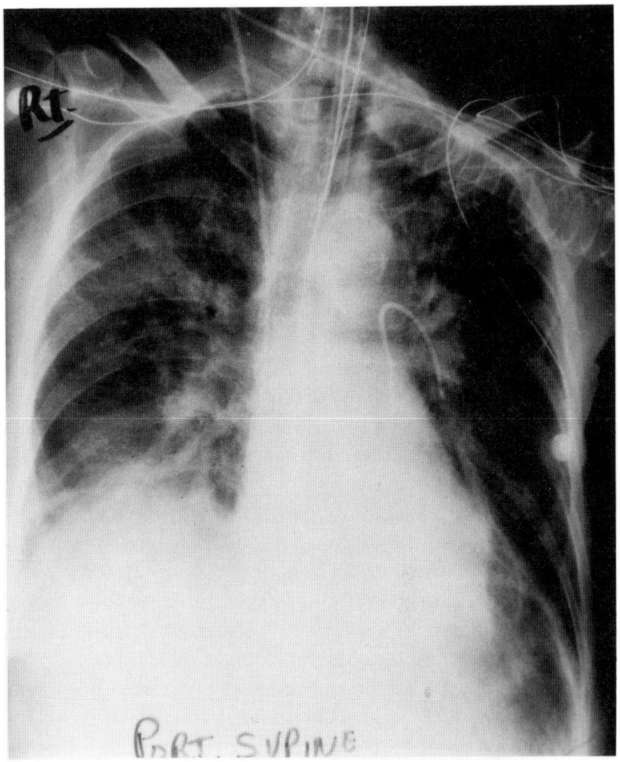

FIGURE 84-5 Significant clearing of pulmonary edema is seen radiologically with same PAWP as that in Fig. 84-4.

secretions were aspirated from her endotracheal tube. An arterial blood-gas determination on 100% oxygen showed a P_{O_2} of 68, P_{CO_2} of 40, and pH of 7.38. The patient was admitted to the surgical ICU where a chest x-ray was done (Fig. 84-4); this showed florid pulmonary edema. A Swan-Ganz catheter was inserted and yielded the following results: cardiac output, 4.2 L/min; mean pulmonary artery pressure, 30 mmHg; and mean PAWP, 10 mmHg. Furosemide, 40 mg, was administered with prompt diuresis, and her arterial blood-gas values 4 h later were: P_{O_2}, 87; P_{CO_2}, 34; and pH, 7.44 on an F_{IO_2} of 0.4. Her cardiac output at this time was 4.4 L/min with a pulmonary artery pressure of 26 mmHg and a PAWP of 10 mmHg. A repeat chest x-ray at this time (Fig. 84-5) showed significant clearing of the pulmonary edema. Weaning parameters done at this time showed a VC of 400, an inspiratory effort of 10 cmH_2O, and a tidal volume of 250 mL. She had been maintained on intravenous morphine, 2 to 4 mg every hour prn for pain control.

She was gradually weaned off the respirator over the next 48 h, and her VC improved from the original 400 to 1100 mL with an inspiratory effort of 25 cmH_2O. Postextubation blood-gas values on room air were: P_{O_2}, 58; pH 7.38; and P_{CO_2}, 42. She was placed on supplemental nasal oxygen. Over the next 3 days the oxygen was discontinued, and she was discharged from the hospital 2 weeks after surgery.

CASE DISCUSSION

The patient's history of chronic smoking and her age were causes for concern regarding operative risk. Since the operation was planned on a semielective basis, it was possible to assess her respiratory function preoperatively. Although the chest x-ray was normal, spirometry indicated significant reactive airway disease which responded to bronchodilator. Although it was planned to repeat her respiratory function prior to surgery, this was not possible because she presented to the emergency room prior to her planned surgery. However, it is probably safe to assume that there was significant improvement in her respiratory status because of her cessation of smoking and the use of bronchodilator therapy following her preoperative respiratory assessment.

Although cimetidine was used initially to treat her ulcer, this had the additional benefit of increasing gastric pH so that if there were any aspiration, the effect on the lung would be minimized. The placement of a nasogastric tube also decreased the likelihood of further gastric acid aspiration.

Judging from the CVP measurement in the operating room this patient probably received more volume infusion than required. She did not have a Swan-Ganz catheter inserted in the operating room, and it is possible that her CVP of 14 may have been a reflection of her chronic pulmonary disease and, therefore, it could not be used as an index of her volume status. The focus on urine output without regard to central pressure monitoring resulted in overtransfusion. This may be related to the effects of ADH and aldosterone which result in conservation of water and oliguria in the presence of adequate hydration.

On examining the patient's postoperative chest x-ray it was evident that she had significant pulmonary edema. It was not clear whether this was capillary leak pulmonary edema or high pressure pulmonary edema. The PAWP of 10 mmHg was regarded as evidence of capillary leak pulmonary edema. However, the rapid clearing of her pulmonary edema with diuresis without any change in the PAWP suggests that the PAWP may have been transiently elevated and at the time of the chest x-ray, there was still the lag phase of pulmonary edema present with a lower PAWP. The lag phase between the chest x-ray and the improvement in gas exchange is also demonstrated in this case. The temporal relationship of the PAWP measurement and the appearance of pulmonary edema radiologically as well as clinically should always be noted to arrive at the appropriate diagnosis and treatment in these patients.

The patient's initial VC in the surgical ICU was depressed despite apparent adequate pain control. A decreased respiratory effort was also demonstrated by the low maximum inspiratory force generated by the patient. This may be attributed to some degree of diaphragmatic dysfunction or narcotic depression of respiratory drive.

Physiotherapy with encouraging deep breathing and coughing as well as bronchodilator therapy were continued in the postoperative period to deal with the patient's reactive airway disease as well as to prevent the accumulation of secretions and the development of a pneumonic or atelectatic process.

This case demonstrates the importance of preoperative assessment of pulmonary function, the identification of correctable pulmonary abnormalities, close monitoring of fluid requirements, using central hemodynamic monitoring, and the role of analgesics, physiotherapy, and mechanical ventilation in supporting patients who may develop respiratory failure in the perioperative period.

References

1. Chung HM, Rudiger K, Schrier RW, Anderson RJ: Postoperative hyponatremia; a prospective study. Arch Intern Med 146:333, 1986.
2. Giesecke AH Jr, Egbert LD: Perioperative fluid therapy, in Miller RD (ed): *Crystalloids in Anaesthesia.* 2d ed. New York, Churchill Livingstone, 1986, p 3132.
3. Colice GL, Matthay MA, Bass E, Matthay RA. Neurogenic pulmonary edema. Am Rev Respir Dis 130:941, 1984.
4. Ali J, Duke K: Decreasing hydrostatic pressure does not uniformly decrease high pressure pulmonary edema. Chest 91(4):588, 1987.
5. Wood LDH, Prewitt RM: Cardiovascular management in acute hypoxemic respiratory failure. Am J Cardiol 47:963, 1981.
6. Ali J, Wood LDH: Pulmonary vascular effects of furosemide on gas exchange in pulmonary edema. J Appl Physiol 57(1):160, 1984.
7. Matthay MA, Chatterjee K: Bedside catheterization of the pulmonary artery: Risks compared with benefits. Ann Intern Med 109:826, 1988.
8. Brismar B, Hedenstierna G, Lundquist H, et al: Pulmonary densities during anesthesia with muscular relaxation—A proposal of atelectasis. Anesthesiology 62:422, 1985.
9. Tokics L, Hedenstierna G, Brismar B, et al: Thoracoabdominal restriction in supine men: CT and lung function measurements. J Appl Physiol 64(2):599, 1988.
10. Craig DB, Wahba WM, Don HF, et al: "Closing volume" and its relationship to gas exchange in seated and supine positions. J Appl Physiol 31:717, 1971.
11. Alexander JI, Horton, PW, Millar WT, et al: The effect of upper abdominal surgery on the relationship of airway closing point to end tidal position. Clin Sci 43:137, 1972.
12. Hoeppner VH, Cooper DM, Zamel N, et al: Relationship between elastic recoil and closing volume in smokers and nonsmokers. Am Rev Respir Dis 109:81, 1974.
13. Warner MA, Divertie MB, Tinker JH: Preoperative cessation of smoking and pulmonary complications in coronary artery bypass patients. Anesthesiology 60(4):380, 1984.
14. Johnson KD, Cadambi A, Seibert AB: Incidence of adult respiratory distress syndrome in patients with multiple musculoskeletal injuries: Effect of early operative stabilization of fractures. J Trauma 25:375, 1985.
15. Ali J, Weisel RD, Layug AB, et al: Consequences of postoperative alterations in respiratory mechanics. Am J Surg 128:376, 1974.
16. Hedenstierna G: Mechanisms of postoperative pulmonary dysfunction. Acta Chir Scand (suppl) 550:152, 1989.
17. Ali J, Yaffe C, Serrette C: The effect of transcutaneous electric nerve stimulation on postoperative pain and pulmonary function. Surgery 89(4):507, 1981.
18. Simonneau G, Vivien A, Sartener R, et al: Diaphragm dysfunction induced by upper abdominal surgery. Am Rev Respir Dis 128:899, 1983.
19. Ford GT, Whitelaw WA, Rosenal TW, et al: Diaphragm function after upper abdominal surgery in humans. Am Rev Respir Dis 127:431, 1983.
20. Road JD, Burgess KR, Whitelaw WA, Ford GT: Diaphragm function and respiratory response after upper abdominal surgery in dogs. J Appl Physiol 57(2):576, 1984.
21. Ford GT, Grant DA, Rideout KS, et al: Inhibition of breathing associated with gall bladder (GB) stimulation in dogs. J Appl Physiol 65(1):72, 1988.
22. Ali J, Khan TA: The comparative effects of muscle transection and median upper abdominal incisions on postoperative pulmonary function. Surg Gynecol Obstet 148:863, 1979.
23. Roussos C: The failing ventilatory pump. Lung 160:59, 1982.
24. Herve P, Simonneau G, Girard P, et al: Hypercapneic acidosis induced by nutrition in mechanically ventilated patients. Glucose vs. fat. Crit Care Med 13:537, 1985.
25. Knill RL, Gelb AW: Peripheral chemoreceptors during anesthesia. Are the watch dogs sleeping? Anesthesiology 57:151, 1982.
26. Brain JD: Anesthesia and respiratory defense mechanisms. Int Anesthesiol Clin 15:169, 1977.
27. Wynne JW, Modell JH: Respiratory aspiration of stomach contents. Ann Intern Med 87:466, 1977.
28. Celli BR, Rodriguez KS, Snider GL: A controlled trial of intermittent positive pressure breathing, incentive spirometry and

deep breathing exercises in preventing pulmonary complications after abdominal surgery. Am Rev Respir Dis 130:12, 1984.
29. Ali J, Serrette C, Wood LDH, Anthonisen NR: Effect of postoperative intermittent positive pressure breathing on lung function. Chest 2:192, 1984.
30. Ali J, Serrette C, Khan TA: The effect of abdominal binders on postoperative pulmonary function. Infections in Surgery 875, November, 1983.
31. Ali MK, Mountain CF, Ewer MS, et al: Predicting loss of pulmonary function after pulmonary resection for bronchogenic carcinoma. Chest 77:337, 1980.
32. Ferguson MK, Little L, Rizzo L, et al: Diffusing capacity predicts morbidity and mortality after pulmonary resection. J Thorac Cardiovasc Surg 96(6):894, 1988.
33. Hall JB, Wood LDH: Liberation of the patient from mechanical ventilation. JAMA 257(2):1621, 1987.

Chapter 85

THE ACUTE ABDOMEN AND INTRAABDOMINAL SEPSIS

R.A. MUSTARD
J.M.A. BOHNEN
B.D. SCHOUTEN

KEY POINTS

- *Acute abdominal problems may present in an occult or unusual fashion in the ICU.*
- *Evaluation frequently requires the conjoint efforts of the intensivist, surgeon, and gastroenterologist.*
- *Prompt diagnosis is the key to successful management.*
- *Computed tomography (CT) scanning or ultrasound should be used liberally in the evaluation of intraabdominal sepsis (IAS).*
- *Complications occur frequently in the postsurgical ICU patient; "stable vitals" does not imply clinical stability.*
- *Postoperative residual or recurrent IAS may not be clinically obvious and may not be demonstrated by a CT scan; cardiorespiratory instability should prompt a high level of suspicion.*
- *The treatment of the febrile postsurgical patient is not simply the administration of further antibiotics.*
- *Acalculous cholecystitis is a treacherous disease which may require urgent treatment despite lack of a definitive diagnosis.*

The diagnosis and management of patients with an "acute abdomen" remains a major clinical problem for surgeons and intensivists. The term "acute abdomen" refers to a patient whose chief presenting symptom is the acute onset of abdominal pain. The vast majority of these patients present in the emergency department and do not require treatment in an ICU. However, the small percentage of patients who do require such treatment constitute a significant fraction of the surgical ICU patients in most general hospitals. Furthermore, the intensivist must be aware that an ICU patient may develop an acute abdomen while being treated for some other condition.

In this chapter, we will first discuss the approach to the ICU patient who develops abdominal pain while undergoing treatment for some other disorder. The bulk of the chapter, however, will be directed to the patient with known IAS who requires intensive care. Emphasis will be placed on the early diagnosis of intraabdominal septic complications.

Evaluation of Acute Abdominal Pain in the ICU Patient

The diagnosis of abdominal pain is heavily dependent on an accurate history and a complete physical examination.[1] Both of these sources of data may be severely limited in the ICU patient. History may be unobtainable because of intubation or a decreased level of consciousness. Physical examination is made difficult by the presence of large numbers of tubes emanating from the patient and may be further compromised by medications such as corticosteroids. Indeed, abdominal pain itself may be masked by narcotics or other painful disease processes. Some physical signs, such as the absence of bowel sounds, which would be considered significant in an otherwise well patient, may not be significant in an ICU patient in whom multiple extraabdominal causes of ileus may be present. Hence, in the ICU setting it is rarely the patient who complains to the physician of abdominal pain, but rather the physician who must infer the presence of an abdominal problem based on nonspecific findings such as unexplained sepsis, hypovolemia, abdominal distention, and so on.

Table 85-1 provides an abbreviated summary of the many causes of acute abdominal pain. Rather than describing a complete algorithm for the diagnosis of these conditions in ICU patients, we will list some important principles.

1. Evaluate the patient in the context of the patient's underlying disorder(s). For example, sudden severe abdominal pain in a patient with congestive heart failure secondary to myocardial infarction is much more likely to be due to mesenteric ischemia than to renal colic.
2. Make liberal use of surgical consultants. A patient with significant unexplained abdominal pain lasting more than 4 h should likely be seen by a surgeon.
3. CT scan or ultrasound of the abdomen are excellent screening tests for acute abdominal problems in patients with unreliable physical examination.

In summary, there is no straightforward approach to the ICU patient who develops an acute abdomen. Indeed, the major problem may be simply determining that the patient

TABLE 85-1 Etiology of Acute Abdominal Pain

1. Inflammatory disorders (e.g., cholecystitis, diverticulitis, perforated peptic ulcer, etc.)
2. Colics
   Biliary
   Renal
   Intestinal obstruction
3. Vascular lesions
   Mesenteric ischemia
   Ruptured abdominal aortic aneurysm
   Intraabdominal or retroperitoneal hemorrhage
4. Urologic or gynecologic disorders
5. Medical disorders (e.g., lupus serositis, sickle cell crisis, etc.)

has an acute abdomen. Successful management of these patients depends on the close collaboration of the intensivist and the surgeon.

The ICU Management of the Patient with an Acute Abdomen

Most patients with an acute abdomen are diagnosed outside the ICU. These patients may require treatment in an ICU for one of four reasons.

1. The patient is very ill but may not require surgical intervention (e.g., severe pancreatitis; see Chap. 165).
2. The patient requires stabilization prior to operation (e.g., septic shock, see Chap. 98).
3. The patient has undergone definitive surgical treatment for the acute abdominal disease but has unrelated medical problems requiring intensive care [e.g., chronic obstructive pulmonary disease (COPD); see Sect. J].
4. The patient has undergone definitive surgical treatment and requires intensive care because of the severity of the abdominal pathology or the occurrence of a postoperative complication such as sepsis.

In this chapter we will consider only patients in the fourth group. This group may be subdivided into septic and nonseptic categories. A common nonseptic acute abdominal condition requiring postoperative ICU care is a ruptured abdominal aortic aneurysm, and the care of these patients is discussed in Chap. 86. Hence, in this chapter, we will consider only the ICU management of patients who have undergone treatment of a septic abdominal disease.

A classification of the sources of IAS is given in Table 85-2. Sepsis resulting from disease originating in the pancreas is discussed in Chap. 165. Also, we will not discuss infections arising in the female reproductive tract (pelvic inflammatory disease) or urinary tract (see Chap. 107). The principles of treatment of IAS are well established. These are

TABLE 85-2 Classification of IAS

Primary Peritonitis
Infected ascitic fluid
Infected peritoneal dialysis catheter
Miscellaneous (e.g., tuberculosis)
Secondary Peritonitis
Intraperitoneal
Biliary tree
Gastrointestinal tract
Female reproductive system
Retroperitoneal
Pancreas
Urinary tract
Visceral abscess
Liver
Spleen

1. Prompt diagnosis and resuscitation
2. Prompt treatment of the underlying pathology and mechanical cleansing of the peritoneal cavity
3. Appropriate antibiotic administration
4. Supportive care of the patient
5. Constant vigilance to detect and treat aggressively any complications arising from the underlying disease or its treatment
6. Close collaboration among all physicians caring for the patient

The importance of prompt diagnosis and treatment cannot be overemphasized. This is one of the few prognostic variables that physicians can control to some extent, and prompt treatment has been repeatedly shown to result in decreased mortality.[2–4]

PRIMARY PERITONITIS

Primary peritonitis is a group of diseases characterized by infection in the peritoneal cavity without an obvious source such as a gastrointestinal tract perforation.[5,6] This most frequently occurs in patients who have ascites secondary to cirrhosis of the liver, congestive heart failure, renal dialysis, and so on. Patients suffering from primary peritonitis rarely require intensive care. However, primary peritonitis may well be present in patients requiring intensive care for other reasons. For example, a cirrhotic patient with portal hypertension and ascites may develop primary peritonitis which precipitates hepatic decompensation leading to variceal bleeding and hypovolemic shock necessitating ICU admission.

The clinical presentation is usually one of fever and physical signs of peritoneal irritation. However, approximately one-third of patients with primary peritonitis will have no signs or symptoms of sepsis referable to the abdomen. Diagnosis is based on clinical suspicion, the patients' presentation, and the Gram stain and culture results obtained from ascitic fluid aspiration. Culture of infected ascitic fluid usually yields aerobic enteric organisms; however, approximately 35 percent of patients with these diseases will have negative ascitic fluid cultures.[6] Blood cultures are also frequently positive in these patients. Primary bacterial peritonitis may be assumed to be present when the ascitic fluid neutrophil count is >250 neutrophils/mm^3. The diagnosis may be confirmed in culture-negative patients by the response to appropriate antibiotic treatment which should be evident within 48 h and is characterized by both clinical improvement and a decrease in the number of white blood cells present in the ascitic fluid.

It is most important to distinguish primary from secondary bacterial peritonitis. *Secondary bacterial peritonitis* is caused by gut luminal contamination and hence multiple organisms are usually found in the ascitic fluid Gram stain or culture. Patients with secondary bacterial peritonitis are unlikely to respond to antibiotic administration alone and usually require surgical treatment.

Antibiotic treatment should be initiated on clinical suspicion of peritonitis and before final culture and sensitivity results are available. Broad-spectrum treatment with either ampicillin and an aminoglycoside or a third generation cephalosporin alone is usually sufficient. The prognosis of these patients depends almost entirely on the underlying liver disease responsible for the ascities.

Patients who develop peritonitis secondary to an infected peritoneal dialysis catheter may or may not respond to antibiotic treatment (usually instilled into the dialysis fluid). Nonresponse requires removal of the catheter and temporary hemodialysis.

BILIARY TRACT SEPSIS

Both sepsis and hyperbilirubinemia are common findings in critically ill patients. When these conditions coexist, the question of biliary tract sepsis arises. However, most jaundiced ICU patients do not have pathology in their biliary trees,[7] and, therefore, before we discuss biliary tract sepsis we will briefly outline the approach to the jaundiced patient.

Infection in the biliary tree results in one or more of three rather different clinical entities. Most commonly infection is only present in the gallbladder and is due to obstruction of the cystic duct by a gallstone. This entity, acute calculous cholecystitis, is usually treated surgically by removal of the gallbladder and only results in ICU admission if the patient has other major medical problems. Of more relevance to the intensivist are the syndromes of acute cholangitis and acute acalculous cholecystitis.

THE JAUNDICED ICU PATIENT

Abnormalities of liver function tests and even clinically evident jaundice are quite common in the ICU patient population. Lamont and Isselbacher, in a classic review article on postoperative jaundice,[7] provide a simple classification: increased pigment load, impaired hepatocellular function, and extrahepatic obstruction. The vast majority of ICU patients with abnormal liver function tests fall into the first two categories. Exclusion of extrahepatic biliary obstruction is best accomplished by[8] history, physical examination, and routine laboratory tests (i.e., the clinical context) and ultrasonography to look specifically for evidence for bile duct dilation. In certain unusual circumstances[8] obstructed bile ducts may not be dilated, and clinical suspicion will require direct visualization of the biliary tree with either endoscopic retrograde cholangiopancreatography (ERCP) or percutaneous transhepatic cholangiography (PTC).

ACUTE CHOLANGITIS

Cholangitis is defined as a bacterial infection within bile ducts. It occurs when bacteria are introduced into a partially or totally obstructed duct system. In this situation the bacteria multiply rapidly within the bile and induce an inflammatory reaction around the small biliary radicles in the liver. When the hydrostatic pressure in the ducts exceeds a certain point, bacteria are literally forced out of the bile canaliculi and into the hepatic sinusoids, resulting in systemic bacteremia. The microbiology of this disease is similar to that of peritonitis caused by gastrointestinal tract perforation. The portal of entry of bacteria into the biliary tree remains a topic of debate.

The clinical presentation is usually obvious, with right upper quadrant abdominal pain, jaundice, and fever (Charcot's triad). Patients may be only mildly ill with bactobilia or critically ill with frank pus under pressure in the biliary tree. Diagnosis may be confirmed with ultrasound, ERCP, or PTC. Treatment consists of biliary decompression and the administration of appropriate broad-spectrum antibiotics to cover both aerobic gram-negative rods and anaerobic gram-negative bacilli. Bile and blood for culture are obtained before antibiotics are started (if possible) to be sure the antibiotic coverage is optimal.

These patients may require intensive care if they develop septic shock either from the disease itself or secondary to bacteremia induced by its treatment. From the intensivists point of view, the management is straightforward—support the cardiorespiratory system until the ducts have been decompressed and the patient is hemodynamically stable and ensure appropriate antibiotics are administered. It must be emphasized that the key to success is adequate biliary decompression. This may be done either surgically (exploration of the common bile duct and insertion of a T tube), endoscopically (nasobiliary drain insertion, sphincterotomy and stone extraction, or placement of an internal stent), or percutaneously (placement of a transhepatic external drain). The adequacy of drainage is confirmed by rapid clinical and biochemical improvement (obvious within 24 to 48 h). A patient with cholangitis who does not improve clinically and may require ongoing cardiopulmonary support must be assumed to have inadequate drainage. In this case it is essential to image the biliary tree to determine the adequacy of the drainage and plan for further decompression. It may also be necessary to obtain a CT scan to look for hepatic abscess(es) induced by the cholangitis.

ACALCULOUS CHOLECYSTITIS

This disease is a child of modern intensive care. It was well summarized in a 1978 article by Long and coworkers:

> Acute acalculous cholecystitis is a treacherous and potentially lethal disease. It may occur in patients without known biliary tract disease who are severely compromised by trauma or gastrointestinal dysfunction and require prolonged intensive care. Its onset is insidious, its presenting symptoms are inconstant, and its neglect can lead to necrosis of the gallbladder with sepsis and death.[9]

This disease occurs in approximately 0.5 to 1.5 percent of long-term (>1 week) ICU patients.[10,11] The etiology of this disease is unknown and hence there are no known ways to prevent it.[12] It appears that in the occasional critically ill patient the gallbladder wall becomes inflamed and infected with enteric organisms. The cystic duct becomes edematous and occluded, but it is not known whether this is the cause or a result of the disease. This may occur at any time during the patient's ICU stay. In about one-third of pa-

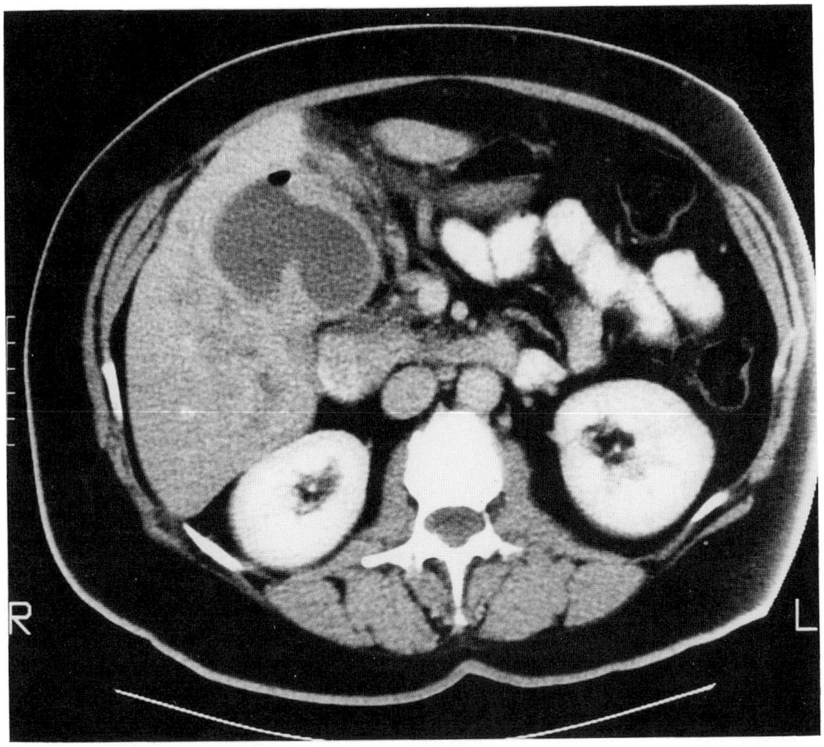

FIGURE 85-1 CT scan diagnostic of acalculous cholecystitis. The patient has an enlarged thick-walled gallbladder with intraluminal gas. The liver around the gallbladder fossa is markedly edematous.

tients, the inflammation has induced partial or complete necrosis of the gallbladder by the time of diagnosis.

The real problem with this disease is the difficulty in achieving a definitive diagnosis without resorting to laparotomy. Attention should be focused on the gallbladder when sepsis or organ failure occurs without a known cause. The patient may have right upper quadrant abdominal tenderness, but an ICU patient can have this sign without cholecystitis. Distention of the liver capsule due to increased venous pressure or sepsis can produce identical physical findings. Liver function tests are not helpful. A biliary radionuclide scan is helpful in that filling of the gallbladder (perhaps with the aid of morphine-induced spasm of the sphincter of Oddi[13]) implies cystic duct patency, which effectively rules out cholecystitis. The most valuable tests are ultrasound and CT scan. Findings of pericholecystic fluid (without ascites), intramural gas, or a sloughed mucosal membrane are virtually diagnostic (Fig. 85-1). Unfortunately, not all patients will have these findings.[11] A thick-walled gallbladder is suggestive, unless the patient has generalized edema. Percutaneous bile aspiration for culture has high false-positive and false-negative rates and is therefore not helpful.

It is our practice to operate on these patients if our clinical index of suspicion is sufficiently high and the patient is deteriorating without obvious cause. About half the patients we operate on for this reason have the disease. These patients are treated with cholecystectomy. The remaining half have a cholecystostomy tube placed to prevent the disease in the future. To date, direct visualization of the gallbladder in the operating room is the only completely accurate method of diagnosis. This can be carried out under local anesthesia but this seems somewhat pointless in the ventilated patient. In the rare patient who is felt to be "too sick to undergo laparotomy" percutaneous transhepatic drainage of the gallbladder may result in significant clinical improvement.[14] This procedure can be carried out at the bedside under ultrasound guidance. It is our experience, however, that these patients should later undergo cholecystectomy before the drainage tube is removed.

SECONDARY BACTERIAL PERITONITIS

In this section we will discuss the ICU management of patients with secondary bacterial peritonitis defined as the presence of pus or gastrointestinal contents in the peritoneal cavity. This may be either localized (abscess) or diffuse (generalized peritonitis). Patients with physical signs of peritoneal irritation due to localized gastrointestinal tract infections are discussed in Chap. 108.

Patients with secondary bacterial peritonitis requiring intensive care form a significant fraction both of all surgical ICU admissions and of all patients with peritonitis. For example, at our hospital, 300 patients with generalized peritonitis or abdominal abscess were treated in the last 5 years. Of these patients, 107 (mean APACHE II score 19.3) required posttreatment ventilatory support for an average of 9.6 days (78 treated surgically, 29 treated percutaneously). One hundred and ninety-three patients (mean APACHE II score 10.4) did not require ventilation (137 treated surgically, 56 treated percutaneously). Patients requiring postoperative ventilatory support were severely ill and had a 64 percent mortality rate compared to patients not requiring such treatment who had only an 11 percent mortality rate. The need for mechanical ventilation may, therefore, be a marker for general severity of illness which results in a poor prognosis.

TABLE 85-3 Anatomic Sites of Bacterial Infection in Postoperative Peritonitis

Intraabdominal	Extraabdominal
Peritoneal fluid	Soft tissue infection
Peritoneal fibrin	Pneumonia
Extraperitoneal tissues (e.g., hepatic macrophages)	Urosepsis
Visceral abscess	Intravascular catheter infection
Within the gastrointestinal tract lumen ("tertiary" peritonitis, *Clostridium difficile* colitis)	Disseminated candidiasis
Infected prosthetic vascular graft	
Acalculous cholecystitis	

PATHOPHYSIOLOGY AND TREATMENT

Generalized peritonitis is usually caused by either bowel infarction (see Chap. 167), or more commonly, bowel perforation. Occasionally, generalized bacterial peritonitis may result from perforation of an infected gallbladder, infected pancreatic pseudocyst, or other rare disease. We shall restrict our attention in this chapter to the vast majority of cases which are due to gastrointestinal tract perforation.

Patients with generalized peritonitis may become very ill because of the anatomy of the peritoneal cavity. Its large surface area permits massive loss of fluids into the abdomen and rapid absorption of bacteria, endotoxin, and inflammatory mediators into the systemic circulation. The hemodynamic effects of generalized peritonitis have been compared with a 50 percent body surface area burn.[15]

Treatment of this disease is well established.[15] Following rapid fluid resuscitation and the initiation of antibiotic therapy, patients undergo laparotomy to close the perforation (or resect, exteriorize, etc.) and remove as much of the contaminating material and inflammatory exudate as possible. Broad-spectrum antibiotics are used to eliminate residual bacterial contamination after laparotomy and because septicemia is common in these patients. The gold standard in antibiotic therapy is the combination of an aminoglycoside and an antianaerobe agent such as metronidazole or clindamycin. To avoid nephrotoxicity, aminoglycosides should not be given to patients with significantly decreased glomerular filtration rates (e.g., elevated serum creatinine, advanced age, hypotension). Single agent treatment with a second generation cephalosporin (cefoxitin) is equally efficacious.[16] Since the administration of broad-spectrum antibiotics may lead to systemic candidiasis, pseudomembraneous colitis, and the selection of multiply resistant organisms, the drugs should be discontinued as soon as the acute episode of abdominal infection has subsided. Unfortunately, there is no straightforward guide to antibiotic discontinuation. The conventional criteria of clinical improvement, no fever, and no leukocytosis have an exceedingly small relapse rate of peritoneal infection but may never be achieved in many ICU patients.[17] In this group, we believe that it is reasonable to stop antibiotics when the patient no longer has physical signs of peritonitis or ileus. If the patient still has fever or leukocytosis, a CT scan should be obtained to rule out intraabdominal abscess. If no abscess is found, antibiotics can be stopped and a search begun for an extraperitoneal source of infection.

The mortality rate of generalized peritonitis is about 30 percent. Known prognostic factors include age, preexisting disease, severity of physiologic derangement at the time of diagnosis, steroid dependency, and peritonitis occurring in the postoperative period.[18] Interestingly, the site of perforation is not a determinant of mortality (with the exception of perforated appendicitis). Perforated peptic ulcers are just as deadly as perforated colons. The cause of death is usually uncontrolled sepsis. Of our 107 ICU patients with peritonitis, 68 died. IAS was considered the main cause in 37 patients (55 percent) and was a contributing cause in 24 patients (35 percent). Only 7 patients (10 percent) suffered a nonseptic death. Essentially all the septic deaths were due to multisystem organ failure (MSOF).

It is widely assumed that the cause of MSOF in these patients is bacterial infection. (It is also possible that the uncontrolled infections are just another result of MSOF caused by an unknown disorder of immunologic regulation—see Chap. 53). When considering treatment of these patients, it is helpful to classify the possible anatomic sites of bacterial infection (Table 85-3). At the present time we do not have specific treatments for all intraabdominal sites of infection. The prevention and treatment of infection in fibrin deposits, tissues, or the gut lumen is a very active research field at this time. For example, many postoperative abscesses likely start as small collections of fibrin-encased bacteria. Intraperitoneal instillation of tissue plasminogen activator may, in the future, prevent many such abscesses.[19] Bacterial overgrowth in the gut lumen may be prevented with appropriate enteral nutrition (see Sect. G).

THE INTENSIVIST'S ROLE. It is the intensivist's role to support these patients postoperatively and be aware of the possible need for further surgical intervention as well as the potential for a large variety of possible complications. Close collaboration between the intensivist and the surgeon is essential for the optimal management of the patient. Supportive treatment is usually straightforward and includes hemodynamic support (recovery from shock), respiratory support, nutritional support [usually with total parenteral nutrition (TPN)], administration of antibiotics, and if necessary, renal support with dialysis or hemofiltration. Complications, however, are many and varied and include complications of the supportive care (e.g., nosocomial infection), complications which may occur in any surgical patient (e.g., pulmonary embolus), and complications which are specific to the patient treated surgically for peritonitis. We will only consider this latter group of problems (Table 85-4).

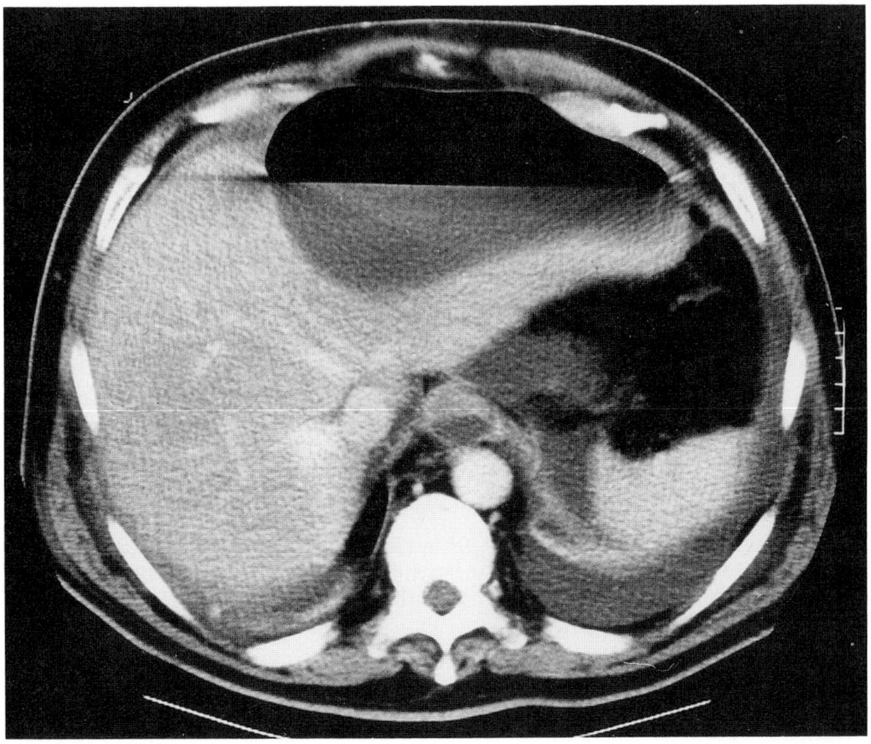

FIGURE 85-2 CT scan demonstrates massive left subphrenic abscess. The patient developed septic shock 11 days after total gastrectomy for adenocarcinoma of the stomach. Following resuscitation in the ICU, this scan was obtained and the abscess was drained percutaneously. The anastomotic leak was later repaired surgically.

These patients must be examined daily by the intensivist, as well as the surgeon, with this list of complications in mind. First, all dressings covering the abdomen should be removed and the wound examined. The skin incision is usually packed open at operation to minimize the incidence of wound infection.[20] Fascial dehiscence may be observed. This complication is not rare and should prompt an immediate surgical consultation. Dehiscence occurred in 17 of our 107 ventilated peritonitis patients. Dehiscence is most common on postoperative days 4 to 8 but may occur at any time. It is heralded by the drainage of serosanguinous fluid through the incision. The diagnosis is confirmed by palpation of the wound (if the skin incision was closed) or the observation of intraabdominal contents in the wound (if the wound was packed open). The presence of loops of bowel in the wound poses the acute risk of evisceration. In some patients with particularly severe peritonitis, it is not technically possible to reapproximate the fascial edges at the end of the surgical procedure. The surgeon then sutures an artifical mesh to the fascia to prevent postoperative evisceration, and the wound is packed with saline-soaked gauze.[21] These patients are particularly prone to forming enterocutaneous fistulae at the surface of their open wounds, and this complication is easily diagnosed by inspection.[22] Finally, all tubes or drains should be inspected to make sure that they have not been dislodged and are functioning as intended. For example, sump drains should be checked to make sure that the air inlet ports are not occluded.

TABLE 85-4 Postoperative Complications Specifically Related to the Surgical Treatment of Peritonitis

Wound Complications	*Complications Arising in the Peritoneal Cavity*
Wound infection	Abscess formation
Necrotizing soft tissue infection	Intraabdominal bleeding
Fascial dehiscence/evisceration	*Miscellaneous*
Gastrointestinal Tract Complications	Postoperative pancreatitis
Ileus	Septicemia
Mechanical obstruction	Acalculous cholecystitis
Enterocutaneous fistula	
Gastrointestinal bleeding	
Anastomotic disruption or perforation	
Ischemic bowel	
Antibiotic-associated colitis	

Secondly, the intensivist needs to determine whether the gastrointestinal tract is functioning adequately to allow enteral feeds. This is sometimes very difficult to predict in the sedated ventilated patient, and it is frequently necessary to challenge the patient by starting tube feeds and simply check the gastric residual volume every 4 h. As will be discussed in Sect. G, enteral feeding is preferred over parenteral feeding in this patient population, if technically feasible.

Thirdly, the intensivist must determine if the patient is septic and if the septic focus is intraabdominal. The most common IAS complication is abscess formation, which occurred in 21 of 107 peritonitis patients who required postoperative ventilation in our series. It is often difficult to determine when the patient's original septic response is abating and a new septic response is being mounted.[23] In general, if the patient is not steadily improving following surgery or if the patient begins to deteriorate in any way, a CT scan of the abdomen should be obtained to identify and localize a possible abscess (Fig. 85-2). However, it is usually not fruitful to scan the patient sooner than 5 to 7 days after laparotomy. Patients in this early postoperative period frequently have multiple intraabdominal fluid collections, most of which are sterile. The patient who is deteriorating in the first week following surgery for peritonitis and who is felt to have persistent or recurrent peritoneal infection usually requires repeat laparotomy. Beyond this early phase, when abscesses are better formed and sterile collections have been resorbed, percutaneous drainage offers a safe and effective method of abscess diagnosis and control.[24] (See Chap. 20.)

OPEN ABDOMEN TREATMENT. In certain circumstances patients with peritonitis require "open abdomen" treatment. These patients fall into two categories—the patient whose fascia could not be closed for technical reasons but who is otherwise stable and the patient whose peritonitis is so severe that in the surgeon's opinion the abdomen should be left open to facilitate repeated laparotomies for peritoneal toilet. The latter group presents a major problem to the intensivist and the ICU nursing staff. These patients undergo laparotomy (through the mesh) every 1 to 3 days until the surgeon feels that the peritoneal cavity is sufficiently "clean." Weaning from ventilatory support is almost always impossible until after the last "scheduled re-laparotomy."[25] Furthermore, during this period of repeated laparotomies large quantities of proteinaceous fluids are lost through the open abdominal wound, and the patients therefore require support with plasma as well as TPN. Fortunately, such drastic treatment for peritonitis is rarely required and has not yet been proven to be more efficacious than conventional management.

VISCERAL ABSCESS

Pyogenic liver abscess is a rare condition which can occur in an ICU patient. Almost any bacterium may be cultured. A wide variety of conditions may give rise to an hepatic abscess (Table 85-5), but it should be noted that at least 20 percent of cases are cryptogenic.[26]

Patients with hepatic abscess usually present with sepsis associated with right upper quadrant pain and occasionally peritoneal findings such as an enlarged liver. Liver function test results are frequently abnormal. The diagnosis is confirmed by CT or ultrasound examination (Fig. 85-3).

The preferred treatment of hepatic abscess is percutaneous drainage for large abscesses. Note that the presence of more than one large abscess does not necessitate open surgical treatment. Antibiotics should be administered as de-

TABLE 85-5 Etiology of Hepatic Abscess

Trauma
Perihepatic sepsis
Systemic bacteremia
Portal bacteremia
Cholangitis
Cryptogenic

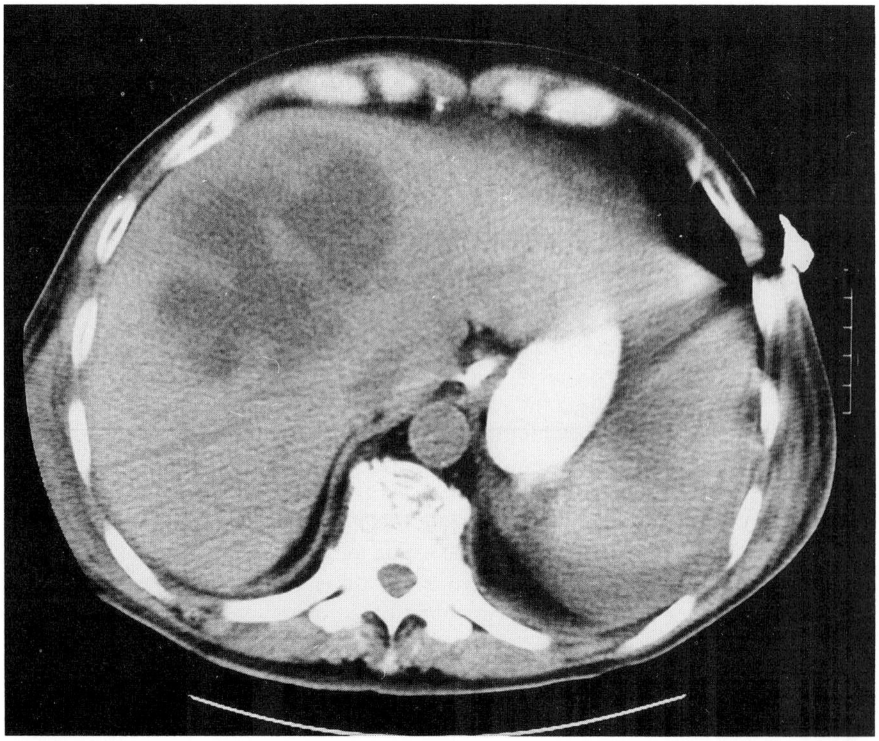

FIGURE 85-3 CT scan demonstrates large pyogenic liver abscess. The patient presented with septic shock and abnormal liver function tests. Following resuscitation in the ICU, an ultrasound was obtained which failed to support the clinical diagnosis of acute cholangitis. This CT scan was therefore carried out and the abscess drained percutaneously. No cause for the abscess was found.

scribed for patients with peritonitis. This may be the only treatment required for patients with multiple small abscesses, usually secondary to cholangitis, after bile duct drainage has been established.

Splenic abscess formation is rare. It may be due to trauma, direct extension of a septic process such as pancreatic abscess, infection of a splenic infarct, or secondary to bacteremia. These patients present with left upper quadrant abdominal pain, left pleural effusion, or sepsis of unknown etiology, and the diagnosis is established by CT or ultrasound examination of the abdomen. The optimal treatment is splenectomy, but percutaneous drainage may be used as a temporizing maneuver.[27]

The Abdomen as a Source of Occult Sepsis

A frequent clinical problem in the ICU is the patient with "a septic picture" or MSOF (or both) with no obvious etiology. Line sepsis, soft tissue infection, foreign body infection, *Candida* septicemia, endocarditis, pneumonia, and urosepsis can often be ruled out. Attention then focuses on the abdomen even if the patient had no known preexisting gastrointestinal pathologic condition. A CT scan of the abdomen is an excellent screening test in this patient group. However, a negative CT scan or ultrasound does not absolutely rule out peritoneal infection.

There are a number of causes of occult IAS (Table 85-6). Acute acalculous cholecystitis was discussed previously. Intraabdominal abscesses which are too small to be seen on CT scan or ultrasound or are hidden between loops of bowel (interloop abscess) are a second well-recognized cause. These can only be diagnosed by laparotomy prompted by clinical suspicion and exclusion of other causes of sepsis. Rarely, a short segment of ischemic or necrotic bowel may be very difficult to detect. If the segment is in the small bowel, the patient will usually have a clinical picture of mechanical small bowel obstruction. However, if the segment is in the left colon, the patient may have no other obvious symptoms. Colonoscopy is the diagnostic method of choice if this is suspected.

Finally, experimental evidence suggests that the gastrointestinal tract itself may be the source of systemic endotoxemia or bacteremia in some ICU patients.[28] It has been hypothesized that the patient's initial critical illness may result in increased gut mucosal permeability with resultant bacterial translocation eventually leading to portal vein bacteremia. MSOF which is triggered by the initial insult may then be perpetuated by this mechanism. Furthermore, as a result of the use of broad-spectrum antibiotics and potent inhibitors of gastric acid production, blood cultures may grow organisms not usually associated with the gastrointestinal tract such as *Staphylococcus epidermidis* or *Candida* species. Clearly, diagnosis of this condition (usually called *tertiary peritonitis*) can be made only by exclusion of other causes of sepsis. Treatment (and prevention) consists of stopping all unnecessary antibiotics and initiating enteral feeds if at all possible. Food in the lumen of the gut is a major stimulant of mucosal growth which preserves mucosal integrity.[29]

TABLE 85-6 Occult Sources of IAS

Acalculous cholecystitis
Small intraabdominal abscess(es)
Ischemic bowel—short segment
"Tertiary" peritonitis

When all attempts at determining a definite etiology for the patient's septic state have failed, the intensivist is often tempted to recommend laparotomy as a diagnostic tool. However, laparotomy in the absence of clinical or laboratory findings pointing to a specific etiology or location of infection is rarely helpful in preventing mortality.[30] Finally, it must be noted that once MSOF is far advanced, even definitive treatment of the underlying intraabdominal source rarely succeeds in reversing this lethal syndrome.[31,32]

CASE PRESENTATION

S.A., a 41-year-old woman, was transferred to The Wellesley Hospital on December 21, 1987 because of peritonitis. This patient had had many medical problems in the past. Twenty years prior to this admission she was found to have systemic lupus erythematosus and required glucocorticoid treatment. Seventeen years prior to admission she became paraplegic, secondary to transverse myelitis. Shortly thereafter her bladder ruptured, and she required an ileal conduit. Three years prior to admission she suffered from a perforated duodenal ulcer which was treated with an omental patch. One year prior to admission she perforated a gastric ulcer and underwent vagotomy and Bilroth II gastrectomy.

On this occasion, she awoke with crampy abdominal pain and vomiting. She was taken to her local hospital where an upright x-ray of the abdomen demonstrated free air.

On arrival at The Wellesley Hospital, <24 h after the onset of her symptoms, she was found to have severe generalized peritonitis. Her blood pressure was not obtainable by palpation. She was given fluids, antibiotics, and steroids in the emergency department and immediately taken to the operating room.

Laparotomy revealed a perforated gangrenous cecum within an incarcerated paraileostomy hernia. Generalized peritonitis was caused by the spread of liquid feces throughout the peritoneal cavity. The cecum was resected and an ileostomy and mucous fistula formed. The peritoneal cavity was lavaged with large quantities of saline. The hernia about her ileal conduit was repaired and the abdominal wound closed using Teflon mesh to prevent undue tension on her fascia. She required infusions of dopamine and epinephrine to maintain a systolic blood pressure between 80 and 110 mmHg during her surgery.

Postoperatively she was cared for in the ICU. A Swan-Ganz catheter was inserted. Twelve hours after the end of the surgical procedure she remained in severe septic shock. She required dopamine (20 μg/kg/min), dobutamine (20 μg/kg/min), and epinephrine (12 μg/min) to maintain a systolic blood pressure of 50 mmHg despite a pulmonary artery wedge pressure of 19 mmHg. Her cardiac output was high (9 L/min) and her systemic vascular resistance very low (350 dyne · sec/cm^5). However, she continued to have a good urine output (100 mL/h) and was relatively easy to oxygenate (P_{O_2} 100; F_{IO_2} 0.35). Antibiotic treatment consisted of 2 g cefoxitin intravenously every 6 h. She had a positive fluid balance of 9 L in the first 24 h of her stay at The Wellesley Hospital.

Four days after operation, she was weaned off all inotropic support. On postoperative day 6 she was started on enteral feeds through a nasogastric tube. Cefoxitin administration was stopped on postoperative day 8. Ten days after the surgical procedure, an abdominal CT scan was performed because of persistent leukocytosis. This demonstrated a right lower quadrant abscess, and a percutaneous drain was inserted and 50 mL pus aspirated. Antibiotics were not restarted. She was extubated the following day and transferred to the ward 24 h later.

Nineteen days after laparotomy, the mesh was removed from the abdominal wall. The granulating wound was covered with a split-thickness skin graft 1 month later. Three months after her perforation, she was returned to the operating room and the ileostomy closed. She recovered well from this procedure but 2 weeks later suffered a sudden cardiac arrest on the ward and could not be resuscitated. No autopsy was performed, and the cause of death was suspected to be a massive pulmonary embolus.

CASE DISCUSSION

This patient provides a classic example of the critically ill patient with IAS. Multiple previous medical problems and the need for steroids had set the stage for the development of the ventral hernia and the resultant sepsis.

The transition, in a period of 24 h, from a state of well-being to severe septic shock is not unusual. The patient had a massive spill of liquid feces into the peritoneal cavity, rapid absorption of nonadherent bacteria across the diaphragmatic lymphatics, and subsequent gram-negative bacteremia.

She required immediate surgery to stop the ongoing contamination of her peritoneal cavity and to reduce, as much as possible, the residual bacterial load her compromised immune system would have to deal with. Note that no attempt was made to completely resuscitate the patient prior to surgery. She was "too sick *not* to operate upon." A similar situation might be the trauma patient with sudden massive hemorrhage in whom it is impossible to transfuse blood as rapidly as it is being lost.

From the technical point of view, her laparotomy was straightforward. The site of the perforation was resected, and the peritoneal cavity was cleansed as much as possible. Primary closure of her fascial wound would have resulted in undue tension on the fascial sutures because of the hernia repair and abdominal distention secondary to tissue edema. The steroid-induced loss of fascial strength necessitated closure without tension using artificial mesh.

Following surgical control of her infection, 4 days elapsed before her state of septic shock had abated to the point that she no longer required inotropic support. The large quantity of fluids (9 L) required for initial resuscitation and the 4-day period of septic shock is quite typical for the patient with severe generalized peritonitis. Considering the severity of her septic state, it is interesting to speculate why she did not develop MSOF. Her previous bouts of peritonitis may have led to the development of anti-endotoxin antibodies which have been shown to be protective in such patients.[33] The corticosteroids she received postoperatively may have damped her nonspecific immune response sufficiently to prevent organ damage without significantly impairing neutrophil bactericidal function.

With respect to her antibiotics, she was treated with cefoxitin rather than an aminoglycoside because hypotension potentiates aminoglycoside nephrotoxicity. Antibiotic administration was stopped 8 days after her surgery when she was afebrile, doing well clinically, and without ileus. A persistent leukocytosis was investigated with a CT scan and a small intraabdominal abscess was found and drained. Antibiotics were not restarted at this time because the patient was clinically well.

She was ventilated for a total of 11 days but did not develop adult respiratory distress syndrome or nosocomial pneumonia. Her need for ventilatory support was mainly due to respiratory muscle weakness presumed to be secondary, in part, to steroid myopathy. Her subsequent hospital course was prolonged primarily because of her paraplegia.

References

1. Silen W: *Cope's Early Diagnosis of the Acute Abdomen,* 15th ed. New York, Oxford University Press, 1979.
2. Stephen M, Loewenthal J: Generalized infective peritonitis. Surg Gynecol Obstet 147:231, 1978.
3. Bohnen J, Boulanger M, Meakins JL, et al: Prognosis in generalized peritonitis. Arch Surg 118:285, 1983.
4. Pitcher WD, Musher DM: Critical importance of early diagnosis and treatment of intra-abdominal infections. Arch Surg 117:328, 1982.
5. Crossly IR, Williams R: Spontaneous bacterial peritonitis. Gut 26:325, 1985.
6. Levison ME, Bush LM: Peritonitis and other intra-abdominal infections, in Mandell GL, Douglas RG, Bennett JE (eds): *Principles and Practice of Infectious Diseases,* 3d ed. New York: Churchill, Livingstone, 1990, p 638.
7. LaMont JT, Isselbacher KJ: Current concepts: Postoperative jaundice. N Engl J Med 288:305, 1973.
8. Scharschmidt BF, Goldberg HI, Schmid R: Current concepts in diagnosis: Approach to the patient with cholestatic jaundice. N Engl J Med 308:1515, 1983.

9. Long TN, Heimbach DM, Carrico CJ: Acalculous cholecystitis in critically ill patients. Am J Surg 136:31, 1978.
10. Savino JA, Scalea TM, Del Guercio LRM: Factors encouraging laprotomy in acalculous cholecystitis. Crit Care Med 13:377, 1985.
11. Cornwell EE, Rodriguez A, Mirvis SE, et al: Acute acalculous cholecystitis in critically injured patients: Ann Surg 210:52, 1989.
12. Parry SW, Pelias ME, Browder W: Acalculous hypersensitivity cholecystitis: Hypothesis of a new clinicopathologic entity. Surgery 104:911, 1988.
13. Flanchbaum L, Alden SM, Trooskin SZ: Use of cholescintigraphy with morphine in critically ill patients with suspected cholecystitis. Surgery 106:668, 1989.
14. McGahan JP, Lindfors KK: Percutaneous cholecystostomy: An alternative to surgical cholecystostomy for acute cholecystitis? Radiology 173:481, 1989.
15. Ahrenholz DH, Simmons RL: Peritonitis and other intra-abdominal infection, in Howard RJ, Simmons RL (eds): *Surgical Infectious Diseases,* 2d ed. Norwalk, CT: Appleton & Lange, 1988, p 605.
16. Malangoni MA, London RE, Spiegal CA: Treatment of intra-abdominal infections is appropriate with single agent or combination antibiotic therapy. Surgery 98:648, 1985.
17. Stone HH, Bourneuf AA, Stinson LD: Reliability of criterion for predicting persistent or recurrent sepsis. Arch Surg 120:17, 1985.
18. Bohnen J, Mustard R, Oxholm S, et al: Apache II score and abdominal sepsis: A prospective study. Arch Surg 123:225, 1988.
19. Rosenthal GA, Quinto J, Kao J, et al: Prevention of intra-abdominal abscesses with fibrinolytic agents. Can J Surg 31:98, 1988.
20. Edlich RF, Rodeheaver GT, Thacker JG: Technical factors in the prevention of wound infections, in Howard RJ, Simmons RL (eds): *Surgical Infectious Diseases,* 2d ed. Norwalk, CT: Appleton & Lange, 1988, p 340.
21. Walsh GL, Chiasson P, Hedderich G, et al: The open abdomen. The marlex mesh and zipper technique: A method of managing intraperitoneal infection. Surg Clin North Am 68:25, 1988.
22. Mastboom WJB, Kuypors HHC, Schoots FJ, et al: Small bowel perforation complicating the open treatment of generalized peritonitis. Arch Surg 124:689, 1989.
23. Machiedo GW, Suval WD: Detection of sepsis in the postoperative patient. Surg Clin North Am 68:215, 1988.
24. VanSonnenberg E, Mueller PR, Ferrucci JT: Percutaneous drainage of 250 abdominal abscesses and fluid collections. Part 1: Results, failures, and complications. Radiology 151:337, 1984.
25. Teichmann W, Wittmann DH, Andreone PA: Scheduled reoperations (Etappenlavage) for diffuse peritonitis. Arch Surg 121:147, 1986.
26. Hau T: Infections of the liver and spleen, in Howard RJ, Simmons RL (eds): *Surgical Infectious Disease,* 2d ed. Norwalk, CT: Appleton & Lange, 1988, p 659.
27. Gleich S, Wolin DA, Herbsman H: A review of percutaneous drainage in splenic abscess. Surg Gynecol Obstet 167:211, 1988.
28. Deitch EA: Does the gut protect or injure patients in the ICU? Perspect Crit Care 1 (2):1, 1988.
29. Wilmore DW, Smith RJ, O'Dwyer ST, et al: The gut: A central organ after surgical stress. Surgery 104:917, 1988.
30. Sinanan M, Maier RV, Carrico CJ: Laparotomy for intra-abdominal sepsis in patients in an intensive care unit. Arch Surg 119:652, 1984.
31. Norton LW: Does drainage of intra-abdominal pus reverse multiple organ failure? Am J Surg 149:347, 1985.
32. Darling GE, Duff JH, Mustard RA, et al: Multiorgan failure in critically ill patients. Can J Surg 31:172, 1988.
33. Ziegler EJ, McCutchan JA, Fierer J, et al: Treatment of gram-negative bacteremia and shock with human antiserum to a mutant *Escherichia coli.* N Engl J Med 307:1225, 1982.

Chapter 86

MANAGEMENT OF THE CRITICALLY ILL VASCULAR SURGERY PATIENT

GIANCARLO PIANO
JOHN ALVERDY
CHRISTOPHER ZARINS

KEY POINTS

- *Risk stratification, cardiac evaluation, and specific anesthetic modifications achieve the best outcome for patients.*
- *Treating coexistent coronary artery disease (CAD) can improve survival.*
- *Vascular reconstructions often cause significant ischemia in critical circulations such as the renal and splanchnic beds.*
- *Understanding the physiologic alterations during surgery permits rapid assessment and prevention of potential postoperative complications.*
- *The goal of invasive monitoring is anticipation and prevention of unexpected hemodynamic alterations.*
- *Attention should be directed to decreasing myocardial oxygen demand while providing adequate myocardial oxygen delivery*
- *Combined vascular procedures, repairs of thoracoabdominal aneurysms, and thrombolytic therapy are being performed with increasing frequency. Management of these complex procedures requires a working understanding of cardiovascular physiology.*

Vascular surgery continues to develop and evolve as a distinct specialty characterized by a unique body of scientific knowledge, precise diagnostic techniques, and effective therapeutic interventions. The practice of vascular surgery encompasses the entire spectrum of care of venous and arterial diseases. Highly successful operative procedures have evolved to correct aneurysmal and occlusive disease throughout the body. Venous reconstructive surgery, although diagnostically and technically demanding, rarely requires the special setting of an ICU. In contrast, perioperative intensive care is a requirement for patients undergoing arterial reconstructive surgery. Therefore, the scope of this chapter will be limited to the care of patients undergoing arterial reconstructions with an emphasis on critical care issues.

Atherosclerotic arterial disease constitutes a major world health problem. It is a leading cause of death in the United States and many other countries. Currently the disease affects one in four Americans with mortality rates exceeding those for all other diseases combined.[1] The physical disability from the disease is likewise staggering. It is estimated that Americans suffer 600,000 strokes and 1.5 million myocardial infarctions each year and that 60,000 undergo major amputations for ischemic limbs. It was estimated that in 1990 more than 900,000 vascular surgical operations were performed.

The situation is further complicated because these diseases primarily affect the elderly who frequently have chronic medical problems, limited physiologic reserves, and limited socioeconomic support. A significant percentage of the elderly population experiences some degree of peripheral vascular disease. Health care strategists forecast that there will be a 34 percent increase in the population older than 65 years by the year 2010, while the total population will increase by only 19 percent. As the population ages, a steady increase in the prevalence of peripheral vascular disease will occur. Although the risk factors for cardiovascular diseases have been identified, preventing arterial diseases will be a long, arduous process. Patients are reluctant to stop smoking, change diets, take medications, and alter sedentary life-styles. Consequently, today's vascular surgeons and critical care physicians will be managing complex vascular problems during their entire careers.

Preoperative Management of the Vascular Patient

The common illnesses associated with atherosclerotic arterial diseases include hypertensive cardiovascular disease, chronic obstructive airway disease, diabetes mellitus, and chronic renal insufficiency. Before major reconstructive vascular surgery, an assessment of health problems and anesthetic risk is performed. The goal is to identify, treat, and closely monitor concurrent medical conditions, thereby reducing perioperative morbidity and mortality. In selected patients, the risks may be prohibitive and require an adjustment in surgical strategy.

INDICES OF ANESTHETIC RISK

Surgery and anesthesia create hemodynamic and metabolic stress for the vascular patient. Determining the probability that this stress will lead to perioperative morbidity or death is the process of risk assessment. In 1963 the American Society of Anesthesiologists (ASA) adopted the DRIPPS modification of Physical Status Class to predict operative risk in surgical patients. The ASA classification is based on a simple clinical assessment of a patient's general physical condition and is currently used as an index of surgical risk because of its close correlation with mortality outcome. However, its usefulness is limited for assessing vascular patients because it is not specific enough for patients with critical levels of disease.[2]

CARDIAC RISK

The operative mortality for elective vascular reconstructive surgery ranges from 2 to 6 percent. Cardiac complications (perioperative myocardial infarction, arrhythmias, heart failure) account for more than 50 percent of the perioperative mortality.[3,4] Because peripheral vascular disease is itself a marker for CAD, the value of screening studies depends on the incidence of angiographically confirmed disease that is functionally significant. Based on numerous studies, the coexistence of CAD in patients with peripheral vascular disease is well established. In a review of 1000 patients undergoing mandatory coronary angiography before peripheral vascular reconstruction at the Cleveland Clinic, mild to severe CAD was discovered in 92 percent, with advanced disease demonstrated in 60 percent. Severe but surgically correctable CAD was demonstrated in 34 percent of patients with a positive cardiac history or an abnormal electrocardiogram (ECG), but more importantly was also detected in 14 percent of patients without cardiac history or an abnormal ECG.[5,6]

Since not all patients have CAD sufficient to warrant coronary artery bypass graft (CABG) or percutaneous transluminal coronary angioplasty (PTCA), several screening methods have been used to identify patients at risk.[4,5,7,8] Methods to assess cardiac risk include clinical indices, ECGs, exercise testing, radionuclide angiography (MUGA scan), echocardiography, various forms of thallium scanning, and routine coronary angiograms. All these methods have shortcomings. Each method suffers from either a lack in sensitivity, specificity, or both, and therefore their discriminate value for predicting outcome may not always be reliable. Even with coronary angiography it is difficult to relate anatomic findings to surgical risk.[9]

Although these methods are discussed in detail elsewhere in this text, their use in a vascular practice merits individual discussion.

CLINICAL INDICES. Specific clinical risk factors predictive of postoperative cardiac complications following vascular surgery include a history of previous myocardial infarction, congestive heart failure, prior stroke, abnormal ECG, angina pectoris, arrhythmias, advanced age, and diabetes mellitus. A classification applying similar clinical risk factors reasonably predicted cardiac complications in 1.3 percent of low-risk patients versus 23.2 percent of high-risk patients.[10] Certain patients are at high risk for life-threatening or fatal cardiac complications; these high-risk factors are myocardial infarction in the last 6 months, unstable angina pectoris, symptomatic aortic valvular stenosis, uncompensated congestive heart failure, and chronic atrial or ventricular arrhythmias. Recent myocardial infarction is the most predictive cardiac risk factor.

In 1977 Goldman and coworkers published a cardiac risk index.[7] A multivariate analysis was applied to 1001 patients undergoing noncardiac procedures. This index uses nine independent risk factors that were identified to represent significant cardiac risk (see Chap. 81). Efforts have been made to validate the Goldman Risk Index in several large prospective series of surgical patients.[11] However, it underestimates cardiac complications in vascular patients. Even using a recent modification of the Goldman Index, death was predicted in only 50 percent of the cases.[12] Although clinical criteria appear to identify patients at obvious risk for perioperative cardiac events, it should be apparent that clinical criteria alone are not sufficiently accurate to predict all of these events.

A 12-lead ECG is commonly abnormal (ST-T wave changes, signs of left ventricular hypertrophy, Q waves) in patients undergoing major vascular surgery. Despite the widespread use of the screening ECG, only a few studies have prospectively evaluated its predictive value. In a study of 200 patients, specific preoperative ECG abnormalities (ST-T waves, ischemic or nonspecific changes, and intraventricular conduction delays) were independent predictors of adverse cardiac outcomes.[13] In contrast, Goldman concluded that ECG abnormalities including old Q waves, ST-T wave changes, or bundle branch block had no significant predictive value.[14] Further study of the ECG's discriminant value for patients undergoing vascular procedures is therefore necessary.

EXERCISE TESTING. Lack of an accurate predictive test has driven the search for a test that studies the patient's capacity to tolerate exertion. Using exercise treadmill testing, patients with a low exercise capacity (maximum heart rate <75 percent of predicted) and a positive ischemic response (ST segment depression of >1 mm) were found to be at highest risk for postoperative myocardial infarctions.[15] Similarly, a recent study of 100 patients using either treadmill testing or arm ergometry showed that patients who were able to achieve 85 percent of maximum predicted heart rate were less likely to have a perioperative myocardial infarct. This was true regardless of the degree of ST segment depression.[16] Unfortunately, many vascular surgery patients are unable to participate in exercise stress testing because they are debilitated from chronic disease, previous strokes, amputations, arthritis, or claudication and therefore cannot exercise adequately.

Intraoperative Management of the Vascular Patient

Successful postoperative management of the complex vascular patient requires an understanding of the intraoperative events that have taken place. The specific postoperative physiologic alterations depend on the particular vascular bed involved and the extent of the underlying illnesses as well as the effects of anesthesia. An understanding of these issues permits rapid assessment and prevention of potential postoperative complications. The decision on how best to monitor the vascular patient is as important as the selection of the operation and depends on the particular organ involved.

GENERAL CONSIDERATIONS

The primary objective for the intraoperative management of the vascular patient is cardiopulmonary protection. Because intraoperative hypotension and hypoxemia are independent predictors of postoperative morbidity and mortality, their avoidance is imperative.[17] This is best achieved by invasive cardiac and pulmonary monitoring. The extent of invasive monitoring should be determined by the magnitude of the operation and the patient's general medical condition. For major vascular reconstructive surgery such as aortic, cerebrovascular, renal, or mesenteric surgery, adequate vascular access including two large bore peripheral venous catheters, continuous ECG monitoring, intraarterial blood pressure monitoring, and placement of a urinary catheter for hourly urine output are minimum requirements. Our experience dictates that continuous pulse oximetry, frequent blood-gas analysis, and end-tidal CO_2 measurements offer added protection against unexpected hypoxemia.

Intraoperative hypotension in the vascular patient is a frequent problem, despite fastidious attention to blood loss and vital signs. Causes include cardiovascular effects of anesthetic agents, inadequate maintenance of intravascular volume, rapid and excessive blood loss, primary myocardial ischemia, and factors that decrease systemic vascular resistance (SVR) (vide infra).

Controversy continues over which patients should undergo invasive monitoring using a pulmonary artery catheter. There is general agreement that the pulmonary artery wedge pressure (Ppw) is a more reliable measure of the left ventricular end-diastolic volume (preload) than central venous pressure. In addition thermodilution cardiac output can be measured and the relationship between preload and stroke volume can be established. Consequently, patients considered in the high-risk category for vascular surgery should be monitored using this technique. One established limitation of pulmonary artery catheter use is the unreliability of this technique in the detection of myocardial ischemia.[18] Transesophageal echocardiography (TEE) offers a more sensitive method for the early detection of wall motion abnormalities which may represent local areas of myocardial ischemia (see Chap. 22).[19] It is our practice to use TEE during selected cases of high-risk vascular surgery. Specific indications for this technique are discussed elsewhere in this text.

AORTIC SURGERY

Modern experience in aortic surgery has demonstrated that improved outcomes can be achieved when operative dissection and blood loss are minimized. For example, the earlier technique of aneurysmectomy has been abandoned in favor of the graft inclusion technique (aneurysmorrhaphy) because the latter technique results in less disruption of periaortic tissues and consequently less blood loss. Recently the technique of retroperitoneal exposure of the aorta has been repopularized. Compared to the transperitoneal approach, this technique is associated with less blood and fluid requirements, less intraoperative hemodynamic fluctuation, and a shorter postoperative ileus.[20] Although definitive data have not clearly demonstrated the superiority of the retroperitoneal approach, it is our preferred method in selected patients.

The clamping and unclamping of the aorta during aortic surgery are crucial events during which meticulous management of blood pressure and cardiac function is critical to minimize stress to the patient. Additionally, because aortic surgery results in the greatest blood loss of all vascular procedures, autotransfusion techniques are used to reduce reliance on banked blood. Expeditious, planned procedures tend to minimize ischemia to critical organ beds such as the kidneys, heart, and gastrointestinal tract during aortic surgery and are important determinants of outcome.

During aortic cross-clamping acute rises in both the afterload and preload are observed.[21] Myocardial ischemia may occur if treatment is delayed. Use of nitroprusside for afterload reduction and nitroglycerin for preload reduction may be required. Another undesirable effect of aortic cross-clamping is a decrease in renal cortical blood flow, which can occur during infrarenal or suprarenal clamping.[22] Renal cortical flow during clamping is often difficult to predict and therefore clamp time must be kept to a minimum. Several therapeutic options are used alone or in combination to treat and prevent renal ischemia. Low dose dopamine (3 to 5 μg/kg/min) infusion, 10 to 20 mg furosemide, or 25 g mannitol may be used to promote tubular flow and diuresis. These agents should be used well in advance of aortic clamping.

Aortic unclamping can result in "declamping shock," thought to occur as vasoactive products of ischemia are released from underperfused beds (such as the lower extremities and the gastrointestinal tract). These toxic products of ischemia and reperfusion can cause both myocardial depression as well as a fall in SVR resulting in profound, recalcitrant hypotension.

Prevention is the best treatment for declamping hypotension. This can be accomplished by avoidance of rapid declamping, judicious volume expansion before declamping, and discontinuation of all myocardial depressants and vasodilators. If acidosis or hypotension persist, $NaHCO_3^-$ and $CaCl_2$ may be used to treat the acidosis and myocardial depression associated with declamping.

Significant bleeding may occur at various times during aortic surgery. Inadequate hemostasis at suture lines due to poor technique, unexpected venous injuries, dilutional coagulopathies, and hypothermia are but a few causes of bleeding following aortic surgery. Immediate recognition of these causes of hemorrhage is essential for treatment. With few exceptions, patients undergoing aortic surgery are fully anticoagulated with heparin, 100 U/kg. Because the half-life of heparin is 90 min, reversal of anticoagulation is usually unnecessary. Occasionally, protamine sulfate (1.5 mg/100 U heparin) is given to reverse the effect of heparin (see Chap. 119). Overzealous use of protamine can result in coagulopathy, hypotension, and bradycardia; therefore, its use should be clearly indicated.

CEREBROVASCULAR SURGERY

Carotid endarterectomy (CEA) has become one of the most commonly performed vascular operations. To achieve low combined morbidity and mortality rates (<5 percent) and a permanent neurologic deficit rate of <2 percent, detailed attention must be paid to appropriate patient selection, thorough preoperative evaluation, anesthetic management, and technical aspects of the operation.[23]

Three anesthetic techniques are commonly used. We prefer a general anesthetic with endotracheal intubation and continuous electroencephalographic (EEG) monitoring to detect cerebral ischemia. Other options include local anesthesia with intravenous sedation or regional nerve blockade, both of which permit awake evaluation of cerebral function.

Cerebral blood flow is determined by many factors including the Pa_{O_2}, Pa_{CO_2}, and the cerebral perfusion pressure (CPP) (Chap. 4). In the patient with diseased cerebral vasculature, normal vascular autoregulatory capacity may be lost. CPP becomes the primary determinant of cerebral blood flow and depends on the mean arterial pressure (MAP) and the intracranial pressure (ICP) or central venous pressure (CVP). Specifically, CPP = MAP − ICP, which underscores the importance of avoiding swings in blood pressure both during and after operations involving the cerebral vasculature. Hypoxemia and hypercapnia result in significant vasodilation of the cerebral vasculature and may increase brain blood volume and adversely alter regional intracerebral blood flow. Therefore, maintaining adequate gas exchange is critical for the management of these patients.

MESENTERIC AND RENAL RECONSTRUCTION

A number of surgical approaches have been described to revascularize mesenteric and renal arteries obstructed by atherosclerosis. These patients require special attention to intravascular volume due to major extracellular fluid shifts. The pathophysiologic alterations which occur during these revascularization procedures demand special considerations with respect to fluid resuscitation and use of vasoactive agents.

Atherosclerotic occlusive disease of the celiac and superior mesenteric artery is the most common cause of chronic intestinal ischemia (see Chap. 167). Various operations have been performed successfully, including endarterectomy and aortomesenteric bypass.[24] Extensive exposure of the upper abdominal aorta is usually achieved from a transperitoneal or thoracoabdominal approach. Dissection of the aorta requires wide exposure and significant retraction of the abdominal viscera, thereby resulting in substantial fluid sequestration. Judicious volume expansion should take place before operation and during vascular occlusion of the mesenteric circulation. Patients with abdominal angina and those with intestinal viability in jeopardy should be rapidly hydrated and given intravenous glucagon (0.06 mg/kg/h). Glucagon reduces splanchnic vascular resistance and may improve marginal collateral flow.[25] This regimen should be maintained for 36 to 48 h postoperatively to ensure high flow rates in the splanchnic bed. Without such intervention, marked mesenteric vasoreactivity may occur, which can produce flow-limiting increases in mesenteric resistance and increase the potential for thrombosis. Mannitol is used frequently to induce a diuresis. Prolonged ischemia of the intestines may occur during the course of mesenteric arterial reconstruction and can lead to the release of toxic oxygen radicals during reperfusion and translocation of gut flora and endotoxins. This may result in a hyperdynamic circulatory response characterized by high cardiac output and low SVR similar to sepsis.[26] Continued circulatory support with vasoactive agents and broad-spectrum antibiotics are warranted until complete resolution is clinically evident. Intravenous glucagon, as mentioned, is an important adjunctive drug during the perioperative period for counterregulatory control of the mesenteric circulation if vasoactive agents are necessary. The best treatment, however, is adequate volume expansion to obviate the need for vasopressors.

INFRAINGUINAL VASCULAR SURGERY

Chronic lower limb ischemia is the most common indication for infrainguinal vascular reconstructions.[27] Patients generally have diffuse, multilevel disease that often requires a combination of procedures, including iliac percutaneous transluminal angioplasty, aortofemoral bypass, femoral-femoral bypass prior to distal reconstruction. This group of patients is generally older, has associated severe CAD and cerebrovascular disease, and often has diabetes.[28] With this level of concomitant disease, the life expectancy is notably lower than for patients with aortoiliac disease. Despite these obstacles, aggressive efforts to save limbs are effective and worthwhile. Functional limb salvage can be achieved in 85 percent of patients until they die, with a procedural mortality rate of 3 percent.[27] Operative mortality rates can be minimized by strict adherence to the principles outlined in previous sections and which are summarized by compulsive preoperative management, careful anesthesia, and surgical precision.

Postoperative Management of the Vascular Patient

GENERAL CONSIDERATIONS

Most life-threatening complications in vascular surgery occur in the early postoperative period. This situation warrants ICU monitoring for most patients undergoing major reconstructive procedures. The general parameters to monitor are continuous arterial pressure using an indwelling catheter, continuous ECG, hourly urine volumes, continuous arterial oxygen saturation, frequent blood-gas analysis, daily weight, and accurate fluid balance. Baseline measurement of hematocrit, electrolytes including ionized and total calcium, blood urea nitrogen, serum creatinine, prothrombin and partial thromboplastin time, and platelet count should be performed.

Of special importance in the vascular patient is the circulatory assessment of the reperfused vascular bed. For example, following cerebrovascular surgery, close neurologic observation is required. Following aortic, mesenteric, or renal revascularization distal pulses, abdominal examination, and renal function must be evaluated repeatedly.

Analgesia must be adequately provided to the vascular patient. If regional anesthesia has been delivered via an indwelling epidural catheter, subsequent narcotic and anesthetic agents can be delivered safely into these systems throughout the postoperative period for up to 48 h. Analgesia and sedation may pose significant obstacles when neurologic evaluation is necessary. It is therefore important to use short-acting sedative agents such as midazolam (2 to 5 mg intravenously) and reversible short-acting narcotic agents such as fentanyl (see Chap. 82).

Mucosal erosions and gastritis can develop within hours of a severe catabolic stress such as occurs following major vascular reconstruction. Prophylaxis against gastric stress erosion should be delivered; H_2 antagonists, antacids, and cytoprotective agents such as sulcralfate or Cytotec have been efficacious. The best index of response to both H_2 blocker and antacids is gastric pH monitoring when available.

Despite intraoperative attempts at thermal conservation using passive external warming (blankets, thermal reflectants, warm intravenous fluids, etc) and active core rewarming (inhalational hyperthermia, warm irrigation fluids), hypothermia can occur following vascular surgery. Hypothermia must be immediately treated to avoid its well-documented untoward effects such as myocardial depression, platelet dysfunction, and shivering, which increases cardiopulmonary work and can cause respiratory embarrassment.

MANAGEMENT OF THE CARDIOPULMONARY SYSTEM

As previously mentioned, cardiac and pulmonary complications are the principle causes of morbidity and mortality following vascular surgery. A rational approach to preventing cardiopulmonary complications during the postoperative period is required. The value of invasive monitoring, particularly with the pulmonary artery catheter, lies in anticipating and preventing hemodynamic alterations and should be viewed as useful even in the stable patient. Patients undergoing vascular surgery often have underlying CAD and, therefore, myocardial protection and avoidance of myocardial ischemia may be best realized with invasive monitoring.

Myocardial ischemia is the result of a complex interplay between the determinants of myocardial oxygen demand and myocardial oxygen supply. End points for minimizing the myocardial risk to patients following vascular surgery include **1.** optimizing oxygen tension ($Pa_{O_2} > 75$ mmHg); **2.** improving oxygen content (hemoglobin >10 g/dL); **3.** achieving adequate MAP; **4.** achieving pharmacologic coronary artery vasodilation; **5.** maintaining the lowest left ventricular end-diastolic pressure consistent with the best stroke volume; and **6.** controlling heart rate. Myocardial demand reduction decreases the potential for myocardial ischemia and can be achieved by decreasing contractility, heart rate, and left ventricular wall stress (lowering the Ppw). However in the early postoperative period, whole body oxygen demands are increased, creating a dichotomy for the clinician. How can systemic oxygen delivery be maintained without precipitating myocardial ischemia? It is our belief that these goals cannot be balanced without the use of the pulmonary artery catheter. Measurement of mixed venous oxygen content is useful in these patients.[29] If a high oxygen extraction ratio exists (oxygen consumption/oxygen delivery) despite normal to high cardiac output, then transfusion is indicated. If the pulmonary capillary wedge pressure (Ppw) is elevated, stroke volume is low, but cardiac output is normal, then oxygen delivery is maintained at the expense of a high heart rate, a situation which may precipitate myocardial ischemia. The use of agents that provide inotropy and afterload reduction may be indicated. Because vascular patients often require volume loading to promote a diuresis, especially in the case of mesenteric or renal reconstruction, exceedingly high filling pressures increase myocardial wall tension and may impair myocardial blood flow.[30] Thus, it can be seen that effective strategies for hemodynamic management in the postoperative patient must optimize oxygen transport and at the same time limit myocardial demand in high-risk patients. This is best achieved using invasive monitoring techniques such as pulmonary artery catheterization.

Postoperative hypertension occurs in up to 50 percent of patients following aortic reconstruction and extracranial carotid bypass. Multiple etiologies may be responsible for postoperative hypertension and include increased sympathetic tone and catecholamine release, postoperative pain, hypervolemia, myocardial ischemia, and activation of the renin-angiotensin axis. Uncontrolled hypertension can result in excessive cardiac work (stroke volume × heart rate × systolic blood pressure) and extreme anastomotic wall tension.

The first step in the treatment of postoperative hypertension is adequate pain control. This can be accomplished with small doses of intravenous opiates. Expanded intravascular volume may also contribute to postoperative hypertension. For example, epidural anesthesia results in loss of sympathetic tone, often requiring volume expansion to maintain the MAP. As this effect resolves, hypertension can be a result of an expanded intravascular volume. Postoperative volume depletion may result in high SVR in an effort to maintain MAP. These dichotomous situations require clinical assessment of intravascular volume (urine volume, urine specific gravity, measurement of cardiac output, stroke volume, and SVR) to direct either diuresis or volume expansion.

Once pain and volume have been addressed, persistent hypertension (>115 percent of preoperative pressure) is treated pharmacologically. The following drugs offer good results in our experience. Labetalol, a noncardioselective β blocker, is useful when given intravenously at doses of 15 to 25 mg every 5 to 15 min until the desired decrease in blood pressure is observed. Intravenous nitroprusside is a potent vasodilator with a short duration of action and offers rapid and reversible control of hypertension. Coronary and cerebral artery "steal" phenomena are theoretical disadvantages to nitroprusside.[31] Reflex tachycardia and cyanide accumulation should restrict its use to short-term control of hypertension. Continuous intravenous nitroglycerin has several advantages over nitroprusside for treating hypertension especially in patients with CAD, angina, or congestive heart failure. These include reduction of collateral resistance in the coronary circulation, reduction of preload, and control of pulmonary artery hypertension in patients with acute respiratory failure. Nifedipine, a calcium channel blocker, is a useful agent for postoperative hypertension. Nifedipine can be administered using the "bite and swallow" route of administration. Its onset of action is within 20 min.

Postoperative blood pressure instability often occurs following CEA and can manifest as either hypertension or hypotension. Hypertension, as mentioned, can occur from a variety of causes, but may also be due to a disturbance of the carotid body baroreceptor reflex.[32] After CEA the newly formed carotid bulb may be subjected to increased circumferential wall stretch with resultant baroreceptor overactivity and reflex hypotension. The blood pressure should be supported with intravenous ephedrine (25 mg intravenously) until this response is attenuated.

Tachycardia is a common finding in the early postoperative period and has various causes including pain, volume depletion, hypoxemia, anemia, and myocardial ischemia or failure. If no cause for tachycardia is found, it should be treated in the vascular patient to minimize the increase in myocardial oxygen demand. We prefer intravenous esmolol (20 mg intravenous push test dose, 10 to 30 μg/kg/min continuous drip) due to its short duration of action (1 to 2 min) and easy reversibility. Persistent tachycardia can be treated with metoprolol (50 mg orally), which is efficacious in reducing postoperative cardiac ischemic episodes in the vascular patient.[33] Asthma is a relative contraindication to the use of β blockers; however, their bronchoconstrictive actions can be offset with β-adrenergic inhalational therapy.

Ventilatory support may be necessary for several hours to days following major vascular reconstruction, especially after abdominal and thoracic procedures. During this period, ventilation is inadequate because general anesthesia impairs pulmonary gas exchange by decreasing ventilatory drive, functional residual capacity, and pulmonary compliance with an overall increase in the work of breathing. Perioperative mechanical support minimizes these effects and improves patient recovery. Once extubation is successful, pulmonary mechanics are optimized by proper patient positioning (up in chair, head elevation) and aggressive pulmonary toilet (deep breathing exercise, incentive spirometry).

RENAL FUNCTION

Postoperative renal failure, once a common occurrence following vascular surgery, portends a poor outcome. The high mortality rate for acute renal failure (ARF) following vascular surgery, reported to be as high as 50 to 75 percent, is felt to be due to the factors relating to the cause of ARF or to complications of multiple organ failure.[34]

Maintenance of renal blood flow, glomerular filtration rate (GFR), and urine output is essential for the prevention of ARF. Renal blood flow and GFR are best maintained with adequate cardiac output and intravascular volume. The gold standard for hourly assessment of renal function is urine volume; however, several points with respect to urine volume in the vascular patient deserve mention. First, it is common practice to perform arteriography before, during, and after vascular surgery. Contrast dyes are hyperosmolar solutions and promote a brisk diuresis. Failure to recognize this situation may lead to unrecognized volume depletion and worse ARF. The duration of effect of a contrast-induced diuresis may be determined by measuring urine specific gravity, which can exceed 1.050 when dye is still present. Second, vascular patients may be volume depleted due to glycosuria secondary to diabetes and diuretic use due to chronic hypertension. It may be difficult in these situations to rely on the urine output as a valid indicator of intravascular volume. Finally, intraoperative mannitol administration may produce a forced diuresis and may lead to volume depletion if the urine volume is not replaced.

Prevention of renal impairment following vascular surgery can be achieved by focusing on two specific goals: **1.** maintaining renal blood flow and GFR by ensuring adequate cardiac output, MAP, and intravascular volume and **2.** maintaining a brisk diuresis (1 to 1.5 mL/kg/h), thereby preventing tubular occlusion from desquamated tubular epithelial cells. These goals can be achieved by the use of low dose dopamine, loop diuretics such as furosemide, and volume expansion with crystalloids, colloids, and mannitol. Mannitol may be used both during and following vascular reconstructions and its mechanism of action is thought to be due to its multiple effects as a diuretic, volume expander, oxygen radical scavenger, and thromboxane A_2 inhibitor (see Chap. 153).

Reperfusion of an ischemic muscular bed can lead to production of toxic oxygen metabolites that may have untoward effects on renal function.[35] In addition, myoglobin may be released if prolonged ischemia of skeletal muscle has occurred. Urine should be microscopically examined for the presence of tubular casts and urine myoglobin and serum creatine kinase measured. A "myonephropathic syndrome" is characterized by progressive rhabdomyolysis and renal failure and is associated with a >50 percent mortality rate.[36] Treatment consists of prompt recognition, mannitol administration, and alkalinization of the urine with $NaHCO_3$ (see Chap. 154).

If oliguric or anuric renal failure occur, continuous arteriovenous hemofiltration (CAVH) should be instituted. Use of CAVH is associated with an improved outcome in patients with postoperative oliguric ARF. Administration of important fluids, such as intravenous hyperalimentation solutions, is not limited by the oliguria when CAVH is used.

ASSESSMENT OF THE PERIPHERAL VASCULATURE

The extremities distal to the reconstruction should be evaluated immediately on arrival to the ICU. This is best achieved by combining palpation of the pulses with Doppler signals. If pulses are present distal to the reconstruction, they can be used alone to follow vessel patency. If no pulses are palpable, a Doppler-obtained ankle-brachial pressure index should be recorded and followed at hourly intervals. Monophasic or absent Doppler signals indicate a failing graft or distal thromboembolism. Although vasoconstriction from hypothermia may result in absence of Doppler signals, any ambiguity in adequacy of the circulation distal to the reconstruction should be communicated to the surgeon.

Some degree of leg edema is usually present following reperfusion of an ischemic limb. The major etiologic factor underlying leg edema is a disruption of lymphatics; however, increased arterial pressure, altered capillary permeability, and loss of vascular autoregulation all may play a role.[37] Other important causes of postoperative leg swelling are deep venous thrombosis (DVT), compartment syndrome, and tense wound hematomas. Postoperative leg swelling due to the revascularization will usually resolve with leg elevation alone. DVT rarely occurs in the immediate postoperative period. If clinical suspicion arises, then duplex scanning can be performed (see Chap. 23). Tense wound hematomas should be surgically evacuated in the operating suite with bleeding sites identified and controlled.

INFECTION

Prophylactic antibiotics are efficacious in decreasing the incidence of graft and wound infections.[38] First generation cephalosporins are preferred for routine prophylaxis. Antibiotics should be continued through the postoperative period until the threat of infection to the wound and graft no longer exists. This includes patients with indwelling arterial, venous, and bladder catheters.

Early postoperative wound infections may pose a significant threat to both life and limb. Failure to appropriately treat wound infections may result in graft sepsis leading to major amputation or death. Rubor, calor, dolor, and loss of function should alert the clinician to the possibility of infection; empirical use of intravenous antibiotics is mandatory. *Staphylococcus aureus* or *Staphylococcus epidermidis* are the most common organisms involved in an early postoperative infection.[39] Antibiotic selection should be directed against these pathogens before culture results are available. Broader antibiotic coverage may be necessary in complicated wounds involving the extremities where aerobic and anaerobic organisms may be present.

Because fresh prosthetic grafts are susceptible to endogenously or exogenously derived bacteremias, routine surveillance of all indwelling devices should be performed. Empirical removal of all indwelling intravascular devices should occur every 3 days.

Persistent occult sepsis in the vascular patient is an uncommon problem. Multiple organ failure states can develop and are usually preceded by a period of hypoperfusion. The presence of common infections such as pneumonia, urinary tract infections, wound infections, and phlebitis should be thoroughly investigated. In their absence, persistent sepsis may be a result of acalculous cholecystitis, ischemic pancreatitis, ischemic colitis, or intestinal infarction. Acalculous cholecystitis, a surgical emergency, occurs in 1 percent of patients following aortic reconstruction.[40] Clinical manifestations include fever, leukocytosis, elevated bilirubin, and right upper quadrant tenderness. Diagnosis is made using bedside ultrasonography and Tc-HIDA scanning. Treatment is immediate cholecystectomy or cholecystostomy. Ischemic pancreatitis has been described following vascular surgery and can present as a fulminant disease similar to alcoholic pancreatitis.[41] High serum amylase and lipase levels, hyperdynamic circulation, abdominal pain, and ileus occur. Bowel rest with total parenteral nutrition, nasogastric suction, and antibiotics are recommended. Splanchnic ischemia can occur either during or following aortic, renal, or mesenteric vascular reconstruction.[42] Gastrointestinal mucosal ischemia may be one of the earliest manifestations of impaired core tissue perfusion in the critically ill.[43] Ischemia of the sigmoid colon has been reported to occur in 5 to 10 percent of patients undergoing abdominal aortic aneurysm surgery, leading to transmural infarction in 1 to 2 percent. The clinical manifestations of small bowel or colon ischemia are protean, and classically described clinical signs such as pain, bloody diarrhea, tachycardia, and fever are often absent. If there is persistent culture-negative sepsis, immediate investigation for gut ischemia should begin. Rigid or flexible proctosigmoidoscopy is the first step in diagnosis and can detect areas of ischemia or infarction in the left colon. Computed tomography (CT) scan of the abdomen with contrast can detect venous thrombosis or air within the intestinal wall or periportal area. Arteriography may be performed but often is difficult to interpret because atherosclerotic lesions in the mesenteric circulation are often present in these patients. However, if previous arteriography is available and new occlusions are present, this modality becomes useful. Finally a thorough effort should be made to search for antibiotic-associated enterocolitis by assay of *Clostridium difficile* enterotoxin. Treatment consists of oral vancomycin or intravenous metronidazole. Once colon ischemia has been identified, immediate treatment is required. If minimal signs of sepsis are present and proctosigmoidoscopy clearly excludes transmural infarction, then a short period of expectant observation with antibiotics directed at the enteric flora is appropriate. However, unstable patients or those with early signs of rapidly progressing sepsis (altered mental status, hyperglycemia, hypoxemia, partial or compensated metabolic acidosis, increasing fluid sequestration, etc.) should undergo immediate surgical exploration.

NUTRITION

Postoperative nitrogen loss is inevitable following major vascular surgery. Cumulative nitrogen losses can be excessive if oral intake is not possible due to a prolonged postoperative ileus. Erosion of lean body mass, impairment of lymphocyte and neutrophil function, and impaired wound healing can occur as a result of inadequate nutrition during the postoperative period and may predispose the patient to development of potentially preventable complications. Nutritional support within the first 24 to 48 h following major vascular surgery is usually unnecessary because of the underutilization of exogenous nitrogen and calorie sources, which occurs from high levels of circulating counterregulatory hormones and cytokines. Once the severe catabolic response is diminished and the patient is hemodynamically stable, if >5 days of inadequate nutritional intake is anticipated, then enteral or parenteral nutritional support should be begun. If, during surgery, the patient is anticipated to require postoperative nutritional support, a nasoenteric feeding tube can be placed intraoperatively and positioned beyond the ligament of Treitz. Elemental feeding can be administered as early as 12 h postoperatively, the presence of clinical ileus notwithstanding. This has been proved to be both safe and efficacious.[44] If enteral access is not available, then parenteral nutrition can be administered through a central venous catheter (see Chap. 92).

Critical Illness and Vascular Disease—Special Considerations

COMBINED CORONARY ARTERIAL AND CEREBROVASCULAR DISEASE

Because atherosclerosis is a systemic disease with focal manifestations, it is not surprising that patients often have synchronous lesions of the carotid and coronary arteries.[45] Patients with coexistent disease present a spectrum of clinical problems. Treatment priorities are usually focused on the most threatening problem: usually either cerebral symptoms or angina. Although patients undergoing coronary revascularization have been found to have severe carotid artery disease in 2 to 12 percent of cases, combined procedures have not been shown to be of benefit.[46] Conversely patients undergoing CEA have a high incidence of CAD. However, we do not subject every patient to simultaneous carotid-coronary surgery. Following appropriate preoperative and anesthetic management, patients with mild to moderate CAD can safely undergo CEA. Situations remain where combined carotid-coronary disease is severe and symptomatic and though a slightly higher risk of stroke has been reported, combined surgery is warranted.[47]

MANAGEMENT OF RUPTURED ABDOMINAL AORTIC ANEURYSM

Despite continued reduction in the mortality rates for elective aortic aneurysm repair, ruptured aortic aneurysms carry a mortality rate as high as 50 percent. Following prompt diagnosis, the preoperative management is identical to any patient with life-threatening hemorrhage: volume resuscitation, blood replacement, and expeditious surgery. The primary determinants of the high mortality rate associated with ruptured abdominal aortic aneurysm are the depth and duration of preoperative shock and the development of hypothermia, coagulopathy, myocardial depression, infection, and other organ failures, which are the result of massive blood transfusion.[48]

Postoperative complications are common and to be expected. Cardiac and respiratory insufficiency are frequent and may require prolonged ventilatory and hemodynamic support. Hypothermia and significant fluid sequestration are invariably present. Patients should remain intubated, mechanically ventilated, and pharmacologically sedated and paralyzed until normothermia and cardiorespiratory stability are achieved.

Renal dysfunction may occur in the immediate postoperative period, and aggressive treatment with either hemodialysis or CAVH is recommended (see Chap. 155). Early intervention can avoid complications by treating volume overload, allowing administration of adequate nutritional support, and limiting the effects of excessive fluid administration from multiple medications common to many of these patients.[49]

Paraplegia occurs in 2 percent of patients following repair of a ruptured abdominal aortic aneurysm, usually as a result of prolonged shock with ischemia to the spinal cord.[50] Once other causes of paraplegia have been eliminated (such as epidural hematoma or herniated disc), high dose steroids should be administered. Although several other treatment options have been proposed, including spinal fluid drainage and glycerol or dextran administration to reduce cord swelling, variable results with each have been reported.[51]

THORACOABDOMINAL ANEURYSM REPAIR

Thoracoabdominal aneurysm (TAA) repair is one of the most complex procedures performed by vascular surgeons. It is associated with significant mortality and formidable morbidity primarily related to underlying diseases such as coronary artery stenosis, renal insufficiency, cerebrovascular disease, and chronic airway disease.[52] The usual surgical approach requires a left lateral thoracoabdominal incision with circumferential division of the left hemidiaphragm. These patients need chest tube placement and aggressive pulmonary toilet. Because of the problems of postoperative pulmonary atelectasis and pain, general and epidural anesthesia combinations are useful. In this manner postoperative pain management can be treated without respiratory compromise.

Most TAA repairs require visceral artery reimplantation (celiac, superior mesenteric, and renal arteries) and will involve long periods of ischemia to these organs. Fastidious attention to cardiopulmonary parameters, urine output, and intravenous fluids is required. It is our practice to titrate multiple vasoactive agents such as low dose dopamine (2.5 μg/kg/min), nitroglycerin (0.25 to 0.50 μg/kg/min), and esmolol (10 to 30 μg/kg/min), to achieve maximum oxygen delivery without excessive cardiac work. Paraplegia is discussed in the section on ruptured aneurysms. It deserves further mention here because it occurs with increased frequency following TAA repair—at variable rates ranging from 0.5 to 40 percent depending on numerous factors. A particularly frustrating aspect of the problem is its relative unpredictability. Clinical manifestations can occur in the immediate postoperative period or days later.[53] Although various techniques have been attempted, complete prevention of neurologic deficits following TAA repair is virtually impossible.

VASCULAR EMERGENCIES ARISING IN THE ICU

Acute limb ischemia can occur in the ICU and usually can be attributed to thrombosis of native arteries or grafts during a low flow state, thromboembolic phenomena from indwelling vascular devices, a hypercoaguable state, or overzealous use of vasopressor agents. Because the physical findings overlap, making a precise diagnosis may be difficult. All patients admitted to the ICU must have initial documentation of all extremity pulses. If palpable pulses cannot be obtained, then Doppler pulse examination should be performed. Hypothermia, central cyanosis, or use of pressor agents can make the physical examination of an extremity difficult to interpret, and noting a change from the initial examination can be critical in initiating evaluation. The management of acute arterial occlusion consists of identifying the cause and initiating immediate anticoagulation. Low cardiac output states should be treated and indwelling devices should be removed.

DRUGS COMMONLY USED IN VASCULAR SURGERY

HEPARIN. Heparin is frequently used during and following vascular surgery. A broad discussion of heparin pharmacology is covered elsewhere and is beyond the scope of the present discussion (see Chap. 119). Certain complications particular to the vascular patient with regard to heparin deserve mention.

Overanticoagulation and bleeding represent the most common complication of heparin. Clinical manifestations of excessive anticoagulation and nonsurgical bleeding are unexplained anemia, persistent requirement for blood, and microvascular hemorrhage from raw surface areas. Frequent sites of blood loss are puncture sites of indwelling catheters, incisions, soft tissue dissection planes (retroperitoneum), and the nasal and orotracheal mucosa. Heparin should be immediately withheld and a prothrombin time, partial thromboplastin time, and platelet count determined. Other causes of bleeding in the vascular patient include hypothermia, dilutional coagulopathy from massive blood loss, and platelet dysfunction.

Another preventable complication of heparin is thrombocytopenia (see Chaps. 119 and 146). Heparin-induced thrombocytopenia is a well-recognized entity that can result in both hemorrhage and arterial thrombosis. It has been reported following extremely small doses of heparin as may be administered during routine flushing of lines; however, it is more commonly manifested following full heparin doses with prolonged continuous infusion. Heparin-induced thrombocytopenia should be included in the differential diagnosis of any patient who develops unexplained bleeding or arterial thrombosis. Routine platelet counts are mandatory for all patients receiving heparin regardless of dosage and route.

DEXTRAN. Continuous intravenous dextran infusion during and after lower extremity bypass grafting has been efficacious in selected cases for the prevention of early thrombosis. This polysaccharide of varying molecular weight exerts its antithrombotic actions via three distinct mechanisms: increasing antiplatelet activity by reducing von Willebrand's factor, increasing clot lysis by altering fibrin polymerization, and promoting blood flow as a volume expander.[54] Hypersensitivity reactions to dextran can occur and are avoided by initial test dosing. Pulmonary edema can also occur; however, this is only seen in patients with limited cardiac function or in renal failure.

MANNITOL. Mannitol is used as a diuretic, thromboxane inhibitor, and an oxygen radical scavenger. The most common pitfall during mannitol administration is the creation of a hyperosmolar state with resultant osmotic diuresis and volume depletion. Although occasional hypersensitivity reactions occur, appropriate central venous monitoring avoids most complications of mannitol.

THROMBOLYTIC AGENTS. Thrombolytic agents such as urokinase and streptokinase have been used for various disorders such as arterial thrombosis, pulmonary emboli, venous thrombosis, and thrombolysis of clotted intravascular catheters. Advances in our understanding of thrombosis have led to a growing acceptance of intraarterial thrombolytic therapy as an important adjunctive treatment of peripheral vascular disease. Currently the most common preoperative indication for intraarterial thrombolysis is acute and subacute thrombosis of suprainguinal and infrainguinal extremity vessels.[55] However, its use has been expanded recently to include intraoperative and postoperative administration. The most undesirable complication following thrombolytic therapy is bleeding and is seen in 7 to 10 percent of patients. Bleeding sites include catheter insertion sites, gastrointestinal tract, genitourinary tract, and most catastrophically, the central nervous system. Although several tests examining the coagulation cascade have been proposed to predict bleeding complications, none reliably predict bleeding. Bleeding at an invaded site (wound; arterial, venous, or urinary catheter insertion site) appears to be an adequate warning sign to a dangerous systemic fibrinolytic state. Intraarterial thrombolysis should be administered with the cooperation of a vascular surgeon, radiologist, and intensive care specialist. This team approach is mandatory for successful and safe thrombolytic therapy.

CASE PRESENTATION

A 60-year-old woman was admitted directly to the ICU with an 8-h history of sharp midscapular and right upper quadrant pain, tachycardia, severe hypertension, and diaphoresis. The patient had an abdominal aneurysm repair 8 years prior to admission and a recent CT scan demonstrated a 6-cm TAA extending from the mid descending thoracic aorta to the proximal infrarenal aortoiliac anastomosis. Medications at the time of admission were furosemide 20 mg daily and hydralazine 10 mg daily. Physical examination was remarkable for a blood pressure of 210/120, pulse 100 regular, and a II/VI holosystolic ejection murmur. Pulses in the upper extremities were normal. The right femoral pulse was present, the left femoral pulse was absent, and all distal pulses were absent. A thoracoabdominal CT scan revealed a contained rupture of the TAA.

A pulmonary artery catheter was placed and revealed a cardiac output of 6.5 L/min, stroke volume of 58 mL, a Ppw of 15 mmHg, and an SVR of 2200 dyne · s/cm^5. Hemoglobin at the time of admission was 12 g/dL and $S\bar{v}_{O_2}$ was 75% with a $P\bar{v}_{O_2}$ of 40 mmHg and an oxygen delivery of 950 mL/min. The patient was placed on nitroprusside titrated to an MAP of 85 to 95, nitroglycerin to reduce the Ppw to 7, and esmolol to decrease the heart rate to 90. Fluid was administered to increase the Ppw to 10 and the stroke volume to 80 mL. Urine output was 50 mL/h and heart rate was 80 to 90 beats/min.

Following induction of general and epidural anesthesia, a transesophageal echo probe was placed. Exposure of the aneurysm was achieved using a thoracoabdominal incision through the ninth intercostal space identifying a contained rupture of the posterior and medial supradiaphragmatic aorta. Prior to aortic cross-clamping 50 g mannitol was administered. Heparin was not given. Nitroprusside, nitroglycerin, and isotonic fluids were administered during the aortic clamping to achieve adequate cardiac output as determined by pulmonary artery thermodilution and to prevent ventricular overdistention and wall motion abnormalities by continuous two-dimensional TEE. The aneurysm was repaired using the endoaneurysmorrhaphy technique; flow to the celiac, superior mesenteric, and renal arteries was provided by suturing a continuous circumferential anastomosis performed around the orifices from within the aneurysm (Carrel patch). Cross-clamp time was 48 min. Blood loss was estimated to be 5000 mL. Fluids administered were 10 L lactated Ringer's solution, 8 U homologous PRBCs, 6 U processed autologous blood, and 8 U fresh frozen plasma.

The patient arrived back in the ICU with a pressure of 110/70, pulse of 100, temperature of 34.5°C (94.1°F), and urine volume of 28 to 30 mL/h. Peripheral vascular examination demonstrated that the right femoral pulse was present, the left femoral pulse was absent, and all distal pulses were absent similar to the preoperative examination. Muscle relaxation was not reversed and ventilatory support of IMV of 12, tidal volume of 800 mL, F_{IO_2} of 50%, PEEP of 5 cmH_2O was provided yielding a peak airway pressure of 35 cmH_2O. Drips included phenylephrine at 2 μg/min, dopamine at 30 μg/kg/min, nitroglycerin at 30 μg/min, and 200 mL colloids and crystalloids per hour. Hemoglobin was 8.0 g/dL. ABGs revealed pH 7.25, P_{CO_2} 32, Pa_{O_2} 110, Sa_{O_2} of 96%. Cardiac output was 7.5 L/min, Ppw 12, and stroke volume 75 mL. Despite a $P\bar{v}_{O_2}$ of 38, the $S\bar{v}_{O_2}$ was 57% due to a rightward shift in the venous oxygen dissociation curve from a metabolic acidosis. The extraction ratio was 40 percent and the oxygen delivery was 771 mL/min. Two units of PRBCs were administered and the extraction ratio was 28 percent with an oxygen delivery of 1061 mL/min. Repeat hemoglobin was 10.8 g/dL. The patient's blood pressure remained labile for the next 24 h primarily from changes in SVR. Because cardiac output remained elevated with adequate stroke volumes, swings in resistance were attributed to reperfusion metabolites and were treated with phenylephrine and volume. No evidence of ischemia was noted on ECG or by enzyme analysis. Pharmacologic paralysis slowly resolved and the patient was found to be neurologically intact, moving all four extremities. During the second postoperative day progressive oliguria developed despite high cardiac output (9.0 L/min), normal Ppw, and several attempts at diuresis. Metolazone and Lasix were given and produced a mild diuresis (30 mL/h for 3 h). However, this effect was short-lived and the patient progressed to severe oliguria/anuria over the next 48 h.

The patient remained in a hyperdynamic state (cardiac output 8 L/min, SVR 600 dyne · s/cm^5) for 5 days postoperatively requiring continuous phenylephrine and nitroglycerin. Esmolol was used during this period to suppress bouts of tachycardia. Enteral and parenteral nutrition were begun on postoperative day 3 and daily hemodialysis was initiated. Two liters of diarrhea per day developed 2 days following initiation of enteral elemental feedings. Prompt endoscopy of the sigmoid colon was performed. The mucosa appeared slightly red and was friable but was otherwise normal. *C. difficile* toxin and Hemoccult tests were negative. Due to profound hypoalbuminemia (1.4 g/dL), 75 g/day of albumin was added to the TPN. Enteral nutrition was continued at 50 mL/h. Total caloric intake was 2400 calories/day with 1.3 g protein/kg/day. Cumulative inputs and outputs on postoperative day 14 revealed the patient was near or at fluid balance and close to her preoperative weight. The chest x-ray was clear and the patient was successfully extubated. Daily dialysis was continued; the patient was tolerating oral intake but still required nutritional support and was having semisolid bowel movements.

On postoperative day 16, during a bowel movement, the patient had a cardiopulmonary arrest preceded by a bradycardic rhythm. She was resuscitated successfully following 10 min of advanced cardiac life support protocol, and 2 days later was extubated. The patient's physical examination revealed her to be neurologically intact; pulses were at baseline and cardiac enzymes were normal. The patient was continued on dialysis for the next 4 weeks with gradual return of renal function sufficient to discontinue dialysis. Four weeks following discontinuation of dialysis her renal function had returned to its preoperative baseline with a discharge creatinine level of 1.4; she was voiding 1200 mL/day.

CASE DISCUSSION

This case illustrates the complexity of the postoperative management of a patient following major aortic reconstructive surgery. Of note is that cardiopulmonary support may be required for a significant period of time during the postoperative period. Hyperdynamic, low resistance states can persist and require ongoing assessment. Following end points such as mixed venous saturation, stroke volume, ECGs, and cardiac enzymes ensures the intensivist that the treatment protocols do not result in ischemia to critical organ beds. ARF in this case was successfully managed by early dialysis. This aggressive approach precluded the deleterious effects of persistent volume overload, chronic ventilator dependence, and inability to provide adequate nutritional support. Of particular note is the prolonged course of renal failure, which ultimately resolved.

References

1. National Center for Health Statistics: Health, United States 1988. DHHS Publication No. (PHS) 89-1232. Public Health-Service, Washington, US Government Printing Office, March 1989, pp 10–17, 66, 67, 100, 101.
2. Hertzer NR et al: The risk of vascular surgery in a metropolitan community: With observations on surgeon experience and hospital size. J Vasc Surg 1:13, 1984.
3. Yeager RA, Moneta GL, McConnell DB, et al: Analysis of risk factors for myocardial infarction following carotid endarterectomy. Arch Surg 124:1142, 1989.
4. Eagle KA, Coley CM, Newell JB, et al: Combining clinical and thallium data optimizes preoperative assessment of cardiac risk before major vascular surgery. Ann Intern Med 110:859, 1989.
5. Hertzer NR, Beven EG, Young JR, et al: Coronary artery disease in peripheral vascular patients: A classification of 1000 coronary angiograms and results of surgical management. Ann Surg 199:223, 1984.
6. Taylor PC: Evaluation and surgical management of patients with severe combined coronary artery disease and peripheral vascular atherosclerosis. Cleve Clin Q 48:172, 1981.
7. Goldman L, Caldera DL, Nussbaum SR, et al: Multifactorial index of cardiac risk in noncardiac surgical procedures. N Engl J Med 297:845, 1977.
8. Carliner NH, Fisher ML, Plotnick GD, et al: Routine preoperative exercise testing in patients undergoing major noncardiac surgery. Am J Cardiol 56:51, 1985.
9. Blombery PA, Ferguson IA, Rosengarten DS, et al: The role of coronary artery disease in complications of abdominal aortic aneurysm surgery. Surgery 101:150–155, 1989.
10. Cooperman M, Pflug B, Martin EW Jr, Evans WE: Cardiovascular risk factors in patients with peripheral vascular disease. Surgery 84:505, 1978.
11. Detsky AS, Abrams HB, McLaughlin JR, et al: Predicting cardiac complications in patients undergoing noncardiac surgery. J Gen Intern Med 1:211, 1986.
12. Johnston KW: Multicenter prospective study of nonruptured abdominal aortic aneurysm. Part II. Variables predicting morbidity and mortality. J Vasc Surg 9:437, 1989.
13. Carliner NH, Fisher ML, Plotnick GD, et al: The preoperative electrocardiogram as an indicator of risk in major noncardiac surgery. Can J Cardiol 2:134, 1986.
14. Goldman L, Caldera DL, Nussbaum SR, et al: Multifactorial index of cardiac risk in noncardiac surgical procedures. N Engl J Med 297:845, 1977.
15. Cutler BS, Wheeler HB, Paraskos JA, Cardullo PA: Applicability and interpretation of electrocardiographic stress testing in patients with peripheral vascular disease. Am J Surg 141:501, 1981.
16. Leppo J, Plaja J, Gionet M, et al: Noninvasive evaluation of cardiac risk before elective vascular surgery. J Am Coll Cardiol 9:269, 1987.
17. Rao TLK, Jacobs KH, El-Etr AA: Reinfarction following anesthesia in patients with myocardial infarction. Anesthesiology 59:499, 1983.
18. Kalman PG et al: Cardiac dysfunction during abdominal aortic operation: The limitations of pulmonary wedge pressures. J Vasc Surg 3:773, 1986.
19. Gewertz BL et al: Transesophageal echocardiographic monitoring of myocardial ischemia during vascular surgery. J Vasc Surg 5(4):607, 1987.
20. Sicard GA, Freeman MB, Van Der Woude JC, Anderson CB: Comparison between transabdominal and retroperitoneal approach for reconstruction of the infrarenal abdominal aorta. J Vasc Surg 5:19, 1987.
21. Lunn JK, Dannemiller FJ, Stanley TH: Cardiovascular responses to clamping of the aorta during epidural and general anesthesia. Anesth Analg 58:372, 1979.
22. Abbott WM, Cooper JD, Austen WG: The effects of aortic clamping and declamping on renal blood flow distribution. J Surg Res 14:385, 1973.
23. Hertzer NR, Arison R: Cumulative stroke and survival ten years after carotid endarterectomy. J Vasc Surg 2:661, 1985.
24. Rapp JH, Reilly LM, Qvarfordt PG, et al: Durability of endarterectomy and antegrade grafts in the treatment of chronic visceral ischemia. J Vasc Surg 3:799, 1986.
25. Shapiro DM, Crounenwett JL, Lindenauer SM, et al: The effect of glycogen and prostacyclin in acute occlusive and postocclusive mesenteric ischemia. J Surg Res 36:535, 1984.
26. Bounous G: The intestinal factor in multiple organ failure and shock. [Editorial, The Montreal General Hospital, Montreal, Quebec, Canada Department of Surgery]. Surgery 107(1):118, 1989.
27. Veith FJ et al: Changing arteriosclerotic disease patterns and management strategies in lower-limb threatening ischemia. Ann Surg 212(4):402, 1990.
28. Andros G, Harris RW, Salles-Cunha SX, et al: Bypass grafts to the ankle and foot. J Vasc Surg 7:785, 1988.
29. Nelson LD: Continuous venous oximetry in critically ill surgical patients. Ann Surg 203:329, 1986.
30. Lumb PD, Wysham DG: Preoperative preparation of high-risk surgical patient. Perspect Crit Care 2(2):33, 1989.
31. Capurro NL, Kent KM, Epstein SE: Comparison of nitroglycerin, nitroprusside, and phentolamine-induced changes in coronary collateral function in dogs. J Clin Invest 60:295, 1977.
32. Bove EL, Fry WJ, Gross WS, Stanley JC: Hypotension and hypertension as consequences of baroreceptor dysfunction following carotid endarterectomy. Surgery 85(6):633, 1979.
33. Pastermack PF, Grossi EA, Baumann FG, et al: Beta blockade to decrease silent myocardial ischemia during peripheral vascular surgery. Am J Surg 158:113, 1989.

34. Bush HL Jr: Renal failure following abdominal aortic reconstruction. Surgery 93:107, 1983.
35. Perry MO, Fantini G: Ischemia: Profile of an enemy. Reperfusion injury of skeletal muscle. J Vasc Surg 6:231, 1987.
36. Haimovici H: Muscular, renal and metabolic complications of acute arterial occlusions: Myonephropathic-metabolic syndrome. Surgery 85:461, 1979.
37. Schubart PJ, Porter JM: Leg edema following femorodistal bypass, in Bergan JJ, Yao JST (eds): *Reoperative Arterial Surgery.* Orlando, Grune & Stratton, 1986, pp 311–330.
38. Kaiser AB, Clayston KR, Mulberin JL, et al: Antibiotic prophylaxis in vascular surgery. Ann Surg 188:283, 1976.
39. Bergamini TN, Bandyk DF, Govostis D, et al: Identification of staphylococcus epidermidis vascular graft infection: A comparison of culture techniques. J Vasc Surg 9:665, 1989.
40. Ouriel K, Ricotta JJ, Adams JT, et al: Management of cholelithiasis in patients with abdominal aortic aneurysm. Ann Surg 198:717, 1983.
41. Warshaw AL, O'Hara PJ: Susceptibility of the pancreas to ischemic injury in shock. Ann Surg 188:197, 1978.
42. Ernst CB: Intestinal ischemia following abdominal aortic reconstruction, in Bernhard VM, Towne JB (eds): *Complications in Vascular Surgery.* 2nd ed. Orlando, Grune & Stratton, 1985, pp 325–350.
43. Fiddian-Green RG, Grantz NM: Transient episodes of sigmoid ischemia and their relation to infection from intestinal organisms after abdominal aortic operations. Crit Care Medicine 15(9):835, 1987.
44. Riley KS, White JL, et al: Immediate postoperative enteral feeding. Surg Forum 31:103, 1980.
45. Hertzer NR, Lees CD: Fatal myocardial infarction following carotid endarterectomy. Three hundred thirty-five patients followed 6–11 years after operation. Ann Surg 194:212, 1981.
46. Brener BJ, Brief DK, Alpert J, et al: The risk of stroke in patients with asymptomatic carotid stenosis undergoing cardiac surgery. A follow-up study. J Vasc Surg 5:269, 1987.
47. Hertzer NR, Loop FK, Beven EG, et al: Surgical staging for simultaneous coronary and carotid disease. A study including prospective randomization. J Vasc Surg 9:455, 1989.
48. Wakefield TW, Whitehouse WM Jr, Wu S-C, et al: Abdominal aortic aneurysm rupture: Statistical analysis of factors affecting outcome of surgical treatment. Surgery 91:586, 1982.
49. Sapir DG, Dandy WE Jr, Whelton A, Cooke CR: Acute renal failure after ruptured abdominal aortic aneurysm: An improved clinical prognosis. Crit Care Med 7:59, 1979.
50. Szilagyi DE, Hageman JH, Smith RF, Elliott JP: Spinal cord damage in surgery of the abdominal aorta. Surgery 83:38, 1978.
51. Crawford ES, Svensson LG, Hess KR, et al: A prospective randomized study of cerebrospinal fluid drainage to prevent paraplegia after high-risk surgery on the thoracabdominal aorta. J Vasc Sur 13(1):36, 1991.
52. Crawford ES, Crawford JL, Safi JH et al: Thoracoabdominal aortic aneurysms: Preoperative and intraoperative factors determining immediate and long-term results of operations in 605 patients. J Vasc Sur 3:389, 1986.
53. Hollier LH, Symmonds JB, Pairolero PC, et al: Thoracoabdominal aortic aneurysm repair. Analysis of postoperative morbidity. Arch Surg 123:871, 1988.
54. Rutherford RB, Jones DN, Bergentz SE, et al: The efficacy of dextran-40 in preventing early postoperative thrombosis following difficult lower extremity bypass. J Vasc Surg 1:765, 1984.
55. McNamara TO, Bomberger RA, Merchant RF: Intra-arterial urokinase as the initial therapy for acutely ischemic lower limbs. Circulation 83 2(supp.I):I-106, 1991.

Chapter 87

CARDIAC SURGERY

JOSEPH P. COYLE
THOMAS L. HIGGINS

KEY POINTS

- *The postoperative course is determined by intraoperative events.*
- *Management in the early postoperative period is determined by the multisystem effects of cardiopulmonary bypass (CPB).*
- *Maintaining cardiovascular function is key to recovery in other systems.*
- *Respiratory care is directed at restoring lung volume and minimizing lung water.*
- *Preservation of renal function is essential in minimizing postoperative morbidity.*
- *Coordination of care is required to facilitate timely interventions and to incorporate input from surgeons, anesthesiologists, cardiologists, intensivists, and consultants.*

More than 300,000 cases involving CPB are performed each year, and all these patients require postoperative intensive care. Unique considerations in the cardiac surgical patient include the multisystem effects of CPB, myocardial recovery from a period of global ischemia during aortic cross-clamping, and the obligate need for invasive monitoring as hemodynamic and ventilatory support are gradually weaned in the early postoperative period. These patients tend to be unstable, with a propensity for rapid physiologic change that can be catastrophic if not avoided or immediately recognized and treated. Since many of the problems presenting in the postoperative ICU reflect decisions and interventions made in the operating room, it is important for the intensivist to have a basic understanding of what has transpired in the operating room to anticipate problems in the recovery period.

As our ability to support the circulation has expanded, so have the indications for cardiac surgery. Though coronary artery bypass grafting (CABG) still comprises the bulk of adult open heart surgical procedures, a large number of patients present for valve repair or replacement, dysrhythmia surgery, thoracic aortic aneurysms, heart transplants, and a growing number of reoperations and combined procedures. The clinical profile of the patient undergoing CABG is changing, with significant increases in the presence of congestive heart failure, advanced age, extensive coronary artery disease, and incidence of concurrent medical problems.[1] Percutaneous transluminal coronary angioplasty (PTCA) has grown exponentially since its introduction in 1977, and this option selects out lower risk patients resulting in sicker, older patients presenting for initial coronary surgery. In the Coronary Artery Surgery Study (CASS), the risk of operative mortality was shown to increase with advanced age, emergency operation, and evidence of left ventricular (LV) dysfunction (congestive failure, rales, LV wall motion abnormalities, increased heart size).[2] Other studies have confirmed these findings and pointed out the additional risk of preoperative renal dysfunction and repeat operation.[3,4] The result of these trends is a persistent increase in the severity of illness in the patient population, which results in higher morbidity and a longer ICU stay due to low output syndrome, respiratory problems, and neurologic complications.[3]

As cardiac surgery has evolved, patients have a higher degree of illness, procedures are more complex and varied, and sophisticated means to provide multiorgan system support have been created. This presents a spectrum of new challenges in the cardiac surgical ICU which are not encountered in other areas of critical care medicine. The cardiac intensivist will be called on to manage critically ill patients who have undergone a wide variety of complex procedures and must have an understanding not only of the specific postoperative considerations of those techniques but of the more general physiologic changes common to all cardiac surgical patients.

Intraoperative Management

THE PREBYPASS PERIOD

MONITORING

An understanding of intraoperative events is essential to an appreciation of the early postoperative course in the cardiac surgical patient. In this section we will discuss the selection of monitors, anesthetic management before bypass based on pathophysiologic state, the elements of CPB, and separation from bypass. The sequence for placement of lines and selection of monitors differs somewhat from institution to institution; however, little controversy exists about the need for large bore intravenous access, direct arterial pressure monitoring, continuous electrocardiography (ECG) with views of V_5 and the limb leads, and central venous access to allow for administration of vasoactive drugs and monitoring of central venous pressure (CVP). Much has been written about the indications for the use of a pulmonary artery (PA) catheter in cardiac surgery; yet, to date, no prospective randomized trials of PA catheters versus central venous catheters have been done. Advocates of PA catheterization claim it is an early sensitive indicator of myocardial ischemia and that CVP alone may be a poor indicator of preload in the patient with global or regional ischemia.[5,6] The use of a PA catheter improves the anesthesiologist's ability in the early detection of hemodynamic abnormalities during coronary surgery, and aggressive management based on hemodynamic parameters derived from the PA catheter has been credited with a marked reduction in the incidence of reinfarction in the perioperative period in patients with coronary artery disease undergoing noncardiac surgery.[7] In a recent, prospective, unrandomized study evaluating the utility of PA catheters versus

CVP in 1094 patients undergoing cardiac surgery, the routine use of a PA catheter did not significantly affect outcome.[6] This study has been criticized on a number of grounds, but it underscores the importance of considering the need for PA catheterization in each individual patient based on the cardiac pathophysiology, coexisting medical problems, procedure, and practice patterns of the physicians and institution providing care.

The advent of two-dimensional transesophageal echocardiography (TEE) has expanded our ability to monitor for ischemia and assess basic hemodynamic parameters in a relatively noninvasive fashion. The development of regional wall motion abnormalities has been shown to be an early sensitive indicator of myocardial ischemia,[8] and the addition of color flow Doppler makes TEE an excellent tool for defining the nature of valvular pathology and adequacy of valve repair in selected patients. To the experienced echocardiographer, TEE can also yield valuable information regarding ventricular volumes and contractility, and it is extremely sensitive in the detection of residual intracardiac air. TEE is an expensive technology with considerable training required to obtain the appropriate views and interpret the findings; a larger experience will be needed before its role in cardiac surgery is clearly defined.

HEMODYNAMIC MANAGEMENT PREBYPASS

The hemodynamic goals in the prebypass period are determined by the underlying cardiac pathophysiology. Anesthetic medications, vasoactive drugs, and intravascular volume are titrated to create favorable conditions, maintain tissue perfusion, and preserve myocardial function until surgical correction can be accomplished. The major stresses during this time are anesthetic induction, laryngoscopy and intubation, sternotomy, and cannulation of the aorta and right atrium. A variety of factors can complicate the prebypass period, such as the need for femoral cannulation in certain cases, the potential for injury to the heart or great vessels with reoperation, or the need to dissect one or both internal mammary arteries (IMAs). The problems encountered at this time vary greatly depending on the lesion to be corrected and other associated medical conditions; some of the more common scenarios are outlined below.

CORONARY ARTERY SURGERY. The major objective in the prebypass period for the patient with coronary artery disease is the detection, prevention, and prompt treatment of myocardial ischemia. A study of over 1000 patients undergoing coronary revascularization in 1985 found a 37 percent incidence of prebypass ischemia which was associated with a threefold increase in the incidence of perioperative myocardial infarction (MI).[9] This was confirmed in a later study by the same group. In both these studies over half the episodes were hemodynamically silent; the remaining episodes correlated with hemodynamic abnormalities, particularly tachycardia, with the quality of the anesthesia care apparently playing a large role in determining outcome. Anesthesia care is directed at controlling the factors that determine the balance between myocardial oxygen consumption and delivery of oxygen to the heart. Myocardial oxygen consumption is minimized by keeping wall tension low and avoiding increases in contractility secondary to release of endogenous catecholamines with surgical stimulation. Myocardial oxygen delivery is maintained by keeping arterial oxygen content high while preserving coronary perfusion pressure, and by avoiding tachycardia which compromises diastolic time for perfusion of the LV. The most common approach to achieve these goals is the use of high doses of the synthetic narcotics fentanyl and sufentanil, which blunt the catecholamine response to stimulation, decrease heart rate, preserve systemic vascular resistance (SVR) without depressing the myocardium. The choice of anesthetic, however, does not appear to play a large role in determining outcome,[10,11] substantiating the observation that it is not what anesthetic is given, but how the patient is managed overall that makes a difference.

VALVULAR SURGERY. In aortic stenosis, LV hypertrophy resulting from chronically elevated afterload leads to a markedly reduced compliance requiring higher filling pressures for a given level of preload and renders these patients very sensitive to small changes in intravascular volume. As a result of decreased compliance, the LV is more dependent on atrial systole for filling, and loss of atrial booster function can lead to significant compromise. This can occur when atrial dysrhythmias are triggered during atrial cannulation. These patients are also more prone to ischemia by virtue of myocardial hypertrophy with decreased coronary reserve, increased wall tension, and high intramyocardial pressures which can compromise subendocardial perfusion.[12] In addition, these patients do not tolerate myocardial depression, since high peak LV intracavitary pressures must be achieved to eject across the stenotic valve.

In chronic aortic insufficiency the LV is usually dilated, with the regurgitant fraction determined by diastolic time and the aortic diastolic pressure (which is a function of SVR). The primary goals with a regurgitant aortic valve are to keep afterload down, maintain heart rate, and avoid myocardial depression in these patients with increased ventricular volume and high wall stress.[12]

Both mitral stenosis and insufficiency result in high pulmonary vascular pressures and subsequent right ventricular (RV) hypertrophy or dysfunction. Much of the perioperative management will be directed to maximizing RV performance and avoiding those things which might further increase pulmonary vascular resistance, such as hypoxemia, acidosis, and drugs which cause pulmonary vasoconstriction. In mitral stenosis it is important to prevent tachycardia to allow adequate time for LV filling.[12] The LV has a chronically decreased preload and increasing preload is best accomplished by keeping heart rate down, maintaining atrial booster function, if present, and keeping left atrial pressure up by maximizing RV function. Left atrial or pulmonary capillary wedge pressure (PCWP) will be a function more of the size of the mitral orifice and the flow across the valve than LV end-diastolic volume. With mitral insufficiency systemic afterload is best reduced to minimize the degree of mitral regurgitation.[12] Systemic vasodilation, either as a result of anesthetics or vasodilators, reduces the

TABLE 87-1 Postoperative Morbidity Associated with Prolonged CPB

Cardiac Dysfunction	*Infection*
Low output syndrome	Mediastinitis
Right heart failure	Sternal wound
IABP requirement	Pneumonia
Neurologic Dysfunction	*Metabolic*
Global	Catecholamine release
Focal	Bradykinin levels
Delirium	Complement activation
Respiratory Problems	*Renal Failure*
Delayed extubation	*Gastrointestinal Complications*
ARDs	Hepatic dysfunction
Coagulopathy	Pancreatitis
Platelet dysfunction	Gastrointestinal bleeding
Fibrinolysis	
Dilutional coagulopathy	

impedance to forward ejection, thus increasing forward flow and reducing the regurgitant fraction. Loading conditions must be taken into account when interpreting the severity of regurgitation with TEE.

MANAGEMENT OF CPB

Despite our best efforts, CPB is still a very abnormal physiologic perfusion state with obligate anticoagulation, hemodilution, hypothermia, loss of pulsatile perfusion, and trauma to the cellular elements of the blood from exposure to air, tubing, filters, and suction. The effects of CPB are responsible in large part for many of the clinical management problems encountered in the postoperative care of the cardiac surgical patient. The systemic response to CPB is characterized in part by markedly elevated catecholamines,[13] complement activation,[14] release of bradykinin,[15] loss of platelet number and function, hemolysis, neutrophil sequestration in the lungs,[15,16] loss of T lymphocytes, loss of renal function, and capillary closure in the cerebral microcirculation.[17] Almost all of the common complications of cardiac surgery have been shown to increase in frequency with increasing pump time over 150 to 180 min (Table 87-1).

The patient is prepared for CPB by the placement of a venous drainage cannula in the right atrium and an aortic inflow cannula in the aortic root. In certain circumstances the vena cavae may be selectively cannulated to allow opening the atria; femoral cannulation may be performed in procedures involving the thoracic aorta or when standard approaches are not possible for other reasons. A prerequisite to initiating CPB is full systemic anticoagulation. This is accomplished with heparin in doses of 300 to 400 U/kg body weight with verification of anticoagulation most commonly using activated coagulation time (ACT) >400 to 480 s.[18] Occasional patients may demonstrate resistance to heparin, particularly when there is a history of previous recent exposure to heparin.[18] Oxygenation and removal of carbon dioxide are accomplished with either a bubble or membrane oxygenator, with the latter growing in popularity due to less disruption of platelets and red cells. Controversy exists regarding the optimal pressures, flows, and acid-base regulation to use on bypass with the issue being how best to maintain cerebral perfusion and minimize neurologic complications[19] while providing the best operating conditions and least trauma to blood.

After CPB is initiated, the patient is cooled and after the heart fibrillates, the aortic cross-clamp is applied. Cardioplegia is given to protect the heart during the ischemic period needed for the surgical repair. Myocardial protection during the cross-clamp period can be provided in a number of ways including topical and systemic hypothermia, and hyperkalemic blood or crystalloid cardioplegia usually delivered into the aortic root proximal to the cross-clamp.[20] There is considerable variation in the contents of cardioplegic solutions in different institutions, and this can have a significant effect on electrolytes in the early postoperative period particularly in regard to potassium and magnesium balance.[21] The longer the cross-clamp time required for the surgical procedure the greater the incidence of myocardial dysfunction on separation from CPB. The global ischemic injury is characterized by decreased ventricular function and compliance with contraction bands and edema seen in the involved myocardium on microscopy.[22] The need for pharmacologic or mechanical support for the heart increases with cross-clamp times in excess of 120 min, although this depends a great deal on the effectiveness of measures to preserve the heart,[23,24] the quality of surgical repair, and the base-line cardiac function.

Certain procedures, such as repair of arch aneurysms and some pediatric procedures, may require the interruption of CPB utilizing deep hypothermia and circulatory arrest.[25] In these situations the patient's temperature is decreased to below 20°C (68°F) on CPB, the head is packed in ice, and the pump is turned off for the minimum time needed to accomplish the repair. Arrest times of up to 45 min are generally well tolerated in these conditions with the frequency of neurologic injury increasing with longer times.[25] The profound hypothermia can result in marked decreases in the number of platelets and white cells[26] and a longer period of rewarming is required to restore temperature in all tissues.

Separation from CPB is attempted after the surgical repair has been accomplished, the patient is thoroughly rewarmed, hematocrit, electrolyte, and acid-base status are corrected, and the lungs are being ventilated.[27] A normal rhythm and conduction frequently return or are easily restored with defibrillation as reperfusion takes place and cardioplegic solution is washed out of the myocardium. Occasional patients will require placement of epicardial pacing wires for atrial or atrioventricular pacing for transient conduction abnormalities.[28] In some institutions epicardial wires are placed routinely in the event of the development of heart block in the early postoperative period. The decision for inotropic support is based on the preexisting cardiac function, duration of cross-clamp time, and visual inspection of the heart in the surgical field. Selection of inotrope will depend on many factors including the degree of functional impairment, the SVR, heart rate, and the practice patterns of the surgeon and anesthesiologist. Calcium is frequently used at the time of separation from CPB since ionized calcium is frequently low after CPB and the inotropic effect of calcium is accentuated in the postischemic myocardium. In addition, calcium counters the residual effects of the hyperkalemic cardioplegia on the conducting system. Once the rhythm and inotropic state have been addressed, the venous drainage to the pump is gradually occluded, resulting in filling of the heart and ejection as manifested by return of PA then systemic arterial pulse pressure. After the venous drainage is completely occluded, the remaining volume in the pump is transfused into the patient through the aortic line as needed until the aortic cannula is removed. LV dysfunction is managed by addressing the determinants of myocardial function including rhythm, coronary perfusion, preload, afterload, and contractility. Intra-aortic balloon counterpulsation (IABP) should be considered in patients who require large doses of potent inotropes (epinephrine, norepinephrine, and isoproterenol), show persistent signs of ischemia, or have refractory ventricular dysrhythmias.[29] In patients with severe ventricular dysfunction a combination of drugs may ultimately be required to successfully separate from bypass using β and α agonists and vasodilators or inotropes with different mechanisms of action titrated to a specific effect. In addition to β agonists, contractility may be improved by phosphodiesterase inhibitors such as amrinone,[30] α agonists,[31] or augmentation of cellular substrate with the infusion of glucose, insulin, and potassium.[32] A small subgroup of patients will not respond to the measures outlined above and may benefit from mechanical assistance to unload the heart, allow time for reperfusion injury to resolve, restore high-energy substrates, and reduce edema. Temporary assistance can be provided for either or both ventricles with the use of ventricular assist devices, usually in the form of a centrifugal pump without a reservoir which does not require anticoagulation.[33] When ventricular function is restored, the patient is returned to the operating room for separation from the assist device, removal of the cannulae, and closure of the chest.

Transient ischemia may develop prior to or shortly after separation from CPB, particularly in the distribution of the right coronary artery, when small bubbles of air embolize down the native coronaries or grafts. This is frequently managed by administering nitroglycerin and increasing perfusion pressure and may necessitate a return to bypass. Persistent ischemia may be an indicator of graft occlusion or spasm and may require topical papaverine or sublingual nifedipine.[34] IMA grafts are dynamic conduits that respond to exogenous catecholamines and vasodilators in a unique fashion. Although experimental studies have not been able to demonstrate a relationship between pressure and flow in these grafts,[35] it has been our experience that patients with IMA grafts will frequently require perfusion pressures in excess of 70 mmHg to normalize ST segments in the early postoperative period.

RV dysfunction is relatively common after cardiac surgery particularly in patients with preexisting pulmonary hypertension or RV dysfunction. The RV, by virtue of its anterior position, is more difficult to protect during the procedure and is more subject to surgical manipulation and trauma.[36] In addition, the right coronary ostium is anterior and therefore, superior in the supine position making the right coronary more prone to air embolism when residual air is present in the aortic root. Management of RV failure after bypass is directed at inotropic support, pulmonary vasodilation, prevention of overdistention of the RV, and maintenance of perfusion pressure (usually with norepinephrine). Refractory RV failure may require selective infusion of norepinephrine through a left atrial line[37] and right atrial infusion of pulmonary vasodilators, such as amrinone and prostaglandin E_1.[38] The use of an intraaortic balloon pump is useful in maintaining RV perfusion pressure when ischemia is present and in severe RV failure a right ventricular assist device may be required to successfully separate from bypass.[39]

The period of time in the operating room after separation from bypass is characterized by achieving hemostasis surgically and with restoration of coagulation (initially with protamine). Protamine binds heparin and removes it from the circulation. Protamine should be administered carefully, because it can produce a number of untoward hemodynamic effects[40] such as vasodilation, myocardial depression, and, rarely, anaphylactoid reactions characterized by pulmonary vasoconstriction, systemic hypotension, and bronchospasm.[41] The coagulopathy that accompanies CPB is characterized by loss of platelets, degranulation of remaining platelets, and decreased platelet aggregation, as well as local and systemic fibrinolysis which produces fibrin degradation products that further interfere with coagulation.[42] The use of desmopressin has been advocated to decrease bleeding after cardiac surgery because of its ability to induce factor VIII release and improve platelet function.[43] ϵ-amino-caproic acid (EACA, Amicar) has also been used to improve coagulation after cardiac surgery by preventing fibrinolysis.[44] Finally, specific blood product support may be required depending on length of bypass, amount of blood transfused, and preexisting platelet function or factor levels.

Postoperative Management

Immediate postoperative goals in all cardiac surgery patients include restoration of normal body temperature and monitoring of hemodynamics, respiratory function, fluid-electrolyte status, and blood loss from mediastinal and pleural drains. Timely intervention may be required to manage shivering or agitation as the patient emerges from anesthesia or to correct inadequate perfusion pressure, low cardiac output, arrhythmias, and ischemia. Cardiac tamponade or excessive bleeding may necessitate emergent return to the operating room for reexploration, and cardiac arrest that does not respond to initial closed chest cardiopulmonary resuscitation (CPR) may require rapid opening of the chest and return to the operating room. This process may be facilitated or hindered by the physical locations of the operating room and ICU, availability of equipment, and, most importantly the training, experience, and division of responsibility of the patient care team.[45]

ROUTINE MANAGEMENT

BLEEDING

Persistent bleeding after cardiac surgery is one of the most common problems in the early postoperative period. The causes of postoperative bleeding are legion and include heparin rebound, acquired platelet defects due to CPB and drugs, dilutional thrombocytopenia and factor deficiency, local and systemic fibrinolysis, disseminated intravascular coagulation (DIC), and preexisting coagulopathies.[42] Laboratory assessment of coagulation status is often not helpful, since the lag time between sampling and results is generally longer than the window of opportunity for corrective action. Quick assessment of coagulation status can be done by observing for clot in the mediastinal tubes, noting oozing from puncture sites, checking ACT,[46] and drawing a blood sample in a clot tube to assess time for clot development and lysis. The use of thromboelastography has been expanding, since it is helpful in defining common problems such as residual heparin, platelet defects, or fibrinolysis. It has been shown to be a better predictor of the need for postoperative reexploration for bleeding than ACT or clotting profile.[47] The initial management of bleeding is more often based on empirical trials than laboratory data; however, it is usually best to draw studies before intervening so that reliable information is available if initial therapy fails. Base-line studies should include prothrombin time, partial thromboplastin time, platelet count, fibrinogen, and fibrin split products (usually modestly elevated after CPB). Since heparin rebound is not uncommon, a trial of 50 to 100 mg protamine is usually given in patients who have not had significant protamine reactions. Desmopressin (DDAVP) may be given slowly in a dose of 3 μg/kg to augment plasma level of von Willebrand factor and to restore platelet function.[43] It must be administered slowly, since rapid administration may induce hypotension.[48] EACA, by virtue of inhibiting fibrinolysis, has been recommended by some authorities to reduce postoperative bleeding[44] and is usually given in a loading dose of 5 g with a continuous infusion of 1 g/h. Blood product support of coagulation starts with platelet infusion, since defects in platelet function are common after CPB.[49] The use of platelets must be weighed against the potential risks of blood-borne infection. Use of fresh frozen plasma, cryoprecipitate, and other blood products is best guided by appropriate laboratory tests if the clinical circumstances permit. Positive end-expiratory pressure (PEEP) has been advocated to compress small mediastinal or chest wall vessels and reduce bleeding, but its use is controversial[50] and hemodynamic depression from PEEP can be significant in the hypovolemic patient. PEEP may be applied to decrease bleeding in increments up to 12 cmH_2O with careful attention to its effect on chest tube output and hemodynamics, with prompt discontinuation if it is ineffective or deleterious.

Transfusion of red blood cells should be guided by the hematocrit, the rate of blood loss, underlying medical problems in the patient, and indicators of oxygen delivery to tissues. In younger patients with a good hemodynamic outcome and no major coexisting medical problems, hematocrits in the low 20s are well tolerated and can usually be expected to gradually increase with diuresis in the early postoperative period. Patients more likely to need transfusion are the elderly, those undergoing reoperation, and those with low preoperative total red cell volumes. The need for transfusion of packed cells can be minimized by autotransfusion of shed mediastinal blood, using a sterile collection circuit consisting of chest tubes and the cardiotomy reservoir, and a peristaltic pump to return the blood to the venous circulation.[51] Reinfusion of unwashed shed mediastinal blood increases levels of fibrin split products[52] and activated complement,[53] though the implications of these effects have not been fully evaluated. The surgical decision to reexplore for bleeding is based on many factors including details of the surgical procedure, hemodynamic stability, volume and rate of blood loss, and coagulation status. The presence of mediastinal blood loss of more than 300 mL in the first hour, 250 mL in the second hour, or 150 mL thereafter has been correlated with surgically correctable bleeding.[54] Early return to the operating room may avert catastrophic hemodynamic collapse, decrease transfusion requirements, and decrease the incidence of wound infection. In one study, sternal wound complications were minimized when patients were explored if blood loss exceeded 200 mL/h for 4 h.[55] During reexploration often no discrete bleeding site is found but evacuation of clot and cauterization of smaller bleeding sites is corrective.

ANESTHETIC EMERGENCE

Ideally the intraoperative anesthetic management is tailored such that the patient remains quiet and comfortable in the ICU until adequately rewarmed, hemodynamically stable, blood loss is minimal, and the patient is ready to begin weaning from mechanical ventilation. The most common technique in cardiac anesthesia uses high dose narcotics which have minimal hemodynamic effects (fentanyl and sufentanil) and muscle relaxants which are not reversed such that emergence is gradual. Problems encountered can include patients who awaken before the relaxant wears off, patients who awaken abruptly with agitation and hemodynamic sequelae, and patients in whom emergence is delayed for a number of reasons. The time between arrival and awakening varies with the anesthetic technique used, but it is not unusual for a patient to awaken from narcotic anesthesia within 2 h of arrival and to be ready for extubation within 12 h. Unless the type, dose, and timing of muscle relaxant is carefully chosen, the patient may awaken while still "paralyzed" from neuromuscular blockade. This will manifest as hypertension, tachycardia, sweating, or nonsustained floppy movements characteristic of residual relaxant. Options for resedation include narcotic analgesics, benzodiazepines,[56] and newer sedative agents such as propofol.[57] The choice of drug depends on the relative contribution of pain, anxiety, and delirium to the clinical presentation. Reassurance and gentle handling of the patient can do a great deal to make therapy more effective and decrease drug requirements. All agents must be used in reduced dosage and carefully titrated, since residual anesthetic agents are present and patients are frequently hypovolemic and thus predisposed to the untoward hemodynamic effects of these drugs.

Delayed respiratory depression may occur after anesthesia with high dose opioids such as fentanyl and sufentanil, particularly when the patient is unstimulated. Residual narcotic has been reported to cause late truncal rigidity, decreased chest wall compliance, hypoventilation, and respiratory acidosis from depressed central ventilatory drive.[58] This complication is most likely to be encountered when patients are extubated early, with low core temperature, and when rewarming and acidosis occur in the postoperative period. Management includes stimulating the patient who is modestly hypoventilating and judicious administration of naloxone (40- to 100-μg increments followed by an infusion of 50 to 100 μg/h) when respiratory depression is more severe. The use of naloxone in this setting can be complicated by severe hypertension precipitating hemorrhage, ventricular failure, pulmonary vasoconstriction, or arrhythmias, and in many situations reintubation and ventilation may be preferable to narcotic reversal.

SHIVERING

The early period after CPB is characterized by a progressive temperature drop that occurs as the warmer richly perfused tissues equilibrate with less perfused tissues, not thoroughly rewarmed at the termination of CPB. Shivering commonly occurs in the early postoperative period as patients actively rewarm after the effect of muscle relaxants has waned. Once temperature begins to increase it does so rapidly although peak temperature may not occur until 8 h after ICU admission.[59] Shivering interferes with the efficiency of mechanical ventilation and may result in respiratory acidosis as a result of increased carbon dioxide production with a subsequent need for higher minute ventilation. Shivering also increases myocardial work and oxygen consumption, placing increased demands on the heart recovering from the effects of cross-clamping and CPB. Since both oxygen consumption and CO_2 production are increased, minute ventilation should be appropriately increased and extubation delayed until the patient is thermally stable. Vasodilation and increased need for intravascular volume are seen in this phase of recovery and may contribute to hemodynamic instability.

Therapy of shivering depends on the severity and the level of consciousness of the patient. When shivering is modest and the patient is responsive and hemodynamically stable, meperidine (25-mg increments) is useful in attenuating the response and increasing patient comfort. Meperidine's use in this setting has not been studied, although it has been used to stop shaking chills and fever in other settings.[60] With severe shivering or when there is hemodynamic instability, use of a muscle relaxant (pancuronium 0.1 mg/kg or vecuronium 0.1 mg/kg) is effective in stopping shivering and allowing the patient to rewarm passively. Care should be taken to be certain that the patient is not awake and paralyzed without sedation or reassurance.

COMPLICATIONS OF CARDIAC SURGERY BY SYSTEMS

CARDIOVASCULAR

For the uncomplicated patient with relatively normal preoperative LV function the tendency is toward a slow increase in SVR in the early postbypass period.[61] During this time, the patient may require vasodilation and will usually require some augmentation of intravascular volume as well. As the patient warms, there is a tendency toward venous and arterial vasodilation, which results in further volume requirement. With increased preload and decreased afterload, cardiac output may increase and reach or exceed preoperative values.[62] The importance of maintaining adequate cardiac output is emphasized by the increased frequency of complications seen in patients with low output syndrome, specifically renal failure, respiratory failure, DIC, central nervous system (CNS) dysfunction, and gastrointestinal bleeding.[63] The exact etiology of multisystem organ failure (MSOF) after open heart surgery has not been elucidated, but may relate to release of vasoactive substances in areas that are not adequately perfused on CPB or in the early postoperative period. No single measure of perfusion is adequate, since regional abnormalities of blood flow can occur even with an overall adequate cardiac output. By the same token, lower than normal cardiac index is not universally associated with poor outcome. Most clinicians consider a cardiac index of 2.1 L/min/m^2 to be adequate, but this number should be interpreted in the light of the patient's age, preoperative status, and organ system function as manifest by adequacy of mental function, signs of peripheral hypoperfusion (mottled skin, low toe temperature), acid-base status, lactate production, mixed venous saturation, and urine output.

DYSRHYTHMIAS. Dysrhythmias are common in the early postoperative period, as the result of electrolyte shifts, myocardial ischemia (due to insufficient myocardial protection or inability to revascularize), acid-base abnormalities, hypothermia, catecholamines, conduction abnormalities, and surgical trauma. Detailed descriptions of ventricular dysrhythmias and their therapy are covered elsewhere in this book, so comments will be limited to unique considerations in the open heart patient. When either supraventricular or ventricular dysrhythmias occur, consideration should be given to contributing factors such as hypokalemia, hypomagnesemia, hypothermia, acidosis, hypoxemia, and ischemia, which frequently are contributory if not causative.

Supraventricular dysrhythmias occur in 20 to 50 percent of patients after cardiac surgery.[64] Although these dysrhythmias may be seen in the early postoperative period, they are also common within the first week after surgery, mandating continued ECG surveillance when patients are discharged from the ICU to the step-down floor. Therapy with β-adrenergic blockers has been shown to be effective in both preventing and treating these events.[64] However, use of β blockers does entail the risk of producing myocardial depression. Esmolol, a short-acting β_1-blocking agent, is especially useful when high sympathetic tone is contributing to the tachydysrhythmias. It is effective in rapidly controlling heart rate and will often convert sinus tachycardia, atrial fibrillation, and atrial flutter to normal sinus rhythm.[65] Esmolol is usually given in 10- to 20-mg increments until appropriate rate control is attained. Then it can be used as an infusion at 50 to 300 μg/kg/min. Although hypotension may limit the use of esmolol, the short half-life allows any adverse effects to be simply treated by stopping the infusion. Verapamil is also useful in this setting with doses of 2.5 to 5.0 mg titrated to effect; hypotension with verapamil can be reversed by administering calcium.[66] It is generally not advisable to combine the use of β blockers and calcium channel blockers, since their combined effects on conduction and contractile function may be accentuated. In patients with atrial pacing wires in place, atrial flutter is effectively treated with rapid overdrive atrial pacing.[67]

Hypokalemia and hypomagnesemia are common after cardiac surgery due to preexisting deficiencies, urinary losses with diuresis, and intracellular shifts in response to circulating catechols. Hypomagnesemia has been implicated in producing dysrhythmias, coronary spasm, and in precipitating hypokalemia. In one study of patients undergoing coronary revascularization without cardioplegic arrest, those given magnesium chloride had a lower incidence of ventricular dysrhythmias.[68] The type of cardioplegic solution administered produces a large difference in postoperative magnesium levels. The use of inotropes seems to play a role, since patients receiving inotropic support have over eight times the risk of developing hypomagnesemia, and those who drop their magnesium levels have higher potassium requirements and greater incidence of dysrhythmias.[21]

TAMPONADE. Signs and symptoms of cardiac tamponade in the postoperative cardiac patient may be markedly different from those seen after chest trauma or as a complication of constrictive or restrictive diseases of the pericardium. A major difference is that the pericardial sac is generally left open after open heart procedures, thus altering the compliance of the cavity. Thus, the classic physical signs of tamponade may not be evident. Surface echocardiography can be difficult due to bandages, edema, and positive-pressure ventilation. The diagnosis should always be suspected when hemodynamic status deteriorates and does not respond to interventions, particularly when accompanied by elevation and equalization of end-diastolic pressures[69] or markedly decreased chest tube output. Diagnosis can be further clouded by the possibility of isolated tamponade of either the left or right atrium.[70] The cause of mediastinal tamponade following heart surgery is generally excessive postoperative bleeding, with accumulated blood and clot producing cardiac compression. While pericardiocentesis is lifesaving in nonsurgical tamponade, it is rarely useful in the postbypass patient since clot cannot be aspirated, and the procedure runs the risk of disrupting newly placed grafts. The usual course is to transport the patient back to the operating room when there is a high index of suspicion, open the chest under minimal anesthesia, at which point hemodynamic improvement occurs so that additional anesthetic can be administered.

LOW OUTPUT SYNDROME. Low output syndrome, defined as a cardiac index of <2.2 L/min/m^2, is associated with a high incidence of postoperative respiratory, renal, hepatic, and CNS failure, gastrointestinal bleeding, DIC, and death. Acute LV dysfunction may develop in the early postoperative period or during later periods of stress such as weaning from mechanical ventilation.[71] As in all patients with shock, treatment depends on diagnosis, provision of adequate filling pressure, and then appropriate inotropic support (see Chaps. 114 and 115). Specific considerations with cardiac surgery patients, however, include the effect of vasoactive agents on coronary blood and graft flow, avoidance of tachydysrhythmias with β-adrenergic stimulation, the possibility of "down-regulation" of receptors from prior catecholamine therapy, and specific maneuvers for treatment of RV failure. Amrinone, a phosphodiesterase inhibitor, is useful as an adjunct to adrenergic support after open heart surgery.[35] The combination of high dose amrinone and dopamine has been successful in a small number of patients with moribund cardiogenic shock after open heart surgery.[72] Heroic doses of vasoactive drugs are sometimes necessary, far exceeding the usual clinical recommendations. IMA grafts retain vascular innervation and thus respond in a dynamic manner, whereas saphenous vein grafts (SVG) are passive. This difference in responsiveness leads to unpredictable effects when using vasoactive substances. In animal studies, epinephrine and nitroglycerin increase IMA flow, but decrease SVG flow.[35] In contrast, nitroprusside decreases IMA flow and increases SVG flow. Phenylephrine decreases flow in both types of grafts, while norepinephrine increases flow, but at the expense of an increase in LV dv/dt.[35] Since mixed use of IMA and SVG grafts is typical, the clinical utility of this information may be limited to changing drugs if ischemia occurs in the distribution of one or the other grafts. In our experience, maintaining mean arterial pressure over 70 mmHg is important in sustaining flow in IMAs and α agonists can be safely used to accomplish this, although careful attention must be paid to cardiac index and signs of ischemia. Measures to treat ischemia in the early postoperative period are similar to those outlined above; however, consideration should be given to potential spasm of grafts or native coronaries and acute occlusion of grafts due to surgically correctable problems. Many factors can affect ST segments other than ischemia, but ischemic changes in the presence of significant ventricular dysfunction or dysrhythmias may warrant TEE or emergent coronary angiography to further define the problem.

The type of surgical lesion corrected plays a large role in determining postoperative hemodynamic management and outcome. Valve replacement patients, in general, are more at risk than those undergoing CABG, and patients with mitral insufficiency seem to be at highest risk for postoperative complications, followed by those with aortic stenosis or regurgitation, and finally mitral stenosis (Higgins TL, unpublished data). Correction of mitral insufficiency results in markedly increased afterload with loss of ejection into the left atrium, and the LV may already be distended as the result of chronic volume overload. These patients frequently require afterload reduction and inotropic support to sustain adequate output. Mitral insufficiency patients are at high risk of postoperative complications, including infection. Patients who undergo aortic valve replacement for stenosis are frequently hypertensive in the early postoperative period, and this can be a particular threat to the aortic suture line. The LV is still hypertrophic and therefore LV compliance is decreased, producing labile hemodynamics with volume shifts and a greater need for atrial booster function. The degree of reversibility of LV function in patients with aortic stenosis may be predicted by a preoperative history of paroxysmal nocturnal dyspnea.[73] After aortic valve replacement for insufficiency, the LV continues to be somewhat dilated and ventricular function may continue to be impaired. After valve surgery, and particularly after reoperation, pacing may be needed for transient or permanent complete heart block.

IABP is indicated for preoperative stabilization of refractory angina pectoris, for stabilization after MI when inotropic support alone is ineffective, and for intractable cardiac failure after CPB. Early survival after IABP can be predicted by near-normal cardiac index that improves, continued high urine output, and high-normal SVR and PCWP.[74] Nonsurvivors present with lower initial cardiac index that fails to improve to normal, accompanied by elevated PCWP and SVR and declining urine output. If the IABP has been inserted percutaneously, a period of groin compression should follow balloon removal. In most cases, it is best to leave a patient ventilated until after this period of compression, since the supine position makes it more difficult to cough and clear secretions. However, patients with excellent ventilatory parameters and no other systemic problems can occasionally be weaned from mechanical ventilation while on IABP support.

POSTOPERATIVE HYPERTENSION. Significant hypertension develops in up to 40 percent of patients undergoing various types of cardiac surgery.[75] The etiology of this postoperative hypertension is multifactorial; common causes include hypoxia, hypercapnia, ventilatory difficulties, hypothermia with shivering, arousal from anesthesia, and surgical manipulation of the great vessels.[76] Increases in mean arterial pressure correlate with changes in plasma catecholamine levels, suggesting increased sympathetic tone. This concept is supported by the ability of stellate ganglion block, which interrupts sympathetic afferents from the heart, great vessels or coronary arteries, to ablate the hypertensive response.[77] In animal experiments, a cardiogenic hypertensive chemoreflex can be elicited by injecting small amounts of serotonin into the left atrium and can be blocked by vagotomy or cyproheptadine. Small chemoreceptors lying between the aorta and PA are thought to be the source of the reflex, and since they receive their blood supply from the proximal left coronary artery, they are implicated in the new hypertension seen with angina pectoris, acute MI, and after CABG.[78] Sodium nitroprusside is the mainstay of treatment for postoperative hypertension, although response to this agent is nearly universal and does not elucidate underlying mechanisms. Other peripheral vasodilators (hydralazine, prazosin) and antihypertensives (clonidine, captopril, nifedipine) have also been used to control the blood pressure elevation after coronary surgery.

Labetalol is effective in lowering elevated blood pressure after CABG, primarily by reducing cardiac output with little change in SVR. In a comparison of intravenous labetalol with sodium nitroprusside for treatment of postbypass hypertension, labetalol caused significant reductions in heart rate and cardiac index, while sodium nitroprusside caused significant increases in heart rate and cardiac index, with stroke volume remaining unchanged in either group.[79] Since the lower heart rate observed with labetalol may improve myocardial oxygen balance, it may be preferable to nitroprusside in those with hyperdynamic circulation and adequate cardiac output. However, nitroprusside would remain the drug of choice when cardiac output is borderline and accompanied by increased SVR. Esmolol, while indicated primarily for treatment of supraventricular tachycardias, is also effective at reducing blood pressure by depressing a hyperdynamic circulation after open heart surgery.[65] It has the advantage of a short half-life, so that if unacceptable hypotension or depression of cardiac index is encountered, the situation can be restored by simply stopping the infusion. Caution must be exercised with the application of esmolol or other β-blocking drugs in the patient whose cardiac index is already low.

NEUROLOGIC COMPLICATIONS

Potential neurologic problems following CABG include focal cerebral lesions resulting in gross sensory-motor abnormalities (hemiparesis, aphasia), severe global encephalopathy (failure to awaken, seizures), peripheral nerve injury (limb palsies and diaphragmatic paralysis), or more subtle neuropsychiatric findings. Reported incidence varies by institution[80] and between retrospective and prospective evaluations. In a prospective study of CABG patients at our institution, new focal findings were noted in 5 percent, and were severe in 2 percent. Prolonged encephalopathy occurred in almost 12 percent, but resolved in all but 2 percent by discharge. Peripheral nerve injuries in this same group of 421 patients included 28 upper extremity deficits, 24 lower extremity mononeuropathies, prolonged hoarseness or vocal cord paresis in 7, phrenic nerve injury in 4, and 1 each of isolated seventh nerve palsy and Horner's syndrome.

Risk factors for CNS injury include emergency operation, severe LV dysfunction, advanced age, presence of peripheral vascular disease, necessity for IABP support, prolonged bypass time (>142 min), and associated valvular procedures or ventriculotomy. The presence of carotid bruits increases the risk of stroke following CABG, comparable in magnitude to the risk reported from carotid endarterectomy.[81] Air or particulate matter originating within the heart or at the cannulation site appears to be a major cause of postoperative cerebral dysfunction.[82] Management should include careful attention to minimize entrainment of air during cannulation and decannulation and removal of air introduced with ventriculotomy or other open procedure. In a recent study, patients undergoing open ventricle procedures were given thiopental in large doses from the time of cannulation to separation from bypass, and had a lower incidence of neurologic sequelae than the control group; however, they required more inotropic support and pacing than the control group.[83] In the patient who fails to awaken appropriately on the first postoperative day, all sedatives, narcotics, and muscle relaxants are withheld and assessment of peripheral neuromuscular function is done using a nerve stimulator. Patients are sent for computed tomography (CT) scanning if unresponsiveness persists to rule out structural problems or cerebral edema. In the unusual situation in which elevated intracranial pressure is suspected, an intracranial pressure monitor is placed to facilitate management with hyperventilation and diuretics. An electroencephalogram is usually done to assess level of activity and rule out seizure activity. The patient with a focal or global neurologic injury is unfortunately usually diagnosed too late for interventions to affect outcome; the prevention of these injuries and the development of monitoring that permits early recognition are challenging areas for future work.

Transient postoperative delirium is seen in approximately 7 percent of patients on the first postoperative day, but resolves either spontaneously or after appropriate medical-surgical intervention in most patients by day 6.[84] Initial management of agitation involves reassurance and orientation of the patient, relief of mechanical problems if present (e.g., full bladder), and treatment of pain or anxiety, if present. If the patient remains agitated, intravenous haloperidol is useful to control agitation and protect the patient from self-harm.

Spinal ischemia can occur after cross-clamping of the thoracic aorta for descending aneurysm repair and result in postoperative paraplegia. Encouraging results have been reported with both intraoperative drainage of cerebrospinal fluid and injection of intrathecal papaverine.[85] Rib resection, during a thoracotomy, rarely can produce a hematoma compressing the thoracic spinal cord. Since this is a treatable, reversible lesion, presence of typical Brown-Séquard neurologic deficit or otherwise unexplained paraplegia should be investigated with either CT or magnetic resonance imaging scanning, and the compression relieved surgically before permanent damage results.

RESPIRATORY CARE

The major goals and objectives of postcardiac surgery respiratory care are provision of adequate oxygenation and ventilation during recovery from anesthesia and surgery, while preserving hemodynamic stability and reducing cardiac workload. Secondary goals include avoidance of barotrauma or infection and maintenance of airway control in the event of hemodynamic instability or neurologic dysfunction. Weaning and extubation can usually be safely accomplished when the patient is awake and responsive, warm, hemodynamically stable, chest tube output is minimal, and oxygenation is acceptable on levels of inspired oxygen that can be provided by mask. Routine weaning and extubation can be hindered by a number of common respiratory problems after CPB including atelectasis, pleural effusions, pulmonary edema, phrenic nerve dysfunction, and loss of lung volume resulting in impaired cough and secretion clearance.

The most common pathophysiologic abnormality in the lungs after cardiac surgery is loss of lung volume with a marked propensity toward subsegmental, segmental, and lobar atelectasis (see Chap. 84). Expected changes in pulmonary function after median sternotomy and CPB include a reduction in vital capacity (VC) of approximately 50 percent, which reaches a nadir on the second and third postoperative day.[86] Functional residual capacity (FRC) is also reduced in the early postoperative period with changes persisting as late as the seventh postoperative day. Radiographic evidence of atelectasis can be found in up to 98 percent of patients.[87] This occurs most commonly in the left lower lobe, although it may be bilateral in as many as 70 percent of patients.[87] The etiology of atelectasis in this setting is multifactorial with contributions from anesthetics, lack of lung inflation on CPB, surgical compression, diaphragmatic dysfunction, undrained pleural effusions or blood, splinting with pain, and decreased surfactant production as a result of hypothermia and injured alveolar epithelial cells.[87] Harvesting of an IMA graft is accompanied by greater impairment in pulmonary function than when SVGs alone are used, independent of age, sex, number of grafts, aortic cross-clamp time, duration of bypass and postbypass fluid gradient.[88] Removal of mediastinal and pleural chest tubes results in improvement of VC, forced expiratory volume at 1s (FEV_1), and peak expiratory flow, possibly related to decreased pain with deep breathing.[89] Decreased VC and maldistribution of ventilation can lead to impaired secretion clearance and further loss of lung volume. This loss of lung volume and atelectasis leads to hypoxemia due to areas of low ventilation/perfusion matching and shunt; the effect of shunt on oxygenation will be magnified in the presence of venous desaturation or agents that interfere with hypoxic pulmonary vasoconstriction such as vasodilators and beta agonists.

The otherwise uncomplicated patient at the authors' institution will be placed on 60% fraction inspired oxygen (F_{IO_2}) with 5 cm PEEP, intermittent mandatory ventilation (IMV) rate of 8 and tidal volume of 12 to 15 mL/kg upon ICU arrival. Auscultation of the chest and a portable chest x-ray are performed immediately, and arterial blood-gas samples drawn after 20 to 30 min of stabilization, and then every 4 h or as clinically indicated. The chest x-ray is essential to check placement of devices (endotracheal tube, PA catheter, IABP, and mediastinal and pleural tubes) as well as to rule out pneumothorax, atelectasis, pleural effusions, and pulmonary edema.

The initially high F_{IO_2} is chosen to protect against possible hypoxemia during hemodynamic instability or shivering, and it is gradually decreased in the first few hours based on blood-gas results or continuous pulse oximetry. PEEP of 2 to 5 cmH_2O is usually provided to maintain lung volume, but it should be used cautiously in the patient with hypovolemia.

Mechanical ventilation can be weaned by a number of different, acceptable approaches, most commonly via progressive decrease in IMV rate. With a high dose narcotic technique, time between ICU arrival and return of consciousness is typically 1.8 h for sufentanil and 2.1 h for fentanyl. The corresponding times to extubation in this small population of relatively healthy patients undergoing first-time CABG were 4.6 and 4.8 h, respectively, with approximately 20 percent of all the patients remaining intubated beyond 8 h.[90] Narcotic disposition is affected by a variety of factors, including age,[91] chronic β-blocking therapy,[92] alcohol use, and genetic differences in drug metabolism. Expected times to awakening and extubation will also be longer with more complex operations (including valve replacement) and with addition of other anesthetic agents such as benzodiazepines or barbiturates. In our experience, unselected patients average 15.5 h of postoperative ventilation, longer if they are over age eighty. Criteria for weaning include a P_{O_2} of at least 70 mmHg on F_{IO_2} of 0.4 or less, with 5 cm or less of PEEP, minute ventilation of <10 L/min, dead space of less than 0.6, and presence of spontaneous respiratory effort. Before extubation, the patient should be awake and able to cooperate, have stable hemodynamics, minimal chest tube drainage, and no ongoing problems such as acute renal failure, that will compromise fluid balance. Criteria for extubation include spontaneous respiratory rate <20 while on continuous positive airway pressure (CPAP) at 40% F_{IO_2}, ability to generate 25 cm of maximal inspiratory pressure, and VC of 12 to 15 mL/kg. Extubation within 4 h of ICU arrival is possible in the stable patient who meets the above criteria, but risky in more complex patients, particularly those with total bypass times >100 min.[87]

We routinely instruct all patients preoperatively in the use of the incentive spirometer and deep breathing techniques. Postoperatively, tracheal suctioning is carried out every 4 h until the patient is able to cough and mobilize secretions spontaneously. Despite a lack of literature support for the use of intermittent positive-pressure breathing (IPPB) treatments, we find it of value in patients who are unable to effectively perform incentive spirometry. Mask CPAP has been used in a similar fashion after extubation to restore lung volume. Inhaled bronchodilators and mucolytics are added when necessary, and aminophylline is added if wheezing is evident or the patient has regularly received bronchodilators preoperatively. Aminophylline improves diaphragmatic contractility and renders it less susceptible to fatigue, making it particularly useful in the long-term patient with poor nutritional status and chronic respiratory failure.

Prolonged postoperative ventilation is more common in elderly, debilitated patients, those undergoing valve operation (particularly mitral procedures), patients requiring reexploration for bleeding or tamponade, those with significant preoperative pulmonary dysfunction as manifest by multiple bronchodilator or home oxygen use and as a manifestation of LV dysfunction[71] (Tables 87-2 and 87-3). Critical factors in weaning these patients from mechanical ventilation include presence of sufficient CNS function to allow clearing of secretions and limited cooperation with the weaning program, a resting minute ventilation of <10 L/min with integrity of the phrenic nerve, diaphragm and respiratory muscles, absence of ongoing infection, hemodynamic stability, adequate nutrition, and either sufficient renal function to facilitate fluid removal or institution of dialytic support (see Chap. 155). Criteria developed for discontinuing prolonged ventilation in medical-surgical patients do not necessarily apply to the cardiac surgery population. A prospective evaluation of the factors that differentiated the ability to wean from mechanical ventilation after open heart surgery found dynamic and static compliance, absence of congestive failure, heart rate < 120 beats/min, $F_{IO_2} < 0.4$, and absence of significant hepatic or renal dysfunction to be the best predictors.[93] Our approach is to provide full ventilatory support when it is apparent that the patient is not ready to wean as a result of inadequate nutrition, cardiovascular instability, infection, or other major systemic disturbance. Appropriate nutritional, hemodynamic, antibiotic, and dialytic support is instituted. Weaning in these patients is directed toward restoring respiratory muscle strength and function through a program of alternating periods of respiratory work with rest on full mechanical ventilation. The work intervals usually take the form of CPAP or CPAP with pressure support to maintain gas exchange with a respiratory rate <30 breaths/min. The length and frequency of work intervals is increased as the patient tolerates. The role of tracheostomy in postoperative cardiac surgical patients is similar to that in other clinical settings of respiratory failure except that consideration must be given to the proximity of the mediastinal wound to the tracheostomy site and the potential for contamination. When the mediastinal wound is well healed and the potential for mediastinitis is considered low, tracheostomy is frequently helpful when it is apparent that weaning will not be completed by 3 weeks postoperatively. Tracheostomy increases patient comfort, assists in clearing secretions, and theoretically helps limit damage to the upper airway, although the last point remains controversial.

TABLE 87-2 Factors Predisposing to Prolonged Ventilation after Open Heart Surgery

Stormy postoperative course (IABP)
Reexploration for bleeding or tamponade
Emergency procedure
Valve operation
LV dysfunction
Renal failure
Fluid overload
Infection (sepsis, mediastinitis, pneumonia)
Malnutrition
Bronchospasm
Phrenic nerve injury
Pulmonary hypertension
MSOF
Advanced age
Neurologic injury (stroke, encephalopathy)

TABLE 87-3 Respiratory Complications after Open Heart Surgery

	Isolated CABG	AVR, MVR or Both	Isolated Mitral Stenosis	Isolated Mitral Insufficiency	Age 80+	All Open Heart Surgery
n	4376	869	64	213	97	6111
Ventilated >48 h %	6.8	17.7	17.1	15.4	24.7	10.1
Any reintubation %	3.9	9.3	3.1	11.7	19.6	5.6
Reintubated for pulm cause %	1.6	4.8	3.1	5.7	14.4	2.4
Tracheostomy %	0.6	3.1	0	3.3	6.2	1.2

SOURCE: Cleveland Clinic Cardiothoracic Database 7/86 through 6/88

Pulmonary edema and pleural effusions are frequent after cardiac surgery for a variety of reasons. The most common cause of pulmonary edema in this setting is cardiogenic from elevated pulmonary vascular pressures due to LV dysfunction. This generally resolves fairly quickly as LV function is improved with appropriate use of vasodilators and inotropes. In the first few hours after cross-clamping LV compliance is often decreased due to myocardial edema and possible reperfusion injury. As a result, higher filling pressures may be required to adequately load the ventricle at end diastole. This can contribute to the development of pulmonary edema particularly when there is a component of alveolar capillary leak.

Occasional patients will develop acute LV dysfunction as a result of fluid shifts or inadequate myocardial blood flow during the increased work imposed by weaning. Dyspnea without blood gas perturbations, falling cardiac output, desaturation of mixed venous blood or ECG changes during weaning suggest this etiology. Treatment options include diuresis, use of afterload-reducing agents, improved inotropy, and more gradual transitions between controlled and spontaneous ventilation using pressure support ventilation.

The development of noncardiogenic pulmonary edema after cardiac surgery is well documented although relatively uncommon. There are a number of possible causes for developing adult respiratory distress syndrome (ARDS) after CPB, including activation of complement and other immune system activation, protamine reactions, allergic reactions to other drugs, leukoagglutinin reactions with transfusion of blood products, splanchnic ischemia, pancreatitis, and sepsis.[94] Management in this setting is similar to management of ARDS in other settings (see Chaps. 127 and 128). The hemodynamic effects of PEEP may be accentuated in these patients particularly those with right heart failure, and circumstances may dictate a lower level of PEEP at the expense of a higher concentration of inspired oxygen.

The reported incidence of phrenic nerve injury varies greatly after cardiac surgery. The phrenic nerve can be injured both transiently and permanently at a number of points as it traverses the thoracic cavity. Injury may occur from topical cooling of the heart transmitted through pericardium,[95] from dissection of either IMA at the base of the pedicle,[96] or from transection of the nerve when dissecting in a reoperation or during thoracic aortic surgery. Injury to the intercostal nerves may also occur as the result of chest retraction. Presence of either or both of these nerve injuries can diminish the strength of respiratory efforts and contribute to postoperative ventilator dependency in the patient with borderline preoperative pulmonary function. Many cases of unilateral phrenic nerve injury result only in mild decrease in VC, left lower lobe atelectasis, or immobility of the left hemidiaphragm and are thus clinically silent, not affecting postoperative recovery. Diaphragmatic paralysis is uncommon, and the incidence appears to be maximal in the early postoperative period, resolving in some patients in a week, but persisting for as long as 70 weeks in others.[96] Diaphragmatic paralysis is suspected if there is tachypnea with paradoxical abdominal motion early during weaning efforts, lower than expected VC, or elevation of one hemidaphragm on postoperative chest x-ray. A marked difference between supine and sitting respiratory mechanics (tidal volume, forced VC, and negative inspiratory force) or failure of the diaphragm to move on fluoroscopic examination ("sniff test") or ultrasonic examination confirms the diagnosis. Electrophysiologic evaluation of the phrenic nerves has been studied,[96] but we rarely find it necessary or helpful in making the diagnosis. Our management approach to diaphragmatic paralysis is to provide full ventilatory support to the patient, supply adequate nutrition, and gradually begin weaning from the respirator by increasing daily increments of time on "flow-by," CPAP, or CPAP with pressure support. Weaning is best attempted when the patient is out of bed sitting in a chair or upright in bed. The patient is rested upon demonstrating signs of inspiratory muscle fatigue,[97] and the patient is usually rested between trials and overnight on full ventilatory support. The duration of the weaning interval or the respiratory workload is gradually increased as the patient tolerates, with arbitrary limits set on the patient's respiratory rate to avoid excessive fatigue. The amount of pressure support is gradually withdrawn and the amount of time extended until the patient can tolerate a full day on T piece or tracheostomy collar. Nighttime ventilation is continued to allow adequate rest, until the patient demonstrates sufficient reserve to breathe independently "round-the-clock." When the patient can breathe on his or her own for 6 h or more, a fenestrated tracheostomy tube is placed to allow communication and use of the upper airway during the day, and full ventilatory support (with sedation as needed) to secure a good night's sleep, while resting the diaphragm completely. At

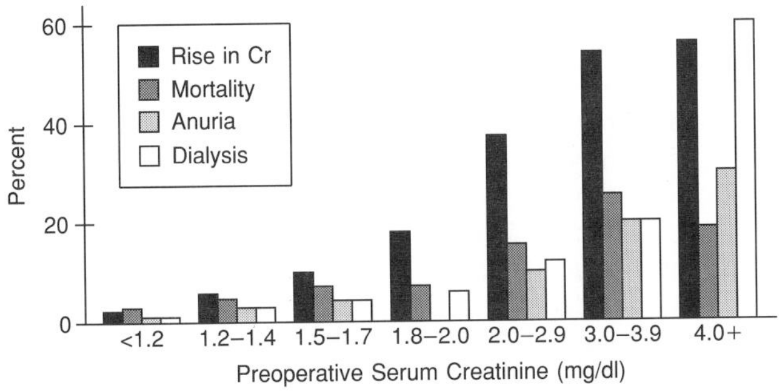

FIGURE 87-1 Renal system complications after CABG. (From Cleveland Clinic Foundation, 1986–1988 (n = 4351).)

this stage, patients may be transferred to a regular nursing floor for the final weeks of rehabilitation, and most are discharged ventilator free, with the tracheostomy tube removed.

RENAL FAILURE

Renal failure after open heart surgery is a serious problem with oliguric failure or anuria reported in 0.7 to 4.3 percent, and an increase in serum creatinine concentration in 2 to 30 percent.[98,99] The incidence of creatinine elevation, anuria, need for dialysis, and complications including mortality, rises when preoperative serum creatinine is >1.7 mg/dL.[100] Mortality in those developing anuric or oliguric renal failure ranged up to 82 percent in older reports, but some evidence indicates that early dialysis may reduce this rate substantially. Since the occurrence of oliguric renal failure with fluid overload also commonly precipitates respiratory failure, there has been a trend toward early application of continuous arteriovenous hemofiltration (CAVH) to remove excess fluid and decrease catecholamines.[101]

A number of univariate risk factors for postoperative renal failure have been identified, including low cardiac output at the end of CPB, age, preoperative elevation of creatinine (Fig. 87-1), preoperative cardiac failure, need for postoperative circulatory support, blood transfusion, and time on bypass.[102] While patients at risk for postoperative renal failure can be identified, evidence is lacking for maneuvers to prevent occurrence of renal failure. Careful attention should be paid to urine output during the procedure, particularly during the CPB. Most centers use mannitol as part of the pump prime, and many clinicians advocate treating those at risk with low dose dopamine (0.5 to 3.0 μg/kg/min). Although there is no prospective study to support this prophylactic use, dopamine has been shown to produce functional improvement in the setting of acute oliguria after CPB.[103] Dopamine has also been shown to preferentially increase renal blood flow in the setting of α-adrenergic drug use, and we routinely add low dose dopamine whenever using norepinephrine.

When renal failure occurs, it generally follows one of the three well-defined patterns.[104] The first pattern, *abbreviated acute renal failure,* occurs after an isolated insult at the time of surgery, results in a peak in serum creatinine level around the fourth postoperative day and prompt recovery if no other events occur. In the second pattern, *overt renal failure,* the acute insult is accompanied by prolonged circulatory failure (pressor use, IABP support), and runs a longer course, with recovery typically occurring in the second or third week after injury, accompanied by improvement of other organ systems. The final pattern, *protracted acute renal failure,* begins like the second, but as recovery occurs, a second insult (sepsis, massive gastrointestinal bleeding, MI) occurs, and permanent failure may result. This pattern is typically accompanied by development of MSOF or ARDS.

Oliguria may ensue from prerenal causes, parenchymal renal damage, or postrenal obstruction. Appropriate diagnostic measures include fluid challenge, monitoring cardiac output and intravascular pressures, and bladder catheterization. In the setting of low cardiac output, compensatory vasoconstriction may occur, resulting in prerenal azotemia. Initial treatment includes volume expansion, afterload reduction, and augmentation of cardiac output to preserve renal blood flow and prevent progression to renal failure. Direct renal parenchymal damage may occur from hemoglobin, myoglobin, or intravenous contrast dye, and alkalinization of the urine may limit renal tubular damage in this setting. Obstructive renal failure is rare in the open heart population after operation, but a renal flow scan or ultrasound can help differentiate between parenchymal and obstructive failure. Once the etiology has been established and corrective measures taken, an aggressive therapeutic approach is needed. Adequate cardiac output should be assured and renal blood flow further increased with dopamine. Diuretics may not modify the course of renal failure, but do assist in fluid management and may delay the urgency of dialysis from the standpoint of fluid overload. Our current practice is to start CAVH or hemodialysis (CAVHD) early, to control fluid balance and electrolytes, and to allow provision of adequate volumes of total parenteral nutrition to meet caloric needs. We suspect, although proof is lacking, that early supportive therapy speeds the return of spontaneous renal function, and anecdotally several patients treated with dialysis or ultrafiltration for anuria have recovered most or all of their renal function.

INFECTIOUS COMPLICATIONS

Pneumonia, sepsis, wound infections, mediastinitis, and urinary tract infections are frequent complications after open heart surgery. The organisms seen in this population are influenced by the type of antibiotic prophylaxis chosen and the portal of entry. While prevailing opinion is that a single dose of cefazolin or vancomycin should suffice for prosthetic valve and other open heart surgery, cefamandole and cefuroxime are reportedly associated with fewer wound infections than cefazolin.[105] Since antibiotic prophylaxis is usually in the form of a broad-spectrum penicillin or cephalosporin, superinfections are frequently with resistant organisms such as *Pseudomonas aeruginosa, Klebsiella, Serratia,* and *Providencia.* Treatment of the first round of infection, usually with a penicillinase-resistant penicillin and aminoglycoside, in the complicated patient, is commonly followed by a second round of infection with more unusual organisms—commonly yeast (*Candida albicans* and others).

Sternal wound infections occur in about 1 percent of patients undergoing median sternotomy.[106,107] Predisposing factors for wound complications after open heart surgery include diabetes, low cardiac output, use of bilateral IMA grafts, and reoperation for excessive postoperative bleeding. Special attention should be paid to the possibility of mediastinitis, particularly in the patient who is a week or more postoperative and has suffered multiple complications during the ICU stay. Mediastinal infection may be manifest by unexplained fever, failure to wean from the ventilator, or an unstable sternum. Confirmation is often difficult, since bone scanning will often be positive with a healing sternum, and surgical exploration and drainage of the wound may be necessary to obtain adequate culture material. Risk factors for suppurative mediastinitis include chronic obstructive pulmonary disease (COPD), repeat operation, pyuria, low ejection fraction, high LV end-distolic pressure, valve or aortic aneurysm repair, prolonged bypass time or return to bypass, prolonged surgery, surgical reexploration, CPR, or mechanical ventilation for longer than 48 h.[108]

GASTROINTESTINAL PROBLEMS

Gastrointestinal complications after CPB occur at a low frequency (1 to 2 percent) but are associated with high mortality.[109] The most frequently encountered complications are postoperative ileus and upper gastrointestinal bleeding. Pancreatitis, cholecystitis, hyperbilirubinemia, bowel perforations, and infarctions are also seen, particularly in high-risk patients. Risk factors for gastrointestinal complications include prolonged bypass time, concurrent renal failure, and length of ventilatory support. The incidence of gastrointestinal bleeding can be minimized by antacid therapy, antihistamine therapy, or barrier protection agents, but evidence is accumulating to suggest that barrier protectors such as sucralfate are associated with lower incidence of nosocomial pneumonia than H_2 blockers.

Jaundice occurs in approximately 20 percent of patients undergoing CPB and is a risk factor for subsequent mortality.[110] While jaundice after CPB is associated with multiple valve replacement, higher transfusion requirements, and longer times on CPB, it also occurs after uncomplicated operations, and may be related to a defect in hepatic excretion of bilirubin.[111]

Acute pancreatitis occurs rarely after bypass but also carries with it a poor prognosis. It is often seen in the setting of MSOF. Although the clinical incidence of pancreatitis by enzyme evidence is <2 percent, evidence of pancreatitis is found on autopsy in up to 25 percent of patients dying after open heart surgery.[112] Several patterns of severe pancreatic injury occur, including acute fulminating pancreatitis leading to death, less severe pancreatitis with abscess formation, and mild chemical pancreatitis manifest by elevations of amylase and lipase without clinical sequelae.[113] Transient elevations of amylase may occur after cardiac surgery unrelated to pancreatic injury, making serum lipase a useful addition to make the diagnosis.

A pattern of mesenteric ischemia can evolve in the early postoperative period related to low perfusion or embolization of atheroma from aortic manipulation. These patients may have marked lactic acidosis and a low SVR. The pattern frequently resolves during the first 10 to 12 h in the ICU but can progress to mesenteric infarction.

The gastroepiploic artery is occasionally used as a conduit for revascularization. These patients appear to be prone to development of postoperative ileus, and we routinely leave an orogastric or nasogastric tube in place until bowel activity is assured.

Risk Factors Predicting Morbidity and Mortality

In our discussions above, we have considered individual complications and the risk factors that predispose to their occurrence. A number of multivariate analyses have delineated risk factors for mortality after open heart surgery. Factors commonly cited as risks for operative mortality following CABG include advanced age, female gender, congestive heart failure, LV dysfunction, left main coronary disease, emergency operation, and reoperation.[2,3,114,115] Factors predisposing to morbidity and mortality after valve surgery include advanced age, endocarditis, female gender, impaired LV function, concurrent ischemic disease, mitral regurgitant lesions, the need for tricuspid annuloplasty, previous operation, diabetes, and ascites.[116] At present, there is no simple, widely accepted method of risk stratification of patients that takes into account the relative importance of each of the factors shown to be significant in influencing outcome. The ability to generate a numerical score, either preoperatively or on ICU admission, would be helpful in assessing quality of care and in focusing attention on patients most likely to have stormy postoperative courses. A three-level (normal, increased, or high-risk) scoring system was developed at the Montreal Heart Institute,[117] but has not become widely utilized. APACHE-II, in common use for noncardiac ICU patients, generates a score between 0 and 71 based on the degree of a patient's physiologic derangement.[118] Since many of these factors (temperature, heart rate, arterial and central venous pressures, arterial pH, electrolytes, hematocrit) are deliberately controlled in the cardiac patient, and the degree of physiologic derangement is rapidly reversible, application of the unmodified APACHE-II score to open heart surgery patients may be relatively insensitive and may overestimate risk of death, although this has not been formally evaluated. The methodology currently in use by the Health Care Financing Administration (HCFA) to adjust reporting data has been criticized as lacking sufficient sensitivity to allow valid inferences about quality of care.[119]

A severity scoring system, based on multivariate analysis of factors contributing to morbidity and mortality after open heart surgery, has been developed at our institution. In the initial version, a score was generated on ICU arrival.[14] The sensitivity and specificity of this system by ROC

TABLE 87-4 Points Assigned for Preoperative Factors

Emergency case	5	COPD or prior lung surgery	2
LV dysfunction	3	Prior vascular surgery	2
psCr > 2.0 mg/dL	4	Mitral insufficiency	2
psCr 1.8–1.9 mg/dL	2	Mitral stenosis	1
psCr 1.6–1.7 mg/dL	1	Aortic insufficiency	1
pHct < 34%	2	Aortic stenosis	1
Age < 75 years	2	History of MI and congestive heart failure	1
Age 65–74 years	1	Female gender	1
Prior heart surgery	2	Diabetes mellitus	1
Weight <65 kg	1		

Scoring system for patients undergoing CABG. Relationship of total score to outcome is displayed in Fig. 87-2.

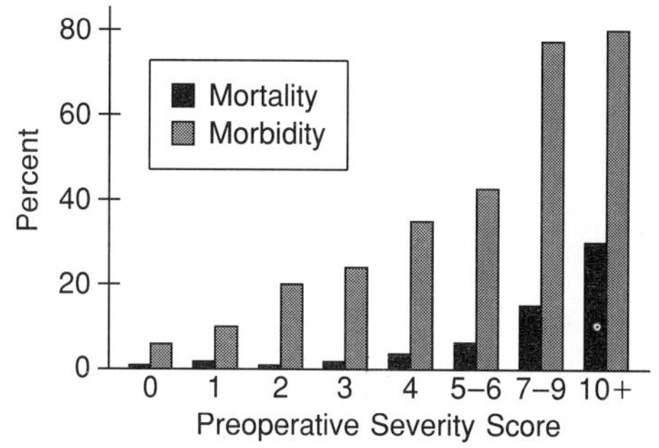

FIGURE 87-2 Morbidity and mortality by preoperative severity score; 5033 patients undergoing CABG. Morbidity and mortality increase with higher severity scores, calculated by adding point values from Table 87-4. Morbidity includes: stroke, ventilation >72 h, renal failure, serious infection, low cardiac output for >4 h, or death. (From Cleveland Clinic Foundation, 1986–1988.)

analysis is similar to that reported for APACHE-II for its population[118] and superior to the HCFA method.[119] A revised model based entirely on preoperative factors is under development.[120] The revised scoring system assigns points for emergency operation, LV dysfunction, preoperative renal failure, preoperative anemia, age over 65, repeat cardiac procedure, weight <65 k, COPD, prior vascular surgery, valvular heart disease, congestive heart failure in presence of prior MI, diabetes mellitus, and female gender (Table 87-4). Patients with no risk factors have an expected mortality rate of <1 percent, while those with multiple factors have a predicted mortality rate of >20 percent (Fig. 87-2). Application of this system will require prospective validation at a variety of institutions to ensure general applicability. We expect that some method of severity scoring will become increasingly important in assessing quality of care, for research, and possibly for realistic preoperative estimates of risk and benefit of surgical versus alternative therapies.

CASE PRESENTATION

A 77-year-old man was admitted with increasing fatigue and pedal edema. Past medical history included mitral valve prolapse, streptococcal endocarditis treated 12 years prior to admission, paroxysmal tachydysrhythmias, hypertension, and recurrent ureteral calculi. Medications at the time of admission were 80 mg propanolol every day, 5 mg zaroxolyn twice daily, 400 mg tocanide three times daily, 0.25 mg digoxin every day, 20 mg furosemide daily, and potassium supplements. The patient was allergic to procainamide and quinidine. Physical examination was remarkable for a grade III/VI midsystolic decrescendo murmur at the left lower sternal border. Echocardiographic examination disclosed mild left atrial enlargement, mildly dilated LV with normal systolic function, bileaflet mitral valve prolapse with 3+ mitral regurgitation and mild mitral annular calcification, and trivial aortic regurgitation. Cardiac catheterization confirmed 3+ mitral regurgitation with prolapse and disclosed presence of a 90 percent diagonal coronary artery lesion, and 40 percent stenosis of the circumflex and posterior descending arteries. LV function was reported as normal. Preoperative BUN level was 34 mg/dL and creatinine content 1.5 mg/dL. The creatinine level rose to 1.8 mg/dL postcatheterization. Because of the perceived risk of renal failure resulting from the dye study, the patient was started on dopamine at 5 μg/kg/min on arrival in the operating room. Anesthesia was then induced with fentanyl and pancuronium, and a stable blood pressure was maintained until onset of CPB. Crystalloid cardioplegia was used, and the mitral lesion was repaired with shortening of the chordae tendineae and quadrilateral resection of the posterior leaflet, mitral annuloplasty, and debridement of the posterior mitral annulus. Total pump time was 1 h and 13 min. The patient was initially stable in the ICU but returned to the operating room for control of bleeding from the atrial cannulation site 4.5 h after arrival. Ventricular dysrhythmias were noted in the early postoperative period, and the patient was slow to awaken. Urine output during the first 48 h was consistently less than intake from vasoactive drugs and medications. The patient awoke on the second postoperative day confused and extubated himself but required immediate reintubation. On reintubation, ranitidine was started as prophylaxis against stress ulceration. Accelerated ventricular rate resulting from atrial fibrillation was successfully treated with digoxin after repeated attempts to convert to sinus by DC cardioversion were unsuccessful. On the seventh postoperative day, a new cardiac murmur was noted on examination and repeat echocardiogram showed a normal repaired mitral valve. Sputum had become thick and yellow, and a fever to 38°C (100.4°F) had developed. The patient was empirically started on ceftazidime for suspected *Klebsiella* pneumonia based on sputum Gram stain findings. On the eighth postoperative day, *Enterobacter* was identified from the sputum and the antibiotic was switched to imipenem based on sensitivity results. On the tenth postoperative day, the patient developed melanotic stools with a fall in hematocrit from 35 to 24 percent. Emergency endoscopy was carried out, and three fresh ulcers were seen in the duodenal bulb although active bleeding had stopped. Two days later, an enteral feeding tube was inserted for nutrition and potentially additional protection against further gastrointestinal bleeding. On the next day, further upper gastrointestinal bleeding occurred requiring endoscopic coagulation of a proximal duodenal ulcer. During the next month, the patient was unable to wean from mechanical ventilation due to poor respiratory mechanics: tidal volume and VC were both low (<200 mL), maximal inspiratory pressure was <24 cmH_2O, and the patient was unable to cooperate with respiratory care. A trial of spontaneous respiration CPAP resulted in respiratory rates of 40 breaths/min even with addition of 8 cm pressure support. Supine and sitting tidal volumes differed by 150 mL; however, fluoroscopy failed to confirm presence of diaphragmatic weakness. The respiratory muscle weakness was attributed to nutritional status. Three weeks postoperatively, tracheal secretions were cultured and revealed *P. aeruginosa* despite the continuing imipenem therapy. Antibiotics were changed to gentamicin, piperacillin, and vancomycin, and the imipenem was discontinued. Fever persisted despite antibiotic therapy. The patient's mental status was noted to worsen late in the day with frank psychosis requiring haloperidol to control agitation on several nights. The patient was started on 25 mg amitriptyline at bedtime for improved nighttime sleep and to relieve chronic depression; marked improvement in mental status was noted after the third night of uninterrupted sleep. The patient began to make progress in weaning from mechanical ventilation. BUN and creatinine values fell to 48 and 1.0, respectively, and the patient was ultimately weaned from mechanical ventilation via pressure support and then on/off trials, and discharged from the hospital.

CASE DISCUSSION

This case illustrates the effect of a preoperative event (rise in creatinine following dye studies) on the need for postoperative care. Despite "prophylactic" use of dopamine in the operating room, postoperative azotemia and oliguria developed. Maintenance of continued urine output, however, was essential in making progress with weaning from mechanical ventilation. Though it is difficult to prove that such prophylactic therapy affects outcome, it is clear the patients who develop full-fledged oliguric renal failure have a worse outcome than those with simply oliguria or a rise in creatinine concentration. Understanding the potential for bleeding from the atrial cannulation site was important in the decision to return the patient to the operating room for control of bleeding in the first 5 h after arrival. Knowledge of the prolonged pump run, with its concomitant risk of later gastrointestinal bleeding, contributed to the decision to start prophylactic ranitidine on the second day of mechanical ventilation. Despite this, the patient still suffered a late complication: gastrointestinal bleeding. (Current practice would be to use sucralfate rather than ranitidine in view of recent evidence that the nosocomial infection rate is increased with H_2 blockers.) The multiple complications in this patient required vigorous follow-up and correction as each occurred. This is typical of the complicated postoperative patient and several of the diagnostic and therapeutic choices involved decisions that require balancing immediate concerns against potential long-term problems (i.e., nephrotoxic antibiotic use to treat an active infection despite compromised renal function). Balancing conflicting priorities is an important part of critical care in general, and particularly in the patient with multisystem failure.

References

1. Naunheim KS, Fiore AC, Wadley JJ, et al: The changing profile of the patient undergoing coronary artery bypass surgery. J Am Coll Cardiol 11:494, 1988.
2. Kennedy JW, Kaiser GC, Fisher LD, et al: Multivariate discriminant analysis of the clinical and angiographic predictors of operative mortality from the Collaborative Study in Coronary Artery Surgery (CASS). J Thorac Cardiovasc Surg 80:876, 1980.
3. Cosgrove DM, Loop FD, Lytle BW, et al: Primary myocardial revascularization. J Thorac Cardiovasc Surg 88:673, 1984.
4. Higgins TL, Estafanous FG, Loop FD, Blum JM: A severity score for cardiac surgery patients. Crit Care Med 17:S39, 1989.
5. Kaplan JA, Wells PH: Early diagnosis of myocardial ischemia using the pulmonary arterial catheter. Anesth Analg 60:789, 1981.
6. Tuman KJ, McCarthy RJ, Spiess BD: Effect of pulmonary artery catheterization on outcome in patients undergoing coronary artery surgery. Anesthesiology 70:199, 1989.
7. Rao TLK, Jacobs KH, El-Etr AA: Reinfarction following anesthesia in patients with myocardial infarction. Anesthesiology 59:499, 1983.
8. Smith JS, Cahalan MK, Benefiel DJ: Intraoperative detection of myocardial ischemia in high-risk patients: Electrocardiography versus two-dimensional transesophageal echocardiography. Circulation 72:1015, 1985.
9. Slogoff S, Keats AS: Does perioperative myocardial ischemia lead to postoperative myocardial infarction? Anesthesiology 62:107, 1985.
10. Tuman KJ, McCarthy RJ: Does choice of anesthetic agent significantly affect outcome after coronary artery surgery? Anesthesiology 70:189, 1989.
11. Slogoff S, Keats AS: Randomized trial of primary anesthetic agents on outcome of coronary artery bypass operations. Anesthesiology 70:179, 1989.
12. Jackson JM, Thomas SJ, Lowenstein E: Anesthetic management of patients with valvular heart disease. Semin Anesth 1(3): 1982.
13. Hine I, Wood W, Mainwaring-Burton R, et al: The adrenergic response to surgery involving cardiopulmonary bypass, as measured by plasma and urinary catecholamine concentrations. Br J Anaesth 48:355, 1976.
14. Kirklin JK, Westaby S, Blackstone EH, et al: Complement and the damaging effects of cardiopulmonary bypass. J Thorac Cardiovasc Surg 86:845, 1983.
15. Kirklin JK: The postperfusion syndrome: Inflammation and the damaging effects of cardiopulmonary bypass, in Tinker JH (ed): *Cardiopulmonary Bypass: Current Concepts and Controversies*. Philadelphia, Saunders, 1989, pp 131–146.

16. Westaby S: Organ dysfunction after cardiopulmonary bypass. A systemic inflammatory reaction initiated by the extracorporeal circuit. Intensive Care Med 13:89, 1987.
17. Murkin JM, Farrar JK, Tweed WA, et al: Cerebral autoregulation and flow/metabolism coupling during cardiopulmonary bypass: The influence of PaC_{O_2}. Anesth Analg 66:825, 1987.
18. Esposito RA, Culliford AT, Colvin SB, et al: The role of the activated clotting time in heparin administration and neutralization for cardiopulmonary bypass. J Thorac Cardiovasc Surg 85:174, 1983.
19. Govier AV: Central nervous system complications after cardiopulmonary bypass, in Tinker JH (ed): *Cardiopulmonary Bypass: Current Concepts and Controversies.* Philadelphia, Saunders, 1989, pp 41–68.
20. Buckberg GD: Strategies and logic of cardioplegic delivery to prevent, avoid, and reverse ischemic and reperfusion damage. J Thorac Cardiovasc Surg 93:127, 1987.
21. Coyle JP, Kamath G, Licina MG, Higgins TL: Factors affecting magnesium levels after cardiac surgery. Anesthesiology 71:A192, 1989.
22. Buckberg GD: A proposed "solution" to the cardioplegic controversy. J Thorac Cardiovasc Surg 77:803, 1979.
23. Kirklin JW, Conti VR, Blackstone EH: Prevention of myocardial damage during cardiac operations. N Engl J Med 301:3, 135, 1979.
24. Buckberg GD: Recent progress in myocardial protection during cardiac operations. Cardiovasc Clin 17(3):291, 1987.
25. Hickey PR, Andersen NP: Deep hypothermic circulatory arrest: A review of pathophysiology and clinical experience as a basis for anesthetic management. J Cardiothorac Anesth 1(2):137, 1987.
26. Shenaq SA, Yawn DH, Saleem A, et al: Effect of profound hypothermia on leukocytes and platelets. Ann Clin Lab Sci 16(2):130, 1986.
27. Moyers JR, Tinker JH: Emergence from cardiopulmonary bypass: Controversies about physiology and pharmacology, in Tinker JH (ed): *Cardiopulmonary Bypass: Current Concepts and Controversies.* Philadelphia, Saunders, 1989, pp 109–129.
28. Baerman JM, Kirsh MM, deBuitleir M, et al: Natural history and determinants of conduction defects following coronary artery bypass surgery. Ann Thorac Surg 44:150, 1987.
29. Maccioli GA, Lucas WJ, Norfleet EA: The intra-aortic balloon pump: A review. J Cardiothorac Anesth 2(3):365, 1988.
30. Goenen M, Pedemonte O, Baele P, Col J: Amrinone in the management of low cardiac output after open heart surgery. Am J Cardiol 56:33B, 1985.
31. Colucci WS, Wright RF, Braunwald E: New positive inotropic agents in the treatment of congestive heart failure. N Engl J Med 314:290, 1986.
32. Coleman GM, Gradinac S, Taegtmeyer H, et al: Efficacy of metabolic support with glucose-insulin-potassium for left ventricular pump failure after aortocoronary bypass surgery. Circulation 80(3):I-91–96, 1989.
33. Schoen FJ, Palmer DC, Bernhard WF, et al: Clinical temporary ventricular assist. J Thorac Cardiovasc Surg 92:1071, 1986.
34. Eide TR, Katz RJ, Poppers PJ: The effect of sublingual nifedipine on coronary venous graft resistance immediately following cardiopulmonary bypass. Anesth Analg 68:462, 1989.
35. Jett GK, Arcidi JM, Dorsey LMA, et al: Vasoactive drug effects on blood flow in internal mammary artery and saphenous vein grafts. J Thorac Cardiovasc Surg 94:2, 1987.
36. Fisk RL, Guilbeau EJ: Perioperative right heart failure: Etiology and pathophysiology. Cardiovasc Clin 17:219, 1987.
37. Coyle JP, Carlin HM, Lake CR, et al: Left atrial infusion of norepinephrine in the management of right ventricular failure. J Cardiothorac Anesth 4(1):80, 1990.
38. D'Ambra MN, LaRaia PJ, Philbin DM, et al: Prostaglandin E_1—A new therapy for refractory right heart failure and pulmonary hypertension after mitral valve replacement. J Thorac Cardiovasc Surg 89:567, 1985.
39. Dembitsky WP, Daily PO, Raney AA, et al: Temporary extracorporeal support of the right ventricle. J Thorac Cardiovasc Surg 91:518, 1986.
40. Horrow JC: Protamine: A review of its toxicity. Anesth Analg 64:348, 1985.
41. Weiss ME, Nyhan D, Peng Z, et al: Association of protamine IgE and IgG antibodies with life-threatening reactions to intravenous protamine. N Engl J Med 320:886, 1989.
42. Bick RL: Hemostasis defects associated with cardiac surgery, prosthetic devices, and other extracorporeal circuits. Semin Thromb Hemost 11:249, 1985.
43. Salzman ED, Weinstein MJ, Weintraub RM, et al: Treatment with desmopressin acetate to reduce blood loss after cardiac surgery: A double-blind randomized trial. N Engl J Med 314(22):1402, 1986.
44. Del Rossi NJ, Cernaianu AC, Botros S, et al: Prophylactic treatment of postperfusion bleeding using EACA. Chest 96:27, 1989.
45. Bazaral MG, Petre J, Cosgrove D, Estafanous FG: Operating room design at the Cleveland Clinic Foundation. Cleve Clin J Med 55:267, 1988.
46. Young JA, Kisker CT, Doty DB: Adequate anticoagulation during cardiopulmonary bypass determined by activated clotting time and the appearance of fibrin monomer. Ann Thorac Surg 26(3):231, 1978.
47. Spiess BD, Tuman KJ, McCarthy RJ, et al: Thromboelastography as an indicator of post-cardiopulmonary bypass coagulopathies. J Clin Monit 3:25, 1987.
48. D'Alauro FS, Johns RA: Hypotension related to desmopressin administration following cardiopulmonary bypass. Anesthesiology 69:962, 1988.
49. Harker LA, Malpass TW, Branson HE, et al: Mechanism of abnormal bleeding in patients undergoing cardiopulmonary bypass: Acquired transient platelet dysfunction associated with selective-granule release. Blood 56(5):824, 1980.
50. Zurick AM, Urzua J, Ghattas M, et al: Failure of positive end-expiratory pressure to decrease postoperative bleeding after cardiac surgery. Ann Thorac Surg 34(6):608, 1982.
51. Cosgrove DM, Amiot DM, Meserko JJ: An improved technique for autotransfusion of shed mediastinal blood. Ann Thorac Surg 40(5):519, 1985.
52. Griffith LE, Billman GF, Daily PO, Lane TA: Apparent coagulopathy caused by infusion of shed mediastinal blood and its prevention by washing of the infusate. Ann Thorac Surg 47:400, 1989.
53. Orr MD, Riester DE: Complement activation in shed blood release of C3a and C5a. Anesthesiology 71:A552, 1988.
54. Michelson EL, Torosian M, Morganroth J, MacVaugh H: Early recognition of surgically correctable causes of excessive mediastinal bleeding after coronary artery bypass graft surgery. Am J Surg 139:313, 1980.
55. Talamonti MS, LoCicero J, Hoyne WP, et al: Early reexploration for excessive postoperative bleeding lowers wound complication rates in open heart surgery. Am Surg 2:102, 1987.
56. Westphal LM, Cheng EY, White PF, et al: Use of midazolam infusion for sedation following cardiac surgery. Anesthesiology 67:257, 1987.
57. Grounds RM, Lalor JM, Lumley J, et al: Propofol infusion for

sedation in the intensive care unit: Preliminary report. Br Med J 294:(6569):397, 1987.
58. Caspi J, Klausner JM, Safadi T, et al: Delayed respiratory depression following fentanyl anesthesia for cardiac surgery. Crit Care Med 16(3):238, 1988.
59. Sladen RN: Temperature and ventilation after hypothermic cardiopulmonary bypass. Anesth Analg 64:816, 1985.
60. Burks LC, Aisner J, Fortner CL, Wiernik PH: Meperidine for the treatment of shaking chills and fever. Arch Intern Med 140:483, 1980.
61. Estafanous FG, Urzua J, Yared JP, et al: Pattern of hemodynamic alterations during coronary artery operations. J Thorac Cardiovasc Surg 87:175, 1984.
62. Urzua J, Zurick AM, Starr NJ, et al: Enhanced cardiac performance following cardiopulmonary bypass. J Cardiovasc Surg 26:53, 1985.
63. Kumon K, Tanaka K, Hirata T, et al: Organ failures due to low cardiac output syndrome following open heart surgery. Jpn Circ J 50:329, 1986.
64. White HD, Antman EM, Glynn MA, et al: Efficacy and safety of timolol for prevention of supraventricular tachyarrhythmias after coronary artery bypass surgery. Circulation 70:479, 1984.
65. Gray RJ, Bateman TM, Czer LSC, et al: Esmolol: A new ultrashort acting beta adrenergic blocking agent for rapid control of heart rate in postoperative supraventricular tachyarrhythmias. J Am Coll Cardiol 5:1451, 1985.
66. Haft JI, Habbab MA: Treatment of atrial arrhythmias: Effectiveness of verapamil when preceded by calcium infusion. Arch Intern Med 146:1085, 1986.
67. Rettig SSG, Frohlig G, Doenecke P, et al: Sustained atrial flutter after cardiac surgery: Successful termination by rapid atrial pacing. Thorac Cardiovasc Surg 32:41, 1984.
68. Harris MNE, Crowther A, Jupp RA, Aps C: Magnesium and coronary revascularization. Br J Anaesth 60:779, 1988.
69. Weeks KR, Chatterjee K, Block S, et al: Bedside hemodynamic monitoring. J Thorac Cardiovasc Surg 71:250, 1976.
70. Bateman T, Gray R, Chaux A, et al: Right atrial tamponade complicating cardiac operation. J Thorac Cardiovasc Surg 84:413, 1982.
71. Lemaire F, Teboul J-L, Cinotti L, et al: Acute left ventricular dysfunction during unsuccessful weaning from mechanical ventilation. Anesthesiology 69:171, 1988.
72. Olsen KH, Kluger J, Fieldman A: Combination high dose amrinone and dopamine in the management of moribund cardiogenic shock after open heart surgery. Chest 94:503, 1988.
73. Rediker DE, Boucher CA, Block PC, et al: Degree of reversibility of left ventricular systolic dysfunction after aortic valve replacement for isolated aortic valve stenosis. Am J Cardiol 60:112, 1987.
74. Norman JC, Cooley DA, Igo SR, et al: Prognostic indices for survival during postcardiotomy intra-aortic balloon pumping. J Thorac Cardiovasc Surg 77:709, 1978.
75. Estafanous FG, Tarazi RC: Systemic arterial hypertension associated with cardiac surgery. Am J Cardiol 46:685, 1980.
76. Fouad FM, Estafanous FG, Bravo EL, et al: Possible role of cardioaortic reflexes in postcoronary bypass hypertension. Am J Cardiol 44:866, 1979.
77. Tarazi RC, Estafanous FG, Fouad FM: Unilateral stellate block in the treatment of hypertension after coronary bypass surgery. Am J Cardiol 42:1013, 1978.
78. James TN: A cardiogenic hypertensive chemoreflex. Anesth Analg 69:633, 1989.
79. Cruise CJ, Skrobik Y, Webster RA, et al: Intravenous labetalol versus sodium nitroprusside for treatment of hypertension postcoronary bypass surgery. Anesthesiology 71:835, 1989.
80. Breuer AC, Furlan AJ, Hanson MR, et al: Central nervous system complications of coronary artery bypass graft surgery: Prospective analysis of 421 patients. Stroke 14:682, 1983.
81. Reed GL, Singer DE, Picard EH: Stroke following coronary-artery bypass surgery. N Engl J Med 319:1246, 1988.
82. Slogoff S, Girgis KZ, Keats AS: Etiologic factors in neuropsychiatric complications associated with cardiopulmonary bypass. Anesth Analg 61:903, 1982.
83. Nussmeier NA, Arlund C, Slogoff S: Neuropsychiatric complications after cardiopulmonary bypass: Cerebral protection by a barbiturate. Anesthesiology 64:165, 1986.
84. Calabrese JR, Skwerer RG, Gulledge AD, et al: Incidence of postoperative delirium following myocardial revascularization. Cleve Clin J Med 54:29, 1987.
85. Svensson LG, Steward RW, Cosgrove DM, et al: Intrathecal papaverine for the prevention of paraplegia after operation on the thoracic or thoracoabdominal aorta. J Thorac Cardiovasc Surg 96:823, 1988.
86. Coyle JP, Steele J, Cutrone F, Higgins TL: Patient controlled analgesia after cardiac surgery. Anesth Analg 70:S1, 1990.
87. Matthay MA, Wiener-Kronish JP: Respiratory management after cardiac surgery. Chest 95:424, 1989.
88. Berrizbetia LD, Tessler S, Jacobowitz IJ, et al: Effect of sternotomy and coronary bypass surgery on postoperative pulmonary mechanics. Chest 96:873, 1989.
89. Higgins TL, Barrett C, Riden DJ, et al: Influence of pleural and mediastinal chest tubes on respiration following coronary artery bypass grafting (CABG). Chest 96:237S, 1989.
90. deLange S, Boscoe MJ, Stanley TH, Pace N: Comparison of sufentanil-O_2 and fentanyl-O_2 for coronary artery surgery. Anesthesiology 56:112, 1982.
91. Bentley JB, Borel JD, Nenad RE, Gillespie TJ: Age and fentanyl pharmacokinetics. Anesth Analg 61:968, 1982.
92. Roerig DL, Kotrly KJ, Ahlf SB, et al: Effect of propranolol on the first pass uptake of fentanyl in the human and rat lung. Anesthesiology 71:62, 1989.
93. Higgins TL, Kraenzler EJ, Blum JM: Evaluation of criteria for discontinuing mechanical ventilation following open heart surgery. Chest 94:40S, 1988.
94. Maggart M, Stewart S: The mechanisms and management of noncardiogenic pulmonary edema following cardiopulmonary bypass. Ann Thorac Surg 43:231, 1987.
95. Large SR, Heywood LJ, Flower CD, et al: Incidence and aetiology of a raised hemidiaphragm after cardiopulmonary bypass. Thorax 40:444, 1985.
96. Abd AG, Braun NMT, Baskin MI, et al: Diaphragmatic dysfunction after open heart surgery: Treatment with a rocking bed. Ann Intern Med 111:881, 1989.
97. Cohen CA, Zagelbaum G, Gross D, et al: Clinical manifestations of inspiratory muscle fatigue. Am J Med 73:308, 1982.
98. Bhat JG, Gluck MC, Lowenstein J, Baldwin DS: Renal failure after open heart surgery. Ann Intern Med 84:677, 1976.
99. Hilberman M, Myers BD, Carrie BJ, et al: Acute renal failure following cardiac surgery. J Thorac Cardiovasc Surg 77:880, 1979.
100. Higgins TL, Paganini EP, Noor FA, Blum J: Postoperative course of patients undergoing coronary artery bypass grafting (CABG) with elevated preoperative serum creatinine. Abstract presented at the Society of Cardiovascular Anesthesiologists Annual Meeting, 1990. Manuscript in preparation.
101. Coraim FJ, Coraim HP, Ebermann R, Stellwag FM: Acute respiratory failure after cardiac surgery: Clinical experience with

the application of continuous arteriovenous hemofiltration. Crit Care Med 14:714, 1986.
102. Koning HM, Koning AJ, Leusink JA: Serious acute renal failure following open heart surgery. Thorac Cardiovasc Surg 33:283, 1985.
103. Davis RF, Lappas DG, Kirklin JK, et al: Acute oliguria after cardiopulmonary bypass: Renal functional improvement with low-dose dopamine infusion. Crit Care Med 10:852, 1982.
104. Myers BD, Moran SM: Hemodynamically mediated acute renal failure. N Engl J Med 314:97, 1987.
105. Slama TG, Sklar SJ, Misinski J, Fess SW: Randomized comparison of cefamandole, cefazolin, and cefurozime prophylaxis in open-heart surgery. Antimicrob Agents Chemother 29:744, 1986.
106. Grossi EA, Culliford AT, Krieger KH, et al: A survey of 77 major infectious complications of median sternotomy: A review of 7,949 consecutive operative procedures. Ann Thorac Surg 40:214, 1985.
107. Sarr MG, Gott VL, Townsend TR: Mediastinal infection after cardiac surgery. Ann Thorac Surg 38:415, 1984.
108. Newman LS, Szczukowski LC, Bain RP, Perlino CA: Suppurative mediastinitis after open heart surgery. Chest 94:546, 1988.
109. Hanks JB, Curtis SE, Hanks BB, et al: Gastrointestinal complications after cardiopulmonary bypass. Surgery 92:394, 1982.
110. Sanderson RG, Ellison JH, Benson JA, Starr A: Jaundice following open-heart surgery. Ann Surg 165:217, 1967.
111. Collins JD, Ferner R, Murray A, Bassendine MF, et al: Incidence and prognostic importance of jaundice after cardiopulmonary bypass surgery. Lancet May 1119, 1983.
112. Haas GS, Warshaw AL, Daggett WM, Aretz HT: Acute pancreatitis after cardiopulmonary bypass. Am J Surg 149:508, 1985.
113. Rose DM, Ranson JHC, Cunningham JN, Spencer FC: Patterns of severe pancreatic injury. Ann Surg 199:168, 1984.
114. Pierpont GL, Kruse M, Ewald S, Wier K: Practical problems in assessing risk for coronary artery bypass grafting. J Thorac Cardiovasc Surg 89:673, 1985.
115. Foster ED, Fisher LD, Kaiser GC, et al: Comparison of operative mortality and morbidity for initial and repeat coronary artery bypass grafting: The coronary artery surgery study (CASS) registry experience. Ann Thorac Surg 38:563, 1984.
116. Lytle BW, Cosgrove DM, Taylor PC, et al: Reoperations for valve surgery: Perioperative mortality and determinants of risk for 1,000 patients, 1958–1984. Ann Thorac Surg 42:632, 1986.
117. Paiement B, Pelletier C, Dyrda I, et al: A simple classification of the risk in cardiac surgery. Can Anaesth Soc J 30:61, 1983.
118. Knaus WA, Draper E, Wagner DP, Zimmerman JE: APACHE II: A severity of disease classification system. Crit Care Med 13:818, 1985.
119. Green J, Wintfeld N, Sharkey P, Passman LJ: The importance of severity of illness in assessing hospital mortality. JAMA 263:241, 1990.
120. Higgins TL, Estafanous MD, Loop FD, et al: Stratification of risk with coronary artery bypass grafting (CABG). Abstract. 3d International Symposium on Anesthesia for Cardiac Patients.

Chapter 88

CRITICAL ILLNESS IN PREGNANCY

MARY E. STREK
JESSE HALL

KEY POINTS

- *Understanding the normal physiology of pregnancy is essential to evaluate cardiopulmonary function in the critically ill gravid woman.*
- *Pregnancy results in an increased cardiac output, which in late pregnancy may be diminished in the supine position by vena caval compression from the enlarged uterus.*
- *The decrease in functional residual capacity (FRC) and increase in oxygen consumption found in normal pregnancy put the pregnant woman at risk for hypoxemia during intubation and in the event of apnea.*
- *Hyperventilation during pregnancy results in a primary respiratory alkalosis and a compensatory metabolic acidosis with the following typical arterial blood-gas values:* $P_{O_2} >$ *100 mmHg,* P_{CO_2} *27 to 32 mmHg, and serum bicarbonate 18 to 21 meq/L.*
- *Fetal viability depends on adequate oxygen delivery. Due to the dilutional anemia of pregnancy, cardiac output becomes the critical determinant of fetal oxygen delivery and must be maintained.*
- *Hemorrhage in pregnancy may be massive and require extraordinary fluid resuscitation.*
- *Vasoactive drugs should be used with caution in the pregnant patient, since they may reduce uterine blood flow.*
- *Sodium nitroprusside should be used only for imminently life-threatening conditions, since cyanide toxicity may result in fetal injury or demise.*
- *Preeclampsia-eclampsia is a multisystem disorder manifest by hypertension, central nervous system dysfunction, coagulopathy, pulmonary edema, renal failure, and liver function abnormalities.*
- *Cardiopulmonary resuscitation must be modified in pregnancy and includes emergent cesarean section in selected patients.*
- *Pregnancy may represent a state of increased risk of pulmonary edemagenesis; acute hypoxemic respiratory failure is most often due to tocolytic therapy and usually resolves with supportive care.*
- *Successful management of critical illness in pregnancy requires continuous integration of the intensive care team with obstetric and neonatal consultants; mechanisms should exist for emergent involvement of the appropriate personnel.*

Pregnancy greatly complicates critical illness since assessment, monitoring, and treatment must take into account both maternal and fetal well-being. Knowledge of the normal changes in maternal respiratory, cardiac, and acid-base physiology in pregnancy is essential to distinguish between adaptive and pathologic changes.

This chapter begins with an overview of the changes in cardiovascular and respiratory physiology in normal pregnancy. Next, the determinants of fetal oxygen delivery are reviewed. The remainder of the chapter focuses on the disorders that can result in critical illness in pregnancy and the appropriate management of each. Finally, the importance of acid-base homeostasis, prophylaxis to prevent gastrointestinal bleeding, and early nutrition are discussed.

In many ways our understanding of the complex interaction between disease state and maternal/fetal physiology is incomplete. Thus, we rely on an approach that assumes that measures which optimize maternal well-being are usually most beneficial to the fetus as well. Nonetheless, throughout critical illness, monitoring and management decisions must take into account fetal as well as maternal parameters. This is best achieved by an expansion of the typical critical care team consisting of nurse, respiratory therapist, and intensivist to include obstetrician and neonatologist as well.

Cardiopulmonary Physiology of Pregnancy

ADAPTATION OF THE CIRCULATION

In pregnancy, numerous circulatory adjustments occur which ensure adequate oxygen delivery to the fetus (Table 88-1). Early in pregnancy maternal blood volume increases, reaching a level 40 percent above base line by the thirtieth week.[1] Blood volume expands in part from a 20 to 40 percent increase in the number of erythrocytes, but to a greater extent from a 40 to 50 percent increase in plasma volume, which results in a mild dilutional anemia.[1] The magnitude of the increase in blood volume is greater with multiple births. This extracellular volume expansion is associated with parallel decreases in colloid osmotic pressure and serum albumin concentration; both plateau at 26 weeks and then decline even further immediately postpartum.[2]

Coincident with the change in maternal blood volume is a 30 to 45 percent increase in cardiac output, the greatest part of which occurs in the first trimester.[2,3] The augmented cardiac output results from an increase in both stroke volume and heart rate, with heart rate reaching a maximum of 15 beats/min above resting nonpregnant levels.[2] Stroke volume rises, both from increased preload due to augmented venous return and decreased afterload due to a fall in systemic vascular resistance. The fall in systemic vascular resistance is attributed to increased synthesis of the vasodilator prostacyclin[2] and arteriovenous shunting to the placental bed. Since the left ventricular end-diastolic pressure remains normal,[1,2] despite a rise in left ventricular

TABLE 88-1 Circulatory Changes in Pregnancy

Parameter	Direction	Time Course
Heart rate	↑	1st and 2d trimesters
Blood pressure	↓	Falls in 1st and 2d trimesters, to return to base line in 3d trimester
Cardiac output	↑	Increases to as much as 40% above pre-pregnancy value by 20th wk
Stroke volume	↑	Increase peaks at 16–24 wk
Systemic vascular resistance (SVR)	↓	Reaches nadir by midpregnancy

TABLE 88-2 Typical Arterial Blood-Gas Values

	P_{O_2}	P_{CO_2}	pH	$(A-a)\ O_2$	S_{O_2}, %
Nonpregnant	98	40	7.40	2	98
Term pregnancy, seated	101	28	7.45	14	98
Term pregnancy, supine	95	28	7.45	20	97

$(A-a)\ O_2$ is the difference between the predicted alveolar P_{O_2} and the measured arterial P_{O_2}, assuming a respiratory quotient of 0.8. Normally this is <10 mmHg. S_{O_2} is the saturation of hemoglobin with oxygen.

SOURCE: Reprinted with permission from Schmidt GA, Hall JB: Pulmonary diseases in pregnancy, in Barron W, Lindheimer M (eds): *Medical Disorders during Pregnancy*. St. Louis, Mosby Yearbook, 1991.

end-diastolic volume,[1,3] ventricular diastolic compliance may be increased. At least one echocardiographic study has suggested that left ventricular performance improves during pregnancy.[1] The exact contributions of increased heart rate, loading conditions, and ventricular performance to the increase in flow are uncertain.

During the course of pregnancy, cardiac output becomes more dependent upon body position, since the gravid uterus can cause significant obstruction of the inferior vena cava with reduced venous return. This effect is most notable in the third trimester. Vena caval obstruction is maximal in the supine position and much less pronounced in the left lateral decubitus position.[1] During labor, uterine contraction can increase cardiac output 10 to 15 percent over resting pregnant levels, by increasing blood return from the contracting uterus.[2] This effect on cardiac output, however, may be tempered by blood loss during delivery.

Blood pressure decreases early in pregnancy, due to peripheral vasodilation perhaps mediated by increased synthesis of prostacyclin and progesterone. Maximal decrements in systolic and diastolic pressures average 5 to 9 and 6 to 17 mmHg, respectively, and occur at 16 to 28 weeks.[4] Blood pressure then increases gradually to return to prepregnancy levels shortly after delivery. A recent review of hypertension in pregnancy suggests that diastolic levels of 75 mmHg in the second and 85 mmHg in the third trimester should be considered the upper limits of normal.[4]

ADAPTATION OF THE RESPIRATORY SYSTEM

Oxygen consumption increases 20 to 30 percent in normal pregnancy;[5] during labor there is a further rise in oxygen consumption to levels 40 to 100 percent above the nonpregnant base line.[6] The increase in oxygen consumption occurs because of fetal and placental needs, as well as for maternal requirements resulting from increased cardiac output and work of breathing.[7] Maternal arterial P_{O_2} is marginally increased by virtue of augmented ventilation but does not contribute significantly to an increase in oxygen delivery. Nonetheless, mild hypoxemia can be induced in gravid patients by the supine position and the alveolar-to-arterial oxygen gradient is often slightly abnormal.[5] Because of this positional hypoxemia during pregnancy, arterial blood-gas samples should be obtained with the patient in the seated position.

Increased oxygen consumption is associated with increased carbon dioxide production, requiring greater alveolar ventilation. Alveolar ventilation, however, is increased above the level needed to eliminate carbon dioxide and P_{CO_2} falls to a partial pressure of 27 to 32 mmHg throughout pregnancy. The augmented alveolar ventilation is attributed to increased circulating progesterone and results from a substantial increase in tidal volume while respiratory rate remains unchanged.[5] Renal compensation, however, results in a maternal pH that is only slightly alkalemic, ranging between 7.40 and 7.45, with serum bicarbonate decreasing to 18 to 21 meq/L[5] (Table 88-2).

FRC and expiratory reserve volume (ERV) decrease about 20 percent during gestation because of increased abdominal pressure from the enlarged uterus which results in decreased chest wall recoil.[5] Conflicting data exist as to whether closing capacity (CC) is elevated in pregnancy. A few studies have documented an increase in the actual volume at which airway closure occurs, while others have shown no change in CC, only a decrease in the difference between FRC and CC due mainly to a decrease in FRC.[5] Nonetheless, the decreased FRC (and perhaps increased CC), when combined with the increased oxygen consumption found in pregnancy, leaves the pregnant woman (and her fetus) more vulnerable to hypoxia in the event of apnea. This is an important consideration during endotracheal intubation. Because inspiratory capacity (IC) actually increases, total lung capacity (TLC) is maintained.[8]

Despite increases in levels of many hormones known to affect smooth muscle, the function of large airways does not appear to be altered in pregnancy. Forced expiratory volume in 1 s (FEV_1), the ratio of FEV_1 to forced vital capacity (FVC), and specific airways conductance are unchanged during pregnancy. That flow volume loops are also unaffected by pregnancy is further evidence of normal airway function.[9]

FETAL OXYGEN DELIVERY

Oxygen delivery to the fetal tissues depends on the oxygen content of uterine artery blood as determined by maternal P_{O_2}, hemoglobin concentration and saturation, and uterine artery blood flow as determined by maternal cardiac output.[2] The small increases in arterial P_{O_2} attributable to hyperventilation have minimal effect on oxygen content since hemoglobin saturation is only marginally increased. The anemia of pregnancy, which reduces oxygen content by 20 to 25 percent, makes the critically ill pregnant patient more dependent than the nonpregnant individual on cardiac output for maintenance of oxygen delivery. Fetal death and congenital heart disease are increased in infants born to mothers with left ventricular outflow obstruction, which confirms the importance of maternal cardiac output in the outcome of the fetus.[2]

Fetal oxygen delivery can be decreased by uterine artery vasoconstriction. Maternal alkalosis can elicit uterine artery vasoconstriction.[2] This effect may be compounded by the resulting leftward shift of the maternal oxyhemoglobin saturation curve, which increases oxygen affinity thereby reducing P_{O_2} in the uterine vein and decreasing the gradient driving oxygen across the placenta. Exogenous or endogenous sympathetic stimulation and maternal hypotension also elicit uterine artery vasoconstriction.[2]

The uterine vasculature may be near maximally dilated under normal conditions and, therefore, unable to adapt to stress by further increases in flow by local vascular adjustment. This notion is supported by investigations in a gravid ewe model of progressive anemia where hematocrit was lowered from 31 to 8 percent. Augmentation of flow to either the uterine or placental beds did not occur, resulting in a progressive decline in oxygen delivery to the fetus.[10] This suggests that the uterine bed is not readily able to increase fetal oxygen delivery by vascular autoregulation.

Compensatory mechanisms do exist, however, to maintain fetal oxygen delivery. At all levels of P_{O_2}, fetal hemoglobin has a higher affinity for oxygen than maternal hemoglobin. Since the normal fetal umbilical vein P_{O_2} is 30 mmHg, aerobic metabolism normally takes place under relatively hypoxic conditions, and fetal tissue hypoxia does not occur until dramatic (by adult criteria) hypoxemia is present. In a primate model, brain injury did not occur until fetal P_{O_2} fell to 9 to 14 mmHg.[11] Protective mechanisms may also exist, at the level of the fetal circulation or peripheral tissues, in response to hypoxic stress. It is estimated that there is 40 mL of available oxygen in fetal blood and tissue stores at term and that oxygen consumption is 20 mL/min. Nonetheless, conditions such as total placental abruption or complete umbilical cord compression, which may completely disrupt oxygen delivery, do not result in hypoxic injury within 2 min. This suggests that compensations such as fetal redistribution of blood flow to vital organs, decreased oxygen consumption in response to hypoxic stress, and successful prolonged dependence of certain tissue beds on anaerobic metabolism may occur.[12]

In summary, during pregnancy oxygen delivery to maternal and fetoplacental tissue beds is highly dependent on adequate blood flow. Maternal oxygen consumption increases progressively during gestation and rises dramatically in labor. In late pregnancy or near term, the fetoplacental unit is unable to increase oxygen delivery by local vascular adjustment. The fetus, however, is protected from hypoxic insult by the avidity of fetal hemoglobin for oxygen relative to maternal hemoglobin, the tolerance of fetal tissues to low P_{O_2}, and perhaps by *fetal* circulatory autoregulation in response to hypoxic insult. These general physiologic characteristics of pregnancy have the following implications for management of critical illness:

1. Assessment of the adequacy of maternal blood flow must be made with an understanding that base-line flow is substantially increased, especially during active labor or with fever, infection, or pain.
2. Diminished placental blood flow represents a threat to fetal well-being and viability, especially if superimposed on anemia or hypoxemia or both. Maternal hypoxemia can be particularly damaging if it elicits vasodilation of nonplacental beds as this results in redistribution of flow from the fetoplacental unit.
3. Although continuous measurement of transcutaneous P_{O_2} in the fetus is feasible, interpretation of this value is difficult and the low base-line value does not provide a wide margin for identifying evolving hypoxia. Measurement of fetal heart rate is a useful but nonspecific indicator of well-being and a late sign of inadequate oxygen delivery. In general, the routinely obtained parameters of oxygen delivery and acid-base status in the mother are the best measures of adequacy of oxygen delivery for both the fetus and the mother.
4. Labor represents a tremendous "aerobic load" to the mother. The clinician must judge if labor should be avoided or postponed during periods of critical illness in which oxygen delivery is marginal.
5. One effective way to reduce aerobic requirements in the critically ill gravid patient is to assume the work of breathing in evolving respiratory failure. Thus, elective intubation and mechanical ventilation may be required early in selected patients.

Circulatory Disorders of Pregnancy

In pregnancy, circulatory impairment may be life-threatening given maternal and fetal dependence on cardiac output for oxygen delivery. In this next section, common causes of hypoperfusion, such as hemorrhage, cardiac dysfunction, trauma, and sepsis, will be discussed. Preeclampsia-eclampsia, which may occur as a result of uteroplacental ischemia, will also be explored. Finally, modifications to cardiopulmonary resuscitation algorithms, made necessary by pregnancy, will be considered.

HYPOPERFUSED STATES

The initial approach to the critically ill hypoperfused gravida is to distinguish between low flow states, caused by inadequate circulating volume, cardiac dysfunction, or trauma and high flow states such as septic shock, while taking into account the physiologic alterations associated with pregnancy. Most often the state of perfusion of the critically ill gravid patient can be determined by bedside assessment. Occasionally, the adequacy of intravascular volume will remain obscure despite careful history, physical examination, and review of routine laboratory data. Other patients will be encountered with obvious ventricular failure requiring vasoactive drug use or respiratory failure requiring careful fluid management. In these instances (Table 88-3), right heart catheterization should be considered. When necessary, this procedure should be performed through the internal jugular vein in the pregnant individual to reduce the incidence of pneumothorax associated with other approaches. If injury or obesity have obscured neck landmarks or made jugular venipuncture impossible, subclavian vein catheterization is an alternative choice. Femoral vein catheterization is relatively contraindicated because of vena caval obstruction by the uterus and the possible need for emergent delivery. In the healthy pregnant woman, right ventricular, pulmonary artery, and pulmonary capillary wedge pressures are unchanged from prepartum values.[2,13]

HEMORRHAGIC SHOCK

Low flow states in pregnancy usually result from blood loss or left ventricular dysfunction. The common causes of hemorrhagic shock in pregnancy are listed in Table 88-4. When hemorrhage occurs in pregnancy it can be massive and swift, requiring immediate intervention. The intensivist may be expected to assist in the management of the following causes of antepartum hemorrhage: premature separation of the normal placental attachment site (placental abruption), disruption of an abnormal placental attachment (placenta previa), and spontaneous uterine rupture. The management of traumatic uterine rupture is discussed later in this chapter.

TABLE 88-3 Relative Indications for Right Heart Catheterization

Routine operative or labor/delivery monitoring
Severe pulmonary hypertension
Significant valvular heart disease
Class III or IV congestive heart failure
Hypertensive crises if complicated by
Pulmonary edema
Heart failure
Oliguric renal failure
Shock, if
Etiology obscure
Volume resuscitation fails
CVP is high
Vasoactive drugs are used
Acute respiratory failure
Accompanied by shock
Requiring mechanical ventilation and PEEP
To determine cause of pulmonary edema

TABLE 88-4 Etiology of Hemorrhagic Shock in Pregnancy

Early	Late (3d Trimester)
Trauma	Trauma
Ectopic or abdominal pregnancy	Placenta previa
Abortion	Placental abruption
DIC	DIC
Hydatidiform mole	Uterine rupture
	Marginal sinus rupture

Placental abruption occurs in 1/77 to 1/250 pregnancies, with an increased incidence in patients with hypertension, high parity, and previous abruption.[14,15] Maternal mortality, usually from hemorrhage, ranges from 0 to 5.2 percent while fetal mortality is higher.[14] The initial event may be a vascular rhexis of the spiral arterioles with formation of a hematoma which then separates the placenta from its site of attachment.[15] The severity of maternal blood loss is correlated with the extent and duration of abruption and fetal demise. Blood loss averages 2 to 3 L when abruption results in fetal death and much of it can remain concealed within the uterus.[14] Severe disseminated intravascular coagulation (DIC) occurs in 30 percent of patients with fetal death.[14] Patients initially present with painful vaginal bleeding and may be misdiagnosed as having premature labor. The diagnosis is a clinical one, although ultrasound may be helpful; elevated fibrin degradation products may predict postpartum hemorrhage.[16]

Placenta previa occurs in approximately 1/200 pregnancies and does not frequently cause massive hemorrhage. Nonetheless, if vaginal examination results in disruption of the placenta over the cervical os, or if invasion of trophoblastic tissue into the myometrium (placenta previa et accreta) occurs, the patient is at risk for massive hemorrhage at delivery.[15] Placenta previa, more common in mutiparous, older patients, also has a tendency to recur in subsequent pregnancies. Fetal mortality is 5 to 10 percent, but can be much higher if maternal shock occurs.[17] The diagnosis is usually made with ultrasound.

Spontaneous uterine rupture occurs in approximately 1/2000 pregnancies.[15] The most common setting in which rupture occurs spontaneously is in the multipara with protracted labor. In overt rupture peritoneal signs may be observed. Nonetheless, substantial blood loss can occur in the absence of significant physical findings.

Common causes of postpartum hemorrhage include uterine atony following placental separation, surgical obstetric trauma, uterine inversion, and coagulopathies due to DIC or amniotic fluid embolism.[15]

MANAGEMENT. Patients at increased risk of bleeding should be identified early, in which case intravenous access and blood typing already will be accomplished. When massive hemorrhage occurs, the initial management of the patient is similar to that of the nonpregnant patient and two or three large bore (16 gauge or larger) venous catheters should be in place. Immediate volume replacement with either crystalloid or colloid should be instituted until blood is available. It is beneficial to position the patient in the left lateral decubitus position to exclude vena caval obstruction from contributing to the already diminished venous return which results from massive hemorrhage.

If shock is not immediately reversed by volume resuscitation or is accompanied by respiratory dysfunction, elective intubation and mechanical ventilation should be performed since hypoxemia superimposed on low flow is particularly injurious to fetus and mother. Military antishock trousers (MAST) can be used in the most profusely bleeding patients to maintain blood pressure until adequate venous access has been secured and large volumes administered. They should not be applied, however, to patients with pulmonary edema. This is merely a temporizing measure and limits access to pelvic and abdominal structures.[18] In antepartum hemorrhage, only the leg compartments should be used. The abdominal compartment should not be inflated in the gravid patient. The leg compartments should be inflated separately to 5 mmHg pressure, followed by the abdominal compartment (in postpartum patients only). Increases of 5 to 10 mmHg pressure are made at 5- to 10-min intervals until bleeding is controlled. The MAST suit should be in place only as long as necessary to initiate definitive therapy and should be deflated one compartment at a time, in reverse order of inflation, with 5 mmHg pressure decrements each 15 min.

Blood replacement with packed red blood cells should begin immediately. Massive obstetric hemorrhage is one setting in which initial resuscitation may require use of unmatched type-specific blood until more complete cross-matching of subsequent units has been accomplished (see Chap. 35). Because critical illness in pregnancy is frequently associated with DIC, massive bleeding should prompt a search for a coagulopathy. If the peripheral blood smear, platelet count, prothrombin time (PT), partial thromboplastin time (PTT), or fibrinogen level suggest excessive factor consumption (DIC), measurement of fibrin degradation products and specific factor levels should be performed (see Chap. 146). Massive blood loss can result in a secondary thrombocytopenia. Prophylactic platelet transfusion is not recommended unless platelet counts fall to 20,000/mm^3 or bleeding persists despite platelet counts of 20 to 50,000/mm^3. Fresh frozen plasma should be used only to correct measured clotting abnormalities, not prophylactically in anticipation of clotting factor depletion.

Surgical evaluation is performed coincident with the initial resuscitation. As circulatory stability returns, a decision is made as to whether surgical intervention, continued conservative management, or angiographic localization and embolization of bleeding sites is most appropriate.[19]

CARDIAC DYSFUNCTION

Hypoperfusion from cardiac dysfunction is most often caused by congestive heart failure due to either preexisting myocardial or valvular heart disease or to a cardiomyopathy arising de novo (1/1300 to 1/4000 deliveries).[20] Prior subclinical heart disease may manifest itself for the first time during pregnancy due to the physiologic changes of pregnancy described earlier. The prevalence of heart disease during pregnancy ranges from 0.4 to 4.1 percent, with a maternal mortality rate of 7 percent in patients with class III or IV heart failure.[1] Patients with severe mitral or aortic stenosis, Eisenmenger's or Marfan's syndromes, or pulmonary hypertension have an even higher mortality rate (25 to 50 percent).[21]

MANAGEMENT. The initial management of the hypoperfused cardiac patient should focus on volume status, and hypovolemia should be excluded as a cause of the low flow state. Right heart catheterization and echocardiography may be helpful in this regard as well as in the further management of cardiogenic shock. Metabolic disturbances can worsen ventricular function in underlying cardiomyopathies; therefore, hypocalcemia, hypophosphatemia, acidosis, and hypoxemia should be avoided. Vasoactive drugs are reserved for circumstances in which hypovolemia has been corrected and maternal perfusion remains inadequate. If cardiogenic shock persists despite adequate preload, dobutamine is the drug of choice. Dobutamine, however, should be reserved for life-threatening conditions because, at least in animal models, it reduces placental blood flow.[22] Concomitantly, infusion of dopamine in low doses (2 to 3 μg/kg/min) should be considered to preserve splanchnic and renal perfusion. Its use in pregnancy, however, has been limited. We advocate the use of dopamine only in situations in which renal function is compromised.[23] When cardiogenic shock is complicated by pulmonary edema, parenteral furosemide should be given; right heart catheterization is necessary to titrate therapy.

When cardiogenic shock persists despite inotropic drug support, afterload reduction with either intravenous sodium nitroprusside or nitroglycerin should be considered. *Because fetal cyanide poisoning has been described in experimental animal models, this agent should be used in the management of cardiogenic shock in pregnancy only when the circulation cannot be stabilized with volume and inotropic drugs.*[4] The dose and duration of therapy should be minimized and the patient converted to oral agents such as hydralazine as soon as possible to avoid nitroprusside toxicity. Converting-enzyme inhibitors should be avoided in pregnancy, because they have been noted to cause anuric renal failure in human neonates exposed in utero and high rates of fetal death in animals.[4]

The hemodynamic alterations of labor and delivery, when imposed on those of pregnancy, make this an especially dangerous time for women with cardiac disease. The optimal method of delivery is an assisted vaginal delivery in the left lateral decubitus position. Epidural anesthesia will ameliorate tachycardia in response to pain, and its vasodilatory actions may be of benefit.[1] Since decreased systemic vascular resistance (SVR) may lead to further decompensation in patients with aortic stenosis, hypertrophic cardiomyopathy, or pulmonary hypertension, general anesthesia may be preferred in these patients.[1] The current consensus is that cesarean section should be reserved for obstetric complications and fetal distress,[20,21] although with improved surgical techniques and close hemodynamic monitoring, cesarean sections may be safer than in the past.[1] Invasive monitoring is required to follow shifts in volume status that occur from the tremendous "autotransfusions" produced by each uterine contraction and blood loss that occurs with delivery.

TRAUMA

During pregnancy, hypoperfusion and shock may occur due to injury from motor vehicle accidents, falls, and assaults.[24] The gravid woman is at greater risk of hemorrhage after trauma, as blood flow to the entire pelvis is increased. Some injuries are unique to pregnancy, including amniotic membrane rupture, placental abruption, uterine rupture, premature labor, and fetal trauma.[24] In a recent series of blunt abdominal trauma in late pregnancy, the most serious complications were placental abruption and uterine rupture.[25] Rapid deceleration injury can cause placental abruption. In the majority of cases, vaginal bleeding will be present when abruption has occurred, although there are reports of "occult" abruption without vaginal bleeding following traumatic injury.[25] Abruption can be rapidly complicated by DIC; therefore, all severely injured gravid patients should have coagulation profiles monitored. Displacement of abdominal contents cephalad increases the risk of visceral injury from penetrating trauma of the upper abdomen. The urinary bladder is a target for injury, because it is displaced into the abdominal cavity beyond 12 weeks of gestation.

The physiologic changes of pregnancy may make evaluation and treatment of the gravid patient more difficult following trauma. Borderline tachycardia and supine hypotension (from vena caval obstruction by the uterus in late pregnancy) may be attributable to pregnancy itself, as opposed to indicating loss of blood volume. Clinical signs of hypovolemia are not observed in trauma victims until intravascular volume is reduced 15 to 20 percent. When hypovolemia is clinically evident in gravid patients, it signifies enormous blood loss, as blood volume has expanded by as much as 40 to 50 percent by the thirtieth week of gestation. Pregnancy may mask findings of peritoneal irritation. In one series of 12 gravid patients receiving peritoneal lavage for evaluation of blunt abdominal trauma, only 2 of these patients exhibited abnormal abdominal signs or symptoms. Nonetheless, 8 had positive lavage with confirmation of intraabdominal bleeding or injury at laparotomy.[26]

Fetal injuries are uncommon in blunt trauma. Fetal skull fracture occurs most often in the third trimester, when the engaged fetal head is at risk of injury from maternal pelvic fractures.[24] Fetal mortality is usually secondary to maternal shock, whether or not trauma involves the uterus. Death from accidents is a leading cause of nonobstetric maternal mortality.

MANAGEMENT. Initially, maternal cardiorespiratory function and the extent of injury should be assessed. If emergent intubation is required, it should be performed by a skilled individual because of the increased risk of aspiration during pregnancy. Since maternal shock is the most likely cause of fetal demise, ensuring the adequacy of the maternal circulation is paramount. If significant hemorrhage is obvious, aggressive fluid replacement as discussed above for hemorrhagic shock is appropriate. Use of the MAST suit may be considered for shock unresponsive to early fluid resuscitation. Once the cervical spine is cleared, the patient should be placed in lateral recumbancy and uterine lift performed if shock is present. Pelvic examination should be performed, as long as overt vaginal bleeding is not present, to look for blood, urine, and amniotic fluid. Nitrazine paper can identify amniotic fluid and confirm rupture of the amniotic membranes. Because needle paracentesis is difficult in the second and third trimester, open peritoneal lavage is advised for assessing severe blunt abdominal trauma. The diagnosis of pelvic or abdominal bleeding can usually be made by ultrasound, computed tomography (CT), or lavage. Once the mother is stabilized, cardiotocographic monitoring including Doppler measurement of fetal cardiac activity and measurement of uterine activity should be performed for 4 h after the injury. When used in trauma patients beyond the 20th week of pregnancy, cardiotocographic monitoring can identify placental abruption, fetal distress, and uterine contractions.[24] Fetomaternal hemorrhage may be identified by the Kleihauer-Betke test; this may be important if the patient is Rh negative and may signal potential fetal exsanguination.[24]

If maternal death occurs despite aggressive resuscitation and the fetus is alive and undelivered, a postmortem cesarean section should be considered. A review of over 150 cases revealed that outcome was crucially related to the duration of time between maternal death and delivery.[27] If <5 min passed, fetal prognosis was excellent; 5 to 10 min good; 10 to 15 min fair; 15 to 20 min poor; and >29 min, fetal survival was unlikely.

SEPTIC SHOCK

Sepsis is another important cause of hypoperfusion in pregnancy, accounting for about 15 percent of maternal deaths.[28] The diagnosis of sepsis in the febrile gravid patient can be confounded by the normal hemodynamic changes of pregnancy (i.e., increased cardiac output, decreased SVR). Awareness of the usual settings and patients at risk for sepsis will increase recognition of this life-threatening state. Animal data suggest that an increased vulnerability to the systemic effects of bacteremia and endotoxemia may exist during pregnancy.[29]

Patients appear to be at the greatest risk of sepsis in the peripartum and postabortion periods. Urinary and genital tract infections from uterus, vagina, and episiotomy site are the most common sources.[28] Clinical settings which increase the risk of sepsis include cesarean section, prolonged rupture of membranes, retained products of conception, poor progress in labor, and prior instrumentation of the genitourinary tract.[28,29] Patients who develop septic shock frequently have a preceding postpartum endometritis or chorioamnionitis.[29] Patients with endometritis present with fever, abdominal pain and tenderness, and purulent lochia.[28] Life-threatening necrotizing fasciitis occurs rarely after cesarean section or episiotomy.[28] Septic abortion is more often seen in countries where access to abortion is limited. The bacterial organisms which must be considered include *Staphylococcus aureus* and *epidermidis;* groups A, B, and D streptococci; *Escherichia coli; Proteus mirabilis; Enterobacter; Klebsiella; Pseudomonas;* anaerobic streptococci and bacteriodes; and rarely *Clostridium perfringens.*[30]

Right heart catheterization of septic pregnant patients usually reveals a high cardiac index and heart rate with a low blood pressure.[30] Based on analysis of left ventricular function curves, some patients may have evidence of myocardial depression despite an increased cardiac index.[30] Systemic vascular resistance index (SVRI) is decreased. In one study of septic shock in pregnancy, the greatest improvement in SVRI occurred in the eight surviving women; their initial SVRI was 885 ± 253 dyne-s/cm^5-m^2 versus 1672 ± 413 dyne-s/cm^5-m^2 following resolution of their hyperdynamic state.[30] It is important to remember that pregnancy itself results in a 25 percent decrease from the prepregnancy vascular resistance of 900 to 1500 dyne-s/cm^5, a decrease in blood pressure, and a 20 percent increase in heart rate. Thus, three useful signs of sepsis—tachycardia, hypotension, and low SVR—must be interpreted with caution in the gravid patient, particularly in the third trimester. Rapid change in hemodynamic parameters, however, suggests infection. Complications of sepsis in pregnancy include pulmonary capillary leak with subsequent adult respiratory distress syndrome (ARDS) and DIC.[30]

MANAGEMENT. The septic gravid patient requires thorough culturing and evaluation of pelvic sites. Empirical antibiotic therapy, to cover what is typically a polymicrobial infection with gram-positive, gram-negative, and anaerobic organisms as discussed earlier, should be given until specific bacteriologic cultures are available. Reasonable regimens include cefoxitin, ampicillin-sulbactam, and clindamycin-gentamicin,[28] although if possible it is best to avoid aminoglycosides due to their potential fetal oto- and nephrotoxicities. Surgical drainage of appropriate pelvic and abdominal sources may be required.

Patients who have evidence of adequate tissue perfusion and oxygen delivery may not require fluid or vasoactive drugs to treat tachycardia and moderate hypotension. Lactic acidosis or end-organ dysfunction is an indication for volume loading, but given the risk of precipitating low pressure pulmonary edema, right heart catheterization should be performed to allow titration of volume therapy. Mechanical ventilatory support should be instituted if needed. If hypoperfusion persists despite volume replacement, the use of inotropic agents such as dobutamine to increase forward flow may be of value in patients who have markedly abnormal ventricular performance. Since there are no clear benefits to using inotropic agents in patients with high flow states whose cardiac function is near normal, one should be willing to withdraw these drugs if adverse effects are noted. Elevated temperature should be controlled with acetaminophen and a cooling blanket, because fever has adverse effects on the fetus.

Although high dose corticosteroids and naloxone have not proven useful in septic shock, recent trials of immunotherapeutic agents directed against bacterial antigens or exotoxins show promise. One study investigated the effects of freeze-dried human plasma rich in antilipopolysaccharide (anti-LPS) immunoglobulin G administration to obstetric and gynecologic patients with sepsis and hypotension.[31] Mortality in anti-LPS–treated patients was 7.1 percent as compared to 47.4 percent in untreated patients, with mean arterial blood pressure rising from 45.1 ± 7.4 to 69.1 ± 9.1 mmHg within 75 min of administration of this preparation. Monoclonal antibodies to bacterial antigens or to endogenous cytokines are currently undergoing clinical evaluation and will likely play a role in the treatment of septic shock in the future (see Chap. 98).

PREECLAMPSIA-ECLAMPSIA

Preeclampsia is a fairly common disorder occurring in 5 to 10 percent of all pregnancies.[4] It occurs primarily in primigravidas after the 20th week of gestation, most often near term. It is characterized by hypertension, proteinuria, and generalized edema. Edema, however, may not be essential to the diagnosis because 30 percent of normal pregnant women may have generalized edema, whereas many of those who progress to eclampsia will not.[4] Coagulation or liver function abnormalities may be noted. Preeclampsia may progress to a convulsive and potentially lethal phase, termed eclampsia, without warning. Eclampsia occurs in 0.05 to 0.2 percent of all deliveries, with an incidence of 1.5 percent in twin deliveries.[32] In one large study fetal mortality was 13 percent, with placental abruption accounting for four of the six deaths; there were no maternal deaths.[32]

Although the exact etiology of preeclampsia is unknown, knowledge of common pathophysiologic features will assist in its management. The hypertension observed in preeclampsia is very labile and is characterized by an increased vascular sensitivity to angiotensin, catecholamines, and vasopressin.[4] Hemoconcentration, in part from increased vascular permeability to macromolecules, occurs along with decrements in placental and renal perfusion. The reduction in placental perfusion occurs before the onset of clinical disease and suggests that uteroplacental ischemia may cause the hypertension and other manifestations of the disease.[4] Some investigators speculate that altered prostaglandin synthesis may mediate these hemodynamic alterations, since low dose aspirin may decrease the incidence of preeclampsia in high-risk populations.[33] Right heart catheterization of 44 untreated preeclamptic patients revealed low normal right atrial and pulmonary capillary wedge pressures (Ppw), a reduced cardiac output, and a markedly elevated SVR.[4] A more recent study of 41 preeclamptic patients, noted a normal Ppw, normal to high cardiac index, and mildly elevated SVR compared to historical controls.[34]

Markers of disease severity that should alert the physician to the increased risk of convulsions include systolic or diastolic pressures >160 and 110 mmHg, respectively (especially after 24 h of hospitalization), pulmonary edema, cyanosis, marked hemoconcentration, and heavy proteinuria or oliguria.[4] Infrequently, patients may develop microangiopathic hemolytic anemia, abnormal liver function tests, and thrombocytopenia known as the HELLP syndrome (*h*emolysis, *e*levated *l*iver enzymes, *l*ow *p*latelets),

TABLE 88-5 Approach to CPR during Pregnancy

Time	Resuscitative Action	Diagnostic Action	Pharmacologic Action
0	Chest thump Ventilation (mouth-to-mouth) External cardiac massage Defibrillate	Electrocardiography for rhythm Check for pulses and perfusion	Intravenous fluids
	Intravenous access: central line	Determine gestational age	Ventricular fibrillation—lidocaine Supraventricular tachyarrhythmia—digitalis/β-blocker as appropriate
1–2 min	Endotracheal intubation plus ventilation with oxygen	Measure arterial blood gases Check for pulses and perfusion Check fetal heart rate, sonography	pH < 7.3—sodium bicarbonate Asystole/bradyarrhythmia—atropine Pulmonary edema—furosemide
2–5 min	Defibrillate as needed	Electrocardiography for rhythm	Ventricular fibrillation—lidocaine
	Position to move uterus to left	Electrocardiography for rhythm Quick measure of blood pressure, pulses, perfusion	Ventricular fibrillation—bretylium Electromechanical dissociation—epinephrine (one time only), isoproterenol
		Measure arterial blood gases	pH < 7.3—sodium bicarbonate
5–10 min	Continue ventilation plus external massage Begin preparation for operative procedure as appropriate Arterial line	Check fetal heart rate, sonography Check for tension pneumothorax, cardiac tamponade, hypovolemia	
	Defibrillate as needed	Measure arterial blood gases	pH < 7.3—sodium bicarbonate
15 min	Open-chest cardiac massage and/or emergency cesarean section as appropriate	Continue as above	Continue as above

SOURCE: Modified and reproduced with permission from Ref. 36.

which is a sign of life-threatening disease.[4] Patients with the HELLP syndrome may have significant liver tenderness, with signs suggesting an acute abdomen. This is important to recognize since inappropriate surgical intervention can be catastrophic and management should focus on the underlying preeclampsia.

Especially worrisome symptoms and signs in any patient with preeclampsia include headache, blurred vision, scotomata, epigastric pain, clonus, increasing serum creatinine level, consumptive coagulopathy, and even mildly elevated liver function tests.[4] Although the risks of eclampsia are higher when the above markers of disease severity are present, up to 25 percent of eclamptics may have minimal elevations of blood pressure prior to convulsing.[4] Eclampsia has been reported to occur up to several weeks postpartum.[33]

MANAGEMENT. Delivery is the therapy of choice in preeclamptic patients who are beyond the 36th week of pregnancy, have evidence of advanced disease such as thrombocytopenia or elevated liver function tests, or have signs of impending eclampsia.[4] Hypertension (diastolic pressure > 105 mmHg) is an indication for treatment with hydralazine, which has a record of safety and efficacy in pregnancy. Nifedipine, labetalol, and diazoxide are second-line agents and should be reserved for patients who do not respond to hydralazine. *Nitroprusside is relatively, and converting-enzyme inhibitors are absolutely, contraindicated in pregnancy.* Diuretics should not be used as they may aggravate the reduced intravascular volume that is often seen in preeclampsia. Magnesium sulfate should be instituted to prevent eclamptic convulsions. Some investigators speculate that volume expansion may reduce blood pressure in preeclampsia by decreasing SVR; however, the increased risk of pulmonary or cerebral edema and lack of proven benefit from volume expansion suggests that it should be avoided and instituted only with a right heart catheter in place.[33]

CARDIOPULMONARY RESUSCITATION

Pregnancy limits the ability to adequately perform cardiopulmonary resuscitation (CPR). If cardiopulmonary arrest does occur, the physiologic changes of pregnancy must be taken into account when performing CPR. The gravid uterus may impede venous return and distal arterial perfusion by compressing the inferior vena cava and aorta. In late pregnancy, the gravid uterus acts like an abdominal binder; the resultant elevation of intrathoracic pressure may limit the ability to create forward flow during CPR. One study described a patient in whom blood pressure could not be achieved during cardiac massage until the uterus was evacuated, after which an immediate pulsatile blood pressure was observed.[35]

These considerations have prompted some modifications to the usual approach to CPR in the pregnant patient. The most thorough review of the subject offers an approach outlined in Table 88-5.[36] The key modification of routine CPR is that the pregnant patient should receive standard CPR while being placed in the left lateral decubitus position to decrease aortocaval compression by the uterus. If standard closed-chest CPR cannot generate a pulse, especially in late pregnancy, open-chest massage and emergency cesarean section should be considered. To facilitate this plan, obstetric, internal medicine, and anesthesiology staff need to be appraised early of any acute deterioration in the circulation of a critically ill gravida.

Respiratory Disorders of Pregnancy

During pregnancy, ventilatory failure may occur from chronic lung disease or asthma and require mechanical ventilation. A more common cause of respiratory compromise in pregnant women is acute hypoxemic respiratory failure. This section will focus on the management of both ventilatory and hypoxemic respiratory failure in the gravid patient.

VENTILATORY FAILURE

With improved medical care, patients with chronic lung diseases such as cystic fibrosis are surviving to childbearing age, presenting new management problems for the intensivist. Asthma, however, remains the most common pulmonary problem encountered in pregnancy, affecting 1 percent of all gravidas. When these conditions require mechanical support, ventilator management necessitates careful attention to the special needs of mother and fetus.

TABLE 88-6 Problems with Airway Management in Pregnancy

Upper airway edema
Diminished airway caliber
Propensity for hemorrhage
Increased risk of aspiration

MECHANICAL VENTILATION

If ventilatory failure is imminent, intubation and mechanical ventilation should be performed electively. Several difficulties in airway management should be anticipated in the critically ill pregnant patient (Table 88-6). Pharyngeal, laryngeal, and vocal cord edema are common, and the highly vascular upper airway may bleed from even minor intubation-related trauma.[37] Consequently, relatively small endotracheal tubes (6 to 7 mm) may be required. An increased risk of aspiration may exist due to delayed gastric emptying, increased intraabdominal pressure, and diminished competence of the gastroesophageal sphincter.[38] Use of cricoid pressure to minimize pulmonary aspiration is advised. Forty percent of maternal deaths associated with general anesthesia in England and Wales from 1976 to 1978 were related to difficulties with endotracheal intubation.[39] Control of the airway should be achieved in an early and elective fashion by a skilled individual.

The initial ventilator settings should be aimed at achieving eucapnea, which in this patient population is a P_{CO_2} of 28 to 35 mmHg. A number of studies in animal models suggest that excessive positive-pressure ventilation resulting in acute respiratory alkalosis can cause fetal asphyxia, presumably from decreased uteroplacental flow in response to the alkalosis or diminished maternal venous return or both. Thus, respiratory alkalosis should be avoided.[40] This usually can be accomplished with tidal volumes in the range of 10 mL/kg and respiratory rates of 15 to 18 breaths/min. In the asthmatic patient (vide infra), lower tidal volume and rate minimize the adverse effects of intrinsic positive end-expiratory pressure (PEEP) (see Chap. 130). The patient with acute pulmonary edema (vide infra) should be ventilated with small tidal volumes (7 to 8 mL/kg) and high rates of 24 to 30 breaths/min. The low tidal volume is preferred because lung stiffness caused by pulmonary edema, as well as the abdominal factors of pregnancy, will result in high airway pressures, increasing the risk of barotrauma. When a diffuse lung lesion is present and toxic levels of oxygen are required, sufficient PEEP should be added to correct arterial hypoxemia on a nontoxic fraction of inspired oxygen ($F_{IO_2} < 0.6$). In the pregnant patient we aim to keep $Pa_{O_2} > 90$ mmHg, a value higher than in the nonpregnant patient, to prevent fetal distress. To minimize the decrease in venous return that occurs with positive-pressure ventilation, it is important that the pregnant patient be managed in a lateral position whenever possible. Measures to avoid atelectasis in the ventilated gravid patient include PEEP, sighs, and alternating the lateral position.

In patients with severe lung lesions requiring toxic concentrations of oxygen and high levels of PEEP or hemodynamic instability, muscle relaxation and sedation will decrease oxygen consumption and assist in stabilization. Pancuronium bromide and morphine sulfate are without adverse fetal effects with short-term use.[2] Benzodiazepines may increase the risk of cleft palate when used early in pregnancy. These agents all cross the placenta; therefore, if given near the time of delivery, immediate intubation of the neonate will be required.

Fetal viability can be maintained throughout pregnancy with mechanical ventilation, even when maternal death occurs. We feel that mechanical ventilation is most appropriate when instituted early in the course of progressive ventilatory failure, to stabilize mother and fetus and then permit identification of reversible factors to allow either safe withdrawal of mechanical support or controlled delivery. These complex decisions are best made in conjunction with the critical care physician, obstetrician, and neonatologist.

CHRONIC LUNG DISEASE

Most chronic pulmonary diseases that can result in ventilatory failure, such as cystic fibrosis, kyphoscoliosis, neuromuscular diseases, pulmonary fibrosis, and chronic obstructive pulmonary disease (COPD), are uncommon in pregnancy. Despite the increased ventilatory demands which occur in pregnancy, ventilatory failure is rare. In one study, several women with a preconception 40 to 75 percent reduction in vital capacity (VC) due to lung resection carried their pregnancy to term and had few respiratory symptoms.[41] Although several authorities suggest that a VC of at least 1 L is essential for a safe and successful pregnancy, one patient has been reported to have completed pregnancy with a VC of only 0.8 L.[42] Thus, severely reduced lung volume alone, to a level compatible with impairment of ventilatory function in the nonpregnant individual, does not preclude a successful conception and pregnancy.

Patients with severe restrictive lung disease and progressive ventilatory insufficiency during pregnancy may benefit from nocturnal positive-pressure ventilation and oxygen administration. One patient with severe kyphoscoliosis and a forced VC of 580 mL, a P_{O_2} of 59 mmHg, and a P_{CO_2} of 52 mmHg at 25 to 28 weeks' gestation, avoided mechanical ventilation by using nocturnal positive-pressure ventilation with a tight fitting mask during weeks 30 to 34 of pregnancy until delivery could be accomplished by cesarean section.[43] This novel approach may be applicable to other pregnant patients with chronic ventilatory impairment. Pulse oximetry should be used to screen patients with marginal ventilatory function for nocturnal hypoxemia.

ASTHMA

In most gravid asthmatic subjects pregnancy does not alter their asthma; however, both improvement and worsening of airflow obstruction have been noted.[37] Early reviews on the outcome of pregnancy in asthmatic women note an increase in the incidence of fetal prematurity and perinatal and maternal mortality.[2] More recent studies, however, have reported no adverse effects on fetal or maternal well-being, unless the asthma is poorly controlled. This suggests that control of asthma and prevention of acute exacerbations are crucial to an improved outcome.[2]

MANAGEMENT. The management of the pregnant patient with status asthmaticus is similar to that of the nonpregnant patient with a few exceptions. Even the usually mild hypoxemia seen in asthma should be avoided in the gravid patient because it is detrimental to the fetus. Oxygenation, therefore, should be assessed even in mild attacks. Since base-line P_{CO_2} is decreased in pregnancy and probably falls further with an acute asthma attack, an arterial blood-gas determination which shows a $P_{CO_2} > 35$ mmHg during status asthmaticus should alert the clinician to impending ventilatory failure. Experience with nonpregnant patients with status asthmaticus and mild hypercapnia, however, has suggested that many can be managed without mechanical ventilatory support.

Most drugs used to treat asthma are considered safe for use during pregnancy. Inhaled bronchodilators are standard therapy. A recent study of inhaled β-agonists in 259 pregnancies (most subjects used metaproterenol), noted no increase in the incidence of congenital malformations, prematurity, low birth weights, Apgar scores, perinatal complications, or mortality.[44] Use of parenteral β-agonists should be limited to situations in which inhaled agents have been ineffective, since epinephrine causes vasoconstriction of the uteroplacental circulation in monkeys and a slight increase in congenital malformations in human beings, and terbutaline may inhibit labor and precipitate pulmonary edema if given near term.[5] Theophylline has an extensive safety record in pregnancy, with the only fetal risk being neonatal theophylline toxicity when given at the time of delivery.[2] Pregnancy decreases theophylline clearance in the third trimester so doses may require adjustment.[37] Patients who do not respond to the above measures should receive parenteral steroids. The increased incidence of spontaneous abortion, placental insufficiency, and cleft palate observed in rodents given corticosteroids during gestation has not been corroborated in human beings.[2] Although the potential risk of fetal adrenal insufficiency exists, this is a rare occurrence.[5] There are case reports of dramatic improvement in bronchospasm following termination of pregnancy.[45] There is no definitive evidence, however, to suggest that termination of pregnancy per se improves maternal outcome in asthma, since anesthesia given for cesarean section may have elicited the bronchodilation noted.

ACUTE HYPOXEMIC RESPIRATORY FAILURE

Pregnancy predisposes to acute hypoxemic respiratory failure from a variety of disorders including those that result in pulmonary edema such as amniotic fluid embolism, β-adrenergic tocolytic therapy, and aspiration. Other causes of hypoxemic respiratory failure include venous air embolism and respiratory infections.

AMNIOTIC FLUID EMBOLISM

Amniotic fluid embolism occurs in 1/10,000 to 1/30,000 pregnancies[37] and is estimated to account for 11 to 13 percent of all maternal deaths.[2] In one large series the mortality rate was 86 percent.[46] Although this series included many cases which predate modern intensive care techniques, one-fourth of the deaths occurred within 1 h of the onset of symptoms, which suggests that even with modern intensive care management mortality will remain substantial.

Various risk factors have been reported: **1.** advanced maternal age; **2.** multiparity; **3.** amniotomy; **4.** cesarean section; **5.** insertion of intrauterine fetal or pressure monitoring devices; and **6.** term pregnancy in the presence of an intrauterine device. The use of uterine stimulants, tumultuous labor, intrauterine death, and meconium in the amniotic fluid have not been substantiated as important risk factors.[2] It is also important to note that this entity has been reported after normal labor and delivery and may occur as early as 20 weeks of gestation in the absence of labor.[2]

The mechanisms of respiratory and circulatory failure in amniotic fluid embolism remain controversial. Amniotic fluid and particulate matter (lanugo hairs, meconium, fat, fetal squames) may enter the maternal venous circulation via endocervical veins, uterine tears, or at the placental site itself and result in pulmonary hypertension.[5] In some animal studies, filtered amniotic fluid is relatively innocuous in less than massive amounts. This suggests that cellular and other debris present in the fluid embolism may be the cause of either mechanical obstruction to the maternal pulmonary vasculature or the trigger to a maternal systemic reaction.[5] Others believe that vasoconstrictor arachidonic acid metabolites present in the amniotic fluid itself may elicit pulmonary hypertension.[37] Circulatory failure has been ascribed to various pathophysiologic processes and may vary over time. Some authors contend that the principal cause is acute right heart strain from acute pulmonary hypertension. The observed acute elevation of pulmonary artery and central venous pressures with subsequent hypoperfusion supports this contention.[47] Others insist that left ventricular failure is the only hemodynamic abnormality consistently observed in human beings, citing data showing elevation of Ppw, minimal increase in the pulmonary vascular resistance, and depressed left ventricular performance.[46] Whatever the true hemodynamic picture, a component of pulmonary capillary leak must exist as severe pulmonary edema occurs at a Ppw < 19 mmHg.[46]

The classic presentation of amniotic fluid embolism is the abrupt onset of severe dyspnea, tachypnea, and cyanosis during labor or soon after delivery and characterizes more than 50 percent of the cases.[2] Shock and bleeding each are the initial presentation in 10 to 15 percent of the cases. Amniotic fluid embolism is frequently complicated by pulmonary edema; it was found in 70 percent of the cases in one autopsy review.[2] Bleeding secondary to DIC occurs in up to 50 percent of patients who survive the first 30 to 60 min. Most of the remaining patients will have evidence for DIC by screening laboratory tests.[2]

MANAGEMENT. The treatment of patients with amniotic fluid embolism and cardiovascular collapse is supportive and aimed at ensuring adequate oxygenation, stabilizing the circulation, and controlling bleeding. The initial management should include intubation, administration of 100% oxygen, and mechanical ventilation with a small tidal volume (8 mL/kg) and rapid rate (24 breaths/min). Often, early sedation and muscle relaxation allow complete rest of the respiratory muscles and confer hemodynamic stability. PEEP is then added to achieve a $Pa_{O_2} > 90$ mmHg on a $FI_{O_2} < 0.6$. Pulmonary artery catheterization allows measurement of the cardiac output and Ppw, followed by hemodynamic adjustments seeking the least Ppw (to reduce vascular leak) providing an adequate cardiac output. Pulmonary arterial blood can be examined cytologically for evidence of abnormal amniotic fluid components—fetal squamous cells, lanugo hairs, etc. Demonstration of these amniotic fluid elements in the maternal pulmonary circulation, however, is not sufficient to make this diagnosis since they have been observed in patients without clinical evidence for amniotic fluid embolism.[16] Vasoactive drugs are frequently required to reverse hypotension. Once DIC is established, factor replacement and heparin therapy, which are controversial, should be undertaken only in conjunction with a hematology consultant.[14,16]

TOCOLYTIC THERAPY

Pulmonary edema associated with β-adrenergic agents given to inhibit preterm labor is seen in as many as 4.4 percent of patients receiving these drugs.[48] Most of the reported cases have resulted from use of intravenous β-mimetics such as ritodrine, terbutaline, isoxuprine, or salbutamol. There is an increased incidence in women with twin gestations,[48] and half the patients in one small series had concurrent evidence of infection, such as fever, elevated white blood cell count, or amnionitis.[2] Most women have intact membranes at the time of presentation. When pulmonary edema develops postpartum, the vast majority of cases are encountered within 12 h of delivery. Pulmonary edema develops acutely, within 30 to 72 h of the initiation of therapy.[2] The development of pulmonary edema more than 24 h after the discontinuation of these drugs suggests another cause.

The pathogenesis of this disorder remains unknown. Pulmonary edema has never been associated with similarly high doses of β-adrenergic agonists during the treatment of asthma. Therefore, some alteration related to pregnancy may predispose women to this complication. Left ventricular function was normal in those patients assessed with echocardiography and invasive monitoring.[48] Observation of normal Ppw in most patients who have pulmonary artery catheters placed has led to speculation that these drugs produce a pulmonary capillary leak.[48] Volume overload may also play a major role since: **1.** large volumes of crystalloid are often given in response to the reflex tachycardia resulting from sympathomimetic drugs; **2.** the intravascular volume expansion and reduced colloid oncotic pressure noted in pregnancy increase susceptibility to hydrostatic edema formation; **3.** sodium and water excretion may be impaired in the supine pregnant patient; **4.** tocolytic agents may increase arginine vasopressin secretion and thus impair water balance; and **6.** the response to diuresis is prompt in these patients.[48]

Most patients complain of chest discomfort and dyspnea, manifest tachypnea and tachycardia with crackles on lung auscultation, and will have pulmonary edema on chest radiography (Table 88-7). Positive fluid balance is often noted in the hours to days preceding the onset of symptoms. In the largest collected series, the mean arterial P_{O_2} on room air was 50.4 ± 2.9 mmHg with a P_{CO_2} of 28.1 ± 2.1 mmHg. The history and clinical findings should help to distinguish this disorder from acute thromboembolic disease, acid aspiration, and amniotic fluid embolism.

MANAGEMENT. The course of this disease is usually benign, and invasive hemodynamic monitoring is usually not required. In a large series there were only two maternal deaths (3 percent); fetal survival was 95 percent.[48] Treatment should consist of discontinuation of tocolytic therapy, oxygen administration, and diuresis. Response is usually rapid, with resolution of tachypnea and hypoxemia often occurring within hours.

ASPIRATION

Aspiration is an uncommon but well-described and ominous complication of the peripartum period, accounting for 2 percent of maternal deaths.[2] Factors that increase the risk of aspiration in the pregnant woman include the increased intragastric pressure which results from external compression by the enlarged uterus, relaxation of the lower esophageal sphincter due to progesterone, delayed gastric emptying during labor, and depressed mental status and vocal cord closure from analgesia.[37] Injury due to aspiration of gastric contents is related to the volume of aspirated material, its acidity, the presence of particulate material, the bacterial burden of the aspirated material, and host resistance to subsequent infection. The early injury results from a chemical pneumonitis, the extent of which is determined primarily by acidity and volume of aspirate. Diffuse lung injury with the development of ARDS may occur early in the course. A late complication of aspiration is the evolution to bacterial pneumonia, which tends to be focal and polymicrobial and occurs 24 to 72 h after the event.

TABLE 88-7 Features of Tocolytic-Induced Pulmonary Edema

Most common cause of pulmonary edema in pregnancy
Associated with β-adrenergic agonist use
Dyspnea, tachypnea, and crackles are typical
Usually occurs shortly after beginning these agents; consider another diagnosis if pulmonary edema occurs >24 h after stopping tocolytic agents
Usually responds promptly to oxygen and diuretics

MANAGEMENT. Prevention of this dread complication should be the primary goal of all physicians assessing and managing the patient's airway. Once aspiration has occurred, treatment is supportive and similar to that of the nonpregnant individual, as discussed elsewhere in this textbook (see Chap. 136). Antibiotics should be given only if bacterial pneumonia develops.

VENOUS AIR EMBOLISM

Although a rare occurrence, venous air embolism may account for 1 percent of all maternal deaths.[2] It occurs during normal labor, delivery of women with placenta previa, criminal abortions using air, orogenital sex, and insufflation of the vagina during gynecologic procedures.[2] Air is thought to enter subplacental venous sinuses, then to embolize through the venous circulation, and finally to obstruct pulmonary blood flow when the air reaches the right ventricle. Two further mechanisms may be important in the pathophysiology of this disorder. They include obstruction of pulmonary arterioles by fibrin microemboli produced at the turbulant air-blood interface and polymorphonuclear leukocyte recruitment and activation by aggregated proteins at the air-blood interface.[2] Symptoms include cough, dyspnea, dizziness, tachypnea, tachycardia, and diaphoresis. Sudden hypotension is usually followed by respiratory arrest. A "mill-wheel murmur" or bubbling sound is occasionally heard over the precordium.[2] Right heart strain, ischemia, and arrhythmias have been noted on the electrocardiogram (ECG). Patients who survive the initial cardiopulmonary collapse may develop noncardiogenic pulmonary edema.

MANAGEMENT. When venous air embolism is suspected, the patient should be placed immediately in the left lateral decubitus position. Aspiration of air from the right heart or pulmonary outflow tract should be attempted with a pulmonary artery catheter.[2] The patient should be ventilated with 100% oxygen in an effort to decrease the size of the embolism by removing nitrogen.[2] Hyperbaric therapy is a time-honored effective way to treat air embolism in diving medicine. Anticoagulation with heparin to treat fibrin microemboli and high dose corticosteroids to decrease pulmonary edema formation have been proposed, but their usefulness in this disorder remains untested.[2]

RESPIRATORY INFECTIONS

The spectrum of organisms that result in bacterial pneumonia is similar to that in the nonpregnant population.[37] In a recent retrospective review of pneumonia during pregnancy, 20 percent of the cases had respiratory failure requiring mechanical ventilation and 44 percent had preterm labor; maternal mortality was 4 percent while fetal mortality was 12 percent.[49] An increased incidence of influenza pneumonia was noted among pregnant patients during the 1918–1919 and 1957–1958 influenza pandemics. Autopsy reports noted the cause of death as respiratory insufficiency from fulminant influenza pneumonia, rather than from secondary bacterial infection as is usually the case in the nonpregnant population.[2] Pregnancy, however, has not been demonstrated to be a risk factor for severe influenza infection except during these pandemic years. Primary varicella zoster infections progress to pneumonia more often in adults than in children. Some have noted an increased progression to pneumonia and an increased mortality in pregnant patients, but the validity of this claim has not been proven conclusively. Coccidioidomycosis is the fungal infection most commonly associated with increased risk of dissemination during pregnancy especially if contracted in the second or third trimester.[5]

MANAGEMENT. The choice of antibacterial agents to treat pneumonia during pregnancy should include consideration of potential fetal toxicity. The penicillins, cephalosporins, and erythromycin (except for the estolate which increases the risk of cholestatic jaundice in pregnancy) are felt to be safe.[2] Tetracycline is contraindicated, and sulfa-containing regimens should be avoided near term.[37] Amantidine has been shown to be teratogenic at very high but not lower doses in animals; its use has not been studied in pregnant women.[2] Favorable results have been obtained using acyclovir to treat pregnant women with varicella pneumonia.[37] No teratogenic effects have been noted in animal studies of acyclovir.[2] It is important to initiate therapy with acyclovir early to affect outcome favorably. Thus, acyclovir should be started at the first sign of respiratory system involvement in pregnant patients with cutaneous varicella infection.[2] Amphotericin B should be used to treat disseminated coccidioidal infections in pregnancy, with ketoconazole reserved for cases in which amphotericin cannot be used due to hypersensitivity.[2] No reports of adverse effects on the fetus have been reported with amphotericin. Ketoconazole has not been studied in pregnancy.

Maintenance of the Internal Environment

While early mortality can be reduced in the critically ill gravid patient by institution of the therapies outlined above, malnutrition, nosocomial infection, renal failure, and gastrointestinal hemorrhage often complicate a prolonged ICU stay and account for much of the later morbidity and mortality. Several of these issues will be discussed below with the aim of establishing the appropriate milieu in which recovery from critical illness can occur.

ACID-BASE STATUS

As previously discussed, pregnancy results in a compensated respiratory alkalosis in which P_{CO_2} and bicarbonate average 30 mmHg and 18 to 20 meq/L, respectively. During labor this respiratory alkalosis worsens due to maternal hyperventilation. Nonetheless, current evidence suggests that the resulting alkalemia is not clinically relevant. In one study, fetal oxygen delivery was not impaired when mothers hyperventilated in labor, as fetal P_{O_2} decreased by only 4 mmHg despite significant increases in maternal and fetal plasma pH.[50] Fetal compensation may result from the fact that alkalosis-induced leftward shift of the fetal hemoglobin saturation curve may preserve fetal oxygen-carrying capacity and carbon dioxide diffuses rapidly across the placenta, allowing quick reestablishment of acid-base homeostasis. Unlike spontaneous hyperventilation, however, respiratory alkalosis from excessive mechanical ventilation can cause fetal asphyxia in animal models as a result of decreased uteroplacental blood flow.[40] Furthermore, maternal metabolic alkalosis has been shown in animal models to significantly decrease placental blood flow and fetal carotid P_{O_2}.[51] Since severe respiratory and metabolic alkaloses in the critically ill are often a result of medical treatment—excessive mechanical ventilation, nasogastric suction, diuretic use, and corticosteroid administration—close monitoring of maternal acid-base status should allow prevention or early correction of the alkalosis.

Acidosis may be detrimental to the fetus and should be avoided. Decreased ventilation, with elevation of P_{CO_2} even to prepregnancy levels, will result in respiratory acidosis. Early intubation and mechanical ventilation are indicated in gravidas prior to the development of hypercapnia and severe respiratory acidosis.

Maternal metabolic acidosis occurs in normal labor and delivery, presumably as a result of hyperventilation and other muscle activity.[52] Lactic acid is produced and these maternal fixed acids pass rapidly to the fetus. In early labor fetal pH averages 7.30 and P_{CO_2} 45 mmHg, with a fall in pH to 7.20 immediately after delivery.[53] The pH falls secondary to a metabolic acidosis, which resolves over the first 60 min of neonatal life. When a maternal metabolic acidosis develops as a result of illness, treatment should be directed at the underlying process after a distinction is made between increased and normal anion gap acidosis. The use of bicarbonate to correct pH is controversial for both pregnant and nonpregnant patients as is discussed in Chap. 158. When bicarbonate is given, serum carbon dioxide levels rise and rapidly diffuse across the placenta. A slower rise of fetal bicarbonate levels occurs because of slower equilibration of charged species. Thus, infused bicarbonate may increase acidosis intracellularly or in fetal tissue beds. For this reason, if correction of an underlying acidosis or delivery are likely to be achieved within hours, treatment with bicarbonate is not recommended. Controlled mechanical ventilation to correct metabolic acidosis is indicated in those circumstances in which the patient is not able to generate sufficient respiratory compensation or the work of breathing will further aggravate the acidosis. This should permit the physician to guarantee an adequate level of ventilation to minimize the extent of acidosis.

PREVENTION OF GASTROINTESTINAL HEMORRHAGE

Pregnancy is not known to result in abnormal gastric acid secretion nor to vulnerability of the upper gastrointestinal mucosa to ulceration, but critical illness is often complicated by gastric erosion and severe bleeding. A number of interventions are currently used as prophylaxis against this common complication. All of them have at least theoretical problems for use in the critically ill pregnant patient.

Antacids and sucralfate act by mixing with and neutralizing gastric contents or by direct coating of the gastric mucosa. Because the enlarging uterus may divide the stomach into antral and fundal pouches, complete mixing of gastric contents is unlikely.[54] These agents, therefore, may fail as prophylaxis against gastric ulceration. Histamine-receptor blockers such as cimetidine and ranitidine have had limited use in pregnancy but appear safe for life-threatening situations. Cimetidine, but not ranitidine, has been shown to have antiandrogen activity and to cause fetal feminization in animals.[55] In a recent study of ulcer prophylaxis in postoperative patients the authors concluded that agents which neutralize gastric pH (histamine blockers and antacids) result in colonization of the upper gastrointestinal tract with nosocomially acquired gram-negative organisms. The increased risk of pneumonia noted in this group was not observed in patients treated with sucralfate.[56]

It is apparent that no agent is ideal. Nonetheless, a safe approach is to begin treatment with either sucralfate or antacids via nasogastric tube to obtain a $pH > 6$ and no accumulation of gastric residuals. The nasogastric tube should not routinely be hooked to suction. In patients unable to receive antacids or sucralfate, therapy with ranitidine should be considered, especially if the patient is near term. Since this therapy is likely to be given for a relatively brief period of time, the benefits of reduction of risk of gastrointestinal hemorrhage are likely to outweigh fetal risks.

NUTRITION

Total parenteral nutrition (TPN) has been used in pregnant patients for extended periods of time for disorders such as inflammatory bowel disease, esophageal stricture, and malignancy. Its use in acute malnutrition associated with critical illness is less well described.[57] During starvation the mother is favored over the fetus in animal studies and in human beings maternal body stores are maintained at the expense of fetal growth during semistarvation.[2] For these reasons aggressive and early nutritional support should be instituted. Patients who have not resumed normal oral intake within 3 days of the onset of critical illness should receive nutritional support. The gut should be used if possible and feedings given as a bolus by nasogastric tube or infusions by a soft duodenal feeding tube. Pregnancy will result in calorie requirements close to 40 kcal/kg/day. Sepsis, trauma, burns, and recent surgery are likely to increase this requirement. If severe liver disease is not present, 1.5 g/kg/day of protein and approximately 20 percent of calories administered as lipids are recommended. A variety of enteral feeding supplements will achieve these goals with tolerable infusion rates. Finally, electrolyte disorders are common in these patients and careful attention must be paid to serum calcium, phosphate, and magnesium levels with additional supplements given as necessary.

Patients who do not tolerate enteral feeding will require TPN. The same guidelines for total calories and distribution of calories as lipids, carbohydrates, and protein can be used. Theoretical concerns about the use of intravenous fat emulsions in pregnancy exist regarding possible placental infarction secondary to fat emboli.[58] Such complications have not been reported, however, and fat emulsions are used in our institution.

FDA DRUG CLASSIFICATION

Since pregnant patients being treated for critical illness may require multiple pharmacologic interventions, it is useful for the American intensivist to be aware of the Federal Drug Administration use-in-pregnancy ratings. Category A drugs are those that have undergone adequate controlled studies in pregnant women which failed to demonstrate risk to the fetus. Category B drugs are those with no evidence of fetal risk in human beings (if animal studies demonstrate risk, human findings do not; or if human studies are inadequate, animal findings are negative). Category C agents are those in which risk cannot be ruled out (human studies are lacking, and animal studies are either positive for fetal risk or lacking; still, potential benefits may outweigh risk). Category D refers to agents with positive evidence of fetal risk by virtue of investigational or postmarketing human data (still, in critical illness potential benefits may outweigh risks). Category X includes those drugs which are contraindicated in pregnancy.

CASE PRESENTATION

C.S., a 23-year-old gravida 1, para 0 presented to a local hospital at 25 weeks' gestation with fever, malaise, dyspnea, and a vesicular rash of 2 days' duration. She also noted nausea, vomiting, chest pain, and abdominal tightness. Physical examination revealed a temperature of 39°C (102.2°F) and a diffuse vesicular skin rash. The room air arterial blood-gas determination revealed a P_{O_2} 66 mmHg, P_{CO_2} 26 mmHg, and pH 7.49 with a saturation of 93%. Chest x-ray showed fluffy nodular infiltrates that were greatest at the bases. A diagnosis of acute varicella pneumonia was made, and she was begun on intravenous acyclovir. Progressive hypoxemia (arterial hemoglobin saturation 85% on 100% face mask) prompted intubation and transfer to the University of Chicago Medical Center.

On presentation to our hospital she was an anxious, intubated young woman. She was febrile with a temperature of 38.9°C (101.9°F), pulse of 122 beats/min, blood pressure 110/60, and she was breathing 30 times/min. Skin examination again revealed diffuse vesicular lesions covering the entire body. Her lungs were clear. Cardiovascular examination was remarkable for a hyperdynamic precordium. Her abdominal examination was notable for a uterus that was soft and nontender at 25 cm. The cervix was 1 cm dilated and 30 percent effaced, membranes were intact, and the fetal heart rate was 150 beats/min. There was radiographic evidence of diffuse, bilateral interstitial infiltrates. The arterial blood-gas values on a F_{IO_2} of 0.5 and 5 cmH_2O of PEEP were P_{O_2} 108 mmHg, P_{CO_2} 28 mmHg, and pH 7.45. The hematocrit was 32 percent and the white blood cell count 8800 with

40 percent polymorphonuclear leukocytes, 45 percent bands, 10 percent lymphocytes, and 5 percent monocytes. Her coagulation profile was normal, as were kidney function studies. Her liver function studies showed an elevated aspartate aminotransferase of 79, an alanine aminotransferase of 44, a lactic dehydrogenase of 282, with a normal alkaline phosphatase and total bilirubin. Her urinalysis showed many polymorphonuclear leukocytes and bacteria.

The admission diagnosis was ARDS due to acute varicella pneumonia. Immediately after transfer, progressive severe hypoxemia developed requiring a F_{IO_2} of 1.0, tidal volume 500 mL, rate of 25 breaths/min, and PEEP 15 cmH_2O. Muscle relaxation and sedation were achieved with pancuronium and lorazepam. Fever was controlled with acetaminophen and a cooling blanket. Pulmonary artery catheterization was performed to assess fluid status and permit measurement of cardiac output and intrapulmonary shunt fraction. Her initial Ppw was 15 mmHg, with a cardiac output of 6.5 L/min, a narrow $(A - V)_{O_2}$ content difference, and an intrapulmonary shunt of 43 percent. Furosemide, in doses of 10 to 20 mg, was given intravenously to reduce intravascular volume, reduce lung liquid, and thus permit tapering of potentially toxic ventilator therapy. When her Ppw was decreased to 8 mmHg, her cardiac output fell to 5.0 L/min and dobutamine in low doses (3 μg/kg/min) was begun with improvement in cardiac output to 7.1 L/min. Her oxygenation quickly improved, and her F_{IO_2} was decreased to 60%.

Immediately on transfer to our hospital, conjoint consultation of the critical care service, obstetrics, and neonatology occurred. Coincident with the deterioration in oxygenation, preterm labor began. Continuous external fetal heart rate monitoring was performed, and magnesium sulfate was given intravenously for tocolysis.

Preterm labor was arrested. She continued on acyclovir for the active varicella infection, cefazolin for an *E. coli* urinary tract infection, and enteral nutrition via a duodenal feeding tube was begun. Sucralfate was given as gastrointestinal bleeding prophylaxis.

Over the course of the next week her skin lesions resolved, she became afebrile, her oxygenation improved, and her shunt decreased to 13 percent. She was placed on 40% continuous positive airway pressure (CPAP) with excellent oxygenation. Preterm labor continued to progress despite the magnesium sulfate tocolysis, and tocolysis with ritodrine was begun. Eight hours later she became febrile and developed a new lung lesion with four quadrant filling on the chest radiograph and a deterioration in oxygenation requiring 100% F_{IO_2} and PEEP 10 cmH_2O. Right heart catheterization data showed no change in the Ppw of 10 mmHg, but a new shunt of 41 percent. Cardiac output was 10.4 L/min. Ritodrine was stopped and furosemide given with brisk diuresis and improvement in oxygenation.

Vaginal examination later that day revealed some bleeding, and a nitrazene test was positive for amniotic fluid. Labor was induced with Pitressin because of evidence for amnionitis. Ampicillin and gentamicin were begun after cultures were obtained. Coagulation parameters were monitored because of evidence for abruption.

Eight hours later the patient delivered a 1040-g male infant in the ICU, with Apgar scores of 4 and 5 at 1 and 5 min, respectively. The infant was intubated immediately and lavaged with artificial surfactant before being transferred to the neonatal ICU. During labor, oxygen delivery was maximized by ensuring adequate oxygenation ($P_{O_2} > 90$ mmHg) and cardiac output. Oxygen consumption was reduced with intravenous midazolam, fentanyl, and pancuronium. Despite this, during the most active stage of labor her $(A - V)_{O_2}$ content difference widened to 5.5 vol %.

Her subsequent course was one of progressive improvement, and she was extubated 2 days after delivery. Her infant did not develop respiratory distress but required 10 days in the neonatal ICU because of initial muscle paralysis and subsequent difficulties with feeding and requirement for oxygen therapy. Both mother and child were eventually discharged home with normal cardiopulmonary and neurologic function.

CASE DISCUSSION

This case exhibits many of the features of critical illness in pregnancy and highlights a number of management issues. Intubation and mechanical ventilation were carried out early in this patient's course to ensure adequate oxygen delivery to maternal and fetal tissues. The patient was transferred to a facility where the full complement of subspecialists necessary to address the myriad problems arising in such a case were available.

Early ventilator management of acute hypoxemic respiratory failure entailed low tidal volumes and PEEP to achieve a nontoxic F_{IO_2}. Throughout the period of mechanical ventilation the patient was managed, when possible, in the lateral decubitus position, and fetal heart rate was monitored. Labor was avoided with magnesium sulfate infusion during the period of early respiratory failure. Initial hemodynamic data were typical of pregnancy, with a high cardiac output. The pulmonary capillary leak was reduced by diuresis and fluid reduction. Dobutamine was used to maintain an adequate cardiac output at a lower Ppw.

Following an initial improvement in gas exchange, tocolysis with ritodrine was undertaken since preterm labor progressed despite magnesium sulfate. It seems likely that this β-adrenergic agonist contributed to edemagenesis, although her lung function worsened coincident with the development of fever and bacteremia. The patient improved quickly with diuresis as is typical of tocolytic-associated pulmonary edema.

Subsequent delivery of her infant was accomplished on the ventilator. She received muscle relaxation to minimize aerobic requirements by other tissue beds during this period of stress. The infant's initial low Apgar scores were likely a result of the action of these agents, which freely cross the placenta, illustrating the importance of considering both the fetal and maternal consequences of all interventions, particularly drug administration. The ultimate excellent outcome for mother and infant is a tribute to the coordination and efforts of the intensive care, obstetric, neonatal, and anesthesia staff involved in their care.

References

1. Sullivan JM, Ramanathan KB: Management of medical problems in pregnancy—Severe cardiac disease. N Engl J Med 313:304, 1985.
2. Hollingsworth HM, Pratter MR, Irwin RS: Acute respiratory failure in pregnancy. J Intens Care Med 4(1):11, 1989.
3. Capeless EL, Clapp JF: Cardiovascular changes in early phase of pregnancy. Am J Obstet Gynecol 161:1449, 1989.
4. Barron WM, Murphy MB, Lindheimer MD: Management of hypertension during pregnancy, in Laragh JH, Brenner BM (eds): *Hypertension: Pathophysiology, Diagnosis, and Management*. New York, Raven Press, 1990.
5. Weinberger SE, Weiss ST, Cohen WR, et al: State of the art: Pregnancy and the lung. Am Rev Respir Dis 121:559, 1980.
6. Gemzell CA, Robbe H, Stern B, Strom G: Observations on circulatory changes and muscular work in normal labour. Acta Obstet Gynecol Scand 36:75, 1957.
7. Pernoll ML, Metcalfe J, Schlenker TL, et al: Oxygen consumption at rest and during exercise in pregnancy. Respir Physiol 25:285, 1975.
8. Gilroy RJ, Mangura BT, Lavietes MH: Rib cage and abdominal volume displacements during breathing in pregnancy. Am Rev Respir Dis 137:668, 1988.
9. Baldwin GR, Moorthi DS, Whelton JR, et al: New lung functions and pregnancy. Am J Obstet Gynecol 127:235, 1977.
10. Edelstone DI, Paulone ME, Maljovec JJ, et al: Effects of maternal anemia on cardiac output, systemic oxygen consumption, and regional blood flow in pregnant sheep. Am J Obstet Gynecol 156:740, 1987.
11. Adamson K, Myers RE: Perinatal asphyxia—Causes, detection, and neurologic sequelae. Pediatr Clin North Am 20:465, 1973.
12. Parer JT: Uteroplacental circulation and respiratory gas exchange, in Shnider SM, Levinson G (eds): *Anesthesia for Obstetrics*. Baltimore, Williams & Wilkins, 1981.
13. Clark SL, Cotton DB, et al: Central hemodynamic assessment of normal term pregnancy. Am J Obstet Gynecol 161:1439, 1989.
14. Finley BE: Acute coagulopathy in pregnancy. Med Clin North Am 73:723, 1989.
15. Hayashi RH: Hemorrhagic shock in obstetrics. Clin Perinatol 13:755, 1986.
16. Weiner CP: The obstetric patient and disseminated intravascular coagulation. Crit Care Obstet 13(4):705, 1986.
17. Naeye RL: Abruptio placentae and placenta previa: Frequency, perinatal mortality, and cigarette smoking. Obstet Gynecol 55:701, 1980.
18. Gunning JE: For controlling intractable hemorrhage: The gravity suit. Contemp Obstet Gynecol 22:23, 1983.
19. Rosenthal DM, Colapinto R: Angiographic arterial embolization in the management of postoperative vaginal hemorrhage. Am J Obstet Gynecol 151:227, 1985.
20. Homans DC: Peripartum cardiomyopathy. N Engl J Med 312:1432, 1985.
21. Gianopoulos JG: Cardiac disease in pregnancy. Med Clin North Am 73:639, 1989.
22. Fishburne JL, Meis PJ, Urban RB, et al: Vascular and uterine responses to dobutamine and dopamine in the gravid ewe. Am J Obstet Gynecol 137:944, 1980.
23. Kirshon B, Lee W, Mauer MB, et al: Effects of low-dose dopamine therapy in the oliguric patient with preclampsia. Am J Obstet Gynecol 159(3):604, 1988.
24. Pearlman MD, Tintinalli JE, Lorenz RP: Blunt trauma during pregnancy. N Engl J Med 323:1609, 1990.
25. Williams JK, McClain L, et al: Evaluation of blunt abdominal trauma in the third trimester of pregnancy: Maternal and fetal considerations. Obstet Gynecol 75:33, 1990.
26. Rothenberger D, Quattlebaum FW, et al: Diagnostic peritoneal lavage for blunt trauma in pregnant women. Am J Obstet Gynecol 129:479, 1977.
27. Weber CE: Postmortem cesarean section: Review of the literature and case reports. Am J Obstet Gynecol 110:158, 1971.
28. Gibbs RS: Severe infections in pregnancy. Med Clin North Am 73:713, 1989.
29. O'Brian WF, Golden SM, Davis SE, et al: Endotoxemia in the neonatal lamb. Am J Obstet Gynecol 151:651, 1985.
30. Lee W, Clark SL, Cotton DB: Septic shock during pregnancy. Am J Obstet Gynecol 159:410, 1988.
31. Lackman E, Pitsoe SB, Gaffin SL: Anti-lipopolysaccharide immunotherapy in management of septic shock of obstetric and gynaecological origin. Lancet 1:981, 1984.
32. Sibai BM, McCubbin JH, Anderson GD, et al: Eclampsia. I. Observations from 67 recent cases. Obstet Gynecol 58:609, 1981.
33. Lindheimer MD, Katz AI: Preeclampsia: Pathophysiology, diagnosis, and management. Ann Rev med 40:233, 1989.
34. Mabie WC, Ratts TE, Sibai BM: The central hemodynamics of severe preecplamsia. Am J Obstet Gynecol 161:1443, 1989.
35. DePace NL, Betesh JS, Kotler MN: Postmortem cesarean section with recovery of both mother and offspring. JAMA 248:971, 1982.
36. Lee RV, Rodgers BD, White LM, et al: Cardiopulmonary resuscitation of pregnant women. Am J Med 81:311, 1986.
37. Noble PW, Lavee AL, Jacobs MM: Respiratory diseases in pregnancy. Obstet Gynecol Clin North Am 15:391, 1988.
38. Baggish MS, Hooper S: Aspiration as a cause of maternal death. Obstet Gynecol 59:33S, 1982.
39. Tomkinson J et al: 1982: Report on confidential enquiries into maternal deaths in England and Wales 1976–1978. Department of Health and Social Security, Report on Health and Social Subjects No. 26. London, Her Majesty's Stationery Office.
40. Levinson G, Shnider SM, deLorimier AA, et al: Effects of maternal hyperventilation on uterine blood flow and fetal oxygenation and acid-base status. Anesthesiology 40(4):340, 1974.
41. Gaensler EA, Patton WE, et al: Pulmonary function in pregnancy: III. Serial observations in patients with pulmonary insufficiency. Am Rev Respir Dis 67:779, 1953.
42. Hung CT, Pelosi M, Langer A, et al: Blood gas measurements in the kyphoscoliotic gravida and her fetus: Report of a case. Am J Obstet Gynecol 121:287, 1975.
43. McKim DA, Dales RE, Lefebvre GG, et al: Nocturnal positive-pressure nasal ventilation for respiratory failure during pregnancy. Can Med Assoc J 139:1069, 1988.
44. Schatz M, Zeiger RS, Harden KM, et al: The safety of inhaled beta-agonist bronchodilators during pregnancy. J Allergy Clin Immunol 82:686, 1988.
45. Gelber M, Sidi Y, Gassner S, et al: Uncontrollable life-threatening status asthmaticus—An indicator for termination of preg-

nancy by cesarean section. Respiration 46:320, 1984.
46. Clark SL, Montz FJ, Phelan JP: Hemodynamic alterations associated with amniotic fluid embolism: A reappraisal. Am J Obstet Gynecol 151:617, 1985.
47. Clark SL: Amniotic fluid embolism. Crit Care Obstet 13(4):801, 1986.
48. Pisani RJ, Rosenow EC: Pulmonary edema associated with tocolytic therapy. Ann Int Med 110(9):714, 1989.
49. Madinger NE, Greenspoon JS, Ellrodt AG: Pneumonia during pregnancy: Has modern technology improved maternal and fetal outcome? Am J Obstet Gynecol 161:657, 1989.
50. Miller FC, Petrie RH, Arce JJ, et al: Hyperventilation during labor. Am J Obstet Gynecol 120:489, 1974.
51. Ralston DH, Shnider SM, deLorimier AA: Uterine blood flow and fetal acid-base changes after bicarbonate administration to pregnant ewe. Anesthesiology 40(4):348, 1974.
52. Albright GA, Ferguson JE, Joyce TH, et al: *Anesthesia in Obstetrics: Maternal, Fetal, and Neonatal aspects.* Boston, Butterworth Publishers, 1986, Chap. 3.
53. Eguiluz A, Lopez Bernal A, McPherson K, et al: The use of intrapartum fetal blood lactate measurements for the early diagnosis of fetal distress. Am J Obstet Gynecol 147:949, 1983.
54. Holdsworth JD, Johnson K, Mascall G, et al: Mixing of antiacids with stomach contents. Anaesthesia 35:641, 1980.
55. Parker S, Schade RR, Pohl CR, et al: Prenatal and neonatal exposure of male rats to cimetidine but not rantidine adversely affect subsequent adult sexual functioning. Gastroenterology 86:675, 1984.
56. Driks MR, Craven DE, Celli BR, et al: Nosocomial pneumonia in intubated patients given sucralfate as compared with antacids or histamine type 2 blockers. N Engl J Med 317:1376, 1987.
57. Lee RV, Rogers BD, Young C, et al: Total parenteral nutrition during pregnancy. Obstet Gynecol 68(4):563, 1986.
58. Heller L: Parenteral nutrition in obstetrics and gynecology, in Greep JM et al (eds): *Current Concepts in Parenteral Nutrition.* The Hague, Martinus Nijhoff, 1977.

Chapter 89

HYPERSENSITIVITY REACTIONS DURING ANESTHESIA AND CRITICAL CARE

MICHAEL F. ROIZEN
JERROLD H. LEVY
JONATHAN MOSS

KEY POINTS

- *Antigen interaction with mast cell or basophil IgE immunoglobin or direct drug actions cause mast cell or basophil release of mediators of anaphylactic and anaphylactoid reactions.*
- *Common causes of hypersensitivity reactions are antibiotics, radiocontrast materials, muscle relaxants, colloids, preservatives, protamine, and narcotics.*
- *Histamine, eosinophilic chemotactic factor of anaphylaxis (ECF-A), slow reacting substance of anaphylaxis (SRS-A), platelet activating factor (PAF), prostaglandins, and kinins are the six known major pharmacologic mediators released in anaphylactic and anaphylactoid reactions.*
- *Symptoms caused by these mediators are usually immediate but may be delayed 2 to 15 min or, in rare cases, as long as 2.5 h after the parenteral injection of antigen.*
- *Since this reaction includes vasodilation and translocation of fluid from capillaries and postcapillary venules (resulting in loss of fluid and colloid from intravascular spaces), effective plasma volume and systemic vascular resistance is reduced followed by shock.*
- *The* sine qua non *of anaphylaxis is severe cardiovascular or respiratory compromise; most conscious patients sense impending doom before the clinical event occurs.*
- *Although various drugs are used to treat anaphylactic and anaphylactoid reactions, cessation of the offending drug, maintenance of the airway, administration of oxygen, blood volume expansion, and administration of titrated doses of epinephrine (very large doses may be needed) are the mainstays of therapy.*
- *Anaphylactic and anaphylactoid reactions are acute, potentially fatal events, but their morbidity and mortality can be reduced by preparation; drills, such as those done for cardiopulmonary resuscitation (CPR); prompt recognition; and aggressive treatment.*

Life-threatening hypersensitivity or pseudoallergic reactions to exogenously derived and administered agents in critical care environments can be, and usually are, successfully treated by a prepared intensivist.[1] These reactions are anaphylactic if immunologically mediated or anaphylactoid if chemically mediated. Rapid recognition and treatment of such reactions can prevent much of the morbidity and mortality that would otherwise occur.

Life-Threatening Hypersensitivity Reactions

Anaphylaxis is a life-threatening, allergic, or immunologically mediated reaction. The term "allergic" applies to immunologically mediated reactions, as opposed to those caused by pharmacologic idiosyncrasy, direct toxicity, drug overdose, or drug interactions.[2] Anaphylactoid reactions produce the same clinical syndrome but are not immunologically mediated. Antigen interaction with mast cell IgE immunoglobin or direct drug actions cause mast cell release of mediators of anaphylactic and anaphylactoid reactions (Fig. 89-1). Vasoactive mediators of these reactions include histamine, ECF-A, SRS-A (a mixture of three leukotrienes, including a potent coronary vasoconstrictor), PAF, kinins, and prostaglandins (see Fig. 89-1). Symptoms usually occur within 15 min of parenteral injection of the causative agent, though they may be delayed. The net effect of these agents is a marked decrease in systemic vascular resistance and the leakage of fluid from the capillaries and postcapillary venules. This reduction in effective plasma volume can result in shock. Thus, volume replacement and administration of epinephrine are therapeutic mainstays. Common causes of such reactions are antibiotics, muscle relaxants, colloids, preservatives, chymopapain, protamine, and radiocontrast materials.

The introduction of chymopapain into the armamentarium of the physician treating herniated nucleus pulposus taught us a great deal about anaphylactic reactions and their treatment. Prior to the introduction of immunoglobulin E (IgE) screening, there was a relatively high incidence of anaphylactic reactions associated with chymopapain administration. We speculate that physicians could reduce by more than 90 percent the morbidity and serious neurologic consequences associated with anaphylactic reactions if they understood the pathophysiology of such reactions. This speculation is based on the following data. In Australia and Britain, mortality rates from anaphylaxis are 3.4 and 4.35 percent, respectively, with an additional 5.6 percent of patients suffering irreversible brain damage.[3,4] In the United States, in a series of cases of anaphylaxis after chymopapain where physicians were aggressively educated and prepared for such reactions in advance, only 3 of 252 (<1.2 percent) patients died or had permanent sequelae.[5] This aggressive education and preparation involved knowledge of immunology, inflammatory mediators, and the therapy for shock, as well as pretreatment with H_1 and H_2 antagonists. Such a therapeutic plan minimizes the consequences of anaphylactic reactions.

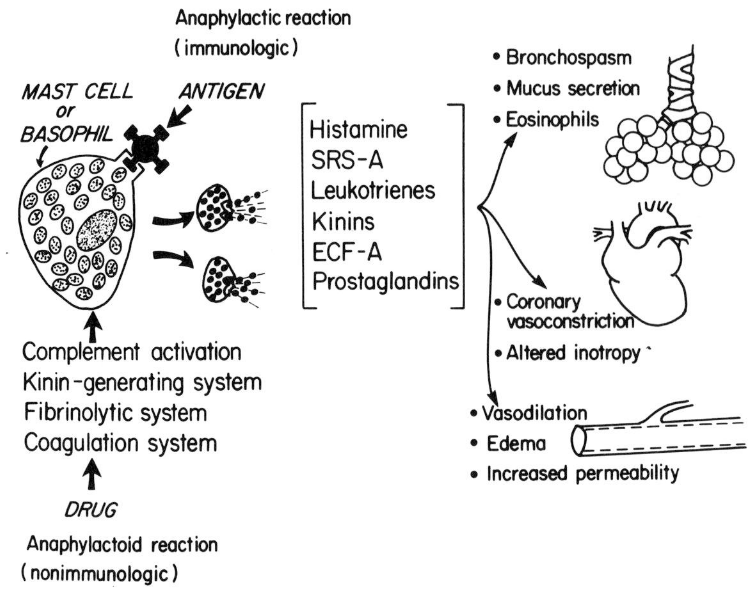

FIGURE 89-1 A summary of the pathophysiologic changes in anaphylactic and anaphylactoid reactions. Anaphylactic reactions (*top*). The allergen enters the body, combines with IgE antibodies on the surface of mast cells and basophils. The mast cells and basophils degranulate, releasing mediators (histamine, SRS-A, leukotrienes, kinins, ECF-A, prostaglandins, PAF, and others). The release of these substances is associated with the signs and symptoms of anaphylaxis—bronchospasm; pharyngeal, glottic, and pulmonary edema; vasodilation; hypotension; decreased cardiac contractility and arrhythmias; subcutaneous edema; and urticaria. Anaphylactoid reactions (*bottom*). The offending agent enters the body and works by nonimmunologically activating systems that cause degranulation of mast cells and basophils. The systems that can be activated to cause release of mediators from basophils and mast cells include the complement system, the coagulation and fibrinolytic system, and the kinin-generating system. Activation of these systems can result in the release of the same mediators from basophils and mast cells and in a syndrome that is clinically indistinguishable from anaphylaxis.

CLINICAL PRESENTATION

The end-organ effects of the mediators noted above produce the clinical syndrome, anaphylaxis. In a sensitized individual, the onset of the signs and symptoms caused by these mediators is usually immediate but may be delayed 2 to 15 min or, in rare cases, as long as 2.5 hours after the parenteral injection of antigen (Fig. 89-2).[6] After oral administration, manifestations may occur at unpredictable times. True anaphylaxis requires immunologically mediated release of some or all of these vasoactive mediators. In contrast, other mechanisms can liberate the vasoactive substances that produce this clinical syndrome. Patients with anaphylactic or anaphylactoid reactions may manifest some or all of the following signs and symptoms.[6,7]

RESPIRATORY SYSTEM

Patients may complain of nasal stuffiness or itching, difficulty in breathing, or retrosternal tightness. Coughing, wheezing, tachypnea, laryngeal stridor, and cyanosis are other manifestations, as are acute respiratory distress and pharyngeal, epiglottic, or glottic edema.

CARDIOVASCULAR SYSTEM

Patients may complain of dizziness or changes in consciousness. They may also complain of chest tightness, sometimes due to myocardial ischemia. A total loss of pulse indicates profound hypotension. Electrocardiographic (ECG) changes can vary from tachyarrhythmias and nonspecific changes of the ST segment or T wave, to ventricular fibrillation, electromechanical dissociation, and asystole.

SKIN

Complaints may range from itching, warmth, and minor swelling of the face or an extremity, to itching of the eyes and nonpitting deep edema in the cutaneous tissue. Patients may manifest the characteristic urticaria or flare of histamine release.

OTHER REACTIONS

Perhaps most impressive in the awake patient is the expression of a sense of doom. Fourteen of 16 conscious patients experiencing an anaphylactic or anaphylactoid reaction attended by the authors have said something like, "I feel horrible" or "I'm going to die" before any hemodynamic or pulmonary symptoms or signs were evident.

An anaphylactic or anaphylactoid reaction may involve any combination of the above symptoms; however, the sine qua non of anaphylaxis is severe cardiovascular or respiratory compromise. Since this reaction includes vasodilation and translocation of fluid from capillaries and postcapillary venules (resulting in loss of fluid and colloid from intravascular spaces), there is a reduction in effective plasma volume and systemic vascular resistance followed by shock.

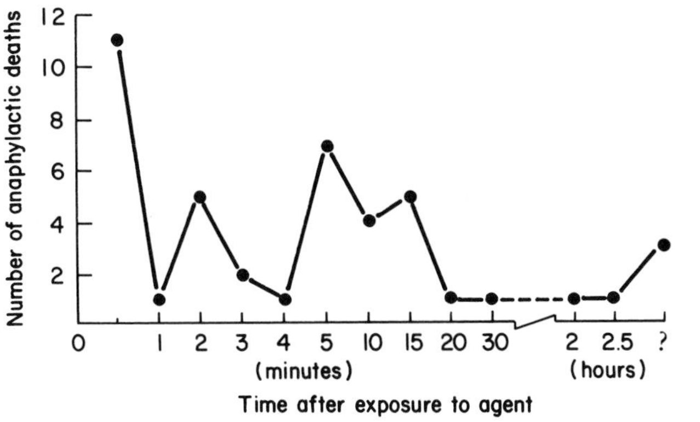

FIGURE 89-2 Interval between exposure and reaction to the allergen in 43 cases of anaphylactic death. Adapted from Reference 15.

Thus, fluid resuscitation is a first priority in treating this syndrome.

The most severe life-threatening reactions result from laryngeal edema, bronchospasm, and vascular collapse, probably end-organ responses secondary to the release of vasoactive substances. The full variety of vasoactive mediators of anaphylactic and anaphylactoid reactions is not known. Understanding the known pharmacologic mediators, however, helps explain the clinical manifestations and rationale for therapy of anaphylaxis.

MEDIATORS OF ANAPHYLACTIC REACTIONS

HISTAMINE

Histamine is a low molecular weight amine stored predominantly in tissue mast cells and circulating basophils. It dilates capillaries and venules and promotes vascular permeability. Its actions on the H_1 and H_2 receptors are thought to be responsible for both decreased systemic vascular resistance and increased permeability in venules.[8] Through H_1-mediated effects, histamine is also a potent coronary vasoconstrictor.[9] Vascular responses of vasodilation and local cutaneous reactions (wheal and flare) are mediated by both H_1 and H_2 receptors. H_2 receptors mediate chronotropic responses.

EOSINOPHILIC CHEMOTACTIC FACTOR OF ANAPHYLAXIS

ECF-A, an acidic peptide with a molecular weight of 500 to 600 daltons, is stored in mast cell granules. It is chemotactic for eosinophils. The exact role of the eosinophil in the allergic response is unclear. During phagocytosis, eosinophils release histaminase, phospholipase D, and arylsulfatase, enzymes that can inactivate histamine and SRS-A.

PLATELET ACTIVATING FACTOR

PAF, acetylglyceryl ether phosphorylcholine, causes platelet aggregation and bronchoconstriction, increases vascular permeability, and modulates leukocyte function.

SLOW REACTING SUBSTANCE OF ANAPHYLAXIS

SRS-A is synthesized in response to antigens and is not stored intracellularly. SRS-A is a mixture of products of the oxidative metabolism of arachidonic acid through the lipooxygenase pathway and is composed of three members of a class of compounds known as leukotrienes (leukotrienes C_4, D_4, and E_4).[10] End-organ effects include potent constriction of bronchial smooth muscle. On a molar basis, SRS-A is 4000 times more potent than histamine in causing bronchoconstriction in normal human beings. Other systemic effects of leukotrienes include cutaneous inflammation, chemotaxis of polymorphonuclear leukocytes, and promotion of lysosomal enzyme release from leukocytes.

PROSTAGLANDINS

Prostaglandins are unsaturated fatty acids synthesized at the time of the inflammatory stimulus. They are also products of the metabolism of arachidonic acid but through the cyclooxygenase pathway. Their biologic activities are specific to the target organ on which they act. Prostaglandins are potent mediators of the inflammatory response and can increase capillary permeability, bronchospasm, pulmonary hypertension, and peripheral vasodilation.

KININS

Kinins are low molecular weight peptides which enhance capillary permeability, dilate certain blood vessels, contract certain smooth muscles, and are perhaps leukotactic. Several processes independent of IgE can generate kinins.

SYSTEMS THAT CAN GENERATE ANAPHYLACTOID REACTIONS

Histamine, ECF-A, SRS-A, PAF, prostaglandins, and kinins are the six known major pharmacologic mediators released by interactions between an antigen and IgE, that is, true anaphylaxis. These vasoactive substances can be liberated independently of IgE by other mechanisms (i.e., anaphylactoid reactions) to produce the same clinical syndrome. There are multiple processes by which biologically active mediators can be generated to produce an anaphylactoid reaction; activation of the blood coagulation and fibrinolytic systems, the kinin-generating sequence, or the complement cascade can produce the same inflammatory substances as are produced in an anaphylactic reaction (see Fig. 89-1).

Histamine can be liberated independently of immunologic reactions. Mast cells and basophils release histamine in response to chemicals or drugs.[11] Most narcotics in high doses can release histamine,[12] producing an anaphylactoid reaction. Such high doses are rarely administered fast enough to release histamine except when given to induce anesthesia. Sedative doses of narcotics or slowly administered anesthetic doses usually do not release appreciable quantities of histamine. Radiographic contrast media and *d*-tubocurarine can also liberate histamine to produce anaphylactoid reactions.[13] Why some patients are prone to histamine release in response to drugs is unknown, but hereditary and environmental factors may play a role.

DETERMINING THE CAUSE OF ANAPHYLACTIC REACTIONS

Frequently, several drugs are administered in a short time, making it difficult to ascertain the drug responsible in an anaphylactic reaction. The course of events will often provide the answer, but if more than one drug has been injected or absorbed, various tests are available to identify the allergen. Skin testing is the most widely used, least expensive, and easiest to perform technique for evaluating sensitivity to an allergen. One of the problems associated with skin testing is false-positive results. In addition, reexposure to an agent that has produced serious adverse effects in the past may provoke another reaction.

Although complement levels may be unchanged and IgE may decrease after an anaphylactic reaction, these conditions do not prove immunologic involvement. As a test, patients have been given the suspected drugs intravenously, after which IgE levels have been observed. This procedure, however, can be life-threatening.

Antigen-specific IgE antibody can be measured using the radioallergosorbent tests (RAST).[14] In the RAST, a complex of a known antigen bound to an insoluble matrix is incubated with the patient's serum. The amount of immunospecific IgE antibody is determined by further incubation of the complex and serum with 125-labelled anti-IgE. Bound radioactivity reflects antigen-specific antibody and is compared with a reference system.

The RAST has demonstrated immunospecific IgE against such diverse agents as insulin, Hymenoptera extracts, and the penicilloyl derivatives of penicillin. A falsely positive RAST is rare, occurring in fewer than 0.5 percent of healthy, nonallergic human beings. Although the sensitivity and predictive positive value of RAST have been questioned, this relatively new test is promising. Specific matrices for most drugs remain to be developed.

If a patient must have a drug that is likely to trigger an anaphylactic or anaphylactoid reaction, several steps should be taken. First, an allergist should be consulted. Second, repeated injections of small amounts of antigen or offending hapten may be given, since this procedure decreases the amount of specific IgE antibody produced and may stimulate T suppressor cells. At the same time, this procedure usually increases the amount of competitive IgG antibody (i.e., blocking antibody). This blocking antibody can compete with IgE for receptors on the surface of basophils and mast cells to decrease the mediators released from these cells.

COMMON CAUSES OF ANAPHYLACTIC AND ANAPHYLACTOID REACTIONS IN CRITICAL CARE OR OPERATING ROOM ENVIRONMENTS

ANTIBIOTICS

Of all parenteral medications, penicillin causes the highest incidence (0.7 to 10 percent) of allergic reactions. However, the fatality rate from shock after administration of penicillin is 0.0015 to 0.002 percent. Retrospectively, penicillin accounted for 75 percent of all fatal anaphylactic reactions.[15] For this reason, penicillin should be administered carefully and with full knowledge of the patient's allergic history to it. Patients who are allergic to penicillin also have a 5 to 30 percent incidence of cross-reactivity with cephalosporins. Hypersensitivity to penicillin has been well-established as an IgE-mediated reaction to one of several moieties, the most common of which is the penicilloyl derivative of the molecule. Other antibiotics may cause anaphylactoid reactions. For example, when administered rapidly, vancomycin causes hypotension and flushing by a direct, pharmacologic effect.[16]

RADIOCONTRAST MATERIALS

Anaphylactoid reactions during radiocontrast material infusions occur in 1 to 2 percent of procedures.[17] The mechanism of such reactions remains unknown. These reactions have proved a fertile ground for retrospective analysis of the benefits of premedicants. When repeated infusions of radiocontrast materials were given to patients with a history of an immediate anaphylactoid reaction to them, the incidence of repeat reactions was 17 to 35 percent. In one study, pretreatment with prednisone and diphenhydramine was associated with subsequent hypotension in 3 of 415 previously reactive patients. But 0 of 180 and 0 of 100 previously reactive patients were hypotensive after pretreatment with prednisone, diphenhydramine, and ephedrine or pretreatment with prednisone, diphenhydramine, ephedrine, and cimetidine, respectively. Although these numbers are of necessity small, they seem to indicate that pretreatment with steroids, histamine receptor-blocking drugs, and sympathomimetics decreases hypotension without a significant risk of adverse effects.

CHYMOPAPAIN

Chymopapain, an agent used to treat herniated nucleus pulposus enzymatically, is associated with a 0.3 to 2 percent incidence of anaphylactic and anaphylactoid reactions. From the release of chymopapain by the Food and Drug Administration (FDA) in November 1982 until September 1983, the incidence of anaphylactic reactions was similar to that in the Phase II trial (i.e., approximately 0.4 percent in men and 1.3 percent in women for the first 30,000 patients treated).[5] Then the incidence decreased significantly (0.25 percent in men and 0.7 percent in women). The mortality rate from such anaphylaxis also decreased from 2 of 13 to 3 of 252. We believe that this successful outcome is attributable to awareness of the pathophysiology of such reactions, vigilance during administration of the drug, and pretreatment of the patient. Although prophylactic administration of antihistamines may not significantly reduce the overall rate of anaphylaxis, it may be a significant factor in reducing mortality attributable to anaphylactic reactions. Alternatively, increased physician awareness and treatment of anaphylaxis may be a significant factor in decreased mortality rates.

LOCAL ANESTHETICS

True allergy to the para-aminobenzoic ester agents, such as procaine, is well documented, but documented allergic re-

TABLE 89-1 Incidence of Anaphylactoid Reactions to Colloid Volume Expanders

Colloid	Incidence (%)
Plasma protein	
Plasma protein derivative	0.019
Human serum albumin	0.011
Dextran	
Dextran 60/75	0.069
Dextran 40	0.007
Starch	
Hydroxyethyl starch	0.085

SOURCE: Adapted from Reference 21.

actions to the amide local anesthetics are rare.[18] Methylparaben, a derivative of para-aminobenzoic acid and a preservative used in many multidose vials of local anesthetics, may well be the offending agent in anaphylactic reactions. If true allergy to one amide local anesthetic agent occurs, a potential for cross-reactivity exists. Although skin testing is used to identify safe local anesthetic agents, there is no support for applying this technique to human beings. Clinical history appears a good discriminator. Most "reactions" in the dental chair appear to result from anxiety or epinephrine responses. For example, in a series of 71 patients having a history of possible allergic reaction to local anesthetics, only 15 percent had a history of clinical manifestations that indicated a hypersensitivity response (i.e., urticaria, wheezing, or facial swelling).[19]

VOLUME EXPANDERS

Colloid

Anaphylactoid reactions to the clinically used colloids have been studied extensively in Europe (Table 89-1).[20,21] Because of kinin contaminants, the purified protein fractions (PPF) are associated with a higher incidence of reactions than are other colloids. The complex polysaccharides can activate the complement system. These reactions do not depend on prior sensitization. The reported incidence of anaphylactoid reactions after PPF varies from 0.007 to 0.085 percent.

Blood Products

Transfusion reactions can be classified as hemolytic or nonhemolytic. Hemolytic reactions result from ABO-antigen incompatible transfusions in which IgG or IgM antibodies from the donor or recipient react with red blood cells, complement is fixed and activated, and lysis of the cells and liberation of complement anaphylatoxins occur.[22] Urticaria, hypotension, and bronchospasm can occur along with activation of the clotting cascade. In a sedated and/or paralyzed patient, bleeding or severe hypotension may be the only sign of a transfusion reaction. The most common allergic reactions to transfusions are nonhemolytic, febrile reactions from leukoagglutinins. Unlike red blood cells, leukocytes and platelets contain HLA antigens of the human histocompatibility system. Antibodies of the IgG or IgM class to these antigens are known as leukoagglutinins. The precise relationship of leukoagglutinins to anaphylactoid reactions remains unclear. Patients who lack serum IgA will generate antibodies to IgA and may have a severe anaphylactoid reaction on transfusion of IgA-replete normal blood.[23] In most cases of transfusion reaction, the magnitude of cell lysis, hypotension, bronchospasm, and increased capillary permeability probably relates directly to the rate and extent of complement activation.

PROTAMINE. A number of case reports and studies have provided evidence that protamine reversal of the effects of heparin can cause a severe life-threatening reaction with generation of anaphylatoxins (C5a) and thromboxane.[24] It remains unclear whether these reactions are immune-mediated, caused by some other mechanism, or are a combination of immune-mediated reactions and those mediated by the freeing of vasoactive compounds with the displacement of vasoactive substances by protamine. Protamine is derived from salmon sperm—thus the theoretical possibility of antigenic crossover with fish allergy. Diabetics who have received protamine zinc insulin (PZI, 25 U contains 0.7 mg protamine) appear to have an increased incidence of this reaction as well as antibodies to protamine.[24,25] More than one mechanism may be involved; production of C5a anaphylatoxins by any mechanism generates thromboxane A_2, which causes pulmonary vasoconstriction, bronchoconstriction, and systemic hypotension. Substitutes for both heparin and protamine are being developed so that patients with known risk factors will be able to undergo safe cardiopulmonary bypass. Until then, dose modification, obtaining hexadiomethine (polybrene) via investigational drug request from the FDA, or using prostaglandin I_2 for cardiopulmonary bypass remain options.

NARCOTICS. Most narcotics (with the possible exception of the fentanyl family) may cause direct release of histamine, urticaria along the vein of administration, and vasodilation. Bronchospasm and angioedema have not been reported, even when large doses of these agents are used for anesthesia before cardiac procedures.[26] Codeine has been implicated in several cases of anaphylactoid reactions, but in all of the reported instances, more than one drug was used simultaneously. An anaphylactoid reaction to morphine and an inordinate sensitivity to histamine release have been reported, but skin testing in this patient produced negative results.[27] Meperidine is the only narcotic to which IgE antibodies have been demonstrated by RAST testing.[28]

THERAPY FOR ANAPHYLAXIS

Sometimes a patient with a history of an anaphylactic or anaphylactoid reaction must receive a substance suspected of producing such a reaction (e.g., iodinated contrast material). Also, some patients have a higher than average likelihood of a reaction (e.g., the atopic woman working in a

TABLE 89-2 Possible Therapy for a 70-kg Individual in the Event of an Anaphylactic or Anaphylactoid Reaction

1. Pretreatment
   A. Consider desensitization.
   B. Administer 50 mg diphenhydramine every 6 h for 24 h, 300 mg cimetidine every 6 h for 24 h, or 150 mg ranitidine every 9–12 h for 24 h; and 2 g hydrocortisone IV 1–6 h before anticipated exposure.
   C. Establish large bore IV and prehydrate patient with maintenance fluid and perhaps 500 mL more.
2. Plan for the worst and assign tasks in advance (e.g., who starts extra IV, who turns patient, who gets crash cart, who draws blood gases).
3. Initial therapy
   A. Stop administration of allergen.
   B. Maintain airway with 100% O_2.
   C. Stop negative inotropic and vasodilating agents.
   D. Expand blood volume.
   E. If indicated, administer 0.05–0.1 mg epinephrine (0.5–1 mL of 1:10,000 solution) every 1–5 min up to a total of 1–2 mg over 1 hr.
4. Secondary therapy (if indicated)
   A. Administer antihistamines (50 mg diphenhydramine, 300 mg cimetidine).
   B. Administer 5–9 mg/kg aminophylline over 20–30 min.
   C. Drip infusion of catecholamines.
   D. Administer steroids (2 g hydrocortisone IV).
5. Evaluate airway for edema before extubating the trachea.

meat tenderizer factory who is about to receive chymopapain). In such instances, pretreatment and therapy for possible anaphylactic and anaphylactoid reactions should be carefully planned (Table 89-2). Although virtually all "evidence" on these subjects is anecdotal, there is enough consistency throughout the literature to justify proposing an optimal approach to these problems.

First, predisposing factors should be sought, and the patient with a history of atopy or allergic rhinitis should be suspected as at risk. Because anaphylactic and anaphylactoid reactions to chymopapain occur five to ten times more frequently in women than in men, one might consider giving patients both H_1- and H_2-receptor antagonists for 16 to 24 h before exposure to a suspected allergen. Perhaps large doses of steroids (2 g hydrocortisone) should also be administered to women before exposure to agents associated with a high incidence of anaphylactic or anaphylactoid reactions.[29] Older patients present a special problem. They are more at risk of complications from both pretreatment (especially vigorous hydration and steroid administration) and therapy for anaphylactic reactions. Drugs likely to trigger anaphylactic or anaphylactoid reactions in this group should be avoided and treatment protocols altered.

Second, and most important, the treatment plan for an anaphylactic or anaphylactoid reaction should be reviewed with other physicians and nurses caring for the patient, and specific tasks should be assigned in advance (e.g., who starts the second intravenous infusion, who turns the patient supine). The slight probability of a serious reaction does not justify lack of planning. If the worst is expected and planned for, adverse outcomes of anaphylactic and anaphylactoid reactions can probably be reduced.

Although various drugs are used to treat anaphylactic and anaphylactoid reactions, cessation of the offending drug, maintenance of the airway, administration of oxygen, blood volume expansion, and administration of epinephrine are the mainstays of therapy (see Table 89-2). These procedures are necessary to treat the sudden hypotension and hypoxia that result from vasodilation, increased capillary permeability, and bronchospasm. Establishing a plan beforehand for the successful therapy of these reactions will diminish unfavorable outcomes. Although a dogmatic treatment protocol is not warranted by the data, data are consistent enough to justify a proposed treatment protocol. Anaphylactic and anaphylactoid reactions are triggered by different mechanisms, but the mediators released and the treatment for these severe reactions are indistinguishable.

INITIAL THERAPY

1. *Discontinue suspected allergen.* This prevents further recruitment of mast cells and release of mediators.
2. *Maintain airway and administer 100% oxygen.* Severe mismatching of ventilation and perfusion may occur from bronchospasm, pulmonary hypertension, and pulmonary capillary leakage.[30] These changes can persist for several hours during anaphylactic reactions, thereby producing hypoxemia. Therefore, the airway should be maintained and supplemental oxygen (we recommend 100%) should be administered until the situation improves. Intubation of the trachea should be considered if not already done.
3. *Discontinue all sedative, vasodepressant agents.* Agents that may have negative inotropic properties or that may decrease systemic vascular resistance should be discontinued since they may contribute to decreased vascular compensation and often interfere with the body's compensatory response to cardiovascular problems. Thus we believe that these agents should be discontinued to avoid hypotension.
4. *Expand blood volume.* Because up to 40 percent of intravascular volume is rapidly lost into the interstitial spaces in an acute anaphylactic reaction during anesthesia,[31] effective therapy consists of rapid replacement of blood volume.[32] Rapid fluid loss and successful treatment with fluid replacement have been documented with an anaphylactic reaction incidentally observed by transesophageal echocardiography.[33] Evidence does not indicate that colloid is more effective than crystalloid. Rapid administration of 1 to 2 L lactated Ringer's solution or normal saline is important in the initial therapy for these reactions. Further blood volume expansion may be necessary if hypotension persists.
5. *Administer epinephrine.* Epinephrine is a mainstay of therapy in acute anaphylaxis for several reasons. Its α-adrenergic effects make it useful for treating hypotension. Its β-adrenergic effects inhibit bronchoconstriction and the release of mediators from stimulated mast cells or basophils by stimulating the production of intracellular cyclic adenosine monophosphate (AMP).[34] For hypo-

tension, 0.05 to 0.1 mg epinephrine (0.5 to 1 mL of a 1:10,000 solution) should be given initially as an intravenous bolus and repeated every 1 to 5 min up to 0.015 mg/kg (or 10 mL of a 1:10,000 solution) for a 70-kg patient, as needed. If cardiac arrest or a total loss of blood pressure or pulse occurs, full cardiopulmonary resuscitative doses of epinephrine are indicated (0.01 mg/kg, not to exceed 1.0 mg total) along with rapid volume expansion. Larger, even massively larger, doses have been needed when titrated to effect, but we do not recommend them as initial doses, since hypertension and tachycardia resulting in myocardial cell death have been reported in such situations. Intramuscular or subcutaneous administration of epinephrine may be unreliable in a hypotensive patient who requires immediate therapy. Interactions with propranolol are possible, and care must be taken not to overdose the patient with epinephrine to the point of severe hypertension (unopposed α-adrenergic effects) and its consequence. Overdose can occur in the absence of propranolol as well. The major threat from chronic β-adrenergic blockade appears to be insufficient responses to epinephrine to terminate the reaction, and increased doses of epinephrine may be required.[35] We believe that any amount of epinephrine is appropriate when *titrated* to effect; the doses indicated above provide a starting point.

SECONDARY TREATMENT

If the above treatment does not result in resolution of symptoms and signs, further treatment with antihistamines, aminophylline, catecholamines, corticosteroids, calcium, and endotracheal intubation may be indicated.

Antihistamines

Histamine is one of the major mediators of the acute manifestations of anaphylactic and anaphylactoid reactions. Because the vasodilatory effects are mediated by both H_1 and H_2 receptors, both receptor sites must be blocked if all potentially harmful cardiovascular effects of histamine are to be antagonized. Studies involving the pretreatment of patients prior to histamine release demonstrate the effectiveness of preventing or blunting adverse cardiopulmonary responses when both H_1- and H_2-receptor antagonists are used.[36] Although histamine is only one of the mediators released in anaphylactic and anaphylactoid reactions, it may account for many of the initial adverse manifestations. No clinical evidence indicates that administration of antihistamines is effective in treating anaphylaxis once mediators have been released. Intact H_2-receptor blockade theoretically may facilitate the release of histamine and potentiate anaphylaxis. Administration of antihistamines is therefore recommended only as secondary treatment in acute reactions. (Suggested doses are 1 mg/kg diphenhydramine or 0.1 mg/kg chlorpheniramine, as H_1 blockers, and 4 mg/kg cimetidine, as an H_2 blocker.)

Aminophylline

If bronchospasm persists (and hemodynamic function is stable), aminophylline may be administered as a bronchodilator. (The initial "loading" dose is 7 to 9 mg/kg, which should be given over 20 to 30 min.)

Catecholamines

ISOPROTERENOL. If bronchospasm persists, isoproterenol may be useful as a pure β-adrenergic agonist and bronchodilator. This drug may also prove useful when combined with epinephrine in the patient taking β-adrenergic receptor blocking drugs. The β_2-adrenergic effects of isoproterenol cause vasodilation and possible hypotension, especially in patients already experiencing vasodilation or depletion of blood volume. Tachycardia is another possible unwanted effect. Because isoproterenol dilates the pulmonary artery, it may be useful in treating the increased pulmonary vascular resistance of severe anaphylactic reactions when oxygenation is a problem or right ventricular dysfunction occurs. (Starting doses for persistent bronchospasm are 0.5 to 1 μg/min/70 kg.)

EPINEPHRINE. When hypotension and bronchospasm persist, an intravenous epinephrine drip may be given after blood volume expansion and the administration of boluses of epinephrine. The starting dose of epinephrine is 1 to 2 μg/min/70 kg and should be titrated to the desired effect.

NOREPINEPHRINE (LEVOPHED). Blood pressure can be maintained in a hypotensive patient with norepinephrine until adequate volume expansion has been achieved. Although α-adrenergic drugs may theoretically potentiate the release of mediators, hypotension is deleterious to both cerebral and coronary perfusion and must be treated aggressively.

Steroids

Although corticosteroids are important drugs to consider and should be given in severe reactions, such as shock with refractory bronchospasm and hypotension, there is no evidence to suggest an appropriate dose or preparation.[29,37] We believe 2 g hydrocortisone phosphate (or its equivalent) is appropriate for severe cardiopulmonary dysfunction. Large doses of methylprednisolone (35 mg/kg) have been shown to inhibit complement-induced polymorphonuclear cell aggregation and lysosomal enzyme release in vitro. Corticosteroids may decrease release of vasoactive mediators and metabolites of arachidonic acid in anaphylaxis by stabilizing membrane phospholipids or by generating macrocortin, which inhibits phospholipid turnover.

Airway Evaluation

Laryngeal edema may occur in anaphylactic reactions, and swelling can persist.[38] If laryngeal edema has occurred, these structures can be examined on extubation.

Calcium

Since release of mediators is a calcium-dependent process, theoretic and experimental evidence indicates that its administration may worsen an anaphylactic condition.[39]

Further study is necessary to confirm the effects of trauma and sedative-hypnotics on immunity and the mech-

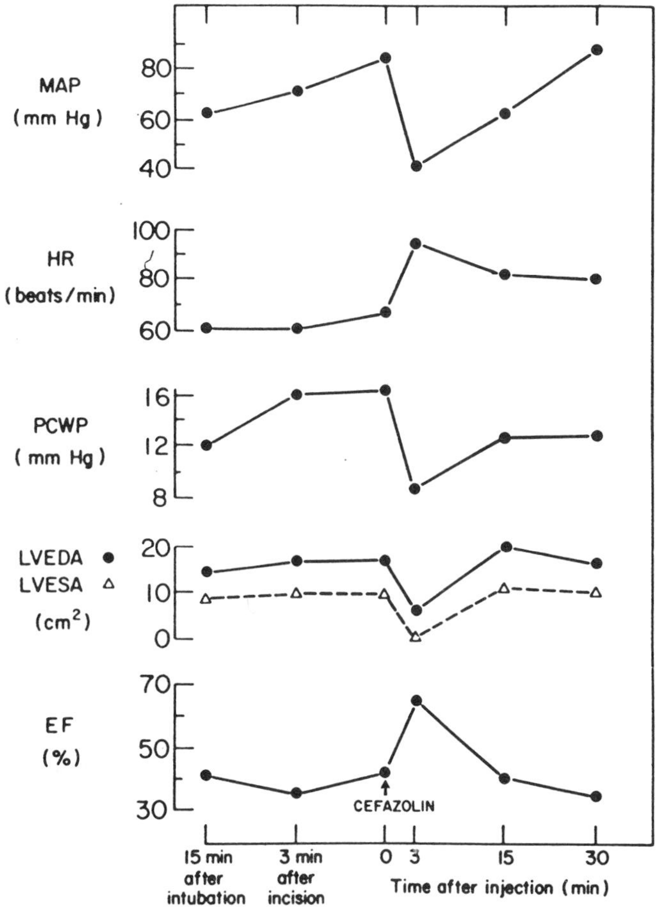

CI ($LITERS \cdot MIN^{-1} \cdot M^{-2}$)	1.88	2.17	1.95	3.69	2.75	2.89
SI ($ML \cdot BEAT^{-1} \cdot M^{-2}$)	30.8	35.6	28.7	38.4	32.3	36.2
SVRI ($DYNE \cdot S \cdot CM^{-5} \cdot M^{2}$)	1056	1081	1532	350	750	1077
PVRI ($DYNE \cdot S \cdot CM^{-5} \cdot M^{2}$)	187	117	89	43	59	252

FIGURE 89-3 Hemodynamic and echocardiographic changes before, during, and after an anaphylactic reaction to cefazolin. MAP, mean arterial blood pressure; HR, heart rate; PCWP, pulmonary capillary wedge pressure; LVEDA and LVESA, left ventricular end-diastolic and end-systolic cross-sectional areas; EF, ejection fraction (LVEDA − LVESA)/LVEDA; CI, cardiac index; SI, stroke index; SVRI, systemic vascular resistance index; and PVRI, pulmonary vascular resistance index. From Reference 33.

anism of this alteration. For now we know that the perioperative period interferes with innate immunity (by mucous and skin membrane transgressions, for example), but it is not clear how much of a role altered acquired immunity plays. Our responses to the altered acquired immunity do, we believe, play a major role in patient outcome after such a reaction.

CASE PRESENTATION

A 60-year-old, 82.5-kg man was admitted to our hospital because of the acute onset of numbness and weakness in his legs. Absence of pulses in the legs led to the diagnosis of aortic occlusion. An aortogram revealed occlusion of the left renal artery and both femoral arteries by a thrombus, and blood flow to the legs and right kidney was minimal. An echocardiogram revealed a large pedunculated thrombus in the left ventricle and pronounced abnormalities in anteroseptal and lateral wall motion. A cardiac surgeon advised against immediate removal of the left ventricular mass, but because of the threatened loss of the lower extremities and impending renal failure, an aortobifemoral bypass graft, right renal revascularization, and left nephrectomy were planned.

The patient's medical history included many years of poorly controlled hypertension and severe coronary artery disease. Four years before this admission, he required a four-vessel coronary artery bypass. Within a year, however, an anteroseptal myocardial infarction occurred. Two years before admission, he had a second infarction (inferior wall of the left ventricle), this time complicated by congestive heart failure and residual exertional angina. Although 40 years before admission, facial and laryngeal edema had occurred after he had ingested aspirin, 10 years after that, penicillin was administered without incident. His current medications consisted of digoxin, furosemide, 1/2-inch 2% nitroglycerin ointment every 6 h, and sublingual nitroglycerin as needed.

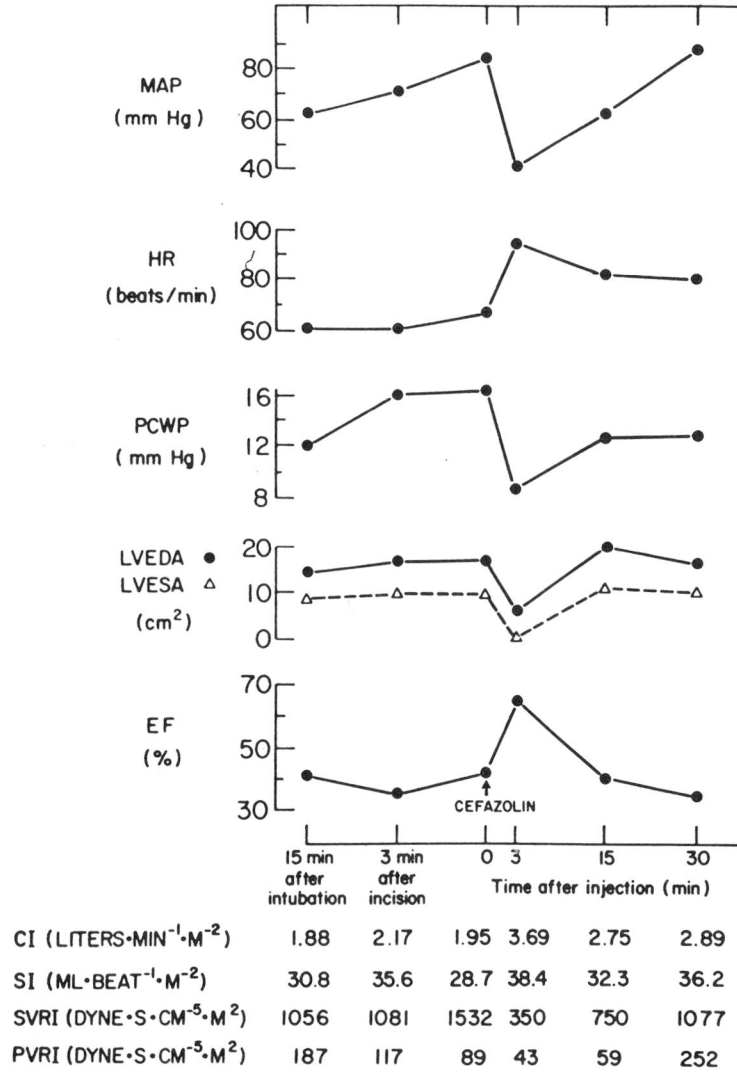

The night before surgery, the patient consented to participate in a study comparing two primary anesthetic agents, sufentanil, a new synthetic narcotic, and isoflurane. Because this patient was the second case of the day, his intravenous lines were begun in the ICU. At that time his pulmonary capillary wedge pressure (PCWP) was 12 mmHg, heart rate was 82 beats/min, and mean arterial pressure (MAP) was 100 mmHg. Prophylactic antibiotic was begun 1 h before his anticipated skin incision. Within 3 min of receiving 300 mg sodium cefazolin, heart rate increased from 67 to 96 beats/min, the patient thought he was going to die, and he complained of severe air hunger. An intense red discoloration covered his entire body, and MAP decreased from 95 to 42 mmHg, despite rapid infusion of 60 mL Ringer's lactate per minute for 15 min; 100% oxygen was administered via face mask. Over the next 15 min, MAP gradually increased to 63 mmHg. Total fluid administered in 15 min was 900 mL. The cefazolin was stopped at the first sign of red discoloration, and 1 mL of a 1/10,000 solution of epinephrine was titrated IV. No further epinephrine was judged to be needed. After a 2-h delay, the patient's course (including operative course) was uneventful. The hemodynamic changes are summarized in Fig. 89-3.

CASE DISCUSSION

This case demonstrates several aspects of an immediate hypersensitivity reaction (type 1), which is produced by the IgE-mediated release of pharmacologically active substances. Anaphylactic reactions can occur when an antigen interacts with IgE to cause degranulation of tissue mast cells and basophils, resulting in the liberation of histamine, prostaglandins, kinins, and SRS-A into circulation. Histamine and kinins have profound effects on the circulation, and histamine and SRS-A directly affect the myocardium. Because a component of SRS-A, leukotriene D_4, is a potent coronary vasoconstrictor, the hypotension of anaphylaxis may be due in part to myocardial ischemia. In animals, leukotriene D_4 has profound systemic effects similar to those of norepinephrine, resulting in increased systemic vascular resistance and MAP. These increases could cause further deterioration in myocardial function. However, we found no evidence of myocardial ischemia. The pronounced hypotension that occurred during this reaction appeared to have been caused by alteration in the loading conditions of the left ventricle and not by a deterioration in myocardial performance. The most pronounced hemodynamic effects concerned venous and arterial vasomotor tone. Values for PCWP, PVRI, SVRI, LVEDA, and MAP decreased at least 50 percent within 3 min of cefazolin administration. These changes probably are due to the early histamine release documented in human beings, because histamine is a potent vasodilator and has direct antidromic, inotropic, and chronotropic action when administered directly into heart muscle.

In this patient, who had preexisting left ventricular dysfunction and severe coronary artery disease, hypotension could have been expected to lead to decreased left ventricular performance. By the same reasoning, if leukotriene D_4 were a major influence in this setting, one would expect evidence of myocardial ischemia, left ventricular failure, or systemic pressor effects. However, no evidence of left ventricular dysfunction occurred during this anaphylactic reaction. Both PCWP and LVEDA decreased (the echocardiography monitor just happened to be present in the patient's ICU room), while stroke index, cardiac index, and ejection fraction increased. Furthermore, no changes indicating ischemia were seen on the V_5 ECG monitor, and no new abnormalities in wall motion were observed on the echocardiogram.

During an anaphylactic reaction, the temptation to administer vasopressors is strong. However, our patient responded to fluid therapy and 100% oxygen with only minimal amounts of epinephrine. Lack of need for epinephrine is unusual; usually epinephrine is titrated until blood pressure is increased. Its major effect may be in stopping degranulation. Data for our patient showed that within 20 min of fluid resuscitation, MAP and heart rate had returned to prereaction levels. We hypothesize that, in the controlled setting of the ICU, with three prepared physicians already at the patient's bedside, treatment of this man's anaphylaxis could focus on ensuring adequate oxygenation and replacing fluids. In many patients it is also appropriate to use epinephrine early in the therapy for anaphylaxis to prevent further degranulation of mast cells. Using a "pure" vasoconstrictor (i.e., norepinephrine) or myocardial stimulant (i.e., isoproterenol or dopamine) in these patients theoretically might increase myocardial work, induce myocardial ischemia, and precipitate arrythmias.

We were able to use volume alone in resuscitating our patient, who responded well. There was thought to be no advantage to adding antihistamines or corticosteroids. Thus, the mild episode of anaphylaxis, its prompt recognition and discontinuation of the offending agent, and our fortuitous monitors allowed us to use volume and only minimal epinephrine as treatment. This allowed us to proceed with the planned procedure without further delay. In other anaphylactic events, volume alone might not suffice and prompt treatment with larger titrated doses of epinephrine would be necessary.

References

1. Levy JH, Roizen MF, Morris JM: Anaphylactic and anaphylactoid reactions: A review. Spine 11:282, 1986.
2. Parker CW: Drug allergy. N Engl J Med 292:511, 732, 957, 1975.
3. Fisher MM: The epidemiology of anaesthetic anaphylactoid reactions in Australasia. Klin Wochenschr 60:1017, 1982.
4. Clarke RSJ, Dundee JW, Garrett RT, et al: Adverse reactions to intravenous anaesthetics: A survey of 100 reports. Br J Anaesth 47:575, 1975.
5. Moss J, Roizen MF, Nordby EJ, et al: Decreased incidence and mortality of anaphylaxis to chymopapain. Anesth Analg 64:1197, 1985.
6. Smith PL, Kagey-Sobotka A, Bleecher ER, et al: Physiologic manifestations of human anaphylaxis. J Clin Invest 66:1072, 1980.

7. Austen KF: Systemic anaphylaxis in the human being. N Engl J Med 291:661, 1974.
8. Plaut M: Histamine, H_1 and H_2 antihistamines, and immediate hypersensitivity reactions. J Allergy Clin Immunol 63:371, 1979.
9. Bristow MR, Ginsburg R, Harrison DC: Histamine and the human heart: The other receptor system. Editorial. Am J Cardiol 49:249, 1982.
10. Goetzl EJ: Mediators of immediate hypersensitivity derived from arachidonic acid. N Engl J Med 303:822, 1980.
11. Lorenz W, Doenicke A, Schöning B, Neugebauer E: The role of histamine in adverse reactions to intravenous agents, in Thornton JA (ed): *Adverse Reactions of Anaesthetic Drugs.* Amsterdam, Elsevier/North Holland Biomedical Press, 1981.
12. Rosow CE, Moss J, Philbin DM, Savarese JJ: Histamine release during morphine and fentanyl anesthesia. Anesthesiology 56:93, 1982.
13. Moss J, Rosow CE, Savarese JJ, et al: Role of histamine in the hypotensive action of *d*-tubocurarine in humans. Anesthesiology 55:19, 1981.
14. Wide L: Clinical significance of measurement of reaginic (IgE) antibody by RAST. Clin Allergy 3:583, 1973.
15. Delage C, Irey NS: Anaphylactic deaths: A clinicopathologic study of 43 cases. J Forensic Sci 17:525, 1972.
16. Newfield P, Roizen MF: Hazards of rapid administration of vancomycin. Ann Intern Med 91:581, 1979.
17. Greenberger PA, Patterson R, Tapio CM: Prophylaxis against repeated radiocontrast media reactions in 857 cases: Adverse experience with cimetidine and safety of beta-adrenergic antagonists. Arch Intern Med 145:2197, 1985.
18. Fisher MM, Pennington JC: Allergy to local anaesthesia. Br J Anaesth 54:893, 1982.
19. Incaudo G, Schatz M, Patterson R, et al: Administration of local anesthetics to patients with a history of prior adverse reaction. J Allergy Clin Immunol 61:339, 1978.
20. Ring J, Stephan W, Brendel W: Anaphylactoid reactions to infusions of plasma protein and human serum albumin. Clin Allergy 9:89, 1979.
21. Ring J, Messmer K: Incidence and severity of anaphylactoid reactions to colloid volume substitutes. Lancet 1:466, 1977.
22. Barton JC: Nonhemolytic, noninfectious transfusion reactions. Semin Hematol 18:95, 1981.
23. Schmidt AP, Taswell HF, Gleich GJ: Anaphylactic transfusion reactions associated with anti-IgA antibody. N Engl J Med 280:188, 1969.
24. Stoelting RK: Allergic reactions during anesthesia. Anesth Analg 62:341, 1983.
25. Stewart WJ, McSweeney SM, Kellett MA, et al: Increased risk of severe protamine reactions in NPH insulin-dependent diabetics undergoing cardiac catheterization. Circulation 70:788, 1984.
26. Lowenstein E, Hallowell P, Levine FH, et al: Cardiovascular response to large doses of intravenous morphine in man. N Engl J Med 281:1389, 1969.
27. Fahmy NR: Hemodynamics, plasma histamine, and catecholamine concentrations during an anaphylactoid reaction to morphine. Anesthesiology 55:329, 1981.
28. Levy JH, Rockoff MA: Anaphylaxis to meperidine. Anesth Analg 61:301, 1982.
29. Schreiber AD: Clinical immunology of the corticosteroids. Prog Clin Immunol 3:103, 1977.
30. Pavek K, Wegmann A, Nordström L, Schwander D: Cardiovascular and respiratory mechanisms in anaphylactic and anaphylactoid shock reactions. Klin Wochenschr 60:941, 1982.
31. Fisher M: Blood volume replacement in acute anaphylactic cardiovascular collapse related to anaesthesia. Br J Anaesth 49:1023, 1977.
32. Fisher MM: The management of anaphylaxis. Med J Aust 1:793, 1977.
33. Beaupre PN, Roizen MF, Cahalan MK, et al: Hemodynamic and two-dimensional transesophageal echocardiographic analysis of an anaphylactic reaction in a human. Anesthesiology 60:482, 1984.
34. Winslow CM, Austen KF: Enzymatic regulation of mast cell activation and secretion by adenylate cyclase and cyclic AMP-dependent protein kinases. Fed Proc 41:22, 1982.
35. Jacobs RL, Rake GW Jr, Fournier DC, et al: Potentiated anaphylaxis in patients with drug-induced beta-adrenergic blockade. J Allergy Clin Immunol 68:125, 1981.
36. Philbin DM, Moss J, Akins CW, et al: The use of H_1 and H_2 histamine antagonists with morphine anesthesia: A double-blind study. Anesthesiology 55:292, 1981.
37. Halevy S, Altura BT, Altura BM: Pathophysiological basis for the use of steroids in the treatment of shock and trauma. Klin Wochenschr 60:1021, 1982.
38. James LP Jr, Austen KF: Fatal systemic anaphylaxis in man. N Engl J Med 270:597, 1964.
39. Tanz RD, Kettelkamp N, Hirschman CA: The effect of calcium on cardiac anaphylaxis in guinea pig Langendorff heart preparations. Agents Actions 16:415, 1985.

SECTION G

NUTRITION

Chapter 90

FUEL UTILIZATION IN CRITICAL ILLNESS

DAVID H. ELWYN
JEFFREY ASKANAZI

KEY POINTS

- *Injury and sepsis increase energy expenditure (EE) and tissue catabolism in proportion to their severity.*
- *Increased substrate cycling (turnover) of proteins, fats, and carbohydrates is characteristic of the metabolic response to injury.*
- *Hyperglycemia, hyperinsulinemia, and increased gluconeogenesis are key parts of the metabolic response to critical illness.*
- *Fatty acid concentrations are normal, glycerol concentrations are increased, and ketogenesis is inhibited in injury and sepsis.*
- *There is a shift from glucose to fat oxidation in insulin-sensitive tissues.*
- *In stressed patients, brain requirements for glucose remain high, even during fasting.*
- *High concentrations of cortisol, glucagon, and catecholamines can largely account for the metabolic response to injury.*
- *The effects of the wound or sepsis are mediated by the afferent nervous system and by cytokines.*
- *The metabolic effects of malnutrition are opposite to those of injury and sepsis.*
- *EE of critically ill patients is difficult to predict; whenever possible it should be measured.*
- *Energy requirements of severely ill patients are 3000 to 3500 kcal/day; this is 150 percent of measured EE or twice predicted normal EE.*
- *Nitrogen (N) requirements of the severely ill patient are about 14 g/day; if the patient is also malnourished, N intake should be increased.*
- *Hyperglycemia may be an adaptive response to the high glucose requirements of the wound.*
- *No effort should be made to reduce plasma glucose concentrations below 250 mg/dL in severely injured or septic patients.*

Physical injury, burn injury, and sepsis effect similar changes in fuel utilization, the extent and duration depending on the severity of the insult. EE and tissue catabolism and mobilization or turnover of protein, fat, and carbohydrate are increased, and there is a shift from carbohydrate to fat oxidation associated with glucose and insulin resistance. Protein-energy malnutrition, a frequent accompaniment of critical illness, changes fuel utilization independently of these other effects, usually in the opposite direction. These changes can markedly affect nutritional requirements and can make it difficult to estimate EE. Whenever possible, EE should be measured in critically ill patients as a guide to nutritional requirements.

Tissue Catabolism

NITROGEN BALANCE IN ACUTE ILLNESS

Any kind of injury or sepsis will cause an increase in N excretion as compared to normal values. Typical increases in N excretion for a variety of conditions are shown in Fig. 90-1.[1] Since diet is the main determinant of N excretion, the values in Fig. 90-1 were measured during infusion of 5% dextrose (D_5W) as the only source of energy.[1] Under these conditions, N excretion is exactly equal to negative N balance. In normal subjects, negative N balance was about 4 g/day; with severe burns this rose to 27 g N/day, corresponding to 169 g/day of protein or about 850 g body cell mass. This is a daily loss of more than 2 percent of body cell mass, a rate that will produce severe malnutrition in 1 to 2 weeks. In the absence of any nutrients, N excretion in normal subjects roughly doubles and would be expected to also increase in burned patients. N losses with severe accidental injury are less than for burns, though still very large (see Fig. 90-1). N losses during elective surgery are less than for accidental injury and depend on the severity of the operation, being less for total hip replacement than for bladder cystectomy. In the particular group of moderately septic patients shown,[2] N losses were about the same as for the cystectomy patients. With more severe sepsis, N losses will be higher but are generally lower than are found with severe trauma or burns. N excretion in the malnourished patients (see Fig. 90-1) was higher than for normals and much higher than for fasted normal subjects, indicating substantial underlying stress, characteristic of hospitalized malnourished patients.

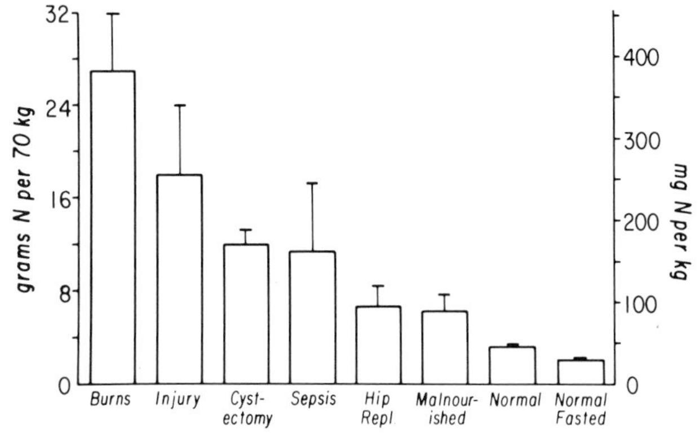

FIGURE 90-1 Total N excretion during 5% dextrose infusion in injured, septic, burned, or malnourished patients and normal subjects. Reproduced from Reference 1 with permission of Critical Care Clinics.

TABLE 90-1 Energy Intakes, Nitrogen Intakes, and Nitrogen Balances in Stressed Patients

Type of Patient	Time of Study	INTAKE N (g/day)	INTAKE Total Energy (kcal/day)	N Balance (g/day)
1. Severe multiple trauma	Immediate postinjury	14	1780	−11
2. Multiple trauma and	Immediate postinjury	0	3170	−13
burns >30%		24	3530	−6
3. Brain injury-Glasgow	Postinjury	13	2300	−11
Coma Score 4–9		17	2990	−8
		21	3450	−3
4. Multiple trauma and	Immediate postinjury	0	3300	−14
burns		7	3300	−6
		14	3300	−4
		21	3300	−3.5
5. Sepsis, moderate	Immediate postinjury	12.7	2290	−0.7
		24.3	2220	0.5
6. Burns, average 56%	4 weeks postinjury	23	3850	2

Adapted from Reference 3.

RESPONSE TO NUTRITIONAL SUPPORT IN STRESSED PATIENTS

Normal subjects given energy equal to expenditure and a protein intake above 5 g N/day will achieve zero N balance. Injured or septic patients are much more resistant to nutrients. They cannot achieve zero N balance at zero energy balance regardless of the N intake.[3] Data for severe injury or burns (Table 90-1) indicate that in the immediate postinjury period, which may last as long as 3 weeks, energy intakes of 3300 to 3500 kcal and N intakes above 14 g/day are associated with N balances of −3 to −6 g/day. At lower energy intakes negative N balance increases. When patients with severe multiple trauma received 1780 kcal/day (see Table 90-1), approximately equal to resting energy expenditure (REE) in normal subjects but about 33 percent below REE in these hypermetabolic patients, N balance averaged −11 g/day for the first 2 weeks postinjury.[4] This indicates a loss of nearly 5 kg (12 percent) of body cell mass in this period notwithstanding nutrient intake which is adequate in health. Other studies shown in Table 90-1 suggest that increasing N intake above 14 g/day has little effect on N balance in stressed patients.

This information indicates that severely injured patients require about 3500 kcal/day, roughly 50 percent above their greater than normal EE, to reduce N losses to an acceptable level of 3 to 6 g/day. When the stress is not great, zero N balance may be achieved within the first week. Even with severe burns, zero or positive N balance can be achieved in time (see item 6, Table 90-1). Elective surgery is associated with obligatory N losses for approximately 3 days postoperatively.[5] In some studies, enteral feeding is more effective in reducing N losses than parenteral feeding.[5] Other studies, of severe burns in both human beings and guinea pigs, indicate that immediate, full-strength enteral feeding reduces the metabolic response to injury and improves N balance compared to intravenous feeding.[3] This is attributed to protection of the intestinal mucosa, providing a barrier to invasion of the body by intestinal microorganisms or their products.

DISTRIBUTION OF TISSUE LOSS FROM MALNUTRITION

Autopsy studies indicate that all organs contribute more or less proportionally to N losses, except for the brain and nervous tissue which undergo little if any loss.[6] There is essentially no loss of N from extracellular tissues.[3] Since skeletal muscle comprises about 70 percent of body cell mass, most of the loss of protein during underfeeding and gain during nutritional repletion must occur in muscle. This has been confirmed by several studies measuring amino acid output of the leg or splanchnic region during starvation and refeeding.[3] There is no preferential sparing of either weight or function of the respiratory muscles, and malnutrition can result in significant loss of pulmonary function.[7] These processes in human beings are quite distinct from those in the laboratory rat, in which N losses during fasting occur mainly in the internal organs and losses from muscle are small.[8]

RESPONSE TO NUTRITIONAL SUPPORT IN STARVED PATIENTS

Malnourished patients are more receptive to nutrients than are injured or even normal subjects.[9] Unlike either of the latter groups, they can achieve markedly positive N balance at zero energy balance (Fig. 90-2). Nevertheless, they require 120 mg N/kg, at zero energy balance, to maintain N equilibrium, which is 50 percent higher than for normal subjects; this is likely related to underlying illness in these hospitalized malnourished patients who require parenteral nutrition. Increasing either energy or N intake will increase

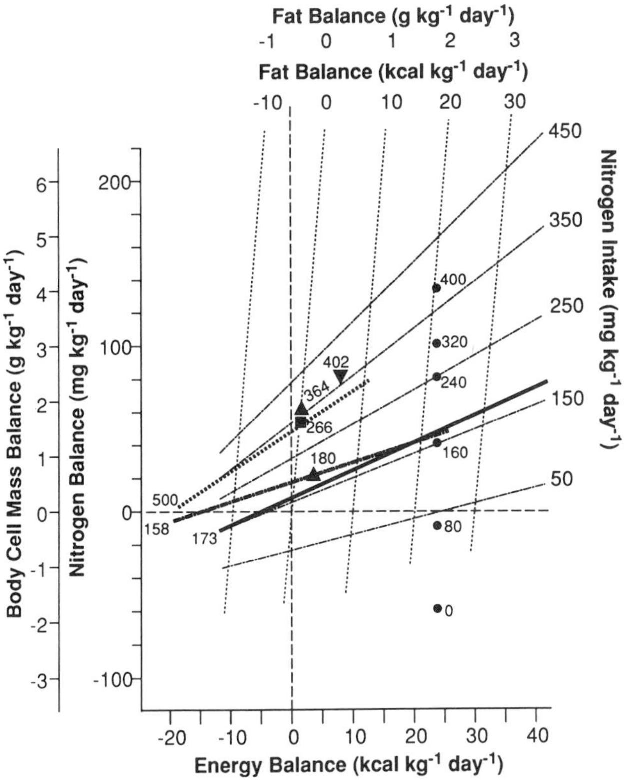

FIGURE 90-2 Schematic relation between nitrogen balance (ordinate), energy balance (abscissa), nitrogen intake (diagonal dashed lines), and fat balance (nearly vertical dashed lines) in malnourished hospitalized adult patients receiving parenteral nutrition. Derivation of grid as previously reported.[9]

N balance, and the effects of the two are synergistic (see Fig. 90-2).

However, the effects on fat balance are very different. Increasing energy intake increases fat balance, but increasing N intake has a slight negative effect on fat balance. At low N intakes, about 150 mg kg^{-1} day^{-1}, the ratio of body cell mass to fat restored is about 0.5:1; at much higher N intakes, around 400 mg kg^{-1} day^{-1}, the ratio ranges from 2:1 to 4:1. This makes it possible to influence the composition of restored tissue to conform to the composition of the tissue which was lost. With chronic starvation, characteristic of anorexia nervosa or chronic obstructive pulmonary disease, with intakes just below EE, the ratio of body cell mass to fat that is lost is about 0.5:1; with rapid weight loss, as occurs with fasting, or with injury or sepsis, the ratio is in the range of 2:1 to 4:1.[3] Nitrogen intakes up to 500 mg kg^{-1} day^{-1} appear to be well tolerated in malnourished patients who have adequate kidney function.[10] Many critically ill patients are malnourished, often seriously so. Patients who are both malnourished and injured appear to have the increased nutrient requirements of the injured patient, together with a response to increasing energy and N intake similar to the malnourished patient.

GLUTAMINE

Glutamine and alanine are the major carriers of amino groups in amino acid transport. Glutamine is also a preferred if not required fuel for rapidly dividing tissues, such as white blood cells (WBCs) and intestinal mucosa.[3,11,12] Immediately after injury or fasting there is a drop of 50 percent or more in muscle glutamine concentration[13] equivalent to some 8 g N. Although glutamine is not an essential amino acid in the usual sense, it appears that after trauma and in the absence of the usual dietary supply of glutamine, the rate of synthesis of glutamine becomes limiting even though there is a great increase in glutamine synthesis and export by muscle.[3,14] This increase in glutamine synthesis in muscle, after trauma, requires N derived from amino acids released by net degradation of protein. The most important N donors appear to be glutamate, serine, and aspartate. Although there has been much speculation on the importance of the branched-chain amino acids as N donors in this process, their actual contribution is relatively minor.[3,14] In support of the concept that glutamine synthesis is limiting after injury are findings that intravenous infusion of the stable peptide, alanyl glutamine, increases N balance, and muscle glutamine concentration in patients after abdominal surgery.[15] Although much research is in progress, commercial preparations of glutamine or its peptides are not yet available for intravenous feeding.

Increased Energy Expenditure in Critical Illness

REE increases up to 30 percent with accidental injury, up to 60 percent with sepsis, and up to 100 percent with severe burns.[16] Malnutrition may decrease REE as much as 40 percent. Mean values of REE (±SEM) for normal subjects and malnourished, postoperative, septic, or accidentally injured patients are shown in Fig. 90-3. These are presented either in kcal kg^{-1} day^{-1}, as measured, or as a ratio to predicted values as estimated by the Harris-Benedict equations (see Chap. 91). The effects of diet on EE are clearly shown for all patient groups. When compared to the predicted values of the Harris-Benedict equation, EEs for the injured and septic patients range from 5 to 25 percent above normal. However, compared to the normal subjects, who were maintained from 4 to 9 days on hypocaloric diets, they are 21 to 42 percent higher. Since patients are usually kept for several days on hypocaloric diets, this latter comparison gives a better indication of the effects of disease state on EE.[17] Many of the septic patients were also malnourished, accounting for the lower values found here than in previous reports.[16] The 95 percent confidence limits of the mean values for the patients average about ±25 percent, indicating a wide range of individual values. The relatively high values for the nutritionally depleted patients indicate considerable underlying disease. Burn patients, not included in this study, would have considerably higher values for EE. Other studies of ICU patients show great individual

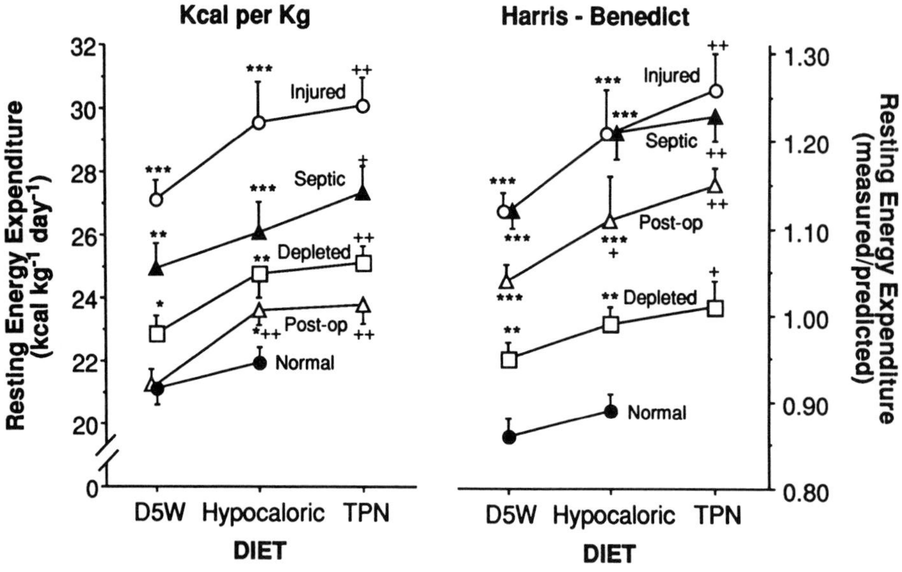

FIGURE 90-3 REE of 43 injured, 31 septic/depleted, 96 postoperative, 67 nutritionally depleted, and 37 normal subjects given intravenous diets. Data presented as kcal kg^{-1} day^{-1} or as percent of predicted values according to the Harris-Benedict equation. Energy intake, as a fraction of REE, averaged 0.31 with D_5W administration, 0.46 with the hypocaloric diet, and 1.35 with TPN. N intake averaged, in mg/kcal REE, 6.4 on the hypocaloric diet, and 10.2 with TPN. Means ± SEM. Differs from normal, $^*p < .05$, $^{**}p < .01$, $^{***}p < .001$; differs from D_5W, $+p < .05$, $++p < .01$, $+++p < .001$. Adapted from Shaw-Delanty, et al.[17]

variability and average values ranging from 5 to 40 percent above predicted, consistent with the data in Fig. 90-3. A large part of this increased EE results from the increased turnover or substrate cycling of protein, carbohydrate, and fat, which are energy-producing processes.[3]

Carbohydrate and Fat Metabolism

GLUCOSE METABOLISM

Both injury and sepsis cause increases in blood glucose concentration despite concomitant increases in insulin concentration.[3] Thus, traumatized patients are insulin resistant. They are also glucose resistant in the sense that, although glucose administration causes greater than normal increases in insulin concentration, the effects of this increased insulin are attenuated. The increased blood glucose level is due primarily to increased production from protein.[18,19] Unlike normal subjects, in whom gluconeogenesis is completely suppressed by administration of D_5W, gluconeogenesis in injured or septic patients is not suppressed until glucose intakes are >600 g/day.[20] Conversion of glucose to lactate and back, variously referred to as the Cori cycle, or turnover or substrate cycling of glucose, is also markedly increased with trauma.[18,19] The burn wound has been shown to use large amounts of glucose and to convert it quantitatively to lactate.[21] Extrapolated to a body burn of 40 percent, the wound can require as much as 300 g glucose daily.[3] Oxidation of glucose, as measured with isotopic tracers, also increases in response to injury,[18,19] but not to the same extent as glucose production or turnover. However, this includes glucose produced from protein and fat. Oxidation of glucose derived only from preformed carbohydrate, i.e., glycogen or dietary carbohydrate, as measured by indirect calorimetry, is reduced with injury or sepsis as compared to normal subjects under the same dietary conditions.

This is illustrated in Fig. 90-4 for injured, septic, or normal subjects given glucose as sole energy source for 3 days. At glucose intakes of either 0.35 × REE, equivalent to infusion of D_5W, or 1.2 × REE, glucose oxidation is less, and fat or protein oxidation is greater in the injured or septic patients as compared to the normal subjects. At a glucose intake of 1.2 × REE, fat oxidation accounts for almost 50 percent of EE in the septic patients, even though glucose has been given in excess of EE for 3 days. A corollary of decreased glucose oxidation at constant intake is that glycogen deposition must be greater than normal in the injured and septic patients.[3] The data in Fig. 90-4 show that the effects of trauma to cause hypercatabolism and glucose/insulin resistance are not always proportional. The septic patients were more insulin and glucose resistant than the injured patients, as shown by higher rates of fat oxidation and lower rates of glucose oxidation (see Fig. 90-4), and also by higher circulating concentrations of both glucose and insulin.[22] However, they were less hypercatabolic, as shown by lower rates of protein oxidation (see Fig. 90-4).

FAT METABOLISM

Concentrations of fatty acids are not increased with trauma and are little affected by increasing glucose intake or insulin concentrations.[3] Turnover of fatty acids is increased with injury or sepsis, and the normal linear relation between fatty acid turnover and concentration is lost.[23]

Glycerol concentrations increase with injury and, as in normal subjects, decrease in response to increases in glucose intake or insulin concentration.[22,24] The increase in glycerol turnover with injury or sepsis is much greater than the increase in fatty acid turnover, which is in turn greater than the increase in fat oxidation.[22,24,25] Glycerol turnover represents, to a first approximation, the amount of triglyceride hydrolysis (lipolysis) taking place in adipose tissue and muscle, which contain no glycerol kinase, and there-

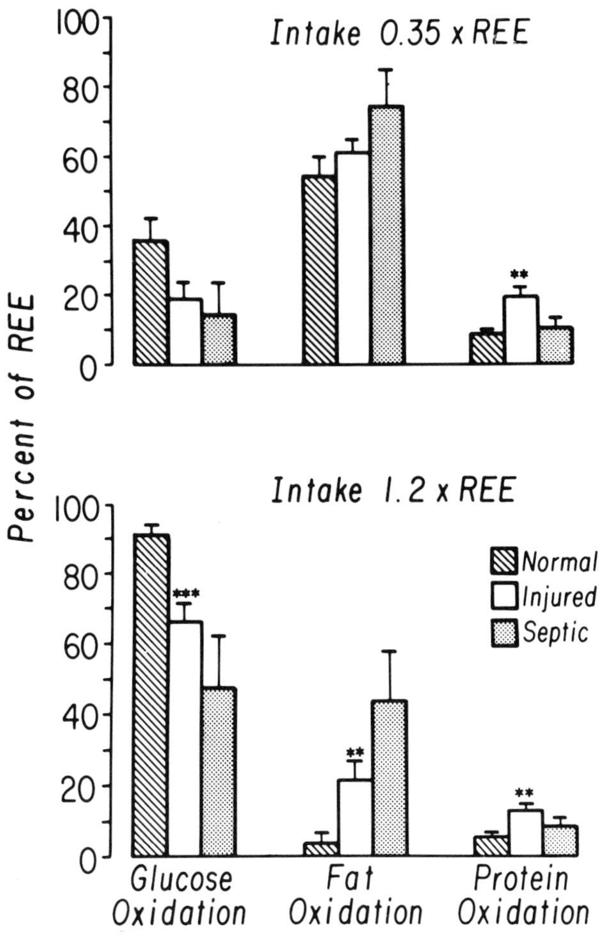

FIGURE 90-4 Glucose, fat, and protein oxidation in normal subjects and injured or septic patients given low or high glucose intakes as sole energy source for 3 days. All data have been normalized to glucose intakes of 0.35 or 1.25 × REE. Differs from normal: $^{**}p < .01$, $^{***}p < .005$. Reproduced from Reference 22 with permission of *Critical Care Medicine.*

fore, cannot reutilize glycerol, which is transported to liver and other tissues which contain glycerol kinase. The difference between glycerol release or turnover and fat oxidation represents the amount of fatty acids, formed by lipolysis, which are reesterified, constituting a substrate cycle. This substrate cycle is greatly increased with trauma or sepsis, much of it taking place within adipose tissue as an intraorgan cycle, but part of it taking place in the liver, thereby effecting an interorgan cycle.[3,22,24,25]

KETOGENESIS

Conversion of fatty acids to ketone bodies is decreased in injured or septic patients as compared to normal subjects on similar diets. The extent of the decrease is proportional to the severity of the insult.[26] As a result, ketone body production in the fasting traumatized patient is not enough to substantially reduce the brain's requirement of 100 to 150 g glucose/day, which must be supplied by net degradation of muscle protein instead.

Neuroendocrine Mediators of the Metabolic Response to Injury

There are two major pathways by which the body senses the presence of injury or infection. The first is the afferent nervous system, which is most important immediately after injury. Spinal analgesia during operation,[27] or severance of the afferent nerve fibers at or before injury[28] will prevent the appearance of the metabolic response in the first few hours after injury. The second pathway, which may be more important subsequently, is elaboration of cytokines by WBCs at the site of injury or infection. These act locally, but also have systemic hormonal effects. The best characterized of these cytokines are interleukin-1 and tumor necrosis factor or cachectin. Both the afferent nerve signals and the cytokines stimulate the hypothalamus, which acts through the sympathetic system and the pituitary to direct a concerted metabolic response. The cytokines also act on target organs such as muscle and liver. While both the afferent nervous system and the cytokines have the potential to effect all the changes seen after injury or sepsis, the exact quantitative contribution of each has not been determined.[3]

The major hormonal changes involve increases in cortisol, glucagon, epinephrine, and norepinephrine levels, the latter mainly representing increased sympathetic activity. In a report of severe burns, increases above normal for blood concentrations were two-fold for glucagon, four-fold for cortisol, eleven-fold for epinephrine, and eight-fold for norepinephrine.[25] Characteristically, insulin also increased by nearly two-fold. The extent of these hormonal changes will vary with the severity of the insult. Infusion of cortisol, glucagon, and epinephrine into normal subjects, at a rate to give plasma concentrations in the range seen with injury, can produce all the metabolic changes seen in stressed patients, including the increase in insulin concentration.[29,30] Thus, it would appear that these three counterregulatory hormones are the major endocrine mediators of the metabolic response to injury.

Why the Metabolic Response to Injury?

The metabolic response to injury may be perceived as a beneficial adaptation to provide an optimal supply of nutrients for wound healing and host defense under conditions in which food is not available; the nutrients must, therefore, be supplied from the body's own tissues. A key feature is maintenance of hyperglycemia. This is required to provide the poorly vascularized wound with large amounts of glucose which are not oxidized but glycolized, returning lactate to the circulation to be resynthesized to glucose in the liver. At normal fasting glucose concentrations, it is unlikely that the wound would be able to extract sufficient glucose for its needs. Since glycogen stores are limited, the glucose is obtained primarily from breakdown of muscle protein. The increase in muscle proteolysis is minimized because there is a shift from glucose to fat oxidation by insulin-sensitive tissues, mediated by increased concentrations of the counterregulatory hormones and increased sympathetic activity, and which occurs despite hyperglycemia and hyperinsulinemia. However, glucose and insulin concentrations are sufficiently high, despite the increases in cortisol, glucagon, and catecholamines, to markedly reduce the increase in ketogenesis normally associated with fasting. As a result, the brain must still obtain almost all of its energy from glucose oxidation, requiring 100 to 150 g glucose daily, which must be obtained by breakdown of 200 to 300 g protein. Thus, although the wound itself has no net requirement for glucose, its requirement for hyperglycemia means that the brain must obtain its glucose from breakdown of muscle protein, producing the hypercatabolism characteristic of injury and sepsis. Since the neuroendocrine changes are due to the wound or sepsis, they do not respond normally to food intake, and the wounded subject is resistant to nutrients.

If the hyperglycemia of injury is a beneficial response, the aim of nutritional therapy should be to maintain a reasonable level of hyperglycemia, not of course to the point of inducing untoward hyperosmolarity, rather than returning glucose concentrations to normal levels. In practice, no attempt should be made to reduce plasma glucose concentrations below 250 mg/dL. If concentrations rise higher than this, they should be controlled by reducing glucose intake, not by giving exogenous insulin. Since stressed patients are insulin resistant, exogenous insulin is ineffective; it also may cause severe hypoglycemia if the patient takes a sudden turn for the better.

CASE PRESENTATION

A 59-year-old man was admitted to the hospital with intermittent rectal bleeding. Past medical history included cigarette smoking at 1 pack/day for 40 years and symptoms of 4 to 5 block claudication in both legs. Findings on admission included blood pressure of 150/80 mmHg, pulse of 80 beats/min, breathing rate of 16/min. A sessile mass was palpated on rectal examination, and proved, on biopsy, to be invasive adenocarcinoma. He underwent an abdominal-perineal resection. On the eighth day after operation, he developed fever and signs of peritonitis and underwent exploratory laparotomy. At operation, the distal portion of the colostomy was seen to be necrotic. Surgical revision was performed. Ten days following the second operation, a third operation was performed due to peritonitis secondary to a necrotic colostomy cuff and multiple intraabdominal abcesses. The colostomy was taken down, a transverse loop colostomy was created, a feeding jejunostomy was placed, and the abcesses were drained.

Due to a jejunal-cutaneous fistula and continuing loss of weight, to 60 kg from 79.3 kg at admission, the patient was referred to the nutrition service for total parenteral nutrition (TPN) 38 days after admission. At this point his problems were probable ongoing sepsis with a persistent low-grade fever and rising WBC count and probable enteric fistula at the site of the jejunostomy. On the day of referral he received 5% dextrose solution as sole caloric intake. Vital signs were stable: blood pressure of 110/60 mmHg, pulse of 100 beats/min, respiratory rate of 28/min, and T_{max} of 101.4°F (38.4°C). His chest was clear to percussion and auscultation. The WBC count was 29,700 and hematocrit 34.1 percent. Plasma concentrations were: Na, 134 meq/L; K, 4.2 meq/L; Cl, 92 meq/L; urea N, 12 mg/dL; glucose, 203 mg/dL. REE was 1700 kcal/day, oxygen consumption ($\dot{V}_{O_2}$) was 368 L/day, carbon dioxide production ($\dot{V}_{CO_2}$) was 276 L/day, respiratory quotient (RQ) was 0.75, N balance was −10 g/day.

The patient was placed on a high calorie TPN regimen providing 2700 kcal/day as 85 g amino acids (340 kcal, 12.8 g N), 100 mL 10% fat emulsion (100 kcal), and 663 g dextrose (2260 kcal). Twenty-four hours after starting TPN he became gradually more tachypneic and complained of shortness of breath. Arterial blood-gas measurements were: pH, 7.51; P_{CO_2}, 26; P_{O_2}, 97; base excess, 0; bicarbonate, 20.5. Minute ventilation ($\dot{V}_E$) was 11 L/min. A chest x-ray was normal. A lung scan showed multiple focal defects in both right and left lung fields consistent with, but not diagnostic of, pulmonary embolism. Due to acute onset of symptoms and associated left calf pain, pulmonary embolism was considered likely. A pulmonary angiogram was negative, however.

By the fourth day of TPN, there were marked increases in REE to 2200 kcal/day, $\dot{V}_{O_2}$ to 452 L/day, $\dot{V}_{CO_2}$ to 416 L/day, and plasma glucose to 297 mg/dL. The RQ was 0.92; $\dot{V}_E$ was 16 L/min; glucose oxidation was 1536 kcal/day; fat oxidation was 368 kcal/day; and positive N balance averaged 1 g/day over the 4-day period. On day 5 glucose intake was reduced by 1000 to 1260 kcal/day, with a total intake of 1700 kcal/day. His dyspnea disappeared within 12 h.

By the sixth day REE had decreased to 1900 kcal/day, $\dot{V}_{O_2}$ to 400 L/day, $\dot{V}_{CO_2}$ to 340 L/day, and plasma glucose to 225 mg/dL. The RQ was 0.85; $\dot{V}_E$ was 12 L/min; glucose oxidation was 844 kcal/day; fat oxidation was 706 kcal/day; and N balance was −2.5 g/day. Over the next few days the sepsis resolved; WBC count and temperature returned to the normal range. After 7 days on the low calorie diet, REE was further reduced to 1800 kcal/day, $\dot{V}_{O_2}$ was 370 L/day, $\dot{V}_{CO_2}$ was 343 L/day, and plasma glucose had fallen to 140 mg/dL. The RQ rose to 0.93; $\dot{V}_E$ remained at 12 L/min. Glucose oxidation was 1270 kcal/day; fat oxidation was 206 kcal/day; and N balance was positive at 1 g/day. At this point the patient was returned to the high calorie TPN (2700 kcal/day) with no recurrence of dyspnea. Mean daily values for the following 7 days were: REE, 1900 kcal/day; $\dot{V}_{O_2}$, 373 L/day; $\dot{V}_{CO_2}$, 401 L/day; plasma glucose, 143 mg/dL; RQ, 1.08; $\dot{V}_E$, 13 L/min; glucose oxidation and conversion to fat, 2260 kcal/day; fat synthesis, 630 kcal/day; N balance positive at 3 g/day; fat balance 78 g/day.

Subsequent recovery was uneventful. The patient returned to full oral feeding 4 weeks later and was discharged from the hospital after another week.

CASE DISCUSSION

This patient combines severe malnutrition, 24 percent weight loss, with moderately severe sepsis, as indicated not only by fever and elevated WBC count, but also by the high plasma glucose level and REE which was 23 percent above that predicted by the Harris-Benedict equation. The response to high glucose hypercaloric TPN was characteristic; a 29 percent increase in REE, a 23 percent increase in $\dot{V}_{O_2}$, a 51 percent increase in $\dot{V}_{CO_2}$, and a 46 percent increase in plasma glucose level. Although glucose plus amino acid intake was in excess of energy expenditure, the RQ remained well below 1.0 and there was substantial oxidation of fat. Glucose oxidation remained well below intake, indicating substantial glycogen deposition. This response was complicated by development of tachypnea. Although there was reason to suspect a lung embolism as the cause of the dyspnea, this does not seem to have been the case. Rather, the dyspnea appeared to be due to the marked increases in $\dot{V}_{O_2}$ and $\dot{V}_{CO_2}$, and the associated increase in $\dot{V}_E$ to 16 L/min. That this respiratory load caused dyspnea indicates a low pulmonary reserve. The blood-gas measurements, showing Pa_{O_2} of 97 and respiratory alkalosis, indicate that the ventilatory response was excessive, a not unusual finding after interventions which increase $\dot{V}_{CO_2}$.

Reduction of glucose intake by 1000 kcal/day lowered $\dot{V}_{CO_2}$ and $\dot{V}_E$ sufficiently that the dyspnea disappeared. REE decreased with the lower intake, though glucose oxidation remained substantially below intake. With the resolution of sepsis, there was a further drop in REE, glucose oxidation rose to equal intake, and there was a marked drop in fat oxidation. When glucose intake was increased to a higher level once more, the RQ rose above 1, there was no net fat oxidation but rather a synthesis of fat from glucose. This was further confirmation that the sepsis was resolved.

N balance was barely positive on the initial high calorie regimen, but had the patient not been malnourished it would probably have been negative. When glucose intake was reduced, N balance became negative, but with resolution of sepsis it was again slightly positive even though total energy intake was less than expenditure. With return to the high energy regimen, N balance improved to 3 g/day and the ratio of body cell mass: fat restored was about 1.2. It is probable that, had the initial high energy diet contained fat and glucose in equicaloric amounts, no dyspnea would have occurred and there would have been no need to reduce energy intake. However, the effect on cumulative N balance would have been small, on the order of 10 to 15 g N over the 7-day period of reduced intake. In retrospect, N balance might have been substantially improved if N intake had been increased to 20 to 24 g/day after resolution of sepsis. Of course, more detailed nutritional evaluation and therapy earlier in the patient's course would have been appropriate.

References

1. Elwyn DH: Protein requirements in the critically ill patient. Crit Care Clin 3:57, 1987.
2. Greig PD, Elwyn DH, Askanazi J, et al: Parenteral nutrition in septic patients: Effect of increasing nitrogen intake. Am J Clin Nutr 46:1040, 1987.
3. Goldstein SA, Elwyn DH: The effects of injury and sepsis on fuel utilization. Annu Rev Nutr 9:445, 1989.
4. Francois G, Bouffier C, Dumont JC, et al: Protein catabolism in trauma patients. Ann Fr Anesth Reanim 2:238, 1983.
5. Rowlands BJ, Giddings AEB, Johnston AOB, et al: Nitrogen-sparing effect of different feeding regimes in patients after operation. J Anaesth 49:781, 1977.
6. Grant JP: Clinical impact of protein malnutrition on organ mass and function, in Blackburn GL, Grant JP, Young VR (eds): *Amino Acids: Metabolism and Medical Applications*. Littleton, MA, Wright PSG, 1983, p 347.
7. Arora NS, Rochester DF: Respiratory muscle strength and maximal voluntary ventilation in undernourished patients. Annu Rev Resp Dis 126:5, 1982.
8. Goodman MN, Larsen PR, Kaplan MM, et al: Starvation in the rat. II. Effect of age and obesity on protein sparing and fuel metabolism. Am J Physiol 239:E277, 1980.
9. Shaw SN, Elwyn DH, Askanazi J, et al: Effects of increasing glucose intake on nitrogen balance and energy expenditure in nutritionally depleted adult patients receiving parenteral nutrition. Am J Clin Nutr 37:930, 1983.
10. Forse RA, Elwyn DH, Askanazi J, et al: The effects of glucose on nitrogen balance at high nitrogen intake in malnourished patients. Clin Sci 78:273, 1990.
11. Newsholme EA, Crabtree B, Ardawi MS: Glutamine metabolism in lymphocytes: Its biochemical, physiological, and clinical importance. Q J Exp Physiol 70:473, 1985.
12. Souba WW, Scott TE, Wilmore DW: Intestinal consumption of intravenously administered fuels. J P E N 9:18, 1985.
13. Askanazi J, Carpentier YA, Michelsen CB, et al: Muscle and plasma amino acids following injury: Influence of intercurrent infection. Ann Surg 192:78, 1980.
14. Pearl RH, Clowes GHA, Hirsch EF, et al: Prognosis and survival as determined by visceral amino acid clearance in severe trauma. J Trauma 25:777, 1985.
15. Stehle P, Zander J, Mertes N, et al: Effect of glutamine peptide supplements on muscle glutamine loss and nitrogen balance after major surgery. Lancet i:231, 1989.
16. Kinney JM, Duke JH Jr, Long CL, et al: Tissue fuel and weight loss after injury. J Clin Pathol 23(suppl 4):65, 1970.
17. Shaw-Delanty SN, Elwyn DH, Askanazi J, et al: Resting energy expenditure in injured, septic and malnourished adult patients on intravenous diets. Clin Nutr 9:305, 1990.
18. Long CL, Spencer JL, Kinney JM, et al: Carbohydrate metabolism in man: Effect of elective operations and major injury. J Appl Physiol 31:110, 1971.
19. Wolfe RR, Durkot MJ, Allsop JR, et al: Glucose metabolism in severely burned patients. Metabolism 28:1031, 1979.
20. Elwyn DH, Kinney JM, Jeevanandam M, et al: Influence of increasing carbohydrate intake on glucose kinetics in injured patients. Ann Surg 190:117, 1979.
21. Wilmore DW, Aulick LH, Mason AD Jr, et al: Influence of the burn wound on local and systemic responses to injury. Ann Surg 186:444, 1977.
22. Jeevanadam M, Grote-Holman AE, Chikenji T, et al: Effects of glucose on fuel utilization and glycerol turnover in normal and injured man. Crit Care Med 18:125, 1990.
23. Nordenström J, Carpentier YA, Askanazi J, et al: Free fatty acid mobilization and oxidation during total parenteral nutrition in trauma and infection. Ann Surg 198:725, 1983.
24. Carpentier YA, Askanazi J, Elwyn DH, et al: Effects of hypercaloric glucose infusion on lipid metabolism in injury and sepsis. J Trauma 19:649, 1979.
25. Wolfe RR, Herndon DM, Jahoor F, et al: Effect of severe burn injury on substrate cycling by glucose and fatty acids. N Engl J Med 317:403, 1987.

26. Smith R, Fuller DJ, Wedge JH, et al: Initial effect of injury on ketone bodies and other blood metabolites. Lancet i:1, 1975.
27. Kehlet H, Moller IW: The effects of regional anaesthesia on the endocrine-metabolic response to surgery and infection, in Oyama T (ed): *Endocrinology and the Anaesthetist: Monographs in Anaesthesiology*. Amsterdam, Elsevier, 1983, p 23.
28. Egdahl RH: Pituitary-adrenal response following trauma to the isolated leg. Surgery 46:9, 1950.
29. Shamoon H, Hendler R, Sherwin R: Synergistic interactions among anti-insulin hormones in the pathogenesis of stress hyperglycemia in humans. J Clin Endocrinol Med 52:1235, 1981.
30. Bessey PQ, Watters J, Aoki TT, Wilmore DW: Combined hormone infusion simulates the metabolic response to injury. Ann Surg 200:264, 1984.

Chapter 91

EVALUATION OF METABOLIC REQUIREMENTS

SIMON BURSZTEIN
JEFFREY ASKANAZI

KEY POINTS

- *Nutrition is an essential component in the management of the critically ill.*
- *Energy expenditure (EE) can be calculated from measurements of oxygen consumption ($\dot{V}_{O_2}$) and carbon dioxide production ($\dot{V}_{CO_2}$).*
- *Instruments for measuring on-line EE can be used readily at the bedside of critically ill patients breathing spontaneously or mechanically ventilated.*
- *Estimation of EE from empirical equations in critically ill patients is unreliable for both evaluation of the degree of hypermetabolism and for determination of nutritional requirements.*
- *For clinical purposes, nutrition may be supplied without precise measurements.*
- *There is a correlation between cumulative negative caloric balance and mortality rate in critically ill patients.*

All vital functions depend on energy supply. In most instances, nutrition is supplied to the different types of patients based on an empirical evaluation of their energy requirements. The purpose of this chapter is to describe the means of evaluating energy requirements by noninvasive methods to allow a more rational approach to nutritional management in the critically ill.

A normal man of 70 kg has a pool of about 174,000 kcal for his energetic use (Table 91-1), as well as nitrogen (N) reserves enabling him to survive periods of starvation up to 70 days.[1,2] Injured, septic, traumatized, and surgical patients usually have increased energy demands and higher rates of protein breakdown, thereby decreasing their ability to endure the added metabolic stress caused by starvation. It has also been recognized that malnourished patients have inadequate tissue repair mechanisms associated with depression of the immune system. These abnormalities, together with those caused by the underlying disease, render the stressed or malnourished patient susceptible to severe infectious complications which may compromise survival. Observations made more than 20 years ago indicated an increased incidence and severity of postoperative complications in patients who were protein deficient[3] or who had lost more than 20 percent of their total body weight.[4] Nutritional support is now an essential part of the management of the critically ill.

TABLE 91-1 Caloric Stores in a Normal 70-kg Man

Fuel	Kg	Amount of Calories (kcal)
Fat	16	149,000
Proteins (mobilizable)	6	24,000
Carbohydrates (glycogen)	0.25	1,000
Total		174,000

To evaluate the metabolic requirements of critically ill patients, we shall describe how nutrients are used during a 24-h period of fasting, during prolonged starvation, and in hypermetabolic states. In the latter part of the chapter we shall discuss the basic principles of indirect calorimetry and other methods of evaluating energy requirements.

Energy Metabolism and Fuel Utilization during Fasting

During fasting, the body draws energy in part from stores of protein and glycogen, but fat represents the largest energy reservoir.[5–7] During the first days, both liver and muscle retain some glycogen, the actual amount depending on previous dietary intake. In this early period, liver glycogen and muscle glycogen both supply about 30 g glucose/day. However, brain glucose requirements of approximately 90 g/day are much greater than can be supplied by glycogen stores alone; the rest is obtained from hepatic gluconeogenesis. Gluconeogenesis uses amino acids, primarily from breakdown of muscle protein, and glycerol, derived from lipolysis of adipose tissue. Lactate and pyruvate, produced by red and white cells and other glycolyzing tissues, such as the kidney medulla and lens of the eye, are also substrates for glucose production in the liver. However, an equal amount of glucose is reconverted to lactate and pyruvate in these tissues, thereby constituting a metabolic cycle (called the Cori cycle) in which there is no net gain or destruction of glucose. A small amount of energy is also supplied to the brain from oxidation of ketone bodies even at this early stage of fasting. The proportions of glucose and ketone bodies used by the brain depend on their relative concentrations in the blood. After a few weeks, concentrations of ketone bodies are higher than those of glucose, and they provide more than one-half the brain requirements. At these high concentrations, ketone bodies are excreted in the urine; fasting of more than 3 or 4 days is therefore associated with metabolic acidosis, which will be partially corrected by the excretion of ketone bodies in the urine.

During fasting or starvation, an almost equal decrease in weight and intracellular N content is observed in most organs and tissues. These values remain nearly invariable in the brain and nervous tissues. Muscle, as the main component of body cell mass, is the major contributor of the 75 g protein provided during a 24-h fast. After 24 h, oxidation of protein and glycogen account for about 500 kcal/day, while the remaining energy, approximately 1300 kcal/day, is supplied by the oxidation of triglycerides from the adipose tissue.

After 4 or 5 days of fasting, the glycogen stores are completely depleted, and glucose and insulin concentrations are at minimum levels. An increasing fraction of gluconeogenesis takes place in the kidney, while EE is lowered by about 20 percent, from 1800 to 1500 kcal/day. Glycogen provides no further contribution, while protein supplies only about 80 kcal (correlating to breakdown of approximately 20 g protein). The remainder is derived from catabolism of approximately 150 g fat. More than one-half the brain's energy is furnished by ketone bodies. Except for the glycolyzing tissues and protein oxidation in the liver, other organs obtain all of their energy requirements from fatty acids. The adaptation to fasting, which consists mainly in minimizing glucose oxidation by the brain and replacing it with ketone body oxidation, permits a reduction in protein loss from 75 g at the onset of fasting to 20 g/day after several weeks. This is reflected in a decrease in urea excretion to nearly zero. Twenty grams protein corresponds to 90 g body cell mass. Since almost all the muscle mass, approximately 28 kg, can be lost before death, it should be theoretically possible to fast for about 200 days if loss of muscle were the limiting factor. However, fat stores are more limiting, and fasts of 60 days usually end in death.

Energy Metabolism and Fuel Utilization during Hypermetabolic States

Severe injury, burns, and infection are usually accompanied by marked alterations in energy metabolism and response to nutrients. EE is increased by about 10 percent after simple elective surgery, by 10 to 30 percent after trauma, by 30 to 50 percent with sepsis, and up to 100 percent with severe burns.[8] Starvation can reduce EE up to 40 percent. Because injured or septic patients are often starved to some extent, their change in EE will be the sum of the two effects. Indeed, EE in the critically ill can range from about 40 percent below to 60 percent above normal values.[9]

The injured, septic, or burned patient is hypercatabolic, as indicated by increased protein breakdown with increased N excretion, as well as hypermetabolic, as indicated by increased EE. As in fasting normal subjects, the bulk of N loss comes from skeletal muscle. As with EE, the extent of the N loss depends on the previous nutritional status and on the severity of stress. In fasting patients, it can exceed 30 g N or 150 g protein daily.

Most critically ill patients have hyperglycemia (termed insulin-resistant diabetes of critical illness). The glucose values vary from just above normal after elective surgery to as high as 800 mg/dl or more in severe cases. The hyperosmolarity associated with these very high glucose concentrations can have adverse consequences, with coma and brain injury among the most dire outcomes. Glucose turnover in trauma and sepsis results from both glucose oxidation and anaerobic glycolysis in wounds or infected tissues. In sepsis, white blood cells at the site of infection use glucose for glycolysis rather than oxidation. This is also true in injury or burn. Wound requirements have been measured[10] in severely burned patients in whom one leg was either severely burned (50 percent) or lightly burned (10 percent). Blood flow and O_2 consumption were measured for the whole body and for a single leg. Glucose consumption and lactate production were also measured in the leg. Leg blood flow, glucose consumption, and lactate production were much higher with the larger leg burn, but there was little difference in O_2 consumption. Almost all the glucose consumed was recovered as lactate. Thus, the major difference between the large and small burns was due to a difference in the amount of glucose used for glycolysis, not for oxidation. The energy derived from glycolysis of glucose is about twenty times lower than that obtained from oxidation of glucose, or 0.2 kcal/g instead of about 4.0 kcal/g. Thus, although the glucose requirements of the wound are very large, the energy delivered to the wound itself is relatively low.

Fat oxidation tends to be higher in hypermetabolic patients than in normal or malnourished subjects. This increase in fat mobilization is accompanied by marked increases in plasma concentrations of glycerol, but not fatty acids. Although fat metabolism and oxidation are increased with stress, ketogenesis is decreased compared to normal fasting subjects.[11] A major difference from normal patients is a significant increase in glucose production used mainly for glycolysis in the wound. However, glycogenolysis is suppressed, and most of the glucose comes from gluconeogenesis. Since ketogenesis is partly inhibited by high glucose and insulin concentrations, all the brain requirements in hypercatabolic-hypermetabolic patients are met by glucose. This increased glucose utilization is derived almost entirely from degradation of muscle protein which attains 2.5 times the rate observed in normal subjects.

Empiricism or Measurement in Nutritional Support?

Providing artificial enteral or parenteral nutrition to critically ill and other patients unable to feed themselves has greatly reduced morbidity and mortality in a number of pathologic conditions. The earliest applications of total parenteral nutrition (TPN) involved children with malabsorption syndromes, but nutritional support has now been demonstrated to benefit a wide range of patients, with significant impact on outcome, infection rate, and duration of hospitalization.[12–15] Much of this therapy has been applied using empirical assessment of caloric needs. While instances of overfeeding have likely occurred and some adverse consequences of excessive calorie administration have recently been described, the overall effect of heightened awareness of need for nutritional support has likely improved patient survival and reduced morbidity. However, although it is possible to manage many patients clinically with empirical assessment of caloric need, it is useful for the intensivist to understand the principles underlying measurement of metabolic requirements and to begin to approach patients selectively in terms of need for monitoring these parameters.

Evaluation of Metabolic Requirements

EE can be assessed accurately by measuring heat loss, a method termed *direct calorimetry*. However, the method of choice for most patients, especially acutely ill patients connected to respirators, infusion pumps, and other devices is *indirect calorimetry*. This approach relies on measurement of heat production from $\dot{V}_{O_2}$, $\dot{V}_{CO_2}$, and nitrogen excretion (NM). Indirect calorimetry is based on two principles: **1.** the law of conservation of energy, and **2.** the energy produced in the body from the oxidation of foodstuffs is equivalent to the energy produced by the combustion of these foodstuffs in the bomb calorimeter. While the end products of combustion of fat and carbohydrate in the bomb calorimeter and in the body are the same (H_2O and CO_2), producing 9.5 kcal/g and 4.17 kcal/g (3.74 kcal/g for glucose), respectively, this is not true for protein. In the body, the end products of protein metabolism are mainly urea, with some other constituents including creatinine, uric acid, ammonia, and 3-methylhistidine, with a production of about 4.4 kcal/g. In the bomb calorimeter, proteins are totally oxidized to CO_2, H_2O, SO_4, and NO_2, with production of about 5.7 kcal/g. Equations can be derived from these measurements for oxidation of carbohydrate (dCH), protein (dP), and fat (dF).[16]

Carbohydrate:

$$1\text{ g dCH} + 0.829\text{ L } O_2 \longrightarrow 0.829\text{ L } CO_2 + 0.67\text{ g } H_2O + 4.17\text{ kcal} \quad (91\text{-}1)$$

Protein:

$$1\text{ g dP} + 0.966\text{ L } O_2 \longrightarrow 0.782\text{ L } CO_2 + 0.41\text{ g } H_2O + 4.4\text{ kcal} \quad (91\text{-}2)$$

Fat:

$$1\text{ g dF} + 2.019\text{ L } O_2 \longrightarrow 1.427\text{ L } CO_2 + 1.07\text{ g } H_2O + 9.3\text{ kcal} \quad (91\text{-}3)$$

Equations (91-1), (91-2), and (91-3) represent fuel oxidation in the body. The three nutrients are probably metabolized simultaneously in different proportions according to the patient's condition and to many other factors, most of which are not well known.

The oxygen consumed in a given period of time is the amount required for oxidation of carbohydrate, protein, and fat. These nutrients use 0.829 L, 0.966 L, and 2.019 L oxygen, respectively, per gram of metabolized food. Simultaneously, carbon dioxide is produced in the amounts of 0.829 L, 0.782 L, and 1.427 L/g carbohydrate, protein, and fat, respectively. When the three nutrients are being metabolized, there is also heat production of 4.17 kcal for each gram of carbohydrate, 4.4 kcal for each gram of protein, and 9.3 kcal for each gram of fat. The above-mentioned facts are expressed by Eqs. (91-4), (91-5), and (91-6), representing events happening in the same period of time. Thus, they can be considered as a system of three equations with four unknowns. To solve these equations for dCH, dP, dF, and EE, one derives the value of dP from the urea excretion in the 24-h urinary output. Since 1 g metabolized nitrogen (NM) is produced by 6.25 g protein, the system of three equations with four unknowns becomes a system of four equations with four unknowns that can therefore be solved:

$$\dot{V}_{O_2}\text{ (L)} = 0.829\text{ dCH} + 0.966\text{ dP} + 2.019\text{ dF} \quad (91\text{-}4)$$
$$\dot{V}_{CO_2}\text{ (L)} = 0.829\text{ dCH} + 0.782\text{ dP} + 1.427\text{ dF} \quad (91\text{-}5)$$
$$\text{EE (kcal)} = 4.17\text{ dCH} + 4.4\text{ dP} + 9.3\text{ dF} \quad (91\text{-}6)$$
$$\text{dP (g)} = 6.25\text{ NM} \quad (91\text{-}7)$$

Since the amount of metabolized protein (dP) is already known from the measured urea or N in the urine, as shown in Eq. (91-7), the resolution of this system of equations allows the calculation of EE, dCH, and dF as a function of $\dot{V}_{O_2}$, $\dot{V}_{CO_2}$, and NM, as shown in Eqs. (91-8), (91-9), and (91-10).

$$\text{EE (kcal)} = 3.586\,\dot{V}_{O_2} + 1.443\,\dot{V}_{CO_2} - 1.180\text{ NM} \quad (91\text{-}8)$$
$$\text{dCH (g)} = 4.113\,\dot{V}_{CO_2} - 2.907\,\dot{V}_{O_2} - 2.544\text{ NM} \quad (91\text{-}9)$$
$$\text{dF (g)} = 1.689\,(\dot{V}_{CO_2} - \dot{V}_{O_2}) - 1.943\text{ NM} \quad (91\text{-}10)$$

Although $\dot{V}_{O_2}$ and $\dot{V}_{CO_2}$ may be measured by the Fick method, metabolic measurements are usually performed by noninvasive methods, by measuring volumes and concentrations of respiratory gases, thus:

$$\dot{V}_{O_2} = (\dot{V}_I \times F_{I_{O_2}}) - (\dot{V}_E \times F_{E_{O_2}}) \quad (91\text{-}11)$$
$$\dot{V}_{CO_2} = (\dot{V}_E \times F_{E_{CO_2}}) - (\dot{V}_I \times F_{I_{CO_2}}) \quad (91\text{-}12)$$

where: $\dot{V}_I$ and $\dot{V}_E$ are the inspired and the expired respiratory volumes, respectively, (over a determined period of time), $F_{I_{O_2}}$ and $F_{E_{O_2}}$ are the inspired and expired concentrations of oxygen, and $F_{I_{CO_2}}$ and $F_{E_{CO_2}}$ are the inspired and expired concentrations of carbon dioxide. In Eq. (91-12) the second term is usually neglected, since $F_{I_{CO_2}}$ is close to zero. NM can be derived from measurements of urea in the 24-h urinary excretion. While $\dot{V}_{O_2}$ and $\dot{V}_{CO_2}$ correspond directly to the O_2 consumed and to the CO_2 produced by the oxidation of nutrients during the measurement, the N measured in the urine does not correspond to the protein breakdown during the same period of time. There are indeed great variations in hourly urea excretions in a single day, and therefore the determination of protein breakdown from N excretion has to be performed over a 24-h period. It has to be emphasized that for EE measurement the factor NM may be neglected.

If we look at Eq. (91-8):

$$\text{EE (kcal)} = 3.586\,\dot{V}_{O_2} + 1.443\,\dot{V}_{CO_2} - 1.180\text{ NM} \quad (91\text{-}8)$$

and assuming a $\dot{V}_{O_2}$ of 0.250 L/min, a $\dot{V}_{CO_2}$ of 0.225 L/min, and an NM of 0.01 g/min, (which are within normal range for these values), EE is 1775.52 kcal/day. A 10 percent error in $\dot{V}_{O_2}$ would cause a 7 percent error in EE; a 10 percent error in $\dot{V}_{CO_2}$ would cause a 3 percent error in EE, whereas a 100 percent error in NM would cause only a 1 percent error in EE. For acutely ill patients with hypercatabolism and large and variable levels of protein breakdown, EE can be calculated from $\dot{V}_{O_2}$ and $\dot{V}_{CO_2}$ only (with a maximum error of no more than 2 percent), by using Eq. (91-13).[17]

$$\text{EE (kcal/day)} = 3.586\ \dot{V}_{O_2}\ \text{(L/day)} + 1.443\ \dot{V}_{CO_2}\ \text{(L/day)} - 21.5 \quad (91\text{-}13)$$

Although total EE can be accurately measured without measuring N excretion, this information is crucial for evaluating the magnitude of protein breakdown and for estimating the daily requirements of N. Today several instruments for measuring on-line EE are available and can be used readily at the bedside of critically ill patients breathing spontaneously or mechanically ventilated.[16]

Evaluation of Energy Expenditure from Cardiac Output and Arteriovenous Oxygen Content Difference

For those critically ill patients who have pulmonary artery and arterial catheters in place, drawing additional small blood samples for measurement of $\dot{V}_{O_2}$ represents no additional risk and may be used for evaluating EE. Cardiac output ($\dot{Q}_T$) is generally considered a necessary part of patient care, and $\dot{V}_{O_2}$ is calculated by the following equation:

$$\dot{V}_{O_2}\ \text{(mL/min)} = \dot{Q}_T\ \text{(mL/min)} \times [\ (a - v)_{O_2}]/100 \quad (91\text{-}14)$$

where $(a - v)_{O_2}$ is the arteriovenous difference of O_2 in mL/100 mL blood. With this method, the accuracy of $\dot{V}_{O_2}$ depends on the accuracy of measurements of $\dot{Q}_T$ and of arterial and venous O_2 content. An error of 2 percent of $\dot{Q}_T$ will give an error of 2 percent in $\dot{V}_{O_2}$. Errors of 2 percent in O_2 content are magnified because we are looking at the arteriovenous difference. In the example cited above, if the arterial (Ca_{O_2}) and venous content (Cv_{O_2}) of oxygen were respectively 21 and 15 mL/100 mL, an error of 2 percent in each determination translates into an error of about 8 percent for the difference of 6 mL/100 mL. Critically ill patients usually have much lower hematocrits; Ca_{O_2} and Cv_{O_2} being thus smaller, errors of 2 percent in each determination translate into smaller errors and are acceptable for clinical use (they can even be reduced by multiple sampling which is quite feasible). Furthermore, values for Ca_{O_2} and Cv_{O_2} are readily available in the ICU, since most automatic blood-gas analyzers calculate and display Ca_{O_2} and Cv_{O_2} as part of routine blood analysis. Thus, with a few sequential blood samples it is possible to obtain $\dot{V}_{O_2}$, with an accuracy of better than 5 percent. The approximate amount of calories produced when 1 L oxygen is consumed by a subject on a normal mixed diet is 4.80 kcal. This figure of 4.80 kcal is the mean caloric equivalent of 1 L oxygen when consumed by the three nutrients. By multiplying the $\dot{V}_{O_2}$ obtained from $\dot{Q}_T$ and $(a - v)_{O_2}$ by 4.80, an error of 5 percent on $\dot{V}_{O_2}$ will give a 10 percent error on EE, which is acceptable for clinical use.

Estimation of Energy Expenditure from Empirical Formulas

Since the necessary equipment to perform EE measurements is still expensive and not always available, many dieticians and nutritionists will estimate EE from standard empirical formulas, such as the Harris and Benedict equations which take into account sex, weight in kg (W), height in cm (H), and age in years (A) as follows:

Men:

$$\text{EE} = 66.5 + 13.7\ \text{W} + 5.00\ \text{H} - 6.78\ \text{A} \quad (91\text{-}15)$$

Women:

$$\text{EE} = 655.0 + 9.56\ \text{W} + 1.85\ \text{H} - 4.68\ \text{A} \quad (91\text{-}16)$$

The values for EE obtained by these formulas are considered the basal metabolic rate (BMR) or the basal energy expenditure (BEE) for normal individuals. They were established from measurements performed in 1919 on 136 normal men, 103 normal women, and 94 infants.[18] For normal individuals the values obtained with this method are within approximately 10 percent of measured values. When applied to different pathologic states, and especially to the critically ill, special correcting factors are used (Table 91-2).[19] These correcting factors are often difficult to apply in critically ill patients, since conditions vary so widely from day to day.[20,21] Even the Harris-Benedict BEE is difficult to determine in the critically ill because of large changes in body weight during the course of critical illness, much of which relates to water loss or gain. A better estimation might be reached by taking into account the lean body mass, though this is not commonly known during critical illness. Estimated EE, even if corrected according to a patient's condition, is thus an unreliable way of monitoring metabolic response in critical illness for evaluating the degree of hypermetabolism or for determining nutritional requirements.

TABLE 91-2 Correction Factors to the Calculated Resting Energy Expenditure for Different Pathologic Conditions

Pathologic Conditions	Correcting Factors (%)
Starvation	−10 to − 30
Elective surgery	+10 to + 20
Injury	+10 to + 30
Sepsis	+30 to + 60
Severe burns	+50 to +120

Practical Implications of $\dot{V}_{O_2}$, $\dot{V}_{CO_2}$, Respiratory Quotient, and Energy Expenditure Measurements

For many years, the usual way to evaluate EE was to multiply a measured value of $\dot{V}_{O_2}$ by 4.80, which is approximately the amount of calories produced when 1 L oxygen is consumed by a subject on a normal mixed diet. The value of 4.80 is the mean caloric equivalent of 1 L oxygen when consumed by the three nutrients (Table 91-3). When $\dot{V}_{O_2}$ is measured with an accuracy of 5 percent, EE can be obtained with an error of about 10 percent. Another way of obtaining EE from $\dot{V}_{O_2}$ is to use nomograms, as suggested by Wilmore, which give an estimation of EE as a function of $\dot{V}_{O_2}$ and body surface area.[22] While a single measurement of $\dot{V}_{O_2}$ over a period of 20 min can provide this rough evaluation of EE, the utility of on-line measurements and displays of $\dot{V}_{O_2}$ in life-threatening situations remains to be investigated. The variations in $\dot{V}_{O_2}$ tend to correlate with changes in EE in all situations, except after a load of carbohydrates, where an excess of lipogenesis over lipolysis, or a net positive fat balance, may produce increased EE without a parallel increase in $\dot{V}_{O_2}$.[17] Even if the error in $\dot{V}_{CO_2}$ measurement is smaller than the error made in $\dot{V}_{O_2}$ measurement, calculating EE from $\dot{V}_{CO_2}$ alone may cause a greater error. The caloric value of 1 L CO_2, if calculated as the mean of the calories produced by each of the nutrients, would be 4.33 kcal. While the range of caloric values for 1 L oxygen is narrow (4.486 kcal/L oxygen for protein and 5.047 kcal/L oxygen for carbohydrate), the range is much wider for CO_2 (5.047 kcal/L CO_2 for carbohydrate and 6.63 kcal/L CO_2 for fat). This explains the inaccuracy in deriving EE from $\dot{V}_{CO_2}$ alone (see Table 91-3).

Thus, the $\dot{V}_{CO_2}$ measurement alone should not be used for EE evaluation, since it has a much greater variability related to food intake than $\dot{V}_{O_2}$. It is well known that carbohydrate administration increases $\dot{V}_{CO_2}$ substantially and that in borderline respiratory failure patients, the increased demand on alveolar ventilation and work of breathing can prolong mechanical support. Also, since the body stores of CO_2 are much greater than those of O_2, there may be a large discrepancy between the CO_2 produced metabolically and the measurement of exhaled CO_2 in the nonsteady state. When both $\dot{V}_{O_2}$ and $\dot{V}_{CO_2}$ can be measured, more reliable metabolic data can be derived as described previously. Finally, the on-line measurement of respiratory quotient (RQ) can also provide us with some important information about the patient's metabolic condition. The values for RQ in the steady state are well known for the different nutrients (Table 91-4). When amino acids are converted to glucose by the process of gluconeogenesis, the RQ is equal to 1, while when fatty acids are converted into ketone bodies, the RQ is 0. It is obvious that myriad metabolic patterns occur at the same time and in different proportions with complex effects on the measured value of RQ. As a generalization, when RQ is close to 1.0, it indicates that the main nutrient utilized is carbohydrate, when it is close to 0.7, it indicates that the main nutrient utilized is fat, and if it is below 0.7, it indicates formation and excretion of incompletely oxidized products such as ketone bodies. An RQ around 0.8 will be difficult to interpret, since it may be due to utilization of protein as the main nutrient or to balanced utilization of all three nutrients. When RQ is above 1.0 (again, in the steady state), we may assume that the patient is in net positive fat balance or that lipogenesis from sugar is greater than the degree of lipolysis.

Little information is available on the pattern of hypermetabolic patients becoming suddenly or progressively hypometabolic and how they respond to different kinds of nutritional treatments. Although critically ill and even multiple organ failure patients need nutritional support, they often seem resistant to nutrition. There is a correlation between cumulative negative caloric balance and mortality rate in multiple organ failure patients. Indeed, patients that present a cumulative negative caloric balance of 10,000 kcal over 4 to 6 days have a very high mortality rate. This degree of negative caloric balance is often seen in postinjury or surgical patients kept in semistarvation.[23]

TABLE 91-3 Heat Production by the Different Foodstuffs during the Utilization of 1 L O_2 and during the Production of 1 L CO_2 (Caloric Equivalent of O_2 and CO_2)

	Caloric Equivalent of 1 L O_2 (kcal/L)	Caloric Equivalent of 1 L CO_2 (kcal/L)
Carbohydrate	5.047	5.05
Protein	4.486	5.68
Fat	4.690	6.63

TABLE 91-4 Respiratory Quotient Values for Some Nutrients

Nutrient	RQ
Carbohydrate	1.0
Protein	0.8
Fat	0.7
Conversion of carbohydrate to fat	8.0
Pyruvic acid, glycuronic acid	1.2
Ethyl alcohol	0.667

CASE PRESENTATION

A 55-year-old man with a prior history of chronic obstructive pulmonary disease (COPD) was referred for evaluation of jaundice. The patient had noticed a weight loss of about 8 to 10 lb over the last 6 months, and painless jaundice for the last 2 weeks associated with vague symptoms of gastric irritability. Laboratory data were consistent with obstructive jaundice. No stones were visible on ultrasound, though a space-occupying lesion in the midepigastrium was noted. A computed tomography scan showed a 5 × 7 cm mass at the head of the pancreas. Preoperative pulmonary function indicated a compensated respiratory acidosis with a Pa_{CO_2} of 50 and Pa_{O_2} of 69 on room air. The forced vital capacity (FVC) was

1.6 L, and the forced expiratory volume in 1 s (FEV_1) 800 mL. The patient was begun on bronchodilator therapy and discontinued tobacco use. Since the patient had lost weight and presented with a serum albumin of 2.9 g/dL, preoperative hyperalimentation was undertaken to reduce postoperative complications. Since the patient's estimated EE according to the modified Harris-Benedict formula was 2000 kcal, he received 2500 kcal/day with 120 g protein and the remaining calories divided evenly between carbohydrates and lipids. After 10 days his general condition improved; he increased his weight by no more than 2 lb, but the total protein and the serum albumin increased to 6.2 g/dL and 3.2 g/dL, respectively.

The patient was brought to the operating room, and after an uneventful Whipple procedure was admitted, intubated, to the ICU. For the first 24 h the patient required full ventilatory support while pain control, theophylline levels, and inhaled bronchodilators were optimized. Caloric supply was increased to 3000 kcal/day, in anticipation of increased requirements of the postoperative state.

Over the next several days repeated attempts were made to diminish mechanical ventilatory support, but on each occasion the patient developed dyspnea and worsened hypercapnia. There was no indication of infection and airflow obstruction, as judged by airway pressures, was not extreme. The patient's respiratory muscle strength did not explain his failure to assume a greater amount of spontaneous ventilation. Despite adjustment of nutritional support to maximize calories delivered as fat, the patient failed to progress to liberation from the ventilator.

On the fifth postoperative day indirect calorimetry measurements were performed. These tests revealed an EE of 2100 kcal. With this data, the patient had his caloric support diminished. On the seventh hospital day, the return of bowel function permitted conversion to enteral feedings. With diminished calorie administration and ongoing management of his underlying lung disease, the patient was able to have mechanical ventilation discontinued over 2 days. On the ninth postoperative day, he was discharged from the ICU.

CASE DISCUSSION

A rough estimation of this patient's nutritional requirements was initially made by empirical assessment. In view of his malnutrition and hypoalbuminemia, supportive therapy was appropriately begun preoperatively to minimize perioperative complications. Such routine preoperative assessment conducted conjointly by the surgical, nutrition, and critical care teams is valuable in mapping postoperative treatment plans.

Empirical formulas were continued postoperatively to assess caloric requirements, but the patient's COPD and failure to tolerate discontinuation of mechanical ventilation, despite optimization of other factors, made measurements by indirect calorimetry a reasonable approach to better define EE. Surprisingly, this was quite different than predicted, a common finding in complex patients encountered in the critical care environment. When adjustments in nutritional support were made in accord with this more accurate assessment of nutritional requirement, it likely resulted in diminished carbon dioxide production, diminished work of breathing, and this facilitated liberation from mechanical ventilation. Indirect calorimetric measurements permitted rational decreases in nutritional support, without risk of inducing postoperative malnutrition.

References

1. Benedict FG: *A Study of Prolonged Fasting.* Washington, DC, Carnegie Institute, 1915 (Publication No. 203).
2. Cahill GF: Starvation in man. N Engl J Med 282:668, 1970.
3. Cannon PR, Wissler RW, Woolridge RL: The relationship of protein deficiency to surgical infection. Ann Surg 120:514, 1944.
4. Studley HO: Percentage of weight loss: A basic indicator of surgical risk in patients with chronic peptic ulcer. JAMA 106:458, 1936.
5. Cahill GF Jr, Herrera MG, Morgan AP: Hormone-fuel interrelationships during fasting. J Clin Invest 45:1751, 1966.
6. Owen OE, Felig P, Morgan AP, et al: Liver and kidney metabolism during prolonged starvation. J Clin Invest 48:574, 1969.
7. Owen OE, Morgan AP, Kemp HG, et al: Brain metabolism during fasting. J Clin Invest 46:1589, 1967.
8. Kinney JM, Duke JH Jr, Long CL, et al: Tissue fuel and weight loss after injury. J Clin Path 23(suppl 4):65, 1970.
9. Weissman C, Kemper M, Askanazi J, et al: Resting metabolic rate of the critically ill patient: Measured versus predicted. Anesthesiology 61:673, 1986.
10. Wilmore DW, Aulick LH, Mason AD Jr, et al: The influence of the burn wound on local and systemic responses to injury. Ann Surg 186:444, 1977.
11. Carpentier YA, Askanazi J, Elwyn DH, et al: The effect of carbohydrate intake on the lipolytic rate in depleted patients. Metabolism 29:974, 1980.
12. Dudrick SJ, Wilmore DW, Roades JE: Can intravenous feeding as the sole means of nutrition support growth in the child and restore weight loss in an adult? An affirmative answer. Ann Surg 169:974, 1969.
13. Mullen JL, Buzby GP, Matthews DC, et al: Reduction of operative morbidity and mortality by combined preoperative and postoperative nutritional support. Ann Surg 192:604, 1980.
14. Buzby GP, Mullen JL, Matthews DC, et al: Prognostic nutritional index in gastrointestinal surgery. Am J Surg 139:160, 1980.
15. Askanazi J, Hensle TW, Starker PA, et al: Effect of immediate postoperative nutritional support on lengths of hospitalization. Ann Surg 203:236, 1986.
16. Bursztein S, Elwyn DH, Askanazi J, et al: The theoretical framework of indirect calorimetry and energy balance, in Bursztein S, Elwyn DH, Askanazi J, Kinney JM (eds): *Energy Metabolism, Indirect Calorimetry and Nutrition.* Baltimore, Williams & Wilkins, 1989, pp. 27–80.
17. Bursztein S, Elwyn DH, Saphar P, Singer P: A mathematical analysis of indirect calorimetry measurements in acutely ill patients. Am J Clin Nutr 50:227, 1989.
18. Harris JA, Benedict FG: A biometric study of basal metabolism of normal individuals. Carnegie Inst Wash Publ 279:266, 1919.

19. Elwyn DH: Nutritional requirements of adult surgical patients. Crit Care Med 8:9, 1980.
20. Kinney JM: The application of indirect calorimetry to clinical studies, in Kinney JM (ed): *Assessment of Energy Expenditure in Health and Disease.* Columbus, Ross Laboratories, 1980, pp. 489–501.
21. Rutten P, Blackburn GL, Flatt JP, et al: Determination of optimal hyperalimentation infusion rate. J Surg Res 18:477, 1975.
22. Wilmore DW, Goodwin CW, Aulick LH, et al: Effect of injury and infection on visceral metabolism and circulation. Ann Surg 192:491, 1980.
23. Barlett RH, Dechert RE, Mault JR, et al: Measurement of metabolism in multiple organ failure. Surgery 92:771, 1982.

Chapter 92

GUIDELINES FOR ENTERAL AND PARENTERAL NUTRITION FOR CRITICALLY ILL PATIENTS

PIERRE SINGER
SIMON BURSZTEIN
JEFFREY ASKANAZI

KEY POINTS

- *The main nutritional goals in intensive care are to match protein-calorie utilization and to minimize negative nitrogen (N) balance.*
- *The gut should be used whenever possible; even if total support is not attainable by enteral route, partial feedings may help maintain gut mucosal integrity.*
- *Avoid overfeeding; this is best done by measurement of energy requirements by indirect calorimetry or using lower estimates (35 to 40 kcal/kg/day) of caloric need.*
- *Use a balanced caloric intake, enterally or parenterally, giving fat and carbohydrates as 50 and 50 percent of the nonprotein caloric intake every day.*
- *Most patients require 120 to 150 kcal/g N administered.*
- *Remember: 30 g muscle contains 6.25 g protein which contains 1 g N which is then metabolized to 1 g urine urea N.*
- *Measurement of serum glucose and electrolytes two to three times a day prevents or detects early the complications of seeking adequate nutrition in critically ill patients.*

Reaching a Positive Energy Balance

PREDICTED AND MEASURED ENERGY EXPENDITURE

Though there is little doubt about the indication for nutritional support in critically ill patients,[1–3] caloric requirements are not well defined. Early application of hyperalimentation utilized as much as 5000 kcal/day. Subsequent approaches[4] titrated nutritional support against urinary urea N. To achieve a positive N balance, 1.75 to 2 times the resting energy expenditure (REE) was administered. Some have recommended up to 8000 kcal/day for burn patients. One common method of estimating EE uses multiple regression equations described by Harris and Benedict in 1919.[5] They found that in normal, resting, awake subjects, basal energy expenditure (BEE) was related to sex, age, height, and weight. Others added stress factors to estimate energy requirements in illness.[6,7] Specific nutrients used, fever, trauma, or surgery were typically weighted factors. Others have advocated a simple system with modifications based on low, moderate, or severe stress.[8]

Bedside indirect calorimetry has been very helpful in assessing actual EE in critically ill patients. Importantly, large differences have been shown between estimated and measured EE. As a rule, measured EE is greater than BEE, but much lower than predicted EE using stress factors.[9,10] While measuring EE is more accurate than most empirical calculations, day-to-day variabilities in EE (ranging between 4 and 56 percent) have been noted.[11] This high variability seems to be linked to temperature and clinical instability. In a stable patient, one measurement seems to be enough for a few days. In unstable patients, a nutritional regimen needs either repeated EE measurements or acceptance that variability in the degree of match between delivered and needed calories will exist.

MUSCLE ENERGY BALANCE

When compared to brain, liver, or kidney, muscle is relatively more resistant to modifications in cellular energy metabolism. However, when muscle biopsies have been taken from patients with severe trauma, sepsis, malnutrition, or after surgery, changes have been noted. In severe malnutrition, adenosine triphosphate (ATP) and adenosine diphosphate (ADP) reserves are decreased and adenosine monophosphate (AMP) levels increased as compared to normal subjects. After 3 weeks of nutritional therapy, the pattern is normalized.[12] In severe trauma or severe sepsis, a tremendous decrease in muscle energy-rich phosphates is found, persisting as long as 30 days after injury. Nutritional support with even small amounts of glucose blunts these changes.

Of the total pool of muscle intracellular amino acids, glutamine represents about 60 percent. During severe stress, a 50 percent reduction of this pool occurs. This reduction is not reversible with nutrition composed of amino acids without glutamine.[12] Although large infusions of amino acids tend to normalize the nonessential amino acid pool, the muscle glutamine pool remains low.[13] In addition, several investigators have shown that in the early stage of critical illness, N balance remains negative, despite large amounts and various types of amino acid administration.[14,15]

CALORIE REQUIREMENT

Ideally, a measurement of EE would assess the REE and allow the provision of adequate nutrition. Positive energy balance can be achieved when providing 1.33 times the measured REE. If no measurement can be performed, providing 2500 kcal/day is appropriate for approximately 85 percent of ICU patients, under- or overnourishing the remainder. Administration of nutrients in excess of metabolic rate of oxidation results in accumulation of the nutrient and

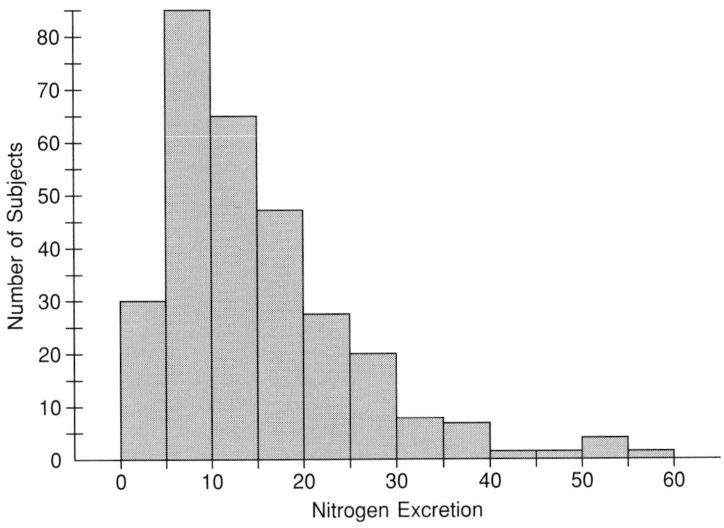

FIGURE 92-1 Nitrogen excretion distribution, expressed in g/day in 300 consecutive critically ill patients. (From Bursztein S, Saphar P, Singer P, Elwyn DH: Am J Clin Nutr 50:227, 1989, with permission.)

possible complications. Excessive nutrients may be converted to fat and accumulate in the liver, thereby causing steatosis. This possibility is suggested by elevations of serum transaminases, total and direct bilirubin, or alkaline phosphatase levels, which should be followed during nutritional support. In patients with compromised respiratory function, glucose overload can increase carbon dioxide production, leading to hypercapnia and respiratory acidosis. Arterial blood-gas monitoring is recommended in these cases. Since the maximal glucose disposal rate in stressed patients is rarely above 7 mg/kg/min, infusion rates should not exceed this level in most circumstances.[16]

Delay in initiation of nutritional support causes muscle atrophy, weaning failure, negative N balance, gastrointestinal atrophy and enteral feeding intolerance, and even heart failure. A refeeding syndrome has been described in patients not fed for a long time. It is characterized by progressive rises in cardiac and respiratory rates, body core temperature, and metabolic rate.[17] When this is noted, a reduction in caloric support, followed by a very gradual increase with close monitoring is mandatory. Fluid overload may also induce congestive heart failure or pulmonary edema, mainly in patients with cardiac wasting. Therefore, nutritional support has to be adjusted for each patient according to specific diseases, metabolic substrate utilization, and development of side effects.

Reaching Positive Nitrogen Balance

ALTERATIONS IN PROTEIN METABOLISM

N excretion is increased in severe illness. In severe trauma and burns, it can reach 40 g/day (Fig. 92-1). The urinary output of N is roughly equivalent to the expected negative N balance, since intestinal losses are minimal if the gastrointestinal tract is intact. Muscle is the major site of protein breakdown and this breakdown provides amino acids for gluconeogenesis.[18] Protein breakdown also occurs in the heart, liver, kidneys, gastrointestinal tract, and lungs.

PROTEIN REQUIREMENTS

Although it is difficult to achieve positive N balance in the patient under stress, one can often minimize negative balance.[19] A loss of 3 to 4 g/N/day for 2 weeks will not cause severe malnutrition. However, a loss of 150 to 250 g N (corresponding to a loss of 14 to 23 percent of the body cell mass) in 10 days can result in significant complications. Therefore, if energy supply is slightly above E, N should be given at rates of not more than 200 mg/kg/day. A 1 g N:120- kcal ratio is suggested as an estimated starting point. In stable patients, a 1:200 ratio is perhaps wiser, whereas for the most severely ill, a 1:100 ratio should be considered. It is useful to remember that 30 g muscle contains 6.25 g protein and 1 g nitrogen, which then metabolizes to 1 g of urine urea N; accordingly, urine urea N of 10 g/24 h predicts a protein requirement of 62.5 g/day to approach N balance.

Specific Nutrients

CARBOHYDRATES

Glucose, with an N sparing effect greater than fat, has traditionally been considered an efficient source of calories.[20] Stressed patients not receiving glucose have decreased concentrations of high energy phosphates on muscle biopsy; the greater the stress, the more glucose is required to prevent this depletion.[21] Following major surgery, wound fibroblasts, brain, and blood cells use a total of about 250 g glucose daily. Therefore, administration of even this small amount has an N sparing effect. Glucose utilization has been studied in stressed patients by glucose-insulin clamp technique, and a maximal utilization of 5 to 7 mg/kg/min has been demonstrated.[22] In sepsis, in trauma, and in the postsurgical period, glucose intolerance may be greater. Excessive glucose administration may also induce hepatic steatosis and respiratory complications such as CO_2 retention.

During stress, in contrast to the normal response, ele-

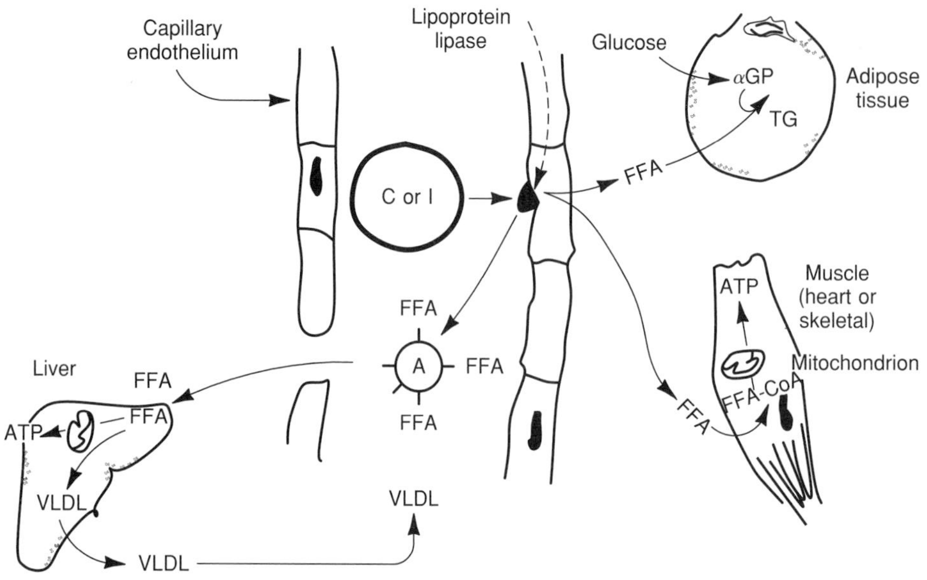

FIGURE 92-2 Pathways of fat metabolism. VLDL, very low density lipoproteins; FFA, free fatty acids; CoA, acetylcoenzyme A; TG, triglyceride; αGP, α glycopeptide. (From Bryan H, Shennan A, Griffin E, et al: Pediatrics 58:787, 1976.)

vated plasma glucose concentrations do not decrease hepatic glucose production. Thus, hyperglycemia is due to an increase of glucose production rather than to a decrease in utilization.[21] Turnover is high. In injury and sepsis, there is also a failure to respond to insulin, most probably because of a postreceptor defect. Moreover, increased catecholamines induce lypolysis, and increased fatty acids compete with glucose as a primary fuel.[23] These phenomena do not contraindicate nutritional support but require that large amounts of insulin be used to avoid severe hyperglycemia and a hyperosmolar state. During sepsis, blood glucose levels should be followed at least every 6 to 8 h to identify mismatching of carbohydrate and insulin administration.

Given intravenously over a prolonged period, glucose can suppress fatty acid release and result in fatty acid deficiency. This is related to the persistent high levels of insulin during intravenous glucose administration. Fat oxidation persists in these cases, despite dextrose infusion; in sepsis, there is even preferential fat oxidation.[23]

Glycerol is a sugar alcohol existing naturally in food. Its metabolism is closely associated with that of fat and carbohydrates. It is a precursor of glycerophosphate, providing the carbon skeleton for gluconeogenesis, taking an important part in oxidative phosphorylation and incorporating into lipid molecules.[24] Glycerol has been used in nutritional support of multiple trauma patients.[25] Glucose and triglyceride levels are significantly decreased during glycerol infusion as compared to glucose administration. Cumulative N balance is similar during glycerol or glucose administration. The administration of glycerol may be of importance in stressed patients with high levels of glycemia and insulin resistance.

LIPIDS

Fats and cardohydrates are interchangeable as a source of calories. Dextrose (as glucose monohydrate), when fully oxidized, gives 3.4 kcal/g, while fat gives 9 kcal/g. The minimal requirement of fat in human beings is 3 to 20 g linoleic acid daily.[26] Continuous infusions of glucose induce high insulin levels, thereby preventing fatty acid mobilization. Therefore, patients should receive at least 1 to 3 g/kg/day of long-chain triglycerides to prevent essential fatty acid deficiency. Moreover, the use of more fat and less carbohydrate seems to decrease the incidence of hepatic steatosis and the production of CO_2, as discussed further below.

INTRAVENOUS FAT EMULSION (IVFE). Two main classes of lipids should be considered. Figure 92-2 shows the metabolism of fat from the bloodstream to the tissue. The fat emulsions used can be categorized in two classes: the long-chain triglycerides (LCT) and the medium-chain triglycerides (MCT) (Table 92-1). A third class of structured lipids is obtained by mixing LCTs and MCTs in specific proportions.[27] The mixture is hydrolyzed and then transesterified randomly, giving MC fatty acids for the energy requirements and LC fatty acids to ensure that essential fatty acid needs are met. This lipid mixture should be considered experimental.

Table 92-1 shows the composition of several LCT and MCT preparations. Concentrations range from 10 to 30%. IVFE effects on the lungs have been the source of concern for their use in critically ill patients.[28] Lung impairment seems to be caused by an IVFE-related increase in prostaglandin production. We observed that slow infusion (0.06 g/kg/h) of Intralipid 20% was associated with an increase in metabolites of prostaglandin I_2 and an increase in intrapulmonary shunt in patients with acute respiratory failure.[29] Thus, slow infusion of IVFE has effects similar to prostacyclin infusions. Although this phenomenon has not yet been proven to be of clinical importance, we recommend slow infusion of lipids in patients with severe hypoxemia.

MCT fat emulsions are not stored in the body as LCT emulsions are.[30] They do not overload the reticuloendothelial system. They are completely oxidized, providing en-

TABLE 92-1 Ten Percent Fat Emulsions

	LCT		MCT/LCT
Lipids	Intralipid	Liposyn II	Lipofundin
Linoleic acid	54%	65.8%	27%
Oleic acid	26%	13%	13%
Palmitic acid	9%	7%	4.5%
Linolenic acid	8%	4.2%	4%
Stearic acid	3%	2.5%	1.5%
Caproic acid			1.5%
Octanoic acid			27.5%
Capric acid			20%
Lauric acid			1%
Egg yolk phosphatide	1.2%	1.2%	0.75%
Glycerol	2.25%	2.5%	2.5%
kcal/mL	1.1	1.1	0.65
Osmolarity	280	300	320

LCT, long-chain triglycerides; MCT, medium-chain triglycerides
SOURCE: Adapted from Kinsella, et al: Nutr Int 6:24, 1990.

ergy quickly. It should be noted that if infused alone, MCTs are ketogenic. Concomittant infusion of glucose decreases lipid oxidation and prevents ketogenesis. From preliminary studies, MCT/LCT mixtures may have more N sparing effect than LCTs alone.

ENTERAL USE OF LIPIDS. If there is normal liver function, pancreatic lipase and colipase activity, and sufficient small intestinal absorption, LC fatty acids can be given enterally. If there is malabsorption or liver dysfunction, MCTs should be used. MCTs are absorbed directly into the portal circulation and oxidized in the liver without need of carnitine. They can be added in a modular enteral feeding regimen.

PROTEINS

The optimal balanced amino acid formula has not been defined. Carbohydrates may not be replaced as a source of glucose for the brain. In burn patients, N loss is eight times greater than in normal subjects and in multiple trauma, six times greater. For most critically ill patients, this hypercatabolic state is uncorrectable, but transient, lasting from days to weeks. Its magnitude can be reduced and partially compensated by administration of protein. As soon as the patient improves, body cell mass can be improved by the appropriate calorie and protein administration.

AMINO ACID COMPOSITION. N balance depends on the amount and the composition of N source administered. Most of the crystalline amino acid solutions available for parenteral use have the same nonessential amino acid composition. Essential amino acids for human beings are valine, leucine, isoleucine, methionine, threonine, lysine, phenylalanine, and tryptophan. Because of chemical instability and rapid conversion to glutamate and ammonia, glutamine has not been used in these solutions. However, its marked intracellular reduction in stressed patients has been noted above (Fig. 92-3). Studies have demonstrated that the synthetic L-alanine-L-glutamine dipeptide can be safely and efficiently administered as a source of glutamine in parenteral nutrition (PN).[31] Unfortunately, it is not yet generally available. Glutamine is of critical importance for the enterocyte,[32] supporting gut mucosal metabolism, structure, and function. It is the principal fuel utilized by the mucosa of the small intestine, lymphocytes, and the kidney (see Fig.

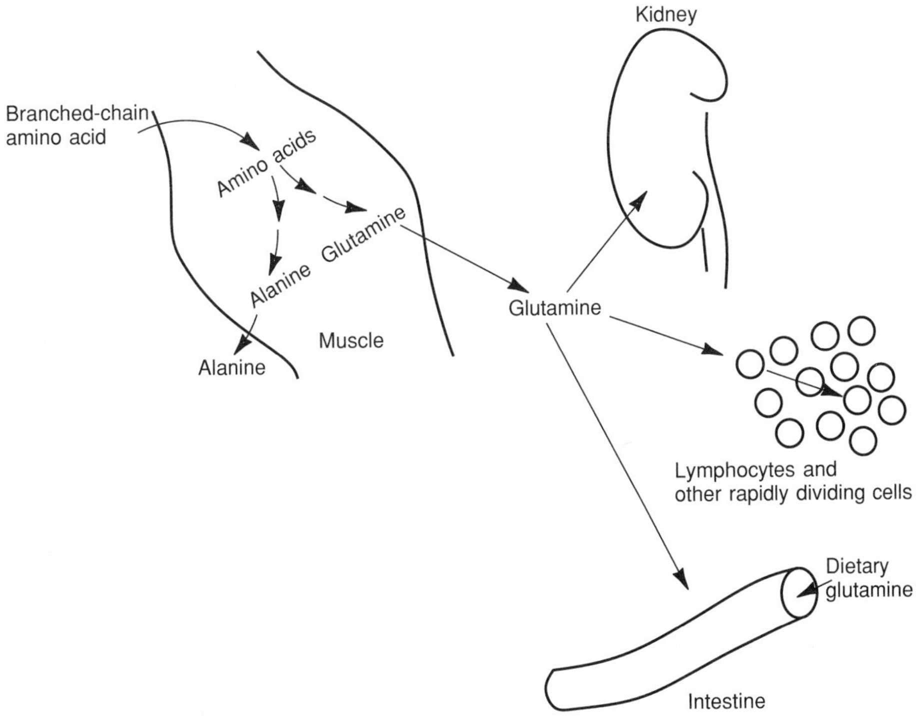

FIGURE 92-3 Combined metabolism of branched-chain amino acids, glutamine, and alanine in the muscle, gut, and in the kidney. (From Reference 47, with permission.)

92-3). When administered enterally, it seems to prevent bacterial translocation.[33] Glutamine is still used experimentally parenterally but is available for enteral use.

Branched-chain amino acids have been advocated for hypercatabolic states, since they are largely metabolized in muscle, and muscle is the major site of protein breakdown during stress. Their metabolism and clinical utility have been reviewed recently.[34] They increase the rate of hepatic and acute phase protein synthesis in septic and severely ill patients. They may be helpful in preventing septic encephalopathy by increasing the aromatic:branched chain amino acid ratio. Despite these theoretical advantages, their clinical effects are controversial, clouded by the heterogenous nature of the patients studied. Though some have demonstrated improved N balance with branched-chain amino acids,[34] others have not.[34,35]

Arginine has been reported to act as a limiting amino acid in burns. It has also been demonstrated to augment T lymphocyte response to mitogens, improve N balance and wound healing, and experimentally improve survival in burns when administered as 1 to 2 percent of the total energy intake.[37] The mechanisms of action on the immune system are unclear.

Protein sources administered enterally include amino acids, short-chain and long-chain peptides from caseinate, soy protein isolates, egg albumin, or lactalbumin. High concentrations of amino acids result in high osmolality. High branched-chain, low aromatic amino acid formulas for chronic liver failure have been tested.[38] Essential amino acid- and histidine-enriched formulas have been suggested for renal failure patients. With the addition of proteins to standard formulas (modular feeding), a more appropriate N:calorie ratio can be reached.

Enteral Feeding

Enteral feeding is nutritionally and metabolically equivalent to parenteral feeding in the severely injured patient.[39,40] If the gastrointestinal tract is functional, enteral feeding is preferred, because it is easier, safer, less expensive, and prevents intestinal mucosal atrophy and stress-induced gastritis. The gastrointestinal tract has been implicated as a source of sepsis in many conditions. Some data[40] suggest that enteral feeding reduces infection in the critically ill, although some studies have not confirmed this finding.[41]

RULES OF ADMINISTRATION

Polyurethane tubes are much more comfortable to the patient. They are introduced nasally. A nasogastric or nasoenteral tube can be left in place for several weeks. When longer support is necessary, gastrostomy or jejunostomy is recommended (see Chap. 95).

Full-strength enteral feeding can be initiated safely as soon as the patient has been stabilized, although some will not tolerate this and require dilution.[42] The feeding is administered continuously by pump or intermittently by gravity or pump over 30 to 60 min every 3 to 6 h. The patient should be kept in a half-sitting position to diminish the risks of aspiration.

Many formulas are available (Table 92-2). They vary in osmolality, amount of calories/mL, and relative composition. When more specific nutritional support has to be administered, a modular diet can be prescribed, using Polycose (Ross Lab) or Moducal (Mead-Johnson) for carbohydrates, Microlipid (Sherwood Med) for fats, and Casec (Mead-Johnson) for protein.

COMPLICATIONS

The complications occurring during enteral feeding are mechanical, gastrointestinal, metabolic, and pharmacologic. The mechanical complications are related to misplacement of the tube (most commonly in the bronchial tree). Nasogastric tube insertion is contraindicated in multiple trauma patients with suspected cribriform plate fracture. Epistaxis, sinusitis, and ruptured esophageal varices have also been associated with introduction of nasogastric tubes. Proper placement of any tube has to be confirmed radiologically before enteral feeding is started.

Nausea and vomiting can occur and are related to fast infusion rate, large volumes, or delayed gastric emptying. Metoclopramide can be used to enhance gastric emptying. Rate and volume of administration must be carefully followed. Aspiration can be a tragic complication. Prevention is achieved by placing the patient in a sitting position, checking the tube position before any administration, monitoring the volume and rate of administration, as well as gastric residuals, and giving metoclopramide when necessary. However, silent aspirations can occur, even with an inflated endotracheal cuff. Transpyloric feeding has decreased aspiration rates.[43] Diarrhea is a common finding in enterally fed patients. The volume of administration, its concentration and osmolality, bacterial contamination and presence of lactose, fat, or gluten are the main causes, together with hypoalbuminemia.[44] Continuous enteral feeding, dilution to reduce osmolality, or addition of pectin often minimize this problem. Addition of loperamide or psyllium hydrophilic mucilloid is effective in some cases. Recently, feeding formulas including dietary fiber have been introduced (Ross Lab).

ELECTROLYTE DEFICIENCIES

Even when serum concentrations of potassium, phosphate, and magnesium are normal in malnutrition and starvation, significant total body content decreases can occur. During refeeding, carbohydrate and water flux moves them into the intracellular space. Their serum concentrations then fall and clinically detectable deficiency syndromes appear. If the patient is severely malnourished, daily monitoring of potassium, phosphate, and magnesium levels is mandatory. In addition sodium, blood urea nitrogen (BUN), glucose, and presence of glycosuria are monitored. If anabolism is achieved, additional supplements will be needed, reaching 60 to 150 meq/day for potassium, 20 to 60 mmol/day for phosphorus, and 15 to 25 meq/day for magnesium.

Hypokalemia can lead to ectopic atrial impulses, electro-

TABLE 92-2 Some of the Polymeric, Semielemental, and Elemental Formulas Available

Formula	Caloric Density (kcal/mL)	Protein g/L (% kcal)	Fat g/L (% kcal)	Carbohydrate g/L (% kcal)	mO/kg
Polymeric					
ISOCAL	1.06	34	44	132	
(Mead-Johnson)		13%	37%	50%	300
OSMOLITE HN	1.06	42	35	134	
(Ross)		14%	31%	55%	300
IMPACT[a]	1.0	59	28	130	
(Sandoz)		24%	25%	51%	<700
PULMOCARE	1.5	63	92	102	
(Ross)		17%	55%	28%	490
HEPATIC-AID	1.1	44	36	169	
(Kendall-McGaw)		15%	28%	57%	500
Semielemental					
VITAL	1.0	42	11	185	
(Ross)		17%	9%	74%	460
CRITICARE HN	1.06	37	3	222	
(Mead-Johnson)		14%	3%	83%	650
Elemental					
VIVONEX HN	1.0	46	1	210	
(Norwich-Eaton)		18%	1%	81%	810

[a]Only formula containing arginine, yeast RNA, and fish oil.

cardiographic changes, muscle weakness, hyporeflexia, paresthesia, and gastrointestinal ileus. When phosphate concentration falls below 1.0 mg/dL, paresthesias, areflexia, muscle weakness, hyperventilation, and even rhabdomyolysis can appear. Refeeding hypophosphatemia can also lead to a pseudo-Guillain-Barré syndrome, but this is uncommon. Inadequate replacement, peritoneal dialysis with hypertonic dextrose solutions, or aggressive use of aluminum-containing antacids all potentiate hypophosphatemia. Finally, hypomagnesemia is very common, mainly in ventilated patients receiving diuretics. It manifests as paresthesias, weakness, and muscle fasciculation. Tetany can also be observed.

During discontinuation of mechanical ventilation, potassium, phosphate, and magnesium levels should be followed closely. Phosphate content of most enteral formulas reaches 75 to 100 percent of the US daily requirements and 90 percent is absorbed by a normal gastrointestinal tract.

The high incidence of metabolic complications (30 to 40 percent) is mainly related to hyponatremia, hyperglycemia, and hypophosphatemia.[45] Fluid and electrolyte management must be followed very closely. Head trauma patients can develop hyponatremia from inappropriate secretion of antidiuretic hormone; cirrhotic and heart failure patients cannot handle large amounts of water and salts.

Interferences between drug metabolism and enteral feeding occur. Decreased absorption of phenytoin,[46] and decreased efficacy of warfarin with vitamin K-containing formulas have been described. Moreover, some formulas may impair hepatic drug metabolism.[47] It seems that the presence of lipid in the enteral preparation may be of importance in maintaining normal hepatic drug metabolism.

Parenteral Nutrition

RULES OF ADMINISTRATION

PN can be administered peripherally or through central access. The peripheral nutrition is suitable for short-term nutritional support in patients who require supplementation of deficient oral or enteral nutrition or when increasing the load on gastrointestinal tract may lead to complications. When longer periods of PN support are necessary or if the patient is seriously ill, PN is administered through a central line.

Dextrose, together with amino acids and fat, may be administered in a triple admixture bag, together with the electrolytes, vitamins, and trace elements required (Table 92-3). Alcoholics require specific additional supplementation of vitamins B_1, B_6, and K. Trace elements, mainly zinc, are mandatory in patients with burns, severe diarrhea, or draining wounds. In other cases, overtreatment could be deleterious.

METABOLIC COMPLICATIONS

Hyperglycemia, sometimes leading to hyperosmolarity, is the most common metabolic disturbance observed in critically ill patients receiving PN. High doses of insulin are required and if severe hyperglycemia evolves, PN may need to be temporarily discontinued.

Hyperlipidemia is common during IVFE infusion and is cleared in a few hours. Lipid disappearance from the plasma is not related to its rate of oxidation.[48] To detect lipid intolerance, serum cholesterol and triglyceride levels

TABLE 92-3 Vitamins and Trace Elements Required in the Critical Care Patient

Vitamin	A	D	E	K	B_1	B_2	B_6
Requirements	2500 IU	400 IU	50 IU	10 mg	5 mg	5 mg	5 mg
MVI-12/mL	600 IU	40 IU	2 IU		0.6 mg	0.7 mg	.08 mg

Vitamin	B_{12}	Folate	Vit C	Niacinamide	Penthotenic	Biotin
Requirements	12 μg		5 mg	500 mg	50 mg	60 μg
MVI-12/mL	1 μg	0.8 mg	100 mg	8 mg	3 mg	12 μg

SOURCE: From Mills CB, et al: 1985.

should be measured 24 h after the first administration and, if normal, followed twice a week. If high levels are reached, infusion rate or dose should be reduced or stopped. Lipid intolerance is more frequent in cirrhotic and multiple system organ failure patients. Abnormal liver function tests have been observed in patients receiving PN. In many cases, these abnormalities are normalized with a decrease of the carbohydrate load and replacement by fat calories. In many cases the liver abnormalities are most probably related to underlying disease and not PN.[49] Coagulation profile should be followed twice a week, because thrombocytopenia and hypercoagulable states have been described.

Finally, electrolytes should be monitored frequently. Calcium, magnesium, but mainly phosphorus have been shown to be depleted in critically ill patients. Hypophosphatemia can induce muscle weakness, weaning failure, arrhythmias, and decreased myocardial function. Decreased sensitivity to vasopressors is many times related to hypocalcemia or hypophosphatemia.

Organ Failure and Specific Nutrition Approaches

RESPIRATORY FAILURE

The interaction of nutrition and the respiratory system is described in Chap. 94. Since carbohydrates are oxidized with a higher respiratory quotient (RQ) than fat and can promote lipogenesis with even greater RQ, patients with borderline ventilatory function may deteriorate with excess CO_2 production from glucose administration. A substitution of fat for part of the carbohydrate decreases ventilatory demand.[50,51] Successful discontinuation of mechanical ventilation seems to be related in part to work of breathing. Muscle fatigue occurs when carbohydrate stores are depleted and when lipid substrates cannot fulfill energy requirement. Thus, nutritional supplements should not be so reduced in the interest of reducing $\dot{V}_{CO_2}$ that energy supplies are inadequate. This balance between too little energy and too much carbohydrate is best titrated in patients having reduced ventilatory reserve by measuring the $\dot{V}_{CO_2}$; if it exceeds expectations, reduce the carbohydrate load and repeat the measurement.

As described previously, the lung effect of IVFE administration seems to be related to the effect on prostaglandin metabolism more than to increased triglyceride synthesis. When used in patients with acute hypoxemic respiratory failure, infusions should be slow and lung shunt followed closely. If infusions are associated with unacceptable deterioration of lung function, they should be withheld until gas exchange improves.

RENAL FAILURE

Considerable evidence has accumulated to suggest that high amino acid loads increase renal plasma flow and glomerular filtration rate in normal subjects and in chronic renal failure patients.[52] Prostaglandins, as well as glucagon, insulin, and growth hormone may play a role as modulators in this process. In acute renal failure, amino acid supplementation has changed survival.[53] High N intake may improve survival only by achieving positive N balance. However, the true impact of protein load on renal function remains unknown. We observed in a small group of patients with acute nonoliguric renal failure that high amino acid load was able to reduce the furosemide dosage by 35 percent and to achieve positive N balance.[54] Therefore, our suggestion is to administer approximately 150 g amino acids to patients with high output renal failure.

HEPATIC FAILURE

Despite the publication of many randomized trials, the value of branched-chain amino acids in management of hepatic encephalopathy remains unclear. Restoration of a normal aromatic:branched-chain amino acid ratio seems a logical goal, but branched-chain amino acids often produce only minor improvements in hepatic encephalopathy.[38] Enteral nutrition and PN have been used in acute liver failure, without showing significant modifications in outcome. We recommend a diet that includes 40 percent carbohydrate, 40 percent fat (MCT and LCT), and 20 percent protein in these patients.

IMMUNE SUPPRESSION

It has only recently been postulated that specific nutritional supplementation could be used to manipulate the immune system. Arginine is a key compound promoting macrophage cytotoxic action.[37] Ribonucleic acid and its metabolites play a critical role in T cell response.[55] Polyunsaturated fatty acids produce a variety of mediators, including prostaglandins and leukotrienes, with a number of effects on immune function and inflammatory response.[56]

Patients with the acquired immunodeficiency syndrome (AIDS) often present with signs of malnutrition. Enteral when possible, or parenteral feeding is mandatory, since the wasting syndrome observed in AIDS is reversible in most cases.[57] Lipid infusion administered in these patients does not modify their immune function.

HEAD TRAUMA

While paraplegic and barbiturate coma patients have low REE, head trauma patients have very high REE with increased protein wasting.[58] Delayed nutritional support because of poor gastric emptying has to be avoided. PN should be started as soon as the patient is stabilized. Enteral feeding will be started with delay in comparison with other trauma patients.

CASE PRESENTATION

A 54-year-old man was admitted for multiple trauma after a motor vehicle accident. He was suffering from subdural hematoma, chest trauma with left pneumothorax, splenic rupture, and fracture of the left femur. After drainage of the subdural hematoma, laparotomy, and splenectomy, he was transferred to the ICU where he was ventilated and monitored for the first 24 h. His intracranial pressure remained around 13 mmHg. He required hyperventilation, antiepileptic therapy, and mannitol administration. His gastric output was 1200 mL for the first day.

According to an indirect calorimetry measurement, the patient's REE was 2200 kcal/day. He was excreting 640 mg/dL of urea in 4500 mL urine/day, so his urine urea N (14.4 g/day) predicted catabolism of 90 g protein/day. TPN was started through a central line. The total calorie intake was 1.33 × 2200 kcal, or about 3000 kcal, divided as 40 percent carbohydrates, 40 percent fat, and 20 percent protein. Glucose (350 g) was administered as 1160 mL $D_{30}W$, 120 g in 650 mL as a 20% fat emulsion, and 1000 mL amino acid solution at 10%. Accordingly, 2400 nonprotein kcal accompanied 100 g protein (16 g N) to give a calorie:N ratio of 150. Electrolytes, vitamins, and trace elements were added to the triple admixture as followed: NaCl 6 g, KCl 4 g, $MgSO_4$ 2 g, $CaCl_2$ 1 g, MVI 2 mL, MTE 3 mL, folic acid 1 mg. Glucosuria was checked regularly four times a day, and electrolytes were checked daily. After 4 days of TPN, the gastric residual decreased to 500 mL, peristaltism was present, and enteral feeding was started with a full-strength commercial regimen, using a continuous feeding pump. After 9 days the patient was extubated and continued to receive enteral feeding until he was able to receive oral nutrition.

CASE DISCUSSION

This multiple trauma patient was expected to be critically ill more than 3 to 5 days and therefore required full nutritional support as soon as he was stabilized. Since he presented with an ileus, a balanced TPN regimen was administered. N loss in the urine was 14.4 g/day. N intake was around 16 g/day, likely resulting in slight negative balance. However, further N loss evaluation was not conducted and should have been repeated, particularly after the shift to enteral support. Moreover, since mannitol was used, osmolality should have been checked daily, and if found to be elevated, TPN should have been stopped or free water access liberalized. As soon as enteral nutrition was possible, it was started at full strength and without complications.

References

1. Apelgren KN, Rombeau JL, Twoney PL, Miller RA: Comparison of nutritional indices and outcome in critically ill patients. Crit Care Med 10:305, 1982.
2. Mullen JL, Buzby GP, Matthews DC, et al: Reduction of operative morbidity by combined preoperative and postoperative nutritional support. Ann Surg 192:604, 1980.
3. Dudrick SJ, Wilmore DW, Vaes HM, Rhoades JE: Can intravenous feeding as the sole means of nutrition support growth in the child and restore weight loss in the adult? An affirmative answer. Ann SUrg 169:974, 1969.
4. Rutten P, Blackburn GL, Flatt JP, et al: Determination of optimal hyperalimentation rate. J Surg Res 18:477, 1975.
5. Harris JA, Benedict FG: Biometric studies of basal metabolism in man. Carnegie Inst Wash 279:266, 1919.
6. Kinney JM, Duke JH Jr, Long CL, Gump F: Tissue fuel and weight loss after injury. J Clin Path 23:65, 1970.
7. Elwyn DH: Nutritional requirements of adult surgical patients. Crit Care Med 8:9, 1980.
8. Cerra FB: *Pocket Manual of Surgical Nutrition.* St. Louis, Mosby, 1984.
9. Cortes V, Nelson LD: Errors in estimating energy expenditure in critically ill surgical patients. Arch Surg 124:287, 1989.
10. Singer P, Elwyn DH, Irving CS, et al: The reliability of estimated energy expenditure in critically ill patients. Crit Care Med. (In press)
11. Vermeij CG, Feenstra BWA, Van Lanschot JB, Bruining HA: Day-to-day variability of energy expenditure in critically ill patients. Crit Care Med 17:623, 1989.
12. Furst P: Intermediary energy metabolism for catabolic state with special regard to muscle tissue, in Wilkinson AW, Cuthbertson DP (eds): *Metabolism and the Response to Injury.* London, Pitman Medical 1976, pp 94–112.
13. Askanazi J, Furst P, Michelsen CB, et al: Muscle and plasma amino acid infusion. Ann Surg 191:465, 1980.
14. Elwyn DH: Protein metabolism and requirements in the critically ill patient. Crit Care Clin 3:57, 1987.
15. Shigzal HM, Forse RA: Protein and caloric requirements with total parenteral nutrition. Ann Surg 192:562, 1980.
16. Black PR, Brooks DC, Bessey PQ, et al: Mechanisms of insulin resistance following injury. Ann Surg 196:420, 1982.
17. Solomon SM, Kirby DF: The refeeding syndrome, a review. JPEN 14:90, 1990.
18. Pearl RH, Clowes GHA, Hirsch EF, et al: Prognosis and survival as determined by visceral amino acid clearance in severe trauma. J Trauma 25:777, 1985.
19. Bursztein S, Elwyn DH: Nitrogen balance, in *Energy Metabolism, Indirect Calorimetry and Nutrition.* Bursztein S, Elwyn DH,

Askanazi J, Kinney JM (eds): Baltimore, Williams & Wilkins, 1989, pp 85–118.
20. Long JM, Wilmore DW, Mason AD Jr, Pruitt BA Jr: Effect of carbohydrate and fat intake on nitrogen excretion during total intravenous feeding. Ann Surg 185:417, 1977.
21. Elwyn DH: The unique role of glucose in artificial nutrition. Impact of injury and malnutrition. Clin Nutr 7:195, 1988.
22. Wolfe RR, Herndon DN, Jahoor F, et al: Effect of severe burn injury on substrate cycling by glucose and fatty acids. N Engl J Med 317:403, 1987.
23. Long CL: Fuel preferences in the septic patient. Glucose or fat? JPEN 11:333, 1987.
24. Tao RC, Kelley RE, Yoshimura NN, Benjamin F: Glycerol. Its metabolism and use as an intravenous energy source. JPEN 7:479, 1983.
25. Singer P, Bursztein B, Elwyn DH, et al: Glycerol as a fuel substrate in multiple trauma patients. Anesthesiology. 73:A260, 1990.
26. JeeJeebhoy KN: Total parenteral nutrition. Annu Rev Coll Phys Surg Can 9:287, 1976.
27. Bach A, Babayan VK: Medium-chain triglycerides. An update. Am J Clin Nutr 36:950, 1982.
28. Skeie B, Askanazi J, Rothkopf MM, et al: Intravenous fat emulsions and lung function. A review. Crit Care Med 16:183, 1988.
29. Singer P, Venus B, Bursztein S, et al: Intravenous fat emulsion infusion in acute respiratory failure. JPEN (Submitted)
30. Bach AC, Frey A, Lutz O: Clinical and experimental effects of medium-chain triglyceride-based fat emulsions. A review. Clin Nutr 8:223, 1989.
31. Stehle P, Zander J, Mertes N, et al: Effect of parenteral glutamine peptide supplements on glutamine loss and nitrogen balance after major surgery. Lancet 1:231, 1989.
32. Souba WW, Smith RJ, Wilmore DW: Glutamine metabolism by the intestinal tract. JPEN 9:608, 1985.
33. Salloum RM, Souba WW, Klimberg S, et al: Glutamine is superior to glutamate in supporting gut metabolism, stimulating intestinal glutamase activity, and preventing bacterial translocation. Surg Forum 10:6, 1989.
34. Skeie B, Kvetan V, Gil KM, et al: Branched chain amino acids: Their metabolism and clinical utility. Crit Care Med 18:549, 1990.
35. Cerra FB, Mazuski J, Teasley K, et al: Nitrogen retention in critically ill patients is proportional to the branched chain amino acid load. Crit Care Med 11:775, 1983.
36. Wounde PV, Morgan RE, Kosta JM: Addition of branched chain amino acids to parenteral nutrition of stressed critically ill patients. Crit Care Med 14:685, 1986.
37. Barbul A: Arginine: Biochemistry, physiology and therapeutic implications. JPEN 10:277, 1986.
38. Erikson LS, Conn HO: Branched-chain amino acids in the management of hepatic encephalopathy: An analysis of variants. Hepatology 10:228, 1989.
39. Grote AE, Elwyn DH, Takala J, et al: Nutritional and metabolic effects of enteral and parenteral feeding in severely injured patients. Clin Nutr 6:161, 1987.
40. Moore FA, Moore EE, Jones TN, et al: TEN versus TPN following major abdominal trauma-reduced septic morbidity. J Trauma 29:916, 1989.
41. Cerra FB, McPherson JP, Konstantinides FN, et al: Enteral nutrition does not prevent multiple organ failure syndrome (MSOF) after sepsis. Surgery 104:727, 1988.
42. Keohane PP, Atrill H, Love M, et al: Relation between osmolality of diet and gastrointestinal side effects in enteral nutrition. Br Med J, 288:678, 1984.
43. Hinsdale JG, Lipkowitz GS, Pollock TW, et al: Prolonged enteral nutrition in malnourished patients with nonelemental feeding. Am J Surg 149:334, 1985.
44. Ford EG, Jennings LM, Andrassy RJ: Serum albumin (oncotic pressure) correlated with enteral feeding tolerance in the pediatric surgical patient. J Pediatr Surg 22:597, 1987.
45. Vanlangingham S, Simpsons, Daniel P, et al: Metabolic abnormalities in patients supported with enteral tube feeding. JPEN 5:332, 1981.
46. Saklad J, Graves RH, Sharp WP: Interaction of oral phenytoin with enteral feedings. JPEN 10:322, 1986.
47. Knodell RG: Effects of formula composition on hepatic and intestinal drug metabolism during enteral nutrition. JPEN 14:34, 1990.
48. Nordenstrom J, Carpentier YA, Askanazi J, et al: Free fatty acid mobilization and oxidation during total parenteral nutrition in trauma and sepsis. Ann Surg 198:725, 1983.
49. Wolfe BM, Walker BK, Shaul DB, Ruebner BH: Effect of total parenteral nutrition into hepatic histology. Arch Surg 123:1084, 1988.
50. Askanazi J, Nordenstrom J, Rosenbaum SH, et al: Nutrition for the patient with respiratory failure. Glucose versus fat. Anesthesiology 54:373, 1981.
51. Shikora SA, Bistrian BR, Borlosa BC, et al: Crit Care Med 18:157, 1990.
52. Ando A, Kawata T, Hara Y, et al: Effects of dietary protein intake on renal function in humans. Kidney Int 36:864, 1989.
53. Abel RM, Beck CH, Abbott WM, et al: Improved survival from acute renal failure after treatment with intravenous essential L-amino acids and glucose. N Engl J Med 288:695, 1973.
54. Singer P, Bursztein S, Segal A, et al: Reduced morbidity in acute renal failure with high rates of amino acid (AA) infusion. Clin Nutr 9:523, 1990.
55. Van Buren CT, Kulkarni AD, Schandle VP, et al: The influence of dietary nucleosides on cell-mediated immunity. Transplantation 36:350, 1983.
56. Kinsella JE, Lokesh B, Broughton S, Whelan J: Dietary polyunsaturated fatty acids and eicosanoids; potential effects on the modulation of inflammatory and immune cells; an overview. Nutr Int 6:24, 1990.
57. Singer P, Rothkopf MM, Askanazi J: Nutritional aspects of the AIDS. Am J Gastroenterol 1991. (In press)
58. Clifton GL, Robertson CS, Grossman RG, et al: The metabolic response to severe head injury. J Neurosurg 60:687, 1985.

Chapter 93

THE ROLE OF BRANCHED-CHAIN AMINO ACIDS IN CRITICAL ILLNESS

BJÖRN SKEIE
ELDAR SÖREIDE
JEFFREY ASKANAZI

KEY POINTS

- *Providing branched-chain amino acids (BCAA) in higher amounts (45 percent) than the normal diet (20 to 25 percent) provides benefit to selected critically ill patients.*
- *The hypermetabolic response to stress (injury, surgery, sepsis) causes negative nitrogen balance which is not ameliorated by BCAA supplementation in most controlled studies; patient selection and more sensitive end points of protein metabolism may modify this conclusion in the future.*
- *BCAA-enriched solutions increase hepatic protein synthesis, acute phase proteins, lymphocyte count, and cutaneous hypersensitivity in septic and injured patients; these clinical observations predict improved healing, tolerance to infection, and survival in patients as already observed in animal models of sepsis and injury treated with BCAA.*
- *Patients with hepatic encephalopathy (HE) recover from coma faster when treated with BCAA-enriched solutions than with no amino acids, but improvement in survival has not been demonstrated.*
- *Tryptophan-mediated behavioral functions (sleep, mood, appetite, nociception, ventilation) may be modulated by BCAA.*

Many controversies about the metabolism and use of BCAA in clinical practice still exist. Most total parenteral nutrition (TPN) regimens contain approximately the average intake of BCAA in a Western diet. Therefore, the question is not whether to provide BCAA, but rather, if BCAA given in higher amounts than normal are useful to achieve suggested metabolic and pharmacologic effects. We recently reviewed several aspects of these controversies.[1] This chapter updates our previous review with special emphasis on the role of BCAA in metabolic stress states, hepatic failure, central nervous system (CNS) dysfunction, heart and renal failure, and the cachexia of malignancy. We put forward the hypothesis that a major role of the increased net rates of protein degradation in muscle during metabolic stress is to provide amino acids, especially the BCAA which donate nitrogen, for the synthesis of glutamine.[1] This glutamine, after release by the muscle, is essential for the functioning of cells of the immune system, cells involved in repair, and for the kidney to combat acidosis. This new hypothesis explains why there is such a large increase in protein degradation in skeletal muscle during injury, sepsis, and burns and indicates that it is an adaptive process and should not be considered as necessarily detrimental to the patient.[1]

The BCAA, valine, leucine, and isoleucine, are among the nine essential amino acids in human beings. The substantial requirement for BCAA is reflected in their abundance in proteins: they account for 35 percent of the essential and 14 percent of the total amino acids in skeletal muscle. The standard balanced amino acid solutions used in intravenous nutrition contain 19 to 25 percent BCAA, while the commercially available BCAA-enriched solutions have about 45 percent of the amino acids as BCAA.[1] BCAA account for about 40 to 45 percent of the total amino acid requirement in human beings.[1] Furthermore, they have metabolic properties and metabolic effects that are unique in several aspects. First, their initial metabolism occurs chiefly in skeletal muscle rather than in the liver. Perhaps surprisingly, this may be of particular importance not so much for muscle but for other tissues and organs in the body. Secondly, one or more of the BCAA may exert a specific regulatory effect on the rates of protein turnover by mechanisms other than their role as precursors for protein synthesis. Thirdly, BCAA are transported into the brain via the same carrier that transports the aromatic amino acids (AAA). Consequently, competition for entry into the brain between BCAA and AAA may influence the rate of synthesis of some monoamine neurotransmitters and, therefore, the level of such neurotransmitters. In this way BCAA could influence behavior.

These various features of the metabolism of BCAA have led to suggestions that they might have therapeutic uses that are pharmacologic, in addition to being components of complete mixtures of amino acids for protein synthesis. No therapeutic uses of BCAA-enriched mixtures have been firmly established, even though the unique metabolic effects of the BCAA suggest that they might be effective in a variety of disorders. This suggests that our interpretation of the metabolism of these amino acids may be oversimplified. Beneficial effects of BCAA-enriched solutions have been demonstrated in treatment of hepatic failure with encephalopathy and in chronic renal failure. Their effects in hepatic encephalopathy, when considered with the effects on respiratory drive and appetite, suggest that stimulation of CNS function occurs. Use of mixtures enriched with BCAA have not clearly been shown to improve nitrogen balance in injured or septic patients. However, nitrogen balance may be an insensitive index for the beneficial effects of BCAA in such patients. Further studies of protein metabolism in the stressed state are required, with special regard to the role of muscle and its metabolism in the immune system, via provision of glutamine for the lymphocytes, macrophages, and tissue repair cells. The variability in clinical results obtained could be explained on the basis of factors which affect the conversion of BCAA to glutamine.[1] Hence, future research should consider whether some patients may be "responders" as opposed to "nonresponders" toward BCAA administration. Analysis of all patients as one population in a disease state such as sepsis may obscure a benefit to select subsets. Recently, the possibility of providing increased glutamine to the stressed patient (as L-alanyl-L-glutamine) as part of parenteral nutrition has been raised.[2] This may have an important impact on the clinical utility of BCAA in stress and septic states.

BCAA as Markers and Therapy for Metabolic Stress States

Sepsis and stress are associated with changes in metabolism that result in net proteolysis and negative nitrogen balance. In addition, amino acid concentrations in plasma change. BCAA may serve as a caloric source, promote synthesis of muscle and visceral protein, and reduce the breakdown of muscle protein. Because of these potential benefits, several trials have been undertaken to study nitrogen balance, morbidity, and mortality in patients receiving BCAA-enriched solutions. A number of studies in human beings and experimental animals have suggested beneficial effects of the use of BCAA solutions in trauma, injury, and sepsis. However, controversy still exists over whether BCAA supplementations are more beneficial for patients with trauma and sepsis than the standard balanced amino acid solutions.

METABOLIC ALTERATIONS IN STRESS

Surgery, trauma, sepsis, or burns result in negative nitrogen balance, due largely to an increased net rate of skeletal muscle breakdown.[1,3] The degree of the catabolic response depends on the severity and duration of the trauma or stress. After an uncomplicated surgical procedure in an otherwise healthy patient, the catabolic response persists for about a week with a net nitrogen loss. These mild nitrogen-losses are well tolerated and readily replaced by subsequent oral feeding. By contrast, the fasting patient suffering from severe trauma or sepsis catabolizes considerably more lean body mass and fat.

The metabolic response can be viewed as a mobilization of body protein, fat, and carbohydrate stores to maintain optimal metabolic conditions for wound repair and host defense when dietary intake is limited or absent. The increased availability of plasma amino acids occurs predominantly at the expense of skeletal muscle protein.[3] Several suggestions have been put forward to explain the increased net rate of protein degradation in skeletal muscle under these conditions:

1. it provides amino acids for the protein synthesis required by the repair processes and by cells of the immune system;
2. it provides amino acids that can act as precursors for hepatic gluconeogenesis;
3. the glucose is required for nervous tissue and cells involved in repair and the immune system; and
4. it provides BCAA which will be oxidized by muscle and hence will provide an energy source for the muscles.

Hyperglycemia occurs in these conditions and may be important in the response to trauma. This is supported by the fact that the rate of gluconeogenesis is increased even in the presence of high plasma levels of glucose. Fatty acids are mobilized from adipose tissue and are used for the energy needs of cardiac, skeletal, and respiratory muscles. Despite the hyperglycemia and the hyperinsulinemia, the muscles of the stressed patient utilize fatty acids instead of glucose. This is a very important role of the glucose/fatty acid cycle; it allows glucose to be spared for tissues that specifically require it, such as the CNS, the immune system, and the healing wound. The hormonal changes include increased levels of adrenal glucocorticoids, glucagon, and catecholamine.[1] The response is probably mediated by afferent nervous pathways and by cytokines and lymphokines, such as interleukin-1.[4]

There is no consensus as to whether changes in plasma amino acid profiles and ratios are specific in sepsis and stress. Some authors report hypoaminoacidemia; others observe no changes or an increase in total amino acid concentration.[1,5] Many authors have reported plasma amino acid profiles that were claimed to be specific for sepsis. Most authors find an increased plasma level of AAA; this may be due to some hepatic dysfunction induced by the septic process.[1,5] The plasma concentrations of the BCAA are most often decreased, but normal or increased concentrations are also described.[1] A specific sepsis pattern, as opposed to a metabolic stress pattern, has not been identified, but with increasing time and severity, the decrease in BCAA concentrations tends to be more pronounced.[6] In both liver failure and severe sepsis, therefore, the changes in the plasma levels of AAA and BCAA result in an increase in the AAA:BCAA concentration ratio.[1,7] Thus, if the change in ratio is severe, it may result in encephalopathy, which is sometimes seen in severe sepsis. The explanation would, therefore, be identical to that suggested for hepatic or other encephalopathies (vide infra).[5,8]

GLUTAMINE FORMATION IN SKELETAL MUSCLE DURING METABOLIC STRESS

Under metabolic stress the muscle and plasma concentrations of glutamine decrease, and yet, the rate of glutamine release by skeletal muscle is increased.[1] Furthermore, it has been shown that the isolated incubated epitrochlearis muscle from thermally injured rats releases glutamine at a greater rate than that from control animals. In addition, the maximum activity of glutamine synthetase is increased by at least 50 percent in the injured animals. On this basis, an hypothesis can be put forward. Increased net rates of protein degradation in muscle provide BCAA within the muscle which can donate their nitrogen for the synthesis of glutamine in the muscle. After release by the muscle, this glutamine is essential for the functioning of the cells of the immune system, those involved in repair, and for the kidney to combat the acidosis which can occur in this condition (Fig. 93-1). More specifically, the increased net rate of protein degradation in skeletal muscle may be essential to provide glutamine for the markedly increased number of cells

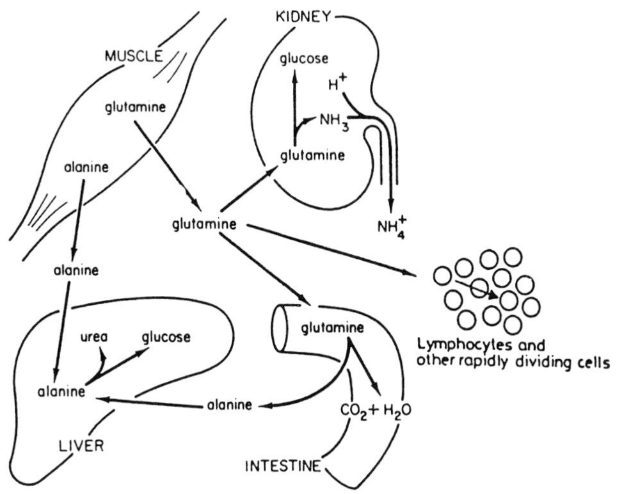

FIGURE 93-1 Interrelationship of organs in glutamine metabolism. For discussion, see text.

involved in cell division (e.g., lymphocytes, fibroblasts, endothelial cells), and for ammonia formation in the kidney.

If glutamine utilization is already higher than required in cells of the immune system, why should it increase further in conditions of sepsis, trauma, burns, or surgery? In all of these conditions, the number of cells of the immune system is increased and their immune "activity" is also increased. The above hypothesis should not imply that the rate of glutaminolysis is in excess in these cells, but that a greater rate of glutaminolysis is required to provide optimal conditions for metabolic control than would be needed solely for energy production. This is a similar situation to that found for the effects of physical training on skeletal muscle. The activities of enzymes that catalyze near-equilibrium reactions, which appear to be present in excess, are increased to a similar extent to those of the key enzymes that catalyze nonequilibrium reactions. This is to preserve the structure of the metabolic pathway which is important in control.

It is important to appreciate that this hypothesis does not necessarily invalidate the basis of previous hypotheses. For example, in skeletal muscle in man, the further oxidation of the keto acids derived from transamination of the BCAA provides some energy; the fate of the glutamine utilized by the cells of the immune system is glutamate, aspartate, and lactate, and all of these can be used as gluconeogenic precursors by the liver. Nonetheless, it is suggested that these are coincidental effects and should not obscure our view that an important if not primary role for muscle BCAA metabolism is to provide nitrogen for the formation of glutamine, which is then used to allow the cells of the immune and repair systems to perform their normal functions. This new hypothesis explains why there is such a large increase in protein degradation in skeletal muscle during injury, sepsis and burns, and indicates that it is essential for the survival of the animal under normal conditions. This point receives support from the observation that the muscle concentration of glutamine was considerably lower in patients who did not survive severe abdominal sepsis in comparison to those who did survive, despite the fact that the rates of muscle protein degradation appeared to be higher in the nonsurviving patients.[9] The new hypothesis should permit discussion of possible means of attempting to artificially improve the provision of glutamine for these cells of the immune system in trauma, sepsis, and burns with more precise knowledge of the metabolic interrelationships between the tissues and of the role of muscle and its metabolism in the immune response.

RATIONALE AND INVESTIGATION OF BCAA IN METABOLIC STRESS STATES

BCAA may inhibit muscle protein degradation and stimulate muscle protein synthesis. Conceivably, infusion of solutions containing BCAA may decrease nitrogen wasting associated with conditions of trauma, surgery, sepsis, or burns, and help provide glutamine for the immune system, the intestine, and the kidney.[1] An accelerated hepatic protein synthesis during sepsis aids survival,[10] probably reflecting increased production of acute phase proteins. Protein turnover in liver may be regulated by BCAA and other amino acids, as protein synthesis in incubated liver slices was stimulated by leucine.[1] In vivo administration of the individual BCAA to rats increased hepatic protein synthesis. Furthermore, protein synthesis was accelerated by various amino acid mixtures, and BCAA-enriched solutions increase the rate of hepatic protein synthesis and acute phase proteins in critically ill and septic patients.[1,11] Acute phase proteins are essential for immunodefense, and consequently, are important in host defense mechanisms against infection. Administration of solutions containing a high proportion of BCAA may thus improve the chances of survival for such patients via this mechanism.[11,12] The BCAA may also correct the increase in the AAA:BCAA concentration ratio in sepsis and could thus be helpful in preventing metabolic encephalopathy.

Several animal studies have indicated that the use of BCAA solutions in injured and septic animals improves nitrogen balance.[1] The most optimistic results have been found in studies where the effects of BCAA have been compared with those obtained with hypocaloric infusions of energy substrates alone or with isonitrogenous infusions of alanine. One study compared hepatic protein synthesis rates in three groups of septic rats that received infusion of dextrose alone, a balanced amino acid solution, or a BCAA-enriched solution.[13] All solutions were isocaloric, and the amino acid solutions were isonitrogenous. There were no differences in hepatic protein synthesis rates among the three groups. The negative nitrogen balance seen in the dextrose-infused animals was reversed to the same degree by the two different amino acid solutions. Conceivably, the ratio of the individual BCAA or the amount of leucine is at least as critical to nitrogen-sparing effect as the percentage of total BCAA infused.[14]

In recent years, many studies concerning the efficacy of BCAA on protein metabolism in catabolic patients have been carried out (Table 93-1). Most studies deal with pa-

TABLE 93-1 Studies of Nitrogen Balance with BCAA Supplementation in Patients with Surgical Stress and Sepsis

Study	Patient Profile	Control/Study BCAA, %	Preferred Therapy	Remarks
Freund[15]	Laparotomy	0/22 0/33 0/100	BCAA	5% dextrose as calorie source All BCAA concentrations supported nitrogen retention equally
Bower[11]	ICU/septic	25/45	BCAA (marginal benefit)	No difference in outcome 25% calories as fat Higher plasma short-turnover proteins in BCAA group
Daly[16]	Gastrectomy/ ileal conduit	25/45	NS*	Dextrose 5%; no fat
Cerra[17]	Laparotomy/ trauma	4 groups with different %BCAA	BCAA	Increased nitrogen-retention with increasing BCAA doses, effect started at 0.5 g/BCAA/day
Cerra[18]	Surgery/multi trauma/sepsis	24/45	BCAA	BCAA: 0.7 g/kg/day Improved nitrogen-retention at the end of the 7-day study with BCAA Improved immunologic function?
Cerra[19]	Laparotomy/ trauma	15.5/50	BCAA	35 kcal/kg/day (dextrose 25%) Positive nitrogen-balance at day 3 with BCAA, at day 6 in control group
Pelosi[20]	Multiple trauma	25/43	BCAA	10-day study
Nuwer[12]	ICU	25/43	BCAA	7-day study Improved immunologic tests
Bonau[14]	Cystectomy/ ileal conduit	0/25 0/45 (leucine low) 0/45 (leucine high)	?	More positive nitrogen-balance with BCAA 25% and 45% (high leucine) than BCAA 45% (low leucine)
van der Wounde[21]	ICU	19/45	NS	4-day study 30 kcal/kg/day; lipid 30%
van Way[22]	ICU	25/45	NS	14-day study
Okada[23]	Gastrectomy:	22/36		7-day study
	subtotal (87 pts)		NS	40 kcal/kg/day; no fat
	total (86 pts)		BCAA	Nitrogen-balance positive after 3 days with BCAA and after 6 days standard solution (total gastrectomy)

*NS, not significant.

tients with severe stress or sepsis due to trauma or major operations. The overall conclusions are clouded by the variability of stress, the number of septic patients included, and the relatively small number of patients. Not much information is given regarding the clinical characteristics of the population under study. It is, therefore, difficult to ascertain whether the improvements are due to the BCAA enrichment or are the result of clinical differences between the groups. This also makes it difficult to demonstrate a clinical benefit regarding morbidity and mortality. In the studies reported, protein intake varies from 1 to 1.5 g/kg/day. Nonprotein calories have been given as glucose only (30 to 40 kcal/kg/day), or in a combination with fat.

In a prospective, randomized trial, infusion of a standard amino acid solution was compared to two BCAA solutions, one of which was enriched primarily with valine, whereas the other was enriched with leucine.[11] The study contained 37 patients who received an isocaloric, isonitrogenous dextrose solution infused within 24 h of the onset of major operation, injury, or sepsis. Marginal improvement in nitrogen retention was demonstrated in the BCAA groups, but cumulative nitrogen retention was not improved. The patients receiving the leucine-enriched solution appeared to maintain a higher rate of hepatic protein synthesis, since the plasma concentration of short-turnover proteins was higher. However, there was no difference in the outcome. When cystectomy and ileal conduit was the surgical insult, there was no difference in the cumulative nitrogen balance when comparing two solutions of 25% and 45% BCAA.[16] Other studies have suggested an advantage for the BCAA.[17–20] In a prospective, controlled trial of nutritional effects of BCAA-enriched solution in 173 surgical patients with gastric cancer, the group receiving a solution high in BCAA demonstrated a statistically significant improvement in nitrogen balance on days 2 and 3 after total gastrectomy.[23] A significant increase in absolute lymphocyte count and delayed cutaneous hypersensitivity occurred in the groups of patients receiving BCAA-enriched solutions,[12,18] as did a significant increase in short half-life plasma proteins such as transferrin and prealbumin.[11,18] Several noncontrolled studies in postoperative patients using hypocaloric nutritional support supplemented with BCAA have reported nitrogen sparing effects, but other studies have not found any difference in nitrogen retention between solutions containing standard or high content of BCAA.[21,22]

Most of the studies showing promotion of nitrogen balance with enriched BCAA solutions have not used a balanced substrate for nonprotein caloric support, though a balanced TPN regimen itself can lead to a positive nitrogen balance.[24] In one study where a balanced substrate for nonprotein caloric support was used (carbohydrate:lipid calorie ratio 7:3), no significant difference was found in nitrogen balance when a 44.6% BCAA solution was compared to standard TPN (19% BCAA).[21] The lack of difference in this study may be due to effective utilization of lipid as a fuel source by both groups. Conceivably, there is an increased dependence on lipids as a fuel source in the septic patient compared to the nonseptic patient;[25] with a mixed fuel source, a BCAA-enriched regimen was associated with a rapid rise in fibrin, transferrin, ceruloplasmin, and α-antitrypsin, as well as platelets.[26] These data suggest that perhaps nitrogen balance alone is a poor index of success or failure of nutritional support in stress conditions.

The in vitro studies that have suggested a beneficial effect of the BCAA on protein turnover have not been performed in models or preparations representing states of trauma or sepsis; however, it is in these states that most investigators feel there may be a clinical benefit associated with the use of BCAA. A failure of the various studies to uniformly detect benefit from BCAA in patients may have several explanations. The control of muscle protein turnover may be modified in sepsis so that much higher levels of leucine may be required to influence protein synthesis in comparison to the normal condition. Secondly, nitrogen balance may be the least sensitive index with which to investigate the efficacy of BCAA. If plasma or muscle glutamine levels are important in facilitating the response to stress, then these levels should be measured in carefully planned experiments. Thus, if protein degradation is designed to provide, in a controlled fashion, sufficient BCAA for glutamine formation in muscle, as suggested above, then nitrogen balance per se may not be a sensible index to measure the usefulness of amino acid infusions. Finally, it is possible that some patients may suffer a limitation in the conversion of BCAA to glutamine in muscle and, if the above discussions have any physiologic validity, they would not benefit from BCAA administration. Inclusion of such patients could complicate the interpretation of results and might explain some of the variability in the results reported. This argument underlines the need to carry out a systematic study into the mechanisms by which the rate of formation of glutamine in muscle is controlled, especially in patients suffering from trauma, sepsis, burns, or surgery. Application of metabolic control-logic to the problem could clarify much of the present discussion and controversy.[1]

BCAA in Hepatic Failure

Several factors contribute to the compromised nutritional status in patients with severe chronic liver disease: poor diet, reduced intake secondary to anorexia, malabsorption, hypercatabolism, and dietary protein restriction. Of all the factors currently known to influence liver regeneration (steroids, triiodothyronine, insulin, glucagon, and other factors), nutrition is the easiest one to manipulate. Parenteral feeding permits selective delivery of necessary nutrients and is, therefore, attractive in this setting. However, the administration of adequate amounts of nutrients to these patients is made difficult by the presence of profound metabolic alterations which impair substrate utilization. In compromised hepatic function, the peripheral plasma levels of glucagon and insulin are elevated, probably due to decreased rates of hepatic degradation.[27] The hyperglucagonemia has also been correlated with portosystemic shunting,[27] and it is likely that the increased insulin results from the same mechanism. The increase in level of glucagon is greater than that of insulin. A reduced insulin activity similar to that observed in type II diabetes mellitus has been reported.[28] The net result is a decreased insulin:glucagon ratio which favors catabolism. Skeletal muscle proteolysis associated with cirrhosis liberates BCAA.[29] Thus, in cirrhotic patients there exists an increased rate of muscle protein degradation coupled with impaired liver function. This induces a profound alteration of the plasma amino acid profile, which probably plays a key role in the pathogenesis of HE (vide infra) and is most likely responsible for the protein intolerance with resultant encephalopathy seen in patients with liver failure. At the same time, there are alterations in supply and utilization of fat and carbohydrates as energy substrates.[28] Impaired glucose and fat utilization are mainly responsible for the energy deficiency and the hypercatabolic state which characterizes advanced cirrhosis.

PLASMA AMINO ACIDS AND HEPATIC ENCEPHALOPATHY

HE is a neuropsychiatric syndrome associated with acute or chronic parenchymal liver disease. HE is due to the failure of the liver to remove an endogenously produced toxic substance or substances from the circulation. The observations that protein and certain other nitrogenous substances in the colon exacerbated hepatic encephalopathy, whereas broad-spectrum antibiotics such as neomycin caused significant amelioration suggested an intestinal origin for the causal substance(s). It is thus thought that the toxic metabolite(s) is able to reach the brain because of defective hepatic metabolism.[30] Ammonia was the earliest candidate for the toxic metabolite in HE. It is produced by bacterial action in the gut and is largely metabolized by the liver to glutamate and urea. It has been demonstrated that ammonia can induce many of the clinical signs of HE, but blood levels of ammonia correlate only approximately with the depth of coma and are not elevated in all patients with HE.[31] Furthermore, ammonia does not appear to produce coma directly; the clinical picture of coma due to ammonia toxicity differs somewhat from that of hepatic encephalopathy. Other toxic substances produced in the gut might act synergistically to cause altered cerebral metabolism. Such substances include mercaptans, short- and medium-chain fatty acids, and phenol. Several of these toxins may be simultaneously responsible.[1]

Hepatic failure is also associated with considerable changes in the plasma concentrations of amino acids, and much attention has been given to the possible role of the amino acid changes in the pathogenesis of the encephalopathy.[32] The hypothesis indicated that accumulation of "false" neurochemical transmitters was important in the pathogenesis of HE. Several biogenic amines, primarily octopamine and phenylethanolamine (both metabolites of tyrosine and phenylalanine), can be stored in nerve terminals in place of true neurotransmitters, norepinephrine, and dopamine. The serum levels of the AAA (phenylalanine, tyrosine, and tryptophan) are elevated considerably, whereas levels of BCAA are markedly reduced.[39] The increase in the levels of the AAA is thought to be due to reduced rate of hepatic metabolism. Since the BCAA are metabolized by muscle, there is a decrease in the BCAA relative to the AAA. Decreases in the levels of the BCAA may also be facilitated due to hyperinsulinemia (decreased hepatic insulin clearance), which would enhance BCAA uptake into muscle. Since BCAA compete with AAA for entry into the brain, these changes would cause increases in the entry of the AAA, especially tryptophan, into the brain so that brain levels of serotonin and other neurotransmitters might increase. This could then contribute to the coma of hepatic failure. Although the reduced ratio of BCAA to large neutral amino acids has been confirmed in cirrhosis, there appears to be no difference in the ratio between patients with and without HE.[34]

If this hypothesis for the etiology of hepatic coma were correct, treatments which reduced rates of brain serotonin formation might be of use (Fig. 93-2). Since increased brain serotonin formation was thought to be due to an increase in the tryptophan level in the brain, treatments to normalize the plasma amino acid pattern, such as infusions of BCAA, were attempted.[1] Although initial results of such treatments were encouraging, more recent studies including randomly assigned control groups have been unable to demonstrate significant benefits (vide infra). The use of BCAA has indicated that muscle protein degradation is excessive in such patients. Consequently, the rationale for using BCAA has shifted toward emphasis on the effects of these compounds on protein turnover in peripheral tissues.[1]

RATIONALE AND INVESTIGATION OF BCAA IN LIVER DISEASE

Patients with liver disease are catabolic. They have smaller stores of glycogen, are insulin resistant, and have a decreased rate of hepatic ketogenesis from fatty acids. Thus, BCAA might be useful in liver disease as an energy source that can be utilized by peripheral conversion. In addition to the use as an energy source, the BCAA effects on protein turnover may decrease muscle breakdown and promote protein synthesis. All of these effects might potentially ameliorate the whole body catabolic state. Furthermore, the increased AAA:BCAA ratio in plasma found in HE can be lowered by the administration of BCAA.[35] The normalization of BCAA and AAA in plasma may lower the penetration of AAA across the brain barrier with normalization of neurotransmitters synthesis (vide supra). Theoretically, peripheral catecholamine synthesis may also be normalized by having a more normal precursor amino acid pool in plasma.

Prior to testing in man, solutions enriched in BCAA underwent extensive testing in dogs and monkeys. An end-to-side portocaval shunt offered a model of HE with an amino acid pattern similar to that seen in man with hepatic failure. The results clearly indicated that a BCAA-enriched solution was superior to amino acid solutions with standard BCAA content in achieving positive nitrogen balance and normalizing neurologic symptoms.[1,35] Encouraged by these promising reports, numerous anecdotal studies were published in which BCAA-enriched amino acid solutions were given with hypertonic dextrose to patients with liver disease,[1,36] producing dramatic effects on arousal from encephalopathy and on the improvement of consciousness in cirrhotic patients. Conclusions of efficacy, however, cannot be drawn from these uncontrolled reports. In a disease as variable as hepatic failure, only randomized and prospective studies can be accepted as showing efficacy.

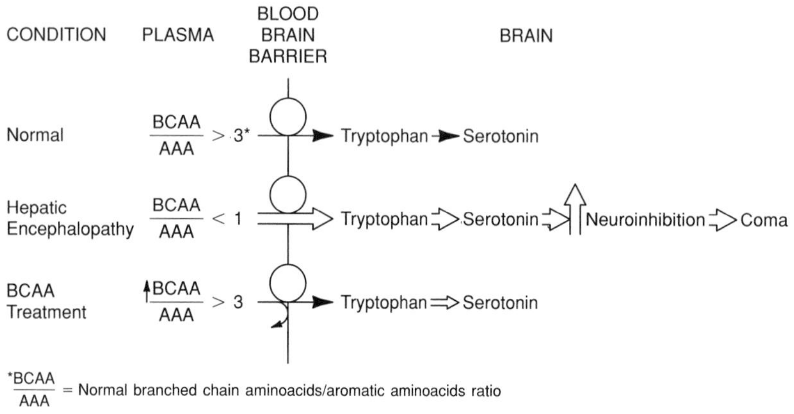

FIGURE 93-2 Overall scheme of the BCAA:AAA ratio in health, hepatic coma, and postulated results of treatment. (Reproduced with permission from Alexander WF, Spindel E, Harty RF, et al: The usefulness of branched chain amino acids in patients with acute or chronic hepatic encephalopathy. Am J Gastroenterol 84:91, 1989.)

TABLE 93-2 Studies of BCAA versus Standard Amino Acids as Nutritional Therapy in Patients with Liver Disease.[a]

Study	No. of Patients	Patient Profile	Preferred Treatment	Measure of Efficacy
Muto[37]	8	Hospitalized cirrhotics	BCAA	Nitrogen balance
Rocchi[38]	36	Stable cirrhotics	Standard amino acids	Nitrogen balance
Okuno[39]	61	Postoperative cirrhotics	Standard amino acids	Nitrogen balance
Kanematsu[40]	56	Postoperative cirrhotics	No difference	Mortality/mental status

[a] SOURCE: From McCullough AJ, Mullen KD, Smanik EJ, et al: Nutritional therapy and liver disease. Gastroenterol Clin North Am 18:619, 1989, reprinted with permission.

Only four studies have compared BCAA-enriched solutions with the standard amino solutions as nutritional therapy in chronic liver disease[37–40] (Table 93-2). The type of patient populations, route, and type of amino acid administration differed between the studies, but all four studies used nitrogen balance as the measure of efficacy. The conclusion of these studies is that BCAA-enriched mixtures provided no improved benefit over standard formulations regarding nitrogen balance. In fact, in two of the studies, the BCAA formulations were inferior to standard amino acid mixtures in achieving nitrogen balance.[38,39]

There have been six controlled randomized clinical studies using intravenous BCAA in patients with acute HE.[41–46] As can be seen in Table 93-3, disagreement concerning their efficacy regarding mortality and improving encephalopathy exists. It should be emphasized that in most of these studies the control group did not receive any amino acids or protein. The first randomized controlled trial of BCAA therapy in acute HE tested the efficacy of BCAA in patients with severe HE.[41] Forty patients with HE were randomly assigned to receive oral lactulose with hypertonic dextrose or 60 g BCAA in isoenergetic hypertonic dextrose. Patients were treated for at least 4 days. Wakeup occurred in 70 percent of the patients receiving BCAA and in 47 percent of those who received lactulose, but the difference was not statistically significant. Intravenous BCAA were thus found to be at least as effective as lactulose in reversing hepatic coma. Blood BCAA levels in patients receiving BCAA were increased at the time of mental recovery as compared to control values before initiation of therapy, but subsequently returned to base line when treatment was discontinued, despite continued improvement in mental state. There were no changes in blood amino acids in patients receiving lactulose, no difference in survival, and nitrogen balance studies were not done. In another trial, the patients were randomized into three groups: group A received lactulose alone plus hypertonic dextrose; group B received a BCAA-enriched solution with hypertonic dextrose; and group C received both lactulose and the BCAA-hypertonic dextrose mixture.[43] Sixty-two percent of the patients in group A, 94 percent in group B, and 100 percent in group C "came out of coma" after 7 days of therapy, and treatments B and C were significantly better than treatment A. In the United States multicenter trial, 75 patients received either oral neomycin and 25 percent dextrose solution intravenously or an isocaloric dextrose solution enriched with BCAA.[44] Wake-up time was significantly shorter and nitrogen balance better in the BCAA-dextrose group as compared with the neomycin-dextrose group. Survival was improved in the group receiving BCAA-dextrose, 85 percent as opposed to 55 percent in the neomycin-dextrose group. The improved survival may, however, be a result of the nutritional support in these patients with severe illness rather than the BCAA mixture in itself.

These studies seem to indicate that BCAA are of value in treatment of HE when given with hypertonic dextrose as an energy source; patients in hepatic coma awoke at least as quickly in response to administration of BCAA and hypertonic dextrose solution as they did in response to the conventional treatment with starvation and neomycin/lactulose therapy, and both regimens worked much more quickly than placebo.[41,43,44,46] The exceptions to this trend have used fat as the major energy source[42,45] and have failed to show that BCAA-enriched solutions are preferable to a standard amino acid solution in HE. No difference in the rate of awakening was found between a group receiving conventional amino acid solution and the other group receiving a 35% BCAA mixture.[45] In both groups, 60 percent of the energy was given as fat. A multicenter study conducted in France and Sweden also failed to confirm any efficacy for the BCAA solution.[42] Fifty patients with cirrhosis and acute HE were randomized to receive 5 days of either 30 kcal/kg/day by amino acid-free TPN or isocaloric TPN with 40 g BCAA/day added. They showed a clinical improvement in HE in 56 percent of patients receiving the BCAA-enriched solution with glucose and fat, but this was not significantly different from 48 percent improvement in the control group receiving the isoenergetic solution of glucose and fat. Fifty percent of the energy was given as fat. Mortality was not significantly different between the two groups. In the opinion of some authors, the high lipid intake would not constitute a source of energy in hepatic failure and could possibly worsen the patient's condition.

It is clear from the trials under review that BCAA enrichment does not further deteriorate HE and that arousal is as fast or faster in a large proportion of the patients than in the control group receiving conventional treatment.[7,48] It is troublesome, however, that in only one study a control group received isonitrogenous amounts of a conventional amino acid mixture;[45] no difference was observed between

TABLE 93-3 Studies of BCAA on Mental Recovery and Mortality in Hepatic Encephalopathy

			PREFERRED TREATMENT	
Study	No. of Patients	Control Treatment	Encephalopathy	Mortality
Rossi-Fanelli[41]	34	Lactulose	ND	ND
Fiaccadori[43]	48	Lactulose	BCAA	ND
Cerra[44]	75	Neomycin	BCAA	BCAA
Strauss[46]	29	Neomycin	BCAA	ND
Michel[45]	47	Standard amino acids	ND	ND
Wahren[42]	50	Glucose	ND	ND

ND = No significant difference between treatments.

the two amino acid mixtures. It should, therefore, be concluded that parenteral amino acid solutions allow a wake-up response which is favorable or better than with conventional treatment. It is not certain, however, that this is due to the BCAA content of the amino acid mixtures. The studies to date do not permit an unqualified conclusion in favor of use of BCAA solutions for patients with HE. Although a beneficial effect on mental status is demonstrable, the impact on mortality is discrepant across trials. Given the uncertainty about effects on mortality and short follow-up times in all studies, a confirmatory randomized controlled trial with longer follow-up periods is warranted.

The primary goal of nutritional support in hepatic failure should be to prevent further injury to the liver cells and to promote their regeneration. When examining amino acid requirements, the approach in the nonencephalopathic patient would be to start with a relatively low intake of a standard amino acid solution at ~0.6 g/kg body wt/day (14 to 23% BCAA) and to increase it stepwise until a goal of between 1.2 and 1.5 g/kg body wt/day is obtained, provided encephalopathy does not occur. Should encephalopathy develop, a BCAA-enriched formula could be substituted to provide ~50 percent of the total amino acid mixture. If, on the other hand, the patient is encephalopathic at the outset, evidence would support the initial use of BCAA-enriched solution together with overall attention to general nutritional, metabolic, and electrolyte requirements. Since no evidence exists at present to suggest that the BCAA-enriched formula should be continued after encephalopathy subsides, conversion to a standard formula should be attempted.[49] Whether it is only the initial concentration of BCAA that improves encephalopathy remains unknown.

Effects of BCAA on Tryptophan-Mediated Behavioral Function

This section emphasizes the importance of the concentrations of plasma amino acids in influencing the concentration of brain amines and the possible behavioral importance of this. Since the entry of tryptophan into the brain is particularly affected by the BCAA, we focus on tryptophan and 5-hydroxy-tryptamine (5-HT). Relevant aspects of metabolic control logic, 5-HT synthesis in the brain, regulation of amino acid levels, and transport of amino acids into the brain are discussed elsewhere.[1] Nerve cells communicate with one another via synapses. Although transient changes in electrical potential convey information along the axons of nerve cells, the transmission of such information across synapses is brought about chemically by neurotransmitters. An increasing number of compounds (>40) is believed to function as neurotransmitters in the CNS, including the catecholamines (noradrenaline, dopamine), acetylcholine, the amino acids glutamate, aspartate, glycine, and taurine, the amines 5-HT and 4-aminobutyrate, and also many peptides.[50] Accordingly, as well as being neurotransmitters in their own right, amino acids are also precursors for many of the neurotransmitters (e.g., the catecholamines, 5-HT, histamine, and the peptide neurotransmitters).

For tryptophan, an hypothesis has been put forward as follows.[1] An increased concentration of this amino acid in plasma will increase the level in the brain. In turn, this will increase the rate of synthesis and brain concentration of 5-HT, and so increase the rate or amount of release of the neurotransmitter into the synapse, causing a change in behavior. The precise behavioral change may depend on the area(s) in the brain in which a change in 5-HT level occurs.

SLEEP AND MOOD

A substantial amount of evidence indicates that 5-HT neurons are involved in the control of sleep. Controlled studies indicate that tryptophan administration can increase sleep duration or drowsiness in normal subjects.[1,51] Differences in the results obtained in various studies can usually be attributed to differences in the dose of tryptophan or the degree of insomnia of the subjects. In subjects with "mild insomnia" or in normal subjects with long sleep latencies, the results appear to be almost always positive. However, in entirely normal subjects or in patients with more severe insomnia, the results are mixed and less clear.[1]

Tryptophan consumption significantly increased self-reported fatigue.[52] Conceivably, biochemical changes brought about by exercise may cause mood changes in normal subjects due to effects on brain tryptophan levels; exercise can lead to mood elevation in normal subjects and can have an antidepressant effect in clinically depressed patients.[1] The feeling of well-being following exercise has been linked to the increased synthesis of endorphins, and

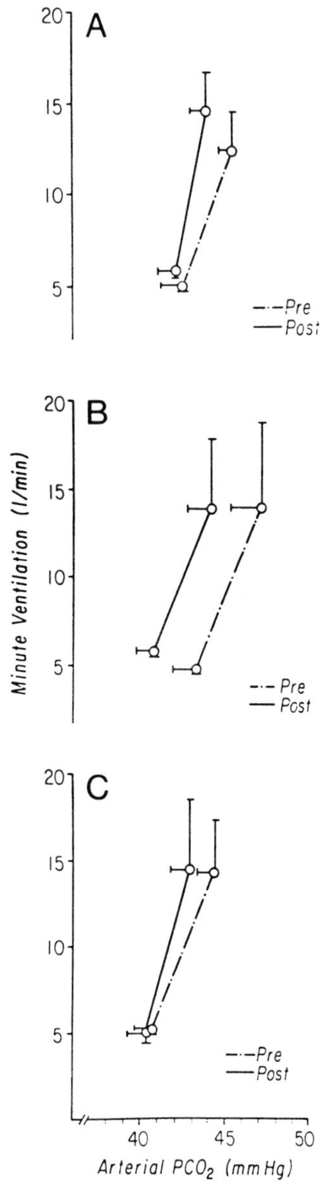

FIGURE 93-3 Ventilatory responses to carbon dioxide before and after 4-h infusion. The points of each line represent the mean values of minute ventilation and the corresponding arterial carbon dioxide tension while breathing room air and 4% carbon dioxide. The bars represent one standard error of the mean. *a*. BCAA-enriched solution; *b*. standard amino acid solution; *c*. Ringer's lactate. (Reproduced with permission from Takala J, Askanazi J, Weissman C, et al: Changes in respiratory control induced by amino acid infusions. Crit Care Med; 16:465, 1988.)

increases in plasma endorphin levels have often been observed following exercise. However, endorphins do not cross the blood-brain barrier and administration of the opiate antagonist naloxone has not prevented the improvement in mood caused by exercise. Exercise has been found to cause significant decreases in the plasma concentrations of BCAA but no change in the total (free plus bound to albumin) concentration of tryptophan.[53] The plasma concentration of free tryptophan measured in marathon runners increased 2.4-fold during the race, probably due to a pronounced elevation in the concentration of plasma free fatty acids during exercise, since these are known to displace tryptophan from albumin. The resulting increase in the plasma concentration of free tryptophan:BCAA ratio should increase the rate of synthesis of 5-HT in the brain. An elevated concentration of 5-HT in specific areas of the brain may be responsible, at least in part, for the development of physical or mental fatigue during prolonged exercise. The hypothesis can be further tested by examining the effect of administration of BCAA on physical and mental fatigue during prolonged exercise.[1]

NOCICEPTION AND VENTILATION

Pain sensitivity is thought to be one of the brain functions influenced by brain 5-HT levels. Tryptophan-enriched diets have been found to potentiate electrically induced endorphin analgesia and to increase pain tolerance in patients with chronic, disabling pain.[54] Furthermore, it has been shown that, in rats, tryptophan-poor corn diets decrease pain thresholds. Single intravenous injections of tryptophan into these animals were able to reverse the increased pain sensitivity, presumably by restoring brain 5-HT levels to normal.

Infusion of a standard amino acid solution stimulates ventilation;[55] the ventilatory response following amino acid infusion exceeded the increase in metabolic rate, suggesting that amino acids specifically increase ventilatory drive. The responses of ventilatory drive did not parallel the changes in $\dot{V}_{O_2}$, but did parallel the change in the ratio of tryptophan to the amino acids that compete with tryptophan for transport across the blood-brain barrier.[1] This decrease in the ratio of tryptophan to its competitors for uptake (val + leu + ile + tyr + phe) led to the hypothesis that the increased ventilatory sensitivity was mediated through inhibition of central 5-HT synthesis resulting from a rise in the amino acids that oppose tryptophan uptake across the blood-brain barrier. 5-HT inhibits respiration,[56] and infusion of a solution consisting primarily (85 percent) of BCAA increased the ventilatory response to CO_2 inhalation[57] (Fig. 93-3). The difference in ventilatory drive is unlikely to be of clinical significance in patients with normal ventilatory reserves, but further studies are necessary to evaluate the possible clinical implication in patients with limited reserve.[57]

APPETITE AND FOOD INTAKE

The relationship between plasma and brain amino acid patterns and feeding behavior demonstrates suppression of food intake when serotonin receptors have been activated directly or indirectly.[58] An increase in food intake resulting from an inhibition of 5-HT metabolism or blockade of receptors has also been reported.[59] It seems that manipulations of 5-HT metabolism can produce changes in food intake, food preferences, and body weight. We have suggested that it may be possible to increase appetite and food intake by giving BCAA-enriched solutions. The hypothesis is that elevated plasma levels of BCAA will decrease the transport of tryptophan across the blood-brain barrier. The resulting decreased 5-HT activity in brain may decrease the anorexic action of 5-HT. TPN with standard amino acid solutions reduces appetite and food intake by an amount that closely compensates for the infused calories.[60] This loss in appetite and food intake may prolong the transition from intravenous to oral feeding in patients who need nutritional support. The reduction in food intake previously seen when TPN is administered does not seem to occur, or at least is less pronounced, when the amino acid solution contains a high proportion of BCAA.[60] If this regimen really decreases the TPN-related reduction in appetite and food intake, BCAA-enriched solutions may play a useful role in the transition from TPN to oral feeding or in increasing the total (intravenous + oral) energy intake.

CASE PRESENTATION

A 38-year-old man with chronic renal failure (CRF), treated with hemodialysis (HD) three times a week, agreed to undergo nocturnal polysomnography and was studied on two nights prior to HD on the following day. He was overweight (150 percent of ideal body weight). The patient had severe sleep apnea and abnormal sleep pattern. Because of continuous arousals in connection with the apneas, his sleep was scored as transitional sleep, type non-REM and REM. He received BCAA (60 mg/kg/h = 1.4 mL/kg/h) or saline solution, intravenously, for 7 h on two different nights. The infusions were started 1 h before habitual bedtime. With BCAA there was an increased ventilation with a decrease (11 percent) in mean end-tidal CO_2 during the 7-h infusion. The BCAA night in this patient was associated with a large decrease in the total number of apneas (from 323 to 94). Furthermore, no central apneas occurred that night. While the apneas on the saline night were associated with regular desaturations from a base line of 95% decreasing to about 40%, the hypopneas and majority of the apneas seen on the BCAA night only caused desaturation down to around 70%. The patient also increased the amount of REM sleep from 12 to 18 percent. Despite improvements with BCAA, the severity of his sleep apnea made this patient a candidate for trial of nocturnal continuous positive airway pressure mask and he was referred for this.

CASE DISCUSSION

Sleep apnea is a common problem in CRF patients with an incidence close to 10 percent. In approximately half the patients, the sleep apneas are primarily of the obstructive type. In the rest, the apneas and hypopneas are of central origin. The infusion of BCAA appeared to stimulate respiration as evidenced by lowering of end-tidal CO_2. In our patient with severe obstructive sleep apnea, BCAA also reduced both the total number of apneas and the severity of oxygen desaturation. This case report suggests BCAA to be useful in the treatment of sleep apnea in CRF patients. Presently, the use of respiratory stimulants in sleep apnea is controversial. Besides the high incidence of toxic side effects, the main critique of pharmacologic interventions in sleep apnea has been concurrent worsening of sleep quality. Previously, use of respiratory stimulants has been associated with increased light and unsteady non-REM sleep, thereby counteracting the other positive effects on sleep apnea. Importantly, this was not the case with BCAA. The increased amount of REM sleep in our patient is thus an aspect that needs further consideration.

The mechanism of the augmented respiratory effects and changes in sleep pattern seen with BCAA infusion is unknown. Elevation of BCAA, which compete for transportation across the blood-brain barrier with amino acids that act as precursors for neurotransmitters, has been proposed as a mechanism. In CRF patients this hypothesis may be of particular relevance because both serum BCAA depletion and specific changes in cerebral uptake of amino acids have been associated with CRF.

References

1. Skeie B, Kvetan V, Gil K, et al: Branched-chain amino acids: Their metabolism and clinical utility. Crit Care Med 18:549, 1990.
2. Stehle P, Zander J, Mertes N, et al: Effect of parenteral glutamine peptide supplements on muscle glutamine loss and nitrogen balance after major surgery. Lancet 1:231, 1989.
3. Kinney JM, Elwyn DH: Protein metabolism and injury. Ann Rev Nutr 3:433, 1983.
4. Baracos V, Rodemann HP, Dinarello CA, et al: Stimulation of muscle protein degradation and prostaglandin E_2 release by leukocytic pyrogen (interleukin-1). A mechanism for the increased degradation of muscle proteins during fever. N Engl J Med 308:553, 1983.
5. Cerra FB, Siegel JH, Border JR, et al: The hepatic failure of sepsis: Cellular versus substrate. Surgery 86:409, 1979.
6. Vente JP, von Meyonfeldt MF, van Eijk HMH, et al: Plasma amino acid profiles in sepsis and stress. Ann Surg 209:57, 1989.
7. Cerra FB, Siegel JH, Coleman B, et al: Septic autocannibalism. A failure of exogenous nutritional support. Ann Surg 192:570, 1980.
8. Rossi-Fanelli F, Freund H, Krause R, et al: Induction of coma in normal dogs by the infusion of aromatic amino acids and its prevention by the addition of branched chain amino acids. Gastroenterology 83:664, 1982.
9. Roth E, Funovics J, Muehlbacker F, et al: Metabolic disorders in severe abdominal sepsis: Glutamine deficiency in skeletal muscle. Clin Nutr 1:25, 1982.
10. Clowes GHA, Hirsch E, George BC, et al: Survival from sepsis: The significance of altered metabolism regulated by proteolysis inducing factor. Ann Surg 202:446, 1985.
11. Bower RH, Muggia-Sullam M, Vallgren S, et al: Branched chain amino acid enriched solutions in the septic patient. A randomized, prospective trial. Ann Surg 203:13, 1986.
12. Nuwer N, Cerra FB, Shronts EP, et al: Does modified amino acid total parenteral nutrition alter immune-response in high level surgical stress? JPEN 7:521, 1983.

13. Pedersen P, Shujun L, Hasselgren PO, et al: Administration of balanced or BCAA-enriched amino acid solution in septic rats. Ann Surg 201:714, 1988.
14. Bonau RA, Ang SD, Malayappa J, et al: High-branched chain amino acid solutions: Relationship of composition of efficacy. JPEN 8:622, 1984.
15. Freund H, Hoover MC Jr, Atamian S, et al: Infusion of the branched chain amino acids in postoperative patients. Am Surg 190:18, 1979.
16. Daly JM, Mihranian MH, Kehoe JE, et al: Effects of postoperative infusion of branched chain amino acids on nitrogen balance and forearm muscle substrate flux. Surgery 94:151, 1983.
17. Cerra FB, Mazuski J, Teasley K, et al: Nitrogen retention in critically ill patients is proportional to the branched chain amino acid load. Crit Care Med 11:775, 1983.
18. Cerra FB, Mazuski JE, Chuter E, et al: Branched chain metabolic support: A prospective, randomized, double-blind trial in surgical stress. Ann Surg 199:286, 1984.
19. Cerra FB, Upson D, Angelico R, et al: Branched chains support postoperative protein synthesis. Surgery 92:192, 1982.
20. Pelosi G, Proietti R, Magalini SI, et al: Anticatabolic properties of branched chain amino acids in trauma. Resuscitation 10:153, 1983.
21. van der Wounde, P, Morgan RE, Kosta JM, et al: Addition of branched-chain amino acids to parenteral nutrition of stressed critically ill patients. Crit Care Med 14:685, 1986.
22. van Way CW, Moore EE, Allo M, et al: Comparison of total parenteral nutrition with 25 percent and 45 percent branched chain amino acids in stressed patients. Am Surg 51:609, 1985.
23. Okada A, Mori S, Totsuka M, et al: Branched-chain amino acids metabolic support in surgical patients: A randomized, controlled trial in patients with subtotal or total gastrectomy in 16 Japanese institutions. JPEN 12:332, 1988.
24. Kirkpatrick JR, Dahn M, Lewis L: Selective versus standard hyperalimentation. A randomized prospective study. Am J Surg 141:116, 1981.
25. Nanni GA, Siegel JH, Coleman B, et al: Increased lipid fuel dependence in the critically ill septic patient. J Trauma 24:14, 1984.
26. Chiarla C, Siegel JH, Kidd S, et al: Inhibition of post-traumatic septic proteolysis and ureagenesis and stimulation of hepatic acute-phase protein production by branched-chain amino acid TPN. J Trauma 28:1145, 1988.
27. Sherwin R, Joshi P, Hendler R, et al: Hyperglucagonemia in Laennec's cirrhosis. The role of portal-systemic shunting. N Engl J Med 290:239, 1974.
28. Riggio O, Merli M, Cangiano C, et al: Glucose intolerance in liver cirrhosis. Metabolism 31:6, 1982.
29. Marchesini G, Zoli M, Angiolini A, et al: Muscle protein breakdown in liver cirrhosis and the role of altered carbohydrate metabolism. Hepatology 1:294, 1981.
30. Zieve L: The mechanism of hepatic coma. Hepatology 1:360, 1981.
31. Hensen DM: Portal-systemic encephalopathy and hepatic coma. Med Clin North Am 70:1081, 1986.
32. James JH, Ziparo V, Jeppsson B, et al: Hyperammonaemia, plasma aminoacid imbalance, and blood brain aminoacid transport: A unified theory of portal-systemic encephalopathy. Lancet 2:772, 1979.
33. Fischer JE: Amino acids in hepatic coma. Dig Dis Sci 27:97, 1982.
34. Morgan MY, Milsom JP, Sherlock S: Plasma ratio of valine, leucine and isoleucine to phenylalanine and tyrosine in liver disease. Gut 19:1068, 1978.
35. Rosen HM, Soeters PB, James JH, et al: Influences of exogenous intake and nitrogen balance on plasma and brain aromatic amino acid concentrations. Metabolism 27:393, 1978.
36. Okada A, Kamata S, Kim CW, et al: Treatment of hepatic encephalopathy with BCAA-rich amino acid mixture, in Walser M, Williamson R (eds): *Metabolism and Clinical Implications of Branched Chain Amino and Ketoacids*. New York, Elsevier-North Holland, 1981, pp 447–452.
37. Muto Y, Yoshida T: Effect of oral supplementation with branched-chain amino acid granules on improvement in decompensated liver cirrhosis: a cross-over controlled trial, in Ogoshi S, Okada A (eds): *Parenteral and Enteral Hyperalimentation*. New York, Elsevier, 1984, pp 280–292.
38. Rocchi E, Casaanelli M, Gilbertini P, et al: Standard or branched-chain amino acid infusions as short-term nutritional support in liver cirrhosis. JPEN 9:447, 1985.
39. Okuno M, Nagayama M, Takai T, et al: Postoperative total parenteral nutrition in patients with liver disorders. J Surg Reg 39:93, 1985.
40. Kanematsu T, Kioyanagi N, Matsumata T, et al: Lack of preventive effect of branched-chain amino acid solution on postoperative hepatic encephalopathy in patients with cirrhosis: A randomized prospective trial. Surgery 104:482, 1988.
41. Rossi-Fanelli F, Riggio O, Cangiano C, et al: Branched chain amino acids vs lactulose in the treatment of hepatic coma: A controlled study. Dig Dis Sci 27:929, 1982.
42. Wahren J, Denis J, Desurmont P, et al: Is intravenous administration of branched chain amino acids effective in the treatment of hepatic encephalopathy? A multicenter study. Hepatology 3:475, 1983.
43. Fiaccadori F, Ghinelli F, Pedretti G, et al: Branched chain amino acid enriched solutions in the treatment of hepatic encephalopathy: A controlled trial, in Capocaccia L, Fischer JE, Rossi-Fanelli (eds): *Hepatic Encephalopathy in Chronic Liver Failure*. New York, Plenum Press, 1984, pp 323–333.
44. Cerra FB, Cheung NK, Fischer JE, et al: Disease specific amino acid infusion (F080) in hepatic encephalopathy: A prospective, randomized, double-blind, controlled trial. JPEN 9:288,1985.
45. Michel H, Bories P, Aubin JP, et al: Treatment of acute hepatic encephalopathy in cirrhotics with a branched-chain amino acids enriched versus a conventional amino acids mixture. Liver 5:282, 1985.
46. Strauss E, dos Santos WR, da Silva EC, et al: Treatment of hepatic encephalopathy: A randomized clinical trial comparing a branched-chain enriched amino acid solution to oral neomycin. Nutritional Support Services 6:18, 1986.
47. Rossi-Fanelli F, Cangiano C, Cascino A, et al: Branched chain amino acids in the treatment of severe hepatic encephalopathy, in Capocaccia L, Fischer JE, Rossi-Fanelli F (eds): *Hepatic Encephalopathy in Chronic Liver Failure*. New York, Plenum Press, 1984, pp 335–344.
48. Naylor CD, O'Rourke K, Detsky AS, et al: Parenteral nutrition with branched-chain amino acids in hepatic encephalopathy: A meta-analysis. Gastroenterology 97:1033, 1989.
49. Blackburn GL, O'Keefe SJD: Nutrition in liver failure. Gastroenterology 97:1049, 1989.
50. Iversen LL: Neurotransmitters and CNS disease. Introduction. Lancet 2:914, 1982.
51. Greenwood MH, Friedel J, Bond AJ, et al: The acute effects of intravenous infusion of L-tryptophan in normal subjects. Clin Pharmacol Ther 16:455, 1974.
52. Wurtman RJ: Behavioral effects of nutrients. Lancet 1:1145, 1983.
53. Blomstrand E, Celsing F, Newsholme EA: Changes in plasma

concentrations of aromatic and branched-chain amino acids during sustained exercise in man and their possible role in fatigue. Acta Physiol Scand 133:115, 1988.
54. King RB: Pain and tryptophan J Neurosurg 53:44, 1980.
55. Askanazi J, Weissman C, LaSala PA, et al: Effect of protein intake on ventilatory drive. Anesthesiology 60:106, 1984.
56. Lundberg DB, Mueller RA, Breese GR: An evaluation of the mechanism by which serotonergic activation depresses respiration. J Pharmacol Exp Ther 212:397, 1980.
57. Takala J, Askanazi J, Weissman C, et al: Changes in respiratory control induced by amino acid infusions. Crit Care Med 16:465, 1988.
58. Harper AE, Peters JC: Amino acid signals and food intake and preference: Relation to body protein metabolism. Experientia (suppl) 44:107, 1983.
59. Blundell JE: Serotonin and appetite. Neuropharmacology 23:1537, 1984.
60. Gil K, Skeie B, Kvetan V, et al: Parenteral nutrition and oral intake: Effect of branched-chain amino acids. Nutr Int 6:291, 1990.

Chapter 94

NUTRITION AND THE RESPIRATORY SYSTEM

SIMON BURSZTEIN
NICOLA P. D'ATTELLIS
JEFFREY ASKANAZI

KEY POINTS

- *Postoperative respiratory complications can be reduced by appropriate nutritional support.*
- *Increased carbon dioxide production during nutritional support may precipitate ventilatory failure.*
- *Increases in carbon dioxide production may be minimized by increasing the proportion of calories delivered as fat.*
- *Malnutrition results in respiratory muscle wasting with adverse consequences for ventilatory function.*
- *Trauma and sepsis alter the response to nutritional support; positive nitrogen (N) balance is difficult or impossible to achieve without enormous calorie loading.*
- *Catabolism after trauma or during sepsis can still be reduced to an acceptable level by rational nutritional support.*

The interaction between nutritional status, nutritional supply, and respiratory function is important in the management of the critically ill. The reduction in postoperative respiratory complications from 24 to 9 percent in malnourished patients fed preoperatively is an important illustration of this interaction and our ability to effect a salubrious outcome.[1] To clarify this interrelationship, the following aspects of the interaction between ventilation and nutrition will be discussed: metabolic demand, ventilatory drive, respiratory and lung function, and practical implications for weaning.

Metabolic Demand

Energy expenditure (EE) in the critically ill patient is determined by either empirical approximation (such as those based on the Harris-Benedict formula, with various adjustments for associated critical illness) or by indirect calorimetric measurement (see Chap. 91). Regardless of approach, it is clear many critically ill patients have substantial elevation of EE. Any increase in EE causes an increase in oxygen consumption ($\dot{V}_{O_2}$), carbon dioxide production ($\dot{V}_{CO_2}$), and work of breathing. Consequently, these increases impose a load and added stress on the respiratory system.

Many injured or septic patients have an increased metabolic rate of approximately 30 to 35 percent. If the resting energy expenditure (REE) is assumed to be about 2000 kcal/day, one may decide to provide a trauma or infected patient with an additional 700 kcal/day. If these additional calories are broadly distributed as carbohydrates, protein, and fat (Table 94-1), during their oxidation within the body about 122 L CO_2 is produced; if supplied as a supplement over a 24-h period, this will increase $\dot{V}_{CO_2}$ by 85 mL/min, representing a substantial increase in respiratory load. In healthy subjects this is not a problem, but in patients with reduced ventilatory reserve of any cause this increase in $\dot{V}_{CO_2}$ may be sufficient to cause respiratory acidosis and acute respiratory failure requiring intubation and mechanical ventilation or to prevent discontinuation of mechanical support.

Different types of nutrients influence respiratory function in different ways and to different degrees, and different types of patients will behave differently to the same nutrient. Septic or injured patients receiving total parenteral nutrition (TPN) increase their $\dot{V}_{O_2}$ and $\dot{V}_{CO_2}$ but usually remain unable to increase their respiratory quotient (RQ) above 1, demonstrating an inability to be in net positive fat balance. On the other hand, normal or depleted patients receiving similar nutrition are capable of increasing their RQ above 1, placing them in net positive fat balance and giving them the ability to synthesize fat from glucose (Fig. 94-1).[2] Importantly, replacing carbohydrates by fats as the fuel source reduces CO_2 production and minute ventilation ($\dot{V}_E$) requirement.[3–5] In the ventilated patient, discontinuation of mechanical support may be made easier by replacing glucose with fat.

Ventilatory Drive

Starvation is associated with a decrease in metabolic rate and a decrease in $\dot{V}_E$. In addition, ventilatory response to hypoxia may be altered. In one study, administration of hypocaloric feedings (500 kcal/day) to normal volunteers for 10 days was associated with a 42 percent reduction in the ventilatory response to hypoxia.[6] In the same study, an amino acid infusion administered after hypocaloric feeding increased neuromuscular drive by decreasing the CO_2 res-

TABLE 94-1 Production of 700 kcal

Foodstuff	Energy (cal)	$\dot{V}_{O_2}$(L)	$\dot{V}_{CO_2}$(L)	H_2O (mL)	R
Carbohydrate 50g	205	41.45	41.45	30	1
Protein 30g	123	28.98	23.46	12.3	0.809
Fat 40g	372	80.76	57.08	42.4	0.707
Total	700	151.19	121.99	84.7	0.806

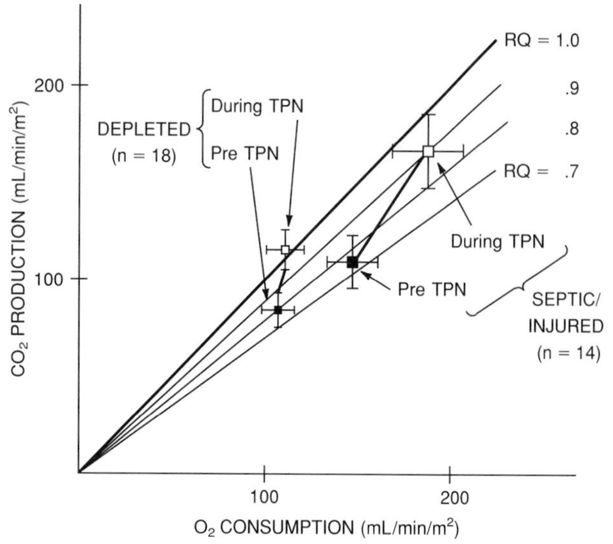

FIGURE 94-1 Response to TPN in two categories of patients. Depleted patients can increase the RQ above 1.0, but have a small increase in $\dot{V}_{O_2}$. Septic and injured patients cannot increase the RQ above 1.0, but show a greater increase in $\dot{V}_{O_2}$. (Reprinted with permission from Reference 2).

piratory threshold. Since CO_2 production remained relatively unchanged during the amino acid infusion, increased CO_2 production could not have accounted for the increase in $\dot{V}$E. Rather, it appears that chemoreceptor threshold response is 'reset' to a lower Pa_{CO_2}, with a leftward shift of the $\dot{V}$E/Pa_{CO_2} relationship. A similar change in ventilatory drive has been noted by comparing patients receiving either 5% dextrose solution or amino acids.[7] These findings are of unclear clinical relevance but may indicate that spontaneously breathing critically ill patients are at risk for development of hypoxia during periods of starvation, particularly in view of the other factors which may blunt ventilatory drive during ICU management. In addition, patients undergoing nutritional support which includes amino acid infusion may have an increased ventilatory load due to a shift in the threshold response to Pa_{CO_2}.

Malnutrition and Lung Function

Specific effects of malnutrition on the respiratory muscles were first described in 1916. Results were obtained from a large necropsy study, in which diaphragm weight loss was plotted against body weight loss. In this study, normally nourished subjects had mean body weights of 59 kg with corresponding diaphragm weights of 246 g; depleted subjects had mean body weights of 45 kg with mean diaphragm weights of 191 g. The results demonstrated the existence of a linear relationship between mean body weight loss and diaphragm weight loss since a mean body weight loss of 23 percent corresponded to a 22 percent loss in mean diaphragm weight. In a more recent study,[8] for a body weight loss of 31 percent, the corresponding weight loss of the diaphragm reached 43 percent. Respiratory muscle weight loss has an immediate effect on respiratory muscle strength, which decreased from 96 percent of normal in a control group to 37 percent in undernourished patients; the vital capacity (VC) in underweight patients decreased to 63 percent of the normal value. In the same group of patients, the maximum voluntary ventilation decreased from 80 percent of predicted in the control group to 41 percent of predicted in the underweight patients.[9]

Other effects of nutritional deprivation on respiratory physiology have been described.[10] Normal subjects on a semistarvation diet for 24 weeks lose 24 percent of their body weight and show a simultaneous progressive decline in respiratory function (measured as VC and resting VE). Both VC and VE return to normal after 12 weeks of refeeding. The reduction in respiratory function is probably due to respiratory muscle weakness. Observations of the same type in patients with anorexia nervosa confirm the relationship between body weight loss and respiratory function.

A significant number of patients (40 percent) suffering from chronic obstructive pulmonary disease (COPD), undergo substantial and progressive weight loss. In COPD, weight loss can be attributed to both the increase in REE secondary to the increase cost of breathing[11] and to a reduced caloric intake secondary to the efforts required for food intake.[12] A recent study in a group of COPD patients showed that a mean body weight loss of 13 percent was associated with an increase in metabolic rate of 10 percent.[13] Furthermore, it has been demonstrated that body weight loss in COPD patients carries a poor prognosis and is associated with increased morbidity and mortality.[12]

Starvation has been demonstrated to cause atrophy of diaphragmatic muscle fibers. However, not all fibers undergo atrophy to the same extent.[14] When diaphragm muscle fibers have been examined in hamsters subjected to undernutrition, type IIa and type IIb (fast twitch) fibers undergo atrophy, but not type I (slow twitch) fibers. This study demonstrated a 25 percent reduction in the diagmeter of fast twitch fibers, but no change in the diameter of slow twitch fibers. The greatest effect on fast fibers as compared to slow fibers may in part explain the decrease in contractile force seen in reponse to maximum tetanic stimulation at 100 Hz, and the relative increase seen during stimulation at 10 to 20 Hz.[16] These results may explain changes in absolute muscle force, fatigability, and muscle relaxation time, all of which have been shown to improve during adequate nutritional repletion.[16–18]

In addition to structural and functional changes of respiratory muscles, lung morphology is also affected by malnutrition. Alteration of terminal air spaces, as in emphysema, has been documented in undernourished animals.[19] Altered surfactant metabolism has also been demonstrated.[20] Conceivably, these changes impair efficient gas exchange and promote alveolar instability and atelectasis in malnourished patients.

Practical Implications for Nutrition and Weaning

When hyperalimentation is administered to patients with COPD or to any patient with reduced respiratory function, ventilatory load increases relatively more than in subjects with normal respiratory function. Improving nutritional status, assessed by increased serum albumin levels, improves respiratory function and facilitates weaning from mechanical ventilation. Thus, nutritional support has two contradictory but distinct effects on ventilation: **1.** short-term, it increases $\dot{V}_{CO_2}$ and ventilatory drive, representing a load on the respiratory system and making weaning difficult, and **2.** long-term, it increases serum albumin levels, reduces extravascular lung water, and improves respiratory muscle function, with a favorable effect on lung parenchyma and on surfactant metabolism, which makes weaning easier. Thus, a very fine line exists between acute ventilatory loads from nutritional support and long-term benefits. In addition, uncomplicated malnourished patients likely differ from trauma or septic patients in response to different nutrients. Thus, to recommend nutritional support, one must consider different categories of patients separately.

Nutritional Support for Injured and Septic Patients

For previously well-nourished patients who have suffered trauma, burns, or elective surgery, or for those with sepsis, the goal of nutritional therapy is to prevent or minimize loss of lean body mass. Since N losses can reach up to 15 to 40 g/day in severely stressed patients, full enteral or parenteral nutrition (PN) should be provided for patients who are not expected to return to adequate oral intake within a day or two. It is important to note that trauma and septic patients are resistant to nutrients, particularly proteins and carbohydrates. Some investigators have found[21] that at least 200 mg N/kg (about 1.4 g protein/kg body weight) results in maximum protein sparing but that above this, further increases in N intake have little further effect. In contrast to N intake, increasing energy intake improves N balance. Even the most severely traumatized patients can probably reach zero N balance if given two to three times their energy expenditure. However, fat deposition becomes enormous.

The thermic effects of both proteins and carbohydrates are of the order of 30 percent or more when given in excess, so that enormous amounts of nutrients can raise EE by 50 percent or more. Therefore, carbohydrates given in excess increase ventilation and work of breathing, but also sympathetic activity, lipogenesis, fatty liver, and liver dysfunction. For these reasons and to avoid undesirable side effects, the quantity of carbohydrates given should never be so great that the energy supplied by carbohydrates and proteins is equal to or greater than EE. Thus, the question remains, how does one pick the appropriate amounts? In the study cited above, daily energy intake was 45 to 50 kcal/kg, about 50 percent above the estimated EE. N balance, at N intakes above 200 mg/kg, was −3.5 g N/day. Losses of this magnitude can be tolerated even for weeks in previously well-nourished patients.[21] In another study of severely injured multiple trauma patients, 200 mg N/kg and 25.5 kcal/kg/day were provided.[22] This level of energy intake was probably 10 to 20 percent below EE. These patients were in daily negative N balances of −10 g in the first week, −11 g in the second, −7 g in the third, and −5 g in the fourth week. Such losses can result in severe morbidity, and it would seem worthwhile to increase energy intakes above this level. Thus, if one chooses an energy intake of 1.33 times REE, one may more closely approximate acceptable N balances.[21] The recommendations for septic or injured patients are:

1. If EE is measured (indirect calorimetry), provide energy (carbohydrate, fat, and protein) at 1.33 times REE with the nonprotein calories given as 50 percent carbohydrate and 50 percent fat, with a calorie:N ratio of 150 kcal/g N.
2. If EE is not measured, provide 2800 kcal/day or 40 kcal/kg/day, with a calorie:N ratio of 150 kcal/g N.

Nutritional Support for Malnourished Patients

Uncomplicated malnourished patients tolerate nutrients with less difficulty than either stressed patients or even normal subjects. Importantly, they can achieve positive N balance at zero energy balance. Most acutely malnourished patients have lost body cell mass (BCM) in the ratio of two parts BCM to one part fat. To restore tissue in this proportion, N intake must be in the range of 300 to 350 mg/kg/day. Since the average REE of malnourished patients is about 26 kcal/kg/day,[23–25] and their weights average close to 60 kg, about 1600 kcal/day per subject is necessary. To restore some fat, administer nutrition at 25 percent above REE to bedridden patients, and at 50 percent above REE to ambulatory patients to compensate for activity energy expenditure (AEE).[25]

The recommendations for malnourished patients are:

1. If EE is measured, provide energy at 1.25 times REE for bedridden patients and 1.5 times REE for ambulatory patients, with a calorie:N ratio of 100 kcal/g N.
2. If EE is not measured, provide 2000 kcal/day or 32 kcal/kg/day to bedridden patients and 2400 kcal/day or 39 kcal/kg/day to ambulatory patients, with the calorie:N ratio of 100 kcal/g N, providing 20 g N/day to bedridden patients and 24 g N/day to ambulatory patients.

A particularly difficult problem is posed by patients who are both malnourished and septic or injured. These patients are more catabolic than the malnourished patients but respond better to nutrients than do the well-nourished stressed patients. Theoretically, they should be given energy at the rates recommended for injured and septic patients, but with a calorie:N ratio of 100. It is important to remember that it is impossible to maintain, much less to restore, lean body mass in these patients.

These recommendations should be used only as guidelines. Obviously, if there are contraindications, such as high blood urea levels or reduced ventilatory reserve, one should reduce the rates of administration of either energy, N, or both. In patients with respiratory failure or reduced pulmonary reserve, the proportion of carbohydrate should be reduced and during the weaning procedure nutrition should be at a minimum level. Though these recommendations seem reasonable to us on general physiologic and nutritional grounds, they are arbitrary, and other arbitrary recommendations may seem equally reasonable. Much larger amounts of nutrients have been given by many intensivists with great success. Until we have prospective trials on the effects of various amounts of nutrients on morbidity and mortality, uncertainty as to optimal amounts will exist. What is less uncertain is that adequate nutrition should always be supplied on a daily basis early in the illness, except when oral feeding is expected within 2 to 3 days.

CASE PRESENTATION

A 58-year-old man with a 45 pack-year smoking history was admitted to the emergency room with multiple trauma following a motor vehicle accident. He arrived intubated, was placed on mechanical ventilation, and was in shock. Further evaluation revealed bilateral pulmonary contusion and a right pneumothorax, a fracture of the right femoral neck, and a tender abdomen. A right No. 34 French chest tube was placed. Arterial blood-gas samples taken thereafter were pH, 7.27; P_{CO_2}, 45; P_{O_2}, 60; Sa_{O_2}, 93%; HCO_3, 19. The patient was placed on positive end-expiratory pressure (PEEP) of 10 cmH_2O and fractional inspired O_2 (F_{IO_2}) of 1.0. The patient was then brought to the operating room for an exploratory laparotomy and open reduction with internal fixation of the femoral fracture. A peritoneal tap and lavage demonstrated an increase in WBC count and amylase, and at laparotomy an anterior jejunal rupture was discovered which was repaired primarily. No other intraabdominal injuries were present.

On the second postoperative day, the patient was started on hyperalimentation. He was given a regimen of 2700 kcal/day, consisting of 50 percent carbohydrate, 50 percent fat, and 120 g protein. The estimated amount of kilocalories was calculated according to the Harris and Benedict formula and corrected according to the Kinney scale. On the fifth day following surgery, the patient's general condition improved, and his pulmonary injury was improved by chest radiography and blood-determination although his $\dot{V}_E$ requirement to maintain a Pa_{CO_2} of 40 was 11 L/min, and the peak-to-pause difference on the ventilator pressure gauge was 16 cmH_2O. It was impossible to disconnect him from the ventilator without marked respiratory distress.

Theophylline and inhaled β-agonist bronchodilators were initiated. Indirect calorimetry measurements of EE showed an expenditure of 2200 kcal/day, following which hyperalimentation was lowered from 2700 to 2000 kcal/day, and the carbohydrate load decreased from 50 to 30 percent. Twelve hours later, the $\dot{V}_{CO_2}$ dropped from 265 mL/min to 220 mL/min; the $\dot{V}_E$ required for eucapnia was now 7 L/min, in part because $\dot{V}_{CO_2}$ decreased and in part because the dead space: tidal volume ratio decreased from 0.58 to 0.45. The patient was successfully weaned and extubated on the sixth postoperative day.

CASE DISCUSSION

After initial evaluation it was evident that pulmonary and abdominal complications of trauma were the most serious injuries requiring modification of supportive therapy. The bilateral pulmonary contusion and single-sided pneumothorax compounded prior obstructive lung disease to decrease pulmonary reserve to the point that postoperative extubation became a major endeavor. In addition, the small bowel injury delayed the onset of enteral intake. Nutrition had to be supplied by a parenteral route. The unsuccessful attempts at extubation, in a patient showing a reasonable improvement of pulmonary status, raised the question whether the prescribed nutritional regime was appropriate, whether airflow obstruction needed bronchodilators, or both. Decreasing caloric load and the proportion of carbohydrate to 30 percent decreased CO_2 production and facilitated discontinuation of mechanical ventilation and the successful extubation of the patient aided in part by reduced dead space and work of breathing effected by bronchodilators. On the seventh day after surgery, the patient was discharged from the ICU. Two days later, the patient was started on an oral diet. Two weeks after his accident, he was admitted to an orthopedic rehabilitation center.

References

1. Mullen JL, Buzby GP, Matthews DC, et al: Reduction of operative morbidity and mortality by combined preoperative and postoperative nutritional support. Ann Surg 192:604, 1980.
2. Askanazi J, Carpentier YA, Elwyn DH, et al: Influence of total parenteral nutrition on fuel utilization in injury and sepsis. Ann Surg 191:40, 1980.
3. Askanazi J, Elwyn DH, Silverberg PA, et al: Respiratory distress secondary to high carbohydrate load: A case report. Surgery 87:597, 1980.
4. Covelli HD, Black JW, Olsen MV, et al: Respiratory failure precipitated by high carbohydrate loads. Ann Intern Med 95:579, 1981.
5. Askanazi J, Nordenstrom J, Rosenbaum SH, et al: Nutrition for the patient with respiratory failure: Glucose versus fat. Anesthesiology 54:373, 1981.
6. Doekel RC Jr, Zwilich CW, Scoggin, et al: Clinical semi-starvation: Depression of hypoxic ventilatory response. N Engl J Med 295:358, 1979.

7. Askanazi J, Weissman C, Lasala P, et al: Effects of increasing protein intake on ventilatory drive. Anesthesiology 60:107, 1984.
8. Arora NS, Rochester DF: Effect of body weight and muscularity on human diaphragm muscle mass, thickness and area. J Appl Physiol 52:63, 1982.
9. Arora NS, Rochester DF: Respiratory muscle strength and maximal voluntary ventilation in undernourished patients. Am Rev Respir Dis 126:5, 1982.
10. Keys A, Brozek J, Henschel A, et al: *Biology of Human Starvation.* Minneapolis, Univ Minnesota, 1950, pp 601–606.
11. Vandenbergh E, Van de Woestijne KP, Gyselen A: Weight changes in the terminal stages of chronic obstructive pulmonary disease: Relation to respiratory function and prognosis. Am Rev Respir Dis 95:557, 1967.
12. Openbrier DR, Irwin MM, Dauber JH, et al: Factors affecting nutritional status and the impact of nutritional support in patients with emphysema. Chest 85:675, 1984.
13. Goldstein MS, Askanazi J, Weissman C, et al: Energy expenditure in patients with chronic obstructive pulmonary disease. Chest 91:222, 1987.
14. Rowe RWD: Effects of low nutrition on size of striated muscle fibers in the mouse. J Exp Zool 167:353, 1968.
15. Kelsen SG, Ference M, Kapoor S: The effects of prolonged undernutrition on the structure and function of the diaphragm. J Appl Physiol 58:1354, 1985.
16. Lopes J, Russell DM, Whitwell J, et al: Skeletal muscle function in malnutrition. Am J Clin Nutr 36:602, 1982.
17. Russell DM, Prendergast PJ, Darby PL, et al: A comparison between muscle and body composition in anorexia nervosa: The effect of refeeding. Am J Clin Nutr 38:229, 1983.
18. Kelly SM, Rosa A, Field S, et al: Inspiratory muscle strength and body composition in patients receiving total parenteral therapy. Am Rev Respir Dis 130:33, 1984.
19. Kerr JS, Riley DJ, Lanza-Jacobi S, et al: Nutritional emphysema in the rat: Influence of protein depletion and impaired lung growth. Am Rev Resp Dis 131:644, 1985.
20. Rubin JW, Clowes GHA Jr, Macnicol MF, et al: Impaired surfactant synthesis in starvation and severe non thoracic sepsis. Am J Surg 123:461, 1972.
21. Larsson J, Martenson J, Vinnars E: Nitrogen requirements in hypercatabolic patients. Clin Nutr (special suppl) 4:0.4, 1984.
22. Francois G, Bouffier C, Dumont JC, et al: Protein catabolism in trauma patients. Ann Fr Anesth Reanim 2:387, 1983.
23. Nordenstrom J, Askanazi J, Elwyn DH, et al: Nitrogen balance during total parenteral nutrition. Ann Surg 197:27, 1983.
24. Chikenji T, Elwyn DH, Gil KM, et al: Effect of increasing glucose intake on nitrogen balance and energy expenditure in malnourished adult patients receiving parenteral nutrition. Clin Sci 72:489, 1987.
25. Elwyn DH, Gump FE, Munro HN, et al: Changes in nitrogen balance of depleted patients with increasing infusions of glucose. Am J Clin Nutr 32:1597, 1979.

Chapter 95

CHOICE AND CARE OF NUTRITIONAL ACCESS SITE

SYLVIE ANNE BURSZTEIN-DE MYTTENAERE
JEFFREY ASKANAZI

KEY POINTS

- *Twenty-five to 30 percent of hospitalized patients develop malnutrition; this complication can be prevented by effective early nutrition often including total parenteral nutrition (TPN) in critically ill patients.*
- *Infection, mostly due to gram-negative and staphylococcal bacteria, represents a major complication of TPN; its prevention relies on rigorous aseptic techniques.*
- *Enteral alimentation by oral, gastric, or jejunal feeding should begin as early as possible.*
- *Cologastric paresis should not be regarded as a contraindication to effective jejunal feeding.*
- *Improper technique should be counted among causes of enteral feeding failure.*

In critically ill patients the provision of nutritional support is essential for the healing process and for prevention or correction of malnutrition. The adequate amount and kind of nutrients may be provided by enteral or parenteral routes. The routes of delivery will be dictated by the patient's pathology and the risks inherent to the parenteral and enteral feeding techniques.

Parenteral Route

The use of long-term intravenous therapy has led to the search for safe methods of vascular access. Also, better care techniques have been introduced to prevent complications and to keep catheters safely in place for longer periods of time. Intravenous lines lasting from a few days to a few weeks are commonly used to provide TPN in the ICU setting until the resumption of enteral alimentation. Cannulations for longer periods of time, however, must be considered in patients whose gastrointestinal tract function is expected to have a long recovery or remain inadequate. Long-term cannulation implies the use of special intravenous devices.

VASCULAR ACCESS

Large veins with high flow rate are required to infuse TPN solutions, since the osmotic strength and low pH of these solutions predispose smaller veins to thrombophlebitis. TPN solutions are thus infused directly into the superior vena cava through a catheter inserted through one of the great veins of the thorax. Catheter insertion techniques have evolved in two directions: from cutdown to percutaneous techniques, and from "through the needle" to Seldinger techniques. External jugular, internal jugular, or subclavian veins are commonly used. The approach is chosen according to the patient's anatomy and the physician's experience.

Internal jugular and supraclavicular subclavian catheters are prone to movement to-and-fro at the insertion site due to head movements, thereby increasing the risk of contamination by microorganisms of cutaneous origin. Subcutaneous tunnelling may obviate this inconvenience.[1] Catheters placed by infraclavicular subclavian cannulation are easier to fix and are also better isolated from tracheostomy or open cervical wounds. On the other hand, in patients with lung disease, internal jugular cannulation is preferred because it is less likely to cause a pneumothorax. Even in experienced hands the risk of pneumothorax exists. Catheters should always be inserted on the side of the more damaged lung or an already existing chest tube. Severe coagulation disorders are a relative contraindication for percutaneous central catheterization at these sites. After factor replacement, we use the infraclavicular route because accidental arterial punctures are less frequent than accidental punctures through the supraclavicular or internal jugular routes. Access to the superior vena cava via long catheters inserted from the antecubital fossa provides another safe alternative. Femoral catheters are prone to infection and thrombosis and should be used only for emergency resuscitation.

Peripheral veins may occasionally be used when hyperalimentation is limited to a few days or given as a supplement to oral alimentation. Thrombophlebitis is a common complication of peripheral alimentation. Only low osmolar solutions (<600 mO/L) should be used in peripheral veins. Since lipid solutions are isoosmolar, at physiologic pH, and rich in calories, a lipid-based alimentation represents the regime of choice for peripheral hyperalimentation. A typical protocol of peripheral hyperalimentation consists of the simultaneous administration of 500 mL 10% Intralipids, with 500 mL of a 5.9% solution of crystalline amino acids in 10% glucose solution. This regime provides 250 calories in carbohydrates, 500 calories in lipids, and 59 g amino acids/L hyperalimentation. Unfortunately, this solution has an osmolarity of about 900 mO/L and provides calories in a lipid:carbohydrate ratio above 50 percent.

Since the ability of patients to clear lipids is highly variable, and these high osmolarity solutions cause vascular injury, we prefer to use two distinct peripheral veins: one for the administration of 2.5 L 10% dextrose with electrolytes (505 mO/L), and one for simultaneous administration of 0.5 L 20% Intralipids with 0.5 L 8.5% amino acids (575 mO/L). This provides 1000 carbohydrate calories and 1000 lipid calories, with 42.5 g amino acids all at relatively low osmotic pressure. The site of cannulation must be changed every 48 to 72 h.

COMPLICATIONS AND CARE OF THE SHORT-TERM CANNULATION

Devices used for short-term cannulation are available in a wide range of forms. The catheters differ by size, length, ratio between internal and external diameter, material, stiffness, lumen number, and technique of insertion. Since complications and their prevention are closely related, they will be considered together in this chapter.

Technical Complications

These tend to be inversely related to the physician's experience with the technique. These complications consist mainly of pleural and mediastinal injury either directly due to the needle, to a stiff catheter, or to the improper use of the flexible guidewire when Seldinger technique is used (advance against resistance or introduction of the nonflexible end).[2] Early diagnosis is important. Proper placement should be verified by free backflow of blood and chest radiograph before infusion of hypertonic fluids. The tip of the catheter should lie in the superior vena cava at the level of the carina. Placement of the catheter into the cardiac chambers may induce ventricular premature contractions and may result in perforation and cardiac tamponade. Misdirection of the catheter to the contralateral side or to the head is also common. This occurs mostly on the right side when a subclavian catheter migrates to the ipsilateral jugular vein because of the abrupt angle between the subclavian vein and the superior vena cava. Misplaced catheters or catheters coiled in the lumen have been associated with a higher incidence of thrombosis and should be redirected using a guidewire.[3]

Infection

The infection rate associated with parenteral nutrition ranges from 2.8 to 27 percent.[4,5] Introduction of organisms during insertion, catheter care, or administration of solutions may result in sepsis, but the catheter itself remains the most common source of infection during TPN. Three mechanisms are involved in catheter colonization. Colonization most often occurs from accumulation of skin organisms along the subcutaneous tract formed around the catheter.[6] Colonization of the hub or of the intraluminal segment of the catheter may also occur when infected solutions are infused. Although fungi may survive in TPN solutions, they do not usually grow to large numbers because of the inhibiting effect of acid pH and hyperosmolarity of crystalline amino acid-dextrose solutions. On the other hand, lipid solutions are isoosmolar and at physiologic pH, favoring both bacterial and fungal growth. In the recently introduced 3-in-1 mixtures, microbial growth is less than in lipid solution alone, though higher than in crystalline amino acid-dextrose solutions.[7] Colonization of the hub or of the intraluminal part of the catheter is usually due to manipulations of the catheter system for drawing blood, piggyback infusion, or pressure measurements. In a prospective study of 200 patients, Ryan and coworkers reported a 20 percent infection rate in general use catheters but only a 3 percent infection rate for catheters used exclusively for TPN.[8] Seeding from distant sources of bacteremia, like surgical wounds or urinary tract infections, is a third mechanism by which catheters may become infected. During bacteremia, the risk of catheter colonization has been estimated at 20 percent.

The risk of infection is increased by several factors and is directly related to the length of time of catheterization. The type of catheter influences bacterial affinity. Colonization is greater with polyvinylchloride (PVC) catheters than with Teflon catheters,[9] while multilumen catheters show a higher incidence of infection compared to single-lumen catheters. This is probably due to the fact that more ports are subject to possible contamination.[10]

To ensure an acceptably low level of infection during TPN, some technical aspects related to catheter insertion, dressing changes, and solution administration should be kept in mind (Table 95-1).

1. Catheter insertion is an elective procedure requiring aseptic conditions. In view of the cutaneous organisms frequently found as catheter contaminants, scrubbing of

TABLE 95-1 Procedural Recommendations for Catheter Insertion and Dressing

Position the patient head down at 15°.
Identify surface markings to minimize skin manipulations afterward.
Scrub patient's skin with antimicrobial soap and allow to dry.
Scrub hands with an antimicrobial soap, dry hands, and wear gloves, surgical gowns, caps, and mask.
Prepare skin:

- With a skin disinfectant (tincture of iodine 2%-alcohol 70%, or povidone-iodine solution, or chlorhexadine 0.5%-alcohol 70%)
- By circular motion from insertion site to periphery
- Using instruments and pad from sterile tray (exclude these instruments from sterile tray once used)

Change gloves if skin-glove contact occurred during skin preparation.
Drape insertion site field with sterile towels.
Apply sterile iodophore-impregnated film on the skin (optional).
Infiltrate with local anesthetic agent.
Puncture the vein with minimal contact between gloves and skin.
Avoid multiple manipulation during introduction of the guidewire (flexible end leading) and threading of the catheter over it.
Secure catheter to prevent motion at the cutaneous exit site (sutures or subcutaneous tunnel).
Clean blood from site, dry, and apply topical ointment (optional).
Apply occlusive gauze dressing (to be changed every other day), or semipermeable transparent dressing (to be changed once a week).
Connect tubing to exposed hub to allow tubing change every 48–72 h without dressing disruption.

the physician's hands and the patient's skin is the first step in catheter placement.

2. The use of acetone to prepare the site is controversial and can by itself cause skin irritation. The insertion site may be prepared with tincture of iodine, chlorhexidine gluconate, or povidone-iodine. All three solutions are bactericidal and fungicidal.
3. The physician should avoid contact between gloves and the patient's skin during initial preparation or change gloves afterward. Even during catheter insertion the contact of the gloves with the skin should be minimized to reduce bacterial contamination. Indeed, after catheterization of the internal jugular vein, contamination of glove tips has been found to be as high as 83 percent, with 13 percent of catheters contaminated as well. When a sterile iodophore-impregnated film was applied on the skin after the initial preparation, both glove and catheter contamination was eliminated.[11]
4. Changes over guidewires of malfunctioning catheters has recently gained increasing popularity because it significantly reduces mechanical complications. This technique has also been proposed to treat catheter-related septicemia.[12] However, when a removed catheter demonstrates significant bacterial growth, the catheter inserted by guidewire almost always becomes infected. Catheter change by guidewire should therefore not be performed when septicemia is confirmed or even strongly suspected. Discontinued catheters should be semiquantitatively cultured,[13] and if the removed catheter is proven to be infected, the catheter inserted over a guidewire should be promptly removed.[14] The risk of technical complications in experienced hands is substantially lower than the risk of sepsis due to catheter change over a guidewire. Therefore, an insertion of a new catheter in a different and clean site is preferable in almost all circumstances.
5. Careful suturing or subcutaneous tunneling is essential to minimize catheter motion at the site of insertion. Suture abscess may compromise catheter sterility and should be searched for at the time of dressing changes.
6. The use of ointment at the time of catheter insertion and at each dressing change remains controversial. Povidone-iodine and triple antibiotic ointment are most commonly used. When studied, triple antibiotic ointment showed either no change or slight decrease in catheter related-infection. However, an increased incidence of *Candida albicans* catheter infection was noted, probably due to alteration in the normal skin flora by the antibiotic ointment.[15] There was no significant decrease in infection rate when povidone-iodine ointment was applied instead of antibiotic ointment.[16] Jarrard and colleagues have suggested that the use of a skin preparation containing antiseptic solution, at the time of dressing changes, might be more beneficial than skin ointment application.[17] In their prospective study of 23 patients, four different ointments and a simple preparation with 10% polyvinyl-povidone were studied. The same rate of skin infection was observed in all groups.
7. Gauze and tape dressings are usually changed every other day. In patients with higher risk for sepsis, dressings are often changed daily. Such intensive protocols are time-consuming and expensive. Some have advocated the use of transparent plastic dressings which are left in place for several days and which allow direct visualization of the catheter insertion site. Studies comparing traditional dressing (every 48 h) with weekly changes of semipermeable transparent dressings have been equivocal in demonstrating statistical differences in skin flora growth or sepsis rate.[18,19] Recently, the duration of application of a clear polyurethane dressing (OpSite, Smith & Nephew) has been prolonged to 10 days without evidence of higher skin colonization and catheter sepsis. Advocates note that clear polyurethane dressings changed every week are cost effective, since they reduce both material and nursing time. However, they also advocate that this protocol not be used unless strict aseptic conditions are observed.[20] Dressing changes should be performed by a specialized team aware of the need for rigorous aseptic technique.
8. Since the tubing-catheter connections may be a major source of contamination, simple systems should be used and connection sites should be cleaned with povidone-iodine and then swabbed with alcohol at the time of tubing changes. Tubing changes every 48 h have been recommended by the Centers for Disease Control. Intervals of 72 h have been shown to be just as safe.[21]

THROMBOSIS AND OCCLUSION. The incidence of formation of a "sleeve" clot around indwelling central lines may be as high as 40 percent and is probably due to coating of foreign material by thrombocytes and fibrin. Catheter occlusion, vein thrombosis, pulmonary embolism, and infection may subsequently occur. There is a wide range of thrombogenicity between different types of catheters. Polyethylene catheters are more thrombogenic than polyurethane or silastic devices. At the present time silicone catheters are considered the least thrombogenic. The incidence of asymptomatic subclavian thrombosis with silicone catheters was 11.5 percent compared to 46 percent with PVC catheters (mean intravenous stay of 12.8 days).[22] Catheters coated with heparin, urokinase, or hydromer are under evaluation. Although heparin-bonded catheters reduce the incidence of catheter occlusion, in terms of clinical thrombophlebitis and degree of thrombus there is no difference between coated and uncoated materials. Recently, the thrombogenic effect of TPN solutions has been studied in vitro and in vivo. Hypertonic TPN solutions are potent inducers of monocyte and endothelial cell procoagulant activity. The procoagulant molecules produced by these cells in response to amino acid solutions and hypertonic dextrose are inhibited by lipid emulsions, suggesting a beneficial effect of coadministration of lipid and crystalloid solutions to reduce TPN-induced thrombosis.[23,24] Some authors have proposed right-sided cannulation rather than left, claiming that the incidence of thrombosis is less because of the shorter intravascular segment.

LONG-TERM CANNULATION

Devices Used for Long-Term Cannulation

In 1973 Broviac advocated the use of a cuffed silicone catheter for prolonged parenteral nutrition.[25] A further modification consisting of a larger internal diameter to allow easier infusion of various solutions and blood drawing was proposed by Hickman.[26] These catheters are introduced into a central vein and passed through a subcutaneous tunnel to exit at a distant site. They have a Dacron sheath incorporated into the tunnel to prevent progression of infection from the skin to the vein. Single- and double-lumen Hickman catheters are available. The double-lumen catheter facilitates administration of both TPN and drugs or blood products and is thus often preferred for oncologic patients.

Local skin infection and sepsis associated with the use of externalized catheters have been partially solved by the introduction of totally implantable catheters. These are made of silicone and are connected to a conical chamber with a self-sealing silicone rubber septum, placed under the skin and into a pocket created in the subcutaneous tissue. For injection into the port a special 22 gauge Huber needle is used to preserve the septum integrity. Placed under local anesthesia, these systems have a long mean duration with low complication rate. They need minimal care—proper skin disinfection before infusion and flushing with heparinized saline at completion of infusion. Unlike the Hickman or Broviac catheters, there is no need for periodic flushes with saline if the port is not used. Since implantable catheters are completely under the skin, they do not require daily dressing changes and do not limit the patient's physical activities. They have a lower rate of infection than Hickman catheters. Major complications include thrombotic events and, in obese patients, loss of access to the reservoir.

Complications and Care in Long-Term Cannulation

Complications associated with the use of these catheters are essentially the same as in short-term catheterization: mechanical complications, infection, and occlusion. However, the need for continuous vein access in patients with a limited number of central venous access sites has brought a very conservative approach in the care of these catheters.

INFECTION. The development of sepsis in association with catheter use ranges from 10 to 25 percent. If the necessity for ongoing venous access is questionable, if infection is obvious at the site of the catheter (pain, cellulitis, pus expressed by milking), or if the clinical situation of the patient deteriorates (chills, fever, septic shock), the foreign body should be removed rapidly and its tip sent for semiquantitative culture. Central and peripheral blood cultures should be performed and appropriate antibiotic therapy started. If catheter-associated infection is suspected because of fever, leukocytosis, or increase in immature polymorphonuclear leukocytes without any other detectable source of infection, an attempt to treat infection is reasonable. Blood cultures must be obtained simultaneously from central line and peripheral sites. Some studies, mostly performed on the pediatric population, have shown that catheter-related infection can be treated without removal of the catheter. A response rate of about 80 percent has been noted.[27] Gram-positive or gram-negative organisms are common etiologic agents of catheter infections. Sepsis by coagulase-negative *Staphylococcus* has emerged in recent years with increasing frequency. The sensitivity of this organism is variable, but until now it has always been sensitive to vancomycin. Therefore, a combined regimen of vancomycin and an aminoglycoside is reasonable until a bacteriologic profile is established. Antibiotic treatment is usually given for 2 to 3 weeks. Catheter-related sepsis has also been treated successfully by an antibiotic-lock technique. Highly concentrated antibiotic solution locked within the catheter for 12 h/day controlled 90 percent of catheter sepsis, avoiding complications of systemic antibiotic therapy and reducing cost and hospital stay.[28] If the infection fails to respond clinically after 48 to 72 h of antibiotic therapy through the catheter or if positive in-line blood cultures persist until day 7 of therapy, then removal is advisable. Failure to respond to treatment is usually due to the presence of undiagnosed abscess or thrombophlebitis necessitating further surgical exploration, or to infections due to *Pseudomonas aeruginosa* or *C. albicans*. Fungal infection always requires catheter removal.

THROMBOSIS AND OCCLUSION. Catheter occlusion occurs in up to 25 percent of patients. It may result from malposition, kinking, clotting, or fibrin sleeve formation around the tip of the catheter. Manifestations of occlusion are either obvious due to limitation or prevention of infusion or should be suspected when blood cannot be aspirated. In case of occlusion, the correct location of the tip of the catheter should first be confirmed by radiograph. If malposition and kinking can be excluded, an infusion of 2 to 3 mL 1000 USP U/mL heparin should be attempted and left in place for 2 to 6 h. If blood return still fails, radiopaque dye studies under fluoroscopy should be performed to exclude a clot or a sheath at the tip of the catheter. Either of these obstructions can produce a ball-valve effect, thereby allowing liquids to enter the catheter but occluding it when negative pressure is applied. This might appear as contrast tracking back along the catheter or as a saclike accumulation at the catheter tip. Thrombolytic treatment has been used with more than 90 percent success in this setting. Both streptokinase and urokinase can be used either by continuous or intermittent injection. The intermittent use of streptokinase, based on a half-life of 18 min, requires dilution of 50,000 U streptokinase in 10 mL saline solution, with bolus injection of 2 mL of the solution into the lumen left in place for 20 min. Aspiration should then demonstrate adequate blood return. The procedure should be repeated until successful. Blood is then cleared from the catheter by continuous saline infusion or by use of a heparin-lock.[29] Good results have also been obtained by infusion of 3000 U streptokinase/h for 12 h. The low cost of streptokinase and its efficacy make it the thrombolytic agent of choice, except in streptokinase-allergic patients who should be treated with urokinase (see Chap. 119). Both drugs restore catheter patency with minimal bleeding complications. In our experience, catheter occlusion is more common since the introduction of all-in-one TPN mixes. Waxy material found in the lumen of the catheter or in the chamber of totally implantable systems has been attributed to lipid aggregation by di- and trivalent ions. This type of occlusion, usually resistant to urokinase treatment, may be successfully cleared by introduction of 2 to 3 mL 70% ethanol in water left in situ for 1 h and then flushed with saline solution and heparin.[30] Hydrochloric acid 0.1 *N* (0.2 to 1 mL) has been successfully used to clear drug and calcium salt obstructions that have a concentration and pH-dependent solubility.[31]

Enteral Routes of Nutritional Access

There is no evidence to suggest that TPN offers any advantage to enteral feeding when the gastrointestinal tract functions properly. If the gastrointestinal tract is even partially functional, it should be used preferentially to feed the patient. Enteral alimentation is easier and cheaper to perform, leads to fewer complications, might be of some value in prophylaxis of gastrointestinal bleeding, prevents intestinal mucosal atrophy, and may decrease the risk of bacterial translocation. It may be administered by mouth, through a gastric tube, or by enterostomy.

GASTRIC FEEDING

Nasogastric Intubation

This approach was first used in 1598 in Venice by Capivacceus. Until recently, stiff No. 14 to 16 French tubes made from polyethylene, PVC, or silicone were used. The latter is considered less damaging to the gastric mucosa. Complications encountered with nasogastric tubes include gastroesophageal reflux, aspiration, pulmonary atelectasis, esophageal stricture, intestinal obstruction and perforation, oropharyngeal mucosal injury, rhinitis and sinusitis, pharyngitis, otitis media, and parotitis. These tubes are particularly uncomfortable for patients and are associated with significant morbidity. When prolonged enteral alimentation is anticipated, alternatives should be considered. Progress in the development of liquid diets has enabled the use of fine nasogastric tubes. Small bore nasogastric tubes, No. 8 to 10 French, are better tolerated by patients, are easier to pass into the duodenum, have a low incidence of esophageal or gastric erosion, and are associated with minimal or no gastroesophageal reflux, thereby carrying less risk of aspiration. A number of these feeding tubes are available. They are made from PVC, silicone, or polyurethane and are passed with the aid of a stylet to keep them rigid during their introduction. Most of the tubes are weighted at their tip with mercury or tungsten to facilitate passage into the duodenum. Feeding tubes with metallic weights at their tips and stiffened by a guidewire can lead to perforation, even when minimal force is exerted. It is therefore recommended that the stylet be used to pass the level of the nasopharynx and then removed so as to reduce the possibility of esophageal or bronchial perforation. Plain x-ray or fluoroscopy are advised to verify the correct position of the tube. The incidence of radiographically detected abnormal position, often into the tracheobronchial tree, is reported to be as high as 1.3 percent, mostly occuring in neurologically impaired patients.[32] Radiologic confirmation of position may not be necessary in awake and cooperative patients. If correct positioning is indicated by auscultation of air entry in the upper left quadrant, within an interval of 24 to 48 h, 85 percent of tubes pass spontaneously into the duodenum.[33] Complications of small bore feeding tubes include tracheal intubation, transbronchial insertion into the pleural space causing pneumothorax (sometimes delayed until after the removal of the misplaced catheter, leaving the bronchial tear open) or hydrothorax, esophageal perforation, dislodgment, and clogging (Table 95-2). The small caliber of the feeding tube might impede the rate of delivery of the diet and limit its use to commercial liquid diets.

TABLE 95-2 Complications of Small Bore Feeding Tubes

Tracheal intubation
Transbronchial perforation (pneumothorax, hydrothorax)
Esophageal perforation (mediastinitis)
Dislodgement
Clogging

Gastrostomy

Patients with head, facial, neck, or esophageal injury, patients with prolonged neurologic impairment, or patients with repeated aspirations are best managed with feeding enterostomy. In these situations, gastrostomy or jejunostomy, the most common sites for enterostomy, should be considered as alternatives. Gastrostomy might be performed surgically in a traditional way, or percutaneously, using endoscopic or radiologic techniques. These techniques differ by their rate of success, cost, and complications.

SURGICAL GASTROSTOMY. The three most commonly used techniques for surgical gastrostomy are the *Stamm gastrostomy,* inserting a tube in the gastric lumen through the anterior wall; the *Witzel gastrostomy,* constructing a serosal tunnel from the gastric wall to prevent leakage; and the *Depage gastrostomy,* constructing a tunnel from a full flap of the anterior gastric wall. The latter technique is used for permanent gastrostomy feeding. Surgical gastrostomy has a significant morbidity and mortality; the complication rate is reported to be as high as 15 percent with a mortality rate of 6 percent. Complications of surgical gastrostomy (Table 95-3) include leakage of the stoma, stenosis or closure of the stoma, wound dehiscence, hemorrhage, skin irritation, cellulitis, wound abcess, misplacement of the tube into the peritoneal cavity and peritonitis, feeding tube migration with gastric outlet obstruction, gastric dilation, and aspiration.[34] The procedure requires laparotomy and

TABLE 95-3 Complications of Surgical Gastrostomy

Stoma stenosis and leakage
Wound dehiscence, hemorrhage, and abscess
Skin irritation and cellulitis
Dislodgement (peritonitis, gastric outlet obstruction)

may be performed under local or general anesthesia, though patients, often in poor condition, are considered to be at high risk for general anesthesia, while local anesthesia often results in poor exposure and patient discomfort. Furthermore, surgical gastrostomy is expensive when compared to nonoperative techniques.

NONOPERATIVE TECHNIQUES. Approaches include fluoroscopic and endoscopic percutaneous gastrostomy. After sonography to exclude solid or hollow viscera that might lie between the anterior abdominal wall and the stomach and after insufflation of the stomach with air through a nasogastric tube, the stomach is punctured under fluoroscopic guidance. Injection of a small quantity of contrast media confirms entry into the stomach. A guidewire is placed, the needle removed, and the tract progressively dilated until it permits insertion of the desired feeding catheter (No. 8 to 10 French). Dislodgement is prevented by using a catheter that forms a loop in the gastric fundus, thereby allowing anterior retraction, or by advancing the catheter distally.[35]

This technique, of course, cannot be used if sonography demonstrates that the stomach is surrounded by other viscera that cannot be displaced. In this case, endoscopy-assisted percutaneous gastrostomy may be performed.[36] An endoscope is inserted to inflate the stomach and to bring the gastric wall to the anterior wall of the abdomen where, by transillumination, a point of puncture is chosen. A needle with a thread of silk is introduced and grasped by the endoscope, then retrieved through the mouth. A mushroom feeding tube (No. 18 French de Pezzer type) is then attached to the silk thread, pulled down the esophagus to the stomach and out through the abdominal wall. The endoscope is then reinserted to verify the position of the feeding tube and to secure it to the stomach wall by apposition of an external and internal crossbar. A single endoscopy technique has also been used where puncture is performed after proper positioning under endoscopy. Under direct vision, a guidewire is then advanced through the needle and into the stomach, over which a peel-away catheter is placed and then replaced by a No. 14 French catheter, with an inflatable balloon of the Foley type pulled against the gastric wall.[37] A comparison of the two percutaneous endoscopic gastrostomy methods found the "push" and "pull" techniques equally efficient, successful, and associated with an acceptable rate of complications.

The success rate for percutaneous gastrostomy is >90 percent. These endoscopic techniques are advantageous in that they can be performed at the bedside of patients on ventilators or on other life-support systems. The operative time is short and requires minimal or no sedation. Also, there is no opening of the peritoneal cavity and the tract between the skin and the stomach is small. Feeding can be started very soon after insertion (6 to 24 h) due to minimal interference with peristalsis. When the patient improves, removal of the feeding tube is easy and does not lead to gastrocutaneous fistula. On the other hand, this technique cannot be used if upper mechanical obstruction (e.g., esophageal stenosis) prevents the free passage of the endoscope to the stomach or if the anterior wall of the stomach cannot be apposed to the abdominal wall. It is relatively contraindicated in obesity and should be avoided when coagulopathy, ascites, or intrabdominal infection are present. The size of the catheter introduced is smaller than that introduced by surgical gastrostomy, and the type of diet given to the patient should, therefore, be taken into account. Potential complications of percutaneous gastrostomy are similar to those for surgical gastrostomy. Although a complication rate of around 10 percent has been reported, many series are rather small. Most studies retrospectively compare surgical and percutaneous techniques. Ho and coworkers reviewed data on 233 patients after surgical and fluoroscopic percutaneous gastrostomy.[38] No statistical difference was found in mortality, though surgical (intraperitoneal leak, wound infection, and aspiration) and nonsurgical complications were significantly higher in surgical gastrostomies. Leakage and infection at the stoma site occurred in 14 percent of the surgically treated patients compared to 0.7 percent of the patients treated by percutaneous gastrostomy. Stiegmann and colleagues compared both techniques in a randomized prospective study in 51 patients and noted little or no difference in morbidity or mortality.[39] Percutaneous technique did permit earlier initiation of feeding and was cost effective.

Percutaneous endoscopic gastrostomy remains a semiblind technique requiring a skilled operator and proper technique and material. The stomach must be sufficiently inflated to displace surrounding organs, thereby preventing injury to liver or colon. Necrosis of the skin has resulted from excessive traction exerted on the external crossbar of the feeding tube. Pneumoperitoneum may occur but usually resolves rapidly and without treatment. Failure of adhesion between the gastric serosa and the abdominal wall can cause gastric defects and intraperitoneal contamination and may lead to death in some patients. Accordingly, replacement of a tube extruded within the first weeks must be followed by confirmation of the correct position in the gastric cavity. If a tube is displaced within days of placement, the entire endoscopic procedure will have to be repeated. Leakage is unusual with percutaneous gastrostomy.

CARE OF GASTROSTOMIES.[40] Granulation tissue formation around the stoma is common and responds well to early treatment with silver nitrate application. Overlooking this problem may lead to more serious difficulties since granulation enhances skin irritation and results in leakage. Skin irritation, with granulation, is probably one of the most common problems of gastrostomy. The skin should be cleaned with soap and water and kept perfectly dry. No occlusive dressing should be applied, since it can increase local moisture and favor moniliasis. Skin irritation is made worse by leakage of gastric fluid around the stoma. This usually results from improper surgical technique or from the use of too large and loose a catheter moving into the stoma and dilating it. Avoiding moisture is the most important point in skin healing. Early protection of the skin against the acid gastric secretion is necessary and obtained by a variety of specialized ostomy dressings. The use of a thinner and well-anchored catheter will allow progressive closure of the stoma around the catheter. When this method fails, a new gastrostomy site must be considered. Catheter length outside the abdominal wall has to be checked on a regular basis. It helps to detect early internal or external migration of the feeding tube. A rubber bumper will prevent catheter movement away from the abdominal wall. Internal migration may lead to intestinal obstruction and vomiting and is more often seen when a Foley catheter is used. The use of air instead of water to inflate the balloon makes it lighter than gastric fluid and less affected by peristaltic movement. External migration has to be diagnosed early since the gastrostomy tract may close in a few hours, thereby preventing the insertion of a new catheter. Migration is suspected when the catheter does not move easily in the gastrostomy tunnel or when the inflow is limited.

ENTERAL ALIMENTATION THROUGH THE STOMACH. When correct position of the gastric tube has been checked, no signs of gastric retention are observed, and the patient has been examined for proper bowel sounds, 5% glucose solution or tap water is started at a slow infusion rate for 1 or 2 h. If no residual gastric fluid is found, then enteral alimentation can follow. The stomach will dilute a hyperosmotic alimentation fluid. Therefore, there is no need for dilution of the enteral formula before use. Elevating the head of the bed at least 30° during the infusion, until 1 h after the end of it, will help to prevent esophageal reflux and decrease the risk of aspiration. Enteral alimentation should begin by slow continuous infusion, increasing progressively to prevent gastric retention or diarrhea. Gastric residual is checked every few hours. After a few days of continuous feeding the regimen may be switched to intermittent feeding. Crushed medications should be replaced by liquid preparations to prevent clogging of the feeding tube. Flushing the tube after meals or medications with 25 or 50 mL water helps to maintain patency. At comparable size the lumen of the de Pezzer catheter is larger than the Foley catheter, thereby decreasing the risk of clogging. Small bore feeding tubes are particularly prone to occlusion. About 6 percent occlude and have to be replaced. Numerous digestive and proteolytic enzymes have been tested for declogging these tubes. None has been effective, and prevention of clogging remains the better treatment. Diet has to be chosen according to the caliber of the feeding tube. Blenderized food should not be used through percutaneous catheters at the beginning.

Duodenal Feeding

Disturbed gastric motility is a common finding in ICU patients. Thus, some clinicians prefer duodenal to gastric feeding. A potential risk of aspiration still exists, however. Simultaneous gastric decompression may obviate this complication but is quite uncomfortable for the patient. Furthermore, continuous duodenal feeding maintained gastric pH > 5 in only 23 percent of patients compared to 75 percent during continuous gastric feeding. This raised the question of the need for additional stress ulcer prophylaxis.[41] Duodenal feeding is usually delivered through a fine bore catheter weighted at its tip, allowing free migration into the duodenum or placement with endoscopy. Right lateral decubitus position and metoclopramide may favor the migration of the catheter into proper position. Complications encountered with small bore catheter placement have already been considered.

Jejunal Feeding

There are several situations in which jejunostomy should be used instead of gastrostomy. These include absolute indications, such as gastric outlet obstruction and duodenal obstruction, and relative indications, such as gastrointestinal fistula, gastroparesis, enhanced gastroesophageal reflux with repeated aspiration, pancreatitis, and major procedures of the upper gastrointestinal tract.

NASOJEJUNAL INTUBATION. Small bore nasojejunal feeding tubes are used in patients prone to gastroesophageal reflux. These are placed by gravitation or endoscopic techniques and, like duodenal tubes, are prone to dislodgement, especially in vomiting patients.

JEJUNOSTOMY. There are three standard types of surgical jejunostomies, as described by Stamm, Witzel, and Marwedel. However, since 1976 feeding by way of needle-catheter jejunostomy has gained wide acceptance. The needle-catheter is introduced by way of a submucosal tunnel into the lumen of the first loop of the jejunum, which is fixed to the anterior wall of the abdomen to avoid volvulus and catheter dislodgement.[42] Needle-catheter jejunostomy is often performed as a secondary procedure after major upper gastrointestinal operations (total gastrectomy, Whipple operation, esophagectomy). It allows feeding in the immediate postoperative period (in a few hours). Indeed, the small bowel regains its motility and ability to absorb nutrients before the stomach and colon have recovered. It also offers a possibility of prolonged enteral alimentation in cases of surgical complication.

Fluoroscopic or endoscopic percutaneous jejunostomy is also possible. Percutaneous gastrostomy is used to introduce and manipulate a guidewire under fluoroscopy through the pylorus into the duodenum, advancing a catheter along it to the duodenojejunal junction, and thereby obtaining a percutaneous feeding jejunostomy. Using these techniques, gastrostomies are converted to jejunostomies, or jejunostomies placed adjacent to existing gastrostomies to allow both gastric decompression and jejunal feeding. Fluoroscopic techniques to replace a needle-catheter jejunostomy that has been discontinued prematurely or dislodged have also been developed.[43] Complications from jejunostomy include gastrointestinal disturbances, hemorrhage, infection, catheter dislodgement, leakage, small bowel obstruction, ischemia, and perforation. The complication rate for needle jejunostomy ranges from 8 to 65 percent. Catheter-related complications may be reduced by use of appropriate technique and material. Feeding-related complications account for approximately 30 percent of complications in jejunostomies. They consist largely of abdominal pain, distention, and diarrhea. Fatal cases due to vomiting and aspiration, as well as fatal outcome due to small bowel ischemia, have been described. Intestinal ischemia may be enhanced by bowel distention. The role of intestinal bacterial proliferation and of luminal content on gut function has not yet been defined.[44]

ENTERAL ALIMENTATION THROUGH A JEJUNOSTOMY. Nutrition is usually provided by continuous feeding. A gradual increase in flow rate and in concentration of the diet solution is essential. Most of the gastrointestinal symptoms observed during feeding (abdominal distention, pain, and diarrhea) follow too rapid progression of osmotic content and rate of administration. The small bowel, unlike the stomach, is unable to dilute a hyperosmolar load. These symptoms usually resolve with dilution, reduction, or cessation of feeding. If jejunal feeding is continued, the patient must be monitored for severe distention, intestinal pneumatosis, and perforation.

Small peptide-based diets are better used in patients with a normal pancreatobiliary system because of their low osmolality; low molecular elemental diets should be reserved for patients with biliary diversion or pancreatic insufficiency. Lactose-free diets are also preferred because depletion of dissacharidase is often observed in critically ill patients suffering from malnutrition. Special care should be taken to maintain the sterility of the solutions infused into the jejunum, since the physiologic barrier of gastric acidity is bypassed and subsequent intestinal bacterial proliferation may be deleterious. The main disadvantage of a feeding jejunostomy relates to the small caliber of the catheter (No. 8 to 10 French) and its length, since it can plug easily if percutaneously introduced from the stomach. This may be prevented by regular flushing with water. Medications should be soluble (not crushed). Furthermore, occluded or dislodged jejunostomies can only be replaced by surgical procedure.

Coordinating Enteral and Parenteral Nutrition

Parenteral and enteral nutrition are equally effective in maintaining and restoring nutritional state. Enteral alimentation is of course the more physiologic way of feeding patients. Enteral alimentation also maintains the intestinal mucosa in a normal morphology and functional state. Enteral alimentation, if properly conducted, causes only few complications. Diarrhea is the most common symptom. Several factors, including hypoalbuminemia, enzyme deficiency, and antibiotic therapy have been implicated as possible causes of this problem. In most cases, however, diarrhea is due to improper technique of enteral feeding: too rapid an administration, too concentrated a solution, too cold a solution, or inappropriate enteral formula. Proper diagnosis and careful application of the right technique of diet administration usually result in a patient's improved tolerance and in successful enteral feedings.

The efforts aimed at enteral feeding must not compromise or impair the nutritional state of the patient. Early institution or reinstitution of TPN may help as an intermediary stage until resumption of normal gastrointestinal function. Also, TPN may be used as a supplement when oral food intake is too low. It has to be kept in mind, however, that the very administration of TPN may cause a delay in resuming normal alimentation. Patients receiving TPN often complain of fullness and nausea when started on enteral alimentation. Indeed, TPN decreases oral food intake and delays the rate of gastric emptying in both moderately and critically ill patients.[45,46] This compromises their ability to ingest enough food to maintain or restore their body weight. Administration of branched-chain amino acids has been demonstrated to stimulate gastric emptying when compared to standard parenteral nutrition regimens.[47] Substitution of branched-chain amino acids for standard amino acids, at the transition period from TPN to oral alimentation, may therefore be of potential benefit in reducing symptoms of gastric discomfort and in improving oral intake.

CASE PRESENTATION

A 54-year-old woman was admitted to the ICU for developing fever and ileus on the ninth day following an anteroperitoneal resection. At relaparotomy, peritonitis due to leakage of the small bowel was diagnosed. However, the site of leak could not be identified because of multiple adhesions. The abdomen was left open with tubes for irrigation and drainage. The early postoperative period was complicated by respiratory failure, ongoing sepsis, hypovolemia, and peripheral edema with total plasma protein content of 5.2 g/dL (albumin 2.6 g/dL). Urinary urea/24 h was 42 g. The fistula appeared after 24 h to be a high output fistula of more than 2000 mL/24 h at pH 8. Blood cultures were positive for *Staphylococcus* coagulase-positive and methicillin-resistant (MRSA). The patient received antibiotic therapy with vancomycin and ciprofloxacin.

Selective digestive decontamination was started early. Losses through the fistula were replaced with fluids and electrolytes. Local irrigation with lactic acid was started to buffer the leaking intestinal fluid and the skin was protected with Karaya. Central TPN was started on the first postoperative day via infraclavicular cannulation of the subclavian vein with a single-lumen catheter. The patient was weaned from the ventilator after 2 weeks, after her septic and metabolic state began to improve. Bowel movements returned after 1 week, so a way to provide enteral alimentation was sought. By day 10, a small orifice in the small bowel became apparent and a silicone feeding tube, No. 12 French, was introduced through the descending limb into the jejunum. Enteral alimentation was started with Osmolyte. TPN was simultaneously administered for 10 more days since complaints of nausea and bloating delayed full enteral therapy.

Because of local cellulitis, the TPN catheter was replaced on day 18 by a contralateral subclavian catheter. A blood culture through the catheter, a culture of the catheter tip, and a local skin swab were all negative. During the next night, multiple ventricular premature contractions and episodes of supraventricular tachycardia occurred. Serum potassium concentration was within normal limits and the patient was put on a lidocaine drip until the following morning. On chest x-ray, the catheter appeared to be in the right ventricle. Its retrieval allowed cessation of antiarrhythmic drugs. Sepsis was cured and antibiotics were stopped soon after enteral alimentation was started. The metabolic state of the patient improved with a further course of 6 weeks of enteral alimentation: gain in weight, normalization of protein level, improvement of albumin : globulin ratio, and local granulation tissue covering the intestine. At this time the surgeon decided that the feeding tube should be pulled out to allow complete closure of the fistula. The patient was switched to TPN, and 2 weeks later closure was obtained without further complications.

CASE DISCUSSION

Enteral alimentation was obviously impossible initially due to peritonitis and high small bowel fistula. Although the patient was septic, TPN was not delayed because it was clear that the patient had massive nutritional requirements (postoperative septic state in a cancer patient maintained for 10 days on 5% dextrose). It was clear too that the patient would be deprived of food for a long period. Thus, we chose to provide TPN by central venous route. Infraclavicular cannulation of the subclavian vein was performed, since sterile occlusive dressings can be easily maintained over this site with minimal movements of the catheter and minimal contamination from airway secretions. Also, it is more comfortable for the patient. In view of the large amount of fluids and electrolytes required to compensate the output of the fistula and the need for antibiotics and TPN administration, we considered the use of a multilumen catheter. However, because of the potential for infection with multiple lumen catheters, we chose to administer TPN through a single-lumen catheter. We did not attempt to use a Broviac or Hickman catheter because these catheters should be reserved for patients requiring long-term treatment after intraabdominal sepsis is resolved. Thus, a special silicone "nutricath" considered less thrombogenic was inserted and used exclusively for TPN. There was no routine change of the central venous catheter.

Local signs of inflammation or general symptoms of infection not attributable to another obvious source of infection may require catheter replacements. It has to be emphasized that any catheter placement has to be checked by chest x-ray, which not only discloses pneumothorax but also ensures proper catheter placement. In this septic patient we wanted to remove the central venous catheter and TPN as fast as possible. One of our major concerns was to find a way to provide enteral alimentation. We also hoped to preserve mucosal integrity and prevent bacterial colonization and translocation in a patient receiving systemic antibiotics. This required placement of a feeding tube at least 40 cm beyond the orifice of the fistula. Commercial weighted feeding tubes have a maximal length of 125 cm. This length was insufficient to cover the distance between the nose and the point we wanted to reach in the small bowel. Fortunately, the orifice of the fistula became apparent and we were able to introduce a small bore silicone feeding tube into the descending limb of the jejunum. Although enteral alimentation was administered by continuous drip and progressively increased, the patient experienced episodes of nausea and bloating, requiring reduction in feeding volume and solution osmolarity. At this point TPN was used as a supplement to enteral feeding so as not to further compromise the nutritional state of the patient. As enteral feeding increased, TPN was progressively decreased. For the last 2 days we switched to peripheral venous alimentation. Six more weeks of enteral alimentation provided good conditions for healing of the fistula in a patient cured from her sepsis.

References

1. Benotti PN, Bothe A, Miller J, et al: Safe cannulation of the internal jugular vein for long term hyperalimentation. Surg Gynecol Obstet 144:574, 1977.
2. Hoshal VL: The consequences of a cavalier approach to central venous catheterization. Acta Anaesth Scand 81(suppl):11, 1985.
3. Johnson CL, Lazarchick J, Lynn HB: Subclavian venipuncture: Preventable complications, report of two cases. Mayo Clin Proc 45:712, 1970.
4. Padberg FT, Ruggiero J, Blackburn GL, Bistrian BR: Central venous catheterization for parenteral nutrition. Ann Surg 193:264, 1981.
5. Keohane PP, Attrill H, Northoven J: Effect of catheter tunnelling and a nutrition nurse on catheter sepsis during parenteral nutrition: A control trial. Lancet 2:1388, 1983.
6. Williams WW: Infection control during parenteral nutrition therapy. JPEN 9:735, 1985.
7. Gilbert M, Gallagher SC, Eads M, Elmore MF: Microbial growth patterns in a total parenteral nutrition formulation containing lipid emulsion. JPEN 10:494, 1986.
8. Ryan JA, Abel RM, Abbott WM, et al: Catheter complications in total parenteral nutrition: A prospective study of 200 consecutive patients. N Engl J Med 290:757, 1974.
9. Sheth NK, Franson TR, Rose HD, et al: Colonization of bacteria on polyvinyl chloride and Teflon intravascular catheters in hospitalized patients. J Clin Microbiol 18:1061, 1983.
10. McCarthy MC, Shives J, Robison RJ, et al: Prospective evaluation of single and triple lumen catheters in total parenteral nutrition. JPEN 11:259, 1987.
11. Levy JH, Nagle DM, Curling PE, et al: Contamination reduction during central venous catheterization. Crit Care Med 16:165, 1988.
12. Bozetti F, Terno G, Bonfanti G, et al: Prevention and treatment of central venous catheter sepsis by exchange via a guide-wire. A prospective controlled trial. Ann Surg 198:48, 1983.

13. Maki DG, Weise CE, Sarafin HW: A semiquantitative culture method for identifying intravenous-catheter-related infection. N Engl J Med 296:1305, 1977.
14. Armstrong CW, Mayhall CG, Miller KB, et al: Prospective study of catheter replacement and other risk factors for infection of hyperalimentation catheters. J Infect Dis 154:808, 1986.
15. Norden CW: Application of antibiotic ointment to the site of venous catheterization: A controlled trial. J Infect Dis 120:611, 1969.
16. Maki DG, Band JD: A comparative study of polyantibiotic and iodophor ointments in prevention of vascular-related infection. Am J Med 70:739, 1981.
17. Jarrard MM, Freeman JB: The effects of antibiotic ointment and skin flora beneath subclavian catheter dressings during intravenous hyperalimentation. J Surg Res 22:521, 1977.
18. Vasquez RM, Jarrard MM: Care of the central venous catheterization site: The use of a transparent polyurethane film. JPEN 8:181, 1984.
19. Andersen PT, Herlevsen P, Schaumburg H: A comparative study of "Op-site" and "Nobecutan gauze" dressings for central venous line care. J Hosp Infect 7:161, 1986.
20. Young GP, Alexeyeff M, Russell D, Thomas RJ: Catheter sepsis during parenteral nutrition: The safety of long-term OpSite dressings. JPEN 12:365, 1988.
21. Syndman DR, Donnelly-Reidy M, Perry LK: Intravenous tubing containing burettes can be safely changed at 72 hour intervals. Infect Control 8:113, 1987.
22. Bozetti F, Scarpa D, Terno G, et al: Subclavian vein thrombosis due to indwelling catheters: A prospective study on 52 patients. JPEN 7:560, 1983.
23. Wakefield A, Cohen Z, Craig M, et al: Thrombogenicity of total parenteral nutrition solutions: I. Effect on induction of monocytes/macrophage procoagulant activity. Gastroenterology 97:1210, 1989.
24. Wakefield A, Cohen Z, Craig M, et al: Thrombogenicity of total parenteral nutrition solutions: II. Effect on induction of endothelial cell procoagulant activity. Gastroenterology 97:1220, 1989.
25. Broviac JW, Cole BS, Scribner BH: A silicone rubber atrial catheter for prolonged parenteral alimentation. Surg Gynecol Obstet 136:602, 1973.
26. Hickman RO, Buckner CD, Clift RA, et al: A modified right atrial catheter for access to the venous system in marrow transplant recipients. Surg Gynecol Obstet 148:871, 1975.
27. Nahata MC, King DR, Powell DA, et al: Management of catheter-related infections in pediatric patients. JPEN 12:58, 1988.
28. Messing B, Peitra-Cohen S, Debure A, et al: Antibiotic-lock technique: A new approach to optimal therapy for catheter-related sepsis in home-parenteral nutrition patients. JPEN 12:185, 1988.
29. Schneider TC, Krzywda E, Andris D, Quebbeman EJ: The malfunctioning silastic catheter—Radiologic assessment and treatment. JPEN 10:70, 1986.
30. Pennington CR, Pithie AD: Ethanol lock in the management of catheter occlusion. JPEN 11:507, 1987.
31. Shulman RJ, Reed T, Pitre D, Laine L: Use of hydrochloric acid to clear obstructed central venous catheters. JPEN 12:509, 1988.
32. McWey RE, Curry NS, Schabel SI, Reines HD: Complications of nasoenteric feeding tubes. Am J Surg 155:253, 1988.
33. Ramos SM, Lindine P: Inexpensive, safe and simple nasoenteral intubation—An alternative for the cost conscious. JPEN 10:78, 1986.
34. Wasiljew BK, Ujiki GT, Beal JM: Feeding gastrostomy: Complications and mortality. Am J Surg 143:194, 1982.
35. Wills JS, Oglesby JT: Percutaneous gastrostomy. Radiology 149:449, 1983.
36. Ponsky JL, Gauderer MWL: Percutaneous endoscopic gastrostromy: A non operative technique for feeding gastrostomy. Gastrointest Endosc 27:9, 1981.
37. Russell TR, Brotman M, Norris F: Percutaneous gastrostomy: A new simplified and cost-effective technique. Am J Surg 148:132, 1984.
38. Ho CS, Yee ACN, McPherson R: Complications of surgical and percutaneous nonendoscopic gastrostomy: Review of 233 patients. Gastroenterology 95:1206, 1988.
39. Stiegmann G, Goff J, VanWay C, et al: Operative versus endoscopic gastrostomy. Preliminary results of a prospective randomized trial. Am J Surg 155:88, 1988.
40. Gauderer MW, Stellato TA: Gastrostomies: Evolution, techniques, indications and complications. Curr Probl Surg 23:657, 1986.
41. Valentine RJ, Turner WW, Borman KR: Does nasoenteral feeding afford adequate gastrointestinal stress prophylaxis? Crit Care Med 14:599, 1986.
42. Delany HM, Carnevale NJ, Garvey JW: Jejunostomy by a needle catheter technique. Surgery 73:786, 1973.
43. Lambiase RE, Dorfman GS, Cronan JJ, et al: Percutaneous alternatives in nutritional support: A radiologic perspective. JPEN 12:513, 1988.
44. Smith-Choban P, Max MH: Feeding jejunostomy: A small bowel stress test? Am J Surg 155:112, 1988.
45. Skeie B, Gil K, Friedman MI, et al: Effects of branched chain amino acids enriched PN solution on voluntary food intake. Clin Nutr 6(suppl):15, 1987.
46. MacGregor IL, Wiley ZD, Lavigne ME, Way LW: Slowed rate of gastric emptying of solid food in man by high caloric parenteral nutrition. Am J Surg 138:652, 1979.
47. Bursztein-De Myttenaere S, Gil K, Heymsfield S, et al: Postabsorptive control of food intake in healthy humans. FASEB J 2:A1975, 1988.

SECTION I

INFECTIOUS DISORDERS IN THE CRITICALLY ILL

Chapter 96

PRINCIPLES OF ANTIMICROBIAL THERAPY

FRED Y. AOKI

KEY POINTS

- *Antimicrobial prophylaxis against bacterial infections is indicated in selected patients undergoing surgical procedures as well as in those with cardiac valvular disease.*
- *Rational antibiotic use requires the most specific diagnosis that can be made, knowledge of commonly used antimicrobial agents, and appropriate monitoring of drugs.*
- *When suspected infection threatens life or major organ function, antimicrobial therapy should be directed at all infectious possibilities of more than trivial probability until the results of definitive investigations are available.*
- *Knowledge of the clinical pharmacology of antibiotics commonly prescribed in the ICU is essential for the intensivist.*

Antimicrobial Use in the Critically Ill

The importance of antimicrobial drugs in the management of patients admitted to the ICU is beyond question. Bacterial, fungal, or viral infections are frequently suspected or documented as diseases that necessitate admission to the ICU or complicate the care of patients admitted initially for management of other problems. The prevention and treatment of infections in ICU patients pose formidable challenges despite advances in our understanding of the pathophysiology of specific infections, the availability of more rapid, sensitive, and specific diagnostic tests, and the development of an array of potent, antimicrobial agents.

PROPHYLAXIS OF INFECTIOUS DISEASES IN ICU PATIENTS

The usefulness of short-term parenteral antibacterial administration to prevent wound and operative site infections after surgery was revitalized by investigations that established the principles of successful preventive therapy. The antibacterial agent must have activity against specific pathogenic agents that cause the infection and be administered just before surgery to achieve therapeutic concentrations in the operative site at the time the incision is made. The efficacy of short-term perioperative prophylaxis is now well established and it is imperative that it be applied, when appropriate, in the management of ICU patients. Details of recommended drugs, doses, and duration of prophylaxis for some specific surgical procedures are described in Table 96-1.

Unlike perioperative antimicrobial prophylaxis in the prevention of wound infection, the efficacy of antibiotics to prevent bacterial endocarditis has not been established by controlled trials and it appears unlikely that such data will ever be available. Nevertheless, the Committee on Rheumatic Fever, Endocarditis and Kawasaki Disease of the Council on Cardiovascular Disease in the Young of the American Heart Association[2] has recommended that to prevent bacterial endocarditis patients with valvulopathy (congenital or acquired) or prosthetic valves (bioprosthetic and homograft valves) be given antimicrobial prophylaxis. The following tables indicate the cardiac conditions for which endocarditis prophylaxis is recommended (Table 96-2), the surgical procedures for which antibacterial prophylaxis is recommended (Table 96-3), and the recommended injectable drugs and doses (Tables 96-4A and 96-4B), all of which are adapted from Reference 2.

In contrast, the utility of antimicrobial agents to prevent infections other than endocarditis and infections unrelated to surgery in ICU patients remains limited or controversial. Two general approaches have been evaluated. In one, antibiotics are applied to sterile sites or clean skin wounds to prevent local infection; in the other, antibiotics are used to selectively eradicate the potentially pathogenic bacteria of the gastrointestinal tract while preserving the anaerobic "nonpathogenic" flora. The former approach includes endotracheal administration of nonabsorbable antibacterial drugs, such as the aminoglycosides, instillation of antibiotics into the urinary bladder, and the covering of wounds by creams mixed with antibacterial agents. With the exception of topical use of sulfonamide creams in the management of burned patients, all these methods have been associated with inconsistent prophylactic effects coupled with a high incidence of relapse, resistance, and superinfection that renders this strategy unacceptable.

The second approach is referred to as selective decontamination of the digestive tract (SDD).[3] The strategy of SDD is based on the hypothesis that eradication of selected components of the oropharyngeal or gastrointestinal tract bacterial and fungal flora can reduce the risk of infection by augmenting the natural defense of these mucosal surfaces conferred by the anaerobic flora. Selective eradication of potentially pathogenic aerobic bacteria in these sites is initially attempted by short-term parenteral antibiotic administration, usually with cefotaxime. Thereafter, acquisition of similar organisms plus yeast is prevented by administering nonabsorbable agents, usually in combination. One regimen uses polymyxin E, tobramycin, and amphotericin B. The antibiotics are administered for the entire duration of the critical illness and, in this respect, SDD clearly differs from short-term perioperative surgical prophylaxis. The role of SDD in the management of patients in the ICU is unclear at present. Evidence that SDD is unequivocally effective in preventing infection is currently lacking and it seems appropriate, therefore, to restrict this approach to research studies.

TABLE 96-1 Recommended Antibiotic Prophylaxis for Some Commonly Performed Surgical Procedures

Surgical Procedure	Recommended Prophylactic Regimen[a]
Gynecologic surgery	
Cesarean section	Cefazolin (1 g IV) after clamping the cord and 6 and 12 h later. Prophylaxis is not indicated in uncomplicated elective procedures. Uterine irrigation with antibiotics may be comparable to systemic therapy. If irrigating antibiotics are used, 2 g cefoxitin in 1 l normal saline is effective. In patients with a β-lactam allergy, metronidazole (500 mg IV) after cord clamping is effective.
Hysterectomy, abdominal or vaginal	Cefazolin (1 g IV) preoperatively and 6 and 12 h later. Second or third generation cephalosporins have not proved to be more effective. In patients with a β-lactam allergy, doxycycline (200 mg IV) preoperatively (1 dose) is effective in vaginal hysterectomy.
Orthopedic surgery	
Arthroplasty of joints, including replacement	For major joint (hip or knee) repair, cefazolin (1 g IV) preoperatively and every 6 h (3 doses) is recommended. A higher dose of cefazolin (2 g) should be considered in knee replacement when a tourniquet is used. Data on prophylaxis in arthroscopic surgery are not available.
Open reduction of fracture	Cefazolin (1 g IV) preoperatively and every 6 h (3 doses). Complex (open) fractures are considered contaminated and cefazolin therapy (1 g every 8 h for 10 days beginning on admission) is indicated.
Laminectomy and spinal fusion	Prophylactic antimicrobials have not proved to be beneficial.
Amputation of lower limb	Cefoxitin (2 g IV) preoperatively and every 6 h (4 doses).
Ophthalmic surgery	
Extraction of lens, including insertion of prosthesis	There are no adequately controlled trials in ophthalmic surgery. A retrospective review of data suggests that antibiotics or topical antiseptics may be effective, but there is no consensus regarding efficacy or choice of therapy.
General surgery	
Cholecystectomy	Cefazolin (2 g IV) preoperatively in "high-risk" patients—i.e., those older than 60 years and those with previous biliary surgery, a history of acute symptoms, or jaundice. In patients with a β-lactam allergy, gentamicin (80 mg IV) preoperatively and every 8 h (3 doses) is effective.
Colon surgery	Neomycin and erythromycin base, 1 g of each orally at 1, 2, and 11 PM on the day before surgery. For emergency colon surgery or situations precluding preoperative oral prophylaxis, cefoxitin (2 g IV) preoperatively and every 4 h (3 doses) is effective. In patients with a β-lactam allergy, metronidazole (500 mg IV), and gentamicin (1.7 mg/kg IV) preoperatively and every 8 h postoperatively (3 doses) are effective.
Primary appendectomy	Cefoxitin (2 g IV) preoperatively and every 6 h (3 doses) in nonperforated appendixes; in perforated appendixes, therapy is continued for 3–5 days. Although combined aerobic and anaerobic coverage appears to be preferable, in patients with a β-lactam allergy, metronidazole (500 mg IV) preoperatively is effective. With perforated appendixes this is continued every 8 h (in either IV or oral administration) for 3–5 days.
Gastric resection	Cefazolin (1 g) preoperatively in "high-risk" patients only—those with a bleeding gastric or duodenal ulcer, an obstructive duodenal ulcer, a gastric ulcer, gastric cancer, or morbid obesity (prophylaxis is not indicated for cases of chronic uncomplicated duodenal ulcers). In patients with a β-lactam allergy, 1 preoperative IV dose of gentamicin (120 mg) and clindamycin (600 mg) may be effective, but data are limited.

TABLE 96-1 (Continued)

Surgical Procedure	Recommended Prophylactic Regimen[a]
Surgery for penetrating abdominal trauma	Cefoxitin (2 g IV) on admission to the hospital. For patients with an intestinal perforation, 2 g cefoxitin IV every 6 h for 2–5 days is effective.
Urologic surgery	
Prostatectomy, transurethral and peritoneal	Antimicrobial prophylaxis is not recommended in patients with sterile preoperative urine cultures. Prophylactic antibiotics have not proved to be effective in transperitoneal needle biopsies of the prostate when the preoperative cultures are sterile.
Surgery on nose, mouth, and pharynx	
Major head, neck, and oral surgery	In major surgical procedures involving an incision through oral or pharyngeal mucosa, a combination of gentamicin (1.7 mg/kg) and clindamycin (300 mg IV) preoperatively and every 8 h (2 doses) is recommended. Cefazolin and third generation cephalosporins have also demonstrated effectiveness when given over a 24-h period perioperatively.
Rhinoplasty and repair of nose	Prophylactic antimicrobials have not proved to be effective.
Cardiothoracic and vascular surgery	
Median sternotomy, coronary artery bypass grafting, and valve surgery	Cefazolin (1 g IV) preoperatively and every 6 h for 48 h. In patients with a β-lactam allergy, vancomycin (15 mg/kg IV) preoperatively, after initiation of bypass (10 mg/kg), and every 8 h postoperatively for 48 h may be effective.
Pacemaker insertion	Cefazolin (1 g) as above; in patients with a β-lactam allergy, no prophylaxis may be a reasonable alternative, given the low incidence of infection.
Thoracic surgery procedure including lobectomy and pneumonectomy	Cefazolin (1 g) preoperatively and every 6 h postoperatively for 24 h. The optimal duration of postoperative prophylaxis has not been established. In penetrating thoracic trauma and in the placement of chest tubes in trauma management, prophylactic antibiotics have not been effective.
Peripheral vascular surgery	Cefazolin (1 g) preoperatively and every 6 h postoperatively for 24 h. The usefulness of antibiotic prophylaxis in carotid artery surgery has not been established, but when infection rates are high, cefazolin should be used as described above.
Neurosurgical procedures	
Cerebrospinal fluid shunting procedures	Antibiotic prophylaxis is not indicated in institutions with low infection rates (<10%). Trimethoprim (160 mg) plus sulfamethoxazole (800 mg) IV preoperatively and every 12 h (3 doses) may be beneficial in institutions with high infection rates (>20%).
Craniotomy	For high-risk procedures (e.g., reexploration and microsurgery), clindamycin (300 mg IV) preoperatively and at 4 h has been effective, as has vancomycin (1 g IV) plus gentamicin (80 mg IM) preoperatively.

[a] Unless otherwise noted, the preoperative dose of intravenous (IV) antibiotic should be administered at about the time of the operative incision. Preoperative intramuscular (IM) antibiotic should be administered 30 min to 1 h before the incision.

SOURCE: Reproduced, with permission, from Kaiser AB: N Engl J Med 315:1129, 1986.

TABLE 96-2 Endocarditis Prophylaxis: Cardiac Conditions

Prophylaxis Recommended
Prosthetic cardiac valves, including bioprosthetic and homograft valves
Previous bacterial endocarditis, even in the absence of heart disease
Most congenital cardiac malformations
Rheumatic and other acquired valvular dysfunction, even after valvular surgery
Hypertrophic cardiomyopathy
Mitral valve prolapse with valvular regurgitation
Prophylaxis Not Recommended
Isolated secundum atrial septal defect
Surgical repair without residua beyond 6 months of secundum atrial septal defect, ventricular septal defect, or patent ductus arteriosus
Previous coronary artery bypass graft surgery
Mitral valve prolapse without valvular regurgitation
Physiologic, functional, or innocent heart murmurs
Previous Kawasaki disease without valvular dysfunction
Previous rheumatic fever without valvular dysfunction
Cardiac pacemakers and implanted defibrillators

SOURCE: Reproduced, with permission, from Dajani AS, et al: JAMA 264:2919, 1990. Copyright 1990, American Medical Association.

TABLE 96-3 Endocarditis Prophylaxis: Surgical Procedures

Prophylaxis Recommended
Tonsillectomy and/or adenoidectomy
Surgical operations that involve intestinal or respiratory mucosa
Bronchoscopy with a rigid bronchoscope
Sclerotherapy for esophageal varices
Esophageal dilation
Gallbladder surgery
Cystoscopy
Urethral dilation
Urethral catheterization if urinary tract infection is present
Urinary tract surgery if urinary tract infection is present[a]
Prostatic surgery
Incision and drainage of infected tissue[a]
Vaginal hysterectomy
Vaginal delivery in the presence of infection[a]
Prophylaxis Not Recommended[b]
Tympanostomy tube insertion
Endotracheal intubation
Bronchoscopy with a flexible bronchoscope, with or without biopsy
Cardiac catheterization
Endoscopy with or without gastrointestinal biopsy
Cesarean section
In the absence of infection for urethral catheterization, dilation and curettage, uncomplicated vaginal delivery, therapeutic abortion, sterilization procedures, or insertion or removal of intrauterine devices

[a] In addition to prophylactic regimen for genitourinary procedures, antibiotic therapy should be directed against the most likely bacterial pathogen.
[b] In patients who have prosthetic heart valves, a previous history of endocarditis, or surgically constructed systemic-pulmonary shunts or conduits, physicians may choose to administer prophylactic antibiotics even for low-risk procedures that involve the lower respiratory, genitourinary, or gastrointestinal tracts.
SOURCE: Reproduced, with permission, from Dajani AS, et al: JAMA 264:2919, 1990. Copyright 1990, American Medical Association.

TABLE 96-4A Endocarditis Prophylaxis Regimens for Oral and Upper Respiratory Tract Procedures in Patients Who Are at Risk

Drug	Dosing Regimen
Ampicillin	IV or IM administration of ampicillin, 2.0 g, 30 min before procedure; then IV or IM administration of ampicillin, 1.0 g, or oral administration of amoxicillin, 1.5 g, 6 h after initial dose
Ampicillin/Amoxicillin/Penicillin-Allergic Patients	
Clindamycin	IV administration of 300 mg 30 min before procedure and IV or oral administration of 150 mg 6 h after initial dose
Patients Considered High Risk and Not Candidates for Standard Regimen	
Ampicillin, gentamicin, and amoxicillin	IV or IM administration of ampicillin, 2.0 g, plus gentamicin, 1.5 mg/kg (not to exceed 80 mg), 30 min before procedure; followed by amoxicillin, 1.5 g, orally 6 h after initial dose; alternatively, the parenteral regimen may be repeated 8 h after initial dose
Ampicillin/Amoxicillin/Penicillin-Allergic Patients Considered High Risk	
Vancomycin	IV administration of 1.0 g over 1 h, starting 1 h before procedure; no repeated dose necessary

SOURCE: Reproduced, with permission, from Dajani AS, et al: JAMA 264:2919, 1990. Copyright 1990, American Medical Association.

THERAPY OF INFECTIOUS DISEASES IN ICU PATIENTS

Rational antibiotic use requires a systematic approach to the assessment of suspected infection that leads to the most accurate, specific diagnosis possible, knowledge of commonly used agents, and appropriate selection and monitoring of drugs.

Regardless of whether infection is suspected in an ICU patient because of the development of florid cardinal symptoms and signs of inflammation (rubor, calor, dolor, tumor, functio laesa) or subtle deterioration such as in the level of consciousness[4] or gas exchange, the same thorough, systematic evaluation is required in assessing the patient. In this evaluation, the first question to be addressed is whether infection can be reasonably inferred to be present. Does the history reveal systemic or local symptoms of inflammation? Are signs of inflammation present? Can other causes of inflammation such as tissue injury because of drug toxicity, immunologic diseases, physical agents (thermal energy, electromagnetic irradiation), and chemical agents such as extravasated cytotoxic drugs, be excluded as a cause of inflammation? Finally, is there laboratory evi-

TABLE 96-4B Endocarditis Prophylaxis Regimens for Genitourinary/Gastrointestinal Procedures

Dose	Dosage Regimen
Standard Regimen	
Ampicillin, gentamicin, and amoxicillin	IV or IM administration of ampicillin, 2.0 g, plus gentamicin, 1.5 mg/kg (not to exceed 80 mg), 30 min before procedure; followed by amoxicillin, 1.5 g, orally 6 h after initial dose; alternatively, the parenteral regimen may be repeated once 8 h after initial dose
Ampicillin/Amoxicillin/Penicillin-Allergic Patient Regimen	
Vancomycin and gentamicin	IV administration of vancomycin, 1.0 g, over 1 h plus IV or IM administration of gentamicin, 1.5 mg/kg (not to exceed 80 mg), 1 h before procedure; may be repeated once 8 h after initial dose
Alternate Low-Risk Patient Regimen	
Amoxicillin	3.0 g orally 1 h before procedure; then 1.5 g 6 h after initial dose

SOURCE: Reproduced, with permission, from Dajani AS, et al: JAMA 264:2919, 1990. Copyright 1990, American Medical Association.

dence of inflammation—frank pus or polymorphonuclear leukocytes in microscopic examinations of body fluids?

The second question for the intensivist is: What is the infectious disease that is occurring? Is this meningitis, pneumonitis, intraabdominal sepsis, intravascular catheter-related bacteremia, or some other process? This question must be answered as specifically as possible because an accurate diagnosis will logically lead to collection of proper specimens for microbiologic testing before antibiotic therapy is initiated, and an appropriate working conclusion about the probable etiologic agents involved.

An outline of the investigation of particular infections is beyond the scope of this chapter and is detailed elsewhere in the text. Contemporary intensivists have access to a wide range of noninvasive radiologic imaging techniques that have been invaluable in confirming the diagnosis of deep visceral infections and assisting in their repeated evaluation during treatment. Occasionally, however, the patient will be too ill to tolerate the most appropriate diagnostic evaluation, which will necessarily limit the accuracy of the initial assessment, but must not delay initiation of antimicrobial therapy. It is axiomatic in the critically ill patient, particularly in those in whom infection or suspected infection threatens life or major organ functions, that antimicrobial therapy directed at all infectious possibilities of more than trivial probability should be given until the results of definitive investigations are available.

Ideally, the choice of antibiotic agent(s) for the treatment of a specific infectious disease in a given host in the ICU should be based on unequivocal results from rigorous, controlled clinical trials. With a few exceptions, such data do not exist. Therefore, the selection of the proper antimicrobial agent depends on careful consideration of the known or likely susceptibility patterns of the putative pathogen in this specific type of patient at this particular institution, the natural history of the infection, and finally, the spectrum of agents likely or known to be effective for treatment of this type of infection. The two former areas are reviewed in other sections of this book and will not be elaborated on here. This chapter emphasizes the importance of a knowledge of the clinical pharmacology of antibiotics as one critical element in the rational use of drugs for treatment of infectious disease in the ICU patient.

The selection of the proper drug is essential to minimize toxicity and maximize efficacy. The following key steps relative to knowledge of the antimicrobial agents in man should be systematically considered in the selection process. In fact, they are essential to the rational use of any drug.

A. *Individualize* the treatment by considering the following in choosing drugs and designing dosage regimens.
- **1.** Processes that alter the pharmacokinetics of the drug
  - a. Physiologic
    - Extremes of age
    - Pregnancy
    - Barriers to drug penetration (e.g., blood-brain barrier, intraocular humors)
  - b. Disease-induced
    - Barriers to drug penetration (avascular abscess wall, infarcts, burn eschar, wet gangrene, etc.)
    - Changes in drug clearance because of hepatic, renal, or other disease (e.g., enhanced aminoglycoside clearance in burned patients, penicillins in cystic fibrosis patients)
  - c. Drugs administered concurrently
    - Chemical interaction (e.g., penicillins inactivate aminoglycosides in azotemic plasma)
    - Enhanced metabolism
    - Competitive inhibition of renal or metabolic clearance in kidney or liver
    - Displacement of highly bound drug from plasma protein
- **2.** Processes that alter the pharmacodynamics of the drug
  - a. Allergy to the drug
  - b. Other (e.g., reduced seizure threshold)

B. *Select* and *monitor* therapeutic end points.
- **1.** Clinical symptoms and signs of infection
- **2.** Laboratory measures of
  - a. Efficacy (e.g., leukocyte concentration, erythrocyte sedimentation rate; serial imaging results such as brain abscess shrinkage on serial computed tomography scans)
  - b. Toxicity (e.g., creatinine concentration and urinalysis in patients receiving aminoglycosides)
- **3.** Microbiologic (e.g., serial cultures, serum bactericidal titers)
- **4.** Pharmacologic—serum concentrations of drugs

Selecting the proper antimicrobial agent, skillfully individualizing the dose regimen, and choosing the appropriate parameters to monitor for beneficial and adverse effects of drugs are closely related to knowledge of the pharmacologic effects of antimicrobial agents in man. The remainder of this chapter reviews these aspects of many classes of antimicrobial agents from the intensivist's perspective.

Antibacterial Agents

In this section, selected aspects of commonly used groups of antimicrobial agents are reviewed, emphasizing the clinical pharmacology of the drugs rather than their molecular pharmacology and mechanisms of action. In addition, antimicrobial drugs most likely to be prescribed by intensivists are discussed.

PENICILLINS

MECHANISM OF ACTION. The penicillins are natural and semisynthetic compounds that have in common a thiazolidine ring connected to a β-lactam ring to which is attached a side chain of variable composition. Although the side chain has been ingeniously and successfully manipulated to alter the antibacterial spectrum of the penicillin molecule, the β-lactam ring itself is essential for the antibacterial activity of the penicillins. Hence, its enzymatic hydrolysis by β lactamases is the most important mechanism of bacterial resistance to penicillins.

Penicillins are generally bactericidal. The first step in the antibacterial effect of penicillins involves binding to penicillin-binding proteins (PBPs), which are peptidases in the cell wall of susceptible bacteria.[5] The PBPs account for 1 percent of the cell membrane proteins and are located in or near the rigid peptidoglycan layer of the cell wall. In gram-positive bacteria this layer is 50 to 100 molecules thick and located on the outside of the cell, whereas in gram-negative bacteria it is 1 to 2 molecules thick and located under the outer external lipopolysaccharide layer. There are a variety of PBPs in different bacterial species. High activity of penicillins against susceptible bacteria correlates with high affinity binding to certain PBPs, especially PBPs 1, 2, and 4. Modifications in the penicillin side chain of some semisynthetic penicillins have enhanced their antibacterial activity against gram-negative bacteria by increasing their ability to pass through the lipopolysaccharide outer layer to reach PBP ligands in the peptidoglycan layer, and less importantly, by increasing their resistance to β lactamases, which these organisms all contain in small amounts in the periplasmic space between the inner and outer membranes.

Penicillin binding to PBPs inhibits the enzymatic catalysis of peptidoglycan assembly and cross-linking. The resulting structural defects may prove lethal in some bacteria, but in others cell lysis is the result of secondary events unleashed by the inhibition of cell wall assembly during which endogenous autolysins (peptidoglycan hydrolases) are activated and cause cell death. In some bacteria, penicillins cause morphologic dysgenesis that is not lethal: inhibition of PBP-2 in *Escherichia coli*, for example, results in the production of stable round forms that continue to grow for several generations before lysis ultimately occurs.[6] The knowledge that different penicillins (and cephalosporins) may thus have different mechanisms of action provides a rational basis for combining two or more of these agents to achieve additive or synergistic antibacterial effects.

The antibacterial effect of the penicillins when susceptible organisms are exposed to intermittent doses of the drugs is determined by composite events occurring during three time periods:[7] the time during which the antibacterial drug exerts its maximal effect, the time during which the drug is present at concentrations that have a definite but lesser bactericidal effect, and the period after which concentrations have fallen to levels that are not bactericidal but during which some bacteria continue to die at a faster rate than the surviving cells can multiply (now known as the period of the postantibiotic effect or PAE).[8]

Bacterial killing during exposure to penicillins in vitro occurs most rapidly when exposure occurs during the logarithmic phase of bacterial growth. The killing effect of penicillin during this phase shows little dependence on concentration in excess of minimal inhibitory levels. Beyond this fact, the relationship between penicillin concentration and bacterial killing is complex even in vitro and, more so, in patients in whom host factors contribute to the antibacterial effect. It has been difficult to use these observations to optimize the way we give penicillins to patients—by intermittent administration or continuous infusion. In the final analysis, it is probable that penicillin concentration need not be maintained in excess of in vitro inhibitory levels continuously to effect cure. The maximum length of time that concentrations may be permitted to fall below bactericidal concentrations in vitro and still be associated with a net reduction in bacterial counts (PAE) varies between organisms. However, because the concentrations at the site of infection cannot be predicted, it is conventional to administer penicillins in relatively high doses at frequent intervals, or else continuously, to ensure the maximal antibacterial effect.[9] It should be recognized, however, that the effectiveness of this strategy depends more on the duration that penicillin concentrations exceed the inhibitory level, than on the increased ratio of the penicillin concentration to the minimal inhibitory concentration (MIC). In fact, extremely high peak concentrations may only increase the susceptibility to some of the concentration-related adverse effects of penicillins (vide infra).

The PAE of the penicillins usually lasts 1 to 3 h against gram-positive coccal bacteria and 1 h against susceptible Enterobacteriaceae and other enteric gram-negative bacteria. The duration of the PAE is more closely related to the duration of exposure to inhibitory concentrations of penicillin than to concentration per se. This is another reason why large increases in dose administered cannot be expected to produce linearly related increments in antibacterial therapeutic effects with this group of antibiotics.

MECHANISMS OF RESISTANCE. Although enzymatic hydrolysis of the β-lactam bond by β lactamases is the most important mechanism of bacterial resistance to penicillins, the foregoing description of the sequence of steps involved in the antibacterial effect of penicillins indirectly identifies other sites and mechanisms of resistance. Many gram-negative bacteria are not susceptible to penicillins because the penicillins cannot diffuse through the lipopolysaccharide layer to interact with PBPs. Mutations in genes encoding PBPs may yield altered transpeptidases that no longer bind penicillins. Finally, mutant streptococci have been described in which exposure to penicillins triggers synthesis of inhibitors of autolysins.

CLASSIFICATION. In view of the central role of penicillins in antimicrobial therapeutics, intensivists must be knowledgeable about this class of drugs. As with all antimicrobial agents, it is prudent to be conversant with a limited number of prototypical agents of each class, rather than to attempt to master them all. The penicillins can be divided into five classes based on their clinically most important antibacterial activity, notwithstanding substantial degrees of overlap demonstrable in vitro.

Natural penicillins—Penicillin G, the prototypical member of this group, is the drug of choice for infections caused by susceptible streptococci, staphylococci, *Clostridia* and *Neisseria* species and oral anaerobes including *Bacteroides melaninogenicus*.

Aminopenicillins—Ampicillin is the only member of this group, which includes amoxicillin, and bacampicillin among others, that can be administered parenterally. It is the drug of initial choice for the treatment of community-acquired meningitis in adults and, when combined with an aminoglycoside, for the therapy of subacute bacterial endocarditis in individuals with native valves and pyelonephritis in otherwise healthy adults with community-acquired infection. Although ampicillin was widely used in the past for treatment for *Haemophilus influenzae* infections, 13 to 20 percent of *H. influenzae* type B bacteria causing respiratory infection in adults are now resistant to ampicillin, usually by virtue of producing β lactamase.[10] A small proportion, approximately 1 percent, of nontypable *H. influenzae* are ampicillin-resistant, non–β-lactamase-producing strains. Accordingly, in the seriously ill patients in whom *H. influenzae* is a potential pathogen, it is prudent to use a drug other than ampicillin until the organism can be shown to lack β lactamase by in vitro testing.

Penicillinase-resistant penicillins such as cloxacillin and nafcillin are the antibacterial drugs of choice for therapy of suspected or proved *Staphylococcus aureus* infection in areas where methicillin-resistant *S. aureus* (MRSA) is not prevalent.

Antipseudomonal penicillins—Carbenicillin and ticarcillin are used to treat patients with suspected or proved infection due to *Pseudomonas aeruginosa*. It is almost exclusively a nosocomial pathogen in one of four settings: patients with extensive second or third degree burns, granulocytopenic cancer patients, adults with cystic fibrosis, and other patients, usually hospitalized and previously treated with antibacterials, who have become colonized with this opportunistic pathogen. The activity of these drugs against *Proteus vulgaris, Proteus rettgeri,* and *Morganella morganii* exceeds that of ampicillin but against other enteric aerobic gram-negative bacilli their potency is not different from ampicillin. Most strains of *P. aeruginosa* that are ticarcillin-resistant owe their resistance to a permeability barrier. Because development of resistance during therapy can be a problem, carbenicillin and ticarcillin are generally used together with an aminoglycoside when *P. aeruginosa* sepsis is suspected or diagnosed.

Extended-spectrum penicillins—Piperacillin, azlocillin, and mezlocillin inhibit *P. aeruginosa* similarly to the antipseudomonal penicillins but in addition have considerably more clinically useful activity against a number of other enteric gram-negative aerobic and anaerobic organisms. Mezlocillin is more active than carbenicillin or ticarcillin against most Enterobacteriaceae but many strains are resistant by production of β lactamases. It is active against oropharyngeal gram-negative anaerobic bacilli but *Bacteroides fragilis* group organisms are not uniformly susceptible. It is highly active against *H. influenzae, meningococci* and gonococci, Streptococci (including *S. faecalis*) and pencillin-sensitive *S. aureus* strains. Azlocillin's chief advantage compared to mezlocillin is its superior activity against *P. aeruginosa.* However, piperacillin is at least as active and often twice so, against *P. aeruginosa* strains compared to azlocillin. Because of this characteristic, it is the antipseudomonal penicillin of choice.

The extended-spectrum penicillins have largely replaced ticarcillin and carbenicillin because of their greater potency and because ticarcillin and carbenicillin may interfere more with platelet formation, an undesirable liability in critically ill patients with thrombocytopenia or other potential causes of hemorrhage (e.g., stress ulcers). As already noted, within this group, the agent of choice is piperacillin.

CLINICAL PHARMACOLOGY. The absorption of orally administered penicillins is sufficiently variable among even ambulatory patients that for this reason alone, in the critically ill patient with multiorgan dysfunction, these drugs are administered only intravenously. The range of doses recommended for some penicillins in adult patients with moderate to severe infection, with normal and severely impaired renal function (<10 mL creatinine clearance), is shown in Table 96-5. Also shown are doses for individuals undergoing dialysis.

In the circulation, pencillins are bound to plasma proteins, chiefly albumin, to varying degrees, ranging from a low of 18 percent for ampicillin to 96 percent for dicloxacillin, the most highly bound penicillin. Although protein-bound antibiotic is not pharmacologically active,[11] serum protein binding of penicillins has not proved to be clinically important because the binding is loose and rapidly reversible in vivo, and the doses used in clinical practice greatly exceed the capacity of the plasma proteins to bind drug. The clinical relevance of diminished binding due to hypoalbuminemia or coadministration of drugs that may compete for the same albumin-binding sites as penicillins is unclear. However, an effect of altered protein binding is likely only to be demonstrable when binding exceeds 90 percent.[12]

TABLE 96-5 Recommended IV Doses of Selected Penicillins for Adult Patients with Moderate to Severe Infection and Normal or Impaired Renal Function or Undergoing Dialysis

	CREATININE CLEARANCE (mL/min)				DOSE IF END-STAGE RENAL FAILURE REQUIRING	
	>60	40–59	10–39	<10	Peritoneal Dialysis	Hemodialysis
Natural						
Penicillin G	1–3 million U/4 h	up to 2 million U/4 h	up to 1 million U/4 h	up to 1 million U/8 h	As for creatinine clearance <10 mL/min	500,000 U/6 h during dialysis
Amino						
Ampicillin	1–3 g/6 h	No change	No change	2–6 g/12 h	As for creatinine clearance <10 mL/min	0.5 g/6 h
Penicillinase-resistant						
Cloxacillin	1.5–3 g/6 h	No change	No change	1–2 g/12 h	?	?
Nafcillin	1.5–3 g/6 h	No change	No change	No change	No change	No change
Antipseudomonal						
Ticarcillin	2–3 g/3 h	No change	3 g initial dose then 2 g/8 h	3 g initial dose then 2 g/12 h	As for creatinine clearance <10 mL/min	3 g after dialysis then 2 g/12 h
Azlocillin	3–5 g/6 h	No change	5 g/12 h	5 g initial dose then 2.5 g/12 h	3 g/12 h	5 g after dialysis then 2.5 g/12 h
Extended-spectrum						
Piperacillin	2–4 g/4 h	No change	2–4 g/8 h	4 g/12 h	2 g after dialysis then 2 g/12 h	2–4 g after dialysis then 4 g/12 h
Mezlocillin	3–4 g/6 h	5 g/12 h	5 g/24 h	5 g/48 h	3 g/12 h	Normal doses

The apparent volume of distribution (AVD) is the theoretical calculated volume in which drug must be uniformly distributed if present at the concentration measured in plasma.[13] AVD is usually expressed as liters per kg of body weight (L/kg). The AVD of penicillins is approximately inversely related to the degree of protein binding, ranging from 9 percent of the body weight for dicloxacillin to 41 percent for ampicillin. The effect of inflammation on the AVD of penicillins has not been comprehensively described, but it is clear that inflammation permits wider anatomic distribution of antibiotics. Elevated temperature from the inflammatory process itself also alters drug distribution.[14] This may result in attainment of therapeutically effective concentrations of penicillins in otherwise relatively pharmacokinetically isolated organs and fluid such as the cerebrospinal fluid (CSF), bronchial secretions, and aqueous or vitreous humor of the eye. Some noninflammatory diseases can adversely affect the penetration of penicillins into tissue with potential compromise of their therapeutic effect. For example, biliary obstruction may be associated with reduced biliary concentrations of penicillins and renal disease with diminished renal parenchymal and urinary concentrations of these drugs. However, administering large doses can overcome, in part, the potential limiting effects of these processes on the treatment outcome.

Pencillins are largely eliminated from the body as unchanged drug by renal proximal tubular secretion and glomerular filtration, but some metabolic transformation occurs varying considerably among penicillins. Accordingly, though metabolic transformation assumes greater importance with increasing degrees of renal failure, the need to reduce doses in that situation varies also. For example, in anuric patients, the plasma elimination $t_{1/2}$ of penicillin G is increased from 0.5 to 10 h and doses must be reduced to obviate dose-related toxic effects (vide infra). On the other hand, the serum elimination $t_{1/2}$ of cloxacillin only increases threefold, to 1.5 h and no dose reduction is required.

Probenecid, an organic acid like the penicillins, competitively inhibits renal tubular secretion of penicillins. Coadministration results in an array of pharmacologic and pharmacokinetic effects including increased plasma concentrations (double in the case of penicillin G), higher concentrations in the CSF because of inhibition of penicillin secretion from CSF into blood by the choroid plexus, and higher free drug concentrations in plasma because of displacement from albumin. The magnitude of these effects is greatest for those penicillins primarily eliminated by secretion of drug from the blood into the nephron lumen fluid by epithelial cells of the proximal renal tubule.

Various other organic acids also compete with penicillin

for secretion by renal tubular cells and produce probenecid-like effects on penicillin disposition. These include aspirin, phenylbutazone, sulfonamides, indomethacin, thiazide diuretics, furosemide, and ethacrynic acid, all drugs that may be concurrently administered to ICU patients being treated with penicillins. The clinical importance of concurrent administration of these drugs on the antibacterial effects of penicillin is not known but is unlikely to be significant.

ADVERSE DRUG REACTIONS. Adverse drug reactions (ADR) include all unwanted effects of drugs. They are classified into those which are immunologically mediated (hypersensitivity or allergic reactions) or dose or concentration related. For antibiotics, the latter class would also include all unwanted or undesired complications arising from perturbations in the normal microbiologic flora (e.g., pseudomembranous colitis and yeast vaginitis), as well as superinfections caused by agents resistant to the antibiotics being administered to the patient. A third class comprises ADR for which the mechanism is not understood. This includes anaphylactoid reactions (similar clinically to anaphylaxis but without a demonstrated immunologic basis) and idiosyncratic effects. ADR to penicillins mostly are of the first two classes. Although they may rarely be fatal (1/100,000 cases treated), hypersensitivity reactions are much more important than dose-related penicillin ADR in the ICU because such intolerance precludes the ready use of this most useful class of drugs (densensitization is possible, vide infra). Allergic reactions to penicillins are not uncommon.[15] The overall incidence in different studies ranges from 0.7 to 10 percent. In order of decreasing frequency, hypersensitivity reactions to penicillins include urticaria, fever, bronchospasm, vasculitis, serum sickness, exfoliative dermatitis, and anaphylaxis. Hypersensitivity reactions may be induced by any of the members of this group and cross-reactions must be anticipated. Anaphylaxis has been reported more commonly with penicillin G than with other members of the penicillin group, but this probably reflects the frequency of its use. Anaphylaxis and accelerated urticarial reactions, rash, and serum sickness are triggered by immunobinding of penicillin antigens to IgE, IgM, and IgG antibodies, respectively.[16] Atopic individuals are not more prone to have allergic reactions to penicillins. About 75 percent of persons without medical exposure to penicillins have IgM antibody to penicilloyl, the most important penicillin antigen produced by breakage of the β-lactam ring. It acts as a hapten by covalently binding to plasma proteins. The formation of another antigen, penicilloic acid, is accelerated in alkaline carbohydrate solution even at room temperature, resulting simultaneously in a loss of microbiologically active drug.[17] Penicillanic acid is yet another product of β-lactam ring breakdown. Its production is accelerated by prolonged maintenance of penicillins in acidic aqueous solutions. Thus, 0.15 M NaCl and 5% dextrose in water with a pH of 5.5 and 4.0, respectively, will increase the speed of penicillanic acid formation. Together, penicilloic and penicillanic acids are known as major determinants because 95 percent of tissue-bound penicillin is in the form of penicilloyl and penicillanic acid conjugates with body proteins. IgG and IgM antibodies to these moieties occur in the majority of patients treated with penicillins, but the allergic reactions that occasionally result are generally limited to skin rash rather than accelerated phenomena. The term *penicillin minor determinants,* on the other hand, refers to benzylpenicillin itself, sodium benzyl penicilloate, and penilloate. IgE-mediated reactions to minor determinants are responsible for the majority of anaphylactic reactions due to penicillins.

Interstitial nephritis associated with methicillin may be a delayed-type hypersensitivity reaction in which the drug induces autoimmunity to renal tubular basement membranes. This unusual immunologically mediated ADR is most commonly seen in patients treated with methicillin for extended periods in large doses, but it has been reported after therapy with most other penicillins and some cephalosporins.

The most important aspect of management of patients with hypersensitivity to penicillins is to avoid causing reactions. A reliable story of anaphylaxis or an accelerated reaction to any member of this group of drugs [or a cephalosporin or carbapenem (imipenem)] is an absolute contraindication to their use. A history of any other form of hypersensitivity reaction should be given appropriate weight in the therapeutic decision-making process and, in particular, should be balanced against the fact that there are no infectious diseases for which penicillins are absolutely the only effective antibacterial available. If it is decided to administer penicillins to a person with a history of a hypersensitivity reaction, skin testing is advised to identify those with severe hypersensitivity. Practically, only one standardized, nonimmunogenic test reagent, benzylpenicilloyl-polylysine, is available. Use of solutions of the parent drugs as reagents is inadvisable because they may both trigger reactions and induce sensitivity; minor determinant mixture is not commercially available. If skin testing is negative, 97 percent of hypersensitive patients will have been excluded, but unfortunately, many of those most likely to experience severe reactions (those with IgE-mediated allergy to the minor determinant) will not have been identified.

Skin testing for penicillin allergy is neither indicated nor of prognostic or diagnostic value for identifying patients with a history of only non–IgE-mediated allergic reactions (i.e., morbilliform skin rash). The information obtained from skin testing must be used within 72 h and repeated if penicillin is used again. A protocol for penicillin allergy skin testing is shown in Table 96-6.[16]

If no reaction to skin test reagent is observed, severe reactions are unlikely, but it is prudent to administer the first dose with epinephrine and resuscitation equipment at hand, and to inject only a fraction of the initial dose. Then wait 15 to 30 min for any acute reaction to appear. If none occurs, the remainder of the initial dose may then be administered. If a reaction occurs during skin testing, desensitization with escalating doses can be effected with appropriate precautions in readiness for dealing with a severe

TABLE 96-6 Penicillin Allergy Skin Testing

Reagents

Benzylpenicilloyl-polylysine (major, Pre-Pen {Taylor Pharmacal Co., Decatur, Illinois}, 6×10^{-5}M)
Benzylpenicillin (10^{-2}M or 6000 U/mL)
If available
Benzylpenicilloic acid (10^{-2}M)
Benzylpenilloic acid (10^{-2}M)
Positive control (histamine 1.0 mg/mL)
Negative control (buffered saline solution)
Dilute the antigens 100-fold for preliminary testing if there has been an immediate generalized reaction within the past year

Procedure

Epicutaneous (scratch or prick) test: examine for 15 min; if there is no significant wheal (4 mm or greater) proceed to intradermal test
Intradermal test: inject 0.02 mL intradermally with a 27-gauge short-bevelled needle; observe for 20 min

Interpretation

Conclusions are only possible if the negative control is negative and the positive control is positive.
Positive test: a wheal >4 mm in mean diameter to any penicillin reagent; erythema must be present.
Negative test: the wheals on the penicillin reagents are equivalent to the negative control.
Indeterminate: all other results

SOURCE: Reproduced, with permission, from Saxon A, et al: Ann Intern Med 107:207, 1987.

reaction. A protocol for penicillin allergy desensitization trial dosing challenge is shown in Table 96-7.[16]

Rashes caused by ampicillin should be distinguished from those caused by other penicillins. They occur in 7 to 8 percent of patients, an incidence three times greater than with all other penicillins and are not considered to be immunologically mediated. Certain patients are more prone to experience ampicillin-induced skin reactions: females, hyperuricemic patients receiving allopurinol, individuals with acute mononucleosis due to Epstein-Barr virus (EBV) or cytomegalovirus (CMV), and those with lymphocytic leukemia, reticulosarcoma, and other lymphomas. The rashes typically are morbilliform, appear 4 to 5 days after initiation of therapy, are not accompanied by other signs of allergy, and will usually subside during continued therapy. Skin testing with ampicillin and major and minor penicillin determinants will be negative. Such rashes, finally, should not be considered a contraindication to subsequent therapy with one of the other penicillins.

Other adverse reactions to penicillins are due to unknown mechanisms but are neither immunologically mediated nor dose related. Neutropenia occurs in about 15 percent of patients treated with methicillin and somewhat less commonly with other penicillins. It generally occurs 10 to 20 days after initiation of therapy and resolves rapidly on discontinuation of therapy. Reversible thrombocytopenia and bone marrow suppression have also been described in patients receiving penicillins.

Four dose-related side effects of the penicillins are uncommon but may be clinically important. First, undesirable augmentation of body sodium or potassium content can occur in patients with salt and water overload (e.g., congestive heart failure or renal failure) who are treated with large doses of penicillins because the penicillins are formulated for injection as salts of one of these cations. Intensivists should specifically select the cationic formulation appropriate for their patient (Table 96-8). On the other hand, hypokalemia has been described in up to 81 percent of patients without significant renal dysfunction treated with methicillin or carbenicillin. The mechanism of this ADR is unclear. While these two penicillins likely behave like a nonabsorbable anion in the distal renal tubule, increasing passive potassium urinary excretion, others have proposed that the hypokalemia may instead be due to an intracellular shift of potassium because of a membrane-altering effect.

Second, penicillins may cause neurotoxic effects including seizures. This is related to an innate pharmacologic effect of the molecule and, hence, to the concentration of drug in the body. Penicillin G is the most inherently epileptogenic of the group. Seizures will usually only be seen in patients with impaired renal function given large doses. Impairment of the blood-brain barrier due to meningeal inflammation, uremia, and cardiopulmonary bypass may contribute to the effect as may hyponatremia or concomi-

TABLE 96-7 Penicillin Allergy Desensitization Trial-Dosing Challenge

Be prepared for a serious generalized reaction
IV access
Premedication with antihistamines and corticosteroids
Resuscitation equipment immediately available
Do epicutaneous (prick or scratch) tests with serial tenfold dilutions beginning at concentration that induced a positive diagnostic test
Do an intradermal test with a solution 10-fold less concentrated than that producing a positive epicutaneous test
After 15 min, inject twice the skin test amount subcutaneously
Proceed at 15-min intervals doubling the dose with subcutaneous injections
Repeat any poorly tolerated dose
Oral "desensitization" is effective, and some think it is safer

SOURCE: Reproduced, with permission, from Saxon A, et al: Ann Intern Med 107:209, 1987.

TABLE 96-8 Cation Content of Some Penicillins

	Sodium Content
Penicillin G[a]	2 meq/million U
Ampicillin	2.6 meq/g
Cloxacillin	2.3
Nafcillin	2.9
Ticarcillin	5.9
Azlocillin	2.2
Piperacillin	2.0
Mezlocillin	1.9

[a] Potassium penicillin G = 1.7 meq/million U

tant probenecid therapy that blocks penicillin excretion from CSF. Neurotoxicity manifests initially as muscular irritability with choreiform, involuntary twitching or myoclonic jerking that will progress to a depressed level of consciousness and ultimately seizures, unless penicillin administration is halted. Penicillin concentrations in lumbar sac CSF in excess of 5 mg/L have been associated with seizures,[18] but the critical concentration in the CSF contiguous with cortical neurons has not been described. This toxic effect of penicillins will resolve with discontinuation of therapy and elimination of penicillin. Unfortunately, in those most predisposed to this ADR (patients with severe renal failure),[19] penicillin clearance will be slower than in those with normal renal function.

A third dose-related side effect of penicillins is impaired platelet aggregation that may lead to clinically important bleeding. Ticarcillin and carbenicillin are the most potent in this regard although piperacillin and mezlocillin as well as penicillin G can induce this defect.[20] The effect is due to a concentration-dependent blocking of receptor sites on platelet membranes, interfering with adenosine-induced aggregation. The defect may persist for up to 12 days after drug discontinuation, suggesting an effect on megakaryocytes as well as circulating platelets. This ADR can be avoided by selecting other potentially effective antibiotics and limiting dose size, especially in patients with other conditions or factors predisposing to hemorrhage, such as thrombocytopenia or severe hepatic dysfunction.

A fourth category of ADR caused by penicillin are those related to suppression of indigenous bacterial flora. The most important example is *Clostridium difficile* toxin-induced pseudomembranous colitis or diarrhea. As a group, the penicillins (and cephalosporins) rank close behind clindamycin as the most common antibacterials causing this undesirable and potentially life-threatening complication.

CEPHALOSPORINS

The cephalosporins resemble the penicillins structurally as well as in their mode of action, versatility, and general lack of toxicity. They possess a β-lactam structure in which the thiazolidine ring characteristic of penicillins is replaced by a six-member dihydrothiazine ring. Modification in the side chains at the 3 and 7 positions of the nucleus has yielded molecules with different pharmacokinetic and pharmacodynamic characteristics, respectively.[21] Side chain modifications at position 7 alter and extend the spectrum of antibacterial activity but also, in some cases, cause unusual adverse pharmacologic effects such as inhibition of vitamin K-dependent hepatocyte synthesis of clotting factors II, VII, IX, and X and induction of antabuse-like reactions in individuals ingesting or being treated with alcohol concurrently.

The potency of cephalosporins against a wide range of clinically important bacteria, together with a general lack of serious toxicity, has led to an emerging consensus that certain members of this group, the third generation drugs, are drugs of first choice for a number of severe, gram-negative bacterial infections, especially nosocomial ones, including meningitis, pneumonitis, bacteremia, and urinary tract infections.[22] This is particularly true for infection caused by multiply resistant organisms and for initial, empirical therapy in the ICU setting. The first and second generation cephalosporins, on the other hand, are not drugs of first choice for any acute life-threatening infectious disease that might be seen in ICU patients. All things considered, cephalosporins rank a close second to the penicillins in importance as antibiotics for use by intensivists.

MECHANISM OF ACTION. The mechanism of action of the cephalosporins is identical to that of the penicillins and involves binding to, and inactivation of, PBPs in the inner aspect of the cell wall of susceptible bacteria. As in the case of the penicillins, inactivation of certain PBPs leads to lethal structural defects in the cell wall; inhibition of others causes nonlethal anomalies with a resulting bacteriostatic effect only, the phenomenon called *tolerance.*

MECHANISM OF RESISTANCE. Resistance to cephalosporin antibiotics is also mediated by mechanisms that confer resistance to penicillins. Cephalosporins may not penetrate through the protein-lined channels, called *porins,* in the lipopolysaccharide cell wall, to the site of the PBPs. This may be an intrinsic characteristic of a bacterium or be acquired as a result of exposure to the antibiotic. The cephalosporin may be inactivated by β lactamases. Finally, although disputed, substantial evidence indicates that exposure to some third generation cephalosporins may induce synthesis of large amounts of β lactamase with high affinity for the cephalosporins. As a result, the antibiotic is avidly bound by the enzyme and unable to interact with PBPs.[23] This is hypothesized to be the mechanism of resistance observed in *Enterobacter, Serratia, Citrobacter,* and *Pseudomonas* species exposed to third generation cephalosporins.

CLASSIFICATION. Cephalosporins are arbitrarily classified as belonging to one of three generations. This classification is based solely on the spectrum of antibacterial activity (Table 96-9). None of the cephalosporins is useful for infections caused by *Streptococcus faecalis,* methicillin-resistant *Staphylococcus epidermidis* and *aureus* (MRSA) and penicillinase-producing *Streptococcus pneumoniae.* They are useful antibacterials, however, for treatment of a wide range of infections and for surgical prophylaxis.[24]

The *first generation cephalosporins* are potent inhibitors of aerobic gram-positive cocci such as *S. aureus* and *S. pneumoniae,* with moderate activity against a limited number of aerobic gram-negative bacilli including *E. coli, Klebsiella pneumoniae,* and indole-negative proteus. They are active against anaerobic gram-positive and gram-negative oropharyngeal organisms, as is penicillin G, but are not consistently effective against *B. fragilis* group and other fecal anaerobic organisms. Cefazolin has emerged as the prototypical agent of this group, which are the most active cephalosporins against susceptible gram-positive cocci.

The *second generation cephalosporins* as a group exhibit enhanced potency against *E. coli, K. pneumoniae* and indole-negative proteus, compared to first generation agents. Indi-

TABLE 96-9 Recommended IV Doses of Selected Cephalosporins for Adult Patients with Moderate to Severe Infection and Normal or Impaired Renal Function or Undergoing Dialysis

	CREATININE CLEARANCE (mL/min)				DOSE IF END-STAGE RENAL FAILURE REQUIRING	
	>60	40–59	10–39	<10	Peritoneal Dialysis	Hemodialysis
First generation						
Cefazolin	0.5–2 g/8 h	0.5 g initial dose then 0.5–2 g/12 h	0.5 g initial dose then 0.25–1 g/24 h	0.5 g initial dose then 0.1–0.5 g/24 h	As for creatinine clearance <10 mL/min	As for creatinine clearance <10 mL/min plus 0.25 g after dialysis
Second generation						
Cefuroxime	0.75–1.5 g/8 h	No change	0.75 g/12 h	0.75 g/24 h	?	0.75 g after each dialysis and each 24 h
Cefoxitin	1–2 g/6–8 h	Same dose at interval of 8–12 h	Same dose at interval of 12–24 h	Same dose at interval of 24–36 h	As for creatinine clearance <10 mL/min	1–2 g after each dialysis and each 72 h
Cefamadole	0.5–4 g/8 h	1–2 g/8 h	0.5–1 g/8 h	0.5–1 g/12 h	As for creatinine clearance <10 mL/min	As for creatinine clearance <10 mL/min
Third generation						
Ceftriaxone	1–4 g/24 h	No change	No change	No change	No change	1 g/24 h
Cefotaxime	0.5–2 g/4–8 h	No change	0.5–2 g/6–8 h	0.5–2 g/8–12 h	As for creatinine clearance <10 mL/min	As for creatinine clearance <10 mL/min plus 0.5–2 g after each dialysis
Ceftazidime	0.5–2 g/8 h	0.5–1.5 g/12 h	0.5–1.5 g/24 h	0.5–1 g/24 h	0.5 g/24 h plus 0.5 g after dialysis	0.25–0.5 g/24 h plus 0.5–1 g after dialysis
Cefoperazone	0.5–2 g/6–12 h	No change	No change	No change	No change	No change

vidual members of this class have clinically important antibacterial activity against β–lactamase-producing *H. influenzae* (cefamandole, cefuroxime, and cefotetan), *B. fragilis* group organisms (cefoxitin, cefotetan), *Neisseria meningitidis* and *gonorrhoeae,* and some species of enteric gram-negative bacilli. However, activity against the last group of organisms is sufficiently variable that knowledge of susceptibility is required to permit use of these agents in nosocomial infections in ICU patients; where such information is not available, it is more appropriate to prescribe a third generation cephalosporin or aminoglycoside initially. The extended spectrums of some of these second generation agents have made them drugs of importance, albeit not first choice, in some serious infections: mixed aerobic/anaerobic bacterial pulmonary, gastrointestinal, and genital tract infections such as aspiration pneumonia, intraabdominal and pelvic peritonitis, pelvic inflammatory disease, and diabetic foot infection (cefoxitin), and pneumonia due to an exacerbation of chronic bronchitis (cefuroxime).

The *third generation cephalosporins* are particularly noteworthy for their potency against aerobic gram-negative bacilli, which they inhibit in concentrations 10 to 100 times less than required for aminoglycosides. They inhibit a wide range of this group of bacteria that are resistant to first and second generation cephalosporins as well as extended-spectrum penicillins and aminoglycosides. Their lack of inherent toxicity also is an advantage in treating ICU patients with multisystem dysfunction, especially renal failure. Two of the third generation cephalopsorins, cefoperazone and particularly, ceftazidime, have clinically useful activity against most strains of *P. aeruginosa,* although susceptibility may differ substantially between institutions. Third generation cephalosporins are not more resistant to penicillinase produced by *S. aureus*, nor are they more active against this organism, than are the penicillinase-resistant penicillins or first generation cephalosporins, which are preferred for therapy of such infections.

Recommended intravenous doses of selected cephalosporins for adult patients with moderate to severe infection and normal or impaired renal function or undergoing dialysis are shown in Table 96-9.

CLINICAL PHARMACOLOGY. Like the penicillins, the cephalosporins are variably bound to plasma proteins [range 15 (cephalexin) to 84 percent (cefazolin)] with AVD 0.10 (cefoxitin) to 0.30 (cefuroxime) L/kg. These characteristics are independent of the generation to which the agent belongs. They differ from the penicillin group pharmacokinetically. **1.** Hepatic biotransformation is a significant route of elimination for some members of this group. Moreover, with cefotaxime, hepatic biotransformation yields metabolites with antibacterial activity that contribute to the overall antibacterial effect although their precise contribution is unclear. **2.** Some have prolonged plasma $t_{1/2}$. For example, the extended plasma $t_{1/2}$ of 8 h for ceftriaxone has made once-to-twice daily dosing feasible without a loss in efficacy. **3.** Some are readily able to cross the blood-brain barrier. Therefore, unlike the first and second generation cephalosporins, the third generation drugs predictably attain therapeutic concentrations in the CSF and are efficacious for treatment of meningitis. In addition to the CSF, therapeutic concentrations of cephalosporins are not attained in the aqueous and vitreous humors of the eye, where only subconjunctival or intraocular injection or topical instillation of antibiotic, respectively, yield effective concentrations.

Probenecid inhibits proximal renal tubule secretion of cephalosporins just as for penicillins, but no advantage of concurrent probenecid therapy in acute serious infection in the ICU patient, compared to administration of larger doses of cephalosporins used alone, has been demonstrated.

Moderate to severe renal dysfunction necessitates reduction in the doses of some of the cephalosporins (see Table 96-9). Hemodialysis or peritoneal dialysis may remove sufficient drug (see Table 96-9) that additional postdialysis doses are required in treating patients with renal failure. Only cefoperazone doses must be reduced in patients with moderate to severe hepatic dysfunction.

ADVERSE DRUG REACTIONS. Hypersensitivity reactions to the cephalosporins qualitatively similar to those produced by penicillins are the most common adverse effect.[16] They are no more common with any single cephalosporin or generation of cephalosporins and probably are related to the shared bicyclic nuclear structure. However, cephalosporins lose both their ring structures when exposed to β lactamases in contrast to penicillin degradation. Thus, molecules unique to cephalosporins that may function as haptens are generated. This probably accounts in part for the lack of predictable cross-allergenicity between penicillins and cephalosporins. Haptenic activity of acyl side chains at position 7 of the β-lactam ring further complicates the predicting of reactions induced by cephalosporins in individuals with a history of penicillin intolerance. However, cross-reactions do occur in penicillin-sensitive patients treated with cephalosporins. The frequency of such cross-reactions is probably low, 5 to 10 percent, but great enough that the risk of a reaction, especially if of the immediate or accelerated type, precludes use of cephalosporins in penicillin-allergic patients. No established testing methods identify cephalosporin allergy.

Dose-related side effects from cephalosporins are different from those induced by penicillins. The likelihood of cation overloading even with large doses of cephalosporins is small. Although they are mostly sodium salts containing up to 3.6 meq Na^+/g (ceftriaxone), even with very large doses of 8/g day, the total sodium load administered is just 28 meq, an amount unlikely to be clinically important except in rare patients with severe sodium and water overload. The epileptogenic potential of the cephalosporins is also substantially less than that of the penicillins. Even in the presence of a blood-brain barrier impaired by meningitis, cefotaxime, which, with ceftriaxone, is the cephalosporin most commonly used to treat this infection, has not been reported to cause myoclonus or convulsions. All cephalosporins in high concentration except cephaloridine are similar to penicillins in interfering with platelet aggregation.

Modifications induced by altering the side chain on the dihydrothiazine ring at position 3 have created cephalosporins with unusual pharmacologic side effects: cefamandole, cefoperazone, cefotetan, and moxalactam all have a methyltetrazolethiol sidechain that provokes a disulfuram-like reaction in patients ingesting or receiving ethanol and causes, in part, hypoprothrombinemia.[25] Pretreatment with the antibiotic at least 3 h before alcohol ingestion (or in the ICU, ethanol infusion therapeutically) appears necessary to precipitate the reaction. Inhibition of hepatic aldehyde dehydrogenase with accumulation of acetaldehyde during metabolism of alcohol is the presumed mechanism. The reaction, consisting of flushing, headache, hypotension, nausea, and vomiting may begin within 5 to 10 min after ethanol exposure. It can be severe and last for hours, clearly something to be avoided in critically ill patients. These four agents may also predispose the patient to bleeding because of interference with synthesis of vitamin K-dependent clotting factors in addition to their inhibition of platelet aggregation. Bleeding may only occur in patients whose oral intake of vitamin K or synthesis of endogenous vitamin K by colonic flora is impaired concomitantly.

Superinfections are surprisingly uncommon given the wide antibacterial spectrum of third generation cephalosporins, occuring in from 1 percent of cefotaxime recipients up to 3 to 5 percent for cefoperazone-treated patients.[26] Superinfections in patients treated with moxalactam have been observed to frequently be caused by *S. faecalis*. Otherwise, superinfection caused by resistant aerobic enteric gram-negative bacilli, *Clostridia* species, and yeast have been the most common.

Adverse effects of cephalosporins on the kidney are rare with two exceptions: cephaloridine in doses > 4 to 6 g/day causes acute tubular necrosis; cephalothin appears to enhance the nephrotoxic effect (but not vestibular- or cochlear toxic effects) of gentamicin and tobramycin.

OTHER β-LACTAM DRUGS

Carbapenems and monobactams are two new classes of β-lactam antibiotics of importance to intensivists (Table 96-10).

CARBAPENEMS

Carbapenems possess novel stereochemical characteristics that distinguish them from the other bicyclic β-lactams, the penicillins, and cephalosporins. Imipenem, the only carbapenem currently licensed, has the widest spectrum of any β-lactam antibiotic studied to date. It is a potent inhibitor of nearly all common bacterial pathogens, including those resistant to aminoglycosides and newer cephalosporins, in concentrations as low as, or lower than, any other β lac-

TABLE 96-10. Recommended IV Doses of Selected Carbapenems, Monobactams, and Combinations of a β-Lactam Antibiotic with a β-Lactamase Inhibitor for Adult Patients with Moderate to Severe Infection and Normal or Impaired Renal Function or Requiring Dialysis

	CREATININE CLEARANCE (mL/min)				DOSE IF END-STAGE RENAL FAILURE REQUIRING	
	>60	40–59	10–39	<10	Peritoneal Dialysis	Hemodialysis
Carbapenem						
Imipenem	0.25–1 g/6 h	No change	0.5/8–12 h	0.5 g/12 h	?	As for creatinine clearance <10 mL/min plus 0.5 g after dialysis
Monobactam						
Aztreonam	1–2 g/6–12 h	0.75–1.5 g/6–12 h	0.5–1 g/6–12 h	0.25–0.5 g/6–12 h	?	?
β-Lactamase inhibitor plus β-lactam antibiotic						
Clavulanate-ticarcillin	3 g + 0.2 g[a]/3–6 h	3 g + 0.2 g/6 h	3 g + 0.2 g/12 h	2.0 g + 0.13 g/12 h	3 g + 0.2 g/12 h	2 g + 0.13 g/12 h plus 3 g + 0.2 g after dialysis

[a]Use 3 g + 0.1 g combination for kidney infection.

tams. It binds primarily to PBP-2 and is not hydrolyzed by most β lactamases, penicillinases, or cephalosporinases. The wide spectrum of activity appears to be related to the ability of this relatively compact β-lactam molecule to diffuse readily through porin channels of gram-negative enteric bacilli, plus β-lactamase resistance conferred on the molecule by the unusual transconformation related to the hydroxethyl sidechain. Tolerance is not observed when bacteria are exposed to imipenem (that is, there is no major discrepancy between inhibitory and bactericidal concentrations), and, unique among β lactams, imipenem exerts a marked postantibiotic effect on both gram-positive and gram-negative bacteria.

Imipenem inhibits gram-positive cocci other than *E. faecium,* and MRSA, most Enterobacteriaceae and gram-negative bacilli including *P. aeruginosa* but excluding most *Pseudomonas cepacia* and *maltophilia* strains, and all oral and most fecal anaerobic bacteria. There is no cross-resistance between imipenem and other β lactams.

The place of imipenem in the therapy of infection in ICU patients is not yet established. Generally, it is most appropriate for indications such as those for which extended-spectrum cephalosporins would be used. In one controlled trial, it was more effective than clindamycin combined with tobramycin for treatment of seriously ill patients with nosocomial intraabdominal infections,[27] although at least five other studies have not shown it to be superior in other populations with intraabdominal infection.[28] It should not be used as monotherapy of *P. aeruginosa* infections because of the risk of resistance. Its greatest value may be that the breadth of its spectrum permits it to be used conveniently in place of multiple drug regimens for polymicrobial infections, with an attendant reduction in the risk of adverse reactions and the number being administered. Recommended intravenous doses of imipenem, aztreonam, and ticarcillin-clavulanic acid for adult patients with moderate to severe infections and variable renal function are shown in Table 96-10.

CLINICAL PHARMACOLOGY. Imipenem is destroyed by gastric acid and therefore is available only in a parenteral formulation. It is 20 percent protein bound and penetrates into a wide variety of tissues but poorly into cells other than brain cells. This latter characteristic makes it unsuitable for treatment of infections caused by bacteria that are primarily intracellular pathogens and may account in part for its epileptogenic potential.

It is not secreted into bile, which probably accounts for its minimal impact on gut flora. It is eliminated from plasma by a first-order process with a mean $t_{1/2}$ of 1 h, primarily by glomerular filtration; renal tubular secretion is minimal so that, as expected, probenecid does not affect imipenem renal clearance.

Although imipenem is remarkably stable to bacterial β lactamases, it is susceptible to metabolic degradation in man, primarily by peptidases in the brush border of renal tubular epithelial cells. Inhibition of these enzymes (by cilastatin, vide infra) increases urinary recovery of undegraded imipenem from 7 to 38 percent up to 70 to 85 percent.

Like cephaloridine, imipenem is toxic to proximal renal tubule epithelial cells. The toxic moiety appears to be a hydrolysis product, the formation of which can be safely blocked by coadministration of cilastatin, which blocks the catalytic effect of dehydropeptidase I in the brush border on imipenem and completely eliminates renal tubular damage without affecting the plasma $t_{1/2}$ of imipenem. A ratio of 1:1

imipenem: cilastatin is optimal and imipenem is marketed in this fixed combination.[29]

ADVERSE DRUG REACTIONS. Imipenem has been generally well tolerated like other β lactams. Major adverse effects such as diarrhea, superinfection, or pseudomembranous colitis are infrequent. Allergic reactions, including rashes and drug fever, occur in 2 to 3 percent of subjects and cross-allergenicity to penicillins has been observed. The incidence of seizures, 0.2 percent in series of patients treated with imipenem,[30] is unique among β-lactam antibiotics; preexisting central nervous system (CNS) disease, old age, and renal insufficiency predispose patients to this serious but reversible side effect. Seizures ought to be preventable by appropriate dose reductions in patients with renal disease, a maneuver of particular importance in patients with CNS disease.

MONOBACTAMS

Aztreonam is the first marketed member of a new completely synthetic class of monocyclic β-lactam antibiotics called monobactams. Aztreonam has no clinically important activity against gram-positive or anaerobic bacteria because of failure to bind to PBPs of these organisms. It binds primarily to PBP-3 in Enterobacteriaceae, *P. aeruginosa* and other gram-negative aerobic bacteria and thereby has a bactericidal effect; its narrow spectrum of activity most resembles that of the aminoglycosides. When combined with other β-lactam antibiotics to treat gram-negative aerobic bacterial infections, the net effect is unpredictable. It is more predictably synergistic, or at least additive, with aminoglycosides.[31] Lack of susceptibility is due to failure of aztreonam to cross the outer cell wall and failure to bind to PBPs. Aztreonam is stable in the presence of a wide variety of β lactamases[32] so that inactivation by this process is less important as a mechanism of bacterial resistance than for other β-lactam antibacterial agents.

The exact niche of aztreonam in the treatment of gram-negative aerobic bacterial infections in ICU patients is unclear at present. The most logical, albeit rare, circumstance for which it could be used would be in treating patients with significant allergy to β-lactam antibiotics (vide infra) in whom its combination with another agent, such as an aminoglycoside to obtain a synergistic or additive effect, is deemed necessary. It could also be used alone in such patients if an aminoglycoside were considered contraindicated, but its relative utility compared to aminoglycosides and other alternatives such as quinolones and trimethoprim-sulfamethoxazole (TMP-SMX) has not been described.

CLINICAL PHARMACOLOGY. Aztreonam is poorly absorbed after enteral administration because of intragastric hydrolysis and hence must be administered either intramuscularly or intravenously. After such injection, it distributes widely and achieves therapeutic concentrations in all body tissues and fluids except perhaps the vitreous humor. Metabolism has a minimal effect on aztreonam clearance in healthy individuals; the sole metabolite is devoid of antibacterial activity. Unchanged drug is primarily eliminated by renal filtration and tubular secretion but some excretion in bile into the gut occurs.[33] Elimination is a first-order process with a plasma $t_{1/2}$ of 1.7 h that is inversely related to glomerular filtration rate and increases to 6 h in anephric patients. The usual dose, 1 to 2 g every 6 to 12 h (maximum 8 g/day), should be reduced in patients with renal insufficiency (see Table 96-10). The drug is removed by both hemodialysis and peritoneal dialysis. Although the amount of drug removed depends on the specific type of dialysis coil used, duration of dialysis and flow rates, etc., generally, a 3.5 mg/kg supplemental dose of aztreonam is required after hemodialysis only. Patients requiring peritoneal dialysis need not receive an extra dose postdialysis but rather only a regular dose of 30 mg/kg/day.

ADVERSE DRUG REACTIONS. Aztreonam shares the general safety profile of other β-lactam antibiotics. Up to 7 percent of patients experience rash, diarrhea, nausea or vomiting, and isolated elevations of serum transaminase concentrations. It is unique among β lactams in being weakly immunogenic and not cross-allergenic with other penicillins or cephalosporins.[16] It has been administered safely to penicillin-allergic patients, including those with positive skin test results. This unique property appears to be due to the fact that aztreonam lacks the allergenic bicyclic nuclear structure of penicillins, cephalosporins, and carbapenem β-lactam antibiotics.

β-LACTAMASE INHIBITORS

Clavulanate and sulbactam are β-lactam compounds that possess weak, insignificant antibacterial activity but are clinically useful because they extend the spectrum of activity of many β-lactam antibiotics by inhibiting β lactamases. They share a common mechanism of action that involves binding to susceptible β lactamases with initial competitive inhibition followed by noncompetitive inactivation of the enzyme by acylation.[34] β lactamases differ in their susceptibility to inhibition: clavulanate and sulbactam inactivate similar types of chromosomal and plasmid-coded, inducible, and constitutive enzymes. *S. aureus* β lactamase is readily inhibited as are the plasmid-mediated enzymes prevalent among Enterobacteriaceae, *P. aeruginosa, H. influenzae, N. gonorrhoeae,* and *Branhamella catarrhalis.* Chromosomally encoded enzymes of *K. pneumoniae, Proteus mirabilis, P. vulgaris,* and *B. fragilis* are all susceptible. Chromosomally encoded β lactamases of *M. morganii, P. rettgeri, Serratia marcescens, Enterobacter* species, and *P. aeruginosa* are relatively nonsusceptible to clavulanate and sulbactam inhibition. These are inducible, important enzymes conferring resistance to third generation cephalosporins.

Clavulanate and sulbactam will enhance the antibacterial effect of many β-lactam antibiotics. However, they have been marketed only in two fixed combinations with amoxicillin and ticarcillin (both with clavulanate) and ampicillin (sulbactam). In the United States and Canada, only ticarcillin-clavulanate is available for intravenous injection, limiting the usefulness of amoxicillin-clavulanate or ampicillin-sulbactam for therapy of seriously ill patients in the ICU.

Combining amoxicillin or ticarcillin with a β-lactamase inhibitor does not sufficiently extend the spectrum of these antibacterials to permit their use for the initial empirical therapy of ICU patients with presumed serious gram-negative or gram-positive infections. Unless in vitro susceptibility testing results are known, they have a similarly restricted role even in patients with infections of established etiology. The lack of an injectable formulation of amoxicillin or ampicillin combined with β-lactamase inhibitor and some noteworthy clinical pharmacokinetic differences in the β-lactam antibiotics and the inhibitors further limits their use (vide infra).

Ticarcillin-clavulanate is available in vials containing 3 g ticarcillin and 0.1 g or 0.2 g clavulanate. The usual dose, based on ticarcillin content, is 3 g every 3 to 6 h (see Table 96-10). Amoxicillin-clavulanate is marketed in fixed combination tablets containing 250 or 500 mg amoxicillin plus 125 mg clavulanate.

CLINICAL PHARMACOLOGY. Coadministration of clavulanate and sulbactam with β lactams does not alter the pharmacokinetics of either component. The plasma $t_{1/2}$ of clavulanate and sulbactam are both approximately 1 h. Approximately half a clavulanate dose is metabolized to inactive metabolites; the remainder is eliminated by glomerular filtration but without significant renal tubule epithelial cell secretion, so that probenecid does not affect clavulanate elimination. Sulbactam elimination parallels that of ampicillin, mediated primarily by renal secretion with a lesser contribution by glomerular filtration and hepatic inactivation. Probenecid interferes with sulbactam renal clearance and prolongs the plasma $t_{1/2}$ by 40 percent.

In patients with renal failure, sulbactam disposition also parallels that of ampicillin so that no dose alterations are required for the two components individually, although the dose of both should be reduced in patients with severe renal insufficiency (see ampicillin). The plasma $t_{1/2}$ of sulbactam in patients with creatinine clearances $<$10 mL/min is 20 h.

Currently available amoxicillin-clavulanate formulations cannot be administered confidently to patients with severe renal insufficiency because the extrarenal elimination of clavulanate in such patients greatly exceeds that of amoxicillin. Clavulanate plasma $t_{1/2}$ in patients with creatinine clearance $<$10 mL/min only increases to an average of 3.8 h from 1 h, whereas that of amoxicillin increases to 16 h from 1 hour. Although not described, the same disparity is likely to occur for clavulanate compared to ticarcillin and this may affect the resulting antibacterial activity.

ADVERSE DRUG REACTIONS. Clavulanate and sulbactam cause slight increments in the frequency of nausea, vomiting, and diarrhea over that caused by the penicillins alone. Duodenojejunal manometric recordings demonstrate that oral amoxicillin-clavulanate causes disturbances in small bowel motility, as observed with erythromycin. This probably accounts for the increased frequency of gastrointestinal symptoms associated with this combination. Whether these changes in motility occur with parenteral administration of ticarcillin-clavulanate has not yet been described.

AMINOGLYCOSIDE ANTIBIOTICS

One or more of the aminoglycoside antibiotics (streptomycin, kanamycin, gentamicin, tobramycin, netilmicin, amikacin, and neomycin) has been a mainstay of our antibacterial armamentarium since the discovery of streptomycin in 1943. Streptomycin today is limited to use in the combination therapy of tuberculosis and for the treatment of brucellosis.

Neomycin is too toxic for systemic use, but is still administered orally for the treatment of portosystemic encephalopathy. The remaining agents—kanamycin, gentamicin, tobramycin, netilmicin, and amikacin—are first-line drugs for the treatment of serious infection caused by Enterobacteriaceae and *Pseudomonas* and *Serratia* species. The importance of these bacterial species as causes of nosocomial infection has progressively increased in the antibacterial era and the importance of the aminoglycosides has increased in parallel. Their utility in the therapy of patients with significant infection in the ICU has been limited by their inherent toxic effects on the proximal tubule epithelial cells of the kidney, the hair cells of the cochlea, saccule, and utricle and by the emergence of strains reisistant to one or more of the members of this group.

MECHANISMS OF ACTION. The aminoglycosides are rapidly bactericidal in contrast to β-lactam antibacterial drugs, which cause bacterial cell death only after a lag period.[9] Although their mode of action has been extensively studied,[35] the precise mechanism(s) of their lethal effect remains unclear. It is generally accepted that they interfere with bacterial protein synthesis by binding to the 30S subunit of bacterial ribosomes, resulting in misreading of mRNA codons and synthesis of faulty bacterial proteins, but the resulting alterations in protein molecules are not considered sufficient by themselves to cause cell death. Aminoglycosides bind to the cell wall and cytoplasmic membrane of susceptible bacteria by an energy-independent electrostatic process and pass into the cell through porins passively. The next phase involves binding to membranous structures and respiratory quinones followed by energy-dependent transport into the cell. The third stage is also energy dependent and involves binding to higher affinity binding sites on membrane-associated ribosomes, resulting in even more rapid transport of the drug into the cell. Aminoglycoside uptake by bacteria depends on energy derived from aerobic metabolism. Thus, all of these agents are inactive under anaerobic conditions because intracellular transport of aminoglycoside is markedly impaired in the absence of oxygen.

MECHANISMS OF RESISTANCE. Aminoglycoside resistance is an intrinsic characteristic of strictly anaerobic bacteria such as clostridia, which do not possess respiratory quinones. Among aerobic organisms, resistance is primarily due to aminoglycoside-inactivating enzymes.[36] Less commonly, ribosomal mutation and diminished permeability of bacterial cells to aminoglycoside molecules account for resistance. High level resistance of some Enterobacteriaceae and other gram-negative aerobic bacilli attributable to aminoglycoside-modifying enzymes is most commonly related to acquisition of R-plasmids. This usually occurs in the setting of heavy and widespread use of these agents (antibiotic selection pressure).[37] Genes coding for these enzymes may be found on plasmids, transposons, bacterial chromosomes, and possibly, bacteriophage genomes. Different enzymes may acetylate, adenylate, or phosphorylate aminoglycosides and by these changes, preclude binding of the drug to ribosomes. The different aminoglycosides vary considerably in their susceptibility to enzymatic modification. For example, although gentamicin is susceptible to modification by at least five different enzymes elaborated by gram-negative bacilli, amikacin is susceptible only to an acetyltransferase found in some *P. aeruginosa* and *Acinetobacter* species strains. As a result, gentamicin resistance emerging under antibiotic selection pressure in institutions is more common than resistance of bacteria to amikacin; resistance of bacteria to tobramycin, netilmicin, and kanamycin is of intermediate prevalence. Although aminoglycoside resistance is, as noted, to some extent a function of use, this association is not entirely predictable because other factors are probably involved.[38]

Compelling in vitro and correlative in vivo data from studies of the antibacterial and therapeutic effects of the aminoglycosides provide strong support for the current practice of treating patients with large doses intermittently to optimize efficacy and minimize toxicity; some have argued for once daily dosing in individuals with normal renal function.[39] These in vitro effects include the marked concentration-dependent aminoglycoside antibacterial effect and PAE. In vitro studies demonstrate that aminoglycosides produce marked, rapid, concentration-dependent bactericidal effects against both gram-positive aerobic cocci and bacilli. This effect is demonstrable over a wide range of concentrations beginning at the MIC and extending beyond therapeutic postdose serum concentrations to levels that are too toxic to be achieved in patients. This observation, which has been corroborated in animals with experimental infection, provides the rationale for attempting to achieve high aminoglycoside concentrations in plasma and at the site of infection.

Aminoglycosides consistently produce a concentration dependent PAE which is probably of therapeutic importance.[39] For both gram-positive and gram-negative aerobic bacteria, it is demonstrable in vitro over a wide range of concentrations, but PAE induced by aminoglycosides persists longer (>3 h) for gram-negative aerobic bacilli than for gram-positive aerobic bacteria (usually <2 h.) The mechanism of the PAE of aminoglycosides is unclear, but is likely related to the time required for organisms to resynthesize proteins essential for replication. In animals with experimental infection and in patients, the PAE is directly related to both the aminoglycoside concentration and time of exposure, as represented directly by the area under the concentration versus time curve at the site of infection or, indirectly, in the plasma. Based on this consideration, it would be anticipated that dose schedules involving intermittent high doses would be most effective. A few clinical studies have confirmed this expectation; most aminoglycosides have proved to be more efficacious and probably less toxic when administered in high doses infrequently rather than in smaller divided doses given frequently or by constant infusion.

Kanamycin, gentamicin, tobramycin, netilmicin, and amikacin are primarily active against aerobic gram-negative bacilli and *S. aureus*. Anaerobic bacteria and facultative anaerobes growing under anaerobic conditions are resistant as are some aerobic gram-positive cocci such as *S. aureus* or *S. pneumoniae*. Streptomycin is the most potent of the aminoglycosides against *Mycobacterium tuberculosis* and is also the drug of choice for *Francisella tularensis* and *Yersinia pestis* infection and brucellosis. Kanamycin utility has been limited by widespread resistance among many Enterobacteriaceae and innate inefficacy against *P. aeruginosa*. Gentamicin, tobramycin, amikacin, and netilmicin share similar spectrums of activity with the following caveats. Tobramycin is twice as potent as gentamicin or netilmicin in inhibiting *P. aeruginosa* in vitro, although the clinical relevance of this superiority is not clear. Netilmicin is the most potent inhibitor of *S. epidermidis*. As noted previously, amikacin is the most resistant to aminoglycoside-inactivating enzymes. As a result, many enteric bacilli resistant to kanamycin, gentamicin, and netilmicin remain susceptible to amikacin.

CLINICAL PHARMACOLOGY. The aminoglycosides are polycations whose polarity is responsible in part for many of their shared clinical pharmacokinetic characteristics. They are poorly absorbed after oral administration, have an apparent volume of distribution that is mathematically similar to the extracellular fluid volume, are excluded from the normal subarachnoid space, vitreous humor and prostatic fluid, and are eliminated almost exclusively by the kidney.[40]

After intramuscular administration, the aminoglycosides are rapidly and completely absorbed. Their apparent volume of distribution is equal to 25 to 30 percent of ideal body weight. The AVD is approximately 25 percent less in obese than nonobese individuals and approximately 20 percent greater in patients with protein-calorie malnutrition. This information must be used to calculate the initial dose, which is a function of the desired plasma concentration multiplied by the AVD. For gentamicin, tobramycin, and netilmicin, the MIC of most susceptible aerobic enteric gram-negative bacilli is 2 to 4 mg/L and toxicity has been shown to increase to unacceptable levels at concentrations in excess of 10 mg/L. It is therefore conventional to prescribe an initial dose to attain a plasma concentration (Cp) of 7 mg/L, which for a 70-kg adult would be 7 mg/L × [70 kg × 25%] = 120 mg. For kanamycin and amikacin, for which desired Cp values are 25 to 30 mg/L, the initial dose, similarly calculated, would be 500 mg.

It has been argued that the more appropriate way to aminister aminoglycosides, at least to patients with normal renal function, is to give the entire daily dose in one infusion.[39] However, no data from a comparative trial have directly evaluated the safety and efficacy of this approach compared to the conventional 8 hourly dosing schedule. Accordingly, it seems prudent to not yet change to this approach as the standard one for aminoglycoside dosing.

Aminoglycosides are actively concentrated in the endolymph of the cochlea, saccule, and utricle and in epithelial cells of the proximal renal tubule, a fact important in the production of aminoglycoside toxicity. Toxicity may be due to inhibition of microsomal protein synthesis, which can be demonstrated in mammalian cells at aminoglycoside concentrations approximating those accumulated in the renal cortex and the perilymph bathing the membranous labyrinth. The nephrotoxic effect may also be due in part to inhibition of synthesis of vasodilatory prostaglandins with resultant unopposed effects of vasoconstrictor prostaglandins and consequent reductions in glomerular filtration. A direct relationship between renal and cochlear-vestibular accumulation of aminoglycosides, the trough serum concentration and toxicity has been proposed by some[39] but denied by others.[41] Less than 1 percent of an injected dose appears in the feces and none in saliva.

Aminoglycosides are eliminated exclusively by glomerular filtration. An inverse realtionship exists between the plasma $t_{1/2}$ and the creatinine clearance as a measure of glomerular filtration rate. At creatinine clearance rates >100 mL/min, the plasma $t_{1/2}$ averages 2 h.[42] As the creatinine clearance declines, the plasma $t_{1/2}$ increases but at a rate out of proportion to the decline in creatinine clearance. Nevertheless, as a first estimate, the plasma $t_{1/2}$ calculated from the serum creatinine concentration can be used to estimate appropriate intervals for administration of maintenance doses.[40] It is probable that an effect of variable aminoglycoside resorption with sequestration in proximal renal tubule epithelial cells and increasing AVD in patients with renal insufficiency contributes to the weakening of the correlation between serum creatinine concentration and aminoglycoside plasma $t_{1/2}$.

One method of prescribing maintenance doses is to replace the initial dose at intervals of three times $t_{1/2}$. Theoretically, in three times $t_{1/2}$ 87.5 percent of the previous dose will have been eliminated so that little (12.5 percent of the dose) remains, and minimal accumulation will occur if the same dose is readministered at this interval. For kanamycin and gentamicin, the plasma $t_{1/2}$ (h) approximates [serum creatinine (μM/L)/22.4]. The appropriate dose interval is three times [plasma $t_{1/2}$]. For tobramycin, netilmicin, and amikacin, a similar assumption about the relationship between plasma $t_{1/2}$ and serum creatinine can be used to simplify their prescription using the same formula.

An alternative method to prescribe aminoglycosides to patients with significant renal insufficiency and prolonged aminoglycoside plasma $t_{1/2}$ is to maintain the interval at the conventional 8 h but to reduce the dose administered proportionately[42] (e.g., if the calculated dose interval is 16 h, one could administer 50 percent of the dose at 8 hourly intervals instead). Such a dose regimen will result in a lower peak plasma aminoglycoside concentration but comparable trough plasma concentrations to those achieved by maintaining the dose (mg/kg) constant and increasing the dose interval (vide supra). The clinical advantage of the former approach has been reviewed and promoted in respect of once daily aminoglycoside dosing,[39] but its superiority and safety in patients with renal insufficiency is not known. Thus, if possible, it is preferable to use antibiotics other than aminoglycosides in patients with renal insufficiency. If aminoglycosides must be used, serum aminoglycosides measurements should be used to maximize efficacy and minimize toxicity (vide infra). The importance of serum aminoglycoside measurements is greater when renal function is fluctuating or when disease or other drugs may be affecting aminoglycoside disposition. For example, in burned and febrile patients aminoglycoside pharmacokinetics are altered and larger doses will be required. In patients with renal failure given both aminoglycosides and penicillins in high doses, aminoglycosides are inactivated. The rate and extent of the inactivation depend on the concentration of the penicillin. Kanamycin, gentamicin, and tobramycin are most susceptible to inactivation in this manner and amikacin the least with netilmicin of intermediate susceptibility.

The Cp versus time curve following intravenous administration of an aminoglycoside dose is affected by the preexisting Cp, the dose administered, and the method of administration (intramuscular or intravenous injection, bolus, or infusion and the rate of infusion). These variables particularly affect the time and magnitude of peak Cp. Trough Cp is less affected by these factors. This variability has made it more difficult to define the relationship between postdose aminoglycoside concentration and therapeutic effect than that between trough Cp and toxic effects. Although incontrovertible data do no exist, other data demonstrate that Cp measured 60 min after intramuscular or 15 min after an intravenous infusion of the aminoglycoside is related to efficacy. For gentamicin, a postdose Cp of 8 mg/L or greater is associated with a better outcome than lower Cp in patients being treated for gram-negative aerobic bacillary pneumonia, whereas concentrations of at least 5 mg/L are associated with a better outcome in patients being treated for nonpneumonia, non-CNS, gram-negative aerobic bacillary infections.[43] It is assumed that the same realtionship holds for netilmicin and tobramycin. For amikacin and kanamycin, postdose Cp values of 20 to 40 mg/L are desirable.

A direct relationship between predose or trough aminoglycosides Cp and toxicity was first demonstrated in 1950 for streptomycin.[44] Trough Cp >3 mg/L during once-daily intramuscular administration of streptomycin for therapy of tuberculosis was associated with an increased risk of dizziness, presumably due to vestibulotoxicity. Old age was also a factor. At other times Cp values were much more variable, and often higher, but did not correlate with this toxic effect. Subsequent studies have suggested an increased risk of gentamicin nephrotoxicity, evidenced by a rise in serum creatinine concentration, when trough gentamicin Cp exceeds 2 mg/L.[39,45] This interpretation is supported by studies in animals.[39]

ADVERSE DRUG REACTIONS. All aminoglycosides share three dose-related, largely reversible toxic effects, although quantitative differences exist between members of this family. The three adverse effects are neuromuscular paralysis, nephrotoxicity, and cochleovestibular toxicity. The mechanism(s) of the unwanted effects are not well characterized, but an interaction of the cationic aminoglycoside molecule with calcium, magnesium, and membrane phospholipids[46] may be common to all. These effects of aminoglycosides are a result of their inherent pharmacologic properties occuring at doses close to those required for treatment. As such, they are not likely completely avoidable.

Neuromuscular paralysis of clinical consequence is not commonly seen but may be serious. Skeletal muscle paralysis involves both inhibition of acetylcholine release and blockade of acetylcholine receptors. Presynaptic inhibition is manifest more by neomycin or tobramycin than streptomycin, whereas the postsynaptic inhibitory effect is manifest more by streptomycin or netilmicin than neomycin. The neuromuscular paralysis is directly related to high concentrations of aminoglycoside at the neuromuscular end plate. As such, it is only observed when the antibiotic is injected rapidly as a bolus or when large quantities of aminoglycoside are administered and absorbed (e.g., by injection in the pleural or peritoneal cavity). The inhibitory effect is accentuated by an additive effect of other neuromuscular blocking agents such as the curariform drugs and succinylcholine or diseases such as botulism intoxication or myasthenia gravis. The effect can be avoided by slow intravenous administration over 30 to 60 min or intramuscular injection. It can be reversed by calcium injection.

Aminoglycoside nephrotoxicity spans a wide spectrum ranging from asymptomatic, increased urinary excretion of renal tubular epithelial cell brush border enzymes to overt renal failure necessitating dialysis. In between is diminished creatinine clearance evidenced by elevated serum creatine concentration. Enzymuria is almost universally demonstrable in patients receiving therapeutic doses of aminoglycosides, whereas oliguric renal failure is rare. Elevated serum creatinine concentration is observed in 5 to 25 percent of treated patients.

The nephrotoxic effect is associated with accumulation of aminoglycoside inside proximal renal tubule epithelial cells with resultant cell damage and, possibly, inhibition of synthesis of vasodilatory prostaglandins resulting in renal afferent arteriolar vasoconstriction and diminished glomerular filtration. Renal injury manifest as elevations in serum creatinine concentration usually occurs several days after initiation of therapy and is largely reversible because of epithelial cell regeneration. Animal and clinical studies indicate that neomycin is the most nephrotoxic and amikacin the least nephrotoxic of currently used aminoglycosides. Gentamicin is more nephrotoxic than tobramycin.

The nephrotoxic effect of aminoglycosides in animal studies is related directly to the height of the trough serum aminoglycoside concentration and the area under the serum concentration-time curve, which in turn are the important determinants of aminoglycoside uptake and sequestration in proximal tubule epithelial cells. This leads to the recommendation that trough serum aminoglycoside concentrations should be as low as possible.[39] For gentamicin, levels <3 mg/L at trough are recommended.[45] Intuitively, the same level would seem to be appropriate for tobramycin and netilmicin, which have similar pharmacokinetic properties and antibacterial potency to gentamicin. The appropriate trough Cp for amikacin is 5 to 10 mg/L.

Additional risk factors for nephrotoxicity include older age, female sex, concomitant liver disease, and hypotension at the time aminoglycoside therapy is initiated. Concomitant drug therapy with cephalothin, cisplatin, amphotericin B, and cyclosporine may add to the nephrotoxic effect of aminoglycosides.

Ototoxic effects of aminoglycoside include hearing loss caused by cochlear injury and vertigo caused by vestibular damage. Neither has been as well studied as has nephrotoxicity because of difficulties in assessing cochlear and vestibular funtion in critically ill patients. Nevertheless, available data suggest that all the injected aminoglycosides can cause both types of injury. There are not consistent differences between injectable aminoglycosides in current use.

The incidence of clinically detectable hearing loss ranges from 0.5 to 5 percent and of vestibular dysfunction causing vertigo or nystagmus, 0.4 to 4 percent. Auditory toxicity is due to selective destruction of the outer hair cells of the organ of Corti, especially at the basal turn with subsequent retrograde degeneration of the associated fibers of the auditory nerve. The vestibular toxicity is due to similar injury to hair cells of the ampullae cristae. Because these are both highly differentiated cells that do not regenerate if destroyed, ototoxicity is irreversible. As in the case of the renal injury caused by aminoglycosides, animal and some clinical data suggest that their ototoxic effects are also related to selective concentration and trapping of the cation aminoglycoside molecules in the perilymph and endolymph of the cochlea and vestibular apparatus and this in turn, to high trough serum aminoglycoside concentrations[44,47] although contrary data show no relationship.[48] Renal insufficiency is the most important risk factor,[48] but dose is important in patients with normal renal function; duration of therapy and older age are of variable pertinence. Concomitant ethacrynic acid, but not furosemide therapy, increases the risk of ototoxicity.

Other adverse effects of aminoglycosides are uncommon: pseudomembranous colitis due to *C. difficile* toxin and hypersensitivity reactions such as rash, fever, and Stevens-Johnson syndrome have been described rarely in recipients of almost all the aminoglycosides. A case of delirium was likely caused by tobramycin.

Although dose-related toxic effects of aminoglycosides may be unavoidable despite assiduous attention to dose selection, the small risk of what are generally reversible toxic effects should not engender use of small, potentially inefficacious doses of these drugs in critically ill ICU patients.

POLYMYXIN B AND E (COLISTIN)

The polymyxins are a group of basic polypeptide antibiotics that inhibit only aerobic gram-negative bacteria. Their antimicrobial action is due to binding to phospholipids in the cytoplasmic membrane with immediate disruption of membrane permeability, macromolecular and ion disequilibrium, and cell lysis. Intrinsic resistance is due in part to inability of the drug to gain access to the cytoplasmic membrane; acquired resistance is rarely observed. Their potency and spectrum of activity against bacteria such as *Enterobacter, E. coli, Klebsiella, Salmonella, Shigella, and Pseudomonas* species are similar to the aminoglycosides. However, because of more marked nephrotoxicity, all but two members of this group, polymyxin B and E (colistin) have been abandoned. Polymyxin B continues to be used in topical or oral formulations from which it cannot be absorbed. Thus, polymyxin B has been administered by mouth to suppress the aerobic gram-negative members of the intestinal flora in immunocompromised patients. Polymyxin E (colistin) alone, or combined with another antibiotic, has a limited but definite role as a parenteral agent for the treatment of infection caused by multiply resistant, nosocomial pathogens for which no less toxic agents are available. Polymyxin has been administered together with rifampicin to treat multiresistant nosocomial *S. marcescens* infection[49] and with cotrimoxazole, to treat *P. cepacia* and *S. marcescens* infections successfully.[50,51] Because it is structurally distinct, it is unaffected by enzymes that degrade β-lactam and aminoglycoside antibiotics.

CLINICAL PHARMACOLOGY. Like aminoglycosides, polymyxins are eliminated unchanged by glomerular filtration. The plasma elimination $t_{1/2}$ of colistin is 1.6 to 3 h. No reliable data exist on the relationship between serum concentrations and either therapeutic or toxic effects. Accordingly, in those uncommon instances when polymyxin E is administered parenterally, avoidance of drug toxicity depends solely on clinical evaluation, urinalysis, and measurement of changes in glomerular filtration rate. In the critically ill ICU patient, the confounding effect of concurrent changes due to disease and other drugs makes this more difficult than usual.

The usual dose of polymyxin E is 2.5 to 5.0 mg/kg/day as two or four divided intramuscular or intravenous doses, or a continuous intravenous infusion at a rate of 5 to 6 mg/h. Polymyxin E accumulates in patients with renal failure so that the total daily dose should be reduced:

Creatinine Clearance (mL/min)	Dose
>20	Standard dose
5–19	25.0% of standard dose every 12 h
<5 and hemodialysis and peritoneal dialysis	15% of standard dose every 12 h

ADVERSE DRUG REACTIONS. Adverse reactions after topical or oral administration are uncommon although nausea, vomiting, and diarrhea are caused by administration of large doses (600 mg or more) by mouth. After parenteral administration, side effects are similar to those caused by aminoglycosides. Reversible dizziness, paresthesias especially affecting the face, incoordination caused by vestibulotoxicity and proteinuria, microscopic hematuria, and progressive azotemia or acute tubular necrosis may occur. Respiratory paralysis due to neuromuscular blockade occurs rarely; unlike that due to aminoglycosides, it cannot be reversed by neostigmine.

VANCOMYCIN

Vancomycin is a unique glycopeptide antibiotic unrelated structurally to any other antibacterial agent. Its antibacterial activity is essentially restricted to gram-positive bacteria. It is the drug of first choice for initial therapy of MRSA and *S. epidermidis* infection.[22] *S. epidermidis* infection is a common bacteremic complication of prolonged catheterization of arteries and veins used to monitor and treat ICU patients. *S. aureus, S. epidermidis,* streptococci, and *Corynebacterium* and *Clostridium* species are almost uniformly sensitive to concentrations of vancomycin (<5 mg/L) that can be safely achieved in the plasma. However, in the face of increasing vancomycin use, strains of vancomycin-resistant staphylococci are being reported. Fortunately, their prevalence has not yet significantly compromised the utility of vancomycin as initial therapy for infections suspected to be caused by these organisms. In addition to its activity as a single agent, in combinations with gentamicin or tobramycin, vancomycin synergically inhibits *S. aureus* strains including those resistant to methicillin and nearly all strains of *S. faecalis*.

MECHANISMS OF ACTION AND RESISTANCE. Vancomycin is bactericidal, in part by inhibition of an early stage in the formation of the peptidoglycan of the cell wall. Resistance to it, at least in enterococci, is associated with synthesis of a plasmid-encoded protein that reduces access of vancomycin to its site of action on the cytoplasmic side of the developing cell wall.

CLINICAL PHARMACOLOGY. Vancomycin is poorly absorbed after oral administration. For systemic therapy it must be injected intravenously because intramuscular injection causes marked discomfort and possibly tissue necrosis. It is 30 to 55 percent protein bound and distributes widely into inflamed tissues and spaces in effective concentrations, including the subarachnoid space in patients with meningitis and the peritoneal cavity in renal failure patients with peritonitis complicating chronic peritoneal dialysis. The AVD is approximately 40 percent of total body weight. It may be 50 percent less on average in morbidly obese patients, but the implication of this for dose calculation is unclear. The drug is eliminated primarily unchanged by glomerular filtration. The plasma elimination $t_{1/2}$ varies widely, with a range of 3 to 13 h (average 6 h) even in patients with normal renal function. Plasma $t_{1/2}$ is prolonged with renal insufficiency, and may be as much as 17 days in anuric patients. In patients with liver disease without concomitant renal dysfunction, plasma $t_{1/2}$ is also increased and has been reported to be as long as 37 h. This observation, as well as the incomplete recovery of injected vancomycin in urine collections from healthy volunteers, indicates that vancomycin is partly eliminated by a nonrenal, presumably hepatic, route.

Vancomycin Cp is directly proportional to dose. The Cp 2 h after infusion of 0.5, 1.0, and 2.0 g in adult volunteers averages 2 to 10, 25, and 45 mg/L, respectively. The mean Cp 6 h after infusion of 0.5 g is 6 mg/L and 12 h after 1.0 g, 5 mg/L.

The usual adult vancomycin dose is 6.5 to 8 mg/kg administered every 6 h or 15 mg/kg every 12 h, given in a relatively dilute solution infused over 60 min. More rapid infusion is frequently associated with the occurrence of the *red-man syndrome,* an important adverse reaction (vide infra). In adults with impaired renal function, dose reductions are recommended to avoid ototoxic, and purportedly, nephrotoxic side effects (vide infra). One nomogram that permits calculation of the appropriate dose interval is shown in Fig. 96-1.[52]

In patients with fluctuating renal function and those with clinically important liver disease, dose intervals should be based on vancomycin concentrations in serum after the usual initial dose. Although the data demonstrating a relationship between serum vancomycin concentration and beneficial or toxic effects are not robust (vide infra), it is conventional to avoid maximum concentrations after the distribution phase is complete (30 min after the end of infusion) of >30 mg/L to avoid ototoxicity and perhaps the red-man synrdrome, as well as trough concentrations >10 mg/L, to avoid nephrotoxicity. If a continuous infusion of vancomycin is administered, the target Cp should be 15 mg/L.

In functionally anephric patients who are being dialyzed, 1 g vancomycin infused weekly yields maximum Cp values of 40 to 50 mg/L that are usually well tolerated and still therapeutic after 7 days (Cp 5 to 7 mg/L). Thus, once weekly vancomycin infusions are a practical and convenient method for treating serious infection in patients requiring dialysis. Hemodialysis does not remove significant amounts of vancomycin so that no supplemental doses need be administered after completion of dialysis.

Vancomycin administered by mouth is effective for therapy of pseudomembranous colitis.[53] It is considered the drug of choice for severe cases, whereas metronidazole is no less effective for mild to moderately severe disease.[54] The recommended dose is 125 mg administered four times per day; the maximum dose is 500 mg administered four times per day. In patients with adynamic ileus, the optimal therapy for pseudomembranous colitis is unknown. Some experts recommend vancomycin administration both intravenously and by nasogastric tube. When cholestyramine is administered by mouth for treatment of pseudomembranous colitis, coadministration of vancomycin should be avoided because it will be inactivated by binding to the resin. In patients with severe pseudomembranous colitis and moderate to severe renal dysfunction treated with vancomycin by mouth, vancomycin concentrations have been reported to reach peak concentrations as high as 13 mg/L depending on the dose given.[55] It was estimated that only an average of 4.0 percent of oral doses were absorbed and that the accumulation of vancomycin in serum was primarily a function of concurrenct renal insufficiency in these patients. Monitoring of serum vancomycin concentrations has been recommended if such therapy is prolonged (>28 days) or involves higher than conventional doses (>2 g/day).

Vancomycin administered intraperitoneally in dialysis fluid is the preferred mode for treatment of gram-positive coccal peritonitis complicating peritoneal dialysis. This choice is predicated on the knowledge that peritonitis in such patients is a superficial and localized infection of the serosal surface of the peritoneum. Both absence of fever in 80 to 90 percent of milder cases and the rarity of bacteremia support this view. Vancomycin moves readily bidirectionally across the inflamed peritoneal lining into the blood stream and vice versa. Accordingly, the Cp ultimately attained approaches that in the peritoneal fluid. One vancomycin treatment schedule for peritonitis begins with a dose of 1 g in the initial dialysate, followed by 50 mg maintenance doses in subsequent exchanges. On such therapy, mean serum vancomycin concentration rises to 9 mg/L at

FIGURE 96-1 Dosage nomogram for vancomycin in patients with various degrees of renal function. The creatinine clearance can be estimated by a formula using the patient's age, sex and serum creatinine as follows:

In males, creatinine clearance (mL/min) =

$$\frac{\text{wt(kg)} \times (140 - \text{age [years]})}{0.81 \times (\text{serum creatinine } [\mu\text{M/L}])}$$

Females = 0.85 × above value

SOURCE: Reproduced, with permission, from Matzke GR, et al: Antimicrob Ag Chemother 25:433, 1984.

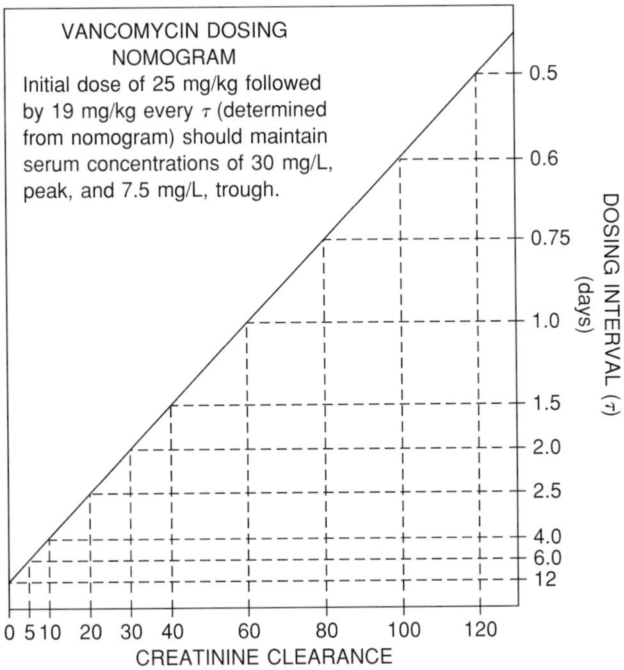

5 h and averages 6 to 9 mg/L during subsequent dwell periods. In patients with severe peritonitis, it is not certain that concomitant intravenous therapy alters the outcome, but vancomycin may be administered by both routes. In such patients, the need for frequent measurement of serum vancomycin concentration to avoid excessively high levels becomes more acute.

ADVERSE DRUG REACTIONS. The red-man syndrome is the most important immediate adverse effect of vancomycin infusion. It appears to be due to histamine release. The reaction may begin within minutes of starting the infusion or shortly after its completion and definitely occurs more commonly with rapid infusions. Generally, tingling and flushing of the neck, face, and thorax develop during the course of a rapid infusion, sometimes with progression to hypotension and shock. The flushed appearance usually resolves over several hours. Antihistamines can prevent vancomycin-induced hypotension in man[56] but their value for treating hypotension after the onset of the reaction is unclear. Nevertheless, treatment with fluid administration, antihistamines, and steroids has been advocated for severe reactions. Many, but not all, occurrences of the syndrome can be prevented by following the manufacturer's strong recommendation that vancomycin be infused over at least 60 min. A maximum rate of administration of 10 mg/min may further reduce the risk of hypotension, as demonstrated in a study in volunteers.[57]

A maculopapular rash (sometimes accompanied by pruritus, fever, and rigors), not dissimilar to the cutaneous flushing seen as a component of the red-man syndrome, may occur in up to 3 percent of patients treated with vancomycin. This adverse effect appears to be an allergic reaction so that intensivists may have to decide whether to risk readministration of the antibiotic in such patients. In those in whom the reaction is part of a typical red-man syndrome, continued therapy with cautious, slower administration has been advocated, but if allergy is diagnosed, use of alternative agents is more prudent.

Ototoxicity due to vancomycin does not appear to be common, but definitive data are lacking. In one prospective study, reversible tinnitus and dizziness occurred in 2 of 34 patients.[58] However, tinnitus may herald high frequency hearing loss and deafness that will progress despite discontinuation of vancomycin therapy. Ototoxicity is probably due to injury to the hair cells of the cochlea, a toxic effect identical to that caused by aminoglycoside antibiotics. It is therefore not surprising that vancomycin ototoxicity is more likely when aminoglycosides are administered concomitantly. Ototoxicity is also more frequent in elderly patients and those with renal failure. It is associated with peak vancomycin serum concentrations of >80 mg/L, but is infrequent if drug is administered so peak and trough serum concentrations are <30 and <10 mg/L, respectively.

The nephrotoxic potential of vancomycin administered alone or in combination with an aminoglycoside is not clear despite several careful prospective observational studies. Nephrotoxicity evidenced by a rise in serum creatinine concentrations has been reported in 5 to 75 percent of patients treated with vancomycin alone and 0 to 22 percent of patients treated with vancomycin plus an aminoglycoside. In one study, trough serum vancomycin concentrations >30mg/L were associated with nephrotoxicity.[59] Renal dysfunction developing during vancomycin therapy is usually mild and reversible, but as many as 9 percent of patients may have persisting evidence of diminished renal function.[60]

Even though the nephrotoxicity of vancomycin is debated, until the issue is clarified, serum creatinine levels should be monitored in patients being treated with vancomycin and doses adjusted to obtain peak and trough serum concentrations of <30 and 10 mg/L, respectively. Combination therapy with an aminoglycoside plus vancomycin requires even more careful attention to these measures.

SULFONAMIDES

The discovery of the antibacterial action of sulfonamides in the 1930s and the administration of these agents systemically to prevent and cure bacterial infections represented a revolutionary breakthrough in medicine and opened the chemotherapeutic era. When first introduced for general use, this group of antibiotics was effective against a wide range of infections caused by aerobic gram-positive and gram-negative bacteria, actinomycetes (*Nocardia* and *Actinomyces*), protozoa (*Pneumocystis carinii, Toxoplasma gondii,* and malarial parasites), and *Chlamydia trachomatis.* Since that time, their usefulness has declined markedly because of a number of factors: the advent of a wide range of alternate agents, the frequent emergence of resistance to sulfonamides in many formerly susceptible microorganisms, an awareness of the frequency and severity of ADR caused by some sulfonamides, and the relative unavailability of parenteral formulations.

CLASSIFICATION. Sulfonamides may be classified as follows:

1. *Sulfonamides rapidly absorbed and eliminated after oral administration.* Sulfisoxazole is the prototypical agent; sulfamethoxazole and sulfadiazine are other widely used members of this class.
2. *Poorly absorbed orally administered sulfonamide.* Sulfasalazine is used to treat ulcerative colitis and Crohn's disease. About 20 percent of an oral dose is absorbed in the small intestine, of which a small portion (about 10 percent) is excreted into urine while the rest is secreted in bile and enters the enterohepatic circulation.[61] This portion plus unabsorbed drug passes into the colon where it is split into two metabolites, sulfapyridine and 5-aminosalicylic acid. The former is absorbed, partly acetylated or hydroxylated in the liver, or conjugated with glucuronic acid and is responsible for most of the toxic effects of sulfasalazine.[62] A small portion of the 5-aminosalicylic acid is absorbed, acetylated, and excreted into the urine. Substantial evidence indicates that unabsorbed 5-aminosalicylic acid accounts for the therapeutic effect of sulfa-

salazine in inflammatory bowel disease, but the mechanism of the beneficial effect is not clear. It may be due to a combination of anti-inflammatory, immunosuppressive, and bacteriostatic effects.

3. *Sulfonamides for topical use.* Sulfacetamide is approximately 90 times more soluble in aqueous solution than sulfadiazine at neutral pH and is nonirritating to the eye. It is formulated as 30% and 10% ophthalmic solutions and a 10% ointment. Ocular fluids and tissues are thus exposed to high concentrations of antibiotic during topical ophthalmic application. However, topical ophthalmic use is associated with a risk of sensitization and this consideration plus the insensitivity of most nosocomial bacteria to sulfonamides limits the usefulness of sulfacetamide for treatment of bacterial conjunctivitis and keratitis in the ICU.

   Two sulfonamides have an established place in the ICU for the topical therapy of patients with second and third degree burns. Silver sulfadiazine is relatively insoluble. It reacts with chloride and protein components of tissue exudate to form silver chloride, silver protein complexes, and sodium sulfadiazine. The relative contributions of each of these products to the potent inhibitory effect of silver sulfadiazine on the growth of a broad spectrum of microorganisms is unclear but inhibition of growth of bacteria, including some species resistant to sulfonamides and fungi,[63] is observed. This suggests that inhibition other than by interference with folate synthesis (vide infra) contributes to the antibiotic effect.

   Mafenide is a sulfonamide marketed as 8.5% cream. Like silver sulfadiazine, it is effective for the prevention of colonization of burns by a large variety of gram-negative and gram-positive bacteria, including some anaerobes. However, *Candida* species are not inhibited as they are by silver sulfadiazine. Mafenide is rapidly absorbed and converted to a nontoxic metabolite, p-carboxybenzenesulfonamide, which is excreted in urine. Unlike all other sulfonamides, mafenide is active in the presence of blood, pus, and serum.

4. *Long-acting sulfonamides.* Sulfadoxine has a singularly long half-life, 7 to 9 days. This has made it an attractive choice for malaria prophylaxis in combination with pyrimethamine (Fansidar®) for the prevention and treatment of illness due to chloroquine-resistant strains of *Plasmodium falciparum.* It has no uses as an antibacterial agent.

MECHANISM OF ACTION. Sulfonamides are structural analogues of para-aminobenzoic acid (PABA). They exert a bacteriostatic effect by competitively inhibiting dihydropteroate synthetase. This enzyme catalyzes the synthesis of dihydropteroic acid, the immediate precursor of folic acid, from PABA. Folic acid is required for 1-carbon transfer reactions for purine synthesis. Most bacterial cells are impermeable to folic acid, in contrast to mammalian cells. These facts concerning the mechanism of action of sulfonamides on susceptible cells account for the selective toxicity of sulfonamides for bacterial but not mammalian cells, the mechanism of bacterial resistance to sulfonamides, inhibition of sulfonamide action in sites of tissue necrosis, and, as will be discussed later, synergistic inhibition of some bacteria by a combination with dihydrofolate reductase inhibitors such as TMP or pyrimethamine.

Because mammalian cells are permeable to folic acid, sulfonamides do not cause dose-related or concentration-related adverse effects on cellular metabolism in man. Side effects are predominantly idiosyncratic or allergic (vide infra).

MECHANISMS OF RESISTANCE. Acquired bacterial resistance to sulfonamides arises by random mutation and selection or by transfer of resistance by plasmids. Such resistance is a stable characteristic whose cumulative prevalence now precludes the use of sulfonamides as initial therapy for all but a few serious infections such as brucellosis, nocardiosis and infection caused by *B. catarrhalis.* Sulfonamide resistance may be mediated by an alteration in the affinity of dihydrofolate reductase for sulfonamide, utilization of alternative pathways for purine and pyrimidine synthesis, and compensatory overproduction of the natural substrate, PABA. Acquired resistance to silver sulfadiazine cream in burn units has been reported and necessitated use of alternative therapy such as silver nitrate and chlorhexidine cream.[64]

CLINICAL PHARMACOLOGY. Most orally administered sulfonamides are rapidly absorbed from the stomach and small intestine, but the efficiency of this process in acutely ill patients has not been described. Absorbed sulfonamides bind to serum proteins, particularly albumin, from 20 percent to over 90 percent and affect disposition. High protein binding of sulfadoxine (97 percent) accounts in part for its long disappearance $t_{1/2}$ from plasma. High protein binding of other sulfonamides administered to neonates can contribute to the development of kernicterus because of bilirubin displacement from albumin binding sites. The lipid-soluble sulfonamides diffuse readily into both inflamed and noninflamed tissues and body fluids including pleural, peritoneal, and ocular fluids and the CSF. They readily cross the placenta and enter the fetal circulation in sufficient concentration to exert both antibacterial and toxic effects.

A varying proportion of sulfonamide is acetylated in the liver or inactivated by other metabolic pathways. The rate of acetylation is genetically determined and slow acetylators are more likely to experience certain side effects than are rapid acetylators (vide infra). Unchanged non–protein-bound sulfonamides as well as metabolites are excreted mainly by glomerular filtration into urine. Different agents are reabsorbed to different degrees in the renal tubules. In the case of sulfadoxine, resorption is so extensive and efficient that this contributes to its long $t_{1/2}$ of 7 to 9 days.

The pH of the urine influences urinary excretion of sulfonamides because they are weak acids. Thus, their clearance is enhanced in the presence of alkaline urine. Generally, however, sufficient free drug reaches the urine to make them effective agents for therapy of urinary tract infections caused by susceptible organisms. In patients with significant renal insufficiency, too little sulfonamide reaches the urine to be effective. Doses must be reduced if they are used to treat nonrenal or nonurinary infection. In burned patients with renal failure, mafenide should be used with caution (vide infra).

ADVERSE DRUG REACTIONS. Overall, sulfonamides cause ADR in about 5% of recipients. The types and severity of ADR are quite varied. They are due largely to allergy and only occasionally to direct dose-related toxic effects.

The best understood dose-related toxic effects include renal colic, urethral pain, hematuria and obstruction due to crystalluria, and hemolysis in patients (and fetuses) with glucose-6-phosphate dehydrogenase deficient erythrocytes. Pseudocyanosis due to methemoglobinemia or sulfhemoglobinemia was seen with earlier sulfonamide formulations; it is rarely seen now. Mafenide causes a unique dose-related toxic effect. Mafenide and its metabolite inhibit carbonic anhydrase, which results in a metabolic acidosis usually compensated for by hyperventilation. In patients with significant renal dysfunction, high concentrations of mafenide and its metabolite will accumulate and exaggerate this effect.

The slow acetylator phenotype is associated with severe, delayed hypersensitivity reactions to sulfonamides.[65] These reactions occur much less commonly than typical exanthematous or urticarial rashes caused by sulfonamides, which resolve rapidly on discontinuation of therapy. They occur late in the course of sulfonamide therapy and are typically heralded by the onset of high fever followed by development of a skin rash such as erythema multiforme. Patients with the slow acetylator phenotype are postulated to have more parent sulfonamide available for oxidative metabolism to intermediates that have been shown to mediate those adverse reactions.[66] The slow acetylator phenotype is also associated with the common side effects of sulfasalazine therapy: nausea, vomiting, anorexia, and headache are related to serum sulfapyridine concentrations >20 mg/L,[62] which are more commonly observed in slow acetylators given the standard dose of sulfasalazine.

Sulfonamides may also cause ADR because of interactions with other drugs being administered concurrently. Sulfadiazine, sulfamethizole, and sulfaphenazole may impair hepatic metabolism of phenytoin and warfarin. Cotrimoxazole may cause an exaggerated hypoprothrombinemic effect in patients taking warfarin if their warfarin dose requirements are high and the plasma albumin level is low (vide infra).

Allergic and idiosyncratic reactions to sulfonamides are relatively common, may occasionally be severe, and rarely are fatal. Skin rashes are fairly frequent, usually occur after about a week's treatment, and may be maculopapular or urticarial. Erythema nodosum and erythema multiforme and, rarely, Stevens-Johnson syndrome may occur. The risk of developing Stevens-Johnson syndrome is increased by prior sulfonamide therapy (because of the risk of sensitization) and administration of long-acting sulfonamides. Cross-allergy between sulfonamides makes it unwise to administer another agent from this group. Moreover, cross-allergy with other non-antibacterial sulfonamide drugs may occur: diuretics (azetazolamide, thiazides, bumetanide, and furosemide), oral hypoglycemic agents, and antithyroid drugs (propylthiouracil). There is no skin test for sulfonamide allergy.

Idiosyncratic reactions include acute agranulocytosis. This rare reaction is usually due to oral sulfonamides and is reversible on cessation of administration. However, leukopenia is seen in as many as 3 to 5 percent of burned patients treated with silver sulfadiazine, usually within 2 to 4 days of initiation of therapy. It is usually self-limiting even with continued use of the drug. Fatal aplastic anemia has been described with sulfonamides, but less commonly than with chloramphenicol; megaloblastic anemia responsive to folic acid in patients with inflammatory bowel disease treated with sulfasalazine and thrombocytopenia have been reported.

Hepatotoxicity is a rare idiosyncratic hypersensitivity reaction to sulfasalazine administration. The toxic effect appears to be due to sulfapyridine, the major absorbed metabolite of sulfasalazine breakdown by colonic bacteria. That this reaction is due to hypersensitivity is suggested by additional features such as rash, lymphadenopathy, arthralgia, and eosinophilia with onset 2 to 4 weeks after initiation of therapy. Drug interactions involving sulfonamides may cause ADR because of interference of hepatic metabolism of the concomitantly administered drug by sulfonamide and displacement of drug from plasma protein by highly bound sulfonamides. For example, tolbutamide, phenytoin, and warfarin metabolism are inhibited by usual therapeutic doses of sulfaphenazole, sulfadiazine, and sulfamethizole. Sulfamethoxazole may displace warfarin from plasma albumin and predispose the patient to an exaggerated anticoagulant effect (interference with hepatic metabolism of warfarin is more important, however).

TRIMETHOPRIM COMBINED WITH SULFAMETHOXAZOLE

Trimethoprim (TMP) is marketed commercially alone and in combination with sulfamethoxazole (SMX) in oral and parenteral formulations in a fixed ratio of 1:5. Due to its greater lipid solubility, TMP distributes more rapidly and widely than the sulfonamide, yielding a plasma TMP:SMX ratio approximately 1:20 throughout the dose interval, the optimal ratio for in vitro synergistic antibacterial effects. This ratio is maintained relatively constant because the two agents have similar elimination $t_{1/2}$ of about 10 h in persons with normal renal function.

MECHANISM OF ACTION. TMP inhibits dihydrofolate reductase of bacteria about 50,000 times more efficiently than that of mammalian cells. It interferes with purine synthesis in the same pathway that sulfonamides act. The combination, therefore, produces synergistic inhibition of replication in certain bacteria.

Trimethoprim is more active than sulfonamide against many bacterial species except *Nocardia, Neisseria,* and *Brucella* species. The net inhibitory effect of the combination of TMP-SMX against bacteria is not consistently predictable. However, a synergistic effect is likely when a bacterium is sensitive to both agents. Moreover, when synergy is demonstrable in vitro, the net antibacterial effect may be bactericidal although the component agents alone are only bacteriostatic.

The clinical advantage of prescribing TMP-SMX together to achieve a synergistic therapeutic effect or to minimize the emergence of resistant isolates during therapy is debated. For example, in urinary tract infection, the activity of TMP greatly exceeds that of the SMX and the potential synergy expected is not observed.[67] Resistance to TMP is increased by TMP use, but its adminsitration together with SMX has not been shown to substantially reduce this occurence.[68]

Trimethoprim enhances the antibacterial activity of antibiotics other than sulfonamides. It enhances the inhibitory effect of rifampin against *H. influenzae* and *Brucella* species. In combination with carbenicillin and rifampicin, it is often synergistic against *P. maltophilia,* a frequently multiply resistant, nosocomial pathogen.[69] The potential utility of these combination therapies in critically ill patients with resistant infections should not be overlooked, but appropriate *in vitro* testing will be necessary to permit confident administration of these combinations.

MECHANISMS OF RESISTANCE. Resistance to TMP is most commonly associated with acquisition of a plasmid that codes for an altered dihydrofolate reductase enzyme. Some species have acquired resistance as a result of the selection of mutants that do not use the tetrahydrofolate pathway to synthesize thymidine. It is not uncommon for 30 to 40 percent of aerobic gram-negative enteric bacteria in hospitals to be TMP, and usually, also SMX, resistant.

CLINICAL PHARMACOLOGY. TMP is a lipid-soluble, weak base. Its AVD, 1.8 L/kg body weight, greatly exceeds that of SMX, 0.24 L/kg body weight. It diffuses freely into most tissues and body fluids and concentrates in prostatic and vaginal fluids, which are more acid than plasma. TMP is eliminated primarily by glomerular filtration as unchanged drug, with a small amount eliminated via the bile. Approximately 10 percent of drug in the urine is inactive metabolites formed in the liver. The elimination $t_{1/2}$ of TMP from plasma is approximately 10 h in patients with normal renal function, but increases with diminished renal function. In severe renal failure, the serum $t_{1/2}$ of SMX is increased slightly more than that of TMP, to a range of 22 to 50 and 14 to 46 h, respectively. This is attributable to the more efficient clearance of TMP than SMX by nonrenal mechanisms.

The usual adult dose for those with normal renal function is 160 to 240 mg TMP and 800 to 1200 mg SMX infused intravenously every 6, 8, or 12 h, depending on the severity of the infection. The dose should be diluted to minimize phlebitis: each 5-mL ampule (TMP 80 and SMX 400 mg) should be diluted in a minimum of 75 mL of D5W, 0.15 *M* NaCl, or Ringer's solution. Extravasation causes local irritation and inflammation. In patients with renal dysfunction, a modified dose is advised: for patients with creatinine clearance >25 mL/min, no reduction in the standard dose; for those with creatinine clearance 15 to 24 mL/min, give one-half the usual dose; below 15 mL/min, use is not recommended.

No published data relate TMP-SMX therapeutic antibacterial effects to Cp, but for *P. carinii* infection, doses should be adjusted to achieve TMP concentrations 1.5 to 2 h after administration of 3 to 10 mg/L (or SMX concentrations of 100 to 150 mg/L).[70] These concentrations are usually achieved with oral or intravenous doses of TMP and SMX of 20 and 100 mg/kg/day in three to four divided doses, respectively, using the fixed dose formulation of TMP with SMX. However, in one study the TMP dose had to be reduced from 15 to 12 mg/kg/day during therapy to maintain these concentrations.[71]

ADVERSE DRUG REACTIONS. In many cases, it is difficult to separate side effects caused by the components of TMP-SMX. TMP causes fewer reactions than the combination, but it is not known whether the combination causes a "synergistic" increase in adverse effects.

Although interference with folic acid metabolism and hence, erythropoiesis, can be demonstrated with high TMP concentrations in normal human bone marrow cells cultured in vitro, concentrations observed during therapy in man do not attain these levels, nor produce such impairment, and this is corroborated by clinical experience. However, in individuals with preexisting megaloblastic anemia, TMP can aggravate neutropenia and thrombocytopenia and interfere with the therapeutic response to either vitamin B_{12} or folic acid. The drug is, therefore, relatively contraindicated in patients with megaloblastic anemia or in those who may be predisposed to this—pregnant women, patients on anticonvulsant drugs (phenytoin, primidone, or barbiturates) and those with macrocytic erythrocytes. For these individuals, regular blood cell counts are advised if prolonged therapy is prescribed.

Combination TMP-SMX may cause an apparent dose-related impairment of renal function in renal transplant patients or individuals with preexisting renal insufficiency, especially if inappropriately high doses of TMP-SMX are used. TMP-SMX should be prescribed cautiously to such patients. It should be noted, however, that TMP-SMX administration may cause a temporary rise in serum creatinine concentration not due to a reduction in glomerular filtration rate. This has been attributed to TMP competitive inhibition of creatinine secretion by the renal tubular cation transport system.

Gastrointestinal reactions are the most common side effects of oral TMP-SMX therapy: 3 percent of recipients experience nausea, vomiting, and anorexia and approximately 0.5 percent, diarrhea. *C. difficile* toxin-induced diarrhea and pseudomembranous colitis have both been reported in patients treated with these agents.

Skin rashes occur in 1.6 to 8 percent of patients treated with TMP-SMX. Most of these are probably caused by the sulfonamide, but TMP occasionally causes rashes when administered alone. The rashes usually present as morbilliform eruptions, less frequently as urticarial or vasculitic processes.

QUINOLONES

The quinolone antibiotics fall into two relatively distinct generations of drugs. The first generation quinolones, nalidixic acid, oxolinic acid, and cinoxacin, achieve effective concentrations only in urine, limiting their usefulness to the oral therapy of uncomplicated urinary tract infection. The second generation quinolones, norfloxacin, ciprofloxacin, pefloxacin, ofloxacin, enoxacin, and fleroxacin, are 4-fluorinated analogues of nalidixic acid with potent, broad-spectrum antibacterial activity and potential utility for the therapy of a wide range of visceral infections. Additional differences include a greater propensity for resistance to emerge during therapy with agents of the nalidixic acid-cinoxacin-oxolinic acid group than the second generation agents. This discussion is limited primarily to two fluorinated quinolones, norfloxacin and ciprofloxacin, which are the only currently available agents of this group.

MECHANISM OF ACTION. The fluorinated quinolones exert a bactericidal effect by interfering with the enzyme DNA gyrase. Human cells do not contain DNA gyrase but do contain an enzyme, topoisomerase, that subserves the same function, namely, to enzymatically cut segments of replicating DNA strands to prevent tangling. DNA gyrase is inhibited by concentrations of 5 to 10 mg/L, which can be achieved during therapy; topoisomerase inhibition requires concentrations 10 to 20 times greater.

The fluorinated quinolones are particularly noteworthy for their antibacterial effect against aerobic gram-negative bacilli. Ciprofloxacin, and to a lesser degree, norfloxacin, inhibits most strains of *P. aeruginosa,* including strains resistant to aminoglycosides. *P. cepacia* and *P. maltophilia* are not uniformly susceptible. Ciprofloxacin is generally more potent than norfloxacin against most bacterial species. In this regard, the second generation fluoroquinolones provide the intensivist with a third group of drugs, after the aminoglycosides and third generation cephalosporins, with predictable, potent inhibitory effects against a wide range of community- and hospital-acquired enteric bacillary pathogens. *H. influenzae* and *N. gonorrhoeae,* including β-lactamase-producing strains, are extremely sensitive to ciprofloxacin and norfloxacin. On the other hand, their effect against gram-positive aerobic organisms such as pneumococci, streptococci, and staphylococci is less striking, and many important anaerobic bacterial pathogens are resistant. Intracellular bacteria inhibited by concentrations achieved during therapy include *Chlamydia, Legionella, Brucella,* mycoplasma, and certain mycobacteria, but clinical experience in the treatment of infections caused by these agents is too limited to support their use except in unusual circumstances.

MECHANISMS OF RESISTANCE. Resistance, particularly of *P. aeruginosa* emerges during therapy with ciprofloxacin. Such strains are usually completely cross-resistant to other quinolones. Mutation in the gene that encodes the DNA gyrase accounts in part for resistance. Increasing resistance of *S. aureus* to both quinolones and methicillin has been reported since the introduction of ciprofloxacin.[72]

CLINICAL PHARMACOLOGY. From 70 to 80 percent of ciprofloxacin and 30 to 40 percent of norfloxacin oral doses are absorbed. The drugs are distributed widely into normal tissues and inflammatory exudates as evidenced by an average AVD of 1.8 and 3.2 L/kg body weight, respectively. Both agents are primarily eliminated into urine by glomerular filtration and probenecid-sensitive tubular secretion. Mean elimination $t_{1/2}$ is 5 and 4 h, respectively, in healthy adults. As expected, the plasma $t_{1/2}$ increases with reductions in renal function. Hepatic biotransformation with urinary excretion of metabolites account for 15 percent of ciprofloxacin elimination, but <5 percent of norfloxacin elimination. Biliary excretion accounts for inconsequential amounts of norfloxacin elimination but somewhat more ciprofloxacin clearance. About 30 percent of doses of both agents administered orally appears in feces as unchanged, presumably unabsorbed, drug.

The quinolones and fluoroquinolones attain therapeutically active concentrations in the urine in patients with moderately severe renal failure. However, nalidixic acid should not be prescribed to patients with renal failure because full doses are required to be effective and these are associated with accumulation of inactive metabolites that may contribute to toxicity. Norfloxacin and ciprofloxacin doses should be halved in patients on dialysis, but supplemental doses are not required after hemodialysis or peritoneal dialysis, because neither drug is substantially removed by these treatments. In the elderly, elimination of both drugs is similar to that observed in young adults so that dose reduction is not required. Antacids containing magnesium or aluminum interfere with ciprofloxacin absorption so their concurrent administration should be avoided. Whether a similar interaction occurs with norfloxacin and antacid is not established.

Ciprofloxacin should be administered intravenously to any seriously ill patient. About 60 percent of an intravenous dose is recovered in urine as unchanged drug during the first 12 h, a figure that exceeds substantially the 30 to 45 percent level observed after oral dosing. The recommended adult dose for patients with urinary tract infection of mild to moderate severity is 200 mg every 12 h. For severe or complicated urinary tract infection, 400 mg every 12 h is recommended. The recommended dose for adult patients with soft tissue or bone or joint infection is 400 mg every 12 h. For patients with impaired renal function, ciprofloxacin doses should be reduced. For those with creatinine clearance of 30 mL/min or greater, no dose reduction is recommended. For those with creatinine clearance 5 to 29 mL/min, 200 to 400 mg every 18 to 24 h is recommended. Appropriate doses for patients with significant hepatic disease have not yet been proposed and validated.

ADVERSE DRUG EFFECTS. Quinolones and fluorinated quinolones are generally well tolerated. Gastrointestinal symptoms including nausea, anorexia, vomiting, and diarrhea occur in <5 percent of patients. Both first and second generation quinolones on the market cause neurologic symptoms whose pathogenesis is unclear. Dizziness and headache are the most common, being reported in 2 percent of patients. Giddiness, excitation or depression, visual disturbances, lethargy, agitation, somnolence, syncope, and, rarely, convulsions and acute psychosis have been reported with the first generation quinolones and norfloxacin but not ciprofloxacin. These effects may be more common in patients given higher doses in the presence of renal dysfunction. Some quinolones interfere with the inhibitory neurotransmitter γ-aminobutyric acid but no clear relationship exists between this characteristic of the quinolones and their propensity to cause neurotoxic symptoms. Nevertheless, the quinolones should be used with caution in patients with CNS disease or renal impairment.

Hypersensitivity reactions are uncommon, but urticarial rash with eosinophilia has been reported in patients treated with first generation quinolones. Of ciprofloxacin-treated patients, 1 percent develop such rashes; with norfloxacin, the frequency is probably half that of ciprofloxacin.

Rare side effects observed with nalidixic acid that intensivists should note because it is not clear whether they may occur with second generation quinolones include intracranial hypertension, lactic acidosis, and hemolytic anemia.

Drug interactions include enhancement of warfarin activity because of displacement from albumin by nalidixic acid, elevated plasma theophylline concentrations caused by impairment of metabolism by ciprofloxacin, and increased risk of CNS toxic effects in patients given nonsteroidal, anti-inflammatory drugs and ciprofloxacin concurrently.

METRONIDAZOLE

Metronidazole is one of a group of 5-nitroimidazoles including tinidazole, nimorazole, carnidazole, and secnidazole, which possess a broad spectrum of antiprotozoal and antibacterial activity. Other than metronidazole, these are only available outside North America. The following comments pertain to metronidazole only and its antibacterial action.

The clinically important antibacterial activity of metronidazole is restricted to obligate anaerobic bacteria. In vitro, metronidazole is a potent bactericidal antimicrobial against anaerobic gram-negative and gram-positive organisms. Resistant anaerobic organisms include *Proprionobacterium species*, many strains of *Bifidobacterium*, *Actinomyces* and *Arachnia*. *Lactobacillus species* and aerobic and microaerophilic streptococci are also resistant.

Administered alone, it is the drug of choice for the therapy of *C. difficile* toxin-associated diarrhea and colitis.[54] For this purpose, it is best administered orally. Administered together with penicillin, metronidazole is the drug of choice for the treatment of brain abscess originating from paranasal sinusitis, which is caused primarily by nonaerobic streptococci, particularly *Streptococcus milleri*, together with β-lactamase producing *Bacteroides species*, which are resistant to penicillin. It is used similarly as one component in the combined antibacterial therapy of temporal lobe brain abscesses of otitic origin from which anaerobic bacteria, particularly *B. fragilis* and aerobic enteric bacilli, are frequently isolated. Favorable results of controlled trials attest to the efficacy of metronidazole combined with an aminoglycoside antibiotic drug for therapy of mixed aerobic-anaerobic infections of the peritoneal cavity and female genital tract. In general, this combination is not different in efficacy from clindamycin, ticarcillin, cefoxitin, or chloramphenicol combined with the aminoglycoside.[73] Advantages arise from differences in the frequency, nature, and severity of adverse effects.

MECHANISM OF ACTION. The mechanism of action of the antibacterial effect of metronidazole has not been fully elucidated. It has been demonstrated that metronidazole is rapidly bactericidal by an immediate inhibition of DNA synthesis. What is unclear is the identity of the metronidazole metabolite(s) that mediate(s) this effect; unchanged metronidazole does not interact with the DNA. It is hypothesized that the drug diffuses into bacterial cells where the nitro group is reduced to an unstable, and as yet, unidentified, reactive intermediate by bacterial nitroreductases.

MECHANISM OF RESISTANCE. Acquired resistance to metronidazole occurs extremely rarely. Isolated reports have documented resistance to metronidazole associated with clinical failure in *B. fragilis* strains. Resistance appeared to be related to a reduced rate of metronidazole uptake and reduction, possibly due to decreased nitroreductase activity.

CLINICAL PHARMACOLOGY. The clinical pharmacology of metronidazole and its two principal metabolites has been studied extensively. It can be administered intravenously, orally, and rectally as a suppository to treat bacterial infection. The absolute bioavailability of orally administered metronidazole approaches 100 percent although the speed of absorption, reflected in the time to peak plasma metronidazole concentrations, varies between individuals. After intravenous administration of 500 mg over 20 min to ill adult patients, the mean metronidazole serum concentration 30 min after the completion of infusion was 27 mg/L and the trough concentration, 16 mg/L.[74] After rectal administration of a 500-mg suppository, mean peak serum concentration after about 3 h was 19 mg/L with the level remaining above 10 mg/L over the next 8 h.[75] These data suggest excellent systemic availability of metronidazole administered rectally and support this route of administration for treatment of infections in those with postoperative ileus. In plasma, <15 percent is bound to plasma proteins. The drug diffuses widely throughout the body: concentrations in saliva and breast milk are comparable to those in the serum; CSF concentrations in normal volunteers average 43 percent of the simultaneous Cp and are therapeutic; urine concentrations range from 76 to 115 mg/L after a 0.5-g dose. The AVD averages 0.74 L/kg body weight. Only about 14 percent of an orally administered dose of metronidazole is excreted in the feces, but concentrations in feces are attained that are much greater than the MIC of metronidazole for *C. difficile,* which is 4 mg/L or less.

Metronidazole undergoes extensive metabolism, probably in the liver, to two oxidation products—an "alcohol" and a "hydroxy" metabolite.[76] The latter is produced in larger amounts, can be readily detected in the plasma of patients with normal renal function, and accumulates in the plasma of those with renal insufficiency. The metabolites possess 5 and 30 percent, respectively, of the antibacterial activity of the parent compound so that they probably contribute in part to the therapeutic effect of metronidazole, particularly in patients with renal failure. Of 500 mg metronidazole administered intravenously to healthy volunteers, 44 percent was recovered in the urine, consisting of parent drug (8 percent), the hydroxy (24 percent), and alcohol (12 percent) metabolites. The mean plasma $t_{1/2}$ of metronidazole is 8.5 h.

In patients with renal insufficiency, metabolites accumulate but the parent compound does not. It is conventional not to reduce the dose of metronidazole for such patients, including those undergoing peritoneal dialysis or hemodialysis. Severe hepatic disease would be expected to reduce the metabolism of metronidazole, but its disposition in such patients and the need for dose reduction has not been described.

Interactions of metronidazole have been described in adults with phenytoin and barbiturates which induce its metabolism. Phenobarbital decreased the plasma $t_{1/2}$ of metronidazole to 3.5 h.

ADVERSE DRUG EFFECTS. In experimental nonhuman systems, metronidazole is teratogenic, mutagenic, and carcinogenic. Comparable effects have not been demonstrated in man, but it is considered prudent to avoid its use during the period of organogenesis in the first trimester of pregnancy. Metronidazole is generally well tolerated. Gastrointestinal side effects occur occasionally. These include a metallic taste, furred tongue, and nausea. Paradoxically, pseudomembranous colitis has been described in patients receiving only metronidazole, although only two confirmed reports exist. In one, this side effect appeared to be caused by a metronidazole-resistant strain of *C. difficile*[77] but in one, the organism was susceptible. Transient reversible leukopenia occurs uncommonly, but it is the most common hematologic side effect. Peripheral neuropathy manifesting as sensory impairment has been described in a number of patients receiving high doses of metronidazole for prolonged periods of time. The cause is not known. One child developed seizures during metronidazole therapy that ultimately resolved completely.

Interactions of metronidazole with a few other drugs are well documented; it can produce an antabuse-like reaction after alcohol ingestion. This is probably due to inhibition of hepatic alcohol metabolism resulting in accumulation of acetaldehyde, which causes the adverse symptoms. Metronidazole augments the hypoprothrombinemic effect of coumadin due to a stereoselective inhibition of the S(−)-moiety (levowarfarin).

ERYTHROMYCIN, CLINDAMYCIN AND LINCOMYCIN

Erythromycin and the lincosamide antibiotics, clindamycin and lincomycin, are considered together because they share similar mechanisms of action and resistance, antibacterial activity, and clinical pharmacologic properties.

ERYTHROMYCIN

Erythromycin is produced by *Streptomyces erythreus.* It is the most important of the macrolide group of antibacterial compounds, which also includes spiramycin (used in Europe to treat *T. gondii* infection), and clarithromycin (a potent inhibitor of *Mycobacterium avium-intracellulare* complex of potential value in AIDS patients[78]), among other experimental agents. The following pertains only to erythromycin.

Erythromycin base is poorly soluble in water, has a pKa of 8.8, and is rapidly inactivated by gastric acid. Many alternative oral formulations have therefore been developed to enhance oral bioavailability over that of the base. Two water-soluble salts, erythromycin-gluceptate and erythromycin-lactobionate, have been developed for intravenous administration. In ICU patients, only the intravenous formulation can ensure adequate systemic delivery of drug, so this discussion does not include the characteristics of the oral products.

In vitro, erythromycin has a broad spectrum of antimicrobial activity that includes bacteria (including chlamydia), mycoplasma, spirochetes *(Treponema pallidum),* ureaplasmas, and some strains of rickettsias. Its useful antibacterial activity includes gram-positive organisms *(S. aureus, S. pyogenes, S. pneumoniae,* and viridans group streptococci, *Corynebacterium diphtheriae, Clostridium perfringens, Listeria monocytogenes),* some gram-negative organisms *(B. pertussis, H. influenzae, N. gonorrhoeae, N. meningitidis,* and *B. catarrhalis), Legionella pneumophila, Mucoplasma pneumoniae, Ureaplasma urealyticum* and *C. trachomatis.*

Clinically, erythromycin is the drug of choice for *M. pneumoniae* and *L. pneumophila* infection. It is the alternative drug of choice for *C. trachomatis* infection of pregnant women and children who cannot be treated with tetracycline and for *C. diphtheriae* infection in penicillin-allergic patients. Although formerly used as the alternative to penicillin in allergic patients with *T. pallidum, B. catarrhalis* and *L. monocytogenes* infection, its use in these infections has been largely superceded by other agents.

MECHANISM OF ACTION. Erythromycin and the other macrolide antibiotics inhibit bacterial growth by interfering with protein synthesis on ribosomes. The erythromycin receptor is a 23S tRNA on the 50S subunit. Erythromycin binding blocks the aminoacyl translocation reaction essential for formation of initiation complexes and elongation of the peptide chain.

In vitro, in low concentration, erythromycin is bacteriostatic; at high concentrations, especially against rapidly dividing cells, a bactericidal effect is observed. However, in patients with endocarditis in whom only bactericidal agents are curative, erythromycin used alone has either failed or been associated with apparent clinical cure but subsequent relapse. Accordingly, in man, erythromycin is likely only bacteriostatic.

MECHANISM OF RESISTANCE. Gram-negative enteric bacilli are uniformly resistant to erythromycin. This is probably due to inability of the drug to penetrate the cell wall to reach the ribosomal site of action, since L-forms of species such as *P. mirabilis,* which have no cell wall, are highly susceptible. In certain other resistant bacteria, a mutational change in the 50S subunit, methylation of the tRNA erythromycin receptor, precludes erythromycin binding. This has been observed in formerly susceptible species such as *Legionella* and appears to be plasmid-mediated. Two other plasmid-mediated mechanisms confer erythromycin resistance on bacteria: diminished permeability of the cell envelope of gram-positive bacteria as occurs with *S. epidermidis* and production of an esterase that hydrolyzes erythromycin observed in some Enterobacteriaceae.

Overall, however, development of erythromycin resistance has neither increased rapidly nor necessitated major changes in the way clinicians use this agent.

CLINICAL PHARMACOLOGY. After intravenous injection, erythromycin has an ADV equal to 0.78 L/kg body weight. Therapeutic concentrations are attained in all sites except the brain and subarachnoid space. Although inflammation enhances erythromycin penetration into brain tissue and CSF, this effect is unpredictable, and erythromycin is thus relatively contraindicated for therapy of brain abscess and meningitis. Protein binding averages 85 percent. Disappearance from plasma is first order with $t_{1/2}$ 1.6 h. Approximately 15 percent of an injected dose appears as unchanged drug in the urine; high concentrations of drug are observed in bile, but the overall contribution of this route of drug clearance to erythromycin elimination is not known. A large proportion of injected erythromycin cannot be accounted for by drug in urine or bile so that extensive biotransformation, probably in the liver, is hypothesized.

The normal plasma $t_{1/2}$ of 1.6 h is only prolonged to 4.8 to 5.8 h in anuric patients. Nevertheless, no dose reduction in such patients is necessary in view of the low risk of any dose-related ADR. In patients with alcoholic liver disease and ascites, plasma $t_{1/2}$ was increased to an average of 1.6 h compared to 1.3 h in concurrently studied healthy controls.[79] Therefore, in such patients, even though this difference in plasma $t_{1/2}$ is statistically significant, it is not likely to be biologically important. Dose reduction is not necessary. In those with more severe liver disease, however, dose reduction would appear prudent, with dose adjustments based on serum concentration monitoring: Cp values of approximately 5 to 10 mg/L are achieved after intravenous injection of 500 to 1000 mg erythromycin in normal individuals and these would seem to be reasonable concentrations to emulate with reduced doses in patients with severe liver disease.

ADVERSE DRUG EFFECTS. Erythromycin is one of the safest antibacterial agents in clinical use, but tolerance is limited by the frequent occurrence of irritative side effects. Firstly, abdominal cramps, dyspepsia, nausea, vomiting, and diarrhea occur, which probably are due, in part, to a direct smooth muscle-stimulating effect of erythromycin.[80] They are observed in patients being treated with drug administered intravenously as well as orally. Although the smooth muscle-stimulating effect can be inhibited in vitro by the antimuscarinic agent atropine, this strategy has not been studied in man. Secondly, the drug predictably causes phlebitis, which can only be partly ameliorated by slow infusion of drug diluted in large volumes of intravenous fluid.

Tinnitus and reversible severe deafness have been described in patients given large intravenous doses of erythromycin.[81] Old age, renal failure, and hepatic insufficiency appear to predispose to this unusual adverse effect. The mechanism of this reaction is not known. Pseudomembranous colitis has been reported in patients treated with erythromycin. Hypersensitivity reactions such as skin rash, fever and eosinophilia are rare.

Cholestatic jaundice caused by erythromycin estolate (and rarely by the stearate) appears to be specifically related to the propionyl ester linkage of the 2′ position so that cross-sensitivity is said not to occur.[82] Thus, a history of cholestatic jaundice during therapy with oral erythromycin estolate is not an absolute contraindication to intravenous therapy with erythromycin gluceptate or lactobionate.

In some individuals, erythromycin can inhibit elimination of methylprednisolone, theophylline, carbamazepine, warfarin, and cyclosporine with significant clinical consequences. The need for vigilance during concurrent therapy with erythromycin and one of these drugs is self-evident; the unpredictability of the interaction necessitates extra attention.

CLINDAMYCIN AND LINCOMYCIN

Lincomycin was isolated from a strain of *Streptomyces lincolnensis* and marketed only for oral administration. A search for better agents by chemical modification of lincomycin led to the development of clindamycin. Clindamycin is available for oral administration as the hydrochloride salt, as well as intravenous injection as the phosphate ester. It is superior in activity to lincomycin and this additional characteristic has led to the exclusive use of clindamycin in critically ill patients. Accordingly, only clindamycin will be reviewed here.

In vitro, the antibacterial spectrum of clindamycin is similar to that of erythromycin with some differences of clinical importance as follows: resistance of *S. aureus* to clindamycin is less common (4 percent) than to erythromycin (9 percent). Clindamycin is inactive against *H. influenzae* and *N. meningitidis* in concentrations attainable in patients. It is much more potent than erythromycin against species of the *B. fragilis* group. However, from 5 percent of *B. fragilis* strains up to 15 percent of *Bacteroides vulgatus* strains are relatively resistant to clindamycin. Nevertheless, this degree of activity against enteric gram-negative anaerobic bacilli is exceeded only by metronidazole. *C. difficile* strains are resistant but other species such as *Clostridium welchii* and *Clostridium tetani* are sensitive. *M. pneumoniae* is resistant.

Clindamycin is arguably the antibiotic of first choice in combination with an aminoglycoside[73] for the therapy of serious mixed aerobic-anaerobic enteric bacterial infection of the abdomen and pelvis (some data demonstrate superiority of imipenem-cilastatin for such infections,[27] but total experience is still limited with this new carbapenem). In similar infections of the soft tissues and skin of the feet of diabetic patients, this combination is also highly efficacious. Clindamycin alone is superior to penicillin as a single agent for treatment of serious anaerobic lung infection,[83] but their combined use for treatment of such infections is now recommended. It is also considered to be as effective as penicillins for the therapy of nonendocarditis infections caused by *S. aureus, S. pyogenes,* and *S. pneumoniae,* and as effective as a single injection of benzathine penicillin in eradicating *C. diphtheriae* from the nasopharynx of asymptomatic arriers. It is an acceptable alternative to penicillin for treatment of cervicofacial actinomycosis. Incidentally, clindamycin and quinine sulfate are extremely effective for treatment of *Falciparum malaria* infection.

Absolute indications for clindamycin do not exist for use as a single drug or in combination with another agent. However, it is a valuable alternative to penicillin in patients who are allergic to the β-lactam agents and is a first-line agent, when combined with an aminoglycoside, for intra-abdominal and pelvic infection and, with penicillin, for anaerobic-aerobic lung infection.

MECHANISM OF ACTION. The mechanism of action of clindamycin is identical to that of erythromycin and both are bacteriostatic in the clinical setting. The clindamycin receptor in bacteria is either identical to the 23S ribosomal RNA target of erythromycin, or overlaps with it, because they interfere with each other in in vitro culture systems.

MECHANISM OF RESISTANCE. Clindamycin resistance in *S. aureus, S. pyogenes,* and *S. pneumoniae* strains is uncommon but can emerge during therapy. Among *S. aureus,* the probability of clindamycin resistance emerging during therapy is greater in those strains that are erythromycin resistant. Resistance is due to modification of the intracellular target of clindamycin. Some authorities state that clindamycin is relatively contraindicated for treatment of infection due to such erythromycin-resistant *S. aureus* strains. Clindamycin-resistant *S. aureus* strains are usually resistant to erythromycin.

Clindamycin resistance in *B. fragilis* group organisms is due to at least two different mechanisms, one of which is plasmid mediated.

CLINICAL PHARMACOLOGY. After intravenous injection, clindamycin distribution is analagous to that of erythromycin. It does not predicably attain therapeutic concentrations in the fluids of the eye, the cavity or wall of brain abscess, or the CSF even in patients with meningitis. High concentrations are demonstrable in bone, but the relevance of this observation to treatment of osteomyelitis is not clear. High concentrations are attained in polymorphonuclear leukocytes, which may contribute to enhanced killing of phagocytosed bacteria. Plasma protein binding is 60 percent.

The elimination of clindamycin is incompletely understood but probably similar to that of lincomycin, which has been more extensively documented. After intravenous injection, approximately 30 percent appears in urine and 5 to 15 percent in feces as unchanged drug and metabolites (n-demethyl clindamycin, clindamycin sulfoxide, and others). The remainder is considered to be metabolized to inactive compounds. The mean plasma $t_{1/2}$ is normally 3 h. Severe renal failure is associated with a doubling of peak Cp and on this basis, halving of the usual dose is recommended. Neither hemodialysis nor peritoneal dialysis enhances its clearance from plasma. The effect of liver disease on clindamycin clinical pharmacokinetics is not clear. Increases in plasma $t_{1/2}$ from 40 to 500 percent have been described. Extrapolating from data indicating the importance of presumed hepatic inactivation and biliary secretion in the elimination of clindamycin, it would seem reasonable to reduce clindamycin doses in patients with severe liver disease. If attempts are made to simulate Cp seen in patients without liver disease, it should be noted that maximum serum concentrations after 300 and 600 mg clindamycin range from 3 to 26 and 6 to 30 mg/L, respectively.

ADVERSE DRUG EFFECTS. Intravenous clindamycin commonly causes local phlebitis, which can be reduced by slow infusion of dilute solutions. The manufacturer recommends dilution to a concentration of 12 mg/L or less and infusion over not <10 min (preferably more than 25 min). The usual dose for adults with moderate to severe infection is 900 to 2400 mg/day in two or three divided equal intravenous doses.

The most important adverse effect of clindamycin administration is diarrhea. This occurs in 2 to 20 percent of treated patients and varies in severity. Clindamycin is the most likely of all antibiotics to cause diarrhea, although other drugs such as ampicillin also are frequently associated with this adverse effect. The precise pathogenesis of diarrheal illness associated with clindamycin is not known. However, in that subgroup of patients in whom diarrhea, and, in florid cases, pseudomembranous colitis, is associated with production of enterotoxin by *C. difficile* in the colon, a direct toxic effect on the colonic mucosa is responsible. *C. difficile* toxin-associated diarrhea has been described in patients receiving clindamycin only by the intravenous route so that a direct local effect of unabsorbed, orally administered drug is not essential to its occurrence. Continuation of clindamycin will intensify the severity of the colitis. However, where clindamycin cannot be discontinued, concomitant oral administration of metronidazole or vancomycin permits safe continuation of the clindamycin.

Hypersensitivity reactions caused by clindamycin occur occasionally. Rash may occur and in one study was observed in 10 percent of treated patients. Drug fever and eosinophilia as described with erythromycin has also been reported during clindamycin therapy.

It is worth reiterating that no cross-allergenicity exists between clindamycin and penicillin.

Unlike erythromycin, clindamycin does not cause clinically important interactions with other drugs.

Antiviral Drugs

Virus infections may cause acute organ failure that necessitates admisssion of adult patients to the ICU or may complicate their management. Occasionally, nosocomial viral infections occur in ICU patients that may be amenable to, and require, specific therapy. Drugs that specifically and selectively inhibit virus replication now have an established role in the management of a small but important and increasing number of serious, acute infections caused by DNA and RNA viruses in both immunocompetent and immunocompromised hosts. Currently available agents include vidarabine, acyclovir, amantadine, ribavirin, zidovudine, and ganciclovir.

All these agents are virustatic only, which partly explains their limited value or failure in patients with defective immune responses.

VIDARABINE

Vidarabine (ara-A) was the first antiviral drug administered parenterally to man whose efficacy was demonstrated unequivocally in a controlled trial (in patients with herpes simplex encephalitis).

In vitro, ara-A inhibits replication of a wide range of DNA viruses [herpes simplex type 1 (HSV-1) and 2 (HSV-2), varicellazoster (VZV), EBV, CMV, adenoviruses, vaccinia, hepatitis B (HBV)] and a single RNA virus, Rous sarcoma. Ara-A inhibits in vitro replication of acyclovir-resistant strains of HSV and VZV. Although ara-A is therapeutic in animals with experimental infections caused by a number of these viruses, in patients it has only been shown to be of value against HSV-1, HSV-2, and VZV infection. Data, however, suggest that ara-A may ameliorate CMV and chronic HBV infections. Its value in treating HSV and VZV infections in patients who have failed to respond to acyclovir due to acyclovir resistance is not yet established.

Ara-A is approved for the treatment of HSV-1 encephalitis. Controlled trials have demonstrated that it is efficacious for the therapy of otherwise healthy neonates with HSV infection (mostly HSV-2) and immunocompromised patients with chickenpox, as well as localized herpes zoster of <72 h duration. It hastens resolution of local pain and discomfort in immunocompromised patients with mucocutaneous HSV infection. Ara-A produces variable results when administered to patients with chronic hepatitis associated with HBV. Reductions in plasma HBV-DNA polymerase and plasma concentrations of HBsAg and HBeAg were observed in some patients.

Ara-A has been used to treat neonates with congenital CMV infections (transient suppression of viruria during therapy was observed) and bone marrow transplant recipients with CMV pneumonitis (no benefit and neurotoxicity in 29 percent of recipients).

MECHANISM OF ACTION. Ara-A is an analogue of adenine deoxyribonucleoside. After administration to man, it is rapidly converted to arabinosyl-hypoxanthine (ara-Hx),[84] whose antiviral activity is significantly less than that of the parent compound (e.g., it is 30 times less potent against HSV). The catalytic enzyme mediating conversion of ara-A to ara-Hx, adenine deaminase, is primarily found in erythrocytes. Ara-A and ara-Hx may act synergistically.[85]

Ara-A selectively inhibits viral DNA synthesis. Its triphosphate metabolite inhibits viral DNA polymerase, ribonucleotide reductase, and DNA chain elongation after incorporation into viral DNA in different experimental systems. The precise mechanism of action in man and relative contribution of ara-Hx to both the therapeutic and toxic effects are unknown. However, it is likely that ara-Hx accounts for most of the antiviral activity. This is supported by the observation that inhibitors of adenine deaminase can markedly enhance the antiviral activity of ara-A in vitro.

MECHANISM OF RESISTANCE. Resistance to ara-A develops in HSV passaged in vitro in the presence of increasing concentrations of ara-A. Although failure of ara-A therapy in immunocompromised hosts infected with HSV has been observed, it is not clear that emergence of resistance to ara-A or ara-Hx is responsible for the inefficacy.

Resistance of other viruses to ara-A, either natural or acquired during therapy, has not been described.

CLINICAL PHARMACOLOGY. Ara-A is relatively insoluble in water, 0.45 mg being the maximum amount that can be dissolved in 1 mL. As a result, unpredictable absorption, pain, and muscle necrosis occur after intramuscular or subcutaneous injection and it cannot be administered by these routes. Crystallization occurs even in solutions containing submaximal concentrations of ara-A, necessitating intravenous infusion through a micropore (0.45 μm) in-line filter.

Ara-A is administered in a dose of 15 mg/kg/day infused over 12 h. During intravenous infusion, ara-A is rapidly converted to ara-Hx, which has a plasma $t_{1/2}$ of 3.5 h in adults with normal renal function. The primary route of elimination of ara-Hx is renal, with 40 to 53 percent of the total daily dose recovered in urine as ara-Hx and 1 to 3 percent as ara-A. The fate of the remainder of the drug remains unknown. Limited data from studies in patients with impaired renal function suggest that ara-Hx accumulates[84] and may account for the exaggerated neurotoxic adverse effects observed in such patients (vide infra).

For patients with severe renal insufficiency, a dose reduction of 25 percent has been suggested, but neither the efficacy nor safety of this reduced dose has been rigorously tested. Ara-Hx is readily removed from plasma by hemodialysis (50 percent over 6 h) so that one-half the usual daily dose of ara-A should be administered after dialysis.

ADVERSE DRUG REACTIONS. In animals, ara-A is teratogenic and may be oncogenic so that it is relatively contraindicated in pregnant patients. In man, ara-A produces significant side effects whose frequency appears related to higher Cp of ara-A or ara-Hx as a result of higher doses (>15 mg/kg/day),[86] renal insufficiency,[87] hepatic insufficiency (chronic HBV), or an interaction during concomitant administration of interferon (in patients with chronic HBV[88]). Mild to moderately severe anorexia, nausea, vomiting, and diarrhea occur in 15 percent of patients but do not usually necessitate discontinuation of treatment. Reversible myelosuppression with anemia, granulocytopenia, and thrombocytopenia has been described. Neurotoxicity evidenced by tremors, myoclonus, dizziness, confusion, psychosis, ataxia, aphasia, dysarthria, neuralgia, seizures, and coma can occur. Death has occurred in five patients but the contribution of underlying diseases has been difficult to determine.

Allopurinol and ara-A administered concomitantly to patients with normal renal function were associated with tremors and impaired cognition that were attributed to allopurinol-induced inhibition of xanthine oxidase with resultant accumulation of ara-Hx.

Finally, water intoxication associated with the administration of large volumes of intravenous fluids needed to deliver ara-A has been a particular concern in patients with HSV encephalitis.

Most of these untoward effects of ara-A therapy are not observed during acyclovir therapy, which has largely replaced this agent for herpesvirus infections.

ACYCLOVIR

Acyclovir is a synthetic, acyclic, purine nucleoside analogue of guanine in which the deoxyribose moiety has been replaced by a hydroxyethoxymethyl substituent. It is a valuable antiviral agent whose therapeutic antiviral effect includes HSV, VZV, and CMV infections. Its effect on acute EBV infection is not clinically significant. It is recommended for prevention and treatment of herpesvirus simiae infection but its actual efficacy in this rare disease remains unknown.

In vitro, acyclovir inhibits HSV-1 and HSV-2 equally in concentrations 10 to 100 times less than are required with ara-A. VZV is 10 times less sensitive than HSV and the susceptibility of VZV to ara-A and acyclovir is similar. EBV is again 10 to 20 times less sensitive than VZV, and CMV 10 times less than EBV, to acyclovir. Acyclovir has demonstrable but minimal inhibitory activity against other viruses (adenoviruses and RNA viruses such as rhinovirus, measles, respiratory syncytial, and HBV).

Acyclovir is approved for the treatment of initial and recurrent mucocutaneous HSV infections in immunocompromised children and adults and severe initial episodes of genital herpes in the normal host. It is the drug of choice for treatment of HSV encephalitis[89] and in neonates with perinatal HSV infection in whom it is no more effective than ara-A but in whom it is more acceptable because it can be administered in smaller volumes of intravenous fluid. It is also the drug of choice for the treatment of VZV skin infections, both primary (chickenpox)[90] and recurrent,[91] in immunocompromised patients. In them, acyclovir both accelerates resolution of the cutaneous eruption as well as prevents cutaneous and visceral dissemination. Acyclovir would be expected to be effective in serious, nonneurologic HSV infections in normal and immunodeficient hosts (esophagitis, hepatitis, etc.), but its efficacy for such infections has only been reported in case reports, not controlled trials. Similarly, acyclovir may be of value in noncutaneous VZV infections.

Cytomegalovirus infections do not respond in a predictable manner to acyclovir because of the relative nonsusceptibility of CMV to acyclovir and to the host immunodeficiency commonly present. In renal transplant recipients, acyclovir has been reported to be more effective than placebo in accelerating resolution of CMV pneumonia, enteritis, hepatitis, nephritis, and retinitis, but its antiviral effect was limited.[92] CMV viremia but not viruria or CMV excretion in the throat was suppressed during therapy. These results give reason for some optimism about the possible role of acyclovir in CMV infection in immunosuppressed hosts. However, they require confirmation. Until that is forthcoming, most clinicians would prescribe ganciclovir (vide infra). Acyclovir transiently suppressed viruria in pediatric patients with congenital CMV infection. No consistent benefit was observed in bone marrow transplant recipients with CMV pneumonitis.[93]

Infectious mononucleosis in normal hosts is favorably affected by acyclovir,[94] but steroids are more likely to be useful to treat oropharyngeal airway obstruction due to lymphatic hyperplasia and hypertrophy. The usefulness of intravenous acyclovir to treat life-threatening EBV complications such as hepatitis or polyclonal B cell lymphoproliferative disease in immunodeficient individuals (X-linked lymphoproliferative syndrome, renal transplant patients, those with severe combined immunodeficiency and ataxia telangiectasia) is unclear, although some favorable effects have been observed.

Acyclovir inhibits HBV in vitro but intravenous acyclovir was of no significant benefit in a small controlled trial in patients with chronic hepatitis.

Herpesvirus simiae, also called herpes B virus, commonly causes infection in Old World monkeys. In rare instances, infection had been transmitted to monkey handlers and laboratory workers manipulating simian tissue. Infection usually presents as severe, fatal encephalomyelitis. If an animal handler is scratched or bitten by a monkey suspected or known to be carrying B virus, an experimental study has suggested that intravenous, but not topical, acyclovir can prevent infection.[95] Its value in patients with established neurologic infection is less clear but its use would seem reasonable.[96]

MECHANISM OF ACTION. Acyclovir inhibits herpesviruses with low toxicity for uninfected host cells. Its therapeutic:toxic ratio in vitro is 30:300. Acyclovir acts as a prodrug that diffuses freely into and out of host cells. In herpesvirus-infected cells, viral thymidine kinase phosphorylates acyclovir to a monophosphate nucleotide. This conversion selectively traps the drug and accounts in large part for its lack of toxicity for uninfected cells. Cellular enzymes convert the monophosphate form to di- and triphosphate nucleotides. Acyclovir triphosphate mediates the antiviral effect by inhibiting viral DNA polymerase and by inserting into DNA, precluding further addition of bases to the DNA strand, a process known as chain termination.

Because EBV possesses little thymidine kinase and CMV none, acyclovir lacks a similar inhibitory effect on these two herpesviruses.

MECHANISM OF RESISTANCE. Strains of HSV relatively resistant to acyclovir in vitro exist in nature and may comprise up to 10 percent of HSV viruses.[97] In addition, acyclovir-resistant strains may be selected in vitro and in animals and patients during therapy. However, in patients, acyclovir inefficacy associated with emergence of strains of reduced susceptibility to the drug is almost exclusively observed in immunocompromised hosts.[97] Acyclovir-resistant strains remain susceptible to ara-A and foscarnet in vitro and these agents have been reported to be effective when acyclovir is not.[98] Acyclovir resistance of VZV has not yet been a clinical problem although in vitro resistant isolates can be selected during serial passage of VZV in cell culture in the presence of drug.

Acyclovir resistance in both HSV and VZV is mediated by genetic alterations that result in production of thymidine kinase defective mutants (mostly) and DNA polymerase-insusceptible mutants (less commonly).[99]

CLINICAL PHARMACOLOGY. Acyclovir is available in topical, oral, and intravenous formulations. Although it is freely soluble in water, solutions have a high pH of 9 to 11 so it is not recommended for intramuscular or subcutaneous injection because it causes tissue inflammation and pain. After intravenous injection, its AVD is comparable to total body water; concentrations in CSF and aqueous humor are 35 to 50 percent of those in the plasma. Binding to plasma proteins is relatively low (9 to 22 percent) so that adverse interactions due to displacement by other drugs have, as expected, not been described.

The elimination $t_{1/2}$ of acyclovir from plasma is directly related to renal function because it is eliminated by both glomerular filtration and renal tubular secretion. The latter mechanism is dominant as evidenced by mean acyclovir clearance that is four to six times greater than creatinine clearance and elevated Cp and prolonged $t_{1/2}$ values in patients given probenecid concurrently. The plasma elimination $t_{1/2}$ ranges from 2.5 in adults with normal renal function to 18 h in those who are anuric. Nonrenal elimination of acyclovir contributes minimally to acyclovir clearance except in the presence of severe renal insufficiency. Up to 14 percent of a dose is eliminated as a glucuronide metabolite in urine; <2 percent appears in feces.

Mean acyclovir plasma $t_{1/2}$ during hemodialysis is approximately 5 h which reflects removal of about 50 percent of drug during 6-h dialysis.

The usual doses of acyclovir are 5 mg/kg for patients with mucocutaneous HSV infection and 10 mg/kg for patients with HSV encephalitis or VZV infection. The dose is repeated at intervals inversely related to creatinine clearance:

Creatinine Clearance (mL/min)	Dose Interval (h)
> 50	8
25–50	12
10–25	24
0–10	24–48

Hemodialysis patients should be given a standard initial dose that is repeated every 48 h and after each dialysis.

ADVERSE DRUG REACTIONS. Acyclovir is relatively free of serious toxicity.

Crystalluria with renal tubular obstruction and elevated serum creatinine concentration can be avoided by not exceeding the recommended doses and by not administering a dose over <60 min. Phlebitis can be avoided by infusing acyclovir in concentrations of <10 mg/mL. Tissue inflammation will develop if drug extravasates during infusion.

Gastrointestinal side effects including nausea, vomiting, abdominal pain, and myelosuppression, which have been previously reported during early studies with doses larger than those currently used, are no longer seen with currently recommended doses.

Neurotoxic symptoms of lethargy, agitation, tremor, disorientation, or transient paraesthesias have been observed in bone marrow transplant recipients during prolonged intravenous acyclovir therapy.[100] They resolved on withdrawal of therapy, but their relation to acyclovir dose, duration of therapy, or plasma or CSF concentrations remains unknown. Psychiatric side effects including hallucinations and depression have been observed in patients with renal failure given doses in excess of those currently recommended, suggesting a dose-related effect.

Serious adverse effects of acyclovir are likely to occur primarily in individuals with renal insufficiency in whom they can probably be largely avoided by careful attention to dose and frequency of administration.

AMANTADINE

Amantadine is a synthetic, tricyclic, basic amine antiviral agent with clinical utility limited to the prevention and treatment of influenza A virus infection.

In vitro, it inhibits influenza A viruses in low concentrations of 0.2 to 0.4 mg/L.[101] This effect has been uniformly demonstrable against all three major pandemic strains of influenza A virus and their subtypes, with hemagglutinin and neuraminidase antigens H1N1 [Spanish influenza virus including HSW1N1 (Swine influenza virus) as a variant], H2N2 (Asian), and H3N2 (Hong Kong).

Amantadine is approved as an antiviral agent for the prevention and treatment of influenza A virus infection. In ICU patients, it will probably be more useful for prevention than for treatment because it has been demonstrated to be efficacious in preventing nosocomial influenza A infection in patients in acute general hospital wards.[102] Evaluation of its therapeutic efficacy has been limited to controlled studies in otherwise healthy, young adults with uncomplicated influenza illness in whom it accelerates resolution of systemic symptoms and some respiratory tract symptoms by 50 percent and hastens the resolution of increased peripheral airways resistance that is presumably related to inflammatory narrowing of small and medium bronchioles. In addition, it reduces the frequency and duration of virus shedding. Unfortunately, no data demonstrate that similar beneficial effects could be achieved by amantadine therapy in ICU patients with influenza A infection complicating severe obstructive airways disease or other severe underlying parenchymal lung disease, or even patients with primary influenza A pneumonia in the absence of preexisting lung disease. Nevertheless, given the unavailability of any other specific, proved anti-influenza drugs, amantadine is worth considering for treating severe influenza A virus infection in ICU patients.

For prophylaxis, amantadine should be administered to susceptible patients if epidemic influenza A infection is present in the community. Susceptible patients will include all those not immunized in the past 6 to 8 months with a vaccine containing strain(s) closely related to, or identical to, the one(s) currently causing outbreak illness or all individuals, if the current epidemic strain is markedly different antigenically from the one(s) contained in the vaccine—an antigenic mutation change called antigenic shift. All patients given prophylactic amantadine should be immunized with the current vaccine simultaneously if the epidemic strain(s) is identical to, or closely related to, the vaccine strain(s). Amantadine should be stopped 10 to 14 days after immunization, by which time vaccine-induced immunity can be expected to have developed. In instances in which a suitable vaccine is not available, contraindicated (severe chicken or egg allergy), or highly likely to not be immunogenic (profoundly immunosuppressed patients), amantadine prophylaxis should be continued until public health authorities signal that the epidemic has ended (usually 2 to 4 weeks).

MECHANISM OF ACTION. Amantadine inhibits replication of influenza A virus by interfering with uncoating of the virus and release of the RNA genome in lysosomes. This effect requires that drug be present continuously in the extracellular milieu. Thus, the prophylactic or therapeutic effect is rapidly lost as drug is excreted from the body following discontinuation of drug administration.

MECHANISM OF RESISTANCE. Susceptibility to the antiviral effect of amantadine is influenced by the virion M2 protein which is found in close proximity to the inner layer of the lipid bilayer component of the influenza virion envelope that is derived from the host cell membrane.[103] Even single amino acid changes in M2 reduce susceptibility to amantadine.

Resistance to amantadine is readily selected for in vitro and during passage in mice experimentally infected with influenza A virus and treated with amantadine. Resistant strains have been recovered from untreated as well as amantadine-treated patients. More studies are required to define the clinical relevance of these observations.

CLINICAL PHARMACOLOGY.[104] Amantadine is highly water-soluble with a pKa of 11. Its utility in the ICU setting is limited by its availability only in enteral forms as capsules of 100 mg or a syrup containing 10 mg/mL. Although data from studies in experimentally infected mice and patients with severe natural infection suggest that inhalation of amantadine as an aerosol may be more effective for influenza therapy than administration enterally, no formulation suitable for aerosol administraion is available. For healthy adults <65 years of age, the recommended amantadine dose is 200 mg/day; for those over age 65, 100 mg/day.

In healthy adults including the elderly, amantadine is slowly (time to peak Cp of 6 to 12 h after ingestion) but virtually completely absorbed, but no data confirm that similar results occur in acutely ill ICU patients. It is widely distributed with a mean AVD of 6.6 L/kg that probably decreases with old age. As expected, the consequences of this pharmacokinetic characteristic are two. First, Cp values are low, averaging 0.5 to 0.8 μg/L at peak and 0.3 μg/L at trough at steady state in young, healthy adults ingesting 200 mg/day and elderly men with normal serum creatinine concentration, ingesting 100 mg/day. Second, negligible amounts are removed by hemodialysis. Amantadine is found in highest concentration in brain, liver, lung, and kidneys in treated animals; a similar localization in man could explain the propensity of this drug to cause CNS side effects (and, in part, ameliorate symptoms of Parkinson's disease). Nasal mucus concentrations of amantadine only approximate concurrent Cp. This may explain the superiority of administration of amantadine as an aerosol for therapy of influenza A in experimentally infected mice and volunteers because aerosol administration of amantadine results in volunteers' mean nasal washing fluid (and presumably mucus and respiratory epithelial cell) concentration of 66 ± 58 μg/L after chronic oral ingestion of 200 mg/day and 30,300 to 111,300 μg/L after inhalation of aerosol generated from a reservoir containing 10 g/L amantadine.[104]

Elimination is a first-order process with a plasma $t_{1/2}$ averaging 14 h in healthy, young adults and 28 h in healthy, elderly men (and presumably, women). Renal clearance exceeds creatinine clearance by approximately three times, implying significant renal tubular secretion of amantadine in addition to elimination by glomerular filtration. The plasma $t_{1/2}$ is inversely related to creatinine clearance and this fact led to the following recommendation for dose modification in patients with stable renal dysfunction:

Creatinine Clearance (mL/min/1.73 m^2 surface area)	Amantadine Dosage
≥ 80	200 mg/day
60–80	200–100 mg alternate days
40–60	100 mg/day
30–40	200 mg twice weekly
20–30	100 mg thrice weekly
10–20	200–100 mg alternate weeks

In patients on hemodialysis, a single 200-mg loading dose should be sufficient. The plasma $t_{1/2}$ of amantadine may be as long as 30 days in such individuals.

ADVERSE DRUG REACTIONS. Amantadine is generally well tolerated. Mild, amphetamine-like adverse symptoms occur in 1 to 10 percent of young adults, manifesting as insomnia, difficulty concentrating, nightmares, jitteriness, and depression. They are rapidly reversible on discontinuation of drug administration. Rarely, severe neurotoxic adverse symptoms ranging from seizures (in those with underlying convulsive disorders), psychosis, and convulsions occur. These generally occur in patients given excessive doses or with renal insufficiency. Amantadine Cp values are usually >1 mg/L in these individuals.

Isolated instances of congestive heart failure, vision loss, and urinary retention have been reported. Livedo reticularis and peripheral edema during chronic therapy have been described.

Anticholinergic and antihistamine drugs may increase amantadine adverse effects. A diuretic containing triamterene and hydrochlorothiazide was associated with neurotoxicity and increased amantadine Cp due to reduced renal clearance. Because amantadine is a cationic drug, its renal tubular secretion would be expected to be reduced by concurrent administration of other basic drugs such as quinidine, nicotine, and TMP. The possibility of such concomitant therapy increasing the frequency or severity of amantadine side effects requires further study.

GANCICLOVIR

Ganciclovir is a synthetic, acyclic, nucleoside analogue of guanine that differs from acyclovir only in possessing a hydroxymethyl group on the ribose remnant. This modest structural alteration nevertheless profoundly affects its antiviral potency and its cellular toxicity. Compared to acyclovir, ganciclovir in vitro is on average 3 times less potent against HSV-1 and HSV-2, 10 times less potent against VZV, similarly potent against EBV, and 10 to 100 times more potent against CMV (0.2 to 2.8 mg/L is inhibitory). Ganciclovir concentrations of approximately 0.6 mg/L are toxic to human bone marrow progenitor cells compared to concentrations in excess of 20 mg/L for acyclovir. The clinically important feature of ganciclovir is its antiviral effect against CMV, but its therapeutic: toxic ratio is 1 or less.

In addition to its low therapeutic: toxic ratio, ganciclovir is mutagenic, teratogenic, and carcinogenic in laboratory animals. Accordingly, its use is limited to patients with serious CMV infections, almost all of whom are immunoincompetent due to iatrogenic factors, such as immunosuppressive drug therapy in transplant recipients, or disease, such as human immunodeficiency virus infection. No controlled clinical trials have demonstrated ganciclovir efficacy and evaluated toxicity, but substantial accumulated data from observational studies of large numbers of patients have supported its utility in CMV infections. These data, using historical controls, are most persuasive for its value in controlling CMV retinitis in HIV-infected individuals.[105] Less substantive data suggest that it can improve 65 percent of HIV-infected patients with CMV enteritis, esophagitis, wasting illness, and possibly, pneumonitis.[106] Controlled trials in bone marrow transplant recipients with CMV pneumonitis have demonstrated that ganciclovir is inefficacious when administered alone or in combination with corticosteroids. However, ganciclovir administered with CMV hyperimmune globulin reduces mortality in some bone marrow transplant recipients with CMV pneumonitis.

Intravitreal ganciclovir appears to be effective for treatment of CMV retinitis in HIV-infected patients and to obviate the toxicity observed with intravenous therapy.

MECHANISM OF ACTION. Ganciclovir inhibits viral DNA replication after intracellular conversion to the triphosphate nucleotide form. Because CMV does not specify a thymidine kinase like HSV, the formation of the monophosphate nucleotide is thought to be catalyzed by cellular kinases. This fact probably accounts, in part, for its less selective accumulation in, and toxicity for, unifected host cells, unlike acyclovir. Ganciclovir-triphosphate acts like acyclovir-triphosphate in selectively inhibiting viral DNA polymerase; its incorporation into viral DNA causes a slowing of DNA chain elongation and ultimately effects chain termination of the viral DNA strand. However, because it possesses two hydroxyl groups on the acyclic side chain, ganciclovir can be incorporated into host and viral DNA without abruptly interfering with chain elongation like acyclovir-triphosphate.

MECHANISM OF RESISTANCE. Ganciclovir-resistant CMV strains have been selected during serial passage of virus in the laboratory in the presence of the drug. Resistance was associated with reduced intracellular accumulation of ganciclovir in infected cells, but the molecular basis of resistance was not further defined. Resistance associated with failure of ganciclovir therapy has been reported in immunocompromised patients. Foscarnet was effective in two such patients.[107]

Acyclovir-resistant thymidine-kinase deficient strains of HSV are susceptible to ganciclovir, but concentrations up to 40 times greater than are required to inhibit the parent strains are needed. Nevertheless, ganciclovir may be a viable therapeutic alternative in such individuals.

CLINICAL PHARMACOLOGY. Ganciclovir is so poorly absorbed (3 to 5 percent of a dose) after oral administration that therapeutic use requires intravenous infusion. The AVD, 1.2 L/kg body weight, indicates extensive extravascular binding in tissues. Ganciclovir diffuses into lungs, liver, aqueous and vitreous humor, and CSF.

Elimination from plasma is by a first-order process with a $t_{1/2}$ of 2.5 to 3.6 h that is inversely related to creatinine clearance because it is excreted as unaltered drug. Even mild impairment of renal function reduces renal clearance of ganciclovir.

The recommended dose of ganciclovir for adults with normal renal function is 5 mg/kg infused intravenously over 1 h every 12 h. For patients with impaired renal function, the dose or interval should be adjusted as follows:

Creatine Clearance (mL/min)	Ganciclovir Dose (mg/kg)	Ganciclovir Dose Interval (h)
≥80	5.0	12
59–79	2.5	12
25–49	2.5	12
<25	1.25	24

Hemodialysis for 4 h removes an average of 53 percent of the body load of ganciclovir; one-half (2.5 mg/kg body weight) the standard dose should be administered after each dialysis.

ADVERSE DRUG REACTIONS. Given its low therapeutic: toxic ratio primarily because of incorporation in replicating host DNA, it is not surprising that ganciclovir causes significant toxic effects in rapidly proliferating tissues and organs. Thus, in laboratory animals, ganciclovir causes hemopoietic, gonadal, and gastrointestinal toxicity.

In man, hemopoietic toxicity has been the most common adverse side effect observed. Neutropenia and thrombocytopenia have been observed in 40 and 20 percent of patients, respectively. Concomitant administration of zidovudine and ganciclovir increased the frequency of neutropenia. Neutropenia and thrombocytopenia are almost always promptly reversible when ganciclovir is discontinued. Frequent measurement of neutrophil and platelet concentrations permits early detection of hematologic toxicity and interruption of therapy if necessary. As with the other antiviral nucleosides, acyclovir and ara-A, ganciclovir causes CNS toxicity ranging from headaches to behavioral changes, psychosis, convulsions, and coma in up to 15 percent of patients. The mechanism is not known. Close observation for CNS toxicity is required during therapy but may be difficult to differentiate from CNS dysfunction due to concurrent disease and other drug therapy in seriously ill patients.

Anemia and phlebitis due to the alkaline pH of the solution have also been reported.

RIBAVIRIN

Ribavirin is a synthetic analogue of guanosine. In vitro, it inhibits the replication of a wide range of RNA and DNA viruses. Clinically, its value in the management of ICU patients is limited to the treatment of individuals with influenza A, B, or respiratory syncytial virus respiratory tract infection with aerosolized drug and the intravenous therapy of patients with Lassa fever, an enzoonotic infection of rodents in West Africa that may be imported in returning travellers and be transmitted from patients to health care workers.

Ribavirin has a broad spectrum of antiviral activity. In vitro, it inhibits a number of RNA and DNA virus in nontoxic concentrations. Susceptible RNA viruses include influenza A and B, respiratory syncytial, parainfluenza, and measles virus; some arenaviruses (Lassa fever and others), bunyaviruses (Hantaan virus plus others), and togaviruses including the alphaviruses (Eastern, Western and Venezuelan equine encephalitis) as well as rabies virus and HIV. Susceptible DNA viruses include HSV-1 and HSV-2 and vaccinia.

In clinical trials, ribavirin has been efficacious when administered as an aerosol to children and adults with respiratory syncytial virus infection and otherwise healthy adults with uncomplicated influenza A or B virus infection. Intravenous ribavirin reduces mortality in patients with Lassa fever. A rigorous evaluation failed to demonstrate any beneficial effect of intravenous plus intracerebroventricular ribavirin in an adult with symptomatic rabies encephalomyelopathy. Its utility for therapy of alphavirus encephalitides has not been reported.

MECHANISM OF ACTION. The precise molecular basis of the antiviral effects of ribavirin is not known. It is probable that multiple mechanisms are involved with differences between RNA and DNA viruses and virus-specific differences within each of these two groups.

Within cells, ribavirin behaves in part like an adenosine analogue, being phosphorylated to its mono-, di- and triphosphate nucleotide forms by cellular adenosine kinase. Ribavirin-5′-phosphate seems to be the principal metabolite mediating the antiviral effect of ribavirin on influenza replication by inhibition of cellular inosine monophosphate dehydrogenase resulting in guanosine depletion and inhibition of viral RNA synthesis. This antiviral effect can be reversed by exogenous guanosine. Ribavirin 5′-triphosphate, on the other hand, also selectively inhibits influenza RNA polymerase, suggesting another locus for the antiviral effect of ribavirin on influenza replication. The multiple modes of action of ribavirin may account for the absence of reports of ribavirin resistance in clinical isolates.

CLINICAL PHARMACOLOGY. Ribavirin is a water-soluble agent that has been administered to patients by aerosol, mouth, and intravenous line.

For aerosol administration to patients with viral pulmonary infection, the drug has been prepared as a solution containing 20 g/L, which must be aerosolized in a special generator to yield particles of about 1.4 μm diameter that will reach terminal airways and alveoli. The estimated dose delivered by such therapy is 0.8 mg/kg body weight/h but is probably highly dependent on tidal volumes and the presence of inflammatory narrowing of small airways, which will affect distribution of airflow. Mean maximum respiratory tract secretion ribavirin concentrations attain 1000 mg/L. A variable amount of ribavirin is absorbed into the circulation, either through the respiratory tract epithelial lining or after ingestion of drug in secretions. Serum concentrations can attain 1 to 3 mg/L.

Oral ribavirin is approximately 45 percent bioavailable. Intravenous administration yields Cp values of 17 and 24 mg/L after doses of 500 or 1000 mg, respectively. These are approximately 10-fold higher than after comparable oral doses. Ribavirin distributes widely throughout the body. It accumulates within erythrocytes due to trapping by phosphorylation. CSF concentrations average 50 to 65 percent of concurrent plasma levels. The drug undergoes extensive hepatic biotransformation as evidenced by recovery of only 24 percent of an intravenous dose as unchanged drug in urine. Elimination from plasma is a triphasic process with half-times of 0.2, 2, and 36 h. Attainment of plateau concentrations in plasma will take 1 to 2 weeks.

The effect of concomitant hepatic or renal disease or other drugs on ribavirin dispostion remains largely unstudied.

ADVERSE DRUG REACTIONS. After administration by aerosol, ribavirin has been generally well tolerated except for mild conjunctival irritation. Wheezing and cough have been observed in patients with asthma or mild chronic obstructive airway disease. These adverse effects were reversible either by discontinuation of aerosol therapy or administration of aerosolized β agonist.[108] When administered to intubated patients by mechanical ventilator, ribavirin aerosol droplets deposit on the tubing and hoses, absorb water due to their hygroscopic nature, and thereby interfere with efficient ventilation. The use of in-line filters, modified circuitry, and careful attention to pressure buildup can minimize deleterious effects on pulmonary gas exchange.

Ribavirin given intravenously for Lassa fever therapy only caused reversible anemia not requiring transfusion, as a side effect.

Chronic oral ribavirin therapy causes CNS and gastrointestinal complaints including headache, lethargy, fatigue, insomnia, anorexia. A dose-dependent, macrocytic hemolytic anemia with a contribution from myelosuppression in those receiving higher doses commonly occurs.

Adverse interactions of ribavirin with other drugs or diseases have not been described.

In view of possible ribavirin teratogenic and embryotoxic effects in man like those observed in small laboratory animals, pregnant nursing staff are advised to avoid protracted exposure to ribavirin aerosol.

ZIDOVUDINE

Zidovudine (azidothymidine, AZT) is a synthetic thymidine nucleoside in which the 3′-hydroxyl group of the deoxyribose moiety has been replaced by an azido group. It is the only agent approved for the treatment of HIV infection, which causes AIDS. As with all other currently available antiviral drugs, it exerts only a virustatic effect and for this reason, therapy must be continued indefinitely.

In vitro, AZT has different effects in different HIV-infected cell substrates. Low concentrations of <2 mg/L inhibit the replication of HIV-1 in exogenously infected cells. Higher concentrations are required to inhibit replication in chronically infected cells, but such concentrations do not inhibit HIV spread through syncytium formation or replication in T cell lines or human macrophage-monocytes; the latter may serve as the cellular reservoir of HIV in man. AZT inhibits EBV replication at concentrations one-third to one-half of maximum Cp observed during oral therapy with 1500 mg/day. Many Enterobacteriaceae are inhibited by AZT at concentrations <1 mg/L, but the clinical relevance of this observation is not known.

In controlled clinical trials, chronic oral AZT therapy reduced mortality and morbidity in AIDS patients and patients with AIDS-related complex (ARC), in large part by reducing the frequency of opportunistic infections.[109] Surrogate markers such as CD4 cell concentrations rose and p24 antigenemia declined. Initial studies evaluated the effect of 1500 mg AZT/day. Subsequent studies with doses as low as 600 mg/day have demonstrated beneficial effects on surrogate markers comparable to those seen with 1500 mg/day in patients with AIDS[110] and 300 mg/day[111] in patients with ARC. Based on these studies and the high frequency of serious hematologic toxic effects of the higher dose, current practice is to administer 500 mg/day to AIDS patients and 300 to 500 mg to ARC patients.[112] In asymptomatic HIV-infected patients, 500 mg AZT/day produces comparable benefits to 1500 mg/day with a much lower frequency of hematologic side effects.[113]

In uncontrolled studies, oral AZT, 1500 mg/day, ameliorated the encephalopathic effects of HIV as evidenced by improvements in both symptoms and signs and brain metabolism assessed by nuclear magnetic resonance spectroscopy.[114] HIV-associated thrombocytopenia and lymphocytic interstitial pneumonia have similarly been reported to respond to AZT therapy.

Intravenous AZT has produced improvement in neurodevelopmental abnormalities in children with HIV infection in an uncontrolled study.

In ICU patients who require AZT (e.g., for severe HIV encephalopathy or thrombocytopenia) and in whom gastrointestinal absorption may be unpredictable, AZT may be administered intravenously. An intravenous dose of 2 mg/kg in an adult, infused over 1 h every 4 h, produces a Cp profile similar to that seen in adults ingesting 200 mg every 4 h. To emulate the Cp-time profile observed with 600 mg/day orally, presumably the dose should be halved.

MECHANISM OF ACTION. AZT is phosphorylated by cellular kinases in both infected and uninfected cells to mono-, di- and triphosphate nucleotide forms. AZT-triphosphate inhibits HIV replication by competitively inhibiting HIV-DNA polymerase (reverse transcriptase) and by being incorporated into the growing DNA chain of the virus to act as a chain terminator. Incorporation into cellular DNA of AZT-triphosphate as a thymidine substitute probably accounts for the toxic effect of AZT on myeloid and erythroid precursors.

MECHANISM OF RESISTANCE. AZT-resistant strains have been recovered from patients during long-term therapy. It is probable that this phenomenon accounts for therapeutic failure of AZT in some patients. AZT-resistant isolates remain susceptible to other retrovirus inhibitors such as dideoxycytidine and foscarnet.[115]

CLINICAL PHARMACOLOGY. From 63 to 95 percent (mean 90 percent) of an oral dose of AZT is absorbed. However, because of first-pass metabolism, the average oral bioavailability is 65 percent (range 52 to 75 percent). Absorption is rapid with peak Cp appearing within 30 to 90 min after ingestion. The effect of gastrointestinal disease including HIV enteropathy on AZT absorption has not been described. The drug distributes widely throughout the body. Concentrations in CSF average 15 to 64 percent of concurrent Cp. AZT is rapidly inactivated to a nontoxic metabolite by hepatic glucuronidation with a plasma elimination $t_{1/2}$ of approximately 1 h for the parent compound. Both AZT and its glucuronide metabolite are eliminated primarily through the kidneys, contributing 14 and 74 percent, respectively, to urinary recovery. Renal elimination is by both glomerular filtration and renal tubular secretion. Probenecid interferes with glucuronidation of AZT and inhibits renal excretion of the nontoxic glucuronide. In anuric patients, the plasma $t_{1/2}$ of AZT increased to only 1.4 h compared to 1 h for controls with normal renal function. However, the plasma $t_{1/2}$ of the principal metabolite (glucuronyl AZT) increased from 1 h to 8 h, with as yet incompletely understood clinical consequences. Hemodialysis has a negligible effect on AZT removal but accelerates clearance of the metabolite. Thus, AZT doses need not be adjusted for patients with renal disease, including those undergoing dialysis.

The effect of hepatic disease on AZT disposition has not been described. AZT accumulation to levels greater than that seen in subjects with normal liver function would be expected. Until more data permit development of validated dose schedules for patients with hepatic disease, one might try the following strategies for minimizing dose-related toxicity: use of lower doses (e.g., 300 mg/day) and frequent assessment of reticulocytes, hemoglobin, and neutrophil concentrations, because these appear to be the most sensitive to AZT toxic effects. Measuring Cp of AZT has no established place in this setting and may be impractical.

ADVERSE DRUG REACTIONS. In adults with HIV disease, ADR observed during AZT therapy were more common in those with more advanced HIV disease and were more common in those receiving larger AZT doses. In all placebo-controlled studies, anemia and granulocytopenia were the most common ADR observed: anemia (hemoglobin value <75 g/L) was observed in 0 to 5 percent of volunteers with asymptomatic and advanced HIV disease [CD4 <200 cells/mm^3 ($<0.2 \times 10^9$ cells/L)] treated with placebo and 1 percent (500 mg/day) or 6 percent (1500 mg/day) up to 29 percent (1500 mg/day) in the same two groups, respectively, treated with AZT. Similarly, granulocytopenia [<750 cells/mm^3 ($<0.75 \times 10^9$/L)] was observed in 2 to 10 percent of subjects in the two groups treated with placebo and 2 (500 mg/day) or 6 percent (1500 mg/day) up to 47 percent (1500 mg/day) in the two groups, respectively, treated with AZT. These hematologic toxic effects generally only appeared after 4 to 6 weeks of therapy and reversed on reduction of AZT doses or temporary discontinuation.

Other ADR intensivists may see include severe headache (42 percent of AZT recipients; 37 percent of placebo-treated subjects), nausea (46 to 61 percent and 18 to 41 percent, respectively, in severe and asymptomatic HIV infection), vomiting (25 percent and 13 percent, respectively), insomnia (5 percent of AZT recipients versus 1 percent of placebo-treated subjects), and myalgia (8 percent versus 2 percent, respectively).

Although many other apparent ADR were reported by subjects in the controlled trials, the high prevalence of the same symptoms in placebo-recipients and the small sample sizes for uncommon ADR meant that the actual spectrum of uncommon AZT ADR remains to be elucidated.

Considering the number of drugs administered concomitantly to HIV-infected patients receiving AZT, a paucity of clinically important interactions have been described. Ganciclovir and AZT produce synergistic suppression of myeloid precursors with granulocytopenia, acetaminophen may inhibit AZT metabolism and increase its Cp, and dapsone plus AZT causes an increased risk of anemia. Ribavirin antagonizes the anti-HIV effect of AZT by inhibiting its phosphorylation to AZT phosphate.

FOSCARNET

Foscarnet (trisodium phosphonoformate hexahydrate) is a relatively insoluble [aqueous solubility 5 percent (wt/wt)] antiviral drug with potential utility for therapy of herpesvirus, HIV, and severe HBV infection. No controlled studies have yet evaluated its efficacy or acceptability relative to other antiviral drugs for these infections. It is not yet available for general use.

Uncontrolled studies suggest that intravenous foscarnet is of potential value for CMV infections (retinitis, pneumonitis, encephalitis) in immunocompromised patients (HIV infected, renal and bone marrow transplant recipients). It is active in vitro against acyclovir-resistant HSV and ganciclovir-resistant CMV and has been reported to be useful for treatment of such infections. Six patients with fulminant hepatitis due to hepatitis B or concomitant Delta virus infection survived in association with intravenous foscarnet therapy. Although the number of patients studied was small and historical controls were used to analyze therapeutic benefit, foscarnet may have an important role in fulminant hepatitis B infection because no other specific treatment for this infection is currently available.

Although the precise role of foscarnet in antiviral chemotherapy remains unclear, it may acquire a place in the treatment of CMV infections, especially in individuals unable to be treated with ganciclovir and patients with acyclovir-resistant HSV and ganciclovir-resistant CMV infections and serious hepatitis B infection. However, much remains to be known about the clinical pharmacology of this drug and optimal regimens for its administration.

In vitro, foscarnet inhibits some DNA and RNA viruses at noncytotoxic concentrations. Susceptible DNA viruses include the human herpesviruses (HSV, CMV, EBV, VZV) and hepatitis B virus. All the herpesviruses are inhibited by concentrations of 45 to 60 mg/L or less except CMV which requires 90 mg/L. Hepatitis B is inhibited by mean foscarnet concentrations of 6 mg/L. Susceptible RNA viruses include Visna virus, some influenza A strains, which are inhibited by 120 mg/L, and HIV which is inhibited 50 percent by 40 mg/L. HIV replication was inhibited by concentrations from 40 to 200 mg/L in different in vitro systems. Cellular cytotoxicity is observed at concentrations of 150 to 300 mg/L, yielding toxic:therapeutic ratios ranging from 1 to 7:1.

Removal of foscarnet up to 15 days after treatment of CMV-infected cell culture resulted in regrowth of virus, attesting to the virustatic effect of the drug. However, HIV inhibition was irreversible after exposure to 200 mg/L but reversible after exposure to 40 mg/L. This suggested virucidal effect needs to be confirmed.

MECHANISM OF ACTION. Foscarnet is an analogue of pyrophosphate, a metabolite of nucleic acid synthesis. It acts by inhibiting DNA and RNA polymerases, including HIV reverse transcriptase. Foscarnet inhibits DNA polymerase activity noncompetitively by binding at the pyrophosphate binding site. Purified DNA polymerase of HSV and CMV are inhibited by concentrations <0.3 mg/L and hepatitis B DNA polymerase by 6 mg/L. HIV reverse transcriptase (DNA polymerase) is inhibited 50 percent by 0.03 mg foscarnet/L. Similarly, noncompetitive inhibition of influenza A RNA polymerase by foscarnet mediates its anti-influenza effect. DNA polymerase from a variety of cells is inhibited by 15 to >150 mg foscarnet/L.

MECHANISM OF RESISTANCE. Foscarnet-resistant strains of HSV-1 and HSV-2 mutants as well as non-HIV retroviruses have been cultivated in in vitro experimental systems, and these mutants have DNA polymerase resistant to foscarnet. However, resistance development has not been observed either during foscarnet therapy of experimental herpesvirus infection in laboratory animals or during clinical trials in patients with HSV or CMV infection. Naturally occurring foscarnet-resistant HSV strains seem rare (1 of 41 HSV isolates in one study).

Resistance appears to be mediated by a mutational change in the foscarnet binding site on the DNA polymerase. Some but not all of these foscarnet-resistant strains exhibited diminished susceptibility to nucleoside analogues such as ara-A, suggesting that the mutational alteration affected a binding site on the enzyme common to both drugs. In addition, an acyclovir-resistant HSV-1 strain with intact thymidine kinase probably mutated at the DNA polymerase exhibited increased sensitivity to foscarnet and ara-A, suggesting that a change in the acyclovir triphosphate binding site affected the interaction of foscarnet and the ara-A triphosphate metabolite with the polymerase.

CLINICAL PHARMACOLOGY.[116] Foscarnet oral bioavailability is low with only 12 to 22 percent of oral doses being absorbed. The combination of poor oral bioavailability and the high doses required (100 to 200 mg/kg/day) even when it is given intravenously suggest that oral therapy will be impractical. Intravenous regimens used to treat CMV infections consist of an initial dose of 20 mg/kg over 30 min followed by continuous infusion of 230 mg/kg/day or 60 mg/kg three times per day, aimed at achieving a target Cp of 45 to 135 mg/L, based on in vitro data. Infusion requires several hours because the maximum concentration of drug recommended for intravenous administration is 2000 mg/L. Steady-state plasma foscarnet concentrations range from 40 to 400 mg/L (mean 100) with a peak Cp of approximately 150 mg/L.

After intravenous administration, the drug disappears from plasma in a triexponential manner with $t_{1/2}$ of 0.5, 3, and 18 h. The long terminal $t_{1/2}$ probably reflects the accumulation and slow release of foscarnet from bone, analagous to the slow release of aminoglycosides from renal cortex.

The kinetic AVD is about 0.6 to 0.7 L/kg. Plasma protein binding is 17 percent. CSF concentrations average 43 percent (range 13 to 68 percent) of simultaneous Cp. Penetration into the retina seems sufficient to inhibit CMV replication and ameliorate retinitis. Knowledge of foscarnet distribution in man is otherwise incomplete. In animals, forcarnet is incorporated, being a phosphate analogue, into the mineral matrix of bone. Foscarnet does not undergo metabolic transformation. It is eliminated unchanged into the urine. Renal clearance averages 130 to 175 mL/min/1.73 m^2 surface area, suggesting that renal tubular secretion and glomerular filtration both contribute to foscarnet elimination.

The kinetics of foscarnet in patients undergoing dialysis require further study. Available data indicate that its Cp declines rapidly during hemodialysis. This is consistent with the knowledge that it is a small molecule (molecular weight 300) that is minimally protein bound. However, its tissue binding will likely preclude extensive removal by dialysis. This facet of foscarnet disposition and its implications for dosing require further study. However, one recommendation suggests reducing the foscarnet dose by 30 mg/kg/day for each 20 μM rise in serum creatinine above 70 μM.[117]

ADVERSE DRUG EFFECTS. Although foscarnet causes biochemical evidence of toxicity (anemia, leukopenia, thrombocytopenia, and elevation in serum creatinine and others), symptomatic toxicity is uncommon. Hallucinations and a flapping tremor, temporally directly related to foscarnet therapy, were associated with a relatively high foscarnet Cp of 449 mg/L and disappeared when foscarnet was discontinued; these were therefore considered to represent direct toxic effects of the drug.

Anemia without alterations in white blood cell count or platelet concentration and mild elevations in the serum creatinine level occur in 15 to 50 percent of patients, but the contribution of concurrent other drugs (e.g., cyclosporine) and underlying disease has been difficult to exclude. Hypercalcemia occurs in about 20 percent of patients and abnormal transaminase in 5 to 10 percent. Local phlebitis is uncommon. Adverse interactions of foscarnet with other drugs have not been described.

Antifungals

Despite its inherent toxicity and the continuing development of new, potent imidazole antifungal drugs, amphotericin B administered alone or in combination with another antifungal agent remains the standard therapy for serious systemic mycoses. Although the arbitrary distinction between antifungal drugs used exclusively for topical therapy of superficial infection or for treatment of mycotic infections of viscera (deep mycoses) is becoming blurred with the development of the newer imidazoles, this discussion is limited to those agents that are, or will soon be, licensed for therapy for deep mycoses: amphotericin B, 5-fluorocytosine, and some of the imidazoles (ketoconazole) and structurally related N-substituted triazoles (fluconazole and itraconazole).

AMPHOTERICIN B

Amphotericin A and B are antifungal antibiotics produced by *Streptomyces nodosus*. They are members of the macrolide polyene family of antibiotics, characterized structurally by a series of conjugated double bonds (polyene) and a large cyclic ring moiety (macrocyclic or macrolide). Amphotericin B is more active than A and therefore used clinically. It exhibits amphoteric behavior, forming relatively soluble salts in basic or acid aqueous media but being extremely insoluble in aqueous solutions at physiologic pH. Accordingly, for clinical use, amphotericin B is formulated for intravenous administration as a colloidal suspension using the bile salt deoxycholate and sodium phosphate buffer. Recently, interest has focused on the encapsulation of amphotericin B in liposomes to reduce its toxic effects.

In vitro susceptibility testing of fungi and yeasts, as with viruses, remains an inexact science. Although improvements are being made in all facets of standardization of techniques and interpretation, published data from different laboratories are difficult to compare. Notwithstanding this fact, there is general agreement that an inverse relationship exists between concentrations of antifungal agents required to inhibit growth in vitro and their therapeutic efficacy. The following yeasts and fungi have MIC values of <1 mg/L to amphotericin B and are considered highly sensitive to this drug: *Cryptococcus neoformans, Blastomyces dermatitidis, Histoplasma capsulatum, Coccidioides immitis, Sporotrichum schenckii, Candida albicans, Paracoccidioides brasiliensis,* and the zygomycoses *(Mucor, Rhizopus, Absidia,* and *Cunninghamella). Aspergillus species* are usually sensitive. The causative agents of chromomycosis *(Phialophora species* and *Cladosporidium carrionii)* are usually resistant to amphotericin B alone but can be effectively inhibited by amphotericin B in combination with 5-fluorocytosine. *Prototheca species,* which cause chronic persistent granulomatous skin and visceral infections, are usually sensitive to amphotericin B. *Naegleria fowleri,* a fresh water ameboflagellate, causes primary amebic meningoencephalitis in man; it is sensitive to amphotericin B.

The effects of combining amphotericin B with antibacterial drugs in vitro, in vivo in animals with experimental fungal infections, or in patients remain of uncertain value. Antibacterial agents such as rifampicin and tetracycline, which are normally without antifungal activity, act additively or synergistically when combined with amphotericin B. This has been attributed to enhanced penetration of the fungal cell because of alterations in permeability caused by amphotericin B. However, data from studies of animals with experimental fungal infections do not suggest a consistent, predictable additive or synergistic effect of the combinations sufficient to warrant their use in patients.

Combining amphotericin B with other antifungal agents in vitro and the results of in vivo studies in animals with experimental fungal infections have demonstrated effects that are at least additive and have been borne out in studies of some infections in patients. Amphotericin B combined with 5-fluorocytosine is at least additive in vitro and in animals with experimental candida and cryptococcal infections. This has permitted the use of lower doses of amphotericin B with lesser attendant toxicity in patients with cryptococcal meningitis and perhaps candidal meningitis and arthritis. In a murine model of systemic aspergillosis, these two drugs produced better results than either agent administered alone and some clinicians recommend their combined use in patients with serious aspergillus infection, especially with significant immunosuppression, although the advantage of combination treatment over amphotericin B alone is not clear.

Results have been conflicting when amphotericin B is combined with imidazole antifungal drugs. Indifference, synergy, and antagonism have all been observed in studies in vitro and in vivo in animals with experimental mycoses. One study suggested antagonism between miconazole and amphotericin B against *C. albicans* in vitro. In view of the unpredictable effects of combining imidazoles and amphotericin, intensivists should be careful about the use of combined therapy unless supported by appropriate in vitro studies indicating absence of antagonism or warranted by the gravity of the situation.

Specific recommendations for the treatment of deep mycoses are found in Chap. 99, 100, and 102. Amphotericin B alone is the drug of choice for some *C. albicans* infections (esophagitis, peritonitis complicating peritoneal dialysis, fungemia, and endophthalmitis), coccidioidomycosis (progressive pulmonary infection and meningitis), histoplasmosis, zygomycoses, and sporotrichosis (systemic, articular, or pulmonary). Amphotericin B combined with 5-fluorocytosine is recommended for therapy of cryptococcal meningitis or disseminated infection especially in the immunocompromised host, systemic candidiasis except as noted above, *Candida* (formerly *Torulopsis*) *glabrata* endocarditis, invasive aspergillosis, and chromomycosis.

MECHANISM OF ACTION. The antifungal action of amphotericin B is complex and largely dependent on its interaction with sterols, primarily ergosterol, in the cytoplasmic membrane of sensitive fungi.[118] The drug appears to form channels or pores that lead to leakage of essential metabolites and eventually, lysis of the cell. In low concentrations, the effect is reversible and the result is inhibition of fungal cell growth. However, at higher concentrations, the effect is irreversible and the drug, therefore is fungicidal.

Amphotericin B potentiates the antifungal effect of 5-fluorocytosine and other agents by enhancing their entry into fungal cells.[119]

MECHANISM OF RESISTANCE. Identification of resistance in vitro depends on the techniques used, but both natural and acquired resistance to amphotericin B during therapy with clinical failure have been considered to be uncommon and not a clinical problem.[120] However, in one survey, 7 percent of 747 strains of *C. albicans, Candida tropicalis,* and *C. glabrata* were resistant to amphotericin B. Resistance was only observed in isolates obtained from oncology patients. These data suggested, contrary to general opinion, that resistance may not be as uncommon as thought and that selection pressure from extensive amphotericin B use in oncology patients in association with granulocytopenia may contribute to resistance development. It is postulated that a major reason why *C. albicans* resistance to amphotericin B antibiotics is uncommon is because it lacks a haploid sexual stage in its life cycle.[120] Thus, the frequency of mutational events that will alter the specific locus where amphotericin B acts will be low. This would also explain the higher frequency of resistance observed with *C. glabrata,* which is haploid.

CLINICAL PHARMACOLOGY. Absorption of amphotericin B after oral administration is negligible. It may be administered intravenously, intrathecally, or intraarticularly into the infected urinary bladder, and in dilute solution, into the peritoneal cavity of patients with fungal peritonitis.

After intravenous infusion, the drug is released from its complex with deoxycholate in the blood, binds extensively (90 percent) to plasma proteins (mostly β lipoprotein) and distributes widely throughout the body but not into CSF or the vitreous humor. Even in patients with cryptococcal meningitis, amphotericin B concentrations in CSF were <10 percent of serum values. The AVD is 4 L/kg but with wide variation. This is consistent with the observed, extensive binding of biologically active amphotericin B in tissues, particularly to sterols in hepatocytes and erythrocytes, in which the concentration is up to 30 times greater than in plasma. The Cp of amphotericin B declines in a biexponential manner after intravenous infusion. There is a rapid initial phase of decline with $t_{1/2}$ of 24 to 48 h and a slow terminal phase of 15 days. Kinetically, this biphasic pattern is consistent with amphotericin B infusion into a central compartment and its equilibration rapidly into two peripheral compartments. The rapid decline in plasma amphotericin B represents equilibration into the former and the phase of slow decline its slow release back into the central compartment from which it is eliminated.

Approximately 2 to 5 percent of a dose is recovered as unchanged drug in the urine. From 16 to 94 percent (median 33 percent) of injected doses can be recovered unchanged by extraction of tissues. The remainder is assumed to be metabolized, but data are not available on this aspect of its disposition. Blood levels are unaffected by hepatic or renal failure. Dose modifications are not required in patients with renal failure to compensate for any effect of oliguria on amphotericin B disposition, but doses may be reduced to mitigate further nephrotoxic effects of the drug. Hemodialysis does not enhance amphotericin B clearance so that such patients do not require alterations in the standard dose. At steady state, plasma amphotericin B concentrations after infusion of 0.5 mg/kg are 1.0 to 1.5 mg/L with reductions to 0.5 to 1.0 mg/L 24 h later. Hyperlipidemic and dyslipidemic states, such as occur in animals with uncontrolled experimental diabetes, alter the distribution of amphotericin B with reduced liver and kidney concentrations, diminished nephrotoxicity, and reduced clearance, associated paradoxically with a fourfold increase in apparent volume of distribution. The clinical implications of such altered disposition of amphotericin B remain to be elucidated.

The disposition of amphotericin B administered other than intravenously has not been extensively studied. Limited data on the decline in amphotericin B concentrations in CSF after instillation of drug into the lumbar sac or cerebral ventricle have been published. Intrathecally administered amphotericin B (0.3 mg) produces peak concentrations of 0.6 to 0.8 mg/L, which decline to 0.2 to 0.3 mg/L after 24 h. Amphotericin B injected into a cerebral ventricle (0.5 mg) yielded mean ventricular CSF concentrations of 1.7, 0.27, and 0.16 mg/L at 4, 24 and 48 h, respectively, after injection. For treatment of yeast peritonitis in renal failure patients undergoing chronic dialysis, amphotericin B is diluted to yield a final dialysate concentration of 1 mg/L. Between dialysis sessions, 25 mg amphotericin B is instilled in 250 mL 5% dextose in water solution with 25 mg hydrocortisone every 48 h. With this regimen, peritoneal fluid predose concentration increased from 1.6 to 2.2 mg/L and concentrations 4 h after instillation, from 2.5 to 3.6 mg/L. Concurrent serum amphotericin B concentrations were 15 to 33 percent as high. These data suggested amphotericin B was sequestered in the peritoneal cavity as the diluent solution was absorbed and that little diffused into serum.

The clinical pharmacokinetics of liposome encapsulated amphotericin B have not been described. In mice and rabbits, liposomal amphotericin B distribution is primarily to organs rich in reticuloendothelial cells, including liver, spleen, and bone marrow. A pharmacokinetic study in mice revealed a reduced area under the serum concentration-time curve for liposomal compound compared to colloidal amphotericin B. It was suggested that liposomal amphotericin B was sequestered in tissues until the vesicles were removed from the circulation by phagocytic cells in the liver and other organs.

ADVERSE DRUG REACTIONS. The inherent toxicity of amphotericin B is evidenced by a high frequency of adverse effects whether the drug is administered intravenously or by any other route. This propensity to cause side effects is compounded by the need, in most patients, for prolonged therapy.

Some patients may tolerate full intravenous doses of amphotericin B without difficulty, but acute and chronic side effects frequently necessitate dose reductions or interruptions in therapy. Acute intolerance manifest by fever, chills, malaise, muscle and joint pain, nausea, vomiting, and hypotension often begins within 1 to 2 h after initiation of therapy and lasts 2 to 4 h. Antipyretic, antiemetic, and antihistaminic drugs may provide some symptomatic relief, but controlled trials reveal little support for these practices.

Therapy should be initiated with a test dose of 1 mg in 20 mL 5% dextrose in water infused over 20 to 30 min, followed by a dose of 0.3 mg/kg infused over 2 to 3 h. Thereafter, to minimize infusion-associated adverse effects, the dose should be gradually increased, if the acuity and severity of the illness permits, to the usual dose of 0.5 mg/kg/day. The maximum recommended dose is 1.5 mg/day. There is, however, not proof from controlled trials that this regimen reduces infusion-related adverse effects of which one or more were observed in 71 percent of patients in one large survey.[121]

Some prophylactic measures have been demonstrated to be efficacious in controlled trials.

1. Ibuprofen, 10 mg/kg, a potent inhibitor of prostaglandin synthesis, administered orally 30 min before initiation of

amphotericin B infusion reduced the frequency of chilling from 87 percent in placebo recipients to 49 percent.[122]
2. Hydrocortisone, 25 mg, injected directly into the intravenous tubing at the start of amphotericin B therapy reduced the frequency of fever and chills from 78 percent in placebo recipients to 56 percent. However, the severity of chills and the level of fever were not less in the hydrocortisone-treated group. Hydrocortisone 50 mg was suggestively more effective than 25 mg (reactions reduced from 36 percent to 22 percent). Hydrocortisone, 50 mg, was not different from pretreatment with 900 mg ASA plus 50 mg diphenhydramine.[123]
3. Meperidine in an average intravenous dose of 45 mg (range 25 to 60 mg) stopped shaking chills induced by amphotericin B in 11 min, whereas interruption of amphotericin B resulted in cessation of the reaction spontaneously in an average of 38 min (range 8 to 95 min).[124]
4. No more effective in preventing infusion-related toxicity was intravenous administration of amphotericin B in 4 versus 1 h, although toxic reactions occurred earlier with the latter (at approximately 2 to 3 versus 1 to 2 h, respectively).[125]

Nephrotoxicity is the most important adverse effect of amphotericin B therapy. The creatinine clearance falls by about 40 percent soon after commencing therapy in all patients and usually stabilizes at 20 to 60 percent of normal thereafter during continued treatment. The appearance of red and white blood cells, albumin, and casts in the urine usually accompanies the decline in the glomerular filtration rate. Thus, no nonnephrotoxic therapeutic dose of amphotericin B exists. However, evidence indicates that the severity of the renal injury is increased by larger doses so the manufacturer recommends an absolute limit of 1.5 mg/kg/day. The nephrotoxic effect of amphotericin B appears related to induction of renal vasoconstriction and cortical ischemia. In experiments in dogs and patients, pretreatment by infusion of 0.15 M NaCl aqueous solution reduced the nephrotoxic effect of amphotericin B. Administration of 1 L physiologic saline prior to administration of the daily dose of amphotericin B, where the patient's condition permits, has been recommended.[126] In some patients, amphotericin B causes a syndrome similar to renal tubular acidosis with its attendant risk of nephrocalcinosis and renal failure. Early recognition and alkali therapy may help avert or minimize irreversible renal injury. In about one-quarter of patients being treated with amphotericin B, hypokalemia and mild to moderate hypomagnesemia from renal potassium and magnesium wasting, respectively, occur and require careful monitoring and replacement.

Amphotericin B administration can be made more convenient by giving 2 days' total dose on alternate days, providing the dose to be infused is <1.5 mg/kg. This strategy does not affect efficacy if the alternate dose is twice the daily dose nor does it reduce the nephrotoxic ADR. Animal studies demonstrating that intravenous mannitol could attenuate amphotericin B nephrotoxicity were not borne out in a controlled study in patients. Other nephrotoxic drugs such as the aminoglycosides and cyclosporine can add to the adverse effect of amphotericin B on the kidney and should be avoided.

If the patient's serum creatinine level increases from the normal range to 170 μM/L or more, amphotericin B should be stopped for 2 to 5 days until the creatinine concentration falls below that level. However, the severity of the fungal infection may necessitate continuing therapy at a reduced dose despite evidence of mild to moderate renal dysfunction. This appears acceptable because the renal dysfunction usually resolves after completeion of a full course treatment unless the total dose exceeds 4 to 5 g.

A reversible normochronic, normocytic anemia occurs in most patients during amphotericin B therapy; the hematocrit frequently declines to stable levels of 22 to 35 percent. Anemia appears to be due to a suppressive effect of amphotericin B on erythroprotein production. Leukopenia and thrombocytopenia are rarely observed.

Hepatic dysfunction is rare; anaphylaxis and hypersensitivity rashes are uncommon.

Extravasated drug may cause cellulitis. It is unclear whether this is due to the polyene drug or the deoxycholate. A similar reaction probably accounts for the arachnoiditis commonly observed with intrathecal injection. This chemical meningitis can cause nerve palsies, manifest as difficulty in voiding, impaired vision, paraplegia, and convulsions.

An adverse interaction of amphotericin B with leukocyte transfusion, causing acute dyspnea, hypoxemia, and interstitial infiltrates has been described by one group but challenged by at least four other groups. However, since amphotericin B can cause polymorphonulcear leukocytes to aggregate in vitro, the possibility that such an adverse interaction occasionally occurs cannot be discounted by the limited negative studies.

Liposomal amphotericin B has been demonstrated in animals with experimental fungal infections and small numbers of patients to have a better therapeutic index than the colloidal formulation available commercially. Both acute infusion-related and chronic renal toxicity side effects were less frequent and severe and liposomal amphotericin B appeared to be effective in patients unresponsive to colloidal amphotericin B.[127] This has been hypothesized to be due to specific delivery of amphotericin B to fungal cells, often in the reticuloendothelial system, by selective transfer to sterols in fungal cells from the vesicles localized in the same site. Recently a patient with hepatosplenic candidiasis complicating cytotoxic therapy for a lymphoma developed acute, reversible, reproducible hypoxemia, elevated pulmonary artery pressure, and depression of cardiac output.[128] The mechanism of this heretofore unreported acute toxic effect of liposomal amphotericin B infusion and its incidence require further study. Nevertheless, the potential advantages of liposomal amphotericin B warrant intensive further evaluation.

5-FLUOROCYTOSINE

5-Fluorocytosine is a fluorinated analogue of cytosine. It is an oral, narrow-spectrum, synthetic antifungal drug usually used in combination with amphotericin B.

In vitro, 5-fluorocytosine inhibits *C. neoformans*, *Candida species* such as *C. krusei*, *C. tropicalis*, and *C. parapsilosis*, *C. glabrata* and the agents of chromomycosis. The MICs of susceptible fungi are usually 6.25 mg/L or less; resistant species have MICs >25 mg/L. *Aspergillus species* are generally moderately to highly resistant. Other causes of deep mycoses such as *B. dermatitidis* and *H. capsulatum* are resistant to 5-fluorocytosine in vitro and clinically.

Clinically, 5-fluorocytosine has a beneficial effect in cryptococcosis, candidiasis, and chromomycosis. However, as a single agent, it is only the drug of choice for the latter disease because its efficacy in the former two is inferior to that of amphotericin B, largely because of the rapid emergence of drug resistance.

MECHANISM OF ACTION. 5-Fluorocytosine inhibits growth of susceptible fungi by at least two mechanisms. It is taken up by susceptible cells and rapidly converted by cytosine deaminase to 5-fluorouridine triphosphate, which is then incorporated in place of uracil into replicating fungal RNA, causing mistranslation and cessation of growth. Another metabolite of 5-fluorocytosine, 5-fluorodeoxyuridine monophosphate interferes with thymidylate synthesis and thereby inhibits DNA synthesis.

The effect of 5-fluorocytosine can be either fungistatic or fungicidal depending on the experimental system used. The synergistic effect of 5-fluorocytosine with amphotericin B against some fungi results from enhanced penetration of 5-fluorocytosine because of alteration of cell membrane permeability caused by the amphotericin B.

MECHANISM OF RESISTANCE. Naturally occurring resistance to 5-fluorocytosine is not uncommon.[120] With *C. neoformans*, it is of the order of 1 to 2 percent. Resistance among *Candida species* is more variable, being demonstrable in from 1 to 37 percent of isolates.

5-Fluorocytosine-resistant strains of *Candida species* and *C. neoformans* can be readily induced in vitro by serial passage in the presence of increasing concentrations of the drug. Such secondary resistance has also been demonstrated in patients with cryptococcal, candidal, and torulopsis infections being treated with this agent. In one study, two-thirds of isolates recovered from patients being treated with 5-fluorocytosine were resistant.

Resistance is associated with loss of the membrane permease that transports cytosine (and 5-fluorocytosine) into the cell, diminished activity of cytosine deaminase or uridine monophosphate pyrophosphorylase that catalyzes conversion to 5-fluorodeoxyuridine. In the majority of *C. albicans* strains resistant to 5-fluorocytosine, resistance results from a deficiency of uridine monophosphate pyrophosphorylase.[120] The loss of the enzyme does not alter the pathogenicity of the resistant strains. On the contrary, 6 to 10 strains of *C. glabrata* resistant to 5-fluorocytosine had lost the enzyme cystosine permease that mediates entry of the drug into the yeast cell.

CLINICAL PHARMACOLOGY. Only an oral formulation is available. In healthy volunteers, more than 90 percent of an oral dose is absorbed, but absorption in critically ill ICU patients may be markedly less. Protein binding in plasma is negligible. 5-Fluorocytosine distributes widely throughout all organs and fluids. Concentrations in CSF are 71 to 85 percent of concomitant serum levels and those in the aqueous humor, 10 to 40 mg/L, which in one study was 20 percent of concomitant serum concentrations. The AVD approximates that of the total body water. Elimination is a first-order process directly related to creatinine clearance and by inference, glomerular filtration. The plasma $t_{1/2}$ is 3 to 6 h in normal individuals and inversely related to creatinine clearance. In functionally anephric patients, plasma $t_{1/2}$ approaches 85 h. A small amount of drug in the body is converted to 5-fluorouracil (5-FU). This is hypothesized to be due to conversion of drug in the bowel by bacteria. This metabolite may account for the hematologic and gut toxicity of 5-fluorocytosine.

The effect of urinary acidification and alkalinization on 5-fluorocytosine in man has not been described but in other species, prolongation and shortening, respectively, of the plasma $t_{1/2}$ of 5-fluorocytosine has been observed. The effect of fluctuating pH in critically ill patients would further reinforce the need to monitor serum concentrations in ICU patients.

5-fluorocytosine is cleared by dialysis; after hemodialysis, a supplemental dose of 37.5 mg/kg is recommended. Patients with serum creatinine concentrations >150 μM/L usually require dose reduction. The following reduced doses should be administered every 6 h: creatinine clearance 40 to 49 mL/min, 5-fluorocytosine 27.5 mg/kg; 20 to 29 mL/min, 18.5 mg/kg; and <10 mL/min, 9.5 mg/kg.

Abnormal liver function appears neither to alter 5-fluorocytosine disposition nor to necessitate dose adjustments. In view of the unpredictable effects of altered gastrointestinal absorption and fluctuating renal function on 5-fluorocytosine kinetics in ICU patients, serum 5-fluorocytosine concentrations should be measured frequently to maintain levels in the effective and nontoxic range.

The recommended daily dose is 50 to 150 mg/kg administered in four equal portions. Effective Cp values range from 35 to 70 mg/L; concentrations >100 mg/L are associated with an increased risk of toxicity.

ADVERSE DRUG REACTIONS. 5-Fluorocytosine causes myelosuppression and enterocolitis. The risk of these side effects correlates with serum concentrations >100 mg/L.

Hematologic side effects of 5-fluorocytosine occur more commonly in patients with disease such as leukemia or drug or radiation therapy that has affected marrow reserves. In extreme instances, fatal bone marrow aplasia has been reported. More commonly observed are leukopenia and thrombocytopenia, which are reversible if 5-fluorocytosine can be removed rapidly. Accordingly, in anephric patients with serum 5-fluorocytosine concentrations of 100 to 150 mg/L in whom elimination will be prolonged, urgent dialysis to remove drug is recommended. The myelosuppressive effect is mediated by direct cytotoxic effects of 5-fluorocytosine on granulocyte and erythroid progenitor cells, as demonstrated in culture systems ex vivo. However, 5-FU, as noted previously, may contribute to the hematologic toxicity of 5-fluorocytosine.

Gastrointestinal side effects (nausea and diarrhea) are uncommon. More severe symptoms including vomiting, abdominal pain, and copious diarrhea warrant careful reevaluation because they may reflect acute mucositis, resembling acute ulcerative colitis.

Hypersensitivity rashes are rare. In 5 percent of patients, hepatotoxicity, as evidenced by mild elevations of serum transaminase concentrations, occurs. These patients should be monitored closely and serum 5-fluorocytosine concentration measured because the hepatotoxic effect may be dose and concentration related.

IMIDAZOLES AND TRIAZOLES

Imidazoles and the structurally related N-substituted triazoles are considered together because they share similar broad spectra of antifungal activity and the same mechanism of action. Their potency and high therapeutic indices suggest that they may ultimately displace amphotericin B as the standard therapy for many serious fungal infections.

Ketoconazole is the prototypical imidazole for therapy of deep mycoses. It is limited in being only available for oral administration, being erratically bioavailable after oral administration, and by inhibiting cytochrome P-450 in a variety of human tissues, being prone to interfere with steroidogenesis and to inhibit the metabolism of other drugs administered concurrently.

N-substitution of the imidazole ring has given rise to a second generation of derivatives called triazoles that have the same antifungal spectrum as ketoconazole but less effect on steroid metabolism. This discussion will be limited to a description of two that are, or shortly will be, licensed for use, fluconazole and itraconazole.

KETOCONAZOLE

Ketoconazole is a weak dibasic synthetic compound soluble in aqueous solution only at pH <3. Consequently, sufficient gastric acid is a prerequisite for adequate dissolution and absorption of this compound, a requirement commonly absent in ICU patients being treated with antacids or H_2-blocking drugs to prevent stress-induced gastric bleeding. Thus, although it is currently the drug of choice to treat some uncomplicated deep mycoses in immunocompetent patients who are not gravely ill, it has a limited role in the therapy of fungal infections in ICU patients.

In vitro, ketoconazole is a potent inhibitor of a wide variety of fungi. Although MIC results from such studies do not correlate uniformly with susceptibility in man, especially for some *C. albicans* strains, the following organisms are susceptible both in vitro and in vivo: *Candida* species including *C. krusei, C. tropicalis, C. albicans, C. parapsilosis,* and *C. glabrata, Sporothrix schenckii, B. dermatitidis, C. immitis, H. capsulatum,* and *P. brasiliensis.*

Pseudallescheria boydii, C. neoformans, Aspergillus species, and the agents of mucormycosis are variably susceptible to ketoconazole in vitro. Ketoconazole is not uniformly effective in infections caused by these agents.

Data are conflicting on the effects of ketoconazole combined with amphotericin B in vitro and currently no evidence indicates a beneficial effect when these agents are combined.

Ketoconazole is the current drug of choice for treatment of mild to moderately severe nonmeningeal blastomycosis, histoplasmosis, coccidioidomycosis, pseudoallescheriasis, and paracoccidioidomycosis in immunocompetent patients. It is also the drug of choice for therapy of oral and esophageal candidiasis and chronic mucocutaneous candidiasis.

MECHANISM OF ACTION. The molecular mechanisms of the antimycotic action of all imidazoles, including ketoconazole, are complex with no single primary target responsible for all observed effects. However, at least two mechanisms of action have been described. At low concentrations, ketoconazole and the other imidazole agents exert a fungistatic effect on susceptible fungi. It inhibits 14-α-demethylation of lanosterol by binding to the cytochrome P-450 enzyme C14 demethylase. This results in accumulation of 14-α-methylsterols and reduced concentrations of ergosterol, which is essential for normal fungal cytoplasmic membrane synthesis.

At high concentrations in vitro,which cannot probably be attained in human tissues, imidazoles are fungicidal to susceptible fungi. This effect is due to direct cell membrane damage with leakage of essential components from the cells, an effect similar to that caused by amphotericin B.

MECHANISM OF RESISTANCE. Acquired resistance to ketoconazole in formerly susceptible fungi appears to be rare. This probably reflects in part the fact that multiple mechanisms of inhibition are involved in the antimycotic effect. As with the polyene agent, amphotericin B, emergence of strains of at least *C. albicans* resistant to ketoconazole (and other imidazole drugs) has not proved to be a clinical problem. Diminished susceptibility of some *C. albicans* strains isolated during chronic suppressive therapy in children with chronic mucocutaneous candidiasis has been reported. Resistance development in other susceptible fungi has also been reported rarely. It is associated with diminished uptake of ketoconazole at the cytoplasmic membrane since there was no diminution in sensitivity with respect to sterol biosynthesis in cell-free systems.

CLINICAL PHARMACOLOGY. After oral administration, in the presence of sufficient hydrochloric acid, ketoconazole is transformed into the hydrochloride salt, which is absorbed rapidly. Peak Cp after administration of 200 to 800 mg increases as a function of dose but the disproportionate prolongation of the time to maximal Cp at doses of 800 mg suggests saturation of enzymes responsible for presystemic elimination of ketoconazole. In dogs, the absolute bioavailability of oral ketoconazole was 50 to 57 percent compared to intravenous doses, but the comparable study has not been described in man. Food does not affect the absorption of ketoconazole. If H_2-blocking drugs or antacids must be administered to patients receiving ketoconazole, they should be given 2 h after the antifungal agent. However, given the prolonged inhibition of gastric HCl secretion produced by H_2 blockers given orally or intravenously, it is speculative whether this strategy will permit ketoconazole to be adequately absorbed.

After absorption into the circulation, ketoconazole is more than 95 percent bound to plasma proteins. Its Cp declines biexponentially. The mean $t_{1/2}$ of ketoconazole in the initial distribution phase is 1 to 2 h. The mean elimination phase $t_{1/2}$ was dose dependent after single oral doses of 100, 200, or 400 mg, being 6.5, 8.1, and 9.6 h, respectively.

Ketoconazole, being a lipophilic drug, distributes widely with an average AVD of approximately 2.4 L/kg. Limited studies in man confirm the wide distribution of ketoconazole observed in animals: detectable concentrations have been measured in almost all fluids and tissues although CSF concentrations are low, consistent with its inefficacy in fungal meningitis.

The major route of elimination of ketoconazole is via metabolic pathways involving hepatic biotransformation and excretion via the biliary tract into the gastrointestinal tract. The major metabolic pathways involve oxidation and degradation of the imidazole ring, O-dealkylation and aromatic hydroxylation to inactive metabolites. Clearance of ketoconazole declines out of proportion to dose over the range of 200 to 800 mg, suggesting that ketoconazole undergoes first-pass metabolism.

Ketoconazole kinetics are not affected by renal insufficiency, but, as expected, significant hepatic insufficiency affects its elimination. Strategies for adjusting ketoconazole doses in patients with liver disease have not been described.

Plasma concentrations of 3 to 5 mg/L were observed during long-term therapy with 200 mg/day. In another study, mean steady-state Cp values were 2.7, 3.4, and 4.8 mg/L during daily therapy with 200, 400, and 600 mg/day. Although a direct relationship has not been demonstrated between serum ketoconazole concentration and efficacy, therapeutic failure has been associated with low serum ketoconazole concentrations. It has been suggested, therefore, that serum ketoconazole concentrations should be monitored in patients not responding to therapy. However, the clinical utility of this strategy has not been confirmed.

ADVERSE DRUG REACTIONS. Ketoconazole at low doses is a drug of comparatively low toxicity but at higher doses, more side effects may be observed. The usual dose is 200 mg once or twice daily, but doses of 800 mg/day have been used with a higher frequency of side effects.

The most common adverse effects are dose-dependent anorexia, nausea, and vomiting, which occur in about 20 percent of patients receiving 400 mg/day. Administration with food may improve tolerance without affecting bioavailability.

Hepatitis evidenced by asymptomatic elevation of serum transaminases affects a few percent of patients with return to normal without interruption of therapy. More severe, occasionally fatal, hepatitis occurs in about 1 in 12,000 recipients. This appears to be an idiosyncratic, hence unpredictable, reaction. Nevertheless, liver function should be assessed before initiation of ketoconazole therapy, and the potential benefits of treatment carefully weighed against the risk of further liver damage.

Ketoconazole at doses of 800 mg/day or more significantly interferes with normal steroid metabolism. Testosterone synthesis is blocked with the possibility of gynecomastia, diminished libido, oligospermia, and hair loss; in women, menometrorrhagia has been observed although the mechanism is not clear; cortisol secretion and the response to adrenocorticotropin may be suppressed. All these effects are not only dose related but reversible by stopping ketoconazole therapy or reducing the dose.

Interactions with other drugs may be clinically important. Administration of ketoconazole with cyclosporine results in increased cyclosporine concentrations and its attendant risk of nephrotoxicity, presumably because of interference with hepatic cyclosporine metabolism. Rifampin coadministration reduces serum ketoconazole levels, presumably by induction of cytochrome P-450 metabolism of the antifungal drug.

Ketoconazole is not thought to potentiate the anticoagulant action of coumadin like miconazole, another imidazole drug, but this is debated. It would seem prudent to monitor the prothrombin time frequently in patients receiving ketoconazole and coumadin until the data are more clear.

ITRACONAZOLE

Itraconazole is a triazole antifungal drug which differs from ketoconazole in several respects. It is more potent in vitro than ketoconazole and more lipophilic, because of which it possesses significantly different clinical pharmacokinetic properties. Its niche in the armamentarium of antifungal drugs for therapy of deep mycoses appears similar, however, to that of ketoconazole except that some anecdotal reports suggest it may be useful to treat sporotrichosis and invasive aspergillosis.

In vitro, the antifungal activity of itraconazole is greater than that of ketoconazole in both its potency and spectrum of action. Unlike ketoconazole, itraconazole also is active against *Aspergillus fumigatus* and *S. schenckii.*

The mechanism of action of itraconazole is identical to that of ketoconazole. Clinical experience to date has been too limited to permit an adequate assessment of primary and secondary resistance.

CLINICAL PHARMACOLOGY.[129] The clinical pharmacokinetic characteristics of itraconazole differ significantly from those of ketoconazole. It is a weak base that is highly ionized and poorly absorbed at the pH of gastric juice. It is insoluble in water and this has largely precluded the development of an injectable formulation.

The absolute bioavailability of itraconazole is approximately 50 percent in dogs; the comparable kinetic parameter in man is not known. The usual adult dose is 200 to 400 mg/day. Ingestion of itraconazole with food doubles its absorption as evidenced by the increase in area under the Cp-time curve. Itraconazole should be taken immediately after a meal to ensure optimal oral bioavailability. As in the case of ketoconazole, oral bioavailability appears to be enhanced at higher doses (>50 mg). This augmented oral bioavailability at higher doses likely is due to transient saturation of metabolic processes in the liver. Plasma protein binding of itraconazole is 99 percent, mainly to albumin. It distributes widely and, as is characteristic of lipophilic drugs, possesses a large AVD, which is 20 times greater than that of ketoconazole and reflects extensive tissue sequestration. However, it has negligible CSF penetration.[130]

The metabolic fate of itraconazole has only been studied in detail in laboratory animals. However, its metabolic fate in man is expected to be comparable to that in animals. Itraconazole undergoes extensive biotransformation, presumably in the liver. More than 30 metabolites have been identified, none of which has antifungal avtivity. About 54 percent of an oral dose is secreted via the bile into the feces and 35 percent into urine primarily as inactive metabolites.

The mean elimination $t_{1/2}$ from plasma ranges from 13 to 18 h. Itraconazole peak Cp attains steady state after about 2 weeks and averages 0.4 to 0.6 mg/L.

In uremic patients with creatinine clearance <12 mL/min, not yet on maintenance hemodialysis, and in volunteers with cirrhosis, itraconazole kinetics were not different from those in normal volunteers. Thus, dose alterations are not recommended for such patients.

In view of the high level of protein binding of itraconazole, it is not surprising that other drugs with similar high level affinity for albumin can displace it and increase its free concentration in plasma. High phenytoin concentrations caused a 17 percent increase in free itraconazole in plasma, but the clinical effect of this increase was deemed insignificant. No alteration of phenytoin or warfarin binding was produced by 2 mg/L concentrations of itraconazole.

ADVERSE DRUG REACTIONS. Like ketoconazole, itraconazole is reasonably well tolerated; 10 to 15 percent of patients experience nausea or vomiting but the intensity does not usually require interruption of therapy.

Unlike ketoconazole, itraconazole appears neither to cause hepatitis, to alter steroidogenesis nor to alter the metabolism of other drugs that are biotransformed by the hepatic cytochrome P-450 oxidase system of man. Because the binding of itraconazole to human cytochrome P-450 is much weaker than that of ketoconazole, it does not interfere with drug metabolizing enzymes even at high doses. This minimizes the risk of adverse interactions with other drugs given concomitantly, as well as the perturbing effect of itraconazole on cytochrome P–450-dependent pathways of steroid hormone metabolism.

No significant effect of itraconazole on the metabolism of coumarin or cyclosporine has been reported. Interaction with a single dose of rifampin, a potent inducer of hepatic drug-metabolizing enzymes, causes a biphasic effect. Initially, inhibition of itraconazole metabolism is followed for at least 3 days by increased clearance (metabolism). The net effect of chronic dosing is hard to predict based on these limited data.

For most therapeutic indications, monitoring of plasma itraconazole concentrations seems unnecessary. In some situations, such as those where absorption may be unpredictable as in ICU patients, or where potentially interacting drugs such as rifampicin are coadministered, measuring plasma levels may be useful in optimizing therapy. However, the published high performance liquid chromatography and bioassays are somewhat complex for this purpose and more importantly, only scant data exist on what desired concentrations ought to be.

FLUCONAZOLE

Fluconazole is a novel, low molecular weight antifungal with two azole rings. Its development provides intensivists with a potent, injectable, broad-spectrum antifungal of the imidazole and triazole class that is unique pharmacokinetically in penetrating readily into CSF across even uninflamed meninges and being eliminated primarily as unchanged drug directly into the urine to yield high bioactive antifungal activity therein.

In vitro, the spectrum of action of fluconazole is comparable to that of ketoconazole as is the scope of resistance (uncommon to rare) and its basis (diminished uptake by fungal cell membranes).

It is efficacious in animal models of several deep fungal infections in both normal and immunocompromised hosts. However, at this time, its relative utility compared to amphotericin B for serious visceral fungal infections is still being evaluated and the definite assessment of this agent is still to be formulated.

Clinically, in addition to being injectable, it has two potential advantages over ketoconazole, which mirror its distinctive kinetic properties. It may be valuable for treatment and chronic suppression of fungal meningitis in immunosuppressed patients such as those with AIDS, and secondly, it may be effective for treatment of fungal urinary tract infection.

CLINICAL PHARMACOLOGY. Fluconazole is highly soluble in water so that both injectable and oral formulations are available. The usual daily adult dose in patients with normal renal function ranges from 100 to 400 mg. Peak Cp values average 4 to 8 mg/L after repetitive doses of 100 mg/day.

After oral administration, more than 90 percent is absorbed although it is unclear whether this occurs in seriously ill ICU patients. Oral bioavailability is not affected by food or gastric pH.[131] Fluconazole is <15 percent bound to plasma protein so that adverse interactions with other drugs due to displacement from plasma proteins is unlikely to be observed. CSF concentrations average 50 (range 74 to 89) percent,[132] respectively, of concurrent Cp in patients with normal and inflamed meninges. Elimination is primarily by glomerular filtration into urine as unchanged drug so that high, therapeutic antifungal concentrations are attained therein. The plasma $t_{1/2}$ in adults with normal renal function is approximately 30 h, making once-daily dosing appropriate. In adults with creatinine clearance <10 mL/min, fluconazole plasma $t_{1/2}$ is 48 h, so that a 50 percent reduction in dose seems prudent. The effect of dialysis or severe hepatic disease on fluconazole disposition and the details of associated dose adjustments needed in such patients remain to be defined.

ADVERSE DRUG REACTIONS. Initial studies suggest that fluconazole shares the same safety profile as itraconazole: gastrointestinal upset is the most common side effect. Transient elevations in serum transaminases have been described. No interference with steroid hormone synthesis has been observed.

Unlike itraconazole, fluconazole administered concurrently with other drugs can affect their metabolism. Addition of fluconazole causes Cp values of phenytoin, sulfonylureas, warfarin, and cyclosporine to increase, presumably by interference with their hepatic metabolism by the cytochrome P-450 oxidation system.

It is expected that renal dysfunction will reduce fluconazole clearance and cause total body content and fluconazole Cp to rise if doses are not reduced. However, the clinical importance of these increased fluconazole Cp values has not yet been demonstrated. It would seem prudent to reduce fluconazole doses as renal function declines.

Fluconazole shows great promise as a potent, safe, single agent for the treatment of fungal meningitis.[132] Its potential compared with amphotericin B for management of this and other deep mycoses remains to be elucidated in controlled trials.

References

1. Kaiser AB: Antimicrobial prophylaxis in surgery. N Engl J Med 315:1129, 1986.
2. Dajani AS, Bisno AL, Chung KJ, et al: Prevention of bacterial endocarditis. Recommendations of the American Heart Association. JAMA 264:2919, 1990.
3. van Saene HKF, Stoutenbeeck CP, Zandstra DF: Concept of selective decontamination of the digestive tract in the critically ill, in van Saene HKF, Stoutenbeeck CP, Lawin P, Ledingham IMcA (eds): *Update in Intensive Care and Emergency Medicine.* Berlin, Springer-Verlag, 1989, p 88.
4. Young GB, Bolton CF, Austin TW, et al: The encephalopathy associated with septic illness. Clin Invest Med 13:297, 1990.
5. Tomasz A: Penicillin-binding proteins in bacteria. Ann Intern Med 96:502, 1982.
6. Curtis NAC, Orr D, Ross GW, Boulton MG: Affinities of penicillins and cephalosporins for the penicillin-binding proteins of *Escherichia coli* K-12 and their antibacterial activity: Antimicrob Agents Chemother 16:533, 1979.
7. Eagle H: Speculations as to the therapeutic significance of the penicillin blood level. Ann Intern Med 28:260, 1948.
8. Craig WA, Vogelmann B: The postantibiotic effect. Ann Intern Med 106:900, 1987.
9. Drusano GL: Role of pharmacokinetics in the outcome of infections. Antimicrob Agents Chemother 32:289, 1988.
10. Tremblay LD, L'Ecuyer J, Provencher P, Bergeron MG, Canadian Study Group: Susceptibility of *Haemophilus influenzae* to antimicrobial agents used in Canada. Can Med Assoc J 143:859, 1990.
11. Wise R: The clinical relevance of protein binding and tissue concentrations in antimicrobial therapy. Clin Pharmacokinet 11:470, 1986.
12. Barza M, Cuchural G: General principles of antibiotic tissue penetration. J Antimicrob Chemother 15(suppl A):59, 1985.
13. Apparent volumes of distribution, in Gibaldi M, Perrier D (eds): *Pharmacokinetics.* New York, Marcel Dekker, 1975, p 175.
14. Ballard BE: Pharmacokinetics and temperature. J Pharmaceut Sci 63:1345, 1974.
15. Isbister T: Penicillin allergy: A review of the immunological and clinical aspects. Med J Austral 1:1067, 1971.
16. Saxon A, Beall GN, Rohr AS, Adelman DC: Immediate hypersensitivity reactions to beta-lactam antibiotics. Ann Intern Med 107:204, 1987.
17. Simberkoff MS, Thomas L, McGregor D, et al: Inactivation of penicillins by carbohydrate solutions at alkaline pH. N Engl J Med 283:116, 1970.
18. Smith H, Lerner PI, Weinstein L: Neurotoxicity and "massive" intravenous therapy with penicillin. Arch Intern Med 120:47, 1967.
19. Bloomer HA, Barton LJ, Maddock RJ Jr: Penicillin-induced encephalopathy in uremic patients. JAMA 200:121, 1967
20. Editorial: Antimicrobials and hemostasis. Lancet I:510, 1983.
21. Mandell GL, Sande MA: Antimicrobial agents: Penicillins, cephalosporins, and other beta-lactam antibiotics, in Gilman AG, Rall TW, Nies AS, Taylor P (eds): *The Pharmacological Basis of Therapeutics.* New York, Pergamon Press, 1990, pp 1086-1087.
22. The choice of antimicrobial drugs: Med Lett Drugs Ther 32:41, 1990.
23. Sanders CC, Sanders WE Jr: Microbial resistance to newer generation β-lactam antibiotics: Clinical and laboratory implications. J Infect Dis 151:399, 1985.
24. The choice of cephalosporins. Med Lett Drugs Ther 32:107, 1990.
25. Shevchuk YM, Conly JM: Antibiotic-associated hypoprothrombinemia: A review of prospective studies, 1966–1988. Rev Infect Dis 12:1109, 1990.
26. Neu HC: Third-generation cephalosporins: Safety profiles after 10 years of clinical use. J Clin Pharmacol 30:396, 1990.
27. Solomkin JS, Dellinger EP, Christon NV, Busutlil RW: Results of a multicenter trial comparing imipenem/cilastatin to tobramycin/clindamycin for intraabdominal infections. Ann Surg 212:581, 1990.
28. Kager I, Nord CE: Imipenem/cilastatin in the treatment of intraabdominal infections: A review of worldwide experience. Rev Infect Dis (suppl 3)7:S518, 1985.
29. Norrby SR: Imipenem/cilastatin: Rationale for a fixed combination. Rev Infect Dis (suppl 3)7:S447, 1985.
30. Calandra GB, Brown KR, Grad LC, et al: Review of adverse experiences and tolerability in the first 2,516 patients treated with imipenem/cilastatin. Am J Med 78(suppl 6A):73, 1985.
31. Aronoff SC, Klinger JD: In vitro activities of aztreonam, piperacillin and ticarcillin combined with amikacin against amikacin-resistant *Pseudomonas aeruginosa* and *P. cepacia* isolates from children with cystic fibrosis. Antimicrob Agents Chemother 25:279, 1984.
32. Sykes RB, Bonner DP, Bush K, Georgopapadakou NH: Aztreonam (Sq 26, 776) a synthetic monobactam specifically active against aerobic gram-negative bacteria. Antimicrob Agents Chemother 21:85, 1982.

33. Swabb EA: Review of the clinical pharmacology of the monobactam antibiotic aztreonam. Am J Med 78(2A):11, 1985.
34. Reading C, Farmer T, Cole M: The beta-lactamase stability of amoxycillin with the beta-lactamase inhibitor, clavulanic acid. J Antimicrob Chemother 11:27, 1983.
35. Bryan LE, Kwan S: Role of ribosomal binding, membrane potential, and electron transport in bacterial uptake of streptomycin and gentamicin. Antimicrob Agents Chemother 23:835, 1983.
36. Davies JE: Resistance to aminoglycosides: Mechanisms and frequency. Rev Infect Dis 5(suppl 2):261, 1983.
37. Price KE, Kresel PA, Farchione LA, et al: Epidemiological studies of aminoglycoside resistance in the USA. J Antimicrob Chemother 8(suppl A):89, 1981.
38. Weinstein RA, Nathan C, Gruensfelder R, Kabins SA: Endemic aminoglycoside resistance in gram-negative bacilli: Epidemiology and mechanisms. J Infect Dis 141:338, 1980.
39. Gilbert DN: Once-daily aminoglycoside therapy. Antimicrob Agents Chemother 35:399, 1991.
40. Pechere J-C, Dugal R: Clinical pharmacokinetics of aminoglycoside antibiotics. Clin Pharmacokinet 4:170, 1979.
41. Dulon M, Aran J-M, Zajic G, Schacht J: Comparative uptake of gentamicin, netilmicin and amikacin in the guinea pig cochlea and vestibule. Antimicrob Agents Chemother 30:96, 1986.
42. Cutler RE, Gyselynck A-M, Fleet WP, Forrey AW: Correlation of serum creatinine concentration and gentamicin half-life. JAMA 219:1037, 1972.
43. Noone P, Parsons TMC, Pattison JR, et al: Experience in monitoring gentamicin therapy during treatment of serious gram-negative spesis. Br Med J I:477, 1974.
44. Line DH, Poole GW, Waterworth PM: Serum streptomycin levels and dizziness. Tubercle, Lond 51:76, 1950.
45. Dahlgren JG, Anderson ET, Hewitt WL: Gentamicin blood levels: A guide to nephrotoxicity. Antimicrobial Agents Chemother 8:58, 1975.
46. Weiner ND, Schact J: Biochemical model of aminoglycoside-induced hearing loss, in Lerner SA, Matz GJ, Hawkins JE Jr (eds): *Aminoglycoside Toxicity*. Little Brown, 1981, pp 113–122.
47. Nordstrom L, Banck G, Belfrage S, et al: Prospective study of the ototoxicity of gentamicin. Acta Path Microbiol Scand Section B, 81(suppl 241):58, 1973.
48. Jackson GG, Arcieri G: Ototoxicity of gentamicin in man: A survey and controlled analysis of clinical experience in the United States. J Infect Dis 124(suppl):S130, 1971.
49. Traub WH, Kleber I: In vitro additive effect of polymyxin B and rifampin against *Serratia marcescens*. Antimicrob Agents Chemother 7:874, 1975.
50. Noriega ER, Rubinstein E, Simberkoff MS, Rahal JJ Jr: Subacute and acute endocarditis due to *Pseudomonas cepacia* in heroin addicts. Am J Med 59:29, 1975.
51. Thomas FE Jr, Leonard JM, Alfred RH: Sulfamethoxazole-trimethoprim-polymyxin therapy of serious multiple drug-resistant serratia infections. Antimicrob Agents Chemother 9:201,1976.
52. Matzke GR, McGory RW, Halstenson CE, Keane WF: Pharmacokinetics of vancomycin in patients with various degrees of renal function. Antimicrob Agents Chemother 25:433, 1984.
53. Keighley MRB, Burdon DW, Arabi Y, et al: Randomized controlled trial of vancomycin for pseudomembranous colitis and postoperative diarrhea. Br Med J II:1667, 1978.
54. Teasley DG, Gerding DN, Olson MM, et al: Prospective radomized trial of metronidazole versus vancomycin for *Clostridium difficile*-associated diarrhoea and colitis. Lancet II:1043, 1983.
55. Matzke GR, Halstenson CE, Olson PL, et al: Systemic absorption of oral vancomycin in patients with renal insufficiency and antibiotic associated colitis. Am J Kidney Dis 9:422, 1987.
56. Sahai J, Healy DP, Garris R, et al: Influence of antihistamine pre-treatment on vancomycin-induced red-man-syndrome. J Infect Dis 160:876, 1989.
57. Newfield P, Roizen MF: Hazards of rapid administration of vancomycin. Ann Intern Med 91:581, 1979.
58. Lindholm DD, Murray JS: Persistence of vancomycin in the blood during renal failure and its treatment by hemodialysis. N Engl J Med 274:1047, 1966.
59. Farber BF, Moellering RC Jr: Retrospective study of the toxicity of preparations of vancomycin from 1974 to 1981. Antimicrob Agents Chemother 23:138, 1970.
60. Mellor JA, Kingdom J, Cafferkey M, Keane CT: Vancomycin toxicity: A prospective study. J Antimicrob Chemother 15:773, 1985.
61. Peppercorn MA: Sulfasalazine: Pharmacology, clinical use, toxicity and related new drug development. Ann Intern Med 101:377, 1984.
62. Cowan GO, Das KM, Eastwood MA: Further studies of sulphasalazine metabolism in the treatment of ulcerative colitis. Br Med J 2:1057, 1977.
63. Speck WT, Rosenkranz HS: Activity of silver sulfadiazine against dermatophytes. Lancet ii:895, 1974.
64. Lowbury EJL, Babb JR, Bridges K, Jackson DM: Topical chemoprophylaxis with silver sulfadiazine and silver nitrate chlorhexidine creams: Emergence of sulfonamide-resistant gram-negative bacilli. Br Med J 1:493, 1976.
65. Rieder MJ, Shear NH, Kanee A, et al: Prominence of slow acetylator phenotype among patients with sulfonamide hypersensitivity reactions. Clin Pharmacol Ther 49:13, 1991.
66. Rieder MJ, Utrecht J, Shear NH, et al: Diagnosis of sulfonamide hypersensitivity reactions by in vitro "rechallenge" with hydroxylamine metabolite. Ann Intern Med 110:286, 1989.
67. Lacey RW: Do sulfonamide-trimethoprim combinations select less resistance to trimethoprim than the use of thimethoprim alone? J Med Microbiol 15:403, 1982.
68. Huovinen P, Mattila T, Kiminki O, et al: Emergence of trimethoprim resistance in fecal flora. Antimicrob Agents Chemother 28:354, 1985.
69. Yu VL, Felegie TP, Yee RB, et al: Synergistic interaction in vitro with use of three antibiotics simultaneously against *Pseudomonas maltophilia*. J Infect Dis 142:602, 1980.
70. McLean I, Lucan CR, Mashford ML, Harman PJ: Modified trimethoprim-sulfamethoxazole doses in *Pneumocystis carinii* peneumonia. Lancet ii:857, 1987.
71. Sattler FR, Cowan R, Nielsen DM, Ruskin J: Trimethoprim-sulfamethoxazole compared with pentamidine for treatment of *Pneumocystis carinii* pneumonia in the acquired immunodeficiency syndrome. A prospective, noncrossover study. Ann Intern Med 109:280, 1988.
72. Shalit I, Berger SA, Gorea A, Frimerman H: Widespread quinolone resistance among methicillin-resistant *Staphylococcus aureus* isolated in a general hospital. Antimicrob Agents Chemother 33:593, 1989.
73. Harding GKM, Nicolle LE, Haase DA, et al: Prospective, randomized comparative trials in the therapy for intraabdominal and female genital tract infections. Rev Infect Dis 6(suppl 1):S283, 1984.
74. Eykyn SJ, Phillips I: Metronidazole and anaerobic sepsis. Br Med J 2:1418, 1976.
75. Ioannides L, Somogyi A, Spicer J, et al: Rectal administration of metronidazole provides therapeutic plasma levels in post-operative patients. N Engl J Med 305:1569, 1987.

76. Houghton GW, Smith J, Thorne PS, Templeton R: The pharmacokinetics of oral and intravenous metronidazole in man. J Antimicrob Chemother 5:621, 1979.
77. Saginur R, Hawley CR, Barltett JG: Colitis associated with metronidazole therapy. J Infect Dis 141:772, 1980.
78. Fernandes PB, Hardy DJ, McDaniel D, et al: In vitro and in vivo activities of clarithromycin against *Mycobacterium avium*. Antimicrob Agents Chemother 33:1531, 1989.
79. Krobath PD, Brown A, Lyon JA, et al: Pharmacokinetics of single-dose erythromycin in normal and alcohol liver disease subjects. Antimicrob Agents Chemother 21:135, 1982.
80. Tomomasa T, Kuroume T, Arai H, et al: Erythromycin induces migrating motor complex in human gastrointestinal tract. Digest Dis Sci 31:157, 1986.
81. Van Marion WF, Van der Meer JWM, Kalff MW, Schnicht SM: Ototoxicity of erythromycin. Lancet ii:214, 1978.
82. Tolman KG, Sannella JJ, Freston JW: Chemical structure of erythromycin and hepatotoxicity. Ann Intern Med 81:58, 1974.
83. Levinson ME, Mangura CT, Lorber B, et al: Clindamycin compared with penicillin for the treatment of anaerobic lung abscess. Ann Intern Med 98:466, 1983.
84. Kinkel AW, Buchanan RA: Human pharmacology, in Pavan-Langston D, Buchanan RA, Alford CA Jr (eds): *Adenine Arabinoside: An Antiviral Agent*. New York, Raven Press, 1975, p 197.
85. Champney KJ, Lauter CB, Bailey EJ, Lerner AM: Anti-herpes virus activity in human sera and urines after administration of adenine arabinoside. J Clin Invest 62:1142, 1978.
86. Lauter CB, Bailey EJ, Lerner AM: Microbiologic assays and neurological toxicity during use of adenine arabinoside in humans. J. Infect Dis 134:75, 1976.
87. Sacks SL, Smith JL, Pollard RB, et al: Toxicity of vidarabine. JAMA 241:28, 1979.
88. Sacks SL, Scullard GH, Pollard RB, et al: Antiviral treatment of chronic hepatitis B virus infection. 4. Pharmacokinetics and side-effects of interferon and adenine arabinoside alone and in combination. Antimicrob Agents Chemother 21:93, 1982.
89. Whitley RJ, Alford CA Jr, Hirsch MS, et al and the NIAID Collaborative Antiviral Study Group: Vidarabine versus acyclovir therapy in herpes simplex encephalitis. N Engl J Med 314:144, 1986.
90. Prober CG, Kirk LE, Keeney RE: Acyclovir therapy of chickenpox in immunosuppressed children—a collaborative study. J Pediatr 101:622, 1982.
91. Shepp DH, Dandliker PS, Meyers JD: Treatment of varicella-zoster virus infection in severely immunocompromised patients. A randomized comparison of acyclovir and vidarabine. N Engl J Med 314:208, 1986.
92. Balfour HH Jr, Bean B, Mitchell CD, et al: Acyclovir in immunocompromised patients with cytomegalovirus disease. A controlled trial at one institution. Am J Med 73(Acyclovir Symposium):241, 1982.
93. Wade JC, Hintz M, McGuffin RW, et al: Treatment of cytomegalovirus pneumonia with high-dose acyclovir. Am J Med 73(Acyclovir Symposium):249, 1982.
94. Andersson J, Sköldenberg B, Ernberg I, et al: Acyclovir treatment in primary Epstein-Barr virus infection. A double-blind, placebo-controlled study. Scand J Infect Dis (suppl)47:107, 1985.
95. Boulton EA, Thornton B, Bauer DJ, Bye A: Successful treatment of experimental B virus *(Herpesvirus simiae)* infection with acyclovir. Br Med J 280:681, 1980.
96. Artenstein AW, Hicks CB, Goodwin BS Jr, Hilliard JK: Human infection with B virus following a needlestick injury. Rev Infect Dis 13:288, 1991.
97. Dekker C, Ellis MN, McClaren C, et al: Virus resistance in clinical practice. J Antimicrob Chemother 12(suppl B):137, 1983.
98. Birch CJ, Tachedjian G, Goherty RR, et al: Altered sensitivity to antiviral drugs of herpes simplex virus isolates from a patient with the acquired immunodeficiency syndrome. J Infect Dis 162:731, 1990.
99. Coen DM: General aspects of virus drug resistance with special reference to herpes simplex virus. J Antimicrob Chemother 18(suppl B):1, 1986.
100. Wade JC, Meyers JD: Neurologic symptoms associated with parenteral acyclovir treatment after marrow transplantation. Ann Intern Med 98:921, 1983.
101. Hayden FG, Cote KM, Douglas RG Jr: Plaque inhibition assay for drug susceptibility testing of influenza viruses. Antimicrob Agents Chemother 17:865, 1980.
102. O'Donoghue JM, Ray CG, Terry DW Jr, Beaty HN: Prevention of nosocomial influenza infection with amantadine. Am J Epidemiol 97:276, 1973.
103. Hay AJ, Zambon MC, Wolstenholme AJ, et al: Molecular basis of resistance of influenza A viruses to amantadine. J Antimicrob Chemother 18(suppl B): 19, 1986.
104. Aoki FY, Sitar DS: Amantadine hydrochloride. Clin Pharmacokinet 14:35, 1988.
105. Jabs DA, Enger C, Bartlett JG: Cytomegalovirus retinitis and acquired immunodeficiency syndrome. Arch Ophthalmol 107:75, 1989.
106. Jacobson MA, Mills J: Serious cytomegalovirus disease in the acquired immunodeficiency syndrome (AIDS). Ann Intern Med 108:585, 1988.
107. Parenti DM, Drew WL, Geinberg JE, et al: Treatment of ganciclovir-resistant CMV[GCV] retinitis with foscarnet [PFA]. Abstract in: *Program and Abstracts:* VI International Conference on AIDS, San Francisco, June, 1990.
108. Light RB, Aoki FY, Serrette C: Tolerance of ribavirin aerosol inhaled by normal volunteers and patients with asthma or chronic obstructive airways disease, in Smith RA, Knight V, Smith JAD (eds): *Clinical Applications of Ribavirin*. Orlando, Academic Press, 1984, p 97.
109. Fischl MA, Richman DD, Grieco MH, et al: and the AZT Collaborative Working Group: The efficacy of azidothymidine (AZT) in the treatment of patients with AIDS and AIDS-related complex. N Engl J Med 317:185, 1987.
110. Fischl MA, Parker CB, Pettinelli C, et al: and the AIDS Clinical Trial Group: A randomized controlled trial of a reduced daily dose of zidovudine in patients with the acquired immunodeficiency syndrome. N Engl J Med 323:1009, 1990.
111. Collier AC, Bozzette S, Coombs RW, et al: A pilot study of low-dose zidovudine in human immunodeficiency virus infection. N Engl J Med 323:1015, 1990.
112. Volberding PA: Clinical applications of antiviral therapy: Use of zidovudine, in Cohen PT, Sande MA, Volberding PA (eds): *The AIDS Knowledge Base*. Waltham, Mass., The Massachussetts Medical Society Publishing Group, 1990, p 4.2.5.
113. Volberding PA, Lagakos SW, Koch MA, et al: and the AIDS Clinical Trials Group of the National Institute of Allergy and Infectious Diseases: Zidovudine in asymptomatic human immunodeficiency virus infection. A controlled trial in persons with fewer than 500 CD4-postitive cells per cubic millimeter. N Engl J Med 322:941, 1990.
114. Yarchoan R, Brouwers P, Spitzer AR, et al: Response of human-immunodeficiency-virus-associated neurological disease to 3′-azido-3′-deoxythymidine. Lancet i:132, 1987.

115. Larder BA, Darby G, Richman DD: HIV with reduced sensitivity to zidovudine (AZT) isolated during prolonged therapy. Science 243:1731, 1989.
116. Gambertoglio JG, Aweeka F, Hassanzadeh-Khayyat M: Pharmacokinetics of foscarnet, in Mills J, Corey L (eds): *Antiviral Chemotherapy. New Directions for Clinical Application and Research.* Vol 2. New York, Elsevier Science Publishing Co, 1989, p 219.
117. Walmsley SL, Chew E, Read Se, et al: Treatment of cytomegalovirus retinitis with trisodium phosphonoformate hexahydrate (Foscarnet). J Infect Dis 157:569, 1988.
118. Palacios J, Serrano R: Proton permeability induced by polyene antibiotics: A plausible mechanism for their inhibition of maltose fermentation in yeast. FEBS Letters 91:198, 1978.
119. Kwan CN, Medoff G, Kobayashi S: Potentiation of the antifungal effects of antibiotics by amphotericin B. Antimicrob Agents Chemother 2:61, 1972.
120. Kerridge D, Nicholas RO: Drug resistance in the opportunistic pathogens *Candida albicans* and *Candida glabrata*. J Antimicrob Chemother 18(suppl B):39, 1986.
121. Grasela TH Jr, Goodwin SD, Walawander MK, et al: Prospective surveillance of intravenous amphotericin B use patterns. Pharmacotherapy 10:341, 1990.
122. Gigliotti F, Shenep JL, Lott L, Thornton D: Induction of prostaglandin synthesis as the mechanism responsible for the chills and fever produced by infusing amphotericin Br J Infect Dis 156:784, 1987.
123. Tynes BS, Utz JP, Bennett JE, Alling DW: Reducing amphotericin B reactions. A double-blind study. Am Rev Respir Dis 87:264, 1963.
124. Burks LC, Aisner J, Fortner CL, Wiernik PH: Meperidine for the treatment of shaking, chills and fever. Arch Intern Med 140:483, 1980.
125. Oldfield EC III, Garst PD, Hostettler C, et al: Randomized, double-blind trial of 1- versus 4-hour amphotericin B infusion durations. Antimicrob Agents Chemother 34:1402, 1990.
126. Branch RA: Prevention of amphotericin B-induced renal impairment. Arch Intern Med 148:2389, 1988.
127. Wiebe VJ, DeGregorio MW: Lipsome-encapsulated amphotericin B: A promising new treatment for disseminated fungal infections. Rev Infect Dis 10:1097, 1988.
128. Levine SJ, Walsh TJ, Martinez A, et al: Cardiopulmonary toxicity after liposomal amphotericin B infusion. Ann Intern Med 114:664, 1991.
129. Heykants J, Michiels M, Meuldermans W, et al: The pharmacokinetics of itraconazole in animals and man: An overview, in Fromtling RA (ed): *Recent Trends in the Discovery, Development and Evaluation of Antifungal Agents.* Barcelona, JR Prous Science Publishers, 1987, p 223.
130. Perfect JR, Durack DT: Penetration of imidazoles and triazoles into cerebrospinal fluid in rabbits. J Antimicrob Chemother 16:81, 1985.
131. Blum RA, D'Andrea DT, Florentino BM, et al: Increased gastric pH and the bioavailability of fluconazole and ketoconazole. Ann Intern Med 114:755, 1991
132. Tucker RM, Willim PL, Arathoon EG, et al: Pharmacokinetics of fluconazole in cerebrospinal fluid and serum in human coccidioidal meningitis. Antimicrob Agents Chemother 32:369, 1988.

Chapter 97

APPROACH TO SEPSIS OF UNKNOWN ORIGIN

R. BRUCE LIGHT

KEY POINTS

- *Consider and critically evaluate the possibility that infection is contributing to the patient's illness at the time of admission and every day in intensive care thereafter.*
- *If infection is suspected but the source is not evident, systematically reexamine the evidence against the common infections in intensive care patients: (i) pneumonia, (ii) vascular catheter infection or phlebitis, (iii) intraabdominal infection, (iv) soft tissue—infected decubitus ulcer or wound infection, and (v) urinary tract infection.*
- *Establish the particular risk factors for infection in the patient in question and systematically search for features of infections for which there is increased risk.*
- *Prescribe empiric antimicrobial therapy for all patients in whom survival or major organ system function is threatened by presumed sepsis. Antimicrobial coverage should be directed at all potential sources of sepsis of more than trivial probability.*

Serious infections are among the most common illnesses leading to admission to an intensive care unit and are by far the most common complications of critical illness in patients admitted for treatment of other diseases. Most often, the nature of the infectious process is evident from the usual basic clinical and laboratory investigation. However, not infrequently infection is suspected in a critically ill patient on the basis of a constellation of clinical features consistent with sepsis (Table 97-1) but without an immediately obvious focus.[1] The intent of this chapter is to outline an approach to the problem of clinically suspected sepsis for which a convincing diagnosis is not evident after the usual initial evaluation. The focus will be primarily on differential diagnosis and presumptive antimicrobial therapy, since details of definitive diagnosis and therapy for specific infections are fully covered elsewhere in this book. Two broad categories of patient presentation can be defined:

TABLE 97-1 Clinical Features Associated with Sepsis

Clinical examination	
	Fever or hypothermia
	Unexplained tachypnea, respiratory alkalosis, or hypoxemia
	Tachycardia and hypotension (low systemic vascular resistance, if calculated)
	Oliguria
	Confusion, mental obtundation
Laboratory examination	
	Leukocytosis or left-shifted leukopenia
	Thrombocytopenia
	Mild to moderate cholestasis or elevation of hepatic transaminases
	Hyperglycemia
	Lactic acidosis

1. *Primary sepsis:* This is acute *sepsis syndrome* or septic shock leading to intensive care admission in a patient without an obvious source of infection. In many such cases the admission to intensive care is for management of acute on chronic organ system failure in which an unidentified infection is a potential factor in precipitating acute decompensation (e.g., acute on chronic respiratory or cardiac failure, diabetic ketoacidosis or acute hyperosmolar state, hepatic encephalopathy, acute on chronic renal failure, etc.)
2. *Secondary sepsis:* This refers to newly developing or persistent hemodynamic instability or features of the sepsis syndrome in a patient already being treated for a serious illness in the intensive care unit.

Approach to Primary Sepsis

SEPSIS DUE TO BACTERIAL INFECTIONS

In the patient without a previous history of significant disease a serious infection leads to the need for intensive care admission for one of three reasons. The first is stupor or coma, usually attributable to meningitis, encephalitis, or an acute parameningeal suppurative process such as brain abscess or subdural empyema. The second is acute respiratory failure, usually due to pneumonia (see Chap. 102) but sometimes caused by the adult respiratory distress syndrome due to sepsis at another site. The third is hypotension, which does not respond promptly to plasma volume expansion. This can be caused by serious infection at any body site. However, the common causes in addition to those mentioned above include acute pyelonephritis, cellulitis, the acute abdomen (including appendicitis, diverticulitis, mesenteric ischemia, suppurative processes of the female genital tract, etc.), and primary bacteremia or endocarditis. These diagnoses account for the majority of cases of clinically apparent sepsis,[2,3] and most will be detected by a thorough general physical examination and the basic laboratory investigation listed in Table 97-2. When this evaluation does not establish a diagnosis to guide therapy, the intensivist must systematically reevaluate the evidence bearing in mind the possibility that the patient may have one of the above-noted common causes of sepsis which has been missed, an infection which may not manifest bedside or laboratory findings specific to one organ system, or a systemic inflammatory process which is not infectious.

Hypotension or frank shock with features of sepsis (fever, elevated or left-shifted white blood cell count, hyperdynamic circulation, confusion, tachypnea) in the absence of localizing findings is the usual problem confronting the intensivist in this patient population. The first

TABLE 97-2 Basic Initial Investigation for Suspected Sepsis in Seriously Ill Patients

Basic initial investigation
- History and physical examination
- Complete blood cell count
- Chest radiograph
- Urinalysis and urine culture
- Blood culture

Additional investigation (where indicated)
- Intracranial infection suspected: lumbar puncture, preceded by computed tomography (CT) scan of head if indication is other than meningismus
- Respiratory infection suspected: sputum or endotracheal secretions for gram stain and culture; radiograph of nasal sinuses (followed by needle aspiration if sinusitis demonstrated); needle aspirate of pleural fluid
- Wound infection or intraabdominal infection suspected: gram stain and culture of wound drainage, needle aspirate of peritoneal fluid collection or abscess; imaging of abdominal contents (ultrasound or CT depending on suspect organ—see Chap. 85)
- Bone or joint infection suspected: radiograph and/or bone scan; needle aspiration for gram stain and culture of suspect joint
- Complicated urinary tract infection suspected: ultrasound or CT scan of kidneys and perinephric space (see Chap. 107)
- Primary bacteremia suspected: remove and culture semiquantitatively all indwelling vascular catheters; cardiac ultrasound (transesophageal approach preferred for suspect endocarditis)

management consideration is to achieve circulatory and respiratory stability and to establish monitoring at a level appropriate to the situation (see Chaps. 98 and 114). The next is a prompt but detailed review of the physical examination, history, and basic laboratory data with attention to a rather long list of diagnoses which are difficult to make at presentation but for which authors of reviews always seem to have a "high index of suspicion."

First, think about a common problem presenting in an uncommon manner. Acute bacterial pneumonia can occasionally present as sepsis without obvious respiratory tract findings and without pulmonary infiltrates on chest radiography. This is usually attributable to severe intravascular volume depletion delaying appearance of the infiltrate or to a poor radiograph. If the x-ray is of insufficient quality to convincingly exclude pneumonia, it should be repeated. In adult populations, central nervous system infections usually manifest nuchal rigidity, headache, or impaired level of consciousness, but confusion or moderate obtundation are occasionally the only findings, particularly in the elderly. Accordingly, in this setting a lumbar puncture (preceded by a CT scan of the head when the clinical indication is other than meningismus) is warranted except in the alert patient without symptoms. Urinary tract infection with sepsis occasionally occurs without localizing symptoms, again particularly in the elderly, and absence of significant pyuria can occur in mishandled urine specimens, with dilute urine, in pyelonephritis with ureteric obstruction, in perinephric abscess, and in prostatitis (see Chap. 107). Finally, many intraabdominal inflammatory processes may not be easily identifiable at the time of the initial evaluation. This is particularly true of acute mesenteric ischemia, in which abdominal findings early in the course are not prominent, the main early clue being sepsis syndrome with progressive metabolic acidosis out of proportion to the apparent inadequacy of systemic oxygen delivery. The most important early diagnostic tool here is repeated physical examination of the abdomen at frequent intervals during the early hospital course until the diagnosis is established either by demonstration of unequivocal physical findings or using an imaging method appropriate to the suspected infective focus. In the clinical setting of unexplained serious sepsis, even relatively subtle abdominal findings should prompt the intensivist to obtain abdominal radiographs [supine anteroposterior (AP) and upright or lateral decubitus] and consultation with a general surgeon. An ultrasound examination is useful for suspected biliary tract disease, peri- and intrahepatic infections, pancreatitis, appendicitis, and suppurative processes involving the kidneys. Abdominal CT is also useful for most of these diagnoses and is more helpful in detecting inflammatory processes associated with the bowel and female genital tract. Angiography is often the only definitive means of establishing or excluding the diagnosis of mesenteric ischemia.

In the absence of one of the initially missed diagnoses noted above, sepsis in previously well individuals is most commonly due to one of the primary bacteremia syndromes or to acute bacterial endocarditis.

Staphylococcus aureus BACTEREMIA

This organism remains the most common cause of primary sepsis in most hospitals. Although something over half of all cases of staphylococcal bacteremia can be attributed to an infected source such as cellulitis, septic arthritis, osteomyelitis, septic phlebitis or infected vascular catheter, or acute endocarditis, the presentation is often sepsis syndrome without a clinically evident source.[4] Several chronic medical illnesses are associated with increased risk of this infection, particularly diabetes mellitus and chronic renal failure. Cutaneous ulcers, parenteral drug abuse, and impetiginized dermatitides also increase risk by providing portals of entry for the organism.

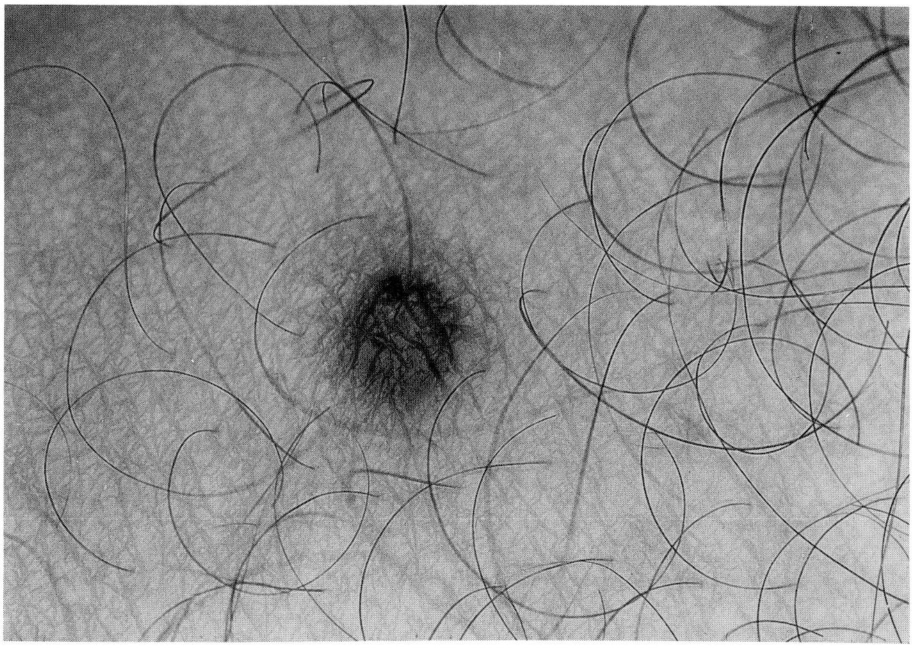

FIGURE 97-1 ***S. aureus*** **bacteremia: one of many nascent pustules in a patient with bacteremia (see Plate 40).**

Clues to the diagnosis from the physical examination mainly come from skin or eye findings (Fig. 97-1; Plate 40) suggestive of bacteremia (petechiae, purpura, pustular papules with or without necrotic changes, subconjunctival or retinal hemorrhages), or localized inflammatory findings suggesting a source of infection or a metastatic focus. Endocarditis must always be considered in staphylococcal bacteremia since this diagnosis has major implications for the nature and duration of therapy as well as prognosis (see Chap. 101). Because of its frequency and poor prognosis if untreated, empiric antimicrobial therapy for life-threatening sepsis of unknown origin should always include coverage for this organism.

MENINGOCOCCEMIA

Meningococcal bacteremia with sepsis may present early in the course without the usual associated findings of petechiae, ecchymoses, or meningismus, though these usually develop quickly thereafter.[5] The diagnosis is established by culture of the organism from blood or cerebrospinal fluid (CSF). Antigen detection tests on CSF can be useful for early diagnosis if positive, but they have not proved sensitive enough to exclude the diagnosis if negative.

PNEUMOCOCCAL BACTEREMIA

Bacteremia without a clinically evident focus occurs with increased frequency in patients with splenectomy[6] and in patients with moderate or severe humoral immunodeficiency (hypogammaglobulinemia, nephrotic syndrome) but is occasionally seen in normals, particularly children and the debilitated elderly. Rapidly progressive and intractable shock and disseminated intravascular coagulation are avoided only by early appropriate antimicrobial therapy. A clinically indistinguishable syndrome is also produced by *Hemophilus influenzae,* which should also be included in the antimicrobial coverage in populations at risk.

SALMONELLA BACTEREMIA

Typhoid fever and enteric fever caused by other Salmonella species may present without prominent abdominal findings. The evanescent "rose spots" on the trunk are often not seen, and most of the other features are shared with other causes of acute sepsis. One diagnostic clue is the dissociation between pulse rate and fever. Endemic foodborne salmonellosis with bacteremia is the more frequent syndrome in most areas, and bacteremia may lead to a secondary focal infection in almost any organ.[7] Since diarrhea may be absent, the only diagnostic clue before the positive blood culture is available may be the dietary history: ingestion of improperly cooked or stored poultry or eggs is probably the most common story, and there may be other affected individuals with varying severity of illness associated with the bacteremic case.

NONBACTERIAL CAUSES OF SEPSIS

Most of the nonbacterial pathogens causing a primary sepsislike syndrome leading to intensive care admission occur in geographically definable areas. Early and effective diagnosis and therapy therefore depend on a knowledge of which of these pathogens are locally endemic and on a careful travel history from the patient or the family.

MALARIA

Most cases of malaria requiring intensive care are due to *Plasmodium falciparum*. Since this is not a relapsing form of malaria, the main diagnostic clue is recent travel to an endemic area. Severe symptomatic *Pl. falciparum* malaria can occur as soon as a few days and as late as a few months after exposure (if the infection was being suppressed with chloroquine). Occasional cases occurring after blood transfusion continue to be reported from nonendemic areas as well. The early presentation may be simply fever with associated symptoms and signs of sepsis, while the manifestations of hepatosplenomegaly, neurologic abnormalities, pulmonary edema, renal failure, and hemolysis occur later in the course. The diagnosis, once entertained, is made by repeated examination of the blood smear for malarial parasites over a period of a few days (see Chap. 112).

ROCKY MOUNTAIN SPOTTED FEVER

Fatalities from this disease are usually in part attributable to delay in initiation of treatment.[8] This is often because the initial presentation was a febrile illness with nonspecific features progressing to shock and major organ-system failure but without the characteristic rash and in the absence of a history of tick-bite. Since confirmation of the diagnosis is generally retrospective, the decision to treat is made on clinical grounds (see Chap. 111).

VIRAL INFECTIONS

Although reasonably common in tropical areas, viral infections are infrequent causes of nonlocalizing sepsis syndrome in temperate countries. Imported cases of viral hemorrhagic fevers occur occasionally and are reviewed in detail in Chap. 112. Severe myocarditis/pericarditis due to enteroviruses can present with fever, hypotension, and prostration. The hypotension, however, is generally associated with a low cardiac output, signs of congestive cardiac failure, an enlarged cardiac silhouette on a chest radiograph, and obvious electrocardiographic changes.[9] Acute viral hepatitis, particularly type B, rarely presents with high fever and the appearance of sepsis in the pre–icteric stage of the disease. This may be associated with a serum-sickness-like illness with urticarial or macular-papular skin rash as well as fever.[10] The subsequent development within a few days of tender hepatomegaly, elevated transaminases, and jaundice makes the diagnosis obvious. Influenza can also present with prominent systemic symptoms which can mimic sepsis; respiratory symptoms are usually a prominent part of the presentation but may be attributed to another process such as congestive heart failure in the elderly and debilitated patient most likely to be severely affected by this virus. Finally, in the severely immunocompromised individual there is ample evidence that a full-blown septic shock picture can be caused by herpes viruses, most typically severe cytomegalovirus (CMV) infection in bone marrow transplant recipients.[11] Severe CMV disease is usually associated with prominent respiratory findings due to diffuse pneumonitis, but viremia does sometimes occur without obvious respiratory disease.

NONINFECTIOUS CAUSES OF APPARENT SEPSIS

Noninfectious systemic inflammatory disorders, toxin exposures, and drug withdrawal may all occasionally be confused with sepsis when they manifest fever associated with hypotension or central nervous system changes (see Table 97-3). *Anaphylaxis* or unusually severe *drug fever* can usually be suspected from the history of exposure to a potential allergen and findings consistent with these diagnoses on physical examination (hives and airway obstruction for anaphylaxis, macular or maculopapular rash for drug fever). Rarely, systemic vasculitides such as *acute hypersensitivity vasculitis, systemic lupus erythematosis* (SLE), or *polyarteritis nodosa* will present with features similar to sepsis; serologic markers are available for SLE, but for most of the others early diagnosis depends on biopsy of an involved site, usually the skin in systemic small-vessel vasculitis. *Acute drug intoxications*, particularly those involving prominent sympathomimetic effects (e.g., acute cocaine overdose), anticholinergic effects (e.g., phenothiazines), or cholinesterase blockade (organophosphate poisoning) can also be misdiagnosed as sepsis if history is unavailable and if physical signs suggestive of drug abuse or of the particular intoxication are missed. *Drug withdrawal syndromes*, particularly from alcohol, opiates, and barbiturates, are also considerations, as is *neuroleptic malignant syndrome*. Finally, *heat stroke* will present with marked pyrexia, prostration, hypotension, and confusion or coma. Historical clues include hot weather exposure in elderly debilitated patients receiving drugs which depress sweating and those with severe underlying cardiac disease or heavy exertion in a hot environment with limitation of water intake in otherwise well individuals (see Chap. 73).

OCCULT SEPSIS IN PATIENTS WITH UNDERLYING MEDICAL ILLNESSES

The patient's underlying medical illness is often the single most important determinant of the clinical approach to sep-

TABLE 97-3 Noninfectious Causes of Apparent Sepsis in Critically Ill Patients

Drug-related syndromes
Acute intoxications and poisonings: cocaine, phenothiazines, organophosphates
Drug withdrawal syndromes
Neuroleptic malignant syndrome
Allergic drug reactions
Anaphylaxis
Systemic vasculitides
Hypersensitivity angiitis
Systemic lupus erythematosus
Polyarteritis nodosa
Acute pancreatitis
Extensive tissue injury
Crush injury
Rhabdomyolysis
Vascular occlusion with tissue necrosis
Heat stroke

sis of unknown origin, affecting both the content and order of the differential diagnosis and the choice of empiric therapy. Briefly discussed below are some of the potentially occult infection syndromes associated with a number of the more common chronic diseases. Not included are illnesses with truly major infection risk, such as human immunodeficiency virus infection and granulocytopenia, which are discussed more fully in Chapters 99 and 100.

DIABETES MELLITUS

Hyperglycemia is both a risk factor in the genesis of a wide range of bacterial and fungal infections and a manifestation of infection in that diabetic ketoacidosis or less severe hyperglycemia in diabetes may have infection as an inciting event.[12] The acutely ill diabetic may not be able to provide history to guide investigation, so in most cases it is prudent to look systematically for infection. Physical examination will generally reveal the soft tissue infections common in this population. The ears, sinuses, and nose should be examined carefully for evidence of otitis media, sinusitis, and the rare but important syndrome of rhinocerebral mucormycosis. A chest radiograph to exclude lower respiratory infections is usually warranted, bearing in mind that in severely dehydrated patients both physical examination and radiographic findings of pneumonia may be minimal. Abdominal examination is complicated by the fact that ketoacidosis itself can produce paralytic ileus and abdominal pain and tenderness, while on the other hand acutely ill diabetics may not fully manifest physical findings associated with an acute surgical abdomen or pyelonephritis. Repeated examination is therefore needed as fluid resuscitation and treatment of the hyperglycemia proceeds. A blood culture, urinalysis, and culture of urine are indicated in virtually all cases. Absolute white blood cell count is generally not helpful since it is usually elevated, but a differential count demonstrating increased numbers of young polymorphs suggests infection.

Staphylococcal bacteremia is probably more frequent in diabetics than in others, both as primary bacteremia and from soft tissue, bone, or joint sources. Gram-negative sepsis from the urinary tract and from soft tissue infections also is more common. Rhinocerebral mucormycosis, a severe fungal infection of the paranasal sinuses producing adjacent periorbital cellulitis, dysfunction or destruction of multiple cranial nerves and depressed level of consciousness due to contiguous central nervous system (CNS) spread, occurs mainly in patients with diabetic ketoacidosis (see Chap. 105). In addition, symptomatic candida urinary tract infection occasionally with candidemia is mainly a disease of diabetics in the absence of urinary tract instrumentation or serious immune dysfunction.

CHRONIC RENAL DISEASE

Staphylococcal bacteremia is also more frequent in patients with chronic renal insufficiency and on hemodialysis, probably related to uremia-induced phagocytic cell dysfunction, high rates of skin colonization with the organism, and repeated skin punctures for vascular access.[13] Patients with nephrotic syndrome may have a degree of hypogammaglobulinemia and loss of other filterable opsonins contributing to an increased incidence of pyogenic infection and primary bacteremia, primarily with encapsulated organisms such as pneumococcus and *H. influenzae.*

HUMORAL IMMUNODEFICIENCY

In addition to common variable hypogammaglobulinemia, reduced humoral immunity occurs in *multiple myeloma, chronic lymphocytic leukemia, and protein-losing enteropathy.* All of these conditions are associated with an increased incidence of pyogenic infections and primary bacteremia, particularly with pneumococcus and *H. influenzae.*

ASPLENIA

Splenectomy is strongly associated with increased risk of primary bacteremia, particularly due to pneumococcus, *H. influenzae,* and to a lesser extent meningococcus and *Staph. aureus.*[14] Functional asplenia in *sickle cell anemia* also increases risk of primary sepsis with these organisms and also with Salmonella.

IMMUNOSUPPRESSIVE DRUG THERAPY

Although it is generally agreed that corticosteroids and cytotoxic immunosuppressive agents used in the treatment of immunologically mediated disease and neoplasms contribute to an increase in the frequency and severity of infections in general, there are really no specific infection syndromes sufficiently characteristic to be useful in differential diagnosis. The important points to note are, first, that serious infections may present with limited physical findings and systemic inflammatory response and, second, that the range of potential pathogens is widened to include bacteria with little propensity to cause disease in normals and fungi such as *Candida* spp.

EMPIRIC ANTIMICROBIAL THERAPY

Suspected infection producing life-threatening illness leading to intensive care admission is an exception to the general rule that antimicrobial therapy should be prescribed only after a presumptive diagnosis has been made. Early and effective antimicrobial therapy for such patients is of critical importance in avoiding septic shock and its complications.[15] In most cases, the basic medical evaluation outlined above will point in the direction of one or more of the categories shown in Table 97-4, and based on this, an antimicrobial regimen can be selected.

When a probable source of sepsis is not found and the illness is such that empiric therapy must be prescribed, the selected regimen should always provide coverage for *Staph. aureus,* the more usual enteric gram-negative bacilli such as *Escherichia coli* and *Klebsiella* spp., group A β-hemolytic streptococci, *Strep. pneumoniae,* and *Neisseria meningitidis.* A second or third generation cephalosporin is generally advised for this purpose.[16] Extension of this basic regimen can then be considered by answering these four questions: **1.** Is CNS infection a possibility? If suspected, this would require use of drugs with good CNS penetration and covering a somewhat different range of organisms (see Table 97-4).

TABLE 97-4 Antimicrobial Therapy for Sepsis of Unknown Etiology

Suspected Source of Sepsis	Usual Pathogens	Suggested Antimicrobial Regimens	Alternative Antimicrobial Regimens
None evident			
Normal host	*Staph. aureus*, streptococci, Enterobacteriaceae, meningococci	Cefuroxime 1.5 g IV q8h and gentamicin 1.5 mg/kg IV q8h or cefotaxime 2 g IV q6h or ceftriaxone 2 g IV q24h	Imipenem/cilastatin 1 g IV q6h or chloramphenicol 750 mg IV q6h
Immunocompromised host	Enterobacteriaceae, *Pseudomonas* spp., *Staph. aureus*, *Staph. epidermidis*, streptococci	Piperacillin 3 g IV q4h and gentamicin 1.5 mg/kg q8h	Ceftazadime 2 g IV q8h and vancomycin 500 mg IV q6h
Skin: (cellulitis, IV drug abuse)	*Staph. aureus*, streptococci, *Pseudomonas* spp.	Nafcillin 2 g IV q4h and gentamicin 1.5 mg/kg IV q8h	Clindamycin 600 mg IV q8h or vancomycin 500 mg IV q6h and gentamicin 1.5 mg/kg IV q8h or ceftazadime 2 g IV q8h
Lung	*Streptococcus pneumoniae*, *Staph. aureus*, Enterobacteriaceae, *Legionella pneumophila*	Cefuroxime 1.5 g IV q8h or cefotaxime 2 g IV q6h or ceftriaxone 2 g IV q24h and erythromycin 1 g IV q6h	Cotrimoxazole: 2.5 mg/kg TMP + 12.5 mg/kg SMX IV q6h and erythromycin 1 g IV q6h
Intracranial			
Meningitis	*Strep. pneumoniae*, meningococcus, *Listeria monocytogenes*, *H. influenzae*, Enterobacteriaceae	Ampicillin 2 g IV q4h	Ceftriaxone 2 g IV q12h or cefotaxime 2 g IV q6h
Abscess	*Bacteroides* spp. and other anaerobes, Enterobacteriaceae, *Staph. aureus*	Metronidazole 500 mg IV q8h and ceftriaxone 2 g IV q24h	Chloramphenicol 750 mg IV q6h
Intraabdominal and female genital tract	Enterobacteriaceae, *Bacteroides fragilis* and other anaerobes	Metronidazole 500 mg IV q8h and ampicillin 2 g IV q6h and gentamicin 1.5 mg/kg IV q8h or clindamycin 600 mg IV q8h and gentamicin 1.5 mg/kg IV q8h or ceftriaxone 2 g IV q24h	Imipenem/cilastatin 1 g IV q6h
Urinary tract	Enterobacteriaceae, enterococcus, coagulase negative, staphylococci	Ampicillin 1 g IV q4h or cefazolin 2 g IV q8h and gentamicin 1.5 mg/kg IV q8h	Cotrimoxazole 2.5 mg/kg TMP + 12.5 mg/kg SMX IV q6h or cefotaxime 2 g IV q6h
Nonbacterial Sepsis Suspected	Rocky Mountain spotted fever	Doxycycline 100 mg IV q12h (see Chapter 111)	Chloramphenical 750 mg IV q6h
	Viral sepsis		
	Herpes viruses	Acyclovir or ganciclovir (see Chapters 99, 100)	
	Hemorrhagic fever	Ribavirin (see Chapter 112)	
	Influenza	Ribavirin (see Chapter 102)	
	Malaria	Quinine (see Chapter 112)	

NOTE: Abbreviations: q4h, q6h, q8h, q12h, q24h, every 4, 6, 8, 12, or 24 h.

2. Is involvement of *B. fragilis* and other anaerobic bacteria in the infectious process likely? Examples are sepsis from necrotizing cellulitides, intraabdominal infection, infected decubitus ulcers, and female genital tract infections. All require inclusion of an effective antimicrobial for *B. fragilis* such as metronidazole, clindamycin, cefoxitin, ampicillin/sulbactam, chloramphenicol, or imipenem/cilastatin.[17] **3.** Is the patient at special risk of being infected with a relatively resistant gram-negative bacillus such as *Pseudomonas* spp.? Prolonged hospitalization, chronic complicated urosepsis, severe immunosuppression, and recent broad spectrum antimicrobial treatment are all examples of this. Antimicrobials useful in this setting include ceftazadime (together with other agents effective against *Staph. aureus* and anaerobes where indicated), ciprofloxacin (with an anaerobic agent where indicated), and imipenem/cilastatin. **4.** Is the patient at special risk for infection with an organism not susceptible to conventional antimicrobials, mandating addition of erythromycin (*Legionella* spp., mycoplasma), a tetracycline (*Francisella tularensis, Coxiella burnettii*, chlamydia, and rickettsia) or quinine (*Pl. falciparum*).

Local differences in antimicrobial susceptibility of organisms must be considered in the selection of specific agents. In many hospitals gentamicin and netilmicin are no longer effective against most Enterobacteriacae and *Pseudomonas aeruginosa* and cannot be recommended for empiric use in seriously ill patients. If other aminoglycosides such as tobramycin or amikacin remain effective, they can be substituted for gentamicin in the suggested regimens. Susceptibilities of Enterobacteriacae to the various β-lactam antibiotics also vary widely in different hospitals, making the choice of which one to use necessarily a local one. *Staph. aureus* is frequently resistant to β-lactam antibiotics in some hospitals but is almost universally susceptible to these drugs in others.[18] Vancomycin must be included in most sepsis of unknown origin treatment regimens in areas where resistance is common.

Approach to Secondary Sepsis

PERSISTENT FEVER IN PATIENTS ON ANTIMICROBIAL THERAPY

Many critically ill patients are admitted to an intensive care unit with an infectious diagnosis such as pneumonia or intraabdominal sepsis for which surgical and antimicrobial therapy have been initiated. Persistent fever despite this therapy is a common problem which requires a systematic approach.

The infectious disease consultants adage, "the second antibiotic always works better," is rooted in impatience to see objective improvement. Prompt defervescence with treatment is always gratifying and is often seen, particularly after surgical drainage of an abscess or similar process. On the other hand, when the infection involves a large mass of inflamed tissue (e.g., severe pneumonia, extensive cellulitis), fever may take much longer to resolve even with highly effective antimicrobial treatment. Fever due to infected intravascular catheters usually resolves within 24 h of catheter removal and institution of appropriate therapy. With pneumonia of moderate severity, fever usually resolves, or at least substantially improves, within 48 to 72 h but in severe cases may take 4 to 6 days to respond. Acute pyelonephritis patients generally defervesce in 48 to 72 h. With severe systemic infections such as staphylococcal endocarditis, fever frequently persists for 5 to 7 days;[19] the same is true of extensive soft tissue infections of limbs. In general, the greater the extent of the infection, the longer it takes to resolve the fever. Only fever or other evidence of sepsis persisting beyond what can reasonably be expected, particularly if there is not even a downward trend or if the fever develops a recurrent spiking pattern, constitutes evidence of failure of the initial therapeutic regimen. Further, before concluding that the initial antimicrobial choice is failing, the clinician should reevaluate all the manifestations of sepsis present, including directional trends in the white blood cell count, platelet count, temperature, level of consciousness, hemodynamic stability, and clinical findings at the site of the infection. This evaluation should also include consideration of potential noninfectious causes of fever and the possibility of a new infection at another site (see below).

Failure of antibiotic therapy to control an infection can be due to incorrect initial choice of drugs (i.e., original infection due to antimicrobial-resistant organism), development of secondary antimicrobial resistance, or failure of the antimicrobial to reach the site of the infection. The treatment regimen initially selected is usually empiric, so an assessment of antimicrobial failure begins with a reevaluation of all available microbiology results and antimicrobial susceptibilities, looking for potentially important pathogens inadequately covered by the initial regimen. If there is no demonstrated resistant pathogen and if the original regimen chosen was in fact appropriate to the clinical situation (see Table 97-3 and other chapters regarding specific infections), it is generally not useful to simply change to different drugs; they are at least as likely to be the wrong ones as the initial choice. Obtaining repeat bacteriology from the site of the infection to guide antimicrobial therapy is usually a better approach.

Antimicrobial resistance appearing secondarily during antimicrobial therapy which initially appeared appropriate is an increasingly recognized phenomenon which occurs by several mechanisms. One is selection and proliferation of resistant organisms which initially were only minor constituents of a polymicrobial infection. This occurs most frequently in complicated intraabdominal sepsis. Typically, after the initial surgical treatment and clinical improvement with the usual antibiotic treatment, fever and other signs of sepsis recur and persist. In the absence of an abscess, which is the most common cause of this sequence of events, infection due to a relatively resistant organism is often found. Review of earlier operative cultures may reveal a relatively resistant *B. fragilis* or a resistant aerobic gram-negative bacillus such as *Ps. aeruginosa* requiring modification of the treatment regimen.[20] Culture of *Candida* spp. from a peritoneal or abscess specimen is more problematic. It often represents simply contamination of the wound rather than infection requiring treatment[21] but, in patients with persistent sepsis without an abscess or other potential resistant pathogen present, may be an invasive pathogen requiring at least short-term systemic treatment.[22] Culture of these resistant organisms from draining wounds also presents problems in interpretation, since these organisms are often cultured from open wounds and from surgical drains even in patients who are doing well (and can be safely ignored in most such cases). However, persistent and copious purulent drainage demonstrating resistant pathogens in a patient with signs of sepsis and without a localized suppurative complication is generally sufficient evidence to warrant a change in antimicrobial therapy.

Another mechanism of late antibiotic failure is in situ microbial mutation. Although not a common event, it does occur with increased frequency when microbial populations are very large and when antimicrobial concentration at the infection site is relatively low; it is also somewhat more common with particular antimicrobials: rifampin and deoxyribonucleic acid– (DNA) gyrase inhibitors such as norfloxacin and ciprofloxacin. Still another mechanism is β-lactamase induction in organisms already preadapted for this. The most clinically important examples of this are *Enterobacter cloacae,* some related enterobacteriacae, and *Pseudomonas* spp., which, although they may initially appear susceptible to cephalosporin antibiotics in vitro, frequently possess inducible β-lactamase, which can lead to development of resistance and therapeutic failure.[23]

However, the most important cause of antimicrobial treatment failure is lack of penetration of the antimicrobial to the site of the infection. Examples include the poor penetration of aminoglycosides into lung tissue and the poor CNS penetration of cefazolin, cefoxitin, clindamycin, and others. But the most important factor, affecting all drugs, is absence of blood supply to the site of infection as occurs with abscess, necrotic tissue, and bony sequestra. Accordingly, apparent antibiotic failure should prompt a careful reevaluation for these entities. This almost always involves repeated imaging procedures such as conventional radiography, ultrasound, or CT.

INFECTIOUS COMPLICATIONS OF CRITICAL ILLNESS

In patients already receiving care in the intensive care unit the possibility of an infectious complication is usually raised by the onset of a new fever, an increase in the white blood cell count, or new onset of hemodynamic instability. In most instances this is accompanied by obvious clinical or laboratory findings indicating the site of the infection; the most common such infections are listed in Table 97-5. Some of these infections have full chapters devoted to them elsewhere in this book.

The clinical approach to diagnosis of such infections involves the usual complete physical examination and basic laboratory investigation. However, there are a number of infections which are either peculiar to the critical care unit or particularly difficult to diagnose in the critically ill. These require a systematic and directed approach to examination and investigation which only comes from specifically considering these entities and excluding them in turn.

NOSOCOMIAL SINUSITIS

This infection is probably substantially underdiagnosed in most intensive care units, mainly because patients with reduced level of consciousness may not complain of sinus pain, the nose and face are often not examined carefully, and radiologic examination of the sinuses is infrequently performed. Patients with large-bore nasogastric (NG) or nasotracheal tubes are at risk due to obstruction of sinus drainage.[24] Nasotracheally intubated head-injured patients seem to be at particular risk.[25] The frontal and maxillary sinuses are most frequently involved. In a patient with a nasal tube, look for purulent nasal discharge on the same side as the tube. Most intensive care units cannot be made dark enough for successful sinus transillumination. However, if the patient is reasonably awake, sinus tenderness can often be demonstrated by pressure over or percussion of the involved sinus. With practice, acceptable radiographs of the sinuses can be made in bed in the unit. Computed tomography of the sinuses is also useful. For details of the bacteriology and approach to treatment see Chap. 105.

SUPPURATIVE PAROTITIS

Painful swelling of the parotid gland with overlying erythema is usually obvious in an awake patient but may be missed in the elderly, severely debilitated, frequently dehydrated patient with reduced level of consciousness who is at greatest risk for this infection.[26] Look for erythema and tender swelling in the preauricular area partly overlying the mandible. On the buccal mucosa, purulent discharge from Stensen's duct may be seen. See Chap. 105 for a discussion of diagnosis and management.

PNEUMONIA

The diagnosis of pneumonia may be obscure in patients who have preexisting pulmonary infiltrates related to pulmonary edema or atelectasis. Even in the absence of clear-cut increases in the extent of the pulmonary infiltrate on chest radiography, the diagnosis should be seriously considered when there is an increase in the amount and purulence of respiratory secretions or an increase in oxygen requirement to maintain arterial oxygenation in association with systemic signs of infection. While these findings often signal pneumonia, it is also true that noninfectious processes such as atelectasis and chemical pneumonitis can produce them as well. Fiber-optic bronchoscopy with quantitative bacteriology of lower respiratory tract specimens can be very useful in establishing or excluding pneumonia when the diagnosis remains unclear (see Chap. 102).[27] In patients already being treated for pneumonia, empyema is sometimes missed, particularly when the pleural fluid is posterior and only AP chest radiographs have been made. Clinical examination findings suggesting pleural fluid may be sufficient to suggest the diagnosis and guide diagnostic thoracentesis, but where this is difficult or uncertain, bedside ultrasonography is helpful and thoracic CT is usually definitive.

URINARY TRACT INFECTION

Urosepsis may be clinically occult for several reasons, first among them being depression of the patient's level of consciousness, impeding detection of renal pain or tenderness. Ureteric obstruction may result in absence of inflammatory cells on urinalysis. In addition, the source of sepsis may not be the kidney but rather the prostate in men or simply mucosal disruption of an infected bladder by the urinary catheter. The evaluation is further complicated by the fact that most critically ill patients have indwelling urinary catheters, most develop bacterial or fungal colonization of the urinary tract within a few days of admission, and this colonization usually does not lead to serious infection. When

TABLE 97-5 Major Nosocomial Infections Complicating Intensive Care for Critical Illness

Site	Diagnosis	Usual pathogens	Predisposing factors
Head and neck	Maxillary or frontal sinusitis	*Staph. aureus,* Enterobacteriaceae, *H. influenzae*	Nasotracheal endotracheal tube, large-bore NG tube, facial trauma
	Suppurative parotitis	*Staph. aureus,* Enterobacteriaceae	Dehydration, poor oral hygiene
	Intracranial pressure monitor infection	Coagulase negative staphylococci, *Staph. aureus*	Long-duration intracranial pressure monitoring, frequent line manipulation
Chest	Pneumonia	Enterobacteriaceae, *Staph. aureus, Pseudomonas* spp.	Endotracheal intubation, depressed level of consciousness, use of antacids or H_2 blockers, aspiration
Skin and Vascular access sites	Vascular catheter infection and suppurative phlebitis	Coagulase negative staphylococci, *Staph. aureus,* Enterobacteriaceae	Poor aseptic technique; occlusive site dressing; frequent catheter manipulation; location: groin, axilla, antecubital fossa; skin infection/contamination: burns, impetiginized rash.
	Wound infection		
	Clean surgery	*Staph. aureus, Strep. pyogenes,* coagulase negative staphylococci, *Candida* spp.	Protracted surgery; aseptic technique breaks; hematoma, prostheses
	Contaminated abdominal surgery	Enterobacteriaceae, *B. fragilis* and other anaerobes	Gross contamination, no antibiotic prophylaxis, inadequate drainage/ debridement, malnutrition
	Infected decubiti	Enterobacteriaceae, *B. fragilis* and other anaerobes, *Staph. aureus*	fecal soilage, poor perfusion or venous stasis, necrotic tissue not debrided
Abdomen	Pseudomembranous colitis	*Clostridium difficile*	Prior antimicrobial therapy
	Acalculous cholecystitis	Enterobacteriaceae, group D streptococci, *B. fragilis* and other anaerobes	Protracted critical illness
	Intraabdominal abscess	Enterobacteriaceae, *B. fragilis* and other anaerobes	Perforated viscus, contaminated abdominal surgery, pancreatitis, malnutrition
Musculoskeletal	Posttraumatic osteomyelitis	*Staph. aureus,* Enterobacteriaceae, mixed anaerobic bacteria	Compound fracture, frank wound contamination, foreign body, poor arterial perfusion, prostheses used for fixation within contaminated wound
	Septic arthritis	*Staph. aureus,* Enterobacteriaceae	Prior bacteremia, overlying cellulitis or skin breakdown, joint surgery or prosthesis in place
Urinary tract infection	Acute pyelonephritis	Enterobacteriaceae, enterococcus	Indwelling urinary catheter, diabetes mellitus, anatomic urologic abnormality or nephrolithiasis

otherwise unexplained sepsis is accompanied by bacteriuria associated with pyuria, the intensivist is usually obliged to treat this with antibiotics which, in the absence of other presumptive infectious diagnoses, should be as specific as possible. Suspicion of ureteric obstruction arising from a deterioration in renal function or poor response to antimicrobial therapy should prompt ultrasonographic imaging of the kidneys. Distinguishing fungal colonization from infection presents even more formidable problems; an approach to this is detailed in Chap. 107.

INTRAABDOMINAL SEPSIS

Abdominal distension with either absence of bowel movements or diarrhea, poorly localized tenderness or discomfort, and quiet or absent bowel sounds due to paralytic ileus of metabolic or systemic cause are all common occurrences in critically ill patients, and their presence does not reliably indicate the presence of an intraabdominal inflammatory process. But these patients are also at increased risk for a number of difficult-to-diagnose intraabdominal infections including biliary tract sepsis (*acute cholecystitis, choledocholi-*

thiasis with cholangitis), intraabdominal *abscess* (particularly in patients with prior abdominal surgery or intestinal perforation), and *ischemic bowel*. *Pseudomembranous colitis* due to *Cl. difficile* can usually be suspected in the context of diarrhea with systemic symptoms following antimicrobial therapy but will sometimes present with sepsis in the absence of diarrhea; there may be abdominal tenderness over the descending colon or blood *per rectum*.[28]

A more detailed approach to the problem of occult intraabdominal sepsis is found in Chap. 85. However, the basic approach centers around repeated examination of the abdomen looking for persistent findings of localized pain, tenderness, or guarding, and any of these should prompt consultation with a general surgeon. Ultrasound examination is of most value in detecting biliary tract disease and inflammatory processes or abscesses of the liver,[29] perihepatic region, pancreas, retroperitoneum, and the pelvis. CT scanning will also detect most of these and is of greater value in detecting abscesses or inflammatory masses associated with the bowel.[30] In the presence of diarrhea, culture of stool for *Cl. difficile* and assay for its toxin is helpful; where there is no diarrhea but there is suspicion of colitis (bloody stool, pain, or tenderness over colon), sigmoidoscopy or colonoscopy may be diagnostic.

PRIMARY BACTEREMIA/FUNGEMIA

An infected intravascular catheter is by far the most common cause of bacteremia or candidemia without obvious source.[31,32] It is also a frequent cause of fever or apparent sepsis without demonstrable bacteremia. Daily patient care routine should include a review of all intravascular catheters in place, noting the conditions under which they were placed, the length of time they have been in place, the appearance of the skin entry site (erythema, tenderness, purulent exudate), the continued need for the catheter, and the availability of alternate sites for catheter placement or route of delivery of therapy. In general, catheters which were inserted with poor aseptic technique, as often occurs during urgent resuscitation, should be removed and replaced at a different site as soon as this is practical. Catheters with local signs of infection should also be removed. When there is fever or sepsis of unknown source, removal or replacement of all indwelling vascular catheters in place for more than 48 h is advisable, performing semiquantitative culture of the intracutaneous portion of the catheters as well as blood cultures obtained by venipuncture.[33] When removal of a central vascular catheter is deemed impractical because of limited vascular access, it is probably reasonable to replace the catheter through the existing puncture site by passing a guide-wire through the catheter, removing it, and placing a new catheter over the wire; even when the semiquantitative culture of the first catheter indicates infection, the infection may not recur. However, if systemic signs of infection persist, removal of the second catheter is usually necessary.[34]

Central venous catheters with extended subcutaneous tunnels designed for longer term use are being used with increasing frequency, particularly for vascular access in treatment of malignancy and for total parenteral nutrition. Bacteremia associated with these catheters is more frequently due to intraluminal infection than is the case with conventional catheters, in which infections more often involve the outside of the catheter along the short tract between the skin and the vein. Accordingly, it may be worthwhile to obtain cultures of blood drawn through the long-stay central vascular catheter and to attempt to treat the infection with antibiotics without catheter removal (see Chap. 101).[35]

NONINFECTIOUS CAUSES OF FEVER OR SEPSIS SYNDROME

Probably the most common noninfective cause of persistent low-grade fever, elevation of the white blood cell count, and mild-to-moderate "septic" hemodynamics is the host response to tissue injury. Large hematomas, traumatic injury to soft tissue, tissue ischemia without infection (particularly limb ischemia), and pulmonary contusion, atelectasis, or chemical pneumonitis are examples of this. Subarachnoid hemorrhage can produce a particularly severe febrile response, usually a few days following the acute bleed. However, the attribution of fever or apparent sepsis to any of these is always a diagnosis of exclusion which follows a careful evaluation for infection, and the diagnosis must be reconsidered at least daily. If correct, the pyrexia and other signs are generally low grade to begin with, and there is a stable elevation of temperature (rather than a hectic pattern) which gradually resolves without antimicrobial therapy.

Drug fever may also be a diagnosis of exclusion, but supporting evidence may be found if looked for carefully. Consideration of this possibility begins with an examination of the patient's medication list, looking for agents known to be more frequently associated with febrile reactions (see Table 97-6).[36,37] Next look for evidence of allergy or inflammatory changes in organ systems most frequently involved in adverse drug reactions. These include skin rashes, unexplained liver enzyme elevations, nephritis (active urinary sediment, unexplained serum creatinine increase, urinary eosinophilia), and hemolytic anemia or unexplained thrombocytopenia. When no other convincing explanation of pyrexia can be found and drug fever is suspected, withdrawal of the drug is usually the best course, substituting a chemically unrelated alternative if the original treatment indication remains.

EMPIRIC ANTIMICROBIAL THERAPY

As in primary sepsis, presumed infection threatening life or major organ function is an indication for empiric therapy. In sepsis occurring in hospitalized patients there is almost always one or more candidate sources for the sepsis, and organisms most frequently involved in infections from those sources should be included in the antimicrobial coverage. This will almost always include *Staph. aureus* and enteric aerobic gram-negative bacilli regardless of the suspected source of sepsis, while coverage for other bacteria

TABLE 97-6 Relative Frequency of Agents Implicated in Etiology of Drug Fever

Class of agents	Frequent	Infrequent or rare
Antimicrobials	β-Lactam agents, sulfonamides and cotrimoxazole, vancomycin, quinine, isoniazid, pyrazinamide, rifampin, amphotiricin B	Aminoglycosides, chloramphenicol, erythromycin, tetracyclines, clindamycin, metronidazole
Inotropic and vasoactive drugs	Hydralazine, methlydopa, amrinone	Digoxin, nitroprusside, nitrates, IV adrenergic agents
Antiarrhythmics	Quinidine, procainamide, amiodarone, atropine	Lidocaine, bretylium, β blockers
Antiepileptics analgesics and sedatives	Phenytoin, barbiturates, phenothiazines, salicylates (at toxic levels only)	Benzodiazepines, acetaminophen, opiates
Miscellaneous agents	Cytotoxic drugs, propylthiouracil, iodides (including IV contrast agents), histamine type 2 blockers	Corticosteroids, theophylline, inhaled bronchodilators, insulin

(anaerobes, *Legionella* spp., relatively resistant gram-positive bacteria, etc.) will depend on the suspected sources of sepsis. Entirely empiric therapy for fungi is generally not warranted except in neutropenic patients in whom antibacterial therapy is failing or in cases in which there is some evidence to support a diagnosis of invasive fungal infection.

More commonly, sepsis syndrome in patients already being treated in intensive care develops more insidiously. In these instances empiric therapy should be more specifically directed and only be undertaken after basic investigations have been performed and a working diagnosis made. This reduces the likelihood of making the major error of undertreating a serious undiagnosed infection and the perhaps less serious error of treating a noninfectious fever or minor infection with expensive and potentially toxic broad spectrum intravenous antimicrobials.

CASE PRESENTATION

A 46-year-old woman was admitted to hospital with acute upper gastrointestinal bleeding due to diffuse erosive gastritis and duodenitis related to ethanol abuse. The bleeding stopped with conservative management only and her condition stabilized. However, it was noted that she had symptoms of ethanol withdrawal and also that she had mild jaundice. The liver was large on examination and the abdomen slightly distended but without evidence of ascites. The serum bilirubin was elevated at 103 μmol/L, and all measured hepatic enzymes were moderately elevated. On the basis of the history and a CT scan of the abdomen confirming diffuse hepatic enlargement, the jaundice was attributed to alcoholic hepatitis.

On the fourth day following admission the patient developed an increased respiratory rate (35/min). Previously alert to slightly agitated, she became confused and drowsy. The temperature increased to 38.2°C. Blood pressure fell to 90/40 but rose to 120/70 after 1.5 L of saline was given intravenously. The abdomen remained distended and was slightly tender diffusely but was not felt to represent an acute abdomen. Chest examination and radiograph were not remarkable. Blood cultures and other repeat blood work were drawn and empiric intravenous clindamycin and gentamicin were begun.

The following day she remained tachypneic at 40/min. Her temperature rose to 39.5°C and her level of consciousness deteriorated; she now opened her eyes to a loud voice and localized pain only. The chest remained clear to examination but the abdomen was somewhat more distended. The white blood cell count was 18.0×10^9/L and the platelet count was 119×10^9/L. Prothrombin time was 13.1 s (control 11.1 s) and the glucose was 21 mmol/L. The bilirubin and hepatic enzymes had declined substantially from the previous values. The blood culture drawn the previous day demonstrated gram-negative bacilli.

Over the next few hours the blood pressure again became unstable and urine output ceased. The patient was then admitted to an intensive care unit. An endotracheal tube was inserted because of persistent hypotension and labored respiration and for airway protection. Mechanical ventilatory support was begun. Large-volume intravenous fluid resuscitation achieved a blood pressure of only 90/50 mmHg and urine output remained low. Dopamine was then infused through an internal jugular vein catheter and titrated to 12 μg/kg/min to achieve a mean blood pressure of 70 mmHg, which was associated with an increase in urine output to 60 mL/H. A pulmonary artery catheter was placed and demonstrated a cardiac output of 10.2 L/min and wedge pressure of 12 mmHg. Physical examination had changed only in that her distended, moderately tender abdomen now had easily demonstrable ascites. Paracentesis revealed purulent fluid with gram-negative bacilli on gram stain which subsequently proved to be *E. coli*, the same organism recovered from the blood. Repeat CT scan of the abdomen revealed only the enlarged liver and ascitic fluid. With a working diagnosis of alcoholic hepatitis with ascites complicated by spontaneous *E. coli* peritonitis, intravenous ampicillin and gentamicin were given. Paralytic ileus precluded enteral nutrition, so total parenteral nutrition was provided through a dedicated central venous catheter. Over the next 5 days the patient's condition gradually improved.

On the eleventh hospital day the temperature again rose to 39.5°C, heart and respiratory rates again increased, and mental obtundation, which had almost cleared, returned. A few hours later the blood pressure began to drop, requiring repeated infusions of intravenous fluid. Examination revealed only increased ascites and mild diffuse abdominal tenderness. Repeat paracentesis showed gram-negative bacilli but later grew out two different strains of *E. coli*. Repeat abdominal CT was unrevealing. Ampicillin and gentamicin were continued and metronidazole, 750 mg every 8 h, added. The following day *C. albicans* was detected on blood cultures and amphotericin B was added to the regimen. A clinically evident source for the fungemia other than the abdomen was not identified.

Two days later the abdominal signs persisted, mental obtundation and fever were not improved, the white blood cell count rose to 29×10^9/L, and the platelet count fell to 65×10^9/L. In addition there was recurrence of upper gastrointestinal bleeding. Contrast was placed in the stomach via the nasogastric tube and abdominal radiographs made at intervals to visualize the upper gastrointestinal tract. The contrast did not demonstrate a perforation. However, extraintestinal gas bubbles were seen in the left upper quadrant of the abdomen. Yet another abdominal CT was done, this time demonstrating a left upper quadrant abscess. The patient then went to laparotomy, which demonstrated a perforation of the descending colon with an adjacent jejunal perforation, necrotic pancreatic tail, and walled-off abscess in the left retroperitoneal area. The abscess was debrided and drained, the jejunal perforation closed, and a colostomy with Hartmann's procedure performed. Culture of the contents of the abscess yielded *E. coli, Peptostreptococcus* spp., *B. fragilis*, and *C. albicans*, so ampicillin, gentamicin, metronidazole, and amphotericin B were continued.

On the first two postoperative days the patient remained febrile and obtunded. She required intravenous dopamine and norepinephrine to maintain an acceptable blood pressure, and with this treatment had a good urine output. Cardiac output was 13 L/min. Moderate interstitial and alveolar pulmonary edema with an increase in oxygen requirement to maintain arterial oxygenation was managed with 7.5 cm H_2O positive end-expiratory pressure (PEEP). The white blood cell count remained elevated, and platelets fell as low as 15×10^9/L. The patient's condition then began to slowly improve. The platelet count first began to rise gradually, followed by a decrease in vasopressor requirement leading to their discontinuation 8 days after surgery. The pulmonary edema cleared, weaning from the ventilator begun at day 10 postsurgery, leading to extubation and transfer to a general ward service 5 days later. Fever began to decline at day 4 but was not absent until day 21. Antimicrobials were stopped 3½ weeks after surgery. All drains were removed, oral feeds successfully begun, and the patient discharged from hospital 77 days from admission.

CASE DISCUSSION

This case illustrates the diverse manifestations of sepsis and also how these manifestations can be used by the clinician as an indicator of patient progress and the need for further investigation. Following admission for upper gastrointestinal bleeding, the patient developed florid manifestations of sepsis leading to investigation and treatment for spontaneous bacterial peritonitis. Initially improving on this therapy, the patient again developed features of sepsis: fever, obtundation, tachypnea, hypotension, oliguria, and thrombocytopenia. Quite correctly, the persistence of these findings in the face of apparently appropriate antimicrobial therapy for aerobic and anaerobic bacteria and fungi did not lead simply to unsupported changes in antimicrobial therapy, but rather led to the persistence of efforts to establish a diagnosis, eventually leading to the correct diagnosis and definitive surgical therapy. In her postoperative course the patient took several days to improve. However, the trend toward overall improvement in the many features of the sepsis syndrome helped avoid unnecessary further investigation and shifts in antimicrobial therapy.

As seen in this case, features of the sepsis syndrome must be carefully looked for in critically ill patients and, when detected, must lead to systematic investigation for a source as well as empiric antimicrobial therapy and intensive supportive measures. Once therapy is instituted, these same features guide the clinician regarding the adequacy of the treatment regimen. Finally, the case illustrates that when the infectious source requires surgical drainage or debridement, sustained improvement is unlikely until definitive surgical treatment is completed; instability related to sepsis must not delay definitive therapy.

References

1. Harris RL, Musher DM, Bloom K, et al: Manifestations of sepsis. Arch Intern Med 147:1895, 1987.
2. Ziegler EJ, McCutchan JA, Fierer J, et al: Treatment of gram-negative bacteremia and shock with human antiserum to a mutant *Escherichia coli*. N Engl J Med 307:1225, 1982.
3. Veterans Administration Systemic Sepsis Cooperative Study Group: Effect of high-dose glucocorticoid therapy on mortality in patients with clinical signs of systemic sepsis. N Engl J Med 317:659, 1987.
4. Sheagren JN: *Staphylococcus aureus:* The persistent pathogen. N Engl J Med 310:1368, 1984.
5. Apicella MA: Neisseria meningitidis, in Mandell GL, Douglas RG Jr, Bennett JE (eds): *Principles and Practice of Infectious Diseases*, 3rd ed. New York, Churchill Livingstone, 1990, pp 1600–1613.
6. Bisno AL, Freeman JC: The syndrome of asplenia, pneumococcal sepsis and disseminated intravascular coagulation. Ann Intern Med 72:389, 1970.

7. Cohen JI, Bartlett JA, Corey GR: Extra-intestinal manifestations of salmonella infections. Medicine 66:349, 1987.
8. Hattwick MAW, Retailliau H, O'Brien RJ, et al: Fatal Rocky Mountain Spotted Fever. Arch Intern Med 240:1499, 1978.
9. Sainani GS, Dekate MP, Rao CP: Heart disease caused by coxsackie virus B infection. Br Heart J 37:819, 1975.
10. Gocke DJ: Extrahepatic manifestations of viral hepatitis. Am J Med Sci 270:49, 1975.
11. Okrent DG, Winston AE: Cardiorespiratory patterns in viral septicemia. Am J Med 83:681, 1987.
12. Allen JC: The diabetic as a compromised host, in Allen, JC (ed): *Infection and the Compromised Host. Clinical Correlations and Therapeutic Approaches,* 2nd ed. Baltimore, Williams & Wilkins, 1981, pp 229–270.
13. Yu VL, Goetz A, Wagener M, et al: *Staphylococcus aureus* carriage and infection in patients on hemodialysis. N Engl J Med 315:91, 1986.
14. Schwartz PE, Sterioff S, Mucha P, et al: Post-splenectomy sepsis and mortality in adults. J Am Med Assoc 284:2279, 1982.
15. Bryan CS, Reynolds KL, Brenner ER: Analysis of 1186 episodes of gram-negative bacteremia in non-university hospitals: The effects of antimicrobial therapy. Rev Infect Dis 5:629, 1983.
16. Smith CR, Ambinder R, Lipsky JJ, et al: Cefotaxime compared with nafcillin plus tobramycin for serious bacterial infections. Ann Intern Med 101:469, 1984.
17. Tally FP, Gorbach SL: Therapy of mixed anaerobic-aerobic infections. Am J Med 78:145, 1985.
18. Brumfitt W, Hamilton-Miller J: Methicillin-resistant *Staphylococcus aureus.* N Engl J Med 320:1188, 1989.
19. Douglas A, Moore-Gillon J, Eykyn S: Fever during treatment of infective endocarditis. Lancet 1:1341, 1986.
20. Heseltine PNR, Yellin AE, Appleman MD, et al: Perforated and gangrenous appendicitis: An analysis of antibiotic failures. Rev Infect Dis 148:322, 1983.
21. Rutledge R, Mandel SR, Wild RE: Candida species: Insignificant contaminant or pathogenic species. Ann Surg 52:299, 1986.
22. Bayer AS, Blumenkrantz MJ, Montgomerie JZ, et al: Candida peritonitis: Report of 22 cases and review of the English literature. Am J Med 61:832, 1976.
23. Sanders WE, Sanders CC: Inducible β-lactamase: Clinical and epidemiological implications for use of newer cephalosporins. Rev Infect Dis 10:830, 1988.
24. O'Reilly MJ, Reddick EJ, Black W, et al: Sepsis from sinusitis in nasotracheally intubated patients. Am J Surg 147:601, 1984.
25. Grindlinger GA, Niehoff J, Hughes SL, Humphrey MA, Simpson G: Acute paranasal sinusitis related to nasotracheal intubation of head-injured patients. Crit Care Med 15:214, 1987.
26. Raad II, Sabbagh MF, Caranasos GJ: Acute bacterial sialadenitis: A study of 29 cases and review. Rev Infect Dis 12:591, 1990.
27. Meduri GU: Ventilator-associated pneumonia in patients with respiratory failure: A diagnostic approach. Chest 97:1208, 1990.
28. Fekety R: Antibiotic-associated colitis, in Mandell GL, Douglas RG, Jr, Bennett JE (eds): *Principles and Practice of Infectious Diseases,* 3rd ed. New York, Churchill Livingstone, 1990, pp 863–869.
29. Marton KI, Doubilet P: How to image the gallbladder in suspected cholecystitis. Ann Intern Med 109:722, 1988.
30. Lundstedt C, Hederstrom E, Brismar J, Holmin T, Strand S-E: Prospective investigation of radiologic methods in the diagnosis of intra-abdominal abscess. Acta Radiol Diag 27:49, 1986.
31. Maki DG: Nosocomial bacteremia: An epidemiological overview. Am J Med 70:719, 1981.
32. Harvey RL, Myers JP: Nosocomial fungemia in a large community teaching hospital. Arch Intern Med 147:2117, 1987.
33. Maki DG, Weise CE, Sarfin HW: A semiquantitative culture method for identifying intravenous catheter-related infections. N Engl J Med 296:1305, 1977.
34. Bozzetti F, Terno G, Bonfanti G, et al: Prevention and treatment of central venous catheter sepsis by exchange via a guidewire: A prospective controlled trial. Ann Surg 198:48, 1983.
35. Flyn PM, Shenep JL, Stokes DC, Barrett FF: In situ management of confirmed central venous catheter-related bacteremia. Pediatr Infect Dis J 6:729, 1987.
36. Lipsky BA, Hirschmann JV: Drug fever. J Am Med Assoc 245:851, 1981.
37. Cunha BA: Drug fever: The importance of recognition. Postgrad Med 80:123, 1986.

Chapter 98
SEPTIC SHOCK

R. BRUCE LIGHT

KEY POINTS

- *Sepsis is the most common cause of shock in most ICUs and is a leading cause of death.*
- *Effective management requires prompt recognition that shock is present based mainly on clinical criteria—evidence of inadequate major organ perfusion (mental obtundation, confusion, or oliguria) associated with hypotension and a potential source of sepsis.*
- *Attribution of a shock state to sepsis is based on recognition of features of the sepsis syndrome (mental changes; hyperventilation; hyperdynamic circulation; elevated, reduced, or left-shifted white blood cell (WBC) count; thrombocytopenia; elevated or reduced temperature) in addition to a potential source of infection.*
- *Immediate resuscitation and cardiorespiratory stabilization are the first priority in septic shock. This usually requires infusion of large volumes of fluid intravenously, infusion of vasoactive drugs when fluid is insufficient, and often endotracheal intubation for mechanical ventilation.*
- *Intravenous empirical antimicrobial therapy directed at all potential infectious sources of more than trivial probability should be given as early as possible. Coverage should always include* Staphylococcus aureus *and the common facultatively aerobic enteric gram-negative bacilli.*
- *Initial basic investigation should always include a thorough physical examination, chest x-ray, and cultures of blood, sputum, and urine. As soon as cardiorespiratory stability is achieved, further investigations needed to establish a source of sepsis should proceed expeditiously, based on the results of the initial evaluation.*
- *Infectious processes requiring surgical drainage or debridement should be surgically treated promptly. Cardiorespiratory instability is usually not an acceptable reason to delay surgical treatment if persistent sepsis is the cause of the instability.*
- *Careful attention to metabolic homeostasis and nutrition is essential to maximize the likelihood of healing and to avoid complications and progressive multisystem organ failure.*

Serious bacterial infection at any body site, with or without bacteremia, is usually associated with important changes in the function of every organ system of the body, changes which are mostly mediated by elements of the host defense system against infection. Among the most important of these changes are the hemodynamic consequences of systemic vasodilation resulting in hyperdynamic circulation, widened pulse pressure, tachycardia, and hypotension. In the great majority of cases administration of additional intravenous fluids, together with efforts to localize and treat infection, results in maintenance of adequate blood pressure and tissue perfusion. Shock is deemed to be present when such volume replacement fails to increase blood pressure to acceptable levels and there is clinical evidence of inadequate perfusion of major organ systems with progressive failure of organ system function. Even with the best modern intensive care supportive methods, more than half the patients meeting this clinical definition of septic shock die, either immediately because the shock cannot be reversed or later because of the ongoing systemic effects of serious infection or the underlying disease. Intensive care management of septic shock, like the management of other forms of shock, demands a rapid but thorough early clinical evaluation and urgent immediate resuscitative efforts carried on in parallel with efforts to determine the source of the sepsis and properly directed empirical antimicrobial therapy. When initial resuscitation has been accomplished and the diagnosis established, definitive medical and surgical management of the infectious problem follows, with continued careful attention to organ system dysfunctions which develop as a result of sepsis. Probably no other entity in critical care practice demands as much from the intensivist in clinical management skills since exemplary care involves both rapid stabilization of the patient from an immediately life-threatening situation and meticulous longer term attention to the many system dysfunctions which develop during sepsis, informed empirical treatment measures along with thoughtful differential diagnosis and progress toward definitive specific therapy, and the coordination of the efforts of the frequently numerous subspecialists which become involved in the care of these patients.

Pathogenesis

A more detailed review of the pathogenesis of the sepsis syndrome can be found in Chap. 55. The fundamental event leading initially to sepsis syndrome and subsequently to shock relates primarily to an interaction between elements of the host immune system and macromolecular constituents of the infecting bacteria. Mononuclear phagocytes coming in contact with such microbial macromolecules are known to release important cytokines, among them interleukin-1 (IL-1) and cachectin, which act as hormones mediating changes in the metabolic and physiologic function of cells throughout the body. Fever, WBC activation and release from bone marrow, changes in hepatic synthetic function, changes in patterns of energy utilization, and increased vascular permeability are all among the effects mediated by these compounds.[1,2] Elevated blood levels of both cachectin and IL-1 are known to be present in many patients with septic shock and have been linked to both the shock state and to severity of illness.[3,4]

The most important mediator effects in the pathogenesis of shock are those that lead to reduced effective circulating blood volume and vasodilation. Cachectin, for example, is known to directly and indirectly cause damage to endothelial surfaces of capillaries resulting in loss of intravascular fluid into the extracellular space, and it is also known to modify cell membrane function in skeletal muscle such that fluid is sequestered within cells. In addition to these important cytokine effects, bacterial macromolecules interact directly with humoral components of the host immune system and the coagulation cascade. Complement may be activated both by antibody-antigen interactions with bacterial constituents or directly by the alternate complement activation pathway. Activated locally at the site of an infection, the complement system leads to chemotaxis for polymorphonuclear leukocytes, activation of these leukocytes, and release of a variety of mediators of inflammation producing increased capillary permeability and vasodilation. Interaction between microbial cell wall constituent antigens and Hageman factor leads to activation of the coagulation system, the fibrinolytic system, and production of active mediators from the kinin system, notably bradykinin, a potent vasodilator.[5] These local consequences of serious bacterial infection may become systemically manifest in one of two ways. First, when the local inflammation is intense, cytokines and other inflammatory mediators from the local inflammatory process may spill over into the systemic circulation. Alternatively, penetration of the locally invading bacteria into the vascular system may lead to bacteremia or fragments of partially destroyed bacteria may be absorbed into the systemic circulation producing antigenemia or toxemia, in either case leading to systemic activation of these inflammatory responses.

Pathophysiology

As noted above, the pathogenetic events leading to shock due to sepsis revolve around vasodilation and reduction in effective circulating plasma volume. An additional effect, with an as yet ill-defined pathogenesis, is relative depression of myocardial contractility. In the early phases of septic shock the hemodynamic consequences of reduced circulating blood volume and vasodilation predominate.[6,7] This is illustrated in Fig. 98-1. Vasodilation on the arterial side of the circulation leads to a decline in systemic vascular resistance (SVR). With the decline in SVR, blood pressure falls unless cardiac output increases enough to maintain blood pressure despite the fall in resistance. In early sepsis and in the presence of otherwise normal cardiovascular function, cardiac output generally does increase and blood pressure is initially maintained, the main manifestations of the reduced arterial resistance being a widened pulse pressure and clinically hyperdynamic circulation. Cardiac output in this phase is relatively well maintained because a fall in the resistance of the peripheral circulation at large leads to an increase in venous return despite a fall in the pressure in systemic capacitance blood vessels caused by the systemic vasodilation and loss of plasma volume to the extravascular space. Hypotension results when cardiac output is not maintained at an adequately increased level in the face of a reduced SVR. This occurs when venous return is compromised by excessive vasodilation or loss of circulating plasma volume or when inadequate myocardial reserve makes it impossible for the host to increase cardiac output sufficiently. Hypotension due to inadequate venous return in the early stages of sepsis is usually readily reversed by plasma volume expansion. When such volume replacement alone does not reverse the hypotension, septic shock is said to be present.

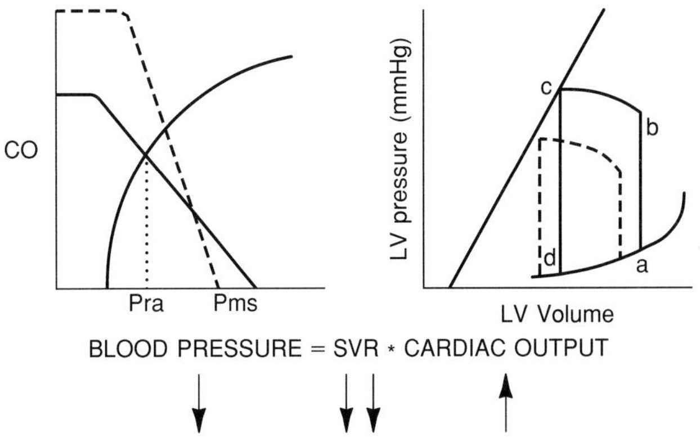

FIGURE 98-1 Cardiovascular changes of early sepsis. In the left-hand panel a cardiac function curve relating cardiac output (or venous return [VR]) to right atrial pressures (Pra) is shown, together with curves relating venous return to the difference between mean systemic pressure (Pms) and right atrial pressure. Pms, the intercept of the venous return line on the Pra axis, is the mean systemic pressure in the body's capacitance vessels, itself determined by the blood volume and the compliance of capacitance blood vessels. The inverse of the slope of the venous return line is called the resistance to venous return (RVR = [Pms − Pra]/VR), determined by the caliber and capacitance of venous vessels and the distribution of cardiac output, which are mainly a function of vasomotor tone. Normal values are illustrated by the solid lines, early sepsis by the interrupted line. Note that sepsis reduces Pms (because of vasodilation and extravascular fluid sequestration) but at the same time reduces RVR. This leads to an increase in cardiac output with a modest increase in Pra. If the cardiac function curve were shifted to the left, which it may be in sepsis because of adrenergic stimulation and reduced vascular resistance to ventricular ejection, the elevated cardiac output is associated with a reduced Pra.

In the right-hand panel, a left ventricular pressure-volume plot is shown, the solid lines illustrating the normal end-systolic pressure volume relationship which defines ventricular contractility (straight line), the normal diastolic pressure-volume relationship (curved line) and a single cardiac cycle beginning at the end-diastolic pressure volume point (a) which is approximately the pulmonary wedge pressure, proceeding to the end of isovolumic ventricular contraction (b), end systole (c) and the end of isovolumic relaxation (d). In sepsis (interrupted lines), arterial vasodilation reduces end-systolic pressure which tends to increase stroke volume (distance b–c on the LV volume axis). In addition, reduced RVR increases venous return, maintaining near-normal end-diastolic pressure and volume, and tending to increase stroke volume, pulse pressure, and cardiac output, especially when heart rate is also increased via baroreceptor reflexes. Hypotension results when the increase in cardiac output is insufficient to compensate for the effect of the low SVR.

Even in these earliest stages of septic shock, it is now known that depression of myocardial function contributes in some measure to the failure of volume repletion to lead to an increase in cardiac output sufficient to reverse hypotension.[8] However, because the cardiac output in this stage is usually high, myocardial dysfunction is not seen as the chief problem. In later stages of sepsis, myocardial depression becomes increasingly prominent, eventually leading to a decline in cardiac output to normal or below normal levels, intractable hypotension, inadequate perfusion of major organ systems, progressive anoxic-ischemic damage to tissues, and death.

Even in the presence of a clinically acceptable blood pressure and cardiac output, there is abundant evidence that systemic distribution of blood flow is abnormal and that energy substrate and oxygen utilization may be impaired.[9,10] Although the pathogenesis of this phenomenon has yet to be fully worked out, it is likely that systemic vasodilation with impairment of the ability of local microvasculature to optimally distribute arterial blood flow is a major factor. This results in the passage of oxygenated arterial blood to tissues which do not require this blood flow to sustain metabolism (which has been termed "nonnutrient blood flow"), while at the same time other tissues, possibly with damaged or plugged microvasculature, are receiving inadequate nutrient blood flow to sustain aerobic metabolism. Overall, this is manifest as a high cardiac output with above normal delivery of oxygenated blood to the body associated with a high mixed venous oxygen tension ($C\bar{v}_{O_2}$) (indicating low extraction of oxygen) together with clinical evidence of inadequate perfusion of some organ systems and systemic lactic acidosis[10–12] (Fig. 98-2). An alternative or additional potential explanation for the failure of body tissues to extract and use oxygen in the face of an above normal supply is the notion of a "metabolic block" due to sepsis. The evidence supporting this possibility is that excess blood lactate in sepsis may be associated with a high blood pyruvate and a normal lactate:pyruvate ratio, an observation compatible with the absence of anaerobic metabolism.[13] Occurring mostly in more chronic sepsis and in the absence of acidemia, this may imply that low fractional extraction of oxygen by tissues can simply be a consequence of the high cardiac output, while excess lactate accumulation can be due to a direct metabolic effect unrelated to inadequate tissue oxygen delivery (see Chap. 56). However, oxygen delivery inadequacy must be regarded as the principle abnormality underlying lactic acidosis in most acutely septic patients, since lactic acidosis generally does improve when oxygen delivery is increased.[11,12]

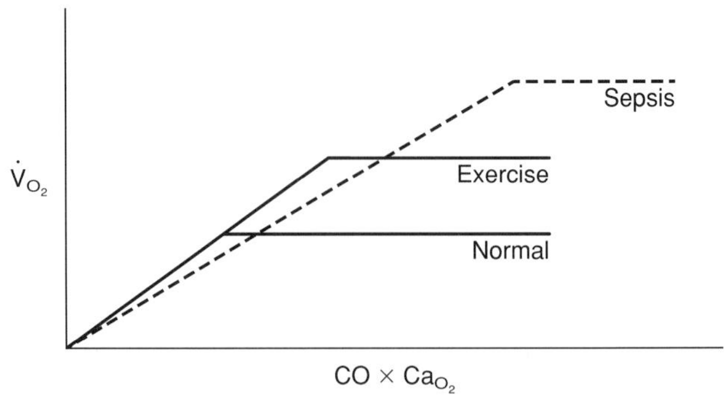

FIGURE 98-2 Relationship between whole body oxygen consumption ($\dot{V}_{O_2}$) and oxygen delivery, the product of cardiac output (CO) and arterial oxygen content (Ca_{O_2}). Normally, $\dot{V}_{O_2}$ is unrelated to CO and Ca_{O_2} over a wide range but begins to fall when either CO or Ca_{O_2} (or both) are insufficient to maintain aerobic metabolism. During exercise both $\dot{V}_{O_2}$ and O_2 delivery increase and the anaerobic threshold for O_2 delivery is also increased. Sepsis also increases $\dot{V}_{O_2}$, but extraction of oxygen from the arterial blood by tissues is impaired. This "flattens" the slope of the relationship (i.e., higher O_2 delivery needed to maintain a given $\dot{V}_{O_2}$) and further increases the anaerobic threshold.

Diagnosis

HIGH CARDIAC OUTPUT HYPOTENSION—THE HEMODYNAMIC DIAGNOSIS

A systolic blood pressure <90 mmHg with evidence of inadequate organ perfusion is termed septic shock when the hypotension is primarily attributable to sepsis-induced vasodilation and when hypotension does not reverse with acute plasma volume expansion of at least 1 L, usually more. The clinical diagnosis is frequently straightforward, particularly when an evident serious infection such as pneumonia, acute pyelonephritis, or an acute abdomen is associated both with shock and the typical clinical features of the sepsis syndrome: fever or hypothermia, mental obtundation, hyperventilation, hot flushed skin, and a wide pulse pressure.[14] The absence of some or all of these features may make the diagnosis more difficult. Elderly, debilitated, or immunosuppressed patients may present without obvious features of a localized infection and may not exhibit a fever. In addition, patients with poor cardiac function or who are more severely volume depleted may have sepsis-induced hypotension but with low pulse volume and cold mottled skin similar to that seen in cardiogenic or hypovolemic shock. Because other forms of shock also produce oliguria and mental obtundation, these are not specific for sepsis unless the mental obtundation or confusional state precedes the onset of severe hypotension. Acute hyperventilation can also be an early clue to the onset of sepsis.

Basic laboratory investigations can be helpful in suggesting sepsis as the etiology of a shock state. The WBC count is usually elevated and left shifted; when the WBC count is low in septic patients in the absence of prior cytotoxic therapy peripheral WBCs are almost all young or immature forms. Thrombocytopenia is frequently seen. Even in the absence of clinically obvious hyperventilation, arterial blood-gas values often demonstrate a respiratory alkalosis, sometimes with mild hypoxemia. Metabolic acidosis with an elevated blood lactate concentration is usual prior to adequate resuscitation.

The differential diagnosis of septic shock includes the other nonseptic causes of hypotension associated with a low SVR, and the forms of shock generally associated with a vasoconstricted peripheral circulation: an obstructed circulation due to an embolism or tamponade, cardiogenic shock, and hypovolemic shock. Hypotension associated with a low SVR is common in severe liver disease and can be produced by allergic reactions to food or drugs, overdosage with drugs with vasodilator properties, toxic shock syndrome, primary or secondary adrenal insufficiency, arteriovenous fistula, and rarely, severe thiamine deficiency or thyroid storm. Anaphylaxis is generally also associated with bronchospasm or laryngeal edema and allergic skin manifestations, while toxic shock syndrome has several relatively specific differentiating findings (see Chap. 113). The history of drug ingestion or exposure usually identifies those patients with vasodilator drug overdose, while overdose with sedative-hypnotic drugs, which may be complicated by hypotension, is usually evident from the presence of a severely depressed level of consciousness.

When the origin of the shock state remains unclear after careful clinical evaluation or when the shock is felt to be multifactorial in origin, pulmonary artery catheterization is frequently helpful in establishing the diagnosis and guiding subsequent therapy. The major forms of shock have relatively characteristic patterns of hemodynamic measurements detailed elsewhere (see Chap. 114). For septic shock, following adequate fluid resuscitation marked by a pulmonary wedge pressure of >10 mmHg, the cardiac output is generally above normal while the blood pressure is below normal, yielding a low calculated SVR. Typically, the arteriovenous oxygen content difference $(a - v)_{O_2}$ is also low and the mixed venous oxygen tension is high, generally above 35 mmHg. There are two main pitfalls to be aware of. First, virtually all of the causes of low SVR noted above will also be associated with these hemodynamic and arteriovenous oxygen patterns. Other diseases associated with shunting of arterial blood directly into the venous circulation can also produce these patterns. These include arteriovenous fistulae, intracardiac left-to-right shunts due to atrial or ventricular septal defects, and Paget's disease of bone. Secondly, patients with hypotension attributable to multiple causes may exhibit a hemodynamic pattern which is not typical of any one entity. The most common such circumstance is serious compromise of cardiac function associated with sepsis. In such cases, the SVR is either low or simply lower than expected in a patient with cardiac dysfunction. The cardiac output, on the other hand, is neither as high as would be expected for septic shock nor as low as expected for cardiogenic shock.

DIAGNOSIS OF THE ETIOLOGY OF SEPTIC SHOCK

The history and physical examination, together with a few basic laboratory investigations, usually yield a presumptive diagnosis of the source of sepsis. For practical purposes, these include **1.** central nervous system (CNS) infection, **2.** chest infections, **3.** intraabdominal sepsis, **4.** skin or soft tissue infections, or **5.** primary bacteremia syndromes. In each of these categories, it is mainly those infections which are most extensive or most likely to produce bacteremia that are implicated in septic shock (Table 98-1).

The CNS infection most often associated with shock is acute bacterial meningitis, usually with bacteremia. Community-acquired meningitis with shock is almost always due to *Streptococcus pneumoniae* or *Neisseria meningitidis.* Most such patients have nuchal rigidity and depressed level of consciousness as well. Bacteremia with shock due to *S. pneumoniae* can precede clinically obvious meningitis, but may be associated with pneumonia evident on the chest radiograph. Meningococcemia can also present with shock without meningismus. The major diagnostic clue in these cases is the petechial rash prominent in most (see Plate 34). In hospitalized patients who have undergone a neurosurgical procedure or who have a basal skull fracture with cerebrospinal fluid (CSF) leak, *S. aureus* or enteric gram-negative bacilli are also important causes of meningitis; however, presentation primarily with a shock syndrome is unusual. Brain abscess, subdural or epidural empyema, and viral CNS infections may all cause critical illness mainly due to direct CNS effects, but are also seldom associated with shock as part of the initial presentation.

In the thorax, the major entities commonly leading to septic shock are acute bacterial pneumonia, generally due to highly invasive pyogenic organisms such as *S. pneumoniae, S. aureus,* enteric gram-negative bacilli or *Legionella pneumophila,* empyema, usually caused by similar pathogens, and mediastinitis due to esophageal perforation. The physical examination and chest radiograph virtually always suggest the diagnosis of pneumonia or empyema in cases of sufficient severity to cause shock. The diagnosis of esophageal perforation is usually suggested by the clinical context—an episode of vomiting or swallowing a sharp or pointed object in outpatients, vomiting or recent esophagoscopy with mucosal injection or esophageal dilation in patients already being treated for an esophageal abnormality. The chest radiograph may show mediastinal air, suggesting the diagnosis, which can usually be established by a contrast esophogram.

Intraabdominal processes, as a group, account for the largest number of cases of septic shock and most are causes of an acute surgical abdomen (see Chap. 85). In the biliary tree, suppurative cholangitis and empyema of the gallbladder are the main considerations. Perforation of the bowel (particularly the colon) with fecal peritonitis and mesenteric ischemia are the more common entities involving the bowel. In the female, septic abortion and postpartum endometritis/myometritis are additional potential sources of sepsis in the abdomen. Acute pancreatitis, even without active infection, can mimic septic shock and later in the course when secondary infection is present is an important cause of septic shock. For all of these, potentially involved bacteria include the facultatively aerobic enteric gram-negative bacilli, aerobic and microaerophilic streptococci, and mixed enteric anaerobic bacteria including *Clostridia* and *Bacteroides fragilis* group. Acute pyelonephritis can also occasionally present with shock; ureteric obstruction with pyonephrosis is often present in such cases. The bacteria involved are usually enteric gram-negatives such as *Escherichia coli*

TABLE 98-1 Major Bacterial Infection Syndromes Associated with Septic Shock

Infection Syndrome	Common Bacterial Pathogens
Primary Bacteremia	
Community-acquired infection in the normal host	*Staphylococcus aureus* *Streptococcus pneumoniae* *Neisseria meningitidis* *Salmonella species*
IV drug abusers, infected IV access in hospital and granulocytopenia	*S. aureus* *Pseudomonas aeruginosa* *Enterobacteriaceae*
Bacteremic Meningitis	*N. meningitidis* *S. pneumoniae*
Acute Bacterial Pneumonia	
Community-acquired	*S. pneumoniae* *S. aureus* *Enterobacteriaceae* *Legionella pneumophila*
Hospital-acquired	*Enterobacteriaceae* *P. aeruginosa* *S. aureus* *Legionella species*
Mediastinitis	Mixed aerobic and anaerobic bacteria
Intraabdominal Sepsis	
Suppurative cholangitis and cholecystitis Peritonitis (from perforation) Mesenteric ischemia Abscess (peritoneal, pancreatic, perihepatic etc) Septic abortion, endometritis	Mixed enteric aerobic and anaerobic bacteria, including *Enterobacteriaceae,* streptococci and *Bacteroides fragilis* group.
Pyelyonephritis, pyonephrosis, renal and perinephric abscess	*Enterobacteriaceae* *Enterococcus* *Pseudomonas species*
Skin and Soft Tissue Infections	
Simple cellulitis or erysipelas with bacteremia	*S. aureus* *Streptococcus pyogenes*
Cellulitis in IV drug users	*P. aeruginosa* *S. aureus*
Necrotizing cellulitides and fasciitis	Mixed enteric aerobic and anaerobic bacteria

but may be streptococci, especially enterococci. When any of these diagnoses are suspected on the basis of the physical examination, the next step following basic resuscitation is generally an imaging procedure for confirmation. Flat and upright radiographs of the abdomen are useful to detect free air associated with perforation. Abdominal ultrasound is the initial procedure of choice for suspect biliary tract sepsis, perihepatic or pancreatic abscess, or pyonephrosis. Computed tomography (CT) is also useful for these diagnoses and is more useful in defining intraabdominal abscesses. Angiography is usually necessary to exclude or demonstrate suspect mesenteric ischemia.

The major skin and soft tissue infections associated with shock are the various forms of cellulitis. Most common is cellulitis due to *S. aureus* or *Streptococcus pyogenes.* In intravenous drug abusers, soft tissue infections may also be due to aerobic gram-negative bacilli, particularly *Pseudomonas species.* Cases with shock are usually clinically obvious, extensive, and associated with bacteremia. Seemingly minor staphylococcal infections complicated by shock may represent toxic shock syndrome (see Chap. 113). Necrotizing soft tissue infections, generally due to mixed aerobic and anaerobic bacteria of enteric origin are also important causes of shock; these are reviewed in detail in Chap. 106.

Septic shock without findings suggestive of meningitis or intrathoracic, intraabdominal, or soft tissue infection may be due to a septic process in one of these areas that has been missed on the initial evaluation, a primary bacteremia or endocarditis syndrome, or to nonbacterial or noninfectious causes. In outpatients presenting with apparent sepsis without localizing findings, the most common primary bacteremia is caused by *S. aureus. S. pneumoniae* and *N. meningitidis* are also occasional causes in the apparently nonimmunocompromised host, while *Haemophilus influen-*

zae and *Salmonella species* are additional important pathogens in patients with an absent or dysfunctional spleen. In intravenous drug abusers, *Pseudomonas aeruginosa* bacteremia or endocarditis is seen. In hospitalized patients, bacteremia due to an infected intravascular catheter is a major cause of sepsis, as is primary bacteremia from the gastrointestinal mucosa in granulocytopenic patients undergoing chemotherapy for malignancy. Nonbacterial and noninfectious causes of apparent sepsis of unclear origin are reviewed in more detail in Chap. 97.

The basic investigation for the etiology of septic shock begins with the physical examination, with emphasis on detecting or excluding the diagnoses noted above. Some clues to diagnosis may be available from the basic laboratory investigation performed as part of the initial evaluation. Granulocytopenia or marked leftshift of the WBC count suggests severe sepsis with bacteremia, unless the granulocytopenia is due to underlying marrow suppression, in which case the possibility of a primary bacteremia with an enteric organism is more strongly considered. Elevated serum bilirubin, alkaline phosphatase, and γ-glutaryl transferase levels suggest biliary obstruction. An elevated serum creatinine content early in the course raises the possibility of pyelonephritis or pyonephrosis, as do pyuria or WBC casts on urinalysis. Respiratory alkalosis and a degree of metabolic acidosis are usual in all forms of sepsis; however, progressive and severe acidosis out of proportion to the apparent deficit in peripheral perfusion is a marker for mesenteric ischemia. A chest radiograph is part of the basic investigation in all patients, as is a flat and upright abdominal radiograph except in patients with a completely benign abdomen or an obvious alternate source of sepsis.

Bacterial cultures of blood and urine should be obtained in all septic patients. Gram staining and culture of respiratory secretions are obtained as well unless the chest radiograph convincingly excludes a pulmonary infiltrate. Needle aspirates for Gram stain and aerobic and anaerobic bacterial culture should also be obtained from all other suspect sites, including pleural or peritoneal fluid, if present, abscess or sinus drainage, joint effusions, and clinically evident soft tissue infections. A lumbar puncture for CSF examination and culture is indicated in patients with nuchal rigidity and those with headache or mental obtundation in whom another septic focus is not identified.

Many patients will already have been given antimicrobial therapy when first seen, particularly if they have been transferred from another hospital or service or if they are postoperative. Although this may somewhat reduce the yield of subsequent cultures, in most infections some days are required to sterilize infected sites, and the intensivist should not be dissuaded from obtaining all the appropriate specimens. Commercially available devices to remove antimicrobials from blood samples are widely used to try to increase the yield from blood cultures in patients already receiving antibiotics; however, there is little evidence that they are more effective than simply repeating conventional blood cultures.

A Gram stain of material from the infected site is generally the only immediately available laboratory test useful in selecting antimicrobial therapy. It can be considered virtually diagnostic when a purulent specimen obtained from a normally sterile site is seen to contain large numbers of a single typical bacterial morphotype. Examples include pneumococci or meningococci seen on Gram stain of CSF, staphylococci seen in pus from an abscess cavity or empyema fluid, large gram-positive bacilli consistent with *Clostridia* from a needle aspirate of a necrotizing fasciitis, or gram-negative bacilli typical of Enterobacteriaceae from a nephrostomy placed to drain a pyonephrosis. However, in most cases a diagnostic Gram stain will not be available. Empirical antimicrobial therapy will usually have to be selected based on the differential diagnosis and clinical setting, awaiting the results of cultures. Most pyogenic bacteria grow relatively quickly on artificial media; it is, therefore, worthwhile for the clinician to communicate with the microbiology laboratory 24 h after cultures are sent, since potentially useful preliminary results may be available at this time. Definitive organism identification and antimicrobial susceptibilities generally require a further 24 h, while results of cultures for anaerobic bacteria often take 72 h or more.

Management

INFECTION MANAGEMENT

EMPIRICAL ANTIMICROBIAL THERAPY. All patients with compromised cardiorespiratory status related to serious infection should receive empirical intravenous antimicrobial therapy immediately. Agents should be selected which provide coverage for organisms likely to cause infection at all identified potential infection sites of more than trivial probability, since it is known that patients with septic shock who receive what later proves to be inadequate antimicrobial therapy are much less likely to survive than if the initial regimen covers the infecting organism.[15,16] Specific recommendations for antimicrobial selection can be found in the chapters relating to the specific infections, and suggested empirical regimens for presumptive therapy of patients with septic shock are shown in Table 98-2. In virtually all cases of septic shock the empirical antimicrobial regimen should be administered intravenously and should include coverage for *S. aureus* and the common facultatively aerobic enteric gram-negatives such as *E. coli* and *Klebsiella species.* A third generation cephalosporin such as cefotaxime, ceftriaxone, or ceftizoxime is usually chosen for this purpose and is given at a dose at the higher end of the suggested dose range for the drug.[17] These agents will also effectively cover the common community-acquired bacteremic CNS infections. Third generation cephalosporins are also reasonable coverage for most causes of acute bacterial pneumonia; however, most clinicians add an intravenous aminoglycoside in severe cases to ensure excellent gram-negative coverage and at least consider the addition of erythromycin for *L. pneumophila.* Mediastinitis due to esophageal perforation, intraabdominal sepsis originating from bowel, the biliary tract or the female genital tract, fulminant hospital-acquired

TABLE 98-2 Empirical Antimicrobial Therapy for Septic Shock

Suspected Source of Sepsis	Recommended Antimicrobial Regimen	Alternative Agents
Primary Bacteremia (no source evident)		
Normal host	Third generation cephlosporin: cefotaxime 2 g IV q6h or cefriaxone 2 g IV q12h or ceftizoxime 2 g IV q8h	Nafcillin and gentamicin, Chloramphenicol and gentamicin, imipenem
IV drug user	Ceftazadime 2 g IV q8h and Nafcillin 2 g IV q4h	Piperacillin and gentamicin, imipenem
Immunocompromised host	Piperacillin 3 g IV q4h and Gentamicin 1.5 mg/kg IV q8h	Ceftazadime and nafcillin, imipenem and gentamicin
Bacteremic Meningitis	Third generation cephalosporin as above	Ampicillin
Cellulitis/Erysipelas	Nafcillin 2 g IV q4h	Cefazolin, vancomycin, clindamycin
Acute Bacterial Pneumonia		
Community-acquired	Third generation cephalosporin as above ± erythromycin 1 g IV q6h	Clindamycin and cotrimoxazole, imipenem ± erythromycin
Hospital-acquired	Third generation cephalosporin as above and gentamicin 1.5 mg/kg IV q8h ± erythromycin 1 g IV q6h	As above
Mixed Aerobic/Anaerobic Infections		
Intraabdominal infections Mediastinitis Fulminant aspiration pneumonia Necrotizing cellulitides and fasciitis Septic abortion, endometritis	Third generation cephalosporin and clindamycin 600 mg IV q8h OR Metronidazole 500 mg IV q8h and ampicillin 2 g IV q4h and gentamicin 1.5 mg/kg IV q8h	Imipenem and gentamicin, piperacillin and gentamicin, cefoxitin and gentamicin, clindamycin and cotrimoxazole
Urinary Tract Infection	Ampicillin 2 g IV q4h and gentamicin 1.5 mg/kg IV q8h	Third generation cephalosporin, ± gentamicin

aspiration pneumonia, and necrotizing cellulitides all require the addition of antimicrobial coverage for anaerobic bacteria, particularly *B. fragilis* group, in addition to agents for aerobic staphylococci, streptococci, and enteric gram-negatives. A variety of regimens are effective. Examples include clindamycin, metronidazole, or chloramphenicol with a third generation cephalosporin; metronidazole with ampicillin and an aminoglycoside; clindamycin, cefoxitin, or imipenem and an aminoglycoside; and clindamycin with intravenous cotrimoxazole or ciprofloxacin.

Some patients are predictably at special risk for infection with organisms known to be relatively resistant to antimicrobials. Patients at risk for infection with resistant gram-negatives such as *P. aeruginosa* include intravenous drug abusers, hospitalized patients who have already been treated with antimicrobial agents, granulocytopenic patients receiving chemotherapy for malignancy, and patients being cared for in units with an endemic or epidemic infection problem with a resistant strain (e.g., burn units, many ICUs). Addition of an agent likely to be effective against these pathogens is advisable. Piperacillin with an aminoglycoside is widely used in this setting, as is ceftazadime combined with other agents to cover staphylococci and anaerobes as indicated; however, the regimen selected must be designed based on knowledge of local resistance patterns. Methicillin-resistant *S. aureus* is also a major problem in many hospitals, mandating the addition of intravenous vancomycin in most cases of septic shock which might involve this organism.

SURGICAL MANAGEMENT. More than half of all cases of septic shock seen in most ICUs are due to infections requiring urgent surgical management. These include infections associated with an obstructed hollow viscus such as suppurative cholangitis or pyonephrosis with ureteric obstruction, abscesses, and infections associated with tissue necrosis such as bowel infarction due to mesenteric ischemia or necrotizing soft tissue infections. Although some of these infections (e.g., suppurative cholangitis) may stabilize initially with supportive measures and antimicrobial therapy and permit later elective surgical management, in most cases surgical treatment should proceed as soon as basic resuscitation has been completed. When a relatively limited procedure, such as ultrasound or CT-guided percutaneous drainage of an infected site can achieve effective drainage, this is generally the procedure of choice (see Chapter 20). More extensive operative procedures are generally required for infections involving necrotic tissue. Continued cardiorespiratory instability due to uncontrolled sepsis in the face of supportive measures and appropriate antimicrobial therapy is not a reason to delay surgical therapy. Rather, this is an indication for prompt drainage or debridement of the source of the infection causing the continued instability.

IMMUNOTHERAPY. Several clinical trials have shown that plasma containing antibody against gram-negative lipopolysaccharide (endotoxin) reduces mortality when given as adjunctive therapy for septic shock due to aerobic gram-negative organisms.[18,19] Monoclonal antibodies against endotoxin have also recently been developed and the results of early clinical trials in septic patients are encouraging.[20] While not generally available at the time of this writing, it is to be expected that antiendotoxin monoclonal antibodies will soon be available for treatment of presumed gram-negative sepsis. It is known that stored plasma from blood banks and immune serum globulin preparations also contain significant titers of naturally occurring antibodies to gram-negative endotoxin as well as other bacterial constituents, and it has been suggested that these products may have therapeutic value in patients with sepsis. Unfortunately, this possibility has not been tested in clinical trials and is, therefore, difficult to advocate at this time.

INITIAL RESUSCITATION FROM SEPTIC SHOCK

Immediate resuscitation and stabilization of the cardiovascular and respiratory systems are the first management considerations in a patient with septic shock, as in shock of other etiologies. Oxygen should be administered immediately by mask if the patient is sufficiently alert to maintain a patent airway and appears to be breathing adequately. If the patient's airway does not appear to be secure or if respirations are ineffective, an endotracheal tube should be placed immediately and assisted ventilation with supplemental oxygen provided. Patients with hypotension not responding promptly to acute volume expansion should also be intubated to avoid respiratory arrest from rapid development of respiratory muscle fatigue caused by failure to adequately perfuse working respiratory muscles.[21,22] In all hypotensive patients except those with clinically obvious volume overload, intravenous fluids are given rapidly. This is best done by quickly infusing 0.5 L normal saline solution or lactated Ringer's solution, repeating this as needed every 5 to 10 min. The physician should remain at the bedside during this initial fluid resuscitation, closely following the patient's mentation, respiration, blood pressure, pulse rate, skin perfusion, and jugular venous pressure, to establish whether the patient is responding to fluid resuscitation. In most cases an indwelling urinary catheter should be placed to permit an ongoing assessment of urine output. Fluid challenges should be repeated until an adequate blood pressure and clinical evidence of reasonable tissue perfusion are achieved or until it is established that the patient's circulatory status is unresponsive to volume resuscitation. If the patient's circulatory status fails to improve with 2 to 3 L of volume infusion or if there are signs of fluid overload, such as elevated jugular venous pressure or pulmonary edema, an infusion of dopamine is added. In addition to improving perfusion pressure this may help preserve renal function in low doses (2 to 5 μg/kg/min). If necessary, the dose can be increased or norepinephrine added and titrated upward from low doses to whatever is required to achieve a mean blood pressure of at least 60 mmHg (Table 98-3). Since beneficial effects of vasoconstrictor therapy remain to some extent controversial and adverse effects abound (digital or gut ischemic necrosis, worsening lactic acidosis), a slow hand in initiating such therapy is warranted, and careful titration of the infusion to the needs of the individual patient is needed to minimize the potential for harm. A 20-year-old previously healthy patient will generally tolerate a lower blood pressure than a 60-year-old patient with peripheral vascular disease. Those who do not respond to moderate fluid challenges alone and require vasoactive drugs should have arterial and pulmonary artery catheters placed as soon as possible to establish whether adequate fluid resuscitation has been given and to guide the titration of the vasoactive drugs.

These initial management measures and basic laboratory investigation (vide infra), which should be accomplished in <1 h, generally will result in a resuscitated patient who is adequately oxygenated and ventilated and has an acceptable blood pressure associated with evidence of adequate tissue perfusion as marked by an improved sensorium, well-perfused skin, and a urine output of 1 mL/kg/h or greater. Attention is then directed toward empirical antimicrobial management, establishing an infectious diagnosis to guide definitive therapy decisions, and optimizing supportive management.

MEASUREMENTS AIDING THE TITRATION OF SUPPORTIVE CARE

Hemodynamic and laboratory monitoring of progress is an important part of the initial resuscitation from shock and subsequent supportive therapy. Blood for the laboratory can be obtained, radiographs made, and vascular and urinary catheters established as the resuscitation proceeds. The key point here is to focus on rapid stabilization of the patient's cardiorespiratory status as a priority; "putting in the lines" to obtain hemodynamic data should not be allowed to delay achievement of this goal.

If it is not already available, the basic laboratory investigation establishing base lines for major organ function and blood electrolyte composition should be obtained. These include a complete blood count, prothrombin time and partial thromboplastin time, serum electrolytes (including magnesium, calcium, and phosphate), serum glucose, liver enzymes and serum bilirubin, and serum creatinine. Serum lactate concentration is also worth measuring, if the test is available. The required frequency for repeated measurement of these tests depends on the patient's progress and which major abnormalities are detected; however, in most patients requiring ongoing intensive care support the basic hematologic and electrolyte measurements should be repeated at least twice daily, whereas less labile measurements (calcium, magnesium, phosphate, liver enzymes) are done about every other day, reducing frequency as the patient improves. The blood lactate concentration, if elevated, should be measured more frequently (every 2 to 4 h) until it is in the normal range. Arterial blood-gas values should also be repeated early in the resuscitation to ensure adequate oxygenation and to detect worsening respiratory failure or metabolic acidosis.

An electrocardiogram and chest radiograph should be obtained in all patients as soon as is practical. An indwelling urinary catheter to monitor hourly urine output should also be placed immediately. Blood pressure can be mea-

TABLE 98-3 Vasoactive and Inotropic Drugs in Sepsis

Drug	Dose[a]	USUAL HEMODYNAMIC EFFECTS[b] Pw	CO	BP	SVR	Comments
Dopamine	2.5–20 μg/kg/min	↑	↑	↑	↑↔	Usual first-line agent to maintain renal cortical perfusion. At higher doses (>10 μg/kg/min) acts like norepinephrine.
Norepinephrine	0.05–2 μg/kg/min	↑	↑	↑↑	↑↑	Useful for increasing BP when dopamine is inadequate. Should not be used to maintain BP caused by low CO due to inadequate blood volume except during acute resuscitation.
Epinephrine	0.05–2 μg/kg/min	↑↔	↑↑	↑↑	↑	Effects and indications similar to norepinephrine.
Phenylephrine	2–10 μg/kg/min	↑	↓	↑↑	↑↑	Increase in BP and SVR purely by peripheral vasoconstriction may reduce CO. Best used for severe hypotension when cardiac index is >5L/min/m².
Dobutamine	2.5–10 μg/kg/min	↓	↑	↑↔	↓	Most useful when low BP is associated with lower CO, normal or high SVR, high Pw (i.e., cardiac dysfunction). Peripheral vasodilation effect may cause decreased BP.
Naloxone	30 μg/kg bolus then 0.5 μg/kg/min infusion	↔	↔	↑	↑	Can be used to reduce vasopressor requirement in patients poorly responsive to these drugs. Not a first-line agent and relatively contraindicated when opiates required for pain relief.

[a]Dose of all agents is generally titrated upward from the lower range until the clinically desired hemodynamic effect is achieved.
[b]Pw, pulmonary wedge pressure; CO, cardiac output; BP, blood pressure; SVR, septemic vascular resistance.

sured repeatedly by sphygmomanometer (every 5 to 15 min) in the initial stages; however, in patients requiring more than simple plasma volume expansion an arterial catheter should be placed to facilitate repeated blood sampling and continuous monitoring of arterial pressure.

Patients in shock should have at least two large bore intravenous catheters in place for administration of fluids and vasoactive drugs. Early placement of a central venous catheter is advisable, permitting safer use of vasoactive drugs and measurement of central venous pressure. Insertion of a flow-directed thermal-dilution pulmonary artery catheter should be considered in patients requiring vasoactive drugs for therapy, those in whom the adequacy of volume resuscitation is in doubt and those with ongoing hemodynamic instability. Generally, placement of this catheter can wait until after basic resuscitation has been achieved.

CARDIORESPIRATORY SUPPORT

Plasma volume expansion alone with crystalloid solutions will achieve an acceptable blood pressure and tissue perfusion in many patients. However, because of the increased vascular permeability associated with sepsis, fluid redistribution from the intravascular space to extravascular space occurs even more rapidly than under normal circumstances and leads to an increased need for continued crystalloid infusions to maintain effective circulating blood volume. Continued positive fluid balance may eventually lead to development of substantial edema in soft tissues. While this is not a major problem if only of moderate degree, severe soft tissue edema may contribute to difficulty with vascular access, impairment of wound healing, gut edema with impairment of function, and to the development of pulmonary edema. Administration of colloid solutions in the form of 5% or 25% albumin or 6% hetastarch will usually permit maintenance of effective circulating blood volume with substantially less need for crystalloid infusion. Stored plasma can be substituted if there is evidence of depletion of coagulation factors (elevated prothrombin time or partial thromboplastin time). Packed red blood cells (RBCs) can also be given if the blood hemoglobin concentration is 100 g/L or less.

As noted above, vasoactive drugs will frequently be required in managing septic shock and should be selected with a knowledge of their different specific actions and the goals of therapy in mind (see Table 98-2). In adequately resuscitated patients who remain hypotensive despite an elevated cardiac output, dopamine or norepinephrine are generally the vasoactive drugs of choice and are used to increase the blood pressure to acceptable levels while maintaining the cardiac output preferably above normal levels. Dopamine is usually tried first, followed by norepinephine if dopamine doses of up to 20 μg/kg/min do not achieve the desired effect.[23,24] Epinephrine is also effective,[25] but only rarely improves the hemodynamic situation when the initial approaches have failed. In occasional cases, where the cardiac output is extremely high (cardiac index >5 L/min/m^2) phenylephrine infusion is a useful agent. In other cases in which compromised cardiac function is prominent, marked by an elevated pulmonary wedge pressure with relatively low cardiac output (<2.5 L/min/m^2), dobutamine is an appropriate choice for initial therapy.

Occasionally, the blood pressure may be difficult to increase to acceptable levels despite adequate volume resuscitation and very high doses of intravenous vasoactive drugs. The pathogenesis of this phenomenon is not well established but may relate to downregulation of adrenergic receptors.[26,27] Some evidence suggests that infusion of naloxone may be useful in this circumstance, increasing blood pressure and reducing vasopressor requirement over a 2 to 4 h period.[28] However, the absence of any immediate efficacy[29,30] and the relative contraindication in patients needing opiates for pain relief limit its utility.

The role for other noncatecholamine vasoactive and inotropic drugs in sepsis is not well established. Phosphodiesterase inhibitors (amrinone, milrinone) have significant inotropic effects but, like dobutamine, are arterial vasodilators. Their use in sepsis cannot be recommended at this time. There is limited evidence that digoxin can improve hemodynamics in sepsis, particularly when myocardial dysfunction is contributing to hypotension;[31] however, in the absence of an independent indication for its use (i.e., atrial fibrillation), the potential for toxicity would generally outweigh the unlikely possibility that a greater enhancement of cardiac contractility would be achieved than that provided by dobutamine infusion. It should also be remembered that ionized hypocalcemia is relatively common in septic patients and is associated with both reduced myocardial performance and a poor outcome.[32,33] It is probably advisable to look for ionized hypocalcemia routinely in critically ill septic patients, correcting it by calcium infusion when it is detected.[34]

There is evidence that critically ill septic patients who can maintain an acceptable blood pressure in the face of a reduced SVR by increasing cardiac output above usual normal values are more likely to survive than those who cannot.[35–37] Although this is almost certainly largely due to differences between patients in underlying cardiovascular reserve and therefore not easily amenable to therapeutic measures, it has been suggested that cardiovascular management of septic shock should include among its goals a higher than normal cardiac output (cardiac index >4.5 L/min/mm^2) and oxygen delivery.[37] Some have even suggested that oxygen delivery (product of arterial oxygen content and cardiac output) and body oxygen consumption should be measured repeatedly, attempting to increase cardiac output until oxygen consumption increases no further. Unfortunately, these measurements are difficult to make with sufficient accuracy to be useful in monitoring.[38] In addition, there is evidence that vasoactive drugs can change body oxygen consumption directly as well as by altering oxygen delivery[11] and that increasing cardiac output and systemic oxygen delivery does not increase body oxygen consumption in patients who do not have a lactic acidosis.[11,12] Accordingly, there is still room for debate concerning the goals of cardiovascular support. Reasonable goals for the present are to attempt to achieve cardiac output and oxygen delivery values which provide an acceptable blood pressure, associated with evidence of adequate organ perfusion and oxygenation. Some suggested goals are found in Table 98-4.

GENERAL SUPPORTIVE MEASURES

Although cardiorespiratory supportive measures are the major focus of attention during the initial resuscitation from septic shock, a wide range of abnormalities in many other organ systems is also common in septic shock and demands attention.

BODY TEMPERATURE CONTROL IN SEPTIC SHOCK. Hypothermia is usually of relatively mild degree and can be managed by covering the patient. Fever requires no treatment in most patients. Exceptions are patients who have extremely limited cardiovascular reserve or hypoxemia such that oxygen delivery to tissues is compromised and may be made worse by the increased metabolic expenditure related to fever and patients with a temperature >41°C (105.8°F). Fanning with tepid sponging or cooling blankets may be used to acutely lower temperature; however, it must be remembered that this may produce shivering and further increased metabolic demand. Antipyretic drugs such as acetaminophen should also be given, along with drugs to inhibit shivering such as meperidine (25 to 50 mg intravenously or intramuscularly). In occasional cases, mechanically ventilated patients with marked pyrexia may require the use of muscle relaxants such as pancuronium or vecuronium to control shivering and rigors (preceded by adequate sedation with benzodiazepines and opiates).

TABLE 98-4 Clinical and Hemodynamic Goals of Cardiorespiratory Management of Septic Shock

Hemodynamic Goals
Pulmonary wedge pressure >10 but <20 mmHg.
Mean blood pressure >60 mmHg.
Cardiac index >3 L/min/m^2
Oxygen Delivery Adequacy
Arterial oxyhemoglobin saturation >95%
Hemoglobin concentration >100 g/L
Mixed venous P_{O_2} >30 mmHg
Blood lactate concentration <2 mM/L
Organ Perfusion
CNS—Improved sensorium
Skin—Warm, well perfused
Renal—Urine output >1 mL/kg/h

ABNORMALITIES OF GLUCOSE AND ELECTROLYTES. Hyperglycemia is common in septic shock and should be treated with insulin infusion if the glucose concentration exceeds 15 mM/L. Eliminating glucose from the intravenous fluid being administered will also aid in controlling hyperglycemia. Electrolyte abnormalities are also common in sepsis and frequently require correction. Hypokalemia, hypomagnesemia, and hypophosphatemia should be looked for early in the course of sepsis and corrected by infusion of the deficient electrolyte. Hyponatremia is most often due to water excess rather than sodium losses; an approach to this problem can be found in Chap. 156. Hypocalcemia is often largely attributable to hypoalbuminemia with reduced protein-bound calcium, but, as noted above, when ionized hypocalcemia is detected it should be corrected by infusion of calcium chloride.

DISORDERS OF BLOOD COMPONENTS. Anemia does not always require correction with infusion of packed RBCs. Hemoglobin values as low as 80 g/L are well tolerated by patients with good cardiovascular reserve and who are not hypoxemic. However, in patients who are unable to generate the high cardiac output needed to maintain aerobic metabolism in sepsis or in patients with significant arterial hypoxemia, packed RBCs should be given to maintain the hemoglobin level between 100 and 120 g/L. Thrombocytopenia is common in sepsis but is not usually associated with significant bleeding problems. Infusion of platelet concentrates may also be relatively ineffective in increasing the blood platelet count since platelet survival is greatly reduced in septic shock. Platelet transfusion should therefore be reserved for patients with active clinical bleeding and platelet counts below 40×10^9/L or patients without significant bleeding with platelet counts below 20×10^9/L.

RENAL DYSFUNCTION. Urine output and renal function must be closely monitored in all septic patients. Rising serum creatinine concentrations or significant oliguria should prompt immediate attention to the adequacy of the circulating blood volume or vasoactive drug support being given, since inadequate renal perfusion associated with low blood pressure or inadequate cardiac output are the most frequent causes of oliguria. The importance of maintenance of renal function in septic shock is difficult to overstate, since oliguria greatly complicates management of fluid balance and nutritional support and will eventually mandate dialysis. A more detailed guide to management of oliguria in shock and the diagnosis of renal failure can be found in Chap. 153.

NUTRITIONAL SUPPORT. Early attention to nutritional support is of critical importance in septic patients. If the source of sepsis does not involve the gastrointestinal tract, every effort should be made to provide nutrition by the enteral route. This may prove difficult, since critically ill patients are frequently receiving high dose opiates for pain relief or sedation, which will impair gut motility, and adynamic ileus of other causes is also common. If failure of gastric emptying impedes provision of enteral nutrition, administration of a gastrointestinal motility-altering agent such as domperidone or sisapride may be worthwhile. If this fails, and the ileum and colon remain functional, passing a feeding tube through the duodenum to the jejunum under fluoroscopic control may permit enteral feeding to proceed. If the enteral route cannot be used, total parenteral nutrition should be provided (see Chap. 92). In patients with poor urine output who are relatively unstable hemodynamically, this may mean that more frequent dialysis is required; however, adequate nutritional support is sufficiently important to justify doing this.

ADJUNCTIVE THERAPY. Many other adjunctive therapies for septic shock have been suggested over the years, but in the absence of reasonable data study in human beings cannot yet be recommended. Therapeutic approaches currently undergoing investigation in the laboratory or in clinical trials include use of antibodies against lipopolysaccharide and cachectin, drugs blocking the production or effects of prostaglandins, leukotrienes, platelet activating factor, and other mediators, as well as the different approaches to managing hemodynamic and oxygen delivery variables noted above. The need for adequate studies in human beings before embracing new therapeutic approaches is best exemplified by the recent considerable enthusiasm for high dose corticosteroid therapy of septic shock. This was largely based on encouraging results from animal experimentation, but in the face of compelling negative results in large scale trials in septic patients,[39–41] steroids have now been abandoned except in physiologic doses for suspected adrenocortical insufficiency.

Prognosis Assessment

In large published series of patients fulfilling the clinical criteria for septic shock, mortality averages 40 to 75 percent overall.[18,39–41] Poorer prognosis is associated with advanced age, infection with relatively antimicrobial-resistant organisms such as *P. aeruginosa,* impaired host immune status, and poor patient functional status prior to the onset of sepsis. Once septic shock is established, harbingers of a poor outcome include intractable hypotension requiring high doses of vasoactive drugs, leukopenia, disseminated intravascular coagulation, and deteriorating myocardial performance. Particularly ominous is sequential organ system failure despite adequate antimicrobial and surgical therapy and optimal supportive management.

CASE PRESENTATION

A 35-year-old woman, a known insulin-dependent diabetic, was found by a friend unconscious in her apartment and brought to the emergency department by ambulance. On initial evaluation she was comatose, responding to but not localizing pain in all four limbs, hypotensive with a blood pressure of 65 mmHg systolic by palpation only and hypothermic at 34°C (93.2°F). Respirations were deep and rapid and the heart rate 160 beats/min. The neck was supple and the chest was clear to examination. The abdomen was difficult to examine but note was made of vague right-sided abdominal tenderness. The extremities were cool and clammy with mottling of the skin on the lower limbs.

Arterial blood-gas determinations revealed normal arterial oxygenation, hypocapnia, and a profound metabolic acidosis. The serum glucose level was 31 mM/L and the blood β-hydroxybutyrate level markedly elevated. Serum sodium content was 135 mM/L and the potassium 3.5 mM/L. The WBC count was 35×10^9/L with 15 percent young neutrophils and the platelet count 75×10^9/L. The hemoglobin value was 170 g/L.

Normal saline solution (3L) was given over the first one-half hour and a high infusion rate of normal saline solution continued subsequently. Insulin infusion was given at 1 U/h. An infusion of potassium chloride was given at 20 mM/h. Supplemental oxygen was given by face mask. With these measures the patient's blood pressure increased to 70/40 mmHg, skin perfusion improved dramatically, pulse volume improved and became bounding, and the patient's level of consciousness improved somewhat.

Following this initial fluid resuscitation, it was noted that the patient's circulation appeared to be hyperdynamic, and hypotension persisted at 70/40 mmHg despite a clinically adequate circulating blood volume. In addition, while the patient continued to hyperventilate, respirations had become increasingly labored and she remained oligoanuric. An endotracheal tube was then inserted and mechanical ventilation with supplemental oxygen initiated. Norepinephrine was infused through an internal jugular central venous catheter and titrated upward until a mean arterial pressure of 70 mmHg was achieved. With this increase in blood pressure, urine output began to increase and the patient's level of consciousness improved to the point that she would respond to voice with eye opening and would localize pain.

A pulmonary artery catheter was then inserted and demonstrated a cardiac output of 14 L/min, a pulmonary artery pressure of 25/10 mmHg and a wedge pressure of 9 mmHg. The $(a - v)_{O_2}$ was 30 mL/L and the $C\overline{v}_{O_2}$ 38 mmHg. Blood lactate concentration, which was 9 mM/L just prior to instituting vasoactive drug therapy fell to 5 mM/L 2 h later.

During the initial period of resuscitation several investigations with respect to possible sepsis had been carried out. The chest x-ray following endotracheal intubation showed clear lung fields and a normal cardiac silhouette. A lumbar puncture showed only normal CSF parameters. Urinalysis, in addition to heavy ketone bodies, showed 50 WBCs per high power field. Blood, urine, and CSF were sent for bacterial culture. Following these investigations the patient was given ceftriaxone, 2 gm intravenously and clindamycin 600 mg every 8 h intravenously.

Over the ensuing hours the patient received additional intravenous fluids and 5 percent albumin solution until the pulmonary wedge pressure reached 15 mmHg. Despite this, the patient continued to require an infusion of norepinephrine to maintain a mean arterial pressure > 60 mmHg. The blood glucose and β-hydryoxybutyrate levels fell progressively with insulin therapy and fluid resuscitation, and urine output increased to an average of 75 mL/h. The WBC count remained elevated at 40×10^9/L with 15 percent young neutrophils and the platelets fell further to 60×10^9/L. With the patient's improving level of consciousness, the physical examination was more revealing. Examination of the abdomen revealed definite right-sided abdominal tenderness both anteriorly and posteriorly. No mass could be appreciated clinically, but there was considerable abdominal guarding. An ultrasound examination of the abdomen was obtained immediately. This revealed a normal gallbladder and biliary tree and a dilated renal pelvis and calyceal system on the right.

A consultation with a urologist was obtained. This led to placement of a nephrostomy tube later the same day with drainage of grossly purulent urine from the right renal pelvis. Gram stain of this material revealed heavy gram-negative bacilli. The following day blood, bladder urine, and the nephrostomy tube drainage demonstrated *E. coli* susceptible to all tested antimicrobials.

Broad-spectrum antimicrobial therapy was then discontinued and intravenous ampicillin 2 g every 4 h given. Over the ensuing 72 h the patient's level of consciousness improved steadily and hemodynamic status improved to the point that norepinephrine infusion could be discontinued. The following day the patient was transferred to a ward urologic service for continued treatment of the urinary tract infection and definitive surgical management of the ureteric obstruction.

CASE DISCUSSION

This patient presented with apparent hypovolemic shock due to diabetic ketoacidosis but with relatively limited evidence of sepsis as the underlying cause of the problem. As the initial resuscitation and investigation went on, features of the sepsis syndrome became more prominent: hypothermia, hyperdynamic circulation with persistent hypotension after volume expansion, persistent mental obtundation, left-shifted leukocytosis, and thrombocytopenia. These features appropriately led to more intensive measures to stabilize the patient's cardiorespiratory status, including endotracheal intubation for mechanical respiratory support and norepinephrine infusion to support the blood pressure and maintain urine output. Basic investigations and physical examination excluded many potential sources of sepsis (cellulitis, meningitis, pneumonia) and pointed to an intraabdominal or renal process. Accordingly, broad-spectrum antimicrobials were given, selected to cover *S. aureus*, aerobic gram-negative bacilli and, because of the potential source in the abdomen, anaerobes including *B. fragilis*.

After ensuring basic cardiorespiratory stability and starting empirical antimicrobials, the next steps in management are optimizing supportive therapy and establishing a definitive diagnosis to guide specific therapy. In this case a pulmonary artery catheter was placed to monitor cardiovascular supportive therapy, giving assurance that norepinephrine was not being used to treat hypotension due to relative hypovolemia. Placement of this catheter was probably not essential in the management of this case, since pulmonary edema limiting fluid therapy was not present and there was clinical evidence of much improved systemic perfusion; however, the information it provided did permit precise management of fluids and vasoactive drugs. Investigation to define the source of the infection was prompt, in this case an abdominal ultrasound examination, and led to immediate surgical drainage of the source of sepsis.

The main points illustrated by the case include the importance of early recognition of the sepsis syndrome in a complex shock presentation and the principle that immediate supportive measures for cardiorespiratory failure and widely directed empirical antimicrobial therapy must be followed by a thorough but rapid evaluation for surgically correctable sources of sepsis.

References

1. Tracey KJ, Lawry SF, Cerami A: Cachectin: A hormone that triggers acute shock and chronic cachexia. J Infect Dis 157:413, 1988.
2. Dinarello CA: Interleukin-I and the pathogenesis of the acute-phase response. N Engl J Med 311:1413, 1984.
3. Marks JD, Marks CB, Luce JM, et al: Plasma tumor necrosis factor in patients with septic shock. Am Rev Respir Dis 141:94, 1990.
4. Calandra T, Baumgartner J-D, Grau GE, et al: Prognostic values of tumor necrosis factor/cachectin, interleukin-1, interferon-α, and interferon-γ in the serum of patients with septic shock. J Infect Dis 161:982, 1990.
5. Colman RW: Contact systems in infectious diseases. Rev Infect Dis 11:S689, 1989.
6. Hess ML, Hastillo A, Greenfield LJ: Spectrum of cardiovascular function during gram-negative sepsis. Prog Cardiovasc Dis 23:279, 1981.
7. Bressack MA, Raffin TA: Importance of venous return, venous resistance and mean circulatory pressure in the pathophysiology and management of shock. Chest 92:906, 1987.
8. Parillo JE, Burch C, Shelhamer JH, et al: A circulating myocardial depressant substance in humans with septic shock. J Clin Invest 76:1539, 1985.
9. Duff JH, Groves AC, McLean APH, et al: Defective oxygen consumption in septic shock. Surg Gynecol Obstet 128:1051, 1969.
10. Nishijima H, Weil MH, Shubin H, et al: Hemodynamic and metabolic studies on shock associated with gram-negative bacteremia. Medicine (Baltimore) 52:287, 1973.
11. Gilbert EM, Haupt MT, Mandanas RY, et al: The effect of fluid loading, blood transfusion, and catecholamine infusion on oxygen delivery and consumption in patients with sepsis. Am Rev Respir Dis 134:873, 1986.
12. Vincent J-L, Roman A, DeBacker D, Kahn RJ: Oxygen uptake/supply dependency: Effects of a short-term dobutamine infusion. Am Rev Respir Dis 142:2, 1990.
13. Cerra FB: Hypermetabolism—Organ system failure: A metabolic response to injury. Crit Care Clin 5:289, 1989.
14. Harris RL, Muscher DM, Bloom K, et al: Manifestations of sepsis. Arch Intern Med 147:1895, 1987.
15. Kreger BE, Craven DE, McCabe WR: Gram-negative bacteremia IV. Re-evaluation of clinical features and treatment in 612 patients. Am J Med 68:344, 1980.
16. Bryan CS, Reynolds KL, Brenner ER: Analysis of 1186 episodes of gram-negative bacteremia in non-university hospitals: The effects of antimicrobial therapy. Rev Infect Dis 5:629, 1983.
17. Smith CR, Ambinder R, Lipsky JJ, et al: Cefotaxime compared with nafcillin plus tobramycin for serious bacterial infections. Ann Intern Med 101:469, 1984.
18. Zeigler EJ, McCutchan JA, Fierer J, et al: Treatment of gram-negative bacteremia and shock with human antiserum to a mutant *E. coli*. N Engl J Med 307:1225, 1982.
19. Baumgastner J, McCutchan JA, Melle G, et al: Prevention of gram-negative shock and death in surgical patients by antibody to endotoxin core glycolipid. Lancet 2(8446):59, 1985.
20. Ziegler EJ, Fisher CJ Jr, Sprung CL, et al: Treatment of gram-negative bacteremia and septic shock with HA-1A human monoclonal antibody against endotoxin. N Engl J Med 324:429, 1991.
21. Roussos C, Macklem PT: The respiratory muscles. N Engl J Med 307:786, 1982.
22. Hussain SNA, Roussas C: Distribution of respiratory muscle and organ blood flow during endotoxin shock in dogs. J Appl Physiol 59:1802, 1985.
23. Desjars P, Pinaud M, Potel G, et al: A reappraisal of norepinephrine therapy in human septic shock. Crit Care Med 15:134, 1987.
24. Schreuder WO, Schneider AJ, Groeneveld ABJ, Thijs LG: Effect of dopamine vs norepinephrine in septic shock: Emphasis on right ventricular performance. Chest 95:1282, 1989.
25. Bollaert PE, Bauer P, Audibert G, et al: Effects of epinephrine on hemodynamics and oxygen metabolism in dopamine-resistant septic shock. Chest 98:949, 1990.
26. Parrat JR: Myocardial and circulatory effects of *E. coli* endotoxin; modification of responses of catecholamine. Br J Pharmacol 47:12, 1973.
27. Forse RA, Leibel R, Askanazi J, et al: Adrenergic control of adipocyte lipolysis in trauma and sepsis. Ann Surg 206:744, 1987.
28. Roberts DE, Dobson KE, Hall KW, et al: Effects of prolonged nalaxone infusion in septic shock. Lancet 2:699, 1988.
29. Bonnet F, Bilaine J, Lloste F, et al: Naloxone therapy of human septic shock. Crit Care Med 13:972, 1985.
30. Rock P, Silverman H, Plump D, et al: Efficacy and safety of naloxone in septic shock. Crit Care Med 13:28, 1985.
31. Nasraway SA, Rackow EC, Astiz ME, et al: Inotropic response to digoxin and dopamine in patients with severe sepsis, cardiac failure and systemic hypoperfusion. Chest 95:612, 1989.
32. Zaloga GP, Chernow B: The multifactorial basis for hypocalcemia during sepsis. Ann Intern Med 107:36, 1987.
33. Lang RM, Fellner SK, Neumann A, et al: Left ventricular contractility varies directly with blood ionized calcium. Ann Intern Med 108:524, 1988.
34. Zaloga GP, Chernow B: Hypocalcemia in critical illness. JAMA 256:1924, 1986.
35. Bland RD, Shoemaker WC, Abraham E, et al: Hemodynamic and oxygen transport patterns in surviving and nonsurviving patients. Crit Care Med 13:85, 1985.
36. Russell JA, Ronco JJ, Lockhat D, et al: Oxygen delivery and consumption and ventricular preload are greater in survivors than in nonsurvivors of the adult respiratory distress syndrome. Am Rev Respir Dis 141:659, 1990.
37. Shoemaker WC, Appel PL, Kram HB, et al: Prospective trial of supranormal values of survivors as therapeutic goals in high-risk surgical patients. Chest 94:1176, 1988.

38. Vermeij CG, Feenstra BWA, Bruining HA: Oxygen delivery and oxygen uptake in postoperative and septic patients. Chest 48:415, 1990.
39. Sprung CL, Caradis PV, Marcial EH, et al: The effects of high-dose corticosteroids in patients with septic shock. N Engl J Med 311:1137, 1984.
40. Bone RC, Fisher CJ Jr, Clemmer IP, et al: A controlled clinical trial of high-dose methylprednisolone in the treatment of severe sepsis and septic shock. N Engl J Med 317:653, 1987.
41. VA Systemic Sepsis Cooperative Study Group. Effect of high-dose corticosteroid therapy on mortality in patients with clinical signs of systemic sepsis. N Engl J Med 317:659, 1987.

Chapter 99

APPROACH TO INFECTION IN PATIENTS RECEIVING CYTOTOXIC CHEMOTHERAPY FOR MALIGNANCY

ERIC J. BOW

KEY POINTS

- *Risk of infection increases as the circulating absolute neutrophil count (ANC) declines below 1.0×10^9/L. The greatest risk of bacteremic infection occurs when the ANC is $< 0.1 \times 10^9$/L.*
- *Cytotoxic therapy for remission-induction therapy for acute myeloid leukemia or conditioning therapy for bone marrow transplantation (BMT) is associated with periods when the ANC is $< 0.1 \times 10^9$/L for 14 to 21 days. The time to marrow recovery (ANC $> 0.5 \times 10^9$/L) can vary from 21 to 42 days.*
- *Intermittent administration of cytotoxic therapy for solid tissue malignancies or lymphoreticular malignancies is often associated with a neutrophil nadir at 10 to 14 days from beginning treatment and with periods of neutropenia (ANC $< 0.5 \times 10^9$/L) of < 5 to 7 days. This pattern of neutrophil recovery influences the natural history of febrile neutropenic episodes.*
- *Febrile episodes during neutropenia are defined by an oral temperature of > 38.3°C (100°F) in the absence of other noninfectious causes of fever such as administration of blood products or pyrogenic drugs (e.g., cytotoxic therapy, amphotericin B), the underlying disease, thromboembolic or thrombophlebitic events, or hemorrhagic events.*
- *A single neutropenic episode may be characterized by one or more febrile episodes of which one or more may represent infections.*
- *Body sites most often associated with infection in the neutropenic patient are those associated with integumental surfaces (skin, upper and lower respiratory tract, and upper and lower gastrointestinal tract).*
- *Antibacterial prophylaxis with oral agents such as cotrimoxazole, norfloxacin, or ciprofloxacin can reduce the frequency of febrile episodes and bacteremic events in patients with protracted neutropenia.*
- *Patients undergoing remission-induction for AML or BMT with a history of herpetic stomatitis or who are IgG seropositive for herpes simplex virus (HSV) are at risk for severe herpetic mucositis. Such patients should be given acyclovir prophylaxis.*
- *Empirical antimicrobial therapy for suspected infection in the febrile neutropenic patient usually is composed of a broad-spectrum antibacterial regimen of an antipseudomonal penicillin or third generation cephalosporin plus an aminoglycoside. Modification of the empirical regimen is often required to optimize the coverage for particular clinical circumstances.*
- *Neutropenic patients responding to empirical antibacterial therapy generally require 4 to 5 days for the response to be observed. Patients remaining febrile at 3 days should be systematically reevaluated, while consideration of modification of the antimicrobial regimen can be made at day 4 or 5, unless clinical deterioration is evident.*

Critical care physicians are often called on to provide metabolic, hemodynamic, and respiratory support for patients with various inherited or acquired defects in host defense that render them susceptible to potentially lethal infections. Patients with single host defense system defects, such as those with inherited immune deficiency syndromes like congenital agammaglobulinemia, are susceptible to particular encapsulated respiratory pathogens such as *Streptococcus pneumoniae* that require the presence of opsonizing antibody for clearance. In contrast, cancer patients undergoing potentially curative high intensity, myeloablative, cytotoxic therapy acquire defects in multiple host defense systems that lead to increased susceptibility to different groups of pathogens normally contained and controlled by the absent or damaged systems. Four broad categories of defects in host defense are clinically relevant: disruption of the integrity of the integumental surfaces; quantitative neutrophilic phagocyte defects; diminished B lymphocyte (humoral) function; and diminished T lymphocyte system function. A working knowledge of the sources of failure in these host defense systems is particularly important for predicting the types of offending pathogens likely to be involved in the kind of life-threatening infections requiring the services of the critical care team. This, in turn, provides a basis for a rational approach to the choice of antimicrobial therapy. This chapter reviews the approach to managing suspected or proven infection in patients with multiple defects in host defense systems, with a particular emphasis on patients undergoing active myelosuppressive cytotoxic therapy since this represents the largest group of immunocompromised patients who will require critical care services. Infections in patients with the acquired immunodeficiency syndrome (AIDS) are discussed in Chap. 100 and in those with organ or marrow transplantation in Chaps. 77 and 150; the problem of lung infiltrates in immunocompromised patients is covered in Chap. 102.

Hematologists and oncologists have long recognized the existence of the direct relationship between dose and response in cancer therapy. Over the last 10 to 15 years the supportive care strategies for cancer patients undergoing remission-induction or salvage therapy have improved sufficiently to permit the extension of dosing to the very limits of toxicity and beyond. For many malignant diseases this has translated into significantly higher response rates and disease-free survival. Cure is now a goal that can be realistically adopted for many more patients with these diseases.

Despite these encouraging results, newer dose-intensive therapeutic approaches render patients highly susceptible to life-threatening infection, which in itself or in association with tumor-related end-organ damage may be accompanied by multisystem failure. The rates of mortality are highest (~80 percent) when cancer patients admitted to ICUs develop respiratory failure. One of the most important negative predictors of outcome for these patients is dysfunction in increasing numbers of organ systems.[1,2] The involvement of three or more organ systems has been strongly associated with hospital death. Further need for critical care services beyond 14 days has been associated with a 100 percent hospital mortality rate in a number of studies.[1,2] Factors such as persistent severe neutropenia and the progress of the underlying malignancy also represent independent variables predictive of outcome. The critical care consultant must give careful consideration to these factors to estimate the probability that a critically ill febrile neutropenic patient will survive the episode long enough for the antineoplastic treatments to have their desired effect

Deficits in Host Defenses Related to Cancer Chemotherapy

MYELOSUPPRESSION AND NEUTROPENIA

The absolute number of circulating segmented neutrophils represents the most important single parameter predictive of the risk for life-threatening infection.[3] An ANC of 1.5 to 8.0×10^9/L can be considered normal for adults. As the ANC declines below 1.0×10^9/L the risk of infection increases, with greatest risk for bacteremic infection at neutrophil counts below 0.1×10^9/L. Figure 99-1 illustrates the relationship between the neutrophil count and infection for a series of patients undergoing remission-induction therapy for acute leukemia.

The ANC is calculated by multiplying the proportion of white blood cells (WBCs) that are segmented neutrophils on a Romanovsky-stained blood smear by the total number of WBCs in a specified volume of blood measured in an automated blood cell counter. Since neutropenic patients with acute leukemia undergoing cytotoxic therapy frequently have total WBC counts of $< 0.5 \times 10^9$/L, neutrophils may be difficult to detect on a manually reviewed stained smear; accordingly, the range of error for the procedure increases dramatically. Further, automated blood cell counters may give misleading results when abnormal cells such as leukemic blasts of similar size as segmented neutrophils are present in the circulation. This should dissuade the clinician from relying too heavily on a single ANC to judge the risk of infection. Rather, the clinical relevance of the ANC lies in the recognition of the range associated with a specific infection risk.

The pattern of change of the ANC also has a significant independent influence on infection risk. In one study, 29 percent of the bacteremic episodes occurred as the neutrophil count was falling, but before the ANC fell below 0.5×10^9/L.[4] Therefore, with a falling neutrophil count, multiple observations over time are necessary to establish a pattern for the neutrophil profile and to estimate the relative infection risk. Survival of an infection during severe neutropenia is also intimately linked to marrow recovery and recovery

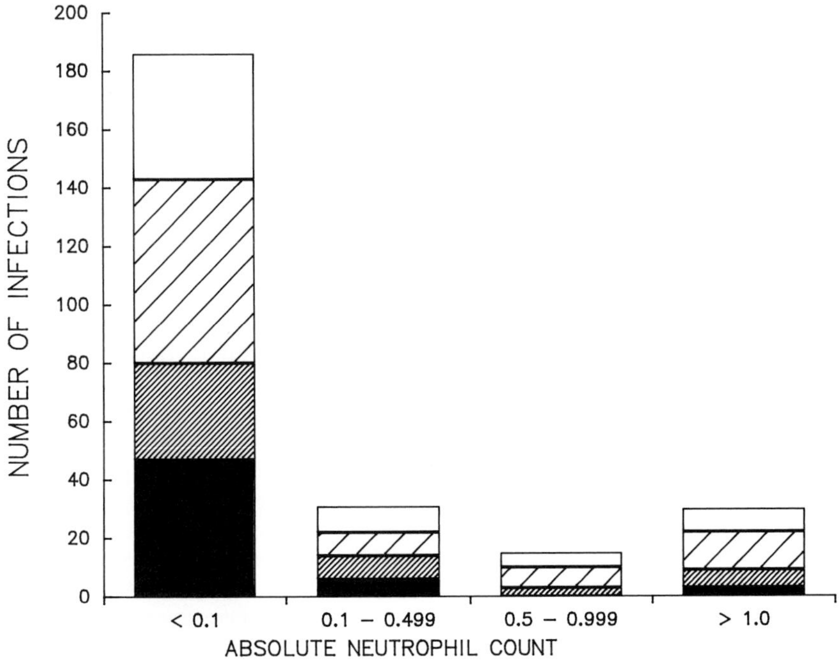

FIGURE 99-1 The relationship of the ANC and occurrence of infection in 98 patients undergoing remission-induction therapy for AML. The proportions of the infections classified as possible infection, clinical infections, nonbacteremic microbiologically documented infection and bacteremic infection are shown. The greatest risk for infection occurs when the ANC is $<0.1 \times 10^9$/L. □, Possible infections; ▨, clinical infections; ▨, nonbacteremic microbiologically documented infections; ■, bacteremia.

of the circulating neutrophil count.[5,6] The poorest outcomes for the infectious episodes occur among patients in whom the ANC continues to decline or fails to increase.[7,8]

The duration of severe neutropenia (ANC $<0.5 \times 10^9$/L) is also related directly to infection risk. The duration of neutropenia is related to the degree of hemopoietic stem cell damage caused by the underlying disease process and by myelosuppressive regimens. Following stem cell suppression, the peripheral neutrophil count falls at a rate inversely proportional to the size of the circulating and marginated peripheral neutrophil pools and the size of the marrow storage pool of mature segmented neutrophils. Marrow recovery follows the recruitment of committed stem cells that are the precursors of granulocytic, monocytic, erythroid, and megakaryocytic cell lines from the resting pluripotential stem cell pool. These hemopoietic stem cells must be able to proliferate to increase their numbers and then differentiate to provide the functional effector cell populations.

Patients receiving pulse doses of chemotherapy for solid tissue malignancies or lymphoreticular malignancies sustain only temporary damage to the hemopoietic stem cell pool. The expected circulating neutrophil nadir occurs generally between day 10 and 14. Although the neutrophilic nadirs may be $<0.5 \times 10^9$/L, the duration of neutropenia is rarely longer than 5 to 7 days. For example, a patient receiving doxorubicin and cyclophosphamide on day 1 and day 8 of a 28-day cycle of a treatment regimen for an intermediate to high grade non-Hodgkin's lymphoma might develop a febrile episode on day 12 in association with an ANC of 0.1×10^9/L. The patient's neutrophil count would be expected to have reached its nadir, and a rise in circulating neutrophils would be predicted to occur between day 15 and 21. The likelihood that this prediction is correct is increased if a relative monocytosis is observed on the differential WBC count. The recovery of peripheral blood monocytes precedes that of circulating neutrophils in chemotherapy-induced aplasia and often heralds the recovery of the ANC.

In general, the more dose-intensive myelosuppressive regimens are associated with more hemopoietic stem cell damage and longer durations of neutropenia. Standard remission-induction regimens for AML are composed of anthracycline drugs such as daunorubicin administered in intravenous doses of 30 to 60 mg/m^2 daily over 3 days and an antimetabolite, cytarabine, administered as an intravenous bolus or as a continuous infusion at doses of 100 to 200 mg/m^2 daily over 5 to 7 days. These regimens predictably produce periods of profound myelosuppression, in which a median of 24 days passes until the circulating neutrophil count rises above 0.5×10^9/L.[9] If more than one cycle of therapy is required to achieve a complete remission, then the median time until marrow recovery may be significantly prolonged by as long as 6 weeks. This additional period of myelosuppression is associated with a significant increase in infectious morbidity.[10]

More intensive regimens using high dose cytarabine (HDARA-C) in doses 15 to 30 times that for standard induction regimens have been successful for salvage therapy of relapsed or resistant leukemia, for initial remission-induction therapy, and for postremission consolidation therapy for acute leukemia. The median time until neutrophil recovery ($>0.5 \times 10^9$/L) following administration of HDARA-C (3.0 g/m^2 infused over 1 h every 12 h for 12 consecutive doses) is 25 to 30 days. Surprisingly this period of myelosuppression is not substantially longer than for standard induction regimens. However, the period of risk for infection can be significantly longer (e.g., extending the time to neutrophil recovery to >40 to 60 days) for heavily pretreated patients where there may be more prolonged direct effects of cytoxic therapy on the marrow stem cell pool or the marrow microenvironment.

OTHER IMMUNOSUPPRESSIVE EFFECTS OF CYTOTOXIC THERAPY

The remission-induction regimens commonly used for acute leukemia have important immunosuppressive effects in addition to the myelosuppressive effects discussed above. Anthracyclines and similar agents (e.g., doxorubicin, daunorubicin, idarubicin, epirubicin, amacrine, mitoxantrone, rubidazone), antimetabolites (e.g., cytarabine, methotrexate, thioguanine, mercaptopurine), and alkylating agents (e.g., cyclophosphamide, ifosfamide, melphalan, busulfan, platinum analogues) have profound suppressive effects on the numbers of circulating T and B lymphoid cells which parallel the acquired functional defects in cell-mediated and humoral immune mechanisms. At the clinical level the consequences of those effects are reflected by an increased susceptibility to pathogens normally controlled by these mechanisms. The ultimate impact on immune responsiveness appears to depend on the schedule of administration.

T LYMPHOCYTE FUNCTION. Indications from in vitro testing of lymphoid cell responsiveness to mitogen-induced blastogenesis suggest that T cell function may be moderately depressed in patients with acute leukemia. Among patients undergoing remission-induction therapy for acute leukemia, decreased cell-mediated immune responsiveness can be detected for up to 6 months following chemotherapy-induced remission.[11,12] Immune function has been observed in some patients to decline once again as a herald to relapse.[11]

The clinical consequences of T cell dysfunction vary with the underlying disease and the cytotoxic regimen. For example, *Pneumocystis carinii* infection is an uncommon phenomenon among adult patients undergoing remission-induction for AML but relatively common among children undergoing consolidation and maintenance phase chemotherapy for acute lymphoblastic leukemia (ALL).[13] An intermediate degree of risk for pneumocystosis appears to be present in those undergoing bone marrow allografting or autografting. The immunosuppressive potential of the conditioning regimens for BMT appears to be greater than that associated with AML-induction regimens. Accordingly, most centers managing these patients recommend administering primary prophylaxis for *P. carinii* in BMT recipients or patients with ALL. These infections rarely occur during the primary period of myelosuppressive therapy-induced neutropenia.

B LYMPHOCYTE FUNCTION. Modern cytotoxic therapy for acute leukemia appears to have a more profound effect on humoral immune competence than on T lymphocyte function. Serum immunoglobulin concentrations and the efficiency of new antigen-induced immunoglobulin synthesis have been observed to decline following institution of remission-induction therapy reaching a nadir at approximately 5 weeks. It has been difficult to separate the effects of the underlying malignant disease from the effects of the cytotoxic therapy. There does not appear to be a prognostically useful parameter of T or B cell function that predicts infection risk in neutropenic patients analogous to the predictive value of the ANC for pyogenic bacterial or fungal infection. However, presence of hypogammaglobulinemia may help identify increased risk of infection by encapsulated bacteria.

INTEGUMENTAL BARRIERS

Integumental barriers represent one of the most important and most often damaged defense system for cancer patients. These barriers include the epithelial surfaces of the skin, the upper and lower respiratory tract, the upper and lower gastrointestinal tract, and the mucosal surfaces lining the genitourinary tract. In critically ill patients, the barrier function of these surfaces may also be compromised by procedures such as percutaneous intravenous catheterization, endotracheal intubation, endoscopic procedures, nasogastric intubation, and indwelling urinary catheterization (Table 99-1).

Integumental damage secondary to cytotoxic therapy has become more prevalent as the dose intensity of the remission-induction regimens has increased. The epithelial surfaces of the gastrointestinal tract appear to be at greatest risk. The antiproliferative effect of therapy prevents cell recruitment into mucosal areas denuded by erosion or by cellular attrition, resulting in the appearance of superficial erosion and ulceration. The absorptive capacity of the gastrointestinal mucosa may also be impaired significantly among recipients of regimens such as HDARA-C, and both anatomic mucosal disruption and absorptive dysfunction appear to temporally parallel that of the neutrophil profile.

TABLE 99-1 Integumental Defects

Damage to Mucosal Surfaces
- Endotracheal Tube
- Nasogastric tube
- Cytotoxic agent-induced damage to gastrointestinal and respiratory epithelial barriers
- Endoscopic diagnostic procedures

Damage to Skin and Supporting Structures
- IV catheters
  - Peripheral IV lines
  - Indwelling central venous catheters
- Indwelling urinary catheters
- Biopsy sites
  - Bone marrow
  - Lymph nodes
  - Skin

A high proportion of patients receiving cytoreductive therapy also experience painful, often debilitating, inflammatory lesions within the oral cavity.[14] The tissues of the periodontium, gingival surfaces, and oral mucosa are affected. Cytotoxic regimens affect the developing basal epithelial cells of the oral mucosa in a manner that parallels the effect on the marrow system cell pool[14] and the intestinal mucosal surface. Mucosal atrophy, cytolysis, and denudation of the mucosal surface result in the typical painful foci of local ulceration typically observed 4 to 7 days after the administration of the cytotoxic agents, and which usually resolve spontaneously between day 14 and 21.[14]

The time of maximum damage to mucosal surfaces appears to be between day 10 and day 14 and, since these areas represent portals through which surface-colonizing microorganisms can gain access to the submucosal tissues and systemic circulation for subsequent dissemination, this is also the time at which primary bacteremia from these sites is most commonly observed. To a limited extent, the type of pathogens recovered in bacteremic infections can be predicted from the pool of microorganisms colonizing damaged mucosal surfaces. Oral mucosal ulceration, particularly that involving periodontal tissues, is often associated with viridans group streptococcal bacteremia. Colonic mucosal damage is more likely to be associated with aerobic gram-negative bacillary infection with *Escherichia coli*, *Klebsiella* species, or *Pseudomonas aeruginosa* when these pathogens are colonizing the lower gastrointestinal tract.

Approach to Fever Associated with Neutropenia

Fever is the hallmark of infection for most patients during periods of prolonged severe neutropenia. The definition of what constitutes a febrile episode due to suspected infection in a neutropenic patient has varied greatly in different studies; but in most a sustained oral temperature of >38°C (100.8°F) or a single value >38.3°C (101°F) has been used. In several studies, authors have qualified the definition of fever by stipulating that the febrile episode must occur in the absence of other noninfectious causes of fever. The Infectious Disease Society of America has suggested that a single oral temperature of >38.3°C (101°F) in the absence of other obvious environmental causes would be a reasonably safe working definition for an infection-related fever in neutropenic patients.[15]

The extent to which characteristics of the febrile episode predict a bacteremic event has been somewhat variable in different studies; however, most agree that patients with initial oral temperatures of >39°C, (102.2°F), shaking chills, clinical shock, initial ANC of $<0.1 \times 10^9$/L, and initial platelet count of $<10 \times 10^9$/L are to some degree predictive of gram-negative bacteremia.[4,16] The duration of fever prior to evaluation, however, does not appear to influence the risk of gram-negative bacteremia.[4]

The neutropenic period may be punctuated by one or more febrile episodes and a single febrile neutropenic episode may represent more than one infectious process. For example, a febrile neutropenic episode associated with a viridans group streptococcal bacteremia may not be seen to defervesce promptly despite the administration of appropriate antibacterial therapy and despite the documentation of a microbiologic cure on the basis of subsequent sterile blood cultures. This phenomenon of a persistent febrile state may occur in association with the concomitant administration of pyrogenic blood products, the presence of a coexisting infection such as an HSV mucositis or a possible fungal superinfection. It is frequently impossible to distinguish clinically the boundaries defining separate sequential infectious processes by the pattern of fever unless a clear pattern of defervescence is seen between one infection and the next. This is particularly frustrating for clinicians managing febrile neutropenic patients without a defined clinical focus of infection or a defined pathogen.

DIAGNOSIS

Most febrile neutropenic episodes are assumed to represent infection. The diagnosis of a febrile state in a neutropenic patient requires a complete but directed clinical history and physical examination designed to identify potentially infected foci for which those patients are at special risk.

Important historical facts may be obtained from the patient, from significant others, and from the patient's medical record. The physician must verify that the patient is neutropenic, the degree of neutropenia, and when the patient is a recipient of cytotoxic therapy, the day of the chemotherapy cycle. The latter is determined relative to the first day of the last cycle of chemotherapy or, in the case of BMT recipients, the day of the BMT.

To avoid omitting the consideration of other noninfectious causes of fever in neutropenic patients, the clinical evaluation should include questions pertaining to the temporal association of the febrile episode to the administration of blood products, to a history of fever associated with the underlying disease, to the administration of chemotherapeutic agents or amphotericin B, to the presence of thrombophlebitis, and to the possible association of the febrile episode to thromboembolic or hemorrhagic events. For example, in a series of neutropenic patients undergoing remission-induction therapy for acute leukemia recently observed by the author,[6] 26 of 72 (36 percent) febrile episodes were due to noninfectious causes (blood products in 33 percent; underlying disease or cytotoxic drugs in 15 percent; unexplained causes in 47 percent). However, the majority of these patients had further febrile episodes for which a diagnosis of infection could not confidently be excluded.

The physical signs of inflammation and infection are influenced by the ANC. The incidence and magnitude of localizing findings such as exudate, fluctuance, ulceration, or fissure formation are reduced in a direct relationship to the ANC.[17] Other localizing findings, such as erythema and focal tenderness, appear to remain as useful and reliable signs of infection regardless of the ANC.

The body systems most often involved with infection in neutropenic patients are those associated with integumental surfaces; that is, the upper and lower respiratory tracts, the upper and lower gastrointestinal tracts and the skin.[18] Table 99-2 lists the pertinent historical and physical clues to be sought in the clinical evaluation of a febrile neutropenic patient.

Examination of the head and neck area should include eyegrounds external auditory canals and tympanic membranes, the anterior nasal mucosa, the vermilion border of the lips, and the mucosal surfaces of the oropharynx. The eyeground examination should seek evidence of retinal hemorrhages as evidence of a bleeding diathesis and of retinal exudates (often described as "cotton wool") that would suggest endophthalmitis associated with disseminated candidiasis. Examination of the external auditory canals and tympanic membranes for erythema or vesicular lesions can implicate this as a focus for infection by respiratory pathogens or herpes group viruses. The anterior nasal mucosal surfaces should be examined for ulcerated lesions that might suggest the presence of a local filamentous fungal infection such as that due to *Aspergillus* species. The skin of the external nares should be examined for vesicular or crusted lesions that would suggest HSV infection. Nasal stuffiness and tenderness over maxillary sinuses suggest that sinusitis is the infectious problem.

The oropharyngeal examination consists of inspection of the dentition; gingival surfaces; mucosal surfaces of the cheeks, hard and soft palate; tongue surfaces; and posterior pharyngeal wall. The presence of decaying teeth and gingival hyperemia implicates those sites as possible sources of bacteremic infection. The presence of shallow, painful mucosal ulcers on an erythematous base suggests herpes mucositis. Progression of this kind of lesion with local tissue necrosis can suggest a polymicrobic infection due to oropharyngeal anaerobic bacteria (e.g., *Fusobacterium nucleatum, Bacteroides melaninogenicus,* peptostreptococci), particularly if cultures for HSV are negative or if such lesions develop during prophylactic or therapeutic administration of acyclovir. Oral thrush or pseudomembranous pharyngitis evolves from an overgrowth of opportunistic yeasts such as *Candida* species. These lesions are characterized by a thick creamy pseudomembrane consisting of masses of fungi existing in both the yeast and mycelial phases. The distribution may be patchy, confluent, or discrete. The pseudomembrane is frequently closely adherent to the underlying mucosal surface such that attempts at removal reveal an erythematous or hemorrhagic base. The diagnosis is suspected by the clinical appearance and confirmed by the demonstration of the pathogen in culture and by the microscopic appearance of budding yeast and pseudohyphae on a Gram's stain or potassium hydroxide preparation.

Chest examination should emphasize evaluation of the lower respiratory tract and central venous catheter sites. The typical signs of pulmonary consolidation may be

TABLE 99-2 Clinical Evaluation of the Febrile Neutropenic Patient

	FINDINGS TO BE SOUGHT	
Body System	Historical	Physical
Eye	Blurring of vision Double vision Loss of vision Pain	Scleral abnormalities Icterus Hemorrhage Local swelling Conjunctival abnormalities Focal erythema Petechiae Retina Hemorrhage "Cotton wool" exudates (e.g., candidal endophthalmitis)
Skin	Skin rash Pruritus (Focal or Diffuse) History of drug reactions Focal pain/swelling IV catheter site(s)	Central venous catheters Insertion site erythema/pain Tunnel site erythema/pain Exit site erythema/pain/exudate Peripheral IV catheters Focal tenderness Focal erythema Exudate at the insertion site Skin rash Papular/macular/vesicular Ulceration Focal areas of necrosis (e.g., ecthyma gangrenosum) Distribution
Upper Respiratory	Painful ear Nasal stuffiness Sinus tenderness Epistaxis	External auditory canals Tympanic membrane erythema
Lower Respiratory	Cough Increased respiratory secretions Dyspnea Hemoptysis Chest pain	Tachypnea Tachycardia Hyperpnea Localized crepitations Consolidation
Upper Gastrointestinal	Odynophagia Dysphagia History of denture use History of herpes stomatitis	Gingival bleeding Pseudomembranous exudate over buccal and gingival surfaces and tongue Mucosal erythema Mucosal ulceration Focal pain Pre-existing periodontitis
Lower Gastrointestinal	Abdominal pain Constipation Diarrhea +/- bleeding Perianal pain with defecation Jaundice	Focal abdominal pain Right upper quadrant (e.g., biliary tree) Right lower quadrant (e.g., cecum/ascending colon) Left lower quadrant (e.g., diverticular disease) Perianal abnormalities Focal tenderness Focal/diffuse erythema Fissures Ulcerations Hemorrhoidal tissues

muted or absent in neutropenic patients; however, localized crepitation on auscultation often precedes the appearance of pulmonary infiltrates radiologically and thus often represents the earliest clue (and often the only clue) to a developing pneumonia in a neutropenic patient. Purulent sputum is similarly reduced in incidence and amount. The neutropenic patient with a developing pneumonia, therefore, may manifest only as febrile illness associated with an increased respiratory rate and a few localized crepitations, with or without an associated cough or radiologic changes.[19] The clinician must search for additional differential diagnostic clues such as the origin of the suspected pneumonia (community or hospital-acquired), the tempo of the illness, the association of the illness with other potentially noninfectious factors such as pulmonary edema, exposure to certain chemotherapeutic agents associated with lung injury (bleomycin, busulfan, cytarabine), radiation therapy, pulmonary thromboemboli, pulmonary hemorrhage, or hyperleukocytosis. The physical assessment of the chest can do little to differentiate infectious or noninfectious causes of pulmonary findings, but it can help identify the lower respiratory tract as the potential infected focus.

The symptoms and signs of an intraabdominal infection may be obvious or muted, focal, or diffuse. The most important finding is focal tenderness.[17] For example, tenderness in the right lower quadrant might suggest neutropenic enterocolitis (typhlitis); right upper quadrant tenderness a biliary tract focus or hepatomegaly; epigastric pain, an upper gastrointestinal focus; left lower quadrant tenderness might suggest colitis or diverticular disease. It is important to examine the perianal tissues for signs of excoriation, local erythema, swelling, tenderness, fissure formation, or hemorrhoidal tissues since this area is frequently the site of major life-threatening infection in neutropenic patients. Digital examination of the rectum is not recommended in neutropenic patients because of the additional risk of tissue damage, bleeding, and infection. A light perianal digital examination can, however, be informative about focal areas of cellulitis without increasing the risk of bacteremic infection.

The examination of the skin should consist of a thorough search for focal areas of pain, swelling, or erythema especially in association with indwelling vascular access devices. Particular attention should be paid to the venous insertion, tunnel, and exit sites associated with central venous catheters. In contrast, nonspecific local pocket tenderness may be the only clue to infection associated with the totally implantable venous access port-reservoir systems.

Skin rashes are a common phenomenon among neutropenic patients. The differential diagnosis must include both infectious and noninfectious causes. Among the former group are focal ulcerative and necrotic lesions caused by metastatic pyogenic bacterial infection such as that associated with bacteremic *P. aeruginosa* or *Staphylococcus aureus* (infections causing ecthyma gangrenosum; see Plate 35) or by disseminated angioinvasive filamentous fungi such as that due to *Aspergillus* species, *Pseudallescheria boydii* or *Fusarium* species (Fig. 99-2). Pustular erythematous lesions diffusely distributed over the skin surface suggest the possibility of disseminated fungal infection such as that caused by *Candida tropicalis* (see Plate 36). Vesicular skin lesions suggest the possibility of infection due to HSV or herpes zoster virus.

The list of possible noninfectious causes of skin rash is long. The three most important considerations are hemorrhagic petechial or ecchymotic rashes associated with profound thrombocytopenia; hypersensitivity rashes associated with specific drugs such as β-lactam antibacterial drugs, allopurinol or trimethoprim-sulfamethoxazole (TMP/SMX); and specific chemotherapy regimen-related rash syndromes (for example, the exfoliative palmar/plantar syndrome associated with high dose cytarabine; Fig. 99-3). These skin rash syndromes may coexist simultaneously. For example, experience has shown that patients undergoing remission-induction therapy with high dose cytarabine for AML may develop hemorrhagic petechial rashes due to thrombocytopenia, palmar/plantar erythema and edema due to cytarabine, macular penicillin-related hypersensitivity rash, and hemorrhagic cutaneous infarcts secondary to angioinvasive bacteremic or fungemic infection all simultaneously. Only careful attention to the pertinent details of history and thorough laboratory investigations can increase the likelihood that the correct diagnosis and therapeutic decisions will be made.

Once the relevant historical details and physical findings are established, the complete evaluation of the febrile neutropenic patient should include a series of laboratory and radiologic investigations designed to complement the clinical examination. Specimens of body fluids such as blood, urine, cerebrospinal fluid, and lower respiratory secretions should be submitted to the clinical microbiology laboratory for culture and antimicrobial susceptibility testing where appropriate. At least two sets of blood cultures should be obtained, at least one of which should be taken from a peripheral venous site. Further, it has been recommended that for patients with multilumen indwelling central venous catheters in situ, each lumen of the catheter should be sampled in addition to blood from the peripheral venous site.[15]

Tissue obtained by biopsy of infected sites can be important in the diagnostic evaluation. Biopsied material should be submitted to the clinical microbiology laboratory for culture and to the pathology laboratory for histopathologic or etiologic evaluation. Remember, it is common for pathogens to be observed histopathologically in infected tissue specimens without recovery of the organism by culture. Such is the case in the syndrome of hepatosplenic candidiasis where budding yeasts and pseudohyphae observed in liver biopsy specimens frequently fail to grow in microbiologic cultures. Skin biopsies are often helpful to distinguish drug-related lesions from those caused by specific pathogenic microorganisms. Although ideally desirable for a complete evaluation, tissue biopsies of suspect sites in neutropenic thrombocytopenic patients carry the additional risks of further infection and bleeding. In addition to skin, the body sites most often considered for biopsy are esophagus (to differentiate mucositis secondary to fungi, pyo-

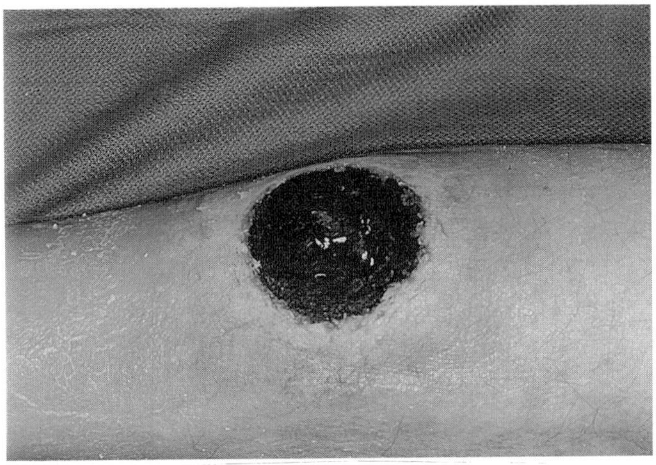

a

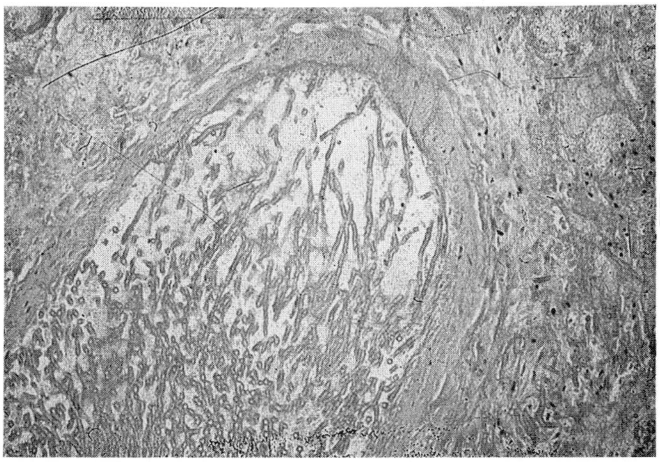

b

FIGURE 99-2 *a*, Necrotic ulcerated skin lesion in a 53-year-old man at day 15 of remission-induction therapy for AML. This lesion was caused by skin infarction secondary to angioinvasive infection due to *Aspergillus flavus*. *b*, Periodic acid-Schiff stain of a biopsy from this lesion demonstrates the invasion of broad, acutely branching septate hyphae into blood vessels.

genic, microorganisms, herpes group viruses or chemotherapeutic agents), liver (to evaluate hepatic lesions due to fungi, herpes group viruses, pyogenic bacteria and drug-related or disease-related hepatic damage), and lung (to evaluate the etiology of progressive infiltrates). Institutions caring for these patients should have a protocol for specimen collection and handling developed in consultation with the appropriate laboratories, the operating theaters, and surgical services.

The basic radiologic investigation is the chest radiograph

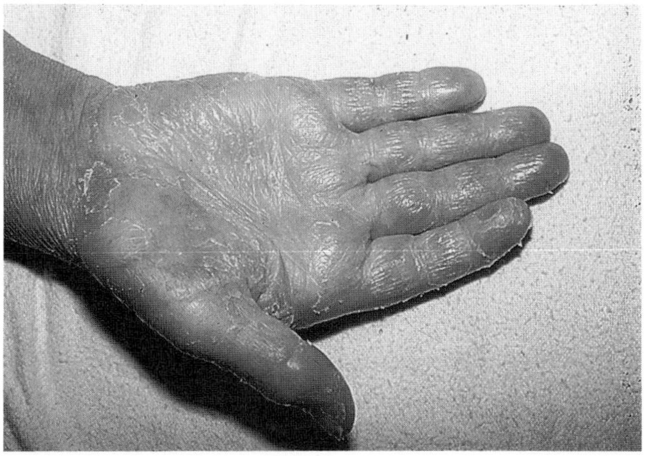

FIGURE 99-3 Palmar/plantar desquamation occurring on day 9 of treatment in a patient receiving high dose cytarabine.

(posterior/anterior and lateral views). When suggested by clinical clues, sinus radiographs are useful for detecting sinus opacification or fluid levels. Panorex radiographs can be helpful for evaluating periodontal infection. Computered tomography (CT) of the abdomen or hepatic ultrasonography is valuable for assessing the significance of abnormalities in cholestatic enzymes γ-glutamyltransferase [GGT] and alkaline phosphatase). This is particularly important if the possibility of hepatosplenic candidiasis exists.

EMPIRICAL ANTIMICROBIAL THERAPY

The empirical initial therapy for suspected infection in febrile neutropenic patients is based on two assumptions:

1. the majority of infections are due to bacteria and
2. the principal pathogens are aerobic gram-negative bacilli (*E. coli*, *Klebsiella pneumoniae*, and *P. aeruginosa*). Accordingly, the antibiotic regimens currently recommended for empirical therapy are designed to have excellent activity against these pathogens. With the recognition of various factors favoring infection with gram-positive organisms, the addition of agents with an improved spectrum of activity against these pathogens when appropriate has also been recommended.

Three classes of effective empirical regimens are available for neutropenic patients: β-lactam plus aminoglycoside combinations; double β-lactam combinations; and monotherapy (Table 99-3). β-Lactam antibacterial agents may be categorized into extended-spectrum antipseudomonal penicillins (for example, carbenicillin, ticarcillin with or without clavulinic acid, piperacillin, azlocillin, or mezlocillin) or third generation antipseudomonal cephalosporins (for example, ceftazidime or cefoperazone). A variety of aminoglycoside antibiotics have proven roles for use with β-lactam antibiotics in neutropenic patients, namely, gentamicin, netilmicin, tobramycin, and amikacin. The choice of aminoglycoside must be based on local institutional bacterial susceptibility patterns, the availability of a mechanism for serum aminoglycoside concentration monitoring, and drug cost. β-Lactam/aminoglycoside combinations offer several potential advantages such as synergistic potential against some aerobic gram-negative bacilli and the prevention of the development of resistance. Depending on circumstances, these advantages may be offset by certain disadvantages such as a relative lack of activity against certain gram-positive cocci, an increased risk of nephrotoxicity and ototoxicity, and the increased costs associated with serum concentration monitoring. Monotherapy with either aminoglycosides or extended-spectrum antipseudomonal penicillins is not recommended.

TABLE 99-3 Antimicrobial Therapy Used for Therapy in Febrile Neutropenic Patients

β-Lactam Antibiotics	
Ticarcillin, Piperacillin, Azlocillin, Mezlocillin	200–300 mg/kg/day IV 4–6 divided doses daily
Cefoperazone	2 g q12h IV
Ceftazidime	2 g q8h IV
Imipenem/cilastatin	500 mg q6h IV
Aminoglycosides	
Gentamicin, Netilmicin, Tobramycin	1.5–2.0 mg/kg q8h IV
Amikacin	7.5 mg/kg q12h IV
Other Agents	
Vancomycin	1.0 g q12h IV
Metronidazole	500 mg q8h IV/PO
Erythromycin	0.5–1.0 g q6h IV
TMP/SMX	10–20 mg/50–100 mg/kg/day in 4 divided doses
Acyclovir	250–500 mg/m^2 q8h IV
Ganciclovir	5 mg/kg q8–12 IV
Amphotericin	0.5–1.5 mg/kg/day IV
5-FC	150 mg/kg/day PO in 4 divided doses

Double β-lactam-containing regimens are safe and effective but costly alternatives to β-lactam/aminoglycoside antibiotic regimens. These regimens consist of an extended-spectrum antipseudomonal penicillin together with a third generation cephalosporin. Cost, hypokalemia, selection of bacterial resistance, and antagonism have been cited as potential disadvantages. The major role for these regimens may be in the setting of preexisting renal insufficiency, or where the patient is receiving potentially nephrotoxic agents concomitantly (for example, cyclosporin A- or cisplatin-containing chemotherapeutic regimens) and where gram-positive organisms such as viridans streptococci are suspected.[7,15]

The intrinsic activity of many of the third generation cephalosporins (e.g., ceftazidime) and carbapenem agents (e.g., imipenem/cilastatin) against aerobic gram-negative bacilli is high. Accordingly, these agents have been used as single agents for empirical treatment of suspected infection. Empirical monotherapy should probably be reserved for patients in whom the expectation for the total period of neutropenia is <1 week. The experience to date suggests that single-agent empirical regimens will require modification, usually by the addition of other antimicrobials, in over two-thirds of patients with neutropenic periods in excess of 1 week.[20,21]

The choice of the type of empirical regimen should be influenced by a number of considerations (Table 99-4), particularly the presence of or potential for renal insufficiency, the expected pathogens, the in situ presence of indwelling central venous access devices, and the suspicion of penicillin hypersensitivity. Renal insufficiency or concomitant use of cyclosporin A, amphotericin B, or cisplatin may lead to a consideration of a double β-lactam combination, or monotherapy, or of the use of a β-lactam/aminoglycoside combination together with intensive aminoglycoside concentration monitoring. If the expected pathogens are *P. aeruginosa* or *Enterobacter* species, a β-lactam/aminoglycoside combination is preferred. Where gram-positive organisms are suspected, particularly among patients who are receiving oral

TABLE 99-4 Considerations Governing the Choice of Empirical Antibacterial Regimen

β-Lactam + Aminoglycoside	Risk of *P. aeruginosa* infection Nosocomial infection Prolonged severe neutropenia
Double β-Lactam	Patients with renal impairment Recipients of other nephrotoxic agents Mild to moderate neutropenia
Monotherapy	Patients with renal impairment Recipients of other nephrotoxic agents Short-term neutropenia
Other Agents	
Vancomycin	Suspect staphylococcal infection Suspect vascular catheter infection Skin or soft tissue infection
Metronidazole	Suspect intraabdominal infection Necrotizing gingivitis Severe oral mucositis Suspect perianal infection

quinolone antibacterial prophylaxis or among patients with indwelling central venous access devices, the addition of increased gram-positive coverage with vancomycin should be considered. Combination regimens are recommended for patients with longer periods of neutropenia such as those undergoing remission-induction for acute leukemia or BMT. Monotherapy with agents such as ceftazidime, cefoperazone, or imipenem/cilastatin may best be reserved for patients with only brief periods of neutropenia, as occurs in patients receiving cytotoxic therapy for solid tissue malignancies or lymphoreticular malignancies.

The time until response to empirical antibacterial therapy varies with the underlying causes of neutropenia.[6,21,22] Among patients with a short duration of neutropenia (<7 days), the median time to defervescence is 2 days (range, 1 to 7 days). Among patients with a prolonged duration of neutropenia (>7 days), the median time to defervescence is 4 to 5 days (range 1 to 14 days). Patients with fever persisting beyond 72 h or broad-spectrum antibiotic therapy should be reevaluated carefully. Table 99-5 lists several of the possible explanations for this. A nonbacterial etiology for the febrile episode should be considered. The various noninfectious causes have already been discussed. Factors such as localized tenderness, change in sensorium, hyperventilation, hypotension, progressive renal insufficiency and acidosis suggest an infectious cause. The reevaluation should include a thorough examination to identify a focus. Cultures of blood (one set from each lumen of the central venous catheter and one set from a peripheral vein), urine, and other potentially infected sites should be submitted to the clinical microbiology laboratory. Repeat chest radiography or diagnostic imaging studies (e.g., ultrasonography or CT) may be performed when abnormalities suggest a specific organ as a potential site for infection. When reevaluation fails to identify the etiology of the persistent fever, the clinician may elect either to continue the initial empirical antibacterial regimen if the patient's condition shows no clinical change or deterioration or to modify the empirical regimen appropriate to the findings of the reevaluation (Table 99-6). If, however, defervescence has not occurred by day 7, the empirical administration of parenteral amphotericin B has been recommended based on the observation that approximately one-third of febrile neutropenic patients unresponsive to 7 days of broad-spectrum antibacterial therapy have fungal superinfection.[15,23] Surveillance cultures for detecting potential fungal pathogens have had some limited usefulness for predicting fungal infection. The recovery of filamentous fungi (e.g., *Aspergillus* species) in a nasopharyngeal surveillance culture in the clinical setting of a persistently febrile profoundly neutropenic patient receiving broad-spectrum antibiotics and who develops new focal pulmonary infiltrates can be, to some extent, predictive of *Aspergillus* pneumonia.[24] The recovery of *Candida albicans* from oropharyngeal, rectal, or urine surveillance cultures has had a positive predictive value of 10 to 15 percent for systematic candidiasis. The recovery of other nonalbicans *Candida* species such as *C. tropicalis*, particularly from

TABLE 99-5 Differential Diagnosis of Fever > 72 h Despite Broad-spectrum Antibacterial Therapy

- Fever is due to a nonbacterial process.
  - Viral infection (HSV,CMV)
  - Fungal infection (candidiasis, invasive aspergillosis)
  - Noninfectious fever (blood products, drugs etc.)
- Bacterial infection is resistant to the antibiotic regimen.
- Second or subsequent infection has developed.
- Bacterial infection is not responding because of inadequate antibiotic serum/tissue levels.
- Infection is associated with an undrained focus (e.g., abscess or prosthetic material [IV catheters])

TABLE 99-6 Considerations for Regimen Modification: Day 5

Progressive necrotising mucositis/gingivitis	⟶	Anaerobic coverage (metro nidazole)
Progressive ulcerating mucositis/gingivitis	⟶	Antiviral therapy (acyclovir)
Dysphagia	⟶	Antifungal (+/− antiviral) therapy if pseudomembranous pharyngitis
Cellulitis or inflammatory changes at venous access sites	⟶	Antistaphylococcal therapy (vancomycin)
Interstitial pulmonary infiltrates	⟶	TMP/SMX +/− erythromycin Consider bronchoalveolar lavage
Focal pulmonary infiltrates	⟶	Observe if ANC is recovering Consider lung biopsy Empirical amphotericin
Abdominal foci	⟶	Typhlitis, Diverticular disease, Perirectal focus } Anaerobic coverage

multiple sites, has had a positive predictive value of over 70 percent for systemic infection. In contrast, the failure to recover *Candida* species in surveillance culture has been associated with a negative predictive value of over 90 percent for invasive disease from *C. albicans* or *C. tropicalis*.[25] This experience suggests that clinicians cannot use surveillance cultures to predict the presence of a candidal infection (except perhaps for *C. tropicalis*). The clinician may be reassured, however, by negative surveillance cultures, properly obtained and processed, that antifungal therapy may not be indicated.[15]

Once a bacterial pathogen is recovered after the initial assessment, the continuation of broad-spectrum coverage is recommended, particularly for patients with prolonged periods of neutropenia, since experience has shown that among patients with gram-positive infection for whom antibacterial therapy is narrowed to be specific for the pathogen recovered, almost half develop a subsequent gram-negative infection.[26] Further, a higher proportion of patients receiving pathogen-specific therapy appear to require modification of the empirical regimen during the course of therapy. Narrowing the spectrum of the empirical regimen once initial evaluation revealed no evidence for pathogens such as *P. aeruginosa* also appears to be unsatisfactory.[27]

The optimal duration of antibacterial therapy is unknown. It is generally recommended that febrile neutropenic patients receive at least 1 week of antibacterial therapy or, after fever resolves, be treated until afebrile for at least 5 days. For severely neutropenic patients (ANC $<0.5 \times 10^9$/L), antibacterial therapy should probably be continued until marrow recovery (e.g., ANC $>0.5 \times 10^9$/L observed on consecutive days). It is not known whether the systemic parenterally administered agents must be continued or whether orally administered agents used for selective gut decontamination may be substituted. If it is decided that antibiotic therapy may be discontinued, patients must be observed closely for recrudescence of fever, in which case systemic antimicrobials are immediately reinstituted. The approach outlined above has been regarded by the Infectious Diseases Society of America as a reasonable strategy for managing patients with neutropenia and fever.[15]

Specific Infection Syndromes in Patients Undergoing Cytotoxic Chemotherapy

Infections occur at a limited number of body sites in febrile neutropenic patients and usually involve the microorganisms colonizing those sites. The three systems most commonly involved are the gastrointestinal tract (oropharynx, gingiva and teeth, esophagus, the gut and perirectal tissues), the respiratory system (sinuses, middle ear, nasopharynx, the tracheobronchial tree, and the pulmonary parenchyma), and the skin (including biopsy sites and sites of vascular access such as indwelling central venous catheter exit sites, tunnel sites, or insertion sites).

OROPHARYNGEAL MUCOSAL AND ESOPHAGEAL INFECTIONS

The natural history of oral mucositis is influenced by the cytotoxic therapy-induced neutropenia, which plays a permissive role in the clinical expression of acute on chronic periodontal infections.[28] This process usually reaches its maximum intensity at the time of neutrophilic nadir, approximately day 10 to 14.[14] At this time polymicrobic infection becomes superimposed on the chemotherapy-induced mucositis. This, in turn, extends the morbidity into the third and fourth week following the commencement of chemotherapy. Although oropharyngeal bacterial flora (viridans group streptococci, anaerobic gram-negative bacilli, and anaerobic gram-positive cocci) probably contribute to disease in most cases of simple mucositis, in several studies, fungi (e.g., *C. albicans*) have played important pathogenetic roles in up to 60 percent of the oral infections among patients with acute leukemia.[29] In addition, reactivated latent HSV infections of the oral cavity have been reported in 50 to 90 percent of seropositive patients undergoing remission-induction therapy or BMT with a median onset between 7 and 11 days.[30] Acute exacerbations of preexisting, asymptomatic, chronic periodontitis occurred in 59 percent of one series of adult patients undergoing remission-induction therapy for acute leukemia.[28] These infections typically occurred when the ANC was $<0.1 \times 10^9$/L. The severity and duration of chemotherapy-associated mucositis correlates to some degree with the extent of preexisting dental plaque and periodontal disease.[31]

CLINICAL APPROACH. Herpetic infections of the oropharynx and esophagus may be anticipated in patients with a history of herpetic stomatitis or in those known to possess IgG antibodies to HSV indicating infection in the past. Although the typical discrete vesicular lesions on an erythematous base may be observed in neutropenic patients, herpetic infections may also manifest as areas of painful ulcerations over a diffusely erythematous base. Such lesions must be distinguished from a typical presentation of oropharyngeal candidiasis or cytotoxic therapy-induced mucositis. Pseudomembranous pharyngitis suggests yeast infection. A thorough examination of the gingival and periodontal tissues for focal areas of pain, erythema, swelling, and bleeding can suggest the periodontium as a potential focus of infection (particularly as a source of bacteremic infection) by viridans streptococci and oropharyngeal gram-negative anaerobic bacilli.[32]

Laboratory aids include virus culture techniques, direct fungal stains, direct electron microscopic examination for virus particles, cytologic examination of cellular material from the base of the ulcer (e.g., Tzanck preparation for the detection of multinucleated giant cells and intranuclear inclusions), or direct herpes simplex antigen detection techniques. The material from a specific lesion should be submitted to the clinical microbiology laboratory for culture and for direct examination. Routine Gram's stain can be helpful in demonstrating the presence of budding yeasts and pseudohyphae suggestive of *Candida* species. A potassium hydroxide mount (to digest extraneous unwanted cellular material) can also provide a clue to this diagnosis by demonstrating the presence of these structures.

MANAGEMENT. The morbidity associated with oropharyngeal or esophageal mucositis can be life-threatening, particularly when local pain interferes with an adequate nutritional intake. Pain control becomes a high priority. Topical anesthetics such as lidocaine in a 2% water-soluble gel of 5% water-insoluble ointment have been widely used with inconsistent success. Continuous intravenous morphine infusions have been successful for symptom control among BMT recipients with cytotoxic therapy-induced mucositis or acute oral graft-versus-host disease. Herpetic mucositis involving the oropharynx or esophagus should be treated with acyclovir. Intravenous acyclovir (250mg/m^2 every 8 h) may be administered for severe cases until oral administration (200 mg every 4 h) can be tolerated for a total course of 7 days. Pseudomembranous candidiasis involving the oropharynx or esophagus may be treated with various approaches. Topical therapy with oral nystatin suspension (2 to 30 million units daily in four divided doses) remains a popular first-line approach. Many physicians prefer to prescribe orally absorbed azole antifungal agents such as ketoconazole (200 to 600 mg daily) or fluconazole (50 to 400 mg daily). It is important to remember that the efficacy of ketoconazole may be compromised by concomitant use of antacid therapy or in the setting of gastric achlorhydria. Invasive candidal esophagitis should be treated with intravenous amphotericin B to a cumulative dose of 500 to 1500 mg (approximately 15 mg/kg), while oropharyngeal candidiasis has been successfully treated with cumulative doses of about 500 mg (5 mg/kg). Necrotizing polymicrobial anaerobic mucositis responds well to metronidazole (500 mg orally or intravenously every 8 h).

Evidence is accumulating that much of the extra morbidity caused by these infections superimposed on chemotherapy-induced mucositis can be significantly reduced by the prophylactic use of antiviral agents such as acyclovir among HSV-seropositive individuals,[33] antiseptics such as chlorhexidine,[34] and antifungal agents such as oral azoles.[35] Further work is required to determine the optimal dose schedules and routes of administration for these agents.

ENTERIC INFECTIONS

Invasive enteric bacterial infections of the gut due to *Salmonella* or *Shigella* species are relatively uncommon in neutropenic patients. Two clinical entities, however, must be considered in febrile neutropenic patients with abdominal pain and diarrhea, toxigenic enterocolitis due to the toxin elaborated from an overgrowth of *Clostridium difficile* and neutropenic enterocolitis (typhlitis).

Clostridium difficile ENTEROCOLITIS. Enterocolitis due to the toxin elaborated by *C. difficile* is a relatively common problem among neutropenic patients receiving broad-spectrum antibiotic therapy, particularly those who are recipients of antibacterial agents with high biliary excretion rates and that are active against intestinal anaerobic bacteria. This problem must be considered when such patients develop abdominal pain in association with watery diarrhea with or without blood. The differential diagnosis includes other infectious (cytomegalovirus [CMV] enterocolitis, typhlitis) and noninfectious (cytotoxic therapy-induced mucosal damage, peptic ulcer disease) causes. Protozoa and helminths are unlikely causes of this syndrome unless there is an associated history of travel to or immigration from areas where pathogens such as *Giardia lamblia* or *Strongyloides stercoralis* are endemic. Diarrheal stools should be submitted to the clinical microbiology laboratory for bacterial culture (to rule out the remote possibilities of salmonellosis, shigellosis, and *Campylobacter* or *Yersinia* infection); examination for ova and parasites (unless this has been done earlier in the patient's course); and culture for *C. difficile* and the detection of *C. difficile* toxin. If *C. difficile* is cultured or the toxin detected, this is sufficient to warrant therapy with either metronidazole (500 mg orally every 8 h for 10 days) or vancomycin (125 to 250 mg orally every 6 h for 10 days) without a sigmoidoscopic examination for detection of the pseudomembranous changes associated with this infection. In patients with a sufficiently typical clinical presentation, it is also reasonable to begin therapy empirically before laboratory confirmation is available.

TYPHLITIS. Typhlitis, also called neutropenic enterocolitis, necrotizing enterocolitis, or ileocecal syndrome, is a serious, potentially life-threatening infection of the bowel wall seen in up to 32 percent of patients undergoing remission-induction therapy for acute leukemia.[36–39] The cecum appears to be favored for the development of this syndrome, possibly related to its relatively tenuous blood supply. Bacterial invasion through an ischemic gut wall in the setting of neutropenia and cytotoxic therapy-induced mucosal surface damage is the probable pathogenesis.[36,37] The syndrome presents a spectrum of severity from mild self-limiting cecal inflammation to fulminant bowel wall necrosis with perforation. The clinical syndrome is typically characterized by abdominal pain and fever in the setting of cytotoxic therapy-induced neutropenia. Abdominal distention, nausea, vomiting, and diffuse watery or bloody diarrhea are also commonly observed. Bacteremia with enteric microorganisms (*E. coli, Klebsiella* species) and *P. aeruginosa* is associated with typhlitis in up to 28 percent of cases.[36] Clinical examination usually reveals a diffusely tender abdomen; however, localization to the right lower or upper quadrants is not uncommon. Ultrasonographic or CT imaging of the abdomen frequently demonstrates thickening and edema of the cecal and right colonic walls with or without inflammatory changes in the surrounding periocolic tissues (Fig. 99-4). Gas in the intestinal wall or an inflammatory phlegmon may also be seen.

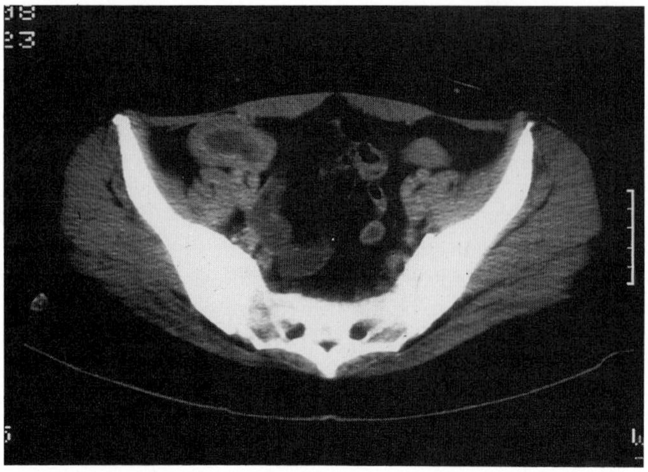

FIGURE 99-4 CT scan of the abdomen of a woman receiving high dose cytarabine for acute leukemia who complained of severe right lower quadrant pain. The wall of the cecum is thickened and edematous consistent with typhlitis.

Management consists of early recognition, bowel rest with nasogastric decompression, intravenous fluid replacement, blood product transfusion and broad-spectrum antibacterial agents directed against the aerobic, microaerophilic and anaerobic enteric microflora (e.g., an antipseudomonal penicillin or third generation cephalosporin plus an aminoglycoside plus an agent effective against obligate anaerobic bacteria). Although surgical consultation early in the evolution of the syndrome is recommended so that all potential management strategies can be planned before an intraabdominal catastrophe occurs, medical management is recommended for the majority of patients who do not have evidence of a major intraabdominal catastrophe. Surgical intervention with right hemicolectomy or local resection of necrotic segments of bowels with anastomosis or diverting ileostomy or colostomy should only be considered in the setting of cecal perforation, massive uncontrollable gastrointestinal bleeding, uncontrollable sepsis, complete bowel obstruction or pneumatosis cystoides intestinalis.[38] Despite optimal management, however, the mortality rate still exceeds 50 percent.[36] The optimal outcome for these patients appears to require a high index of suspicion for the syndrome, aggressive supportive care, and marrow recovery. It is important to recognize the high risk of recurrence (up to two-thirds of cases) with subsequent cycles of cytotoxic therapy.[37]

PERIRECTAL INFECTIONS. Infections of the perirectal tissues may be life-threatening in neutropenic patients. The majority of cancer patients with this complication have received cytotoxic therapy for leukemia or lymphoreticular malignancy within the preceding month and are severely neutropenic (ANC $<0.5 \times 10^9$/L) at the time of presentation.[40] Although the presence of neutropenia may preclude the development of frank suppuration, perirectal infection must be suspected if there is focal tenderness, perirectal induration, or erythema with or without fluctuance or tissue necrosis.[17] Although some cases may be associated with a preexisting pathologic process such as an anal fissure or thrombosed hemorrhoidal tissues, most patients present no obvious predisposing factor. Conceivably, small abrasions or tears in the rectal mucosa may be the primary event allowing tissue invasion by the microflora colonizing the rectum, anus, and perineum. The most common microorganisms associated with perirectal infections are enteric gram-negative bacilli (e.g., *E. coli, Klebsiella* species, *Enterobacter* species), *P. aeruginosa,* obligately anaerobic gram-negative bacilli (e.g., *Bacteriodes* species), enterococci and peptostreptococci. Wound aspirates from these patients most commonly demonstrate polymicrobic infections with *E. coli,* enterococci, and anaerobic bacteria.[40] Recurrent episodes of infection are frequent (up to 26 percent of episodes in one series) among patients recovering from one perirectal infection and receiving subsequent cycles of cytotoxic therapy.[40] The optimal approach to management is controversial. In general, neutropenic patients should be managed medically unless local care, systemic antimicrobics and blood product support fail to contain the infection and if an obvious inflammatory collection must be surgically drained. The likelihood of medical management success is increased if the antimicrobial regimen contains both an aminoglycoside and an agent effective against anaerobic bacteria (e.g., clindamycin or metronidazole). Current standards suggest that an appropriate regimen should consist of a broad-spectrum antipseudomonal penicillin (e.g., carbenicillin, ticarcillin, piperacillin, azlocillin, or mezlocillin) or a third generation antipseudomonal cephalosporin (e.g., cefoperazone or ceftazidime) plus an aminoglycoside (e.g., gentamicin, netilmicin, tobramycin, or amikacin) and an antianaerobic agent (e.g., clindamycin or metronidazole). Further, vancomycin may be added if despite these antimicrobials the cellulitis appears to progress. Early detection and aggressive medical management with antimicrobials have significantly decreased the infection-related mortality rate from >50 percent to <20 percent.[40]

INVASIVE FUNGAL INFECTIONS

OPPORTUNISTIC YEAST INFECTIONS. This group of opportunistic unicellular fungal organisms of the form-class Blastomycetes and form-family Cryptococcaceae includes six genuses: *Cryptococcus* (e.g., *Cryptococcus neoformans,* the agent of cryptococcal meningitis), *Malassezia* (e.g., *Malassezia furfur,* the agent of pityriasis versicolor), *Rodotorula* (e.g., *Rodotorula rubra,* an agent causing pulmonary and systemic infections), *Candida* (e.g., *C. albicans,* the commonest cause of candidiasis), *Trichosporon* (e.g., *Trichosporon beigelii,* the agent of white piedra and systemic infections in compromised hosts), and *Torulopsis* (e.g., *Torulopsis glabrata,* now reclassified under the genus *Candida*). *Candida albicans, C. tropicalis, C. glabrata,* and *Trichosporon* species are part of the normal microflora of the mouth, colon, and vagina. Consequently, it is not surprising to find those agents involved in the pathogenesis of infections among immunocompromised patients with damaged mucosal and integumantel surfaces.

Invasive candidiasis encompasses deep infections of various organ sites with *Candida* species. *Candida albicans* is the most commonly observed; however, *C. tropicalis, C. glabrata, C. parapsilosis, C. krusei,* and *C. guilliermondii* are causal agents of infection in neutropenic patients as well. When multiple organ sites are involved, the term *disseminated candidiasis* may be more appropriate. The most common forms of invasive candidiasis encountered in neutropenia patients are candidemia with or without associated central venous catheter infection, chronic systemic candidiasis (hepatosplenic candidiasis), endophthalmitis, hematogenously spread skin infection and renal candidiasis. The pathogenesis is the invasion of damaged integumented surfaces by colonizing yeasts during severe immunosuppression and myelosuppression.

Candidemia without evidence of metastatic infection is frequently associated with indwelling central venous catheters. Such patients should have the catheter removed and, if febrile with constitutional symptoms of infection, receive treatment with antifungal therapy.[41] An accepted approach would be to administer amphotericin B intravenously to a total dose of 500 to 1000 mg. Patients with evidence of dissemination to other end-organs should be treated with amphotericin B to total doses of 15 to 30 mg/kg (1 to 3 g.). Patients with central nervous system involvement should probably also receive 5-flucytosine (5-FC). Imidazoles such as ketoconazole or miconazole are not recommended. The role of the newer triazole, fluconazole, in the treatment of invasive candidiasis in neutropenic patients, although promising, is as yet unproven.

Chronic systemic candidiasis, also referred to as granulomatous hepatitis, focal hepatic candidiasis, or hepatosplenic candidiasis, has emerged as a significant problem among recipients of high dose cytotoxic therapy.[42–46] The typical clinical presentation is a patient who has received HDARA-C, followed by a febrile illness, which persists despite broad-spectrum antimicrobial therapy and recovery of the circulating neutrophil count. There may be associated right upper quadrant tenderness, hepatomegaly, splenomegaly, and elevated serum alkaline phosphatase and GGT levels. The diagnosis may be established by imaging studies of the abdomen using ultrasonography or CT showing multiple abscesses in the liver and splenic parenchyma (Fig. 99-5). Where possible, a tissue biopsy should be considered for histopathologic and microbiologic confirmation. Biopsy of these lesions demonstrates the presence of necrotizing granulomata, frequently (but not uniformly) containing budding yeasts and pseudohyphal elements consistent with *Candida* species. Liver biopsy specimens should be submitted in a dry sterile container to the clinical microbiology laboratory and processed for pyogenic bacteria, mycobacteria, viruses, and fungi. Specimens for histopathologic evaluation may be submitted to the pathology laboratory in fixative and processed for staining with hematoxylin and eosin, with periodic acid-Schiff (PAS), with an acid-fast stain, and with methenamine silver. Multiple sections through the paraffin-embedded tissue fragments may be necessary to detect the pathogens. In the author's experience, open liver biopsy is the most reliable means of definitively establishing the diagnosis. The pathogen is often not grown despite appropriate culture of the tissue specimen. The determination of a correct diagnosis becomes an im-

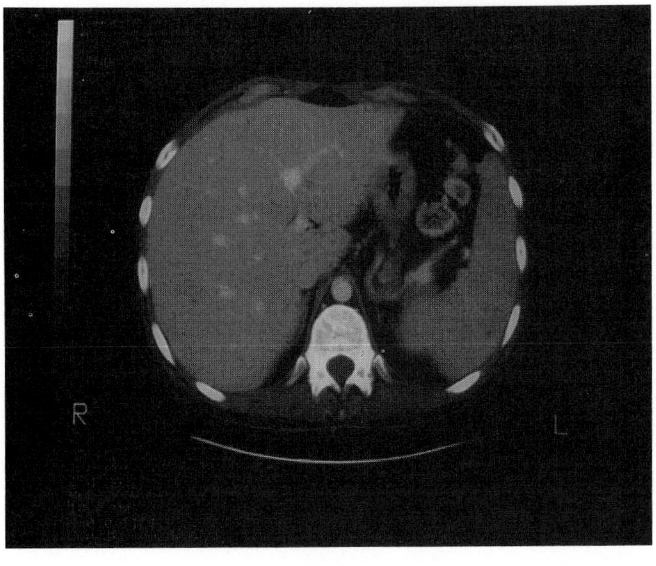

FIGURE 99-5 CT scan of the abdomen in a 22-year-old male recipient of high dose cytarabine for relapsed high grade non-Hodgkin's lymphoma. Multiple areas of decreased attenuation are noted in the hepatic and splenic parenchyma consistent with hepatosplenic candidiasis.

portant factor contributing to the planning of potentially curative postremission therapeutic strategies.

About half the patients respond to systemic amphotericin B (with or without 5-FC) in cumulative doses as high as 9 g. However, even in those who respond, the difficulty with diagnosis and the requirement for prolonged antifungal therapy frequently results in failure to complete planned postremission therapeutic regimens for the underlying malignancies, leading to shortened disease-free survival. The toxicities of prolonged systemic amphotericin B (anemia, renal insufficiency, hypokalemia, fever, chills, nausea) and 5-FC (myelosuppression) are also limiting. More recently, experience with the newer triazole antifungal agent, fluconazole, has suggested that this may be a useful approach for patients unable to tolerate or failing amphotericin B-containing regimens.

OPPORTUNISTIC FILAMENTOUS FUNGAL INFECTIONS. Opportunistic filamentous fungal infections are frequently life-threatening complications among neutropenic patients undergoing remission-induction treatment for AML or BMT. These infections are most often caused by *Aspergillus* species (e.g., flavus, fumigatus, niger) and the Zygomyctes (e.g., *Absidia, Rhizopus, Rhizomucor, Mucor*). They produce similar clinical syndromes in compromised hosts, including necrotizing nasal mucosal infection, sinusitis, endophthalmitis, cerebral parenchymal infection, pulmonary parenchymal infection, cutaneous infection, typhlitis, hepatosplenic abscesses, osteomyelitis, and intravascular infections. They are characterized by blood vessel invasion resulting in thrombosis and blood vessel obstruction which, in turn, causes ischemia and infarction of the distal tissues. This is the mechanism for the clinical manifestations such as pulmonary cavitary disease, hemoptysis, cutaneous infarcts (see Fig. 99-2), strokelike syndromes due to intracranial infection (Fig. 99-6) and parenchymal hepatic infarction (Fig. 99-7). Infection occurs following the germination of inhaled conidia on the respiratory epithelium with the production of invasive hyphae.

Another group of emerging pathogens in immunocompromised patients are the agents of the *hyalohyphomycoses*, a term encompassing all opportunistic mycoses caused by nondematiaceous molds. Examples of pathogens in this group are species of *Fusarium, Penicillium, Scopulariopsis, Acremomium, Geotrichum,* and *P. boydii.* These agents often appear in tissue as hyaline septate branching hyphae and may be angioinvasive. Little differentiates them morphologically from species of *Aspergillus.* Many species are not susceptible to amphotericin B, which is of clinical importance.

These microorganisms are ubiquitous and present in a wide variety of natural and synthetic materials such as soil, decaying vegetation, fireproofing materials, water, and air. *Aspergillus* species have been frequently detected in the air of hospital rooms and, in particular, in circumstances associated with construction and renovation.[47] The management of leukemia and BMT patients in specialized self-contained hospital nursing units outfitted with high-efficiency particulate air filtration (HEPA) has significantly reduced the incidence of invasive aspergillosis.[47]

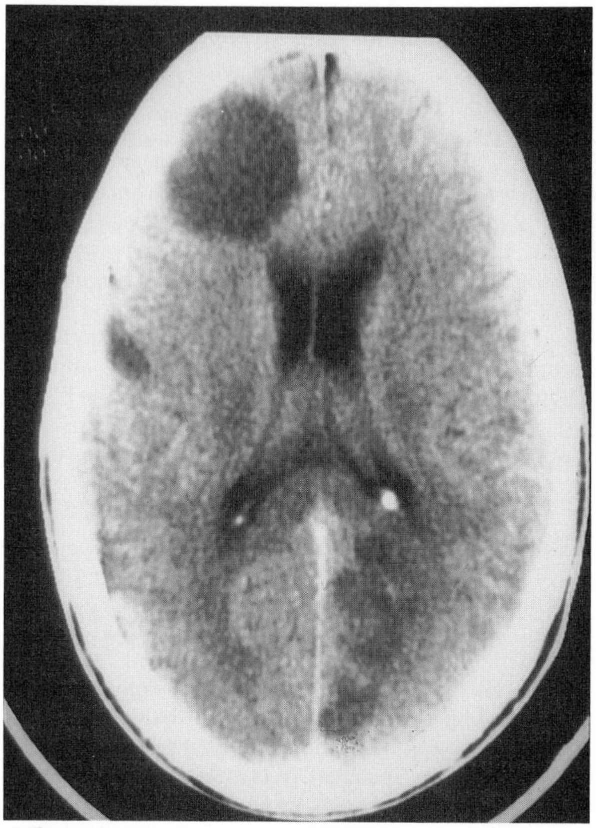

FIGURE 99-6 CT scan of the brain shows an intracerebral infarct in a 27-year-old man being treated for AML complicated by disseminated aspergillosis.

Invasive aspergillosis in leukemia and BMT patients has been reported to have mortality rates in excess of 90 percent almost regardless of treatment.[48] The risk of this infection increases with the duration of neutropenia to a plateau of 70 to 80 percent at 5 weeks.[49] Marrow recovery represents the single most important factor relating to survival of invasive fungal infection in neutropenic patients.[5,50]

The clinical findings relate to the infected organ site. Fever is almost invariably present. Evidence of tissue ischemia and infarction may provide clues to the diagnosis. The most common presentation is that of focal pulmonary infiltrates in a persistently febrile severely neutropenic patient unresponsive to broad-spectrum antibacterial therapy. It has been widely accepted that nasal cultures positive for *Aspergillus* species in this setting can be highly predictive (~90 percent) of invasive aspergillosis.[24] Positive cultures from other respiratory specimens such as sputum, bronchial brushings, or bronchoalveolar lavage fluid can predict invasive aspergillosis in high-risk patients.[51] These observations, however, have not been universal. Among 200 neutropenic inpatients recently reviewed by the author, serial nasal surveillance cultures showed that the predictive

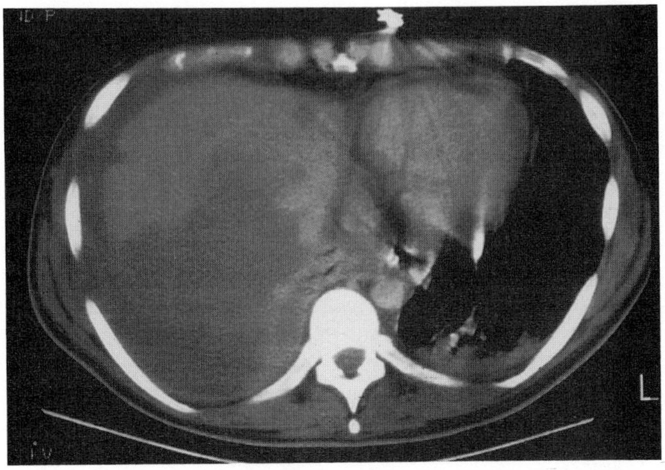

FIGURE 99-7 CT scan of the abdomen in a patient with AML shows massive hepatic infarction secondary to disseminated aspergillosis.

value for invasive aspergillosis of a positive nasal culture for *Aspergillus* species was only 9 percent. This suggests that the predictive value of a positive nasal culture may be sufficiently high to be of clinical use only in the presence of other factors highly associated with invasive pulmonary aspergillosis, that is, focal or nodular pulmonary infiltrates appearing in a febrile patient during profound prolonged neutropenia despite broad-spectrum antibacterial therapy. Based on multivariate analysis of patients with acute leukemia, a number of factors predictive of invasive opportunistic fungal disease have been identified by different investigators.[52–54] In each of these studies the duration of neutropenia was the most important independent variable. Other related variables were the duration of cytotoxic therapy (which gives rise to prolonged neutropenia), the duration of neutropenia associated with antibacterial therapy, and colonization by fungi at surveillance culture sites.

The definitive diagnosis of invasive aspergillosis usually requires a biopsy of involved tissue. The demonstration of dichotomously branching septate hyphae at acute angles in methenamine silver- or PAS-stained tissue sections suggests the diagnosis; however, these morphologic characteristics in stained tissue sections are also shared by species of *Fusarium* and *P. boydii*. Microbiologic identification in culture is required to confirm the diagnosis. This is important since organisms such as *P. boydii* are not susceptible to amphotericin B.

In leukemia patients the mortality rate from invasive pulmonary aspergillosis has ranged between 13 and 100 percent whereas in BMT patients the mortality rate approaches 100 percent.[48] Aspergillosis evolves and progresses despite the concomittant administration of amphotericin B at daily doses of 0.5 mg/kg.[55] Improved responses and survival rates for leukemia patients have been reported with the use of high dose amphotericin B (1.0 to 1.5 mg/kg/day in contrast to a more standard dose of 0.5 to 0.7 mg/kg/day) without serious or permanent renal damage.[55] Anecdotal reports and studies in animal models support the use of 5-FC with amphotericin B.[48] Doses of 5-FC of 100 to 150 mg/kg daily in four divided doses orally usually result in serum levels of 50 to 100 mg/L. There is an increased risk of excess myelosuppression with serum levels above these values. Since 5-FC is excreted predominantly in the urine and concominant amphotericin B therapy is almost always associated with a significant decline in renal function, regular monitoring of 5-FC levels and appropriate adjustment of dose to maintain levels in this range are mandatory.

There is a high risk of relapse (>50 percent) in cancer patients surviving an initial episode of invasive aspergillosis during subsequent cytotoxic treatments.[56] A combination of high dose amphotericin B (1.0 mg/kg/day) and 5-FC (100 mg/kg/day) has been used successfully to protect leukemia patients who developed invasive pulmonary aspergillosis during initial remission-induction against reactivation of the infection during subsequent cycles of cytotoxic therapy and without delay of marrow recovery.[57] This seems to be a rational approach for leukemic patients but its validity for BMT patients remains to be proved. The role of combinations of amphotericin with other agents such as rifampin or the azoles remains unclear and cannot be recommended at the present time.

A promising development for reducing toxicity has been the use of liposome-encapsulated amphotericin B.[58] Early reports have suggested a reduction in toxicity without reduction in efficacy. Although this has permitted the administration of higher doses of amphotericin B, it is unclear whether this is accompanied by an increased efficacy, which, in turn, would have a major impact on the outcome of high-risk leukemia and BMT patients.

INTRAVENOUS CATHETER INFECTIONS

Peripheral intravenous catheters have long been recognized as a source of sepsis for critically ill patients. Venous and arterial cannulae physically disrupt the integrity of the skin and blood vessels, thus providing an avenue for ingress of bacteria or fungi colonizing the skin surfaces at the site of cannula placement. Factors associated with intravenous cannula infection include the type of cannula, the duration of use, the technique of skin preparation for insertion, and the use of venotoxic infusates. The most common microorganisms associated with intravenous site infection are gram-positive organisms such as *S. aureus,* the coagulase-negative staphylococci, *Corynebacterium* JK; gram-negative bacilli such as the Enterobacteriaceae, *P. aeruginosa* and *Acinetobacter anitratus;* and fungi such as *Candida* species. Erythema, swelling, exudate, and focal tenderness associated with a peripheral intravenous catheter site should always alert the clinician to these etiologic possibilities. Suspect catheters should be promptly and carefully removed using aseptic technique and submitted to the clinical microbiology laboratory in a sterile dry container for microbiologic evaluation.

Venous access is a major problem for patients with complex multi-system problems. The need for repeated blood sampling for monitoring and for the administration of different therapies has led to the widespread use of indwelling tunneled central venous catheters. These devices provide a reliable access for venous blood sampling and administration of chemotherapy, blood products, antimicrobial agents, total parenteral nutrition, crystalloids, and vasoactive agents. Infection associated with these devices may occur at the exit site (the point at which the catheter exits the skin), the tunnel site (that portion of the catheter buried subcutaneously extending from the exit site to the insertion site), and the insertion site (that site, often associated with an infraclavicular or small lateral neck incision, where the catheter is inserted into a large central vein, such as the subclavian or internal jugular vein).

Erythema, exudate, and focal tenderness at the exit site suggest, but do not prove, the presence of infection. A quantitative increase in bacterial colony counts in culture swab from the exit site has been associated with an increased possibility that central venous catheter infection is present.[59,60] *Staphylococcus epidermidis* and *Corynebacterium* JK are the most commonly isolated colonizing microorganisms at the exit site and represent the most common etiologic agents associated with catheter sepsis in cancer patients.[61,62] Catheter-related sepsis is suspected if bacteremia or fungemia are present unassociated with any other site of suspected infection. The predominant mechanism of infection appears to be bacterial migration from the exit site along the outside surface of the catheter. Suspected catheter exit site infection, with or without associated bacteremia, may be treated with antimicrobials without removing the line.[63] Unless exit site surveillance cultures dictate otherwise, the empirical antibacterial therapy should include an agent such as vancomycin, which is active against *S. epidermidis* and *Corynebacterium* JK in addition to *S. aureus* and streptococci. Infection of the subcutaneous tunnel site is more difficult to control with antimicrobial agents alone and often requires catheter removal. Catheter removal is also often recommended in the setting of bacteremia due to more highly pathogenic organisms such as *S. aureus, P. aeruginosa,* or *Serratia marcescens,* catheter-related fungemia, or persistent catheter-related bacteremia that has not responded to appropriate antibacterial therapy.

Infection Prevention in the Neutropenic Host

ANTIBACTERIAL PROPHYLAXIS

Antibacterial chemoprophylaxis is widely used for preventing or modifying the etiology of bacterial infection in patients for whom the expected duration of neutropenia is longer than 7 days. Oral nonabsorbable antimicrobial regimens consisting of agents such as aminoglycosides (e.g., neomycin, gentamicin, or tobramycin), vancomycin, polymyxin B, colistin, and nystatin have not been consistently effective for reducing the incidence of infection. In addition, they are unpalatable and costly. On the other hand, oral absorbable antibacterial regimens consisting of TMP/SMX or a fluroquinolone agent (e.g., norfloxacin or ciprofloxacin) have proved useful, although investigators have cautioned that efficacy appears to be intimately linked with compliance,[64] personal hygiene, the spectrum of antimicrobial activity of the regimen,[65] the cytotoxic potential of the antineoplastic regimen, and the timing of the administration of the regimen relative to the onset of the neutropenia-related risk for bacterial infection.[6,66]

The experience with oral quinolones has shown a significant reduction in the morbidity and mortality due to infection by aerobic gram-negative bacilli compared to TMP/SMX.[6,67] The "trade-off" for this appears to be an increase in the risk of infection due to gram-positive organisms such as coagulase-negative staphylococci, enterococci, and viridans group streptococci. The presence of a tunneled indwelling central venous catheter adds to the risk for infections due to coagulase-negative staphylococci,[68] whereas severe mucositis and periodontal disease appear to predispose to viridans streptococcal infection.[32] A syndrome of viridans streptococcal bacteremia has been recognized among high dose cytarabine or BMT recipients, which is often associated with pulmonary infiltrates and hypotension.[69] The pathogenesis is believed to involve severe cytotoxic therapy-induced intestinal mucosal damage in the setting of severe prolonged neutropenia and gastrointestinal lumenal colonization by these organisms. Quinolones may select for these microorganisms. Of clinical importance is the inconsistent susceptibility of these organisms to penicillin G and the apparent need to modify the empirical antibacterial regimen by the addition of intravenous vancomycin to improve the likelihood of a successful outcome for the febrile neutropenic episode. Bacterial infections among TMP/SMX recipients have been due to coagulase-negative staphylococci, viridans streptococci, and TMP/SMX-resistant aerobic gram-negative bacilli such as *P. aeruginosa.*[66]

Knowledge of the chemoprophylactic regimen used and the degree of patient compliance may aid the physician in predicting the likely pathogen involved in the febrile neutropenic episode. Infection occurring in a quinolone recipient should be considered for early gram-positive coverage, whereas infection occurring in a TMP/SMX recipient should be considered for broad-spectrum coverage that includes *P. aeruginosa.*

ANTIFUNGAL PROPHYLAXIS

The major goals of antifungal prophylaxis are to reduce the morbidity and mortality of superficial and invasive opportunistic fungal infections and to reduce the use of toxic antifungal therapy such as amphotericin B. Prophylactic strategies should be applied with a clear understanding of the pathogenesis of the microorganisms involved.

FILAMENTOUS FUNGI. Filamentous fungi such as *Aspergillus* species, Zygomycetes, and *P. boydii* are acquired by inhalation of spores called conidia. The conidia germinate on the respiratory epithelium to produce invasive hyphae. There are three possible ways to prevent this. First, patients may be managed in nursing units outfitted with a HEPA filtration system. This reduces the concentration of airborne conidia and the risk of patient exposure. Although this approach is effective for reducing the risk of filamentous fungal infection, it is expensive and has no impact for patients exposed to airborne conidia outside the nursing unit or for those who are already infected before entering the unit. Second, topical agents such as amphotericin B sprayed by aerosol into the nares theoretically might reduce the risk of conidial germination. One randomized study from the Institute Jules Bordet in Brussels[58] evaluated the use of intranasal amphotericin B (5 mg/mL in sterile water with a total daily dose of 10 mg in three divided doses) in 90 neutropenic episodes. There was no significant difference in the empirical use of intravenous amphotericin B (35 versus 27 percent); however, only 1 of 46 recipients of aerosolized amphotericin B developed suspected or proven invasive aspergillosis compared to 7 of 44 controls. Although this is encouraging, intranasal amphotericin cannot be accepted as a satisfactory alternative to air filtration until further studies are done. Third, systemic antifungal therapy might prevent the progression of hyphal growth once germination occurs. Systemic amphotericin B plus 5-FC has been used successfully to prevent reactivation of previously documented invasive pulmonary aspergillosis among leukemia patients undergoing further postremission cytotoxic therapy.[57] This approach is potentially toxic and probably should be reserved for those in whom opportunistic filamentous fungal infection has been proved by microbiologic or histopathologic methods. The role of newer approaches such as liposomal amphotericin B or the triazole antifungal agents such as fluconazole or itraconazole with greater in vitro activity against *Aspergillus* species is unknown at this time. Several studies are underway to address this issue.

OPPORTUNISTIC YEASTS. Yeast infections, primarily *Candida* species, colonize the patient and cause infection by invading damaged integumental surfaces. HEPA filtering plays no role in the prevention of these infections. The use of topical agents such as nystatin or amphotericin B has had a small impact on colonization profiles but no significant impact on the incidence of invasive fungal infection or the need to use empirical systemic amphotericin B for suspected invasive fungal infection. Topical chlorhexidine mouth rinses (0.12% chlorhexidine digluconate three times daily) have been effective for reducing the morbidity of oropharyngeal candidiasis in a series of marrow allograft recipients.[34] Further, a reduction in candidemia was also noted (0 versus 19 percent, $p < .03$), suggesting the oropharynx as a possible source for these events. The overall value of this strategy must be evaluated in further trials in different populations at risk.

Systemic antifungal therapy for the prevention of opportunistic yeast infections remains controversial. Published studies using the imidazoles, ketoconazole, clotrimazole, and miconazole have demonstrated a reduction of yeast colonization but have failed to demonstrate a consistent reduction in clinical disease or the need to use empirical systemic amphotericin B. There has also been a selection for more resistant yeasts such as *Candida krusei* and *Candida glabrata* in the surveillance cultures of ketoconazole recipients. The newer triazole antifungal agents are now under study and appear promising for the reduction of oropharyngeal candidiasis and perhaps even invasive disease. How and where these agents should be used must be based on definitive clinical trials. No firm recommendations can be made at this time.

ANTIVIRAL PROPHYLAXIS

Reactivation of HSV infection is one of the most common causes of oropharyngeal and esophageal mucositis in patients undergoing remission-induction for leukemia or BMT.[70] This complication is painful and can substantially impair adequate nutritional intake and drug administration. Herpes mucositis stomatitis and esophagitis can largely be prevented by prophylactic use of acyclovir. Patients at risk for these infections are those with a history of previous herpetic infection. They may be reliably identified by a clear history of the typical vesicular lesions of herpetic stomatitis or by the identification of IgG antibodies against HSV in patients' sera. Between 60 and 80 percent of HSV-seropositive patients will reactivate during cytotoxic therapy.[33,70] It has been recommended that patients undergoing remission-induction therapy, consolidation therapy, or salvage therapy for acute leukemia and those undergoing bone marrow allografting or autografting who are IgG seropositive for HSV-1 are candidates for acyclovir prophylaxis.[33] Oral and intravenous routes of administration have been studied and found effective. It remains unclear whether oral administration is as effective as intravenous administration in patients receiving regimens highly toxic to intestinal mucosal surfaces such as high dose cytarabine or etoposide-containing regimens or BMT conditioning regimens. Acyclovir in doses of 250 mg/m^2 administered intravenously every 12 to 8 h or oral acyclovir administered in doses of 200 to 400 mg four to five times daily has successfully prevented HSV mucositis.[33] Prophylaxis for 1 month or less from initiation of treatment has been associated with recurrences in 58 to 70 percent of patients after the acyclovir was discontinued. Accordingly, it has been recommended that prophylaxis be continued for 6 weeks from the beginning of induction or conditioning [33] or up to 6 weeks following marrow recovery in BMT recipients. Acyclovir doses of 800 mg every 12 h orally appears to be effective for this. We currently recommend prophylaxis with acyclovir for HSV-seropositive patients undergoing BMT or induction for acute leukemia. BMT recipients and those patients receiving gut mucosa-damaging high dose cytarabine receive acyclovir 250 mg/m^2 intravenously every 12 h until marrow recovery then oral acyclovir 800 mg every 12 h for a total of 6 weeks. Patients receiving less gut-damaging regimens are given acyclovir 800 mg orally every 12 h for 6 weeks.

CASE PRESENTATION

A 38-year-old woman was admitted to hospital for a second cycle of postremission therapy for acute nonlymphocytic leukemia in first remission. Her admission Karnofsky performance status was 100 percent. Physical examination revealed no abnormalities. Her temperature on admission was 36.8°C (98.1°F); WBC count, 8.5 × 10^9/L; ANC, 6.29 × 10^9/L; and platelet count, 162 × 10^9/L. On the day following admission she began postremission therapy with cytarabine 1.5 g/m^2 (2.5 g/dose) infused over 1 h every 12 h for 12 consecutive doses on days 1 through 6. On the seventh day she received etoposide 1.2 g/m^2 by continuous infusion and on days 8, 9, and 10 she received daunorubicin intravenously, 45 mg/m^2/dose. A bone marrow examination prior to the consolidative course of treatment revealed no evidence of leukemia. Chest x-ray performed at the time of admission revealed no evidence of any abnormalities. A central venous catheter had been implanted in the right subclavian vein and the tip was present in the distal superior vena cava. On the day following admission selective gut decontamination with TMP/SMX 160/800 mg administered orally every 12 h was started.

The patient remained well until day +10 of therapy at which time her oral temperature increased to 38.3°C (101°F) and remained persistently elevated. At the same time, the patient developed severe crampy abdominal pain with localization in the right lower quadrant in association with profuse watery diarrhea. Associated with this she became hypotensive with a blood pressure of 80/40 mmHg. Her ANC was 0.02 × 10^9/L. An abdominal ultrasonographic examination demonstrated thick-walled bowel in the right lower quadrant. CT examination of the abdomen on the same day showed moderate thickening of the wall of the intestine in the right lower quadrant consistent with typhlitis.

The patient became increasingly toxic with persistent fever, tachycardia, hypotension, and poor urinary output. On day +11 she was transferred to the ICU for monitoring, for volume resuscitation, and for intravenous pressor therapy. Following three sets of blood cultures, she was empirically started on intravenous broad-spectrum antibacterial therapy consisting of ceftazidime, vancomycin, and amikacin. Metronidazole was added to the regimen because of the right lower quadrant pain and the abdominal ultrasonographic and CT evidence of typhlitis. The following day the three sets of blood cultures grew *K. pneumoniae* susceptible to ceftazidime and amikacin but resistant to TMP/SMX.

The patient was treated in the ICU between day +11 and day +15 for gram-negative bacillary septic shock. Plasma volume was expanded using crystalloid solutions and albumin; however, infusion of dopamine and later norepinephrine was required to maintain an acceptable blood pressure. Although her temperature remained between 38° and 39°C (100.4° and 102.2°F), she subjectively and objectively improved in response to the supportive treatments. By the time she was ready for discharge from the ICU on day +15 her temperature had fallen to 38°C, (100.4°F), her right lower quadrant pain had disappeared, and her cardiopulmonary status had stabilized. At this point her ANC was 0 and remained <0.1 × 10^9/L until day +33. A follow-up CT examination of the abdomen on day +26 revealed complete resolution of the cecal wall thickening.

On day +20 the patient's temperature again rose to 39.8°C (105.6°F) in association with oropharyngeal ulcerating mucositis. Subsequent viral cultures revealed the presence of HSV. Further, on day +20 the patient's oropharyngeal examination also revealed white pseudomembranous changes in addition to the ulcerating mucositis. Gram's stain of the pseudomembranous material revealed budding yeasts and pseudohyphae. A subsequent culture revealed *C. albicans*. The patient also complained of pain on swallowing, suggesting esophagitis. With clinical diagnoses of HSV and *C. albicans* mucositis as well as probable invasive esophageal candidiasis, the patient was treated with both intravenous acyclovir and with systemic amphotericin B. Acyclovir was given in a dose of 5 mg/kg every 8 h for 10 days, and systemic amphotericin B was given from day +20 through to day +42 to a total dose of 660 mg. The oral ulceration and odynophagia rapidly resolved. Vancomycin was discontinued on day +20; however, she continued to receive the combination of ceftazidime plus amikacin. Her temperature gradually fell to a low-grade fever between 37.5°C (100.1°F) and 38.6°C (102.7°F). During this time the ANC remained at 0.

On day +29 her temperature once again rose abruptly to 39.2°C (104.3°F) in association with a chill. Blood cultures obtained peripherally and from the central venous catheter on that day both grew *S. epidermidis* and a viridans streptococcus within 24 h. Vancomycin was administered intravenously, and by day +34 (day 4 of vancomycin therapy) her temperature was 37.4°C (99.5°F). Coincident with this, the ANC reached levels above 0.1 × 10^9/L, and her subsequent hospital course was uneventful.

CASE DISCUSSION

This case illustrates several important points in the management of the febrile neutropenic patient. The patient received high dose cytotoxic chemotherapy resulting in profound life-threatening neutropenia lasting 24 days during which time four microbiologically documented infections occurred. The sequence of infectious complications observed in this patient is fairly typical of what is seen in this group of patients. The initial bacteremic infection associated with typhlitis occurred relatively early during a protracted period of profound neutropenia. Subsequently, into the second and third week, severe mucositis associated with HSV infection and invasive candidiasis were prominent, and still later in the course a superinfection of the central venous catheter developed due to gram-positive cocci colonizing the skin of the catheter exit site. This patient further illustrates that these infections are usually due to pathogens colonizing the surfaces associated with the infection. In this case, the infections were derived from the lower gastrointestinal tract, the oropharyngeal mucosal surfaces, and the skin.

The first infection was a gram-negative bacteremia due to a TMP/SMX-resistant *K. pneumoniae* in association with cecal typhlitis. This led to septic shock requiring ICU admission for monitoring, volume expansion, and blood pressure support with vasoactive drugs. The patient responded to the appropriate broad-spectrum combination antibacterial regimen. Cecal typhlitis represents one of the major gastrointestinal complications that can be associated with high dose cytarabine chemotherapy. It is likely that the gastrointestinal tract was the portal of entry for the *K. pneumoniae,* which likely colonized that site despite the administration of TMP/SMX. If gut surveillance cultures had demonstrated colonization by this microorganism, which was not susceptible to the selected gut decontaminating regimen, it might have led to a substitution with another decontaminating agent such as one of the oral quinolones. Bacteremic events due to TMP/SMX-resistant colonizing gram-negative bacilli are becoming an increasing problem among neutropenic patients for whom TMP/SMX is being prescribed.

The initial empirical antibacterial therapy for septic shock consisted of three drugs—a broad-spectrum antipseudomonal third generation cephalosporin, ceftazidime; a broad-spectrum aminoglycoside, amikacin; and an agent effective against gram-positive organisms, vancomycin. The combination gram-negative coverage with ceftazidime and amikacin was important for the potential synergistic effect that the combination would have against a gram-negative bacillary pathogen, to provide broad-spectrum activity against the potential pathogens colonizing the cytotoxic therapy-induced damaged gastrointestinal mucosal surfaces and, lastly, to prevent the development of resistance. Because the source of sepsis was believed to be the lower gastrointestinal tract, metronidazole was added to cover anaerobic bacteria as well. It is controversial whether vancomycin is required as part of the empirical antibacterial regimen. Recent studies have suggested that the administration of vancomycin may be safely delayed until diagnostic cultures reveal the presence of a gram-positive organism. This may be related to the relatively lower virulence of many of the gram-positive organisms associated with infections in neutropenic patients. This is illustrated by the course of this patient who developed a polymicrobic gram-positive central venous catheter-related bacteremia 9 days following the discontinuance of vancomycin. She responded promptly to the readministration of vancomycin without necessitating the removal of the central venous catheter. This polymicrobial gram-positive bacteremia occurred while the patient was still receiving ceftazidime plus amikacin. Although this regimen has a high degree of activity against aerobic gram-negative bacillary pathogens, it is not thought to be optimal for the treatment or prevention of infection due to gram-positive cocci.

The patient developed two simultaneous oropharyngeal and esophageal infections subsequent to the first bacteremic event: an HSV ulcerating mucositis and a *C. albicans* pseudomembranous pharyngitis and esophagitis. These responded appropriately to the administration of systemic antiviral and antifungal therapy. The treatment of oropharyngeal and esophageal candidiasis with relatively low total doses of amphotericin B (that is, 10 to 15 mg/kg total dose) appears to be quite successful. Although amphotericin B remains the standard treatment, other agents may be equally as effective for treating these superficial opportunistic fungal infections. Imidazole antifungal drugs such as ketoconazole or triazole antifungals such as fluconazole may be equally as effective without the potential toxicities of amphotericin B. Further studies are needed to clarify this question.

The last infectious complication occurred on day +29 of the cycle: a central venous catheter infection due to two gram-positive cocci, *S. epidermidis* and a viridans group streptococcus. These were effectively treated with vancomycin, which was chosen because of the high prevalence of methicillin-resistant coagulase-negative staphylococci in the institution. Further it was felt that vancomycin would offer satisfactory coverage for both microorganisms.

The recovery from the final infectious episode was paralleled by the recovery of the patient's bone marrow, and as is usual no further infectious complications were seen. Achievement of such a successful outcome, as illustrated by this case, requires constant vigilance for infections throughout the period of chemotherapy-induced neutropenia and integumental disruption, with a prompt and aggressive diagnostic and therapeutic approach for each episode as it arises. Bear in mind that while infectious complications are often multiple and diverse they are to some extent predictable from their time of onset after chemotherapy, the severity of immunosuppression and tissue injury, and the prior use of antimicrobial prophylaxis and therapy.

References

1. Lloyd-Thomas AR, Dhaliwal HS, Lister TA, Hinds CJ: Intensive therapy for life-threatening medical complications of haematological malignancy. Intensive Care Med 12:317, 1986.
2. Torrecilla C, Cortes JL, Chamorro C, et al: Prognostic assessment of the acute complications of bone marrow transplantation requiring intensive therapy. Intensive Care Med 14:393, 1987.

3. Schimpff SC: Dilemmas and choices in infection management of the cancer patient. Eur J Cancer Clin Oncol 25:1351, 1989.
4. Pizzo PA, Robichaud KJ, Wesley R, Commors JR: Fever in the pediatric and young adult patients with cancer. Medicine 61:153, 1982.
5. Bow EJ, Louie TJ: Changes in endogenous microflora among febrile granulocytopenic patients receiving empiric antibiotic therapy: Implications for fungal superinfection. Can Med Assoc J 137:397, 1987.
6. Bow EJ, Rayner E. Louie TJ: Comparison of norfloxacin with cotrimoxazole for infection prophylaxis in acute leukemia. Am J Med 84:847, 1988.
7. Feld R, Louie TJ, Mandell 1, et al: A multicenter comparative trial of tobramycin and ticarcillan versus moxalactam and ticarcillin in febrile neutropenic patients. Arch Intern Med 145:1083, 1985.
8. EORTC International Antimicrobial Therapy Cooperative Group: Ceftazidime combined with a short or long coursè of amikacin for empirical therapy of gram-negative bacteremia in cancer patients with granulocytopenia. N Engl J Med 317:1692, 1987.
9. Bow EJ, Kilpatrick M, Scott BA, Clinch J: AML in Manitoba: Observations on the use of "3:7" induction regimens. Clin Invest Med 13 (suppl):B48, 1990.
10. Kurrle E, Dekker AW, Gaus W, et al: Prevention of infection in acute leukemia: A prospective randomized study of the efficacy of two different drug regimens for antimicrobial prophylaxis. Infection 14:226, 1986.
11. Hersh EM, Gutterman JU, Mauligit GM, et al: Serial studies of immunocompetance of patients undergoing chemotherapy for acute leukemia. J Clin Invest 54:401, 1974.
12. Dupuy JM, Kourilsky FM, Fradelizzi D, et al: Depression in immunologic reactivety of patients with acute leukemia. Cancer 27:323, 1971.
13. Walzer PD, Perl DP, Krogstad DJ, et al: *Pneumocystis carinii* pneumonia in the United States. Epidemiological, diagnostic and clinical features, in Robbins JB, DeVita VT Jr, Dutz W (eds): *Symposium on Pneumocystis carinii infection.* NCI Monograph #43. Washington DC, National Cancer Institute, 1976, pp 55–63.
14. Lockhart PB, Sonis ST: Relationship of oral complications to peripheral blood leukocyte and platelet counts in patients receiving cancer chemotherapy. Oral Surgery 48:21, 1979.
15. Hughes WT, Armstrong D, Bodey GP, et al: Guidelines for the use of antimicrobial agents in neutropenic patients with unexplained fever. J Infect Dis 161:381, 1990.
16. Bates DW, Cook EF, Goldman L, Lee TH: Predicting bacteremia in hospitalized patients. Ann Intern Med 113:495, 1990.
17. Sickles EA, Greene WH, Wiernik PH: Clinical presentation of infection in granulocytopenic patients. Arch Intern Med 135:715, 1975.
18. Walsh TJ: The febrile granulocytopenic patient in the intensive care unit. Crit Care Clin 4:259, 1988.
19. Rubin RH, Greene R: Etiology and management of the compromised patient with fever and pulmonary infiltrates, in Rubin RH, Young LS (eds): *Clinical Approach to Infection in the Compromised Host.* New York, Plenem, 1988, pp 131–163.
20. Pizzo PA, Hathorn JW, Hiemenz J, et al: A randomized trial comparing ceftazidime alone with combination antibiotic therapy on cancer patients with fever and neutropenia. N Engl J Med 315:552, 1986.
21. dePauw BE, Feld R, Deresinski S, et al: Multicentre, randomized comparative study of ceftazidime versus piperacillin plus tobramycin as empirical therapy for febrile granulocytopenic patients, in *6th International Symposium on Infections in the Immunocompromised Host,* Peebles Scotland, June 1990, Abstract #116.
22. Rubin M, Hathorn JW, Pizzo PA: Controversies in the management of febrile neutropenic cancer patients. Cancer Invest 6:167, 1988.
23. Pizzo PA, Robichaud KJ, Gill FA, Witebsky FG: Empiric antibiotic and antifungal therapy for cancer with prolonged fever and granulocytopenia. Am J Med 72:101, 1982.
24. Aisner J, Murillo J, Schimpff SC, Steere AC: Invasive aspergillosis in acute leukemia: Correlation with nose cultures and antibiotic use. Ann Intern Med 90:4, 1979.
25. Sandord GR, Merz WG, Wingard JR, et al: The value of fungal surveillance cultures as predictors of systemic fungal infection. J Infect Dis 142:503, 1980.
26. Pizzo PA, Ladisch S, Robichaud K: Treatment of gram-positive septicemia in cancer patients. Cancer 45:206, 1980.
27. Riben PD, Horsman GB, Rayner E, et al: Emergence of tobramycin-resistant *S. epidermidis* possessing aminoglycoside modifying enzymes and bacteremia superinfection during empiric therapy of febrile neutropenia episodes. Clin Invest Med 8:272, 1985.
28. Overholser CD, Peterson DE, Williams LT, Schimpff SC: Periodontal infection in patients with acute nonlymphocytic leukemia, prevalence of acute exacerbations. Arch Intern Med 142:551, 1982.
29. DeGregorio MW, Lee WMF, Ries CA: Candida infections in patients with acute leukemia: Ineffectiveness of nystatin prophylaxis and relationship between oropharyngeal and systemic candidiasis. Cancer 50:2780, 1982.
30. Montgomery MT, Redding WS, LeMaistre CF: The incidence of oral herpes simplex virus infection in patients undergoing cancer chemotherapy. Oral Surg, Oral Med, Oral Pathol 61:238, 1986.
31. Lindquist SF, Hickey AJ, Drane JB: Effect of oral hygiene on stomatitis in patients receiving cancer chemotherapy. Prost Dent 40:312, 1978.
32. Peterson DE, Minah GE, Overholser CD, et al: Microbiology of acute periodontal infection in myelosuppressed cancer patients. J Clin Oncol 5:1461, 1987.
33. Gold D, Corey L: Acyclovir prophylaxis for herpes simplex virus infection. Antimicrob Agents Chemother 31:361, 1987.
34. Ferretti GA, Ash RC, Brown AT, et al: Control of oral mucositis and candidiasis in marrow transplantation: A prospective, double-blind trial of chlorhexidine digluconate oral rinse. Bone Marrow Transpl 3:483-493, 1988.
35. Brammer KW: Management of fungal infection in neutropenic patients with fluconazole. Haematol Blood Transfusion 33:546, 1990.
36. Schamberger RC, Weinstein HJ, Delorey MJ, Levey RH: The medical and surgical management of typhlitis in children with acute nonlymphocytic (myelogenous) leukemia. Cancer 57:603, 1986.
37. Keidan RD, Fanning J, Gatenby RA, Weese JL: Recurrent typhlitis; a disease resulting from aggressive chemotherapy. Dis Colon Rectum 32:206, 1989.
38. Moir CR, Scudamore CH, Benny WB: Typhlitis: Selective surgical management. Am J Surgery 151:563, 1986.
39. Kunkel JM, Rossenthal D: Management of the ileocecal syndrome. Neutropenic enterocolitis. Dis Colon Rectum 29:196, 1986.
40. Glenn J, Cotton D, Wesley R, Pizzo P: Anorectal infectious in patients with malignant diseases. Rev Infect Dis 10:42, 1988.
41. Crislip MA, Edwards JE: Candidiasis. Infect Dis Clin North Am 3:103, 1989.

42. Bodey GD, Anaussie EJ: Chronic systemic candidiasis. Eur J Clin Microbiol Infect Dis 8:855, 1989.
43. Jones JM: Granulomatous hepatitis due to candida albicans in patients with acute leukemia. Ann Intern Med 94:475, 1981.
44. Tashjian LS, Abramson JS, Peacock JE: Focal hepatic candidiasis: A distinct clinical variant of candidiasis in immunocompromised patients. Rev Infect Dis 6:689, 1984.
45. Haron E, Feld R, Tuffnell P, et al: Hepatic candidiasis; an increasing problem in immunocompromised patients. Am J Med 83:17, 1987.
46. Thater M, Pastakia B, Shawker TH, et al: Hepatic candidiasis in cancer patients: The evolving picture of the syndrome. Ann Intern Med 108:88, 1988.
47. Sherertz RJ, Belani A, Kramer BJ et al: Impact of air filtration on nosocomial aspergillus infections. Am J Med 83:709, 1987.
48. Denning DW, Stevens DA: Antifungal and surgical management of invasive aspergillosis: Review of 2121 published corres. Rev Infect Dis 12:1147, 1990.
49. Gerson SL, Talbot GH, Hurwitz S, et al: Prolonged granulocytopenia: The major risk factor for invasive pulmonary aspergillosis in patients with acute leukemia. Ann Intern Med 100:345, 1984.
50. Albelda SM, Talbot GH, Gerson SL, et al: Pulmonary cavitation and massive hemoptysis in invasive pulmonary aspergillosis. Influence on bone marrow recovery in patients with acute leukemia. Am Rev Respir Dis 131:115, 1985.
51. Letitz SM: Aspergillosis. Infect Dis Clin North Am 3:1, 1989.
52. Schwartz RS, Mackintosh R, Schrier SL, Greenberg PL: Multivariate analysis of factors associated with invasive fungal disease during remission induction therapy for acute myelogenous leukemia. Cancer 53:411, 1984.
53. Wiley JM, Smith N, Leventhal BG, et al: Invasive fungal disease in pediatric acute leukemia patients with fever and neutropenia during induction chemotherapy: A multivariate analysis of risk factors. J Clin Oncol 8:280, 1990.
54. Tollemar J, Ringden O, Bostrom L, et al: Variables predicting deep fungal infections in bone marrow transplant recipients. Bone Marrow Transpl 4:635, 1989.
55. Burch PA, Karp JE, Merz WG, et al: Favorable outcome of invasive aspergillosis in patients with acute leukemia. J Clin Oncol 5:1985, 1987.
56. Robertson MJ, Larson RA: Recurrent fungal pneumonias in patients with acute nonlymphocytic leukemia undergoing multiple courses of intensive chemotherapy. Am J Med 84:233, 1988.
57. Karp JE, Burch PA, Marz W: An approach to intensive antileukemia therapy in patients with previous invasive aspergillosis. Am J Med 85:203, 1988.
58. Meunier F: New methods for delivery of antifungal agents. Rev Infect Dis 11(suppl 7):S1605, 1989.
59. Conly JM, Grieves K, Peters B: A prospective randomized study comparing transplant and dry gauze dressings for central venous catheters. J Infect Dis 159:310, 1965.
60. Armstrong CW, Mayhall CG, Miller KB, et al: Clinical predictors of infection of central venous catheters used for parenteral nutrition. Infect Control Hosp Epidemiol 11:71, 1990.
61. Landoy Z, Rotstein C, Lucey J, Fitzpatrick J: Hickman-broviac cathether use in cancer patients, J Surg Oncol 26:215, 1984.
62. Lowder JN, Lazarus HM, Herzig RH: Bacteremias and fungemias in oncology patients with central venous catheters: Changing spectrum of infection. Arch Intern Med 142:1456, 1982.
63. Benezra D, Kiehn TE, Gold JWIM, et al: Prospective study of infections in indwelling central venous catheters using quantitative blood cultures. Am J Med 85:495, 1988.
64. Pizzo PA, Robichaud KJ, Edwards BK, et al: Oral antibiotic prophylaxis in patients with cancer: A double-blind randomized placebo controlled trial. J Pediatr 102:125, 1983.
65. Bow EJ, Rayner E, Scott BA, Louie TJ: Selective gut decontamination with nalidixic acid or trimethoprim/sulfamethoxazole for infection prophylaxis in neutropenic cancer patients: Relationship of efficacy to antimicrobial spectrum and timing of administration. Antimicrob Agents Chemother 31:551, 1987.
66. Bow EJ, Louie TJ: Emerging role of quinolones in the prevention of gram-negative bacteremia in neutropenic cancer patients and in the treatment of enteric infections. Clin Invest Med 12:61, 1989.
67. Dekker AW, Rosenberg-Arska M, Verhoef J: Infection prophylaxis in acute leukemia: A comparison of ciprofloxacin with trimethoprim/sulfamethoxazole and colistin. Ann Intern Med 106:7, 1987.
68. Wade JC, Schimpff SC, Newman KA: Staphylococcus epidermidis: An increasing cause of infections in patients with granulocytopenia. Ann Intern Med 97:503, 1982.
69. Weisman SJ, Scoopo FJ, Johnson GM, et al: Septicemia in pediatric oncology patients: The significance of viridans streptococcal infections. J Clin Oncol 8:453, 1990.
70. Saral R, Ambinder RF, Burns WH, et al: Acyclovir prophylaxis against herpes simplex virus infection in patients with leukemia. Ann Intern Med 99:773, 1983.

Chapter 100

AIDS IN THE INTENSIVE CARE UNIT

JULIO S.G. MONTANER
PETER PHILLIPS
JAMES A. RUSSELL

KEY POINTS

- *The acquired immunodeficiency syndrome (AIDS) is caused by chronic infection with the human immunodeficiency virus (HIV), which causes progressive depletion of T helper lymphocytes leading to severe cellular immunodeficiency.*
- *After a median incubation of approximately 12 years, infected subjects develop multiple opportunistic infections and/or neoplasms characteristic of AIDS. At present, AIDS carries a 100 percent mortality.*
- *HIV transmission is currently limited to sexual exposure (homosexual or heterosexual), exposure to blood or blood products (including transplanted organs), and perinatal exposure (transplacentally, at the time of delivery or through lactation).*
- *HIV cannot be transmitted through casual contact. Universal precautions, however, should be implemented and enforced to minimize the risk of occupational exposure to HIV as well as other infectious agents. The rate of seroconversion following a single accidental needle stick or mucous membrane exposure appears to be well below 1%.*
- *Zidovudine (Azidothymidine, AZT, Retrovir) has been shown to prolong survival of selected groups of HIV-infected patients. Anemia, macrocytosis, reticulocytopenia, and leucopenia of varying severity are characteristic bone marrow effects of zidovudine therapy.*
- *ddI (Didanosine, 2'3'-Dideoxyinosine) is an experimental nucleoside widely used in North America for the treatment of advanced HIV disease clinically resistant to AZT or when intolerance precludes AZT use. Pancreatitis, peripheral neuropathy, seizures, hyperuricemia, and even gout have been reported to occur with increased frequency among ddI-treated patients. Bone marrow suppression, on the other hand, rarely occurs as a result of ddI therapy.*
- *Acute respiratory failure (ARF) secondary to* Pneumocystis carinii *pneumonia (PCP) is the most frequent cause of ICU admission among HIV-infected individuals.*
- *PCP is usually diagnosed in the ICU using bronchoalveolar lavage (BAL). BAL fluid should always be appropriately processed to allow identification of* P. carinii, *other fungi, common bacteria, mycobacteria, and viruses.*
- *PCP-related ARF should be aggressively treated with specific antimicrobials, adjunctive systemic corticosteroids, and oxygenation support.*
- *The mortality of PCP-related ARF has significantly decreased with the use of adjunctive systemic corticosteroids. Patients developing ARF despite corticosteroid treatment, however, continue to have a dismal prognosis.*
- *The issue of life support should be discussed early and reassessed frequently with the HIV-infected individual. ICU admission and life support, however, should be discouraged for patients with multiple life-threatening complications for which there is no effective therapy. Because the outlook of AIDS and its related diseases is changing rapidly, rigid policies regarding ICU eligibility should be discouraged.*

Human Immunodeficiency Virus Infection

The acquired immunodeficiency syndrome (AIDS) is caused by chronic infection with the human immunodeficiency viruses (HIV-1, HIV-2, and possibly others). These retroviruses have a tropism for helper T lymphocytes that leads to their dysfunction and gradual depletion.[1,2] It is now known that HIV can infect other cells including macrophages and B lymphocytes.[3,4] Eventually, this results in the development of the otherwise unusual opportunistic infections and neoplasms characteristic of AIDS.

Since initially described, AIDS has reached pandemic proportions. The World Health Organization (WHO) estimated that, by early 1990, over 220,000 cases of AIDS had been reported in over 150 countries. The dimension of the problem can be better appreciated by knowing that there are an estimated 5 to 10 million HIV-infected people and that the most conservative forecasts predict not less than 1 million AIDS cases worldwide during the years 1990 to 1995.

Although the proportion of AIDS cases requiring intensive care unit (ICU) admission has generally been small, the actual number of AIDS-related ICU admissions has been rising steadily over the last decade. Furthermore, we anticipate that this trend may be accentuated as new therapeutic developments continue to change the natural history of AIDS from a rapidly lethal to a relatively chronic and manageable disease.

TRANSMISSION

The most common route of transmission of HIV remains sexual intercourse. It must be emphasized that homosexual and heterosexual transmission occur and in both cases bidirectional transmission is possible.[5] The second most prevalent form of transmission is through exposure to infected blood or blood products, including transplanted organs. Since the widespread adoption of HIV screening of donated blood, however, parenteral transmission of HIV is limited almost exclusively to intravenous drug use.[6] Finally, the infection can also be transmitted perinatally. This refers to infection of the offspring transplacentally, at the time of delivery or through lactation.[7]

PLATES

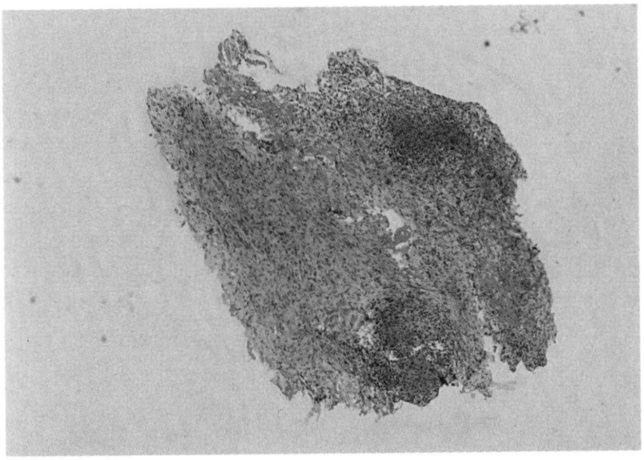

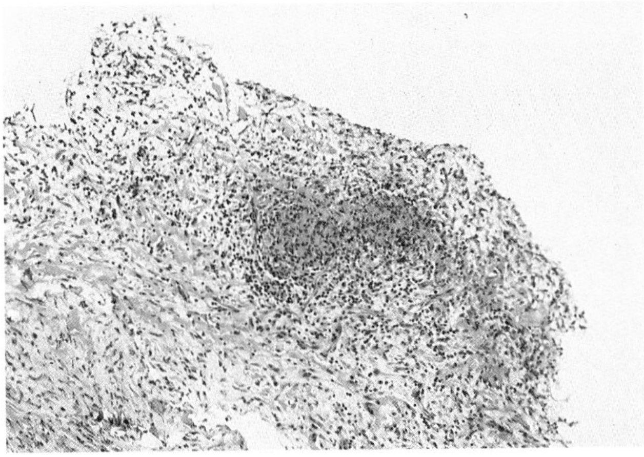

A B

PLATE 1 Pleural biopsy at low (*a*) and high (*b*) power magnification reveals epithelioid granulomas typical of pleural tuberculosis. Cultures were positive for *Mycobacterium tuberculosis.*

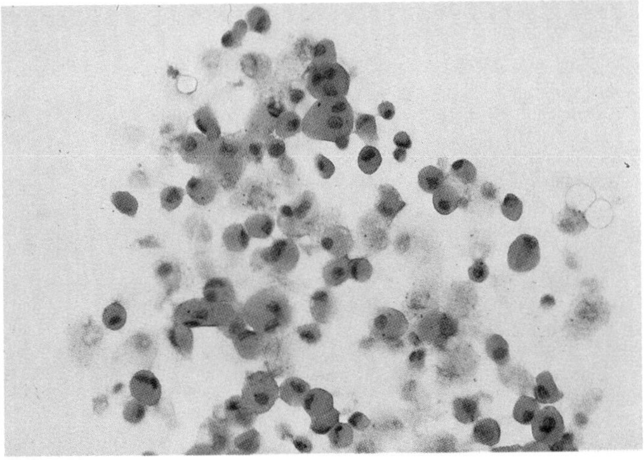

PLATE 2 Adequate induced sputum specimen showing alveolar macrophages [hematoxylin and eosin (H&E) ×100].

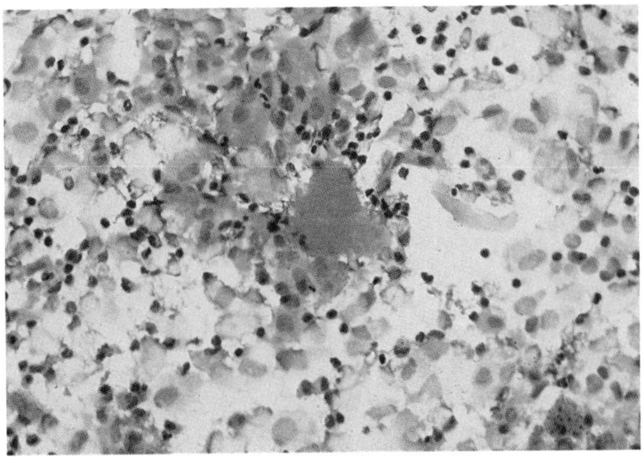

PLATE 3 BAL specimen showing characteristic granular material found in pneumocystis pneumonia infection (H&E ×100).

PLATE 4 Cup-and-saucer–shaped *Pneumocystis* organisms seen on BAL (GMS ×100).

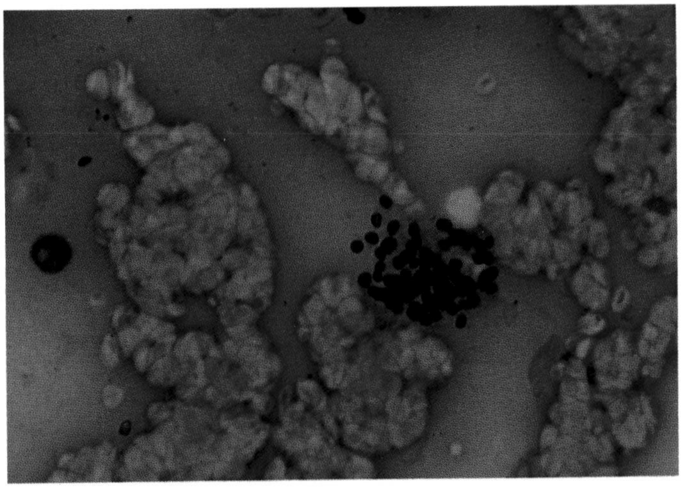

PLATE 5 Hyphae of aspergillus seen on BAL preparation (GMS ×100).

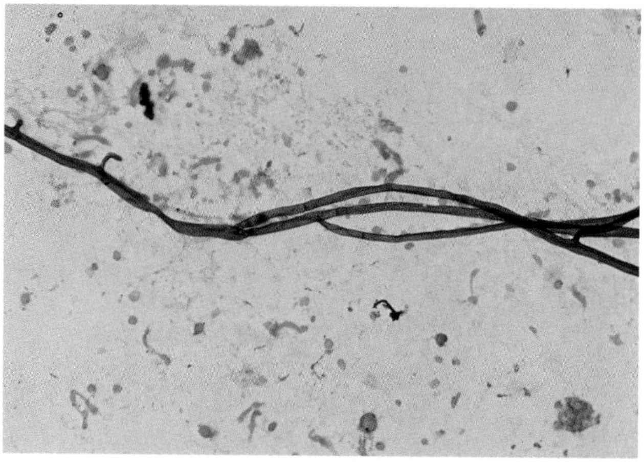

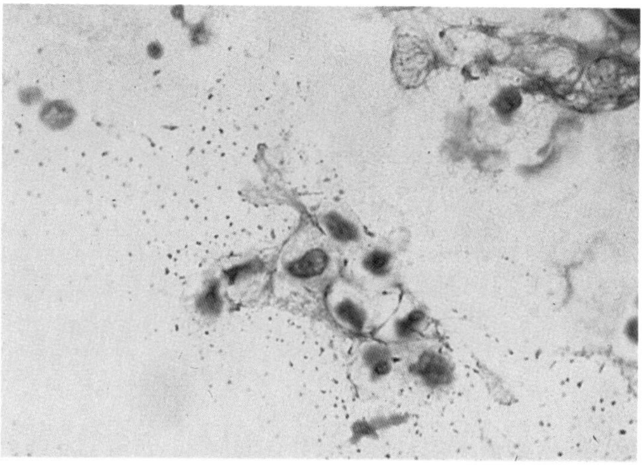

PLATE 6 *Mycobacterium tuberculosis* seen in bronchoalveolar lavage specimen (Ziehl-Neelsen stain ×100).

PLATE 7 Transbronchial biopsy showing recurrence of leukemia in the lung (H&E ×100).

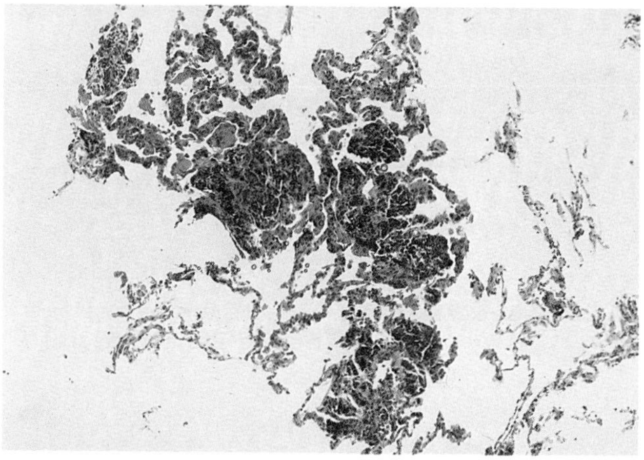

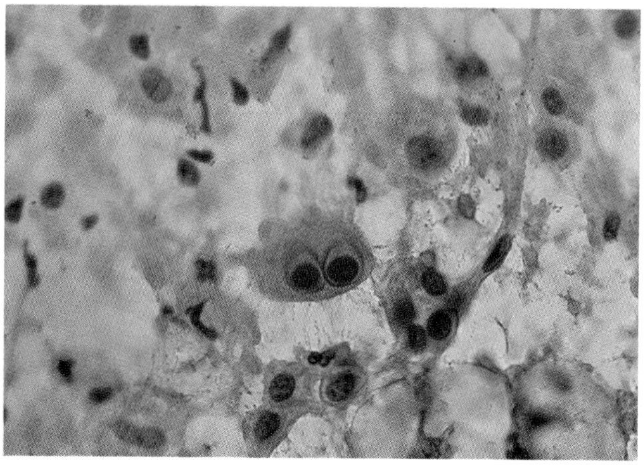

PLATE 8 Scrimp preparation of open lung biopsy showing characteristic intranuclear and intracytoplasmic inclusions of CMV (H&E ×100).

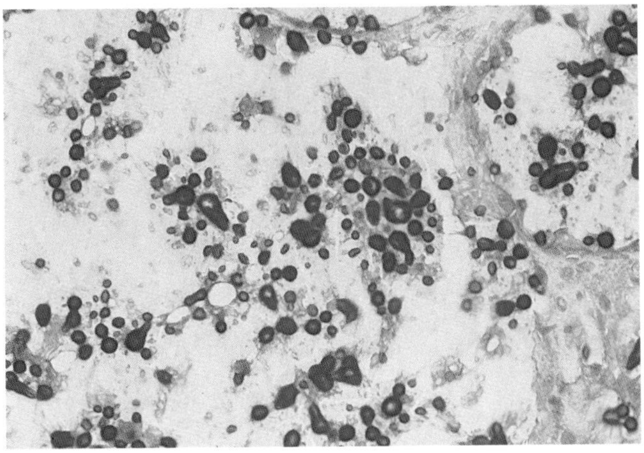

PLATE 9 Budding yeasts showing mucin positive capsule characteristic of cryptococcosis (mucicarmine stain ×100).

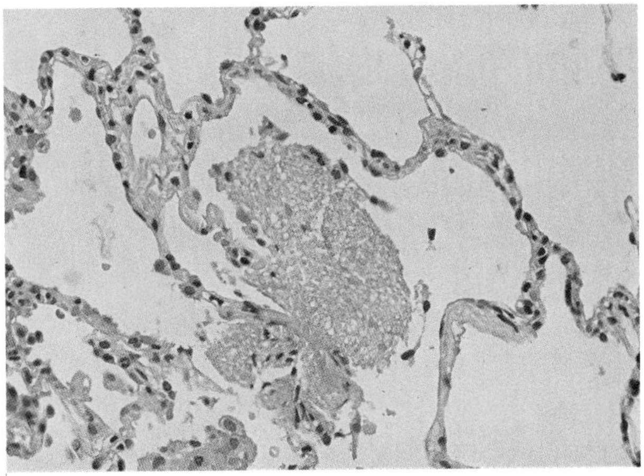

PLATE 10 Characteristic foamy honeycomb material seen in alveolar spaces in pneumocystis pneumonia (H&E ×100).

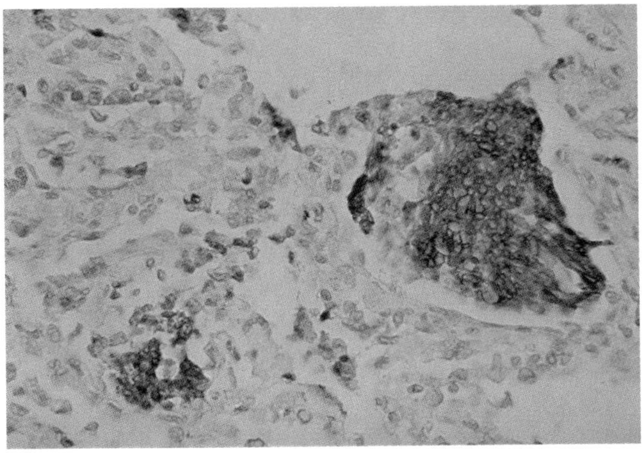

PLATE 11 Monoclonal antibody staining of *P. carinii* (immunohistochemical staining ×100).

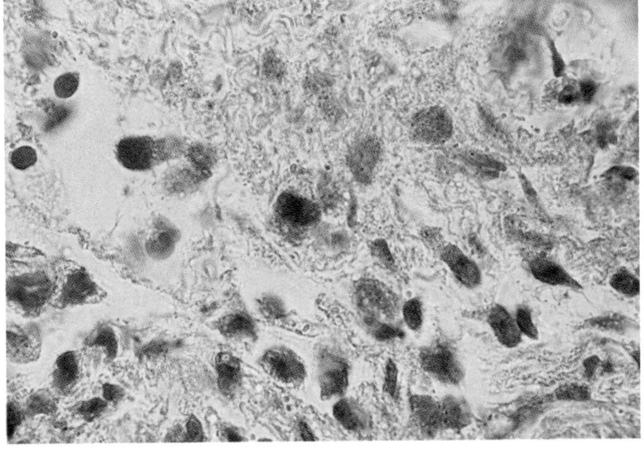

PLATE 12 Monoclonal antibody staining of CMV (immunohistochemical stain ×100).

PLATE 13 Stop frame two-dimensional echocardiographic and color flow Doppler images of the long axis view of the left ventricle (LV) and left atrium (LA) obtained from the left parasternal window. In this patient inferior wall myocardial infarction resulted in necrosis of the posteromedial papillary muscle, disruption of some of the chordal attachments of the posterior mitral leaflet, and mitral regurgitation in association with a flail mitral valve. *Right.* In systole, the posterior mitral leaflet fails to coapt normally with the anterior leaflet, and the flail segment (arrow) prolapses into the left atrium. *Left.* In this systolic color flow Doppler stop frame image, a heterogenous mosaic of colors (aqua and yellow predominantly) originates from the mitral orifice and spreads through the left atrium under the anterior mitral leaflet. This abnormal Doppler signal represents the anteriorly directed flow disturbance of mitral regurgitation resulting from the flail posterior mitral leaflet. In the absence of mitral regurgitation, no color flow Doppler signals would be detected in the left atrium in systole except for the relatively homogenous red signals in the posterior left atrium which are attributed to pulmonary venous return.

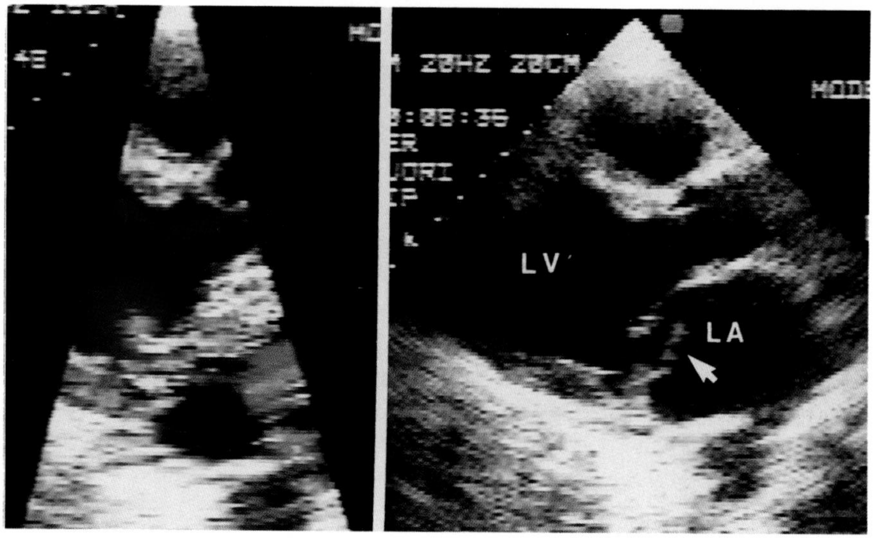

PLATE 14 Stop frame color flow Doppler echocardiograms in systole (*left*); and diastole (*center*) of the long axis view of the left ventricle (LV) and atrium (LA) obtained from the parasternal window. The schematic drawing (*right*) illustrates the location of the aortic valve (AV) within the aorta (Ao) and the mitral valve (MV) within the LV inflow tract. *Left.* In systole an aqua mosaic Doppler signal of disturbed flow velocities originating from the mitral orifice and spreading into the LA signifies mitral regurgitation. *Center.* In diastole the same patient now has an abnormal heterogenous color Doppler signal originating from the AV and extending into the LV outflow tract representing aortic regurgitation.

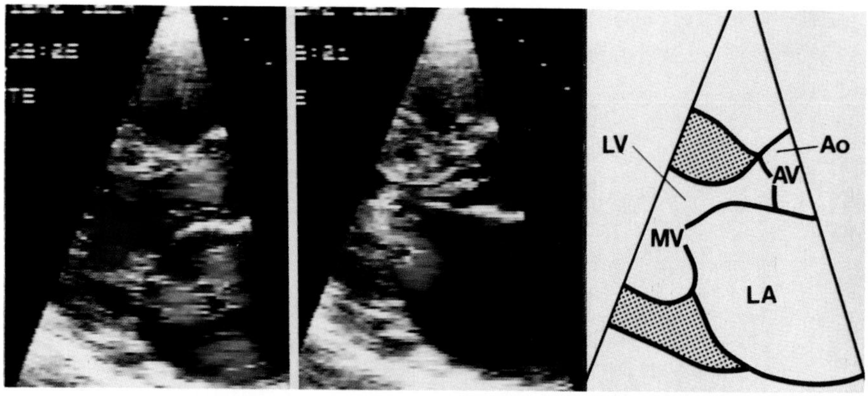

PLATE 15 Systolic stop frame color flow Doppler echocardiogram of the four chamber view of the heart obtained with the transducer at the left ventricular apex along with schematic drawing. Mitral regurgitation is represented by the heterogenous mosaic of colors originating from the orifice of the mitral valve (MV) and spreading to fill approximately two-thirds of the left atrium (LA). Secondary tricuspid regurgitation is depicted by the abnormal color flow Doppler signals originating from the orifice of the tricuspid valve (TV) and extending to fill a large portion of the right atrium (RA). Figure 21-14 (see page 288) illustrates the continuous wave Doppler measurements obtained from these regurgitant flow velocity disturbances (LV = left ventricle, RV = right ventricle).

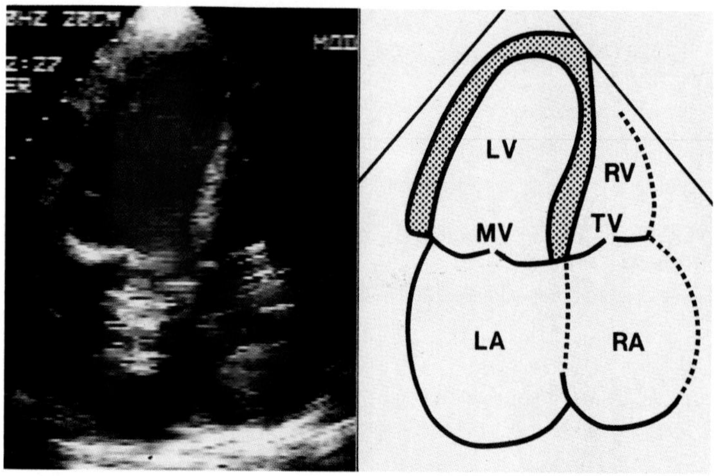

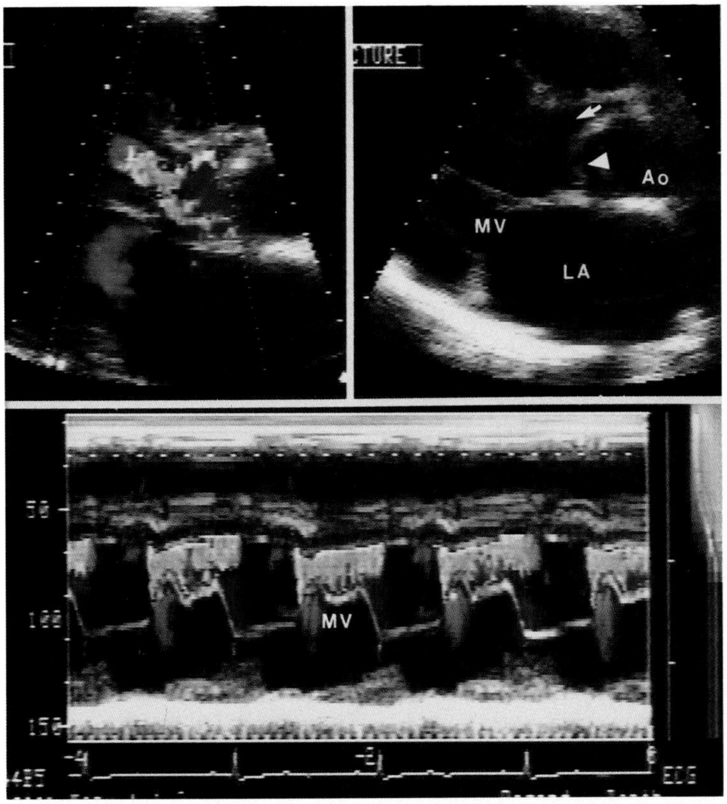

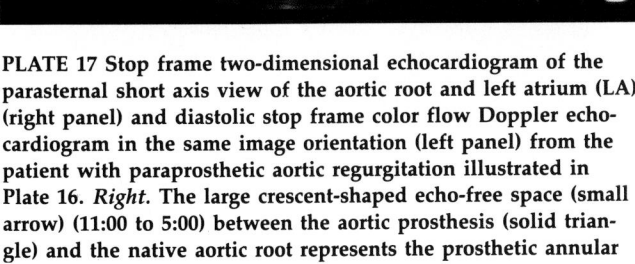

PLATE 16 Stop frame two-dimensional echocardiogram of the parasternal long axis view of the mitral valve (MV), left atrium (LA) and aorta (Ao) (top right panel), diastolic stop frame color flow Doppler echocardiogram with the same image orientation (top left panel), and accompanying color flow Doppler M-mode echocardiogram (bottom panel) from a patient with paraprosthetic aortic regurgitation. *Top right.* The center of the prosthesis is indicated by the solid triangle. An echo-lucent channel (small arrow) between the native aortic root tissues (anteriorly) and the annulus of the aortic prosthesis represents the anatomic path for paravalvular regurgitation. *Top left.* Superimposed on the two-dimensional echocardiographic anatomy, this diastolic stop frame image from the patient's color flow Doppler echocardiogram illustrates two distinct mosaic patterned (aqua colored) flow disturbances in the left ventricular outflow tract proximal to the prosthetic aortic valve. An anterior paraprosthetic regurgitant jet and a posterior paravalvular regurgitant jet coalesce to form a single regurgitant disturbance anterior to the mitral valve. *Bottom.* The M-mode echocardiogram of the anterior mitral valve (MV) leaflet is displayed along with the ECG below. During diastole (just prior to the QRS of the ECG), the aqua color is mapped on the M-mode echocardiogram anterior to the anterior mitral leaflet. In the tachycardic patient, color Doppler M-mode echocardiography can be extremely useful for precisely timing transient color flow disturbances seen during real time playback of the two-dimensional color flow Doppler study.

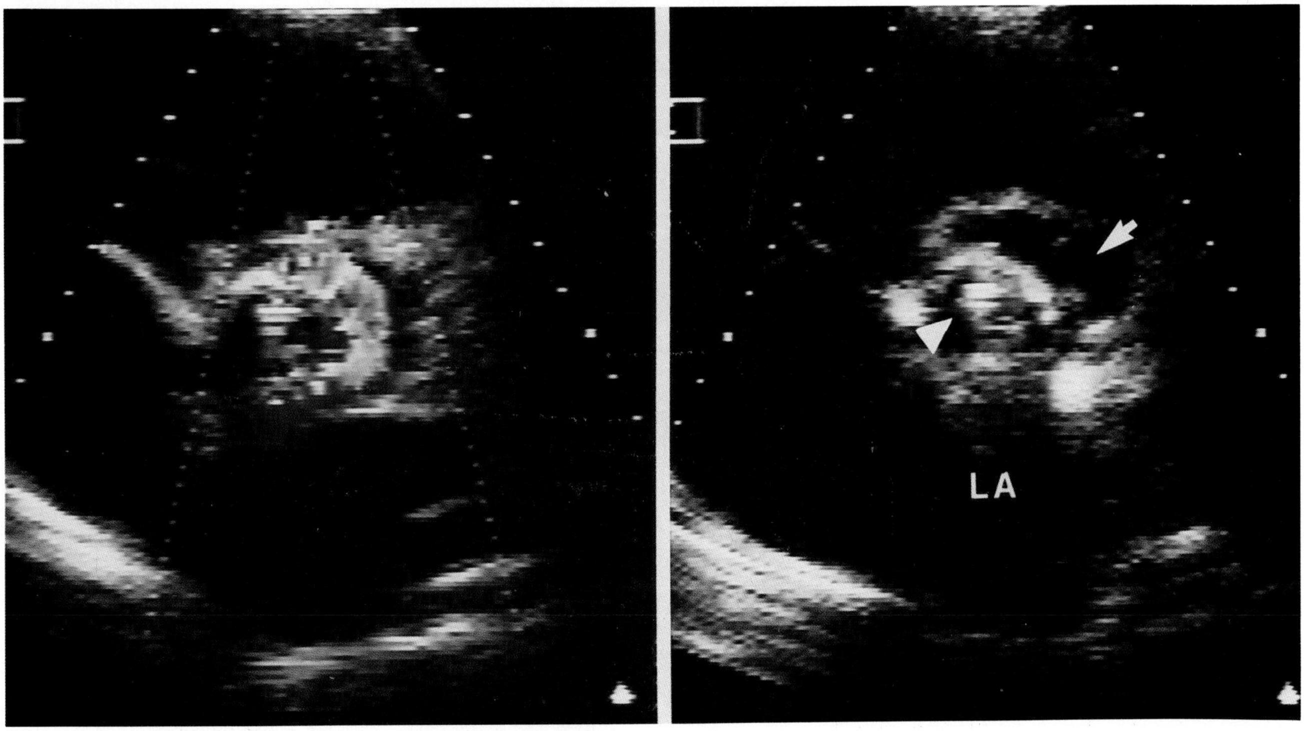

PLATE 17 Stop frame two-dimensional echocardiogram of the parasternal short axis view of the aortic root and left atrium (LA) (right panel) and diastolic stop frame color flow Doppler echocardiogram in the same image orientation (left panel) from the patient with paraprosthetic aortic regurgitation illustrated in Plate 16. *Right.* The large crescent-shaped echo-free space (small arrow) (11:00 to 5:00) between the aortic prosthesis (solid triangle) and the native aortic root represents the prosthetic annular dehiscence and the path for paravalvular aortic regurgitation. *Left.* The diastolic stop frame color flow Doppler image maps the paraprosthetic aortic regurgitation to the dehiscence channel as a variegated aqua color Doppler signal. The two paravalvular regurgitant jets imaged in Plate 16 represent transection of the anterior and posterior limbs of this crescent-shaped flow disturbance in the long axis plane which is orthogonal to this image.

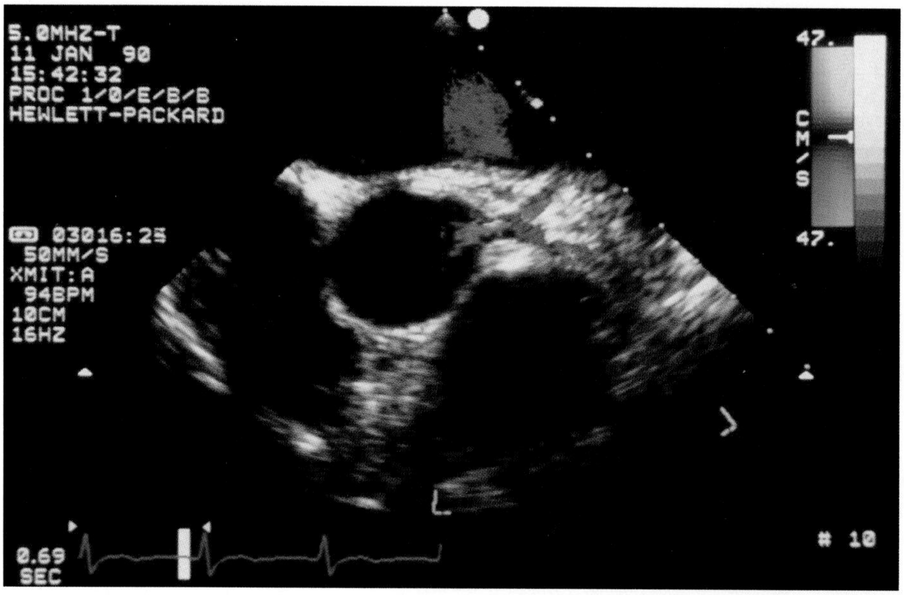

PLATE 18 The left main coronary artery and the bifurcation of the left anterior descending and circumflex coronary arteries. TEE enables both morphologic examination and color Doppler interrogation of the proximal coronary arteries. (Figure courtesy of Hewlett-Packard, Andover, MA.)

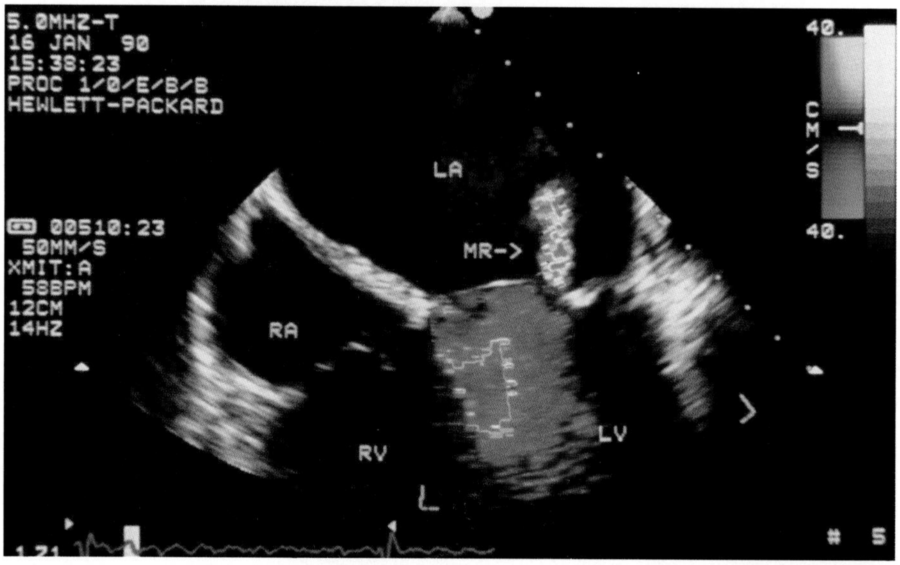

PLATE 19 A jet of mitral regurgitation is seen in the left atrium. The mosaic color of the jet is caused by the high velocities typical of mitral regurgitation. Mapping of the atrium throughout systole is necessary to determine the severity of the mitral regurgitation. (Figure courtesy of Hewlett-Packard, Andover, MA.)

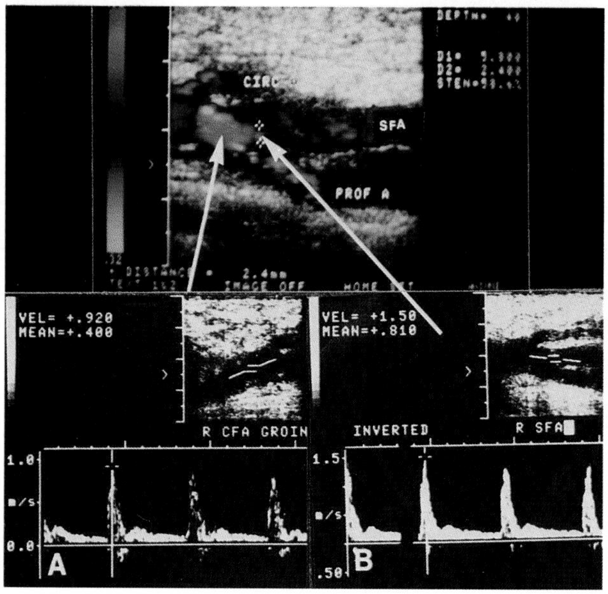

PLATE 20 Color duplex ultrasonography of the common femoral bifurcation. A 50 percent diameter stenosis in the proximal superficial femoral artery is demonstrated. Pulsed Doppler spectral analysis of flow at the stenosis (B) demonstrates significant flow acceleration to 1.5 m/sec and spectral broadening compared to the common femoral artery.

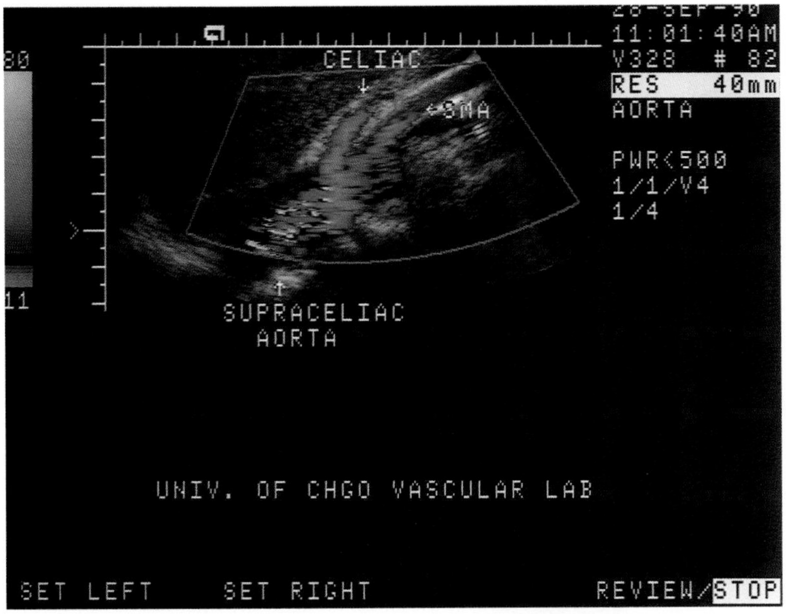

PLATE 21 Color duplex ultrasonography of a normal supraceliac aorta, proximal celiac and superior mesenteric arteries (SMA).

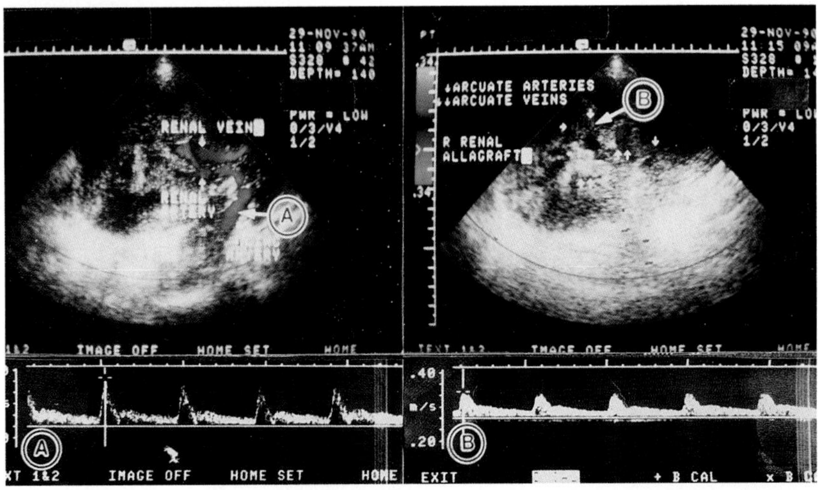

PLATE 22 Color duplex ultrasound of (*a*) renal allograft hilum. The external iliac, donor renal artery and vein are visualized; pulsed Doppler spectral analysis reveals a normal biphasic waveform with continuous flow in diastole. (*b*) Arcuate arteries and veins of the same allograft; a similar flow pattern is observed.

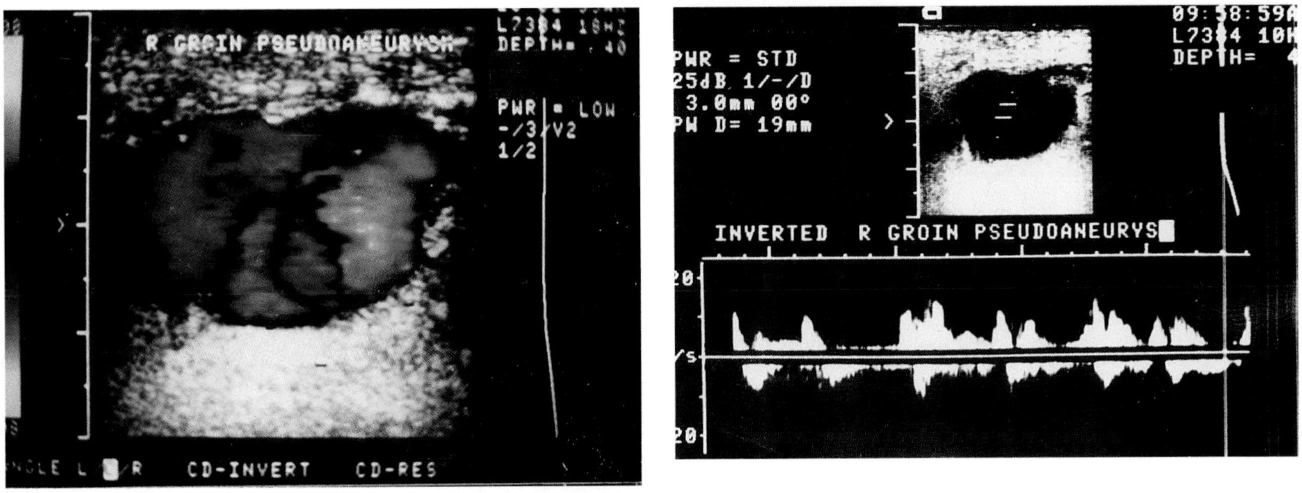

PLATE 23 Color duplex ultrasonography of a right femoral pseudoaneurysm. To and fro flow is represented by red (to) and blue (fro). Pulsed Doppler spectral analysis reveals an erratic bidirectional flow pattern.

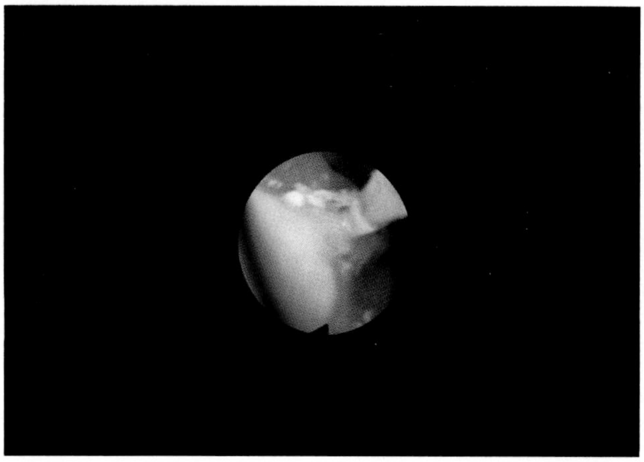

PLATE 24 Injection needle (yellow) embedded into esophageal varix during sclerotherapy.

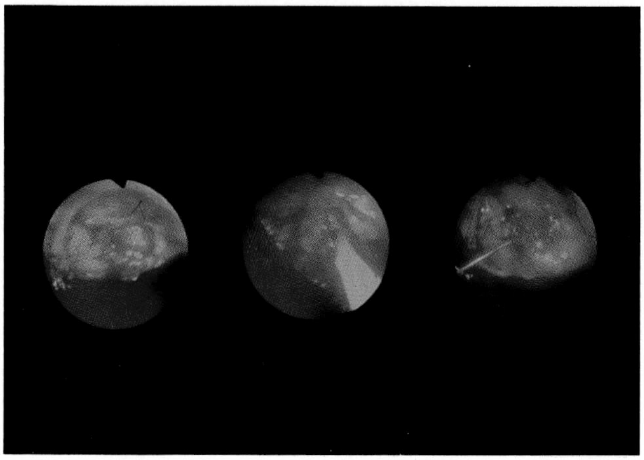

PLATE 25 Injection therapy for visible vessel. A spurting artery in a gastric ulcer (left) is treated by injection therapy (center) resulting in immediate cessation of bleeding (right). (Photo courtesy of Dr. Paul Kortan, University of Toronto.)

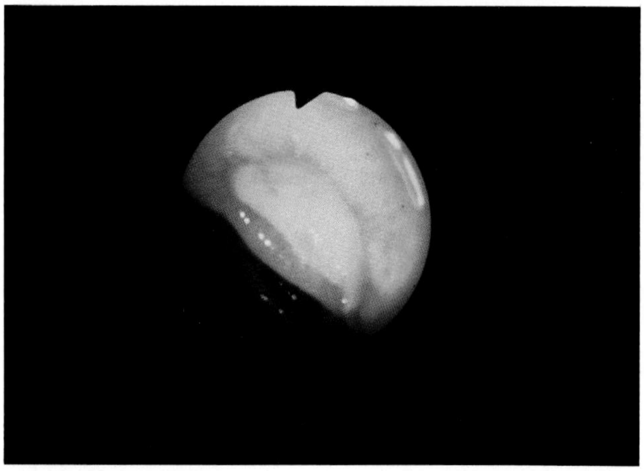

PLATE 26 "Clean based" gastric ulcer. A gastric ulcer without an adherent clot or visible vessel will have a recurrent bleeding incidence of only 10 percent.

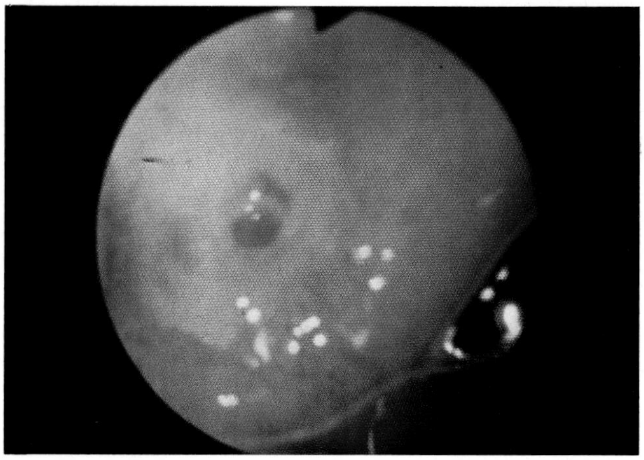

PLATE 27 Visible vessel within a duodenal ulcer. A nonbleeding visible vessel, often seen as a red "spot" within an ulcer, carries a 50 percent incidence of rebleeding.

PLATE 28 Erythema multiforme: typical "target" lesions on legs with central necrosis and peripheral erythema.

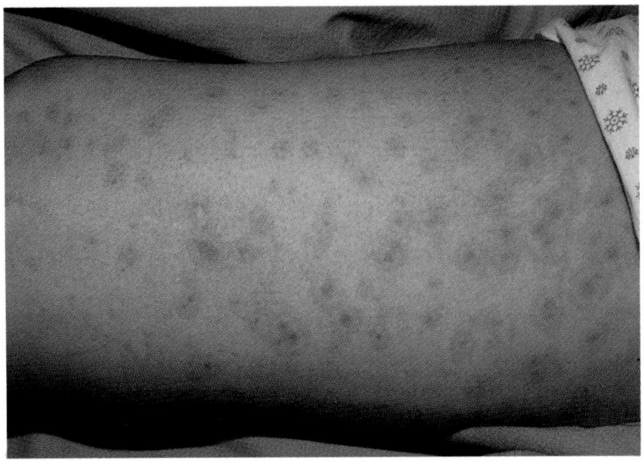

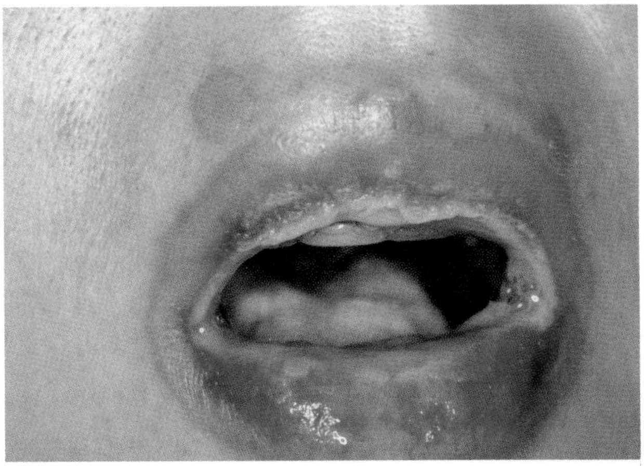

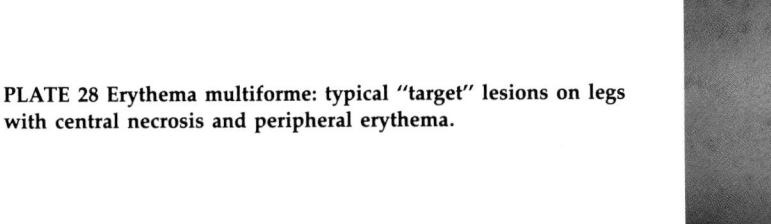

PLATE 29 Stevens-Johnson syndrome: erosive involvement of lips and oral mucosa.

PLATE 30 Decubitus ulceration: superficial necrosis and erythema in a lesion of unknown depth.

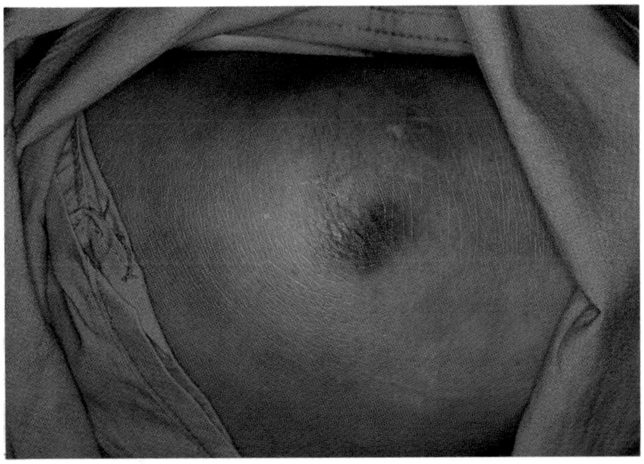

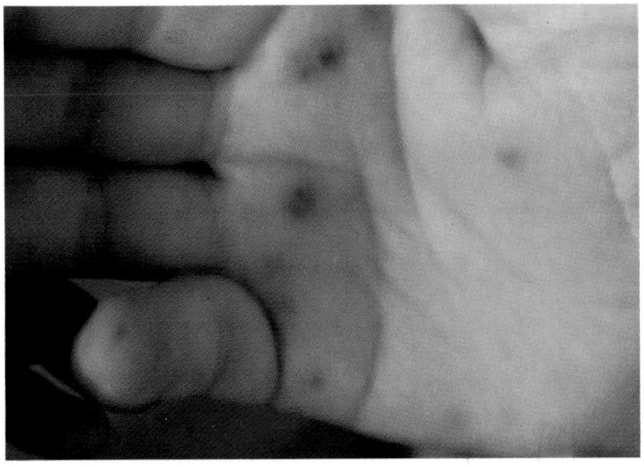

PLATE 31 Osler's nodes: randomly distributed tender nodules on the palm of the hand in a patient with *Staphylococcus aureus* endocarditis.

PLATE 32 Subacute bacterial endocarditis: nontender, purpuric macules with irregular borders scattered on the toes (Janeway lesions).

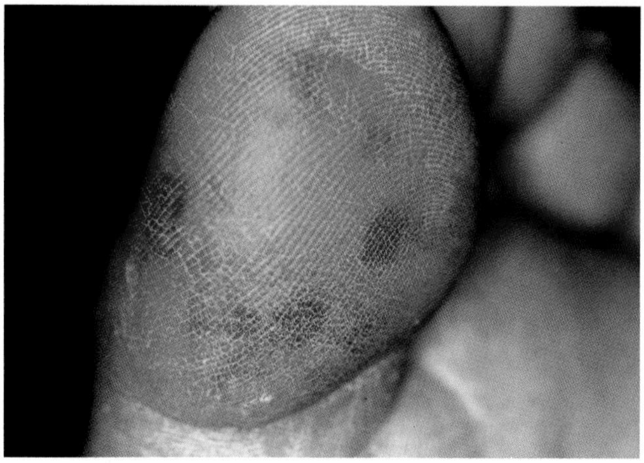

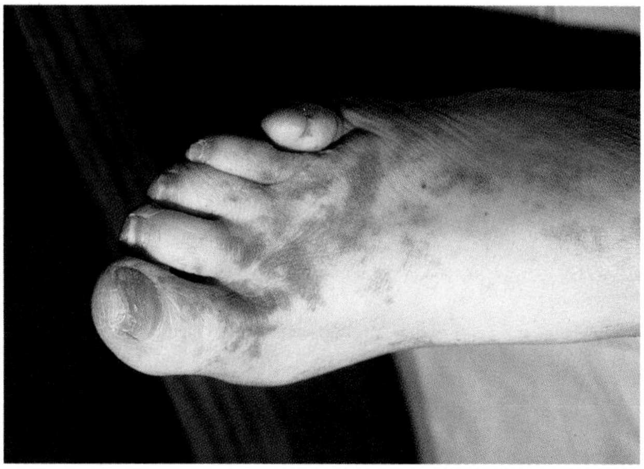

PLATE 33 Meningococcemia: purpuric lesions with irregularly angulated borders.

PLATE 34 Meningococcemia: petechiae of the bulbar and palpebral conjunctivae.

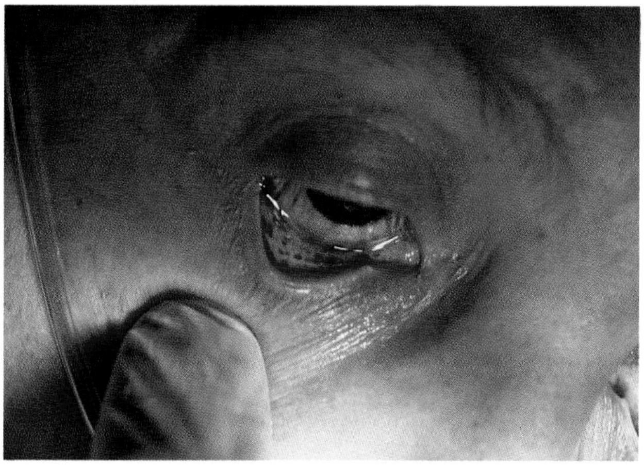

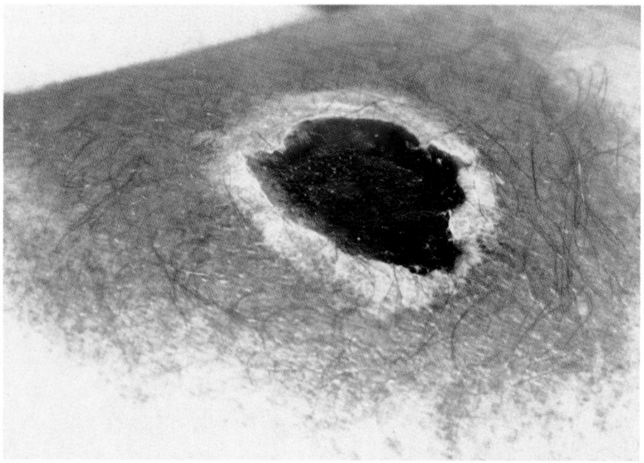

PLATE 35 Ecthyma gangrenosum: necrosis and eschar formation on an erythematous base.

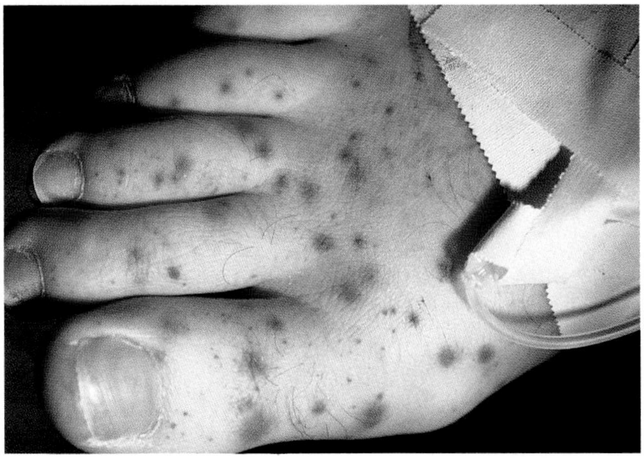

PLATE 36 Candida sepsis: scattered papules, many of which progressed to pustules.

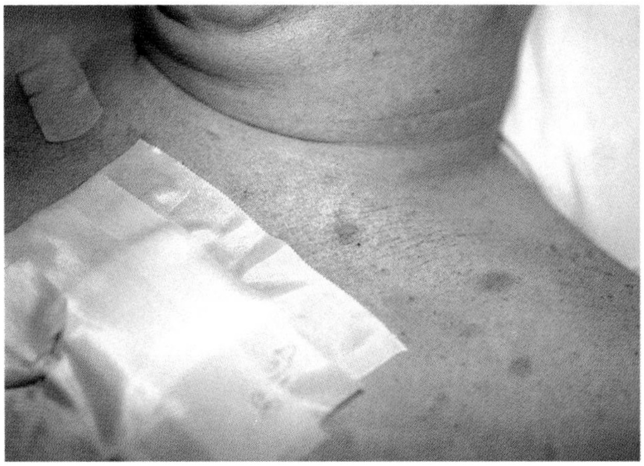

PLATE 37 Leukemia cutis: soft, plum-colored nodules.

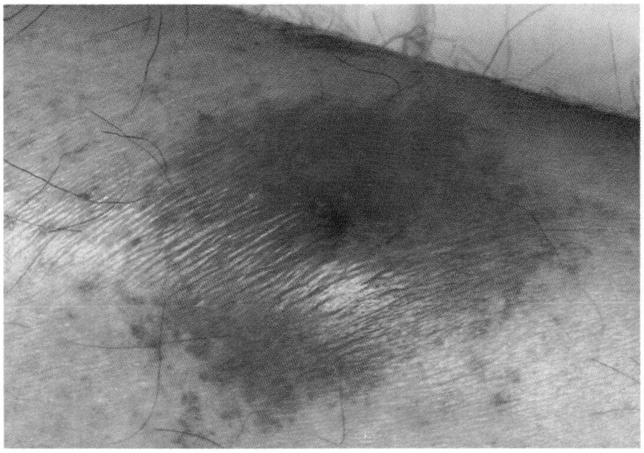

PLATE 38 Vasculitis: erythema with nodular, grey, necrotic center.

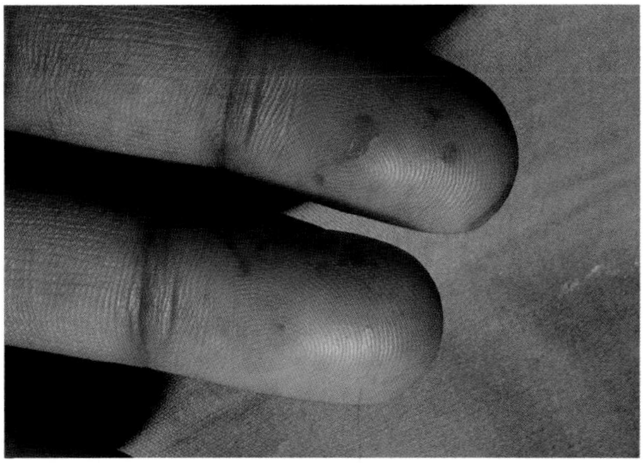

PLATE 39 Systemic lupus erythematosus: irregularly distributed and shaped erythematous, macular, digital infarcts.

PLATE 40 *Staphylococcus aureus* bacteremia: one of many nascent pustules in a patient with bacteremia.

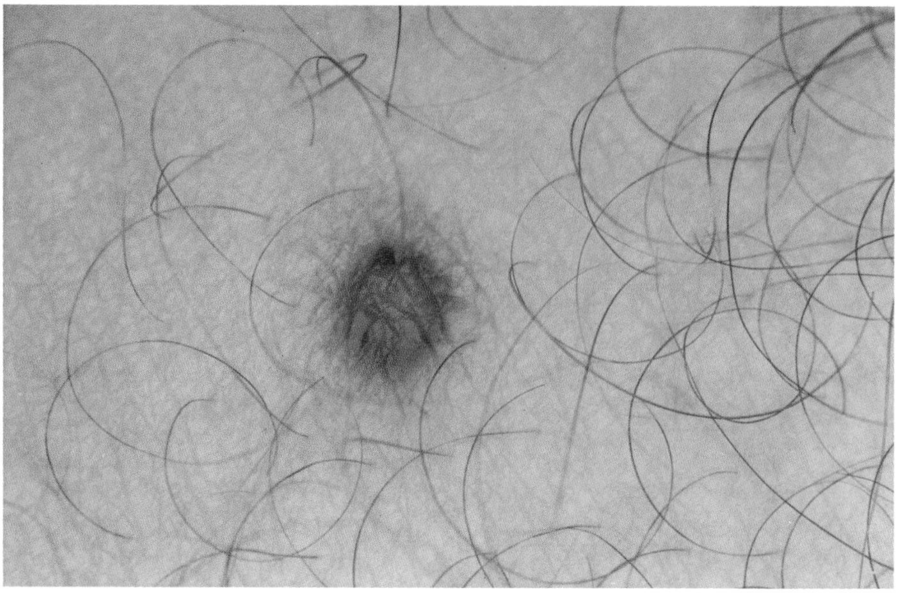

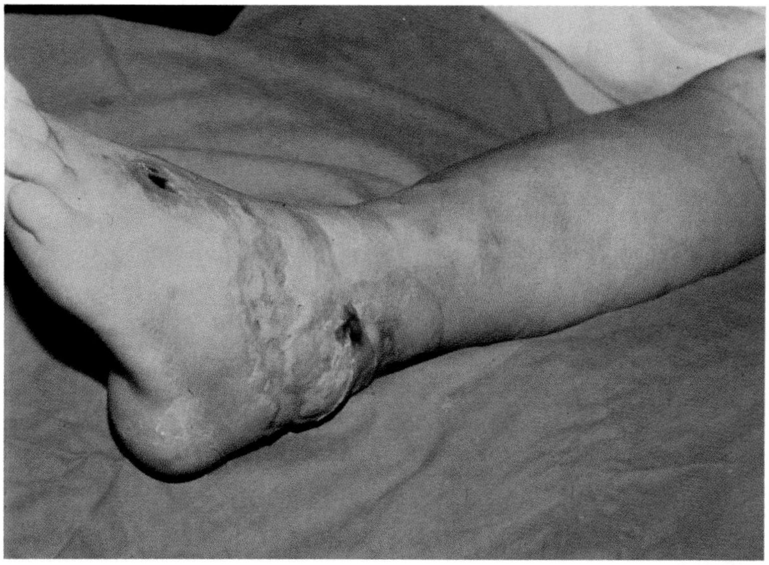

PLATE 41 Necrotizing fasciitis of the lower leg. Dusky erythema is present with blistering and small patches of dermal gangrene.

PLATE 42 Postoperative appearance of the lower leg illustrated in Plate 41. All necrotic subcutaneous tissue was excised.

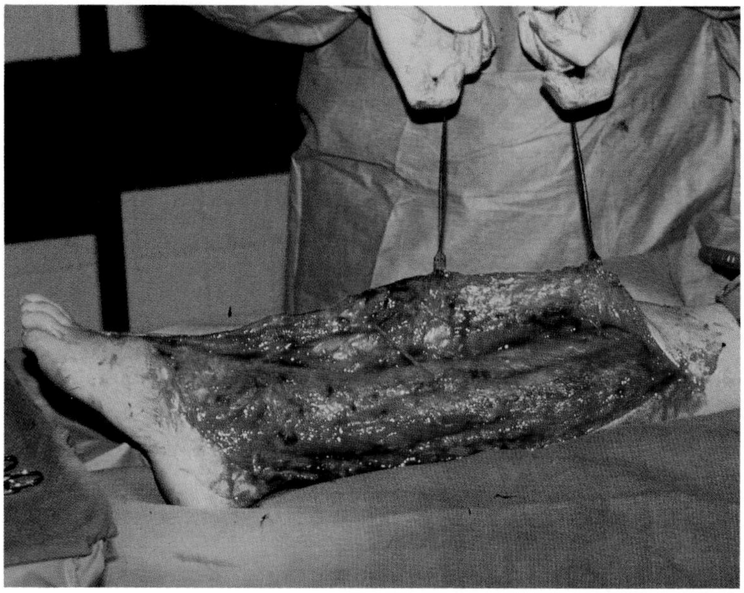

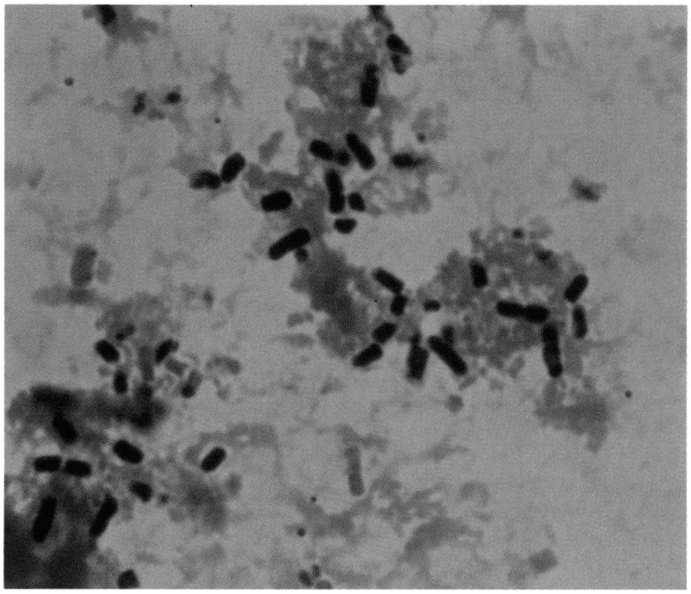

PLATE 43 Gram stain of *Clostridium perfringens.*

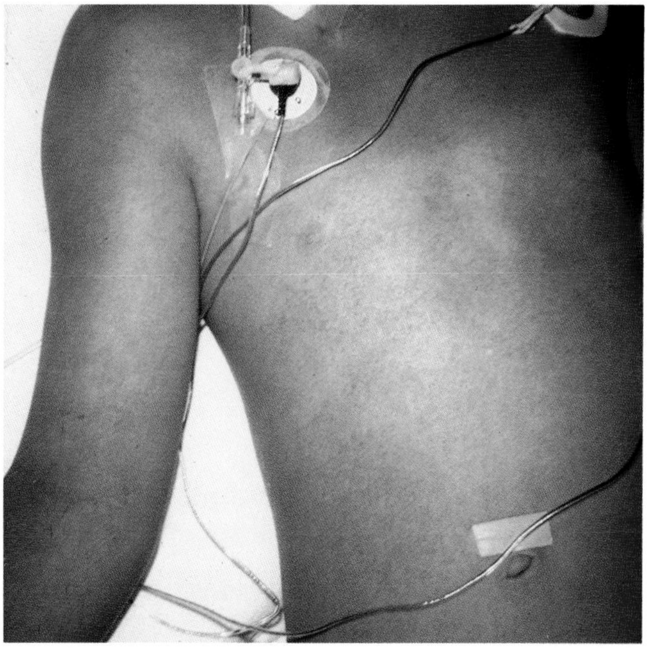

PLATE 44 This photograph shows the diffuse erythroderma on the trunk and arm of a 10-year-old female with toxic shock syndrome.

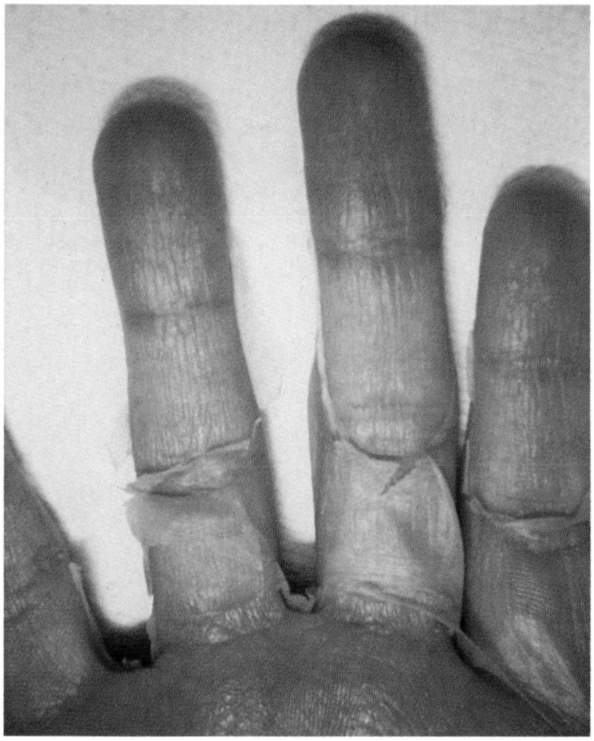

PLATE 45 Full-thickness desquamation of the fingers 10 to 14 days after the onset of symptoms of toxic shock syndrome.

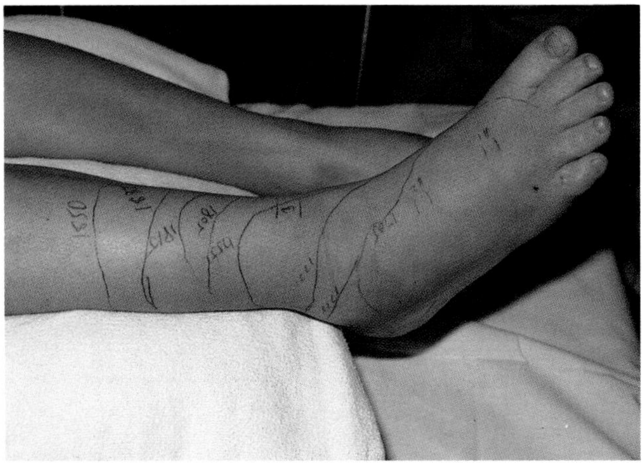

PLATE 46 Local manifestations of *Crotalus atrox* envenomation. This seven-year-old patient demonstrates two puncture wounds at the base of the little toe. A surrounding area of ecchymosis is evident. The lines represent serial markings of the advancing edge of swelling (using visual evaluation and palpation of induration). Circumferential measurements of the swelling were also followed at the sites marked #1, #2, and #3. Measurements were made every 15 to 30 min.

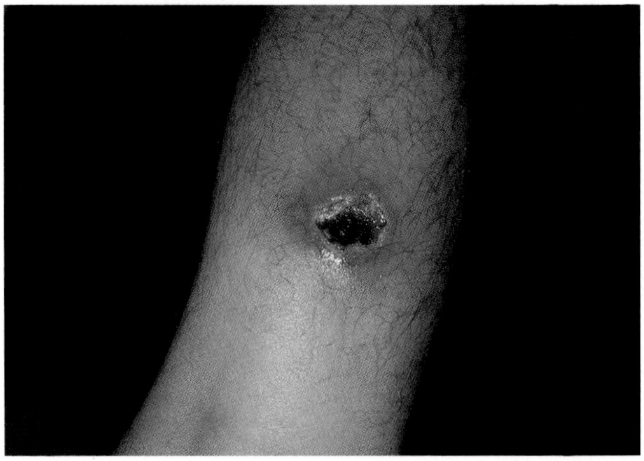

PLATE 47 Necrotic arachnidism of the calf. This patient represents a typical presentation of presumed necrotic arachnidism. He presented to the emergency department on the third day after developing a systemic syndrome consisting primarily of weakness, malaise, and a feverish feeling in conjunction with the development of an enlarging leg lesion which later ulcerated. Systemic complications did not occur. Healing over the next 2 months resulted in a scarred area the size of the original lesion. Brown spiders as well as wolf spiders were found in the home.

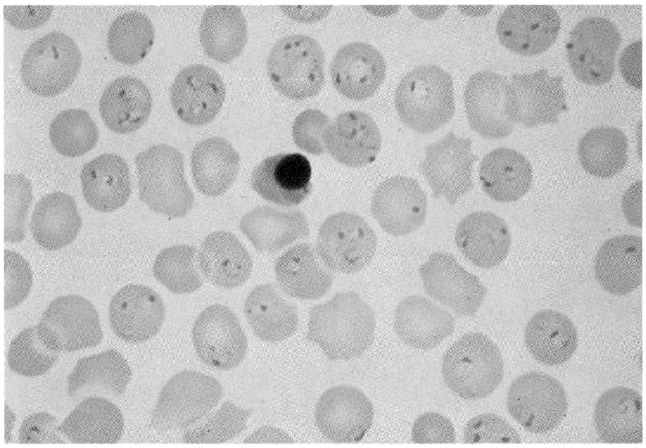

PLATE 48 *Plasmodium falciparum* hyperparasitemia in a thin blood film from a patient with cerebral malaria. *(Copyright DA Warrell.)*

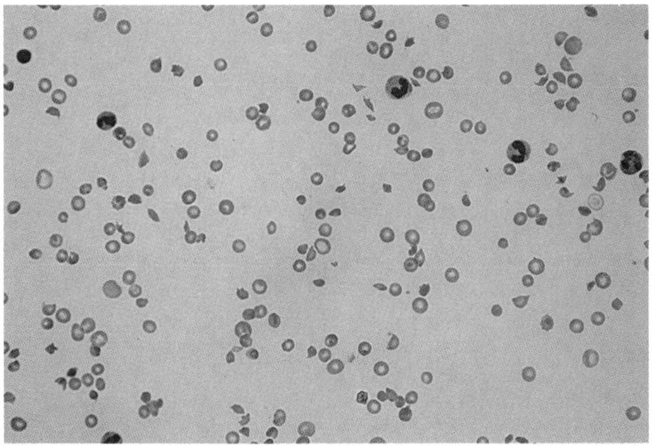

PLATE 49 Admission (hospital day 1) peripheral blood smear (Wright-Giemsa stain) of patient B.B. showing characteristic RBC morphology of microangiopathic hemolytic anemia (MAHA). Magnification ×350.

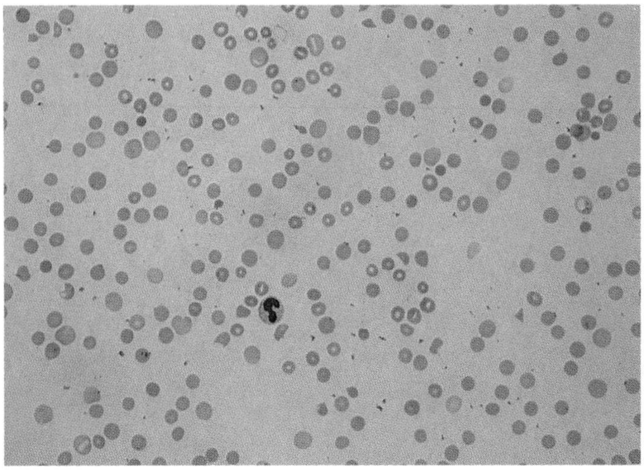

PLATE 50 Same as Plate 49, hospital day 3. B.B. has undergone one plasma exchange prior to this blood smear. Microangiopathic changes are much less severe. The spherocytes are secondary to transfused blood. Polychromatophilia is also seen, demonstrating increased bone marrow production.

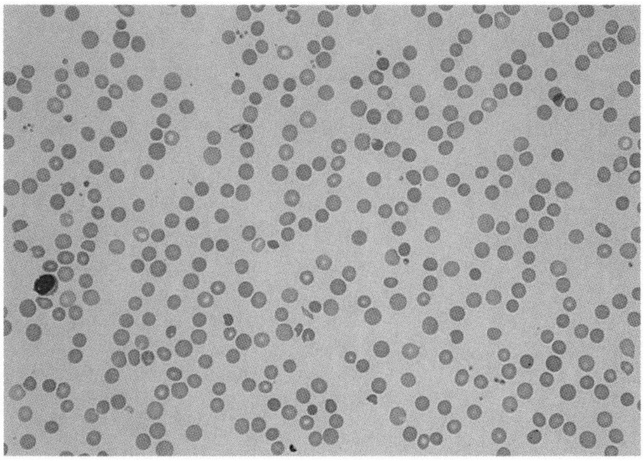

PLATE 51 Same as Plate 49, hospital day 6. Patient B.B. after four plasma exchanges. Microangiopathic RBC changes show continued improvement.

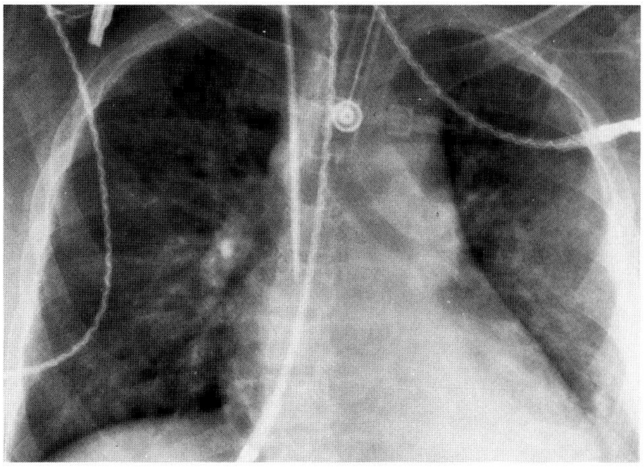

PLATE 52 Portable chest x-ray of an obese patient obtained with a 6:1 grid at 90kV demonstrating mild edema, left lower lobe consolidation, a central line, and an endotracheal tube. Note excellent mediastinal detail, including bronchi and catheter, which cannot be achieved with non-grid technique, except in very small adults and children.

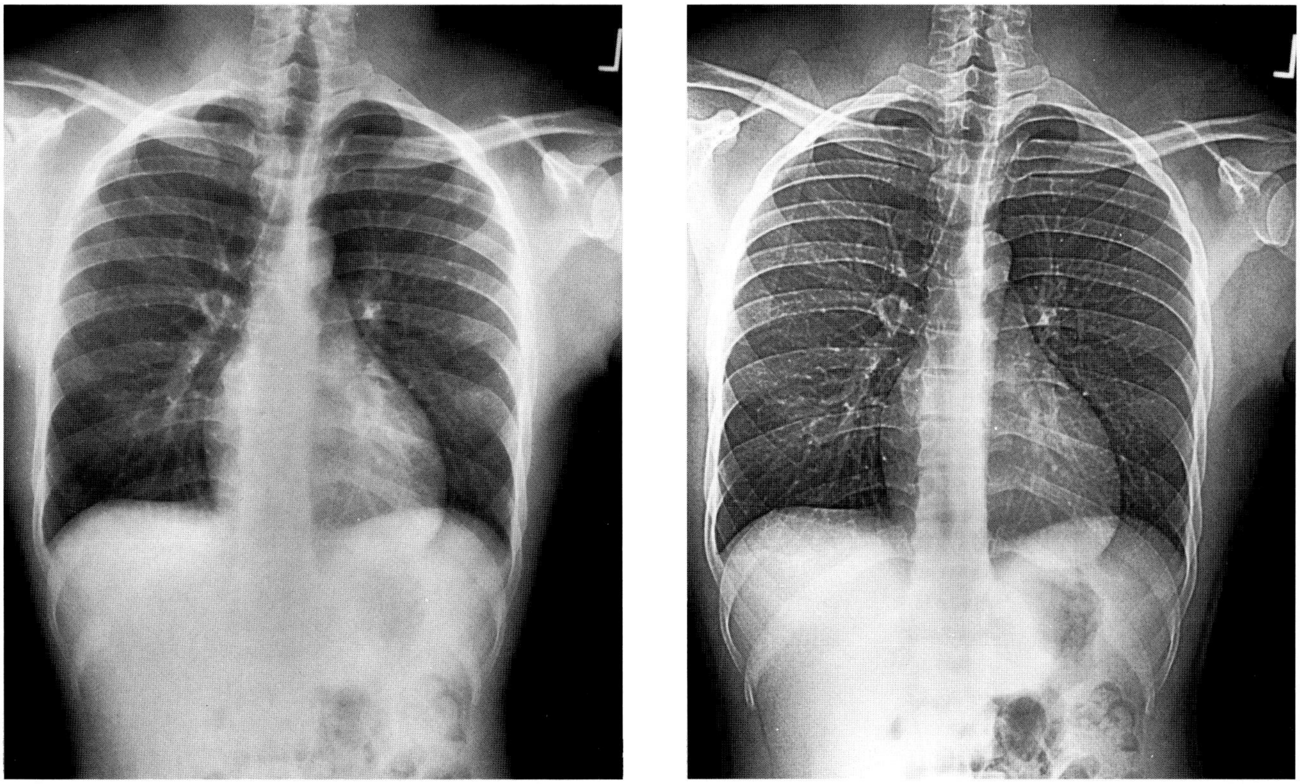

A *B*

PLATE 53 Storage phosphor digital radiograph of the chest. *a:* Mild digital processing (enhancement) provides a conventional-appearing image. *b:* Heavier processing enhances mediastinal structures, as well as bones and soft tissues.

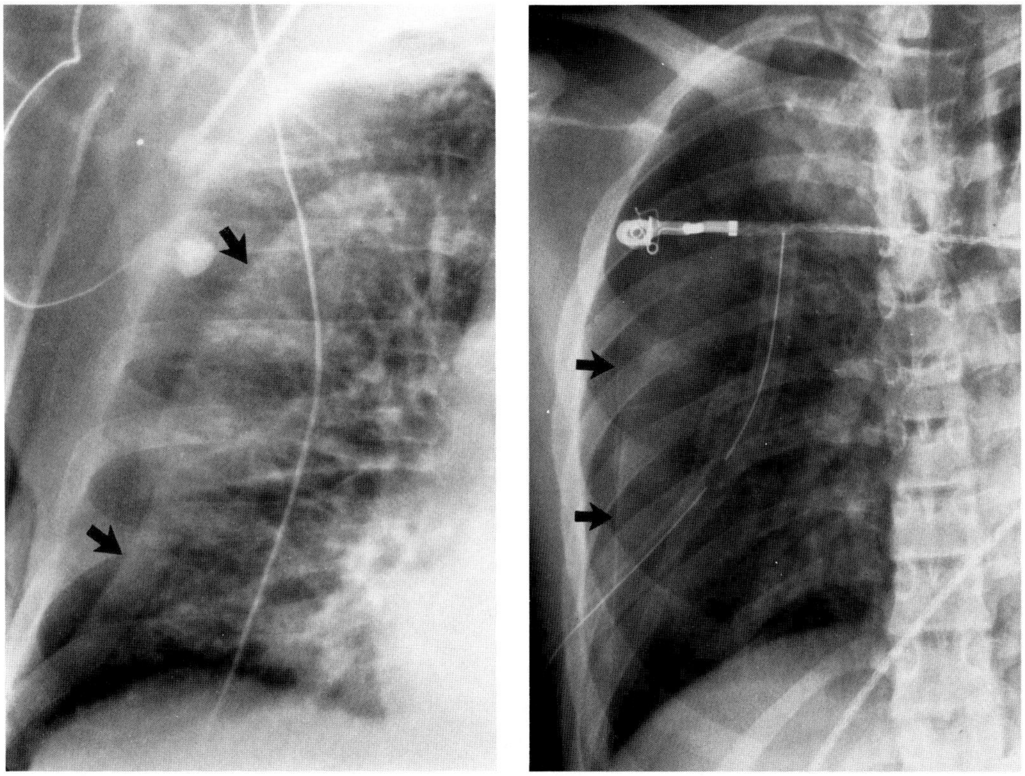

A *B*

PLATE 54 Skinfold. *a:* Skinfolds (arrows) may closely mimic a pneumothorax but are often multiple and bilateral, in addition to other characteristic features (see text). *b:* A true pneumothorax (arrows) typically appears as a very fine linear opacity, which represents the visceral pleura, lateral to which lung markings are absent.

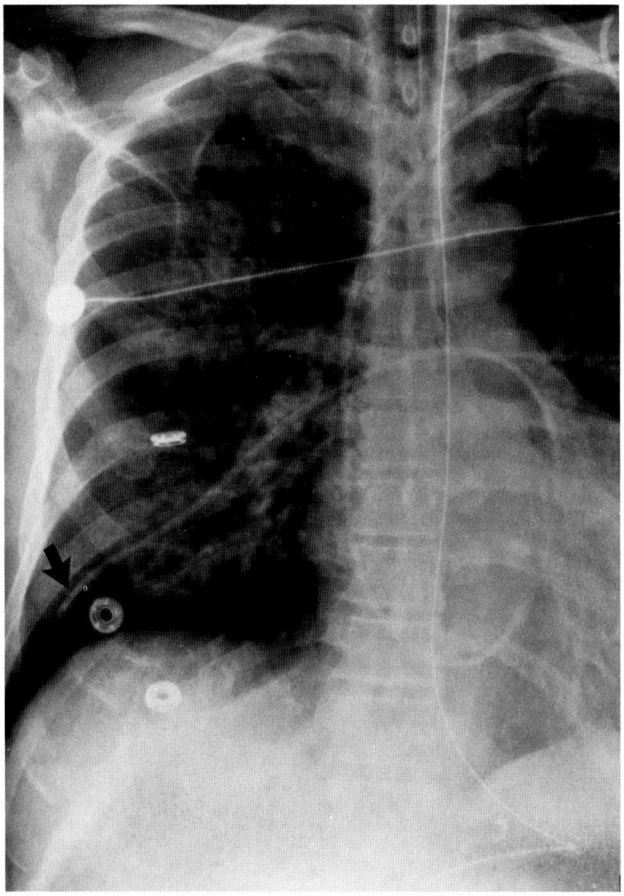

PLATE 55 Swan-Ganz catheter extends far peripherally in the right lung (arrow). Excessively distal positioning may lead to pulmonary infarction.

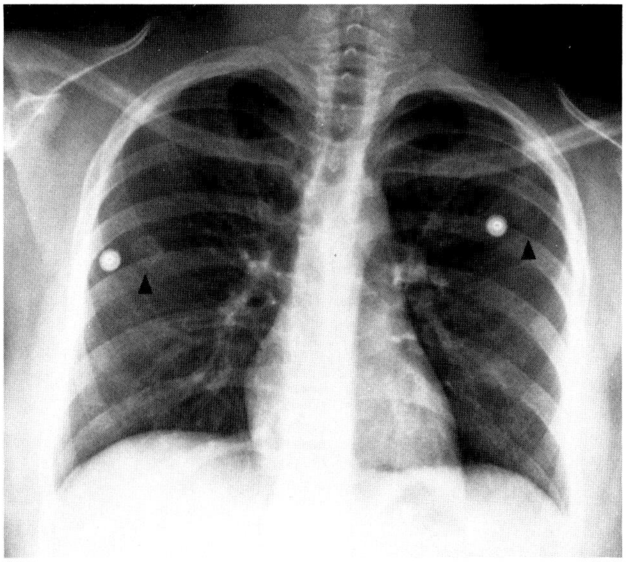

PLATE 56 EKG lead artifacts. The metallic densities seen over both lungs are the metallic portions of adhesive EKG electrodes. The fainter nodular densities adjacent to them (arrowheads) are caused by silver nitrate gel used to ensure good skin contact. These artifacts, which may be mistaken for pulmonary nodules, can only be distinguished by their positional relation to the metallic device.

It is important to emphasize that HIV is not transmitted through casual contact. After a single accidental needle stick or mucous membrane exposure to contaminated material, the rate of seroconversion is approximately 3 per 400 exposures, or 0.76 percent. This is particularly reassuring for the families and health care providers of AIDS patients. In the ICU setting, the so-called universal precautions recommended for patients infected with the hepatitis B virus are sufficient to deal appropriately with HIV.[8] Nevertheless, the risk of acquiring HIV infection in the workplace is real;[9] this issue, therefore, should not be hidden but openly discussed, and health care institutions should adopt exemplary policies to deal fairly and compassionately with such occurrences.

PATHOPHYSIOLOGY

HIV preferentially infects T lymphocytes bearing the surface marker CD4 or OKT4, the so-called helper T cells or T4 cells. This tropism is mediated through a specific interaction between GP160, a viral envelope glycoprotein, and the CD4 molecule itself. HIV is also capable of infecting a number of other bone-marrow-derived cells including monocytes/macrophages, Langerhan-dendritic cells, microglial cells, B lymphocytes and, bone marrow stem cells.[10,11]

Once within the cell, the viral ribonucleic acid (RNA) and reverse transcriptase are released. The reverse transcriptase generates a deoxyribonucleic acid (DNA) sequence complementary to the viral RNA, which then integrates into the host cell's genome to produce new viral particles, which in turn will infect other susceptible cells. As a result of direct and indirect viral effects, T4 cell dysfunction and cell death occurs.[11]

These events correlate with a progressive decrease in the absolute lymphocyte count, the percentage of T4 cells, and the T4/T8 ratio, also known as helper-suppressor, or H-S, ratio. Increases in erythrocyte sedimentation rate (ESR), immunoglobulins, and immunocomplexes are also characteristic. In fact, different combinations of the above markers have been proposed to enhance the ability of the CD4 count to stage the disease.[12] A number of other surrogate markers (including P-24 antigen, P-24 antibody, β_2 microglobulin, and neopterin) have been found useful in the assessment of HIV disease.[13]

NATURAL HISTORY

Infection by HIV can be associated with an acute syndrome that is retrospectively identified in 20 to 30 percent of patients. This is usually a nonspecific "flulike" illness often confused with acute infectious mononucleosis and characterized by marked debilitation, sore throat, skin rash, fever, lymphadenopathy, and less commonly dysphagia. This usually benign and self-limited syndrome, also known as seroconversion illness, is believed to be an immune-complex-mediated phenomenon resulting from the early antibody response to the infection by HIV. Typically, after a variable period of time (median 12 years) with little or no symptoms, progressive immunodeficiency develops rendering the individual susceptible to the development of opportunistic infections, wasting, and/or neoplasms characteristic of AIDS. Currently, AIDS carries a 100 percent mortality.

ANTIRETROVIRAL TREATMENT

To date, only one chemotherapeutic agent, zidovudine (also known as AZT, Azidothymidine or Retrovir) has been definitely shown to be effective in decreasing mortality and disease progression in patients with advanced HIV disease.[14] More recently, prolongation of the disease-free interval has been documented in asymptomatic individuals with T4 cells ≤500 cells/mm^3 treated with 500 mg/per day of zidovudine.[15] The long-term benefit of such treatment remains to be proven.[16]

In the ICU particularly, it is important to be aware of the hematologic effects of zidovudine, which can vary from mild anemia to severe bone marrow suppression. In general, zidovudine produces a predictable mild macrocytic anemia and reticulocytopenia, usually stable after the first 18 weeks of treatment. Mild leukopenia, although frequent, is rarely a problem. Bone marrow studies usually demonstrate mild to moderate dysplastic and megaloblastoid changes.[17] Occasionally severe bone marrow suppression develops. This is usually rapidly reversible upon discontinuation of therapy unless an underlying bone marrow insult (opportunistic infection, malignancy, chemotherapy) precludes its recovery. Whenever zidovudine therapy is discontinued, however, the relative benefit of this decision must be weighed against the fact that this can lead to a rise in P24 antigenemia, a marker of viral replication.[18]

Recently, ddI (also known as Didanosine, or 2′,3′-Dideoxyinosine) has been reported to have promising effects in vitro and in phase I trials. It is anticipated that an increasing number of patients will continue to be treated with this form of therapy in the foreseeable future. To date, it appears that this agent has a beneficial effect on the course of HIV disease, as suggested by its effect on CD4 lymphocytes and P-24 antigenemia. In addition, this new nucleoside appears to be seldom associated with the hematologic toxicity characteristic of AZT. Clinical improvement (resolution of hairy leukoplakia, weight gain, and increased level of energy) have also been reported with this agent. The major limiting toxicities of ddI appear to be painful peripheral neuropathy and pancreatitis. Often hypertriglyceridemia, hyperamylasemia, and hyperuricemia occur as a consequence of ddI administration. These are generally felt to precede the clinical onset of pancreatitis or gout. Diarrhea and gastrointestinal upset, although relatively frequent, are generally of less clinical importance. A limited number of patients have developed seizures while on ddI. However, it is not clear at this time if this represents a direct effect of the drug or simply undiagnosed central nervous system (CNS) complications of HIV disease.[19–22]

It is likely that in the near future, several new chemotherapeutic agents will be added to our therapeutic armamentarium, and these will hopefully continue to change the prognosis and natural history of this disease.

THE SPECTRUM OF DISEASE IN THE ICU

Although HIV-infected individuals may develop many medical complications, the causes leading to their ICU admission are generally quite limited. These may be divided according to their relationship to the HIV infection. Causes of ICU admission unrelated to the HIV infection are generally similar to those found in non-HIV-infected individuals of comparable age and risk groups (i.e., young intravenous drug users or homosexual males in North America), and since HIV infection is generally asymptomatic early in its course, many patients with clinically unsuspected HIV infection are treated in ICUs and emergency rooms. Patients with these conditions usually respond to standard management, and their prognosis appears to be similar to that of non-HIV-infected patients who have the same condition unless there is concomitant severe immunodeficiency, in which case the prognosis tends to be determined by the severity of the immunodeficiency.

Of the causes of ICU admission related to the HIV infection, acute respiratory failure (ARF) secondary to *Pneumocystis carinii* pneumonia (PCP) is by far the most important due to its high frequency and its potentially high mortality. The other conditions listed in Table 100-1 are relatively uncommon causes of ICU admission. However, they should be kept in mind to avoid potentially fatal mistakes.[23] Less frequently, a person with AIDS may be admitted to the ICU without knowledge of the HIV status. Obviously, the presence or history of minor or major opportunistic infections, wasting, otherwise unexplained extensive herpes zoster or persistent generalized lymphadenopathy combined with a history (or clinical evidence) of high-risk activities will necessitate consideration of HIV infection and related diseases in the differential diagnosis. A number of laboratory features commonly found among HIV-infected individuals can provide the initial basis for considering HIV infection within the differential diagnosis. Among them lymphopenia, decreased CD4 count, anemia, thrombocytopenia, hypergammaglobulinemia, and increased immunocomplexes or β_2 microglobulin are the most characteristic. It must be emphasized however, that HIV infection should not be diagnosed unless this has been confirmed using specific serologic tests [i.e., enzyme-linked immunosorbent assay (ELISA) and Western blot].

TABLE 100-1 ICU Admissions in HIV-infected Individuals* (St. Paul's Hospital, 1985–1990)

PCP	92%
Cerebral toxoplasmosis	3%
Bacterial pneumonia	2%
Gastrointestinal bleeding	2%
Kaposi's sarcoma	3%
Lymphoma	2%
Cardiomyopathy	2%

*More than one condition may be present at any given time.

Respiratory Disease Complicating HIV Infection

Acute respiratory failure secondary to PCP remains the most frequent cause of ICU admission among HIV-infected individuals in most centers across North America (Table 100-1). Despite this, the initial diagnostic workup of patients with acute pulmonary disease should always consider less frequent etiologies, among them common bacteria, other fungi, mycobacteria, and viruses. Although Kaposi's sarcoma (KS) can result in ARF, it is highly unlikely that this will occur in the absence of overt mucocutaneous disease. Progression to ARF in KS patients is usually a reflection of overwhelming disease that is unlikely to respond to currently available chemotherapeutic modalities in any significant way.

From a laboratory standpoint, patients present with varying degrees of hypoxemia, hypocarbia, and other nonspecific abnormalities related to the underlying HIV disease, as discussed above. If available, the CD4 count can aid in the differential diagnosis as it would be unusual for PCP to occur when the CD4 count is greater than 250 cells/mm^3.[24] An elevated lactic dehydrogenase (LDH) in a patient with known HIV infection and respiratory distress is characteristic of PCP, and its level tends to correlate with the severity of the episode; furthermore, changes in the LDH level tend to parallel the course of PCP.[25] It must be emphasized, however, that an elevated LDH cannot be interpreted as diagnostic of PCP since this enzyme can also be elevated due to pulmonary embolism, lymphoma, megaloblastic anemia, liver infiltration or dysfunction, and hemolysis (commonly seen among patients receiving dapsone prophylaxis for PCP) or during long-term AZT therapy.

By the time ARF requiring ICU admission develops, the radiologic picture has usually evolved to a diffuse alveolar pattern characteristic of the adult respiratory distress syndrome (ARDS). However, a careful review of previous chest x-rays can, at times, aid in the differential diagnosis, as shown in Table 100-2.[26,27] The clinical, laboratory, and radiologic pattern is seldom specific enough to establish the diagnosis, which should be confirmed using appropriate

TABLE 100-2 Major Radiologic Differential Diagnosis of Lung Involvement in AIDS*

Normal chest x-ray: PCP, CMV, MAC
Diffuse or localized interstitial pattern: PCP, CMV, MAC, MTb
Diffuse alveolar pattern: PCP, cardiogenic pulmonary edema
Miliary pattern: MTb
Consolidation: common bacteria, MTb, PCP, KS
Nodular opacity: PCP, common bacteria, KS
Upper lung field involvement: PCP, MTb
Pneumothorax: PCP
Cavity: MTb, PCP, bacteria
Pleural effusion: KS, common bacteria, mycobacteria

*Abbreviations: PCP, *Pneumocystis carinii pneumonia;* CMV, *cytomegalovirus;* MAC, *Mycobacterium avium complex;* MTb, *M. tuberculosis;* KS, *Kaposi's sarcoma.*

laboratory examinations. This is particularly important when the patient does not yet carry a diagnosis of AIDS, because of the serious prognostic and therapeutic implications of this diagnosis. If sputum is available, this should be screened for common bacteria and mycobacteria. Blood cultures should also be obtained, particularly in febrile patients. The key to the etiologic diagnosis relies on obtaining tracheobronchial secretions.[28] In the ICU setting, particularly in the ventilated patient, bronchoscopic bronchoalveolar lavage (BAL) is the preferred approach. Bronchoscopy should be performed using appropriate cardiorespiratory monitoring, including pulse oximetry and an electrocardiogram (ECG).

The sensitivity of BAL for *P. carinii* and other treatable pathogens commonly found in AIDS patients exceeds 95 percent. BAL specimens should be concentrated to increase sensitivity. Aliquots should be referred for viral, bacterial, fungal, and mycobacterial studies. *P. carinii* screening should be specifically requested as this is not routinely performed in most laboratories. Sputum induction and transbronchial biopsies, although valuable techniques in the routine evaluation of these patients, are not recommended in the critically ill and ventilated patient. In the few cases in whom the initial BAL does not provide a diagnosis, an open lung biopsy should be considered. This decision will be influenced by the general status of the patients as well as the likelihood of diagnosing a treatable condition.[28,29]

Pneumocystis carinii PNEUMONIA

Pneumocystis carinii, recently reclassified as a fungus, is a ubiquitous organism that produces human disease throughout the world, usually in the setting of severe immunosuppression. Asymptomatic primary infection generally occurs early in life. Rarely *P. carinii* can be found incidentally at autopsy in the absence of symptoms. It is not clear whether this represents late infection or early disease not yet manifested clinically.

PCP was the index disease that facilitated the clinical recognition of AIDS. Since then, it has also become the first major AIDS-related opportunistic infection for which development of effective therapy has led to important improvement in survival. Despite these advances, PCP remains the most frequent serious opportunistic infection among those infected with HIV. In North America, PCP represents the AIDS index disease in 65 percent of cases and will eventually affect over 85 percent of patients during their lifetime.[29–31] PCP is generally a late event in the evolution of HIV infection as demonstrated by a CD4 count usually below 250 cells/mm^3.[24] Therefore, it is recommended that all HIV-infected individuals with CD4 counts below 250 cells/mm^3 or those who have had an episode of PCP should receive life-long PCP prophylaxis.[24]

CLINICAL AND RADIOLOGIC FEATURES

Dyspnea, nonproductive cough, and fever are the classical features of PCP. In critically ill patients, the physical examination demonstrates evidence of acute respiratory distress, with surprisingly few adventitious sounds on auscultation of the chest. Acute hypoxemic respiratory failure requiring mechanical ventilation has been reported to occur in as many as 20 percent of hospitalized patients.[32] Most often this occurs within the first 3 days of starting antimicrobial therapy; less frequently acute hypoxemic respiratory failure develops as a complication of diagnostic bronchoscopy and rarely as the initial presentation to the emergency room.[33]

Clinically overt PCP usually develops over a period of several days to weeks, and in this time the radiologic picture tends to progress from a normal chest x-ray to a diffuse bilateral interstitial pattern. Varying degrees of alveolar involvement can be seen; even frank consolidation may occur, as seen in Figs. 100-1 to 100-3. A number of atypical radiologic presentations have been described, including cystic changes, pneumothoraces (Fig. 100-4), nodular or masslike opacities, and even cavities.[26] Upper lung field involvement, as seen in Fig. 100-5, has also been increasingly recognized, particularly (but not exclusively) in the context of aerosol pentamidine prophylaxis.[27] To what extent aerosol pentamidine prophylaxis is responsible for the apparent increased frequency of PCP-related pneumothoraces remains controversial.

DIAGNOSIS

As discussed above, given the nonspecific nature of the clinical, laboratory, and radiologic picture of PCP, diagnostic confirmation is desirable. BAL is a rapid, safe, and effec-

FIGURE 100-1 Posteroanterior chest x-ray of PCP demonstrating interstitial disease preferentially localized to the right hilum and lower lung zone.

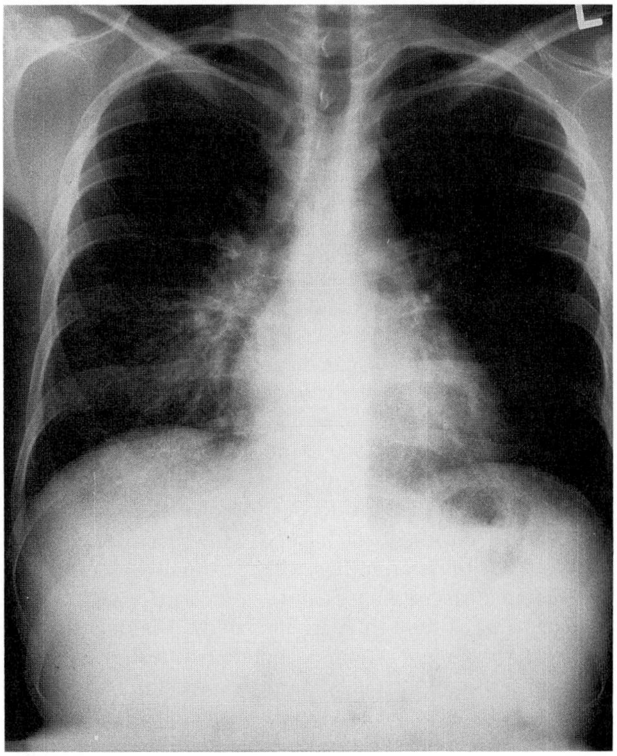

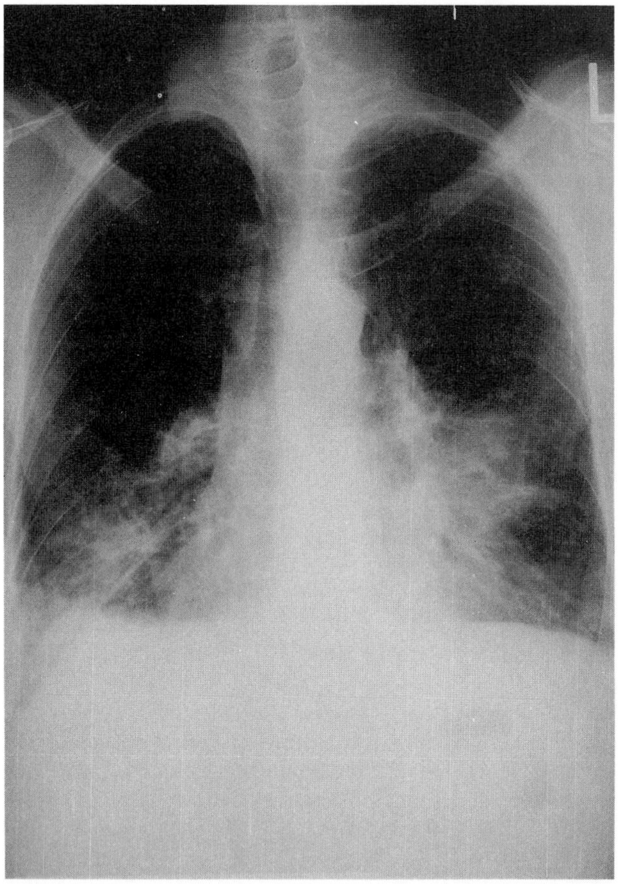

FIGURE 100-2 Posteroanterior chest x-ray of PCP demonstrating extensive bilateral basilar lung involvement.

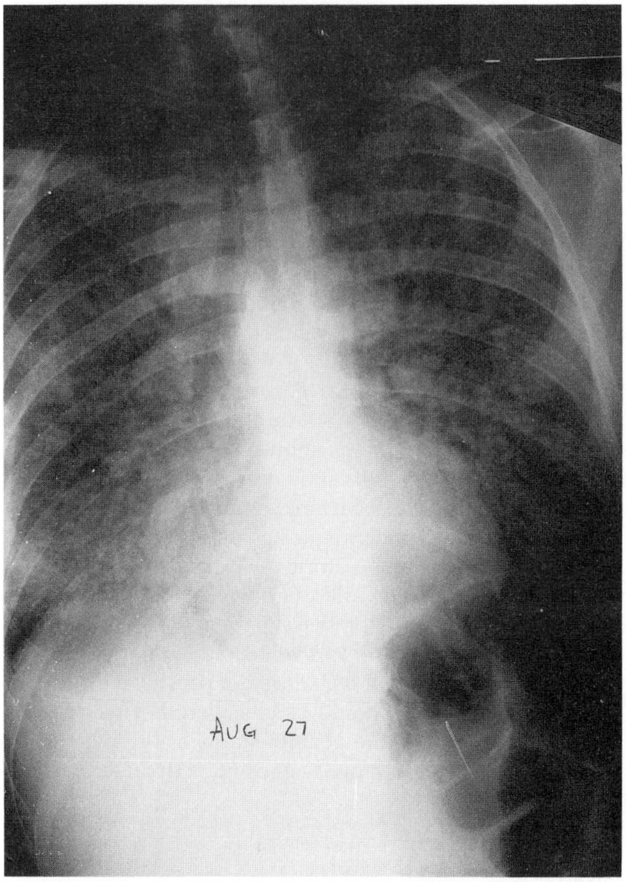

FIGURE 100-3 Anteroposterior chest x-ray demonstrating diffuse bilateral lung disease secondary to PCP in a patient with respiratory failure immediately prior to intubation. Air bronchograms can be seen throughout the lung, particularly in the upper lung fields bilaterally.

tive means of obtaining tracheobronchial secretions to provide an adequate diagnostic specimen. Lung biopsy is exceptionally required to confirm the diagnosis of PCP. As seen in Plate 10 (Fig. 18-9), the usual pathologic picture of PCP consists of a mild to moderate interstitial inflammatory reaction with predominance of lymphocytes and alveolar macrophages and the presence of a classic foamy alveolar exudate (as seen with hematoxylin-eosin, H&E). The foamy appearance of the alveolar exudate is due to the presence of the cystic form of the organism, which is not stained with H&E but can be easily recognized using readily available special stains (Plate 4; Fig. 18-3). As seen in Plate 3 (Fig. 18-2), BAL allows clear identification of the organism if the specimen is appropriately concentrated and stained.[28,29] The composition of the alveolar exudate has not been conclusively established. However, BAL studies suggest that this is an inflammatory exudate rich in immunoglobulins, macrophages, and suppressor/cytotoxic lymphocytes.[34,35] Although *P. carinii* infection is usually confined to the lungs, systemic pneumocystosis (involving liver, spleen, lymph nodes, adrenals, and eyes), has been recently reported with increasing frequency.[36]

MANAGEMENT

Trimethoprim-sulfamethoxazole (TMP-SMX) is effective against *P. carinii* as well as many gram-negative and gram-positive organisms. TMP-SMX is administered intravenously or orally at a dose of 20 and 100 mg/kg daily, respectively, in four divided doses for not less than 14 days. Poor tolerance of TMP-SMX among HIV-infected patients is a significant problem, with adverse drug reactions occurring in 60 to 100 percent of patients. These include rash, fever, liver dysfunction, renal dysfunction, leukopenia, thrombocytopenia, hyponatremia, anemia, and gastrointestinal upset. Less common but at times severe are mucocutaneous reactions, occurring generally at the end of the first week of treatment. A number of reports have documented successful desensitization of TMP-SMX-sensitive patients using progressively larger doses of the drug. Hypersensitivity-type reactions such as fever or rash can also be treated with diphenhydramine or corticosteroids.[37–39]

Pentamidine isethionate was initially used for the treatment of African trypanosomiasis. Since 1958, it has been known to be effective against *P. carinii*. Pentamidine is usu-

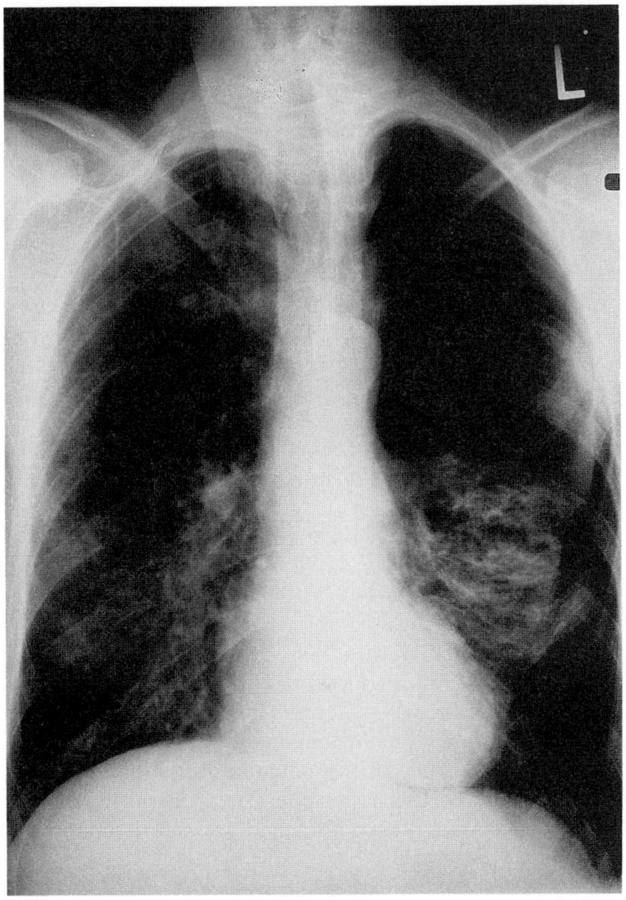

FIGURE 100-4 Posteroanterior chest x-ray of a patient with PCP who presented with a left-sided pneumothorax.

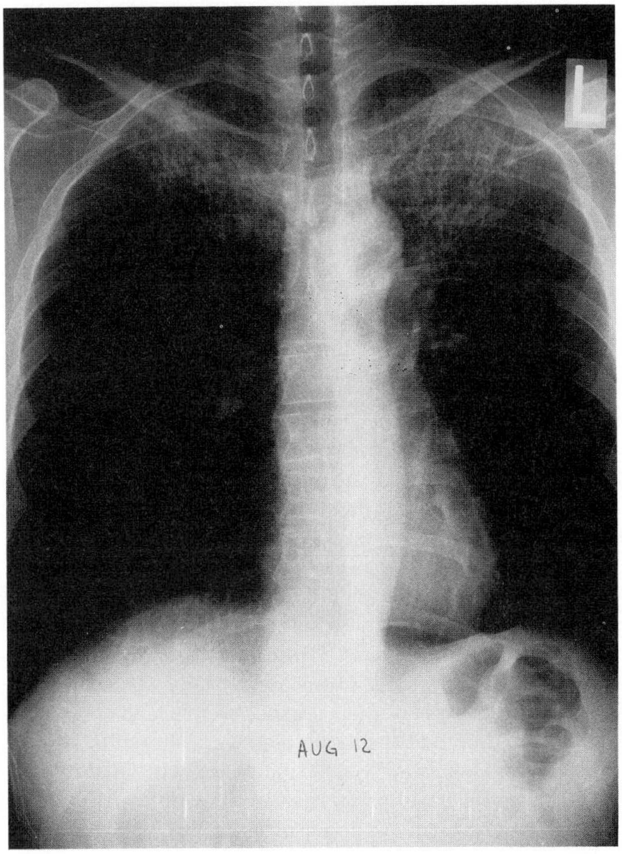

FIGURE 100-5 Posteroanterior chest x-ray of PCP presenting as bilateral upper lung disease.

ally administered intravenously once daily at a dose of 4 mg/kg diluted in 250 mL of 5% dextrose and water for not less than 14 days. Adverse reactions are common, occurring in up to 100 percent of patients in some series. Common adverse drug reactions are renal and liver dysfunction, neutropenia, thrombocytopenia, hyponatremia, rash, fever, and gastrointestinal upset. Hypotension is commonly associated with pentamidine infusion. This can be minimized by administering the drug slowly over several hours; if severe or long-lasting hypotension occurs, this should be treated supportively as it is readily reversible. Occasionally, carbohydrate metabolism abnormalities (hypo- or hyperglycemia) may develop including insulin-dependent diabetes mellitus. Ventricular arrhythmias and pancreatitis have also been reported. Finally, preliminary observations suggest an increased risk of pancreatitis among patients receiving ddI and systemic pentamidine concomitantly. Coadministration of these two drugs is currently contraindicated. Because adverse reactions to pentamidine are related to its systemic concentration and because of its poor absorption through the alveolar surface, aerosol therapy has been investigated.[37,38] In a recent pilot study, a high cure rate with no significant systemic toxicity was achieved using 5 mg/kg daily via a nebulizer in a highly selected group of patients with mild PCP. The only reported adverse effects were cough and bronchospasm in the majority of patients; however, these adverse effects were easily prevented by premedication with a β_2 agonist bronchodilator. Because of contradictory results and increasing concern regarding the possibility of uneven drug distribution, early relapse, and systemic pneumocystosis, aerosol pentamidine therapy should be reserved as a prophylactic regimen, and it should not be recommended as standard therapy at this time[40–42] and particularly not in critically ill patients.

Dapsone (DPS), a sulfone, used for the treatment of leprosy and dermatitis herpetiformis, has been shown to be effective against *P. carinii* particularly when DPS, 100 mg by mouth OD is combined with trimethoprim (TMP) by mouth 20 mg/kg daily in four divided doses. Recently, DPS-TMP has been shown to have similar efficacy and better tolerability than TMP-SMX.[43] Based on this data, DPS-TMP has become the preferred choice for the treatment of patients with mild to moderate PCP in the ambulatory setting. Adverse reactions are common, including hemolytic anemia with methemoglobinemia, thrombocytopenia, neutropenia, liver dysfunction, pancreatitis, rash, and gastrointestinal upset which often interferes with oral administration. The DPS-induced methemoglobinemia and hemolytic anemia are particularly severe among individuals with glucose-6-dehydrogenase deficiency. It is also important to note that the hemolytic anemia will produce an increase in LDH that should not be misinterpreted as a sign of worsening PCP.[25] Among the remaining therapeutic alternatives, trimetrexate has failed to find a place in our therapeutic armamentarium despite early favorable reports.[44] Clindamycin-primaquine[45] and 566C80 (a newly developed 1,4-hydroxynaphthoquinone),[46] on the other hand, are promising antimicrobials currently undergoing clinical testing.

Recently, attention has focused on the role of corticosteroids as an adjuvant therapy for PCP. Corticosteroid use was initially reported to be associated with increased survival in a number of retrospective studies, particularly among patients with severe PCP requiring mechanical ventilation.[32] Recently, a prospective, randomized placebo-controlled study demonstrated a beneficial short-term effect of adjunctive corticosteroid therapy,[25] preventing the characteristic early deterioration in gas exchange seen in the untreated patients and resulting in a faster resolution of the episode (as measured by respiratory rate, temperature, heart rate, Pa_{O_2}, and LDH). More recently Gagnon et al. reported the results of their prospective placebo-controlled trial where adjuvant corticosteroids were shown to significantly decrease mortality among patients with PCP-related ARF.[47] On the basis of the available evidence,[25,32,47,48] a panel convened under the auspices of the National Institutes of Health (NIH) and the University of California recently recommended that systemic corticosteroids be used routinely as adjuvant therapy of moderate and severe PCP if no contraindications are present.[49] Although the exact dose, regimen, duration of treatment, and threshold at which adjuvant corticosteroids should be started have not yet been definitively established, a regimen consisting of prednisone 40 mg by mouth twice daily for the initial 7 days followed first by 40 mg by mouth OD for 7 days and then by 20 mg by mouth OD for the final 7 days was adopted.[49] According to these recommendations, corticosteroids should be started early in the course of the disease, and to this end a Pa_{O_2} threshold of 70 mmHg has been proposed.[49] It must be emphasized that adjuvant corticosteroid therapy should be continued while on anti-PCP antimicrobials to avoid the rapid deterioration often seen following the premature discontinuation of adjuvant corticosteroids.

The initial selection of the antimicrobial agent for the treatment of a PCP episode generally lies outside the ICU. Patients with mild to moderate PCP are generally started on DPS-TMP orally. If there is a concern regarding superimposed bacterial infection, TMP-SMX would be a better choice given its broader antimicrobial spectrum. Pentamidine should be generally reserved for in-patients with microbiologically proven PCP and documented sulfa drug intolerance. If the patient is first diagnosed in the ICU, TMP-SMX or pentamidine intravenously will generally be used as the initial antimicrobial. Corticosteroids should be started at once in any patient whose Pa_{O_2} is below 70 mmHg while breathing room air unless there is an absolute contraindication for their use. Response to antimicrobials is generally slow, and significant improvement usually does not occur until after 5 to 7 days.[38] With the use of adjunctive corticosteroids, however, significant improvement can be observed within the first 3 days of treatment.[25] Patients who fail to improve within the first 5 days of therapy should be thoroughly reviewed to rule out potential intercurrent infections or other complications. Although *P. carinii* resistance to the antimicrobials has not been documented, lack of improvement within 7 days of therapy is generally interpreted as a failure of treatment and therefore an indication for a trial of the alternative agent. A change in antimicrobial would also be warranted if severe adverse reactions develop despite the use of adjunctive corticosteroids. It must be emphasized that although there is no evidence of increased efficacy when combining TMP-SMX with pentamidine, there is, however, evidence of increased toxicity.

If possible, antiretroviral therapy should be continued during the acute PCP episode. Usually this is feasible if AZT is used in lower doses (i.e., 300 mg daily), which have also been shown to have at least some antiviral effect in recently published studies.[50] If adverse reactions develop, AZT can be discontinued for a brief period of time until the adverse reaction resolves. It must be noted that ddI should not be used at this time in combination with sulfa drugs or pentamidine because of the potential for additive toxicity (including pancreatitis or peripheral neuropathy) and that a brief drug holiday is recommended prior to reinitiation of ddI therapy.

PROGNOSIS

Untreated, PCP is universally fatal. With the use of appropriate antimicrobials mortality is below 10 percent. However, this clearly increases with the severity of the episode.[32,33,49] The expected mortality of a mild first episode of PCP, therefore, is usually negligible. In addition, young age and early diagnosis have been correlated with better outcome.[32,33] Respiratory failure requiring mechanical ventilation, as discussed above, was initially reported to have a mortality greater than 80 percent in most series.[51,52] More recently, with the addition of systemic corticosteroids, mortality has been reduced to less than 50 percent.[32,47,49] It appears, however, that if PCP-related acute respiratory failure develops, despite early intervention with corticosteroids and appropriate antimicrobial agents, the prognosis is dismal.[53]

Mycobacterium tuberculosis (MTb)

Tuberculosis (Tb) occurs with varying degrees of frequency among HIV-infected individuals, reaching 20 percent in some series. Because the risk of developing Tb is proportional to the risk of developing it prior to the acquisition of HIV, its incidence in North America is greatest among intravenous drug users, blacks, and Latin Americans. Tb usually develops within the year prior to the diagnosis of other AIDS-defining conditions. It must be noted, however, that disseminated Tb in an HIV-infected individual is diagnostic of AIDS according to the Centers for Disease Control (CDC) classification of HIV disease.

The symptoms of Tb in the context of HIV are generally nonspecific. This is particularly the case because "classic" Tb symptoms such as fatigue, malaise, weight loss, fever, and night sweats are extremely common, even in moderately advanced stages of HIV disease. Unlike in the immunocompetent host, in the context of HIV disease Tb usually has radiologic features similar to those of primary Tb, including hilar and/or mediastinal adenopathy, mid and lower lung infiltrates, pleural effusions, or a miliary pattern. Apical infiltrates or cavities are only seen in a minority of patients. As many as 10 percent of cases have a normal chest x-ray with a positive sputum culture for MTb. Furthermore, PCP is simultaneously diagnosed in as many as 25 percent of the cases of Tb. Prospective tuberculin skin testing (PPD) is useful among HIV-infected individuals, as Tb develops more frequently in patients known to have a previously positive test; however, at the time of diagnosis of AIDS at least 30 percent of patients are anergic. MTb can usually be easily diagnosed with smear and culture of sputum or BAL. Of particular note is the high diagnostic yield of blood (42 percent) and stool cultures (40 to 50 percent).

According to the American Thoracic Society (ATS) and the CDC, Tb in HIV-infected adults should be treated with isoniazid (INH) 300 mg daily and rifampin 600 mg daily (or 450 mg for patients weighing less than 50 kg). Pyrazinamide 20 to 30 mg/kg daily should be added for the initial 2 months of therapy. Ethambutol 25 mg/kg daily should also be added if INH resistance is suspected or if CNS disease or dissemination are present. Treatment should be continued for a minimum of 9 months and not less than 6 months after documented culture conversion.[54]

Mycobacterium avium COMPLEX (MAC)

The number of cases of MAC-related disease continues to increase among HIV-infected individuals, particularly since AIDS patients live longer and other opportunistic diseases are more effectively treated. Disease caused by MAC is usually clinically nonspecific. Fever, anorexia, wasting, malaise, and night sweats are frequently present. Unlike Tb, disease due to MAC occurs late in the course of HIV infection, usually following other opportunistic infections. Despite frequent pulmonary involvement, specific respiratory signs and symptoms are usually absent. The same can be said with regard to the radiologic involvement of the lung.

The diagnosis is generally made by recovery of the organism from sputum, BAL, lymph node, liver, bone marrow, bowel, stool, or blood specimens. Treatment of MAC disease remains largely unrewarding. Combination therapy (Table 100-3) has been used with limited success.[54,55] Given the poor prognosis of MAC disease at this time, the patients' eligibility for ICU care should be carefully reassessed when that is felt to be the principal cause of their critical illness. Whether or not new experimental regimens will improve survival remains to be seen. At present, patients who have failed or cannot tolerate the above-mentioned chemotherapy often find symptomatic relief with corticosteroid therapy.

TABLE 100-3 Antimicrobial Therapy of Common Infections in AIDS Patients

Infection	Drug of Choice	Total Daily Dose	Dose Interval	Route	Usual Duration	Alternative Therapy
Protozoa						
Toxoplasmosis (*Toxoplasma gondii*)	Pyrimethamine[1]	200 mg loading dose, then 1.0–1.5 mg/kg (usually 75–100 mg)	Daily	PO	4–6 weeks[2]	Pyrimethamine *plus* clindamycin 900–1200 mg IV[3] q6–8 h until marked improvement, then 450–600 mg PO q6h
	plus Sulfadiazine	4–6 g	6 h	PO	4–6 weeks	
	Maintenance therapy: Pyrimethamine[1]	25–50 mg	Daily	PO	Indefinitely	Pyrimethamine 25–50 mg/d PO *plus* clindamycin 300–450 mg PO q6h
	plus Sulfadiazine	2 g	6 h	PO	Indefinitely	
Cryptosporidiosis (*Cryptosporidium*)	Spiramycin[4]	3 g	8 h	PO	3 weeks	
Giardiasis (*Giardia lamblia*)	Quinacrine	300 mg	8 h	PO	5 d	Metronidazole 250 mg tid for 5 d *or* tinidazole

TABLE 100-3 Antimicrobial Therapy of Common Infections in AIDS Patients (Continued)

Infection	Drug of Choice	Total Daily Dose	Dose Interval	Route	Usual Duration	Alternative Therapy
Amebiasis *(Entamoeba histolytica)*	Metronidazole[5]	2.25 g	8 h	PO, IV	10 d	Dehydroemetine[6] 1–1.5 mg/kg/d IM (maximum 90 mg/d) for up to 5 d followed by a luminal agent (e.g., iodoquinol, diloxanide furoate, or paromomycin)
	followed by Iodoquinol	1.95 g	8 h	PO	20 d	
Isosporiasis *(Isospora belli)*	Trimethroprim-sulfamethoxazole	640 mg 3200 mg	6 h	PO, IV	10 d[7]	Metronidazole or quinacrine
Fungi						
Pneumocystosis *(P. carinii)*	Trimethoprim-sulfamethoxazole	20 mg/kg 100 mg/kg	6 h	IV, PO	14–21 d	Pentamidine 4 mg/kg/d IV, IM[8] *or* Trimethoprim 20 mg/kg/d divided q6h PO *plus* dapsone 100 mg PO daily
Candidiasis:						
Oropharyngeal	Clotrimazole	50 mg (10 mg troche 5 times/d)	4 h	Dissolve in mouth	7–14 d[9]	Nystatin vaginal tablets 100,000 units dissolve in mouth tid (ketoconazole 200 mg/d or fluconazole 50–100 mg/d if refractory to topical therapy)
Esophageal	Ketoconazole	200–400 mg	Daily	PO	3–4 weeks[9]	Topical therapy as for oropharyngeal candidiasis *or* amphotericin B 0.3–0.6 mg/kg IV daily for 7–14 d
	or Fluconazole	200 mg loading dose then 50–100 mg	Daily	PO	3–4 weeks[9]	
Focal invasive or disseminated	Amphotericin B[10]	0.5–1.0 mg/kg	Daily	IV	Until total dose at least 1–2 g	Fluconazole 400 mg loading dose PO, IV then 200–400 mg/d[11]
Cryptococcosis *(Cryptococcus neoformans)*	Amphotericin B	0.4–0.8 mg/kg	Daily	IV	2–10 weeks[12]	Fluconazole 400 mg loading dose PO, IV, then 200–400 mg daily for 10 weeks
	with/without 5-Flucytosine	100–150 mg/kg	6 h	PO, IV	2–10 weeks	
	Maintenance therapy: fluconazole	200 mg	Daily	PO	Indefinitely	Amphotericin B 1 mg/kg IV, once or twice weekly indefinitely
Histoplasmosis *(Histoplasma capsulatum)*	Amphotericin B	0.5–1.0 mg/kg	Daily	IV	Until total dose 1–2 g[13]	—

TABLE 100-3 Antimicrobial Therapy of Common Infections in AIDS Patients (Continued)

Infection	Drug of Choice	Total Daily Dose	Dose Interval	Route	Usual Duration	Alternative Therapy
	Maintenance therapy: amphotericin B	1 mg/kg	Weekly	IV	Indefinitely	Itraconazole 400 mg/d *or* ketoconazole 400 mg/d indefinitely
Coccidioidomycosis: *(Coccidioides immitis)*						
Extrameningeal	Amphotericin B	0.5–1.0 mg/kg	Daily	IV	Until total dose 1–2 g[13]	Fluconazole 400 mg/d PO, IV *or* ketoconazole 400 mg/d
	Maintenance therapy: ketoconazole	400 mg	Daily	PO	Indefinitely	Amphotericin B 1 mg/kg weekly *or* fluconazole 400 mg/d
Meningitis	Amphotericin B	0.5–1.0 mg/kg	Daily	IV	Until total dose 1–2 g IV	Ketoconazole 400–1200 mg/d PO *plus* IT[14] amphotericin *or* fluconazole 400 mg/d PO, IV
	plus Amphotericin B	0.1–0.3 mg	3 times per week	IT[14]	Long term[15]	
Viruses						
Herpes simplex						
Mucocutaneous	Acyclovir	1 g (200 mg 5 times/d)	4 h	PO	10 d[16]	Foscarnet 60 mg/kg IV q8h[17] *or* vidarabine 15 mg/kg/d IV
		or 15 mg/kg	8 h	IV	10 d	
Visceral or disseminated	Acyclovir	30 mg/kg	8 h	IV	10 d	Vidarabine 15 mg/kg/d IV *or* foscarnet 60 mg/kg IV q8h
Herpes zoster						
Dermatomal	Acyclovir	4 g (800 mg 5 times/d)	4 h	PO	5–7 d	
		or 36 mg/kg	8 h	IV	7 d	Vidarabine 15 mg/kg/d 5–7 d
Disseminated	Acyclovir	36 mg/kg	8 h	IV	7 d	Vidarabine 15 mg/kg/d *or* foscarnet 60 mg/kg q8h
CMV (cytomegalovirus)	Ganciclovir[18]	10 mg/kg	12 h	IV	14 d	Foscarnet 60 mg/kg IV q8h
	Maintenance therapy[19]: ganciclovir	5 mg/kg	Daily	IV	Indefinite	Foscarnet 90–120 mg once daily IV
HIV	Zidovudine[20]	300–600 mg	4–8 h	PO	Indefinite	Dideoxyinosine (ddI)
Bacteria						
Streptococcus pneumoniae:						
Uncomplicated pneumonia	Penicillin G[21]	1.2 million units	12 h	IM	7–10 d	Cephalosporin (e.g., cefuroxime 0.75–1.5 g IV q8h) *or*

TABLE 100-3 Antimicrobial Therapy of Common Infections in AIDS Patients (Continued)

Infection	Drug of Choice	Total Daily Dose	Dose Interval	Route	Usual Duration	Alternative Therapy
Streptococcus pneumoniae (cont.)						erythromycin 500 mg PO, IV q6h
Empyema or hypotensive	Penicillin G	5–10 million units	6 h	IV	7–10 d	Cephalosporins
Staphylococcus aureus						
Pneumonia, bacteremia	Cloxacillin *or* nafcillin *or* oxacillin[22]	8–12 g	4–6 h	IV	14 d	Vancomycin 15 mg/kg IV q12h
Hemophilus influenzae						
Pneumonia	Ceftriaxone	1–2 g	Daily	IV	10–14 d	Ampicillin 1–2 g IV q6h (if sensitive) *or* cefotaxime 1–2 g IV q6–8 h *or* cefuroxime 0.75–1.5 g IV q8h
Salmonella bacteremia	Ampicillin	8–12 g	6 h	IV	3–4 weeks[23]	Cefotaxime 1–2 g IV q6–8 h, *or* ceftriaxone 1–2 g IV daily, *or* ciprofloxacin 500–750 mg PO q12h
Listeria meningitis	Ampicillin	200 mg/kg	4 h	IV	2–4 weeks	Trimethoprim-sulfamethoxazole (dosage as for PCP)
	plus Gentamicin[24]	4.5–6 mg/kg	8 h	IV	2–4 weeks	
Syphilis						
Early (primary, secondary and latent <1 yr)	Benzathine[25] penicillin G	2.4 million units	once	IM		Doxycycline 100 mg PO bid for 2 weeks[26] *or* tetracycline 500 mg PO qid for 2 weeks[26]
Late[27] (>1 yr duration) and neurosyphilis	Aqueous crystalline penicillin G	12–24 million units	4 h	IV	10 d	Ceftriaxone 1 g IM or IV daily for 14 d *or* procaine penicillin G 2.4 million units IM daily *plus* probenecid 1 g PO daily for 10 d *or* amoxicillin 3 g + 0.5 g probenecid PO bid for 15–30 d[28]
	followed by benzathine penicillin G	2.4 million units	weekly	IM	3 weeks (3 doses)	
Mycobacteria						
Mycobacterium tuberculosis	Isoniazid[29]	300 mg	Daily	PO	9 months[30]	If drug toxicity or drug resistance, then alternative drugs include streptomycin, para-aminosalicylic acid (PAS), ethionamide, cycloserine, kanamycin, dapsone, clofazamine, rifabutine, and ciprofloxacin
	Rifampin[31]	600 mg	Daily	PO, IV	9 months	
	Pyrazinamide	20–30 mg/kg	Daily	PO	2 months	
	Ethambutal[32]	25 mg/kg	Daily	PO	2 months	

TABLE 100-3 Antimicrobial Therapy of Common Infections in AIDS Patients (Continued)

Infection	Drug of Choice	Total Daily Dose	Dose Interval	Route	Usual Duration	Alternative Therapy
M. avium complex *(MAC)*	Amikacin[33]	7.5 mg/kg	Daily	IV	4 weeks	Alternatives include rifabutine, clofazamine, ethionamide, clarithromycin
	Ethambutal	15 mg/kg	Daily	PO	indefinite[33]	
	Rifampin[31]	600 mg	Daily	PO	indefinite[33]	
	Ciprofloxacin	1.5 g	12 h	PO	indefinite[33]	

Abbreviations: PO, by mouth; IV, intravenous; IT, intrathecal; IM, intramuscular; d, days; q6h, every 6 h; tid, three times per day; qid, four times per day.

NOTES:
[1]Pyrimethamine should be used in conjunction with folinic acid (10–50 mg/d for primary therapy, 10–20 mg/d for maintenance therapy) in order to minimize hematologic toxicity (anemia, leukopenia, thrombocytopenia). AZT should be used with caution or withheld during the acute phase of treatment of toxoplasmosis.
[2]Primary therapy for toxoplasmosis should be continued until complete resolution or marked improvement has occurred clinically and radiologically (usually 4–6 weeks).
[3]The dosage of clindamycin for toxoplasmosis has not been established but suggested as outlined. (See Ref. 62).
[4]The efficacy of spiramycin has not been established for cryptosporidiosis.
[5]Indicated for intestinal disease and/or liver abscess. Asymptomatic cyst passers may be treated with a luminal agent, e.g., iodoquinol 650 mg tid for 20 d (alternative: diloxanide furoate 500 mg tid for 10 d or paromomycin 25–30 mg/kg/d divided in 3 daily doses for 7 d). Chloroquine phosphate 600 mg base (1 g)/d for 2 d, then 300 mg base (500 mg)/d for 2–3 weeks may be used in the management of amebic liver abscess.
[6]Because of the potential for cardiotoxicity, patients receiving dehydroemetine should remain sedentary and have electrocardiographic monitoring.
[7]Continue treatment for 3 more weeks with trimethoprim (160 mg)-sulfamethoxazole (800 mg) PO, bid.
[8]Intramuscular pentamidine has been associated with sterile abscess formation. The preferred route is slow IV infusion over 2–4 h.
[9]Mucosal candidiasis in HIV patients has a high relapse rate. Intermittent or continuous maintenance therapy (systemic or topical) may be required.
[10]Consider addition of 5-flucytosine in patients with overwhelming infection or local involvement with meningitis or endophthalmitis.
[11]The duration of fluconazole therapy is not established. A minimum duration of 1–2 months is recommended.
[12]Patients should receive amphotericin B with or without 5-flucytosine until significantly improved and stable, at which time treatment can be continued with fluconazole 400 mg/d PO, IV to complete a 10-week course of treatment. Patients treated initially with amphotericin B (without 5-flucytosine) may have a better clinical response rate with higher dosage of amphotericin B (e.g., 0.7–0.8 mg/kg/d).
[13]Treatment with amphotericin B is continued until there is significant clinical improvement.
[14]IT amphotericin B (cisternal, cervical, ventricular, or lumbar) should be started at a low dose (0.01–0.025 mg) and increased gradually as tolerated to a dose of 0.1–0.3 mg 3 times weekly. The best intrathecal route of administration is cisternal.
[15]IT amphotericin B 3 times per week for 3 months then 1–2 times per week for several months. Further dosage tapering is based upon clinical course and spinal fluid parameters.
[16]Long-term suppressive therapy (acyclovir 200 mg 2–5 daily) may be required to control frequent relapses.
[17]Foscarnet or vidarabine may be used to treat acyclovir-resistant (thymidine-kinase-deficient) herpes simplex infection.
[18]AZT should be discontinued during ganciclovir treatment in most cases because of additive hematologic toxicity (granulocytopenia). If long-term ganciclovir is indicated, then consider ddI.
[19]Maintenance therapy is mandatory for CMV retinitis but not always required for gastrointestinal involvement. A dosing schedule of 6 mg/kg/d for 5 d per week has also been used.
[20]AZT is indicated in the following patients: AIDS, ARC, HIV-associated thrombocytopenia, HIV neurologic disease, CD4 200–500/mm^{m3} if symptomatic or at greater risk of disease progression in the near future (e.g., thrush, rapidly falling CD4 count, P24 antigenemia, or elevation in β_2-microglobulin, IgA, or circulating immune complexes) (see Ref. 16).
[21]Empiric therapy for acute bacterial pneumonia in HIV-infected patients may be provided with trimethoprim-sulfamethoxazole (activity against pneumococcus, *H. influenza,* and *Branhamella* in addition to *P. carinii*). Sulfa-allergic patients may be treated empirically with cefuroxime or ampicillin (unless ampicillin-resistant *H. influenzae* is a concern).
[22]Vancomycin is the drug of choice for empiric therapy in areas where methicillin-resistant *S. aureus* is encountered.
[23]3–4 weeks of treatment to try and reduce likelihood of relapse, need not all be given by IV route.
[24]Some authors also recommend IT gentamicin.
[25]Some authorities advise CSF examination and/or treatment with a regimen appropriate for neurosyphilis for all patients coinfected with syphilis and HIV, regardless of the clinical stage of syphilis. HIV-infected patients should have frequent follow-up and serologic testing at 1, 2, 3, 6, 9, and 12 months. Any patient without a 4-fold decline in nontreponemal serology by 3 months for primary or secondary syphilis, or 6 months in early latent syphilis, or a 4-fold rise in titer at any time should have a CSF examination and be treated with the neurosyphilis regimen unless reinfection can be established as the cause of the increased titre (see Ref. 63).
[26]Treponema-cidal antibiotics (e.g., penicillin) are preferred for syphilis in HIV-infected patients.
[27]HIV-infected patients who have late syphilis should undergo cerebrospinal fluid examination. Those patients who have a normal spinal fluid examination (including negative CSF VDRL) do not require high-dose IV penicillin therapy and should receive benzathine penicillin G 2.4 m.u. IM weekly for 3 doses.
[28]Efficacy of the alternative regimens for syphilis is not clearly established.
[29]Isoniazid: higher dose of 10 mg/kg recommended for tuberculous meningitis until clinical response observed.
[30]Antituberculous therapy should be continued for 9 months or at least 6 months after conversion to culture negative state.
[31]Rifampin dose of 10 mg/kg if body weight below 50 kg.
[32]Ethambutal not required unless drug resistance or disseminated disease known or suspected.
[33]In a nonrandomized prospective study, this four-drug regimen was associated with a reduced mycobacterial burden and improvement in systemic symptoms (see Ref. 55). The duration of therapy has not been established, but the usual recommendation in non-AIDS patients has been 18–24 months.

CYTOMEGALOVIRUS (CMV)

The pathogenic importance of CMV in the lungs in the context of AIDS remains controversial. CMV isolation from pulmonary secretions in AIDS patients appears to have little prognostic value. In fact, despite the addition of corticosteroids to the treatment of PCP, we have failed to identify the once much feared rise in the frequency of CMV pneumonitis. On the other hand, the prominent role of CMV as a gastrointestinal or ocular pathogen among these patients is clearly recognized.

CMV pneumonitis in the context of AIDS should be diagnosed only if hypoxemia and diffuse pulmonary infiltrates coexist with evidence of CMV cytopathic effect (i.e., intranuclear and intracytoplasmic inclusions) in lung tissue and with histologic absence of other likely cause to explain the pulmonary disorder.[56] CMV disease is usually treated with ganciclovir (DHPG) as outlined in Table 100-3. Long-term maintenance therapy is required for CMV retinitis but may not always be needed in gastrointestinal disease. In the context of AIDS, CMV disease tends to occur at a late stage, and whether or not patients respond to specific therapy, survival following an episode of CMV is generally poor.

OTHER CAUSES OF PULMONARY INFILTRATES

Bacterial pneumonias tend to occur with increased frequency among HIV-infected individuals. Community-acquired pneumonias are usually due to *Streptococcus pneumoniae, H. influenza, and S aureus. Legionella* pneumonitis, contrary to early reports, occurs rarely among HIV-infected individuals. Clinical features of community-acquired bacterial pneumonia are indistinguishable from those described in the immunocompetent host. Chest x-rays usually demonstrate segmental or lobar consolidation. Sputum culture is often diagnostically helpful. If this is not the case, bronchoscopic studies will generally identify the etiologic agent.[57]

Nosocomial pneumonias among HIV-infected individuals are indistinguishable from those occurring in other hospitalized patients. These are usually caused by gram-negative organisms and tend to have a high mortality despite adequate therapy.[57]

Fungal pneumonias (other than PCP) are a rare cause of respiratory failure among HIV-infected individuals. Often they represent the pulmonary epiphenomenon of disseminated infection. Among them *C. neoformans, H. capsulatum,* and *C. immitis* are the most frequently encountered. *Aspergillus* has only occasionally been found to produce pneumonia in these patients. Candidiasis of the trachea, bronchii, or lungs, despite being recognized by the CDC as an AIDS-defining condition, is not a significant problem among these patients. This is particularly surprising as oral and esophageal candidiasis are extremely common. Treatment of fungal diseases is outlined in Table 100-3; once again, long-term maintenance therapy is required.[57]

Kaposi's sarcoma (KS) involves the lungs in up to 25 percent of patients with mucocutaneous KS. Clinically significant pulmonary KS without obvious mucocutaneous involvement is exceptionally rare. Pulmonary KS is often indistinguishable from other HIV-related pulmonary diseases. Cough and dyspnea are commonly the presenting features. Fever, wheezing, hoarseness, and even upper airway obstruction can occur. Sputum production is usually not present. Hemoptysis, on the other hand, is relatively frequent. Chest x-ray usually shows nodular opacities of varying sizes coexisting with varying degrees of interstitial disease. Pleural and nodal involvement are also frequent. Bronchoscopic evaluation usually helps to rule out a superimposed treatable HIV-related disease in patients with pulmonary KS. It also may allow visualization of the characteristic red-violaceous lesions in the endobronchial tree. Although biopsy of these lesions at times can provide diagnostic confirmation, this is rarely required. No definitive therapy is currently available for the treatment of systemic KS. Interferon has been used with some limited success for the treatment of early disease. Radiation therapy or chemotherapy have had some limited success in providing short-term palliation. Given the poor prognosis of KS-related ARF at this time, these patients are unlikely to benefit from ICU support.[58]

Neurologic Complications in HIV-infected Patients

Neurologic disease secondary to opportunistic infection or neoplasm may be associated with a depressed level of consciousness and occasionally precipitate ICU consultation and care. More often the neurologic disease may be a concomitant problem in patients requiring ICU care for other reasons.

The most frequently encountered neurologic syndromes in HIV-infected patients are meningitis, dementia, encephalopathy, focal neurologic deficits, myelopathy, peripheral neuropathy, and myopathy.[59,60] The various etiologic agents responsible for these syndromes in addition to key points of clinical presentation and diagnostic evaluation are summarized in Table 100-4. In general, most of the treatable infections complicating AIDS produce either meningitis or progressive focal neurologic deficits due to localized inflammatory lesions in the brain, and both of these syndromes are usually associated with headache. On the other hand, most of the causes of diffuse brain involvement are not associated with headache. A suggested sequence of investigations in the HIV-infected patient with headache or CNS dysfunction is outlined in Fig. 100-6. Antimicrobial therapy is outlined in Table 100-3.

MENINGITIS

The clinical presentation of both acute and chronic meningitis is little different in the AIDS patients from that seen in the immunocompetent host; these include headache, fever, and nuchal rigidity of variable duration and severity.

The most important treatable cause of meningitis in the HIV-infected patient is *C. neoformans.* Other treatable but

TABLE 100-4 Neurologic Complications in HIV-infected Patients

Neurologic Syndrome	Etiologic Agents	Clinical Presentation	Diagnostic Evaluation
Meningitis	*C. neoformans*	Often headache, fever, and vomiting; sometimes confusion, seizure, meningismus, cranial nerve palsies; may be asymptomatic meningitis and present with fevers, fungemia and/or extrameningeal lesion (e.g., skin, pneumonia)	CSF white blood count usually <20/mm^3; CSF, glucose, and protein often normal; cryptococcal antigen positive >90% in CSF and 99% in serum; positive India Ink 50–90%; fungal cultures (blood, CSF, urine)
	Aseptic (?HIV)	Headache, meningismus, and fever (all less common in chronic cases), with/without cranial neuropathies (V, VII, VIII); may occur with seroconversion, but more common in advanced HIV	CSF examination: mild mononuclear pleocytosis, protein elevated, glucose normal (differential diagnosis also includes syphilis and lymphomatous meningitis)
	M. tuberculosis	Usually subacute-chronic meningitis. Headache, fever, with/without meningismus, and cranial nerve palsies	CSF Exam: lymphocytic pleocytosis, low glucose, and increased protein; smear for acid fast bacilli insensitive; cultures for *M. tuberculosis*
	C. immitis	Fever, headache, with/without meningismus, confusion (consider if travel/residence history for endemic zone: e.g., southwestern U.S.)	Serology (antibody detection) for serum and CSF; any positive CSF titre usually diagnostic of meningitis; lymphocytic pleocytosis usually >50 cells/cmm^3, elevated protein, low glucose; fungal cultures of blood and CSF
	Bacterial (pneumococcus, meningococcus, *Listeria, H. influenzae*)	Fever, headache, meningismus with/without confusion, seizures; bacterial meningitis rare in HIV-infected patients	CSF exam: polymorphonuclear pleocytosis, high protein, low glucose, with/without positive gram stain and/or bacterial antigens (pneumococcus, meningococcus, *H. influenzae*); bacterial cultures of blood and CSF
Diffuse Brain Disease			
AIDS dementia complex	HIV	Usually alert, but impaired cognition, behavior, and motor function; sometimes organic psychosis or mania	Abnormalities on neuropsychologic testing; non-specific CSF abnormalities including elevated protein and IgG but usually no pleocytosis; CT/MRI: atrophy
Diffuse encephalopathies	Toxic/metabolic disorders (e.g., hypoxia, sepsis, drugs), CNS toxoplasmosis, CNS lymphoma, occasionally viral infection (HSV, CMV)	Impaired alertness and cognition, with/without focal neurologic deficits	Blood chemistry to exclude metabolic causes, with/without drug levels, serology for toxoplasmosis; CT head scan with contrast (or MRI): focal lesions in toxoplasmosis, lymphoma, herpes simplex encephalitis
Focal Brain Disease			
Toxoplasmosis	*Toxoplasma gondii*	Headache, progressive focal deficit(s) over days-weeks, fever with/without altered mental status, with/without seizure	CT scan (with contrast) or MRI: ring-enhancing lesion(s) in cortex, thalamus, or basal ganglia; may have atypical CT appearances; toxoplasma serum serology positive; possible brain biopsy.
Lymphoma	no agent has been discovered	Headache, with/without progressive focal deficit(s), confusion, lethargy, seizure; more slowly progressive than toxoplasmosis	CT scan (with contrast) or MRI: usually 1–2 lesions in white matter, may mimic toxoplasmosis but enhancement usually weaker and homogenous; possible brain biopsy

(Continued)

TABLE 100-4 Neurologic Complications in HIV-infected Patients (Continued)

Neurologic Syndrome	Etiologic Agents	Clinical Presentation	Diagnostic Evaluation
Progressive multifocal leukoencephalopathy	JC virus (papovavirus)	Slowly progressive focal deficits (over weeks), or altered mental status.	CT scan (with contrast) or MRI: nonenhancing white matter lesions without mass effect; possible brain biopsy
Neurosyphilis	*Treponema pallidum*	Focal neurologic deficit (vascular involvement), Bell's palsy or optic neuritis; occasionally meningitis	Positive serum VDRL, and FTA-abs; CSF exam: mononuclear pleocytosis, elevated protein, with/without positive VDRL; CSF profile (if VDRL negative) is indistinguishable from CSF abnormalities due to HIV
Myelopathy			
Subacute, chronic	HIV (vacuolar), HTLV-1	Slowly progressive, painless ataxia and spasticity; bowel-bladder dysfunction occurs late; often coexistent with dementia	CT scan, or MRI, with/without myelography; with/without HTLV-1 serology
Acute, subacute (transverse myelitis)	Varicella zoster, lymphoma, cytomegalovirus	More rapid onset of myelopathy than for HIV	CT scan or MRI, myelography
Peripheral Neuropathy			
Axonal neuropathy	? HIV	Distal, mainly sensory, painful ("burning feet"), symptoms more prominent than signs	With/Without nerve conduction studies
Toxic axonal neuropathy	ddI, 2-,3-dideoxycytidine, others	As for axonal neuropathy	With/Without nerve conduction studies
Acute-chronic demyelinating neuropathy	? Autoimmune response to HIV	Similar to Guillain-Barré syndrome; occurs during early or latent period of HIV infection	Nerve conduction studies; CSF: elevated protein, and mild pleocytosis
Radiculopathies	Varicella zoster virus	*Herpes zoster* dermatomal vesicular lesions, painful lesions	Clinical diagnosis, with/without Tzanck smear, viral culture
	Cytomegalovirus	Subacute and progressive ascending polyradiculopathy with sensory loss, urinary retention, and flaccid paraparesis	CSF: Polymorphonuclear pleocytosis, elevated protein, low glucose, with/without CSF culture positive for CMV; rule out bacterial and tuberculous meningitis
Myopathy	AZT	Ranges from asymptomatic elevation of CPK to progressive myalgia, atrophy, and weakness (especially proximal leg muscles)	Consider muscle biopsy (mitochondrial abnormalities with/without inflammatory cell infiltrates) if persists after stopping AZT
	HIV?	As for AZT-induced myopathy	Consider muscle biopsy: myopathic changes (variable fiber size, vacuolar change and fiber destruction), with/without inflammatory infiltrates; ultrasound if localized inflammation to rule out pyomyositis

uncommon etiologies include MTb, *C. immitis*, *T. pallidum* (syphilis), *L. monocytogenes*, and the usual causative agents of bacterial meningitis (pneumococcus, meningococcus, *H. influenzae*). Antimicrobial therapy is outlined in Table 100-3. Treatment of HIV-related aseptic meningitis has not been established.

DIFFUSE BRAIN DISEASE (dementia and encephalopathy)

AIDS dementia complex appears to be due to chronic HIV infection of the CNS. Patients with AIDS dementia complex manifest varying degrees of impaired cognition, behavior, and motor function but usually remain alert. In contrast, the diffuse encephalopathies associated with toxic and metabolic disorders, CNS toxoplasmosis, lymphoma, or viral infection (e.g., herpes simplex or CMV) usually result in impairment of cognition associated with a disturbance in the level of consciousness. Patients with AIDS dementia complex should be treated with AZT, which has been associated with sustained improvement in neurologic performance in up to 50 percent of patients.[61] Whether ddI can have a similar beneficial effect on neurologic performance remains to be determined.

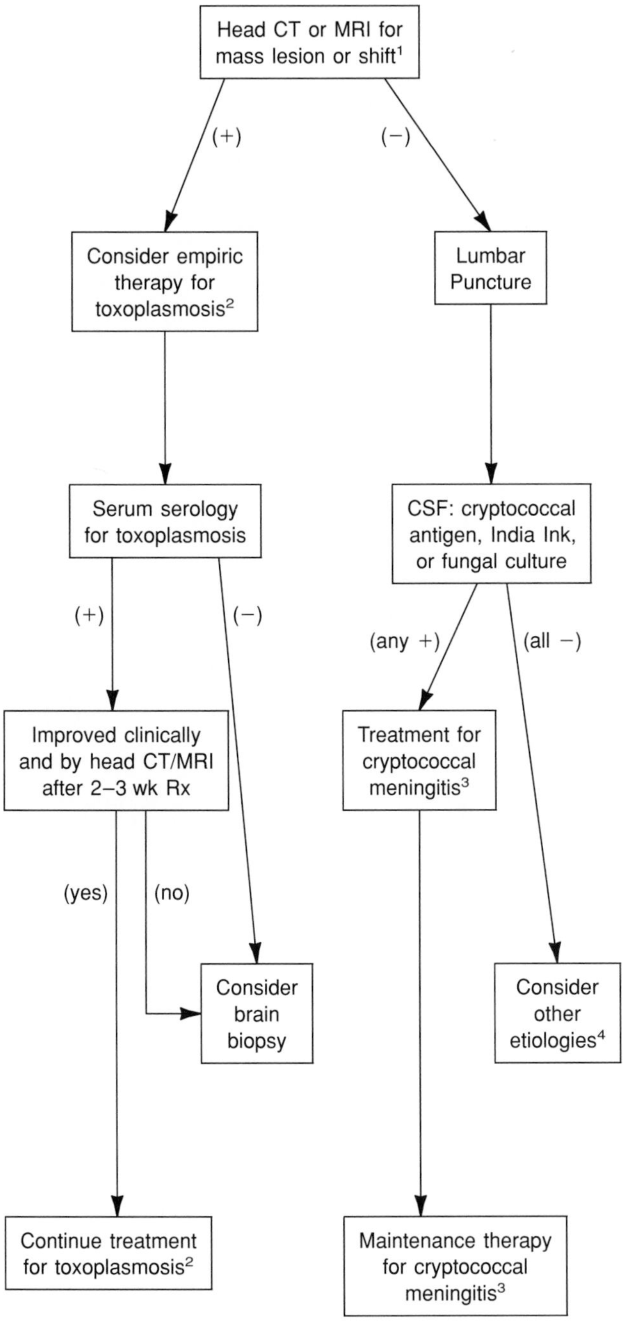

FIGURE 100-6 An approach to the management of new or worsening headache or CNS dysfunction in the HIV-infected patient.
(1) CT (preferably enhanced) or magnetic resonance imaging (MRI) should be done urgently, particularly in patients with focal neurologic findings, papilledema, or seizures. Those presenting with an acute onset of symptoms associated with neck stiffness (compatible with acute bacterial meningitis) should have a lumbar puncture performed as the initial investigation provided there are no contraindications (e.g., papilledema or focal neurologic deficit). Delays involved in obtaining CT or MRI in such patients before lumbar puncture and the initiation of empiric antimicrobial therapy may adversely affect outcome. Patients presenting with headache alone or in association with lethargy and confusion should have CT or MRI as the initial investigation. However, if unacceptable delays (as judged by the urgency of the clinical situation) are involved in obtaining CT or MRI, then lumbar puncture should be considered provided there are no contraindications. Sinusitis is common in HIV-infected individuals and may often be asymptomatic. Radiologic findings of sinusitis may be incidental in the HIV-infected patient with headache, and coexistent (unrelated) intracranial pathology may still need to be excluded. The serum cryptococcal antigen assay (CRAG) is a rapid, accurate, and noninvasive method for identifying cases of cryptococcal meningitis among HIV-infected patients presenting with headache or other neurologic symptoms and signs. Results of serum CRAG may be available well before CT/MRI and lumbar puncture. Acutely ill patients with a positive serum cryptococcal antigen may be started on systemic antifungal therapy if significant delays are anticipated in completing other investigations (CT/MRI and lumbar puncture) since CSF cultures and antigen titers usually remain positive during the first few days or weeks of treatment.
(2) If clinical presentation and CT (enhanced) or MRI are compatible with a diagnosis of CNS toxoplasmosis, then empiric therapy should be started as outlined in Table 100-3. Serum cryptococcal antigen testing should be done in patients with focal lesion(s) on CT head scan which are atypical for toxoplasmosis, or if not responding to empiric therapy for toxoplasmosis since cryptococcal meningitis may be associated with cryptococcoma.
(3) See Table 100-3 for treatment of cryptococcal meningitis.
(4) Tuberculous meningitis, bacterial meningitis (including *Listeria monocytogenes*), aseptic meningitis (HIV), neurosyphilis, HIV dementia, herpes simplex encephalitis, metabolic encephalopathy, and thrombotic thrombocytopenic purpura.

FOCAL NEUROLOGIC DISEASE

Patients presenting with progressive focal neurologic deficit(s) should have an urgent computed tomography (CT) head scan with contrast (Figs. 100-7 and 100-8), which will usually yield evidence of CNS toxoplasmosis (Fig. 100-7), lymphoma (Fig. 100-8), or progressive multifocal leukoencephalopathy (PML). Patients with a CT head scan compatible with toxoplasmosis should be treated empirically (see Table 100-3). Those who do not respond to empiric therapy, particularly when serum serology for toxoplasmosis is negative, should be considered for brain biopsy.[62] Although less responsive to therapy, some patients with CNS lymphoma may have a significant response to radiotherapy and chemotherapy. At this time, there is no known effective treatment for PML. Neurosyphilis is only occasionally responsible for focal neurologic deficit(s), but it is important to consider this diagnosis as this represents a readily treatable condition.[63,64] Occasional cases of focal brain disease may be due to cryptococcoma, tuberculoma, vascular disorders, and herpes simplex encephalitis.

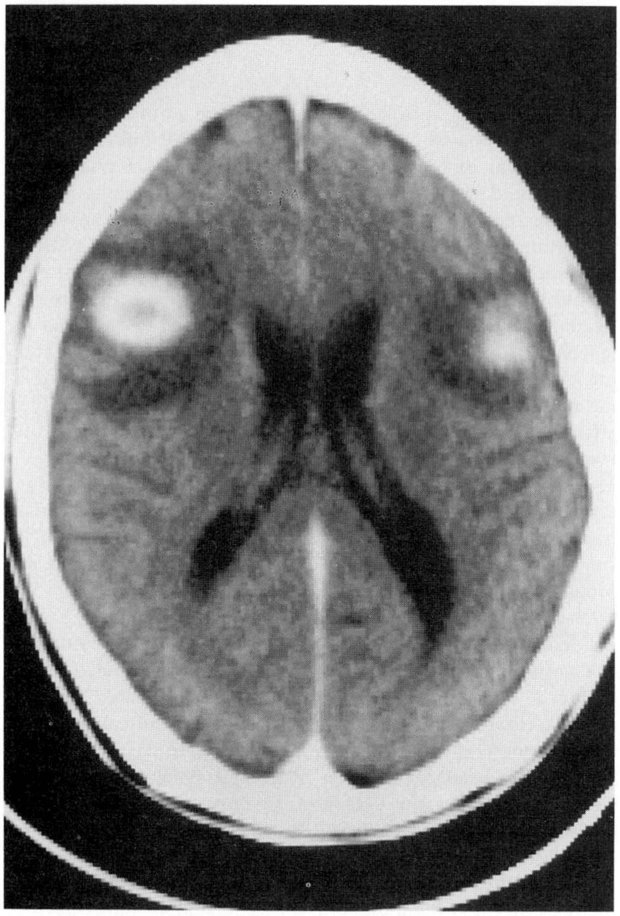

FIGURE 100-7 Double-dose delayed CT scan of the head demonstrating two lesions of cerebral toxoplasmosis. Note the ring-enhancing appearance of the right cerebral lesion.

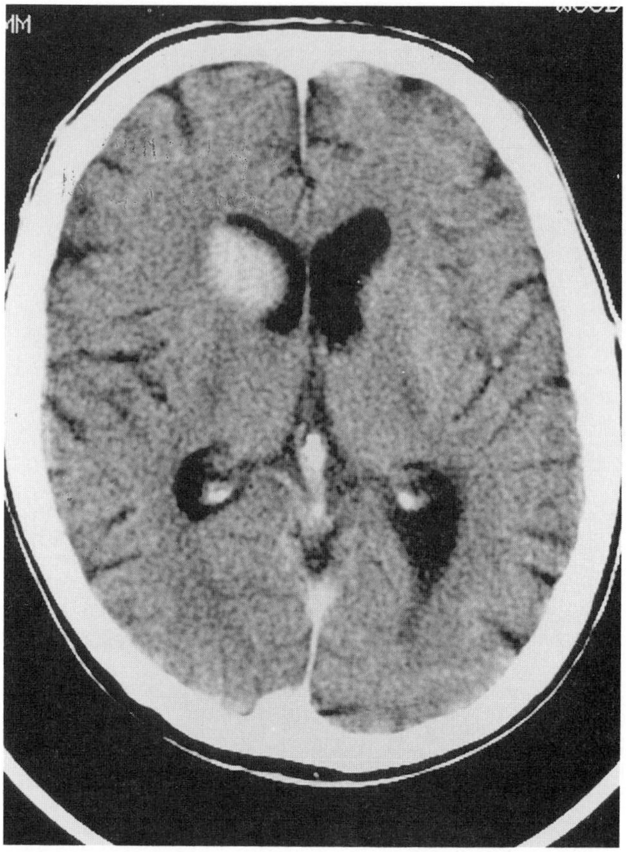

FIGURE 100-8 Double-dose delayed CT scan of the head demonstrating a lesion of cerebral lymphoma in a patient with HIV infection. Note the subependymal localization of the lesion, which is common in cerebral lymphoma.

MYELOPATHY, PERIPHERAL NEUROPATHY, AND MYOPATHY

A slowly progressive vacuolar myelopathy may occur in HIV-infected individuals. This should be differentiated from the more rapid onset of myelopathy associated with lymphoma, herpes zoster, or CMV. CMV may occasionally cause a subacute progressive polyradiculopathy[65] that presents with sacral sensory loss, urinary retention, and flaccid paraparesis within days to weeks. The cerebrospinal fluid (CSF) is markedly abnormal in CMV polyradiculopathy with a polymorphonuclear pleocytosis, hypoglycorrhachia, and elevated protein. CMV may be cultured from the CSF, but treatment should be started empirically with ganciclovir. Herpes zoster may result in a painful radiculopathy that persists long after resolution of the dermatomal vesicular lesions. However, postherpetic neuralgia is less common in HIV-infected patients.

Peripheral neuropathy may occur at any time during the course of HIV infection. During the early or latent period there may be an inflammatory demyelinating neuropathy with a presentation similar to that of the Guillain-Barré syndrome. This may respond to corticosteroids or plasmapheresis. Later in the course of HIV infection, an axonal neuropathy (possibly due to HIV) results in a painful, distal neuropathy that is mainly sensory. Treatment is symptomatic with analgesics or pain-modifying agents (e.g., amitriptyline or carbamazepine). A similar picture may be caused by drugs, particularly ddI.

AZT has been associated with myopathy, which may present with asymptomatic elevation in creatine kinase (CK), or progressive myalgia and weakness, particularly in the proximal leg muscles. AZT should be discontinued in symptomatic patients, and clinical improvement as well as a decrease in CK usually occur within 2 weeks. Patients who have improved after a drug-free interval can be restarted at lower doses under close medical supervision.[66] Muscle biopsy should be considered if the myopathy persists after withdrawal of AZT. If muscle biopsy shows significant inflammatory infiltrates but no opportunistic pathogens or mitochondrial changes, then an immune-mediated myopathy should be suspected. HIV-1-associated myopathy may be mediated by an immune mechanism; and some patients have responded to corticosteroids.[66]

Fungal Infections (Other Than PCP) in the HIV-infected Patient

CANDIDIASIS

Although candidiasis is the most common opportunistic fungal infection in AIDS, the vast majority of such cases are limited to mucosal disease involving the oropharynx, esophagus, or vagina. Treatment is therefore aimed at control of symptoms as outlined in Table 100-3. Deep candida infections (e.g., endophthalmitis or vertebral osteomyelitis) or disseminated candidiasis are rarely encountered in the setting of HIV infection, and in such instances risk factors for invasive candidiasis can often be identified. These include granulocytopenia, immunosuppressive therapy, prolonged vascular catheterization, recent surgery (e.g., gastrointestinal, cardiac), broad-spectrum antibiotics, and intravenous drug abuse. Management of candidemia includes removal of any potentially infected vascular catheters and careful assessment for the presence of metastatic sites of infection such as endophthalmitis. Candidemic patients should receive a course of amphotericin B totaling at least 500 mg. Fluconazole is an alternative to amphotericin B for treatment of candidemia or focal invasive or disseminated candidiasis, as outlined in Table 100-3.

CRYPTOCOCCOSIS

Cryptococcosis occurs in approximately 5 to 10 percent of individuals at some point during the course of HIV infection. Cryptococcal disease in AIDS usually presents as a subacute to chronic meningitis. The duration of symptoms before presentation varies from a few days to several weeks. It is important to note that the diagnosis may be overlooked because headache and other neurologic symptoms may be mild or absent. Furthermore, meningeal signs are present in only a minority of cases. Other presentations of cryptococcosis include pneumonia, skin lesions, and fever.[67]

An elevated opening pressure at lumbar puncture is common in cryptococcal meningitis., However, the abnormalities in spinal fluid cell count, glucose, and protein may be minimal or absent despite positive results for India ink smear, fungal culture, and cryptococcal antigen. The spinal fluid white blood cell count is usually less than 20 mm^3 and predominantly lymphocytic. The CSF glucose is usually normal but may be low. The serum cryptococcal antigen provides a rapid, noninvasive test that is particularly helpful in identifying the HIV-positive patient with cryptococcal disease.[67] The organism may be cultured from spinal fluid, blood, urine, sputum, and skin lesions. Patients with *C. neoformans* isolated from an extraneural site should be investigated for the presence of disseminated disease, including a lumbar puncture even in the absence of headache or neurologic symptoms.

A suggested sequence of investigations in the HIV-infected patient with headache or CNS dysfunction is outlined in Fig. 100-6. An HIV-infected patient presenting with an illness compatible with cryptococcosis and whose serum cryptococcal antigen is positive may be started on antifungal therapy before completion of the investigations should there be delays involved in obtaining a CT head scan (or MRI) or contraindications to performing a lumbar puncture (e.g., mass lesion on CT head scan or coagulopathy). Optimal treatment of AIDS-related cryptococcal meningitis has not been determined (see Table 100-3); however, it appears that a higher initial response rate may be achieved with amphotericin B 0.7 mg/kg daily plus oral 5-flucytosine rather than with fluconazole as initial treatment.[68,69] The role of flucytosine in the management of AIDS-related cryptococcal meningitis remains controversial.[67,68] Long-term maintenance therapy to prevent relapse is both better tolerated and more effective with fluconazole 200 mg per day than with amphotericin B 1 mg/kg once weekly.[70]

HISTOPLASMOSIS

In North America, histoplasmosis is usually geographically restricted to the endemic zone extending from Mexico and Texas up through the central United States (especially the Mississippi valley area) and into eastern Canada. Most patients with histoplasmosis will have a history of exposure to endemic areas. Histoplasmosis occurs in less than 0.5 percent of AIDS patients.

Histoplasmosis in the context of AIDS is usually a disseminated infection. The clinical presentation is usually that of a nonspecific febrile illness often accompanied by one or more of hepatosplenomegaly, pulmonary infiltrates, lymphadenopathy, anemia, leukopenia, and thrombocytopenia.[71] A rapid presumptive diagnosis can be obtained by demonstrating the organism in a buffy coat smear, bone marrow biopsy, or occasionally other tissues. The small intracellular yeast forms are present within leukocytes. The diagnosis is confirmed by fungal culture (blood, bone marrow, respiratory tract specimens, lymph node, or skin biopsy), which may take several weeks. Complement fixation titres may be negative in up to 30 percent in non-AIDS patients with histoplasmosis. Similarly, in AIDS patients, a negative serology for histoplasmosis does not reliably exclude the disease. Histoplasma antigen detection in body fluids remains investigational. Initial therapy is with amphotericin B until a cumulative dose of 1 to 2 g is reached. Maintenance therapy is required with either once weekly amphotericin B or daily ketoconazole or itraconazole (see Table 100-3).

COCCIDIOIDOMYCOSIS

Coccidioidomycosis is an endemic mycosis that is restricted epidemiologically in North America to the southwestern United States and northern Mexico. This infection should be considered in HIV-infected individuals who have history of exposure to endemic areas and who present with a compatible illness. Clinical features of coccidioidomycosis are nonspecific; they include one or more of fevers, dyspnea, diffuse reticulonodular pulmonary infiltrates, focal pulmonary lesions, meningitis, skin lesions, arthritis, and lymphadenopathy. Some patients may have fevers and weight loss with no focal lesions.[72] The diagnosis is made by histologic examination and fungal culture of respiratory secretions, tissue biopsies (skin or lymph node), spinal fluid, and blood. The characteristic coccidioidal spherules may be identified using lactophenol cotton blue, Gomori's silver methenamine, or Papanicolaou's stains. The spinal fluid characteristics in coccidioidal meningitis usually include a pleocytosis of greater than 50 cells/mm^3 which are predominantly lymphocytes. The CSF glucose is low and the protein is elevated. Serum serology for coccidioidomycosis is positive in approximately 90 percent of HIV-related cases. Positive spinal fluid serology (complement fixation) for *C. immitis* usually indicates the presence of coccidioidal meningitis. Therapy is outlined in Table 100-3.

Supportive Care for the AIDS Patients in the ICU

Resuscitation and supportive care of the AIDS patient in the ICU includes airway protection, respiratory support, cardiovascular monitoring and support, gastrointestinal and nutritional management, and psychologic supportive care. Airway assessment is important in patients who have depressed level of consciousness, usually because of neurologic problems or systemic sepsis, and in patients who have acute respiratory failure. Detailed discussion of the management of acute hypoxemic respiratory failure is presented in Chap. 128. In general, patients with arterial hypoxemia require supplemental high-flow, high-concentration oxygen. If hypoxemia is refractory to supplemental oxygen, then mask continuous positive airway pressure (CPAP) of 5 to 10 cmH_2O may improve arterial hypoxemia and decrease respiratory rate in alert patients who are able to protect their airway.[73] Mask CPAP has been used for up to 11 days. Pneumothorax occurs infrequently, in approximately 5 percent of patients.[73] Mask CPAP also allows speech and therefore ongoing discussion regarding prognosis and therapeutic options. Endotracheal intubation and mechanical ventilation are indicated in patients who require airway protection, in patients who are hypercarbic, and in patients who do not respond to CPAP. Assist-control ventilation with positive end-expiratory pressure is usually necessary for PCP patients who require mechanical ventilation.

AIDS patients who are critically ill may develop cardiovascular instability. Systemic arterial catheterization is appropriate for continuous arterial pressure monitoring and arterial blood gas determinations. Hypotension may be caused by hypovolemia, autonomic neuropathy, pentamidine, or sepsis syndrome. Hypovolemia may be caused by increased insensible fluid losses, diarrhea, and inadequate intake. Autonomic neuropathy occurs in some AIDS patients and appears to explain sudden, occasionally fatal hypotension and bradycardia.[74] The hypotension that may occur during infusion of pentamidine can be minimized by infusion of pentamidine slowly over 4 h, as described above. Hypotension in critically ill AIDS patients may be a complication of sepsis syndrome secondary to bacterial sepsis (e.g., pneumococcus, *H. influenzae*, *Staphylococcus*, or enteric gram-negative bacilli), PCP, or other systemic fungal infection such as histoplasmosis. Patients who have PCP, similar to patients who have bacterial sepsis, have tachycardia, decreased systemic vascular resistance, increased cardiac output, and hypotension.[75] The clinical approach to management is similar to that for other critically ill patients, detailed in Chaps. 98 and 114.

Enteropathy, malnutrition, and weight loss are very common gastrointestinal problems in AIDS patients. Up to 30 percent of AIDS patients have multiple gastrointestinal pathogens.[76] The causes of common gastrointestinal problems in AIDS patients are listed in Table 100-5 and their treatment is outlined in Table 100-3. Esophagitis may be caused by *Candida*, CMV, and HSV. Candida esophagitis usually presents with dysphagia, but marked odynophagia suggests either HSV or CMV esophagitis. Oropharyngeal and esophageal candida infection rarely give rise to deep visceral involvement or disseminated candidiasis. Diarrhea occurs in about 50 percent of AIDS patients and is caused by gastrointestinal infections, AIDS-associated enteropathy, and much less commonly by gastrointestinal neoplasms. Gastroenteritis may be secondary to *Cryptosporidium*, *Giardia*, *Isospora*, *Salmonella*, MAC, Tb, and CMV. *Cryptosporidium*, an intestinal protozoan, is one of the most common causes of severe diarrhea. Therapy for *Cryptosporidium* remains experimental and not very effective. Enterocolitis may be the result of infection with *Shigella*, *Campylobacter*, *E. histolytica*, and CMV. Finally, sexually transmitted proctitis caused by gonorrhea, syphilis, *Chlamydia*, or HSV may produce severe rectal symptoms accompanied by frequent small-volume stools associated with blood and mucus. *Clostridium difficile* colitis should also be considered in patients recently treated with antibacterial agents. Many AIDS patients have diarrhea due to AIDS-associated enteropathy.[77] AIDS-associated enteropathy, by definition, is not caused by the recognized infections already mentioned but may represent an unidentified infectious cause, possibly HIV or an autoimmune disorder.

Investigation of critically ill AIDS patients with esophagitis usually includes esophagoscopy and biopsy. Investigation of diarrhea includes examination of stool for ova and

TABLE 100-5 Causes of Common Gastrointestinal Problems in AIDS Patients

Problem	Organisms
Esophagitis	Candida, CMV, HSV
Gastroenteritis	Cryptosporidium, *G. lamblia*, *I. belli*, Salmonella, *MAC*, tuberculosis, CMV
Enterocolitis	Shigella, *Campylobacter*, *Entamoeba*, *CMV*, *Cryptosporidium*, MAI
Venereal proctitis	Gonorrhea, chlamydia, syphilis, HSV

*Abbreviations: CMV, cytomegalovirus, HSV, herpes simplex virus; MAC, *mycobacterium avium* complex; MAI, *M. avium*-intracellulare.

parasites, stool culture including mycobacteria, and occasionally flexible sigmoidoscopy[78] and *C. difficile* toxin assay. The treatment of critically ill AIDS patients who have diarrhea includes bowel rest, antimicrobial therapy (Table 100-3), intravenous fluid and electrolytes, symptomatic antidiarrheal therapy (e.g., diphenoxylate hydrochloride 5 mg orally three to four times daily or loperamide hydrochloride 4 mg initially then 2 mg after each diarrheal stool to 16 mg daily maximum), and nutritional therapy. Antimotility agents should be avoided when certain enteric pathogens (e.g., *Salmonella, Shigella, E. histolytica,* and *C. difficile*) are suspected. Total parenteral nutrition will almost always be necessary in critically ill patients who have significant diarrhea because enteral nutrition is seldom tolerated and usually exacerbates diarrhea. Malnourished AIDS patients who are critically ill and do not have diarrhea often respond adequately to enteral nutrition supplemented as appropriate with potassium, magnesium, calcium, and phosphate.

AIDS patients and their loved ones may also suffer important emotional and psychologic problems that require counseling, psychologic support, and the empathy of health care workers. In many communities with a high prevalence of AIDS patients, there are active peer support groups that may be extremely helpful. In addition, family physicians and referring specialists who have long-term care relationships with patients and their loved ones can provide valuable support to the critical care team.

ICU Eligibility of the AIDS Patient

The two fundamental issues determining ICU eligibility in patients with AIDS are the patient's prognosis and the patient's wishes regarding life support. Concerning prognosis, it is necessary to assess both the prognosis of the acute illness necessitating life support and the prognosis of the underlying HIV disease. Prior to the development of AIDS, the prognosis of HIV disease is generally dictated by the CD4 count. It must be recognized, however, that at any given CD4 count, the presence of the so-called minor opportunistic infections (particularly oral candida, hairy leukoplakia, and tuberculosis) worsens the prognosis significantly. Recently, a prognostic staging system has been suggested for patients who have AIDS.[79] The presence of each of the following abnormalities is scored one point: severe diarrhea or serum albumin $\leq$2.0 g/dL, any neurologic deficit, Pa_{O_2} $\leq$50 mmHg, hematocrit <30 percent, lymphocyte count <2500/mL, white blood cell count <2500 and platelets <140,000. Patients are divided into stages I to III according to their scores (0 points, 1 point, and 2 to 7 points, respectively). In the original study 1-year survivals were 50, 30 and 8 percent for stages I to III, respectively. Although this prognostic score has not been extensively validated, it suggests that the overall survival of AIDS patients decreases sharply with increasing organ system involvement, similar to patients with acute respiratory failure. This information can be extremely useful in assisting in the assessment of eligibility of AIDS patients for life support in the ICU.[80]

As in any other critical illness, it is of utmost importance to involve the patient or those close to the patient, whenever possible, in discussions regarding the appropriateness of ICU admission and life support. Often the issue of life support has been previously considered, and the patient has already made his or her wishes known to the primary physicians, friends, or relatives.[80,81] ICU admission and life support are generally inappropriate for patients with multiple life-threatening complications for which there is no particularly effective therapy (e.g., lymphoma). It is reasonable, however, to offer ICU admission and life support to patients with a reasonable quality of life who have a potentially reversible acute illness.[82] In every instance, clear goals of ICU admission should be established with the patient, family, and treating physicians. Obviously, a lucid, well-informed patient and the family may refuse life support. Finally, it must be emphasized that the outlook of AIDS and its related conditions is changing rapidly.[83] For this reason, rigid policies regarding ICU admission are undesirable,[81] and detailed evaluation of each situation on a case-by-case basis is required.

CASE PRESENTATION

A 29-year-old white, homosexual male was admitted through the emergency department because of fever, cough, and dyspnea. He had been known to be HIV positive for 3 years prior to admission; the date of his seroconversion was unknown. Five days prior to admission the patient developed cough, initially dry, subsequently productive of small amounts of white sputum accompanied by increasing dyspnea on exertion, malaise, fever (39.4°C), and chills. Review of systems was remarkable only for occasional red blood on stool secondary to an anal fissure.

Physical examination revealed a pleasant young male in minimal distress without evidence of malnutrition. Heart rate was 98/min, blood pressure 140/90 mmHg, respiratory rate 36/min, and temperature 38.9°C. There was erythema with white patches in the posterior oropharynx consistent with oral candidiasis. There were multiple mobile 1- to 2-cm lymph nodes in the supraclavicular fossae, axillary, and inguinal regions. Chest examination revealed inspiratory crackles in both bases. The rest of the examination was normal. Pertinent investigations included white cell count 11.4×10^9/L, with 63% neutrophils, 13% young PMNS, and 17% lymphocytes. An arterial blood gas on room air demonstrated pH 7.48, P_{CO_2} 36 mmHg, P_{O_2} 59 mmHg, bicarbonate 27 mmol/L. Chest x-ray showed bilateral interstitial infiltrates that were more pronounced in the lower lung zones. The serum LDH was elevated at 419 U/L (normal 60 to 200), serum glutamic-oxaloacetic transaminase 68 U/L (normal 0 to 40), while the bilirubin was normal. Serum quantitative immunoglobins showed increased IgA at 487 mg/dL (normal 70 to 310). The T cell helper-suppressor ratio was 0.13 (normal 0.95 to 3.4) and the absolute helper T cell was reduced at 70/mm^3 (normal 430 to 1360).

The patient was admitted to hospital and given 40% oxygen by face mask with achievement of acceptable arterial oxygen saturation. He underwent flexible fiberoptic bronchoscopy the following morning, which was tolerated well. Bronchoscopy BAL fluid revealed *P. carinii* organisms on toluidine blue stain. Ziel Nielsen stain and subsequent cultures for tuberculosis were negative. There were scant growths of *S. pneumoniae* and *H. influenzae,* and the patient was treated with intravenous pentamidine 260 mg over 2 h daily and oral ketoconazole for oral candidiasis. Despite these measures, the patient remained febrile and developed chills, diaphoresis, and increasing dyspnea. By the fourth hospital day, the chest x-ray showed increasing interstitial infiltrates with consolidation of the left lower lobe. Arterial blood gases on high-flow 100% oxygen by face mask showed a pH of 7.45, P_{CO_2} 35 mmHg, P_{O_2} 104 mmHg, bicarbonate 24 mmol/L, with an O_2 saturation of 97%. The patient was admitted to the ICU. Intravenous ampicillin 2 g intravenously every 4 h was initiated because of the previous positive sputum culture and left lower lobe consolidation on chest roentgenogram. Hydrocortisone 250 mg intravenously every 6 h was added.

The following day the patient was afebrile, the respiratory rate had fallen to 25 from 40/min, and there was less respiratory distress, so he was transferred back to the medical ward. However, 48 h later, the patient again became increasingly dyspneic. Arterial blood gases breathing 40% oxygen by mask showed pH of 7.54, P_{CO_2} 34 mmHg, P_{O_2} 41 mmHg, bicarbonate 30 mmol/L, and arterial O_2 saturation of 84%. The patient was readmitted to the ICU and oxygen was increased to 100% by face mask, which initially achieved acceptable arterial oxygenation. However, oxygenation continued to deteriorate rapidly and the respiratory rate rose to 48/min, necessitating urgent but elective endotracheal intubation and mechanical ventilation with 10 cmH_2O positive end-expiratory pressure. Arterial blood gases on 50% oxygen showed pH 7.48, P_{CO_2} 41 mmHg, P_{O_2} 69 mmHg, bicarbonate 30 mmol/L, and O_2 saturation of 95%. A nasogastric feeding tube was inserted and continuous enteral feeding was started. Twelve hours after intubation, the patient was changed to CPAP at 10 cmH_2O without ventilatory assist and tolerated this well, maintaining acceptable arterial blood gases. He remained afebrile. Over the next 3 days, the chest x-ray gradually improved, CPAP was gradually reduced to 5 cmH_2O, and the patient was successfully extubated. He was transferred back to the medical ward on hydrocortisone, pentamidine, ampicillin, oral ketoconazole, and 40% oxygen. Hydrocortisone was tapered to 400 mg daily.

Two days later, the patient had a syncopal episode and shortly thereafter was found to have a pulse of 72/min, blood pressure 140/90 mmHg, and a low potassium level at 2.8 mmol/L. An ECG showed ventricular premature beats and marked QT prolongation. This lead to admission to the coronary care unit for continuous ECG monitoring, and while there he was started on lidocaine 2 mg/min for frequent PVCs. The patient had several episodes of polymorphic ventricular tachycardia over the next 48 h as well as sinus bradycardia to 35/min, which was treated with continuous isoproterenol infusion. Lidocaine was discontinued and magnesium sulfate was infused intravenously. Pentamidine was discontinued and intravenous TMP-SMX was substituted. Subsequently, isoproterenol was discontinued, sinus rhythm at 70 to 80/min was maintained, and there were no further episodes of ventricular tachycardia or syncope. The patient continued to improve and was discharged home.

Following discharge from hospital the patient was followed and subsequently treated with AZT and then ddI in addition to aerosol pentamidine for secondary PCP prophylaxis. He has had subsequent problems including CMV retinitis eventually resulting in blindness despite treatment with ganciclovir; *Staphylococcus epidermidis* bacteremia secondary to permanent Hickman catheter, treated with removal of the intravenous access and systemic antibiotics; drug-induced neutropenia treated with granulocyte-macrophage colony-stimulating factor (GM-CSF); and vitritis treated with posterior subtenons injection of steroid. Four years after his ICU admission for PCP he remains alive with a quality of life he considers acceptable.

CASE DISCUSSION

This patient's presentation was typical for PCP with cough, fever, and progressive dyspnea accompanied by signs of some respiratory distress but with only a few crackles at the bases. His chest x-ray showed typical bilateral symmetric interstitial infiltrates with normal pleura and normal heart size. Advanced immunodeficiency was confirmed by the markedly decreased helper cell count. In this case, pentamidine was initiated only after the diagnosis of PCP was confirmed. However, today most clinicians, including ourselves, would initiate therapy on admission in a case with such a typical presentation, performing bronchoscopy to confirm the diagnosis within 24 to 48 h. The case further illustrates the excellent diagnostic yield of BAL for PCP.

Initial management included oxygen and pentamidine on the medical ward. Typically patients often deteriorate in the first few days after admission, as in this case, and develop worsening respiratory symptoms, hypoxemia, and pulmonary infiltrates. At the time this patient was seen in 1986, the role of corticosteroids in PCP was uncertain so corticosteroids were instituted as a salvage therapy, only after the patient developed acute respiratory failure. In 1990, the role of corticosteroids is well established for treatment of moderate and severe PCP, and in cases like this they would be initiated immediately after admission to reduce the risk of early deterioration and acute respiratory failure.

The patient required intubation and mechanical ventilation for acute hypoxemic respiratory failure but very quickly could be managed with CPAP alone. An alternative management strategy would be initiation of mask CPAP up to 10 cmH_2O. Should this approach fail to achieve acceptable arterial oxygenation and patient comfort, endotracheal intubation and mechanical ventilation could then be used.

After discharge to the medical ward, the patient developed syncope, which was found to be caused by ventricular tachycardia with a *torsade de pointes* pattern. This was treated with intravenous magnesium sulfate, intravenous isoproterenol, and discontinuation of pentamidine. Recognition of this unusual complication of pentamidine illustrates the importance of maintaining a broad perspective regarding clinical aspects of therapy in patients with AIDS.

The patient required only 4 days of CPAP, a course typical for patients who are going to survive mechanical ventilation for PCP and acute respiratory failure. His young age, good nutritional status, and the use of corticosteroids also contributed to his favorable outcome. Long-term follow-up reveals that the patient remains alive approximately 4 years after the initial episode of acute respiratory failure secondary to PCP. Although he has also suffered numerous subsequent important complications of HIV disease including KS, CMV retinitis leading to blindness, bone marrow depression, and bacterial sepsis, most of these have been managed as an outpatient, and he remains grateful for the institution of mechanical ventilation and intensive care for the treatment of his life-threatening acute respiratory failure.

References

1. Barre-Sinoussi F, Chermann JC, Rey F, et al: Isolation of a new T lymphotropic retrovirus from a patient at risk for acquired immune deficiency syndrome (AIDS). Science 110:868, 1983.
2. Gallo RC, Salahuddin SZ, Popovic M, et al: Frequent detection and isolation of cytopathic retroviruses (HTLV-III) from patients with AIDS and at risk for AIDS. Science 224:500, 1984.
3. Montagnier L, Gruest J, Chamaret S, et al: Adaptation of lymphadenopathy associated virus (LAV) to replication in EBV-transformed B lymphoblastoid cell lines. Science 225:63, 1984.
4. Gartner S, Markovits P, Markovitz DM, Kaplan MH, Gallo RC, Popovic M: The role of mononuclear phagocytes in HTLV-III/LAV infection. Science 233:215, 1986.
5. Johnson AM, Laga M: Heterosexual transmission of HIV. AIDS 2(1):S49, 1988.
6. Des Jarlais DC, Friedman SR. HIV and intravenous drug use. AIDS 2(1):S65, 1988.
7. Anderson RM, Medley GF. Epidemiology of HIV infection and AIDS: Incubation and infection periods, survival and vertical transmission. AIDS 2(1):S57, 1988.
8. CDC: Guidelines for prevention of transmission of human immunodeficiency virus and hepatitis B virus to health-care and public-safety workers. MMWR 38:1, 1989.
9. Kelen GD, Fritz S, Qaqish B, et al: Unrecognized human immunodeficiency virus infection in emergency department patients. N Engl J Med 318:1645, 1988.
10. Folks TM, Kessler SW, Orenstein JM, Justement JS, Jaffe ES, Fauci AS: Infection and replication of HIV-1 in purified progenitor cells of normal human bone marrow. Science 242:919, 1988.
11. Levy JA: The human immunodeficiency virus and its pathogenesis. Infectious Dis Clin of N Am 2:285, 1988.
12. Schechter MT, Craib KJP, Le TN, et al: Progression to AIDS and predictors of AIDS in seroprevalent and seroincident cohorts of homosexual men. AIDS 3:347, 1989.
13. Moss AR: Predicting who will progress to AIDS. BMJ 297:1067, 1988.
14. Fischl MD, Richman DD, Grieco MH, et al: The efficacy of azidothymidine (AZT) in the treatment of patients with AIDS and AIDS-related complex: A double-blind, placebo-controlled trial. N Engl J Med 317:185, 1987.
15. Volberding PA, Lagakos SW, Koch MA, et al: Zidovudine in asymptomatic human immunodeficiency virus infection: A controlled trial in persons with fewer than 500 CD4-positive cells per cubic millimeter. N Engl J Med 322:941, 1990.
16. Ruedy J, Schechter MT, Montaner JSG; Zidovudine for early human immunodeficiency virus (HIV) infection: Who, when, and how? Ann Int Med 112:721, 1990.
17. Gelmon K, Fanning M, Falutz J, Montaner JSG, Tsoukas C, O'Shaughnessy M, Wainberg M, Ruedy J: Nature, time course and dose dependence of zidovudine related side effects. Results from the Multicentre Canadian Aziothymidine Trial. AIDS 3(9):555, 1989.
18. Wainberg M, Falutz J, Fanning M, et al: Cessation of zidovudine therapy may lead to increased replication of HIV-1. JAMA (261)6:869, 1989.
19. Lambert JS, Seidlin M, Reichman RC, et al: 2',3'-Dideoxyinosine (ddI) in patients with the acquired immunodeficiency syndrome or AIDS-related complex. N Engl J Med 322(19):1333, 1990.
20. Cooley TP, Kunches LM, Saunders CA, et al: Once-daily administration of 2', 3'-Dideoxyinosine (ddI) in patients with the acquired immunodeficiency syndrome or AIDS-related complex. N Engl J Med 322(19):1340, 1990.
21. Fauci AS: ddI—a good start, but still phase I. N Engl J Med 322:1386, 1990.
22. Yarchoan R, Pluda JM, Thomas RV, et al: Long-term toxicity/activity profile of 2',3'-dideoxyinosine in AIDS or AIDS-related complex. Lancet 336:526, 1990.
23. Flora GS, Modilevksy T, Antoniskis D, Barnes PF: Undiagnosed tuberculosis in patients with human immunodeficiency virus infection. Chest 98:1056, 1990.
24. CDC. Guidelines for prophylaxis against *Pneumocystis carinii* pneumonia for persons infected with human immunodeficiency virus MMWR 38(5S):1, 1989.
25. Montaner JSG, Lawson LM, Levitt N, Belzberg A, Schechter MT, Ruedy J: Corticosteroids prevent early deterioration in patients with moderately severe AIDS-related *Pneumocystis carinii* pneumonia and the acquired immunodeficiency syndrome (AIDS). Ann Int Med 113(1):15, 1990.
26. Golden JA, Sollitto RA: The radiology of pulmonary disease. Clin Chest Med 9:481, 1988.
27. Abd AG, Neirman DM, Ilowite JS, Pierson RN, Loomis Bell AL, Jr: Bilateral upper lobe *Pneumocystis carinii* pneumonia in a patient receiving inhaled pentamidine prophylaxis. Chest 94(2):329, 1988.
28. Clement MJ, Luce JM, Hopewell PC: Diagnosis of pulmonary diseases. Clin Chest Med 9:497, 1988.
29. Levine SJ, White DA: *Pneumocystis carinii.* Clin Chest Med 9(3):395, 1988.
30. Murray JF, Felton CP, Garay SM, et al: Pulmonary complications of the acquired immunodeficiency syndrome: Report of a National Heart, Lung and Blood Institute Workshop. N Engl J Med 310:1682, 1984.
31. Murray JF, Garay SM, Hopewell PC, Mills J, Snider GL, Stover DE: Pulmonary complications of the acquired immuno-

deficiency syndrome: An update. Am Rev Respir Dis 35:504, 1987.
32. Montaner JSG, Russell JR, Lawson LM, and Ruedy J: Acute respiratory failure secondary to *Pneumocystis carinii* pneumonia in the acquired immunodeficiency syndrome: A potential role for systemic corticosteroids. Chest 95(4):881, 1989.
33. El-Sadr W, Simberkoff MS: Survival and prognostic factors in severe *Pneumocystis carinii* pneumonia requiring mechanical ventilation. Am Rev Respir Dis 137:1264, 1988.
34. Young KR, Rankin JA, Naegel GP, Reynolds HY: Bronchoalveolar lavage cells and proteins in patients with acquired immunodeficiency syndrome. Ann Intern Med 103:522, 1985.
35. White DA, Gellene RA, Gupta S, Cunningham-Rundles C, Stover DE: Pulmonary cell populations in immunosuppressed patients. Chest 88:352, 1985.
36. Telzak EE, Cote RJ, Gold JWM, Campbell SW, Armstrong D: Extrapulmonary *Pneumocystis carinii* infections. Rev Infect Dis 12(3):380 1990.
37. Wofsy CB: *Pneumocystis carinii* pneumonia, in Leong G, Mills J (eds): *Opportunistic Infections in Patients with the Acquired Immunodeficiency Syndrome.* New York, Marcel Dekker, 1989, pp 317–340.
38. Wharton BM, Coleman DL, Wofsy CB, Luce JM, Blumenfeld W, Hadley WK, Ingram-Drake L, Volberding PA: Prospective randomized trial of trimethoprim-sulfamethoxazole versus pentamidine for *Pneumocystis carinii* pneumonia in the acquired immunodeficiency syndrome. Ann Intern Med 105:37, 1986.
39. Gordin FM, Simon GL, Wofsy CB, Mills J: Adverse reactions to trimethoprim-sulfamethoxazole in patients with acquired immunodeficiency syndrome. Ann Intern Med 100:495, 1984,
40. Leoung GS, Feigal DW, Montgomery AB, et al: Aerosolized pentamidine for prophylaxis against *Pneumocystis carinii* pneumonia: The San Francisco Community Prophylaxis Trial. N Engl J Med 323:769, 1990.
41. Montaner JSG, Lawson LM, Gervais A, et al: Aerosol pentamidine for the secondary prophylaxis of AIDS-related *Pneumocystis carinii* pneumonia: A placebo-controlled study. Ann Intern Med 114:948, 1991.
42. Armstrong G, Bernard E: Aerosol pentamidine. Ann Intern Med 109:852, 1988.
43. Medina I, Mills J, Leoung G et al: Oral therapy for *Pneumocystis carinii* pneumonia in the acquired immunodeficiency syndrome. A controlled trial of trimethoprim-sulfamethoxazole versus trimethoprim-dapsone. N Engl J Med 323(12):776, 1990.
44. Allegra CJ, Chabner BA, Tauzon CV, et al: Trimetrexate for the treatment of *Pneumocystis carinii* pneumonia in patients with the acquired immunodeficiency syndrome. N Engl J Med 317:978, 1987.
45. Toma E, Fournier S, Poisson N, et al: Clyndamycin with primaquine for *Pneumocystis carinii* pneumonia. Lancet I:1046, 1989.
46. Hughes WT, Gray V, Gutteridge WC, Latter VS, Podney M. A hydroxynapthoquinone, 566́ C80 is effective in experimental *Pneumocystis carinii* pneumonitis. Antimicrob Agents Chemother 34:225, 1990.
47. Gagnon S, Boota AM, Fischl MA, Baier H, Kirksey OW, La Voie L: Corticosteroids as adjunctive therapy for severe *Pneumocystis carinii* pneumonia in the acquired immunodeficiency syndrome: A double-blind placebo-controlled study. N Engl J Med 323:1444, 1990.
48. Bozette SA, Sattler FR, Chiu J, et al: A controlled trial of early adjunctive treatment with corticosteroids for *Pneumocystis carinii* pneumonia in the acquired immunodeficiency syndrome. N Engl J Med 323:1451, 1990.
49. Consensus statement on the use of corticosteroids as adjunctive therapy for pneumocystis pneumonia in the acquired immunodeficiency syndrome. N Engl J Med 323:1500, 1990.
50. Collier AC, Bozzette S, Coombs R, et al: A pilot study of low dose zidovudine in human immunodeficiency virus infection. N Engl J Med 323:1015, 1990.
51. Wachter MW, Luce JM, Turner J, et al: Intensive care of patients with the acquired immunodeficiency syndrome. Outcome and changing patterns of utilization. Am Rev Respir Dis 134:891, 1986.
52. Steinbrook R, Lo B, Moulton J, et al: Preferences of homosexual men with AIDS for life-sustaining treatment. N Engl J Med 314:457, 1986.
53. Quieffen J, Ronco JJ, Russell JA, Lawson LM, Schechter MT, Ruedy J, Montaner JSG: Worsening survival of mechanically ventilated acute respiratory failure secondary to AIDS-related PCP. Clin Invest Med B21:123, 1990.
54. Pitchenick AE, Fertel D, Bloch AB: Mycobacterial disease: Epidemiology, diagnosis, treatment and prevention. Clin Chest Med 9:524, 1988.
55. Chiu J, Nussbaum J, Bozzette S, et al: Treatment of disseminated Mycobacterium avium complex infection in AIDS with Amikacin, Ethambutol, Rifampin, and Ciprofloxacin. Ann Intern Med 133:358, 1990.
56. Jacobson MA, Mills J: Cytomegalovirus infection. Clin Chest Med 9:443,1988.
57. Fels AOS: Bacterial and fungal pneumonias. Clin Chest Med 9:449, 1988.
58. Ognibene FP, Shelhamer JH: Kaposi's sarcoma. Clin Chest Med 9:459, 1988.
59. McArthur JC: Neurologic manifestations of AIDS. Medicine (Baltimore) 66:407, 1987.
60. Price RW, Brew B: Management of neurologic complications of HIV-1 infection and AIDS, in Sande MA, Volberding PA (eds): *The Medical Management of AIDS.* Philadelphia, W. B. Saunders, 1990, pp 161–181.
61. Yarchoan R, Thomas R, Grafman J, Wichman A, Dalakas M, McAtee N, Berg G, Fischl M, Perno CF, Klecker RW, Buchbindinder A, Tay S, Larsen S, Myers CE, Broder S: Long-term administration of 3′-azido-2′,3′-dideoxythymidine to patients with AIDS-related neurologic disease. Ann Neurol 23 (suppl):582, 1988.
62. Israelski DM, Dannemann BR, Remington JS: Toxoplasmosis in patients with AIDS, in Sande MA, Volberding PA (eds): *The Medical Management of AIDS.* Philadelphia, W. B. Saunders, 1989, pp 241–264.
63. CDC. 1989 sexually transmitted diseases treatment guidelines. MMWR 38:5, 1989.
64. Zenker PN, Rolfs TR: Treatment of syphilis, 1989. Rev Infect Dis 12:S590, 1990.
65. Miller RG, Storey JR, Greco CM: Ganciclovir in the treatment of progressive AIDS-related polyradiculopathy. Neurology 40:596, 1990.
66. Till M, MacDonell KB: Myopathy with human immunodeficiency virus type 1 (HIV-1) Infection: HIV-1 or zidovudine. Ann Int Med 113:492, 1990.
67. Chuck SL, Sande MA: Infections with *Cryptococcus neoformans* in acquired immunodeficiency syndrome. N Engl J Med 321:794, 1989.
68. Larsen RA, Leal MAE, Chan LS: Fluconazole compared with amphotericin B plus flucytosine for cryptococcal meningitis in AIDS: A randomized trial. Ann Int Med 113:183, 1990.
69. Dismukes W, Cloud G, Thompson S, et al: Fluconazole vs. amphotericin B therapy of acute cryptococcal meningitis. Abstract 1065, 29th Interscience Conference on Antimicrobial Agents and Chemotherapy, Houston, 1989.

70. Powderly W, Saag M, Cloud G, Dismukes W, Meyer R, Robinson P: Fluconazole vs. amphotericin B as maintenance therapy for prevention of relapse of AIDS-associated cryptococcal meningitis. Abstract 1162, Interscience Conference on Antimicrobial Agents and Chemotherapy, Atlanta, October 1990.
71. Graybill JR: Histoplasmosis in AIDS. J Infect Dis 158:623, 1988.
72. Galgiani JN, Ampel NM: Coccidioidomycosis in human immunodeficiency virus-infected patients. J Infect Dis 162:1165, 1990.
73. Gregg RW, Friedman BC, Williams JF, McGrath BJ, Zimmerman JE: Continuous positive airway pressure by face mask in *Pneumocystis carinii* pneumonia. Crit Care Med 18:21, 1990.
74. Craddock C, Pasvol G, Bull R, Protheroe A, Hopkin J: Cardiorespiratory arrest and autonomic neuropathy in AIDS. Lancet 2:16, 1987.
75. Ronco JJ, Montaner JSG, Fenwick JC, Ruedy J, Russell JA: Pathologic dependence of oxygen consumption on oxygen delivery in acute respiratory failure secondary to AIDS-related *Pneumocystis carinii* pneumonia. Chest 98:1463, 1990.
76. Smith PD, Lane HC, Gill VJ, et al: Intestinal infections in patients with the acquired immunodeficiency syndrome: Etiology and response to therapy. Ann Intern Med 108:328, 1988.
77. Kotler DP, Gaetz HP, Lange M, Klein EB, Holt PR: Enteropathy associated with the acquired immunodeficiency syndrome. Ann Intern Med 101:421, 1984.
78. Johanson JR, Sonnenberg A: Efficient management of diarrhea in the acquired immunodeficiency syndrome (AIDS). Ann Int Med 112:942, 1990.
79. Justice AC, Feinstein AR, Wells CK: A new prognostic staging system for the acquired immunodeficiency syndrome. N Engl J Med 320(21):1388, 1989.
80. Wachter RM, Luce JM, Lo B, Raffin TA: Ethics in cardiopulmonary medicine: Life-sustaining treatment for patients with AIDS. Chest 95:647, 1989.
81. Smedira NG, Evans BH, Grais LS, Cohen NH, Lo B, Cooke M, Schecter WP, Find C, Epstein-Jaffe E, May C, Luce JM: Withholding and withdrawal of life support from the critically ill. N Engl J Med 322:309, 1990.
82. Bone RC, Rackow EC, Weg JG, members of the ACCP/SCCM Consensus Panel: Ethical and moral guidelines for the initiation, continuation, and withdrawal of intensive care. Chest 97:949, 1990.
83. Luce JM, Wachter RM, Hopewell PC: Editorial: Intensive care of patients with the acquired immunodeficiency syndrome: Time for a reassessment? Am Rev Respir Dis 137:1261, 1988.

Acknowledgment

This work was supported in part by the National Health and Research Development Programme, Health and Welfare, Ottawa, Canada.

Chapter 101

ENDOCARDITIS AND OTHER INTRAVASCULAR INFECTIONS IN THE CRITICALLY ILL

C. GLENN COBBS
MARK B. CARR

KEY POINTS

- *The possibility of intravascular infection should be considered in all critically ill patients with:*
  - *bacteremia or fungemia of uncertain origin, particularly when there are known intravascular or endocardial abnormalities or intravascular devices*
  - *fever or hemodynamic instability of unclear origin*
  - *signs of inflammation related to an indwelling intravascular device*
- *Blood cultures are the most important diagnostic test for this group of infections, because most intravascular infections will result in persistent bacteremia or fungemia.*
- *Successful therapy often requires prolonged administration of microbicidal agents plus removal of devices.*
- *Certain microbes including staphylococci, enterococci, aerobic gram-negative bacilli, and yeasts are especially likely to cause intravascular infectious disease.*

Patients hospitalized in ICUs may have an intravascular infectious disorder as their primary problem, as a complication of their main disorder, or as a nosocomial infection occurring during their stay. Violation of anatomic barriers by indwelling intravascular devices and by surgery, as well as impairment of cellular or humoral immune function related to critical illness, contribute to invasion by a variety of microbial pathogens. Infections of intravascular foreign bodies or native vascular structures themselves are likely to be associated not only with symptoms and signs of local inflammation but also evidence of disseminated disease due to metastatic spread of infectious agents. The purpose of this chapter is to provide the clinician caring for patients in an ICU with an approach to the patient with suspected or proven intravascular infectious disorders. We will emphasize the underlying clinical situations that predispose to intravascular infection, the pathogenesis of the disorders, the symptoms and signs of disease, and the appropriate diagnostic procedures, particularly those that provide assistance in choice of antimicrobial therapy and selection of ancillary medical and surgical procedures. Tables 101-1 and 101-2 list the intravascular infections of native vessels and those associated with intravascular devices, respectively.

Intravascular Infections in the Absence of Any Foreign Device

INFECTIVE ENDOCARDITIS ON A NATIVE VALVE

PATHOGENESIS. The pathogenesis of infective endocarditis (IE) usually involves transient bloodstream invasion by microorganisms followed by adherence of the organism to the endocardial surface and multiplication of the microorganism within a layer of platelets and fibrin, which is relatively inaccessible to host phagocytic defenses. The likeli-

TABLE 101-1 Intravascular Infection in Native Vessels

Site	Infectious Disorder	Comment
Medium and large arteries	Mycotic aneurysm	Abdominal aortic aneurysms Various sites complicating endocarditis
Intracranial cavernous sinus	Cavernous sinus thrombosis	Follows facial cellulitis *Staphylococcus aureus* common etiology
Heart	Native valve endocarditis	Usually occurs at site of prior endocardial damage
Head and neck venous structures	Postanginal sepsis	Fusobacterium, Bacteroides common. Metastatic disease frequent.
Pelvic veins	Pelvic vein thrombophlebitis	Following septic abortion, pelvic inflammatory disease in women.
Portal veins	Pylephlebitis	Complication of intra-abdominal abscess; perforated appendix, peridiverticular abscess, etc.

TABLE 101-2 Infections of Intravascular Devices

Location	Device	Comment	Percent Infected
Heart	Prosthetic valve Patch	Risk of infection on mitral valve equals aortic valve	2% NR
Great veins and heart	Pacemaker (permanent)	Transvenous and epicardial employed	Transvenous—2% Sutureless epicardial—4% Sutured epicardial—5%
	Pulmonary arterial catheter	Swan-Ganz; plastic, triple-lumen catheter	Colonization of tip—8% Bacteremia—2%
Great veins alone	Broviac catheter	Cuffed, tunneled silicone elastomer catheter	6%[a]
	Hickman catheter	Cuffed, tunneled silicone elastomer catheter	12%[a]
	Mediport	Subcutaneous device	NR
	Subclavian and internal jugular	Plastic, single- vs triple-lumen	11.6% (single) 35.7% (triple)
	Hemodialysis catheter	Plastic double-lumen catheter, subclavian vein	10%
Peripheral veins	Plastic IV line	e.g., Jelco, Angiocath	Phlebitis—25% Bacteremia—5%
	Steel needles	Phlebitis more common than bacteremia; rarely last longer than 48 h	Phlebitis—5–20%[a]
	Scalp vein needle		Phlebitis—4% Bacteremia—0%
Aorta and peripheral arteries	Arterial line pressure monitoring device	Bacteremia may reflect contamination by monitoring device	NR
	Vascular grafts	Increase in infection if graft crosses groin	2%

[a]Included all forms of infection

hood that a patient with or without underlying valvular heart disease may develop IE depends on the species and concentration of microorganisms in the blood, the presence or absence of antimicrobial agents in serum at the time of bacteremia/fungemia, and the characteristics of the endocardium. Clearly, some microorganisms are much more likely to adhere to endocardium than others. *Staphylococcus aureus*, enterococci, and other streptococci are most adherent. Enteric gram-negative bacilli and anaerobic microorganisms are less so. Since *S. aureus* is also commonly found on the skin and is frequently involved in minor infections of the skin, which can result in transient bacteremia, this organism is a common cause of acute bacterial endocarditis, particularly in patients without significant underlying valvular heart disease. Viridans-type streptococci, which constitute normal flora of the upper airway, may gain access to the bloodstream from trauma to the teeth or gingiva (as in dental work) and constitute a common cause of infection presenting subacutely, nearly always in a patient with a significant predisposing valvular abnormality. Admittedly, many of the distinctions between acute and subacute endocarditis are blurred in the modern era. Enteric gram-negative organisms, being much less adherent to endocardium, cause many fewer cases of endocarditis relative to the frequency of bacteremia caused by these organisms. However, gram-negative organisms which have a greater propensity to adhere to surfaces, such as *Pseudomonas aeruginosa,* and which can gain access to the circulation via contaminated intravenous injections (as in drug abusers) or infection at other body sites produce a significant proportion of cases. The most common nosocomial pathogenesis of IE in critically ill patients involves cellulitis at peripheral vascular access sites with resultant transient bacteremia/fungemia and localization of microorganisms on a previously damaged heart valve.

CLINICAL AND LABORATORY FEATURES. Table 101-3 lists the most common signs and symptoms encountered in patients with native valve IE. Table 101-4 lists the most common laboratory abnormalities encountered. Because most reports stress community-acquired disease, patients developing IE while hospitalized in an ICU may not manifest identical findings. Nevertheless, fever and a heart murmur are the most common findings in IE, with both being found in at least 80 percent of cases.

A number of peripheral manifestations may be present in patients with IE. A variety of skin lesions occur, petechiae being most common. These are 1- to 2-mm red, nonblanching macules which turn brown and fade within 2 to 3 days. They are especially prominent over the upper trunk, extremities, conjunctiva, and soft palate. Vascular hemorrhages in the optic fundus are called Roth spots. Splinter

TABLE 101-3 Frequency of Symptoms and Signs at Presentation of Infective Endocarditis

Symptoms	Frequency (%)	Signs	Frequency (%)
Fever	85	Fever	95
Malaise	25	Murmur	85
Myalgias/arthralgias	25	Petechiae	35
Headache	20	Osler's nodes	10
Back pain	25	Hemiparesis	10
Delirium	10	Coma	5

hemorrhages are vascular hemorrhages occurring under the nails but are often difficult to distinguish from traumatic lesions. Osler's nodes are erythematous, tender, subcutaneous papules that occur on the finger pads (Plate 31). They are 2 to 5 mm in diameter and may be multiple. Janeway lesions are painless, erythematous macules, larger than Osler's nodes, which occur on the palms and soles (Plate 32).

Systemic emboli occur in approximately 40 percent of patients with left-sided valvular infection. In the central nervous system (CNS), embolic occlusion of peripheral arteries results in the stroke syndrome. Emboli to the spleen and kidney often cause abdominal pain. Emboli to mesenteric arteries may cause ischemic bowel disease or frank infarction of small bowel. Emboli to muscles are common but usually clinically inapparent.

Patients with IE may also present with heart failure due to valve malfunction, embolic myocardial infarction, myocarditis, or systemic toxicity due to "sepsis." Renal failure is also a prominent sequela of untreated IE, whether occurring on a native or prosthetic valve.

Disorders of the CNS are prominent in patients with IE. As many as 50 percent of patients with IE will have some neurologic abnormality. Mental status changes such as confusion, delirium and psychosis are most common. Focal neurologic symptoms and signs may be caused by an embolic stroke, a bleeding mycotic aneurysm, meningitis, or cerebral artery vasculitis. Overall, approximately 30 percent of patients with IE will have evidence of a focal neurologic event during their illness.

Anemia is common in patients with IE. Leukocytosis occurs in about 40 percent of patients. Changes in the renal sediment, particularly proteinuria and microscopic hematuria, are usually present in patients with endocarditis. In long-standing disease rheumatoid factor is present in about one-half of patients.

TABLE 101-4 Frequency of Various Laboratory Abnormalities in Infective Endocarditis

Laboratory Finding	Frequency (%)
Anemia	80
Thrombocytopenia	20
Leukocytosis	30
Increased erythrocyte sedimentation rate	95
Hypergammaglobulinemia	25
Hematuria	40
Proteinuria	60

DIAGNOSIS. Blood cultures are the most important laboratory tests in the diagnosis of IE. The vast majority of blood cultures obtained when a patient is not receiving antimicrobial therapy will be positive. In approximately 5 to 10 percent of patients with presumed IE, no etiologic organism is initially isolated. The causes of culture-negative endocarditis are prior antibiotics and endocarditis due to fastidious organisms, including anaerobes, nutritionally deficient streptococci, *Coxiella burnetti, Legionella pneumophila, Chlamydia psittaci,* members of the HACEK group, and various fungi. HACEK is an acronym for a group of small, fastidious, gram-negative bacilli, which includes *Haemophilus* species, *Actinobacillus actinomycetemcomitans, Cardiobacterium hominis, Eikenella corrodens* and *Kingella kingae.* Longer incubation of cultures, special culture techniques to aid in isolation of fastidious microorganisms and the use of serologic studies for coxiella, chlamydia, and histoplasma may aid in diagnosis.

Echocardiography is useful in identifying vegetations or local complications of IE but cannot be used to exclude the diagnosis. Transthoracic echocardiography has a 60 to 80 percent sensitivity in detecting vegetations in IE. Transesophageal echocardiography is useful when image quality with standard echocardiography is inadequate.

MANAGEMENT. Patients encountered in the ICU with fever, cardiac murmurs, or other findings suggesting the possibility of IE should always be evaluated for the possibility of valve infection; this generally involves multiple blood cultures and echocardiography. While this evaluation proceeds, two central questions arise: which clinical situations warrant empirical antimicrobial therapy and which do not, and what empirical therapy should be selected. In general, physicians managing patients with *possible* IE should initiate therapy when one of the following situations is present: **1.** the patient is critically ill; **2.** antimicrobial therapy will be necessary for some other infectious disorder; **3.** early valve replacement is contemplated because of valve malfunction; **4.** IE is clinically suspected and one or more blood cultures are positive for an etiologic microorganism that can cause IE.

In patients with undiagnosed fever or other findings which make IE a diagnostic consideration but without any of these indications for immediate therapy, it is reasonable to withhold antimicrobials until blood cultures and the results of other investigations provide support for the diagnosis.

Empirical therapy in this critically ill patient group requiring immediate treatment should be selected to cover *S. aureus,* streptococci including enterococcus, and, particularly in patients at special risk for these organisms, enteric gram-negative bacilli. Intravenous nafcillin, 2 g every q4 h with 2 g ampicillin intravenously every 4 h and gentamicin, 1.5 mg/kg intravenously every 8 h (with appropriate adjustment for abnormal renal function) is a reasonable empirical regimen in most cases, pending the results of blood cultures.

In patients with an established diagnosis of IE, management entails a careful choice of antimicrobial therapy based on identification and characterization of the etiologic microorganism and ongoing consideration of surgical measures which may be necessary for cure. Table 101-5 lists the most common etiologic microorganisms causing IE and the frequency of valvular involvement in native valve IE. Staphylococci, various streptococci, "diphtheroids," gram-negative aerobic bacilli, and yeasts are the most common microorganisms responsible for nosocomial IE. Table 101-6 describes the recommended antimicrobial regimens for treatment of IE. Certain principles are followed when treating patients with IE. Parenteral antibiotics are preferred over oral agents because of more sustained antibacterial activity associated with intravenous antibiotics and erratic absorption associated with many oral drugs. Bacteriocidal agents are superior to bacteriostatic drugs. Long-term antimicrobial therapy is almost always required to cure the infection. Finally, in vitro testing of the microorganism's susceptibility to the antimicrobial agents chosen may be useful in predicting clinical outcome. Minimal inhibitory concentrations (MICs) and minimal bacteriocidal concentrations (MBCs) of antimicrobial agents used to inhibit and kill the microorganism, respectively, are useful in choosing treatment regimens. The serum bacteriocidal test (Schlicter test) is a measurement of antibacterial activity of the patient's serum, at peak and trough antimicrobial concentrations, against the patient's microorganisms. This test remains somewhat controversial primarily because of lack of standardization; however, many feel that a peak serum inhibitory concentration (SIC) of 1:8 is associated with successful treatment of IE at least 80 percent of the time.

TABLE 101-5 Etiology and Valve Involvement in Native Valve Endocarditis

Microorganism	Percentage
Streptococci	55%
Enterococci	7%
Staphylococcus aureus	25%
Staphylococcus epidermidis	6%
Gram-negative bacilli	6%
Fungi	1%
Culture negative	7%
DISTRIBUTION OF VALVULAR LESIONS	
Aortic	35–50%
Mitral	50%
Tricuspid	10%
Pulmonic	1%

Valve replacement may be lifesaving in patients with IE. Indications for urgent valve replacement include severe heart failure, valvular obstruction, fungal endocarditis, ineffective antimicrobial therapy, and the presence of an unstable prosthetic device.[1] A point system to aid in evaluation of the need for surgical intervention in IE has been described.[2] The various complications that develop during IE are assigned a weighted point value according to their importance as indicators for valve replacement. A total of 5 or more points indicates the need for urgent surgery. Table 101-7 lists the conditions associated with need for valve replacement and their relative point rating. Severe heart failure is considered heart failure that does not respond to maximal medical therapy (see Chap. 122). Moderate heart failure is failure that is still present after routine but not maximal medical therapy.

PROGNOSIS. The outcome of treatment for IE is heavily influenced by the relative pathogenicity of the infecting organism, the location of the infected valve, and the presence of complications of the infection. *S. aureus* typically produces a severe and destructive endocarditis that is fatal in about 50 percent of cases when the infection occurs on the aortic or mitral valve. However, if the infection is of the tricuspid valve, as typically occurs in intravenous drug users, the prognosis is substantially better. Gram-negative IE, particularly due to *P. aeruginosa,* also carries a relatively poor prognosis largely related to the limited activity of available antimicrobials against this organism. In the absence of major complications, lower grade infections such as *Streptococcus viridans* infection tend to do well with medical therapy alone, although some patients will require surgical intervention. Complications associated with worse prognosis include severe cardiac failure or shock, major arterial emboli, myocardial abscess formation, and associated major organ system failure.

ANTIMICROBIAL PROPHYLAXIS. Prevention of IE in susceptible individuals has been emphasized for many years because of the significant morbidity and mortality associated with the disease. Prophylactic antimicrobial therapy is based on the knowledge that bacteremia commonly occurs during certain medical procedures and that certain cardiac abnormalities place patients at an increased risk for the development of IE following bacteremia. The procedures most frequently associated with bacteremia include dental extraction, periodontal surgery, lower gastrointestinal procedures, and genitourinary procedures. Bronchoscopy, endoscopy and barium enemas are also associated with bacteremia but to a lesser degree. Most of the common procedures carried out in ICUs, including endotracheal intubation, urethral catheterization, and insertion of central vascular catheters percutaneously, pose little risk of bacteremia and do not require prophylaxis.

TABLE 101-6 Antimicrobial Therapy for Infective Endocarditis and Other Intravascular Infections[a]

Organism	Recommended Therapy	Penicillin Allergic
1. Penicillin sensitive streptococci ($MIC \leq 0.1$)	Penicillin G 10–20 million U IV qd for 4 weeks plus [c]Aminoglycoside for first 2 weeks: (Streptomycin 7.5 mg/kg (≤500 mg) IM q12h or gentamicin 1.0 mg/kg (≤80 mg) IM/IV q8h)	Cephalothin 2.0 g IV q4h for 4 weeks[b] plus Aminoglycoside for 4 weeks
2. Relatively "resistant" streptococci (Penicillin MIC 0.2–0.5)	Pen G 20 million U/d for 4 weeks plus Aminoglycoside[d] for 4 weeks	Cephalothin 2.0 g IV q4h for 4 weeks[b] plus Aminoglycoside for 4 weeks
3. Resistant streptococci ($MIC > 0.5$) (includes enterococci)	Penicillin G 20–30 million U IV qd for 6 weeks (Ampicillin 12 g IV qd is alternative) plus Aminoglycoside[d] for 6 weeks	Vancomycin 30 mg/kg (<2 g) q day for 6 weeks plus Aminoglycoside[d] for 6 weeks
4. Staphylococci (penicillin-sensitive)	Penicillin G 20 million U IV qd for 6 weeks	Cephalothin 2.0 g IV q4h for 6 weeks[b]
5. Staphylococci (methicillin-sensitive)—in absence of prosthetic valve	Nafcillin 1.5–2.0 g IV q4h for 4–6 weeks[e]	Cephalothin 2.0 g IV q4h for 4–6 weeks[b]
6. "Methicillin-resistant" staphylococci	Vancomycin 30 mg/kg IV (<2 g) per day +/− Rifampin 300 mg po q8h for 6 weeks	Same
7. Staphylococci (methicillin sensitive)—in presence of prosthetic valve	Nafcillin 2.0 g IV q4h for 6–8 weeks plus rifampin 300 mg[f] plus Aminoglycoside for 2 weeks	Cephalothin 2 g IV[b] q4h for 6–8 weeks plus rifampin[f] plus Aminoglycoside for 2 weeks
8. Staphylococci (methicillin resistant) in presence of prosthetic valve	Vancomycin 30 mg/kg/24h IV (<2 g) for 6–8 weeks, rifampin 300 mg for 6–8 weeks[f] plus Aminoglycoside for 2 weeks	
9. Corynebacterium	Penicillin G 20–30 million IV qd for 6 weeks plus Aminoglycoside for 6 weeks	Vancomycin 30 mg/kg (<2 g) qd IV for 6 weeks
10. Gram-negative bacilli		
a. Enterobacteriaceae	Therapy should be directed by in vitro susceptibilities.	Same
b. Pseudomonas	Therapy should be directed by in vitro susceptibilities though usual regimen includes tobramycin (8 mg/kg/day) plus extended spectrum penicillin.	Same though ceftazidime plus tobramycin (8 mg/kg/d) frequently used
c. HACEK group	Ampicillin 2.0 g IV q4h is commonly used though therapy should be directed by in vitro susceptibilities (aminoglycoside frequently used in combination).	Choice directed by in vitro susceptibilities
11. Rickettsia		
Coxiella burnetti	Tetracycline 500 mg po q6h for at least 1 year plus trimethoprim 480 mg plus sulfamethoxazole 2400 mg qd until there is no evidence clinically of disease or phase I antibody titer is <1:128.	Same
12. Fungal	Amphotericin B plus surgery	Same
13. Culture-negative endocarditis	Penicillin G 20 million U IV qd for 6 weeks plus an aminoglycoside for 2 weeks	Cephalothin 2.0 g IV[b] q4h for 6 weeks

[a]Duration of treatment given applies to native valve infective endocarditis only.
[b]If patient sensitivity to penicillin is of the immediate hypersensitivity type, vancomycin is recommended.
[c]Aqueous crystalline penicillin G should be used alone in patients over 65 years of age or who have renal disease or hearing impairment.
[d]Choice of aminoglycoside should depend on in vitro susceptibilities.
[e]Addition of an aminoglycoside is optional.
[f]Use of rifampin in coagulase-negative staphylococcal infection is recommended. The value of rifampin in coagulase-positive staphylococcal infections is controversial.

TABLE 101-7 Point System for Assessing the Need for Cardiac Surgery in Infective Endocarditis

	Point Rating[a]	
Complication	Native Valve IE	Prosthetic Valve IE
Heart failure		
Severe	5	5
Moderate	3	5
Mild	1	2
Fungal etiology	5	5
Persistent bacteremia	5	5
Organism other than streptococci	1	2
Relapse after medical therapy	2	3
Single major embolus	2	2
Two or more emboli	4	4
Vegetations by echocardiography	1	1
Early close of mitral valve by echocardiography	2	NA
Ruptured chordae tendineae or papillary muscle	3	NA
Heart block	3	3
Rupture of sinus of Valsalva or ventricular septum	4	4
Unstable prosthesis	NA	5
Early prosthetic valve endocarditis	NA	2
Periprosthetic leak	NA	2
Valvular obstruction	5	5

[a] Accumulation of 5 or more points implies need for valve replacement.
NA, not applicable.
SOURCE: Adapted from Reference 2.

Cardiac abnormalities that predispose patients to IE include aortic and mitral valve disease, ventricular septal defects, patent ductus arteriosus, coarctation of the aorta, prosthetic valves, and valves which previously have been infected. Patients with atrial septal defects, cardiac pacemakers, and atherosclerotic lesions are not felt to require prophylaxis. Mitral valve prolapse with redundancy of the valve seen on echocardiogram or evidence of mitral regurgitation is an indication for prophylaxis.

The specific antimicrobial agents chosen for prophylaxis are dependent on the specific procedure to be performed, the cardiac abnormality present and the presence or absence of penicillin allergy (Table 101-8). In critically ill patients with underlying cardiac abnormalities who are un-

TABLE 101-8 Endocarditis Prophylaxis

Procedure	Standard Regimen	Standard Oral Regimen for PCN Allergic Patients	Alternative Parenteral Regimens
Dental or respiratory tract procedure	Amoxicillin 3.0 g po 1 h before, then 1.5 g 6 h later.	Erythromycin, 1.0 g po 2 h before, then 500 mg 6 h later *OR* Clindamycin 300 mg po 1 h before, then 150 mg 6 h later.	Ampicillin 2.0 g IV or IM 30 min before, then 1.0 g 6 h later *OR* Clindamycin 300 mg IV 30 min before, then 150 mg 6 h later *OR* Vancomycin 1.0 g IV over 1 h starting 1 h before procedure; no repeat dose necessary.
Gastrointestinal or genitourinary tract procedure	Ampicillin, 2.0 g IV or IM, plus gentamicin 1.5 mg/kg body weight IV or IM given 30 min before, repeat 8 h later.		Vancomycin, 1.0 g IV, slowly over 1 h, plus gentamicin, 1.5 mg/kg body weight IV or IM, given 1 h before, repeat 8 h later.

dergoing procedures with a risk of bacteremia, a parenteral regimen is usually appropriate.

MYCOTIC ANEURYSM

PATHOGENESIS AND MICROBIAL ETIOLOGY. Mycotic aneurysms are aneurysmal dilations of arteries, caused by infection of the vessel wall with consequent weakening of the vessel's structure. They occur most commonly in patients with infective endocarditis and in that instance usually involve vessels of smaller calibre. The pathogenesis probably involves embolic localization of a valvular vegetation with extension of suppuration from the lumen circumferentially into the vessel wall. Another proposed mechanism is embolization of the vasa vasorum by infected material from the valve. In the absence of underlying IE, mycotic aneurysm may occur following transient bacteremia with seeding of a previously damaged site in a large artery, most commonly an ulcerated atherosclerotic plaque in the abdominal aorta. Mycotic aneurysms may also occur in intravenous drug abusers who both damage and contaminate the wall of a large artery by direct intraarterial injections of drugs; mycotic aneurysms of the lower extremity, particularly the femoral artery, are most common in this population.

Endocarditis-associated mycotic aneurysms are caused by the same microorganisms causing the IE; streptococci, staphylococci, and occasionally gram-negative enteric bacilli, the latter being more common among drug abusers. *S. aureus* and *Salmonella* species are the most frequent causes of mycotic aneurysms of the abdominal aorta and are not usually associated with IE.

CLINICAL FEATURES. Intracranial mycotic aneurysms are most commonly encountered in patients who already carry a diagnosis of IE. These aneurysms are usually asymptomatic unless they rupture. In that circumstance symptoms and signs are consistent with subarachnoid or intracerebral hemorrhage with sudden onset of severe headache, decrease in level of consciousness, and focal neurologic signs. Mycotic aneurysms of visceral arteries have a variable presentation based on the organ involved. In the case of the small bowel, there may be colicky abdominal pain and symptoms of small bowel obstruction. In the case of hepatic arterial aneurysms, an important differential diagnostic consideration is ascending cholangitis because of fever, right upper quadrant pain, and jaundice. Mycotic aneurysms of the external iliac artery may present with pain in the lower anterior abdomen, quadriceps wasting, diminished deep tendon reflexes, and arterial insufficiency of the ipsilateral lower extremity.[3]

Patients with mycotic aneurysms of the abdominal aorta present with pain and fever, often of weeks' or months' duration. In as many as one-third of patients with abdominal aortic aneurysms there is extension into the lumbar or thoracic vertebrae with resultant osteomyelitis. Aortoenteric fistula may occur if an aneurysm erodes into bowel lumen. On physical examination, in addition to fever, there may be a palpable mass in the abdomen.

DIAGNOSIS. In patients with IE clinical suspicion of a mycotic aneurysm usually arises after an episode of new neurologic symptoms in the case of intracranial aneurysms or local findings suggestive of aneurysms as noted above. Clinical suspicion of a leaking intracerebral aneurysm should prompt infused and uninfused computed tomography (CT) examinations initially; however an angiogram is generally necessary to exclude or confirm the diagnosis. The diagnosis of mycotic aneurysm of the abdominal aorta is also made on the basis of clinical suspicion, demonstration of bacteremia, and radiologic examination. CT of the abdomen may indicate a perivascular collection of fluid or actual blood in an aneurysm or pseudoaneurysm. Arteriography may also be helpful in demonstrating an aortic mycotic aneurysm and bone films may show erosion of adjacent vertebral bodies.

MANAGEMENT. The management of mycotic aneurysm depends on the organ involved. In the case of intracranial mycotic aneurysms there is debate regarding the most appropriate therapy. For peripheral intracranial aneurysms, clipping is probably indicated. For deep lesions, for which a surgical approach is felt to be hazardous, antimicrobial therapy alone is advisable because many aneurysms will resolve spontaneously with medical treatment. A history of bleeding, large aneurysm size, and persistence of the aneurysm following antimicrobial therapy are all factors that increase the advisability of surgery for accessible lesions. In the case of abdominal aortic aneurysms, surgical resection of the involved aorta is almost always necessary. Antimicrobial therapy for mycotic aneurysms and other intravascular infections without foreign bodies is outlined in Tables 101-6 and -9.

TABLE 101-9 Recommended Duration of Antimicrobial Therapy for Patients with Various Intravascular Infections

Patients without Intravascular Foreign Bodies	
Infectious Disorder	Duration of Treatment
Cavernous sinus thrombosis	2 weeks following the resolution of all signs of the disease (usually 4 weeks)
Mycotic aneurysm	4–6 weeks; 2–4 weeks after resection of the aneurysm
Postanginal sepsis	4 weeks or 10 days following resolution of local symptoms and signs
Pelvic vein thrombophlebitis	4 weeks (consider anticoagulation)
Pylephlebitis	4–6 weeks. If associated with liver abscess consider additional treatment until abscess is resolved.

CAVERNOUS SINUS THROMBOSIS

Cavernous sinus thrombosis usually results from direct spread of bacteria from a contiguous focus of infection. Extension of bacteria may occur by several routes including septic thrombophlebitis of the angular and ophthalmic veins from facial cellulitis, along the lateral sinus and petrosal sinuses from middle ear infections, via the pterygoid venous plexus from a peritonsillar abscess, following a dental infection from osteomyelitis of the maxilla or from a cervical abscess, and along the venous plexus surrounding the internal carotid artery from the middle ear or jugular bulb.

S. aureus is the cause of cavernous sinus thrombosis in about 50 percent of cases. Streptococci, anaerobes, and other aerobes account for most of the rest.[4] Patients with cavernous sinus thrombosis generally present with the early onset of external ophthalmoplegia with decreased sensation around the eye. The physical examination reveals periorbital edema and chemosis, and, as the illness develops, meningismus, altered mental status and cranial nerve palsies especially of III, IV, V, and VI become evident. Examination of the fundus often reveals striking venous congestion. The differential diagnosis of cavernous sinus thrombosis includes orbital cellulitis and rhinocerebral phycomycosis (mucormycosis). The distinction between cavernous sinus thrombosis and orbital cellulitis is sometimes difficult. Bilateral involvement, as well as fifth nerve palsy, a fixed, dilated pupil and signs of meningitis are all more likely in cavernous sinus thrombosis than orbital cellulitis.

Although the diagnosis may be evident on clinical grounds alone, several imaging modalities can be useful. Ultrasound examination of the orbit can be useful in defining periorbital abscess formation which may require surgical intervention. CT examination with contrast will also aid in this, as well as being useful in demonstrating sinusitis or underlying osteomyelitis, and may establish the diagnosis of cavernous sinus thrombosis as well. Carotid angiography and orbital venography have also been used to establish the diagnosis but are not recommended since they are unlikely to influence management. Following CT, a lumbar puncture is warranted, but it is usually sterile with a parameningeal inflammatory pattern: pleocytosis and elevated protein without significant hypoglycorrhachia. Blood cultures are mandatory and are often positive; if sinus or abscess drainage is performed, fluid should be cultured for both aerobic and anaerobic bacteria. When rhinocerebral mucormycosis is a consideration, usually in a diabetic with blackish nasal discharge in addition to the rest of the syndrome, surgical exploration with biopsy and histologic examination for fungi is needed to establish the diagnosis.

Successful management of cavernous sinus thrombosis depends on early, effective antimicrobial therapy. Even with the best medical and surgical therapy the outcome is often unsatisfactory. For this reason, adjunctive therapies such as corticosteroids and anticoagulation have been tried, but without success and they cannot be recommended. The regimens shown in Tables 101-6 and 101-9 can be used when a bacterial etiology has been established. Prior to bacteriologic confirmation, empirical therapy depends on the underlying infection suspected.

POSTANGINAL SEPSIS

In 1936, in an article entitled "On Certain Septicemias Due to Anaerobic Organisms," Lemierre described a group of patients with pharyngitis complicated by bacteremia due to anaerobic microorganisms.[5] Subsequently, this disorder, usually referred to as "postanginal sepsis," has been described frequently.[6] The pathogenesis is thought to involve bacterial invasion of the mucosa of the posterior pharynx with extension of suppurative thrombophlebitis (ST) into the internal jugular veins. Bacteremic spread of the infection is common, with lung, liver, and joints the most common sites of metastatic disease. Clinically, the patients present with sore throat, chills, fever, and occasionally jaundice. On physical examination, in addition to the toxicity and fever, there may be palpable tender thrombosis of the jugular vein as well as evidence of septic arthritis, pleuropulmonary disease, or jaundice. An enhanced CT scan will usually demonstrate internal jugular vein thrombophlebitis, and is useful to localize purulent collections requiring drainage. Chest radiograph may show scattered infiltrates due to septic pulmonary emboli. *Fusobacterium necrophorum* has most commonly been isolated from blood, although *Bacteroides fragilis* and other mouth anaerobes have been reported as well.

Management includes early recognition and treatment of the disorder with effective antimicrobial therapy. Antibiotics should be directed against anaerobic bacteria, with drugs such as metronidazole, chloramphenicol, imipenem-cilastatin or ticarcillin/clavulanic acid. Prompt surgical intervention to drain any purulent material present locally or distantly is required in addition to antibiotics.

SEPTIC PELVIC VEIN THROMBOPHLEBITIS

Pelvic vein thrombophlebitis most often develops 1 to 2 weeks after delivery or gynecologic surgical intervention or in the setting of pelvic suppuration, such as following septic abortion or postcesarean section endometritis.

Symptoms include fever, chills, anorexia, nausea, vomiting, and abdominal pain.[7] On physical examination, there may be tenderness in the lower quadrants, and tender venous structures may be palpated in one-third of patients.[8] Eighty percent of pelvic vein thromboses complicating pregnancy and delivery occur on the right side, perhaps because of compression of the right ovarian vein at the pelvic brim by the enlarged uterus. In 5 percent of episodes thrombosis is apparent only on the left and in 14 percent it is bilateral. Spread distally to femoral veins is unusual.

The most serious complication of suppurative pelvic vein thrombosis is pulmonary embolization. When this occurs the patient presents with respiratory distress associated with pulmonary opacities which are often pleural-based. Even though the process is associated with thrombosis and bacterial suppuration in the venous lumen, bacteremia is unusual with an overall prevalence of only 30 percent. Microorganisms isolated from the blood, or from the veins if surgery is carried out, include those which are normally present in the pelvis, particularly *Peptostreptoccus* species,

Peptococcus species, *Bacteroides fragilis,* aerobic gram-negative bacilli such as *E. coli,* klebsiella, and enterobacter, group A and group B beta-hemolytic streptococci and, rarely, staphylococci.

The diagnosis can be difficult since the findings are similar to a wider range of other pelvic and lower abdominal inflammatory conditions. Probably the best imaging modality to support the diagnosis is contrast-enhanced computed tomography; ultrasound examination may also be useful if the intravascular thrombus can be demonstrated.

Successful treatment frequently requires both antimicrobial therapy and heparinization; indeed, in the appropriate clinical context fever which is failing to respond to apparently appropriate antimicrobials and which responds to addition of intravenous heparin can be regarded as support for the diagnosis.[9] Complications are mainly those related to suppurative pulmonary emboli.

PYLEPHLEBITIS

Pylephlebitis is septic thrombosis of the portal vein and its branches. It is a complication of intra-abdominal suppuration and was first described in patients with appendicitis or diverticulitis. The illness evolves in three phases. In the first phase symptoms and signs of the original intraabdominal disorder such as acute appendicitis or perforated diverticulum predominate. The second phase involves portal bacteremia, with resultant invasion and thrombosis of portal veins. In the third phase, abscess formation in the liver occurs as a result of proximal spread of the suppurative material. Late signs and symptoms include fever, abdominal pain, jaundice and right upper quadrant tenderness. The liver is enlarged in one-half of patients. Laboratory studies reveal an elevated white blood cell count with increased numbers of immature granulocytes, and abnormal liver function tests, particularly elevations of the alkaline phosphatase and aspartate aminotransferase (AST). Bacteremia is not a consistent finding. CT is especially useful in demonstrating this disorder, showing clot in the portal veins and occasionally gas in portal vein radicles in the liver. The microorganisms responsible reflect large bowel flora and include aerobic gram-negative bacilli such as *Escherichia coli, Klebsiella,* and *Enterobacter,* anaerobic microorganisms such as *Peptococcus, Peptostreptococcus, B. fragilis, Fusobacterium* and gram-positive aerobic species such as staphylococci and enterococci.

Successful therapy requires surgical correction of the primary problem as well as high-dose antibacterial therapy directed against the offending pathogens. Pyogenic liver abscesses resulting from this disorder are usually best treated with prolonged medical therapy alone, unless they are few and relatively large, in which case percutaneous drainage may be useful. Surgical drainage of multiple small abscesses is very difficult, often requires a transperitoneal approach, and is not recommended. The effectiveness of antibacterial therapy may be judged by physical examination, resolution of fever and leukocytosis, and improvement of abnormalities demonstrated by ultrasound or contrast studies.

Infections of Intravascular Prosthetic Devices

PROSTHETIC VALVE ENDOCARDITIS

PATHOGENESIS AND MICROBIOLOGY. Prosthetic heart valves may become infected early following implantation or later during the life of the device. Overall, about 2 percent of patients with prosthetic heart valves become infected, one-third in the first few months after valve implantation and two-thirds later. In early prosthetic valve endocarditis (PVE) the presumed pathogenesis involves inoculation of the operative site at the time of surgery or the localization of microorganisms on the new device following transient bacteremia associated with indwelling lines used in the perioperative period. Factors associated with an increased risk of PVE include IE of the native valve prior to valve resection and replacement, use of a mechanical valvular device in contrast to a tissue heterograft or homograft, a history of intravenous drug abuse, male gender (possibly because of the greater likelihood of superficial cellulitis as a result of shaving prior to surgery), and longer cardiopulmonary bypass time.[10]

In late PVE, (i.e., disease appearing more than 60 days after replacement) the pathogenesis more closely resembles that of native valve disease.[11] Extension of local tissue disease via lymphatics to the bloodstream or direct inoculation of microorganisms via capillary beds, as occurs during dental work, results in transient bacteremia with localization on the prosthetic device.

Microorganisms most commonly responsible for PVE are listed in Table 101-10. *Staphylococcus epidermidis* is the most common cause of early PVE. *S. aureus* and gram-negative bacilli are also prominent etiologic microorganisms during this time period. Other less commonly encountered microorganisms are enterococci, other streptococci, and yeast. Microorganisms found in patients with late PVE tend to be similar to those seen in native valve disease. Viridans streptococci are common, as is *S. aureus; S. epidermidis* and gram-negative bacilli are less common.

CLINICAL FEATURES: The signs, symptoms, and clinical laboratory abnormalities seen in prosthetic valve endocarditis are generally similar to those encountered in patients with native valve endocarditis, except that patients with PVE have a higher prevalence of cardiac complications. Clinical evidence of these cardiac complications may include new and changing regurgitant murmurs caused by paravalvular leak from dehiscence of the valve ring, intraventricular and atrioventricular conduction defects resulting from extension of a paravalvular abscess into the interventricular septum, and muffling of prosthetic heart sounds or new stenotic murmurs related to malfunction of the valve caused by a vegetation.

DIAGNOSIS: Diagnostic difficulty arises in the immediate postoperative period when bacteremia occurs in a patient with a new prosthetic valve. In this setting, blood cultures yielding staphylococci, "diphtheroids" and yeasts are more likely to represent true prosthetic valve infection than is gram-negative bacilli bacteremia, which is more likely due to indwelling venous catheter infection.

In patients with late prosthetic valve endocarditis caused by staphylococci or streptococci, bacteria are usually recovered consistently from blood cultures providing the patient has not received prior antimicrobial therapy. Generally, three sets of blood cultures obtained over a brief period of time from different venipuncture sites are sufficient to identify the etiology of prosthetic valve infection. The echocardiogram and the cinefluoroscopic examination may be of some help in patients with prosthetic valve endocarditis. Echocardiography helps identify vegetations and local suppurative complications as well as determine ventricular function and valvular integrity, although the metallic devices tend to result in distorted echo signals which confuse the interpretation. A cinefluorogram which reveals more than a 7° rocking of the prosthesis is very suggestive of valve dehiscence. Patients with neurologic symptoms associated with PVE should also undergo a CT of the head to detect embolic hemorrhagic infarcts and abscess. Since CT does not reliably exclude mycotic aneurysm, cerebral angiography may also be indicated when CT findings do not adequately explain the neurologic symptoms.

MANAGEMENT. The same principals described for treatment of native valve endocarditis apply for treatment of PVE.[12] The antimicrobial agents used in the treatment of PVE are outlined in Table 101-6. In general, initial antimicrobial therapy is chosen on the basis of identification and susceptibility tests of the infecting microorganism. When the infecting microorganism has not been identified, initial therapy should include vancomycin and gentamicin to cover the likely possibilities of *S. epidermidis*, *S. aureus*, and streptococci. Ill, bacteremic patients who may have IE should be treated without delay. In addition, if heart surgery is scheduled because of valve deterioration or antimicrobial therapy is required for some other indication in a patient with suspected endocarditis, therapy should be initiated without waiting for the results of blood cultures. Relative indications for valve replacement in PVE include early PVE, nonstreptococcal late PVE, and periprosthetic leak. Patients with PVE should be treated for 6 to 8 weeks in most instances whether or not the valve is removed. If microorganisms can be cultured at the time of valve replacement, we recommend 6 to 8 additional weeks of therapy beginning at that time.

TABLE 101-10 Etiology of Prosthetic Valve Endocarditis

Microorganism	Early PVE	Late PVE
Staphylococci		
S. epidermidis	30%	20%
S. aureus	20%	11%
Streptococci		
Group D streptococci	5%	12%
Viridans streptococci	4%	25%
Gram-negative bacilli	20%	12%
Corynebacterium		
(Not *C. diphtheriae*)	8%	3%
Fungi	10%	5%
Other or		
culture negative	3%	12%

CARDIAC PACEMAKER INFECTIONS

Four major varieties of pacemakers are presently in use: transvenous and epicardial temporary pacemakers with external generators and transvenous and epicardial pacemakers of the permanent variety with implanted generator boxes. The pathogenesis and management of infections of temporary transvenous pacemakers is essentially identical to that for other percutaneous central vascular catheters and is not discussed further here (see Chap. 24). The most common complication affecting permanently implanted pacemakers is mechanical failure (failure to pace or sense correctly), but infection is the next most common. Approximately 4 percent of pacemakers become infected at some point after placement. Generator box infections, infection of the electrode along its subcutaneous course, and bacteremic infection of the intravascular portion of the electrode, with or without associated endocarditis, each contribute approximately one-third to the overall infection problem. Diabetes mellitus, cancer, and corticosteroid therapy have all been noted to predispose to infection of the device. Skin erosion adjacent to a generator pouch also predisposes to direct invasion of the apparatus. As with PVE, pacemaker infections can be classified as early or late; early ones are those occurring in the first 3 to 6 months. Early infections can generally be attributed to wound contamination by skin organisms at the time of implantation, whereas late infection, particularly of the intravascular electrode, is often due to transient bacteremia with adherence of organisms to the surface of the device. Particularly in the case of staphylococcal infections, adherence to the foreign material is facilitated by an exopolysaccharide glycocalyx produced by the organism. This material also forms a protective layer over the biofilm on the foreign body, contributing to impairment of the local antibacterial activity of polymorphonuclear leukocytes and reducing the effectiveness of antimicrobial therapy.

Staphylococcus epidermidis and *S. aureus* are the most common microorganisms isolated from patients with generator pocket or electrode infections. In one large study of pacemaker infections, *S. epidermidis* accounted for 44 percent of episodes and *S. aureus*, 29 percent.[13] They are also the most common organisms isolated from the blood of patients with pacemaker infections in the absence of obvious generator pocket or electrode disease. Other etiologic microorganisms which have been reported include *Corynebacterium* species, gram-negative aerobic bacilli, and occasionally fungi.

Chills, fever, and other constitutional symptoms without another evident source is the usual presentation of pacemaker infection. The diagnosis is made by inspecting the generator pocket and the subcutaneous electrodes along with obtaining blood cultures. Generator pocket and subcutaneous electrode infections usually evidence local inflammation without bacteremia or with transient bacteremia. Persistent bacteremia in a patient with an intravascular pacemaker suggests intravascular electrode infection or IE. Since most pacemakers are implanted in the right ventricle, the associated endocarditis is usually not accompanied by systemic embolic phenomena but may produce septic pulmonary emboli or multifocal pneumonia, as in right-sided endocarditis of other causes. Echocardiography has been of limited utility in diagnosis because of the confounding signals generated by the foreign body.

There are three main considerations in developing a therapeutic plan for management of pacemaker infection. One is the identity of the suspected or proven infecting microorganisms, second is the particular component of the apparatus that is involved, and the third is the presence or absence of bacterial infection at sites other than the pacemaker itself. Infected pacemakers must be removed when the generator box is infected, when there is persistent bacteremia, and when there is evidence of IE. A few authors have suggested that patients with permanent transvenous pacemakers that have been present for a long duration, and who have bacteremia without evidence of generator box infection or IE, can be tried on antibacterial therapy in the hope that the infection on the device may be cured without replacement. If treatment of pacemaker infection is attempted without removal of the device, 4 to 6 weeks of intravenous antimicrobial therapy is probably necessary as an initial trial. In the case of fungal agents or mycobacteria, a longer duration of therapy is necessary and is more likely to be unsuccessful. If the decision is made to remove the pacemaker then the new transvenous generator should be located in a deeper pocket. Antimicrobial therapy is chosen on the basis of the microorganism isolated from the skin and subcutaneous tissue or bloodstream and is described in Tables 101-6 and 101-11. Two weeks of antimicrobial therapy after removal of the device is probably sufficient in the case of most generator pocket infections due to pyogenic microorganisms unless there is metastatic disease or secondary native valve IE in which case the usual duration of treatment for native valve endocarditis is used after the device is removed. Transvenous lead infections also require device removal and parenteral antimicrobial therapy. It is sometimes difficult to extricate the transvenous electrode tip from the right heart. Tricuspid valve or ventricular wall tears have occurred. If percutaneous electrode removal is impossible, thoracotomy is required.

TABLE 101-11 Recommended Duration of Antimicrobial Therapy for Infections of Intravascular Devices

Infectious Disorder	Recommended Duration of Treatment
Pacemaker infection, generator box, and/or bacteremia	2 weeks after device removed, 4–6 weeks if not removed
Hickman, Broviac, Mediport catheter infection	
A. Exit site infection	2 weeks
B. Tunnel infection	2 weeks after device removal
C. Bacteremia	2 weeks and reculture; consider venogram/fibrinolytic therapy
Central and peripheral lines	7–10 days after device removal (see text); 2 weeks for *S. aureus* bacteremia
Prosthetic heart valves	6–8 weeks
Arterial vascular grafts	6–8 weeks

PERIPHERAL INTRAVENOUS LINES

Almost all patients in an ICU will have devices for administering intravenous fluids or for monitoring vascular pressures. These intravenous lines are suspect in any febrile patient. Chemical thrombophlebitis, catheter-associated bacteremia, and septic thrombophlebitis (ST) are specific complications that may involve these devices. So-called chemical thrombophlebitis or sterile thrombophlebitis of peripheral veins occurs frequently in hospitalized patients; the incidence may be as high as 33 percent, depending on how long the device has been present.[14] Factors associated with chemical thrombophlebitis include the use of hypertonic infusion solutions, polyethylene catheters, prolonged venous catheterization, and manipulation of the catheter. Clearly, it is difficult or impossible to distinguish a sterile chemical phlebitis from an infection on examination alone, so this determination generally depends on catheter removal followed by microbiologic examination of the blood and the catheter itself as outlined below.

An infected catheter may also serve as a source of bacteremia in the absence of obvious local inflammation. Mild inflammatory changes may be present adjacent to the device or there may be ST, a situation in which the lumen of the vein is occluded by infected clot. In this instance, following removal of the device, frank pus can often be expressed from the exit site. ST accounts for approximately 10 percent of hospital-acquired infections with an incidence of about one-half of a percent in the general hospital population and about 8 percent in patients with serious burns.[15] In patients with burns, morbidity and mortality is especially high, not only because of the patient's injury, but because ST is often masked by the extensive tissue destruction present. In burn patients, infection may also develop after the intravenous line has been removed, with a latent period ranging from 2 to 10 days.[16] In one series, less than one-half of the cases were diagnosed antemortem.[17] In another series, fever was present in 70 percent of patients, but local signs and symptoms were present in only one-third.[18] Bacteremia complicated ST in 80 percent of patients and septic emboli to the lung were apparent in 40 percent. The mean duration of venous cannulation prior to the development of ST is 5 days. Therefore, a high index of suspicion for this diagnosis should be maintained when dealing with burn patients.

The microbial etiology of peripheral intravenous catheters is extremely variable, involving both the usual organisms colonizing normal skin, such as *S. aureus*, coagulase-negative staphylococci and streptococci, and enteric organisms originating from the patient or from the environment which may colonize body surfaces in critically ill patients (e.g., *E. coli, Enterobacter, Pseudomonas, Acinetobacter* species, etc). Yeasts, particularly *Candida albicans,* also cause a significant proportion of these infections.

The management of patients with suspected or proved infection of a peripheral intravenous catheter first requires removal of the catheter. Blood cultures should be drawn by venipuncture from another site and the removed catheter should be cultured semiquantitatively.[19] If pus can be expressed from the puncture site this should be Gram stained and cultured. It is sometimes useful to obtain blood cultures before and immediately after the line is removed to determine if an infecting microorganism can be isolated from blood prior to device removal and if the infecting microorganism persists in the blood after device removal. In patients whose main manifestations of infection are mild or moderate local inflammation without findings of septic thrombophlebitis, immediate antimicrobial therapy is generally unnecessary. In some cases simple catheter removal will result in resolution of local findings. If signs or symptoms persist and culture of blood or the catheter reveals a pathogen, then specific therapy can be begun. In more severely ill patients with a strong suspicion of sepsis from the intravenous catheter, empirical antimicrobial therapy in addition to catheter removal may be warranted. Initial choice of antimicrobial therapy may be guided by Gram stain of pus expressed from the site. Usually antistaphylococcal therapy and therapy directed against prevalent gram-negative aerobic bacilli is chosen initially when the Gram stain is indeterminate, and adjusted subsequently when an etiologic diagnosis is established. Dosage and duration are indicated in Tables 101-6 and 101-11. Treatment of ST often requires a combination of both antimicrobial therapy and incision and drainage. The procedure of choice is venotomy, with excision of the involved segment proximally as far as suppuration and clot is encountered. Patients with an infected plastic intravenous line, steel needle, or scalp vein needle associated with bacteremia are treated at least 5 to 7 days after the device is removed. In the case of *S. aureus* bacteremia from a peripheral venous line, even in the absence of obvious clinical findings it is difficult to be certain there is no metastatic spread of infection, so 2 weeks of parenteral therapy is the minimal duration of therapy recommended. Some authors recommend additional oral therapy even in instances where there is no documented metastatic disease.

INFECTIONS IN CENTRAL VENOUS DEVICES

Percutaneously introduced central venous catheters are subject to the same range of infectious complications as peripheral intravenous catheters. The incidence of bacteremia complicating central venous cannulation varies greatly depending on the type of catheter and the length of time it has been in place, but is generally about 5 percent. Venous thrombosis without infection has also been reported to occur in about 5 percent of longer-term central venous catheters, although a degree of asymptomatic thrombosis has been observed in as many as one-half.[20] Extensive thrombosis with infection, ST, remains fortunately uncommon. Local symptoms and signs are not common in central venous device infection since the vein is generally well below the skin and subcutaneous tissue layers. Fever may be the only evidence of infection. Occasionally there may be edema of the supraclavicular area at the site of the device as well as prominence of superficial veins on the upper torso on the ipsilateral side. An elevated and left-shifted white blood cell count may be present. Blood cultures are usually positive in such patients if no prior antibiotics have been administered.

Pulmonary artery catheters may be complicated by the same infectious problems seen with central venous catheters.[21] In addition, inflammation of the tricuspid and pulmonic valve due to the foreign body may predispose to localization of microorganisms which transiently gain access to the circulation and thereby lead to right-sided IE. In one study 4 percent of patients with pulmonary artery catheters had positive blood cultures attributable to the catheter.[22] This was especially common when devices had been left in place for longer than 4 days. Another complication is septic pulmonary embolization.

Broviac and Hickman catheters are specialized central venous devices used when venous access is needed for a prolonged period of time. They are fabricated from a silicone elastomer material in contrast to polyethylene, which is used in many peripheral and central venous devices. The silicone elastomer is less susceptible to colonization or invasion by microorganisms and may also be less thrombogenic.[23] Infection may involve the skin at the exit site only, the subcutaneous tunnel extending from the exit site to the vein entry site, or the intravascular lumen. Exit site infection is defined as infection of the exit site with extension <2 cm from that site. Tunnel infection is defined as evidence of inflammation >2 cm from the exit site. In one study of Hickman catheter complications, exit site infections occurred in 3 percent, tunnel infections in 6 percent, and isolated bacteremia in 3 percent. A rare patient develops ST of the central vein. Venography is useful in suspected Hickman and Broviac catheter infections to identify a thrombin sheath within the device, which would suggest the possibility of an infectious complication. However, a thrombin sheath may also occur without microbial colonization.

Microorganisms responsible for central venous line infection include staphylococci, gram-negative aerobic bacilli, streptococci, enterococci, corynebacterium ("diphtheroids"), and occasionally yeasts (Table 101-12).

The approach to suspected or proved percutaneous central vascular infection is in most respects similar to that outlined for peripheral intravenous catheter infections. Diagnosis hinges on local inspection, blood cultures, and semiquantitative culture of the intracutaneous portion of the suspect catheter after removal. Empirical therapy, based on a Gram stain if possible, is given when the infection is associated with evidence of frank systemic sepsis. Because of the substantial frequency of unexplained fever in critically ill patients and the paucity of local findings as-

TABLE 101-12 Microorganisms Responsible for Infections of Intravascular Devices

Organisms	PVE[a] (%)	Pacemaker (%)	CVL[b] (%)	Hickman Line (%)	Vascular Graft (%)
S. epidermidis	27	42	30	35	10
S. aureus	14	35	8	5	15
Streptococci (includes enterococci)	26	—	3	5	30
Gram-negative rods	14	—	18	25	30
Diphtheroid and gram-positive rods	7	—	2	21	3
Fungi	9	—	24	7	2
Unknown	3	23	15	2	10

[a]Prosthetic valve endocarditis
[b]Central venous line

sociated with infection of central vascular catheters, these catheters must often be removed on the basis of suspicion alone and often they prove not to be the culprit. When the indication for the central venous catheter is still present and additional sites for catheter placement are scarce, it is probably acceptable to change the catheter over a guidewire, awaiting the result of the semiquantitative catheter culture and blood culture to determine whether the site can continue to be used.[24]

In general, proved infection of a percutaneous central vascular line should be managed with both catheter removal and specific antimicrobial therapy (described in Tables 101-6 and 101-11). Exit site infections and bacteremia from tunneled central vascular catheters can sometimes be managed by antimicrobial therapy alone without catheter removal. However, when there is a tunnel infection or evidence of ST, the device must be removed. It has been suggested that infection with gram-positive microorganisms may be easier to eradicate than with gram-negative ones, but others have been unable to confirm this. Patients with a Hickman catheter, a Broviac catheter, or Mediports are treated for 2 weeks if the device is not removed, preferably with bacteriocidal or fungicidal agents. If relapse occurs, the device should be removed and an additional 2 weeks of therapy administered. If the device is removed initially then treatment is continued for at least 1 week and until the infection is clinically resolved.

An additional modality of treatment of infected devices such as the Hickman, Broviac, or Mediport has been the utilization of thrombolytic agents to try to lyse fibrin sheaths, which occur in the lumen and seem to predispose to and perpetuate infection. Several methods are described in Chap. 119. The success of the thrombolytic therapy can be judged by comparing pre- and posttreatment venogram studies. Finally, some advocate the use of heparin in addition to antibiotics when there is evidence of venous thrombosis or when signs of infection persist despite adequate antibacterial therapy.

ARTERIAL GRAFTS

Arterial grafts have an infection rate that has varied between 2 percent and 6 percent in different studies[25–27] with a mortality rate as high as 50 percent. The pathogenesis of graft infection is analogous to that of prosthetic valve disease, with some patients presumably developing infectious disorders of the graft as a result of inoculation of microorganisms at the time of surgery and others developing infection later due to adherence of microorganisms that have gained access to the circulation. Grafts remain susceptible to infection for a rather long period of time due to the slow process of pseudointima formation in the graft lumen. Overall, graft infections present a mean of 8 months after implantation but late disease may occur as long as 7 to 10 years after graft placement.[28] Autogenous vein grafts are the least susceptible to infection. Knitted Dacron grafts appear to be more susceptible and woven Dacron grafts have a risk of infection somewhere in between. Grafts which cross the femoral area seem to be at greatest risk for infection, possibly due to contamination by bowel flora at the time of implantation.

The microbial etiology of vascular graft infection is shown in Table 101-12. Gram-positive microorganisms, particularly *S. aureus*, are the most common cause of graft infections, particularly in the groin or popliteal area. Gram-negative enteric microorganisms such as *E. coli*, proteus, or pseudomonas are more often the cause of abdominal graft suppuration.

Graft infections generally present with variable systemic constitutional symptoms, non-specific laboratory evidence of an inflammatory process (leukocytosis, elevated ESR), and findings at the graft site which vary depending on the location of the graft. Intraluminal infection may present as fever and nonspecific constitutional complaints due to bacteremia. Patients with a vascular graft who have persistent bacteremia with no other known source must be approached as if they have a graft infection. Extraluminal infection may present with evidence of local graft infection with erythema, tenderness and swelling over the graft site, with systemic inflammatory symptoms without definite localizing findings, or with graft occlusion. Rapid swelling suggests disruption of the suture line with bleeding and false aneurysm formation and almost always implies graft infection. The most common presentation of groin or leg graft site infection is a localized abscess or draining sinus. Graft thrombosis should be suspected when signs and symptoms of peripheral arterial insufficiency develop. Exteriorization of the graft secondary to breakdown of tissue overlying the graft is pathognomonic of infection.

With infection of abdominal aortic grafts, swelling of tissues surrounding the graft may produce a mass effect, sometimes with evidence of ureteral obstruction or hydronephrosis. In addition, symptoms and signs of lower extremity ischemia may occur. The development of an aortoduodenal fistula between an infected aortic graft and the duodenum is a catastrophic complication. Patients in this group present with hematemesis or circulatory collapse.

Not infrequently a diagnosis of graft infection must be based predominantly on the clinical features noted above if blood cultures are negative. The most useful imaging procedure is scanning with indium or technetium-labelled white blood cells, which can demonstrate the inflammatory process along the course of the vascular graft.[29] CT scanning is perhaps preferable if soft tissue edema due to infection surrounding the graft or false aneurysm formation can be demonstrated. When the graft is removed for presumed infection, the graft itself and swabs from the graft bed should be cultured for both aerobes and anaerobes and examined for fungi.

Management of an infected intravascular graft almost always requires specific antimicrobial therapy chosen on the basis of the presumed or demonstrated infecting microorganism as well as graft removal. When antimicrobial therapy alone is attempted, graft infection usually persists. If a graft provides the only blood supply to a distal organ or extremity, then some variety of revascularization must be carried out at the time of graft removal. An example is the utilization of an axillofemoral graft to bypass an infected aortic bifurcation prosthesis.

Specific antimicrobial regimens and suggested duration of therapy are indicated in Tables 101-6 and 101-11.

ARTERIAL PRESSURE MONITORING DEVICES

The most common intraarterial monitoring device used in patients hospitalized in ICUs is the indwelling radial arterial catheter. Generally, the infection rate is low. In one series, 23 of 95 patients with 130 arterial lines revealed evidence of local inflammation;[30] however, bacteremia or fungemia was demonstrated in only 5. Arterial catheters at other sites, particularly the groin, have both higher infection rates and higher incidence of later complications such as false aneurysm formation. These catheters are usually placed under emergent circumstances because of absent radial pulses; they should be removed and replaced at another site at the earliest opportunity and observed closely for signs of infection while they remain in place. The microorganisms isolated directly from infected arterial lines or from the bloodstream in patients with them have generally been gram-positive cocci including *S. aureus, S. epidermis,* and enterococci, as well as gram-negative aerobic bacilli. Polymicrobial bacteremia may be slightly more common in arterial line infections. In addition to invasive microorganisms from skin, outbreaks of arterial line infections have been caused by contamination of fluid used in the strain gauge monitoring system.[31] *Flavobacterium, Serratia,* and *Enterobacter* species were recovered in these outbreaks. The approach to diagnosis and management is identical to that for percutaneous central venous catheters. Successful management of infected arterial lines requires removal of the device and specific antimicrobial therapy. Usually patients do well and chronic suppuration at the arterial line site is unusual following removal.

An Approach to Patients with Fever and Suspected Intravascular Infection

Intravascular infection is usually suspected in a critically ill patient when fever or other clinical or laboratory features of sepsis are present without a satisfactory alternative explanation. Blood cultures are mandatory in all such patients as an initial step, and all permanent or temporary intravascular devices should be carefully inspected for local evidence of infection.

Patients with otherwise unexplained positive blood cultures in the presence of an intravascular device must be presumed to have an infection of the device. When the device is a temporary one, such as a peripheral intravenous line, central venous catheter, or temporary pacemaker, it should be removed. In most cases intravenous antimicrobials appropriate for the organism should be given for 1 to 2 weeks. If pus can be expressed from the puncture site or there is persistent bacteremia, surgical exploration of the peripheral veins is indicated. As noted earlier, tunnelled central venous catheters call for a more selective approach, summarized in Fig. 101-1. When positive blood cultures are attributed to an infected permanent intravascular device, the initial clinical decision is whether or not the device should be removed. Indications for "permanent" intravascular device removal depend on the variety of the device and have been discussed previously.

Positive blood cultures in the absence of an intravascular device and without an evident infection such as cellulitis, pneumonia, severe urinary tract infection, cholangitis, or intraabdominal abscess predisposing to bacteremia are most commonly due to an occult abscess or to intravascular suppuration. When sufficient clinical suspicion suggests the possibility of an intravascular infection such as a mycotic aneurysm, native valve endocarditis, postanginal sepsis, pelvic vein thrombophlebitis, or pylephlebitis, appropriate special diagnostic studies outlined earlier should be promptly performed and appropriate antimicrobial therapy for the bacteremia initiated. In addition, when the diagno-

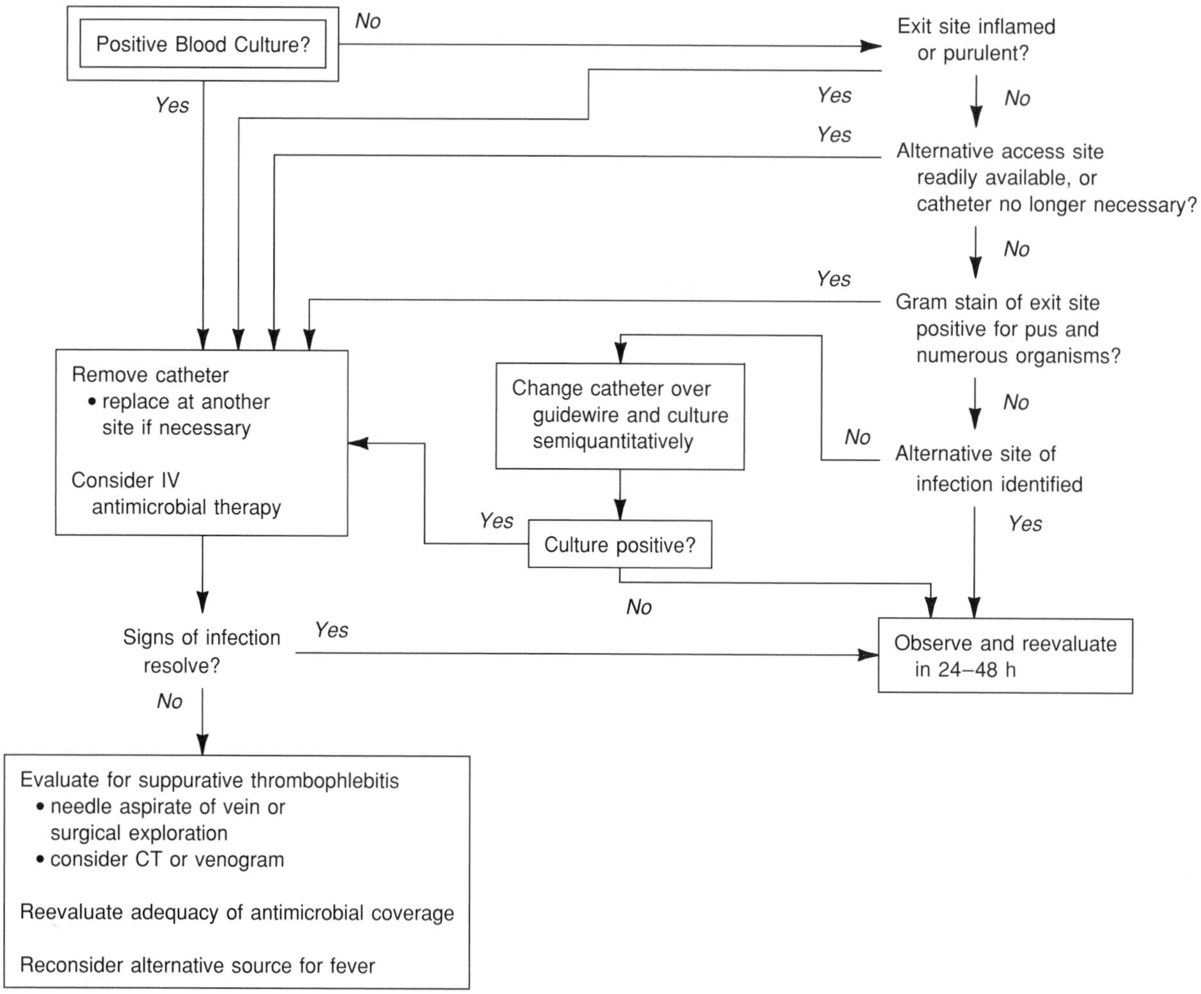

FIGURE 101-1 Approach to bacteremia caused by an infected temporary intravascular device.

sis has been established, appropriate surgical intervention is often required as noted above.

Another group of critically ill patients in whom intravascular infection must be considered are those with fever and persistently sterile blood cultures, either while receiving antimicrobial therapy or not. When antimicrobial agents are being administered for some other reason, it may be especially difficult to make a diagnosis of the precise etiology of intravascular infection. Even if antimicrobial therapy can be discontinued, it may still take as long as 2 weeks for blood cultures to become positive again. In the patient with a prosthetic heart valve, blood culture-negative IE is a consideration. In those with permanent pacemakers or vascular grafts, infection with a fastidious organism which is difficult to detect by usual methods is also a possibility, as is infection of a part of the device which is extravascular. The approach to these infections involves blood cultures designed to detect more fastidious organisms (vide supra), serologic studies for infections not detected by culture, and imaging studies aimed at acquiring nonmicrobiologic support for the diagnosis of infection. An echocardiogram demonstrating a vegetation on a valve, or an arteriogram showing a mycotic aneurysm, or a scan with labelled white blood cells demonstrating increased uptake around a vascular graft may be sufficient to raise the index of suspicion high enough to proceed to more definitive therapy.

Patients with fever, negative blood cultures, and temporary devices in place should be examined carefully for evidence of local inflammation at the site of the device and if present, the device should be removed and cultured semiquantitatively: a colony count of <15 when the intracutaneous portion of a vascular catheter is rolled on an agar plate virtually excludes sepsis due to infection of that line, whereas higher bacterial counts provide some support for the diagnosis.[19]

A fairly common practice in some centers involves changing the central venous line over a guidewire in the febrile patient whose central vascular catheter exit site does not look infected and who is not bacteremic; if the line tip culture is positive then the central venous line is replaced in a sterile site. Data to support or refute this practice is not compelling; therefore, one must weigh the risk of the catheter being the source of sepsis against the risk associated with placement of a new catheter or doing without it. An algorithmic approach to diagnosis and management of suspected central vascular catheter infection is given in Fig. 101-2.

Finally, even in the patient with fever of unknown source, negative blood cultures, and no intravascular device in place, an intravascular infection remains an important diagnostic consideration. Mycotic aneurysms, culture-negative native valve endocarditis, pelvic vein septic thrombophlebitis, or pylephlebitis are all examples of this. The key points in diagnostic approach are a careful history and physical examination and consideration of the clinical context. Examples include a woman with fever without bacteremia following delivery, where a pelvic vein thrombophlebitis must be considered, new or previously demonstrated pathologic heart murmur, raising the possibility of culture-negative IE, or known intravenous drug abuse suggesting the possibility of mycotic aneurysm.

Duration of Antimicrobial Treatment

Table 101-6 lists the appropriate antibiotics and duration of therapy for endocarditis based on the microorganisms isolated. Tables 101-9 and 101-11 indicate the recommended duration of antimicrobial therapy for patients with and without intravascular foreign bodies, respectively. Patients with PVE should be treated for 6 to 8 weeks in most instances whether or not the valve is removed. If microorganisms are culturable at the time of valve replacement, we recommend 6 to 8 additional weeks of therapy. In patients with pacemakers that are removed, 2 weeks of parenteral antibacterial therapy is recommended unless there is evidence of secondary native valve endocarditis, in which case the usual duration of treatment for native valve endocarditis is used after removal of the device. If treatment of pacemaker infection is attempted without removal of the device, 4 to 6 weeks is probably necessary as an initial trial. Patients with uncomplicated Hickman catheter, Broviac catheter, or Mediport-associated bacteremia are treated for 2 weeks if the device is not removed. Plastic intravenous line, steel needle, or scalp vein needle infections are treated at least 5 to 7 days after the device is removed. In the case of *S. aureus* bacteremia complicating peripheral venous lines, a careful search for metastatic spread is mandatory and 2 weeks' parenteral therapy is probably the minimal duration of therapy. Some authorities recommend additional oral therapy even in instances where there is no documented metastatic disease. In a patient with a peripheral device and ST, surgical venectomy is recommended.

CASE PRESENTATION

A 70-year-old white man was admitted to the coronary ICU because of dyspnea. The patient had had a mitral valve prosthesis implanted 18 months previously for mitral valve disease with mitral insufficiency. Because of a chronic dilated cardiomyopathy as a result of the longstanding mitral regurgitation, the patient's heart failure persisted after valve replacement and he was being managed with digitalis and diuretics. Two weeks prior to admission, he began to notice increasing shortness of breath, which progressed until the time of admission. His vital signs were unremarkable except for tachypnea and the physical examination confirmed acute pulmonary edema. He was managed in the ICU with diuretic therapy and careful monitoring.

Approximately 3 days after admission to the ICU, at a time when the patient was improving, an erythematous, painful cellulitis became apparent at the site of an intravenous catheter. The catheter was removed and cultured. *S. aureus* was recovered from the catheter tip as well as from blood cultures obtained simultaneously. The patient was begun on intravenous nafcillin, but 2 days later remained febrile. Blood cultures drawn at that time were also positive for *S. aureus*. A new mitral insufficiency murmur was heard. Cinefluoroscopic examination of the mitral valve prosthesis revealed >7° of motion during systole, a finding consistent with valve dehiscence. Cardiovascular surgeons were asked to see the patient but felt that he was too ill for valve replacement. The

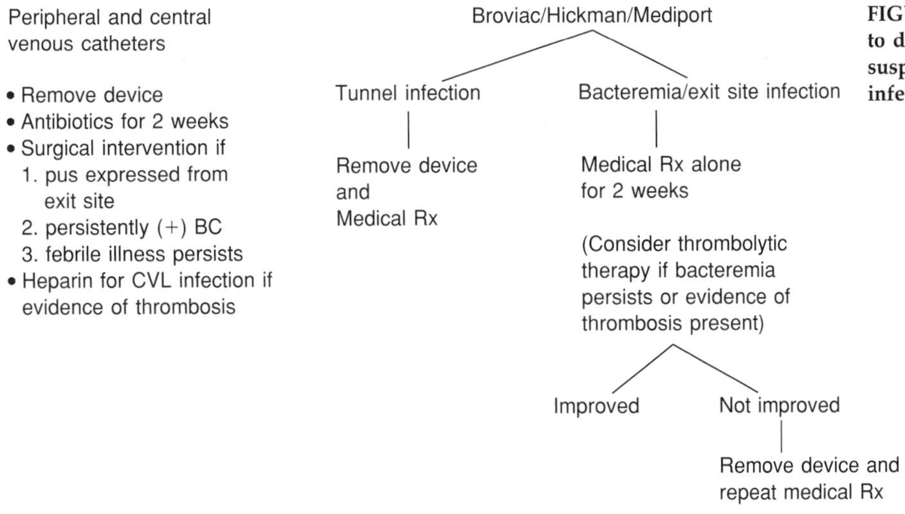

FIGURE 101-2 Algorithmic approach to diagnosis and management of suspected central vascular catheter infection.

patient died from persistent bacteremia and progressive heart failure on the tenth hospital day.

CASE DISCUSSION

This case is an example of an infected intravenous catheter leading to staphylococcal bacteremia with seeding of a prosthetic device. In this particular case, since the patient presented with worsening cardiac failure, it is also conceivable that he had IE at presentation. However, even in retrospect there was little to indicate this; there was no fever, leukocytosis, or new cardiac murmur at presentation. Had any of these been present, then blood cultures at the time of admission would have been mandatory.

Since the intravenous catheter had been inserted under usual sterile conditions and had been present for only 3 days, the resulting cellulitis and bacteremia must be regarded as simply one of the usual risks taken when using intravenous therapy. Even though the infected catheter was removed and the patient started on intravenous nafcillin as soon as the cellulitis was recognized, IE still resulted. Once IE was established, the infection pursued a course typical of the rapidly progressive and destructive infection produced by *S. aureus*.

The decision to withhold surgical treatment deserves comment. While the surgical opinion offered was that the patient was too sick to operate on, it is also true that in staphylococcal PVE complicated by valve dehiscence, cardiac failure, and uncontrolled infection, survival without surgery would be extremely unusual with each of these being an unequivocal indication for surgery in PVE (see Table 101-7). It remains possible that early surgical intervention with valve replacement might have led to a better outcome.

References

1. Dinubile MJ: Surgery in active endocarditis. Ann Intern Med 96:650, 1982.
2. Alsip SG, Blackstone EH, Kirk JW, et al: Indications for cardiac surgery in patients with active infective endocarditis. Am J Med 78(suppl 6B):138, 1985.
3. Feinsod FM, Norfleet RG, Hoehn JL: Mycotic aneurysm of the external iliac artery. A triad of clinical signs facilitating early diagnosis. JAMA 238(3):245, 1977.
4. Shaw RE: Cavernous sinus thrombophlebitis: A review. Br J Surg 40:40, 1952.
5. Lemierre A: On certain septicemias due to anaerobic organisms. Lancet 1:701, 1936.
6. Sinave CP, Hardy GJ, Fardy PW: The Lemierre syndrome: Suppurative thromophlebitis of the internal jugular vein secondary to oropharyngeal infection. Medicine 68(2):85, 1989.
7. Josey WF, Staggers SR: Heparin therapy in septic pelvic thrombophlebitis: A study of 46 cases. Am J Obstet Gynecol 120:228, 1974.
8. Munster AM: Septic thrombophlebitis: A surgical disorder. JAMA 230:1010, 1974.
9. Josey WE, Cook CC: Septic pelvic thrombophlebitis: Report of 17 patients treated with heparin. Obstet Gynecol 35(6):891, 1970.
10. Ivert TSA, Dismukes WE, Cobbs CG, et al: Prosthetic valve endocarditis. Circulation 69(2):223, 1984.
11. Karchmer AW, Dismukes WE, Buckley MJ, et al: Late prosthetic valve endocarditis: Clinical features influencing therapy. Am J Med 64:199, 1978.
12. Mayer KH, Schoenbaum SC: Evaluation and management of prosthetic valve endocarditis. Prog Cardiovasc Dis 25(1):43, 1982.
13. Bluhm G: Pacemaker infections in a clinical study with special reference to prophylactic use of some isoxozolyl penicillins. Acta Med Scand (suppl) 699:1, 1985.
14. Johnson RA, Zajae RA, Evans ME: Suppurative thrombophlebitis: Correlation between pathogen and underlying disease. Infect Control 7:582, 1986.
15. Berkowitz FE, Argent AC, Baise T: Suppurative thrombophlebitis: A serious nosocomial infection. Pediatr Infect Dis J 6(1):64, 1987.
16. O'Neill JA, Pruitt BA, Foley FD, et al: Suppurative thrombophlebitis—A lethal complication of intravenous therapy. J Trauma 8:250, 1968.
17. Stein J, Pruitt BA: Suppurative thrombophlebitis: A lethal iatrogenic disease. N Engl J Med 282:1452, 1970.
18. Pruitt BA, Stein J, Foley FD, et al: Intravenous therapy in burn patients. Suppurative thrombophlebitis and other life-threatening complications. Arch Surg 100:399, 1970.
19. Maki DG, Weis CE, Sarafin HW: A semiquantitative culture method for identifying intravenous-catheter-related infection. N Engl J Med 296(23):1305, 1977.
20. Brismar B, Hardstedt C, Molmborg AS: Bacteriology and phlebography in catheterization for parenteral nutrition. Acta Chir Scand 115, 1980.
21. Michel L, Marsh HM, McMichan JC, et al: Infection of pulmonary artery catheters in critically ill patients. JAMA 245(10):1032, 1981.
22. Katz JD, Cronau LH, Barash PG, et al: Pulmonary artery flow-guided catheters in the perioperative period: Indications and complications. JAMA 237(26):2832, 1977.
23. Jacobs MB, Yeager M: Thrombotic and infectious complications of Hickman-Broviac catheters. Arch Intern Med 144:1597, 1984.
24. Bozzetti F, Terno G, Bonfanti G, et al. Prevention and treatment of central venous catheter sepsis by exchange via a guidewire: A prospective controlled trial. Ann Surg 198:48, 1983.
25. Wolma FJ, Derrick JR, McCoy J: Management of infected arterial grafts. Am J Surg 126:798, 1973.
26. Goldstone J, Moore WS: Infection in vascular prostheses: Clinical manifestations and surgical management. Am J Surg 128:225, 1974.
27. Ilgenfritz FM, Jordan FT: Microbiological monitoring of aortic aneurysm wall and contents during aneurysmectomy. Arch Surg 123:506, 1988.
28. Willwerth BM, Waldhausen JA: Infection of arterial prostheses. Surg Gynecol Obstet 139:446, 1974.
29. Rubin RH, Fischman AJ, Callahan RJ, et al: ^{111}In-labeled nonspecific immunoglobulin scanning in the detection of focal infection. N Engl J Med 321:935, 1989.
30. Band JD, Maki DG: Infections caused by arterial catheters used for hemodynamic monitoring. Am J Med 67:735, 1979.
31. Weinstein RA, Stamm WE, Kramer L, et al: Pressure monitoring devices: Overlooked source of nosocomial infection. JAMA 236(8):936, 1976.

Chapter 102 PNEUMONIA

R. BRUCE LIGHT

KEY POINTS

- *Pneumonia is one of the leading causes of respiratory failure leading to intensive care unit (ICU) admission, and is by far the most common nosocomial infection in critically ill patients. Mortality exceeds 50 percent for severe community-acquired pneumonia requiring ICU admission, and varies from 30 to 60 percent in nosocomial cases.*
- *The initial approach to diagnostic testing and empiric therapy is guided by an assessment of the nature of the clinical pneumonia syndrome present. These include:*

  Community-acquired pneumonia
  - *Acute bacterial pneumonia*
  - *Atypical pneumonia syndrome*
  - *Aspiration pneumonia/lung abscess*
  - *Chronic pneumonia syndrome*

  Nosocomial pneumonia

  Pulmonary infiltrate in immunocompromised host
- *Investigation of acute pneumonia syndromes should always include a blood culture and Gram stain and culture of lower respiratory tract secretions. Smear and culture for* Legionella *spp. and serologic testing for other atypical pathogens should be done when atypical pneumonia features are present, and in otherwise undiagnosed cases of severe pneumonia.*
- *Fiberoptic bronchoscopy with quantitative bacteriology of a protected brush specimen or bronchoalveolar lavage specimen is the procedure of choice for diagnosis of acute community-acquired and nosocomial pneumonias that respond poorly to treatment and resist diagnosis by noninvasive means.*
- *Empiric intravenous antimicrobial therapy should be begun immediately in all critically ill patients with acute pneumonia syndromes. Antimicrobial coverage should include all pathogens of more than trivial probability and should always include* Streptococcus pneumoniae, Staphylococcus aureus, *and* Enterobacteriaceae. *In atypical cases or fulminant pneumonia of unknown cause, erythromycin should be added to cover* Legionella *spp.*
- *Empiric antimicrobial therapy can be initially withheld in less severely ill patients in whom the diagnosis of infectious pneumonia is in doubt and in patients with a chronic pneumonia syndrome, pending definitive diagnosis.*
- *Pulmonary infiltrates in an immunocompromised host may be due to any of the infectious agents affecting the normal population, to opportunistic infections, or to noninfectious processes. The required approach combines empiric therapy, selected on the basis of the particular infectious agents for which the patient is at special risk, with a timely stepwise diagnostic approach that moves from noninvasive testing to fiberoptic bronchoscopy to open lung biopsy at a rate determined by the rate of progression of the patient's undiagnosed pneumonia.*

Pneumonia remains the leading infectious cause of death in the developed world. It is also the most frequent infection leading to admission to most ICUs and, by far, the most important nosocomial infection complicating the treatment of patients admitted to ICUs for other problems. Between 20 and 30 percent of all patients in most general ICUs have pneumonia at some point in their hospital course. Nosocomial pneumonia is associated with a mortality rate of between 30 and 60 percent, depending on the virulence of the infectious organism and the underlying state of the patient.[1–5] Mortality for community-acquired pneumonia patients requiring ICU admission may be even higher—50 to 70 percent in different series.[6,7] A systematic approach and an aggressive attitude toward diagnosis and treatment of pneumonia is therefore fundamental to good critical care practice.

The discussion that follows categorizes the major pneumonia syndromes as **1.** community-acquired pneumonia, **2.** nosocomial pneumonia, and **3.** pulmonary infiltrates in the immunocompromised host. While the etiologies of pneumonia in these three categories overlap to some degree, the underlying pathogeneses, etiologic differential diagnoses, and approaches to empiric antimicrobial therapy differ considerably.

Community-Acquired Pneumonia

Pneumonia in patients presenting from outside of hospital can lead to ICU admission for a variety of reasons: hypoxemic or hypercapnic respiratory failure, depressed level of consciousness due to hypoxia or sepsis, or hypotension related to relative hypovolemia or septic shock. While supportive management for all of these problems is generally similar for all types of pneumonia, and the principles of circulatory and respiratory management are little different from those for shock and respiratory failure of other causes, there are major differences between the different forms of pneumonia in the approach to diagnosis and empiric antimicrobial therapy. The great majority of community-acquired pneumonias are due to common bacterial pathogens such as *Streptococcus pneumoniae, Staphylococcus aureus,* and *Haemophilus influenzae.* However, in all unselected series of pneumonia a significant minority of cases are caused by a large number of less common pathogens with widely differing antimicrobial susceptibilities,[6,8,9,10] nearly all of which can cause pneumonia of sufficient severity to require intensive care. Approximate percentages for the major causes of community-acquired pneumonia are shown in Table 102-1; the distribution of etiologies, however, varies widely among different geographic areas.

TABLE 102-1 Infectious Etiologic Agents Implicated in Severe Community-Acquired Pneumonia Requiring Intensive Care Support

Etiologic Agent	% of Cases Admitted*	
Acute bacterial pneumonia	65	
Streptococcus pneumoniae		40
Haemophilus influenzae		5
Staphylococcus aureus		10
Enterobacteriaceae		10
Atypical pneumonia	20	
Legionella pneumophila		10
Mycoplasma pneumoniae		5
Chlamydia psittaci		2
Coxiella burnetii		1
Viral		2
Aspiration pneumonia/lung abscess	10	
Chronic pneumonia syndrome	5	
Mycobacterium tuberculosis		3
Endemic dimorphic fungi		2

*The percentages shown are approximate only, based on published studies from different geographic locations and population bases. Because these percentages represent cases requiring hospital admission and ICU care, pneumonias that more commonly cause severe illness (*Staphylococcus aureus*, enteric gram-negative bacilli, *Legionella* spp. etc.) are over-represented compared to unselected community-acquired pneumonia. Also note that most published series include 20–50% for which no etiologic diagnosis was made and which are not included in this table.

PATHOGENESIS

Pathogenic mechanisms of pneumonia vary greatly among the different etiologic agents, depending on the relative virulence of the organism, which host defenses are most important in preventing infection with that organism, and the common route of entry of the organism into the lung. The three major routes of entry are *aspiration* of oropharyngeal or gastric contents into the lung, *inhalation* of aerosols or particles containing organisms, and *hematogenous* spread of organisms into the lung from another infected site.

Aspiration accounts for the vast majority of pulmonary infections, the particular clinical syndrome being determined by the quantity of material aspirated, the nature of the bacteria in the aspirated material, and the efficiency of the host's pulmonary defense mechanisms. The upper airway of normal human beings is frequently colonized by *Streptococcus pneumoniae, Haemophilus influenzae,* and, occasionally, *Staphylococcus aureus,* in addition to the normal microflora consisting of mixed aerobic and anaerobic bacteria. Colonization by enteric gram-negative bacilli, such as *Escherichia coli* or *Klebsiella pneumoniae,* is much less frequent, occurring in fewer than 1 percent of persons in the community at large—although it is more frequent in alcoholics, persons with poor oral hygiene, and the institutionalized elderly.[11,12] Even people who have normal upper airway reflexes aspirate small quantities of oropharyngeal material during sleep.[13] Normally the organisms so aspirated are cleared by the bronchial mucociliary clearance mechanism, while any residual debris is cleared by the phagocytic cells present in alveoli and on the bronchial mucosa. However, if the aspirate contains organisms with significant potential for virulence, and if the aspiration occurs in a human host with impaired pulmonary clearance mechanisms, the organism can proliferate in the pulmonary parenchyma and cause pneumonia. Pneumonia due to relatively high-grade pathogens such as *Streptococcus pneumoniae, Staphylococcus aureus,* and enteric gram-negative bacilli generally occurs as an acute infection without clinically obvious major aspiration (i.e., the aspiration is subclinical) but in patients with damaged or deficient host defenses. Examples include pneumonia following a viral respiratory infection (which impairs ciliary clearance mechanisms), pneumonia in alcoholics or others with intermittently depressed level of consciousness (greater opportunity for subclinical aspiration), and pneumonia in patients with impaired mucociliary clearance (chronic obstructive pulmonary disease [COPD], chronic bronchitis) or relative immunologic impairment (diabetes mellitus, uremia, hypogammaglobulinemia).

The normal microflora of the upper airway has limited virulence and therefore causes pulmonary infection mainly when aspiration is more florid, when the aspirated oropharyngeal material is present in greater quantity, or when there is severe local impairment of tracheobronchial clearance. Examples of these conditions include risk factors for major aspirations, such as uncontrolled epileptic seizures or abnormal motor control of the upper airway; periodontal disease; and bronchial obstruction due to foreign body aspiration or neoplasm. The infection produced by these relatively nonpathogenic bacteria is usually an indolent one producing a subacute, but necrotizing, pneumonia with eventual liquefaction of pulmonary parenchyma and abscess formation.

Because the numbers of microorganisms reaching the lung usually are extremely small when the route of entry is inhalation, only organisms that are highly efficient pathogens produce infection by this mechanism. This does not include most of the common bacterial pathogens, but does include most respiratory viruses, *Legionella* spp., *Mycoplasma pneumoniae, Chlamydia* spp., *Coxiella burnettii, Mycobacterium tuberculosis,* and most of the endemic fungal pneumonias. These pathogens are inhaled and deposited within alveoli, evading tracheobronchial mucociliary clearance. For the most part they share the ability either to resist phagocytosis or to survive intracellularly within phagocytes, requiring the development of a humoral and cell-mediated immune response to limit infection.

For hematogenous spread of infection to the lung the organisms must gain access to the venous circulation, which carries the organisms to the lung; there they lodge in the pulmonary microvasculature and proliferate. The pneumonia is usually diffuse or multinodular throughout both lung fields. In most cases either there is an established infection elsewhere, which is then carried to the lung, or organisms are injected directly into the blood stream, as in intravenous drug abusers and persons given contaminated intravenous fluid infusions. The common pathogens are *Staphylococcus aureus* and aerobic gram-negative bacilli such as *Pseudomonas aeruginosa*. A few rare pulmonary infections due to very virulent organisms that gain entry directly through damaged skin are also transmitted to the lung hematogenously; such pulmonary involvement may occur in tularemia, brucellosis, and melioidosis.

PATHOPHYSIOLOGY

The proliferation of microorganisms within the pulmonary parenchyma elicits the host's full acute inflammatory response, with exudation of protein-rich fluid and influx of large numbers of phagocytic cells into alveoli and airways. The local mechanical consequences of this include impaired distribution of ventilation and a decrease in lung compliance, both contributing to increased work of breathing and the symptom of dyspnea. Ventilation/perfusion ($\dot{V}/\dot{Q}$) mismatch is increased somewhat, particularly in predominantly interstitial pneumonias, but in most acute bacterial pneumonias the major mechanism for arterial hypoxemia is intrapulmonary shunt due to maintenance of pulmonary arterial blood flow to consolidated lung.[14,15] There is also evidence that metabolically active inflammatory cells within the consolidated lung consume oxygen, further reducing pulmonary venous oxygen content and arterial oxygenation.[14,16,17]

The local inflammatory response includes activation of mononuclear phagocytic cells, which are the main source of interleukin-1, cachectin, and other cytokines that act as hormones mediating the acute phase response. These effects result in fever, leukocytosis, and the many other metabolic changes of infection described in more detail in Chap. 55. In more severe cases, bacteremia or microbial antigenemia may activate the inflammatory response systemically, leading to frank septic shock (see Chap. 98).

CLINICAL AND RADIOGRAPHIC FEATURES

The basic features common to most forms of pneumonia include **1.** the presence of a systemic inflammatory response manifest as fever, elevation of the white blood cell count, and, in severe cases, other features of the sepsis syndrome (see Chap. 55); **2.** pulmonary symptoms such as cough, sputum production or hemoptysis, dyspnea, and pleuritic chest pain (if the pleura is involved); **3.** physical findings consistent with an inflammatory pulmonary parenchymal process, such as tachypnea, rales, or signs of consolidation (bronchial breathing, dullness to percussion, increased vocal fremitus over the consolidated lung region); **4.** evidence of abnormal lung function, such as arterial hypoxemia, and either hypocapnia (in a hyperventilating, dyspneic patient) or hypercapnia (in a patient with acute or chronic respiratory failure); and **5.** a radiographic pulmonary infiltrate consistent with pneumonia.

There are major differences in the time course, frequency, and pattern of all of these findings among the many forms of pneumonia caused by the multiplicity of etiologic agents. The author finds that a syndromic approach, based on the clinical, epidemiologic, and radiographic features—information generally available for most patients when they are initially seen—is a useful starting point in the assessment of pneumonia. These clinical syndromes include:

1. Acute bacterial pneumonia
2. Atypical pneumonia
3. Aspiration pneumonia
4. Chronic pneumonia

Not all patients' stories fit comfortably into these categories, but in most cases the attempt to categorize the syndrome is a useful guide to further investigation and selection of antimicrobial therapy.

ACUTE BACTERIAL PNEUMONIA SYNDROME

The typical history for community-acquired bacterial pneumonia is acute onset of fever, with chills or rigors, associated with dyspnea and a cough productive of purulent or bloody sputum—sometimes with pleuritic chest pain. Patients with no chronic underlying disease often report a preceding upper respiratory tract infection, but most pneumonias occur in the presence of a predisposing illness, such as alcohol abuse, chronic lung disease, chronic cardiac or renal failure, or malignancy. In more severely debilitated patients or the institutionalized elderly, specific history may be unavailable; new or worsened confusion and tachypnea noted by attendants is often the only history in these instances.

Physical examination reveals a tachypneic, apprehensive patient with tachycardia, fever, and diaphoresis. Crackles are heard over the involved lung fields on auscultation. There may be signs of pulmonary consolidation (bronchial breathing, dullness to percussion, increased tactile fremitus).

The chest radiograph will usually demonstrate air space consolidation with either a lobar or a bronchopneumonic pattern. A dense lobar infiltrate, particularly with an air bronchogram, very strongly suggests acute bacterial pneumonia (see Fig. 102-1); bronchopneumonic and patchy infiltrates are less specific. Interstitial infiltrates virtually exclude the usual bacterial pneumonias, although diffuse reticulonodular patterns or multicentric pneumonia sometimes occur with hematogenous pneumonia—e.g., in intravenous drug abusers (see Fig. 102-2).

The polymorphonuclear leukocyte count is usually elevated and shifted leftward, but may be depressed in severely ill patients with shock, or may even be within the normal range in debilitated or elderly patients.

ATYPICAL PNEUMONIA SYNDROME

The term *atypical pneumonia syndrome* was coined to describe the pneumonia syndrome caused by *Mycoplasma pneumoniae*, a pneumonia usually occurring in people in the second and third decades of life without major underlying disease predisposing to acute bacterial pneumonia. The clinical syndrome consists of a prodromal upper respiratory tract

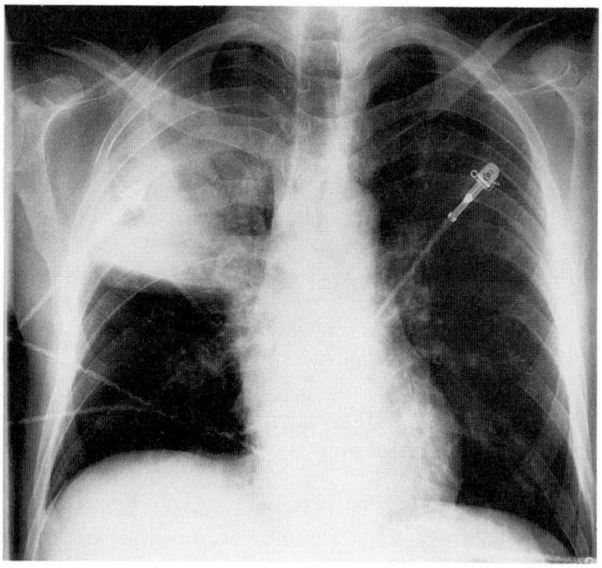

FIGURE 102-1 Dense localized infiltrate consistent with acute bacterial pneumonia. Note the air bronchogram, the downward-bulging transverse fissure and the cavitation within the infiltrate, suggesting necrotizing infection with a mucoid organism such as *Klebsiella pneumoniae*, which did prove to be the pathogen in this case.

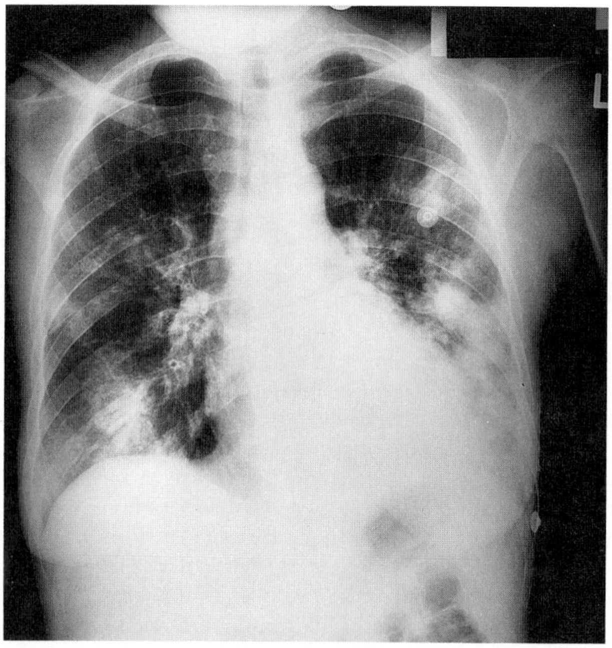

FIGURE 102-2 Multicentric hematogenous *Staphylococcus aureus* pneumonia in an intravenous drug abuser with severe cellulitis at an injection site. Note the multicentric regions of air space consolidation.

infection followed by an increasingly persistent dry cough associated with low-grade fever—frequently with extrapulmonary symptoms, such as diarrhea, myalgia, arthralgia, and skin rash. In severe cases the patient is tachypneic and cyanotic, but examination of the chest generally reveals only widespread crackles without signs of pulmonary consolidation. The pharynx may be red; bullous myringitis is occasionally present, and a rash is sometimes seen. The chest radiograph most typically shows a unilateral segmental infiltrate, but may show patchy or interstitial infiltrates bilaterally. In patients requiring intensive care for respiratory failure due to this infection, diffuse bilateral interstitial and alveolar infiltrates are usual (see Fig. 102-3). Other extrapulmonary features can also lead to the need for intensive care, particularly encephalomyelitis or myocarditis (manifest more commonly as prolonged Q-T interval or ventricular arrhythmias than as congestive heart failure). A moderately "septic" appearance and hemodynamic assessment is usual; however, frank septic shock is not, and hypotension is more often due to volume depletion.

In the more severe cases seen in the ICU the polymorphonuclear leukocyte count is elevated and shifted leftward. Hemolytic anemia may be present, because of the presence of high-titer cold agglutinins—which may also produce erroneous red cell indices or "error flags" on automated cell counters, because of red cell agglutination. Moderate elevation of hepatic transaminase levels is common. While most patients do not produce sputum, in those who do it is usually purulent both grossly and on microscopic examination; organisms are conspicuously absent on Gram stain.

Several other pulmonary infections that share "atypical" features with *Mycoplasma pneumoniae* pneumonia are usefully placed in this category (see Table 102-2). Although they vary considerably in many respects, they have in common several key features: **1.** epidemiologic clues to diagnosis different from usual acute bacterial pneumonia are often present; **2.** extrapulmonary features are common; **3.** diagnosis is primarily by serologic methods rather than direct smear or culture of respiratory specimens; and **4.** treatment with conventional antimicrobials for acute bacterial pneumonia is ineffective.

Legionnaire's Disease

While early descriptions of community-acquired Legionnaire's disease emphasized the many atypical features that set it apart from usual bacterial pneumonia,[18] we now

TABLE 102-2 Atypical Pneumonia Syndrome: Infectious Agents that May Produce Severe Pneumonia with an Atypical (Nonbacterial) Clinical Presentation

Mycoplasma pneumoniae
Legionella pneumophila
Chlamydia psittaci
Coxiella burnetii
Viral Pneumonia (influenza A & B, varicella-zoster, RSV, E-B virus, adenovirus)
Francisella tularensis
Pneumocystis carinii

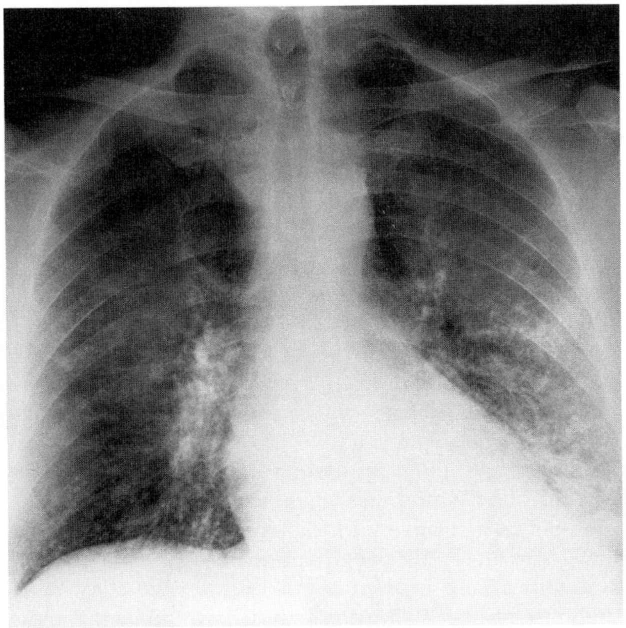

FIGURE 102-3 Diffuse interstitial and alveolar infiltrates in a patient with acute *Mycoplasma pneumoniae* pneumonia complicated by acute respiratory failure.

know that it can present in ways clinically indistinguishable from disease due to pneumococcus.[19] Clinical features that may suggest the diagnosis include dry cough, preceding diarrhea or other gastrointestinal (GI) symptoms, and encephalopathy not explained by other features of the illness. Epidemiologic clues include exposure to aerosols generated by cooling towers or to sites of soil excavation, underlying chronic lung disease, and immunologic impairment, particularly that due to corticosteroid therapy.[20] In patients requiring intensive care, the course is usually one of rapidly progressive pneumonia, sometimes with the aforementioned atypical features or extrapulmonary involvement, complicated by acute hypoxemic respiratory failure. The radiologic abnormalities are variable; most characteristic is peripheral rounded air space consolidation with ill-defined margins (see Fig. 102-4); however, patchy infiltration is also common.[21]

There is usually a leftward-shifted leukocytosis and, in severe cases, thrombocytopenia. Acute renal failure occurs occasionally, and an active urinary sediment is common. A variety of electrolyte abnormalities are seen, and elevated hepatic transaminase levels are common; however, these are not useful in differential diagnosis.

Chlamydia psittaci

The major epidemiologic clue to psittacosis is exposure to infected birds—often pets (budgerigars, etc., which may or may not be visibly ill) in homes or pet stores, or commercial birds, such as turkeys, which may shed the organism when

FIGURE 102-4 *a:* Ill-defined, large air space density in the left lower lobe of a patient with community-acquired *Legionella pneumophila* pneumonia. *b:* As often occurs in this disease, despite appropriate IV antimicrobial therapy, new infiltrates appeared and progressed in the right lung over the initial 24–48 h.

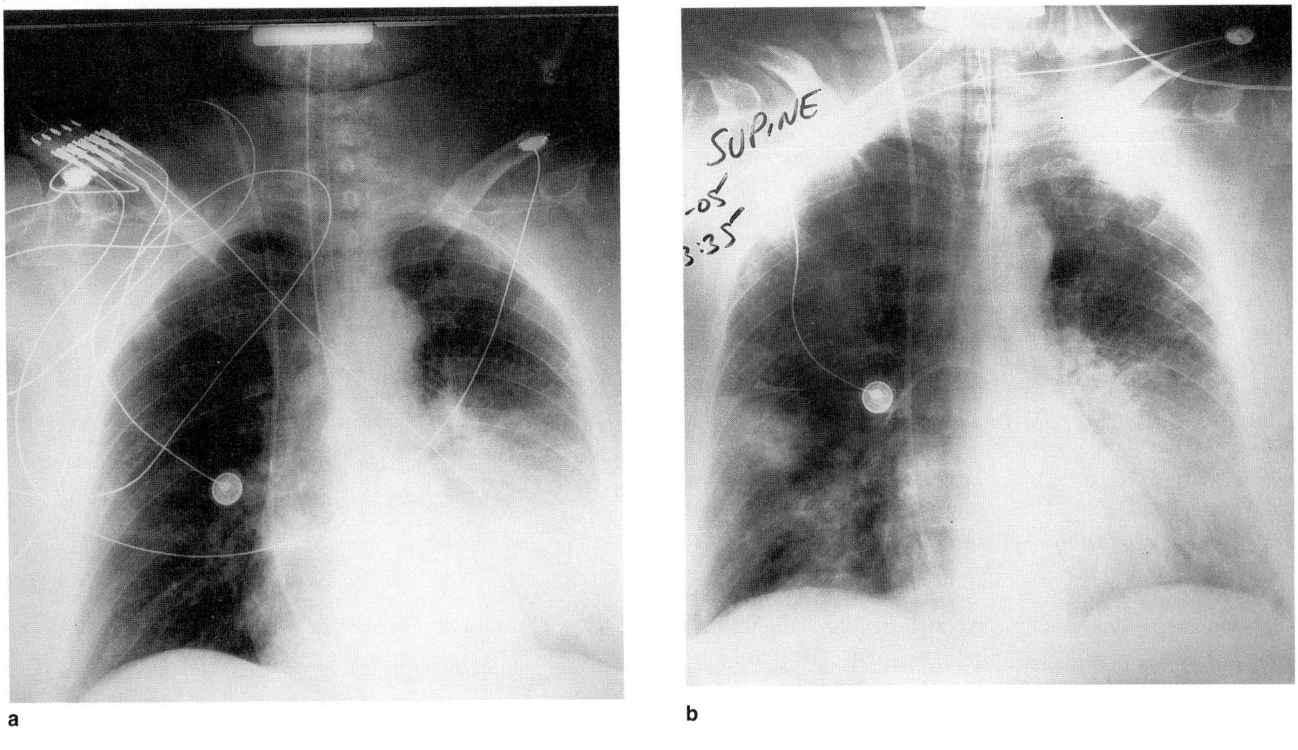

killed and eviscerated in processing plants. The pneumonia follows exposure by 1 to 2 weeks. High fever and a persistent dry cough are frequently associated with a variety of atypical features: myalgias, headache, GI symptoms, and occasionally a macular rash. As in other atypical pneumonias, crackles over involved lung regions, *without* signs of pulmonary consolidation, are usual. Extrapulmonary physical findings are not infrequent: hepatomegaly, splenomegaly, pleural and pericardial friction rubs, and—in the rare case with complicating endocarditis—pathologic cardiac murmurs. In severe cases dyspnea and hypoxia are prominent; encephalopathy, with confusion, obtundation, or even coma, may occur. The pulmonary infiltrate is generally a patchy infiltrate in all lung fields, with lower lobe predominance; but this is too variable to be a major differential point. Other routine laboratory studies are equally nonspecific, demonstrating only the usual hematologic and biochemical changes common in patients with serious infections.

Other *Chlamydia* species may also cause pneumonia (*Chlamydia pneumoniae* commonly, *Chlamydia trachomatis* rarely) but generally do not cause acute community-acquired pneumonia sufficiently severe to require intensive care, unless they occur in patients with severe underlying debility.

Q Fever Pneumonia

Coxiella burnetii is a rickettsia-like organism that is transmitted to human beings by inhalation of aerosols or suspended particulate matter from a wide variety of domestic and wild animals, including sheep, goats, cattle, domestic fowl, mice, rabbits, and parturient cats. Usually the infected animal is not ill. The illness begins with fever and chills, associated with myalgia and severe diffuse headache in most cases. A minority of persons with Q fever have GI symptoms. Cough is usually not severe, and is nonproductive; but in cases likely to be referred for intensive care, dyspnea and hypoxemia are prominent. Peripheral segmental infiltrates or rounded opacities are the most common radiographic findings, but no radiologic pattern excludes the diagnosis. Leukocytosis, elevated hepatic transaminase levels, and electrolyte disturbances are common but not specific.

Viral Pneumonia

In adults, the major viral causes of pneumonia that produce illnesses severe enough to lead to ICU admission are influenza viruses A and B. Rarely, severe pneumonia can be caused by respiratory syncytial virus (RSV) in the debilitated elderly or the immunocompromised; by varicella-zoster virus (VZ) in healthy adults with primary chicken pox, or secondary to disseminated herpes zoster in the immunocompromised; Epstein-Barr virus in non-immunocompromised adults with unusually severe infectious mononucleosis; or adenovirus in susceptible young adults in close contact (e.g., military recruits). Severe influenza occurs during epidemic periods of the year ("flu season," usually winter or early spring), particularly in non-immunized patients who are elderly or have significant underlying disease. A "flu-like" illness, with fever, myalgia, headache, sore throat, and harsh cough with burning retrosternal chest pain, is followed by increasing dyspnea and prostration. Physical findings include pharyngitis, crackles and wheezes in all lung fields, tachypnea, and cyanosis. The chest x-ray generally shows diffuse interstitial infiltrates (see Fig. 102-5) unless there is a complicating acute bacterial pneumonia as well—a common circumstance.

Pneumocystis carinii Pneumonia (PCP)

Although this infection has long been thought of primarily as an opportunistic pathogen of the severely immunocompromised, the recent increase in the prevalence of the human immunodeficiency virus (HIV) among otherwise previously well young adults has changed all that. PCP represents the initial presenting illness in as many as 65 percent of HIV-infected individuals developing AIDS. It presents as a relatively insidious illness characterized by low-grade fever, dry cough and increasing dyspnea, usually with diffuse interstitial infiltrates on the chest radiograph (see Chap. 100). Although PCP would be the immediate consideration with this presentation in a patient with established AIDS, the diagnosis is less obvious when a diagnosis of AIDS has not yet been made, particularly when the patient is not known to be at increased risk for HIV infection (high-risk sexual activity, prior transfusion with potentially HIV-contaminated blood products, illicit intravenous drug use, or exposure to multiply-used non-sterile needles, etc.). Accordingly, the diagnosis of PCP should be at least considered in cases of diffuse atypical pneumonia, the appropriate history taken to establish HIV infection risk, and other clinical features which may suggest HIV infection sought (see Chap. 100).

FIGURE 102-5 Diffuse interstitial infiltrates due to influenza A pneumonia in an elderly, but otherwise well, individual.

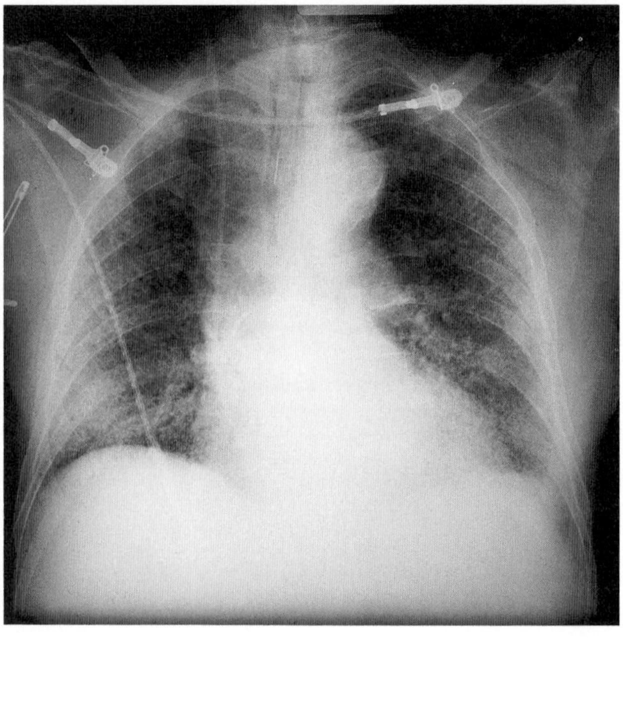

ASPIRATION PNEUMONIA SYNDROMES

Frank aspiration of oropharyngeal or gastric contents can produce any of a number of different clinical presentations, depending on the amount and nature of the material aspirated.[22] Large-particle aspiration causes airway obstruction with acute asphyxia (the "cafe coronary"), atelectasis, unilateral or localized hyperinflation, or—subacutely—bacterial pneumonia or lung abscess due to impaired mucociliary clearance in the airway obstructed by a foreign body. Small-particle or liquid aspiration usually causes a low-grade chemical pneumonitis, with a pulmonary infiltrate that clears over a few days without treatment. When the aspirated liquid is gastric acid a more severe chemical burn results, with rapid exudation of fluid into the lung. Consequences can include acute hypovolemic hypotension and, if the region of damaged lung is relatively large, acute hypoxemic respiratory failure.

In most cases of witnessed pulmonary aspiration the number and pathogenicity of aspirated bacteria is low, and no infection requiring immediate antimicrobial therapy is present. In addition, there is no evidence that administering antimicrobials at this point reduces the risk of subsequent infective pneumonia, which, when it occurs, becomes evident 3 days to 1 week after the episode of aspiration.[22,23] A major exception to this rule is aspiration of gastric contents which have become heavily contaminated with mixed enteric organisms. This occurs in the setting of bowel obstruction with accumulation of large amounts of feculent upper gastrointestinal fluid, which may be aspirated. It may also occur after upper abdominal surgery or in the presence of upper GI bleeding or paralytic ileus, particularly when there is absence of the normal low gastric pH on account of achlorhydria or treatment with antacids or histamine-blocking agents. Aspiration of feculent gastric contents can result in a fulminant necrotizing pneumonia due to mixed aerobic and anaerobic enteric bacteria. Prompt broad-spectrum antimicrobial therapy is mandatory.

A much more common syndrome related to pulmonary aspiration is pneumonia or lung abscess due to the predominantly anaerobic normal microflora of the mouth. Persons at particular risk are those who have a propensity toward aspiration because of continuously or intermittently depressed level of consciousness (alcohol or drug abuse, epileptic seizures, stupor or coma of any cause), an impaired swallowing mechanism (esophageal or neurologic disease), or an impairment of tracheobronchial clearance mechanisms (endobronchial lesion or foreign body). Following the aspiration episode, a low-grade pneumonia, manifest as cough, fever, and malaise, begins within a few days to 1 week. A chest radiograph at this time will usually reveal a patchy infiltrate, which may be unilateral or bilateral, occurring a little more commonly in the right lung and predominantly in lung zones that would be dependent in the supine patient (posterior segments of the upper and lower lobes). If the patient does not seek medical attention at this stage, the illness evolves over 1 to 4 weeks, with a persistent fever with night sweats; malaise; anorexia; and weight loss. The onset of production of large amounts of foul-smelling, watery sputum signals the development of a lung abscess, manifest on the chest radiograph as a cavity (or multiple smaller cavities), often with an air-fluid level, surrounded by a pulmonary infiltrate (see Fig. 102-6). Involvement of the pleura often results in empyema, evidenced by clinical examination and x-ray findings consistent with a pleural effusion related to the region of pulmonary consolidation. Most patients with this syndrome are subacutely, rather than acutely, ill, but very large empyema collections or relatively extensive pneumonia can produce respiratory failure. In particular, the onset of respiratory insufficiency due to reexpansion pulmonary edema after drainage of large empyemas may require intensive supportive therapy.

Leukocytosis may be mild or marked; many patients are anemic, especially those with a more protracted course. Electrolyte disturbances, particularly hyponatremia, are common. A variety of biochemical abnormalities related to lengthy illness and malnutrition may be present, including hypoalbuminemia, hypophosphatemia, and hypomagnesemia. None of these is particularly valuable in categorizing the syndrome.

CHRONIC PNEUMONIA SYNDROME

Pneumonia in intensive care practice is predominantly an acute problem; in a significant minority of cases, however, a chronic progressive pulmonary process presents with impending or established respiratory failure or with circulatory consequences of the inflammatory process. It is critically important to recognize the presentation as chronic, because the approaches to both diagnosis and empiric therapy are entirely different from those employed in patients with acute pneumonia syndromes. Because the differential diagnosis of this syndrome can be extremely large, including many relatively exotic infectious diseases as well as a number of noninfectious entities, a systematic and aggressive diagnostic approach is more rewarding than wide-spectrum empiric therapy, the initial approach generally adopted for acute pneumonias.

The usual definition of the syndrome is progressive pulmonary symptoms (cough, dyspnea, pain) for a period of 3 weeks to several months, associated with radiographic evidence of an inflammatory pulmonary parenchymal process. The patient generally appears chronically, rather than acutely, ill, and is often malnourished or cachectic. Hematologic and routine biochemical testing reveals the usual evidence of a long-standing inflammatory process: mild leukocytosis, lymphopenia, and anemia, more often with thrombocytosis than with thrombocytopenia; hypoalbuminemia; and multiple mild electrolyte abnormalities. Depending on the cause of the process and the specific other organs involved, a wide variety of other findings may be present.

DIAGNOSIS

Pneumonia is often an obvious diagnosis, particularly when respiratory symptoms associated with a new pulmonary infiltrate and systemic signs of infection occur in a pre-

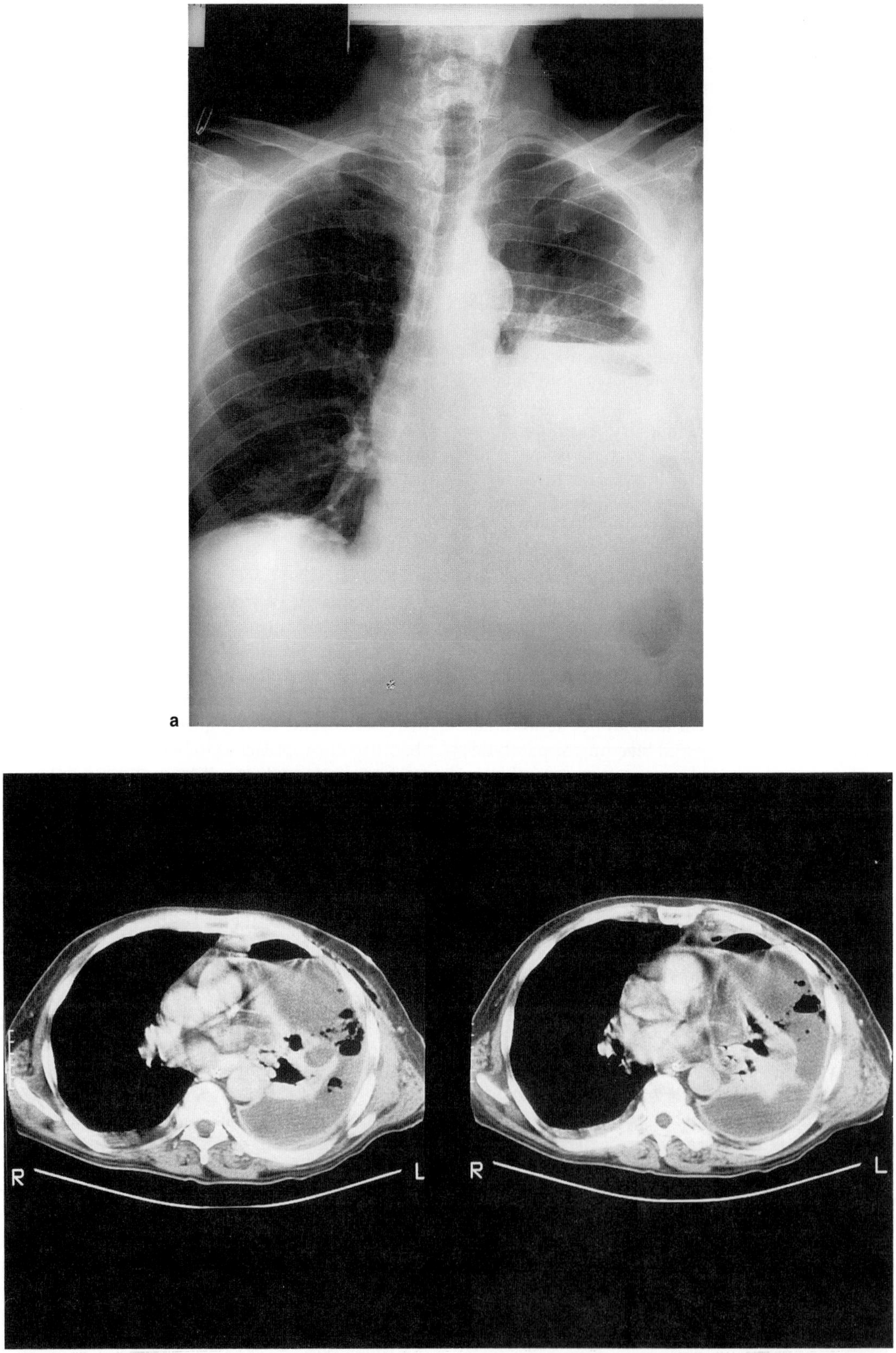

a

b

FIGURE 102-6 Aspiration-associated anaerobic pneumonia and empyema. *a:* The chest radiograph demonstrates multiple fluid levels with incompletely drained empyema fluid, and underlying atelectasis or consolidation. *b:* A CT scan of the thorax reveals the multiple loculations of empyema fluid and, predominantly, atelectasis of the underlying lung. This patient required decortication to achieve adequate drainage and reexpansion of the lung.

viously well patient. However, in patients with underlying lung or cardiac disease the diagnosis may be more difficult. Increased dyspnea and cough with low-grade fever in a patient with an underlying chronic lung disease associated with chronic chest radiograph abnormalities may be due to pneumonia, but may also represent a viral bronchitis, or even an infection or inflammatory process elsewhere in the body. In a patient with known congestive cardiac failure, respiratory deterioration with a moderate leukocytosis and asymmetric radiographic findings of pulmonary edema may be due simply to heart failure; but the radiographic asymmetry may be due to an underlying pneumonia. These less certain situations can be approached in either of two ways, depending on a clinical assessment of the relative likelihood that superimposed pneumonia is present, the severity of the illness, and the potential consequences of a wrong judgement. When pneumonia seems less likely and the patient is relatively stable, it is often reasonable to treat the underlying condition, withholding antimicrobial therapy with the expectation that the patient will improve without it. In the patient with congestive heart failure, steady clearing of the pulmonary edema, including the asymmetric region, without increasing systemic signs of infection helps to exclude the diagnosis of pneumonia; but failure of the local infiltrate to clear with diuresis, persistent productive cough, fever, and leukocytosis mandate further investigation and empiric treatment for pneumonia. In a more severely ill patient, in whom it is felt that any delay in treatment for pneumonia would adversely affect outcome, it is more prudent to initiate empiric antimicrobial therapy at the outset, and to stop it later if the clinical course does not support the initial impression of possible pneumonia.

Cough with sputum production, fever, and leukocytosis without a convincing pulmonary infiltrate on chest radiograph is usually due to viral bronchitis; or, in the patient with chronic lung disease, to an exacerbation of chronic bronchitis due to a viral infection or to increased endobronchial bacterial microflora. However, in occasional cases pneumonia may be present but not yet manifest on the radiograph. This is usually due to intravascular volume depletion's delaying the appearance of the infiltrate (see Fig. 102-7) or to a technically inadequate radiograph. Repeating the radiograph with better technique or after volume resuscitation will usually clarify these situations.

When one has made a clinical diagnosis of pneumonia, the next major issues are making an etiologic diagnosis and prescribing antimicrobial therapy. This is made more difficult by the fact that while most pneumonias are caused by a small number of common pathogens, a significant minority are caused by a wide range of less common pathogens that require differing approaches to investigation and treatment. The differential diagnosis also includes a large number of noninfectious causes of pulmonary infiltrates associated with an acute inflammatory response. For acute pneumonias these include pulmonary atelectasis, chemical pneumonitis from aspiration or toxic inhalation, pulmonary infarction from pulmonary embolism, lung contusion in trauma cases, and a range of immunologically mediated acute pneumonitis syndromes. Noninfectious causes of subacute and chronic pneumonias are even more common.

FIGURE 102-7 An example of delay of radiologic diagnosis of pneumonia attributable to volume depletion. These chest radiographs were obtained just 4 h apart. At the time the radiograph on the right was obtained, the patient had severe dyspnea, crackles in the right lung, and hypoxemia requiring urgent intubation; until then she had been treated vigorously with diuretics for presumed cardiac failure, although no radiologic evidence for this, and only equivocal clinical evidence, was present. After fluid resuscitation for hypotension (and demonstration of a low pulmonary wedge pressure), extensive pulmonary infiltrates quickly became evident in the right lung (left-hand panel). These were attributed to acute *Escherichia coli* nosocomial pneumonia.

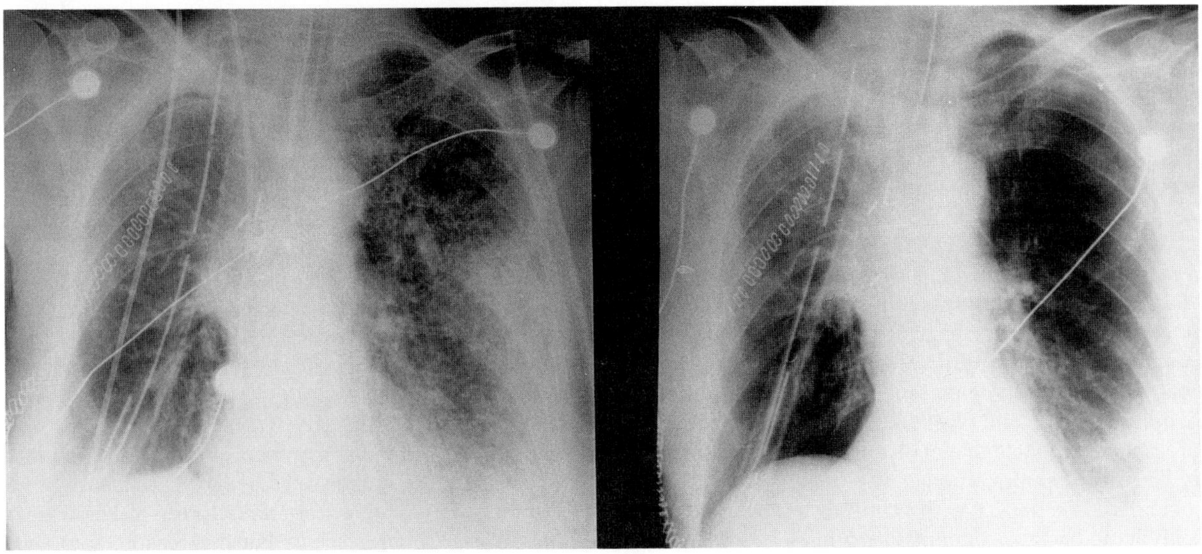

Many of these diagnoses can be suspected on the basis of the clinical context; but in severe cases otherwise consistent with an infectious etiology, it is usually best to proceed with investigation and initial empiric therapy for infection until such an etiology is excluded.

The first step in the diagnostic assessment is to try to categorize the pneumonia as one of the four syndromes listed under Clinical and Radiographic Features, above. The diagnostic and immediate therapeutic approach to each is different: Presumed acute bacterial pneumonia mandates empiric antibacterial therapy and investigation directed at isolating the offending bacterium; atypical pneumonia requires empiric therapy with entirely different antimicrobials for the predominantly nonbacterial pathogens and mainly serologic investigation for the involvement of these organisms; aspiration pneumonia/lung abscess is generally treated empirically with agents directed at the predominantly anaerobic normal oral microflora, with investigation aimed mainly at uncovering an underlying anatomic cause for the pneumonia; and, finally, the chronic pneumonia syndrome, which has an extremely large differential diagnosis including infectious and noninfectious entities, usually does not require empiric therapy but does mandate a systematic and often invasive approach to establishing the diagnosis.

ACUTE BACTERIAL PNEUMONIA SYNDROMES

All patients with a clinical diagnosis of pneumonia leading to ICU admission should have a blood culture and a Gram stain and culture of lower respiratory tract secretions. In non-intubated patients the immediately available lower respiratory tract sample is sputum, which is a mixture of materials from the lung and the upper respiratory tract and which has many well-known limitations in diagnosis: The patient may not be able to produce a good specimen; the specimen may contain potentially pathogenic organisms that come from the upper respiratory tract but are not the cause of the pneumonia; and contaminating organisms from the upper airway may overgrow the real pathogen on the culture plate and prevent its detection. Despite these problems, sputum examination remains a good place to start, mainly because in a significant minority of cases—and particularly in the most severe cases of bacterial pneumonia—the Gram stain, with subsequent confirmation by culture, can be diagnostic.

The utility of the Gram stain can be maximized by microscopic evaluation of the degree to which the sample is contaminated by upper respiratory secretions.[24] A specimen with large numbers of polymorphonuclear leukocytes (more than 25 per high-power field) and few large epithelial cells (fewer than 10 per hpf) is reasonably likely to represent a good-quality lower respiratory tract specimen and can usefully be examined further to determine the predominant bacterial morphotype present. Those with large numbers of epithelial cells and few leukocytes are mostly saliva; they are unlikely to yield useful diagnostic information and should be discarded after another and better specimen has been obtained. In a patient with a clinical syndrome consistent with acute bacterial pneumonia, a microscopically acceptable specimen that contains large numbers of bacteria of a single morphotype, and few bacteria of other types, is strong evidence that this is the cause of the pneumonia. A fairly definitive result such as this occurs in fewer than one-third of cases; however, it occurs more commonly in the most severe cases—those with extensive pneumonia due to *Streptococcus pneumoniae, Staphylococcus aureus,* and enteric facultatively aerobic gram-negative bacilli—and in cases where an endotracheal tube has been placed, permitting the collection of a less heavily contaminated lower respiratory tract specimen.

Preliminary results of blood and sputum cultures are usually available at 24 to 48 h. While a positive blood culture for a recognized pneumonia pathogen is definitive, positive sputum cultures must be interpreted in light of the original Gram stain of the specimen, bearing in mind that potential pathogens grown from a specimen that contained mainly upper respiratory tract material may not be the cause of the pneumonia.

In most cases of acute bacterial pneumonia the investigations noted above are all that is needed. Patients with severe bacterial pneumonia leading directly to ICU admission nearly always have positive blood or respiratory secretion cultures, while those that are less ill at the time of hospital admission usually improve with empiric antimicrobial therapy (whether or not a positive culture is obtained). Further investigation is needed in patients whose condition deteriorates or fails to improve and in whom the initial investigation has failed to provide an etiologic diagnosis to guide changes in therapy. The first step in a newly intubated patient is to repeat the Gram stain and culture of lower respiratory tract secretions. In deteriorating non-intubated pneumonia patients the procedure of choice is fiberoptic bronchoscopy using a protected brush to collect a specimen from the consolidated lung segment, or bronchoalveolar lavage of the region. Since many of these patients have significantly compromised respiratory function, the procedure should be performed by an experienced bronchoscopist with other personnel present to continually monitor the patient's respirations, blood pressure and pulse, and oxygenation. A pulse oximeter to monitor arterial oxygen saturation continuously is strongly advised. In patients who have significant arterial hypoxemia to begin with, it is usually best to insert an endotracheal tube and provide both supplemental oxygen and assisted ventilation to facilitate bronchoscopy. The specimens obtained should be Gram-stained and cultured quantitatively for conventional bacteria; the finding of more than 10^5 colony-forming units, per mL, of a recognized pathogen is diagnostic of infection.[25,26] The specimen should also be stained and cultured for *Legionella* spp. and sent for smear and culture for mycobacteria and fungi. In most cases it is also wise to do cytologic examination of the specimen (see Chap. 17 for details).

ATYPICAL PNEUMONIA SYNDROMES

Among the pathogens grouped as "atypical pneumonia," the one with the greatest propensity to present with an illness indistinguishable from usual acute bacterial pneumonia is *Legionella pneumophila*. For this reason, some hospital laboratories in areas of high prevalence routinely culture all submitted lower respiratory tract secretions for this organism. If this is not done routinely, it should be ordered specifically for all patients in whom an etiologic diagnosis is not immediately evident from the Gram stain. A direct fluorescent antibody stain for *Legionella* is also available. This can be done on sputum, endobronchial aspirates, or bronchoscopy specimens; but it must be remembered that, particularly with sputum, the sensitivity of the test is not high, and false-positives can result from cross reaction of the fluorescent antibody with other gram-negative species.

When atypical pneumonia is suspected on clinical grounds (see above), additional investigations should be ordered according to the epidemiologic features of the case. Acute and 14-day blood specimens for serologic examination will establish the diagnosis in *Mycoplasma pneumoniae, Chlamydia psittaci, Coxiella burnetii,* and influenza A and B infections. Marked elevation of serum cold agglutinins may help support an initial diagnosis of *Mycoplasma* infection, but low levels do occur with a variety of other infections as well. Serology is also valuable in diagnosing some rare bacterial infections that may mimic atypical pneumonia: *Francisella tularensis* pneumonia and brucellosis. Legionnaire's disease can be detected serologically as well, but because the antibody response to the organism may be slow, convalescent blood specimens should be drawn at 6 weeks as well as at 2 weeks.

Suspicion of *Pneumocystis carinii* pneumonia, generally based on the clinical and radiographic features and history of factors placing the patient at increased risk of HIV infection, should prompt early consideration of fiberoptic bronchoscopy with bronchoalveolar lavage. Serologic testing for HIV is usually also a part of this investigation.

ASPIRATION PNEUMONIA SYNDROMES

The approach to aspiration-associated acute bacterial pneumonia due to the usual pyogenic aerobic organisms is the same as that for pneumonia due to subclinical aspiration. However, most community-acquired aspiration pneumonias, and particularly those progressing to lung abscess, are caused by organisms constituting the normal flora of the oropharynx. These are predominantly anaerobic. Culture of sputum or endotracheal aspirates will always demonstrate some of these organisms, because of the inevitable contamination of these specimens with saliva; and the microbiology laboratory will report the result of aerobic cultures as containing "normal flora." Anaerobic culture of such specimens is not worthwhile, because they too would demonstrate "normal flora" in virtually all patients whether or not these organisms were pathogenically important. When the clinical presentation suggests aspiration pneumonia and conventional sputum or endobronchial aspirate cultures reveal only "normal flora," in most cases it is reasonable to make a clinical diagnosis of pneumonia due to mixed oropharyngeal anaerobic bacteria, and to treat accordingly. In less obvious cases, in which bronchoscopy is done to establish an etiologic diagnosis, it is reasonable to perform both aerobic and anaerobic cultures on protected brush or bronchoalveolar lavage specimens, because they are less likely to be contaminated by saliva. Bronchoscopy at some time in the treatment course is indicated in many patients with anaerobic pneumonia or lung abscess—particularly those with no clear-cut increased risk of significant aspiration—in order to exclude a predisposing endobronchial lesion.

CHRONIC PNEUMONIA SYNDROMES

Some of the many infectious and noninfectious diseases that may present as a chronic pneumonia syndrome are listed in Table 102-3. Patients with undiagnosed chronic pneumonia syndrome are less common in the ICU environment, because the chronicity of progressive symptoms usually leads patients to seek medical attention before intensive care is required. In those who do present already in respiratory failure there are usually extensive bilateral pulmonary infiltrates, and the radiologic pattern is sometimes helpful in suggesting the diagnosis. However, almost every "characteristic" radiologic pattern can be caused by several different disease processes. Among infectious causes, reactivating pulmonary fibrocaseous tuberculosis generally demonstrates characteristic upper lobe predominance, with cavities and pleural thickening and scarring; miliary tuberculosis and chronic hematogenous tuberculosis usually present with a diffuse miliary or reticulonodular pattern (see Chap. 109). But other infections can mimic upper lobe tuberculosis reactivation—particularly chronic necrotizing bacterial pneumonia (usually due to *Klebsiella pneumoniae*, occasionally to *Pseudomonas aeruginosa* or *Staphylococcus aureus*), melioidosis, and some fungal infections. A miliary

TABLE 102-3 Infectious and Noninfectious Etiologies of the Chronic Pneumonia Syndrome

Bacterial and mycobacterial infections
Tuberculosis
Chronic cavitary bacterial pneumonia (*Klebsiella pneumoniae, Pseudomonas aeruginosa,* others)
Actinomycosis
Nocardiosis
Melioidosis
Aspiration-induced anaerobic pneumonia and lung abscess
Fungal infections
Blastomycosis
Coccidiodomycosis
Paracoccidioidomycosis
Histoplasmosis
Cryptococcosis
Chronic necrotizing aspergillosis
Noninfectious causes
Systemic vasculitides
Malignancy
Interstitial pneumonitis (fibrosing alveolitis) and other idiopathic infiltrative pulmonary diseases
Bronchiolitis obliterans with organizing pneumonia (BOOP)
Lymphomatoid granulomatosis
Sarcoidosis
Toxic exposures and drug reactions

reticulonodular pattern can also be caused by disseminated fungal infections, malignancy, and noninfectious granulomatous diseases.

Lower respiratory tract secretions should be sent for routine Gram stain and culture for bacteria, and several specimens should be examined and cultured for mycobacteria and fungi. In patients who have spent time in the Far East, examination for ova and parasites should be done to exclude infection with *Paragonimus westermani*. Cytologic studies for malignancy should be done in most cases. If sputum or endobronchial secretions are used, these should be sent repeatedly (3 to 5 specimens) to maximize yield. In patients from whom satisfactory secretions cannot be obtained, fiberoptic bronchoscopy with bronchoalveolar lavage is most satisfactory.

Other noninvasive tests for infectious agents, such as serologic testing and skin tests, which are often of some diagnostic value in less severely ill patients, are not helpful in critically ill patients. On the other hand, for some of the noninfectious diseases—particularly systemic vasculitides and other immunologically mediated diseases with pulmonary involvement—testing for the specific autoantibodies associated with these syndromes can be very useful (see Chaps. 126 and 137).

Many of the causes of the chronic pneumonia syndrome also cause extrapulmonary manifestations. The nature of these associated findings is frequently of considerable help in suggesting the correct diagnosis; examples include skin or bone involvement with pulmonary blastomycosis, sinusitis with Wegener's granulomatosis, lymphocytic meningitis with coccidiodomycosis or tuberculosis, granulomatous oral lesions with paracoccidioidomycosis and glomerulonephritis with Goodpasture's syndrome and other immunologically mediated systemic diseases. When other organ systems are involved, it is often less risky for a patient with significantly compromised respiratory function to undergo biopsy of the extrapulmonary site of involvement rather than of the lung.

If a diagnosis is not promptly established by the initial examination of lower respiratory tract secretions, if the clinical constellation of findings is not characteristic enough to establish a diagnosis on these grounds, and if no extrapulmonary site of involvement suitable for biopsy is present, most critically ill patients with chronic pneumonia syndrome should go immediately to open lung biopsy. The range of potential diagnoses and risks associated with empiric therapy for most of the diagnostic entities is simply too great to attempt management without establishing a definitive diagnosis. In a patient who has reached a stage of the disease requiring intensive care, the necessary time for further observation of the course or attempts at empiric trials of therapy is lacking.

ANTIMICROBIAL THERAPY

BACTERIAL PNEUMONIA

When a specific etiologic diagnosis for bacterial pneumonia has been established on the basis of the blood culture or the respiratory tract secretion Gram stain and culture, antimicrobial therapy directed specifically at that pathogen can be prescribed (see Table 102-4). The regimens suggested here are applicable when in-vitro testing demonstrates that the organism is susceptible to the listed antimicrobial; resistant strains would require appropriate alternative therapy. However, in most cases of pneumonia the etiologic diagnosis is not available at the outset, and empiric therapy must be directed at the most probable bacterial etiologies in the particular patient being treated. Since patients requiring intensive care are usually in a relatively precarious state that makes the consequences of undertreatment unacceptable, it is a principle of therapy in this class of patient that antimicrobial treatment should be very conservative; that is, it should cover all etiologic possibilities except the quite remote ones. Some suggested empiric regimens are shown in Table 102-5.

ASPIRATION PNEUMONIA SYNDROMES

Most cases of witnessed or otherwise recent aspiration of oropharyngeal or gastric contents associated with a new pulmonary infiltrate represent an acute chemical pneumonitis rather than an infection. These will usually resolve without antimicrobial therapy, with deep breathing and coughing; or with chest physiotherapy when required. There is no convincing evidence that early administration of antimicrobials reduces later incidence of complicating bacterial pneumonia, although there is evidence that such treatment is often associated with subsequent pneumonia caused by a relatively antimicrobial-resistant organism.[22,23] Aspiration that has resulted in pneumonia, lung abscess, or empyema due to oropharyngeal anaerobic bacteria has usually been treated, at least initially, with penicillin. In a critically ill patient with this syndrome, however, therapy should usually begin with either penicillin 2 million U IV q 4 h and metronidazole 750 mg IV q 6 h, or clindamycin 900 mg q 8 h. Aspiration can also be complicated by later development of aerobic acute bacterial pneumonia; in these cases the regimens listed in Tables 102-4 and 102-5 apply. Much less commonly, aspiration can produce an acute, rapidly progressive necrotizing pneumonia. This infection usually involves both anaerobes and facultatively aerobic enteric gram-negative bacilli. The clinical context is often major aspiration in a patient without gastric acid (and therefore a large gastric bacterial population), or with an accumulation of feculent material in the stomach due to adynamic ileus, upper gastrointestinal bleeding, or bowel obstruction. Treatment must include adequate coverage for anaerobes, including *Bacteroides fragilis*, and aerobic gram-negative organisms. As in other acute gram-negative pneumonias, it is unwise to rely on an aminoglycoside alone for aerobic gram-negative coverage. Acceptable initial regimens include piperacillin 3 g IV q 4 h with gentamicin 1.5 mg/kg IV q 8 h, clindamycin 900 mg IV q 8 h with cefotaxime 2 g IV q 6 h, and imipenem 750 mg IV q 8 h with gentamicin 1.5 mg/kg IV q 8 h.

ATYPICAL PNEUMONIA

Erythromycin has become the drug of choice for the less severely ill patient with suspected atypical pneumonia.

TABLE 102-4 Antimicrobial Therapy for Acute Bacterial or Atypical Pneumonia of Known Etiology in Critically Ill Patients

Acute Bacterial Pneumonia	Recommended Antimicrobial Therapy*	Alternative Antimicrobial Agents
Streptococcus pneumoniae and other streptococci	Penicillin G 1 million U IV q 4 h	Cefazolin, clindamycin, or vancomycin
Staphylococcus aureus		
Methicillin-sensitive	Nafcillin 2 g IV q 4 h	Cefazolin, clindamycin, or vancomycin
Methicillin-resistant	Vancomycin 500 mg IV q 6 h	—
Haemophilus influenzae		
β-Lactamase–negative	Ampicillin 2 g IV q 6 h	Cefuroxime, co-trimoxazole
β-Lacatamase–positive	Cefuroxime 1.5 g IV q 8 h	Co-trimoxazole, chloramphenicol
Moraxella (Branhamella catarrhalis)	Cefuroxime 1.5 g IV q 8 h	Co-trimoxazole
Enterobacteriaceae (*Klebsiella, E. coli, Enterobacter* spp., etc.)	Cefotaxime 2 g IV q 6 h and gentamicin 1.5 mg/kg IV q 8 h	Imipenem, co-trimoxazole, ciprofloxacin
Pseudomonas aeruginosa	Piperacillin 3 g IV q 4 h and tobramycin 1.5 mg/kg IV q 8 h	Imipenem and tobramycin, ciprofloxacin
Anaerobic pneumonia/ lung abscess	Penicillin 2 million U IV q 4 h and metronidazole 750 mg IV q 8 h	Clindamycin, chloramphenicol
Legionella pneumophila	Erythromycin 1 g IV q 6 h and rifampin 600 mg IV daily	Co-trimoxazole and rifampin
Mycoplasma pneumoniae	Erythromycin 1 g IV q 6 h	Tetracycline
Chlamydia psittaci	Tetracycline 500 mg IV q 6 h	Erythromycin
Coxiella burnetii	Tetracycline 500 mg IV q 6 h ± rifampin 600 mg IV daily	Chloramphenicol
Yersinia pestis	Streptomycin 30 mg/kg IM OD	Chloramphenicol, tetracycline
Francisella tularensis	Gentamicin 1.5 mg/kg IV q 8 h	Chloramphenicol, tetracycline
Influenza A or RSV (severe with respiratory failure)	Ribavirin aerosol 1 g/day over 12–18 h	—
Varicella-zoster	Acyclovir 10 mg/kg IV q 8 h	

*Note that all drug dosages cited are for patients with normal renal function; dosage adjustment for renal insufficiency is required for a number of the agents listed. Monitoring of blood drug levels is strongly advised for the aminoglycosides, vancomycin, and chloramphenicol.

This is because it is effective against the two most common causes of the syndrome, *Mycoplasma pneumoniae* and *Legionella pneumophila*, and is also effective against the most common cause of community-acquired bacterial pneumonia, *Streptococcus pneumoniae*. In the critically ill patient, erythromycin 1 g IV q 6 h is given when the clinical presentation suggests the possibility of *Mycoplasma* or *Legionella* infection, and also in any case of severe pneumonia of unknown cause. In this patient population, treatment for bacterial pneumonia, as outlined above, should also be given until the diagnosis is established. Tetracycline is also effective against *Mycoplasma;* but it is not a drug of first choice for atypical pneumonia, because of limited activity against *Legionella*. However, when the clinical context suggests the possibility of infection due to *Coxiella burnetii* or *Chlamydia psittaci* tetracycline 500 mg IV q 6 h is the agent of choice. Rifampin 600 mg IV or PO should be added for patients with fulminant atypical pneumonia, and for patients with pneumonia due to *Legionella pneumophila* or Q fever that is responding poorly to the initial treatment regimen.

CHRONIC PNEUMONIA SYNDROME

Empiric therapy is seldom indicated for cases of chronic pneumonia syndrome. The pace of the illness is generally such that a delay of hours or a few days in establishing the diagnosis is not critical, and the large differential diagnosis makes empiric treatment selection difficult. One occasional exception to this rule is extensive pneumonitis or pulmonary hemorrhage in a patient with sufficient extrapulmonary evidence to support a clinical diagnosis of a systemic

TABLE 102-5 Empiric Antimicrobial Therapy for Critically Ill Patients with Acute Community-Acquired Pneumonia

Clinical Setting	Recommended Antimicrobial Therapy*	Alternative Agents
Acute bacterial pneumonia syndrome (including patients with COPD or alcohol abuse)	Cefuroxime 1.5 g IV q 8 h	3d-generation cephalosporin, co-trimoxazole
Institutionalized elderly	Cefotaxime 2 g IV q 6 h	Imipenem, co-trimoxazole
Atypical pneumonia syndrome	ADD TO ABOVE: Erythromycin 1 g IV q 6 h	—
Anaerobic aspiration pneumonia/lung abscess	Penicillin G 2 million U IV q 4 h and metronidazole 750 mg IV q 8 h	Clindamycin, imipenem, chloramphenicol
Fulminant pneumonia	Cefotaxime 2 g IV q 6 h and gentamicin 1.5 mg/kg IV q 8 h and erythromycin 1 g IV q 6 h	Imipenem and erythromycin

*Note that dosages cited are for patients with normal renal function; dosage adjustment for renal insufficiency is required for several of these agents. Monitoring of blood levels is strongly advised for aminoglycosides and chloramphenicol.

inflammatory disease such as lupus erythematosus, Goodpasture's syndrome, polyarteritis, or Wegener's granulomatosis (see Chap. 126 and 137). A full discussion of specific therapies for all of the infectious and noninfectious causes of the chronic pneumonia syndrome is beyond the scope of this chapter; however, treatment regimens for the more common fungal pneumonias are listed in Table 102-6, and therapy for tuberculosis is detailed in Chap. 109.

SUPPORTIVE THERAPY

In most aspects, supportive therapy for patients with pneumonia is similar to that for other patients with infections requiring intensive care. It is mainly in the approach to cardiovascular and respiratory supportive therapy that pneumonia differs to some degree. Most patients are intravascularly volume-depleted at presentation and require some intravenous volume expansion with crystalloid solutions. While it is imperative to ensure adequate circulating blood volume, it must also be borne in mind that pneumonia represents inflamed tissue within the lung, which is a site of localized "permeability edema" that may worsen with excessive volume expansion.[27] Septic pneumonia patients are also at increased risk of developing more generalized pulmonary edema (as in adult respiratory distress syndrome (ARDS)—see Chap. 54). Hypotension that does not respond to reasonable volume expansion is usually due to septic shock, the management of which is detailed in Chaps. 98 and 114.

TABLE 102-6 Treatment Regimens for Fungal Pneumonia Associated with Critical Illness in the Non-Immunocompromised Host

Etiologic Agent	Recommended Antimicrobial Therapy
Blastomyces dermatitidis	Amphotericin B 0.5–0.8 mg/kg IV OD to total dose of 2–2.5 g
Histoplasma capsulatum	as above
Coccidioides immitis (without CNS involvement)	Amphotericin B 0.5–0.8 mg/kg IV OD to total dose of 3–4 g
Cryptococcus neoformans	Amphotericin B 0.3–0.5 mg/kg IV OD and flucytosine 150 mg/kg daily in 4 divided doses, for 6 weeks

The most frequent reason for a patient with pneumonia to require intensive care is respiratory failure. An approach to management of this problem is detailed in Chaps. 127 and 128. In patients with chronic lung disease especially, the most usual form of respiratory failure is acute-on-chronic hypercapnic respiratory failure, requiring a period of mechanical ventilatory support until the infection is controlled. Hypoxemic respiratory failure is the more common reason for admission in patients without underlying chronic lung disease. Immediate management of the respiratory failure depends on the severity of the presentation. Some patients require immediate endotracheal intubation and ventilatory support. This includes all those with a depressed level of consciousness or an otherwise poorly protected airway; those with arterial hypoxemia not immediately reversible with oxygen administration, progressively increasing hypercarbia, or other signs of impending respiratory arrest (see Chap. 133); and those with hypotension not immediately reversible by volume expansion.

In the awake, hemodynamically stable patient with effective respirations but with significant arterial hypoxemia, the first step is oxygen administration. This should be given using a high-flow mask with a reservoir attached. Adequate arterial oxygenation (Pa_{O_2} greater than 60 mmHg and O_2 saturation greater than 90%) should then be established by repeating the arterial blood gas measurement or by pulse oximetry. However, because intrapulmonary shunt is the primary mechanism for hypoxemia in pneumonia, oxygen therapy is sometimes ineffective in correcting the hypoxemia. If the patient is otherwise stable, a trial of continuous positive airway pressure (CPAP) by face mask can be tried. If this does not correct the hypoxemia or if it is poorly tolerated because of discomfort produced by the mask, abdominal distention with gas, or increased difficulty in breathing—endotracheal intubation is indicated.

Some special considerations apply to the use of both CPAP and positive end-expiratory pressure (PEEP) therapy to improve oxygenation in patients with pneumonia. There is evidence both from animal models of pneumonia[28] and from studies of human beings[29] that gas exchange may not improve, or may even deteriorate, with PEEP. This is because the positive airway pressure, in addition to recruiting alveoli in consolidated lung and improving gas exchange, can compress alveolar blood vessels in relatively normal lung more than in consolidated lung, resulting in a redistribution of pulmonary blood flow away from normal lung and toward lung involved in the pneumonia. CPAP and PEEP are therefore used cautiously in this population, to ensure that when one of these techniques is used it will result in improved, rather than worsened arterial oxygenation. In patients with extremely poor arterial oxygenation that cannot be corrected by ventilation with oxygen and PEEP, the main remaining avenue of therapy is to attempt to optimize oxygen delivery by transfusing the patient with packed red blood cells to establish a hemoglobin level of about 12.0 g/dL and using careful infusion of volume expanders and vasoactive drugs to achieve a relatively high cardiac index (4 L/kg per m^2, or more). This approach should also involve putting the patient entirely to rest with sedation and controlled ventilation and controlling the body temperature with antipyretics, in order to minimize unnecessary oxygen consumption. These measures may permit maintenance of aerobic metabolism at arterial oxygen saturation values that would ordinarily be considered unacceptable. Careful monitoring of blood pH, mixed venous oxygen tension, serum lactate level, cardiac output, and organ system function are needed to ensure adequacy of oxygen delivery under these circumstances (see Chap. 128). Improvement of $\dot{V}/\dot{Q}$ matching by placing the patient with the "good" lung dependent does improve arterial oxygenation,[30] but it is relatively impractical to keep a patient in this position continuously. Improved arterial oxygenation, also due to improved ventilation/perfusion matching, has been reported after cyclooxygenase blockade with acetylsalicylic acid or indomethacin, but these therapies must still be regarded as experimental.[31,32] In occasional cases, particularly those with marked right-left asymmetry of disease and severe refractory hypoxemia, it may be reasonable to institute separate ventilation of the two lungs (see Chap. 10). This involves substantial risks associated with placement and maintenance of the tube, as well as problems with tracheobronchial toilet and the need for continuous deep sedation, but has been apparently lifesaving in some cases.[33]

Clearance of respiratory secretions is frequently a problem in critically ill patients with pneumonia. In many, the increased secretions and failure to clear them effectively may be the major factor mandating endotracheal intubation. Chest physiotherapy with posturing, percussion, and vibration has been shown to help mobilize secretions in this patient population,[34] and can improve gas exchange[35] and reduce atelectasis; therefore it is worth prescribing for most patients with pneumonia in critical care areas. Bronchoscopy has been used to facilitate secretion clearance as well, but there is little evidence of greater efficacy than is achieved with physiotherapy.

As in other critically ill patients, a multiplicity of metabolic, hematologic, and blood electrolyte abnormalities occur and may require correction. Especially important in the pneumonia patient is hyponatremia due to inappropriate vasopressin secretion, leading to impaired water excretion by the kidney; this is common and makes administration of hypotonic intravenous solutions potentially hazardous.[36] The correction of metabolic alkalosis of any cause may also be important, since this may be associated with an improvement in arterial oxygenation due to improved $\dot{V}/\dot{Q}$ matching related to potentiation of regional hypoxic pulmonary vasoconstriction.[37]

Nosocomial Pneumonia

Nosocomial pneumonia differs significantly from community-acquired pneumonia in aspects of pathogenesis and in the range of usual microbial pathogens seen. Approaches to diagnosis are generally similar to those for community-acquired pneumonia; however, the approach to antimicrobial therapy differs considerably, reflecting the different spectrum of pathogens. In addition, since nosocomial pneumonia by definition occurs in patients already under medical care for illnesses requiring hospitalization, the possibility of preventing its occurrence exists and is an important aspect of the day-to-day care of the critically ill patient.

PATHOGENESIS AND MICROBIOLOGY

The most common microbial causes of nosocomial pneumonia are listed in Table 102-7. This table has been constructed from data gathered in a number of surveys of different patient populations, and it must be emphasized that hospital populations are not identical with respect to risk for pneumonia caused by each of these pathogens. As in community-acquired pneumonia, the basic event leading to pneumonia is usually subclinical aspiration of oropharyngeal material, an event for which hospitalized patients are at increased risk on account of disease and medical intervention. These include depressed level of consciousness due to head injury, metabolic disease, or sedative and anesthetic drugs; and impaired laryngeal reflexes and esophageal sphincter function due to neurologic disease or instrumentation of the airway or esophagus. Although endotracheal intubation with a cuffed tube may prevent frank aspiration of gastric contents, it is no barrier to the minor degrees of aspiration required to transfer potential pathogens from the upper to the lower respiratory tract. The patient's ability to deal effectively with contamination of the lower respiratory tract may also be compromised. Mucociliary clearance may be impaired by damage to the tracheal mucosa by endotracheal tubes, metabolic disease, or drugs; and immunologic defenses may be impaired by underlying disease or by immunosuppressive therapy.

The explanation for the nature of the common pneumonia pathogens is the pattern of colonization of the upper airway, which determines which organisms gain access to the lung when aspiration occurs. In previously well patients admitted to ICUs with acute illness that compromises airway defenses, pneumonia in the few days following admission is most often due to organisms that are frequent colonizers of the upper airway in normal persons: *Staphylococcus aureus*, *Streptococcus pneumoniae*, and, to a lesser extent, *Haemophilus influenzae* and *Branhamella catarrhalis*.[38] Patients with underlying chronic lung disease are frequently colonized with these same pathogens, but non-typable *Haemophilus influenzae* and *Moraxella* (*Branhamella*) *catarrhalis* are more frequent in patients with underlying lung disease than in normal persons and therefore cause early nosocomial pneumonia more frequently in these patients.[39,40] Patients who have other chronic debilitating diseases, those who have been in the hospital for a number of days, and those who have been previously treated with antimicrobials are at greatly increased risk of having upper airway colonization and subsequent pneumonia due to enteric facultatively aerobic gram-negative bacilli such as *Klebsiella pneumoniae*, *Escherichia coli*, *Enterobacter* spp., and *Pseudomonas aeruginosa*.[1–5]

In patients already being treated in an ICU environment who are receiving mechanical ventilatory support, it is also known that the stomach is an important colonization reservoir leading to subsequent upper airway and endobronchial colonization and infection.[41] Neutralization of normal gastric acidity by antacids and histamine blockers given to prevent gastric erosion and bleeding contributes to this colonization by allowing organisms to survive and grow in the stomach.[42,43] Tube feeding also keeps stomach acid neutralized and permits gastric colonization.[44]

The only important nosocomial pathogen from the atypical pneumonia group is *Legionella pneumophila*. The pathogenesis of this infection in hospitalized patients is inhalation of aerosols containing the organism. In outbreak situations this can usually be traced to presence of the organism in hospital water supplies, with dissemination by showers and baths and the like, or to cooling tower contamination. Ground excavation near an outside air intake has also been implicated. It is likely that many hospitalized patients are exposed to *Legionella*, given its widespread presence in hospital water supplies; however, most cases continue to occur among the immunosuppressed hospitalized population, particularly those on corticosteroid treatment for prevention of organ transplant rejection.[20] This is presumably because a patient with suppressed cell-mediated immunity has a reduced capacity to clear even small inhaled inocula of this intracellular pathogen, with which a patient with intact cell-mediated immunity can cope easily.

TABLE 102-7 Bacterial Causes of Nosocomial Pneumonia in Patients Requiring Intensive Care

Organism	Frequency (% of Cases)*
Enterobacteriaceae (*Klebsiella*, *E. coli*, *Enterobacter*, *Proteus*, *Acinetobacter*, *Serratia*, etc.)	30–50
Staphylococcus aureus	10–30
Pseudomonas aeruginosa	10–20
Streptococci (including *Streptococcus pneumoniae*)	10–15
Legionella spp.	5–15
Haemophilus influenzae	2–10
Moraxella (*Branhamella*) *catarrhalis*	2–10
Anaerobes	2–5

*Ranges shown are derived from a number of studies from different geographic areas and different patient populations. Incidence of each infection varies greatly depending on local circumstances.

DIAGNOSIS

The clinical features and radiographic findings associated with nosocomial pneumonia are similar to those of community-acquired pneumonia, but may be greatly confounded by other disease processes common in hospitalized patients, particularly those in intensive care. The diagnosis is suggested by the presence of a pulmonary infiltrate consistent with pneumonia on chest radiograph, increased amount and purulence of lower respiratory tract secretions (sputum or endobronchial aspirates), deterioration in gas exchange and increased dyspnea, and an increase in temperature or leukocyte count. There are problems with both sensitivity and the specificity of this clinical definition. Postmortem studies of critically ill patients with extensive lung disease of other causes have indicated that many patients had clinically unsuspected bacterial pneumonia at the time of death.[45] On the other hand, several studies have indicated that in the general ICU patient population other processes, such as chemical pneumonitis due to aspiration, atelectasis, and purulent tracheobronchitis, can produce many or all of the same clinical findings as pneumonia, and that pneumonia can be significantly overdiagnosed in this context.[46]

One approach to establishing that pneumonia is present, and at the same time determining the causative agent, is fiber-optic bronchoscopy with protected brushing or bronchoalveolar lavage (BAL) of the suspect lung region coupled with quantitative bacteriology of the specimen obtained. In nonintubated patients culture of 10^5 colony-forming units per mL, and in intubated patients 10^3 colony-forming units per mL, of a particular pathogen from a telescoping plugged catheter (TPC) specimen vortexed in 1.0 mL of saline solution (both 10^3 and 10^5 colony-forming units per mL have been used for BAL specimens) establishes the diagnosis; counts below this level reliably exclude it.[25,26,46–48] However, a significant false-positive rate has been noted in some series,[48] and in others the TPC and BAL results have not agreed consistently.[47] It must also be pointed out that because the organism implicated in the pneumonia by bronchoscopy is usually also cultured from endobronchial aspirates, the main utility of bronchoscopic methods with quantitative bacteriology is in excluding pneumonia in a patient with clinical criteria for the diagnosis and positive conventional tracheobronchial cultures. However, in most cases with negative bronchoscopic cultures in these series the endobronchial aspirate cultures were also negative for convincing pathogens.[47] Therefore, while it can be concluded that these bronchoscopic methods are both sensitive and fairly specific for the diagnosis of bacterial pneumonia in hospitalized patients, it is not clear that all patients with suspected nosocomial pneumonia require bronchoscopy for diagnosis.

At present a careful clinical approach to the diagnosis of nosocomial pneumonia, both in ward patients and in intubated ICU patients, remains a reasonable first approach. Some patients have clinical presentations with such marked pyrexia, leukocytosis, deterioration in lung function, and advancing infiltrates that the diagnosis is not reasonably in question. It remains only to obtain the appropriate specimen to establish the etiology; in most such cases this is sputum or endobronchial aspirates and a blood culture. It is mainly in patients with less florid presentations, with marginal changes in the major diagnostic parameters and with infiltrates that could be either atelectasis or pneumonia, that the diagnosis is substantially in doubt. In these cases the usual best policy is to obtain endobronchial secretions for Gram stain and culture, provide chest physiotherapy and/or frequent posturing of the patient and endobronchial suctioning, and withhold antimicrobial treatment initially. Over the ensuing hours to days the result of the culture will become available; the additional information regarding the progress of the pulmonary process, the systemic inflammatory response without antimicrobial treatment, and the initial cultures will aid in making the judgement about whether an infection requiring antimicrobial treatment is present. In cases where substantial uncertainty remains, fiberoptic bronchoscopy, with a protected specimen brush, or BAL with quantitative bacteriology is a reasonable next step.

MANAGEMENT

The principles of supportive management for nosocomial pneumonia are identical to those outlined above for community-acquired pneumonia. However, there are several differences in antimicrobial therapy, because of the considerably different range of etiologic agents seen. Atypical pneumonia is much less common in hospitalized patients, and, when it occurs, is most often caused by *Legionella* spp. Bacterial pneumonias make up the vast majority of cases and, as noted above, are much more likely to be caused by *Staphylococcus aureus* or enteric gram-negative bacilli—and, in particular subgroups of patients, by relatively antimicrobial-resistant gram-negative bacilli. Suggested empiric antimicrobial regimens for hospital-acquired pneumonia are listed in Table 102-8, and those for specific proven pathogens in Table 102-4.

The pathogens causing hospital-acquired pneumonia are much more likely to cause a destructive necrotizing pneumonia than are the common community-acquired pathogens, and therefore are more likely to result in formation of abscesses and empyema, pneumothorax, and permanent fibrosis of involved lung regions. They also are more difficult to eradicate permanently from the lung with antimicrobial therapy. Accordingly, duration of antimicrobial therapy is generally longer—usually at least 3 weeks to as much as 6 or 8 weeks, depending on the initial response, presence of abscess cavities, and susceptibility of the organism. Treatment should always be parenteral initially, and for most enteric gram-negative organisms should usually include two different agents effective against the pathogen. After 10 to 14 days, if a good clinical response has been observed, completion of the treatment course with an appropriate oral agent is reasonable. Oral agents suitable for this use include co-trimoxazole, amoxicillin/clavulanic acid, and, for resistant organisms such as *Pseudomonas* spp., ciprofloxacin.

As in outpatients, pulmonary aspiration in hospital patients can result in a simple chemical pneumonitis or atelectasis that does not require antimicrobial therapy. Hospitalized patients are much more likely to have been receiving antimicrobial agents for other indications, agents that reduce gastric acidity, and are more likely to have conditions predisposing to development of large numbers of pathogenic bacteria in the oropharynx and the stomach (e.g., recent surgery, adynamic ileus, tube feeding, etc.). This increases the risk of an acute necrotizing bacterial pneumonia in these patients. Accordingly, if there is evidence to support an active infectious process following presumed or witnessed aspiration, antimicrobial therapy directed at both gastrointestinal anaerobes and relatively resistant enteric gram-negative bacilli should be given.

Antimicrobial selection for hospital-acquired pneumonia, to a much greater extent than that for community-acquired pneumonia, must be based on knowledge of which pathogens are prevalent in the environment in a particular hospital—or even in a particular unit within the hospital, since antimicrobial resistance patterns vary greatly in different locations. The recommendations listed in the tables must therefore be used with caution and with knowledge of local conditions.

PREVENTION

The considerable mortality associated with nosocomial pneumonia, particularly in critically ill patients, has led to much interest in developing methods to prevent these infections. Prevention would clearly depend on breaking the pathogenetic chain leading from colonization of the upper respiratory and gastrointestinal tract with potential pathogens to aspiration of these colonizers into the respiratory tract; establishment of lower respiratory tract colonization;

TABLE 102-8 Empiric Antimicrobial Therapy for Nosocomial Pneumonia Associated with Critical Illness

Clinical Setting	Recommended Antimicrobial Therapy*	Alternative Antimicrobial Therapy
Acute nosocomial pneumonia (postoperative or complicating medical illness)	Cefotaxime 2 g IV q 6 h and gentamicin 1.5 mg/kg IV q 8 h	Co-trimoxazole IV
Nosocomial pneumonia with increased risk of resistant aerobic gram-negatives (i.e., prior broad-spectrum antibiotics, acute leukemia, endemic resistant organisms, etc.)	Piperacillin 3 g IV q 4 h and gentamicin 1.5 mg/kg IV q 8 h	Imipenem, ciprofloxacin IV and ampicillin
Fulminant pneumonia following aspiration	Clindamycin 900 mg IV q 8 h and cefotaxime 2 g IV q 6 h	Clindamycin and co-trimoxazole IV, metronidazole and ampicillin and gentamicin
Suspect legionellosis (endemic, organ transplant, steroid use) or undiagnosed fulminant pneumonia	ADD Erythromycin 1 g IV q 6 h to one of above regimens	—

*Doses cited are for patients with normal renal function; dosage adjustments for renal insufficiency are required for a number of the listed agents. Monitoring of blood drug levels is strongly advised for aminoglycosides and choramphenicol.

and then failure of the pulmonary clearance mechanisms and immune system to contain the organism, leading to invasion of the pulmonary parenchyma. Attempts to break the chain at each of the points mentioned has been tried by various investigators, with limited success.

Prevention of upper airway and gastric colonization by enteric gram-negative bacilli has received the most attention in recent years. There is now reasonably compelling evidence that stomach acid helps minimize such colonization and that administration of H_2 blockers or antacids for prophylaxis against upper gastrointestinal bleeding increases it.[41–43] Use of sucralfate, an agent that protects the mucosa and prevents bleeding without increasing stomach pH, successfully preserves the antibacterial effects of stomach acidity, with a reduction in the rate of nosocomial pneumonia in some studies.[43] If bleeding prophylaxis is used, sucralfate may be preferable to an H_2 blocker or antacid, except in patients with known peptic ulcer disease.

Unfortunately, stomach acid is also neutralized by tube-feed preparations,[44] and all critically ill patients who can tolerate enteral feeding are fed enterally as early in their course as is practical. This limits the usefulness of sucralfate in this population. One suggested, but so far untested, approach is to place the feeding tube distal to the duodenum; advantages include reduced gastric emptying problems and aspiration risk, and maintenance of gastric acidity. However, in the absence of convincing data this cannot be strongly recommended, except for patients with substantial gastric emptying problems. Another suggested approach is administration of tube feeding intermittently rather than continuously, allowing gastric acidity to return during a 4- to 8-h interval of enteral feeding and reduce bacterial populations. This has been reported to reduce pneumonia rates in one study[49]—unfortunately, one with a relatively nonrigorous experimental design. Nevertheless, this is a relatively easy and inexpensive intervention based on tenable reasoning, and it may be prudent to use enteral feeding in this way while waiting for more definitive experimental work to be completed.

A variety of prophylactic antimicrobial regimens, both topical and systemic, have also been used to prevent colonization and pneumonia. Most of these studies have been able to demonstrate that colonization can indeed be limited and the rate of pneumonia in ICU patients reduced.[50–53] However, some authors have also found that universal use of a prophylactic agent eventually led to an increase in the rate of pneumonia due to bacteria that were highly antimicrobial-resistant and were associated with an increased mortality rate,[54] and in most other studies the reduced rate of pneumonia was not associated with a reduction in mortality or in use of ICU resources. This is important, since for most of these regimens the daily cost of prophylaxis greatly exceeds the cost of intravenous treatment for an established infection. For these reasons, none of the currently available prophylactic antimicrobial regimens can be recommended, except for short-term application to control an outbreak situation.[55]

Reducing the risk of aspiration in seriously ill patients involves mainly common-sense measures. For a non-intubated patient who has difficulty in swallowing or reduced level of consciousness, nursing the patient on his or her side with the head slightly down may be helpful. Frequent and careful suctioning and mouth care are also important. In patients with nasogastric tubes, and those with otherwise disturbed esophageal sphincter function, the upright position and sleeping with the head of the bed up reduces the risk of gastroesophageal reflux and aspiration. When the nasogastric tube is in place solely for feeding purposes, and it has been established that gastric emptying is adequate, the large-bore tube can be changed to a soft small-bore tube, which is less likely to interfere with the esophageal sphincter and is also more comfortable.

For intubated patients, exemplary nursing care can have a substantial role in reducing pneumonia risk. Good mouth care, suctioning of the oropharynx before endotracheal tube cuff deflation or before turning of the patient, no-touch sterile suctioning technique, careful monitoring of endotracheal tube cuff seal and pressure, and early detection and correction of gastroesophageal reflux problems are all measures that have yet to be studied in a systematic way with regard to infection rate; but they almost certainly account for much of the extremely wide variation in nosocomial pneumonia rates in different ICUs.

Pulmonary Infiltrates in the Immunocompromised Host

Immunocompromised patients with fever and new pulmonary infiltrates usually come to the attention of the intensive care physician when they develop imminent or established acute respiratory failure, or when a period of endotracheal intubation with mechanical ventilatory support is needed to facilitate an invasive diagnostic procedure. That both of these events occur relatively frequently says a great deal about the many special problems posed by this group of patients: the differential diagnosis of pulmonary inflammatory processes is wide, establishing a definitive diagnosis is often difficult, empiric antimicrobial therapy is often ineffective, and the patient's condition can deteriorate rapidly.

The nature of the immunologic abnormality that is present in a given case has a major bearing on the nature of the infective processes likely to be present. The major categories of immunologic abnormality include: **1.** Deficient humoral immunity. (These are patients with agammaglobulinemia and multiple myeloma or chronic lymphocytic leukemia [without intensive chemotherapy]). **2.** Deficient phagocytic cell function or number. (Patients with chemotherapy-induced granulocytopenia make up the majority in this group.) **3.** Deficient cell-mediated immune function. (This includes patients on corticosteroids or other immunosuppressive drugs for control of a variety of inflammatory diseases, control of rejection after organ transplantation, and less intensive chemotherapy for a variety of malignancies. It also includes acquired immunodeficiency syndrome (AIDS), which is discussed elsewhere in more detail in Chap. 100.) Many patients have mixed immune dysfunction, especially those on rigorous chemotherapeutic regimens for cancer. In Table 102-9 are listed the major pulmonary infections most strongly associated with each type of immune dysfunction.

CLINICAL FEATURES

In addition to the information regarding the nature of the immunodeficiency noted above, clues to the etiologic diagnosis may be available from details of the history and physical examination.

The timing of the onset of the illness, with respect to previous chemotherapy and duration of immunosuppression, is often very helpful. Following cytotoxic chemotherapy resulting in granulocytopenia, acute bacterial infections predominate in the first 2 to 3 weeks. Subsequently, especially with illnesses occurring in the face of broad-spectrum antimicrobial therapy, opportunistic fungal infections are

TABLE 102-9 The More Common Opportunistic Pulmonary Infections of the Immunocompromised Host

Predominant Immunodeficiency*	Most frequent Pulmonary Infections	Clinical Setting
Humoral immunodeficiency	Pyogenic bacterial pneumonias	Hypogammaglobulinemia Chronic lymphocytic leukemia Multiple myeloma
Phagocytic cell deficiency	Bacterial pneumonia Fungal pneumonias Aspergillosis Candidemia with pulmonary involvement Cryptococcosis	Chemotherapy-induced granulocytopenia Acute myelogenous leukemia
Cell-mediated immunodeficiency	*Pneumocystis carinii* pneumonia Legionellosis Nocardiosis CMV pneumonia Cryptococcosis Mycobacteriosis	Lymphoma or acute lymphocytic leukemia undergoing chemotherapy High-dose corticosteroid therapy Organ transplantation AIDS

*Note that these categories are not mutually exclusive. Bone marrow transplant recipients, for example, suffer mainly from bacterial and fungal infections associated with phagocytic cell deficits early after transplant; but after marrow recovery mainly develop infections related to chronic suppression of cell-mediated immunity.

increasingly common. After bone marrow and other transplantation procedures, bacterial infections also predominate early, with viral and fungal infections occurring weeks to months later. In this patient population cytomegalovirus (CMV) pneumonia is of particular importance, occurring with increased frequency in patients known to be CMV-seropositive; in bone marrow recipients CMV pneumonitis also frequently follows acute graft-versus-host disease.[56] Some noninfectious causes of pulmonary infiltrates also follow a somewhat predictable time course: radiation pneumonitis usually occurs 4 to 10 weeks after treatment; pulmonary edema due to acute toxic myocarditis after high-dose doxorubicin therapy usually occurs a few days to a few weeks after treatment, while the cardiomyopathy from both doxorubicin and daunorubicin is increasingly frequent with increasing cumulative dose; and interstitial pneumonitis due to bleomycin is common at cumulative doses of more than 450 U, although damaging pulmonary reactions to this cytotoxic drug and to others can occur with much lower doses.[57]

Although the pace at which the pulmonary process progresses is to some degree characteristic for each etiologic agent, this is highly variable and greatly dependent on the nature and severity of the underlying immunologic deficit. *Aspergillus* spp., for example, produce an indolent localized pneumonia in patients treated with immunosuppressive drugs and corticosteroids if phagocytic cell function is relatively preserved[58]; but in patients with severe combined immunodeficiency, and in some with long-term granulocytopenia from chemotherapy for myelogenous leukemia, the illness may be fulminant.[59] *Pneumocystis carinii* causes a severe, rapidly progressive diffuse pneumonia in patients with lymphoma or leukemia, but usually an insidious illness in those with AIDS. It is also worth bearing in mind that an apparent change in the pace of progression of disease may signal the presence of more than one process—e.g., an acute bacterial infection superimposed on a more slowly progressive disease, such as interstitial pneumonitis.

The physical examination is only occasionally revealing in this patient group. Examination of the chest almost never adds to the radiologic assessment. However, extrapulmonary findings may be very helpful in differential diagnosis as well as provide a potential alternative site for diagnostic testing. Central nervous system involvement (meningitis or encephalitis) points to systemic fungal infections, tuberculosis, bacteremia with metastatic foci, or disseminated viral infections, and mandates CT scanning of the brain followed by lumbar puncture. Disseminated aspergillus infection, in addition to involving the lung and brain, may produce necrotizing skin lesions. Ecthyma gangrenosum (see Plate 35) signals bacteremia—usually with *Pseudomonas aeruginosa,* and usually producing a diffuse multinodular pneumonia. Staphylococcal bacteremia and pneumonia may be associated with widespread cutaneous pustules, while the rare case of disseminated candidiasis with pulmonary involvement may be associated with a papular rash, myalgias, or "cotton wool" exudates on funduscopic examination.

RADIOGRAPHIC FEATURES

The chest x-ray appearance of the pulmonary infiltrate can be a useful guide to differential diagnosis, but is seldom specific enough to establish the diagnosis by itself. The most important differentiation to be made is whether the infiltrate is a localized process or a diffuse one.

Diffuse infiltrates, if they are of infectious origin, imply infection with a pathogen that has reached the lung hematogenously in large numbers or has spread rapidly along the respiratory mucosa early in the course of the infection. Examples include viral infections such as CMV, which is actually a systemic infection; hematogenous bacterial pneumonia (*Pseudomonas aeruginosa* most commonly); miliary or chronic hematogenous tuberculosis; and candidemia with secondary candidal pneumonitis. *Pneumocystis carinii* pneumonia (PCP) is typically a diffuse pneumonia as well (see Fig. 102-8), but for less well-understood reasons, since the pathogenesis of the infection remains relatively unclear. Noninfectious processes producing diffuse infiltrates are those in which the entire lung is exposed equally to the damaging agent, either through the bloodstream or via lymphatics (see Table 102-10). Examples include drug-associated lung injury, leukemic infiltration or lymphangitic carcinomatosis of the lung, and idiopathic interstitial pneumonitis.

Localized infiltrates due to infectious causes are generally those in which the organism has gained access to the lung by aspiration of oropharyngeal material or by inhalation of the pathogen. Examples include most cases of acute bacterial pneumonia, including nocardial pneumonia and *Legionella pneumophila* pneumonia, and most cases of opportunistic fungal pneumonia, such as those caused by *Aspergillus, Mucor,* and *Cryptococcus* spp. The appearance of the infiltrate sometimes provides a diagnostic clue. *Legionella pneumophila* often produces air space consolidation with a peripheral, ill-defined, rounded density, often with rapid subsequent progression (see Fig. 102-4).[21] Localized infiltrates due to aspergillus usually begin as enlarging nodular infiltrates or patchy bronchopneumonia in the granulocytopenic patient (see Fig. 102-9), with the development of central necrosis, cavitation, and "air crescent" signs associated with marrow recovery.[60] Hematogenous spread of infection causing a localized infiltrate also occurs occasionally, although this most often produces multiple locally spreading infiltrates that may not be anatomically adjacent; hematogenous bacterial infections, especially septic thromboemboli, are examples of this. The major noninfectious entities producing localized infiltrates are atelectasis, pulmonary embolism with infarction, and metastatic neoplastic disease.

APPROACH TO DIAGNOSIS AND MANAGEMENT

Diagnosis and management must be considered together, particularly for patients requiring support in an ICU. There are usually two phases to the approach. In the first phase a presumptive diagnosis or group of potential diagnoses is formulated and empiric therapy begun while relatively

TABLE 102-10 Noninfectious Causes of Pulmonary Infiltrates in the Immunocompromised Host and the Clinical Settings in Which They Are Most Frequently Seen

Noninfectious Diagnosis	Clinical Settings
Diffuse pulmonary infiltrates	
Interstitial pneumonitis due to cytotoxic drug therapy	Bleomycin (>150 mg total) or non-dose-related reaction to bleomycin, cyclophosphamide, methotrexate, and others
Cardiogenic pulmonary edema	Preexisting cardiac disease Chemotherapy with daunorubicin or doxorubicin
Lymphangitic carcinomatosis	Carcinoma poorly responsive to therapy
Leukemic infiltration of lung	Uncontrolled acute leukemia
Acute low-pressure pulmonary edema (diffuse alveolar damage)	Leukemic cell lysis after chemotherapy Leukoagglutination reaction following transfusion
Focal pulmonary infiltrates	
Pulmonary metastasis	Untreated or poorly responsive primary carcinoma
Atelectasis	Endobronchial lesion Chest wall or upper abdominal pain Depressed cough or respiration (narcotics)
Pulmonary infarction (pulmonary thromboembolism)	Hypercoagulable state due to carcinoma or paraproteinemia, immobility, venous obstruction
Radiation pneumonitis	Recent (4–12 weeks) radiotherapy with lung exposure

noninvasive diagnostic testing is implemented. Many patients respond to initial therapy or, if they do not, have a tenable diagnosis established on the basis of the initial investigation, leading to a revision of the initial therapeutic regimen. In the second phase, the onset of which is marked by the emerging opinion that a definitive diagnosis is necessary because of the failure of empiric therapy or the pace and severity of progression of disease, increasingly invasive diagnostic testing is performed until the diagnosis is established and definitive therapy begun. The key to appropriate management is to take great care neither to abandon the frequently correct initial diagnosis and treatment too soon (and thereby subjecting many patients to the risk of an unnecessary lung biopsy), nor to wait too long to proceed to a definitive diagnostic procedure (making the diagnosis too late to reverse the disease).

The major considerations governing the initial empiric antimicrobial approach and the selection of diagnostic procedures are **1.** the underlying disease, and the timing of the pulmonary process with respect to it; **2.** the presence of major clues to the diagnosis from the initial clincal evaluation; **3.** the radiologic pattern; and **4.** the physiologic stability of the patient and the rate of progression of the disease. Patients with pulmonary infiltrates that fit a commonly seen clinical and radiologic pattern quite well, and who are physiologically stable, can be treated empirically pending the results of initial diagnostic testing. Those who have a less certain clinical and radiologic pattern, and who are unstable or getting worse quickly, require prompt and definitive diagnostic testing.

Patients with diffuse infiltrates should receive intravenous wide-spectrum antimicrobials directed at hematogenous bacterial pneumonia, at least until initial culture results are available. Piperacillin 3 g IV q 4 h and gentamicin 1.5 mg/kg IV q 8 h is usually acceptable. Erythromycin 1 g IV q 6 h and co-trimoxazole (20 mg/kg trimethoprim with 100 mg/kg sulfamethoxazole per day in four divided doses) are given to cover *Pneumocystis carinii* (unless the patient has been receiving co-trimoxazole prophylaxis, in which case the diagnosis is essentially excluded), as well as most conventional bacteria and atypical pneumonia pathogens. Investigations include blood cultures, respiratory and stool specimens for viral culture, culture of blood for CMV, respiratory secretions for Gram stain and culture, and examination for acid-fast bacilli and fungi. In patients with predominant CMI impairment (lymphoma, steroid or immunosuppressive drug therapy, or organ transplant) who have not received co-trimoxazole and have negative blood

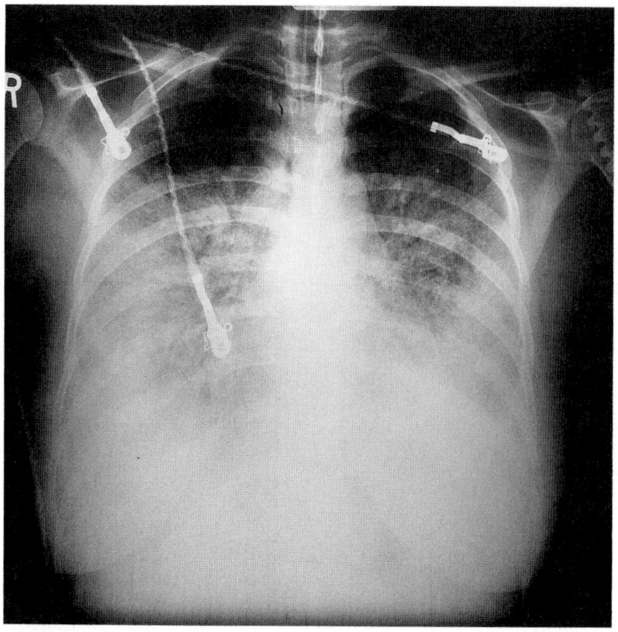

FIGURE 102-8 Severe *Pneumocystis carinii* pneumonia in a patient with acute myelogenous leukemia undergoing induction chemotherapy. Note the lower lobe and perihilar predominance of the mainly alveolar infiltrate, with areas of frank consolidation and, in the right lower lobe, an air bronchogram.

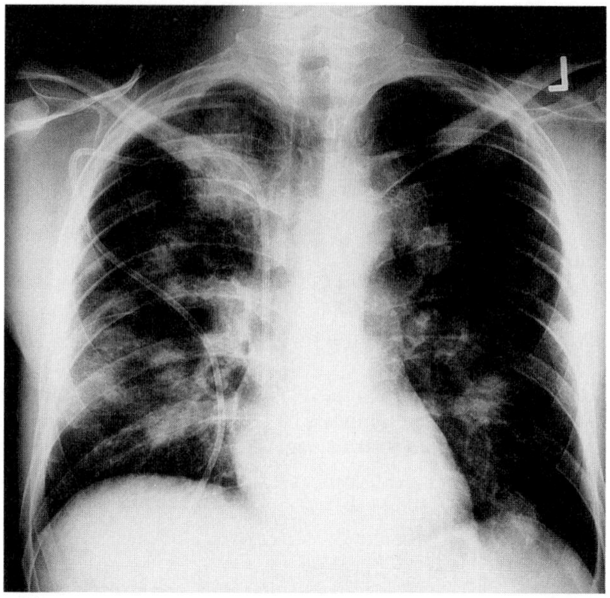

FIGURE 102-9 Pulmonary aspergillosis in a patient with acute myelogenous leukemia and protracted granulocytopenia. Note the multiple dense alveolar infiltrates forming large expanding nodules.

cultures, PCP is usually the leading infectious possibility, followed by CMV. Unlike what is seen in AIDS patients with PCP, the number of organisms in the lung is not large; hence sputum examination for the organism is not useful. Early bronchoscopy with BAL or a protected specimen brush is advised. The specimen obtained should be examined for the full range of pathogens mentioned above. Cytologic examination of cells for evidence of CMV, and culture of respiratory secretions and blood for CMV, will help in establishing that diagnosis. Bronchoscopic methods have excellent diagnostic yield for infectious diagnoses in this setting, but are much less useful in defining noninfectious etiologies for diffuse infiltrates.[61,62] Accordingly, for patients who are at lesser risk for PCP and CMV, for those in whom the initial investigation excludes these possibilities, and for those with rapidly progressive diffuse lung disease, open lung biopsy should be considered. Open lung biopsy remains controversial in this setting; although a definitive diagnosis can be established in most patients and therapy adjusted appropriately, in severely ill patients this most often does not lead to survival, because of current therapeutic limitations[63]; further, significant morbidity due to the procedure is not uncommon.[64] Nevertheless, it is the author's opinion that in selected cases open biopsy can be very useful, offering the best chance of survival to the minority of patients with reversible disease. In the face of progressing disease, if a biopsy is to be done it is important to make the decision to proceed before the patient has progressed to frank respiratory failure.

The diagnosis of localized pulmonary infiltrates due to conventional bacterial pneumonia can usually be established with sufficient certainty by blood cultures, respiratory secretion Gram stain and culture, direct fluorescent antibody (DFA) staining and culture of respiratory secretions for *Legionella pneumophila,* and the clinical response to empiric antimicrobial therapy—usually piperacillin 3 g IV q 4 h and gentamicin 1.5 mg/kg IV q 8 h, unless it is known that the patient is colonized with a pathogen resistant to these antimicrobials. Consideration should be given to adding erythromycin 1 g IV q 6 h for legionellosis in all cases where the pneumonia has atypical features, especially in hospitals where cases are being seen. If the diagnosis is not immediately forthcoming or the patient does not respond promptly to empiric therapy, bronchoscopy should be done and BAL or protected brush specimens sent for examination for bacteria, acid-fast bacilli; DFA and culture for *Legionella;* fungal elements; and cytologic examination. If there is no contraindication (see Chap. 17), transbronchial biopsy may increase the yield for invasive fungal infection and for malignancy. However, as many as 50 percent of cases of invasive fungal infection may not be detected by bronchoscopic methods and require open lung biopsy for diagnosis.[65] Culture of aspergilli from nasal scrapings or sputum can be helpful in this regard. Though culture of aspergilli is not indicative of disease in normal persons, in severely immunocompromised patients with granulocytopenia and acute leukemia such positive cultures are strongly associated with invasive disease.[66,67]

When the diagnosis has been established definitive therapy is begun, and other agents started empirically are discontinued unless other indications for their use remain. A discussion of the full range of therapies for noninfectious etiologies of pulmonary infiltrates is beyond the scope of this chapter; drug regimens for the major infectious causes of opportunistic pneumonia are shown in Table 102-11.

CASE PRESENTATION

Mr. R.S., a 55-year-old man with a 5-year history of chronic lymphocytic leukemia under good control with chronic prednisone and chlorambucil therapy, presented to hospital with fever, malaise, and cough productive of large amounts of yellow sputum. He said that he had initially developed an upper respiratory tract infection with a mild cough about 4 weeks earlier. Oral erythromycin was prescribed for 7 days; he improved and was well for about a week. His cough then returned and was associated with moderate dyspnea and low-grade fever. He took oral erythromycin for a further 5 days without obvious effect, and therefore discontinued it. Over the next 4 days he became increasingly febrile and dyspneic and began to cough up increasing amounts of colored sputum.

He was admitted and started on intravenous co-trimoxazole (20 mg/kg trimethoprim and 100 mg/kg sulfamethoxazole per day). Physical examination showed him to be diaphoretic and dyspneic, using accessory muscles of respiration. There were no extrapulmonary findings. The white cell count was elevated, at 15×10^9 cells per L, and shifted leftward. The chest radiograph demonstrated a diffuse reticular infiltrate with a small nodular component most prominent in the right lower lobe. Sputum Gram stain showed heavy pus but no organisms. Examination of sputum for acid-fast bacilli and fungal elements was negative. Arterial blood gases showed a respiratory alkalosis and marginally acceptable arterial oxygenation with the patient breathing oxygen through a face mask at 10 L/min.

A bronchoscopy with BAL done on the second hospital day was unrevealing, showing the same results as the sputum study. Erythromycin 1 g IV q 6 h was added on the fourth hospital day; however, by this time the radiograph showed worsening infiltrates. The patient now had an arterial P_{O_2} of only 48 mmHg with maximum deliverable oxygen by face mask and nasal prongs. The patient was electively intubated awake with topical upper airway anesthesia, and mechanical ventilation with 5 cm H_2O PEEP instituted, achieving a P_{O_2} of 75 mmHg at an F_{IO_2} of 0.6. Rifampin 600 mg IV OD was added to the antimicrobial regimen. An open lung biopsy was then performed. The lung histology revealed sheets of polymorphonuclear leukocytes in alveoli consistent with an acute infection, but no organisms were seen, despite examination for bacteria, acid-fast bacilli, fungi, and *Pneumocystis carinii*.

Supportive respiratory therapy and antimicrobials were continued. Over the next 5 days the patient gradually improved, with a fall in temperature to the normal range, gradual improvement in gas exchange, and clearing of the pulmonary infiltrates. With PCP and bacterial pathogens excluded by the biopsy, co-trimoxazole was discontinued. The patient was extubated 8 days after the biopsy and sent to the ward the following day, where he convalesced uneventfully. An IgM titer against *Myco-*

TABLE 102-11 Antimicrobial Therapy for Opportunistic Lung Infections in Critically Ill Immunocompromised Patients

Pulmonary Infection*	Antimicrobial Regimen
Pneumocystis carinii pneumonia	Co-trimoxazole 5 mg/kg TMP† and 25 mg/kg SMX† IV q 6 h *or* Pentamidine 4 mg/kg IV q 24 h
Nocardia asteroides pneumonia or abscess	Sulfonamide 2 g q 6 h (IV if available) *or* Co-trimoxazole (as above) ±amikacin 5 mg/kg IV q 8 h
Aspergillosis	Amphotericin B 0.6–1.0 mg/kg IV q 24 h to total dose of 2.0 g *and,* if permitted by degree of myelosuppression, flucytosine 150 mg/kg IV or PO per day initially, reducing dose to achieve 1 h pre-dose blood levels of 50–75 μg/mL
Candidal pneumonia due to associated candidemia	Amphotericin B 0.3–0.6 mg/kg IV q 24 h *or* Fluconazole 400 mg IV q 24 h
CMV pneumonia	Ganciclovir 2.5 mg/kg IV q 8 h *and* CMV immune globulin 400–500 mg/kg on alternate days (4–10 doses)
Varicella-zoster, disseminated, with pneumonia	Acyclovir 10 mg/kg IV q 8 h

*Treatment regimens for the more common acute bacterial pneumonias are shown in Tables 102-4 and 102-6, and for the dimorphic fungi in Table 102-6. Antituberculous drug regimens are given in Chap. 109.
†TMP = trimethoprim, SMX = sulfamethoxazole.

plasma pneumoniae, consistent with recent acute infection, was reported the day after transfer to the ward. A 3-week course of erythromycin was completed with oral therapy at home.

CASE DISCUSSION

This case exemplifies many of the dilemmas facing the intensivist in the diagnosis and therapy of severe life-threatening pneumonia. Although this patient was immunocompromised to a degree, he ultimately proved to have an unusually severe case of a common community-acquired atypical pneumonia. Although this possibility had been dismissed at the time of his hospital admission, it was later reconsidered, on the basis of the evidence that he had apparently responded—at least transiently—to oral erythromycin; the radiologic pattern, which suggested an atypical pneumonia; and the presence of copious amounts of purulent sputum without organisms on Gram stain.

The question facing the medical staff at the end of the first 4 days in hospital, at which time the patient had life-threatening respiratory failure, was whether simply to continue with empiric antimicrobial therapy, on the assumption that he had erythromycin-responsive disease that had worsened because the drug had not been given, or to proceed to a definitive biopsy procedure to ensure that other treatable diagnoses were not missed before the patient became irretrievably ill. In a non-immunocompromised patient atypical pneumonia would be the overwhelmingly probable diagnosis, and in retrospect it would appear that since this was the diagnosis the biopsy was unnecessary. In this patient, however, undiagnosed tuberculosis, disseminated fungal disease, and idiopathic or drug-associated interstitial pneumonitis were also considerations, in view of his underlying disease. The biopsy therefore served the purpose of excluding other potentially treatable diagnoses, limiting the necessary breath of empiric treatment.

Some errors in management in this case are worth pointing out. First, if the diagnosis of community-acquired atypical pneumonia had been more strongly considered at the time of hospital admission and erythromycin given, the patient might have improved and been spared the rigors of his subsequent hospital course. Even in immunocompromised patients, the first pathogens to consider are those common in the normal population. With predominantly diffuse infiltrates (and the other "atypical pneumonia" features) the addition of erythromycin to the empiric antimicrobial regimen should always be considered. Second, since this patient had been ill about 3 weeks prior to his hospital admission, it is conceivable that if a convalescent serum for atypical pneumonia pathogens had been sent and tested immediately at the time of admission the diagnosis could have been established noninvasively much earlier.

The more exemplary features of the case are that after initial noninvasive diagnostic testing and empiric treatment proved unsuccessful, the patient underwent bronchoscopy and then open lung biopsy in rapid succession, each accomplished before the patient became "too sick" to proceed. Together with the escalating diagnostic testing, empiric therapy was widened to include the major conventional pneumonia pathogens and atypical pneumonia pathogens. As is usual practice, empiric therapy for tuberculosis, fungi, and other exotic pathogens was not added, nor was intensified immunosuppressive treatment for noninfectious inflammatory processes; instead the invasive diagnostic approach was relied on to detect or exclude them.

References

1. Craven DE, Kunches LM, Kilinsky V, et al: Risk factors for pneumonia and fatality in patients receiving continuous mechanical ventilation. Am Rev Respir Dis 133:792, 1986.
2. Langer M, Mosconi P, Cigada M, et al: Long-term respiratory support and risk of pneumonia in critically ill patients. Am Rev Respir Dis 140:302, 1989.
3. Torres A, Aznar R, Gatell JM, et al: Incidence risk, and prognosis factors of nosocomial pneumonia in mechanically ventilated patients. Am Rev Respir Dis 142:523, 1990.
4. Bryan CS, Reynolds KL: Bacteremic nosocomial pneumonia: Analysis of 172 episodes from a single metropolitan area. Am Rev Respir Dis 129:668, 1984.
5. Celis R. Torres A, Gatell JM, et al: Nosocomial pneumonia: A multivariate analysis of risk and prognosis. Chest 93:318, 1988.
6. Marrie TJ, Durant H, Yates L: Community-acquired pneumonia requiring hospitalization: 5-year prospective study. Rev Infect Dis 11:586, 1989.
7. Hook EW, Horton CA, Schaberg DR: Failure of intensive care unit support to influence mortality from pneumococcal bacteremia. JAMA 249:1055, 1983.
8. Research Committee of the British Thoracic Society and the Public Health Service: Community-acquired pneumonia in adults in British hospitals in 1982–1983: A survey of aetiology, mortality, prognostic factors and outcome. Q J Med 62:195, 1987.
9. Pachon J, Prados MD, Capote F, et al: Severe community-acquired pneumonia: Etiology, prognosis and treatment. Am Rev Respir Dis 142:369, 1990.
10. Yu VL, Kroboth FJ, Shonnard J, et al: Legionnaires' disease: New clinical perspective from a prospective pneumonia study. Am J Med 73:357, 1982.
11. Mackowiak PA, Martin RM, Jones SR, Smith JW: Pharyngeal colonization by gram-negative bacilli in aspiration-prone persons. Arch Intern Med 138:1224, 1978.
12. Valenti WM, Trudell RG, Bently DW: Factors predisposing to oropharyngeal colonization with gram-negative bacilli in the aged. N Engl J Med 298:1108, 1978.
13. Huxley EJ, Viroslav J, Gray WR, Pierce AK: Pharyngeal aspiration in normal adults and patients with depressed consciousness. Am J Med 64:564, 1978.
14. Davidson FF, Glazier JB, Murray JF: The components of the alveolar-arterial oxygen tension difference in normal subjects and in patients with pneumonia and obstructive lung disease. Am J Med 52:754, 1972.
15. Light RB, Mink SN, Wood LDH: Pathophysiology of gas exchange and pulmonary perfusion in pneumococcal pneumonia in dogs. J Appl Physiol 50:524, 1981.
16. Light RB: Intrapulmonary oxygen consumption in experimental pneumococcal pneumonia. J Appl Physiol 64:2490, 1988.

17. Fritts HW Jr, Strauss B, Wichern W, Cournand A: Utilization of oxygen in the lungs of patients with diffuse, nonobstructive pulmonary disease. Trans Assoc Am Physicians 76:302, 1963.
18. Miller AC: Early clinical differentiation between legionnaires' disease and other sporadic pneumonias. Ann Intern Med 90:526, 1979.
19. Woodhead MA, MacFarlane JT: Legionnaires' disease: A review of 79 community-acquired cases in Nottingham. Thorax 41:635, 1986.
20. Cordes LG, Fraser DW: Legionellosis: Legionnaires' disease; Pontiac fever. Med Clin North Am 64:395, 1980.
21. Dietrich PA, Johnson RD, Fairbank JT, Walke JS: The chest radiograph in Legionnaires' disease. Radiology 127:577, 1978.
22. Wynne JW, Modell JH: Respiratory aspiration of stomach contents. Ann Intern Med 87:466, 1977.
23. Bynum LJ, Pierce AK: Pulmonary aspiration of gastric contents. Am Rev Respir Dis 114:1129, 1976.
24. Murray PR, Washington JA: Microscopic and bacteriologic analysis of expectorated sputum. Mayo Clin Proc 50:339, 1975.
25. Thorpe J, Baugham R, Frame PT, et al: Bronchoalveolar lavage for diagnosing acute bacterial pneumonia. J Infect Dis 155:855, 1987.
26. Khan FW, Jones JM: Diagnosing bacterial respiratory infections by bronchoalveolar lavage. J Infect Dis 155:862, 1987.
27. Hanly P, Light RB: Plasma volume expansion and PEEP in a canine model of acute *Pseudomonas* pneumonia. Lung 167:285, 1989.
28. Mink SN, Light RB, Cooligan T, Wood LDH: Effect of PEEP on gas exchange and pulmonary perfusion in canine lobar pneumonia. J Appl Physiol 50:517, 1981.
29. Kanarek DJ, Shannon DC: Adverse effect of positive end-expiratory pressure in refractory hypoxemia. Am Rev Respir Dis 112:457, 1975.
30. Remolina C, Khan AU, Santiago TV, Edelman NH: Positional hypoxemia in unilateral lung disease. N Engl J Med 304:523, 1981.
31. Light RB: Indomethacin and acetylsalicylic acid reduce intrapulmonary shunt in experimental pneumococcal pneumonia. Am Rev Respir Dis 134:520, 1986.
32. Hanly PJ, Roberts D, Dobson K, Light RB: Effect of indomethacin on arterial oxygenation in critically ill patients with severe bacterial pneumonia. Lancet i:351, 1987.
33. Carlon GC, Ray C, Klein R, et al: Criteria for selective positive end-expiratory pressure and independent synchronized ventilation of each lung. Chest 74:501, 1978.
34. Rossman CM, Waldes R, Sampson D, Newhouse MT: Effect of chest physiotherapy on the removal of mucus in patients with cystic fibrosis. Am Rev Respir Dis 126:131, 1982.
35. Holody B, Goldberg HS: The effect of mechanical vibration physiotherapy on arterial oxygenation in acutely ill patients with atelectasis or pneumonia. Am Rev Respir Dis 124:372, 1981.
36. Dreyfuss D, Leviel F, Paillard M, et al: Acute infectious pneumonia is accompanied by a latent vasopressin-dependent impairment of renal water excretion. Am Rev Respir Dis 138:583, 1988.
37. Brimioulle S, Kahn RJ: Effects of metabolic alkalosis on pulmonary gas exchange. Am Rev Respir Dis 141:1185, 1990.
38. Langer M, Cigada M, Mandelli M, et al, (Intensive Care Unit Group of Infection Control): Early onset pneumonia: A multicenter study in intensive care units. Intensive Care Med 13:342, 1987.
39. Simon HB, Southwick FS, Moellering RC, Sherman E: *Haemophilus influenzae* in hospitalized adults: Current perspectives. Am J Med 69:219, 1980.
40. Hager H, Verghese A, Alvarez S, Berk SL: *Branhamella catarrhalis* respiratory infections. Rev Infect Dis 9:1140, 1987.
41. Atherton ST, White DJ: Stomach as source of bacteria colonizing the respiratory tract during artificial ventilation. Lancet i:968, 1978.
42. duMoulin GC, Paterson DG, Hedley-Whyte J, Lesbon A: Aspiration of gastric bacteria in antacid-treated pateints: A frequent cause of postoperative colonization of the airway. Lancet i:242, 1982.
43. Driks MR, Craven DE, Celli BR, et al: Nosocomial pneumonia in intubated patients given sucralfate as compared with antacids or histamine type 2 blockers. N Engl J Med 317:1376, 1987.
44. Pingleton S, Hinthorn DR, Liu C: Enteral nutrition in patients receiving mechanical ventilation. Am J Med 80:827, 1986.
45. Bell RC, Coalson JJ, Smith JD, Johanson WG Jr: Multiple organ system failure and infection in adult respiratory distress syndrome. Ann Intern Med 99:293, 1983.
46. Fagon JY, Chastre J, Hance AJ, et al: Detection of nosocomial lung infection in ventilated patients: Use of a protected specimen brush and quantitative culture techniques in 147 patients. Am Rev Respir Dis 138:110, 1988.
47. Torres A, De La Bellacasa JP, Xaubet A, et al: Diagnostic value of quantitative cultures of bronchoalveolar lavage and telescoping plugged catheters in mechanically ventilated patients with bacterial pneumonia. Am Rev Respir Dis 140:306, 1989.
48. Chastre J, Viau F, Brun P, et al: Prospective evaluation of the protected specimen brush for the diagnosis of pulmonary infections in ventilated patients. Am Rev Respir Dis 130:924, 1984.
49. Lee B, Chang RWS, Jacobs S: Intermittent nasogastric feeding: A simple and effective method to reduce pneumonia among ventilated ICU patients. Clin Intens Care 1:100, 1990.
50. Klick JM, duMoulin GC, Hedley-Whyte J, et al: Prevention of Gram-negative bacillary pneumonia using polymyxin aerosol as prophylaxis. II. Effect on the incidence of pneumonia in seriously ill patients. J Clin Invest 55:514, 1975.
51. Stoutenbeek CP, van Saene HK, Miranda DR, Zandstra DF: The effect of selective decontamination of the digestive tract on colonisation and infection in multiple trauma patients. Intensive Care Med 10:185, 1984.
52. Ledingham IM, Alcock SR, Eastaway AT, et al: Triple regimen of selective decontamination of the digestive tract, systemic cefotaxime, and microbiological surveillance for prevention of acquired infection in intensive care. Lancet i:785, 1988.
53. Kerver AJH, Rommes JH, Mevissen-Verhage EAE, et al: Prevention of colonization and infection in critically ill patients: A prospective randomized study. Crit Care Med 16:1087, 1988.
54. Feeley TW, du Moulin GC, Hedley-Whyte J, et al: Aerosol polymyxin and pneumonia in seriously ill patients. N Engl J Med 293:471, 1975.
55. Brun-Buisson C, Legrand P, Rauss A, et al: Intestinal decontamination for control of nosocomial multiresistant gram-negative bacilli: Study of an outbreak in an intensive care unit. Ann Intern Med 110:873, 1989.
56. Meyers JD, Flournoy N, Thomas ED: Risk factors for cytomegalovirus infection after human marrow transplantation. J Infect Dis 153:478, 1986.
57. Cooper JAD, White DA, Matthay RA: Drug-induced pulmonary disease. Part 1: Cytotoxic drugs. Am Rev Respir Dis 133:321, 1986.
58. Binder RE, Faling J, Pugatch RD, et al: Chronic necrotizing pulmonary aspergillosis: A discrete entity. Medicine 61:109, 1982.
59. Gerson SL, Talbot GH, Hurwitz S, et al: Discriminant scorecard for diagnosis of invasive pulmonary aspergillosis in patients with acute leukemia. Am J Med 79:57, 1985.

60. Albelda SM, Talbot GH, Gerson SL, et al: Pulmonary cavitation and massive hemoptysis in invasive pulmonary aspergillosis. Am Rev Respir Dis 131:115, 1985.
61. Stover DE, Zaman MB, Hajdu SI, et al: Bronchoalveolar lavage in the diagnosis of diffuse pulmonary infiltrates in the immunocompromised host. Ann Intern Med 101:1, 1984.
62. Williams DE, Yungbluth M, Adams G, Glassroth J: The role of fiberoptic bronchoscopy in the evaluation of immunocompromised hosts with diffuse pulmonary infiltrates. Am Rev Respir Dis 131:880, 1985.
63. Warner DO, Warner MA, Divertie MB: Open lung biopsy in patients with diffuse pulmonary infiltrates and acute respiratory failure. Am Rev Respir Dis 137:90, 1988.
64. Potter DP, Pass HI, Brower S, et al: Prospective randomized study of open lung biopsy versus empirical antibiotic therapy for acute pneumonitis in non-neutropenic cancer patients. Ann Thorac Surg 40:422, 1985.
65. Albelda SM, Talbot GH, Gerson SL, et al: Role of fiberoptic bronchoscopy in the diagnosis of invasive pulmonary aspergillosis in patients with acute leukemia. Am J Med 76:1027, 1984.
66. Aisner J, Murillo J, Schimpff SC, Steere AC: Invasive aspergillosis in acute leukemia; Correlation with nose cultures and antibiotic use. Ann Intern Med 90:4, 1979.
67. Yu VL, Muder RR, Poorsattar A: Significance of isolation of aspergillus from the respiratory tract in diagnosis of invasive pulmonary aspergillosis: Results from a three year prospective study. Am J Med 81:249, 1986.

Chapter 103

BACTERIAL INFECTIONS OF THE CENTRAL NERVOUS SYSTEM

ALLAN R. TUNKEL
W. MICHAEL SCHELD

KEY POINTS

- *More than 85 percent of adults with bacterial meningitis present clinically with fever, headache, meningismus, and signs of cerebral dysfunction; elderly patients, however, may present with insidious disease manifested only by lethargy or obtundation, variable signs of meningeal irritation, and no fever.*
- *Occasionally, a patient with acute bacterial meningitis may have a low cerebrospinal fluid (CSF) white cell count despite high bacterial concentrations in cerebrospinal fluid; therefore a Gram stain and culture should be performed on every CSF specimen even if the cell count is normal.*
- *A latex agglutination test should be performed on every CSF specimen taken from a patient in whom bacterial meningitis is suspected; a* Limulus *lysate assay is useful when gram-negative meningitis is possible.*
- *Neuroimaging techniques have little role in the diagnosis of acute bacterial meningitis. However, a computed tomography (CT) scan should be performed prior to lumbar puncture when a space-occupying lesion of the central nervous system (CNS) is suspected.*
- *Empiric antimicrobial therapy, based on the patient's age and underlying disease status, should be initiated as soon as possible in patients with presumed bacterial meningitis; therapy should never be delayed while awaiting diagnostic tests such as CT.*
- *Adjunctive dexamethasone therapy has been shown to reduce morbidity in infants and children with acute* Haemophilus influenzae *type b meningitis; further studies are needed before this form of therapy can be recommended in adult patients.*
- *Only about one-half of patients with brain abscess present with the classic triad of fever, headache, and focal neurologic deficit; the clinical presentation of brain abscess in immunosuppressed patients may be masked by the diminished inflammatory response.*
- *The diagnosis of brain abscess has been revolutionized by the development of CT; magnetic resonance imaging (MRI) may offer advantages over CT in the early detection of cerebritis, cerebral edema, and satellite lesions.*
- *Aspiration of brain abscess by stereotaxic CT guidance is useful for microbiologic diagnosis, drainage, and relief of increased intracranial pressure.*
- *A short course of corticosteroids may be useful in patients with brain abscess who have deteriorating neurologic status and increased intracranial pressure.*
- *Cranial subdural empyema should be suspected in patients with headache, vomiting, fever, change in mental status, and rapid progression of focal neurologic signs.*
- *Spinal epidural abscess may develop acutely or chronically with symptoms and signs of focal vertebral pain, nerve root pain, motor or sensory defects, and paralysis; the transition to paralysis may be rapid, indicating the need for emergent evaluation, diagnosis, and treatment.*
- *Surgical therapy is essential for the management of subdural empyema and epidural abscess, because antibiotics do not reliably sterilize these lesions.*
- *Lateral gaze palsy may be an early clue to the diagnosis of cavernous sinus thrombosis, because the abducens nerve is the only cranial nerve traversing the interior of the cavernous sinus.*
- *The noninvasive diagnostic procedure of choice for suppurative intracranial thrombophlebitis is MRI, which can differentiate between thrombus and normally flowing blood.*

Bacterial infections of the CNS are frequently devastating. The brain possesses several defense mechanisms (e.g., intact cranium and blood-brain barrier) to prevent entry of bacterial species; but once microorganisms have gained entry to the CNS, host defense mechanisms are inadequate to control the infection. Antimicrobial therapy is limited by the poor penetration of many agents into the CNS as well as by the ability of antibiotics to induce inflammation in the CNS via their bacteriolytic action, thereby contributing to brain damage. Here we review meningitis, brain abscess, subdural empyema, epidural abscess, and intracranial thrombophlebitis, emphasizing recent developments in diagnosis and therapy as they pertain to the care of the critically ill patient.

Meningitis

EPIDEMIOLOGY AND ETIOLOGY

The rates of morbidity and mortality from bacterial meningitis remain unacceptably high despite the availability of effective antimicrobial therapy. The overall annual attack rate for bacterial meningitis is approximately 3.0 cases per 100,000 population in the United States, although there is some variability according to geographic area, sex, and race.[1] Incidence and mortality rates in the United States for the various meningeal pathogens are shown in Table 103-1, which reflects a study of the surveillance of cases of bacterial meningitis in 27 states from 1978 to 1981.

Haemophilus influenzae is isolated in 48.3 percent of all cases of bacterial meningitis in the United States. About 40 to 60 percent of cases are seen in children from 2 months to 6 years of age; of these 90 percent are due to capsular type b strains. Disease is most likely initiated after nasopharyngeal acquisition of a virulent organism with subsequent

TABLE 103-1 Incidence and Mortality Rates for Bacterial Meningitis in the United States, 1978–1981

Organism	Percentage of Total Cases	Mortality Rate (%)
Haemophilus influenzae	48.3	6.0
Neisseria meningitidis	19.6	10.3
Streptococcus pneumoniae	13.3	26.3
Streptococcus agalactiae	3.4	22.5
Listeria monocytogenes	1.9	28.5
Other*	7.5	33.7
Unknown	5.9	16.4

*Includes *Escherichia coli*, other Enterobacteriaceae, staphylococci, *Pseudomonas* species, and other streptococcal and *Haemophilus* species.
SOURCE: Adapted from Schlech WF et al.[1]

systemic invasion. *H. influenzae* accounts for only about 5 percent of total isolates after age 6 years; isolation of the organism in this older age group should suggest the possible presence of certain predisposing factors, including sinusitis, otitis media, epiglottitis, pneumonia, head trauma with CSF leak, diabetes mellitus, alcoholism, splenectomy or asplenic states, and immune deficiency (e.g., hypogammaglobulinemia).[2]

Meningitis due to *Neisseria meningitidis* is most often found in children and young adults and may occur in epidemics. Here again nasopharyngeal carriage of virulent organisms accounts for initiation of infection.[3] Infection is more likely in persons who have deficiencies in the terminal complement components (C5, C6, C7, C8, and perhaps C9)—the so-called membrane attack complex, in which there is a greater than 8000-fold increase over normal incidence of neisserial infections.[4]

Pneumococcal meningitis is most frequently observed in adults (over age 30 years), and is often associated with distant foci of infection, such as pneumonia, otitis media, mastoiditis, sinusitis, and endocarditis. Serious pneumococcal infections may be observed in persons with predisposing conditions such as splenectomy or asplenic states, multiple myeloma, hypogammaglobulinemia, and alcoholism. *Streptococcus pneumoniae* is the most common meningeal isolate in head trauma patients who have suffered basilar skull fracture with subsequent CSF leak.[5]

Listeria monocytogenes accounts for only about 1.9 percent of all cases of bacterial meningitis, but carries a high mortality rate. Infection with *Listeria* is more likely in neonates, the elderly, alcoholics, cancer patients, and immunosuppressed adults (e.g., renal transplant patients).[6] However, up to 30 percent of adults, and 54 percent of children and young adults with listeriosis have no apparent underlying condition. Listeriosis has been associated with several food-borne outbreaks involving contaminated cole slaw, milk, and cheese.

Meningitis due to aerobic gram-negative bacilli is observed in specific clinical situations.[7] *Escherichia coli* is isolated in 30 to 50 percent of infants with bacterial meningitis under 2 months of age. *Klebsiella* species, *E. coli*, and *Pseudomonas aeruginosa* may be isolated in patients who have had head trauma or neurosurgical procedures; in the elderly; in immunosuppressed patients; and in patients with gram-negative septicemia. Despite the low frequency of meningitis due to this group of organisms, the mortality rates are very high (around 84 percent with *P. aeruginosa*, until recently).

Specific clinical situations also predispose to the development of meningitis due to staphylococcal species.[8] *Staphylococcus epidermidis* is the most common cause of meningitis in persons with CSF shunts. Meningitis due to *Staph. aureus* is frequently found in the early post-neurosurgical period. Underlying diseases among persons with no prior CNS disease who develop *Staph. aureus* meningitis include diabetes mellitus, alcoholism, chronic renal failure requiring hemodialysis, and malignancies. Conditions that increase *Staph. aureus* nasal carriage rates (e.g., intravenous drug abuse, insulin-requiring diabetes, hemodialysis) may also predispose to staphylococcal infection of the CNS.

CLINICAL PRESENTATION

The classic clinical presentation in adults with bacterial meningitis includes fever, headache, meningismus, and signs of cerebral dysfunction[9]; these symptoms and signs are found in more than 85 percent of cases. Also common are nausea, vomiting, rigors, profuse sweating, weakness, myalgias, and photophobia. The meningismus may be subtle or marked, accompanied by Kernig's and/or Brudzinski's signs.[10] Kernig's sign is elicited by flexing the thigh on the abdomen with the knee flexed; the leg is then passively extended, and if there is meningeal inflammation the patient resists leg extension. Brudzinski's sign is present when passive flexion of the neck leads to flexion of the hips and knees. However, these signs are elicited in only about 50 percent of cases of bacterial meningitis in adults. Cerebral dysfunction is manifested by confusion, delirium, or a declining level of consciousness ranging from lethargy to coma. Cranial nerve palsies (especially involving cranial nerves III, IV, VI, and VII) and focal cerebral signs are uncommon (10 to 20 percent of cases). Seizures occur in about 30 percent of all cases. Papilledema is rare (fewer than 1 percent) and should suggest an alternate diagnosis, such as an intracranial mass lesion. Late in the disease patients may develop signs of increased intracranial pressure, including coma, hypertension, bradycardia, and IIId-nerve palsy; these findings are ominous prognostic signs.

Certain symptoms and signs may suggest an etiologic diagnosis in patients with bacterial meningitis. Persons with meningococcemia present with a prominent rash, principally on the extremities (about 50 percent of cases).[11] Early in the disease course the rash may be erythematous and macular; but it quickly evolves into a petechial phase, with further coalescence into a purpuric form. The rash often matures rapidly, with new petechial lesions appearing during the physical examination. A petechial, purpuric, or ecchymotic rash may also be seen in other forms of meningitis (i.e., those due to ECHO virus type 9, *Acinetobacter* species, *Staph aureus*, and, rarely, *Strep. pneumoniae* or *H. influenzae*), in Rocky Mountain spotted fever or *Staph.*

aureus endocarditis, and in overwhelming sepsis (due to *Strep. pneumoniae* or *H. influenzae*) in splenectomized patients. An additional suppurative focus of infection (e.g., otitis media, sinusitis, or pneumonia) is present in 30 percent of patients with pneumococcal or *H. influenzae* meningitis, but is rarely found in meningococcal meningitis. Meningitis due to *Strep. pneumoniae* is relatively likely after head trauma in persons who have suffered basilar skull fractures in which a dural fistula is produced between the subarachnoid space and the nasal cavity, paranasal sinuses, or middle ear.[5] These persons commonly present with rhinorrhea or otorrhea due to a CSF leak; a persistent defect is a common explanation for recurrent bacterial meningitis.

Certain subgroups of patients may not manifest the classic signs and symptoms of bacterial meningitis. Usually in a neonate there is no meningismus or fever, and the only clinical clues to meningitis are listlessness, high-pitched crying, fretfulness, refusal to feed, and/or irritability. Elderly patients, especially those with underlying conditions such as diabetes mellitus or cardiopulmonary disease, may present with insidious disease manifested only by lethargy or obtundation, variable signs of meningeal irritation, and no fever. In this subgroup, altered mental status should not be ascribed to other causes until bacterial meningitis has been excluded by CSF examination. A post-neurosurgical patient or a patient who has undergone head trauma also presents a unique clinical situation, since these patients already have many of the symptoms and signs of meningitis from their underlying disease processes.[5,12] One must observe a low threshold for CSF examination in these patients should they develop any clinical deterioration.

DIAGNOSIS

The diagnosis of bacterial meningitis rests on the CSF examination. The opening pressure is elevated in virtually all cases; values over 600 mmH_2O suggest cerebral edema, presence of intracranial suppurative foci, or communicating hydrocephalus. The appearance of the fluid may be cloudy or turbid if the white blood cell count is elevated (more than 200 cells per mm^3). If the lumbar puncture is traumatic the CSF may appear bloody initially, but it should clear as flow continues. Xanthochromia—a pale-pink to yellow-orange color of the supernatant of centrifuged CSF—is found in patients with subarachnoid hemorrhage, usually within 2 h post-hemorrhage.

The CSF white cell count is usually elevated in untreated bacterial meningitis, ranging from 100 to 10,000 cells per mm^3, with a predominance of neutrophils. About 10 percent of patients present with a lymphocytic predominance (greater than 50 percent) in CSF. Some patients may have a very low CSF white cell count (0 to 20 cells per mm^3) despite high bacterial concentrations in CSF; these patients have a poor prognosis. Therefore, a Gram stain and culture should be performed on all CSF specimens, even with a normal cell count. A CSF glucose concentration less than 40 mg/dL is found in about 60 percent of patients with bacterial meningitis, and a CSF:serum glucose ratio less than 0.31 is observed in 70 percent of cases. The CSF glucose level must always be compared to a simultaneous serum glucose concentration. The CSF protein concentration is elevated in virtually all cases of bacterial meningitis, presumably because of disruption of the blood/brain barrier.

CSF examination by Gram stain permits a rapid, accurate identification in 60 to 90 percent of cases of bacterial meningitis. False-positive findings may occur as a result of contamination either in the collection of tubes or in staining. Cultures of CSF are positive in 70 to 80 percent of cases. These percentages may decrease in patients who have received prior antimicrobial therapy.

Several rapid diagnostic tests have been developed to aid in the diagnosis of bacterial meningitis.[13,14] Counterimmunoelectrophoresis (CIE) detects specific antigens in CSF due to meningococci (serogroups A and C), *H. influenzae* type b, pneumococci (representing 83 serotypes), type III group B streptococci, and *E. coli* K1. Sensitivity ranges from 62 to 95 percent, but the test is highly specific. Newer tests employing staphylococcal coagglutination or latex agglutination are more rapid and sensitive than CIE. However, none of the tests detects antigens of group B meningococci. One of these rapid diagnostic tests (preferably latex agglutination) should be performed on all CSF specimens from patients in whom bacterial meningitis is suspected when the Gram stain is negative. The *Limulus* lysate test is useful in cases of gram-negative meningitis in which a positive test (indicating the presence of endotoxin) indicates that a gram-negative organism is the cause of the meningitis, although it does not distinguish between types of gram-negative organisms that may be present (i.e., low specificity).

Neuroimaging techniques have little role in the diagnosis of acute bacterial meningitis, except to rule out the presence of other pathologic conditions or to identify a parameningeal source of infection. However, CT or MRI may be useful in patients with prolonged fever several days after initiation of antimicrobial therapy, prolonged obtundation or coma, new or recurrent seizure activity, signs of increased intracranial pressure, or focal neurologic deficits. MRI is better than CT for evaluation of subdural effusions, cortical infarctions, and cerebritis, although it is more difficult to obtain an MRI scan in a critically ill patient—which limits its usefulness in many patients with meningitis.

TREATMENT

ANTIMICROBIAL THERAPY

The initial approach to the patient with suspected bacterial meningitis is to perform a lumbar puncture to determine whether the CSF findings are consistent with that diagnosis. Patients should receive empiric antimicrobial therapy based on their age and underlying disease status if no etiologic agent is identified by Gram stain or rapid diagnostic tests. In patients with a focal neurologic examination, a CT scan should be performed immediately to exclude an intracranial mass lesion, since lumbar puncture is relatively contraindicated in that setting. However, since obtaining a CT scan generally entails some delay, empiric antimicrobial therapy should be started immediately and before the CT scan and lumbar puncture, because of the high mortality in patients with bacterial meningitis in whom antimicrobial therapy is delayed. Our choices for empiric antibiotic therapy in patients with presumed bacterial meningitis, based on age, are shown in Table 103-2.[15] For neonates aged from 0 to 3 weeks, the most likely infecting organisms are *E. coli, Strep. agalactiae,* and *L. monocytogenes;* for ages 4 to 12 weeks, infection may be due, in addition, to either *H. influenzae* or *Strep. pneumoniae.* In both of these age groups, empiric therapy with ampicillin plus a third-generation cephalosporin (cefotaxime or ceftriaxone) should be initiated. From age 3 months to 6 years, *H. influenzae* is by far the most common etiologic agent of bacterial meningitis, and from 6 to 18 years the pneumococcus and the meningococcus are also possibilities; empiric therapy with a third-generation cephalosporin should be used pending culture results. In adults aged 18 to 50 years, most cases of meningitis are due to *N. meningitidis* and *Strep. pneumoniae,* and penicillin G or ampicillin should be empirically used. In older adults (50 years of age and older), the meningococcus and the pneumococcus are possible causes, as well as *L. monocytogenes* and gram-negative bacilli. Empiric therapy should consist of ampicillin in combination with a third-generation cephalosporin, because of the increased frequency of aerobic gram-negative bacillary meningitis in this age group. One other situation deserves comment: In postneurosurgical patients or patients with CSF shunts or foreign bodies, likely infecting organisms include staphylococci (either *Staph. epidermidis* or *Staph. aureus*), diphtheroids, and gram-negative bacilli (including *P. aeruginosa*). Antimicrobial therapy in these situations should consist of vancomycin plus ceftazidime pending culture results.

Once an infecting microorganism has been isolated, antimicrobial therapy can be modified for optimal treatment.[15] Our antibiotics of choice are shown in Table 103-3. Dosages for adults are listed in Table 103-4. For bacterial meningitis due to *Strep. pneumoniae* or *N. meningitidis,* penicillin G and ampicillin are equally efficacious. However, while pneumococci have been uniformly susceptible to penicillin [minimal inhibitory concentration (MIC) less than, or equal to, 0.06 μg/mL] in past years, reports from several centers have now documented both relatively and highly resistant strains of pneumococci with MICs of 0.1 to 1.0 μg/mL and 2 μg/mL and above, respectively. In view of these recent trends, susceptibility testing should be performed on all CSF isolates. For relatively resistant strains, a third-generation cephalosporin (e.g., cefotaxime or ceftriaxone) should be used; for highly resistant strains, vancomycin is the antimicrobial agent of choice. Meningococcal strains that are relatively resistant to penicillin have also been reported from several areas (particularly Spain); but most patients harboring these strains have recovered with standard penicillin therapy, so their clinical significance is unclear.

Treatment of *H. influenzae* type b meningitis has been hampered by the emergence of β-lactamase-producing strains of the organism, which now account for approximately 25 percent of all isolates in the United States.[1] Chloramphenicol resistance has also been reported in the United States (fewer than 1 percent of isolates) and Spain (50 percent, or more, of isolates). In addition, a recent study found chloramphenicol to be bacteriologically and clinically inferior to certain β-lactam antibiotics (ampicillin, ceftriaxone, and cefotaxime) in childhood bacterial meningitis, in which the majority of cases were due to *H. influenzae* type b.[16] From the above findings and other studies, the third-generation cephalosporins (e.g., cefotaxime and ceftriaxone) seem to be at least as efficacious as ampicillin plus chloramphenicol for therapy of *H. influenzae* meningitis. Cefuroxime, a second-generation cephalosporin, has also been evaluated for therapy of *H. influenzae* meningitis. Although initial studies documented an efficacy for this drug similar to that of ampicillin plus chloramphenicol, recent case reports have documented delayed CSF sterilization and the development of epiglottitis in patients receiving cefuroxime for meningitis. In addition, a recent prospective randomized study of ceftriaxone and cefuroxime for the treatment of childhood bacterial meningitis documented the superiority of ceftriaxone; patients receiving this drug had milder hearing impairment and more rapid CSF sterilization than those receiving cefuroxime.[17] We currently recommend a third-generation cephalosporin for empiric therapy when *H. influenzae* is considered a likely infecting pathogen.

The treatment of bacterial meningitis in adults that is

TABLE 103-2 Empiric Therapy of Purulent Meningitis

Age	Standard Therapy	Alternative Therapies
0–3 weeks	Ampicillin plus a third-generation cephalosporin*	Ampicillin plus an aminoglycoside†
4–12 weeks	Ampicillin plus a third-generation cephalosporin*	Ampicillin plus chloramphenicol
3 months–18 years	Third-generation cephalosporin*	Ampicillin plus chloramphenicol; cefuroxime
18–50 years	Penicillin G or ampicillin	Third-generation cephalosporin*
>50 years	Ampicillin plus a third-generation cephalosporin*	Ampicillin plus an aminoglycoside;† trimethoprim-sulfamethoxazole

*Cefotaxime or ceftriaxone.
†Gentamicin, tobramycin, or amikacin.

TABLE 103-3 Antimicrobial Therapy of Bacterial Meningitis

Organism	Antibiotic of Choice
Neisseria meningitidis	Penicillin G or ampicillin
Streptococcus pneumoniae	Penicillin G or ampicillin
Haemophilus influenzae (β-lactamase–negative)	Ampicillin
Haemophilus influenzae (β-lactamase–positive)	Third-generation cephalosporin*
Enterobacteriaceae	Third-generation cephalosporin*
Pseudomonas aeruginosa	Ceftazidime†
Streptococcus agalactiae	Penicillin G or ampicillin†
Listeria monocytogenes	Ampicillin or penicillin G†
Staphylococcus aureus (methicillin-sensitive)	Nafcillin or oxacillin
Staphylococcus aureus (methicillin-resistant)	Vancomycin
Staphylococcus epidermidis	Vancomycin‡

*Cefotaxime or ceftriaxone.
†Addition of an aminoglycoside should be considered.
‡Addition of rifampin may be indicated.

caused by gram-negative enteric bacilli has been revolutionized by the third-generation cephalosporins,[15] with cure rates of 78 to 94 percent. One agent, ceftazidime, is also active against *P. aeruginosa* meningitis; this agent, alone or in combination with an aminoglycoside, resulted in cure of 19 of 24 patients with *Pseudomonas* meningitis in one report.[18] Intrathecal or intraventricular aminoglycoside therapy should be considered if there is no response to systemic therapy, although this therapy is now rarely needed. The quinolones (e.g., ciprofloxacin or pefloxacin) have been used in some patients with gram-negative bacillary meningitis,[19] but at this time can be considered only for patients with meningitis due to multidrug resistant gram-negative bacilli, or for patients in whom conventional therapy has failed.

TABLE 103-4 Recommended Doses of Antibiotics for Intracranial Infections in Adults with Normal Renal Function

Antibiotic	Total Daily Dose in Adults (Dosing Interval)
Penicillin G	24 million U (q 4 h)
Ampicillin	12 g (q 4 h)
Nafcillin, oxacillin	9–12 g (q 4 h)
Chloramphenicol	4–6 g* (q 6 h)
Cefotaxime	8–12 g (q 4 h)
Ceftriaxone	4–6 g† (q 12 h)
Ceftazidime	6–12 g‡ (q 8 h)
Vancomycin	2 g (q 12 h)
Gentamicin, tobramycin	3–5 mg/kg (q 8 h)
Amikacin	15 mg/kg (q 8 h)
Trimethoprim-sulfamethoxazole	10 mg/kg§ (q 12 h)
Metronidazole	30 mg/kg (q 6 h)

*Higher dose recommended for pneumococcal meningitis.
†Actual dose studied was 50 mg/kg every 12 h.
‡Not enough patients studied to make firm recommendations.
§Dosage based on trimethoprim component.

The third-generation cephalosporins are inactive against meningitis caused by *L. monocytogenes*, an important meningeal pathogen; this is a major drawback of these agents. Therapy in this situation should consist of ampicillin or penicillin G; addition of an aminoglycoside should be considered in documented infection, at least for the first several days of treatment.[6] Alternatively, trimethoprim-sulfamethoxazole can be used.[20] Patients with *Staph. aureus* meningitis should be treated with nafcillin or oxacillin, with vancomycin reserved for patients allergic to penicillin and patients with disease caused by methicillin-resistant organisms.[8] Infection with *Staph. epidermidis*, the most likely isolate in a patient with a CSF shunt, should be treated with vancomycin, with rifampin added if the patient fails to improve. Shunt removal is often essential to optimize therapy.

The duration of therapy for bacterial meningitis should be 10 to 14 days for most causes of nonmeningococcal meningitis, and 3 weeks for meningitis due to gram-negative enteric bacilli.[21] Seven days of therapy appears adequate for meningococcal meningitis; several reports have suggested that 7 days of therapy is efficacious also for *H. influenzae* meningitis. However, therapy must be individualized, and on the basis of clinical response some patients may require longer courses of treatment.

ADJUNCTIVE THERAPY

Despite the availability of effective antimicrobial therapy, the morbidity and mortality from bacterial meningitis remain unacceptably high. Recent studies have focused on the pathogenesis and pathophysiology of bacterial meningitis, in the hope of developing innovative strategies for adjunctive treatment.[15] Recent work in experimental animal models of meningitis has suggested a potentially useful role for anti-inflammatory agents (e.g., corticosteroids and nonsteroidal anti-inflammatory agents) in decreasing the inflammatory response in the subarachnoid space, which may be responsible for the development of neurologic sequelae. Adjunctive dexamethasone therapy has recently been evaluated in a double-blind placebo-controlled trial in 200 infants and children with bacterial meningitis.[22] The patients who received dexamethasone and antibiotics, in comparison to those who received antibiotics plus placebo, became afebrile sooner and were significantly less likely to acquire moderate-to-severe bilateral sensorineural hearing loss. These findings were significant only for meningitis due to *H. influenzae* type b. In another study, of children and adults, there was a significant reduction in case fatality rates and overall neurologic sequelae in patients with pneumococcal meningitis who received dexamethasone in addition to antibiotics.[23] Concerns have been raised about the routine use of dexamethasone therapy in all patients with bacterial meningitis,[24] but it appears likely that this agent will prove useful as adjunctive therapy in children and possibly in adults, pending results of ongoing studies. If dexamethasone is to be used, however, it should be administered concomitantly with, or just before, antibiotic therapy, to attenuate the CSF inflammatory response. Close monitoring of the hematocrit, and of the stool guaiac (for occult blood), is essential during therapy, since gastrointestinal hemorrhage has been reported.

Other adjunctive therapies may be useful in critically ill patients with bacterial meningitis. Patients with signs of increased intracranial pressure (e.g., altered level of consciousness; dilated, poorly reactive—or nonreactive—pupils; and ocular movement disorders) who are stuporous or comatose, precluding assessment of worsening neurologic function, may benefit from the insertion of an intracranial pressure monitoring device. A detailed discussion of the management of raised intracranial pressure will be found in Chap. 34. Seizures must be treated promptly to avoid status epilepticus, which might lead to anoxic brain injury (see Chap. 142). Another important adjunctive measure in patients with bacterial meningitis is fluid restriction to combat hyponatremia caused by excess secretion of antidiuretic hormone—although this is not appropriate in the presence of shock or dehydration, since hypotension may predispose to cerebral ischemia. Many patients, particularly children, with bacterial meningitis are hyponatremic (serum sodium level less than 135 meq/L) upon presentation; the degree and duration of hyponatremia may contribute to neurologic sequelae. If the patient is not hypotensive, fluids should be restricted to one-half maintenance level; the serum sodium level will normalize in most patients. The management of hyponatremia is discussed in greater depth in Chap. 156.

PREVENTION

A final point concerns chemoprophylaxis of contacts of meningitis cases, which is indicated for contacts of patients with either *N. meningitidis* or *H. influenzae* type b meningitis. For contacts of a patient with meningococcal meningitis, chemoprophylaxis usually is administered only to intimate contacts (e.g., family or roommates); it is not indicated for other groups (e.g., office co-workers or classmates) unless there has been intimate contact.[11] However, one study has suggested that school-aged children may be at increased risk of secondary infection where classrooms are crowded, or contact during lunch or recess is frequent, or both. Prophylaxis is not necessary for medical personnel caring for cases unless there has been intimate contact (e.g., mouth-to-mouth resuscitation). All contacts (both children and adults) of a case of *H. influenzae* meningitis should receive chemoprophylaxis if exposure has occurred in a household or day care center containing children 4 years of age or younger (other than the index case), provided that the exposure to *H. influenzae* type b was in the week prior to prophylaxis.[25] The drug of choice for chemoprophylaxis, for contacts of both types of meningitis, is rifampin. For contacts of patients with *H. influenzae* meningitis, rifampin at a daily dose of 20 mg/kg (not exceeding 600 mg) for 4 consecutive days is most effective. For contacts of meningococcal cases, one rifampin dose of 10 mg/kg (not exceeding 600 mg) twice a day for 2 days is effective.[11] One dose of ciprofloxacin (500 or 750 mg) may also be efficacious in eradication of the meningococcal nasopharyngeal carrier state.

Brain Abscess

EPIDEMIOLOGY AND ETIOLOGY

Brain abscess is one of the most serious complications of head and neck infections. Even in the antibiotic era, mortality from brain abscess was not appreciably different from that in the preantibiotic era (about 40 to 60 percent), until the past decade, when mortality decreased to between 5 and 10 percent.[26] This improvement is likely due to recent developments in diagnosis and treatment, which are discussed below. There is a large geographic variability in the incidence of brain abscess, with about 4 to 10 cases seen annually on active neurosurgical services in developed countries.

Bacteria can reach the brain by several different mechanisms. The factors predisposing to brain abscess and the etiologic agents in each circumstance are shown in Table 103-5.[27] The most common pathogenic mechanism of brain abscess formation is spread from a contiguous focus of infection, most often in the middle ear, mastoid cells, or paranasal sinuses. Early studies reported that 40 percent of brain abscesses were associated with otitis media, but this has been decreasing in recent years. However, if antibiotic therapy of otitis is neglected, there is an increased risk of intracranial complications. Brain abscess secondary to otitis media is bimodally distributed, with peaks in the pediatric age group (acute otitis media) and after age 40 years (chronic otitis media). Most cases of brain abscess due to otitis media occur in the temporal lobe and cerebellum. The etiologic agents in brain abscess secondary to otitis media include a broad range of bacterial species, including streptococci, *Bacteroides fragilis*, and members of the Enterobacteriaceae family.

Paranasal sinusitis continues to be an important condition predisposing to brain abscess, most commonly in persons between 10 and 30 years of age. The frontal lobe is the predominant site of abscess localization, although when brain abscess complicates sphenoid sinusitis the temporal lobe or sella turcica is usually involved.[27] Streptococci are the predominant bacterial species involved in brain abscess secondary to sinusitis, although anaerobes, *Staph. aureus*, and gram-negative bacilli have also been isolated.

Brain abscess occurs less commonly from dental infections, but, when present, appears more likely following infection of the molar teeth. The frontal lobe is usually involved, but temporal lobe extension has also been described.

A second mechanism of brain abscess formation is hematogenous dissemination to the brain from a distant focus of infection. These abscesses are usually multiple and multiloculated, and have a higher mortality rate than abscesses that arise secondary to contiguous foci of infection.[26–28] The most common sources in adults are chronic pyogenic lung diseases—especially lung abscess, bronchiectasis, empyema, and cystic fibrosis. Anaerobes (*Fusobacterium* and *Bacteroides* species) and streptococci are likely infecting pathogens in this situation, as are *Nocardia* and *Actinomyces*

TABLE 103-5 Predisposing Conditions and Microbiology in Brain Abscess

Predisposing Condition	Usual Bacterial Isolates
Otitis media or mastoiditis	Streptococci (anaerobic or aerobic), *Bacteroides* sp., Enterobacteriaceae
Sinusitis (frontoethmoidal or sphenoidal)	Streptococci, *Bacteroides* sp., Enterobacteriaceae, *Staphylococcus aureus, Haemophilus* sp.
Dental sepsis	Mixed *Fusobacterium, Bacteroides,* and *Streptococcus* sp.
Penetrating trauma or post-neurosurgery	*Staphylococcus aureus,* streptococci, Enterobacteriaceae, *Clostridium* sp.
Congenital heart disease	Streptococci, *Haemophilus* sp.
Lung abscess, empyema, bronchiectasis	*Fusobacterium, Actinomyces,* and *Bacteroides* sp.; *Nocardia asteroides*; streptococci
Bacterial endocarditis	*Staphylococcus aureus,* streptococci
Immunosuppressed host	*Nocardia,* Enterobacteriaceae

SOURCE: Adapted from Wispelwey B, Scheld WM.[27]

species. Brain abscess may also occur hematogenously from wound and skin infections, osteomyelitis, pelvic infection, cholecystitis, and other intraabdominal infections. Another predisposing factor leading to hematogenously acquired brain abscess is cyanotic congenital heart disease (accounting for 5 to 10 percent of all brain abscess cases, with higher percentages in some pediatric series), most commonly due to tetralogy of Fallot and transposition of the great vessels.[29] Brain abscess is rare after bacterial endocarditis (fewer than 5 percent of cases in most series), despite the presence of persistent bacteremia. Hereditary hemorrhagic telangiectasia is a predisposing factor almost always observed in patients with coexistent pulmonary arteriovenous malformations; perhaps it allows septic emboli to cross the pulmonary circulation without capillary filtration. Brain abscesses have also developed following esophageal dilatation and sclerosing therapy for esophageal varices.

Trauma is a third pathogenic mechanism in the development of brain abscess, whether secondary to an open cranial fracture with dural breech, or post-neurosurgical, or secondary to foreign body injuries (especially in children).[5] The incidence of brain abscess formation after head trauma ranges from 3 to 17 percent in military populations, where it is usually secondary to retained bone fragments or contamination of initially "sterile" missile sites with bacteria from skin, clothes, and the environment. Predisposing traumatic conditions in the civilian population include compound depressed skull fractures, dog bites, rooster pecking, and, especially in children, injury from lawn darts and pencil tips. Likely infective microorganisms after trauma include staphylococci, streptococci, gram-negative bacilli, and anaerobes.

Finally, brain abscess is cryptogenic in about 20 percent of patients.[27] Many of these cases are secondary to unrecognized dental foci of infection. In this subgroup of patients, broad antimicrobial therapy is indicated pending culture results (see Treatment, below).

Overall, the most commonly isolated bacterial species in brain abscess are streptococci (aerobic, anaerobic, and microaerophilic), present in 60 to 70 percent of cases.[27] These bacteria (especially the *Strep. milleri* group) normally reside in the oral cavity, appendix, and female genital tract, and have a proclivity for abscess formation. *Staph. aureus,* which was isolated in 25 to 30 percent of cases in the pre-antibiotic era, now accounts for 10 to 15 percent of isolates, although the frequency of isolation of *Staph. aureus* is increased in certain clinical situations (e.g., cranial trauma, endocarditis). Attention to proper culture techniques has increased the isolation of anaerobes, with *Bacteroides* species isolated in 20 to 40 percent of cases—often in mixed culture.[27] Enteric gram-negative bacilli (*Proteus* species, *E. coli, Klebsiella* species, and *Pseudomonas* species) are isolated in 23 to 33 percent of patients. Other bacterial species occur less commonly (in fewer than 1 percent of cases) and include *H. influenzae, Strep. pneumoniae, L. monocytogenes,* and *Nocardia asteroides* (*Nocardia* is more often isolated in patients with T-lymphocyte or mononuclear phagocyte defects). Nocardial brain abscesses have increased in incidence with the increasing numbers of immunosuppressed patients, although up to 48 percent of patients with nocardiosis have no underlying conditions. Brain abscesses due to *Actinomyces* species are commonly associated with pulmonary and odontogenic infections.

CLINICAL PRESENTATION

The clinical course of brain abscess may be indolent or fulminant; three-quarters of patients have symptoms for less than 2 weeks. Most of the clinical manifestations are due to the presence of space-occupying lesions within the brain.[27,28,30] The most common symptom is headache, present in more than 70 percent of patients. The headache is usually moderate-to-severe and hemicranial, but may be generalized. Other findings include nausea and vomiting (about 50 percent of cases), nuchal rigidity (about 25 percent), and papilledema (about 25 percent). Mental status changes ranging from lethargy to coma occur in the majority of cases. Seizures, usually generalized, occur in 25 to 35 percent of patients. Fever appears in only 45 to 50 percent of cases; afebrile patients tend to be older, have a longer duration of illness, and have a higher mortality rate. Only about one-half of patients present with the classic triad of fever, headache, and focal neurologic deficit. Patients with frontal lobe abscess often present with headache, drowsiness, inattention, and deterioration in mental status; the most common focal neurologic signs are hemiparesis, with unilateral motor signs, and a motor speech disorder. The clinical presentation of cerebellar abscess may include ataxia, nystagmus, vomiting, and dysmetria. Persons with abscess of the temporal lobe may present with ipsilateral headache and aphasia, if the lesion is in the dominant hemisphere. A visual field defect (e.g., an upper homonymous quadrantanopia) may be the only presenting sign of a temporal lobe abscess. Persons with brain stem abscesses usually present with facial weakness, fever, headache, hemiparesis, dysphagia, and vomiting. Clues as to the site of the infection's origin should also be sought; these include otorrhea, orbital cellulitis, purulent nasal discharge, dental sepsis, and postoperative or posttraumatic cranial infection; such findings occur in about 60 percent of cases. Finally, it is important to note that the clinical presentation of brain abscess in immunosuppressed patients may be masked by the diminished inflammatory response.

DIAGNOSIS

The diagnosis of brain abscess has been revolutionized by the development of CT, which not only is an excellent means to examine the brain parenchyma, but is superior to standard radiologic procedures for examination of the paranasal sinuses, mastoid cells, and middle ear. The sensitivity of CT is 95 to 99 percent for brain abscess; it also yields information concerning the extent of surrounding edema, presence or absence of a midline shift, presence of hydrocephalus, and possibility of imminent ventricular rupture.[31,32] The characteristic appearance of brain abscess on CT scanning is a hypodense center with a peripheral uniform ring enhancement following the injection of contrast material; this is surrounded by a variable hypodense area of brain edema. A similar appearance is seen with neoplasms, granulomas, cerebral infarction, or resolving hematoma. Contrast enhancement of the ependymal lining suggests ventriculitis. Other CT findings include nodular enhancement and areas of low attenuation without enhancement; this latter finding is observed during the early cerebritis stage, prior to abscess formation; as the abscess progresses, contrast enhancement is observed. In later stages, as the abscess becomes encapsulated, contrast no longer differentiates the lucent center, and the CT appearance is similar to that in the early cerebritis stage. The use of delayed films may be helpful, because the presence of contrast material in the center of the lesion suggests cerebritis. The absence of contrast material likely indicates a well-encapsulated lesion. This difference is important therapeutically, since cerebritis may respond to medical therapy alone, whereas most encapsulated lesions require surgical intervention. CT scanning is also useful for following the course of brain abscess—although after aspiration, improvement in CT appearance may not be seen for up to 5 weeks or longer. Complete resolution may take 4 to 5 months.

Scintigraphy with ^{111}In-labeled leukocytes has also recently been evaluated in the diagnosis of brain abscess.[33] Radiolabeled leukocytes migrate to, and accumulate in, an area of active inflammation, thereby differentiating brain abscess from other cerebral mass lesions—although false-positive scans can be observed in necrotic tumors, and false-negative scans in patients receiving corticosteroids. This modality is most useful as a complementary test to CT scanning.

The role of MRI in the diagnosis of brain abscess has not been extensively evaluated.[34] Preliminary data indicate that MRI may offer advantages over CT in the early detection of cerebritis; in the detection of cerebral edema, where it heightens the contrast between edema and adjacent brain, and makes more conspicuous the spread of inflammation into the ventricles and subarachnoid space; and in earlier detection of satellite lesions. Contrast-enhanced MRI scanning, using the paramagnetic agent gadolinium diethylenetriamine penta-acetic acid (Gd-DTPA), has the advantages of clearly differentiating the central abscess, surrounding contrast-enhancing rim, and cerebral edema surrounding the abscess. These data are encouraging. MRI may become the diagnostic procedure of choice for brain abscess, although it is not always feasible in critically ill patients.

A major advance in the use of CT scanning is the availability of stereotaxic CT-guided aspiration of the abscess to facilitate bacteriologic diagnosis. However, aspiration during the early cerebritis stage may be complicated by hemorrhage. At the time of aspiration, a specimen should be sent for Gram stain (and other special stains—e.g., Ziehl-Neelsen, modified acid-fast, and silver stains, where appropriate), routine culture, and anaerobic culture. The use of this modality in the treatment of brain abscess is discussed under Surgical Therapy in the section Treatment, below.

Lumbar puncture is contraindicated in patients with suspected or proven brain abscess, because of the risk of life-threatening cerebral herniation after removal of CSF. When lumbar puncture is performed the CSF profile is nonspecific, with a predominantly mononuclear pleocytosis and an elevated protein concentration. Hypoglycorrhachia is present in only 25 percent of cases, and fewer than 10 percent of CSF cultures are positive.[28] Microorganisms usually are not demonstrated on Gram stain, unless the abscess has ruptured into the subarachnoid space or there is accompanying meningitis.

TREATMENT

ANTIMICROBIAL THERAPY

Due to the alteration of the blood/brain barrier in the area of the brain abscess, there is increased penetration of normally excluded antibiotics into the brain. However, the increased penetration does not predict antibiotic entry into cerebral abscesses. Brain abscess concentrations of antibiotics have been measured, and several generalizations can be made[26,27]: (1) metronidazole can be expected to achieve inhibitory levels for sensitive anaerobic microorganisms; (2) chloramphenicol concentrations in the brain are likely to be satisfactory; and (3) concentrations of various penicillins and cephalosporins in brain tissue and abscess are usually poor—although, when given in large parenteral doses, these agents achieve therapeutic concentrations for sensitive microorganisms.

When a diagnosis of brain abscess is made, either presumptively, by radiologic studies, or by aspiration of the abscess, antimicrobial therapy should be initiated. Aspiration may provide an etiologic diagnosis on Gram stain examination, but when aspiration is either impractical or delayed we recommend empiric therapy based on the likely etiologic agent, if a predisposing condition can be identified (see Table 103-6). Because of the high rate of isolation of streptococci (particularly the *Streptococcus milleri* group) from brain abscesses of various etiologies (see Table 103-5), high-dose penicillin G (20 to 24 million U/day), or another drug (e.g., a third-generation cephalosporin, either cefotaxime or ceftriaxone) that is active against this organism, should be included in initial therapeutic regimens.[27] Penicillin is also active against most anaerobic species, with the notable exception of *B. fragilis,* which is isolated in a high percentage (20 to 40 percent) of brain abscess cases. When *B. fragilis* is suspected, we recommend the addition of metronidazole (7.5 mg/kg every 6 h) and reserve chloramphenicol for cases where metronidazole cannot be used. The advantages of metronidazole over these other agents include its bactericidal activity against *B. fragilis* (the others are frequently bacteriostatic) and the high concentrations it attains in brain abscess pus, even with concomitant corticosteroid administration. In addition, one retrospective review has suggested that metronidazole may improve mortality rates in patients with brain abscess.[35] In cases in which *Staph. aureus* is a likely infecting pathogen (e.g., cranial trauma or post-neurosurgery), nafcillin should be used. Vancomycin, which penetrates well into brain abscess fluid,[36] is reserved for patients allergic to penicillin or cases where methicillin-resistant organisms are likely or have been isolated. The penetration of clindamycin, erythromycin, and the first-generation cephalosporins into brain abscesses is usually inadequate to achieve therapeutic concentrations, precluding their use in this setting. For empiric therapy when members of the Enterobacteriaceae family are suspected (e.g., in cases of abscess of otitic origin), either a third-generation cephalosporin or trimethoprim-sulfamethoxazole should be used.

One regimen that has theoretical advantages and covers a broad range of possible infecting bacterial pathogens is metronidazole, nafcillin, and a third-generation cephalosporin (either cefotaxime or ceftriaxone) (see Table 103-6). In addition to activity against gram-negative bacilli, these third-generation cephalosporins have excellent antistreptococcal activity and possess antistaphylococcal action. However, it is important to note that there are no clinical trials comparing this regimen to traditional penicillin-containing formulas. If *P. aeruginosa* is a likely infecting pathogen, ceftazidime is the third-generation cephalosporin of choice. However, if ceftazidime is the third-generation cephalosporin used in empiric therapy of brain abscess, the regimen must also include penicillin G to treat a possible streptococcal infection, since ceftazidime has unreliable gram-positive activity.

Once an infecting pathogen is isolated, antimicrobial therapy can be modified (see Table 103-7). Antimicrobial therapy with high-dose intravenous antibiotics should be continued for 4 to 6 weeks and is often followed by oral antibiotic therapy for 2 to 6 months, if an appropriate agent is available. Shorter courses (3 to 4 weeks) may be adequate for patients undergoing excision of the abscess. Surgical therapy (see below) is often required for treatment of brain abscess, although certain subgroups of patients can be managed without surgery.[37] These include patients with medical conditions that increase the risk of surgery; patients with multiple abscesses, or abscesses in a deep or dominant location; patients with concomitant meningitis or ependymitis; patients with early abscess reduction with clinical improvement after antimicrobial therapy; and patients with abscess size under 3 cm.

SURGICAL THERAPY

Most patients require surgical management for optimal treatment of brain abscess. The two procedures judged equivalent by outcome are aspiration of the abscess after

TABLE 103-6 Empiric Antimicrobial Therapy for Brain Abscess

Predisposing Condition	Antimicrobial Regimen
Otitis media or mastoiditis	Metronidazole plus a third-generation cephalosporin*
Sinusitis	Nafcillin or vancomycin† plus metronidazole plus a third-generation cephalosporin*
Dental sepsis	Penicillin plus metronidazole
Cranial trauma or post-neurosurgery	Vancomycin plus a third-generation cephalosporin*
Congenital heart disease	Penicillin plus a third-generation cephalosporin*
Unknown	Nafcillin or vancomycin† plus metronidazole plus a third-generation cephalosporin*

*Cefotaxime or ceftriaxone; ceftazidime is used if *P. aeruginosa* is suspected.
†Vancomycin is used in the penicillin-allergic patient or when methicillin-resistant *Staph. aureus* is suspected.

TABLE 103-7 Antimicrobial Therapy for Brain Abscess

Organism	Standard Therapy	Alternative Therapies
Streptococcus milleri and other streptococci	Penicillin G	Third-generation cephalosporin,* vancomycin
Bacteroides fragilis	Metronidazole	Chloramphenicol, clindamycin
Fusobacterium sp., *Actinomyces*	Penicillin G	Metronidazole, chloramphenicol, clindamycin
Staphylococcus aureus	Nafcillin	Vancomycin
Enterobacteriaceae	Third-generation cephalosporin*	Aztreonam†
Haemophilus sp.	Third-generation cephalosporin*	Aztreonam†
Nocardia asteroides	Trimethoprim-sulfamethoxazole	Ampicillin, erythromycin, amikacin, imipenem (all †)

*Cefotaxime or ceftriaxone.
†Limited data available for use of these agents; firm recommendations are not possible at this time.

burr hole placement, and complete excision after craniotomy.[28,38,39] Drainage and marsupialization are now rarely used. The choice of procedure must be individualized for each patient. Aspiration may be performed by stereotaxic CT guidance, affording the surgeon rapid, accurate, and safe access to virtually any intracranial point. Aspiration can also be used for swift relief of increased intracranial pressure. Incomplete drainage of multiloculated lesions is a major disadvantage of aspiration; these lesions frequently require excision. Other risks of aspiration are that it may allow the abscess to rupture into the ventricle, and that pus may leak into the subarachnoid space, resulting in ventriculitis or meningitis.

Complete excision after craniotomy is most often employed in patients in a stable neurologic condition. Surgery is also indicated for abscesses exhibiting gas on radiologic evaluations, and for posterior fossa abscesses. In the patient with worsening neurologic deficits, including deteriorating consciousness or signs of increased intracranial pressure, surgery should be performed emergently. Excision is contraindicated in the early stages, before a capsule is formed.

ADJUNCTIVE THERAPY

Intracranial pressure monitoring has become important in the management of brain abscess patients in the intensive care unit who have cerebral edema[26] (see Chap. 34). The use of these monitoring devices has diminished the likelihood of transtentorial herniation, brain stem compression, and further injury from cerebral ischemia.

Corticosteroids have been used as one method to manage increased intracranial pressure, although their use remains controversial.[27] These agents may retard the encapsulation process, reduce antibiotic entry into the CNS, increase necrosis, and alter the appearance of ring enhancement on CT as inflammation subsides, thereby obscuring information from sequential studies. Steroids (dexamethasone dosage in adults, 4 to 6 mg every 6 h) are most useful, however, in the patient with deteriorating neurologic status and increased intracranial pressure, where they may prove lifesaving. When used to treat cerebral edema, steroids should be used for the shortest time possible. The management of increased intracranial pressure is discussed in Chap. 34.

Subdural Empyema and Epidural Abscess

EPIDEMIOLOGY AND ETIOLOGY

The term *subdural empyema* refers to a collection of pus in the space between the dura and arachnoid. This type of infection accounts for about 20 percent of all localized intracranial infections.[40–42] The disease was essentially lethal prior to the advent of antimicrobial therapy; but with current methods of diagnosis and treatment, mortality rates range from 10 to 20 percent. The most common predisposing conditions are otorhinologic infections—especially infection of the paranasal sinuses, which are affected in 50 to 80 percent of cases.[40,41,43] The pathogenesis involves spread of infection to the subdural space via valveless emissary veins in association with thrombophlebitis, or via extension of an osteomyelitis of the skull with accompanying epidural abscess. The mastoid cells and middle ear are the source in 10 to 20 percent of patients, especially in geographic areas (e.g., Sri Lanka) where many cases of otitis media are not treated promptly with antibiotics. Other predisposing conditions include skull trauma,[5] neurosurgical procedures, and infection of a preexisting subdural hematoma. The infection is metastatic in a minority of cases (about 5 percent), principally from the pulmonary system. A number of different bacterial species have been isolated from cranial sub-

TABLE 103-8 Bacteriology of Cranial Subdural Empyema and Spinal Epidural Abscess

Organism	Cranial Subdural Empyema	Spinal Epidural Abscess
Staphylococci (including *Staph. aureus* and *Staph. epidermidis*)	15	65
Streptococci (aerobic, anaerobic, and microaerophilic)	36	8
Aerobic gram-negative bacilli	3	17
Other anaerobes	18	2
Other	8	2
Unknown	20	6

SOURCE: Data summarized from references 42–44, 47, 48.

dural empyemas,[42,44] (see Table 103-8), including streptococci (35 to 40 percent of cases), staphylococci (about 15 percent), aerobic gram-negative bacilli (about 3 percent), and anaerobes (33 to 100 percent, when careful culturing is performed); these organisms make up the microbial flora frequently isolated from patients with chronic sinusitis and cranial abscesses.

Spinal subdural empyema is a rare condition occurring secondary to metastatic infection from a distant site.[45] *Staph. aureus* is the most frequent isolate, whereas streptococci are found less frequently.

The term *epidural abscess* refers to a localized infection between the dura mater and the overlying skull or vertebral column. Cranial epidural abscess can cross the cranial dura along emissary veins, so subdural empyema often is also present.[40] Therefore, the etiology, pathogenesis, and bacteriology of intracranial epidural abscess are usually identical to those described for subdural empyema (see above), with the initial focus of infection in the middle ear, paranasal sinuses, or mastoid cells.

Spinal epidural abscess, on the other hand, usually follows hematogenous dissemination from foci elsewhere in the body to the epidural space, or, by extension, from vertebral osteomyelitis.[46,47] Hematogenous spread occurs in 25 to 50 percent of cases, secondary to infections of the skin (furuncles, cellulitis, infected acne), urinary tract infections, periodontal abscesses, pharyngitis, pneumonia, or mastoiditis. Mild blunt spinal trauma may provide a devitalized site susceptible to transient bacteremia. Infection of the epidural space has also been reported following penetrating injuries; extension of decubitus ulcers or paraspinal abscesses; back surgery; lumbar puncture; and epidural anesthesia. Bacteremia may be an important predisposing factor, since the incidence of spinal epidural abscess is increased in patients who use intravenous drugs[48] or have intravenous catheters. The infecting microorganism in the vast majority of cases is *Staph. aureus* (range of 50 to 95 percent in various series)[5] (see Table 103-8). Other isolates include aerobic and anaerobic streptococci (about 8 percent of cases) and gram-negative aerobic bacilli (about 18 percent), especially *E. coli* and *P. aeruginosa*.

CLINICAL PRESENTATION

Persons with subdural empyema can present in a rapidly progressive, life-threatening clinical condition.[40–42] Symptoms and signs relate to the presence of increased intracranial pressure, meningeal irritation, or focal cortical inflammation. In addition, 60 to 90 percent of patients have evidence of the antecedent infection (e.g., sinusitis or otitis). Headache, initially localized to the infected sinus or ear, is a prominent complaint, and can become generalized as the infection progresses. Vomiting is common as intracranial pressure increases. Early in the infection about one-half of patients have altered mental status, which can progress to obtundation if the patient is not treated. Fever above 39°C is present in most cases. Focal neurologic signs appear in 24 to 48 h, progressing rapidly, with eventual involvement of the entire cerebral hemisphere. Hemiparesis and hemiplegia are the most common focal signs, although ocular palsies, dysphasia, homonymous hemianopsia, dilated pupils, and cerebellar signs have also been observed. Seizures (either focal or generalized) are observed in more than 50 percent of cases. Signs of meningeal irritation (e.g., meningismus) are found in about 80 percent of patients, although fewer have either Kernig's or Brudzinski's signs. If the patient remains untreated, neurologic deterioration rapidly occurs, with signs of increased intracranial pressure and cerebral herniation. Papilledema develops in fewer than 50 percent of patients. This fulminant picture may not be seen in patients with subdural empyema following cranial surgery or trauma; in patients who have received prior antimicrobial therapy; in patients with infected subdural hematomas; or in patients with infections metastatic to the subdural space.

Spinal subdural empyema usually manifests itself as radicular pain and symptoms of spinal cord compression, which may occur at multiple levels.[45] Clinically, this lesion is difficult to distinguish from a spinal epidural abscess (see Diagnosis, below).

The onset of symptoms in cranial epidural abscess may be insidious and overshadowed by the primary focus of infection (e.g., sinusitis or otitis media).[40] Headache is a usual complaint, but the patient may otherwise feel well unless the clinical course is complicated (e.g., by development of subdural empyema or involvement of deeper intracranial structures). Because the dura is closely apposed to the inner surface of the cranium, the abscess usually enlarges too slowly to produce sudden major neurologic deficits (in contrast to subdural empyema) unless there is deeper intracranial extension. However, there may eventually be development of focal neurologic signs and either focal or generalized seizures. Without treatment, papilledema and other signs of increased intracranial pressure develop as the abscess enlarges. An epidural abscess near the petrous bone may present as Gradenigo's syndrome, characterized by involvement of cranial nerves V and VI, with unilateral facial pain and weakness of the lateral rectus muscle.[49]

Spinal epidural abscess may develop within hours to days (after hematogenous seeding), or may pursue a chronic course over months (associated more often with vertebral osteomyelitis).[46–50] Most abscesses pass through the following stages: focal vertebral pain; root pain; defects of motor, sensory, or sphincter function; and paralysis. Pain is the most consistent symptom and is accompanied by local tenderness at the affected level in over 90 percent of cases. Subsequently, radicular pain develops; it is followed by progression to weakness and paralysis. Fever occurs in most patients during the course of the illness. Headache and neck stiffness may also occur. Respiratory function may be impaired if the cervical spinal cord is involved. The usually irreversible manifestations of cord involvement include muscle weakness, sensory deficits, and disturbances of sphincter control. At this juncture there may be rapid transition to paralysis (usually within 24 h from onset of weakness), indicating the need for emergent evaluation, diagnosis, and treatment.

DIAGNOSIS

Subdural empyema should be suspected in any patient with meningeal signs and a focal neurologic deficit. Lumbar puncture is contraindicated in this setting, because of the risk of cerebral herniation. When lumbar puncture is performed, however, CSF findings are nonspecific and include elevated opening pressure, moderate neutrophilic pleocytosis, and an increased protein concentration. Unless the course is complicated by bacterial meningitis, CSF Gram stain and cultures are negative. Skull radiographs may demonstrate evidence of concurrent sinusitis or osteomyelitis.

The diagnostic procedure of choice is either CT, with contrast enhancement, or MRI.[40,51] The typical CT appearance is a crescentic or elliptically shaped area of hypodensity below the cranial vault or adjacent to the falx cerebri. Loculations may also be seen. Depending on the extent of disease, there is often associated mass effect with displacement of midline structures. After the administration of contrast material, a fine, intense line of enhancement can be seen between the subdural collection and the cerebral cortex. However, false-negative CT scans do occur. MRI provides greater clarity of morphologic detail and may detect empyema not clearly seen on CT; it is of particular value in identifying subdural empyemas located at the base of the brain, along the falx cerebri, or in the posterior fossa. On the basis of signal intensity, MRI can differentiate extraaxial empyemas from most sterile effusions and chronic hematomas. Both CT and MRI are also useful for demonstrating sinusitis and otitis, although CT is superior to MRI in bone imaging and should be used in cases of penetrating injury and of osteomyelitis. Cerebral arteriography should be utilized on an emergent basis when MRI is unavailable and subdural empyema is suspected despite a normal CT scan. Arteriography can establish the presence of a subdural avascular mass and detect spread of the mass to the contralateral or parafalx subdural space.

MRI is the diagnostic procedure of choice for spinal subdural empyema, because it gives more accurate information as to the extent of the lesion than does CT.[49,50] Myelography should be performed when neither MRI nor CT is available. It is important to note that *myelography may not detect the entire length of the empyema if complete blocks are present at multiple levels.* Both MRI and myelography detect cord compression, block, or multiple extraaxial defects.

CT and MRI are also the diagnostic procedures of choice for cranial epidural abscess, demonstrating a superficial, circumscribed area of diminished density.[40] The possibility of adjacent subdural empyema or other intracranial involvement can also be assessed. MRI or CT should be performed in cases of suspected spinal epidural abscess, with myelography reserved for use in locations where neither MRI nor CT is available.

TREATMENT

The therapy of subdural empyema and epidural abscess optimally requires a combined medical-surgical approach. Surgical therapy is essential, because antibiotics do not reliably sterilize these lesions without concurrent drainage; because cultures of purulent material guide antimicrobial therapy; and because surgical decompression is useful in controlling increased intracranial pressure.

ANTIMICROBIAL THERAPY

Once purulent material is aspirated, antimicrobial therapy should be initiated; it should be based on a Gram stain and on the site of primary infection[40,52] (see Table 103-9). For suspected *Staph. aureus,* nafcillin (1.5 g every 4 h) should be used, with vancomycin (1.0 g every 12 h) reserved for patients allergic to penicillin and for cases where methicillin-resistant organisms are suspected. Metronidazole (15 mg/kg loading dose, then 7.5 mg/kg every 6 h) is used when anaerobes (e.g., *B. fragilis*) are suspected. For aerobic gram-negative bacilli, a third-generation cephalosporin (cefotaxime or ceftriaxone) should be used, with ceftazidime reserved for cases in which *P. aeruginosa* is likely. Parenteral antibiotics should be continued for 3 to 6 weeks, depending on the patient's clinical response. Longer periods of intravenous therapy (and perhaps oral therapy) may be required if an associated osteomyelitis is present.

Presumptive antimicrobial therapy for spinal epidural abscess must include a first-line antistaphylococcal agent (nafcillin or vancomycin); coverage for gram-negative organisms should be included for any patient with a history of a spinal procedure or of intravenous drug abuse.[47,49] In addition, pending culture results, empiric antimicrobial therapy in patients who have undergone a spinal procedure should include vancomycin for presumed involvement by *Staph. epidermidis.*

SURGICAL THERAPY

The optimal surgical approach for subdural empyema is controversial, and there are several unanswered questions with regard to management.[40] First, should drainage be performed by craniotomy or via burr holes? (Previous studies documented a lower mortality rate in patients undergoing craniotomy, although it may be that a larger percentage of gravely ill patients were treated with burr holes because

TABLE 103-9 Empiric Antibiotic Therapy for Subdural Empyema, Epidural Abscess, and Septic Intracranial Thrombophlebitis

Condition	Site of Primary Infection	Antibiotics
Cranial subdural empyema, cranial epidural abscess, or septic intracranial thrombophlebitis	Paranasal sinusitis, otitis media, or mastoiditis	Nafcillin or vancomycin† plus metronidazole plus a third-generation cephalosporin*
	Cranial surgery	Nafcillin or vancomycin† plus a third-generation cephalosporin*
	Hematogenous from distant and/or unknown site	Nafcillin or vancomycin† plus metronidazole plus a third-generation cephalosporin*
Spinal epidural abscess or spinal subdural empyema	Extension of osteomyelitis or paravertebral infection	Nafcillin or vancomycin† plus a third-generation cephalosporin*
Spinal epidural abscess	Hematogenous spread	Nafcillin or vancomycin† plus a third-generation cephalosporin*
Spinal subdural empyema	Hematogenous spread	Nafcillin or vancomycin†

*Cefotaxime or ceftriaxone should be used. If *Pseudomonas aeruginosa* is suspected, ceftazidime is indicated instead.
†Vancomycin is indicated in the penicillin-allergic patient or when methicillin-resistant *Staph. aureus* is suspected.
SOURCE: Modified from Greenlee JE.[52]

of the greater surgical risk. Burr hole therapy may be more efficacious in the early stages of subdural empyema, when the pus is liquid, since thickening occurs as the disease progresses, making aspiration more difficult. If burr holes are to be placed, they should be multiple, allowing extensive irrigation. Craniotomy, however, may be essential for posterior fossa subdural empyema, and is also needed in 10 to 20 percent of patients initially treated with trephination. Thus, burr hole drainage, even with catheter irrigation, may not adequately drain the empyema. When craniotomy is performed, wide exposure should be afforded to allow adequate exploration of all areas where subdural pus is suspected.) Second, should antibiotics be instilled locally to irrigate the subdural space? (Although antibiotic irrigation has become common, there are no data on the potential benefits of this practice.) Third, should drains, or catheters, be left in the subdural space? (This decision is best made by the neurosurgeon intraoperatively; however, with drains in place the risk of nosocomial superinfection must be kept in mind.) Finally, surgical correction of the antecedent otorhinologic infection may also be necessary. In patients with spinal epidural abscess, laminectomy with decompression and drainage must be performed as a surgical emergency in order to minimize the likelihood of permanent neurologic sequelae. Some patients (those with an unacceptably high surgical risk or without neurologic deficits) have been treated with antibiotics alone; however, these patients must be followed carefully by clinical examination and with serial CT scanning or MRI.

ADJUNCTIVE THERAPY

Patients may also require various adjunctive measures to control increased intracranial pressure. Preoperative use of mannitol, hyperventilation, and/or dexamethasone may be effective in controlling intracranial pressure prior to surgical decompression. Corticosteroids, however, should be tapered rapidly after surgical therapy, because of the increased risk of secondary infection. We believe a short course of corticosteroids is appropriate in cases where surgical intervention is delayed or contraindicated. Anticonvulsants should be used in patients with seizures.

Suppurative Intracranial Thrombophlebitis

EPIDEMIOLOGY AND ETIOLOGY

Septic intracranial thrombophlebitis involves both venous thrombosis and suppuration.[53] It may begin within veins and venous sinuses, or may follow infection of the paranasal sinuses, middle ear, mastoid, face, or oropharynx; and may involve additional vessels by propagation or discontinuous spread. Septic thrombophlebitis may also occur in association with epidural abscess, subdural empyema, or bacterial meningitis. Occasionally, there may be metastatic spread from distant sites of infection. Conditions that increase blood viscosity or coagulability—including dehydration, polycythemia, pregnancy, oral contraceptive use, sickle cell disease, malignancy, and trauma—increase the likelihood of thrombosis.

The antecedent conditions that predispose to the development of intracranial venous sinus thrombosis depend on the close proximity of various structures to the dural venous sinuses[54,55] (see Fig. 103-1). The usual predisposing conditions for cavernous sinus thrombosis are paranasal sinusitis (especially frontal, ethmoidal, or sphenoidal), or infection of the face or mouth. Likely infecting bacterial pathogens depend on the initial source: staphylococci, streptococci, gram-negative bacilli, and anaerobes if the antecedent condition is sinusitis, and predominantly *Staph. aureus* secondary to facial infections. Otitis media and mastoiditis are infections associated with lateral sinus thrombosis and infection of the superior and inferior petrosal sinuses. Infections of the face, scalp, subdural space, and epidural space, and meningitis, are associated with suppu-

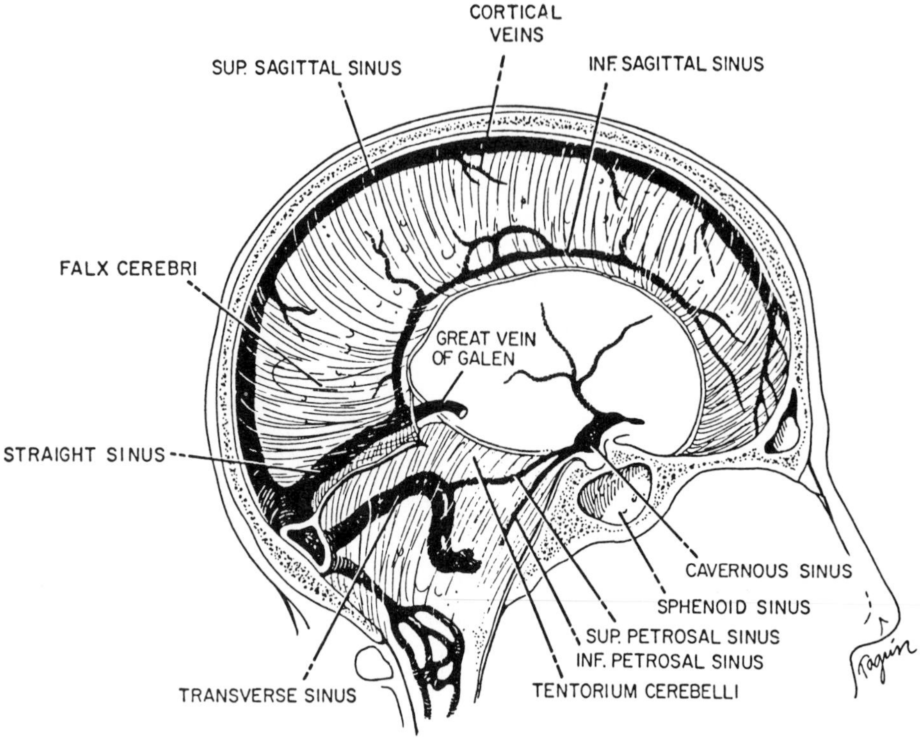

FIGURE 103-1 Lateral cross section of the skull, demonstrating the major dural venous sinuses. Note that the cavernous sinus is in close proximity to the sphenoid air sinus, and that the anterior segment of the superior sagittal sinus is near the frontal air sinus. Reprinted, with permission, from Southwick FS, Richardson EP Jr, Swartz MN: Septic thrombosis of the dural venous sinuses. Medicine 65:82, © by Williams & Wilkins, 1985.

rative thrombophlebitis of the superior sagittal sinus. Again, the likely infecting microorganisms depend on the associated primary condition (see Table 103-5).

In cavernous sinus thrombosis, *Staph. aureus* is the most important infecting microorganism, isolated in over two-thirds of cases. This relates to the importance of this organism in infections of the face and scalp, and in acute sphenoid sinusitis. Less common isolates include streptococci (isolated in about 17 percent of cases), pneumococci and gram-negative bacilli (5 percent each), and *Bacteroides* species (2 percent).

CLINICAL PRESENTATION

The clinical manifestations of suppurative cortical thrombophlebitis depend on the location of involvement. With involvement of the cortical venous system, the appearance of neurologic deficits depends on the adequacy of collateral venous drainage.[56] Persons with inadequate collateral flow present with impairment of consciousness, focal or generalized seizures, symptoms of increased intracranial pressure, and focal neurologic signs (e.g., hemiparesis). Aphasia is common if the dominant cerebral hemisphere is involved.

The findings in dural venous sinus thrombosis also depend upon location.[54,55] In cavernous sinus thrombosis, the most common complaints are periorbital swelling (73 percent of cases) and headache (52 percent). Headache is more common if the antecedent condition is sinusitis rather than a facial infection. Other symptoms include drowsiness, diplopia, eye tearing, photophobia, and ptosis. Fever is present in over 90 percent of patients. Other common signs are proptosis, chemosis, periorbital edema, and weakness of the extraocular muscles (due to involvement of cranial nerves III, IV, and VI). Since the abducens nerve is the only cranial nerve traversing the interior of the cavernous sinus, a lateral gaze palsy may be an early neurologic finding. Papilledema, or venous engorgement, and change in mental status are observed in 65 percent and 55 percent of patients, respectively. Meningismus is present in about 40 percent of cases, usually secondary to retrograde spread of the thrombophlebitis. About 25 percent of patients have dilated or sluggishly reactive pupils, decreased visual acuity (frequently progressing to blindness), and dysfunction of cranial nerve V. As the infection spreads to the opposite cavernous sinus through the intercavernous sinuses, findings are duplicated in the opposite eye. Persons with septic cavernous sinus thrombosis may present with either acute or chronic illness.[55] In the acute presentation (generally secondary to facial infection), the onset between primary infection and cavernous sinus thrombosis is short (less than 1 week), in which the patient appears in quite a toxic state, with rapid development of the symptoms and signs described above; there is also rapid progression to bilateral eye signs. In contrast, there is a more indolent form of cavernous sinus thrombosis, usually secondary to dental infection, otitis media, or paranasal sinusitis. In these patients, the orbital manifestations are often unimpressive, and involvement of the contralateral eye is a late and inconsistent finding.

Patients with septic lateral sinus thrombosis complain predominantly of headache (more than 80 percent of cases); earache, vomiting, and vertigo also may occur, since otitis media is a common predisposing condition.[53,54,56] Fever and abnormal ear findings are observed in the majority of patients (79 percent and 98 percent, respectively), and there may also be VIth nerve palsy, facial pain and altered facial sensation, papilledema, and mild nuchal rigidity. Thrombosis of the superior sagittal sinus produces an abnormal mental status, motor deficits, nuchal rigidity, and papilledema. Seizures occur in over half of patients. Patients with sinusitis as a predisposing condition tend to have a subacute onset of symptoms. Involvement of the inferior petrosal sinus may produce ipsilateral facial pain and lateral rectus muscle weakness (Gradenigo's syndrome).

DIAGNOSIS

The noninvasive diagnostic procedure of choice for suppurative intracranial thrombophlebitis is MRI.[57] This technique visualizes blood vessels and differentiates between thrombus and normally flowing blood. It can also reveal the evolution and resolution of the entire veno-occlusive process. CT scanning, with and without intravenous contrast material, also permits diagnosis of venous sinus thrombosis,[58] although it is considerably less sensitive and reliable than MRI. CT usually reveals unilateral or bilateral multiple irregular filling defects in the enhancing cavernous sinus, with or without orbital inflammatory change. An additional benefit of both MRI and CT is the ability to evalute fully the paranasal sinuses and to provide information concerning subdural and epidural infection, cerebral infarction, cerebritis, hemorrhage, and cerebral edema. In cases in which MRI or CT is negative but suspicion of septic thrombophlebitis is high, carotid arteriography with venous phase studies should be performed. In cavernous sinus thrombosis, arteriography reveals narrowing of the intracavernous segment of the carotid artery.[56] Orbital venography may also be useful, and is the most definitive method of demonstrating cavernous sinus thrombosis.[55]

Other laboratory studies are usually nonspecific.[54,55] Lumbar puncture demonstrates a mild pleocytosis (either mononuclear, neutrophilic, or mixed) and an elevated protein concentration (consistent with a parameningeal focus of infection), although in septic thrombosis of the superior sagittal sinus there may be findings consistent with frank meningitis; often the causative organism is isolated on CSF culture. Blood cultures may be positive, especially in patients with a rapidly progressive course. Chest radiographs may reveal evidence of septic pulmonary emboli following propagation of thrombus into the inferior petrosal sinus and jugular vein. Sinus radiographs may document involvement of the paranasal sinuses, although conventional radiographs are inferior to MRI and CT in the detection of sphenoid sinusitis.

TREATMENT

ANTIMICROBIAL THERAPY

Appropriate antimicrobial therapy of septic intracranial thrombophlebitis depends on the antecedent clinical condition. The likely organisms are similar to those observed in cranial subdural empyema and epidural abscess; empiric antibiotic therapy should be directed toward those organisms[56] (see Table 103-9). If the antecedent condition is paranasal sinusitis, empiric therapy should be directed toward gram-positive organisms (staphylococci and streptococci), aerobic gram-negative bacilli, and anaerobes. In cavernous sinus thrombosis, an antistaphylococcal agent should always be included (because of the high incidence of *Staph. aureus* isolates) in the empiric therapeutic regimen pending culture results. Nafcillin should be used, with vancomycin reserved for penicillin-allergic patients and cases where methicillin-resistant organisms are suspected.

SURGICAL THERAPY

Surgical intervention may be required for optimal therapy. Certainly, surgical drainage of infected sinuses is necessary when antimicrobial therapy alone is ineffective. This is especially important in patients with cavernous sinus thrombosis secondary to sphenoid sinusitis; some authors have recommended operative intervention for patients who develop cavernous venous thrombosis as a complication of sinusitis. Internal jugular vein ligation has been utilized for lateral sinus vein thrombosis, and thrombectomy has also been used in some situations, but the efficacy of these procedures is poorly defined. Surgical therapy may also be required for other infections (e.g., dental abscess).

ADJUNCTIVE THERAPY

The use of anticoagulants (e.g., heparin) is controversial, although there is literature to support their use in prevention of the spread of thrombus from the cavernous sinus to other dural venous sinuses and cerebral veins.[54] Recent evidence indicates that anticoagulation (in combination with antibiotics) reduces mortality and is most beneficial early in the treatment of cavernous sinus thrombosis, to reduce morbidity among survivors.[59] However, the hazards of intracranial hemorrhage (bleeding from sites of cortical venous infarction or from sites on the intracavernous walls of the carotid artery) must be recognized. In the absence of specific contraindications, anticoagulation is most likely to be useful early in the course of cavernous sinus thrombosis. Anticoagulation is not recommended for septic lateral sinus vein thrombophlebitis, because cortical veins overlying the infected mastoid may become occluded, resulting in small venous hemorrhagic infarcts. Such infarcts make the risk of intracerebral hemorrhage following anticoagulation prohibitively high.

CASE PRESENTATION

Ms. S.S., a 33-year-old white female, was admitted because of a change in mental status. The patient had no significant past medical history until 7 years prior to admission, when a diagnosis of Hodgkin's disease was established. Evaluation at that time included a staging laparotomy with splenectomy. The disease was localized above the diaphragm and the patient was treated with radiotherapy.

She did well until 2 days prior to this admission, when she went to her local physician with complaints of headache and stiff neck. Examination at that time revealed a temperature of 38°C and mild resistance to neck flexion. No mental status or neurologic deficits were noted. The physician diagnosed the "flu" and prescribed acetaminophen. She returned to the physician the next day with worsening symptoms, predominantly a diffuse headache and stiff neck. On examination her temperature was 38.5°C with otherwise normal vital signs. She exhibited moderate resistance to neck flexion. Funduscopic exam revealed no papilledema. Examination of the extremities showed a bluish discoloration of several toes of both feet. She was mildly lethargic, but had no focal neurologic deficits. Her physician prescribed erythromycin and she was sent home. Early the next morning, she was found at home lying on the floor and screaming; she was totally disoriented. Her family brought her to the emergency room.

On physical examination, her temperature was 40°C, pulse 120, respirations 34 per minute, and blood pressure 80/50 mmHg. The head was atraumatic and the pupils were equal, round, and reactive to light. The funduscopic exam was normal. Severe pain was elicited on any neck movement. Examinations of the chest and heart were normal. Abdominal examination revealed a left upper quadrant scar without other abnormalities. There was peripheral gangrene of the fingers and toes. The patient was obtunded, thrashing about the bed, and could follow no commands. No focal neurologic abnormalities were appreciated. Babinski responses were present bilaterally.

Laboratory evaluation demonstrated a hemoglobin concentration of 10.1 g/dL with a hematocrit of 30.4. The white blood cell count was 24,300 cells per mm^3, with 80 neutrophils, 15 bands, and 5 lymphocytes. The platelet count was 149,000 per mm^3. Electrolyte measurements were sodium, 130 meq/L; potassium, 3.4 meq/L; chloride, 95 meq/L; and bicarbonate, 10 meq/L. The BUN and creatinine levels were 30 mg/dL and 2.0 mg/dL, respectively. The PT was 15.5 (control of 11) seconds, and the PTT 44 (control of 40) seconds. An arterial blood gas measurement taken with the patient breathing ambient air showed a pH of 7.38, P_{O_2} of 85 mmHg, and P_{CO_2} of 23 mmHg. The chest radiograph revealed no abnormalities.

Clinical Course

In the emergency room, an intravenous line was started and infusion of normal saline solution begun. The patient received 2 g each of cefotaxime and ampicillin intravenously and was sent for an emergency noncontrast CT scan of the head, which revealed no abnormalities. Lumbar puncture revealed an opening pressure of 280 mmH_2O. The CSF had a cloudy appearance. The white cell count was 12 cells per mm^3, all of which were neutrophils. The CSF glucose level was 3 mg/dL; CSF protein level, 398 mg/dL. Gram stain of CSF showed sheets of gram-positive diplococci, which were also observed on a Gram stain smear of a drop of peripheral blood. The patient was admitted to the intensive care unit (ICU).

Upon admission to the ICU, the patient suffered a grand mal seizure. Intravenous diazepam was administered, and seizure activity terminated after a total dose of 10 mg. She then received phenytoin with a total loading dose of 1 gram, followed by 300 mg/day.

Antimicrobial therapy was initiated with intravenous penicillin G at a dosage of 4 million U every 4 h. The blood pressure responded to intravenous fluids. By the next day, the patient began to exhibit some improvement in mental status—she was able to state her name, although she was not oriented to time or place. CSF and blood cultures grew *Strep. pneumoniae,* and susceptibility testing revealed that the organism was susceptible to penicillin (minimal inhibitory and bactericidal concentrations to penicillin G, 0.06 μg/mL).

Over subsequent days the patient continued to improve and became totally oriented. Her serum and coagulation studies normalized, and she remained afebrile. However, three toes on her right foot began to exhibit evidence of necrosis and eventually required amputation. Upon discharge she received vaccination with the 23-valent pneumococcal vaccine.

CASE DISCUSSION

This case illustrates many of the concepts of acute bacterial meningitis. With her history of splenectomy, this patient was at risk for overwhelming infection with several encapsulated bacterial pathogens, including *Strep. pneumoniae, N. meningitidis,* and *H. influenzae* type b. In addition, she was at increased risk for infection with *L. monocytogenes* because of her prior history of Hodgkin's disease. Clinical evaluation initially revealed only minor symptoms of headache and neck stiffness, but there was rapid progression to a fulminant course. Laboratory evaluation revealed a leukocytosis with a left shift; the electrolyte concentrations and arterial blood gas analysis were consistent with a combined metabolic acidosis and respiratory alkalosis.

The management of acute bacterial meningitis is illustrated by the institution of antimicrobial therapy (ampicillin plus cefotaxime) prior to CT scanning, to cover the likely bacterial pathogens in this immunosuppressed patient. One treatment dose of each antibiotic will not alter the CSF profile significantly when the lumbar puncture is performed soon after the CT. The CSF formula revealed an increased opening pressure, relatively low cell count, decreased glucose level, and markedly elevated protein level. The low neutrophil response is associated with overwhelming sepsis and a poor prognosis. Once an infecting pathogen was isolated, therapy was modified to target the specific infectious agent.

Adjunctive therapy was needed only to control seizure activity. Had the patient's condition continued to deteriorate, an intracranial monitoring device would have been placed to measure intracranial pressure. Therapies, including mannitol and hyperventilation, would have been instituted if appropriate. This patient did not receive corticosteroids since, at present, little information is available to recommend their routine use in meningitis in adults. These recommendations may change, pending ongoing clinical studies.

Acknowledgments

We gratefully acknowledge Eve Lorraine Schwartz for her secretarial assistance. This work supported in part by a research grant (RO1-AI17904) and a training grant (T32-AI07046) from the National Institute of Allergy and Infectious Diseases. W.M.S. is an established investigator of the American Heart Association.

References

1. Schlech WF, Ward JI, Band JD, et al: Bacterial meningitis in the United States, 1978 through 1981. The national bacterial meningitis surveillance study. JAMA 253:1749, 1985.
2. Spagnuolo PT, Ellner JJ, Lerner PI, et al: *Haemophilus influenzae* meningitis: The spectrum of disease in adults. Medicine 61:74, 1982.
3. McGee ZA, Stephens DS, Hoffman LH, et al: Mechanisms of mucosal invasion by pathogenic *Neisseria.* Rev Infect Dis 5:S708, 1983.
4. Ross SC, Densen P: Complement deficiency states and infection: Epidemiology, pathogenesis and consequences of neisserial and other infections in an immune deficiency. Medicine 63:243, 1984.
5. Tunkel AR, Scheld WM: Acute infectious complications of head trauma, in Braakman R (ed): *Handbook of Clinical Neurology, Head Injury.* Amsterdam, Elsevier, 1990, p 317.
6. Gellin BG, Broome CV: Listeriosis. JAMA 261:1313, 1989.
7. Cherubin CE, Marr JS, Sierra MF, Becker S: *Listeria* and gram-negative bacillary meningitis in New York City, 1972–1979. Frequent causes of meningitis in adults. Am J Med 71:199, 1981.
8. Schlesinger LS, Ross SC, Schaberg DR: *Staphylococcus aureus* meningitis: A broad-based epidemiologic study. Medicine 66:148, 1987.
9. Carpenter RR, Petersdorf RG: The clinical spectrum of bacterial meningitis. Am J Med 33:262, 1962.
10. Verghese A, Gallemore G: Kernig's and Brudzinski's signs revisited. Rev Infect Dis 9:1187, 1987.
11. Scheld WM: Meningococcal diseases, in Warren KS, Mahmoud AAF (eds): *Tropical and Geographical Medicine,* 2d ed. New York, McGraw-Hill, 1990, p 798.
12. Schoenbaum SC, Gardner P, Shillito J: Infections of cerebrospinal fluid shunts: Epidemiology, clinical manifestations, and therapy. J Infect Dis 131:543, 1975.
13. Martin WJ: Rapid and reliable techniques for the laboratory detection of bacterial meningitis. Am J Med 75(1B):119, 1983.
14. Saubolle MA, Jorgensen JH: Use of the *Limulus* amebocyte lysate test as a cost-effective screen for gram-negative agents of meningitis. Diagn Microbiol Infect Dis 7:177, 1987.
15. Tunkel AR, Wispelwey B, Scheld WM: Bacterial meningitis: Recent advances in pathophysiology and treatment. Ann Intern Med 112:610, 1990.
16. Peltola H, Anttila M, Renkonen OV, The Finnish Study Group: Randomised comparison of chloramphenicol, ampicillin, cefotaxime, and ceftriaxone for childhood bacterial meningitis. Lancet 1:1281, 1989.
17. Schaad UB, Suter S, Gianella-Borradori A, et al: A comparison of ceftriaxone and cefuroxime for the treatment of bacterial meningitis in children. N Engl J Med 322:141, 1990.
18. Fong IW, Tomkins KB: Review of *Pseudomonas aeruginosa* meningitis with special emphasis on treatment with ceftazidime. Rev Infect Dis 7:604, 1985.
19. Scheld WM: Quinolone therapy for infections of the central nervous system. Rev Infect Dis 11:S1194, 1989.
20. Levitz RE, Quintiliani R: Trimethoprim-sulfamethoxazole for bacterial meningitis. Ann Intern Med 100:881, 1984.
21. Radetsky M: Duration of treatment in bacterial meningitis: A historical inquiry. Pediatr Infect Dis J 9:2, 1990.
22. Lebel MH, Freij BJ, Syrogiannopoulos GA, et al: Dexamethasone therapy for bacterial meningitis. Results of two double-blind placebo-controlled trials. N Engl J Med 319:964, 1988.
23. Girgis NI, Farid Z, Mikhail IA, et al: Dexamethasone treatment for bacterial meningitis in children and adults. Pediatr Infect Dis J 8:848, 1989.
24. Täuber MG, Sande MA: Dexamethasone for bacterial meningitis: Increasing evidence for a beneficial effect. Pediatr Infect Dis J 8:842, 1989.
25. Peter G: Treatment and prevention of *Haemophilus influenzae* type b meningitis. Pediatr Infect Dis J 6:787, 1987.
26. Kaplan K: Brain abscess. Med Clin North Am 69:345, 1985.
27. Wispelwey B, Scheld WM: Brain abscess. Clin Neuropharmacol 10:483, 1987.
28. Chun CH, Johnson JD, Hofstetter M, Raff MJ: Brain abscess. A study of 45 consecutive cases. Medicine 65:415, 1986.
29. Saez-Llorens XJ, Umaña MA, Odio CM, et al: Brain abscess in infants and children. Pediatr Infect Dis J 8:449, 1989.
30. Brewer NS, MacCarty CS, Wellman WE: Brain abscess: A review of recent experience. Ann Intern Med 82:571, 1985.
31. Wheelan MA, Hilal SK: Computed tomography as a guide in the diagnosis and follow-up of brain abscesses. Radiology 135:663, 1980.
32. Weisberg L: Clinical–CT correlations in intracranial suppurative (bacterial) disease. Neurology 34:509, 1984.
33. Rehncrona S, Brismar J, Holtas S: Diagnosis of brain abscesses with indium-111 labeled leukocytes. Neurosurgery 16:23, 1985.
34. Haimes AB, Zimmerman RD, Morgello S, et al: MR imaging of brain abscess. AJR 152:1073, 1989.
35. Alderson D, Strong AJ, Ingham MR, Selkon JB: Fifteen year review of the mortality of brain abscess. Neurosurgery 8:1, 1981.
36. Levy RM, Gutin PH, Baskin DS, Pons VG: Vancomycin penetration of a brain abscess: Case report and review of the literature. Neurosurgery 18:632, 1986.
37. Boom WH, Tuazon CU: Successful treatment of multiple brain abscesses with antibiotics alone. Rev Infect Dis 7:189, 1985.
38. Stephanov S: Surgical treatment of brain abscess. Neurosurgery 22:724, 1988.
39. Mampalam TJ, Rosenblum ML: Trends in the management of bacterial brain abscesses: A review of 102 cases over 17 years. Neurosurgery 23:451, 1988.
40. Silverberg AL, DiNubile MJ: Subdural empyema and cranial epidural abscess. Med Clin North Am 69:361, 1985.
41. Coonrod JD, Dans PE: Subdural empyema. Am J Med 53:85, 1972.
42. Kaufman DM, Miller MH, Steigbigel NH: Subdural empyema: Analysis of 17 recent cases and review of the literature. Medicine 54:485, 1975.
43. Kaufman DM, Litman N, Miller MH: Sinusitis: induced subdural empyema. Neurology 33:123, 1983.
44. Yoshikawa TT, Chow AW, Guze LB: Role of anaerobic bacteria in subdural empyema. Report of four cases and review of 327 cases from the English literature. Am J Med 58:99, 1975.
45. Dacey RG, Winn HR, Jane JA, Butler AB: Spinal subdural empyema: Report of two cases. Neurosurgery 3:400, 1978.

46. Baker AS, Ojemann RG, Swartz MN, Richardson EP Jr: Spinal epidural abscess. N Engl J Med 293:463, 1975.
47. Danner RL, Hartman BJ: Update of spinal epidural abscess: 35 cases and review of the literature. Rev Infect Dis 9:265, 1987.
48. Koppel BS, Tuchman AJ, Mangiardi JR, et al: Epidural spinal infection in intravenous drug abusers. Arch Neurol 45:1331, 1988.
49. Greenlee JE: Epidural abscess, in Mandell GL, Douglas RG Jr, Bennett JE (eds): *Principles and Practice of Infectious Diseases*, 3d ed. New York, Churchill Livingstone, 1990, p 791.
50. Lasker BR, Harter DH: Cervical epidural abscess. Neurology 37:1747, 1987.
51. Weingarten K, Zimmerman RD, Becker RD, et al: Subdural and epidural empyemas: MR imaging. AJR 152:615, 1989.
52. Greenlee JE: Subdural empyema, in Mandell GL, Douglas RG Jr, Bennett JE (eds): *Principles and Practice of Infectious Diseases*, 3d ed. New York, Churchill Livingstone, 1990, p 788.
53. DiNubile MJ: Infections of the cranial dura and dural sinuses, in Harris AA (ed): *Handbook of Clinical Neurology*, vol 52, *Microbial Disease*. Amsterdam, Elsevier, 1988, p 167.
54. Southwick FS, Richardson EP Jr, Swartz MN: Septic thrombosis of the dural venous sinuses. Medicine 65:82, 1985.
55. DiNubile MJ: Septic thrombosis of the cavernous sinuses. Arch Neurol 45:567, 1988.
56. Greenlee JE: Suppurative intracranial phlebitis, in Mandell GL, Douglas RG Jr, Bennett JE (eds): *Principles and Practice of Infectious Diseases*, 3d ed. New York, Churchill Livingstone, 1990, p 793.
57. Macchi PJ, Grossman RI, Gomori JM, et al: High field MR imaging of cerebral venous thrombosis. J Comput Assist Tomogr 10:10, 1986.
58. Goldberg AL, Rosenbaum AE, Wang H, et al: Computed tomography of dural sinus thrombosis. J Comput Assist Tomogr 10:16, 1986.
59. Levine SR, Twyman RE, Gilman S: The role of anticoagulation in cavernous sinus thrombosis. Neurology 38:517, 1988.

Chapter 104

ENCEPHALOMYELITIS

JOHN C. GALBRAITH
D. LORNE TYRRELL

KEY POINTS

- *Herpes simplex virus (HSV) is the most common cause of fatal sporadic encephalitis. Early recognition and early treatment with acyclovir significantly improves outcome.*
- *A diagnosis of encephalomyelitis should be suspected in patients with fever, headache, behavioral changes, unexplained focal neurologic signs or seizures, or altered mental status without an obvious alternative explanation.*
- *Focal neurologic abnormalities are demonstrable either clinically or with neurodiagnostic evaluation in >90 percent of cases of herpes simplex virus encephalitis (HSVE).*
- *Definitive diagnosis of HSVE requires brain biopsy; however, treatment must be commenced with acyclovir as soon as the diagnosis is clinically suspected.*
- *If focal neurologic signs are present, computed tomography (CT) or magnetic resonance imaging (MRI) scanning should be performed prior to lumbar puncture. Diagnostic imaging is helpful in ruling out other treatable causes of altered mental status and also may identify patients with increased intracranial pressure (ICP) in whom lumbar puncture may be dangerous.*
- *Unless contraindicated, an early lumbar puncture should be performed. This is especially important to rule out bacterial meningitis.*
- *The cerebrospinal fluid (CSF) is almost always abnormal in encephalomyelitis, usually demonstrating increased leukocytes generally between 10 and 500/mm^3. The CSF glucose value is usually normal and the protein content is usually normal or slightly elevated. Although a completely normal CSF does not rule out encephalomyelitis, it should heighten suspicion for a toxic or metabolic encephalopathy.*
- *Arboviruses are the most common cause of encephalitis worldwide. Their frequency varies dramatically depending mainly on the season and geographic locale.*
- *Although viruses are the most common cause of encephalomyelitis, nonviral causes should be carefully ruled out because they are often readily treatable.*
- *Intensive supportive care is indicated in patients with encephalitis because these patients may make remarkable recoveries even after prolonged periods of unconsciousness.*

Encephalitis and myelitis refer to inflammation of the brain and spinal cord, respectively. These processes may occur together, often with meningeal involvement, hence the terms *meningoencephalitis* and *meningoencephalomyelitis*. Encephalomyelitis may result from direct invasion of a microorganism into the central nervous system (CNS) or as a result of a demyelinating autoimmune process triggered by a recent vaccination or infection. Up to 20 percent of all encephalitides result from this latter autoimmune hypersensitivity reaction and have been variously termed *postinfectious, parainfectious,* and *postvaccinial.* Strictly speaking, postinfectious refers to neurologic syndromes following an infection, whereas parainfectious describes those occurring simultaneously with an infection. Postvaccinial refers to the encephalomyelitis which follows immunization. Regardless of the exact pathogenesis, the clinical manifestations and differential diagnosis of these processes overlap to such a degree that they may be considered together.

In this chapter the approach to the patient with suspected encephalitis will first be outlined. This will be followed by a more detailed discussion of selected infectious etiologies highlighting pathogenesis, epidemiology, clinical features, diagnostic evaluation, treatment, and prognosis. The chapter will conclude with a brief summary of the supportive care in the ICU after which an illustrative case will be presented and discussed.

Approach to the Patient with Suspected Encephalomyelitis

There are a multiplicity of etiologies for encephalomyelitis[1] (Table 104-1). Unfortunately, most patients do not present with symptoms and signs pathognomonic of a certain cause, but rather with nonspecific problems of fever, headache, and behavioral changes or altered mental status. One must, therefore, have a clear approach in the workup of such patients. As with other areas of medicine, the approach should begin with a careful history and physical examination. The clinical features alone are not generally sufficient to establish an etiologic diagnosis but do influence the likelihood of some diagnoses. For instance, age can be a factor in that neonates are the group at highest risk for meningoencephalitis from HSV type 2 (HSV-2). Enteroviruses and bacterial infections, including group B streptococcus and *Listeria monocytogenes,* should also be considered in the differential diagnosis of progressive encephalitis in neonates.

Beyond the neonatal period, the setting of disease may provide helpful clues. Arbovirus encephalitis is more or less likely depending on the season, locale, degree of insect exposure, and current prevalence of disease in a given community. Most outbreaks of Eastern equine encephalitis are preceded by enzootics of disease in local horses and pheasants. Likewise, epidemics of St. Louis encephalitis are often preceded by serologic changes in chickens. Tick exposure in specific geographic areas should heighten the suspicion for Lyme disease, Rocky Mountain spotted fever, or ehrlichiosis. Similarly, exposure to certain animals may be suggestive for rabies or leptospirosis.

The progression of disease often suggests certain causes. Encephalitis developing 1 to 2 weeks following immunization or a viral syndrome is more likely postinfectious,

TABLE 104-1 Causes of Encephalomyelitis

Viral	
Herpetoviridae	Herpes simplex
	Varicella zoster
	Epstein-Barr
	Cytomegalovirus
Togaviridae	Alphaviruses
	Eastern equine
	Western equine
	Venezuelan equine
	Rubivirus
	Rubella
Flaviridae	St. Louis
	Murray Valley
	Japanese B
Bunyaviridae	California (La Crosse)
Picornaviridae	Echovirus
	Coxsackievirus
	Poliovirus
Arenaviridae	Lymphocytic choriomeningitis
Rhabdoviridae	Rabies
Retroviridae	Human immunodeficiency virus
	Human T cell lymphotropic virus (myelitis)
Paramyxoviridae	Measles
	Mumps
Myxoviridae	Influenza
Adenoviridae	Adenovirus
Nonviral	
Bacterial meningitis, brain abscess	
Parameningeal infection	
Infective endocarditis	
Mycoplasma	
Mycobacterium	
Rickettsia	
Borrelia (Lyme disease)	
Leptospira	
Treponema pallidum	
Nocardia	
Actinomycosis	
Cryptococcus	
Coccidioides	
Mucormycosis	
Histoplasma	
Toxoplasma	
Plasmodium falciparum	
Trypanosomiasis	
Acanthamoeba	
Naegleria	
Connective tissue diseases, vasculitis	

NOTE: Conditions which may resemble encephalitis include tumor, toxic or metabolic encephalopathy, intracranial hemorrhage/hematoma, cerebrovascular disease.

whereas an acute fulminant course is more in keeping with HSVE. A slowly progressive neurologic disease is characteristic of "slow virus infections," including Creutzfeldt-Jacob disease, subacute sclerosing panencephalitis (SSPE) and acquired immunodeficiency syndrome (AIDS) encephalopathy. A chronic or fluctuating course suggests mycobacterial or fungal infections. The diagnosis of CNS tuberculosis is difficult and requires a high index of suspicion. A subacute meningoencephalitis with certain associated systemic symptoms may suggest immunologic disorders (e.g., systemic lupus erythematosus or sarcoidosis) or, alternatively, neoplastic disease such as lymphoma, leukemia, or breast or lung cancer.

The immune status of the patient is also important when considering the various etiologic possibilities. Patients who are immunocompromised frequently develop unusual forms of encephalitis. Hypogammaglobulinemic patients may develop a chronic encephalitis with enteroviruses. Rhinocerebral mucormycosis most often occurs in diabetics with ketoacidosis and in neutropenic leukemics who have been on broad-spectrum antibiotics. Toxoplasmosis is the most common cause of encephalitis in AIDS patients. Other causes of encephalitis in AIDS include cytomegalovirus (CMV) and other herpes viruses, fungi (especially cryptococcus), mycobacterium, and uncommon pathogens like *Nocardia, Listeria, Acanthamoeba* and papovavirus.

Physical examination lends little to the diagnostic approach except in cases where a characteristic rash is present, such as in varicella, measles, Lyme disease, or Rocky Mountain spotted fever. Evidence of disease outside the CNS can suggest certain causes. For example, most patients with CNS disease associated with *Mycoplasma pneumoniae* have antecedent or concurrent respiratory tract infection. A thorough neurologic examination is important since the presence of focal neurologic signs heightens the likelihood of treatable infectious etiologies and mandates the commencement of empirical antimicrobial therapy. Although it is noteworthy that encephalitis caused by HSV is associated with focal neurologic findings in 85 percent of patients, these findings are nonspecific. Even when present in patients with fever, they could represent other CNS diseases such as parameningial infection, subdural empyema, brain abscess, hemorrhage, vascular disease, or tumor.

The presence of focal neurologic abnormalities clearly mandates urgent diagnostic imaging with either CT scanning or MRI. Although the sensitivity of these techniques is limited in diagnosing encephalitis, they are essential and invaluable in ruling out other CNS processes which could be clinically confused with encephalitis and which require alternative specific therapy. In addition, the CT or MRI scans can identify patients with increased ICP in whom lumbar puncture is contraindicated.

A lumbar puncture is an important step in the diagnostic evaluation of encephalitis and should be performed early unless there is a specific contraindication. It is especially important to rule out bacterial meningitis. If there is concern for increased ICP and possible herniation, a cisternal puncture should be considered. CSF should be sent for cell count, chemistry, virus isolation, and stains and culture for fungi and bacteria (including mycobacteria). A completely normal lumbar puncture significantly reduces the likelihood of encephalitis and raises the possibility of toxic or metabolic encephalopathy. Reye's syndrome must be distinguished from encephalitis. This syndrome has been associated with several viral infections, especially influenza and varicella zoster. It occurs most often in children who are usually afebrile, but have altered mental status along with hepatomegaly. CSF protein and cell counts are normal, but the blood ammonia level is almost always elevated. Other clues to the diagnosis of Reye's syndrome include elevated liver enzyme levels in serum and hypoglycemia. Patients with normal CSF examinations should be monitored carefully, and if the index of suspicion for encephalitis remains high, further neurodiagnostic evaluation, including a second lumbar puncture, should be considered. Further evaluation of all patients with encephalitis includes neurodiagnostic evaluation with an electroencephalogram (EEG) and a CT scan or MRI scan. Ancillary studies such as serology should be performed depending on the specific characteristics of each case. If no specific diagnosis is established, then brain biopsy should be considered. As will be discussed later in the chapter under HSVE, some physicians prefer a trial of empirical treatment with acyclovir in those patients with clinical pictures compatible with HSVE prior to brain biopsy. Ongoing surveillance for alternative diagnoses must be maintained and, if the clinical response is unfavorable, then brain biopsy should be performed. If brain biopsy fails to ascertain the diagnosis and the encephalitis remains clinically compatible with HSVE, then the full course of acyclovir should be completed.

AIDS patients are unique. The approach to management in these patients again requires a complete neurodiagnostic assessment along with toxoplasma serology. If the encephalitis is compatible with toxoplasmosis, then empirical treatment with pyrimethamine and sulfadiazine is begun. Clinical and radiographic improvement is anticipated to occur within 10 days of commencing therapy. However, if there is evidence of disease progression, then brain biopsy for definitive diagnosis should be performed. More than one pathogen may occasionally be isolated in AIDS patients with CNS disease.

Myelitis

The diagnostic and therapeutic approach to myelitis without encephalitis is somewhat different. Polio should be suspected in cases where there is a history of recent immunization or contact with a recently immunized individual. The pattern of myelitis caused by polio and other enteroviruses is primarily lower motor neuron disease; characteristically there is an asymmetric flaccid paralysis with preserved sensation and bladder function. The diagnosis is established by viral isolation from stools, throat, or CSF along with serologic confirmation.

Patients with transverse myelitis usually present with limb weakness and a sensory level along with loss of bowel and bladder control. This syndrome may result from a variety of infectious diseases; however, in most cases, there is no identifiable cause. It is important to exclude the potentially treatable causes such as tuberculosis, syphilis, herpes zoster, schistosomiasis, and human immunodeficiency virus (HIV). The numerous parainfectious etiologies of transverse myelitis include measles, mumps, rubella, influenza, and *M. pneumoniae,* and the management of these causes is strictly supportive. Regardless of the exact etiology, early neurodiagnostic evaluation with myelography and CT or MRI scanning is important to rule out spinal cord compression, epidural abscess, or hemorrhage.

A syndrome known as tropical spastic paraparesis (TSP) is associated with human T-lymphotropic virus type I (HTLV-I) infection. TSP is characterized by spastic paraperesis or paraplegia with pyramidal signs, occasional mild distal sensory loss, and occasional sphincter incontinence. HTLV-I is endemic in certain geographic regions including Africa, southern Japan, and the Caribbean basin.

Herpes Simplex Virus Encephalitis

EPIDEMIOLOGY AND PATHOGENESIS

HSVE is the most common fatal nonepidemic encephalitis, accounting for between 5 to 10 percent of all reported cases.[2] The exact incidence is unknown but it has been estimated to occur in 1/250,000 of the population per year.[3] It is seen in all ages, in both sexes, and in all seasons.[4] The patient is seldom immunocompromised and one cannot predict who is at risk for HSVE. HSVE is particularly important because untreated it has a very high mortality rate. Recent developments in antiviral therapy have significantly improved the outcome.[5]

A temporal lobe syndrome is the most common clinical presentation for HSVE, but atypical presentations may occur with involvement of parietal or frontal lobes. The predilection for frontal or temporal lobes has led to the speculation that HSVE results from the retrograde spread of infection from the nasopharynx along the olfactory pathway to the basal portion of the frontal and temporal lobes. Alternatively, latent virus in the trigeminal ganglia may become activated and may reach the CNS along a neurotropic route.[6] Either of these pathogenetic mechanisms may explain why HSV-1 more commonly causes adult encephalitis than HSV-2. Serologic evaluation indicates that approximately 70 percent of HSVE is due to reactivation of latent HSV, whereas approximately 30 percent is due to primary infection. The median age for patients developing primary HSVE is 15 years, whereas the median age for recurrent infection is 50 years.[5]

CLINICAL AND LABORATORY FEATURES

There are no pathognomonic clinical symptoms or signs of HSVE that distinguish it from encephalitis of other etiologies.[4] The clinical presentation may be abrupt or insidious. There may be an influenza-like prodrome. Clinical findings include fever (90 percent), headache (81 percent), alteration of consciousness (97 percent), personality changes (85 percent), dysphasia (76 percent), autonomic dysfunction (60 percent), ataxia (40 percent), hemiparesis (38 percent), seizures (38 percent), cranial nerve defects (32 percent), visual field loss (14 percent), and papilledema

(14 percent). Eighty-five percent of patients have clinical findings indicative of focal neurologic disease.[4]

Adult HSVE may occur in the presence or absence of mucocutaneous HSV lesions. Although a history of recurrent HSV lesions was obtained in 22 percent of patients with HSVE, this history was also found with equal frequency in patients with encephalitis of other etiologies.[4]

The laboratory investigations are not diagnostic short of a brain biopsy. However, a number of investigations support the clinical impression of HSVE and provide useful information to support the decision to proceed to a biopsy.

Examination of the CSF reveals an abnormality in 90 to 97 percent of cases.[4,7] Usually there is a lymphocytic predominance with between 10 and 500 leukocytes/mm^3, although early in the course of illness, polymorphonuclear cells (PMNs) may predominate. Seventy-five to 80 percent of samples have red blood cells (RBCs) indicating the hemorrhagic nature of this encephalitis. The glucose level is generally normal and the protein content is only moderately elevated. Viral cultures are almost always negative. Intrathecal antibody production and HSV antigen detection in CSF have not proven useful in the early diagnosis, but may be helpful in making a retrospective diagnosis.[8,9] Recently, Rowley and coworkers reported the detection of HSV DNA in CSF using the polymerase chain reaction.[10] This technique may prove very valuable as an early noninvasive diagnostic test to confirm HSVE. However, in this first report, the CSF samples were not taken early in the disease and further studies to confirm its usefulness are required.

Neurodiagnostic tests such as EEG, brain scan, CT scan, and MRI are useful in confirming and localizing the CNS lesion. EEG has been shown to be more sensitive than brain scan or CT scans early in the course of HSVE.[4] In 80 to 90 percent of cases, the initial EEG is abnormal, with predominantly spiked and slow wave patterns localized to the area of the brain involved. Paroxysmal lateral epileptiform discharges (PLEDs) are characteristic of HSVE, but are neither pathognomonic nor common.[11,12] Although EEG may be the earliest localizing laboratory test, specificity is lacking. Sodium pertechnetate ^{99}Tc brain scans are only abnormal in about half the cases of HSVE and demonstrate radionuclide uptake in the involved area of the brain.[4] Similarly, CT scans are abnormal early in the course of illness in about half the cases of HSVE. Abnormalities include localized edema, low density lesions, mass effect, contrast enhancement, and hemorrhage (Fig. 104-1).[4] More recently, MRI has become available and may be the most sensitive neurodiagnostic test owing to its high sensitivity to changes in brain water content and excellent delineation of the temporobasal lobe of the brain[13] (Fig. 104-2). MRI may be more specific than the EEG[14] and has been advocated by some as the first diagnostic step in the evaluation of suspected HSVE; however, the clinical experience with MRI in this disease remains limited.

DIAGNOSIS AND MANAGEMENT

At the present time, brain biopsy is the only rapid and reliable way to diagnose HSVE. However, the necessity of a brain biopsy remains controversial. Several authors favor empirical treatment without biopsy in suspected HSVE.[8,15] There are several arguments against a brain biopsy to confirm the diagnosis.

1. Since only 5 to 10 percent of patients presenting with encephalitis have HSV as the cause, if all patients with encephalitis are biopsied, many unnecessary brain biopsies would be performed.
2. Although the biopsy may establish another diagnosis, in many cases these other diagnoses can be made without a biopsy.
3. There is potential for morbidity and mortality with biopsy.
4. The toxicity of acyclovir, the drug of choice in the treatment of HSVE, is very minimal.
5. A brain biopsy may yield a false-negative result in up to 5 percent of cases.
6. Improvements in diagnostic neuroradiology, such as MRI, will likely improve the selection of patients for treatment with acyclovir.

Some authors have supported brain biopsy in patients suspected of having HSVE.[2,16] Several arguments for biopsy are advocated.

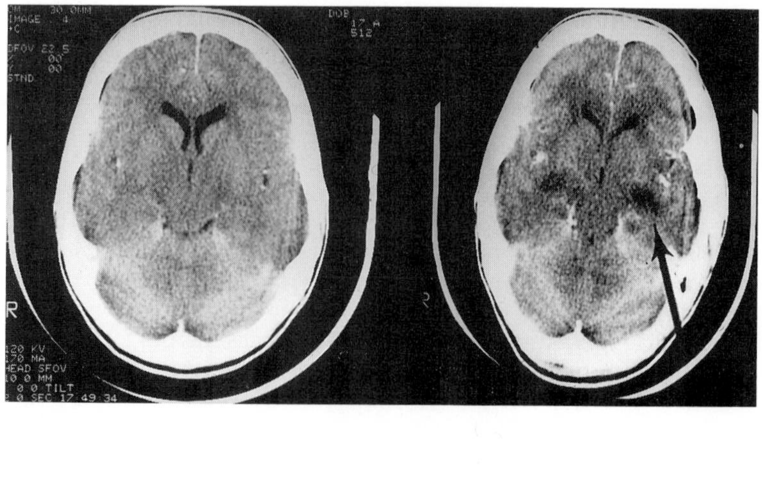

FIGURE 104-1 CT scan of the head in a patient with HSVE demonstrating bilateral hippocampal hypodensities. Involvement of the temporal lobes is classic for HSVE.

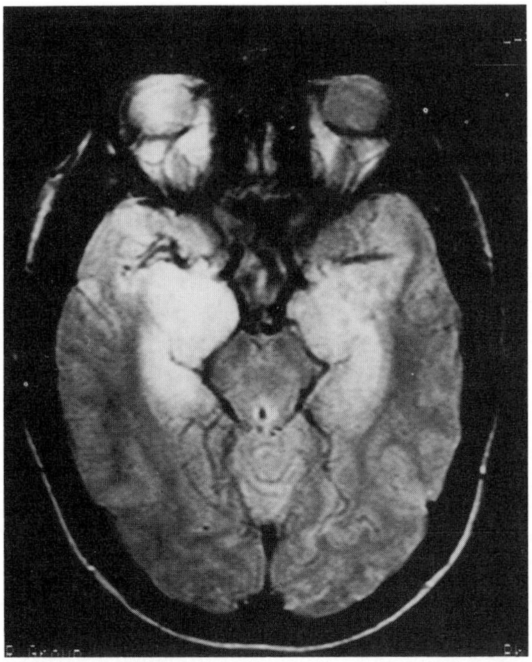

FIGURE 104-2 T2 weighted MRI of the head demonstrating increased signal intensity involving the medial aspects of the temporal lobes in the region of the hippocampus bilaterally more marked on the right than the left. These appearances are highly suggestive for HSVE.

1. Optimal patient management occurs with early definitive diagnosis.
2. A significant percentage (9 percent) of patients that present with a clinical picture compatible with HSVE have an alternative treatable disease diagnosed on biopsy.
3. The morbidity associated with brain biopsy is low although this varies depending on the center;[17,18] the NIAID collaborative antiviral study group reported a morbidity rate of 1.4 percent.[16]

We endorse the principle of obtaining a definitive diagnosis; however, the availability of an experienced neurosurgeon who is willing to perform the procedure is often the deciding variable. We emphasize the importance of early therapy; treatment with acyclovir should not be delayed while a brain biopsy is being organized.

If a brain biopsy is not performed, the patient must complete a full course of therapy with ongoing investigation and surveillance to rule out other diseases mimicking HSVE such as bacterial abscess, tuberculosis, cryptococcosis, toxoplasmosis, rickettsial infections, and neoplastic or vascular diseases. When a brain biopsy specimen is taken, the pathology and microbiology laboratories should be notified. Specimens should be submitted for viral isolation, culture for fungal, mycobacterial and bacterial pathogens, and pathology. Early detection of viral antigens is most important, and the specimen should be examined by immunofluorescence, immunoperoxidase, or an enzyme-linked immunosorbent assay (ELISA) procedure for sensitive detection of herpes antigen. In HSVE, HSV-1 frequently grows in 24 to 48 h and is nearly always positive by day 5. The histologic findings of HSVE include perivascular mononuclear cell cuffing, and frequently there is a prominent PMN infiltration. The classic finding is eosinophilic intranuclear inclusions (Cowdry's type A).[12] These histologic changes have a sensitivity of 56 percent and a specificity of 86 percent. Electron microscopy for HSV has a sensitivity of 45 percent and a specificity of 98 percent.[6] However, antigen detection tests such as ELISA, immunofluorescence, or immunoperoxidase staining are rapid, sensitive (>70 percent) and specific.

The recommended treatment of HSVE is acyclovir at a dose of 10 mg/kg every 8 h for 10 to 14 days. Clinical trials have clearly demonstrated that vidarabine is more effective than placebo[19] and acyclovir more effective than vidarabine.[5,20] It should be emphasized that early treatment is important and influences prognosis. Unfortunately, brain biopsy has a false-negative rate of up to 5 percent. For this reason we advocate that acyclovir should be continued for a full 10 days in the absence of an alternative diagnosis or contraindications to its use.

The toxicity of acyclovir is minimal. Uncommonly, precipitation of crystals in renal tubules can occur in poorly hydrated patients. This is manifest by a rise in serum creatinine and blood urea nitrogen (BUN) levels which can be reversed by increased hydration, dosage adjustment, or discontinuation of therapy. Patients at a higher risk of nephrotoxicity include those with preexisting renal disease or receiving concommittant nephrotoxic drugs. The dosage of acyclovir should be adjusted in renal failure[21] (Table 104-2).

Patients who receive acyclovir for suspected HSVE should also receive broad-spectrum antibiotics, such as cloxacillin, cefotaxime, and metronidazole for the first 48 to 72 h until CSF and brain biopsy cultures for bacteria are reported negative.

The precise factors that determine the therapeutic response are unknown. Patients who are younger than 30 years and present with a Glasgow coma score of >10 have the best outcome.[5] Patients who present with a Glasgow coma score of <6, irrespective of age, have a very poor prognosis. Other markers of poor outcome include bilateral

TABLE 104-2 Dosage of Intravenous Acyclovir for Herpes Simplex and Varicella-Zoster Encephalitis According to Renal Function

Creatinine Clearance ($mL/min/1.7\ m^2$)	Dosage Schedule
>50	10 mg/kg every 8 h
25–50	10 mg/kg every 12 h
10–25	10 mg/kg every 24 h
0–10	5 mg/kg every 24 h
Hemodialysis (3 times/week)	5 mg/kg every 24 h
Postdialysis	6.0 mg/kg after dialysis

SOURCE: Adapted from Reference 21.

abnormalities on the EEG as well as the presence of identifiable lesions on the original CT scan.[12]

Long-term complications of HSVE infection are common and include residual dysphasias, paresis, paresthesias, behavioral changes, and a Korsakoff-like amnesia. HSVE is a serious illness. Even with acyclovir treatment the mortality rate is 28 percent and only 38 percent of patients recover with minor or no residuum.[5]

HERPES SIMPLEX VIRUS TYPE 2 (HSV-2)

HSV-2 as a cause of encephalitis is seen primarily, although not exclusively, in neonates. In adults it is more frequently seen as a cause of aseptic meningitis concurrent with primary genital infection.

Neonatal infection occurs with the frequency of 26/100,000 deliveries and although infection may be localized to the skin, it is more often disseminated.[22] Infection is acquired by passage of infants through the birth canal of infected mothers, especially those with primary infection. It is recommended that all women in labor be examined for genital HSV-like lesions and if present (and if the membranes are intact) a cesarean section should be performed.[23] Unfortunately, most neonatal exposure to HSV results from excretion of virus by asymptomatic mothers at delivery. One cannot, therefore, predict nor prevent these exposures. Because HSV-2 causes 90 percent of primary genital herpes and 99 percent of recurrent infections, neonatal HSV infections are usually caused by HSV-2. HSV-2 causes more morbidity than HSV-1 in neonatal encephalitis.[24] Approximately 50 percent of neonates with encephalitis are premature and typically clinical illness begins 1 to 3 weeks after birth. Although CNS disease might occur in isolation, more commonly there is evidence of diffuse disease with accompanying skin lesions, hepatitis, pneumonitis, or a disseminated intravascular coagulation.[6]

The diagnosis should be suspected in any infant becoming ill during the first weeks of life. The skin vesicles are the easiest source of viral isolation and confirmation of diagnosis, but up to 20 percent of newborns with HSV infection never have skin involvement.[25] These infants often excrete virus from peripheral sites in the absence of skin lesions, and hence conjunctival, throat, and CSF specimens should be submitted for viral isolation. Further diagnostic evaluation may include EEG, brain scan, CT scan, ultrasound, and MRI, alone or in combination, depending on the circumstances. Occasionally, brain biopsy may be necessary for the diagnosis. Early empirical treatment with acyclovir is important in reducing mortality and morbidity. Without treatment, mortality is 50 to 85 percent and morbidity is 100 percent. With antiviral therapy the mortality is reduced to 10 to 57 percent but up to 86 percent still suffer neurologic sequelae.[22]

Varicella-Zoster Virus (VZV)

Primary VZV infection (chickenpox) may rarely be complicated by encephalitis, transient focal neurologic changes, aseptic meningitis, transverse myelitis, or Guillain-Barré syndrome. Viral replication in the CNS may contribute to the neurologic complications, but the pathogenesis is not well defined. There are two forms of encephalitis.[26] The cerebellar form is seen in children and occurs with a frequency of 0.1 to 0.75 percent of cases of chickenpox. It is characterized by ataxia, nystagmus, headache, nausea, vomiting, and nuchal rigidity. This illness is usually self-limited, lasting 2 to 4 weeks, and the majority of children have a complete recovery. The mortality rate is only 0.5 percent. The adult form is more severe and is usually manifested by altered sensorium, seizures, and focal neurologic signs, and has a mortality rate up to 35 percent.

After chickenpox, the virus becomes latent, but may erupt later in the form of shingles. Encephalitis, myelitis or both may accompany shingles. Evidence for direct viral invasion of the CNS is lacking and hence some have speculated that the encephalitis or myelitis is immunopathologically mediated.[26] It can occur between 30 days before onset of the rash to as late as 10 months afterward, although usually the neurologic symptoms present within the first 2 weeks of the exanthem. Patients who are immunosuppressed, including those with AIDS, or those who have disseminated zoster or a trigeminal distribution of zoster are at higher risk for developing encephalitis. The mortality rate of encephalitis is 10 to 20 percent; however, most survivors recover completely.

Diagnosis may usually be established on the basis of the characteristic lesions of chickenpox or zoster. The virus may be identified from vesicular scrapings on immunofluorescence, electron microscopy or culture.[22] The virus grows slowly, usually requiring 2 to 3 weeks for a positive culture. Serologic recognition of the presence of specific IgM may be useful for diagnosing primary chickenpox. Like HSVE, acyclovir is the drug of choice for this encephalitis, at doses of 10 mg/kg every 8 h. In vitro studies have demonstrated that the concentration of acyclovir required to inhibit VZV is considerably higher than that for HSV.[26]

Cytomegalovirus

Cytomegalovirus encephalitis (CMVE) is not uncommon in immunocompromised patients.[27] The presentation is typically subacute with disorientation, paresthesia, psychotic behavior, and mental obtundation being prominent clinical features.[6] Diagnosis can be extremely difficult because viral cultures even from the brain may be negative. The diagnosis may have to be made on the basis of histology and the isolation of CMV from multiple peripheral sites.[22] In AIDS patients, where CMV infection is common, the diagnosis is especially challenging because the presentation may be quite variable, ranging from ascending myelitis to apathy and dementia. CSF viral cultures have been positive on occasion but are usually negative. Even the histologic appearances are variable and sometimes viral inclusions are lacking. CMV infects all cell types in the CNS with microglial nodules being the most common resulting lesion. Necrotizing lesions may also be seen. CMVE has occurred together with HSVE in AIDS patients.[27]

CMVE is rare in immunocompetent individuals but has been reported.[28] Patients tend to be relatively young, aged 20 to 52 years. The pathogenesis is unclear. The typical clinical picture is similar to HSVE with severe headache, fever, and focal neurologic signs. CSF examination reveals a mild pleocytosis and the EEG may be markedly abnormal. Differentiation from HSVE requires specific virologic studies. In contrast to AIDS patients where progressive deterioration is the rule, immunocompetent patients with CMVE usually recover but may have long-term sequelae.

Ganciclovir, an acyclovir analogue, is a promising antiviral agent with activity against CMV.[21] Currently, clinical trials are underway to evaluate its efficacy in treating CMV infections in immunocompromised hosts. The standard dose is 5.0 mg/kg intravenously every 12 h, administered as a 1-h infusion and given for 2 to 3 weeks. Dosage must be altered downward in renal dysfunction. Possible adverse effects include granulocytopenia, thrombocytopenia, anemia, and elevated serum concentrations of bilirubin, alkaline, phosphatase, and creatinine.

Epstein-Barr Virus (EBV)

Neurologic complications occur in <1 percent of cases of mononucleosis, but are the leading cause of death in EBV infections.[6] CNS manifestations can include aseptic meningitis, Guillain-Barré syndrome, Bell's palsy, transverse myelitis, or encephalitis.[22] EBV encephalitis (EBVE) typically is acute in onset and may be diffuse or focal with abnormalities localized usually to the cerebellum or temporal lobe. Diagnosis may be readily evident if the encephalitis occurs in the setting of fever, pharyngitis, lymphadenopathy, and positive EBV serology. In children, the monospot is frequently negative, but the diagnosis can be confirmed by detection of specific IgM to EBV capsid antigen. CSF changes usually reveal a mononuclear pleocytosis with fewer than 200 cells/mm^3. Atypical lymphocytes may be seen in the CSF. The protein content may be normal or mildly elevated and the glucose level is usually normal.[22] Although EBVE may be severe, it is usually self-limited and almost all survivors recover without sequelae.

Arboviruses

Arboviruses are a group of enveloped RNA viruses that are transmitted by insects. Eighteen viruses in this group are known to cause encephalitis and together they are the most common cause of encephalitis worldwide.[6] The relative predominance of the different arboviruses varies depending on the geographic locale, season, and weather conditions (Table 104-3). In temperate climates infections tend to be seasonal, occurring mainly in the summer when arthropod populations are high. Human beings are incidental hosts and do not play a part in the natural history of the arboviruses that cause encephalitis. Asymptomatic and mild infections are most common. Serologic evidence indicates that the proportion of infections manifested as disease varies depending on the specific virus as well as on the age of the host. In Eastern equine encephalitis, 1/10 to 40 infections results in encephalitis, whereas in Murray Valley encephalitis, only 1/1000 infections results in encephalitis.

The pathogenesis of arbovirus encephalitis is believed to begin with an initial viremia followed by localization in the CNS. The virus likely crosses the blood-brain barrier via infected cells that migrate through the blood vessels of the brain. Once within the CNS the virus may replicate in neurons or glial elements.

The clinical features of the different arbovirus encephalitides are summarized in Table 104-4. Generally, arbovirus encephalitides follow the typical pattern of acute onset fever, headache, and meningismus with progression to an alteration in mental status. Examination of the CSF

TABLE 104-3 Epidemiology of the Major Arboviruses

Disease	Virus	Vector	Reservoir	Geographic Location	Approximate No. of cases in US/Year
1. Eastern equine encephalitis	Toga (alpha)	Mosquito	Birds	North, Central and South America (especially Atlantic and Gulf states)	0–12
2. Western equine encephalitis	Toga (alpha)	Mosquito	Birds	North, Central and South America (in US in regions west of Mississippi; in Canada in prairie provinces)	3–50
3. Venezuelan equine encephalitis	Toga (alpha)	Mosquito	Horses	Florida, Texas, Central and South America	0–5
4. St. Louis encephalitis	Flavi	Mosquito	Birds (esp. chickens)	North, Central and South America	20–2500
5. Japanese B encephalitis	Flavi	Mosquito	Pigs and birds	Asia (esp. southern and eastern Asia)	0
6. Murray Valley encephalitis	Flavi	Mosquito	Birds	Australia, New Guinea	0
7. California (La Crosse) encephalitis	Bunya	Mosquito	Rodents	Midwestern US	50–200

TABLE 104-4 Clinical Aspects of Arbovirus Infection

Disease	Clinical Features	Morbidity and Mortality in Patients Who Develop Encephalitis
1. Eastern equine encephalitis (EEE)	Mainly affects children and the elderly Abrupt onset with fulminant course Seizures are common; diffuse signs	50–75% mortality; 30% of survivors have severe sequelae: mental retardation, behavior changes, seizures, and paralysis
2. Western equine encephalitis	Mainly affects infants and the elderly Subclinical infections are common Similar to EEE but milder (except in infants)	3–7% mortality; sequelae less than with EEE
3. Venezuelan equine encephalitis	Many subclinical infections <4% develop encephalitis Myalgias are prominent	10–20% mortality
4. St. Louis encephalitis	<1% of infected people develop encephalitis Most severe in elderly May have tremor, seizures, paresis, syndrome of inappropriate antidiuretic hormone, urinary symptoms	5–15% mortality; mortality increases with age Neurasthenia may be a persistent problem
5. Japanese B encephalitis	Most common arbovirus worldwide Mainly among children <2% of infected develop encephalitis A vaccine is available	10–50% mortality especially among children Up to 70% of survivors have neuropsychiatric sequelae
6. Murray Valley encephalitis	Patients frequently present in coma Rapid disease progression in infants	20–50% mortality 40–100% of survivors have neurologic sequelae
7. California (La Crosse) encephalitis	Mainly affects boys (ages 3–10 years) Fulminant onset with seizures Rapid recovery after 2–5 days	<2% mortality Up to 15% have behavioral problems or recurrent seizures

usually shows fewer than 500 leukocytes and the majority are mononuclear although early on there may be a PMN predominance. The protein content is usually normal or slightly elevated. The glucose level is characteristically normal. Virus isolation is rare; hence, distinguishing between the different viruses requires careful consideration of epidemiologic and clinical variables together with serology.[29–33] At present, there is no effective antiviral therapy and management is strictly supportive. The mortality and morbidity vary depending on the specific arbovirus and the age and health of the patient.

Enteroviruses

Enteroviruses are very common causes of meningitis but only cause a small proportion of encephalitis. They rank behind arboviruses, HSV, and lymphocytic choriomeningitis (LCM) virus as causes of encephalitis that are proven to be viral in the United States. Enteroviruses are distributed worldwide and infections are most prevalent in the summer and autumn months in the temperate climates. At least 50 to 80 percent of nonpolioenteroviral infections are completely asymptomatic.[34] When encephalitis does develop it may vary from lethargy, drowsiness, and personality changes to seizures, paresis, and coma. The clinical findings suggest generalized involvement in most cases, but focal abnormalities including partial motor seizures, hemichorea, and acute cerebellar ataxia have been reported. Enteroviral encephalitis can mimic HSVE.

CSF findings typically reveal between 10 to 500 leukocytes/mm^3 with a lymphocytic predominance although neutrophils may predominate early. The CSF protein content is normal or slightly elevated and the glucose level is normal. Diagnosis is best established by virus isolation from the CSF; however, CSF viral cultures may be negative and the diagnosis may be inferred from isolation of virus from nonneurologic sites such as throat washings or feces. Although primary serologic diagnosis is not practical because of the number of serotypes, a demonstration of increasing titers of neutralizing antibodies to throat or feces isolates is useful in establishing the etiologic role of these nonneurologic isolates.

The course of illness is generally benign and treatment is supportive. However, neonates may develop a severe illness culminating in death and infants <1 year often have persistent neurologic sequelae. In addition, patients with antibody deficiencies may have severe infection. A syndrome of chronic enteroviral meningoencephalitis occurs in agammaglobulinemia.[35] Thirty percent of these patients present with edema or a dermatomyositis-like syndrome.[22] The course is prolonged and clinical manifestations may include headaches, seizures, hearing loss, lethargy or coma, weakness, ataxia, paresthesias, diminished intellectual acuity, development delay, hemiparesis, cranial nerve palsies, episodic confusional states, symptoms consistent with transient ischemic episodes, personality changes, dysarthria, hepatitis, and arthritis. In this syndrome the mortality rate is high and the only therapeutic modality with efficacy is the administration of specific neutralizing antibody, usually as part of a mixed immunoglobulin preparation.[35,36]

Polio is a neurotropic enterovirus, but due to the widespread use of polio vaccines its incidence has dramatically declined. Poliomyelitis still occurs in patients who have not received the vaccine and is common in underdeveloped countries. Rarely paralytic polio may develop in association with the use of the vaccine. Paralysis occurs in 0.1 percent of all poliovirus infections. In adults poliomyelitis often begins with muscle pain particularly involving the neck or lumbar region. This pain may be relieved by motion. Subsequently there is progression to weakness and paralysis, usually over 2 to 3 days. A characteristic feature of the paralysis of poliomyelitis is its asymmetric distribution. Another key point to note in the clinical diagnosis of poliomyelitis is that sensation is usually preserved. If sensory loss is present then an alternate diagnosis such as Guillain-Barré syndrome should be considered. Poliomyelitis very rarely takes the form of encephalitis.[34] When it does occur, it is seen principally in infants. It is manifested primarily by confusion and disturbances in consciousness. In addition, seizures and spastic paralysis may be seen. The illness is not distinguishable clinically from encephalitis due to many other viruses. The diagnosis is established when virus is isolated from the CSF. Unfortunately, unlike other enteroviruses, isolating polio viruses from the CSF is rare; therefore, throat and stool cultures should be taken in addition to acute and convalescent sera.[22]

Enterovirus 71 is a picornavirus which can cause an epidemic paralytic disease indistinguishable from poliomyelitis. Like other enteroviruses it may cause hand-foot-mouth disease. Paralysis may be accompanied by encephalitis or cranial nerve involvement. The diagnosis is established when enterovirus 71 is isolated from vesicle fluid, feces, oropharyngeal sections, urine, or CSF. The treatment is supportive but the mortality rate may be as high as 65 percent in patients with bulbar disease.[34]

Lymphocytic Choriomeningitis Virus

LCM virus is an arenavirus which is endemic in mice and can be transmitted to human beings.[37] LCM virus infection may occur worldwide but has only been demonstrated in Europe and the Americas. Human infection is most commonly seen in young adults although all ages may be affected. Most cases occur outside of summer months. The exact mode of transmission is not known but may be related to aerosols, direct contact with rodents, or rodent bites. The incubation period is usually from 5 to 10 days. The illness typically has an influenza-like prodrome followed later by a severe headache. A few patients go on to develop a clinical picture of encephalomyelitis, with confusion, psychosis, paraplegia, or disturbances of cranial, sensory, or autonomic nerve function. Other occasional complications include orchitis, myopericarditis, arthritis, and alopecia. Laboratory findings show a leukopenia and thrombocytopenia. The CSF typically reveals several hundred lymphocytes/mm^3 with a normal to elevated protein level and a normal to reduced glucose content. Infection is usually diagnosed by a fourfold rise in complement-fixing antibodies or virus isolation.[22] The treatment is supportive and rarely is the illness fatal.

Rabies Virus

Rabies virus is the only rhabdovirus which can affect human beings. It is transmitted to human beings virtually always by the bite of an infected mammal, although infection by the respiratory route may also occur. In countries where domestic animal rabies is well controlled most disease is associated with wild animal infection. Human disease is rare in the United States with only 50 cases being reported to the Centers for Disease Control from 1960 to 1987.[38] In countries where domestic animal rabies has not been controlled, it remains a significant problem. In 1985, 25,000 deaths were reported to the World Health Organization, but because this reporting is voluntary, it is an underestimation of the actual number of cases.[39] The incubation period is usually 20 to 90 days although in reported cases it has varied from 4 days to 19 years. During the incubation period the patient is well. A prodrome of 2 to 10 days which may include paresthesia at the bite site is followed by evidence of CNS infection which may include hyperactivity, bizarre behavior, seizures, nuchal rigidity, or paralysis. The mental status gradually deteriorates with disorientation, stupor, and coma.[40] The case fatality rate is virtually 100 percent. No tests are currently available to diagnose rabies infection before the onset of clinical disease. Rabies should be suspected in any case of encephalitis, especially if there is a history of an animal bite. Diagnosis can be established rapidly using immunofluorescent procedures to detect viral antigens on either biopsy of the skin of the posterior neck or conjunctival smears.[22] Rabies is a disease which is much easier to prevent than cure. However, cases have occurred even in patients receiving optimal prophylaxis. Patients should be isolated, recognizing that rabies virus may be present in saliva, tears, urine, CSF, and other body fluids or tissues.

Treatment is supportive but the outcome is dismal. High dose passive rabies immunogloblin has been used in some cases with no clear benefit.[41]

Two survivors in a review of 38 human rabies cases in the United States both received rabies vaccine before the onset of their illness and intensive supportive care after the onset of illness.[40]

Human Immunodeficiency Virus

HIV is a neurotropic pathogen which may cause CNS disease varying from aseptic meningitis to an encephalitis resulting in dementia and death (see Chap. 100 for more details). Postmortem studies of patients dying of HIV-related complications have suggested that CNS infection is always present even when it is not clinically apparent. The diagnosis should be suspected in patients with encephalitis who have risk factors for or clinical evidence of HIV infection. Serology is used to confirm HIV infection, but there are no good means at present of antemortem diagnosis of CNS disease.[22]

Measles

Measles is an acute infection caused by a paramyxovirus. This virus is highly contagious and causes infections with a worldwide distribution. It remains a significant problem, especially in unimmunized children and adults. Measles encephalomyelitis is one of the most common complications of measles. Although it is rare in children <2 years old, it complicates approximately 1/1000 measles infections in older children. The mortality rate is 10 to 20 percent and the majority of survivors have neurologic sequelae.[42]

Acute postinfectious encephalomyelitis probably has an autoimmune pathogenesis.[43] The illness is of abrupt onset and typically begins a week after the onset of the rash. However, it has been reported to have occurred prior to the onset of the rash or weeks after. The illness is manifest by recurrence of fever, seizures, motor abnormalities, and a depressed level of consciousness. The abrupt onset of the encephalomyelitis in the setting of the typical exanthem is a characteristic feature which helps to differentiate postinfectious encephalomyelitis from other forms of viral encephalitis that have a more gradual onset. The CSF is normal in approximately one-third of patients. However, it typically shows a lymphocytic pleocytosis with a normal or slightly elevated CSF protein. It is noteworthy that up to 50 percent of patients with measles have detectable EEG abnormalities.[44] The severity of the initial illness does not correlate with the severity or type of sequelae. Treatment is supportive but, unfortunately, a high proportion of those who recover are left with a significant neurologic deficit.

A less common complication of measles infection is subacute sclerosing panencephalitis (SSPE). SSPE occurs from weeks to months to years after measles and although the exact pathogenesis is unknown, it appears that persistent infection results from defective viral production of membrane or envelope proteins which allow the virus to escape immunosurveillance.[45] The disease is progressive, usually fatal, and occurs most often in children. This illness has been clinically divided into four stages:

1. cerebral signs;
2. convulsive and motor signs;
3. coma and opisthotonus;
4. mutism, loss of cerebrocortical function, and myoclonus.[46]

The most useful laboratory findings in SSPE include an abnormal EEG with the typical pattern consisting of well-defined periodic bursts of high voltage activity with an interval between bursts of usually 3 to 5 s and increased levels of γ globulin and measles antibody in CSF.[47] The presence of complement-fixing measles antibody in the CSF is a valuable test for establishing the diagnosis.[48] Biopsy is not considered necessary for the diagnosis since the clinical findings combined with the finding of measles antibody in the CSF are sufficient to establish the diagnosis in essentially all cases. Brain tissues of patients with SSPE typically demonstrate intranuclear inclusions containing paramyxovirus nucleocapsids on electron microscopic examination. The presence of measles antigen in the brain tissue may be demonstrated by either measles-specific fluorescence or measles-specific immunoperoxidase labeling. There is no well-established effective treatment for this condition; however, isoprinosine (inosiplex) has been reported to produce remission for >2 years in 5 of 15 patients in one study.[49] Other reports describe mixed benefits with isoprinosine and further evaluation is required.[50–52]

Mumps

Meningitis occurs in 15 percent of mumps cases, although CSF abnormalities may occur in up to 50 percent. Meningitis is a common benign condition to be distinguished from encephalitis which is rare and more serious. Encephalitis occurs in approximately 1/6000 cases of mumps.[53] There is bimodal distribution of illness: an early onset illness which coincides with parotitis and represents damage to neurons directly due to viral invasion and a more common late onset illness that develops 7 to 10 days after the onset of parotitis and is a postinfectious demyelinating process because of the host response to infection.

The clinical features are a diffuse encephalitis with fever, marked change in level of consciousness, seizures, paresis, aphasia, and involuntary movements. The CSF examination reveals the typical viral meningoencephalitis picture with a lymphocytic pleocytosis and a normal or slightly elevated CSF protein. There may, however, be a PMN cell predominance and hypoglycorrhacia. No rapid procedures are available for diagnosing mumps.[22,54] Virus may be isolated from CSF on tissue culture. Serology may be used to confirm the diagnosis. Encephalitis may occur secondary to mumps in the absence of clinical meningitis or parotitis. The treatment is supportive and sequelae of psychomotor retardation and convulsive disorders have been reported. The mortality rate is 1.4 percent.[55] Other neurologic syndromes rarely associated with mumps include deafness, cerebellar ataxia, facial palsy, transverse myelitis, ascending polyradiculitis, and a poliomyelitis-like syndrome.

Rubella

Encephalitis is a rare postinfectious complication of rubella. It occurs with a frequency of approximately 1/5000. It occurs more frequently in adults than in children. The symptoms are similar to but milder than those seen with measles. Diagnosis is established on the basis of serology and the treatment is supportive. The overall mortality rate is 20 percent.[56] A rubella SSPE-like syndrome is well described, usually in young adults as opposed to measles associated SSPE which tends to occur in children.

Mycoplasma pneumoniae

M. pneumoniae is a frequent cause of upper and lower respiratory tract infections in otherwise healthy people. In hospitalized patients with *M. pneumoniae* respiratory disease, up to 10 percent have complicating CNS disease.[57,58] The pathogenesis of the CNS disease is unclear; however, it has been postulated that the disease may result from direct invasion by the organism, a neurotoxin elaborated by the organism, or an autoimmune reaction precipitated by the *Mycoplasma* infection (i.e., parainfectious).[59,60] Multiple patterns of CNS involvement associated with *M. pneumoniae* have been reported. These include meningitis, encephalitis, psychosis, cerebellar ataxia, hemiplegia, transverse myelitis, and polyradiculitis. The encephalitis may be focal, mimicking HSVE, or nonfocal. Most patients have antecedent respiratory symptoms or signs. In one series, the mean interval between the onset of respiratory symptoms and the onset of neurologic disease was 10 days, with a range of 3 to 23 days. In encephalitis, the CSF usually reveals a lymphocytic predominance combined with a moderate elevation of the protein content and a normal glucose level. *M. pneumoniae* has rarely been identified histologically or recovered from biopsy specimens. The diagnosis is established by serology. The treatment is mainly supportive and no controlled prospective trials have evaluated the role of antibiotics. However, intravenous tetracycline would seem to be an appropriate agent. Unfortunately, a significant number of patients are left with long-term neurologic sequelae, especially patients who have focal encephalitis or high CSF protein content and pleocytosis.

Rocky Mountain Spotted Fever

Encephalitis may occur as a complication of Rocky Mountain spotted fever. This disease is caused by *Rickettsia rickettsii* and is transmitted by the bite of an infected tick (see Chap. 111). It is seen most frequently in the eastern United States, especially in younger people. The illness is characterized by the sudden onset of fever, malaise, headache, chills, and conjunctival injection. This is followed 2 to 3 days later by a maculopapular rash that appears first on the wrist and ankles, but rapidly spreads to the rest of the body including the palms and soles. The rash is often petechial or may become confluent and hemorrhagic. Routine laboratory tests for rapid diagnosis early in the illness are not readily available. A fourfold rise in antibody titer between acute and convalescent phase sera is considered diagnostic. The treatment of choice is chloramphenicol. Unfortunately, neurologic involvement with this disease is associated with a bad prognosis. Among 37 patients followed for 1 to 8 years after acute Rocky Mountain spotted fever, 21 had residual neurologic abnormalities.[62]

Lyme Disease

Lyme disease is the most common vector-borne infection in North America and Europe. It is a multisystem disease which results from infection with the spirochete *Borrelia burgdorferi* transmitted by a tick bite. Neurologic involvement occurs in 15 to 25 percent of patients, usually occurring weeks to months after infection. The typical pattern is fluctuating symptoms of meningitis with superimposed cranial or peripheral radiculoneuropathies. Acute or chronic encephalomyelitis may also occur. In patients with CNS involvement, the CSF may show a lymphocytic pleocytosis with elevated protein levels. Unfortunately, a test that uniformly indicates active infection in the CNS is lacking. The diagnosis is established when patients with a clinically compatible illness are demonstrated to have positive serology. In patients who have Lyme disease with neurologic abnormalities, the recommended treatment is ceftriaxone 2 g daily for 14 days.[63] The wide spectrum of neurologic involvement that may occur over time with Lyme disease is worth emphasizing.

Leptospirosis

Leptospirosis is a multisystem disease that may involve the CNS.[64] It is caused by spirochetes of the genus *Leptospira* and is a zoonosis of worldwide distribution. Man becomes infected via either direct or indirect contact with infected animals. Subclinical infection occurs commonly. Clinical infection is more commonly mild and anicteric; however, there is a severe icteric form. Leptospirosis is typically a biphasic illness beginning with a septicemic phase characterized by an abrupt onset of fever, headache, myalgias, and nausea and vomiting. This persists for 4 to 7 days and is followed by a second or immune phase where fever is usually low grade or absent. The headache during this stage is characteristically intense and may be accompanied by mild delirium. Common physical findings include muscle tenderness, conjunctival suffusion, adenopathy, hepatosplenomegaly, and rashes. Examination of the CSF reveals a mild mononuclear pleocytosis with a normal or slightly elevated protein. In this milder form of leptospirosis, focal neurologic signs and evidence of encephalitis are uncommon.

In icteric leptospirosis, the illness is more severe and is characterized by impaired renal and hepatic function, hemorrhage, myocarditis, and severe alterations in consciousness. The definitive diagnosis requires isolation of the organism or seroconversion. The organisms can be isolated from the blood or CSF during the first 10 days of the illness. Subsequently they may be isolated from the urine. Treatment of very severely ill patients consists of intravenous penicillin along with general supportive therapy to manage the life-threatening complications of renal failure, hypotension, and hemorrhage. The mortality rate in the more severe cases is between 5 and 10 percent.

Cryptococcus neoformans

Cryptococcosis is a systemic infection caused by the ubiquitous yeast-like fungus *C. neoformans*. Infection most frequently occurs in patients who are immunocompromised, especially those with AIDS. Infection tends to localize to the CNS. Onset may be abrupt in patients receiving corticosteroid therapy or those receiving treatment for lymphoreticular malignancies, but most frequently it is insidious with mild and nonspecific complaints such as headache, irritability, somnolence, and clumsiness. Often there are behavioral changes. On physical examination the patient is frequently afebrile with minimal or no nuchal rigidity. Papilloedema is noted in about one-third of cases and cranial nerve palsies are seen in about one-fifth.[65] CSF examination may reveal an elevated opening pressure with elevated protein content, decreased glucose level, and small numbers of leukocytes. It should be emphasized that in AIDS patients there are minimal or no abnormalities of the CSF, but cryptococci grow in culture. In 50 percent of patients with cryptococcal meningoencephalitis, the organism may be identified in India ink smears of CSF. Latex agglutination detects antigen in CSF, but positive tests must be confirmed by cultures before a definite diagnosis of cryptococcosis can be made. The recommended treatment is a combination of amphotericin B 0.3 mg/kg body weight daily intravenously plus flucytosine 37.5 mg/kg body weight every 6 h by mouth for 6 weeks.[66] Amphotericin may cause an impairment in renal function which results in a secondary rise in flucytosine levels, which must be monitored regularly. Eradication of infection seldom, if ever, occurs in AIDS patients. Excluding AIDS patients, the mortality rate in treated cryptococcal meningoencephalitis is approximately 25 to 30 percent.[67]

Toxoplasma Gondii

T. gondii is the causative agent in toxoplasmosis. It is a worldwide, obligate, intracellular, protozoan parasite that infects virtually all mammalian species. Toxoplasmic encephalitis was historically a relatively rare disease seen sporadically in immunocompromised patients particularly those with malignancies of the reticuloendothelial system as well as organ transplant recipients. However, this disease has risen to prominence in association with AIDS. It occurs in between 3 and 40 percent of patients with AIDS and is now recognized as the most common cause of intracerebral mass lesions in AIDS patients.[68] It is believed that toxoplasmic encephalitis results from reactivation of chronic latent infection. Clinically the CNS manifestations of toxoplasmosis are nonspecific and highly variable. They may take the form of cerebral mass lesions, meningoencephalitis, or diffuse encephalitis. Focal abnormalities are common, and they include focal seizures, hemiparesis, hemiplegia, hemisensory loss, cerebellar tremor, homonymous hemianopsia, cranial nerve palsies, diplopia, blindness, personality changes, and severe headache. Generalized abnormalities may also occur, and they include weakness, myoclonus, confusion, lethargy, disorientation, and coma. Immunocompromised patients with toxoplasmosis have predominantly CNS manifestations; however, extraneural manifestations of the disease include chorioretinitis, pneumonitis, myocarditis, orchitis, and peritonitis.

CSF examination of patients with toxoplasmic encephalitis generally reveals an elevated protein content with a mononuclear pleocytosis of up to several hundred cells. The glucose level is normal or slightly depressed. However, CSF analysis may be completely normal. CT scanning of the brain in AIDS patients with cerebral toxoplasmosis reveals abnormalities in >90 percent.[69,70] Most commonly the lesions are in the region of the basal ganglia, midbrain, or brain stem and are rounded and hypodense with peripheral "ring" enhancement, but may show diffuse or no contrast enhancement. Lesions may be single or multiple with multiple lesions being more specific for toxoplasmosis. MRI is reportedly more sensitive than CT for subdural abnormalities.[71] The abnormalities demonstrated on either MRI or CT are not pathognomonic; however, multiple hypodense ring-enhancing lesions in an HIV-infected individual are nearly so.

The diagnostic serologic changes associated with toxoplasmosis infection in immunocompetent individuals are seldom seen in AIDS patients with toxoplasmic encephalitis. Moreover, although negative toxoplasmosis serology in AIDS patients reduces the likelihood of toxoplasmosis infection, there are several reports of false-negative tests.[72,73] Local antibody production to *T. gondii* in the CSF is specific but lacks sensitivity, and therefore is of limited diagnostic usefulness. Unfortunately, antigen detection methods in the CSF have not yet proven helpful in the diagnosis.[68]

In AIDS patients with suspected toxoplasmic encephalitis, it is desirable to have a confirmed diagnosis since similar lesions may be due to tuberculosis, other bacteria, fungi, or lymphoma. However, not unlike the controversy surrounding brain biopsy in HSVE, many neurosurgeons as well as physicians are reluctant to perform or request open brain biopsy. Hence, AIDS patients who have encephalitis that is clinically and radiographically compatible with toxoplasmosis are usually given a therapeutic trial with pyrimethamine and sulfadiazine. Biopsy is reserved for patients who fail to respond to therapy or if the patient's neurologic status is rapidly deteriorating. Clinical and radiographic responses to therapy should be seen within 10 days of starting therapy. The recommended dose of pyrimethamine is 75 to 100 mg/day. Sulfadiazine is given at 100 mg/kg/day (maximum of 8 g/day) in two divided doses.[74] This therapy is continued for 4 to 6 weeks after resolution of all signs and symptoms. In AIDS patients, discontinuation of therapy has been frequently associated with relapse of toxoplasmic encephalitis. The overall prognosis of AIDS patients with CNS toxoplasmosis has been poor, with a median survival time of 4 months.

Acanthamoeba

Granulomatous amebic encephalitis (GAE) is caused by *Acanthamoeba castellani, A. culbertsoni*, and *A. astronyxis*. These are free-living ameba that have been isolated from soil, water, and air from diverse geographic locations. GAE is a subacute opportunistic infection that spreads hematogenously from pulmonary or skin lesions to the CNS. It occurs predominantly in debilitated or immunosuppressed individuals. Typically these patients present with mental status abnormalities, seizures, fever, headache, and hemiparesis. They may also demonstrate meningismus, visual disturbances, or ataxia. The diagnosis is frequently made postmortem. Brain biopsy is the only way to make the diagnosis antemortem. Little is known about the treatment of GAE; however, it has been recognized that the diamidine derivatives (pentamidine) have the greatest activity against *Acanthamoeba*.[75]

Naegleria

Naegleria fowleri is another free-living ameba that causes primary amebic meningoencephalitis (PAM). This ameba has been isolated from soil, river, and lake water and is especially prominent in warmer thermally polluted fresh water lakes. PAM appears primarily in healthy children and young adults who have a history of recent swimming in warm fresh water. The illness is characterized by abrupt onset of fever, nausea and vomiting, headache, and meningismus. The encephalitis is fulminant and in most patients progresses to coma and death. CSF examination typically reveals a neutrophilic pleocytosis, elevated protein level, and normal or reduced glucose value. Gram stain reveals pus cells, but no bacteria. However, if a wet mount is made of the CSF, motile trophozoites of *N. fowleri* may be seen. Only two patients are known to have survived PAM and they both had received high dose systemic and intrathecal amphotericin B.[75]

Supportive Therapy in the ICU

Intensive supportive care is indicated in patients with encephalitis, because these patients may make remarkable recoveries even after prolonged periods of unconsciousness.

The usual first principles of establishing and maintaining airway patency, oxygenation, and adequate ventilation in patients with disordered CNS function should be applied. A poor gag reflex or ineffective cough are markers of the need for airway protection. Special care must be taken in the intubation of patients with suspected encephalomyelitis to prevent potentially catastrophic increases in ICP. Intubation should be performed early in an elective fashion by an experienced person (see Chap. 6). Hypotension is also dangerous for patients with increased ICP and if present it should be treated with intravenous fluids and slight elevation of legs.

Strict monitoring of fluid, electrolyte, and glucose balance is necessary because of the possibility of hypothalamic involvement in the encephalitic process. Moreover, depending on the specific etiologic agent of encephalitis, there may be concurrent dysfunction of other organ systems compromising the patient's normal mechanisms of autoregulation and homeostasis. Nutrition must be maintained, preferably with enteral alimentation, but parenteral nutritional support may be necessary. Routine skin and eye care should not be neglected.

Although controversial, ICP monitoring is advocated by some for adults with severe encephalitis. Treatment of increased ICP has been required in up to 75 percent of patients in some series.[5] Major rises in ICP may lead to further neurologic compromise or death. Elevated ICP has been associated with a poor prognosis.[76] Therapy for raised ICP includes optimizing head position, hyperventilation to maintain a P_{CO_2} at 25 to 30 mmHg, osmotic agents such as mannitol (100 g in 500 mL D_5W) infused intravenously over 10 to 20 min every 4 to 6 h as needed in an effort to keep the ICP <20 mmHg (see Chap. 34).

Seizures are also a recognized complication of encephalitis and are best managed by phenytoin at a loading dose of 15 to 18 mg/kg. This should be infused at a rate not exceeding 50 mg/min in a glucose-free solution to prevent precipitation. Transient hypotension and heart block can occur during intravenous phenytoin administration and thus blood pressure and electrocardiographic monitoring are required. A therapeutic plasma level of 10 to 20 mg/mL is usually achieved with a daily maintenance dose of phenytoin of 300 to 500 mg (4 to 8 mg/kg). This may be given intravenously or orally. The half-life of phenytoin is long (36 h); therefore, a steady state is not achieved until 5 to 7 days have elapsed.

If seizures persist despite loading with phenytoin then phenobarbital may need to be added (see Chap. 142). One should not assume that the seizures are secondary to the encephalitis until other treatable precipitating causes such as structural or metabolic abnormalities have been ruled out. Complications of prolonged seizures may include cerebral edema, aspiration, rhabdomyolysis, myoglobinuria, hyperthermia, and hypoxia. These should be treated as they arise. Extreme hyperthermia may develop secondary to the encephalitis itself and be an aggravating cause of seizures. It should be controlled by appropriate cooling measures. Medical and nursing staff frequently ask questions about contagiousness. Except for a very few causes of encephalomyelitis, there is very little risk of disease transmission. Enteric precautions should be exercised when caring for patients with suspected enteroviral (including polio) infection. Isolation precautions against respiratory secretions should be taken in patients with suspected tuberculosis, rabies, measles, mumps, or LCM infection. Secretions from lesions of patients with VZV are potentially infectious and appropriate precautions should be applied. Finally, universal precautions including masks, gowns, gloves, and eye protection should be worn by all personnel participating in acute resuscitation, especially those involved in endotracheal intubation.

CASE PRESENTATION

A 59-year-old woman was admitted to a tertiary care hospital with mental obtundation. The history began approximately 2 weeks prior to admission when she had complaints of depression which were felt to be reactive to the recent death of her husband. Four days prior to admission she developed symptoms of headache along with nausea and vomiting. She was admitted to her local hospital and was noted to be withdrawn and lethargic. She was treated with chlorpromazine and dimenhydrinate for presumed diagnosis of migraine and depression with some apparent improvement in her headache. However, the following day she was noted to be disoriented with dysphasia and subsequently had a witnessed generalized seizure lasting approximately 3 min. Following this she was hemodynamically stable but neurologically unresponsive. She was then transferred urgently to the tertiary care hospital. Two hours prior to her seizure she had been given an 800-mg dose of ibuprofen. The referring physician wondered if she had developed a toxic confusional state secondary to the ibuprofen or if she had had a stroke.

On physical examination in the emergency room the patient was noted to be afebrile but had prominent meningismus. She was responsive only to pain, but there was no papilledema and no focal neurologic signs were elicited. Complete blood count, serum biochemistry, urinalysis, and chest x-ray were all normal. A lumbar puncture was performed and this revealed a normal opening pressure. CSF examination revealed an elevated WBC count of $101/mm^3$ with a lymphocytic predominance. The RBC count was $224/mm^3$ and the protein level was elevated at 1.01 g/L. The CSF glucose value was 3.8 mM/L (with a concurrent serum glucose value of 5.7). No bacteria were seen on Gram stain.

The patient was given acyclovir 10 mg/kg intravenously every 8 h (serum creatinine level was 54 mM/L) along with broad-spectrum antibiotics (cloxacillin + ceftriaxone + metronidazole). In addition, the patient was loaded with phenytoin and an urgent CT scan was arranged. The CT scan revealed only slight venticular enlargement.

The patient was admitted with a presumptive diagnosis of HSVE. Early in her hospital course, her neurologic status deteriorated and her gag reflex was noted to be absent. Concern regarding her ability to protect her airway led to her transfer to the ICU and intubation. An EEG was done and demonstrated PLEDs from the left temporal area with diffuse slowing of the background. Eventually, cultures from CSF, sputum, and urine specimens returned negative. Similarly, AFB stains and mycobacterial cultures from these specimens were negative. The patient's antibiotics were discontinued and acyclovir maintained. Over the next 48 h the patient's neurologic status gradually improved and she was subsequently extubated. She was transferred to the medical ward where she completed the 10-day course of acyclovir. Her neurologic status markedly improved over the course of her hospitalization, but at discharge and subsequent follow-up, she had a residual dysphasia.

CASE DISCUSSION

This case illustrates several points in the diagnosis and management of encephalomyelitis. Although most cases of encephalitis exhibit the triad of fever, headache, and altered mental state, it is not invariable. The diagnosis was delayed in this case, perhaps in large measure because of the absence of fever. Clearly, in any patient who presents with altered mental status or personality change, one should consider the possibility of an infectious etiology regardless of the absence of fever or the presence of a normal WBC count. In retrospect, it is easy to point out how dangerous it is to attribute a severe headache with vomiting and personality change to migraine and depression.

Speech abnormalities are seen in 76 percent of patients with HSVE and hence are a helpful clue to the diagnosis. Seizures are another frequent accompaniment of HSVE (38 percent), as well as other causes of encephalitis, and should serve as an alarm to heighten the suspicion for encephalitis. The referring physician's concerns regarding a toxic effect of a drug or of a vascular event contributing to this patient's symptomatology were not unreasonable, and this emphasizes the broad scope of the differential diagnosis in patients presenting with symptoms referable to the CNS.

Meningismus was demonstrated in this patient; however, it is worth emphasizing that signs of meningeal irritation are frequently not present in patients with encephalitis, particularly those who are severely mentally obtunded. Despite the fact that this patient was markedly obtunded, there were no focal neurologic signs nor papillidema; hence, the patient underwent a lumbar puncture. In patients in whom there is concern regarding elevated ICP, a lumbar puncture should be deferred until after CT or MRI scanning has been done. However, any delays in arranging diagnostic tests including scans or brain biopsy should *not* result in a delay in the institution of antimicrobial therapy.

The CSF almost always reveals an abnormality in patients with encephalitis. In this patient the results were typical of acute viral encephalitis with a mildly elevated WBC count with a predominance of lymphocytes combined with a modest elevation of protein content and a normal glucose level. These findings are nonspecific; for example, paraspinal or epidural abscess could yield similar results. The RBCs in the CSF could represent a traumatic tap, but in this case are in keeping with the hemorrhagic nature of HSVE. Viral cultures in HSVE are almost always negative but newer diagnostic modalities, such as the polymerase chain reaction, may ultimately help in providing a definitive diagnosis of HSVE without a brain biopsy.

The CT scan did not reveal a focal abnormality in this case. The sensitivity of the CT scan or radionuclide brain scan is approximately 50 percent in early disease. The EEG is more sensitive and in this case was helpful in that it demonstrated PLEDs which are characteristic but not pathognomonic of HSVE. MRI potentially may be a more sensitive and specific neurodiagnostic test and some have advocated it as the first step in the assessment of patients with suspected HSVE.

Patients with HSVE may develop severe neurologic compromise and require airway protection. Intubation should proceed ideally in a controlled, planned, elective fashion by an experienced person to ensure that precipitous and dangerous rises in ICP are avoided. Finally, this case emphasizes the serious nature of HSVE in that although the patient recovered, she was left with some residual neurologic deficit.

References

1. Griffin DE, Johnson RT: Encephalitis, myelitis and neuritis, in Mandell GL, Douglas RG, Bennett JE (eds): *Principles and Practice of Infectious Diseases.* 3d ed. New York, Churchill Livingstone, 1990; pp 762–769.
2. Hanley DF, Johnson RT, Whitley RJ: Yes, brain biopsy should be a prerequisite for herpes simplex encephalitis treatment. Arch Neurol 44:1289, 1987.
3. Whitley RJ: Herpes simplex virus infections of the central nervous system. Am J Med 85(S2A):61, 1988.
4. Whitley RJ, Soong S-J, Linneman C Jr, et al: Herpes simplex encephalitis. JAMA 247:317, 1982.
5. Whitley RJ, Alford CA, Hirsch MS, et al: Vidarabine versus acyclovir therapy in herpes simplex encephalitis. N Engl J Med 31:144, 1986.
6. Ho DD, Hirsch MS: Acute viral encephalitis. Med Clin North Am 69:415, 1985.
7. Koskiniemi M, Vaheri A, Taskinen: Cerebrospinal fluid alterations in herpes simplex virus encephalitis. Rev Infect Dis 6:608, 1984.
8. Wasiewski WW, Fishman MA: Herpes simplex encephalitis: The brain biopsy controversy. J Pediatr 113:575, 1988.
9. Nahmias AJ, Whitley RJ, Visintine AN, et al: Herpes simplex encephalitis: Laboratory evaluations and their diagnostic significance. J Infect Dis 145:829, 1982.
10. Rowley AH, Whitley RJ, Lakeman FD, Wolinsky SM: Rapid detection of herpes simplex virus DNA in cerebrospinal fluid of patients with herpes simplex encephalitis. Lancet 335:440, 1990.
11. Ch'ien LT, Boehm RM, Robinson H, et al: Characteristic early electroencephalographic changes in herpes simplex encephalitis. Arch Neurol 34:361, 1977.
12. Kohl S: Herpes simplex encephalitis in children. Pediatr Clin North Am 35:465, 1988.
13. Schroth G, Gawehn J, Thron A, et al: Early diagnosis of herpes simplex encephalitis by MRI. Neurology 37:179, 1987.
14. Schroth G: Reply to letter. Neurology 38:335, 1988.
15. Fishman RA: No, brain biopsy need not be done in every patient suspected of having herpes simplex encephalitis. Arch Neurol 44:1291, 1987.
16. Whitley RJ, Cobbs CG, Alford CA, et al: Diseases that mimic herpes simplex encephalitis. JAMA 262:234, 1989.
17. Morawitz RB, Whitley RJ, Murphy DM: Experience with brain biopsy for suspected herpes encephalitis: A review of 40 consecutive cases. Neurosurgery 12:654, 1983.
18. Kaufman HH, Catalano LW: Diagnostic brain biopsy: A series of 50 cases and a review. Neurosurgery 4:129, 1979.
19. Whitley RG, Soong S-J, Dolin R: Adenine arabinoside therapy of biopsy-proved herpes simplex encephalitis: National Institute of Allergy and Infectious Diseases Collaborative Antiviral Study. N Engl J Med 297:289, 1977.
20. Sköldenberg B, Alestig K, Burman L: Acyclovir versus vidarabine in herpes simplex encephalitis. Lancet 2:707, 1984.
21. Deeter RG, Khanderia U: Recent advances in antiviral therapy. Clin Pharm 5:961, 1986.
22. Chonmaitree T, Baldwin CD, Lucia HL: Role of the virology laboratory in diagnosis and management of patients with central nervous system disease, in Morello JA (ed): *Clinical Microbiology Reviews.* Chicago, American Society of Microbiology, 1989, pp. 1–11.
23. Prober CG, Hensleigh PA, Boucher FD, et al: Use of routine viral cultures at delivery to identify nenoates exposed to herpes simplex virus. N. Engl J Med 318:887, 1988.
24. Corey L, Stone ET, Whitley RJ, et al: Difference between herpes simplex type I and type II neonatal encephalitis in neurological outcome. Lancet 1:1, 1988.
25. Whitley RJ, Nahmias AJ, Visintine AM, et al: The natural history of herpes simplex virus infection of mother and newborn. Pediatrics 66:489, 1980.
26. Straus SE, Ostrove JM, Enchauspé G, et al: Varicella-zoster virus infections. Ann Intern Med 108:221, 1988.
27. Morgello S, Cho ES, Nielsen S, et al: Cytomegalovirus encephalitis in patients with acquired immunodeficiency syndrome. Hum Pathol 18:289, 1987.
28. Siegman-Igra Y, Michaeli D, Doron A, et al: Cytomegalovirus encephalitis in a noncompromised host. Isr J Med Sci 20:163, 1984.
29. Kaplan MH: Central nervous system infections. Curr Opinion Infect Dis 2:287, 1989.
30. Monath TP: Flavivirus, in Mandell GL, Douglas RG, Bennett JE (eds): *Principles and Practice of Infectious Disease.* 3d ed. New York, Churchill Livingstone, 1990, pp 1248–1251.
31. Hirsch MS: Acute viral central nervous system diseases, in Rubenstein E, Federman DD (eds): *Scientific American Medicine,* New York, Scientific American Inc., 1988, 7; XXVII; pp 1–5.
32. Monath TP: Alphavirus, in Mandell GL, Douglas RG, Bennett JE (eds): *Principles and Practice of Infectious Diseases.* 3d ed. New York, Churchill Livingstone, 1990, pp 1241–1242.
33. Johnson KM: California encephalitis and bunyaviral hemorrhagic fevers, in Mandell GL, Douglas RG, Bennett JE (eds): *Principles and Practice of Infectious Diseases.* 3d ed. New York, Churchill Livingstone, 1990, pp 1326–1329.
34. Modlin JF: Picornaviridae, in Mandell GL, Douglas RG, Bennett JE (eds): *Principles and Practice of Infectious Diseases.* 3d ed. New York, Churchill Livingstone, 1990, pp 1352–1379.
35. McKinney RG, Keitz SL, Wilfert CM: Chronic enteroviral meningoencephalitis in agammaglobulinemic patients. Rev Infect Dis 9:334, 1987.
36. Kondoh H, Kobayashi K, Sugioo Y, Haydshi T: Successful treatment of echovirus meningoencephalitis in sex-linked agamma-globulinaemia by intrathecal and intravenous injection of high titre gammaglobulin. Eur J Pediatr, 146:610, 1987.
37. Johnson KM: Lymphocytic choriomeningitis virus, Lassa virus (Lassa fever) and other arenaviruses, in Mandell GL, Douglas RG, Bennett JE (eds): *Principles and Practice of Infectious Diseases.* 3d ed. New York, Churchill Livingstone, 1990, pp 1329–1336.
38. Fishbein DB, Dobbins JE, Bryson JH, et al: Rabies surveillance, United States, 1987. MMWR 37:1, 1988.
39. Bernard KW, Fishbein DB: Rabies virus, in Mandell GL, Douglas RG, Bennett JE (eds): *Principles and Practice of Infectious Diseases.* 3d ed. New York, Churchill Livingstone, 1990, pp 1291–1303.
40. Anderson LJ, Nicholson KG, Tauxe RV, Winkler WG: Human rabies in the United States, 1960 to 1979: Epidemiology, diagnosis and prevention. Ann Intern Med 100:728, 1984.
41. Hattwick, MAW, Corey L, Creech WB: Clinical use of human globulin immune to rabies virus. Abstract. J Infect Dis 133 (suppl):226, 1976.
42. Johnson RT, Griffin DE, Hirsch RL, et al: Measles encephalo-

myelitis—clinical and immunologic studies. N Engl J Med 310: 137, 1984.
43. Moench TR, Griffen DE, Obriecht CR, et al: Acute measles in patients with and without neurologic involvement: distribution of measles virus antigen and RNA. J Infect Dis 158:433, 1988.
44. Gibbs FA, Gibbs EL, Carpenter PR, et al: Electroencephalographic changes in uncomplicated childhood diseases. JAMA 171:1050, 1959.
45. Dhib-Jalbut S, McFortand HF, Mingidie ES, et al: Humoral and cellular immune responses to matrix protein of measles virus in subacute sclerosing panencephalitis. J Virol 62:2483, 1988.
46. Jabbour JT, Garad JH, Lemmi H, et al.: Subacute sclerosing panencephilitis. A multidisciplinary study of eight cases. JAMA 207:2248, 1969.
47. Sever JL: Persistent measles infection of the central nervous system: Subacute sclerosing panencephalitis. Rev Infect Dis 4:467, 1983.
48. Sever JL, Krebs H, Ley A, et al: Diagnosis of subacute panencephalitis. The value and availability of measles antibody determinations. JAMA 228:604, 1974.
49. Huttenlocher PR, Mattson RH: Isoprinosine in subacute sclerosing panencephalitis. Neurology 29:763, 1979.
50. Jones CE, Dyken PR, Huttenlocher PR, et al: Inosiplex therapy in subacute sclerosing panencephalitis. Lancet 1:1034, 1982.
51. DuRant RH, Dyken PR: The effect of inosiplex on the survival of subacute sclerosing panencephalitis. Neurology 33:1053, 1983.
52. Noetzel MJ, Dodson WE: Progressive CT abnormalities despite clinical improvement in SSPE treated with inosiplex. Ann Neurol 13:457, 1983.
53. Baum SG, Litman N: Mumps virus, in Mandell GL, Douglas RG, Bennett JE (eds): *Principles and Practice of Infectious Diseases.* 3d ed. New York, Churchill Livingstone, 1990, pp 1260–1265.
54. Grandien M, Olding-Stenkvist E: Rapid diagnosis of viral infections in the central nervous system. Scand J Infect Dis 16:1, 1984.
55. Centers for Disease Control. Mumps surveillance, January 1977–December 1982. MMWR 1984.
56. Heggie, AD, Robbins FC: Natural rubella acquired after birth. Am J Dis Child 118:12, 1969.
57. Lassell GH, Cole BC: Mycoplasmas as agents of human disease. N Engl J Med 304:80, 1981.
58. Ponka A: The occurrence and clinical picture of serologically verified *Mycoplasma pneumoniae* with emphasis on central nervous system, cardiac, and joint manifestations. Ann Clin Res 24:1, 1979.
59. Hodges GR, Fass RJ, Saslaw S: Central nervous system diseases associated with *Mycoplasma pneumoniae* infection. Arch Intern Med 130:277, 1972.
60. Lever RJ, Kalavsky SM: Central nervous system disease associated with *Mycoplasma pneumoniae* infection: Report of five cases and review of the literature. Pediatrics 52:658, 1973.
61. Westenfelder GO, Akey DT, Corwin SJ, Vick NA: Acute transverse myelitis due to *Mycoplasma pneumoniae* infection. Arch Neurol 38:317, 1981.
62. Rosenblum MJ, Masland RL, Harrell TG: Residual effect of rickettsial disease on the central nervous system. Arch Intern Med 90:444, 1952.
63. Steere AC: Lyme disease. N Engl J Med 321:586, 1989.
64. Farrar WE: Leptospira species (Leptospirosis), in Mandell GL, Douglas RG, Bennett JE (eds): *Principles and Practice of Infectious Diseases.* 3d ed. New York, Churchill Livingstone, 1990, pp 1813–1816.
65. Diamond RD: *Cryptococcus neoformans,* in Mandell GL, Douglas RG, Bennett JE (eds): *Principles and Practice of Infectious Diseases.* 3d ed. New York, Churchill Livingstone, 1990, pp 1980–1989.
66. Bennett JE, Dismukes WE, Duma RJ, et al: A comparison of amphotoericin B alone and combined with flucytosine in the treatment of cryptococcal meningitis. N Engl J Med 301:126, 1979.
67. Diamond RD, Bennett JE: Prognostic factors in cryptococcal meningitis. A study of 111 cases. Ann Intern Med 80:176, 1974.
68. Luft, JL, Remington JS: Toxoplasmic encephalitis. J Infect Dis 157:1, 1988.
69. Post, MJD, Kursunoglu SJ, Hensley GT, et al: Cranial CT in acquired immunodeficiency syndrome: Spectrum of diseases and optimal contrast enhancement technique. AJR 145:929, 1985.
70. Levy, RM, Rosenbloom S, Perrett LV: Neuroradiologic findings in AIDS: A review of 200 cases. AJR 147:977, 1986.
71. Ramsey RG, Gerenia GK: CNS complications of AIDS: CT and MR findings. AJR 151:449, 1988.
72. Wanke C, Tuazon C, Kovacs A, et al: Toxoplasma encephalitis in patients with acquired immune deficiency syndrome: Diagnosis and response to therapy. Am J Trop Med Hyg 36:509, 1987.
73. Gotzsche PC, Bygbjerg IC, Olesen B, et al: Yield of diagnostic tests for opportunistic infections in AIDS: A survey of 33 patients. Scand. J Infect Dis 20:396, 1988.
74. McCabe RE, Remington JS: *Toxoplasma gondii,* in Mandell GL, Douglas RG, Bennett JE (eds): *Principles and Practice of Infectious Diseases.* 3d ed. New York, Churchill Livingstone, 1990, pp 2090–2103.
75. Petri WA, Ravdin JI: Free living amebae, in Mandell GL, Douglas RG, Bennett JE (eds): *Principles and Practice of Infectious Diseases.* 3d ed. New York, Churchill Livingstone, 1990, pp 2049–2056.
76. Barnett GH, Ropper AH, Romeo J: Intracranial pressure and outcome in adult encephalitis. J Neurosurg 68:585, 1988.

Chapter 105

LIFE-THREATENING INFECTIONS OF THE HEAD, NECK, AND UPPER RESPIRATORY TRACT

ANTHONY W. CHOW

KEY POINTS

- *A thorough knowledge of the fascial relationships and the potential anatomic routes of infection is a prerequisite to optimal management of deep neck infections.*
- *The microbic etiology of deep infections of the head and neck is complex and typically polymicrobial in nature. Anaerobes generally outnumber aerobes by a factor of 10:1.*
- *The development of marked asymmetry in the course of a submandibular space infection should be viewed with great concern since it may be indicative of extension to the lateral pharyngeal space.*
- *In immunocompromised patients, the classical manifestations of infection are often altered, and features of systemic toxicity may be absent.*
- *Penicillin remains the antibiotic of choice for odontogenic deep neck infections, but immunocompromised patients require a broader spectrum against organisms such as Staphylococcus aureus and enteric gram-negative rods.*
- *Chronic sinusitis, otitis, and mastoiditis are the most important causes of parameningeal infection and intracranial suppuration. Computed tomography is the single neuroimaging technique proven to be the most useful for the diagnosis of these conditions.*

Life-threatening infections of the head, neck, and upper respiratory tract have become less common in the postantibiotic era. Consequently, many physicians are unfamiliar with these conditions. Furthermore, with widespread use of antibiotics and profound immunosuppression in some patients, the classical manifestations of these infections are often altered. Features of systemic toxicity, such as chills and fever, and local signs, such as edema and fluctuance, may be absent. Thus, physicians unfamiliar with these entities may underestimate their extent and severity. The gravity of this dichotomous situation is accentuated in that these infections often have a rapid onset and may progress to fatal complications. In this chapter, the key clinical manifestations of several life-threatening infections of the head, neck, and upper respiratory tract are highlighted, and the critically important anatomic relationships that underlie their diagnosis and management are emphasized.

General Anatomic Considerations

Life-threatening infections of the head, neck, and upper respiratory tract most commonly originate from suppurative complications of dental, oropharyngeal, or otorhinolaryngeal infections. From these sites, infection may extend along natural fascial planes into deep cervical spaces or vascular compartments (Fig. 105-1). The deep cervical fascia ranges from loose areolar connective tissue to dense fibrous bands. It invests muscles and organs, thus forming planes and spaces. Notably, these fascial planes both separate and connect distant areas, thereby both limiting and directing the spread of infection. These infections may be fatal either by local airway occlusion or by direct extension to vital structures such as the mediastinum or carotid sheath. Otorhinocerebral infections may cause intracranial suppuration such as cerebral or epidural abscess, subdural empyema, and cavernous or cortical venous sinus thrombosis (Fig. 105-2). A thorough knowledge of the fascial relationships and the potential anatomic routes of infection is a prerequisite to understanding the etiology, manifestations and complications of deep neck infections. Such knowledge will not only provide valuable information on the nature and extent of infection but will also suggest the optimum surgical approach for effective drainage.

Microbic Etiology and Pathogenesis

The microbic etiology of deep infections of the head and neck is complex and typically polymicrobial in nature. As a rule, it reflects the autochthonous microflora of the contiguous mucosal surfaces from which the infection originated. Due to the close anatomic relationship, the resident flora of the oral cavity, upper respiratory tract, and certain parts of the ears and eyes share many common organisms (Fig. 105-3).[3] Anaerobes generally outnumber aerobes at all sites by a factor of 10:1.[4] Although less is known about the pathogenic potential of individual species, it is clear that as a group these organisms are structural opportunists and invade deep tissues when normal mucosal barriers are broken (such as during pharyngitis, odontogenic infections, or direct trauma). Invasiveness is often influenced by synergistic interactions of multiple species, both aerobic and anaerobic. Moreover, certain species or combinations may be more invasive or more resistant to therapy than others.

Bacteria most commonly isolated from deep space infections include *Bacteroides, Peptostreptococcus, Veillonella, Actinomyces, Fusobacterium,* and microaerophilic streptococci. The majority are sensitive in vitro to penicillin G, but an increasing number of species (e.g., 40 percent or more of *Bacteroides melaninogenicus* in certain geographic areas) are now resistant[5]. The importance of this in vitro finding in the treatment of such polymicrobial infections is largely unknown. While anaerobes are likely to be involved in

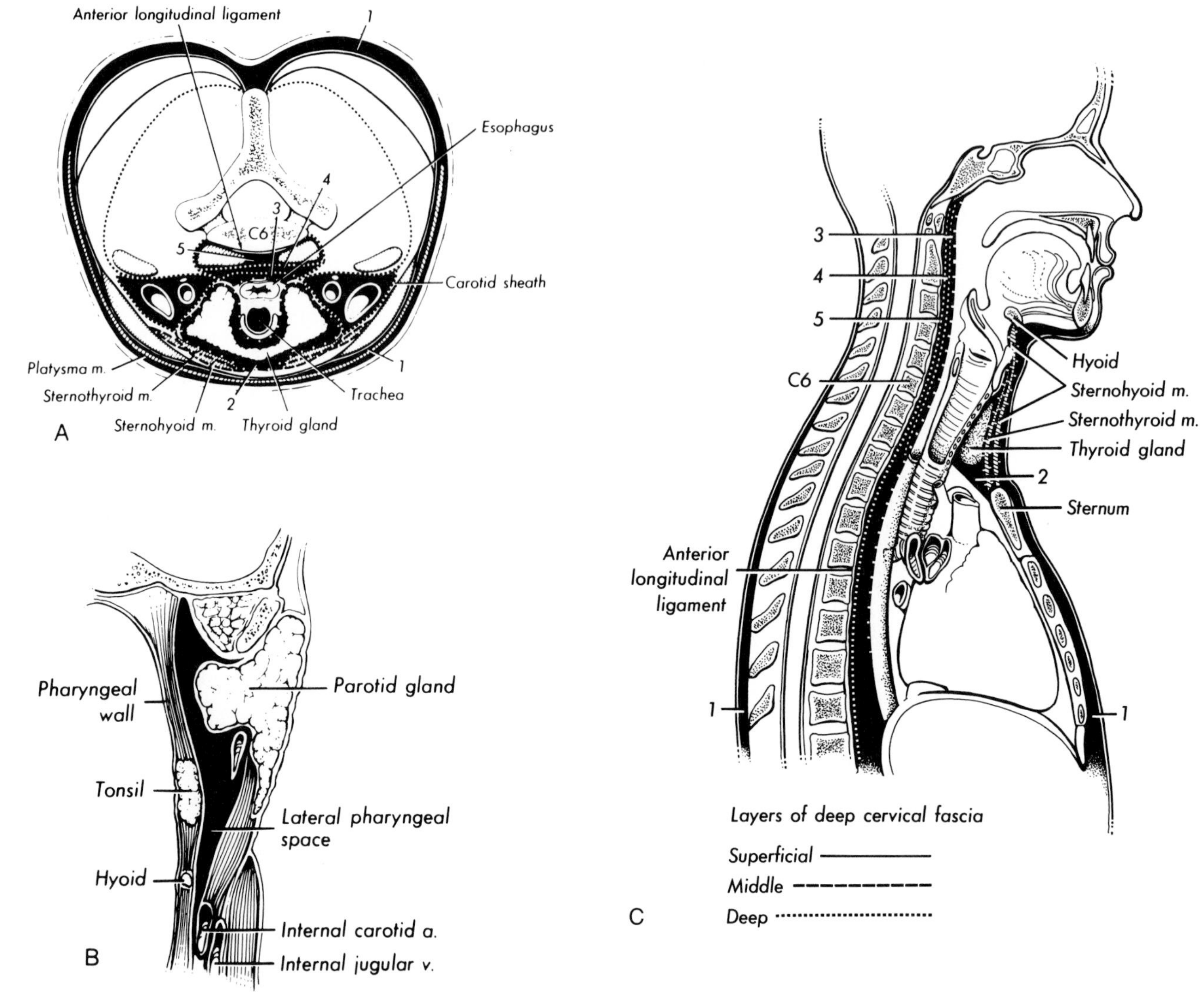

FIGURE 105-1 Relation of lateral pharyngeal, retropharyngeal, and prevertebral spaces to the posterior and anterior layers of deep cervical fascia: 1, superficial space; 2, pretracheal space; 3, retropharyngeal space; 4, "danger" space; 5, prevertebral space. (*a*) Cross section of the neck at the level of thyroid isthmus. (*b*) Coronal section in the suprahyoid region of the neck. (*c*) midsagittal section of the head and neck. Reproduced with permission from Chow.[1]

most head and neck infections, a small but significant proportion of cases will also contain other pathogens such as *Staphylococcus aureus* and facultative gram-negative rods including *Pseudomonas aeruginosa*.

Clinical Syndromes

CERVICAL FASCIAL SPACE INFECTIONS

Deep fascial space infections of the head and neck are most frequently odontogenic in origin (Fig. 105-4).[1,6,7] The potential pathways of extension of these infections from one space to another are illustrated in Fig. 105-5. Cervical fascial space infections considered to be "life threatening" include those of the submandibular, lateral pharyngeal, and retropharyngeal-danger-prevertebral spaces. Their salient clinical features are summarized in Table 105-1. The approach to radiographic and microbiologic diagnosis is discussed toward the end of this chapter. Recommended antimicrobial regimens for initial empiric therapy are summarized in Table 105-2.

SUBMANDIBULAR SPACE INFECTIONS

The prototypical infection of this space is known as Ludwig's angina. In 1836, von Ludwig described five patients with "gangrenous induration of the connective tissues of the neck which advances to involve the tissues that cover the small muscles between the larynx and the floor of the mouth". It is characteristically an aggressive, rapidly spreading "woody" or brawny cellulitis involving the submandibular space. Although the submandibular space is further divided by the mylohyoid muscle into the sublin-

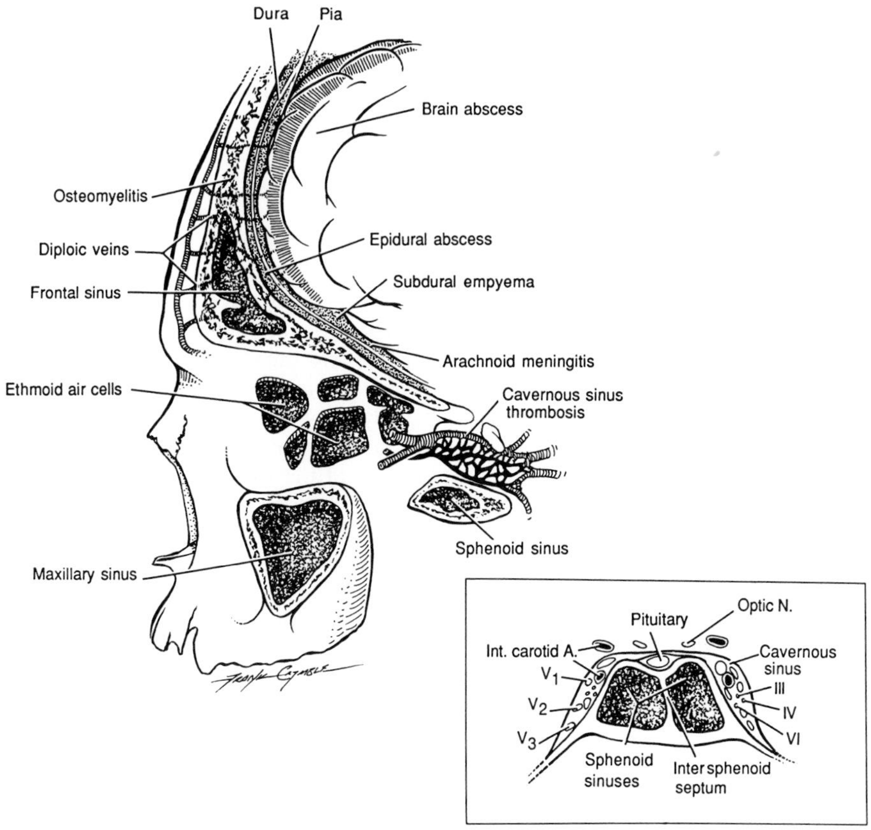

FIGURE 105-2 Major routes for intracranial extension of infection either directly or via the vascular supply. The coronal section demonstrates the structures adjoining the sphenoid sinus. Reproduced with permission from Vortel and Chow.[2]

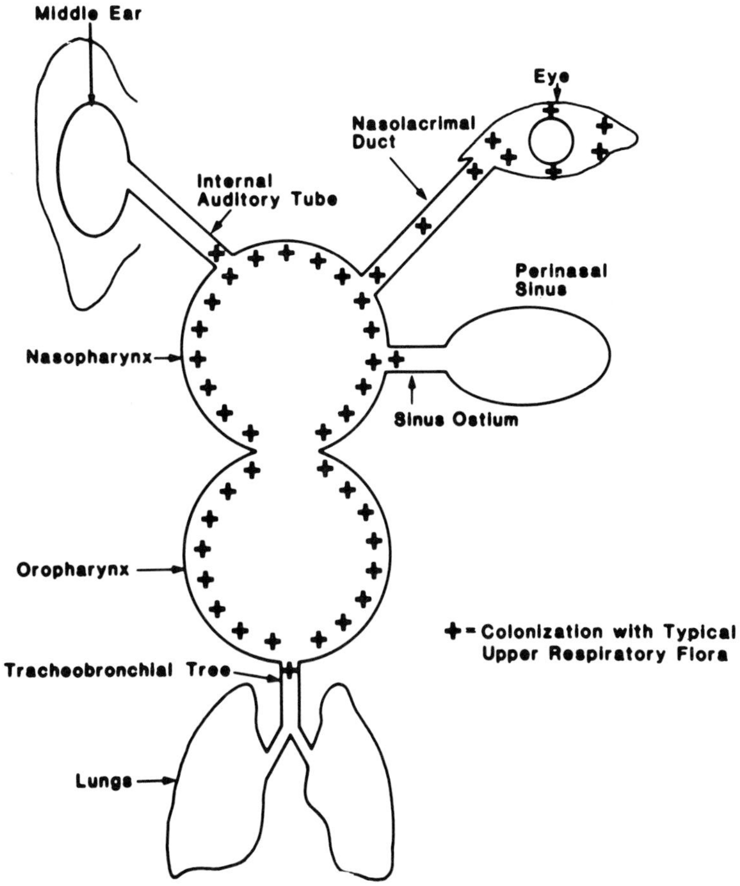

FIGURE 105-3 Diagrammatic illustration of the anatomic relationship of head and neck structures and distribution of the indigenous flora. Reproduced with permission from Todd.[3]

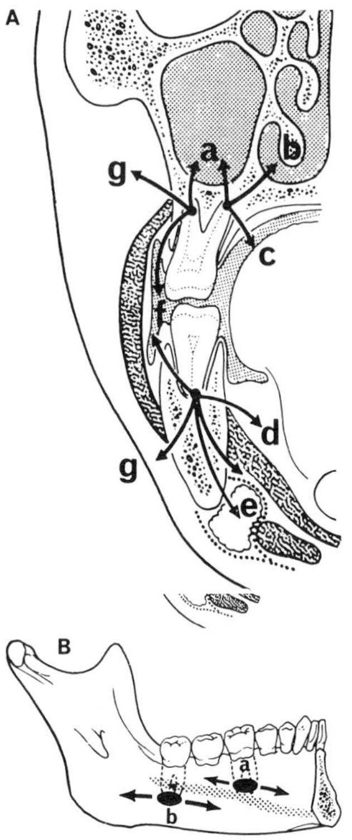

FIGURE 105-4 Routes of spread of odontogenic infections. **(*a*) Coronal section at first molar teeth: a, maxillary antrum; b, nasal cavity; c, palatal plate; d, sublingual space (above mylohyoid space); e, submylohyoid space; f, intraoral presentation with infection spreading through the buccal plates inside the attachment of the buccinator muscle; and g, extraoral presentation to buccal space with infection spreading through the buccal plates outside the attachment of the buccinator muscle. (*b*) Lingual aspect of the mandible: a, tooth apices above the mylohyoid muscle with spread of infection into sublingual space; b, tooth apices below the mylohyoid muscle with spread of infection into submylohyoid space. Reproduced with permission from Chow, Roser, and Brady.[6]**

gual space above and the submylohyoid space below (Fig. 105-6), it can be considered as a single unit due to a direct communication around the posterior aspect of the mylohyoid muscle. Ludwig's angina most commonly follows infection of the second or third mandibular molar teeth (70 to 85 percent of cases). The submylohyoid space is initially involved, as the roots of these teeth are located below the attachments of the mylohyoid muscle to the mandible (Fig. 105-4B). Also, since the lingual aspects of periodontal bone around these teeth are thinner, medial spread of infection is facilitated. Infection extends contiguously (rather than by the lymphatics, which would limit the infection to one side) to involve the sublingual and thus the entire submandibular space in a symmetrical manner. Less commonly, an identical process initially involving the sublingual space can arise from infection of the premolars and other teeth or from trauma to the floor of the mouth. Once established, infection can evolve rapidly. The tongue may enlarge to two or three times its normal size and distend posteriorly into the hypopharynx, superiorly against the palate, and anteriorly out of the mouth. Immediate posterior extension of the process will directly involve the epiglottis (Fig. 105-6). There exists a little regarded dangerous connection between the submandibular and lateral pharyngeal spaces known as the buccopharyngeal gap. This is created by the styloglossus muscle as it leaves the tongue and passes between the middle and superior constrictor muscles to attach on the styloid process. Thus, cellulitis of the submandibular space may spread directly into the lateral laryngeal space and thereby to the retropharyngeal space and mediastinum (Fig. 105-6).

Clinically, the patient is febrile and complains of mouth pain, stiff neck, drooling, and dysphagia, leaning forward to maximize the airway diameter. A tender, symmetrical and indurated swelling, sometimes with palpable crepitus, is present in the submandibular area. The mouth is held open by lingual swelling. Respirations are usually difficult, while stridor and cyanosis are considered as ominous

TABLE 105-1 Comparative Clinical Features of Deep Fascial Space Infections

Space	Pain	Trismus	Swelling	Dysphagia	Dyspnea
Submandibular	Present	Minimal	Mouth floor; submylohyoid	Present if bilateral involvement	Present if bilateral involvement
Lateral pharyngeal					
Anterior	Severe	Prominent	Anterior lateral pharynx; Angle of jaw	Present	Occasional
Posterior	Minimal	Minimal	Posterior lateral pharynx (hidden)	Present	Severe
Retropharyngeal (and danger)	Present	Minimal	Posterior pharynx	Present	Present
Masticator					
Masseteric and pterygoid	Present	Prominent	May not be seen	Absent	Absent
Temporal	Present	None	Face, orbit	Absent	Absent
Buccal	Minimal	Minimal	Cheek	Absent	Absent
Parotid	Severe	None	Angle of jaw	Absent	Absent

SOURCE: Megran, Scheifele, and Chow.[8]

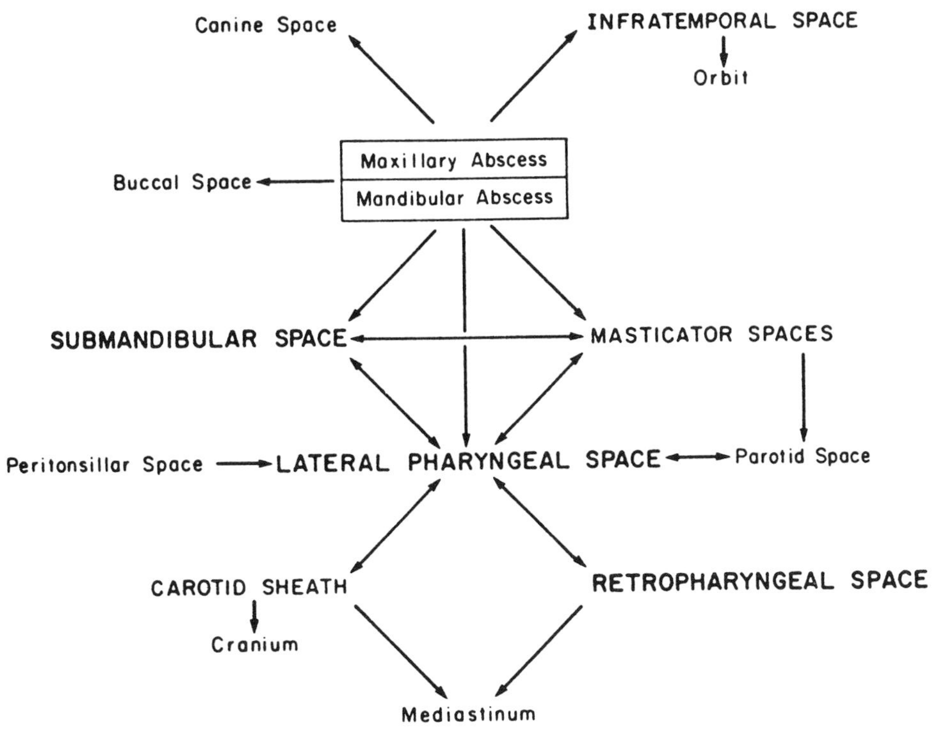

FIGURE 105-5 Potential pathways of extension in deep fascial space infections. Reproduced with permission from Blomquist and Bayer.[7]

signs. Radiographic views of the teeth may indicate the source of infection, and lateral views of the neck will demonstrate the degree of soft tissue swelling around the airway and possibly submandibular gas. The development of significant asymmetry of the submandibular area should be viewed with great concern since it may be indicative of extension to the lateral pharyngeal space. Well-timed surgical drainage will reduce the risk of spread to this space and subsequently to the superior mediastinum.[9]

The therapy of Ludwig's angina has undergone a number of modifications since its initial description.[10] While maintenance of an adequate airway is the primary concern and may necessitate urgent tracheostomy, most cases can be managed initially by close observation and intravenous antibiotics. If cellulitis and swelling continue to advance rapidly or if dyspnea occurs, artificial airway control should be gained immediately, before stridor, cyanosis, and asphyxia require that it be done under emergency conditions. There is general agreement that blind oral or nasotracheal intubation is both traumatic and unsafe in advanced Ludwig's angina because of the potential for induction of severe laryngospasm. A recommended approach is to use a flexible fiberoptic scope to assess the airway and to aid in inserting an endotracheal tube. Tracheostomy is still the

TABLE 105–2 Alternative Empiric Antibiotic Regimens for Life-threatening Infections of the Head, Neck, and Upper Respiratory Tract

	ANTIBIOTIC REGIMENS*	
Infection	Normal Host	Compromised Host
Submandibular, lateral pharyngeal, and retropharyngeal infections	Penicillin G, 2–4 MU IV q4–6h; and clindamycin, 600 mg IV q8h; or cefoxitin, 1–2 g IV q6h; or metronidazole, 500 mg IV q8h	Cefotaxime, 2 g IV q6h; or ceftizoxime, 4 g IV q8h; or piperacillin, 3 g IV q4h; or imipenem 500, mg IV q6h
Peritonsillar abscess	Penicillin G, 2–4 MU IV q4–6h; and clindamycin, 600 mg IV q8h; or cefoxitin, 1–2 g IV q6h	Cefotaxime, 2 g IV q6h; or ceftizoxime, 4 g IV q8h; or piperacillin, 3 g IV q4h
Pharyngeal diphtheria	Penicillin, 1–3 MU IV q4–6h; or erythromycin, 0.5–1 g IV q6h	Same as normal host
Acute epiglottitis	Ampicillin, 1–2 g IV q6h, plus chloramphenicol, 0.5 g IV q6h; or cefuroxime, 2 g IV q8h	Cefotaxime, 2 g IV q6h; or ceftriaxone, 1 g IV q12h; or cefotetan, 2 g IV q12h

*Abbreviations: MU, million units; IV, intravenous; q4h; q6h, etc., every 4 h, every 6 h, etc.

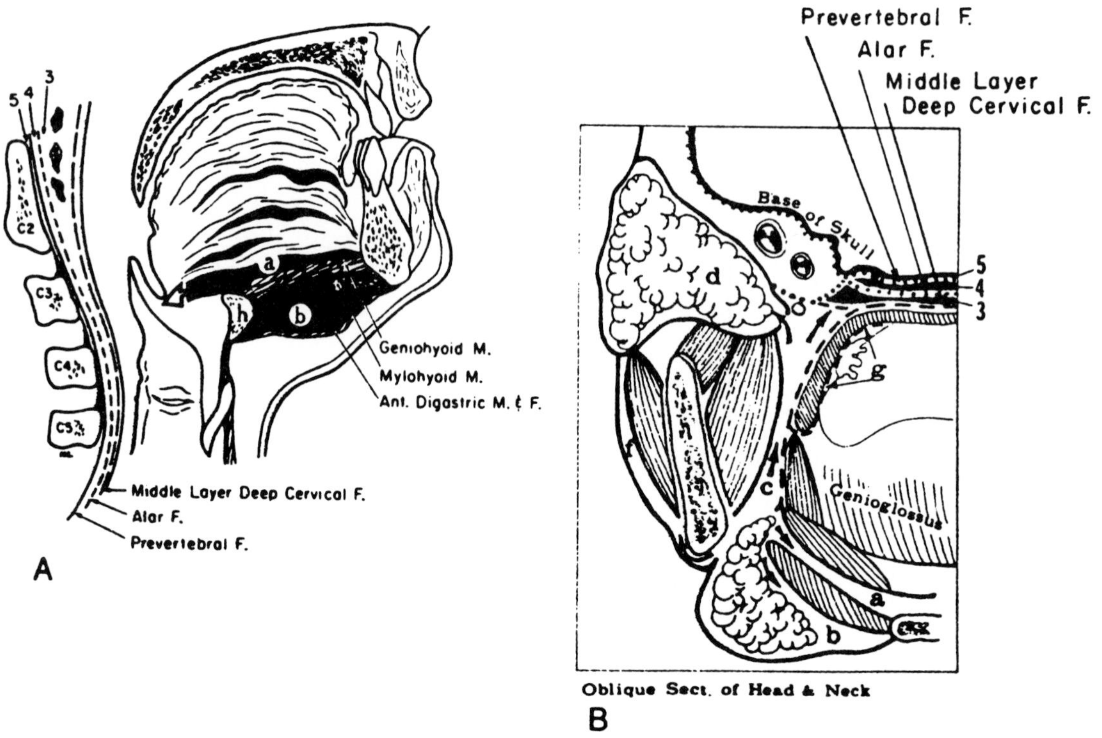

FIGURE 105-6 Anatomic relationships in Ludwig's angina. Sagittal (*a*) and oblique (*b*) sections of head and neck: a, sublingual space; b, submylohyoid space; c, lateral pharyngeal space; d, parotid gland; f, masticator space; g, peritonsillar space; h, hyoid bone; 3, retropharyngeal space; 4, danger space; 5, prevertebral space. Reproduced with permission from Blomquist and Bayer.[7]

most widely recommended means of airway control, although cricothyroidotomy is advocated by some experts because of a lower complication rate.

Penicillin G is the antibiotic of choice, but immunocompromised patients require a broader spectrum of antibiotic coverage against organisms such as facultative gram-negative rods and *S. aureus.* Early surgical decompression, much advocated in the preantibiotic era, is unlikely to locate pus and at best may only moderately improve the airway. Pus collections develop relatively late (not usually present in the first 24 to 36 h) and are sometimes difficult to detect clinically. If the patient is not responding adequately to antibiotics alone after this initial period or if fluctuance is detectable, needle aspiration or a more formal incision and drainage procedure under general anaesthetic should be performed. Preferably, this should be done with a cuffed tracheostomy in place. Additionally, the infected teeth implicated in the sepsis should be extracted.

With the combined use of systemic antibiotics and aggressive surgical intervention, the mortality rate for Ludwig's angina has declined dramatically from over 50 percent in the preantibiotic era to 0 to 4 percent currently.

LATERAL PHARYNGEAL SPACE INFECTIONS

These infections are potentially life threatening because of involvement of vital structures within the carotid sheath and a tendency to bacteremic dissemination. Anatomically, the lateral pharyngeal space (also known as the pharyngomaxillary space) is shaped like an inverted cone in the lateral neck, with its base at the skull and its apex at the hyoid bone (Fig. 105-1B). Its medial wall is continuous with the carotid sheath, and anteriorly it lies between the superior pharyngeal constrictor muscle medially and the internal pterygoid muscle, mandibular ramus, and parotid gland laterally (Fig. 105-7). It is divided into an anterior (prestyloid or muscular) compartment and a posterior (retrostyloid or neurovascular) compartment by the styloid process and its attached muscles, the stylomandibular ligament, and the insertion of these structures into the hyoid bone. The anterior compartment contains no vital structures, but only fat, lymph nodes, connective tissue, and muscle. It is the compartment most closely related to the tonsillar fossa and the internal pterygoid muscle. The posterior compartment contains the ninth to twelfth cranial nerves, the carotid sheath and its contents, and the cervical sympathetic trunk. Infections of the lateral pharyngeal space may arise from sources throughout the neck. Dental infections are most common, followed by peritonsillar abscess (postanginal sepsis) and rarely parotitis, otitis, or mastoiditis (Bezold's abscess).

Infection of the anterior compartment is often suppurative. Since most patients are already compromised by infection elsewhere, diagnosis of lateral pharyngeal involvement is often delayed. The cardinal clinical features, in order of importance, are (1) trismus; (2) induration and swelling below the angle of the mandible; (3) systemic tox-

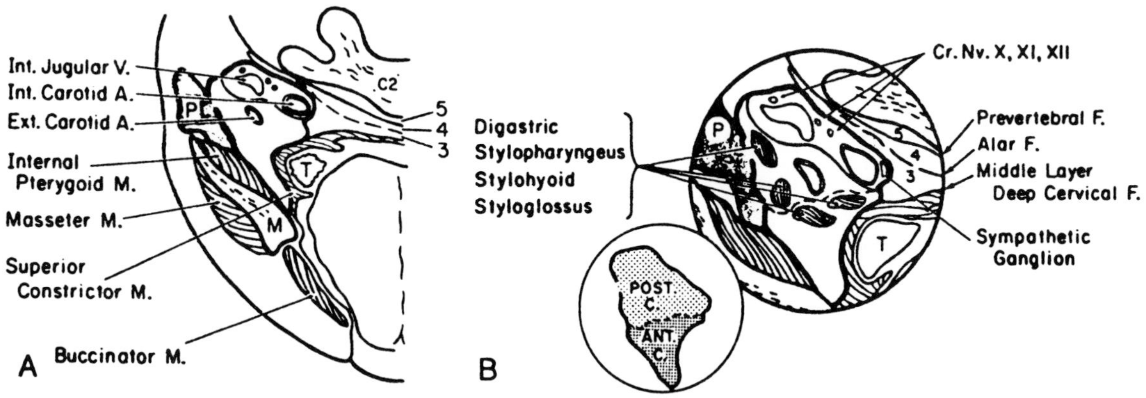

FIGURE 105-7 Cross sections of the lateral pharyngeal space: P, parotid gland; T, tonsil; M, mandible; 3, retropharyngeal space; 4, danger space; 5, prevertebral space; Inset, anterior and posterior compartments of lateral pharyngeal space. Reproduced with permission from Blomquist and Bayer.[7]

icity with fever and rigors; and (4) medial bulging of the pharyngeal wall. Although not prominent, dyspnea can occur. Suppuration may advance quickly to other spaces, particularly to the retropharyngeal space and the mediastinum, or spread to involve the posterior compartment of the lateral pharyngeal space. In these cases, timely surgical incision and drainage is of utmost importance.

Postanginal sepsis can involve either the anterior or the posterior compartment, but as lymphatic drainage is the most important mechanism of spread, it most often involves the carotid sheath alone. A history of sore throat, while usually present on admission, is not invariable, it may only be mild or unilateral, and there may be a latent period of up to 3 weeks before manifestations of deep infection develop. The patient presents either in a toxic condition or insidiously with a fever of undetermined origin. Trismus is absent, and signs of local suppuration may be subtle clinically because of the tight connective tissue around and within the carotid sheath. This confines the infection and may limit it to only the internal jugular vein. Dyspnea may be prominent as edema and swelling descend directly to involve the epiglottis and larynx. Swelling of the pharyngeal wall, if present, will be behind the palatopharyngeal arch and is easily missed.

Suppurative jugular thrombophlebitis is the most common vascular complication of lateral pharyngeal space infection.[25] An indurated swelling of a few centimeters in length may be palpable behind the sternocleidomastoid muscle or may be found more deeply behind the palatopharyngeal arch. Trismus is minimal and may be absent. Vocal cord paralysis or other neurologic signs representing lower cranial nerve involvement may be present. These signs are frequently missed (detected in only 20 percent of cases antemortem in one series) unless specifically sought and may be transient. The patient may thus present as an obscure septicemia (50 percent of cases). Metastatic abscesses are common, characteristically involving the lungs, bones, and joints or other sites. There may be retrograde spread of infection with cerebral abscess or meningitis. A diagnosis of right-sided bacterial endocarditis may be considered. In common with other anaerobic septicemias, hepatic enlargement, tenderness, abnormal liver function tests, and even frank jaundice may be present, which may misdirect investigations and further delay diagnosis.[11] Positive gallium or white-cell-labeled indium uptake in the neck is a useful diagnostic aid in these cases. Rarely, the carotid artery is involved, leading to an arteritis, aneurysm formation and eventually rupture. This complication is usually heralded by several minor bleeds before a major hemorrhage occurs and signals the need for urgent surgical intervention. Such bleeding may involve the oral cavity, nose, or ear or appear as ecchymosis in the neck and surrounding tissues. An ipsilateral Horner's syndrome, or otherwise unexplained ninth to twelfth cranial nerve palsies, are additional premonitory syndromes of carotid sheath involvement.

Treatment of lateral pharyngeal space infection initially depends on whether local suppuration is present, but often this is difficult to determine. Computed tomography (CT) scanning, careful needle aspiration, or more definitive incision and drainage may be required. Most cases of postanginal sepsis with suppurative jugular thrombophlebitis can be managed medically without the need for ligation or surgical resection of the infected vein. Prolonged courses of intravenous antibiotics (3 to 6 weeks) will be required. Since anaerobic bacteremia caused by *Bacteroides* species or *Fusobacterium necrophorum* is frequently present,[12] and penicillin resistance among these organisms is increasingly recognized, therapy may require addition of metronidazole, clindamycin, or β-lactamase-stable cephalosporins. Fever may be slow to resolve, even in cases successfully treated, particularly if there is metastatic involvement. Anticoagulants have sometimes been used in this setting, but efficacy is unconfirmed. Surgical ligation of the internal jugular vein, the only available therapeutic option in the preantibiotic era, is now required only in the rare patient who fails to respond to antibiotic therapy alone. When there is impending or frank rupture of the carotid artery, this must be ligated immediately, paying special attention to the airway and restoration of blood volume. Predictably, morbidity (e.g., stroke) and mortality are high (20 to 40 percent). In all such cases, early surgical intervention is the key to a successful outcome.

RETROPHARYNGEAL, DANGER, AND PREVERTEBRAL SPACE INFECTIONS

The retropharyngeal, danger, and prevertebral spaces all lie between the deep cervical fascia surrounding the pharynx and esophagus anteriorly and the vertebral spine posteriorly (Fig. 105-1A). The retropharyngeal space is bound anteriorly by the constrictor muscles of the neck and their fascia and posteriorly by the alar layer of the deep cervical fascia, extending from the base of the skull to the level of the superior mediastinum where the two fascial layers fuse. The "danger" space is interposed between the retropharyngeal space anteriorly and the prevertebral space posteriorly. It extends from the base of the skull and descends freely through the entire posterior mediastinum to the diaphragm. The prevertebral space is bound by the prevertebral fascia, which originates posteriorly on the spinous processes and encircles the splenius, erector spinae, and semispinalis muscles. Prior to completing its circle anterior to the vertebral bodies, it fuses to the transverse processes. At this point it is split into two layers: the more anterior alar fascia and the prevertebral fascia. The prevertebral space extends from the base of the skull to the coccyx, thus allowing infectious spread as far down as the psoas muscle sheath.

Retropharyngeal abscesses are among the most serious of deep space infections, since infection can extend directly into the anterior or posterior portions of the superior mediastinum or into the entire length of the posterior mediastinum via the "danger" space (Fig. 105-1A).

Retropharyngeal infections may occur in both children and adults. In young children, infection usually reaches this space within lymphatic channels, most commonly as complications of suppurative adenitis following infections of the upper respiratory tract. The onset may be insidious, with little more than fever, irritability, drooling, or possibly nuchal rigidity. More acute symptoms include dysphagia and dyspnea. The latter may be either due to a local mass effect or secondary to laryngeal edema. Generally there is little pain, but the neck may be held rigid and tilted to the unaffected side. Definite bulging of the posterior pharyngeal wall is usually seen but may need careful palpation to be appreciated. The main dangers are severe laryngeal edema with airway obstruction and abscess rupture with consequent aspiration pneumonia or asphyxia. Many cases will respond to antibiotic therapy alone if treatment precedes the development of frank suppuration.

In adults, infection may reach the retropharyngeal space from either local or distant sites. The former usually results from penetrating trauma (e.g., from chicken bones or following instrumentation); in such cases, presence of a sore throat or difficulty in swallowing or breathing may be the first indications of infection. More distant sources include odontogenic sepsis and peritonsillar abscess (now a rare cause). Infection from these sources may often obscure the diagnosis because of associated trismus, which makes direct examination of the posterior pharyngeal wall difficult. In this setting, radiographic views of the lateral neck are especially helpful and may demonstrate cervical lordosis with swelling and gas collections in the retropharyngeal space, causing anterior displacement of the larynx and trachea. Radiographs may also help to differentiate this infection from prevertebral space sepsis arising from cervical osteomyelitis. Once a diagnosis is made, surgical exploration and wide drainage should be carried out without delay.

Acute necrotizing mediastinitis is the most feared complication of retropharyngeal space infections.[13] The onset is rapid and is characterized by the following: (1) widespread necrotizing process extending the length of the posterior mediastinum, occasionally into the retroperitoneal space; (2) rupture of mediastinal abscess into the pleural cavity with empyema or development of loculations; and (3) pleural or pericardial effusions, frequently with tamponade. Aspiration pneumonia is also a significant problem (50 percent of cases) and may be secondary to impairment of swallowing or spontaneous rupture of the abscess into the airway. As to be expected, the mortality in adults is high (25 percent), even when appropriate antibiotics are administered. Early diagnosis and timely debridement are the mainstays of successful treatment. Mediastinal drainage may be attained by either the cervicomediastinal or the transthoracic approach. Although the cervical approach may be effective in early mediastinitis, thoracotomy is generally indicated once the necrotizing process has entered the danger space. In patients who are recovering, it is important to restrict all oral intake until the swallowing impairment, which may have a prolonged course, has resolved completely.

SUPPURATIVE PAROTITIS

Acute bacterial parotitis is a specific clinical entity primarily affecting the elderly, malnourished, dehydrated, or postoperative patient. Ductal (Stensen's) obstruction secondary to sialolithiasis appears to be a major predisposing condition. Other predisposing factors include sialogogic drugs and trauma. Clinically, there is sudden onset of firm, erythematous swelling of the pre- and postauricular areas extending to the angle of the mandible. This is associated with exquisite local pain and tenderness but without trismus. Systemic findings of high fevers, chills, and marked toxicity are generally present. Septicemic spread may lead to osteomyelitis of the adjacent facial bones. Staphylococci have been the predominant isolates, and empiric antibiotic therapy should include an antistaphylococcal agent. Early surgical drainage and decompression of the gland are generally required, since spontaneous drainage is uncommon. Because of its close relationship with the posterior aspect of the lateral pharyngeal space, progression of infection into the parotid space may lead to massive swelling of the neck with respiratory obstruction and has the added potential risk of direct extension into the danger and visceral spaces and hence to the posterior mediastinum (Fig. 105-1).

PERITONSILLAR ABSCESS AND PHARYNGEAL DIPHTHERIA

PERITONSILLAR ABSCESS

This condition, also known as *quinsy,* is a suppurative complication of acute tonsillitis involving the peritonsillar space. The latter consists of loose areolar tissue overlying the tonsil surrounded by the superior pharyngeal constrictor muscle and the anterior and posterior tonsillar pillars. Peritonsillar abscesses may affect patients of all ages but are most common among young adults between the ages of 15 and 30 years. The patient appears ill with fever, sore throat, dysphagia, trismus, pooling of saliva, and a muffled voice. The abscess is usually unilateral, with associated cervical lymphadenitis. Examination of the pharynx in the majority of cases reveals swelling of the anterior pillar and the soft palate and, less commonly, the middle portion or lower pole of the tonsil. Initially, needle drainage in the Trendelenburg position should be attempted and the patient closely monitored and managed with intravenous antibiotics alone. Failure to obtain pus is an indication for surgical incision and more formal exploration. Delays increase the risk of spontaneous rupture. Aspiration of purulent material is the main hazard, particularly in the sleeping patient. More serious complications include (1) airway obstruction, especially with bilateral disease or when laryngeal edema develops; and (2) lateral dissection (usually from infections of the middle or lower portions of the tonsil) through the superior pharyngeal constrictor muscle to involve the lateral pharyngeal space (Fig. 105-6B). Continued signs of sepsis after drainage of the peritonsillar space usually indicate concomitant, undrained lateral pharyngeal space infection. Fatalities associated with peritonsillar abscess (over 50 percent in the preantibiotic era) were largely due to this complication.

Ideally antibiotics should be tailored according to the results of cultures of aspirated pus, but these are infrequently performed. Also, results are unlikely to be helpful unless specimens are collected without oropharyngeal contamination and are transported in appropriate media. Group A β-hemolytic streptococci (often as part of a mixed flora containing anaerobes) are most commonly isolated. Occasionally other β-hemolytic streptococci, *Haemophilus influenzae, S. aureus,* or anaerobes alone are cultured. Penicillin G, however, is effective therapy in most cases. Bilateral tonsillectomy should be performed once the patient has recovered to avoid recurrences. Interim antibiotic prophylaxis should be considered in high-risk cases.

PHARYNGEAL DIPHTHERIA

Widespread immunization has substantially reduced infections caused by toxigenic strains of *Corynebacterium diphtheriae.* Yet local outbreaks of infection continue to occur sporadically, where reservoirs of infections (e.g., nasopharyngeal carriage) and suboptimal levels of immunization exist. All age groups, irrespective of immunization status, may develop diphtheria, but the majority are usually children and young adolescents. Those previously immunized are more likely to have milder or asymptomatic infections. Tonsillitis is the commonest manifestation, but any site in the upper airway can be infected. Nasopharyngeal involvement usually occurs by contiguous spread from the tonsils. In these patients, local symptoms of sore throat and dysphagia frequently follow a prodrome of fever, malaise, headache, nausea, and vomiting. While infection is limited to the mucosal epithelium (toxin absorption is responsible for systemic complications), the tonsils, uvula, and pharynx may swell considerably, sometimes sufficiently to suggest the presence of a peritonsillar or retropharyngeal collection. Furthermore, a brawny nonpitting edema or "bull neck" may develop secondary to reactive cervical lymphadenopathy. With nasopharyngeal infection, cervical lymphadenopathy may be marked. Diphtheria is known for the formation of a tenacious membrane, but this is not an invariable finding and may be confined to the tonsillar mucosa. It may be produced by other infections, but the typical membrane of diphtheria quickly becomes discolored and necrotic (Fig. 105-8). Bleeding may occur following attempts to remove it and may sometimes be severe. Airway obstruction by membrane and local swelling may complicate severe tonsillar and nasopharyngeal infection but is more likely when the larynx is primarily involved. Urgent tracheostomy may then be required, and if this fails to bypass the obstruction, bronchoscopy to remove any membrane present in the lower airways should be considered.

Circulating toxin is responsible for the neurologic and cardiac manifestations of diphtheria (peripheral neuropathy and myocarditis). These manifestations develop after a latent period of 1 to 2 weeks or more and are influenced by the rate of toxin production (increased by more available iron) and absorption (greater in the nasopharynx). Gravis, intermedius, and mitis variants of *C. diphtheriae* are similarly toxigenic, and their distinction is primarily of epidemiologic importance. Of the neurologic complications, palatal, ocular, or ciliary paralysis are the earliest to develop and may be followed by motor or sensory changes in the limbs; but these symptoms are all reversible.[14] Myocarditis may develop acutely or insidiously, with a gradually rising serum aspartic transaminase level. Manifestations include shock, heart failure, arrhythmias, and various conduction disturbances. The prognosis for cardiac disease is guarded, but complete recovery is the rule for those who survive.

For immediate treatment, equine diphtheria antitoxin should be given whenever clinical evidence of diphtheria exists, as early administration reduces the risk of myocarditis. The dose depends on the site and severity of the infection. Testing for hypersensitivity to horse protein (and desensitization if necessary) of all patients is mandatory. Diagnostic confirmation requires culturing *C. diphtheriae,* which must then be shown to be toxigenic. The organism is sensitive to a number of antibiotics, including penicillin G

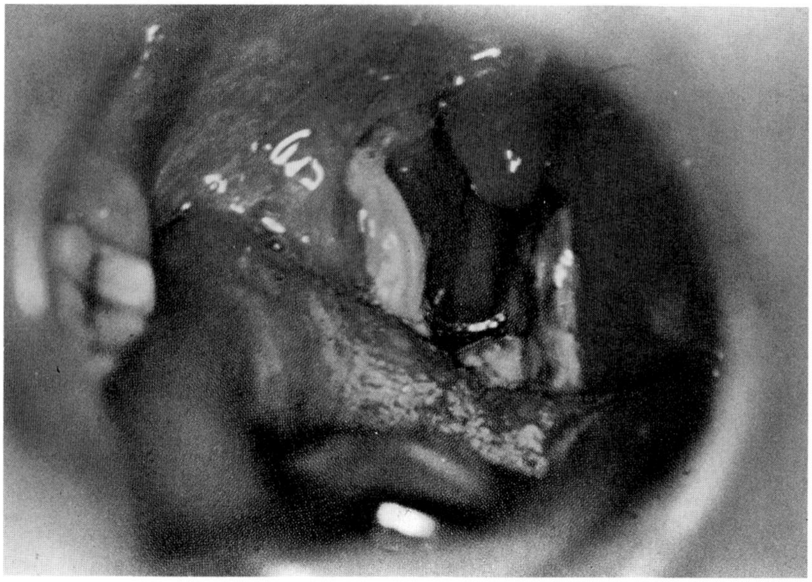

FIGURE 105-8 Tonsillar diphtheria with characteristic grayish green *membrane* overlying the right tonsil. Reproduced with permission from Whiting and Chow.[14]

and erythromycin. These agents are equally effective and are used for treating clinical cases as well as carriers and contacts.

ACUTE EPIGLOTTITIS AND LARYNGOTRACHEOBRONCHITIS

ACUTE EPIGLOTTITIS

Acute epiglottitis is caused by nonsuppurative inflammatory edema involving the supraglottic structures and the epiglottis, predominantly from infection by *H. influenzae* type b. Other bacteria, such as *Streptococcus pneumoniae, S. aureus,* and *H. parainfluenzae,* are implicated in a minority of cases. Because of the relatively small size of the supraglottic larynx in children, even small degrees of swelling may rapidly lead to complete respiratory obstruction.[15] While the incidence of deep space infection has fallen, acute epiglottitis remains one of the most common of these life-threatening infections. This in part may be attributed to the continued high prevalence and susceptibility among preschool children to *H. influenzae* type b. While children remain most susceptible, some adults are also affected, and therefore all physicians should be familiar with this condition.

In older children and adults, the chief initial complaint is a sore throat and later odynophagia; but in younger children, the physician has to rely on clinical findings. Typically, the triad of fever, stridor, and drooling are present, and the patient tends to sit up and remain quiet, leaning forward to facilitate breathing. The voice is muffled rather than hoarse. Inspiration tends to draw down the epiglottis and further obstruct the airway, so that respirations are deliberately slow rather than rapid. Cyanosis, pallor, or bradycardia are late signs of severe airway obstruction and signal the urgent need to establish an artificial airway.[16]

Once suspected, confirmation of the diagnosis will depend on the condition of the patient, bearing in mind that this can change rapidly and unexpectedly. Two aspects relevant to emergency management warrant emphasis: (1) the need for highly experienced personnel in all stages of treatment and (2) even when there is close monitoring, there may be an abrupt change in the clinical course, and resuscitation measures in a proportion of such cases may still be unsuccessful. An orderly airway insertion, on a prophylactic basis, is a much safer measure, avoiding the problems of emergency intubation. There is some controversy over whether nasotracheal intubation is the safer and more appropriate measure, although this will depend on personal preferences and specific clinical setting in a given patient. It is recommended that direct visualization and intubation be performed in the operating room, under general anaesthesia, by a skilled anaesthetist. Equipment necessary for emergency tracheostomy and a bronchoscope should be immediately available. Attempted visualization of the cherry-red epiglottis by direct laryngoscopy in an awake patient may itself precipitate acute airway obstruction, either by dislodging a mucus plug or causing the patient to gag, and is discouraged. Radiographic views of the lateral neck usually show an enlarged epiglottis, with edematous supraglottic structures and ballooning of the hypopharynx (Fig. 105-9). However, when clinical signs point toward the diagnosis of epiglottitis, radiologic investigation should not precede airway management to avoid further delay in treatment.

Additional laboratory data may indicate a moderate leukocytosis with left shift and positive cultures of blood and epiglottis. A concurrent pneumonia may be demonstrated on chest x-ray in about 25 percent of cases. Antibiotic treatment may be initiated with a combination of both ampicillin and chloramphenicol or with a β-lactamase-resistant cephalosporin such as cefuroxime, cefotaxime, or ceftriaxone.

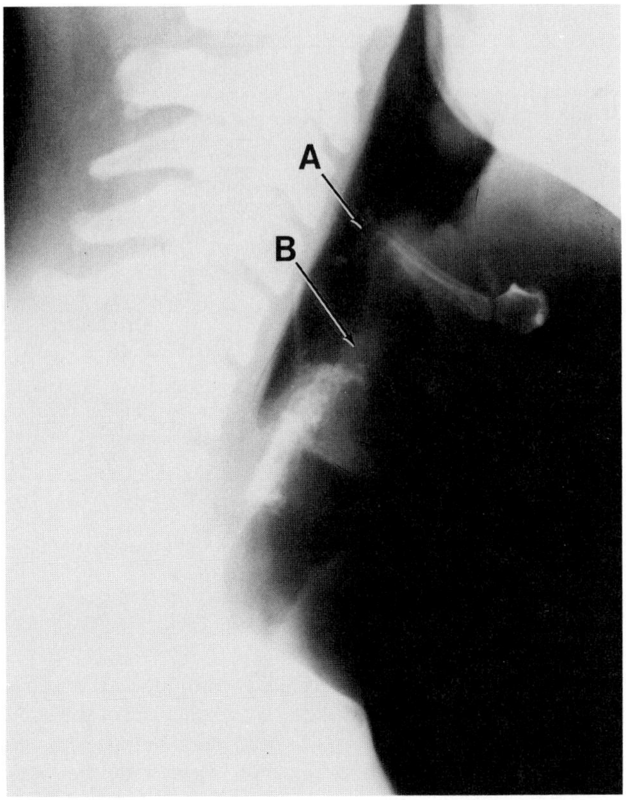

FIGURE 105-9 Lateral view of the neck in an adult with acute epiglottitis, showing soft tissue swelling of the epiglottis (*a*) and aryepiglottic folds (*b*). Reproduced with permission from Chow, Bushkell, Yoshikawa, et al.[17]

Culture and sensitivity results will dictate the ultimate choice of antibiotic that should be continued for 7 to 10 days. When *H. influenzae* infection is demonstrated, prophylactic rifampin should be provided for *all* household contacts when the household contains other contacts less than 4 years old. It remains to be determined if the recently developed vaccines (e.g., *H. influenzae* type B polysaccharide or conjugate vaccines and pneumococcal polysaccharide vaccine) will be efficacious in reducing the incidence of this dreaded complication.

LARYNGOTRACHEOBRONCHITIS, OR CROUP

This condition primarily affects young children following a viral upper respiratory infection caused by influenza, parainfluenza, respiratory syncytial virus, adenovirus, and occasionally *Mycoplasma pneumoniae*.[24] Inflammation results in edematous swelling of the conus elasticus with narrowing of the infraglottic structures. Unlike bacterial epiglottitis, laryngotracheobronchitis follows a more gradual course that may be either self-limiting or progress to respiratory obstruction. Clinical findings include a "brassy" or "barking" nonproductive cough associated with varying degrees of inspiratory stridor, hoarseness, and respiratory distress. Respirations are noisy, often accompanied by chest wall retractions and inspiratory and expiratory wheezing. Nasal discharge and pharyngeal injection are common, but the epiglottis and supraglottic structures appear normal. Fever and malaise are present as part of the upper respiratory viral syndrome. A lateral radiograph of the neck can be helpful by showing the characteristic infraglottic narrowing. Management is similar to that in supraglottic laryngitis, which includes humidification, hydration, oxygen, and antibiotic therapy for secondary bacterial infection. Use of sedatives and narcotics, which suppress the cough reflex, is to be avoided. The role of steroids remains unclear. Occasionally, an artificial airway may be required for 2 to 5 days or more. Extubation may sometimes be difficult because of additional edema secondary to the endotracheal tube itself. It seems reasonable that if the patient fails extubation, a tracheostomy should then be considered rather than reintubation.

PERICRANIAL INFECTIONS AND INTRACRANIAL SUPPURATION

SINUSITIS, OTITIS, AND MASTOIDITIS

Fortunately, suppurative and life-threatening complications of acute and chronic sinusitis have become relatively infrequent in the postantibiotic era. However, because of the unique pericranial location of these air spaces and the rich vascular supply in this region, contiguous spread of infection may extend intracranially via the diploic veins and result in serious complications such as meningitis, brain abscess, subdural or epidural empyema, osteomyelitis of the skull, and cavernous and other cortical venous sinus thrombosis.[18] The clinical spectrum of such complications may be quite varied (Table 105-3).[15] Since the roof of the frontal and ethmoidal sinuses forms the anterior cranial fossa, infection within either sinus may produce a frontal epidural abscess, subdural empyema, or a frontal lobe brain abscess (Fig. 105-2). Frontal sinusitis may also result in thrombosis of the superior sagittal sinus, which arises in the roof of the frontal air sinuses. Extension of infection into bone can lead to "Pott's puffy tumor," while an orbital extension may lead to periorbital cellulitis. The ethmoidal sinuses are separated from the orbital cavity by a papery thin orbital plate. Perforation of the plate allows direct spread of infection into the retro-orbital space. Ethmoidal sinusitis can also spread to the superior sagittal vein or the cavernous venous sinus (Fig. 105-2). The sphenoid sinus occupies the body of the sphenoid bone in close proximity to the pituitary gland above, the optic nerve and optic chiasma in front, and the internal carotids, the cavernous sinuses, and the temporal lobes of the brain on each side (Fig. 105-2). Thus sphenoid sinusitis can spread locally to cause cavernous sinus thrombosis, meningitis, temporal lobe abscess, and orbital fissure syndromes.[18,23] The superior orbital fissure syndrome, characterized by orbital pain, exophthalmos and ophthalmoplegia, is due to involvement of the abducens, oculomotor, and trochlear nerves and the ophthalmic division of the trigeminal nerve as they pass through the orbital fissure.[2] Extension of infection from the maxillary sinus into the adjacent structures may result in

TABLE 105-3 The Clinical Spectrum and Investigation of Intracranial Complications

Complication	Clinical Signs	Cerebrospinal Fluid	COMPUTED TOMOGRAPHY	
			Plain	With Contrast
Meningitis	Headache, fever,$^{++}$ stiff neck, lethargy,$^{++}$ rapid course	High PMNs* and protein; low sugar	Normal	Diffusely enhanced
Osteomyelitis	Pott's puffy tumor^{+-}	Normal	Bony defect	Bony defect
Epidural abscess or mucocele	Headache,$^{+-}$ fever^{+-}	Normal	Lucent area	Biconvex capsule
Subdural empyema	Headache,$^{+-}$ convulsions,$^{+-}$ hemiplegia,$^{+-}$ rapid course^{+-}	High PMNs and protein; normal sugar	Lucent area	Crescent shaped enhancement
Cerebral abscess	Convulsions,† headache,† personality change†	Lymphocytosis; normal sugar	Lucency with mass effect	Capsule
Venous sinus thrombosis (cavernous)	"Picket-fence" fever,$^{++}$ rapid course^{++} (orbital edema,$^{++}$ ocular palsies^{++})	Normal or high PMNs	Nonspecific	Enhancing lesion

*PMNs: polymorphonuclear leukocytes.
$^{++}$Characteristically seen.
$^{+-}$May or may not be seen.
†Frequently seen.
SOURCE: Fairbanks and Milmoe.[15]

osteomyelitis of the facial bones, including prolapse of the orbital antral wall with retro-orbital cellulitis, proptosis, and ophthalmoplegia. Direct intracranial extension from the maxillary sinus is rare, except in rhinocerebral mucormycosis and other invasive fungal sinusitis. Infections of the middle ear or mastoid within the petrous bone may extend into the middle fossa to involve the temporal lobe or into the posterior fossa to involve the cerebellum or brain stem. The skull overlying the dura of the cerebrum is covered extracranially by the galea aponeurotica. Pericranial infections, secondary either from head trauma or a craniotomy, may result in a subgaleal abscess and cranial osteomyelitis, with possible retrograde spread through the emissary veins to the epidural, subdural, and subarachnoid spaces.

Sinusitis occurring after prolonged nasotracheal intubation is a recognized complication among critically ill patients.[19] The reported incidence ranges from 2 to 5 percent among patients with nasotracheal intubation longer than 5 days. Whether the use of nasogastric, soft feeding tubes, or the Sengstaken-Blakemore tube carries a similar risk is currently unknown. This event is probably secondary to local trauma and edema within the intubated nasal cavity and is further promoted by limited head mobility, resulting in impaired drainage of the sinuses through the natural ostia. In contrast to community-acquired sinusitis, nosocomial sinusitis in the critically ill is often clinically silent, except for unexplained fever and leukocytosis. Purulent rhinorrhea and opacification or air-fluid level on sinus roentgenograms or CT scans may suggest the diagnosis. The sequelae of unrecognized infection can be catastrophic, with intracranial extension and fulminant sepsis. A high percentage of nosocomial sinusitis is polymicrobial (42 percent in one series), and the majority of patients may be receiving broad spectrum antibiotics at the time of diagnosis. The use of antral puncture for drainage and specimen collection for gram stain and culture is strongly recommended. Antimicrobial therapy should be guided by gram stain of the aspirate and culture results. Broad spectrum coverage of *S. aureus* and enteric gram-negative bacilli is generally required.

RHINOCEREBRAL MUCORMYCOSIS AND MALIGNANT OTITIS EXTERNA

Rhinocerebral mucormycosis is a progressive and destructive infection of the paranasal sinuses caused by the Mucoraceae fungal family: *Absidia, Mucor, Rhizomucor,* and *Rhizopus.* It occurs primarily in debilitated patients with uncontrolled diabetes and ketoacidosis, in profoundly dehydrated children, and in neutropenic patients receiving cytotoxic therapy. The infection begins in the nose or nasopharynx and spreads through the sinuses into the orbit or central nervous system. It may extend through the cribriform plate to involve the meninges and the adjacent frontal lobe and cranial nerves or it may extend through the nasolacrimal duct to involve the orbit, producing panophthalmitis. These fungi have a predilection for the walls of arteries and infection spreads by this route, causing thrombosis and tissue infarction. The internal carotid artery or its major branches may be involved, as may the cavernous sinus. Clinically, black necrotic lesions may be found on the nasal mucous membranes or the soft palate. When orbital involvement is seen, there is proptosis, ophthalmoplegia, blindness, chemosis, and corneal anaesthesia. Extension into the cranial cavity is manifested by headache, meningismus, trigeminal or facial cranial nerve palsy, seizures, and other focal neurologic signs. Progressive obtundation is seen, culminating in coma. The diagnosis is confirmed by the presence of broad nonseptate hyphae in biopsy specimens and a positive culture. Treatment requires aggressive surgical debridement and systemic amphotericin B. With early diagnosis, control of the underlying condition, and appropriate antimicrobial therapy, long-term survival has been reported in 85% of cases.

Malignant otitis externa is a progressive and necrotizing infection of the external ear caused by *P. aeruginosa,* with spread through the cartilaginous and bony canal to the base of the skull. Affected patients are usually debilitated and often have poorly controlled diabetes mellitus. The infection is associated with severe otalgia, hearing loss, purulent discharge, edema, and granulation tissue or "polyp" in the cartilaginous portion of the external ear canal. Three stages of progression are recognized clinically: (1) locally invasive disease; (2) disease associated with facial palsy; and (3) disease associated with multiple cranial nerve palsies. In the latter stages, infection may involve the infratemporal fossa by extension into the temporal or occipital bone. Prolonged medical therapy in conjunction with local debridement of granulation tissue and infected cartilage is effective in the majority of patients. In patients with more extensive disease involving the base of the skull and multiple cranial nerve palsies, results of therapy are not as successful and up to 20 months of antimicrobial treatment may be required to achieve eradication of infection without relapse.

INTRACRANIAL SUPPURATION

These dreaded complications, which most commonly arise from chronic sinusitis, mastoiditis, or deep fascial space infections, are only briefly reviewed here. Readers are referred to Chap. 103 for a more comprehensive description of these entities.

Brain Abscess

Most brain abscesses occur in association with three identifiable clinical settings: (1) contiguous focus of infection, particularly sinusitis, otitis, or mastoiditis; (2) cranial trauma or postcraniotomy; and (3) hematogenous spread from an extracranial focus of infection, especially the lung and heart valves. Otogenic (e.g., temporal lobe or cerebellum) and sinusitis-related (e.g., frontal lobe) brain abscess account for approximately 50 percent of all pericranial sources of infection.[20] Hematogenous brain abscesses are frequently multiple and in the distribution of the middle cerebral artery (i.e., posterior frontal or parietal lobes). The clinical presentations of brain abscesses are quite variable and appear to be primarily influenced by their anatomic location, proximity to the ventricles, cisterns or dural sinuses, and major alterations in the intracranial pressure dynamics secondary to the mass effect. Thus, a pontine abscess may bulge posteriorly and block the aqueduct of Sylvius acutely to cause obstructive hydrocephalus. An occipital lobe abscess could rupture or leak into the ventricular system, causing ventriculitis, or it could involve the transverse sinus and cause septic thrombophlebitis or a subdural empyema. Four distinctive clinical presentations of a brain abscess can be recognized, based on the unique pathophysiologic events implicated: (1) rapid focal mass expansion; (2) intracranial hypertension; (3) diffuse brain destruction; and (4) focal neurologic deficit. In the last category, the temporal progression of infection is so slow that it is often misdiagnosed as a neoplasm. Fever is present in only 45 to 50 percent of patients; therefore, absence of fever should not be used to exclude the diagnosis of brain abscess.

Subdural Empyema and Cranial Epidural Abscess

Intracranial subdural empyema in the adult usually results from a suppurative infection of the paranasal sinuses, mastoid, or middle ear. An acute flare-up with local pain and increase in purulent nasal or aural discharge and onset of generalized headache and high fevers are the first indications of intracranial spread. They are followed within days by focal neurologic findings such as unilateral motor seizures, hemiplegia, hemianesthesia or aphasia, and signs of increased intracranial pressure with progressive lethargy and coma. The neck is stiff, but cerebrospinal fluid (CSF) examination is more consistent with an aseptic meningitis syndrome. In infants and young children, however, an intracranial subdural empyema is almost invariably a complication of bacterial meningitis. Early signs such as irritability, poor feeding, or increased head size are nonspecific, but hemiparesis, convulsions, stupor, and coma may rapidly ensue. *Streptococcus pneumoniae, S. agalactiae,* and *H. influenzae* are the most common causes.

Cranial epidural abscess is usually associated with a postcraniotomy infection or a cranial osteomyelitis secondary to chronic sinusitis or middle ear infection. The onset of symptoms may be insidious and overshadowed by the localized inflammatory process. Focal neurologic findings are less common than in subdural empyema. Rarely, a fifth and sixth cranial nerve palsy may develop in association with infections of the petrous portion of the temporal bone (Gradenigo's syndrome).

Septic Intracranial Thrombophlebitis and Mycotic Aneurysm

Septic intracranial thrombophlebitis most frequently follows infection of the paranasal sinuses, middle ear, mastoid, or oropharynx. If collateral venous drainage is adequate, septic venous thrombosis may produce only transient neurologic findings or may be silent. If the thrombus outstrips collateral flow, however, progressive neurologic deficits will result with impairment of consciousness, focal or generalized seizures, and increased intracranial pressure. The clinical findings vary with the location of cortical veins or dural sinuses involved. Cavernous sinus thrombosis is characterized by abrupt onset with diplopia, photophobia, orbital edema, and progressive exophthalmos. Involvement of cranial nerves III, IV, V, and VI produces ophthalmoplegia, a midposition fixed pupil, loss of corneal reflex, and diminished sensation over the upper face. Obstruction of venous return from the retina results in papilledema, retinal hemorrhage, and visual loss. Thrombosis of the superior sagittal sinus produces bilateral leg weakness and may cause communicating hydrocephalus. Occlusion of the lateral sinus produces pain over the ear and mastoid and may cause edema over the mastoid (Griesinger's sign). Involvement of cranial nerves V and VI produces ipsilateral facial pain and lateral rectus weakness (Gradenigo's syndrome). Intracranial mycotic aneurysm usually results from septic embolization as a complication of bacterial endocarditis. This produces infection and necrosis in the arterial wall, which leads to dilation and possible rupture. Mycotic aneurysms can be multiple and are usually found on distal branches of the middle or anterior cerebral arteries. The early clinical manifestations are similar to those of cerebral emboli and infarction. The weakened vessel may be visualized to progressively increase in size on serial angiograms. Since the clinical course of a mycotic aneurysm is quite variable and the risk of rupture with catastrophic cerebral hemorrhage cannot be predicted even after successful therapy of the underlying endocarditis, early surgical intervention is advised.

Diagnostic Considerations

MICROBIOLOGIC TECHNIQUES

It is imperative that clinical specimens for the diagnosis of deep head and neck infections are obtained without contamination by the resident oronasopharyngeal flora. This is best accomplished using a needle and syringe for aspiration of loculated pus through an extraoral approach. After cleansing the skin, pus is aspirated into the syringe. All air is carefully expressed, and the needle tip is inserted into a rubber stopper. This allows the exclusion of air, and the specimen can then be transported directly to the laboratory. This method of specimen collection is superior to using swabs. If a swab is used, it should be saturated with purulent material and inserted into a commercially available transport tube specifically designed to transport swabs under anaerobic conditions. An additional swab should be taken for gram stain. The gram stain is particularly useful in the assessment of head and neck infections because anaerobic bacteria may require 48 h or longer for growth, and the morphology of some of the bacteria may be characteristic enough to suggest a provisional diagnosis and, ultimately, therapy. Infected tissues obtained intraoperatively are also suitable for anaerobic and aerobic processing, provided that care is taken to preclude contamination by the normal resident flora.

IMAGING TECHNIQUES

Radiography is a sensitive method for the diagnosis of acute sinusitis in adults and children over the age of 1 year. Ultrasonography is no better than radiography. The presence of abnormal radiographic findings (e.g., complete opacification, air-fluid level, or mucosal thickening of 4 mm or more in children and 5 mm or more in adults) is predictive of infection as determined by sinus puncture in 75 percent of cases, while a normal radiograph correlates with a normal aspirate in 80 percent of cases. Four standard radiographic views are used: occipitomental (Waters') projection for the maxillary sinus, posteroanterior (Caldwell's) projection for the ethmoidal and frontal sinuses, and lateral and submental-vertex projections for the sphenoid sinus. Radiographic examination is less useful in chronic sinusitis because of persistent abnormalities and in children under the age of 1 year because of redundant sinus mucosa and asymmetry of facial bone or sinus development. An orthopantomogram is indicated if an odontogenic infection is suspected.

For deep fascial space infections and retro-orbital cellulitis, CT scanning is extremely sensitive and accurate for localization of infection.[21] If a retropharyngeal infection is suspected, radiographic views or CT scans of the lateral neck can help determine if the infection is in the retropharyngeal space or the prevertebral space. The former suggests an odontogenic source, while the latter suggests involvement of the cervical spine.[22] For investigation of cranial or cervical osteomyelitis, conventional radiographs are relatively insensitive. The combination of CT scanning with technetium bone scans and gallium or white-cell-labeled indium scans has greatly improved the diagnostic yield.

CT scanning is the single neuroimaging technique that has most consistently advanced the diagnostic accuracy of intracranial infections such as brain abscess, subdural empyema, and epidural abscess. The typical CT findings in brain abscess are an area of decreased attenuation surrounded by a "ring" of enhancement following injection of contrast. CT will also detect cerebral edema, hydrocephalus, an associated mass effect, and presence of extracranial infection. In subdural empyema, CT reveals inward displacement of cerebral substance due to an extracerebral mass. In epidural abscess, CT demonstrates a thick and circumscribed area of diminished density associated with extracerebral displacement and contiguous cranial osteomyelitis. Radionuclide brain scans and cerebral angiography remain useful as complementary procedures for the localization of certain central nervous system infections, particularly posterior fossa lesions and demonstration of mycotic aneurysms. It remains to be seen if newer techniques such as magnetic resonance imaging and positron emission tomography will further improve the diagnostic yield in early pericranial or intracranial infections.

Therapeutic Considerations

Although resuscitation and surgical measures are of primary importance in the initial management of these life-threatening infections, appropriate antibiotics are essential for a successful outcome. Empiric antimicrobial regimens for head and neck and upper respiratory tract infections are summarized in Table 105-2. Recommendations for intracranial suppurative complications are discussed in Chap. 103. Maximum doses of systemic antimicrobials should be administered in order to optimize penetration of bone and the blood-brain barrier. Therapy should be continued for 2 to 3 weeks. Intracranial and vascular or bone infections may require at least 6 to 8 weeks of intravenous antibiotics. Where anaerobes are implicated, penicillin G remains the antibiotic of first choice. Clindamycin or chloramphenicol are useful alternatives in the penicillin allergic patient and have the advantage of more effective coverage against β-

lactamase-producing anaerobes. Metronidazole may also be considered in this setting, particularly when *Bacteroides melaninogenicus, B. fragilis,* or *Fusobacterium necrophorum* is suspected. Its lack of activity against gram-positive anaerobic cocci such as *Peptostreptococcus* and facultative organisms such as streptococci and *S. aureus* is a disadvantage that precludes monotherapy of head and neck infections with metronidazole alone. Combination of penicillin or clindamycin with metronidazole may be an alternative. For immunocompromised and critically ill patients, broad spectrum coverage for aerobic gram-negative rods, *S. aureus,* as well as anaerobes (e.g., cefotaxime, ceftizoxime, or imipenem) is indicated (Table 105-2). The final selection of antimicrobial therapy should be guided by culture results and susceptibility data.

While considerable advances have been made in our understanding of these life-threatening oropharyngeal and otorhinolaryngeal infections, vigilance in terms of both diagnosis and management are required to avoid the high mortality associated with this important group of conditions.

CASE PRESENTATION

A 67-year-old man was admitted to the surgical intensive unit following trauma to the head, chest, and abdomen sustained in a motor vehicle accident. Extensive facial and periorbital swelling was present due to superficial lacerations and blunt injury, but there were no orbital or maxillofacial fractures. He was comatose but had no focal neurologic findings. CT scan of the head indicated cerebral edema but no subdural hematoma or cranial fractures. He required nasotracheal intubation and ventilatory support because of a flail chest and lung contusion. Hemodynamic status was maintained. He was placed on cefotaxime, 2 g IV every 6 h, for suspected aspiration and possible pneumonia. His clinical condition stabilized, and he began to awake and respond to verbal commands. However, on the sixth hospital day, he developed spiking fevers to 40°C despite continuation of antibiotics. Nasotracheal suctions were unremarkable while chest findings showed improvement of infiltrates radiographically. Facial swelling had subsided considerably, and all sutured sites appeared clean. The abdomen was benign. The Foley catheter was removed. Blood and urine cultures were negative, and all intravenous and arterial lines were changed and catheter tips cultured. Blood work revealed marked leukocytosis with a total white cell count of 24,000/mm^3 and left shift. On the tenth day, the fever persisted and he became increasingly obtunded with slight nuchal rigidity. The blood pressure remained normal. Funduscopic examination revealed bilateral retinal venous congestion but no papilladema. Neurologic examination revealed bilateral orbital swelling with exophthalmos and presence of ophthalmoplegia, a midposition fixed pupil, and loss of corneal reflex in the left eye, suggestive of a left third, fourth, and sixth cranial nerve palsy. The remainder of the general physical examination was unchanged. A lumbar puncture revealed clear CSF with opening pressure of 300 mm^3 H_2O, cell count of 25 leucocytes/mL (all lymphocytes), and normal protein and glucose content. Gram stain and culture of the CSF were negative. A CT scan with contrast revealed no intracranial lesions, but the sphenoid and maxillary sinuses were opacified. There was also haziness within both cavernous sinuses. Intravenous antibiotics were changed to imipenem, 500 mg every 6 h, and cloxacillin, 1.5 g every 6 h, and dexamethaxone, 1 g, was administered. Surgical drainage of the sphenoid and maxillary sinuses was performed 2 days later. He awoke on the fourth day postoperatively, steadily improved, and was eventually discharged without neurologic sequelae after completing 3 weeks of antimicrobial therapy.

CASE DISCUSSION

This patient developed acute nosocomial sinusitis secondary to nasotracheal intubation. A maxillary sinusitis eventually progressed to sphenoidal involvement resulting in cavernous sinus thrombosis. The initial clinical presentation was relatively silent except for high spiking fevers and marked leukocytosis suggestive of a deep-seated abscess. Routine investigation of potential sources of persistent fever were unrewarding. If the neurologic findings indicative of cavernous sinus thrombosis had not been noted and the CT scan was not repeated, the primary source of infection might have remained undiagnosed. Nosocomial sinusitis should be considered as a potential source of unexplained fever in the critically ill patient who has received prolonged nasotracheal or nasogastric intubation. Patients with orofacial and head injury are particularly at risk. Trauma to the nasal mucosa from repeated invasive instrumentation, sedation, sinus hematoma, and immobilization of the head may obstruct the sinus ostia, impair sinus drainage, and promote suppurative infection. Nosocomial sinusitis is characterized by resistant aerobic gram-negative bacilli and *S. aureus* as well as streptococci and anaerobes. Broad spectrum antibiotic coverage is required. Since paranasal sinus suppuration may behave as a closed space infection, systemic antibiotics alone without surgical drainage may be ineffective. Treatment failure is tolerated particularly poorly in this population. Since nosocomial sinusitis is often clinically inapparent, its presence must be sought aggressively. The clinician must not limit the investigation of the source of a persistent fever only to the common and clinically accessible sites such as the sputum, urine, blood, wound, and intravenous catheters. Routine and careful examination of the nasal turbinates may reveal purulent discharge. When the diagnosis is suspected, CT scanning is invaluable and should be obtained early. Since hospital-acquired antibiotic-resistant pathogens are frequently encountered and infection often persists despite antibiotic therapy, treatment should be guided by culture and sensitivity testing of isolates recovered by antral aspiration. The nasotracheal tubes should be replaced orally. Successful therapy is usually attended by prompt defervescence of fever.

References

1. Chow AW: Infections of the oral cavity, neck and head, in Mandell LA, Douglas RG, Bennett JE (eds): *Principles and Practice of Infectious Diseases*, 3rd ed., New York, Churchill Livingstone, 1990, pp 516–529.
2. Vortel JJ, Chow AW: Sinus infections, in Gorbach SL, Bartlett JG, Blacklow NR (eds): *Infectious Diseases in Medicine and Surgery*. Philadelphia, WB Saunders, in press.
3. Todd JK: Bacteriology and clinical relevance of nasopharyngeal and oropharyngeal cultures. Ped Infect Dis 3:159, 1984.
4. Roscoe DL, Chow AW: Normal flora and mucosal immunity of the head and neck. Infect Dis Clin N Am 2:1, 1988.
5. Edson RS, Rosenblatt JE, Lee DT, McVey EA: Recent experience with antimicrobial susceptibility of anaerobic bacteria: Increasing resistance to penicillin. Mayo Clin Proc 57:737, 1982.
6. Chow AW, Roser SM, Brady FA: Orofacial odontogenic infections. Ann Intern Med 88:392, 1978.
7. Blomquist IK, Bayer AS: Life-threatening deep fascial space infections of the head and neck. Infect Dis Clin N Am 2:237, 1988.
8. Megran DW, Scheifele DW, Chow AW: Odontogenic infections. Ped Infect Dis 3:257, 1984.
9. Finch RG, Snider GE, Sprinkle PM: Ludwig's angina. JAMA 243:1171, 1980.
10. Patterson HC, Kelly JH, Strome M: Ludwig's angina: An update. Laryngoscope 92:370, 1982.
11. Baddour IM, Land MA, Barrett FF, Rivara FP, Bruce WM, Bisno AL: Hepatobiliary abnormalities associated with postanginal sepsis: Common manifestations of an uncommon disease. Diag Microbiol Infect Dis 4:19, 1986.
12. Seidenfeld SM, Sutker WL, Luby JP: Fusobacterium necrophorum septicemia following oropharyngeal infection. JAMA 248:1348, 1982.
13. Toews A, De La Rocha AG: Oropharyngeal sepsis with endothoracic spread. Can J Surg 23:256, 1980.
14. Whiting JL, Chow AW: Life-threatening infections of the mouth and throat. J Crit Illness 2:36, 1987.
15. Fairbanks DNF, Milmoe GJ: Complications and sequelae: An otolaryngologist's perspective. Ped Infect Dis 4(Suppl 6):s75, 1985.
16. Bass JW, Steele RW, Wiebe RA: Acute epiglottitis: A surgical emergency. JAMA 229:671, 1974.
17. Chow AW, Bushkell LL, Yoshikawa, TT, et al: Haemophilus parainfluenzae epiglottis with meningitis and bacteremia in an adult. Am J Med Sci 267:365, 1974.
18. Kaplan RJ: Neurological complications of infections of the head and neck. Otolaryngol Clin N Am 9:729, 1976.
19. Linden BE, Aguilar EA, Allen SJ: Sinusitis in the nasotracheally intubated patient. Arch Otolaryngol Head Neck Surg 114:860, 1988.
20. Yoshikawa TT, Quinn W: The aching head: Intracranial suppuration due to head and neck infections. Infect Dis Clin N Am 2:265, 1988.
21. Salit IE: Diagnostic approaches to head and neck infections. Infect Dis Clin N Am 2:35, 1988.
22. Bryan CS, King BG, Bryant RE: Retropharyngeal infection in adults. Arch Intern Med 134:127, 1974.
23. Lew D, Southwick FS, Montgomery WW, Weber AL, Baker AS: Sphenoid sinusitis: A review of 30 cases. N Engl J Med 309:1149, 1983.
24. Muszynski MJ, Marks MI: Epiglottis, croup, and laryngitis, in Schlossberg D (ed): *Infections of the Head and Neck*. New York, Springer-Verlag, 1987, pp 133–147.
25. Willis PI, Vernon RP: Complications of the space infections of the head and neck. Laryngoscope 91:1129, 1981.

Chapter 106
SOFT TISSUE INFECTIONS

JOHN CONLY

KEY POINTS

- *Soft tissue infections characterized by extensive necrosis of subcutaneous tissue, fascia, or muscle are uncommon, but mandate prompt recognition and urgent surgical treatment.*
- *The classic hallmarks of virulent soft tissue infections are extensive involvement of the subcutaneous tissues and a relative paucity of cutaneous involvement until late in the course of the infection.*
- *Most persons with rapidly spreading soft tissue infections present acutely with extreme systemic toxicity.*
- *Successful management of these critically ill patients depends on prompt diagnosis by clinical and radiologic means.*
- *The principles of management include fluid resuscitation, hemodynamic stabilization, broad-spectrum antimicrobial administration, and early surgical intervention.*
- *Prompt surgery in which a definitive diagnosis is reached, and all necrotic tissue debrided, should be considered the mainstay of treatment.*
- *The highest mortality rate occurs when the diagnosis is delayed or initial surgical treatment is limited.*

Classification of Soft Tissue Infections

In severe soft tissue infections the initial presentation may be obscure; it often belies the relentless progression of subcutaneous tissue necrosis and dissection that remains unrecognized beneath a normal-appearing skin. Successful management depends on early recognition that a virulent soft tissue infection is present, followed by prompt investigation to establish a specific diagnosis. To accomplish this, a clear understanding of the classification of these entities is required. Unfortunately, the published literature on the subject can be quite confusing, because of a lack of uniformity in descriptive terminology and in the use of differing classification schemes, which may be based on either clinical or bacteriologic findings. The problem is further compounded by the fact that certain clinical entities may involve one or more anatomic planes within the subcutaneous tissue, and one or more bacterial species may be responsible for the same or different clinical entities. Although classification schemes based on microbial etiology may be most complete, they offer little to the clinical diagnostic process necessary to expedite appropriate management.[1] To place a useful clinicoanatomic classification into perspective, an understanding of the basic anatomy and microbial ecology of the skin and subcutaneous tissues is necessary.

NORMAL ANATOMY AND MICROBIAL ECOLOGY OF THE SKIN AND SOFT TISSUES

The skin is a two-layered membrane consisting of an outer layer, the *epidermis,* and an inner layer, the *dermis.* The skin resides on a fibrous connective tissue layer, the *superficial fascia.* Beneath this, the avascular *deep fascia* overlies and separates muscle groups and acts as a mechanical barrier to the spread of infections from superficial layers to the muscle compartments. Between the superficial and deep fascia lies the *fascial cleft,* which is mainly composed of adipose tissue and contains the superficial nerves, arteries, veins, and lymphatics that supply the skin and adipose tissue. Infections of the fascial cleft do not involve the blood vessels of the skin until later in the course of the process, when direct involvement of the blood vessels of the superficial fascia occurs.

Normally the skin has a resident and a transient flora. The resident, or normally occurring, flora includes *Corynebacterium* species, coagulase-negative staphylococci, and *Micrococcus* species. *Staphylococcus aureus* is not considered part of the resident flora, but colonization rates of 10 to 30 percent in the anterior nares, axillae, groins, and perineum may be noted. Hospitalized patients and health care workers tend to have higher rates of colonization of *Staph. aureus.* Gram-negative bacilli are not considered part of the normal resident flora, although they may occasionally be found in the moist intertriginous areas, such as the toe webs, groins, and perineum. The transient flora is made up of bacteria that are collected from extraneous sources and colonize the cutaneous surface for only a short period (hours to days). These organisms are highly variable, but are often pathogenic gram-negative bacilli such as *Escherichia coli, Proteus* species, *Pseudomonas aeruginosa,* and other gram-negative bacilli.[2] Critically ill patients frequently have compromised natural defense barriers, with concomitant increases in transient flora colonization.

CLINICOANATOMIC CLASSIFICATION

Most classification schemes for soft tissue infections are based on clinical presentation or microbiologic etiology. Figure 106-1 shows a practical approach to the classification that is based on the affected anatomic plane of the soft tissues, the most commonly encountered clinical terms, and microbial etiology. The terms used in this chapter and a partial listing of frequently encountered synonyms are given in Table 106-1.

The *common superficial pyodermas* include erysipelas, impetigo, ecthyma, furunculosis, and carbunculosis. These entities do not extend beyond the skin or its appendages and will not be discussed further.

The *cellulitides* include what we commonly refer to as cellulitis, anaerobic (or gangrenous) cellulitis, and the clinically distinctive variant of gangrenous cellulitis called *progressive bacterial synergistic gangrene (Meleney's gangrene).*

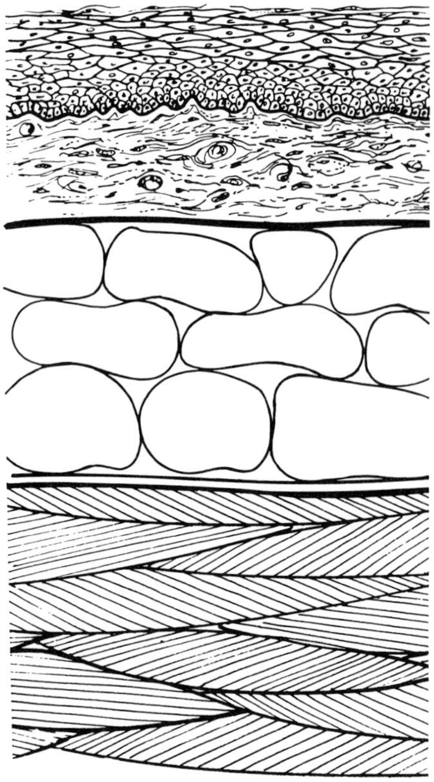

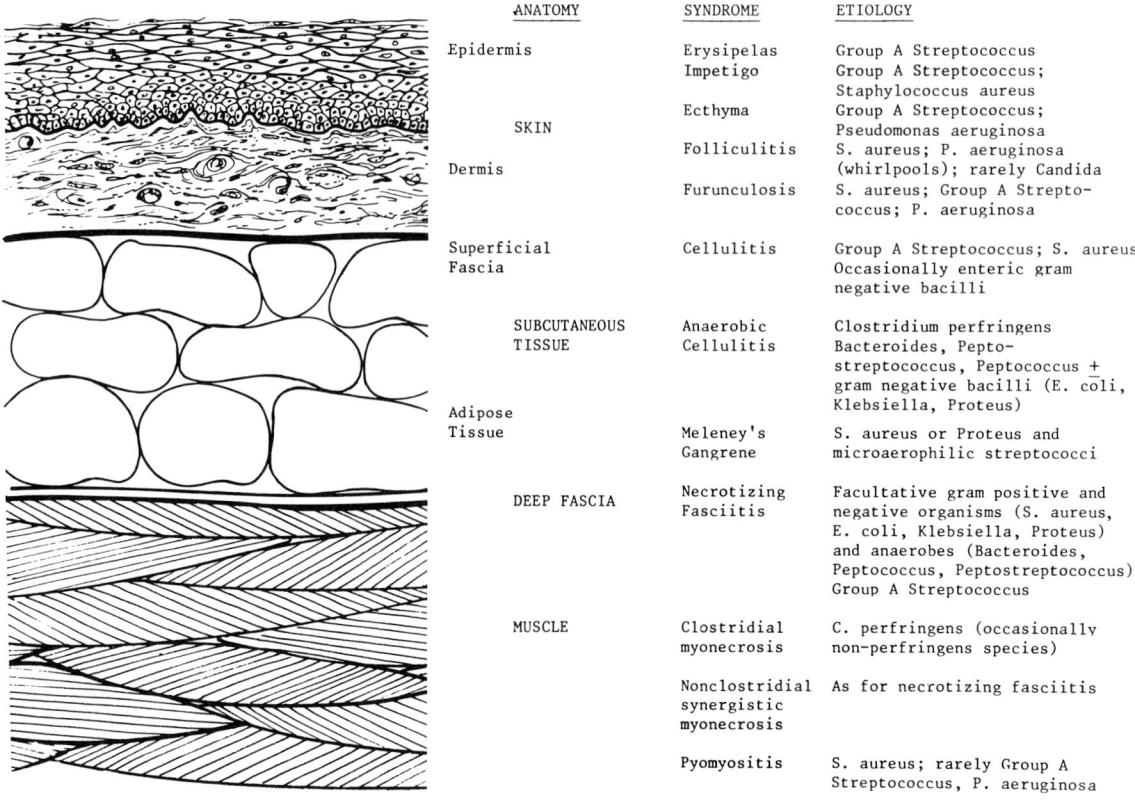

ANATOMY	SYNDROME	ETIOLOGY
Epidermis	Erysipelas	Group A Streptococcus
	Impetigo	Group A Streptococcus; Staphylococcus aureus
SKIN	Ecthyma	Group A Streptococcus; Pseudomonas aeruginosa
	Folliculitis	S. aureus; P. aeruginosa (whirlpools); rarely Candida
Dermis	Furunculosis	S. aureus; Group A Streptococcus; P. aeruginosa
Superficial Fascia	Cellulitis	Group A Streptococcus; S. aureus Occasionally enteric gram negative bacilli
SUBCUTANEOUS TISSUE	Anaerobic Cellulitis	Clostridium perfringens Bacteroides, Peptostreptococcus, Peptococcus ± gram negative bacilli (E. coli, Klebsiella, Proteus)
Adipose Tissue	Meleney's Gangrene	S. aureus or Proteus and microaerophilic streptococci
DEEP FASCIA	Necrotizing Fasciitis	Facultative gram positive and negative organisms (S. aureus, E. coli, Klebsiella, Proteus) and anaerobes (Bacteroides, Peptococcus, Peptostreptococcus); Group A Streptococcus
MUSCLE	Clostridial myonecrosis	C. perfringens (occasionally non-perfringens species)
	Nonclostridial synergistic myonecrosis	As for necrotizing fasciitis
	Pyomyositis	S. aureus; rarely Group A Streptococcus, P. aeruginosa

FIGURE 106-1 Clinicoanatomic classification of soft tissue infections.

Cellulitis is an acute spreading infection of the skin extending below the superficial fascia to involve the upper subcutaneous tissues—usually their upper third. These infections do not involve the deep fascial layer. The production of gas by anaerobic organisms and the subsequent presence of soft tissue gas, either palpable or demonstrable radiographically, and the propensity to produce necrosis in the subcutaneous tissue (and eventually in the skin) are major differentiating features of anaerobic and classic cellulitis. *Progressive bacterial synergistic gangrene* was the original term used to describe a distinct form of cellulitis often occurring postoperatively.[3] Gangrenous changes of the skin, with subsequent necrotic ulcer formation in the center of the cellulitic area, are characteristic of this entity.

Necrotizing fasciitis is an acute infection involving the deep fascia, subcutaneous tissue, and superficial fascia to variable degrees. The muscle tissue beneath the deep fascia is unaffected. The skin may not be involved early in the course of the infection, but as the process continues the skin becomes involved. Fournier's syndrome (or gangrene) is a form of necrotizing fasciitis that affects the scrotum and genitalia.[4] In this setting, because there is virtually no subcutaneous fat between the epidermis and dartos fascia, cutaneous gangrene readily develops.

The *myonecroses* include clostridial myonecrosis (otherwise known as gas gangrene), nonclostridial myonecrosis [which has also been termed "synergistic necrotizing cellulitis" (a misnomer)], pyomyositis, and vascular gangrene. Rapid necrosis of the muscle and, later, of the overlying subcutaneous tissue and skin are characteristic of the myonecrotic syndromes. Pyomyositis, an exception, is a rare acute bacterial infection localized to the muscle, usually occuring after penetrating trauma. Abscess formation, rather than necrosis, occurs. Vascular gangrene occurs in a limb devitalized by arterial insufficiency.

Major Soft Tissue Infections

CELLULITIS

PATHOGENESIS

Cellulitis most often occurs in a setting of previous trauma of the skin, with local inoculation of microorganisms; or secondary to an underlying skin lesion or a postoperative wound infection; or as contiguous spread from another suppurative infection of other soft tissues or bone. However, cellulitis may also occur in the absence of any obvious local trauma. Following inoculation of microorganisms into the subcutaneous tissues and skin, an acute inflammatory response is seen in the epidermis, dermis, adipose tissue, and superficial fascia, to varying degrees. The inflammatory response consists of predominantly polymorphonuclear leukocytes without necrosis.

TABLE 106-1 Necrotizing Soft Tissue Infections—Clinical Entities and Synonyms

Clinical Entity	Synonyms
Anaerobic cellulitis (clostridial and nonclostridial)	Clostridial cellulitis, gangrenous cellulitis, epifascial gangrene, gas abscess, localized gas gangrene, crepitant cellulitis
Progressive bacterial synergistic gangrene	Meleney's gangrene, bacterial synergistic gangrene, postoperative progressive gangrene, Meleney's ulcer, chronic burrowing ulcer
Necrotizing fasciitis	Hospital gangrene, acute infective gangrene, necrotizing erysipelas, suppurative fasciitis, hemolytic streptococcal gangrene, acute dermal gangrene, necrotizing genital infection, Fournier's syndrome, synergistic gangrene of the scrotum
Clostridial myonecrosis	Gas gangrene
Nonclostridial myonecrosis	Nonclostridial gas gangrene, synergistic anaerobic myonecrosis, crepitant myositis, synergistic necrotizing cellulitis, necrotizing cutaneous myositis

ETIOLOGY

The most common organisms causing classic cellulitis are *Streptococcus pyogenes* and *Staph. aureus.* Less commonly encountered organisms include *Strep. pneumoniae,* other streptococci, and gram-negative bacilli. Cellulitis due to gram-negative bacilli occurs primarily in immunosuppressed or granulocytopenic patients. A severe form of cellulitis may occur in individuals exposed to *Aeromonas hydrophila* in fresh water; the organism gains access through lacerations during swimming or wading. A severe and fulminant form of cellulitis that rapidly progresses to necrosis and bacteremia may be caused by *Vibrio* species, especially *V. vulnificans,* acquired by exposure of a traumatic wound to salt water or raw seafood drippings.[5]

PRESENTATION

Classic cellulitis is characterized by erythema, pain, edema, and local tenderness involving an area of the skin with ill-defined borders. The area of initial cutaneous involvement expands rapidly. Occasionally there is lymphangitis and regional lymphadenopathy. Systemic manifestations include fever, malaise, and rigors. With untreated or rapidly progressive cellulitis, the process may spread to involve an entire extremity, producing increasingly severe systemic toxicity. Dehydration, mental apathy or obtundation, disseminated intravascular coagulopathy, respiratory failure, and septic shock may follow, necessitating intensive care management.

MANAGEMENT

Appropriate laboratory diagnostic studies should be performed prior to institution of antimicrobial therapy. Any skin abrasions or draining sites should be swabbed for immediate Gram stain and culture. The stain is examined for both the presence and the morphologic appearance of the microorganisms, and the number and types of cells. Needle aspiration after injection of 0.5 mL of nonbacteriostatic saline into the leading edge of the cellulitis may be attempted; potential pathogens have been isolated in 10 to 38 percent of cases.[6,7] A combination of needle aspiration, skin biopsy, and blood cultures results in isolation of pathogens in about 25 percent of cases.[8]

For severe infections where both streptococci and staphylococci are considered, parenteral administration of a high-dose penicillinase-resistant penicillin (nafcillin, cloxacillin) in doses of 8 to 12 g/day, in 4 or 6 divided doses, is most appropriate. Alternate agents include a first-generation cephalosporin, such as cefazolin or cephalothin (6 to 8 g/day); vancomycin (2 g/day); and clindamycin (1200 to 2400 g/day). If the etiologic agent proves to be streptococcal, penicillin G should be substituted (6 to 12 million U/day). In the immunocompromised host, or in the presence of a rapidly progressive cellulitis developing following a fresh- or salt-water injury, an aminoglycoside (gentamicin, tobramycin), 3 to 5 mg/kg in 3 or 4 divided doses, should also be administered.

Local care of cellulitis includes immobilization and elevation of the affected area. These measures are most appropriate when an extremity is affected. Analgesic drugs are administered as necessary. Application of cool compresses may aid in the reduction of pain. The extent of the cellulitis should be outlined on the skin with a felt-tip marker at the time of admission to facilitate objective daily assessments of the extent of spread. Frequent inspection of the involved area is necessary to detect any areas of crepitus or suppuration, which would require surgical drainage. Abscesses of the subcutaneous tissue are not infrequent after extensive cellulitis; judicious use of repeated needle aspiration may be necessary. Failure to achieve defervescence and a decrease in systemic toxicity within 48 to 72 h after institution of appropriate antimicrobial therapy should arouse suspicion of suppuration or a more virulent soft tissue infection, such as necrotizing fasciitis or myonecrosis.

ANAEROBIC CELLULITIS

PATHOGENESIS

The term used for this type of cellulitis is not properly descriptive, but persists due to common usage. Other terms for this process include *gas abscess, gangrenous cellulitis, localized gas gangrene,* and *epifascial gangrene.* The process usually represents infection of already devitalized subcutaneous tissue. The deep fascia is not involved. Microorganisms are introduced into the subcutaneous tissues from an operative or accidental wound or from a preexisting local infection. The groin and perineal regions are especially susceptible to this type of infection because of their proximity to the fecal flora. The subcutaneous tissues are devitalized from a local injury, an inadequately debrided wound, or a metabolic disturbance that might compromise vascular supply (e.g., diabetes mellitus). Usually the infectious process is not invasive, but remains localized within the area of devitalized tissue.[9] Extensive gas formation and suppuration, usually limited to the area of devitalized tissue, is present. Anaerobic cellulitis is several times more common than anaerobic myonecrotic syndromes.

ETIOLOGY

Anaerobic cellulitis may be clostridial or nonclostridial. *Clostridium perfringens* is the most commonly isolated clostridial species, followed by *C. septicum*. Gram-negative rods, staphylococci, or streptococci may occasionally be present, but are not the predominant isolates. The nonclostridial form of anaerobic cellulitis is essentially the same process as clostridial cellulitis, but has a different microbiologic etiology. Obligate anaerobes represent the predominant isolates, with *Bacteroides fragilis* "group," *Bacteroides* species, *Peptostreptococcus*, and *Peptococcus* encountered most frequently. Other bacteria that may be present include the gram-negative enteric bacilli *(E. coli, Klebsiella)*, staphylococci, and streptococci.

PRESENTATION

The clinical pictures of both clostridial and nonclostridial anaerobic cellulitis are very similar and may be discussed together. Since this infection represents the local invasion of already devitalized tissue, the process does not generally have a virulent progressive course. The onset is gradual, with mild-to-moderate local pain and only mild-to-moderate tissue swelling. Constitutional symptoms are not prominent; the relative paucity of symptoms is helpful in distinguishing this entity from myonecrotic infections. A thin, dark, malodorous discharge from the wound or inoculation site, sometimes containing fat globules, with extensive and prominent gas formation, is characteristic. There may be a dusky erythema present, with extensive crepitus in the involved area. Although not initially invasive beyond the area of devitalized tissue, the condition must not be considered benign. If it is inadequately managed, spread of the infection will eventually occur and lead to a rapid and extensive undermining of the skin similar to that seen in necrotizing fasciitis, with corresponding systemic toxicity.

A distinctive variant of gangrenous cellulitis was described and named by Meleney several decades ago.[3] It has been called *progressive bacterial synergistic gangrene, postoperative progressive gangrene, Meleney's gangrene*, and—if associated with burrowing necrotic tracts producing distant lesions—*Meleney's ulcer*. The process usually begins postoperatively, particularly after abdominal or thoracic surgery. Pain and erythema appear at the wound site or about the sutures 1 to 2 weeks after surgery. This slowly develops into a shaggy ulcer with a gangrenous center surrounded by an inner zone of purple discoloration, which in turn is surrounded by an outer zone of erythema. Without treatment, the course is one of relentless indolent extension, but without significant systemic toxicity. Satellite lesions may occur; they represent tracts of burrowing subcutaneous infection that surface to produce a gangrenous ulcer on the skin. Pathologically the process is usually limited to the upper third of the subcutaneous fat, but occasionally it extends down to fascia. The lesion was originally thought to be caused by a synergistic interaction between microaerophilic streptococci and *Staph. aureus*, but recently other microorganisms, including *Proteus* species and other gram-negative enteric bacilli, have been implicated.

MANAGEMENT

Drainage from the wound or site of local injury should be sent for immediate Gram stain and culture. The optimal method for obtaining anaerobic cultures is to use a needle and syringe to aseptically aspirate the crepitant area at a site removed from the wound. After aspiration, all air is carefully expressed, the needle removed, and a rubber cap placed on the tip of the syringe. Alternatively, the needle's tip may be inserted into a rubber stopper. If a swab is used, contact with normal flora should be avoided and a commercially available transport medium should be used. Blood cultures should also be obtained. Radiologic examination should be performed to assess the presence and extent of soft tissue gas.

Initial antimicrobial selection is guided by the Gram stain of the purulent drainage. If only large "boxcar-shaped" gram-positive bacilli are present, the causative microorganism is *Clostridium*, and moderate-to-high doses of parenteral penicillin G (10 to 20 million U/day in 6 to 8 divided doses) are indicated. If multiple organisms of differing morphology are present on the Gram stain then one may assume that the process is polymicrobial, and an empiric broad-spectrum antimicrobial regimen should be instituted. An aminoglycoside (gentamicin or tobramycin, 3 to 5 mg/kg per day in 3 divided doses) and clindamycin (1200 to 2400 mg/day in 3 or 4 divided doses), with or without penicillin G (10 to 20 million units/day in 6 to 8 divided doses), would be appropriate. In patients with impaired or changing renal function, a third-generation cephalosporin, such as cefotaxime or ceftazidime, can be used instead of an aminoglycoside. An alternate single agent is imipenem.

The major conditions to be differentiated from anaerobic cellulitis are necrotizing fasciitis and the myonecrotic syndromes.[10] Distinguishing between clostridial myonecrosis and anaerobic cellulitis is necessary to avoid unnecessary extensive debridement. The definitive differentiation occurs at the time of surgery, which is mandatory to establish the diagnosis. The involved soft tissue must be laid open widely, devitalized tissue debrided, suppurative foci drained, and all involved fascial planes opened. The deep fascia and muscle must be carefully examined; if they are healthy, no further surgery is necessary. Further debridement may be necessary, depending on the amount of devitalized tissue present. The management of Meleney's gangrene includes wide excision of the lesion plus antimicrobials dictated by the culture results.

NECROTIZING FASCIITIS

PATHOGENESIS

Necrotizing fasciitis is an uncommon but severe infection involving the subcutaneous tissue and the deep fascia. It spreads rapidly in the fascial cleft, sparing the overlying skin until the later stages. Extensive undermining of the skin is the hallmark of this infection. It may affect persons of all ages, but is more common in middle-aged and elderly adults. The infections may occur anywhere, but infections in the perineal region and in the extremities are most commonly reported.

The most common initiating injury leading to infection is minor trauma (about 80 percent of reported cases); operative wounds and decubitis ulcers account for most remaining cases. Presentation is usually acute or subacute, ranging from 3 to 14 days after the injury. In a minority of cases the onset is very sudden, proceeding in dramatic fashion from a tiny abrasion to septic shock, with massive subcutaneous necrosis, within 24 h. Most patients have underlying chronic illnesses.[11,12] Diabetes has been found in 20 to 50 percent of patients in most series, often with varying degrees of ketoacidosis; severe arteriosclerosis has been noted in another 20 to 33 percent. Cardiovascular or renal disease is present in 50 percent. Nutritional status is also an important consideration, with either marked obesity or marked wasting noted in the majority of cases. Other associated factors have been hepatic disease and metastatic carcinoma.

After the initial bacterial invasion the infection spreads rapidly along fascial planes and subcutaneous fat, with ischemic tissue facilitating spread of the necrotizing process. At an early stage, histologic examination of full-thickness skin biopsies reveals no abnormality. However, the subcutaneous fat and fascia show a contiguous nonspecific inflammatory reaction, with fibrinoid arteriolitis and thrombosis of vessels, and subsequent necrosis. If the condition is left untreated, the overlying skin becomes extensively necrotic because of thrombotic occlusion of the venules and arterioles supplying it.

It has been shown that traumatic surgical and vascular injuries generate areas of relative tissue anoxia, with the result that carbohydrate and protein metabolism proceed anaerobically, generating lactic acid. Buffer systems become depleted and acidosis develops, causing lysosomal disruption, which causes local autolysis and destruction. This environment provides an ideal milieu for anaerobic growth. Whether actual infection evolves is determined by several factors, including method and amount of inoculum, altered host defense mechanisms, and virulence of the bacteria.[13] Little is known about the method or amount of inoculum. Altered host defenses play an important role in propagation of the infection. High blood alcohol levels, steroids in high doses, and metabolic acidosis inhibit adherence of phagocytes. Patients with cirrhosis and metastatic carcinoma have poor phagocyte chemotaxis. The virulence of the bacteria is determined, to some extent, by their capabilities to produce various enzymes—e.g., hemolysins, fibrinolysin, hyaluronidase, and collagenase. Synergistic action of different bacterial species has also been postulated on the basis of evidence from clinical experience and from experimental infections in animals.[14] An example of this is the production of necrotic abdominal wall lesions in mice with fusobacteria and a streptococcus. Gas production in the soft tissues is through anaerobic metabolic pathways by anaerobes or facultative bacteria. It is commonly assumed that aerobic organisms assist the growth of anaerobes by using oxygen, diminishing redox potential, and supplying catalase. Local ischemia and reduced host defense mechanisms in the presence of virulent pathogens combine to produce a milieu that is responsible for the alarmingly rapid spread (see Fig. 106-2).

ETIOLOGY

Necrotizing fasciitis is most often a synergistic polymicrobial bacterial infection in which at least one anaerobic organism (usually a *Bacteroides, Peptostreptococcus,* or *Peptococcus* species) is isolated in combination with one or more facultative organisms (usually non–group A streptococci, *E. coli, Klebsiella* or *Proteus* species, or *Staph. aureus*).[15] The majority of cases have multiple organisms present, with an average of 3 to 4 isolates per patient. It is important to note that group A streptococcus alone may also cause necrotizing fasciitis; some authors distinguish acute streptococcal necrotizing fasciitis as a separate entity. *Vibrio vulnificus* has also been reported to cause a particularly virulent form of necrotizing fasciitis.

PRESENTATION

With necrotizing fasciitis, there is often a trivial injury followed by the onset of pain and swelling, after several hours or days, with chills and fever. There may be considerable pale erythema in the involved area; brown-to-bluish skin discoloration is not uncommon later in the course of the illness (Fig. 106-3 and Plate 41). If the condition is left to progress, frank cutaneous gangrene may be seen. Pain is gradually replaced by numbness or analgesia as a result of

FIGURE 106-2 The pathogenic process in necrotizing fasciitis.

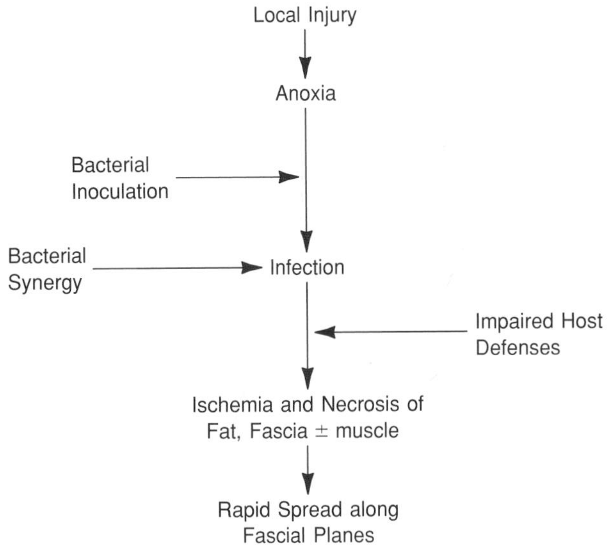

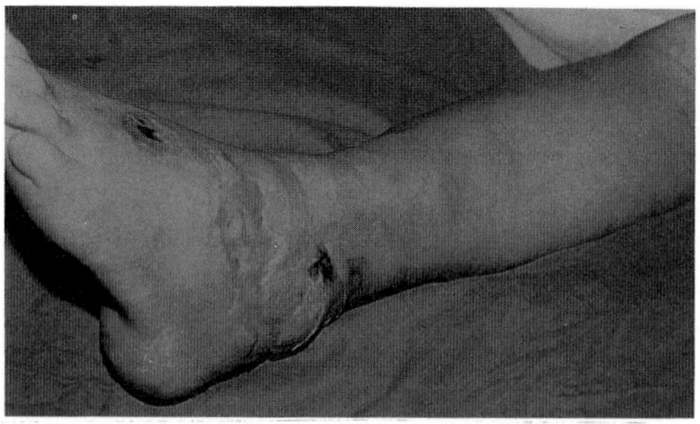

FIGURE 106-3 Necrotizing fasciitis of the lower leg. Dusky erythema is present with blistering and small patches of dermal gangrene. See Plate 41.

compression and destruction of cutaneous nerves. Hypoesthesia of the affected area may be a useful sign of the extensive undermining that occurs. Edema is present in most patients. Crepitation is not usual, but may be found in patients seen later in the course of the illness. Fluid-filled vesicles may appear in the area of erythema, often quickly followed by frank cutaneous gangrene. If an exudate is present it is described as serosanguineous and foul-smelling. Systemic toxicity with disorientation is often severe. Large extracellular fluid shifts, hypotension, shock, and jaundice may follow. Bacteremia has been reported in as many as one-third of patients.

A significant manifestation of necrotizing fasciitis is extensive undermining of the skin (Fig. 106-4 and Plate 42) associated with subcutaneous fat and deep fascial necrosis.[16] The undermining can be demonstrated by passing a sterile instrument along the plane just superficial to the deep fascia (see Fig. 106-5); the instrument cannot be passed with ordinary cellulitis.

FIGURE 106-4 Postoperative appearance of the lower leg illustrated in Fig. 106-3 (Plate 41). All necrotic subcutaneous tissue was excised. See Plate 42.

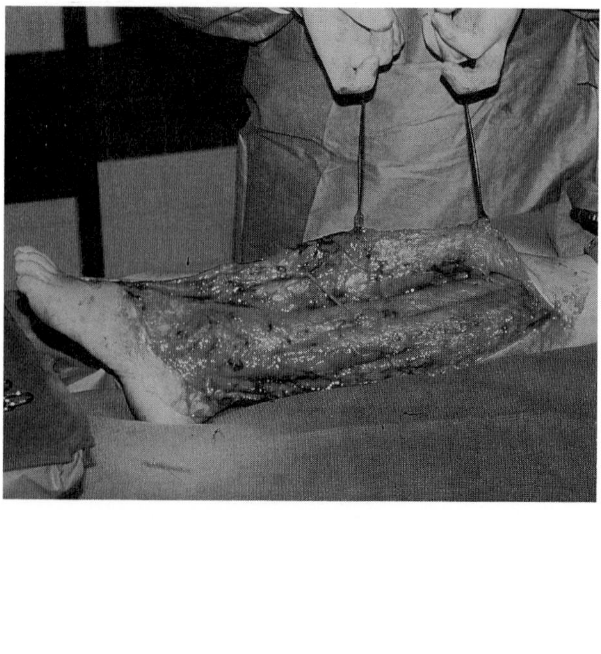

MANAGEMENT

Prior to institution of antimicrobial therapy, direct needle aspiration of the involved area for immediate Gram stain, and for aerobic and anaerobic cultures, should be obtained. Probing the lesion through an existing drainage site or through a small skin incision will reveal the characteristic undermining of skin seen in necrotizing fasciitis. The use of full-thickness skin biopsy with frozen section may aid the diagnosis.[17]

The principles of management include general supportive measures, antimicrobial administration, and definitive surgery. General measures include the placement of central venous and arterial monitoring catheters, administration of intravenous fluids to correct dehydration, maintenance of adequate oxygenation, treatment of any underlying diseases (e.g., correction of ketoacidosis or congestive heart failure), and attention to the patient's nutritional needs. Total parenteral or enteral nutrition is required in the postoperative state to meet the dramatically increased nitrogen requirements associated with tissue repair, hyperthermia, sepsis, and vital organ needs. Antibiotic selection should be guided by initial Gram stain. Coverage should be broad spectrum and include coverage for anaerobes, especially *B. fragilis.* An aminoglycoside (gentamicin, tobramycin), 3 to 5 mg/kg per day in 3 divided doses, plus clindamycin, 1200 to 2400 mg/day in 3 to 4 divided doses, is adequate initial therapy. If large gram-positive rods are noted, suggesting clostridia, penicillin G should be added (20 to 24 million U/day in divided doses). In penicillin-allergic patients, chloramphenicol and metronidazole are useful as alternate agents. In patients with impaired or rapidly changing renal function due to underlying disease or acute tubular necrosis, a third-generation cephalosporin, such as cefotaxime or ceftazidime, can be used in place of the aminoglycoside. An alternate single agent is imipenem. The mainstay of management is surgical exploration, debridement, and drainage, which should be done as soon as possible. Debridement and excision of all necrotic subcutaneous adipose tissue and fascia is required. The wound is packed open. Daily exploration under general anesthesia is indicated for truncal or perirectal infections and for all patients who remain in a toxic condition. Frequent dressing changes are performed after suitable analgesia, and are continued until healthy granulation tissue appears. Careful and regular reinspection of the wound is necessary, because initial debridement is seldom complete, and small foci of infection and necrotic tissue often lead to further progression. It must be emphasized that *conservative surgery leads to relapse of the process.* In the pelvic and upper thigh regions, a hip disarticulation or hemipelvectomy may be required.

Mortality is extremely variable, ranging from 4 to 74 percent. High APACHE (Acute Physiology and Chronic Health Evaluation) scores on admission, age greater than 50 years, diabetes, truncal disease, and failure of adequate initial debridement are associated with high mortality rates.[18]

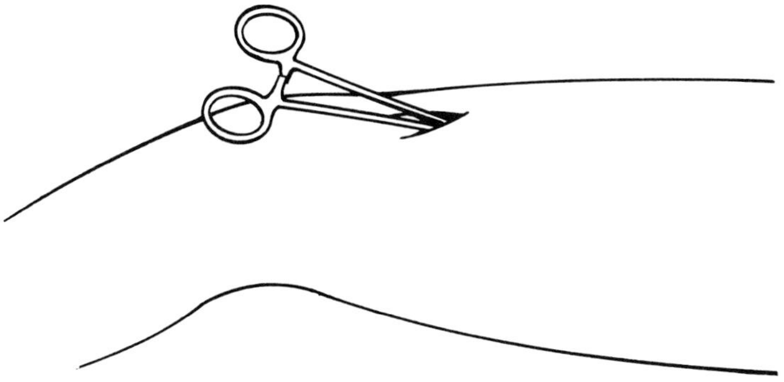

FIGURE 106-5 Necrotizing fasciitis with unopposed passage of a blunt instrument along the fascial cleft, indicating the characteristic undermining between the subcutaneous tissue and deep fascia.

MYONECROSIS

PATHOGENESIS

The bacterial myonecrotic syndromes all involve bacterial invasion of previously undamaged healthy muscle, resulting in its rapid destruction. The process often referred to as *gas gangrene* is a fulminant life-threatening infection that mandates early diagnosis and intervention. Bacterial myonecrotic syndromes may be of clostridial or nonclostridial origin. Both entities have a similar pathogenesis, clinical presentation, and management.[16] Clostridial myonecrosis occurs in the setting of muscle injury and concomitant soil or foreign body inoculation with clostridial spores. Although most commonly encountered in penetrating war wounds, it is seen now in the following settings: (1) trauma, especially motor vehicle or agricultural accidents involving open fractures; (2) the postoperative period, especially after bowel or biliary surgery; (3) malignancy, especially colorectal tumors; (4) arterial insufficiency in an extremity; (5) septic abortion; (6) occasionally in burn wounds; and (7) rarely, after intravascular or intramuscular injections. Although colonization of a traumatic wound by clostridia is common, the frequency of clostridial myonecrosis is only about 1 percent. In an animal model, the minimal dose of *Clostridium perfringens* required to produce a fatal infection is reduced by a factor of 10^6 when the organism is injected into devitalized, as opposed to normal, muscle. Clinically, however, clostridial myonecrosis does occasionally occur even in the absence of devitalized muscle. Once the clostridia begin to proliferate, several potent exotoxins are produced that have the capacity to destroy host tissue. At least 17 toxins are produced by *C. perfringens*, including alpha-toxin, a phospholipase that disrupts cell membranes and results in hemolysis, platelet destruction, widespread capillary damage, and myofibril destruction. Mu-toxin, a hyaluronidase, facilitates tissue spread and is thought to be responsible for the massive edema associated with this condition. As the process spreads, the involved muscle undergoes rapid destruction. Early pallor, edema, and loss of elasticity give way to a discolored, noncontractile muscle, which eventually becomes friable and disintegrates. The histologic findings are of coagulation necrosis.

Myonecrosis due to organisms other than clostridia has a pathogenesis not unlike that of necrotizing fasciitis. The infection is introduced via a break in the skin—through intravenous injection of illicit drugs, a surgical wound or enterostomy, a decubitis ulcer, or a fistula. Predisposing factors include diabetes mellitus, obesity, advanced age, renal disease, and local trauma; diabetes mellitus is reported most commonly. In drug addicts, infections of the extremities are more common, whereas perineal and buttock infections are more common in other populations. The synergism between the multiple microorganisms responsible for the myonecrosis likely facilitates the spread. Presumably the facultative bacteria assist the growth of anaerobes by using available oxygen and destroying tissue (reducing the redox potential), which in turn promotes a favorable milieu for the proliferation of anaerobic organisms. The process often involves muscle and fascia extensively, and may secondarily involve areas of subcutaneous tissue and skin. It should be noted that necrotizing fasciitis will ultimately involve muscle as well, if left to progress.

ETIOLOGY

C. perfringens is the most common cause of clostridial myonecrosis, producing 80 to 95 percent of cases (Fig. 106-6 and Plate 43). *C. novyi* and *C. septicum* are responsible for 5 to 20 percent with other species implicated rarely. Nonclostridial myonecrosis is usually polymicrobial, although group A streptococcus may be the sole causative agent. Most commonly, a mixture of facultative bacteria (*E. coli, Klebsiella* species, *Enterobacter* species, *Proteus* species, *Staph. aureus*) and anaerobic bacteria (*Bacteroides* species, *Peptostreptococcus* species, *Peptococcus* species) is found—an etiology similar to that seen in necrotizing fasciitis. *Aeromonas hydrophila* has also been described as causing severe myonecrosis after penetrating muscle injury in a fresh-water environment.

PRESENTATION

The incubation period of clostridial myonecrosis, from time of injury to appearance of symptoms, is usually 2 to 3 days, but may be as little as 6 h. Intense pain, out of proportion to the extent of injury, is characteristic. The pain rapidly progresses in intensity and distribution. Fever is not present until later in the course. Within hours there appear signs of

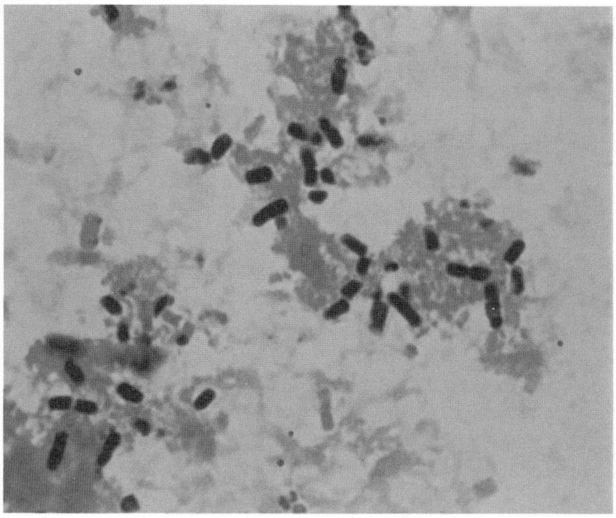

FIGURE 106-6 Gram stain of *Clostridium perfringens*. See Plate 43.

severe systemic toxicity—mental confusion, irritability, marked tachycardia, tachypnea, sweating, pallor, and hypotension. Delirium and stupor may supervene, although a period of intense mental alertness may occur prior to the onset of delirium. Renal failure, progressive hypotension and septic shock, intravascular hemolysis, and disseminated intravascular coagulopathy may ensue. Bacteremia occurs in only 10 to 15 percent of cases. Profound metabolic acidosis is common and can overwhelm compensatory hyperventilation, causing respiratory failure. Examination of the wound may initially show only tense edema and mild erythema. Later a spreading zone of woody edema appears, along with a characteristic bronzing of the skin. A thin, watery, brownish discharge with a sickly sweet odor may be present. Gas bubbles may be present in the discharge. Crepitus is usually present, but is not a prominent feature. Tense blebs containing a thin serosanguineous fluid develop in the overlying skin, and areas of cutaneous necrosis appear in later stages. If an open wound is present, edematous muscle may herniate through the wound to the skin surface.

In nonclostridial myonecrosis, the process has its onset over several days. The port of entry is usually evident in the vicinity of the area of involvement. Pain of moderate-to-severe intensity, and erythema, rather than edema, are more prominent. Progression is rapid, and systemic toxicity is severe; it may progress to shock and multisystem organ failure. Local crepitus may be present, as may a characteristic "dirty dishwater" discharge. Progression of the infection is rapid and may involve fascia and subcutaneous tissues.

MANAGEMENT

Early diagnosis is critical; its importance cannot be overemphasized. Confusion about the types of gas gangrene, failure to recognize that the infection does not have the usual signs of pyogenic inflammation, and failure to recognize that clostridial infections can develop without a history of recent trauma can all create diagnostic difficulties. The major considerations are other gas-forming infections of the soft tissues, including anaerobic cellulitis and necrotizing fasciitis. The severe toxemia, limited crepitus, tense edema, and characteristic bronzing of the skin are suggestive, but not definitive, evidence of clostridial myonecrosis. Similarly, areas of cutaneous necrosis in a severely ill patient with a "dirty dishwater" discharge suggest a nonclostridial myonecrosis. Adjunctive diagnostic tools include the Gram stain and radiography. A Gram stain of the discharge or of soft tissue aspirate in clostridial myonecrosis reveals large gram-positive bacilli with blunt ends, but few or no pus cells (which are destroyed by the clostridial lecithinase). A mixed flora is seen with nonclostridial myonecrosis. Precautions should be taken to ensure that anaerobic specimens are appropriately collected and promptly transported to the laboratory. A radiograph of the involved area may reveal gas that is not palpable and will also give an indication of the distribution of such gas.

The principles of management include general supportive measures, antimicrobials, and surgery. Surgical exploration is definitive and is mandated by the mere suspicion of either clostridial or nonclostridial myonecrosis. More important than the label placed on a given case is the need for urgent surgical intervention, which is the ultimate diagnostic and therapeutic maneuver. Bacterial myonecrosis is characterized by a darkened, "cooked" appearance of the muscle, which does not contract on stimulation and bleeds very little on incision. Excision of involved muscles—or amputation, if necessary—and decompressive fasciotomies are the mainstays of surgical treatment. Any necrotic fascia or subcutaneous tissue should be debrided. General supportive therapy includes insertion of appropriate monitoring lines, administration of isotonic crystalloid to maintain blood pressure, maintenance of adequate oxygenation, correction of severe acidosis, and maintenance of electrolyte balance. Blood should be given sparingly during the acute stages if evidence of extensive hemolysis is present. Nutritional support is necessary in these critically ill patients, especially in the postoperative period.

For clostridial myonecrosis the antimicrobial treatment of choice is high-dose penicillin G, 20 to 24 million U/day in 6 to 8 divided doses. The dosage must be appropriately reduced if significant degrees of renal failure are present. Chloramphenicol, 1 to 2 g/day in 4 divided doses, is a good alternate choice in the penicillin-allergic patient. In the presence of a mixed flora on Gram stain, the antimicrobial selection should include an aminoglycoside (gentamicin, tobramycin), 3 to 5 mg/kg per day in 3 divided doses, plus clindamycin, 1200 to 2400 mg/day in 3 to 4 divided doses. If clostridia are present on Gram stain then penicillin should also be added to the regimen, since some clostridia are resistant to clindamycin.[19] A third-generation cephalosporin, such as cefotaxime or ceftazidime, may be used in place of the aminoglycoside. Imipenem is a useful alternative as a single agent in nonclostridial myonecrosis.

Hyperbaric oxygen has been advocated as an adjunctive measure in patients with clostridial myonecrosis, but its role is still controversial.[20] Controlled trials have not been done and are unlikely to be done, because of the limited number of cases that might be seen at a given institution and ethical considerations in the randomization of critically ill patients. Evidence supporting the use of hyperbaric oxygen comes from animal experiments, case reports, and uncontrolled small series. Its role at present appears to be in the management of selected patients with extensive involvement in whom extensive surgical debridement would be so mutilating as to threaten life or limb.

CASE PRESENTATION

Mr. R.H., a 27-year-old previously healthy single man, was admitted to the hospital with a 2-day history of edema and pain in the right leg. Four weeks previously, in a motor vehicle accident, he had sustained a comminuted compound fracture of the midshaft of the right tibia and fibula, which had been managed by debridement, open reduction, and external fixation. The hospital course had been complicated by necrosis of a 3- by 5-cm area of skin over the fracture site, requiring debridement, muscle flap, and skin graft to cover the defect. The postdischarge course was uneventful until 48 h prior to admission, when the patient noted pain and edema in the right leg, maximal over the site of the skin graft. The pain and edema progressed to involve the entire leg; on the day of admission, a thin, seropurulent, malodorous discharge was noted along the inferior border of the skin graft site. Fever, rigors, and general malaise were also present.

Examination revealed a moderately ill–appearing young man with a temperature of 39.4°C, a respiratory rate of 16, a heart rate of 100, and a blood pressure of 170/80 mmHg. The patient was anxious but cooperative. The right leg was grossly edematous and tense, with a glistening appearance of the skin. The popliteal pulse was present, but the posterior tibial and dorsalis pedis pulse were not palpable, although they were audible by Doppler examination. The point of maximal tenderness was over the site of the graft. Motor and sensory exams of the right lower extremity were normal. Moderate pain was elicited on forced dorsiflexion. The remainder of the examination was unremarkable.

The hemoglobin concentration was 13.9 mg/dL, with a hematocrit of 41. The white blood cell count was 19,700 cells per mm^3. The levels of electrolytes, urea, and creatinine were within normal limits. The electrocardiogram and chest x-ray were unremarkable. Two views of the right tibia and fibula revealed the comminuted fracture of the tibia, with two screws present through the fracture site, marked soft tissue edema, and a small amount of gas in the soft tissues. A Gram stain of the purulent drainage revealed moderate numbers of white blood cells and a few gram-positive cocci. The patient was started on intravenous fluids; gentamicin, 120 mg every 8 h, and clindamycin, 600 mg every 6 h, was instituted. A presumptive diagnosis of necrotizing fasciitis was made. The patient was taken to the operating room for debridement and decompressive fasciotomy. The previously grafted muscle was necrotic and was excised. The deep fascia was edematous but not necrotic. Frank pus was encountered upon entering the posterior compartment. The distal portions of the muscles in all four leg compartments were found to be necrotic and were excised until bleeding viable muscle was encountered. Immediate Gram stain of the debrided tissue revealed small-to-moderate numbers of pus cells, moderate numbers of gram-positive cocci, and some large gram-positive bacilli. Penicillin G, 3 million U every 3 h, was added to the antimicrobial regimen. Tissue was sent for aerobic and anaerobic cultures. Over the next 24 h, although the patient remained afebrile, there were noted confusional episodes, marked diaphoresis, increasing hypotension (80 mmHg systolic), tachycardia (120 beats per min), and tachypnea (24 respirations per min). The right foot was noticeably cool, and the pedal pulses were no longer audible by Doppler examination. The lower thigh was now edematous and indurated. The patient was transferred to the intensive care unit (ICU). A right internal jugular central venous catheter was inserted, and revealed a central venous pressure of 2 cm H_2O. A right radial anterial line was inserted, and revealed a mean arterial pressure of 60 mmHg. A urinary catheter was inserted to monitor hourly urine output.

Laboratory findings at this time revealed a hemoglobin level of 11.0 mg/dL, and a white blood cell count of 39,000 cells per mm^3 with a marked left shift. The arterial blood gases on room air revealed a P_{O_2} of 78 mmHg (saturation 93%); P_{CO_2} of 32 mmHg; HCO_3 concentration of 13 meq/L; and pH of 7.22. The initial culture results revealed *Staph. aureus*, a hemolytic group C streptococcus, and an unidentified *Clostridium* species. A bolus of 1 L of normal saline solution increased the systolic blood pressure to 100 mmHg. Urine output was 80 to 100 mL/h. An emergency angiogram visualized the posterior tibial artery to the ankle, but the anterior tibial and pereoneal arteries were not visualized beyond the tibial fracture site.

Following hemodynamic stabilization, the patient was immediately returned to the operating room for further exploration. The proximal muscles in the posterior compartment were found to be necrotic, and a through-knee amputation was performed. Medial and lateral incisions extending up the thigh were made, and extensive necrotic fascia and adipose tissue were noted posterolaterally to the mid-thigh level. A small amount of necrotic subcutaneous tissue and fascia was found medially. The underlying muscle was normal. After extensive debridement the wounds were packed with bulky dressings.

Postoperatively the systolic blood pressure dropped to 60 mmHg and only partially responded to fluid replacement. A dopamine infusion was started at 5 μg/kg per min, to maintain a systolic blood pressure of 90 mmHg. Over the next 36 h the dopamine was weaned and the patient stabilized with a sustained systolic blood pressure of 110 mmHg. On the second ICU day the patient was returned to the operating room for inspection of the thigh wound; only minor debridement was required. The encephalopathy and metabolic acidosis settled, and the patient was transferred back to the ward after a 3-day ICU stay. Final tissue cultures revealed *Staph. aureus*, group G streptococci, and *Clostridium sordellii*. The gentamicin was discontinued.

CASE DISCUSSION

This case illustrates a typical presentation of a necrotizing soft tissue infection. The predisposing factor was the contaminated wound, which occurred at the time of the compound fracture. The incubation period was somewhat prolonged, but presumably there was a delayed germination of clostridial spores within the previously damaged muscle. A diagnosis of necrotizing fasciitis was entertained, but the findings were of a myonecrosis. Although all nonviable muscle was excised, a compartment syndrome caused vascular insufficiency, which likely caused further muscle ischemia, with further myonecrosis—which precipitated the deteriorating clinical course. Interestingly, a necrotizing fasciitis was also found at the time of the second operation.

The case illustrates the need for urgent surgical intervention to make a definitive diagnosis, and for constant monitoring for progression of the process after the initial surgery; it also illustrates the dramatic speed at which these virulent infections may progress. Although the outcome was fortunate in this case, it is easy to see how significant underlying medical problems and delayed surgical intervention would have produced a higher risk of mortality.

References

1. Baxter CR: Surgical management of soft tissue infections. Surg Clin North Am 52:1483, 1972.
2. Simmons RL, Ahrenholz DM: Infections of the skin and soft tissues, in Howard RJ, Simmons RL (eds): *Surgical Infectious Diseases*, 1st ed. New York, Appleton-Lange, 1982, p 507.
3. Meleney FL: Bacterial synergism in disease processes with confirmation of synergistic bacterial etiology of certain types of progressive gangrene of the abdominal wall. Ann Surg 94:961, 1931.
4. Rudoph R, Soloway M, DePalma RG, Persky L: Fournier's syndrome: Synergistic gangrene of the scrotum. Am J Surg 129:591, 1975.
5. Tacket CO, Brenner F, Blaker PA: Clinical features and an epidemiologic study of *Vibrio vulnificus* infections. J Infect Dis 149:558, 1984.
6. Newell PM, Norden CW: Value of needle aspiration in bacteriologic diagnosis of cellulitis in adults. J Clin Microbiol 26:401, 1988.
7. Kielhofner MA, Brown B, Dall L: Influence of underlying disease process on the utility of cellulitis needle aspirates. Arch Intern Med 148:2451, 1988.
8. Hook EW III, Hooton TM, Horton CA, et al: Microbiologic evaluation of cutaneous cellulitis in adults. Arch Intern Med 146:295, 1986.
9. George WL: Other infections of skin, soft tissue, and muscle, in Finegold SM, George WL (eds): *Anaerobic Infections in Humans*. San Diego, Academic Press, 1989, p 485.
10. Feingold DS: The diagnosis and treatment of gangrenous and crepitant cellulitis, in Remington JS, Swartz MN (eds): *Current Clinical Topics in Infectious Diseases*. New York, McGraw-Hill, 1981, p 259.
11. Rea WJ, Wyrick WJ: Necrotizing fasciitis. Ann Surg 172:957, 1970.
12. Gozal D, Ziser A, Shupak A, et al: Necrotizing fasciitis. Arch Surg 121:233, 1986.
13. Tehrani MA, Ledingham IMcA: Necrotizing fasciitis. Postgrad Med J 53:237, 1977.
14. Roberts DS: Synergic mechanisms in certain mixed infections (editorial). J Infect Dis 120:720, 1969.
15. Giuliano A, Lewis F Jr, Hadley K, Blaisdell FW: Bacteriology of necrotizing fasciitis. Am J Surg 134:52, 1977.
16. Ahrenholz DH: Necrotizing soft-tissue infections, in Howard RJ (ed): *The Surgical Clinics of North America*. Philadelphia, WB Saunders, 1988, p 199.
17. Stamenkovic I, Lew DP: Early recognition of potentially fatal necrotizing fasciitis. N Engl J Med 310:1689, 1984.
18. Pess ME, Howard RJ: Necrotizing fasciitis. Surg Gynecol Obstet 161:357, 1985.
19. Rosenblatt JE: Antimicrobial susceptibility testing of anaerobic bacteria. Rev Infect Dis 6:S242, 1984.
20. Finegold SM: Therapy and prognosis of anaerobic infections, in Finegold SM, George WL (eds): *Anaerobic Infections in Human Disease*. San Diego, Academic Press, 1989, p 793.

Chapter 107

URINARY TRACT INFECTIONS

GERARD J. SHEEHAN
GODFREY K.M. HARDING

KEY POINTS

- *All patients with severe urosepsis should have ultrasound examination of the kidneys [and consideration of other imaging procedures such as computed tomography (CT) scan], since suppurative complications such as pyonephrosis or intrarenal or perinephric abscess are common.*
- *In critically ill patients who are unstable because of complicated urosepsis, drainage is a priority.*
- *Both ureteric stents and percutaneous drainage can be used to definitively drain or temporarily stabilize a patient with suppurative complications.*
- *Empiric antimicrobial therapy for acute complicated urosepsis should include combination therapy such as ampicillin plus an aminoglycoside.*
- *Widespread use of urinary catheters leads to a high incidence of bacteriuria, about 5 percent per day. Fifty percent become infected by 10 days. Patients are also predisposed to candiduria.*
- *Asymptomatic bacteriuria should be treated in all patients prior to instrumentation to avoid the development of gram-negative bacteremia and subsequent sepsis.*
- *If a urinary catheter is inserted in a patient in the intensive care unit (ICU), its usefulness needs to be regularly reassessed.*
- *Treatment of bacteriuria without local signs of infection should be considered in patients with fever or sepsis only after a careful search for other potential sites of infection.*

Septicemia and septic shock can arise even from a first urinary tract infection (UTI) or following instrumentation of the urethra or bladder. Urinary tract infection is thus an important initiating event for ICU admission. In addition, because of the frequent need for urinary catheterization in critically ill patients, UTI is a common sequela of intensive care. Finally, bacteriuria acquired through catheterization comprises a reservoir of antimicrobial-resistant hospital pathogens.

Bacteriuria simply means the presence of bacteria in the urine. Significant bacteriuria implies the presence of 10^5 organisms or more per milliliter by a quantitative method. However, it has been demonstrated that a count of 10^2 aerobic gram-negative organisms or more per milliliter from a woman with pyuria and symptoms of lower UTI represents true infection.[1] Low-level bacteriuria (or candiduria) of any quantity in a hospitalized, catheterized patient rapidly advances to significant bacteriuria, provided the patient is not receiving antimicrobial agents to which the organism is susceptible.[2] Thus any level of bacteriuria in a catheterized ICU patient is worthy of consideration as a cause of sepsis.

Pyuria means the presence of white blood cells in urine. This is most commonly measured by determining the number of cells per microscopic high-power field in a centrifuged urine specimen. Using the commonly applied criterion of 5 cells per microscopic high-powered field, pyuria, when present, is a reliable indicator of UTI, especially when cells greatly exceed this number. However, the sensitivity is not high, and the absence of such pyuria does not reliably exclude UTI.

Acute Pyelonephritis

MICROBIOLOGY

The vast majority (90 percent) of community-acquired UTIs in females are due to *Escherichia coli. Staphylococcus saprophyticus* is the second commonest pathogen.[3] Other enterobacteria (e.g., *Proteus* spp., *Klebsiella* spp., *Enterobacter* spp.) are also encountered. In male patients *E. coli* is also the commonest community-acquired urinary pathogen, but other enterobacteria and *Enterococcus* spp. are more commonly encountered.

For both men and women the spectrum of pathogens changes in the hospital environment.[4] *E. coli* is still common, but a high frequency of *Pseudomonas* spp., *Enterococcus* spp., coagulase-negative staphylococci, and *Candida* spp. is encountered. The latter more resistant pathogens are especially prevalent in the catheterized patient who is receiving antimicrobial agents.

Persistent or relapsing bacteriuria due to *Proteus mirabilis* should prompt a search for a staghorn calculus. Isolation of *Staphylococcus aureus* in a urine culture is uncommon and should always raise the possibility of seeding of the urinary tract through the bloodstream. Such patients should be reviewed for evidence of intravascular cannula infections ("line sepsis"), endocarditis, osteomyelitis, and pneumonia. A cortical renal abscess (renal carbuncle) may be present.

PATHOGENESIS

E. coli causes most UTIs, and within this species only a few serotypes are usually implicated (01, 02, 04, 06, 07, 075). Patients with recurrent UTIs often have vaginal epithelial cells and periurethral cells to which *E. coli* adhere more readily as compared to control subjects who do not experience UTIs.[5,6] Furthermore a majority of *E. coli* producing UTI have several virulence factors.[7,8] These include P-fimbriae, hemolysin production, possession of certain O and K serotypes, increased amount of K antigen (capsular polysaccharide), resistance to serum bactericidal activity, and the capacity to cause hemagglutination which is D-mannose resistant. Thus certain strains are "selected out" of the fecal floral and are capable of causing UTI (uropathogenic *E. coli*). These various factors allow adhesion to periurethral cells, ascent of the ureters, and multiplication in the renal tissue despite normal host defenses. They are operative in patients who have infection of an anatomically normal urinary tract. In contrast *E. coli* causing infection of the urinary tract of patients with reflux nephropathy or obstruction are not uropathogenic.[8]

Urine itself will inhibit the growth of microorganisms. Anaerobes can only multiply in the urinary tract under very special circumstances where the oxygen tension is low such as in scar tissue, tumors, and necrotic tissue. High osmolarity, acid pH, and urea all inhibit bacterial growth. Glucose provides a better medium for multiplication of *E. coli.*

Tamm-Horsfall protein, secreted by the loop of Henle, contains mannose residues which bind to type 1 fimbriae on *E. coli* and aggregate the organism preventing uroepithelial attachment and ascent against the urinary flow.[9] The majority of *E. coli* contain type 1 fimbriae. Those that contain P-fimbriae instead have a selective advantage. Voiding of the bladder is the most important host defense mechanism. Similarly the flow of urine washes bacteria downward. Vesicoureteric reflux frustrates this defense and allows establishment of upper urinary tract infection. The medulla and papillae of the kidney are prone to infection because of hyperosmolality and low blood flow. During pyelonephritis an acute inflammatory exudate develops which limits infection but also contributes to scarring.

DIAGNOSIS

Acute pyelonephritis is a syndrome of fever along with evidence of renal inflammation such as costovertebral angle tenderness or flank pain. There are often signs of systemic toxicity and sometimes bacteremia. However, infection of the upper urinary tract may occur silently or with only subtle manifestations.[10] Silent pyelonephritis (also called subacute or occult pyelonephritis) is present in up to 30 to 50 percent of patients with clinical cystitis in primary care settings. Such subclinical pyelonephritis may produce minimal symptoms and smoulder on for long periods.

Patients requiring ICU admission will sometimes have been admitted to the ward with a classic history of acute pyelonephritis. Subsequent deterioration should prompt a search for urinary tract obstruction such as calculus or renal papillary necrosis, or for a suppurative focus in or around the kidney (intrarenal or perinephric abscess, vide infra). If therapy has relied on ampicillin alone, then resistance of the organism may explain the deterioration. Features which suggest obstruction include classic renal colic or severe costovertebral angle tenderness, a palpable kidney due to hydronephrosis, and lack of clinical response to antimicrobial therapy.

Gram's stain of a drop of unspun urine can provide rapid, specific information. It may show gram-negative bacilli, gram-positive cocci in clumps, gram-positive cocci in chains, large gram-positive yeasts, or, much less often, a polymicrobial pattern. It can be valuable for distinguishing the less common etiologies (*S. aureus, S. saprophyticus, Enterococcus faecalis, Candida* spp., and polymicrobial-anaerobic) from the aerobic gram-negative bacilli that comprise the vast majority of pathogens. When repeated after the initiation of therapy, the disappearance of bacteria gives some assurance that the antimicrobial agents are effective in vivo.[9]

A urine culture should always be obtained prior to therapy. It usually identifies the infecting organism(s) unless the patient has received prior antimicrobial agents or has complete obstruction or a perinephric abscess. Blood cultures should also always be obtained in the acutely septic patient since patients may have concomitant bacteremia with metastatic infection or the primary source of the organism may have been elsewhere with seeding to the kidneys.

ANTIMICROBIAL THERAPY

A number of regimens are appropriate as empiric therapy of acute pyelonephritis. These include an aminoglycoside combined with ampicillin, cefazolin, or trimethoprim-sulfamethoxazole. An aminoglycoside combined with a ureidopenicillin such as piperacillin may be preferred for hospital-acquired infection, where *P. aeruginosa* and *E. faecalis* are more likely to be encountered. Initial reliance on a single agent is unwise as the patient may succumb to overwhelming septic shock during the 48 h required for antimicrobial susceptibility results to become available. Approximately 30 percent of *E. coli* isolates from community-acquired infections are ampicillin resistant. Approximately 10 percent of such isolates are resistant to first-generation cephalosporins and trimethoprim-sulfamethoxazole, and less than 2 percent are resistant to aminoglycosides. The prevalence of resistance to a given agent will vary from community to community. Such rates are invariably higher for nosocomial isolates and in patients with a prior history of antimicrobial exposure. Approximately 40 percent of nosocomial aerobic gram-negative urinary isolates are resistant to first-generation cephalosporins.[11] Therefore, one should always be aware of the antimicrobial susceptibilities of isolates from one's own geographic location because this information enables one to select empiric therapy in a particular ICU or hospital more appropriately.

In patients with a higher risk of aminoglycoside toxicity such as those with prior renal impairment, liver dysfunction, advanced age, shock, or oliguria, consideration should be given to a third-generation cephalosporin such as cefotaxime, ceftriaxone, ceftizoxime, or ceftazidime; a monobactam such as aztreonam; a carbapenem such as imipenem in combination with cilastatin; a ureidopenicillin such as piperacillin, ticarcillin in combination with clavulanic acid, or a parental quinolone such as ciprofloxacin. All these agents and those mentioned previously achieve high levels in the urine, as glomerular filtration is their chief mode of excretion. Once the organism is isolated and identified, then the antimicrobial regimen should be promptly adjusted. Once systemic toxicity and fever have resolved, an oral regimen can be started. Agents which inhibit cell wall synthesis, such as the β-lactams, may be less effective.[12,13] The hypertonic renal medulla may allow residual bacteria to survive as L-forms (cell wall deficient protoplasts), despite the presence of these antimicrobial agents. Most often trimethoprim-sulfamethoxazole or a quinolone such as norfloxacin or ciprofloxacin are used as oral therapy. Lack of response manifested by hemodynamic instability or continued fever should prompt immediate investigation to discover obstruction or suppurative complications. Some patients may be admitted to the ICU in septic shock (see Chap. 98).

RADIOLOGIC INVESTIGATIONS

Ultrasound has displaced intravenous urography (IVU) as the initial investigation for patients with upper urinary tract infection and suspected obstruction. It has the advantage of being portable and can be carried out at the bedside obviating the need for transport of an unstable patient out of the ICU. It is inexpensive and safe in pregnancy. It will reliably diagnose most causes of obstruction and perinephric collections. The results, however, are dependent on the skill and persistence of the operator. Both IVU and nuclear medicine techniques will give an assessment of the excretory function of each kidney which is not available by ultrasound. CT scanning more accurately defines the anatomy of the renal parenchyma than ultrasound and gives a clear cross-sectional view of the surrounding anatomy. Complications of upper urinary tract infection such as cortical abscess, acute focal bacterial nephritis (AFBN), and perinephric abscess can be distinguished more readily by CT scan. Accurate placement of percutaneous drains into suppurative collections may require CT scanning to delineate all structures precisely.[14] Despite this, ultrasound is the investigation of choice for patients with pyelonephritis because of its lack of toxicity, ease of applicability, and low cost. An ultrasound and a plain radiograph of the kidneys, ureters, and bladder (KUB) will detect almost all correctable lesions.

CT scanning is indicated in a patient with an upper urinary tract infection with persistent sepsis in whom an ultrasound does not reveal an explanation. Further studies will be indicated in a minority of patients to more accurately delineate abnormalities detected by ultrasound. It may also be useful in selected patients where the ultrasound has revealed a suspected parenchymal suppurative lesion but has not distinguished AFBN from suppuration. The accuracy of the CT scan is enhanced by intravenous contrast material which can also reveal information about the excretory function of each kidney. Such contrast material can cause adverse reactions such as anaphylaxis and acute renal failure. Risk factors for the latter include dehydration, diabetes mellitus, prior renal impairment, and multiple myeloma.[15]

IVU has a limited role. It is effective at excluding obstruction. A totally obstructed kidney will be revealed by lack of excretion on the affected side, so little further information may be apparent about the cause of the obstruction or about debris or calculi within the hydronephrotic pelvicaliceal system. IVU is superior at demonstrating the collecting system and thus at confirming a diagnosis of papillary necrosis with characteristic medullary cavities and filling defects within the renal pelvis. Other unsuspected diagnoses may also be revealed by IVU such as tuberculosis, or renal scarring due to childhood reflux nephropathy.

Retrograde urography carried out in conjunction with cystoscopy will demonstrate the anatomy of the collecting system in a nonexcreting kidney. A variety of adverse effects can rarely result from the passage of the ureteral catheters or stents including hemorrhage, perforation, or septicemia. However, this procedure may permit relief of obstruction by passage of a stent or manipulation of a calculus. The accurate and safe passage of percutaneous nephrostomy tubes requires the prior demonstration of the anatomy of the collecting system. This can be done by ultrasound, IVU, or retrograde studies.

Radionuclide scanning has a limited role in the assessment of patients with UTI. While scanning for gallium citrate (^{67}Ga citrate) accumulation in areas of inflammation has seen the widest use, it has substantial limitations. Radiolabeled endogenous leukocytes reinjected into the patient offer advantages over gallium scanning. Technetium is now displacing the more difficult ^{111}Indium as the labeling agent. White blood cell scanning is more specific for infection, the result is available within 4 h, and interpretation is not obscured by normal excretion into the kidney and gastrointestinal tract. These investigations are particularly useful when the clinical findings are nonspecific in a patient with an undiagnosed fever or in establishing a diagnosis of cyst infection in a patient with polycystic kidneys.[16]

Cortical scintigraphy with technetium-^{99m} glucoheptonate (^{99m}TcGH) or ^{99m}Tc dimercaptosuccinic acid (^{99m}TcDMSA) yields images of the renal parenchyma related to perfusion. Patients with upper urinary tract infection may show focal defects that probably correspond to areas of AFBN that are detectable by CT scan. However, studies to correlate these investigations have not been done. Cortical scintigraphy may be useful in establishing whether the renal parenchyma is infected or not. Furthermore, obstruction of the tract can be diagnosed by the administration of furosemide and the use of delayed images.[17]

Acute Focal Bacterial Nephritis (Acute Focal Lobar Nephronia)

Human kidneys consist of from five to eleven lobes (usually eight) each of which contains a conical medullary pyramid whose apex converges into a renal papilla projecting into a calyx. Each pyramid is capped by cortical tissue to form a renal lobe and is separated from other lobes by a renal column containing the interlobar arteries and veins.[18] With the advent of CT scanning there has been increasing recognition of AFBN. This is analogous to lobar pneumonia as the abnormalities are limited to one or more renal lobes. Patients manifest the usual features of acute pyelonephritis but do not respond with defervescence within 48 h, prompting investigation for obstruction or suppurative focus. IVU is usually normal. Ultrasound may be normal or may reveal a solid, hypoechoic, poorly defined mass without evidence of liquefaction.

Noncontrast CT scanning, like ultrasound, is frequently normal. With intravenous contrast enhancement the nephrogram invariably reveals one or more wedge-shaped areas of decreased density. Such lesions may be demonstrated in a significant proportion of patients with acute pyelonephritis. The differential diagnosis of AFBN includes neoplasm, evolving renal infarct, and abscess. Demonstration of enhancing tissue within the mass on delayed CT images excludes cancer and abscess. AFBN resolves on antimicrobial therapy, but scarring and atrophy may result. Histopathology shows intense polymorphonuclear leukocyte infiltration without liquefaction, so neeedle aspiration or percutaneous drainage is not indicated. *E. coli* is the most common organism isolated from patients with AFBN.[9,19,20]

Renal Abscess

AFBN may progress to suppuration especially when associated with obstruction. The abscess may drain spontaneously into the calyxes,[21] or may rupture through the renal capsule to form a perinephric abscess. The usual pathogens are enterobacteria (*E. coli, K. pneumoniae,* and *Proteus* spp.). These organisms which arise by the ascending route are now commoner than cortical abscess arising from hematogenous spread. The latter was the commonest form of renal suppurative infection in the preantibiotic era and is usually due to *S. aureus*. In such patients there is frequently a preceding history of a cutaneous staphylococcal infection such as a furuncle.[22]

The clinical features of either form of renal abscess can be subtle. The patient often has chills and fever along with back or abdominal pain. Costovertebral angle tenderness, a flank mass, or involuntary guarding of the upper lumbar and paraspinal muscles may point to the diagnosis. Prominent abdominal features such as nausea, vomiting, and abdominal guarding may suggest another intraabdominal cause. Clinical features at other sites due to hematogenous dissemination of *S. aureus* may be found such as endocarditis, osteomyelitis, or lung abscess.

IVU is abnormal in the majority of patients but is nonspecific, with an intrarenal mass effect seen in only a minority of patients. Ultrasound usually demonstrates an ovoid mass of decreased attenuation within the parenchyma. This may initially mimic AFBN, a cyst, or a tumor. Dependent echoes changing with position represent shifting debris within the abscess cavity. Gas within the abscess can be recognized. Definitive characterization of fluid within the mass is done by demonstration of enhanced transmission of the beam through the mass and refraction of the beam at the fluid-solid interface. The presence of debris within a cyst or an abscess is a strong indication of infection. The diagnosis can be confirmed by gallium scan, white blood cell scan, or needle aspiration. Since hemorrhage within a cyst or necrotic debris within a tumor can occasionally mimic an abscess, confirmation by aspiration or nuclear medicine scanning is usually necessary. Alternatively, serial scanning until resolution while the patient is receiving antimicrobial therapy may suffice.[14]

Ultrasound can be technically inadequate because of obesity, overlying bowel gas, subcutaneous emphysema, wounds, or dressings. CT scanning shows a distinctly marginated low attenuation (0 to 20 Hounsfield units) mass that fails to enhance. Sharp demarcation is demonstrated between the mass and surrounding normal enhancing renal tissue. There may be a surrounding rim of increased enhancement (the ring sign). The CT scan is more sensitive than ultrasound for small lesions (<2 cm diameter) and for gas.[14]

The classic therapy of intrarenal abscess is incision and drainage with a nephrectomy if necessary for larger abscesses. It is now clear that a trial of intravenous antimicrobial therapy will succeed in the majority of patients once microbial etiology is established by urine, blood, or aspirate culture. This is especially true when the pathogen is *S. aureus*.[22] Close monitoring of the response, including disappearance of fever and leukocytosis and diminution of size as assessed by ultrasound or CT, is necessary. Percutaneous drainage using ultrasound or CT guidance is another alternative to surgery and should be tried as initial therapy when the abscess cavity is large.[23]

Emphysematous Pyelonephritis and Pyocystis

Gas within the urinary tract has three possible origins: **1.** atmospheric gas introduced during diagnostic procedures or during trauma, **2.** as a result of a fistula with a hollow organ, **3.** from multiplying, gas-producing organisms such as enterobacteria or anaerobes. Emphysematous pyelonephritis is a disease characterized by gas formation in the renal parenchyma and surrounding tissues. It is a fulminant disorder with a high mortality. The majority of patients have uncontrolled diabetes mellitus and obstruction of the urinary tract. *E. coli* and other enterobacteria account for the majority of pathogens with the rest being polymicrobial anaerobes. The pathology reveals extensive necrotizing pyelonephritis with abscess formation, papillary necrosis, intrarenal vascular thrombi, and even sloughing of the entire kidney. The differential diagnosis includes **1.** gas in a renal tumor, which can occur after embolization, and **2.** evolving traumatic renal infarct.[24]

The diagnosis is made radiologically. Plain radiographs may show diffuse mottling of the parenchyma as an early sign. More advanced cases show extensive bubbles in the parenchyma and a gas crescent surrounding the kidney within the perinephric space. Both ultrasound and CT are much more sensitive than plain films at detecting gas. CT identifies the gas clearly and unambiguously. Ultrasound identifies gas by the artifacts produced. These include an intense band of echoes distant to the gas and "dirty shadowing" distally with poorly defined margins and many echoes. This must be distinguished from the shadows associated with calculi which produces "clean shadows" with sharply defined margins.[14]

A review of the case reports in the literature prior to 1982 suggests that surgical intervention within 48 h combined with antimicrobial therapy is associated with improved outcome. Although relief of obstruction may be sufficient, nephrectomy is frequently necessary. The possible involvement of the contralateral kidney needs to be borne in mind. General supportive measures, including control of hyperglycemia, may also affect the outcome.[24]

Pyocystis (pus in the urinary bladder) with or without gas-forming organisms can present with features of sepsis, lower urinary tract signs, and pneumaturia. Patients with chronic oliguria on dialysis or those who have had diversion of urine away from the bladder (e.g., ileal conduit) are especially predisposed. Antimicrobial therapy and bladder irrigations may be sufficient therapy, but necrosis of the bladder wall as revealed by gas in the muscular layers on CT will require surgical resection.[25]

Perinephric Abscess

The perinephric space contains the kidney, the renal fat pad, and the adrenal gland. It is conical and open at the bottom allowing the ureters to exit.[18] Previously the perinephric space was depicted as a featureless, fat-filled region. However, it is now clear that bridging septa exist within it which act as lamellar barriers to the spread of infection or hematoma. Multiple loculations may arise causing difficulty with percutaneous drainage.[26]

Perinephric abscess generally arises from an intrarenal abscess. The majority are due to enterobacteria (*E. coli, K. pneumoniae, Proteus* spp.) and a minority to *S. aureus*. Polymicrobial mixed aerobic and anaerobic bacteria are also common. Documentation of a polymicrobial anaerobic cause should prompt a search for either a gastrointestinal tract source or ureteric obstruction. Perinephric abscess is usually confined by the renal fascia. Perforation is possible leading to anterior retroperitoneal space infection, peritoneal infection, posterior retroperitoneal infection, and retrofascial space infection. The latter may lead to a psoas abscess presenting in the groin.[27]

Perinephric abscess is an insidious disease that has a 50 percent mortality due to delay in diagnosis.[28] Most patients have fever and chills. Other features may include weight loss, nausea, vomiting, dysuria, flank pain, abdominal pain, pleuritic chest pain, and pain in the thigh or groin. Symptoms are usually of at least 2 weeks duration and often extend for months.[29] The patient may present for investigation of fever of unknown origin. Other patients are given an initial diagnosis of acute pyelonephritis. Flank mass or renal tenderness will be present in the majority of patients.

With the ready availability of ultrasound and CT the diagnosis is now made earlier. Ultrasound demonstrates fluid that may contain debris or gas. The CT shows loculated collections with decreased attenuation (0 to 20 Hounsfield units). The abscess wall may show increased attenuation after intravenous contrast material. Thickening of the renal fascia (Gerota's fascia) and unilateral enlargement of the kidney or psoas muscle may also be seen. The diagnosis can be confirmed by aspiration of the pus with a 20-gauge needle.[14]

Most patients can be treated by a combination of intravenous antimicrobial agents and percutaneous drainage. Even for those who require open surgical drainage there may be initial benefit from percutaneous drainage to allow for better preoperative stabilization.[29] A combination of clindamycin along with either an aminoglycoside or a third-generation cephalosporin is appropriate as initial empiric therapy if it is suspected that polymicrobial aerobic and anaerobic or *S. aureus* organisms are the cause of the abscess.

Pyonephrosis

Pyonephrosis arises when infection develops proximal to an obstruction of a hydronephrotic kidney. The underlying cause may be a calculus, stricture, neoplasm, or congenital anomaly. Unilateral loss of renal function is present along with infection of the renal parenchyma. Intrarenal or perinephric abscess may also be present. Clinical presentation is similar to perinephric abscess and may be insidious. Initial investigations should include a plain abdominal radiograph to look for calculi. Ultrasound will reveal a distended upper urinary tract. Specific features of pyonephrosis that allow distinction from simple hydronephrosis include sedimented echoes and dispersed internal echoes within the dilated collecting system. These findings are present in a minority of patients with pyonephrosis.[30] In a septic patient with hydronephrosis, either a gallium scan, white blood cell scan, or direct aspiration is indicated. CT is more sensitive for detecting radiolucent calculi and will also establish if there is accompanying infection in the tissues around the kidney. Once the diagnosis is made, a nephrostomy tube should be used to drain the infection. It will also allow subsequent contrast pyelography and stone removal.

Infected Cysts

Dependent debris can be demonstrated in a renal cyst by ultrasound or CT and suggests infection. Absence of such a finding, however, does not exclude a pyocyst. Aspiration of cyst fluid for Gram's stain and culture will establish the diagnosis. Assessment is much more problematic in polycystic renal disease. Pyocysts may arise from ascending infection or by hematogenous seeding. In the presence of uremia, systemic responses to infections such as fever and leukocytosis are often blunted. Infected cysts may manifest as persistent sepsis unresponsive to intravenous antimicrobial agents such as a combination of ampicillin and gentamicin. Delineation of the infected cyst as the cause usually requires white blood cell scanning. A positive result can allow attempted percutaneous drainage of the particular cyst. Alternatively, unilateral nephrectomy can be carried out with preservation of the uninfected kidney. A trial of antimicrobial therapy should first be carried out if the patient is stable. Lipophilic agents such as trimethoprim-sulfamethoxazole, chloramphenicol, or ciprofloxacin are more likely to succeed. Lipophobic agents such as β-lactams and aminoglycosides penetrate cysts poorly if at all.[31,32]

Urinary Tract Infection due to Candida

Candida species are normal gastrointestinal tract commensals of humans whose numbers are usually suppressed by the bacterial flora. They are gram-positive organisms encountered as ovoid unicellular forms. Special fungal media are unnecessary for their recovery as they grow readily on routine blood agar plates and in vented blood culture bottles.[33] Quantitative methods are commonly applied to *Candida* in urine cultures; 10^4 colony forming units per milliliter has been associated with renal infection and should be regarded as indicating at least infection of the bladder.

Disseminated candidiasis may originate in the urinary tract or secondarily seed it. Microabscesses form diffusely in the kidney and in other parenchymal organs. The skin, bones, spleen, eyes, liver, endocardium, myocardium, and central nervous system are typical sites of seeding, but the kidneys are almost universally affected. Renal failure may develop from bilateral parenchymal renal involvement. Neutropenia, loss of mucous membrane integrity due to chemotherapy, burns, steroid use, diabetes mellitus, total parental nutrition, and upper gastrointestinal tract surgery all predispose to invasive candidiasis. Overgrowth on superficial tissues such as skin, mucous membranes, and the gastrointestinal tract frequently precedes invasion and is often associated with prolonged broad-spectrum antibacterial therapy. Although there may be extensive tissue involvement, direct evidence of such deep *Candida* infection is frequently lacking. Blood cultures are positive in only half the cases.

Primary infection of the urinary tract is generally associated with prolonged placement of a urinary catheter along with broad-spectrum antibacterial systemic agents. Candiduria confined to the bladder is usually present for a variable period prior to renal infection.

Candiduria should be assumed to reflect renal infection if the patient has any of the predispositions to invasive candidiasis listed above, is receiving broad-spectrum antibacterial therapy, and continues to have features of sepsis such as fever or leukocytosis. Isolation of *Candida* from other sites such as respiratory secretions, wound exudate, or throat swabs should heighten suspicion of systemic candidiasis. A search should be made for specific features of disseminated candidiasis such as white "cotton wool" exudates in the retina, nodular skin lesions, bone lesions, and blood culture negative endocarditis. Unilateral or bilateral hydronephrosis should raise suspicion of a fungus ball. Microscopic examination of the urinary sediment may reveal *Candida* casts.[34] A careful evaluation of these clinical and laboratory data should allow selection of those patients who require early empiric amphotericin B therapy. Consideration should be given to such therapy in patients who have persistent fever despite broad-spectrum antimicrobial agents without another explanation.

Renal or disseminated infection requires systemic amphotericin B therapy in a dose of 0.6 mg/(kg · day) with its attendant toxicities.[35] Amphotericin B is usually continued until an accumulated dose of 1 gm is achieved. Fluconazole and 5-fluorocytosine are alternative, less reliable therapies. Ketoconazole is not acceptable as it is not appreciably excreted through the kidney. Hydronephrosis caused by a fungus ball should be relieved by percutaneous nephrostomy tubes. Irrigation of the ureter with an amphotericin B solution is effective in some cases. Lack of response radiologically should prompt surgical excision.[36]

A more commonly encountered situation is that of the stable ICU patient who has persistent candiduria. For such a patient amphotericin B bladder irrigation (50 mg of amphotericin B in 1000 mL of sterile water administered over 24 h by a three-way catheter) for 5 days should be considered.[37] This will cure candiduria confined to the bladder. Daily urine cultures should be done immediately upon stopping. Immediate relapse of candiduria is indirect evidence for renal infection and should prompt initiation of systemic amphotericin B therapy and investigations for a fungus ball.

Prostatic Infections

The prostatic infection syndromes which most likely result in a patient being admitted to the ICU are acute bacterial prostatitis and chronic bacterial prostatitis which has been surgically manipulated or instrumented with resultant bacteremia.[38] Acute bacterial prostatitis may present with the sudden onset of high fever up to 40°C, chills and malaise which are soon followed by irritative symptoms such as urgency, frequency, and dysuria. These may be associated with difficulty voiding or acute retention of urine. Usually there is a dull, aching pain in the perineum, rectum, or sacrococcygeal region. Rectal examination reveals a very tender, swollen, and warm prostate.

Since there is usually a concomitant bladder infection with the identical pathogen, the offending organism can be isolated from a culture of urine. Prostatic massage for culture should be avoided because it may be very painful and may induce bacteremia in patients with acute bacterial prostatitis. Gram-negative enteric organisms are now the most frequent pathogens. *Enterococcus fecalis* may also be responsible.

The regimen used for the treatment of acute pyelonephritis can also be used for the treatment of acute bacterial prostatitis. Because of the intense inflammatory response in acute bacterial prostatitis, most antimicrobial agents cross the prostatic epithelium effectively. Only a few antimicrobial agents such as trimethoprim and the newer quinolones, such as norfloxacin and ciprofloxacin, cross the uninflamed prostatic epithelium well. Therefore, patients should be initially treated with a regimen such as ampicillin and an aminoglycoside.

Because of the severity of the acute inflammation, after collection of the appropriate urine and blood specimens for culture, the parenteral antimicrobial regimen should be started. If the patient responds appropriately, the parenteral antimicrobial therapy can be continued for 7 days. Since very rarely a patient with acute prostatitis may develop chronic infection, it may be prudent to continue with an oral antimicrobial agent such as trimethoprim-sulfamethoxazole, norfloxacin, or ciprofloxacin for a further 5 weeks to eradicate all the organisms from the prostate.

When a patient with acute bacterial prostatitis or a UTI develops a spiking fever in spite of adequate antimicrobial treatment and fluctuation of the prostate is present on rectal examination, a prostatic abscess should be suspected. If not appropriately treated, prostatic abscesses may rupture into the rectum, urethra, or perineum. Transrectal ultrasonography and CT are very helpful in the preoperative diagnosis of prostatic abscess.[39] As with an abscess anywhere in the body, the definitive therapy of an acute prostatic abscess includes surgical drainage in addition to antimicrobial therapy. This can be adjusted according to the results of aerobic and anaerobic culture of abscess contents. Transurethral resection of the prostate with unroofing or perineal aspiration of pus guided by transrectal ultrasonography usually provide adequate drainage.[39]

Catheter-Associated Bacteriuria

Prior to the 1960s urinary catheters had "open" drainage systems, with a significant bacteriuria prevalence of 100 percent within 4 days of continuous use. The principal route of acquisition was intraluminal. The widespread introduction of closed urinary drainage systems has significantly reduced these high rates. The prevalence of catheter-associated bacteriuria is time dependent. One percent of patients will acquire bacteriuria from single "in-out" catheterizations.[40] The per day risk of developing bacteriuria is about 5 percent; thus about 40 percent of patients catheterized for 10 days will have acquired significant bacteriuria.[41]

Factors associated with a higher prevalence of catheter-associated bacteriuria include increasing age and female sex.[42] Systemic antimicrobial agents protect against catheter-associated bacteriuria during the first 5 days of catheterization.[42] Subsequently, however, organisms manifesting extensive antimicrobial resistance become prevalent such as enterococci, coagulase-negative staphylococci, *Candida* spp., and *Pseudomonas* spp. Ascent of bacteria to the bladder occurs predominantly outside the lumen when a closed drainage system is used. The space between the catheter and the urethral mucous membrane is filled by a variable amount of fluid, mucus, and inflammatory exudate. This is static and lacks inhibitory factors against bacterial proliferation. A progressive multiplication of organisms originating from the meatus occurs which accounts for the time-dependent acquisition and for the higher rates associated with the female urethra.[43]

In 15 to 20 percent of patients the organism originates from the collecting bag and ascends intraluminally. Contamination of the collecting bag occurs in association with disconnections of the distal catheter or during emptying of the bag near the drainage port. Organisms have been carried on the hands of personnel or in the collecting urinal from one source patient to the collecting bags of others.[44] Thus, intraluminal spread is the mechanism associated with most epidemics of catheter-associated bacteriuria.[45]

Catheterization of the bladder is unavoidable in most patients in the ICU. Indications include the monitoring of urine output in patients with shock, hemodynamic instability, or polyuric renal failure and the relief of lower urinary tract obstruction. Less justifiable is its routine use to avoid incontinence and contamination of the perineal skin in the stable patient. The difficulty of maintaining continence is compounded by the high prevalence of disturbed consciousness and the frequent need for sedation. Nevertheless, the almost universal use of urinary catheters in most ICUs can be reduced by early withdrawal of catheters in selected patients. These include alert and stable patients who can maintain continence, patients with anuric renal failure for whom once-a-day catheterization will suffice, and male patients with an intact voiding mechanism who can be managed with condom drainage. Intermittent catheterization can be utilized in stable patients with neurogenic bladders and in some patients with disturbed consciousness.[46] The necessity for the catheter should be frequently questioned and a trial of removal attempted when feasible. Once in place there is no need for regular scheduled replacements of the catheter, which can be left indefinitely provided it is functioning well and there are no encrustations.[47]

Bacteremia arises uncommonly in any given patient with catheter-associated bacteriuria.[48] However, such episodes collectively account for 30 to 40 percent of all cases of hospital-acquired bacteremia. They frequently are associated with manipulation or instrumentation including passage of a new urinary catheter. Therefore, all patients with bacteriuria with or without pyuria should have their bacteriuria treated prior to instrumentation of the urinary tract.

In the ICU, where hospital-acquired bacteriuria is commonly identified early because of routine surveillance, single-dose therapy with an agent such as trimethoprim-sulfamethoxazole, an aminoglycoside, a third-generation cephalosporin, extended spectrum penicillin, or quinolone to which the organism is susceptible may be appropriate in selected female patients provided that the urinary catheter has been removed and there is no clinical suspicion of sepsis[49]. This approach is only appropriate when the infection is confined to the lower urinary tract. Infection suspected or proven to be in the upper urinary tract such as clinical pyelonephritis, relapse of bacteriuria after short-course therapy, bacteriuria detected in a patient with structural renal disease, or bacteriuria detected in urine directly from the ureters or renal pelvis requires 2 weeks of therapy. Relapse of such infection requires 6 weeks of therapy.[12,50]

CASE PRESENTATION

A 26-year-old female was admitted to a medical ward because of 24 h of fever and right costovertebral angle tenderness. There was a preceding history of intermittent dysuria and frequency for 7 days.

Past history revealed recurrent UTIs in childhood. Physical examination revealed a tender right kidney and a temperature of 39°C. Urinalysis showed 100 white blood cells per microscopic high-powered field. She received intravenous ampicillin 1 g intravenously every 6 h. Thirty-six hours later she had a fever of 40°C with rigors, respiratory rate of 45 per minute, sinus tachycardia of 140 beats per minute, systolic blood pressure of 70 mmHg by palpation, and was peripherally vasoconstricted. She was confused and exquisitely tender on percussion over the right costovertebral angle. Arterial blood gases revealed hypoxemia and metabolic acidosis (pH 7.25, P_{CO_2} 29, P_{O_2} 55 on 5 L O_2 per minute by nasal prongs). She was intubated and transferred to the ICU where she required 12 L of crystalloid over the next 24 h along with 5 mcg/(kg · min) dopamine to maintain hemodynamic stability.

Urine cultures taken at admission grew 10^5 *E. coli* organisms per milliliter which were resistant to ampicillin but susceptible to cefazolin, trimethoprim-sulfamethoxazole, and gentamicin. Two blood cultures taken at admission also grew the same *E. coli* in both vials. Ampicillin was discontinued, and she was started on cefazolin 1 g every 8 h and gentamicin 80 mg every 8 h intravenously. Ultrasound of the abdomen showed a hydronephrotic right kidney. Gram stain of a percutaneous aspirate showed 4+ pus cells and 3+ gram-negative bacilli. Immediate nephrectomy was considered but rejected because of her unstable hemodynamics and a coagulopathy. Cystoscopic retrograde pyelography revealed a ureteric stricture. A ureteric stent was passed through the stricture and drained frank pus.

She then became hemodynamically stable and afebrile. On the fourth day of ICU admission fever returned. CT scan with contrast enhancement showed that the hydronephrosis had subsided. The renal parenchyma was atrophic and shrunken. A parenchymal ovoid nonenhancing lesion 4 cm in diameter of low intensity was also demonstrated. This contained debris and had the appearance of an abscess. Fluid was also demonstrated in the perinephric space. Both of these collections were aspirated and showed 3+ pus cells and 3+ gram-negative bacilli on Gram stain. Using a modified Seldinger technique, size eight pig-tail catheters were inserted into the parenchymal abscess and the perinephric space. The patient subsequently became afebrile. She was discharged from the ICU and completed a 14-day course of oral trimethoprim-sulfamethoxazole 160/800 mg twice a day. Bacteriuria due to *E. coli* with the same antibiogram was detected 5 days after stopping this therapy. The ureteral stent remained in place. An IVU showed no function on the right side and normal excretion and anatomy on the left. The absent function was confirmed by a renal scan with ^{99m}TcDMSA which demonstrated no excretion on the right side. An elective nephrectomy was done. Pathologic examination showed that the perinephric and parenchymal abscesses had resolved. The kidney was contracted and severely scarred. The parenchyma was thinned and contained microabscesses. The tissue contained patchy infiltrates of polymorphonuclear leukocytes with dense infiltrates of lymphocytes and plasma cells.

CASE DISCUSSION

This patient's course illustrates some significant points about urinary tract infection in the ICU. Only a small minority of patients with pyelonephritis are likely to progress to renal suppuration and septic shock.

1. It is the patient with a history of recurrent infections in childhood that is more likely to have chronic renal scarring related to childhood reflux nephropathy or another lesion such as a ureteric stricture.
2. A significant proportion of *E. coli* isolates even from the community may be ampicillin resistant (approximately 30 percent in some studies); therefore, broader empiric antimicrobial coverage while awaiting the results of cultures and sensitivities is needed. Had she received gentamicin, she might not have developed septic shock.
3. Ultrasound is a reliable means of detecting obstruction in these patients and can be applied in the ICU setting without the necessity of transporting an unstable patient. All patients with urinary tract infection requiring ICU support should have this investigation early in their course.
4. Both ureteric stents and percutaneous drainage can be used to either definitively drain or temporarily stabilize a patient with suppurative complications.
5. A "test of cure" culture is indicated after antimicrobial therapy of acute pyelonephritis. Relapse in this patient indicated continued infection of the affected kidney. This could have been dealt with by a longer course (6 weeks) of antimicrobial therapy or by indefinite suppression preferably with a non-cell-wall active agent. Absent function demonstrated by IVU and renal scan meant that there was little to be gained by this.

This case is not typical of most patients with pyelonephritis but is illustrative of many of the issues that become important for the minority who deteriorate to the point of requiring ICU admission.

References

1. Stamm WE, Counts GW, Running KR, et al.: Diagnosis of coliform infection in acutely dysuric women. N Engl J Med 307:463, 1982.
2. Stark RP, Maki DG: Bacteriuria in the catheterized patient. N Engl J Med 311:560, 1984.
3. Latham RH, Running K, Stamm WE: Urinary tract infections in young adult women caused by *Staphylococcus saprophyticus*. JAMA 250:3063, 1983.
4. Turck M. Stamm W: Nosocomial infection of the urinary tract. Am J Med 70:651, 1981.
5. Schaeffer AJ, Jones JM, Dunn JK: Association of in vitro *Escherichia coli* adherence to vaginal and buccal epithelial cells with susceptibility of women to recurrent urinary-tract infections. N Engl J Med 304(18):1062, 1981.
6. Kozody NL, Harding GKM, Nicolle LE, et al.: Adherence of *Escherichia coli* to epithelial cells in the pathogenesis of urinary tract infection. Clin Invest Med 8(2):121, 1985.

7. Stamm WE, Hooton TM, Johnson JR, et al.: Urinary tract infections: From pathogenesis to treatment. J Infect Dis 159(3):400, 1989.
8. Lomberg H, Hellstrom M. Jodal U, et al.: Virulence-associated traits in *Escherichia coli* causing first and recurrent episodes of urinary tract infection in children with or without vesicoureteral reflux. J Infect Dis 150(4):561, 1984.
9. Sobel JD: Pathogenesis of urinary tract infections. Infect Dis Clinics North Am 1(4):751, 1987.
10. Komaroff AL: Acute dysuria in women. N Engl J Med 310:368, 1984.
11. Platt R: Diagnosis and empiric therapy of urinary tract infection in the seriously ill patient. Rev Infect Dis 5:S65, 1983.
12. Stamm WE, McKevitt M, Counts GW: Acute renal infection in women: Treatment with trimethoprim-sulfamethoxazole or ampicillin for two or six weeks. Ann Intern Med 106:341, 1987.
13. Preiksaitis JK, Thompson L, Harding GKM, et al.: A comparison of the efficacy of nalidixic acid and cephalexin in bacteriuric women and their effect on fecal and periurethral carriage of Enterobacteriaceae. J Infect Dis 143:603, 1981.
14. Piccirillo M, Rigsby C. Rosenfield AT: Contemporary imaging of renal inflammatory disease. Infect Dis Clin North Am 4:927, 1987.
15. Parfrey PS, Griffiths SM, Barrett JB, et al.: Contrast material—induced renal failure in patients with diabetes mellitus, renal insufficiency or both. A prospective controlled study. N Engl J Med 320:143, 1989.
16. Bretan PN, Price DC, McClure RD; Localization of abscess in adult polycystic kidney by indium-111 leukocyte scan. Urology 32:169, 1988.
17. Conway JJ: The role of scintigraphy in urinary tract infection. Semin Nucl Med 18:308, 1988.
18. Williams PL, Warwick R, Dyson M, Bannister LH (eds.): The urogenital system, in *Gray's Anatomy*, 37th ed, Churchill Livingstone, Norwich, England, 1989, p 1396.
19. Meyrier A, Condamin MC, Fernet M, et al.: Frequency of development of early cortical scarring in acute primary pyelonephritis. Kidney Int 35:696, 1989.
20. Soulen MC, Fishman EK, Goldman SM, et al.: Bacterial renal infection: Role of CT. Radiology 171:703, 1989.
21. Soulen MC, Fishman EK, Goldman SM: Sequelae of acute renal infections: CT evaluation. Radiology 173:423, 1989.
22. Patterson JE, Andriole VT: Renal and perirenal abscesses. Infect Dis Clin North Am 4:927, 1987.
23. Sacks D, Banner MP, Meranze SG, et al.: Renal and related retroperitoneal abscesses: Percutaneous drainage. Radiology 167:447, 1988.
24. Michaeli J, Mogle P. Perlberg S, et al.: Emphysematous pyelonephritis. J Urol 131:203, 1984.
25. Lees JA, Falk RM, Stone WJ, et al.: Pyocystis, pyonephrosis and perinephric abscess in end stage renal disease. J Urol 134:716, 1985.
26. Kunin M: Bridging septa of the perinephric space: Anatomic, pathologic, and diagnostic considerations. Radiology 158:361, 1986.
27. Heseltine PNR, Appleman MD: Retroperitoneal infections, in Finegold SM, George WL (eds): *Anaerobic Infections in Humans*. Academic Press, San Diego, 1989, p 385.
28. Thorley JD, Jones SR, Sanford JP: Perinephric abscess. Medicine (Baltimore) 53:441, 1974.
29. Sheinfeld J, Erturk E. Spataro RF, et al.: Perinephric abscess: Current concepts. J Urol 137:191, 1987.
30. Vehmas T, Paivansalo M, Taavitsainen M, et al.: Ultrasound in renal pyogenic infection. Acta Radiol 29:675, 1988.
31. Schwab SJ, Bander SJ, Klahr S: Renal infection in autosomal dominant polycystic kidney disease. Am J Med 82:714, 1987.
32. Sklar AH, Caruana RJ, Lammers JE, et al.: Renal infections in autosomal dominant polycystic kidney disease. Am J Kidney Dis 10:81, 1987.
33. Crislip MA, Edwards JE: Candidiasis. Infect Dis Clin North Am 3:103, 1989.
34. Gregory MC, Schumann GB, Schumann JL, et al.: The clinical significance of candidal casts. Am J Kidney Dis 4:179, 1984.
35. Fisher MA, Talbot GH, Maislin G, et al.: Risk factors for amphotericin B-associated nephrotoxity. Am J Med 87:547, 1989.
36. Leiter E, Whitehead ED, Desai SB: Fungus balls in renal pelvis. NY State J Med, 82:64, 1982.
37. Wise GJ, Wainstein S, Goldberg P, et al.: Candidal cystitis. J Urol 116:718, 1976.
38. Meares EM: Acute and chronic prostatitis: Diagnosis and treatment. Infect Dis Clin North Am 1(4):855, 1987.
39. Weinberger M, Cytron S, Servadio C, et al.: Prostatic abscess in the antibiotic era. Rev Infect Dis 10(2):239, 1988.
40. Kass EH: Asymptomatic infections of the urinary tract. Trans Assoc Am Physicians 69:56, 1956.
41. Warren JW, Platt R, Thomas RJ, et al.: Antibiotic irrigation and catheter-associated urinary-tract infections. N Engl J Med 299(11):570, 1978.
42. Garibaldi RA, Burke JP, Dickman ML, et al.: Factors predisposing to bacteriuria during indwelling urethral catheterization. N Engl J Med 291:215, 1974.
43. Garibaldi RA, Burke JP, Britt MR, et al.: Meatal colonization and catheter-associated bacteriuria. N Engl J Med 303(6):316, 1980.
44. Marrie TJ, Major H, Gurwith M, et al.: Prolonged outbreak of nosocomial urinary tract infection with a single strain of *Pseudomonas aeruginosa*. Can Med Assoc J 119:593, 1978.
45. Stamm WE: Nosocomial urinary tract infections, in Bennett JV, Brachman PS (eds): Hospital Infections, 2d ed, Little, Brown, Boston, 1986, p 375.
46. Guttmann L, Frankel H: The value of intermittent catheterization in the early management of traumatic paraplegic and tetraplegia. Paraplegia 4:63, 1966.
47. Kunin CM: Care of the urinary catheter, in Kunin CM (ed): *Detection, Prevention and Management of Urinary Tract Infections*, 3d ed. Lea and Febiger, Philadelphia, 1987, p 153.
48. Krieger JN, Kaiser DL: Urinary tract etiology of bloodstream infections in hospitalized patients. J Infect Dis 148(1):57, 1983.
49. Harding GKM, Nicolle LE, Ronald AR, et al. How long should catheter-acquired urinary tract infection in women be treated? Ann Intern Med. 114:713, 1991.
50. Ronald AR: Optimal duration of treatment for kidney infection. Ann Intern Med 106:467, 1987.

Chapter 108

GASTROINTESTINAL INFECTIONS

THOMAS BUTLER

KEY POINTS

- *Intestinal infections usually present as diarrhea, with or without fever, and with dehydration as a major clinical feature. However, some infections present as ileus, abdominal distention, acute abdomen, or generalized peritonitis.*
- *The stool should be examined for fecal leukocytes: positive leukocytes denote an inflammatory, invasive pathogenesis, while negative leukocytes denote noninflammatory or toxigenic etiologies.*
- *Culture of the stool for enteric pathogens and microscopic examination for parasites are useful diagnostic procedures for community-acquired infections but should be omitted for hospital-acquired infections.*
- *Colonoscopy is a useful diagnostic procedure in some patients with bloody diarrhea and suspected colitis.*
- *The wide use of antibiotic therapy in critically ill patients predisposes them to pseudomembranous colitis. Testing the stool for toxin of* Clostridium difficile *is helpful.*
- *Therapy for intestinal infections includes rehydration with isotonic fluids and appropriate antimicrobial therapy for identified or suspected pathogens.*
- *Empiric antimicrobial therapy for diarrheal pathogens is advised only in septic patients or in patients strongly suspected of having enteric fever. In patients with evidence of an acute surgical abdomen, empiric therapy should also include coverage for enteric facultatively aerobic gram-negative organisms and anaerobes, including* Bacteroides fragilis.
- *Surgical intervention is required when intestinal perforation or gangrene is suspected and when purulent material from an abscess or peritonitis needs to be removed and cultured for bacterial pathogens.*

Clinical Approach to Intestinal Infections in Critical Care

Intestinal infections can result in the need for intensive care management when severe diarrhea leads to intravascular volume depletion and shock or when invasive bacterial infection leads to sepsis with cardiorespiratory instability. Regardless of diagnosis, the first priority in the patient with an intestinal infection with one of these complications is resuscitation and cardiorespiratory stabilization (see Chaps. 47 and 114).

The next priority is detection of serious septic complications of the intestinal infection and consideration of major alternative diagnoses. Seriously ill patients with diarrhea should have an abdominal x-ray (flat and upright) to detect ileus, megacolon, peritoneal fluid, and free peritoneal air. In patients with suspected focal infections or abscess, ultrasonography and computerized tomographic (CT) examination are useful. In some patients with inflammatory diarrhea or suspected colitis, colonoscopy and biopsy will be revealing. If intestinal ischemia is suspected, mesenteric angiography may be necessary. All patients with abdominal findings suggestive of any of these entities should be assessed by a general surgeon early in the hospital course.

At this stage, the need for early empiric antimicrobial therapy should be considered. For diarrheal syndromes complicated by volume depletion alone, antimicrobial therapy is generally not indicated until a specific diagnosis is established. However, in patients with clinical evidence of sepsis or with suspected peritonitis, abscess, intestinal perforation, or gangrene, intravenous antimicrobial therapy directed at enteric gram-negative bacilli and anaerobes, including *Bacteroides fragilis,* should be initiated.

The diagnostic approach to the patient with community-acquired diarrhea begins with microscopic examination of the stool. This examination, often called the *fecal leukocyte test,* should be performed with a portion of liquid stool that preferably contains mucus or blood. A drop of stool is placed on a slide, mixed thoroughly with two drops of methylene blue, and covered with a coverslip. The presence of abundant polymorphonuclear leukocytes should help diagnose inflammatory diseases, such as dysentery and antibiotic-associated colitis. Furthermore, it should help distinguish these diseases from noninflammatory diarrheal syndromes caused by viruses and enterotoxigenic bacteria. Amebic dysentery is detected by the presence of trophozoites in fresh stool under microscopic examination. The stool should be cultured for bacterial pathogens and examined for ova and parasites. Particularly in patients previously treated with antimicrobials, *Clostridium difficile* cytotoxin should be looked for in the stool as well.

The stool leukocyte test is also useful in patients with hospital-acquired diarrhea. However, cultures and parasitic examinations should be omitted since they so rarely give positive results in developed countries.[1] Instead, stool should be tested for *C. difficile* cytotoxin.

Noninfectious causes of diarrhea also need to be considered. In patients receiving tube feedings and elixir medications, osmotic diarrhea can be detected and evaluated by measuring the stool osmotic gap.[2] If the stool osmotic gap (stool osmolality minus 2 times the sum of stool sodium concentration and stool potassium concentration) is greater than 100 meq/L, the diarrhea is probably osmotic in nature. Therefore, osmotic stimulation to the intestine should be removed by modifying the osmolality of the tube feedings and elixir medications (especially those containing sorbitol). Other medications that are often implicated in causing diarrhea include magnesium-containing antacids, cimetidine, potassium and phosphorous supplements, laxatives, lactulose, quinidine, and antibiotics.[3] Other noninfectious factors that may cause diarrhea include partial obstruction of the intestine and hypoalbuminemia.

Therapeutic approaches to patients with intestinal infections vary according to diagnostic categories, as discussed in following sections. All patients need to be monitored for rehydration with isotonic fluids and for electrolyte balance and acid-base status. Antimicrobial drugs should be used selectively in patients with diagnosed infections (Table 108-1). Surgical intervention is reserved for patients with suspected peritonitis, abscess, intestinal perforation, or intestinal gangrene.

Noninflammatory Diarrheas

CHOLERA

Cholera is the prototype of watery diarrheal syndromes in which intestinal fluid loss is so copious that hypovolemic shock with profound acidosis may ensue. Cholera is termed "noninflammatory" because the intestinal epithelium remains structurally intact and leukocytes are absent from tissues and stool. Although cholera is rare in developed countries, a few cases have occurred on the southern coast of the United States, near the Gulf of Mexico.[4]

PATHOPHYSIOLOGY

The diarrhea associated with cholera is caused by an exotoxin called cholera toxin and secreted by *Vibrio cholerae.* This enterotoxin is a protein with a molecular weight of 84,000 and a subunit structure consisting of the A subunit (enzymatically active) and the B subunit (binding). Cholera toxin produces enzymatic changes in epithelial cells in the small intestine, leading to an intracellular increase in concentration of cyclic adenosine monophosphate (cAMP) and a resultant active secretion of chloride ions by these cells. Inhibition of normal absorption of sodium and chloride also occurs and leads to losses of isotonic fluid from the extracellular space into the intestinal lumen. The electrolyte composition of stool in adults is, approximately (in meq/L), sodium 120, potassium 24, chloride 95, and bicarbonate 52. The blood pH in severe cases is about 7.2 due to stool losses of bicarbonate. Despite large losses of potassium in stool, hypokalemia may not be initially present due to metabolic acidosis, which causes a shift of intracellular potassium into extracellular fluid.[5]

CLINICAL PRESENTATION

Following an incubation period of 1 to 2 days, in severe cholera there is a sudden onset of painless watery diarrhea. The diarrhea may be preceded momentarily by epigastric gurgling sounds and sensations of bloating, nausea, and vomiting. In some cases, vomiting is frequent and severe and accompanies the diarrhea. Fever is usually absent. Muscle cramps, especially in the calves, are a common complaint. The watery diarrhea is passed frequently and often gives a sense of relief from abdominal bloating and cramping. Each bowel movement may amount to about a cupful of liquid and may be repeated several times an hour. In adults with severe cholera, the rate of purging can average nearly half a liter per hour, with some patients purging more than a liter an hour. Over a period of 4 to 12 hours, the typical patient develops severe dehydration. If not rehydrated, patients may die as soon as 6 h after the onset of diarrhea.[6,7]

For any given patient with cholera who has not received rehydration therapy, the clinical picture depends directly on the quantity of liquid stool that has been passed into the intestinal lumen (Table 108-2). In patients with severe de-

TABLE 108-1 Antimicrobial Treatment of Selected Gastrointestinal Infections

Cholera	Tetracycline 500 mg 4 times a day (50 mg/kg/day in children) for 3 days. For children less than 10 yr and in pregnancy, furazolidone 5 mg/kg/day in 4 divided doses for 3 days.
Shigellosis	Trimethoprim-sulfamethoxazole, 160 and 800 mg, respectively, 2 times a day (10 and 50 mg/kg/day, respectively, in 2 divided doses for children) for 3 days
Campylobacteriosis	Erythromycin 500 mg 4 times a day or, in children, 50 mg/kg/day in 4 divided doses for 5 days
Enteric fever	Chloramphenicol 50–60 mg/kg/day in 4 divided doses until defervescence, then 30 mg/kg/day in 4 divided doses to complete 14-day course. Alternatives: trimethoprim sulfamethoxazole (same dose as for shigellosis) for 14 days or ceftriaxone 2–4 g each day (75 mg/kg/day in children) for 7 days.
C. difficile colitis	Vancomycin 125 mg orally 4 times a day for 7–10 days or metronidazole 500 mg orally or intravenously 3 times a day for 7–10 days or cholestyramine 4 g 3 or 4 times a day for 7–10 days
Amebiasis	Metronidazole 750 mg 3 times a day for 10 days
Giardiasis	Metronidazole 250 mg 3 times a day for 5 days
Cryptosporidiosis	Spiramycin 1 g orally 3 times a day for at least 14 days
Salmonellosis	Most patients do not require antibiotic. For suspected extraintestinal infection, ampicillin 100 mg/kg/day for 7–10 days.
Yersiniosis	Streptomycin 30 mg/kg/day for 7–10 days

TABLE 108-2 Symptoms and Signs of Cholera Correlated with Severity of Dehydration

	Mild (1–4%)	Moderate (5–7%)	Severe (≥ 8%)
Symptoms	Thirst	Thirst, weakness, lethargy, shortness of breath	Prostration, obtundation, labored breathing
Signs of dehydration	None	Dry mucous membranes, loss of skin turgor	Marked dryness of mucous membranes, loss of skin turgor
Pulse rate	Normal	Increased	Very increased
Blood pressure	Normal	Diminished with orthostatic changes	Frank hypotension
Respirations	Normal	Hyperpnea	Kussmaul respirations

NOTE: The percentage of dehydration is estimated from the weight of fluid lost divided by the body weight times 100.

hydration (fluid loss exceeding 8 percent of total body weight), the mucous membranes of the eyes and mouth are dry, the skin appears wrinkled, and the eyes appear sunken. One can assess loss of skin turgor by grasping a fold of abdominal skin between one's fingers, releasing it, and checking to see if the skin retains its ridged shape for an abnormally long period. The patient's voice will sound faint or high pitched due to dryness of membranes in the respiratory tract and the breathing pattern will be deep and rapid due to metabolic acidosis. Additionally, the pulse will be rapid and weak and the blood pressure often unobtainable.

Severe cholera causes hemoconcentration and metabolic acidosis. The acute contraction of extracellular fluid volume leads to hematocrits in excess of 55% and total serum protein concentrations of greater than 10 g/100 mL. Concentrations of sodium, potassium, and chloride are usually close to normal, but bicarbonate concentrations can be reduced to 10 meq/L or lower. An increased serum anion gap is due to increases in anionic protein concentration, lactic acidemia, and hyperphosphatemia.[8] With correction of the acidosis, the serum potassium will decrease markedly. Consequently, potassium needs to be replaced during correction of the acidosis. Increases in serum urea nitrogen and creatinine concentrations that occur during severe cholera are usually mild and rapidly corrected after rehydration. Elevations of serum calcium and magnesium concentrations are likewise mild. Furthermore, since total serum proteins are increased, concentrations of free ionic calcium and magnesium are likely to be normal.

DIAGNOSIS

Rapid presumptive identification of *V. cholerae* can be accomplished by placing a drop of liquid stool on a microscope slide overlaid with a coverslip. Rapid linear motility of the organism, under a dark field or phase contrast microscope, is characteristic. The addition of 01 antiserum to the stool preparation will result in loss of this motility.

V. cholerae grows well on most bacteriologic media but is inhibited on selective agars such as MacConkey's agar. The preferred selective media for culturing stool include thiosulfate-citrate-bile salts-sucrose agar (TCBS), on which the organism produces yellow colonies, and taurocholate tellurite gelatin agar (TTGA), on which the organism produces black colonies.

MANAGEMENT

The proper management of cholera includes prompt rehydration by replacing the estimated prior fluid loss and maintenance of hydration by quantitatively replacing any continuing fluid losses. To accomplish this, diarrhea fluid should be collected and measured at regular intervals. Ringer's lactate is the best commercially available intravenous solution, though fluids especially developed for severe diarrhea are optimal. One such fluid is *Dhaka solution,* which contains (in meq/L) sodium 133, potassium 13, chloride 98, and acetate 48. Normal saline is inferior to the polyelectrolyte solutions since it does not correct the acidosis or replace the potassium. Five percent dextrose and water (D5W) should not be used in cholera since it will not restore the volume deficit and may lead to hyponatremia. For patients who are alert and well enough to take fluids by mouth, oral rehydration fluid may be used to quantitatively replace lost diarrhea fluid. Oral fluid should have glucose or sucrose with the following composition (per L): sucrose 40 g, sodium 90 meq, potassium 20 meq, chloride 80 meq, and bicarbonate 30 meq.

Antibiotics should be given to shorten the course of the disease and decrease the total purging volume, thus lessening the requirements for rehydration fluids (Table 108-1). All antibiotics can be given orally. There is no advantage to the parenteral route, but intravenous tetracycline or trimethoprim-sulfamethoxazole can be given to complicated patients who are unable to take or absorb orally administered antibiotics.

COMPLICATIONS
Complications are rare if dehydration is corrected and hydration is maintained with a suitable polyelectrolyte solution. Most complications are the result of underhydration or use of inappropriate solutions. If rehydration is inadequate, acute renal failure can occur, especially in patients who are given volumes sufficient to maintain life but insufficient to restore circulation. Myocardial infarction and cerebrovascular thrombosis have been described as rare complications in adults. Hypokalemia occurs if rehydration fluids contain insufficient potassium. It may be manifested by abdominal distention, paralytic ileus, urinary retention, muscular weakness, cardiac arrhythmias, and even death. Acute pulmonary edema can occur with overreplacement of intravenous fluids, especially if the fluids have not corrected the acidosis. Mild asymptomatic hypoglycemia occurs commonly in children during rehydration. Severe hypoglycemia occurs only occasionally and may manifest as seizures and coma. If these should occur during therapy, intravenous glucose should be given immediately while awaiting a blood glucose determination. Pregnant women frequently abort if severely dehydrated; principles of treatment are the same as with other patients. Important determinants of mortality in cholera are hypoglycemia, pneumonia, septicemia, and preexisting malnutrition.[9]

OTHER NONINFLAMMATORY DIARRHEAS

Other noninflammatory infections include enterotoxigenic *Escherichia coli* (ETEC), *Aeromonas hydrophilia,* and the viruses rotavirus and Norwalk agent. These may mimic cholera in their presentation but are generally less severe.

PATHOPHYSIOLOGY
In ETEC infections, there are two major groupings of enterotoxins produced by given strains of *E. coli:* a heat-labile toxin (LT), which resembles cholera toxin, and a heat-stable toxin (ST). LT acts like cholera toxin on the small intestinal epithelium to raise intracellular cAMP concentrations. ST acts to raise intracellular levels of a different cyclic nucleotide, cyclic guanosine monophosphate, with similar results as LT: isotonic fluid is secreted from the extracellular space into the intestinal lumen. The viral infections of the intestine have a different pathophysiology that does not involve enterotoxins. Virus particles enter the epithelial cells on the tips of villi in the small intestine. Structural changes that ensue include shortening of villi and appearance of mononuclear leukocytes in the adjacent lamina propria. Ulceration of the mucosa does not occur, but epithelial cells on the absorptive villus tips die at a faster than normal rate. The lost villus epithelial cells are replaced by the migration of crypt epithelial cells. Since crypt epithelial cells are more active in secretion and have insufficient time to mature into normal absorptive function, the epithelial surface shifts toward net secretion and consequent diarrhea.

CLINICAL PRESENTATION
The clinical presentation is usually liquid stools, abdominal cramps, and dehydration. Vomiting often precedes or accompanies the diarrhea. Fever is usually mild or absent in enterotoxic infections but may be prominent in viral infections. Acidosis and hypokalemia will develop in proportion to the quantity of fluid lost from the body's extracellular space.

DIAGNOSIS
The presence of red cells or leukocytes in the stool is evidence against the diagnosis of noninflammatory infection. Bacterial cultures of stool should be performed. A heavy growth of *E. coli* suggests the diagnosis of ETEC infection. However, confirmation of this diagnosis requires demonstration of toxin by a specialized research laboratory or by the Centers for Disease Control in Atlanta, Georgia. Viral infections cannot be identified by routine methods, but enzyme-linked immunoassays (ELISAs) are commercially available for rotavirus (such as Rotazyme). For the Norwalk agent, electron microscopy of the stool is required and is appropriate mainly in the research setting.

MANAGEMENT
The principles of management are the same as for cholera. Lost fluid volume should be replaced quantitatively with an isotonic solution such as Ringer's lactate. Careful attention should also be paid to replacing potassium and correcting acidosis. These forms of infectious diarrhea are self-limited and do not require antibiotic treatment.

Dysentery

Acute dysentery is a syndrome consisting of fever, abdominal pain, and frequent passage of stools containing blood and mucus. The most common causes are bacterial infections with species of *Shigella, Campylobacter, Salmonella, E. coli,* and *Yersinia* and the parasitic infection *Entamoeba histolytica* (amebiasis). Serious complications are more common than with noninflammatory diarrheas because of the invasive and inflammatory destructive character of the disease. Accordingly, intensive care is sometimes required in serious cases, especially when patients present with septic manifestations, toxic megacolon, colonic perforation, or hemolytic-uremic syndrome.

PATHOPHYSIOLOGY

Shigellosis is the prototype of the acute bacillary dysenteries, but in recent decades in developed countries, these infections have declined in incidence and have been surpassed by *E. coli* 0157:H7 and *Campylobacter* infections. Four species of shigellae are recognized on the basis of antigenic and biochemical properties: *Shigella dysenteriae* (group A), *S. flexneri* (group B), *S. boydii* (group C), and *S. sonnei* (group D). There are over 40 serotypes among these species, each of which is designated by the species name followed by a specific Arabic number. *S. dysenteriae* 1 is called the Shiga bacillus and causes epidemics with higher mortality than other serotypes.[10]

Serotypes are determined by the 0 polysaccharide side chain of the lipopolysaccharide (endotoxin) in the cell wall. Endotoxin is detectable in the blood of severely ill patients and may be responsible for the complication of the hemolytic-uremic syndrome. To be virulent, shigellae must be able to invade epithelial cells, as tested in the laboratory by keratoconjunctivitis in the guinea pig (Sereney test) or HeLa cell invasion. Shiga toxin is produced by *S. dysenteriae* 1 and in lesser amounts by other serotypes. Shigalike toxin, or verotoxin, is produced by *E. coli* 0157:H7. Both toxins act by inhibiting protein synthesis.[11]

Since the microorganisms are relatively resistant to acid, shigellae pass the gastric barrier more readily than other bacteria, and as few as 200 ingested bacilli can initiate disease in healthy adults. In contrast, typhoid or cholera bacilli require much larger numbers to produce disease in normal individuals. During the incubation period, usually 12 to 72 h, the organisms traverse the small bowel, penetrate colonic epithelial cells, and multiply intracellularly. An acute inflammatory response ensues in the mucosa, resulting in superficial ulcerations and shedding of shigella organisms into stools and attendant prodromal symptoms (Table 108-3). Advancing inflammation causes edematous narrowing of crypt gland necks, leading to the formation of crypt abscesses. Initially the inflammation is confined to the rectosigmoid colon, but after about 4 days of illness it may advance to involve the proximal colon. In severe cases, there may be pancolitis with extension of inflammation into the terminal ileum, and pseudomembranous types of colitis may develop. Diarrhea results because of impaired absorption of water and electrolytes by the inflamed colon.[12]

Although the colonic inflammation is superficial, bacteremia occurs occasionally, especially in *S. dysenteriae* 1 infections. Susceptibility of organisms to serum complement–mediated bacteriolysis may explain the infrequency of bacteremia and disseminated infection. Colonic perforation is a rare complication, typically superimposed on toxic megacolon.

Patients with severe colitis due to *S. dysenteriae* 1 or *E. coli* 0157:H7 are prone to develop the hemolytic-uremic syndrome. Treatment of uncomplicated dysentery with trimethoprim-sulfamethoxazole and treatment of ampicillin-resistant infections with ampicillin have been shown to be associated with development of hemolytic-uremic syndrome. In this complication, fibrin thrombi are deposited in the renal glomeruli, causing cortical necrosis and fragmentation of red cells.[13]

CLINICAL PRESENTATION

Most patients with dysentery begin their illness with a nonspecific prodrome (Table 108-3). The height of the temperature varies, and children commonly exhibit febrile convulsions. The initial intestinal symptoms soon follow as cramps, loose stools, and watery diarrhea, which usually precede the onset of dysentery by one or more days. The dysentery consists typically of flecks and small clots of bright red blood and mucus in stools that are small in volume. Frequency of passage is often as high as 20 to 40 times a day and is accompanied by excruciating rectal pain and tenesmus during defecation. Some patients develop rectal prolapse during severe straining. The amount of blood in stools varies widely but is usually small because of the superficial colonic ulcerations. Abdominal tenderness is often most marked in the left lower quadrant over the sigmoid colon but may also be generalized. The fever is likely to abate after a few days of dysentery, making afebrile bloody diarrhea an occasional clinical presentation. After 1 to 2 weeks of untreated disease, some patients with unrelenting symptoms will have progressed to a serious illness requiring intensive care.

Complications include dehydration, which can be a cause of death, especially in children and the elderly. Shigella septicemia occurs mainly in children with *S. dysenteriae* 1 infections who are malnourished.[14] The leukemoid reaction and hemolytic-uremic syndrome may develop later in the course, after antibiotic treatment and once dysentery has started to improve. The hemolytic-uremic syndrome is characterized by the triad of hemolytic anemia, thrombocytopenia, and renal failure (see Chap. 147). Toxic megacolon develops in some patients and is characterized by abdominal distention, decreased bowel sounds, high fever, and an x-ray depicting dilation of the colon with air. Neurologic

TABLE 108-3 Evolution of Clinical Syndromes in Shigellosis

Stage	Time of Appearance after Onset of Illness	Symptoms and Signs	Pathology
Prodrome	Earliest	Fever, chills, myalgias, anorexia, nausea, vomiting	None or early colitis
Nonspecific diarrhea	0–3 days	Abdominal cramps, loose stools, watery diarrhea	Rectosigmoid colitis with superficial ulceration
Dysentery	1–8 days	Frequent passage of blood and mucus, tenesmus, rectal prolapse, abdominal tenderness	Colitis extending sometimes to proximal colon, crypt abscesses, inflammation in lamina propria
Complications	3–10 days	Dehydration, seizures, septicemia, leukemoid reaction, hemolytic-uremic syndrome, ileus, peritonitis	Severe colitis, terminal ileitis, endotoxemia, intravascular coagulation, toxic megacolon, colonic perforation

manifestations can be striking and include delirium, seizures, and nuchal rigidity.

DIAGNOSIS

Dysentery should be considered in any patient with acute onset of fever and diarrhea. Examination of the stool is essential. Blood and pus are grossly apparent in severe bacillary dysentery; even in milder forms of the disease, microscopic examination of the stool often reveals numerous leukocytes and erythrocytes. The peripheral white cell count is of little diagnostic value, since it may range from less than $3000/mm^3$ to more than $30{,}000/mm^3$. Sigmoidoscopic examination reveals diffuse erythema with a mucopurulent layer and friable areas of mucosa, with shallow ulcers to 3 to 7 mm in diameter.

Definitive diagnosis depends upon isolating causative bacteria by selective media. A rectal swab, a swab of a colonic ulcer obtained by sigmoidoscopic examination, or a freshly passed stool specimen should be inoculated immediately on culture plates or into carrying media. Since isolation rates of shigellae from freshly passed stools of patients with shigellosis may be as low as 67 percent, culturing for 3 successive days is recommended. Stool cultures are generally positive within 24 h after onset of symptoms and may remain positive for several weeks in the absence of antimicrobial therapy. Appropriate culture media include blood, MacConkey, desoxycholate, and salmonella-shigella (S-S) agars.

TREATMENT

The effectiveness of antimicrobial agents in treating shigellosis has been well established. Appropriate antimicrobial therapy instituted early may decrease the duration of symptoms by 50 percent and decrease the duration of excretion of shigellae (an important factor for nosocomial transmission) by a far greater percentage. Infection by *S. dysenteriae* 1 may result in a 10 to 30 percent mortality rate in the absence of antimicrobial therapy. Therefore, appropriate antimicrobials are mandatory with this pathogen (Table 108-1). Because of the increasing frequency of plasmid-mediated antimicrobial resistance to *Shigella* infections, drug susceptibility testing is important. Certain drugs that appear effective in vitro, including amoxicillin and nonabsorbable antimicrobials such as neomycin or kanamycin, are not effective in vivo. Trimethoprim-sulfamethoxazole is effective therapy against infection caused by susceptible strains of *Shigella*. However, the association of usage of trimethoprim-sulfamethoxazole and development of hemolytic-uremic syndrome in *E. coli* 0157:H7 infections should deter physicians from using this drug in suspected *E. coli* infections. In patients with dysentery due to *Campylobacter*, *Salmonella*, and *Yersinia*, antibiotics have not been shown to have any beneficial effects on the course of the intestinal disease. However, antibiotics may be advised in severe cases and in most critically ill patients because of the possibility of bacteremia and other extraintestinal manifestations.

Fluid losses in shigellosis are qualitatively similar to those in other infectious diarrheal diseases. The patient should be treated with appropriate intravenous fluids in quantities adequate to correct clinical signs of saline depletion. The requirement for fluids is generally small, but fluid repletion will be lifesaving in exceptional cases. Agents that decrease intestinal motility should not be used. Such preparations as diphenoxylate and paregoric may exacerbate symptoms, presumably by retarding intestinal clearance of the microorganisms. There is no convincing evidence that pectin- or bismuth-containing preparations are helpful.

MANAGEMENT OF COMPLICATIONS

Toxic megacolon is suspected because of abdominal distension and a massively dilated colon on x-ray. In toxic megacolon, the therapeutic aims are to decompress the colon by inserting a rectal tube and to try to restore intestinal motility by achieving good electrolyte balance. Because these patients are at risk for peritonitis and generalized sepsis originating from the colon, broad spectrum antibiotic treatment with a regimen such as clindamycin or a ureidopenicillin (piperacillin or mezlocillin) with an aminoglycoside should be instituted (see Chap. 166).

Perforation of the colon may result after development of toxic megacolon or from a deeply ulcerated colonic mucosa. Perforation is suspected in patients with a tender abdomen, septic appearance, and evidence of peritoneal air or fluid on x-ray. This complication is usually catastrophic, with rapid evolution of septic shock. Emergency surgery is indicated as soon as the perforation is detected.

The hemolytic-uremic syndrome typically follows the onset of acute dysentery by about 1 week. Although fatalities have been reported from this complication, the majority of patients have reversible renal failure and will recover following appropriate intensive care. Some patients with profound anemia require transfusion, while patients with serum creatinine concentrations in excess of 4 mg/100 mL require hemodialysis.

Necrotizing Enteritis (Pig Bel)

Necrotizing enteritis is an acute and often fatal complication of infectious diarrhea and usually occurs in children in developing countries. This intestinal disease is a recently recognized entity, which has been reported as identical clinical syndromes or closely related variants under the names *segmental infarcts of the small intestine* and *acute segmental ischemic enteritis* in Thailand; *acute segmental necrotizing enteritis* and *acute ischemic enteritis* in India; *necrotizing enterocolitis* in Kuwait; *necrotizing enteritis* in Sri Lanka; and *enteritis necroticans* (pig bel) in New Guinea. Patients with this illness are likely to need intensive care because they are frequently septic or in shock and often show signs of an acute abdomen.[15,16]

PATHOPHYSIOLOGY

An investigation of an outbreak of this disease (following ingestion of pork contaminated with *Clostridium perfringens*) in New Guinea suggests that the disease results from an acute infection and that necrosis is due to the beta toxin produced by this organism. It has been further suggested that the digestive enzyme trypsin, which degrades the beta toxin, may be inhibited by dietary substances in sweet potatoes or by intestinal worms, thus allowing the toxin to be active in causing the disease. However, not all patients are infected with *C. perfringens,* and other factors appear to be important in pathophysiology. Circulatory insufficiency to the small intestine occurs and causes ischemic necrosis of the mucosa and, sometimes, of the deeper layers of the intestinal wall in a segmental distribution.[17] The histopathological features include mucosal necrosis, edema of the submucosa, and air in the submucosa (pneumatosis intestinalis). These lesions are similar to those seen in neonatal necrotizing enterocolitis (NEC). One difference is that in NEC the anatomic distribution of the disease is most commonly in the terminal ileum and proximal colon, in contrast to its distribution in the jejunum in necrotizing enteritis.[18]

CLINICAL PRESENTATION

Patients who develop necrotizing enteritis have a preceding acute illness characterized by fever, vomiting, and diarrhea. This may last a few days until the onset of abdominal pain or distention with ileus and the passage of bloody stools. Some patients are hypotensive and septic in appearance, and some show signs of intestinal perforation and generalized peritonitis. The white blood cell count may be elevated and serum protein concentrations decreased.

DIAGNOSIS

The diagnosis should be suspected in a patient with bloody diarrhea, ileus, and clinical appearance of sepsis. An abdominal x-ray may reveal paralytic ileus and pneumatosis intestinalis. Culture of the stool for *C. perfringens* should be considered, but the identification of beta toxin is available only in certain research laboratories.

MANAGEMENT

Restoration of effective perfusion of the intestine by treating shock may reverse early lesions and prevent progression of this disease to frank intestinal gangrene. Standard therapy of shock, using plasma-expanding isotonic intravenous fluid and broad spectrum antibiotics, gives the critically ill patient the best chance of recovery. The dilated bowel should be decompressed by nasogastric intestinal intubation and suction. Resection of gangrenous bowel should be attempted in patients who fail to improve with medical therapy or who show signs of perforation or acute peritonitis. Mortality rates in this disease usually exceed 50 percent regardless of whether medical or surgical treatment is employed.

Enteric Fever

Enteric fever is a bacterial disease caused by *Salmonella typhi* that is characterized by prolonged fever, abdominal pain, diarrhea, delirium, rose spots, and splenomegaly. It is complicated sometimes by intestinal bleeding and perforation.[19] Enteric fever is synonymous with typhoid fever, which is occasionally caused also by *Salmonella enteritidis* bioserotype paratyphi A or B. Infection is transmitted by ingestion of bacteria via contaminated water and food, and chronic asymptomatic fecal carriers are an important reservoir of infection. Antimicrobial treatment reduces mortality to less than 5 percent of cases. Intensive care may be required for the patients who develop intestinal bleeding, perforation, delirium, coma, or septic shock.

PATHOPHYSIOLOGY

Salmonella typhi is a motile gram-negative rod in the family Enterobacteriaceae and belongs to serogroup D1. The polysaccharide side chain of its 0 antigen confers serologic specificity to the organism and is essential in virulence because *Salmonella* other than *S. typhi* and *S. enteritidis* bioserotype paratyphi A or B do not produce enteric fever in human beings. These antigens play critical roles in permitting the organisms to invade lymphoid tissue from the gut lumen and to multiply within macrophages. Large numbers of bacteria in the lymphoid tissues of the intestine (Peyer's patches), liver, spleen, and bone marrow cause inflammation in these sites. Hyperplasia of Peyer's patches sometimes causes intestinal bleeding and perforation.[20]

CLINICAL PRESENTATION

The evolution of disease syndromes occurs stepwise over 1 to 3 weeks (Table 108-4) but may be variable in the time of appearance. The early symptoms of fever, abdominal pain, and prostration tend to persist throughout the illness, which in untreated cases last a month or longer. Abdominal pain occurs in more than half of patients and is frequently diffuse or located in the right lower quadrant over the terminal ileum. Diarrhea occurs in about a third of patients and consists of either watery stools or semisolid stools described as "pea soup"; melena occurs less commonly. Patients are rarely jaundiced. Rose spots occur in more than half of light-skinned individuals but are often not visible in dark-skinned patients. The rash is seen most commonly on the shoulders, thorax, and abdomen and rarely on the extremities. The lesions are erythematous macules or papules about 1 to 5 mm in diameter, which typically blanch with pressure but may become hemorrhagic in nature. They fade quickly after a few days of treatment. Many patients display abnormal behavior or altered mental status that may be out of proportion to the severity of the systemic illness. Among the common presentations are "toxic" staring, delirium, aphonia, and coma. Seizures are common in children.[21,22]

TABLE 108-4 Evolution of Typical Symptoms and Signs of Typhoid Fever

Disease Period	Symptoms	Signs	Pathology
First week	Fever, chills gradually increasing and persisting; headache	Abdominal tenderness	Bacteremia
Second week	Rash, abdominal pain, diarrhea or constipation, delirium, prostration	Rose spots, splenomegaly, hepatomegaly	Mononuclear cell vasculitis of skin, hyperplasia of Peyer's patches, typhoid nodules in spleen and liver
Third week	Complications of intestinal bleeding and perforation, shock	Melena, ileus, rigid abdomen, coma	Ulcerations over Peyer's patches, perforation with peritonitis
Fourth week and later	Resolution of symptoms, relapse, weight loss	Reappearance of acute disease, cachexia	Cholecystitis, chronic fecal carriage of bacteria

In about 5 percent of patients, the complications of intestinal bleeding and intestinal perforation will occur, usually after the second week of illness. These complications occur more often in adolescents and adults than in children. Bleeding occurs from ileal ulcers and may present as melena or bright red blood in stools. Brisk bleeding develops rarely, though it is an occasional cause of death. Intestinal perforation presents as the sudden development of more severe abdominal pain, distention, and tenderness. Bowel sounds are diminished, and abdominal x-ray usually reveals free air. Perforation most often occurs unexpectedly, after a few days of treatment when a patient has begun to improve. Other complications of typhoid fever include myocarditis, acute cholecystitis, meningitis, and pneumonia, which develops as a superinfection due to other bacteria.

DIAGNOSIS

The preferred method of diagnosis is isolation of *S. typhi* from a blood culture. The blood culture is positive in most patients during the first 2 weeks of illness. Urine and stool cultures are positive less frequently but should be taken to increase the diagnostic yield. The bone marrow culture is the most sensitive test, positive in nearly 90 percent of cases, and can be used when a bacteriologic diagnosis is crucially needed or in patients who have been pretreated with antibiotics. The Widal test for agglutinating antibodies against the somatic (0) and flagellar (H) antigens of *S. typhi* is widely used for retrospective serodiagnosis but is not helpful in acute management.[23]

TREATMENT

Chloramphenicol has remained the drug of choice since its introduction in 1948 because no other drug has been demonstrated to cause more rapid or consistent improvement of disease (Table 108-1). Resistance to chloramphenicol mediated by plasmid R factors has been reported only occasionally in patients who acquired infections in Mexico, India, and Thailand. In patients unable to take oral medication, the same dosage should be given intravenously until the patient can take capsules.[24,25]

Alternative drugs should be considered when *S. typhi* resistant to chloramphenicol is isolated or strongly suspected. Since alternative drugs are nearly equal to chloramphenicol in clinical efficacy, a physician may choose to use another drug for a patient in whom bone marrow suppression is undesired. Trimethoprim-sulfamethoxazole is effective in a standard adult dose of 160 mg trimethoprim–800 mg sulfamethoxazole given orally or intravenously twice a day for 14 days. Other drugs that are effective include ampicillin (intravenously), amoxicillin, cefoperazone, and ceftriaxone.

Patients who are dehydrated, are anorectic, or have diarrhea should receive intravenous saline with attention to electrolyte and acid-base disturbances. Patients with brisk intestinal bleeding will require blood transfusion. It is very rare that bleeding will persist in quantities great enough to require surgical intervention. Patients with suspected perforation should have abdominal and upright chest x-rays to look for free air and peritoneal fluid. Laparotomy should be undertaken as early as possible to suture the perforation, and gentamicin should be added to broaden coverage for polymicrobial peritonitis. Ileal resection has been required in some cases in which inflammatory destruction of the ileum was too advanced to permit successful closure of localized perforations.

Pseudomembranous Colitis

Among seriously ill patients in intensive care units, frequent antibiotic usage makes the side-effects of antibiotic-associated diarrhea and pseudomembranous colitis common iatrogenic problems. Although these conditions can be serious, mortality can be averted by early recognition and appropriate treatment.

PATHOPHYSIOLOGY

Virtually all antibiotics, except for vancomycin, have the potential to cause this disease. Antibiotics most associated with this complication are clindamycin, ampicillin, and cephalosporins. Estimates of the incidence of antibiotic-associated diarrhea with these drugs are 5 to 25 percent, with higher risk occurring in older patients and with more prolonged use of antibiotics. The cause of this complication is suppression of the normal colonic bacterial flora with resultant overgrowth of *C. difficile.*[26] This organism produces toxins, including toxin A (enterotoxin) and toxin B (cytotoxin), that damage the colonic epithelial cells and result in inflammation and impairment of normal fluid absorption by the colon.[27,28]

CLINICAL PRESENTATION

The most common presentation is watery diarrhea in a patient receiving an antibiotic, though in some patients diarrhea starts after the antibiotic is discontinued. More severe cases will have fever, abdominal pain, and passage of bloody stools. Diarrhea may be absent when patients have ileus. The worst cases of pseudomembranous colitis result in toxic megacolon, perforation, and generalized peritonitis. There is evidence that sudden deaths among elderly institutionalized patients are associated with toxin of *C. difficile* in the stool.[29] Not all patients with *C. difficile* toxin in the stool present with diarrhea, however, and many toxin-positive patients have only mild disease.

DIAGNOSIS

Stool examination often reveals leukocytes and red cells. Assay of stool for *C. difficile* toxin has become the best diagnostic test. However, false-positive results of latex agglutination tests for toxin have been reported and indicate that test results need to be correlated with clinical findings to be useful.[30] Sigmoidoscopy should be done in suspected cases and reveals a spectrum of mucosal changes from mild erythema to a granular, friable, or hemorrhagic mucosa or the presence of a pseudomembrane. Culture of the stool for *C. difficile* is not practical since this organism is part of the normal flora. However, culture of the stool for other enteropathogens should be done.

TREATMENT

Discontinuation of the offending antibiotics, when feasible, is appropriate; the symptoms will promptly disappear in many cases. However, in critically ill patients who require antibiotics, an alternative antibiotic regimen should be considered with the hope that other antibiotics will not allow the toxin-mediated disease to be further propagated. Specific treatment should be given to patients with moderate or severe symptoms due to pseudomembranous colitis and to patients with positive stool toxin assays whose diarrhea persists after discontinuation of the antibiotic (Table 108-1).[31]

CASE PRESENTATION

An 86-year-old woman is transferred from a local nursing home with fever, abdominal pain, and obtundation. Her medical history is notable for peptic ulcer disease, strokes, and mild dementia. At baseline, she is unable to ambulate and is incontinent of urine and stool but enjoys her interactions with family members and other nursing home residents.

On examination in the emergency room, the blood pressure is 70/40, the heart rate 115, the respiratory rate 40, and the temperature 39.0°C. The patient is electively intubated, a large-bore intravenous catheter is placed, and she is resuscitated with normal saline. The white blood cell count is 17,000/mm^3 with 30 percent band forms. An upright chest x-ray reveals free air beneath the diaphragm. She is given clindamycin, ampicillin, and gentamicin intravenously and taken to the operating room where a perforated peptic ulcer is discovered. The perforation is oversewn and a vagotomy performed, and she is transferred to the intensive care unit.

Parenteral nutrition, cimetidine, and subcutaneous heparin are begun immediately postoperatively. Antibiotics are continued. Over the first 3 days, she becomes hemodynamically stable, her mental status improves, fever resolves, and white cell count normalizes. Weakness and abdominal distention prevent early liberation from the ventilator.

On the fifth hospital day, bowel sounds return, and the nurse notes that the patient is incontinent of liquid stool. Enteral feeding is begun through a soft tube. The abdomen becomes softer and the medical team anticipates that a trial of spontaneous breathing will soon be successful. The following morning, the patient seems comfortable on a T-piece, but the nurse requests a rectal tube for increasing diarrheal stool. By afternoon, the temperature rises to 38.5°C, and the respiratory rate is 44. The abdomen is moderately distended and diffusely, mildly tender. Enteral feeding is discontinued and acetaminophen given. On the seventh hospital day, fever persists, abdominal pain has worsened, and the white cell count has risen to 20,000. A CT scan of the abdomen, ordered in search of an abdominal abscess, shows only postoperative changes. Cultures of blood, urine, and stool are requested.

Increased intravenous fluids are required to match stool output. Cimetidine is discontinued. Finally, microscopic examination of the stool with methylene blue reveals large numbers of fecal leukocytes. An assay for *C. difficile* toxin is positive. Clindamycin is discontinued and intravenous metronidazole given. Over the next 2 days, diarrhea resolves, fever abates, and the patient is extubated. On the fourteenth day, she returns to her home, eating a normal diet.

CASE DISCUSSION

This case illustrates the development of pseudomembranous colitis superimposed on critical illness. Predisposing factors included advanced age and treatment with broad spectrum antibiotics. In this case, the diagnosis was difficult since stool incontinence raised little concern in an elderly, demented patient. When stool volume increased remarkably, the response was to insert a rectal tube rather than to consider the cause. Even when it became impossible to ignore the diarrhea, there were so many likely culprits (enteral feeds, cimetidine, antibiotics, vagotomy-induced dysmotility, intraabdominal abscess) that the true diagnosis remained obscure. Had a fecal leukocyte examination been performed early, revealing an inflammatory diarrhea, each of these potential causes could have been excluded. Indeed, when fecal leukocytes were discovered, the newly focused differential diagnosis promptly led to the cause of illness.

In critically ill patients, new diseases may present insidiously, their manifestations attributed to a preexisting condition. In this woman, the risk of postoperative abscess was real. Nevertheless, the delay in considering a diagnosis of pseudomembranous colitis likely prolonged both the need for mechanical ventilation and the intensive care stay.

Ideally, when a diagnosis of pseudomembranous colitis is made, all antibiotics should be discontinued. As is typical in critically ill patients, however, this was thought to be unwise because of recent peritonitis. Therefore, substituting metronidazole for clindamycin both preserved anaerobic coverage and removed a likely offending agent.

References

1. Siegel DL, Edelstein PH, Nachamkin I: Inappropriate testing for diarrheal diseases in the hospital. JAMA 263:979, 1990.
2. Edes TE, Walk BE, Austin JL: Diarrhea in tube-fed patients: Feeding formula not necessarily the cause. Am J Med 88:91, 1990.
3. Heimburger DC: Diarrhea with enteral feeding: Will the real cause please stand up? Am J Med 88:89, 1990.
4. Blake PA, Allegra DT, Snyder JD, Barrett TJ, McFarland L, Caraway CT, Feeley JC, Craig JP, Lee JV, Puhr ND, Feldman RA: Cholera—a possible endemic focus in the United States. N Engl J Med 302:305, 1980.
5. Carpenter CCJ: The pathophysiology of secretory diarrheas. Med Clin North Am 66:597, 1982.
6. Speelman P, Butler T, Kabir I, et al: Colonic dysfunction during cholera infection. Gastroenterol 91:1164, 1986.
7. Rabbani GH: Cholera. Clin Gastroenterol 15:507, 1986.
8. Wang F, Butler T, Rabbani GH, Jones PK: The acidosis of cholera. Contributions of hyperproteinemia, lactic acidemia, and hyperphosphatemia to an increased serum anion gap. N Engl J Med 315:1591, 1986.
9. Butler T, Islam M, Azad AK, Islam MR, Speelman P: Causes of death in diarrheal diseases after rehydration therapy: An autopsy study of 140 patients in Bangladesh. Bull Wld Hlth Org 65:317, 1987.
10. Levine MM: Bacillary dysentery. Mechanisms and treatment. Med Clin North Am 66:623, 1982.
11. Keusch GT: Shigella infections. Clin Gastroenterol 8:645, 1979.
12. Butler T, Speelman P, Kabir I, Banwell JG: Colonic dysfunction during shigellosis. J Infect Dis 154:817, 1986.
13. Koster F, Levin J, Walker L, Tung KSK, Gilman RH, Rahaman MM, Majid MA, Islam S, Williams RC: Hemolytic-uremic syndrome after shigellosis. Relation to endotoxemia and circulating immune complexes. N Engl J Med 298:927, 1978.
14. Struelens MJ, Patte D, Kabir I, Salam A, Nath SK, Butler T: Shigella septicemia: Prevalence, presentation, risk factors, and outcome. J Infect Dis 152:784, 1985.
15. Murrell TGC, Roth L, Egerton J, Samels J, Walker PD: Pig-bel: Enteritis necroticans. Lancet 1:217, 1966.
16. Johnson S, Echeverria P, Taylor DN, Paul SR, Coninx R, Sakurai J, Eampokalap B, Jimakorn P, Cooke RA, Lawrence GW, Walker PD: Enteritis necroticans among Khmer children at an evaluation site in Thailand. Lancet 2:496, 1987.
17. Bounous G: Acute necrosis of the intestinal mucosa. Gastroenterol 82:1457, 1982.
18. Butler T, Dahms B, Lindpaintner K, Islam M, Azad MAK, Anton P: Segmental necrotizing enterocolitis: Pathological and clinical features of 22 cases in Bangladesh. Gut 28:1433, 1987.
19. Butler T, Knight J, Nath SK, Speelman P, Roy SK, Azad MAK: Typhoid fever complicated by intestinal perforation: A persisting fatal disease requiring surgical management. Rev Infect Dis 7:244, 1985.
20. Edelman R, Levine MM: Summary of an international workshop on typhoid fever. Rev Infect Dis 8:329, 1986.
21. Butler T, Islam A, Kabir I, Jones PK: Patterns of morbidity and mortality in typhoid fever dependent on age and gender: review of 552 hospitalized patients with diarrhea. Rev Infect Dis 13:85, 1991.
22. Thisyakorn U, Mansuwan P, Taylor DN: Typhoid and paratyphoid fever in 192 hospitalized children in Thailand. Am J Dis Child 141:862, 1987.
23. Murphy JR, Baqar S, Munoz C, Schlesinger L, Ferreccio C, Lindberg AA, Svenson S, Losonsky G, Koster F, Levine MM: Characteristics of humoral and cellular immunity to *Salmonella typhi* in residents of typhoid-endemic and typhoid-free regions. J Infect Dis 156:1005, 1987.
24. Hornick RB: Selective primary healthcare: Strategies of control of disease in the developing world. XX. Typhoid fever. Rev Infect Dis 7:536, 1985.
25. Hoffmann SL, Punjabi NH, Kumala S, Moechtar A, Pulungsih SP, Rivai AR, Rockhill RC, Woodward TE, Loedin AA: Reduction of mortality in chloramphenicol-treated typhoid fever by high dose dexamethasone. N Engl J Med 310:82, 1984.
26. Bartlett JG, Chang TW, Gurwith M, Gorbach SL, Onderdonk AB: Antibiotic-associated pseudomembranous colitis due to toxin producing clostridia. N Eng J Med 298:531, 1978.
27. Rolfe RD, Finegold SM (eds): *Clostridium difficile:* Its role in intestinal disease. San Diego, Academic Press, Inc., 1988.
28. Rolfe RD: Role of anaerobic bacteria in other bowel pathology, in Finegold SM, George WL (eds): *Anaerobic Infections in Humans.* San Diego, Academic Press, Inc., 1989, pp 679–690.
29. Bender BS, Bennett R, Laughon BE, Greenough WB III, Gaydos C, Sears SD, Forman MS, Bartlett JG: Is *Clostridium difficile* endemic in chronic care facilities? Lancet 2:11, 1986.
30. Qadri SMH, Akter J, Ostrawski S, Qadri SGM, Cunha BA: High incidence of false positives by a latex agglutination test for the diagnosis of *Clostridium difficile* associated colitis in compromised patients. Diagnostic Microbiol Infect Dis 12:291, 1989.
31. Teasley DG, Gerding DN, Olson MM, Peterson LR, Gebhard RL, Schwartz MJ, Lee JT, Jr: Prospective randomized trial of metronidazole versus vancomycin for *Clostridium difficile*-associated diarrhea and colitis. Lancet 2:1043, 1983.

Chapter 109

CRITICAL ILLNESS DUE TO *Mycobacterium tuberculosis*

RICHARD LONG

KEY POINTS

- Mycobacterium tuberculosis *rarely causes acute life-threatening illness; it is a slow-growing pathogen (doubling time, 12 to 18 h) against which antituberculous drugs are highly effective.*
- *Acute respiratory failure may result when a large quantity of heavily infected liquid caseum ruptures into the bronchial tree or vasculature.*
- *When mycobacteria infect the pericardium, meninges, or adrenal glands, critical illness may result by virtue of the location of the active tuberculous process.*
- *Delay in instituting therapy is the major obstacle to recovery from the life-threatening complications of tuberculosis.*
- *Corticosteroids, in addition to an effective regimen of antituberculous drugs, may reverse the toxicity and reduce the exudative reaction associated with the tuberculous inflammatory response.*
- *Relatively early in the course of human immunodeficiency virus (HIV) infection, tubercle bacilli dormant in the host may reactivate and disseminate. Such disease may present with unusual features, but usually responds well to treatment.*

When tubercle bacilli enter the host for the first time—nearly always by inhalation into the lung—they are ingested by macrophages and transported to regional lymph nodes. If spread is not contained at the level of regional lymph nodes, organisms reach the bloodstream and widespread dissemination occurs. Such primary infection and dissemination is usually asymptomatic; lesions heal spontaneously, although dormant viable bacilli may remain and be potential foci for later reactivation (postprimary disease). Rarely the primary lesion in the lung progresses directly to active disease, or the disseminated foci go directly on to active disease—e.g., miliary or meningeal tuberculosis. During the 2 to 8 weeks that follow primary infection, cell-mediated immunity and delayed hypersensitivity develop in the infected host. These inflammatory responses benefit the host by localizing and destroying substantial numbers of bacteria, but they also cause tissue destruction and may contribute to the development of critical illness.

The above sequence of events is also seen in illnesses caused by nontuberculous mycobacteria; however, these organisms are less virulent and are rarely encountered except in patients with significant underlying chronic lung disease or HIV infection. With few exceptions, the lack of effective antibiotics poses the greatest problem in the management of patients with nontuberculous mycobacterial disease.

Acute Respiratory Failure

PATHOGENESIS

Significant hypoxemia is a rare complication of fibrocaseous pulmonary tuberculosis. It is reported to occur in fewer than 2 percent of cases in the antibiotic era.[1] Angiographic and histologic studies report parallel involvement of lung parenchyma and vasculature, thereby limiting major ventilation/perfusion ($\dot{V}/\dot{Q}$) mismatches. Rarely, however, the liquid contents of a tuberculous cavity or caseous lymph node may flood contiguous or noncontiguous regions of normal lung, producing acute air space disease (tuberculous pneumonia). Experimental evidence suggests that hypersensitivity to tuberculoprotein contributes to the genesis of this lesion. The resulting gas exchange defect is due to intrapulmonary shunt localized to lung parenchyma involved in the pneumonia.

Unlike tuberculous pneumonia, where heavily infected liquid caseum enters the bronchial tree, in miliary tuberculosis organisms enter the bloodstream either directly or indirectly, via lymphatics. Most patients with miliary tuberculosis and a miliary pattern on chest radiograph are not critically ill. They have pulmonary function abnormalities characteristic of interstitial lung disease.[2] The occasional development of respiratory failure under these circumstances, with the adult respiratory distress syndrome (ARDS), probably depends on the dose and type of bacillary antigen entering the bloodstream, as well as on the state of the host's cell-mediated immunity and possible delayed hypersensitivity.[3] No endotoxin or exotoxin has ever been identified in the tubercle bacillus. Although disseminated intravascular coagulation (DIC) has been associated with miliary tuberculosis complicated by ARDS, the weight of evidence suggests that DIC is not the cause of the respiratory failure but is itself secondary to thrombosis of small vessels in the region of the tubercles, or to a tuberculous arteritis.[4,5] DIC in association with ARDS due to miliary tuberculosis signals a poor prognosis.

CLINICAL MANIFESTATIONS

In fibrocaseous pulmonary tuberculosis, local and constitutional symptoms are nonspecific but are important for their chronicity. Coughing to clear cavitary secretions may become much more bothersome when bronchial involvement becomes extensive. In general, physical findings underestimate the extent of illness; despite extensive disease, they may be minimal until bronchogenic spread occurs and the patient develops respiratory failure. The presence of chronic cavitary pneumonia with acinar shadows on chest radiograph (Fig. 109-1) is characteristic.

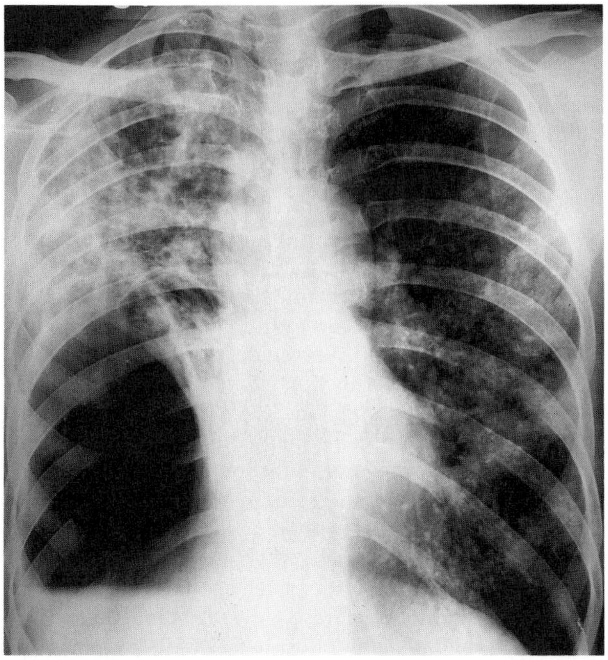

FIGURE 109-1 Tuberculous pneumonia. Fairly discrete acinar shadows are present in the left lung, remote from the confluent air space disease on the right.

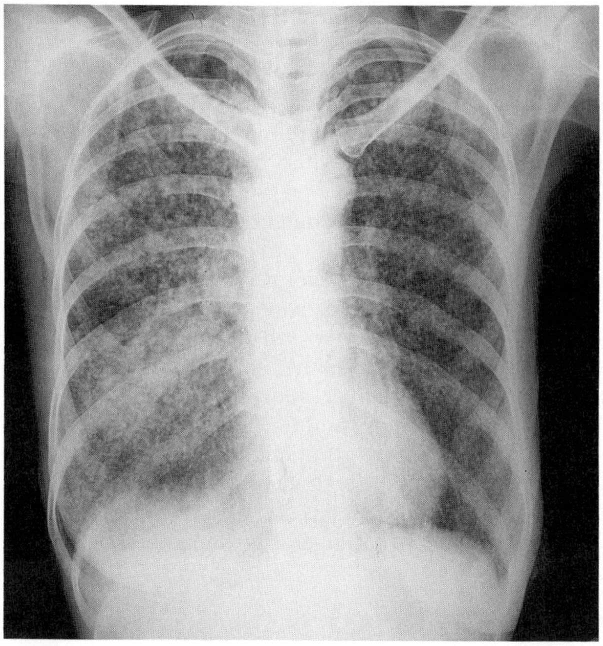

FIGURE 109-2 Miliary tuberculosis. Discrete small nodules 1 to 3 mm in size, uniformly distributed throughout the lungs.

Most patients with respiratory failure due to miliary tuberculosis have ARDS. Diagnostic difficulty arises mainly because of failure to consider miliary tuberculosis in someone who presents with ARDS of unknown etiology. Typically these patients are middle-aged or older and come from a population in which tuberculosis is endemic or one that is at increased risk of progressive disease (e.g., HIV infection). Often they are subacutely or chronically ill (with symptoms that have lasted over 2 weeks), with fever and weight loss, before they develop hematogeneous dissemination and respiratory failure.[6–13] Without treatment, most patients with miliary tuberculosis will die of respiratory failure.[14]

There may be a classic miliary pattern on chest radiograph (Fig. 109-2), but it is important to appreciate that no such pattern need be present. The earliest histologic finding in miliary tuberculosis is a focal exudative reaction involving two to five alveolar air spaces.[15] This lesion develops into a caseous or noncaseous tubercle that is thought to become radiographically discernible at about 6 weeks after the acute dissemination. Still later, as the cellular foci are transformed into hyaline connective tissue, the lesion shrinks in size and disappears from the radiograph. Multiple hematogenous seedings may occur in the same patient. Rarely, when the host is severely immunocompromised, an acute malignant form of miliary tuberculosis may occur. This has been called *nonreactive miliary tuberculosis,*[16] because the lesions are mainly necrotic, with few typical granulomas, and are teeming with tubercle bacilli. On other occasions, lymphatic involvement in the lung may predominate and result in a reticular network of thin, dense lines on chest radiograph—*lymphangitis reticularis tuberculosa.*[17]

Respiratory failure in both fibrocaseous and miliary tuberculosis may be complicated—and occasionally caused—by nonmycobacterial sepsis, massive hemoptysis, pneumothorax, and upper airway obstruction.

A wide variety of hematologic disturbances, including leukopenia, have been described in tuberculosis. These, together with alterations in local lung defense mechanisms, may contribute to the development of nonmycobacterial sepsis and a failure of the patient to respond to antituberculous therapy alone.[18]

Advanced fibrocaseous disease may be associated with massive hemoptysis, but this is not common. When aspirated, the blood may cause air space disease radiographically similar to tuberculous pneumonia. As with massive hemoptysis of other etiologies, urgent steps to localize and control the bleeding must be taken—bearing in mind that nonbronchial systemic collaterals may be the source (see Chap. 137).

As is the case with any necrotizing lung infection, pneumothorax, with possible bronchopleural fistula, is a recognized complication. Endobronchial disease may lead to air trapping (compounding the risk of barotrauma) and cause significant resistance to airflow.

DIAGNOSIS

Acid-fast bacilli are usually readily identifiable in the sputum of patients with tuberculous pneumonia. Unfortunately, significant hypoxemia may actually delay consideration of tuberculosis as a possible etiology of the pneumonia by suggesting a nontuberculous bacterial cause.[19] The relatively normal total leukocyte count found in tuberculosis may provide a clue that the pneumonia is not due to infection with pyogenic bacteria. The differential diagnosis includes nontuberculous chronic cavitary pneumonias such as those due to fungal disease, nocardiosis, melioidosis, and chronic cavitary *Klebsiella pneumoniae* infection.

Smear and culture of sputum or endotracheal secretions for acid-fast bacilli are negative in most cases of miliary tuberculosis, but should be performed repeatedly in any case. The tuberculin skin test is of extremely limited value in this context and is probably not worth doing. Diagnosis usually requires an invasive procedure, such as bone marrow biopsy, liver biopsy, lumbar puncture, or fiberoptic bronchoscopy with brushings and transbronchial biopsy. In the absence of an obvious extrapulmonary source for specimens we proceed from bone marrow biopsy to fiberoptic bronchoscopy with brushings and biopsy. The presence of caseation or acid-fast bacilli strongly suggests tuberculosis.

MANAGEMENT

DRUG ADMINISTRATION

The early administration of effective antituberculous drugs in adequate dosage is absolutely critical to recovery. If a tuberculous etiology of respiratory failure is strongly suspect, it is advisable to initiate therapy even before the results of diagnostic procedures are available. Although nontuberculous mycobacteria may cause similar disease, treatment should be directed at *M. tuberculosis* pending culture results. At least three drugs are recommended: isoniazid (INH) with pyridoxine (50 mg daily), rifampin (RIF), and streptomycin (SM). If possible, it is desirable to include a fourth: pyrazinamide (PZA). The use of such a four-drug regimen minimizes the chances that patients with drug-resistant *M. tuberculosis* will receive inadequate treatment. Drug resistance should be suspected in all immigrants from countries with a high prevalence of drug resistance; in all patients thought to have acquired their infection from a known resistant case; and in all patients from socioeconomically deprived groups, such as aboriginal peoples. The daily dose, route of administration, side effects, and monitoring of the five first-line drugs are outlined in Table 109-1. Ethambutol (EMB) may substitute for SM, but neither it nor PZA is available for parenteral use in North America. This may be an important consideration. INH and RIF may be delivered intravenously; experience with their prolonged administration by this route has recently been reported.[20]

DRUG TOXICITY

INH, RIF, PZA, and, rarely, EMB have all been reported to cause hepatitis. Moreover, they are frequently being administered to patients with underlying alcoholic liver disease as well as varying degrees of involvement of the liver by tuberculous infection. Fortunately, jaundice or significant hepatocellular dysfunction is uncommon from miliary tuberculosis alone, though in 90 to 100 percent of cases there is microscopic involvement of the liver. It is important, nevertheless, that liver function be monitored.

Most antituberculous drug–induced liver disease occurs within the first 3 months of therapy and is age-related; frequency increases substantially after age 35. We recommend at least weekly monitoring of liver enzymes, in particular the aspartate aminotransferase (AST), alanine aminotransferase (ALT), and alkaline phosphatase (AP) levels, as well as the liver function tests; serum albumin, bilirubin, and prothrombin time. If the liver enzymes rise to levels in excess of 3 times normal (especially if the ALT level is greater than 100 U/L), with or without new symptoms that may be ascribed to hepatobiliary disease (nausea, vomiting, vague abdominal discomfort), we are very concerned about liver toxicity and repeat the tests within 72 h. However, when the diagnosis of tuberculosis is certain and the patient is critically ill, continued treatment is essential. If levels remain stable we simply watch, as they may return to normal within 1 to 2 weeks. If, however, they continue to rise, we stop the INH, since it is by far the most likely offending agent.[21] Patients who have abnormalities in these measurements before treatment (e.g., those with alcoholic liver disease) who are asymptomatic to begin with but become symptomatic on therapy, or show evidence of deterioration in their enzyme levels or liver function tests on therapy, represent another group in which we would stop INH. It is probable that the toxicity of INH is enhanced by alcoholism. Cautious reintroduction of this agent may be attempted when enzymes or liver function tests return to

TABLE 109-1 First-Line Drugs in the Treatment of Tuberculosis

Drug	Daily Dose	Route	Side Effects	Monitoring
Isoniazid	5–10 mg/kg up to 300 mg	PO, IM, IV	Peripheral neuritis, hepatitis, hypersensitivity	ALT/AP/AST
Rifampin	10–20 mg/kg up to 600 mg	PO, IV	Hepatitis, febrile reaction, purpura (rare)	ALT/AP/AST
Pyrazinamide	15–30 mg/kg up to 2 g	PO	Hyperuricemia, hepatotoxicity	Uric acid, ALT/AP/AST
Streptomycin	15–30 mg/kg up to 1 g	IM	Cranial nerve VIII damage, nephrotoxicity	Vestibular function, audiograms, BUN, creatinine
Ethambutol	15 mg/kg	PO	Optic neuritis (reversible with discontinuation of drug; very rare at 15 mg/kg); skin rash	Red-green color, visual acuity

normal. So as not to lose track of these measurements, it is worthwhile to adopt the habit of plotting them on a graph.

CORTICOSTEROIDS

Provided the patient is receiving effective antituberculous drug therapy, it is our policy to administer pharmacologic doses of corticosteroids (methylprednisolone 125 mg IV twice daily) to all patients with acute respiratory failure due to tuberculosis unless there is a strong suspicion of coincident bacterial sepsis. Before this is done, a sample of blood for random serum cortisol determination should be sent. If the adrenal glands are functioning properly, a stress level should be recorded; however, it is not necessary to wait for this result before instituting systemic steroids. This approach is advised for the following reasons: **1.** It is often unclear whether adrenocortical insufficiency is present and contributing to the patient's instability—an uncertainty that may be compounded by the use of RIF, since this drug is known to induce hepatic microsomal enzymes and hence reduce the half-lives and clinical efficacy of corticosteroids[22]; **2.** Corticosteroids are acknowledged to reduce the exudative reaction and systemic toxicity in severe tuberculosis[23]; and **3.** corticosteroids have been demonstrated to hasten the resolution of tuberculous pneumonia.[24] It should be emphasized that these compounds can be administered safely provided the patient is taking an effective regimen of antituberculous drugs; generally we discontinue the steroids over a period of 1 to 6 weeks.

OTHER MANAGEMENT CONCERNS

Several related problems may require identification and treatment. Tuberculosis can deplete both visceral and skeletal muscle protein, potentiating cardiac and respiratory muscle dysfunction. Hyponatremia due to the syndrome of inappropriate antidiuretic hormone (SIADH) has also been described. And coexistent pericardial disease (see below) may also result in high left and right heart pressures, contributing to respiratory insufficiency and hepatic dysfunction.

PREVENTION

Public health measures must not be forgotten in the ICU. Ideally, all patients with smear-positive pulmonary tuberculosis should be isolated, regardless of whether they have an endotracheal tube in place or not. Ventilation should meet or exceed current published standards,[25] and, where possible, ultraviolet light should be added to further reduce the risk to personnel. Unfortunately, ordinary clinical masks are ineffective protection for those attending the patient; specifications for an alternate mask that is both effective and acceptable have yet to be established. Whenever possible, disposable circuitry should be used during mechanical ventilation, and a breathing circuit filter should be placed in the expiratory line. The circuitry and the filter should be changed every 12 h. If nondisposable equipment is used, it must be gas-sterilized before being reused.

Tuberculous Pericarditis

PATHOGENESIS AND CLINICAL MANIFESTATIONS

Although *M. tuberculosis* may infect the myocardium, the likelihood of this infection causing significant cardiac dysfunction is extremely remote. On the other hand, involvement of the pericardium, with the potential for cardiac tamponade or effusive-constrictive pericarditis, is not uncommon. Pericardial involvement is most often due to rupture of an adjacent caseous node into the pericardial sac. Less commonly it is part of a progressive hematogenous dissemination, often with involvement of other serosal surfaces.

Although the patient may present with fever and precordial pain, the onset is often subtle, dominated by the cardiovascular consequences of effusion. Cardiac compression with progressive impairment of diastolic filling results from rapidly evolving small-volume effusions or slowly evolving large-volume effusions—in accordance with the pressure-volume characteristics of the pericardium. Early on, compression is due to fluid alone; with time an effusive-constrictive process develops. From then on, cardiac compression will persist, as reflected in a persistently elevated jugular venous pressure, even though the effusion is removed and intrapericardial pressure reduced to normal by pericardiocentesis. When decompensated, the patient will present with low cardiac output, blood pressure, and pulse pressure, together with high jugular venous pressure and systemic vascular resistance.

DIAGNOSIS

The anatomic diagnosis of pericarditis with effusion is usually quickly made on the basis of physical findings and laboratory examinations—particularly cardiac ultrasound—but etiologic diagnosis is often difficult. The tuberculin test is usually, but not always, positive, and evidence of extrapericardial tuberculosis is usually lacking. Fever is usual but not invariable and also occurs with pericarditis of other etiologies. Routine hematologic and blood chemistry evaluation is not helpful except to detect or exclude abnormalities that may be associated with other causes of pericarditis. Fluid obtained by pericardiocentesis is similar to the fluid of tuberculous pleurisy (exudate with a lymphocyte pleocytosis), but a positive acid-fast smear is very uncommon, and culture is positive in only 25 to 50 percent of cases. We therefore limit pericardiocentesis to a therapeutic role and, in the absence of associated extrapericardial tuberculosis, favor pericardial biopsy for definitive diagnosis. Included in the differential diagnosis are granulomatous pericarditis secondary to rheumatoid arthritis or sarcoidosis, and malignant pericardial disease (see Chap. 121).

MANAGEMENT

Pericarditis with apparent circulatory compromise due to cardiac compression mandates urgent therapeutic and diagnostic pericardiocentesis, or subxiphoid pericardiostomy if there is a significant pericardial effusion present on echocardiography (see Chap. 27). Until this can be determined, cardiac output and blood pressure should be maintained by administration of intravenous fluids (see Chap. 121). Should the right atrial or central venous pressure remain elevated and cardiac output and blood pressure fail to respond after the intrapericardial pressure has been returned to normal, or should there be no pericardial effusion on echocardiography, the next step is urgent pericardiectomy.

All patients are treated with antituberculous drugs as for pulmonary tuberculosis. Unless otherwise contraindicated, we also administer prednisone, 60 to 80 mg/day, and taper the dosage over 6 weeks. Patients not requiring pericardiectomy at the outset should be followed clinically and with repeat echocardiography over a period of 6 to 8 weeks. Those developing constrictive pericarditis during this time undergo pericardiectomy; those not developing it appear to do well.[26]

Tuberculous Meningitis

PATHOGENESIS AND CLINICAL MANIFESTATIONS

Tuberculous meningitis is usually due to rupture of a subependymal tubercle into the subarachnoid space, rather than direct hematogenous seeding of the meninges themselves; this accounts for the observation that when meningitis complicates miliary disease it generally develops after several weeks of illness. The brunt of the pathologic process falls on the basal meninges, where a thick gelatinous exudate accumulates, obliterating the pontine and interpeduncular cisterns and extending to the meninges around the medulla, the floor of the third ventricle and subthalamic region, the optic chiasm, and the undersurfaces of the temporal lobes. By comparison, the convexities are little involved. The exudate also surrounds the spinal cord. Unlike the pyogenic meningitides, the inflammatory exudate is not confined to the subarachnoid space but frequently spreads along the pial vessels and invades the underlying brain. Cranial nerves are involved by the inflammatory exudate as they traverse the subarachnoid space. Arteries become inflamed and occluded, with infarction of brain. Blockage of the basal cisterns frequently results in a meningeal obstructive hydrocephalus. Hydrocephalus due to marked ependymitis with blockage of cerebrospinal fluid (CSF) in the aqueduct or fourth ventricle is a less common occurrence.

DIAGNOSIS

Tuberculous meningitis can be strongly suspected when meningeal signs are associated with active extrameningeal tuberculosis, but the cornerstone of diagnosis is examination of the CSF. In one recent series,[27] 65 percent of cases demonstrated between 100 and 500 cells per mm^3, 14 percent contained between 0 and 99, and the remainder between 500 and 1500; the protein concentration was 100 to 500 mg/dL in 65 percent of cases but under 100 mg/dL in 25 percent; and the CSF sugar content, said to be characteristically low, was less than 45 mg/dL in only 17 percent of cases. Lymphocytes were the preponderant cells in 73 percent of patients, the remainder demonstrating a majority of polymorphonuclear leukocytes, usually early in the course. Acid-fast bacilli were visible on the stained CSF sediment in a minority of cases in the initial examination; but importantly, when the fluid from four serial spinal taps was examined, the organisms were seen in 87 percent. Because poor prognosis is directly related to delayed diagnosis, treatment should commence as soon as a presumptive diagnosis is made, without waiting for bacteriologic confirmation. In a patient suspected of having tuberculous meningitis, computed tomography (CT) and nuclear magnetic resonance imaging (MRI) may provide useful diagnostic and prognostic information by defining the presence and extent of basilar arachnoid meningitis, the presence of cerebral infarction, and the presence and course of hydrocephalus.[28] The differential diagnosis includes viral meningitis and other chronic inflammatory processes.

MANAGEMENT

INH, RIF, and PZA are recommended. With meningeal inflammation the concentration of INH and CSF equals that in the blood. Doses of 10 mg/kg daily are advisable until a favorable course has been established; thereafter the usual doses suffice. RIF also penetrates the blood/brain barrier fairly well, reaching a concentration, on average, half as high as that in the blood but well above the minimal inhibitory concentration for *M. tuberculosis.* PZA is also recommended in all cases, as it reaches concentrations in the CSF equal to those in serum and significantly adds to the early bactericidal activity of INH and RIF.

Most authorities advise the adjunctive use of corticosteroids in patients with **1.** confusion or the presence of focal signs such as cranial nerve palsies or hemiplegia, or **2.** stupor or dense paraplegia or hemiplegia.[29]

Tuberculous Adrenocortical Insufficiency

PATHOGENESIS AND CLINICAL MANIFESTATIONS

In classic Addison's disease the tuberculosis is inactive and the adrenocortical tissue is replaced with granulomas, often partially calcified. Reactivation of tuberculosis, either in a localized form (e.g., in an area of lung) or in a disseminated miliary form, may occur in such patients, resulting in symptoms and signs of active tuberculosis as well as chronic adrenal insufficiency. Miliary tuberculosis may also involve the adrenals incidentally, producing random granulomas that do not cause functional impairment; or massively, resulting in acute or subacute adrenal failure.[30]

DIAGNOSIS

The diagnosis may be suggested when a patient with suspected or proven tuberculosis develops hypotension refractory to volume and vasoactive drugs. The finding of bilaterally enlarged, calcified adrenals on CT of the abdomen[31] may further support the diagnosis. It is important to be aware that the random cortisol level may still be in the normal range; the diagnosis of adrenal insufficiency is then confirmed by an absence of response to intravenous corticotropin (see Chap. 160).

TREATMENT

Adrenocortical insufficiency secondary to active tuberculosis necessitates the administration of stress levels of glucocorticoids (hydrocortisone 100 mg bolus, repeated every 6 to 8 h) and maintenance doses of mineralocorticoids (fludrocortisone acetate 0.05 to 0.1 mg orally per day), in addition to antituberculous drugs as for pulmonary disease.

Tuberculosis and HIV Infection

Tuberculosis is an especially common opportunistic infection in HIV-infected persons from populations with a high background prevalence of tuberculous infection—e.g., intravenous drug abusers, and immigrants from Africa and Central America. The presentation may be unusual; there is a greater frequency of extrapulmonary disease, and pulmonary disease may be noncavitary, involve any lung zones, and be associated with intrathoracic adenopathy—features atypical of postprimary disease in non-HIV-infected persons.

Invasive procedures may be necessary for diagnosis; however, the yield of a positive sputum smear from persons with pulmonary tuberculosis and HIV infection is only slightly less than that in patients with pulmonary tuberculosis alone. Immunosuppression may reduce the likelihood of seeing granulomas on biopsy.

Just as tuberculosis should be considered in any HIV-infected individual also at risk for tuberculous infection, HIV infection must be considered in any tuberculous patient from a high-risk group for HIV infection. The implications of co-infection relate to public health, safety of health care workers, and the possibility that vital organ dysfunction is not purely related to *M. tuberculosis* but may also be due to other HIV-related opportunistic infections or malignancies. Tuberculosis in HIV–co-infected persons appears to respond well to the usual antituberculous drugs; a minimum of 9 months and at least 6 months of therapy following documented culture conversion is recommended.

CASE PRESENTATION

A 24-year-old Native American woman was referred with a 3-week history of fever and cough. Her symptoms had begun within hours of delivery of her first child. Her pregnancy and past health had been unremarkable except for ethanol abuse. The cough was productive of yellowish, occasionally blood-tinged, sputum. No acute process was seen on chest radiograph. Routine culture of sputum and urine had not identified a specific pathogen, and there was no evidence of genital tract infection. The fever had not responded to broad-spectrum antibiotics. On the day of her referral she had become dyspneic; upon admission she was tachypneic (respiratory rate 36) and her lips and nail beds were cyanotic. Bronchial breathing was heard over both lungs posteriorly. The jugular venous pressure was within normal limits. The liver span was 12 cm. A spleen tip, but no lymphadenopathy, was felt. A room air arterial blood gas analysis revealed a Pa_{O_2} of 37 mmHg, a Pa_{CO_2} of 28 mmHg, and a pH of 7.50. A chest radiograph revealed a miliary pattern with some volume loss in the left lower lobe. The total leukocyte count in peripheral blood was 8000/mm^3, with 35 percent mature and 51 percent young polymorphonuclear leukocytes. The serum albumin level was 2.4 g/dL. A urinalysis was reported as showing 100 pus cells, many erythrocytes, and no bacteria. A Mantoux test was negative; however, a Mantoux test performed 6 years earlier, because of a family history of tuberculosis, had been positive, with 20 mm of induration. A presumptive diagnosis of miliary tuberculosis was made, antituberculous drugs were begun, and sputum and urine were sent for acid-fast smear and culture. Supplemental oxygen was delivered by face mask. On the night of the patient's admission her blood pressure fell to 75 mmHg systolic during sleep. Intravenous saline solution was administered, a random serum cortisol was sent, and the patient was begun on intravenous cortisone acetate. An echocardiogram was reported as normal. There was no clinical or laboratory evidence of DIC, nor of HIV infection. Her blood pressure improved but she became increasingly dyspneic so that intubation and mechanical ventilation became necessary. A pulmonary artery catheter was inserted. The shunt fraction was 28 percent, cardiac output 17 L/min., arterial-venous content difference 2.7 vol %, pulmonary capillary wedge pressure 18 mmHg, systemic arterial pressure 160/60 mmHg. The systemic vascular resistance was estimated to be 440 dyn · s/cm^5. Systemic steroids were continued, fluid restricted, antituberculous drugs given parenterally, and enteral feeding begun. The patient's hemodynamic and gas exchange abnormalities improved dramatically over the next 24 to 48 h (cardiac output 5 to 10 L/min, pulmonary capillary wedge pressure 5 to 10 mmHg) and it was possible to extubate her within 5 days. The serum cortisol measurement performed prior to intubation revealed a stress level of circulating cortisol. Sputum and urine were positive for acid-fast bacilli on smear, and ultimately were positive for *M. tuberculosis* on culture. A bone marrow examination performed on the first day of the patient's admission revealed granulomas.

CASE DISCUSSION

This patient's clinical course is typical of the patient who develops respiratory failure from miliary tuberculosis. The classic presentation—coming from a population in which the disease is endemic and having a prolonged febrile illness, a normal total leukocyte count, and a miliary pattern on chest radiograph—permitted a rapid diagnosis of tuberculosis at the referral center. Antituberculous drugs were begun empirically, with no waiting for confirmation of the diagnosis. Upon arrival at the referral hospital the patient was in hypoxemic respiratory failure but compensated. During the first night her condition deteriorated. A low blood pressure was probably secondary to a low systemic vascular resistance as well as volume depletion. Hypoadrenalism, cardiac compression or dysfunction, and blood loss were ruled out. Increasing dyspnea was probably secondary to an increased work of breathing as well as possibly deteriorating gas exchange secondary to increased lung water after vigorous volume replacement. The rapid improvement in hemodynamics and gas exchange is not explainable on the basis of antituberculous drug effects or nutritional support alone. Volume restriction and suppression of the inflammatory response appeared to be major contributors to the patient's early recovery.

Acknowledgment

The author wishes to thank Heather Smith for her preparation of this chapter.

References

1. Agarwal MK, Muthuswamy PP, Banner AS, et al: Respiratory failure in pulmonary tuberculosis. Chest 72:605, 1977.
2. Williams MH Jr, Yoo OH, Kane C: Pulmonary function in miliary tuberculosis. Am Rev Respir Dis 107:858, 1973.
3. Dannenburg AM Jr: Immune mechanisms in the pathogenesis of pulmonary tuberculosis. Rev Infect Dis II:S369, 1989.
4. Goldfine ID, Schachter H, Barclay WR, Kingdon HS: Consumption coagulopathy in miliary tuberculosis. Ann Intern Med 71:775, 1969.
5. Krauss JS, Walter DH: Miliary tuberculosis and consumption of clotting factors by multifocal vasculopathic coagulation. South Med J 72:1479, 1979.
6. Huseby JS, Hudson LD: Miliary tuberculosis and adult respiratory distress syndrome. Ann Intern Med 85:609, 1976.
7. Murray HW, Tuazon CU, Kirmani N, Sheagren JN: The adult respiratory distress syndrome associated with tuberculosis. Chest 73:37, 1976.
8. Hsu JT, Padula JP, Ryan SF: Miliary tuberculosis and respiratory distress syndrome. Ann Intern Med 89:140, 1978.
9. Fieber SS, Cohn JD, Jacobs FM: Adult respiratory distress syndrome secondary to activated miliary tuberculosis following surgery. J Med Soc NJ 76:357, 1979.
10. Dee P, Teja K, Korzeniowski O, Suratt PM: Miliary tuberculosis resulting in adult respiratory distress syndrome: A surviving case. AJR 134:569, 1980.
11. So SY, Yu D: The adult respiratory distress syndrome associated with miliary tuberculosis. Tubercle 62:49, 1981.
12. Dyer RA, Chappell WA, Potgieter PO: Adult respiratory distress syndrome associated with miliary tuberculosis. Crit Care Med 13:12, 1985.
13. Piqueras AR, Marruecos L, Artigas A, Rodriguez C: Miliary tuberculosis and adult respiratory distress syndrome. Intensive Care Med 13:175, 1987.
14. Chapman CB, Whorton CM: Acute generalized miliary tuberculosis in adults. N Engl J Med 235:239, 1946.
15. Auerbach O: Acute generalized miliary tuberculosis. Am J Pathol 20:121, 1944.
16. O'Brien JR: Non-reactive tuberculosis. J Clin Pathol 7:216, 1954.
17. Price M: Lymphangitis reticularis tuberculosa. Tubercle 49:377, 1968.
18. Agarwal MK, Muthuswamy PT, Banner AS, Addington WW: Septicemia: Occurrence with bacteriologically positive pulmonary tuberculosis. JAMA 238:2297, 1977.
19. Heffner JE, Strange C, Sahn SA: The impact of respiratory failure on the diagnosis of tuberculosis. Arch Intern Med 148:1103, 1988.
20. Koestner JA, Jones LK, Polk WH, Sawyers JL: Prolonged use of intravenous isoniazid and rifampin. DICP, Ann of Pharm 23:48, 1989.
21. Maddrey WC: Isoniazid-induced liver disease. Semin Liver Dis 1:129, 1981.
22. Edwards OM, Galley JM, Courtenay-Evans RJ, et al: Changes in cortisol metabolism following rifampicin therapy. Lancet 7:549, 1974.
23. Horne NW: A critical evaluation of corticosteroids in tuberculosis. Adv Tuberc Res 15:1, 1966.
24. McLean RL, Ward A, Wilborn JW Jr, Burton ZC Jr: Early corticosteroid effect on acute tuberculous pneumonia. Twenty-second Research Conference in Pulmonary Diseases. Veterans Adm Med Bull 97, 1963.
25. Nardell EA: Dodging droplet nuclei, Am Rev Respir Dis 142:501, 1990.
26. Long R, Younes M, Patton N, Hershfield E: Tuberculous pericarditis: Long term outcome in patients who received medical therapy alone. Am Heart J 117:1133, 1989.
27. Kennedy DH, Fallon RJ: Tuberculous meningitis. JAMA 241:264, 1979.
28. Bhargava S, Gupta AK, Tandon PN: Tuberculous meningitis: A CT study. Br J Radiol 55:189, 1982.
29. O'Toole RD, Thornton GF, Mukherjee MK, Nath RL: Dexamethasone in tuberculous meningitis: Relationship of cerebrospinal fluid effects to therapeutic efficacy. Ann Intern Med 70:39, 1969.
30. Sadler de CMR, Beresford OD: Miliary tuberculosis associated with Addison's disease. Tubercle 52:298, 1971.
31. Wilms GE, Baert AL, Kint EJ, et al: Computed tomographic findings in bilateral adrenal tuberculosis. Radiology 146:729, 1983.

Chapter 110
TETANUS

PERRY GRAY
DANIEL ROBERTS

KEY POINTS

- *Tetanus is a toxin-mediated disease caused by* Clostridium tetani *and characterized by trismus, dysphagia, and localized muscle rigidity near a site of injury, often progressing to severe generalized muscular spasms complicated by respiratory failure and cardiovascular instability.*
- *The diagnosis of tetanus is made on clinical grounds alone. A clinical diagnosis of presumed tetanus is sufficient to initiate treatment.*
- *Patients with tetanus should be managed in an intensive care unit. In severe cases, the first priority is control of the airway to ensure adequate ventilation and correction of hypotension related to hypovolemia and/or autonomic instability.*
- *Antitoxin therapy with human tetanus immune globulin is given intramuscularly (3000 to 6000 I.U.) as early as possible. In cases that have not yet progressed to generalized spasms, 250 I.U. given intrathecally by lumbar puncture is advised.*
- *Treatment to limit continued production and absorption of toxin includes surgical debridement of the site of injury and antimicrobial therapy with intravenous penicillin or metronidazole.*
- *Muscle rigidity and spasms are treated with high dose diazepam and morphine. In some cases, addition of a nondepolarizing muscle relaxant is also needed.*
- *Cardiovascular instability due to autonomic dysfunction is managed by ensuring normovolemia, diazepam, and morphine therapy and magnesium sulfate infusion when needed.*
- *Supportive measures include early provision of nutrition, correction of electrolyte disturbances, subcutaneous heparin administration for prophylaxis of deep venous thrombosis, and prompt antimicrobial therapy for nosocomial infection.*
- *With meticulous management of the manifestations of this disease and careful attention to prevention of its major complications, complete recovery is possible in most cases.*

Tetanus is one of the best examples of a disease for which modern intensive care can offer a truly major improvement in long-term useful survival. Often a disease of otherwise healthy active people, the fully developed form is frequently rapidly fatal unless the patient is supported through a lengthy period of painful muscle spasms complicated by respiratory failure, cardiovascular instability, and increased risk of pulmonary embolism and nosocomial infection. However, if all of these problems are meticulously managed, complete recovery can be expected. In developed countries, this disease is likely to remain an uncommon but challenging problem that demands an alert and aggressive approach to initial diagnosis and management coupled with careful attention to supportive care and avoidance of complications over a period of weeks to months to achieve the eventual excellent outcome possible in most cases.

Pathogenesis

Although tetanus is primarily a disease of underdeveloped countries, there are approximately 100 cases per year reported in the United States.[1,2] The male–female ratio is approximately 3:1, representing a greater incidence of tetanus prone wounds in males. Because preformed circulating antibody to tetanospasmin can completely prevent development of the disease, tetanus occurs primarily in nonimmunized or inadequately immunized patients. However, in rare instances tetanus has developed in patients who had received their primary series, as well as proper "booster" doses of toxoid,[3,4] so a history of proper immunization does not entirely exclude the diagnosis of tetanus.

The disease is caused by *Clostridium tetani,* an anaerobic bacterium that exists in both vegetative and sporulated forms and has been isolated from soil, feces of humans and animals, dust, wounds, intact skin, catgut, and talcum powder. During unfavorable conditions the organism exists in the sporulated form, which can remain viable for several months. It is resistant to boiling and antiseptics but is killed by autoclaving at 121°C for 15 min. *Clostridium tetani* is not locally invasive and does not provoke an inflammatory response, and inoculation of spores into viable tissue does not produce tetanus. However, tissue necrosis, foreign bodies, or concurrent anaerobic or facultative anaerobic infections lower the normal oxidation-reduction potential of the tissue, which allows conversion to the vegetative form with subsequent toxin formation. The toxins produced include *tetanolysin,* which causes in vitro hemolysis but plays no role in the development of the disease, and *tetanospasmin,* which is a potent neurotoxin responsible for the clinical disease state. Toxin formed in a skin wound enters the underlying muscle and may spread to adjacent muscles. It then accumulates in the nerve endings of motor fibers. Retrograde transport of the toxin then occurs via intraaxonal and periaxonal pathways from nerve endings to the ventral horns of the spinal cord or motor nuclei of the cranial nerves. If toxin is produced in larger amounts, it also accumulates in the lymphatic system of the invaded muscle, enters the blood stream via the thoracic duct, and is disseminated throughout the body. Toxin passing from blood to skeletal muscle then accumulates in the nerve endings of the motor fibers and proceeds to the ventral horns (or cranial nuclei) or is taken up by the lymphatic system and recirculated in the blood. The rate of accumulation of toxin in the ventral horns of the spinal cord depends on the length of the neural pathway and the activity of the muscles involved.[5] Since jaw muscles and spinal postural muscles have short neural pathways to the ventral horns and are continually active in the awake human, this is the likely explanation for trismus and neck stiffness early in the course of the illness.

In the anterior horn or cranial nerve nuclei the toxin accumulates in the presynaptic apparatus and impairs spontaneous secretion and evoked release of neurotransmitter. Because inhibitory synapses are more sensitive to the effects of tetanus toxin than excitatory synapses, impaired inhibition of motoneurons and interneurons results in enhanced excitation and muscular rigidity. Disruption of the inhibitory interneurons within the propriospinal connections results in enhanced excitation such that stimulation from the periphery, such as light touch or visual or auditory stimuli from the reticular formation, can result in the generalized spasms seen in tetanus.

The effect of tetanus toxin on the neuromuscular junction is presynaptic inhibition of acetylcholine release, which can result in paralysis of muscles. Paralysis is less frequent and usually localized to areas of high toxin concentration because the neuromuscular junction is not as sensitive to tetanus toxin as the inhibitory neurons.

Autonomic dysfunction in severe tetanus is well described but poorly understood. Whether this dysfunction represents a direct effect of the toxin or a secondary response to factors arising during the development of tetanus is not clear.

Classification

There are three clinical forms of tetanus; generalized, local, and cephalic. Generalized tetanus is the most common form and is characterized by diffuse muscle rigidity. Localized tetanus is characterized by rigidity of a group of muscles in close proximity to the site of injury. Cephalic tetanus, which is a variant of local tetanus, is defined as trismus plus paralysis of one or more cranial nerves.[6] It is important to realize that both local and cephalic tetanus may progress to generalized tetanus, the latter occurring in approximately 65 percent of cases.

Clinical and Laboratory Manifestations

The most common means by which *C. tetani* enters the human host is through lacerations, especially if associated with tissue necrosis or foreign body. Tetanus can also follow burns or animal bites, septic abortion complicated by gangrene of the uterus and, rarely, after otherwise uncomplicated abdominal surgery.[7] Untreated middle ear infections account for up to 30 percent of the cases of tetanus in India.[8] Intravenous drug users can develop tetanus associated with skin infections caused by use of inadequately sterilized needles.[9] However, in 15 to 25 percent of cases a portal of entry cannot be determined *(cryptogenic tetanus)*.[3,8,9]

The interval between injury and onset of clinical symptoms is usually from 3 days to 3 weeks but occasionally is as long as several months. Cephalic tetanus after scalp or facial injury tends to occur earlier with an incubation period of 1 day to 2 weeks.[6] In general, the shorter the incubation period, the more severe the disease. However, a long incubation does not guarantee a mild attack.

Muscular rigidity is the most prominent early symptom of tetanus. Rigidity of the masseter muscle (trismus) results in difficulty opening the mouth and chewing. Rigidity of the facial muscles gives the characteristic smile of tetanus *(risus sardonicus)*. Opisthotonos is caused by rigidity of the vertebral muscles and antigravity muscles. Abdominal muscle rigidity may simulate peritonitis. Nuchal rigidity may simulate meningitis. In the Edmonson and Flowers series of 100 patients,[3] trismus and dysphagia (described as sore throat) were the presenting symptoms in 75 cases and neck and back stiffness in 14 cases. However, in 91 cases, it was possible to demonstrate trismus on initial physical examination.

The period of onset of the disease is defined as the interval between the first symptom and the first generalized muscular spasm. Approximately 75 percent of patients with tetanus will have spasms. A shorter period of onset is usually predictive of a severe attack.

Spasms are initially tonic, followed first by high-frequency and then low-frequency clonic activity. In very severe tetanus, spasms may occur so frequently that status epilepticus may be suspected and may be forceful enough to cause fractures of long bones and of the spine. Spasm-induced damage to muscles can also result in rhabdomyolysis complicated by acute renal failure.[10] They may be initiated by touch, noise, lights, and swallowing, even in the sleeping patient. Spasms severe enough to require treatment may persist for up to 6 weeks.

In addition to being extremely painful, spasms can produce a variety of significant secondary effects. Apnea occurs when spasms involve the respiratory muscles or larynx. Paralysis of skeletal muscle may occur following periods of sustained spasms due to presynaptic inhibition of acetylcholine release at the neuromuscular junction. Similarly, paralysis of urinary bladder musculature together with spasm of perineal muscles have been implicated in causing acute urinary retention. In pregnancy, spasms can cause abortion or miscarriage, although the fetus is not directly affected since the toxin does not cross the placenta. Inadequately treated spasms can also produce fever, although secondary infection and direct and indirect actions of toxin on hypothalamic temperature regulation are often implicated.

The autonomic nervous system dysfunction of severe tetanus usually occurs 1 to 2 weeks after the onset of the disease but may occur earlier.[11] Manifestations of impaired sympathetic inhibition include tachycardia, labile hypertension alternating with hypotension, peripheral vasoconstriction, fever, and profuse sweating. Overactivity of the parasympathetic nervous system causes increased bronchial and salivary gland secretions, bradycardia, and sinus arrest.[12]

A complete blood count will usually show a leukocytosis with a left shift and, less frequently, a lymphocytosis. Examination of urine may reveal proteinuria and leukocytes thought to be due to accumulation of tetanus toxin in the kidneys.[8] Other nonspecific laboratory abnormalities include elevation of serum transaminases, increased catecholamine levels in serum and urine and decreased serum cholinesterase level. Creatine phosphokinase (CPK) is usually normal initially but generally rises with the onset of muscular spasms. Although the cerebrospinal fluid (CSF) in tetanus has frequently been said to be normal,[1–3] Idoko reported elevated CSF protein levels ranging from 540 to 4000 mg/L in 12 out of 15 patients with tetanus.[13]

Complications of tetanus are numerous and frequent. The need for long-term endotracheal intubation and ventilatory support coupled with increased risk of aspiration may result in bacterial pneumonia. Other nosocomial infections also occur, as in many patients requiring long-term stay in an intensive care unit (ICU). These may include infections of vascular access catheters, catheter-related urosepsis, and infected decubitus ulcers. Protracted immobilization places the patient at risk for deep venous thrombosis and pulmonary thromboembolism, which is not infrequently reported as a cause of death.

Diagnosis

The diagnosis of tetanus is based on clinical manifestations rather than laboratory tests. Tissue cultures are positive in less than 50 percent of patients.[14] Since the organism is noninvasive, blood cultures are of little value except in diagnosing secondary infection. The major clinical features on which the diagnosis of tetanus is based are listed in Table 110-1 along with the features of other conditions with which it can be confused. Strychnine poisoning may present with trismus, risus sardonicus, extensor spasms, opisthotonos, hyperflexia, stiffness, and myalgia. Symptoms usually begin 5 to 60 min after ingestion and resolve after 6 h, although the hyperflexia, stiffness, and muscle pains may last 3 to 7 days. The short duration of the disease allows differentiation from tetanus. Trismus, dysphagia, oculogyric crisis, involuntary contractions of muscle groups, and opisthotonos are all signs of an acute dystonic reaction caused by neuroleptic drugs. Stiff-man syndrome is characterized by initially intermittent followed by continuous spasms of limb and trunk muscles that disappear during sleep. Rabies may present with hyperexcitability, dysphagia, dyspnea, respiratory muscle spasms, and opisthotonos. However, trismus, facial palsy, nuchal rigidity, and continuous muscle rigidity are not seen in rabies. Cutaneous hyperaesthesia is quite marked in rabies, as are disturbances in mentation, and both are absent in tetanus. Isolated paralysis of the facial nerve may be due to Bell's palsy or an early manifestation of cephalic tetanus.[8] Patients with meningitis have nuchal rigidity but not trismus. However, examination of CSF is mandatory if the diagnosis is unsure. Determination of serum calcium will rule out hypocalcemic tetany. Unlike trismus owing to these processes, tetanic trismus becomes more pronounced as the jaw is forced open.[8] Isolated trismus may be due to subluxation or arthritis of the temporomandibular joint or any inflammatory process involving teeth, mouth, tonsils, or pharynx.

Treatment

Patients with a presumptive diagnosis of tetanus should be admitted to an ICU.[3,14–16] Since the period of onset of the disease ranges from less than 1 to 12 days, even patients with mild tetanus (trismus, dysphagia, and localized rigidity) should be observed in an ICU for at least 1 week (2 weeks if no resolution of symptoms is noted). Patients with incubation periods of greater than 20 days who have only localized rigidity can be safely discharged to the ward after a few days of observation provided no progression of the disease has occurred.

The principles of initial treatment of tetanus consist of airway management, sedation, treatment of the portal of entry, antitoxin therapy, administration of appropriate antibiotics, and general supportive measures.[3,8,14–16] Drugs commonly used in the management of tetanus are listed in Table 110-2 together with their indications and usual doses.

Appropriate management of the airway is the first priority. Patients with trismus and localized rigidity with no evidence of respiratory compromise do not require prophylactic endotracheal intubation. Patients with diffuse rigidity, especially if unresponsive to benzodiazepine therapy, should be intubated, even in the absence of respiratory compromise. Intubation should be performed in all patients who have already had a generalized spasm or in any patient with evidence of respiratory compromise, including patients with severe dysphagia who are in danger of aspiration. The preferred route (nasotracheal vs. orotracheal) and method (awake vs. anesthetized) of intubation depends on

TABLE 110-1 Differential Diagnosis of Tetanus: Clinical Features

	Tetanus	Strychnine	Neuroleptics	SMS*	Rabies	Meningitis
Trismus	+	+	+	+	−	−
Nuchal Rigidity	+	+	+	+	−	+
Risus Sardonicus	+	+	−	−	−	−
Opisthotonus	+	+	+	−	+	−
Muscle Rigidity Continuous	+	+	+	−	−	−
Muscle Rigidity Intermittent	−	−	−	+	+	−
Encephalopathy	−	−	−	−	+	+
Rapid Course	−	+	+	−	−	−

*Stiff-man syndrome.

TABLE 110-2 Drugs Used in Medical Management of Tetanus

Medication	Indication	Dose*
hTIG†	Local or cephalic tetanus	250 I.U. intrathecal
hTIG	Generalized tetanus	3000–6000 I.U. intramuscular
Penicillin G	Toxin production (given in all cases)	1×10^6 units IV q6h for 10 days
Diazepam	Cardiovascular instability and sedation	2.5–20 mg IV q2–6h
Morphine	Sedation and analgesia	2.0–10 mg IV q1h or 1.0–2.0 mg/kg IV q12h
Magnesium sulfate	Cardiovascular instability	70 mg/kg IV load; then 1–3 g IV q1h
Vecuronium	Neuromuscular blockade for severe muscle spasms	3–4 mg/h IV

*Abbreviations: q1h, q2h, etc.: every 1 h, every 2 h, etc.
†Human tetanus immune globulin.

the clinical situation. Ideally intubation should be performed by an anesthesiologist. An emergency cricothyroidotomy tray should be at the bedside prior to attempted intubation. If paralysis is required to facilitate intubation, a nondepolarizing agent should be used as depolarizing neuromuscular blocking agents (i.e., succinylcholine) may cause hyperkalemia and cardiac arrest in patients with tetanus.[17]

Patients with muscular rigidity should be sedated with intravenous diazepam and morphine. The doses should be titrated to reduce rigidity and provide adequate analgesia, respectively. Tetanic spasms are treated using a combination of intubation and ventilation, sedation, and neuromuscular blockers.[3,8,14,18] Pancuronium,[8] atracurium,[19] and vecuronium[18] have been reported as being safe and effective in controlling tetanic spasms. Vecuronium has no cardiovascular side effects, which may be advantageous in treating patients with autonomic dysfunction.[18]

Aggressive surgical treatment of tetanus-producing wounds results in improved survival. The wound should be excised with a 2-cm margin.[2] If gangrene is present, amputation of the extremity at least one uninvolved joint proximal to the wound should be performed.[2] The decision to perform a hysterectomy on a patient who develops tetanus following induced abortion or in the postpartum period should be based on the presence of associated invasive bacterial sepsis, gangrene of the uterus, or uterine injury. Tetanus is not an indication for hysterectomy.[8,16]

Several studies comparing mortality rates of patients with tetanus treated with and without antitoxin have produced conflicting results. However, the importance of answering this question has been markedly reduced by the availability of hTIG, which has no serious adverse effects. It is now generally agreed that patients with tetanus should be treated with antitoxin as soon as possible.[3,8,14,16] However, controversy persists regarding the preferred route and dosage of antitoxin. There is evidence that in patients who have not yet progressed to generalized rigidity and spasms, intrathecal hTIG is more effective than intramuscular hTIG in preventing generalization, and can reduce the mortality rate.[20] Conversely, once generalization has occurred, the administration of intrathecal hTIG has failed to improve survival.[21] It is currently recommended that all patients with tetanus that is not yet generalized receive a single dose of intrathecal hTIG (250 I.U.) via lumbar puncture. Ideally, preparations containing no preservatives should be used for intrathecal injections. Preparations containing thiomersol as a preservative result in a higher incidence of vomiting. However, no more serious side effects have been reported to date. Intramuscular doses of hTIG ranging from 3000 to 6000 I.U. have been suggested.[14,16] It is important to administer antitoxin prior to debridement because the toxin may be introduced into the blood stream during manipulation.[1,4]

Antibiotics are generally given both to treat infection at the injury site and to eliminate continued toxin production. Penicillin G, 1 million units intravenously (IV) every 6 h for 10 days is the antibiotic of first choice for *C. tetani*.[14,16] Metronidazole, tetracycline, erythromycin, and chloramphenicol are also effective.[14,16,22]

General supportive measures include establishing intravenous access to maintain adequate fluid and electrolyte balance. A Foley catheter should be inserted in all but the mildest cases to prevent urinary retention. Sulcralfate should be given prophylactically for stress ulcers. Muscular spasms and increased catecholamine release have been implicated in producing a hypermetabolic state with consequent rapid development of nutritional deficiency.[23] Therefore, early provision of adequate nutrition is a priority. Ideally, intubated patients should be fed using the nasojejunal route to minimize the possibility of aspiration. Subcutaneous heparin is given to prevent deep venous thrombosis. Physiotherapy prevents contractures in patients treated with neuromuscular blockers.

Arterial and pulmonary artery catheterization may be required to manage the autonomic dysfunction of severe tetanus.[1] The cardiac output may be low or normal but is more commonly elevated.[24,25] The pulmonary capillary wedge pressure and central venous pressure are usually normal but may be low in patients with severe spasms and diaphoresis, which have led to hypovolemia. It is important to ensure that hypovolemia is promptly corrected, since this will substantially increase the potential for immediately life-threatening hypotension in the presence of the autonomic instability. Treatment of cardiovascular instability consists of deep sedation, which, if not successful, is followed by high-dose magnesium sulfate infusions.[24–26] Diazepam, in doses up to 20 mg/h IV should be tried initially, followed by morphine using doses of up to 10 mg/h. Alternately, successful control of autonomic dysfunction has been achieved using intermittent boluses of morphine, 1 to 2 mg/kg IV over 15 min every 12 h.[25] If magnesium sulfate is used, it is important that diazepam and morphine be continued.[26] A loading dose of 70 mg/kg IV over 5 to 20 min is followed by a continuous infusion titrated to maintain serum magnesium levels between 2.5 and 4.0 mmol/L. This usually requires infusion rates of 1 to 3 g/h.[24] Serum calcium and magnesium levels should be measured every 4 h. Calcium supplements may be required to maintain serum calcium levels above 1.7 mmol/L.[24] Any magnesium-induced cardiac arrhythmias should also be treated with IV calcium. Epidural bupivacaine has also been successfully used to control autonomic dysfunction.[27] In the past, β blockers have been used. However, there is now evidence that their use is associated with a significant risk of death due to cardiac arrest,[12,28–30] and they are no longer recommended.

Prognosis

With modern intensive care management, mortality ranges from 10 to 15 percent overall and is no longer influenced by age.[31] In areas where such care is not available, mortality rates of between 25 and 50 percent are usual.[1,3,15,32]

Finally, it is important to remember that recovery from tetanus does not guarantee natural immunity.[8] Patients should begin their primary immunization series prior to leaving hospital; indeed, since passive immunization with hTIG does not interfere with successful active immunization, the series can begin even before the patient leaves the ICU.

CASE PRESENTATION

A 69-year-old woman with a past medical history of severe rheumatoid arthritis treated with ASA and prednisone 5 mg by mouth and severe but medically controlled hypertension suffered an acute collapse at home. Ambulance attendants called to the scene described her as unconscious and cyanosed, rigid all over, with ineffective respirations but with a strong pulse. She was resuscitated by hand ventilation with oxygen through a mask; no airway could be passed because her mouth could not be opened. On arrival at hospital another apneic episode led to nasotracheal intubation using a fiberoptic bronchoscope. Following transfer to a tertiary care hospital, she was alert and responsive but was stiff in all four limbs with painful generalized spasms after loud noises or other stimulation. Additional history obtained from family members revealed that she had suffered a pretibial laceration from the edge of a car door 10 days previously. This had been sutured at a physician's office at which time tetanus toxoid was given. There was no history of previous immunization. Over the 5 days preceding admission the patient had complained of difficulty swallowing, pain in the throat and neck, and difficulty opening the mouth. Based on the history of a laceration, absence of previous tetanus immunization, dysphagia, trismus, muscular rigidity, and spasms followed by respiratory arrest, a clinical diagnosis of severe generalized tetanus was made. Immediate management included administration of 5000 units of hTIG intramuscularly followed by debridement of the laceration despite the fact that it did not appear infected. A lumbar puncture was performed and 250 units of hTIG was given intrathecally.

Hypoxemic respiratory failure was a major problem in the initial hospital course. Initial arterial blood gases showed a Pa_{O_2} of 125 mmHg, P_{CO_2} of 27 mmHg, and pH 7.51 ventilated at an FIO_2 of 1.0. Chest radiograph demonstrated bilateral upper lobe infiltrates consistent with pulmonary aspiration or bacterial pneumonia. Penicillin, 2 million units every 4 h, and gentamicin, 70 mg every 4 h, were given, and chest physiotherapy and endotracheal suctioning were begun. Gas exchange improved over the first 48 h, permitting ventilation at an FI_{O_2} of 0.6, but the chest radiograph deteriorated with development of left lower lobe atelectasis. A tracheostomy was performed on the fifth day and improved tracheobronchial toilet led to better gas exchange and radiographic clearing of infiltrates and atelectasis.

The muscle spasms present at admission became progressively more severe and frequent over the first 48 h. Diazepam was given intravenously beginning with 2.5 to 5 mg every 1 to 2 h as needed, increasing to as much as 10 to 20 mg every 2 h to control spasms. Pain was controlled with morphine, 5 mg every 2 to 4 h. Despite large doses of diazepam, spasms persisted and required addition of pancuronium, 4 mg IV given every 4 to 6 h as needed, and this was continued from the third to the eighth day. With control of the muscle spasms a fever of 39.5°C disappeared, and initially markedly elevated CPK levels fell to a moderately elevated range. Because of the high CPK values, initial management also included intravenous rehydration and maintenance of a urine output over 100 mL/H, and no problems with renal insufficiency developed.

Hemodynamic instability characterized by wide swings in blood pressure developed on the second hospital day and persisted for about 2 weeks. These were managed primarily with additional diazepam and morphine for hypertensive periods and with volume expansion for hypotensive episodes. A pulmonary arterial catheter was placed to aid management during the five most unstable days early in the course. Crystalloid and albumen solutions were used to keep the P_w between 10 and 15 mmHg, which appeared to reduce the frequency of periods of extreme hypotension. Hypertension was not well controlled with the initial measures and blood pressure often reached mean values of 150 mmHg. This led to addition of propranolol, 0.5 to 1.0 mg IV every 4 to 6 h. Later, when hypotensive episodes had ceased but hypertension persisted, hydralazine, 25 mg every 6 h, was also added. After the tenth day of treatment cardiovascular instability was no longer a problem, but antihypertensive therapy was still required.

Other treatment measures included administration of cortisone acetate, 100 mg IV every 6 h, because of the patient's long-standing prednisone use; heparin, 5000 units subcutaneously every 8 h, for prevention of venous thrombosis; and nasojejunal enteral feeding beginning on the second hospital day and continuing until extubation. A new fever of unclear origin developed at day 20. Despite repeated examination and culture of blood, urine, and tracheal secretions, a convincing source was not initially evident, although there was some redness and purulence around the tracheostomy site. All vascular catheters were changed and cultured. *Enterobacter cloacae* was grown from both the tracheostomy site and in large numbers from an internal jugular catheter. The fever resolved with a 10-day course of IV gentamicin.

All sedative drugs and muscle relaxants had been discontinued by the tenth day. However, the patient remained in an unresponsive state without localizing neurologic signs. This was attributed, apparently correctly, to benzodiazepine accumulation and encephalopathy associated with critical illness, since her level of consciousness steadily improved over the next 2 weeks. Weaning from respiratory support was begun at day 40. She no longer needed ventilator support by day 55 and was discharged from the ICU to a medical ward 1 week later. She required rehabilitation in hospital for a further 2 months before discharge home. Prior to discharge an additional dose of tetanus toxoid was given to be followed by another in 1 year.

CASE DISCUSSION

The presentation and course of disease in this patient is entirely typical of severe tetanus in the developed world: a minor injury occurring in an unimmunized individual followed in a few days by trismus and dysphagia, shortly thereafter by generalized tetanus with rigidity, muscle spasms, respiratory failure, and cardiovascular instability due to autonomic dysfunction. These severe manifestations improved by the second and third week, but recovery required a total of 9 weeks of intensive care and a further lengthy period of rehabilitation, in this case likely partly attributable to the patient's age and other medical conditions.

The initial management was generally appropriate with intramuscular hTIG given prior to debriding her wound to avoid facilitating further toxin absorption. The dose given was within recommended guidelines, although there are data indicating that much lower doses may be equally effective. The use of intrathecal hTIG in this case is controversial, since it is unlikely to be effective after fully developed generalized tetanus is present. If the disease had been recognized several days earlier, its use might have been associated with a less severe course.

The management of the muscle spasms and cardiovascular instability were typical of what is usually required, with reliance primarily on benzodiazepines and morphine, with a nondepolarizing muscle relaxant when needed for control of spasms. The use of propranolol for control of hypertension here can be questioned, since this has been associated with death related to hypotension and bradycardia, but perhaps can be justified in this case by the presence of severe underlying hypertension, particularly later in the course when hypotension was less of a problem.

The case also illustrates the careful attention to supportive care required for a successful outcome in tetanus: prophylaxis against thrombosis, nutritional support, treatment for underlying medical conditions, tracheobronchial toilet and respiratory support, and prompt recognition and treatment of nosocomial infection. In addition, many weeks of convalescence and rehabilitative care may be needed to achieve full recovery. Finally, note that tetanus toxoid was given before discharge since the disease itself does not generate a protective immune response.

References

1. Center for Disease Control: Tetanus; United States 1985–1986. MMWR 36(29):477, 1987.
2. Percy AS, Kukora JS: The continuing problem of tetanus. Surg Gynecol Obstet 160(4):307, 1985.
3. Edmondson RS, Flowers MW: Intensive care in tetanus: Management, complications and mortality. Br Med J 1(6175):1401, 1979.
4. Passen EL, Andersen BR: Clinical tetanus despite a protective level of toxin-neutralizing antibody. JAMA 255(9):1171, 1986.
5. Kaeser HE, Saner A: The effect of tetanus toxin on neuromuscular transmission. Eur Neurol 3(4):193, 1970.
6. Jagoda A, Riggio S, Burguieres T: Cephalic tetanus: A case report and review of the literature. Am J Emerg Med 6(2):128, 1988.
7. Lennard TWJ, Gunn A, Sellers J, Stoddart JC: Tetanus after elective cholecystectomy and exploration of the common bile duct. Lancet 1(8392):1466 (Letter), 1984.
8. Veronesi R. (ed): *Tetanus, Important New Concepts*. Excerpta Medica, 1981.
9. Cherubin CE: Epidemiology of tetanus in narcotic addicts. NY State J Med 70(2):267, 1970.
10. Raman GV, Lee HA: Tetanus and renal failure. Br J Clin Pract 38(7–8):275, 1984.
11. Kerr JH, Corbett JL, Prys-Roberts C, Smith AC, Spalding JM: Involvement of the sympathetic nervous system in tetanus. Studies on 82 cases. Lancet 2(562):236, 1968.
12. Wright DK, Lalloo UG, Nayiager S, Govender P: Autonomic nervous system dysfunction in severe tetanus: Current perspectives. Crit Care Med 17(4):371, 1989.
13. Idoko JA, Akpam JE, Anjorin FI: Cerebrospinal fluid (CSF) changes in tetanus. Trans Roy Soc Trop Med Hyg 80(1):168 (Letter), 1986.
14. Alfrey D, Rauscher LA: Tetanus: A review. Crit Care Med 7(4):176, 1979.

15. Trujillo MH, Castillo A, Espana J, Manzo A, Zerpa R: Impact of intensive care management on the prognosis of tetanus. Analysis of 641 cases. Chest 92(1):63, 1987.
16. Weinstein L: Tetanus. N Engl J Med 289(24):1293, 1973.
17. Azar I: The response of patients with neuromuscular disorders to muscle relaxants. Anesthesiology 61(2):173, 1984.
18. Powles AB, Ganta R: Use of vecuronium in the management of tetanus. Anesthesia 40(9):879, 1985.
19. Peat SJ, Potter DR, Hunter JM: The prolonged use of atracurium in a patient with tetanus. Anesthesia 43(11):962, 1988.
20. Gupta PS, Kapoor R, Goyal S, Batra VK, Jain BK: Intrathecal human tetanus immunoglobulin in early tetanus. Lancet 2(8192):439, 1980.
21. Vakil BJ, Armitage P, Clifford RE, Laurence DR: Therapeutic trial of intracisternal human tetanus immunoglobulin in clinical tetanus. Trans Roy Soc Trop Med Hyg 73(5):579, 1979.
22. Ahmadsyah I, Salim A: Treatment of tetanus: An open study to compare the efficacy of procaine penicillin and metronidazole. Br Med J 291(6496):648, 1985.
23. O'Keefe SJD, Wesley A, Jialal I, Epstein S: The metabolic response and problems with nutritional support in acute tetanus. Metabolism 33(5):482, 1984.
24. James MFM, Manson EDM: The use of magnesium sulphate infusions in the management of very severe tetanus. Int Care Med 11(1):5, 1985.
25. Rie MA, Wilson RS: Morphine therapy controls autonomic hyperactivity in tetanus. Ann Int Med 88(5):653, 1978.
26. Lipman J, James MFM, Erskine J, et al: Autonomic dysfunction in severe tetanus: Magnesium sulfate as an adjunct to deep sedation. Crit Care Med 15(10):987, 1987.
27. Southorn PA, Blaise GA: Treatment of tetanus-induced autonomic nervous system dysfunction with continuous epidural blockade. Crit Care Med 14(3):251, 1986.
28. Wesley AG, Hariparsad D, Pather M, Rocke DA: Labetalol in tetanus. Anesthesia 38(3):243, 1983.
29. Buchanan N, Smit L, Cane RD, De Andrade M: Sympathetic overactivity in tetanus fatality associated with propranolol. Br Med J 22(6132):254, 1978.
30. Dundee JW, Morrow WFK: Labetalol in severe tetanus. Br Med J 1(6171):1121, 1979.
31. Jolliet P, Magnenat J-L, Kobel T, Chevrolet J-C: Aggressive intensive care treatment of very elderly patients with tetanus is justified. Chest 97(3):702, 1990.
32. Udwadia FE, Lall A, Udwadia ZF, Sekhar M, Vora A: Tetanus and its complications: Intensive care and management experience in 150 Indian patients. Epidemiol Infect 99(3):675, 1987.

Chapter 111

ROCKY MOUNTAIN SPOTTED FEVER

LISA G. KAPLOWITZ
DAVID H. WALKER

KEY POINTS

- *The diagnosis of Rocky Mountain spotted fever (RMSF) must be considered in the differential diagnosis of febrile illnesses—particularly those associated with gastrointestinal or neurologic symptoms and/or rash—in endemic areas during the summer months.*
- *Treatment with tetracycline or chloramphenicol must be initiated on the basis of reasonable clinical suspicion of RMSF without awaiting confirmation, since most deaths result from treatment delay.*
- *Rocky Mountain spotted fever is a vasculitic illness with multiorgan involvement in its advanced stages, which may require circulatory, respiratory, and other supportive measures.*
- *The diagnosis of RMSF may be established early by skin biopsy if a rash is present, with demonstration of the organism by immunofluorescent antibody staining. Serologic diagnosis can be made after the first week of illness.*

Epidemiology

Rocky Mountain spotted fever (RMSF) is the most prevalent rickettsial infection in the United States. The causative organism, *Rickettsia rickettsii,* is transmitted by a number of tick vectors, most commonly the dog tick *(Dermacentor variabilis)* and the wood tick *(Dermacentor andersoni).* While this disease was initially described and studied in the Rocky Mountain states of Idaho and Montana, the largest numbers of cases in the past 40 years have been reported from the Piedmont Plateau region, from Maryland south through Georgia; significant numbers of cases have also been reported from Oklahoma, Tennessee, Arkansas, and Kansas in recent years.[1,2] Smaller endemic foci have been reported from other areas of the country, including a small park in New York City.[3]

Even in endemic areas, only a small percentage of ticks carry *Rickettsia rickettsii.* Further, each infected tick must feed for a prolonged period—usually 2 to 24 h—before the rickettsial organisms are activated and inoculated into the host. Consequently, the risk of acquiring disease from any single tick bite is small, even in endemic areas.

Most cases are diagnosed between April and October, with the largest numbers reported between June and August; these times correspond to periods of peak tick activity. All age groups are affected, though the largest numbers of cases are reported in children and adolescents.[4] The incidence of this infection in the United States increased in the 1960s and 1970s, peaking around 1980; annual reported cases have decreased since then. In 1989 there were 603 cases reported to the Centers for Disease Control, for an annual incidence of 0.25 per 100,000 population.[1]

Rickettsemia occurs soon after a tick bite has transmitted the organism, and is followed by rickettsial invasion of vascular endothelial cells. The organisms proliferate within the cytoplasm and nucleus of endothelial and smooth muscle cells of the capillary bed, eventually resulting in a diffuse necrotizing vasculitis.[5] Cellular damage appears to result directly from rickettsial parasitization; there is no evidence of toxin production. Vasculitis and increased vascular permeability resulting from localized rickettsial proliferation can occur in any organ system; this accounts for the systemic nature of the disease.

Clinical Findings

EARLY CLINICAL MANIFESTATIONS

The incubation period from the time of the tick bite to the onset of clinical symptoms ranges from 3 to 14 days. Only about 75 percent of patients report a history of a tick bite, which is virtually always painless and only rarely results in an eschar. The severity of clinical illness ranges from mild to severe with a fatal outcome in some cases. The initial symptoms of RMSF are relatively nonspecific and include malaise, myalgias, headache that can be quite severe, and fever that often is as high as 102 to 104°F. Gastrointestinal symptoms occur frequently; approximately 75 percent of patients report symptoms of nausea, vomiting, diarrhea, or abdominal pain within the first 3 to 5 days of illness. Neurologic symptoms are not infrequent in early or moderately advanced disease, and can include lethargy and mental status changes.[6]

Although the presence of a rash is considered a hallmark of RMSF, the rash usually does not appear until 3 to 6 days into the illness, and at least 10 percent of patients never develop a rash.[6] The rash often begins on the extremities, around the wrists and ankles, but can involve any area of the body. The initial lesions are macular or maculopapular; they progress to petechial or purpuric lesions in more advanced disease. With progressive disease, the rash frequently involves the palms of the hands and soles of the feet.

MANIFESTATIONS OF ADVANCED DISEASE

Most patients do not develop evidence of advanced RMSF until late in the first week and into the second week of illness. Most deaths occur in the second week of illness, because the diagnosis was not considered and appropriate antibiotic therapy not instituted early in the course of the disease.[7] Increased mortality has been reported in persons over 40 years of age and in males, particularly black men. Fulminant disease, with death occurring within a few days of the onset of illness, has been reported in a few black men with glucose-6-phosphate dehydrogenase (G6PD) deficiency, and on that basis it has been postulated that hemolysis may contribute to fulminant illness.[8] Consequently, it is important to consider a diagnosis of RMSF in any black male with a fulminant vasculitic illness in the appropriate setting (summer months in endemic areas), so that appropriate antibiotics can be initiated promptly.

As the illness progresses, increasing signs of a systemic vasculitis become evident; eventually there is multiorgan involvement. Seizures and coma can occur as manifestations of central nervous system vasculitis and rickettsial encephalitis. Other neurologic manifestations of advanced disease include muscular twitching, tremors, rigidity, tardive dyskinesia, and hyperesthesia; focal neurologic deficits and ataxia are less common, but have been reported.[9] Papilledema due to retinal vasculitis has been reported, with normal cerebrospinal fluid pressure recorded; anterior uveitis has also been reported with RMSF.[10]

Hypovolemia can occur, because of the diffuse vasculitis and leakage of intravascular fluid into the interstitial space, often resulting in hypotension and edema. Renal failure can also occur in advanced disease and is invariably due to either hypotension and prerenal azotemia, or shock and acute tubular necrosis.[11] Pneumonitis is another manifestation of advanced disease and is due to rickettsial injury to the pulmonary vasculature, and resulting interstitial edema.[12,13] While pathologic evidence of nonnecrotizing mononuclear myocarditis has been documented, cardiogenic pulmonary edema is an infrequent consequence of RMSF.

Vasculitis has been documented as involving the abdominal viscera as well, accounting for severe abdominal pain mimicking an acute surgical abdomen in occasional cases.[14] Mild-to-moderate elevations in liver transaminase levels have been reported in RMSF; pathologic studies reveal portal vasculitis and triaditis, and focal hepatocellular necrosis. Myositis, with marked elevations in serum creatine phosphokinase (CPK) levels, has also been reported as a manifestation of advanced disease.[15]

Coagulopathy due to RMSF has been noted to occur in advanced disease. Clinical bleeding is associated with a circulating anticoagulant and elevated levels of fibrin split products, but only rarely with low fibrinogen levels.[6] There is evidence of activation of platelets, coagulation pathways, and the fibrinolytic system that is initiated early in the course of disease and is related to endothelial cell damage.[16] Associated thrombocytopenia can contribute to the bleeding diathesis in such cases.

Skin necrosis and gangrene of the extremities also occur in advanced disease, often without evidence of coagulopathy. Localized vasculitis and resulting small vessel thrombosis appear to account for these complications of RMSF.

Diagnosis

While one definitive method of diagnosis of rickettsial disease is isolation and identification of the etiologic organism from the patient's blood or tissues, this is seldom performed. Virtually no hospital laboratories, and only a few reference laboratories, attempt the isolation of rickettsiae, because of the fear of the biohazard involved in isolation techniques.[17]

Serologic tests remain the major means of making a diagnosis of RMSF, though they do not become diagnostic until 7 to 10 days after the onset of clinical disease. Consequently, serologic tests are not useful in making an early diagnosis of RMSF. In the appropriate clinical situation, antirickettsial therapy should not be withheld until diagnostic serologic test results have been reported. At present, the most accurate serologic tests include the indirect immunofluorescent antibody (IFA), indirect hemagglutination (IHA), and latex agglutination (LA) techniques, with sensitivities of 94 to 100 percent, 91 to 100 percent, and 71 to 94 percent, respectively; the specificities of all three tests range from 96 to 100 percent.[18] Antibodies to Weil-Felix antigens, such as OX-19 and OX-2, are nonspecific, and complement-fixing antibodies are insensitive; neither test should be used clinically at present. For a definitive diagnosis of RMSF, a fourfold rise in a serologic test specific for spotted fever–group rickettsiae between acute and convalescent serum samples should be documented.

Biopsy of skin lesions, with staining of the tissue with an immunofluorescent antibody stain specific for spotted fever–group rickettsiae, can provide a rapid diagnosis when the test is positive. This test provides the only method for a rapid early diagnosis of RMSF and is performed on biopsies of skin lesions obtained with a 3-mm punch. Failure to biopsy a rickettsial cutaneous lesion, or to obtain sections through the center of the lesion, can result in false-negative results. Biopsy specimens should be obtained as soon as possible, though therapy should not be withheld while a biopsy is arranged. Treatment with antirickettsial drugs for over 48 h will substantially reduce the number of rickettsiae seen in biopsy specimens. Immunofluorescent stain of rickettsiae in skin biopsy specimens has a sensitivity of 70 percent and a specificity of 100 percent[18]; negative results, therefore, do not exclude the diagnosis. The immunofluorescent antibody stain for spotted fever–group rickettsiae can also be performed on tissue obtained at surgery or at autopsy; organisms within vascular endothelial cells will stain positive if rickettsial vasculitis is present. This technique can also be useful in making a postmortem diagnosis of RMSF.

Laboratory abnormalities are not uncommon in advanced disease, though none are specific for RMSF. The white blood cell count is often normal, but frequently there is a marked rise in the percentage of immature neutrophils.[6] Thrombocytopenia is a common manifestation of advanced disease with diffuse vasculitis. Hyponatremia can occur, and has been shown to be due to antidiuretic hormone secretion that occurs in response to hypovolemia and hypotension.[19] As has been mentioned, elevations of liver transaminase levels are not uncommon in advanced disease, with the serum aspartate aminotransferase (AST) level usually substantially higher than that of serum alanine aminotransferase (ALT). An increased AST level may also be due to an associated myositis; marked elevations in CPK levels have been reported in some patients.

The differential diagnosis of RMSF is extensive. The early symptoms are nonspecific; often a diagnosis of viral syndrome, gastroenteritis, or bronchitis is made in the first few days of illness.[6] Later in the course of the illness, the differential diagnosis includes a wide range of vasculitides. The early rash may be simulated by atypical measles.[20] The advent of petechiae or purpura often results in consideration of meningococcemia or other bacterial septicemia.[21,22] The presence of thrombocytopenia may result in consideration of thrombotic thrombocytopenic purpura.[23]

Management

The only antibiotics proven effective for the treatment of RMSF are the tetracyclines and chloramphenicol—both rickettsiostatic agents. There is no documented difference in efficacy between these agents for treatment of this infection. Antibiotic therapy should be initiated as early as possible. Initiation of appropriate antibiotic therapy prior to the sixth day of illness usually results in complete recovery. Most deaths from RMSF occur in the second week of illness, typically because the correct diagnosis was not considered and initiation of appropriate therapy was delayed.

In patients with moderate-to-severe disease, intravenous antibiotics should be initiated as soon as the diagnosis of RMSF is considered. Chloramphenicol can be administered intravenously at a dose of 50 to 100 mg/kg per day, in 4 divided doses. The major toxicity of chloramphenicol is hematologic—either a rare idiosyncratic aplastic anemia developing weeks to months after administration of the drug, or a more common dose-related suppression of the bone marrow that is reversible upon stopping the drug. Chloramphenicol is the drug of choice for pregnant women with RMSF, because tetracyclines are contraindicated in pregnancy.[24] It is also frequently used to treat young children, because of concern about the staining of teeth with tetracycline therapy.

Doxycycline, a long-acting tetracycline, is preferred to generic tetracycline for intravenous administration. The drug is administered twice a day; it can be given to patients with renal insufficiency, because excretion is predominantly nonrenal. The intravenous dose is 100 mg twice a day, after an initial loading dose of 200 mg. Often the diagnosis of RMSF is only presumptive, and broad-spectrum antibiotic therapy is appropriate because of other differential diagnosis considerations, such as meningococcemia or other bacteremias. It is important to recognize, however, that most broad-spectrum antibiotic regimens considered for patients with clinical sepsis—such as the broad-spectrum cephalosporins, penicillins, or aminoglycosides—have virtually no activity against *Rickettsia rickettsii* and will not be effective in treating RMSF.

It often requires a number of days for antibiotic therapy to result in clinical improvement, especially in advanced disease. Supportive care must focus on the specific organ systems most severely affected by the vasculitis. As mentioned previously, hypotension occurs frequently in advanced disease as a consequence of diffuse vascular injury and leakage of intravascular fluid into the interstitial space, and is associated with peripheral and/or periorbital edema in many cases. Prompt intravascular volume repletion with intravenous fluids can prevent the development of acute tubular necrosis and renal failure. Renal insufficiency is a poor prognostic indicator, and may progress to renal failure in spite of intravenous rehydration.

Hypotension and hypovolemia may result in increased secretion of antidiuretic hormone and the development of hyponatremia.[19] This is not an example of the syndrome of inappropriate antidiuretic hormone secretion, since hypotension and hypovolemia are appropriate stimuli of antidiuretic hormone secretion. The management of hyponatremia associated with RMSF is intravenous hydration to correct hypovolemia; fluid restriction in this situation can be disastrous. The serum sodium level is rarely low enough to be life-threatening, and adequate volume repletion usually results in correction of the serum sodium level within 48 h.

Interstitial pulmonary edema can occur as a result of rickettsial infection of the pulmonary vasculature; in most cases it is noncardiogenic. Placement of a pulmonary artery catheter for measurement of pulmonary vascular pressure may be essential for optimal fluid management, since interstitial pulmonary edema may occur in the face of hypovolemia. Frequently, interstitial pulmonary edema first appears after intravenous hydration has been initiated. Pulmonary and peripheral edema will resolve gradually after institution of appropriate antirickettsial therapy.

Seizures are a not-infrequent complication of advanced rickettsial vasculitis involving the central nervous system. Antiseizure medication should be instituted to control seizures once they have occurred. The onset of seizures is a very poor prognostic sign. Once recovery from the infection has occurred, there are seldom permanent neurologic sequelae; usually continuation of antiseizure medication is not necessary.

As mentioned previously, coagulopathy and thrombocytopenia are manifestations of disseminated vasculitis; both indicate a poor prognosis. While heparin and dextran therapies have been used in the management of severe coagulopathy, there is no indication of their effectiveness in this setting, and these therapies are not recommended. Platelet transfusions may be warranted if thrombocytopenia is severe or the patient has significant bleeding. Steroid therapy has also been employed for patients with advanced disease, but again, there are no controlled studies to support this treatment.

In summary, management of advanced RMSF must include prompt initiation of appropriate intravenous antibiotic therapy. Careful management of intravascular volume is essential, especially in the management of renal insufficiency and pneumonitis. Multiorgan failure is not uncommon once disseminated vasculitis has developed; at this stage of illness, mortality is quite high. Initiation of appropriate antirickettsial therapy based on a presumptive diagnosis of RMSF is essential if significant morbidity and mortality are to be avoided.

CASE PRESENTATION

A 42-year-old white man was admitted to a hospital in late May with a 6-day history of fever, nausea, headache, muscle aches, and confusion. He had been in good health except for mild hypertension controlled with diuretic medication. He had no history of tick bite, but had worked in his yard in central North Carolina about 3 days prior to the onset of illness. He had seen his private physician 4 days prior to admission, complaining of 2 days of fever as high as 103°F, headache, nausea, and myalgias. His physician diagnosed a viral illness and prescribed acetaminophen and bed rest; a complete blood cell count and platelet count were normal. His fevers and headache continued, and on the morning of admission his wife noted that he was very weak and confused. On admission he was noted to have a faint macular rash on his chest, but no rash on his extremities; he was disoriented and had a blood pressure of 80/60. He had thrombocytopenia, renal insufficiency, and hyponatremia, with a normal white blood cell count, though there were 40 percent bands. He was treated with a cephalosporin and an aminoglycoside for presumed sepsis, and received intravenous hydration. Six hours after hospitalization, he had difficulty breathing; a chest x-ray revealed diffuse interstitial infiltrates. In the next 12 h he had progressive respiratory difficulty and required intubation and ventilator support. Thirty-six hours after hospitalization, he had a seizure and developed diffuse purpura; he also required increased intravenous fluid and blood product support, plus pressors, because of severe hypotension. Though the diagnosis of RMSF was considered at this point, and chloramphenicol therapy initiated, the patient died 12 h later with intractable hypotension and cardiac arrest. Immunofluorescent staining of a skin biopsy specimen of his purpuric rash was positive for *Rickettsia rickettsii*.

CASE DISCUSSION

The severe manifestations and fatal outcome of RMSF in this patient were the result of delay in suspecting the diagnosis. While early clinical manifestations were nonspecific, clues to the diagnosis included a febrile illness in an endemic area of the country during the late spring. At the time of admission, however, many of the symptoms, physical signs, and laboratory findings of this infection were present, including fever, marked persistent headache, confusion, hypotension, thrombocytopenia, hyponatremia, renal insufficiency, and a marked left shift in the neutrophil count. The rash present at the time of admission was not typical of RMSF, but was an important clinical sign. While bacterial sepsis was a reasonable consideration, RMSF should also have been considered and appropriate antibiotic therapy (doxycycline or chloramphenicol) added to the coverage for bacteremia.

During his 48-h stay in the hospital the patient required multiple supportive measures, including ventilator, blood volume, and pressor support but died in spite of them. A skin biopsy obtained earlier might have established the diagnosis; but in cases such as this the diagnosis must be considered early and appropriate therapy initiated presumptively to avoid a fatal outcome. This case illustrates the need to suspect the diagnosis of RMSF on the basis of clinical findings and the appropriate epidemiologic setting.

References

1. Centers for Disease Control: Rocky Mountain spotted fever and human ehrlichiosis—United States, 1989. MMWR 39:281, 1990.
2. Taylor JP, Istre GT, McChesney TC: The epidemiology of Rocky Mountain spotted fever in Arkansas, Oklahoma and Texas, 1981 through 1985. Am J Epidemiol 127:1295, 1988.
3. Salgo MP, Telzak EE, Currie B, et al: A focus of Rocky Mountain spotted fever within New York City. N Engl J Med 318:1345, 1988.
4. Wilfert CM, MacCormack N, Kleeman K, et al: Epidemiology of Rocky Mountain spotted fever as determined by active surveillance. J Infect Dis 150:469, 1984.
5. Walker DH: Pathology and pathogenesis of the vasculotropic rickettsiosis, in Walker DH (ed): *Biology of Rickettsial Diseases*. Boca Raton, CRC Press, 1988, p 115.
6. Kaplowitz LG, Fischer JJ, Sparling PF: Rocky Mountain spotted fever: A clinical dilemma, in Remington JS, Swartz MN (eds): *Current Clinical Topics in Infectious Diseases*, vol 2. New York, McGraw-Hill, 1981, p 89.
7. Hattwick MAW, Retailliau H, O'Brien RJ, et al: Fatal Rocky Mountain spotted fever. Arch Intern Med 240:1499, 1978.
8. Walker DH, Kirkman HN: Rocky Mountain spotted fever and deficiency in glucose-6-phosphate dehydrogenase. J Infect Dis 142:771, 1980.
9. Massey EW, Thames T, Coffey E, Gallis HA: Neurologic complications of Rocky Mountain spotted fever. South Med J 78:1288, 1985.
10. Duffey RJ, Hammer ME: The ocular manifestations of Rocky Mountain spotted fever. Ann Ophthalmol 19:301, 1987.
11. Walker DH, Mattern WD: Acute renal failure in Rocky Mountain spotted fever. Arch Intern Med 139:443, 1979.
12. Lankford HV, Glauser FL: Cardiopulmonary dynamics in a severe case of Rocky Mountain spotted fever. Arch Intern Med 140:1357, 1980.
13. Sacks HS, Lyons RW, Lahiri B: Adult respiratory distress syndrome in Rocky Mountain spotted fever. Am Rev Respir Dis 123:547, 1981.
14. Walker DH, Lesesne HR, Varma VA, Thacker WC: Rocky Mountain spotted fever mimicking acute cholecystitis. Arch Intern Med 145:2194, 1985.
15. Krober MS: Skeletal muscle involvement in Rocky Mountain spotted fever. South Med J 71:1575, 1978.
16. Rao AK, Schapira M, Clements ML, et al: A prospective study of platelets and plasma proteolytic systems during the early stages of Rocky Mountain spotted fever. N Engl J Med 318:1021, 1988.
17. Oster CN, Burke DS, Kenyon RH, et al: Laboratory-acquired Rocky Mountain spotted fever. N Engl J Med 297:859, 1977.
18. Walker DH: Diagnosis of rickettsial diseases. Pathol Annu 23 (part 2):69, 1988.
19. Kaplowitz LG, Robertson GL: Hyponatremia in Rocky Mountain spotted fever: Role of antidiuretic hormone. Ann Intern Med 98:334, 1983.

20. Horwitz MS et al: Atypical measles mimicking Rocky Mountain spotted fever. N Engl J Med 289:1203, 1973.
21. Siegel DM, Freeman RG: Pseudomonas endocarditis with embolic phenomena and a false positive Weil-Felix titer. Arch Dermatol 122:711, 1986.
22. Milunski MR, Gallis HA, Fulkerson WJ: *Staphylococcus aureus* septicemia mimicking Rocky Mountain spotted fever. Am J Med 83:801, 1987.
23. Turner RC, Chaplinski TJ, Adams HG: Rocky Mountain spotted fever presenting as thrombotic thrombocytopenic purpura. Am J Med 81:153, 1986.
24. Gallis HA, Agner RC, Painter CJ: Rocky Mountain spotted fever in pregnancy. N C Med J 45:187, 1984.

Chapter 112

MALARIA AND VIRAL HEMORRHAGIC FEVERS IN RETURNED TRAVELERS

DAVID A. WARRELL

KEY POINTS

- *Consider the diagnosis of malaria in any ill, febrile patient with a history of travel to a malarious area or of a blood transfusion.*
- *Transfer the patient to an intensive care unit and make a rapid clinical assessment, including spot measurement of blood glucose.*
- *If the diagnosis of severe falciparum malaria is proved or suspected, initiate antimalarial chemotherapy using optimal doses of an appropriate agent (quinine or quinidine) administered by controlled-rate intravenous infusion, using a loading dose. Monitor the clinical and parasitologic responses.*
- *Prevent, or detect early and treat, the numerous complications (especially generalized convulsions, hypoglycemia, and hyperpyrexia).*
- *Ensure correct fluid, electrolyte, and acid-base balance. Control fluid replacement to prevent circulatory overload and pulmonary edema.*
- *Expert nursing care (of the unconscious patient) is essential.*
- *Avoid the use of potentially harmful ancillary treatments of unproven benefit, such as corticosteroids, heparin, and epinephrine.*
- *Consider the diagnosis of viral hemorrhagic fevers in patients with fever, pharyngitis (Lassa fever), hemorrhagic shock, jaundice, and elevated serum hepatic enzyme concentrations, if there is an appropriate travel history and special risk of exposure.*
- *Isolate the patient and isolate or keep under surveillance their primary contacts. Handle all specimens with caution and be sure to exclude other treatable diseases, especially severe falciparum malaria, typhoid, and meningococcemia.*
- *Attempt virologic confirmation of the diagnosis.*
- *Give specific antiviral treatment: ribavirin for Lassa fever, hemorrhagic fever with renal syndrome, and Congo-Crimean hemorrhagic fever; hyperimmune serum for Argentine hemorrhagic fever, Ebola virus disease, and Congo-Crimean hemorrhagic fever.*
- *Give appropriate supportive treatment for shock and other complications.*
- *Give special attention to educating and protecting medical and nursing staff and primary contacts.*

Malaria

PARASITES AND LIFE CYCLES

Malaria is a mosquito-borne protozoal infection caused in humans by four species of *Plasmodium*—*P. falciparum, P. vivax, P. malariae,* and *P. ovale.* Only *P. falciparum* causes potentially life-threatening malaria, but other species can cause severe illness in debilitated individuals. Sporozoites are inoculated by female *Anopheles* mosquitoes while feeding. The sporozoites of all the human malarias invade hepatocytes where they develop into schizonts and, after 6 to 16 days, rupture to release merozoites into the bloodstream. Some sporozoites of *P. vivax* and *P. ovale* remain dormant in the liver for months or years in the form of hypnozoites. *P. falciparum* and *P. malariae* may persist as inapparent low-grade parasitemias to cause symptomatic recrudescences. However, these species do not persist in the liver. The erythrocytic cycle consists of invasion, development from rings to mature pigmented multinucleated schizonts, and rupture with release of merozoites. These invade erythrocytes to produce repeated cycles of infection or develop into male and female gametocytes. Merozoites cannot reinvade the liver from the blood. Erythrocytes containing mature trophozoites and schizonts of *P. falciparum* are sequestered in the tissues. Gametocytes taken up by mosquitoes complete a sexual cycle producing sporozoites which are injected with the mosquito's saliva during a blood meal. The intervals between the mosquito bite and the appearance of parasitemia are 10 days for *P. falciparum,* 8 to 13 days for *P. vivax,* 9 to 14 days for *P. ovale,* and 15 to 16 days for *P. malariae.* Intervals between the bite and first symptom (incubation period) are a few days longer.

EPIDEMIOLOGY

Malaria is endemic in the tropics except in the islands of the South Central Pacific Ocean (Fig. 112-1). *P. falciparum* is the commonest cause of malaria in Africa, Haiti, many parts of South America, southeast Asia, and Papua New Guinea but is absent from the eastern Mediterranean. *P. vivax* has been the dominant species in most parts of the Indian subcontinent, but there is now a resurgence of *P. falciparum;* it is replaced by *P. ovale* in West Africa but occurs with varying frequency throughout other parts of the malaria endemic area. *P. malariae* infections are widespread but usually infrequent.

Children who grow up in holoendemic areas are frequently infected and eventually acquire immunity to symptoms and severe manifestations of malaria. In these regions, severe disease is confined to infants and young children. This immunity lapses in those who move outside the endemic area for several years. Thus, Asian or African immigrants living in Europe or North America may become susceptible to symptomatic malaria by the time they return home on vacation. Outside the endemic areas, autochthonous malaria may occur in those living around international airports. Malaria can be transmitted by blood transfusion, contaminated needles (for example, among

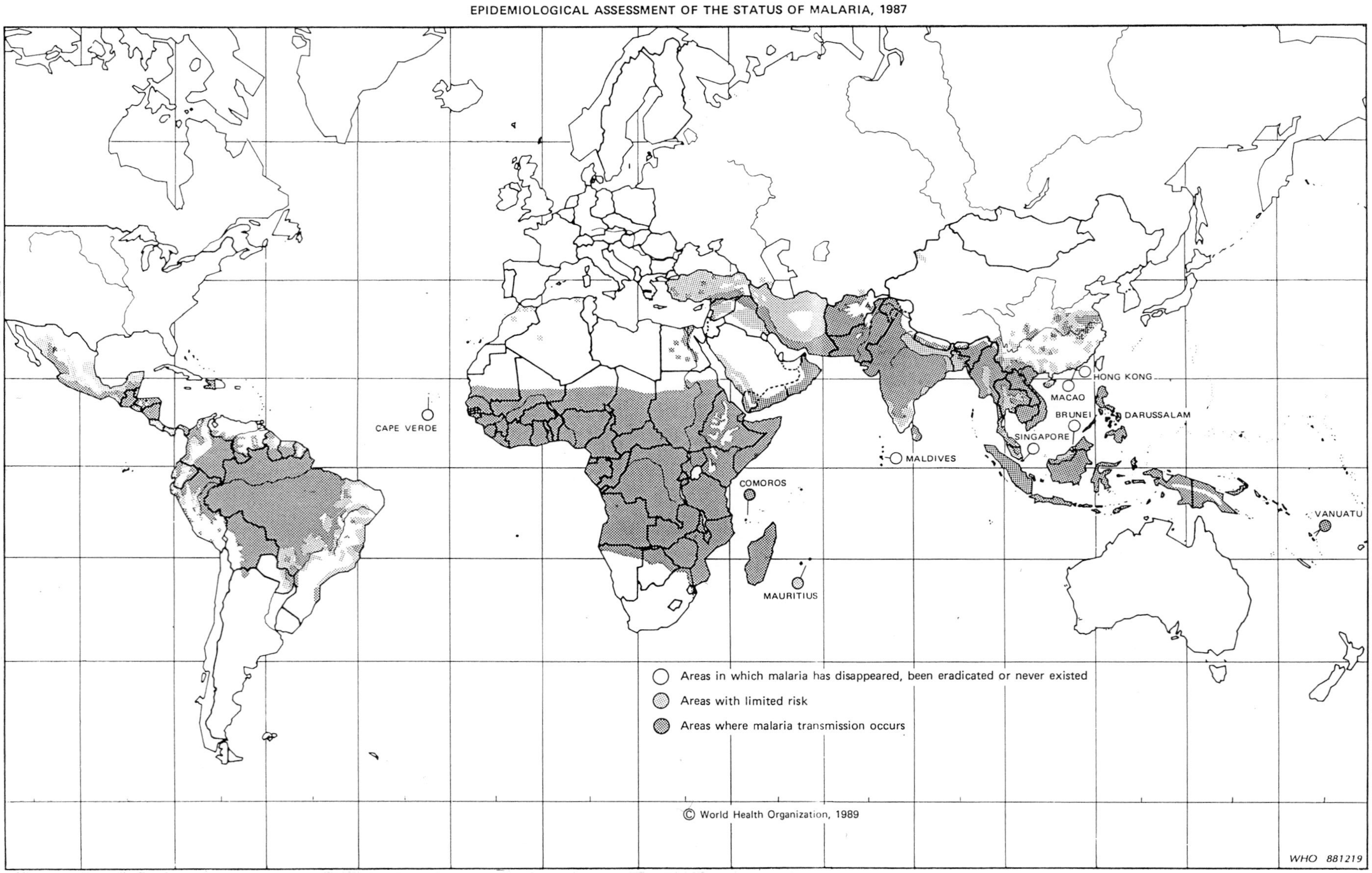

FIGURE 112-1 Distribution of malaria in the world. *(Reproduced by permission of the WHO.)*

intravenous and subcutaneous drug abusers), by marrow and tissue transplants, and transplacentally (congenital malaria).

PATHOPHYSIOLOGY: GENERAL[1]

Symptoms and pathologic changes are attributable to the asexual erythrocytic parasites and to secondary effects on macrophages and the immune system. Schizogony stimulates macrophages to release interleukin-1, tumor necrosis factor (TNF), and other cytokines. Cytoadherence to the wall of venules by erythrocytes containing mature trophozoites and schizonts is now thought to play the major role in producing organ and tissue dysfunctions. The molecular basis of cytoadherence is the binding of malarial antigens expressed on the erythrocyte surface (possibly $PfEMP_1$) to endothelial receptors such as intracellular adhesion molecule 1 (ICAM-1),[2] membrane glycoprotein CD36,[3] or the multifunctional adhesive glycoprotein, thrombospondin.[4] Sequestration of parasitized erythrocytes is most marked in brain, kidney, gut, placenta, skeletal muscle, liver, bone marrow, and retina.[5] The resulting stagnation of blood flow causes hypoxia and anaerobic glycolysis with increased lactic acid production.[6]

PATHOPHYSIOLOGY OF SPECIFIC ORGAN AND TISSUE DYSFUNCTIONS

Anemia results principally from hemolysis of parasitized erythrocytes. Enhanced splenic removal of nonparasitized erythrocytes and dyserythropoiesis may contribute, but the role of immune hemolysis remains controversial. *Intravascular hemolysis and hemoglobinuria* in patients with inherited erythrocytic enzyme defects such as glucose-6-phosphate-dehydrogenase deficiency is commonly associated with the use of oxidant antimalarial drugs such as primaquine and chloroquine. Classical *blackwater fever* has been attributed to quinine-related immune hemolysis, but the evidence is inconclusive. *Thrombocytopenia* results from splenic sequestration or immune destruction; there is no evidence of reduced marrow production. The full picture of *disseminated intravascular coagulation* (DIC) is uncommon. Neurologic symptoms *(cerebral malaria)* are attributable to sequestration of parasitized erythrocytes in small blood vessels. There is no histopathologic evidence that inflammation or immune complex damage is involved in the pathogenesis of human cerebral malaria, but plasma concentrations of TNF correlate with severity and are highest in fatal cases.[7] In human cerebral malaria there is no demonstrable increase in permeability of the blood-cerebrospinal fluid barrier, and cerebral edema is found as a terminal phenomenon in a minority of cases.[8] *Acute pulmonary edema* may be precipitated by fluid overload but is more commonly associated with normal or low pulmonary artery wedge pressures and resembles adult respiratory distress syndrome. There is sequestration of leukocytes in the pulmonary capillaries as in experimental "endotoxin lung." *Hypoglycemia* may result from quinine- or quinidine-induced hyperinsulinemia or from inhibition of hepatic gluconeogenesis by TNF, in association with low plasma insulin concentrations appropriate to the degree of hypoglycemia. *Renal and hepatic dysfunction* have been attributed to vasoconstriction but could also result from vascular obstruction by sequestered parasitized erythrocytes.[9] *Shock (algid malaria)* is frequently associated with secondary gram-negative rod septicemia but may also arise in patients with acute pulmonary edema, dehydration, lactic acidosis, hypoglycemia, and hemorrhagic shock following gastrointestinal hemorrhage or splenic rupture.

CLINICAL FEATURES

FALCIPARUM MALARIA[10]

The shortest interval between the infecting mosquito bite and the first symptom is 7 days, a fact which may be useful in excluding the diagnosis of malaria in patients who fall ill less than a week after entering a malarial endemic region. More than 80 percent of patients with imported falciparum malaria present with symptoms within 1 month of leaving the endemic area, while only a few percent present between 3 and 12 months or longer after leaving. None of the symptoms of malaria is specific. The illness may start with headache, a fever, or chill or a feeling of lethargy. Other frequent symptoms are backache, myalgias, postural syncope, prostration, vomiting, and diarrhea. Physical signs include anemia, jaundice, and tender hepatosplenomegaly. The absence of focal symptoms, lymphadenopathy, and rash (other than herpes labialis) may be helpful in distinguishing malaria from some other fevers. The classical tertian or subtertian fever (a fever spike every 36 or 48 h) is now rarely allowed to manifest itself, and even the dramatic cycle of chill, hot phase, and diaphoresis is uncommon.

Severe life-threatening falciparum malaria is defined by the presence of any of the features listed in Table 112-1.[11] There are age and geographic variations in the frequency of these different features.[12] In most parts of the world, cerebral malaria is the commonest manifestation of severe malaria in adults; but jaundice is more common in Vietnam, and renal failure in Papua New Guinea.

Cerebral malaria should be considered in any febrile patient who has been exposed to *P. falciparum* infection who develops impairment of consciousness of any degree. A trial of antimalarial chemotherapy may be warranted in such patients even if parasitemia is not evident in the peripheral blood smear. A strict definition of cerebral malaria demands unrousable coma, the demonstration of asexual *P. falciparum* parasitemia, and the exclusion of other causes of coma, especially of bacterial meningitis and locally prevalent viral encephalitides.[13,14] Clinical features of cerebral malaria other than coma include generalized convulsions, dysconjugate gaze, forcible jaw closure and tooth grinding (bruxism), signs of a symmetrical upper motor neuron lesion and extensor posturing. Retinal hemorrhages and, rarely, exudates carry a severe prognosis in patients with cerebral malaria and indicate impending coma in those who are still conscious. After a few days of febrile symptoms, coma may develop insidiously or suddenly with a generalized convulsion. Survivors recover consciousness within a

TABLE 112-1 Severe Manifestations and Complications of Falciparum Malaria

Defining Criteria of Severe Disease	Other Manifestations
1. Cerebral malaria (unrousable coma)	1. Impaired consciousness but rousable
2. Severe normocytic anemia	2. Prostration, extreme weakness
3. Renal failure	3. Hyperparasitemia
4. Pulmonary edema	4. Jaundice
5. Hypoglycemia	5. Hyperpyrexia
6. Circulatory collapse, shock	
7. Spontaneous bleeding or disseminated intravascular coagulation	
8. Repeated generalized convulsions	
9. Acidemia or acidosis	
10. Macroscopic hemoglobinuria	

few days and are usually free of neurologic sequelae. Psychiatric manifestations (brief reactive psychosis) and focal convulsions without loss of consciousness are uncommon.

Renal functional impairment of some degree occurs in about a third of adult patients with severe falciparum malaria. Acute tubular necrosis develops in a minority. Acute renal failure is often associated with classical blackwater fever.

Acute pulmonary edema is a serious and often fatal development associated with hyperparasitemia, renal failure, lactic acidosis, use of excessive parenteral fluid replacement, and in peripartum pregnant women.[15]

Hypoglycemia is an increasingly recognized complication of falciparum malaria and its treatment. Symptoms of hypoglycemia may be confused with those of malaria itself, and so hypoglycemia must be specifically excluded in all patients with impaired consciousness, extensor posturing, convulsions, shock, and in pregnant women in whom there is evidence of fetal distress. The most common clinical settings in which hypoglycemia develops are chemotherapy with cinchona alkaloids (quinine and quinidine), which are known to induce hyperinsulinemia even in the convalescent phase and particularly in pregnant women; in pregnant women in general, even if they appear asymptomatic; and in adults and children with hyperparasitemia and other evidence of severe disease.

Shock (algid malaria) may complicate severe malaria itself or be a result of simple dehydration or acute hemorrhage, but in many patients the clinical impression of gram-negative septicemia is confirmed by blood culture. Cardiac arrhythmias and myocardial failure are extremely rare.

Bleeding, coagulopathy, and DIC are clinically significant hemostatic abnormalities which seem to be relatively common among nonimmune travelers with severe falciparum malaria. Thrombocytopenia is common in both falciparum and vivax malarias, and its degree is not related to prognosis.

Acidosis, usually resulting from lactic acid accumulation, presents with rapid deep respirations in severely ill patients.

Massive intravascular hemolysis and hemoglobinuria in patients with normal erythrocyte enzymes has been termed "blackwater fever." This puzzling syndrome is associated with intermittent use of quinine, mild or absent parasitemia and fever, loin pain, vomiting, diarrhea, polyuria followed by oliguria and passage of black urine, tender hepatosplenomegaly, profound anemia, and deep jaundice.

Hepatic dysfunction is manifested by deep jaundice with a major component of conjugated bilirubin, prolonged prothrombin time, increased concentrations of serum aminotransferases (rarely more than three to five times greater than normal), and a low or falling serum albumin.

The mortality of severe falciparum malaria ranges from 10 to 50 percent. In adults, impaired consciousness alone, without any evidence of other organ or tissue dysfunctions, carries an excellent prognosis.[13]

OTHER MALARIAS

Initial febrile and influenza-like symptoms are as unpleasant as in falciparum malaria. The fever in untreated vivax and ovale malarias has a tertian periodicity (fever spike every 48 h), and in *P. malariae* infection has quartan periodicity (every 72 h). Vivax and ovale malarias may relapse for 8 years or longer after the initial infection, and malariae infection may recrudesce for 50 years or more. Splenic rupture in vivax malaria has proved fatal, and some debilitated children or adults have died of severe anemia. *P. malariae* malaria may prove severe or even fatal in immunocompromised patients who acquire the infection by transfusion. *P. malariae* infection is thought to be an important cause of nephrotic syndrome especially in Africa.

DIAGNOSIS

Malaria must be included in the differential diagnosis of any severely ill and febrile patient. A detailed travel history is essential. It must include information about stopovers in malarious areas even if the ultimate destination was malaria-free. One patient was infected during a 1-h stop at the international airport outside Abidjan, Ivory Coast. Routes of infection other than mosquito bites must be considered, such as blood transfusions and needlestick injuries. A diagnosis of malaria is more likely if the patient took no precautions against mosquito bites and no antimalarial chemoprophylaxis, or if they took their drugs irregularly or stopped prematurely. The differential diagnosis of malaria includes other infections which cause *chills and rigors,* especially those which do not cause focal signs or symptoms (e.g., influenza, enteric fevers, brucellosis); *jaundice* (e.g., viral hepatitis, leptospirosis, yellow fever, and relapsing fevers); *hemorrhage* (e.g., viral hemorrhagic fevers, hepatic failure); *hyperpyrexia* (e.g., heatstroke, malignant hyperthermia), *gastrointestinal symptoms* (e.g., gastroenteritis, traveler's diarrhea, salmonellosis); and *encephalopathy* (e.g., viral, bacterial, fungal, protozoal).

Microscopic diagnosis is achieved by examining conventional hematologic thin blood smears and thick films, preferably made at the bedside using blood straight from the patient which has not been stored with anticoagulant. Wright's, Field's, Leishman's, and Giemsa stains are suitable [Fig. 112-2 (Plate 48)]. Parasites should be counted in relation to erythrocytes or leukocytes in the same field, and the parasite concentration (per microliter) calculated from total erythrocyte or leukocyte counts. Blood examinations should be repeated at 12-h intervals as parasitemia may fluctuate. They need not be timed to coincide with a fever spike or paroxysm. There is no advantage in using venous or arterial blood instead of blood obtained by finger prick. Nail bed puncture is less painful than the more usual pulp puncture. Blood smears should be examined at 12 hourly intervals after starting treatment until parasitemia has disappeared for at least 24 h. Peripheral parasitemia may sometimes be undetectable in patients subsequently found (at autopsy) to have parasitized erythrocytes sequestered in their brains, and so a therapeutic trial of antimalarial drugs should be considered if there is clinical suspicion of severe malaria. The presence of gametocytes indicates recovery from infection; their morphology distinguishes falciparum from other malarias. Neutrophil leukocytosis is found in severe falciparum malaria. Thrombocytopenia is common in falciparum and vivax malarias.

MANAGEMENT OF SEVERE MALARIA

Severe malaria is nearly always the result of *P. falciparum* infection. Because the disease can evolve rapidly, with sudden clinical deterioration and with involvement of many vital organs and tissues, severe falciparum malaria is a medical emergency which should, ideally, be managed in an intensive care unit.

INITIAL CLINICAL ASSESSMENT AND MANAGEMENT (Table 112-2)

The clinical history, taken from the patient or accompanying friends and relatives, should include precise details (times, places) of travel to the tropics, preventive methods, recent antimalarial therapy, and previous attacks of malaria. A history of ominous events such as convulsions, diminishing urine output, black urine, and psychosis should be elicited. It is important to know whether a female patient is pregnant. In severely ill patients, a rapid initial examination should be carried out to exclude other diagno-

TABLE 112-2 Initial Management of Patients with Severe Malaria

1. Clear and maintain airway.
2. Position semiprone or on side.
3. Weigh the patient, calculate dosage.
4. Start antimalarial chemotherapy.
5. Make rapid clinical assessment.
6. Take blood for diagnostic smear, monitoring of blood sugar (rapid "stix" method), hematocrit and other laboratory tests.
7. Exclude or treat hypoglycemia.
8. Assess state of hydration.
9. Give prophylactic anticonvulsant (phenytoin) and consider need for additional drugs (antimicrobials, vitamin K, etc.).
10. Measure and monitor urine output. If necessary, insert urethral catheter. Measure urine specific gravity and sodium concentration.
11. Plan first 8 h intravenous fluids—including diluent for antimalarial drug, glucose therapy, and blood transfusion.
12. Consider inserting central venous pressure or pulmonary artery catheter to monitor fluid replacement.
13. If rectal temperature exceeds 39°C, remove patient's clothes, tepid sponge, fan, use hypothermia mattress, and consider antipyretic (paracetamol/acetaminophen).
14. Do lumbar puncture to exclude meningitis. Consider other infections.

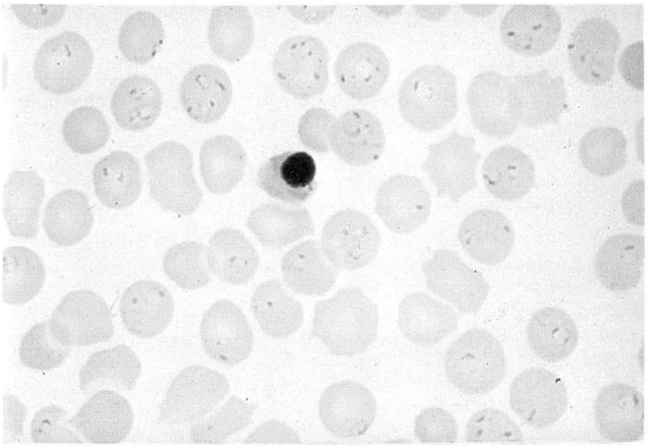

FIGURE 112-2 ***Plasmodium falciparum*** **hyperparasitemia in a thin blood film from a patient with cerebral malaria. See Plate 48.** ***(Copyright DA Warrell.)***

ses (e.g., meningitis) and to detect life-threatening complications such as pulmonary edema, renal failure, shock, and hypoglycemia. In patients with malarial parasitemia, the physician must keep an open mind about other disease processes, especially in residents of the malarious zone in whom parasitemia may be irrelevant to their current illness. Initial investigations must include a parasite count (which is of prognostic importance), hematocrit, full blood count, and measurement of electrolytes, blood urea, and creatinine. Frequent measurement of the blood glucose concentration is most important. It can be checked rapidly and repeatedly at the bedside using one of the many commercially available methods. The blood should be cultured. In patients with respiratory distress, arterial pH, blood gas tensions, bicarbonate, and lactic acid concentrations should be measured. In patients with impaired consciousness and other neurologic signs, lumbar puncture is important to exclude treatable meningoencephalitides. The usual precautions should be observed before carrying out a lumbar puncture: search for clinical evidence of raised intracranial pressure, lateralizing neurologic signs, and signs of imminent coning, local skin sepsis, etc. If there is any doubt, a computed tomography (CT) scan should be performed first. The overwhelming global experience is that lumbar puncture is safe in *adult* patients with cerebral malaria. However, Kenyan children may show progressive signs of cerebral compression and raised intracranial pressure.[16] In cerebral malaria the cerebrospinal fluid (CSF) is usually normal. However, a mild lymphocyte pleocytosis (up to about 15 cells per microliter) and mildly raised total protein concentration is found occasionally. Low or undetectable CSF glucose concentration indicates hypoglycemia. CSF opening pressure was normal in 80 percent of Thai adults with cerebral malaria[8] but was elevated in Kenyan children.[16]

ANTIMALARIAL CHEMOTHERAPY

In patients with proven or suspected severe falciparum malaria, appropriate chemotherapy (usually with quinine) must be started immediately. Delay in diagnosis and treatment and the use of inappropriate antimalarial drugs accounts for most cases of fatal imported malaria. Recommended parenteral regimens for treatment of severe malaria are summarized in Table 112-3.

CINCHONA ALKALOIDS (QUININE AND QUINIDINE)

Quinine is the drug of choice for severe falciparum malaria, unless it is certain that the infection was acquired in an area where the strains of *P. falciparum* have not developed resistance to chloroquine (December 1990: Dominican Republic, Haiti, Central America west and north of the Panama Canal, the Middle East, Egypt, Gambia). Even if the patient acquired the infection in an area where *P. falciparum* remains sensitive to chloroquine, this drug should not be considered for therapy if the infection has developed in the face of weekly chloroquine prophylaxis. If quinine for intravenous administration is not immediately available [for example, in the United States where it is supplied by the Centers for Disease Control, Atlanta, Georgia—24-h Malaria Hotline telephone number *(404) 332-4555*], quinidine gluconate injection may be available for the treatment of cardiac arrhythmias and can be used to initiate treatment.[17,18] Quinine and quinidine should never be given by intravenous "push" or bolus injection but should be administered by slow, controlled rate intravenous infusion using an intravenous drip with a metered chamber or an infusion pump. Unless the patient has been given quinine, quinidine, or mefloquine within the previous 24 h, an initial loading dose should be used so that therapeutic blood concentrations can be achieved rapidly.[19,20] The initial dose

TABLE 112-3 Severe Falciparum Malaria: Antimalarial Chemotherapy

1. *Quinine:* 7 mg dihydrochloride *salt*/kg (loading dose) IV by infusion pump over 30 min followed immediately by 10 mg/kg (maintenance dose) diluted in 10 mL/kg isotonic fluid by IV infusion over 4 h, repeated every 8 h until the patient can swallow, then quinine tablets approx. 10 mg salt/kg every 8 h to complete 7 days of treatment.

   OR

2. *Quinine:* 20 mg *salt*/kg (loading dose) by infusion over 4 h, then 10 mg/kg over 4 h, every 8 h until patient can swallow, then quinine tablets to complete 7 days of treatment.

   OR

3. *Quinidine:* 10 mg gluconate *base*/kg (loading dose) by infusion over 1 to 2 h, followed by 0.2 mg/(kg · min) by infusion pump for 72 h or until the patient can swallow, then quinine tablets to complete 7 days of treatment.

   OR

4. *Quinidine:* 15 mg gluconate *base*/kg (loading dose) by IV infusion over 4 h, then 7.5 mg/kg over 4 h, every 8 h until patient can swallow, then quinine tablets to complete 7 days of treatment.

Loading dose should not be used if patient received quinine, quinidine, or mefloquine within the preceding 24 h. For infections acquired in areas of quinine resistance (e.g., Thailand) add an oral course of tetracycline 250 mg every day for 7 days except in children under 8 years and in pregnant women.
In patients requiring more than 48 h of parenteral therapy reduce the quinine maintenance dose to one-half (i.e., 5 mg salt/kg every 8 h).

should not be reduced in pregnant women or in patients with renal and hepatic dysfunction, but the maintenance dose should be halved after 48 h of parenteral treatment, unless the patient can continue treatment by the oral route. The dose should also be reduced if, at any stage, the plasma concentration exceeds 15 mg/L (45 μmol/L). In patients treated with quinidine, the electrocardiogram (ECG) should be monitored continuously and blood pressure measured every 30 min during the initial loading dose infusion.

TOXICITY OF CINCHONA ALKALOIDS

Plasma concentrations of these drugs above about 5 mg/L are associated with "cinchonism": giddiness, tinnitus, high tone deafness, tremors, blurred vision, nausea, and vomiting. Concentrations above 20 mg/L may cause blindness, deafness, hypotension, ECG abnormalities, and central nervous system depression. However, patients with malaria are more tolerant of high plasma concentrations than uninfected patients who take overdoses of these drugs. This may be explained by increased binding of quinine by acute phase reactive proteins, especially α_1 acid glycoprotein. Quinidine more than quinine causes prolongation of the QT_c interval and QRS complex, but this is rarely associated with dysrhythmia or hypotension unless the drugs are given too rapidly. The most frequent important side effect of quinine and quinidine is hypoglycemia which may occur at any stage of treatment and may cause recurrent neurologic symptoms in patients who appear to have recovered from cerebral malaria. Normal therapeutic doses can be used safely even in the third trimester of pregnancy.[21] In these patients it is important to assess uterine activity and fetal condition before the start of quinine treatment to avoid confusion of the effects of malaria and high fever *per se* from those of the drug.[21] In patients with severe quinine toxicity (following oral or parenteral administration), quinine elimination can be increased by oral or nasogastric administration of activated charcoal.[22]

CHLOROQUINE

This drug should be given by slow, controlled rate intravenous infusion.[23,24]

Chloroquine Toxicity

Plasma concentrations above 250 ng/mL may cause dizziness, diplopia, difficulty with visual accommodation, dysphagia, nausea, and vomiting. Much higher concentrations may cause vasodilation, hypotension, cardiotoxicity, and death. Severe chloroquine toxicity can be treated with diazepam and isoprenaline under intensive care unit conditions.[25] Pruritus is a common complication of chloroquine in Africans and some other black-skinned races.

TREATMENT OF SEVERE FALCIPARUM MALARIA WITH OTHER ANTIMALARIAL DRUGS

Intravenous administration of quinine, quinidine, or, where appropriate, chloroquine is currently the optimal treatment for severe falciparum malaria. However, in an emergency, if these drugs are not available, mefloquine suspension could be given by nasogastric tube[26] or sulfadoxine-pyrimethamine (Fansidar) by intramuscular injection. Resistance to Fansidar is widespread in southeast Asia, South America, and East and Central Africa.

SUPPORTIVE CARE OF PATIENTS WITH SEVERE FALCIPARUM MALARIA

HYPERPYREXIA

This may be responsible for febrile convulsions in children, fetal distress in pregnant women, and, when sustained at core temperatures in excess of 40°C, may cause irreversible neurologic damage. Core temperature should be monitored, and, when necessary, the patient should be tepid-sponged and fanned, placed on a hypothermia mattress, or given an antipyretic (e.g., acetaminophen).

CEREBRAL MALARIA

More than 50 percent of adults and even more children with cerebral malaria suffer one or more generalized convulsions. These must be controlled rapidly and, ideally, prevented as they may be followed by persistent neurologic deterioration (deepening coma) and often complicated by aspiration pneumonia. In patients with cerebral malaria, a loading dose of phenytoin should be given followed by maintenance doses adjusted according to blood level measurements. Treatments for cerebral edema are unnecessary in the majority of adult patients with cerebral malaria.[8,27] In Kenyan children with cerebral malaria there was evidence of raised intracranial pressure which could be reduced by intravenous infusion of mannitol 1 g/kg over 20 min.[16] A number of ancillary treatments for cerebral malaria have been advocated in the past but are no longer recommended. Most have potentially dangerous side effects and are contraindicated. For example, dexamethasone in doses of approximately 2 mg/kg and 11 mg/kg did not improve the mortality of cerebral malaria in two double-blind placebo controlled trials.[13,28] Dexamethasone prolonged unconsciousness and was associated with an increased incidence of secondary bacterial infections and gastrointestinal hemorrhage. Immunosuppressant treatment has been attempted in cerebral malaria, based on the unlikely hypothesis that it is an immunopathy. A recent double-blind placebo controlled trial of cyclosporine A [5 mg/(kg · day) for 5 days] in patients with cerebral malaria in Ho Chi Minh City, Vietnam suggested that this drug was deleterious in the highest-risk group of patients (Trinh-Kim-Anh et al. unpublished).

ANEMIA

Significant anemia is an inevitable accompaniment of severe malaria. If transfusion becomes necessary for severe anemia, packed red blood cells should be transfused while the patient is carefully monitored for evidence of incipient pulmonary edema. Diuretics, such as intravenous furosemide, may be required during the transfusion to reduce the risk of fluid overload. In malaria endemic areas such as Africa, patients may present in anemic "cardiac failure" (high output state with generalized edema) especially in pregnancy. In such patients, and in those with incipient pulmonary edema, exchange transfusion may be the safest way of correcting severe anemia. Blood transfusion may have little permanent effect in raising the hematocrit of patients with severe malaria because of the greatly reduced survival of even nonparasitized erythrocytes.[29] Although some physicians have suggested that this may be caused by quinine-induced hemolysis, continuation of quinine therapy is nevertheless absolutely essential.

HYPOGLYCEMIA

The possibility of hypoglycemia in patients with severe or deteriorating symptoms must constantly be borne in mind. Frequent monitoring of the blood glucose is essential. Intravenous 50% dextrose (25 to 50 mL) should be tried if hypoglycemia is suspected or proved. If hypoglycemia is persistent or recurrent, and further infusions of hypertonic glucose seem undesirable because of incipient pulmonary edema, fluid overload, or hypokalemia, release of pancreatic insulin by cinchona alkaloids can be blocked by the somatostatin analogue Sandostatin (SMS201-995). This can be administered by continuous intravenous infusion pump (50 μg/h) or, more conveniently, as a single subcutaneous dose of 50 μg. Glucagon (1 mg subcutaneously) must be given, as somatostatin also blocks glucagon release.[30]

METABOLIC (LACTIC) ACIDOSIS

This results from impaired tissue perfusion caused by hypovolemia and microvascular obstruction, reduced hepatic clearance of lactate, and, in patients with a large parasite burden, from the parasites' lactic acid production. Tissue perfusion and oxygenation should be improved by correcting hypovolemia, clearing the airway, increasing inspired oxygen concentration (and considering mechanical ventilation), and the treatment of gram-negative bacteremia, a frequently associated complication. (For treatment of lactic acidosis see Chap. 158.)

DISSEMINATED INTRAVASCULAR COAGULATION

Severe DIC with spontaneous bleeding and fibrin deposition in the lungs and other tissues is an unusual complication of severe falciparum malaria but appears to be relatively more common in nonimmune travelers. (For treatment of DIC see Chap. 146.)

DISTURBANCES OF FLUID AND ELECTROLYTE BALANCE

Patients with severe falciparum malaria are commonly dehydrated and hypovolemic on admission to the hospital as a result of decreased fluid intake, increased insensible losses through sweating and hyperventilation during febrile episodes, gastrointestinal fluid losses (vomiting and diarrhea), and sometimes during the diuretic phase of recovery from acute renal failure. If these patients are denied parenteral fluid replacement, they are at high risk of developing hypotension, shock, inadequate tissue perfusion, lactic acidosis, and renal failure. On the other hand, excessive fluid replacement in the presence of hypoalbuminemia and neutrophil-mediated increases in pulmonary capillary permeability may lead to acute and catastrophic pulmonary edema. Thus, fluid balance and functional intravascular volume must be carefully assessed, and when doubt exists about the adequacy of the intravascular volume or if there is hemodynamic instability or pulmonary edema, a central venous or pulmonary artery catheter should be inserted. (For correction of hyponatremia, hypocalcemia, hypophosphatemia, and hyper- or hypokalemia see Chap. 156.)

PULMONARY EDEMA

This may be associated with high central venous and pulmonary wedge pressures (caused by volume overload and/or anemia) or with low pressures as in adult respiratory distress syndrome (ARDS) of other causes. See Chaps. 54 and 128 for a discussion of the management of these complications.

RENAL FAILURE

Oliguria may be prerenal, caused by volume depletion, or attributable to acute renal failure (see Chap. 153).

HEMOGLOBINURIA AND BLACKWATER FEVER

Intravascular hemolysis may be associated with acute renal failure. Some nephrologists believe that "pigment nephropathy" can be prevented by the use of mannitol and bicarbonate. Packed red blood cells should be transfused to maintain the hematocrit above 20 percent. Despite the suggestion that quinine-related hemolysis may be responsible for blackwater fever, treatment with cinchona alkaloids in patients with severe falciparum malaria should not be stopped unless an effective alternative drug is available. If renal dialysis is indicated (Chap. 155), hemodialysis or hemofiltration are preferable to peritoneal dialysis since there may be impairment of peritoneal perfusion and acute malaria is a hypercatabolic state.

HYPERPARASITEMIA

Mortality generally increases with parasitemia, exceeding 50 percent at parasitemias above 500,000 per microliter. It has been suggested that exchange transfusion, by reducing the burden of parasitemia more rapidly than does chemotherapy alone, might reduce this appalling mortality. Other advantages of exchange transfusion might be the removal of harmful metabolites, toxins, and mediators and the restoration of normal red blood cell mass, platelets, clotting factors, and other depleted substances. However, these advantages must be weighed against the potential dangers and difficulties of the procedure. These include electrolyte disturbances (hypocalcemia), cardiovascular complications, and infection by retroviruses and other pathogens. The supply of blood screened for human immunodeficiency virus (HIV) and hepatitis B is becoming extremely difficult in tropical countries such as those of Africa. In more than 70 reported cases, red blood cell exchange achieved rapid reduction in parasitemia which, in some cases, was accompanied by evidence of clinical improvement.[18,31] Partial exchange, using only 1 or 2 L of blood, which is much more practicable in the tropical endemic area, has also produced encouraging results.[31] Exchange transfusion should probably be considered in nonimmune travelers who are severely ill, who have deteriorated on conventional chemotherapy, and who have parasitemias above 10 percent. Exchange can be achieved by alternately venesecting and transfusing the patient, or by continuous cell separation (hemopheresis). Arterial and central venous or pulmonary wedge pressure must be measured frequently during exchange transfusion. If possible, plasma concentrations of the antimalarial drug (usually quinine or quinidine) should be measured at the end of the procedure in case additional treatment is needed.

RUPTURED SPLEEN

This is the only life-threatening complication which is more common in vivax than falciparum malaria. It must be suspected and excluded in patients who develop abdominal pain and shock. Ultrasound is useful for detecting free blood in the peritoneum and a tear in the splenic capsule. Invasive techniques such as needle aspiration of the peritoneal cavity, laparoscopy, or laparotomy may be required. Because of the risks of susceptibility to pneumococcal and other infections, overwhelming postsplenectomy sepsis, and the appreciable mortality and complications of splenectomy itself, there is an increasing tendency to attempt conservative treatment for splenic rupture. This involves bed rest and close observation for at least a week in case of sudden deterioration requiring urgent surgical intervention.

CASE PRESENTATION

In 1979, a 54-year-old English woman, who had been living in Zambia for 24 years but had never taken antimalarial chemoprophylaxis, became unwell with nausea and vomiting for 1 week before flying home to England. On arrival she was seen by a general practitioner who diagnosed "flu or a gastric upset" for which antacid was prescribed. The next day she noticed headache and fever and was seen again by the general practitioner. Her condition deteriorated so that by the evening of her admission to the hospital 5 days after returning to England she was unable to speak. She was found to be irritable and dysphasic. Her pupils were equal and small, the tendon reflexes were symmetrical, and the plantar responses extensor. Her oral temperature was 37.2°C. She was jaundiced and her skin was cool and clammy. Her blood pressure was 70/60 mmHg, and the pulse rate was 120 per minute. Auscultation of the heart and lungs was normal. Hemoglobin was 15.5 g/dL, total white blood cell count was 9900 per microliter, plasma sodium was 137, urea was 8.4, and glucose was 5.3 (mmol/L). Twenty percent of peripheral erythrocytes were parasitized with *P. falciparum.* She was started on chloroquine, given by slow intravenous infusion. (In 1979, Zambian strains of *P. falciparum* were fully sensitive to chloroquine.) Later she developed apneic episodes with Cheyne-Stokes respiration and was transferred to the intensive care unit. At this stage she was unrousable and had nonpurposive responses to painful stimuli. Her breathing was irregular, and she had one grand mal convulsion lasting 30 s controlled by diazepam, after which her pupils became dilated. She had two further grand mal convulsions and was started on phenytoin. Mechanical ventilation was started because of deteriorating arterial oxygen tension. She was in early pulmonary edema and was treated with diuretics. Parasitemia cleared quickly, but 5 days after admission her blood urea had risen and peritoneal dialysis was started. She was digitalized because of a high pulse rate and episodes of supraventricular tachycardia. Twenty-four hours later there were signs of improvement, oxygenation had improved, and she was extubated. However, an aspiration pneumonia, attributed to *Staphylococcus aureus,* developed 3 days later; she developed respiratory distress and had to be reintubated, and a tracheostomy was performed. Her serum albumin had fallen, and she was becoming generally edematous. *Pseudomonas* was grown from the peritoneal dialysate, and she was started on amikacin and ticarcillin. Low-dose dopamine was given to improve her urine output. After 2 weeks of mechanical ventilation, she was again extubated. She was by now fully conscious but was not moving her limbs. She was being fed via nasogastric tube. There was slow neurologic improvement, and 1 month after her admission peritoneal dialysis was stopped and her tracheostomy tube was removed. She was finally discharged from the hospital 36 days after admission, and, when followed up 8 weeks after the start of her illness, was found to be psychologically intact.

CASE DISCUSSION

This case makes a number of very important points. Although the patient had been living in a malarious area and not taking precautions, malaria was not initially suspected by the general practitioner when she arrived back in England with headache, fever, and gastrointestinal symptoms. Although chloroquine was the treatment of choice for falciparum malaria acquired in Zambia in 1979, this drug would not now be used for the treatment of severe falciparum malaria because of the extensive spread of chloroquine-resistant strains. In patients with cerebral malaria, the risk of generalized convulsions with subsequent neurologic deterioration and the risk of aspiration is so high that phenytoin prophylaxis is recommended as soon as the diagnosis has been made. For the treatment of acute renal failure developing in patients with severe falciparum malaria, hemofiltration or hemodialysis is preferred to peritoneal dialysis because of questionable circulation to the peritoneum and the hypercatabolic state associated with this infection. Early nutritional support is extremely important to compensate for this state. Secondary bacterial infections were a major problem. The pneumonia was probably attributable to aspiration during her grand mal convulsions.

Viral Hemorrhagic Fevers

At least 12 viruses, most of them tropical and zoonotic, can cause severe febrile illnesses in humans, characterized by varying degrees of shock, hemorrhage, and hepatic, myocardial, and renal damage (Table 112-4).[32] Imported cases in travelers are extremely rare, but because of the exotic nature, potential infectivity, and high mortality of the diseases, these incidents usually cause a disproportionate amount of public alarm and media attention.

EPIDEMIOLOGY AND TRANSMISSION (Table 112-4)

Mosquito transmission from mammals to humans is responsible for jungle yellow fever and Rift Valley fever (RVF), and from human to human for urban yellow fever and dengue. Primary dengue is an uncomfortable infection but is not dangerous. However, secondary infection in children with a different serotype may cause dengue shock syndrome or dengue hemorrhagic fever. Inhalation or ingestion by humans of virus excreted by rodents in their urine causes hemorrhagic fever with renal syndrome (HFRS)[33] and the Arenavirus infections. Ticks transmit Omsk hemorrhagic fever, Kyasanur forest fever, and Congo-Crimean hemorrhagic fever (CCHF) from mammals to humans, but the arthropod vectors of Marburg and Ebola virus diseases (MEVD) are unknown. A new Filovirus which shows some crossreactivity with Ebola virus was recently discovered in cynomolgus monkeys imported to the United States from the Philippines. Although it causes fatal disease in monkeys, seroconversion in monkey handlers was asymptomatic.[34]

CLINICAL FEATURES

Knowledge of incubation period (Table 112-4) is important as it may exclude the diagnosis in patients who develop symptoms too long after leaving or too soon after entering the endemic area. For example, a patient who becomes febrile more than 3 weeks after leaving west Africa is unlikely to be suffering from Lassa fever.

FEVER

This is the usual early symptom. It starts suddenly in HFRS, RVF, and MEVD but insidiously in Lassa fever. In primary dengue, the fever is characteristically diphasic or "saddleback" in contour, falling on the third day and returning with the rash a day or two later.

TABLE 112-4 Viral Hemorrhagic Fevers

	Geographic Distribution	Mammalian Host	Arthropod Vector	Incubation Period, (Days)	Mortality, %
		Flaviviridae			
Yellow fever	Africa, South America	Monkeys	*Aëdes*, etc., mosquitoes	3–6	20–50 (jaundice)
Dengue hemorrhagic fever	Global tropics, subtropics	—	*Aëdes* mosquitoes	5–8	5–20
Kyasanur Forest disease	Karnataka State, India	Monkeys	Ticks	3–8	5–10
Omsk hemorrhagic fever	Siberia, USSR	Muskrats, domestic animals	Ticks	2–9	?
		Bunyaviridae			
Hemorrhagic fever with renal syndrome	Asia, Europe	Rodents	—	8–35	3–5
Congo Crimean hemorrhagic fever	Africa, Middle East, Eastern Europe	Mammals, birds	Ticks	~3	15–40
Rift Valley fever	Sub-Saharan Africa	Domestic animals	*Culex* mosquitoes	2–6	5–10
		Arenaviridae			
Lassa fever	West Africa	Multimammate rat	—	7–20	1–20
Argentine hemorrhagic fever	Northeastern Argentina	Small rodents	—	5–19 (Argentine and Bolivian)	10–20
Bolivian hemorrhagic fever	Eastern Bolivia	Small rodents	—		10
		Filoviridae			
Marburg and Ebola virus disease	East, central, southern Africa	African monkeys	?	Marburg 3–8 Ebola 4–16	30–90

HEMORRHAGE

This is extremely variable in its incidence and severity in the various viral hemorrhagic fevers.[35] Spontaneous bleeding from the gums and nose, into the conjunctivae, skin (as petechiae or large ecchymoses), lungs and gastrointestinal tract may be sufficiently severe to cause hemorrhagic shock. It is worst in yellow fever, MEVD, Argentine hemorrhagic fever (AHF), and Bolivian hemorrhagic fever (BHF). Hemorrhagic infarction of the anterior pituitary was reported in patients with the Korean form of HFRS.[36]

SHOCK

This is usually attributable to hypovolemia resulting from increased capillary permeability. Shock usually develops after a few days of illness and is preceded by a rise in hematocrit and fall in serum protein with appearance of proteinuria.[36,37] Some patients show clinical evidence of leakage of plasma into the tissues: periorbital, facial, or sometimes conjunctival edema in the Korean form of HFRS and Lassa fever; serous effusions in dengue shock syndrome and intense retroperitoneal edema in the Korean form of HFRS. Pulmonary edema (ARDS) is a feature of many of the hemorrhagic fevers and may be precipitated by excessive fluid replacement.

MYOCARDITIS

Clinical, ECG, and histopathologic evidence of myocarditis has been found in AHF, BHF, and in the Korean form of HFRS. In particular, ECG changes are present in more than 70 percent of cases of AHF.

HEPATIC DYSFUNCTION

Biochemical evidence of hepatitis is common in CCHF, MEVD, and Arenavirus infections, but jaundice and hepatic failure are most unusual. Liver damage may be very severe in yellow fever and RVF: patients become progressively jaundiced and develop hepatic failure and massive spontaneous hemorrhage, usually from the gastrointestinal tract.[38]

RENAL FAILURE

This is a central feature of HFRS, and "hepatorenal syndrome" is seen in yellow fever and CCHF.

ENCEPHALOPATHY

This is particularly common in the Korean form of HFRS, RVF, Kyasanur Forest disease, AHF, and BHF. It is less common in Lassa fever.

DISSEMINATED INTRAVASCULAR COAGULATION

This may occur in dengue hemorrhagic fever, yellow fever, HFRS, and the Arenavirus infections.[35]

RASHES

A perifollicular maculopapular rash on the trunk, back, and shoulders which appears on the fourth to seventh day of illness is typical of MEVD. A macular erythematous rash is typical of primary dengue. Petechial rashes are seen in dengue hemorrhagic fever, HFRS, RVF, AHF, and BHF.

OTHER FEATURES

Conjunctivitis, retrosternal pain, and a painful, exudative pharyngitis, without coryza or rhinorrhea, are common in the early stages of Lassa fever. Sensorineural deafness develops in a third of patients during convalescence. One to three weeks after the acute symptoms of RVF, about 1 percent of patients develop a severe retinal vasculitis with exudates, hemorrhage, and edema. Severe gastrointestinal symptoms, nausea, vomiting, diarrhea, are common in MEVD.[39]

LABORATORY INVESTIGATIONS

Specimens from patients with suspected viral hemorrhagic fevers should be handled with great caution.[39,40] However, it is essential that a specific diagnosis be confirmed (see below) and that other treatable conditions be excluded.[41] Investigations should include examination of thick and thin blood smears for malaria; full blood count; blood cultures; culture of throat swab, urine, and stool (depending on the patient's symptoms); and storage of acute and convalescent sera for retrospective serology. Initially, leukopenia (absolute lymphopenia and neutropenia) is common, but the white blood cell count may rise later in the illness. Neutrophil leukocytes showing a failure of nuclear segmentation are seen in MEVD (acquired Pelger-Huët anomaly). The nuclei are round, bilobed, or dumbbell-shaped. Concentrations of serum enzymes, especially aspartate aminotransferase (AST, SGOT), are raised. In Lassa fever the concentration of serum AST has prognostic significance: levels of other serum hepatic enzymes may also be grossly elevated in the absence of jaundice.[42] Hyperbilirubinemia is most marked in yellow fever in which the serum bilirubin may reach 48 mg/dL. Coagulopathy (prolonged clotting times and evidence of increased fibrinolysis) results from hepatic necrosis and disseminated intravascular coagulation. Hemoconcentration, hypoalbuminemia, and proteinuria are associated with clinical evidence of increased capillary permeability and the development of shock. Blood urea and creatinine concentrations are raised in dehydrated patients and in those who develop acute tubular necrosis with HFRS, yellow fever, and RVF.

DIAGNOSIS

Virologic diagnosis is made in a high containment (P3) laboratory.[32] In most of the viral hemorrhagic fevers, isolation of virus is attempted from the blood, especially in the early days of the illness, using Vero cells and other cell lines and inoculation into rodents. Diagnostic viral morphology may be seen on electron microscopy of formalin-fixed liver (e.g., in MEVD) or other tissues, or there may be a diagnostic histologic appearance (e.g., Councilman and Torres bodies in hepatocytes in yellow fever). Viruses are identified in human tissues and in tissue cultures using indirect fluorescent antibody assays (IFA), in some cases employing monoclonal antibodies to viral antigens (e.g., Lassa fever). Various serologic techniques are also available including detection of specific IgM.

CLINICAL DIFFERENTIAL DIAGNOSIS

This includes all those tropical febrile illnesses characterized by prostration, shock, hemorrhage, encephalopathy, and renal and hepatic dysfunction in varying degrees. Severe falciparum malaria is the most important entity to be excluded. Other conditions which may be confused with viral hemorrhagic fever include other viral causes of hepatitis (HAV, HBV, HCV, HDV, HEV, HFV) and encephalitis, leptospirosis, relapsing fevers, typhoid, typhus, meningococcemia, and other septicemic conditions complicated by DIC.[40] If there is jaundice and hepatic failure, acute hepatic necrosis from poisons and the fulminant fatty hepatic necrosis of pregnancy must be considered. The acute painful exudative pharyngitis of Lassa fever must be distinguished from streptococcal sore throat, infectious mononucleosis, and other viral upper respiratory tract infections.[42] Diagnosis can be helped by up-to-date knowledge of current epidemics (e.g., by reading the Centers for Disease Control's *Morbidity and Mortality Weekly Report (MMWR)* or the World Health Organization's *Weekly Epidemiological Report*). The possibility of yellow fever will be excluded in those who have been adequately vaccinated. A detailed history will often help to establish the risk of a particular viral hemorrhagic fever. For example, many are localized to particular habitats or occupations at particular seasons of the year. Medical staff and those receiving injections through unsterilized needles were at high risk of MEVD and Lassa fever, contact with African and Asian monkeys and their tissues has been responsible for MEVD, while contact with animals' blood is important in RVF and Omsk hemorrhagic fever.

MANAGEMENT

SPECIFIC TREATMENT

Ribavirin (Tribavirin), a purine nucleoside analogue with antiviral activity against some RNA viruses, has proved effective in the treatment of Lassa fever and Hantaan virus infection (HFRS).[40,41] In Lassa fever, ribavirin is given by intravenous injection in a loading dose of 30 mg/kg followed by 16 mg/kg every 6 h for 4 days, and then 8 mg/kg every 8 h for 6 days, completing a total of 10 days' treatment.[43] A similar regimen has proved effective in HFRS in China.[44] Preclinical data suggest that ribavirin might also be effective in AHF, RVF, and CCHF. Convalescent (hyperimmune) human plasma reduced the mortality of AHF but caused some late neurologic complications.[45,46] Convalescent plasma (250 to 300 mL) did not prove beneficial in human patients with Lassa fever[43] but deserves reevaluation in view of its efficacy in combination with ribavirin in monkeys.[47] Plasma containing Ebola virus specific neutralizing antibodies was used in one proven case of Ebola virus infection. Viremia decreased within the next 12 h.[48] An intravenous infusion of 250 to 500 mL is recommended. This might lead to persistent excretion of virus. Hyperimmune human immunoglobulin for CCHF (CCHF-Venin) produced by the Institute of Infectious and Parasitic Diseases, Sofia, Bulgaria, has been used in patients with severe CCHF with encouraging results.[49]

SUPPORTIVE TREATMENT

Patients with suspected or proven viral hemorrhagic fever should be isolated in accommodation where they can receive close clinical supervision, the necessary laboratory investigations, and if necessary intensive care.[50] Primary contacts should also be observed in isolation,[37] or under surveillance,[42] depending on the virus involved. Ribavirin prophylaxis is recommended in some cases (see below). Treatment of the various complications of these syndromes including fluid and electrolyte disturbances, shock, hemorrhage and DIC, pulmonary edema and renal and hepatic failure is not substantially different from that in other diseases (the reader is referred to other chapters for discussions of the management of these problems). In dengue shock syndrome, correction of hypovolemia with isotonic saline, plasma expander or packed red blood cells, as appropriate, and pressor agents are effective.[51] Studies of Korean HFRS indicated that shocked patients with a warm periphery and bradycardia responded to intravenous noradrenaline (norepinephrine). Those with cold periphery, tachycardia, increased peripheral resistance, and marked hypovolemia responded better to plasma expanders.[36,37] Corticosteroids were not beneficial in HFRS or dengue hemorrhagic fever.[52,53]

PROTECTION OF MEDICAL AND NURSING STAFF AND CONTACTS[39,40,42,50]

All staff coming into contact with the patient should be fully briefed about the nature of the disease and the mode of transmission. In the case of suspected yellow fever, only immunized staff should be allowed near the patient. Prophylactic oral ribavirin in an *adult* dose of 500 to 600 mg every 6 h for 7 to 10 days is recommended for high-risk contacts of patients with Lassa fever, HFRS, and CCHF. This regimen may result in mild anemia.[42,54] Primary contacts of Lassa fever cases should be kept under surveillance for 21 days. It is reassuring that none of the medical staff or contacts of 20 well-documented cases of imported Lassa fever were infected.[54] Some progress has been reported in the development of a vaccine against Lassa fever.[55] Ideally, patients should not be moved from the hospital where they are originally diagnosed.

References

1. Warrell DA: Pathophysiology of severe falciparum malaria in man. Parasitology 94(suppl):S53, 1987.
2. Berendt AR, Simmons DL, Tansey J, et al.: Intercellular adhesion molecule-1 is an endothelial cell adhesion receptor for *Plasmodium falciparum*. Nature 341:57, 1989.
3. Oquendo P, Hundt E, Lawler J, et al.: CD36 directly mediates cytoadherence of *Plasmodium falciparum* parasitized erythrocytes. Cell 58:95, 1989.
4. Tandon NN, Kralisz U, Jamieson GA: Identification of glycoprotein IV (CD36) as a primary receptor for platelet-collagen adhesion. J Biol Chem 264(13):7576, 1989.
5. MacPherson GG, Warrell MJ, White NJ, et al.: Human cerebral malaria: a quantitative ultrastructural analysis of parasitized erythrocyte sequestration. Am J Pathol 119:385, 1985.

6. Warrell DA, White NJ, Veall N, et al.: Cerebral anaerobic glycolysis and reduced cerebral oxygen transport in human cerebral malaria. Lancet ii:534, 1988.
7. Kwiatkowski D, Hill AVS, Sambou I, et al.: TNF concentration in fatal cerebral, non-fatal cerebral and uncomplicated *Plasmodium falciparum* malaria. Lancet 336:1201, 1990.
8. Warrell DA, Looareesuwan S, Phillips RE, et al.: Function of the blood-cerebrospinal fluid barrier in human cerebral malaria: rejection of the permeability hypothesis. Am J Trop Med Hyg 35(5):882, 1986.
9. Molyneux ME, Looareesuwan S, Menzies IS, et al.: Reduced hepatic blood flow and intestinal malabsorption in severe falciparum malaria. Am J Trop Med Hyg 40(5):470, 1989.
10. Bradley DJ, Newbold CI, Warrell DA: Malaria, in Weatherall DJ, Ledingham JGG, Warrell DA (eds): *Oxford Textbook of Medicine.* Oxford, Oxford University Press, 1987, p 5.474.
11. Warrell DA, Molyneux ME, Beales PF (eds): Severe and complicated malaria. World Health Organization Malaria Action Programme: Second Edition Trans R Soc Trop Med Hyg 84(suppl): June 1990.
12. Molyneux ME, Taylor TE, Wirima JJ, et al.: Clinical features and prognostic indicators in paediatric cerebral malaria: a study of 131 comatose Malawian children. Q J Med 71(265):441, 1989.
13. Warrell DA, Looareesuwan S, Warrell MJ, et al.: Dexamethasone proves deleterious in cerebral malaria. A double-blind trial in 100 comatose patients. *N Engl J Med* 306(6):313,1982.
14. Warrell DA: Editorial. Cerebral malaria. Q J Med 71(265):369, 1989.
15. Charoenpan P, Indraprasit S, Kiatboonsri S, et al.: Pulmonary edema in severe falciparum malaria. Hemodynamic study and clinicophysiologic correlation. Chest 97:1190, 1990.
16. Newton CRJC, Kirkham FJ, Winstanley PA, et al.: Raised intracranial pressure in African children with cerebral malaria. Lancet, in press.
17. Phillips RE, Warrell DA, White NJ, et al.: Intravenous quinidine for the treatment of severe falciparum malaria. Clinical and pharmacokinetic studies. N Engl J Med 312(20):1273, 1985.
18. Miller KD, Greenberg AE, Campbell CC: Treatment of severe malaria in the United States with continuous infusion of quinidine gluconate and exchange transfusion. N Engl J Med 321(2):65, 1989.
19. White NJ, Looareesuwan S, Warrell DA, et al.: Quinine loading dose in cerebral malaria. Am J Trop Med Hyg 32(1):1, 1983.
20. Davis TME, Supanaronond W, Pukrittayakamee S, et al.: A safe and effective consecutive-infusion regimen for rapid quinine loading in severe falciparum malaria. J Infect Dis 161:1305, 1990.
21. Looareesuwan S, Phillips RE, White NJ, et al.: Quinine and severe falciparum malaria in late pregnancy. Lancet ii:4, 1985.
22. Prescott LF, Hamilton AR, Heyworth R: Treatment of quinine overdosage with repeated oral charcoal. Br J Clin Pharmacol 27:95, 1989.
23. White NJ, Watt G, Bergquist Y, et al.: Parenteral chloroquine for treating falciparum malaria. J Infect Dis 155(2):192, 1987.
24. White NJ, Miller KD, Churchill FC, et al.: Chloroquine treatment of severe malaria in children: pharmacokinetics, toxicity and revised dosage recommendations. N Engl J Med 319(23):1493, 1988.
25. Riou B, Barriot P, Rimailho A, et al.: Treatment of severe chloroquine poisoning. N Engl J Med 318(1):1, 1988.
26. Chanthavanich P, Looareesuwan S, White NJ, et al.: Intragastric mefloquine is absorbed rapidly in patients with cerebral malaria. Am J Trop Med Hyg 34(6):1028, 1985.
27. Looareesuwan S, Warrell DA, White NJ, et al.: Do patients with cerebral malaria have cerebral oedema? A computed tomography study. Lancet i:434, 1983.
28. Hoffman SL, Rustama D, Punjabi NH, et al.: High-dose dexamethasone in quinine-treated patients with cerebral malaria: a double-blind placebo-controlled trial. J Infect Dis 158(2):325, 1988.
29. Looareesuwan S, Merry AH, Phillips RE, et al.: Reduced erythrocyte survival following clearance of malarial parasitaemia in Thai patients. Br J Haematol 67:473, 1987.
30. Phillips RE, Warrell DA, Looareesuwan S, et al.: Effectiveness of SMS201-995, a synthetic, long-acting somatostatin analogue, in treatment of quinine-induced hyperinsulinaemia. Lancet i:713, 1986.
31. Looareesuwan S, Phillips RE, Karbwang J, et al.: *Plasmodium falciparum* hyperparasitaemia. Use of exchange transfusion in seven patients and a review of the literature. Q J Med 75:471, 1990.
32. McCormick JB, Fisher-Hoch S: Viral haemorrhagic fevers, in Warren KS, Mahmoud AAF (eds): *Tropical and Geographical Medicine.* New York, McGraw-Hill, 1990, p 700.
33. Pon E, McKee KT, Diniega BM, et al.: Outbreak of hemorrhagic fever with renal syndrome among US marines in Korea. A J Trop Med Hyg 42:612, 1990.
34. Centers for Disease Control: Filovirus infections among persons with occupational exposure to nonhuman primates. MMWR 39:266, 1990.
35. Cosgriff TM (ed): International Symposium on haemostatic impairment associated with haemorrhagic fever viruses. Rev Infect Dis 11(suppl):S669, 1989.
36. Symposium on Epidemic Hemorrhagic Fever. Am J Med 16:619, 1954.
37. Entwisle G, Hale E: Haemodynamic alterations in haemorrhagic fever. Circulation 15:414, 1957.
38. Monath TP: Yellow fever: a medically-neglected disease. Report on a seminar. Rev Infect Dis 9(1):165, 1987.
39. Simpson DIH: Marburg and Ebola virus infections: a guide for their diagnosis, management and control. *WHO Offset Publication,* No. 36. Geneva, 1977.
40. Centers for Disease Control: Management of patients with suspected viral haemorrhagic fever. *MMWR* 37(suppl):S3, 1988.
41. Warrell DA: Imported virus disease: the clinical diagnosis of Lassa fever and Marburg and Ebola virus diseases, in Weatherall DJ (ed): *Advanced Medicine 14.* London, Pitman Medical, 1978, p 255.
42. Holmes GP, McCormick JB, Trock SC, et al.: Lassa fever in the United States. Investigation of a case and new guidelines for management. N Engl J Med 323:1120, 1990.
43. McCormick JB, King IJ, Webb PA: Lassa fever, effective therapy with ribavirin. N Engl J Med 314:20, 1986.
44. Huggins JW: Prospects for treatment of viral haemorrhagic fevers with ribavirin, a broad spectrum antiviral drug. Rev Infect Dis 11(suppl):S750, 1989.
45. Maiztegui JI, Fernandez NJ, de Damilano AJ: Efficacy of immune plasma in treatment of Argentine haemorrhagic fever and association between treatment and a late neurological syndrome. Lancet ii:1216, 1979.
46. Enria DA, Franco SG, Ambrosio A: Current status of the treatment of Argentine haemorrhagic fever. Med Microbiol Immunol (Berl) 175:173, 1986.
47. Jahrling PB, Peters CJ, Stephen EL: Enhanced treatment of Lassa fever by immune plasma combined with ribavirin in cynomolgus monkeys. J Infect Dis 149:420, 1984.
48. Emond RTD, Evans B, Bowen ETW, et al.: A case of Ebola virus infection. *Br Med J* 2:541, 1977.
49. Vassilenko SM, Vassilev TL, Bozadjiev LG, et al.: Specific intravenous immunoglobulin for Crimean-Congo haemorrhagic fever (letter). Lancet 335:791, 1989.
50. Fisher-Hoch SP, Price MJ, Craven RB: Safe intensive care man-

agement of a severe case of Lassa fever using simple barrier nursing techniques. Lancet ii:1227, 1985.
51. World Health Organization: Dengue haemorrhagic fever: diagnosis, treatment and control. Geneva, WHO, 1986.
52. Sayer WJ, Entwistle G, Uyeno B, et al.: Cortisone therapy of early epidemic haemorrhagic fever: a preliminary report. Ann Intern Med 42:839, 1955.
53. Sumarmo, Talago W, Asrin A: Failure of hydrocortisone to affect outcome in dengue shock syndrome. Pediatrics 69:45, 1982.
54. Johnson KM, Monath TP: Imported Lassa fever—reexamining the algorithms. N Engl J Med 323:1139, 1990.
55. Fisher-Hoch SP, McCormick JB, Auperin D, et al.: Protection of rhesus monkeys from fatal Lassa fever by vaccination with a recombinant vaccinia virus containing the Lassa virus glycoprotein gene. Proc Natl Acad Sci USA 86:317, 1989.

Chapter 113
TOXIC SHOCK SYNDROME

P. JOAN CHESNEY

KEY POINTS

- *Risk factors for toxic shock syndrome (TSS) include damage to skin or a mucous membrane colonized by* Staphylococcus aureus, *insertion of a foreign body, and deep tissue infection with* S. aureus.
- *TSS is caused by circulating toxin(s) of* S. aureus *and not by circulating bacteria.*
- *Disease onset and progression may be extremely rapid and fulminant, even when the site of infection does not appear inflamed.*
- *Predictable manifestations of TSS that are not seen in septic shock include generalized erythroderma, intense mucous membrane erythema, myalgias, a profound secretory diarrhea, and early-onset acute renal failure.*
- *A profound decrease in systemic vascular resistance and massive capillary leak syndrome (CLS) result in hypotension and organ ischemia.*
- *Multisystem organ involvement and, ultimately, failure are always present in moderate-to-severe disease. Specifically, hypocalcemia and hypophosphatemia are common, despite acute renal failure.*
- *The most common causes of death are intractable adult respiratory distress syndrome (ARDS), arrhythmias, and bleeding.*
- *Because of the ongoing CLS, maintenance of an adequate cardiac output may require administration of fluids far exceeding usual baseline requirements needs. Such fluid replacement will markedly increase the lung edema due to ARDS.*
- *It is imperative to identify and drain the focus of infection and to remove any associated foreign bodies. Continued toxin production will thwart all other management efforts.*
- *Intravenous immune globulin (IVIG) has a high titer of antibody to one of the identified toxins, toxic shock syndrome toxin 1 (TSST–1). Use of IVIG and corticosteroids should be considered in severe cases.*

Nonmenstrual toxic shock syndrome (TSS) is now as common as menses-associated TSS. Thus, in the intensive care unit there will be as many children, males, and nonmenstruating females with TSS related to one of the risk factors in Table 113-1 as women with menses-associated TSS. As outlined in Table 113-1, TSS may occur in association with any deep tissue *S. aureus* infection, with a foreign body insertion, or with trauma to skin or to a mucous membrane normally colonized with *S. aureus,* such as the upper respiratory tract or the female genital tract.[1,2]

TABLE 113-1 Risk Factors for Toxic Shock Syndrome (TSS)

NONMENSTRUAL TSS
Skin trauma
Postoperative skin infection
Posttraumatic skin abrasion or bite
Needle injection or aspiration; ear piercing
Insect bite
Burns—chemical, scald, or fire
Dermatitis
Foreign body insertion
Augmentation mammoplasty
Septorhinoplasty with Teflon splint insertion
Orthopedic prosthetic devices
Barrier contraceptive use—diaphragm or sponge
Sutures
Peritoneal dialysis and central venous catheters
Insulin pump
Mucous membrane trauma
Respiratory
Mechanical injury
Surgical trauma
Infection: Sinusitis, tracheitis, croup, influenza, pneumonia, dental infections, pharyngitis
Genitourinary tract
Postpartum, postoperative
Gastrointestinal tract
Enterocolitis, peritonitis
Deep tissue Staphylococcus aureus *infection*
Pyomyositis, osteomyelitis, endometritis, pyarthrosis, abscess, endocarditis, pneumonia, postoperative, etc.
MENSTRUAL TSS
Associated with tampon use
No tampon use
NO OBVIOUS FOCUS
TSS with no identifiable focus

Pathogenesis

Following bacterial replication at the initial site of infection, toxin (but not bacteria) is disseminated throughout the body. Although TSST-1 is associated with more than 90 percent of *S. aureus* strains isolated from patients with menstrual TSS, it is associated with only 66 percent of strains isolated from foci of infection associated with nonmenstrual TSS.[3] Thus, the toxin "causing" at least one-third of cases of nonmenstrual TSS is not yet known.

TSST-1 is not itself damaging to most cells in vitro. It is, however, a very potent stimulus in vitro for the release of both interleukin-1 (IL-1) and tumor necrosis factor (TNF) from macrophages. Thus it has been suggested that the clinical manifestations of TSS may rather result from extensive endogenous mediator release than represent the direct effects of TSST-1 or other toxins themselves.[4]

Pathophysiology

The changes induced by the toxins or mediators involve almost every tissue and organ. Histopathologically, the two most prominent changes are a mild lymphocytic perivasculitis and an extensive interstitial edema in every organ, including the heart and brain.[5,6] The edema appears to be a result of both the generalized loss of vascular tone, resulting in peripheral congestion, and the capillary leak syndrome (CLS)—both of which are induced by the toxins or mediators. The situation does not appear to be quite this simple, however, since the same mediators are released in a number of unrelated severe illnesses that do not resemble TSS.

Unique features of TSS suggesting a yet-unidentified toxin include the erythroderma of skin and mucous membranes; subscleral hemorrhages; myalgias; and often-profound secretory diarrhea. Additional unique features include accelerated renal failure, hypocalcemia with elevated serum levels of a calcitonin-like molecule, mucous membrane ulcerations, and bullae with a characteristic cleavage between the dermis and epidermis.[7]

Clinical Manifestations

The onset is usually abrupt, with symptoms of chills and fever, headache, sore mouth and throat, nausea, vomiting, generalized myalgias with tender and weak muscles, abdominal pain, malaise, and profuse diarrhea. Within the next 24 to 48 h, generalized edema, arthralgias, erythroderma, conjunctival injection, cough, orthostatic dizziness or syncope, oliguria, and incontinence may develop (see Fig. 113-1 and Plate 44). The patient then begins to manifest symptoms of a diffuse encephalopathy, and may become obtunded.[1,7]

On examination of a moderately or severely ill patient, the most striking findings are fever; agitation or disorientation; generalized erythroderma (if the patient is not in shock) and myalgias; cyanotic, poorly filling nailbeds; and mottling of the extremities, superimposed on edematous facies and extremities. The conjunctivae and all mucous membranes are intensely red and may be ulcerated. Abdominal tenderness and nuchal rigidity may be present, because of severe myalgias. Dehydration, due to prolonged fever, vomiting, diarrhea and decreased fluid intake, as well as the loss of vascular tone and CLS, will be manifest as tachycardia, tachypnea, hypotension, poor capillary refill, and oliguria or anuria. Suspected foci of infection will probably not appear inflamed.[8,9]

FIGURE 113-1 This photograph shows the diffuse erythroderma on the trunk and arm of a 10-year-old female with toxic shock syndrome. See Plate 44.

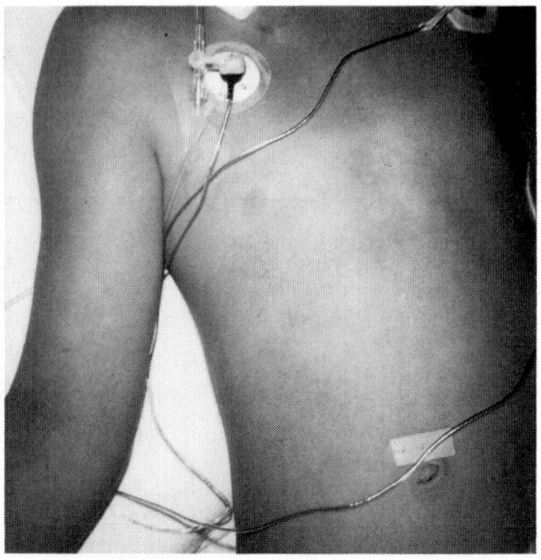

Laboratory

The laboratory changes outlined in Table 113-2 are those expected in an acutely ill, febrile, dehydrated person with poor organ perfusion. Several aspects of this profile deserve comment. The hypocalcemia, which may result in tetany, is due in part to the hypoproteinemia; it is also thought to be related to the high levels of a circulating calcitonin-like molecule. The hypophosphatemia, which may be profound, persists despite the presence of renal failure and is of unknown cause. Hyperbilirubinemia and liver function abnormalities are the result of a toxic triaditis, not of an ischemic centrilobular necrosis. Hypoproteinemia is probably secondary to the CLS, while the pyuria and cerebrospinal fluid (CSF) pleocytosis appear to be related to the generalized mucositis and serositis.

Although the leukocytosis is not usually impressive,

TABLE 113-2 Distinctive Laboratory Profile in Toxic Shock Syndrome

Metabolic Changes	
Hypocalcemia	Lactic acidosis
Hypophosphatemia	Azotemia
Hypoproteinemia	↑ Serum creatine kinase
Hypoalbuminemia	↑ Myoglobinemia
Hyponatremia	Hyperbilirubinemia
Hypocholesterolemia	↑ Liver enzymes
Hypoferremia	
Hypomagnesemia	
Impaired renal concentrating ability	
Hematologic Changes	
Anemia	Lymphopenia
Leukocytosis	Thrombocytopenia
Marked left shift	Occasional DIC
Many immature neutrophils	
Mucositis and Serositis	
Pyuria	
Cerebrospinal fluid pleocytosis	
Microbiology	
Staphylococcus aureus in pure culture from a normally sterile site, or present in a site of mixed flora. Negative blood, urine, CSF cultures	

there are almost always more than 90 percent immature and mature neutrophils. The elevated creatine phosphokinase (CPK) level and myoglobinemia may reflect IL-1–induced proteolysis. The elevated blood urea nitrogen (BUN) and creatinine levels are due initially to prerenal azotemia, and later to acute tubular necrosis. The lactic acidosis reflects generalized organ ischemia secondary to dehydration, organ edema, and a decreased circulating blood volume.[7] The clinical manifestations required to fulfill the case definition for moderate and severe disease are outlined in Table 113-3.

Differential Diagnosis

The diseases listed in Table 113-4 include the syndromes of fever, rash, or apparent multisystem disease most often confused with TSS. A TSS–like syndrome associated with group A beta-hemolytic streptococci may be caused by the erythrogenic toxins and may be indistinguishable from that due to *S. aureus*.[15]

TABLE 113-3 Toxic Shock Syndrome Case Definition

Fever
- Temperature ≥38.9°C

Rash
- Diffuse macular erythroderma

Desquamation
- 1–2 weeks after onset of illness—particularly of palms, soles, fingers, and toes

Hypotension
- Systolic blood pressure ≤90 mmHg for adults; for children, <5th percentile for age, for ages <16 years
- Orthostatic syncope or orthostatic dizziness*

Involvement of 3 or more of the following organ systems:
- Gastrointestinal: vomiting or diarrhea at onset of illness
- Muscular: Severe myalgia or CPK level greater than twice the upper limit of normal
- Mucous membrane: Vaginal, oropharyngeal, or conjunctival hyperemia
- Renal: BUN or serum creatinine greater than twice the upper limit of normal: or, ≥5 white blood cells per high-power field in the absence of a urinary tract infection
- Hepatic: Total bilirubin, SGOT, or SGPT greater than twice the upper limit of normal
- Hematologic: Platelets ≤100,000/mm^3
- Central nervous system: Disorientation or alterations in consciousness without focal neurologic signs when fever and hypotension are absent

Negative results on the following tests, if obtained:
- Blood, throat, or cerebrospinal fluid cultures. Blood cultures may be positive for S. aureus*
- Serologic tests for Rocky Mountain spotted fever, leptospirosis, or measles

*Modifications: Toxic Shock Syndrome, United States 1970–1982. *MMWR* 31:201, 1982.

SOURCE: Centers for Disease Control Follow-up on Toxic-shock Syndrome. *MMWR* 29:441, 1980.

TABLE 113-4 Differential Diagnosis of TSS Including Diseases Associated with Fever, Exanthem, and Multisystem Organ Involvement

Meningococcemia
TSS-like illness due to group A beta-hemolytic streptococci
Measles
Septic shock
Rocky Mountain spotted fever
Kawasaki disease
Staphylococcal scarlatiniform eruption (scalded skin syndrome)
Severe drug eruption (Stevens-Johnson syndrome or toxic epidermal necrolysis)
Enteroviral syndrome with myocarditis
Leptospirosis
Salmonella infection
Systemic lupus erythematosus
Reye syndrome
Urinary tract infection
Secretory gastroenteritis

Management

Following the initial evaluation, if the patient is hypotensive or has orthostatic hypotension, laboratory studies should be obtained while the administration of intravenous (IV) fluids is being initiated. As the ultimate course is unpredictable in the early stages, close observation and monitoring are mandatory, except in the mildest cases. Initial studies should include all of the blood studies described in Table 113-3 as well as a urinalysis, chest x-ray, ECG, and cultures of blood and urine.

While IV fluids are being administered, possible foci of infection should be identified (Table 113-1), foreign bodies (including sutures) removed, gram stains and cultures obtained, and drainage and irrigation accomplished, if possible. Failure to identify and adequately drain the source of the toxin will thwart all subsequent therapy.

The severity and duration of hypotension are probably the most important determinants of whether acute renal failure (ARF) and life-threatening arrhythmias occur. Rapid reversal of hypotension is therefore imperative. Infusion of large volumes of fluid, up to 20 L per 24 h in an adult, may be necessary to maintain adequate cardiac output, venous return, and blood pressure. Subcutaneous edema, ARDS, and myocardial failure may all be continuing manifestations of the CLS and not of fluid overload. Thus the vascular volume status should be assessed independently on the basis of the central venous pressure, blood pressure, capillary refill, and urine output—assuming that diuretics and overt renal failure are not present.[1] While it is critical to avoid hypovolemia, excessive volume administration is also counterproductive. Fluid administration should be guided by the endpoint of adequacy of cardiac output as judged by mentation, urine output, arteriovenous oxygen content difference, etc. (see Chap. 114).

Antistaphylococcal β-lactamase–resistant antibiotics should be given intravenously in maximal recommended doses. This is particularly important in nonmenstrual cases, which may be associated with a deep tissue infection or bacteremia. Vancomycin should be initiated if there is reason to suspect a methicillin-resistant organism.[4]

In one retrospective study, 25 patients given a total dose of 38 ± 30 mg/kg of a prednisone equivalent over 3.4 ± 0.4 days were compared to 20 patients who received no corticosteroids. Corticosteroids were reported to have a beneficial effect on the severity of illness and duration of fever when given early in the illness.[10] Unless there is evidence of adrenal insufficiency, however, it may be appropriate to use corticosteroids only in patients in whom the hypotension does not respond, within the first few hours, to adequate fluid administration, antimicrobials, and drainage of the infected focus; or in patients in whom the infected focus cannot be drained such as pneumonia.

Commercial preparations of intravenous immunoglobulins (IVIG) contain high levels of antibody to TSST-1, and potentially to other, yet-unidentified, toxins. Administration of IVIG for toxin neutralization has been shown to be beneficial in a rabbit model of TSS.[11] Although IVIG has not yet been systematically tested in human beings with TSS, it might also be considered for the same patients as may be eligible for corticosteroid administration.[4] Ongoing research includes investigations into the use of monoclonal antibodies to IL-1, TNF, and TSST-1.

In the most severely ill patients, particularly those who do not respond to the initial therapy described above, the mortality rate resulting from ARDS and arrhythmias is high.[5,6] The ARDS becomes most severe following fluid resuscitation for the CLS; the arrhythmias may be associated with a toxic cardiomyopathy. When managed aggressively and early, the ARDS usually responds to mechanical ventilation and positive end-expiratory pressure (PEEP).

Hemodynamic monitoring in severely ill patients has demonstrated three stages in severe disease: the hyperdynamic, decompensated, and recovery stages.[12] The initial, hyperdynamic, stage is associated with decreased blood pressure, decreased systemic vascular resistance, increased cardiac index, and normal pulmonary capillary wedge pressure (PCWP). In the decompensated stage the blood pressure may be unchanged, but myocardial dysfunction is evident as measured by a decrease in the cardiac index and an increase in the PCWP, with left atrial and ventricular end-diastolic diameters at the upper limits of normal. IV dobutamine has been beneficial to patients in this stage.[12] In the recovery stage, echocardiograms return to normal. Thus a reversible toxic cardiomyopathy is probably an important cause of cardiorespiratory failure in TSS.[13,14]

Other important aspects of management include the symptomatic therapy of acid-base and electrolyte disorders, including hypocalcemia, disseminated intravascular coagulation (DIC), acute renal failure, and increased intracranial pressure.

Antibiotic therapy should be given for as long as the underlying infection dictates, but in no case for less than 10 to 14 days. Oral therapy with dicloxacillin may be considered once the patient is clearly improved and taking fluids by mouth if the focus of infection is small enough and superficial enough that IV antibiotics are no longer required.

Assays for the production of TSST-1 by *S. aureus* isolates, and for the serum antibody titers to TSST-1, are available in specialized research laboratories. Detection of TSST-1 in tissues or body fluids is difficult and is available only in research laboratories.[1,4,7]

Since at least one-third of *S. aureus* isolates from nonmenstrual cases do not make TSST-1, absence of detectable toxin does not exclude the diagnosis. Indications for performing toxin testing are therefore extremely limited.

CASE PRESENTATION

A healthy 16-year-old male had a small lipoma of the arm removed under local anesthesia, with placement of polyglycolic (Dexon) sutures. Within 14 h he experienced nausea, vomiting, watery diarrhea, myalgias, chills, and fever. Within 24 h of the procedure he was admitted to the hospital with mental confusion, fever, hypotension (systolic blood pressure of 60 mmHg), erythroderma, and markedly injected mucous membranes, including the conjunctivae. The biopsy site appeared normal, but was opened. The sutures were removed and the site was drained of a serous fluid, which had gram-positive cocci in clusters on Gram stain and which grew *S. aureus*. The initial laboratory data are outlined in Table 113-5.

Despite the administration of nafcillin, an aminoglycoside, dexamethasone (10 mg), and 6 L of crystalloid in the first 3 h of hospitalization, the patient's systolic blood pressure remained at 60 to 90 mmHg; 3 h later he had a cardiorespiratory arrest. Electric countershock was required for ventricular tachycardia, and mechanical ventilation was initiated. Renal, respiratory, and hepatic failure were complicated by DIC, gastritis, and neurologic dysfunction following the arrest. Hemodialysis was required for 40 days. Positive end-expiratory pressure and 100 percent fraction of inspired oxygen were needed initially to maintain adequate oxygenation.

Cryoprecipitate, fresh frozen plasma, blood, and platelets were required for the DIC and thrombocytopenia. Over the ensuing 3 weeks, invasive monitoring, vasoactive drugs, total parenteral nutrition, and steroids were used. Desquamation of the palms, soles, fingers, and toes occurred (see Fig. 113-2 and Plate 45). The patient

TABLE 113-5 Serum and Arterial Blood* Laboratory Studies on Admission

Na = 134 meq/L	Ca = 5.3 mg/dL
K = 4.3 meq/L	TP = 2.8 g/L
CL = 108 meq/L	Alb = 1.3 g/L
CO_2 = 11 meq/L	Bilirubin = 3.0 mg/dL
Creat = 3.9 mg/dL	CPK = 9,320
WBC 14,600 mm^3	Hct = 34%
PMN = 35%	Plats = 200,000/mm^3
Bands = 36%	pH = 7.21*
Monos = 3%	P_{CO_2} = 20 torr*
Meta = 10%	Pa_{O_2} = 234 torr*
Myelo = 13%	BE = −15 meq/L*
Atyp = 3%	

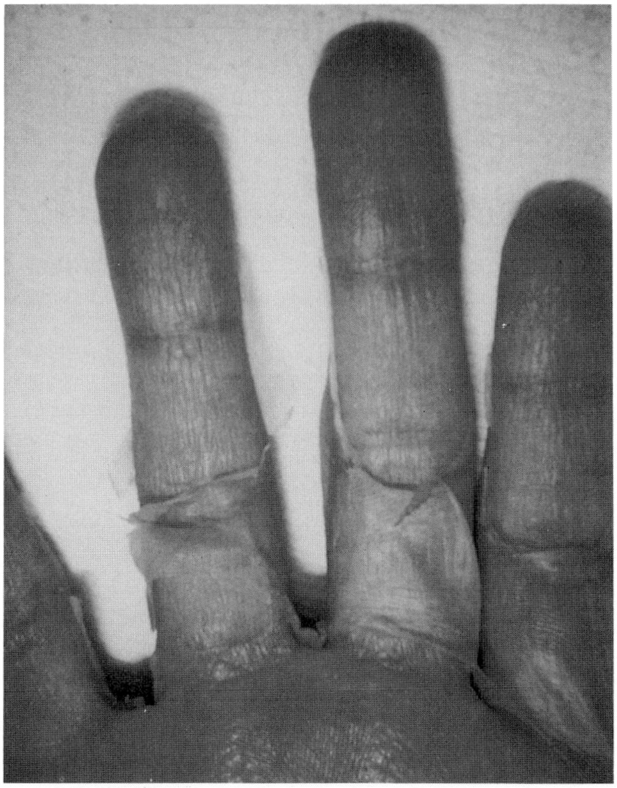

FIGURE 113-2 Full thickness desquamation of the fingers 10–14 days after the onset of symptoms. See Plate 45.

was discharged after 50 days of hospitalization, still weak but able to walk, and with no obvious central nervous system residua.

The *S. aureus* isolated from the wound produced only staphylococcal enterotoxin B (SEB) in vitro. The patient had a fourfold increase in antibody to SEB during hospitalization.

CASE DISCUSSION

This patient's presentation and course illustrate several important principles in the diagnosis and management of TSS. Surgical trauma to an area of the body frequently colonized by *S. aureus* allowed entry of the toxin-producing organism into an area rich in nutrients, with ideal conditions for toxin production. Toxin dissemination occurred rapidly, inducing the unique manifestations of TSS—erythroderma, myalgias, a secretory diarrhea, and injected mucous membranes. Other manifestations characteristic of TSS (Tables 113-2, 113-3) and of the loss of vascular tone and CLS were also present 24 h after the procedure, reflecting the multisystem organ failure.

The biopsy site appeared normal or uninflamed, as is usually the case for infected foci in TSS. Quite correctly, however, the site was opened, the sutures removed, and the serous fluid Gram stained and cultured. The rapid administration of a β-lactamase–resistant penicillin, corticosteroids, and fluids was too late to reverse toxin- or endogenous mediator–induced CLS in the lungs and heart.

The life-threatening arrhythmia required electric countershock; the ARDS was managed with prolonged positive-pressure ventilation with PEEP. The anoxic/ischemic multiple organ damage did not reverse immediately, and the patient continued to require invasive monitoring, vasoactive drugs, mechanical ventilation, blood and platelets, hemodialysis, intensive fluid and electrolyte management, and total parenteral nutrition (TPN) for several weeks. Prophylactic intubation should be considered in the management of such severely ill patients, as eventual cardiorespiratory arrest (related to the excessive work of breathing in the face of hemodynamic instability) can be anticipated.

The use of corticosteroids in TSS is controversial and is based on one retrospective study, described above. The anticipated beneficial effects of corticosteroids in vivo are based on in-vitro observations of their effects on lysosomal membrane stabilization and on mediator production, release, and metabolism.[10] As the authors of that study caution, however, there may be detrimental effects of such therapy including well-described complications, such as gastritis, as well as the potential for impairing the immune response, which may increase the rate of recurrence. Since no prospective controlled trials of the use of corticosteroids for TSS have been performed, most physicians reserve their use for severe cases that have not responded to most other management strategies, particularly cases where the focus of infection cannot be drained and continued short-term toxin production is anticipated.

IVIG was not used in this patient, but might have helped to neutralize circulating toxin. The sites of toxin breakdown, conjugation, and elimination are not known; but if both renal failure and hepatic biliary stasis are present, it seems that there may be inefficient toxin removal, and that IVIG might act to modify this process. The patient's *S. aureus* isolate did not make TSST-1, as is characteristic of 33 percent of such strains from nonmenstrual cases.[3]

The patient appeared to have no neurologic sequelae on discharge, but did have the prolonged and predictable sequelae of muscle pain and tenderness. The vast majority of previously healthy patients recover from TSS without long-term sequelae; this underlines the importance of aggressive early and anticipatory management.

Acknowledgement

The author expresses her gratitude to Ms. Shirley Elam for her skillful preparation of the manuscript.

References

1. Todd JK: Toxic shock syndrome. Clin Microbiol Rev 1(4):432, 1988.

2. Reingold AL, Hargrett NT, Dan BB, et al: Nonmenstrual toxic shock syndrome: A review of 130 cases. Ann Intern Med 96:871, 1982.
3. Garbe PL, Arko RJ, Reingold AL, et al: Staphylococcus aureus isolates from patients with nonmenstrual toxic shock syndrome. Evidence for additional toxins. JAMA 253:2538, 1985.
4. Parsonnet J: Mediators in the pathogenesis of toxic-shock syndrome: Overview. Rev Infect Dis 11(S1):S263, 1989.
5. Paris AL, Herwaldt LA, Blum D, et al: Pathologic findings in twelve fatal cases of toxic-shock syndrome. Ann Intern Med 96:852, 1982.
6. Larkin SM, Williams DN, Osterholm MT, et al: Toxic shock syndrome: Clinical, laboratory, and pathologic findings in nine fatal cases. Ann Intern Med 96:858, 1982.
7. Chesney PJ: Clinical aspects and spectrum of illness of TSS: Overview. Rev Infect Dis 11(S1):S1, 1989.
8. Dorman KJ, Thompson DM, Conn AR, et al: Toxic shock syndrome in the postoperative patient. Surg Gynecol Obstet 154:65, 1982.
9. Bartlett P, Reingold AL, Graham DR, et al: Toxic shock syndrome associated with surgical wound infections. JAMA 247:1448, 1982.
10. Todd JK, Ressman M, Caston SA, et al: Corticosteroid therapy for patients with toxic shock syndrome. JAMA 252:3399, 1984.
11. Melish ME, Frogner K, Hirata S, Murata MS: Use of IVGG for therapy in the rabbit model of TSS (abstract). Clin Res 35(1):220A, 1987.
12. Fisher CJ Jr, Horowitz A, Albertson TE: Cardiorespiratory failure in toxic shock syndrome: Effect of dobutamine. Crit Care Med 13:160, 1985.
13. Burns JR, Menpace FJ: Acute reversible cardiomyopathy complicating toxic shock syndrome. Arch Intern Med 142:1032, 1982.
14. Fitz JD, Weeks KD, Duff P: Left ventricular dysfunction in a patient with toxic shock syndrome. Am J Obstet Gynecol 146:467, 1983.
15. Stevens DL, Tanner MH, Winship J, et al: Severe group A streptococcal infections associated with a toxic shock–like syndrome and scarlet fever toxin A. N Engl J Med 321:1, 1989.

SECTION I

CARDIOVASCULAR DISORDERS IN THE CRITICALLY ILL

Chapter 114

SHOCK

KEITH R. WALLEY
LAWRENCE D.H. WOOD

KEY POINTS

- *Shock is present when there is evidence of multisystem organ hypoperfusion; it often presents as reduced mean blood pressure.*
- *Initial resuscitation aims to establish an adequate airway, breathing, and circulation; a working diagnosis or clinical hypothesis of the cause of inadequate circulation should always be made immediately by physical examination and clinical presentation before treatment is initiated.*
- *The most common causes of shock are high cardiac output hypotension, or* septic shock, *reduced pump function of the heart, or* cardiogenic shock, *and reduced venous return despite normal pump function, or* hypovolemic shock. *Overlapping etiologies can confuse the diagnosis, as can a short list of other less common etiologies, which are often separated by echocardiography and right heart catheterization.*
- *Initial cardiovascular therapeutic interventions are volume infusion for hypovolemic shock or inotropic and vasodilating drugs for cardiogenic shock; each should be regarded as testing the clinical hypothesis concerning the etiology of shock and therefore requires careful evaluation before and soon after implementation.*
- *Identify and correct early all factors aggravating shock; these include suboptimal ventilator therapy, infections, arrhythmias, acidosis, and hypothermia.*
- *Because shock affects organ systems and therapy, and organ system function and therapy affect shock, these interactions need to be considered in interpreting data and choosing therapeutic interventions.*
- *Urgent discontinuation of excessive invasive measurements and therapy should follow hemodynamic stabilization of the patient.*

Shock is a common critical illness necessitating admission to the ICU or occurring in the course of critical care. Because shock may be due to a wide variety of disease states, an adequate discussion must include a broad differential diagnosis of the many etiologies of shock, each requiring separate discussion of how the condition proceeds to a hypoperfusion state in order to present rational therapy. Yet the effective initial diagnosis and treatment follows a less detailed path at a rapid pace at the bedside of the patient in shock, based in large part on understanding cardiovascular pathophysiology described in Chap. 2. This chapter discusses shock the way that problem should be approached in each patient: first with an early working diagnosis, then an approach to urgent resuscitation, which confirms or changes the etiology, followed by a pause to ponder the broader differential diagnosis of the types of shock. Then we consider the goals of therapy in more detail and conclude with a discussion of the interactions among shock, organ system dysfunction, and therapy. In this way, we hope to provide both an effective approach to the early diagnosis and treatment of shock and a scholarly discussion of the topic in a format that allows early diagnosis and treatment to proceed urgently by referring the reader to details of pathophysiology (see Chap. 2) and of other disease states later in this chapter.

Establishing a Working Diagnosis of the Cause of Shock

DEFINITIONS OF SHOCK

Shock is present if evidence of multisystem organ hypoperfusion is apparent. Evidence of hypoperfusion obtained during the rapid initial clinical evaluation of a patient in shock may include tachycardia, low mean blood pressure, altered mental status, and decreased urine output. Hypotension has special importance because it commonly occurs during shock, blood pressure is easily measured, and because extreme hypotension always results in shock. Important caveats are that even modest hypotension (mean < 60 mmHg, systolic < 90 mmHg) is not always associated with shock and shock can occur despite elevated blood pressure, as illustrated in the case presentation at the end of the chapter. Furthermore, cuff blood pressure measurements may markedly underestimate central blood pressure in low flow states.[1]

Many other definitions of shock of varying complexity have been proposed, reflecting the diverse, complex, and incompletely understood pathophysiology of shock. One important manifestation of hypoperfusion is tissue hypoxia, often indicated by lactic acidosis and other metabolic abnormalities (see Chaps. 55 through 57). Determining what type of shock is present is important for implementing effective initial therapy and setting the tempo of therapy. Indeed, it is appropriate for the initial working definition to change in each patient as therapy is initiated and as more patient data become available allowing incorporation of further pathophysiologic concepts. For example, if a pulmonary artery catheter is inserted, then shock may be diagnosed by concurrently finding that lactate levels are elevated and that changes in oxygen consumption depend on

TABLE 114-1 Early Formulation of a Working Diagnosis of the Etiology of Shock

Shock Features	Septic	Cardiogenic	Hypovolemic
Blood pressure	↓	↓	↓
Heart rate	↑	↑	↑
Respiratory rate	↑	↑	↑
Mentation	↓	↓	↓
Urine output	↓	↓	↓
Arterial pH	↓	↓	↓
Is Cardiac Output Reduced?	No	Yes	Yes
Pulse pressure	↑	↓	↓
Diastolic pressure	↓ ↓ ↓	↓	↓
Extremities/digits	Warm	Cool	Cool
Nailbed return	Rapid	Slow	Slow
Heart sounds	Crisp	Muffled	Muffled
Temperature	↑ or ↓	↔	↔
White cell count	↑ or ↓	↔	↔
Site of infection	++	−	−
Is the Heart Too Full?	No	Yes	No
Symptoms/clinical context	Sepsis/liver failure	Angina/ECG	Hemorrhage/dehydration
Jugular venous pressure	↓	↑	↓
S_3, S_4, gallop rhythm	−	+++	−
Respiratory crepitations	−	+++	−
Chest radiograph	Normal	Large heart ↑ upper lobe flow Pulmonary edema	Normal
What Does Not Fit?			
Overlapping etiologies (septic + cardiogenic, septic + hypovolemic, cardiogenic + hypovolemic)			
Short list of other etiologies	*High output hypotension*	*High right atrial pressure hypotension*	*Nonresponsive hypovolemia*
	Thyroid storm Arteriovenous fistula Paget's disease	Cardiac tamponade Right ventricular infarction Pulmonary hypertension	Adrenal insufficiency Anaphylaxis Spinal shock
Get more information	Echocardiography, right heart catheterization		

changes in oxygen delivery.[2] Taken to a level of sophistication currently not feasible, if tissue adenosine triphosphate (ATP) and other high energy phosphate stores are assessed, then shock could be diagnosed using a biochemical definition.

A QUESTIONING APPROACH TO THE INITIAL CLINICAL EXAMINATION

A much less sophisticated working definition of shock is helpful in the initial diagnosis and management of the hypotensive patient (see discussion of Table 2-2 in Chap. 2). This approach acknowledges that shock is identified in most patients by hypotension, and that mean blood pressure is the product of cardiac output and the systemic vascular resistance (SVR). Accordingly, hypotension may be due to reduced cardiac output or reduced SVR. Initial examination of the hypotensive patient seeks to answer the question; *is cardiac output reduced or not?* High cardiac output hypotension is most often signaled by a large pulse pressure, a low diastolic pressure, warm extremities with good nailbed return, fever (or hypothermia), and leukocytosis (or leukopenia); these clinical findings strongly suggest a working diagnosis of septic shock, the initial treatment for which is thoughtful antibiosis combined with adequate but not excessive expansion of the vascular volume (Table 114-1).

By contrast, low cardiac output is signaled by a small pulse pressure and cool extremities with poor nailbed return. In this case, clinical examination turns to a second question; *is the heart too full or not?* A heart which is too full in a hypotensive patient is signaled by elevated jugular venous pressure (JVP), peripheral edema, crepitations on lung auscultation, a large heart with extra heart sounds (S_3, S_4), chest pain, ischemic changes on the electrocardiogram (ECG), and a chest radiograph showing a large heart with dilated upper lobe vessels and pulmonary edema. These findings suggest cardiogenic shock, most often due to ischemic heart disease, and are generally absent when the low cardiac output is due to hypovolemia (see Table 114-1). Then, clinical examination reveals manifestations of blood loss (hematemesis, tarry stools, abdominal distention, reduced hematocrit, trauma), or manifestations of dehydration (reduced tissue turgor, vomiting or diarrhea, negative fluid balance). This distinction between cardiogenic and hypovolemic shock allows initial therapy to focus on vasoactive drugs or on volume infusions, respectively.

Whenever the clinical formulation is not obvious after answering the first two questions, the intensivist may find it helpful to ask a third; *what does not fit?* Most often, the answer is that the hypotension is due to two or more of these commonest etiologies of shock; viz., septic shock complicated by myocardial ischemia or hypovolemia, cardiogenic shock complicated by hypovolemia or sepsis, and hypovolemic shock masking sepsis or ischemia heart disease. At this time, more data is frequently needed, especially aided by echocardiography and right heart catheterization. Interpretation of the data and response to initial therapy frequently confirm the multiple etiologies or lead to a broader differential diagnosis of the etiologies of shock (vide infra). A short list of common etiologies other than septic, cardiogenic, or hypovolemic shock can be grouped as they present (see Table 114-1)—high cardiac output hypotension which does not appear due to sepsis or liver failure, high right atrial hypotension not due to left ventricular ischemia, and poorly responsive hypovolemic shock.

Urgent Initial Resuscitation

During the first hour the urgent initial resuscitation aims to avoid later sequelae of organ system hypoperfusion by rapidly restoring an adequate circulation. Effective therapy is based on the working diagnosis established by a systematic survey and confirmed or changed by the response to therapy. During this time, additional data are obtained from catheterization and special tests to titrate therapy toward the goal of correcting the hypoperfusion state with minimal complications. This stage ends with a careful reconsideration of what happened to set the goals of longer term therapy or to obtain additional diagnostic tests appropriate to evaluate further the type of shock.

PRIMARY SURVEY

No specific therapy has been demonstrated to be uniformly successful in managing shock and mortality rates remain high. However, it is clear that, if untreated, shock will lead to death; irreversible organ system damage often develops rapidly. Therefore, we believe that early institution of aggressive resuscitation will improve a patient's chances of survival. To improve efficiency at the necessarily rapid tempo a systematic approach to initial evaluation and resuscitation is useful as it is during cardiac emergencies (ACLS) and trauma (ATLS). In analogy to these systematic "ABC" approaches, a primary survey of a critically ill patient in shock should include assessing and, if necessary, establishing an airway; evaluating breathing and considering mechanical ventilator support; and resuscitating the inadequate circulation.

AIRWAY AND BREATHING. Most patients in shock have one or more indications for airway intubation and mechanical ventilation, which should therefore be instituted early. Although a few patients in shock can be managed safely without airway intubation and mechanical ventilation, these should be thought of as the exception. Significant hypoxemia (even if suspected before the results of a blood-gas analysis are available) is one indication for airway intubation and mechanical ventilation because external masks and other devices may not reliably deliver an adequate fraction of inspired oxygen ($F_{I_{O_2}}$). Initially a high $F_{I_{O_2}}$ (100%) is used until blood-gas analysis allows titration of the $F_{I_{O_2}}$ down, toward less toxic concentrations, while maintaining adequate arterial oxygenation. Ventilatory failure is another indication for airway intubation and mechanical ventilation. Elevated and rising Pa_{CO_2} reliably establishes the diagnosis of ventilatory failure, but this is often a late finding. Young, previously healthy patients, in particular, are able to defend P_{CO_2} and pH up until a precipitous respiratory arrest. Therefore, clinical signs of respiratory muscle fatigue or subtle evidence of inadequate ventilation are more important early indicators.[3] For example, a patient in shock with a Pa_{CO_2} of 30 and a pH of 7.2 has inadequate respiratory compensation for the metabolic acidosis indicating ventilatory failure. Such a patient may be much more acidotic at the tissue level, as evidenced by a much greater mixed venous P_{CO_2} associated with the large arteriovenous difference in CO_2 which occurs in low cardiac output states.[4]

It is often useful to ask the patient who is working hard to ventilate whether he is tiring. Responses, ranging from no response to long cogent replies, are useful in deciding to initiate airway intubation and mechanical ventilation. Whatever the response, tachypnea >30/min, abdominal paradoxical respiratory motion, accessory muscle use, or other manifestations of labored breathing should lead to early elective intubation and ventilation of the patient in shock (see Chap. 133). In addition to treating hypoxemia and ventilatory failure, airway intubation and mechanical ventilation with sedation and, if necessary, muscle paralysis will decrease oxygen demand of the respiratory muscles allowing improved oxygen delivery to other hypoperfused tissue beds.[5] This is important in shock where the respiratory muscles consume a disproportionate share of the whole body oxygen delivery,[6] particularly because patients are frequently hyperventilating in response to acidosis, sepsis, or pain. Airway intubation may benefit even slightly obtunded patients who may inadequately protect their airways at this time of increased ventilatory drive and anxiety. In shock, airway intubation and mechanical ventilation should precede other complicated procedures, such as central venous catheterization, or complicated tests that require transportation of the patient, because these procedures and tests restrict the medical staff's ability to continuously assess the airway and ensure adequacy of ventilation. Whenever shock is accompanied by arterial hypoxemia, increased $F_{I_{O_2}}$ and positive end-expiratory pressure (PEEP) can correct arterial saturation in the ventilated patient. Note that intubation and positive-pressure ventilation frequently reduce venous return in the patient with hypovolemic shock, so greater volume resuscitation needs to be anticipated, and selecting an adequate but small tidal volume (8 mL/kg) minimizes this problem. On the other hand, the hypotension is often ameliorated by ventilation in the patient having adequate circulating volume, especially the patient in cardiogenic shock (vide infra).

CIRCULATION. The initial working definition we propose emphasizes that shock is most commonly a circulatory disorder. Accordingly, rapid cardiovascular resuscitation is the cornerstone of management. Yet, it is important to recognize that cardiovascular resuscitation means much more than simply restoring a normal blood pressure. That is, if there is evidence of tissue hypoperfusion then oxygen delivery to the tissues is inadequate to maintain normal aerobic metabolism and function at any measured blood pressure. Oxygen delivery is the product of cardiac output, oxygen-carrying capacity of the blood, and arterial oxygen saturation. It follows that the product of the three components is more important than any one in isolation.[7] Therefore, cardiovascular resuscitation is closely tied to correcting hemoglobin concentration and saturation (see Chap. 1).

Equally important is the obvious but frequently bypassed concept that effective cardiovascular resuscitation aims to reverse the cause of shock; hence, the emphasis on establishing a working diagnosis before urgent resuscitation. From the clinical hypothesis concerning the etiology, it follows that a patient in hypovolemic shock should receive aggressive intravascular volume expansion until the hypoperfusion state is corrected without vasoactive drugs, while the patient with cardiogenic shock and a gallop rhythm or elevated JVP needs vasoactive drug therapy without volume expansion. Yet diagnostic uncertainty and the need for urgent resuscitation often combines these therapies during this first hour—a practice which inadvertently delays correct diagnosis and subsequent effective resuscitation for the apparent gain of raising blood pressure sooner (vide infra).

The goal of cardiovascular resuscitation is to attain an adequate cardiac output and oxygen delivery to correct organ system hypoperfusion. After the shock state is improved with adequate vascular volume expansion, the lowest left ventricular filling pressure needed to maintain adequate cardiac output and oxygen delivery is sought.[8] This approach minimizes the complications of pulmonary edema or ventricular dysfunction (or both) due to excessive ventricular preload; if shock is not corrected by adequate circulating volume, then inotropic agents are indicated and will be more effective when the circulation is full. The rationale does not target specific values of pulmonary vascular pressures or cardiac output; rather it implies that management of the patient in shock involves repeated assessment to answer the question—is the heart too full or not? Based on the initial assessment of the patient in shock, the clinician makes an initial judgment that cardiac output and oxygen delivery are inadequate and that they will be improved by a selected intervention. If the heart is not too full, the indicated intervention is a volume challenge conducted in such a way as to ensure that improved output is detected (increased blood and pulse pressures), or the heart is observed to become too full (rising JVP, gallop, crepitations). Accordingly, this intervention is not only regarded as therapy but also as the test of the theme of resuscitation in deciding whether the therapy has been "too little versus too much." Resuscitation of the circulation particularly consists of reevaluation before and after stepwise therapeutic intervention; as soon as it becomes clear that the volume replacement is "too much" because the heart is too full in the hypotensive patient, inotropic drug therapy begins and is increased until it becomes too much or the combined volume and inotropic drug therapy corrects the shock.

For example, for a patient in shock with clinical evidence of hypovolemia, 1 or 2 L (or more) of warmed crystalloid solution (normal saline or Ringer's lactate) can be infused as fast as possible (<10 min) followed by immediate reevaluation. Therapy has quickly been instituted and the clinical evaluation of intravascular hypovolemia is tested leading to the next clinical evaluation that there is still evidence of tissue hypoperfusion (or not) and the patient is hypovolemic, euvolemic, or hypervolemic. Initial cardiovascular resuscitation may also use blood, blood products, colloid solutions, and inotropic or vasoactive drugs. Like the fluid infusion example given above, all of the interventions should be regarded as treatment and as tests of the initial clinical evaluation. Therapy does not begin with inotropic or other vasoactive agents when the circulatory volume is inadequate because these drugs often obscure shock by raising blood pressure without correcting the low cardiac output state (vide infra).

CATHETERS AND FREQUENT MEASUREMENTS DURING INITIAL RESUSCITATION

After an airway is established and breathing ensured, correction of the circulatory abnormality always requires good intravenous access. For large volume administration two peripheral intravenous catheters of gauge 16 or larger are required. Alternatively or additionally, a large bore central venous catheter may be used to infuse volume or vasoactive drugs and to facilitate early insertion of a right heart catheter if it is required; this central catheter should be connected to a pressure transducer for early recording of the central venous pressure (CVP) to evaluate its response to volume challenges. ECG monitoring is easily accomplished and usefully measures heart rate and rhythm to detect early, and so facilitate rational treatment of, tachy- or brady-arrhythmias aggravating the low flow state.

The urinary bladder should be catheterized to measure urine output and to facilitate urine sampling. A nasogastric or orogastric tube to decompress the stomach and later to deliver medication and nutrition is useful in the intubated patient. Measuring arterial pressure using a peripheral arterial or femoral arterial catheter is useful because in the patient in shock with low cardiac output or low blood pressure, cuff pressures may be inaccurate.[1] Arterial blood-gas and other blood samples are then readily obtained. Early echocardiography can be used to distinguish poor ventricu-

TABLE 114-2 Urgent Resuscitation of the Patient with Shock; Intravenous Volume and Vasoactive Drug Therapy

Hemorrhagic Shock including Trauma, Ruptured Aneurysms	Nonhemorrhagic Hypovolemia including Septic Shock	Cardiogenic Shock due to Myocardial Ischemia
	Volume therapy	
Elevate legs, MAST Access/infuse emergency blood Group/match/administer warmed blood/components >3 L/20 min warmed saline Equal volumes of colloid or substitutes (albumin, dextran, hetastarch) Continue aggressive volume infusion until blood pressure normal Consider early surgical hemostasis	Elevate legs 3 L/20 min warmed saline Group/match packed RBCs and plasma re dilutional anemia Continue aggressive volume infusion until blood pressure normal or heart "too full" Detect and treat tamponade with pericardiocentesis, thoracostomy, peritoneal drainage, or reduced PEEP	When heart is "too full," ↓ blood volume (rotating tourniquets, phlebotomy, nitroglycerin, morphine, diuretics). If the heart is not "too full," or blood pressure ↓ with above interventions, 5% NaCl 250 mL/20 min Repeat if blood pressure ↑ until heart too full
	Vasoactive drug therapy	
Awaiting adequate volume repletion, institute multipurpose agent (*dopamine* or *epinephrine*) and increase dose from 1 toward 10 (μg/kg/min for dopamine; μg/min for epinephrine) as needed to maintain blood pressure. If higher doses are needed, add *norepinephrine* (2–20 μg/min). Discontinue these drugs as urgently as volume repletion and hemostasis allow (see second column).	Avoid vasoactive drugs until heart "too full." Except *dopamine* (2–5 μg/kg/min) for renal perfusion early. Nitroglycerin and nitroprusside are contraindicated. Vasoconstrictors delay adequate volume repletion (see left column). In right heart overload with shock *norepinephrine* (2–20 μg/min) may help by maintaining RV perfusion; in septic shock, vasoconstrictors may help when adequate volume replacement provides inadequate perfusion pressure (see text).	*Dobutamine* (5–15 μg/kg/min) to enhance contractility without excess tachycardia, arrhythmia, or vasoconstriction; higher doses dilate skeletal vascular bed. *Dopamine* (2–5 μg/kg/min) to preserve renal cortical blood flow; at higher dose (4–12 μg/kg/min), increases heart rate, contractility, venous tone, and preload, like *epinephrine*. *Nitroglycerin* (25–250 μg/min) for venodilation with minimal arterial dilation except for the coronary circulation. *Sodium nitroprusside* (0.1–5 μg/kg/min) for arterial dilation to reduce afterload and allow greater ejection from a depressed left ventricle or regurgitant aortic/mitral valve.

lar pumping function from hypovolemia; a good study can exclude or confirm tamponade, pulmonary hypertension, or significant valve dysfunction, all of which influence therapy and can replace the more invasive right heart catheterization.

EARLY DEFINITIVE THERAPY

The initial hour of urgent resuscitation must implement and evaluate therapy directed at the working diagnosis. Such early definitive therapy aims to provide adequate but not excessive circulating volume, followed by rational vasoactive agents to raise blood flow or redistribute it favorably in the patient with hypotension despite a full circulation (Table 114-2). Simultaneously, detection and treatment of other factors aggravating the hypoperfusion state are aided by a systematic review to ensure that such "secondary" conditions are not overlooked during volume and vasoactive drug resuscitation (see Table 114-3).

RATIONALE FOR VOLUME EXPANSION. In this book addressing the common manifestations of critical illness for intensivists having different backgrounds and practice patterns, it is important to label some preconceptions in approaching the initial cardiovascular management of shock. The cardiologist-intensivist is most often diagnosing and treating hypotension in patients with disordered ventricular pumping function; hypovolemia is considered cautiously as an occasional contributor to shock because volume resuscitation has adverse effects in aggravating myocardial dysfunction since the heart in cardiogenic shock is often too full. Consequently, the early resuscitation of hypotensive patients by physicians trained by cardiologist-intensivists (often this includes internal medicine residents and in-hospital cardiopulmonary resuscitation teams) includes one 18 gauge intravenous line with dextrose/0.5 *N* saline running to keep the vein open while central lines are inserted for appropriate vasoactive drugs needed to enhance contractility, adjust preload and afterload, or to control arrhythmias. Not infrequently, volume infusion awaits right heart catheterization after an array of vasoactive drugs fails to restore normal blood pressure.

By contrast, the surgical and anesthesiology intensivists are often treating hypotension in traumatized or hemorrhaging perioperative patients where the initial resuscitation focuses appropriately on correcting hypovolemia by rapid infusion of blood products through two 14 gauge central lines until evidence of hypervolemia is clear or the hypotension is corrected. Not infrequently, "pressor agents" accompany volume therapy to raise blood pressure more quickly, such that a confusing array of pharmacologic agents confounds evaluation of the end point of volume resuscitation.

Although both approaches are appropriate "preconceptions" in such "specialized" circumstances, they each leave too many hypotensive patients with inadequate circulating volume long after the first hour of urgent resuscitation. We encourage an early check on the assumed cause of shock for all patients, in part because many hypoperfusion states fall between these extremes. That is, all hypotensive patients require an adequate circulating volume, so volume infusion should be pushed until a discernable "too much" as evidenced by clinical examination revealing a heart which is too full; then positive inotropic drugs (dobutamine) can be effective in increasing output from the heart with adequate preload but poor pump function.

The rate and composition of volume expanders must be adjusted in accord with the working diagnosis (see Table 114-2), but for all diagnostic categories the infusion must be sufficient to test the clinical hypothesis by effecting a short-term end point indicating benefit (increased blood pressure and pulse pressure) or complication (increased JVP, new gallop or extra heart sounds, pulmonary edema). Absence of either response indicates an inadequate challenge, so the volume administered in the next interval must be greater than the last. In obvious hemorrhagic shock, blood must be obtained early, warmed and filtered; blood substitutes are administered in large amounts (plasma, albumin, hetastarch, dextran and saline) until the blood pressure rises or the heart becomes too full. At the other extreme, a working diagnosis of cardiogenic shock without obvious fluid overload requires a smaller volume challenge (250 mL NaCl in 20 min). In each case, and in all other types of shock, the next volume challenge depends on the response to the first; it should proceed soon after the first so that the physician does not miss the diagnostic clues evident only to the examining critical care team at the bedside during this urgent resuscitation.

RATIONALE FOR VASOACTIVE DRUG THERAPY FOR SHOCK. Too often, the blanket coverage of "pressor agents" is used early in all types of shock. Because some positive inotropic drugs can cause venoconstriction to increase cardiac output by endogenous volume shifts (dopamine, epinephrine), there is a rationale [like that of raising the patient's leg or applying military antishock trousers (MAST)] for the common practice of starting these agents in some hypotensive patients while the volume resuscitation proceeds. Yet, this often confounds the determination of an adequate circulating volume as well as the diagnosis of the etiology of shock. This diagnostic confusion is even greater when arteriolar constricting agents are used to raise the blood pressure (norepinephrine, phenylephrine, metaraminol, methoxamine), for the clinical signs are obscured which separate a too low cardiac output from a high output; furthermore, the end points of volume infusion up to a heart "too full" are lost by the induced increase in SVR, which rarely improves the hypoperfusion state.

Accordingly, we discourage use of the term "pressor" drugs to avoid the confusion as to how vasoactive agents affect shock; instead, we encourage the early volume resuscitation to a heart which is "too full," followed by rapid titration of a positive inotropic agent (dobutamine 2 to 10 μg/kg/min) to enhance myocardial contractility, and a mesenteric vasodilator (dopamine 2 to 5 μg/kg/min) to preserve renal function—arteriolar vasoconstrictors are rarely indicated in the early resuscitation (see Table 114-2). This approach avoids persistent hypovolemia as the cause for prolonged hypotension, at the risk of causing pulmonary edema or aggravating the pumping dysfunction of the ischemic myocardium. We are not cavalier about fluid overload—indeed, just as soon as the heart becomes evaluated as "too full," we shift goals to aim for the lowest circulating volume which still provides adequate perfusion and O_2 delivery[8]—but we emphasize that rational diagnosis and early resuscitation from shock requires an adequate circulating volume before vasoactive drugs can be effective. Of course, the discerning intensivist is aware that the initial evaluation of some hypotensive patients reveals a heart "too full," so vasoactive therapy starts immediately, but this should not translate into a "shock protocol" that initiates vasoactive drugs before ensuring adequate volume resuscitation (see Chap. 125 for a more detailed discussion).

CORRECTING CONTRIBUTING CAUSES OF SHOCK. The rapid initial assessment of the patient in shock and initial therapy aimed at supporting respiration and circulation is a busy and action-packed time. It is important to consider early institution of other definitive therapy and the potential benefit of early input from consultant experts. For example, in suspected septic shock institution of antibiotic therapy for infection should not be overlooked in the first hour (Table 114-3). Early surgical consultation for potential surgical problems (abdominal sepsis or other abscesses, gastrointestinal hemorrhage, thoracostomy for pneumothorax) should be obtained. Bradycardia requires atropine, isoproterenol, and/or a paced rhythm; tachyarrhythmias merit lidocaine (ventricular), digoxin (supraventricular), or defibrillation (Table 114-3 and Chap. 120). Expert cardiology consultation is helpful early especially where invasive reperfusion of the coronary circulation, transvenous pacemakers, or pericardiocentesis needs consideration.

Continuous and early application of techniques to anticipate, prevent, or correct hypothermia prevents secondary coagulopathy, coma, and nonresponsiveness to volume and pharmacologic resuscitation (see Table 114-3). The diagnosis and correction of acidemia rely on ventilator therapy to keep Pa_{CO_2} (hence tissue P_{CO_2}) low while confirming the presence and magnitude of anion gap acidosis without the osmolar gap of exogenous poisons (methanol, ethylene glycol). Concurrent exclusion of ketoacidosis (alcoholic or diabetic) suggests the commonest cause in shock—lactic acidosis. Beyond reestablishing perfusion and oxygen delivery, describing intercurrent liver dysfunction or ischemic

TABLE 114-3 Urgent Resuscitation of the Patient with Shock; Managing Factors Aggravating the Hypoperfusion State

Respiratory Therapy
Protect the airway—consider early elective intubation.
Prevent excess respiratory work—ventilate with small volumes
Avoid respiratory acidosis—keep Pa_{CO_2} low
Maintain oxygen delivery—FI_{O_2}, PEEP, hemoglobin
Infection in Presumed Septic Shock—(see Chaps. 97 and 98)
Empirical rational antibiosis for all probable etiologies
Exclude allergies to antibiotics
Search, incise, and drain abscesses (consider laparotomy)
Arrhythmias Aggravating Shock (see Chap. 120)
Bradycardia (rate <80/min in shock)
Correct hypoxemia—FI_{O_2} = 1.0
Atropine 0.6 mg, repeat x2 for effect
Increase dopamine to 10 μg/kg/min
Add isoproterenol (1–10 μg/min)
Consider transvenous pacer
Ventricular ectopy, tachycardia
Lidocaine
Detect and correct K^+, Ca^{2+}, Mg^{2+}
Detect and treat myocardial ischemia
Supraventricular tachycardia
Consider defibrillation early
Digoxin for rate control of atrial fibrillation
Sinus tachycardia >140/min
Detect and treat pain and anxiety
Midazolam/fentanyl drip
Morphine
Detect and treat hypovolemia
Metabolic (Lactic) Acidosis
Characterize to confirm anion gap without osmolal gap
Rule out or treat ketoacidosis, aspirin intoxication
Hyperventilate to keep $Pa_{CO_2} \approx 25$ mmHg
Calculate bicarbonate deficit and replace half if pH < 7.0
Correct ionized hypocalcemia
Consider early dialysis
Hypothermia
Maintain skin dry and covered with warmed blankets
Warm vascular volume expanders
Aggressive rewarming if temperature <35°C (95°F)

organs as sources of reduced clearance or increased production are important adjuncts to early assessment of the severity and prognosis of lactic acidosis. Legitimate uncertainty exists concerning the treatment of lactic acidosis with intravenous $NaHCO_3$, in part because intracellular acidosis may be made worse, lactic acid production may increase, and ionized hypocalcemia may depress cardiovascular function.[9] Our approach is to hyperventilate the patient to Pa_{CO_2} equalling 25 mmHg and to measure ionized calcium; if it is reduced, we administer calcium. When pH remains <7.0, we calculate the HCO_3 deficit and administer half the correcting dose of $NaHCO_3$ with more calcium. If the correction is much less than expected, we institute a further search for the source of excess lactate production and consider early hemodialysis against a bicarbonate bath with high ionized calcium. The evidence for these preferences is not conclusive (see Chaps. 3 and 158).

WHAT JUST HAPPENED?

During the urgent initial resuscitation, the physician attempts to solve complex physiologic problems which, a priori, have unknown solutions, using therapeutic interventions with complex and often competing effects. A rational approach to this seemingly impossible task is to use the same approach employed by research scientists confronting other problems with unknown solutions—repeated hypothesis testing. Hypothesis testing refers to the process whereby the physician evaluates the patient; first to determine the most likely etiology of the shock state; then to estimate what the best therapeutic intervention is to correct the hypothesized abnormality; and finally to reevaluate the patient after the intervention to confirm that the shock is improved. The outcome dictates the next therapeutic intervention or invites a refined or alternative explanation for the hypoperfused state. For example, the physician evaluating a patient in shock finds evidence of hypovolemia, a thready pulse, and cool extremities; he formulates the hypothesis that hypoperfusion is present due to a reduction of intravascular volume. He treats the patient and tests the hypothesis by rapidly infusing 3 L warmed saline. Repeat examination demonstrates improved perfusion confirming the initial hypothesis when the blood pressure normalizes; if the same patient remained hypotensive but now with a large pulse pressure and warm extremities, formulation of a refined hypothesis is invited (septic shock) leading to the next therapeutic intervention (antibiosis, search for source of sepsis), which is also a test of the refined hypothesis. On the other hand, persistent hypotension with a thready pulse, cool extremities, elevated JVP, gallop rhythm, and lung crepitations now suggests cardiogenic shock requiring vasoactive therapy.

Accurate formulation of clinical hypotheses leads to more rapid and efficient patient care. Accurate hypothesis formulation depends on understanding the pathophysiology of the different types of shock, especially when the outcome of the initial therapy did not fit with the working diagnosis. Then, overlapping etiologies of shock or special types of pathophysiology must be considered during this pause at the end of the urgent resuscitation (see Table 114-1). The move to a search for new etiologies is aided when the interventions were adequate to test the initial hypothesis. During the same period of reconsideration, therapies initiated in haste can be reduced to the minimum required to maintain their end point, while the physician reconsiders the ongoing diagnosis and treatment in the light of the broader differential of the types of shock. These numerous possibilities are best approached in categories of presentation (Table 114-4). For high right atrial pressure-hypotension not obviously due to left ventricular ischemia, cardiac tamponade, acute pulmonary hypertension, and right ventricular infarction must be excluded; for nonresponsive hypovolemia, Addison's disease, anaphylaxis, and neurogenic shock should be considered in the appropriate clinical context; and high cardiac output hypoperfusion which may not be due to sepsis or liver failure is occasionally due to thyroid storm, Paget's disease, or other

TABLE 114-4 Causes of and Contributors to Shock

Decreased Pump Function of the Heart—Cardiogenic Shock	Decreased Venous Return with Normal Pumping Function—Hypovolemic Shock
Left ventricular failure	Cardiac tamponade (increased right atrial pressure—central hypovolemia)
Systolic dysfunction—decreased contractility	Pericardial fluid collection
Myocardial infarction	Blood
Ischemia and global hypoxemia	Renal failure
Cardiomyopathy	Pericarditis with effusion
Depressant drugs: β blockers, calcium channel blockers, antiarrhythmics,	Constrictive pericarditis
Myocardial contusion	High intrathoracic pressure
Respiratory acidosis	Tension pneumothorax
Metabolic derangements: acidosis, hypophosphatemia, hypocalcemia	Massive pleural effusion
Diastolic dysfunction—increased myocardial diastolic stiffness	Positive-pressure ventilation
Ischemia	High intraabdominal pressure
Ventricular hypertrophy	Acites
Restrictive cardiomyopathy	Massive obesity
Consequence of prolonged hypovolemic or septic shock	Post extensive intraabdominal surgery
Ventricular interdependence	Intravascular hypovolemia (reduced mean systemic pressure)
External compression (see cardiac tamponade below)	Hemorrhage
Greatly increased afterload	Gastrointestinal
Aortic stenosis	Trauma
Hypertrophic cardiomyopathy	Aortic dissection and other internal sources
Dynamic outflow tract obstruction	Renal losses
Coarctation of the aorta	Diuretics
Malignant hypertension	Osmotic diuresis
Valve and structural abnormality	Diabetes (insipidus, mellitus)
Mitral stenosis, endocarditis, mitral/aortic regurgitation	Gastrointestinal losses
Obstruction due to atrial myxoma or thrombus	Vomiting
Papillary muscle dysfunction or rupture	Diarrhea
Ruptured septum or free wall	Gastric suctioning
Arrhythmias	Loss via surgical stomas
Right ventricular failure	Redistribution to extravascular space
Decreased contractility	Burns
Right ventricular infarction, ischemia, hypoxia, acidosis	Trauma
Greatly increased afterload	Postsurgical
Pulmonary embolism	Sepsis
Pulmonary vascular disease	Decreased venous tone (reduced mean systemic pressure)
Hypoxic pulmonary vasoconstriction, PEEP, high alveolar pressure	Drugs
Acidosis	Sedatives
ARDS, pulmonary fibrosis, sleep disordered breathing, chronic obstructive pulmonary disease	Narcotics
Valve and structural abnormality	Diuretics
Obstruction due to atrial myxoma, thrombus, endocarditis	Anaphylactic shock
Arrhythmias	Neurogenic shock
	Increased resistance to venous return
	Tumor compression or invasion
	Venous thrombosis with obstruction
	PEEP
	Pregnancy
High Cardiac Output Hypotension	**Other Causes of Shock with Unique Etiologies**
Septic shock	Thyroid storm
Sterile endotoxemia with hepatic failure	Myxedema coma
Arteriovenous shunts	Adrenal insufficiency
Dialysis	Hemoglobin and mitochondrial poisons
Paget's disease	Cyanide
	Carbon monoxide
	Iron intoxication

arteriovenous fistulas. When these possibilities are considered, it is often essential to obtain more hemodynamic data via echocardiography and right heart catheterization.

Types of Shock

A number of classifications of shock are possible, in part dependent on the exact definition of shock; here we initially emphasize inadequate organ system perfusion and hypotension. Inadequate perfusion can result primarily from decreased pump function of the heart, decreased venous return of blood to the heart, or reduced arterial tone, possibly associated with abnormal blood flow distribution, such that blood pressure is reduced and some capillary beds may not be adequately perfused even when total cardiac output is normal or elevated (see Table 114-4). Shock due to decreased pump function of the heart is commonly cardiogenic shock due to left ventricular ischemia. Other causes of decreased pump function include right ventricular ischemia, dysfunction of heart valves, or greatly elevated pulmonary arterial pressure. Decreased venous return when pump function is normal is most commonly due to hemorrhagic or dehydration hypovolemia, but we emphasize other mechanisms including decreased venous tone due to drugs or neurologic injury. Of course, right atrial pressure may be increased by abnormal pressures surrounding the heart in the absence of ventricular dysfunction, so our etiologic classification includes these various causes of tamponade within the group having reduced venous return as the primary mechanism; note that these conditions associated with high right atrial pressure and systemic hypotension might have been classified as cardiogenic shock (see Table 114-1). Septic shock is the most common cause of shock resulting from abnormal arterial tone and blood flow distribution, although other causes such as severe liver failure, peripheral shunts, and even anaphylactic shock share this mechanism. Defining shock as anaerobic metabolism of multiple organ systems, often signaled by lactic acidosis, allows classification of the shock state associated with metabolic poisons, such as carbon monoxide, which results in histotoxic hypoxia due to an inadequate uptake of oxygen by the mitochondria (see Table 114-4). Other shock states, particularly septic shock, may also involve an inability of tissues to extract delivered oxygen, but we note that the lactic acidosis of sepsis is not necessarily due to anaerobic metabolism (vide infra).

In describing and distinguishing between the types of shock, it is helpful to call to mind the Starling relationships between left ventricular stroke volume and left atrial pressure (see discussion of Fig. 2-4 in Chap. 2). When cardiac output and stroke volume are reduced, a low pulmonary wedge pressure (Ppw approximately equal to left atrial pressure) signals hypovolemic shock, but a high Ppw signals cardiogenic shock. With the caveats discussed in Chap. 2, the mechanisms underlying these interpretations of Starling curves are revealed by diastolic and systolic volume-pressure relationships (see discussion of Figs. 2-4 through 2-7 in Chap. 2). In all hypotensive states, baroreceptor reflexes are stimulated to raise cardiac output via venoconstriction, to raise blood pressure via arterial constriction, and to increase heart rate and contractility. Distinguishing types of shock is further aided by understanding venous return curves, especially as they are coupled with cardiac function curves (right atrial pressure versus cardiac output; see discussion of Figs. 2-9 through 2-16 in Chap. 2). Accordingly, we use these relationships in the following discussion to compare and contrast cardiovascular mechanisms responsible for cardiogenic shock (Fig. 114-1), hypovolemic shock (see Fig. 114-2), and septic shock (see Fig. 114-3). Separating these from other etiologies of shock is aided by considering their typical hemodynamic measurements (see Table 2-3 in Chap. 2). Our goal is to link pathophysiology of the circulation to the broader differential diagnosis of the types of shock in Table 114-4 to facilitate the accurate etiologic diagnosis and management based on additional hemodynamic measures as required by the response to urgent resuscitation.

DECREASED PUMP FUNCTION—CARDIOGENIC SHOCK

Pump function is measured as the output of a pump for a given input. The diagnosis of decreased pump function as the cause of shock is made by finding evidence of inappropriately low output (cardiac output) despite normal or high input (right atrial pressure). Cardiac output is the most important "output" of the heart and is clinically assessed in the same way that perfusion was assessed on the urgent initial examination. Better estimates are later obtained by thermodilution measurement using a pulmonary artery catheter, nuclear medicine scans, and Doppler echocardiographic techniques. Right atrial pressure is the most easily measured "input" of the whole heart and is initially assessed by examination of jugular veins. Following catheter insertion, CVP can be measured accurately. Other outputs, such as stroke work or left ventricular ejection fraction, and other inputs, such as left ventricular end-diastolic pressure (LVEDP) or volume (LVEDV), are useful to determine the specific cause and to quantify decreased pump function. Left and right ventricular dysfunction can each be caused by decreased systolic contractility, increased diastolic stiffness, greatly increased afterload (including obstruction), valvular dysfunction, or abnormal heart rate and rhythm.

CAUSES OF LEFT VENTRICULAR FAILURE. Acute or acute on chronic left ventricular failure resulting in shock is the classic example of cardiogenic shock and is identified as a subset of decreased pump function by finding evidence of a low cardiac output in relation to high left ventricular filling pressures. Clinical findings of low cardiac output and increased left ventricular filling pressures include, in addition to assessment of perfusion, pulmonary crackles in dependent lung regions, presence of a third heart sound, absence of crisp heart sounds, and clinical evidence of ventricular dilation. These findings are not always present or unambig-

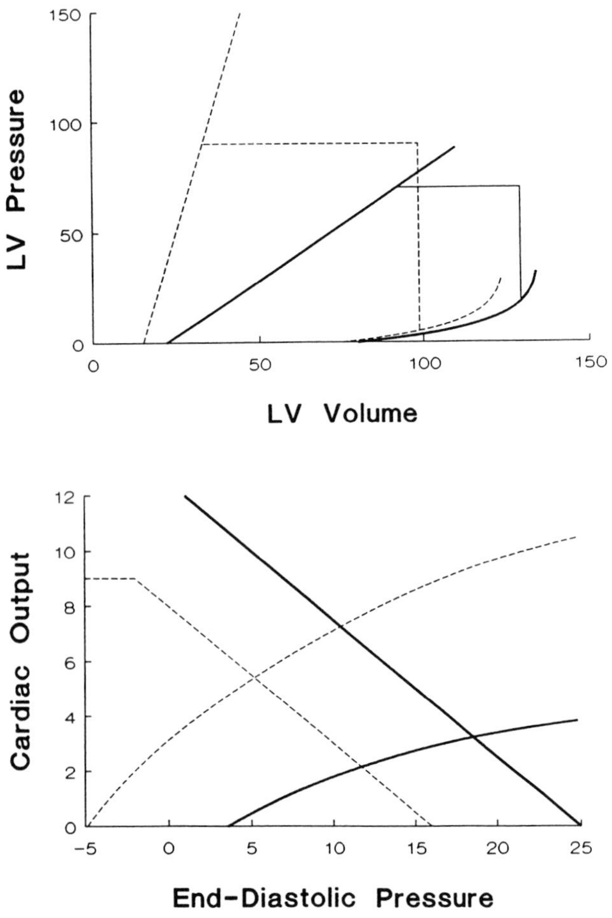

FIGURE 114-1 Cardiovascular mechanics in cardiogenic shock. The upper panel compares the abnormalities of systolic and diastolic left ventricular pressure (ordinate)-volume (abscissa) relationships during cardiogenic shock (continuous) with normal pressure-volume relationships (dashed lines). The primary abnormality is that the end-systolic pressure-volume relationship (sloped straight lines) is shifted to the right mainly by a marked reduction in slope (decreased contractility). As a result, at similar or even lower systolic pressures the ventricle is not able to eject as far so that end-systolic volume is greatly increased and stroke volume is therefore decreased. To compensate for the decrease in stroke volume the curvilinear diastolic pressure-volume relationship shifts to the right, which indicates decreased diastolic stiffness (increased compliance). To maximize stroke volume, diastolic filling increases even further, associated with an increase in end-diastolic pressure.

Why end-diastolic pressure increases is determined from the "pump function" and "venous return" curves illustrated in the bottom panel as a plot of cardiac output (ordinate) versus right atrial end-diastolic pressure (abscissa). The decrease in contractility from the top panel results in a shift of the curvilinear cardiac function curve from its normal position (dashed curve, *bottom panel*) down and to the right (continuous curve, *bottom panel*). Since end-diastolic pressure and cardiac output are determined by the intersection of the cardiac function curve (curvilinear relationships, *bottom panel*) with the venous return curve (straight lines, *bottom panel*), the shift of the cardiac function curve immediately results in a decrease in cardiac output and an increase in end-diastolic pressure. Compensatory mechanisms (fluid retention by the kidneys, increased sympathetic tone) act to maintain venous return by increasing mean systemic pressure (Pms, the venous pressure when cardiac output = 0) from 16 to 25 mmHg as indicated by the rightward shift from the dashed straight line to the continuous straight line in the bottom panel. The effect is that end-diastolic pressure increases so that stroke volume (*upper panel*) and cardiac output (*bottom panel*) are increased toward normal.

uous. Therefore, pulmonary artery catheterization is helpful and often essential in establishing the diagnosis and titrating therapy. Cardiogenic shock then is usually associated with a cardiac index <2.2 L/min/m^2 when the pulmonary artery occlusion pressure has been raised to more than 18 mmHg.[10]

Systolic dysfunction. Figure 114-1 illustrates the pathophysiologic abnormalities of cardiogenic shock due to decreased left ventricular contractility. The primary abnormality is that the end-systolic pressure-volume relationship is shifted down and to the right (see Fig. 114-1, *upper panel*) so that, at the same afterload, the ventricle cannot eject as far (decreased contractility). The result of this is that left ventricular pump function is reduced. That is, the pump function curve is also shifted down and to the right (see Fig. 114-1, *lower panel*) so that at similar preloads cardiac output is reduced. Three mechanisms which counter the fall in cardiac output are illustrated. The diastolic ventricle becomes more compliant possibly from stress relaxation of the pericardium and myocardium so that stroke volume increases at the same end-diastolic pressure (rightward shift of the diastolic pressure-volume relationship in *upper panel*). Afterload decreases resulting in increased stroke volume (see Fig. 114-1, *upper panel*). Finally, mean systemic pressure (Pms) rises (see Fig. 114-1, *lower panel*) aided by avid fluid retention by the kidneys and by increased venous tone mediated by the sympathetic nervous system and the associated increase in circulating catecholomines. Accordingly, the Frank-Starling mechanism of increasing cardiac output by increasing diastolic filling is used.

As a result of a decrease in contractility the patient presents with elevated left and right ventricular filling pressures and a low cardiac output. Mixed venous oxygen saturation may be well below 50% because cardiac output is low. In the presence of physiologic pulmonary shunt that accompanies pulmonary edema, the low saturation of mixed venous blood shunting by the lung contributes to substantial arterial desaturation. Accordingly, arterial desaturation aggravates the low oxygen delivery due to reduced cardiac output, as does intercurrent anemia.

Acute myocardial infarction or ischemia is the most common cause of left ventricular failure leading to shock. The principle effect of myocardial infarction is to depress systolic contractility, which in completely infarcted areas becomes zero or even negative (paradoxical regional wall motion). Shock has occurred in 10 to 20 percent of patients with transmural myocardial infarction.[11] However, the recent use of fibrinolytic therapy and the possible beneficial effects of early surgical revascularization have reduced the incidence of cardiogenic shock to approximately 5 percent.[12,13] Infarction of >40 percent of the myocardium is often associated with cardiogenic shock;[14] anterior infarction is more likely to lead to shock than inferior or posterior infarction. Details of the diagnosis and management of ischemic heart disease are discussed in Chap. 116; other causes of decreased left ventricular contractility in critical illness are discussed in more detail in Chap. 115, as each may contribute to shock.

Diastolic dysfunction. Increased left ventricular diastolic stiffness contributing to cardiogenic shock occurs during myocardial ischemia, and in a range of less common disorders including late stages of hypovolemic shock and septic shock (see Table 114-4); note that all causes of tamponade listed in Table 114-4 need to be considered in a systematic review of causes of diastolic dysfunction.[15] Cardiac function is depressed since stroke volume is decreased by decreased end-diastolic volume due to increased diastolic stiffness. Diastolic dysfunction in a hypotensive patient with low cardiac output and high filling pressures is often identified by a small (rather than large) LVEDV by bedside echocardiography. Conditions resulting in increased diastolic stiffness are particularly detrimental when systolic contractility is decreased because decreased diastolic stiffness (increased compliance) (see Fig. 114-1, *upper panel*) is a normal compensatory mechanism (contrast the diastolic mechanisms in Fig. 114-1, *upper panel* with Fig. 2-8 in Chap. 2). Establishing the diagnosis of increased diastolic stiffness is often difficult, and is best identified by echocardiography as contributing to hypotension in patients with low cardiac output and high ventricular diastolic pressures by a small diastolic volume and a good ejection fraction with very small end-systolic volume.

Increased diastolic stiffness is difficult to treat[15] except when it is due to an acute reversible cause such as ischemia (or the causes of tamponade listed in Table 114-4). Fluid infusion results in large increases in diastolic pressure without much increase in diastolic volume. Positive inotropic agents are associated with the development of histologic contraction band changes which may worsen diastolic compliance.[16] Afterload reduction when systolic function is normal decreases blood pressure without increasing cardiac output, except when nitroprusside corrects the diastolic stiffness.[17] Indeed, if conventional therapy of cardiogenic shock aimed at improving systolic function is ineffective, then increased diastolic stiffness should be strongly considered as the cause of decreased pump function.

Valvular dysfunction. Acute mitral regurgitation, because of rupture of cordae or the papillary muscle or papillary muscle dysfunction, most commonly is due to ischemic injury. The characteristic murmur and the presence of large *v* waves on the pulmonary artery occlusion pressure trace suggest significant mitral regurgitation, which may be quantified using Doppler echocardiographic examination. Rupture of the ventricular septum with left-to-right shunt is detected using Doppler echocardiographic examination or by observing a step-up in oxygen saturation of blood from the right atrium to the pulmonary artery.[18] Acute obstruction of the mitral valve by left atrial thrombus or myxoma may also result in cardiogenic shock. These conditions are generally surgical emergencies.

More commonly, valve dysfunction aggravates other primary etiologies of shock. Aortic and mitral regurgitation reduces forward flow and raises LVEDP whatever the state of contractility, and this regurgitation is ameliorated by effective arteriolar dilation, as by nitroprusside infusion. Note that vasodilator therapy can effect large increases in cardiac output without much change in the systemic mean blood pressure, pulse pressure or diastolic pressure, so right heart catheterization and repeat echocardiography to confirm increased cardiac output and reduced valvular regurgitation are essential to titrating effective vasodilator doses. By contrast, occasional patients are noted to decrease their blood pressure and cardiac output on inotropic drugs like dobutamine; then excluding dynamic ventricular outflow obstruction by echocardiography or treating it by increasing preload, afterload and end-systolic volume are essential.

Cardiac arrhythmias. Not infrequently, arrhythmias aggravate hypoperfusion in other shock states. Ventricular tachyarrhythmias are often associated with cardiogenic shock; sinus tachycardia and atrial tachyarrhythmias are often observed with hypovolemic and septic shock (see Table 114-3). Specific therapy of tachyarrhythmias depends on the specific diagnosis as discussed in Chap. 120. Inadequately treated pain and unsuspected drug withdrawal should be included in the ICU differential diagnosis of tachyarrhythmias; whatever their etiology, the reduced ventricular filling time can reduce cardiac output and so aggravate shock. Bradyarrhythmias contributing to shock may respond acutely to atropine or isoproterenol infusion and then pacing; hypoxia or myocardial infarction as the cause should be sought and treated. Symptomatic hypoperfusion resulting from bradyarrhythmias, even in the absence of myocardial infarction or high degree atrioventricular (AV) block, is an important indication for temporary pacemaker placement that is sometimes overlooked.

Treatment of left ventricular failure. Management of patients with cardiogenic shock requires repeatedly testing the hypothesis of "too little versus too much." Clinical examination is not accurate enough so that a pulmonary artery catheter is almost always required. Initial therapy for cardiogenic shock follows from consideration of the pathophysiology illustrated in Fig. 114-1 and includes optimizing filling pressures, increasing contractility by improving the ratio of myocardial oxygen supply to demand or by using inotropic drugs, and optimizing afterload. Temporary mechanical support with an intraaortic balloon pump (IABP) is often extremely useful in cardiogenic shock and should be considered early on as a support device in patients who may benefit from later surgical therapy.[19] Important additional therapy includes early institution of thrombolytic therapy in acute coronary thrombosis[12] and revascularization or surgical correction of other anatomic abnormalities where appropriate. Cardiac transplantation and mechanical heart implantation are considered when other therapy fails.

Filling pressures are optimized to improve cardiac output but avoid pulmonary edema. Depending on the initial presentation, cardiogenic shock frequently spans the spectrum of hypovolemia (so that fluid infusion helps) to hypervolemia with pulmonary edema (where reduction in intravascular volume results in substantial improvement).[8] If gross fluid overload is not present, then a rapid fluid bolus should be given. In contrast to patients with hypovolemic or septic shock, a smaller bolus (250 mL) of crystalloid solution should be infused as fast as possible. Immediately after infusion the patient's circulatory status should be reassessed. If there is improvement but hypoperfusion persists, then further infusion with repeat examination is indicated to attain an adequate cardiac output and oxygen delivery while seeking the lowest filling pressure needed to accomplish this goal. If there is no improvement in oxygen delivery and evidence of worsened pulmonary edema or gas exchange, then the limit of initial fluid resuscitation has been defined. Crystalloid solutions are used particularly if the initial evaluation is uncertain because crystalloid solutions rapidly distribute to the entire extracellular fluid compartment. Therefore, after a brief period of time only one-quarter to one-third remains in the intravascular compartment and evidence of intravascular fluid overload rapidly subsides.

Contractility increases if ischemia can be relieved by decreasing myocardial oxygen demand or by improving myocardial oxygen supply by increasing coronary blood flow (coronary vasodilators, thrombolytic therapy, surgical revascularization, IABP counterpulsation) or by increasing the oxygen content of arterial blood. Inotropic drug infusion attempts to correct the physiologic abnormality by increasing contractility (see Fig. 114-1). However, this occurs at the expense of increased myocardial oxygen demand.[20] Afterload is optimized to maintain arterial pressures high enough to perfuse vital organs (including the heart) but low enough to maximize systolic ejection. When systolic function is normal, afterload reduction often reduces blood pressure with little increase in cardiac output; when systolic function is much reduced, vasodilator therapy may improve systolic ejection and increase perfusion, even to the extent that blood pressure rises.[21] In patients with very high blood pressure, the end-systolic volume increases considerably such that stroke volume and cardiac output fall unless LVEDV and LVEDP are greatly increased; this sequence is reversed by judicious afterload reduction.

DIAGNOSIS AND MANAGEMENT OF RIGHT VENTRICULAR FAILURE. Right ventricular failure as a cause of cardiogenic shock is often identified by finding elevated right atrial pressure and low cardiac output not explained by left ventricular failure or cardiac tamponade. The most common causes of shock due to right ventricular failure are right ventricular infarction and pulmonary embolism resulting in greatly increased right ventricular afterload.

Right ventricular infarction is found in approximately half of inferior myocardial infarctions and is complicated by shock only 10 to 20 percent of the time.[22] Isolated right ventricular infarction with shock is uncommon.[23] The hemodynamic findings of right ventricular infarction must be distinguished from cardiac tamponade and constrictive pericarditis[24] and include Kussmaul's sign, low cardiac output, high filling pressures, and often equalization of right atrial, right ventricular diastolic, pulmonary artery diastolic, and pulmonary artery occlusion pressures. Pulmonary crackles are classically absent. Therapy includes fluid infusion and dobutamine.[25] Because bradyarrhythmias are common and AV conduction is frequently abnormal, AV sequential pacing often dramatically improves cardiac output and blood pressure in shock due to right ventricular infarction.[26] IABP counterpulsation may also be useful as are early fibrinolytic therapy and angioplasty when indicated (see Chap. 116).

Right ventricular ischemia, with or without coronary artery disease, probably is a more important cause of right ventricular dysfunction than generally recognized. In shock states systemic arterial pressure is often low and right ventricular afterload (pulmonary artery pressure) may be high due to emboli, hypoxemia, acidosis, sepsis, or adult respiratory distress syndrome (ARDS). Therefore, right ventricular perfusion pressure is low leading to right ventricular ischemia and decreased contractility which, in the face of normal or high right ventricular afterload, results in right ventricular dilation. Subsequent right-to-left shift of the interventricular septum limits left ventricular filling. Cardiac output is then limited by right ventricular systolic ejection and left ventricular diastolic filling.

Therapy of right ventricular failure due to decreased right ventricular perfusion and increased afterload is evolving. Recent animal studies suggest that, acutely, in right ventricular shock due to pulmonary embolism interventions such as norepinephrine infusion may increase systemic arterial pressure more than pulmonary arterial pressure resulting in improved right ventricular perfusion.[27] Improved right ventricular function and total cardiac function may result. This approach has not been carefully tested in patients in shock due to right ventricular failure. Established approaches include verifying that pulmonary emboli are present and initiating therapy with anticoagulation, fibrinolytic agents, or surgical embolectomy, as necessary. Hypoxic pulmonary vasoconstriction may be reduced by improving alveolar and mixed venous oxygenation by increasing $F_{I_{O_2}}$ or increasing oxygen delivery by other means such as blood transfusion. Pulmonary vasodilator therapy may be useful in some patients if pulmonary artery pressures can be lowered without significantly lowering systemic arterial pressures. Prostaglandin E_1 and many other agents have been variably successful. Measurements of pulmonary artery pressure, systemic pressure, cardiac output, and oxygen delivery before and after a trial of a specific potential pulmonary vasodilator are essential (see Chap. 117).

DECREASED VENOUS RETURN—HYPOVOLEMIC SHOCK

The pressure driving venous return back to the right atrium was described in Chap. 2 as mean systemic minus right atrial pressure, where the mean systemic pressure is determined by the vascular volume and by the unstressed volume and capacitance of the systemic vessels. Venous return to the heart when right atrial pressure is not elevated may be inadequate due to decreased intravascular volume (hypovolemic shock), due to decreased tone of the venous capacitance bed so that mean systemic pressure is low (e.g., neurogenic shock), and occasionally due to increased resistance to venous return (e.g., obstruction of the inferior vena cava). In the presence of shock, decreased venous return is determined to be a contributor to shock by finding low left and right ventricular diastolic pressures, often in an appropriate clinical setting such as trauma or massive gastrointestinal hemorrhage. Venous return may also be reduced when right atrial pressure is much increased despite normal ventricular pumping function, as when the pressure surrounding the heart is much increased.

COMPRESSION OF THE HEART BY SURROUNDING STRUCTURES. Compression of the heart (cardiac tamponade) limits its diastolic filling and can result in shock with inadequate cardiac output despite very high right atrial pressures. Diagnosis of cardiac tamponade is made physiologically using right heart and pulmonary artery catheterization to demonstrate a low cardiac output and elevated and approximately equal right atrial, right ventricular diastolic, pulmonary artery diastolic, and pulmonary artery occlusion pressures (particularly their waveforms). The diagnosis is often best confirmed anatomically using echocardiographic examination demonstrating pericardial fluid, diastolic collapse of the atria and right ventricle, and right-to-left septal shift during inspiration. Septal shift during inspiration and increased afterload that accompany decreased intrathoracic pressure during inspiration account for the clinically observed pulsus paradoxus.[28] Although pericardial tamponade by accumulation of pericardial fluid is the most common cause of cardiac tamponade, other structures surrounding the heart may also produce tamponade. Tension pneumothorax tamponades the heart so that the patient is hypotensive and in shock despite distended jugular veins. Massive accumulations of pleural fluid may also occasionally tamponade the heart. Pneumopericardium may occasionally result in cardiac tamponade and shock in adults but this complication is more common in infants. Greatly elevated abdominal pressures may elevate the diaphragm and raise intrathoracic pressure enough to impair diastolic filling (see Chap. 121).

Decreasing the pressure of the tamponading chamber by needle drainage of the pericardium, pleural space, and peritoneum can rapidly and dramatically improve venous return, blood pressure, and organ system perfusion. Therefore the goal of therapy is to accomplish this decompression as rapidly and safely as possible. In patients who are hemodynamically stable, fluid infusion is a temporizing therapy which increases mean systemic pressure so that venous return increases even though right atrial pressure is high. In hemodynamically stable patients if it is safe to take the time needed to get ultrasonic guidance for needle aspiration or surgical drainage then this should be done. Otherwise, in an emergency, blind needle drainage is necessary (see Chap. 27).

HYPOVOLEMIC SHOCK. Hypovolemia is the most common cause of shock due to decreased venous return and is illustrated in Fig. 114-2. Intravascular volume is decreased so that the venous capacitance bed is not filled, leading to a decreased pressure driving venous return back to the heart. This is seen as a left shift of the venous return curve in Fig. 114-2, *lower panel*, so that cardiac output decreases at a low end-diastolic pressure (intersection of the venous return curve and cardiac function curve). Endogenous catecholamines attempt to compensate by constricting the venous capacitance bed and thereby raising the pressure driving venous return back to the heart so that 25 percent reductions in intravascular volume are nearly completely compensated for. Orthostatic decrease in blood pressure by 10 mmHg or increase in heart rate of more than 30 beats/min[29] may detect this level of intravascular volume reduction. When approximately 40 percent of the intravascular volume is lost, sympathetic stimulation can no longer maintain mean systemic pressure resulting in decreased venous return and clinical shock.

After sufficient time (more than 2 h) and severity (>40 percent loss of intravascular volume), patients often cannot be resuscitated from hypovolemic shock.[30,31] This observation highlights the urgency with which patients should be resuscitated. It also points out that the pathophysiology of hypovolemic shock is more extensive than just the volume deficit. A "no reflow" phenomenon is described so that after stagnation, neutrophils become adherent to endothelial surfaces and even after adequate fluid resuscitation, may block capillary beds[32] so that tissue hypoxia is not alleviated. Gut ischemia and systemic release of inflammatory mediators contribute to the pathophysiology.[33] Additionally, reduction in cardiac function (the rightward shift of the cardiac function curve in Fig. 114-2, *lower panel*) is observed so that even after restoration of left and right atrial pressures, cardiac output remains low.[16] This reduced cardiac function is due to increased diastolic stiffness developing during hypovolemic shock, which impairs ventricular filling as illustrated by the left shift of the diastolic pressure-volume relationship in Fig. 114-2, *upper panel*.[34]

Shock following trauma is a form of hypovolemic shock where extensive pathophysiologic abnormalities, in addition to intravascular volume depletion, are present (see Chap. 59). Intravascular volume may be decreased due to loss of blood and significant redistribution of intravascular volume to other compartments, i.e., "third spacing." Release of inflammatory mediators may result in pathophysiologic abnormalities resembling septic shock. Cardiac dysfunction may be depressed from direct damage from myocardial contusion, from increased diastolic stiffness, from right heart failure, or even circulating myocardial depressant substances. Shock related to burns similarly is multifactorial with a significant component of intravascular hypovolemia (see Chap. 68).

Other causes of shock due to decreased venous return include severe neurologic damage or drug ingestion resulting in hypotension due to loss of venous tone. As a result of decreased venous tone, the mean systemic pressure falls, thereby reducing the pressure gradient driving blood flow back to the heart so that cardiac output and blood pressure fall. Obstruction of veins due to compression, thrombus formation, or tumor invasion increases the resistance to venous return and may occasionally result in shock.

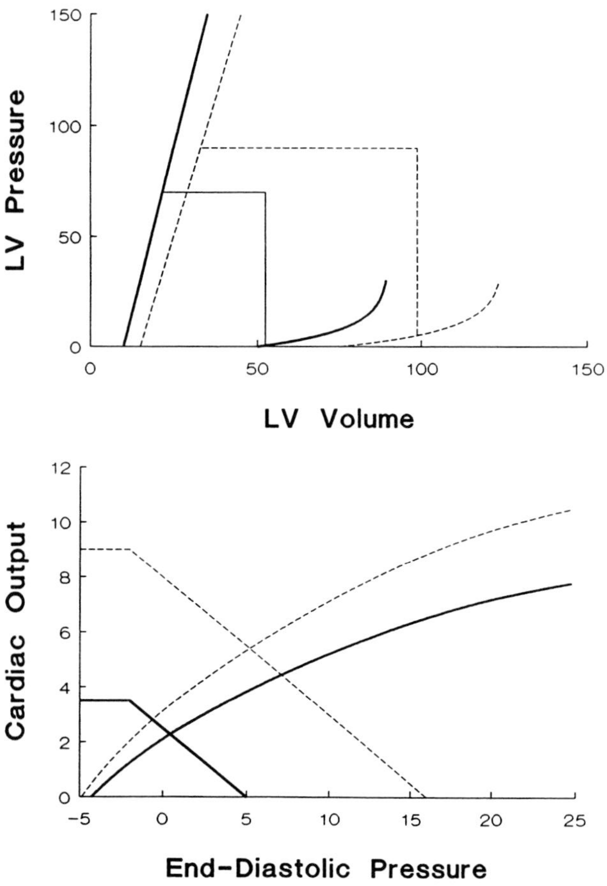

FIGURE 114-2 Cardiovascular mechanics in hypovolemic shock (axes labeled as in Fig. 114-1). During hypovolemic shock the primary abnormality is a decrease in the intravascular volume so that mean systemic pressure decreases as illustrated by a shift of the venous return curves from the normal relationship (straight dashed line, *lower panel*) leftward (straight continuous line, *lower panel*). This hypovolemic venous return curve now intersects the normal cardiac function curve (dashed curvilinear relationship, *lower panel*) at a much lower end-diastolic pressure so that cardiac output is greatly reduced.

In the upper panel, the increased sympathetic tone accompanying shock results in a slight increase in contractility, as illustrated by the slight left shift of the left ventricular end-systolic pressure-volume relationship (from the dashed straight line to the solid straight line in the upper panel). However, since the slope of the end-systolic pressure-volume relationship is normally quite steep, the increase in contractility cannot increase stroke volume or cardiac output much and is therefore an ineffective compensatory mechanism in patients with normal hearts.

If volume resuscitation to correct the primary abnormality is delayed for several hours, the diastolic pressure-volume relationship shifts from its normal position (dashed curve, *upper panel*) resulting in increased diastolic stiffness (continuous curve, *upper panel*). Increased diastolic stiffness results in a decreased stroke volume and therefore a depressed cardiac function curve (continuous curve, *lower panel*) compared to normal (dashed curve, *lower panel*). This decrease in cardiac function due to increased diastolic stiffness probably accounts for "irreversibility" of severe prolonged hypovolemic shock.

The principal therapy of hypovolemic shock and other forms of shock due to decreased venous return is rapid initial fluid resuscitation.[30] Warmed crystalloid solutions are readily available. Colloid-containing solutions result in a more sustained increase in intravascular volume. However, in the setting of demonstrated or potential leaking endothelial surfaces (e.g., ARDS) the colloid rapidly redistributes into the entire extravascular water compartment. Pulmonary edema and tissue edema may be aggravated.[30] The role of hypertonic saline and other resuscitation solutions is currently uncertain. Alternatively, transfusion of packed red blood cells increases oxygen-carrying capacity and expands the intravascular volume and is therefore a doubly useful therapy. In an emergency, initial transfusion often begins with type-specific blood before a complete crossmatch is available. An optimum hematocrit has not yet been defined and certainly varies for varying clinical problems. Blood viscosity starts to rise rapidly as hematocrit rises above 45 percent. Therefore, in patients who may have an inadequate oxygen delivery, it is reasonable to transfuse blood to raise the hematocrit toward this level. After a large stored red blood cell transfusion, clotting factors, platelets, and serum ionized calcium decrease and therefore should be measured and replaced if necessary.

As additional support to fluid resuscitation, catecholamines such as dopamine and epinephrine increase venous tone, mean systemic pressure, and venous return at doses $< 10\ \mu g/kg/min$ for dopamine and $<10\ \mu g/min$ for epinephrine (see Table 114-2); at higher doses, these agents increase arterial resistance. Infusion of these agents may aid in quickly restoring blood pressure. However, this apparently salutary effect of catecholamines is not due to increased cardiac contractility during hypovolemic shock in an otherwise healthy person. Continued administration of these agents is inappropriate and dangerous because the problem is inadequate fluid administration, not decreased ventricular contractility.

Recognizing inadequate venous return as the primary abnormality of hypovolemic shock alerts the physician to several commonly encountered and potentially lethal complications of therapy. Airway intubation and mechanical ventilation increase negative intrathoracic pressures to positive values and thus raise right atrial pressure. The already low pressure gradient driving venous return to the heart worsens, resulting in marked reduction in cardiac output and blood pressure. Yet ventilation treats shock by reducing the work of respiratory muscle, so it should be implemented early with adequate volume expansion. Sedatives and analgesics are often administered at the time of airway intubation, resulting in reduced venous tone because of direct relaxing effect on the venous capacitance bed or because of a decrease in circulating catecholamines. Thus, the pressure gradient driving venous return falls. Therefore, in the hypovolemic patient these medications may markedly

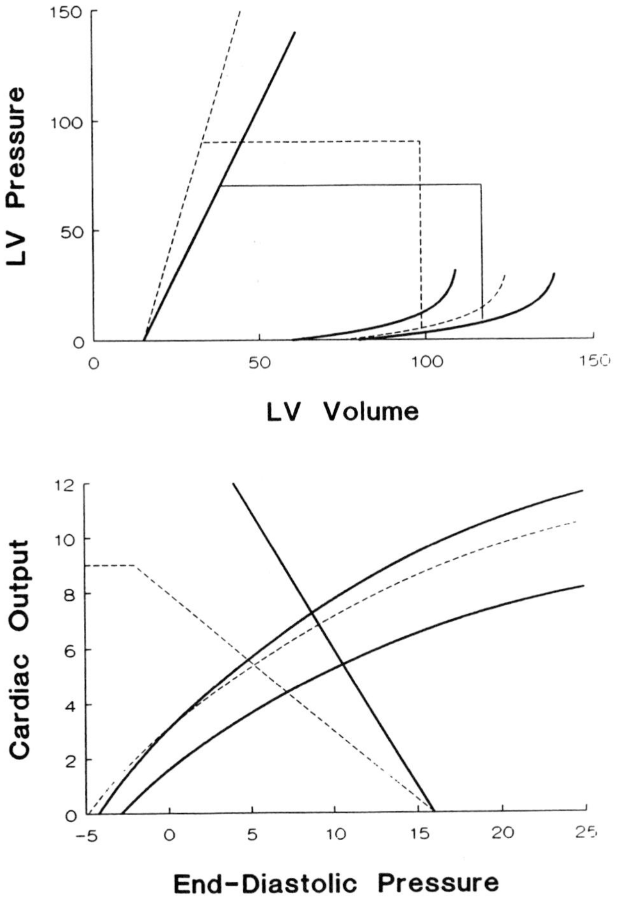

FIGURE 114-3 Cardiovascular mechanics in septic shock (axes labeled as in Fig. 114-1). Septic shock has important independent effects on left ventricular pressure-volume relationships, on the venous return curve, and on the arterial vascular resistance. Depressed systolic contractility indicated by a decreased slope of the left ventricular end-systolic pressure-volume relationship from normal (dashed sloped line, *upper panel*) to sepsis (continuous sloped line, *upper panel*) is caused in part by a circulating myocardial depressant factor; yet the end systolic volume remains about normal due to the reduced afterload. Survivors of septic shock have a large end-diastolic volume even at reduced diastolic pressure associated with dilation of their diastolic ventricles indicated by a shift of the normal diastolic pressure-volume relationship (dashed curve, *upper panel*) to the right (right hand continuous, *upper panel*). As a result, stroke volume is increased. However, in nonsurvivors stroke volume falls because of a leftward shift of the diastolic pressure-volume relationship (left hand continuous curve, *upper panel*) indicating increased diastolic stiffness and impaired diastolic filling.

The cardiac function curve illustrated in the bottom panel for survivors is normal (dashed curvilinear relation) or slightly increased (continuous curvilinear relation due to reduced afterload). The peripheral circulation during septic shock is often characterized by high flows and low vascular pressures. It follows that the resistance to venous return is decreased as indicated by a steeper venous return curve (continuous straight line, *lower panel*) compared to normal (straight dashed lines, *lower panel*). This accounts for the high venous return and so large end-diastolic volumes and stroke volumes. As with other interventions, resistance to venous return may be decreased in part by redistribution of blood flow to vascular beds with short time constants. However, the nonsurvivors may have significantly depressed cardiac function (downward shifted continuous curve, *lower panel*) because of the additive effects of decreased systolic contractility and impaired diastolic filling. Depending on the relative contribution of the abnormalities of ventricular mechanics and peripheral vascular changes, cardiac output is usually normal or high even at relatively normal end-diastolic pressures until diastolic dysfunction limits cardiac output by reducing diastolic volume even at high diastolic pressures.

reduce cardiac output and blood pressure and should be used with caution and with ongoing volume expansion.

HIGH CARDIAC OUTPUT HYPOTENSION—SEPTIC SHOCK

Septic shock is the most common example of shock that may be primarily due to reduced arterial vascular tone and reactivity, often associated with abnormal distribution of blood flow. Gram-negative bacilli are the cause in approximately two-thirds of the cases and approximately one-third of patients with gram-negative bacteremia develop septic shock.[35] Evidence of end-organ hypoperfusion and dysfunction may be present at low, normal, and high cardiac outputs and oxygen deliveries. During evaluation and resuscitation, normal or increased cardiac output with low SVR hypotension is manifested by a large pulse pressure, warm extremities, good nailbed capillary filling, and a low diastolic and mean blood pressure. This high cardiac output hypotension is often accompanied by an abnormal temperature and white blood cell count and differential and an evident site of sepsis. However, the diagnosis is sometimes initially unclear when septic shock is combined with cardiogenic or hypovolemic shock, which limit the usual increase in cardiac output, oxygen delivery, and mixed venous oxygen saturation.

A number of pathophysiologic mechanisms contribute to inadequate organ system perfusion in septic shock. There may be abnormal distribution of blood flow at the organ system level, within individual organs, and even at the capillary bed level. The result is a mismatch between oxygen supply and demand (see discussion of Fig. 1-4 in Chap. 1). Some organs, tissues, or capillary beds receive more flow and oxygen delivery than required so that oxygenated blood is functionally shunted by them while other organs, tissues, or capillary beds have an inadequate oxygen delivery and therefore are unable to maintain aerobic metabolism and normal function. In addition, there may be a cellular defect in metabolism so that even cells exposed to adequate oxygen delivery may not maintain normal aerobic metabolism. It should be noted that the evidence for tissue hypoxia in septic shock is not conclusive (see Chaps. 56 and 57); so many other abnormalities of oxygen and substrate metabolism exist and contribute to the abnormality of septic shock, that it is a naive assumption that increasing cardiac output and oxygen delivery further will have a beneficial effect.

The cardiovascular abnormalities of septic shock, as illustrated in Fig. 114-3, are extensive and include systolic and diastolic abnormalities of the heart, abnormal arterial tone, abnormalities of capillary flow, and altered tone of the venous bed. Depressed systolic contractility illustrated as a rightward shift of the end-systolic pressure-volume relationship in Fig. 114-3, *upper panel,* has been shown to occur in septic shock,[36] leading to a renewed focus on therapy for associated heart failure.[37] At least part of the depression in systolic contractility is due to a circulating myocardial depressant factor of sepsis[38] that may be dialyzable. Part of the depression of contractility may be related to a change in oxygen and substrate metabolism. The heart extracts less oxygen, which could indicate a defect in its ability to extract oxygen;[39,40] if so, that decreased oxygen consumption in the face of continued oxygen demand may result in depressed systolic contractility.[41] Additionally, the metabolic substrate for myocardial metabolism changes so that free fatty acids are no longer the prime substrate and more lactic acid is metabolized.[40] Decreased systolic contractility associated with septic shock is reversible over 5 to 10 days as the patient recovers.[36]

Despite this clear evidence of decreased contractility in sepsis, its contribution to the pathophysiology and treatment of septic shock is not so clear. Note that these "depressed" ventricles often pump cardiac outputs >10 L/min with normal values of preload, so this amount of systolic dysfunction is probably a minor contributor to the hypoperfusion state of sepsis. Further, inotropic therapy[37] may be responsible for subsequent diastolic dysfunction observed in hypovolemic shock.[16,34] Ventricles of survivors of septic shock dilate during diastole as is the normal response to decreased ventricular contractility. However, ventricles of nonsurvivors do not dilate, suggesting that they are stiffer than ventricles of the survivors.[42] Stroke volume and therefore cardiac output may decrease because of impaired diastolic filling in the later stage of septic shock; a recent hypothesis links its diastolic dysfunction to contraction bands associated with excessive emptying of the ventricle driven by endogenous catecholamine release or by inotropic therapy against the much reduced afterload.[34]

Decreased arterial resistance is almost always observed in septic shock.[43] Early in septic shock a high cardiac output state exists with normal or low blood pressure. The low arterial resistance is associated with impaired arterial autoregulation. Redistribution of blood flow to low resistance, short time constant, vascular beds (such as skeletal muscle) results in decreased resistance to venous return as illustrated in Fig. 114-3, *lower panel,* by a steeper venous return curve. As a result, cardiac output may be increased even when cardiac function is decreased (see Fig. 114-3, *lower panel*) due to decreased contractility (see Fig. 114-3, *upper panel*). Hypovolemia, due to redistribution of fluid out of the intravascular compartment and to decreased venous tone, impedes venous return during septic shock. The microcirculation is also affected so that capillary blood flow is abnormal with increased numbers of leukocytes adhering to endothelial surfaces and altering red blood cell distribution.

Initial therapy of septic shock is fluid administration to correct any intercurrent component of hypovolemia. While fluid resuscitation is ongoing, the lowest filling pressures compatible with an adequate cardiac output and oxygen delivery are sought, yet it is hard to know what is adequate. ARDS or increased pulmonary capillary permeability edema may be associated with sepsis so that pulmonary edema may occur at much lower pulmonary artery occlusion pressures. In this setting colloid infusion should be avoided since it will likely worsen the pulmonary edema. Blood transfusion is a useful therapy as it will expand the intravascular space and increase the oxygen-carrying capacity of the blood and therefore increase oxygen delivery via two mechanisms. Early institution of antibiotic therapy is central to successful therapy (see Table 114-3). Initially the antibiotic choice is not specific and is based in part on the potential pathogens (see Chap. 98). As microbiology data become available, the antibiotic regimen should be made more specific; not infrequently, sterile endotoxemia or gut-derived transient bacteremia mimics the hemodynamics of septic shock, especially in patients with hepatic failure or multisystem organ failure (MSOF) (see Chap. 53).

Other therapeutic interventions are of less certain value. Steroid therapy had previously been proposed as therapy of septic shock; however, several studies have convincingly demonstrated no benefit.[44,45] Treatment with endorphin antagonists, usually naloxone, may be of benefit in some patients, although this benefit may not become evident for many hours.[46] In septic shock where ongoing endotoxemia is suspected to be contributing to shock, antiendotoxin antibodies have been tested with potential for future success.[47] Because tumor necrosis factor levels rise very early in sepsis and may mediate the pathophysiologic abnormalities of sepsis, the development of nontoxic therapies that can be administered prophylactically has been proposed.[48] Because some of the mediators of septic shock may be dialyzable, dialysis or a variant of hemofiltration may prove useful. Therapy aimed at preventing tissue damage caused by mediators of inflammation (using ibuprofen), by oxygen radicals (using N-acetyl cysteine), and by intracellular calcium overload (using verapamil) has been proposed (see Chaps. 55 and 98). Accordingly, current effective therapy for septic shock includes rational early antibiosis and adequate expansion of the circulating volume.

OTHER TYPES OF SHOCK

As detailed in Table 114-4, there are many less common etiologies of shock, and the diagnosis and management of several causes of high right atrial pressure hypotension are discussed elsewhere in this book (see Chaps. 115, 117, 118, 120 through 122). A few other types of hypovolemic shock merit early identification by their characteristic features and lack of response to volume resuscitation. Anaphylactic shock results from the effects of histamine and other mediators of anaphylaxis on the heart, circulation, and the peripheral tissues (see Chap. 89). Despite increased circulating catecholamines and the positive inotropic effect of cardiac H_2 receptors,[49] histamine may depress systolic contractility via other mediators of anaphylaxis.[50] Marked arterial vasodilation results in hypotension even at normal or increased cardiac output. Like septic shock, blood flow is redistributed to short time constant vascular beds. The endothelium becomes more permeable so that fluid may shift out of the vascular compartment into the extravascular and intracellular compartments, resulting in intravascular hypovolemia. Venous tone and therefore venous return are reduced, so the mainstay of therapy of anaphylactic shock is fluid resuscitation of the intravascular compartment, and includes epinephrine and antihistamines as adjunctive therapy.[51,52]

Neurogenic shock is uncommon. In general, in a patient with neurologic damage that may be extensive, the cause of shock is usually associated with blood loss, but many patients with neurogenic shock develop decreased vascular tone, particularly of the venous capacitance bed, which results in pooling of blood in the periphery. Therapy with fluid will increase mean systemic pressure. Catecholamine infusion will also increase mean systemic pressure and stimulation of α receptors will increase arterial resistance, but these are rarely needed once circulation volume is repleted, and this use often delays adequate volume expansion.

A number of endocrinologic conditions may result in shock. Addison's disease or other disorders with inadequate catecholamine response may result in shock or may be an important contributor to other forms of shock.[53] Whenever it is suspected, diagnosis should be established by measuring serum cortisol and conducting a corticotropin stimulation test while presumptive therapy proceeds by dexamethasone (see Chap. 160). Hypothyroidism and hyperthyroidism may in extreme cases result in shock;[54] thyroid storm is an emergency requiring urgent therapy with Lugol's solution, propylthiouracil, steroids, propranolol, fluid resuscitation, and identification of the precipitating cause (see Chap. 162). Pheochromocytoma may lead to shock by markedly increasing afterload and by redistributing intravascular volume into extravascular compartments.[55] In general, the therapeutic approach involves treating the underlying metabolic abnormality, resuscitating with fluid to produce an adequate cardiac output at the lowest adequate filling pressure, and infusing inotropic drugs, if necessary, to improve ventricular contractility if it is decreased. Details of diagnosis and therapy of shock associated with poisons (carbon monoxide, cyanide) are discussed in Chaps. 175 and 176.

Goals of Therapy of Shock

The goal of therapy is to reverse the pathophysiologic abnormalities of shock with adequate therapeutic intervention but to avoid adverse consequences of excessive therapy. This involves continuously testing the clinical hypothesis of "too little versus too much." There are no specific "numbers" to aim for although evaluation of the type of shock and clinical assessment of the pathophysiologic abnormalities aids the physician in choosing the best therapeutic intervention that, when administered, will act as a test of the clinical assessment. Tables of normal hemodynamic values are frequently misleading because an appropriate value for one patient in shock or recovering from shock is often inappropriate for another patient in shock—and usually well outside the normal range. For example, a normal cardiac output in a septic patient may be inappropriately low so that there is continued evidence of tissue hypoperfusion. On the other hand, vigorous resuscitation with fluid and vasoactive drugs to achieve a normal blood pressure may be excessive. At a lower blood pressure, a patient with sepsis may have no evidence of ongoing tissue hypoperfusion and fluid administration to increase the blood pressure to a numerical goal may result in tissue and pulmonary edema that may be disadvantageous. Vasoconstrictors to maintain a normal blood pressure at a numerical goal may result in worsened distribution of cardiac output and increase oxygen demand of tissues so that some vital tissue beds may become even more hypoxic. Accordingly, we encourage the urgent restoration of an adequate circulating volume to restore cardiac output and O_2 delivery, aided if necessary by vasoactive drugs, and complemented by respiratory therapy to rest respiratory muscles and effect saturation of an adequate circulatory hemoglobin; then, we encourage an equally urgent reduction of each of these many interventions to the least level effecting the same goals of respiratory and cardiovascular management aided by diminishing ancillary measurements as uncertainty decreases concerning etiology and management of shock.

GOALS OF RESPIRATORY MANAGEMENT

The initial goal of airway intubation and mechanical ventilation is to correct inadequate oxygenation and ventilation and to rest the respiratory muscles so to limit their need for the limited blood flow. Initially a high F_{IO_2} is chosen and mechanical ventilation attempts to do all of the work of breathing so that respiratory muscle oxygen consumption is minimized. Often this is best accomplished using a controlled mechanical ventilation mode with a low trigger threshold to allow patient-initiated assisted breaths; delivering an adequate minute ventilation to reduce ventilatory drive; using a high enough inspiratory flow rate to rapidly unload and relax any contracting inspiratory muscles; and administering adequate doses of sedatives and analgesics. If the patient continues to work hard on the mechanical ventilator then muscle paralysis may improve the efficiency of mechanical ventilation and speed resolution of the acute shock state.

Immediately after initiating mechanical ventilatory support the goal of minimizing therapeutic intervention (reducing toxic F_{IO_2}, lowering PEEP, liberating the patient from mechanical ventilation), while ensuring that the pathophysiologic abnormalities are reversed, starts in earnest.[5] When blood-gas data are available, the least toxic F_{IO_2} consistent with adequate arterial oxygenation is sought. The least PEEP consistent with adequate arterial saturation of sufficient circulatory hemoglobin on a nontoxic F_{IO_2} is used. Although PEEP can reduce venous return in the patient in shock, it is helpful to note that PEEP often increases output in patients with cardiogenic shock and pulmonary edema[56] so the physician should not delay trying PEEP to fix the hypoxemia. Similarly, when septic or hypovolemic shock is complicated by pulmonary vascular leak, these patients often tolerate PEEP to correct hypoxemia without reducing their cardiac output or blood pressure provided their vascular volume is adequate.

Reversing the reasons for airway intubation and mechanical ventilation is the most important aspect of the process of liberating the patient from mechanical ventilation. For example if a patient has been paralyzed and sedated to decrease the oxygen demand of the respiratory muscles and the reason for increased demand (e.g., shock and acidosis) has been reversed then paralysis should quickly be discontinued and the patient allowed to trigger the ventilator. Indeed, if the indication for assisted ventilation is gone, and frequently this happens quickly, then the patient should be allowed to do as much of the work of breathing as is consistent with useful exercise of the respiratory muscles without fatigue. Specific ventilator modes which facilitate this are considered in detail in Chap. 127. Intubation and mechanical ventilation should be discontinued as rapidly as is safely possible because intubation and mechanical ventilation are associated with significant ongoing risk.

GOALS OF CARDIOVASCULAR MANAGEMENT

Cardiovascular management aims to maintain a cardiac output and oxygen delivery adequate to reverse tissue hypoperfusion but avoid adverse effects of excessive therapy by seeking the lowest ventricular filling pressures and lowest vasoactive drug infusions required to achieve this goal.[8] The hypothesis testing approach to volume resuscitation and vasoactive drug infusion applies in all shock states as we have described. The value of distinguishing between shock states is that it leads to more accurate prediction of the outcome of an intervention and therefore leads to less overshoot and undershoot of therapeutic interventions. For example, in the absence of pulmonary edema, fluid infusion may be useful in cardiogenic shock but this must be tested with small volumes of crystalloid to avoid dangerous excessive fluid overload that may occur. In contrast, if the clinical assessment clearly identifies marked intravascular hypovolemia, for example after a motor vehicle accident and brisk hemorrhage, then extremely rapid fluid infusion of several liters of solution, including blood and colloid, is appropriate therapy and is unlikely to overshoot toward hypervolemia.

Cardiovascular resuscitation often includes "inotropic" or "vasoactive" agents such as dobutamine and dopamine. The clinical assessment of the mechanism of shock is again important in choosing the specific agent. For example, dopamine beneficially increases contractility in some shock states, but it also increases venous return by constricting the capacitance veins even in hypovolemic shock and may acutely appear beneficial. The continued use of these agents in hypovolemic shock, masking inadequate fluid resuscitation, is dangerous. Dobutamine increases ventricular contractility and reduces afterload, which may result in increased cardiac output and oxygen delivery in cardiogenic shock. However, if contractility is already good so that it cannot be increased much further, then dobutamine may only serve to decrease afterload and preload which, in the hypovolemic patient, may result in hypotension leading to worsened perfusion. Dopamine can redistribute blood flow toward and away from vital organs depending on dose and on the specific shock state. That is, dopamine in the range of 0.5 to 5 μg/kg/min may selectively improve renal and mesenteric blood flow (see Chap. 125). In high cardiac output hypotensive septic shock, norepinephrine may improve renal blood flow[57] by increasing arterial pressure above a critical threshold required to perfuse the kidneys. However, at higher doses, dopamine may redistribute blood flow away from the kidney and gut, and in any other clinical setting noradrenaline reduces renal, cardiac, and brain blood flow. Thus, depending on the mechanism of shock, specific vasoactive agents may be beneficial or detrimental (for further discussion, see Chap. 125).

FREQUENT MEASUREMENTS

The goals of therapy involve continued hypothesis testing, which can only be achieved by repeated evaluation of the patient. This is the basis for frequent repeated measurements—often called monitoring. Of course, monitoring implies that an alarm will sound when the recorded variable (like the ECG) is detected to be aberrant; it is helpful to note that most hemodynamic measures are not alarmed, except for the answer they provide to a specific question.[58] If a question that a vascular pressure, flow, or image can answer is not asked or if the answer to that question will not alter therapy, then the catheter or other transducer should be discontinued since it will most likely only contribute to confusion and complications. Indeed, we encourage the same urgency in discontinuing invasive hemodynamic measurements when answers to diagnostic and therapeutic questions are already evident as we encourage the early implementation of these measures. For example, one helpful test of the continued need for right heart catheter measurements is to ask whether a new catheterization is warranted to obtain the information revealed by the current catheter; if not, remove it!

Repeated physical examination is often the most effective monitoring that can be done. Other frequent measurements, usually instituted early, include continuous ECG, urine output, arterial pressure, and CVP. Using the ventilator and other devices, extensive measurements of pulmonary mechanics and function can occur in intubated patients including respiratory rate, tidal volume, $F_{I_{O_2}}$, peak, mean, and end-expiratory airway pressures, static end-inspiratory and end-expiratory airway pressures, end-tidal CO_2 concentration, and O_2 consumption and CO_2 production.

Placement of a pulmonary artery catheter allows detailed repeated cardiovascular measurements. CVP, right ventricular pressures, pulmonary artery pressures, Ppw, and thermodilution cardiac output can be measured as frequently as necessary to determine the cardiovascular abnormalities and to measure the effect of therapeutic interventions as tests of clinical hypotheses. Because more pressures, volumes, and flows can be measured with more sophisticated measuring devices, more sophisticated hypotheses may be tested. For example, using a pulmonary artery catheter, following a rapid crystalloid fluid infusion, a small rise in CVP or pulmonary artery occlusion pressure suggests that the ventricle is operating on the compliant-partially full portion of the diastolic pressure-volume relationship. However, a sharp rise in CVP or Ppw suggests that the ventricle is quite full during diastole and that further volume infusion will likely result in marked increases in these pressures and increase the risk of high pressure pulmonary edema. Thus, the hypothesis that the patient remains hypovolemic may be more accurately tested with a pulmonary artery catheter. Because cardiac output can be measured with a thermistor-tipped pulmonary artery catheter, oxygen delivery may be calculated. Therefore, the ability of any given intervention to increase oxygen delivery can be assessed. Right heart thermodilution or volume conductance catheters may allow rapid assessment of stroke volume and right heart ejection fractions allowing specific hypotheses regarding right heart function to be tested.

TEMPO

We believe that rapid initial resuscitation to restore tissue oxygenation and reverse shock will improve patient outcome. We base this on the observation that untreated shock leads quite rapidly to death. Lactic acid levels and tissue damage increase with the duration of tissue hypoperfusion. Tissue damage and organ dysfunction are related to the duration of shock. Therefore, one of the most important contributions the intensivist can make to the care of a shock patient is to establish an appropriately rapid management tempo. Careful evaluation of the need for radiographic examination weighed against the time spent doing these tests away from other care, or determining when the best time is to place a pulmonary artery catheter weighed against the time that it will divert the physician's attention away from other matters, both depend very much on the intensivist's judgment and familiarity with the clinical setting. Frequently, appropriate decision-making regarding sequence and tempo of care can markedly decrease the duration of initial assessment and resuscitation.

The mirror image of urgent implementation is rapid liberation of the resuscitated patient from excessive therapy. It is not uncommon for the patient with hypovolemic or septic shock to stabilize hemodynamically on positive-pressure ventilation with high circulating volume and several vasoactive drugs infusing at a high rate (dopamine 20 μg/kg/min). Too often, hours or days of "weaning" pass, when a trial of spontaneous breathing, diuresis, and sequential reduction of the drug dose by half each 10 min can return the patient to a much less treated stable state within the hour. Of course, this rapid discontinuation may be limited by intercurrent hemodynamic or other instability, but defining each limit and justifying ongoing or new therapy is the essence of titrated care in this postresuscitation period. Utilizing the sophisticated critical care nursing and monitoring of the critical care unit to maintain the tempo of recovery to the preshock state should reduce the duration and complications of critical care.

Important Clinical Interactions

HOW SHOCK AFFECTS ORGAN SYSTEMS

Altered mental status ranging from mild confusion to coma is a frequently observed effect of shock on neurologic function when brain blood flow falls by approximately 50 percent.[59] However, patients recovering from shock infrequently suffer a neurologic deficit unless they have concomitant cerebrovascular disease. One exception is that encephalopathy may follow hypovolemic shock in pediatric patients. Thus, in general, the brain is selectively protected against hypoperfusion compared to other organ systems. The brain, like the heart, maintains a fairly constant oxygen extraction ratio so that to meet its metabolic needs under a wide variety of circumstances, it autoregulates cerebral blood flow. Maximal cerebral vasodilation is reached, and decreased neurologic function is observed, when mean arterial pressure falls below 50 to 60 mmHg in normal individuals (see Chap. 34). However, cerebral blood flow may be adequate at even lower pressures in septic shock and other shock states. In addition, elevated P_{CO_2} dilates and decreased P_{CO_2} constricts cerebral vessels; after a step change in P_{CO_2}, this effect lasts for less than a day, when equilibration restores cerebral vascular resistance at the new P_{CO_2}.[60] Finally, profound hypoxia results in markedly decreased cerebral vascular resistance.

Shock is primarily a cardiovascular disorder so that adverse effects of shock on the cardiovascular system imply a positive feedback loop leading to cardiovascular collapse. Up to the point of cardiovascular collapse, the heart is preferentially protected from the adverse effects of shock, particularly by excellent coronary autoregulation. Coronary autoregulation results in a constant and high (70 percent) myocardial oxygen extraction ratio[41] and is sufficient to maintain adequate coronary blood flow down to very low mean arterial pressures. While myocardial oxygen demand during shock may be elevated due to increased heart rate and increased levels of circulating catecholamines, low afterload and low preloads reduce myocardial oxygen demand. Despite these compensatory mechanisms, myocardial oxygen demand eventually exceeds oxygen supply leading to segmental[61] and global[41] myocardial dysfunction with ST and T wave changes apparent on the ECG.[62] Myocardial perfusion is redistributed away from the endocardium and this maldistribution is further aggravated by circulating catecholamines. If severe hypoxemia or anemia contribute to limited myocardial oxygen delivery then the heart may shift to anaerobic metabolism with a concomitant decrease in systolic contractility and output. Unless quickly reversed, this downward spiral rapidly leads to death.[41] The diffuse systemic inflammatory process accompanying septic shock has additional effects on the heart. The ability of the myocardium to extract oxygen is decreased and the normal metabolic substrate of myocardial metabolism shifts from predominantly free fatty acids to lactate.[40] Circulating myocardial depressant factors contribute to decreased systolic contractility in septic shock and probably in other forms of shock.[38] Metabolic acidosis[63] and respiratory acidosis[64] result in intracellular myocardial acidosis and decreased contractility. As lactic acid levels rise, ionized calcium levels fall and contribute to decreased contractility.[9] During hypovolemic shock[34] and in nonsurvivors of septic shock,[42] increased diastolic stiffness develops, resulting in decreased cardiac pump function. Arrhythmias frequently occur and lead to further reduction in cardiac pump function.

Shock affects the lungs by worsening ventilation perfusion matching and by increasing shunt.[65] Increased ventilation associated with shock results in increased work of breathing to the extent that a disproportionate amount of blood flow is diverted to fatiguing ventilatory muscles.[6,66] Therapy with vasoactive agents may further worsen the shunt.[8,67] Frequently shock leads to overt ARDS,[68] sometimes called "shock lung." The problem of maintaining oxygen delivery, balanced against the need for low pulmonary venous pressures to avoid worsened pulmonary edema, is aggravated.

Autoregulation by the brain and heart may divert blood flow from splanchnic organs resulting in ischemic injury of the liver, pancreas, and gut leading to decreased function and cellular damage. Early in shock increased catecholamines, glucagon, and glucocorticoids increase hepatic gluconeogenesis leading to hyperglycemia. Later when synthetic function fails, hypoglycemia occurs. Clearance of metabolites and immunologic function of the liver are also impaired during hypoperfusion.[69] Typically, centrilobular hepatic necrosis leads to release of transaminases as the predominant biochemical evidence of hepatic damage, and bilirubin levels may be high.[70] Shock may lead to gut ischemia before other organ systems become ischemic even in the absence of mesenteric vascular disease. Mucosal edema, submucosal hemorrhage, and hemorrhagic necrosis of the gut may occur. Importantly, the barrier function of the gut against enteric organisms and their toxic products fails so that the gut becomes a source of toxic mediators[33] (see Chap. 53).

The glomerular filtration rate falls as renal cortical blood flow is reduced by decreased arterial perfusion pressures and also by afferent arteriolar vasoconstriction due to increased sympathetic tone, catecholamines, and angiotensin. Additionally, the ratio of renal cortical to medullary blood flow decreases. Renal hypoperfusion may lead to ischemic damage with acute tubular necrosis while debris and surrounding tissue edema obstruct tubules.[71] Loss of tubular function is compounded by loss of concentrating ability because medullary hypertonicity decreases.

Shock impairs reticuloendothelial system function leading to impaired immunologic function.[72] Coagulation abnormalities and thrombocytopenia are common hematologic effects of shock. Disseminated intravascular coagulation occurs in approximately 10 percent of patients with hypovolemic and septic shock.

HOW ORGAN SYSTEMS AFFECT SHOCK

Organ system hypoperfusion results in functional impairment, which has important effects on the shock state. Altered neurologic function may contribute in simple ways, such as impaired ability to protect the airway, to more complex ways, such as decreased release of corticotropin-releasing factor leading to decreased corticotropin release and relative adrenal insufficiency. Decreased cardiac function directly leads to worsening of the shock state and may form part of a detrimental positive feedback loop as discussed above.

Decreased pulmonary gas exchange leads to hypoxemia, respiratory acidosis, and worsened metabolic acidosis all of which may depress cardiac function or contribute to decreased delivery of oxygen to other vital organ systems.[41,63,64] Stiff lungs or increased pressures in structures surrounding the heart may impair diastolic filling of the ventricle and thereby worsen the shock state; pulmonary hypertension associated with shock, ARDS, and PEEP further impairs cardiac function by increasing right ventricular afterload with concomitant right-to-left septal shift.[8,73] There is little evidence that acute lung injury per se causes ventricular dysfunction.[74]

Decreased hepatic function during shock impairs normal clearance of drugs such as narcotics and benzodiazepines, lactic acid, and other metabolites that may adversely affect the cardiovascular system by decreasing venous return or decreasing cardiac function. Hypoperfusion of the gut has been proposed as a key link in the development of MSOF following shock, particularly when ARDS precedes sepsis,[33] i.e., loss of gut barrier function results in entrance of enteric organisms and toxins into lymphatics and the portal circulation. Since the immunologic function of the liver is impaired,[69] bacteria and their toxic products, particularly from portal venous blood, are not adequately cleared. These substances as well as inflammatory mediators produced by hepatic reticuloendothelial cells are released into the systemic circulation and may be an important initiating event of a diffuse systemic inflammatory process that leads to MSOF[75] or to the high cardiac output hypotension of endotoxemia.[37] Additionally, pancreatic ischemic damage may result in the systemic release of a number of toxic substances including a myocardial depressant factor.[76]

Impaired renal function or renal failure leads to worsened metabolic acidosis, hyperkalemia, impaired clearance of drugs and other substances; all contribute to the poor outcome of patients in shock with renal failure. Decreased renal perfusion pressure results in increased renin, angiotensin, and aldosterone levels with resultant redistribution of blood flow. Other organ systems can have profound effects on the shock state. Shock combined with impaired hematopoetic and immunologic function seen with hematologic malignancies or following chemotherapy is nearly uniformly lethal. Endocrine disorders, from insufficient or ineffective insulin secretion to adrenal insufficiency, adversely affect cardiac and other organ system function. Conceivably, impaired parathyroid function is unable to maintain calcium homeostasis so that ionized hypocalcemia is observed during lactic acidosis or its treatment with sodium bicarbonate infusion[9] as it is following citric acid loads that accompany massive stored red cell transfusions.

HOW SHOCK AFFECTS THERAPEUTIC INTERVENTIONS

Hypoperfusion alters the efficacy of drug therapy by slowing delivery of drugs, altering pharmacokinetics once delivered, and decreasing the clearance of drugs. For example, subcutaneous injection of medications may fail to deliver useful quantities of a drug in the setting of decreased perfusion. When adequate perfusion is reestablished, the drug may be delivered in an unpredictable way at an inappropriate time. Thus, parenteral medications should be given intravenously to patients with evidence of hypoperfusion. In marked hypoperfusion states, peripheral intravenous infusion may also be ineffective and central venous administration may be necessary to effectively deliver medications. Once the drug is delivered to its site of action it may not have the same effect in the setting of shock. For example, catecholamines are less effective in an acidotic or septic state (see Chap. 125). Since there may be significant renal and hepatic hypoperfusion, drug clearance is frequently greatly impaired. With these observations in mind, it is appropriate to consider for each drug, necessary changes in route, dose, and interval of administration in shock patients.

HOW THERAPEUTIC INTERVENTIONS AFFECT SHOCK

Many therapeutic interventions commonly used in the ICU may worsen the shock state. For example, airway intubation and mechanical ventilation using positive airway pressures increase pleural pressure from normal negative values to positive values. Right atrial pressure, therefore, increases to reduce the pressure gradient driving venous return back to the heart.[77] The necessary use of analgesics and sedatives in critically ill patients may have important additional detrimental effects. Analgesics and sedatives may reduce venous tone either directly or by decreasing sympathetic stimulation. As a result cardiac output and oxygen delivery may fall.[8,77] In a patient with already decreased intravascular volume or an impaired ability to mount a further sympathetic response the impediment to venous return resulting from positive-pressure ventilation may result in marked reduction in cardiac output and blood pressure.

The increase in intrapulmonary pressures following intubation and mechanical ventilation are frequently amplified by addition of PEEP, by development of intrinsic PEEP, and by inverse ratio and other modes of ventilation. Increased intrapulmonary pressures expand and recruit alveoli and redistribute alveolar edema to the interstitial space[78,79] improving arterial oxygenation (see discussion of Fig. 1-9 in Chap. 1). However, since the lung is more distended it may become less compliant due to its curvilinear volume-pressure relationship so that, despite no change in tidal volume, mean and peak airway pressures rise leading to barotrauma. In addition, lung previously in West's zone 2 or 3 may now be in West's zone 1 conditions, which means physiologic dead space increases. As a result P_{CO_2} may detrimentally rise at the same minute ventilation (see discussion of Fig. 2-20 in Chap. 2).

Volume resuscitation with electrolyte solutions may worsen tissue edema. If endothelial membranes are leaky, then colloid administration may even be worse. Inotropic and vasoactive drugs may improve blood pressure or cardiac output but may worsen the distribution of blood flow so that perfusion of some vital organs may be decreased. For arrhythmias that impair cardiac function antiarrhythmic agents may be necessary but calcium channel blockers, lidocaine, disopyramide, and others may reduce myocardial contractility and worsen the shock state. In summary, during shock many common therapeutic interventions may have important adverse consequences. This is further reason to regard therapeutic interventions as tests, with clear recognition that if they are not beneficial they will be stopped.

Bicarbonate therapy of metabolic acidosis associated with shock may have adverse consequences. Bicarbonate reduces ionized calcium levels further with potentially detrimental effect on myocardial contractility.[9] Because bicarbonate and acid reversibly form carbon dioxide and water, a high P_{CO_2} is observed. Particularly during bolus infusion, acidotic blood containing bicarbonate may have a very high P_{CO_2} which readily diffuses into cells resulting in marked intracellular acidosis; recall that hypoperfusion already increases tissue P_{CO_2} by carrying off the tissue CO_2 production at a higher mixed venous P_{CO_2} due to reduced blood flow. Intracellular acidosis results in decreased myocardial contractility.[64] These adverse consequences of bicarbonate therapy may account partly for the lack of benefit observed with bicarbonate therapy of metabolic acidosis.[9,80]

Outcome

Untreated, shock leads to death. Even with rapid, appropriate resuscitation shock is associated with a high initial mortality rate, and tissue damage sustained during shock may lead to delayed sequelae. A number of studies have identified several important predictors. Cardiogenic shock is associated with approximately a 90 percent mortality with medical management alone and blood lactate, cardiac output or stroke work, and arterial pressure predict outcome.[81] A blood lactic acid level in excess of 5 mmol/L is associated with 90 percent mortality in cardiogenic shock[82] and high mortality in other shock states. These mortality rates have fallen during the last decade of interventional cardiology (see Chap. 116) and aggressive antibiosis (see Chap. 98). In septic shock a falling cardiac output predicts death[83] and high concentrations of bacteria in blood and a failure to mount a febrile response predict a poor outcome.[33] Age and preexisting illness are important determinants of outcome.[84] MSOF is an important adverse outcome, leading to a mortality rate in excess of 60 percent, as discussed extensively in Chap. 53 through 57.

CASE PRESENTATION

A 61-year-old man collapsed at home and was brought to the hospital. He had been generally unwell and had lost 20 lb over several months. He had a past history of an adenocarcinoma of the lung resected 5 years previously and had an intermittent history of peptic ulcer disease. He was a smoker and had a history of alcohol abuse.

Initial examination showed him to be diaphoretic with cool ashen gray colored skin and central cyanosis. He was obtunded with a Glascow coma score of 9. His heart rate was 120, blood pressure 180/105, temperature 34.5°C (94.7°F), and respiratory rate 28 with a Kussmaul's pattern. His pupils were 2 mm and reactive; his neck was supple. His trachea was midline, and the left lung base was dull to percussion with increased transmission of breath sounds and coarse crackles. Cardiovascular examination revealed thready peripheral pulses despite the measured blood pressure with cold, cyanotic extremities with markedly slowed nail bed capillary refill. His jugular veins were easily seen and flat while he was supine. His heart sounds were normal. Bowel sounds were absent and rectal examination disclosed dark blood in his rectum. Urine output over the first 30 min was 4 mL.

Shortly after clinical examination and after initiating volume resuscitation (vide infra), his hemoglobin was found to be 164 g/L, white blood cell count was 19.8, anion gap was 30, creatinine was 584 mM/L and BUN was 48.4 mM/L. Arterial blood-gases with pH 7.30, P_{CO_2} 28, and P_{O_2} 54 showed metabolic acidosis with incomplete respiratory compensation and hypoxemia. Chest x-ray demonstrated increased opacification of his left lower lobe. ECG was unchanged from 1 year previously and suggested an old anteroseptal infarction.

Despite his high blood pressure he was clearly in shock because he had evidence of multisystem organ hypoperfusion based on cardiovascular and neurologic examinations, skin and extremities, and urine output. Although several types of shock may have been contributing, he was clearly hypovolemic. He was also working hard to breathe probably because he was acidotic, hypoxic, and possibly septic. This evaluation constitutes the clinical hypothesis. Based on this, two large bore peripheral intravenous catheters were inserted, ECG monitoring initiated, he was intubated and mechanical ventilation using 100% oxygen and the assist-control mode was begun. Simultaneously he was given 4 L warmed normal saline over 30 min with repeat physical examination after each liter, which tested and confirmed the primary clinical hypothesis of hypovolemia. His urinary bladder was catheterized and a nasogastric tube was placed. Physical examination was completed. As fluid resuscitation continued, his blood pressure fell to 120/70 and heart rate decreased to 110. Perfusion of his extremities improved and his urine output in the second half hour increased to 55 mL. Laboratory tests and chest x-ray results became available and suggested the possibility of sepsis. Accordingly, early therapy also included broad-spectrum antibiotics including ampicillin for gut organisms, and other interventions included naloxone, thiamine, and urgent surgical consultation regarding possible bowel ischemia.

Following initial resuscitation his acidosis improved but did not resolve and an arterial lactate level was found to be 10 mM/L. To test the clinical hypothesis that he continued to have inadequate organ system perfusion despite a normal blood pressure and evidence of improved peripheral perfusion, a pulmonary artery catheter was inserted. His right atrial pressure was 5, pulmonary artery pressure was 35/15, a pulmonary artery occlusion pressure was 8, cardiac output was 7.5 L/min and cardiac index was 4.2 L/min/m^2; the mixed venous saturation was 78%. Laparotomy disclosed infarcted bowel in the region of the watershed between the superior mesenteric and inferior mesenteric arteries. Blood cultures grew pneumococci.

CASE DISCUSSION

Our synthesis after the first day of therapy was that the patient had developed pneumococcal pneumonia and sepsis. While obtunded at home for some period of time, he became hypovolemic so that he presented with mixed septic and hypovolemic shock. His preexisting vascular disease plus markedly increased sympathetic tone allowed him to maintain a high blood pressure even though his cardiac output was low. Bowel ischemia developed as a result of shock and vascular disease, contributing to septic hemodynamics and lactic acidosis. This case illustrates the common finding that initially shock may be due to several causes; therapy is also a test of the clinical hypothesis and points out the important interaction between shock, organ systems, and therapy.

References

1. Cohn JN: Blood pressure measurement in shock: Mechanism of inaccuracy in auscultatory and palpatory methods. JAMA 199:972, 1967.
2. Fenwick JC, Dodek PM, Ronco JJ, et al: Increased concentrations of plasma lactate predict pathologic dependence of oxygen consumption on oxygen delivery in patients with adult respiratory distress syndrome. J Crit Care 5:1, 1990.
3. Grassino A, Macklem PT: Respiratory muscle fatigue and ventilatory failure. Annu Rev Med 35:625, 1984.
4. Von Planta M, Weil MH, Gazmuri RJ, et al: Myocardial acidosis associated with CO_2 production during cardiac arrest and resuscitation. Circulation 80:684, 1989.
5. Hall JB, Wood LDH: Liberation of the patient from mechanical ventilation. JAMA 257:1621, 1987.
6. Hussain SNA, Roussos C: Distribution of respiratory muscle and organ blood flow during endotoxic shock in dogs. J Appl Physiol 59:1802, 1985.
7. Schumacker PT, RW Samsel: Oxygen delivery and uptake by peripheral tissues: Physiology and pathophysiology. Crit Care Clin 5:255, 1989.
8. Wood LDH, Prewitt RM: Cardiovascular management in acute hypoxemic respiratory failure. Am J Cardiol 47:963, 1981.

9. Cooper DJ, Walley KR, Wiggs BR, Russell JA: Bicarbonate does not improve hemodynamics in critically ill patients who have lactic acidosis: A prospective, controlled clinical study. Ann Intern Med 112:492, 1990.
10. Forrester JS, Diamond G, Chatterjee K, Swan HJC: Medical therapy of acute myocardial infarction by application of hemodynamic subsets. Part I. N Engl J Med 295:1356, 1976.
11. Scheidt S, Ascheim R, Killip T: Shock after acute myocardial infarction: A clinical and hemodynamic profile. Am J Cardiol 26:556, 1970.
12. Chesebro JH, Knatterud G, Roberts R, et al: Thrombolysis in myocardial infarction (TIMI) trial—Phase I: A comparison between intravenous tissue plasminogen activator and intravenous streptokinase: Clinical findings through hospital discharge. Circulation 76:142, 1987.
13. Kennedy JW, Ritchie JL, Davis KB, Fritz JK: Western Washington randomized trial of intra-coronary streptokinase in acute myocardial infarction. N Engl J Med 309:1477, 1983.
14. Page DL, Caulfield JB, Kastor JA, et al: Myocardial changes associated with cardiogenic shock. N Engl J Med 285:133, 1971.
15. Zile MR: Diastolic dysfunction: Detection, consequences and treatment. Mod Concepts Cardiovasc Dis 58:67, 1989, 59:1, 1990.
16. Crowell JW, Guyton AC: Further evidence favoring a cardiac mechanism in irreversible hemorrhagic shock. Am J Physiol 203:248, 1962.
17. Brodie BR, Grossman W, Mann T, et al: Effects of sodium nitroprusside on left ventricular diastolic pressure-volume relations. J Clin Invest 59:59, 1977.
18. Radford MJ, Johnson RA, Daggett WM, et al: Ventricular septal rupture: A review of clinical and physiologic features and an analysis of survival. Circulation 64:545, 1981.
19. Subramanian VA, Roberts AJ, Zema MJ, et al: Cardiogenic shock following acute myocardial infarction: Late functional results after emergency cardiac surgery. NY State J Med 80:947, 1980.
20. Mueller H, Ayres SM, Gregory JJ, et al: Hemodynamics, coronary blood flow, and myocardial metabolism in coronary shock: Response to 1-norepinephrine and isoproterenol. J Clin Invest 49:1885, 1970.
21. Lipkin DP, Frenneaux M, Maseri A: Beneficial effect of captopril in cardiogenic shock. Lancet 2(8554):327, 1987.
22. Cohn JN, Guiha NH, Broder MI, Limas CJ: Right ventricular infarction: Clinical and hemodynamic features. Am J Cardiol 33:209, 1974.
23. Roberts N, Harrison DG, Reimer KA, et al: Right ventricular infarction with shock but without significant left ventricular infarction: A new clinical syndrome. Am Heart J 110:1047, 1985.
24. Lorell B, Leinbach RC, Pohost GM, et al: Right ventricular infarction: Clinical diagnosis and differentiation from cardiac tamponade and pericardial constriction. Am J Cardiol 43:465, 1979.
25. Dell'Italia LJ, Starling MR, Blumhardt R, et al: Comparative effects of volume loading, dobutamine and nitroprusside in patients with predominant right ventricular infarction. Circulation 72:1327, 1985.
26. Love JC, Haffajee CI, Gore JM, Alpert JS: Reversibility of hypotension and shock by atrial or atrioventricular sequential pacing in patients with right ventricular infarction. Am Heart J 108:5, 1984.
27. Ducas J, Prewitt RM: Pathophysiology and therapy of right ventricular dysfunction due to pulmonary embolism. Cardiovasc Clin 17:191, 1987.
28. McGregor M: Pulsus paradoxus. N Engl J Med 301:480, 1979.
29. Knopp R, Claypool R, Leonardt D: Use of the tilt test in measuring acute blood loss. Ann Emerg Med 9:72, 1980.
30. Rackow EC, Falk JL, Fein IA, et al: Fluid resuscitation in circulatory shock; a comparison of the cardiorespiratory effect of albumen hetastarch and saline solutions in patients with hypovolemic and septic shock. Crit Care Med 11:839, 1983.
31. Rush BF: Irreversibility in the post-transfusion phase of hemorrhagic shock. Adv Exp Med Biol 23:215, 1971.
32. Barroso-Aranda J, Schmid-Schonbein GW, Zweifach BW, Engler RL: Granulocytes and no-reflow phenomenon in irreversible hemorrhagic shock. Circ Res 63:437, 1988.
33. Haglund U: The splanchnic organs as the source of toxic mediators in shock. *Perspectives in Shock Research.* New York, Alan R Liss, 1988, pp 135–145.
34. Walley KR, Cooper DJ: Diastolic stiffness impairs left ventricular function during hypovolemic shock in pigs. Am J Physiol 260:H702, 1991.
35. Kreger BE, Craven DE, McCabe WR: Gram-negative bacteremia III: Reassessment of etiology, epidemiology and ecology in 612 patients. Am J Med 68:332, 1980.
36. Parker MM, Shelhamer JH, Bacharach SL, et al: Profound but reversible myocardial depression in patients with septic shock. Ann Intern Med 100:483, 1984.
37. Schremmer B, Dhainault J: Heart failure in septic shock: Effects of inotropic support. Crit Care Med 18:549, 1990.
38. Parrillo JE, Burch C, Shelhamer JH, et al: A circulating myocardial depressant substance in humans with septic shock. J Clin Invest 76:1539, 1985.
39. Cunnion RE, Schaer GL, Parker MM, et al: The coronary circulation in human septic shock. Circulation 73:637, 1986.
40. Dhainaut J-F, Huyghebaert M-F, Monsallier JF, et al: Coronary hemodynamics and myocardial metabolism of lactate, free fatty acids, glucose, and ketones in patients with septic shock. Circulation 75:533, 1987.
41. Walley KR, Becker CJ, Hogan RA, et al: Progressive hypoxemia limits left ventricular oxygen consumption and contractility. Circ Res 63:849, 1988.
42. Russell JA, Ronco JJ, Lockat D, et al: Oxygen delivery and consumption and ventricular preload are greater in survivors than in nonsurvivors of the adult respiratory distress syndrome. Am Rev Respir Dis 141:659, 1990.
43. Winslow EJ, Loeb HS, Rahimtoola SH, et al: Hemodynamic studies and results of therapy in 50 patients with bacteremic shock. Am J Med 54:421, 1973.
44. Bone RC, Fisher CJ, Clemmer TP, et al: A controlled clinical trial of high-dose methylprednisolone in the treatment of severe sepsis and septic shock. N Engl J Med 317:653, 1987.
45. The Veterans Administration Systemic Sepsis Cooperative Study Group. Effect of high-dose glucocorticoid therapy on mortality in patients with clinical signs of systemic sepsis. N Engl J Med 317:659, 1987.
46. Roberts DE, Dobson KE, Hall KW, Light RB: Effects of prolonged naloxone infusion in septic shock. Lancet 2(8613):699, 1988.
47. Ziegler EJ, McCutchan JA, Fierer J, et al: Treatment of gram-negative bacteremia and shock with antiserum to a mutant *Escherichia coli.* N Engl J Med 307:1225, 1982.
48. Marks JD, Marks CB, Luce J, et al: Plasma tumor necrosis factor in patients with septic shock. Am Rev Respir Dis 141:94, 1990.
49. Watkins J, Dargie HJ, Brown MJ, et al: Effects of histamine type 2 receptor stimulation on myocardial function in normal subjects. Br Heart J 47:539, 1982.
50. Cooper DJ, Thompson C, Walley KR, et al: Histamine infusion

decreases left ventricular contractility in humans. Fed Proc 4:A340, 1990.
51. Smith PL, Kagey-Sobotka A, Bleecker ER, et al: Physiologic manifestations of human anaphylaxis. J Clin Invest 66:1072, 1980.
52. Beaupre PN, Roizen MF, Cahalan MK, et al: Hemodynamic and two-dimensional transesophageal echocardiographic analysis of an anaphylatic reaction in a human. Anesthesiology 60:482, 1984.
53. Rao RH, Vagnucci AH, Amico JA: Bilateral massive adrenal hemorrhage: Early recognition and treatment. Ann Intern Med 110:227, 1989.
54. Nicoloff JT: Thyroid storm and myxedema coma. Med Clin North Am 69:1005, 1985.
55. Brunjes S, Johns VJ, Crane MG: Pheochromocytoma: Postoperative shock and blood volume. N Engl J Med 262:393, 1960.
56. Scharf SM, Bianco JA, Tow DE, Brown R: The effects of large negative intrathoracic pressure on left ventricular function in patients with coronary artery disease. Circulation 63:871, 1981.
57. Schaer GL, Fink MP, Parrillo JE: Norepinephrine alone versus norepinephrine plus low-dose dopamine: Enhanced renal blood flow with combination pressor therapy. Crit Care Med 13:492, 1985.
58. Chatterjee K, Parmley WW, Ganz W, et al: Hemodynamic studies: Their uses and limitations. Am J Cardiol 64:30, 1989.
59. Harper AM: Autoregulation of cerebral blood flow: Influence of the arterial blood pressure on the blood flow through the cerebral cortex. J Neurol Neurosurg Psychiatry 29:398, 1966.
60. Muizelarr JP, Van der Poel HG, Li Z, et al: Pial arteriolar vessel diameter and CO_2 reactivity during prolonged hyperventilation in the rabbit. J Neurosurg 69:923, 1988.
61. Thomas F, Smith JL, Orme JF, et al: Reversible segmental myocardial dysfunction in septic shock. Crit Care Med 14:587, 1986.
62. Terradellas JB, Bellot JF, Saris AB, et al: Acute and transient ST segment elevation during bacterial shock in seven patients without apparent heart disease. Chest 81:444, 1982.
63. Teplinsky K, O'Toole M, Olman M, et al: Effect of lactic acidosis on canine hemodynamics and left ventricular function. Am J Physiol 258:1193, 1990.
64. Walley KR, Lewis TH, Wood LDH: Acute respiratory acidosis decreases left ventricular contractility but increases cardiac output in dogs. Circ Res 67:628, 1990.
65. Jardin F, Eveleigh MC, Gurdjian F, et al: Venous admixture in human septic shock. Comparative effects of blood volume expansion, dopamine infusion and isoproterenal infusion on mismatching of ventilation and pulmonary blood flow in peritonitis. Circulation 60:155, 1979.
66. Aubier M, Trippenbach T, Roussos C: Respiratory muscle fatigue during cardiogenic shock. J Appl Physiol 51:449, 1981.
67. Prewitt RM, Wood LDH: Effect of sodium nitroprusside on cardiovascular function and pulmonary shunt in canine oleic acid pulmonary edema. Anesthesiology 55:537, 1981.
68. Rinaldo JE, Rogers RM: ARDS: Changing concepts of lung injury and repair. N Engl J Med 306:900, 1982.
69. Loegerling DJ, Saba TM: Hepatic Kuppfer cell dysfunction during hemorrhagic shock. Circ Shock 3:107, 1976.
70. Birgens HS, Hendriksen J, Poulsen H: The shock liver: Clinical and biochemical findings in patients with centrilobular liver necrosis following cardiogenic shock. Acta Med Scand 204:417, 1978.
71. Solez K: Pathogenesis of acute renal failure. Int Rev Exp Pathol 24:277, 1983.
72. Loegerling DJ: Humoral factor depletion and reticuloendothelial depression during hemorrhagic shock. Am J Physiol 232:H283, 1977.
73. Jardin F, Farcot J, Borsiante L, et al: Influence of positive end-expiratory pressure on left ventricular performance. N Engl J Med 304:387, 1981.
74. Hansen DE, Borow KM, Newmann A, et al: Effects of acute lung injury and anaesthesia on left ventricular mechanics. Am J Physiol 251:1195, 1986.
75. Pinsky MR, Matuschak GM: Multiple systems organ failure: Failure of host defense homeostasis. Crit Care Clin 5:199, 1989.
76. Lefer AM: Pharmacologic and surgical modulation of myocardial depressant factor formation and action during shock. Prog Clin Biol Res 111:111, 1983.
77. Prewitt RM, Oppenheimer L, Sutherland JB, Wood LDH: Effect of positive end-expiratory pressure on left ventricular mechanics in patients with hypoxemic respiratory failure. Anesthesiology 55:409, 1981.
78. Malo J, Ali J, Wood, LDH: How does positive-end expiratory pressure reduce shunt in pulmonary edema? J Appl Physiol 57:1002, 1984.
79. Pare P, Warriner B, Baile EM, Hogg JC: Redistribution of pulmonary extravascular water with PEEP in canine pulmonary edema. Am Rev Respir Dis 127:590, 1983.
80. Morris, LR, Murphy MB, Kitabchi AE: Bicarbonate therapy in severe diabetic ketoacidosis. Ann Intern Med 105:836, 1986.
81. Afifi AA, Chang PC, Liu VY, et al: Prognostic indexes in acute myocardial infarction complicated by shock. Am J Cardiol 33:826, 1974.
82. Weil MH, Afifi AA: Experimental and clinical studies on lactate and pyruvate as indicators of the severity of acute circulatory failure (shock). Circulation 41:989, 1970.
83. Nishijima H, Weil MH, Shubin H, Cavanilles J: Hemodynamic and metabolic studies on shock associated with gram-negative bacteremia. Medicine 52:287, 1973.
84. Kreger BE, Craven DE, McCabe WR: Gram-negative bacteremia IV: Reevaluation of clinical features and treatment in 612 patients. Am J Med 68:344, 1980.

Chapter 115

VENTRICULAR DYSFUNCTION IN CRITICAL ILLNESS

KEITH R. WALLEY
L.D.H. WOOD

KEY POINTS

- *Understanding cardiovascular dysfunction in a critically ill patient requires consideration of both cardiac function and systemic vascular factors controlling venous return.*
- *Cardiac dysfunction may be due to left ventricular dysfunction, right ventricular dysfunction, or external compression (cardiac tamponade).*
- *Decreased ventricular pump function may be due to decreased contractility (dilated cardiomyopathy), increased diastolic stiffness (restrictive or hypertrophic cardiomyopathy), increased afterload, abnormal heart rate and rhythm, or valvular dysfunction.*
- *Management of ventricular dysfunction aims to reverse the cause by optimizing preload and afterload and correcting abnormalities in heart rhythm, valve function, and contractility.*
- *Acute reversible contributions to depressed contractility result from ischemia, hypoxemia, acidosis, ionized hypocalcemia and other electrolyte abnormalities, myocardial depressant factors, and hypo- and hyperthermia.*
- *Prevention and early diagnosis of the common complications of critical illness limit morbidity and mortality in patients whose primary cause for ventricular dysfunction is* not *ischemic heart disease; this approach also aids patients with ischemic heart disease.*
- *Management of acute on chronic heart failure progressively includes: oxygen; optimizing preload with diuretics, morphine, and nitrates or fluid infusion for hypovolemia; afterload reduction; increasing contractility with digoxin, catecholamines, or phosphodiesterase inhibitors; antiarrhythmic drugs; intraaortic balloon counterpulsation; and cardiac transplantation.*

Much has been written and implemented concerning the major cause of ventricular function-ischemic heart disease (see Chap. 116). This chapter reviews the etiology and management of circulatory disturbances arising in critically ill patients whose primary cause for ventricular dysfunction is more related to complications of other multisystem organ failures (MSOF), without diminishing the possibility that occult ischemic heart disease might be unmasked by the stress imposed by MSOF or its diverse treatments. We believe that these causes of ventricular dysfunction are quite common, detectable, and treatable in medical and surgical ICUs, and even influence the outcome of critical care in patients managed in coronary care units. Accordingly, we emphasize how critical illness disturbs both ventricular function and the systemic factors governing venous return, while leaving the detailed diagnosis and management of ischemic heart disease to Chap. 116. To avoid redundancy, we refer liberally to other chapters in this book which discuss mechanisms for ventricular dysfunction in the context of other diseases (see Chaps. 2, 114, 117, 120 through 123).

Assessment of Cardiovascular Dysfunction

The function of any pump can be defined by the relationship of the output of the pump to its input.[1] *Cardiac pump function* can be defined by the relationship of cardiac output to right atrial pressure (Pra). Cardiac output is the most important output of the whole heart and Pra is an easily measured input of the whole heart. Cardiac output is initially assessed as high, adequate, or inadequate by cardiovascular examination and by clinical evaluation of perfusion. Later, after placement of a pulmonary artery catheter or when other tests become available, cardiac output can be more accurately quantitated using the thermodilution technique, nuclear medicine imaging, or Doppler echocardiographic evaluation. Pra is initially evaluated by clinical examination of distention of the jugular veins and later may be more accurately measured as the central venous pressure (CVP). Other outputs, such as stroke work, and other inputs, such as pulmonary artery occlusion pressure (Ppw), serve to quantitate cardiac dysfunction and to determine the specific cause of cardiac dysfunction.

One specific cause of cardiac dysfunction is decreased left ventricular pump function which, after cardiac tamponade is excluded, can be defined as left ventricular end-diastolic pressure (EDP) (a left ventricular input) elevated in relationship to the cardiac output (a left ventricular output). Another specific cause of cardiac dysfunction is decreased right ventricular pump function. The right ventricle, compared to the left ventricle, is a more complex pump whose pump function depends heavily on afterload, interaction with left ventricular function, and right ventricular end-diastolic volume (EDV) (which, for the right ventricle more than the left, is not closely related to EDP). Thus, the best output and input to define right ventricular pump function is uncertain. However, if cardiac tamponade and decreased left ventricular pump function are excluded, right ventricular pump function is depressed if Pra (a right ventricular input) is elevated in relationship to cardiac output (a right ventricular output).

DEFINITION OF CARDIAC FUNCTION AND ITS RELATION TO VENOUS RETURN

The pump function curve of the whole heart is illustrated as the relationship between cardiac output and Pra over a range of values (Fig. 115-1*a*). Sometimes this relationship is

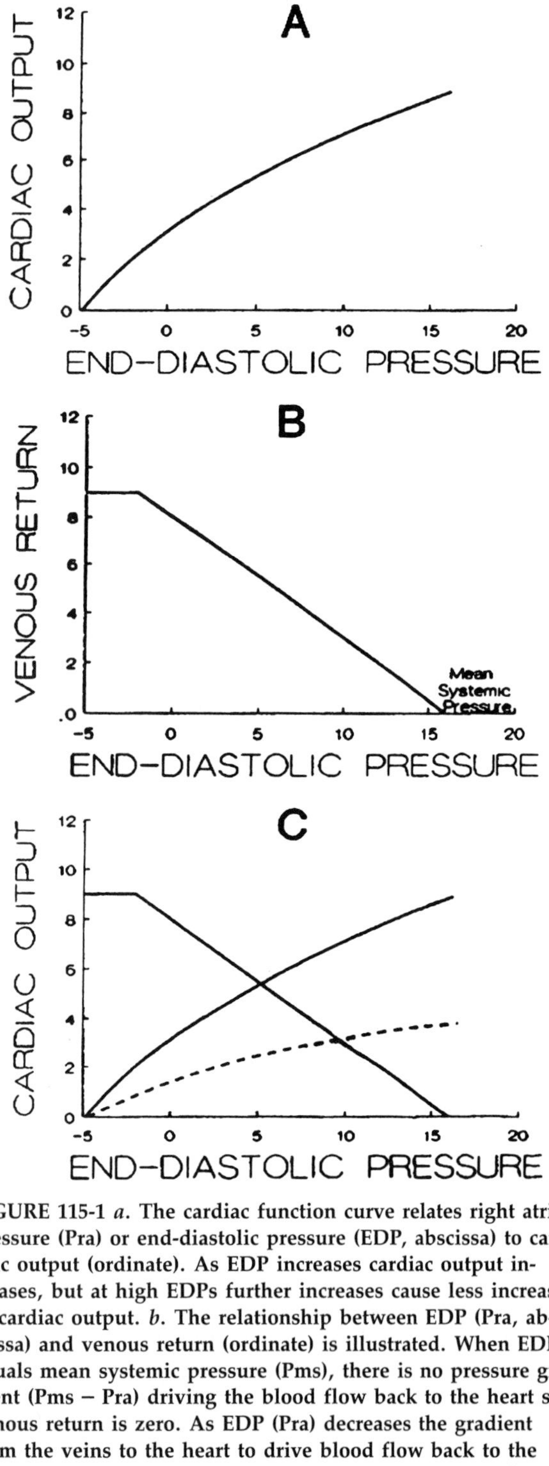

FIGURE 115-1 ***a*****. The cardiac function curve relates right atrial pressure (Pra) or end-diastolic pressure (EDP, abscissa) to cardiac output (ordinate). As EDP increases cardiac output increases, but at high EDPs further increases cause less increase in cardiac output.** ***b*****. The relationship between EDP (Pra, abscissa) and venous return (ordinate) is illustrated. When EDP equals mean systemic pressure (Pms), there is no pressure gradient (Pms − Pra) driving the blood flow back to the heart so venous return is zero. As EDP (Pra) decreases the gradient from the veins to the heart to drive blood flow back to the heart increases so that venous return increases. At very low EDPs (Pra < 0), central veins collapse and act as Starling resistors so that further decreases in EDP do not increase venous return.** ***c*****. The cardiac function curve and the venous return curve are drawn on the same axes (continuous lines). The intersection of the cardiac function curve and the venous return curve defines the operating point of the circulation, here at an EDP (Pra) of approximately 5 mmHg and a cardiac output of approximately 5 L/min. The interrupted cardiac function curve illustrates decreased cardiac function, causing reduced cardiac output (about 3 L/min) at a higher EDP (Pra = 10 mmHg).**

called a Starling function curve although this term has been applied historically to a pump function curve where stroke work is the output.[2] The relationship between cardiac output and Pra importantly illustrates that, as input increases, output increases, but as progressively higher values of input are approached, the slope of this curve decreases. Thus, increasing Pra is more effective in increasing cardiac output at low values of Pra than at high values.

Most physicians are aware that increased contractility improves cardiac and ventricular pump function by shifting the pump function curve upward and to the left so that at the same filling pressure an increased cardiac output is generated. It is equally important to realize that abnormalities in afterload, diastolic stiffness, valve function, and heart rate also can shift this relationship, and these factors are often more important than changes in systolic function in modulating ventricular dysfunction encountered in the noncoronary care ICU.

CONTROL OF VENOUS RETURN BY THE SYSTEMIC VESSELS

Cardiac function is tightly coupled to venous return and many patients with presumed cardiac dysfunction have instead abnormalities of the factors driving venous return. Pra and cardiac output define the cardiac function curve but also define the venous return relationship.[3] Figure 1*b* illustrates that as Pra is decreased venous return increases since the pressure driving venous return back to the heart, mean systemic pressure (Pms) minus Pra, increases (see discussion of Figs. 2-9 through 2-13 in Chap. 2 for details of definition and derivations of these concepts). The factors which determine venous return are Pms, Pra, and the resistance to venous return (RVR). In steady state, the cardiac function curve and the venous return curve are necessarily coupled because cardiac output must equal venous return. Thus, the operating point of the heart is not defined by the cardiac function curve nor by the venous return curve but by the intersection of these two curves (Fig. 1*c*). Accordingly, patients with cardiovascular dysfunction having abnormal values of heart rate, Pra, aortic pressure, and cardiac output may have cardiac dysfunction to account for these abnormalities or may have abnormalities of venous return. It follows that in every patient with suspected abnormal cardiovascular function one should consider both cardiac function and venous return in attempting to understand the abnormality.

In health, cardiac output is controlled by mechanical properties of the systemic vessels adjusted by neurohumoral reflexes; when output and blood pressure fall, baroreceptor reflexes act to increase flow by raising Pms via sympathetic nervous and humoral output (see discussion of Figs. 2-14 through 2-16 in Chap. 2). The importance of factors driving venous return is evident during exercise or even during the act of standing up. Without increased venous tone (as can occur with some spinal cord injuries) or increased muscle activity aided by venous valves, cardiac output and therefore blood pressure fall precipitously in changing from a recumbent to an upright position. As an

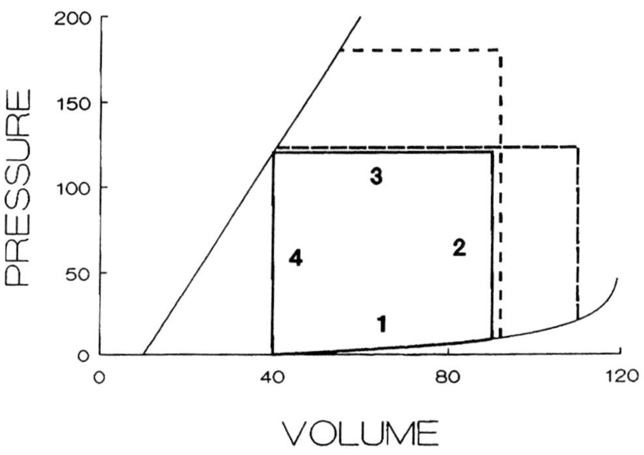

FIGURE 115-2 Left ventricular pressure-volume relationships are illustrated. The continuous thick lines represent a single cardiac cycle as a pressure-volume loop. During diastole the ventricle fills along a diastolic pressure-volume relationship (labelled 1). At the onset of systole left ventricular pressure rises with no change in volume (labelled 2). When left ventricular pressure exceeds aortic pressure, the aortic valve opens and the left ventricle ejects blood (labelled 3) to an end-systolic pressure-volume point. The ventricle then relaxes isovolumically (labelled 4).

At a higher pressure afterload the left ventricle is not able to eject as far (illustrated by the short interrupted lines). Conversely, at a lower afterload the left ventricle is able to eject further so that all end-systolic points lie along and define the end-systolic pressure volume relationship (ESPVR, or Emax). Increased diastolic filling (here illustrated by the long interrupted lines) results in increased stroke volume from the larger EDV to an ESV that lies on the same ESPVR; accordingly, increased afterload reduces stroke volume unless preload increases to compensate.

extension of normal physiology, in critically ill patients without a previous history of cardiac dysfunction the major factor limiting cardiac output is often altered venous return. Only in patients with marked ventricular dysfunction is cardiac output limited by decreased pump function. Knowing this avoids incorrect diagnosis and treatment. For example, positive inotropic drugs (dopamine, epinephrine, dobutamine) usually improve cardiac output even in patients with no ventricular dysfunction. Presumably, their main effect in these patients is to increase venous return by increasing Pms and by decreasing the RVR (by redistributing blood flow to vascular beds with short transit times) as has been demonstrated for epinephrine.[4] This improvement in cardiovascular function is often attributed to improved cardiac function because stroke volume and cardiac output are increased at the same or reduced Pra or left atrial pressure (Pla). Yet the corollary that the prior inadequate cardiovascular dysfunction was due to cardiac dysfunction is not necessarily true and may delay therapy aimed at factors governing venous return such as plasma volume expansion while the vasoactive drugs ineffectively flog the empty heart.

CONTROL OF VENTRICULAR PUMPING FUNCTION

The ventricular pump function curve can be altered by changes in contractility, preload, afterload, heart rate and rhythm, and valvular function (see discussion of Figs. 2-4 through 2-8 in Chap. 2). Consider the pressure-volume relationship of the left ventricle in Fig. 115-2. During diastole the left ventricle fills from end-systolic volume (ESV) to EDV at low pressures along the diastolic pressure-volume relationship. Diastole ends when systolic contraction starts so that left ventricular pressure rises with no change in volume while the aortic and mitral valves are closed. When left ventricular pressure exceeds aortic pressure the aortic valve opens and left ventricular ejects to the end-systolic pressure-volume point. The ventricle then relaxes to complete this cardiac cycle and pressure-volume loop. At increased pressure load during systole (see the short dashed line in Fig. 115-2), it is not surprising that the ventricle does not eject as far; conversely, the ventricle is able to eject further at decreased pressure afterload. All end-systolic pressure-volume points lie along a line, the end-systolic pressure-volume relationship (ESPVR). Ejections from different diastolic volumes still end on the ESPVR.[5] An increase in contractility results in increased ejection at any given afterload so that the ESPVR shifts to the left; conversely a shift to the right of the ESPVR indicates decreased contractility. Because of these characteristics, the ESPVR has been proposed as a good index of ventricular contractility independent of changes in preload and afterload; because this slope is maximal at end systole and has the units of elastance ($E = \Delta P/\Delta V$), it has been denoted Emax.[5]

This pressure-volume representation of ventricular function is related to the ventricular pump function curve in a straightforward manner (Fig. 115-3). To determine the ventricular pump function curve from the ventricular pressure-volume representation one determines the cardiac output for a given filling pressure. First, the EDV for a given filling pressure is determined by the diastolic pressure-volume relationship. Then, the ESV is determined at a given afterload and contractile state from the ESPVR. Stroke volume is simply the difference between EDV and ESV. Finally, cardiac output is heart rate times stroke volume. Therefore, if the diastolic pressure-volume relationship is constant, afterload is constant, and heart rate is constant, an increase in contractility decreases ESV and results in an increased stroke volume and cardiac output at the same filling pressure. Accordingly, an increase in ventricular contractility results in a leftward and upward shift of the ventricular pump function curve. An increase in contractility from a normal steep ESPVR does not decrease ESV much and therefore does not improve the ventricular pump function much. This explains why increased contractility is only a minor contributor to regulation of ventricular function in normal human beings. By contrast, when ventricular contractility is decreased as indicated by a decrease in slope of the ESPVR, an increase in contractility significantly decreases ESV to improve ventricular pump function, explaining why positive inotropic agents are useful in treating dilated cardiomyopathies.

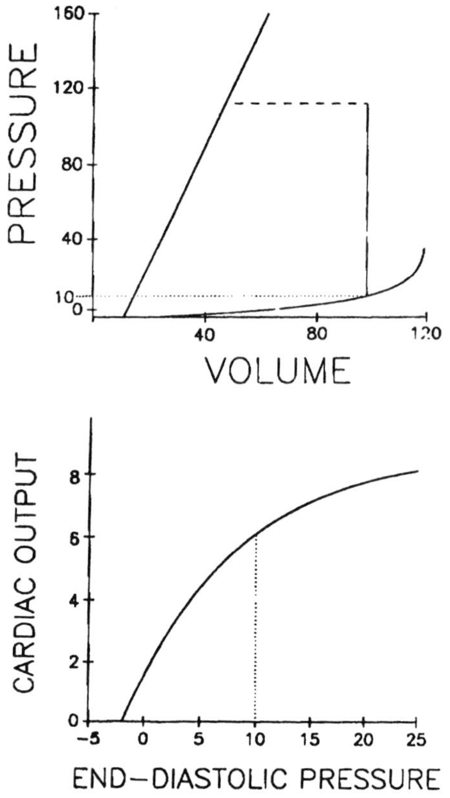

FIGURE 115-3 The cardiac function curve *(bottom panel)* is related to the left ventricular pressure-volume relationships *(top panel)*. In the top panel, stroke volume (horizontal interrupted line) is the difference between ESV and EDV. EDV at end-diastolic pressure (EDP = 10 mmHg) is illustrated on the diastolic pressure-volume relationship; ESV is determined by the end-systolic pressure (ESP) and the ESPVR (Emax). Therefore for any EDP cardiac output can be calculated if heart rate is known. An increase in EDP increases EDV and cardiac output in the bottom panel. At EDP = 10, an increase in contractility would result in an increased stroke volume since the ESPVR shifts to the left, therefore cardiac output increases at the same EDP and the cardiac function curve shifts up. An increase in diastolic stiffness would result in a decrease in EDV and in stroke volume at the same EDP, ESP, and Emax, so increased diastolic stiffness shifts the cardiac function curve down to the right.

When contractility, the diastolic pressure-volume relationship, and heart rate are all constant, a decrease in pressure afterload will result in a decrease in ESV so stroke volume and cardiac output increase.[6] Thus, decreased afterload also improves ventricular pump function by shifting the function curve up and to the left. Normal hearts with steep ESPVRs do not eject substantially further with a decrease in afterload because ESV does not decrease much. This explains the observation that decreasing afterload in normal patients does not substantially increase cardiac function and output but leads to hypotension. However, in patients with depressed contractility as signalled by a decreased slope of the ESPVR, a small decrease in afterload causes greater ejection to a smaller ESV so that stroke volume and cardiac output are substantially increased at the same ventricular filling pressure. Therefore, in patients with depressed systolic contractility afterload reduction is an effective means of improving ventricular pump function.[6]

Independent of contractile state, afterload, and heart rate, increased stiffness of the diastolic pressure-volume relationship reduces stroke volume because EDV is decreased at the same ventricular filling pressure. Therefore, an increase in stiffness of the diastolic left ventricle leads to a rightward and downward shift of the ventricular pump function curve.[7] This may be erroneously interpreted as decreased ventricular contractility when, in this case, depressed ventricular function is completely accounted for by increased ventricular diastolic stiffness (see discussion of Fig. 2-6 in Chap. 2). An increase in heart rate may also shift the ventricular pump function curve to the left and upward. However, when heart rate increases, stroke volume often decreases because there is less time for the ventricle to fill during diastole so that EDV decreases. Ultimately, when there is no other change in the factors driving venous return, heart rate increases cardiac output only slightly at heart rates <100 and at higher heart rates has essentially no effect on cardiac output.[8] At very high heart rates exceeding 150 min^{-1}, diastolic filling becomes markedly impaired and cardiac output decreases as heart rate increases further. When control of heart rate is abnormal due to abnormal pacemaker function or abnormal cardiac rhythm, inappropriately low heart rates do become important and can limit cardiac output. For example, if a patient is hypotensive and critically ill to the extent that heart rate is expected to be 100, yet he is able to generate a heart rate of only 50, then artificially increasing heart rate will substantially improve cardiac output.

In summary, a complete evaluation of the contribution of ventricular dysfunction to the cardiovascular performance in critical illness acknowledges that cardiac output and ventricular filling pressures depend as much on factors driving venous return as they do on cardiac function. In fact, most critically ill patients without a past history of cardiac disease have abnormalities of venous return in excess of abnormalities of cardiac function. Accordingly, cardiac output is limited by the heart only in patients with marked ventricular dysfunction, and the ventricular pump function curve is dependent not only on contractility but also on afterload, the diastolic ventricular pressure-volume relationship, and heart rate.

MEASUREMENT OF VENTRICULAR FUNCTION

Depressed cardiac function may be due to left ventricular dysfunction, right ventricular dysfunction, or external compression (cardiac tamponade). Here we focus on left ventricular and right ventricular dysfunction because cardiac tamponade is discussed in Chap. 121. Yet, in every case one should consider whether the pericardium and other structures surrounding the heart are affecting cardiac function (see discussion of Table 2-1 in Chap. 2). The specific causes of ventricular dysfunction, both right and left, are decreased contractility (a shift down and to the right of the ESPVR), increased diastolic stiffness (a shift up and to the left of the diastolic pressure-volume relationship), increased afterload, a change in heart rhythm and rate, and abnormal valvular function. How can one determine the presence of depressed ventricular pump function, then distinguish between right and left ventricular dysfunction, and finally identify the specific cause?

THE CLINICAL EXAMINATION. Left ventricular dysfunction is characterized by high left ventricular filling pressures in relation to cardiac output. Likewise, right ventricular dysfunction is characterized by high right ventricular filling pressures in relation to cardiac output. Importantly there is a close interaction between the left and right ventricles so that, most commonly, both left and right ventricular dysfunction coexist. Initially, clinical examination attempts to identify the presence and severity of depressed cardiac pump function and attempts to distinguish the contributions of right and left ventricular dysfunction. Evaluations of perfusion and mean blood pressure, pulse pressure, and heart rate give a clinical estimate of whether cardiac output is reduced or not (see Table 114-1). Right ventricular filling pressure may be judged by distention of jugular veins. Evidence of dependent pulmonary crackles on physical examination due to heart failure suggest that left ventricular filling pressures are elevated—usually above 20 to 25 mmHg. The range of Pla associated with pulmonary crackles may allow changes of left ventricular filling pressure to be followed by auscultation of the lungs in the acute setting, but in chronic congestive heart failure, where pulmonary lymphatic drainage increases, crackles may not be present even at filling pressures as high as 30 mmHg. An audible third heart sound (S_3) suggests an elevated Pla in the presence of a dilated left ventricle, but an S_3 may also be heard in restrictive myocardial disease and constrictive pericardial disease when left ventricular EDV is reduced.

RIGHT HEART CATHETER. In severe ventricular dysfunction or in critical illness where even mild ventricular dysfunction contributes significantly to severity of illness, more accurate measures of ventricular function are required than can be determined by clinical examination. Important tools in the ICU are pulmonary artery catheterization, radionuclide ventriculography, and echocardiographic evaluation (see Chaps. 21 and 25). Pulmonary artery catheterization, using a thermistor-tipped catheter with a distal port at the tip and a proximal port 30 cm from the tip, can accurately determine cardiac output using the thermodilution technique. Right ventricular filling pressure can be measured as CVP using the proximal port. Left ventricular filling pressure may be estimated as the Ppw (with important limitations discussed in Chap. 25). Therefore, the separate contributions of right ventricular and left ventricular dysfunction can be estimated by considering the right ventricular function curve (cardiac output versus Pra) and the left ventricular function curve (cardiac output versus Ppw). Right ventricular afterload can be measured as pulmonary artery pressure (Ppa) using the distal port of the pulmonary artery catheter and left ventricular afterload can be measured by measuring systemic arterial pressure. Additionally heart rate and rhythm are evaluated by electrocardiography (ECG).

INTEGRATING HEMODYNAMICS WITH IMAGING STUDIES. When depressed ventricular function is not due to increased afterload or abnormal heart rhythm, the distinction between decreased contractility and increased diastolic stiffness cannot be determined by right heart catheterization alone. Accordingly techniques that image ventricular diastolic and systolic volumes contribute substantially to the information obtained from pulmonary artery catheterization. The presence of enlarged V waves on the Pra trace or on the Ppw trace indicates tricuspid and mitral regurgitation, respectively. However, the size of the V waves depends on a number of factors including compliance of the atria and ventricles so that accurate assessment of valvular dysfunction using a pulmonary artery catheter alone is impossible. Thus, additional imaging techniques are also required to assess valvular function.

The most readily available imaging techniques are gated radionuclide ventriculography and echocardiography. Commonly, the ejection fraction and derived measurements are the only reported results of a gated radionuclide ventriculogram because ejection fraction is more accurately measured than absolute ventricular volumes. In stable patients with primary cardiac disease an ejection fraction <0.4 is generally an excellent indicator of decreased contractility; yet, ejection fraction is very sensitive to changes in preload and afterload so that in critically ill patients who may have very abnormal preloads and afterloads, which may change rapidly, ejection fraction is a much less useful indicator of contractility.[9] In this setting the ejection fraction must be interpreted in conjunction with hemodynamic measurements from a pulmonary artery catheter. Alternatively, gated radionuclide ventriculography can be used to estimate ventricular diastolic and systolic volumes by tracing out regions of increased radioactivity over the diastolic and systolic ventricles. Then one of a number of possible geometric formulas can be used to estimate diastolic or systolic ventricular volume.[10] These measurements may be inaccurate due to incorrect identification of regions which represent the ventricles or due to inaccuracies introduced by the geometric formulas.

Even with these limitations, two distinctions are evident: a small EDV when filling pressures are normal or high indicates that increased diastolic stiffness contributes to decreased ventricular pump function; and a large EDV when afterload is normal or low indicates that depressed contractility contributes to decreased ventricular pump function. Similar conclusions can be made by echocardiography, which also provides several additional evaluations of valvular function (see Chap. 122). Cross-sectional two-dimensional echocardiographic views during diastole and systole allow for calculation of ventricular circumferential fiber shortening. The percent ventricular circumferential fiber shortening is another commonly used index of ventricular function. Percent ventricular fiber shortening, like ejection fraction, suffers from its sensitivity to changes in preload and afterload.[11] Therefore, end-diastolic and end-systolic diameters should also be determined separately and interpreted in the light of measured pressures and flows. One extension of coupling echocardiographic measurements to pressure measurements is to plot rate-corrected velocity of left ventricular circumferential fiber shortening versus end-systolic wall stress.[12] This analysis derives from the ESPVR and therefore provides a relatively preload- and afterload-insensitive index of ventricular systolic contractility. This type of analysis may, therefore, become increasingly important to distinguish decreased systolic function from increased diastolic stiffness as the cause of decreased ventricular pump function.

Doppler echocardiographic examination allows measurement of the velocity of blood flow across valves and in vessels. Because blood flow across valves is turbulent, the pressure gradient across the valve is proportional to velocity squared. In fact, the pressure across the valve is nearly equal to four times velocity squared—a simple formula that contributes to assessment of valve dysfunction. Valvular insufficiency is also identified using Doppler echocardiographic examination and is facilitated by computer enhancement to produce a color Doppler image of blood velocities. The major limitation to conventional echocardiographic examination is that critically ill patients frequently are on positive-pressure mechanical ventilation and have lung disease so that lung shadows obscure echocardiographic views, making accurate examination difficult. Transesophageal echocardiographic examination circumvents this problem and is therefore an important new tool in evaluating ventricular pump function in critically ill patients (see Chap. 22).

Mechanisms and Management of Left Ventricular Dysfunction

Causes of decreased ventricular pump function include decreased contractility, increased diastolic stiffness (so that preload volume is diminished despite high filling pressures), increased afterload, abnormal heart rate and rhythm, and valvular dysfunction. This section addresses the diverse acute and chronic etiologies of left ventricular dysfunction and concludes with principles of management of each.

DECREASED LEFT VENTRICULAR SYSTOLIC FUNCTION

CHRONIC CAUSES. Dilated cardiomyopathies are the most well-known chronic causes of decreased left ventricular contractility.[14] Most frequently, dilated cardiomyopathy is associated with coronary artery disease, presumably due to previous ischemic events and infarctions leading to a dilated, poorly functional left ventricle.[14] This has been given many names including cardiomyopathy resulting from coronary artery disease and ischemic cardiomyopathy. Idiopathic cardiomyopathy is about one-fifth as common. Alcoholic cardiomyopathy is an important cause of chronic dilated ventricular dysfunction to be considered in critically ill patients.[14] Particularly in younger patients, inflammatory cardiomyopathy (myocarditis), usually viral, is an important cause of acute dilated cardiomyopathy that may lead to a chronic dilated cardiomyopathy in 10 percent of cases.[14] Rare causes such as the glycogen storage diseases also may be found in young patients. Multiple less common causes may be encountered (Table 115-1).

TABLE 115-1 Chronic Causes of Decreased Contractility (Dilated Cardiomyopathies)

Coronary artery disease
Idiopathic
Inflammatory (viral, toxoplasmosis, Chagas' disease)
Alcoholic
Postpartum
Uremic
Diabetic
Nutritional deficiency (selenium deficiency)
Metabolic disorder (Fabry's disease, Gaucher's disease)
Toxic (adriamycin, cobalt)

These multiple different etiologies of dilated cardiomyopathy lead to decreased ventricular contractility in a number of ways. Loss of myocardium with and without extensive replacement with fibrous connective tissue leads to decreased contractility.[15] Myocardial noradrenaline stores are depleted and β receptor density is reduced in chronic dilated cardiomyopathy.[16] Biochemical changes that may also contribute to decreased contractility include decreased efficiency of the sarcoplasmic reticulum calcium pump, decreased actinomyosin adenosine triphosphatase (ATPase) activity, and change of myosin isoenzyme composition.[15]

ACUTE CAUSES. In the ICU, acute causes of worsened left ventricular contractility may be more important than a consideration of the causes of chronic depression in left ventricular contractility because the acute causes are potentially

TABLE 115-2 Acute Reversible Contributors to Decreased Contractility

Ischemia
Hypoxia
Respiratory acidosis
Metabolic acidosis
Hypocalcemia
Hypophosphatemia
Possibly other electrolyte abnormalities (Mg^{++}, K^{+})
Exogenous substances (alcohol, β blockers, calcium channel blockers, antiarrhythmics)
Endogenous substances (endotoxin, histamine, tumor necrosis factor, interleukin-1, platelet activating factor)
Hypo- and hyperthermia

reversible (Table 115-2). Acute causes of depressed left ventricular contractility include ischemia, hypoxemia, respiratory acidosis, metabolic acidosis, ionized hypocalcemia, exogenous toxins such as alcohol and drugs, endogenous toxins such as circulating depressant factors of sepsis, and hypo- and hyperthermia.

Myocardial ischemia. Transient ischemic episodes occur frequently in critically ill patients. The onset of ischemia is due to myocardial oxygen demand exceeding the ability of the myocardium to extract oxygen from the oxygen supply (coronary blood flow times arterial oxygen content). Myocardial oxygen demand is increased by increasing heart rate, contractility, afterload, preload, and basal metabolic rate of the myocardium.[17] Many of the underlying illnesses encountered in the critically ill and many of the therapies, including fluid and inotropic or vasoactive drug infusion, contribute to markedly increased oxygen demand. Because of the prevalence of coronary artery disease in older patient populations, ischemia in the ICU is frequently regional with associated wall motion abnormalities. Accordingly, a high index of suspicion and an early aggressive diagnostic approach is indicated and facilitates the early treatment of ischemic coronary artery disease as discussed in more detail in Chap. 116.

Myocardial hypoxia. Critically ill patients may also manifest global left ventricular hypoxia. Hypoxemia and anemia may significantly reduce myocardial oxygen delivery, and myocardial oxygen extraction defects such as are encountered in sepsis[18] may lead to hypoxia of the whole heart or hypoxia of global regions such as the endocardium. When the heart becomes progressively hypoxic, metabolic and functional changes ensue;[19] the extraction ratio of the heart increases but not enough to prevent anaerobic metabolism after coronary blood flow is maximized, so that the heart consumes less oxygen and lactic acid and may become a lactic acid producer (Fig. 115-4*a*). Then, contractility is depressed so that the left ventricle becomes an acutely dilated, poorly functioning pump (Fig. 115-4*b*). If inadequate oxygen delivery in relation to demand is not quickly corrected, then the heart may enter a detrimental positive feedback loop of decreasing contractility, decreasing cardiac output and coronary perfusion, and thereby further decreasing contractility leading to precipitous cardiac arrest.[19] In this canine model this vicious cycle occurred when arterial O_2 saturation (Sa_{O_2}) fell below 75% (Pa_{O_2} = 40 mmHg) when hemoglobin concentration was 14 g/dL. Accordingly, aggressive measures to prevent this level of hypoxemia by keeping Sa_{O_2} >90% is indicated; maintaining a normal hematocrit in hypoxic critically ill patients with risks for myocardial ischemia is part of this therapy.

Myocardial acidosis. Respiratory acidosis and metabolic acidosis are additional derangements of arterial blood-gases and the internal environment, which may lead to depressed left ventricular contractility. Respiratory acidosis results in myocardial intracellular acidosis, and intracellular acidosis decreases the effect of intracellular calcium on the contractile proteins so that contractility is decreased.[20] Decreased contractility due to respiratory acidosis can be countered by infusion of β agonists, which increase the in-

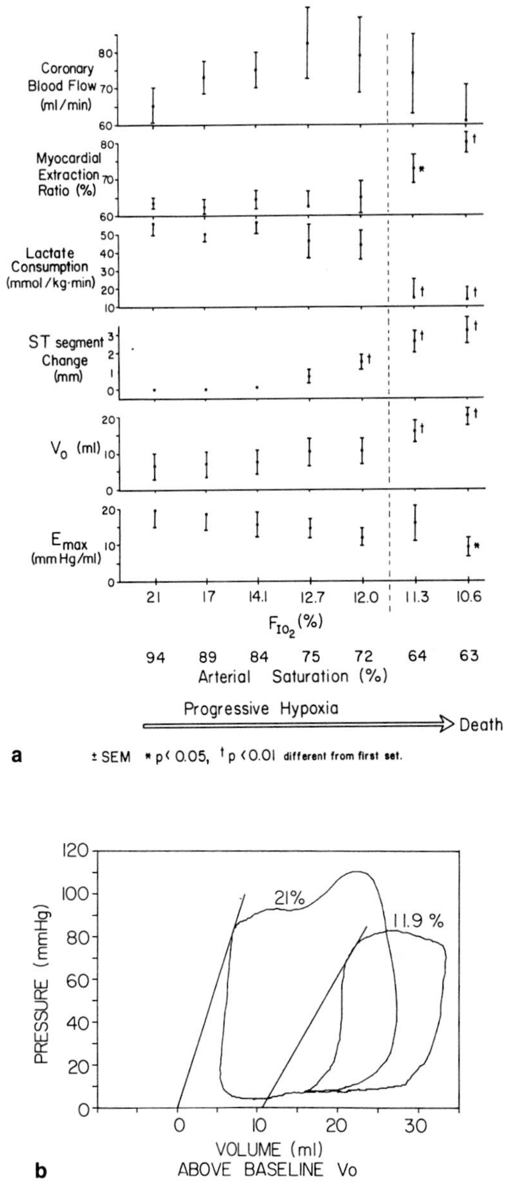

FIGURE 115-4 ***a.*** **Effects of hypoxemia on left ventricular metabolism and contractility. Seven stages of progressively decreasing inspired oxygen fraction (F_{IO_2}) and Sa_{O_2} are shown on the abscissa. Coronary blood flow initially increases to maintain the other displayed variables unchanged. When coronary blood flow can increase no further (and then falls because of decreased blood pressure), myocardial oxygen consumption is decreased, signalled by increased myocardial extraction ratio, reduced lactate consumption, and ST segment elevation; dilated cardiac dysfunction ensues (increased Vo and decreased Emax). All changes occur at approximately the same time, thereby defining two distinct phases, aerobic and anaerobic, as indicated by the dashed line.** ***b.*** **Pressure-volume loops from a typical experiment are illustrated with the ESPVR from vena caval occlusions superimposed. Data are presented from baseline (F_{IO_2}, 21%) and final hypoxic (F_{IO_2}, 11.9%) stages. In all dogs Vo increases with hypoxia. (Reproduced with permission from Reference 19.)**

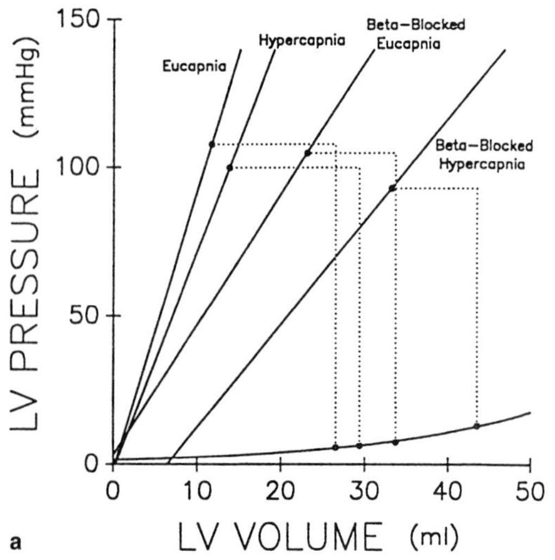

a

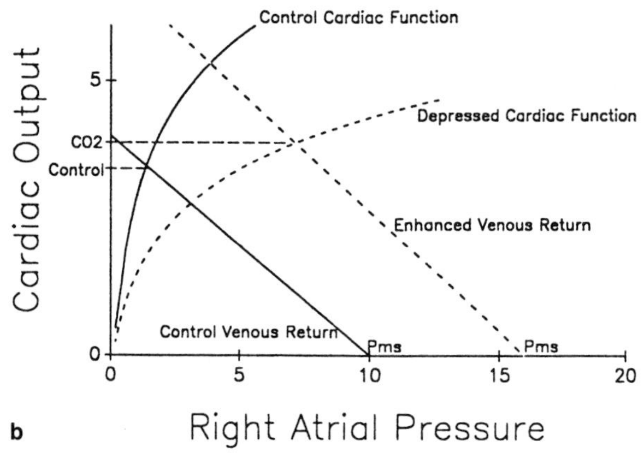

b

FIGURE 115-5 ***a.*** **Effects of respiratory acidosis on left ventricular contractility. Average ESPVRs for all experimental conditions are illustrated as continuous lines, as is the invariant diastolic pressure-volume relation. The interrupted lines connect closed circles, indicating the EDV and ESP for each condition. Before β blockade, respiratory acidosis decreases contractility (reduced Emax with no change in Vo), and ESV increases. Stroke volume is maintained by an equal rise in EDV along essentially the same diastolic pressure-volume relation. After β blockade, respiratory acidosis decreases stroke volume slightly, but both ESV and EDV are markedly increased.** ***b.*** **Schematic cardiac function and venous return curves before β blockade are illustrated for control (continuous lines) and respiratory acidosis (interrupted lines). Respiratory acidosis increases Pms from 10 to 15 mmHg, as occurs during epinephrine infusion, but decreases contractility so that hypercapnic venous return curves intersect the decreased cardiac function curve at a higher cardiac output and Pra than in control conditions. Respiratory acidosis also increases heart rate, which moves the decreased cardiac function curve toward the control position without increasing contractility much, so the increased Pra during respiratory acidosis is ameliorated. (Reproduced with permission from Reference 21).**

tracellular calcium concentration during systole and ameliorate the effect of intracellular acidosis.[21] Indeed, the normal marked sympathetic reflex response to respiratory acidosis ameliorates to some extent depressed contractility due to respiratory acidosis (Fig. 115-5*a*). The increased sympathetic response also increases Pms so that venous return may improve in the face of decreased contractility due to respiratory acidosis (Fig. 115-5*b*); then the stroke volume is maintained or increased by increased EDV and EDP. However, in the absence of a normal sympathetic reflex response, for example due to concurrent therapy with β blockers or due to down regulation of myocardial β receptors in critically ill patients, respiratory acidosis may significantly contribute to depressed contractility and reduced cardiac output despite high preload at P_{CO_2} levels of 60 and certainly by P_{CO_2} levels of 90.[21]

Metabolic acidosis may also decrease left ventricular contractility, but its effects are less marked than respiratory acidosis. Metabolic acidosis defined by measuring arterial blood-gas values reflects the extracellular compartment. The intracellular compartment is affected to the extent that the metabolic acid anion permeates the cell. Common organic acids such as lactic and keto acids have anions that do not easily cross into the intracellular compartment so that a severe metabolic acidosis measured by arterial blood-gas analysis may not be associated with significant intracellular acidosis and therefore may not depress ventricular contractility much. For example, lactic acidosis at a normal P_{CO_2} begins to depress contractility at pH 7.1 to 7.2 but even at a pH of 7.0 the depression in contractility remains quite small.[22]

Ionized hypocalcemia. During septic shock and in patients critically ill from diverse causes, serum ionized calcium levels are often low.[23] Further acute reductions may result in a substantial decrease in left ventricular contractility. Left ventricular myocardial contractility depends on the flux during systole of ionized calcium from the extracellular and sarcoplasmic reticular compartments into the myocardial intracellular compartment. Decreased extracellular ionized calcium concentration results in decreased flux and decreased contractility.[24] Following transfusion of red blood cells stored in standard citrated media, serum ionized calcium levels can fall dramatically because calcium is bound by citric acid. Lactic acid, like citric acid, also appears to bind ionized calcium. Thus, in patients with elevated lactic acid levels, due to shock or for other reasons, ionized calcium progressively decreases as lactate levels increase.[25] Bicarbonate infusion also can rapidly reduce ionized calcium levels and, as a result, may depress ventricular contractility.[26] In addition to ionized hypocalcemia other electrolyte abnormalities including hypophosphatemia, hypomagnesemia, and hypokalemia or hyperkalemia may contribute to decreased contractility, or more importantly, to arrhythmias.

Side effects of common drugs. Exogenous toxins may result in acutely depressed myocardial contractility. Ethanol is a commonly encountered substance that acutely depresses contractility, although in some patients ventricular pump function may be preserved by ethanol's vasodilating effects.[27] Drugs commonly used in the ICU that significantly depress contractility include β blockers, calcium channel blockers, and antiarrhythmics such as disopyramide and lidocaine.

Septic shock and other high output hypotension. In a number of shock states the presence of circulating myocardial depressant factors has been proposed. Serum from patients with septic shock has been shown to contain a factor which decreases contractility in isolated muscle strips.[28] This circulating myocardial depressant factor of sepsis is, to some extent, dialyzable. Depression in contractility has also been shown to be produced by endotoxin, tumor necrosis factor (TNF), interleukin-1 (IL-1), and platelet activating factor.[29] These mediators may be steps on the pathway to generating a single myocardial depressant factor or may themselves be mediators of myocardial depression. Despite the myocardial depression, intensivists should note that the hearts of septic patients in whom this mild reduction in contractility has been demonstrated are pumping 10 L min^{-1} cardiac output when their preload is normal; accordingly, the etiology of their hypoperfusion states likely resides in the septic paralysis of arteriolar (and in part venular) smooth muscle, with a minor contribution from decreased contractility.

Anaphylactic shock may also result in production of circulating myocardial depressant factor or factors. Histamine has multiple effects on contractility, preload, afterload, and heart rate. Accordingly some measurements, such as ejection fraction, may suggest enhanced contractility because afterload is reduced. However, preload- and afterload-insensitive indices demonstrate that histamine depresses left ventricular contractility in human beings,[30] although the primary cause of hypoperfusion is hypovolemia (see Chap. 89). Both hyperthermia and hypothermia may decrease myocardial contractility and contribute to depressed left ventricular function observed during sepsis and other critical illnesses associated with marked abnormalities of body temperature (see Chaps. 72 and 73).

MANAGEMENT OF REDUCED LEFT VENTRICULAR CONTRACTILITY IN CRITICAL ILLNESS. *Identify and correct acute reversible causes.* It is important to identify the multiple different potential causes for depressed contractility in critically ill patients because, while alone they may be insufficient to account for the left ventricular dysfunction, together they may significantly depress function. Importantly, these causes of acute reduction in ventricular contractility may be reversible. The primary treatment is reversal of the cause, if possible. Therefore, if ischemia or hypoxemia is present, aggressive attempts to correct these should be instituted. In the presence of coronary artery disease standard care including coronary vasodilation with nitrates or calcium channel blockers may be helpful. Thrombolytic therapy within 4 to 6 h of acute coronary thrombosis or emergency angioplasty decreases the incidence of congestive heart failure and improves outcome (see Chap. 116). Correction of hypoxemia and anemia may result in substantial improvement in ventricular function. Attention should be paid to decreasing factors that increase myocardial oxygen demand. Therefore, choosing the lowest level of inotropic and vasoactive drugs that produces the desired therapeutic effect will minimize their contribution to myocardial oxygen demand. Likewise, alleviating pain is important to diminish the associated tachycardia and increased sympathetic tone.

In ventilated patients with left ventricular dysfunction, the detrimental effects of respiratory acidosis should be considered and efforts made to increase alveolar ventilation either by decreasing dead space or by increasing minute ventilation; note that mixed venous and so tissue P_{CO_2} is much higher than Pa_{CO_2} when the cardiac output is low. Our approach is to administer greater alveolar ventilation to keep Pa_{CO_2} about 25 mmHg to avoid tissue acidosis, while ensuring that the mechanical effects of increased positive-pressure ventilation do not reduce venous return further. In general, metabolic acidosis should be treated by reversing its etiology. Compensatory respiratory alkalosis by hyperventilation may be a reasonable temporizing measure to treat metabolic acidosis, but this may be limited by the potential for significant cerebral vasospasm, which can occur below a P_{CO_2} of 20 to 25. Since CO_2 is readily diffusible through the cell membrane, partial respiratory correction of the extracellular metabolic acidosis may result in complete correction of the intracellular acidosis. Mounting evidence indicates that alkali therapy for metabolic acidosis is of no benefit and may be dangerous even at pH as low as 7.0 for a number of reasons.[26] Bicarbonate infusion results in an increase in P_{CO_2} due to chemical equilibrium of HCO_3^- with H_2O and CO_2, unless compensatory hyperventilation is also instituted. Particularly during rapid bolus injection, local P_{CO_2} may climb to extremely high values so that myocardial intracellular acidosis may transiently be severe. Just as with respiratory acidosis, high P_{CO_2} from bicarbonate infusion may result in marked depression of left ventricular myocardial contractility.[21] This accounts for the dangerous transient fall in blood pressure and cardiac output often observed when bicarbonate is infused as a bolus. Bicarbonate therapy is associated with an increase in lactic acid production because bicarbonate increases the rate-limiting step of glycolysis. As a result, lactic acid levels are even higher after bicarbonate infusion. Bicarbonate therapy also decreases ionized calcium levels.[25,26]

Decreased contractility due to ionized hypocalcemia can be corrected with an intravenous infusion of calcium. It has been recommended that after approximately 6 U transfusion that ionized hypocalcemia be corrected by infusion of approximately 1 g calcium chloride or calcium gluconate. Contractility will increase following calcium infusion for ionized hypocalcemia during lactic acidosis and following bicarbonate infusion. However, substantial problems arise when infusing calcium in patients with evidence of anaerobic metabolism or ischemia. In the presence of myocardial ischemia, for example, calcium is not adequately pumped out of the intracellular compartment so that systolic relaxation is slowed and active contraction due to the presence of calcium in the intracellular compartment may persist through diastole. The result is increased diastolic stiffness and the potential for formation of myocardial contraction bands (vide infra). The increased intracellular calcium concentration may also contribute to cell death. Therefore, infusion of calcium depends on the physician's assessment of need for increased contractility versus assessment of intracellular hypoxia. Hypophosphatemia, hypomagnesemia, hypokalemia, hyperkalemia, and other metabolic disturbances should also be corrected because they may lead directly or indirectly to altered cardiovascular function.

Treatment of myocardial depression due to circulating myocardial depressant factors has been attempted with antibodies to endotoxin and TNF, naloxone, and dialysis. Whether these therapies are effective is still uncertain. Antibodies to circulating factors appear to be beneficial in some cases[31] but are limited because often the circulating factor (endotoxin, TNF) is only present for brief periods of time early in the course of sepsis.[32] Naloxone administered over short periods is not consistently effective, but longer duration infusions of one or more days may result in improvement of hemodynamic measurements.[33] Dialysis or hemofiltration have not been adequately tested in human septic shock, but animal studies suggest that depressed left ventricular contractility due to a myocardial depressant factor of sepsis is reversed. If these new therapies are used, they should be carefully monitored in each patient for beneficial cardiovascular effect.

Managing the depressed heart. Having reversed the acute contributors to depressed left ventricular contractility, standard therapy of decreased left ventricular contractility includes optimizing of ventricular filling pressure, increasing contractility with inotropic agents, decreasing afterload, and where appropriate intraaortic balloon counterpulsation leading to surgical correction of coronary artery stenosis or other surgically correctable lesions.[34] The ventricular pump function curve illustrates the Frank Starling mechanism, which shows that increased ventricular filling results in increased ejection even when contractility is depressed. The limit to increased ventricular filling is generally set by the onset of pulmonary edema or further aggravation of depressed contractility by excess preload. This latter phenomenon is sometimes attributed to a downslope of the Starling curve, but is better explained by a new depressed curve related to the increased wall stress in the distended left ventricle.

Pulmonary edema fluid enters the lung interstitium according to the Starling equation (see discussion of Fig. 2-21 in Chap. 2). At normal protein osmotic pressures (largely due to albumin) and normal permeability of the pulmonary endothelium ($\sigma = 0.7$), pulmonary edema starts to develop at Ppw values above 20 to 25 mmHg.[35] Some patients in chronic low output congestive heart failure do not develop pulmonary edema until Ppw values exceed 30 mmHg possibly because of improved lymphatic drainage. With this in mind it is appropriate to increase cardiac output by intravascular fluid expansion, searching for the Ppw that produces the highest cardiac output without resulting in substantial pulmonary edema;[34] of course, this search often necessitates preload reduction using venodilating agents like nitroglycerin (Table 115-3). In the presence of decreased oncotic pressure due to decreased albumin or in the presence of leaky pulmonary endothelium, pulmonary edema may form at considerably lower Ppw values,[35] and in adult respiratory distress syndrome (ARDS) or pneumonia, pulmonary edema may form at very low Ppw values.

Inotropic or vasoactive agents are extremely useful in reversing depressed systolic contractility (see Chap. 125). Dobutamine acts mainly on β_1-receptors and results primarily in increased ventricular contractility and in mild peripheral vasodilation.[36] Doses from 2 to 15 $\mu g\ kg^{-1}\ min^{-1}$ are infused in a central venous line. Particularly in the presence of intravascular hypovolemia, dobutamine's vasodilating effect may exceed its effect on increasing cardiac output so that blood pressure may fall unacceptably. Dopamine is also a useful drug and when infused at 0.5 to 5 $\mu g\ kg^{-1}\ min^{-1}$ stimulates dopaminergic receptors resulting in redistribution of blood flow to the kidneys and

TABLE 115-3 Effect of Direct-Acting Vasodilators*

Drug	Route of Administration	Dosage	Onset of Effect	Duration of Effect	Large Arteries	Arterioles	Veins
Sodium nitroprusside (Nipride)	Intravenous	25–400 μg/min	Immediate	—	+	+++	+++
Nitroglycerin (Tridil)	Intravenous	10–200 μg/min	Immediate	—	++	+	+++
Isosorbide dinitrate (Isordil; Sorbitrate, Isobid; Isotrate; Sorate, Sorbide; Dilatrate)	Oral	20–60 mg	30 min	4–6 h	++	+	+++
Hydralazine (Apresoline)	Oral	50–100 mg	30 min	6–12 h	0	+++	±
Hydralazine (Apresoline)	IV or IM	5–40 mg	15 min	4–8 h	0	+++	±
Minoxidil (Loniten)	Oral	10–30 mg	30 min	8–12 h	0	+++	0
Diazoxide (Hyperstat)	Intravenous bolus	100–300 mg	Immediate	4–12 h	0	+++	±
Nifedipine (Procardia)	Oral	10–20 mg	20–30 min	2–4 h	++	+++	±
	Sublingual	10–20 mg	15 min	2–4 h	++	+++	±

*Reproduced with permission from: Cohn JN: Drugs used to control vascular resistance and capacitance, in *The Heart.* (JW Hurst et al, eds.) McGraw-Hill, 1990, p. 1675.

splanchnic bed. Dopamine is predominantly a β agonist in doses of 5 to 10 $\mu g\ kg^{-1}\ min^{-1}$, but at doses exceeding 10 $\mu g\ kg^{-1}\ min^{-1}$ dopamine is an α agonist and therefore increases arterial resistance.[37] Dopamine increases Pms so that venous return increases, resulting in increased left ventricular filling pressures.[38] The increased afterload at high doses and increased filling pressures associated with dopamine are often undesirable in treating decreased contractility. Therapy combining dopamine in the dopaminergic range with dobutamine is often helpful. Amrinone, milrinone, and enoximone are phosphodiesterase inhibitors that probably increase contractility by increasing intracellular calcium during systole (see Chap. 125). These agents may also result in afterload reduction and therefore may be particularly beneficial in treating depressed contractility. Amrinone is often given as a 0.75-mg/kg loading dose followed by an infusion of 5 to 10 $\mu g\ kg^{-1}\ min^{-1}$.[39] The use of digoxin to increase contractility remains controversial in the acute setting.[40]

In general, although positive inotropic agents improve contractility, they do so at the cost of increased myocardial oxygen demand and decreased efficiency of oxygen utilization and therefore may precipitate ischemia. Myocardial oxygen demand increases because of the associated increased heart rate, increased contractility (left shift of the ESPVR), increased preload, increased afterload, and increased basal metabolism. Dopamine has all of these effects. On the average, dobutamine has less of a chronotropic effect and does not increase preload compared to dopamine. Dobutamine also may produce mild arterial vasodilation and therefore afterload reduction. For these reasons, dobutamine at comparable doses may have less of an effect than dopamine on myocardial oxygen demand. Epinephrine increases heart rate but markedly increases myocardial oxygen demand by increasing contractility, preload, afterload, and the basal myocardial metabolic rate. Isoproterenol increases heart rate and myocardial oxygen demand even more than other inotropic agents. Digoxin increases myocardial oxygen demand and intracellular calcium, which may contribute to cell damage during ischemia.

Afterload reduction is an important therapeutic intervention in patients with depressed left ventricular systolic contractility due to a decrease in slope of the ESPVR. Because there is a decrease in slope of this relationship, small reductions in pressure afterload can result in improved ejection to smaller ESVs.[6] The reduction in ESV results in increased stroke volume and also results in substantially decreased end-systolic wall stress since, by the Laplace relationship, wall stress is proportional to the product of cavity pressure and radius. The decrease in wall stress reduces myocardial oxygen demand. Afterload reduction in some critically ill patients may result in unacceptable hypotension. For that reason it is best to start with an easily titratable medication with a very short half-life such as nitroprusside (see Chap. 125). Nitroprusside is infused at an increasing dose while the response of cardiac output and blood pressure is measured repeatedly so that an optimum dose resulting in maximum cardiac output with adequate perfusing pressures is chosen. Nitroprusside and other nitrates may mediate their effects in a way similar to endothelium-derived relaxing factor (EDRF), through the effects of nitric oxide to increase vascular smooth muscle relaxation. Nitroprusside at higher doses can result in significant toxicity with cyanide formation and methemoglobinemia. When circulatory stability is achieved, other longer acting agents are substituted; angiotensin-converting enzyme inhibitors are particularly useful,[42] as are alternative drugs (see Table 115-3).

Temporary support with intraaortic balloon counterpulsation is appropriate when damaged myocardium is expected to recover or as supportive therapy leading to surgical correction of an anatomic abnormality.[43] Balloon inflation during diastole improves diastolic perfusion of the coronary and systemic arterial beds. During systole, deflation of the balloon reduces afterload allowing for increased ejection by a ventricle with markedly decreased contractility. Intraaortic balloon counterpulsation has been found to be most beneficial when it is used as a supportive measure leading to surgery for correctable lesions (see Chap. 116).

INCREASED DIASTOLIC STIFFNESS

In normal hearts and in hearts with depressed ventricular function increasing preload is an important mechanism of increasing cardiac output. For hearts with normal systolic function left ventricular end-diastolic filling pressures are often in the range of 0 to 10 mmHg and result in an adequate cardiac output. For hearts with depressed contractility, higher filling pressures are usually required for an adequate cardiac output. Therefore, there is no uniformly optimum filling pressure. EDV has been proposed as a better definition of preload than EDP but volume is difficult to measure. In fact, consideration of the whole diastolic pressure-volume relationship is required to fully understand preload.[7]

Left ventricular function may be substantially impaired by increased diastolic stiffness of the left ventricle—a shift up and to the left of the diastolic pressure-volume relationship. This is a problem whose importance is equal at least to depressed contractility in the critically ill patient. Depressed systolic function reduces stroke volume because ESV increases; by contrast, increased diastolic stiffness reduces stroke volume because EDV decreases (see Fig. 2-6 in Chap. 2). Increased diastolic stiffness is a relatively frequent problem encountered in critically ill patients. It differs from depressed ventricular contractility because it is much more difficult to treat and does not respond to conventional therapy of decreased left ventricular pump function.[7] In fact, in the absence of an imaging study which demonstrates increased diastolic stiffness (small EDV in relation to the EDP), the diagnosis of increased diastolic stiffness is suggested by finding depressed ventricular pump function unresponsive to fluid loading, inotropic agents, and afterload reduction.

CHRONIC CAUSES. Chronic diseases which increase diastolic stiffness are often referred to as nondilated cardiomyopathies and hypertrophic cardiomyopathies (see Table 2-1 in Chap. 2). These include concentric left ventricular hypertrophy due to hypertensive cardiovascular disease, hypertrophic cardiomyopathy, and restrictive myocardial diseases. In addition, diseases of the pericardium including constriction and effusion, and other processes which increase intrathoracic pressure, result in increased diastolic stiffness, as discussed in Chap. 114 (see Table 114-4). Concentric hypertrophy due to chronic hypertension is very common and, although it seldom primarily accounts for severe depression in ventricular pump function, it may be an important contributor in combination with acute diseases depressing systolic function. Hypertrophic cardiomyopathy results in increased diastolic stiffness and may also result in greatly increased afterload due to dynamic aortic outflow obstruction. Over a period of days and months calcium channel blockers, particularly verapamil, may reduce evidence of increased diastolic stiffness and more rapidly, due to their negative inotropic effect, alleviate dynamic outflow obstruction in patients with hypertrophic cardiomyopathy.[44]

Restrictive cardiomyopathies include amyloidosis, hemochromatosis, sarcoidosis, endomyocardial fibrosis, some glycogen storage diseases, and restriction because of surgical correction of acquired and congenital abnormalities. Amyloidosis is uncommon at age 40 but by age 90 has a prevalence of 50 percent.[7] Clinical examination may reveal a Kussmaul's sign, rapid x and y descents in the jugular venous pressure so that a and v waves are prominent, and an S_3. Hepatojugular reflux may be prominent because the increased venous return produced by this maneuver cannot be accommodated by the stiff heart. Diastolic ventricular pressure measurements may show a "square root sign" which is a rapid early rise in diastolic pressure to a relatively constant plateau. Echocardiographic evaluation may demonstrate rapid early diastolic filling to a relatively fixed diastolic diameter similar to the "square root sign" and increased myocardial echogenicity may be observed in amyloidosis.[7,45]

ACUTE CAUSES. Just as with diseases resulting in depressed left ventricular systolic function, it is also important to consider the acute, potentially reversible causes of increased diastolic stiffness.[46] Regional or global ischemia results in delayed systolic relaxation contributing to increased diastolic stiffness. During ischemia, decreased adenosine triphosphate (ATP) stores limit the rate of calcium uptake by the sarcoplasmic reticulum so that the exponential decay of systolic pressure is delayed. When severe, incomplete systolic relaxation may extend to end diastole. This change in diastolic stiffness usually precedes depressed contractility because the sarcoplasmic reticulum calcium pump has a lower affinity for ATP than do the contractile proteins. In addition, ischemia may result in increased diastolic stiffness by increasing pericardial pressure as a result of increased CVPs.[47] Therefore, in the setting of increased diastolic stiffness, any ischemia should be aggressively treated.[48] Nitrates increase coronary blood flow and also decrease tone in the venous capacitance bed, thereby reducing pericardial pressure; nitroprusside also reduces diastolic stiffness.[49]

Increased intrathoracic or intrapericardial pressure is a common reversible cause of apparent increased diastolic stiffness in critical illness. Intrathoracic pressure is increased by positive-pressure mechanical ventilation and more so by the addition of positive-end expiratory pressure (PEEP). Positive airway pressures and PEEP are variably transmitted to the heart depending on the distensibility of the lungs and chest wall. If the lungs are very distensible and the chest wall is relatively rigid (as with a tense abdomen), then most of an increase in airway pressure will be transmitted to the heart so that to maintain the same chamber volumes the atrial and ventricular pressures have to increase as much; this accounts for part of the reduction in venous return and cardiac output if and when Pms does not increase by a similar amount.[50] A common misconception is that if the lungs are very stiff, as in the early exudative phase of ARDS, then less of an increase in airway pressures will be transmitted to the heart. Yet, because PEEP reduces shunt by reaerating flooded lung regions, the chest wall volume and pleural pressure increase as much or more in ARDS (see discussion of Fig. 1-9 in Chap. 1), so the increase in Pra with PEEP may be just as much as in patients with normal lungs. Increased intrathoracic pressure due to pneumothorax or massive pleural effusion may tamponade the heart and thereby result in apparent increased diastolic stiffness. Greatly increased intraabdominal pressure may elevate the diaphragm and similarly increase diastolic stiffness. Pericardial pressure may be increased by pericardial effusion and rarely by massive pneumopericardium. Because all of these causes of increased intrathoracic or intrapericardial pressure leading to apparent increased diastolic stiffness are treatable, they must be identified or excluded early in critically ill patients.

Hypovolemic shock and septic shock may result in increased diastolic stiffness.[51] The increased diastolic stiffness associated with both of these kinds of shock is associated with irreversibility of the shock state and increased mortality. Over the course of several hours hypovolemic shock results in substantial depression of left ventricular function despite slightly increased systolic contractility. All of the decrease in left ventricular pump function is accounted for by the stiff diastolic left ventricle so that higher filling pressures are required to produce smaller than normal EDVs. The increase in diastolic stiffness is reversible over the course of 7 to 10 days,[52] but when diastolic stiffness becomes severe, the shock state becomes irreversible. Excessive fluid infusion attempting to increase EDV simply results in greatly elevated left ventricular filling pressures resulting in pulmonary edema.

In septic shock, when depressed left ventricular systolic contractility occurs, the response of surviving patients is that of decreased diastolic stiffness or increased diastolic ventricular compliance.[53] This is the usual response to decreased left ventricular systolic contractility seen with other dilated cardiomyopathies.[54] However, in nonsurviving patients with septic shock the diastolic left ventricles do not dilate to increase EDV and thereby do not compensate for the increased ESV due to decreased systolic contractility. The diastolic ventricles of the nonsurvivors are therefore much stiffer than the ventricles of the survivors and in fact may be stiffer than normal ventricles.[55] Infusion of catecholamines and calcium may further contribute to increased diastolic stiffness by contraction band formation.[51]

Hypothermia with body temperature falling below 35°C (95°F) also results in increased left ventricular diastolic stiffness. This is a reversible phenomenon as temperature is increased. This is an important consideration during massive fluid resuscitation and mandates resuscitation with warmed infusions.

MANAGEMENT OF DIASTOLIC DYSFUNCTION. While acute diastolic stiffness due to ischemia, tamponade, and tension pneumothorax are readily treated, and therapy with calcium channel blockers may reduce diastolic stiffness over time in hypertrophic cardiomyopathy, acute therapy to reverse diastolic stiffness in the critical care setting is difficult.[7] Therefore, searching for optimum filling pressure that maximizes ventricular diastolic filling without resulting in substantial pulmonary edema is a critically important component of care in these patients. In addition, hypovolemia and sepsis should be treated aggressively and promptly, inotropic agents should be used at the lowest dose that results in the desired systolic or vascular effect, hypothermia prevented and treated, and tachycardia or atrioventricular (AV) arrhythmias should be treated early (vide infra).

SPECIAL EFFECTS OF ALTERED AFTERLOAD ON VENTRICULAR FUNCTION IN CRITICAL ILLNESS

An increase in afterload decreases left ventricular pump function because stroke volume is reduced as a result of increased ESV (see Fig. 115-2). In malignant hypertension elevated aortic pressure results in decreased cardiac output and elevated left ventricular filling pressures leading to pulmonary edema even if contractility is normal. Antihypertensive therapy results in rapid improvement (see Chap. 123). When contractility is depressed, increased afterload may worsen cardiac function even more. This is particularly important in dilated cardiomyopathies where increased afterload may be observed due to increased sympathetic tone, activation of the renin-angiotensin-aldosterone axis, and abnormally increased vascular smooth muscle tone.

Aortic valvular stenosis or dynamic obstruction of the aortic outflow tract may also increase afterload and contribute to decreased left ventricular pump function (see Chap. 122). Dynamic outflow tract obstruction is most commonly due to hypertrophic cardiomyopathy. However, patients with preexisting concentric hypertrophy due to chronic hypertension who have a decrease in intravascular volume may develop dynamic aortic outflow tract obstruction with the classical findings of systolic anterior motion of mitral valve leaflet, increased ejection velocities signifying increased gradients across the aortic outflow tract, and cavity obliteration at end systole. This appears to occur most commonly in elderly women. Volume infusion to reverse intravascular hypovolemia may prevent left ventricular cavity obliteration and outflow tract obstruction and thereby reduce ventricular afterload. It is important to identify outflow tract obstruction as the cause of increased afterload because this cause of increased afterload is worsened by conventional afterload reduction therapy.

End-systolic pressure is often regarded as the left ventricular afterload.[5] Because the ventricle ejects intermittent pulses of blood into the arterial circulation, it is occasionally important to consider impedance as the afterload to the left ventricle. Phasic pressures and flows varying with heart rate may result in reflected pressure waves altering the contour of the proximal aortic root wave form. In most states only a fraction of the energy output of the left ventricle is contained in the phasic pressure and flow component and the majority of the energy output is contained in the average flow (cardiac output) and mean blood pressure. Yet the effects of altered resistive impedance on the velocity and extent of ventricular shortening has not been completely explained, especially in some critical illness.[6,11,12,56] When afterload is dramatically reduced or when intravascular volumes are expanded, the resulting high cardiac output state is sometimes called high output cardiac failure. Actually cardiac function still lies on a normal cardiac function curve but the greatly increased venous return associated with low afterload results in high right- and left-sided filling pressures with the appearance of right- and left-sided congestion. This is particularly apparent in the presence of AV valvular stenosis which may previously have been occult. Causes of high output failure include anemia, arteriovenous fistulas, hepatic failure, Paget's disease, thyrotoxicosis, pregnancy, carcinoid syndrome, and renal cell carcinoma.

ABNORMAL HEART RATE AND RHYTHM

Normally heart rate and contractile states are matched to venous return and afterload to maximize the efficiency of the cardiovascular system. Even though heart rate is often of lesser importance in trying to increase cardiac output, excessively high or excessively low heart rates may limit cardiac output. Bradycardia is an important abnormal rhythm in a critically ill patient. First it is important to determine if hypoxemia, drugs like acetylcholinesterase inhibitors, or other reversible insults are the cause of bradycardia. In these cases treatment consists of rapid reversal of the cause. In other cases where bradycardia is due to primary cardiac disease including myocardial infarction with involvement of the conducting system, therapy is directed at increasing heart rate by other means. Acutely, bradycardia may be treated with atropine and, if necessary, by isoproterenol infusion titrated to heart rate response. These temporizing measures allow placement of temporary or permanent pacemakers. In addition to the well known indications for temporary pacing following myocardial infarction, it should be recognized that symptomatic bradycardia from any cause is an indication for pacing.

Tachycardia at sufficiently high rates results in an inadequate diastolic filling time so that stroke volume is reduced because adequate diastolic filling does not occur and the contribution to ventricular diastolic filling by the atria is less efficient, particularly in atrial fibrillation. An end-diastolic gradient across the mitral valve develops at high heart rates. Hypoxemia and acidosis encountered in critically ill patients are frequently associated with ventricular and, even more commonly, supraventricular tachyarrhythmias. Hyperkalemia and hypokalemia, hypocalcemia, and hypomagnesemia are common electrolyte disturbances associated with increased incidence of ventricular arrhythmias. Accordingly, management of atrial and ventricular tachyarrhythmias involves correcting these potential contributing abnormalities.

Arrhythmias including atrial fibrillation, atrial flutter, ventricular tachycardia, and ventricular fibrillation should be immediately cardioverted if they are contributing to a shock state. Otherwise rapid heart rate due to atrial fibrillation is slowed with digoxin loading followed by maintenance dose. It has recently been proposed that therapy with verapamil is more effective and that some of the potential detrimental consequences of verapamil, including depressing systolic contractility, may be at least partially ameliorated by infusion of calcium.[57] Paroxysmal supraventricular tachycardia usually reverts following maneuvers to increase vagal tone or following verapamil infusion. Multifocal atrial tachycardia responds to correction of underlying pulmonary disease and also to verapamil.[58] Ventricular premature contractions that contribute to altered hemodynamic function or other ventricular tachyarrhythmias must be treated. Specific management of ventricular arrhythmias is detailed in Chap. 120.

VALVULAR DYSFUNCTION

The valves regulate preload and afterload and are therefore important determinants of left ventricular pump function (see Chap. 122). In critically ill patients the effect of preexisting valvular disease may change with altered hemodynamics or the extent of valvular disease may change primarily. For example, aortic and mitral insufficiency contribute to low cardiac output at high ventricular filling pressures in critical illness, and both respond quickly to afterload reduction; and mitral regurgitation may worsen acutely due to increased EDV and expansion of the mitral annulus. On the other hand, mitral valve prolapse may worsen at low ventricular volumes due to hypovolemia. In high cardiac output states previously insignificant mitral stenosis may result in a high Pla and pulmonary edema. The gradient across the stenotic aortic valve may increase in high flow states and conversely decrease in low flow states so that without considering the flow across the valve an incorrect judgment of the functional significance of the valvular disease may be made. Dysfunction of prosthetic valves is important to identify and may be a surgical emergency.

Mechanisms and Management of Right Ventricular Dysfunction

Right ventricular pump function also depends on contractility, afterload, preload (the diastolic pressure-volume relationship), heart rhythm, and valve function. However, the right ventricle differs from the left ventricle such that the relative importance of each of these components is different. The left ventricle is well designed to generate high pressures. Its thick walls and small chamber volume result in manageable levels of wall stress despite high intracavitary pressures. The helical arrangement of muscle fibers changing from endocardium to epicardium in concentric layers results in a strong wall with an efficient distribution of wall stress.[59] The right ventricle, on the other hand, is a thin-walled pump whose surface has a large radius of curvature so that it is not suited as a high pressure generator. Instead the right ventricle functions as an excellent flow generator at low pressures. Right ventricular contraction moves sequentially from the apex to the pulmonary outflow tract giving it features of a peristaltic volume pump.[60] During diastole the right ventricle at normal diastolic pressure lies below its stressed volume, a feature which allows it to accommodate a large filling volume without an elevation in EDP. Because of these features, volume preload and, most importantly, pressure afterload become even more important determinants of right ventricular function than they are in the left ventricle.

DECREASED RIGHT VENTRICULAR SYSTOLIC FUNCTION

Contractility of the right ventricle is decreased approximately to the same extent as in the left ventricle by the many causes listed for the left ventricle (see Tables 115-1 and 115-2). Occasionally right ventricular contractility is disproportionately reduced as in right ventricular infarction, right ventricular dysplasia, Uhl's anomaly, isolated right ventricular myopathy, and myopathy associated with uncorrected atrial septal defect. Right ventricle ischemia in the absence of coronary artery disease is very important during critical illness. When afterload is elevated, the right ventricle responds along a preload-dependent right ventricular systolic pressure-volume relationship so that right ventricular ESV increases.[61,62] Right ventricular chamber pressures are increased, and the radius of curvature is increased so that the wall stress in the thin right ventricular wall increases dramatically. Therefore, right ventricular myocardial oxygen demand increases proportionately. Supply of oxygen is set by right ventricular coronary blood flow and the oxygen content of the blood. Right ventricular coronary blood flow depends on the gradient between mean aortic pressure and pressures in the right ventricular wall. At increased right ventricular pressures the right ventricular intramural pressure rises so that the gradient for right ventricular coronary blood flow decreases. Oxygen supplied to the right ventricular myocardium may not meet oxygen demand so that contractility decreases, further worsening right ventricular function.[63]

DISORDERS OF RIGHT VENTRICULAR PRELOAD, AFTERLOAD, RHYTHM, AND VALVES

Increasing right ventricular EDV results in an increase in right ventricular stroke volume even though right ventricular EDP may not increase much because normally EDV is below right ventricular diastolic stressed volume. Because of this and because Pra is heavily influenced by intraabdominal, intrathoracic, and intrapericardial pressures, Pra is probably a poor indicator of right ventricular preload.

The afterload of the right ventricle is the Ppa (Table 115-4). This may be chronically elevated by emphysematous destruction of small pulmonary vessels, chronic hypoxic pulmonary vasoconstriction due to obstructive pulmonary disease and restrictive chest wall diseases, recurrent pulmonary embolism, chronically elevated Pla due to mitral stenosis or left ventricular congestive failure, primary pulmonary hypertension, and a number of connective tissue and inflammatory diseases which involve the pulmonary vasculature.[64] Acute causes of pulmonary hypertension are also important to identify as they are more often reversible. In addition, while the right ventricle may hypertrophy and accommodate severe chronically increased afterload, moderate acute pulmonary hypertension may rapidly lead to right ventricular decompensation. Important causes of acute pulmonary hypertension in critically ill patients include pulmonary embolism, hypoxic pulmonary vasoconstriction, acidemic pulmonary vasoconstriction, pulmonary infection, ARDS, sepsis, and acutely elevated Pla (see Chap. 117).

As with the left ventricle, the right ventricle depends on normal rate and rhythm to attain optimum function. Right ventricular valvular disease is less common and less important than left ventricular valvular disease. This is because right ventricular pressures are much less than left ventricular pressures so that gradients across the valves are considerably less. In critically ill patients, tricuspid valve disease with endocarditis is common either as a preexisting condition such as endocarditis or as a result of instrumentation with a pulmonary artery catheter or other right heart catheters.

TABLE 115-4 Causes of Elevated Right Ventricular Afterload

Chronic
Chronic hypoventilation
Recurrent pulmonary emboli
Primary pulmonary hypertension
Associated with connective tissue diseases
Chronically elevated left atrial pressure (mitral stenosis, left ventricular failure)
Acute
Pulmonary embolus
Hypoxic pulmonary vasoconstriction
Acidemic pulmonary vasoconstriction
ARDS
Sepsis
Acute elevation in left atrial pressure
Positive-pressure mechanical ventilation

VENTRICULAR INTERACTION

DIAGNOSIS OF VENTRICULAR INTERDEPENDENCE. Combined pump dysfunction of right and left ventricles is more common than isolated right or left ventricular pump dysfunction. Part of the explanation is that the diseases resulting in decreased pump function more commonly involve both ventricles. However, the right and left ventricles interact in important ways which, when recognized, may lead to a more effective therapeutic approach. The right and left ventricles are contained inside the same pericardial cavity within the chest wall and the right and left ventricles share the intraventricular septum.[65] Accordingly, much of the interaction between the right and left ventricles is mediated via the parallel coupling produced by the pericardium and septal shift. The right ventricle is also connected in series with the left ventricle so that a substantial rise in Pla is transmitted back through the pulmonary vasculature and results in a rise in right ventricular afterload. Additionally, the left ventricle is the pump which perfuses the right and left coronary circulations so that decreased systemic pressure combined with elevated right ventricular pressures may result in hypoperfusion of the right ventricle.

Detrimental ventricular interaction is generally only a problem when right heart and pulmonary circulation pressures are high. A common cause of elevated right heart pressures is elevated Ppa due to increased pulmonary vascular resistance (PVR). Table 115-4 lists a number of important and common causes in critically ill patients. Pulmonary embolus is often missed and difficult to diagnose with radionuclide perfusion scans in patients with coexistent lung disease. Right ventricular pressure and Pra rise. Elevated right ventricular pressure shifts the intraventricular septum from right to left during diastole resulting in increased left ventricular diastolic stiffness (see discussion of Fig. 2-5 in Chap. 2). During systole, left ventricular pressure usually is sufficiently > right ventricular pressure so that the septum shifts back. This systolic shape change means that the myocardium of the left ventricular freewall must shorten even more for less of an ejected stroke volume. The rise in Pra is transmitted through the compliant right atrium to the pericardial space. The rise in pericardial pressure tamponades all other cardiac chambers. When pericardial effusion is present these effects are magnified. When Pla is high due to mitral stenosis or decreased left ventricular pump function, Ppa values rise. Chronically this may additionally result in increased PVR. The resultant right ventricular failure with right-to-left septal shift impairs left ventricular filling, which may be a critical insult in these diseases.

TREATMENT OF VENTRICULAR INTERDEPENDENCE. Management aims to reduce Ppa values and to reduce parallel coupling of the left and right ventricles. Reversible contributions to pulmonary hypertension are treated as outlined in the discussion of right ventricular afterload. Parallel coupling by elevated pericardial pressure is reduced by relieving pericardial tamponade if present; reducing intrathoracic pressures by decompressing thoracic and abdominal fluid and air collections and by airways management to reduce Ppa; and in select patients, by surgically opening or removing the pericardium and by leaving a sternal incision open and only closing the overlying skin.

Unresuscitatable cardiac arrest is a common outcome when perfusion of the right ventricle is threatened because right ventricular pressures are high relative to left ventricular pressures. This happens in massive pulmonary embolism and in cases of severe pulmonary hypertension. Thrombolytic therapy and pulmonary vasodilator therapy attempt to reverse the cause. Animal models of massive pulmonary embolism suggest that successful acute cardiovascular management attempts to raise systemic pressures more than right-sided pressures.[63] Therefore noradrenaline or adrenaline, which have substantial α agonist effect, improve right ventricular perfusion and are more successful in immediate resuscitation than isoproterenol or dobutamine.

Acute on Chronic Heart Failure

Heart failure carries a poor prognosis with a survival rate of only 50 percent after 5 years.[66] Mortality is highest during the first 2 years and increases with worsened functional status so that patients with New York Heart Association class III or IV heart failure have a survival rate of approximately 50 percent after 1 year and 30 percent after 2 years. Mortality is often related to episodes of acute decompensation which punctuate the course of heart failure. Important precipitating causes of acute decompensation are listed in Table 115-5. A review of these reveals why chronic heart failure is often exacerbated in the course of critical illness, so early detection and management of acute on chronic heart failure is an essential component of critical care.

TABLE 115-5 Common Precipitating Factors of Acute on Chronic Heart Failure

Poor compliance with medications
Dietary indiscretion (salt load, alcohol)
Infection
Fever
High environmental temperature
Effect of a new medication (β blocker, calcium channel blocker, antiarrythmic, nonsteroidal anti-inflammatory)
Arrhythmia (typically, new atrial fibrillation)
Ischemia or infarction
Valve dysfunction (endocarditis, papillary muscle dysfunction)
Pulmonary embolism
Surgical abdominal event (cholecystitis, pancreatitis, bowel infarct)
Worsening of another disease (diabetes, hepatitis, hyperthyroidism, hypothyroidism)

PRECIPITATING FACTORS

Poor compliance with medications and new medications are common precipitating events. Dietary indiscretion with increased sodium load or alcohol ingestion leading to a further acute depression in systolic contractility are frequently seen. Intercurrent illness such as a urinary tract infection or viral syndrome, fever, or high ambient temperatures may make greater demands on cardiac output than can be met. Onset may be slow and patients complain of decreased exercise tolerance, dyspnea, paroxysmal nocturnal dyspnea, and swelling of ankles and abdomen worsening over days and weeks. Rapid onset suggests that ischemia or arrythmia may be the cause. Cardiac output may be depressed so that the kidneys are hypoperfused. The response of the kidneys is to avidly retain sodium and water, which may further worsen volume overload. Volume overload leads to elevated venous pressures with subsequent pulmonary edema due to elevated Pla and peripheral edema due to elevated systemic venous pressures. There is an excessive reflex release of catecholamines leading to tachycardia and increased arterial tone so that arterial resistance rises. Increased arterial resistance as afterload may be detrimental to left ventricular pump function. Activation of the renin-angiotensin axis accounts for avid renal absorption of sodium. Vasopressin release increases water retention. Coronary artery disease is common in this population so that decompensation may have followed an acute ischemic coronary event or coronary ischemia may be precipitated by worsened congestive heart failure.

CLINICAL FEATURES

Patients are often anxious, tachycardic, and tachypneic with evidence of hypoperfused extremities and possibly cyanosis. Jugular veins are distended and hepatojugular reflux may be demonstrable on physical examination. Typically the sternal angle is approximately 5 cm above the right atrium when the patient's torso is at a 30° to 45° angle. Right ventricular filling pressure is no higher than 6 to 8 cmH_2O so that jugular venous distention is usually no higher than 1 to 3 cm above the sternal angle in normal patients. An apical impulse lateral to the midclavicular line or >10 cm from the midsternal line is sensitive but not specific in indicating left ventricular enlargement while an apical diameter >3 cm indicates left ventricular enlargement.[67] A sustained apical impulse suggests left ventricular hypertrophy or aneurysm. An S_3 or summation gallop is often present but may be obscured by increased respiratory sounds. Pulse pressure is often reduced so that peripheral pulses are "thready." Crackles are heard in dependent lung fields but, in severe cardiac failure, are heard in all zones. Wheezes and a prolonged expiratory phase may be noted, suggesting edema surrounding the airways. Hepatomegaly, which may be pulsatile particularly with tricuspid valve insufficiency, may be present and there is evidence of dependent edema in the lower extremities and over the sacrum.

Chest x-ray findings suggesting elevated left ventricular filling pressures include upper zone redistribution of vascular markings, septal lines (Kerley B lines), loss of pulmonary vascular definition, perivascular and peribronchial cuffing, perihilar interstitial and then alveolar filling patterns, and pleural effusions. The cardiopericardial silhouette may be enlarged suggesting enlarged cardiac chambers and the azygos vein may be enlarged suggesting elevated Pra.

MANAGEMENT

Therapy of acute on chronic heart failure initially aims to treat intravascular overload and improve gas exchange. Therefore, the patient is positioned with the torso elevated at least 45° and oxygen is administered (indications for intubation are considered in Chap. 114). Good intravenous access, optimally central venous, is established. Furosemide (20 to 40 mg initially followed by increasing doses as required) induces a rapid diuresis. Even before diuresis is established furosemide reduces Pla by a venodilating effect[68] and also reduces intrapulmonary shunt.[69] Titrated morphine doses decrease venous tone and thereby decrease left ventricular filling pressures and improve pulmonary edema. In addition, morphine may make the patient less anxious, thereby decreasing whole body oxygen demand. Nitrates are venodilators that serve to decrease left ventricular filling pressure and mild arterial vasodilators resulting in decreased afterload. Nitrates have the additional benefit of being coronary vasodilators. In cases of severe volume overload and pulmonary edema when fluid cannot be removed from the intravascular compartment quickly enough, rotating tourniquets on the extremities or phlebotomy of 100 to 150 mL blood may result in substantial improvement. Further afterload reduction in critically ill patients starts with an easily titratable vasodilator such as nitroprusside, or in the setting of ischemia, intravenous nitroglycerin. Following stabilization, afterload-reducing agents including angiotensin enzyme inhibitors may be additionally beneficial. Depressed contractility can be treated by stopping medications that tend to depress contractility and by reversing concurrent conditions which depress myocardial contractility. Additionally positive inotropic agents may be used, including dobutamine, dopamine, and phosphodiesterase inhibitors. Dobutamine and phosphodiesterase inhibitors also act as peripheral vasodilators and therefore beneficially also reduce afterload. If acute decompensation leads to cardiogenic shock and recovery is anticipated following medical or surgical intervention, then intraaortic balloon counterpulsation should be instituted.

CASE PRESENTATION

A 39-year-old homosexual male with acquired immunodeficiency syndrome (AIDS) presented with a week history of progressive dyspnea. AIDS had been diagnosed 2 years prior to admission based on *Pneumocystis carinii* pneumonia (PCP) and human immunodeficiency (HIV)-positive serology. Except for one recurrence of PCP he had been relatively well in the past 2 years. One week prior to admission he was seen by his family physician who prescribed erythromycin for his dyspnea. One day prior to admission he was seen again because of worsened symptoms and this time his physician noted an S_3 on cardiac examination and bilateral pleural effusions on chest x-ray. On the day of admission he presented to the emergency room with severe dyspnea.

Initial examination showed him to be in acute respiratory distress. His heart rate was 150, blood pressure 80/60, respiratory rate 40, and he was afebrile. He was alert and oriented, cyanosed, and he was using all accessory muscles of ventilation although there was no paradoxical diaphragmatic movement. Crackles were heard to half way up his chest posteriorly. His jugular veins were distended to the angle of his jaw sitting upright and a gallop rhythm was auscultated. His peripheral pulses were thready and his extremities were cool. He had an enlarged, tender, pulsatile liver.

Initial laboratory data included arterial blood-gases with pH 7.25, P_{CO_2} 15, and P_{O_2} 85 on high flow 100% O_2 facemask. Serum bicarbonate level was 6 mM/L, his anion gap was calculated as 21, and plasma lactate content was 16.8 mM/L. Hemoglobin was 8.8 g/dL, creatine kinase (CK) and CK-MB were not elevated, and an ECG showed low voltages, Q waves anteriorly suggesting a previous anterior myocardial infarction, and nonspecific ST-T wave changes. Chest x-ray showed an enlarged pericardial silhouette, increased interstitial markings, and bilateral pleural effusions.

During the first hour he was intubated and ventilated with 100% oxygen and a tidal volume of 700 mL at 30 min^{-1}; then pH was 7.28, P_{CO_2} was 12, and P_{O_2} was 64 mmHg (O_2 saturation = 85%). Central venous access was immediately established, and dopamine was infused at 10 μg/kg/min resulting in improved blood pressure to 90/65. An echocardiogram showed marked dilation of all four cardiac chambers, global hypokinesis of the left ventricle, and a very small pericardial effusion. A pulmonary artery catheter was inserted, which showed a Pra of 26, Ppa of 50/32, Ppw of 32, a cardiac index of 1.4 L min^{-1} m^2, with a mixed venous oxygen saturation of 35%.

Furosemide (40 mg IV), nitroglycerin (20 μg/min IV), and morphine were administered. When PEEP of 10 cmH_2O was added, O_2 saturation increased to 90%, but blood pressure and cardiac index decreased associated with a fall in Ppw to 24. An infusion of 500 mL saline and reduction of the PEEP to 5 cmH_2O returned blood pressure and cardiac index to their pretreatment values without changing the measured Ppw. PEEP was then increased progressively from 5 to 10 to 15 cmH_2O to increase Sa_{O_2} to 95% without dropping the blood pressure or cardiac index; during this increase of PEEP another 500 mL saline was administered, and Ppw rose to

30 mmHg measured at end expiration when PEEP = 15 cmH_2O.

In the next 4 hours he was treated with dobutamine incremented from 5 to 10 to 15 μg/kg/min, the dopamine infusion was decreased to 3 μg/kg/min, and nitroprusside infusion was initiated while blood pressure and cardiac output were repeatedly measured. Blood pressure was then 100/60, cardiac index was 2.5, mixed venous saturation was 67%, and heart rate was 120/min. Morphine administration continued and furosemide was administered resulting in a sustained diuresis with a net output of 1.3 L; when his Ppw fell to 24 mmHg measured at end expiration while still on PEEP = 15 cmH_2O, he was transfused 2 U packed red blood cells. His $F_{I_{O_2}}$ was reduced stepwise to 40% maintaining an Sa_{O_2} well above 90%.

The next day he had substantially improved. He was alert and oriented, had improved perfusion to his extremities, maintained a good urine output, and his arterial lactate level had fallen to 4.4. In addition to his acid-base status, his oxygenation improved so that his $F_{I_{O_2}}$ was reduced to 30%. On the second day after admission he was successfully extubated. He remained in the ICU for several more days where he was started on captopril and digoxin while dopamine and dobutamine were discontinued. He spent a further 2 weeks on a medical ward prior to his discharge on lasix, captopril, and digoxin with a diagnosis of acute on chronic heart failure.

CASE DISCUSSION

This unfortunate young man presented with biventricular failure of uncertain etiology, complicated by shock and pulmonary edema. Initial dopamine therapy increased blood pressure, presumably by increasing contractility. He was ventilated at high minute volume to rest his respiratory muscles and to maintain respiratory compensation for his lactic acidosis. He was oxygenated to ensure adequate Sa_{O_2}, but when Sa_{O_2} was <90% on 100% O_2, PEEP was added while he was being treated with morphine to reduce discomfort, anxiety, and preload, with furosemide to reduce preload, and with nitroglycerin to reduce preload and minimize any myocardial ischemia contributing to his ventricular dysfunction.

This combined therapy had the unexpected effect of reducing Ppw excessively, associated with an untoward fall in cardiac index and blood pressure. Presumably, the dilation of systemic veins by morphine, nitroglycerin, and furosemide, and the increase in Pra and resistance to venous return effected by PEEP,[50] rendered this patient relatively hypovolemic for his current left ventricular dysfunction. Of several possibilities to explain his critical hypotension, hypovolemia was tested by reducing the PEEP and expanding his circulating volume by infusing saline. When the blood pressure and cardiac output increased again, it was concluded that an optimal preload had been defined. Then PEEP could be increased again to correct desaturation without decreasing venous return. In retrospect, this patient's hypoxic, acidemic left ventricle probably required a transmural Ppw of about 25 mmHg to maintain an adequate cardiac index in the presence of a high systemic vascular resistance; enough venous return to provide adequate preload was maintained by high circulating catecholamines, until vasoactive drugs caused venodilation. Conceivably, withholding nitroglycerin and furosemide until dobutamine had increased cardiac index and blood pressure would have achieved subsequent cardiovascular stability earlier and without the hypotensive interval.

Over a short subsequent period, inotropic therapy was maximized with dobutamine, while dopaminergic doses of dopamine were used to maximize the renal distribution of his low cardiac output. When blood pressure increased sufficiently, afterload reduction was initiated and titrated with increasing doses of sodium nitroprusside until cardiac output peaked at a stable high value of Ppw. Morphine administration was supplemented with furosemide to reduce ventricular preload to the least Ppw maintaining this cardiac index, thereby to minimize wall stress and pulmonary edema; then O_2 transport was improved by transfusing packed red blood cells with careful monitoring of Ppw. The result of these combined acute therapeutic maneuvers was increased stroke volume at reduced Ppw; note that Ppw decreased from 32 mmHg on PEEP = 0 to 24 mmHg on PEEP = 15. This allowed correction of the lactic acidosis by increased cardiac output and hematocrit at reduced heart rate and amelioration of the hypoxia and tachypnea. Intravenous vasoactive drugs were then switched to oral agents before discharge from the ICU for further diagnostic work-up of the etiology of his acute on chronic heart failure.

References

1. Elzinga G, Westerhof N: How to quantify pump function of the heart. Circ Res 44:303, 1979.
2. Sarnoff SJ, Berglund E: Starling's law of the heart studied by means of simultaneous right and left ventricular function curves in the dog. Circulation 9:706, 1954.
3. Goldberg HS, Rabson J: Control of cardiac output by systemic vessels. Am J Cardiol 47:696, 1981.
4. Caldini P, Permutt S, Waddell JA, Riley RL: Effect of epinephrine on pressure, flow, and volume relationships in the systemic circulation of dogs. Circ Res 34:606, 1974.
5. Sagawa K: The ventricular pressure-volume diagram revisited. Circ Res 43:677, 1978.
6. Chatterjee K, Parmley WW: The role of vasodilator therapy in heart failure. Prog Cardiovasc Dis 19:301, 1977.
7. Zile MR: Diastolic dysfunction: Detection, consequences and treatment. Mod Concepts Cardiovasc Dis 58:67, 1989; 59:1, 1990.
8. Cowley AW Jr, Guyton AC: Heart rate as a determinant of cardiac output in dogs with arteriovenous fistula. Am J Cardiol 28:321, 1971.
9. Kass DA, Maughan WL, Zhong MG, et al: Comparative influence of load versus inotropic states on indexes of ventricular contractility: Experimental and theoretical analysis based on pressure-volume relationships. Circulation 76:1422, 1987.
10. Davila JC, Sanmarco ME: An analysis of the fit of mathematical models applicable to the measurement of left ventricular volume. Am J Cardiol 18:31, 1966.

11. Borow KM, Green LH, Grossman W, Braunwald E: Left ventricular end-systolic stress-shortening and stress length relations in humans. Am J Cardiol 50:1301, 1982.
12. Colan SD, Borow KM, Neumann A: Left ventricular end-systolic wall stress-velocity of fiber shortening relation: A load-independent index of myocardial contractility. J Am Coll Cardiol 4:715, 1984.
13. Seward JB, Bijoy K, Khandheria, Oh JK: Transesophageal echocardiography: Technique, anatomic correlations, implementation, and clinical applications. Mayo Clin Proc 63:649, 1988.
14. Johnson RA, Palacios I: Dilated cardiomyopathies of the adult I. N Engl J Med 307:1051, 1119, 1982.
15. Parmley WW: Pathophysiology of congestive heart failure. Am J Cardiol 55:9A, 1985.
16. Bristow MR, Ginsburg R, Minobe W, et al: Decreased catecholamine sensitivity and adrenergic-receptor density in failing human hearts. N Engl J Med 307:205, 1982.
17. Suga H, Yamada O, Goto Y: Energetics of ventricular contraction as traced in the pressure-volume diagram. Fed Proc 43:2411, 1984.
18. Dhainault JF, Hayghebaert MF, Monsallier JF, et al: Coronary hemodynamics and myocardial metabolism of lactate, for fatty acids, glucose and ketones in patients with septic shock. Circulation 75:533, 1987.
19. Walley KR, Becker CJ, Hogan RA, et al: Progressive hypoxemia limits left ventricular oxygen consumption and contractility. Circ Res 63:849, 1988.
20. Steenbergen C, Deleeuw G, Rich T, Williamson JR: Effects of acidosis and ischemia on contractility and intracellular pH of rat heart. Circ Res 41:849, 1988.
21. Walley KR, Lewis TH, Wood LDH: Acute respiratory acidosis decreases left ventricular contractility but increases cardiac output in dogs. Circ Res 67:628, 1990.
22. Teplinsky K, O'Toole M, Olman M, et al: Effect of lactic acidosis on canine hemodynamics and left ventricular function. Am J Physiol 258:H1193, 1990.
23. Desai TK, Carlson RW, Geheb MA: Prevalence and clinical implication of hypocalcemia in acutely ill patients in a medical intensive care setting. Am J Med 84:209, 1988.
24. Lang RM, Fellner SK, Neumann A, et al: Left ventricular contractility varies directly with blood ionized calcium. Ann Intern Med 108:524, 1988.
25. Cooper DJ, Walley KR, Dodek P, Russell JA: Correlation of decreased plasma ionized calcium and increased lactic acidosis may be due to lactate and bicarbonate binding calcium. Am Rev Respir Dis 141:A771, 1990.
26. Cooper DJ, Walley KR, Wiggs BR, Russell JA: Bicarbonate does not improve hemodynamics in critically ill patients who have lactic acidosis. Ann Intern Med 112:492, 1990.
27. Greenberg BH, Schultz R, Runkemeier GL, Giswold H: Acute effects of alcohol in patients with congestive heart failure. Ann Intern Med 97:171, 1982.
28. Parrillo JE, Burch C, Shelhamer JH, et al: A circulating myocardial depressant substance in humans with septic shock. J Clin Invest 76:1539, 1985.
29. Natanson C: Studies using a canine model to investigate the cardiovascular abnormality of and potential therapies for septic shock. Clin Res 38:206, 1990.
30. Cooper DJ, Thompson C, Walley KR, et al: Histamine infusion decreases left ventricular contractility in humans. Fed Proc 4:A340, 1990.
31. Ziegler EJ, McCutchan JA, Fierer J, et al: Treatment of gram-negative bacteremia and shock with human antiserum to a mutant escherichia coli. N Engl J Med 307:1225, 1982.
32. Marks JD, Marks CB, Luce J, et al: Plasma tumor necrosis factor in patients with septic shock. Am Rev Respir Dis 141:94, 1990.
33. Roberts DE, Dobson KE, Hall KW, Light RB: Effects of prolonged naloxone infusion in septic shock. Lancet 8613(2):699, 1988.
34. Katy AM: Changing strategies in the management of heart failure. J Am Coll Cardiol 13:513, 1990.
35. Stein L, Beraud JJ, Morissette M, et al: Pulmonary edema during volume infusion. Circulation 52:483, 1975.
36. Leier CV, Unverferth DV: Dobutamine. Ann Intern Med 99:490, 1983.
37. Goldberg LI, Hsieh Y, Resnekov L: Newer catecholamines for treatment of heart failure and shock: An update on dopamine and a first look at dobutamine. Prog Cardiovasc Dis 19:327, 1977.
38. Carroll JD, Lang RM, Neuman AL, et al: The differential effects of positive inotropic and vasodilator therapy on diastolic properties in patients with congestive cardiomyopathy. Circulation 74:815, 1985.
39. Goldstein RA: Clinical effects of intravenous amrinone in patients with congestive heart failure. Circulation 73(suppl III):191, 1986.
40. Goldstein RA, Passamani ER, Roberts R: A comparison of digoxin and dobutamine in patients with acute infarction and cardiac failure. N Engl J Med 303:846, 1980.
41. Mueller H, Ayres M, Gregory J, et al: Hemodynamics, coronary blood flow, and myocardial metabolism in coronary shock; response to 1-norepinephrine and isoproterenol. J Clin Invest 49:1885, 1970.
42. McAlpine HM, Morton JJ, Leckie B, Dargie HJ: Hemodynamic effects of captopril in acute left ventricular failure complicating myocardial infarction. J Cardiovasc Pharmacol 9(suppl 2):S25, 1987.
43. Schreiber TL, Miller DH, Zola B: Management of myocardial infarction shock: Current status. Am Heart J 117:435, 1989.
44. Borrow RO, Rosing DR, Bacharach SL, et al: Effects of verapamil on left ventricular systolic function and diastolic filling in patients with hypertrophic cardiomyopathy. Circulation 64:787, 1981.
45. Stoddard MF, Pearson AC, Kern MJ, et al: Left ventricular diastolic function: Comparison of pulsed Doppler echocardiographic and hemodynamic indexes in subjects with and without coronary artery disease. J Am Coll Cardiol 13:327, 1989.
46. Gaasch WH, Levine HJ, Quinones MA, Alexander JK: Left ventricular compliance: mechanisms and clinical implications. Am J Cardiol 38:645, 1976.
47. Smiseth OA, Manyari DE, Lima JA, et al: Modulation of vascular capacitance by angiotensin and nitroprusside: A mechanism of changes in pericardial pressure. Circulation 76:875, 1987.
48. Miller RR, DeMaria AN, Amsterdam EA, et al: Improvement of reduced left ventricular diastolic compliance in ischemic heart disease after successful coronary artery bypass surgery. Am J Cardiol 35:11, 1975.
49. Brodie BR, Grossman W, Mann T, McLaurin LP: Effects of sodium nitroprusside on left ventricular diastolic pressure-volume relations. J Clin Invest 59:59, 1977.
50. Fessler HE, Brower RG, Wise RA, Permutt S: Effects of positive-end-expiratory pressure on the gradient for venous return. Am Rev Respir Dis 143:19, 1991.
51. Walley KR, Cooper DJ: Diastolic stiffness impairs left ventricular function during hypovolemic shock in pigs. Am J Physiol 260:H702, 1991.
52. Alyono D, Ring WS, Anderson RW: The effects of hemorrhagic shock on the diastolic properties of the left ventricle in the con-

scious dog. Surgery 83:691, 1978.
53. Parrillo JE, Parker MM, Natanson C, et al: Septic shock in humans. Ann Intern Med 113:227, 1990.
54. Forrester JS, Diamond G, Parmley WW, Swan JC: Early increase in left ventricular compliance after myocardial infarction. J Clin Invest 51:598, 1972.
55. Russell JA, Ronco JJ, Lockhat D, et al: Oxygen delivery and consumption and ventricular preload are greater in survivors than in nonsurvivors of the adult respiratory distress syndrome. Am Rev Respir Dis 141:659, 1990.
56. Prewitt RM, Wood LDH: Effects of altered resistive load on left ventricular systolic mechanics in dogs. Anesthesiology 56:195, 1981.
57. Klein HO, Kaplinsky E: Digitalis and verapamil in atrial fibrillation and flutter. Drugs 31:185, 1986.
58. Scher DL, Arsura EL: Multifocal atrial tachycardia: Mechanisms, clinical correlates, and treatment. Am Heart J 118:574, 1989.
59. Streeter DD Jr, Henry SM, Spotnitz HM, et al: Fiber orientation in the canine left ventricle during diastole and systole. Circ Res XXIV:339, 1969.
60. Meier GD, Ziskin MC, Santamore WP, Bove AA: Kinematics of the beating heart. IEEE Trans Biomed Engin 27:319, 1980.
61. Dell' Italia L, Walsh RA: Right ventricular diastolic pressure-volume relations and regional dimensions during acute alterations in loading conditions. Circulation 77:1276, 1988.
62. Maughan WL, Shoukas AA, Sagawa K, Weisfeldt ML: Instantaneous pressure-volume relationship of the canine right ventricle. Circ Res 44:309, 1979.
63. Ducas J, Duval D, Dasilva H, et al: Treatment of canine pulmonary hypertension: Effects of norepinephrine and isoproterenol on pulmonary vascular pressure-flow characteristics. Circulation 75:235, 1987.
64. Rounds S, Hill NS: Pulmonary hypertensive diseases. Chest 85:397, 1984.
65. Weber KT, Janicki JS, Shroff S, Fishman AP: Contractile mechanics and interaction of the right and left ventricles. Am J Cardiol 47:686, 1981.
66. McFate Smith, W: Epidemiology of congestive heart failure. Am J Cardiol 55:3A, 1985.
67. Eilen SD, Crawford MH, O'Rourke RA: Accuracy of precordial palpation for detecting increased left ventricular volume. Ann Intern Med 99:628, 1983.
68. Dikshit K, Vyden JK, Forrester JS, et al: Renal and extra-renal hemodynamic effects of furosemide in congestive heart failure after acute myocardial infarction. N Engl J Med 288:1087, 1973.
69. Ali J, Wood LDH: Pulmonary vascular effects of furosemide on gas exchange in pulmonary edema. J Appl Physiol 57:160, 1984.

Chapter 116
MYOCARDIAL ISCHEMIA

JOHN T. BARRON
JOSEPH E. PARRILLO

KEY POINTS

- *Myocardial ischemia results from an imbalance between myocardial oxygen demand and supply.*
- *The major determinants of myocardial oxygen requirements are heart rate, contractility, and wall stress (afterload).*
- *Provocative stimuli that increase myocardial oxygen demand should be minimized and factors which enchance oxygen supply maximized.*
- *Unstable ischemia syndromes that are not provoked by exogenous stimuli usually result from acute development of intracoronary thrombosis.*
- *Intravenous nitroglycerin should be administered for refractory anginal chest pain.*
- *Aspirin should be administered to patients with unstable angina; if angina recurs heparinization is indicated.*
- *Acute myocardial infarction (MI) presenting within 6 h of symptoms onset should be treated with thrombolytic therapy.*
- *Coronary angiography is indicated only in patients in whom a coronary revascularization procedure is contemplated.*
- *Cardiogenic shock carries an 80 to 100 percent mortality rate unless coronary perfusion is reestablished.*
- *Urgent coronary revascularization by angioplasty or bypass surgery is indicated in patients with severe coronary disease who remain unstable.*

Myocardial ischemia from compromised coronary blood flow or from an imbalance in the myocardial oxygen supply:demand ratio frequently may go unrecognized in an ICU setting. Signs of myocardial ischemia may be obfuscated by other coexisting illnesses present in the critically ill patient. Physical examination in these patients is often limited or altered by other disease processes, and there may be multiple potential causes for hemodynamic instability. Myocardial ischemia and attendant left ventricular dysfunction may complicate the course and treatment of a particular illness. Conversely, multisystem illness may set the conditions for diminished delivery of oxygen to the heart. It is for these reasons that the critical care physician must maintain a high index of suspicion for myocardial ischemia in the hemodynamically unstable patient in the ICU setting, especially in the patient with a prior history or multiple risk factors for coronary artery disease.

Patients hospitalized for noncardiac reasons who develop chest pain suggestive of myocardial ischemia may have an antecedent history of angina, or no prior history, suggesting that occult coronary artery disease is present. In either case, development of angina is likely the result of increased myocardial demand for oxygen that exceeds the supply, which is limited by obstructive atherosclerotic coronary artery disease. This is not unlike the case of chronic stable angina (or "fixed-threshold" angina), where angina does not occur at rest, but occurs predictably with exertion when the work of the heart and myocardial O_2 requirements increase. With rest, O_2 requirements return to base line and angina resolves.[1]

Myocardial requirement for oxygen, and hence oxygenated blood, is affected by three major variables: heart rate, myocardial wall stress, and contractility. The principal determinants of myocardial wall stress are ventricular preload and afterload; systemic vascular resistance (SVR) is a major component of afterload. It is difficult to enumerate all the factors in critically ill patients that could alter these variables. The simplest approach to treatment is to attempt to decrease the myocardium's requirement for oxygen by withdrawal of provocative stimuli that increase the work of the heart. Alternatively, in other instances, alleviation of myocardial ischemia may simply entail increasing the amount of oxygen dissolved in blood (e.g., in pulmonary disease), or by increasing the hemoglobin concentration (e.g., in profound anemia) that is delivered to the coronary vascular bed. Myocardial ischemia relieved by these measures usually results in prompt restoration of left ventricular function without significant cellular damage since the obstruction to flow is ordinarily fixed and not total.

The pathophysiology of unstable coronary syndromes and MI usually involves dynamic partial or complete occlusion of an epicardial coronary artery because of acute intracoronary thrombus formation.[2] Less commonly, vasospasm of a coronary artery is the cause of occlusion.[3] Identification of exogenous provocative factors, if any, is more difficult. Simply removing or lessening stimuli which increase myocardial oxygen requirements, such as reducing heart rate, may not be sufficient to increase the myocardial oxygen supply: demand ratio, and unless attempts are made to reestablish coronary blood flow significant myocardial damage may ensue.

Recognition of Myocardial Ischemia

SIGNS AND SYMPTOMS OF MYOCARDIAL ISCHEMIA

Myocardial ischemia is most commonly manifested as constant substernal chest tightness or pressure. The pain is typically left-sided and may radiate to the throat and jaw or to the left shoulder and left arm. Angina occasionally may be right-sided, interscapular, or perceived in the epigastrium. It is also often accompanied by acute onset of dyspnea and diaphoresis; these latter signs may be helpful in diagnosis because the critically ill patient may not be able to communicate the presence of pain.

Because other syndromes may mimic angina, it is important to consider these in the differential diagnosis.[4] These

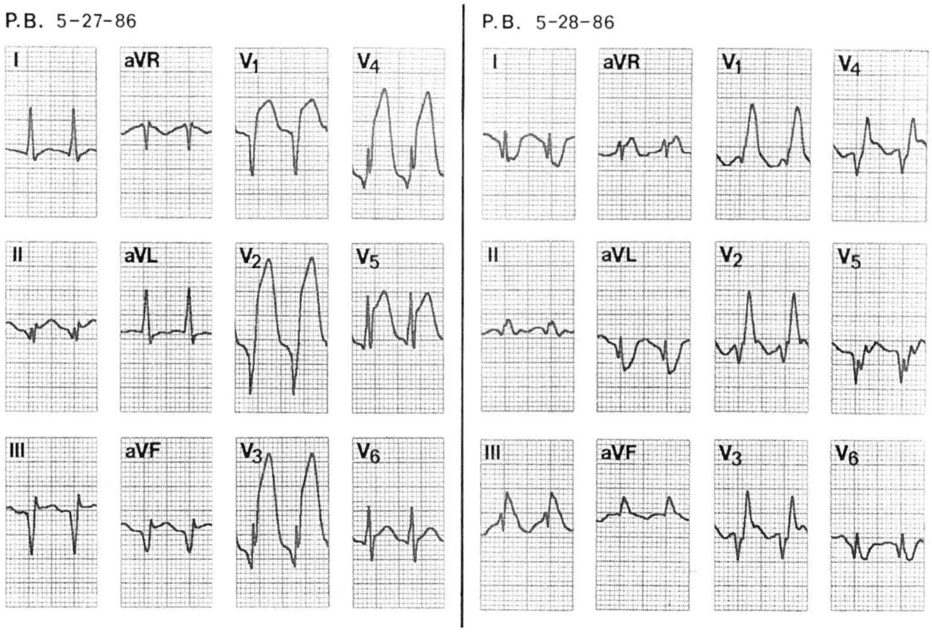

FIGURE 116-1 Serial ECGs from a 54-year-old man who developed acute onset of chest pain, dyspnea, and diaphoresis. *Left.* ECG on first presentation within 4 h of symptom onset showing peaked T waves and hyperacute elevation of ST segments in the anterior precordial leads and inferior limb leads. Q wave development is already evident in these leads. *Right.* ECG obtained 18 h afterward demonstrating MI in evolution with reversion of ST segments and concomitant development of q waves. A bifascicular block (RBBB + LPFB) has also developed.

include pericarditis, pleuritis, dissecting aortic aneurysm, pulmonary embolism, musculoskeletal pain, costochondritis, and pain of gastrointestinal origin. Other heart diseases (valvular heart disease, cardiomyopathies, myocarditides) not attributable to coronary artery stenosis may also cause substernal chest tightness and should also be included in the differential diagnosis.

The physical examination, although perhaps insensitive and nonspecific, especially in the patient with multisystem illness or with preexisting left ventricular dysfunction, may be helpful in confirming the diagnosis.[5] During the ischemic episode, auscultation of the precordium may reveal the presence of a fourth heart sound, indicative of a noncompliant segment of dysfunctional left ventricle. The emergence of a mitral regurgitant murmur attributable to papillary muscle dysfunction may also be heard. A systolic bulge occasionally may be palpated on the precordium, in the area of the apex of the heart, representing contact of an ischemic dyskinetic segment of the left ventricle with the chest wall. With extensive myocardial dysfunction, a third heart sound may be present. Elevated jugular veins signal right ventricular diastolic pressure elevation and appearance of pulmonary crackles (in the absence of pulmonary disease) indicates elevated left ventricular filling pressures secondary to depressed left ventricular function. A chest x-ray may be especially useful in confirming the presence of pulmonary edema or in discerning pulmonary from cardiac causes of chest pain or dyspnea.

THE ISCHEMIC ELECTROCARDIOGRAM

The electrocardiographic (ECG) abnormalities in myocardial ischemia are widely variable and depend in large part on the extent and nature of coronary stenosis and the presence of collateral blood flow to ischemic zones. The first ECG changes demonstrable with acute occlusion of a coronary artery are T wave changes in the leads reflecting the anatomic area of myocardium in jeopardy. If the occlusion is total, the T wave is peaked;[6] if subtotal, the T wave is flattened or inverted. In the presence of preexisting T wave abnormalities, interpretation of T wave changes is less reliable. Previously flattened or inverted T waves may revert upright, masking ischemic changes—the so-called pseudonormalization of T waves.

As total occlusion continues, there is elevation of the ST segments in the same leads (Fig. 116-1). Hyperacute ST elevation is indicative of transmural ischemia of a segment of the left ventricle.[7] While elevation of ST segments usually connotes myocardial injury, if the occluded vessel is opened with a thrombolytic agent or other intervention within 1 to 6 h minimal myocardial cell death may occur, and the ST segments may normalize.

Elevation of ST segments is also seen in pericarditis, but the ST elevation is diffuse and does not develop as acutely as ST elevation due to ischemia. The morphology of the ST segments in pericarditis tends to be concave upward, while that of ischemia is convex. Also, the PR segment in lead aVR may be elevated in pericarditis.[8]

Subtotal occlusion of an epicardial coronary artery may not result in ST elevation, but rather only T wave changes or ST depression in the leads reflecting the involved myocardium. In this circumstance, the mass of myocardium in jeopardy is ordinarily not as extensive as when there is total occlusion of a vessel with associated ST elevation. Alternatively, the mass of myocardium in jeopardy may not be as discretely localized as with ST elevation. As such, infarctions with ST depression may not evolve q waves, which represent discrete regions of irreparably damaged tissue. When infarction is not associated with q waves on the surface ECG, it is termed a "non-q wave" infarct. Evolution of q waves, on the other hand, is typically preceded by ST segment elevation.

Depression of the ST segments and T wave inversions may also be caused by a myriad of factors besides ischemia. These include cardioactive drugs, in particular digoxin, and electrolyte disorders, in particular hypokalemia. Left ventricular hypertrophy and acute left ventricular pressure overload as might occur in hypertensive crisis, may also result in ST depression—the so-called strain pattern. Supraventricular tachycardias have also been shown to result in ST depression, even in the absence of coronary artery disease.

Other more subtle ECG signs of myocardial ischemia are slight prolongation of the QT interval, prolongation of the QRS interval, or diffuse abnormalities of the ST segment and T wave. These abnormalities, however, are not specific to ischemia and may be caused by electrolyte shifts, drugs such as digoxin, and numerous other causes frequently present in patients in the ICU. When these changes are observed, correlation with the clinical status of the patient is required.

Evolution of q waves in acute MI may proceed within a few to several hours after onset of occlusion of an epicardial coronary artery (see Fig. 116-1). They are located in the leads reflecting the wall of the left ventricle affected and correspond to areas of irreparably damaged myocardium. Q waves represent unopposed initial depolarization forces away from the mass of infarcted myocardium, which has lost electrical activity and no longer contributes to the mean QRS voltage vector. Concomitant with formation of q waves is a decrease in the magnitude of the R waves in the same leads, representing diminution of voltage in the mass of infarcted myocardium. Indeed, loss of R wave voltage, when compared with previous ECG tracings, may be the only ECG evidence for the presence of permanent myocardial damage.

An inferior-posterior wall MI frequently reveals itself as enhanced R waves in the anterior chest leads, representing augmented depolarization forces anteriorly, which are now less opposed by posterior forces. Since posterior MI occurs with inferior wall infarction about 30 percent of the time, evidence for inferior wall ischemia and injury, coupled with increased anterior precordial lead R wave voltage, makes the involvement of the posterior wall likely. This not withstanding, isolated posterior wall MI may not have these features, or the anterior lead ECG changes may be very subtle with T wave inversion or ST segment depressions. Infarction of the posterior wall is not readily detected on the standard 12-lead ECG because the electrical activity of the posterior myocardium is in large part masked by the remaining mass of the left ventricle. Placement of posterior chest leads (V_9 to V_{11}) will detect changes from the posterior myocardium and will confirm the presence of posterior wall injury or infarction.

Involvement of the right ventricle in MI is also not readily detected on the standard 12-lead ECG because of the small mass of the right (compared to the left) ventricle and because of the positioning of the standard precordial leads away from the right ventricle. The right ventricular voltage is ordinarily dwarfed by the large voltage of the left ventricle. Therefore, if involvement of the right ventricle is suspected clinically, recordings from right precordial leads (V_3R to V_5R) may be helpful; if the right ventricle is involved, ST segment and evolution of q waves will be demonstrable.[15,16] Right ventricular infarction occurs approximately 30 percent of the time with left ventricular inferior-posterior wall infarctions, so evidence for inferior lead ECG changes are to be expected.

Also frequently overlooked is a high lateral wall MI. The only ECG changes may be T wave inversion or ST elevation in leads I and aVL. Since these leads normally have small physiologic q waves, a pathologic q wave indicative of MI may be discerned with difficulty.

It is important to note that QRS voltage can be affected by multiple factors, such as lead placement, body position, QRS axis shifts, and pericardial and thoracic abnormalities that may shield the electrical activity of the heart. These conditions are frequently encountered in patients in the ICU and should be taken into consideration in interpretation of q waves and R waves.

SILENT ISCHEMIA

Recent interest has focused on the ECG changes associated with "silent" myocardial ischemia, i.e., objective ECG evidence of myocardial ischemia which is not associated with angina or with anginal equivalents.[9] Silent myocardial ischemia may be an incidental observation on a cardiac monitor or on a routine ECG. It consists of transient ST segment depression lasting several minutes to hours.[10] Recurrent ventricular arrhythmias may also be a manifestation of silent ischemia.

The distinction between overt angina and silent myocardial ischemia may be attributable to a difference in the duration of compromised coronary blood flow and also to differential perception of pain. The pathophysiologic basis for silent ischemia is uncertain, but probably resembles that of variant angina wherein coronary vasospasm likely plays a prominent role.[11] As with variant angina, there is usually preexisting coronary artery disease of varying degrees that may be otherwise totally asymptomatic. Alternatively, the patient may have an antecedent history of coronary artery disease, i.e., stable angina or may have had episodes of rest angina. The frequency of episodes of ST segment depression correlates with the severity of coronary artery disease in patients with known coronary artery disease or history of angina.

Associated with episodes of silent ST depression is decreased left ventricular function, which often precedes the ECG changes.[12,13] In patients monitored hemodynamically with pulmonary artery (PA) catheters, silent ischemia may be manifested by gradually increasing pulmonary artery diastolic and wedge pressures, reflecting a rising left ventricular end-diastolic pressure (LVEDP). These signs of left ventricular dysfunction may precede ST segment changes. ECG studies of patients with silent ischemia also confirm the presence of left ventricular dysfunction as suggested by the appearance of transient wall motion abnormalities and evidence of diminished diastolic compliance.

It is important to note that not all episodes of transient ST segment depression are attributable to silent ischemia. In fact, the sensitivity and specificity of this finding for the presence of coronary artery disease is moderate.[14] Nevertheless, should this finding be observed incidentally on the cardiac monitor, especially in association with transient elevation of left ventricular filling pressures, it is prudent to consider the possibility of myocardial ischemia as a potential factor complicating the course of the critically ill patient.

CONDUCTION DISTURBANCES

A variety of conduction disturbances, ranging from prolongation of the PR interval to bundle branch block and complete heart block, may supervene in myocardial ischemia. These may be transient or permanent depending on the involved coronary artery and the nature of the occlusion. Occlusion of the right coronary artery can be associated with first degree atrioventricular (AV) block, sinus or junctional bradycardia, or complete heart block with a narrow QRS complex. These conduction disturbances are associated with right coronary artery occlusion and inferior wall MI[17] because the sinoatrial (SA) and AV nodal arteries are branches of the right coronary artery in the majority of persons.[18,19] The SA and AV nodes consequently become ischemic, resulting in bradyarrhythmias. Also, inferior wall MI may activate the Bezold-Jarisch reflex, resulting in enhanced vagal tone. It is postulated that the Bezold-Jarisch reflex is activated on distention of mechanoreceptors located in regions of the inferior wall and apex. It is enhanced vagal tone in inferior infarcts that may also account for nausea and vomiting commonly associated with inferior infarcts. The occurrence of hypotension that is out of proportion to the extent of myocardial damage in inferior infarcts may also be partly attributed to a vasodepressor reflex mediated by the vagus. Since the bundle branches are not ordinarily supplied by the right coronary artery, the morphology of the QRS complex in right coronary artery occlusion is usually narrow, i.e., conduction distal to the AV node is intact.[20] Occasionally, however, an inferior wall MI can produce a left bundle branch block (LBBB).

With occlusion of the left anterior descending coronary artery resulting in an anterior and anterior septal MI, the bundle of His and bundle branches are in jeopardy and right bundle branch blocks (RBBB) or LBBB or bifascicular blocks may develop. A bundle branch block complicating an anterior wall MI usually signifies that the mass of infarcted myocardium is large. Bundle branch blocks complicating MI usually require transvenous pacing since the risk of progression to advanced AV block is high.[21,22]

ARRHYTHMIAS

Ventricular ectopic beats and ventricular arrhythmias are common during ischemic episodes.[23] Ventricular arrhythmias may be the only ECG manifestation of ischemia. An ischemic myocardium is particularly vulnerable to ventricular fibrillation provoked by a premature ventricular contraction (PVC) falling on the vulnerable period of ventricular repolarization. The more complex (PVCs with more than one morphology) and the more repetitive the ectopy, the greater the probability of sustained ventricular tachycardia or fibrillation.[24]

Supraventricular arrhythmias can also occur in ischemic syndromes. Atrial fibrillation accompanies acute MI approximately 10 to 15 percent of the time[25] either from direct atrial infarction or from increased atrial pressure and distention of the atrial wall as a consequence of elevated LVEDP.

LABORATORY DIAGNOSIS OF ACUTE MYOCARDIAL INFARCTION

Measurement of enzymes released into the serum from necrotic myocardial cells after infarction can aid the diagnosis when ECG changes are nondiagnostic or equivocal.[26,27] Although these tests are useful, the assay time may require several hours or may not be immediately available. Critical therapeutic interventions, therefore, should not be delayed pending assay results. The most useful and reliable enzyme determination for MI is creatine kinase (CK). CK released from the myocardium begins to appear in the plasma within 4 to 8 h after onset of infarction, peaks at 12 to 24 h, and returns to base line at 2 to 4 days. The magnitude, rate of rise, and diminution of serum CK levels is a function of the total mass of myocardium affected, the extent and nature of coronary occlusion (e.g., total or subtotal occlusion), rate of washout from the infarcted myocardium, and clearance from the body. CK is a constituent of many tissues, including skeletal muscle, and therefore, elevated total CK is not specific for MI. Fractionation by gel electrophoresis of CK isoenzymes can identify whether the CK is of myocardial origin. Fourteen percent of myocardial CK is of the MB isoenzyme; the isoenzyme is also present in other tissues, but in much less quantity.

To be diagnostic for MI, the total plasma CK value must be elevated above the upper limit of normal and must be composed of at least 3.0 percent MB fraction. Typically, serum CK and MB fraction are drawn with the first presentation of suspected infarction and every 6 to 8 h thereafter, over the next 24 to 36 h to ensure that the peak release of enzyme is not missed. The total CK appearing in the serum in association with myocardial injury correlates well with the magnitude of infarction size.

In non-q wave MIs, the total serum CK value occasionally may not exceed the upper limits of normal, even though the percent MB fraction is usually above 3 percent. In such circumstances, an elevated CK concentration that is at least double the patient's previously documented level may be considered as evidence for a probable MI, if other clinical indices of infarction are present. Errors in sample collecting or assay may partly account for the low total CK determination in these instances. When CK-MB is elevated, causes of false-positive elevations should be considered when the clinical picture is unclear or when the ECG is nondiagnostic or unchanged. Table 116-1 gives the cardiac and systemic

TABLE 116-1 Causes of Elevated Creatine Kinase (CK-MB) Level Other Than Myocardial Infarction

Myocardial damage
Myocarditis
Pericarditis
Myocardial trauma
Systemic disease with cardiac involvement
Muscular dystrophy
Hypothermia
Hyperthermia
Reye's syndrome
Peripheral source of CK-MB
Myositis
Rhabdomyolysis
Athletic activity
Prostate surgery
Caesarean section
Gastrointestinal surgery
Tumors
Miscellaneous
Renal failure
Subarachnoid hemorrhage
Hypothyroidism

Adapted from Reference 27. Lee TH, Goldman L: Ann Intern Med 105:221, 1986.

causes of elevated CK-MB values in the absence of overt myocardial ischemia.

Serum glutamic-oxaloacetic transaminase (SGOT) and lactic dehydrogenase (LDH) are also released from necrotic myocardial tissue postinfarction. These enzymes are relatively nonspecific for MI since they are present in other tissues. Their usefulness in diagnosing MI derives from their relatively late appearance in the serum after the onset of coronary occlusion. They can be of help when an MI is suspected to have occurred several days before the patient presented or before it was suspected clinically. SGOT content peaks in the serum 36 to 48 h after MI and LDH content peaks at 2 to 4 days. Serum LDH is of more utility than SGOT for diagnosing infarction because the pattern of isoenzymes of LDH appearing in the serum changes when LDH is released from the myocardium. Isoenzyme 1 (LDH_1) content increases and is present in a higher serum concentration than LDH_2 (an isoenzyme inversion or "flip"), the latter being present in greater concentrations than LDH_1 under normal conditions. When indicated, serum LDH and isoenzyme levels should be determined on initial presentation and daily for 2 to 4 days if confirmatory evidence for MI is needed.

OTHER SERUM TESTS

A mildly elevated white blood cell count (12,000 to 15,000/mm^2) and an increased erythrocyte sedimentation rate may also be seen 2 to 4 days after MI. However, these indices are obviously not very specified for infarction, especially in patients with other medical illnesses.

ECHOCARDIOGRAPHY

An emergency portable two-dimensional echocardiogram may aid the diagnosis of MI when other variables are equivocal. The presence of discrete segmental wall motion abnormalities of the left ventricle suggests compromise of blood flow to those segments.[28] Additionally, right ventricular hypokinesis or akinesis, suggestive of right ventricular infarction, may be seen. Infarct segment expansion may also be evident during the acute phase of infarction. A Doppler flow study guided by two-dimensional echocardiography can detect mitral regurgitation secondary to papillary muscle dysfunction.[29]

When the clinical diagnosis of acute MI may be uncertain or equally consistent with other syndromes (e.g., aortic dissection, cardiac tamponade, pericarditis), an echocardiographic study may be particularly useful to determine the need for early interventions such as thrombolysis.

RADIONUCLIDE STUDIES

Technetium pyrophosphate is deposited in irreversibly damaged regions of myocardium.[30] The regions of radioactivity are detected by scintigraphy and appear as "hot spots" on imaging. The period during which technetium pyrophosphate scanning is most sensitive for the detection of infarcted myocardium is approximately 1 to 3 days after MI; a positive scan may remain positive from weeks to months thereafter. Whereas the sensitivity and specificity for detection of a transmural infarct are high with this technique, they are low to moderate for a non-q wave or subendocardial infarct. Therefore, the usefulness of this test is limited for the diagnosis of MIs, especially non-q wave infarcts,[31] since it offers little information unavailable by other means.

Thallium 201 is transported into viable myocardial tissue by adenosine triphosphate (ATP)-dependent processes via the Na^+-K^+-ATPase. Necrotic or scarred myocardial tissue from new or previous MI will appear as a "cold spot" on scintigraphy. The sensitivity of this test for the detection of infarcts is greatest in the first 24 h post infarction and decreases appreciably thereafter.[32] Its sensitivity is best when myocardial damage is discrete and transmural. Furthermore, it cannot distinguish new from old infarcts.

Thallium 201 scintigraphy is most useful in conjunction with exercise stress testing in the noninvasive evaluation for the presence or absence of coronary artery disease. Demonstration of areas of decreased thallium uptake with exercise that normalize with rest is indicative of coronary artery occlusive disease limiting the perfusion of blood in the vessel supplying that region.[32,33] In patients unable to exercise, infusion of dipyridamole in conjunction with thallium scintigraphy may be performed. Dipyridamole will dilate normal coronary arteries more than diseased arteries, thereby producing a coronary steal syndrome. Regions of the left ventricle supplied by the stenotic vessels will become ischemic and not accumulate the isotope.[34]

Radionuclide angiography can be useful in the assessment of global left ventricular function after MI. It provides

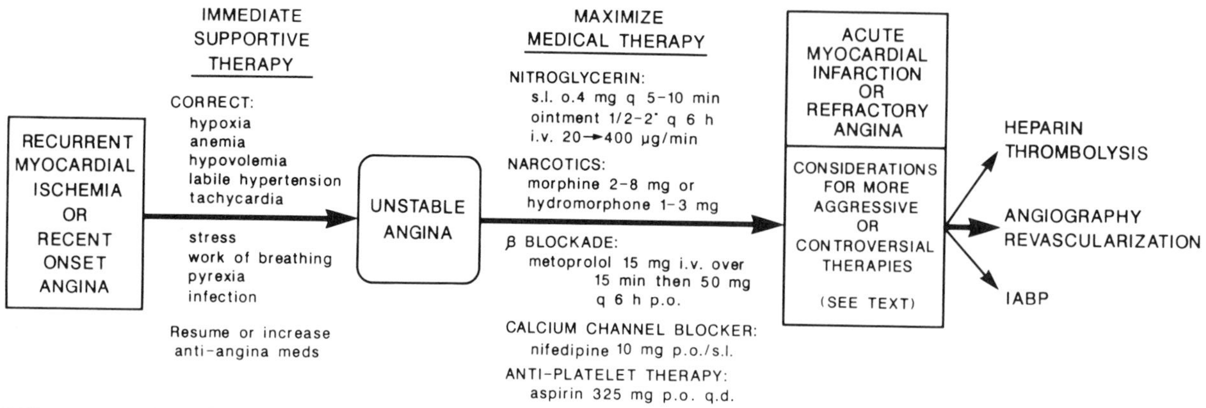

FIGURE 116-2 Timeline of therapeutic modalities for myocardial ischemic syndromes.

an accurate quantitation of left ventricular ejection fraction,[35] even at the bedside. In addition, evaluation of left ventricular regional wall motion can be obtained, although two-dimensional echocardiography may be superior for this purpose. A major use for radionuclide angiography in the setting of MI is in the assessment of suspected right ventricular infarction.[36] The first-pass radionuclide angiogram can provide an adequate quantitation of right ventricular ejection fraction and good assessment of right ventricular wall motion.[36]

Radionuclide angiography may be undertaken in conjunction with exercise stress testing in the evaluation of suspected coronary artery disease in patients able to exercise. Its sensitivity and specificity has been reported to be equal to or exceed that of thallium stress testing for this purpose.

Therapeutic Modalities in the Treatment of Ischemic Syndromes (Fig. 116-2)

STABLE ANGINA

Patients with a history of stable angina who develop chest pain while in the critical care setting are best treated by removal of provocative stimuli that increase myocardial oxygen consumption or lead to compromised coronary blood flow, if these factors can be identified. For example, correction of hypoxia, anemia, hypovolemia, tachycardia, or correction of labile hypertension may be sufficient to control anginal episodes. Often overlooked are fever, infection, anxiety, stress, activity, and work of breathing. If the patient was receiving antianginal medications before hospitalization, these should be continued and the dosages possibly increased.

In instances of refractory angina or where provocative stimuli cannot be ameliorated, it may be necessary to perform coronary angiography and revascularization of the culprit vessels (preferably by percutaneous transluminal coronary angioplasty [PICA]) especially if the myocardial ischemia is complicating further management of the patient.

UNSTABLE ANGINA

When angina is of recent onset (i.e., within the last 48 h) or occurs at rest, especially in the absence of stimuli which increase myocardial oxygen requirements, there is a moderately high probability of the development of a MI within the next few days to weeks. Thus, unstable angina is said to be present.[1,41,42]

NITRATES. Nitroglycerin is a mainstay of therapy for unstable angina because of its efficacy and rapid onset of action. Nitroglycerin is a vasodilator that preferentially dilates venous capacitance vessels, thus decreasing venous return and, therefore, left ventricular preload. The decrease in preload leads to a decrease in left ventricular wall stress, a major determinant of myocardial oxygen consumption. At higher doses in some patients, nitroglycerin relaxes arterial smooth muscle as well, causing a modest decrease in afterload, which also contributes to wall stress.[37] In addition, nitroglycerin will dilate epicardial coronary arteries, including arteries with stenoses, resulting in augmented coronary blood flow. Evidence also indicates that nitroglycerin redistributes coronary blood flow to ischemic regions by dilating collateral vessels.[38]

The quickest mode of administration of nitroglycerin is sublingual. Sublingual doses of 0.4 mg may be administered every 5 to 10 min to a total of three doses, if required to control pain. Because of its hemodynamic actions, systemic blood pressure may fall after administration, so frequent blood pressure checks are required. Hypotension, should it occur, normally resolves by placing the patient in the Trendelenburg position and by giving intravenous saline boluses. Topical transdermal nitrates, such as nitroglycerin ointment, 0.5 to 2 inches every 6 to 8 h may be applied after angina has resolved with conventional sublingual doses.

If sublingual nitroglycerin does not resolve chest pain completely, intravenous nitroglycerin may be initiated starting at a dose of 10 to 20 μg/min. It may be titrated upward as tolerated in increments of 10 to 20 μg/min every 5 to 10 min until pain resolves or until the systemic systolic pressure is 95 to 110 mmHg. An upper limit of 400 μg/min is usually accepted as maximal; above this dose one does not usually see a further clinical response. A further decrease in blood pressure can compromise perfusion of the coronary vascular bed.

NARCOTICS. Persistent angina not responsive to nitroglycerin may be treated with intravenous narcotics. Narcotics may be given as the dose of nitroglycerin is being titrated upward. The initial agent administered is morphine sulfate. In addition to relieving pain, morphine has beneficial effects on improving the myocardial O_2 supply:demand ratio. It produces centrally mediated dilation of venous capacitance vessels and thus, decreases left ventricular preload and decreases myocardial wall tension. It is especially beneficial when there is coexisting pulmonary edema.[39]

Caution should be exercised when administering morphine because of its potential hypotensive effect and because of its ability to enhance vagal tone. As mentioned, patients with myocardial ischemia may have heightened vagal tone, especially when there is involvement of the right coronary artery and the inferior wall of the left ventricle. Administration of morphine in this setting can lead to sinus bradycardia, sinus arrhythmias, and AV nodal conduction disturbances, as well as exacerbation of nausea and vomiting. It is our preference, therefore, to administer 1 to 3 mg hydromorphone under these circumstances to control pain. Hydromorphone is more potent than morphine, and it is our experience that it seems to have less vagotonic and hypotensive effects.

β BLOCKADE. The rationale for administration of intravenous β blockers during ischemic episodes derives from their negative chronotropic and negative inotropic properties. Heart rate and contractility are two of three major determinants of myocardial oxygen consumption. By altering these variables, myocardial ischemia can be significantly attenuated.[40] These agents are particularly effective in patients with angina who remain tachycardic or hypertensive (or both) or in patients with supraventricular tachycardia complicating myocardial ischemia. They are relatively contraindicated in patients with marginal blood pressure, since they may cause further decreases in blood pressure. Other contraindications include preexisting bradycardia, AV nodal conduction disturbances, and evidence for left ventricular failure. Intravenous administration of β blockers, therefore requires continuous ECG monitoring and frequent blood pressure determination because of potential cardiodepressive effects. A short-acting β blocker, such as esmolol, may be the preferred agent in patients who have the potential for hemodynamic instability or who have relative contraindications. Otherwise, in the absence of contraindications, we administer the β_1 selective blocker metoprolol at a dose of 15 mg intravenously over 15 to 20 min until the heart rate is between 60 and 70 beats/min, provided the systolic blood pressure does not fall below 95 mmHg. Thereafter 50 mg every 6 h is given orally.

CALCIUM CHANNEL BLOCKERS. Although most recent evidence indicates that acute formation of thrombus in an epicardial artery is responsible for compromised coronary blood flow in unstable angina, vasospasm of the involved coronary artery may play an important contributing role.[43,44] Vasoactive substances released from the platelet thrombus can aggravate the coronary occlusion. Administration of calcium channel blockers may relieve vasospasm by direct dilatation of coronary vascular smooth muscle.[45] Nifedipine is the calcium channel blocker of choice under these circumstances and when angina persists despite nitrates and narcotics because it has the least cardiodepressant action (along with nicardipine), and it is available in a form that can be administered rapidly. It is available as a liquid contained within a capsule so it may be administered by puncturing the capsule and then swallowing the liquid or by chewing and then swallowing the capsule whole. When given in this form, vasodilation usually ensues within 10 to 20 min with a 10-mg dose. Significant and rapid decrease in blood pressure can occur with nifedipine from marked peripheral vasodilation; hypotension, therefore, should be anticipated.

Vasospasm is the predominant precipitant of angina in patients with Prinzmetal's or variant angina.[3] In contrast to stable fixed-threshold angina, chest pain occurs predominantly at rest without antecedant increases in myocardial oxygen demand as reflected by elevations of heart rate or blood pressure, for example. Factors leading to vasospasm are not clearly identifiable, and it is postulated that at least some patients have a generalized vasospastic disorder. This is supported by the observation that many patients with variant angina have no or only mild coronary artery disease. Other patients may have atherosclerotic coronary stenoses which are subcritical, but serve as sites of vasospasm, possibly as a consequence of abnormalities of the underlying smooth muscle or derangements in endothelial physiology. The illicit use of cocaine is increasingly being recognized as a cause of coronary vasospasm leading to angina and myocardial ischemia. Variant angina attributable to vasospasm responds well to treatment with calcium channel blockers.

It is difficult, if not impossible, to discern whether coronary vasospasm or acute thrombus formation is the predominant factor responsible for compromised coronary blood flow in patients with unstable angina or impending MI. This distinction is not trivial, since there is no compelling evidence indicating that calcium channel blockers are of significant benefit in the early phase of an acute MI.

When coronary vasospasm occurs, there is typically marked ST elevation associated with chest pain, although some patients exhibit ST segment depression. However, these ECG changes are also seen when thrombosis is the

TABLE 116-2 Cardiovascular Effects of Calcium Channel Blockers

	Nifedipine	Nicardipine	Diltiazem	Verapamil
Vasodilation	+++	+++	++	++
Myocardial depression	+	0	++	+++
Depresses AV conduction	0	0	+	++
Depresses SA node	0	0	++	+

Adapted from Med Clin North Am 72:454, 1988 and from Mayo Clin Proc 60:539, 1985.

predominant factor. Nevertheless, vasospasm may be suspected when there is wide and rapid fluctuation of the ST segments (either elevation or depression) on the bedside ECG monitor. Table 116-2 list the calcium channel blockers available and their effects on the heart and peripheral circulation. The selection of calcium channel blocker used for long-term treatment after the patient has been stabilized depends in large part on the status of left ventricular function and on the presence or absence of sinus or AV nodal conduction disturbances (see Table 116-2).

ANTIPLATELET THERAPY. Considerable evidence has accumulated indicating that development of intracoronary thrombus is the principal precipitating event in acute myocardial ischemic syndromes. Acute intracoronary atherosclerotic plaque rupture presumably precipitates thrombus formation by exposing the platelets and other blood elements to thrombogenic substances present locally. Inhibition of thrombus formation, therefore, is a major strategy in the treatment of unstable angina. Several large multicenter trials have established the efficacy of aspirin in the treatment of patients with unstable angina.[46–48] Aspirin, as an inhibitor of platelet cyclooxygenase and, hence, formation of thromboxane A_2, retards platelet aggregability and consequent thrombus formation. Patients presenting with unstable angina who are treated with 325 mg aspirin have a significant reduction in the incidence of refractory angina, MI, and (in some studies) cardiac death.

Aspirin therapy initiated in the early stages of acute MI has also been recently shown to significantly reduce mortality, especially in combination with thrombolytic therapy.[49] Therefore, since aspirin has been clearly proven to be beneficial in acute ischemic syndromes, it should be administered routinely in all patients with unstable angina. A single tablet of 164 mg or 325 mg, taken immediately and daily thereafter is sufficient to effectively inhibit platelet activity.

HEPARIN THERAPY. Intravenous heparin has recently been evaluated for treatment of patients with unstable angina.[48] Heparin was as effective as aspirin for both treating patients with unstable angina and in preventing MI. Heparin was superior to aspirin in reducing the incidence of refractory angina episodes. The combination of heparin and aspirin did not clearly produce added benefit, but did increase the risk of bleeding complications. These results reinforce the notion that anticoagulation is indeed of benefit in unstable angina, but whether heparin has distinct advantages over aspirin, or whether combination therapy has advantage over monotherapy remains to be determined. Nevertheless, should patients with unstable angina treated with aspirin continue to have ischemic episodes despite treatment with aspirin, it may be prudent to initiate full heparin therapy. Heparin is given initially in a bolus of 5000 to 10000 U then 1000 U/h to maintain the activated partial thromboplastin time (PTT) at one and a half to two times the control. It is continued for 3 to 7 days until coronary angiography and possible coronary revascularization is performed, or until ischemic events have clearly subsided, provided no untoward bleeding episodes have occurred. Concomitant aspirin therapy should be continued, probably indefinitely.

The benefits of anticoagulation therapy should be weighed against the risk of bleeding complications, especially in critically ill patients who likely have a propensity to develop thrombocytopenia and coagulopathy.

THROMBOLYTIC THERAPY

Limited information is available on the efficacy of thrombolytic therapy in unstable angina. The studies performed did not demonstrate added benefit over treatment with aspirin alone.[50] As such, because of the significant risk of bleeding with these agents, the routine use of thrombolytic therapy cannot be recommended, until there is evidence to the contrary. The efficacy of thrombolytic therapy in acute MI is discussed below.

CORONARY ANGIOGRAPHY IN UNSTABLE ANGINA

Coronary angiography should generally be reserved for unstable patients in whom a possible revascularization procedure is anticipated in the near future. One must keep in mind that coronary angiography is *not* a therapeutic intervention, but a *diagnostic* test. Angiography is of little tangible value if coronary artery bypass graft (CABG) surgery or angioplasty are not viable options. For example, it may be deemed that a critically ill patient would not tolerate a surgical procedure because of complicating medical condition unrelated to hemodynamic instability imparted by cardiac dysfunction from myocardial ischemia. Percutaneous coronary angioplasty (PTCA) may be performed in such patients, if warranted (vide infra), but it is to be noted that the risk of acute closure of the vessel during the procedure is approximately 2.5 percent, which under normal circumstances would require emergency CABG surgery.[51] Patients who are ordinarily not considered suitable candidates for CABG are generally not suitable candidates for angioplasty as well.

Recommendations for timing of angiography in unstable ischemic syndromes are controversial. Early angiography can identify patients with left main or severe three-vessel disease, in whom early CABG surgery can be lifesaving. An opposing argument is that performance of angiography tends to incline the clinician to a more aggressive approach than is necessarily needed at reestablishing optimal coronary patency.[52] As mentioned, acute intracoronary thrombus formation underlies much of the pathophysiology of unstable ischemic syndromes. With sufficient time, lysis of the thrombus by the patient's intrinsic fibrinolytic system may occur, obviating subsequent angioplasty or CABG surgery.

The decision to perform early angiography should be based on the frequency and severity of angina episodes and the nature and extent of ECG changes. For example, extensive ST depression in the anterior chest leads suggests stenosis of the proximal left anterior descending artery or left main coronary artery, total occlusion of which would result in sudden death. Frequent anginal episodes or episodes that are difficult to control with conventional antianginal medications also presage impending infarction. Under these circumstances, early angiography is indicated. Otherwise, in cases in which the patient stabilizes readily with pharmacologic agents and aspirin/heparin, there is no need for early angiography. Indeed, under these circumstances, an option available is to forego coronary angiography altogether and then evaluate patients several days to weeks later when they are completely stabilized and ambulatory. This can be accomplished by exercise stress testing which can stratify patients according to risk for subsequent cardiac events.[53] Our usual approach, however, is to perform coronary angiography on all patients who are appropriate candidates after they have stabilized but before hospital discharge.

INTRAAORTIC BALLOON PUMP (IABP)

An IABP is a device that is inserted via the femoral artery into the descending thoracic aorta just distal to the aortic arch. A 40-mL balloon at the tip of the catheter is inflated during ventricular diastole by a pneumatic pump in synchrony with closure of the aortic valve, and deflated on opening of the aortic valve. Inflation and deflation are gated to the R and T waves on the ECG or to the arterial pressure tracing recording. By deflating during ventricular systole, ventricular afterload is reduced, resulting in significant decreases in myocardial wall stress and significant decreases in myocardial oxygen requirements.[54] Furthermore, inflation during ventricular diastole increases vascular resistance, resulting in augmentation of coronary blood flow, since perfusion of the coronary vascular bed occurs predominantly during diastole. The predominant effect of an IABP in relieving myocardial ischemia is by decreasing oxygen demand by afterload reduction.[55]

An IABP is indicated in unstable angina when the angina and attendant ECG abnormalities are persistent and refractory to maximal pharmacologic therapy. It is particularly indicated in this situation when coronary angiography or possible revascularization cannot be performed within a reasonably short time or as a method to control progressive unstable angina to allow coronary angiography to be performed safely. It may also be inserted in patients who are stable and have undergone angiography, but in whom precarious coronary lesions (e.g., left main coronary artery stenosis) have been identified. Typically, these patients are maintained on the device while awaiting surgery or angioplasty.

Although insertion of an IABP can result in immediate and dramatic relief of myocardial ischemia, placement of this device can be associated with significant complications. These include aortic dissection, femoral artery lacerations, hematomas, femoral neuropathies, renal failure from renal artery occlusion, arterial thrombi and emboli, limb ischemia, and line sepsis. These potential complications must be weighed in determining that an IABP should be inserted. Once inserted, the patient should be placed on full anticoagulating doses of intravenous heparin by constant infusion. Frequent checks of peripheral pulses and surveillance for other complications should be performed routinely. Also, prophylactic administration of intravenous antibiotics with good gram-positive coverage, such as oxacillin or a cephalosporin, is usually instituted.

CORONARY REVASCULARIZATION FOR UNSTABLE ANGINA

Both CABG surgery and angioplasty can be options when coronary revascularization is considered. In general, CABG surgery is indicated in left main and three-vessel coronary artery disease, with or without preserved left ventricular function.[56,57] Whether revascularization should be undertaken in other scenarios, e.g., single- or double-vessel disease, depends on numerous factors, including the location of the lesions within the vessels, the degree and morphology of the stenoses and size of the vessels, area of myocardium in jeopardy, and importantly, left ventricular function. In the absence of left main or three-vessel disease, the major consideration in deciding whether revascularization is required is if the patient continues to have anginal chest pain. In a stabilized patient who is pain free for several days and who has undergone angiography, the physiologic significance of identified coronary lesions may be decided by having the patient undergo stress thallium testing. Evidence for reversible ischemia by thallium stress testing is cause for the appropriate revascularization intervention.

When a tight stenosis (>80 percent) of the proximal portion of the left anterior coronary artery is identified in a patient with unstable angina, we recommend that the patient be managed aggressively. One should consider early revascularization, regardless of whether the patient may be pain free. That is, we would usually forego additional noninvasive evaluation and proceed directly to either angioplasty or surgery. This is based on the higher risk of untoward cardiac events in this subgroup of patients.[58]

The selection of either angioplasty or surgery, again, depends on multiple factors. Angioplasty is probably the preferred modality in single-vessel disease with proximal lesions. In contrast, surgery is the preferred modality with three-vessel disease. Management of two-vessel disease would depend on coronary anatomy and other factors. The indications for one technique over the other are presently under debate. Firm recommendations cannot be made until the results of multicenter studies presently underway are available.

Acute Myocardial Infarction—Therapeutic Approach

Symptoms suggestive of MI are usually similar to those of ordinary angina, but the intensity and duration of symptoms are greater. Nausea, vomiting, and diaphoresis are usually more prominent features, as are stupor and malaise. The latter may be attributed to low cardiac output ($\dot{Q}_T$).

Compromised left ventricular function may result in pulmonary edema with development of pulmonary bibasilar crackles and jugular venous distention; a fourth heart sound can be present with small infarcts or even mild ischemia, but a third heart sound is usually indicative of more extensive damage.

The initial measures in treatment also entail administration of oxygen, nitrates, and narcotics to relieve pain. Narcotics also reduce anxiety, the salutory effects of which have been known for decades and cannot be underestimated. It is also important to provide reassurance to the patient.

β BLOCKADE

Administration of intravenous β blockers during the early phase of infarction has been advocated for several years, and relatively recent evidence substantiates this recommendation.[53,59] Administration of 15 mg metoprolol intravenously over 15 to 20 min and then 50 mg orally every 6 h thereafter has been shown to reduce mortality and to preserve myocardial function postinfarction. These salutory effects of intravenous β blockers have been demonstrated in q wave infarctions. Patients with non-q wave infarctions apparently do not benefit.

Contraindications to intravenous metoprolol include overt cardiac failure, second degree AV block, hypotension, sinus bradycardia, and of course, cardiogenic shock. A history of bronchospastic pulmonary disease also is a relative contraindication. Acute β blockade is not absolutely contraindicated in patients with insulin dependent diabetes mellities, since blood glucose levels are ordinarily checked frequently and routinely in the ICU (long-term β blockade therapy in the patients may not be desirable, however). If metoprolol is well tolerated, it may be continued at 50 mg every 6 h thereafter. It should be immediately discontinued if any of the above conditions develop.

THROMBOLYTIC THERAPY

Overwhelming evidence from multiple clinical trials documents the ability of thrombolytic agents administered early in the course of an acute MI to reduce infarct size, preserve left ventricular function, and reduce short-term and long-term mortality.[60–62] These benefits from thrombolytic therapy are achieved if it is initiated within 4 to 6 h of symptom onset. Results from one recent large clinical trial using the combination of aspirin and streptokinase (SK) have indicated that reduction in mortality may be obtainable if treatment is initiated even after 6 h (but not after 24 h) of symptom onset.[63]

The benefit from thrombolytic therapy derives from the ability of these agents to lyse intracoronary thrombi and thereby produce coronary patency and reestablish blood flow to affected regions. The two principal thrombolytic agents in wide use today are SK and tissue plasminogen activator (TPA). SK administration can achieve coronary arterial patency approximately 50 to 60 percent of the time, while administration of TPA achieves patency in 70 to 80 percent of cases. The difference in patency rates is the principal difference in clinical efficacy between these two agents. Evaluation of complications due to bleeding, including hemorrhagic stroke, has not shown significant difference between these agents. As for mortality reduction and preservation of left ventricular function, there is no clear benefit of one agent over the other. Large clinical trials with head-to-head comparison of the two agents are presently underway to evaluate relative clinical efficacy. Newer thrombolytic agents are being developed to improve our ability to use thrombolysis safely.

CRITERIA FOR USE OF THROMBOLYTIC AGENTS AND PATIENT SELECTION. Because of the small, but nonetheless significant, complication of bleeding, most notably intracranial hemorrhage, selection of patients with acute MI for a thrombolytic agent should be undertaken with prudence and caution. This is of special importance in ICU patients who may have a predisposition to bleeding complications because of multiple factors. The ideal patient for thrombolytic therapy is a relatively young patient with no history of bleeding, who presents with marked ST elevation in the anterior chest leads within 4 h of symptom onset. Since anterior MI usually involves greater myocardial mass than other infarct locations and is associated with poorer prognosis, it is these patients who derive the most benefit. The benefits, in this case, clearly outweigh the risks.

Thrombolytic therapy should be initiated in appropriate candidates with symptoms of MI not >6 h and at least 20 to 30 min from onset of symptoms. On presentation, angina or anginal equivalent should not totally or near-totally resolve with 2 to 3 sublingual nitroglycerin tablets and there should be firm ECG evidence for infarction: at least 1 to 2 mm ST elevation in at least two contiguous leads.[62] Table 116-3 gives the relative and absolute contraindications to thrombolytic therapy.

Recommendations are less defined for initiation of thrombolytic therapy in patients with suspected infarction

TABLE 116-3 Contraindications to Thrombolytic Therapy

Absolute
Any active or recent bleeding other than menstruation
Intracranial neoplasm, AV malformation, or aneurysm
Stroke or neurosurgery within the past 6 months
Head trauma within 14 days
Relative
Major thoracic or abdominal surgery within 10 days
Diabetic retinopathy
Pregnancy
Coagulation disorders
Bacterial endocarditis
Uncontrolled hypertension (above 200/110 mmHg)
Prolonged or traumatic cardiopulmonary resuscitation

Adapted from Goldhaber SZ, Braunwald E: In Braunwald E (ed): *Heart Disease* Philadelphia, Saunders, 1988, p 1588.

but without classic ST segment elevation, with ST depression, or where ECG changes are diffuse or nonspecific. ST segment depression may be indicative of nontransmural ischemia or necrosis, which may evolve into the so-called non-q wave infarction. Alternatively, ST segment depression may represent occlusion of the left circumflex artery or posterior branches of the right coronary artery which supply regions of myocardium which are relatively electrically silent on the standard 12-lead ECG. As such, ST depression may, in fact, represent reciprocal changes of a region where there is true ST elevation. Placement of leads V_7 to V_{11} may be helpful under these circumstances.

It is also important to keep in mind that diffuse ST elevation may represent pericarditis, not infrequently seen in ICU patients, and diffuse ST depression or new nonspecific ST-T changes can be seen in dissecting anterior aneurysm of the aorta. In such circumstances, administration of thrombolytic agents can be catastrophic.[64] Therefore, where the clinical presentation has atypical features and the diagnosis of MI is in doubt, the performance of emergency echocardiography may be especially helpful. Ultimately, the decision to administer thrombolytic agents must be made on a clinical basis, weighing the risks and benefits.

PROTOCOL FOR TISSUE PLASMINOGEN ACTIVATOR AND STREPTOKINASE ADMINISTRATION

TISSUE PLASMINOGEN ACTIVATOR. A 10-mg bolus is given intravenously followed by 50 mg over the next hour by constant infusion. Then, 20 mg is administered in the second hour, and an additional 20 mg over the third hour, to a total of 100 mg over 3 h. Should significant bleeding or a dramatic change in mental status occur, the infusion should be stopped.

STREPTOKINASE. SK is administered over 1 h to a total of 1,500,000 U by constant infusion. As with TPA, should significant bleeding or mental status changes occur, the infusion should be stopped.

Since SK is derived from bacteria and is therefore potentially antigenic, its administration occasionally results in anaphylactic reactions that range from minor itching or chills to serious hypotension. For this reason, 100 mg hydrocortisone is commonly administered immediately prior to intravenous SK in an attempt to abort or ameliorate potential anaphylactic reactions. TPA does not cause anaphylactic reactions because it is synthesized by recombinant DNA techniques using the human genome.

ADJUNCTIVE THERAPY. A large clinical trial has documented the efficacy of the addition of a single dose of aspirin (160 mg) to a thrombolytic regimen.[49] Therefore, we recommend that 160 to 325 mg aspirin be started concomitantly with thrombolytic therapy. Afterward, 325 mg aspirin should be continued daily.

Heparin is usually initiated either concomitantly with thrombolytic therapy or after the infusion is completed.[61,49] It is ordinarily started as a bolus of 5000 to 10,000 U, followed by 1000 U/h by constant infusion; therapy is aimed at achieving an activated PTT of one and a half to two times control. It is continued for 3 to 7 days or until coronary angiography is performed.

The precise roles and timing of aspirin, heparin, and the combination of the two as adjunctive therapy with thrombolytic therapy in acute MI and in preventing reocclusion postthrombolytic therapy is currently being evaluated in large multicenter trials.

Additional benefit in mortality was reported when intravenous metoprolol was added to the TPA regimen in q wave infarcts.[53] Therefore, in the absence of contraindications, metoprolol should be initiated in concert with thrombolytic therapy according to the protocol previously given.

ANGIOPLASTY IN ACUTE MYOCARDIAL INFARCTION

The role of immediate PTCA in acute MI is controversial. The principal issue is whether emergency angiography and emergency PTCA of the infarct-related artery should be performed in place of treatment with a thrombolytic agent. Proponents of the "direct" angioplasty approach argue that the diagnosis of coronary occlusion is made definitively and that a reperfusion rate approaching 90 to 95 percent can be achieved, which is superior to the 70 to 80 percent reperfusion rate with TPA. Furthermore, with direct PTCA, the bleeding complications of thrombolytic therapy are avoided. Very importantly, PTCA can be feasibly performed in all MI patients, including those who are deemed inappropriate candidates for TPA.[52,64] In this regard, analysis of the reasons for withholding thrombolytic therapy in MI patients indicates that only 37 percent of patients presenting with an acute MI are considered appropriate candidates, given the present guidelines for thrombolytic therapy.[60,61]

Against the strategy of emergency PTCA in lieu of thrombolytic therapy is the higher incidence of abrupt reclosure of a coronary lesion subjected to PTCA, as opposed to thrombolysis.[62,65,66] As mentioned, acute thrombus formation is usually responsible for coronary occlusion and dilation of a lesion containing fresh thrombus that has not had sufficient time to organize leaves greater potential for rethrombosis. Additionally, it is argued that direct PTCA is impractical logistically, even in well-staffed and well-equipped centers. To be optimally effective and to compare favorably with thrombolytic therapy, resources and staff must be mobilized within a very few hours so that reperfusion can be established with speed comparable to that obtained with thrombolytic therapy.

Presently, we recommend that a thrombolytic agent and adjunctive therapy be administered initially to appropriate candidates. If hemodynamic instability ensues or there is refractory chest pain despite therapy, emergency cardiac catheterization and PTCA of the infarct-related vessel should be performed at the earliest possible time. If PTCA is not immediately available, an IABP should be placed until PTCA or CABG surgery is performed.

Patients presenting initially in cardiogenic shock are best managed with emergency PTCA if possible (vide infra). The mortality rate of cardiogenic shock is 80 to 100 percent if treated with conventional pharmacologic therapy alone, so it is important to ensure that reperfusion is established to preserve as much myocardium as possible. Moreover, these patients ordinarily require placement of multiple lines (e.g., transvenous pacemaker, PA catheter) and may suffer cardiac arrests requiring chest compression. The risk of untoward bleeding complications under these conditions is likely high if a thrombolytic agent is administered.

Evolving Myocardial Infarction

Once the period in which either revascularization of the infarct-related artery has been attempted or the period has passed in which tangible benefits are no longer obtainable (i.e., >6 h) the goal of treatment of acute MI is to monitor and prevent lethal ventricular arrhythmias and to prevent hemodynamic instability. Pharmacologic therapy initiated at first presentation should be continued.

We routinely place MI patients on an intravenous nitroglycerin drip beginning at a concentration of 20 μg/min. The dose is titrated upward every 5 to 15 min in increments of 10 to 20 μg/min to achieve a systolic blood pressure of approximately 95 to 110 mmHg or as high as needed (usually 400–600 μg/min maximum) to control recurrent episodes of angina. If angina recurs, intravenous boluses of 200 to 400 μg or 0.4 mg nitroglycerin sublingually may be given followed by increases in the nitroglycerin drip.

Calcium channel blockers may be continued or increased if angina recurs. Among these drugs, nifedipine and nicardipine have the most vasodilating effect and least cardiodepressant effect (see Table 116-2). Diltiazem and verapamil slow conduction in the AV node and therefore should be used cautiously in combination with β blockers and in inferior wall MIs, where vagal tone is exaggerated. Diltiazem can also depress the rate of sinus node discharge.

Diltiazem is the only calcium channel blocker that has been proven to have tangible benefits in the management of MI patients.[67] Its salutory effect appears to be limited to patients with non-q wave MIs, who do not have evidence of congestive heart failure.[68] It is given at a dose of 30 to 60 mg every 6 to 8 h.

Patients with extensive anterior wall MI are prone to formation of aneurysms of the left ventricle and formation of ventricular thrombi. Studies indicate that left ventricular thrombus develops in approximately 30 to 40 percent of anterior wall MIs; 10 to 15 percent of these embolize.[69,70] Left ventricular thrombi appear with highest frequency between the third and fourth day after MI, but can occur as long as 3 months later, as detected by serial echocardiographic studies. Because the appearance of left ventricular thrombi can vary widely, routine use of full anticoagulating doses of intravenous heparin has been advocated in extensive anterior wall MI. Although this recommendation is controversial,[71] in patients with no contraindications to heparin therapy, it is presently our practice to routinely anticoagulate patients with extensive anterior wall MI, even if a thrombus is not demonstrable by echocardiography. Heparin is continued for 7 days and oral coumadin is continued for several weeks thereafter.

ARRHYTHMIA MONITORING. A major purpose for admitting MI patients to the ICU is to monitor and prevent malignant arrhythmias. Ventricular extrasystoles are common after MI and are a manifestation of electrical instability of peri-infarct areas. The incidence of sustained ventricular tachycardia or fibrillation is highest within the first 3 to 4 h, but may occur at any time. Malignant ventricular arrhythmias may be heralded by frequent PVCs (>5 to 6/min), complex ectopy (couplets, multiform PVCs) and salvos of nonsustained ventricular tachycardia. However, malignant arrhythmia may occur suddenly without these preceding "warning" arrhythmias. Therefore, the prophylactic use of intravenous lidocaine has been advocated even in the absence of ectopy.[72] Other authors indicate that such an approach is not warranted since the potential of lidocaine toxicity is not trivial, and patients can be easily cardioverted in the ICU setting in any case. Nevertheless, we favor the prophylactic use of lidocaine in most patients especially in the first 6 h after MI.

In patients older than 70 years or in patients with severe congestive heart failure or liver dysfunction, the dose of lidocaine administered should be reduced since the incidence of toxicity is increased. In the ordinary patient, a loading dose of 50 to 100 mg should be administered, followed by a drip of 1 to 2 mg/min, depending on body weight. If complex ectopy persists, additional boluses may be given to a total of 220 mg, with concomitant adjustment in the drip, to a total of 4 mg/min. At maximal doses of lidocaine, residual ectopy may be tolerated, unless it is particularly frequent or if salvos of nonsustained ventricular tachycardia persist. In such cases, procainamide is added at a loading dose of 1000 mg at a rate of 20 to 50 mg/min followed by a drip of 1 to 4 mg/min. Procainamide is the initial drug of choice if there is coexisting ventricular tachycardia and sustained supraventricular tachycardia. Breakthrough ventricular tachycardia/fibrillation resistant to these drugs should be treated with bretylium, started at a 500-mg loading dose over 30 min followed by a 1 to 4 mg/min drip.

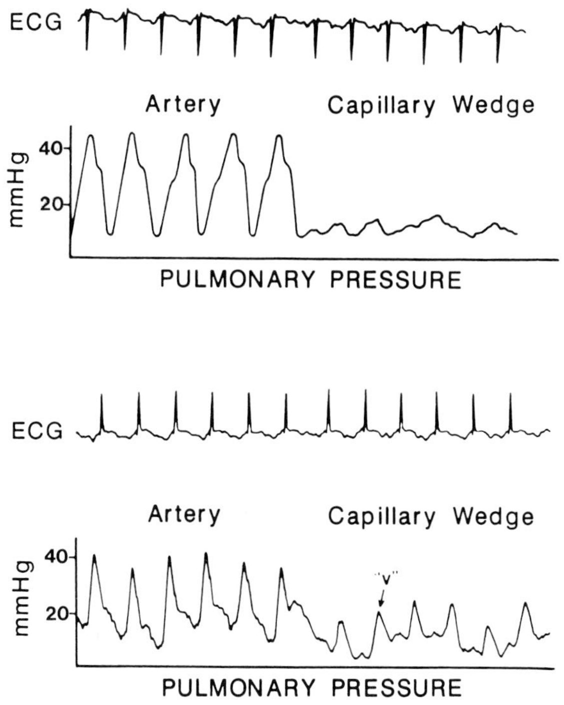

FIGURE 116-3 Pressure tracing obtained from a balloon-floatation catheter in a branch of the pulmonary artery and in the wedge position. *a*. Normal PCWP tracing. *b*. PCWP tracing in a patient with an inferior-posterior MI resulting in posterior papillary muscle dysfunction and attendant mitral regurgitation. Prominent *v* waves reflecting back pressure from regurgitant flow into the left atrium and pulmonary circuit are demonstrable.

Acidosis, hypoxemia, and hypokalemia should always be sought as causes of ectopy. Magnesium depletion is also a frequently overlooked cause of persistent ectopy.[73] It may occur especially in patients on diuretics. The serum magnesium level, even if it is within normal limits, may not reflect myocardial concentrations. We therefore administer 2 to 4 g $MgSO_4$ in divided doses over 24 h when ectopy is particularly difficult to eradicate, provided renal failure is not present.

Accelerated idioventricular rhythm, also called slow ventricular tachycardia, is frequently observed in the period after MI. It represents enhanced automaticity of a parasystolic focus and usually has a rate of 60 to 110 beats/min. This rhythm is ordinarily considered benign and will frequently resolve spontaneously. However, it occasionally can accelerate to frank ventricular tachycardia. Therefore, lidocaine is administered prophylactically when this arrhythmia persists.

HEMODYNAMIC MONITORING. Management of certain subsets of patients with acute MI is optimized by determining hemodynamic variables obtained by right heart catheterization via placement of a PA catheter. Several pieces of important information can be gleaned in complicated MI patients with hemodynamic instability by insertion of this catheter. By measurement of the mean pulmonary capillary wedge pressure (PCWP), $\dot{Q}_T$, and SVR, changes in left ventricular performance can be assessed as therapeutic interventions are made. It is important to have accurate, serial hemodynamic assessments of these patients since interventions based on erroneous clinical information may lead to further instability. The wave form of the PCWP tracing may reveal certain derangements of the left heart. For example, the presence of a prominent *v* wave suggests significant mitral regurgitation. A significant *v* wave is at least 10 mmHg above the mean PCWP (Fig. 116-3). A ventricular septal defect, mitral stenosis, or markedly decreased compliance state of the left ventricle may also produce *v* waves.

Right atrial and right ventricular pressures and waveforms determined on initial insertion can provide valuable diagnostic information when the diagnoses of cardiac tamponade or right ventricular infarction are entertained. Furthermore, right heart chamber hemoglobin O_2 saturation may be obtained when a complicating left-to-right shunt is a possibility, as in a ventricular septal defect.

In general, the placement of a PA catheter is indicated whenever hemodynamic instability is present that does not improve relatively quickly with simple therapeutic manuevers (e.g., saline bolus, intravenous loop diuretics, nitroglycerin). A PA catheter is indicated when pulmonary edema is suspected to be attributable to moderate or severely compromised left ventricular function or when intravenous inotropes or vasodilators for afterload reduction are used. It is also indicated to differentiate cardiac from pulmonary causes of hypoxemia and pulmonic infiltrates on chest x-ray. This is a frequent dilemma in ICU patients. PA catheters are not indicated in uncomplicated MIs or when minor pulmonary edema can be managed with small doses of diuretics and nitrates.

In cases where PA catheters are inserted, insertion of an arterial line is often necessary as well, but may be omitted if frequent and reliable systemic blood pressure readings can be obtained readily. Patients with significant hypoxemia or those on ventilators requiring frequent arterial blood-gas determinations may also require an arterial line to avoid multiple arterial sticks.

In 1967 Killip and Kimball[74] devised a classification of patients with acute MI based on the presence and extent of pulmonary rales and the presence of a third heart sound (Table 116-4). Not surprisingly, there was a progressively greater mortality rate as pulmonary congestion and left ventricular dysfunction supervened. However, with better and wider pharmacologic and interventional modalities available today, these data are probably outdated. This notwithstanding, the Killip classification can be used to guide the decision to insert a PA catheter. Clearly, class III and IV patients require PA catheters, while class I patients do not. Class II patients, if normotensive and not hypoxemic, should be managed with diuretics and nitroglycerin initially. If there is no appreciable response, if the clinical examination worsens or hemodynamic instability ensues, a PA catheter should be inserted to help guide further management.

TABLE 116-4 Killip Classification of Patients with Acute Myocardial Infarction

	Definition	Incidence (%)	Mortality (%)
Class I	No signs of failure	30–40	8
Class II	Mild to moderate failure (bibasilar) rales and S_3)	30–50	30
Class III	Frank pulmonary edema	5–20	44
Class IV	Cardiogenic shock	10	80–100

Adapted from Killip T, Kimball JT: Am J Cardiol 20:457, 1967.

Since many patients with acute MI will have received or are candidates for thrombolytic and intravenous heparin therapy, prudence should be exercised in deciding to perform central venipuncture or to place arterial lines. Should invasive monitoring be required nonetheless, it may be prudent to use insertion sites such as the brachial or femoral vessels, which are easily compressible should significant bleeding occur.

PHARMACOLOGIC SUPPORT FOR THE FAILING LEFT VENTRICLE

Overall treatment of the failing ventricle emphasizes reducing preload, decreasing afterload, and increasing cardiac contractility.

Treatment of low $\dot{Q}_T$ states complicating an MI is directed toward increasing forward flow by reducing afterload of the left ventricle. Afterload is a major determinant of left ventricular performance in normal and failing hearts and significant increases in stroke volume and $\dot{Q}_T$ can be accomplished with afterload reduction. Furthermore, afterload contributes to myocardial wall stress, a major determinant of myocardial O_2 consumption. Afterload reduction, therefore, can ameliorate residual myocardial ischemia, which by itself can improve left ventricular performance. Decreasing resistance to outflow is particularly beneficial in mitral regurgitation and ventricular septal defects. Preload reduction also relieves myocardial ischemia and pulmonary edema by decreasing left ventricular filling pressure. Therefore, by changing the loading conditions of the left ventricle, cardiac performance can be increased appreciably without resorting to positive inotropic intervention and without further requirement of the myocardium for oxygen.

NITRATES. Intravenous nitroglycerin is an ideal agent to use for both preload and afterload reduction. At low doses it preferentially relaxes venous capacitance vessels and thereby decreases preload. In many patients at higher doses it relaxes arterial smooth muscle as well, resulting in a decrease in SVR and afterload.[75] It is administered according to the protocol previously described to maintain a systolic blood pressure of 95 to 110 mmHg or to maintain a PCWP of 15 to 18 mmHg. In complex patients with adult respiratory distress syndrome or those who are mechanically ventilated on positive end-expiratory pressure, the PCWP may not faithfully reflect the filling pressure of the left ventricle. Optimal filling pressures under these circumstances are defined by titration of fluid challenges against observed $\dot{Q}_T$ and other indices of adequate perfusion. In a patient with persistently depressed $\dot{Q}_T$ but elevated SVR, careful additional titration of nitrates upward may lead to further afterload reduction and to an increase in $\dot{Q}_T$, without depressing blood pressure below the target value of 90 to 95 mmHg.

The other intravenous nitrate preparation is nitroprusside,[75] which is a more potent vasodilator than nitroglycerin. The disadvantage to using this agent over nitroglycerin is that because of its very potent vasodilating properties, it may produce a "coronary steal," i.e., it may cause diversion of blood flow from ischemic to nonischemic zones. Also, nitroprusside is metabolized to thiocyanate, a metabolic poison that can accumulate after 48 h of infusion leading to metabolic derangements and mental obtundation. Nevertheless, nitroprusside should be used if nitroglycerin at reasonably high doses (300 to 600 μg/min) does not produce desired hemodynamic effects in reducing SVR. Nitroprusside is started at 0.5 μg/kg/min and most patients respond to 2 μg/kg/min. If needed, one can use infusions as high as 10 μg/kg/min. Serum thiocyanate levels should be determined after 24 h and if found to exceed 10 mg/dL, nitroprusside should be discontinued.

DIURETICS. Pulmonary edema from an elevated PCWP is treated with an intravenous loop diuretic (furosemide, bumetanide, or ethacrynic acid). Diuretics also are used to maintain adequate urine output in low $\dot{Q}_T$ states. When furosemide or bumetanide at high doses (40 to 80 mg every 6 to 8 h for furosemide and 1 to 2 mg every 6 to 8 h for bumetanide) do not produce adequate diuresis, oral doses of metalozone (5 to 10 mg daily) are added or combinations of furosemide and ethacrynic acid or bumetanide and ethacrynic acid are tried. Since these agents also produce kaliuresis, hypokalemia should be expected and corrected with K^+ supplements. These agents also increase urinary excretion of magnesium. As noted, magnesium depletion can also be arrhythmogenic, and magnesium supplementation may be warranted.

It is important to remember that potent loop diuretics can increase urine output even when there is inadequate renal blood flow, so it must not be assumed that a brisk diuresis is evidence for improved hemodynamics.

INOTROPES. In addition to diuretics and vasodilators, intravenous inotropes may also be needed to augment $\dot{Q}_T$ in a damaged left ventricle. Dobutamine is predominantly a β_1 agonist that increases myocardial contractility.[77] It has minimal chronotropic properties and may produce modest decreases in SVR as well. Dobutamine is initiated at 5 μg/kg/min and may be increased to 10 to 20 μg/kg/min. Since adrenergic agonism can be arrhythmogenic, malignant ventricular arrhythmias may occur, in which case it should be discontinued or the dose decreased.

When urine output remains low or is marginal, low dose dopamine (2 to 5 μg/kg/min) may be used as an adjunct or in combination with dobutamine to augment renal blood flow and urine output. Dopamine at low doses exerts this effect by vasodilation of the renal vascular bed mediated by specific dopaminergic receptors.

An alternate inotropic agent is amrinone.[77] Because it increases intracellular cyclic adenosine monophosphate, amrinone also has relaxing effects on vascular smooth muscle and can produce a significant decrease in SVR. Amrinone is started with a loading dose of 0.75 mg/kg over 15 to 30 min, followed by constant infusion at 5 to 15 g/kg/mg. Amrinone can also produce ventricular arrhythmias, so close ECG monitoring is required. Elevation of liver transaminase levels and thrombocytopenia are also not uncommon, so routine serial blood tests should be performed.

Congestive heart failure refractory to either dobutamine alone or amrinone alone occasionally responds to both in combinations.[78]

DIGOXIN. The use of digoxin for congestive heart failure complicating acute MI is controversial. Digoxin produces only modest intropic effects, and its arrhythmogenic potential is not insignificant. Recent evidence, however, reaffirms its safety in acute MI.[79] Moreover, it is unequivocally beneficial in controlling ventricular rate in atrial fibrillation, which occurs approximately 10 to 15 percent of the time in acute MI. For control of ventricular rate in atrial fibrillation, digoxin may be loaded with 0.25 mg to 0.5 mg intravenously initially, followed by an additional 0.5 mg to 0.75 mg in divided doses in the next 24 h. For inotropic support, there is ordinarily no need to rapidly digitalize patients though the above regimen can be used for subacute severe heart failure. In most patients slow digitalization is reasonable using 0.25 mg intravenously every day. The dose should be adjusted if there is renal failure.

HYPOTENSION IN ACUTE MYOCARDIAL INFARCTION: THE USE OF PRESSORS

When MI is complicated by borderline hypotension (85 to 95 mmHg systolic pressures) that is not responsive to saline boluses or discontinuation of nitrates, it is advisable to attempt to elevate blood pressure first by augmenting forward $\dot{Q}_T$ with inotropes such as dobutamine. Administration of vasconstrictors under these circumstances will impose additional afterload on a myocardium that is already failing and may result in elevation of the PCWP and aggravation of pulmonary edema. This is of special consideration when there is significant preexisting mitral regurgitation since increased afterload can exacerbate regurgitation. The left ventricular filling pressure may fall when dobutamine is initiated so it is important to carefully maintain the PCWP at a sufficiently high level so that stroke volume and $\dot{Q}_T$ are optimal yet pulmonary edema is minimal. However, dobutamine may not increase blood pressure in many patients even with optimal left ventricular filling pressure and despite augmentation of $\dot{Q}_T$. Therefore, severe hypotension or hypotension unresponsive to dobutamine should be treated with high dose dopamine starting at 10 μg/kg/min; it may be titrated to as high as 20 μg/kg/min as needed to achieve a systolic blood pressure of 90 to 100 mmHg, so that perfusion to the coronary and systemic vascular beds is maintained. Hypotension refractory to dopamine is treated with norepinephrine starting at 2 to 4 μg/min and titrating upward as subsequently needed.

When systemic vasconstrictors are required to maintain blood pressure, the rationale for using nitrates for reducing afterload of the left ventricle is negated. However, nitroglycerin may still be used under these circumstances for vasodilation of ischemic coronary vascular beds and for reducing preload to relieve pulmonary edema. If high doses of pressors are needed to support blood pressure, serious consideration must be given for placement of an IABP in an effort to increase forward $\dot{Q}_T$ and reduce myocardial oxygen requirements.

CARDIOGENIC SHOCK

Cardiogenic shock is generally characterized by hypotension (<90 mmHg), depressed cardiac index (<2.2 L/min/m^2), elevated PCWP (>18 mmHg), a low urine output (<20 ml/h), and signs of hypoperfusion. These patients are typically hypoxemic from pulmonary edema and have peripheral manifestations of hypoperfusion such as cold, clammy skin that is pale and mottled. Unless hemodynamic decompensation can be relatively quickly reversed, this syndrome carries a mortality rate of 80 to 100 percent. Placement of an IABP is usually indicated in patients not responsive to pharmacologic therapy and in whom there is a potentially correctable lesion. Even though frank hypoxemia may not be present, we recommend that these patients be intubated early and placed on mechanical ventilation to relieve the work of breathing and spare that portion of the $\dot{Q}_T$ ordinarily distributed to the respiratory muscles. It is also important to optimize the oxygen-carrying capacity of the blood by maintaining the hematocrit to at least 35 percent and by raising the fraction inspired oxygen and Pa_{O_2} as required.

Encouragingly, a few recent retrospective reports indicate that emergency CABG surgery or PTCA reduces mortality substantially for patients who are revascularized within 24 h of symptoms onset.[80,81] Hemodynamic instability may not be present initially in some MI patients who ultimately slip into shock several hours to days after onset of infarction. Nevertheless, for patients presenting in shock or in patients with extensive anterior wall infarction in the early stages of instability, it is important to establish reperfusion of the infarct-related artery as quickly as possible. Accordingly, emergency angiography followed by either direct PTCA or emergency CABG surgery should be performed, provided these modalities can be initiated quickly. When time permits or if there is delay in mobilizing the appropriate staff and resources, an IABP should be inserted before transfer to the catheterization laboratory to stabilize the patient and to facilitate the catheterization procedure.

Where catheterization and PTCA or CABG surgery are not available, thrombolytic therapy should be instituted, even perhaps in patients who are at high risk for bleeding complications, since the alternative to no reperfusion is bleak. Before thrombolytic therapy is administered, attempts should be made to exclude causes of shock other than primary myocardial failure, e.g., tamponade, free wall rupture, ventricular septal defect, or rupture of a papillary muscle.

RIGHT VENTRICULAR INFARCTION

The right ventricle is involved to varying extents in inferior-posterior wall MI in about 30 percent of cases. Right ventricular infarction is characterized hemodynamically by an elevated right atrial pressure but a low to normal PCWP. The major hemodynamic derangement is poor contractility of the right ventricle, resulting in inadequate filling of the left ventricle and, therefore, depressed $\dot{Q}_T$.[82] There is also diminished right ventricular compliance or increased diastolic volume resulting in elevated right heart pressures as evidenced by jugular venous distention on physical examination. Tricuspid valve insufficiency from dysfunctional right ventricular papillary muscles is also a common feature.

Because the left heart filling pressures are low, there is ordinarily absence of pulmonary edema, despite jugular venous distention. A clear chest x-ray with jugular venous distention in the face of an inferior wall MI should lead to the suspicion of coexisting right ventricular infarct. The diagnosis is substantiated by demonstration of ST segment elevation in the right precordial leads (V_3R to V_5R). Two-dimensional echocardiography may reveal a dilated right ventricle with right ventricular wall motion abnormalities. A gated first-pass radionuclide angiogram may show a depressed right ventricular ejection fraction.

Administration of even small doses of nitroglycerin to these patients may further decrease preload possibly resulting in hypotension. Marginal hypotension in right ventricular infarct patients usually responds to augmentation of preload with boluses of saline solution. When hypotension exists that is unresponsive to fluid boluses, extensive damage to the inferior-posterior wall of the left ventricle is almost always present.

Treatment of right ventricular infarcts entails administration of fluid to satisfactorily fill the left ventricle. Nitroglycerin may be administered to control recurrent episodes of ischemia, but it should be administered in concert with fluid. Dobutamine is necessary to augment both right and left ventricular forward flow in instances when hypotension is present that is unresponsive to fluid boluses. Occasionally in severe hemodynamic compromise due to right and left ventricular infarction, afterload reduction of the left ventricle with an IABP may be required. With decreased compliance or increased volume of the damaged right ventricle, the contribution of atrial contraction to right ventricular filling assumes greater importance. Therefore, when transvenous pacing is required for a conduction disturbance (vide infra) dual chamber AV sequential pacing affords better right ventricular contraction than does single chamber pacing.

TABLE 116-5 Indications for Transvenous Pacing in Acute Myocardial Infarction

Third or second degree AV block (type I or type II) with slow ventricular response resulting in hemodynamic compromise unresponsive to atropine
Sinus or junctional bradycardia with hemodynamic compromise unresponsive to atropine
Third degree AV block in the presence of anterior-lateral MI
Alternating LBBB and RBBB
New bifascicular block
New RBBB
New first degree AV block + LBBB or RBBB (preexisting or new)
New first degree AV block + preexisting bifascicular block
Type II second degree AV block with wide complex QRS
Controversial indications
New LBBB
Third degree AV block or type II second degree AV block with narrow QRS escape in inferior wall MI that is tolerated well hemodynamically

Adapted from References 21, 22, and 83.

INDICATIONS FOR TEMPORARY PACING IN ACUTE MYOCARDIAL INFARCTION

Damage to the impulse formation and conduction system of the heart from MI can result in bradyarrhythmias and conduction disturbances that do not respond reliably to conventional pharmacologic agents such as atropine or isoproterenol. These disturbances may lead to further hemodynamic compromise and coronary hypoperfusion. Disturbances of conduction distal to the AV node and His bundle, as occurs in complete heart block with a ventricular escape rhythm, are particularly worrisome, even if they are tolerated well hemodynamically. Ventricular foci are unstable and unreliable; their discharge rate may be widely variable, with abrupt acceleration to ventricular tachycardia or deceleration to asystole. It is this characteristic of subsidiary ventricular pacemakers that guides the indication for prophylactic placement of temporary transvenous pacing in acute MI. Table 116-5 gives these indications, which are based on studies documenting the progression to high grade AV block when the indicated conduction disturbances are present. Any bradyarrhythmia unresponsive to atropine that results in hemodynamic compromise requires pacing. Pacing for a LBBB remains controversial because some studies indicate that progression to high grade block is high, while others do not.[83]

CASE PRESENTATION

A 74-year-old white man with a history of ankylosing spondylitis with severe kyphoscoliosis, congestive heart failure with mild to moderate aortic insufficiency, and chronic obstructive pulmonary disease was hospitalized for left upper lobe pneumonia. Sputum culture grew methicillin-resistant *Staphylococcus aureus*. Despite several days of intravenous vancomycin therapy, the patient's respiratory status worsened, and he became frankly hypoxemic requiring intubation and mechanical ventilation. Repeat chest x-ray revealed patchy infiltrates throughout the left lung, with a more localized area in the left upper lobe at the lateral border that was consistent with lung abscess. Sputum samples obtained after intubation were cultured and also grew methicillin-resistant *Staphylococcus.* Because the patient had deteriorated despite appropriate therapy and the lung abscess was located at the lateral lung margin, it was decided to drain the abscess. It was drained through the transthoracic approach and an indwelling drain was placed.

The patient's ICU course on mechanical ventilation was complicated by episodes of oxygen desaturation and hypercapnia thought to be attributed to exacerbation of bronchospastic disease. Additionally, there was accumulation of fluid in the lower extremities and presacral regions and evidence for increasing pulmonary vascular redistribution on serial upright chest x-rays. Administration of loop diuretics for developing heart failure resulted in diuresis but the patient had intermittent episodes of hypotension that would respond subsequently to intravenous saline boluses. Moreover, wheezing, hypercapnia, and O_2 desaturation did not resolve with diuresis. A PA catheter was placed for optimal fluid management and treatment of heart failure. Inhaled bronchodilator and steroid therapy was initiated to treat bronchospasm.

On several occasions, following inhaled bronchodilator therapy, the patient would complain of substernal chest tightness. The ECG showed sinus tachycardia with new 2 to 3 mm ST segment depression in V_4 to V_6 that would resolve with sublingual nitroglycerin tablets. He was given 1 inch of topical nitroglycerin ointment every 6 h. Despite discontinuation of inhaled bronchodilator therapy, he developed paroxysmal atrial flutter, with a ventricular rate of 160 that was accompanied by crushing substernal chest pain and a drop in blood pressure by 30 mmHg to 104/60. The patient was immediately electrically cardioverted to normal sinus rhythm, resulting in resolution of chest pain and restoration of blood pressure. Subsequently, the patient was given loading doses of digoxin and placed on intravenous procainamide to control future bouts of atrial flutter. Diltiazem at 60 mg every 6 h per nasogastric tube was added to the antianginal regimen.

The patient's pneumonia and respiratory status gradually improved with antibiotics, intravenous corticosteroids, and theophylline. During attempts at weaning him off the ventilator, the patient would become tachypneic and diaphoretic with evidence of O_2 desaturation by pulse oximetry. The PCWP was elevated during these episodes, and the bedside ECG monitor showed more pronounced ST segment depression and more frequent PVCs. Chest pain was inconsistent with the above findings. The nitrate regimen was changed and nifedipine was added, but episodes of O_2 desaturation during attempts at weaning persisted. It was felt that the anginal episodes refractory to medical therapy were preventing successful weaning off mechanical ventilation. It was decided, therefore, that coronary angiography would be performed to identify any lesions that would be conducive to angioplasty so that myocardial ischemia and associated left ventricular dysfunction during weaning could be alleviated.

Coronary angiography revealed a left dominant system with a 90 percent narrowing of the proximal to mid left circumflex artery, just distal to the take-off of the first obtuse marginal branch. The remaining vessels had insignificant disease. The circumflex lesion was successfully dilated using balloon angioplasty, and the patient was successfully weaned off mechanical ventilation several days afterward.

CASE DISCUSSION

This case demonstrates how myocardial ischemia can complicate the course and management of another medical illness in a critically ill patient. Tachycardia, induced by an adrenergic bronchodilator, precipitated anginal episodes; angina would subside with nitroglycerin or as the effect of the adrenergic agonist (tachycardia, inotropy) waned. Moreover, attempts at weaning off mechanical ventilation, which necessarily increases the work of breathing, further aggravated the imbalance of myocardial oxygen supply: demand, provoking myocardial ischemia as evidenced by associated ST segment depression and increased frequency of PVCs demonstrable on the bedside ECG monitor.

Left ventricular dysfunction resulting from myocardial ischemia is suggested by the transient elevation of the PCWP and attendant O_2 desaturation. Ischemia will produce reversible depression of both systolic and diastolic function of the left ventricle, resulting in significant elevations of LVEDP, as reflected by the PCWP. As the PCWP rose, the patient would have significant decreases in hemoglobin O_2 saturation, suggesting that transient pulmonary edema was compromising alveolar gas exchange.

Diltiazem was the calcium channel blocker initially chosen because it dilates coronary arterial smooth muscle, decreases AV nodal conduction, and slows the rate of sinus node firing. The latter properties of the drug account for the lack of development of reflex tachycardia seen with nifedipine. Thus, administration of diltiazem would not produce tachycardia-provoking ischemia and if atrial flutter were to redevelop diltiazem would slow the ventricular rate, in conjunction with digoxin. Although verapamil is more effective at slowing AV nodal conduction, it depresses left ventricular contractility more than does diltiazem.

The myocardial ischemia in the patient was refractory to maximal medical therapy. The only alternative was to perform a revascularization procedure, if this patient were to wean successfully from mechanical ventilation. However, the internist did not feel this patient would be an appropriate surgical candidate should CABG surgery be required. Nevertheless, the patient agreed to undergo PTCA without surgical backup.

References

1. Rutherford JD, Braunwald E, Cohn PF: Chronic ischemic heart disease, in Braunwald E (ed): *Heart Disease*. Philadelphia, Saunders, 1988, p 1317.
2. Sherman CT, Livrak, Grundfest W, et al: Coronary angioscopy in patients with unstable angina. N Engl J Med 315:913, 1986.
3. Oliva PB, Potts DE, Pluss RG: Coronary arterial spasm in Prinzmetal angina. Documentation by coronary arteriography. N Engl J Med 288:745, 1973.
4. Hurst JW: Atherosclerotic coronary heart disease: Historical bench marks, methods of study and clinical features, differential diagnosis and clinical spectrum, in Hurst JW (ed): *The Heart*. New York, McGraw-Hill, 1989, p 961.
5. Pasternak RC, Braunwald E, Sobel E: Acute myocardial infarction, in Braunwald E (ed): *Heart Disease*. Philadelphia, Saunders, 1988, p 1222.
6. Dressler W, Roesler H: High T waves in the earliest phase of infarction. Am Heart J 34:627, 1947.
7. Chou T: Myocardial infarction, injury and ischemia, in Chou T: *Electrocardiography in Clinical Practice*. 2d ed. New York, Grune & Stratton, 1986, p 147.
8. Spodick DH: Diagnostic electrocardiographic sequences in acute pericarditis. Significance of PR segment and PR vector changes. Circulation 48:575, 1973.
9. Pepine CJ: Silent myocardial ischemia: Definition, magnitude and scope of the problem. Cardiol Clin 4:577, 1986.
10. Kawanishi DT, Rahimtoola SH: Silent myocardial ischemia. Curr Prob Cardiol 12(9):515, 1987.
11. Maseri A: Role of coronary artery spasm in symptomatic and silent myocardial ischemia. J Am Coll Cardiol 9:249, 1987.
12. Uptan MT, Rerych SK, Newman GE, et al: Detection of abnormalities in left ventricular function during exercise before angina and ST segment depression. Circulation 62:340, 1980.
13. Sugishita Y, Kosek S, Matsuda M, et al: Dissociation between regional myocardial dysfunction and ECG changes during myocardial ischemia induced by exercise in patients with angina pectoris. Am Heart J 106:1, 1983.
14. Crawford MH, Mendoza CA, O'Rourke R, et al: Limitations of continuous ambulatory electrocardiogram monitoring for detecting coronary artery disease. Ann Intern Med 89:1, 1978.
15. Perloff JK. The recognition of strictly posterior myocardial infarction by conventional scalar electrocardiography. Circulation 30:706, 1964.
16. Crof CH, Nicod P, Corbett JR, et al: Detection of acute right ventricular infarction by right precordial electrocardiography. Am J Cardiol 50:421, 1982.
17. Norris RM: Heart block in posterior and an anterior myocardial infarction. Br Heart J 31:352, 1969.
18. Anderson KR, Ho SY, Anderson RH: Location and vascular supply of the sinus node in human heart. Br Heart J 41:28, 1979.
19. Chou T: Atrioventricular block; concealed conduction, in Chou T: *Electrocardiography in Clinical Practise*. 2d ed. New York, Grune & Stratton, 1986 p 493.
20. Puech P: Atrioventricular block; the value of intracardiac recordings, in Kriker DM, Goodwen JF (eds): *Cardiac Arrhythmias: The Modern Electrophysiological Approach*. Phildadelphia, Saunders, 1975 p 81.
21. Hindman MC, Wagner GS, JaRo M, et al: The clinical significance of wide branch block complicating acute myocardial infarction. 1. Clinical characteristics, hospital mortality and one year follow-up. Circulation 58(4):679, 1978.
22. Hindman MC, Wagner GS, Jaro M, et al: The clinical significance of bundle branch block complicating acute myocardial infarction. 2. Indications for temporary and permanent pacemaker insertion. Circulation 58(4):689, 1978.
23. Lown B, Fakhro AM, Hood WB, et al: The coronary care unit: New perspectives and directions. JAMA 199:156, 1967.
24. Campbell RWF, Murray A, Julian DG: Relation of ventricular arrhythmias to ventricular fibrillation. Br Heart J 43:109, 1980.
25. Meltzer LE, Kitchell JB: The incidence of arrhythmias associated with acute myocardial infarction. Prog Cardiovasc Dis 9:50, 1966.
26. Rapaport E: Serum enzymes and isoenzymes in the diagnosis of acute myocardial infarction. Prog Cardiovasc Dis 46:43, 1977.
27. Lee TH, Goldman L: Serum enzyme assays in the diagnosis of acute myocardial infarction. Ann Intern Med 105:221, 1986.
28. Feigenbaum H, Corya BC, Dillon JC, et al: Role of echocardiography in patients with coronary artery disease. Am J Cardiol 37:775, 1976.
29. Feigenbaum H: Coronary artery disease, in Feigenbaum H: *Echocardiography*. 4th ed. Philadelphia, Lea & Febiger, 1986, p 462.
30. Parkey RW, Bonte FJ, Meyer SL, et al: A new method for radionuclide imaging of acute myocardial infarctions in humans. Circulation 50:540, 1974.
31. Massie BM, Botvinick EH, Werner JA, et al: Myocardial scintigraphy with technetium 99m stannous pyrophosphate: An insensitive test for nontransmural myocardial infarctions. Am J Cardiol 43:186, 1979.
32. Wackers FJ, Busemann-Sokole E, Samson G, et al: Value and limitations of thallium-201 scintigraphy in the acute phase of myocardial infarction. N Engl J Med 295:1, 1979.
33. Pohost GM, Alpert NA, Ingwall JS, et al: Thallium redistribution: Mechanism and clinical utility. Semin Nucl Med 10:70, 1980.
34. Gould KL: Noninvasive assessment of coronary stenosis by myocardial perfusion imaging during pharmacologic vasodilation. 1. Physiologic basis and experimental validation. Am J Cardiol 41:267, 1978.
35. Hecht HS, Mirell SG, Robert EL, et al: Left ventricular ejection fraction and segmental wall motion by peripheral first-pass radionuclide angiography. J Nucl Med 19:17, 1978.
36. Tobinick E, Schelbert HR, Henning H, et al: Right ventricular ejection fraction in patients with acute anterior and inferior myocardial infarction assessed by radionuclide angiography. Circulation 57:1078, 1978.
37. Cohn PF, Gorlin R: Physiologic and clinical actions of nitroglycerin. Med Clin North Am 58:407, 1974.
38. Gorlin R, Brachfeld N, Macleod C, Bopp P: Effect of nitroglycerin on the coronary circulation in patients with coronary artery disease or increased left ventricular work. Circulation 19:705, 1959.
39. Zelis R, Mansour EJ, Capone RJ, et al: The cardiovascular effects of morphine: The peripheral capacitance and resistance vessels in human subjects. J Clin Invest 54:1247, 1974.
40. Frishman WH: Multifactorial actions of beta-adrenergic blocking drugs in ischemic heart disease. Curr Concepts Circ 67(suppl):11, 1983.
41. Braunwald E: Unstable angina. A classification. Circulation 80:410, 1989.
42. Hurst JW: The recognition and treatment of four types of angina pectoris and angina equivalents, in Hurst JW: *The Heart*. New York, McGraw-Hill, 1989, p 1048.
43. Hillis LD, Braunwald E: Coronary artery spasm. N Engl J Med 299:695, 1978.

44. Epstein SE, Talbot TL: Dynamic coronary artery tone in precipitation, exacerbation and relief of angina pectoris. Am J Cardiol 48:797, 1981.
45. Mehta J, Conti CR: Calcium channel antagonists in the treatment of unstable angina. Am J Cardiol 50:919, 1982.
46. Lewis HD, Davis JW, Archibald DG, et al: Protective effects of aspirin against acute myocardial infarction and death in men with unstable angina: Results of a Veterans Administration Cooperative Study. N Engl J Med 309:396, 1983.
47. Cairns JA, Gent M, Singer J, et al: Aspirin, sulfinpyrazone, or both in unstable angina. N Engl J Med 313:1369, 1985.
48. Theroux P, Ouimet A, McCans J, et al: Aspirin, heparin, or both to treat acute unstable angina. N Engl J Med 319:1105, 1988.
49. ISIS-2 Collaborative Group: Randomized trial of intravenous streptokinase, oral aspirin, both, or neither among 17,187 cases of suspected acute myocardial infarction. Lancet ii:349, 1988.
50. Topol EJ, Kleinman NS, Joelson JM, et al: Tissue plasminogen activator for unstable angina pectoris. A multicenter, randomized, double blind placebo controlled trial. J Am Coll Cardiol 13:191A, 1989.
51. Murphy DA, Craver JM, Jones EL, et al: Surgical revascularization following unsuccessful percutaneous transluminal coronary angioplasty. J Thorac Cardiovasc Surg 84:342, 1982.
52. Holmes DR, Topol EJ: Reperfusion momentum: Lessons from the randomized trials of immediate coronary angioplasty for myocardial infarction. J Am Coll Cardiol 14(6):1572, 1989.
53. The TIMI Study Group. Comparison of intravenous and conservative strategies after treatment with intravenous tissue plasminogen activator in acute myocardial infarction: Result of the thrombolysis in myocardial infarction (TIMI) phase II trial. N Engl J Med 320:618, 1989.
54. Bolooki H: In *Clinical Application of Intra-aortic Balloon Pump*. Mount Kisco, NY, Futura, 1977.
55. Gewirtz H, Ohley W, William DO, et al: Effects of intra-aortic balloon counterpulsation on regional myocardial blood flow and oxygen consumption in the presence of coronary artery stenosis. Observation in an awake animal model. Am J Cardiol 50:829, 1982.
56. European Coronary Surgery Study Group. Prospective randomized study of coronary bypass surgery in stable angina pectoris. Lancet 2:491, 1980.
57. CASS Principal Investigators and Their Associates: Coronary artery surgery study (CASS): A randomized trial of coronary bypass surgery. Survival data. Circulation 68(5):939, 1983.
58. deZaan C, Bar FW, Janssen JHA, et al: Angiographic and clinical characteristics of patients with unstable angina showing an ECG pattern indicating critical narrowing of the proximal LAD coronary artery. Am Heart J 117(3):657, 1989.
59. The MIAMI Trial Research Group: Metoprolol in acute myocardial infarction: A randomized placebo-controlled international trial. Eur Heart J 6:199, 1985.
60. The ASSET Study Group. Trial of tissue plasminogen activator for mortality reduction in acute myocardial infarction. Lancet ii:525, 1988.
61. Gruppo Italiano per lo Studio della streptochinasi nell' Infarto Miocardico (GISSI): Effectiveness of intravenous thrombolytic treatment in acute myocardial infarction. Lancet ii:397, 1986.
62. The TIMI Study Group. The thrombolysis in myocardial infarction (TIMI) trial. N Engl J Med 312:932, 1985.
63. Blankenship JC, Almquist AK: Cardiovascular complications of thrombolytic therapy in patients with a mistaken diagnosis of acute myocardial infarction. J Am Coll Cardiol 14:1579, 1989.
64. O'Keefe JH, Rutherford BD, McConahay DR, et al: Early and late results of coronary angioplasty without antecedent thrombolytic therapy of acute myocardial infarction. Am J Cardiol 64(19):1221, 1989.
65. The TIMI Research Group. Immediate vs delayed catheterization and angioplasty following thrombolytic therapy for acute myocardial infarction. TIMI II A results. JAMA 260:2849, 1988.
66. Topol EJ, Califf RM, George BS, et al: A randomized trial of immediate vs delayed elective angioplasty often intravenous tissue plasminogen activator in acute myocardial infarction. N Engl J Med 317:581, 1987.
67. Gibson RS, Boden WE, Theroux P, et al: Diltiazem and reinfarction in patients with non Q wave myocardial infarction. N Engl J Med 315:423, 1986.
68. The Multicenter Diltiazem Post Infarction Trial Research Group. The effect of diltiazem on mortality and reinfarction after myocardial infarction. N Engl J Med 319:385, 1988.
69. Chesebro JL, Fuster V: Antithrombotic therapy for acute myocardial infarction: Mechanism and prevention of deep venous, left ventricular, and coronary artery thromboembolism. Circulation 74(suppl III):III-1-10, 1986.
70. Meltzer RS, Visser CA, Fuster V: Intracardiac thrombi and systemic embolization. Ann Intern Med 104:689, 1986.
71. Nihoyannopoulos P, Smith GC, Maseri A, Foale RA: The natural history of left ventricular thrombus in myocardial infarction: A rationale in support of masterly inactivity. J Am Coll Cardiol 14(4):903, 1989.
72. Lie KL, Wellens HJ, VanCapelli FJ: Lidocaine in the prevention of primary ventricular fibrillation. A double blind randomized study of 212 consecutive patients. N Engl J Med 291:1324, 1974.
73. Lauler DP, et al: A symposium: Magnesium deficiency—pathogenesis and strategies for repletion. Am J Cardiol 63(14):1G–45G, 1989.
74. Killip T, Kimball JT: Treatment of myocardial infarction in a coronary care unit. A two year experience with 250 patients. Am J Cardiol 20:457, 1967.
75. Chiariello M, Gold HK, Leinbach RC, et al: Comparison between the effects of nitroprusside and nitroglycerin on ischemic injury during acute myocardial infarction. Circulation 54:766, 1976.
76. Sonnenblick EH, Frishman WH, LeJemtel TH: Dobutamine: A new synthetic cardioactive sympathetic amine. N Engl J Med 300:17, 1979.
77. Alousi AA, Farah AE, Lesher GY, et al: Cardiotonic activity of amrinone. Circ Res 45:666, 1979.
78. Gage J, Rutman H, Lucido D, LeJemtel T: Additive effects of dobutamine and amrinone on myocardial contractility and ventricular performance in patients with severe heart failure. Circulation 74(2):367, 1986.
79. Muller JE, Turi PH, Stone RE, et al: Digoxin therapy and mortality after myocardial infarction. N Engl J Med 314(5):265, 1986.
80. Lee L, Bates ER, Pitt B, et al: Percutaneous transluminal angioplasty improves survival in acute myocardial infarction complicated by cardiogenic shock. Circulation 78:1345, 1988.
81. DeWood MA, Notske RN, Hensley MD, et al: Intra-aortic balloon counterpulsation with and without reperfusion for myocardial infarction shock. Circulation 61:1105, 1980.
82. Iqbal MZ, Liebson PR, Messer JV: Right ventricular infarct. Cardiovasc Rev Rep 1(9):693, 1980.
83. Codini MA: Conduction disturbances in acute myocardial infarction: The use of pacemaker therapy. Clin Prog Pacing Electrophysiol 1(2):142, 1983.

Chapter 117

CRITICAL ILLNESS DUE TO PULMONARY HYPERTENSION AND COR PULMONALE

KENNETH W. PRESBERG
L.D.H. WOOD

KEY POINTS

- *Pulmonary hypertension (PH) occurs late in the course of diverse disease processes when signs of cor pulmonale (CP) are already present; in the ICU, early recognition of PH and CP prevents untoward effects of therapy intended for more common forms of cardiopulmonary failure.*
- *Bedside two-dimensional echocardiography with color-aided Doppler is the most helpful noninvasive evaluation for early, accurate diagnosis of PH and CP; pulmonary artery catheterization affords accurate serial pressure and flow measurement for titration of therapy.*
- *Hypoxic pulmonary vasoconstriction is a reversible contributor to PH due to chronic lung disease; such patients should be evaluated for nocturnal desaturation and sleep-disordered breathing (SDB), because acute or long-term oxygen therapy (LTOT) reduces PH and mortality in this population.*
- *In acute on chronic respiratory failure, correction of hypoxemia and conventional treatment of the exacerbation will reduce pulmonary artery pressure (Ppa) and vascular resistance (PVR) and increase oxygen delivery ($\dot{Q}_{O_2}$); vasodilator therapy can increase cardiac output ($\dot{Q}_T$) and $\dot{Q}_{O_2}$ and decrease PVR in patients on LTOT.*
- *Accurate recognition of chronic major vessel thromboembolism is important because thromboendarterectomy can result in dramatic improvement in those patients who are candidates for surgery.*
- *Left ventricular (LV) dysfunction is common in progressive systemic sclerosis, mixed connective tissue disease, and SDB; however, empirical diuresis and vasodilator therapy for LV dysfunction may precipitate relative hypovolemic hypotension despite high right atrial pressure (Pra) in these patients.*
- *Therapy for acute hemodynamic decompensation requires early correction and prevention of hypoxemia and titration to an optimal circulating volume; if the patient remains hypotensive, dobutamine (5 to 10 μg/kg · min) is the preferred inotropic agent, followed as needed by norepinephrine (1 to 5 μg/min) to increase mean systemic blood pressure (BP) and right coronary perfusion.*
- *Short-acting pulmonary vasodilator therapy can then be considered to reduce RV afterload and increase $\dot{Q}_T$, with pulmonary and systemic arterial catheterization to confirm benefits and to minimize the risk of aggravating systemic hypotension; nitroprusside, isoproterenol, PGE_1, and prostacyclin have been effective in this context.*
- *Supraventricular arrhythmias occur often in this patient population; in the hemodynamically compromised individual expeditious cardioversion is warranted, while short-acting antiarrhythmic agents can be used in less emergent conditions.*
- *Preoperative assessment of the patient with PH provides accurate hemodynamic assessment and optimization, which continues throughout the perioperative period; anesthetics that risk cardiac depression or venodilation must be avoided.*

Pulmonary hypertension (PH) is diagnosed when mean pulmonary artery pressure (Ppa) is >18 mmHg with normal or reduced pulmonary blood flow ($\dot{Q}_T$); the pressure difference between Ppa and the pulmonary wedge pressure (Ppw) should not exceed 9 mmHg, so the pulmonary vascular resistance (PVR) is normally below 2 mmHg/L/min.[1] Most PH can be attributed to vasoconstrictive or obstructive mechanisms secondary to chronic lung or cardiovascular diseases; a minority of patients present with idiopathic or primary pulmonary hypertension (PPH). As these mechanisms raise PVR and Ppa, the right ventricle (RV) dilates and its ejection fraction (RVEF) falls; when chronically exposed to these increased loads, the dilated RV undergoes hypertrophy, systemic venous pressure increases, and a diagnosis of cor pulmonale (CP) or pulmonary heart disease is made. Heart rate often increases as RVEF and stroke volume fall, and hypotension and shock can develop at high right atrial pressure (Pra) because of increasing RV afterload or RV ischemia.

In the ICU, PH often presents as an associated finding during the evaluation and critical care of an exacerbation of the underlying chronic airflow obstruction (Chap. 129), restrictive disease of the lung or chest wall (Chap. 132), or thromboembolic disease (Chap. 118); not infrequently, a diagnostic search reveals a reversible component of sleep-disordered breathing (SDB) or nocturnal desaturation (Chap. 135). Beyond treating the underlying diseases as described in more detail in the other chapters cited above, the intensivist uses oxygen therapy[2] (Chap. 11) and pulmonary vasodilators[3] to reduce PVR. Yet acute therapeutic reduction of PVR confers only a modest improvement on the poor survival of patients with PH and CP, so stabilization should be viewed as a guide to long-term therapy (favorable acute responses of PVR to O_2 or vasodilators predict better long-term benefits) or as a bridge to heart-lung or lung transplantation. In the ICU, early diagnosis of PH and CP permits effective therapy of the hypoperfusion state; too often, other treatments intended for more common causes of cardiopulmonary failure (see Chaps. 114 through 116) aggravate the acute deterioration of these patients. Accordingly, this chapter reviews the pathophysiology, diagnosis, and treatment of PH and CP with a focus on the ICU presentation.

Clinical Presentation and Diagnosis of Pulmonary Hypertension

SYMPTOMS OF PULMONARY HYPERTENSION

Patients can remain relatively asymptomatic with severe elevations in Ppa, so they often present to medical attention late in their disease. Many patients with New York Heart Association functional class III or IV status secondary to PPH have mean Ppa values >50 mmHg.[3,4] Breathlessness and fatigue are the most common limiting symptoms at presentation and can be progressive and severely disturbing to patients' life-styles. Syncope and near-syncope, presumably associated with a low cardiac output state, can plague some patients and can lead to accidents and severe personal injury. Sudden death is also not uncommon in these disorders. Chest pain (which can be anginal in nature), palpitations, and leg edema are also common. Hemoptysis can occur but is usually not massive nor a cause of respiratory compromise by itself. Hoarseness can be a presenting sign as well, secondary to compression of the recurrent laryngeal nerve from an enlarged pulmonary artery. Admissions to the hospital are often precipitated by progression of breathlessness, severe exertional limitation, and marked increases in lower extremity edema. Syncope and other symptoms attributable to hypotension are the most alarming and warrant immediate evaluation. These symptoms are not specific for PH and can be related to other diseases such as obstructive airway disease, left heart failure, and cardiac arrhythmia; accordingly, these disorders must be excluded or evaluated and treated while the diagnosis of PH is pursued.

PHYSICAL SIGNS IN PULMONARY HYPERTENSION

Few findings attributable to PH exist early in the disease process. They are evident in patients with advanced disease or CP who require treatment in the ICU; often, these signs provide the first clues to the existence of PH and CP in a patient without these diagnoses previously established. Absence of these signs cannot rule out PH because they are not sufficiently sensitive. Cardiac examination reveals a narrowly split S_2 with an accentuated P_2 component heard in the "pulmonic area" (left second parasternal intercostal space). The S_2 may later widen and remain fixed when RV dilation develops. This auscultation finding can be accompanied by a pulmonary artery pulsation in the same area. A diastolic murmur in the "pulmonic area" can occur secondary to pulmonary regurgitation associated with a dilated proximal pulmonary artery from increased RV systolic pressure pulsation. This finding has been associated with more severe elevations in Ppa in patients with PPH.[4] An S_4 heard at the left lower parasternal area that increases with inspiration ("right-sided S_4") can also be discerned occasionally. Flow murmurs heard over the lung fields during breath-holding can indicate pulmonary vascular obstruction secondary to chronic major vessel thromboembolism. This has been suggested to be a fairly specific finding when distinguishing chronic major vessel thromboembolism as the cause of severe PH from conditions such as PPH.[5]

The diagnosis of cor pulmonale, or pulmonary heart disease, is usually applied once the right heart and systemic circulation adaptations to PH become clinically apparent. In addition to the signs of PH, other cardiac signs include elevated jugular venous *a* waves when Pra is elevated. An accentuated jugular venous *v* wave, a pulsatile liver, and a holosystolic murmur (best heard at the left lower sternal border radiating to the apex and increasing with inspiration) are a triad of signs indicating tricuspid regurgitation (TR). An S_3 in the same area that may also increase with inspiration indicates a dilated RV. Precordial palpation in the patient with CP can reveal a parasternal lift, which is suggestive of a hyperdynamic RV consistent with RV hypertrophy or an acutely dilated RV. Peripheral edema in CP is due to elevated systemic venous pressures. The systemic circulation undergoes adaptations to maintain venous return (VR) in the setting of elevated Pra by increasing systemic vascular volume and pressure. Marked bilateral peripheral edema in the absence of clear signs of left heart failure and pulmonary edema should alert the physician to the possible presence of isolated right heart failure or a hypoproteinemic state.

NONINVASIVE DIAGNOSIS OF PULMONARY HYPERTENSION

Bedside echocardiographic evaluation can confirm the diagnosis of PH and CP as well as guide treatment. In a study of patients with severe chronic obstructive pulmonary disease (COPD), the echocardiogram detected CP in 25 of 33 patients, whereas clinical criteria inclusive of physical examination, electrocardiography (ECG), and chest x-ray indicated the diagnosis in only 13.[6] Although radiographic and ECG findings of PH and CP are not uniformly present, these noninvasive techniques are readily obtainable and can help establish the diagnosis; however, they contribute less to assessing hemodynamic responses to therapy.

ECHOCARDIOGRAPHY FINDINGS (see Chap. 21). When pulmonary hypertension is severe, the RV is often dilated with paradoxical septal motion toward the LV cavity in diastole to reduce LV dimensions and compliance (see discussion of Fig. 2-5 in Chap. 2). When inferior vena cava dimensions are increased and lose their normal variation with respiration on the subxyphoid view, Pra was shown to exceed 15 mmHg.[7] Combined with an estimate of Pra, Doppler flow analysis allows accurate estimation of Ppa but depends on detectable TR and optimal placement of the sonographic transducer perpendicular to the regurgitant jet; color flow-aided Doppler techniques provide better prediction of pulmonary artery systolic pressures as compared to Doppler alone.[8] When TR exists (as in about 80 percent of patients with PH), the peak RV systolic pressure—which

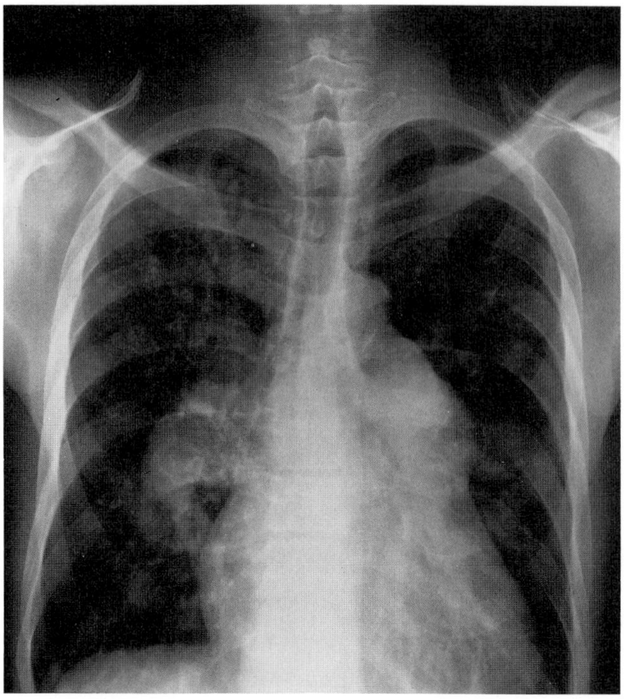

FIGURE 117-1 Posteroanterior chest x-ray from a 52-year-old man with a diagnosis of PPH. Note the markedly enlarged proximal right and left pulmonary arteries and prominent ascending and descending branches of the pulmonary arteries.

corresponds to the pulmonary artery systolic pressure—exceeds Pra by the value calculated from a modified Bernouilli equation; $\Delta P = 4v^2$, where v is the velocity of the regurgitant jet in m/s (see Chap. 21). Right ventricular hypertrophy (RVH) is diagnosed by increased wall thickness, and signals chronic PH (about 10 mmHg/mm RV wall thickness); failure to meet strict criteria for RVH in the setting of PH suggests an acute elevation in Ppa.

CHEST X-RAY. In PH the main pulmonary arteries can be enlarged and can be confused for hilar adenopathy or mass lesions (Fig. 117-1). The right descending branch of the pulmonary artery is often well visualized and should not have a diameter ≥ 16 mm. A greater diameter is a specific marker for PH in patients with COPD and pulmonary fibrosis.[9,10] Peripheral pruning of vessels in the outer lung fields suggests thrombosis or remodeling of the distal pulmonary arteries, which occur in chronic PH.[3] An enlarged azygous vein suggests elevated Pra. Right-sided chamber enlargement can be present with an enlarged cardiac silhouette encroaching on the retrosternal air space on lateral view. Evidence of primary lung disease on chest x-ray can help distinguish the cause of PH, but the quality of the anteroposterior (AP) portable film may limit accurate diagnosis. Careful review of prior posteroanterior and lateral films may disclose evidence of preexisting PH to help distinguish between acute or chronic PH in the acutely ill individual, and so guide diagnostic and therapeutic strategy. In critically ill patients, AP portable chest films with poor resolution may limit the diagnostic utility of these findings.

COMPUTED TOMOGRAPHY. Computed tomography (CT) can aid in the diagnosis of the etiology of PH. Conventional CT scans can provide useful information when mediastinal fibrosis or a mediastinal mass is causing pulmonary venous or other large pulmonary vessel obstruction. High resolution CT scanning can distinguish between various causes of interstitial fibrosis, and this technique can guide lung biopsy when indicated.[11]

ELECTROCARDIOGRAPHY. The ECG findings in PH and CP are discussed in detail in Chap. 30 and summarized in Table 117-1. ECG findings consistent with CP are present in 85 percent of patients with PPH; most of these patients remain in normal sinus rhythm.[3] These findings are present about 50 percent of the time in thromboembolic PH. Obesity (often present in SDB) and hyperinflation in COPD can obscure detection of RVH due to the physical interference to ventricular voltage determinations, rendering this test less sensitive for CP in these conditions. In a large series of patients with COPD, ECG criteria for RVH were present in only 33 percent of the patients who had RVH at autopsy.[9] Figure 117-2 is an ECG from a patient with PPH and CP and demonstrates many of the ECG abnormalities from Table 117-1. Supraventricular arrhythmias are common, and appropriate treatment necessitates accurate recognition of the arrhythmia, especially distinguishing multifocal atrial tachycardia (MAT) from other arrhythmias, and separating supraventricular tachycardia with aberrant conduction from ventricular arrhythmias (see Chaps. 30 and 120).

TABLE 117-1 Electrocardiographic Findings in Pulmonary Heart Disease

Finding (Significance)	Criteria
Right atrial enlargement	"P pulmonale" P wave axis > +70 Tall peaked P waves in limb and right chest leads; qR in V_1
Right ventricular hypertrophy (RVH)	Reversal of precordial pattern—R > S in V_1 and V_2; large S in V_5 or V_6
Severe RVH	RR′ pattern with R > R′ (not RBBB)
Right axis deviation; (RVH or acutely loaded right ventricle)	QRS axis > +90
$S_1Q_3T_3$ pattern (? pulmonary embolism)	S wave in I, Q wave in III and inverted T wave in III
Multifocal atrial tachycardia (MAT)	3 or more P wave morphologies in a single lead with varying PR, PP, RR intervals; Rate >100/min
Supraventricular tachycardia with abberant conduction	See Chap. 30

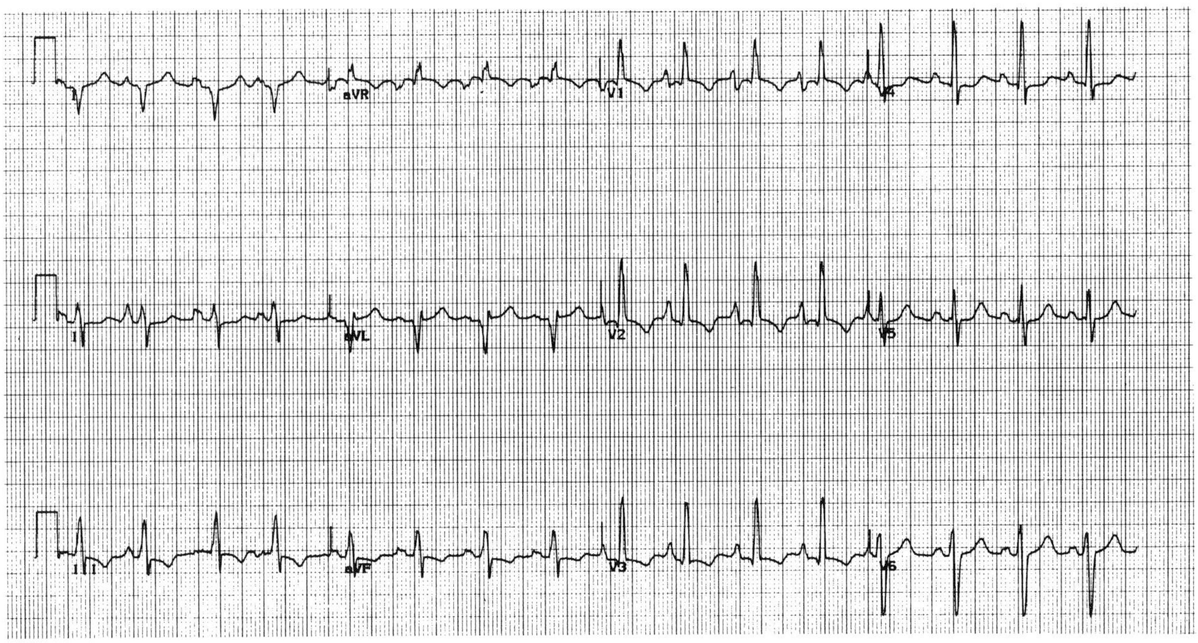

FIGURE 117-2 12-lead ECG from a 28-year-old black woman with PPH. Note the "notched" P waves in the chest leads and the qR in lead V_1 both indicative of right atrial enlargement; there is right axis deviation (ventricular axis = 166°) and severe RVH (R > S and RR′ with R > R′ in leads V_1 and V_2)

VENTILATION/PERFUSION ($\dot{V}/\dot{Q}$) SCANS. $\dot{V}/\dot{Q}$ scans can be obtained at bedside in many institutions to exclude pulmonary embolism in the critically ill patient; a normal scan excludes a large proximal embolus with reasonable certainty. There are very few other reasons to consider a $\dot{V}/\dot{Q}$ scan in the critically ill patient with PH. The deficit on perfusion scan in chronic major vessel thromboembolism often underestimates the degree of vascular obstruction seen on angiogram.[5] A high probability scan in patients with chronic PH is *not* a specific finding for pulmonary embolism and requires confirmation by angiogram before hazardous therapy is initiated or continued.[12] In PPH, $\dot{V}/\dot{Q}$ scans may reveal nonspecific, nonsegmental defects on perfusion scan, perhaps suggesting the microvascular thrombotic subtype of PPH.[4] The macroaggregated albumin or albumin microsphere medium used for perfusion scans has been implicated in the hemodynamic deterioration of patients with initial low flow states and minimal residual unobstructed pulmonary vasculature; with the precautions of using freshly prepared medium and a dose reduction to include no more than 150,000 particles, $\dot{V}/\dot{Q}$ scans are safe if indicated in PH.[12]

INVASIVE DIAGNOSTIC APPROACHES TO PH AND CP

RIGHT HEART CATHETERIZATION. Pressure and thermodilution $\dot{Q}_T$ measurements aid the initial assessment of the patient with suspected RV limitation of $\dot{Q}_T$ and BP, and allow titration of the hemodynamic response to therapy. Oxygen content analysis on traversing the right-sided chambers aids in excluding or locating left-to-right shunts in congenital or acquired septal defects, and provides arteriovenous O_2 content differences to aid evaluation of the hypoperfusion state. Frequently, the indication for right heart catheterization is to confirm or exclude PH as the cause of systemic hypotension in a patient with obviously increased Pra, so the differential diagnoses include myocardial infarction (including RV infarction) and cardiac tamponade (see discussions of Tables 2-2 and 2-3 in Chap. 2). Typical pressure values include high Pra, often with a large *v* wave indicating TR, with a corresponding elevation of RV diastolic pressure. Elevated pulmonary artery systolic pressures approximate RV systolic pressures except in the rare instances of pulmonic stenosis. The pulmonary artery pulse pressure (PP) is often much increased, associated with a diastolic pressure exceeding Ppw. As discussed in Chap. 2, both findings are attributed to the high PVR which impedes the normal transit of each stroke volume through the pulmonary vessels during systole; this necessitates diastolic flow (hence, the diastolic pressure drop between Ppa and Ppw), and causes abnormal systolic distention of the proximal pulmonary arteries (hence the large PP). Mean Ppa is often twice normal (12 to 16 mmHg) despite normal or reduced pulmonary blood flow, so PVR ($[\text{Ppa} - \text{Ppw}]/\dot{Q}_T$) is increased except when PH is due to LV dysfunction characterized by greatly increased Ppw. When the patient with increased PVR is able, a modest exercise test (lifting books in bed) frequently uncovers marked PH when $\dot{Q}_T$ increases slightly; this documentation of exercise PH (and the associated mixed venous O_2 desaturation) is helpful to compare with corresponding values after therapy.

In experienced hands, the complications of bleeding and pneumothorax from a central line placement are infrequent (see Chap. 25). However, in a patient with systemic hypotension and right heart failure these complications may be fatal if they cause further hemodynamic compromise, so a safer approach (brachial or femoral vein) should be considered. Pulmonary artery catheterization can be less than routine in these patients due to the dilated right heart, TR, and low flow state, which impair flow-directed placement of the catheter and maintenance of the catheter in the pulmonary artery. One should anticipate the need for fluoroscopy, aided by catheters with blind end channels for indwelling guide wires to facilitate fluoroscopic manipulation and to maintain the catheter in the correct position.[3] When the catheter cannot be maintained in the pulmonary artery, neither thermodilution nor Fick $\dot{Q}_T$ values are reliable; then $\dot{Q}_T$ can be measured using a thermistor-tipped femoral artery catheter to measure thermal or dye dilution after cold saline or cardiogreen is injected into the right atrium.

Left heart catherization is pursued in patients with PH who are suspected of having congenital heart defects or valvular lesions as the cause of pulmonary hypertension. Technical and diagnostic considerations are discussed in Chaps. 26, 87, and 122.

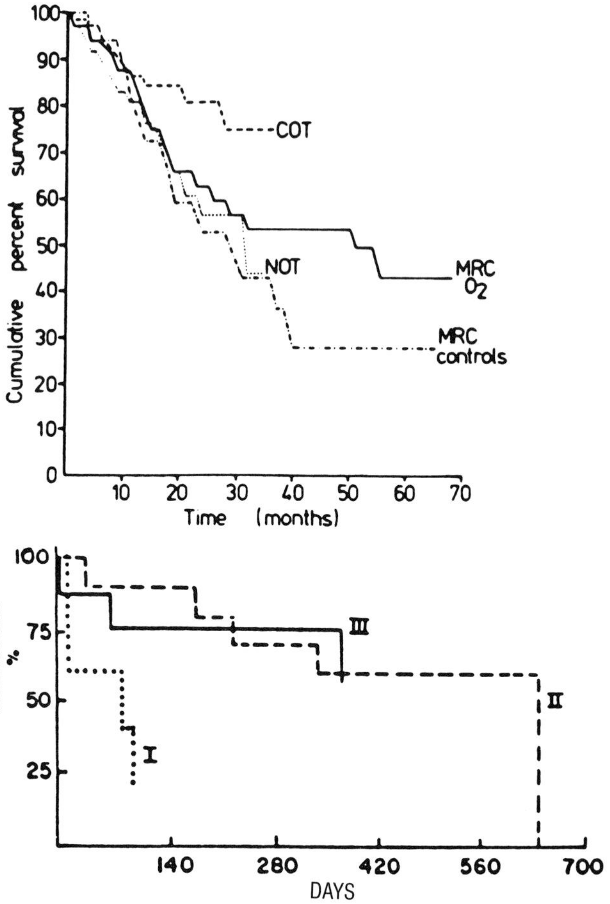

FIGURE 117-3 *Upper panel.* **Survival data for the Medical Research Council (MRC) and North American (NOT, COT) long-term oxygen therapy trials. Note that in the MRC study, patients receiving nocturnal oxygen therapy (NOT) had improved survival over controls receiving none. In the North American trial, patients receiving continuous oxygen therapy (COT) had improved survival over patients receiving only NOT. (From Flenley DC: Long-term home oxygen therapy. Chest 87:99, 1985, with permission)** *Lower panel.* **Correlation between acute response to vasodilators and longer term prognosis. Kaplan-Meier estimate of survival in patients with PPH. Group I: nonresponders; acute PVR response to nifedipine or hydralazine <20 percent reduction (n = 5). Group II: acute responders not given long-term vasodilators (n = 9). Group III: acute responders given long-term vasodilators (n = 9). In this randomized study, long-term vasodilator treatment did not alter survival. (Reproduced from Rich S, Brundage BH: The effect of vasodilator therapy on the clinical outcome of patients with primary pulmonary hypertension. Circulation 71:119, 1985, with permission)**

PULMONARY ANGIOGRAPHY. In the patient with apparent acute PH, or in a patient with known PH and an acute deterioration, pulmonary embolism is invariably suspected. In those patients being considered for thrombolysis, embolectomy, or thromboendarterectomy, pulmonary angiography is essential. When the patient is hypotensive, transport from the ICU to the radiology suite may not be prudent; in some institutions, better critical care is maintained by performing an urgent angiogram in the coronary care unit or in the cardiac catheterization laboratory. If the patient is in a marginal respiratory status, elective intubation and ventilation should be effected before the procedure.

A retrospective study identified patients predisposed to hemodynamic compromise from pulmonary arteriography as those with concomitant RV dysfunction and RV end-diastolic pressure (RVEDP) >20 mmHg; yet many patients with RVEDP values exceeding that "threshold" were studied without incident.[13] Selective angiograms can be accomplished without significant morbidity in patients with acute pulmonary embolism and PH; they have been accomplished without significant adverse effects in other patient populations with severe elevations in Ppa.[4] The safety of pulmonary angiography in this setting is discussed further in Chap. 118.

OPEN LUNG BIOPSY. Lung histology and analysis of pulmonary vascular pathology have been nonspecific in predicting pulmonary vasoreactivity or prognosis in patients with PPH, and open lung biopsy did not provide information that would guide vasoactive drug therapy in the patient with acute hemodynamic compromise.[14] By contrast, pulmonary vascular pathology has been used to determine operability in children with congenital heart disease and left-to-right shunts, by identifying those patients who are likely to experience pulmonary hypertensive crises postoperatively.[15] Lung histology may identify a progressive primary lung disease that may respond to steroids or other drug therapy (see Chap. 132). High resolution CT scanning now enables more accurate diagnosis of the various interstitial lung diseases and may provide sufficient diagnostic information by itself to guide empirical drug therapy or

TABLE 117-2 Chronic Disorders Associated with Pulmonary Hypertension

	PRIMARY MECHANISM OF PULMONARY HYPERTENSION	
Clinical Category	Vasoconstriction	Obstruction
Obstructive Airways Disease		
Emphysema	+	+
Chronic bronchitis	+	
Bronchiectasis	+	
Cystic fibrosis	+	
Thoracic Cage Deformities		
Kyphoscoliosis	+	
Thoracoplasty	+	
Hypoventilation Syndromes		
Neuromuscular diseases	+	
Obesity-hypoventilation syndrome	+	
Obstructive sleep apnea syndrome	+	
Interstitial Fibrosis		
Pneumoconioses	+	+
Sarcoidosis and other granulomatous diseases	+	+
Collagen vascular diseases	+	+
Idiopathic pulmonary fibrosis	+	+
Drug reactions		+
Radiation pneumonitis		+
Thromboembolism/Embolic Disease		
Pulmonary thromboembolism (chronic major vessel)		+
Sickle hemoglobinopathies		+
Foreign body emboli		+
Metastatic carcinoma (tumor embolism)		+
Cardiac Defects		
Congenital disorders with left-to-right shunts		+
Chronic mitral stenosis		+
Chronic Ambient Hypoxic Exposure		
High altitude pulmonary disease	+	
Idiopathic Disorders		
Primary pulmonary hypertension	?	+
Pulmonary venoocclusive disease	?	+
Portal hypertension states	?	+
Diffuse smooth muscle proliferation		+
Fibrosing mediastinitis		+

help disclose the optimal biopsy site.[11] The post thoracotomy changes of open lung biopsy do not exclude future transplantation in many centers[16] (see Chaps. 78 and 79).

Diseases Associated with Chronic Pulmonary Hypertension

Many of the *chronic* disease states associated with PH are listed in Table 117-2 according to familiar clinical categories, with the probable mechanism(s) of increased PVR indicated. Of these disorders, COPD, chronic thromboembolic PH and PPH provide much of the basis for the understanding of the pathophysiology of PH and right heart dysfunction, so many of the safety versus efficacy issues pertaining to the diagnostic and treatment approaches to these disorders are generalized from our knowledge of these diseases. Note that survival is quite short in these conditions and that O_2 therapy and pulmonary vasodilating agents can reduce PVR, associated with improved survival (Fig. 117-3).

CHRONIC OBSTRUCTIVE PULMONARY DISEASE

In patients with severe airflow obstruction, PH is common and is associated with worse prognosis.[9] RVEF is often reduced, though it does not vary inversely with Ppa and PVR as might be expected.[9,17] Decreases in RV function may also be secondary to hypoxemia, hypercapnia, and other factors such as increased intrathoracic pressures and LV dysfunction (see Chap. 115). Occasionally, Ppa and PVR can be elevated in these patients to the severe degree seen in PPH. However, most of the time the elevations in mean Ppa are mild to moderate (<40 mmHg), the resting $\dot{Q}_T$ is within the normal range, and $\dot{Q}_T$ can still be increased as required by exercise or during exacerbations of the COPD. Despite these apparent normal $\dot{Q}_T$ responses, the right-sided hemodynamics may be limiting, insofar as they preclude a sufficient increase in $\dot{Q}_T$ to effect the required oxygen delivery in the face of hypoxemia.[18] Factors that contribute to the development of PH in COPD have not been definitively identified with the exception of chronic hypoxia. Other factors include microvascular obliteration with progressive emphysema; intermittent increases in RV pressure load associated with exercise, exacerbations of respiratory failure, and increased intrathoracic pressure; hypoxemia (with and without Ppa elevation) associated with exercise; and nocturnal oxygen desaturation.

During exacerbations of COPD in patients with CP, Ppa and PVR increase during the acute phase of the illness with significant diminution during recovery.[9,17] Acute oxygen therapy has not consistently decreased Ppa and PVR, suggesting that other factors besides acute hypoxic pulmonary vasoconstriction (HPV) cause the rise in Ppa with exacerbations.[2,9,17] Patients with COPD receiving LTOT have increased survival (Fig. 117-3, *upper panel*). The acute hemodynamic response to 24 h of O_2 therapy predicts response to LTOT, for patients who reduced Ppa more than 5 mmHg had an 85 percent survival rate compared to 22 percent survival in nonresponders.[2] Such findings suggest that LTOT confers survival by ameliorating HPV and reducing PVR, but the improved survival could be due to effects other than the beneficial effect on pulmonary vascular hemodynamics.[2] Increased Ppa during the acute exacerbations of COPD may cause right heart dysfunction and decompensation—usually signalled by peripheral edema. Yet, $\dot{Q}_T$ is often higher in "decompensated" patients, and the edema may be attributed to appropriate increases in systemic venous pressure required to maintain $\dot{Q}_T$ despite increased Pra (see discussion of Fig. 2-12 in Chap. 2).

The abnormal resting $\dot{V}/\dot{Q}$ variance does not increase significantly during exercise, so most exercise desaturation in COPD is due to perfusion of lung units having low $\dot{V}/\dot{Q}$ with mixed venous blood having abnormally low O_2 saturation as a result of their $\dot{Q}_T$ increasing insufficiently for the increase in O_2 consumption.[19] Nocturnal oxygen desaturation may occur during rapid eye movement sleep and is due to hypoventilation and increased $\dot{V}/\dot{Q}$ mismatching in these patients;[2] values of mean Ppa at rest are significantly elevated in these patients versus other COPD patients with similar degrees of airways disease. In addition, the patients with nocturnal desaturation have more pronounced elevations in Ppa with exercise, suggesting that tone or remodeling of the pulmonary vasculature is more marked.[20] Accordingly, nocturnal desaturation may aggravate PH in COPD and should be treated aggressively.[2]

Digoxin in COPD and CP has only improved right heart function in those patients with coexistent left heart failure and is associated with an increase in toxicity in this patient population.[21] Vasodilator therapy has been tried with numerous agents including the newer prostaglandin derivatives; prostacyclin[22] and PGE_1[23] increased $\dot{Q}_T$ and decreased PVR in many patients, while hydralazine seems to be the most beneficial of the other agents tried.[9] Vasodilator therapy can be associated with worsening $\dot{V}/\dot{Q}$ matching and reduced Pa_{O_2} and oxygen delivery, so it should be restricted to those patients with COPD and cardiopulmonary failure whose $\dot{Q}_T$ is limited by right heart dysfunction after first-line therapy has failed, and whose arterial hypoxemia is easily corrected with O_2 therapy; even then, precautions to detect early adverse effects of systemic vasodilation and reduced right coronary perfusion are indicated (vide infra). Phlebotomy from a hematocrit of 61 to 50 percent was associated with a decrease in PVR in patients with COPD and CP, but $\dot{Q}_T$ remained the same and oxygen delivery fell; decreases in hematocrit below 50 percent did not result in any hemodynamic change.[24] Therefore, phlebotomy should be reserved for the rare patient with severe polycythemia whose $\dot{Q}_T$ is severely limited and who is not responsive to other therapy.

PULMONARY FIBROSIS

A correlation exists between the degree of restriction on pulmonary function testing and the development of PH (see Chap. 132). The elevation in Ppa and PVR is due to obliteration of the pulmonary microvasculature and remodeling of the residual vascular bed. The pulmonary vasculature changes are largely fixed, with vasoreactivity contributing only a minor part of the PH; yet many patients with pulmonary fibrosis show acute and chronic amelioration of PH with LTOT.[2] In pulmonary fibrosis, PH is predicted by a decrease in diffusing capacity below 45 percent of the predicted value.[10] Nevertheless, some of the diseases in this category, most notably progressive systemic sclerosis (PSS) and mixed connective tissue disease, often show a disparity between the pulmonary function abnormalities and the degree of PH, and primary pulmonary vascular pathologic changes have been described.[25] Diffusing capacity also predicts prognosis in patients with PSS with a very poor 5 year survival rate when the diffusing capacity is <40 percent predicted.[25] Isolated pulmonary vasculopathy occurs in the CREST variant of PSS, associated with a very poor prognosis.[25] Primary myocardial microvascular abnormalities and fibrosis also uniquely occur in PSS and can cause myocardial ischemia and dysfunction of the RV and LV. This myocardial abnormality is invariably associated with ECG abnormalities and perfusion defects on thallium 201 scanning; these perfusion defects may significantly reverse with nifedipine.[25] Sarcoidosis is not uncommonly associated with isolated decreases in diffusing capacity and the presence of PH out of proportion to the degree of lung fibrosis and restriction.[26] Therefore, the diffusing capacity and signs of PH need to be monitored along with other assessments of pulmonary function in these disorders. Exertional limitation and exercise desaturation are also common in these conditions and treatment with LTOT is strongly suggested for increased exertional tolerance and for prevention of CP.[2] The desaturation with exercise in patients with pulmonary fibrosis is due in large part to the RV limitation of increased $\dot{Q}_T$ with exercise; this causes a fall in mixed venous O_2 in blood perfusing lung units with very low $\dot{V}/\dot{Q}$ to cause most of the arterial desaturation, and to a lesser extent the desaturation is worsened by a small diffusion defect for lung O_2 transfer.[27]

Pulmonary fibrosis causes significant PH and CP late in the course of the disease, so steroids or other drug therapy are not expected to help acutely reverse a hemodynamically compromised state. Nevertheless, steroids are administered empirically in unstable patients with the relative risks, including infection. Vasodilator therapy has not been as extensively tested in these patients, but a significant response occurs in a minority of patients with advanced fibrosis; adverse effects also occur.[28,29] Hydralazine decreased PVR and increased $\dot{Q}_T$ without any change in Ppa in patients with mild elevations in Ppa and normal $\dot{Q}_T$; lung biopsy showed a preponderance of inflammation over fibrosis, so the effect vasodilation will have in the presence of more advanced disease and right heart failure is not known.[28,30] Short-acting vasodilators have been reported to effect vasodilation safely in some cases of secondary PH and hold promise for selecting those patients who may benefit from this therapy.[22]

THORACIC CAGE DEFORMITIES, NEUROMUSCULAR DISEASE, AND SLEEP-DISORDERED BREATHING

Chronic hypoxia secondary to hypoventilation and $\dot{V}/\dot{Q}$ mismatching stimulates HPV to cause PH in restrictive diseases of the thoracic cage[31] (see Chap. 132). Reactive narrowing may occur in the pulmonary vessels over years due to increased flow through the residual vasculature in those conditions with restriction or loss of part of the pulmonary vascular bed, analogous to the vascular narrowing observed in congenital left-to-right shunts. PH can be quite severe in these patients and can often approach the values seen in PPH (Case Presentation, vide infra).

Right heart dysfunction and PH complicate SDB, and are ameliorated in some patients with the correction of apneas and hypoxia[32] (see Chap. 135). Why some patients develop PH in this disorder is no more clear than in other disorders, but some authors have suggested the presence of significant obstructive lung disease and daytime hypoxemia may be key contributing factors.[33] Some patients are significantly hypoxic with hypercapnia during the day and remain so even after correction of obstructive apnea, and this chronic hypoxia can certainly predispose to the development of PH. Therefore, correction of chronic hypoxia and relief of intermittent hypoxia associated with obstructive or central apneas is the first order of therapy.[32] Systemic hypertension is prevalent in this population, and one should be cognizant of possible LV dysfunction on this basis.

THROMBOEMBOLIC DISEASES

Chronic major vessel thromboembolism can lead to PH; less often, other emboli associated with intravenous drug use, metastatic cancer, sickle hemoglobinopathies, and shistosomiasis cause PH. The first disease has received much attention due to the dramatic response to thromboendarterectomy that occurs in most patients who survive the perioperative period.[5] This is not a common disorder since most patients who survive acute pulmonary embolus go on to resolve the embolus. Most patients present with severe exertional limitation along with severe PH and right heart dysfunction. These limiting symptoms often follow a prolonged asymptomatic period subsequent to a retrospectively recalled event suggesting past pulmonary embolism. Physical examination reveals changes consistent with PH and right heart dilation, but also may reveal flow murmurs over the lung fields. These murmurs are reported as high pitched in character and increased with inspiration and may be specific to this disease. Distinguishing diagnostic evaluations include the invariable presence of an abnormal $\dot{V}/\dot{Q}$ scan, so a normal or low probability scan nearly excludes this diagnosis.[5] Pulmonary angiography is essential and often shows significantly more obstruction than that suggested by perfusion scan and permits distinguishing new emboli from chronic unresolved thromboemboli. Pulmonary angioscopy and ultrafast CT scan have also been used to further define the extent of the obstruction prior to surgical intervention. Those lesions amenable to surgical correction with a thromboendarterectomy include lesions of the main, lobar, and segmental arteries. Perioperative mortality is now reported at 12 percent, but survivors of the operation have early functional improvement and most go on to resume normal activities. Anticoagulation prevents recurrent emboli but does not help resolve the well-formed chronic thromboembolus; thrombolytic therapy is, therefore, not useful in this disease either.

Acute pulmonary embolism is discussed in detail in Chap. 118, but several points are worth reinforcing here: early accurate and safe diagnosis and institution of specific therapy is the goal—$\dot{V}/\dot{Q}$ scan and pulmonary angiography are the diagnostic tests, and the risks and benefits of these procedures are discussed above and in Chap. 118; prognosis is good in those patients who survive the acute event and have adequate therapy initiated promptly; early empirical anticoagulation is usually safe, but in those instances where anticoagulation is contraindicated, there should be a low threshold for placement of an inferior vena caval filter; and low dose heparin reduces the risk of pulmonary embolism in patients in the ICU.[34] Adequate control of the circulation and respiration are imperative before the patient is transported from the ICU for an angiogram. Management of hypotension and RV strain from massive pulmonary embolism may be guided by observations in canine models of autologous clot emboli. Hydralazine and isoproterenol decreased Ppa.[35] By contrast, no effect on pulmonary hemodynamics was seen with PGE_1.[36] Thrombolysis is sufficiently risky that it should be reserved for those patients with massive documented embolism who are showing persistent hypoperfusion. Thrombolyisis in this context has been seen to afford hemodynamic improvement, but without documented improved survival in treated patients.[37]

CONGENITAL HEART DISEASES ASSOCIATED WITH LEFT-TO-RIGHT SHUNTS

Patent ductus arteriosus, ventricular septal defect, and atrial septal defect of both the primum and secundum type are the most common causes of pulmonary vascular abnormalities, and the atrial septal defect of the secundum type is the most common of these that can present in adulthood. Surgery is the therapy of choice and early correction affords the best prevention of pulmonary vascular abnormalities that, when severe, preclude surgical correction. Echocardiography with Doppler and agitated saline can provide useful diagnostic information (see Chap. 21). Pulmonary artery catheterization with oxygen content analysis on passing the catheter through the right atrium and RV can detect an oxygen "step-up" suggestive of a septal defect, which can be confirmed by angiography. A recent review discussed the potential mechanisms for the development of PH in these disorders and the diagnostic approach and decision process for surgical correction.[15] After surgical correction these patients may develop a pulmonary hypertensive crisis.

Pulmonary hypertensive crises occur more often after surgery in those patients with more advanced pulmonary vascular changes. The exact etiology is unknown but the interaction between vascular endothelium and circulating blood elements after bypass with hypothermia is postulated to release potent vasoconstrictors derived from eicosanoids.[15] Therapy includes supranormal oxygen, hyperventilation (P_{CO_2} to 25 to 30 mmHg), and vasodilators if needed. Effective pulmonary vasodilation in this condition has been accomplished with prostaglandins PGE_1 and PGI_2 and, previously with the α-adrenergic blocking agent, tolazoline. This latter agent, though, has a number of reported significant side effects. High dose PGE_1 in combination with high dose norepinephrine infusion (to offset the systemic vasodilator effects of PGE_1) was successful in reversing life-threatening pulmonary hypertension and right

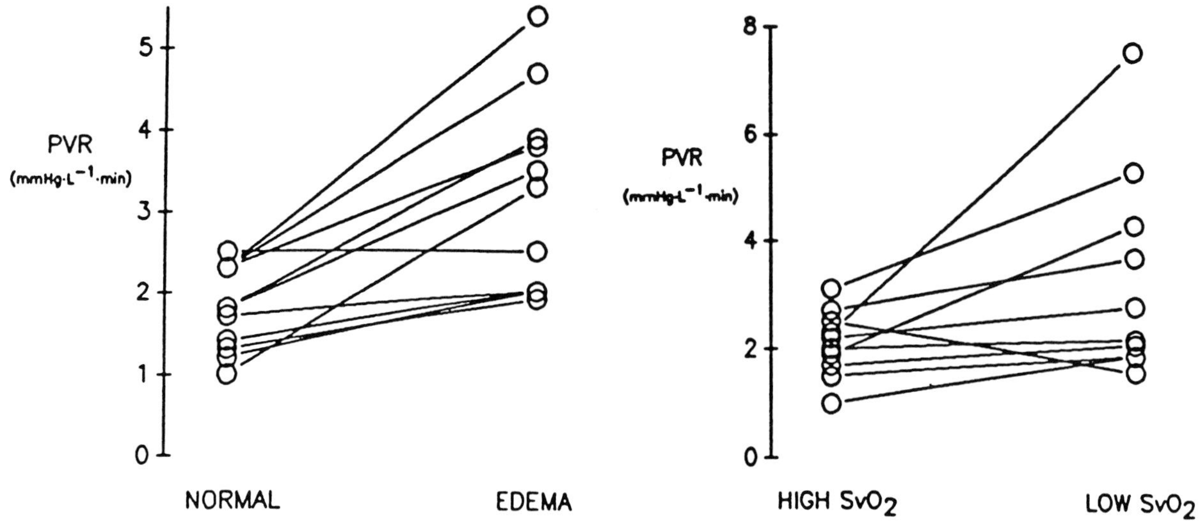

FIGURE 117-4 Acute pulmonary edema induced by oleic acid in 10 dogs increases PVR *(left panel)*, but perfusing the same edematous lungs with ECMO-oxygenated blood (Sv_{O_2} = 90%) returned PVR to the preedema level *(right panel)*. To the extent that these data can be extrapolated to the clinical arena, they suggest that most PH in the early exudative phase of ARDS is due to mixed venous hypoxic pulmonary vasoconstriction, explaining why vasoactive drugs or increased Sv_{O_2} reduces PVR in ARDS. (Reproduced from Reference 40, with permission)

heart failure in five consecutive patients in the immediate postbypass period after mitral valve replacement.[38] There was substantial improvement in the $\dot{Q}_T$ along with a decease in PVR with this therapy and no significant change occurred in the systemic blood pressure. Patients with preoperative PH or congestive heart failure (CHF) are reported to be the most prone to this crisis. PGE_1 has also been very useful in the relief of PH and RV dysfunction in the postcardiac transplant patient.[39]

ADULT RESPIRATORY DISTRESS SYNDROME (ARDS)

In the early exudative phase of ARDS, PH is mild and rarely limits $\dot{Q}_T$. In canine models of acute pulmonary vascular leak, most of the increase in PVR is abolished by perfusing the edematous lungs with fully oxygenated blood (Fig. 117-4), suggesting that HPV is responsible for the PH.[40] Positive end-expiratory pressure (PEEP) also reduces PVR in edematous lungs, perhaps by oxygenating previously flooded alveoli formerly exposed only to mixed venous P_{O_2}.[41] Nitroprusside reduces PVR in edematous lungs by blocking HPV.[40,42] Not infrequently, pulmonary vasodilators reduce PVR and increase $\dot{Q}_T$ in patients with ARDS; although this beneficial effect is confounded in part by the concomitant increase in pulmonary shunt, O_2 delivery is often maintained.[43,44] Accordingly, the manipulation of PVR in early ARDS is recommended as an exercise in titration for extra gains in $\dot{Q}_T$ and $\dot{Q}_{O_2}$ or reductions in PEEP and inspired oxygen fraction ($F_{I_{O_2}}$) after the patient's cardiopulmonary status has been optimized by seeking **1.** the least Ppw providing adequate $\dot{Q}_T$ and $\dot{Q}_{O_2}$, **2.** the least PEEP providing 90% saturation of an adequate hematocrit on nontoxic $F_{I_{O_2}}$, and **3.** the least tidal volume effecting adequate CO_2 elimination (for further discussion, see Chap. 128). Of course, such an exercise in pulmonary vasodilation is fraught with uncertainty concerning effects of pulmonary blood flow distribution on the lung injury or repair. In the absence of convincing clinical data, canine studies suggest that blood pH does not affect PVR, so correction of acidosis is unlikely to reduce PVR,[45] while increasing hematocrit up to 40 percent will increase $\dot{Q}_{O_2}$ without increasing PVR.[46] Later, in the proliferative stage of ARDS, progressive PH is associated with increased dead space, pulmonary fibrosis, vascular remodeling, and a high prevalence of small vessel thrombosis. Prognosis is poor in these patients, and there is little information concerning the contribution of PH or its treatment to outcome (see Chap. 54).

IDIOPATHIC DISORDERS INCLUDING PRIMARY PULMONARY HYPERTENSION

Primary PH is associated with primary pulmonary vascular changes and greatly elevated Ppa and PVR. It is a diagnosis of exclusion once the above causes have been discarded. The clinical findings of this disorder have recently been summarized from the NIH Registry data on these patients.[3,4] Classically, the disease was reported in young adult females, although the disease has been shown to occur in all age groups with a clustering in the 20- to 45-year-old range. Dyspnea and fatigue are the most common symptoms early in the disease and diagnosis is usually established within 3 years of the appearance of symptomatology (mean 2 years), although severe PH is usually already present at this stage. Fatigue and peripheral edema are more common in the more symptomatic patients. Noninvasive studies (echocardiography, chest x-ray, ECG) confirm the diagnosis in the vast majority of patients, although 6

TABLE 117-3 Hemodynamic Responses to the Acute Trial of Vasodilators

Drug and Reference	Number of Patients	Cardiac Output % Change	PA Pressure % Change	TPR or PVR % Change	SYS Pressure % Change
Captopril					
Rich[44]	4	+10	+5	−4	−10
Ikram[18]	5	0	−15	−11	−22
Leier[22]	5	+18	−2	+2	—
Diazoxide					
Wang[56]	3	+78	−14	−52	−23
Honey[17]	9	+74	−4	−44	−26
Hydralazine					
Lupi-Herrera[26]	12	+55	+3	−23	—
Responders[a]	6	+69	−8	−43	—
Packer[31]	11	+35	0	−30	−13
Fisher[9]	5	+33	+2	−24	−26
Rich[41]	16	+30	0	−20	—
Groves[13]	7	+54	+2	−33	−15
Isoproterenol					
Daoud[7]	6	+47	+10	−23	−5
Lupi-Herrera[26]	5	+55	−17	−33	−6
Nifedipine					
Mohiuddin[28]	6	+34	−20	−38	−10
Rubin[47]	9	+47	−3	−36	−14
Packer[31]	11	+7	−23	−38	−20
Olivari[29]	7	+31	−14	−35	−14
Fisher[9]	5	+7	−14	−22	−16
Rich[41]	23	+29	−4	−22	—
Barst[2]	9	+21	−18	−32	−14
Responders[a]	5	+24	−28	−48	−17
High Dose Nifedipine/Diltiazem					
Rich[40]	13	+22	−30	−43	−15
Responders[a]	8	+41	−43	−60	−12
Nitroglycerin					
Pearl[36]	9	+28	−15	−40	−15
Nitroprusside					
Fuleihan[10]	7	+29	−8	−26	−11
Phentolamine					
Levine[23]	4	+25	−4	−28	—
Prostacyclin					
Guadagni[14]	4	+26	−30	−47	−33
Rubin[46]	7	+56	−11	−43	−14
Groves[13]	7	+77	−7	−44	−15
Barst[2]	9	+41	−18	−47	−9
Responders[a]	5	+38	−31	−58	−5
Jones[19]	10	+18	−4	−19	−14
Verapamil					
Landmark[21]	9	+14	−11	−4	—
Packer[31]	12	−12	−25	−20	−15

PA, pulmonary arterial; SYS, systemic arterial; TPR, total pulmonary resistance.
[a]Responders: a subset singled out as having a good hemodynamic response to the vasodilator.
SOURCE: Reproduced with permission from Weir EK: *Acute Vasodilator Testing and Pharmacological Treatment of Primary Pulmonary Hypertension*. All citations refer to reference list in Chap. 37 of Ref. 3.

percent of patients have an essentially normal noninvasive evaluation. Different pathologic subtypes have been described in the registry patients with a recent broader classification including pulmonary arteriopathy with plexiform lesions, thrombotic lesions, isolated medial hypertrophy, intimal fibrosis and medial hypertrophy, and pulmonary venoocclusive disease.[14] Pulmonary artery pressures and resistances were highest with plexiform lesions, and this group along with the pulmonary venoocclusive group exhibited a worse prognosis as compared to the patients with pulmonary arteriopathy with thrombotic lesions. This survival behavior was evident even within the first 6 months of entry into the registry.

Histologic subtype did not predict response to vasodilator therapy; other issues pertaining to evaluation for elective acute vasodilator testing and chronic vasodilator ther-

TABLE 117-4 Intravenous Pulmonary Vasodilating Agents

	Initial Dosage	Incremental	Maximal	$t_{1/2}$	Peak Effect
Short-acting agents					
Nitroprusside	10 μg/min	× 2 every 2 min	4 μg/kg/min	3.5 min	Immediate
Isoproterenol	1 μg/min	1 μg/min every 2 min	5 μg/min	3.8 min	Immediate
PGE_1	30 ng/kg/min	20 ng/kg/min every 10 min	NA	NA	Immediate
Prostacyclin	1 ng/kg/min	1 ng/kg/min every 10 min	24 ng/kg/min	3.0 min	Immediate
Nitroglycerin	10 μg/min	× 2 every 2 min	4 μg/kg/min	2.7 min	Immediate
Selected longer-acting agents					
Nifedipine (p.o.-gel)	10 mg	10 mg every 15 min	30 mg[a]	120 min	25 min
Hydralazine	5 mg (IV)	5 mg every 5 min	20 mg	180 min	45 min

[a]See Reference 49 for recent higher effective doses.
NA Information not available.

apy were recently reviewed.[14,47,48] Many agents increase $\dot{Q}_T$ and reduce PVR without reducing systemic BP during acute trials (Table 117-3); in general, patients with a good response to acute trials do better with long-term vasodilators (see Fig. 117-3, *lower panel*). Accordingly, the intensivist has the opportunity to improve the hemodynamic status of the patient with PPH while collecting data predicting the response to long-term vasodilators during an acute trial of pulmonary vasodilation with short-acting agents (Table 117-4) in a safe environment. This approach should be extrapolated cautiously to patients with PH secondary to chronic lung diseases, but when $\dot{Q}_T$ may be limited by PH, the ICU is a good place for an acute vasodilator trial.[22,28–30] High dose calcium channel blocker therapy and continuous intravenous prostacyclin therapy have shown long-term hemodynamic benefit and regression of right heart changes in a small number of patients with PPH.[49,50] A definitive prospective study of anticoagulation in PPH patients is not available, but retrospective studies suggest a better prognosis in those patients who received anticoagulation so this therapy warrants consideration in PPH.[4] Given that most patients have a poor 5 year survival, heart-lung transplantation and lung transplantation are other therapeutic options being pursued in these patients (see Chaps. 78 and 79).

Pulmonary venoocclusive disease is generally included with PPH, but many consider this to be a distinct entity. Radiologic signs can result from the pulmonary venous obstruction, including Kerley B lines. Pulmonary artery catheterization often reveals a significantly elevated Ppw due to significant pulmonary venous obstruction. Pulmonary arterial lesions similar to those seen in the veins have been present in 50 percent of patients in some series, and these lesions can account for the PH in the absence of significant venous obstruction.[51]

Other disorders associated with an elevated Ppw and PH include mitral stenosis, fibrosing mediastinitis or mediastinal mass lesions impinging on pulmonary venous return, anomalous pulmonary venous return, the rare entity of diffuse smooth muscle proliferation of the lung,[52] and, commonest of all, left heart failure. CT scan of the thorax can disclose the mediastinal lesions and possibly the diffuse smooth muscle proliferation in the lung if high resolution technique is used.

Conditions associated with portal hypertension and cirrhosis have been associated with severe PH. Some debated whether these rare reports represented simply the background occurrence of PPH which coincidentally overlapped with these conditions. Nevertheless, PH associated with these conditions seems independent of PPH and portal hypertension may be the unifying factor predisposing to the pulmonary vascular changes. In a recent comparison of 17 patients with PH associated with portal hypertension (with and without cirrhosis) and 192 patients with PPH in the NIH Registry, it was found that the portal hypertension group was older, less likely to experience Raynaud's phenomenon or syncope, and had significantly decreased PVR and SVR as compared to the NIH group; pulmonary pathologic findings and survival, however, were not significantly different between these groups.[3]

Cardiopulmonary Deterioration in the Patient with Pulmonary Hypertension

Resuscitation of the patient with PH and RV dysfunction who develops refractory hypotension and shock presents a challenging and urgent situation to the critical care physician. Decreases in systemic BP can be followed precipitously by cardiopulmonary arrest and death. This scenario is not uncommon in the most closely monitored patient in the ICU or even in patients undergoing elective pulmonary vasodilator trials. Accordingly, any decline in systemic manifestations of adequate perfusion warrants an expeditious evaluation of the patient and early institution of therapy. This systematic evaluation for reversible causes of hemodynamic compromise should include correcting oxygenation and acid-base status; titrating circulating volume to optimize RV and LV preload; enhancing RV myocardial contractility and reducing RV afterload; establishing and maintaining adequate BP to maintain RV perfusion; and correcting intercurrent LV dysfunction. Figure 117-5 presents a schematic outline of sequential evaluation and resuscitation of the PH patient with hemodynamic compromise as a basis for the following discussion. Successful resuscitation and stabilization provide an opportunity for evaluating the patient as a candidate for lung or heart-lung transplantation (see Chaps. 78 and 79); without transplantation, the long-term prognosis of such a patient is poor.

FACTORS INFLUENCING SYSTEMIC VENOUS RETURN AND OPTIMAL VOLUME RESUSCITATION

The pressure driving VR is the mean systemic pressure (Pms, the zero flow equilibration pressure in the systemic vasculature) minus Pra. The resistance to venous return (RVR) is a flow-weighted average of regional resistances in the systemic circulation from the LV outflow tract to the right atrium, so VR = (Pms − Pra)/RVR. Pms depends on the *stressed vascular volume* (the volume that is associated with a positive transmural pressure change) and *vascular compliance* at volume above the stressed vascular volume. Cardiac function is coupled with the systemic circulation so that VR = $\dot{Q}_T$ at a value of Pra low enough to allow the steady state value of VR, yet high enough to fill the heart sufficiently to eject the steady state value of $\dot{Q}_T$.[53,54] With significant decreases in $\dot{Q}_T$, passive elastic forces of the systemic vasculature and baroreceptor reflex activity mediated by the sympathetic nervous system act to increase Pms, and so increase VR; in animal models, the passive elastic forces of the systemic vasculature contribute at least as much as reflexes to the increased VR.[54] In PH and CP, Pra is often elevated so an increase in Pms is required to maintain VR; if Pms cannot increase sufficiently, $\dot{Q}_T$ becomes inadequate (see Chap. 2 for further discussion).

Primary decreases in Pms can be associated with vascular volume loss from diuresis, hemorrhage, fluid redistribution into extravascular spaces with hypoproteinemic states, postoperative volume fluxes, and vascular leak syndromes. Hence the first step toward resuscitation is ensuring adequate vascular volume and interventions to prevent volume loss. An initial fluid bolus of crystalloid in the amount of 500 mL to 1 L over 10 to 15 min is recommended; when systemic BP rises much more than Pra, relative hypovolemia is responsible for part of the hypotension. Then, further replacement of volume with blood is preferred provided the hematocrit will not exceed 45 percent. Cessation of diuretics and a search for sources of occult blood loss (see

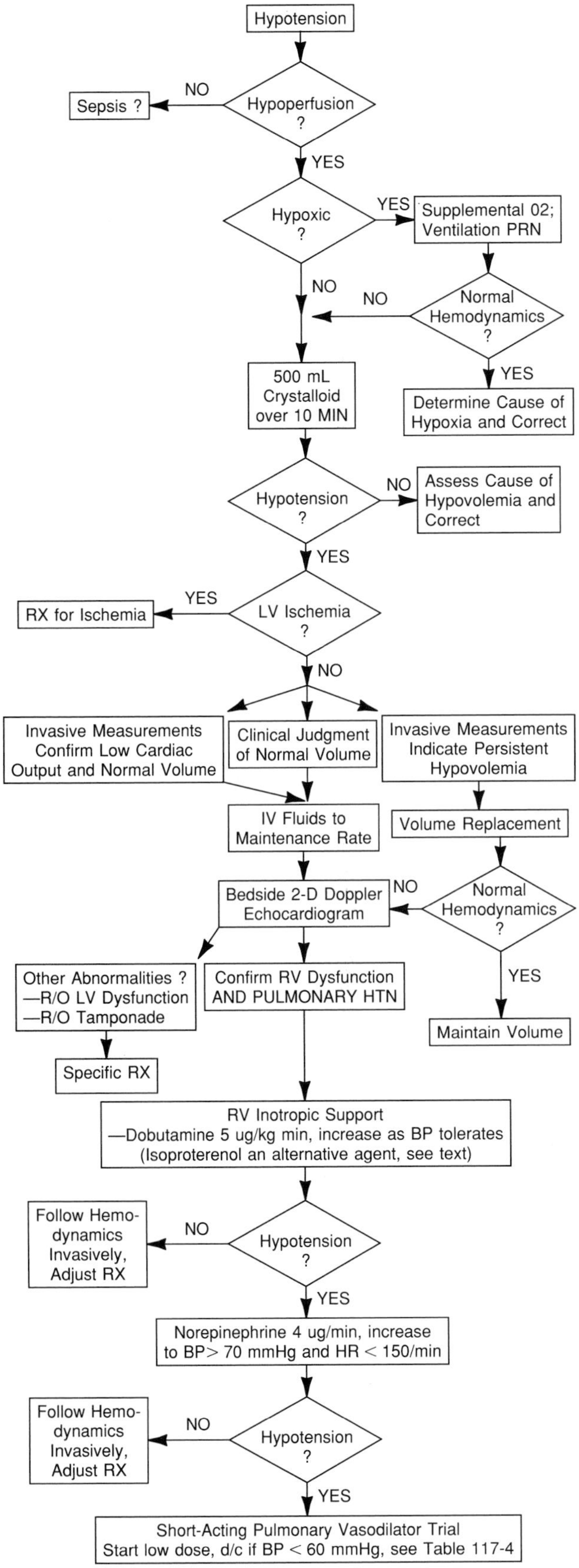

FIGURE 117-5 Flow diagram for systematic and expeditious evaluation and resuscitation of the patient with PH who develops hypotension. Key points of evaluation and judgment include 1. assurance of adequate *oxygenation;* 2. assurance of *adequate vascular volume* and venous return; 3. appropriate *inotropic support* for the dilated, loaded RV; 4. aggressive *vasopressor support* in the persistently hypotensive patient in shock potentially caused by *RV ischemia* from decreased right coronary flow. Note the utility of the two-dimensional bedside echocardiogram if available. Evaluation for pulmonary embolism is directed according to clinical suspicion and when resuscitation allows safe diagnostic studies (see text for discussion).

discussion of Table 114-2 in Chap. 114) or bleeding diatheses are practical early steps. If the initial fluid bolus and further volume resuscitation are not associated with improvement, or even cause a decline in $\dot{Q}_T$ and BP, further volume infusion should be limited to a maintenance rate, and a careful reassessment of volume status, RV afterload, and RV function should be obtained with echocardiography and right heart catheterization. Then vasoactive drug therapy is indicated (vide infra), while further volume loading is avoided because it reduces $\dot{Q}_T$ and BP despite increasing Pra; most often, this is due to detrimental RV-LV interactions or to reduced perfusion of the dilated RV by a hypotensive systemic circulation.

The Pms can also be reduced due to the increase in vascular compliance and unstressed volume as occur with systemic vasodilation secondary to drugs and sepsis. Drugs effecting systemic venodilation lower Pms, especially when the circulating volume is reduced; accordingly, before the administration of such drugs as *morphine, nitroglycerin,* and *furosemide,* adequate vascular volume should be established. *Histamine* also causes venodilation, so intercurrent allergic reactions or side effects of common ICU medications, such as muscle relaxants, should be excluded along with adrenal cortical insufficiency in those patients who may be receiving chronic steroid therapy for their underlying condition associated with PH. Of course, pulmonary vasodilators also have systemic vasodilating effects that significantly limit their use, and they have been reported to precipitate cardiovascular collapse and death.[29,47] The decrease in Pms effected by these agents can be countered by volume infusion and agonists, which constrict systemic vessels and increase blood pressure. Management of septicemic vasodilation in the patient with PH and CP is especially troublesome because of the unusual vulnerability to reduced Pms and to reduced coronary perfusion. Early rational antibiosis must be combined with aggressive volume infusion to the end points described above; then positive inotropic agents (dobutamine 5 to 10 μg/kg/min) and α agonists (norepinephrine 1 to 5 μg/min) should be added to correct hypotension (vide infra).

The Pra is elevated when RV performance deteriorates either due to primary myocardial failure or increased pressure load on the RV leading to decreased RVEF. The right atrial hypertension of PH can be aggravated by increases in pleural (Ppl) and pericardial pressures, and by factors increasing RV afterload. Obstructive airways disease can be associated with increases in alveolar pressure, and hence Ppl, at end expiration (intrinsic PEEP, or $PEEP_i$); $PEEP_i$ can be minimized by optimal bronchodilation and by allowing sufficient time for expiration by using low tidal volumes and the lowest rates which allow adequate CO_2 elimination (see Chap. 127). Vigorous coughing can be associated with syncope, presumably from increases in Ppl, which decrease VR. Patients with obstructive airways disease, hemoptysis, or other endobronchial pathology are the patients most predisposed to paroxysms of coughing, so measures to suppress the cough are reasonable to avoid transient decreases in VR. Mechanical ventilation with positive pressure and PEEP can increase Ppl and Pra, so minimizing PEEP and tidal volume can increase $\dot{Q}_T$.

Pericardial pressures may be increased when excessive cardiac chamber enlargement and loading reach the physical limits of the pericardial space, after which further loading causes an increase in pericardial pressure and Pra (see Chap. 121). Limiting overzealous volume loading and RV pressure afterload may prevent this effect, but finding the balance between providing adequate preload without effecting excess RV dilation requires careful titration in each patient with PH and systemic hypotension.

VENTRICULAR INTERDEPENDENCE

Gross RV enlargement occurs with RV dysfunction and increased pulmonary vascular pressure load, which can be made worse by excessive volume loading. With increasing enlargement, the RV cavity impinges on the LV cavity so that initial interventricular septal flattening is followed by significant septal protrusion into the LV cavity (see discussion of Fig. 2-5 in Chap. 2). This mechanical deformation causes a decrease in the size of the LV and measured LV diastolic compliance decreases in animal models of this condition.[35,55] Furthermore, the limitation of an enclosed pericardial space contributes to the mechanical restriction to filling the LV. These mechanical abnormalities join to decrease LV filling and output. In an animal model of successive autologous clot emboli, volume loading was associated with worse LV mechanical deformation by RV enlargement, and hemodynamics were adversely affected in the most severe pulmonary hypertensive state; hemodynamics did show some correction with volume depletion although direct measurement of $\dot{Q}_T$ was lacking.[55] It is unclear whether the volume loading reduced $\dot{Q}_T$ by the LV deformation, or by aggravating RV dysfunction through increased pulmonary vascular pressure and volume load, so that LV filling is reduced by decreased RV output. The latter possibility is supported by the lack of effect of an intact pericardium on hemodynamics in these animal models of increased RV pressure load and RV failure.[56] Phlebotomy may occasionally increase $\dot{Q}_T$, especially when dilated right-sided chambers cause severe septal shift to the left on echocardiography. Yet, it is not clear at what point further volume loading of a dilated, pressure-loaded RV is deleterious and may warrant volume reduction. Accordingly, small volume challenges or reductions should be tried to determine which increases $\dot{Q}_T$ in each patient.

RIGHT VENTRICULAR DYSFUNCTION

Right ventricular performance may be impaired by RV ischemia and afterload in PH associated with decreased $\dot{Q}_T$ and shock. Output from the normal RV is more dependent on volume than on end-diastolic pressure, so Pra is more important for influencing VR than as an index of preload or an aid in evaluating RV contractility by cardiac function curves. Under increased pulmonary vascular pressure load, the RV becomes more spherical and RVEF decreases, to cause parallel upward shifts in the diastolic pressure-volume relation of the RV; yet, this is not correlated with decreasing $\dot{Q}_T$ as extrapolated from estimates of RV end-systolic and diastolic volumes and heart rate.[57] Accord-

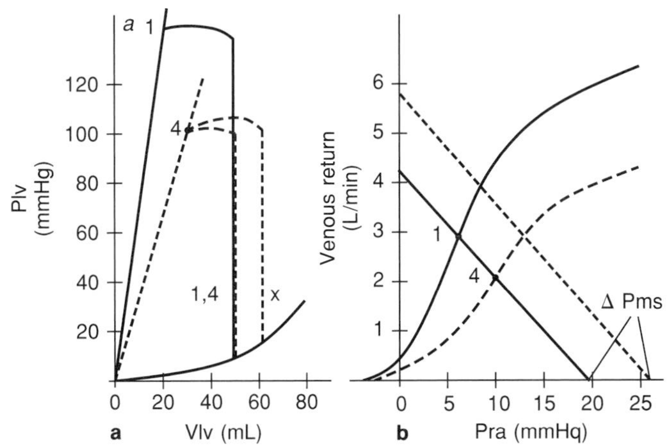

FIGURE 117-6 Panel *a* shows LV systolic mechanics at pH 7.4 (continuous end-systolic line labelled '1') was depressed by intravenous lactic acid infusion to pH 7.2 (dotted end-systolic line labelled '4'). As a result, stroke volume (and so Q̇T) was reduced by lactic acidosis when end-diastolic volume and pressure were similar. Panel *b* shows cardiac function and venous return curves (continuous lines intersecting at '1'—pH 7.4, venous return 2.8 L/min, Pra 6 mmHg); lactic acidosis depressed the cardiac function curve (dotted curve intersecting continuous venous return curve at '4'—venous return = 2 L/min, Pra = 10 mmHg), in part by reducing contractility and in part by increasing Ppa from 20 to 48 mmHg. (Reproduced with permission from Teplinsky K, O'Toole M, Olman M, et al: Effect of lactic acidosis on canine hemodynamics and left ventricular function. Am J Physiol 258:H1193, 1990)

ingly, there is no clear hemodynamic or other diagnostic analysis that accurately reflects the contractile state of the RV.

Optimum RV function depends on adequate myocardial oxygen delivery and therefore coronary perfusion. The pressure driving coronary perfusion of the RV is mean BP minus the mean RV pressure. Right coronary autoregulation is not as efficient as in the left coronary circulation, so systemic BP is a key determinant of right coronary perfusion.[58] In contrast to the left coronary circulation, the right system does not favor subepicardial versus subendocardial regions in the normal and low pressure ranges and is not cardiac cycle dependent—adequate myocardial perfusion occurs in systole as well as diastole in the normal RV.[58] However, in the face of RVH, the subendocardium is more prone to decreases in perfusion with decrements in coronary flow, and myocardial perfusion may become more cardiac cycle dependent with subendocardial perfusion occurring mainly in diastole as in the LV. Whether the hypertrophied right heart is more prone to ischemic injury as has been shown for the hypertrophied LV is not clear. The susceptibility to the increased ischemic insult in the latter case may be more a function of the altered coronary vasomotor response to injury related to factors other than hypertrophy of the ventricle itself.[59] Increases in Ppa cause RV enlargement, increased RV pressure, and commensurate increases in myocardial wall stress and oxygen consumption; coronary blood flow increases with these afterload changes.[60] Therefore, for normal oxygen delivery to the pressure-loaded RV to occur, systemic hemodynamics must provide the driving pressure to support an increase in right coronary flow; hence, function of the loaded RV may deteriorate with systemic hypotension.

Pumping function of the hypertrophied RV may be depressed by several metabolic derangements of critical illness known to depress LV contractility (see Chap. 115). Hypoxemia and respiratory acidosis both reduce LV systolic function and also squeeze systemic veins to increase diastolic volume (see discussion of Fig. 115-4 and 115-5 in Chap. 115). Lactic acidosis also depresses LV contractility (Fig. 117-6*a*); when this was associated with PH, Pra increased and Q̇T decreased (Fig. 117-6*b*). Conceivably, correction of hypoxemia, acidosis, and other metabolic abnormalities is an important adjunctive therapy for RV dysfunction in PH and CP, just as adding dobutamine may enhance the systolic performance of the afterloaded RV. Of course, correction of hypoxemia also reduces HPV to reduce RV afterload, but correction of acidosis probably has no effect on PVR.[45] The left panel of Fig. 117-7 shows the consistent increase in PVR during intravenous infusion of lactic acid to reduce pH to about 7.1, but the right panel shows no increase in PVR during intraarterial infusion to the same pH; it seems that the increased PVR previously ascribed to acidemic pulmonary vasoconstriction is actually microvascular obstruction due to products of intravascular hemolysis or coagulation induced by venous acid infusion.[45]

Right ventricular afterload is more than Ppa and PVR. Impedance to RV output is also influenced by pulmonary vascular compliance and pulsatile flow. In particular, the efficiency of the RV as a pump is significantly influenced by the compliance characteristics of the proximal pulmonary vasculature,[61] and proximal arterial constriction produces a more formidable RV dynamic afterload than lung microvascular injury to a similar pressure elevation.[62] Pulmonary vascular occlusion methods call attention to the alteration of compliances in the different segments of the pulmonary vasculature under various vasomotor stimuli,[63] and studies of remodeling of the pulmonary circulation during PH suggest reduced vascular compliance may play an important role in increasing impedance to RV ejection.[3] These compliance characteristics of the pulmonary vasculature suggest a three-compartment model of the pulmonary circulation, and allow measurement of the longitudinal distribution of compliance and resistance of the pulmonary vascular bed under normal conditions and under various stimuli. These methods offer potential for more insightful understanding of the impedance characteristics of the pulmonary circulation on the RV, and balloon occlusion measurements are obtainable in clinical settings.[64]

INTEGRATED AGGRESSIVE APPROACH TO EARLY RESUSCITATION

When PH is complicated by reduced Q̇T and BP, simultaneous or rapid sequential implementation of positive-pressure ventilation, optimization of circulating volume, inotropic support, systemic vasoconstriction to enhance coronary

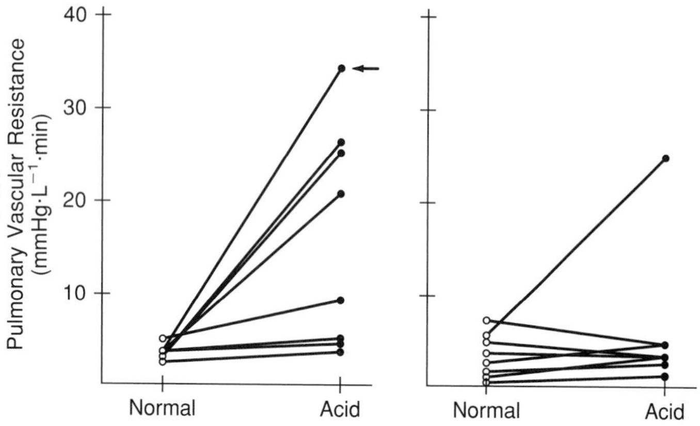

FIGURE 117-7 The effect on PVR (ordinate) of lactic acid infusion to lower pH from 7.4 (normal) to 7.1 (acid) in 18 anesthetized dogs. *Left panel.* Intravenous infusion increased median PVR from 3.6 to 21.7 mmHg/L/min (P < 0.05). *Right panel.* Intraarterial infusion did not significantly increase median PVR (2.7 to 3.5, ns). Reduced pH did not cause pulmonary vasoconstriction, but intravenous acid infusion caused intravascular hemolysis to raise PVR by pulmonary microembolism. (Reproduced with permission from Reference 45)

perfusion, and pulmonary vasodilation probably provides the best short-term resuscitation; with up to five concurrent and potentially antagonistic therapeutic regimes, early detection of adverse effects by continuous bedside hemodynamic measurements is essential.

As in all patients with shock, early implementation of mechanical ventilation effects adequate O_2 saturation and CO_2 elimination while minimizing the work of breathing (see Chap. 114). Initially, FI_{O_2} should be 1.0 to eliminate all HPV and provide complete O_2 saturation. FI_{O_2} can then be reduced to the least value effecting about 100% saturation; note that 90% O_2 saturation (Pa_{O_2} 55 to 65 mmHg) on FI_{O_2} = 0.4 implies that many alveoli have very low values of P_{O_2} which cause HPV, so the FI_{O_2} should be increased to minimize HPV. In PH and CP due to COPD, $PEEP_i$ may impede VR, so ventilator settings should be selected to minimize $PEEP_i$ (the least tidal volume and respiratory rate effecting an acceptable Pa_{CO_2}—see Chaps. 127 and 129); this approach also minimizes the increases in PVR due to alveolar vascular compression. In pulmonary fibrosis or restrictive diseases of the thorax, alveolar pressures are often excessive when conventional tidal volumes are used, so starting with 6 to 8 mL/kg at a rate of 24/min is better (see Chap. 132). Whether to increase or reduce circulating volume in the hypotensive patient with PH and high Pra often requires trial (and error); not infrequently, the initiation of mechanical ventilation provides the correct direction—worse hypotension signals hypovolemia requiring a volume challenge, while increased BP suggests that the patient might benefit from further reduction of circulating volume.

After initial optimization of volume status as discussed above (see Factors Influencing Systemic Venous Return and Optimal Volume Resuscitation), an infusion of dopamine (2 to 4 μg/kg/min) is initiated to minimize renal cortical hypoperfusion (see Chap. 114), and dobutamine (5 μg/kg/min) is started to enhance RV contractility and output. Initial echocardiography or right heart catheterization is helpful in evaluating the responses to volume infusion and dobutamine, but these should not be delayed in a hemodynamically unstable patient while awaiting these diagnostic measures, for BP and Pra changes suffice to get initial therapy directed. Inotropic support of the adequately perfused but abnormally loaded RV has been studied extensively in animal models where the pulmonary vasculature was embolized with autologous clot or foreign body microspheres; when these interventions reduced $\dot{Q}_T$ and RVEF and increased PVR without frank shock, dobutamine was the most effective agent in increasing $\dot{Q}_T$ with little change in PVR and systemic BP.[35] Patients who were in decreased $\dot{Q}_T$ states from massive pulmonary embolism also showed hemodynamic benefit from dobutamine infusion.[65] Isoproterenol is also effective in increasing $\dot{Q}_T$ in these conditions, but with tachycardia and decreases in SVR and in systemic BP.[35] This last effect seems to render isoproterenol less desirable than dobutamine as the first-line inotropic agent for RV failure given the right coronary perfusion dependence on systemic BP; note that dobutamine also causes hypotension when doses exceed 10 μ/kg/min, presumably due to stimulation of peripheral vascular β_2 receptors to cause arteriolar dilation especially in the skeletal muscles. Note further that norepinephrine and dopamine, which have more potent systemic vasoconstrictor effects, did not increase $\dot{Q}_T$ at this level of mild to moderate PH where isoproterenol and dobutamine did increase $\dot{Q}_T$ in the same preparations.[35] Digoxin has been used in patients with PPH without the toxicity reported for the COPD population with CP, but also without documented benefit.[3,48] Since the catecholamine excess and frequent transient metabolic disturbances associated with acute hemodynamic compromise predispose to digoxin-induced toxicity, it should be avoided as a method of acute inotropic support in this situation.[21,48] Volume loading and nitroglycerin have been uniformly ineffective in restoring $\dot{Q}_T$ and BP in these conditions; hydralazine increases $\dot{Q}_T$ but often in association with further tachycardia and decreases in systemic BP.[56]

As RV dysfunction becomes more severe and $\dot{Q}_T$ falls further with commensurate decreases in systemic BP, RV ischemia can contribute to the decrease in RV output. Under these conditions, agents such as norepinephrine, which can increase systemic BP and therefore right coronary perfusion, have been most effective in stabilizing or improving hemodynamics. In fact, most other vasoactive agents and volume loading in these severe conditions have not been able to prevent a rapidly progressive deterioration and death in these animal models. One study suggested a threshold of RV dysfunction where these systemic vasoconstrictors are beneficial in improving RV function over inotropic support with dobutamine alone.[35] Human studies in severe septic shock have documented a beneficial RV hemodynamic response to a short-term infusion of either dopamine or norepinephrine.[66] However, these agents were not continued and they had an indeterminate impact on mortality, which exceeded 75 percent in this group of patients. Low dose dopamine in conjunction with norepinephrine infusion was seen in an animal study to preserve other end-organ perfusion over norepinephrine infusion alone.[67] Intraaortic balloon pump (IABP) has been preliminarily studied in an animal model of thrombin-induced microvascular injury and PH and was not effective in improving hemodynamics or increasing coronary perfusion.[68] However, this technology was applied to a previously normal, acutely loaded RV. Conceivably, the hypertrophied RV will be more cardiac cycle dependent for coronary perfusion, so these data may not preclude a potential benefit of IABP on coronary perfusion in a chronically loaded, hypertrophied RV. Such aggressive intervention may be justified as a bridge of support for someone proceeding expeditiously to transplantation.

Successful resuscitation of the patient in acute RV dysfunction depends on early positive response to the above measures. When there are continuing or progressive signs of inadequate perfusion, a *short-acting* pulmonary vasodilating agent may be of benefit. These agents are potentially harmful in this setting due to their concomitant dilation of the systemic vasculature. For this reason, one should choose a short-acting agent at the lowest starting dose and titrate dosage increases carefully with invasive pulmonary and systemic hemodynamic monitoring; nitroprusside, isoproterenol, PGE_1, and prostacyclin (PGI_2) are reasonable choices (see Table 117-4). In elective pulmonary vasodilator trials, short-acting agents have been useful to determine safety of administration of other vasodilators and to predict the magnitude of the long-term response.[3,47,48] Despite this advantage, PGI_2 and PGE_1 may cause rebound platelet activation on discontinuation so coincident heparin therapy may be recommended; these agents are contraindicated in thromboembolic disease. In contrast to elective pulmonary vasodilator trials that seek to provide evidence for hemodynamic benefit by responses which would be statistically significantly better than spontaneous hemodynamic variations, the simple end point in this hemodynamically unstable and failing situation is the temporary improvement of $\dot{Q}_T$. If measured by the thermodilution method, a response 20 percent above baseline would constitute a positive response in pulmonary blood flow. However, if $\dot{Q}_T$ increases without an appreciable decrease in PVR, Ppa values will rise creating a further increased pressure load on the RV, and the RV may further deteriorate on this basis. If resuscitation does prove to be successful, long-term vasodilator therapy should be tried in carefully monitored conditions.[48]

Supraventricular arrhythmias are common in this patient population. As usual, one should look to rule out hypoxemia or metabolic disturbances as precipitating causes (see Chap. 120). Cardioversion is the first measure of choice for arrhythmias in the patient with PH and a hemodynamically compromised status. In a less emergent setting, drug therapy can be instituted with the caution that the common side effect of hypotension secondary to the usual pharmacologic agents may not be well tolerated in the face of PH and right heart dysfunction. Therefore, one may opt for shorter-acting agents, such as esmolol or adenosine,[69,70] when appropriate, in an attempt to convert the rhythm back to sinus rate with the least risk of prolonged systemic hypotension. Digoxin can be used for responsive arrhythmias, but it has a high risk:effectiveness ratio when used to treat heart failure in PH due to lung disease.[21] MAT is an important rhythm disturbance to recognize due to its association with hypoxemia, metabolic disturbances, and theophylline toxicity along with the known refractoriness to digoxin and cardioversion therapy. Esmolol, selective β_1-blocking agents and verapamil have been the most successful pharmacologic therapies for MAT;[70] the hypotension induced by verapamil is ameliorated by prior administration of calcium gluconate.

PREOPERATIVE ASSESSMENT OF THE HIGH-RISK PATIENT WITH PH AND CP

In a patient with significant PH and CP, surgery and anesthesia may become necessary (see Chap. 81). In these instances close communication with the anesthesiology team helps to avoid cardiac depressants and agents commonly associated with systemic venodilation and hypotension despite values of Pra which are apparently high (but are relatively low for this patient population). Preoperative pulmonary artery catheterization or intraoperative transesophageal echocardiography are helpful for early diagnosis and management of hypotension. Given the occasional technical difficulties involved in the placement of this catheter, this procedure should be performed in the ICU with fluoroscopy available. Local and epidural anesthesia have been used successfully to avoid complications during labor and delivery in pregnant patients with PH.[71] Special perioperative considerations for the patient with PH and CP undergoing heart-lung or lung transplantation are discussed in Chaps. 78 and 79.

CASE PRESENTATION

B.S. is a 57-year-old African-American female who has a history of tuberculosis (TB) treated with left upper lobectomy followed by thoracoplasty of the left thorax 35 years ago. She also reports subsequently receiving a year of "pills" for TB. She has a remote history of hypertension not receiving treatment; there are no other medical problems or use of cigarettes or alcohol. She was doing well up to a year ago when she experienced palpitations, ankle swelling, and mild shortness of breath. She denied any exertional limitations with her usual activities—housework, casual walking, and occasional walking of two flights of stairs. She states she was diagnosed with "heart disease" and was given digoxin and furosemide.

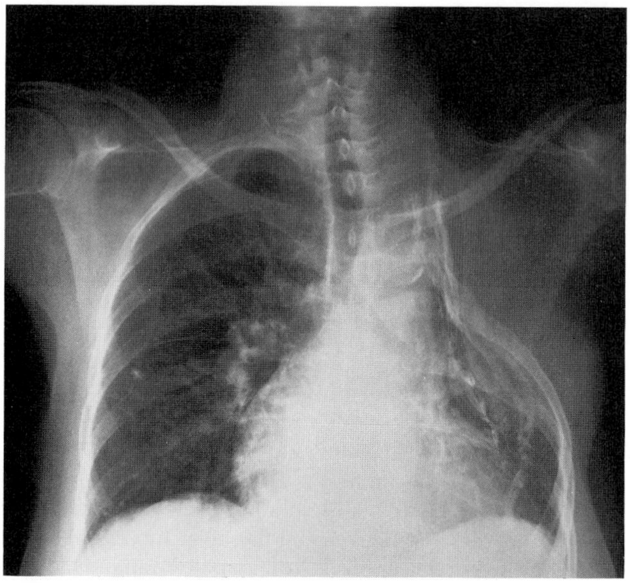

FIGURE 117-8 Posteroanterior chest x-ray from the patient described in the illustrative case. The patient has had a left thoracoplasty and has severe PH. The diameter of the right descending branch of the pulmonary artery measures 19 mm, consistent with PH.

She felt somewhat better until 1 month ago when she was admitted to another hospital with a diagnosis of "bronchitis." Details of this admission were not obtainable, but she was given antibiotics and continued on her heart medications and was discharged in a week. She was not able to ambulate well since that discharge due to shortness of breath and dizziness with walking and progressive swelling of both legs.

Over the few days prior to this admission, she was largely bed bound. She did experience occasional night sweats and reported vague central chest pain; there was no documented fever, productive cough, or hemoptysis. Medications on admission included digoxin 0.25 mg/day, furosemide 40 mg/day, potassium chloride 20 meq/day, and ranitidine 150 mg/day. Other past medical history was unremarkable. Examination revealed a grossly edematous, mildly tachypneic female who appeared fatigued. Vital signs revealed a BP of 110/75, heart rate of 110/min with regular rhythm, respiratory rate of 20/min and temperature of 37.1°C. Chest examination revealed the postthoracoplasty changes on the left and occasional basilar crackles were heard on the right. Cardiac examination revealed jugular venous pulsations up to 10 cm above the sternal notch, 3+ edema to the thighs and over the sacrum, a palpable P_2, and an RV lift which was sustained in character; auscultation revealed that S_1 was normal, the S_2 had a fixed split and the P_2 component was increased, no S_3 was appreciated, and a III/VI holosystolic murmur was heard throughout the mid precordium, which increased with respiration. Abdominal examination was notable for a tender liver but without overt pulsation. Neurologic examination was intact with good cognitive function.

Laboratory data on admission were remarkable for an arterial blood-gas (ABG) on room air showing pH 7.37, P_{CO_2} 56, P_{O_2} 37. Three L/min O_2 therapy by nasal prongs reduced the hypoxemia and pH (pH 7.28, P_{CO_2} 74, P_{O_2} 83). The chest radiograph (see Fig. 117-8) revealed left thoracoplasty changes and scarring in the residual left lower lobe, a normal right lung field, increased diameter of right descending pulmonary artery (19 mm) and right heart enlargement suggested on lateral view. ECG revealed normal sinus rhythm at 98/min with a QRS axis of +105 degrees, P pulmonale and voltage criteria for RV hypertrophy. These were all new findings compared to an ECG obtained 13 years ago. The white blood cell count was 5.5, and hemoglobin and hematocrit were 14.6 and 45.6, respectively. SGOT, bilirubin and LDH were mildly elevated. Electrolytes, albumin, and coagulation studies were within normal limits. A serum digoxin level was 1.2 μg/mL. An echocardiogram obtained the morning of admission documented findings consistent with severe CP with RVH (RV thickness = 8 mm), RV dilation, and right-to-left bowing of the interventricular septum throughout the cardiac cycle. Moderate to severe tricuspid regurgitation was found and peak Ppa by Doppler flow analysis was estimated to be 64 mmHg above Pra; pulmonary outflow tract Doppler exhibited early systolic peaking consistent with PH. LV function was judged to be normal. A $\dot{V}/\dot{Q}$ scan was obtained to rule out the possibility of acute pulmonary embolism; there were no defects in perfusion of the right lung, but there was minimal ventilation and perfusion of the left lung.

Despite these observation, the working diagnosis was CHF due to intercurrent myocardial ischemia, hypoxia, or acidosis; she was admitted to the ICU where 2 inches of nitroglycerin paste was applied cutaneously. Oxygen therapy corrected the hypoxemia with tolerable worsening of hypercapnia. A diuresis was effected with furosemide (40 mg) and digoxin (0.125 mg daily) was continued IV. With this therapy, the patient became obtunded and hypotensive (90/70). She was electively intubated and mechanical ventilation was initiated with a tidal volume of 800 mL (12 mL/kg), assist-control rate of 12, PEEP of 5 cmH_2O and F_{IO_2} of 1.0; this caused peak pressure and pause pressure of 45 and 35 cmH_2O, respectively, with ABG of pH 7.32, P_{CO_2} 42, P_{O_2} 258, and a further reduction in BP (70/55). This new metabolic acidosis was associated with an arterial lactate level of 7 meq/L. The new chest radiograph revealed no changes, and the temperature and white cell count remained normal. The patient became anuric.

An intensive care consultant was asked to see the hypotensive, ventilated patient; she reduced the tidal volume to 400 mL, and increased the rate to 20/min which reduced peak and pause pressures to 28 and 20 cmH_2O, respectively, and increased BP to 80/60 with little change in the ABG. An IV fluid challenge (250 mL saline in 20 min) and a dopamine infusion (3 μg/kg/min) increased the BP further to 90/65, but the patient remained anuric. A right heart catheter was placed, which required fluoroscopic guidance and repetitive positioning due to retrograde looping of the catheter secondary to the severe tricuspid regurgitation. Initial measurements revealed: Pra, 20 mmHg; RV, 90/16 mmHg; Ppa, 90/38 mmHg; Ppw, 17 mmHg; $\dot{Q}_T$, 3.0 L/min; and mixed venous O_2 ($P\bar{v}_{O_2}$), 27 mmHg with a calculated $(a - v)_{O_2}$ content difference of 8.0 mL O_2%. Review of the history, physical examination, and laboratory findings by the intensivist with the admitting physician changed the working diagnosis to acute on chronic respiratory failure in a patient with chronic PH and CP. She was now hypoperfused despite adequate preload, oxygenation, and ventilation, so further vasoactive drug therapy was indicated.

Dobutamine (5 μg/kg/min) was initiated; BP increased to 100/70 and $\dot{Q}_T$ was 3.6 L/min with a small increase in Ppa (95/40) and Pv_{O_2} (32 mmHg). Norepinephrine infusion was added at 8 μg/min in an attempt to restore systemic BP and right coronary perfusion. BP rose to 130/90 and $\dot{Q}_T$ increased to 4.2 L/min (Pv_{O_2}, 35 mmHg). Then isoproterenol was started (1 μg/min) and increased to 4 μg/min in an attempt to augment $\dot{Q}_T$ by reducing PVR. Isoproterenol was discontinued when a 15 mmHg drop in systolic BP and an increase in heart rate from 110 to 130/min were associated with a reduction in $\dot{Q}_T$ (3.8 L/min). The new hypotension was corrected within 10 min of discontinuing the drug. Nitroprusside was then initiated at 0.1 μg/kg/min and increased by five successive doublings of the dose until BP began to decrease at 3.2 μg/kg/min, when the dose was reduced to 2 μg/kg/min; then $\dot{Q}_T$ was 5.2 L/min, BP was 120/60, and Ppa decreased to 80/30 with Ppw of 15 mmHg. Urine output began again, and significant steady diuresis (1500 mL) was accomplished over the next 12 h with this vasoactive therapy and repeated small doses of furosemide. Then, $\dot{Q}_T$ was 6 L/min, Pra was 15, Ppa was 70/25, BP was 100/50, and heart rate decreased to 100/min; the patient regained consciousness and responded appropriately to questions while demonstrating no abnormalities to neurologic examination.

Within 24 h the norepinephrine infusion was discontinued over 30 min by halving the dose three times without a significant reduction in BP or $\dot{Q}_T$. Nitroprusside was then discontinued in the same way with no change in Ppa or $\dot{Q}_T$ and an increase in BP (140/80). Dobutamine was similarly discontinued, and $\dot{Q}_T$ decreased to 5.2 L/min with BP 130/80, Pra 13, Ppa 65/25, and Ppw 13 mmHg. During the liberation of this patient from vasoactive agents, she demonstrated a spontaneous vital capacity of 900 mL, a maximum negative inspiratory pressure at FRC of 38 cmH_2O, and comfortable spontaneous breathing at 24/min with a tidal volume of 330 mL; she was allowed to breathe spontaneously overnight, with careful observation to exclude SDB or nocturnal desaturation on F_{IO_2} of 0.4, and she was extubated successfully early the next morning. Then ABG on room air showed P_{O_2} 64, P_{CO_2} 50, and pH 7.41. After discharge from the ICU a complete sleep study revealed eight desaturations below 80% without apneas during air breathing, but no desaturations during 2 L/min nasal O_2 therapy. She was discharged from the hospital on continuous O_2 therapy without digoxin or furosemide for regular clinic and echocardiographic follow-up; long-term vasodilator therapy was considered but withheld pending reevaluation of right heart function on LTOT.

CASE DISCUSSION

The patient exhibits severe PH and CP with RV dysfunction secondary to an unusual cause of PH—thoracoplasty. Thoracoplasty will result in increased flow through the residual pulmonary vasculature, and chest wall abnormalities cause hypoventilation leading to hypercapnia, hypoxemia, and hypoxic pulmonary vasoconstriction. This would have been evident to informed evaluation a year earlier, when O_2 therapy was indicated. By this admission, tricuspid regurgitation, peripheral edema, and fatigue had progressed in the absence of clinical, radiologic, or echocardiographic evidence of LV dysfunction, so CHF was not the correct diagnosis. Indeed, therapy aimed at CHF (furosemide, nitroglycerin) reduced venous tone, volume, and pressure to precipitate systemic hypotension and a hypoperfusion state due to relative hypovolemia despite a high Pra. Initial resuscitation instituted ventilatory management with a standard tidal volume (12 mL/kg), which was much too large for her restrictive disease of the chest wall, so VR was further reduced until the intensivist reduced the tidal volume.

The immediate increase in BP on reducing ventilation confirmed relative hypovolemia as contributing to the hypotension, so a volume challenge was indicated while low dose dopamine effected better distribution of the presumed low $\dot{Q}_T$ to the renal cortex. By then, right heart catheterization confirmed the clinical diagnosis (CP and PH) and hemodynamic state (low $\dot{Q}_T$ due to right heart overload), so further volume challenge might reduce rather than increase $\dot{Q}_T$. Instead, dobutamine infusion improved output by enhancing contractility, but the patient remained hypotensive. At some risk of adversely affecting peripheral perfusion, a trial of norepinephrine was successful in providing further increase in output. Accordingly, hemodynamic support was applied in appropriate sequential stages to ensure adequate vascular volume, provide inotropic support to the dilated RV with dobutamine, and increase BP with norepinephrine to increase coronary flow—all with temporal but incomplete benefit. Short-acting pulmonary vasodilator trials were a calculated risk aimed to reduce PVR and increase $\dot{Q}_T$ beyond a barely acceptable level in this patient given their risk of further hypotension. Isoproterenol was administered and withdrawn, when its adverse effects dissipated in minutes without further compromise to this patient; by contrast, nitroprusside reduced PVR and increased $\dot{Q}_T$ with decreasing BP. Then vascular volume reduction and longer-term beneficial effects of O_2 facilitated adequate output at reduced right heart pressures until nitroprusside could be withdrawn. Once the shock was corrected, the patient was able to resume spontaneous ventilation and be discharged from the ICU for LTOT.

References

1. Weir EK, Reeves JT: *Pulmonary Hypertension*. Mount Kisco, NY, Futura, 1984.
2. Hall JB, Wood LDH: Oxygen Therapy, in West JB, Crystal RG (eds): *The Lung; Scientific Foundations*. New York, Raven Press, 1990, pp 2143–2154.
3. Fishman AP (ed): *The Pulmonary Circulation: Normal and Abnormal; Mechanisms, Management and the National Registry*. Philadelphia, University of Pennsylvania Press, 1990.
4. Rich S, Dantzker DR, Ayres S, et al: Primary pulmonary hypertension: A national prospective study. Ann Intern Med 107:216, 1987.
5. Moser KM, Auger WR, Fedullo PF: Chronic major-vessel thromboembolic pulmonary hypertension. Circulation 81:1735, 1990.
6. Himelman RB, Struve SN, Brown JK, et al: Improved recognition of cor pulmonale in patients with severe chronic obstructive pulmonary disease. Am J Med 84:891, 1988.
7. Simonson JS, Schiller NB: Sonospirometry: A new method for noninvasive estimation of mean right atrial pressure based on two-dimensional measurements of the inferior vena cava during measured inspiration. J Am Coll Cardiol 11:557, 1988.
8. Hamer HPM, Takens BL, Posma JL, Lie KI: Noninvasive measurement of right ventricular systolic pressure by combined color-coded and continuous wave doppler ultrasound. Am J Cardiol 61:668, 1988.
9. Matthay RA, Niederman MS, Weideman HP: Cardiovascular-pulmonary interaction in chronic obstructive pulmonary disease with special reference to the pathogenesis and management of cor pulmonale. Med Clin North Am 74(3):571, 1990.
10. Panos RJ, Mortenson RL, Niccoli SA, King TE: Clinical deterioration in patients with idiopathic pulmonary fibrosis: Causes and assessment. Am J Med 88:396, 1990.
11. Swensen SJ, Aughenbaugh GL, Brown LR: High resolution computed tomography of the lung. Mayo Clin Proc 64:1284, 1989.
12. Powe JE, Palevsky H, McCarthy KE, Alavi A: Pulmonary arterial hypertension: Value of perfusion scintigraphy. Radiology 164:727, 1987.
13. Perlmutt LM, Braun SD, Newman GE, et al: Pulmonary arteriography in the high-risk patient. Radiology 162:187, 1987.
14. Palevsky HI, Schloo BL, Pietra GG, et al: Primary pulmonary hypertension: Vascular structure, morphometry, and responsiveness to vasodilator agents. Circulation 80:1207, 1989.
15. Rabinovitch M: Problems of pulmonary hypertension in children with congenital cardiac defects. Chest 93:119S, 1988.
16. Nicod P, Moser KM: Primary pulmonary hypertension: The risk and benefit of lung biopsy. Circulation 80:1486, 1989.
17. Macnee W, Wathen CG, Flenley DC, Muir AD: The effects of controlled oxygen therapy on ventricular function in patients with stable and decompensated cor pulmonale. Am Rev Respir Dis 137:1289, 1988.
18. Kawakami Y, Kishi F, Yamamoto H, Miyamoto K: Relation of oxygen delivery, mixed venous oxygenation and pulmonary hemodynamics to prognosis in chronic obstructive pulmonary disease. N Engl J Med 308:1045, 1983.
19. Schumacker PT: Pulmonary gas exchange during exercise, in Leff AR (ed): *Cardio-Pulmonary Exercise Testing*. Orlando, Grune & Stratton, 1986, pp 23–44.
20. Fletcher EC, Luckett RA, Miller T, Fletcher JG: Exercise hemodynamics and gas exchange in patients with chronic obstruction pulmonary disease, sleep desaturation, and a daytime PaO_2 above 60 mmHg. Am Rev Respir Dis 140:1237, 1989.
21. Mathur PN, Powles P, Pugsley SO, et al: Effect of digoxin on right ventricular function in severe chronic airflow obstruction. Ann Intern Med 95:283, 1981.
22. Jones K, Higgenbottam T, Wallwork J: Pulmonary vasodilation with prostacyclin in primary and secondary pulmonary hypertension. Chest 96:784, 1989.
23. Naieje R, Melot C, Mols PL, et al: Reduction in pulmonary hypertension by prostaglandin E_1 in decompensated chronic obstructive pulmonary disease. Am Rev Respir Dis 125:1, 1982.
24. Weisse AB, Moschos CB, Frank MJ, et al: Hemodynamic effects of staged hematocrit reduction in patients with stable cor pulmonale and severely elevated hematocrit levels. Am J Med 58:92, 1975.
25. Owens GR, Follansbee WP: Cardiopulmonary manifestations of systemic sclerosis. Chest 91:118, 1987.
26. Smith LJ, Lawrence JB, Katzenstein AA: Vascular sarcoidosis: A rare cause of pulmonary hypertension. Am J Med Sci 285:38, 1983.
27. Agusti AGN, Roca J, Gea J, et al: Mechanisms of gas exchange impairment in idiopathic pulmonary fibrosis. Am Rev Respir Dis 143:219, 1991.
28. Ohar J, Pollatty C, Robichaud A, et al: The role of vasodilators in patients with progressive systemic sclerosis, interstitial lung disease and pulmonary hypertension. Chest 88:263S, 1985.
29. Packer M, Medina N, Yushak M: Adverse hemodynamic and clinical effects of calcium channel blockade in pulmonary hypertension secondary to obliterative pulmonary vascular disease. J Am Coll Cardiol 4:890, 1984.
30. Lupi-Herrera E, Seoane M, Verdejo J, et al: Hemodynamic effect of hydralazine in interstitial lung disease patients with cor pulmonale. Chest 87:564, 1985.
31. Bergofsky EH: Respiratory failure in disorders of the thoracic cage. Am Rev Respir Dis 119:643, 1979.
32. Hall JB: The cardiopulmonary failure of sleep-disordered breathing. JAMA 255:930, 1986.
33. Bradley TD, Rutherford R, Grossman RF, et al: Role of daytime hypoxemia in the pathogenesis of right heart failure in the obstructive sleep apnea syndrome. Am Rev Respir Dis 131:835, 1985.
34. Pingleton SK, Bone RC, Pingleton WW, Ruth WE: Prevention of pulmonary emboli in a respiratory intensive care unit: Efficacy of low-dose heparin. Chest 79:647, 1981.
35. Prewitt RM: Pathophysiology and treatment of pulmonary hypertension in acute respiratory failure. J Crit Care 2:206, 1987.
36. Ducas J, Light RB, Schick U, Prewitt RM: Effects of prostaglandin E_1 on the pulmonary vascular pressure-flow relationship in canine pulmonary hypertension. J Crit Care 3:24, 1988.
37. Goldhaber SZ: Tissue plasminogen activator in acute pulmonary embolism. Chest 95:282S, 1989.
38. D'Ambra MN, LaRaia PJ, Philbin DM, et al: Prostaglandin E_1: A new therapy for refractory right heart failure and pulmonary hypertension after mitral valve replacement. J Thorac Cardiovasc Surg 89:567, 1985.
39. Armitage JM, Hardesty RL, Griffith BP: Prostaglandin E_1: An effective treatment of right heart failure after orthotopic heart transplant. J Heart Transplant 6:348, 1987.
40. Presberg K, Yanos J, Monk R, et al: The role of mixed venous hypoxemia in the pulmonary hypertension and shunt of canine low pressure pulmonary edema. Am Rev Respir Dis 139:A416, 1989.
41. Ali J, Wood LDH: Factors affecting perfusion distribution in canine oleic acid pulmonary edema. J Appl Physiol 60:1498, 1986.
42. Wood LDH, Prewitt RM: Cardiovascular management in acute

hypoxemic respiratory failure. Am J Cardiol 47:963, 1981.
43. Bihari D, Smithies M, Gimson A, Tinker J: The effects of vasodilation with prostacyclin on oxygen delivery and uptake in critically ill patients. N Engl J Med 317:397, 1987.
44. Melot C, Lejeune P, Leeman M, et al: Prostaglandin E_1 in the adult respiratory distress syndrome. Am Rev Respir Dis 139:106, 1989.
45. Presberg KW, Sznajder JI, Melendres J, et al: Distribution of pulmonary vascular resistance during lactic acid infusion in dogs. J Appl Physiol 68:1328, 1990.
46. Julien M, Hakim TS, Vahi R, Chang HK: Effect of hematocrit on vascular pressure profile in dog lungs. J Appl Physiol 58:743, 1985.
47. Weir EK, Rubin LJ, Ayres SM, et al: The acute administration of vasodilators in primary pulmonary hypertension. Am Rev Respir Dis 140:1623, 1989.
48. Palevsky HI, Fishman AP: The management of primary pulmonary hypertension. JAMA 265:1014, 1991.
49. Rich S, Brundage BH: High-dose calcium channel-blocking therapy for primary pulmonary hypertension: Evidence for long-term reduction in pulmonary arterial pressure and regression of right ventricular hypertrophy. Circulation 76:135, 1987.
50. Rubin LJ, Mendoza J, Hood M, et al: Treatment of primary pulmonary hypertension with continuous intravenous prostacyclin (epoprostenol): Results of a randomized trial. Ann Intern Med 112:485, 1990.
51. Wagenvoort CA, Wagenvoort N, Takahashi T: Pulmonary veno-occlusive disease: Involvement of pulmonary arteries and review of the literature. Hum Pathol 16:1033, 1985.
52. Wagener OE, Roncori AJ, Barcat JA: Severe pulmonary hypertension with diffuse smooth muscle proliferation of the lungs. Chest 95:234, 1989.
53. Goldberg HS, Rabson J: Control of cardiac output by systemic vessels: Circulatory adjustments to acute and chronic respiratory failure and the effect of therapeutic interventions. Am J Cardiol 47:696, 1981.
54. Rothe CF, Gaddis ML: Autoregulation of cardiac output by passive elastic characteristics of the vascular capacitance system. Circulation 81:360, 1990.
55. Belenkie I, Dani R, Smith ER, Tyberg JV: Effects of volume loading during experimental acute pulmonary embolism. Circulation 80:178, 1989.
56. Calvin JE, Langlois S, Garneys G: Ventricular interaction in a canine model of acute pulmonary hypertension and its modulation by vasoactive drugs. J Crit Care 3:43, 1988.
57. Dell'Itallia LJ, Walsh RA: Right ventricular diastolic pressure-volume relations and regional dimensions during acute alterations in loading conditions. Circulation 77:1276, 1988.
58. Yonekura S, Watanabe N, Downey HF: Transmural variation in autoregulation of right ventricular blood flow. Circ Res 62:776, 1988.
59. Harrison DG, Barnes DH, Hiratzka LF, et al: The effect of cardiac hypertrophy on the coronary collateral circulation. Circulation 71:1135, 1985.
60. Brooks H, Kirk ES, Vokonas PS, et al: Performance of the right ventricle under stress: Relation to right coronary flow. J Clin Invest 50:2176, 1971.
61. Piene H, Sund T: Flow and power output of right ventricle facing load with variable input impedance. Am J Physiol 6:H125, 1979.
62. Calvin JE, Baer RW, Glantz SA: Pulmonary artery constriction produces a greater right ventricular dynamic afterload than lung microvascular injury in the open chest dog. Circ Res 56:40, 1985.
63. Linehan JH, Dawson CA, Rickaby DA: Distribution of vascular resistance and compliance in a dog lung lobe. J Appl Physiol 53:158, 1982.
64. Hakim TS, Maarek JI, Chang HK: Estimation of pulmonary capillary pressure in intact dog lungs using the arterial occlusion technique. Am Rev Respir Dis 140:217, 1989.
65. Jardin F, Genevray B, Brun-Ney D, Margairaz A: Dobutamine: A hemodynamic evaluation in pulmonary embolism shock. Crit Care Med 13:1009, 1985.
66. Schreuder WO, Schneider AJ, Groeneveld AB, Thijs L: Effect of dopamine versus norepinephrine on hemodynamics in septic shock: Emphasis on right ventricular performance. Chest 95:1282, 1989.
67. Shaer GL, Fink MP, Parillo JE: Norepinephrine alone versus norepinephrine plus low-dose dopamine: Enhanced renal blood flow with combination pressor therapy. Crit Care Med 13:492, 1985.
68. Qvist J, Mygind T, Crottogini A, et al: Cardiovascular adjustments to pulmonary vascular injury in dogs. Anesthesiology 68:341, 1988.
69. Garratt C, Linker N, Griffith M, et al: Comparison of adenosine and verapamil for termination of paroxysmal junctional tachycardia. Am J Cardiol 64:1310, 1989.
70. Scher DL, Arsurea EL: Multifocal atrial tachycardia: Mechanisms, clinical correlates, and treatment. Am Heart J 118:574, 1989.
71. Sorensen MB, Korshin JD, Fernandes A, Secher O: The use of epidural analgesia for delivery in a patient with pulmonary hypertension. Acta Anaesthesiol Scand 26:180, 1982.

Chapter 118

PULMONARY EMBOLIC DISORDERS: THROMBUS, AIR, AND FAT

GREGORY A. SCHMIDT

KEY POINTS

- *Pulmonary embolism (PE) is common, underdiagnosed, and lethal, yet readily treatable.*
- *Prophylaxis and accurate diagnosis are essential to improving outcome.*
- *The cause of death in PE is circulatory failure (acute cor pulmonale) due to right heart ischemia.*
- *Pulmonary angiography is the gold standard for diagnosis, is relatively safe, and is frequently necessary in critically ill patients.*
- *Most patients can be effectively treated with a 10,000-U bolus of heparin, followed by a continuous infusion to maintain the partial thromboplastin time (PTT) at 1.5 to 2.5 times control.*
- *Critically ill patients may especially benefit from aggressive use of vena caval interruption.*
- *Thrombolytic therapy should be reserved for patients with massive, proven embolism and circulatory instability.*
- *Air and fat embolism usually present as adult respiratory distress syndrome (ARDS), and are managed with mechanical ventilation, oxygen, and positive end-expiratory pressure (PEEP).*

This chapter will cover diseases involving embolism to the pulmonary circulation, including pulmonary thromboembolism, as well as the less common conditions of venous air embolism and fat embolism. Thromboembolism is predominantly an acute circulatory insult, with important but less dramatic consequences for gas exchange. In contrast, both air and fat embolism usually present as acute hypoxemic respiratory failure (AHRF).

Pulmonary Thromboembolism

PE is a dramatic and life-threatening complication of underlying deep venous thrombosis (DVT). Therefore, much of the management of PE is grounded in the prophylaxis, diagnosis, and treatment of DVT. Much of our knowledge about DVT and PE is derived from patients who are not critically ill. When generalizations regarding clinical manifestations, utility of diagnostic tests, and efficacy of therapeutic approaches are extrapolated to the critically ill population, it is with some risk.

Pulmonary thromboembolism is a common, yet underdiagnosed illness, which accounts for substantial morbidity and mortality. It has been estimated that 630,000 persons each year suffer PE in the United States alone, with nearly 200,000 deaths (Fig. 118-1).[1] Thirty percent of untreated patients die, while only 8 percent succumb with effective therapy, so that failure to diagnose PE is a serious management error. Critically ill patients form a unique subset of those at risk. The presence of indwelling lines and forced immobility make these patients particularly susceptible to venous thromboemboli. Diagnosis, which is difficult even in ambulatory patients, is further impeded by barriers to communication and physical examination. Moreover, alternate explanations for hypoxemia, lung infiltrates, respiratory failure, and hemodynamic instability are readily available so that a diagnosis of pulmonary thromboembolism might not be seriously considered. Finally, critically ill patients are likely to have limited cardiopulmonary reserve, so that pulmonary emboli may be particularly lethal.

PATHOPHYSIOLOGY

Venous thrombosis begins with the formation of microthrombi at a site of venous stasis or injury. Thrombosis impedes flow and generates further vascular injury, favoring progressive clot formation. In some patients, clot becomes substantial and propagates to a proximal vein where it has the potential to embolize to the pulmonary circulation. Most clinically relevant pulmonary emboli originate as proximal venous thrombi in the leg or pelvic veins. However, in the ICU, the routine placement of upper body catheters for vascular access, monitoring, drug administration, and nutrition raises the likelihood of important upper body sources of thrombi. How significantly these upper body thrombi contribute to PE in critically ill patients is unknown.

PE occurs when thrombi detach and are carried through the great veins to the pulmonary circulation. Pulmonary vascular occlusion has important physiologic consequences which lead to the manifestations of illness as well as to clues to diagnosis. PE has an impact most notably on gas exchange and the circulation.

GAS EXCHANGE. Physical obstruction to pulmonary artery (PA) flow creates dead space in the segments served by the affected arteries. This creation of dead space has several effects on P_{CO_2} and end-tidal CO_2 (ET_{CO_2}), which can provide clues to diagnosis. If minute ventilation ($\dot{V}_E$) does not change, as occurs in a mechanically ventilated, muscle-relaxed patient, P_{CO_2} will rise. However, most patients augment $\dot{V}_E$ more than necessary to maintain elimination of CO_2, so that P_{CO_2} typically falls with PE. In health, the ET_{CO_2} is nearly the same as arterial CO_2. After pulmonary embolization, since end-tidal gas is a mixture of alveolar gas (in which PA_{CO_2} approximates Pa_{CO_2}) as well as the newly created physiologic dead space gas (in which P_{CO_2} approximates inspired P_{CO_2}, or nearly zero), ET_{CO_2} falls in propor-

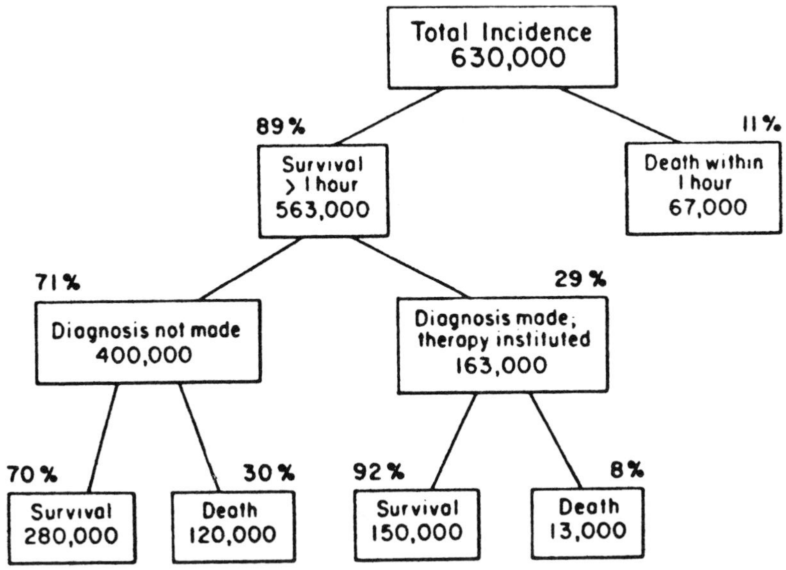

FIGURE 118-1 Natural history of pulmonary embolism based on reasonable extrapolations from known data. Reprinted from Reference 1, with permission.

tion to the degree of dead space and no longer approximates Pa_{CO_2} (Fig. 118-2).

A widened alveolar to arterial gradient for oxygen $(A-a)_{O_2}$ is present in the great majority of patients with PE. However, since hyperventilation is the rule, Pa_{O_2} may not be low. In fact, only 63 percent of patients with proven PE demonstrate a P_{O_2} <70.[2] Therefore, a normal P_{O_2} does not conclusively exclude a diagnosis of PE.

The mechanisms of hypoxemia have been elucidated by applying the multiple inert gas elimination technique (MIGET) to patients with PE.[3,4] Shunt is found in only a few patients. In some, this may be due to opening of a probe patent foramen ovale when right atrial pressure rises following PE (vide infra), with a consequent intracardiac, right-to-left shunt. Since shunt is more likely to be found when patients are studied after some delay, atelectasis due to impaired surfactant production may contribute. In most patients, however, the most important pulmonary derangement is mismatching of ventilation and perfusion. In addition, the fall in cardiac output ($\dot{Q}_T$) that accompanies most pulmonary emboli leads to a fall in mixed venous saturation. This lowered venous saturation magnifies any hypoxemia due to shunt or ventilation/perfusion ($\dot{V}/\dot{Q}$) mismatch (Fig. 118-3).

While impaired oxygenation is important and often provides a clue to the diagnosis of PE, it is typically responsive to modest oxygen enrichment of inspired gas. Similarly, most patients are able to double or triple $\dot{V}_E$ if necessary so that ventilatory failure is uncommon following PE. In fact, the greatest impact of PE is on the circulation, not on gas exchange. Although there are exceptions (e.g., some patients with severe chronic obstructive pulmonary disease [COPD]), morbidity and mortality from PE relate to cardiovascular compromise, not respiratory failure.

CIRCULATION. PE obstructs the pulmonary vascular bed mechanically as well as via presumed humoral and other mechanisms. This increases right ventricular afterload

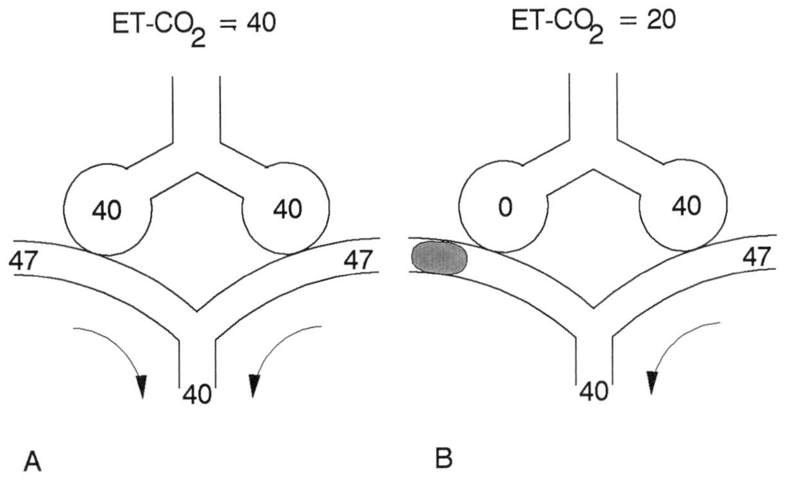

FIGURE 118-2 End-tidal CO_2 in PE. Panel A demonstrates the normal end-tidal CO_2, reflecting the alveolar CO_2 of 40. Panel B illustrates the effect of obstruction of blood flow to half the ventilated alveoli. The end-tidal CO_2 falls in proportion to the fraction of ventilated alveoli which are no longer perfused. All numbers are P_{CO_2}, in mmHg.

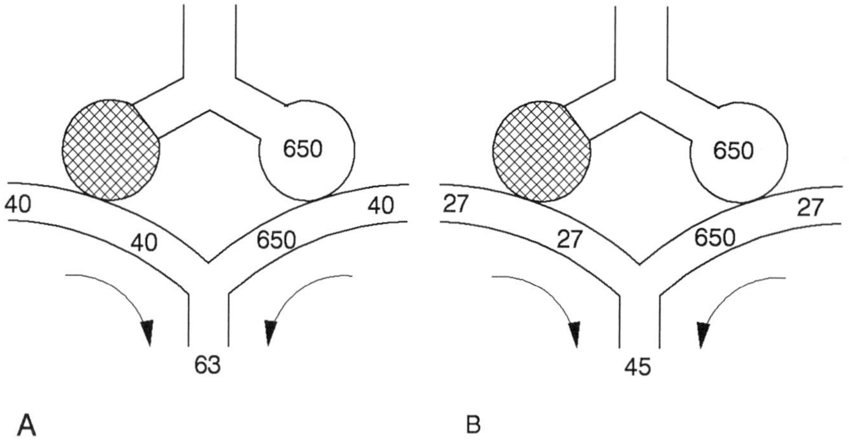

FIGURE 118-3 Effect of the mixed venous oxyhemoglobin saturation on arterial saturation in the setting of venous admixture. Panel A shows the effect of a 50 percent shunt on Pa_{O_2} in a patient breathing 100% oxygen who has a normal mixed venous P_{O_2} of 40 mmHg (75% saturation). Panel B illustrates the same patient after the mixed venous P_{O_2} has fallen to 27 (50% saturation). Note that the Pa_{O_2} and saturation have fallen significantly despite the fact that the $F_{I_{O_2}}$ and the lungs have not changed at all. All numbers are P_{O_2}, in mmHg.

which, compounded by tachycardia, increases right ventricular oxygen consumption. The right ventricle dilates and thins, its wall tension rises, and coronary perfusion is impeded. At the same time, pulmonary vascular obstruction hinders $\dot{Q}_T$ and additionally causes hypoxemia. Therefore, just at the time when the right ventricle needs increased oxygen delivery, the left ventricle may not be able to supply it. The superposition of increased right heart oxygen demand on decreased oxygen supply puts the right ventricle at risk for ischemia, which could lead to failure of the right heart (cor pulmonale). Studies in dogs with acute experimental PE support the hypothesis that ischemia underlies acute cor pulmonale.[5] (See Chap. 117.)

If acute pulmonary vascular obstruction is sufficiently massive to cause mean PA pressure to exceed approximately 40 mmHg to maintain $\dot{Q}_T$, the right heart will abruptly fail. This is the likely cause of sudden death in patients with large PEs. On the other hand, small PEs are unlikely to compromise the circulation (or lead to death), but instead manifest as dyspnea, hypoxemia, or chest pain (or remain undetected).

Of particular interest to the intensivist is the patient with a sublethal, yet large, PE. With increased afterload, the right ventricle dilates to a larger end-diastolic volume. This is associated with elevated right atrial and ventricular pressures and abnormally low $\dot{Q}_T$. One consequence of raised right atrial pressure is the potential for right-to-left shunting across a probe patent foramen ovale. This could allow paradoxical embolization to the systemic circulation as well as contribute to hypoxemia. The increase in right ventricular pressure and volume also affects the left heart. A change in shape of the right ventricle and corresponding shift of the interventricular septum from right to left alters the diastolic pressure-volume characteristics of the left ventricle (Fig. 118-4). The consequent reduction in left ventricular compliance impairs diastolic filling, thereby reducing left ventricular preload and creating yet another obstacle to $\dot{Q}_T$. An alternative explanation for the apparent decrease in left ventricular performance is reduced preload due to a fall in transmural filling pressure. Pericardial constraint might explain the fact that the left ventricular end-diastolic pressure (or wedge pressure) does not fall.[6]

Clinical Manifestations

HISTORY, EXAMINATION, AND LABORATORY DATA

Most patients with PE will complain of dyspnea, chest pain, and apprehension.[7] Less common symptoms are cough, diaphoresis, and hemoptysis. It is notable that most patients will not have symptoms of venous thrombosis. Syncope is uncommon but described in all large series of PE (Table 118-1).

The majority of patients will demonstrate tachypnea and tachycardia. Pleural rub and signs of DVT are seen only occasionally. Fever is more common than is generally appreciated and seen in half the patients.[7] Patients with large emboli may have the typical findings of any patient with low output shock such as hypotension, narrow pulse pressure, and poor peripheral perfusion. Occasionally, unanticipated failure to come off mechanical ventilation or unexplained episodes of respiratory distress may be hints to a diagnosis of PE.

TABLE 118-1 Symptoms and Signs of Pulmonary Embolism

Symptom	Incidence (%)
Dyspnea	80
Pleuritic pain	70
Apprehension	60
Cough	50
Symptoms of DVT	35
Hemoptysis	25
Central chest pain	10
Palpitations	10
Syncope	5
Sign	**Incidence (%)**
Tachypnea	90
Fever	50
Tachycardia	50
Increased P_2	50
Signs of DVT	33
Shock	5

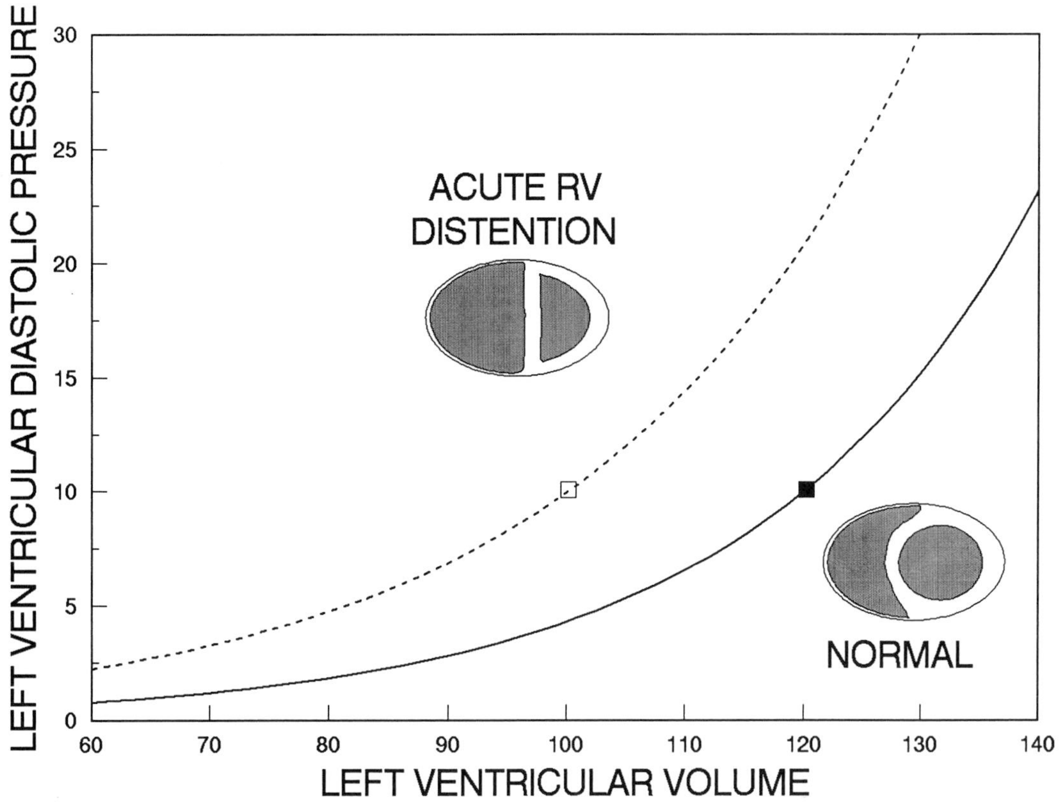

FIGURE 118-4 Left ventricular diastolic pressure-volume (PV) relationship before and after right ventricular dilation. The normal PV relationship (solid line) shows that large increments in diastolic volume are accompanied by small changes in pressure. With right ventricular distention (broken line), increments in volume are associated with relatively greater pressure changes. Note that at the same LV filling pressure of 10 mmHg, the normal ventricle contains 20 mL more blood than following RV distention. This is associated with a correspondingly higher stroke volume and $\dot{Q}_T$. Pressures are in mmHg, and volumes are in mL.

Most patients will demonstrate hypoxemia or at least a widened $(A-a)_{O_2}$. However, since a small but significant fraction will have normal oxygenation,[2] the blood-gas value should not dissuade a physician from considering the diagnosis when the rest of the clinical picture is suggestive. The chest x-ray may demonstrate areas of oligemia (Westermark's sign) and rare patients will develop a pleural based, truncated cone (Hampton's hump); however, most films have only nonspecific findings. In fact, the greatest utility of the chest film is in making (or excluding) alternative diagnoses such as pneumonia, pneumothorax, or aortic dissection. Nevertheless, the typical (albeit nonspecific) findings of basilar atelectasis, elevation of the diaphragm, and pleural effusion should always suggest PE when there is no alternative explanation. Electrocardiography (ECG) may reveal signs of right heart strain such as rightward axis shift, right bundle branch block, or right precordial strain but usually only shows sinus tachycardia.

SIGNS FROM MORE INVASIVE MONITORING

Valuable signs of PE may come from many of the devices used to monitor critically ill patients. The intensivist may derive clues from the ventilator, expired gas analysis, the PA catheter, or incidentally during echocardiography. The sensitivity and specificity of these monitors for the diagnosis of PE are not known. Nevertheless, wise physicians attempt to incorporate all available data into their synthesis of the patient. This is especially important in the ICU where the history and physical examination are difficult or impossible to obtain.

THE VENTILATOR. To maintain P_{CO_2}, the patient with PE must augment the $\dot{V}_E$. Therefore, any unexplained increase in $\dot{V}_E$ should prompt consideration of PE. Of course, any cause of rising dead space (airflow obstruction, hypovolemia, PEEP) or CO_2 production (anxiety, pain, fever, sepsis) will also increase $\dot{V}_E$. However, when none of these is apparent, especially when other clues are evident, PE becomes more likely.

EXPIRED CARBON DIOXIDE. As described above, the increment in dead space after PE causes a detectable fall in ET_{CO_2}. With technologic improvements in these devices, noninvasive assessment of expired CO_2 is becoming increasingly practical in the ICU. A corollary of the fall in ET_{CO_2} with PE is that if $\dot{V}_E$ does not rise (e.g., muscle-relaxed patient), the total excretion of CO_2 (expired CO_2

concentration × VE) must fall. Therefore, Pa_{CO_2} will rise progressively until a new steady state is reached at a higher P_{CO_2}. Again, in the muscle-relaxed patient there are many explanations for a rising CO_2, but if no explanation is forthcoming, consideration of PE is indicated.

PULMONARY ARTERY CATHETER. The most obvious clues from the PA catheter are the elevations in right atrial, right ventricular, and PA pressures and the fall in $\dot{Q}_T$ that occur with PE. Along with the reduced $\dot{Q}_T$ will be seen a widening of the arterial (A) to venous (V) oxygen content difference (Fick principle) and a decrement in the mixed venous oxygen saturation ($S\bar{v}_{O_2}$). Recognition of this may be facilitated with an oximetric catheter. A final clue from the PA catheter may lie in the difference between the PA diastolic pressure and the wedge pressure (Ppw). Normally, flow through the pulmonary circulation is pulsatile, so that by the end of diastole, there is no more flow from the PA to left atrium. Without flow, there can be no pressure gradient from the PA to left atrium. Thus the end-diastolic PA pressure and the Ppw are nearly equal. When there is obstruction of the pulmonary vascular bed, however, flow is not completed by the end of diastole and a pressure gradient remains. A discrepancy between the PA diastolic pressure and Ppw may provide a clue to PA obstruction.

Unfortunately, each of these is certainly nonspecific (and probably not sensitive) so that only rarely do such changes indicate PE. For example, cardiac dysfunction (systolic or diastolic) causes a rise in right heart pressures and a fall in $\dot{Q}_T$; any cause of low $\dot{Q}_T$ causes a widened A − V oxygen content difference; and any cause of tachycardia or increased $\dot{Q}_T$ may raise the PA diastolic to Ppw gradient.

ECHOCARDIOGRAPHY. Echocardiography is increasingly used to assess cardiac function, volume status, and pericardial disease. Occasionally, a study requested for evaluation of a low flow state may unexpectedly reveal findings strongly suggestive of PE. These include a dilated, thin-walled, poorly contracting right ventricle, and bowing of the interventricular septum to the left. Very rarely, echocardiography may demonstrate a thrombus in the right atrium or right ventricle (see Chap. 21).

Diagnosis

SPECIAL PROBLEMS IN THE ICU

The typical critically ill patient is unable to complain of the usual symptoms of PE, has numerous explanations for tachycardia and tachypnea, is hemodynamically unstable, and is a poor candidate for $\dot{V}/\dot{Q}$ lung scanning or leg studies. Therefore, serious consideration of a diagnosis of PE is often tantamount to performing a pulmonary angiogram (vide infra). For that reason, it is important to have a clear sense of the probability of PE in any given patient. Such a judgment is complex, and validated algorithms for determining prior probability in critically ill patients are not available. Synthesis of the patient's cardiopulmonary physiology, combined with an assessment of risk factors, is all the clinician has to go on. Obviously, there is no substitute for experience in managing these very difficult patients. In the following sections, the contribution of various tests in evaluating suspected PE is discussed. An approach to diagnosis is summarized in Fig. 118-5.

RISK FACTORS

Since the symptoms, signs, and laboratory findings of PE are usually nonspecific, to wait for a patient with classic, unmistakable clues before pursuing a diagnosis risks missing the majority of patients with this potentially lethal disease. However, since nonspecific indicators of potential PE are ubiquitous, indiscriminant pursuit of the diagnosis is prohibitively costly and dangerous. Most patients with PE have identifiable risk factors (Table 118-2). Absence of such risk factors should lead the physician to seek alternative explanations for the patient's findings other than thromboembolism. On the other hand, when numerous risk factors are present, the diagnosis should be more seriously considered.

DIAGNOSTIC TESTS

PERFUSION LUNG SCAN. Intravenous injection of radiolabelled colloid leads to embolization of perfused segments of the lungs. Subsequent scanning of the thorax reveals the distribution of pulmonary blood flow. Since this can be performed with portable equipment, it can be used in critically ill patients. A serious limitation of perfusion lung scanning, however, is its lack of specificity. Any cause of decreased perfusion to an area of lung, such as hypoxic vasocontriction or the presence of West zone I, will lead to a perfusion defect indistinguishable from that due to PE. Falsely positive perfusion scans are therefore likely in patients who have asthma, COPD, atelectasis, hypovolemia, or who are on PEEP (or have intrinsic PEEP). Since these conditions are common in critically ill patients, perfusion scans are rarely used. In contrast to an abnormal scan (which is nonspecific), a normal scan can be very useful. Because the perfusion scan is sensitive to PE, a normal scan effectively excludes the diagnosis. This test is most likely to affect management when PE is considered in the setting of a normal chest radiogram and presumed normal lung ven-

TABLE 118-2 Risk Factors for Pulmonary Embolism

Epidemiologic Factors:	Obesity, prior thromboembolism, advanced age, malignancy (especially adenocarcinoma), estrogens
Venous Stasis:	Immobility, paralysis, leg casts, varicose veins, congestive heart failure, prolonged travel and use of muscle relaxants
Injury:	Postsurgical, posttrauma, postpartum
Hypercoagulable States:	Proteins C and S and antithrombin-III deficiency, lupus anticoagulant, polycythemia, macroglobulinemia
Indwelling Lines:	Central venous and pulmonary artery catheters

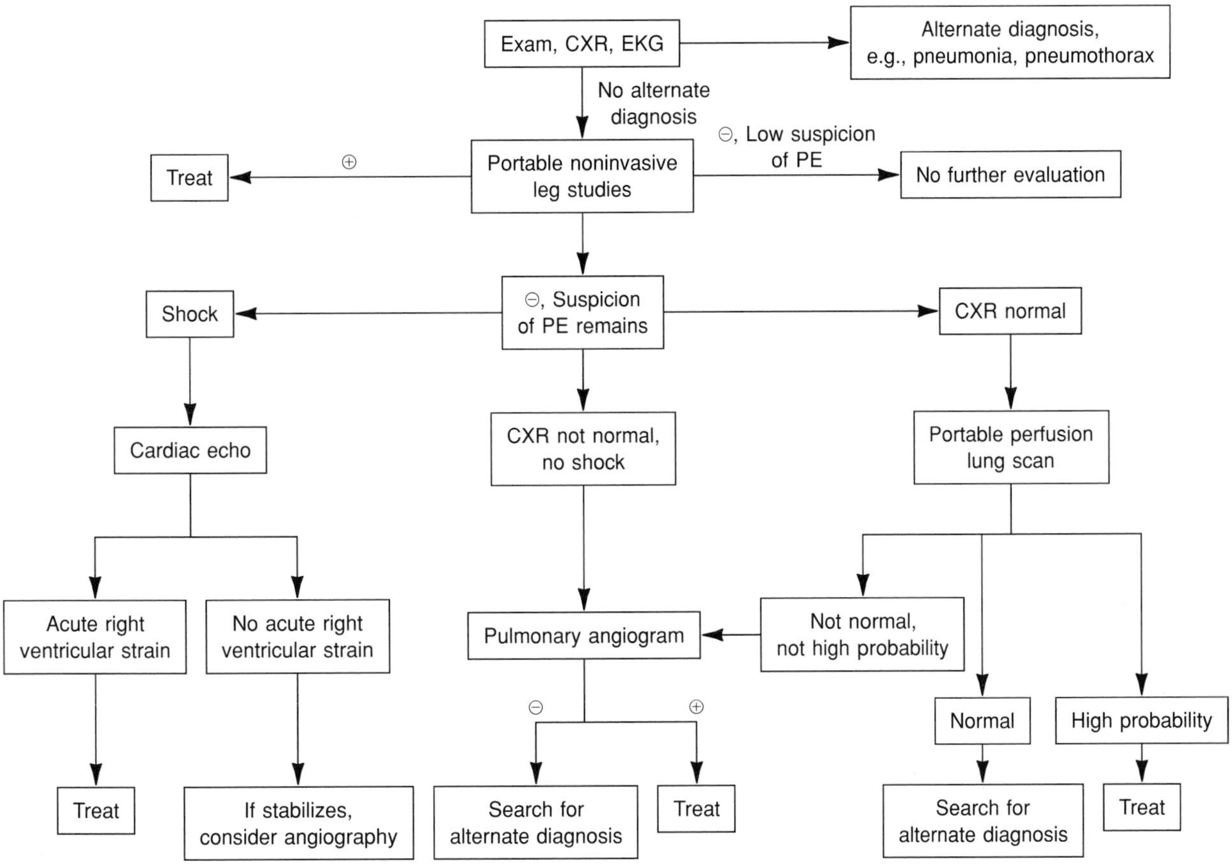

FIGURE 118-5 Algorithm for evaluation of a critically ill patient suspected of having a pulmonary embolus. If alternate diagnoses are not confirmed by examination, chest x-ray and ECG, noninvasive leg studies can be requested. If these are of adequate technical quality and are positive, treatment is indicated. If they are negative and the prior suspicion of PE is very low, no further evaluation for PE is warranted. If the suspicion of PE remains, most patients must undergo angiography. This may not be possible in a patient in shock, in whom echocardiography may provide support for a diagnosis of PE, or alternatively, demonstrate an alternate explanation for shock. Finally, rare patients with normal chest x-rays should have perfusion lungs scans done, since this may exclude PE from consideration. If the scan is not definitive, however, angiography is necessary.

tilation. Some additional limitations and risks are discussed under Ventilation/Perfusion Lung Scan.

VENTILATION/PERFUSION LUNG SCAN. Since most falsely positive perfusion lung scans occur when ventilation abnormalities lead to areas of hypoxic vasoconstriction, it is reasonable to presume that the addition of ventilation scanning will increase the specificity for the diagnosis of PE. In fact, there is wide agreement that $\dot{V}/\dot{Q}$ scan patterns judged to be "high probability" are very useful to the clinician, exhibiting a specificity of 85 percent. Although 15 of 100 patients with "high probability" $\dot{V}/\dot{Q}$ scans will not have PEs, the risk of treating them is felt to be less than the risk and cost of performing pulmonary angiography in all 100 patients. Scans of "indeterminate" (or "intermediate") probability indicate a substantial likelihood of PE (about 40 percent) so that most physicians believe that further evaluation to prove or exclude the diagnosis is imperative.

The area of greatest controversy in the utilization of $\dot{V}/\dot{Q}$ scanning is in the interpretation of "low probability" scans. Early reports generated the belief that patients with "low probability" scans had less than a 5 percent chance of harboring a PE.[8] In fact, two large, prospective trials[9,10] have now confirmed that 16 to 40 percent of patients with "low probability" scans have PE, indicating that the term "low probability" is simply misleading.

The practical application of $\dot{V}/\dot{Q}$ scanning is as follows. Normal scans exclude the diagnosis of PE. "High probability" scans provide sufficient grounds for treatment of PE. All scans which are not normal and not "high probability" should be considered indeterminate.[11] Generally, all such scans should prompt further evaluation (vide infra). Of course there is room for physician judgment. A low prior probability of PE or poor overall patient prognosis may make additional testing unattractive. This approach is summarized in Fig. 118-6.

Unfortunately, there are further problems applying $\dot{V}/\dot{Q}$ scanning to critically ill patients. $\dot{V}/\dot{Q}$ scanning is technically difficult in intubated patients. Moreover, some of the sensitivity and specificity depends on obtaining multiple

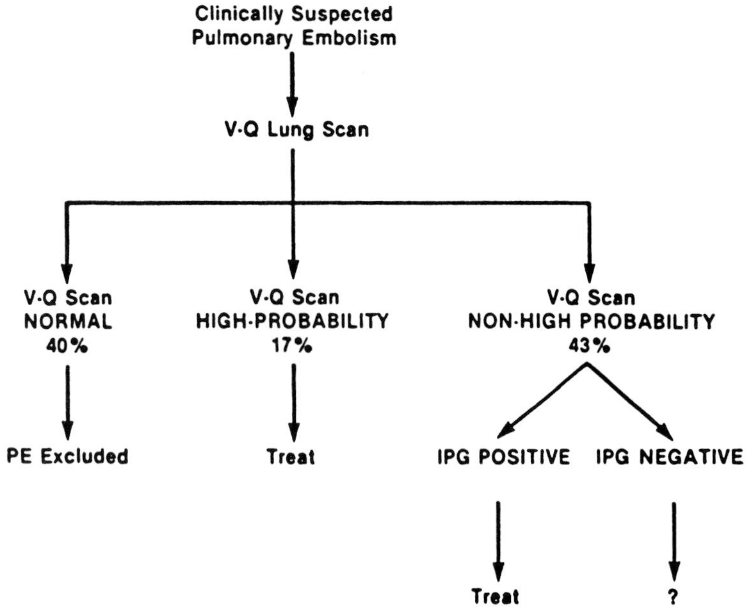

FIGURE 118-6 Utility of the ventilation/perfusion ($\dot{V}/\dot{Q}$) lung scan. Normal and high probability scans allow confident exclusion or inclusion of a diagnosis of PE. All other scan results are unhelpful and mandate further evaluation. The ? indicates that there are insufficient data on which to base recommendation for evaluation or therapy in patients with nondiagnostic scans and negative leg studies. The percentages refer to the proportion of all patients with suspected PE who can be expected to have a given $\dot{V}/\dot{Q}$ scan result. This schema is based largely on patients who are not in ICUs. Reprinted from Reference 11, with permission.

views of high quality. Of course, it may not be possible to get more than a single anteroposterior view when the patient cannot cooperate. Some patients are so likely to have indeterminate results (e.g., those with COPD or status asthmaticus) that scanning serves only to waste time[12] and we proceed with alternate tests. Finally, there is a finite (albeit small) risk when colloidal particles are intentionally embolized to a compromised pulmonary circulation. In normal adults only about 1 percent of the pulmonary arterial bed is occluded during a perfusion scan, which is clearly insignificant. In a patient with a massive embolus and shock (with critical compromise of the right ventricle) only 25 percent of the original vascular bed may be patent. Injection of colloid may reduce this to roughly 24 percent, a decremental insult of 4 percent. The right ventricle may be unable to tolerate this sudden additional load. Anecdotes of sudden death following injection of colloid have been reported.

PULMONARY ANGIOGRAPHY. Pulmonary angiography is the "gold standard" for the diagnosis of PE. Its sensitivity is sufficiently high to detect embolism even weeks to months after its occurrence. The earliest documented resolution of an angiogram to normal following a PE is 7 days. Thus, this test can definitively exclude embolism if a negative study is obtained even a week following the onset of symptoms.[13] Since it is invasive, costly, somewhat riskier than $\dot{V}/\dot{Q}$ scanning, and requires the presence of an interventional radiologist (rather than a technician), many physicians are reluctant to request it. On the other hand, because $\dot{V}/\dot{Q}$ scanning is so often unhelpful (or inapplicable) in critically ill patients, pulmonary angiography can be especially useful.

This test is safer than generally appreciated. The mortality rate is around 0.2 percent as shown in several large series.[14,15] Several patients who have died had severe pulmonary hypertension and cor pulmonale at the time of the procedure. This has led some physicians to conclude that pulmonary hypertension is a contraindication to pulmonary angiography. The degree of risk in patients with pulmonary hypertension was directly addressed in one review of pulmonary angiography.[15] Elevated PA systolic pressure (>70 mmHg) and elevated right ventricular diastolic pressure (>20 mmHg) were identified as risk factors. Even in these sickest patients, however, the mortality rate was only 2 percent. In patients with severe chronic pulmonary hypertension who are being considered for surgical endarterectomy (admittedly a different population) angiography has been performed quite safely.[16] Nonionic, low osmolality contrast agents may be able to reduce risk even further.

Failure to diagnose PE presents substantial risks to patients, especially in the critically ill who may have little cardiovascular reserve. Therefore, when a $\dot{V}/\dot{Q}$ scan is not practical (patient too ill), is unlikely to be helpful (COPD, asthma, ARDS), or has not aided the clinician (low or indeterminate scan), pulmonary angiography may be essential. This invasive procedure may be obviated, however, in some patients by positive results of leg studies.

NONINVASIVE LEG STUDIES. Noninvasive leg studies include impedance plethysmography, phleborrheography, venous Dopplers, and B-mode ultrasound scanning of leg veins. The technical details of these procedures and differences between them are beyond the scope of this chapter, but which particular test to choose is largely a function of local expertise. B-mode ultrasound scanning is an attractive option in critically ill patients since it is easily portable. However, isolated iliac thrombi cannot be seen, the experience with this technique is limited, and its true utility is unknown.[17] It is important to realize that the utility of all of these studies in the diagnosis of venous thrombosis has been validated in patients who are studied in a vascular laboratory, with high quality equipment. The technical quality of portable studies in critically ill patients is rarely optimal. To generalize from the outpatient experience to the ICU is potentially dangerous. Nevertheless, these studies are worth obtaining since they may be definitely positive and form sufficient grounds for anticoagulation. Venography is only very rarely used in the diagnosis of venous thrombosis in critically ill patients and will not be discussed, but the principles of its application to patients with possible PE parallel the use of noninvasive studies.

Noninvasive leg studies cannot make nor exclude the diagnosis of PE. Almost one-third of patients with proven PEs will not have detectable venous thrombosis,[9] and, of course, proven venous thrombosis is no proof that clot has embolized. However, leg studies which reveal venous thrombosis provide a rationale for therapy (typically anticoagulation). This usually makes the question of PE a moot one. Those who have negative leg studies should have further evaluation unless the clinical suspicion of PE is low (see Fig. 118-5).

EMPIRICAL DIAGNOSIS

Occasionally, an empirical diagnosis of PE seems clear cut to the managing physician. No alternative diagnoses may seem plausible, or further diagnostic steps (usually pulmonary angiography) seem too much trouble. Although this approach may appear attractive, it almost never proves correct. First, the clinical diagnosis is simply too unreliable, even for the most experienced clinician. Second, there are always alternative diagnoses. Finally, the doubt which lingers after an empirical diagnosis too frequently haunts subsequent management. Progression of symptoms or signs despite therapy raises questions about failure of treatment or the need for alternative treatments. Complications of treatment (usually hemorrhage due to heparin, occasionally thrombocytopenia) create uncertainty about the necessity of the toxic therapy, or precipitate more diagnostic interventions in a newly unstable state. Since critically ill patients are more likely to have complications of therapy, empiricism is rarely appropriate.

Treatment

The majority of patients with PE will not die from the clot which leads to diagnosis. As long as reembolization is prevented, the patient will survive, while intrinsic fibrinolysis restores pulmonary blood flow. Therefore, the primary goal of all therapies for PE is to prevent reembolization. Some patients, however, survive the initial embolus, yet remain in shock. These patients, who are overrepresented in ICU populations, may succumb to the initial embolus. Additional therapy to hasten clot resolution, aimed at more promptly restoring the circulation, might be useful in such patients. Supportive care, anticoagulation, vena caval interruption, thrombolysis, fluid and vasoactive drug administration, and rarely, surgical embolectomy all must be considered in the treatment of this disease. An integrated approach to the treatment of PE is presented in Fig. 118-7.

SUPPORTIVE CARE

OXYGEN AND BED REST. Patients typically present with hypoxemia which responds well to oxygen therapy since the underlying pathophysiology is usually $\dot{V}/\dot{Q}$ mismatch. Bed rest accomplishes two goals. First, limitation of activity probably reduces the likelihood of dislodging further clots from the presumed leg source. Second, bed rest reduces oxygen consumption ($\dot{V}_{O_2}$), and thereby the demand for $\dot{Q}_T$. Taken to its limit, this might involve muscle relaxation and mechanical ventilation in the patient with shock, to reduce $\dot{V}_{O_2}$ to a minimum.

SPECIFIC THERAPIES

ANTICOAGULATION. Heparin is the mainstay of therapy for PE. It is effective in preventing reembolization while allowing fibrinolysis to proceed. Heparin should be instituted once the diagnosis is seriously considered as long as there is no contraindication to anticoagulation. Treatment begins with an intravenous bolus of 7500 U to 10,000 U, usually followed by a maintenance infusion of heparin. Some evidence supports the use of subcutaneous calcium heparin for continued anticoagulation since therapeutic plasma heparin levels are easily attained.[18] Although this treatment is simpler and cheaper than continuous infusion heparin, it remains insufficiently proven to replace standard care, especially in critically ill patients. Maintenance heparin should be titrated to achieve a PTT of 1.5 to 2.5 times control, or to heparin levels of 0.3 to 0.4 IU/mL plasma using the protamine sulfate neutralization test. This typically requires an infusion rate of 1000 U/h, given intravenously, or 15,000 U twice daily, given subcutaneously. Coumadin anticoagulation should be instituted after 4 or 5 days, although earlier conversion may be safe as well. If the patient is clinically unstable, heparin should probably be continued rather than coumadin, to facilitate rapid adjustment of anticoagulation should that be required. Monitoring and complications of anticoagulation are covered in Chap. 119.

VENA CAVAL INTERRUPTION. Since most thromboemboli originate in the legs, pelvis, or inferior vena cava (IVC),[19] inferior vena caval interruption (VCI) is effective therapy for PE. While this does nothing for the embolized clot, VCI is highly effective in preventing reembolization and death. Several methods have been devised for VCI, including surgical ligation or plication, balloon occlusion, and percutaneous placement of filters. Placement of filters by interventional radiologists and vascular surgeons has replaced all other methods since the new devices are easily placed and maintain caval patency.[20] Conventional indications for the use of VCI in patients with venous thromboembolism have included contraindications to anticoagulation, hemorrhage following anticoagulation, failure of anticoagulation to prevent recurrent embolization, and prophylaxis of extremely high-risk patients.

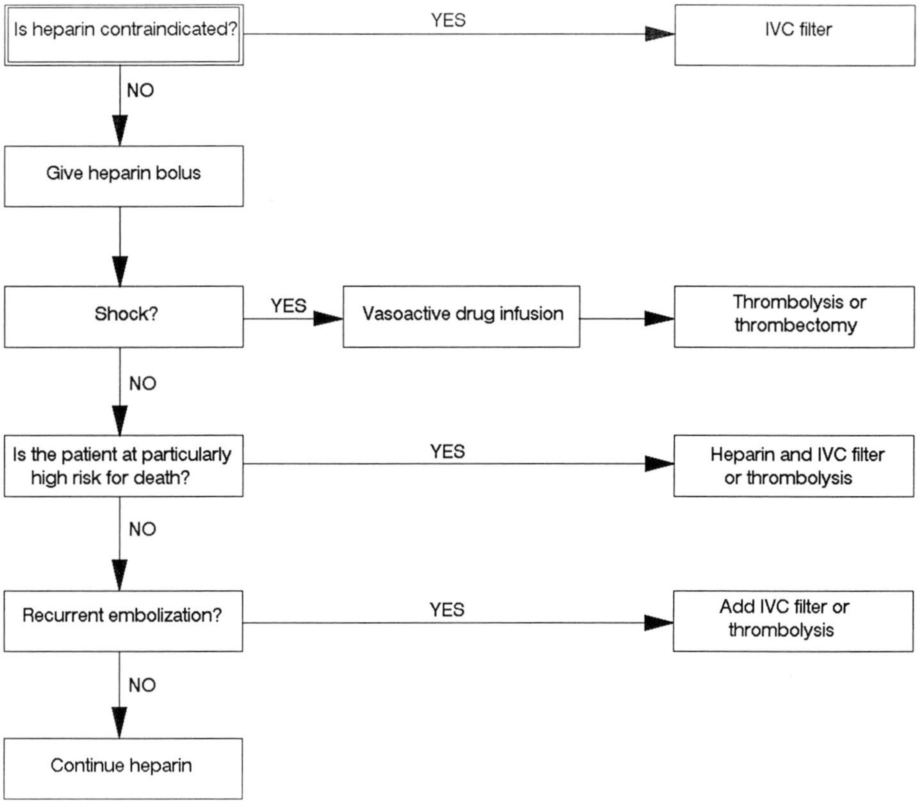

FIGURE 118-7 Treatment of PE in critically ill patients.

As VCI devices have evolved, they have become smaller and more easily placed. As physicians have become more experienced with them, they have become safer as well. In addition, new devices are on the horizon which may be retrievable from the vena cava. It is little surprise then that indications for VCI use are expanding. Even so, caval filters are probably greatly underutilized in the sickest patients. Those with critical cardiopulmonary compromise may least be able to tolerate the admittedly low risk of heparin failure. Patients who survive sublethal embolism but remain hemodynamically compromised may benefit from VCI since recurrent embolism, while unlikely, will be fatal. In addition, some patients have such a predictably high risk of venous thromboembolism that VCI may be indicated even before any thrombosis is detected. For example, we have placed caval filters prophylactically in patients with severe COPD and proximal venous thrombosis and in a woman with Crohn's disease complicated by toxic megacolon and ARDS on her way to the operating room.

The significance of upper extremity sources of thromboemboli in ICU patients, who often have central catheters, is unknown but probably small. Nevertheless, inferior VCI would clearly be ineffective so that when the clinical presentation suggests an upper source, due consideration should precede placement of this device. Filters have been placed in the superior vena cava and in the suprarenal IVC with apparent safety, but the experience is small.

A final point about VCI is that while it prevents recurrent embolization, it does not treat the (presumed) leg source. Therefore, when these devices are used, concomitant anticoagulation is necessary (unless the indication for VCI is contraindication to anticoagulation).

THROMBOLYTIC THERAPY. Potential advantages to thrombolytic therapy over anticoagulation include removal of the thrombotic source, reduction in the postphlebitic syndrome, more rapid restoration of a normal circulation, prevention of chronic pulmonary thromboembolism and pulmonary hypertension, and improved survival. More rapid clot lysis and more prompt reduction of right heart pressures have been unequivocally demonstrated.[21] A long-term beneficial effect on pulmonary diffusing capacity has also been shown.[22] Unfortunately, no impact has been demonstrated on more relevant end points such as mortality or clinical morbidity. Although our increasing experience with thrombolytic therapy has made it progressively safer, it is clearly more risky than standard anticoagulation. It is for these reasons that thrombolysis is not widely accepted for the treatment of PE, whereas it is for acute myocardial infarction.

Some patients may benefit from the proven ability of thrombolytic therapy to rapidly improve right heart pressures. For example, death in the patient with massive embolism and shock is from acute cor pulmonale. Thus, rapid reduction in right heart pressures might allow survival.[23] In addition, such a patient is critically sensitive to even minor

TABLE 118-3 Alternative Thrombolytic Strategies in Acute Massive Pulmonary Embolism

- Urokinase, 4400 U/kg bolus, followed by 4400 U/kg/h for 24 h[21]
- Urokinase, 1,000,000 U bolus over 10 min, followed by 2,000,000 U over 110 min[25]
- Urokinase, 15,000 U/kg bolus over 10 min[26]
- rTPA, 0.6 mg/kg bolus[27]
- Streptokinase, 250,000 U over 30 min, followed by 100,000 U/h for 24 h

recurrent embolism. Removal of the embolic source might therefore confer additional survival benefit. Because these arguments are attractive and since such patients are so likely to die, thrombolytic therapy should be given in the setting of proven massive embolism and shock.[24] However, clear benefit has never been demonstrated in such patients.

The optimal regimen for thrombolytic therapy has not been established. One approach is to give recombinant tissue plasminogen activator (rTPA), 100 mg intravenously over 2 h, followed by heparin when the PTT falls to twice control.[25] Alternative thrombolytic strategies are outlined in Table 118-3.[25–27] There is no advantage to infusing the thrombolytic agent directly into the PA.[28] Monitoring and complications of thrombolytic therapy are covered in Chap. 119.

FLUID AND VASOACTIVE DRUG ADMINISTRATION. Volume administration with saline or colloid has generally been advocated in patients with PE and shock on the grounds that it will increase filling pressures and thereby augment $\dot{Q}_T$. However, in a patient with elevated right heart pressures and a grossly distended right ventricle, it is possible that further distention of the right ventricle during volume administration will increase myocardial oxygen consumption, yet fail to increase $\dot{Q}_T$ and oxygen supply. In addition, to the extent that fluids increase right ventricular end-diastolic volume, the interventricular septum will bulge further to the left, impede left heart filling, and further compromise $\dot{Q}_T$. Experimental studies to determine the effect of fluids have shown a detrimental effect on hemodynamics.[29] Therefore, volume administration should not be routine therapy unless the patient is clearly hypovolemic. When fluids are given, guidance using right heart catheterization and echocardiography is essential.

There is also controversy regarding the use of vasoactive drugs to treat the hypoperfusion caused by PE. Successful use of vasoconstrictors, inotropes, and vasodilators has been reported. Since no controlled studies in patients have been performed it is hard to give firm recommendations. However, the pathophysiology of this form of shock and the results of some animal experiments provide some guidance. When any of these drugs are used, serial assessment of the effect of the intervention is mandatory. Any drug which does not result in the intended salutary effect should be discontinued promptly.

Norepinephrine. The rationale for the use of this vasoconstrictor is based on the assumption that right ventricular ischemia is the fundamental problem leading to shock. A vasoconstrictor which increases systemic arteriolar tone could raise aortic pressure and augment coronary blood flow, without increasing right ventricular load. In animal models of sublethal PE, norepinephrine was shown to be superior to no therapy, to volume administration, and to isoproterenol in the maintanence of $\dot{Q}_T$ as well as in survival time.[30] In the clinical setting, hypoperfusion may have additional contributors such as left ventricular dysfunction or ischemic heart disease, so that a vasoconstrictor might be less beneficial than in controlled animal experiments. Nevertheless, norepinephrine should be the first choice when a vasoactive drug is needed for hypoperfusion. Infusion is initiated at 2 μg/min and adjusted based on the hemodynamic response.

Inotropic Agents. Dopamine, dobutamine, isoproterenol, and epinephrine would all be expected to increase right ventricular oxygen consumption, possibly without improving right ventricular blood flow. Nevertheless, each has been anecdotally reported to be beneficial in severe PE. Isoproterenol has been advocated for its known effect in reducing pulmonary vascular resistance. However, when there is fixed, mechanical obstruction to pulmonary flow, isoproterenol has no effect. None of these drugs is an attractive first choice in shock due to PE. As in any patient with a hypoperfusion state, dopamine can be administered in low doses (2 μg/kg/min) to maintain renal perfusion.

Vasodilators. A drug which caused pulmonary vasodilation without decreasing blood pressure would be attractive. Unfortunately, the pulmonary vascular obstruction after massive PE is largely fixed. In addition, vasodilators selective for the pulmonary vasculature are not yet available. All vasodilators risk reducing systemic vascular resistance in the face of a right heart limitation to $\dot{Q}_T$. Since the resultant hypotension would likely be fatal in the setting of massive PE, vasodilators should not be used.

EMBOLECTOMY. Surgical extraction of PA clot is a dramatic solution to the problem of massive PE. Usually performed under cardiopulmonary bypass, it has the advantages of stabilizing $\dot{Q}_T$ mechanically, quickly removing the problem, and preventing the possibility of chronic pulmonary hypertension. Substantial disadvantages include the risk of induction of anesthesia in an unstable patient, invasiveness, logistical barriers to availability, and cost. It is likely that most times that the procedure would be considered, the patient would be either better or moribund by the time the procedure could be performed. More importantly, simpler, yet effective alternatives are usually available, such as heparin in the majority and thrombolytic therapy for patients in shock. Most physicians consider surgical embolectomy only in patients with proven, massive PE with unstable circulations and contraindications to thrombolytic therapy. Nevertheless, one group has reported excellent results with this procedure and advocate it routinely in all patients with large PEs.[31]

Special Considerations

PREGNANCY

The pregnant woman who may have PE presents unique challenges. Pregnancy is thought to be a risk factor for venous thrombosis, and PE is the second leading cause of death among gravidas (next to trauma.)[32] The addition of the fetus, as well as anatomic considerations, leads to several key differences in management.

DIAGNOSIS. Diagnosis can be more difficult because of reluctance to perform potentially risky procedures, particularly involving diagnostic radiology. However, it is important not to lose sight of the risk of failing to make the diagnosis. Thus, when the diagnosis is seriously considered, it should be pursued. $\dot{V}/\dot{Q}$ scans probably pose little risk to the fetus. The estimated radiation dose is small, and the risk is clearly less than that of missing a diagnosis.[33] Impedence plethysmography is also less useful in pregnancy due to mechanical compression of the IVC by the enlarged uterus, especially in the third trimester. A positive result in the first two trimesters is sufficient basis on which to anticoagulate, but may not be in the last trimester unless the vascular laboratory has particular expertise in pregnancy.[34] The risk of pulmonary angiography is not known, but when indicated, it should not be withheld out of concern of fetal radiation exposure. The maternal risks of undiagnosed and untreated PE are clear.

TREATMENT. Heparin therapy is not different during pregnancy. However, coumadin, which is teratogenic, should not be instituted. Rather, long-term treatment should consist of subcutaneous heparin.[35] Thrombolytic therapy risks spontaneous abortion and uterine bleeding. Nevertheless, several case reports of the successful use of thrombolytic treatment of PE have appeared. Vena caval interruption requires some modification as well. The left ovarian vein (a potential source of clot) drains into the left renal vein. Therefore, when a caval filter is placed, it should be inserted to a suprarenal position, rather than below the renal veins. Again, several cases of successful use of these devices have been described.

CHRONIC OBSTRUCTIVE PULMONARY DISEASE

Patients with COPD are at increased risk for PE. In addition, their preexisting respiratory compromise and abnormal pulmonary vasculature leave them particularly vulnerable to the cardiopulmonary consequences of PE. Ironically, diagnosis of PE in the setting of COPD in unusually difficult. Patients commonly complain of dyspnea, chest pain, cough and anxiety, and occasionally note hemoptysis and leg swelling. Their examinations, chest radiograms, ECGs, and arterial blood-gas values are usually abnormal at base line. $\dot{V}/\dot{Q}$ scans are worthless.

When patients with COPD present with symptoms which are atypical for their usual exacerbation, particularly when the Pa_{CO_2} is reduced from previously elevated values, it is worth considering the diagnosis.[36] Positive leg studies may provide a rationale for anticoagulation and obviate the need for further investigation, although this approach has been called into question.[37] Short of this, however, pulmonary angiography is the only reliable means for establishing a diagnosis. The physician and patient may be in the unfortunate position of having to repeatedly consider an invasive procedure or risk a missed diagnosis. In fact, it is in just this type of situation that PEs go undiagnosed. There is no simple answer to this problem and PEs will continue to be underdiagnosed until better, less invasive tests are available.

PATIENTS WITH COAGULATION OR PLATELET DISORDERS

The risk of venous thromboembolism in patients with chronic liver disease or marked thrombocytopenia is not known. While it seems sensible to conclude that the risk must be lower than if clotting and platelet function were normal, PEs occur even when the bleeding tendency is severe.[38,39] Therefore, when the clinical presentation strongly suggests PE, thrombocytopenia and coagulopathy should provide little reassurance, and diagnostic testing is indicated. Patients with chronic renal failure do seem to be at a remarkably low risk of venous thromboembolism, so that alternative diagnoses should always be sought.

Prophylaxis against Venous Thromboembolism

A discussion of prophylaxis has been left to the end of the chapter because here it is particularly easy to emphasize several points. PE is common, lethal, usually missed, difficult to evaluate, and costly to treat; more so in critically ill patients. Therefore, it is best to *prevent* this disease. A full treatment of prophylaxis is beyond the scope of this chapter, but a few points are worth making.

Prophylaxis, generally using subcutaneous heparin (5000 U twice daily) has been shown to be safe and effective in general medical patients, and in those with stroke or acute myocardial infarction in reducing thromboembolic events.[40] There is overwhelming evidence that routine preoperative minidose heparin saves lives, without serious bleeding.[41] In the absence of a contraindication, nearly all critically ill patients should receive minidose heparin. When heparin is unsafe (e.g., neurosurgical patients), alternative methods of prophylaxis, such as intermittent pneumatic compression cuffs, should be instituted. Finally, although controversial, some patients at extremely high risk of PE should have consideration given to prophylactic insertion of vena caval filters (vide supra).

Air Embolism

The syndrome of air (or gas) embolism results when air enters the vasculature, travels to the pulmonary circulation, and causes circulatory or respiratory embarrassment. It is uncommonly recognized in critically ill patients, but is quite likely underdiagnosed.

PATHOPHYSIOLOGY

The syndrome is triggered when a gas, usually air, enters a vessel, typically a vein. It travels with the venous return to the right heart and lungs, where it may have circulatory or respiratory consequences. Occasionally, air reaches the arterial circulation leading to systemic manifestations.

ENTRY OF AIR INTO THE VASCULATURE. Development of air embolism requires an abnormal communication between air and the blood vessel. In addition, there must be a pressure gradient to favor entry of air into the vessel, rather than bleeding from the vessel. Trauma, surgical incisions, and intravascular catheters create the commonest sources of air entry. In addition, there are more subtle paths through which air can reach the vasculature, such as in damaged, mechanically ventilated lungs of patients with ARDS. The driving gradient for air entry may be provided by air under pressure, as during positive-pressure ventilation or high pressure wound irrigation. Alternatively, the air may be at atmospheric pressure, but the intravascular pressure is subatmospheric. For example, any vein which is above the heart by an amount exceeding the central venous pressure is likely to be at less than atmospheric pressure (and therefore appears collapsed). Table 118-4 lists some of the causes of the air embolism syndrome.

TABLE 118-4 Etiology of Air Embolism

Surgery and Trauma Related	Nonsurgical
Neurosurgery, especially upright	Cardiopulmonary resuscitation
Liver transplantation	Gastrointestinal endoscopy
Total hip replacement	Positive-pressure ventilation
Harrington rod insertion	Infusion computed tomography scan
Spinal fusion	Scuba diving
Pulsed saline irrigation	Self-induced
Removal of tissue expanders	Orogenital sex
Transurethral resection, prostate	
Arthroscopy	
Open heart surgery	
Hysterectomy	
Cesarean section	
Head and neck trauma	
Pacemaker insertion	
Tenkhoff catheter placement	
Intraaortic balloon pump	
Bone marrow harvest	
Epidural catheter placement	
Central line placement	
Percutaneous lung biopsy	
Laser bronchoscopy	
Retrograde pyelography	
Hemodialysis	
Percutaneous lithotrypsy	

CIRCULATORY CONSEQUENCES. Massive air embolization can fill the right heart, impede venous return, and thereby stop circulation. Thus, sudden death is one of the possible outcomes. It is estimated that >100 mL air must be acutely infused to arrest circulation. Most often, however, air passes through the right heart into the lungs. There it raises PA pressure, but has predominantly respiratory consequences.

RESPIRATORY CONSEQUENCES. Air is carried into the pulmonary vasculature where it embolizes in pulmonary arterioles and capillaries. The abnormal air-blood interface is thought to denature plasma proteins, creating amorphous proteinaceous and cellular debris at the surface of air bubbles.[42] This debris attracts and activates white blood cells, facilitating injury to the pulmonary capillaries. Endothelial injury increases capillary permeability, which leads to alveolar flooding. The resulting noncardiogenic pulmonary edema accounts for the majority of symptoms and signs due to air embolism (see Chap. 128). In addition, air embolization leads to bronchoconstriction, a point which may be useful in diagnosis.[43]

Although the dominant gas exchange abnormality is hypoxemia, carbon dioxide elimination is impaired as well. As pulmonary vessels become occluded, alveoli subtended by them are ventilated, but unperfused. This increment in dead space may be signalled by a drop in ET_{CO_2}, if this is being monitored (as in the operating room). In the patient with fixed $\dot{V}E$ (for example, if the patient is muscle relaxed), P_{CO_2} will rise. Either of these may lead to suspicion of the diagnosis.

EXTRATHORACIC MANIFESTATIONS. Air embolism is occasionally accompanied by systemic findings. If air directly enters the pulmonary veins, as may occur in patients being mechanically ventilated with acute lung injury, bubbles pass directly to the arterial circulation. However, since air typically enters a systemic vein, the arterial circulation is protected from embolization by the filtering effect of the pulmonary circulation. Nevertheless, bubbles can pass to the left side of the heart via the foramen ovale, which is probe patent in up to 30 percent of people. This type of foramen ovale does not ordinarily allow right-to-left shunting, due to the higher pressures in the left atrium. After significant embolization to the pulmonary circulation, however, right heart pressures rise, reversing the interatrial gradient. This allows bubbles to pass directly from the right to left atrium, then to the systemic circulation. Even in the absence of a foramen ovale, air can reach the arterial circulation since the lungs do not fully filter air, especially when a large amount is embolized. Air may pass through large extraalveolar vessels or through the pulmonary capillaries themselves. In animal experiments, the threshold rate of venous air infusion which overwhelms pulmonary filtering is 0.30 mL/kg/min.[44] For a 70-kg man, this value translates to only 21 mL/min.

Once air reaches the arterial circulation, peripheral embolization leads to ischemic manifestations in the brain, heart, skin (livedo reticularis),[45] and other organs. Some of

TABLE 118-5 Manifestations of Air Embolism

Dyspnea, hypoxemia
Confusion, stroke, or peripheral embolization
Hypotension, shock
Diffuse alveolar infiltrates
Increment in airway pressures
Increased dead space, rising $\dot{V}_E$
Abrupt fall in ET_{CO_2}
Detection of air by echocardiography, Doppler monitor, or radiography

the ischemic manifestations in the periphery are probably mediated by polymorphonuclear leukocytes and oxygen radicals, as is the injury in the lung.[46]

PRESENTATION

Air embolism is usually recognized when it presents as acute hypoxemic respiratory failure. As noted above, it may also manifest as an acute hypoperfusion state or as peripheral embolization. The chest x-ray shows diffuse alveolar filling. We have seen one case in which intracardiac and intraarterial air was grossly evident on the chest radiograph. Increased dead space may be indicated by increased $\dot{V}_E$, increased P_{CO_2}, or decreased ET_{CO_2}. Rarely, echocardiography will demonstrate residual air (or ongoing embolization) in the heart. Precordial Doppler monitoring during high-risk surgery is well suited for detecting air (Table 118-5).

A diagnosis of air embolism is usually considered when air is witnessed to enter an intravascular catheter. It is also likely to be considered in extremely high-risk settings such as upright neurosurgery. However, if air embolism is only thought of when it is grossly apparent, many episodes will go unappreciated. It should also be included in the differential diagnosis of patients with hypoperfusion, systemic embolization, obtundation, and respiratory failure, especially when more likely causes are lacking.

The differential diagnosis of air embolism includes other forms of noncardiogenic pulmonary edema, as well as cardiogenic edema. Thus, volume overload, sepsis, and gastric acid aspiration must be excluded.

MANAGEMENT

The goals of treatment are to prevent reembolization while supporting respiration and circulation. In most cases, resolution is prompt. The source of air entry should be indentified and closed, if possible. Alternatively, the gradient favoring air entry can be lessened, as for example by saline administration to raise intravascular pressures. When air embolism complicates positive-pressure ventilation, it may be advisable to lower airway pressures by lowering tidal volumes, reducing PEEP, or intentional hypoventilation.

In certain situations, it may be possible to retrieve air from the venous circulation or right heart, especially intraoperatively when a catheter is in place for that purpose. This should not be routinely attempted in other settings, however, because significant amounts of air cannot usually be removed. Positional maneuvers to prevent air from embolizing to the lungs (such as head down left decubitus) are largely unproven. Similarly, the distribution of arterial emboli seems little affected by the Trendelenburg position, since the force of arterial flow greatly outweighs the buoyancy of the bubbles.[47]

Standard treatment is similar to that of any patient with ARDS. Mechanical ventilation to reduce the work of breathing, with oxygen and PEEP to maintain arterial saturation are usually necessary. Although the pulmonary edema is not related to hypervolemia, the degree of lung leak is probably sensitive to filling pressures. Therefore, filling pressures should be reduced to the lowest value that allows an adequate $\dot{Q}_T$ (see Chap. 128).

In animal experiments, corticosteroids given before embolization, or shortly following embolization, reduce the degree of lung injury. In high-risk neurosurgical patients on steroids, the incidence of the syndrome seems less than in similar patients who are not so treated, suggesting a prophylactic benefit in human beings, as well. Nevertheless, no clear role for these agents has been demonstrated, and they should not be routinely given. Potential future therapies include other anti-inflammatory drugs and agents directed against oxygen free radicals.

Hyperbaric treatment is of theoretical benefit since compression reduces the size of bubbles. This reduces the surface area for activation of white blood cells and can thereby limit pulmonary and systemic injury. Such therapy is standard when the mechanism of gas embolism is decompression, such as in professional and recreational divers. It is not routinely used in other critically ill patients, however. Since patients usually respond readily to standard supportive measures, and since the syndrome typically resolves in only 24 to 48 h, there seems little role for hyperbaric treatment. It is probably better to keep patients in the ICU where they remain under the watchful eye of the health care team, rather than to risk transport for an unproven treatment.

Fat Embolism

The fat embolism syndrome (FES) is associated with fat particles in the microcirculation of the lung. It is most common following long bone fractures, typically presenting as dyspnea and confusion. However, FES is seen after other forms of trauma and in several nontraumatic conditions as well. After long bone or pelvic fracture, the incidence of the syndrome is at least 10 percent when evidence for it is prospectively sought.[48] Since the clinical manifestations are usually mild, FES is often unrecognized. Even when lung injury is obvious, its cause may be attributed to infection, aspiration, or traumatic ARDS, rather than to fat embolization. Some of the causes of FES are presented in Table 118-6.

TABLE 118-6 Causes of Fat Embolism Syndrome

Traumatic Fat Embolism
Long bone fracture (especially femur)
Other fractures
Blunt trauma to fatty organs (e.g., liver)
Liposuction
Nontraumatic Fat Embolism
Pancreatitis
Diabetes mellitus
Lipid infusions
Sickle cell crisis
Burns
Cardiopulmonary bypass
Decompression sickness
Lymphangiography
Cyclosporine infusion

PATHOPHYSIOLOGY

NONTRAUMATIC EMBOLISM. Fat globules are seen in pulmonary (and other) vessels at autopsy and can be found in venous blood. In contrast to traumatic embolism, the fat is probably not derived from bone marrow, but rather arises from lipids in the blood. Serum from acutely ill patients has the capacity to agglutinate chylomicrons and very low-density lipoproteins (VLDL), as well as liposomes of nutritional fat emulsions.[49] It has been proposed that C-reactive protein (CRP), which provokes the calcium-dependent agglutination of each of these lipid-containing substances, may underlie nontraumatic FES. Since CRP is dramatically elevated in trauma, sepsis, and inflammatory disorders, this provides a mechanism for fat embolization.

An alternative, but less attractive, hypothesis implicates the liberation of free fatty acids (FFAs) from fat stores. Although FFAs are known to injure the pulmonary vascular endothelium, their concentration in the systemic circulation during critical illness does not rise sufficiently to account for lung injury. An understanding of the pathophysiology is potentially valuable in the search for prophylactic and therapeutic approaches to these patients, since corticosteroids, for example, may ameliorate the toxic effect of embolized fat but act to mobilize FFA.

TRAUMATIC EMBOLISM. Fracture of bone releases neutral fat which embolizes into the pulmonary vasculature. The derivation of this fat from bone is supported by the finding of coincident particles of bone marrow at autopsy in patients with long bone fractures. Local hydrolysis of fat by lung lipase releases toxic FFAs, which generate endothelial injury.

CLINICAL MANIFESTATIONS

Following injury, there is usually a latent interval of 12 to 72 h before the syndrome becomes evident. The dominant findings are related to lung injury. Patients with FES present as ARDS, with dyspnea, hypoxemia, and a diffuse lung lesion. In addition, there is often confusion, obtundation, or coma, signs due to cerebral fat embolism rather than coincident hypoxemia. The typical neuropathologic findings include fat microemboli and diffuse petechial hemorrhagic infarcts. Petechiae are also seen on the skin, particularly over the upper chest, neck, and face. On fundoscopic examination, embolized fat may be detected in retinal vessels (Purtscher's retinopathy). Often thrombocytopenia and anemia are present.

The diagnosis is usually based on the clinical findings in a patient at risk for FES, but can be confirmed by detection of fat globules in the urine.

PROPHYLAXIS AND TREATMENT

The substantial incidence of the syndrome and the large number of patients with a well-defined risk factor (long bone fracture) have provided the opportunity to evaluate prophylactic approaches. The least controversial strategy has involved a shift toward early fixation of long bone fractures, even in patients with multiple trauma. Early fixation decreases the incidence of FES, as well as of ARDS and pneumonia, and reduces length of stay.[50–52] More controversial is the use of prophylactic corticosteroids. Nearly all trials of methylprednisolone, in both high (7.5 mg/kg every 6 h) or low dose (1.5 mg/kg every 8 h), have shown a reduction in the incidence of the FES, as well as less severe hypoxemia.[53,54] Nevertheless, concerns regarding the risk of infection and impairment of wound healing have limited the routine use of these drugs. There are potential roles for glucose and insulin, heparin, ethanol and albumin, but none of established efficacy.

Once the syndrome becomes evident, treatment is that of ARDS (see Chap. 128). Prevention of reembolization by fracture fixation should be attempted, and supportive management with oxygen and PEEP initiated. It has been suggested that corticosteroids may be of benefit, but it is not clear that the benefits outweigh the risks.

CASE PRESENTATIONS

Case 1.

P.E. is a 45-year-old white woman admitted with a history of episodic, colicky, epigastric pain for elective cholecystectomy. She weighed 210 lb although she was otherwise healthy. The procedure was performed without difficulty and she was recovering uneventfully. On the third postoperative day she complained of dyspnea and palpitations. A chest radiogram revealed bilateral lower lung field atelectasis, and the patient was given an incentive spirometer. The following morning she was cyanotic and in marked respiratory distress. The blood pressure was 90/70, the heart rate 130, the respiratory rate 42, and the temperature 37.8°C (100.3°F). An arterial blood-gas sample revealed a P_{O_2} of 53, P_{CO_2} of 30, and pH of 7.41. A spun hematocrit was 44 percent. A repeat chest film showed little change. An ECG was notable for sinus tachycardia and nonspecific T wave changes. She was given oxygen and fluids and moved to the ICU.

A presumptive diagnosis of PE was made and a bolus

of heparin, 10,000 U, was given intravenously. After administration of 2 L saline solution, the blood pressure was 90/72, the heart rate 124, the respiratory rate had increased to 48, and the patient became confused. Nasal intubation was accomplished without the need for drugs, and the patient was sedated, muscle relaxed, and mechanically ventilated. A continuous infusion of heparin was initiated at 1000 U/h. Dopamine was begun at 2 μg/kg/min. Bedside impedance plethysmography failed to establish a diagnosis of venous thrombosis but was technically compromised. The blood pressure had stabilized at 100/70 but urine output was only 20 mL in the first hour. Urgent echocardiography revealed a grossly dilated, thin-walled, poorly contracting right ventricle. The interventricular septum bulged to the left during diastole. She was then taken to the interventional radiology suite where pulmonary angiography confirmed the clinical diagnosis of PE. Thrombolytic therapy was thought to be contraindicated due to the recent laparotomy so an IVC filter was placed below the renal veins. On return to the ICU, the blood pressure remained 100/70. A PA catheter revealed a right atrial pressure of 18 mmHg, right ventricle 48/18, PA 48/23, Ppw 15, and $\dot{Q}_T$ 2.9 L/min. Norepinephrine was instituted at 2 μg/min and increased to 8 μg/min while following the $S\bar{v}_{O_2}$. Repeat hemodynamics included blood pressure 112/72, heart rate 115, and $\dot{Q}_T$ 3.8. Urine output increased to 40 mL/h.

Heparin was adjusted to maintain a PTT of about two times control, maintenance fluids were given and over the next 2 days, it became possible to reduce the norepinephrine infusion without compromising $\dot{Q}_T$. Muscle relaxation was discontinued, the patient allowed to awaken, and over the next 2 days, mechanical ventilation was withdrawn. Coumadin was initiated and she was transferred to the ward after 7 days in the ICU.

Case Discussion

This case illustrates several key points in the management of a critically ill patient with PE. First, preoperative prophylaxis, which was not given here, should be routine. Second, new dyspnea on the third postoperative day was inappropriately dismissed as due to atelectasis. In this setting, PE should have been seriously considered. The diagnosis was considered only after a second embolus, at which time the patient was too sick to cooperate with $\dot{V}/\dot{Q}$ lung scanning. A perfusion scan alone was thought to be unlikely to affect management since the chest film was abnormal. It was reasonable to attempt noninvasive leg studies since a positive result would have provided an indication for anticoagulation while lending support to the clinical impression of PE. However, because a vena caval filter was likely to be indicated if PE were the diagnosis, immediate pulmonary angiography would also have been justified. Alternative diagnoses were appropriately excluded with a spun hematocrit, an ECG, and a chest radiogram.

Since the patient was in shock on presentation to the ICU, subsequent deterioration during transport and diagnostic procedures seemed imminent. Therefore, the circulation was stabilized by instituting mechanical ventilation. This served to reduce $\dot{V}_{O_2}$, and the demand for $\dot{Q}_T$.

Once pulmonary angiography confirmed the diagnosis, a vena caval filter was inserted at the same time to protect against the small possibility of additional emboli. Since echocardiography showed a distended right ventricle, aggressive fluid administration was not continued. Rather, a vasoconstrictor was given to improve right heart perfusion and relieve potential ischemia. This therapy was titrated using physiologic end points of peripheral perfusion and allowed stabilization until clot breakup and lysis could proceed.

Surgical embolectomy was briefly considered but by the time the necessary arrangements could have been made, the patient was substantially improved.

Case 2.

A 30-year-old, previously healthy woman was brought to the ICU following extensive hepatic resection for an invasive sarcoma. The intraoperative period was notable for acute hemodynamic collapse treated with epinephrine and volume administration. After 15 min, she was stabilized and the operation completed. The anesthesiologist had noted an abrupt drop in ET_{CO_2} just before the hypotensive episode. Based on these findings, a diagnosis of tumor embolism was made.

On transfer to the ICU, the blood pressure was 100/70, the heart rate 130, and temperature 36.5°C (97.7°F). The ventilator was set on assist-control with a tidal volume of 600 mL, rate of 26, F_{IO_2} 0.6, and PEEP 5 cm. An arterial blood-gas analysis showed a P_{O_2} of 65, P_{CO_2} 38, pH 7.44. Chest x-ray revealed four quadrant airspace infiltrates. The patient was not awake, not triggering the ventilator, and not shivering. Urine output was only 20 mL/h.

Five hours later, a PA catheter was inserted to exclude hypovolemia as a cause for decreased urine output. Pressure findings included: right atrial, 6 mmHg; right ventricle, 23/6; PA 23/10; Ppw 8; $\dot{Q}_T$ was 5.6 L/min. Subsequently urine output was found to be 70 mL/h and the patient was awake and alert. Repeat arterial blood-gas determinations showed P_{O_2} 310, P_{CO_2} 25, pH 7.53. The following morning, the chest x-ray revealed substantial clearing. The patient was extubated, determined to be neurologically fully intact, and thereafter, transferred to the ward.

Case Discussion

This case illustrates a patient with intraoperative air embolization. The newly created dead space manifested as a drop in ET_{CO_2} and later, as a normal P_{CO_2} despite a relatively high $\dot{V}_E$. The typical picture of hypoxemia and diffuse radiographic edema was apparent in the ICU.

As is common following air embolization, the correct diagnosis was not considered. However, this type of operation (extensive hepatic resection) puts a patient at high risk for entrainment of air at the operative site. Either tumor embolism or thromboembolism could account for the intraoperative course, including the fall in ET_{CO_2}, but both are unlikely given the extremely rapid recovery and the normal pulmonary hemodynamics only hours following nearly lethal embolism.

Once the source of air entry is closed, treatment consists solely of supportive management with mechanical ventilation, oxygen, and PEEP. A prompt recovery can be anticipated.

References

1. Dalen JE, Alpert JS: Natural history of pulmonary embolism. Prog Cardiovasc Dis 17:259, 1975.
2. D'Alonzo GE, Dantzker DR: Gas exchange alterations following pulmonary thromboembolism. Clin Chest Med 5:411, 1984.
3. Huet Y, Lemaire F, Brun-Buisson C, et al: Hypoxemia in acute pulmonary embolism. Chest 88:829, 1985.
4. Manier G, Castaing Y, Guenard H: Determinants of hypoxemia during the acute phase of pulmonary embolism in humans. Am Rev Respir Dis 132:332, 1985.
5. Vlahakes GJ, Turley K, Hoffman JIE: The pathophysiology of failure in acute right ventricular hypertension: Hemodynamic and biochemical correlates. Circulation 63:87, 1981.
6. Belenkie I, Dani R, Smith ER, et al: Ventricular interaction during experimental acute pulmonary embolism. Circulation 78:761, 1988.
7. Stein PD, Willis PW, DeMets DL: History and physical examination in acute pulmonary embolism in patients without preexisting cardiac or pulmonary disease. Am J Cardiol 47:218, 1981.
8. Biello DR, Mattar AG, McKnight RC, et al: Ventilation-perfusion studies in suspected pulmonary embolism. AJR 133:1033, 1979.
9. Hull RD, Hirsh J, Carter CJ, et al: Pulmonary angiography, ventilation lung scanning, and venography for clinically suspected pulmonary embolism with abnormal perfusion lung scan. Ann Intern Med 98:891, 1983.
10. The PIOPED Investigators. Value of the ventilation/perfusion scan in acute pulmonary embolism. JAMA 263:2753, 1990.
11. Hull RD, Raskob GE, Hirsh J: The diagnosis of clinically suspected pulmonary embolism: Practical approaches. Chest 89(suppl):417S, 1986.
12. Smith R, Ellis K, Alderson PO: Role of chest radiography in predicting the extent of airway disease in patients with suspected pulmonary embolism. Radiology 159:391, 1986.
13. Dalen JE, Banas JS, Brooks HL, et al: Resolution rate of acute pulmonary embolism in man. N Engl J Med 280:1194, 1969.
14. Mills SR, Jackson DC, Older RA, et al: The incidence, etiologies, and avoidance of complications of pulmonary angiography in a large series. Radiology 136:295, 1980.
15. Perlmutt LM, Braun SD, Newman GE, et al: Pulmonary angiography in the high-risk patient. Radiology 162:187, 1987.
16. Nicod P, Peterson K, Levine M, et al: Pulmonary angiography in severe chronic pulmonary hypertension. Ann Intern Med 107:565, 1987.
17. Lensing AWA, Prandoni P, Brandjes D, et al: Detection of deep-vein thrombosis by real-time B-mode ultrasonography. N Engl J Med 320:342, 1989.
18. Doyle DJ, Turpie AGG, Hirsh J, et al: Adjusted subcutaneous heparin or continuous intravenous heparin in patients with acute deep venous thrombosis. Ann Intern Med 107:441, 1987.
19. Moser KM: Venous thromboembolism. Am Rev Respir Dis 141:235, 1990.
20. Jones TK, Barnes RW, Greenfield LJ: Greenfield vena caval filter: Rationale and current indications. Ann Thorac Surg 42(suppl): S48, 1986.
21. UPET Study Group. Urokinase pulmonary embolism trial: Phase 1 results. JAMA 214:2163, 1970.
22. Sharma GVRK, Burleson VA, Sasahara AA: Effect of thrombolytic therapy on pulmonary-capillary blood volume in patients with pulmonary embolism. N Engl J Med 303:842, 1980.
23. Come PC, Kim D, Parker JA, et al: Early reversal of right ventricular dysfunction in patients with acute pulmonary embolism after treatment with intravenous tissue plasminogen activator. J Am Coll Cardiol 10:971, 1987.
24. Hirsh J, Hull RD: Treatment of venous thromboembolism. Chest 89(suppl): 426S, 1986.
25. Goldhaber SZ, Kessler CM, Heit J, et al: Randomised controlled trial of recombinant tissue plasminogen activator versus urokinase in the treatment of acute pulmonary embolism. Lancet ii:293, 1988.
26. Petitpretz P, Simmoneau G, Cerrina J, et al: Effects of a single bolus of urokinase in patients with life-threatening pulmonary emboli: A descriptive trial. Circulation 70:861, 1984.
27. Levine MN, Weitz J, Turpie AGG, et al: A new short infusion dosage regimen of recombinant tissue plasminogen activator in patients with venous thromboembolic disease. Chest 97(suppl):168S, 1990.
28. Verstraete M, Miller GAH, Bounameaux H, et al: Intravenous and intrapulmonary recombinant tissue-type plasminogen activator in the treatment of acute massive pulmonary embolism. Circulation 77:353, 1988.
29. Belenkie I, Dani R. Smith ER, et al: Effects of volume loading during experimental acute pulmonary embolism. Circulation 80:178, 1989.
30. Molloy WD, Lee KY, Girling L, et al: Treatment of shock in a canine model of pulmonary embolism. Am Rev Respir Dis 130:870, 1984.
31. Lund O, Nielsen TT, Schifter S, et al: Treatment of pulmonary embolism with full-dose heparin, streptokinase or embolectomy—Results and indications. Thorac Cardiovasc Surg 34:240, 1986.
32. Kaunitz AM, Hughes JM, Grimes DA, et al: Causes of maternal mortality in the United States. Obstet Gynecol 65:605, 1985.
33. Ponto JA: Fetal dosimetry from pulmonary imaging in pregnancy: Revised estimates. Clin Nucl Med 11:108, 1986.
34. Didolkar SM, Koontz C, Schimberg PI: Phleborrheography in pregnancy. Obstet Gynecol 61:363, 1983.
35. Ginsberg JS, Hirsh J: Use of anticoagulants during pregnancy. Chest 95(suppl):156S, 1989.
36. Lippmann M, Fein A: Pulmonary embolism in the patient with chronic obstructive pulmonary disease. Chest 79:39, 1981.
37. Prescott SM, Richards KL, Tikoff G, et al: Venous thromboembolism in decompensated chronic obstructive pulmonary disease. Am Rev Respir Dis 123:32, 1981.
38. Phillips B, Woodring J: Autoanticoagulation does not preclude pulmonary emboli. Lung 165:37, 1987.
39. Needleman SW, Stein MN, Hoak JC: Pulmonary embolism in patients with acute leukemia and severe thrombocytopenia. West J Med 135:9, 1981.
40. Halkin H, Goldberg J, Modan M, et al: Reduction of mortality in general medical in-patients by low-dose heparin prophylaxis. Ann Intern Med 96:561, 1982.
41. Collins R, Scrimgeour A, Yusuf S, et al: Reduction in fatal pulmonary embolism and venous thrombosis by perioperative administration of subcutaneous heparin. N Engl J Med 318:1162, 1988.
42. Albertine KH: Lung injury and neutrophil density during air

embolization in sheep after leukocyte depletion with nitrogen mustard. Am Rev Respir Dis 138:1444, 1988.
43. Sloan TB, Kimovec MA: Detection of venous air embolism by airway pressure monitoring. Anesthesiology 64:645, 1986.
44. Butler BD, Hills BA: Transpulmonary passage of venous air emboli. J Appl Physiol 59:543, 1985.
45. Marini JJ, Culver BH: Systemic gas embolism complicating mechanical ventilation in the adult respiratory distress syndrome. Ann Intern Med 110:699, 1989.
46. Dutka AJ, Kochanek PM, Hallenbeck JM: Influence of granulocytopenia on canine cerebral ischemia induced by air embolism. Stroke 20:390, 1989.
47. Karuparthy VR, Downing JW, Husain FJ, et al: Incidence of venous air embolism during cesarean section in unchanged by the use of a 5 to 10° head-up tilt. Anesth Analg 69:620, 1989.
48. Fabian TC, Hoots AV, Stanford DS, et al: Fat embolism syndrome: Prospective evaluation in fracture patients. Crit Care Med 18:42, 1990.
49. Hulman G: Pathogenesis of non-traumatic fat embolism. Lancet i:1366, 1988.
50. Bone LB, Johnson KD, Wiegelt J, et al: Early versus delayed stabilization of femoral fractures. J Bone Joint Surg 71A:336, 1989.
51. Johnson KD, Cadambi A, Seibert GB, et al: Incidence of adult respiratory distress syndrome in patients with multiple musculoskeletal injuries: Effect of early operative stabilization of fractures. J Trauma 25:375, 1985.
52. Behrman SW, Fabian TC, Kudsk KA, et al: Improved outcome with femur fractures: Early vs. delayed fixation. J Trauma 30:792, 1990.
53. Kallenbach J, Lewis M, Zaltzman M, et al: "Low-dose" corticosteroid prophylaxis against fat embolism. J Trauma 27:1173, 1987.
54. Schonfeld SA, Ploysonsang Y, Dilisio R, et al: Fat embolism prophylaxis with corticosteroids. Ann Intern Med 99:438, 1983.

Chapter 119

ANTICOAGULANTS AND THROMBOLYTIC AGENTS

GREGORY A. SCHMIDT

KEY POINTS

- *Anticoagulants and thrombolytic agents are potentially life-saving drugs when used prophylactically or employed therapeutically in critically ill patients.*
- *Most patients who do not have a contraindication to heparin should be given prophylactic therapy with 5000 U subcutaneously twice daily.*
- *Thrombolytic therapy clearly improves survival and function in selected patients with acute myocardial infarction (AMI). Its role in venous thromboembolism is less well established.*
- *The most serious risk of anticoagulants and thrombolytic drugs is major hemorrhage, which occurs in about 5 (heparin) to 15 percent or more (thrombolytic therapy) of patients in the intensive care unit (ICU).*
- *Hemorrhage can be greatly reduced by avoiding vascular punctures in patients who may receive these drugs.*
- *Intracranial hemorrhage remains an unavoidable complication in approximately 0.6 percent of patients treated with thrombolytic agents.*
- *When acute hemorrhage due to thrombolytic therapy mandates reversal of the fibrinolytic state, cryoprecipitate is the blood product of choice.*

Heparin

Heparin is a naturally occurring mucopolysaccharide extracted from bovine lung or from porcine or bovine gut mucosa. The commercially available preparations consist of a mixture of heparins of differing molecular weights (MW) (average MW = 15,000 to 18,000), related to variable polymerization of the polysaccharide units. Low-molecular-weight heparin fractions (MW = 3000 to 9000) appear to differ in their antithrombotic effects and risk of hemorrhage and are currently the subjects of clinical trials. Heparin is available as the sodium or calcium salt.

ACTIONS

The antithrombotic effect of heparin is incompletely understood, but it is related to heparin's ability to bind to antithrombin III, facilitating the inhibition of clotting factors IIa, IXa, Xa, XIa, and XIIa. Factor Xa, situated at a crucial point in the common pathway of coagulation, is particularly sensitive to the heparin–antithrombin III complex (see Fig. 119-1). Substantially higher levels of heparin are necessary to inhibit thrombin (factor IIa) once it is formed. For this reason, low-dose heparin is effective in prophylaxis against thrombosis, while higher doses are required once clotting is established. Thrombi propagate by continually assimilating new fibrin, even once fibrinolysis of the clot begins. Heparin slows the incorporation of new fibrin, preventing clot extension.

Additional actions of heparin may contribute to its therapeutic efficacy and hemorrhagic tendency. At high concentrations (0.3 U/mL and above), heparin combines with heparin cofactor II to catalyze inhibition of thrombin. This effect may contribute importantly to antithrombotic activity when heparin is used in high doses or following bolus administration (especially since the action of the heparin–antithrombin III complex diminishes at high concentrations).[1] Heparin also influences platelet function and may prolong the bleeding time. Platelet actions probably contribute more to hemorrhagic consequences than to antithrombotic activity. Low-molecular-weight heparins have less impact on platelet function yet retain their antifactor Xa activity. This may explain the increasingly recognized fact that these substances can effectively prevent thrombosis while causing less bleeding.[2]

INDICATIONS AND CONTRAINDICATIONS

Critically ill patients who do not have a contraindication to heparin should be placed on prophylactic minidose heparin to prevent deep venous thrombosis. Although the risk-benefit ratio of prophylactic heparin has never been assessed in this population, benefits have been shown in general medical inpatients over the age of 40 and in patients with nonhemorrhagic stroke and AMI.[3] Minidose heparin should also be given preoperatively to most patients since this approach has been demonstrated to reduce deep venous thrombosis, pulmonary emboli, mortality, and hospital costs, while not causing serious bleeding.[4]

Full-dose heparin is indicated in the treatment of deep venous thrombosis, arterial thrombosis, pulmonary embolism, acute anterior myocardial infarction, unstable angina, valvular heart disease, atrial fibrillation, and following thrombolytic therapy. In patients with pulmonary embolism who are treated with vena caval interruption, heparin should be continued as treatment for the presumed underlying venous thrombosis. Heparin has also been used for nonhemorrhagic stroke, progressing stroke, and transient ischemic attacks, although its efficacy is unproved in these settings. Lower doses are sometimes used to treat patients with disseminated intravascular coagulation (see Chap. 146). Contraindications to anticoagulation are listed in Table 119-1.

DOSING AND MONITORING

Heparin can be given by continuous intravenous infusion, intermittent bolus, or subcutaneous injection. Heparin given subcutaneously is absorbed gradually, with a peak

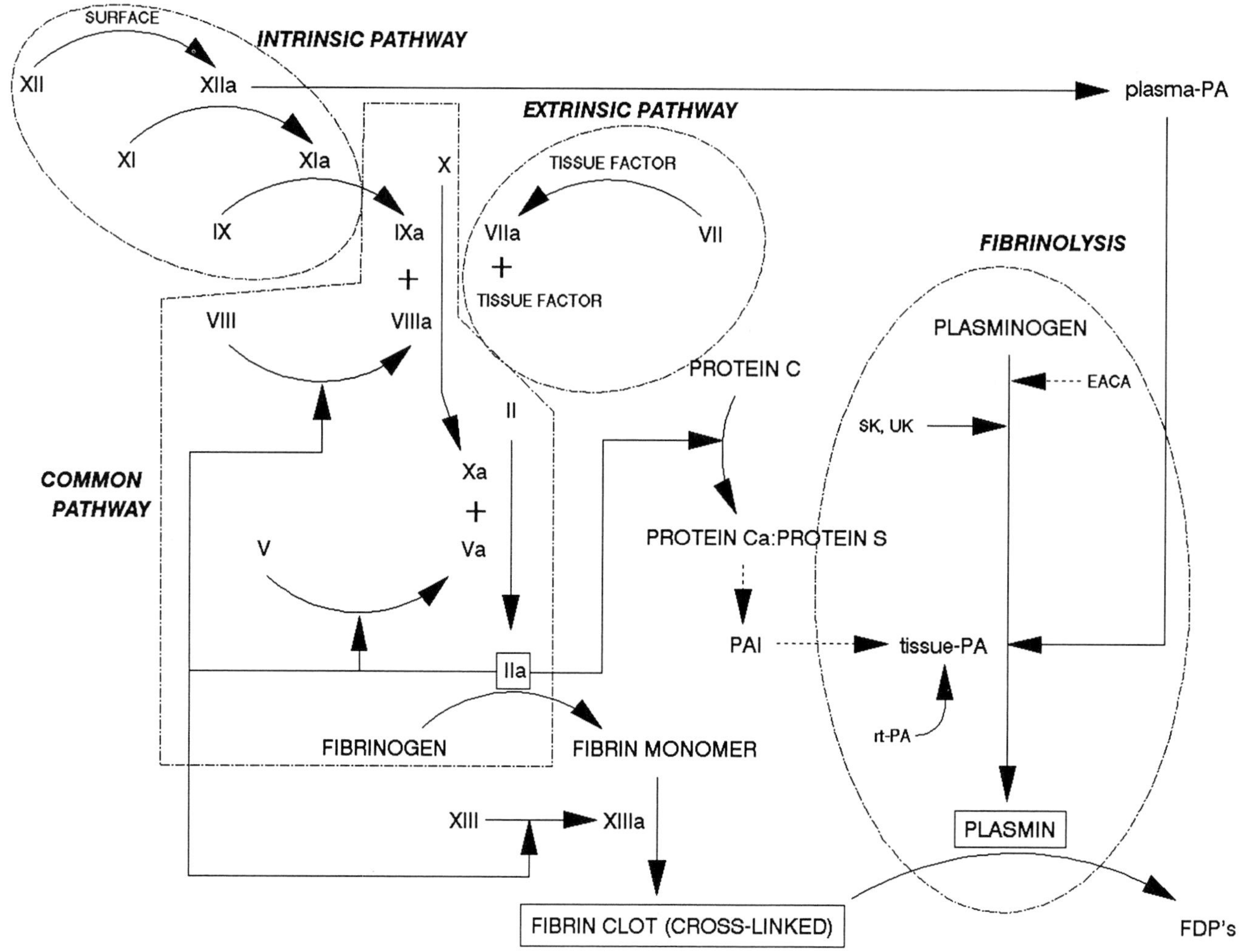

FIGURE 119-1 The coagulation and fibrinolytic pathways. The endpoint of both the intrinsic and extrinsic pathways is to activate factor X. The key step of the common pathway is the generation of thrombin (factor IIa), which has important actions on clotting and fibrinolysis. Thrombin causes the formation of fibrin monomer. At the same time, it feeds back positively to facilitate the common pathway by activating factors VIII and V. It also activates factor XIII, thereby leading to a cross-linked clot. Thrombin initiates fibrinolysis as well, by leading to the formation of the active protein C:protein S complex, which in turn inhibits plasminogen activator inhibitor (PAI). This leaves the action of t-PA unchecked, and plasmin is formed. Plasmin is the final step leading to clot lysis. The sites of action of SK, UK, and rt-PA are noted: all lead to plasmin generation. Epsilon-aminocaproic acid (EACA), an antifibrinolytic agent, inhibits the conversion of plasminogen to plasmin. Solid lines indicate stimulation; dotted lines indicate inhibition. Plasma-PA = plasma plasminogen activator; FDP = fibrin degradation product.

TABLE 119-1 Contraindications to Anticoagulation

Absolute
Active serious hemorrhage
Intracranial bleeding
Recent (<2 weeks) CNS or eye surgery
Relative
Recent major surgery
Uncontrolled hypertension
Large nonhemorrhagic stroke
Bleeding diathesis
Hepatic or renal failure
Heparin-associated thrombocytopenia

effect at 4 h and a duration of 12 h. It can therefore be administered on a twice daily schedule. Given in sufficient doses, full anticoagulant levels can be easily attained. The kinetics of absorption may depend on whether the sodium or calcium salt is used, with the calcium salt yielding therapeutic levels more quickly.[5] Low-molecular-weight heparins are absorbed more readily and have a longer half-life than standard heparin, so they can be given once daily.

Intermittent intravenous bolus use is associated with increased hemorrhagic risk compared to intravenous infusion, so the latter method is preferred. When given intravenously, heparin has an immediate effect and a half-life of approximately 90 min. The therapeutic effect differs markedly between patients and is further modulated by the magnitude of thrombosis. Patients with pulmonary embolism clear heparin more rapidly than normal volunteers or patients with deep venous thrombosis. It is therefore necessary to follow the anticoagulant effect by measuring the partial thromboplastin time (PTT) or heparin levels.

Heparin is usually initiated as a bolus of 5000 to 10,000 U intravenously, followed by a continuous infusion of 1000 U/h. The PTT should not be assessed for 4 to 6 h, since before that it may reflect the bolus rather than the infusion dose. If the PTT is less than 1.5 times control, the infusion should be increased by 100 U/h and then reassessed. Infusions of up to 50,000 U per 24 h are not uncommon. If the PTT is greater than 2.5 times control, the infusion should be stopped for 1 h and then reinstituted at a dose that is 100 U/h less. When given following thrombolytic therapy, heparin is typically begun at 1000 U/h and adjusted to maintain the PTT at 1.5 to 2 times control for 3 to 7 days. Full-dose subcutaneous regimens generally utilize 15,000 U subcutaneously every 12 h, with the PTT assessed midway between doses. By either route, when heparin is given in full therapeutic doses, it is titrated to maintain a PTT of 1.5 to 2.5 times control or to maintain a heparin level of 0.3 to 0.4 U/mL. When continued systemic anticoagulation with warfarin (Coumadin) is required, heparin should be given for 7 to 10 days and overlapped with warfarin (Coumadin) for 5 days.[6]

Minidose heparin (typically 5000 U subcutaneously, given twice daily) does not usually affect the PTT, or does so only minimally, and assessing its activity is generally unnecessary. The PTT is relatively insensitive to low-molecular-weight heparins, so their activity should be followed by measuring heparin levels (anti-factor Xa assay).

COMPLICATIONS

BLEEDING

The most important complication of heparin is bleeding. In a pooled analysis of its use in deep venous thrombosis, major bleeding (bleeding greater than 1 L, bleeding requiring blood transfusion, intracerebral bleeding) was reported in 2 of 59 patients (3 percent).[7] In a group of 121 patients given heparin for all indications, 8 percent developed major hemorrhage (fatal, life threatening, potentially life threatening, leading to reoperation, or requiring at least 3 U of blood).[8] Hemorrhage typically occurs from the gastrointestinal or urinary tract or from surgical incisions. Less common sites of serious bleeding include the retroperitoneum, adrenal glands, soft tissues, nose, and pleural space. Intracranial hemorrhage is very rare in patients anticoagulated with heparin. Bleeding is especially common in patients with comorbid conditions (serious cardiac disease, liver dysfunction, active renal disease, cancer, severe anemia). Those with two or more of these conditions had 20 times the risk of patients who had none of them.[8] The intensity of anticoagulation is also a factor, with the risk of hemorrhage substantially higher when the PTT is more than 3 times control. Additional risk factors include concomitant antiplatelet drug administration, advanced age, unsuspected anatomic lesion (e.g., duodenal ulcer), and invasive procedures.

Occult gastrointestinal tract bleeding related to anticoagulation occurs commonly but should not be attributed solely to the anticoagulant. In a prospective trial of patients given heparin or warfarin, 21 (12 percent) developed occult gastrointestinal tract blood loss. Of the 16 of these patients who underwent diagnostic investigation, a new endoscopic diagnosis was made in 15 (although most were benign and required no change in management).[9]

The approach to treatment of the patient who bleeds on heparin depends on the severity of bleeding. When bleeding is minor, simply stopping the heparin may be sufficient. Bleeding related to needle sticks may respond to sustained direct pressure. When hemorrhage endangers life or organ function, a more aggressive approach is mandatory. Transfusion of fresh frozen plasma is usually ineffective since circulating heparin inhibits the function of transfused factors. Protamine sulfate is an antidote to heparin. The dose of protamine depends on heparin levels and is therefore related to dose, route of administration, and time since the last dose. When hemorrhage immediately follows a bolus of heparin, sufficient protamine to completely neutralize the heparin (1 mg protamine per 100 U heparin) should be administered. In the more usual situation where heparin therapy is ongoing, the dose of protamine should be based on the approximate half-life of heparin (90 min). Since protamine, too, is an anticoagulant, the dose should be estimated to only half correct the estimated circulating heparin. Protamine has been known to cause hypotension, shock, dyspnea, and pulmonary hypertension upon intravenous injection. The incidence is reduced by giving the drug very slowly (no more than 50 mg in 10 min). When protamine is administered, a physician should be present in case of an anaphylactoid reaction.

Alternatives for the treatment of underlying conditions should be considered once heparin is stopped. For example, the patient with pulmonary embolization should have vena caval interruption with a percutaneous filter. If heparin was being used as prophylaxis against deep venous thrombosis in a patient at high risk, intermittent pneumatic compression cuffs can be substituted.

HEPARIN-ASSOCIATED THROMBOCYTOPENIA

Thrombocytopenia is a relatively common complication of heparin administration, typically occurring after several days of therapy. It is more common in patients given bovine lung heparin (10 percent) than in those treated with porcine heparin (<5 percent)[10] and may be related to the heparin lot. The mechanism of thrombocytopenia in most patients is thought to be related to specific IgG directed against heparin. Heparin binds normally to platelets, and in individuals who develop antiplatelet IgG, an IgG: platelet-antigen immune complex forms on the platelet surface. Through the platelet Fc receptor, the immune complex may result in activation and aggregation of platelets.[11] Thrombocytopenia is not seen with highly purified low-molecular-weight heparins, suggesting that higher-molecular-weight components may be responsible. It is also rare in patients given prophylactic minidose heparin, occurring in only 1 of 348 patients.[11] This suggests that heparin-associated thrombocytopenia is also dose related.

The onset of thrombocytopenia is usually on the third to fifteenth day (mean = day 10) but can occur after several hours in patients previously sensitized. The severity of thrombocytopenia is variable (commonly to 50,000) but can be severe (less than 5000). Most patients remain asymptomatic, but some suffer major arterial or venous thrombosis or life-threatening hemorrhage. Rarely, this syndrome is associated with skin bullae which progress to necrosis (heparin necrosis). These may occur at sites of injection or at distant sites. Any time heparin is given, it is prudent to measure platelet counts on a daily basis. An otherwise unexplained drop in platelet count of 30 percent has been suggested as the threshold which should prompt discontinuation of heparin,[11] although there is little on which to base this. Heparin-dependent IgG should be sought in the patient serum, since a positive result may simplify management decisions. None of the available assays are fully sensitive, so a negative test is no guarantee against recurrent thrombocytopenia or thrombosis if the patient is rechallenged with heparin. The ^{14}C-serotonin release assay has been recommended as the most sensitive and specific.[11]

While platelet counts sometimes normalize despite continued heparin administration, the drug should be stopped since potentially catastrophic thrombosis may occur unpredictably. Once the syndrome is initiated, even trivial amounts of heparin can perpetuate it. Heparin-containing flush solutions, indwelling catheters, and even heparin-bonded pulmonary artery catheters have been reported to sustain the syndrome. After discontinuation of all heparin, the platelet count usually rises in 2 or 3 days. Platelet transfusion should be avoided, even if the patient is bleeding, since this may precipitate arterial thrombosis. If continued anticoagulation is necessary, porcine or low-molecular-weight heparin can be substituted, or warfarin treatment begun. Treatment of arterial thrombosis associated with heparin-induced thrombocytopenia is based on anecdotes but has included thrombolytic therapy, antiplatelet agents, and plasmapheresis.[11] When heparin must be administered to a patient who is known to be sensitive (e.g., for coronary artery bypass grafting, hemodialysis), the risk of thrombosis may be reduced by employing low-molecular-weight heparin or giving concomitant antiplatelet agents or iloprost (a prostacyclin analogue).

UNCOMMON COMPLICATIONS

Anaphylaxis is a rare consequence of heparin use. Hypersensitivity may also manifest as a skin rash. Hypoaldosteronism (hyperkalemia) is a rare sequel to its administration, and osteoporosis is seen only with long-term use and is therefore of little relevance in the ICU.

Oral Anticoagulants

Oral anticoagulants are only occasionally used in the ICU. Sometimes the transition to chronic oral therapy is begun before the patient leaves the ICU or must be initiated because of heparin thrombocytopenia. Since oral anticoagulants are widely used in outpatients and result in a substantial incidence of life-threatening hemorrhage, the intensivist can expect to see patients admitted for bleeding or hypotension. Finally, these drugs are sometimes taken in intentional overdoses.

ACTIONS

Factors II, VII, IX, and X, as well as proteins C and S, require the hydroquinone form of vitamin K_1 to attain biological activity. These factors are synthesized as inactive zymogens and require carboxylation of glutamic acid residues for activity. The reduced form of vitamin K_1 is oxidized during these carboxylation reactions and must then be reduced to the active form (the vitamin K cycle). This reduction is accomplished by vitamin K_1 epoxide reductase, an enzyme which is competitively antagonized by warfarin. By preventing the postribosomal modification of the procoagulant factors to their active forms, warfarin acts as an anticoagulant. At the same time, however, it inhibits the synthesis of the naturally occurring anticoagulant substances, proteins C and S, and may thereby be thrombogenic.

DOSING AND MONITORING

Warfarin is rapidly and completely absorbed from the gastrointestinal tract and then circulates almost exclusively bound to albumin. Drugs which displace warfarin from albumin have the potential to promote its anticoagulant effects. Many classes of drugs can enhance or inhibit its actions through various mechanisms (Table 119-2). Peak plasma levels are seen in about 3 h, although the peak effect does not occur until 36 to 72 h later, depending on the

TABLE 119-2 Drugs which Interact with Warfarin (Coumadin)

Increased Effect	Decreased Effect
Allopurinol	Antacids
Amiodarone	Antihistamines
Anesthetics, inhalation	Barbiturates
Cefamandole	Carbamazepine
Chloramphenicol	Corticosteroids
Chlordiazepoxide	Diuretics[a]
Chlorpromazine	Haloperidol
Cimetidine	Methylxanthines
Cotrimoxazole	Paraldehyde
Diazepam	Ranitidine[a]
Diuretics[a]	Rifampin
Methyldopa	Tetracycline
Metronidazole	Vitamin K
Moxalactam	
Neomycin	
Phenytoin	
Quinidine	
Ranitidine[a]	
Sulfonamides	

[a] Both increased and decreased effects are seen.

half-lives of previously synthesized clotting factors. The half-life of warfarin itself is about 35 h. Factor VII levels fall most rapidly, prolonging the prothrombin time (PT), although the full antithrombotic effect is not seen for several days. This provides the rationale for overlapping heparin and warfarin therapies for at least 5 days, even though the PT will rise sooner.

The adequacy of warfarin anticoagulation has generally been assessed by measuring the PT. It has been difficult to compare the degree of anticoagulation between different centers, however, because they employ several different thromboplastins of varying sensitivities. For example, the rabbit brain thromboplastin used in the United States is relatively unresponsive to warfarin's effect. On the other hand, the thromboplastins used in the United Kingdom are much more responsive, while those used in Europe are of intermediate sensitivity. In order to facilitate comparison of anticoagulation, there has been a move to encourage normalization of the reported results by referring to an internationally accepted standard thromboplastin. The degree of anticoagulation should now be expressed in terms of the international normalized ratio (INR), which reports the result as that which would have been obtained had the internationally accepted standard thromboplastin been used.[12]

Warfarin anticoagulation is typically begun at 10 mg/day for 3 days, with a reduction (or augmentation of) the dose after that until the PT (or INR) is prolonged into the desired range. Larger loading doses will not achieve adequate anticoagulation any sooner and are potentially dangerous. The anticoagulant effect of warfarin is assessed by measuring the PT, with the desired level depending on the indication for the drug and the type of PT assay performed. For most conditions, a PT of 1.3 to 1.5 times control (INR = 2.0 to 3.0), using rabbit brain thromboplastin, is the desired effect. When sensitive thromboplastins are used, therapeutic anticoagulation requires a higher PT (2.0 to 3.0). The only conditions for which a PT of 1.5 to 2.0 (rabbit thromboplastin), or an INR of 3.0 to 4.5, is recommended are prevention of systemic embolism in patients with mechanical prosthetic heart valves and prevention of recurrent systemic embolism.[12]

COMPLICATIONS

BLEEDING

As with heparin, the most important side effect of warfarin use is hemorrhage, occurring in 2.4 to 8.1 percent of patients chronically anticoagulated.[13] The risk is dose related and proportional to the prolongation of the PT. Spontaneous hemorrhage during oral anticoagulant therapy should prompt consideration of an underlying structural lesion. The sites of hemorrhage parallel those of patients who bleed while on heparin. In contrast to bleeding due to heparin, hemorrhagic diathesis can be immediately reversed by a transfusion of fresh frozen plasma (2 to 4 U). The use of more concentrated factor products, such as prothrombin complex concentrates, should be reserved for urgent situations unresponsive to fresh frozen plasma. Vitamin K_1 (phytonadione; not vitamin K_3, menadione, or vitamin K_4, menadiol, which are ineffective) can be given to antagonize the effects of warfarin, but its action is delayed for 3 to 6 h, requiring synthesis of new clotting factors by the liver. For this reason, and because it makes reinstitution of warfarin therapy complicated, vitamin K_1 is rarely indicated. It should be given (10 mg subcutaneously or intravenously, or 25 mg orally) in the setting of warfarin overdose since no long-term anticoagulant effect is desired. The half-life of vitamin K_1 is shorter than that of warfarin, so repeat doses will be needed, usually every 6 h. Following the initial dose of vitamin K_1, repeat oral or parenteral doses should be guided by the PT, but therapy is nontoxic and should continue for at least 7 to 10 days. Hastened elimination of warfarin has been reported with administration of cholestyramine.[14]

WARFARIN SKIN NECROSIS

As noted above, one of the early effects of warfarin is to impair the function of protein C in addition to its effects on procoagulant factors. Since the half-life of protein C is very short (similar to that of factor VII), warfarin may cause a paradoxical hypercoagulable state. This can result in thrombosis in the skin, causing necrosis, and occasionally requiring amputation. Patients with congenital deficiencies of protein C may be at particular risk for this rare condition. Warfarin necrosis usually occurs in the first week of therapy and typically manifests in areas with abundant subcutaneous tissue such as the abdomen, breast, and buttocks, or in the periphery (tip of the nose, penis).

TERATOGENESIS

Use of warfarin during the sixth to twelfth weeks of gestation may result in a typical embryopathy consisting of a variety of skeletal abnormalities. Given later in pregnancy, it may cause central nervous system abnormalities and optic atrophy in the fetus. For these reasons, heparin is the anticoagulant of choice during pregnancy.

Dextran

Dextran is glucose polymer, available as 40,000 dalton (dextran 40) and 70,000 dalton (dextran 70) preparations. These agents are used primarily as colloid volume expanders but have a small role as anticoagulant drugs. Dextran interferes with platelet and coagulation factor function. It is effective in reducing the incidence of venous thromboembolism in surgical patients, but it is more dangerous and expensive than the available alternatives. Dextran is not useful for established thromboembolic disease. The usual dose is 50 mL/h of dextran 40, while following urine output and specific gravity.

Side effects include volume overload, osmotic diuresis, renal failure, and anaphylaxis. Dextran is made up of osmotically active particles and is effective in drawing extravascular fluid into the vascular space. This may be the desired effect during resuscitation of hypovolemic patients, but it can lead to volume overload in other settings. The drug is renally excreted and causes an osmotic diuresis, which can lead to hypovolemia. Dextran has been known to precipitate in renal tubules, inducing renal failure. This toxicity is exacerbated by hypovolemia. Finally, the most feared complication of dextran is anaphylaxis, which is seen in up to 5 percent of patients. The reaction is usually noticed early in the infusion and consists of rash, urticaria, bronchospasm, hypotension, and death.

Thrombolytic Agents

The thrombolytic armamentarium consists of five drugs: streptokinase (SK), acylated plasminogen streptokinase activator complex (APSAC), urokinase (UK), single-chain urokinase plasminogen activator (scu-PA), and recombinant tissue-type plasminogen activator (rt-PA). These drugs all convert plasminogen to plasmin, thereby stimulating fibrinolysis. They differ in their mechanism of plasminogen activation, their fibrin specificity, and their pharmacokinetics. The advantage of thrombolytic agents is their ability to lyse clots which have already formed; this same quality also accounts for their hemorrhagic tendency. These drugs have found a significant place in the management of thrombotic disorders, and, when used judiciously, can reduce morbidity and mortality.

INDICATIONS AND CONTRAINDICATIONS

These drugs are indicated for the treatment of selected patients with acute myocardial infarction and pulmonary embolism and may have a role in the treatment of deep venous thrombosis, unstable angina, and peripheral arterial occlusion. Recently they have been employed to clear occluded long-term intravenous catheters. Contraindications are largely related to the risk of hemorrhage and are detailed in Table 119-3.

TABLE 119-3 Contraindications to Thrombolytic Therapy

Absolute
Trauma (including CPR) or major surgery within 10 days
Recent puncture in a noncompressible site
Active or recent internal bleeding
Hemorrhagic diathesis
Recent central nervous system surgery or active intracranial lesion
Uncontrolled hypertension (blood pressure >180/110)
Known hypersensitivity, or for SK, use of SK within 6 months
Diabetic hemorrhagic retinopathy
Acute pericarditis
Recent obstetrical delivery
History of stroke
Relative
Pregnancy
High likelihood of left heart thrombus
Advanced age
Liver disease

ACTIONS AND ADMINISTRATION

The mechanisms of action of this class of drugs can best be understood by reviewing the normal process of intrinsic clot lysis (fibrinolysis) (see Fig. 119-1). The coagulation cascade, which forms and propagates clots, is opposed by fibrinolysis, which dissolves and limits the propagation of clots. Initiation of clotting simultaneously activates fibrinolysis through depression of inhibitors of tissue-type plasminogen activator (t-PA), and possibly through a direct action of factor XIIa on plasminogen. Thrombolytic agents exploit this intrinsic system by converting plasminogen to the active plasmin, thereby spurring fibrinolysis.

Some of the differences in thrombolytic agents relate to their fibrin specificity. Plasmin produced in the bloodstream is rapidly inactivated by α_2-antiplasmin. However, the unleashing of fibrinolysis results in the consumption of available α_2-antiplasmin. Subsequent excess plasmin is not specific for fibrin, but rather it nonspecifically proteolyzes fibrinogen, factor V, factor VIII, and von Willebrand factor as well. This results in a generalized breakdown of hemostasis. Since fibrinogen repletion requires greater than 24 h once these drugs are stopped, the hemorrhagic diathesis is protracted. The advantage of newer thrombolytic agents is that plasmin activation is dependent on fibrin and is therefore relatively more localized to the area of the clot. Nevertheless, even these fibrin-specific drugs generate a systemic lytic state.

SK

SK binds to circulating plasminogen, creating a complex which is then a potent plasminogen activator. This lack of clot specificity accounts for the relative inefficiency of clot lysis and the systemic nature of the lytic state. SK is derived from streptococci and is associated with a significant incidence of febrile reactions. For this reason, pretreatment with acetaminophen, diphenhydramine, and hydrocortisone is advised. Antigenicity precludes retreatment with SK for at least 6 months. For AMI, the drug is given as 1,500,000 U over 1 h. In other conditions, treatment is usually initiated with a bolus of 250,000 U, followed by a continuous infusion of 100,000 U/h. The infusion is continued for 24 h for the treatment of pulmonary embolism (PE), and for 48 to 72 h for deep venous thrombosis (DVT) (see Table 119-4).

APSAC

This drug is formed by combining streptokinase and plasminogen to form the activator complex and then chemically acylating the active site which is responsible for plasminogen activation. In vivo, the inactive drug is slowly converted to the active plasminogen-streptokinase complex. Theoretically, there should be time for the inactive complex to bind to fibrin before deacylation, resulting in clot specificity. However, APSAC generates a profound systemic lytic state, like streptokinase. It also is antigenic, therefore providing no advantages over SK. APSAC is given as a 30-mg bolus for coronary thrombolysis.

TABLE 119-4 Selected Thrombolytic Regimens

Pulmonary embolism
- UK: 4400-U/kg bolus, followed by 4400 U/kg per h for 24 h
- UK: 1,000,000-U bolus over 10 min, followed by 2,000,000 U over 110 min
- UK: 15,000-U/kg bolus over 10 min
- rt-PA: 0.6-mg/kg bolus over 2 min
- rt-PA: 100 mg over 2–3 h
- SK: 250,000 U over 30 min, followed by 100,000 U/h for 24 h

Myocardial infarction
- SK: 1,500,000 U over 1 h
- APSAC: 30-mg bolus over 2–4 min
- rt-PA: 100 mg over 3 h (60 mg first hour, 20 mg each following hour)

Deep venous thrombosis
- SK: 250,000 U over 30 min, followed by 100,000 U/h for 48–72 h
- rt-PA: 0.5 mg/kg over 4–8 h
- rt-PA: 0.05 mg/kg per h for 24 h

Catheter occlusion
- SK: 10,000 U per 2 mL into catheter. Attempt to aspirate every 10 min
- UK: 10,000 U per 2 mL into catheter. Attempt to aspirate every 10 min
- rt-PA: 2 mg per 2 mL into catheter. Attempt to aspirate every 10 min

UK

Urokinase is a serine protease which directly cleaves plasminogen to plasmin. This specificity for plasminogen is beneficial since fibrinogen is not consumed. UK is not antigenic and can therefore be given repeatedly. The optimal regimen for UK infusion has not been determined, and several methods are in use. For acute pulmonary embolism, one approach is to infuse 1,000,000 U as a bolus, followed by 2,000,000 units over 110 min.[15] Alternatives are to give a bolus of 4400 U/kg, followed by 4400 U/kg per h for 12 to 24 h,[16] or simply 15,000 U/kg as a 10-min bolus.[17]

scu-PA

Also known as prourokinase, this substance is a single-chain precursor of urokinase. It is slowly hydrolyzed to urokinase in vivo, and since it has a high affinity for fibrin-bound plasminogen, it appears to be very clot-specific. The dose of this drug has not been determined, but 1-h infusions of 70 mg have been used.[18]

rt-PA

Endothelial cells release the endogenous mediator of thrombolysis, t-PA. A commercial product, produced through recombinant DNA technology, is called recombinant t-PA, or rt-PA. This drug binds to plasminogen on the surface of the clot, thereby producing plasmin locally. This fibrin specificity partly explains the efficacy of rt-PA. A systemic fibrinolytic state is generated, but it is of lesser magnitude than that created by the other thrombolytic drugs. Several therapeutic regimens have been employed, including 100 mg over 2 or 3 h[19,20] and 0.6 mg/kg as a single bolus for pulmonary embolism,[21] and 100 mg over 3 h (60 mg first hour, 20 mg each following hour) for AMI.[22] Longer, lower-dose infusions have been employed for DVT, such as 0.5 mg/kg over 4 to 8 h[23] or 0.05 mg/kg per h for 24 h.[24]

CLEARING OCCLUDED CATHETERS

Thrombolytic agents are commonly used to clear thrombosed central venous catheters (especially chronic indwelling lines) and occluded arteriovenous cannulas. Attempts should always be made to free the line by conventional means (careful syringe technique), since these drugs may induce hemorrhage. Most of these agents have been successfully used in this setting. The least expensive approach is to instill low-dose SK (e.g., 10,000 U per 2 mL) into the catheter, followed in 10 min by attempts to withdraw through the catheter. Repeated attempts to aspirate are made every 10 min for an hour, following which SK is flushed from the lumen. Repeat attempts may increase the likelihood of success. In one group of patients in whom UK failed to establish catheter patency, rt-PA was usually successful (2 mg per 2 mL).[25] It must be emphasized that thrombolytic therapy should only be used for clearing catheters when more usual efforts have failed and the occluded line is truly necessary. Some medical centers have protocols in place to limit the potentially dangerous overuse of lytic therapy in this setting.

MONITORING AND HEPARINIZATION

Our current state of knowledge does not provide useful guidelines for monitoring the degree of lysis. In general, both arterial and venous punctures should be avoided during the use of thrombolytic drugs. Various measures of the lytic state correlate poorly with both efficacy and incidence of bleeding, so outside of clinical research protocols, routine monitoring is not indicated. When SK is given, the manufacturer recommends that the thrombin time be assayed at 4 h to ensure that a lytic state is achieved. This is based on the concern that if plasminogen is fully consumed, none will remain to complex with SK and form the active plasminogen activator. With no residual plasminogen or plasminogen activator present, a paradoxical hypercoagulable state is possible. An adequate lytic state can be assumed if the thrombin time is prolonged above the normal limits of the laboratory or if the fibrinogen level is reduced.

Clinical monitoring should include serial neurologic examinations to detect central nervous system hemorrhage and frequent vital signs to detect gastrointestinal tract or retroperitoneal hemorrhage. Patients who have undergone catheterization should have the groin puncture examined and preferably have repeated measurements of thigh girth. Huge volumes of blood can be lost into the thigh and groin, especially in obese patients, with little external evidence of bleeding. In patients with pulmonary embolism, the adequacy of oxygenation should be assessed using oximetry, rather than arterial blood gases, in order to reduce punctures. In patients with myocardial infarction, additional monitoring for the success of reperfusion and for superimposed arrhythmias is necessary.

Heparin is typically infused beginning after the first hour of rt-PA administration in the setting of AMI, or, following SK or UK administration, when the fibrinogen level rises above 100 mg/dL or the thrombin time falls to 1.5 to 2 times control. Its efficacy has not yet been assessed however, although trials are in progress. Heparin is given without a bolus at 1000 U/h and titrated to a PTT of 1.5 to 2 times control.

COMPLICATIONS

BLEEDING

The greatest limitation of the thrombolytic drugs, and the factor which has limited their acceptance for the treatment of venous thromboembolism, is the consequential incidence of bleeding. In the initial Urokinase Pulmonary Embolism Trial, 45 percent of patients given urokinase suffered serious bleeding, compared with 27 percent of those who received heparin.[16] In contrast, in recent, noninvasive trials using streptokinase in patients with AMI, the incidence of severe bleeding has been only 0.6 to 5.9 percent (see Table 119-5).[26,27] The risk of bleeding has been reduced through the accumulated experience with these drugs, in particular by avoiding vascular punctures. The importance of maintaining vascular integrity is demonstrated by reviewing similarly recent trials in which coronary arteriography was part of the protocol; the incidence of severe bleeding has been about 15 percent.[28] In patients treated for pulmonary embolism, in whom pulmonary angiography is the rule, the risk of hemorrhage is over 20 percent. Those treated for deep venous thrombosis have a somewhat lesser risk (see Table 119-5).

One of the hopes for the second-generation, fibrin-specific thrombolytic agents has been that the risk of serious bleeding would be reduced. While fibrin specificity probably accounts for the improved efficacy of these agents, the risk of hemorrhage is no less than with streptokinase. In the trials of rt-PA in myocardial infarction, most of which have necessitated coronary arteriography, the incidence of major hemorrhage has been about 12 percent.[28] While there is some evidence that hemorrhage is related to the degree of systemic lysis, the relationship is weak. The most important predictors of risk seem to be the number of vascular punctures, the duration of lytic therapy, and the coadministration of antiplatelet drugs or heparin. It is extremely important when anticipating the use of a lytic drug to limit invasive procedures as much as possible. For example, a patient with massive pulmonary embolism might be managed with pulse oximetry and serial examinations rather than arterial blood gases or an arterial catheter. When vascular punctures are necessary, prolonged local compression is mandatory. Future trials will examine the utility of brief, high-dose, bolus infusions as a means of limiting hemorrhagic risk and will attempt to determine the necessity of heparinization following successful lysis.

When serious bleeding occurs, the lytic agent should be immediately discontinued and reliable, multiple, large-bore catheters secured. Direct compression of bleeding vessels may stop or slow ongoing blood loss. If heparin has been given, it too should be stopped and consideration given to reversing heparinization with protamine. Most patients will be adequately managed without the transfusion of clotting factors. If it becomes necessary to reverse the lytic state, cryoprecipitate, which contains fibrinogen and factor VIII (both of which are consumed by plasmin), is the preferred blood product.[29] The initial dose is 10 U, after which the fibrinogen level should be assayed. Fresh frozen plasma (as a source of factors V and VIII), platelets, and fibrinolytic drugs (e.g., ϵ-aminocaproic acid 5 g over 30 min) all may play a role in the critically bleeding patient (see Fig. 119-2).

TABLE 119-5 Hemorrhage in Patients Treated with Thrombolytic Agents

Disease	Drug	Risk of Hemorrhage, %	Intracranial Bleeding, %
MI	SK	1	0.15
MI, invasive	SK	15	0
MI, invasive	rt-PA	12	0.6
PE	SK, rt-PA	20	?
DVT	SK	10	?

Note: ?—numbers too small.
Data taken from Fennerty et al.[28]

ALLERGIC EFFECTS

Allergic reactions, including skin rashes, fever, and hypotension are rare except with SK and APSAC. Mild reactions can be treated with antihistamines and acetaminophen. More severe reactions should prompt the addition of hydrocortisone. Hypotension usually responds to volume administration.

CASE PRESENTATION

A 50-year-old, obese, white woman was admitted with nausea, vomiting, and colicky right-upper-quadrant pain. She was found to have gallstones and choledocholithiasis and was initially treated with intravenous fluids, antibiotics, nasogastric suction, and analgesia. On the second hospital day she was taken for cholecystectomy which was completed without incident. Her postoperative course was remarkable only for abdominal pain for which she continued to receive narcotics. On the third postoperative day, while being assisted to the bathroom, she complained of dyspnea and lightheadedness and slumped to the floor.

On examination, she was in moderate respiratory distress with a rate of 36, her blood pressure was 90/70, heart rate was 125, and she was afebrile. She was confused and diaphoretic. Oxygen was applied, fluids given, and she was transferred to the ICU. The chest radiograph revealed bibasilar atelectasis and a small right pleural effusion. On a 50 percent face mask an arterial blood gas

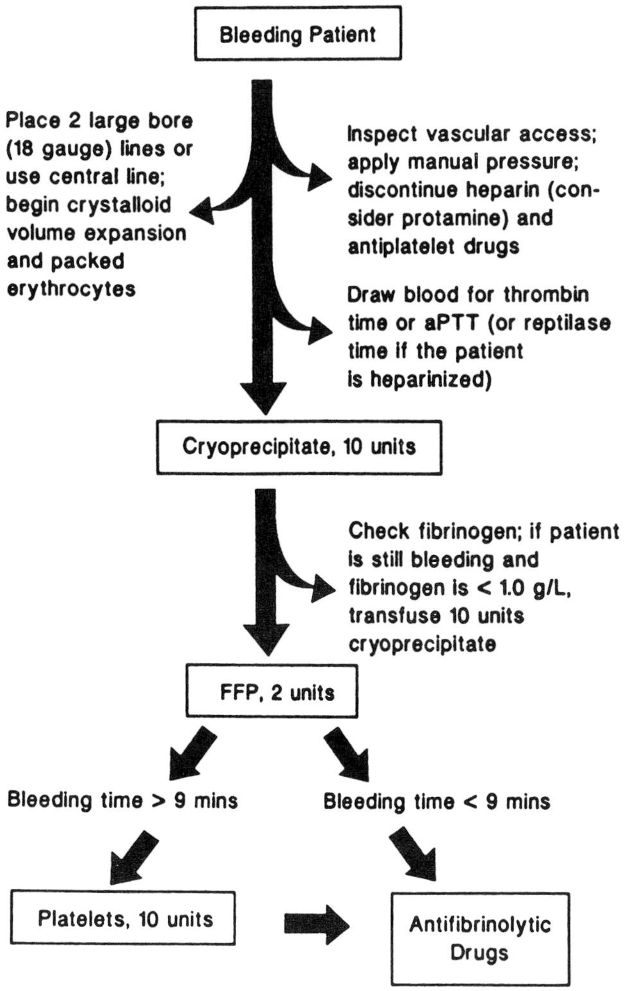

FIGURE 119-2 Strategy for the treatment of hemorrhage complicating thrombolytic therapy. aPTT = activated partial thromboplastin time; FFP = fresh frozen plasma. *(Reproduced from Sane et al.[29] with permission.)*

showed a P_{O_2} of 65 mmHg, P_{CO_2} of 33 mmHg, and pH of 7.32. A bolus of 5000 U of heparin was given on the assumption that this event was a postoperative pulmonary embolism. A duplex ultrasound examination of the lower extremities subsequently revealed occlusion of the left deep femoral and popliteal veins. A bedside perfusion lung scan showed numerous perfusion defects, but a ventilation scan could not be obtained. Heparin anticoagulation was continued at 1000 U/h but required increasing infusion rates to 2000 U/h in order to maintain the PTT at 2 times control. Eight hours following her deterioration, the patient was alert with a blood pressure of 100/70, heart rate of 110, and breathing at 26 breaths per minute. The urine output was 25 mL/h.

Over the next 4 days she gradually improved and the heparin infusion decreased gradually to 1200 U/h to maintain the same PTT. Oral feeding had been resumed successfully. She was preparing to move to the ward when the clinical hematology laboratory called to notify the service that a routine platelet count from that morning was 80,000. Upon review, the count had been 130,000 the day prior, and 420,000 postoperatively. No medications could be implicated, so heparin was immediately discontinued, and a first dose of Coumadin, 10 mg orally, was given. Plans were made to place an inferior vena caval filter later that same morning. The next day the patient was moved to the floor, Coumadin was adjusted to achieve a stable PT of 1.3 times control (INR = 2.0), and she was discharged to home on the fourteenth postoperative day.

CASE DISCUSSION

This case illustrates several issues regarding anticoagulation which are commonplace in the ICU. The first point is that prophylactic, subcutaneous heparin should be given routinely before elective cholecystectomy and most other general surgical procedures since it has been shown to decrease the incidence of DVT, PE, and fatal PE, without undue risk of bleeding. Although this woman's PE was easy to diagnose, it was nearly fatal. Thus prophylaxis is superior to diagnosis and treatment following the event.

In this case a sublethal embolus was felt to be clinically very likely; however, a pulmonary arteriogram or an adequate and high probability ventilation-perfusion scan would have been necessary to conclude this with certainty. Massive PE with shock, as in this patient, is an indication for thrombolytic therapy. However, an absolute contraindication, recent surgery, made this unavailable. Had this embolus occurred in a nonoperative setting, it would have been necessary to confirm the diagnosis of PE with an arteriogram in order to justify the risk of thrombolytic therapy.

The initial infusion rate of heparin (2000 U/h) is rather typical when there is extensive thrombosis, because of the altered kinetics of heparin elimination in this setting. Different dosing requirements are seen in different patients, and even the same patient may need a different infusion rate over time, pointing out the importance of following the PTT.

A complication of heparin therapy, heparin-associated thrombocytopenia (HAT), was likely here since no other drugs seemed likely offenders. The onset on the fourth to fifth day is typical of HAT. More careful review of the daily platelet count, which should be routine in patients on heparin, could have led to discontinuation of heparin at least a day earlier. Since this phenomenon is probably dose related, it would not likely have occurred with prophylactic heparin. While no adverse thrombotic events were seen here, these are unpredictable and potentially devastating. It is essential to stop heparin immediately, even when anticoagulation is required. To prevent potentially fatal recurrent embolism, vena caval interruption was performed. Since this serves to prevent PE, but doesn't treat the underlying DVT, the use of warfarin is necessary for at least several months.

References

1. Ofusu FA, Fernandez F, Gauthier D, et al: Heparin cofactor II and other endogenous factors in the mediation of the antithrombotic and anticoagulant effects of heparin and dermatan sulphate. Semin Thromb Hemost 11:133, 1985.
2. Green D, Lee MY, Lim AC, et al: Prevention of thromboembolism after spinal cord injury using low-molecular-weight heparin. Ann Intern Med 113:571, 1990.
3. Halkin H, Goldberg J, Modan M, et al: Reduction of mortality in general medical in-patients by low-dose heparin prophylaxis. Ann Intern Med 96:561, 1982.
4. Collins R, Scrimgeour A, Yusuf S, et al: Reduction in fatal pulmonary embolism and venous thrombosis by perioperative administration of subcutaneous heparin: overview of results of randomized trials in general, orthopedic, and urologic surgery. N Engl J Med 318:1162, 1988.
5. Doyle DJ, Turpie AGG, Hirsh J, et al: Adjusted subcutaneous heparin or continuous intravenous heparin in patients with acute deep vein thrombosis. Ann Intern Med 107:441, 1987.
6. Hyers TM, Hull RD, Weg JG: Antithrombotic therapy for venous thromboembolic disease. Chest 89(suppl):26S, 1986.
7. Goldhaber SZ, Buring JE, Lipnick RJ, et al: Pooled analyses of randomized trials of streptokinase and heparin in phlebographically documented acute deep venous thrombosis. Am J Med 76:393, 1984.
8. Landefeld CS, Cook EF, Flatley M, et al: Identification and preliminary validation of predictors of major bleeding in hospitalized patients starting anticoagulant therapy. Am J Med 82:703, 1987.
9. Jaffin BW, Bliss CM, Lamont JT: Significance of occult gastrointestinal bleeding during anticoagulation therapy. Am J Med 83:269, 1987.
10. Green D, Martin GJ, Shoichet SH, et al: Thrombocytopenia in a prospective randomized double-blind trial of bovine and porcine heparin. Am J Med Sci 288:60, 1984.
11. Warkentin TE, Kelton JG: Heparin and platelets. Hematol/Oncol Clin North Am 4:243, 1990.
12. Hirsh J, Poller L, Deykin D, et al: Optimal therapeutic range for oral anticoagulants. Chest 95(suppl):5S, 1989.
13. Levine MN, Raskob G, Hirsh J: Hemorrhagic complications of long-term anticoagulant therapy. Chest 95(suppl):26S, 1989.
14. Renowden S, Westmoreland D, White JP, et al: Oral cholestyramine increases elimination of warfarin after overdose. Br Med J 291(ii):513, 1985.
15. Goldhaber SZ: Thrombolysis in venous thromboembolism: an international perspective. Chest 97(suppl):176S, 1990.
16. UPET Study Group: Urokinase pulmonary embolism trial: phase 1 results. JAMA 214:2163, 1970.
17. Petitpretz P, Simmoneau G, Cerrina J, et al: Effects of a single bolus of urokinase in patients with life-threatening pulmonary emboli: a descriptive trial. Circulation 70:861, 1984.
18. Van der Werf F, Vanhaecke J, de Geest H, et al: Coronary thrombolysis with recombinant single-chain urokinase type plasminogen activator in patients with acute myocardial infarction. Circulation 74:1066, 1986.
19. Goldhaber SZ, Kessler CM, Heit J, et al: A randomized controlled trial of recombinant tissue plasminogen activator versus urokinase in the treatment of acute pulmonary embolism. Lancet ii:293, 1988.
20. Wilcox RG: Thrombolysis with tissue plasminogen activator in suspected acute myocardial infarction: the ASSET study. Chest 95(suppl):270S, 1989.
21. Levine MN, Weitz J, Turpie AGG, et al: A new short infusion dosage regimen of recombinant tissue plasminogen activator in patients with venous thromboembolic disease. Chest 97(suppl):168S, 1990.
22. Bates ER, Topol EJ: Thrombolytic therapy for acute myocardial infarction. Chest 95(suppl):257S, 1989.
23. Turpie AGG, Levine MN, Hirsh J, et al: Tissue plasminogen activator (rt-PA) vs heparin in deep venous thrombosis: results of a randomized trial. Chest 97(suppl):172S, 1990.
24. Kessler CM: Anticoagulation and thrombolytic therapy: practical considerations. Chest 95(suppl):245S, 1989.
25. Atkinson JB, Bagnall HA, Gomperts E: Investigational use of tissue plasminogen activator (t-PA) for occluded central venous catheters. J Parenter Enteral Nutr 14:310, 1990.
26. The ISAM Study Group: A prospective trial of intravenous streptokinase in acute myocardial infarction (I.S.A.M.). N Engl J Med 314:1465, 1986.
27. ISIS-2: Randomized trial of intravenous streptokinase, oral aspirin, both, or neither among 17,187 cases of suspected acute myocardial infarction. Lancet ii:349, 1988.
28. Fennerty AG, Levine MN, Hirsh J: Hemorrhagic complications of thrombolytic therapy in the treatment of myocardial infarction and venous thromboembolism. Chest 95(suppl):88S, 1989.
29. Sane DC, Califf RM, Topol EJ, et al: Bleeding during thrombolytic therapy for acute myocardial infarction: mechanisms and management. Ann Intern Med 111:1010, 1989.

Chapter 120

RHYTHM DISTURBANCES

IAN H. SANTORO
JEFFREY S. SOBLE
THOMAS E. BUMP

KEY POINTS

- *Continuous electrocardiographic (ECG) monitoring in ICU patients uncovers a wide range of arrhythmias, many of which do not require therapy.*
- *Recognizing the hemodynamic impact of an arrhythmia is of particular importance in developing an appropriate treatment strategy.*
- *Appropriate management of arrhythmias hinges on identifying and correcting predisposing conditions.*
- *Arrhythmia management requires understanding the appropriate use of multiple modalities, most notably antiarrhythmic drug therapy, cardiac pacing, and electrical cardioversion and defibrillation.*
- *The proarrhythmic potential of antiarrhythmic therapy is important and should not be underestimated.*
- *Consideration of antiarrhythmic drug pharmacokinetics is particularly important in critically ill patients with multisystem organ dysfunction, who are at increased risk of developing drug toxicity.*

Patients in ICUs present a challenging array of arrhythmias. This is partly because continuous cardiac monitoring exposes a variety of benign arrhythmias, which are ubiquitous even in healthy subjects, including sinus tachycardia, sinus bradycardia, type I second degree atrioventricular (AV) block (especially during sleep), and isolated premature atrial and ventricular beats. In addition, critically ill patients are subject to a number of arrhythmogenic stresses that predispose them to various serious arrhythmias such as advanced heart block, atrial flutter and fibrillation, and ventricular tachycardia (VT). Arrhythmia management may be the primary indication for admission to an ICU. Clearly, every intensivist should be skilled in diagnosis and management of arrhythmias.

Successful management of arrhythmias depends on accurate diagnosis. The 12-lead ECG and the adequately long rhythm strip are the premier diagnostic instruments (see Chap. 30). When the nature of an arrhythmia remains obscure even after the surface ECGs have been analyzed, additional information can be gleaned from direct atrial recordings obtained from intracardiac, epicardial, or transesophageal electrodes (Chap. 32). Further diagnostic information may be produced by observing the patient's response to interventions such as carotid sinus massage or adenosine injection.

Accurate assessment of an arrhythmia's hemodynamic impact is also crucial for successful management. Bradycardias cause hemodynamic compromise when the heart cannot produce a compensatory increase in stroke volume to maintain the cardiac output. Hemodynamic compromise is produced by tachycardias through at least five mechanisms (Table 120-1). The individual's response to an arrhythmia also depends on the ability of the peripheral vasculature to compensate for reductions in cardiac output. Hypovolemia, vasodilator therapy, autonomic neuropathy, and increasing age are a few of the factors that can reduce the ability of the peripheral vasculature to adapt to decrements in cardiac output.

The interplay of all the above factors is complex, and the degree of hemodynamic compromise usually cannot be predicted by ECG analysis alone. A patient with a structurally normal heart can tolerate sustained VT, whereas a patient with extensive myocardial damage or valvular disease might suffer a severe drop in cardiac output from ventricular bigeminy. The impact of an arrhythmia on a patient can best be judged by learning the patient's symptoms, examining the patient during the arrhythmia, and evaluating the effect of the arrhythmia on the kidneys and other organ systems. In the ICU, the physician is often handicapped by the impossibility of speaking with patients who are intubated or obtunded; and it will often be difficult to determine if it is the arrhythmia or some nonarrhythmic factor that is compromising organ function. On the other hand, the intensivist may have information not available to physicians in other settings, such as the cardiac output or arterial pressure during the arrhythmia.

Once the arrhythmia has been diagnosed and its effect on the patient assessed, the intensivist must select the appropriate management for the patient, through careful weighing of the risks and potential benefits to that patient of each of the available therapies. Here, the intensivist faces special problems not shared by the cardiologist working in an outpatient clinic. For example, the risks of therapy (e.g., the negative inotropic effects of some of the drugs) are different in the critically ill patient than in the ambulatory patient. Drug metabolism is drastically altered when the kidneys, liver, or both have failed. The automatic implantable defibrillator, which is the most effective available therapy for VT, cannot be used in patients with sepsis, neoplasm, or any of a large number of illnesses commonly encountered in ICU patients. Thus, the intensivist may have to adapt,

TABLE 120-1 Factors Determining the Extent of Hemodynamic Compromise during Tachycardia

Shortening of diastolic filling time
Increase in myocardial oxygen demand with resultant ischemia and left ventricular dysfunction
Loss of AV synchrony
Asynchronous left ventricular contraction (during any rhythm with LBBB or ectopic ventricular activation)
Atrial stretch causing reflex hypotension (Bezold-Jarisch reflex)

not adopt, the algorithms for arrhythmia management found in cardiology textbooks.

Bradycardias

Bradycardia is often defined as any cardiac rhythm that produces a ventricular rate below 60 beats/min. However, this rate is not the boundary between normal and abnormal, for there is no rate that separates physiologic from pathologic. It is perfectly natural for a healthy person to have a sinus rate of 35 to 40 beats/min at rest or especially during rapid eye movement sleep,[1,2] and yet a heart rate of 70 beats/min can be pathologic in a young patient with pneumonia. When made aware of a patient with bradycardia, the physician must first assess the hemodynamic impact of the rhythm. This will dictate whether cardiopulmonary resuscitation must be instituted immediately, or if a more deliberate approach to the problem can be taken. Again, rate alone is not a sufficient guide, for a heart rate of 30 beats/min causes no symptoms in some patients and hemodynamic collapse in others.

The types of bradycardia are sinus bradycardia and AV block.

SINUS BRADYCARDIA

Sinus bradycardia and sinus pauses occur either when the sinus node fails to discharge (depolarize) on time or when a sinus node discharge fails to excite the neighboring atrial myocardium. These phenomena may result from excessive vagal tone, deficient sympathetic tone, or intrinsic dysfunction of the sinus node or perinodal tissue. The latter may include degenerative, ischemic, inflammatory (e.g., myocarditis), or infiltrative processes (e.g., amyloidosis or sarcoidosis). Some causes of sinus bradycardia are easily identified, such as endotracheal suction producing excessive vagal tone, while others are too easily overlooked. Sinus bradycardia may be the only clue to hypothyroidism in the patient who remains ventilator dependent; it may herald rapid cerebral herniation in a patient whose elevated blood pressure is overlooked (Cushing's reflex); it may be the first sign of hyperkalemia; or it may be the first sign of an abdominal catastrophe (due to increased vagal tone from visceral distention) or sepsis in an obtuded patient.

The appropriate diagnostic work-up begins with a physical examination, paying careful attention to the signs of the underlying causes of sinus bradycardia. Often the ICU nurse can document the temporal relation between a procedure and the resultant sinus bradycardia. Medication lists must be checked carefully for iatrogenic causes of sinus bradycardia, such as β blockers, calcium channel blockers, morphine, or amiodarone. If necessary, thyroid function tests to rule out hypothyroidism, Holter monitoring to document sick sinus syndrome, or abdominal films to look for visceral distention or perforation can be ordered.

Management of sinus bradycardia begins with eradicating or treating the underlying cause, if any exists. Other measures to increase the heart rate are unnecessary when the bradycardia has caused no symptoms or signs of hemodynamic compromise, as is the case with most patients. When there is hemodynamic compromise, treatment should be instituted. In emergencies, atropine, β agonists, or temporary transcutaneous pacing (also called noninvasive or external pacing) can be administered. These can be sufficient to tide a patient over a transient bradycardia, or can serve as a bridge for the patient until transvenous pacing can be implemented, in the case of a more persistant bradycardia. Intravenous atropine, 0.5 mg, every 5 min to a total dose of 1.5 to 2.0 mg, rapidly antagonizes cholinergic input to the sinoatrial node and equally rapidly increases the heart rate, to the extent that vagal tone has been contributing to the bradycardia. Patients with intrinsic sinus node dysfunction may not respond to atropine. Unfortunately, atropine is difficult to titrate, and its administration frequently produces a sinus tachycardia, which in patients with myocardial ischemia may be deleterious. Doses >2 mg should be avoided, because excessive atropine can cause delirium or even coma. It may be given endotracheally; the recommended dose is 1.0 to 2.0 mg diluted in 10 mL sterile water or normal saline.

Epinephrine is the catecholamine of choice for the treatment of patients with profound bradycardia and hypotension. It stimulates both α and β receptors and therefore has pressor effects as well as positive chronotropic effects. It has a far shorter half-life than atropine and can be more readily titrated. During cardiopulmonary resuscitation, the recommended dose is 0.5 to 1.0 mg given every 5 min, either intravenously or endotracheally (for the latter route it should be diluted in 10 mL sterile water or normal saline). However, it can also be administered as a continuous infusion by mixing 1 mg in 250 mL 5% dextrose in water and starting with an infusion rate of 2 μg/min.

Isoproterenol is the catecholamine of choice if the patient has bradycardia and hypertension. It is a pure β agonist and has vasodilating rather than vasopressor activity. It can also be administered as a titratable continuous infusion, by mixing 1 mg in 250 mL 5% dextrose in water and infusing at 1 to 2 μg/min up to a dose of 20 μg/min.

β Receptors are more widely distributed in the heart than are the muscarinic receptors that are blocked by atropine. As a result, the β agonists, unlike atropine, can accelerate subsidary pacemakers in the ventricle. This can be beneficial in the patient whose intrinsic sinus node dysfunction precludes any speeding of sinus rate in response to drugs; but there is also considerably more potential for the induction of VT from infusions of β agonists than from atropine.

Cardiac pacing is an important therapeutic modality for patients with sinus bradycardia that is causing hemodynamic compromise. When pacing is required, some patients will benefit from the maintainence of AV synchrony by atrial or AV sequential pacing. Patients who do poorly with ventricular pacing include those whose atrial kick contributes significantly to ventricular filling (e.g., patients with hypertrophic cardiomyopathy, dilated cardiomyopathy with diminished cardiovascular reserve, or right ventricular infarction). Other patients who do poorly with ventricular pacing are those who have intact ventriculoatrial conduction, for during ventricular pacing these patients have a P wave in every ST segment, causing the atria to contract against closed tricuspid and mitral valves. The different techniques of pacing are described in Chap. 32.

ATRIOVENTRICULAR BLOCK

The AV conduction system includes the AV node, His bundle, and bundle branches with their extensive and variable arborization. The left bundle branch usually bifurcates into a left anterior fascicle and a left posterior fascicle, producing a trifascicular infranodal conduction system (the right bundle branch being the third fascicle). Block can occur along any portion of this pathway.

The causes of heart block are numerous (Table 120-2), but many can be rapidly excluded. AV nodal block is classically produced by increased vagal tone (it occurs during sleep in young, healthy people and at rest in athletes), inferior wall myocardial infarction (both because of increased vagal tone and because of AV nodal ischemia), and drugs (digoxin, β blockers, and calcium channel blockers). Infranodal block is classically produced by hypertensive heart disease, anterior wall myocardial infarction, and mitral annular calcification (Lev's disease). AV nodal block is more likely than infranodal block to be transient or reversible. When the cause of block is not obvious, and especially when the block is new, some consideration should be given to obtaining studies to rule out a recent myocardial infarction, an echocardiogram to look for mitral annular calcification, left ventricular hypertrophy, and to assess ventricular function, and a Holter monitor to see if the conduction disturbance worsens at times.

TABLE 120-2 Causes of Heart Block

Myocardial infarction/ischemia	Trauma
Cardiomyopathies	Postcardiac surgery
Hypertensive	Infectious diseases
Ischemic	Endocarditis (usually aortic)
Nonischemic, dilated	Syphilis
Drugs	Tuberculosis
Digitalis	Lyme disease
β Blockers	Diphtheria
Calcium channel blockers	Chagas' disease
Phenytoin	Toxoplasmosis
Tricyclic antidepressants	Mumps
Most antiarrhythmics	Inflammatory diseases
Increased vagal tone	Myocarditis
Visceral distention	Rheumatic fever
Pain	Collagen-vascular diseases
Carotid hypersensitivity	Ankylosing spondylitis
Infiltrative processes	Rheumatoid arthritis
Amylodosis	Polymyositis
Sarcoidosis	Endocrine diseases
Hemochromatosis	Thyrotoxicosis
Gout	Myxedema
Paget's disease	Addison's disease
Tumors	Congenital heart disease
Degenerative disease	Congenital complete heart block
Lev's disease	Poisoning
Lenegre's disease	Lead
Calcific aortic stenosis	Organophosphate
Muscular distrophies	
Friedreich's ataxia	

BUNDLE BRANCH BLOCK. Though bundle branch block can appear in patients with otherwise normal hearts, it often reflects cardiac disease. This is especially true of left bundle branch block (LBBB), which often accompanies left ventricular dysfunction, particularly when there is also leftward axis deviation. Since bundle branch block can reflect underlying heart disease, its discovery should prompt a thorough cardiac evaluation.

In the past, bifascicular block (LBBB, right bundle branch block [RBBB] with left anterior fascicular block, or RBBB with left posterior fascicular block) was feared to reflect impending complete heart block. However, several large prospective studies demonstrated that the annual rate of progression to complete heart block is only 1 percent in patients with *chronic* bifascicular block.[3,4] Other studies have shown that surgery can be performed safely in these patients without backup pacing.[5] The same is true of elective cardioversion of atrial fibrillation in patients with chronic bifascicular block.[6] It has also been demonstrated that Swan-Ganz catheterization can be performed in patients with LBBB with at most a negligible incidence of progression to high degree AV block.[7] Thus, the discovery of bundle branch block should not lead to heightened concerns regarding need for pacing.

The story is considerably different for patients who develop bundle branch block in the setting of acute myocardial infarction. A subset of these patients is at very high risk for developing symptomatic heart block.[8,9] A recent consensus statement proposed that temporary pacing be administered to all patients who develop bifascicular block in the setting of acute myocardial infarction.[10]

FIRST DEGREE AV BLOCK. First degree heart block is defined by a PR interval >200 msec. It is often found in normal persons. In the ICU it can reflect high vagal tone, inferior wall ischemia, myocarditis, or the effect of β blockers, calcium channel blockers, or digitalis on AV nodal conduction. First degree AV block is often transient and always asymptomatic. In the absence of associated bundle branch block, the anatomic site of the disorder is usually the AV node and only very rarely the His bundle. Block in the His bundle carries a worse prognosis; only His bundle recordings can differentiate between block in the AV node and block in the His bundle. When bundle branch block and first degree heart block occur together, the conduction delay responsible for the long PR interval is intranodal in half the patients and infranodal (i.e., reflecting disease in the bundle branch or fascicle which is not blocked) in the other half. Infranodal block carries a worse prognosis.

SECOND DEGREE AV BLOCK. Second degree AV block is of two types, each of which exhibits intermittent failure of supraventricular impulses to conduct to the ventricle.

Mobitz type I second degree AV block conforms to the "rules of Wenckebach": relative stability of duration of the PP interval; progressive elongation of the PR interval with simultaneous progressive shortening of the RR interval until there is failed conduction to the ventricle with an ensuing pause; the RR interval containing the nonconducted supraventricular impulse is < two times the basic PP interval. The anatomic site of this conduction disturbance is most often the AV node. It often occurs during sleep in healthy young people without heart disease.

Isolated Mobitz I AV block usually does not produce hemodynamic compromise and does not require urgent therapy. However, when it is associated with other conduction disturbances in the setting of acute myocardial infarction, temporary pacing may be warranted because of the possibility of progression to complete heart block.[10] The long-term prognosis of patients with persistent Mobitz I AV block has also been found to be improved by permanent pacing.[11]

Mobitz type II second degree AV block exhibits a constant duration of the PR and RR intervals until suddenly a P wave fails to conduct, causing a pause that is exactly twice the RR interval. The anatomic site for this conduction block is usually infranodal and results from extensive damage to the His bundle and fascicles. The marked impairment of conduction pathways necessary to produce this arrhythmia often results from extensive anterior myocardial infarction or the depressant effect of drugs or metabolic imbalances on a degenerated conduction system.

Mobitz type II second degree AV block is widely accepted as an indication for permanent pacemaker placement because it is thought to forbode progression to complete heart block. This has been found to be the case when it occurs in patients with bundle branch block or in the setting of acute myocardial infarction, but there is little evidence to support prophylactic permanent pacing in asymptomatic patients with Mobitz II block who have not had a recent myocardial infarction or bundle branch block.

Some patients with Mobitz II block should receive temporary pacing while they await implantation of a permanent pacemaker. Of course, this is true of patients with symptoms like syncope or near-syncope that might be attributable to episodes of complete heart block with ventricular asystole (i.e., Stokes-Adams attacks). In addition, some asymptomatic patients should receive temporary pacing, including those with acute myocardial infarction, recent cardiac surgery, endocarditis, and myocarditis. These are patients with a rapidly changing myocardial substrate, which increases the chances that sudden exacerbation of their conduction disturbance might occur.

Many patients with *2:1 AV block* develop hemodynamic compromise and require pacing and, in some cases, temporizing therapy with atropine or catecholamines. Some patients, though, are asymptomatic and hemodynamically stable with this rhythm. Tradition holds that urgent prophylactic pacing should be used in asymptomatic patients if there is associated acute myocardial infarction, myocarditis, endocarditis, or recent myocardial infarction or if the heart block appears to be at an infranodal level rather than in the AV node. An infranodal site of block is suggested if conducted beats have bundle branch block, if exercise or atropine fail to increase the percentage of conducted beats, or if at other times the patient has a Mobitz II pattern of conduction. A His bundle recording is the only way to prove the site of block.

THIRD DEGREE AV BLOCK. Third degree, or complete, heart block occurs when there is complete failure of supraventricular impulses to conduct to the ventricles. If available, an escape rhythm (junctional, fascicular, idioventricular) originates below the site of block, producing a narrow QRS complex if from the junction and a wide QRS complex if from the bundle branches or fascicles. The higher anatomically the escape focus in the conduction system, the faster the escape rate, with escape rhythms of 45 to 60 beats/min from the region of the AV node and His bundle and 30 to 40 beats/min from escape foci in the ventricle (idioventricular rhythm). Occasionally in the extremely diseased conduction system, no escape rhythm will supervene and asystole will result.

In third degree heart block, P waves occur independently of and at a faster rate than the QRS complexes of the escape rhythm. This dissociation of the P waves and the QRS complexes will produce a constantly varying PR interval and fluctuating morphology of the ST segment and T wave as the P waves shift their position relative to the QRS complexes.

The most common causes of third degree heart block in the ICU are acute myocardial infarction, endocarditis, postcardiac surgery, trauma, and metabolic and drug-induced suppression of cardiac conduction. Most patients who develop third degree heart block in the ICU become symptomatic from a decrease in cardiac output and require urgent treatment. Even in asymptomatic patients, any prediction of the reversibility of third degree heart block is too tenuous to withhold treatment until such reversal occurs. The only exception to this rule is in asymptomatic patients with congenital complete heart block.

The management of complete heart block is identical to that for profound sinus bradycardia (vide supra): temporizing with atropine, epinephrine, or isoproterenol or temporary transcutaneous pacing, until a transvenous pacing system can be readied. The decision to implant a permanent pacemaker depends on the circumstances and reversibility of the arrhythmia. In acute inferior wall infarction, a permanent pacemaker is not necessary if the heart block spontaneously resolves as it usually does. However, permanent pacing is justified even for transient complete heart block in the setting of acute anterior myocardial infarction, when it evolves from Mobitz II type second degree AV block, and when it is associated with bundle branch block during conducted beats.

Tachycardias and Ectopy

ANTIARRHYTHMIC THERAPY

In the ICU, tachycardia and ectopy are more common than bradycardia. Unlike bradycardias, which nearly always respond to pacing, tachycardias do not respond uniformly well to a single kind of therapy. Instead, the intensivist must be acquainted with different acute therapies including antiarrhythmic drugs, antitachycardia pacing, and electrical cardioversion and defibrillation, as well as more definitive therapies such as catheter ablation, antiarrhythmic surgery, or implantation of antitachycardia devices.

ANTIARRHYTHMIC DRUGS. Antiarrhythmic drugs are often classified according to their presumed mechanism of action (Table 120-3).[12] The sodium channel blocking drugs form the most heterogeneous group and are therefore subclassified into drugs that release quickly from the sodium channel following repolarization (class 1B), drugs which release slowly (class 1C), and drugs which release at an intermediate rate (class 1A). The chief merit of the classification scheme is that it provides a framework for discussing antiarrhythmic drugs. However, the scheme has important limitations. For example, when a patient responds to a drug it does not guarantee that he will respond to other drugs from the same class or subclass.[13,14] Also, some drugs do not fit neatly into one class: for instance, amiodarone has characteristics that could place it in classes 1A, 2, 3, and 4. Quinidine, procainamide, and disopyramide have class 3 properties as well as class 1A properties.

Table 120-3 lists the drugs which have been approved by the United States Food and Drug Administration (FDA) for use against arrhythmias, along with their approved indications. These indications do not accurately reflect clinical practice. For instance, although propranolol and acebutolol are the only orally administered β blockers that have been FDA approved for use against arrhythmias, other β blockers are also commonly used to treat supraventricular arrhythmias and some ventricular arrhythmias. Though diltiazem has not received FDA approval for antiarrhythmic indications, it is widely used for the same purposes as verapamil. Similarly, procainamide, disopyramide, and the class 1C drugs are all widely used for supraventricular arrhythmias, though they have not been approved for this indication.

Even when a drug is said to be effective against an arrhythmia, it does not mean that the drug will always suppress the arrhythmia. Lidocaine is effective <50 percent of the time at terminating episodes of sustained VT, and quinidine is effective <50 percent of the time at terminating episodes of atrial fibrillation. Encainide and flecainide are effective at reducing the frequency of premature complexes, but usually do not completely eradicate them. For most arrhythmias there is no way to predict if a drug will be effective in a particular patient. Ultimately, an element of trial and error always comes into play.

Antiarrhythmic drugs all have the potential to cause considerable toxicity. It is not surprising that drugs which can suppress tachycardias can also suppress normal cardiac rhythm, especially in patients with intrinsic dysfunction of the cardiac conduction system. Thus, virtually every antiarrhythmic drug has been reported to cause sinus bradycardia or heart block. Furthermore, these drugs have become increasingly notorious for their proarrhythmic effect, i.e., their capacity to cause a new tachycardia to appear in a patient or to exacerbate the preexisting arrhythmia by causing it to occur more frequently, be more sustained, or be less well-tolerated.[15,16]

Several different mechanisms for proarrhythmia are likely. Drugs that delay repolarization may contribute to the appearance of early after-potentials, which may underlie rhythms ranging from ventricular extrasystoles to torsade de pointes, a rapid and dangerous form of VT.[17] Digi-

TABLE 120-3 FDA-Approved Antiarrhythmic Drugs with Their Indications

		FDA-Approved Indications
Class 1. Drugs that block the fast inward sodium channel		
Class 1A	Quinidine	Supraventricular and ventricular arrhythmias
	Procainamide	Life-threatening or symptomatic ventricular arrhythmias
	Disopyramide	Premature ventricular beats and episodes of ventricular tachycardia
Class 1B	Lidocaine	Ventricular arrhythmias
	Tocainide	Life-threatening ventricular arrhythmias
	Mexiletine	Symptomatic ventricular arrhythmias
	Moricizine	Life-threatening ventricular arrhythmias
Class 1C	Flecainide	Life-threatening ventricular arrhythmias
	Encainide	Life-threatening ventricular arrhythmias
	Propafenone	Life-threatening ventricular arrhythmias
Class 2. Drugs that block β receptors		
	Propranolol	Supraventricular and ventricular arrhythmias and inappropriate sinus tachycardia
	Acebutolol	Ventricular premature beats
	Esmolol	Control of ventricular rate in atrial flutter and fibrillation and noncompensatory sinus tachycardia
Class 3. Drugs that delay repolarization		
	Bretylium	Ventricular fibrillation and other life-threatening ventricular arrhythmias
	Amiodarone	Life-threatening recurrent ventricular arrhythmias only when other agents have failed
Class 4. Drugs that block calcium channels		
	Verapamil	Control of ventricular rate in atrial flutter and fibrillation; paroxysmal supraventricular tachycardia (SVT)
Unclassified Drugs		
	Digoxin	Control of ventricular rate in atrial flutter and fibrillation; paroxysmal SVT
	Adenosine	Paroxysmal SVT

talis toxicity probably causes arrhythmias by producing late after-potentials.[18] Drugs which slow conduction can stabilize reentry and turn nonsustained tachycardia into sustained.[19] Drugs with negative inotropic effects might reduce a patient's ability to tolerate an arrhythmia and increase the likelihood that the tachycardia will degenerate into a more dangerous form. Amiodarone can lead indirectly to sudden worsening of arrhythmia by causing hyperthyroidism.

Most antiarrhythmic drugs have negative inotropic effects.[20,21] These effects usually are not manifest in patients with normal left ventricular function, but can be devastating in patients with left ventricular dysfunction, particularly those with a left ventricular ejection fraction <30 percent. Disopyramide, class 1C agents, β blockers, and calcium channel blockers are the drugs most notorious for precipitating heart failure in patients with underlying left ventricular dysfunction. Other common side effects of antiarrhythmic drugs are listed in Table 120-4. This is by necessity a partial list; whenever a patient develops a new symptom or laboratory abnormality while taking an antiarrhythmic medication, keep an open mind toward the possibility that the drug is the culprit.

TABLE 120-4 Extracardiac Side Effects of Antiarrhythmic Drugs

Class 1A	
Quinidine	Diarrhea, hypotension, cinchonism, thrombocytopenia
Procainamide	Lupus-like syndrome, agranulocytosis
Disopyramide	Anticholinergic effects (dry mouth, urinary retention, exacerbation of glaucoma)
Class 1B	
Lidocaine	Confusion, seizures, coma
Tocainide	Confusion, seizures, coma, agranulocytosis, pulmonary fibrosis
Mexiletine	Confusion, seizures, coma, nausea
Moricizine	Light-headedness
Class 1C	
Flecainide	Dizziness, headache, visual disturbance
Encainide	Dizziness, headache, visual disturbance
Propafenone	Dizziness, headache, visual disturbance
Class 2	
Propranolol	Exacerbation of asthma, lethargy, exacerbation of periperal vascular disease, masking of hypoglycemia
Acebutolol	Same as propranolol
Esmolol	Same as propranolol
Class 3	
Bretylium	Vasodilation and hypotension, parotid pain
Amiodarone	Intentional tremor and ataxia, pulmonary fibrosis, dermal photosensitivity, constipation, cirrhosis, hypothyroidism or hyperthyroidism
Class 4	
Verapamil	Constipation, vasodilation, hypotension
Unclassified	
Digoxin	Nausea, visual disturbance, confusion
Adenosine	Flushing

Antiarrhythmic drugs usually cause their side effects at serum concentrations only a little higher than their minimum therapeutic concentration. The drugs must be administered in such a way as to produce serum concentrations within a narrow therapeutic window. During chronic maintenance therapy, this is usually accomplished by administering enough drug to offset elimination, at intervals equal to the elimination half-life. When antiarrhythmic therapy is not emergently required, treatment can begin at a low dose, with gradual dose escalation until the desired effect is produced.

In the ICU, it is common for arrhythmias to require urgent therapy. Here the goal is to produce a therapeutic serum concentration quickly, and subsequently to keep the concentration in the therapeutic range. Typically a loading dose is given to raise the serum concentration into the therapeutic range. At the same time, a maintenance dose is started to offset drug elimination. But, if only these steps are taken, the patient is left unprotected for a while following the bolus. This is because most antiarrhythmic drugs obey two-compartment pharmacokinetics, i.e., following a bolus, drugs disappear from the circulation (the central compartment) by two routes: elimination and distribution into adipose tissue and other sites (the peripheral compartment). Drug leaves the central circulation by the latter route until its concentration in the peripheral compartment equals the concentration in the central compartment. To keep the serum concentration of a drug within the therapeutic range following a bolus, the physician should supplement the maintenance dose with additional boluses to offset distribution. In the near future, computerized infusion pumps will facilitate the acute administration of drugs by enabling delivery of exponentially tapering infusions that account for both elimination and distribution.[22]

Dosing schedules have been developed for each antiarrhythmic drug (Table 120-5). Use of these schedules should be tempered by an appreciation of how pharmacokinetics might be altered in the particular patient. The dose of an antiarrhythmic drug should be adjusted with a view to potential interactions with other drugs that the patient might be taking (Table 120-6). Also, various disease states can affect the pharmacokinetic characteristics of drugs. The absorption of oral drugs (i.e., their bioavailability) can be reduced by bowel resection, mesenteric ischemia, or congested intestinal mucosa. On the other hand, bioavailability can be increased by hepatic dysfunction, which reduces the extent to which the liver removes orally administered drugs from the portal circulation (i.e., the first-pass effect). Drug elimination can be reduced or even abolished by hepatic or renal dysfunction, depending on the site of metabolism or elimination of the drug (Table 120-7). Disease states have a variable effect on the size of the central and peripheral compartments, which are critical determinants of the appropriate size of a loading dose.

The usual way to compensate for variability in pharmacokinetics is to monitor for efficacy and side effects and to monitor serum concentrations of drugs. Serum concentrations are useful though the concentrations of active metabolites may not be measured (e.g., 3-hydroxyquinidine and

TABLE 120-5 Doses of Antiarrhythmic Drugs

Drug	Loading Dose	Maintenance Dose	Gastrointestinal Absorption, %	Oral Bio-availability	Therapeutic Plasma Concentration
Digoxin	10–15 μg/kg or 0.5–1.0 mg IV/PO then 0.25 mg prn to total 1.0–2.5 mg	0.125–0.750 mg qd prn IV/PO	75–90	50–80	0.5–2.0 ng/mL
Adenosine	6–12 mg IV	—	—	—	—
Verapamil	2.5–10 mg IV over 2–5 min	2.5–5.0 μg/kg/min or 120–480 mg PO qd	90	10–22	15–100 μg/L
Propranolol	0.5–1.0 mg IV q5 min to 0.1–0.2 mg/kg total dose	10–40 mg PO qid-bid to 320 mg PO total dose	95	20–50	50–100 ng/mL
Atenolol	5 mg IV over 5 min, repeat in 10 min	50 mg PO qd-bid, initiate 10 min after IV dose	50	50	0.2–0.5 μg/mL
Metoprolol	5 mg IV q5min to total dose 15 mg	50 mg PO bid to total dose 450 mg PO qd	95	50	50–100 ng/mL
Labetolol	0.25 mg/kg IV (or 20 mg) over 2 min, repeat 40, 80 mg IV prn	2 mg/min IV or 100–400 mg PO bid	95	25	0.7–3.0 μg/mL
Esmolol	500 μg/kg/min IV	50–300 μg/kg/min IV	—	—	—
Quinidine	5–7 mg/kg IV at 20 mg/min (gluconate) or 600–1000 mg PO (sulfate)	10–30 mg/kg total dose PO divided bid-qid depending on preparation	95	70–80	2.0–5.0 μg/mL
Procainamide	15–20 mg/kg IV at 20 mg/min to total dose 1.0 g or 1000 mg PO (standard preparation)	1–4 mg/min IV or 50–100 mg/kg total dose PO divided tid-qid depending on preparation	70–90	70–90	Procainamide 5–10 μg/mL NAPA 10–30 μg/mL
Disopyramide	300–400 mg PO (standard preparation)	Standard 100–400 mg PO qid; CR 200–300 mg PO bid	80–100	90	3–6 μg/mL
Lidocaine	1.0 mg/kg IV; 0.5 mg/kg in 10 min to total dose 3.0 mg/kg	30–50 μg/kg/min or 1–4 mg/min	—	—	1–5 μg/mL
Encainide	0.6–1.0 mg/kg IV over 15 min	25–50 mg PO tid-qid	95	7–82	1–56 ng/mL
Flecainide	1.5–2.0 mg/kg IV	100–200 mg PO bid	95	95	0.2–1.0 μg/mL
Moricizine	—	200–300 mg PO tid	—	38	0.1–0.3 μg/mL
Mexiletine	0.5–1.5 mg/min IV or 400 mg PO	200–400 mg PO tid	90	88	0.5–2.0 μg/mL
Propafenone	1–2 mg/kg IV or 600–900 mg PO	150–300 mg PO tid	95	25–75	0.5–2.0 μg/mL
Bretylium	5 mg/kg IV; repeat bolus 10 mg/kg q15–30 min to total dose 30 mg/kg	0.5–2.0 mg/min IV	—	—	0.6–20.0 μg/mL
Phenytoin	1.0 g at 20 mg/min	300 mg PO qd	—	57–85	6.0–20 mg/L
Amiodarone	5–10 mg/kg IV over 5–10 min or 800–1600 mg qd PO	200–800 mg PO qd	—	22–88	1.0–2.5 μg/mL

2′-oxoquinidinone). Also, serum concentrations of drugs do not reflect the free or protein-bound fractions. α_1 Acid glycoprotein, the serum protein which binds most antiarrhythmic drugs, is an acute phase reactant and its serum concentration rises during acute myocardial infarction, during renal transplant, with malignancy, in the postoperative period, in old age, and in general as a response to any physical stress.[23] As a consequence, in these situations the percentage of drug available to act on the cardiac membrane can be reduced.

Lidocaine, a prevalent antiarrhythmic drug in the ICU, deserves special consideration as an example of the importance of pharmacokinetics in antiarrhythmic therapy. Lidocaine is almost entirely metabolized in the liver, and its rate of clearance approaches the rate of hepatic blood flow. Impaired clearance can be anticipated in the presence of liver disease, as well as during hypotension, low output states, and in the setting of congestive heart failure—conditions in which hepatic blood flow is reduced. In addition to reducing clearance, congestive heart failure has been found to reduce the central compartment of the volume of distribution by as much as 50 percent,[24,25] and may necessitate reductions in both the loading and the maintainance dose. Lidocaine clearance has also been shown to be reduced in the elderly, during prolonged infusions lasting over 24 h, and by the concommitant administration of β blockers (propanolol, metoprolol) and cimetidine. Signs and symptoms of lidocaine toxicity should be watched for carefully in all patients receiving lidocaine infusion, but in particular in those who are receiving high infusion rates (>2 mg/min), or

TABLE 120-6 Drug-Drug Interactions

Drug	Drugs Causing Increased Level of Antiarrhythmic Agent	Drugs Causing Decreased Levels of Antiarrhythmic Agent
Digoxin	Quinidine, amiodarone, verapamil, nifedipine, propafenone, antibiotics, esmolol, diphenoxylate, propantheline	Neomycin, cholestyramine, sulfasalazine, kaolin-pectate, antacids
Propranolol	Cimetidine, chlorpromazine	Rifampin, phenytoin, phenobarbitol, ethanol, aluminum hydroxide gels
Adenosine	Potentiated by dipyridamole, carbamazepine	Antagonized by methylxanthines
Verapamil	—	Rifampin, phenobarbital
Atenolol	—	—
Metoprolol	—	—
Labetolol	Cimetidine	—
Esmolol	Morphine	—
Quinidine	Amiodarone, verapamil, cimetidine, thiazides, carbonic anhydrase inhibitors	Rifampin, phenobarbital, phenytoin, nifedipine, antacids
Procainamide	Amiodarone	—
Disopyramide	—	Phenytoin
Lidocaine	β Blockers, cimetidine, norepinephrine	Phenobarbital, isoproterenol
Encainide	Cimetidine	—
Flecainide	Propranolol, amiodarone	—
Moricizine	β Blockers, cimetidine	—
Mexiletine	Cimetidine	Cimetidine, rifampin, phenytoin, phenobarbitol
Propafenone	Cimetidine	—
Bretylium	—	—
Phenytoin	Disulfiram, tolbutamide, isoniazid, phenobarbital, diazepam, estrogens, cimetidine, amiodarone, ethosuximide, sulfonamides, acute alcohol intoxication	Carbamazepine, chronic alcohol intoxication
Amiodarone	—	—

who have any of the aforementioned factors predisposing toward lidocaine accumulation. Drug levels should be followed closely in this setting.

Procainamide is also commonly used in the acute management of arrhythmias, and a basic understanding of its metabolism is essential to its safe and effective use. Procainamide is both excreted unchanged in the urine and metabolized in the liver. N-acetylprocainamide (NAPA), its primary metabolite, has antiarrhythmic properties and is eliminated almost entirely by renal excretion. With renal dysfunction or congestive heart failure, procainamide and, in particular, NAPA levels increase and can predispose to significant toxicity. In the acute care setting levels of both procainamide and NAPA should be monitored and the ECG examined for QRS widening and QT prolongation.

When patients fail to respond to drugs, other therapeutic modalities are available. Antitachycardia pacing or direct current shock can be used to terminate episodes of tachycardia, and in some cases pacing can be used to prevent recurrences of tachycardia. These therapies are discussed in Chaps. 31 and 32. Other potentially curative treatments include catheter ablation and cardiac surgery.

Catheter ablation involves the positioning of an electrode catheter so that its tip electrode is adjacent to the arrhythmogenic substrate. Energy is then delivered through the tip electrode to a reference electrode patch on the patient's chest wall. The purpose is to injure the endocardium adjacent to the tip electrode and to destroy the arrhythmogenic substrate. Two forms of energy have been used: direct-current shocks delivered from an external defibrillator and radiofrequency current. The extent of damage produced by direct-current shocks is impossible to titrate and in some patients has been excessive, resulting in bursts of VT, hypotension, and a small incidence of late sudden death.[26] This technique has, therefore, been largely superceded by the radiofrequency technique.

Ablation with radiofrequency current involves the passage through a catheter of up to 50 watts (70 V) of radiofrequency current (150 kHz to 1 MHz) for periods of time ranging up to 60 s. It creates injury by heating and dessicating the neighboring myocardium. The residuum of radiofrequency ablation is a well-demarcated spherical or oval zone of coagulation necrosis, which is less likely to serve as a new focus for arrhythmias than is the heterogeneous, less

TABLE 120-7 Pharmacokinetics and Dose Adjustments of Antiarrhythmic Drugs

Drug	Major Route of Elimination	Elimination Half-life (h) (PO)	Protein-bound, %	Volume of Distribution (Vd), L/kg	Excreted Unchanged in Urine, %	Dose Adjustment	Removed by Dialysis
Digoxin	R (80%) H (20%)	33–44	25	6–15	50–70	RF; hypo-thyroid	No
Adenosine	Erythrocytes, vascular endothelium	10 s	—	—	—	—	—
Verapamil	H	4 min IV 3–7 h PO	90	—	3–4	—	No
Propranolol	H	3.5–6.0	90	3–5	35	HF, CHF	No
Atenolol	R	6–9	5	—	50	RF, CHF	Yes
Metoprolol	H	3–7	12	5.6	5	CHF	No
Labetolol	H	6–8	50	—	60	HF, CHF	No
Esmolol	Erythrocyte esterases	9 min IV	55	—	2	CHF	—
Quinidine	H (60–80%) R (10–50%)	5–9	80	2–4	20–50	RF, HF, CHF	No
Procainamide	R (50–60%) H (10–30%) (NAPA–R)	2.4–4.9	15	1.7–2.5	50–60	RF, CHF	Yes
Disopyramide	R	6–9	40–90	1.0	40–60	RF, CHF (HF)	Yes
Lidocaine	H	0.5–2.0	30	1–2	10	HF, CHF	No
Encainide	Poor metabolizer phenotype H 20%, R 80% Extensive metabolizer H 80%, R 20%	ODE: 2.5–4.0 MODE: 6–14	71–78	2–6	45	RF (HF)	—
Flecainide	H	14–20	35–45	8–10	10–50	RF	No
Moricizine	H	1.5–3.5	95	> 300	1	RF	No
Mexiletine	H	12–16	70	10	10	HF, CHF	—
Propafenone	H	7–12	—	60	18–38	HF	—
Bretylium	R	13.6	0–6	3.5	80–90	RF	Yes
Phenytoin	H	18–36 RF: 8	90	0.5–1.0	—	—	No
Amiodarone	H	13–100 days	95–97	70–150	—	HF, CHF	No

R, renal; H, hepatic; RF, renal failure; HF, hepatic failure; CHF, congestive heart failure; ODE, O-desmethylencainide; MODE, 3-methoxy-O-desmethylencainide

well-defined scar left by direct-current shock. Radiofrequency ablation has virtually none of the adverse sequelae of direct-current shock.

The first application of catheter ablation was for destruction of the AV conduction system at the level of the AV node and His bundle, in patients with refractory supraventricular tachyarrhythmias.[27,28] Ablation of the AV junction is still performed in patients with a rapid ventricular response to atrial fibrillation or flutter when control cannot be achieved with drugs and the patient cannot be kept in sinus rhythm. The drawback is that complete heart block is induced and patients often require a permanent pacemaker, though this can be avoided when the ablation is delivered proximally enough in the AV node that a robust and reasonably rapid junctional escape rhythm remains.

Other forms of supraventricular tachycardia (SVT) can be cured by ablation without destruction of the normal conduction system. In patients with the Wolff-Parkinson-White (WPW) syndrome, accessory pathways can be ablated, removing the substrate of both the reentrant SVT and the rapid ventricular response to atrial fibrillation.[29] In patients with AV nodal reentrant tachycardia, one limb of the reentrant loop can be selectively ablated, leaving the other AV nodal limb intact and sparing AV conduction.[30] Ectopic atrial tachycardias may be curable through ablation of the atrial focus or the critical link of an intraatrial reentrant circuit.

Catheter ablation has also been used to treat VT.[31] To be effective, the catheter tip must be positioned next to a critical link in the reentry circuit.[32,33] This is typically a zone of slow conduction at the border of an aneurysm. Patients with nonischemic dilated cardiomyopathy may have a VT in which the right bundle branch forms one limb of the reentrant circuit and the left bundle branch forms the other limb; in these cases, ablation of the right bundle branch is effective therapy.[34]

Cardiac surgery of various types has been widely used to treat arrhythmias. For example, accessory pathways in patients with the WPW syndrome can be divided by an incision made at the AV groove in the location where the pathway has been localized.[35] An alternative approach which does not require cardiopulmonary bypass is to apply cryosurgery to the site of the pathway.[36] A similar surgical approach has been used for AV nodal reentrant tachycardia.[37] The success rate for these techniques is over 95 percent, and the perioperative mortality is <1 percent. However, catheter ablation will probably render these techniques obsolete.

Surgery can also be used to treat VT. The site from which the VT emerges can be identified through electrophysiologic mapping (it is the earliest part of the ventricle to be activated during VT). Once it is localized, it can be surgically excised or frozen by cryosurgery.[38] An alternative approach is to use visual guidance and remove scarred endocardium, for the reentrant loop seems to pass through endocardial scar in most cases.[39] With either approach the efficacy rate is approximately 75 percent with a perioperative mortality rate of 10 to 15 percent.

Antitachycardia devices, including automatic implantable defibrillators and antitachycardia pacemakers, are invaluable in treating patients with recurrent tachyarrhythmias who have not responded to drug therapy and are not candidates for potentially curative procedures. Antitachycardia pacemakers have primarily been used in patients with SVTs, because pacing stimuli do not reliably terminate VT and, in fact, can cause it to degenerate into ventricular fibrillation (VF). These devices operate by detecting the presence of an episode of tachycardia (for example, when the atrial rate exceeds a specified threshold) and by responding with a short train of pacing stimuli which terminate the arrhythmia (see Chap. 32). Catheter ablation will probably reduce the indications for antitachycardia pacemakers.

The use of automatic implantable defibrillators is rapidly expanding. These devices also monitor the heart rate to detect the presence of an episode of VT or VF. When an episode occurs, these devices deliver shocks of up to 35 J directly to the heart through endocardial or epicardial electrodes. Newer versions can deliver heirarchical therapy: high energy shocks for VF and burst pacing for slow VT. Automatic implantable defibrillators are nearly completely effective at preventing sudden death.[40] However, they are expensive and require major surgery for implantation, with a perioperative morbidity of 1 to 4 percent. Also, they do not always prevent syncope, because it can take 10 to 20 s for the device to complete a cycle of arrhythmia detection, capacitor charging, and shock delivery.

ACUTE MANAGEMENT OF TACHYCARDIAS

Because there are numerous different types of tachycardia, acute or chronic management depends on the mechanism of the tachycardia and the degree to which it is compromising the patient. The mechanism of a tachycardia may be obvious to the physician, because of its appearance on the rhythm strip or ECG, or because the patient has previously undergone a diagnostic evaluation of the same rhythm disorder. On the other hand, the mechanism may at first be inapparent. This is most likely to be the case when there is no prior history of arrhythmia and when P waves are not clearly visible in the ECG during the tachycardia. Here, the initial approach should aim not only to terminate the tachycardia but to collect as much diagnostic information as possible, to aid in further management.

Indications for emergent or urgent treatment of tachyarrhythmias include impairment of consciousness, hypotension, pulmonary edema, and cardiac ischemia. In these situations, there may be little or no opportunity to collect diagnostic information. Direct-current shock is nearly always effective at restoring sinus rhythm at least temporarily in patients with paroxysmal SVT, atrial flutter, atrial fibrillation, VT, and VF. It is ineffective against sinus tachycardia, many cases of ectopic atrial tachycardia, multifocal atrial tachycardia (MAT), and accelerated junctional rhythm. It is contraindicated in patients with digitalis intoxication because it may lead to intractable VF; in this setting resuscitation should include antidigitalis Fab fragments rather than electrical countershock.

In patients who are conscious during tachycardia, direct-current shock should not be first-line therapy.[41] Other approaches are more likely to enable the physician to diagnose the mechanism of tachycardia. First, a 12-lead ECG should be obtained and inspected. Its characteristics may lead to a diagnosis (Chap. 30). Atrial activity should be recorded directly if this is convenient (e.g., if the patient has had temporary epicardial atrial pacing leads left in place during recent cardiac surgery). If the mechanism of tachycardia is still unclear, carotid sinus massage may be used to increase vagal input to the sinus and AV nodes. Before performing carotid sinus massage, the physician should be sure that the patient does not have significant cerebrovascular disease. Carotid sinus massage should not be performed in patients with carotid bruits or in those with an absent carotid pulse. To perform carotid massage, the patient should be placed in the supine position with the neck hyperextended and the head turned slightly away from the side to be massaged. It is important for the patient to be relaxed, so that sympathetic tone is minimized. The carotid pulse at the angle of the jaw is gently found. If slight pressure here has no effect, firm pressure with a rotating massaging motion can then be applied for a maximum of 5 s, first on one side and then the other (never to both sides at once). A continuous rhythm strip should be obtained to collect diagnostic information. In patients with cerebrovascular disease, other vagal maneuvers may be performed—such as the Valsalva maneuver, immersion of the face in ice water, or provocation of the gag reflex. Eyeball massage can elicit heightened vagotonia but should be avoided because it can cause retinal detachment.

Vagal maneuvers have different effects on different types of tachycardia. Sinus tachycardia can be slowed momentarily, with perhaps enough slowing that P waves are no longer hidden within T waves. AV reciprocating tachycardia using a bypass tract or AV nodal reentrant tachycardia may be abruptly terminated by vagal maneuvers. In atrial flutter or atrial tachycardia, the atrial rhythm is usually undisturbed by vagal maneuvers, but the ventricular response can be transiently slowed, with perhaps enough slowing that P waves are clearly visible between consecutive QRS complexes so that the atrial rate can be measured. Except in rare cases, VT is undisturbed by carotid massage.

Vagal maneuvers may fail to perturb the cardiac rhythm, leaving the physician still unsure of the mechanism of the tachycardia. Carotid massage and the Valsalva maneuver are particularly likely to be ineffectual in patients with high sympathetic tone, i.e., in typical ICU patients. Under these circumstances, the next step depends on whether the patient has a narrow QRS (i.e., <120 msec in duration) or wide QRS during tachycardia.

In patients with *narrow QRS tachycardia* of undiagnosed mechanism, the next step is usually to administer adenosine or verapamil, which are more potent than vagal maneuvers at blocking conduction in the AV node. These are almost always effective at terminating AV nodal reentrant tachycardia and AV reentrant tachycardia and in temporarily slowing the ventricular response to atrial tachycardia or atrial flutter, so that a diagnosis can be made. Both medicines can be given by intravenous bolus and produce their effects almost immediately. Adenosine (6 mg rapid intravenous push, followed by 12 mg rapid intravenous push if necessary) is the preferred agent in hypotensive patients, because of its shorter half-life and lesser likelihood of causing problematic hypotension. However, the hypotensive effects of verapamil (2.5 mg intravenously, repeated as necessary to a total dose of 10 mg) can be prevented by pretreatment with 1 g intravenous calcium chloride, which does not interfere with the electrophysiologic effects of the verapamil on the AV node.

If the mechanism of tachycardia is still obscure following verapamil or adenosine, the physician has several options for further diagnostic action. A β blocker can be given, which would slow the rate of most cases of sinus tachycardia, allowing it to be diagnosed. Esmolol is a good choice in acute situations because of its short half-life. The physician should also determine whether it is reasonable to make a direct recording of atrial activity using transesophageal or transvenous electrodes.

The overwhelming majority of *wide QRS complex tachycardias* of undiagnosed mechanism are due to VT (81 percent), with far fewer due to supraventricular tachyarrhythmia with aberrant conduction (14 percent) or antegrade conduction over an accessory pathway (5 percent).[42] The presence of organic heart disease and especially of ischemic heart disease greatly increases the likelihood of VT, whereas a history of long-standing episodes of tachycardia in the absence of organic heart disease increases the likelihood of supraventricular tachyarrhythmia. The presence of AV dissociation (i.e., lack of a relationship between P waves and QRS complexes) proves the diagnosis of VT. Atrial activity can be apparent in the surface ECG, but, if it is not, the physician must decide whether to directly record atrial activity during tachycardia using transesophageal or transvenous electrodes (Chap. 32). When P waves are not apparent on the surface ECG, and a direct recording of atrial activity is not available, indirect evidence of AV dissociation (and therefore proof of the diagnosis of VT) is provided by the presence of capture beats or fusion beats during tachycardia, or by the appearance of intermittent cannon a waves in the jugular venous pulse.

If AV dissociation is absent or cannot be proven, other techniques must be used to establish a diagnosis of the mechanism of tachycardia. Vagal maneuvers or adenosine can be used; a supraventricular origin of the tachycardia would be suggested if the tachycardia is terminated or if AV block is produced. Another potentially diagnostic maneuver is to give a bolus of lidocaine; if the rhythm terminates it is likely to be VT. Verapamil must be avoided because it can cause VT to degenerate into VF. Verapamil and digoxin are also contraindicated in another type of wide QRS tachycardia, namely, atrial flutter or fibrillation conducting antegradely over an accessory pathway in a patient with the WPW syndrome. Both drugs can cause the ventricular rate to increase in these patients and can cause the rhythm to degenerate into VF.

The 12-lead ECG obtained during tachycardia may provide diagnostic clues (Table 120-8). It should be compared with the ECG of the patient during sinus rhythm; if during sinus rhythm the patient has a similar, wide QRS (because of fixed bundle branch block), the likelihood that the tachycardia is supraventricular in origin is increased. ECGs and rhythm strips obtained when the patient is in sinus rhythm should also be searched for the presence of premature atrial beats that conduct with functional bundle branch block; if the QRS morphology of these beats resembles that during tachycardia, then SVT is rendered more likely. If the onset of tachycardia has been captured electrocardiographically, it should be determined whether tachycardia was initiated by a premature atrial beat, which again would favor a supraventricular origin for the tachycardia. The regularity of the rhythm of the tachycardia should be examined. Regularity is a characteristic of both SVTs and VTs, but gross irregularity at rates >200 beats/min favors atrial fibrillation with antegrade conduction over an accessory pathway.

SUPRAVENTRICULAR TACHYCARDIA AND ECTOPY

Tachycardias and ectopy are usually classified as supraventricular or ventricular in origin. Supraventricular tachyarrhythmias are comprised of a wide variety of different ar-

TABLE 120-8 Morphologic Criteria Favoring Ventricular Tachycardia during Wide QRS Complex Tachycardia

QRS duration >140 ms with RBBB morphology
QRS duration >160 ms with LBBB morphology
Positive QRS concordance (predominantly positive QRS in all precordial leads)
Extreme left axis deviation (−90° to ± 180°)
Combined LBBB with right axis deviation
Different QRS pattern during tachycardia than baseline in patients with preexisting bundle branch block

rhythmias including sinus tachycardia, atrial tachycardia, atrial flutter, atrial fibrillation, junctional reciprocating tachycardias, and accelerated junctional rhythm. Each of these has certain ECG features that allow it to be distinguished from other similar arrhythmias (Chap. 30). How the rhythm responds to interventions often permits more precise identification.

SINUS TACHYCARDIA. Sinus tachycardia, defined as a sinus rhythm >100 beats/min, is probably the most frequent rhythm disturbance in the ICU, and the number of potential etiologies is formidable. It may be an early sign of significant problems such as occult hemorrhage, thyrotoxicosis, alcohol withdrawal, cardiac tamponade, pulmonary embolism, or pneumothorax, or it may be attributable to any number of overt causes such as infection, pain, or anxiety. Based on the patient's clinical history and physical examination, the physician should usually be able to attribute the sinus tachycardia to a stimulus and to order the appropriate confirmatory test (e.g., hematocrit, arterial bloodgas, chest x-ray, thyroid function tests, etc.).

Appropriate management of sinus tachycardia begins with removing or treating the underlying cause. This should be sufficient to restore a normal heart rate. Other measures to decrease the heart rate, such as β blockade, are rarely indicated. However, β blockade can be appropriate in the hyperadrenergic patient whose sinus tachycardia may be deleterious, as in thyroid storm, aortic dissection, or acute myocardial infarction with preserved left ventricular function. It can be accomplished with 1 to 3 mg propranolol intravenously every 3 to 5 min as necessary to a total of 0.1 mg/kg, or esmolol by continuous infusion.

Rarely, sinus tachycardia arises from reentry in and around the sinus node. In these cases, the tachycardia starts and stops suddenly. An underlying physiologic stimulus such as anemia or pain is less likely to be found than with typical sinus tachycardia. The tachycardia may respond to vagal maneuvers, β blockers, verapamil, or digoxin, though a class 1A or 1C drug may be required to terminate an episode and to prevent recurrences.

ATRIAL ECTOPY AND TACHYARRHYTHMIAS. Rhythms that arise from the atria include atrial premature beats, atrial tachycardia, atrial flutter, and atrial fibrillation. The atrial tachyarrhythmias are generally separated according to the atrial rate: atrial tachycardias having an atrial rate of up to 250 beats/min, atrial flutter having an atrial rate of 250 to 330 beats/min, and atrial fibrillation having an atrial rate >330 beats/min.

Atrial tachyarrhythmias often occur in patients with structural heart disease or other predisposing condition (Table 120-9) and, in fact, may be the presenting sign of a serious disorder.

Atrial premature beats are common in healthy people and patients in the ICU. They occasionally portend an underlying medical problem and their presence should generate awareness by the physician that any of the causes of atrial ectopy listed in Table 120-9 may be unrecognized; however, an elaborate diagnostic evaluation is not indicated as part of the management of infrequent isolated atrial premature beats. Isolated ectopic atrial beats rarely cause symptoms other than a sensation of "skipped beats," which can be treated in most patients with reassurance alone. In general, antiarrhythmic drugs are unnecessary. However, frequent nonconducted ectopic atrial beats may slow the heart rate enough to compromise cardiac output, causing a need for suppressive treatment. Treatment of nonconducting premature atrial beats consists of a class 1A or 1C antiarrhythmic agent, with full awareness of potential side effects and possible proarrhythmic effect. Treatment of conducting premature atrial beats, when necessary, should begin with drugs which depress the AV node, such as digoxin, β blockers, or calcium channel blockers. If these fail to control the patient's symptoms, class 1A or 1C drugs can be added.

TABLE 120-9 Causes of Atrial Ectopy and Atrial Tachyarrhythmias

Hypertensive heart disease
Hyperthyroidism
Pericarditis
Congestive heart failure
Mitral valve disease (mitral stenosis, mitral regurgitation, mitral valve prolapse)
Postcardiac surgery
Sick sinus syndrome
Myocardial infarction
Pulmonary embolism
COPD
Drugs (catecholamines, theophylline, caffeine, nicotine)
Alcohol (either acute intoxication or withdrawal)
Digitalis toxicity
Cardiac contusion
Idiopathic

Atrial tachycardias are distinguished from sinus tachycardia by virtue of the different ECG morphology of the P wave during tachycardia, indicating an ectopic origin of atrial activation. There are several different types of atrial tachycardia, each with a different mechanism.

Intraatrial reentrant tachycardia (IART) is paroxysmal in nature (i.e., starts and stops suddenly) and is characterized by uniform P waves with at most minor irregularity in rhythm. It usually occurs in the presence of structural heart disease with atrial enlargement, in patients who are also subject to atrial flutter and fibrillation.[43] It is often quite refractory to antiarrhythmic drugs except for amiodarone, which is usually effective.[43] Drugs that depress the AV node (digoxin, β blockers, and calcium channel blockers) have no effect on the atrial rate but may slow the ventricular response by reducing the frequency of atrial beats which propagate to the ventricles. IART can be converted to sinus rhythm by rapid atrial pacing or by direct current shock.

Multifocal atrial tachycardia (MAT) has an incessant quality, i.e., it waxes and wanes rather than starting and stopping suddenly. It is characterized by nonuniform P waves and an irregular atrial rate. It especially tends to occur in patients with pulmonary disease who acquire features predisposing to MAT: right atrial enlargement, hypoxia, hypercapnia, acidosis, electrolyte disturbances (particularly hypokalemia and hypomagnesemia), and therapy with aminophylline and β agonists.[44] Triggered automaticity may be the underlying mechanism of MAT, though the supporting evidence for this is circumstantial.

The mainstay of treatment of MAT is the removal of the pulmonary, cardiac, metabolic, or infectious cause that often underlies the arrhythmia. Correction of hypokalemia and hypomagnesemia are particularly important, and magnesium supplementation has been reported to convert MAT to normal sinus rhythm even in patients with normal magnesium levels. Some patients with MAT respond to calcium channel blockade or β blockade. These therapies can slow the ventricular rate by reducing the fraction of atrial impulses that propagate to the ventricles or by suppressing the ectopic atrial foci. Digitalis is generally not effective in the treatment of MAT. In fact, patients with MAT, who may have hypokalemia, hypomagnesemia, hypoxia, or uremia, are predisposed to digitalis intoxication. Class I antiarrhythmic agents have no role in the treatment of MAT. This tachycardia cannot be terminated by rapid atrial pacing or by direct-current shock.

Automatic atrial tachycardia (AAT) arises from increased abnormal automaticity in an ectopic atrial focus. It is characterized by uniform P waves with a different ECG morphology than sinus P waves, and an atrial rate of 120 to 200 beats/min. It can be seen in acute myocardial infarction, exacerbation of chronic obstructive pulmonary disease (COPD), acute alcohol ingestion, severe metabolic derangements such as hypokalemia, hypomagnesemia, or hypoxemia, and high catecholamine states. Ectopic atrial tachycardia alone or with AV conduction block is common in digitalis toxicity, where the mechanism is probably triggered automaticity due to late after-depolarizations. Finally, AAT sometimes occurs in young, otherwise healthy patients who do not have an identifiable precipitating factor. In these cases, persistent AAT can lead to cardiomyopathy with potentially severe left ventricular dysfunction, which can partially or completely resolve after the tachycardia is controlled.

As with the other atrial tachycardias, AAT responds best to eradication of the systemic illness that has precipitated it (if any). The ventricular rate can sometimes be reduced by blocking AV nodal conduction with digitalis, β blockade, or calcium channel blockade, but 1:1 conduction often persists. It is sometimes possible to convert the atrial rhythm to sinus rhythm using a class 1A or 1C drug or amiodarone. Moricizine has been said to be effective against AAT, even when other drugs have failed. Electrical cardioversion and antitachycardia pacing are ineffective against AAT.

If ectopic atrial tachycardia with AV conduction block is present, digitalis intoxication must be suspected and a digitalis level obtained immediately. Digitalis should be withheld until digitalis toxicity is excluded. Phenytoin is often effective against atrial tachycardia due to digitalis toxicity. Digitalis antibodies should be administered for extreme degrees of digitalis toxicity and to patients who are hemodynamically compromised by their digitalis-induced arrhythmia; otherwise, if the patient is stable, the digitalis level can be followed and allowed to return to normal by endogenous metabolism.

Atrial flutter is a rhythm in which the atria beat at a rate of 250 to 350 beats/min. The mechanism of atrial flutter seems nearly always to be reentrant, with a wavefront that circles around the entrances of the venae cavae into the right atrium. The ECG morphology of the P waves is always very uniform and creates a sawtooth appearance, particularly in the inferior leads (II, III, aVF) and lead V_1. Atrial flutter can have variable AV conduction, but usually occurs with 2:1 AV block, producing a regular ventricular rate of approximately 150 beats/min. This characteristic of atrial flutter justifies the inclusion of atrial flutter in the differential diagnosis of any regular tachycardia with a ventricular rate of 150 beats/min. Slower ventricular rates during atrial flutter can occur with intrinsic dysfunction of AV conduction, with high vagal tone, or with agents or maneuvers that decrease AV nodal conduction. The ventricular rate during atrial flutter can be faster than 150 beats/min in patients with accelerated AV nodal conduction, in the presence of an accessory AV pathway (sometimes called a Kent bundle), or if the patient has been treated with a type I antiarrhythmic agent without prior blockade of AV nodal conduction.

Carotid sinus massage or adenosine can be used diagnostically to increase the degree of AV block and allow better visualization of the atrial flutter waves on the ECG. Other means of improving the detection of atrial flutter waves include recording from electrodes that have been positioned in the esophagus directly behind the atrium, or directly into the atria via a transvenous approach. Temporary epicardial electrodes may be available for recording atrial activity in patients who have undergone cardiac surgery.

In most patients, therapy for atrial flutter starts with control of the ventricular response using digoxin, a β blocker, or a calcium channel blocker. It may be difficult or impossible, though, to produce a heart rate <100 beats/min with these drugs. When the ventricular response cannot be adequately controlled, the next therapeutic step is to convert the atria to sinus rhythm. This can be accomplished with antiarrhythmic drugs, antitachycardia pacing, or electrical cardioversion. Drugs that are at least occasionally effective against atrial flutter include the class 1A and 1C agents and moricizine or amiodarone. However, these drugs often slow the atrial rate without terminating the tachycardia, which can lead paradoxically to a faster ventricular rate because a greater fraction of atrial beats may conduct to the ventricles at slower atrial rates. For example, a patient may experience 2:1 conduction with an atrial rate of 300 beats/min, and 1:1 conduction at an atrial rate of 200 beats/min. Therefore, class 1 drugs should not be used to treat atrial flutter unless the patient's ventricular rate is slow or the patient has been pretreated with digoxin, a β blocker, or a calcium channel blocker.

Antitachycardia pacing or electrical cardioversion can be used in patients who need immediate restoration of sinus rhythm or when drugs have failed to convert the rhythm. Antitachycardia pacing, described in Chap. 32, is especially convenient in patients with temporary epicardial pacing leads in place on the atria following cardiac surgery, but it can also be accomplished through transvenous or transesophageal electrode catheters. Pace termination is preferred to electrical cardioversion in certain situations such as excess digitalization, known severe conduction disease or sick sinus syndrome, fully awake state, or following a recent meal. The risk of systemic embolism during conversion of atrial flutter is low, and patients with atrial flutter do not have to be anticoagulated prior to conversion.

Pace termination of atrial flutter is accomplished by using a special pulse generator capable of rapid pacing rates. A continuous ECG rhythm strip should be obtained during the procedure to ensure, among other things, that the atria and not the ventricles are being paced. Typically, trains of stimuli are delivered to the atria, starting at 125 percent of the unpaced atrial rate and lasting for 20 to 30 s. Pacing is then abruptly terminated or gradually slowed and the rhythm strip inspected for restoration of normal sinus rhythm. Pacing at an insufficiently rapid rate "entrains" the atria (i.e., captures the atria and raises the atrial rate to the rate of the pacing stimuli) but fails to convert the rhythm to normal sinus rhythm. If atrial flutter persists, another attempt at pace termination can be made at a faster rate of stimulation; sometimes rates of up to 450 pulses/min are necessary. Rapid atrial pacing often causes atrial fibrillation, which may revert spontaneously to normal sinus rhythm or else require electrical cardioversion. If atrial flutter persists despite attempts at rapid atrial pacing, short bursts of atrial pacing at 400 to 500 beats/min can be used to precipitate atrial fibrillation, during which the ventricular rate is often easier to control than it is during atrial flutter.

Electrical cardioversion of atrial flutter, described in Chap. 31, should be performed with synchronized shock, which delivers the shock during a QRS complex. The initial shock should have an energy of 20 to 50 J. If atrial fibrillation rather than normal sinus rhythm results after cardioversion, or if atrial flutter persists, further attempts with higher energy levels can be undertaken.

Atrial fibrillation is a rhythm in which atrial activation is disorganized and the atria do not contract effectively. It is probably caused by a variant of reentry in which the activation wavefront travels in an endlessly varying path, giving rise to subsidiary wavelets.[45] Unless the patient has heart block, the ventricular rate is irregularly irregular. It is usually not difficult to diagnose atrial fibrillation though it is occasionally mimicked by MAT or atrial flutter with variable AV conduction; and when there is very rapid conduction during atrial fibrillation, the ventricular rate can be deceptively regular.

Potential complications of atrial fibrillation include hemodynamic compromise from rapid ventricular rate and from loss of atrial contraction. In addition, patients with atrial fibrillation are susceptible to systemic embolism, especially in the presence of rheumatic mitral stenosis, dilated cardiomyopathy, and history of prior embolism. Management of atrial fibrillation includes detection and correction of the underlying cause (if any), ventricular rate control, conversion to sinus rhythm, and anticoagulation.

Atrial fibrillation may be caused by any of the conditions listed in Table 120-9. In addition, it is common in patients with the WPW syndrome (vide infra). If the patient has no obvious cause of atrial fibrillation (e.g., recent thoracic surgery or acute myocardial infarction), thyroid function tests should be performed. In addition, transthoracic or transesophageal echocardiography can be used to identify mitral valve pathology, left ventricular hypertrophy, or evidence for other causes of atrial fibrillation, evaluate left atrial size, and look for left atrial thrombus. Left atrial size is a critical determinant of the likelihood that a patient can be kept in sinus rhythm following conversion; the likelihood is low in patients with left atrial diameters >4.5 cm. Patients with sudden onset of atrial fibrillation and no obvious cause should be evaluated for the possibility of pulmonary embolism. Finally, in patients with risk factors or known coronary artery disease, myocardial ischemia should be considered.

Control of ventricular rate is one of the highest priorities in managing atrial fibrillation. This is usually accomplished with a drug or drugs that prolong AV nodal refractoriness: digoxin, β blockers, or calcium channel blockers. Digoxin therapy has the drawback that there may be a lag of several hours between its administration and the appearance of its therapeutic effects. Also, the AV nodal blocking effects of digoxin and the calcium channel blockers are antagonized by circulating catecholamines. For these reasons, β blockers are comparatively well-suited for ventricular rate control in the ICU, except in patients with bronchospasm or severe left ventricular dysfunction. When there is a question whether a patient can tolerate a β blocker, a trial of esmolol can be attempted fairly safely, because of its short half-life.

The ventricular response can be difficult to control in patients who are hyperadrenergic, hyperthyroid, febrile, or hypoxic. Also, some patients have congenital accelerated AV conduction because of short AV nodal refractory periods or the presence of an accessory AV pathway (also called a Kent bundle or bypass tract). Patients with the latter condition are said to have the WPW syndrome; their diagnosis is recognizable from the irregularly irregular wide and bizarre QRS complexes occurring at a rapid rate. The ventricular rate during atrial fibrillation of patients with WPW cannot be controlled by digoxin or calcium channel blockers. Instead, because accessory pathways are sodium channel dependent, class 1A or 1C drugs must be used to control the ventricular response.

When the ventricular response cannot be controlled or when patients suffer hemodynamic compromise from the loss of atrial contraction, it is reasonable to attempt to restore sinus rhythm. Pharmacologic cardioversion can sometimes be achieved with class 1A or 1C drugs or amiodarone. Drugs are more likely to cardiovert the atria successfully when atrial fibrillation has been present for only a short period of time. Other factors that influence the likelihood of successful pharmacologic cardioversion include atrial size, and whether or not the patient has a persisting cause of fibrillation such as hyperthyroidism or hypoxia.

Direct-current shock may be used to convert the atrium to sinus rhythm, when drugs have failed or when urgent conversion is needed. Cardioversion for atrial fibrillation is detailed in Chap. 31. As with atrial flutter, the shock should be synchronized with the QRS, starting with a dose of 50 J and, if necessary, progressing up to 400 J. Atrial fibrillation is less likely to recur following cardioversion if the patient is pretreated with quinidine or another antiarrhythmic drug. Generally, patients should be cardioverted only if the goal is to keep them in long-term sinus rhythm, although in the ICU setting it may be necessary to obtain short-term improvement during a period of hemodynamic instability. Before starting long-term antiarrhythmic drug therapy, however, the physician should be aware that this course of action may expose a patient to an increased overall mortality risk.[46]

Anticoagulation should be considered in every patient with intermittent or persistent atrial fibrillation. Anticoagulation is strongly indicated in patients with associated rheumatic mitral stenosis, left ventricular dilation, or history of prior systemic embolism. It is also strongly recommended in patients who are to undergo elective cardioversion if atrial fibrillation has been present for more than several days. These patients should be anticoagulated for at least 2 weeks before cardioversion and should continue to be anticoagulated for at least another 2 weeks after conversion because of the potential lag before the full return of atrial contractility.

Anticoagulation also reduces the risk of stroke in patients with atrial fibrillation and no identifiable cause ("lone atrial fibrillation").[47] The long-term benefits of low dose warfarin generally outweigh the risk of serious bleeding in this setting. However, the short-term risk of stroke in patients with nonrheumatic atrial fibrillation is only about 3 percent per year even without anticoagulation, so emergency anticoagulation is not necessary and may be unwise in severely ill patients who have the potential for developing bleeding from any of a number of causes.

JUNCTIONAL TACHYARRHYTHMIAS. Several different types of tachycardia arise from or involve the AV junction, including accelerated junctional tachycardia and the two most common forms of paroxysmal SVT, namely, AV nodal reentrant tachycardia and AV reentrant tachycardia using an accessory pathway.

Paroxysmal supraventricular tachycardia PSVT is a rhythm in which the atria and ventricles beat with a regular rhythm and at the same rate, which is usually between 120 and 250 beats/min. It is named "paroxysmal" because it starts suddenly, rather than gradually speeding up. The two most common forms of PSVT are *AV nodal reentrant tachycardia* and *AV reentrant tachycardia*. These two types of PSVT are also called reciprocating tachycardias. Both often occur without associated heart disease or other predisposing factor; thus, the presence of a reciprocating tachycardia should not prompt a search for an underlying condition. The differential diagnostic list for PSVT also includes two less common arrhythmias, intraatrial reentrant tachycardia and sinoatrial reentrant tachycardia (vide supra).

Atrioventricular nodal reentrant tachycardia arises from the region of the AV node in patients who have at least two pathways through the AV node. Tachycardia occurs when a reentrant wavefront propagates antegradely down one AV nodal pathway and retrogradely back another. The pathways come together distally in the region of the His bundle. Proximally, the atrial insertions of the pathways may be centimeters apart, so that perinodal atrial tissue serves as a link in the pathway. In the usual form of this tachycardia, the atria and ventricles are activated simultaneously and P waves are invisible on the surface ECG because they are buried in the QRS complexes. In the unusual form of AV nodal reentry, inverted P waves (signifying retrograde activation of the atria from the AV node) are seen preceding each QRS complex, with a normal PR interval.

Atrioventricular reentrant tachycardia occurs in patients with accessory AV pathways. These pathways are congenital, not acquired, and may be present anywhere in the mitral or tricuspid anulus. The tachycardia is due to macroreentry in which the reentrant wavefront propagates antegradely down the normal conduction system (AV node, His bundle, and bundle branches), across the ventricle, retrogradely up the extranodal accessory pathway, and across the atrium back to the AV node. The QRS complex is normal during tachycardia, unless functional or preexisting bundle branch block is present, because the ventricles are activated purely via the normal conduction system. During sinus rhythm these patients may have slurring of the upstroke of their QRS complexes (i.e., delta waves) if there is antegrade conduction over the accessory pathway; in such cases the patients are said to have the WPW syndrome. Some patients do not have antegrade conduction over their accessory pathways during sinus rhythm, and therefore do not have slurred QRS upstrokes. These patients are said to have concealed bypass tracts.

Episodes of either type of reciprocating tachycardia can be managed according to the protocol outlined above for the initial management of narrow complex tachycardia. Direct-current shock can be used if hemodynamic compromise is severe. Otherwise, vagal maneuvers should be tried followed by, if necessary, verapamil or adenosine. Both drugs are highly effective when they are administered in appropriate doses, terminating at least 90 percent of episodes of reciprocating tachycardia. The physician should not fall prey to the common misconception that verapamil should not be used to terminate AV reentrant tachycardia in patients with the WPW syndrome. Actually, verapamil is safe and effective against reciprocating tachycardia in these patients, though it and digoxin are contraindicated for the treatment of atrial flutter or fibrillation with rapid conduction over the accessory pathway in these patients.

In the rare instances that reciprocating tachycardia does not respond to verapamil or adenosine, the physician must consider the possibility that the mechanism of tachycardia is something different from AV nodal reentry or AV reentry. At the same time, a β blocker, digoxin, or an antiarrhythmic drug from class 1A or 1C may be tried. Occasionally, it may be helpful to use a temporary atrial pacing lead to record atrial activity to verify the mechanism of tachycardia and to deliver burst pacing to terminate the tachycardia (Chap. 32).

Recurrences of reciprocating tachycardia can be prevented by digoxin, β blockers, calcium channel blockers, or drugs from class 1A or 1C. However, for most of these drugs the efficacy rate is considerably <90 percent. The effects of digoxin on the AV node are counteracted by catecholamines, so the efficacy of digoxin may be limited in hyperadrenergic patients in the ICU. Also, oral verapamil is less effective at preventing episodes of tachycardia than intravenous verapamil is at terminating episodes. The reason for this is unclear but may involve the fact that a much higher plasma concentration of verapamil can briefly be produced by an intravenous bolus than can be maintained indefinitely by oral therapy. The potential risks of class 1 drugs should be remembered and weighed when considering their use for PSVT. Finally, amiodarone is certainly effective against PSVT, but should be used only as a last resort because its potential side effects limit its use to life-threatening arrhythmias.

Accelerated junctional tachycardia, like ectopic atrial tachycardia, is commonly seen in the ICU patient with severe systemic illness. It is particularly associated with digitalis intoxication, theophylline toxicity, or recent thoracic surgery. Its mechanism is increased automaticity of the AV junction. Its usual rate is 70 to 140 beats/min. P waves during tachycardia are inverted in the inferior leads, reflecting retrograde activation of the atria, and appear before or within or immediately after the QRS complexes. Like other SVTs, accelerated junctional tachycardia may appear electrocardiographically either as a narrow QRS complex tachycardia or as a wide QRS complex tachycardia if aberrant conduction is present. When it appears as a rhythm with narrow QRS complexes, it can be difficult to differentiate from AV nodal reentrant tachycardia, except that the latter starts and stops suddenly and responds to drugs which slow conduction through the AV node. Neither of these two characteristics is true of accelerated junctional rhythm, which actually may be quickened by verapamil. When accelerated junctional tachycardia occurs as a wide complex tachycardia (e.g., because of functional bundle branch block), it may closely resemble VT. Unlike either AV nodal reentry or most forms of VT, accelerated junctional tachycardia does not respond to direct-current shock or to antitachycardia pacing.

The treatment of accelerated junctional tachycardia consists primarily of eradicating the underlying cause of heightened junctional automaticity or waiting for resolution of acute myocardial infarction, myocarditis, or the postoperative state. If the underlying problem is digitalis toxicity, treatment should consist of discontinuation of digoxin, correction of hypokalemia, and administration of antidigitalis antibodies if indicated by the presence of hemodynamic compromise.

Children may develop a serious form of accelerated junctional tachycardia in which the ventricular rate can range from 140 to 370 beats/min. This rhythm, called junctional ectopic tachycardia (JET), appears in the first 6 months of life, sometimes without precipitating factors and sometimes following cardiac surgery.[48] The first line of therapy is to maximize vagal tone (for example, by using morphine instead of meperidine or barbiturates, if sedation is necessary) and to minimize sympathetic tone. Lowering body temperature to 33° to 35°C (91.4° to 95°F) may also help.[49] JET does not respond to most antiarrhythmic drugs or to electrical therapy (direct-current shock or antitachycardia pacing). It may respond to amiodarone; when JET is refractory to amiodarone, ablation of the AV junction must be considered.

VENTRICULAR ECTOPY AND VENTRICULAR TACHYCARDIA

Ventricular arrhythmias are extremely common in the ICU. These arrhythmias include premature ventricular complexes (PVCs), accelerated idioventricular rhythm (AIVR), VT, and VF.

PREMATURE VENTRICULAR COMPLEXES. These occur in patients with or without heart disease. Continuous ambulatory monitoring reveals PVCs in at least half the healthy population.[2] Infrequent PVCs should, therefore, cause little or no alarm and should not prompt further diagnostic evaluation or antiarrhythmic therapy. On the other hand, frequent PVCs or PVCs that occur consecutively in couplets or salvos should heighten suspicion of underlying heart disease, electrolyte disorder, drug toxicity, or other problem (Table 120-10).

The management of PVCs depends on the setting in which they occur. Many critically ill patients require no specific therapy other than correction of metabolic abnormalities or treatment of their underlying condition. Occasionally, frequent or consecutive PVCs may cause hemodynamic compromise and thus warrant antiarrhythmic therapy. Frequent PVCs may also hinder effective timing of intraaortic balloon counterpulsation (IABP) and therefore require suppressive therapy.

It is common practice to administer antiarrhythmic drugs for certain types of PVCs in the setting of acute myocardial infarction, in the hope of preventing VT or VF.[10] The following types of PVCs are widely thought to be "warning arrhythmias" that warrant therapy: frequent PVCs (>6/h) closely coupled PVCs (R on T), multiform PVCs, and salvos of consecutive PVCs. The rationale for giving antiarrhyth-

TABLE 120-10 Causes of Ventricular Ectopy

Cardiac ischemia/infarction	Acid-base disorders
Cardiomyopathies	Hypoxemia
Ischemic	Drugs
Nonischemic, dilated	Digitalis
Hypertrophic	Phenothiazines
Restrictive	Antiarrhythmic agents
Arrhythmogenic right ventricular dysplasia	Tricyclic antidepressants
Mechanical irritation (catheter, pacemaker wire)	Excess catecholamine states
Electrolyte disorders	Coronary reperfusion
Hypokalemia	Congenital heart disease
Hypomagnesemia	Mitral valve prolapse
Hypocalcemia	Idiopathic

mic drugs to patients with these arrhythmias has been predicated on several assumptions: **1.** the belief that the presence of these types of PVCs identify patients who are at high risk for developing sustained VT or VF; **2.** the belief that effective suppression of PVCs indicates effective treatment of the arrhythmogenic substrate which predisposes to VT and VF; and **3.** the belief that suppression of VT and VF in the monitored setting translates into an improvement in survival.

These assumptions may not be correct. For example, VF often appears without antecedent ventricular ectopy during acute myocardial infarction.[50] In addition, PVC suppression does not guarantee prevention of VT and VF, at least in outpatients during the first year following myocardial infarction.[51] Finally, though prophylactic lidocaine has been shown to reduce the incidence of VF in the setting of acute myocardial infarction, it has not been shown to improve survival when given to all patients with acute myocardial infarction.[52] Unfortunately, the utility of lidocaine in the subset of patients with warning arrhythmias has never been studied. In our view, lidocaine should be reserved for patients whose ventricular ectopy has caused hemodynamic compromise, or when there is a trend toward worsening frequency and severity of ventricular ectopy which suggests to the physician that the patient is likely to develop life-threatening VT or VF.

ACCELERATED IDIOVENTRICULAR RHYTHM. This is a regular, wide QRS complex rhythm that occurs at rates of 70 to 110 beats/min. It is often seen in the setting of inferior myocardial infarction or as a reperfusion arrhythmia. It is due to enhanced automaticity and is characterized by a "warm up" period during which the idioventricular rhythm gradually accelerates, producing fusion beats prior to its becoming the predominant rhythm. Deceleration of AIVR is likewise accompanied by fusion beats. AIVR can be distinguished from slow VT (based on reentry), in that the latter more often begins abruptly following a PVC, and ends abruptly, rather than displaying the more gradual onset and offset characteristic of AIVR. AIVR requires no treatment and is usually transient.

VENTRICULAR TACHYCARDIA. This is a tachycardia with a rate >120 beats/min and with wide QRS complexes. The causes are similar to those for isolated PVCs (see Table 120-10). In VT, the rhythm may be regular or irregular. The QRS complexes during tachycardia are identical to each other in the case of *monomorphic* VT, or continuously varying in the case of *polymorphic* VT. The term *nonsustained* is usually applied to episodes which terminate spontaneously within 30 s of their onset; and the term *sustained* is usually applied to episodes which last for longer than 30 s or which require therapy for termination.

Ventricular tachycardia arises from a variety of mechanisms. Monomorphic VT occurring in patients with ventricular aneurysms is due to reentry near the border of the scar.[53] The VT arising in the setting of digitalis toxicity is probably due to triggered automaticity arising from late after-depolarizations.[54] Patients with dilated cardiomyopathy are subject to a type of VT that is monomorphic and usually with a LBBB morphology, and is due to macroreentry with a wavefront that travels down the right bundle branch, across the interventricular septum, up the left bundle branch and into the His bundle before starting another circuit.[55] Torsade de pointes, a polymorphic VT which arises in various settings (Table 120-11) is probably caused by triggered automaticity due to early after-depolarizations.[56] Catecholamine-dependent VT, which occurs in patients with structurally normal hearts, may be due to accelerated phase 4 depolarization.[57] Verapamil-sensitive VT, which also occurs in patients with structurally normal hearts, may be caused by triggered activity due to late after-depolarizations.[58]

TABLE 120-11 Causes of the Long QT Syndrome and Torsade de Pointes

Congenital or idiopathic (with or without congenital neural deafness)
Drugs
Type 1A antiarrhythmics (and other antiarrhythmics)
Psychoactive drugs (phenothiazines, tricyclic and tetracyclic antidepressants)
Severe bradycardia
AV block
Marked sinus bradycardia
Metabolic abnormalities
Hypokalemia
Hypomagnesemia
Hypocalcemia
Liquid protein diets/starvation
Neurologic disease
Subarachnoid hemorrhage
Strokes
Encephalitis
Arsenic poisoning
Myocardial infarction and ischemia

Ventricular tachycardia often causes severe hemodynamic compromise and can be lethal. Cardiac arrests from VT or VF must be managed with cardiopulmonary resuscitation including airway management, mechanical ventilation, chest compressions, and electrical defibrillation with 200 J followed, if necessary, by 300 and then 360 J (Chap. 31). If the arrest has been witnessed, a precordial thump may be administered if an electrical defibrillator is not immediately available. If the patient remains in VT or VF despite these measures, 1.0 mg 1:10,000 epinephrine should be given intravenously followed by another attempt at electrical defibrillation. This dose of epinephrine should be repeated every 5 min while the patient remains in pulseless VT or VF. When VT or VF persists, lidocaine (an initial intravenous bolus of 1 mg/kg followed by repeated boluses of 0.5 mg/kg every 8 min to a total of 3 mg/kg) may be given. If the rhythm is refractory to lidocaine, bretylium (10 mg/kg) may be administered. Throughout this process, concerted efforts should be made to identify and correct electrolyte disturbances or acid-base imbalances.

Many episodes of VT do not cause cardiovascular collapse. If the patient is hemodynamically stable, a 12-lead

ECG and rhythm strip should be obtained and the diagnosis of VT confirmed from among the other causes of a wide QRS complex VT. The conscious patient with VT does not need to be electrically cardioverted. Instead, lidocaine can be administered. If it is ineffective, one can try procainamide in the case of patients who are stable with the VT or bretylium for patients who are conscious but unstable. Rarely, the physician may have the option of pace-terminating the episode of VT (e.g., in patients who have temporary ventricular pacing leads in place). The technique of pace termination is discussed in Chap. 32.

Certain types of VT are refractory to electrical shock and to the usual antiarrhythmic drugs. VT from digitalis intoxication may require management with antidigoxin antigen binding fragments (Fab). The dose of antidigoxin Fab to be delivered can be calculated by calculating the total body load of digoxin as the serum concentration of digoxin (in ng/L) multiplied by the volume of distribution (equal to the patient's weight in kilograms multiplied by 5.6 L/kg). The total body load of digoxin is then divided by 600 (the number of nanograms of digoxin bound by each vial) to determine the number of vials which should be administered to the patient. Antidigoxin Fab also binds digitoxin, and the same calculations can be used to determine the number of vials to be given, except that the volume of distribution of digitoxin is 0.56 L/kg. Patients usually respond clinically to the antibody fragments within 30 min of administration.[59] The serum concentration of digoxin climbs after administration of the antibody fragments, because they remove digoxin from extravascular binding sites. The Fab-digitalis complexes are excreted by the kidneys with a half-life of 16 to 20 h in patients with normal renal function. It is not clear how the complexes are eliminated in patients with renal insufficiency; however, such patients have responded well to anti-digoxin Fab.

Torsade de pointes is another type of VT requiring special management. It receives its name, which translates to "twisting of the points," from the manner in which the QRS complexes appear to rotate around the isoelectric baseline, with beat-to-beat variability in axis and morphology. It occurs in the setting of a prolonged QT interval. Other features of torsade include episodes that are generally nonsustained, initiation by a late extrasystole (not uncommonly during short-long-short sequences produced by isolated PVCs), T wave alternans prior to episodes, and occasional degeneration into VF. A recent classification system separates torsade into cases that are pause dependent and those that are adrenergic dependent, based on differences in clinical presentation, inciting factors, and response to therapy.[56] β-Adrenergic blockade is the best therapy of adrenergic-dependent torsade, including most congenital forms and most forms caused by neurologic disorders (subarachnoid hemorrhage, stroke, or encephalitis). Pause-dependent torsade (including most of the commonly acquired forms) is chiefly treated by removal of any offending drugs (e.g., class 1A antiarrhythmics) and correction of electrolyte abnormalities. Episodes of sustained torsade respond to electrical cardioversion. While waiting for the underlying disorder to be corrected, recurrent torsade can be prevented using interventions that shorten the QT interval, such as atrial or ventricular pacing at rates of 90 to 110 beats/min or isoproterenol. Pacing is preferred in patients with concomitant coronary artery disease. Lidocaine is often ineffective in the treatment of torsade, and class 1A antiarrhythmic agents should be avoided because they can further prolong the QT interval. Magnesium sulfate has been reported to abolish torsade with a high rate of success.[60]

Several other types of VT are refractory to direct-current shock or to the usual antiarrhythmic drugs. Extreme hyperkalemia (with serum potassium concentration >8 meq/L) can cause an incessant VT with a sinusoidal morphology. It should be treated with intravenous calcium (10 to 30 mL of 10% calcium gluconate given over 1 to 5 min), hypertonic glucose plus insulin, and sodium bicarbonate (44 to 132 meq, or one to three ampules). Class 1C antiarrhythmic drugs (flecainide, encainide, and propafenone) cause a similar VT, which occasionally responds to lidocaine but can be highly refractory. Theoretically, this arrhythmia might respond best to hypertonic sodium, which would counteract the sodium channel blocking effects of the class 1C agent.[61,62] Another VT refractory to direct-current shock and to class 1 drugs is a rare form of verapamil-responsive VT, which occurs in young patients with no identifiable heart disease.[63] The QRS morphology of this VT resembles RBBB with left axis deviation. This VT provides the exception to the rule that verapamil has no role in the management of VT. Finally, refractory VT or VF can be the terminal event in patients with truly end-stage heart disease in which mechanical cardiac function is so severely diminished that the patient would not survive even if the VT could be terminated. In this situation the arrhythmia is called *secondary* VF (or VT).

Once an episode of VT or VF has been terminated, the physician must turn attention to preventing recurrences. Efforts should be made to identify and treat any of the causes of VT listed in Table 120-10. Careful attention should be paid to the most common precipitants of ventricular ectopy in the ICU setting, including electrolyte disturbances, hypoxemia, cardiac ischemia, intracardiac catheters, and drugs such as digoxin, aminophylline, and adrenergic agents. To prevent recurrences of VT or VF, an infusion of an antiarrhythmic agent should be administered. Typically the chosen drug is the one which successfully terminated the initial episode of VT. The infusion may be necessary for up to 24 to 48 h until the cause of the VT has been fully evaluated and managed. Lidocaine is the most commonly used agent in this setting, though it may be replaced by procainamide or bretylium if either of these two drugs has been more effective for the patient.

Occasionally, VT immediately recurs despite the administration of standard antiarrhythmic agents. In these situations, several options exist. High dose intravenous magnesium has been effective in both hypomagnesemic and normomagnesemic patients with intractable VT and VF, in patients with torsade de pointes, and in patients with digitalis intoxication.[64] The recommended intraveneous dosage is 10 to 15 mL of 20% $MgSO_4$ in 1 min, followed by 500 mL of 2% $MgSO_4$ over 5 h. In patients without digitalis intoxication, this regimen of magnesium administration may produce hypokalemia, necessitating concomitant potassium administration. Contraindications to continued administration include renal failure, a loss of deep tendon reflexes, rise in serum Mg above 5 meq/L, fall in systolic blood pressure below 80 mmHg, or pulse below 60 beats/min.

Amiodarone is another therapeutic option for VT that has been refractory to class 1 agents. High dose oral loading of amiodarone (adjusted to serum levels) has been shown to produce significant suppression of VT within 2 days.[65] Also, IABP can provide dramatic improvement in arrhythmia control, especially in cases where cardiac ischemia underlies refractory VT. VT in the setting of slow intrinsic heart rates (sinus bradycardia or AV block) may respond to measures to increase the heart rate such as atropine, isoproterenol, or pacing.

Many patients with VT do not have an easily identifiable or correctible cause of their arrhythmia. Effective antiarrhythmic therapy for each patient must be identified prior to discharge from a monitored setting. The physician should not take false encouragement from an absence of VT during monitoring after conversion of an episode of sustained VT; it is the nature of some cases of sustained VT to recur after long periods of remission. Treatment options for patients at risk for recurrent VT include chronic oral antiarrhythmic drug therapy, surgical or catheter-mediated ablation of the focus of VT, or implantation of an automatic implantable cardioverter-defibrillator. Invasive electrophysiologic testing is often used to select the appropriate treatment for individual patients who have survived an episode of sustained VT.[66] In patients who have survived an episode of VF, invasive electrophysiologic testing is less useful because it is less predictive than it is in patients who have experienced sustained VT.[67]

VENTRICULAR FIBRILLATION. This is a rhythm with disorganized, chaotic ventricular activity and no discernible QRS complexes on the surface ECG. The ECG fibrillatory waves may have a low enough amplitude to cause VF to be mistaken for asystole.[68] VF is associated with complete loss of cardiac output and is quickly fatal if an adequate rhythm is not rapidly restored. The causes of VF are generally the same as for VT (see Table 120-10), but also include causes such as profound hypothermia and electrical injury. During an acute myocardial infarction, the greatest risk for VF occurs within the first 4 to 6 h and falls off dramatically thereafter.[69]

Treatment of VF consists of *immediate* delivery of high energy electrical countershock, accompanied, if necessary, by cardiopulmonary resuscitation. The principles of defibrillation are detailed in Chap. 31. In general, successful defibrillation is closely correlated to the time to delivery of countershock.[70] The utmost importance must be given to recognizing and correcting metabolic abnormalities, and once an adequate rhythm is restored, evidence for underlying myocardial ischemia or infarction should be sought, because this may dictate the need for specific interventions such as IABP or emergent coronary revascularization.

There has been considerable interest in identifying strategies for preventing VF, especially in the setting of acute myocardial infarction. As discussed above, prophylactic lidocaine reduces the incidence of VF following acute infarction, though it does not improve survival.[52] Acute β blockade in the setting of acute infarction also causes a significant reduction in the incidence of VF and also improves survival, without reducing the frequency of PVCs or nonsustained VT.[71] Ventricular arrhythmias may be prevented by keeping the serum potassium level in the high normal range.[72]

CASE PRESENTATION

A 75-year-old man was admitted to the ICU following respiratory failure requiring endotracheal intubation and mechanical ventilation. He presented with a fever of several days' duration, poor oral intake, and a cough productive of brown sputum. The past medical history was notable for COPD, chronic renal insufficiency, and hypertension. Medications were unknown. Physical examination was notable for a blood pressure of 150/95 mmHg, heart rate 125 beats/min, and labored respirations at 38 breaths/min. Neck veins were distended. Barrel chest was tympanitic to percussion, with focal right lower lung field wheezes and soft breath sounds in the remaining lung fields. The cardiac impulse was barely palpable, and the heart sounds were distant; no murmurs were heard. There was mild pedal edema. Initial laboratory evaluation revealed severe hypoxemia with a P_{O_2} of 45 mmHg; K^+ 3.1 meq/L; Mg^{2+} 1.1 meq/L; Cr 3.2 mg/dL; mildly elevated hepatic transaminases. Chest x-ray showed flattened diaphragms, cardiomegaly, and a right lower lobe infiltrate. ECG revealed sinus tachycardia at 125 beats/min, biatrial enlargement, LBBB with a left axis deviation, and a QRS width of 130 ms.

The admitting diagnosis was respiratory failure in a man with COPD, pneumonia, and congestive heart failure. He was treated with antibiotics, potassium and magnesium replacement therapy, and a single dose of furosemide which produced a brisk 500 mL urine output. Ten cmH_2O of intrinsic positive end-expiratory pressure (PEEPi) was discovered with an expiratory hold maneuver. Soon after admission, ECG monitoring revealed frequent premature atrial and ventricular ectopy followed by a sustained regular wide QRS tachycardia at 150 beats/min. A 12-lead ECG with a long rhythm strip demonstrated a QRS morphology and axis similar but not identical to the baseline QRS, but with a QRS duration of 150 msec, and no evidence of AV dissociation or fusion complexes. The blood pressure decreased to 100/75 mmHg during the arrhythmia and the patient had normal mentation. Arterial blood-gas analysis on 40% O_2 revealed a P_{O_2} 116 mmHg, P_{CO_2} 38 mmHg, pH 7.45.

The rhythm was interpreted as atrial flutter with 2:1 conduction and digoxin, 0.5 mg intravenous push was administered with no response. Carotid massage failed to affect the rhythm. Adenosine, 6 mg rapid intravenous push, and subsequently 12 mg rapid intravenous push, also had no effect on the rhythm. A lidocaine bolus of

100 mg was given followed by an infusion of 2 mg/min and the rhythm converted to sinus tachycardia at 130 beats/min with a QRS morphology and axis similar to the admission ECG. The arrhythmia was reinterpreted as VT.

After conversion to sinus tachycardia, the blood pressure remained low at 95/70 mmHg and a pulmonary artery flotation catheter was placed revealing low filling pressures with a pulmonary capillary wedge pressure of 14 mmHg with a cardiac index of 2.0 L/min/m^2. Administration of fluid and adjustment of mechanical ventilation to minimize PEEPi normalized the cardiac index and blood pressure. A repeat potassium level was 3.2 meq/L and more potassium was given. The patient remained stable for the next 24 h until a nurse noted that he was increasingly agitated. The intern ordered diazepam. Two hours later, the patient seized. The resident ordered a lidocaine level, which was elevated at 8 μg/mL.

CASE DISCUSSION

This case highlights many of the difficulties of arrhythmia interpretation and management in ICU patients with multisystem organ dysfunction. This elderly man presented with multiple reasons for arrhythmias—respiratory failure and hypoxemia due to pneumonia superimposed on COPD; hypokalemia and hypomagnesemia possibly due to medications the patient was taking at home (e.g., diuretics); clinical and radiographic evidence of congestive heart failure; and a conduction abnormality (LBBB) often associated with underlying coronary artery disease. The methodical correction and treatment of each of these problems would decrease the likelihood of arrhythmia occurrence. Despite correct initial treatment, this patient developed a wide QRS complex tachycardia heralded by frequent atrial and ventricular ectopy.

The initial differential diagnosis of the arrhythmia included a worsening sinus tachycardia with LBBB, an SVT superimposed on the baseline LBBB, or VT. The patient was hemodynamically stable with this rhythm abnormality despite mild hypotension, obviating immediate cardioversion. The next step included identifying the arrhythmia and determining the degree to which it contributed to the hypotension. Other factors contributing to mild hypotension included hypovolemia, the result of poor oral intake and furosemide-induced diuresis; and PEEPi, which decreases venous return to the heart and lowers cardiac output, especially with concomitant hypovolemia. The rhythm was misinterpreted as atrial flutter with 2:1 ventricular conduction due to its regularity, the rate of 150 beats/min typical of 2:1 atrial flutter, the absence of AV dissociation and fusion complexes, and the similarity of the QRS complex morphology to the baseline LBBB QRS complex. Despite this, VT remained the most likely diagnosis given the patient's underlying cardiac dysfunction and the lack of specificity of the mentioned features of the arrhythmia for excluding VT. The failure to alter the ventricular response to presumed atrial flutter with carotid massage and adenosine was correctly interpreted as suggestive of VT and for that reason lidocaine was given, which restored sinus tachycardia.

Persistent hypotension following restoration of sinus tachycardia was correctly considered an indication for invasive monitoring of filling pressures and cardiac index, the results of which exposed hypovolemia rather than VT as the major contributor to the hypotension. The repeat low potassium level reinforces the necessity of continued reevaluation in patients with ongoing arrhythmias. The importance of an understanding of antiarrhythmic drug pharmacokinetics in disease is exemplified by the occurrence of a seizure secondary to lidocaine toxicity. This patient had three factors contributing to potential lidocaine toxicity: hepatic dysfunction with elevated transaminases, secondary to either primary hepatic disease or hepatic congestion from congestive heart failure; low cardiac output, secondary to both myocardial dysfunction and hypovolemia; and a prolonged lidocaine infusion, because the half-life of lidocaine increases after infusions of 24- to 48-h duration.

References

1. Guilleminault C, Pool P, Motta J, Gillis AM: Sinus arrest during REM sleep in young adults. N Engl J Med 311:1006, 1984.
2. Brodsky M, Wu D, Denes P, Kanakis C, Rosen KM: Arrhythmias documented by 24 hour continuous electrocardiographic monitoring in 50 male medical students without apparent heart disease. Am J Cardiol 39:390, 1977.
3. McAnulty JH, Rahimtoola SH, Murphy ES, et al: A prospective study of sudden death in "high-risk" bundle-branch block. N Engl J Med 299:209, 1978.
4. Dhingra RC, Palileo E, Strasberg B, et al: Significance of the HV interval in 517 patients with chronic bifascicular block. Circulation 64:1265, 1981.
5. Pastore JO, Yurchak PM, Janis KM, et al: The risk of advanced heart block in surgical patients with right bundle branch block and left axis deviation. Circulation 57:677, 1978.
6. Cascio WE, Foster JR, Sheps DS: Elective cardioversion in the presence of conduction disturbances. J Electrocardiol 1:63, 1984.
7. Morris D, Mulvihill D, Lew WYW: Risk of developing complete heart block during bedside pulmonary artery catheterization in patients with left bundle-branch block. Arch Intern Med 147:2005, 1987.
8. Hindman MC, Wagner GS, JaRo M, et al: The clinical significance of bundle branch block complicating acute myocardial infarction. 1. Clinical characteristics, hospital mortality, and one-year follow-up. Circulation 58:679, 1978.
9. Hindman MC, Wagner GS, JaRo M, et al: The clinical significance of bundle branch block complicating acute myocardial infarction. 2. Indications for temporary and permanent pacemaker insertion. Circulation 58:689, 1978.
10. Gunnar RM, Bourdillon PDV, Dixon DW, et al: Guidelines for the early management of patients with acute myocardial infarction: A report of the American College of Cardiology/American Heart Association Task Force on Assessment of Diagnostic and Therapeutic Cardiovascular Procedures (Subcommittee to Develop Guidelines for the Early Management of Patients with Acute Myocardial Infarction). J Am Coll Cardiol 16:249, 1990.

11. Shaw DB, Kerwick CA, Veale D, et al: Survival in second degree atrioventricular block. Br Heart J 53:587, 1985.
12. Vaughan Williams EM: A classification of antiarrhythmic actions reassessed after a decade of new drugs. J Clin Pharmacol 24:129, 1984.
13. Bauernfeind RA, Swiryn S, Petropoulos AT, et al: Concordance and discordance of drug responses in atrioventricular reentrant tachycardia. J Am Coll Cardiol 2:345, 1983.
14. Hession M, Blum R, Podrid PJ, et al: Mexiletine and tocainide: Does response to one predict response to the other? J Am Coll Cardiol 7:338, 1986.
15. Selzer A, Wray HW: Quinidine syncope. Paroxysmal ventricular fibrillation occurring during treatment of chronic atrial arrhythmias. Circulation 30:17, 1964.
16. Velebit V, Podrid PJ, Lown B, Raeder E: Aggravation and provocation of ventricular arrhythmias by antiarrhythmic drugs. Circulation 65:886, 1982.
17. Brachmann J, Scherlag BJ, Rozenshtraukh LV, Lazzara R: Bradycardia-dependent triggered activity: Relevance to drug-induced multiform ventricular tachycardia. Circulation 68:846, 1983.
18. Hoffman BF, Rosen MR: Cellular mechanisms for cardiac arrhythmias. Circ Res 49:1, 1981.
19. Rinkenberger RL, Prystowsky EN, Jackman WM, et al: Drug conversion of nonsustained ventricular tachycardia to sustained ventricular tachycardia during serial electrophysiologic studies: Identification of drugs that exacerbate tachycardia and potential mechanisms. Am Heart J 103:177, 1982.
20. Gottlieb SS, Weinberg M: Hemodynamic and neurohumoral effects of quinidine in patients with severe left ventricular dysfunction secondary to coronary artery disease or idiopathic dilated cardiomyopathy. Am J Cardiol 67:728, 1991.
21. Ravid S, Podrid PJ, Lampert S, Lown B: Congestive heart failure induced by six of the newer antiarrhythmic drugs. J Am Coll Cardiol 14:1326, 1989.
22. Bump TE, Brown J, Yurkonis C, et al: Optimal control of antiarrhythmic drug infusion, in Ensminger WD, Selam JL (eds): *Infusion Systems in Medicine.* Mount Kisco, NY, Futura, 1987, pp 249–261.
23. Kupersmith J: Monitoring of antiarrhythmic drug levels: Values and pitfalls. Ann NY Acad Sci 432:138, 1984.
24. Thomson PD, Melmon KL, Richardson JA, et al: Lidocaine pharmacokinetics in advanced heart failure, liver disease, and renal failure in humans. Ann Intern Med 78:499, 1973.
25. Kessler KM, Kayden DS, Estes DM, et al: Procainamide pharmacokinetics in patients with acute myocardial infarction or congestive heart failure. J Am Coll Cardiol 7:1131, 1986.
26. Evans GT Jr, Scheinman MM, Zipes DP, et al: The percutaneous cardiac mapping and ablation registry: Summary of results. PACE 9:923, 1986.
27. Scheinman MM, Morady F, Hess DS, Gonzalez R: Catheter-induced ablation of the atrioventricular junction to control refractory supraventricular arrhythmias. JAMA 248:851, 1982.
28. Gallagher JJ, Svenson RH, Kasell JH, et al: Catheter technique for closed-chest ablation of the atrioventricular conduction system: A therapeutic alternative for the treatment of refractory supraventricular tachycardia. N Engl J Med 306:194, 1982.
29. Warin J-F, Haissaguerre M, Lemetayer P, et al: Catheter ablation of accessory pathways with a direct approach. Results in 35 patients. Circulation 78:800, 1988.
30. Haissaguerre M, Warin JF, Lemetayer P, et al: Closed-chest ablation of retrograde conduction in patients with atrioventricular nodal reentrant tachycardia. N Engl J Med 320:426, 1989.
31. Hartzler GO: Electrode catheter ablation of refractory focal ventricular tachycardia. J Am Coll Cardiol 2:1107, 1983.
32. Stevenson WG, Weiss JN, Weiner I, et al: Resetting of ventricular tachycardia: Implications for localizing the area of slow conduction. J Am Coll Cardiol 11:522, 1988.
33. Fitzgerald DM, Friday KJ, Wah JAYL, et al: Electrogram patterns predicting successful catheter ablation of ventricular tachycardia. Circulation 77:806, 1988.
34. Tchou P, Jazayeri M, Denker S, et al: Transcatheter electrical ablation of right bundle branch. A method of treating macroreentrant ventricular tachycardia attributed to bundle branch reentry. Circulation 78:246, 1988.
35. Sealy WC, Hattler BG Jr, Blumenschein SD, Cobb FR: Surgical treatment of Wolff-Parkinson-White syndrome. Ann Thorac Surg 8:1, 1969.
36. Klein GJ, Guiraudon GM, Perkins DG, et al: Surgical correction of the Wolff-Parkinson-White syndrome in the closed heart using cryosurgery: A simplified approach. J Am Coll Cardiol 3:405, 1984.
37. Ross DL, Johnson DC, Denniss AR, et al: Curative surgery for atrioventricular junctional ("AV nodal") reentrant tachycardia. J Am Coll Cardiol 6:1383, 1985.
38. Horowitz LN, Harken AH, Kastor JA, Josephson ME: Ventricular resection guided by epicardial and endocardial mapping for treatment of recurrent ventricular tachycardia. N Engl J Med 302:589, 1980.
39. Kehoe R, Zheutlin T, Finkelmeier B, et al: Visually directed endocardial resection for ventricular arrhythmia: Long term outcome and functional status. J Am Coll Cardiol 5:497, 1985.
40. Echt DS, Armstrong K, Schmidt P, et al: Clinical experience, complications, and survival in 70 patients with the automatic implantable cardioverter/defibrillator. Circulation 71:289, 1985.
41. Kowey PR: The calamity of cardioversion of conscious patients. Am J Cardiol 61:1106, 1988.
42. Akhtar M, Shenasa M, Jazayeri M, et al: Wide complex tachycardia. Reappraisal of a common clinical problem. Ann Intern Med 109:905, 1988.
43. Haines DE, DiMarco JP: Sustained intraatrial reentrant tachycardia: Clinical, electrocardiographic and electrophysiologic characteristics and long-term follow-up. J Am Coll Cardiol 15:1345, 1990.
44. Scher DL, Arsura EL: Multifocal atrial tachycardia: Mechanisms, clinical correlates, and treatment. Am Heart J 118:574, 1989.
45. Waldo AL: Mechanisms of atrial fibrillation, atrial flutter and ectopic atrial tachycardia—A brief review. Circulation 75(suppl III):37, 1987.
46. Coplen SE, Antman EM, Berlin JA, et al: Efficacy and safety of quinidine therapy for maintenance of sinus rhythm after cardioversion. A meta-analysis of randomized controlled trials. Circulation 82:1106, 1990.
47. The Boston Area Anticoagulation Trial for Atrial Fibrillation Investigators. The effect of low-dose warfarin on the risk of stroke in patients with nonrheumatic atrial fibrillation. N Engl J Med 323:1505, 1990.
48. Gillette PC: Diagnosis and management of postoperative junctional ectopic tachycardia. Am Heart J 118:192, 1989.
49. Bash SE, Shah JJ, Albers WH, Geiss DM: Hypothermia for the treatment of postsurgical greatly accelerated junctional ectopic tachycardia. J Am Coll Cardiol 10:1095, 1987.
50. Lie KI, Wellens HJ, Downar E, Durrer D: Observations on patients with primary ventricular fibrillation complicating acute myocardial infarction. Circulation 52:755, 1975.
51. The Cardiac Arrhythmia Suppression Trial (CAST) Investigators. Preliminary report: Effect of encainide and flecainide on

mortality in a randomized trial of arrhythmia suppression after myocardial infarction. N Engl J Med 321:406, 1989.
52. MacMahon S, Collins R, Peto R, et al: Effect of prophylactic lidocaine in suspected acute myocardial infarction: An overview of results from the randomized, controlled trials. JAMA 260:1910, 1988.
53. Harris L, Downar E, Mickleborough L, et al: Activation sequence of ventricular tachycardia: Endocardial and epicardial mapping studies in the human ventricle. J Am Coll Cardiol 10:1040, 1987.
54. Wieland JM, Marchlinski FE: Electrocardiographic response of digoxin-toxic fascicular tachycardia to Fab fragments: Implications for tachycardia mechanism. PACE 9:727, 1986.
55. Caceres J, Jazayeri M, McKinnie J, et al: Sustained bundle branch reentry as a mechanism of clinical tachycardia. Circulation 79:256, 1989.
56. Jackman WM, Friday KJ, Anderson JL, et al: The long QT syndromes: A critical review, new clinical observations, and a unifying hypothesis. Prog Cardiovasc Dis 31:115, 1988.
57. Sung RJ, Shapiro WA, Shen EN, et al: Effects of verapamil on ventricular tachycardias possibly caused by reentry, automaticity, and triggered activity. J Clin Invest 72:350, 1983.
58. Sung RJ, Keung EC, Nguyen NX, et al: Effects of beta-adrenergic blockade on verapamil-responsive and verapamil-irresponsive sustained ventricular tachycardias. J Clin Invest 81:688, 1988.
59. Wenger TL, Butler VP Jr, Haber E, Smith TW: Treatment of 63 severely digitalis-toxic patients with digoxin-specific antibody fragments. J Am Coll Cardiol 5:118A, 1985.
60. Tzivoni D, Banai S, Schuger C, et al: Treatment of torsade de pointes with magnesium sulfate. Circulation 77:392, 1988.
61. Winkelmann BR, Leinberger H: Life-threatening flecainide toxicity. Ann Intern Med 106:807, 1987.
62. Pentel PR, Goldsmith SR, Salerno DM, et al: Effect of hypertonic sodium bicarbonate on encainide overdose. Am J Cardiol 57:878, 1986.
63. German LD, Packer DL, Bardy GH, Gallagher JJ: Ventricular tachycardia induced by atrial stimulation in patients without symptomatic cardiac disease. Am J Cardiol 52:1202, 1983.
64. Iseri LT, Brodsky MA: Magnesium therapy of cardiac arrhythmias in critical-care medicine. Magnes Res 8:299, 1989.
65. Mostow ND, Vrobel TR, Noon D, Rakita L: Rapid suppression of complex ventricular arrhythmias with high-dose oral amiodarone. Circulation 73:1231, 1986.
66. Mason JW, Winkle RA: Electrode-catheter arrhythmia induction in the selection and assessment of antiarrhythmic drug therapy for recurrent ventricular tachycardia. Circulation 58:971, 1978.
67. Poole JE, Mathisen TL, Kudenchuk PJ, et al: Long-term outcome in patients who survive out of hospital ventricular fibrillation and undergo electrophysiologic studies: Evaluation by electrophysiologic subgroups. J Am Coll Cardiol 16:657, 1990.
68. Ewy GA: Ventricular fibrillation masquerading as asystole. Ann Emerg Med 13:811, 1984.
69. Lawrie DM, Higgins MR, Godman MJ, et al: Ventricular fibrillation complicating acute myocardial infarction. Lancet 2:523, 1968.
70. Kerber RE, Sarnat W: Factors influencing the success of ventricular defibrillation in man. Circulation 60:226, 1979.
71. Ryden L, Ariniego R, Arnam K, et al: A double-blind trial of metoprolol in acute myocardial infarction: Effects on ventricular tachyarrhythmias. N Engl J Med 308:614, 1983.
72. Nordrehaug JE, Johannessen KA, von der Lippe G: Serum potassium concentration as a risk factor of ventricular arrhythmias early in acute myocardial infarction. Circulation 71:645, 1985.

Chapter 121

PERICARDIAL INVOLVEMENT IN CRITICAL ILLNESS

KERRY TEPLINSKY

KEY POINTS

- *Pericardial disease should be considered in any patient with a low cardiac output syndrome and elevated right atrial pressures.*
- *Understanding the events of ventricular filling is the key to distinguishing between cardiac tamponade and constrictive pericarditis.*
- *There is no general consensus as to which drainage procedure is best used to treat effusive pericardial disease.*
- *Pericardial disease is not a contraindication to anticoagulation.*
- *Purulent pericarditis is exceedingly uncommon, even in immunocompromised patients.*
- *The echocardiogram is the best noninvasive tool for evaluating the presence and significance of effusive pericardial disease.*

In the critically ill patient with an acute or subacute low cardiac output state, pericardial disease in the form of effusion or constriction must be considered and excluded from other potential etiologies. On the other hand, the potential for pericardial inflammation, infection, or effusion often prompts extensive evaluation and may result in delay of appropriate therapy in situations where the pericardial process contributes little to the patient's instability. Accordingly, it is important not merely to be able to identify pericardial disease, but also to understand the pathophysiology and natural history in the critically ill patient as well. Therefore, rather than provide a catalog of pericardial diseases, the goals of this chapter are to provide the reader with the tools for the following:

1. To evaluate a critically ill patient and determine if pericardial involvement may be contributing to a low output state—specifically, to be able to identify and treat patients with cardiac tamponade, constrictive pericarditis, and effusive-constrictive pericarditis.
2. To evaluate patients with suspected or known pericardial disease and determine whether this may be a potential cause for concern—specifically, to be able to address the issues of anticoagulation, ischemia, and infection in patients with pericardial effusion or acute pericarditis.

Hemodynamic Effects of Pericardial Disease

The hemodynamic effects of pericardial disease result entirely from interference with cardiac filling. The underlying pathologic process can develop rapidly, as in effusive disease, or slowly, as in constrictive disease. However, even with a chronic pericardial process, a patient's clinical condition can deteriorate acutely. As with myocardial, valvular, and pulmonary vascular disease, *pericardial disease must be considered in all patients with low cardiac output syndromes and evidence for high right atrial pressures.*

Understanding the pathophysiology of disordered cardiac filling helps distinguish between cardiac tamponade, constrictive pericarditis, and the hybrid entity called effusive-constrictive pericarditis. The visceral and parietal pericardium encase the atria and ventricles and contribute to the overall compliance of the heart as measured by the pressure-volume relationship.[1] In health there is minimal pericardial fluid, and the pressure within the pericardial space approximates pleural and mediastinal pressures. With inspiration, pleural pressure becomes more negative, venous return to the thorax increases, and filling of the right atrium and ventricle increase. This increased filling causes a higher transmural pressure, yet, we record a fall in right-sided intracavitary pressures because the point of reference, the atmosphere, has not changed, but the more negative pleural pressure is transmitted through the pericardium to the heart.[2] Therefore, right atrial pressure normally falls with inspiration. Examination of the pulsatile atrial and ventricular pressure waves as well as the Doppler estimate of blood flow across the atrioventricular (AV) valve allows us to follow the events of cardiac filling (Fig. 121-1). Beginning with ventricular systole, while the AV valve is closed, venous return increases and atrial pressure increases. This pressure increase inscribes the *v wave* on the atrial pressure tracing. As ventricular pressure falls below atrial pressure, the AV valve opens. *Passive flow* from atrium to ventricle occurs early in diastole and is shown by the first peak in the Doppler velocity signal in Fig. 121-1. The resulting fall in atrial pressure is known as the *y descent* and parallels ventricular pressure in early diastole. As the ventricle fills, the atrial-to-ventricular pressure gradient narrows and flow decreases across the valve, seen as a decrease in Doppler velocity (bold arrow in Fig. 121-1). Then, with atrial systole there is a rapid rise in right atrial pressure *(a wave)* with an increase in flow across the valve as shown by the increase in Doppler velocity. The AV valve closes and ventricular filling stops when ventricular pressure exceeds atrial pressure (thin arrow). This is followed by a fall in right atrial pressure during isovolumic atrial relaxation (*x descent).*

Since pericardial fluid is free flowing, pericardial pressure is distributed among all chambers in a manner which equalizes the intracavitary pressures. This effect is present at all chamber volumes, thereby reducing the gradient for blood flow between the chambers throughout diastole. This

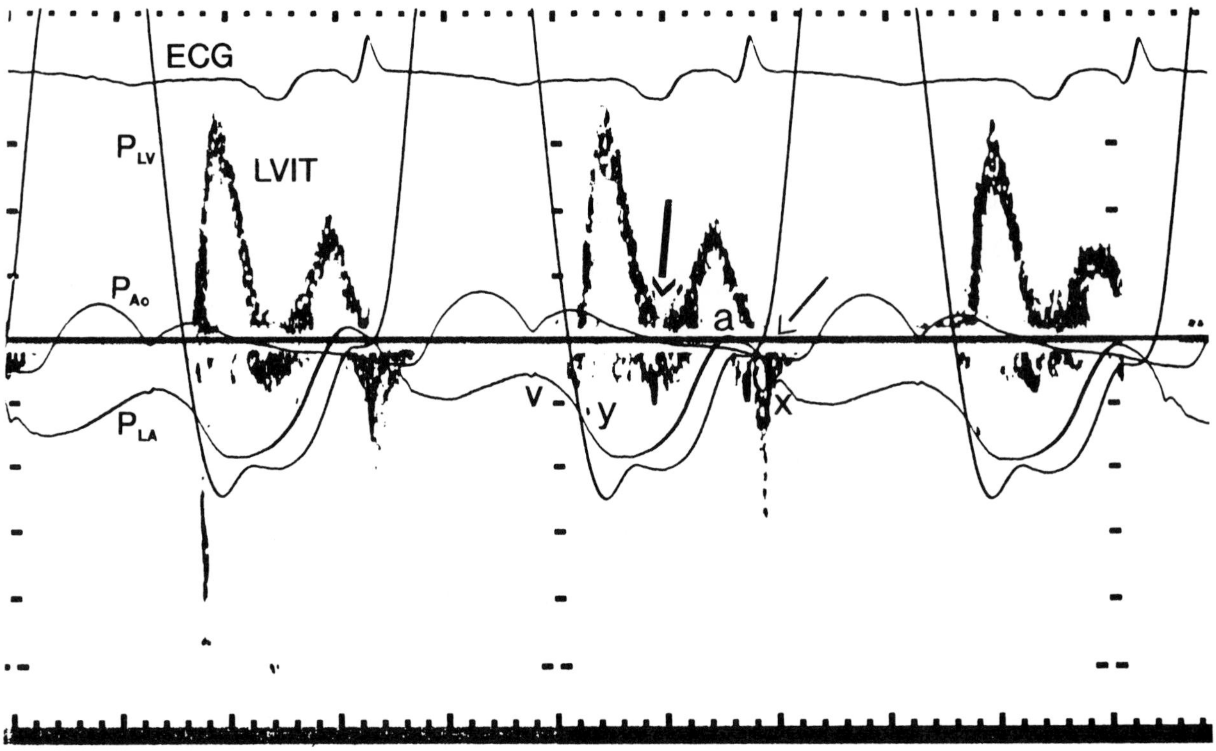

FIGURE 121-1 Simultaneous left atrial, left ventricular, and aortic pressure recordings and ventricular inflow Doppler signal. The bold arrow marks the end of passive ventricular filling when the pressure gradient between atrium and ventricle is small. The thin arrow marks AV valve closure and corresponds to the time when ventricular pressure exceeds atrial pressure and transvalvular flow stops. The *a, v* waves and *x, y* descents are as described in the text. P_{LA}, P_{LV}, and P_{Ao} correspond to left atrial, left ventricular, and aortic pressures. Note that left ventricular and aortic pressures are on different scales.

is inconsequential in small effusions, but becomes hemodynamically important as the size of the effusion increases. In contrast, the thickened pericardium present in constrictive pericarditis does not restrict chamber expansion at low volumes and therefore need not impair ventricular filling early in diastole. However, since the maximum volume in the constricted pericardium is fixed, at higher chamber volumes the limiting constraint is reached, filling is limited, and the pressure in all cardiac chambers will become equal. Therefore, even though both these processes, fluid compression and pericardial constriction, affect all cardiac chambers contained within the pericardium, differences in the filling patterns that result allow us to distinguish between cardiac tamponade and constrictive pericarditis based on the physical examination and catheterization data.

CARDIAC TAMPONADE—HEMODYNAMIC PROFILE

As fluid accumulates in the pericardial space, pericardial pressure rises in accordance with pericardial compliance. If pericardial pressure, which is an external pressure that can be thought of as pushing in on the cardiac chambers, exceeds the pressure acting to distend the chambers, cardiac filling cannot occur. Theoretically, only one cardiac chamber needs to be compressed by fluid to inhibit cardiac filling, but this discussion will assume uniform pressure distribution throughout the pericardial space. Since a catheter located in a chamber measures pressure relative to atmosphere, a given chamber volume will generate a greater intracavitary pressure if it is squeezed externally as in tamponade. Yet, since the actual distending pressure of a chamber is the transmural pressure (intracavitary pressure minus pericardial pressure), the measured increase in intracavitary pressure does not reflect greater chamber distention. Similarly, for a given intracavitary pressure, the actual distending pressure and intracavitary volume will be reduced in the presence of an elevated pericardial pressure. As shown in Fig. 121-2, if the right ventricular diastolic pressure is measured on the manometer as 25 mmHg and the pericardial pressure is 20 mmHg, the distending pressure of the right ventricle is actually 5 mmHg, and the ventricle will be operating on the lowest end of the Frank-Starling curve. With the pathophysiology in mind, analysis of the pressure tracings will be diagnostic. In tamponade there will be equalization of the *diastolic* pressures on *both sides* of the heart. (Note: there is always equalization of diastolic pressures *on each side* of the heart in that the right atrial *a* wave and the right ventricular end-diastolic pressure [RVEDP] are equal except in tricuspid stenosis or pulmonic insufficiency.) In tamponade, the right atrial *a* wave, RVEDP, pulmonary wedge *a* wave, and left ventricular end-diastolic pressure (LVEDP) are all equal. Because the

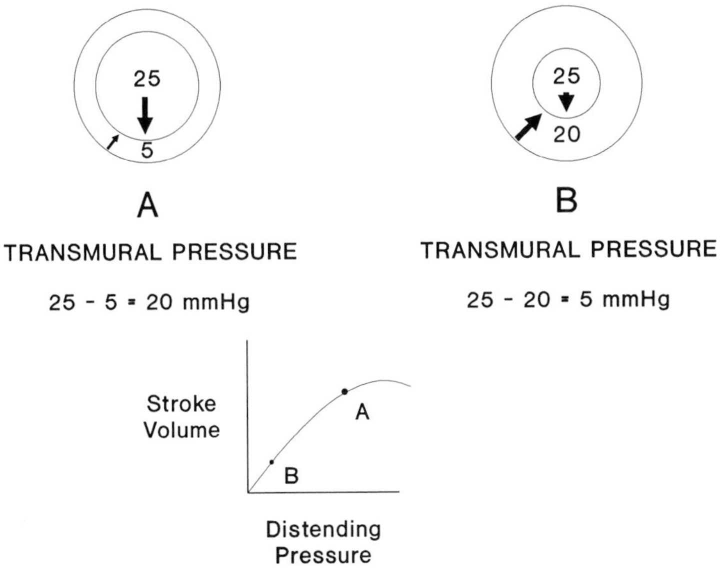

FIGURE 121-2 *Top.* Distending pressure or transmural pressure equals intracavitary minus pericardial pressure. A = in pericardial effusion without compromise, a measured intracavitary pressure of 25 mmHg still amounts to an adequate distending pressure. B = a tense pericardial effusion will cause the same measured intracavitary pressure while the actual distending pressure is only 5 mmHg. *Bottom:* The effect of pericardial fluid on ventricular performance based on the Frank-Starling principle. Note in each case that the measured chamber pressure would be 25 mmHg.

effusion is distributed in a manner which tends to equalize pressure between chambers, no gradient for blood flow appears across the tricuspid valve, except during atrial contraction. Therefore, early diastolic ventricular filling does not occur. This is reflected by the absence of the *y* descent in the atrial tracings (Fig. 121-3) and by the absence of a sharp rise in ventricular pressure early in diastole (Fig. 121-4).

In a spontaneously breathing patient, inspiration will move blood into the thorax, allowing some increased filling of right atrium and ventricle. However, because the negative pleural pressure of inspiration will be transmitted through the pericardial fluid to the chambers, the recorded intracardiac pressure will decrease with inspiration, which is normal. Pericardial compliance is such that cardiac compression develops at pericardial pressures between 15 and 20 mmHg. In this range, pericardial and right atrial pressures will be identical if measured simultaneously.

In summary, the diagnosis of cardiac tamponade is made by **1.** elevated diastolic pressures, **2.** equal *end-diastolic* pres-

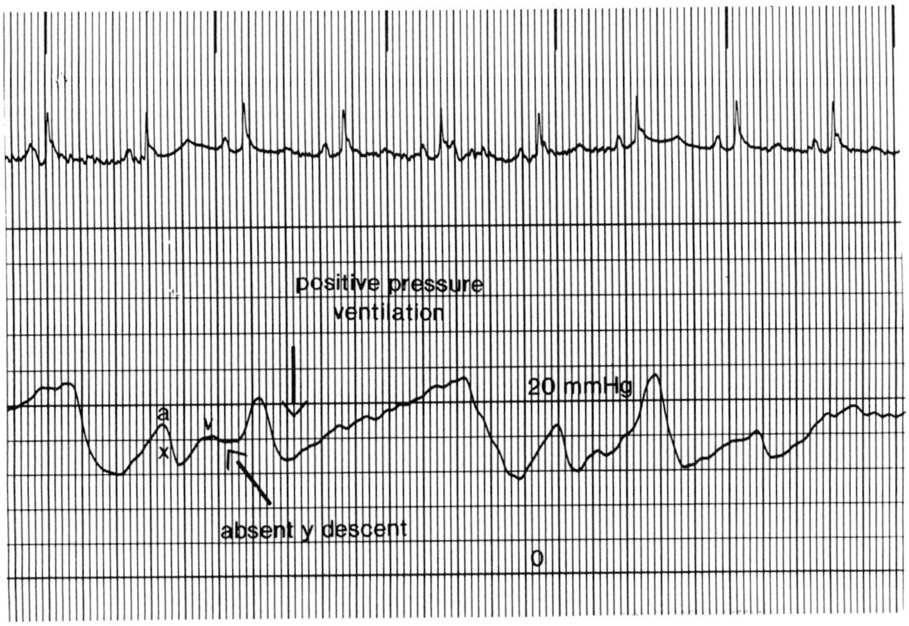

FIGURE 121-3 Right atrial pressure from a patient with cardiac tamponade during mechanical ventilation. Note, the absent *y* descent and the blunting of the waveforms, especially during positive-pressure ventilation.

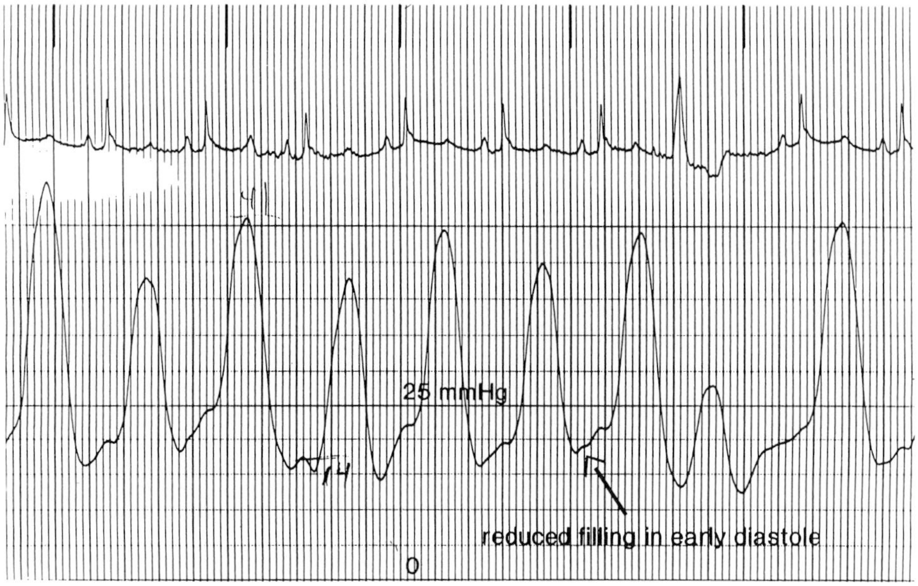

FIGURE 121-4 Right ventricular pressure from a patient with cardiac tamponade. Note the slow rise in ventricular pressure in early diastole, corresponding to reduced passive filling.

sure in the RV and LV (or pulmonary wedge position), **3.** absence of ventricular filling early in diastole, and **4.** absent *y* descent in the atrial tracings.

CONSTRICTIVE PERICARDITIS—HEMODYNAMIC PROFILE

With constriction, the pericardium encases the heart like a rigid box. Filling can proceed only until the limits of distensibility are met, whereupon pressure rises quickly if any more volume enters the chamber. In the right and left ventricles this rapid early diastolic filling and abrupt halt gives rise to the classic *dip and plateau configuration* on the pressure waveform (Fig. 121-5). In the atrial pressure tracing, rapid ventricular filling (passive atrial emptying) results in a rapid *y* descent with an early nadir and sharp rise in atrial pressure as the ventricle cannot expand further. Similarly, following atrial systole the fall in atrial pressure, or *x* descent is rapid, with a quick rise in atrial pressure. These events inscribe the classic *M shape* in the right atrial tracing of constrictive pericarditis (Fig. 121-6). Because the overall volume of the pericardium is fixed, ventricular interdependence will result in identical RVEDP and LVEDP once the limits of chamber enlargement are met (Fig. 121-7). At low chamber volumes the right and left ventricular diastolic pressures may not be identical, because the chambers are not yet encroached upon by the pericardium. However, volume administration will eventually result in increases in and equalization of right and left ventricular pressures as both ventricles develop the same compliance, set by the rigid pericardium.

Normally, during inspiration the increase in venous return results from a fall in intrathoracic pressure. This increase in venous return acts to raise right atrial and ventric-

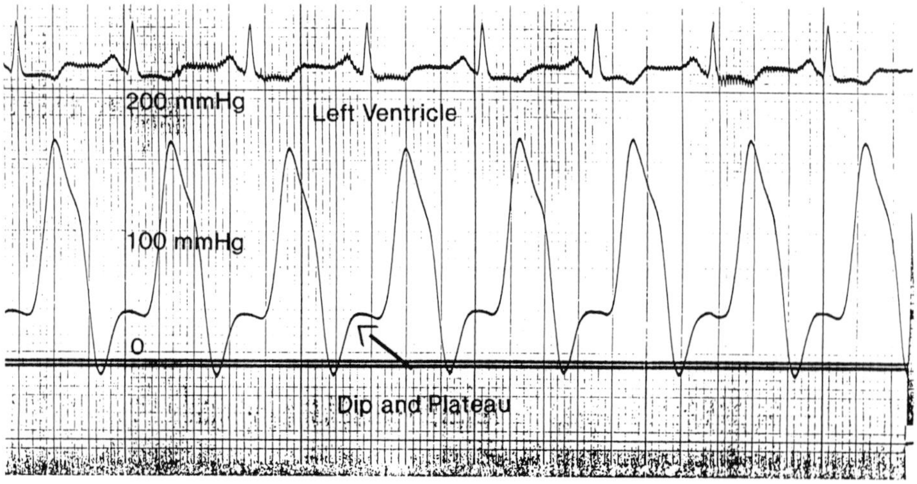

FIGURE 121-5 Left ventricular pressure in a patient with constrictive pericarditis. Note the dip and plateau caused by rapid inflow of blood early in diastole, with very little filling in the last two-thirds.

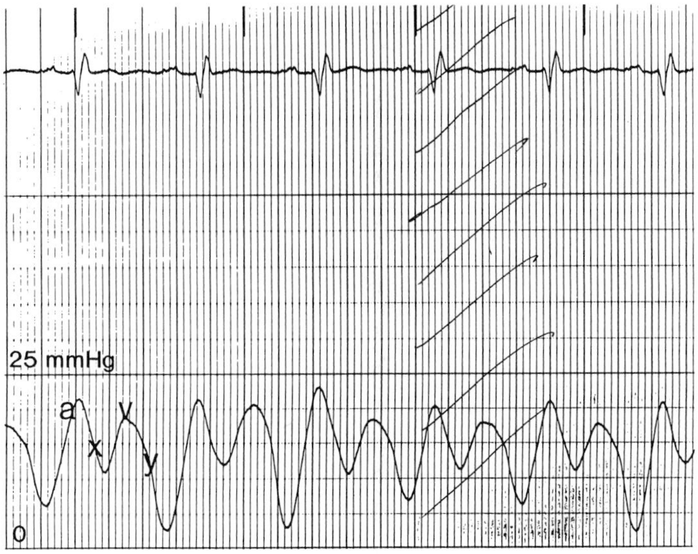

FIGURE 121-6 Right atrial pressure in a patient with constrictive pericarditis. Note the prominent *x* and *y* descents and the M shape. The *a*, *v* waves and *x*, *y* descents are as described in text.

ular pressure in accordance with the compliance of these chambers. Normally, the compliance of these structures is such that the rise in cardiac pressure brought about by increased filling is less than the fall in pleural pressure generated during inspiration, and the net result is a fall in measured chamber pressure with inspiration.

In conditions where the compliance of the heart and pericardium is reduced, the rise in pressure that accompanies venous return is greater than normal. Yet, this rise can never exceed the fall in intrathoracic pressure that accompanies inspiration, or venous return would necessarily stop. If the negative thoracic pressure generated by inspiration were the only force acting to return blood during inspiration, there could never be a rise in venous pressure above what it was when inspiration started. How then does the Kussmaul sign occur? The answer is that abdominal pressure rises with inspiration so that the driving pressure to translocate blood into the thorax during inspiration is negative pleural pressure plus positive abdominal pressure. Indeed, it has been shown in a series of patients with constrictive pericarditis that the rise in right atrial pressure that occurs with inspiration parallels the rise in abdominal pressure.[3] This explanation does not require that the pericardial contents be exempt from the changes in thoracic pressure that accompany respiration, as has been often invoked to explain Kussmaul's sign. It merely requires that the increase in right atrial pressure resulting from the return of a given volume of blood exceed the fall in pressure accompanying inspiration. This can occur only because of abdominal driving pressure. Negative thoracic pressure can be transmitted to the heart, but if the compliance curves of the right atrium and ventricle are steep enough, there will still be a rise in measured right atrial pressure. This is the likely explanation for the observation of Kussmaul's sign in patients with cardiomyopathy, pulmonary embolism, and right ventricular infarction, all conditions in which the pericardium is normal.

If abdominal pressure increases with inspiration, why then does not right atrial pressure always increase with inspiration in a parallel fashion? Conceivably, at low or normal venous pressures, abdominal pressure that develops during inspiration does not result in translocation of enough blood to raise right atrial pressure because the vena cavae are "empty." Therefore, elevated venous pressure is a necessary factor in the genesis of Kussmaul's sign. It is possible that a shape change in the pericardial structures accompanies the downward movement of the diaphragm on inspiration. Such a movement may alter cardiac compliance and explain the rise in atrial pressure which occurs. Though interesting in theory, this is refuted by the observation that

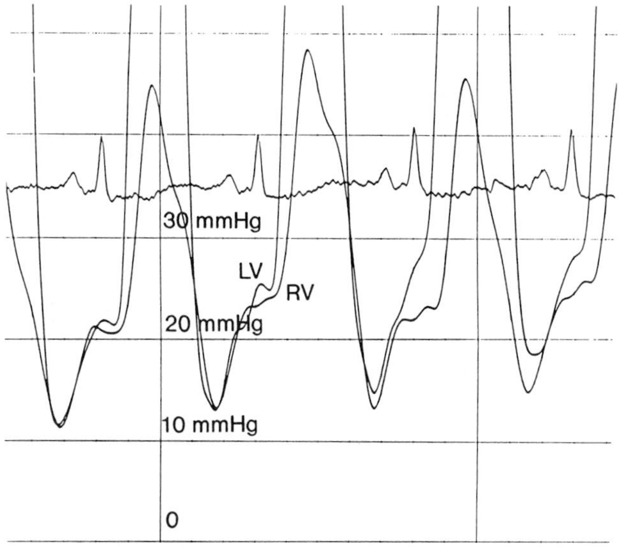

FIGURE 121-7 Simultaneous right and left ventricular pressure in a patient with constrictive pericarditis. The pressures are elevated and near equal with little rise in right ventricular pressure during the last two-thirds of diastole. RV = right ventricle, LV = left ventricle.

external compression of the abdomen *raises* both the diaphragm and the cardiac pressures (hepatojugular reflux).

In summary, the diagnosis of constrictive pericarditis is made by **1.** elevated diastolic pressures, **2.** equal diastolic pressure in right and left ventricles, **3.** completion of ventricular filling early in diastole recognized as the dip and plateau in the ventricular tracing, **4.** rapid x and y descents in the atrial tracings, and **5.** presence of the Kussmaul's sign.

EFFUSIVE-CONSTRICTIVE PERICARDITIS

The entity of effusive-constrictive pericarditis is a combination of these two processes seen most commonly, but not exclusively, in patients treated for malignancy.[4] The hemodynamic presentation is of tamponade, until pericardial fluid is removed, at which time the profile is of constriction with no clinical improvement gained by the removal of pericardial fluid. The case presented later in this chapter illustrates this principle.

TABLE 121-1 Etiology of Pericardial Disease

Etiology	Effusive	Constrictive	Effusive-Constrictive
Idiopathic	X	X	X
Postradiation			
(Early)	X		
(Late)	X	X	X
Postinfarct			
(Early)	X		
(Late)	X	X	
Infection			
(Early)	X		
(Late)	X	X	X
Collagen disease			
(SLE, MCTD, RA)[a]	X	X	
Renal failure	X	X	
Postoperative			
(Early)	X		
(Late)		X	

[a]SLE = systemic lupus erythematosus
MCTD = mixed connective tissue disease
RA = rheumatoid arthritis

Clinical Considerations

In a critically ill patient, history of prior radiation therapy or renal failure can be useful in distinguishing between myocardial, valvular, and pericardial disease. Yet, because many diseases affect both myocardium and pericardium, there may still be confusion over the location of the primary abnormality based on history alone. In addition, because many of the diseases which result in eventual pericardial constriction first cause effusion, the specific pathophysiologic process resulting in patient deterioration is often not discernible from patient history alone. As illustrated in Table 121-1, there is considerable overlap of etiology between different processes, and it may be best to view hemodynamically important pericardial disease as a continuum from effusive to constrictive with combined effusive-constrictive present in some patients.[5] Unfortunately, the time course for the development of these processes varies and, just as cardiac tamponade can develop slowly many months following mediastinal radiation, so can effusive-constrictive disease develop quickly in patients with acute illness. We do not wish to minimize the importance of patient history, for it is recognition of pertinent history that places pericardial disease on the list of considerations. We believe that the important principle here is to know what illnesses pericardial disease is *associated* with and not to concern oneself with whether effusion or constriction is more likely. The diagnosis will become clear soon enough.

Pericardial disease, if not suggested by patient history, should be considered in any patient with a *low cardiac output state who has elevated jugular venous pressure.* In acutely ill patients, this is only rarely associated with hypertension, and serves to distinguish pericardial disease from the deterioration associated with respiratory failure, hypertensive crisis, or primary myocardial failure. However, in patients who slowly develop hemodynamic impairment, the classic acute low output syndrome may not be present, and cases have been reported of patients hypertensive at the time tamponade is diagnosed.

In both tamponade and constriction, stroke volume is low because of inadequate end-diastolic volume, and aortic pulse pressure will usually be $<$40 mmHg. During inspiration patients with cardiac tamponade will have a fall in systolic blood pressure $>$10 mmHg, the *pulsus paradoxus,* which is the result of a fall in left ventricular stroke volume. The mechanism for this has been long debated and probably reflects an increase in venous return during inspiration which acts to distend the right ventricle. In the setting of a fixed pericardial volume, this increase in right ventricular volume causes the interventricular septum to shift leftward, thereby compromising filling of the left ventricle. Figure 121-8 illustrates the nature of this ventricular interaction in a patient with constrictive pericarditis. On inspiration, right ventricular volume and pressure increase, which result in a decrease in the size of the left ventricle (top panel). This decrease in LV chamber size effectively lowers compliance in the ventricle, and inflow decreases substantially, as reflected in the center panel of Fig. 121-8. The resultant contraction generates a smaller pressure which, if small enough, may even fail to open the aortic valve (bottom panel). It should be noted that all that is required for pulsus paradoxus to develop is an increase in venous return with inspiration to a heart that is limited in its ability to expand. When these conditions are met, pulsus paradoxus is observed in severe myocardial failure, effusive-constrictive pericarditis, and constrictive pericarditis.

Tachycardia is present uniformly in patients with cardiac tamponade as well as in patients with constrictive pericarditis who are critically ill. Atrial arrhythmias occur in both but are not useful diagnostically. The hallmark of the physical examination is the jugular venous pressure (JVP). In

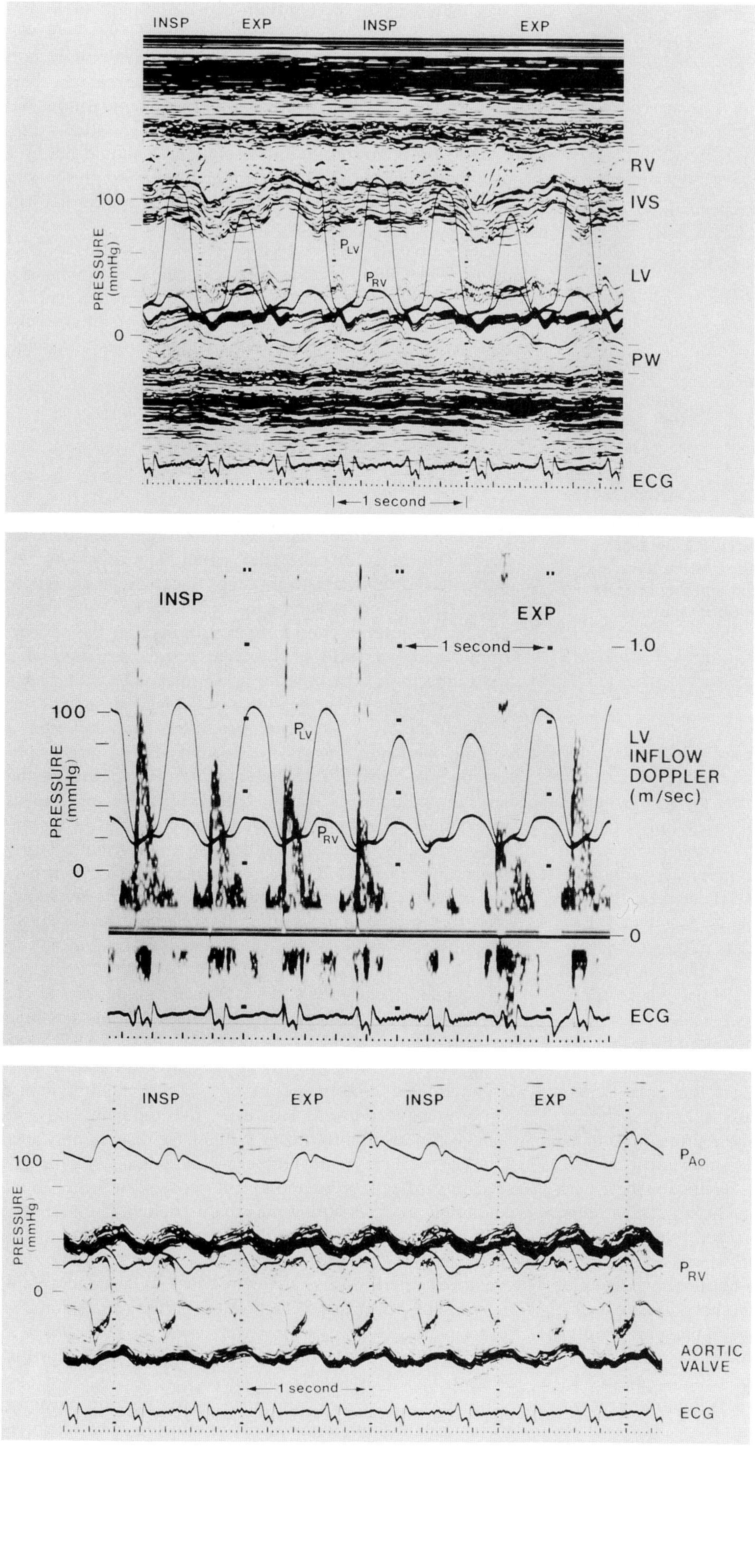

FIGURE 121-8 *Top.* Simultaneous left and right ventricular pressures superimposed on M-mode echocardiogram in a patient with constrictive pericarditis. At end inspiration the interventricular septum shifts leftward, enlarging the right ventricle while the left ventricle is made smaller. Associated with this is a higher right ventricular systolic pressure and a lower left ventricular systolic pressure. *Center.* Simultaneous left and right ventricular pressures superimposed on the left ventricular inflow Doppler signal. Left ventricular inflow velocity falls during inspiration, corresponding to the decrease in left ventricular filling noted in the top panel. This is associated with a decrease in generated left ventricular pressure and a rise in right ventricular pressure. *Bottom.* Aortic pressure superimposed on M-mode through the aortic valve. At end inspiration, aortic valve opening is markedly reduced as is aortic pressure. RV = right ventricle, LV = left ventricle, IVS = interventricular septum, PW = posterior wall, Ao = aorta, INSP = inspiration, EXP = expiration.

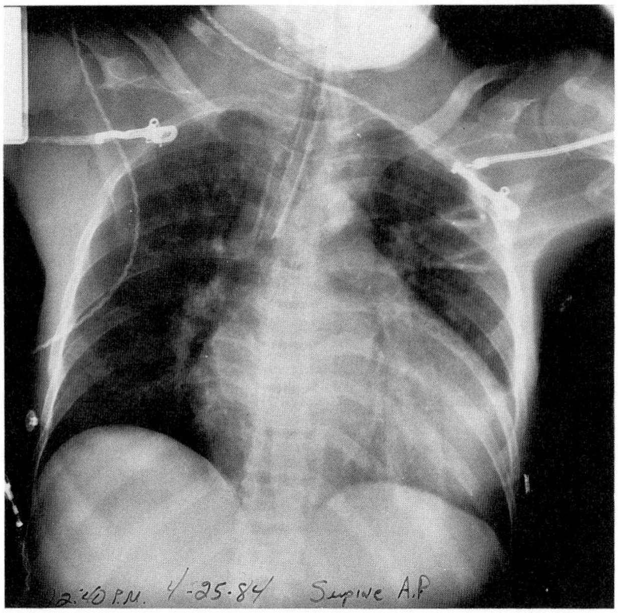

FIGURE 121-9 Chest x-ray (anterior) of a patient with rapidly increasing pericardial effusion and hemodynamic evidence of cardiac tamponade. Note the rounded nature of the lower portion of the cardiac silhouette and the rapid tapering of the silhouette at the base of the heart, giving the appearance of a plastic bag filled with water sitting on a table.

both cardiac tamponade and constrictive pericarditis, the JVP will be at least 18 to 20 cmH_2O (>15 mmHg) and is best observed with the patient lying no flatter than 45°. In tamponade blood flows from atrium to ventricle only in atrial systole because there is no pressure gradient between chambers during the rest of diastole. Therefore, early ventricular filling does not occur. This is reflected by the absence of the *y* descent in the atrial tracings (see Fig. 121-3) and by the absence of a sharp dip and rise in the ventricular tracing early in diastole (see Fig. 121-4). This is in marked contradistinction to constrictive pericarditis, where there will be brisk, easily seen rises and falls in the JVP because of the rapid and abrupt cessation of ventricular filling that occurs early in diastole and during atrial contraction. This often gives a fluttering appearance on the neck veins, which can also be seen in patients with severe myocardial failure or tricuspid regurgitation. When sinus rhythm is replaced by atrial fibrillation, the *a* wave and *x* descent will be lost in the JVP, allowing for easy distinction between tamponade and constriction based on the jugular venous waveforms as the only waveform consistently present will be the *v* wave. Therefore, the jugular venous column will have very little pulsation during atrial fibrillation in the patient with tamponade in contrast to the sharp *v* wave and *y* descent present in the patient with constrictive pericarditis. During inspiration there is a rise in JVP (Kussmaul's sign) observed in constriction which is not usually present in tamponade. This inspiratory increase in JVP will be present independent of rhythm.

Palpation of the precordium can be helpful, with tamponade resulting in a soft, quiet precordium, whereas constriction is often associated with an active dynamic precordium. In constriction auscultation may reveal an early diastolic sound or knock which reflects the rapid inflow and abrupt cessation of blood flow. The heart sounds in tamponade are often muffled and soft. There should not be a third heart sound present in tamponade, so the presence of a diastolic noise speaks for constriction. A pericardial friction rub may be present in both diseases.

Other physical signs which reflect long-standing venous pressure elevation, such as hepatic congestion, venous stasis, or peripheral edema are frequent accompaniments of constrictive pericarditis and slowly developing effusive disease, in contrast to acute tamponade developing as a result of aortic dissection, trauma, or perforation.

Diagnostic Considerations

The *chest x-ray* can be useful in identifying patients with cardiac tamponade, especially when one considers the quiet precordium that accompanies the enlarged silhouette (Fig. 121-9). The characteristic "water bottle" appearance seen on the anterior chest x-ray results because the pericardium covers very little of the great vessels, and there is a rapid tapering of the bulging pericardial silhouette. It has been likened to the appearance of a plastic bag of water sitting on a table. This appearance differs from that seen in volume-overloaded hearts, which may also be grossly enlarged, but which do not have a narrow tapering at the base. In addition, the volume-loaded heart is boot shaped, not rounded like the silhouette in tamponade. In constrictive pericarditis, the cardiac silhouette can be small or large, depending on antecedent heart disease. In excess of 60 percent of cases demonstrate some calcification on x-ray. However, this finding is most often identified on the lateral radiograph, which is usually unavailable in the critically ill patient.

Electrocardiography (ECG) can be useful in identifying patients who have effusive disease, but is neither sensitive nor particularly specific. A reduction in overall QRS voltage is seen in both limb and precordial leads in patients with large effusions, independent of whether hemodynamic compromise is present. However, this reduction in QRS voltage can also be found in pulmonary disease and obesity. Electrical alternans (QRS axis changing beat by beat) is seen in cardiac tamponade and is reported to occur most commonly in cases with a malignant etiology (Fig. 121-10). It is fairly specific for tamponade but is seen in a minority of cases. An ECG is of little diagnostic value in a patient with constrictive pericarditis. There are often T wave abnormalities present, but this is of such a nonspecific nature that it is of no value. As always, however, *when the ECG voltage is inconsistent with the size of the heart on x-ray, a diagnosis of pericardial disease should be considered.*

Two-dimensional echocardiography is the best noninvasive tool for establishing the presence of effusive pericardial dis-

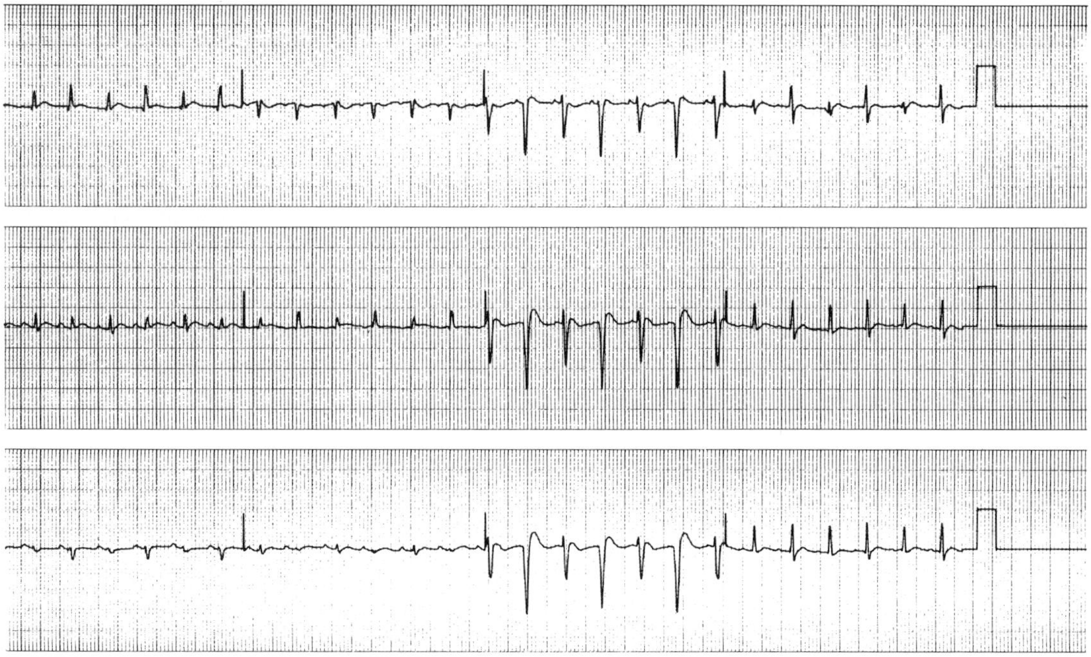

FIGURE 121-10 ECG from a patient with cardiac tamponade demonstrates low voltages in the limb leads and marked electrical alternans.

monary arterial pressure. Although there are two-dimensional echocardiographic signs of constriction, such as abrupt halt in chamber expansion during diastole, these are difficult to quantify and are observer dependent to a large degree. Abnormalities in transvalvular flow patterns dur-

ease and helps establish its hemodynamic importance[6] (see Chap. 21). The classic abnormalities of tamponade include compression of the right atrium throughout the cardiac cycle and compression of the right ventricle during diastole, with the latter being more specific for cardiac tamponade. Other findings seen in tamponade which indicate the hemodynamic importance of the effusion include interventricular septal shift leftward during inspiration, with reduced transmitral flow, reduced aortic valve opening, and reduced transaortic Doppler flow.[7] These likely explain the pulsus paradoxus which is often present, but can also be seen in other conditions with exaggerated ventricular interdependence including constriction and severe myocardial failure. It is important to note that loculated effusions can cause abnormal cardiac filling by compression of a single cardiac chamber, and the diagnosis of tamponade should not be excluded because of the absence of a global pericardial effusion.

There are several echocardiographic signs of constrictive pericarditis, none of which is pathognomonic.[8] The pericardium may appear thickened on M-mode, but this is not usually diagnosed with confidence. However, because passive ventricular filling occurs early and stops abruptly, flattening of the left ventricular free wall is present in the last half of diastole. In addition, as a result of early rapid filling, there is a brisk anterior motion or notching of the interventricular septum as left ventricular volume increases (Fig. 121-11). Another echocardiographic finding of constrictive pericarditis is premature opening of the pulmonic valve which occurs because right ventricular pressure, which rises rapidly during mid diastole, transiently exceeds pul-

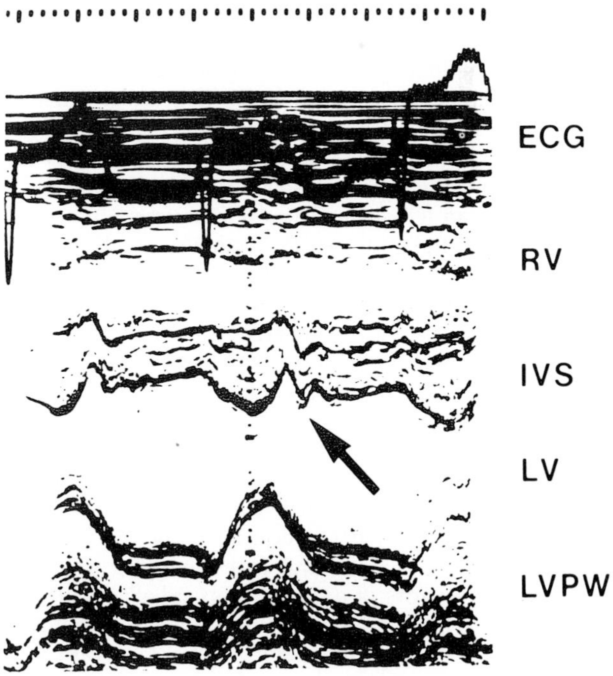

FIGURE 121-11 M-mode echocardiogram from a patient with constrictive pericarditis. Note the flattened posterior wall of the left ventricle during diastole, consistent with little ventricular filling. The early rush of blood into the ventricle results in a shuttering motion of the interventricular septum and creates a notch (arrow). RV = right ventricle, LVPW = left ventricular posterior wall, RV = right ventricle, IVS = interventricular septum.

ing diastole develop in the setting of reduced chamber compliance. Doppler techniques have been the basis for analyzing these abnormalities and may allow for diagnosis of constriction.[9]

Pericardial thickening and pericardial effusion are readily detected by either *computed tomography* (CT) or *magnetic resonance imaging* (MRI) with high sensitivity.[10,11] In addition, since fast CT scanning and MRI are capable of looking at dynamic chamber processes and patterns of filling, they provide physiologic information in addition to anatomic data. The limitations of both techniques are the difficulties encountered in performing these tests on critically ill patients. Therefore, since alternative diagnostic tools are available at the bedside, the utility of these techniques is small in patients with acute deterioration secondary to pericardial disease.

In some instances it will be difficult to distinguish *constrictive pericardial disease* from *restrictive cardiomyopathy* even with echocardiographic and pulmonary artery catheter data available. When this is the case, right and left heart catheterization is needed for simultaneous measurement of right and left ventricular pressures. In constrictive pericarditis, at low diastolic pressures (<10 mmHg), right and left ventricular pressures may be disparate, but they will converge as fluid is administered (<5 mmHg difference). In restrictive cardiomyopathy the limitation to chamber filling is not uniform since it depends on myocardial mass and chamber size. Therefore, at low pressures right and left ventricular pressures may be identical, but they will diverge as pressure increases, with left ventricular pressure rising greater than right ventricular pressure.[12] Therefore, preload augmentation or reduction can be a useful tool in the catheterization laboratory to help distinguish pericardial constriction from restrictive cardiomyopathy if the diagnosis is not evident from initial hemodynamics. Though this can easily be done in a catheterization laboratory, it can also can be performed in an ICU with C-arm fluoroscopy.

In summary, the approach to an underperfused patient involves assessment of JVP. If this is elevated, the waveforms are important in helping to establish a diagnosis. Low voltage or electrical alternans on ECG support effusion, and a chest radiograph with a characteristic appearance is very persuasive. If the clinical diagnosis is still not clear, an appropriate next step is assessment of intracardiac pressures and cardiac output with a pulmonary artery catheter. This usually affords the diagnosis and aids in management of the patient. An alternative approach is to perform combined two-dimensional echocardiographic and Doppler assessments, which are useful in establishing both the presence and severity of effusive, myocardial, or valvular disease. This approach is less useful than invasive monitoring of cardiac pressures in directing subsequent care.

Treatment Options

There is not a consensus as to the best approach to the patient with cardiac tamponade. What is clear is that more patients will die from failure to recognize tamponade than from choosing needle versus surgical drainage. Institutional preference and operator experience are as important in the consideration of therapy as are any available data.

Pericardiocentesis is a lifesaving procedure which can be performed safely and quickly at the bedside. Echocardiography to guide needle placement is extremely useful, because saline can be injected to confirm location in the pericardial space.[13] If a pulmonary artery catheter is in place, simultaneous right atrial and pericardial pressures can be recorded and the diagnosis of tamponade quickly confirmed without moving the patient from the ICU. A multiholed catheter can be left in for drainage purposes, with continuous drainage up to 7 days using slow infusion of heparinized saline to maintain catheter patency.[14]

In patients with large effusions and tamponade, the immediate therapeutic success rate of needle drainage is high when done in a controlled manner. However, up to 50 percent of patients may develop recurrent effusions of importance.[15] As a diagnostic tool, needle drainage has about a 50 percent sensitivity for malignancy and probably lower for other causes. This may be an important consideration in the decision as to which procedure to perform. However, in patients with clear hemodynamic compromise, we believe needle drainage can be performed safely and quickly and is the procedure of choice. After the immediate life threat is removed, consideration of a more definitive option is appropriate.

Subxiphoid pericardiotomy can be performed under local or general anesthesia and has a high therapeutic success rate. Following this procedure, development of recurrent effusion or constriction occurs in about 33 percent of patients, apparently independent of etiology.[16,17] We do not believe that this should deter the use of this procedure in patients after successful needle drainage. Similarly, in the patient who can be transported safely without prior needle drainage, we believe this technique is the treatment of choice. The diagnostic yield from surgical drainage and biopsy is not significantly greater than needle drainage in patients with malignancy and should not, of itself, be the motivation for performing a surgical procedure.[18,19]

There are advocates of *complete pericardial removal* for therapy of tamponade. This clearly increases the short-term risks and provides no clear benefit in our mind. It is established that the long-term survival of patients with tamponade depends on the underlying disease rather than the type of surgical procedure performed.[20] This extensive resection is best reserved for patients with loculated posterior effusions that are not adequately drained by a subxiphoid procedure.

A brief word about *medical management* prior to drainage is needed. Fluid administration is the best treatment option. Ventricular interdependence is accentuated by increases in central blood volume, and the respiratory changes in stroke volume seen in tamponade will be more exaggerated by fluid administration. Yet, the best way to improve stroke volume of *both ventricles* is to increase transmural pressure in each ventricle. This can only occur by increasing central volume. There is no evidence that inotropic agents or vasodilators in any way alter the hemodynamics of tamponade prior to drainage.[21,22]

Rare episodes of pulmonary edema have been reported[23,24] postdrainage and are probably related to the sudden increase in right ventricular output in the patient who has already received large fluid volumes.

Constrictive pericarditis needs to be treated with wide surgical excision. Patients usually improve quickly, although up to 25 percent may have persistence of a low cardiac output state despite complete pericardiectomy.[20] This is thought to be the result of underlying myocardial disease and selects a group with a high mortality. Some degree of diastolic abnormality persists for months as the epicardium begins to remodel and the myocardium improves. Most patients develop a significant improvement in functional class within months of the surgery.

Nonhemodynamic Considerations

ANTICOAGULATION

It is not infrequent that indications for short- or long-term anticoagulation arise in patients with pericardial effusion or pericarditis, particularly in the setting of acute myocardial infarction (MI). Although anecdotal reports of patients with pericarditis or effusion developing tamponade following anticoagulation exist, in certain groups of patients (anterior MI, ventricular thrombus, pulmonary embolism, etc.) the risks of withholding anticoagulation are clearly high. In two large prospective series of patients with acute MI, the incidence of pericarditis[25] and effusion[26] were 6 percent and 25 percent, respectively, during week 1. In these patients anticoagulation was not related to the development of effusion, and no patients in either series developed tamponade. In fact, in the European Cooperative Group Study of thrombolysis in acute infarction, patients treated with plasminogen activator and anticoagulation had a lower incidence of postinfarct pericarditis than the control group given anticoagulants alone.[27] Therefore, it does not appear that systemic anticoagulation can be shown to contribute to hemodynamic decline in any predictable manner.

It has been proposed that pericarditis developing weeks after MI (Dressler's syndrome) may be diminishing in incidence as a result of less aggressive anticoagulation.[25] However, patients today are probably anticoagulated more often (the era of thrombolysis and angioplasty) than ever before, making a decrease in the incidence of Dressler's syndrome more likely related to the increase in aspirin use rather than a decrease in anticoagulation. There are case reports of constrictive pericarditis developing post-MI in patients who developed effusions while anticoagulated, but the incidence of this is very small and of considerably less importance than the complication of postinfarction ischemia. In addition, it should be noted that there is a small, but real incidence of tamponade developing in patients with acute idiopathic pericarditis independent of anticoagulant therapy.[28] Despite this, we believe the presence of an effusion or pericardial rub postinfarct *is not* a contraindication for short- or long-term anticoagulation therapy.

MANAGEMENT OF EFFUSION IN RENAL FAILURE

Up to 40 percent of patients with chronic renal failure will develop pericardial effusions at some point in their course, with a smaller number developing symptoms of pericarditis.[29] This appears to be independent of the etiology of renal disease. Pericardial effusions are not limited to the predialysis phase of renal failure and may develop or worsen during maintenance dialysis. There is some question as to whether heparin contributes to the development of effusion, but patients dialyzed using heparin-free solutions still develop effusions. Since preload is reduced during hemodialysis, the concern of making an asymptomatic effusion into a hemodynamically significant effusion is real. From a standpoint of prognosis, when an effusion exists prior to intensive hemodialysis or develops early in the course (weeks), the chances of clearing the effusion with dialysis are highest.[30] Similarly, the first episode of effusive pericarditis is the most likely to respond to intensive dialysis. Although many other prognostic factors have been examined, the size of the effusion is the single most important determinant of need for therapy. Effusions estimated at 200 to 250 mL by echocardiography (>1 cm on M-mode) should be drained, especially if there is no resolution after 10 to 14 days of intensive hemodialysis (6 h daily). Hemodialysis is more effective than peritoneal dialysis for reducing effusion and should be initiated early if there is evidence of increasing size.

In addition to dialysis, indomethacin and systemic steroid therapy have been tried to halt the progress of effusive pericardial disease in this population. Both have generally failed. Indomethacin is useful for reducing the fever associated with pericardial disease, and steroids have been reported to reduce the effusion in selected cases. The instillation of triamcinolone into the pericardial space at the time of needle or surgical drainage has met with mixed results in uremic pericarditis. We believe prudence dictates that failure to resolve an effusion or progression of effusions while undergoing intense hemodialysis is an indication for drainage. Institutional preferences dictate the type of procedure performed. Pericardiocentesis is safe and effective in experienced hands, but probably has a 50 percent recurrence rate associated with it based on pooled data available.[31] Subxiphoid pericardiotomy can be performed safely in these patients, has a recurrence rate much smaller than needle drainage, and a low risk for the development of constrictive pericarditis. Therefore, in the nonemergent setting, the initial drainage procedure of choice for the enlarging effusion in a patient with renal failure is subxiphoid pericardiotomy. Pericardiectomy, although advocated by some, requires general anesthesia and may expose the critically ill patient to unnecessary risk.

PURULENT PERICARDITIS—WHEN TO WORRY?

Many times patients will be treated for a systemic infection and, during therapy, a pericardial effusion will be detected. Does this imply an infected pericardial space, and do we need to address it specifically? Alternatively, a patient undergoing appropriate treatment for a systemic infection will not improve as quickly as expected. Is an infected pericardial space the reason? These are frequently questions that need to be addressed in the management of critically ill patients. We will attempt to provide a rationale for approaching these questions.

The pericardium is a highly vascular structure, yet, it is rare to find hematogenous dissemination of infection when compared to local spread. The most common settings for purulent pericarditis are in patients with *empyema, mediastinitis, endocarditis, postpericardiotomy,* and *burns.*[32] However, pericardial effusions in any of these instances are still far more likely to be sterile than infected. Therefore, how can we determine which patients in this high-risk group are likely to be infected? ECG, echocardiography, and electrocardiography are generally not useful in this setting. Gallium 67 (^{67}Ga) uptake, when used with single photon emission computed tomographic (SPECT) imaging has been reported to yield resolution allowing distinction between pericardial and myocardial inflammation and may be able to detect inflammation associated with secondary infection of the pericardial space. In addition, several reports of tubercular pericarditis diagnosed by planar ^{67}Ga imaging exist. However, in complex patients who may have multiple areas of ^{67}Ga uptake in the region, simultaneous use of technetium 99 and ^{67}Ga with subtraction imaging has been reported to greatly increase the specificity of the test and may be the best option.[33] These diagnostic tools need only be used when a clinical suspicion exists. Aside from the rare deterioration caused by tamponade in a patient with purulent pericarditis, a rapidly deteriorating clinical course in an infected patient with an effusion is unlikely to be the result of pericardial infection. Knowledge of the organism causing the infection is not helpful in attempting to discern pericardial involvement since pericardial involvement has been reported with a wide range of organisms. However, in the clinical settings discussed above, patients who are clearly worsening for otherwise unexplainable reasons and who have pericardial fluid evident on echocardiography should undergo a more definitive diagnostic procedure, because the mortality rate from purulent pericarditis is high.[34] ^{67}Ga scanning may be useful in ambiguous cases, but the best direct approach is pericardiectomy, because needle drainage and even subxiphoid pericardiotomy usually result in incomplete drainage and fail to resolve infection. Some centers will perform a subxiphoid procedure, and proceed to pericardiectomy via a midline sternotomy if infection is present. It should be kept in mind that the concentration of antibiotics in the pericardial space approaches that of serum and that this infectious process may have developed in the face of appropriate antibiosis. Therefore, short of complete drainage, the hope for improvement is small. Needle drainage, even using echocardiographic guidance, can be dangerous since the amount of fluid is often small. To summarize, *secondary infectious pericarditis* is rare, and need not be pursued in most patients who have effusions. However, in the setting of local infection, the odds increase, and once considered, the diagnosis must be aggressively pursued and the condition treated.

Primary purulent pericarditis is rare, even in the immunocompromised patient, and is often detected fortuitously when a ^{67}Ga scan or echocardiograph shows pericardial involvement in a patient studied for other reasons. Reported cases of gram-positive, gram-negative, fungal, and mycobacterial pericarditis do exist, but in the absence of obvious nearby infection or tumor, no cause will be identified for the presence of a pericardial effusion in most patients. In a series of patients without apparent etiology for pericardial effusion, diagnostic pericardiocentesis and biopsy after 1 to 3 weeks of illness had a yield of <10 percent. The diagnostic yield was higher as the size of the effusion increased. Of note, established infectious etiology represented <10 percent of all cases.[28] In summary, it is extremely rare for purulent pericarditis to present as the cause of fever in an otherwise healthy patient. Therefore, we recommend that it not be pursued as a possible diagnosis until many other considerations have been exhausted.

PERICARDIAL DISEASE FOLLOWING CARDIAC SURGERY

Pericardial abnormalities following a cardiac surgical procedure occur in three distinct times, representing three different, but possibly related processes. In the first few hours following surgery, hemopericardium and hemomediastinum can occur with resultant hemodynamic compromise identical to cardiac tamponade, even though the pericardium is left open. Patients at highest risk for this complication are those who have excessive bleeding associated with previous cardiac surgery, those who have excessive bleeding from previous pericardial inflammation, and patients who have had long bypass times with disruption of coagulation mechanisms. However, some 60 percent of patients have effusions postoperatively, making it difficult to identify truly high-risk patients.[35] Occasionally, hemodynamic collapse will be preceded by a fall in the amount of mediastinal drainage, but often deterioration is rapid in onset. The treatment of choice is reoperation with removal of blood from the mediastinum and identification of the bleeding site. This complication is *very rare* after the first 12 h have passed, and its consideration should not interfere with attempts to diagnose other causes of poor performance postoperatively.

The postpericardiotomy syndrome occurs several weeks postoperatively in 10 to 20 percent of patients and is characterized by fever, chest pain, and presence of a friction rub.[36] In many ways, it is analogous to Dressler's syndrome which occurs weeks postinfarction. Good evidence supports an autoimmune pathogenesis, with anti-heart antibodies and circulating immune complexes present in many patients.[37] ECG changes identical to those seen in acute pericarditis may be present, making the diagnosis of post-

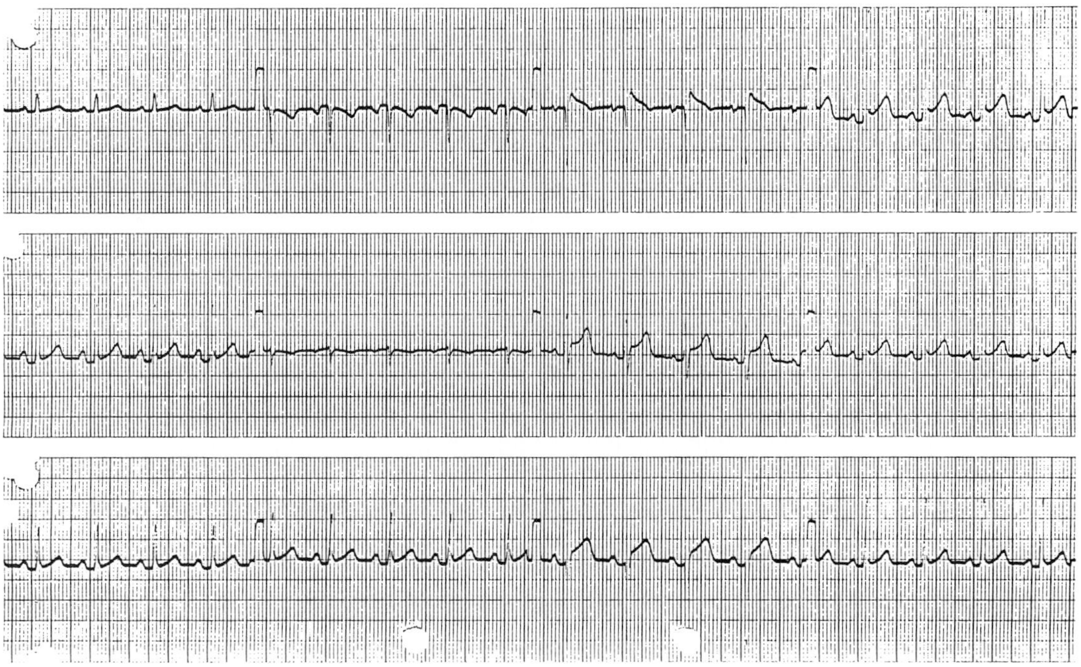

FIGURE 121-12 12-lead ECG of a patient with acute pericarditis. Note PR segment depression prominent in leads 2, 3, aVF. ST segment elevation is present globally (except aVR) and concave upward.

operative ischemia a consideration. Aspirin therapy, if not already present, is the treatment of choice. Corticosteroids are useful in patients who do not respond to aspirin. The incidence is highest in patients undergoing valve surgery, because they may not routinely be treated with aspirin postoperatively.

Constrictive pericarditis is a recognized sequelum of cardiac surgery, occurring in <1 percent of patients.[38] The presenting findings are identical to those in constriction arising de novo and consist of evidence for elevated right-sided pressure with a low cardiac output in a chronically ill patient. The reported time to onset can be as short as 6 weeks or as long as years following surgery. In one series of patients, almost 65 percent of patients with postoperative constriction were felt to have suffered from the postpericardiotomy syndrome earlier in their course.[39] Treatment in the severe case requires pericardial stripping, made more difficult by the presence of bypass grafts.

ACUTE PERICARDITIS OR ISCHEMIA?

Inflammation of the pericardium, regardless of etiology, may result in chest pain which can be confused with that of myocardial ischemia. The list of diseases associated with acute pericarditis is long, and though a history of prior typical angina may be useful in distinguishing ischemia from pericarditis, recurrent acute pericarditis is a well-recognized entity.[40] There may be a prodrome in patients with viral pericarditis, but this will be helpful in a minority of patients. The pain may be pleuritic and reminiscent of pulmonary embolism. Often, but not invariably, fever is present, especially in severe cases. The inflamed pericardium gives rise to a friction rub heard over the precordium, which is pathognomonic for the disease. Although the rub can be fleeting, it is hard to make the diagnosis in the absence of a rub. Leukocytosis and an elevated erythrocyte sedimentation rate may be present. The creatine kinase level may be mildly elevated if significant epicardial involvement is present. The classic ECG findings are *global* ST segment elevation which is concave upward, with ST depression present in leads aVR and V_1. PR segment depression is present in >50 percent of patients and can be useful in distinguishing pericarditis from infarction (Fig. 121-12). Over a several day period, the ST and PR segments will return to normal, following which T wave inversion may develop. Eventually, the T wave abnormalities will return to normal. A distinguishing feature from acute MI or Prinzmetal's angina is the concave nature of the ST segment elevations in pericarditis as opposed to convex elevations in MI or Prinzmetal's. In addition, in MI, as the ST segments normalize and T waves invert, there is not a phase where they pass through "normal." Unlike pericarditis, of course, in acute infarction there may be Q waves present early which will help distinguish between the different causes of chest pain.

CASE PRESENTATION

A 62-year-old woman with a history of intravenous drug use presented with 1 week of fever and chills. On admission blood pressure was 130/90 mmHg, heart rate was 80/min, and temperature was 102.4°F (39°C). Examination revealed a grade 3/6 holosystolic murmur throughout the precordium, as well as a Janeway lesion on the sole. ECG revealed sinus rhythm with normal conduc-

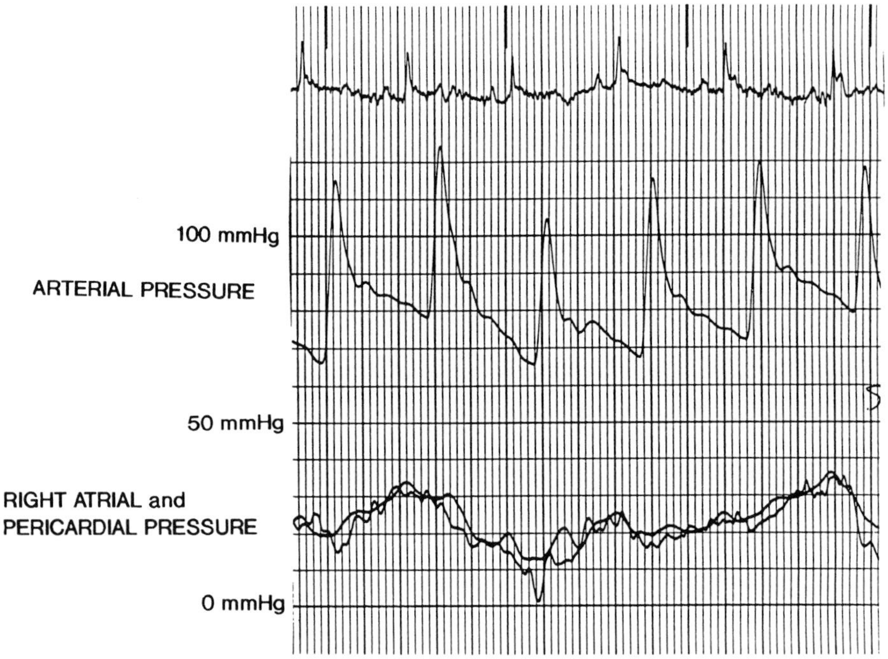

FIGURE 121-13 Simultaneous right atrial, pericardial, and arterial pressure in a patient with effusive-constrictive pericardial disease. Note elevated and equal right atrial and pericardial pressures. Also, note the fall in blood pressure with inspiration brought about by ventricular interdependence.

tion, and chest x-ray revealed bilateral pulmonary infiltrates. The white cell count was elevated at 18,000/mm^3 with 12 percent band forms and 83 percent polymorphonuclear cells. A diagnosis of acute bacterial endocarditis was made, and the patient was treated with intravenous vancomycin and gentamicin with resolution of fever. Blood cultures drawn on admission grew *Staphylococcus aureus* and *Enterococcus.*

On the third hospital day a pericardial friction rub was noted and two-dimensional echocardiography revealed mild mitral and tricuspid regurgitation, likely mitral valve vegetation, and a trivial pericardial effusion. Twenty-four hours later the patient developed acute respiratory failure and hypotension, necessitating ventilatory support. Physical examination suggested low cardiac output with elevated right-sided pressure, but no

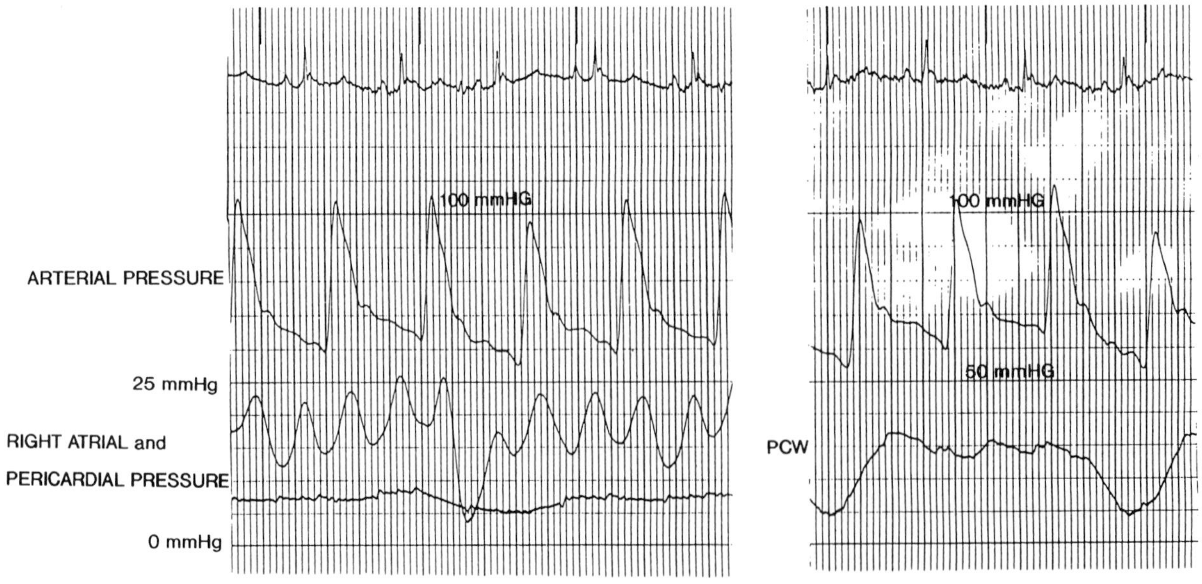

FIGURE 121-14 Hemodynamic pressure measurements after pericardiocentesis in the patient described. Right atrial and pericardial pressures are no longer equal. Right atrial pressure remains elevated and takes on the appearance of constriction. Pulmonary wedge pressure (PCW) remains elevated.

worsening of the regurgitant murmurs. Pulmonary arterial catheterization revealed the following: right atrial mean pressure 18 mmHg with *a* wave 18 mmHg and absent *v* wave and *y* descent; right ventricle 36/16 mmHg (with presence of pulsus alternans); pulmonary artery 36/22 mmHg; pulmonary wedge mean pressure 19 mmHg with no discernible a or v waves. With blood pressure of 90/60 mmHg, thermodilution-determined cardiac output was 2.95 L/min. A diagnosis of cardiac tamponade was made, and the patient was given volume infusion while being prepared for pericardiocentesis. The right atrial and pulmonary wedge pressures rose to 22 and 24 mmHg, respectively, with volume infusion, but there was no improvement in blood pressure or cardiac output. Repeat echocardiogram demonstrated a large increase in the pericardial effusion, some evidence for reduced filling of the right atrium and ventricle, and vigorous performance of a small left ventricle. Pericardiocentesis was performed using ECG guidance with contrast echocardiography to confirm needle placement in the pericardial space. Pericardial and right atrial pressures were identical at 20 to 25 mmHg (Fig. 121-13), and 450 mL serosanguinous fluid was removed. Following removal of the fluid, pericardial pressure decreased to <10 mmHg while the right atrial and pulmonary wedge pressures remained elevated at 22 mmHg with the appearance of sharp *x* and *y* descents in the right atrial tracings (Fig. 121-14). Aortic blood pressure and cardiac output failed to improve following successful pericardiocentesis. Repeat echocardiography confirmed a decrease in the pericardial effusion, absence of right ventricular diastolic collapse, and again demonstrated vigorous left ventricular systolic performance in the absence of significant valvular incompetence (Fig. 121-15). The pericardial fluid contained 190,000 red cells and 77,000 white cells, but failed to grow any organisms while peripheral blood cultures remained positive. Despite aggressive respiratory and circulatory support, the patient continued to manifest a low cardiac output syndrome and died a few days later.

Postmortem examination revealed fibrinous exudate between and attached to the pericardial surfaces and 20 mL serosanguinous fluid. There were mitral and tricuspid valvular vegetations without myocardial abscess formation and multiple bilateral pulmonary infiltrates and abscesses present.

CASE DISCUSSION

Pericarditis is a recognized complication of bacterial endocarditis and usually results in small pericardial effusion without hemodynamic consequence, with subsequent deposition of fibrinous material in the pericardial space. The clinical and pathologic findings in this patient suggest effusive-constrictive pericarditis with features of both cardiac tamponade and pericardial constriction in the presence of acute infective endocarditis.

There was little question of the diagnosis of acute endocarditis on presentation. However, as the patient deteriorated despite antibiotic therapy and in the absence of severe valvular dysfunction, other causes for her failure to improve were considered. The physical examination revealed a low output state with evidence of central venous pressure elevation, but nondistinct jugular waveforms. The low output state was inconsistent with our expectation for an infected patient, and a pulmonary artery catheter was placed for further diagnosis. The initial hemodynamics revealed elevated and equal right atrial and pulmonary wedge pressures, with absent *y* descent diagnostic of tamponade, with low cardiac output and systemic blood pressure. An echocardiogram was obtained to guide pericardiocentesis, which confirmed the presence of a large effusion. On introduction of the needle into the pericardial space, the pericardial and right atrial pressures were elevated and equal, pathognomonic for tamponade (see Fig. 121-13). Following removal of 450 mL fluid, the pericardial pressure fell but the right

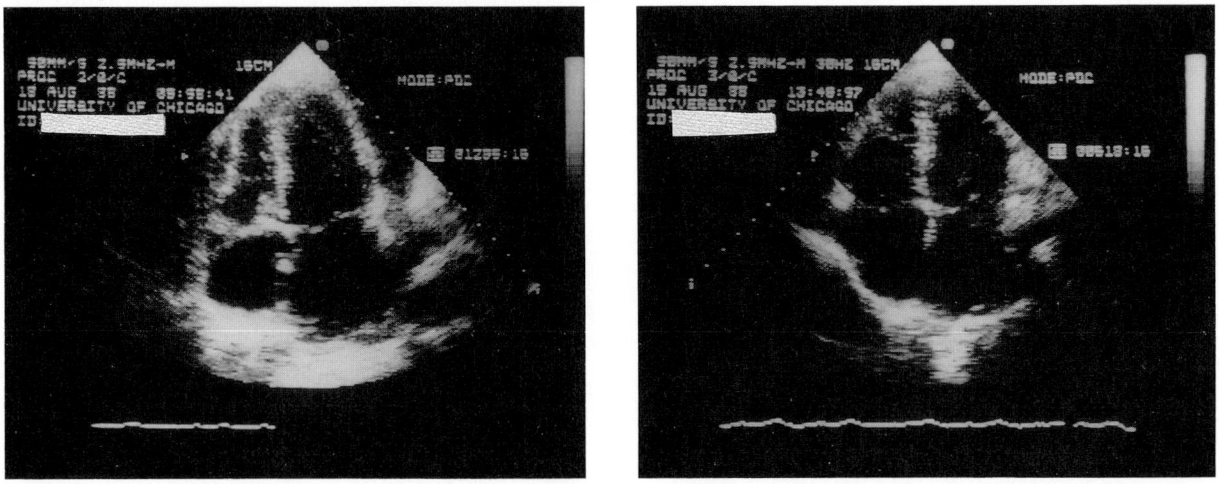

FIGURE 121-15 *Left.* **Two-dimensional echocardiogram shows large pericardial effusion and right ventricular collapse at end diastole.** *Right.* **Postpericardiocentesis the effusion is gone and right ventricular collapse is no longer evident.**

atrial and pulmonary wedge pressures remained elevated and equal at end diastole (see Fig. 121-14). Now however, the right atrial waveforms displayed the classic M shape of constrictive pericarditis, with emergence of steep and rapid x and y descents. M-mode echocardiography revealed flattening of the posterior wall of the left ventricle (see Fig. 121-11) along with notching of the interventricular septum suggesting constrictive pericarditis. The postmortem examination confirmed the presence of pericardial constriction.

This case, though atypical of the clinical setting in which effusive-constrictive pericarditis develops, defines this disorder by virtue of the hemodynamic abnormalities—constrictive pericarditis which is only realized after tamponade is removed. It illustrates the need to search further for explanations when a clinical course is other than expected. Finally, it is illustrative of the importance of recognizing the combination of low cardiac output state and elevated JVP and pursuing the possible causes quickly.

References

1. Janicki JS, Weber KT: The pericardium and ventricular interaction, distensibility, and function. Am J Physiol 238:H494, 1980.
2. Shabetai R, Mangiardi L, Bhargava V et al: The pericardium and cardiac function. Prog Cardiovasc Dis 22:107, 1979.
3. Meyer TE, Sareli P, Marcus RH et al: Mechanisms underlying Kussmaul's sign in chronic constrictive pericarditis. Am J Cardiol 64:1069, 1989.
4. Mann T, Brodie BR, Grossman W et al: Effusive-constrictive hemodynamic pattern due to neoplastic involvement of the pericardium. Am J Cardiol 41:781, 1978.
5. Cameron J, Oesterle SN, Baldwin JC et al: The etiologic spectrum of constrictive pericarditis. Am Heart J 113:354, 1987.
6. Singh S, Wann LS, Schuchard GH et al: Right ventricular and right atrial collapse in patients with cardiac tamponade—A combined echocardiographic and hemodynamic study. Circulation 70:966, 1984.
7. Burstow DJ, Oh JK, Bailey KR et al: Cardiac tamponade: Characteristic Doppler observations. Mayo Clin Proc 64:312, 1989.
8. Schnittger I, Bowden RE, Abrams J, Popp RL: Echocardiography: Pericardial thickening and constrictive pericarditis. Am J Cardiol 42:388, 1978.
9. Hatle LK, Appleton CP, Popp RL: Differentiation of constrictive pericarditis and restrictive cardiomyopathy by Doppler echocardiography. Circulation 79:357, 1989.
10. Isner JM, Carter BL, Bankoff MS et al: Computed tomography in the diagnosis of pericardial heart disease. Ann Intern Med 97:473, 1982.
11. Sechtem U, Tscholakoff D, Higgins CB: MRI of the abnormal pericardium. Am J Radiol 147:245, 1986.
12. Meaney E, Shabetai R, Bhargava V et al: Cardiac amyloidosis, constrictive pericarditis, and restrictive cardiomyopathy. Am J Cardiol 38:547, 1976.
13. Chandraratna PAN, Reid CL, Nimalasuriya A et al: Application of 2-dimensional contrast studies during pericardiocentesis. Am J Cardiol 52:1120, 1983.
14. Patel AK, Kosolcharoen PK, Nallasivan M et al: Catheter drainage of the pericardium. Practical method to maintain long term patency. Chest 92:1018, 1987.
15. Markiewicz W, Borovik R, Ecker S: Cardiac tamponade in medical patients: Treatment and prognosis in the echocardiographic era. Am Heart J 111:1138, 1986.
16. Ghogh SC, Larrieu AJ, Ablaza SG et al: Clinical experience with subxiphoid pericardial decompression. Int Surg 70:5, 1985.
17. Peihler JM, Pluth JR, Schaff HV et al: Surgical management of effusive pericardial disease. Influence of extent of pericardial resection on clinical course. J Thorac Cardiovasc Surg 90:506, 1985.
18. Mills SA, Julian S, Holliday RH et al: Subxiphoid pericardial window for pericardial effusive disease. J Cardiovasc Surg 30:768, 1989.
19. Posner MR, Cohen GI, Skarin AT: Pericardial disease in patients with cancer. The differentiation of malignant from idiopathic and radiation-induced pericarditis. Am J Med 71:407, 1981.
20. McCaughan BC, Schaff HV, Piehler JM et al: Early and late results of pericardiectomy for constrictive pericarditis. J Thorac Cardiovasc Surg 89:340, 1985.
21. Martins JB, Manuel WJ, Marcus ML et al: Comparative effects of catecholamines in cardiac tamponade: Experimental and clinical studies. Am J Cardiol 46: 59, 1980.
22. Kerber RE, Gascho JA, Litchfield R et al: Hemodynamic effects of volume expansion and nitroprusside compared with pericardiocentesis in patients with acute cardiac tamponade. N Engl J Med 15:929, 1982.
23. Vandyke WH, Cure J, Chakko CS et al: Pulmonary edema after pericardiocentesis for cardiac tamponade. N Engl J Med 309:595, 1983.
24. Shenoy MM, Dhar S, Giffin R et al: Pulmonary edema following pericardiotomy for cardiac tamponade. Chest 86:647, 1984.
25. Lichstein E, Arsura E, Hollander G et al: Current incidence of post myocardial infarction (Dressler's) syndrome. Am J Cardiol 50:1269, 1982.
26. Galve E, Garcia-Del-Castillo H, Evangelista A et al: Pericardial effusion in the course of myocardial infarction: Incidence, natural history, and clinical relevance. Circulation 73:294, 1986.
27. Van de Werf F, Arnold AE: Intravenous tissue plasminogen activator and size of infarct, left ventricular function, and survival in acute myocardial infarction. Br Med J 297:1374, 1988.
28. Permanyer-Miralda G, Sagrista-Sauleda J, Soler-Soler J: Primary acute pericardial disease: A prospective series of 231 consecutive patients. Am J Cardiol 56:623, 1985.
29. Frommer JP, Young JB, Ayus JC: Asymptomatic pericardial effusion in uremic patients: Effect of long term dialysis. Nephron 39:296, 1985.
30. Rutsky EA, Rostand SG: Treatment of uremic pericarditis and pericardial effusion. Am J Kidney Dis 10:2, 1987.
31. Kumar S, Lesch M: Pericarditis in renal disease. Prog Cardiovasc Dis 22:357, 1980.
32. Fowler NO, Manifsas GT: Infectious pericarditis. Prog Cardiovasc Dis 16:323, 1973.
33. Karl RD Jr, Hartshorne MF, Cawthon MA et al: Dual isotope scanning with gallium-67 citrate and technetium-99m radiopharmaceuticals. Clin Nucl Med 10:507, 1985.
34. Rubin RH, Moellering RC: Clinical, microbiologic, and therapeutic aspects of purulent pericarditis. Am J Med 59:68, 1975.
35. Stevenson LW, Child JS, Laks H et al: Incidence and significance of early pericardial effusions after cardiac surgery. Am J Cardiol 54:848, 1984.
36. Miller RH, Horneffer PJ, Gardner TJ et al: The epidemiology of the post pericardiotomy syndrome: A common complication of cardiac surgery. Am Heart J 116:1323, 1988.
37. De-Scheerder I, Wulfrank D, Van-Renterghem L et al: Association of anti-heart antibodies and circulating immune complexes

in the post-pericardiotomy syndrome. Clin Exp Immunol 57:423, 1984.
38. Cimino JJ, Kogan AD: Constrictive pericarditis after cardiac surgery: Report of three cases and review of the literature. Am Heart J 118:1292, 1989.
39. Killian DM, Furiasse JG, Scanlon PJ et al: Constrictive pericarditis after cardiac surgery. Am Heart J 118:563, 1989.
40. Fowler NO, Harbin AD: Recurrent acute pericarditis: Follow-up study of 31 patients. J Am Coll Cardiol 7:300, 1986.

Chapter 122

VALVULAR HEART DISEASE

DUANE FOLLMAN
PAUL SOBOTKA

KEY POINTS

- *In valvular heart disease, the clinician must determine the status of the four major hemodynamic parameters: preload, afterload, heart rate, and contractility.*
- *These four parameters must be interpreted based on the pathophysiology of the valvular lesion as well as on the underlying critical illness and then adjusted accordingly.*
- *The more severe a valvular lesion, the narrower the therapeutic window for optimal management.*
- *A subclinical valvular lesion may be asymptomatic until a critical illness supervenes.*
- *If a patient's hemodynamic status appears worse than expected for the level of critical illness, consider valvular heart disease.*
- *In multivalvular disease, the most clinically significant lesion must be treated first.*
- *A mild, acute regurgitant lesion may give more symptoms than a severe, chronic lesion.*
- *All prosthetic valves carry an underlying mild to moderate stenosis.*
- *Endocarditis may easily be masked by an underlying critical illness.*
- *Hypertrophic cardiomyopathy is a therapeutic paradox. Best results are obtained by maximizing loading conditions and minimizing inotropy.*

Valvular heart disease was once synonymous with rheumatic heart disease. There has been a decrease in rheumatic heart disease in the past 25 years, but there has also been an increase in nonrheumatic valvular heart disease. Because of this, valvular heart disease is still a common medical problem. Many patients with valvular heart disease will be seen in the intensive care setting often with a nonvalvular-related illness. The clinical impact of valvular disease is different during critical illness than in the resting state. A valvular lesion which is insignificant at rest may become clinically important under physiologic stress. The focus of this chapter will be on general management principles of patients with critical illness who have valvular heart disease, rather than on the management of pure, isolated valvular heart disease.

In most critically ill patients who are hemodynamically compromised, the overriding goal is improvement in oxygen delivery to the tissues. The determinants of oxygen delivery include hemoglobin concentration, oxygen saturation, and cardiac output. In this chapter, it is assumed that hemoglobin and oxygen saturation have been optimized in accord with the principles outlined in Chap. 1. Therefore, the goals of this chapter are to illustrate the mechanisms of impaired cardiac output in valvular disease and to provide a foundation for management. A fundamental understanding of the four major hemodynamic parameters is essential to the care of patients with valvular heart disease.

Preload is defined as the force which stretches the cardiac muscle to its precontraction volume. Clinically, this is known as the transmural filling pressure of the heart, estimated as the pulmonary capillary wedge pressure or left ventricular end-diastolic pressure. Preload is related to a patient's volume status and the compliance of the ventricle. A poorly compliant (stiffer) chamber will be less full at any given filling pressure than a more compliant ventricle (see Chap. 2). In addition, noncompliant chambers are generally more sensitive to loading conditions than more compliant ones.

Afterload is the force opposing contraction of the stimulated heart muscle, usually estimated clinically as the mean aortic pressure (ignoring the effects of intrathoracic pressure). It is, therefore, largely a function of the systemic vascular resistance in patients without valvular heart disease. In rare circumstances, it is important to consider the effect of intrathoracic pressure on afterload, as in the patient with status asthmaticus. Adjustments in afterload are made with vasodilators, vasoconstrictors, aortic balloon counterpulsation, and, unusually, a change in intrathoracic pressure.

Contractility refers to the intrinsic ability of the heart to generate the force and velocity necessary for contraction. This is adjusted by adding either positive or negative inotropes or by relieving ischemia.

Heart rate is the final relevant parameter in patients with valvular heart disease. This can be adjusted with a pacemaker or with careful use of β blockers and/or calcium channel blockers. Proper management of critically ill patients with valvular heart disease requires optimizing these four variables in a way which maximizes cardiac output within the constraints of the critical illness. The more severe a valvular lesion, the narrower the window for optimal management.

The Pathophysiology of Valvular Disease

Valvular lesions are clinically important because they limit cardiac output, create abnormal chamber pressures, engender rhythm disturbances, provide a nidus for infection, predispose to systemic embolism, or generate ventricular ischemia. The pathophysiology of each specific valvular lesion will be considered shortly. However, certain fundamental principles apply to all valves. Any valvular lesion may be asymptomatic and undetected, becoming manifest only during critical illness. This may be seen as a hemodynamic response to an illness far worse than would be expected from the illness itself. Moreover, valvular lesions may create abnormal chest radiographs, intravascular pressures, or vascular waveforms which are easily misinterpreted if the valvular lesion is not diagnosed. For example, if a patient with respiratory distress is found to have cephalization of blood flow and a pulmonary capillary wedge pressure of 25, most physicians would make a diagnosis of cardiogenic pulmonary edema. If the patient has severe, chronic mitral stenosis, however, these findings do not clearly indicate volume overload and are even consistent with hypovolemia. Obviously, misinterpretation of the hemodynamics might lead to potentially devastating management errors.

In patients with *stenotic lesions,* cardiac output is very dependent on heart rate, preload, and contractility, and less dependent on afterload. Chronic adaptation decreases the upstream chamber's compliance, making the cardiac output very sensitive to changes in preload.

Gorlin and Gorlin[1] utilized mechanical engineering principles to mathematically define the conditions across a stenotic valve. The equation for calculating the valve area is

$$A = \frac{\mathrm{CO/(EP)(HR)}}{44.3CP^{0.5}}$$

where

- CO = cardiac output, mL/min
- A = valve area, cm^2
- C = constant unique to aortic or mitral valve ($C = 1.0$ for aortic, tricuspid, and pulmonic valves and $C = 0.85$ for mitral valves)
- P = transvalvular pressure gradient
- EP = systolic (aortic) or diastolic (mitral) ejection period (sec)
- HR = heart rate (min^{-1})

The Gorlin formula does have its limitations. It assumes a steady axisymmetric flow through a fixed orifice; it neglects the viscous properties of blood; and it is somewhat inaccurate at extreme transvalvular pressure differences and low cardiac outputs. Corrections must be made for valves which are simultaneously stenotic and insufficient where the valve area may be underestimated. The constant is an empirically derived correction factor. Little work has been done to justify this calculation on pulmonic, tricuspid, or aortic valve areas. Despite these limitations, the equation is a reliable method of calculating valve areas and making therapeutic decisions.

Maximal flow (CO) through stenotic valves requires optimizing the ejection period (HR) and pressure gradient (P). The pressure gradient is largely determined by preload and cardiac contractility.

Regurgitant lesions must be defined as acute or chronic. Minor regurgitation in an acute situation is often more catastrophic than major regurgitation in a chronic setting. Chronic lesions allow a chamber to distend and become more compliant, allowing symptoms to appear slowly. In acute lesions, however, chambers have not had time to adequately compensate, making them unable to handle the increase in preload. Regurgitant flow markedly decreases the efficiency of the heart and increases its O_2 consumption. Inotropes with α-adrenergic properties (e.g., dopamine) may increase the regurgitant fraction and worsen the situation, while inotropes with β-adrenergic properties (e.g., dobutamine) generally improve the hemodynamic profile. Intraaortic balloon pumps are absolutely contraindicated in aortic insufficiency because their diastolic augmentation will increase the regurgitant flow.

Control of heart rate in the setting of a regurgitant lesion is particularly important. If the heart rate is too fast, there is too little time for forward flow, and if the heart rate is too slow, there is too much time for regurgitant flow. Decreasing afterload, increasing preload, and optimizing heart rate are the mainstays of treatment for regurgitant lesions.

Mixed lesions are a tremendous clinical challenge. Management requires achieving optimal cardiac output by diagnosing and treating the most clinically significant lesion while closely monitoring the hemodynamic response.[2]

General Principles of Diagnosis and Management

DIAGNOSTIC METHODS

HISTORY AND PHYSICAL EXAMINATION

Frequently the history is nonspecific in patients with chronic valvular disease. Typical symptoms relate to a low cardiac output state, pulmonary congestion, systemic congestion, or chest discomfort. Many patients may be completely asymptomatic, especially with regurgitant lesions. The physical exam is of obvious importance; attention should be directed toward evidence of a low output state or congestion. This has been well reviewed elsewhere.[3]

ELECTROCARDIOGRAPHY

Electrocardiography (ECG) is useful in assessing the cardiac rhythm, chamber enlargement, or chamber hypertrophy. Since the ECG is frequently not sensitive nor specific, it must be interpreted with caution. This is especially important in the acute care setting where large changes in electrolytes, volume status, hemoglobin level, etc., can cause significant ECG changes. Acute valvular problems are notable for usually displaying nonspecific ECG findings unless ischemia is a precipitating factor.

NONINVASIVE IMAGING

The chest x-ray is important in looking for pulmonary vascular redistribution, chamber size, and underlying pulmonary pathology (see Chap. 19).

Echocardiography has revolutionized the noninvasive approach to valvular heart disease. The risk is negligible even in critically ill patients. It is less risky and can easily be performed at the bedside. Echocardiography can quantify regurgitant and stenotic valve lesions, assess left ventricular function, estimate pulmonary artery pressures, visualize the valves, and help direct therapy (see Chap. 21). With the advent of Doppler and transesophageal echocardiography, accuracy correlates well with that of cardiac catheterization. Chamber compliance and loading conditions can be closely estimated with echocardiography. If transthoracic echocardiography is difficult because of concurrent obesity, ventilator management, or lung disease, then transesophageal echocardiography should be performed (see Chap. 22).

Nuclear imaging in the intensive care unit (ICU) setting is logistically difficult. A gallium scan is occasionally helpful in diagnosing and managing bacterial endocarditis, especially in patients with fever of unknown origin. A thallium scan may identify ischemic causes of valve failure. Generally, however, sufficient information can be achieved with echocardiography with less difficulty.

INVASIVE DIAGNOSIS

A pulmonary artery catheter (see Chap. 25) is necessary in managing most patients in the ICU setting who have significant underlying valvular disease. Frequent assessment of cardiac output and pulmonary capillary wedge pressure for loading conditions are all necessary for proper management. Ideally a "paceport" pulmonary artery catheter should be used in case it becomes necessary to adjust heart rate or treat new heart block, a common complication of valvular heart disease.

Left heart catheterization, performed in a cardiac catheterization laboratory, usually is indicated after all medical modalities have been exhausted and a definite surgical intervention or valvuloplasty must be performed (see Chap. 26). The purpose of left heart catheterization is to clarify left ventricular (LV) hemodynamics and LV function. The seriousness of valve stenosis or insufficiency can be well demonstrated. If surgical correction is planned, coronary angiography is necessary in case concurrent coronary bypass grafts are indicated.

GENERAL ASPECTS OF MANAGEMENT

Carefully serial histories and repeated physical examinations are more valuable than high technology. Either may provide clues to subtle valvular deterioration. Management of all valvular lesions during superimposed critical illness requires arterial blood pressure monitoring, pulmonary artery pressure monitoring (see Chap. 25), and utilization of radiology, echocardiography, and other diagnostic modalities. Underlying medical conditions must aggressively be treated since these will directly affect the loading conditions, heart rate, and contractility. In particular, other determinants of oxygen delivery should be maximized and oxygen consumption should be reduced. Lowering oxygen consumption may be as simple as treating fever or controlling agitation. In extreme circumstances, such as critical hemodynamic compromise, even the oxygen consumption of normal movement and breathing must be reduced by initiating muscle relaxation and mechanical ventilation. Finally, patients with valvular disease must have appropriate antibiotic prophylaxis for surgical procedures (see Table 122-1).

TABLE 122-1 Recommendations for Antibiotic Prophylaxis for the Prevention of Bacterial Endocarditis

Upper Respiratory Procedures	
Oral	
Amoxicillin	3 g 1 h before procedure and 1.5 g 6 h later
Penicillin allergy:	
Erythromycin	1 g 2 h before procedure and 500 mg 6 h later
Parenteral	
Ampicillin	2 g IM or IV 30 min before procedure
plus Gentamicin	1.5 mg/kg IM or IV 30 min before procedure
Penicillin allergy:	
Vancomycin	1 g IV infused *slowly* over 1 h beginning 1 h before procedure
Gastrointestinal and Genitourinary Procedures	
Oral	
Amoxicillin	3 g 1 h before procedure and 1.5 g 6 h later
Parenteral	
Ampicillin	2 g IM or IV 30 min before procedure
plus Gentamicin	1.5 mg/kg IM or IV 30 min before procedure
Penicillin allergy:	
Vancomycin	1 g IV infused *slowly* over 1 h beginning 1 h before procedure
plus Gentamicin	1.5 mg/kg IM or IV 30 min before procedure

SOURCE: Adapted from the Medical Letter, vol 31, issue 807, December 15, 1989, p 112.

Aortic Stenosis

Aortic stenosis can involve the supravalvular, valvular, or subvalvular areas. Supravalvular aortic stenosis is a rare congenital disorder. There is also a very rare congenital type of membranous subaortic stenosis. Thus, the vast majority of patients with aortic stenosis have *valvular* stenosis whether from rheumatic heart disease, a bicuspid valve, or calcific valvular disease. Hypertrophic cardiomyopathy is incorrectly known as idiopathic hypertrophic subaortic stenosis; because there is no primary valve abnormality, it best fits in the family of cardiomyopathies. Nevertheless, it will be considered in this chapter.

PATHOPHYSIOLOGY

Obstruction to flow through the aortic orifice limits LV ejection. Therefore, stroke volume, cardiac output, and mean aortic pressure fall, while mean LV systolic pressure rises. Heart rate and contractility typically increase in order to compensate for reduced stroke volume. Finally, the left ventricle dilates (preload increases) in order to create higher intracavitary pressures and thereby generate a higher transvalvular pressure gradient (see Fig. 122-1). This combination of increased preload, afterload, contractility, and heart rate increases myocardial oxygen demand. At the same time, the reduced mean aortic pressure and impaired diastolic filling, compounded by increased LV wall tension, limit LV coronary flow. As stenosis progresses, or as new demands for cardiac output are superimposed by critical illness, myocardial oxygen demands outpace oxygen supply, leading to ischemia, arrhythmia, and death. On this substrate, reduced systemic vascular resistance (SVR), whether due to sepsis or to vasodilating drugs, can be potentially lethal. In contrast to the more usual congestive cardiomyopathy in which vasodilation reduces afterload and improves cardiac output, in the setting of aortic stenosis, the valve lesion prevents any increase in cardiac output. Therefore, the mean aortic pressure simply drops, further reducing myocardial perfusion.

In chronic aortic stenosis, compensatory mechanisms lead to LV dilation and hypertrophy, with a consequent reduction in ventricular compliance. Thus patients become unusually sensitive to small reductions in filling pressure. Further, this impaired compliance (and resulting high filling pressures) leads to atrial hypertension and hypertrophy and, eventually, to pulmonary hypertension.

CLINICAL PRESENTATION

The classic triad of aortic stenosis includes angina, dyspnea on exertion, or syncope. These classic symptoms may be preceded by dizziness or fatigue. Many patients are asymptomatic. Critically ill patients may manifest angina from increased cardiac oxygen consumption, syncope from altered hemodynamics or arrhythmias, and dyspnea from LV dysfunction.

The peripheral pulses (reflecting the reduced stroke volume) are of small amplitude and rise and diminish slowly (pulsus parvus et tardus). The blood pressure is often surprisingly normal but only at the cost of increased SVR. The left ventricle can be easily palpated, occasionally with a systolic thrill. Auscultation reveals an ejection click followed by a crescendo-decrescendo murmur and a faint or absent second heart sound. A fourth heart sound is frequently prominent due to the poorly compliant left ventricle. Concomitant diastolic regurgitant aortic murmurs are not uncommon. LV dysfunction, manifested by a third heart sound or signs of pulmonary edema, is associated with a poor prognosis. Concurrent pulmonary hypertension is an especially foreboding sign.[4]

Aortic *stenosis* can mimic aortic *sclerosis*. Both tend to have prominent fourth heart sounds followed by an aortic ejection click with a 3–4/6 crescendo-decrescendo murmur. Both can have evidence of valvular insufficiency and a systolic thrill. Aortic stenosis is unique clinically by having a sustained LV impulse with an attenuated-delayed carotid upstroke. The carotid upstroke in aortic sclerosis is usually normal. The aortic component of the second heart sound is diminished or absent in aortic stenosis as is the aortic ejection click (in severe disease). Pulmonic valve closure is

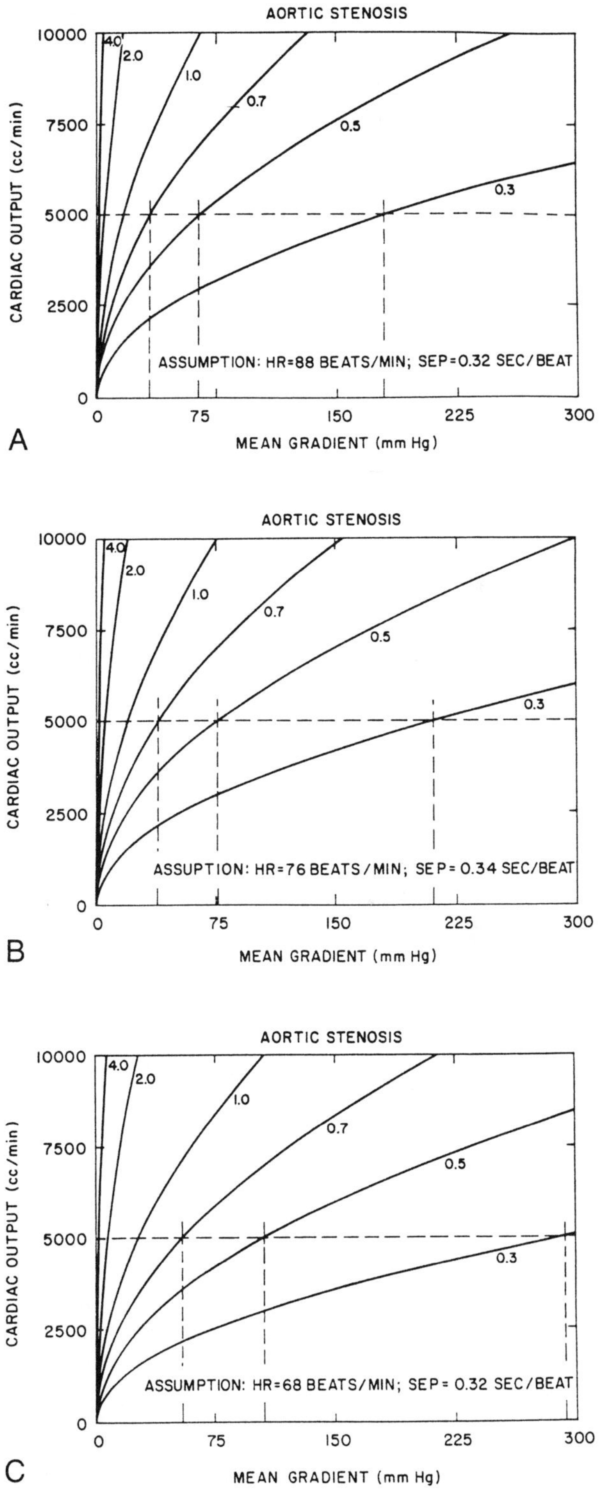

FIGURE 122-1 Relationships between cardiac output and mean aortic systolic pressure gradient in patients with aortic stenosis, calculated using the Gorlin equation. The individual curves represent orifice areas of 4.0, 2.0, 1.0, 0.7, 0.5, and 0.3 cm^2. A, B, and C represent flow-gradient relations at differing heart rates and systolic ejection periods. (From Grossman W: *Cardiac Catheterization and Angiography*, 4th ed. p 159. Philadelphia, Lea and Febiger, 1991. Courtesy of Dr. James J. Ferguson III.)

prominent in aortic stenosis and may be mistaken for A_2, where pulmonic valve closure is normal in aortic sclerosis. Generally, the aortic valve is much more calcified in aortic stenosis. Evidence of pulmonary hypertension is unusual in aortic sclerosis. An echocardiogram should be obtained if the above objective parameters suggest aortic stenosis. If the history includes rheumatic fever, angina, congestive heart failure (CHF), or syncope with an aortic valvular murmur, an echocardiogram is indicated.

DIAGNOSTIC TESTS

The *ECG* usually reveals LV hypertrophy (LVH) with a "strain" pattern. There is often poor R wave progression which may mimic an anterior infarction. Severe disease may lead to left bundle branch block or anterior hemiblock. Atrial fibrillation is uncommon and suggests ischemic heart disease or concomitant mitral valve disease. The *chest x-ray* may be normal or may reveal a large heart. Poststenotic aortic dilation and pulmonary vascular redistribution should be sought.[5] *Echocardiography* is the mainstay of diagnosis. This can reveal valve morphology, valve mobility, LVH, LV function, pulmonary hypertension, and, most importantly, the transvalvular gradient. If aortic stenosis is suspected, an immediate echocardiogram should be performed.[6] Right heart catheterization is not helpful in diagnosing aortic stenosis but is useful in its management (vide infra). It also helps in risk stratification if pulmonary hypertension is found. Low cardiac output suggests a late stage of disease.

MANAGEMENT

Medical management of critically ill patients with aortic stenosis is limited primarily to adjusting preload and contractility. Obviously, any underlying medical condition must be very aggressively treated. Preload should first be optimized with the guidance of a pulmonary artery catheter. The pulmonary capillary wedge pressure should be as high as clinically acceptable. If further medical interventions are needed, contractility may be increased with judicious use of dopamine or dobutamine, optimizing cardiac output to maintain perfusion to vital organs. Efforts should be made to keep the cardiac output at minimal necessary levels when using inotropes. Efforts to go above minimal necessary values will increase oxygen consumption which may lead to ischemia, arrhythmias, or LV dysfunction. Since afterload is fixed by the stenosis, unloading agents [nitroprusside, angiotensin-converting enzyme (ACE) inhibitors] or antianginals (nitrates) must be used with *extreme* caution. They are seldom helpful, and, more importantly, catastrophic hypotension can occur with even small amounts of these agents. Vasoconstrictors may result in chest pain or dyspnea and increase the likelihood of arrhythmias due to increased cardiac oxygen consumption. If serious arrhythmias occur, urgent mechanical interventions (surgical, valvuloplasty, or intraaortic balloon pump) must be considered. If angina occurs, aggressive efforts to intervene must include the judicious use of intravenous nitrates, heparinization, and a reduction in the dose of inotropes. If these measures fail, an intraaortic balloon pump should be inserted and mechanical correction performed without delay. Intraaortic balloon counterpulsation should be an intermediate supportive measure prior to surgery or valvuloplasty. Generally, the aortic valve should be replaced if the aortic valve area is less than 0.75 cm^2 or 0.6 cm/m^2 body surface area (BSA). This may not be the case in the critically ill patient. Moderate aortic stenosis may amplify any symptoms of a supervening critical illness. If symptoms are refractory despite maximal medical management, a moderately stenotic valve should have either a valvuloplasty or be replaced.

Prior to a definitive intervention, a full cardiac catheterization should be performed to assess the transvalvular gradient, LV function, and the coronary anatomy. This will aid in determining the proper procedure. If the risk of coronary disease is low, echocardiography may be sufficient for a preoperative evaluation, although this point remains controversial.[7–9]

Ideally, patients with aortic stenosis refractory to medical management should have a valve replacement, since aortic valvuloplasty has a high short-term (less than 1 year) restenosis rate. However, surgery is often not possible in an unstable patient. The decision for urgent surgery should be based on the underlying illness, the patient's short-term prognosis, LV function, the presence of infection, the patient's age, and complicating medical problems [chronic obstructive pulmonary disease (COPD), cerebrovascular accident (CVA), etc.]. If surgical correction is feasible, immediate surgery should be performed. Generally, a bioprosthetic valve should be used to avoid the need for anticoagulation. This is especially true in the older population. If surgery is not feasible, then valvuloplasty is an excellent short-term (approximately 6 months) temporizing procedure which should allow the patient to recover adequately from the other medical problems (see Chap. 26). Valve replacement can then be done at a later date. Valvuloplasty may improve the hemodynamics enough to allow liberation from a ventilator, decrease the angina enough to minimize antianginal agents, or decrease the marked sensitivity to loading conditions.

Aortic Insufficiency

Aortic insufficiency has multiple etiologies, many of them from systemic disorders. These include the connective tissue abnormalities of Reiter's syndrome, ankylosing spondylitis, Marfan's syndrome, Ehlers-Danlos syndrome, and even rheumatoid arthritis (see Table 122-2). Syphilis and

TABLE 122-2 Etiologies of Aortic Insufficiency

Rheumatic heart disease	Ehlers-Danlos syndrome
Endocarditis	Ankylosing spondylitis
Syphilis	Reiter's syndrome
Dissecting aortic aneurysm	Rheumatoid arthritis
Marfan's syndrome	Bicuspid aortic valve

rheumatic fever are both well-known causes of chronic aortic insufficiency. Acutely, bacterial endocarditis and aortic dissection are the most common causes of aortic insufficiency. Blunt trauma is a rare cause.[10]

PATHOPHYSIOLOGY

Regurgitant flow requires a larger stroke volume to produce an effective cardiac output. This requires more work from the left ventricle during systole, resulting in higher oxygen consumption. Diastole is also compromised in aortic insufficiency. The ventricle receives blood not only from the left atrium but from the regurgitant aortic volume as well. This volume overload demands that the ventricle dilate to optimize Starling forces leading to an increased stroke volume. The ventricle becomes relatively more compliant to handle the larger diastolic volumes, so the LV end-diastolic pressure (LVEDP) initially remains in the normal range. Clinically, this physiologic adaptation results in a relatively high systolic blood pressure and a lower diastolic blood pressure (wide pulse pressure). The severity of regurgitation is dependent upon **1.** the size of the regurgitant orifice, **2.** the pressure difference between aortic and LV diastolic pressures, **3.** the effectiveness of systole (to generate forward flow), **4.** the duration of diastole, and **5.** SVR. Eventually, LVH occurs which increases the stiffness of the ventricle, raising the LVEDP. This leads to impairment of oxygen delivery through the coronary arteries and, combined with the elevated oxygen consumption, results in a chronic, often low-grade ischemia which eventually decreases both systolic and diastolic function. Pulmonary congestion and decreased tissue perfusion then occur. Underlying coronary artery disease only serves to accelerate this process.

In acute aortic insufficiency, the pathophysiology is quite different. The ventricle has not had adequate time to compensate by becoming more compliant. It is unable to dilate to handle the larger regurgitant volumes. The pericardium may limit the amount of dilation of the acutely decompensated ventricle, markedly increasing the EDPs. The size of the ventricle remains relatively normal. The aortic EDP becomes more important in determining ventricular diastolic pressure and may even equalize with the LVEDP in late diastole, a phenomenon known as *diastasis*. Diastasis can also be seen in very severe, chronic aortic insufficiency. Diastasis manifests at slower heart rates or on compensatory pauses after a premature ventricular contraction (PVC), at pressures of about 40 to 60 mmHg (see Figs. 122-2 and 122-3). Severe regurgitation can result in the LVEDP being greater than the left atrial pressure (LAP) causing premature closure of the mitral valve. This serves to protect the pulmonary vasculature from pulmonary edema. In this instance, the LAP, judged by the pulmonary capillary wedge pressure (PCWP), may underestimate the LVEDP. The increased LVEDP and lower aortic diastolic pressure results in diminished myocardial perfusion which limits oxygen delivery to the myocardium. This, in combination with the increased oxygen consumption of the acutely stressed ventricle, can accelerate the patient's hemodynamic demise.

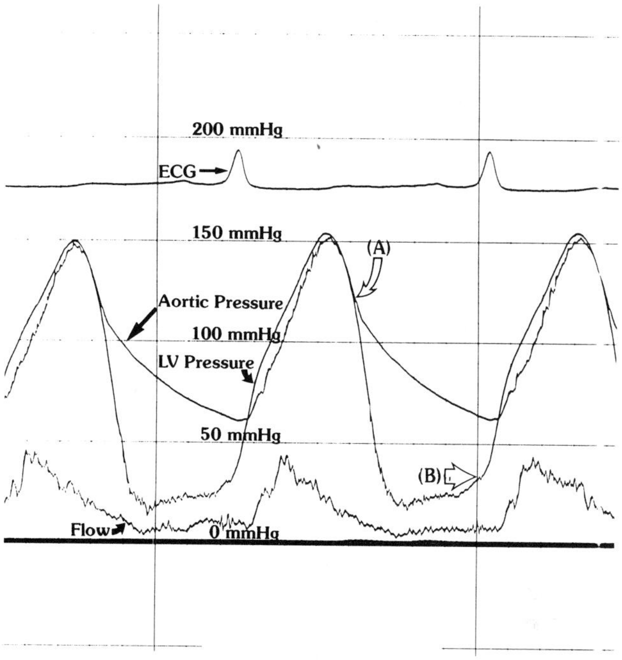

FIGURE 122-2 This tracing represents simultaneous monitoring of the LV and aortic pressure in a patient with severe chronic aortic insufficiency. Note can be made of the wide pulse pressure. Also, the compensatory pause after a premature ventricular contraction yields a longer diastolic filling time. The aortic diastolic pressure equals the left ventricular end-diastolic pressure (point A), a phenomenon known as diastasis. Also, at point B, the shorter diastolic filling time decreases the aortic regurgitant flow resulting in a narrow pulse pressure.

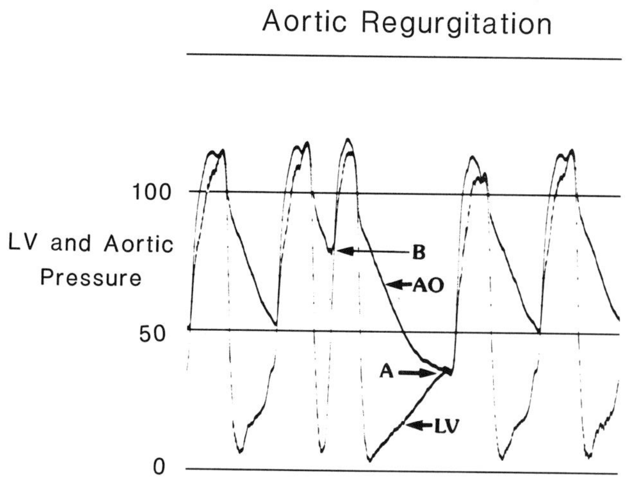

FIGURE 122-3 Simultaneous pressure (and flow) tracing of the left ventricle and aorta in a patient with severe aortic insufficiency. Normally the aortic valve closes at A, but aortic pressure progressively decreases as blood flows retrograde into the ventricle. The aortic diastolic pressure decreases toward the left ventricular end-diastolic pressure (B) (the LV equivalent to the pulmonary capillary wedge pressure). If they equalize, diastasis occurs. The left ventricular end-diastolic pressure is elevated at nearly 30 mmHg suggesting a less compliant ventricle. Notice also the wide aortic pulse pressure.

TABLE 122-3 Comparison of Hemodynamic and Angiographic Findings in Acute and Chronic Aortic Regurgitation*

Datum	Acute Regurgitation	Chronic Regurgitation	*P* Value
Age, year	33 ± 14	40 ± 15	NS†
Regurgitant fraction	0.6 ± 0.1	0.7 ± 0.1	NS
LVEDP, mmHg	41 ± 12	36 ± 13	NS
Ejection fraction	0.6 ± 0.1	0.6 ± 0.1	NS
Heart rate, beats/min	108 ± 15	71 ± 14	<0.0005
Left ventricular volumes, (mL/m^2)			
EDV	146 ± 28	264 ± 64	<0.0005
ESV	57 ± 23	101 ± 42	<0.025
SV	89 ± 22	163 ± 57	<.005
Aortic pressure, mmHg			
Systolic	110 ± 14	155 ± 26	<0.0005
Diastolic	56 ± 11	50 ± 6	NS
Mean	78 ± 12	90 ± 8	<0.025
Pulse pressure, mmHg	55 ± 7	105 ± 22	<0.0005
Systemic vascular resistance (dyn·s·cm^{-5})	1326 ± 372	1341 ± 461	NS

*Mean ±standard deviation. EDV—end-diastolic volume, ESV—end-systolic volume, SV—stroke volume, and LVEDP—left ventricular end-diastolic pressure.
†Not significant.
SOURCE: From Mann T et al.: Assessing the hemodynamic severity of acute aortic regurgitation due to infective endocarditis. N Engl J Med 293:108, 1975.

If an acute event occurs on a chronically insufficient valve, the hemodynamic and clinical consequences will largely be dependent on the level of LV compensation prior to the acute event. Table 122-3 summarizes the hemodynamic differences between acute and chronic aortic insufficiency.

CLINICAL PRESENTATION

Angina may be an early symptom due to the increased myocardial oxygen requirements and the low aortic diastolic pressure. Nevertheless, patients with severe chronic aortic insufficiency may be surprisingly asymptomatic until a critical illness occurs. Typical symptoms of dyspnea and fatigue then occur. Patients are usually sensitive to hypovolemia.[11]

The exam is notable for a hyperdynamic precordium and a wide pulse pressure. The peripheral pulses are brisk with a rapid runoff. There is a systolic (high flow) murmur in the aortic area with a diastolic blowing murmur. The Austin Flint murmur is a diastolic murmur heard near the apex representing regurgitant flow impinging on the mitral valve.

When a critical illness supervenes in a patient with chronic aortic insufficiency, these symptoms and signs are magnified. Dyspnea is especially useful as a clue to decompensation of aortic insufficiency. Any illness which increases afterload increases the regurgitant fraction and will likely worsen the patient's symptoms. Similarly, administration of catecholamines may paradoxically make the patient worse, rather than better. Hypovolemia is also poorly tolerated since a reduction in end-diastolic volume leads to a reduced stroke volume even if the regurgitant fraction doesn't change.

Acute aortic insufficiency is a medical and surgical emergency. Since the ventricle has not had adequate time to compensate, it is relatively stiff (noncompliant). Therefore, the acute increment in end-diastolic volume due to the regurgitant flow causes a dramatic rise in the end-diastolic pressure to nearly aortic diastolic pressure (diastasis), and pulmonary edema ensues. The physical exam is notable for pulmonary edema, hypotension, and clinical shock. The peripheral signs so well demonstrated in chronic aortic insufficiency are not as clinically evident in acute insufficiency.[12]

DIAGNOSTIC TESTS

It is important to determine, as soon as possible, whether aortic insufficiency is acute or chronic. In chronic aortic insufficiency the ECG often shows LVH and left atrial enlargement. If the ECG is normal except for marked sinus tachycardia, an acute lesion is more likely. Heart block is an uncommon finding. Echocardiography is of great assistance since it can assess LV size and function as well as the amount of regurgitation. It also facilitates evaluation of the aortic root, valve morphology, the presence of vegetations, and the stiffness of the ventricle. The echocardiogram also can demonstrate mitral valve preclosure.[13] Right heart catheterization in a patient with chronic, asymptomatic disease will reveal normal pressures and cardiac output. In acute regurgitation, the PCWP will be significantly elevated (greater than 20) with a low cardiac output. Severe chronic aortic insufficiency can mimic acute aortic insufficiency, except the LV is of normal size in the latter.

MANAGEMENT

Management of regurgitant lesions requires improving forward flow while minimizing the regurgitant fraction. In an unstable patient, this therapy should be guided by a pulmonary artery catheter. Afterload reduction is the first intervention and is best accomplished acutely with nitroprusside unless refractory hypotension is present. Oral vasodilators are best avoided in the acute care setting. Pulmonary edema may require a loop diuretic, and early intubation should be considered. If afterload reduction fails to improve cardiac output and pulmonary congestion, an inotrope should be added. Dobutamine is an ideal choice because of its purely beta properties and afterload reduction. Low-dose dopamine should be given as well for its ability to augment renal blood flow. Amrinone is a useful alternative because of its afterload-reducing properties coupled with its ability to increase contractility. However, its half-life is longer, so it may be difficult to titrate. Norepinephrine should be avoided unless complete cardiovascular collapse occurs because it increases systemic vascular resistance and will likely worsen the degree of insufficiency. Intraaortic balloon counterpulsation is contraindicated since it merely serves to increase regurgitation and worsen symptoms.

Care must also be taken to avoid both excessive tachycardia which decreases forward flow, and bradycardia (an uncommon problem in acute aortic insufficiency) which increases regurgitant flow. Tachycardia can be difficult to control, but increases in preload along with cautious use of digoxin (with its indirect vagal effects) may be adequate. Verapamil and β blockers may decrease contractility more than they decrease heart rate and so are unlikely to be of benefit. Aggressive volume administration may be necessary to maximize preload, even if this requires ventilatory assistance. Bradycardia is best avoided by using dobutamine or a pacemaker. Isoproterenol can be considered as a temporizing measure until a pacemaker can be placed, but it is highly arrhythmogenic. Its use is also limited because of its marked vasodilator properties. These vasoactive drugs are adjusted as needed until an optimal cardiac output is obtained. The adjustment must be individualized because of variations in LV function, loading conditions, and the severity of valvular insufficiency.

Ancillary measures applicable in all patients include antibiotic prophylaxis for indicated procedures and aggressive treatment of arrhythmias. Atrial arrhythmias are uncommon, but ventricular arrhythmias occur in the acute setting. Lidocaine and procainamide can be given intravenously and are usually adequate. Digitalis is frequently useful in treating mild heart failure of chronic aortic insufficiency.

If medical management fails, surgery must be recommended. Surgical consultation is best obtained early in the course of management. In chronic lesions, all attempts at medical therapy should be tried. In acute insufficiency, the valve must be replaced at the earliest sign of hemodynamic compromise since further severe compromise may occur with little warning. To delay surgery in an effort to improve the patient's condition usually results in further deterioration, increasing the risk of surgical correction. A cardiac catheterization should be performed (if possible) to assess coronary status and LV function, at least in patients in whom there is a suspicion of coronary artery disease. This may be unnecessary in the younger patient with no risk factors. Early correction can maintain good LV function.[14]

Mitral Stenosis

Mitral stenosis (MS) is simply resistance to diastolic flow through the mitral valve. Its cause is usually rheumatic heart disease, but atrial myxomas, vegetations, and thrombi can also obstruct mitral flow.

PATHOPHYSIOLOGY

Mitral stenosis represents the restriction of blood flow from the left atrium and pulmonary veins into the left ventricle from a narrowed mitral valve. The normal mitral valve area is 4.5 to 6 cm^2. Symptoms usually are not noticed until the valve area is reduced to roughly 1.5 cm^2, and replacement is usually not necessary until it falls further to 1 cm^2 or less. Symptoms are not necessarily proportional to the degree of stenosis. Patients with mitral stenosis require a long diastolic filling period (DFP) to allow blood to maximally fill the left ventricle. Cardiac output is, of course, based on heart rate and stroke volume, and if the DFP is too long, the cardiac output will fall due to a decreased heart rate. If the DFP is too short (as in sinus tachycardia or atrial fibrillation), the cardiac output will drop as well due to inadequate LV filling and small stroke volumes. Thus, patients who are critically ill may paradoxically decrease their cardiac output when a tachycardic response to a physiologic stress occurs. Because of the limited filling of the left ventricle, the pulmonary veins become congested and pulmonary edema occurs. In order to compensate for the inability to increase cardiac output, the arteriovenous oxygen content difference may widen. Over time, the left atrium enlarges and the pulmonary lymphatic drainage increases. The resulting high pulmonary venous pressures eventually lead to pulmonary arterial hypertension. In severe cases, the LAP can reach 25 to 30 mmHg or greater. The atrial contribution to cardiac output can reach as high as 20 percent which can often mean the difference between hemodynamic stability and hemodynamic compromise. In sinus rhythm, the pulmonary capillary wedge pressure shows both prominent a and v waves with a delayed y descent. In irregular rhythms, the PCWP can vary from beat to beat, so an average of many cycles (at least 10) is required for a proper pressure analysis. Pulmonary manifestations of mitral stenosis include increased lung stiffness, decreased lung volumes, and a variable degree of airway obstruction.

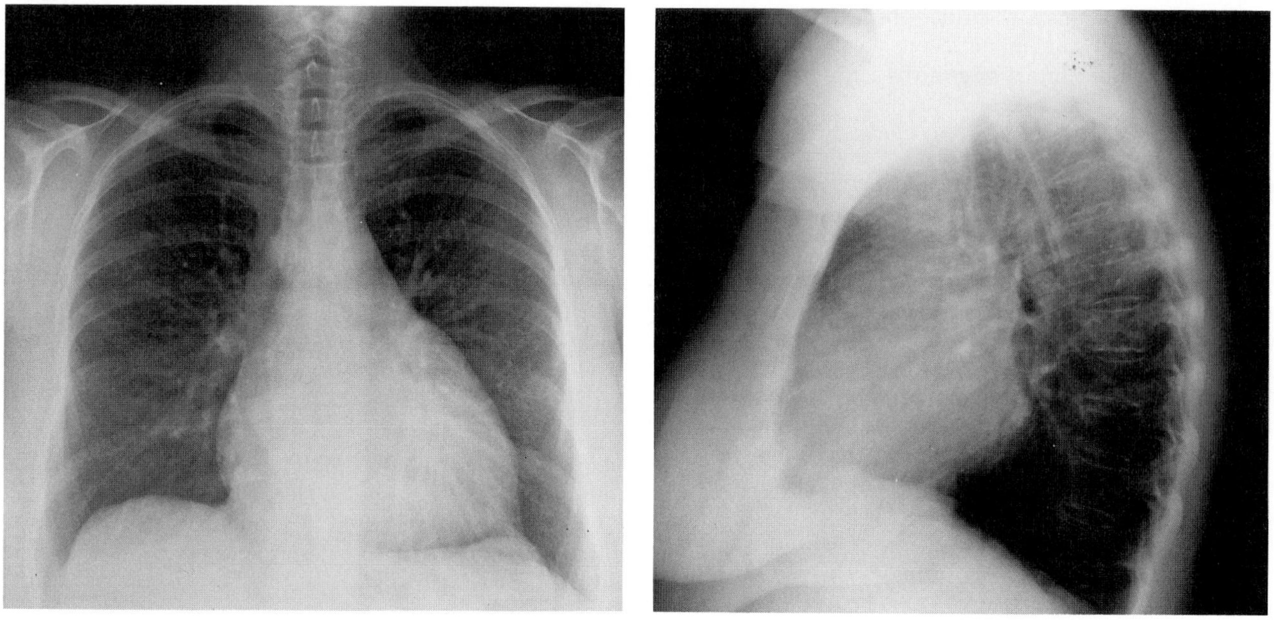

FIGURE 122-4 A chest radiograph in a patient with mitral stenosis revealing the enlarged left atrium and the calcified mitral valve.

CLINICAL PRESENTATION

MS may remain subclinical until an acute illness intervenes. A common presentation is dyspnea, with or without hemoptysis, due to pulmonary edema. Patients may also complain of chest pain or exhibit symptoms of left atrial enlargement such as hoarseness or palpitations. There may be systemic manifestations of clot embolization. The exam is notable for a normal to low blood pressure with an increased S_1, increased P_2, and a prominent opening snap followed by a diastolic murmur with presystolic attenuation. It is the *length* of the murmur, not the loudness, that determines severity. There are signs of pulmonary congestion and pulmonary hypertension in many patients.

DIAGNOSTIC TESTS

The ECG can be helpful by revealing left atrial enlargement or atrial fibrillation with or without right ventricular hypertrophy. The chest x-ray can show the large left atrium with evidence of pulmonary congestion (see Fig. 122-4). A calcified valve may be seen. The echocardiogram is particularly valuable in the diagnosis and management of these patients. It can evaluate left atrial size, valve structure and function, orifice size, presence or absence of vegetations, and the pulmonary artery pressure. Doppler echocardiography can assess the severity of the gradient and estimate cardiac output.[15] The right heart catheterization is helpful both in the diagnosis and management of MS. The pulmonary capillary wedge (PCW) tracing shows an increased *a* wave (if the patient is in sinus rhythm) with a normal to increased *v* wave. The PCW pressures are usually in the 20 to 30 mmHg range. It is important to remember that the PCW pressure reflects left atrial pressure but no longer indicates LVEDP. The PCW pressure is heart-rate dependent (vide supra). In this setting, LV volume (preload) may be inadequate despite a high PCW pressure. It is often necessary to supplement the information obtained from the pulmonary artery catheter with echocardiography. There may be pulmonary hypertension, and the cardiac output is usually normal to decreased. Prolonged balloon inflation can precipitate hemoptysis in patients with MS, so occlusion times should be limited to the minimum necessary for proper evaluation.

MANAGEMENT

Management of critically ill patients with MS is extremely difficult. The controllable factors are preload, heart rate, and, to a small extent, contractility. Patients are extremely sensitive to afterload reduction requiring extreme caution when vasodilators are used. Small increases in preload can lead to pulmonary edema [especially when the lung is damaged, as adult respiratory distress syndrome (ARDS)], while small reductions in preload can precipitate hypotension. Careful diuresis or volume repletion, guided by a pulmonary catheter, echocardiography, and frequent exams is necessary.

As discussed in the pathophysiology section, tachycardia can actually decrease cardiac output. A shortened diastolic filling period does not allow adequate ventricular filling. Alternatively, if the diastolic filling period is too long, the heart-rate contribution to cardiac output is diminished and cardiac output again falls. Most patients have an optimal range of cardiac output, and this must be determined carefully on an individual basis. This will vary with any change in loading conditions or level of cardiac function. Frequent clinical assessments or cardiac output determinations will aid in optimizing heart rate.

To control refractory (supraventricular) tachycardia, careful use of a β blocker or calcium channel blocker is indicated. This is necessary if any supraventricular tachycardia supervenes (atrial fibrillation/flutter, multifocal atrial tachycardia, marked sinus tachycardia) which results in clinical deterioration or a significant decrease in cardiac output. Ideally a short-acting drug should be used because of the inability to predict response, side effects, or changing loading conditions. Esmolol is a good initial choice because of its rapid titration and short duration of action (see Chap. 125). If there is a contraindication to β blockers, cautious administration of verapamil or diltiazem can be attempted, although hypotension may occur. Obviously, aggressive treatment of the underlying disease is preferred over drug therapy. Symptomatic reentrant AV nodal tachycardias can be treated with adenosine which has very good efficacy with a short duration of action. Adenosine is given as a 6-mg rapid intravenous bolus which can be repeated in 2 min with 12 mg if no clinical response occurs. Its short duration of action ($t_{1/2}$ is 10 s) limits side effects. It is ideal to give this via a central venous catheter to optimize its effect and limit dilution. It should not be used if the patient has greater than first-degree heart block unless a pacemaker is present. Intravenous verapamil can also be used, but extreme care must be exercised because of its afterload-reducing qualities. Digoxin is generally not a good medication for controlling the sinus rate but may be helpful for other reasons (vide infra). If medications are not effective or they are contraindicated because of hypotension or LV dysfunction, mechanical correction must occur.

Atrial fibrillation is often a catastrophic complication, so prevention of atrial arrhythmias must be a goal of therapy. Digoxin may aid in the prevention of atrial fibrillation, although this is controversial. At a minimum, it will help prevent the rapid (and life-threatening) ventricular response if atrial fibrillation occurs. We therefore recommend routinely using digoxin in critically ill patients with MS. A type IA antiarrhythmic drug should be strongly considered if rhythm strips reveal frequent premature atrial contractions (PACs) in an unstable patient. Procainamide is an excellent first choice because of the ability to administer it intravenously. Procainamide can be given intravenously at 20 mg/min until **1.** hypotension occurs, **2.** the QRS or QT widen by greater than 50 percent, or **3.** 1 g of procainamide is given (750 mg for small individuals). In emergent situations, 750 mg to 1 g can be *carefully* given over 20 to 30 minutes, monitoring again for the above side effects. A maintenance infusion of 2 to 4 mg/kg/h can then be instituted. The maintenance dose should be reduced by 50 percent if CHF or renal impairment is present. A procainamide and *N*-acetylprocainamide (NAPA) level should be drawn about 12 h later and the dose adjusted accordingly. Procainamide levels should be 4 to 8 mcg/mL and NAPA 7 to 15 mcg/mL. *Do not* use long-acting preparations in the ICU (per nasogastric tube) because breaking the pill will remove its long-acting properties. Other antiarrhythmics (again not long-acting) can be given per nasogastric tube if the patient is absorbing medications properly. If atrial fibrillation occurs and the patient is at all unstable, urgent electrical cardioversion should be performed. Beta blockers or calcium channel blockers may also be helpful in controlling the heart rate of patients who have acceptable LV function.

Another major risk of mitral stenosis is systemic clot embolization. At highest risk are patients with atrial fibrillation or left atrial enlargement. Anticoagulation is mandatory in these patients and highly recommended in those who are at all symptomatic from mitral stenosis. This should include nearly all patients in the ICU setting (see discussion on anticoagulation in valvular heart disease). One caution is that hemoptysis secondary to excessive pulmonary venous pressure may be precipitated or worsened.[16] If hemoptysis is severe, or recurrent emboli occur despite anticoagulation, surgical correction of the stenosis should be performed.

Inotropes may be attempted to increase cardiac output but are usually of little benefit.[17] If medical measures fail to maintain an adequate cardiac output, the stenosis must be repaired. Balloon valvuloplasty should be the first consideration. Patients with mitral valve disease have a much smaller restenosis rate than patients with aortic valve disease, so valvuloplasty is frequently a definitive therapy (see Chap. 26). If there is recurrent embolization or a contraindication to valvuloplasty, then valve replacement must be performed. A cardiac catheterization prior to either procedure can assess the severity of the valvular gradient, LV function, and the status of the coronary arteries. In young patients with no cardiac risk factors, an echocardiographic evaluation may be adequate, and surgical correction performed without coronary angiography.

Antibiotic prophylaxis for procedures must be routine (see Table 122-1). Ancillary measures include careful sedation and the maintenance of a slightly upright posture. Morphine is an excellent medication because it sedates, is vagotonic, decreases pulmonary vascular resistance, and is easily reversed.

Mitral Insufficiency

The fourth major valvular lesion is mitral insufficiency. As in aortic insufficiency, it is useful to distinguish acute from chronic disease. Chronic mitral regurgitation is usually caused by rheumatic fever, mitral valve prolapse, ischemic heart disease, or LV dilation from several etiologies.[18] Less common causes are various connective tissue disorders, chest trauma, and several forms of congenital heart disease. Acute mitral regurgitation usually results from papillary muscle dysfunction due to ischemic heart disease or endocarditis. Valve cusp dysfunction, especially from endocarditis, is frequently seen. Finally, acute mitral insufficiency may be related to prosthetic valve dysfunction (see section on prosthetic valves).

PATHOPHYSIOLOGY

The level of regurgitation depends upon the duration of systole, the relative incompetence of the valve, and the acuteness of the valvular disruption. The loading conditions of the ventricle, the systemic and pulmonary vascular resistances, volume status, and LV function also contribute to the severity of mitral regurgitation. Throughout the hospital stay, the relative level of mitral regurgitation may change on a day-to-day basis. Patients with moderate to severe mitral insufficiency are frequently unable to increase their cardiac output proportionate to their needs.

In chronic mitral insufficiency, the left atrium, left ventricle, and pulmonary vasculature have adequate time to compensate. The left atrium dilates and becomes more compliant, minimizing the hemodynamic stress on the pulmonary vasculature. The left ventricle has to eject a larger volume of blood as well as relax properly to accept the larger diastolic volume. This results in a larger ventricle which has increased compliance. Over time, the ventricle hypertrophies to compensate for ejecting the larger volumes. The left atrium also dilates to accept the larger volumes. As time progresses, the atrium thickens and becomes less compliant. The pulmonary vasculature requires little adaptation early in disease, but as time progresses, it responds to the rising LAP, and pulmonary hypertension ensues. In severe, chronic mitral insufficiency, the left atrium eventually becomes very poorly compliant and left atrial pressure, once normal to slightly elevated, becomes very elevated and pulmonary vascular congestion occurs. Left ventricular function (ejection fraction) appears artificially elevated because of more complete (but retrograde) emptying of the left ventricle. As the disease progresses, the LV systolic function becomes worse, but noninvasive measures will indicate artificially vigorous systolic function.

The PCWP in early, chronic mitral insufficiency is nearly normal with a slightly increased *v* wave. As the left atrium becomes thickened and less compliant, the *v* wave becomes prominent and is usually associated with pulmonary hypertension. Therefore, a large *v* wave is not necessarily diagnostic of severe mitral regurgitation. The cardiac output remains within normal limits.

Acute mitral insufficiency represents a different pathologic process. Regardless of the cause, the left atrium has not had adequate time to become compliant, so it is unable to tolerate the large volumes without increasing pressure. It will be of near normal size on echocardiography. The left ventricle has not been able to adapt by increasing compliance, so ventricular filling is impaired and forward stroke volume is significantly decreased. The pulmonary vasculature and lymphatics have not had time to adapt, and pulmonary edema is an early, rapid consequence. The PCWP is markedly elevated with a *v* wave which can reach 60 to 80 mmHg (which may be approaching the systolic blood pressure) (see the case presentation at the end of this chapter). If the *v* wave is 3 times larger than the mean PCWP, then acute mitral regurgitation can be confidently diagnosed. Lesser elevations are consistent with either an acute, chronic, or acute-on-chronic process. The cardiac output will be markedly diminished despite an artificially good ejection fraction on a two-dimensional echocardiogram.

CLINICAL PRESENTATION

Patients with chronic disease may manifest symptoms only during a critical illness. This is especially true in patients who are vasoconstricted, a situation which encourages regurgitant flow. Deterioration typically causes dyspnea and congestion. Phrenic nerve irritation due to the large left atrium may cause coughing or hoarseness. The exam will usually reveal some pulmonary congestion and neck vein distension. Neither the length nor the intensity of the murmur correlate with its severity.

Patients with acute mitral regurgitation appear critically ill, with pulmonary edema, tachycardia, and hypoperfusion. This again is because the left atrium has not had time to compensate by increasing its compliance nor has the pulmonary vasculature been able to adjust to higher pressures. Acute, moderate regurgitation is usually much more symptomatic than chronic, severe regurgitation.

DIAGNOSTIC TESTS

The ECG may reveal only left atrial enlargement in chronic disease. In acute disease, sinus tachycardia with an acute injury or infarction pattern (in ischemia-related disease) can be seen. The chest x-ray will show a large left atrium in chronic insufficiency and pulmonary edema in acute disease. An acute illness superimposed on chronic disease may cause any of the above scenarios.

Echocardiography is the most important diagnostic tool available. It can assess valve character, function, and extent of insufficiency. A flail mitral leaflet can usually be seen, as can a vegetation. The Doppler study can reveal the severity of the regurgitation and even the relative stiffness of the left atrium. If transthoracic echocardiography produces poor images, transesophageal echocardiography should be performed (see Chap. 22). Nuclear studies should be relegated to assessing the level of ischemia or infarction in acute papillary muscle rupture secondary to a myocardial infarction.[19] A gallium scan may reveal evidence of infection in the heart.

Pulmonary artery catheterization is necessary in assessing the patient's volume status. This is especially important in managing the critical combination of ARDS and mitral regurgitation. When aggressively managing mitral insufficiency, the relative height of the *v* wave in conjunction with cardiac output and blood pressure can help in guiding the efficacy of therapy. If cardiac output is unchanged or improved and the *v* wave decreased, the therapeutic intervention has been successful. A reduction in the *v* wave can also suggest deteriorating ventricular function which will result in hypotension and a decreased cardiac output. The LVEDP (preload) is best represented by the *a* wave in the wedge tracing (see Fig. 122-8).[20] Left heart catheterization should only be needed prior to surgical correction. This is necessary primarily to assess coronary status and may not be necessary in younger individuals with few risk factors.

MANAGEMENT

Hemodynamic management requires encouragement of forward flow and prevention of pulmonary edema.[21–23] This can be achieved by adjusting preload, afterload, and, to some extent, contractility. The first intervention should be to decrease afterload. In the unstable patient, nitroprusside should be used because of its very short half-life, assuming an adequate blood pressure can be maintained. Intravenous enalaprilat (which also has a relatively short half-life) is an alternative, but experience with it is not as extensive. Patients who have another underlying heart disease (e.g., cardiomyopathy, pulmonary hypertension, pericardial disease) in addition to the valve lesion may experience dramatic hypotension in response to afterload reduction. The second major therapeutic endeavor is to optimize preload. If blood pressure and cardiac output are acceptable, then preload *reduction* with intravenous nitroglycerine can be of benefit in reducing pulmonary congestion. Diuretics can be used in those patients with signs of pulmonary congestion with an adequate blood pressure. In severely hypotensive patients, extremely large volumes of fluid may be required to maintain an adequate perfusion pressure at the expense of pulmonary edema. Early ventilatory support should then be initiated.

Inotropic agents must be used with caution. Those which increase systemic vascular resistance will increase the regurgitant volume.[24] Dobutamine is an ideal first drug because of its ability to reduce pulmonary venous pressures, lower systemic vascular resistance, and increase cardiac output. Amrinone is another useful drug because of its afterload reducing ability, but early hypotension is possible. Renal doses of dopamine are usually well tolerated. Intraaortic balloon counterpulsation can also increase forward flow by reducing afterload (as long as aortic insufficiency is not present). It also augments coronary perfusion and decreases oxygen consumption, which avoids ischemia in hypotensive states, especially in patients with coronary disease. Intravenous nitroglycerine and heparin should be added if ischemia is considered the cause of papillary muscle dysfunction. Usually other evidence of ischemia is present such as ischemic ECG changes, chest pain, or evidence of an old myocardial infarction. Urgent surgery must be performed for cases refractory to medical management or if mechanical support is required.

Excessive tachycardia must be avoided and atrial fibrillation prevented. Therefore, digoxin should be given if there are no contraindications, although this remains controversial. If frequent premature atrial contractions occur, a type IA antiarrhythmic should be given (see earlier discussion on mitral stenosis). Procainamide is preferred because it can be given intravenously, but quinidine sulfate or disopyramide may be given if oral or nasogastric intake is not contraindicated. Beta blockers can be used to slow the heart rate to optimal levels, but very short acting drugs such as esmolol should be used. Verapamil should be used with caution because of its hypotensive effects. Adenosine can be used for paroxysmal AV nodal tachycardia (see management in mitral stenosis). Ancillary measures include the aggressive treatment of superimposed critical illness. Antibiotic prophylaxis is necessary prior to all indicated procedures. Finally, systemic anticoagulation should be instituted during atrial fibrillation unless there is a contraindication.

Hypertrophic Cardiomyopathy

Hypertrophic obstructive cardiomyopathy (HOCM) is an autosomal dominant disease which results in an excess of abnormal, disordered myofibrillar tissue usually located in the cardiac septum, resulting in improper cardiac function. HOCM is not really a valvular problem. Further, it is a misnomer to call it "idiopathic hypertrophic subaortic stenosis" because it incorrectly implies that stenosis is a major problem in this disease. This disease is usually confined to the left ventricle, while the right ventricle is rarely involved.

PATHOPHYSIOLOGY

The major hemodynamic abnormality in HOCM is the inability of the ventricular muscle to relax, preventing adequate LV filling (i.e., diastolic dysfunction). Systolic function is relatively preserved but uncoordinated because of the abnormal myofibrillar organization.

Early in systole, the asymmetrically hypertrophied ventricle contracts with unusual strength, promptly ejecting the majority of the stroke volume. For reasons yet unclear, the anterior mitral leaflet moves toward the septum and, instead of closing by moving posteriorly, it moves anteriorly causing systolic anterior motion (SAM) of the leaflet. This is either the result of septal distortion of the papillary muscle or the Venturi effect "pulling" on the anterior leaflet. The consequence is mitral insufficiency, which is very common in HOCM. After systole, the stiff ventricle inhibits diastolic filling. All these problems are magnified by anything that increases contractility or reduces either preload (including volume depletion) or afterload. These all cause earlier obstruction, smaller ejection volumes, and lower cardiac output. Patients are often asymptomatic at rest, but when any stress occurs, the resultant tachycardia, decreased SVR, increased catecholamines, and volume depletion can result in hypotension and pulmonary edema.

Hemodynamically, the arterial tracing may reveal a "spike and dome" contour which represents the early, forceful ejection of blood followed by the slower ejection of blood during the obstruction (see Figs. 122-5 and 122-6). The pulmonary artery catheter usually reveals normal right heart pressures with a normal to slightly decreased cardiac output at rest. The PCWP often is elevated (20 to 30 mmHg) representing the inability of the ventricle to relax. Also the

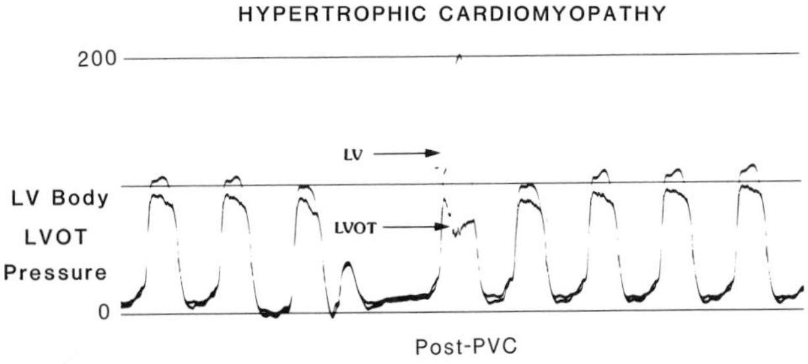

FIGURE 122-5 Tracing of hypertrophic cardiomyopathy revealing the classic spike and dome tracing. LV represents a pressure manometer in the LV body, and LVOT represents a manometer tracing in the left ventricular outflow tract. This is most prominent in a post-PVC tracing. The post-PVC beat also exaggerates the intracardiac gradient.

increased *v* wave represents the mitral insufficiency seen in HOCM.

In a left heart catheterization, the apical portion of the left ventricle can become entrapped by the septum, resulting in very high pressures in that area. The subvalvular portion of the ventricle does not become entrapped and can appear normal. The aortic pressure is either normal or reveals the spike and dome physiology.

CLINICAL PRESENTATION

Clinically, these patients often resemble those with refractory CHF. They often are young patients in whom routine treatment for CHF with diuretics and inotropes results in clinical deterioration. Syncope (or near syncope), chest pain, and dyspnea are common complaints. A positive family history is very important. It can often be missed in the elderly.

The physical exam is notable for an increased *a* wave in the jugular venous waveform and a normal *v* wave. The arterial pulse is brief and abrupt representing the spike and dome physiology. The cardiac impulse is usually lateral and sustained. There is a prominent fourth heart sound. The first heart sound is normal, followed by a late systolic murmur heard in the aortic area. The murmur gets louder with anything that unloads the heart (e.g., standing, nitrates, Valsalva) and softer with anything that increases the loading conditions (squatting, Trendelenburg). A murmur of mitral regurgitation and a third heart sound may be heard as well. The second heart sound is usually normal.

DIAGNOSTIC TESTS

The ECG reveals marked QRS voltage increases, marked T wave inversion, and poor R wave progression. Q waves can be seen in the inferior leads (pseudoinfarction). A diagnosis of LVH with an old inferior infarction suggests HOCM. The chest x-ray appears normal in most cases, but left ventricular or left atrial enlargement can be seen with nuclear studies.

The echocardiogram is the most important noninvasive diagnostic test. The echo will reveal a disproportionately

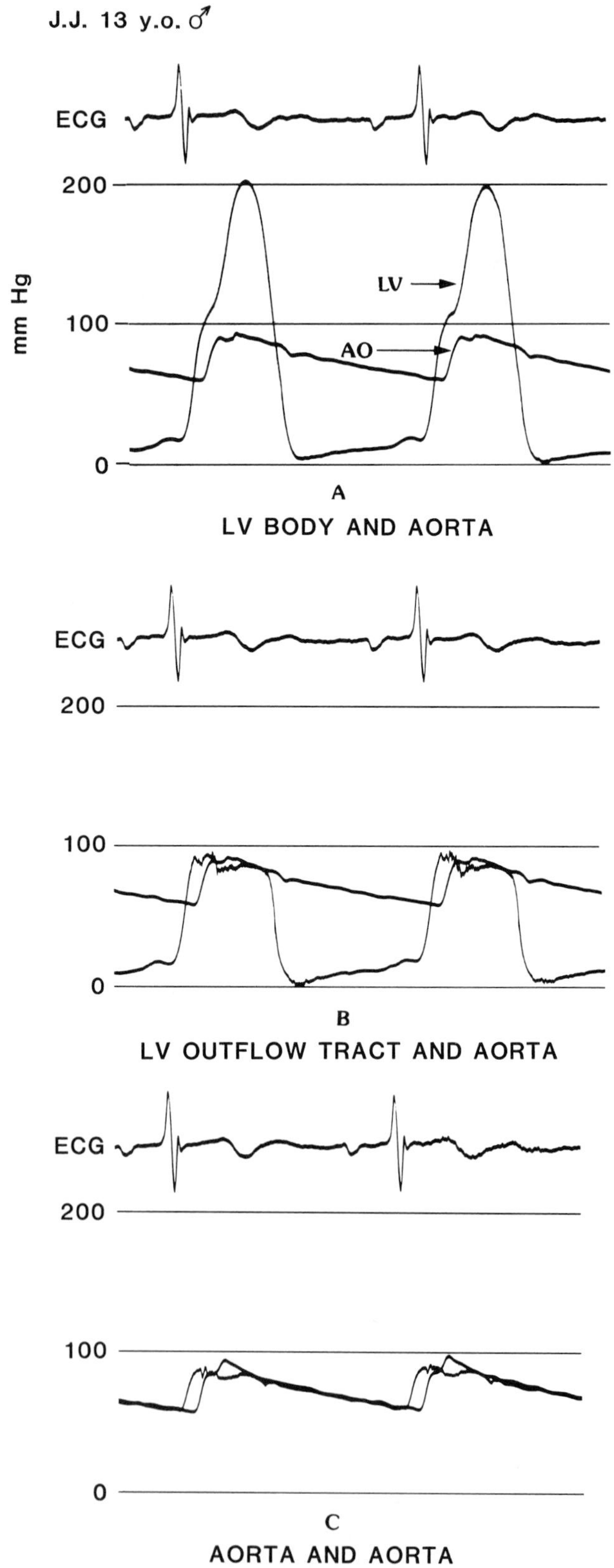

FIGURE 122-6 This tracing represents the classic hemodynamic tracing of hypertrophic cardiomyopathy. LV represents the distal pressure transducer initially in the body of the left ventricle (A), in the LV outflow tract (B), and above the aortic valve in the aorta (C). The intraventricular pressure gradient is easily seen when comparing A and B.

large septum, SAM, mitral regurgitation, a small ventricular cavity, and mitral leaflet dysfunction. Doppler echocardiography can confirm diastolic dysfunction.[25,26] If transthoracic echocardiography is equivocal yet the clinical suspicion remains, a transesophageal echocardiogram should be performed. Gated radionuclide imaging techniques will reveal an abnormally high ejection fraction. Diastolic abnormalities can also be seen on gated studies.

The radial artery waveform may reveal a bisferious pulse during arterial blood pressure monitoring.[27] Catheterization of the right heart typically shows mild pulmonary hypertension and an increased v wave on the pulmonary capillary wedge tracing. The v wave will decrease when loading conditions are increased, since mitral regurgitation is reduced. The cardiac output will decrease when afterload is reduced or when contractility is augmented, a response which will seem paradoxical if the patient is thought to have systolic dysfunction (CHF). Left heart catheterization should only be necessary as a presurgical test or when the diagnosis is equivocal. Catheterization will reveal diastolic dysfunction (a high resting LVEDP), an increased ejection fraction, and the presence of mitral regurgitation. The *intracardiac* pressure gradient will also be seen which confirms the diagnosis. The catheterization laboratory is the safest place to put the patient through any necessary pharmacologic maneuvers (e.g., amyl nitrite, isoproterenol).

MANAGEMENT

Management of patients with HOCM in the ICU is very challenging. It is first imperative to establish the diagnosis. Once confirmed, the principles of management are to minimize contractility and maximize loading conditions. A β blocker in large doses should be the initial drug of choice. This has the added benefit of being antiarrhythmic. If there is a contraindication to β blockers, then a calcium channel blocker, preferably verapamil, should be used.[28,29] These drugs also minimize tachycardia, thereby increasing filling time.[30] Both drugs usually require very high doses for effectiveness. Propranolol with its relatively short half-life is preferred. The experience with esmolol is minimal.

Patients with HOCM who have pulmonary edema usually improve with saline administration and calcium channel or β blockers. This is also true for those who are hypotensive. Compromised patients can tolerate large volumes of saline. While it is tempting to use vasodilators and diuretics, the standards in the treatment of CHF, they should be avoided. Norepinephrine is the preferred drug for refractory hypotension pending surgical correction because of its afterload increasing abilities. Drugs which increase contractility, such as digoxin, epinephrine, dobutamine, and amrinone, should not be used. If a patient complains of chest pain, nitrates should be given with extreme caution because they may cause catastrophic hypotension. Following medical therapy, if a patient still has evidence of congestive heart failure, then surgical correction must be considered. This involves partial septal resection with or without mitral valve replacement. A left heart catheterization usually dictates the type of surgical correction.[31]

Because of diastolic dysfunction, the ventricle is quite dependent on atrial function. Atrial fibrillation can, therefore, be a medical emergency in patients with HOCM. A type IA antiarrhythmic should be instituted for prophylaxis if frequent PACs or short runs of atrial fibrillation are occurring. This may prevent potentially catastrophic atrial fibrillation. Disopyramide is preferred because of its negative inotropic quality. Digoxin should not be used to block the AV node. Atrial flutter or fibrillation should be immediately electrically cardioverted (see Chap. 31).

Ventricular arrhythmias are frequent in these patients. Lidocaine is the drug of choice, but amiodarone, β blockers, or disopyramide can be considered as well. Systemic anticoagulation should be reserved for those patients with atrial fibrillation refractory to cardioversion. Finally, patients with HOCM are at increased risk of endocarditis, so prophylaxis must be instituted prior to indicated procedures (Table 122-1).

Prosthetic Valves

Prosthetic valves present a special problem in the ICU setting. Prosthetic valves can become dysfunctional through mechanical failure, infection, thrombosis, or sewing ring problems. Disease may present as a regurgitant lesion (paravalvular or valvular), a worsening stenotic lesion, a source of recurrent embolization, or a nidus of infection. All prosthetic valves carry a mild to moderate stenosis, a point relevant to management.[32] Obviously one must be aware of the type of valve and its location. If no data are available, a portable chest x-ray can often provide this information.[33,34] Both mechanical and bioprosthetic valves can develop paravalvular leaks due to problems with the sewing ring. Bioprosthetic valves are much more likely than mechanical valves to leak through the valve orifice. Partial detachment of any prosthetic valve can also occur, which presents as valvular insufficiency. Slow leaks can be subclinical until very late, whereas significant tears in the valvular ring can result in symptoms of acute valvular insufficiency. Paraprosthetic leaks occur most commonly within 6 months of the valvular surgery. Whenever any of the above occur, prosthetic valve endocarditis should be considered.

Mechanical valves can exhibit mechanical dysfunction. Discs can become stuck and give a combined stenotic-regurgitant pathophysiology. This usually results in immediate and severe clinical consequences. The clinician should evaluate the valve for a thrombus (via echocardiography) and examine the patient for evidence of embolism.

Mechanical valves also have a higher risk of a thrombus simply occluding the valve. The size and location of the thrombus contribute to the pace and severity of deterioration. Thrombi are much more likely to occur with valves in the mitral position than the aortic. Occasionally, severe hemolysis with mechanical valves requires replacement, but this is fortunately an uncommon phenomenon with the newer valves today. As tissue valves age, many become insufficient and patients must frequently be treated for valvular insufficiency.

All valves carry a high risk of endocarditis, and antibiotic prophylaxis must be used as indicated (see Table 122-1).

CLINICAL PRESENTATION

Historical clues to prosthetic valve dysfunction are vague but are similar to those of any worsening valve lesion. Attention should be directed to the presence of fever, chills, neurologic complaints, or other evidence of embolization. Since all valves have an intrinsic murmur, the focus must be on changing murmurs. A diastolic murmur in the aortic area or a systolic murmur in the mitral area must be taken especially seriously because these suggest insufficiency lesions. Absence of closing sounds may portend critical valve dysfunction, but even normal sounds are sometimes difficult to hear. Evidence for fluid retention, peripheral emboli, or neurologic sequelae must be carefully sought.

DIAGNOSTIC TESTS

The laboratory exam often reveals a mild hemolytic anemia with an increased sedimentation rate even when the valve is functioning normally. The ECG is usually helpful in diagnosing new arrhythmias (e.g., atrial fibrillation) or new conduction defects. Echocardiography is technically more difficult with mechanical valves, but Doppler studies can be done with excellent results.[35,36] Transesophageal echocardiography is especially helpful in this setting, often revealing a previously unseen vegetation or thrombus.[37–39] Right heart catheterization should be performed with special care regarding sterile technique, but subacute bacterial endocarditis (SBE) prophylaxis is not indicated for this procedure. A left heart catheterization may be necessary to diagnose prosthetic valve failure if the clinical exam or echocardiography gives insufficient information. Mechanical valves in the aortic position make assessment of LV hemodynamics difficult, and a transseptal technique may be needed to enter the left ventrical via the left atrium. Cardiac fluoroscopy can be used to assess proper leaflet or ball motion, and angiography can reveal valvular regurgitation. A bedside fluoroscopy unit is sometimes adequate in assessing mechanical valve dysfunction if an urgent assessment is needed.

MANAGEMENT

Medical management of a patient with a properly functioning prosthetic valve is similar to that of a patient with mild valvular stenosis. Tissue valves that are insufficient may be managed similarly to native valves. Management of prosthetic valve malfunction is generally surgical, especially with mechanical valves.

Surgery should be performed if the valve is dysfunctional, infected, a source of recurrent embolization despite anticoagulation, or if a thrombus inhibits proper valve function. The proper timing of surgery is important, and the patient's clinical status, type of valve, and underlying valvular pathology all must be considered. Any acute deterioration demands urgent surgery. A patient with a slowly failing valve may be safely managed while the underlying critical illness is stabilized. At the earliest window of opportunity, surgery must be performed.[40]

Anticoagulation in Valvular Heart Disease

The recommendations for anticoagulation in valvular heart disease are much debated.[41,42] General recommendations cannot be made, but each case must be evaluated on an individual basis. The clinician must frequently weigh the risk of bleeding against the risk of thrombus formation when critical illness supervenes. Those at high risk of thrombosis should be maintained on anticoagulant therapy if possible because of the significant risk of embolization of clot. Those with controversial indications can usually be managed safely off anticoagulation during an acute illness. Generally, anticoagulation is adequate when the partial thromboplastin time (PTT) is 1.5 to 2 times the control value. If there has been recent embolization of a clot (<6 months), then the PTT should be raised to 2 to 2.5 times control.

NATIVE VALVE DISEASE

In patients with mitral stenosis, anticoagulation is recommended in those who have symptoms of CHF, are in atrial fibrillation, or have evidence of a thrombus on echocardiography. Controversial indications include an enlarged left atrium without arrhythmias or asymptomatic patients with mild to moderate mitral stenosis.

Patients with mitral insufficiency usually are at a relatively low risk of embolization as long as they are in sinus rhythm. If atrial fibrillation occurs, systemic anticoagulation is preferred because the risk of thrombus formation increases 2- to 4-fold. Anticoagulation can otherwise be temporarily discontinued during an acute illness unless there is evidence of peripheral embolization or the presence of clot on echocardiography. An echocardiogram is recommended prior to stopping anticoagulation on all patients with mitral valvular disease.

Patients with aortic, pulmonic, and tricuspid valvular disease have a much lower risk of thrombus formation, and anticoagulation is usually not necessary. Many recommend anticoagulation for atrial fibrillation and aortic valvular heart disease, but this too can be withdrawn during an intervening critical illness. If there is evidence of either systemic or pulmonary emboli, then anticoagulation should be implemented.

BIOPROSTHETIC VALVES

Patients with normally functioning bioprosthetic valves can usually be treated like those with a normally functioning native valve (even in the mitral position). If a bioprosthetic

TABLE 122-4 Incidence of Thromboembolic Complications*

Author	Prosthesis	Aortic, %	Mitral, %
Starr	Starr-Edwards		
	1965–1972	4.8	6.6
	1973–1984	1.8	2.9
Baudet	St. Jude	0.3	0.5
Dzer	St. Jude	2.1	1.7
Marshall	Bjork-Shiley	1.0	1.5
Janieson	Carpentier	1.1	1.7
Brais	Ionescu	1.4	4.0
Ionescu	Ionescu	0.6	2.5
Gallucci	Hancock	—	2.1

*The incidence of thromboembolic complications is expressed as the percent of patients experiencing a thromboembolic event within 1 year.

SOURCE: Adapted with permission from Cowan JC: Surgery for valvular heart disease, in Hall RJC and Julian DG (eds): *Diseases of Cardiac Valves*, London, Churchill Livingston, 1989.

valve was placed less than 6 months prior to the present illness, the risk of thrombus formation is higher, and anticoagulation should be initiated if possible. Abnormally functioning bioprosthetic valves should otherwise be anticoagulated like abnormally functioning native valves (vide supra). A patient with a malfunctioning valve and concurrent atrial fibrillation should be anticoagulated.[41–43]

MECHANICAL VALVES

Patients with mechanical valves are at significant risk for embolism and require anticoagulation unless extensive bleeding is present. Valves in the mitral position are at especially high risk for thrombus formation (especially if atrial fibrillation is present), and anticoagulation should be stopped for no more than 48 h for necessary procedures. Mechanical valves in the aortic position usually tolerate a lack of anticoagulation for longer periods, but reinstitution of anticoagulation should be reinstituted at the earliest opportunity (see Table 122-4).

PARTIAL ANTICOAGULATION

Does partial anticoagulation work? Data are scant in this area, but evidence does suggest that partial anticoagulation is more beneficial than none at all in those very high risk patients.[41] It is highly preferable to aggressively treat the underlying hemorrhagic lesion and reinstitute full anticoagulation than to partially anticoagulate and hope no thrombus occurs. Otherwise, the physician is simultaneously undertreating two disorders.

Endocarditis

This topic is covered comprehensively in Chap. 101, but the important cardiologic points will be reviewed here. Endocarditis is particularly foreboding in a patient with another critical illness. Patients may have undiagnosed disease for several days since critical illness can obscure many of the findings of endocarditis. The patient may present with insufficient or stenotic lesions.[44–49] Vegetations (see Fig. 122-7) are not seen by echocardiography in 30 to 40 percent of all patients with endocarditis, so a negative study does not rule out the diagnosis. Transesophageal echocardiography has proven particularly helpful in patients with endocarditis, often revealing a vegetation not shown by a transthoracic study. This is especially true for patients on ventilators or when transthoracic echocardiography is technically difficult.

Hemodynamic management of cardiac complications of endocarditis are similar to those of other valvular diseases. Patients who are asymptomatic can be followed by frequent physical exams. In symptomatic patients, a right heart catheter should be placed to evaluate the cardiac output, loading conditions, and the presence of valvular insufficiency (tricuspid, pulmonic, and mitral). Tricuspid endocarditis is not generally considered a contraindication to right heart catheterization when this procedure is otherwise indicated. Intraarterial blood pressure monitoring is only necessary for patients whose blood pressure is highly labile, who are hypotensive, or who have symptoms of marked CHF. A left heart catheterization is used to define the level of valvular insufficiency, LV function, and coronary status as a prelude to surgery. In aortic valve endocarditis, crossing the aortic valve to enter the left ventricle should be avoided. Immediate surgical consultation must be obtained as soon as the diagnosis is made so that the surgical team is prepared in case an emergency occurs.

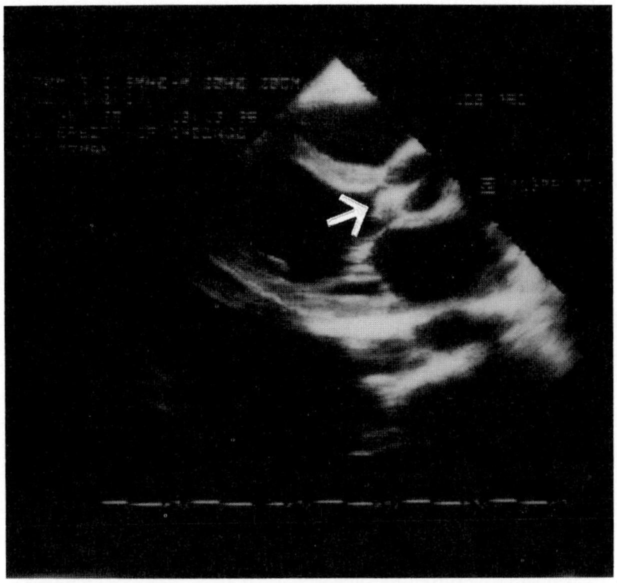

FIGURE 122-7 This is an echocardiographic representation of a large aortic valve vegetation (see arrow) in a patient with aortic valve endocarditis. The size of the vegetation does not necessarily determine the need for emergent replacement.

Generally, the hemodynamic complications of endocarditis are those of acute valvular insufficiency. Medical management of individual valvular disorders is quite similar to that described earlier in this chapter. The focus in patients with endocarditis is the *progression* of disease. If rapid hemodynamic deterioration occurs despite aggressive medical therapy, surgery must be performed as soon as feasible.

Right-sided endocarditis is usually well tolerated without urgent surgical correction. Severely insufficient lesions involving the tricuspid or pulmonic valve are relatively well tolerated. Management requires keeping the right atrial and right ventricular end-diastolic pressures high enough to maintain an adequate cardiac output. Dobutamine can dilate pulmonary vessels and improve right-sided cardiac output. Surgery often involves simple removal of the valve or, on occasion, replacement with a bioprosthetic valve. On the opposite end of the spectrum, progressive aortic incompetence usually bodes a poor medical prognosis, and surgery should be considered as soon as possible. Mitral incompetence is often less predictable and should be managed on an individual basis. In both aortic and mitral endocarditis, if symptoms gradually worsen despite aggressive management and there is a suggestion of a worsening lesion, surgery should be seriously considered.

The indications for surgery must be individualized. Rapid catheterization with urgent surgery should be performed if the patient is at all unstable. The valve involved, the underlying organism, the underlying medical condition of the patient, and the severity of the cardiac lesion must all be taken into account. General indications for surgery are summarized in Table 122-5.

If the patient has recurrent emboli despite aggressive medical management, surgery must be considered. Patients who develop severe heart failure secondary to valvular disruption must undergo surgery if possible. Mild to moderate heart failure may be watched carefully, but any sign of further deterioration often heralds hemodynamic collapse, especially in aortic and mitral endocarditis.

A very serious cardiac complication of endocarditis is the development of a myocardial abscess. This rare complication usually occurs in aortic valve endocarditis and presents as progressive heart block, valvular insufficiency, and occasionally as pericarditis. In contrast to pericarditis in subacute endocarditis (which is often immune-mediated and relatively benign), the pericarditis of acute aortic endocarditis may be purulent, requiring urgent surgery.[50] Extravalvular extension of disease despite antibiotic management is another indication for surgery. Prosthetic valve endocarditis usually requires surgical corrections after several days of antibiotics if the patient is stable.

A final point regards the highly controversial area of anticoagulation for endocarditis. Data are somewhat ambiguous.[41,42,51–55] Anticoagulation in native valve endocarditis has not been shown to have any benefit on the course of endocarditis and can actually increase the risk of intracranial bleeding. The risk of bleeding from a mycotic aneurysm or infarction usually outweighs any benefit of anticoagulation. Valvular disease with evidence of a thrombus on echocardiography or clinical evidence of peripheral emboli probably warrants systemic anticoagulation. The data on prosthetic valve endocarditis suggest that aggressive antibiotic treatment is more important than anticoagulation in preventing neurologic complications of prosthetic valve endocarditis.[56] Nevertheless, anticoagulation should be given to patients with endocarditis of a mechanical valve. The increased risk of intracerebral bleeding must be accepted. Heparin should be used because it is more easily titrated and reversed if urgent intervention is needed. Keeping the PTT around 1.5 times control is usually adequate.[57,58]

TABLE 122-5 Indications for Surgery for Endocarditis

1. Intractable heart failure secondary to valve leaflet compromise
2. Repeated embolic phenomena
3. No response of infection despite 1 week of proper intensive therapy
4. Presence of a septal abscess
   - Development of heart block
   - Aortic valve involvement
   - Presistance of block after 1 week of intensive medical therapy
5. Recurrent endocarditis more than 6 months after a cure unless a different valve is involved
6. Relapse of infection within 3 months
7. Valvular obstruction
8. Ruptured chordae tendineae
9. Periprosthetic leak or unstable prosthesis
10. Endocarditis in the sinus of Valsalva
11. Fungal endocarditis

CASE PRESENTATION

Mr. M is an 82-year-old retired teacher who was admitted for a 2-week history of fevers. He was in very good health until 2 weeks prior to admission when he noticed a progressive increase in fatigue, malaise, anorexia, and a nonproductive cough. Shortly thereafter he noticed low-grade fevers and a cough productive of whitish sputum. He went to see his physician. A murmur was heard in the clinic and his temperature was 38°C, so he was admitted. He had no chest pain or shortness of breath nor had he been recently instrumented.

His past history was notable for prostatic obstruction requiring a transurethral resection 15 years ago. On admission he noted increasing frequency and urgency on urination but had no discharge or burning. He also had had both knees replaced with prostheses 4 years prior to admission for arthritis. There was no history of intravenous drug use. He did not smoke or drink. There was no history of rheumatic fever. His only medication was aspirin.

His exam was notable for mild lethargy. His blood pressure was 125/65 with a heart rate of 100 and a respira-

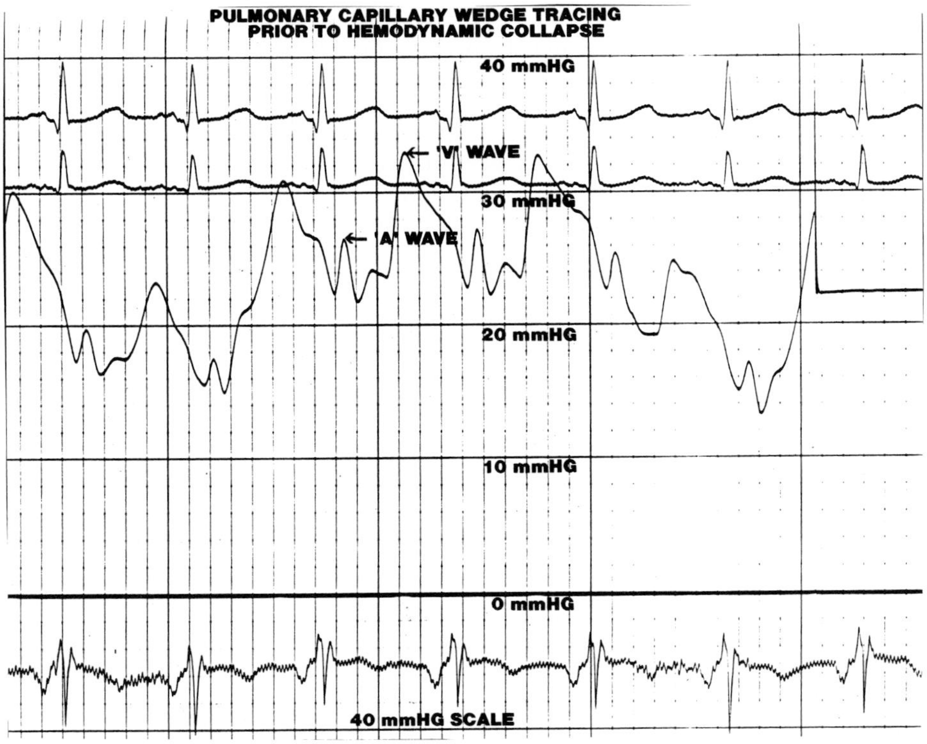

a

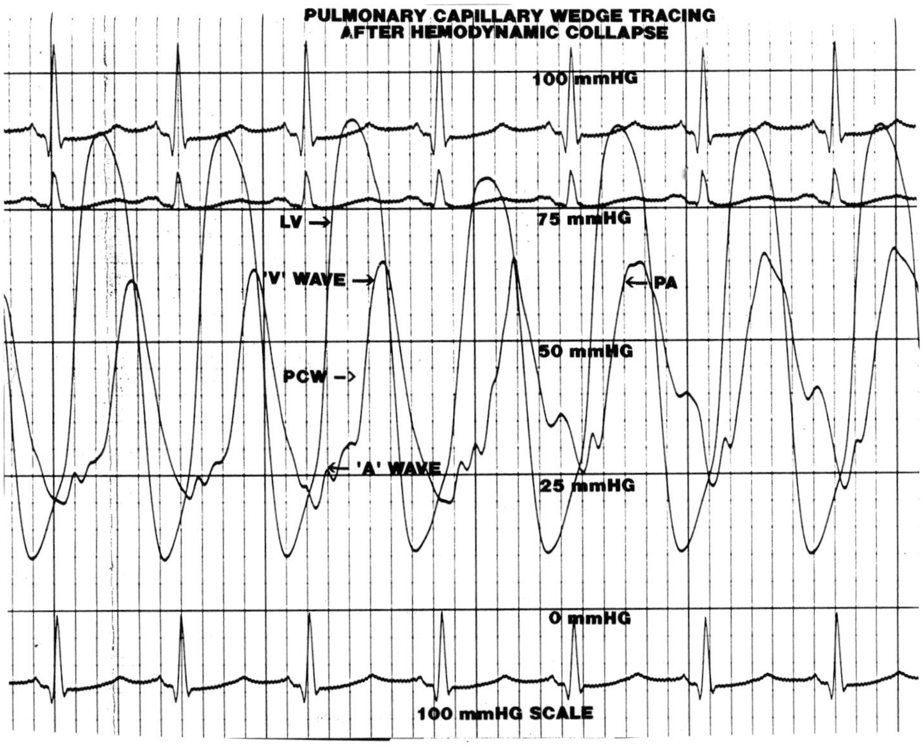

b

FIGURE 122-8 *a*. The hemodynamic tracing prior to cardiovascular collapse. (This is on a 40-mmHg scale.) The *a* wave is roughly 25 mmHg, and the *v* wave is roughly 32 mmHg. The blood pressure at this time was 115/70. *b*. This represents the hemodynamic pressure tracing after cardiovascular collapse. (This is on a 100-mmHg scale during pullback from the PCW pressure to the pulmonary artery pressure.) Note that the systolic blood pressure is roughly 85 mmHg. The PCW pressure tracing reveals a *v* wave which is now nearly 65 mmHg, whereas the *a* wave remains nearly the same. Notice also how subtle the difference is between the *v* wave on the PCW pressure tracing and the pulmonary artery pressure tracing. Differentiation could only be confidently made with careful evaluation of the actual paper tracing.

tory rate of 20. His temperature was 38°C. His dental condition was excellent, and the fundoscopic exam was normal. There were no abnormal skin findings.

His lungs were clear to both auscultation and percussion. The cardiac exam revealed a jugular venous pressure of 2 cm at 30° with a slightly increased *v* wave and a normal *a* wave. The carotid upstroke was slightly diminished with no bruits. There was no S_4, a decreased S_1 with a slightly decreased A_2, and an increased P_2. There was a grade 3/6 holosystolic murmur heard at the left sternal border radiating to the axilla. The abdomen was normal. The rectal exam revealed an enlarged prostate, and the stool was slightly positive for occult blood. The extremities showed no clubbing, cyanosis, or edema. There were no focal neurologic findings.

Significant laboratories on admission were a white blood cell count of 18.8 with 77 neutrophils and 9 bands. The hemoglobin was 11.9 g/dL with a hematocrit of 35. The platelet count was 85,000 with a prothrombin time of 15.5 sec and a normal PTT. His creatinine was 1.3 mg/dL. The ESR was 58. He had an SGOT of 39 IU, SGPT of 58 IU, alkaline phosphate of 94 IU, and a total bilirubin of 1.1 mg/dL. The calcium was 7.8 mg/dL. A room air blood gas revealed a pH of 7.50, a P_{O_2} of 53 mmHg, and a P_{CO_2} of 27 mmHg. The chest x-ray was normal, and the ECG revealed a heart rate of 100 with a nonspecific right ventricular conduction delay.

Because of the fever and heart murmur, he was started on ampicillin and gentamicin and was shortly switched to gentamicin and ceftazidime. Within 48 h, 5/6 blood cultures became positive for an unusual gram-negative bacillus, presumably from the oropharynx or genitourinary tract. An echocardiogram revealed normal LV function, a myxomatous mitral valve with moderate mitral regurgitation, and mild tricuspid regurgitation. There was no evidence for vegetations. An abdominal CT was negative. A 48-h gallium scan showed mild uptake in the right shoulder and moderate uptake in the peritracheal and hilar areas of the chest. A colonoscopy showed only a small nonbleeding polyp.

While on antibiotics, he continued to have a low-grade fever (37.5°C). His hemoglobin decreased to 7.9 g/dL, while the platelet count increased to 115,000. The gram-negative organism had not yet been identified but was found to be sensitive to gentamicin, ceftazidime, and ampicillin. The antibiotics were changed to gentamicin and ampicillin.

On day 9 of his admission, he complained of moderate dyspnea. The exam revealed a heart rate of 115 with a blood pressure of 100/50. He had rales in both lower lung fields. His cardiac exam revealed a slightly worsened murmur in the mitral area. He was electively intubated and taken to the cardiac catheterization area where a right heart catheterization revealed a cardiac output of 4.4 L/min. The PCWP tracing revealed a very large *v* wave (see Fig. 122-8*a*). His mitral valve appeared slightly calcific. His coronaries showed only mild atherosclerosis. Left ventriculography was not done because of his unstable condition.

During the procedure his systolic blood pressure fell to 60 mmHg. An intraaortic balloon pump was inserted and dobutamine was started at 10 μg/kg/min. One liter of saline was given and the blood pressure increased to 110/70. The PCWP tracing showed an even higher *v* wave which was nearly indistinguishable from his pulmonary artery tracing (see Fig. 122-8*b*). He was immediately taken for cardiac surgery where the posterior leaflet of the mitral valve was largely replaced by vegetation, and the posterior papillary muscle was nearly transsected. A Carpentier-Edwards valve was used for replacement. He subsequently has done well.

CASE DISCUSSION

This case demonstrates the rapid deterioration a patient can have with endocarditis. It appears that another strut from the papillary muscle was lost during the catheterization, worsening his condition. Management included encouraging forward flow by inserting an intraaortic balloon pump which also decreased his myocardial oxygen consumption. Unloading agents were not used because of his hypotension. Dobutamine was a good initial choice for inotropic support because it increased contractility while reducing afterload, encouraging forward flow. Early intubation allowed the aggressive administration of fluids despite pulmonary edema to maximize preload and encourage forward flow. It underscores the need for urgent intervention with any sign of deterioration. Any delay in this case would have shortly resulted in death. A very similar course could easily have occurred in a patient with a recent acute myocardial infarction and new hemodynamic collapse from an *ischemic* or *infarcted* papillary muscle. Management would be similar except that coronary artery surgery would likely be necessary in addition to valve replacement.

References

1. Gorlin R, Gorlin SG: Hydraulic formula for calculation of the area of the stenotic mitral valve, other cardiac valves and central circulatory shunts. Am Heart J 41:1, 1951.
2. Terzaki AK, Cokkines DV, Cooley DA, et al.: Combined mitral and aortic valve disease. Am J Cardiol 25:588, 1970.
3. Hurst JW, et al. (eds): *The Heart*, 7th ed. New York, McGraw-Hill, 1990.
4. McHenry MM, Rice N, Matlof HJ, et al.: Pulmonary hypertension and sudden death in aortic stenosis. Br Heart J 41:463, 1979.
5. Szamosi A, Wassberg B: Radiologic detection of aortic stenosis. Acta Radiol Diagn 24:201, 1983.
6. Neumann A, Lang RM, Borow KM: Doppler echo in aortic stenosis. Cardiology 5:120, 1988.
7. St. John Sutton MG, St. John Sutton M, Oldershaw P, et al.: Valve replacement without preoperative cardiac catheterization. N Engl J Med 305:1233, 1981.
8. Roberts WC: No cardiac catheterization before cardiac valve replacement—a mistake. Am Heart J 103:930, 1982.

9. O'Rourke RA: Preoperative cardiac catheterization. Its need in most patients with valvular heart disease. JAMA 248:745, 1982.
10. Hall RJC, Julian DG: *Diseases of Cardiac Valves,* New York, Churchill Livingstone, 1989, pp 120–139.
11. Ricci DR: Afterload mismatch and preload reserve in chronic aortic regurgitation. Circulation 66:826, 1982.
12. Dervan J, Goldberg S: Acute aortic regurgitation: Pathophysiology and management, in Frankl WS, Brest AN (eds): *Valvular Heart Disease: Comprehensive Evaluation and Management,* Cardiovascular Clinics, Philadelphia, FA Davis, 1986, pp 281–288.
13. Perry GJ, Helmcke F, Nanda NC, et al.: Evaluation of aortic insufficiency by Doppler color flow mapping. J AM Coll Cardiol 9:952, 1987.
14. Carroll JD, Gaasch WH, Zile MR, et al.: Serial changes in left ventricular function after correction of chronic aortic regurgitation. Dependence on early changes in preload and subsequent regression of hypertrophy. Am J Cardiol 51:476, 1983.
15. Feigenbaum H (ed): *Echocardiography,* Philadelphia, Lee & Febiger, 1986, pp 249–262.
16. Schwartz R, Meyerson RM, Lawrence LT, et al.: Mitral stenosis, massive pulmonary hemorrhage and emergency valve replacement. N Engl J Med 272:755, 1966.
17. Silverstein DM, Hansen DP, Ojiambo HP, et al.: Left ventricular function in severe pure mitral stenosis as seen at the Kenyatta National Hospital. Am Heart J 99:727, 1980.
18. Sanders CA, Armstrong PW, Willerson JT, et al.: Etiology and differential diagnosis of acute mitral regurgitation. Prog Cardiovasc Dis 14:129, 1971.
19. Kusiak V, Brest AN: Acute mitral regurgitation: Pathophysiology and management, in Frankl WS, Brest An (eds): *Cardiovascular Clinics and Valvular Heart Disease: Comprehensive Evaluation and Management.* Philadelphia, FA Davis, 1986, pp 257–280.
20. Grose R, Strain J, Cohen MV: Pulmonary arterial *v* waves in mitral regurgitation: Clinical and experimental observations. Circulation 69:214, 1984.
21. Giuffrida G, Bonzani G, Betocchi S, et al.: Hemodynamic response to exercise after propranolol in patients with mitral stenosis. Am J Cardiol 44:1076, 1979.
22. Rippe JM, Howe JP III: Acute mitral regurgitation, in Dalen JE, Alpert JS (eds): *Valvular Heart Disease,* 2d ed. Boston, Little, Brown and Company, 1987, pp 151–176.
23. Greenberg BH: Mitral insufficiency: Use of vasodilators. Prim Cardiol 10:155, 1984.
24. Corin WJ, Monrad ES, Murakami T, et al.: The relationship of afterload to ejection performance in chronic mitral regurgitation. Circulation 76:59, 1987.
25. Maron BJ, Gottdiener JS, Arce J, et al.: Dynamic subaortic obstruction in hypertrophic cardiomyopathy: Analysis by pulsed Doppler echocardiography. J Am Coll Cardiol 6:1, 1985.
26. Nishimura RA, Tajik AJ, Reeder GS, et al.: Evaluation of hypertrophic cardiomyopathy by Doppler color flow imaging: Initial observations. Mayo Clin Proc 61:631, 1986.
27. Braunwald E, Lambrew CT, Rockoff SD, et al.: Idiopathic hypertrophic subaortic stenosis: I. A description of the disease based upon an analysis of 64 patients. Circulation 30 (suppl 4): IV3, 1964.
28. Maron BJ, Bonow RO, Cannon RO III, et al.: Medical Progress: Hypertrophic cardiomyopathy: Interrelations of clinical manifestations, pathophysiology and therapy. N Engl J Med 316:(14), p 844, 1987.
29. Chatterjee K: Calcium antagonist agents in hypertrophic cardiomyopathy. Am J Cardiol 59:146B, 1987.
30. Ito I: Impaired left ventricular rapid filling during exercise in patients with hypertrophic cardiomyopathy. Clin Cardiol 10:147, 1987.
31. Duda AM, Gill CC, Kitazume H, et al.: Surgical treatment of idiopathic hypertrophic subaortic stenosis with other cardiac pathology. Cleve Clin Q 51:27, 1984.
32. Rashtian MY, Stevenson DM, Allen DT, et al.: Flow characteristics of four commonly used mechanical heart valves. Am J Cardiol 58:743, 1986.
33. Mehlman DJ, Resnekov L: A guide to the radiographic identification of prosthetic heart valves. Circulation 57:613, 1978.
34. Mehlman DJ: A guide to the radiographic identification of prosthetic heart valves: an addendum. Circulation 69:102, 1984.
35. Daniel WG, Hanrath P, Mugge A, et al.: Assessment of mitral prosthetic valve dysfunction by transesophageal color coded Doppler echocardiography. Circulation 78:2421, 1988.
36. Mahan EF, Nanda NC: Echocardiographic evaluation of prosthetic cardiac valves. Cardiol Clin 8:369, 1990.
37. Cooper DM, Stewart WJ, Schiavone WA, et al.: Evaluation of normal prosthetic valve function by Doppler echocardiography. Am Heart J 114:576, 1987.
38. Mohr-Kahaly S, Erbel R, Kupferwasser I, et al.: Regurgitation of prosthetic heart valves analyzed by transesophageal 2D color Doppler. Eur Heart J 9(suppl II):274, 1988.
39. Khandheria B, Seward J, Oh J, et al.: Mitral prosthesis malfunction: utility of transesophageal echocardiography. J Am Coll Cardiol. 13:69A, 1989.
40. Syracruso DC, Bauman FO, Maim JR: Prosthetic valve reoperation: Factors influencing early and late survival. J Thorac Cardiovasc Surg 77:346, 1979.
41. Levine HJ, Pauker SG, Salzman EW: Antithrombotic therapy in valvular heart disease. Chest 95(suppl):980S, 1989.
42. Sherman DG, Dyken ML, Fisher M, et al.: Antithrombotic therapy for cerebrovascular disorders. Chest 95(suppl):140S, 1989.
43. Chesebro JH, Adams PG, Fuster V: Antithrombotic therapy in patients with valvular heart disease and prosthetic heart valves. J Am Coll Cardiol 8:41B, 1986.
44. Weinstein L, Schlessinger JJ: Pathoanatomic, pathophysiologic and clinical correlations in endocarditis. N Engl J Med 291:832 and 1122, 1974.
45. Weinstein L: Life-threatening complications of infective endocarditis and their management. Arch Intern Med 146:953, 1986.
46. Mills J, Tuley J, Abbott J: Heart failure in infective endocarditis: Predisposing factors, course and treatment. Chest 66:151, 1974.
47. Mann T, McLaurin L, Grossman W, et al.: Assessing the hemodynamic severity of acute regurgitation due to infective endocarditis. N Engl J Med 293: 108, 1975.
48. Roberts WC, Ewy GA, Glancy DL, et al.: Valvular stenosis produced by active infective endocarditis. Circulation 36:449, 1967.
49. Sacks PV, Lakier JB, Barlow JW: Severe aortic stenosis produced by bacterial endocarditis. Br Med J 3:97, 1969.
50. Alsip SG, Blackstone EH, Kirklin JW, et al.: Indications for cardiac surgery in patients with active infective endocarditis. Am J Med 78:138, 1985.
51. Kanis JA: The use of anticoagulants in bacterial endocarditis. Postgrad Med J 50:312, 1974.
52. Wilson WR, Geraci JE, Danielson GK, et al.: Anticoagulant therapy and nervous system complications in patients with prosthetic valve endocarditis. Circulation 57:1004, 1978.
53. Balgado AV, Furlan AJ, Keys TF, et al.: Neurologic complications of endocarditis: A 12-year experience. Neurology 39:173, 1989.
54. Hart RG, Kagan HK, Joerns SE: Mechanisms of intracranial hemorrhage in infective endocarditis. Stroke 18:1048, 1987.
55. Carpenter JL, McAllister CK: Anticoagulation in prosthetic valve endocarditis. South Med J 76:1372, 1983.
56. Fuster V, Badimon L, Badimon JJ, et al.: Prevention of throm-

boembolism induced by prosthetic heart valves. Semin Thromb Hemost 14:50, 1988.

57. Leport C, Vilde Bricaire F, Cohen A, et al.: Fifty cases of late prosthetic valve endocarditis: improvement in prognosis over a 15 year period. Br Heart J 58:66, 1987.

58. Butchart EG, Lewis PA, Grunkemeier GL: Cardiovascular surgery 1987, part 1: Valvular heart disease: Low risk of thrombosis and serious embolic events despite low-intensity anticoagulation: Experience with 1,004 Medtronic Hall valves. Circulation 78(suppl 1):I66, September 1988.

Chapter 123

MALIGNANT HYPERTENSION

WILLIAM J. ELLIOTT

KEY POINTS

- Malignant hypertension *is severely elevated blood pressure with symptoms and/or signs of acute target organ damage.*
- *Signs of malignant hypertension include funduscopic hemorrhages, exudates, or papilledema, encephalopathy, pulmonary edema, gross hematuria, epistaxis, and acute elevations in serum creatinine concentrations.*
- *Blood pressure is acutely reduced so that pressure-flow relationships may be reestablished without dropping flow past the autoregulatory capacity of the vascular bed.*
- *Treatment is promptly initiated with a short-acting, intravenous vasodilator (e.g., sodium nitroprusside at 0.5 μg/kg/min); mean arterial pressure is reduced 10 to 20 percent in the first hour, and 20 to 30 percent thereafter.*
- *The intravenous vasodilator is withdrawn after 6 to 24 h in favor of oral antihypertensive agents.*
- *The prognosis in malignant hypertension depends on the care with which the blood pressure is reduced acutely, the presenting serum creatinine level, and long-term blood pressure control.*

Definitions and Historical Background

Severe elevations of blood pressure, together with evidence of acute target organ damage (e.g., papilledema or bilateral hemorrhages/exudates in the ocular fundi, encephalopathy, acute congestive heart failure, acute renal insufficiency) have long been grouped under "malignant hypertension."[1] Originally proposed in Germany (as "bösartig hypertension"), this nomenclature, along with "accelerated hypertension" (i.e., severely elevated blood pressures with less severe degrees of acute target organ damage), has been commonly used in American medicine since 1928.[2] The World Health Organization still recognizes the utility of the designation, despite recent American recommendations that have reclassified the terminology, perhaps to reflect more positively on our current ability to successfully treat patients with this problem.[3]

"Malignant hypertension" first entered the medical vocabulary when there was no effective treatment for severe hypertension, and the inexorable progression of these patients to death over just a few months led many to feel that the prognosis in the early 1900s was at least no better than that of patients with incurable cancer. In that sense, the term was certainly justified, as the 1 year survival rates in a number of the earliest series (before any therapy was available) were all <22 percent. Despite some mild early success with dietary and a few surgical interventions, the development of effective hypotensive drug therapy has markedly improved the long-term prognosis of patients presenting with complications of such severe degrees of hypertension (Fig. 123-1).

Most American physicians have now become comfortable with the distinction made by the Third Report of the Joint National Committee, in which hypertensive states requiring acute care have been divided into *hypertensive emergencies,* which require lowering of the blood pressure in a matter of minutes to hours to avoid further target organ damage, and *hypertensive urgencies,* which are somewhat less threatening and are most commonly treated by oral medications, as the blood pressure needs to be brought under control in a matter of hours to days.[1] Table 123-1 lists some of the common clinical situations that fall into these two categories. Some patients, of course, could be included in either group, depending on the severity of illness and condition at presentation.

Another major reason for abandoning the distinction between malignant and lesser degrees of severe hypertension (often based solely on the basis of funduscopic examination) is the observation that there is no longer a difference in outcome between patients with papilledema (which can be a subtle physical finding) and those with hemorrhages or exudates. This has been shown in two large series: 200 patients from Birmingham and 139 more from Glasgow.[4,5] An obvious reason for this is that the treatment of malig-

TABLE 123-1 Clinical Settings Requiring Rapid Control of Hypertension

Hypertensive Emergencies (require control of blood pressure in hours)
- Severely elevated blood pressure with:
  - Encephalopathy (blood pressure need not be extraordinary)
  - Acute cerebrovascular accident (especially hemorrhagic, but also including atherosclerotic and embolic disease)
  - Acute aortic dissection
  - Acute left ventricular failure
  - Acute myocardial infarction
  - Bleeding from vascular surgery sites (threatening suture lines), severe epistaxis
  - Acute head injury
  - Excess catecholamines: pheochromocytoma crisis, monoamine oxidase inhibitor crisis

Hypertensive Urgencies (require control of blood pressure in hours or days)
- Severely elevated blood pressure with:
  - Physical signs or laboratory findings suggesting subacute target organ damage
  - Recent discontinuation of antihypertensive drugs (rebound hypertension)
  - Impending or recent surgical procedures:
    - Need for emergent surgery
    - Immediate postoperative period
    - Status post renal transplantation
    - Severe body burns

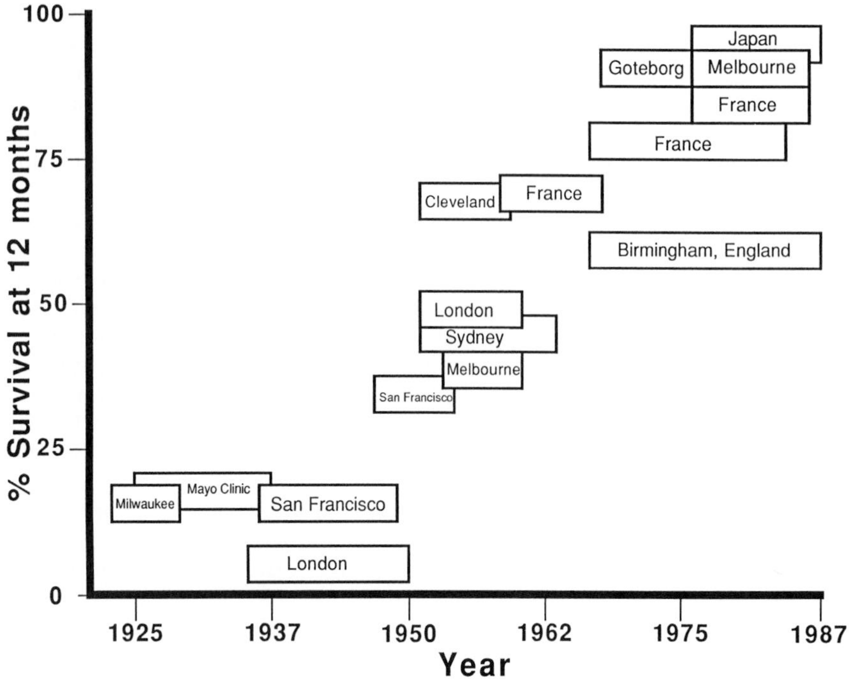

FIGURE 123-1 Improvement in 1 year survival rates in malignant hypertension. Locales of each series are given within a rectangle defined by the beginning and ending year of each study.

nant hypertension has now become so effective at preventing premature death that the condition of the fundi at presentation carries little long-term prognostic significance.

Pathophysiology

Although most patients presenting with malignant hypertension are now promptly and effectively treated, much early investigation in this disease has resulted in two major pathophysiologic contributory factors: disordered autoregulation in important vascular beds, followed by arteritis in the late stages. Figure 123-2 summarizes the data of Strandgaard and coworkers (in 8 hypertensive and 6 normotensive patients), which demonstrate a "shift to the right" of the blood pressure versus cerebral blood flow (autoregulatory curve).[6] These data essentially confirm in human beings much previous work in animal models showing that the intact, untreated organism accommodates slowly to chronic hypertension by "normalizing" cerebral, renal, splanchnic, and sometimes even cardiac blood flow, despite increased blood pressure in those beds. Acute hypertension in the cat has been shown to result in acute vasoconstriction of cerebral arteries (thereby protecting the smaller—and presumably more delicate—arterioles) until "blow-out" of the larger vessels occurs at very high pressures. As elevated arterial pressure is maintained, chronic vasoconstriction leads to hypertrophied muscular intima in the affected arteries, resulting in the characteristic pathologic changes (thickened arterial walls, etc.) seen at autopsy.

The "shift to the right" of the autoregulatory curve has its most important implication in the treatment of the condition (see below). This was recognized years ago by German physicians, who noted that renal function often deteriorated after systemic blood pressure was reduced. This phenomenon eventually led to the name of "essential hypertension," as it was thought that the elevated blood pressure was in fact necessary to keep the renal and other vascular beds properly perfused.

The second major pathophysiologic feature of malignant

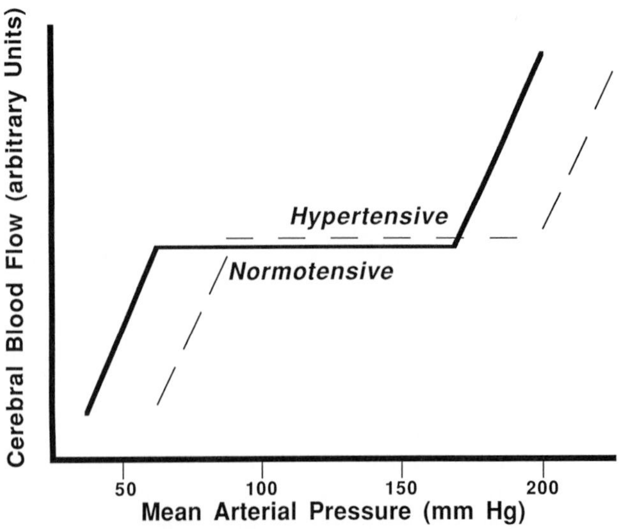

FIGURE 123-2 Autoregulation of cerebral blood flow during varied blood pressure in hypertensive (dashed) and normotensive (solid) persons. Data adapted from Johansson, et al.[6]

hypertension is the necrotizing arteriolitis seen in the later stages of the process. Although primarily recognized by pathologists at autopsy, the vasculitic process seems to occur in many vascular beds (clinically, the optic fundus is the easiest to recognize) and is thought to be related (as both cause and effect) to relative ischemia in the affected areas. This probably has its most important implication in the renal bed, where relative ischemia of the juxtaglomerular apparatus leads to increased production of renin, which typically further elevates the blood pressure via its effects on angiotensin II. This "vicious cycle" probably explains why many patients with true malignant hypertension have elevated plasma renin activity, and why many respond quite remarkably to therapy with angiotensin-converting enzyme (ACE) inhibitors.[7,8] Besides the intravascular volume depletion that is probably renin-mediated, other important clinical consequences of malignant hypertension include thrombocytopenia, intravascular hemolysis, and ischemia in other vascular beds at risk (e.g., cardiac ischemia and failure, diseased peripheral vascular beds, and transient ischemic attacks/strokes).

Epidemiologists have identified several important risk factors for the development of malignant hypertension, some of which may be independent of those that predict bad outcomes in any chronic disease. Socioeconomic factors (e.g., level of schooling, income grouping, social classes) are predictors for poor outcome in severe hypertension, as they are in many treatable chronic illnesses.[9] Many case reports of malignant hypertension are attributed to oral contraceptive pills, with hypertension disappearing after their discontinuation. Cigarette smoking has also been implicated in many epidemiologic surveys.[9,10] The most important factors for preventing malignant hypertension appear to be proper detection of less severe cases of hypertension, adequate medical follow-up, and compliance with pharmacologic therapy. It has been suggested that nearly any type of drug therapy for hypertension will nearly eradicate the emergence of the malignant phase, but this hypothesis is unlikely to be proven in any clinical trial.

Diagnosis

Since even defining malignant hypertension is so difficult, it is not surprising that diagnosing the condition is also problematical. Most authors, however, agree that the diagnosis is most easily made by the association of an extremely elevated blood pressure (actual numbers are of little import) with physical examination or laboratory findings or both, which are indicators of acute target organ damage.

When considering the diagnosis of malignant hypertension, it is important to focus the physical examination on several important organ systems, not only to initiate therapy without delay (if indicated), but also to be certain that no other complicating condition needs concomitant therapy. Certainly the examination begins with the mental status and overall neurologic picture, lest hypertensive encephalopathy go untreated.[11] Hypertensive encephalopathy and a global reduction in consciousness due to an acute cerebrovascular accident with intraventricular bleeding (with elevated blood pressure and reduced heart rate, the so-called Cushing reflex) both require reduction in blood pressure, but there may be important differences in the time taken to lower the blood pressure. The acute diagnosis of hypertensive encephalopathy is often difficult, because headache, altered consciousness, and other less severe degrees of central nervous system (CNS) dysfunction are sometimes associated with elevated blood pressures, often at extreme levels.[11] Although sometimes identifiable by its characteristic appearance on computed tomographic (CT) scans, the diagnosis of hypertensive encephalopathy can often be made by a good examination of the optic fundi (preferably through dilated pupils), which typically show advanced retinopathy (Keith-Wagener-Barker grades III and IV). Improvement in mental status is typically seen after reduction in blood pressure, but this only confirms a diagnosis after therapy is begun.

A thorough examination of the optic fundi is essential, not only because it sometimes allows the diagnosis of malignant hypertension to be made by the recognition of papilledema (when few other signs are present), but it also gives an excellent indication of the duration and severity of the hypertension. Findings in the optic fundus can be good clues leading to the investigation of the patient for secondary forms of hypertension, especially renal artery stenosis (which has been found in up to 58 percent of patients with grade III or IV fundi in one American series)[12] or pheochromocytoma. Patients with Conn's syndrome (primary hyperaldosteronism due to an adrenal adenoma) are unlikely to develop either funduscopic abnormalities or malignant hypertension. Other funduscopic signs helpful in identifying those patients who have already suffered damage to the retina due to severe hypertension are Siegrist's streaks (chains of pigmented spots running alongside an already sclerosed choroidal artery) and Elschnig's spots (acutely, whitish discolorations or chronically, black pigment over a yellow or red halo, due to localized detachment of the retina with intervening serous fluid buildup).

Bedside assessment of cardiac function (râles, effusions in the chest, jugular venous distention, audible third heart sound, ascites, peripheral edema, etc.) is also crucial, in that cardiac decompensation with congestive heart failure ought to be treated not only by reduction in blood pressure, but also with diuresis, afterload reduction, and so on. In addition, studies to rule out a myocardial infarction are usually in order when there is cardiac decompensation associated with severe hypertension, but they may not be indicated with malignant hypertension without heart failure. Physical examination of the abdomen sometimes discloses bruits (which are an important and highly predictive sign for renal arterial disease),[13] palpable kidneys (sometimes due to progressive polycystic kidney disease in the adult), or other masses (e.g., large extraadrenal pheochromocytomas, which are sometimes found in the organ of Zuckerkandl). Inspection of the fingers is sometimes helpful, in that Lindsay's "half-and-half" nails (i.e., pink or white proximal nailbeds; darker red, pink or brownish distal nails; often with loss of the lunula) have been associated with renal dysfunction,[14] and are often noted on physical examination long before other reliable physical signs of renal impairment. Livedo reticularis of the skin has been associated with cerebrovascular disease (especially vasculitis and seizures, i.e., Sneddon's syndrome), and is often seen in patients with vasculitis or collagen-vascular diseases.

Management

The most important first step in the management of severe hypertension is the determination of the urgency of blood pressure reduction. When the patient has true malignant hypertension or one of the other situations found in Table 123-1, the blood pressure must be reduced within hours. Otherwise, the patient may be managed in a much less intense manner and the blood pressure brought under control over the course of the next few hours or days, usually with oral medications (vide infra).

When the patient has a hypertensive emergency, the technical adjuncts to therapy should be minimized in favor of prompt blood pressure reduction. It is not always necessary to have the patient comfortable in an ICU bed, with a calibrated arterial cannula and modern monitoring devices for the electrocardiogram and respiratory systems in place. Instead, beginning therapy with an appropriate intravenously administered, short-acting drug using frequent sphygmomanometric blood pressure measurements is certainly quicker, and assures that a medically sophisticated person will be at the bedside to frequently monitor the patient's status.

The object of the exercise is to lower the patient's blood pressure gradually to a sufficient degree and for a sufficient amount of time so that the "right-shifted" autoregulatory curve moves back toward normal. It is usually wise to use an intravenously administered medication for this purpose, because the dose of a constant infusion can be promptly revised downward if necessary, whereas oral pills cannot be recalled if the blood pressure plummets. Unfortunately, for a given patient, the degree and time of blood pressure lowering that will be deleterious is not known; therefore, only general guidelines can be given. Most authorities and much clinical experience suggest that the mean arterial pressure be reduced only about 15 percent during the first hour, and gradually thereafter to a diastolic blood pressure between 100 and 110 mmHg (or a reduction of 25 percent compared to initial baseline, whichever is higher).[15,16] Gradual reduction of blood pressure to normal (i.e., diastolic <90 mmHg), or even by as little as 35 percent has been associated with major organ dysfunction, coma, and death, as has blood pressure reduction which occurs very quickly (e.g., using bolus diazoxide).

Many complications of blood pressure reduction have been recognized, usually due to an all-too-sudden change in blood pressure which is lower than the threshold of the autoregulatory capacity of the organ system involved (e.g., seizures, coma, or death when cerebral blood flow is precipitously reduced) or to drug-specific side effects (e.g., development of pulmonary edema with labetalol). Many of the reported complications in the treatment of malignant hypertension appear paradoxical in that appropriate drugs cause inappropriate side effects (e.g., nifedipine causing myocardial ischemia). The more commonly reported complications include seizures, blindness, coma, paraplegia, pancreatitis, myocardial ischemia, exacerbations of renal insufficiency (vide infra), acute renal failure, and death.[17]

The choice of intravenous antihypertensive agent is wide, and currently becoming even wider. Most authorities continue to recommend sodium nitroprusside as the drug of choice, because of its short onset time, duration of action, and overall effectiveness.[18,19] Limitations of nitroprusside therapy include its metabolic products (thiocyanate and cyanide), which can accumulate at high doses (>2 μg/kg/min) or during long infusion periods (typically >24 h). These are potentially fatal (especially in patients with renal or hepatic disease and with Leber's optic atrophy) and are often first recognized by the patient (who complains of nausea, fatigue, and muscle spasms) or the physician (widening anion gap, rising lactate level, and disoriented or psychotic patient). Nitroprusside is typically begun at 0.5 μg/kg/min and increased by 0.5 to 1.0 μg/kg/min every 3 to 5 min until the blood pressure reaches the target range. It is seldom necessary to increase the dose beyond 8 to 12 μg/kg/min, which does increase the likelihood of toxicity; often all that is necessary is to raise the patient's head, or dangle the legs over the bedside to allow venous pooling. A temporary dose reduction is recommended before trying either maneuver, because cerebral hypoperfusion is possible in either situation. Another approach to the extremely volume-constricted patient with malignant hypertension (established by elevated urine specific gravity and osmolality; low serum potassium and high aldosterone and peripheral renin activity measurements; and relative refractivity to nitroprusside) is to give intravenous saline solution, but this is seldom necessary. Once the effective dose of nitroprusside has been found, the process of choosing an oral medication to replace nitroprusside should begin.

The other drugs available for infusion are most useful in certain clinical situations. Nitroglycerin (typically begun at 5 μg/min with nonabsorbing infusion sets, with dose increases every 3 to 5 min by 5 to 10 μg/min, as needed) is very useful in the setting of severe hypertension with angina, during coronary artery bypass surgery, or during neurosurgery. Labetalol can be given either as multiple miniboluses (typically escalating in dose at 15-min intervals: e.g., 25 mg, then 50 mg, then 100 mg, then 200 mg, etc.), or as a constant dose infusion. Diazoxide is probably better given as slow, minibolus injections (e.g., 50 mg every 15 min) or by continuous infusion. Trimethaphan and phentolamine are useful mainly for dissecting aortic aneurysms and pheochromocytoma crisis, respectively.

These agents are used less commonly than nitroprusside because of their relative disadvantages. Intravenous nitroglycerin is relatively unstable in solution, tends to "stick" to intravenous lines (and therefore leads to variability in dose administered over time), leads to tolerance during prolonged administration, and can cause profound headache. Labetalol is not always effective in that some patients achieve little improvement in blood pressure, and some develop tachyphylaxis over time. It has been difficult to predict the oral dose necessary for chronic therapy even after successful use of the intravenous preparation. Because it is a more potent β- than α-blocking agent (7:1 ratio when given intravenously to human beings versus 3:1 orally), it carries the restrictions of use of β blockers (e.g., relatively contraindicated in heart failure, asthma, heart block worse than first degree, etc.). Rapidly injected 300-mg boluses of diazoxide can cause precipitous hypotension and acute complications.[17] Its unpredictability in action, striking reflex tachycardia, tendency to exacerbate or cause diabetes mellitus, and retain fluid have since tended to outweigh its formerly touted ability to "reset the barostat," such that it is now only rarely used for hypertensive emergencies.

A number of drugs currently under investigation may improve the therapy of malignant hypertension, especially for specific patient groups. Nicardipine and fenoldopam are both effective, but nicardipine may be more beneficial in patients with subarachnoid hemorrhage or diminished renal function.[20] Fenoldopam has been shown to acutely improve several parameters of renal function in patients with severe, accelerated, and malignant hypertension, and may be preferable for long-term infusions.[21]

One of the most troubling presentations of malignant hypertension is the occasional patient with minor focal neurologic findings, because there is then a conflict regarding diagnosis of the intracerebral process versus prompt treatment of the severe hypertension. In most such instances, a pragmatic approach is to attempt acute blood pressure reduction, but to a somewhat lesser extent (e.g., 10 percent reduction in mean arterial pressure), with a low threshold to diminish or stop the infusion should the neurologic picture worsen. Serial neurologic examinations (preferably with written tasks, e.g., signature, clock-drawing, etc.) should be done to compare and assess the degree of worsening or improvement in this setting. The investigative procedures can (and often do) wait longer than the 10 to 20 min necessary to begin nitroprusside; both head CT scans and lumbar punctures can be performed during nitroprusside infusion. If the neurologic findings disappear completely on lowering the blood pressure, the diagnostic procedures may be less pressing.

There is currently some controversy regarding the effects of different drugs on cerebral blood flow in patients with malignant hypertension. There is concern that those drugs which tend to increase cerebral blood flow may be deleterious, because they may increase cerebral perfusion (and pressure) despite lowering systemic pressures. As there are few studies dealing with drug-induced changes of cerebral perfusion in patients with extremely elevated blood pressures, the hypothesis is difficult to evaluate objectively. Most authorities recommend treatment of the patient with malignant hypertension by lowering blood pressure, regardless of the drug's effect on cerebral perfusion, but allowing the blood pressure to rise somewhat if the patient has problems with CNS dysfunction as the blood pressure is lowered.

The choice of drug to treat the individual patient depends somewhat on the patient's presenting condition. If an aortic dissection is likely, the preferred therapy includes propranolol (or another intravenously given β blocker) to decrease dP/dt and either nitroprusside or trimethaphan for lowering the blood pressure to greater degrees than usually necessary for the treatment of malignant hypertension. When a pheochromocytoma causes major increases in plasma norepinephrine concentration, careful dosing with intravenous phentolamine (5 mg bolus every 10 to 20 min, as necessary) is the recommended therapy. In most other situations when intravenous therapy will be necessary only for a short time (e.g., 12 to 24 h), nitroprusside is widely preferred because of its short plasma half-life (thus allowing quick down-titration should the blood pressure plummet) and prompt onset of action.[22]

Assuming that the patient survives the acute reduction of blood pressure with an intravenously administered agent (which is the norm nowadays), the prognosis in malignant hypertension largely depends on changes in renal function.[23] Patients presenting with malignant hypertension without severe renal dysfunction (i.e., serum creatinine levels <5.0 mg/dL) seldom require acute dialysis, whereas 75 percent of those with creatinine values >10 mg/dL have needed dialysis within several days.[24] Chronic control of blood pressure is important for patients with malignant hypertension who initially require dialysis, as some patients have regained sufficient renal function to "escape" dialysis after months of effective antihypertensive therapy.[25]

The most common problem in the management of patients with malignant hypertension is not substituting an oral medication soon enough after the blood pressure is stabilized with nitroprusside, leading to the accumulation of toxic metabolites. Typically after 6 to 24 h at goal blood pressure on nitroprusside therapy, the more difficult task arises of choosing an appropriate oral agent for the acute control of blood pressure (i.e., so the intravenous agent can be down-titrated). Because many medications currently are available for this (e.g., 57 in the tightly regulated United States alone), distinguishing among the choices can be difficult. It is probably wiser to avoid prodrugs (e.g., those that require conversion by other organs to active drug), agents capable of quickly reducing the blood pressure, or those which can cause precipitous hypotension (e.g., captopril, nifedipine, etc.; vide infra), unless they are given in very small doses. Instead, it may be preferable to use agents which will lower the blood pressure incrementally within a few hours, so that the dose of intravenous medication might be gradually reduced (as necessary) to keep the blood pressure within the target range. The usual considerations of cost, frequency of dosing, anticipated side effects, and concomitant diseases of the individual patient are also important if the agent chosen is to be continued as long-term (i.e., outpatient) antihypertensive therapy. A β blocker with a long half-life or an immediate-release formulation of calcium antagonist is often useful when changing over from an intravenous to an oral regimen. Because even "balanced" vasodilators like nitroprusside can cause fluid and sodium retention, a diuretic (typically of the loop diuretic class) is also often given if the urine output during blood pressure reduction has not been voluminous.

Differential Diagnosis

After the diagnosis of malignant hypertension is made and the patient begun on appropriate therapy, the physician should return to the important issue of what underlying conditions predisposed this individual to enter the malignant phase. The physical examination may already give important clues to this, as noted above. Patients with malignant hypertension have a higher prevalence of secondary causes, but most still have primary (or essential) hypertension. On a population basis, renovascular disease is probably the most common form of secondary hypertension and far exceeds the prevalence of pheochromocytoma, which is still an occasional cause of malignant hypertension (especially when presenting as congestive heart failure). Conn's syndrome very rarely produces either severe (much less, malignant) hypertension or high grade retinopathy. Screening tests for secondary hypertension (e.g., 24-h urine collections for vanillylmandelic acid (VMA) and metanephrines, and renal scans—with captopril if available, or intravenous digital subtraction angiography, where available) are often performed on the second or third hospital day (i.e., after the patient moves out of the ICU), and can be followed up by more formal tests (e.g., clonidine suppression or renal angiography) if indicated.

There is often concern that a patient with malignant hypertension may harbor a pheochromocytoma. The history (especially if it includes headache, hypertension, hyperhydrosis, and hyperglycemia) is often very helpful, but many relatively asymptomatic persons with pheochromocytoma have been described. If the blood pressure is found to vary widely (before or during therapy), if there is inappropriate tachycardia, or if the patient has cutaneous signs of the phakomatoses or familial syndromes known to be associated with pheochromocytoma, the probability is elevated. In such patients, it may be difficult to control the blood pressure with nitroprusside alone, and careful dosing with intravenous phentolamine (2 to 5 mg given slowly to start, followed by 5 to 10 mg every 10 to 20 min, as necessary, until an infusion can be started) can be recommended. Precipitous hypotension is the potential problem and can be avoided by careful and small dosing. In general, the most useful screening test for pheochromocytoma is still the 24-h collection of urine for VMA and metanephrines, but often a plasma sample (taken from an indwelling intravenous line and handled appropriately) obtained while the patient has very high blood pressure can be good evidence against a pheochromocytoma if the plasma catecholamine levels are normal. More formal pharmacologic tests (clonidine suppression, glucagon stimulation) can be performed, if indicated, after acute therapy for malignant hypertension, and usually in the outpatient setting. Localization tests (abdominal CT scan, magnetic resonance imaging, or ^{131}I-monoiodobenzylguanidine scan) are usually performed (again in the outpatient department) before surgery is attempted.

Drug ingestion is becoming an increasingly important cause of severe elevations in blood pressure, sometimes with acute target organ damage. The well-known problem of "rebound" hypertension after cessation of antihypertensive medications is seen most prominently with α agonists (particularly clonidine) and sometimes β blockers, but has been reported with calcium channel blockers and minoxidil as well. Monoamine oxidase inhibitors are rarely used by physicians other than psychiatrists because of the potential for tyramine-induced catastrophe, which can easily be confused with malignant hypertension. Phenylpropanolamines are capable of elevating blood pressure, but the small doses available over-the-counter rarely cause severe hypertension. Young women without previous histories of hypertension have been known to develop malignant hypertension during oral contraceptive therapy. In contrast to many other patients in the malignant phase, such patients often need no further pharmacologic therapy after acute treatment except discontinuing their birth control pills. Drugs of abuse (especially cocaine and phencyclidine) have recently become very prevalent, and can often cause acute hypertension with target organ damage that is very difficult to distinguish from classic malignant hypertension.[26] Other rare and recently recognized causes of malignant hypertension include IgA nephropathy, vasculitides (especially periarteritis nodosa), and 17-α-hydroxylase deficiency.

Certainly many other conditions can present much in the same manner as malignant hypertension. Aside from pseudohypertension (i.e., erroneously elevated blood pressures as measured by cuff and sphygmomanometer, but normal intraarterial pressures, thought to be due to sclerotic arteries),[27] these are most easily grouped by affected organ system: brain, heart, kidneys, etc. Hypertensive encephalopathy is often difficult to separate from subarachnoid hemorrhage, acute cerebrovascular accident, and other less urgent neurologic syndromes (brain tumor, head injury, subdural hematoma, postictal state, cerebral vasculitis associated with collagen-vascular disease, etc.) until the optic fundi are thoroughly examined. Patients with acute pulmonary edema typically have elevated plasma catecholamine levels, and often their blood pressures are raised to very high levels.

Patients with known renal failure are at risk for severe elevations in blood pressure (especially if noncompliant with their antihypertensive therapy) and can mimic malignant hypertension unless the degree of chronic renal insufficiency is known. Two special cases exist when patients are compliant, and these should be recognized by the physician. Recent (re-)institution of antihypertensive therapy often transiently raises the serum creatinine level in patients with chronic renal insufficiency, so the history of exactly when the patient began drug therapy for hypertension is important. The patient who has recently started an ACE inhibitor and has better blood pressure, but an elevated serum creatinine level, should be suspected of having renal artery stenosis. Most patients with acute nephritis have only modest degrees of hypertension despite their hematuria and are therefore unlikely to be confused with those having malignant hypertension. Rarely, patients with acute intermittent porphyria present with severe hypertension, abdominal pain, and abnormally colored urine, which can be confused with malignant hypertension.

Drugs for Hypertensive Urgencies

Compared to several years ago, many drugs are now available for the effective treatment of severe hypertension that does not require reduction within minutes to hours. This task is usually accomplished by oral administration of vasodilators, but can be risky if the dose is inappropriately large or the drug used is a poor match for the individual patient. There is currently controversy as to whether most asymptomatic persons presenting with severe hypertension need be treated as "hypertensive urgencies," as previous experience has indicated that few asymptomatic individuals with diastolic blood pressures as high as 140 mmHg suffer untoward events.[28] This was most convincingly demonstrated in the initial Veterans Administration trial, in which no adverse events occurred in the placebo treated group for the first 2 months after randomization.[29] A similar group of 42 patients with uncomplicated hypertension (diastolic blood pressures up to 160 mmHg) also had no adverse consequences for at least 2 months.[30] A recent randomized trial of "clonidine loading" lowered blood pressures, but no improvements in long-term outcome were detected.[28]

Many physicians have been favorably impressed with nifedipine as treatment for severe hypertension,[31] and only recently have some reports of hypotension and other complications surfaced.[32] The bite-and-swallow technique (i.e., have the patient chew the capsule until it breaks and then wash down the liquid with water) using 10-mg capsules is prompt and effective, whereas the sublingual method (applying the contents of a capsule directly under the tongue, and insisting that the patient not swallow) appears less reliable, especially when patients perform sublingual therapy properly. Administration of a second dose of nifedipine to patients having insufficient lowering of blood pressure 30 min after the first dose is probably preferable to trying to treat acute hypotension due to a larger initial dose. Caution is advised in using nifedipine in the elderly, those with congestive heart failure or acute angina, and those who are intravascularly volume depleted; these caveats apply equally well to all orally administered drugs for the acute therapy of hypertension.

Treatment of severe hypertension with clonidine hydrochloride has been widely adopted (especially by emergency physicians),[28,33] using a protocol of loading with 0.2 mg and followed by a further 0.1 mg/h until the blood pressure goal is reached or 0.6 mg is delivered. This has been effective therapy in nearly all patients so treated, but has two major drawbacks. The first is that there is a high frequency of sedation using these doses of clonidine (which is obviously of major import when serial assessment of the sensorium is important), which affects the ability of the patient to drive home and appear in clinic on the following day. Secondly, clonidine is prescribed as chronic therapy for many patients at the end of the protocol (typically at one-half the required "urgent" dose, taken in divided doses each day). As many patients presenting with "urgent" hypertension have a problem with compliance with medications, it is probably unwise to choose an antihypertensive agent with a strong potential for rebound hypertension when abruptly discontinued.

Captopril and enalaprilate are two available ACE inhibitors also effective in the acute therapy of severe hypertension. They may have a role in the treatment of malignant hypertension (which often does include an activation of the renin-angiotensin-aldosterone system), especially when intravenous therapy with other drugs is insufficient.[34] Some patient groups (especially congestive heart failure, renal insufficiency, and volume depletion) are very sensitive to the blood pressure lowering effects of ACE inhibitors, such that these agents have not yet become first-line therapy, except in certain centers in Brazil.[34] Captopril is typically given in a dose of 6.25–25 mg (crushed tablets hasten oral absorption) and often lowers blood pressure in 15 to 30 min. Enalaprilate is given intravenously beginning at 2.5 mg and also has a short onset of action. These drugs can cause or exacerbate renal insufficiency in those patients with critical renal artery stenosis (although this is rare) and sometimes can precipitate or exacerbate hyperkalemia.

Other oral drugs that are occasionally helpful include nitrates (for the patient with chronic angina), and minoxidil (which is very effective in the uncommon situation of the patient already receiving a β blocker and diuretic).

CASE PRESENTATION

A 56-year-old white male professor sought the attention of an ophthalmologist due to 1 day of blurred vision in the right eye. Because of abnormalities of the retina, he was referred to a retinal specialist, who confirmed the presence of papilledema. Blood pressure, measured by a nurse at that visit, was allegedly 190/110. He was referred to an internist for control of blood pressure and had no complaints other than cold feet for about 12 months, and erectile impotence for 6 months. He took no medications, and aside from a single "120/80" (8 years earlier), had not had his blood pressure measured in 25 years. Six years earlier, his wife had been diagnosed as hypertensive, and since then the diet in the home was remarkably low in sodium. The patient confessed to frequently eating salty soups, sandwiches, and snacks at the Faculty Club, however. He did not smoke and drank only occasional alcohol. On presentation, he had blood pressure 230 to 250/130 to 135 with a regular heart rate at 88; bilateral papilledema, hemorrhages, and exudates in the fundi; a grade

1/6 systolic ejection murmur heard best at the left lower sternal border; no abdominal bruits; and bilaterally poor (1+) pedal pulses. He was quickly admitted to a monitored hospital bed for rapid reduction of blood pressure. Intravenous access was obtained, blood sent for admitting laboratory tests, and nitroprusside begun at 0.5 μg/kg/min. An ECG showed left ventricular hypertrophy with strain, and a chest x-ray displayed left ventricular enlargement and old left apical pleural scarring. Over the next 2 h, the rate of the nitroprusside infusion was incrementally titrated to 2.0 μg/kg/min at 20-min intervals, and the diastolic blood pressure was maintained between 100 and 110 mmHg. Blood counts and serum chemistries were normal except for a BUN of 36 mg/dL, creatinine of 1.9 mg/dL, cholesterol of 294 mg/dL, and LDH of 208 IU. The peripheral smear disclosed schistocytes and polychromasia. The urine contained 2+ protein, 4+ blood, with 3 to 5 red cells and occasional white cells/high power field. During 6 h of nitroprusside therapy (monitored by a physician at the bedside during the infusion), he had no complaints; he was then given 50 mg atenolol, and the nitroprusside weaned off over 2 h, to keep the diastolic blood pressure between 100 and 110 mmHg. During the infusion, he excreted 1.2 L urine (almost doubling his pretreatment urinary flow rate) and temporarily improved his creatinine clearance, from 65 to 99 mL/min. His peripheral renin activity was measured at 5.3 ng Ang II/mL/h (normal 0 to 2), and his 24-h sodium excretion was 360 mEq. He was discharged after plasma samples obtained 3 h after and before 0.3 mg of oral clonidine contained norepinephrine in a ratio <0.5. Six weeks later, he underwent renal angiography as an outpatient (after his serum creatinine level increased to 2.4 mg/dL while taking lisinopril), which disclosed no renal arterial stenoses; renal vein renin activities (in samples taken at the same time as the angiogram) were: 6.2 (left), 6.8 (right), and 5.6 ng Ang II/mL/h (below the renal veins). During 2 years of follow-up, his blood pressures have been well controlled (average 142/88) on lisinopril 20 mg/day and acebutolol 400 mg/day, and his serum creatinine level has decreased to 1.8 mg/dL, with a creatinine clearance of 76 mL/min. His papilledema resolved after 10 days and there are now only a few scattered small choroidal scars where there were once acute hemorrhages.

CASE DISCUSSION

Illustrative points in this case include the fact that the patient was essentially asymptomatic, despite a very elevated blood pressure, which was likely to have been chronic. The patient was admitted to a hospital floor bed with a cardiac monitor because it was the first bed available; it might have been preferable to have been in an ICU, but often (as in this case), this consumes time (to transfer out the patient currently in the bed, clean the room, etc.). A bed with a cardiac monitor and a physician at the bedside to continuously monitor the patient for a few hours surely qualifies as intensive care even if not within the confines of such a unit. Nitroprusside was chosen because of its quick action, both in lowering blood pressure and in being quickly reversible if untoward side effects (e.g., symptoms of cerebral hypoperfusion) occur. Atenolol was given before the nitroprusside was weaned because of the high baseline heart rate; no diuretic was given because his urine output during therapy was acceptable (if not high). Immediate-release verapamil or perhaps high dose diltiazem might have also been acceptable substitutes. ACE inhibitors were avoided acutely, both because of potential renal artery disease (in the setting of poor pedal pulses, elevated creatinine level, and malignant hypertension), and because the pharmacokinetics are not appropriate (captopril and lisinopril can lower blood pressure quickly and precipitously; enalapril requires time to undergo deesterification by the liver).

The search for secondary causes of hypertension in many patients with malignant hypertension is bound to be fruitless, as both pheochromocytoma and renal artery disease are relatively rare in any population of hypertensive patients. Nonetheless, both have a higher incidence in this type of hypertension and even constitute a majority in some series. This patient was screened for both while hospitalized; a clonidine suppression test was done to rule out pheochromocytoma. Because of the increase in serum creatinine concentration after lisinopril (chosen because of the positively charged side chain, and thought to be less likely to cause problems in this professor with thinking and other CNS-related activity), there was further reason to rule out renal artery disease, which was eventually accomplished by a renal angiogram and renal vein renins. Although angiography is hardly indicated in every case of malignant hypertension, the possibility of renal artery disease should not be overlooked.

References

1. Joint National Committee on Detection, Evaluation and Treatment of High Blood Pressure: The 1984 report of the Joint National Committee. Arch Intern Med 144:1045, 1984.
2. Keith NM, Wagener HP, Kernohan JW: The syndrome of malignant hypertension. Arch Intern Med 41:141, 1928.
3. The 1988 Report of the Joint National Committee on the Detection, Evaluation, and Treatment of High Blood Pressure. Arch Intern Med 148:1023, 1988.
4. Ahmed MEK, Walker JM, Beevers DG, Beevers M: Lack of difference between malignant and accelerated hypertension. Brit Med J 292:235, 1986.
5. McGregor E, Isles CG, Jay JL, et al: Retinal changes in malignant hypertension. Brit Med J 292:233, 1986.
6. Johansson B, Strandgaard S, Lassen NA: The hypertensive "breakthrough" of autoregulation of cerebral blood flow with forced vasodilatation, flow increase, and blood-brain barrier damage. Circ Res 34–35 (suppl. I):I167, 1974.
7. Davies DL, Beevers DG, Briggs JD, et al: Abnormal relationship between exchangeable sodium and the renin-angiotensin system in malignant hypertension and in hypertension with chronic renal failure. Lancet 1:683, 1973.

8. Ferguson RK, Vlasses PH, Koplin JR, et al: Captopril in severe treatment-resistant hypertension. Am Heart J 99:579, 1980.
9. Bennett NM, Shea S: Hypertensive emergency: Case criteria, sociodemographic profile, and previous care of 100 cases. Am J Public Health 78:646, 1988.
10. Petitti DB, Klatsky AL: Malignant hypertension in women 15–44 years, and its relation to cigarette smoking and oral contraceptives. Am J Cardiol 52:297, 1983.
11. Healton EB, Brust JC, Feinfeld DA, Thomson GE: Hypertensive encephalopathy and the neurologic manifestations of malignant hypertension. Neurology 32:127, 1982.
12. Davis BA, Crook JE, Vestal RE, Oates JA: Prevalence of renal vascular hypertension in patients with grade III or IV hypertensive retinopathy. N Engl J Med 301:1273, 1979.
13. England WL, Grim CE, Weinberger MH, Roberts SD: Cost-effectiveness in the detection of renal artery stenosis. J Gen Intern Med 3:344, 1988.
14. Lindsay PG: The "half-and-half" nail. Arch Intern Med 119:583, 1967.
15. Ferguson RK, Vlasses PH: Hypertensive emergencies and urgencies. JAMA 255:1607, 1986.
16. Reuler JB, Magarian GJ: Hypertensive emergencies and urgencies: Definition, recognition, and management. J Gen Intern Med 3:64, 1988.
17. Ledingham JGG, Rajagopalan B: Cerebral complications in the treatment of accelerated hypertension. Q J Med 49:25, 1979.
18. Drugs for Hypertensive Emergencies. The Medical Letter 29:18, 1987.
19. Cohn JN, Burke LP: Nitroprusside. Ann Intern Med 91:752, 1979.
20. Wallin JD, Fletcher E, Ram CVS, et al: Intravenous nicardipine for the treatment of severe hypertension: A double-blind, placebo-controlled, multicenter trial. Arch Intern Med 149:2262, 1989.
21. Elliott WJ, Weber RR, Nelson KS, et al.: Renal and hemodynamic effects of intravenous fenoldopam versus nitroprusside in severe hypertension. Circulation 81:970, 1990.
22. Calhoun DA, Oparil S: Current Concepts: Treatment of hypertensive crisis. N Engl J Med 323:1177, 1990.
23. Jespersen B, Eiskjaer H, Christiansen NO, et al: Malignant arterial hypertension: Relationship between blood pressure control and renal function during long-term observation of patients with malignant nephrosclerosis. J Clin Hypertension 3:409, 1987.
24. Isles CG, McLay A, Boulton Jones JM: Recovery in malignant hypertension presenting as acute renal failure. Q J Med 53:439, 1984.
25. Bakir AA, Bazilinski N, Dunea G: Transient and sustained recovery from renal shutdown in accelerated hypertension. Am J Med 80:172, 1986.
26. Mangiardi JR, Daras M, Geller ME, et al: Cocaine-related intracranial hemorrhage: Report of 9 cases and review. Acta Neurol Scand 77:177, 1988.
27. Littenberg B, Wolfberg C: Pseudohypertension masquerading as malignant hypertension: Case report and review of the literature. Am J Med 84:539, 1988.
28. Zeller KR, Von Kuhnert L, Matthews C: Rapid reduction of severe asymptomatic hypertension: A prospective controlled trial. Arch Intern Med 149:2186, 1989.
29. Veterans Administration Cooperative Study Group on Antihypertensive Agents: Effects of treatment on morbidity in hypertension. JAMA 202:116, 1967.
30. Wolff FW, Lindeman RD: Effects of treatment in hypertension. J Chronic Dis 19:227, 1966.
31. Houston MC: Treatment of hypertensive urgencies and emergencies with nifedipine. Am Heart J 111:963, 1986.
32. Wachter RM: Symptomatic hypotension induced by nifedipine in the acute treatment of severe hypertension. Arch Intern Med 147:556, 1987.
33. Houston MC: Treatment of hypertensive emergencies and urgencies with oral clonidine loading and titration: A review. Arch Intern Med 146:586, 1986.
34. Ramos O: Malignant hypertension: The Brazilian experience. Kidney Int 26:209, 1984.

Chapter 124

AORTIC DISSECTION

JOSEPH J. AUSTIN
B. WILLIAM SHRAGGE

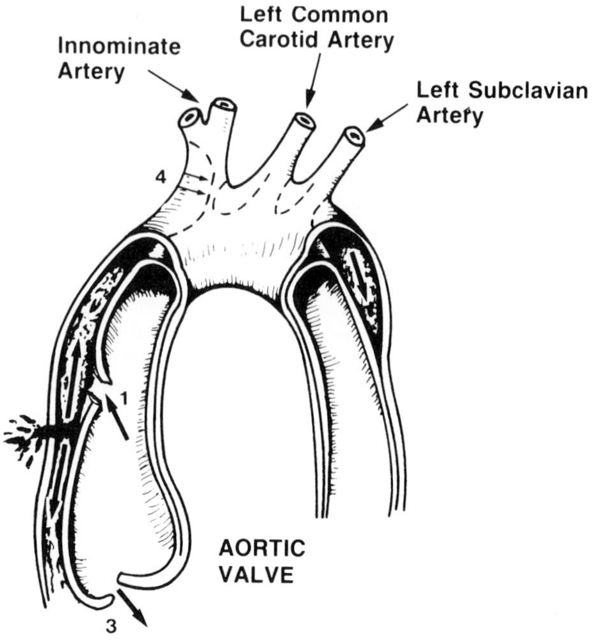

FIGURE 124-1 Aortic dissection begins with an intimal tear (1) leading to a hematoma which separates the layers of the aortic wall. The sequelae are rupture through the adventitia into the pericardium (2); prolapse of the aortic valve cusps leading to aortic insufficiency (3); compression of the aortic branch vessels (4); and aneurysmal dilation of the ascending arch and descending aorta.

KEY POINTS

- *Acute aortic dissection occurs more commonly than ruptured abdominal aortic aneurysm.*
- *The typical pain, poor peripheral perfusion, and evidence of aortic branch occlusion suggest the diagnosis.*
- *Early pharmacologic control of systolic blood pressure and the pulse wave* (dP/dT) *is imperative.*
- *Investigations must be undertaken urgently to confirm the diagnosis and direct definitive treatment.*
- *Emergency surgical repair is indicated for Type A dissections.*
- *Control of blood pressure is important to minimize complications and maximize survival both in the postoperative period and in long-term follow-up.*

Aortic dissection is the most common catastrophe affecting the aorta, occurring two to three times more commonly than acute abdominal aortic aneurysm rupture.[1] The reported incidence is approximately 10 to 20 per million per year.[2] Rarely is the outcome of a cardiovascular disease so dependent on the skills and cooperation of the intensivist and the cardiovascular surgeon as it is with acute dissections of the aorta. Maximal survival is dependent on a high index of suspicion of the diagnosis despite a myriad of different presentations, early pharmacologic intervention for control of blood pressure, rapid diagnosis with appropriate imaging, and then appropriate relegation to medical or surgical management depending on the dissection type. Without treatment, the 3-month mortality is 85 to 90 percent, but with the appropriate treatment survivals of over 80 percent can be expected.

Pathogenesis

Previously, aortic dissections were referred to as *dissecting aneurysms* as originally coined by Laennec. This is a misnomer in that the pathology is a dissecting hematoma which separates the intima and inner layers of the media from the outer medial and adventitial layers (Fig. 124-1). The intima is therefore not aneurysmal and is, if anything, narrowed. Blood invades the media through a tear in the intima and proceeds antero- or retrogradely through the aortic wall forming a false lumen. The hematoma spirals around the right and posterior aspects of the ascending aorta, supraposteriorly along the arch, then down the left and posterior aspects of the descending aorta.[3] The hematoma may then have several serious sequelae. It may rupture into the pericardial space causing tamponade or into the pleural space with exsanguinating hemorrhage or rarely back into the true lumen distally. It may also cause occlusion of aortic branch arteries or prolapse of one or more of the aortic cusps resulting in aortic insufficiency.

Generally, the tear is due to either a weakening of the wall of the aorta or an increase in luminal shear stress or both.[3] Weakening of the aortic wall occurs as the result of "medial degeneration" or iatrogenic injury. Medial degeneration (cystic medial degeneration or necrosis) is manifested by the loss of smooth muscle cells and accumulation of basophilic amorphous material with or without associated "cysts" in the aortic media. This is believed to be due to inborn errors of metabolism (Marfan's or Ehlers-Danlos syndrome). There is a reduction in the cohesiveness of the layers of the aortic wall as a result. Other causes of reduced wall strength causing aortic dissection include annuloaortic ectasia, bicuspid aortic valve, coarctation and pregnancy (especially third trimester).

Iatrogenic injuries occur during open heart surgical procedures at any point where the aorta is invaded such as the aortotomy for an aortic valve replacement or the proximal anastomosis of an aorto–coronary bypass graft.

Stresses applied to the aortic wall increase wall tension and lead to dissections. Most important are intraluminal sheer stresses which are related both to the level of the systolic blood pressure and to the steepness of the aortic pulse wave.[2] This is referred to as dP/dT_{max} and represents the speed with which the maximal systolic pressure is attained in the aortic root. As this increases, so too does the sheer stress on the ascending aorta.

Classification

Dissections are classified by timing and location to identify the morbidity and mortality for the specific lesions.

TIMING

- Acute: Less than 2 weeks.
- Chronic: More than 2 weeks.

Acute dissections are very high risk lesions with the estimated mortality of 50 percent for the first 48 h (or 1 percent per hour).

LOCATION

- Type A: Ascending aorta is involved independent of the site of the intimal tear (since 15 percent of transverse arch and 5 percent of descending aortic tears will involve the ascending aorta).
- Type B: Descending aorta (beyond the left subclavian artery).

This classification system, proposed by Daily and colleagues and popularized by the Stanford group, replaces the original system proposed by DeBakey (Fig. 124-2). Using this classification, 60 percent of all dissections are Type A, involving the ascending aorta, and 40 percent are Type B and affect only the descending thoracic aorta. It is based on the risk of sudden death from the dissection which is highest when the ascending aorta is involved as in Type A. Here the dissection may cause tamponade, severe aortic insufficiency, and congestive heart failure as well as coronary thrombosis. Type B dissections do not have these risks and can generally be approached and managed conservatively. As a result, therapeutic interventions are dependent on location with almost all Type A dissections requiring urgent operative intervention, while Type B dissections are primarily managed pharmacologically with surgery only for specific complications.

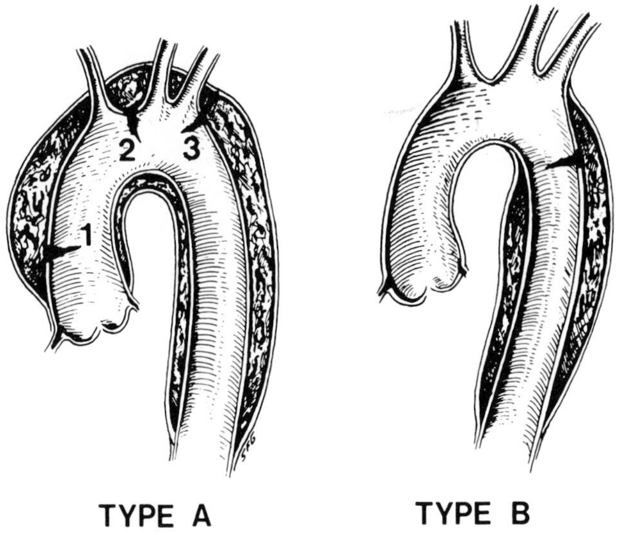

FIGURE 124-2 Classification of aortic dissection based on the presence or absence of ascending aortic involvement. Type A dissections involve the ascending aorta and Type B do not. The intimal tear in Type A dissections may be in the ascending aorta (1), the arch (2), or the descending aorta (3). Type A includes DeBakey types I and II. In Type B dissection the intimal tear is distal to the left subclavian artery origin. Type B dissections correspond to DeBakey's type III. (Reprinted from McGoon C: *Cardiac Surgery*, 2nd ed, AN Brest, Editor-in-Chief, F.A. Davis, Philadelphia, 1987, with permission.)

Clinical Picture

Men, particularly black males, are at two to three times the risk of developing an aortic dissection as women. More than 90 percent will have a history of hypertension requiring treatment. The presentation of an acute dissection can be subtle, demanding great attention to detail to make the diagnosis or it can be classical and obvious. The signs and symptoms are related to the location of the tear and the extent of the hematoma dissection. These are manifested mainly by pain, poor peripheral perfusion despite an increased blood pressure, and aortic branch occlusion signs and symptoms.

PAIN

Typically, the pain is either retrosternal or central, interscapular back pain but may be epigastric. Classically it begins in the chest, moves to the back, and then moves down to the abdomen or lower extremities as the dissection progresses, but this pattern is rarely seen. Patients describe the pain as "sharp," "tearing," or "knifelike" and is most often excruciating in intensity. To differentiate it from angina, the pain is maximal immediately upon onset, and it is difficult to obtain complete relief with opiates alone.

POOR PERFUSION

Often patients present with evidence of shock with a cool clammy periphery, ashen coloring, and depressed level of consciousness and yet markedly elevated systolic blood pressure frequently exceeding 200 mmHg. Most often this is caused by reflex sympathetic discharge from the intense pain. It can occur, however, with myocardial infarction due to coronary artery occlusion by the dissection or from severe aortic insufficiency with congestive heart failure which is present in 30 to 60 percent of patients with Type A dissections. If the blood pressure is depressed, the dissection may have ruptured into the pericardium with tamponade (as occurs in 30 percent of Type A dissections) or into the pleural space (left more often than right) with resulting hypovolemia.

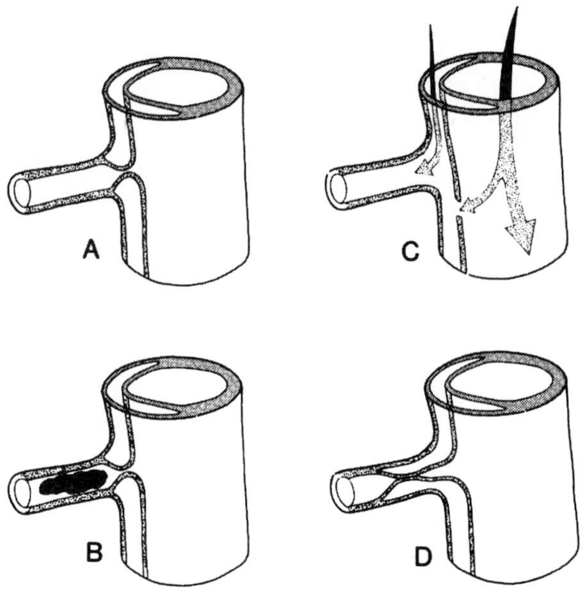

FIGURE 124-3 Aortic branch occlusion mechanisms. (A) Compression of the true lumen by the false lumen with a patent true lumen. (B) Complete occlusion of the true lumen by the false lumen with thrombosis. (C) Complete avulsion of the intima from the origin of the branch vessel with blood flow provided both from the false lumen and the true lumen via distal reentry. (D) Complete occlusion of the true lumen by the false lumen beyond the branch orifice. (Reprinted from Cambria et al[4] with permission.)

AORTIC BRANCH OCCLUSION SIGNS AND SYMPTOMS

Approximately one-third of patients will present with compromised flow to a major branch of the aorta as part of their presentation.[4] The vessel may be sheared off or compressed resulting in occlusion and/or thrombosis or be perfused through the false channel (Fig. 124-3). Table 124-1 lists the vessels affected and their manifestations. The innominate artery and the left renal and iliac arteries are affected most frequently because of the spiral motion of the hematoma as it rounds the arch and descends in the thoracoabdominal aorta. Fortunately the visceral and renal vessels are affected in less than 3 percent of patients as their involvement denotes a very poor prognosis.

TABLE 124-1 Aortic Branch Occlusion

Site	Manifestation
Iliofemoral (35%)	Lower extremity ischemia
Carotid (21%)	Cerebrovascular accident (CVA)
Subclavian (14%)	Upper extremity ischemia
Renal (14%)	Renal Failure or hypertension
Mesenteric (8%)	Intestinal ischemia
Abdominal Aorta (7%)	Aortic aneurysm

NOTE: Peripheral vascular complications listed in decreasing frequency. Overall 8–56% of patients sustain aortic branch complications. Extensive dissections are at higher risk (49–56%) than if isolated to either the ascending or proximal descending aorta (8–13%).

Neurologic sequelae are particularly concerning. Some neurologic dysfunction, such as depressed level of consciousness, dizziness, etc., is said to occur in 30 to 50 percent of patients.[5] Concrete, focal neurologic deficits, however, occur much less frequently (<10 percent overall) and may affect the central nervous system, spinal cord, or peripheral nerves. Central nervous system deficits range from minor transient ischemic attacks to deep coma. Cerebrovascular accidents causing hemiparesis affect 5.5 to 6.7 percent of Type A dissections. They are primarily due to innominate/carotid artery occlusion with the right side affected in two-thirds of cases. They can also be caused by emboli or low flow with thrombosis due to previous carotid stenosis. Paraparesis and paraplegia are fortunately rare (2 percent of Type A) as they portend a very poor prognosis.

Investigations and Diagnosis

LABORATORY

Laboratory data are usually within normal limits in patients with acute dissection. The white blood count may be slightly elevated to 12,000 to 20,000 most likely as a stress response. Electrocardiogram interpretation may show left ventricular hypertrophy due to chronic hypertension, but other changes are rare. Acute ischemic changes should raise the concern of coronary artery involvement by the dissection in the patient with a typical history.

DIAGNOSTIC IMAGING

Diagnostic imaging is the most important investigation for the diagnosis and classification of aortic dissections. Standard anteroposterior and upright lateral chest x-rays often reveal a widened mediastinum, although this may be absent in up to 40 percent of Type A dissections (Fig. 124-4). Classically the aorta bulges to the right with Type A and to the left with Type B dissections. Occasionally a double rim of calcification may be present in the distal aortic arch or a pleural effusion may be present (left more than right) due mainly to a serous sympathetic reaction rather than frank blood from a rupture.

More specific investigations include aortography, computed tomography (CT) scanning, magnetic resonance imaging (MRI), and echocardiography, which are all highly accurate for the diagnosis and classification of dissections. Many authors believe that aortic angiography is the most definitive diagnostic method with sensitivity and specificity of 88 to 90 percent and 90 to 95 percent, respectively.[2,6] In addition to confirming the diagnosis by illustrating the true and false channels, the aortogram can pinpoint the site of intimal tear (Fig. 124-5), establish the extent of the dissection as well as quantitate the severity of aortic insufficiency if present, and identify the presence and degree of aortic branch occlusions. Some authors, however, express concerns over false negative reports due to viewing the flap and both lumens en face with the central beam missing small, localized dissection and possibly missing the flap

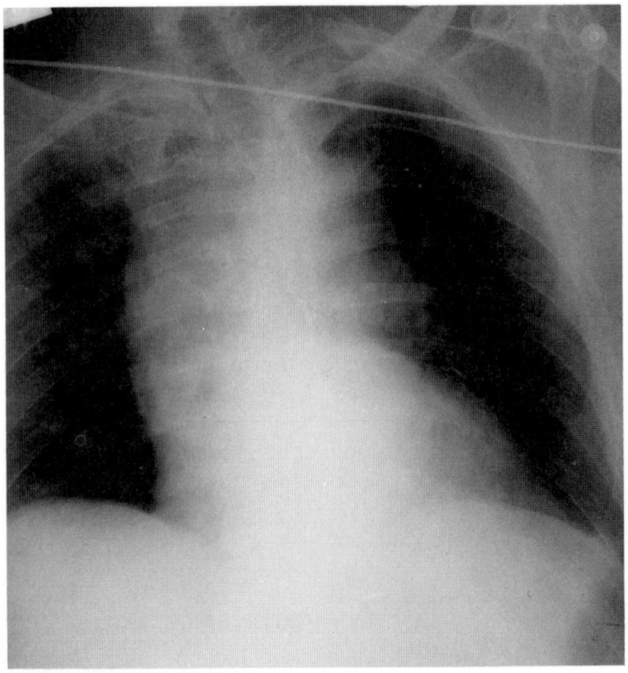

FIGURE 124-4 Chest x-ray illustrating widened mediastinum with blunting of the aortic knob.

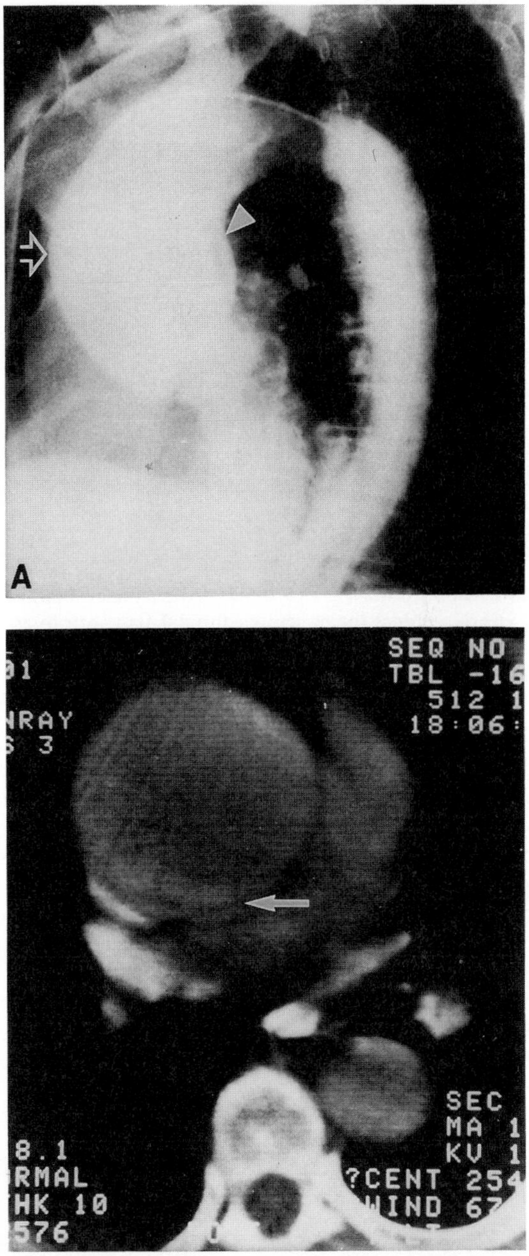

FIGURE 124-5 (A) Aortogram (lateral projection). Grossly dilated ascending aorta (open arrow) with visible intimal flap (solid arrow). Note normal descending aorta. (B) Contrast CT of thorax of same patient. Arrow identifies intimal flap. (Reprinted from Kotler N, Steiner RM: *Cardiac Imaging: New Technologies and Clinical Applications,* AN Brest, Editor-in-Chief, F.A. Davis, Philadelphia, 1986.)

due to simultaneous opacification of both true and false lumens.[7] The procedure is also invasive and requires a contrast load, and so less invasive investigations are preferred.

CT scanning is a noninvasive technique which yields excellent images of dissections, especially Type B. Specific identification of the *true* and *false* lumens with a flap is possible as well as detection of pericardial effusions and accurate depiction of the extent of the dissection (see Fig. 124-6 and 124-7). CT is very specific (~100 percent) for the diagnosis of dissection[6,8] (especially Type B) but is less sensitive than aortography or echocardiography (83 percent). Therefore, if the CT is negative and the suspicion of aortic dissection remains high, other investigations should be done to rule out a dissection. As well as lacking sensitivity, CT does not yield information regarding aortic insufficiency or left ventricular function and requires both contrast administration and exposure to radiation. CT is also inferior to aortography for identifying the site of the intimal tear. Recently, however, this has been shown to have little bearing on the type of dissection or surgical success.

Echocardiography is likely the diagnostic modality of choice for aortic dissections. Both transthoracic and transesophageal two-dimensional echocardiography can accurately evaluate the most important issues of dissections, which are involvement of the ascending aorta, presence and severity of aortic insufficiency, and presence of aortic arch dilation. Two lumens may be seen separated by a flap or there may be central displacement of intimal calcification. The addition of color-coded doppler allows better identification of the true and false lumens even if the false lumen is thrombosed. The presence of a pericardial effusion and any left ventricular wall motion abnormalities may also be accurately assessed.

Transthoracic echocardiography is less accurate than transesophageal in the diagnosis of aortic dissections. It is also frequently technically limited due to chest wall abnormalities, chronic obstructive pulmonary disease, and obesity.

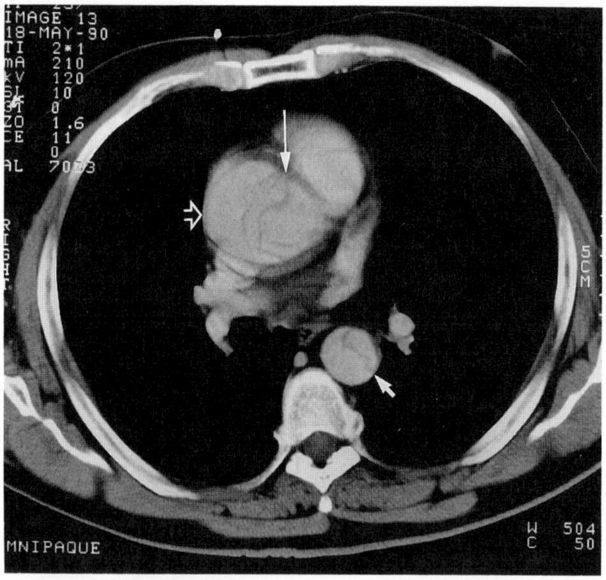

FIGURE 124-6 Contrast CT of thorax. Aneurysmal dilation of aorta clearly evident (open arrow). Intimal flap seen in ascending aorta (long arrow) and continues into descending aorta (short arrow).

Transesophageal echocardiography[9] is the most efficient and accurate diagnostic modality available presently (Figs. 124-8 and 124-9). Its sensitivity and specificity are over 98 percent, and so this technique very accurately identifies the presence or absence of a dissection. Notably, it can be performed in less than 30 min in an emergency room or intensive care unit. The efficiency and mobility are very important in the management of critically ill patients who are best cared for in a well-monitored intensive care unit rather than in the radiology suite. Occasional complications have included transient arrhythmias (atrioventricular block, bradyarrhythmias, and premature ventricular contractions), but generally the procedure is well tolerated.

MRI has been used sparingly to date but does show promise in the investigation of acute dissections.[6,10] It is noninvasive and does not require contrast or ionizing radiation. Excellent contrast can be obtained between extraluminal structures, and it allows the visualization of vascular walls and both clotted and flowing blood. Although diagnostic accuracy is estimated at 90 percent, larger experiences are necessary to confirm its reliability.

The authors presently recommend transesophageal echocardiography as the initial investigation. If this is not immediately available, then CT of the thorax is performed. If negative and there is still a strong suspicion of dissection, then arch angiography may be performed. This approach should, of course, be modified by availability and the local expertise with these imaging techniques at each individual institution.

Natural History

Untreated acute aortic dissections have a uniformly poor prognosis. Fifty percent of patients die within the first 48 h and less than 10 percent will survive 1 month. Poor prognostic variables include aortic branch complications (particularly mesenteric and renal arteries), Type A dissections, associated coronary artery disease (CAD), and neurologic deficits (CVA and paraplegia).[11]

Treatment

To maximize survival, optimal treatment of acute dissections must include early pharmacologic control of blood pressure and pain, often before the definitive diagnosis is made, combined with appropriate surgical intervention. All

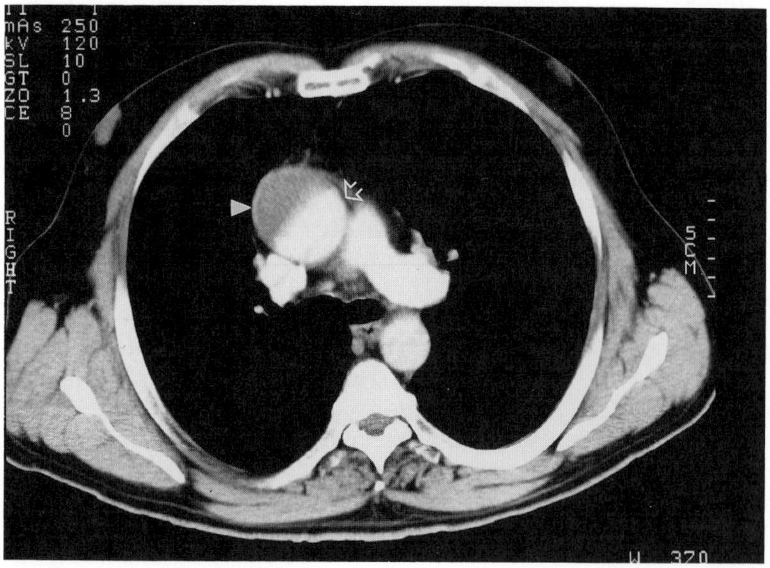

FIGURE 124-7 Contrast CT of thorax. Dilated aortic root and intimal tear present. Contrast fills true lumen first (open arrow). False lumen filling is delayed (solid arrow).

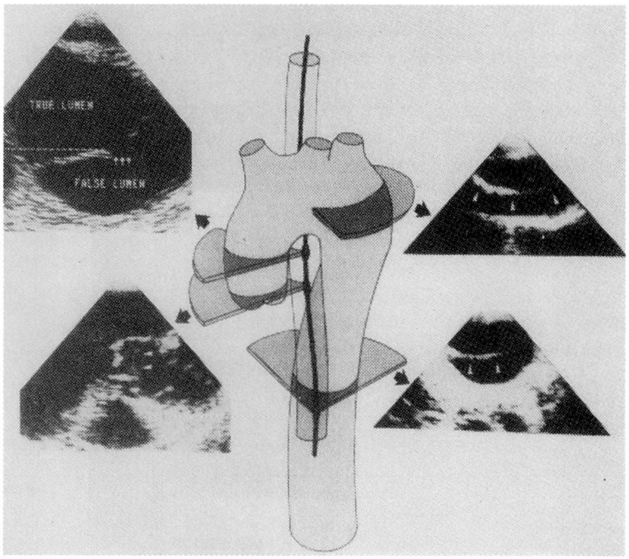

FIGURE 124-8 Transesophageal echocardiogram of Type A dissection. Note clear depiction of true and false lumen as well as intimal flap originating in the ascending aorta (two arrows in bottom left image) and extending into the descending aorta. (Reprinted from Erbel et al[9] with permission.)

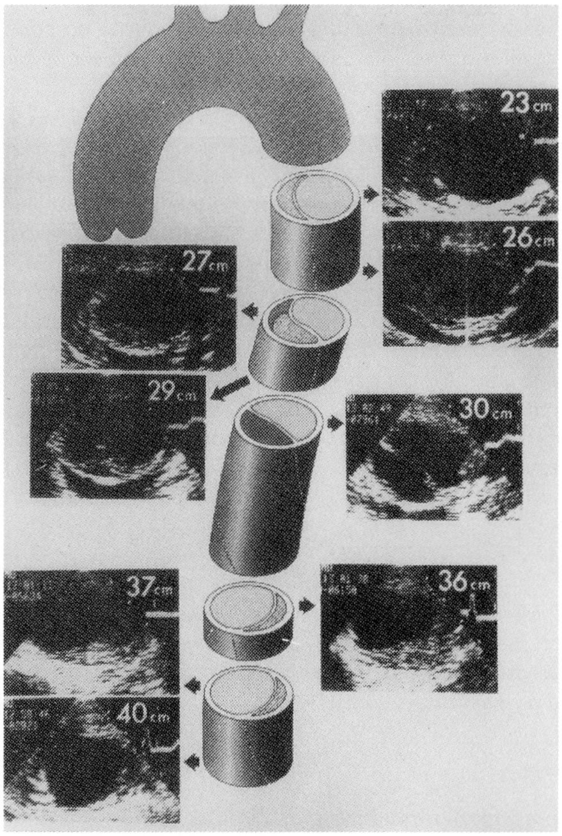

FIGURE 124-9 Transesophageal echocardiogram of Type B dissection. True and false lumens illustrated with spiraling of the dissecting hematoma around the aorta. (Reprinted from Erbel et al[9] with permission.)

patients with aortic dissections must have intensive monitoring in a critical care setting. The patient should be placed on a cardiac monitor and have an intraarterial catheter inserted for ongoing blood pressure monitoring. Central venous pressure and urinary catheters should also be inserted. Blood should be drawn for standard laboratory investigations as well as cross and typing for blood transfusion in case surgery is needed. The patient should be observed closely for any change of hemodynamic parameters or neurologic function and for evidence of organ ischemia.

Pharmacologic Control of Blood Pressure

Intravenous antihypertensive agents are used to reduce the level of systolic blood pressure and the pulse wave (dP/dT_{max}) to halt the progression of the dissecting hematoma. With the hematoma stabilized, pain can usually be controlled with intravenous opiates and the patient further stabilized. Several agents are available for the intensive care unit control of systolic blood pressure and dP/dT_{max} and are listed in Table 124-2 along with their suggested mechanism of action and duration of activity.

Labetolol has arisen as the first choice in antihypertensive agents for aortic dissections. It is a selective alpha$_1$ and nonselective β-adrenoreceptor blocker and so reduces dP/dT_{max} and systolic blood pressure by β-blockade and vasodilation. It can be delivered by bolus or continuous infusion, but most authors prefer the bolus technique. Its peak reduction in systolic blood pressure occurs within 5 min, and its duration of action is 2 to 12 h. It is suitable for long-term control of blood pressure in oral form.

If labetolol is not available, then sodium nitroprusside and propranolol hydrochloride may be used. Propranolol must be given because nitroprusside increases dP/dT_{max} through a sympathetic reflex from its peripheral vasodilatory effects when used alone.

Patients who cannot tolerate β-blockade (chronic obstructive pulmonary disease, congestive heart failure, bradycardia) may be treated with trimethaphan camsylate. In order to adequately reduce the systolic blood pressure, it may be necessary to elevate the head of the bed or dangle the patient's legs over the side of the bed. Occasionally trimethaphan may need to be combined with reserpine or guanethidine. It has many sympathoplegic side effects and can drop the blood pressure quite precipitously. Tachyphylaxis occurs quickly.

Systolic blood pressure should be reduced to levels which will halt the progression of the dissection. Most authors agree that a systolic blood pressure of 90 to 100 mmHg is desirable as long as the patient has adequate organ perfusion as evidenced by a clear sensorium, good urine output, and absence of lactic acidosis.

Definitive Management

Acute aortic dissections are extremely dangerous lesions which may become complicated with rupture and death at

TABLE 124-2 Antihypertensive Agents in Acute Aortic Dissection

Drug	Mechanism	Administration (Intravenous)
Labetolol hydrochloride (Trandate)	α_1 and β_{1+2} adrenergic blocker; decreases peripheral resistance without reflex increase in heart rate and myocardial contractility (dP/dT_{max}); action in 5–10 min; half-life 5–8 h	1. Bolus infusion: 0.25 mg/kg over 2 minutes; may repeat every 10 min 2. Continuous infusion: 1–2 mg/min
Sodium nitroprusside (Nipride)	Direct vascular smooth muscle relaxant; decreases peripheral resistance and preload, may increase dP/dT_{max} when used alone; action in 1–2 min; half-life 3–4 min	Continuous infusion: 0.5–8.0 μg/kg/min
Propanolol hydrochloride (Inderal)	β-adrenergic blocker; decreases myocardial contractility and peripheral resistance; action in 1–2 min; half-life 2–3 h	Bolus infusion: 1–3 mg over 2–3 min; may repeat in 2–3 min
Trimethaphan camsylate (Arfonad)	Autonomic ganglion blocker; direct vascular smooth muscle relaxant; decreases peripheral resistance	Continuous infusion: Begin with 3–4 mg/min

any moment. Pharmacologic control of systolic blood pressure must therefore be instituted as soon as the diagnosis is strongly suspected clinically. Investigations should be performed expeditiously to determine the dissection type and the presence of aortic branch complications. Definitive surgical repair must be undertaken emergently when indicated. Type A dissections should be offered urgent surgical intervention for maximal survival. Relative contraindications to surgery include severe organ dysfunction, such as severe coronary artery disease and chronic obstructive lung disease; old age (i.e., over 80 years old); moribund patient; paraplegia; and CVA. Whether an acute CVA represents a contraindication to surgery is controversial. CVA does represent an independent negative influence on survival. Surgery may make the neurologic deficit worse due to intraoperative bleeding from heparinization, embolization, or reperfusion injury when the occluded carotid is reopened. Without surgery, however, these patients have a near uniformly fatal prognosis. It has been shown that the presence of the CVA does not increase the risk of mortality with surgery. Shumway's group[5] found 85 percent of survivors to be improved or unchanged neurologically and suggested there is no way to predict neurologic outcome from the preoperative neurologic status. A cerebrovascular accident is therefore a relative contraindication to surgery, and only deeply comatose or moribund patients should be refused definitive surgical repair.

Aortic branch complications are best managed by restoring flow to the true lumen by definitive repair of the dissection and postoperative assessment for persistent ischemia.[4] Less than 10 percent of patients will require further surgical procedures for persistent ischemia after definitive repair of the dissection.

Type B dissections of the descending aorta are generally best managed by intensive medical treatment of blood pressure with surgery reserved for complications of the disease. These complications are a result of progression of the dissection despite maximal medical therapy. An increase in size, new aortic insufficiency, and an increase in organ ischemia due to aortic branch occlusion (e.g., abdominal pain, renal dysfunction, or lower extremity ischemia) suggest progression of the dissection and the need for surgical intervention. Intractable pain, evidence of a new pleural or pericardial effusion, acute saccular aneurysms, or a rapid increase in size over a period of hours indicates impending or frank rupture, and emergent surgical repair is imperative for survival.

This approach has been challenged recently.[11] The operative mortality in acute Type B dissections was reported to be reduced from 38 to 13 percent in a small group of patients. This would be an improvement over medical therapy alone, which suffers from a 20 percent mortality. A larger experience is necessary before this aggressive approach is adopted for all Type B dissections.

Type B dissections should be admitted to critical care units for control of their blood pressure and pain and for observation for complications. Close observation with frequent chest x-rays and repeat CT scans or MRI will allow early identification of complications and prompt surgical intervention.

Surgical Intervention

Dr. Michael DeBakey is credited with the initial surgical successes in the treatment of acute aortic dissections. The procedures can be considered as being separate for Type A and Type B dissections.

TYPE A

The surgical procedures for Type A dissections are designed to treat the life-threatening complications in the ascending aorta. There are many factors which are important for deciding the appropriate surgical procedure for each patient. Many of these can be identified preoperatively

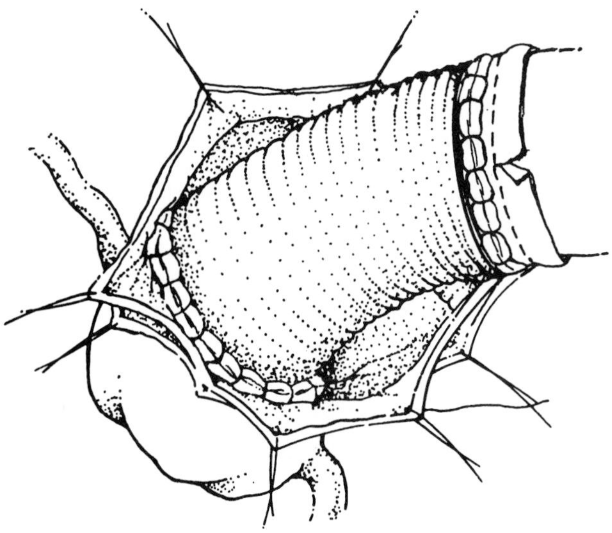

FIGURE 124-10 Suprasinus repair. The ascending aorta is replaced with a Dacron graft. The proximal anastomosis is above the aortic valve and the suture lines are reinforced with felt strips. The distal anastomosis is proximal to the origin of the innominate artery.

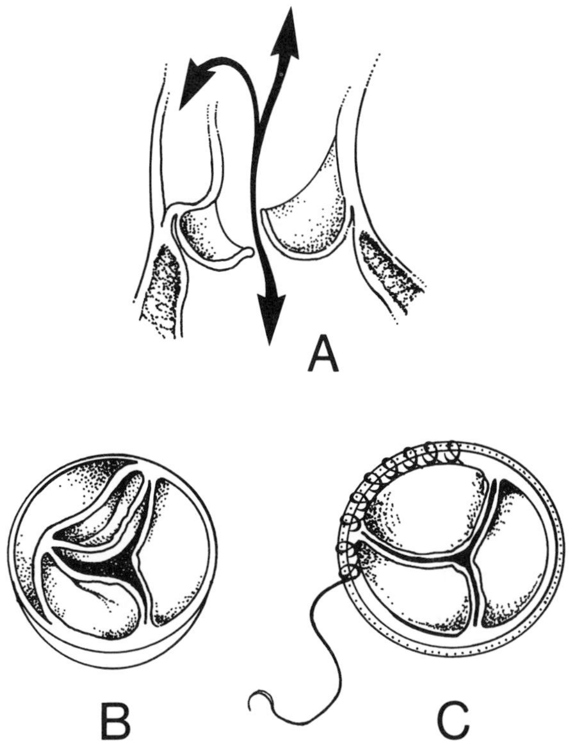

FIGURE 124-11 Resuspension of the aortic valve. The valve cusps are detached from the aortic wall resulting in aortic insufficiency (A and B). The commissures of the aortic valve are sutured back to the outer wall of the aorta to restore the normal relationships of the valve (C). The ascending aorta is replaced with a suprasinus graft.

such as the competency of the aortic valve patency of the coronary arteries, size of the aortic arch, quality of the aortic tissue (e.g., Marfan's, Ehlers-Danlos), and presence or absence of associated aortic branch compromise. The surgical options include simple graft interposition, resuspension of the aortic valve and graft interposition and composite graft insertion.

General preparation of the patient for the procedure includes continuous monitoring of arterial and central venous pressure and often pulmonary artery catheter insertion for pulmonary artery pressure and cardiac output monitoring. The patient is placed on cardiopulmonary bypass (CPB) by inserting the arterial cannula into a femoral artery to leave the ascending aorta and aortic arch clear for surgical repair. Through a median sternotomy, the patient undergoes CPB with either deep hypothermia (15 to 18°C) and total circulatory arrest[12] or continuous CPB with hypothermic cardiac arrest.

Some surgeons prefer to use total circulatory arrest especially for the distal anastomosis. It is usually necessary as well for any repair or replacement of the aortic arch. The time spent with the circulation arrested should ideally be kept to less than 45 min to minimize organ dysfunction. The brain is the most sensitive of the body's organs to prolonged circulatory arrest so this must be kept to a minimum to ensure a good neurologic outcome.

Suprasinus graft interposition is performed for dissections not involving the aortic valve and without gross dilation of the aortic arch. It involves interposing a Dacron tube graft from just above the aortic valve to the innominate artery (Fig. 124-10). The aortic wall may be reinforced with fibrin glue and/or felt to increase the strength of these friable tissues.

Resuspension of the aortic valve with suprasinus tube graft replacement of the ascending aorta is indicated for aortic insufficiency in Type A dissections with otherwise normal aortas. As illustrated in Fig. 124-11, the aortic valve commissures are tacked back to the outer wall of the aorta so as to return the cusps to their normal position and restore competency to the valve. The patient's own aortic valve is preserved and is most often competent.[13] The ascending aorta is replaced with a tube of Dacron to replace the segment of the weakened aorta and prevent later rupture. The inner and outer walls of the aorta are reapproximated at the points the graft is sutured to the aorta. If the aortic arch is not frankly aneurysmal, the graft is sutured to the distal ascending aorta.

Composite grafts consist of a prosthetic valve attached to a Dacron tube graft (Fig. 124-12). This procedure was popularized by Bentall and requires the replacement of the aortic valve and insertion of the coronary arteries into the graft. The Bentall procedure is indicated for underlying disease of the aortic wall where there is high risk of later aneurysmal dilation of the aorta such as in Marfan's, Turner's, and annuloaortic ectasia. It is also indicated for tears arising close to the coronary sinuses or if the native aortic valve is diseased. The prosthetic valve of the composite graft may be either mechanical or bioprosthetic. The most popular mechanical valves are the Bjork-Shiley tilting discs and the St. Jude bileaflet. These are placed primarily in young patients

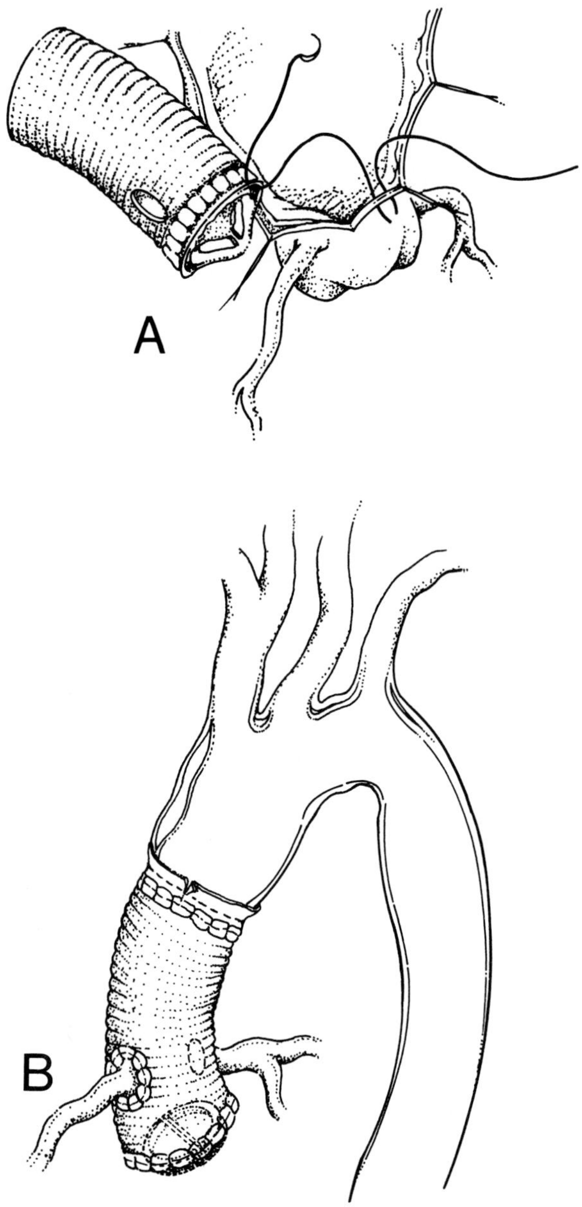

FIGURE 124-12 Composite graft replacement (Bentall). The aortic valve is removed and replaced with a valved conduit (A). The left and right main coronary arteries are reimplanted into the graft (B).

(less than 60 to 65 years old) in whom there are no contraindications to anticoagulation as they require lifelong warfarin therapy. Older patients or those with contraindications to anticoagulation may have a bioprosthetic valved conduit inserted, such as the Carpentier-Edwards porcine valve.

Each of these procedures may involve extension of replacement of the aorta to include the aortic arch in whole or in part. This adds significantly to the risk of the operative procedure, but if the arch is grossly aneurysmal, freedom from late operation and overall survival is increased significantly with immediate repair.[14]

The resolution of aortic branch complications should be assessed at the end of the procedure. Pulses should be checked over both carotids, radial and femoral arteries. If concerns exist for the presence of ongoing ischemia, then immediate surgical revascularization should be undertaken. This usually involves an extraanatomical reconstruction such as axilloaxillary bypass for upper limb ischemia or femorofemoral bypass for unilateral lower ischemia. Aortic fenestration is necessary for bilateral lower extremity ischemia. This involves opening the abdominal aorta and resecting a portion of the inner wall (consisting of intima and part of the media) so as to allow flow through both the true and false lumens to restore blood flow to the lower extremities.

If evidence of renal or visceral ischemia existed preoperatively, then close observation must be maintained postoperatively for their resolution. If ongoing metabolic acidosis or depressed renal function exists, then consideration should be given to urgent surgical exploration. These patients have a very poor prognosis, however, both with and without surgical repair.

TYPE B

Surgical repair of dissections involving the descending thoracic aorta (which may include the transverse arch but not the ascending aorta) is undertaken for failure of medical therapy to control the progress of the dissecting hematoma and for aortic branch compromise. Replacement of the descending thoracic aorta is usually necessary from the left subclavian artery down to mid or lower thoracic levels (Fig. 124-13). The surgery is performed through a left thoracotomy and requires single-lung anesthesia and cross-clamping the aorta at the level of the left subclavian artery. The aorta is opened and replaced with a long Dacron tube. Controversy exists as to protection of the spinal cord during aortic cross-clamp. The concern is to maintain blood flow to the distal aorta and so to the collateral vessels to the cord. Although many options exist, the most popular are some form of CPB (using femorofemoral or atriofemoral bypass); intraluminal shunt (Gott); partial drainage of cerebrospinal fluid; and the simple clamp and sew technique. No technique has been shown to be superior to the others, however, in reducing the high-risk (~40 percent) of paraplegia with surgical repair of acute Type B dissections.

Results

MORBIDITY

Patients undergoing surgical repair of aortic dissections are subject to the same postoperative complications as with any open heart procedure. Early complications include myocardial infarction, low-output syndrome (systolic blood pressure less than 90 mmHg with an elevated left atrial pressure requiring inotropic support), arrhythmia, bleeding, respiratory complications (prolonged ventilation, atelecta-

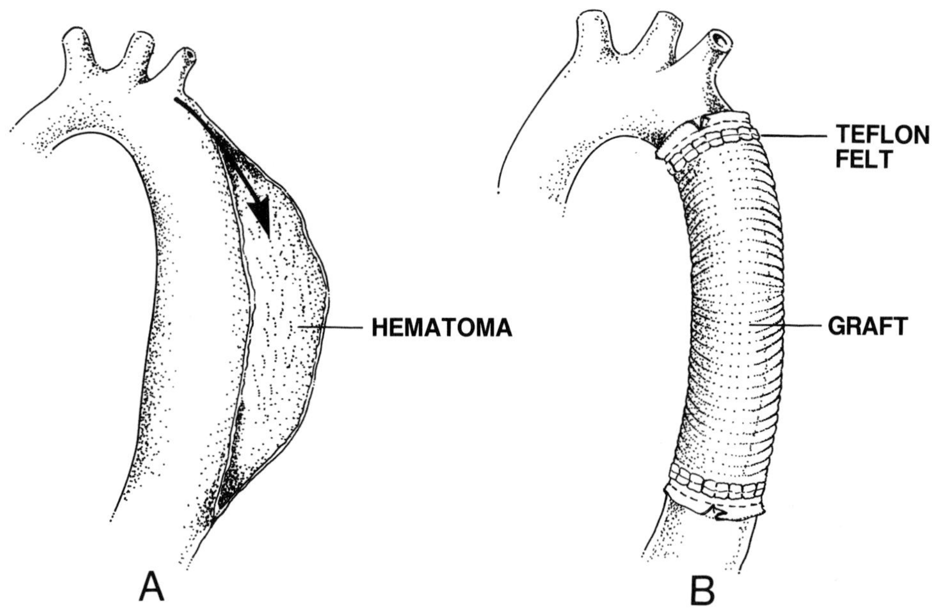

FIGURE 124-13 Repair of Type B dissection. The intimal tear is just distal to the left subclavian artery (A). The descending aorta is replaced with a Dacron graft with felt reinforcement of the suture lines (B).

sis, and effusion), CVA, and renal failure. Complications specific to repair of Type B dissections include paraplegia/paraparesis (up to 40 percent with rupture), renal and intestinal ischemia, recurrent laryngeal nerve palsy, and chylothorax.[15] Important late complications of both Type A and B dissections include late aneurysm formation and redissection of the aorta.

MORTALITY

Acute Type A dissections have an approximate mortality risk of 20 percent with operation (range 7 to 35 percent). The risk is increased with rupture, age greater than 80 years old, and associated illnesses, especially coronary artery disease.

Type B dissections survive with medical therapy in 80 percent of cases. If complications arise requiring surgery, then the mortality increases, reaching 75 percent if renal and visceral artery occlusion is present.

Follow-up

Control of the patient's blood pressure is the single most important variable determining late complications and survival in the management of both Type A and B dissections whether they have undergone surgical repair or not.[2,16,17] In the postoperative period, the systolic blood pressure is maintained at the lowest level capable of sustaining normal organ function as indicated by sensorium, urine output, etc. When the patient is transferred to the ward and onto oral antihypertensives, the type and dose must be modified to prevent orthostatic hypotension and syncope. Some form of β-blocker must be used (unless contraindicated) to control dP/dT_{max} as well as the systolic pressure. The blood pressure control must be maintained lifelong so as to minimize the risk of later aneurysm development or redissection.[16] New aneurysms form because in 85 percent of cases, the false lumen remains patent and so the wall of the aorta is permanently weakened. DeBakey's study[17] highlights the importance of long-term hypertension control. He followed 527 patients for 20 years after surgical repair of dissections and 45.5 percent developed subsequent aneurysms if hypertension was not controlled. If hypertension was controlled, however, only 17.4 percent developed subsequent aneurysms.

CASE PRESENTATION

A previously well 56-year-old patient was sitting at home when he experienced acute retrosternal chest pain. The pain was tearing in quality and was the most excruciating he had ever suffered. The pain radiated through to his back between his scapulae, progressed down his back, through to his abdomen, and finally into his lower extremities. On presentation to the emergency room he complained of some numbness in his left leg. He was ashen in color but alert and oriented. His blood pressure was 210/100 mmHg. Cardiovascular system examination did not reveal evidence of aortic insufficiency, and all pulses were easily palpable. The remainder of the physical examination was unremarkable. The patient had no significant medical or surgical problems in his history and particularly no history of hypertension.

The chest x-ray (Fig. 124-14) demonstrated marked widening of the mediastinum without pleural effusion. The electrocardiogram was normal. On the basis of the history, physical examination, and chest x-ray findings, the diagnosis of acute aortic dissection was tentatively made, and the patient was started immediately on labetolol using 1- to 2-mg boluses intravenously to control his hypertension. Liberal doses of morphine were given intravenously for his pain, which was more easily

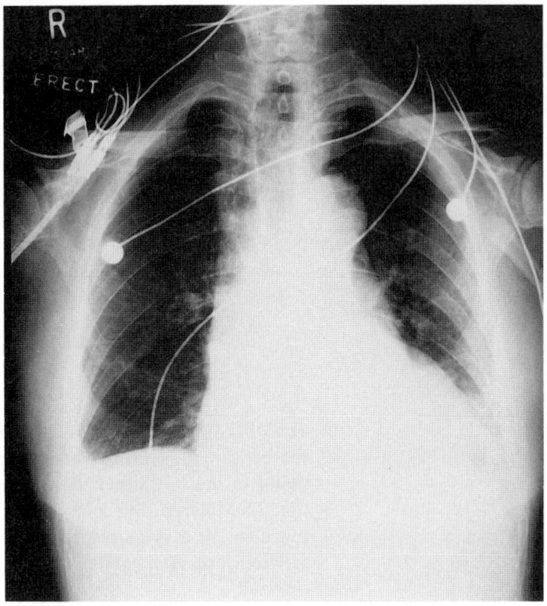

FIGURE 124-14 Chest x-ray illustrating marked widening of the mediastinum.

controlled when his blood pressure was reduced to 110/80 to 120/80 with labetolol.

A CT scan with contrast of the patient's thorax was performed urgently. CT was chosen as transesophageal echocardiography was not immediately available. The CT (Fig. 124-15) clearly demonstrated a dilated aortic root with a Type A dissection involving the entire aorta.

The patient was taken directly to the operating room. From the time of the inception of the patient's pain to his arrival in the operating room, just over 3 h had passed. The patient was placed on CPB using left femoral arterial and right atrial venous cannulation. Blood-tinged fluid was present within the pericardium, and the ascending aorta was dilated to almost 7 cm. The dilation continued into the region of the aortic arch and descending aorta. Profound hypothermia (10°C) with total circulatory arrest was utilized for the distal repair. The distal anastomosis was performed to the aorta at the innominate artery with the graft bevelled so as to replace the inferior portion of the arch as well (Fig. 124-16). The aortic valve was congenitally bicuspid necessitating a Bentall procedure. The patient tolerated the procedure very well.

The patient was maintained on labetolol intravenously during his 48-h intensive care unit admission in order to keep his systolic blood pressure at 90 to 100 mmHg. He was discharged home on the eighth postoperative day on oral antihypertensives. He will be reviewed in clinic at 3, 6, and 12 months and then annually with general history and physical examination as well as CT scan to observe his blood pressure control and the status of his remaining aorta.

CASE DISCUSSION

This case illustrates many of the important issues of aortic dissection. The dramatic presentation in a previously well patient suggested the diagnosis even without further investigation. Chest x-ray and CT were performed to confirm the diagnosis and identify the dissection type so as to determine definitive therapy. Paramount in the patient's management was the early institution of hypertension control and expedient investigation and surgical intervention. The blood-tinged pericardial fluid suggested imminent rupture and should reinforce the need for urgent investigation and treatment of aortic dissections.

Long-term survival is dependent on hypertension control and close follow-up of the remaining aorta for evidence of redissection or aneurysm formation. This patient must therefore be followed every 6 to 12 months to ensure his survival is maximized.

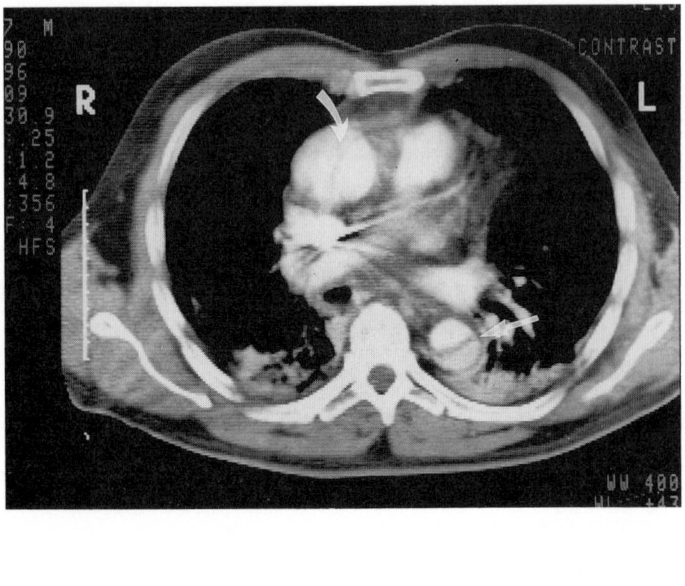

FIGURE 124-15 Contrast CT of thorax. The ascending aorta is dilated with an intimal flap obvious (curved arrow). The dissection extends to the descending aorta (solid arrow).

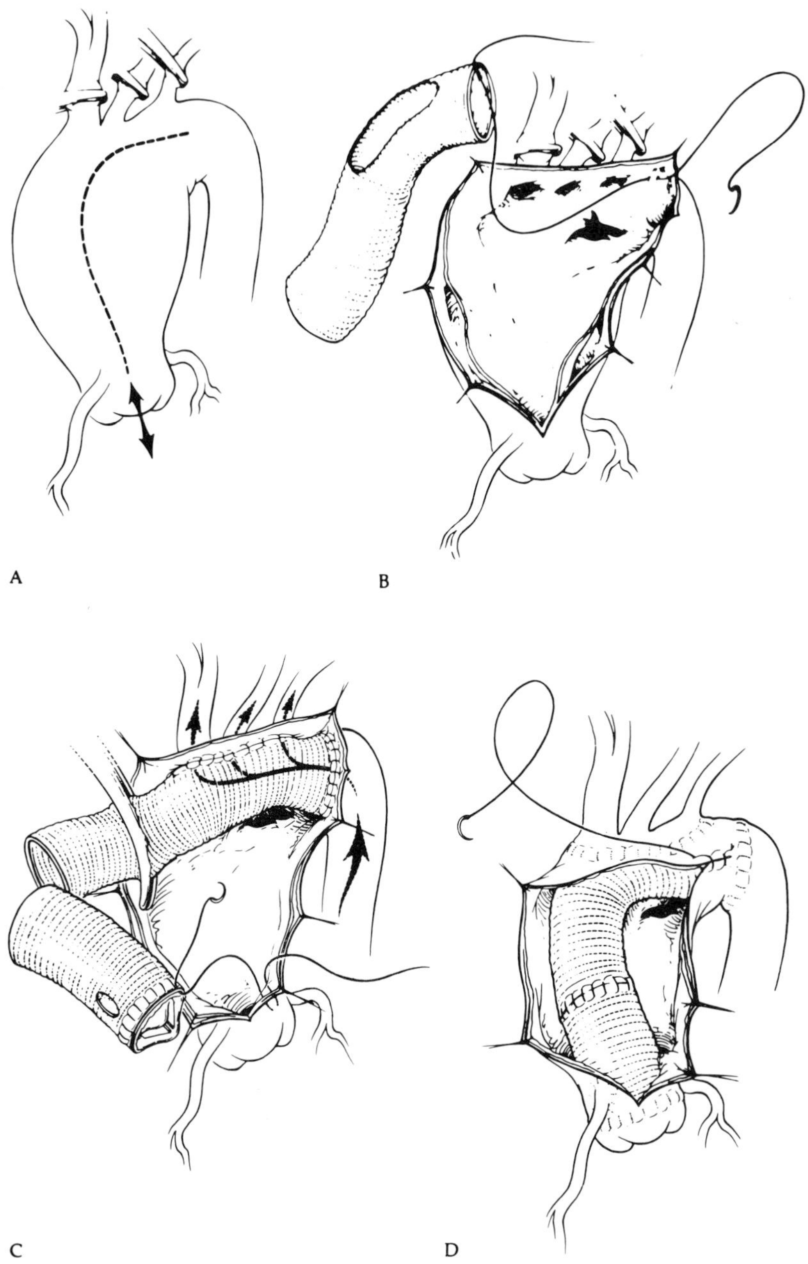

FIGURE 124-16 Repair of Type A dissection. (A) Markedly dilated ascending aorta and arch with aortic insufficiency (arrows). The aorta is opened longitudinally (dotted line). (B) Intimal tear located in aortic arch. Note the separation of the layers of the aortic wall in ascending aorta. The distant anastomosis is to the descending aorta. (C) Cranial vessels anastomosed to graft and circulation restored. Composite graft is sutured into position proximally. Note button holes in graft for anastomosis of coronary arteries. (D) Proximal and distal grafts are joined. Aneurysm sac is closed over the graft. (Reprinted from Graham JM, Stinnett DM: Operative management of acute aortic arch dissection using profound hypothermia and circulation arrest. Ann Thorac Surg 44:192, 1987, with permission.).

References

1. Sorensen HR, Olsen H: Ruptured and dissecting aneurysms of the aorta: Incidence and prospects of surgery. Acta Chir Scand 128:644, 1964.
2. Wheat MW, Jr: Acute dissection of the aorta, in Brest, A (ed): *Cardiovascular Clinics*. Philadelphia, F.A. Davis, 1987, vol. 17, no. 3, pp 241–262.
3. Hirst AE, Gore I: The etiology and pathology of aortic dissection, in Doroghazi RM, Slater EE (eds): *Aortic Dissection*. New York, McGraw-Hill, 1983.
4. Cambria RP, Brewster DC, Gertler J, et al: Vascular complications associated with spontaneous aortic dissection. J Vasc Surg 7:199, 1988.
5. Fann JI, Sarris GE, Miller C, et al: Surgical management of acute dissection complicated by stroke. Circulation 80(Supp I):257, 1989.
6. Wechsler RJ, Kotler MN, Steiner RM: Multimodality approach to thoracic aortic dissection, in Brest A (ed): *Cardiovascular Clinics*, Philadelphia, F.A. Davis, 1986, vol. 17, no. 1, pp 385–408.
7. DeSanctis RW, Doroghazi RM, Austen WG, et al: Aortic dissection. N Engl J Med 31:1060, 1987.
8. Thorsen MK, San Dretto MA, Lawson TL, et al: Dissecting aortic aneurysms; accuracy of computed tomographic diagnosis. Radiology 148:773, 1983.
9. Erbel R, Daniel W, Visser C, et al: Echocardiography in diagnosis of aortic dissection. Lancet 8636:458, 1989.
10. Goldman AP, Kotler MN, Scanlon MH, et al: The complementary role of magnetic resonance imaging, Doppler echocardiography and computed tomography in the diagnosis of dissecting thoracic aneurysms. Am Heart J 111:9, 1986.

11. Miller DC, Mitchell RS, Oyer PE, et al: Independent determinants of operative mortality for patients with aortic dissections. Circulation 70:153, 1984.
12. Graham JM, Stinnett DM: Operative management of acute aortic arch dissection using profound hypothermia and circulatory arrest. Ann Thorac Surg 44:192, 1987.
13. Koster JK, Jr, Cohn LH, Mee RBB: Late results of operation for acute aortic dissection producing aortic insufficiency. Ann Thorac Surg 26:461, 1987.
14. Bachet J: Replacement of the transverse aortic arch during emergency operation for type A acute aortic dissection. J. Thorac Cardiovasc Surg 98:310, 1989.
15. Jex RK, Schaff HV, Piehler JM, et al: Early and later results following repair of dissections of the descending thoracic aorta. J Vasc Surg 3:226, 1986.
16. Doroghazi RM, Slater EE, DeSanctis RW, et al: Long-term survival of patients with treated aortic dissection. J Am Coll Cardiol 3:1026, 1984.
17. DeBakey ME, McCollum CH, Crawford ES, et al: Dissection and dissecting aneurysms of the aorta: Twenty-year follow-up of five hundred and twenty-seven patients treated surgically. Surgery 92:1118, 1982.

Chapter 125

VASOACTIVE DRUGS

WILLIAM J. ELLIOTT
DANIEL D. GRETLER

KEY POINTS

- *Many drugs are useful in improving cardiac contractility; often dobutamine (starting at 1 to 2 μg/kg/min) is used initially, but dopamine, digoxin, and phosphodiesterase inhibitors are sometimes helpful.*
- *Patients with inadequate tissue perfusion are best managed by addressing the underlying cause, ensuring an adequate intravascular volume, and only thereafter instituting therapy with vasoconstrictors (e.g., dopamine, beginning at 1 to 2 μg/kg/min) or positive inotropes (e.g., dobutamine, beginning at 1 to 2 μg/kg/min), guided by frequent hemodynamic measurements.*
- *Currently foremost among the many drugs useful in lowering blood pressure is intravenous nitroprusside (beginning at 0.5 μg/kg/min); when it is begun, thought must be directed immediately to choosing a substitute, as its prolonged or high dose use often leads to toxicity.*
- *Drugs sometimes useful in increasing heart rate include atropine (particularly in inferior myocardial infarction), and isoproterenol, which can be used temporarily until a pacemaker can be placed.*
- *Drugs useful in lowering heart rate include the β blockers (particularly esmolol), verapamil or adenosine (for paroxysmal supraventricular tachycardias), and digoxin (especially useful in controlling ventricular rate in atrial fibrillation/flutter).*

Drugs Useful in Improving Myocardial Contractility

Cardiac output is determined by the product of heart rate and stroke volume. Pharmacologic support of cardiac output is almost always based on an increase in stroke volume. Unless heart rate is exceptionally low (e.g., in sick sinus syndrome or conduction block) and felt to be a major contributing factor to heart failure, an increase in heart rate is usually not recommended. In the occasional case where it appears indicated, it is best achieved with a pacemaker (see Chap. 32). Increasing heart rate carries the risk of precipitating myocardial ischemia and shortens the cardiac cycle and hence, ventricular filling time and preload. This can lead to a decrease in stroke volume and overall cardiac output. In the case of tachyarrhythmias, it may be beneficial to decrease heart rate to restore adequate ventricular filling time, which is especially important if myocardial compliance is low.

Stroke volume is determined by preload, afterload, and the contractile state of the myocardium (see Chap. 2). The modulation of each of these factors is at the basis of most pharmacologic therapy of heart failure. The pharmacologic approach aimed at altering preload and afterload is discussed in Chaps. 114 and 115. Increasing myocardial inotropy might seem the most obvious pharmacologic goal in heart failure. Indeed, the prototype of the positive inotropes, digoxin, has been the mainstay of the pharmacologic treatment of heart failure for over 200 years. However, vasodilator therapy has now become the preferred first-line treatment in many cases.[1] Positive inotropic drugs (Table 125-1) have the disadvantage of greatly increasing myocardial oxygen demand. While this may be especially detrimental in the setting of coronary artery disease, it is of concern in many other critical care situations, where the oxygen supply:demand ratio is frequently compromised. Conversely, an increase in cardiac output may be able to markedly improve the hemodynamic situation, and the decision regarding the use of positive inotropes has to be individualized. Aside from these considerations, hypoxemia, acid-base imbalance, as well as electrolyte abnormalities (especially a low level of ionized calcium) have a negative inotropic effect, and may contribute to hypoperfusion.

If acute positive inotropic effects are deemed necessary in critically ill patients, adrenergic drugs are preferred. They are powerful and rapidly acting, and there has been a vast experience with their use. However, because of the downregulation of β-adrenergic receptors on which they act, their prolonged use is associated with a progressive decline in effectiveness.

DOBUTAMINE

Dobutamine is one of the first-line adrenergic agents used to increase myocardial contractility (Table 125-2). Unlike most other adrenergic agents discussed in this chapter, dobutamine is a synthetic catecholamine and is devoid of potent vasoactive properties.[2,3] Having something of a misnomer, dobutamine has no important activity on dopamine receptors. The commercial formulation is a racemic mixture of two isomers: one activating β-, the other α-, adrenergic receptors. This combination of vasoconstrictor and vasodi-

TABLE 125-1 Summary of Pharmacologic Receptor Selectivity for Commonly Used Adrenergic Drugs

Catecholamine	DA-1	β_1	β_2	α_1	α_2
Dopamine[a]	1+[b]–4+	0–3+	0–2+	0–3+	0–1+
Dobutamine	0	3+	1+	0–1+	0
Norepinephrine	0	2+	1+	3+	3+
Epinephrine	0	3+	3+	3+	3+
Isoproterenol	0	3+	3+	0	0

[a]Dopamine's pharmacologic effects are very much dose related and somewhat variable between patients. Low doses (~1–3 μg/kg/min) stimulate primarily the DA-1 and DA-2 receptors; high doses (>20–50 μg/kg/min) produce mostly α-adrenergic stimulation.
[b]Relative degree of stimulation on 1- to 4-point scale.

TABLE 125-2 Drugs to Increase Cardiac Contractility

Drug Name	IV Dose Range	Oral Dose Range
Dobutamine	2–15 μg/kg/min	NA
Dopamine	0.5–10 μg/kg/min	NA
Isoproterenol	1–8 μg/kg/min	NA
Digoxin	0.25–1.0-mg loading dose, followed by 0.125–0.25 mg/day	Same as IV or slightly higher due to decreased bioavailability
Amrinone	0.75 mg/kg loading dose, then 5–10 μg/kg/min	NA
Milrinone	50 μg/kg over 10 min, then 0.375–0.75 μg/kg/min	7.5–10 mg q.i.d. or q4h

lator compounds essentially produces no net effect on vascular tone, while leaving a strong inotropic effect, presumably mediated by β_1 and α_1 receptors. In practice, it usually decreases ventricular filling pressures and may cause mild vasodilation, with some of the changes in preload and afterload being a reflection of an improved cardiac output.[4] Coronary perfusion improves as a result of the increase in cardiac output. Peripheral perfusion usually improves as well, although this effect is greater in the skeletal musculature, compared to renal and mesenteric beds.[5] It causes less tachycardia than the other adrenergic drugs (including dopamine), which is one of its main advantages. It is most useful when an increase in cardiac output is sought in a patient without significant hypotension, especially when systemic vascular resistance (SVR) is normal or elevated. This is frequently the case in the setting of acute myocardial infarction and heart failure, where dobutamine may be less likely than other agents to worsen ischemia. Because decreased myocardial contractility is a hallmark of septic shock, dobutamine is also used in this setting, where it is frequently combined with dopamine.[6] Typically, cardiac output and oxygen delivery increase approximately one-third, while blood pressure remains unchanged.[7] The reduction in filling pressures seen with dobutamine may offer some advantages for this drug over dopamine. Occasionally, blood pressure may fall when dobutamine is administered. If this is the case, restoring adequate preload with the judicious administration of fluids, with or without a reduction in dose, may be necessary. The drug is usually well tolerated, producing only occasional, dose-related problems related to tachycardia and arrhythmias as well as gastrointestinal irritation.

DOPAMINE

Because of its many pharmacologic effects, dopamine is somewhat less useful, if acutely improving myocardial contractility is the only desired end point,[8] although it is frequently used in many other settings (vide infra and Tables 125-1 through 125-3). Dopamine's positive inotropic action, mediated by the activation of β_1-adrenergic receptors, starts at doses as low as 2 to 5 μg/kg/min and is occasionally sufficient to restore adequate hemodynamics. Most other adrenergic vasopressors, including norepinephrine and epinephrine, also possess inotropic properties, and can increase myocardial contractility. However, their main indication remains peripheral vasoconstriction (vide infra).

Dopamine, when used in high doses (>10 μg/kg/min) leads to vasoconstriction, mediated by activation of α_1-adrenergic receptors. Occasionally, a reduction in blood pressure can be observed when using very low doses (0.5 to 2 μg/kg/min). This phenomenon is due to the activation of vasodilatory ("dopamine-1" or "DA-1") receptors in the renal and splanchnic circulation, as well as perhaps, to a lesser extent, the cerebral and coronary circulation. This effect is responsible for the increase in urinary output observed with low dose dopamine administration.[9] At doses >15 μg/kg/min, these effects on dopamine receptors are overwhelmed, due to widespread α_1-receptor-induced vasoconstriction. The agent also inhibits aldosterone synthesis and secretion and thus has some natriuretic properties.[10] Dopamine-induced catecholamine release from endogenous myocardial stores probably contributes to the positive inotropic and vasoconstrictor effects. Dopamine occasionally causes nausea and vomiting, an effect thought to be due to a central dopamine ("DA-2") effect. Other problems associated with the use of dopamine are similar to those seen with other adrenergic agents, and include dose-dependent tachycardia, arrhythmias, as well as cardiac and other tissue ischemia.

ISOPROTERENOL

Isoproterenol is a powerful inotropic agent, but of limited clinical use for this indication, as it is one of the most potent chronotropic agents available. Its principal pharmacologic action is the activation of β_1- and β_2-adrenergic receptors. The β_1 receptor mediates its positive inotropic effect; the β_2 receptor is responsible for its chronotropic effect, as well as its actions as a vasodilator and bronchodilator. The powerful stimulation of two major determinants of myocardial oxygen demand, heart rate and contractility, has frequently proven detrimental at the bedside. Unlike most other adrenergic agents discussed here, it is a vasodilator and may decrease blood pressure. Unfortunately, it also tends to redistribute blood flow to areas such as the skin and skeletal musculature, while reducing flow to cerebral, myocardial, and renal tissues. Although it may be combined with a vasoconstrictor, other drugs (e.g., dobutamine) are often preferred. Isoproterenol is best reserved for the treatment

TABLE 125-3 Drugs to Increase Systemic Vascular Resistance

Drug Name	IV Starting Dose	Maintenance Dose
Dopamine	1–2 μg/kg/min	0.5–50+[a] μg/kg/min
Norepinephrine	2 μg/kg/min	2–20 μg/kg/min
Epinephrine	0.1–0.25-mg bolus, but may be given by constant infusion (0.01–0.3 mg/min)	0.5–1 mg q 5 min (during CPR)
Metaraminol	0.5 mg over 2–3 min	0.5–5 mg slow IV push over 2–3 min
Phenylephrine	0.5 mg over 2–3 min	0.5–5 mg slow IV push over 2–3 min

[a] At the higher doses of infused dopamine, α-agonism becomes the overwhelming pharmacologic effect. Higher doses are often necessary in patients with congestive heart failure or acidosis. For some physicians, norepinephrine is the α-agonist preferred over dopamine at the higher doses (exceeding 20–50 μg/kg/min).

of hemodynamically significant bradycardia, although a transvenous or external pacemaker is preferable[11] (see Chap. 32).

PHOSPHODIESTERASE INHIBITORS

Newer agents which increase myocardial contractility include amrinone[12,13] and milrinone,[14] of which amrinone is available only in an intravenous formulation (see Table 125-2). The two drugs act by mechanisms entirely different from cardiac glycosides or adrenergic drugs. They inhibit the enzyme phosphodiesterase, thus increasing the cellular availability of cyclic adenosine monophosphate (AMP). While this appears to explain their positive inotropic action at least in part, they also exhibit vasodilatory properties. It is not clear to what extent these contribute to their therapeutic actions. As is the case with the catecholamines, the inotropic effect is seen within minutes of administration. Amrinone usually increases cardiac output without significant effects on heart rate, although higher doses may lead to tachycardia and hypotension.[15] Nevertheless, results with these newer agents have been mixed. Cardiac ischemia may be exacerbated and they exhibit significant side effect profiles, including thrombocytopenia, fever, gastrointestinal irritation, hepatic dysfunction and arrhythmias.[16] Though they are not first-line drugs, they may be tried in selected cases, especially when other drugs have failed or cannot be used.

DIGOXIN

Digoxin is mostly used for the chronic therapy of heart failure. Its mechanism of action is thought to stem from an inhibition of the Na^+/K^+ adenosinetriphosphatase (ATPase) and consequent increase in intracellular sodium, and ultimately, intracellular calcium availability. The value of digoxin in the therapy of shock is limited. It produces only modest improvement in cardiac output in patients with cardiogenic shock and may further elevate afterload. In the ICU, digoxin is most frequently used for the acute control of a rapid ventricular response in atrial tachyarrhythmias. On the other hand, although the onset of the positive inotropic effect is delayed, it is permissible to start digoxin in the ICU, especially if long-term therapy is anticipated. As with chronic therapy, precautions have to be taken to avoid hypokalemia and hypomagnesemia, which increase the drug's propensity to cause arrhythmias (see Table 125-2). Moreover, the caveats regarding the increase in myocardial oxygen demand by positive inotropes apply to digoxin as well. Digoxin toxicity is a frequent occurrence in patients on chronic digitalis therapy, and significant arrhythmias may occur. If supportive care including the correction of electrolyte levels fails to rapidly correct life-threatening arrhythmias, intravenous digoxin-specific F_{ab} antibody fragments are available which bind the drug and rapidly eliminate it renally as a drug-antibody complex.

GLUCAGON

Lastly, glucagon (1 to 3 mg/h intravenously) has also been used to increase contractility. Its effect is independent of β-adrenergic receptor activation and may thus be useful in patients who have received β-blocking agents. However, its modest effect, together with a considerable side effect profile, including tachycardia, make it a less desirable choice. In addition, convincing data supporting its widespread use are lacking.

COMBINATION THERAPY

Although drugs have been discussed individually, the combination of two or more agents is often beneficial in clinical practice.[6,17] This is especially true for inotropic agents in combination with a vasodilator (vide infra) or low dose dopamine used along with another positive inotropic agent (e.g., dopamine at 3 μg/kg/min + dobutamine). While an initial "best guess" can be made when choosing a drug (or drug combination), a fail-safe prediction of each patient's response is impossible. Each administration of the drugs discussed has to be regarded as an "experiment." Most drugs are started at the lower recommended doses and titrated upward, depending on the clinical response. The frequent, systematic reassessment of the clinical picture, including hemodynamic parameters, cannot be sufficiently stressed. Based on the response, decisions are made regarding change in dose, substitution with other drugs or the addition of another agent. Lastly, the weaning of the patient from vasoactive and cardioactive drugs is frequently difficult. It has to occur gradually, with special attention paid to the underlying condition, as well as factors such as the adequacy of intravascular volume, and the respiratory, hormonal, acid-base, electrolyte and nutritional status.

Drugs to Increase Systemic Vascular Resistance

Vasoconstrictors are typically used in severely hypotensive patients to maintain or restore adequate perfusion pressure, especially in the coronary vasculature. This is necessary to interrupt the vicious cycle of a decreased myocardial perfusion leading to a decrease in cardiac output, which further worsens coronary perfusion. However, the use of vasoconstrictors is a double-edged sword, as they have the propensity to decrease peripheral blood flow and worsen tissue ischemia. In addition, as afterload increases, cardiac output may fall. This is especially true when cardiac output is strongly dependent on afterload, as is the case in heart failure. Pharmacologic blood pressure support must be regarded as a temporizing measure, pending the resolution (or correction) of the underlying problem, which has to be identified and addressed as soon as possible[18] (see Chap. 114).

Before starting pharmacologic blood pressure support, the adequacy of intravascular volume must be ensured. The use of vasoconstricting drugs in a hypovolemic patient may increase blood pressure, but will only serve to worsen already compromised tissue perfusion. Volume status in critically ill patients is best determined by invasive means, usually a pulmonary artery catheter.[19] If the exact volume status is in doubt, small (100 to 500 mL) amounts of fluid should be administered. The absence of an increase in pulmonary capillary wedge pressure after such a "fluid challenge" usually indicates intravascular volume deficit. This maneuver may be more useful than the use of absolute pulmonary capillary wedge pressures (e.g., 14 to 18 mmHg), as the absolute pressure also depends on parameters other than volume status (e.g., myocardial compliance; see Chap. 25).

The correction of hypovolemia can be achieved with crystalloids, colloids, or blood (usually in the form of packed red blood cells).[20] Blood is indicated in anemic patients if an increase in tissue O_2 delivery is indicated. Increasing the hematocrit above normal levels is not only wasteful of precious banked blood products, but also detrimental to the microcirculation, because it increases blood viscosity. The decision to use crystalloids versus colloids is more difficult.[21] Theoretically, colloids such as albumin or hetastarch offer the advantage of increasing the oncotic pressure, and they remain in the intravascular space for a longer period of time. Albumin thus would appear to be especially useful in hypoalbuminemic patients and patients with intravascular hypovolemia despite overall fluid overload (e.g., the hypovolemic cirrhotic with ascites). On the other hand, crystalloids are much less expensive and no major study comparing the two has been able to show a significant difference in outcome. More important than the choice of colloids versus crystalloid is undoubtedly the restoration of an adequate intravascular volume. It must be kept in mind that when using crystalloids, the amount needed to produce a volume expansion of a given magnitude is two to four times that of colloids. Volume therapy is optimized by paying careful attention to hemodynamic parameters such as pulmonary capillary wedge pressure and stroke volume.

DOPAMINE

One of the most frequently used pharmacologic agents (summarized in Table 125-3) for circulatory support in critically ill patients is dopamine,[22] which is discussed in detail above. At doses above 10 μg/kg/min, its α-adrenergic vasoconstrictor properties become increasingly evident, whereas lower doses lead to β-receptor stimulation, and still lower doses to specific activation of dopamine receptors. As a vasoconstrictor, high dose dopamine can be combined with a vasodilator such as nitroprusside to improve cardiac output by increasing contractility and decreasing afterload, while preserving the increased blood flow to renal, and perhaps, cerebral and coronary vascular beds.

EPINEPHRINE

Epinephrine is a combined α- and β-adrenergic agent, although mainly α effects are observed at higher doses. It is the drug of choice in cardiopulmonary arrest.[11] During cardiopulmonary resuscitation (CPR) it is administered as an intravenous bolus of 0.5 to 1.0 mg every 5 min. If intravenous access is not available in an emergency, epinephrine can be administered endotracheally, as it is absorbed well through airway mucosa.[23] It is also the drug of choice in anaphylactic shock, where it specifically antagonizes two of the major pathophysiologic mechanisms, vasodilation and bronchoconstriction. Capillary permeability may be reduced, but the clinical importance of this continues to be controversial. The usual dose of epinephrine for this indication is 0.1 to 0.5 mg intravenously as a bolus or a constant infusion (see Table 125-3). Occasionally, it is also used as a vasoconstrictor in hypotensive patients, using a continuous intravenous drip, in situations other than anaphylaxis. However, because of the relative numbers of α_1 and β_2 receptors in different vascular beds, it tends to shunt blood away from vital organs, such as the kidney, and into the skeletal musculature. For the same reason, it is an especially powerful vasoconstrictor in the cutaneous vasculature, frequently causing skin necrosis in the extremities, especially when used in moderate to high doses. Additional adverse effects are similar to those of other adrenergic drugs.

NOREPINEPHRINE

Norepinephrine is one of the most powerful adrenergic vasoconstrictors, because of its potent action on α_1 receptors and lack of effect on vasodilatory β_2 receptors (see Table 125-3).[24] It also activates β_1 receptors, albeit to a lesser degree, and thus may produce a modest increase in myocardial contractility. It has been suggested that coronary and cerebral blood flow may be relatively spared despite global vasoconstriction, because of differences in the distribution of α receptors and because of its greater effect on diastolic blood pressure compared to other agents, such as epinephrine. However, this view remains controversial. Because of the increase in afterload, the drug usually does not increase cardiac output. At times, output may actually decrease in a dose-dependent fashion, with a concomitant increase in left ventricular end-diastolic pressure.[25] Norepinephrine can be used in severely hypotensive patients, especially when other agents have failed. Additionally, it may be helpful in septic shock, when SVR is greatly decreased,[26] as well as in situations with loss of venous tone. Problems related to its use are similar to those discussed with other vasoconstrictors. Additionally, it may cause a vagally mediated reflex bradycardia, which may be poorly tolerated by many patients with compromised cardiac output. While tissue ischemia may be seen with any vasoconstrictor, it is of special concern with norepinephrine. This complication is especially likely when high doses are used for prolonged periods of time, and ischemia frequently is seen in the kidneys, spleen, skin, and muscles. If local extravasation of norepinephrine (or other α_1 adrenergic vasoconstrictors) occurs, local tissue necrosis can be prevented by the local infusion of the α-adrenergic blocker, phentolamine (5 mg in a diluted solution).

OTHER VASOCONSTRICTORS

Less frequently used agents include metaraminol, which has a pharmacologic profile similar to norepinephrine, as well as phenylephrine and methoxamine, which are pure α-adrenergic vasoconstrictors (see Table 125-3). Their main indications include neurogenic shock and hypotension associated with spinal anesthesia, where loss of venous and arterial tone must be addressed simultaneously.

Drugs Useful in Lowering Systemic Vascular Resistance

In the setting of the ICU, the many drugs available to lower SVR are most easily divided into two groups. The smaller number of hypotensive agents are those available for intravenous administration; the larger number of agents includes those which are first delivered into the gastrointestinal tract (Table 125-4).

The major advantages for the use of intravenously delivered hypotensive agents are the wider applicability in a broader range of patients (especially those who have recently had surgery, ileus, diabetic gastroparesis, or other reason to suspect that gastrointestinal absorption is functioning less than perfectly), or those who are nasotracheally intubated, in whom the presence of an orogastric tube or

TABLE 125-4 Drugs to Lower Systemic Vascular Resistance

Drug Name	IV Dose Range	Oral Dose Range
Sodium **nitroprusside**	0.5–8 μg/kg/min	NA
Nicardipine HCl[a]	5–15 mg/h	NA
Fenoldopam mesylate[a]	0.1–1.5 μg/kg/min	NA
Labetalol HCl	10–525 mg, given as minibolus injections	200–800 mg/day
Esmolol HCl	500 μg/kg/min × 4–5 min, then 150–300 μg/kg/min	NA
Metoprolol HCl	5–15 mg q 6–12 h	50–200 mg/day
Atenolol HCl	5–10 mg q 6–12 h	50–200 mg/day
Propranolol HCl	1–5 mg q 4–6 h	20–320 mg b.i.d.
Enalaprilat	1.25–5 mg q 6 h	NA
Verapamil HCl	5–10 mg q 2–6 h	120–480 mg/day
Methyldopa	125–500 mg q 6 h	125–500 mg b.i.d.
Hydralazine	5–20 mg q 6 h	10–100 mg b.i.d
Diazoxide	50 mg every 10 min minibolus injections	NA
Nitroglycerin	5–500 μg/kg/min	0.3–0.8 mg SL
Phentolamine	5–10-mg bolus every 10 min	NA
Trimethaphan camsylate	3–6 mg/min	NA
Nifedipine	5–10 mg "bite and swallow"	10–30 mg q 4–6 h
Clonidine HCl	0.1–0.2 mg q h	0.1–0.3 mg b.i.d.
Captopril	6.25–40 mg q 6–8 h	12.5–75 mg t.i.d.

[a]Investigational agents (awaiting FDA approval) as of December 1, 1990.

contralateral nasogastric tube has not yet been established. Many of the agents available for intravenous administration also have rather short pharmacologic half lives, leading to improved ability to "titrate" the agents more quickly against the appropriate end point: usually the mean arterial pressure in the case of hypotensive agents. This generally can lead to improved "control" of blood pressure, in that nearly any level of blood pressure can be quickly attained and maintained with the shorter-acting intravenous agents.

INTRAVENOUS AGENTS

NITROPRUSSIDE

With few exceptions, the current intravenous "drug of choice" for acutely lowering blood pressure[27] is the nonspecific vasodilator, sodium nitroprusside.[28] The advantages of this agent include a very short time of onset of action (typically, 1 to 2 min), a short elimination half-life (2 to 3 min in patients with normal renal and hepatic function), nearly universal efficacy, and relative ease of administration. The disadvantages, however, are important, because nitroprusside toxicity can be devastating if not recognized, particularly if precautions are not taken to minimize the probability of developing toxicity. In most patients, the toxicity of the compound is directly related to the total administered dose of the drug (i.e., dosage infused multiplied by the time of administration). Symptomatic side effects (flushing, headache, "tingling of the scalp") are particularly common when the drug is given at high doses (>5 μg/kg/min), and are relatively easy to recognize. Fortunately, they are most prominent at the beginning of the infusion of the higher doses, and often decrease in intensity, even when the dosage is not adjusted downward. The more troublesome toxic effects of nitroprusside occur when the drug is given over a prolonged period of time (e.g., >24 h). Since nitroprusside is broken down by red blood cells into the potent inhibitor of oxidative phosphorylation, cyanide, which is then metabolized by the liver to the less toxic thiocyanate, which is then cleared by the kidneys, it is relatively easy to produce toxicity from either or both of these poisons by giving the drug, even at low doses, for a long time. Initial efforts at minimizing toxicity, by concomitant infusion of either hydroxocobalamine[29] or thiosulfate,[30] were moderately successful, but have unfortunately not been routinely put into practice; instead the focus has been on minimizing the total dose. Since the symptoms of cyanide/thiocyanate toxicity (typically restlessness, mental confusion, and hyperreflexia) are not commonly recognized in early stages in many ICU patients, it is important to be alert for an otherwise unexplained metabolic acidosis, which is often the first sign of nitroprusside toxicity.[31] The best confirmatory test for nitroprusside toxicity is a blood cyanide level, but few clinical laboratories are prepared for this analysis. Helpful, but less specific, laboratory abnormalities seen in cyanide toxicity include: elevated lactate level, elevated lactate:pyruvate ratio, and increased mixed venous oxygen concentrations. More commonly available than cyanide levels is a blood thiocyanate concentration, but this determination typically takes longer than a few hours; the best approach is to recognize the possibility of toxicity, send blood for thiocyanate (to be used later as confirmation of toxicity), and withdraw nitroprusside in favor of another vasodilator. Treating nitroprusside toxicity (once diagnosed) is troublesome, as the calculation of the proper dose of each of the available antidotes depends on hours-old concentrations of thiocyanate (or even better, cyanide, when available). Aside from stopping the nitroprusside infusion, hydroxocobalamine (which complexes circulating cyanide to form vitamin B_{12}) is probably the best therapy for nitroprusside toxicity, as it is the least toxic antidote (see Chap. 176). Sodium nitrite, sodium thiosulfate, and particularly methylene blue are themselves capable of toxicity, typically methemoglobinemia; dosage calculations for each are difficult, at best. The use of sodium nitroprusside is contraindicated in patients with Leber's optic atrophy and tobacco amblyopia, neither of which is common enough to seriously restrict its use. Solutions of nitroprusside must be protected from light, which is commonly done by wrapping both the bag and tubing containing nitroprusside in aluminum foil.

Sodium nitroprusside is best administered via a constant-dose infusion of the drug into an intravenous line used solely for nitroprusside. Extension tubing is kept to a minimum, a three-way stopcock is connected directly to the hub of the intravenous cannula, and the third line (i.e., not carrying the nitroprusside from the pump, and not the intravenous cannula) is "off" when the nitroprusside infusion is begun. By using this method, the "dead space" of tubing containing nitroprusside solution is kept to a minimum, and very troublesome "bolus" injections of nitroprusside, which may occur when the "third line" is open, are avoided. The usual starting dose is 0.5 μg/kg/min, which can be increased in increments of 0.25 to 1.0 μg/kg/min every 5 to 10 min as necessary to achieve the desired blood pressure. The most important thing to be considered when beginning sodium nitroprusside is how and when the medication can be stopped, as toxicity is thus minimized. The most common difficulty in using sodium nitroprusside is not how or when to use it, but indeed, in deciding on the agent or agents to replace it.

NICARDIPINE AND FENOLDOPAM

There are at least two investigational compounds (see Table 125-4) which are close to Food and Drug Administration (FDA) approval which will likely make sodium nitroprusside less commonly used, if not obsolete. One of these is the intravenously active and water-soluble dihydropyridine calcium antagonist, nicardipine,[32] which acts by vasodilating the arteriolar smooth muscle cells via the inhibition of the calcium-dependent, slow inward current. Another promising agent is the DA-1 agonist, fenoldopam, which not only lowers blood pressure by direct vasodilation due to stimulation of the DA-1 receptors on the vascular smooth muscle cells, but also seems to have some beneficial effects on renal function, not seen with the direct vasodilator, sodium nitroprusside.[33]

β BLOCKERS

LABETALOL. Several of the β-blocking drugs are available for intravenous use; many of these are perhaps more useful for acutely lowering heart rate (vide infra) than they are for lowering blood pressure. The most commonly used β blocker for lowering blood pressure is labetalol, which contains four diastereomeric compounds with different effects on both α and β receptors.[34] The marketed mixture has the unique properties of being both a nonspecific β blocker, as well as a less potent α_1 blocker. The relative potency of α versus β blockage is somewhat higher (typically 1:3) with the intravenously administered form of the compound (presumably due to differences in stereoselective first-pass metabolism of the various diastereomers when the mixture is given orally, when the relative potency decreases to about 1:7). Thus, the intravenously administered compound is a more potent agent for acutely lowering blood pressure than is oral labetalol. Aside from a tendency to cause orthostatic hypotension, the disadvantages of labetalol are common to all of the β blockers: they should not be used in patients with reactive airways disease or with cardiac conduction disturbances worse than first degree heart block; they are contraindicated in most patients with severe left ventricular dysfunction and congestive heart failure. The side effect profile of labetalol is similar to other vasodilators: flushing, nausea, itching, tingling of the scalp. Labetalol also shares the typical β blocker side effects (precipitation of asthma or congestive heart failure, prolongation of hypoglycemic coma in insulin-dependent diabetics, reduction in exercise capacity, bradycardia, and others), but additionally can cause major orthostatic falls in blood pressure and (like one of its components, dilevalol) has occasionally been implicated in very severe hepatotoxic reactions.

Labetalol is typically administered in ascending "minibolus" intravenous injections, beginning with 10 mg, followed by 25 mg in 10 min if the response was inadequate, followed by doubling the dose at 10- to 20-min intervals (see Table 125-4). Most physicians limit the dose (during the ascending dose phase of acutely reducing the blood pressure) at 525 mg. Once the blood pressure goal has been achieved, it can be given at 4- to 6-h intervals (which is probably more reliable) or by constant dose infusion.

SELECTIVE β_1 BLOCKERS. Esmolol, metoprolol, and atenolol are relatively selective β_1-blocking agents which are sometimes used intravenously to reduce heart rate and blood pressure. Esmolol[35] has the unique property of being hydrolyzed by serum esterases, resulting in a short elimination half-life of about 9 min and a similarly short duration of action (typically 20 to 30 min), whereas the other drugs have longer half-lives, in the 4 to 6 h range. Esmolol is therefore often used during anesthesia and postoperative periods, beginning with a loading dose of 500 μg/kg/min for 4 to 5 min, followed by a constant dose infusion of 150 to 300 μg/kg/min (see Table 125-4). This regimen will often reduce heart rate and blood pressure within the first minute of administration, which can be sustained with the maintenance dose. When used intravenously, metoprolol is usually given 5 to 15 mg every 6 h in the absence of renal failure; atenolol is usually given 5 to 10 mg every 6 to 12 h, but the dose should be adjusted downward (or the dosing frequency lengthened) in the presence of renal insufficiency.

PROPRANOLOL. Propranolol is the original nonselective β blocker, which is also often used via the intravenous route. Propranolol shares all of the caveats of the other β blockers listed above. It is typically administered in 1 to 5-mg doses every 4 to 6 h (see Table 125-4); it is important to remember for all the β blockers that the intravenous dose is only 5 to 20 percent of the usual oral dose, because drug given by the intravenous route avoids hepatic first-pass metabolism, which typically disposes of 80 to 95 percent of the orally administered dose.

OTHER AGENTS

ENALAPRILAT. A new approach to the treatment of hypertension by the intravenous route is now available with the angiotensin-converting enzyme (ACE) inhibitor, enalaprilat.[36] This compound is the des-ethyl hydrolysis product of the commonly used oral agent, enalapril, which undergoes deesterification in the liver when given by mouth. The active compound, enalaprilat, is an effective hypotensive agent when given intravenously, although the efficacy is probably not as high as some of the nonspecific vasodilators. Difficulties in using the drug are sometimes encountered in patients with hyperkalemia, chronic renal insufficiency, and renal artery stenosis. The well-known problems of ACE inhibitors, including angioneurotic edema (particularly important when it involves the larynx), cough, and rash do occur with the intravenously administered agent, although they seem to occur more commonly with chronic administration. Enalaprilat is typically given in doses of 1.25 to 5 mg every 6 h in patients with normal renal function, and the dose must be downwardly adjusted for increasing degrees of renal insufficiency (see Table 125-4). The blood pressure response is variable and often unpredictable; major decreases in blood pressure can be seen as soon as 10 min after administration. Monitoring of renal function and potassium are necessary after the drug is given.

VERAPAMIL. Of the calcium antagonists, only verapamil is currently available for intravenous use, although others are being studied. Intravenous verapamil seems to be a better agent for interruption of supraventricular arrhythmias (vide infra) than for control of blood pressure, perhaps due to the differential effects of the D- and L-enantiomers. Although intravenously administered verapamil does often lower blood pressure (see Table 125-4), the effects on the cardiac conduction system appear to occur earlier and at lower doses, such that intravenous verapamil is not often used to control blood pressure when there are no problems with supraventricular arrhythmias.

METHYLDOPA. Methyldopa, an α_2 agonist, is one of the more traditional antihypertensive agents available for intravenous use. Over the last 30 years, it has been used in many patients with good results, usually at doses starting at 125 to 250 mg every 6 h, with an upper limit of 2 g/day (see Table 125-2). The many disadvantages of methyldopa are well-known, because it has been used for a long time, and include dulling and interference with the sensorium (probably the major reason it has fallen out of favor in ICUs), autoimmune hemolytic anemia, hepatotoxicity, fevers, postural hypotension, and fluid retention. Reserpine is also available through the parenteral route, but is often associated with troublesome side effects in ICU patients, particularly with adversely affecting the mental status.

DIRECT-ACTING VASODILATORS. Three additional direct-acting vasodilators can be used intravenously: hydralazine, diazoxide, and nitroglycerin. Hydralazine has the disadvantage of causing reflex tachycardia in most patients who receive it, which can be a problem in the patient with compromised coronary circulation. It is effective, however, and is given in doses of 5 to 20 mg every 4 to 6 h (see Table 125-4); the effect is typically seen within 10 to 20 min. It is probably best used in young patients (e.g., those with toxemia) or those elderly patients who have diminished baroreflex sensitivity (i.e., those who will not experience reflex tachycardia when challenged with a vasodilator). Diazoxide[37] is a very interesting molecule which was strongly advocated in the late 1970s because of its dilation of resistance arterioles, increase in cardiac output, minimal effect on brain function, and fairly impressive efficacy. The original method of administration was a brisk bolus injection of 300 mg within 30 s, but this occasionally leads to a precipitous fall in blood pressure, which must be just as quickly reversed with saline infusion. It is now advocated to give the drug as "minibolus" infusions of 50 to 100 mg every 5 to 10 min (see Table 125-4), which largely avoids the sudden hypotension. Unfortunately, the major side effects (severe fluid retention, exacerbation of diabetes mellitus, nausea, dizziness, and flushing) make it less attractive than some of the newer agents. Nitroglycerin is a direct-acting vasodilator with a very prompt onset of action, which is sometimes difficult to administer, as it "sticks" to plastic (e.g., intravenous tubing). It is often given in starting doses of 5 μg/min (but doses up to 100 μg/min are often necessary, see Table 125-4), with the typical side effects being headache, flushing, tachycardia, vomiting, and (uniquely) methemoglobinemia (if given for a prolonged period or at high dose). These side effects tend to limit its general clinical utility, unless the patient has ongoing cardiac ischemia.

PHENTOLAMINE AND TRIMETHAPHAN. Two other agents which have been used to lower blood pressure via the intravenous route for a long time are now relegated to rather specific indications. Phentolamine is probably still the best acute therapy for the crisis of pheochromocytoma, since it is specific pharmacologic therapy for the overabundance of catecholamines seen in this disease. It is typically administered as a 5 to 10-mg bolus and can be repeated every 5 to 10 min as necessary; it can also be given by continuous infusion (see Table 125-4). Trimethaphan camsylate is now given nearly exclusively in the setting of its traditional use: patients with dissecting aortic aneurysms (see Chap. 124). Because of its powerful effects as a ganglionic blocking agent, its utility in other settings is often outweighed by the side effects, which include severe orthostatic hypotension, paresis of bowel and/or bladder, blurred vision, and xerostomia. Orthostatic hypotension can sometimes be used therapeutically, for trimethaphan, labetalol, and nitroprusside. If one wishes to give only "low doses" of these drugs, but the hypotensive effect is insufficient, it is often useful to raise the head of the bed or "dangle" the legs over the side of the bed; these maneuvers often will lower blood pressure to the desired levels when either nitroprusside, labetalol, or trimethaphan are being infused.

DIURETICS. Concomitant with the agents given above, there is sometimes a need for diuretic therapy, due to the fluid retention which often accompanies the acute reduction of blood pressure. In these settings, intravenous diuretics are often used as an adjunct to therapy, rather than due to any specific immediate antihypertensive effects of the diuretics themselves. Chlorothiazide (250 to 500 mg) is the most commonly administered intravenous thiazide, although several other oral thiazides are also used. Similarly, the "loop" diuretics, furosemide and bumetanide, are effective diuretics, and typically have a shorter duration of action in the patient with reasonably normal renal function.

ORAL AGENTS

In patients with a functioning and accessible gastrointestinal tract, it is largely preferable to administer hypotensive agents orally. This is done both to minimize the chances for intravenous drug-drug interactions (e.g., mixing problems, pharmacokinetic interactions, and so on) and to minimize cost, as the intravenously administered agents (and the attendant tubing, pumps, and other equipment) are far more expensive in most hospitals than are pills.

The three oral agents with the widest experience for the acute reduction of blood pressure are the three oral drugs discussed for use in hypertensive urgencies in Chap. 123. Many patients, however, do have need of some hypotensive therapy despite not qualifying as a hypertensive urgency, and many of the usual oral drugs for hypertension are useful in this setting.

NIFEDIPINE

Nifedipine has become very widely used for the prompt treatment of hypertension, particularly in hospital settings, where there are no particular concomitant conditions which require attention. Most now advocate giving the 10-mg capsule by the "bite and swallow" technique,[38] which avoids the problem with poor sublingual bioavailability of the nifedipine solution. The only major problem with this is that some patients still experience hypotension,[39] and in many patients "rushing to the bedside" to administer nifedipine for a relatively innocuous degree of asymptomatic hypertension is followed by an even worse period of severe hypotension. If the desired hypotensive effect of nifedipine is not seen after 20 to 30 min, the dose can be repeated; this is probably safer than giving 20 mg to start (see Table 125-4).

CLONIDINE

Oral clonidine has been widely used for hypertensive urgencies. It is effective, relatively prompt in onset, and easily titratable (greater doses usually result in a further hypotensive response). Clonidine has the relative disadvantage of causing dry mouth (often already a problem in awake, intubated patients), rebound hypertension (in noncompliant patients), and changes in mental status, which is probably the major reason both it and methyldopa are not commonly used in ICUs. Clonidine therapy is usually started with 0.1 to 0.2 mg, depending on the age and volume status of the patient, and additional 0.1-mg doses can be administered every hour or two thereafter, depending on the blood pressure result obtained (see Table 125-4). Once the target blood pressure has been achieved, clonidine is usually administered twice a day, in generally half to two-thirds the dose necessary during the initial, acute reduction of blood pressure.

CAPTOPRIL

Captopril was the first ACE inhibitor to be widely used and can reduce blood pressure rather quickly (over 20 to 30 min), particularly when the 25-mg tablet is crushed and administered as either an oral or sublingual powder (see Table 125-4).[40] Acutely, it has essentially the same side effects and contraindications as enalaprilat, discussed above. Like enalaprilat, it can cause particularly disastrous hypotension, especially in volume-depleted patients, or those with congestive heart failure, renal insufficiency, or renovascular hypertension. Like nifedipine and clonidine, frequently repeated doses often do lead to an increased hypotensive effect, but the efficacy of repeated doses is probably less than either of the two other drugs.

MISCELLANEOUS ORAL AGENTS

Other drugs which are often useful in treating the severely hypertensive patient (who typically requires a multiple-drug regimen for adequate control of blood pressure) include the nonspecific vasodilator minoxidil (typically given with a long-acting β blocker and a diuretic in once-daily doses,[41] particularly in patients with renal dysfunction), the α_1 blockers prazosin and terazosin (often in combination with verapamil and a diuretic), and the longer-acting versions of some of the drugs discussed above. These agents are particularly useful when controlling the blood pressure long-term (e.g., in an ICU patient with Guillain-Barré syndrome) or after the patient is transferred from the ICU to a "step-down" unit.

Drugs Useful in Increasing Heart Rate

Bradycardia can have many causes and frequently does not necessitate therapy. On the other hand, since cardiac output is determined by the product of heart rate and stroke volume, excessive bradycardia can occasionally contribute to symptomatic heart failure. This is especially true in patients with compromised systolic cardiac function. Additionally, significant bradycardia may cause serious ventricular ectopy and require treatment for this reason. As always, the underlying problem must be kept in mind, as its correction may result in the normalization of heart rate. Examples include the rewarming of hypothermic patients, the correction of hypothyroidism, or the discontinuation of certain drugs, such as β blockers, clonidine, morphine, or potent vasoconstrictors (e.g., norepinephrine). Sometimes less appreciated is the possibility that severe hypovolemia can be associated with profound bradycardia, in which case fluid administration corrects both problems.[42]

TABLE 125-5 Drugs to Increase Heart Rate

Drug Name	IV Dose Range	Oral Dose Range
Atropine	0.5–1-mg bolus	NA
Isoproterenol HCl	0.5 μg/min (starting dose)	NA

If it is determined that bradycardia is hemodynamically significant in a given patient, therapy aimed directly at increasing heart rate may be indicated (Table 125-5). However, heart rate is a primary determinant of myocardial oxygen demand, a consideration which is especially important in the setting of coronary artery disease. A trial of atropine[43] (0.5 to 1.0 mg) is often warranted in cases of sinus bradycardia, where excessive vagal tone may be the culprit. About 15 percent of patients with inferior wall myocardial infarctions may exhibit this problem, a situation where atropine with or without fluid administration may work quite well. On the other hand, if bradycardia recurs despite repeated doses of atropine, a temporary pacemaker in demand mode is often used for 24 to 48 h.

The overall preferred mode of therapy for most cases of symptomatic bradycardia is electrical pacing (see Chap. 32). Ideally, atrial pacing is performed with an intravenous pacemaker, except in cases of high grade atrioventricular (AV) block, when AV (or ventricular) pacing is used. The initial rate is usually set at 80 to 100 beats/min. In emergency situations, external pacemakers are increasing in popularity, pending the placement of an intravenous device. If electrical pacing is not available in an emergency, an intravenous isoproterenol drip can be used as a temporary measure, titrated to the lowest effective dose. Heart rate should rarely be increased to more than 60 beats/min with isoproterenol, and special attention must be given to the occurrence of arrhythmias and the possible worsening of myocardial ischemia. If the problem persists, a pacemaker should be inserted as quickly as possible, and isoproterenol therapy discontinued.

Drugs Useful in Lowering Heart Rate

In certain ICU situations, lowering heart rate is an acceptable and desirable goal of therapy. Nonvasoactive drug therapy is sometimes required, e.g., analgesics, antipyretics, antithyroid drugs. Several common situations where

TABLE 125-6 Drugs to Decrease Heart Rate

Drug Name	IV Loading Dose Range	Maintenance Oral Dose Range
Esmolol	500 μg/kg/min × 4–5 min	150–300 μg/kg/min (IV)
Atenolol	5–10 mg q 6–12 h	50–200 mg q day
Metoprolol	5–15 mg q 6–12 h	50–200 mg q day
Propranolol	1–5 mg q 4–6 h	20–320 mg b.i.d.
Verapamil	5–10 mg q 10 min	120–480 mg q day
Adenosine	6–12-mg bolus	NA
Digoxin	0.5–1.0-mg loading dose (over 2–24 h)	0.125–0.25 mg q day

control of heart rate (using vasoactive drugs) is important include acute myocardial infarction, supraventricular tachycardia, and atrial fibrillation. The therapy for each of these is usually different and depends totally on the diagnosis in the individual patient.

β BLOCKERS

Perhaps the most effective drugs to lower heart rate (particularly in the ICU, and when no other cardiac rhythm disturbance is present) are the β blockers. They are especially helpful in the setting of acute myocardial infarction, where they have other benefits. Many studies during the last decade have found a reduction in both mortality and cardiac morbidity when intravenously administered β blockers are given when patients are admitted to the ICU with an acute myocardial infarction, especially when there is no acute heart block, pulmonary congestion, or history of asthma. When a short trial of β blockade is desired in an ICU patient, esmolol[35] is often used because it has a very brief time of onset and most importantly, the shortest elimination half-life of all β blockers. The various β blockers (and the differences between those available for either intravenous or only oral use) are summarized above in the section on hypotensive agents (see Tables 125-4 and 125-6).

VERAPAMIL AND ADENOSINE

Two other drugs which are often useful in lowering heart rate, particularly in the setting of the patient with paroxysmal supraventricular tachycardias (PSVT), are verapamil and adenosine.[44,45] Intravenously administered verapamil is over 90 percent effective in terminating episodes of PSVT and is usually given intravenously in doses of 5 to 10 mg, which may be repeated if the first bolus is ineffective (see Table 125-6). The major unwanted side effect of intravenous verapamil is hypotension, which is typically the desired effect when it is given orally. The difference between the two effects (slowing of the cardiac conduction system versus lowering blood pressure) is probably due to stereoselective first-pass hepatic metabolism of the orally administered compound, which reduces the plasma ratio of the D- and L-enantiomers. Since L-verapamil is thought to be more responsible for the effects on the cardiac conduction system, the racemate (equal concentrations of each enantiomer) given intravenously primarily affects the cardiac conduction system, with some patients suffering hypotension. Fortunately, the "antidote" for this side effect, the calcium cation, is available and easily administered, such that most patients are relatively hypotensive only for short periods of time. Adenosine has the advantage of acting and being distributed within the bloodstream and eliminated rather quickly, compared to verapamil, and is equal or better in efficacy for patients with PSVT. Several comparative studies between the two drugs have demonstrated no significant differences in efficacy rates, but the relatively lower incidence of hypotension and other side effects seen with adenosine is balanced by a much higher price, often twenty to fifty times the cost of verapamil. In patients with wide-complex tachycardias, particularly when Wolff-Parkinson-White syndrome is suspected, many recommend the use of adenosine first (rather than verapamil, which may precipitate ventricular fibrillation).[46]

DIGOXIN

Atrial fibrillation with a rapid ventricular response has been successfully controlled by digoxin for over 200 years. Most physicians are quite facile with the loading dose (typically 0.5 mg, given in two divided doses over 30 min, followed by two further 0.25-mg boluses over the next 2 h, depending on the ventricular response rate), and reductions in dose necessary when digoxin is administered in patients with chronic renal insufficiency, or those who are concomitantly given quinidine, verapamil,[47] or many other commonly used drugs. Digoxin levels can sometimes be a guide to further therapy with the drug, but are most useful in the setting of digoxin toxicity, particularly when extremely elevated.[48] Seldom, however, are treatment decisions based on digoxin levels, as the ventricular response rates, cardiac rhythm (beware of accelerated idioventricular rhythm, and situations in which there is obvious atrioventricular block), and patient's symptoms (the classic "yellow-halo around lights" described by Withering is often preceded by gastrointestinal complaints) are often better guides to the dosing of digoxin.

CASE PRESENTATION

A 75-year-old woman with moderate obesity and a history of mild systolic hypertension and mild hypercholesterolemia presented with 26 h of midepigastric pain and "fullness" which was unrelieved by antacids. An ECG demonstrated "hyperacute" T waves and new Q waves in leads II, III, and aVF. Her initial examination was remarkable for a few rales at both bases, and a loud S_3. During her first 6 h in the ICU, she developed progressive sinus bradycardia to 48 beats/min, with occasional sinus nodal arrest, followed by frequent ventricular escape beats. During the seventh hour, she had continuous 2:1 Wenckebach heart block. This initially responded to intravenous atropine (0.5, then 1 mg), but after 2 h, she complained of chest pain; the rhythm was idioventricular at a rate of 30 to 32, which did not respond to atropine. Isoproterenol was given at 0.5 to 1.0 μg/min (adjusted to keep the heart rate at or slightly above 60 beats/min), and a temporary pacemaker was quickly inserted. Her course was uneventful until the second hospital day, when she redeveloped upper abdominal pain, with concurrent dyspnea, diaphoresis, and blood pressures as high as 240/110 (with pain). After refusing cardiac catheterization and possible bypass surgery, she was treated with intravenous nitrates (titrated against pain, but limited to a dose of 15 μg/kg/min because of a severe unrelenting headache) and then sodium nitroprusside (which kept the diastolic blood pressure <95 mmHg), but she continued to have dyspnea at rest. Her chest x-ray and oxygenation deteriorated, and a pulmonary artery catheter was placed. The SVR was 2200 dyne/sec/cm^{-5}, the pulmonary artery wedge pressure 22 mmHg, and the cardiac index (CI) was 1.8 L/min/m^2. This improved to 3.1 L/min/m^2 after the institution of dobutamine, which was increased sequentially from 1 to 6 μg/kg/min, concomitant with a decrease in pulmonary artery wedge pressure to 14 mmHg, and a decrease in SVR to 1400 dyne/sec/cm^{-5}.

On the fifth hospital day, the blood pressure gradually decreased to a nadir of 86/72. CI was 2.1 L/min/m^2; pulmonary artery wedge pressure was initially 8 mmHg, and SVR was 1850 dyne/sec/cm^{-5}. After administration of 2 U packed red blood cells (as her hematocrit had decreased from 42 percent on admission to 28 percent) and 1.25 L normal saline solution over the next 6 h, the wedge pressure increased to 18 mmHg, and increased most after the last 250 mL saline solution. Blood pressure increased only marginally during these maneuvers; CI was 2.3 L/min/m^2, and SVR was 2150 dyne/sec/cm^{-5}. Arterial lactate was measured at 4 mEq/L, and dobutamine was increased to 15 μg/kg/min, resulting in a blood pressure of 118/84, CI of 3.2 L/min/m^2, and a decrease in arterial lactate level to 2 to 2.5 mEq/L. The blood pressure remained near 110/80 over the next 4 days, but resisted attempts to "wean" the dobutamine. On the sixth day of dobutamine administration, her serum sodium and potassium levels were 130 and 5.7 mEq/dL (they were 139 and 4.1 on admission), and the diagnosis of Addison's disease was considered. A plasma cortisol sample was obtained, and 4 mg dexamethasone given intravenously. The blood chemistries and blood pressures returned toward normal, and the dobutamine was successfully discontinued. She was moved to the "step-down" unit on hospital day 17 and discharged on low dose metoprolol and aspirin after a submaximal exercise tolerance test with thallium imaging disclosed evidence of continuing ischemia in the distribution of the right coronary artery.

CASE DISCUSSION

This case illustrates several important points regarding the use of vasoactive drugs in ICU patients. Just after her acute inferior myocardial infarction, the patient developed cardiac conduction disturbances, presumably related to ischemia of the AV node. These were initially treated successfully with atropine, but when angina and severe bradycardia supervened (and when the idioventricular rhythm was unresponsive to further atropine), isoproterenol was used as a temporizing measure until a transvenous pacemaker began functioning. Because of continuing ischemia and pain-associated hypertension, her blood pressure was lowered first with a nitroglycerin infusion (preferred here among the many antihypertensive agents because of its coronary arterial vasodilator properties), and then with nitroprusside (when nitroglycerin did not achieve goal blood pressure without undue symptomatic side effects). Despite this "balanced" approach to reduce preload and afterload, she continued to be dyspneic, and have signs and symptoms of cardiac failure. To aid management, a pulmonary artery catheter was placed and used to guide inotropic support of her failing myocardium, beginning with relatively low dose dobutamine. This drug was chosen because of its ability to increase cardiac contractility, without major effects on heart rate or SVR. Isoproterenol, dopamine, digoxin, and even the phosphodiesterase inhibitors (amrinone or milrinone) were alternatives, but each has significant disadvantages in the setting described: isoproterenol primarily increases heart rate (and myocardial oxygen demand); dopamine often leads to increases in blood pressure and SVR, particularly at doses over 5 μg/kg/min; digoxin has a narrow therapeutic window, often prolongs AV nodal conduction times, and cannot be discontinued abruptly. Because of the high frequency of side effects, the phosphodiesterase inhibitors are typically reserved for situations when other inotropes are not sufficiently helpful.

On the fifth hospital day, when the patient became hypotensive with decreased cardiac output and higher SVR than previously, hypovolemic shock was initially diagnosed, and attention was directed to reestablishing an adequate circulating blood volume. She was given blood (to ensure adequate hemoglobin-carrying capacity of her limited cardiac output), followed by saline solution, with frequent monitoring of the pulmonary artery wedge pressure. Only after no further improvement in these parameters following a 250-mL "bolus" of saline was dobutamine dose increased further. Other drugs which might produce the same effect include dopamine (which can cause peripheral vasoconstriction), norepinephrine (which can worsen pulmonary congestion), epinephrine (which concomitantly increases heart rate), metaraminol, or phenylephrine.

When the patient failed to improve on the sixth day of dobutamine, appropriate reevaluation resulted in the diagnosis of subacute addisonian crisis. This was treated promptly with dexamethasone and followed by a quick ACTH stimulation test; (see Chap. 160), with resultant improvement in efficacy of intravenous inotropes, consistent with the in vitro demonstration of downregulation of β-adrenergic receptors in the absence of corticosteroids. It is likely that the eventual good outcome would not have occurred without attention to *all* the aspects of support of the severely ill patient using vasoactive drugs.

References

1. Katz AM: Changing strategies in the management of heart failure. J Am Coll Cardiol 13:513, 1990.
2. Ruffolo RR Jr: The pharmacology of dobutamine. Am J Med Sci 294:244, 1987.
3. Majerus TC, Dasta JF, Bauman JL, et al: Dobutamine: Ten years later. Pharmacotherapy 9:245, 1989.
4. Liang CS, Wood WB: Dobutamine infusion in conscious dogs with and without autonomic nervous system inhibition: Effects of systemic hemodynamics, regional blood flows and cardiac metabolism. J Pharmacol Exp Ther 229:364, 1984.
5. Vatner SF, McRitchie RJ, Braunwald E: Effects of dobutamine on left ventricular performance, coronary dynamics and distribution of cardiac output in conscious dogs. J Clin Invest 53:1265,1974.
6. Boyd JL, Stanford GG, Chernow B: The pharmacotherapy of septic shock. Crit Care Clin 5:133, 1989.
7. Vincent J-L, Roman A, Kahn RJ: Dobutamine administration in septic shock: Addition to a standard protocol. Crit Care Med 18:689, 1990.
8. Carey RA, Jacob L: The role of dopaminergic agents and the dopamine receptor in treatment for congestive heart failure. J Clin Pharmacol 29:207, 1989.
9. Goldberg LI: Dopamine—Clinical uses of an endogenous catecholamine. N Engl J Med 291:707, 1974.
10. Malchoff CD, Hughes J, Sen S, et al: Dopamine inhibits the aldosterone response to upright posture. J Clin Endocrinol Metab 63:197, 1986.
11. Conference on Standards and Guidelines for CPR and Emergency Cardiac care. Standards and guidelines for cardiopulmonary resuscitation and emergency cardiac care. JAMA 255:2985, 1986.
12. Wood W Jr: Controlled and uncontrolled studies of phosphodiesterase III inhibitors in contemporary cardiovascular medicine. Am J Cardiol 63:46A, 1989.
13. Konstam MA, Cohen SR, Wieland DS, et al: Relative contribution of inotropic and vasodilator effects to amrinone-induced hemodynamic improvement in congestive heart failure. Am J Cardiol 57:242, 1986.
14. DiBianco R, Shabetai R, Kostuk W, et al: A comparison of oral milrinone, digoxin, and their contribution in the treatment of patients with chronic heart failure. N Engl J Med 320:677, 1989.
15. Colucci WS, Wright RF, Braunwald E: New positive inotropic agents in the treatment of congestive heart failure: Mechanisms of action and recent clinical developments. N Engl J Med 314:349, 1986.
16. Franciosa JA: Intravenous amrinone: An advance or wrong step? Editorial. Ann Int Med 102:399, 1985.
17. Löllgen H, Drexler H: Use of inotropes in the critical care setting. Crit Care Med 18:S56, 1990.
18. Houston MC, Thompson L, Robertson DA: Shock—Diagnosis and management. Arch Intern Med 144:1433, 1984.
19. Chatterjee K, Parmley WW, Ganz W, et al: Hemodynamic studies: Their uses and limitations. Am J Cardiol 64:3D, 1989.
20. Rackow EC, Falk JL, Fein IA, et al: Fluid resuscitation in circulatory shock: A comparison of the cardiorespiratory effects of albumin, hetastarch, and saline solutions in patients with hypovolemic and septic shock. Crit Care Med 11:839, 1983.
21. Gammage G: Crystalloid vs. colloid: Is colloid worth the cost? Int Anesthesiol Clin 25:37, 1987.
22. Murphy MB, Elliott WJ: Dopamine and dopamine receptor agonists in cardiovascular therapy. Crit Care Med 18:S14, 1990.
23. Chernow B, Roth BL: Pharmacologic manipulation of the peripheral vasculature in shock. Circ Shock 18:141, 1986.
24. Dasta JF: Norepinephrine in septic shock: Renewed interest in an old drug. Drug Intell Clin Pharm 24:153, 1990.
25. Schremmer B, Dhainaut J: Heart failure in septic shock: Effects of inotropic support. Crit Care Med 18:S49, 1990.
26. Desjars P, Pinaud M, Potel G, et al: A reappraisal of norepinephrine therapy in human septic shock. Crit Care Med 15:134, 1987.
27. Calhoun DA, Oparil S: Current concepts: Treatment of hypertensive crisis. N Engl J Med 323:1177, 1990.
28. Cohn JN, Burke LP: Nitroprusside. Ann Intern Med 91:752, 1979.
29. Cottrell JE, Casthely P, Brodie JD, et al: Prevention of nitroprusside-induced cyanide toxicity with hydroxocobalamine. N Engl J Med 298:809, 1978.
30. Cole PV, Vesey CJ: Sodium thiosulphate decreases blood cyanide concentrations after the infusion of sodium nitroprusside. Br J Anaesthesiol 59:531, 1987.
31. Schulz V: Clinical pharmacokinetics of nitroprusside, cyanide, thiosulphate, and thiocyanate. Clin Pharmacokinet 9:239, 1984.
32. Wallin JD, Fletcher E, Ram CVS, et al: Intravenous nicardipine for the treatment of severe hypertension: A double-blind, placebo-controlled, multicenter trial. Arch Intern Med 149:2262, 1989.
33. Elliott WJ, Weber RR, Nelson KS, et al: Renal and hemodynamic effects of intravenous fenoldopam versus nitroprusside in severe hypertension. Circulation 81:970, 1990.
34. Goa KL, Benfield P, Sorkin EM: Labetalol: A reappraisal of its pharmacology, pharmacokinetics and therapeutic use in hypertension and ischemic heart disease. Drugs 37:583, 1989.
35. Frishman WH, Murthy S, Strom JA: Ultra-short acting intravenous beta blocker for use in critically ill patients. Med Clin North Am 72:359, 1988.
36. Rutledge J, Ayers C, Davidson R, et al: Effect of intravenous enalaprilat in moderate and severe systemic hypertension. Am J Cardiol 62:1062, 1988.
37. Huysmans FTM, Thien RA, Koene RAP: Acute treatment of hypertension with slow infusion of diazoxide. Arch Intern Med 143:882, 1983.
38. Haft JL, Litterer WE III: Chewing nifedipine to rapidly treat hypertension. Arch Intern Med 144:2357, 1984.
39. Wachter RM: Symptomatic hypotension induced by nifedipine in the acute treatment of hypertension. Arch Intern Med 147:556, 1987.
40. Abe I, Kawasaki T, Kawazoe N, Omae T: Acute electrocardiographic effects of captopril in the initial treatment of malignant or severe hypertension. Am Heart J 106:558, 1983.
41. Spitalewitz S, Porush JG, Reiser IW: Minoxidil, nadolol, and a diuretic: Once a day therapy for resistant hypertension. Arch Intern Med 146:882, 1986.
42. Barriot P, Riou B: Hemorrhagic shock with paradoxical bradycardia. Intensive Care Med 13:203, 1987.

43. Das G: Therapeutic review: Cardiac effects of atropine in man: An update. Drug Intell Clin Pharm 27:473, 1989.
44. DeMarco JP, Miles W, Akhtar M, et al: Adenosine for paroxysmal supraventricular tachycardia: Dose ranging and comparison with verapamil. Ann Intern Med 113:104, 1990.
45. Rankin AC, Rae AP, Oldroyd KG, Cobbe SM: Verapamil or adenosine for the immediate treatment of supraventricular tachycardia. Q J Med 74:203, 1990.
46. Sharma AD, Klein GJ, Yee R: Intravenous adenosine triphosphate during wide QRS complex tachycardia: Safety, therapeutic efficacy, and diagnostic utility. Am J Med 88:337, 1990.
47. Klein HO, Kaplinsky E: Verapamil and digoxin: Their respective effects on atrial fibrillation and their interaction. Am J Cardiol 50:894, 1982.
48. Selzer A: Role of serum digoxin assay in patient management. J Am Coll Cardiol 5 (suppl A):106A, 1985.

Chapter 126
RHEUMATOLOGY IN THE ICU

WALTER G. BARR
JOHN A. ROBINSON

KEY POINTS

- *New-onset rheumatic diseases rarely prompt ICU admission in the absence of a revealing prodrome.*
- *In most patients without a previously established collagen vascular disease, suspected vasculitis will be explained by an alternative diagnosis.*
- *Immunoserologic assessment of critically ill patients is a two-edged sword providing both enlightenment and misleading shadows. All immunoserologic testing must be interpreted with a thorough understanding of the patient's clinical condition.*
- *Inability to assign specific diagnostic labels to patients with severe immunoinflammatory disease should not delay therapeutic intervention.*
- *Not all ischemic skin lesions that appear to be vasculitis are. Pseudovasculitis of various causes should always be part of the differential diagnosis.*
- *Empirical trials with corticosteroids can be a rational approach to patient care when such trials are carried out appropriately.*
- *Organic brain syndrome without focal neurologic deficits or evidence of systemic vasculitis is unlikely to be secondary to vasculitis.*
- *Fever in patients with collagen vascular disease should be presumed infectious if accompanied by chills, leukocytosis with a left shift, or hypotension.*
- *Patients who have been treated with significant doses of corticosteroids within the past year may require empirical replacement therapy during critical illness or surgical procedures until adrenal insufficiency can be excluded.*

Rheumatologists seldom lend their expertise to the medical ICU. The tempo and level of intensity of most rheumatic disorders are more suited to outpatient management. Patients with these diseases admitted to the medical ICU most often have problems not directly related to their primary illness. Sepsis, massive gastrointestinal bleeding, and myocardial infarcts may arise secondary to treatment. The major direction of care in these circumstances often comes from the intensivist. Circumstances do arise that require the unique insight of the experienced clinical rheumatologist, who at times, must direct the management of a disease-specific complication. Just as often the rheumatologist is asked to address a diagnostic dilemma spawned by puzzling clinical and laboratory data. This chapter addresses the more common issues that prompt the rheumatologist and the intensivist to collaborate.

Rheumatic Disease-Specific Intensive Care Scenarios

SYSTEMIC LUPUS ERYTHEMATOSUS

FEVER: IS IT THE LUPUS? Fever in the patient with lupus presses the clinician for an urgent answer to the question: is this due to lupus activity or infection? Fever is a common finding in active systemic lupus erythematosus (SLE) affecting more than 80 percent of patients at some time.[1] The lupus fever has no specific pattern and it may respond to the usual antipyretics or require corticosteroids. Single daily morning dose prednisone may not control late afternoon or evening fevers. Leukocytosis and increased bands on peripheral smear are strong presumptive evidence for infection. Complements, including C3 and C4, are acute phase reactants and usually rise with infection. Low levels of complement occur in some but not all patients with active lupus. For unexplained reasons, patients with SLE produce little or no C-reactive protein (CRP) in response to their illness. It has been suggested that high levels of CRP in the lupus patient indicate infection, but exceptions to this rule occur.

In the ICU setting, the febrile patient with SLE is probably best considered infected and treated with broad-spectrum antibiotics pending results of cultures. Infection is most likely to be caused by nonopportunistic organisms and coverage for gram-positive and gram-negative aerobes represents adequate empirical therapy when no obvious source has been recognized.

MYOCARDIAL INFARCT IN THE LUPUS PATIENT: IS IT VASCULITIS? Myocardial infarction makes a major contribution to excessive mortality in SLE. Mortality data suggest a bimodal distribution with many late deaths in SLE secondary to ischemic heart disease. The primary cause of ischemic heart disease in lupus is atherosclerosis. Autopsy studies in young women with lupus with death from any cause show an excessive incidence of atherosclerosis in comparison to age-matched females.[2] The cause is not totally clear but chronic immune complex disease and corticosteroids probably are contributing factors.

Vasculitis in SLE may affect any organ including the heart. Most patients with coronary artery vasculitis have evidence of vasculitis in other organs. Serologic evidence of active lupus and markers of systemic inflammation including low hemoglobin and albumin are likely to be present. Acute therapy would include high dose corticosteroids (vide infra). In the face of widespread vasculitis, additional intervention with parenteral immunosuppressives and plasmapheresis may be indicated.

Corticosteroids are potentially hazardous and high doses may predispose to ventricular rupture. Therefore, they should not be used in the absence of reasonable clinical suspicion for coronary vasculitis. If the lupus patient is in apparent clinical remission without evidence of widespread vasculitis, treatment should be the same as that for the non-lupus patient. Early cardiac catheterization can help clarify the nature of the vascular disease.

RENAL FAILURE: IS IT TREATABLE LUPUS NEPHRITIS? In patients with SLE in the ICU, renal insufficiency may be due to a variety of factors including drugs, especially nonsteroidal anti-inflammatory drugs (NSAIDs), hypovolemia, sepsis, or previous renal disease. In some cases, active lupus nephritis is a contributing factor. A careful examination of the urinary sediment is the most critical diagnostic tool. Proteinuria, casts and red blood cells indicate glomerulitis. Lupus patients with active nephritis are most often hypertensive. Significant renal lupus (other than membranous disease) is often associated with low complement levels and elevation of anti-DNA antibody.

In a patient with a creatinine level above 4.0 mg/dL who has been adequately hydrated, divorced from nephrotoxic drugs, and with evidence of active glomerulitis, the question arises: is more aggressive immunosuppression desirable? The answer to this question depends on the degree of potential disease reversibility. A renal biopsy can help clarify this issue. The presence of significant chronic disease should dampen enthusiasm for aggressive therapy. Review of old records can be enlightening if long-standing loss of renal function is documented.

Clinicians have become increasingly aware that immunosuppression in the lupus patient with advanced renal disease can be more hazardous than progression to complete renal failure. Patients with lupus tolerate dialysis in a fashion comparable to other patients and results of renal transplantation are favorable.[3] Paradoxically, patients with lupus who develop chronic renal failure often enjoy an amelioration of extrarenal symptoms.[4] A few patients have recovered sufficient renal function to allow withdrawal from dialysis. For all these reasons, the overzealous administration of immunosuppression in patients with lupus and advanced renal disease is to be discouraged.

RESPIRATORY FAILURE AND LUNG INFILTRATES: IS IT LUPUS PNEUMONITIS? Respiratory failure in a patient with SLE is an ominous development. A paradigm of a compromised host is a patient with lupus who is on high dose corticosteroid therapy. The usual opportunistic pulmonary infections need to be urgently excluded by bronchoalveolar lavage, bronchoscopic transbronchial biopsy, or open lung biopsy. If no superimposed infections or embolic etiology can be found and treated, lupus-related respiratory failure remains a diagnosis of exclusion and can be due to either lupus pneumonitis or diffuse pulmonary hemorrhage. Acute lupus pneumonitis is characterized by fever, tachypnea, and hypoxemia, which may be accompanied by cough, pleuritic chest pain, and hemoptysis.[5] Radiologic findings are highly variable, but usually bilateral and at least bibasilar. This diagnosis is not only one of exclusion, but unfortunately still rests solely on clinical suspicion.

The other SLE-related cause of respiratory failure is diffuse pulmonary hemorrhage.[6] Although invasive aspergillus or tuberculosis can erode a pulmonary vessel and cause hemorrhage, gross hemoptysis, when present, usually indicates alveolar hemorrhage. Hemoptysis is not usually seen in lupus pneumonitis; unfortunately, this finding is present in <50 percent of patients with alveolar hemorrhage. Blood or hemosiderin-laden macrophages found during bronchoscopy in a patient without heart failure can be helpful findings but are nonspecific. The presence of thrombocytopenia is not helpful, but bleeding sufficient to cause acute respiratory failure almost invariably causes an acute drop in hematocrit. In fact, treatment should not be delayed in order to distinguish between lupus pneumonitis and lupus-associated hemorrhage, because mortality is extremely high in either syndrome and treatment strategies are similar.

Pulmonary hypertension, sometimes severe, is frequently present. Cardiac filling pressures can occasionally be helpful discriminators to exclude acute cardiogenic pulmonary edema. Pulmonary artery thrombosis masquerading as massive pulmonary emboli can occur in patients with pulmonary hypertension or thrombotically active anticardiolipin (ACL) antibodies.

The mortality of lupus pneumonitis is high and treatment should be aggressive. Individual preferences will dictate modes of therapy since no consensus exists on either the etiology of the syndrome or effective treatment. Pulse methylprednisolone, usually 500 to 1000 mg intravenously given for 3 to 5 days, or bolus cyclophosphamide at 0.5 to 1 g/m^2 has been used. The latter will require 7 to 14 days for optimal effect. Plasma exchange may serve as a useful temporizing treatment during the interim.

BRAIN DYSFUNCTION: IS IT LUPUS? A patient with acute, severe neurologic deficits and a history of SLE or a clinical syndrome and laboratory evidence suggestive of systemic vasculitis presents a diagnostic and therapeutic dilemma for the critical care clinician. In the vast majority of instances, involvement of the central nervous system (CNS) in SLE occurs as an organic brain syndrome or seizures in young females with active multisystem disease. Patients with organic brain syndromes manifest psychosis usually early after the onset of SLE. A common dilemma is to differentiate between steroid-induced pseudoorganic brain syndromes and those due to active SLE. Early onset development of psychosis while on low doses of corticosteroids, and fulminant progression usually characterize the CNS disease due to SLE. Depressive syndromes with or without auditory, visual, or even olfactory hallucinations in a patient on a dose of corticosteroids usually higher than 0.5 mg/kg/day are usually drug induced. Because there is little evidence that high dose corticosteroids ameliorate the CNS manifestations of SLE, rapid reduction of corticosteroid dosage is usually the simplest and most direct clinical strategy when a quandary exists as to whether CNS dysfunction is drug induced.

Lupus-induced seizures are usually grand mal, but can be very pleomorphic and usually occur in patients with active SLE.[7] Rapidly progressive, multisystem SLE that is further complicated by early onset of a seizure syndrome usually portends a poor outcome. The development of a seizure disorder in a patient with a long history of inactive SLE or in a patient with SLE entering remission is usually due to something else. There is also little clinical evidence that high dose corticosteroids alone influence the course of seizure disorders in SLE and these patients should be aggressively treated with conventional anticonvulsive therapy. Many rheumatologists will resort to concomitant pulse methlyprednisone, alkylating agents and/or plasma exchange in the setting of fulminant CNS-SLE, but these therapies are of unproven benefit.

Three other CNS manifestations of SLE can be puzzling. A small subset of patients with SLE who have taken NSAIDs, especially ibuprofen, will develop a meningitis-like picture that is characterized by fever, severe headache, nuchal rigidity, and cerebrospinal fluid neutrophilia or pleocytosis.[8] In an immunosuppressed patient, these findings prompt consideration of both common and unusual bacterial and fungal etiologies. The entire syndrome will remit rapidly once the drug is discontinued.

Migraine headaches, some of spectacular intensity, are frequent in SLE.[9] They usually respond to increases in corticosteroid dosage.

Actual paralysis is uncommon in SLE. Rare instances of transverse myelitis occur in the context of active SLE. Until recently this was thought to be secondary to necrotizing vasculitis in the spinal arteries. It is likely, however, that most instances have been secondary to thrombosis associated with high titers of IgG ACL antibodies.[10] This differentiation may be important because the primary treatment of this syndrome is not aggressive immunomodulation of SLE, but appropriate anticoagulation.

SCLERODERMA

PULMONARY HYPERTENSION: CAN ANYTHING BE DONE? Severe pulmonary hypertension in scleroderma is seen in two clinical settings. Patients with diffuse scleroderma may develop pulmonary hypertension due to advanced pulmonary fibrosis. Patients with limited cutaneous disease (CREST) may develop severe pulmonary hypertension in the absence of significant parenchymal lung disease. This often occurs in the second decade of illness. In both settings, the vascular disease is characterized by bland endothelial proliferation and vascular occlusion. The inflammatory infiltrate is sparse and response to steroids or immunosuppression is poor. Therapy of pulmonary hypertension in this setting is most often disappointing. Responsiveness depends on the presence of a residual vasospastic component in addition to the obliterative, nonreversible disease. The common practice of placing a pulmonary artery catheter and trying a sequence of vasodilators is being abandoned by many clinicians because of lack of effectiveness, attendant hazards, and the inability to address the issue of long-term treatment efficacy.[11] These issues are more fully analyzed in Chap. 117. In essence, advanced pulmonary hypertension in scleroderma is now treatable only if the patient is a candidate for transplantation.

HYPERTENSIVE RENAL CRISIS. Until recently, hypertensive renal crisis in patients with scleroderma was the major cause of mortality. It typically develops in patients with diffuse cutaneous disease and rarely in patients with limited cutaneous disease or CREST.[12] Most often, patients have early (<5 years) disease. Patients develop a marked increase in blood pressure that may be accompanied by abnormalities of urinary sediment (erythrocytes) and the peripheral blood smear (fragmented cells). Headache, visual disturbance, and mental status dysfunction may accompany the hypertension.

The pathogenesis of hypertensive renal crisis involves a high renin state. Although combinations of older antihypertensive agents were occasionally successful, the advent of angiotensin-converting enzyme (ACE) inhibitors has revolutionized the outlook for this problem. Rheumatologists have a low threshold for using these agents in scleroderma patients and typically initiate them at the first diagnosis of hypertension.

In the setting of acute hypertensive renal crisis, larger doses of ACE inhibitors should be used. Although captopril and enalapril have both been used, some prefer captopril because of ability to adjust the dose more flexibly. Diuretics (hydrochlorothiazide, furosemide) may potentiate the effect of ACE inhibitors. Nipride can be used for immediate effect.

Some patients may progress to complete renal failure despite blood pressure control. Continued use of ACE inhibitors and dialysis may be required for months prior to recovery of renal function, but the recovery rate may be as high as 50 percent.[13]

POLYMYOSITIS/DERMATOMYOSITIS

DIAGNOSIS IN THE ICU. Very ill patients in the ICU may be weak and have elevations of creatine phosphokinase (CPK). Such clinical data prompt speculation about the presence of immune-mediated myositis. The most common presentation of polymyositis is the insidious onset of proximal muscle weakness, at times associated with myalgia. The acute development of de novo polymyositis in the ICU is unlikely. Similarly, acute fulminant disease requiring ICU admission with subsequent diagnosis is uncommon. Nonetheless, patients with undiagnosed polymyositis may be discovered in the ICU following admission for another reason (e.g., aspiration pneumonia). More likely is the presence of weakness (usually generalized) in combination with a spurious or nonimmune cause of CPK elevation. Intramuscular injections and myonecrosis during severe episodes of hypotension are common causes of increased CPK levels in critically ill patients.

The skin lesions of dermatomyositis are so highly characteristic as to be diagnostic of dermatomyositis when accompanied by weakness and an elevated CPK value. Nearly all patients with active polymyositis will display an elevated CPK or aldolase level, although occasional patients will have normal muscle enzymes.[14] A unilateral electromyogram (EMG) can provide supportive evidence for the presence of myopathy. Fibrillation potentials suggest active inflammation. A bedside EMG can be done in the ICU, although technical artifact may complicate the interpretation.

The EMG should be done unilaterally because EMG needle artifact may be confused with muscle inflammation histologically. Because polymyositis/dermatomyositis is a symmetrical disease, the corresponding maximally affected muscle group can be biopsied on the opposite side. Open biopsy can be done at the bedside preferably by an experienced surgeon to ensure proper handling of muscle tissue. Needle biopsy of muscle using a Polley-Bickel needle is advocated by some and appears suitable for providing confirmation of active muscle inflammation.

RESPIRATORY FAILURE. Patients with polymyositis/dermatomyositis may develop respiratory failure secondary to muscle weakness involving the diaphragm, intercostal, and accessory muscles. If pharyngeal muscles are involved, acute respiratory failure may be precipitated by aspiration pneumonia. Patients with respiratory failure have a poor prognosis.[15] Some patients with dermatomyositis and this type of profound weakness harbor an underlying malignancy.

Steroids are the mainstay of acute management of inflammatory myositis. Prednisone, 1 to 2 mg/kg/day, or its approximate intravenous equivalent of methylprednisolone (in single or divided doses) may be given. In the ventilator-dependent patient, a short trial of pulse steroids may be justified—500 to 1000 mg methylprednisolone intravenously every day for 3 days. Improvement in respiratory muscle strength can be judged by a rise in the maximal inspiratory pressure. Second-line agents in polymyositis/dermatomyositis include methotrexate, azathioprine, and cyclophosphamide. Azathioprine is not useful in the acute setting due to slow onset of action. Methotrexate is most commonly used after corticosteroids. The most experience in myositis is with the intravenous route of administration; the dose is 25 to 75 mg intravenously weekly.

Uncontrolled trials with plasmapheresis and combination plasmapheresis and leukocytapheresis have reported benefits and may be considered in refractory patients.[16,17]

RHEUMATOID ARTHRITIS

METHOTREXATE PNEUMONITIS. Oral low dose methotrexate given intermittently emerged as the major therapeutic innovation in the treatment of rheumatoid arthritis during the 1980s. It is both highly effective and generally well tolerated. The major toxicity is an acute pneumonitis characterized by dyspnea and nonproductive cough.[18] Diffuse pulmonary infiltrates are present at diagnosis or appear within days. Opportunistic infections mimicking this syndrome have only rarely been reported.[19] Patients suffer profound hypoxemia. They appear extremely ill and deaths have been reported. The mechanism is unclear but is presumed to be a hypersensitivity reaction to the drug. Some patients have been rechallenged without developing the syndrome. Reliable predictive markers for this syndrome have not been identified.

Diagnosis depends on the above clinical scenario developing in a patient taking methotrexate at any dose. Duration of treatment prior to symptoms has been variable. Bronchoscopy with brushings and biopsy shows nonspecific inflammation and its main justification is to rule out an opportunistic infection. Because these are rare, it is not unreasonable to forego bronchoscopy initially. Open lung biopsy is unnecessary.

Treatment includes O_2, withdrawal of drug, and corticosteroids. Some have argued that steroids are not critical to recovery. The usual dose is prednisone 1 mg/kg/day or its equivalent in single or divided doses. Most patients will show signs of recovery within a week. Eventually, recovery is typically complete.

CERVICAL SPINE SUBLUXATION. Arthritis commonly affects the cervical spine in rheumatoid arthritis with estimates as high as 80 percent of patients.[20] Subluxation of vertebrae secondary to ligamentous laxity may occur at single or multiple levels. Subluxation of C1 on C2 is particularly dangerous because of the capacity of the odontoid process (or dens) of C2 to compress the anterior spinal cord with motion. Thus, sudden hyperextension of the neck during intubation could result in quadriplegia. In reality, such occurrences are rare. The explanation may, in part, include the fact that progressive resorption of the dens often accompanies the most severely unstable necks. Symptomatic patients can be diagnosed with magnetic resonance imaging (MRI) or myelogram. However, some dramatic subluxations on MRI are not accompanied by neurologic signs or symptoms. Flexion and extension films of the cervical spine may show dynamic instability and subluxation of C1 on C2. There is little data about the specificity or sensitivity of such films to predict a cervical cord catastrophe. Clearly, caution should be exercised in the intubation of patients with rheumatoid arthritis and neck disease; if time allows, nasotracheal or fiberoptically guided endotracheal intubation is preferred. However, when the risk of delayed intubation is sufficiently great, the procedure should not be delayed for radiographic studies, because the risk of cord catastrophe is quite low.

HYPERVISCOSITY SYNDROME. Hyperviscosity syndrome is characterized by visual disturbance, headache, and ischemia. The most common cause is Waldenstrom's macroglobulinemia in which monoclonal production of IgM in gram quantities is caused by clonal expansion of B cells. Patients with rheumatoid arthritis may develop a similar syndrome related to circulating intermediate-size immune complexes.[21] Patients usually have long-standing seropositive disease. Treatment with plasmapheresis acutely reduces levels of immune complexes. Concurrent therapy with cyclophosphamide is necessary for prolonged therapeutic benefit.

Perplexing Cases: Is this a Rheumatic Disease?

FEVER OF UNDETERMINED ORIGIN: RHEUMATIC CAUSES The traditional definition of a fever of undetermined origin (FUO) depicts a patient with a significant fever of 6 weeks' or greater duration and no definable cause. In actual practice, an FUO, depending on the impatience of the attending physician, usually becomes the working diagnosis within 3 to 14 days after a fruitless search for classic causes of pyrexia. By far, the most common causes of FUO are occult infection, drugs, and occasionally malignancy. After those are excluded, one must consider a limited array of rheumatic diseases that could be present in a febrile patient with protracted fever. Because rheumatoid arthritis, scleroderma and its variants, dermatomyositis, polymositis, and polymyalgia rheumatica are not usual causes of significant fever, they need not be strongly considered.

Systemic lupus erythematosus can present with high fevers, either spiking or relatively constant, and leukopenia, hypoalbuminemia, anemia, and elevated erythrocyte sedimentation rate (ESR) but few other overt clinical signs of lupus such as rash or serositis, polyarthritis, or active urinary sediment. Most systemic necrotizing vasculitides will be evident after examination of the skin, chest radiograph, and urinary sediment. Myocardial dysfunction, age, and demographics of the patient with fever may point to either Kawasaki's disease or Lyme disease as the source, while acute valvular dysfunction is being increasingly recognized in SLE and also may be the clue to acute rheumatic fever in an adult.[22] An extremely high ESR is a nonspecific laboratory clue in FUO, but antibodies to relevant antinuclear or streptococcal specifities provide supportive evidence.

A most vexing diagnosis to pin down is that of adult Still's disease. These patients will have relentless spiking fevers, at times a history of FUO in childhood, leukocytosis, mild to moderate hepatic enzyme changes, and an occasional truncal rash.[23] Polyarthritis or arthralgias are not a constant feature early in this syndrome.

In the final analysis, treatment may have to be based on the supposition that the patient has relentless, immunologically driven, noninfectious inflammation that evades specific diagnosis. Blanket suppression of cytokines and white blood cell responses by corticosteroid induction may be necessary. The steroid dose is tailored to control fever and normalize the acute phase response.

MULTIPLE AUTOANTIBODIES AND MULTISYSTEM INFLAMMATORY DISEASE: WHAT NAME DO I GIVE IT? The collagen-vascular diseases are characterized by the presence of sterile inflammation in multiple organs and multiple autoantibodies. The prototype disease is SLE which is characterized by the widest clinical and serologic spectrum. Other diseases include scleroderma, Sjögren's syndrome, polymyositis/dermatomyositis, rheumatoid arthritis, and syndromes with overlapping features (overlap syndrome, undifferentiated connective tissue disease). One subset of the latter group has been called mixed connective tissue disease (MCTD). The clustering of clinical features and the nature and diversity of autoantibodies may strongly suggest one disorder rather than another, but the overlap of clinical, serologic, and pathologic features among these diseases is great. This can lead to considerable consternation for clinicians. Debates about whether a given patient has SLE, primary Sjögren's syndrome, MCTD, or another overlap syndrome are tiring, usually unresolvable, and generally irrelevant. The therapy for the immunologically active phase of these disorders is not disease specific. The absence of a consensus label should not delay therapeutic efforts.

THE ELDERLY PATIENT WITH AN ELEVATED SEDIMENTATION RATE: IS THIS TEMPORAL ARTERITIS? Within the ICU, advanced age, elevation of the ESR, anemia, and various nonspecific clinical features—chiefly fever— may converge to raise the question of temporal arteritis. Temporal arteritis is a granulomatous vasculitis that affects those over age 60 (mean age 70) and has a proclivity to affect extracranial vessels and branches of the aorta. A myriad of uncommon clinical features may occur but headache, polymyalgia rheumatica, visual disturbance, scalp tenderness, and jaw claudication are the common fingerprints of this disease. Treatment is highly effective with prednisone in doses of 40 to 60 mg/day.[24]

The onset of this disease is typically insidious and its complications rarely prompt admission to the ICU. The question is, therefore, more commonly framed in terms of whether the patient has developed new-onset temporal arteritis in the ICU (probably not) or did he have it as a comorbid state at admission. History and old records are critical in this regard.

Physical examination is unreliable. Temporal artery biopsy is the gold standard although sensitivity varies with the institution. A classical clinical scenario that includes headache, visual symptoms, jaw claudication, scalp tenderness, and polymyalgia rheumatica may be sufficiently compelling to prompt treatment. Usually the situation is murkier. There is no substitute for the temporal artery biopsy, which can be done under local anesthesia with little morbidity. A sufficiently large piece (4 to 5 cm) should be obtained and adequate cuts done. Contralateral biopsy is done routinely by some if a first biopsy is negative. That decision will be influenced by the details of the clinical scenario and the risk of an empirical trial with steroids. A negative biopsy in a marginal clinical situation is reasonable grounds to withhold therapy.

ABDOMINAL PAIN AND ELEVATED ERYTHROCYTE SEDIMENTATION RATE: IS THIS VASCULITIS? The clinical presentation of acute abdominal pain is constrained to a limited number of clinical findings, regardless of cause. Unfortunately, there is nothing unique about massive gastrointestinal bleeding or the development of an acute abdomen when a patient has a high ESR and vasculitis is the etiology.

If the patient is already known to have systemic vasculitis, and this is usually the case when the gut becomes involved, the differential diagnosis of the acute abdomen and elevated ESR is a bit more simple. Here, early gastroduodenoscopy and colonoscopy with biopsy and perhaps vascular contrast studies may be necessary. In the rare situation when a patient with no or relatively limited vasculitic findings in skin and renal and pulmonary systems develops fulminant vasculitis of the bowel, diagnosis may remain elusive until arteriography or surgical exploration. Patients on high dose corticosteroid therapy for preexisting systemic vasculitis may develop small bowel or colonic ischemia, or perforation with relatively few physical findings, even in the face of profound intraabdominal sepsis.

Unusual causes of acute abdominal pain in patients with systemic vasculitis include hepatic infarctions, especially in SLE and polyarteritis, which can mimic many other intraperitoneal acute events. In this situation, hepatic computed tomography (CT) or MRI imaging is helpful. Massive bleeding can occur in most forms of systemic vasculitis, especially Henoch-Schönlein purpura, polyarteritis, and mixed cryoglobulinemia. Diarrhea and profound protein-losing enteropathy and acute bowel obstruction secondary to adhesive serositis have occurred rarely in SLE. There is nothing unique about acute pancreatitis in the patient with SLE; appropriate biochemical and imaging assessment will confirm this diagnosis.

The proper perspective must be maintained when the clinician attempts to make the diagnosis of systemic vasculitis involving the gut by analysis of small bowel or colonic tissue since <50 percent of endoscopically obtained biopsies will be helpful in the diagnosis.[25] Although careful circumspection should be exercised before embarking on exploratory laparotomy in patients with SLE or other vasculitis with abdominal pain and suspected perforation, one should err on the side of surgical exploration. More than one-half the patients with SLE and an acute abdomen will die.[26] Surgical exploration will correctly identify the major pathophysiology of the syndrome and dictate appropriate management. Increasing availability of laparoscopes with enhanced optics may obviate the need for laparotomy. The vast majority of patients with polyarteritis nodosa who develop an acute abdomen usually die from extensive bowel ischemia, infarction, and perforation unless early surgical intervention occurs. The contemporary use of alkylating agents, corticosteroids, and other aggressive therapies may reduce this highly fatal complication in this group of vasculitides.

In summary, any patient with vasculitis, especially one with SLE, who develops an acute abdomen is in dire jeopardy. Routine clinical, laboratory, and radiology assessments are not usually helpful. Early endoscopy, biopsy, arteriography in selected instances, and ultimately early surgical exploration are usually necessary.

LUNG INFILTRATES IN RENAL FAILURE: IS THIS AN IMMUNE-MEDIATED PULMONARY-RENAL SYNDROME? When a patient, usually but not always a young male, has abnormalities of renal function and then develops increasing shortness of breath, hemoptysis, and bilateral diffuse infiltrates, an immune-mediated pulmonary-renal syndrome should be strongly considered and ruled out as soon as possible. The clinician must be wary because the symptoms can occur in reverse; that is, increasing compromise of pulmonary function may precede significant changes in renal function.

Hemoptysis has many causes in patients with renal failure. Some examples would include SLE, Wegener's granulomatosis, advanced cardiac failure, polyarteritis nodosa, Henoch-Schönlein purpura, and rapidly progressive glomerulonephritis. The latter disease in actuality is probably one end of the spectrum of a group of diseases mediated by antibodies to epitopes common to both alveolar and glomerular basement membranes (GBM).[27] In its classical expression, anti-GBM disease is called Goodpasture's syndrome.

Most diseases with pulmonary and renal manifestations can be distinguished from the immune-mediated pulmonary renal syndromes by their unique extrarenal characteristics. Once they are excluded, one is then confronted with a patient with glomerulonephritis and pulmonary hemorrhage. The diagnosis of the pulmonary-renal syndrome rests on establishing the presence of antibasement membrane antibodies in the peripheral blood or in situ deposition in a renal biopsy. Characteristic histologic findings in the renal biopsy are those of a diffuse proliferative necrotizing glomerulitis highlighted by a somewhat unique characteristic of rather exuberant crescent formation. Although not well documented by systematic clinical studies, the increasing use of immunohistologic analysis on tissue obtained by the transbronchial route may circumvent the need to obtain diagnostic tissue by renal biopsy.[28] The diagnosis of an immune-mediated pulmonary-renal syndrome is important because efficacious therapy exists, especially when initiated early in the disease. Alveolar GBM antibodies can be rapidly removed by vigorous plasma exchange and then B cell clones with basement membrane specificities can be suppressed or clonally eliminated with cytoreductive therapy.[29] The efficiency of GBM antibody removal can be monitored easily by sequential GBM antibody assays. The approach to a patient in the ICU with hemoptysis and renal failure should include close attention to maintenance of adequate pulmonary function, rapid acquisition of tissue, either renal or pulmonary (or both), and appropriate immunopathologic analysis of any and all biopsy specimens in parallel with serologic assays for circulating GBM antibodies.

CNS DYSFUNCTION: IS THIS CEREBRAL VASCULITIS? Patients with or without connective tissue disease and nonspecific markers of systemic inflammation who develop signs of brain dysfunction are routinely suspected of having CNS vasculitis. Often the likelihood is considered low but addressed in the interests of "not missing anything."

Rarely does CNS vasculitis cause psychosis or coma without focal neurologic signs. Isolated angiitis of the CNS, particularly in early stages, is an exception but would not be expected to give multisystem disease that prompts ICU admission. Finding focal deficits on examination is problematic in the comatose or disoriented patient. A skilled neurologist can contribute more than imaging techniques. MRI and CT scanning may reveal a lesion suggesting an ischemic event. However, no pattern is specific for vasculitis. Angiography is the gold standard, although in small vessel vasculitis it may be nondiagnostic. Mobilization to angiography in the critically ill ICU patient can be problematic. The role for leptomeningeal biopsy is unclear. An empirical trial with steroids may be appropriate.

HYPERSENSITIVITY VASCULITIS: WHAT IS THE CAUSE? The most common form of cutaneous vasculitis in any setting is cutaneous necrotizing venulitis, usually referred to as hypersensitivity vasculitis and recognized clinically as palpable purpura. The palpability of these lesions is caused by inflammatory infiltrates. Other less common expressions include bullous disease and cutaneous ulcers. The lesions have a tendency to occur in dependent areas and in ambulatory patients are found in the legs and buttock area. Localization may be atypical in bedridden ICU patients. By far, the most common cause of new-onset hypersensitivity vasculitis in the ICU patient is drugs. Any drug may be implicated but thiazides, sulfa drugs, and penicillins are common offenders. Clues to nondrug causes would include significant digital involvement including associated nailbed infarcts, ulcerative lesions, significant glomerular inflammation, and any other evidence of extracutaneous vasculitis such as mononeuritis multiplex.

The presence of cryoglobulins or low complement levels suggests a nondrug cause. Skin biopsy can be done early but usually adds no additional diagnostic information. Predominant lymphocytic infiltration may help to support a diagnosis of drug-induced disease.[30] Immunofluorescence on biopsied tissue is rarely helpful, but the presence of IgA is supportive of a diagnosis of Henoch-Schönlein purpura.[31] Progression to major vasculitis does not predictably occur, but hypersensitivity vasculitis may be the presenting manifestation of a major systemic vasculitis such as Wegener's granulomatosis or Churg-Strauss vasculitis. Therapy may be restricted to withdrawal of the most likely offending drug. Refractory cases have been managed with prednisone (0.5 mg/kg/day), colchicine (0.6 mg three times daily), dapsone (150 mg/day), and rarely, cytotoxic agents. Topical therapy adds little in the absence of skin breakdown. Complete resolution may take weeks.

ISCHEMIC DIGITS: IS THIS VASCULITIS? Patients in the ICU may develop ischemic digits. Contributing factors include hypotension, use of radial arterial lines, and vasoconstrictors. Often the issue of vasculitis is raised.

Single extremity involvement speaks strongly against systemic vasculitis as the cause. Similarly, isolated toe involvement is more likely to be due to a combination of noninflammatory vascular disease and diminished blood flow due to hypotension, vasoconstrictors, or cholesterol emboli. The latter may shower from the aorta and create a pseudovasculitic picture, particularly after anticoagulation therapy is initiated or following instrumentation of the aorta.[32] Extreme symmetry of lesions with all digits involved is more suggestive of a generalized low flow state than vasculitis.

Clues to vasculitis as the cause of digital ischemia include the coexistence of a disease associated with digital vasculitis such as SLE or scleroderma, random involvement of multiple limbs, the presence of nailbed infarcts, and other associated cutaneous markers specific to vasculitis such as palpable purpura. Likewise, extracutaneous markers of vasculitis including glomerulitis and patchy neurologic deficits would enhance suspicion for that diagnosis.

Male patients with a history of heavy smoking should be suspected of Buerger's disease (thromboangiitis obliterans). Lupus and other connective tissue disease patients with ischemic digits may have thrombotic complications secondary to ACL antibody and not true vasculitis.[33]

Biopsy of ischemic digits is usually impractical and potentially hazardous. The necessity to amputate a gangrenous digit should prompt careful instruction to the surgeon to be sure to biopsy the digital artery immediately proximal to the gangrene. In this setting, angiography often reveals nonspecific findings of small vessel disease but may suggest emboli and at times reveal the source such as a subclavian plaque. An angiographic pattern suggestive of Buerger's disease has been described.[34]

LUNG INFILTRATES AND ELEVATED SEDIMENTATION RATE: IS THIS VASCULITIS? Frequently elevated ESRs become laboratory aberrations looking for a disease state. The unwary clinician may let an elevated ESR be the driver for a costly and unrewarding work-up. Once it is known that a patient has an elevated ESR and the usual causes for this nonspecific laboratory abnormality have been reasonably excluded, the impulse is to link any and all remaining clinical abnormalities to the abnormal ESR. Unexplained pulmonary infiltrates, a common finding in critically ill patients, are good examples that provoke the question: "Is this a pulmonary vasculitis?" Common sense should prevail and dictate that the diagnosis of pulmonary vasculitis as a principle entity should be one of exclusion. If a young female, on corticosteroids, with a fever, rash, alopecia, and pericarditis develops a pulmonary infiltrate, she should be considered to have an infectious disease or pulmonary embolism until proven otherwise. If a previously bedridden patient with advanced rheumatoid arthritis suddenly develops pulmonary infiltrates and hypoxemia, the etiology should be considered embolic until proven otherwise; and, if a patient with advanced scleroderma that includes the proximal gut develops pulmonary infiltrates, aspiration pneumonia should be strongly considered. Conversely, one can approach the patient with pulmonary infiltrates and an elevated ESR in reductionist fashion.

If a careful search for extrapulmonary evidence of vasculitis is not rewarding, it will be highly unlikely that primary pulmonary vasculitis is present since it is very unusual for vasculitis to involve only the pulmonary tree. There are rare instances when vasculitis can be isolated to the pulmonary tree in a systemic rheumatic disease. Rarely, patients with ACL antibodies may develop pulmonary infiltrates secondary to in situ pulmonary artery thrombosis and/or pulmonary embolism. These patients will simulate a primary vasculitic pulmonary picture, but the primary therapy is anticoagulation.

Interpretation of Rheumatology Laboratory Abnormalities in the ICU: Reading the "Tea Leaves" (Table 126-1)

ERYTHROCYTE SEDIMENTATION RATE

The ESR is an indirect determination of the acute phase response and may be elevated in the setting of infection or active rheumatic disease. Values are higher for women and the elderly. The exact appropriate adjustment for age is not certain. The presence of monoclonal proteins and alterations in size, shape, and number of red blood cells will influence the ESR. ESR rises during normal pregnancy and should not be used to monitor rheumatic diseases under these circumstances. The ESR increases in end-stage renal failure of whatever cause and is not indicative of an underlying rheumatic disorder.[35]

TABLE 126-1 Serologic Tests in Rheumatic Diseases

Antibody	Disorder
A. Tests with high specificity* for collagen vascular disease	
Anti-native DNA	SLE
	Rarely anything else
Anti-Sm (Smith)	SLE
Anti-Ro (SS-A)	Congenital heart block
	Antinuclear antibody-negative lupus
	Subacute cutaneous LE
	Primary Sjögren's syndrome
	SLE
Anticentromere	Limited cutaneous variant of scleroderma (CREST)
Scl-70 (Topoisomerase I)	Diffuse scleroderma
Antineutrophil cytoplasmic antibody	Wegener's granulomatosis
	Microscopic polyarteritis nodosa
	Idiopathic crescentic glomerulonephritis
Anti-ribonucleoprotein	SLE
	Mixed connective tissue disease
	Undifferentiated connective tissue disease
Anti-La (SS-B)	SLE
	Primary Sjögren's syndrome
B. Tests with low specificity for collagen vascular disease	
Antinuclear antibody	SLE
	Other autoimmune diseases
	Normals (usually low titer)
	Drug-induced
	Aging
Rheumatoid factor	Rheumatoid arthritis
	Mixed cryoglobulinemia
	Aging
	Subacute bacterial endocarditis
	Any cause of chronic antigenic stimulation
Anticardiolipin antibody	Anticardiolipin antibody syndrome
	Normals
	Viral illness
	SLE
	Other autoimmune diseases

*Unlikely to be found in normals, with aging, or as a nonspecific immune response to infection.

The level of the rise in ESR correlates imperfectly with disease activity and may at times be normal in patients with active rheumatoid arthritis or SLE. Patients with markedly elevated ESR (MESR) are those with values >100 mm/h. These patients deserve special attention because such elevations are unlikely to be explained by age or normal physiologic state and are a more reliable sickness indicator. The illnesses associated with MESR include infection, malignancy, rheumatic disorders such as vasculitis, connective tissue disease, rheumatoid arthritis, and temporal arteritis as well as end-stage renal failure, nephrotic syndrome, and other inflammatory diseases such as hepatitis and colitis. In most series looking at MESR, 3 to 10 percent of patients will have no diagnosis to explain the abnormal laboratory value.[36] Some of these patients will eventually reveal an underlying pathology while others will demonstrate spontaneous improvement in the ESR.

In the ICU, the ESR is likely to be elevated for multiple reasons. An MESR should not prompt an unreasonable search for vasculitis or other concurrent rheumatic disease, particularly in the presence of renal failure and nephrotic syndrome.

ANTINUCLEAR ANTIBODIES

The presence of antinuclear antibodies (ANA) in high titer provides presumptive evidence for the presence of collagen vascular disease and, in particular, SLE. Lower levels of ANA can be nonspecific, possibly normal, and at times explained by age, prior drug therapy, or a first degree relative with lupus. Low levels of ANA in the elderly can be particularly misleading in the presence of an age-related elevation of the ESR. It has been estimated that 15 to 25 percent of normal, healthy individuals over the age of 60 will have circulating ANA.[37] These data are confounded by a small but definite incidence of new cases of SLE among the elderly.

Screening ANA is typically done by a standard, indirect immunofluorescence (IF) technique. Its development followed the LE cell test, which has now been relegated to historical interest only. The test is now performed most commonly on HEp-2 cells and is sensitive for detecting the presence of SLE, but as noted above, is hindered by the lack of specificity. Interest in specific ANA has spawned a long and at times confusing list of tests of variable utility. A brief overview of the most useful specific ANA follows.

ANTICENTROMERE ANTIBODY: This antibody to the kinetechore of chromosomes is detected by recognition of a particular speckled pattern of IF on HEp-2 cells. It is, in general, the only pattern detected on screening ANA useful for diagnostic purposes. It is found most commonly in the limited cutaneous variant of scleroderma (CREST). In this subset of patients, the test has been positive in 44 to 98 percent of those tested.[38,39] Less commonly, it may be seen in diffuse scleroderma and primary biliary cirrhosis with or without evidence of scleroderma.

ANTIBODIES TO DNA. Antibodies to DNA fall into two major categories by virtue of reacting to antigenic determinants on the phosphate deoxyribose backbone of the DNA helix or determinants on the nucleotide bases. The former represent antibodies to native double-stranded DNA while the latter react with single-stranded DNA.

Antibodies to single-stranded DNA are more common and are found across a spectrum of rheumatic and nonrheumatic disorders. They are of no practical clinical utility.

Antibodies to double-stranded DNA are useful since they have great specificity for SLE and are found in 60 to 70 percent of patients with that disease.[40] Low levels of this antibody have occasionally been found in other connective tissue diseases.

ANTIBODIES TO Sm. This antibody is named after a patient "Smith" in whom it was first described. The antibody has great specificity for SLE and is rarely found in patients with other connective tissue diseases. Sensitivity is only about 30 percent for SLE. It is not to be confused with an antibody to smooth muscle (SM), which is not a marker for collagen vascular disease but is found in patients with chronic liver disease. There is no definite clinical profile of Sm-positive patients with SLE. Titers are not useful for assessment of disease activity.

ANTIBODIES TO nRNP. Antigenic determinants for nuclear ribonucleoprotein (nRNP) may occur in a molecular complex with Sm, and antibodies to Sm and RNP are often found in the same patient. Antibodies to nRNP may be seen in SLE, scleroderma, or overlap syndromes. The presence of overlapping clinical features and high titers of antibody to RNP defines a clinical subset of patients referred to as MCTD.

ANTIBODIES TO SS-A/Ro AND SS-B/La. These antigens were originally described in patients with Sjögren's syndrome (SS) and SLE. They are RNA-protein conjugates. SS-A and Ro have antigenic identity as do SS-B and La. The Ro and La refer to the antigen as localized to the cytoplasm, whereas SS-A and SS-B are nuclear antigens.

Determination of SS-B/La rarely has clinical utility, but in most assays is measured along with SS-A/Ro, which may be very useful. The Ro antibody has been described in 60 percent of so-called "ANA-negative SLE." Anti-Ro antibody is also highly prevalent in the setting of congenital heart block and neonatal SLE.[41] In those cases, the antibody is found in mother and child. Other clinical scenarios associated with anti-Ro antibody include subacute cutaneous lupus and C2 deficiency. Anti-Ro antibody occurs in 25 to 40 percent of unselected patients with SLE.

The major indications for ordering these tests are in a setting in which SLE is strongly suspected but the screening ANA is negative; congenital heart block; neonatal lupus; and the initial evaluation of a patient with a positive ANA.

ANTIBODIES TO SCL-70 (TOPOISOMERASE I). Antibodies to Scl-70 are directed towards DNA topoisomerase I and inhibit its function.[42] They are found in 20 to 40 percent of patients classified as diffuse systemic sclerosis and rarely in patients with limited cutaneous disease or CREST. Determination of this antibody is part of the evaluation of patients suspected of having scleroderma.

ANTINEUTROPHIL CYTOPLASMIC AUTOANTIBODIES (ANCA). The detection of antibodies directed against neutrophil cytoplasmic components now offers a useful serologic tool for the diagnosis and management of a small group of disorders characterized by systemic necrotizing vasculitis and glomerulonephritis.[43] These disorders include Wegener's granulomatosis, microscopic PAN, and idiopathic crescentic glomerulonephritis. The renal lesions in these disorders have in common necrotizing vascular injury and a paucity of immune deposits.

ANCA are found in 90 percent of patients with active, generalized Wegener's granulomatosis and 60 to 70 percent of those with limited disease. The titer often parallels disease activity and may be helpful in distinguishing a disease flare from intercurrent infection or other morbidity in patients with Wegener's granulomatosis.

ANCA can be found in 80 percent of patients with active pauci-immune necrotizing and crescentic glomerulonephritis, which is one of the major causes of rapidly progressing glomerulonephritis (RPGN). Two specific patterns of ANCA have been identified and are referred to as cytoplasmic ANCA (C-ANCA) and perinuclear (P-ANCA). In general, patients with Wegener's granulomatosus have demonstrated C-ANCA, whereas those with idiopathic crescentic glomerulonephritis have demonstrated P-ANCA.[44] Overlap of these patterns occurs.

The clinical scenarios that warrant measurement of ANCA are patients with known or suspected Wegener's granulomatosis and patients with RPGN. These antibodies have also been occasionally identified in Churg-Strauss vasculitis, Takayasu's disease, SLE, relapsing polychondritis, and Behcet's disease.

ANTIBODIES IN POLYMYOSITIS-DERMATOMYOSITIS. In general, serologic testing has been of little practical value in the diagnosis and management of patients with polymyositis or dermatomyositis. Recently, a number of specific ANA have been identified in patients with these diseases and are available commercially. The exact role of these antibodies in the management of patients in unclear, but they may be useful in patients who represent a diagnostic dilemma.

Jo-1 antibody can be found in 20 to 30 percent of patients with polymyositis and, less commonly, in dermatomyositis. The presence of the antibody highly correlates with associated interstitial lung disease. Antibodies to the nuclear antigen Mi occur in about 25 percent of the patients with dermatomyositis and rarely in polymyositis. Antibody to PM-1 or PM-Scl defines a small subset of polymyositis patients (10 percent), half of whom will have accompanying features of scleroderma. Occasionally, patients with scleroderma and no myositis will have this antibody.

RHEUMATOID FACTOR

Rheumatoid factors (RF) are autoantibodies, predominantly IgM isotype, that are directed against multispecies antigenic determinants on the heavy chain of IgG. They are nonspecific, rarely diagnostic and almost never useful in the critical care setting. These autoantibodies can be found in normals and many disease states and have a prevalence that varies directly with age and sex (female preponderance). RF can arise as a epiphenomenon during acute illness or chronic antigenic stimulation of almost any cause. They are present, sometimes in significant titer, in bacterial endocarditis, granulomatous diseases, and most rheumatic diseases at some point in time. The presence of RF, occurring in tandem with significant decreases of serum complement components C3 and C4, may provide a diagnostic clue in rarely encountered clinical syndromes such as rheumatoid vasculitis with cryoglobulins or essential mixed cryoglobulinemia and vasculitis. These syndromes can present with gastrointestinal tract involvement and hemorrhage, compromised renal function or progressive peripheral neuropathy, and skin ulceration. The recognition of these vasculitic syndromes mandates aggressive intervention with cytoreductive therapy—usually cyclophosphamide and therapeutic plasma exchange.[45,46]

COMPLEMENT LEVELS

In theory, the detection of direct (classic) complement pathway activation by the measurement of serum C4 and C3 levels should provide the clinician with laboratory support for using treatment protocols that suppress the sequelae of complement activation. A prototype disease where C4 and C3 changes should be helpful is SLE. Unfortunately, there is an imperfect correlation between clinical activity of any disease, especially SLE, and decreased C3 and C4 levels. In fact, it is now clear that conventional measurements of serum C3 and C4 assays, which supposedly detect immune complex complement activation in the patient, can inappropriately drive therapy decisions toward the use of immunosuppressives or corticosteroids when not indicated.[47]

Moreover, C3 synthesis is increased by acute inflammation of any cause, serving as a classic acute phase reactant. It is easy to visualize a scenario where a patient with SLE being treated with corticosteroids who has increased consumption of C3 may develop secondary bacterial infection, which stimulates the production of C3 in its role as an acute phase reactant. The end result will be a normal serum level of C3, which may engender a false sense of security with regard to SLE disease activity. Conversely, the significantly reduced synthesis of C3 in many hepatic diseases is reflected in low plasma levels that can be misinterpreted. Plasma C4 is a more sensitive indicator of direct pathway activation; but, for many of the same reasons that relate to C3 determinations, a decreased C4 level should never be the sole determinant of intervention with potent immunosuppressive therapy. Patients with SLE or overlap variants may have heterozygous or homozygous defects in C4 production. These patients will always have low C4 levels, regardless of disease activity.

ICU patients admitted with either meningococcemia or gonoccocemia provide one of the rare reasons for the determination of total hemolytic complement level. This assay serves as a screening test that depends on the functional presence of all individual complement components. A significant decrease in hemolytic activity may identify patients with terminal complement component deficiency who are at high risk for recurrent bacteremia. Such patients may require fresh frozen plasma in conjunction with antibiotic therapy and should be immunized with meningococcal vaccine prior to discharge.

In summary, conventional measurements of serum complement levels are not helpful in predicting activation in this complex system. When sensitive assays for activation peptides or complement activation complexes become available, assessment of the complement pathway may become more clinically relevant.

IMMUNE COMPLEX ASSAYS

A multiplicity of biologic and physical assays can detect circulating immune complexes. Whenever a highly diverse panel of assays is available to the clinician, this is usually a clue that the test itself is not helpful in the conduct of clinical care. Indeed, no clinical setting justifies the measurement of circulating immune complexes, for either diagnostic or prognostic purposes. Circulating immune complexes are a normal response of the immune system to antigenic stimulation. They are nonspecific in defining disease etiology and also misleading, especially because current assays measure only the presence of circulating immune complexes and do not directly measure their immunopathologic potential, if any.

CRYOGLOBULINS

Cryoglobulins are monoclonal, oligoclonal, or polyclonal immunoglobulins with a thermal propensity for precipitation at decreased temperatures and subsequent resolubilization with warming. In the vast majority of instances, they occur as acute or chronic phase reactants during bacterial or viral infections and many rheumatic disease syndromes. Plasma cryoglobulins, especially when assessed as cryocrits, are very nonspecific and may simply reflect ongoing antibody formation and subsequent complexing with antigen; indeed, they have been termed "the poor man's immune complex assay." Abnormal elevations of the ESR can be masked by some cryoglobulins that form gels at ambient temperatures and impede the rate of erythrocyte descent. Pseudoleukocytosis can occur when automated cell counting procedures count crystallized cryoproteins as white blood cells. Patients with cryoglobulin-mediated immune complex syndromes should be followed in terms of their clinical activity; clinicians should not rely on cryocrit decreases during therapy. Falls in cryocrits may be misleading because cryoproteins, even at extremely low levels in plasma, can be highly efficient complement activators.

ANTICARDIOLIPIN ANTIBODIES

The ACL antibodies belong to a family of antiphospholipid antibodies (APLAs), including those responsible for the lupus anticoagulant (LA) and biologic false-positive tests for syphilis. These antibodies often, although not always, occur together. The clinical syndromes associated with these antibodies belong to a growing list that can be explained largely by the capacity of these antibodies to induce thrombosis in the venous and arterial circulation. Thrombocytopenia and recurrent fetal loss are the other major consequences of APLAs. The combination of APLAs and one or more of these clinical features has been termed the "antiphospholipid antibody syndrome."

Chronic false-positive serologic tests for syphilis are associated with autoimmune disease, notably SLE, and are found with increased frequency in patients with ACL and LA activity. Lupus anticoagulants are IgG or IgM antibodies that prolong phospholipid dependent tests in vitro by interference with the calcium-dependent binding of prothrombin (factor II) and factor Xa to phospholipids, thus inhibiting the generation of prothrombinase. This usually results in prolongation of the activated partial thromboplastin time (APTT) with or without slight prolongation of the prothrombin time (PT).[33] LA is a common cause of prolongation of the PTT but not the only cause. Most patients with LA do not have SLE.

Usually, ACL antibodies are detected in an enzyme-linked immuno-sorbent assay (ELISA) using bovine cardiolipin as substrate. These are the most commonly detected antiphospholipid antibodies. They are generated transiently in the course of acute infections including mycoplasma and gram-negative infections. These antibodies are usually of the IgM isotype and not associated with thrombosis. IgM ACL as well as the LA may be induced by a variety of drugs including phenothiazines, procainamide, phenytoin, hydralazine, quinidine, and streptomycin. These antibodies are most often not associated with thrombotic events, but exceptions to this rule occur.

ACL antibodies are noted in 2.5 percent of the general population.[33] For most of these patients, the antibodies have no clinical significance. The risk of thrombosis and fetal loss has been generally associated with higher levels of antibody and the IgG isotype. Unfortunately, exceptions occur. Thus, the presence of ACL antibody should not in itself prompt therapeutic intervention.

A myriad of neurologic events including stroke, transient ischemic attacks, and amaurosis fugax have been associated with the presence of LA and ACL antibody. Their presence should be suspected in patients having no risk factors for thrombosis or who have associated autoimmune disease or suggestive screening laboratory abnormalities, including prolonged PTT or false-positive serologic tests for syphilis. Skin lesions secondary to LA/ACL include gangrene, hemorrhage, and purpura. Necrosis may mimic vasculitis.

The vasculopathy of APLA syndrome is not vasculitis but primarily thrombosis of large or small arteries or veins. Steroids may normalize the LA but have little impact on ACL antibody levels. Treatment for major thrombotic complications of this syndrome is heparin and coumadin. Steroids are indicated for associated clinical features related to systemic inflammation.

Use of Corticosteroids, Immunosuppressives, and Anti-inflammatory Drugs in the Critically Ill Patient

CORTICOSTEROIDS

Corticosteroids have potent immunosuppressive and anti-inflammatory properties that, in combination with rapid onset of action, make them the drug of choice for the initial therapy of most acute, life-threatening rheumatic disorders. Even low doses of prednisone (<10 mg/day) have potent anti-inflammatory effects and are being used with increased frequency in patients with rheumatoid arthritis.

For purposes of controlling inflammation and immunomodulation, "short-acting" glucocorticoids with little or no mineralocorticoid activity are preferred. The oral drug of choice is prednisone, which is converted to prednisolone in the liver. While active liver disease impairs that conversion, it appears to be offset sufficiently by decreased rate of elimination of prednisolone to eliminate the need to preferentially use prednisolone in patients with cirrhosis or active liver disease. The intravenous drug of choice is methylprednisolone (Solumedrol). The dose equivalency is 4 mg methylprednisolone to 5 mg prednisone (see Chap. 160).

The dose of prednisone or methylprednisolone is largely empirical. For serious, life-threatening problems, 1 mg/kg/day of prednisone is a good starting point. Dividing the dose into a twice-a-day or other dose-divided schedule may increase efficacy (as well as toxicity) and is recommended by some for initial therapy. Extremely large doses of intravenous methylprednisolone (500 to 1000 mg) daily have been used for brief periods (3 to 5 days) with variable success in a variety of clinical settings, mostly in the context of SLE. In vitro studies suggest that such large doses may produce a qualitatively different response in lymphocyte function.[48] Unique side effects to this form of therapy, including sudden overwhelming sepsis and sudden death, are rare. This form of therapy is generally reserved for patients who have failed conventional high dose therapy with corticosteroids with or without another immunosuppressive agent.

Patient response to corticosteroids varies. Failure to respond is likely due to the nature and severity of the disease. The effectiveness of glucocorticoids may be reduced by simultaneous use of other drugs that induce hepatic microsomal enzyme activity such as phenytoin, barbiturates, and rifampin. Bioavailability of prednisone may be reduced by antacids sometimes prescribed for concurrent use. Cortisol and its synthetic derivatives are bound to corticosteroid-binding globulin and albumin. The bound steroid is not active. Increased frequency of prednisone side effects has been observed at low serum albumin levels,[49] probably reflecting an increase in the unbound, active fraction of the drug.

Patients who are purified protein derivative (PPD) positive and about to undergo corticosteroid therapy (particularly with doses of prednisone of 20 mg/day or greater) should be considered for isoniazid (INH) prophylaxis

(300 mg/day orally). The reported risk of reactivation ranges from low in asthmatics to higher in the elderly and in patients immunosuppressed by virtue of other drugs or their primary disease. The patient with a positive PPD and either a normal chest x-ray or a single calcified nodule probably does not require prophylaxis.[50] If the patient has significant impairment of the immune system or the chest film shows fibronodular scarring, the risk is enhanced considerably and prophylaxis with INH is advisable.[51]

Steroid therapy suppresses cutaneous delayed hypersensitivity responses by inhibiting recruitment of macrophages to the skin test site. This phenomenon is reversible on stopping the drug. In one study, treatment with 10 mg prednisone daily totally inhibited cutaneous tuberculin sensitivity in both active and inactive cases of tuberculosis with a mean reversion time of 13.6 days and reconversion time of 6 days following discontinuation of the drug.[52]

Acute adrenocortical insufficiency may occur in critically ill patients who have been treated with chronic glucocorticoid therapy (see Chap. 160). On the basis of available data, any patient who has received a glucocorticoid at a dose equivalent to 20 to 30 mg prednisone daily should be suspected of having hypothalamic-pituitary-adrenal (HPA) system suppression.[53] At doses closer to but above the physiologic range, a month is probably the minimum duration required for HPA suppression. Patients receiving the equivalent replacement doses of steroid (5 mg prednisone) as single morning dose therapy are at low risk of iatrogenic adrenal insufficiency. In the absence of hemodynamic instability, they do not require full "stress dose" replacement therapy. An ACTH stimulation test can resolve the question of adrenal suppression (see Chap. 160), but the clinical reality usually dictates empirical coverage with "stress doses" of corticosteroids. This can be accomplished with 100 mg hydrocortisone (Solu-cortef) intravenously every 8 h. This is approximately the equivalent of 75 mg prednisone. Higher doses are not necessary and potentially more hazardous.

Use of corticosteroids on alternate days is associated with some decrease in chronic drug morbidity. In the urgent setting of the critically ill patient, the greater effectiveness of daily or split daily doses of steroids recommends such a dosing schedule.

IMMUNOSUPPRESSIVES

CYCLOPHOSPHAMIDE. Cyclophosphamide (Cytoxan) is an alkalating agent with broad immunosuppressive properties. It is generally embraced as the drug of choice for suppression of progressive, life-threatening autoimmune disease unresponsive to corticosteroids alone. Effectiveness has been reported in a broad spectrum of collagen-vascular diseases and primary vasculitides including SLE, Wegener's granulomatosis, polyarteritis nodosa, and polymyositis-dermatomyositis.

Cyclophosphamide causes broad suppression of B and T cell function and acts as a potent inhibitor of antibody production. Anti-inflammatory effects have also been described.

The drug is rapidly absorbed orally. It is inert until metabolized in the liver. Extravasation of the drug is not caustic to soft tissues. Sixty percent of the drug is excreted in the urine in the form of active metabolites. Impaired excretion of these active metabolites because of renal insufficiency can potentiate the therapeutic and toxic effects of a given dose of drug.

The drug can be given orally, usually at a dose of 2 mg/kg/day, or intravenously. To circumvent toxic effects associated with chronic drug exposure, intravenous bolus cyclophosphamide therapy has become an increasingly popular alternative at doses of a 0.5 to 1.0 g/m^2. The onset of immunosuppressive activity of cyclophosphamide is estimated at 10 to 14 days following initiation of therapy. Although unproven in rigorous clinical trials, there is an operational principle that immunosuppression can be achieved more rapidly with intravenous bolus therapy. Hence, bolus cyclophosphamide is most often given in the setting of progressive life-threatening disease requiring immunosuppression. A major short-term side effect of bolus therapy is a predictable white blood cell count nadir 7 to 10 days after drug infusion. Leukocyte count levels typically recover in 2 to 3 days. However, if the patient has a concurrent bacterial infection during the nadir period, the consequences of even transient profound neutropenia can be disastrous. Many of the other side effects of therapy with cyclophosphamide are related to chronic use, including gonadal suppression, oncogenesis, pulmonary interstitial fibrosis, and hypogammaglobulinemia.

A recent report suggests that bolus cyclophosphamide is less effective than oral cyclophosphamide in patients with Wegener's granulomatosis.[54] This study raises questions about the predictable superiority of bolus cyclophosphamide in all clinical situations.

AZATHIOPRINE. Azathioprine is a commonly used drug with mild to moderate immunosuppressive properties, which may in large part be explained by a preferential reduction of natural killer cells. Onset of action is slow, probably taking months. It is often used concurrently with corticosteroids in patients requiring unacceptably high doses of steroids, to reduce the steroid dose. It is not the drug of choice when significant immunosuppressive effect is needed on an urgent basis. Risk for infection is modest in the absence of leukopenia.

Azathioprine is metabolized in the liver to the active metabolite, 6-mercaptopurine, a purine analogue. The drug interferes with purine biosynthesis and is ultimately metabolized by xanthine oxidase. Administration of allopurinol, which inhibits xanthine oxidase, to a patient on a stable dose of azathioprine may result in a fatal drug overdose. The azathioprine dose should be reduced by 50 to 75 percent in the presence of allopurinol.

Dose range for this drug is 1 to 3 mg/kg/day. It is primarily metabolized in the liver, but the need for dose adjustment in the presence of liver disease is variable and may be unnecessary. Drug half-life can increase in renal failure but may not prove clinically significant. Cautious observation for the development of cytopenia is indicated in the presence of hepatic or renal failure. The drug is well absorbed orally and may be given intravenously in doses equivalent to the oral form.

METHOTREXATE. Although methotrexate was introduced for the treatment of rheumatoid arthritis more than 30 years ago, several open trials in the early 1980s resulted in renewed interest in this drug. Low dose oral methotrexate has now replaced gold as the remitting agent of first choice in rheumatoid arthritis for many rheumatologists. The drug is accepted as effective in psoriatic arthritis and Reiter's syndrome as well as polymyositis. Experience is currently being gained with its use in SLE and scleroderma. Use of methotrexate in the critically ill rheumatic disease patient is currently limited to patients with polymyositis-dermatomyositis refractory to corticosteroids.

Methotrexate is a folic acid analogue and the major folic acid antagonist in clinical use. The drug is absorbed after oral ingestion but with significant variability. More predictable serum levels can be achieved by intramuscular or intravenous administration. High dose methotrexate can alter antibody production and cellular immunity. Low dose oral methotrexate (25 mg/week or less) as used in rheumatoid arthritis may be mainly anti-inflammatory or directly inhibiting to synovial lining cells.

Low dose methotrexate is given in rheumatoid arthritis in initial doses of 5 to 7.5 mg and may be gradually increased to levels of 25 mg/week. Methotrexate for rheumatic disorders is delivered on a weekly basis. This regimen is associated with less toxicity than when the drug is given more frequently, particularly a reduction in hepatotoxicity. Most patients will respond at doses between 7.5 and 15 mg. Intravenous methotrexate for myositis is given in doses ranging from 25 to 75 mg weekly. A dose of 1 mg/kg/week has been used in childhood dermatomyositis-polymyositis.[55] Such a dose calculation may be a reasonable first approach in the treatment of adults.

Adverse reactions forcing discontinuation of the drug in short-term trials with rheumatoid arthritis occur in 5 to 31 percent of patients. Most toxicity is relatively minor and associated with advanced age, malnutrition, and impaired renal function. Nausea, vomiting, oral ulcers, rash, leukopenia, thrombocytopenia, and pancytopenia may all occur. Cirrhosis may occur in some patients treated for long periods of time and appears to be related to cumulative dose and probably the nature of the underlying disease being treated. The risk appears to be greater in psoriatic arthritis than rheumatoid arthritis. Ethanol may potentiate the hepatotoxicity of methotrexate. Baseline liver biopsy is not indicated in the absence of risk factors for existing liver disease. Patients with ascites and large effusions are at greater risk for methotrexate toxicity. Folic acid, 1 mg daily, has been recommended as a means of preventing adverse reactions and particularly hematologic side effects in patients treated for rheumatoid arthritis.[56] The use of folic acid does not appear to reduce effectiveness of the drug. In serious episodes of pancytopenia, leucovorin may be used.

Toxicities of particular concern in ICU patients include leukocytoclastic vasculitis, which has been reported with high dose therapy used to treat osteogenic sarcoma as well as low dose therapy for rheumatoid arthritis. Opportunistic infections with herpes zoster and *Pneumocystis carinii* have been reported even with low dose methotrexate although they are uncommon. Finally, an acute hypersensitivity pneumonitis occurs infrequently but may result in profound hypoxemia.

CYCLOSPORINE. The emergency use of cyclosporine outside the setting of clinical transplantation will be a rare event. Urgent therapy for patients with fulminant psoriasis, inflammatory bowel disease, and idiopathic thrombocytopenic purpura (with bleeding) may include the use of cyclosporine. Due to extraordinary interpatient bioavailability differences and unpredictable dose requirements, it is hazardous to rely on the use of standard doses calculated on a mg/kg basis. An efficacious method is to start a patient on 3 to 5 mg/kg/day orally. If the need for rapid achievement of therapeutic blood levels is needed, intravenous doses that are one-third to one-fourth of the calculated oral requirement of cyclosporine should be used. The intravenous route is almost always preferable in young children and patients with hypermotile or malabsorptive gastrointestinal disease. Although there is not any clear evidence linking drug effect to drug level, an empirical therapeutic goal is to achieve a drug trough level of approximately 200 ng/mL of cyclosporine (serum assay; 400 ng/mL in whole blood assays).[57]

A serious side effect of this drug is seizure provocation in children and young adults. Psychosis occurs rarely in any age group, but a propensity for it may be enhanced in an ICU setting. Most cardiac transplant patients will have significant systemic hypertension while taking cyclosporine, but this side effect is less troublesome in patients with autoimmune diseases. A disparate group of drugs affect cyclosporine metabolism and absorption or potentiate its nephrotoxicity. The latter morbidity is frequent in the volume-depleted patient. Constant diligence is necessary to maintain trough levels in the putative therapeutic nontoxic range when patients are critically ill.

HIGH DOSE INTRAVENOUS GLOBULIN. High dose intravenous antibody therapy may be indicated for therapy-resistant immune-mediated thrombocytopenia associated with significant bleeding, especially gastrointestinal, or when there is a need to either transiently elevate platelets or prolong the half-life of transfused platelets prior to splenectomy.[58] These modified, biologically active immunoglobulins are given at approximately a 0.4 g/kg dose and followed by platelet transfusions as indicated. Imaginative uses of these expensive biologics are frequent, usually in disease settings where all else has failed. Appropriate clinical trials are needed before their widespread use. The theoretical risk of generating anaphylatoxins or other complement-derived vasoactive mediators during rapid infusion of modified immunoglobulin preparations has been overstated.

ANTI-INFLAMMATORY AGENTS

NONSTEROIDAL ANTI-INFLAMMATORY DRUGS. The NSAIDs generally have little role to play in the management of patients in the ICU. Ulcerogenesis, hemostatic defects, and impairment of renal function converge as a group of notably unfriendly toxic effects for the critically ill patient. In general, corticosteroids are usually a safer alternative when anti-inflammatory effect is necessary in the ICU. For instance, corticosteroids in low doses can be used to control symptomatic synovitis in the rheumatoid patient and are considerably less hazardous than NSAIDs. Moderate dose oral, parenteral, or intraarticular steroids may be used for gout.

Nonacetylated salicylates (salsalate, choline magnesium trisalicylate) represent a safe class of NSAIDs generally devoid of ulcerogenic or hemostatic complications. Lack of efficacy as anti-inflammatory agents is a problem. In the patient on coumadin, displacement of drug from binding proteins may potentiate the PT in an unpredictable and, at times, dramatic fashion.

In those patients in whom an NSAID is needed, the choice is largely empirical and arbitrary. Several clinical studies have suggested that sulindac may be less nephrotoxic because the active sulphide metabolite is oxidized by the renal cortex to an inactive form of the drug.[59] The renal-sparing effect of sulindac has been challenged and clearly is only partially protective.

Ibuprofen has been reported to cause aseptic meningitis in patients with SLE.[8] Although this complication is rare, the drug should probably be avoided in these patients. Tolmetin and sulindac have also been reported to cause this problem.[60,61]

Indomethacin is a very potent cyclooxygenase inhibitor with potent effectiveness and toxicity (both renal and gastrointestinal). It can be given by rectal suppository.

For patients unable to take oral drugs, an intramuscular NSAID, ketorolac tromethamine (Toradol), is available. Ketorolac, 30 mg intramuscularly, is reported to have analgesic effectiveness comparable to 6 to 12 mg morphine with less drowsiness, nausea, and vomiting. Studies on its use in gout or other rheumatic disorders are unavailable.

Misoprostol (Cytotec) is highly effective as prophylaxis against ulcers caused by NSAIDs. It is more effective in that role than H_2 blockers. For the critically ill patient who needs treatment with an NSAID, concurrent treatment with misoprostol (100 to 200 μg every 6 h) should be initiated unless the patient is pregnant.

COLCHICINE. Colchicine is a highly effective, time-honored therapy for acute gout. Because it is not ulcerogenic, does not inhibit hemostasis, and can be given parenterally, it is a valuable drug for the treatment of acute gout in the ICU. The use of oral colchicine tablets (0.5 or 0.6 mg) for acute gout traditionally calls for one tablet to be given hourly up to ten doses until relief of symptoms or side effects. Cramps and diarrhea can be severe, which accounts for the greater popularity of NSAIDs when oral medicines can be tolerated. A four-times-daily dose for 2 to 3 days followed by a twice-a-day prophylactic dose represents a less effective, but better tolerated, use of oral colchicine.

Intravenous colchicine is rapidly effective particularly when started within 24 h of the onset of the attack. The usual dose is 1 mg mixed in 20 to 50 mL normal saline and infused over 30 to 60 min. The line should be free flowing because extravasated drug is highly irritating. The patient may be reevaluated in 6 to 8 h and the dose repeated as needed. A maximum of 2 mg intravenously in 24 h and 3 mg in 48 h represents a cautious approach to use of this drug. The best case for caution is the knowledge that gout is not fatal and will eventually resolve even in the absence of therapy. The use of intravenous colchicine is more hazardous in patients with renal and hepatic insufficiency, sepsis, the elderly, those previously taking oral colchicine, and those recovering from chemotherapy. Major risks under these circumstances are bone marrow depression with peripheral neutropenia and thrombocytopenia (nadir 3 to 6 days after drug given), shock, peripheral neuritis, and myopathy. Preexisting bone marrow depression, a creatinine clearance <10 mL/min, severe oliguria, severe sepsis, and significant liver disease represent absolute contraindications to intravenous colchicine.[62] In the face of one or more of these contraindications, alternative approaches to treatment include NSAIDs and parenteral or intraarticular steroids.

Therapeutic Pheresis in the Critically Ill Patient with Rheumatic Disease

PLASMAPHERESIS

Therapeutic plasmapheresis can effect rapid removal of circulating antigens, immune complexes, pathologic antibodies, and circulating cytokines and improvement in the function of the fixed monocyte system. Plasmapheresis should be considered for patients with fulminant vasculitis of any cause, drug-resistant thyroid storm, selected poisonings, and a subset of life-threatening pulmonary-renal syndromes. Because cyclophosphamide and azathioprine have at least a 7 to 14-day window prior to a therapeutic effect, plasma exchange can be efficacious as a temporizing measure in many syndromes that will ultimately require such cytoreductive therapy. Plasma exchange is also the treatment of choice for patients with thrombotic thrombocytopenic purpura (TTP), acutely deteriorating myasthenia gravis, and rapidly progressive or severe inflammatory peripheral neuropathies. Therapeutic apheresis also provides an immediate clinical response in many patients with fulminant SLE with severe CNS dysfunction.

The procedure has a wide margin of safety when machines with membrane separation technology are used. The amount of extracorporeal volume, at any point in time, is much less than when the patient is exchanged with equipment that requires centrifuge bowl separation of blood components. Still, patients with decreased effective plasma volume or significant coronary artery disease remain at risk with all plasma-separation technologies available and must be closely monitored during the procedure. The frequency of exchange can be based on the isotype of the putative pathogenic antibody involved and the known kinetics of IgG clearance. Ultimately, however, the frequency and amount of exchange depends on the clinical status of the patient. Plasma volume varies with the height, size, sex, and hematocrit; nomograms are available that should be used for effective calculation. A 1.0 plasma volume exchange will remove approximately 65 percent of intravascular IgG from a patient, a 1.5 plasma volume exchange 78 to 80 percent of IgG. Larger volume removals are associated with increased time on the machine, increased citrate toxicity, and most importantly, only very small incremental increases in IgG removal. A common rationale used to determine the frequency of plasmapheresis is based on "resting" the patient on alternate days to allow reequilibration between extravascular and intravascular IgG. TTP and hyperviscosity syndromes, in which plasma volumes are expanded and the proteins generating hyperviscosity are predominantly within the intravascular space, can be effectively treated by aggressive and daily higher volume exchanges.

Patients with severe hepatic disease cannot metabolize citrate rapidly and plasma exchanges should be done at the lowest possible citrate:plasma ratio. Serious side effects of citrate-induced hypocalcemia are extremely rare when volume replacement is done with calcium-spiked 5 percent albumin. Fresh frozen plasma should never be used for routine replacement unless the patient has TTP or concomitant severe clotting factor deficiencies. Temporary decreases in several clotting factors during plasma removal, reflected by changes in PT and the APTT, are usually transient and not of clinical concern unless the patient has significant associated hemostatic deficiencies or severe hepatic dysfunction.

Because many patients in ICUs will not have suitable antecubital venous access or will be unable to provide arm pumping to generate sufficient venous flow during an apheresis procedure, dual-lumen, polyurethane dialysis/apheresis catheters are usually placed in a femoral vein and will provide high flow access. If subclavian or internal jugular catheters are used, the return port should be in the cava since relatively undiluted citrated blood has, on rare occasion, been thought to precipitate arrhythmias. Most patients undergoing plasma exchange do not require intravenous antibody replacement after each apheresis procedure. Exceptions to this rule are patients with hypoproteinemic states, especially the nephrotic syndrome, those with active infection and those undergoing intensive, daily, high volume therapeutic aphereses.

A standard rule for apheresis treatment of patients with autoaggressive syndromes, especially those with autoimmune antibody production, is that plasma exchange alone, while an effective temporizing measure, will ultimately not be efficacious and theoretically could be deleterious to the patient unless the apheresis treatment is closely linked to the use of an alkylating agent. The theory behind coupled therapy is straightforward.[63] Reduction in levels of pathogenic antibody, regulatory antibody, and regulatory cytokines can induce proliferation of B cells and possibly also T cells. Proliferating cells then become susceptible to alkylation and either clonal abortion or anergy occur when cyclophosphamide is given. The dose of cyclophosphamide ranges from 500 mg to 1 g/m^2 in 5% dextrose and water over a period of 30 to 60 min. Premedication for nausea is given routinely but may be unnecessary in some patients. The alkylating treatment can be given immediately after the last plasmapheresis and up to 48 h thereafter. Protocols for the frequency of apheresis, at least in the treatment of SLE, vary widely, but usually encompass an induction period of 5 to 7 exchanges of 1.0 to 1.5 plasma volume over 7 to 10 days until approximately 250 mL plasma/kg have been removed from the patient. This induction period is followed by some form of immunosuppressive therapy, usually cyclophosphamide.[64]

PROTEIN A COLUMNS

Protein A absorption columns provide on-line removal of IgG antibody and circulating immune complexes; they have the benefit of returning most other plasma components to the patient. Protein A pheresis has been effective in drug-resistant idiopathic thrombocytopenic purpura and cancer chemotherapy-associated TTP/hemolytic uremic syndrome.[65] The efflux of activated inflammatory and vasoactive mediators generated from plasma by the protein A silica absorption vehicle can cause transient shaking chills, fever, and hypotension. This usually occurs at the end or after the termination of the procedure. New protein A membranes with secondary anaphylatoxin traps may obviate this side effect in the near future. Specific secondary membranes with native DNA or acetylcholine receptors may also be available in the future.

LEUKAPHERESIS

Leukapheresis can be performed efficiently on centrifuge belt machines and is highly effective in reducing peripheral blast counts to levels that are less threatening to maintenance of adequate microcirculation and more amenable to chemotherapy. Combination leukaplasmapheresis has been performed in patients with scleroderma and polymyositis/dermatomyositis refractory to conventional management.

Empirical Therapy for Suspected Rheumatic Disease

In puzzling cases, the rheumatologist may discern from the nuances of the clinical examination, serologic testing, and invasive procedures that the patient has rheumatic disease. Sometimes the rheumatologist, like the intensivist, cannot make a definite diagnosis, yet confronts a critically ill patient who *may* have a rheumatic disease. The clinical status of such patients is usually at an unacceptable plateau or even more likely deteriorating. Should that patient be given empirical therapy? Recognition of our shortcomings in diagnosis and the inability of some patients to tolerate a critical invasive test recommends such a course in selected patients.

Prior to initiation of empirical therapy, it is helpful to ask a series of related questions.

1. Has infection been reasonably excluded? Infection and cancer most commonly mimic rheumatic disease. Since empirical therapy usually implies immunosuppressive drugs and most commonly corticosteroids, infection must be ruled out. Here the emphasis should be on "reasonably" making such an assessment. Endless sets of blood cultures should not delay a difficult decision.
2. What do I suspect the patient may have? It should be possible to formulate a plausible if unprovable diagnostic hypothesis. Such a hypothesis is critical to the rest of the experiment. If it is impossible to generate a "working diagnosis," it is doubtful the therapeutic trial will work. Autopsy study of these patients is likely to reveal cancer or no diagnosis.
3. What is adequate therapy for this suspected diagnosis? Treatment for a suspected diagnosis ranges from adequate to aggressive. In the absence of a definite diagnosis, it is reasonable to choose a level of therapeutic intensity that is usually adequate for the suspected disorder. Aggressive treatment approaches to an unconfirmed illness create another set of confounding variables and may place the patient at a further disadvantage.
4. What will I use as my parameters to judge therapeutic success? Empirical therapy should proceed with a clear understanding of the yardsticks that will measure therapeutic responsiveness. These parameters can then be rigorously monitored. Furthermore, blind spots in the baseline data can be addressed before therapy is begun.
5. What is the duration of a reasonable trial for this disorder? Agreement on the duration of a therapeutic trial should precede its initiation. Failure to develop such an end point can result in excessively long and risky therapy on the one hand or a course that falls short of an adequate trial. Furthermore, spontaneous improvement or improvement in response to other therapies may result in prolonged and unnecessary treatment.

The clinician needs to be vigilant to the risks associated with any trial of empirical therapy. However, after addressing the above questions, such a trial may represent both rational and compassionate care.

CASE PRESENTATION

A 43-year-old man was admitted directly to the medical ICU with gross hematuria and hemoptysis. He had been in good health until 8 months prior to admission when he developed a middle ear infection that was recalcitrant to multiple courses of antibiotics and ultimately required tube drainage. In the following months, he developed progressive fatigue, weight loss, headache, ocular inflammation requiring topical steroids, and arthralgia. During the few weeks prior to admission, he noted a quickening of the tempo of his illness, developing red lesions on the legs and culminating in multiple episodes of hemoptysis followed by gross hematuria.

On examination, the patient appeared pale and chronically ill. Septal mucosa of the left nostril was erythematous and ulcerated. The medial perilimbal conjuctiva was slightly injected. Lungs were clear. Heart rate was 98 and regular. Abdomen was benign. There was palpable synovitis at the elbows, right wrist, left fourth metacarpophalangeal joint, and right knee. Examination of the skin revealed nailfold infarcts, petechiae at the fingertips, and multiple petechial lesions on the toes with clustering at the posterior left calf.

Laboratory data revealed a white blood cell count of 14,100 with 87 segs, 12 lymphs, 1 mono. Hemoglobin was 11.1 and platelet count was 394,000. ESR was 70 mm/h. Albumin was 2.6 g/dL, BUN 110 mg/dL, and creatinine 6.5 mg/dL. PT and PTT were normal. Urinalysis showed 2 + proteinuria, 4 + blood and >100 RBCs per high power field with 5–10 WBCs. ANCA determination was 183 units (<22 units = negative) which is in the strongly positive range. ANA, RF, and cryoglobulins were negative. Chest x-ray was normal. ECG showed sinus tachycardia at the rate of 102, but was otherwise within normal limits. Renal biopsy showed necrotizing crescentic glomerulonephritis and was negative for immunofluorescence.

On the evening of admission, a rheumatology consult was called and a preliminary diagnosis of Wegener's granulomatosis was made. Treatment was initiated with 40 mg intravenous methyl-prenisolone twice daily and 150 mg cyclophosphamide intravenously daily. No further hemoptysis was noted during the hospitalization. Arthralgias diminished 24 h after steroid therapy was initiated. The serum creatinine level peaked at 9.3 mg/dL 2 days after admission and declined to 4.0 mg/dL over the next week. The patient's general sense of well-being improved and 10 days after admission to the ICU, he was discharged from the hospital.

CASE DISCUSSION

This case illustrates the dramatic clinical presentation that can accompany immune-mediated pulmonary-renal syndromes. Such cases count among the unusual reasons that patients are directly admitted to the ICU because of a primary rheumatic process. As with most patients in this circumstance, there was a history of prodromal features that pointed toward the diagnosis. These features were partly nonspecific constitutional complaints, but more specific complaints of ocular inflammation, "red spots" on the legs, and arthritis suggested a systemic vasculitis. The history of refractory middle ear infections dictated a working diagnosis of Wegener's granulomatosis on the evening of admission.

The diagnosis of systemic vasculitis can be certified only through biopsy or angiography. Since other diseases may mimic vasculitis but have entirely different therapeutic approaches, the clinician must make every effort to obtain such documentation. Nonetheless, substantial clinical evidence of fulminant vasculitis dictates that therapy be initiated before a diagnosis can be completely substantiated. Hence, this patient was treated for presumed Wegener's granulomatosis on the evening of admission while plans were made for further diagnostic investigation. The patient was treated with a combination of intravenous methlyprednisolone and cyclophosphamide. The methylprednisolone was given at a dose of 1 mg/kg/day and the dose divided to provide greater therapeutic impact in the acute setting. Cyclophosphamide can be given at doses higher than 2 mg/kg/day in the early treatment of severe Wegener's granulomatosis, but the presence of renal failure makes the effective dose higher. Aggressive immunosuppression must be tempered by the potential consequences of a profoundly neutropenic patient in the ICU.

Renal biopsy was performed for two reasons. It offered an option for diagnosis. Although the renal pathology of Wegener's granulomatosis is not completely specific, in this clinical setting it provides data highly supportive of that diagnosis. Secondly, it provides useful information with regard to prognosis of this patient's renal function. If the biopsy had shown mostly fibrotic glomerular crescents, plans for dealing with chronic renal failure would have been made during this admission.

Finally, relatively specific serologic testing for Wegener's granulomatosis now exists. The presence of high titers of ANCA in this patient confirmed the diagnosis of Wegener's granulomatosis and provided a serologic marker for monitoring future disease activity.

References

1. Schur P: Clinical features of SLE, in Kelley WN, Harris ED, Ruddy S, Sledge CB, (eds). *Textbook of Rheumatology,* 3d ed. Philadelphia, Saunders, 1989, pp 1101–1129.
2. Haider TS, Roberts WC: Coronary arterial disease in systemic lupus erythematosus—quantification of degrees of narrowing in 10 necropsy patients. Am J Med 70:775, 1981.
3. Nossent HC, Swaak TJG, Berden JHM, Dutch Working Party on Systemic Lupus Erythematosus: Systemic lupus erythematosus after renal transplantation: Patient and graft survival and disease activity. Ann Intern Med; 114(3):183, 1991.
4. Cheigh JS, Stenzek KH, Rubin AL, et al: Systemic lupus erythematosus in patients with chronic renal failure. Am J Med 75:602, 1983.
5. Lawrence EC: Systemic lupus erythematosus and the lung, in Lahita RG (ed). *Systemic Lupus Erythematosus.* New York, Wiley, 1987, pp 691–708.
6. Millman RP, Cohen TB, Levinson AI, et al: SLE complicated by acute pulmonary haemorrhage: Recovery following plasmapheresis and cytotoxic therapy. J. Rheumatol 8:1021, 1981.
7. McCune WJ, Golbus J: Neuropsychiatric lupus. Rheum Dis Clin North Am 14(1):149, 1988.
8. Widener HL, Littman DH: Ibuprofen induced meningitis in systemic lupus erythematosus. JAMA 239:1062, 1978.
9. Brandt KD, Lessell S: Migrainous phenomenon in systemic lupus erythematosus. Arthritis Rheum 21:7, 1978.
10. Harris EN, Gharavi AE, Hughes GRV: Anti-phospholipid antibodies. Clin Rheumatic Dis 11(3):591, 1985.
11. Silver RM, Miller KS: Lung involvement in systemic sclerosis. Rheum Dis Clin North Am 16(1):199, 1990.
12. Seibold JR: Scleroderma, in Kelly WN, Harris ED, Ruddy S, Sledge CB (eds).: *Textbook of Rheumatology,* 3d ed. Philadelphia, Saunders, 1989, pp 1215–1244.
13. Steen VD, Costantino JP, Shapiro AP, Medsger TA Jr: Outcome of renal crisis in systemic sclerosis: Relation to availability of angiotensin converting enzyme (ACE) inhibitors. Ann Intern Med 113:352, 1990.
14. Bohan A, Peter JB, Bowman RL, Pearson CM: A computer assisted analysis of 153 patients with polymyositis and dermatomyositis. Medicine 56:255, 1977.
15. Medsger TA, Robinson H, Masi AT: Factors affecting survivorship in polymyositis: A life table study of 124 patients. Arthritis Rheum 14:249, 1971.
16. Dau PC: Plasmapheresis in idiopathic inflammatory myopathy: Experience with 35 patients. Arch Neurol 38:544, 1981.
17. Cecere FA, Spiva DA: Combination plasmapheresis/leukocytapheresis for the treatment of dermatomyositis/polymyositis. Plasma Ther Transfus Technol 3:401, 1982.
18. Sostman HD, Matthay RA, Putman CE, Walker Smith GJ: Methotrexate-induced pneumonitis. Medicine (Baltimore) 55:371, 1976.
19. Perrquet JL, Harrington TM, Davis DE: *Pneumocystis carinii* following methotrexate therapy for rheumatoid arthritis Letter. Arthritis Rheum 16:1291, 1983.
20. Hollingsworth JW: *Management of Rheumatoid Arthritis and Its Complications.* Chicago, Year Book, 1978, pp 215–221.
21. Silberman A, Holmes EW, Miller BJ, et al: Serum hyperviscosity associated with rheumatoid arthritis: Description of a case with analysis of intermediate immune complexes in the serum. Ann Clin Lab Sci 16:26, 1986.
22. Pope RM: Rheumatic fever in the 1980s. Bull Rheum Dis 38(3):1, 1989.
23. Elkon KB, et al: Adult onset Still's disease: Twenty year follow-up and further study of patients with active disease. Arthritis Rheum 25:647, 1982.
24. Hunder GG: Giant cell (temporal) arteritis. Rheum Dis Clin North Am 16(2):399, 1990.
25. Camilleri M, Pusey CD, Chadwick VS, Rees AJ: Gastrointestinal manifestations of systemic vasculitis. Q J Med 52:141, 1983.
26. Zizic TM, Classen JN, Stevens MB: Acute abdominal complications of systemic lupus erythematosus and polyarteritis nodosa. Am J Med 73(4):525, 1982.
27. Johnson JP, Moore J, Austin HA, et al: Therapy of antiglomerular basement membrane antibody disease: Analysis of the prognostic significance of clinical, pathologic and treatment factors. Medicine 64:219, 1985.
28. Abboud RT, Chase WH, Ballon HS, et al: Goodpasture's syndrome: Diagnosis by transbronchial lung biopsy. Ann Intern Med 89:635, 1978.
29. Johnson JP, Whitman W, Briggs WA, Wilson CB: Plasmapheresis and immunosuppressive agents in anti-basement membrane antibody-induced Goodpasture's syndrome. Am J Med 64:354, 1978.
30. Massa MC, Su WPD. Lymphocytic vasculitis: A clinical pathologic study. J Cutan Pathol 11(2):132, 1984.
31. Van Hale HM, Gibson LE, Schroeter AL: Henoch-Schönlein vasculitis: Direct immunofluorescence study of uninvolved skin. J Am Acad Dermatol 15:665, 1986.
32. Sigal LH: Pseudovasculitis syndromes, in McCarty DJ (ed).: *Arthritis and Allied Conditions,* 11th ed. Philadelphia, Lea & Febiger, 1989, pp 1189–1196.
33. Bowles CA: Vasculopathy associated with the antiphos-

pholipid antibody syndrome. Rheu Dis Clin North Am 16(2):471, 1990.
34. Joyce JW: Buerger's disease (thromboangiitis obliterans). Rheum Dis Clin North Am 16(2):471, 1990.
35. Bathon J, Graves J, Jens P, et al: The erythrocyte sedimentation rate in end-stage renal failure. Am J Kidney Dis X(1)34, 1987.
36. Connelly CS, Panush RS: Markedly elevated sedimentation rates: What is their clinical significance? in *Postgraduate Advances in Rheumatology*. Berryville, Virginia, Forum Medicum, 1990, IV–VII.
37. Recker DP, Klippel JH: Perplexing antinuclear antibody syndrome (PANAS), in *Postgraduate Advances in Rheumatology*. Berryville, Virginia, Forum Medicum, 1989, IV–III.
38. Cattogio LJ, Bernstein RM, Black CM, et al: Serologic markers in progressive systemic sclerosis: Clinical correlations. Ann Rheum Dis 42:23, 1983.
39. Chorzelski TP, Jablonska S, Beutner EH, et al: Anticentromere antibody: An immunological marker of a subset of systemic sclerosis. Br J Dermatol 113:381, 1985.
40. Harmon CE: Antinuclear antibodies in autoimmune disease. Med Clin North Am 69(3):547, 1985.
41. Ramsey-Goldman R, Hom D, Deng J-S, et al: Anti-SS-A antibodies and fetal outcome in maternal systemic lupus erythematosus. Arthritis Rheum 29:1269, 1986.
42. Jarzabek-Chorzelska M, Blaszczyk M, Jablonska S, et al: Scl 70 antibody—a specific marker of systemic sclerosis. Br J Dermatol 115:393, 1986.
43. Falk RJ, Jennette JC: Anti-neutrophil cytoplasmic autoantibodies with specificity for myeloperoxidase in patients with systemic vasculitis and idiopathic necrotizing and crescentic glomerulonephritis. N Engl J Med 318:1651, 1988.
44. Specks U, DeRemee RA: Granulomatous vasculitis. Rheum Dis Clin North Am 16(2):377, 1990.
45. Scott DG, Bacon PA: Intravenous cyclophosphamide plus methylprednisolone in treatment of systemic rheumatoid vasculitis. Am J Med 76(3):377, 1984.
46. Geltner D, Kohn RW, Gorevic P, Franklin EC: The effect of combination therapy (steroids, immunosuppressives, and plasmapheresis) on 5 mixed cryoglobulinemia patients with renal, neurologic, and vascular involvement. Arthritis Rheum 24(9):1121, 1981.
47. Frank, MM: Complement: A brief review. J Allergy Clin Immunol 84:411, 1989.
48. Kimberly RP: Pulse methylprednisolone in SLE. Clin Rheum Dis 8(1):261, 1982.
49. Lewis GP, Jusko WJ, Burke CW, Graves L, and the Boston Collaborative Drug Surveillance Program: Prednisone side-effects and serum-protein levels, a collaborative study. Lancet 2:778, 1971.
50. Sahn SA, Lakshiminarayan W: Tuberculosis after corticosteroid therapy. Br J Dis Chest 70:195, 1976.
51. Iseman MD: Tuberculosis prophylaxis during corticosteroid therapy-reply. JAMA 258:263, 1987.
52. Bovornkitts S, Kangsadal P, Sathirapat P, Oonsombatti P: Reversion and reconversion rate of tuberculin skin reactions in correlation with the use of prednisone. Department of Medicine, Siriraj Hospital Medical School, XXXVIII:51, 1960.
53. Behrens TW, Goodwin JS: Glucocorticoids, in: McCarty DJ (ed).: *Arthritis and Allied Conditions,* 11th ed. Philadelphia, Lea & Febiger, 1989, pp 604–621.
54. Hoffman GS, Leavitt RY, Fleisher TA, et al: Treatment of Wegener's granulomatosis with intermittent high-dose intravenous cyclophosphamide. Am J Med 89:403, 1990.
55. Fischer TJ et al: Childhood dermatomyositis and polymyositis—treatment with methotrexate and prednisone. Am J Dis Child 133:386, 1979.
56. Morgan SL, Baggott JE, Vaughn WH, et al: The effect of folic acid supplementation on the toxicity of low dose MTX in patients with rheumatoid arthritis. Arthritis Rheum 33(1):9, 1990.
57. Kahay BD: Cyclosporine. N Engl J Med 321:1725, 1989.
58. NIH Consensus Conference. Intravenous immunoglobulin: Prevention and treatment of disease. JAMA 264(24):3189, 1990.
59. Ciabattoni G et al: Effects of sulindac and ibuprofen in patients with chronic glomerular disease. N Engl J Med 310:279, 1984.
60. Ruppert GS, Barth WF: Tolmetin-induced aseptic meningitis. JAMA 245:67, 1981.
61. Ballas ZK, Donta ST: Sulindac-induced aseptic meningitis. Arch Intern Med 142:165, 1982.
62. Terkeltaub RA, Ginsberg MH, McCarty DJ: Pathogenesis and treatment of crystal-induced inflammation, in McCarty DJ (ed).: *Arthritis and Allied Conditions,* 11th ed. Philadelphia, Lea & Febiger, 1989, pp 1691–1710.
63. Schroeder JO, Euler HH, Loffler H: Synchronization of plasmapheresis and pulse cyclophosphamide in severe systemic lupus erythematosus. Ann Intern Med 107:344, 1987.
64. Barr WG, Hubbell EA, Robinson JA: Persistently active systemic lupus erythematosus treated with intermittent plasmapheresis and bolus cyclophosphamide, in Oda T, Shiokawa Y, Inque N (eds).: *Proceedings of the 1st International Congress of the World Apheresis Association.* Cleveland, ISAO Press, 1987, pp 696–700.
65. Snyder HW, Mittelman A, Cochran SK, Balint JP, Jones FR, the PROSORBA Clinical Trial Group: Successful treatment of cancer chemotherapy-associated thrombotic thrombocytopenic purpura/hemolytic uremic syndrome (TTP/HUS) with protein A immunoadsorption. Presented: American Society of Hematology; Boston: Nov 28–Dec 4, 1990.

SECTION J

PULMONARY DISORDERS IN THE CRITICALLY ILL

Chapter 127

MANAGEMENT OF THE PATIENT ON A VENTILATOR

JESSE B. HALL
LAWRENCE D. H. WOOD

KEY POINTS

- *Ventilator parameters should be determined by the pathophysiology underlying the particular form of respiratory failure requiring mechanical support; this approach facilitates stabilization and comfort of the patient on the ventilator, prevention of common complications, and early liberation from this supportive therapy.*
- *All ventilator orders should be accompanied by plans to minimize airway complications, prevent thromboembolic disease and gastrointestinal hemorrhage, and provide adequate nutrition.*
- Whenever *the adequacy of oxygen exchange is in question, the initial fraction of inspired oxygen (F_{IO_2}) on the ventilator should be 1.0; this will be diagnostic as well as therapeutic, since failure to achieve full arterial hemoglobin saturation identifies a significant right-to-left shunt.*
- *Typical ventilator settings for the patient with normal lung mechanics and gas exchange include an F_{IO_2} of .30 to .40, tidal volume of 8 to 12 mL/kg, and respiratory rate of 8 to 12 breaths per min; if mechanical ventilation has been instituted to rest fatigued respiratory muscles, sedation and muscle relaxation may be necessary to completely eliminate respiratory muscle activity.*
- *Atelectasis of dependent lung regions should be prevented by measures to increase end-expired lung volume and to reduce airway closure; this prophylactic regimen should be applied gently to patients with normal respiratory mechanics, and more aggressively to patients with severe airflow obstruction and/or perioperative respiratory failure.*
- *The patient with severe airflow obstruction often develops pulmonary barotrauma and/or hypoperfusion after institution of positive-pressure ventilation; almost invariably this is the result of gas trapping and intrinsic positive end-expiratory pressure (PEEPi) causing hyperinflation, high intrathoracic pressure, and diminished venous return, and responds to vigorous volume resuscitation and reduced minute volume.*
- *The goals of ventilator management in severe airflow obstruction include a peak airway pressure below 55 cmH_2O, PEEPi below 15 cmH_2O, and eucapnea; this can be best achieved with resting the respiratory muscles, high flow rates (60 L/min), low tidal volumes (5 to 7 mL/kg) and respiratory rates of 12 to 18 breaths per min; in some cases intentional hypoventilation is indicated.*
- *Stabilizing the patient with acute-on-chronic respiratory failure on the ventilator entails response to diminished venous return resulting from positive-pressure ventilation, and avoidance of excessive minute ventilation and consequent alkalemia.*
- *The patient with acute hypoxemic respiratory failure (AHRF) resulting from pulmonary edema will require initial ventilator settings of an F_{IO_2} of 1.0, tidal volume of 6 to 7 mL/kg, and respiratory rate of 24 to 28 breaths per min; positive end-expiratory pressure (PEEP) is then added to allow use of a nontoxic (i.e., .60 or lower) F_{IO_2}.*
- *Goals of ventilator management for the patient with AHRF include a peak airway pressure below 45 cmH_2O, the lowest tidal volume providing acceptable Pa_{CO_2}, adequate oxygen delivery to peripheral tissues, and the least PEEP achieving 90% saturation of an adequate arterial hemoglobin on an F_{IO_2} of .60 or less; PEEP does not reduce lung water but merely redistributes it. Circulatory management in these patients can reduce lung water and potentially improve outcome, while measures to reduce oxygen consumption (muscle relaxation, cooling) and enhance cardiac function allow adequate oxygen delivery at lower pulmonary vascular pressures.*
- *In distinctly inhomogeneous lung disease with AHRF (e.g., lobar pneumonia), PEEP may not improve intrapulmonary shunt and should be used only if clear benefit is demonstrated; adjuncts to adequate oxygenation include positioning the diseased lobe(s) uppermost, and split-lung ventilation to apply PEEP to the diseased side only.*
- *While some patients may require sedation and muscle relaxation for initial stabilization on the ventilator, this intervention should not be used to routinely adapt the patient to the machine; rather, ventilator adjustments should be used to stabilize and comfort the patient.*
- *The approach to liberation of the patient from mechanical ventilation is a mirror image of the assessment of the underlying pathophysiology that initially resulted in respiratory failure; a variable period of respiratory muscle rest relieves fatigue and allows the initiation of measures to reduce respiratory load and increase respiratory muscle tone, power, and coordination.*

Too often the management of the patient on a ventilator is guided by (1) prescribed orders widely applied to diverse patients regardless of their underlying lung function, or (2) "mode"-dominated thinking on the part of the physician, by which various microprocessor-controlled machine functions are hoped to have a salutary effect on patient outcome. This chapter offers an alternative approach, in which ventilator parameters are set in accord with the underlying pathophysiology of different forms of respiratory failure. This facilitates early stabilization of the patient on the ventilator in such a way as to optimize carbon dioxide removal and oxygen delivery within the limits of abnormal neuromuscular function, lung mechanics, and gas exchange, all with a minimum of complications. This approach is also useful in setting the stage for liberating the patient from the mechanical ventilator, a process that can be thought of as the mirror image of initial tailoring of ventilator settings to the underlying pathophysiology.[1] Once abnormalities of neuromuscular function, lung mechanics, and gas exchange are identified, their correction at a pace limited only by underlying disease permits the most expeditious withdrawal of this dangerous supportive therapy.

Other chapters of this book are complementary to the information presented here. The pathophysiology of respiratory failure is broadly reviewed in Chap. 1; the details of mechanical ventilator technology are outlined in Chap. 8; and other chapters (e.g., Chap. 84, Perioperative Respiratory Failure, and Chap. 130, Status Asthmaticus) discuss the way in which mechanical ventilatory support fits into general management of specific problems. This monograph will offer broad guidelines for stabilizing patients with various disorders on the ventilator. Of course, each critically ill patient presents myriad problems and challenges that require the crafting of a specific therapeutic regime; but it is possible to identify five "types" of respiratory failure, all sharing common approaches to mechanical ventilation. They are represented by (1) the patient with normal lung mechanics and gas exchange, (2) the patient with severe airflow obstruction, (3) the patient with acute-on-chronic respiratory failure, (4) the patient with acute hypoxemic respiratory failure, and (5) the patient with restrictive lung or chest wall disease. Accordingly, approaches for each class of patient will be discussed. We then comment on techniques for optimizing patient comfort and communication; appropriate responses to "crises" on the ventilator; and indications for discontinuation of mechanical support. Finally, we provide an approach for the "difficult-to-wean" patient.

Guidelines for Stabilizing the Patient on a Ventilator

Concomitant to all ventilator orders should be consideration of (1) a daily inspection and management plan for the artificial airway, to minimize upper airway injury; (2) pharmacologic and/or mechanical prophylaxis against thromboembolic disease; (3) prophylaxis against gastrointestinal hemorrhage; and (4) means of establishing and continuing nutrition. These topics are explored in detail in Chap. 52 and elsewhere in this book.

Most ventilators offer a host of alarm functions to indicate ventilator malfunctions and changes in the patient's condition. Apnea alarms are almost universally present. When the $F_{I_{O_2}}$ is measured along the inspiratory limb of the ventilator, alarm limits are routinely set 5 to 10 percent above and below the desired setting. If expired minute ventilation is monitored, alarm limits set approximately 10 percent above and below the stable and desired level of minute ventilation are appropriate. Low pressure alarms are typically set at 5 to 15 cmH_2O, and normally signal a large inspiratory gas leak. Peak pressure alarms should be determined by individual patient conditions, to be discussed further below.

PATIENTS WITH NORMAL LUNG MECHANICS AND GAS EXCHANGE

Patients with normal lung mechanics and gas exchange can require mechanical ventilatory support (1) because of loss of central drive to breathe (e.g., drug overdose or structural injury to the brainstem); (2) because of neuromuscular weakness (e.g., high cervical spinal cord injury, acute idiopathic myelitis, myasthenia gravis); (3) as an adjunctive therapy in the treatment of shock[2,3]; or (4) in order to achieve hyperventilation (e.g., in the treatment of elevated intracranial pressure following head trauma) (see Table 127-1). Following intubation, initial ventilator orders (see Table 127-1) should be an $F_{I_{O_2}}$ of .40, a tidal volume of 8 to 12 mL/kg, and a respiratory rate of 8 to 12 breaths per min; if hyperventilation is sought, the initial rate should be increased to the range of 18 to 24 breaths per min. It should be noted that this tidal volume recommendation is 50 percent greater than the spontaneous tidal volumes of normal patients (5 to 9 mL/kg), and 50 percent less than that recommended in many other monographs concerning ventilator settings. This two-fold discrepancy arose from the early days of ventilator therapy, when thoughtful physicians asked their ventilated patients whether they were getting enough air; invariably, these patients with polio or chronic obstructive pulmonary disease (COPD) (see Preface) claimed air hunger until tidal volume had been increased from the lowest to the highest levels. We are persuaded that the vast majority of patients with normal gas exchange and lung mechanics are comfortable with an intermediate tidal volume. Early implementation of measures to prevent atelectasis should include the addition of sighs. This is particularly important in patients with neuromuscular diseases requiring a prolonged period of mechanical ventilation, for they tend to develop atelectasis and even lobar collapse. For these patients we use the upper limit of tidal volume (12 mL/kg), a measure that satisfies their air hunger.

All patients should have measures implemented to avoid atelectasis and promote pulmonary toilet. Three-point turning and chest physiotherapy are desirable in all patients unless other conditions preclude such mobilization. A number of rotating beds are currently under evaluation for mechanically ventilated patients to prevent atelectasis and complicating pneumonia.[4] Sighs (given at a frequency of 6 to 12 per h, at a volume of 1.5 to 2 times the tidal volume) or small amounts of PEEP (2.5 to 7 cmH_2O) are useful to increase functional residual capacity (FRC) and prevent alveolar collapse. Many of these measures will be

TABLE 127-1 Mechanical Ventilation of Patients with Normal Lung Mechanics and Gas Exchange

Indications	
	Central nervous system depression
	Neuromuscular weakness
	Adjunctive therapy for shock
	Hyperventilation following brain injury
Settings	
	$F_{I_{O_2}}$ .21–.40
	Tidal volume 8–12 mL/kg
	Rate 12 breaths per min
	Peak flow adjusted to patient comfort
	SIMV or A/C mode with minimal sensitivity
Things to consider	
	Target Pa_{CO_2} of 25 mmHg if goal is reduction of intracranial pressure
	Higher minute ventilation or use of sedation/muscle relaxation in shock
	Measures to prevent atelectasis
	Three-point turning
	Chest physiotherapy
	Sighs
	Low levels of PEEP

SIMV = synchronized intermittent mandatory ventilation; A/C = assist/control.

unnecessary in the young patient receiving tidal volumes of 8 to 12 mL/kg. However, older age, history of smoking, volume overload, and obesity make it more likely that some degree of alveolar collapse will occur without preventive measures. If lobar collapse does occur and lung mechanics are nearly normal, recruitment can be attempted by gradually increasing the tidal volume at the bedside while monitoring the airway pressure. Recruitment of the lobe is signaled by an airway pressure that does not rise, or even falls, with an increment in tidal volume; proof of ventilation to the collapsed lobe can then be sought by examination or chest radiograph. The patient should then be returned to the recommended tidal volume, and the measures that have been put in place to prevent atelectasis should be reviewed. During the use of large tidal volumes to recruit a collapsed lobe, airway pressures should not be allowed to exceed 45 cmH_2O.

Of course, if gas exchange is entirely normal, the $F_{I_{O_2}}$ can likely be decreased further on the basis of pulse oximetry or arterial blood gas determinations the aim being an arterial saturation of more than 90 percent. At the time of securing an artificial airway, misadventures such as right mainstem intubation can occur; for this reason we prefer to begin the patient on mechanical ventilation with the "buffer" of supplemental oxygen. Indeed, if *any* question exists regarding the adequacy of gas exchange, the patient should be ventilated initially with an $F_{I_{O_2}}$ of 1.0; this will be a diagnostic as well as a therapeutic maneuver, since failure to achieve full saturation of arterial blood confirms a significant intrapulmonary shunt (see below). Inspiratory flow for the patient with normal lung mechanics generally can be set at 40 L/min, and adjusted slightly upward if this relieves a sense of dyspnea in the alert patient.[5] Even in most tachypneic patients with underlying lung disease—and certainly in those individuals with normal lung mechanics—inspiratory flow rates in excess of 60 L/min are rarely indicated.[6]

The patient may be allowed to interact with the ventilator in a number of ways. Alert patients with weakness can be placed on a synchronized intermittent mandatory ventilation (SIMV) or assist/control (A/C) mode with a minimal (-2 cmH_2O) trigger sensitivity. This allows the patient to take intermittent small breaths (SIMV) or trigger each breath (A/C); yet, with these initial settings, either mode tends to minimize the patient's work of breathing—which is appropriate to his or her weak, and possibly fatigued, respiratory muscles. Alternatively, neuromuscular disease patients may be maintained with pressure support (PS) ventilation (see Chap. 8 and 9). In this mode, the ventilator, servo-controlled by the monitored proximal airway pressure, varies inspiratory flow as necessary to maintain pressure at the airway opening at a preset level.[7,8] Even weak patients able to initiate breaths can have the PS level adjusted (usually to the range of 10 to 20 cmH_2O) to maintain an adequate tidal volume (500 to 800 mL) without excessive tachypnea (respiratory rate below 25 breaths per min). It is important to realize that PS ventilation is mechanically supported but entirely spontaneous, with no machine "backup," unless mixed with a mode such as SIMV. Thus, early in the course of management, hypoventilation may occur despite use of PS if there is further deterioration of muscle strength or blunting of drive to breathe by disease or drugs. In addition, a variety of different electronic control and mechanical delivery systems exist for pressure support on different ventilators, and inspiratory flow and airway pressure profile may not readily be adapted to achieve patient comfort and minimal effort during early phases of ventilatory support.[9]

Patients with drug overdose or central nervous system injury can be managed in a similar way. Again, an assisted but spontaneous breathing mode, such as PS, should not be used if the drive to breathe is potentially reduced. SIMV or A/C is useful for a comatose patient, particularly to provide patient-initiated breathing as the patient awakens. If hyperventilation is being used to reduce intracranial pressure, the mode of ventilation is largely irrelevant, since the result is likely to be cessation of patient effort as ventilator rate is increased, titrated to give a Pa_{CO_2} of approximately 25 mmHG (see Chap. 34). Some patients with devastating brain stem injury manifest central neurogenic hyperventilation, with large tidal volumes and high respiratory rates. Modification of ventilator settings is not usually effective in eliminating or reducing patient effort; we have encountered patients who overcome low tidal volume settings by triggering the inspiratory valve two or three times on each inspiration. Sedation and muscle relaxation is often necessary to control ventilation, and the prognosis is poor.

Patients with septic or cardiogenic shock that deteriorates despite initial fluid and vasoactive drug resuscitation should be considered for mechanical ventilation, despite normal gas exchange and, typically, a low Pa_{CO_2} associated with their hypoperfusion-related lactic acidosis[2,3] (see Chap. 114). The goals here are to decrease lactate production by the respiratory muscles, allow diversion of respiratory muscle blood flow to other compromised organs, and avert sudden respiratory arrest.[2,3] The respiratory rate in these patients should be gradually increased to 20 to 24 breaths per min, in an attempt to have inspiratory efforts cease, as judged by bedside observation of the patient and the proximal airway pressure gauge; not infrequently, the inspiratory effort is diminished by increasing inspiratory flow. If such adjustments do not diminish breathing effort to an undetectable level, sedation should be attempted. If this does not succeed in cessation of inspiratory efforts and the patient continues to have evidence of hypoperfusion, muscle relaxation should be considered.

While the patient is being placed on the ventilator, a number of things should be monitored. Institution of positive-pressure ventilation may reduce venous return in any patient (see Chap. 2). It is more likely to occur in patients with a low mean systemic pressure (e.g., hypovolemia; vasodilating drugs; or decreased sympathetic tone from sedating drugs, neuromuscular disease, or age-reducing muscle tone) or very high intrathoracic pressures [e.g., in restrictive chest wall disease; during use of PEEP in the treatment of ARDS; or with gas trapping producing intrinsic PEEP (see below)]; but any patient may have an unsuspected degree of hypovolemia that, when combined with the effects of drugs used at the time of intubation, results in hypoperfusion. With marked reduction in venous return with intact cardiovascular reflexes, hypotension and tachycardia will occur. If these changes in blood pressure and heart rate are noted, rapid volume infusion is recommended; simultaneously the patient should be returned to slow bagging with 100% oxygen. If this does not rapidly restore vital signs, another event complicating intubation and stabilization on the ventilator should be considered (e.g., hypoxia, pneumothorax, myocardial infarction).

Soon after the initiation of mechanical ventilation, airway pressures should be assessed (see Chap. 1). To confirm normal lung mechanics, an adult ventilated with an 8-mm or larger endotracheal tube should have a peak-to-pause pressure gradient of 3 to 7 cmH_2O at an inspiratory flow of 40 L/min; with an 800 mL tidal volume, the pause (or inspiratory "hold") pressure should be 15 to 20 cmH_2O or less. Thus, peak airway pressures are typically 18 to 27 cmH_2O. The peak airway pressure alarm can be set at 45 to 50 cmH_2O. Airway pressures that are substantially higher than these should prompt consideration that respiratory system mechanics are deranged; partitioning between peak and pause pressures will allow determination of whether this is an elastic or a resistive abnormality (see Chap. 1).

PATIENTS WITH SEVERE AIRFLOW OBSTRUCTION

Airway disease with large increases in both inspiratory and expiratory resistance occurs in status asthmaticus (see Chap. 130); in inhalation injury with airway edema and mucosal sloughing following thermal insult; and, rarely, with central airway lesions, such as tumor or foreign body, that cannot be bypassed with the endotracheal tube (see Table 127-2). In isolated upper airway injuries assessment of the extent of damage is often possible by bronchoscopy shortly before, or at the time of, intubation. Bronchoscopy should not be performed routinely on patients with asthma.[10]

TABLE 127-2 Mechanical Ventilation of Patients with Severe Airflow Obstruction

Indications
Status asthmaticus
Thermal injury of the upper airway
Mass in the central airways
Tracheal stenosis
Settings
F_{IO_2} .30–.50
Tidal volume 5–7 mL/kg
Rate 15–18 breaths per min
Peak flow 60 L/min
Controlled mechanical ventilation
Things to consider
Diminished venous return is common in this setting and responds to volume resuscitation
Early sedation and muscle relaxation
Maintain peak airway pressure <55 cmH_2O
Maintain PEEPi <15 cmH_2O
Intentional hypoventilation may be preferable to gas trapping and high airway pressures

Patients with severe airflow obstruction requiring mechanical support are usually extremely anxious and distressed. Sedation should be routine; large quantities of benzodiazepines are frequently required. Muscle relaxation is also advised in most cases during initial management. These interventions help to reduce oxygen consumption (and hence carbon dioxide production), to lower airway pressures, and to relieve patient distress.

The gas exchange abnormalities of airflow obstruction are largely limited to ventilation/perfusion mismatch; an F_{IO_2} of .30 to .50 will achieve arterial saturation in the vast majority of patients.[11] Requirements for a higher F_{IO_2} should prompt a search for an alveolar filling process. The initial tidal volume should be small (5 to 7 mL/kg), and the respiratory rate 12 to 15 breaths per min. A peak flow of 60 L/min is recommended.[10,12] The goals are (1) to minimize peak airway pressures (below 55 cmH_2O), facilitated by lower tidal volumes and sedation with muscle relaxation; (2) to minimize gas trapping at end expiration (see Fig. 127-1) (PEEPi below 15 cmH_2O), facilitated by reduced ventilation and higher flow rates to maximize expiratory time; and (3) to achieve adequate ventilation (as judged by a Pa_{CO_2} of 40 mmHg and a pH of 7.40). During initial management the ventilation should be controlled mechanical ventilation (CMV), so either SIMV or A/C can be used at a mandatory rate sufficient to provide adequate ventilation in the absence of patient effort.

If the ventilator settings suggested above achieve a peak airway pressure of less than 55 cmH_2O and a PEEPi below

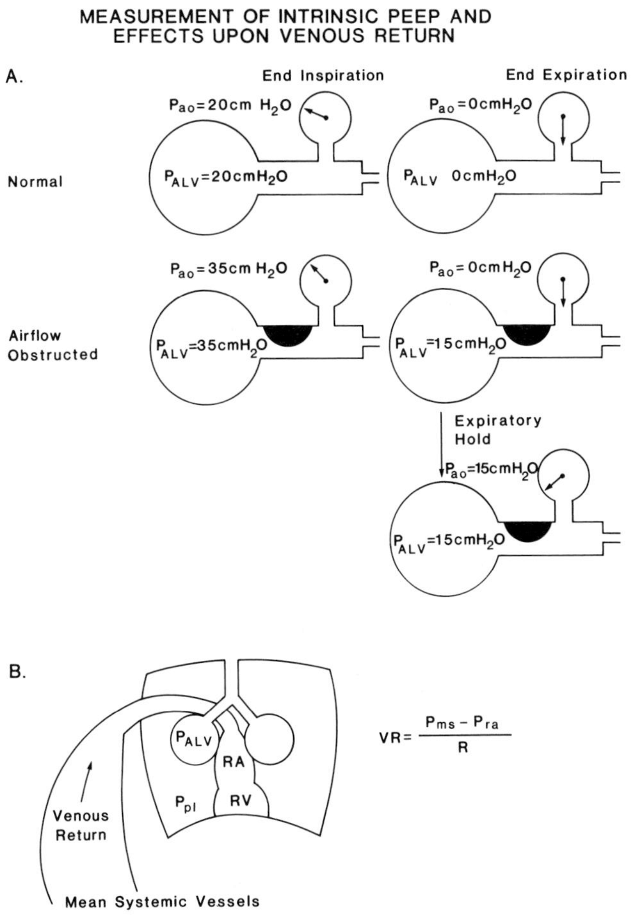

FIGURE 127-1 A. Measurement of intrinsic or "occult" PEEP (PEEPi). During mechanical ventilation of "normal" patients without airflow obstruction, alveolar pressure (Palv) rises during inspiration and, once gas flow ceases at end-inspiration, is equivalent to pressure measured at the airway opening (Pao) and displayed on the ventilator pressure gauge. At end-expiration Palv falls to zero and is equivalent to Pao. With severe airflow obstruction, alveolar emptying is not complete at end expiration and Palv does not fall to zero and is not faithfully measured by Pao. However, prolonging the expiratory period with an expiratory hold maneuver (achieved by occluding the expiratory and inspiratory limbs) will allow continued emptying of alveoli into the central airways. Pao will rise, allowing determination of PEEPi. B. The effects of PEEPi on the circulation. With severe airflow obstruction and gas trapping, PEEPi may be large (>15 cmH_2O), causing an elevation in pleural (Ppl) and right atrial (RA) pressures. Since venous return is determined by the pressure gradient between the systemic vessels and right atrium (Pms − Pra) divided by the resistance to flow (R), substantial elevations of Pra may result in clinically significant reductions of venous return and thus hypoperfusion. This is particularly likely to occur when high levels of minute ventilation are delivered to airway-obstructed patients with either hypovolemia or other causes of low Pms.

15 cmH_2O, barotrauma, in the form of pneumomediastinum, subcutaneous emphysema, and pneumothorax, usually can be avoided. Unfortunately, many patients do not achieve all of the goals outlined. In the face of inadequate ventilation (Pa_{CO_2} much greater than 40 mmHg, with severe acidosis) or excessive gas trapping (PEEPi greater than 15 cmH_2O), it is probably preferable to tolerate higher proximal airway pressures, since in central airway lesions and asthma most of the high pressure dissipates across the relatively robust airways.[10] Thus higher flow rates can be tried in an effort to increase expiratory time (and promote alveolar emptying); or higher tidal volumes can be selected, with lower respiratory rates. Even so, many patients so treated remain hypoventilated. In this setting, intentional hypoventilation may be continued with bicarbonate infusion to correct untoward acidosis (see Chap. 130)—a strategy aimed at avoiding positive-pressure complications, at the cost of inadequate alveolar ventilation.[10]

Since pleural pressure is extremely high in these patients (being proportional to PEEPi plus the effect of each positive-pressure breath), venous return is frequently impaired, with inadequate tissue perfusion (see Fig. 127-1). When this is suspected in a tachycardiac and hypotensive patient, it can be confirmed by disconnecting the sedated and muscle-relaxed patient from the ventilator and noting a flow of gas from the endotracheal tube during the prolonged expiration. This is then associated with a resolution of tachycardia and hypotension over the course of 30 to 60 s. Appropriate circulatory management in these circumstances is massive volume infusion and avoidance of vasodilating drugs (e.g., morphine, nitrates).

Since gas trapping is extreme in these patients, PEEP set on the ventilator confers no benefit and, indeed, has been associated with deterioration of circulatory function.[10,13] Sighs are undesirable. Aggressive chest physiotherapy is mandatory in status asthmaticus, since many patients mobilize mucous plugs during their recovery phase; often these plugs are so large and tenacious as to compromise endotracheal tube patency. Since peak proximal airway pressure is so high in this patient group, upper limit alarms of 55 to as high as 75 cmH_2O (rarely higher) are often required. As noted above, special attention must be paid to inspiratory flow rates and expiratory times in these patients, and the particular flow settings of the ventilator at hand must be carefully monitored. Flow adjustments such as inspiratory flow pattern or inspiratory pause time, which often have minimal effect on the patient without airflow obstruction, can have dramatic impact on this patient group and must not be used in any arbitrary fashion. Inspiratory pause settings should be used *only* when peak and pause pressure measurements are being made in the assessment of lung mechanics. We have encountered inspiratory pauses left in place inadvertently following determination of lung mechanics, with disastrous consequences of worsened hyperinflation and hypoperfusion. Similarly, the descending flow profile commonly used with inverse-ratio ventilation is perverse in reducing the peak-to-pause pressure difference while shortening expiratory time.

PATIENTS WITH ACUTE-ON-CHRONIC RESPIRATORY FAILURE (ACRF)

Acute-on-chronic respiratory failure (ACRF) is a term used to describe the exacerbations of chronic ventilatory failure, often requiring ICU admission, occurring in patients with COPD (see Chap. 129).[14] While most commonly associated with tobacco abuse, irreversible chronic airflow obstruction also occurs in alpha 1 antiprotease deficiency, cystic fibrosis, and, much less commonly, widespread bronchiectasis (see Table 127-3). Unlike patients with status asthmaticus, patients in this population tend to have relatively small increases in inspiratory resistance, with most obstruction occurring with dynamic airway collapse during expiration, although many patients exhibit features of both reversible and irreversible airflow obstruction. As a consequence, in the patient with COPD and minimally reversible airway disease, peak airway pressures on the ventilator tend not to be extraordinarily high, yet dynamic gas trapping, with PEEPi and its consequences, is common (see Fig. 127-1).[15] At the time of intubation and conversion to positive-pressure ventilation, hypoperfusion is common, as manifested by tachycardia and relative hypotension. As in the patient with status asthmaticus, this is almost invariably due to diminished venous return and responds to fluid resuscitation; the fluid requirement in this setting may be substantial.

Since the majority of these patients require mechanical ventilation at a point of worsening hypoventilation—often with clinical evidence of respiratory muscle fatigue—the goal is to rest the patient completely for 36 to 72 h[16] (see Table 127-3). Also, since the patient typically has an underlying compensated respiratory acidosis, eucapnea may range from a Pa_{CO_2} of 45 mmHg to as high as 80 mmHg or more. Excessive ventilation at the time when mechanical support is instituted brings the risk of immediate and severe respiratory alkalosis and, over time, bicarbonate wasting by the kidney, with acid-base homeostasis achieved at a lower Pa_{CO_2} that the patient will be unable to maintain at the time when liberation from mechanical ventilation is sought. The goals of rest and appropriate hypoventilation can usually be achieved with initial ventilator settings of a tidal volume of 6 to 7 mL/kg and a respiratory rate of 24 to 28 breaths per min, with either an SIMV or an A/C mode set on minimal sensitivity. Since gas exchange abnormalities are primarily those of ventilation/perfusion mismatch, supplemental oxygen in the range of an F_{IO_2} of .25 to .40 should achieve better than 90% saturation of arterial hemoglobin. Indeed, gas exchange abnormalities requiring an F_{IO_2} greater than .5 should prompt a search for complicating alveolar filling processes, such as left ventricular failure with pulmonary edema, pneumonia, or lobar collapse. Inspiratory flow rates may be adjusted in accord with resolution of the patient's dyspnea. Measures to prevent atelectasis and its complications (e.g., three-point turning, chest physiotherapy, sighs) are necessary. Since the majority of patients with COPD requiring mechanical ventilatory support have dynamic gas trapping with PEEPi levels of 5 to 10 cmH_2O or higher, there is little benefit to be gained from extrinisic PEEP added as a ventilator intervention to prevent atelectasis. Indeed, even small amounts of extrinsic PEEP have been shown to risk adverse circulatory consequences; this suggests that the distribution of airflow resistances is quite heterogenous, with extrinisic PEEP at levels less than PEEPi causing hyperexpansion of unobstructed lung units.[12,17] However, continuous positive airway pressure (CPAP) may be advantageous during the periods of diminishing ventilator support in this patient group (see below).[18]

The majority of patients with COPD will appear exhausted at the time when mechanical support is instituted and will sleep with minimal breathing efforts. To the extent that muscle fatigue has played a role in a patient's functional decline, rest and sleep are desirable. Two to three days of such rest presumably will restore biochemical and functional changes associated with muscle fatigue (see Chap. 133). Small numbers of patients are difficult to rest on the ventilator, because of continuation of significant effort to trigger breaths. Attempting to trigger all breaths in the face of PEEPi levels of 10 to 15 cmH_2O requires significant patient work, since pleural pressure must be reduced enough to counterbalance the PEEPi level before the patient may trigger a breath.[19] On the other hand, ventilating the patient to a Pa_{CO_2} significantly less than his or her baseline can result in cessation of breathing effort, but causes alkalemia acutely and results in renal bicarbonate wasting—to such an extent that when the patient is finally rested, a protracted period of hypoventilation with gradually increasing bicarbonate stores must be undertaken. This can be a difficult management problem.[20] We advise a careful search for processes that might drive the patient to a respiratory rate higher than is desirable (e.g., hypoperfusion, pleural effusion, pain). Such processes need prompt correction. The ventilator rate should be adjusted to a Pa_{CO_2} resulting in a pH of 7.35 to 7.40. If the patient continues to make significant inspiratory efforts—especially if these efforts are ineffective in actually triggering a machine breath or generating a tidal volume—judicious use of sedation should be considered, although large amounts may be necessary to achieve cessation of respiratory efforts.

TABLE 127-3 Mechanical Ventilation of Patients with Acute-on-Chronic Respiratory Failure

Indications
- Inability to avoid progression to respiratory muscle fatigue

Settings
- F_{IO_2} .25–.40
- Tidal volume 6–8 mL/kg
- Rate 15–18 breaths per min
- SIMV or A/C mode

Things to consider
- Complete rest for 36–72 h
- Diminished venous return with resulting hypoperfusion is common when positive-pressure ventilation is first begun
- Alkalemia from excessive ventilation is common
- Continued effort from triggering the ventilator with PEEPi present may occur and may prevent resolution of fatigue
- PEEP or CPAP may be beneficial at the time the patient begins respiratory muscle exercise

CPAP = continuous positive airway pressure.

PATIENTS WITH ACUTE HYPOXEMIC RESPIRATORY FAILURE (AHRF)

Acute hypoxemic respiratory failure (AHRF) results from diverse processes causing alveolar filling with blood components (see Table 127-4), the end results of which are impaired lung mechanics and gas exchange (see Chap. 128). The gas exchange impairment results from intrapulmonary shunt, is in large part refractory to oxygen therapy, and is the major contributor to respiratory failure requiring mechanical support[21] (see Chaps. 11 and 128).

Patients exhibiting both shock and AHRF at the time that mechanical ventilation is instituted almost always require initial sedation and muscle relaxation. The initial F_{IO_2} should be 1.0. This is necessary in view of the extreme hypoxemia of this patient group, and also confirms the formulation of AHRF, since the initial pulse oximetry or arterial blood gas determinations should reflect a large (i.e., greater than 30 percent) intrapulmonary shunt ($\dot{Q}s/\dot{Q}_T$). The tidal volume should be 6 to 7 mL/kg. The relatively small tidal volume is selected to maintain low ventilating pressures in the face of the restrictive mechanical defect brought on by alveolar filling or collapse, particularly in view of the fact that PEEP will be added to the circuit to achieve a nontoxic F_{IO_2} (see below); recall that these apparently small tidal volumes effect large excursions of the few nonflooded air spaces. There is also experimental evidence that small tidal volumes following acute lung injury may limit further lung injury and intrapulmonary shunt.[22] In order to achieve adequate ventilation, rates of 24 to 28 breaths per min are usually required, as predicted from the tachypnea in these patients. Controlled mechanical ventilation rests the respiratory muscles initially, and can move to either an A/C mode, with low sensitivity (2 cmH_2O), or an SIMV mode after the patient is stabilized.

The majority of patients can be adequately ventilated with marginal, but life-sustaining, oxygen delivery with the mechanical support outlined above. Unfortunately, an F_{IO_2} of 1.0 is toxic itself, causing diffuse alveolar damage akin to that caused by the lesions that require its institution. Therefore, PEEP is added to the ventilator circuit and titrated to a reduction in F_{IO_2} to a nontoxic level (i.e., below .60). We prefer to add PEEP to the circuit with pulse oximetry monitoring in place and following the bedside static lung compliance [C = Tidal Volume/(Pause pressure-PEEP)]. Addition of PEEP results in redistribution of fluid from the alveolar to the interstitial compartment, with recruitment of flooded and collapsed alveoli.[23] This alveolar recruitment results in an increase in lung compliance that parallels the improvement in gas exchange. With each incremental increase in PEEP, alveolar recruitment—and, hence, increment in compliance—tends to occur within 5 to 10 breaths. Thus, we add PEEP in 5-cmH_2O increments while measuring compliance 30 to 60 s following each change. If compliance increases with a given increase in PEEP, indicated by the pause pressure's rising by less than the amount of PEEP added to the expiratory circuit, further increments are made until compliance is noted to "plateau" or fall. This indicates a falloff in alveolar recruitment and lung hyperinflation without improvement in gas exchange. Indeed, at this point increases in pleural and right atrial pressure are often of sufficient degree to compromise venous return and cause hypoperfusion, heralded by tachycardia and hypotension, for which the patient must be monitored throughout the PEEP titration.

This approach has been described by some authors as a means of attaining "best PEEP," defined as the greatest oxygen delivery ($\dot{Q}_{O_2}$).[24] We would modify it further, for the goal is not strictly the PEEP to achieve the best $\dot{Q}_{O_2}$, but rather the least PEEP to achieve 90% saturation on a nontoxic F_{IO_2}; this minimizes airway pressures and lung inflation to prevent diverse forms of barotrauma, and is further aided by reducing further the tidal volume. Note that the distinction here is that "least" PEEP is less than "best" PEEP when a reduction in $\dot{Q}_{O_2}$ below the maximum level is acceptable. Once the "neighborhood" of ideal PEEP has been identified by the bedside compliance measurements described above, the F_{IO_2} can be decreased while following arterial saturation with pulse oximetry. Once an F_{IO_2} of .60 is achieved, PEEP can be decreased to the least amount necessary to maintain an arterial hemoglobin saturation of 90% as determined by arterial blood gases.

These guidelines can usually be met with PEEP levels of 10 to 20 cmH_2O. With the use of small tidal volumes as described above, and in the absence of coincident airway disease (e.g., in a burn patient with both airway thermal injury and inhalation-induced ARDS), peak airway pressures can usually be maintained at 45 cmH_2O or less. In contrast to acceptable peak airway pressures in status asthmaticus (see above), it is important to maintain airway pressures in AHRF at less than 45 to 50 cmH_2O to avoid barotrauma. This is because there is little dissipation of pressure across large airways, and the monitored peak airway pressure reflects closely the pressure and hyperinflation occurring at an alveolar level.

TABLE 127-4 Mechanical Ventilation of Patients with Acute Hypoxemic Respiratory Failure

Indications
- Failure to maintain adequate arterial hemoglobin saturation via O_2 and positive pressure delivered by mask, and/or tachypnea and dyspnea predicting imminent respiratory muscle fatigue

Settings
- F_{IO_2} initially 1.0
- Tidal volume 6–7 mL/kg
- Rate 24–28 breaths per min
- SIMV or A/C with minimal sensitivity
- PEEP titrated at the bedside while following lung compliance, O_2 saturation, and blood pressure

Things to consider
- Least PEEP achieving 90% saturation of an adequate arterial hemoglobin on a nontoxic ($\leq$.60) F_{IO_2}
- Least pulmonary capillary wedge pressure consistent with an adequate cardiac output
- In lobar pneumonia, PEEP may not improve and may increase intrapulmonary shunt

Once specimens have been collected from the airway for microbiologic and other studies, it is useful not to "break" PEEP in patients with ARDS. This is because many patients quickly (even in the course of briefly suctioning the airway) can become extremely hypoxemic. This supports multiple observations that PEEP does not reduce lung water but rather redistributes it at a short distance from alveoli, although sufficiently far from the air-blood interface to improve gas exchange.[23] It is often necessary to inform novice nursing and respiratory therapy staff to resist the temptation to clear the airway and ventilator tubing of the ARDS patient of edema fluid. Each discontinuation of PEEP allows rapid alveolar flooding and, often, airway flooding, thus creating a self-fulfilling prophecy to the care giver attempting to clear edema fluid. A number of modified suctioning adapters are available to provide a route to the airway without removing positive pressure, although most tend to leak at PEEP levels above 15 cmH_2O.

Sighs and other measures to prevent atelectasis are not necessary during the acute phases of AHRF, when PEEP levels are typically in excess of 10 cmH_2O. It should be remembered that these patients are at risk of atelectasis as they improve and PEEP levels are decreased. This is probably due, in part, to surfactant deficiency during the recovery from diffuse alveolar damage, and will certainly be aggravated by the use of small tidal volumes. Strategies to avoid this include increasing the tidal volume as $\dot{Q}s/\dot{Q}_T$ falls below 20 percent and PEEP levels are decreased below 10 cmH_2O. Tidal volumes as high as 12 mL/kg may be used as long as peak airway pressure remains below 45 cmH_2O.

The ventilator management outlined above may be considered routine therapy for AHRF arising from diffuse lung lesions. Circulatory management directed at reducing edemagenesis and decreasing the duration of this supportive therapy is described in Chap. 128.[25,26] Other forms of ventilator management have been proposed by some authors; these include inverse ratio ventilation (IRV—see Chap. 9)[27] and high frequency ventilation (HFV—see Chap. 1). It is not clear if IRV confers any benefit apart from PEEP, which in this mode arises as PEEPi resulting from the shortened expiratory times.[28] As compared to routine ventilator management, HFV[29] or continuous flow ventilation[30] does not allow any reduction in mean lung volume or alveolar pressure for a given reduction in $\dot{Q}s/\dot{Q}_T$. This mode of ventilation does offer the theoretical benefit, however, of causing relatively small pressure oscillations as compared to conventional modes. This may result in less potentiation of lung injury, as discussed above.[22] At the present time, however, it must be viewed as an experimental approach to management of these clinical problems.

While some recent descriptive studies have pointed to a degree of inhomogeneity in ARDS, a number of disease processes producing AHRF are distinctly inhomogeneous—a characteristic that may require modification of ventilator management. Acute bacterial lobar pneumonia is the prototype of such inhomogeneous lung disease. Despite consolidation of a single lobe receiving only 20 percent of ventilation prior to infection, shunts of 40 percent or greater can be encountered, since pulmonary arterial flow to the infected lobe rises almost twofold and the bacteria and neutrophils that are part of the inflammatory infiltrate consume oxygen themselves, further desaturating blood flowing from the lobe.[31] While initial management including an F_{IO_2} of 1.0, small tidal volumes, and rapid ventilatory rates is appropriate in treating these forms of AHRF, a caution should be raised about PEEP therapy: Since the consolidated lung segments have a markedly reduced compliance in comparison to uninvolved lung, addition of PEEP may simply hyperexpand normal lung segments. In fact, it is possible that alveolar pressure in normal lung segments could be increased sufficiently with PEEP therapy to exceed pulmonary arterial pressure, with the potential of blood flow's being further shunted from normally ventilated lung, with further deterioration in gas exchange.[31]

Patients with focal lung disease, such as lobar pneumonia, should have a cautious trial of PEEP, since these lesions are often associated with more diffuse lung edema and atelectasis that may not be completely apparent radiologically. The clinician must be prepared to abandon PEEP therapy, however, if there is no improvement in $\dot{Q}s/\dot{Q}_T$. In these circumstances, positioning of the patient with the lung infiltrate uppermost, and/or hyperventilating the patient to shift the oxyhemoglobin curve to the left, may provide short-term improvement in arterial saturation (see Chap. 11).

PATIENTS WITH OTHER RESTRICTIVE PROCESSES

While homogeneous lung disease producing AHRF, such as ARDS in its early, exudative phase, represents a restrictive mechanical defect of the lung, management is directed largely at the gas exchange abnormality. A number of lung and chest wall diseases, however, can produce a severe restrictive defect that with small additional insults (e.g., pneumonia) can result in respiratory failure requiring mechanical support (see Table 127-5). Lung fibrosis in advanced stages, severe kyphoscoliosis, obesity, and intraabdominal processes such as massive ascites and intraperitoneal hemorrhage are examples of this mechanical load on the respiratory system. The other form of severe restrictive disease commonly encountered by the intensivist is ARDS in its late, proliferative phase. This can develop in as short a time as 10 to 14 days following acute lung injury, and is characterized by pulmonary fibrosis, often with cessation of the initiating pulmonary capillary leak.

These patients are best managed with small tidal volumes (6 to 7 mL/kg) and rapid ventilatory rates (18 to 24 breaths per min). The F_{IO_2} requirement will be determined by the degree of alveolar filling or collapse, if any. On very rare occasions we have encountered patients with enormous restrictive loads from intraabdominal catastrophes (e.g., massive intraperitoneal bleeding following obstetric complications) with large intrapulmonary shunts despite insignificant alveolar flooding present on chest radiograph. We speculate that in such patients large numbers of alveo-

TABLE 127-5 Mechanical Ventilation of Patients with Restrictive Disease

Indications
- Acute insult (e.g., pneumonia), or complicating restrictive lung (e.g., pulmonary fibrosis) or chest wall (e.g., kyphoscoliosis) disease
- Proliferative-phase ARDS
- Rarely, massive and tense fluid collection in the abdomen

Settings
- F_{IO_2} .30–.50
- Tidal volume 6–7 mL/kg
- Rate 18–24 breaths per min
- SIMV or A/C mode

Things to consider
- Measures to relieve restriction (e.g., escharotomy, abdominal tap)
- Benefit of upright posture for intraabdominal processes
- This patient group is prone to increased physiologic dead space if high minute ventilation and PEEP is used and relative hypovolemia exists

lar units may be at a thoracic gas volume below the closing volume of their associated airways throughout the tidal volume range, with these nonventilated units producing a large intrapulmonary shunt.

A number of interventions may be undertaken to correct these restrictive abnormalities. Acute eschar formations of the chest wall resulting in entrapment require emergent escharotomy. Massive free fluid collections in the abdomen may be tapped. Finally, the obese patient may be managed in an upright or semi-upright position to minimize the restrictive effect of abdominal contents on diaphragm excursion.

These patients are particularly prone to creation of physiologic dead space via attempts to increase minute ventilation with increased ventilatory rates or tidal volumes. Alveolar pressures may rise above pulmonary arterial pressure in nondependent portions of the lung during positive-pressure ventilation (particularly if PEEP is also being used) in these patients. The result is increased West Zone I conditions, or physiologic dead space. The same increase in minute ventilation can raise mean intrathoracic pressure to a level that compromises venous return (see Fig. 127-1) with diminished cardiac output. This, in turn, can cause a fall in arterial saturation if mixed venous P_{O_2} falls and substantial ventilation/perfusion mismatch or shunt exists within the lung. In extreme circumstances, increasing tidal volume, rate, and PEEP in these patients causes Pa_{O_2} to fall and Pa_{CO_2} to rise, and eventually leads to hypoperfusion. This circumstance must be recognized, since progressive increases in minute ventilation or PEEP can be life-threatening. The appropriate course is correction of hypovolemia and reduction of minute ventilation and PEEP (see Chap. 52). Right heart catheterization may be indicated in selected patients, to guide fluid and ventilator management.

Facilitating Patient Comfort and Communication

Ideally the mechanically ventilated patient should be alert, comfortable, and capable of communicating with the health care team to provide assessment of neurologic and gastrointestinal function, so that complications of critical illness may be identified at the earliest possible time (see Chap. 52). These desirable goals must be weighed against the need to heavily sedate, and even muscle-relax, some patients with cardiovascular instability, severely compromised oxygen delivery to peripheral tissues, and severe airflow obstruction (see above and Table 127-6).

A number of points regarding the use of sedation and muscle relaxants need to be made. Whenever muscle relaxation is undertaken, the agent should be withdrawn on a daily basis until evidence of neuromuscular transmission and function returns, to prevent excessive drug accumulation. Cases that involve impaired renal and hepatic function call for muscle relaxation with continuous infusions of vecuronium or atracurium; the same approach of the least dose of medication should be pursued. Whenever muscle relaxation is attempted, careful assessment of the level of sedation should be conducted frequently (see Chaps. 82 and 83). This is particularly true when infusions of midazolam or fentanyl are used for a long time, since the adequate dose of medication can be extremely difficult to predict in a given patient.

When patients improve and muscle relaxation is no longer necessary, and underlying gas exchange or ventilatory abnormalities are sufficiently improved to begin assessment for discontinuation of mechanical ventilation, those individuals who have received high doses of sedation for prolonged periods may require a slow taper of medication and, if they are opiate-dependent, institution of methadone. Patients should be kept maximally alert during daylight hours, with sedation limited, if possible, to evening hours. Use of short-acting benzodiazepines or haloperidol may facilitate sleep, keeping the patient maximally rested for efforts directed at discontinuation of mechanical support during the day. Much excessive sedation can be avoided by frequent communication between care giver and patient; frequent reassurance of the patient; and identification of sources of pain and anxiety, with attention di-

TABLE 127-6 Indications for Sedation and Muscle Relaxation During Mechanical Ventilation

- Hypoperfusion with lactic acidosis
- Status asthmaticus or other airway disease with high airway pressures and PEEPi
- Acute hypoxemic respiratory failure with cardiovascular instability and/or toxic F_{IO_2} despite use of PEEP
- Control of central neurogenic hyperventilation
- ACRF with high PEEPi and a struggling patient

ACRF = acute-on-chronic respiratory failure.

rected at specific causes rather than global sedation for apparent agitation.

Response to "Crises" in the Mechanically Ventilated Patient

A vast array of sudden and potentially catastrophic changes in clinical condition can occur in the course of mechanical ventilation. A number of these problems are discussed in Chap. 52. We will focus on two sources of difficulty that are typically signaled not only by patient distress, but by ventilator alarms as well—alarms warning of excessively low or high airway pressures.

In all circumstances in which the function of the ventilator, the position and patency of the airway, or the possibility of air leak have to be determined urgently, the patient must be removed from the ventilator and hand-bagged with 100% oxygen. This point is extremely important, since this maneuver circumvents ventilator malfunction immediately, provides the clinician with direct subjective information concerning any changes in the patient's lung mechanics, focuses attention on the patient and not the machine, and avoids the distractions that even an experienced individual encounters in troubleshooting a complex device.

Low-pressure alarms signal machine malfunction, inadvertent low tidal volume setting, or a leak within the system. Large persistent leaks can occur within the ventilator itself, at the inspiratory outflow port, along the inspiratory tubing, at the connection to the Y-adapter and endotracheal tube, around the endotracheal tube cuff, or through a bronchopleural fistula drained by a chest tube. Removing the patient from the ventilator, attaching an ambu bag directly to the endotracheal tube, and observing normal resistance indicates that neither the patient nor the artificial airway is the source of the leak. While the patient is being ventilated manually, a methodical search will identify the problem within the ventilator or connecting tubing. If hand-bagging indicates minimal resistance and adequate ventilation is difficult to achieve, an endotracheal tube cuff leak or a bronchopleural fistula is suggested. Neck auscultation and a hand placed over the mouth will identify large cuff leaks; failure to achieve a seal with reinflation of the cuff requires urgent reintubation. A large bronchopleural fistula can be identified by inspection of the chest tube and pleural drainage system.

Excluding alarm or gauge malfunction, sudden increases in airway pressure signaled by the machine's alarm indicate obstruction of the artificial airway, obstruction to gas flow through the expiratory limb, patient effort opposing the machine-delivered breath ("bucking" or "fighting" the ventilator), or sudden changes in the mechanics of the respiratory system. Removing the patient from the ventilator for manual ventilation allows appropriate focus on the airway and patient. If bagging is difficult, a suction catheter should be immediately passed through the endotracheal tube. If the catheter cannot be advanced 25 cm or more, obstruction is likely. If changing the head position does not relieve kinking, and obstruction is not due to biting, emergent reintubation is necessary. If the patient is biting an endotracheal tube placed orally, a bite block should be placed and the evaluation of tube patency repeated. If the patient is capable of biting despite a block, a short-acting muscle relaxant should be administered.

If the airway is patent and the patient extremely difficult to ventilate manually, a muscle relaxant should be given if the patient is making strenuous efforts to breathe. If this eliminates the difficulty with bagging, then the cause(s) of the patient's earlier desperate breathing efforts should be sought. Possibilities to be excluded immediately include hypoxemia, hypercapnea, shock, and a new central nervous system process.

Persistent difficulty with bagging in a muscle-relaxed patient with a patent endotracheal tube suggests that a new process in the airway, pleura, lung, or chest wall is raising the resistive or elastic pressures associated with ventilation. Auscultation, palpation, and percussion often identify pneumothorax, or collapse and/or consolidation, on the affected side; early portable chest radiography confirms these diagnoses and/or identifies new etiologies of the crisis (see Chaps. 16 and 19). Placing the patient back on the ventilator and measuring peak and plateau pressures as well as PEEPi will help determine whether the problem is resistive or elastic. A high peak-to-plateau gradient with PEEPi suggests airflow obstruction; bronchospasm or other obstructing process should be considered. A high plateau pressure in this setting suggests a tension pneumothorax or new process in the parenchyma of the lung.

Liberation of the Patient from the Mechanical Ventilator

For purposes of focus, we refer to the process of discontinuation of mechanical ventilatory support not as "weaning"—which connotes the withdrawal of a benign and nurturing life-support system—but rather as "liberation," connoting release from a confining, limiting, and dangerous circumstance.[1] The complications associated with mechanical ventilation are legion, and are best avoided or minimized by aggressive efforts to shorten the duration of this therapeutic intervention.

By use of the pathophysiologic categories given above, it is often possible to make early identification of patients with resolvable underlying problems who can rapidly make the transition to spontaneous breathing. The patient with normal lung function but superimposed transient central nervous system depression (e.g., drug overdose) or transient weakness (e.g., myasthenia gravis) often requires ventilatory support for a short period of time and therefore does not suffer the pulmonary, circulatory, nutritional, and metabolic complications that make a return to spontaneous breathing a protracted endeavor. Thus, when the drive to breathe returns (as signaled by the patient's consistent triggering of the ventilator) or strength becomes adequate (as signaled by a vital capacity in excess of 1 L), spontaneous breathing should be resumed. Of course, decisions to extubate remain apart from discontinuation of the ventilator. Extubation requires sufficient levels of consciousness and strength in the patient to ensure (1) airway reflexes, to prevent aspiration; (2) maintenance of a patent airway; (3) adequate cough; and (4) adequate clearance of secretions.

Similarly, patients ventilated for hypoperfused states (e.g., sepsis, cardiogenic shock) may be returned to spontaneous breathing promptly upon stabilization of the circulation, provided that multiorgan dysfunction has not supervened. When patients who have been hyperventilated for central nervous system injury have stabilized or improved, ventilation should be reduced gradually (e.g., over 2 to 3 days), thus avoiding a rapid increase in Pa_{CO_2} with large increases in cerebral blood flow and the potential for intracranial pressure to rise to undesirable levels. If central nervous system improvement persists over the period of return to normal minute ventilation, and the drive to breathe is intact, then the transition to spontaneous breathing can often be accomplished promptly.

Patients with severe airflow obstruction due to status asthmaticus often improve over 1 to 3 days with bronchodilators, corticosteroids, and clearance of mucous plugs. If neither complicating pneumonia, lobar collapse, nor neuromuscular weakness has occurred, sedation and muscle relaxation should be held as airway pressures fall to 30 to 40 cmH_2O. Very brief trials (20 min) of spontaneous breathing, with either a T-piece, CPAP, or pressure support (PS), are then appropriate, followed promptly by extubation. We prefer not to delay this process, since prolonged breathing through the endotracheal tube can be associated with worsening bronchospasm. Patients with upper airway obstruction secondary to burn injury or mass should have bronchoscopic evaluation. With mass lesions, surgical or laser bronchoscopy may restore the airway luman sufficiently to permit a return to spontaneous ventilation. Again, the fall in proximal airway pressures during mechanical ventilation should help to identify the point at which resistive load has been substantially reduced.

Finally, some patients with acute hypoxemic respiratory failure have a reduction in lung shunt over 1 to 3 days (e.g., by successful circulatory management of ARDS or resolution of lobar pneumonia) to a level such that supplemental oxygen delivered by mask or nasal cannula would be sufficient to maintain arterial hemoglobin saturation at 90% or higher. This usually correlates to an intrapulmonary shunt of 20% or less with the use of PEEP at 5 cmH_2O or less. These patients, too, may have a brief trial of spontaneous breathing with CPAP or PS and then be evaluated for extubation.

MANAGEMENT OF THE "DIFFICULT-TO-WEAN" PATIENT

Most patients with chronic lung disease and superimposed acute lung insult (e.g., ACRF or restrictive lung disease—see above) or acute respiratory failure with more than 3 to 4 days of mechanical ventilatory support require a more gradual return to spontaneous breathing. In the case of chronic lung disease, this is due in part to the markedly reduced pulmonary reserve with which the patient entered the current bout of respiratory failure. In all patients, ongoing ventilator dependence is likely related to cumulative intercurrent complications; the high work of breathing that may exist despite apparently "full" ventilatory support (with the potential for progression to, or failure to recover from, respiratory muscle fatigue); and a component of muscle atrophy that may develop during mechanical support.[20,32]

All such patients benefit from an approach that initially assesses both respiratory load and neuromuscular competence, with a guiding awareness that ongoing ventilator dependence results from weakness relative to the load on the respiratory system. As long as this remains true, the patient requires mechanical support while he or she is being strengthened and while loads are identified and reduced. As the balance tips more favorably, increasing amounts of respiratory effort can be expected of the patient, and thus a program of progressive exercise and conditioning can be fashioned within the limits of the patient's strength and endurance.

The initial conditions that must be met in all patients (see Table 127-7) prior to consideration of "weaning" are acceptable gas exchange (acceptable oxygen saturation with $F_{I_{O_2}}$ 0.5 or less, PEEP 7.5 cmH_2O or less, and acceptable Pa_{CO_2} and pH when minute ventilation is not excessive); adequate drive and ability to breathe (as indicated by regular triggering of the ventilator); and a stable circulation.

The first respiratory "load" to be assessed is the minute ventilation ($\dot{V}_E$) (see Table 127-8). Ideally, $\dot{V}_E$ should be 10 L/min or less; high levels of $\dot{V}_E$ represent a large ventilatory demand, since the relationship of $\dot{V}_E$ to work of breathing is nonlinear. Nonetheless, some patients with excellent respiratory muscle function can be liberated from mechanical ventilation with $\dot{V}_E$ as high as 15 to 20 L/min. $\dot{V}_E$ above 10 L/min should prompt consideration of (1) large dead-space fraction (e.g., emphysema, pulmonary embolus, Zone I lung conditions); (2) high oxygen consumption (e.g., sepsis, fever, overfeeding, excessive muscle activity); (3) high respiratory quotient (e.g., feeding with excessive carbohydrates); or (4) hyperventilation (e.g., metabolic acidosis, pain, anxiety).

For any given $\dot{V}_E$, the patient should then be assessed for the mechanical load imposed by resistive and elastic factors of the respiratory system (see Fig. 127-2).[33] This is easily accomplished by ventilating the patient briefly at a low tidal volume (4 to 6 mL/kg) and a rate slightly above that neces-

TABLE 127-7 Necessary Conditions for Consideration of Discontinuation of Mechanical Ventilation

Stable circulation and absence of myocardial ischemia, sepsis, and uncontrolled acidosis
Adequate pulmonary O_2 exchange as evidenced by Sa_{O_2} >90% with $F_{I_{O_2}}$ <0.5 and PEEP <7.5 cmH_2O
Adequate ability to ventilate spontaneously (V_T >5 mL/kg, VC = 3 × V_T, NIF >30 cmH_2O, and f <36 per min)
Absence of excessive respiratory load

TABLE 127-8 Causes of Increased Minute Ventilation

Large dead space fraction	
	Emphysema
	Pulmonary embolus
	Zone I lung conditions
High oxygen consumption	
	Sepsis
	Fever
	Overfeeding
	Excessive muscle activity
High respiratory quotient	
	Excessive carbohydrate feeding
Hyperventilation	
	Pain
	Anxiety
	Metabolic acidosis

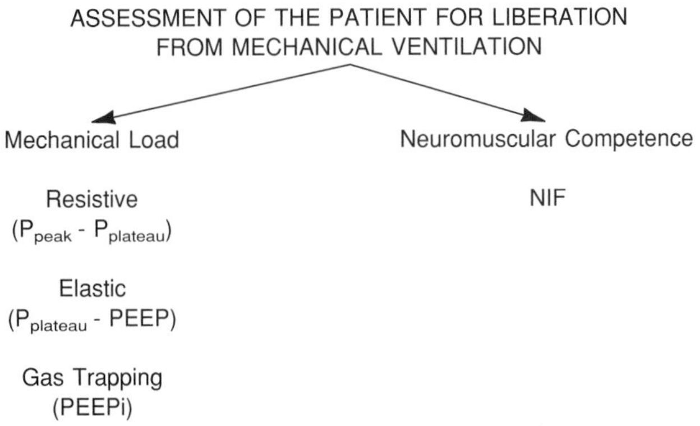

FIGURE 127-2 Assessment of patients for liberation from mechanical ventilation. When gas exchange is suitable, minute ventilation not excessive, and drive to breathe present, it is appropriate to judge neuromuscular competence relative to the mechanical load imposed upon the respiratory muscles. P_{peak} = peak airway pressure measured on the ventilator; $P_{plateau}$ = plateau or static pressure measured at end inspiration; PEEPi = intrinsic PEEP measured with end expiratory hold maneuver; NIF = negative inspiratory force. See text for details.

sary to meet $\dot{V}_E$ and cause inspiratory muscle efforts, as judged at the bedside, to cease. Peak, plateau (end-inspiratory), and PEEPi (end-expiratory) pressure measurements are then made. A high peak-to-plateau pressure gradient indicates a resistive load; attention should be directed toward relief of bronchospasm, treatment of excessive airway secretions, central airway obstructions, congestive heart failure with "cardiac asthma," and the patency of the artificial airway. The latter point is important. Endotracheal tube resistance is directly related to the length of the tube and inversely related to the fourth power of the radius. Despite the fact that large (e.g., 8- to 9-mm) tubes yield a resistance of only a 3 to 7 cmH_2O/L per s when measured in vitro, much higher resistances have been demonstrated in acutely ill patients, presumably because of kinking and encrustation of the tube.[34] This problem can be identified by the airway resistance's varying with head position, or by direct inspection of the airway. If a large resistance is conferred by the airway, changing the endotracheal tube should be considered. In all patients, some degree of pressure support during spontaneous breathing should be considered to overcome this fixed airway resistance.[8,20]

High plateau pressures signal diminished respiratory system compliance and should prompt consideration of lung parenchymal abnormalities (e.g., pulmonary edema, lung fibrosis, infection) or chest wall stiffness (e.g., obesity, splinting, ascites) (see Fig. 127-2). Pulmonary edema often responds to appropriate fluid and diuretic management, and intraabdominal contributions to respiratory system stiffness can be minimized by tapping fluid, controlling pain with splinting, and putting the patient in the upright position.

High PEEPi levels usually signal significant expiratory airflow obstruction, sometimes exacerbated by high $\dot{V}_E$ and active expiratory muscle contraction at end expiration. When PEEPi is very high (10 cmH_2O or higher), airflow obstruction is usually severe enough to preclude efforts at spontaneous ventilation, since the patient must drop pleural pressure by at least this amount before he or she is able to trigger a breath or initiate inspiratory gas flow. The hyperinflation associated with high PEEPi may also contribute to diminished respiratory system compliance and result in diminished inspiratory muscle efficiency. While treatment of the causes of PEEPi is clearly desirable, it is not necessary to eliminate all positive alveolar pressure at end expiration, since it is present in many stable ambulatory patients with COPD.[35] Strategies to decrease PEEPi include treatment of airway disease and prolongation of expiratory time by reducing $\dot{V}_E$ and inspiratory time. During periods of exercise, the adverse effects of PEEPi on energy expenditure may be reduced by using PEEP (in a patient who is triggering the ventilator) or by using CPAP (in a spontaneously breathing patient).[18,20]

Respiratory muscle strength may be assessed by measurement of the negative inspiratory force (NIF) (see Fig. 127-2). This measurement is accomplished by occlusion of the airway with a manometer in place, after informing the patient and coaching him or her as to how to make a maximal inspiratory effort from functional residual capacity. It is often necessary to maintain occlusion of the airway for a prolonged period (up to 30 s) to obtain a maximal patient effort.[36] While some studies have indicated poor reproducibility of this measurement,[37] and its exact relationship to "weaning" is imperfectly understood, we find the trends in an individual patient useful in guiding the health care team through the causes of ventilator dependence. Admittedly, this measurement at best correlates to muscle strength and does not inform one as to endurance. Assessments of respiratory work loads as they relate to the patient's endurance and the likelihood of progressing to fatigue can be made from measurements such as the pressure-time index of the respiratory system, although these parameters are not routinely available at the bedside[20,38] (see Chap. 133). Alternatively, the NIF can be readily measured daily in advance of judgments regarding the level of mechanical support appropriate for a given patient. A markedly reduced NIF (30 cmH_2O or less) should prompt a search for causes of muscle weakness (see Fig. 127-2).

Most often the causes of diminished strength or endurance prove to be multifactorial, but a number of generalizations can be made. Since respiratory muscle function depends on adequate supplies of energy substrates and oxygen, it is important that the patient have adequate perfusion and reasonable arterial oxygen content—particularly if there is underlying muscle weakness and an increased mechanical load upon the respiratory system. We have encountered patients in whom underlying hypoperfusion related to sepsis first manifested itself as failure to tolerate increased work of breathing as ventilatory support was withdrawn, and others in whom severe right or left ventricular dysfunction with an essentially fixed cardiac output became apparent as "weaning" from the ventilator was attempted. In patients with borderline adequacy of perfusion, a rapid deterioration during attempts to diminish mechanical support is often encountered[39] (see Fig. 127-3). Other extremely important causes of muscle weakness include electrolyte disturbances, most prominently hypokalemia, hypocalcemia, hypomagnesemia, and hypophosphatemia.[1,40,41] These abnormalities must be aggressively sought, since they often contribute to weakness, can be corrected relatively quickly, and frequently arise during the course of nutritional support necessary in patients requiring prolonged mechanical ventilation.[42]

Finally, muscle fatigue may contribute to weakness and diminished endurance in these patients well after their initial days on the ventilator. A number of investigations have demonstrated that respiratory muscle contraction is unlikely to cease in most patients receiving mechanical ventilation, despite a variety of ventilator adjustments (see above); indeed, in many modes of ventilation the patient's work of breathing may be substantial.[20,42] Thus it is possible that a weak patient will remain weak, through continued breathing effort, despite the institution of mechanical support.[43] This can be difficult to discern clinically. Clues that this might be occurring include the use of accessory muscles; persistence of a sense of dyspnea, despite mechanical support; and observation of the patient's "sucking down" the measured proximal airway pressure, so that it varies significantly from breath to breath (i.e., by more than 5 cmH_2O) as the patient either assists or resists tidal volume delivery. When this degree of patient effort is noted, interventions that may be helpful are increased inspiratory flow, smaller tidal volumes with higher rates, and, in the patient with PEEPi, use of PEEP or CPAP. When this phenomenon is sufficient to induce weakness, it is often necessary to sedate the patient to allow recovery of respiratory muscle function.

The relationship between the NIF, as a measure of muscle strength, and load upon the respiratory system has been investigated in a limited number of normal individuals in an inspiratory loading model[44] (see Chap. 133). When the pressure cost of breathing is less than 30 to 40 percent of the NIF, normal individuals are able to sustain spontaneous breathing; when the pressure cost of tidal volume generation rises above this level, the time to fatigue progressively shortens. Accordingly, we match the measured NIF against the measured airway pressures, roughly estimating that an NIF 2 to 3 times greater than the peak pressure with each breath will be necessary before spontaneous breathing can be sustained indefinitely. While this approach is somewhat crude, it is certainly readily applied at the bedside on a day-to-day basis. Other measures of patient status during discontinuation of mechanical ventilation, such as occlusion pressure at the airway opening, external pressure–volume work, and oxygen cost of breathing, are relatively difficult to obtain on a routine clinical basis and, for the present, remain largely research tools.[20,45,46]

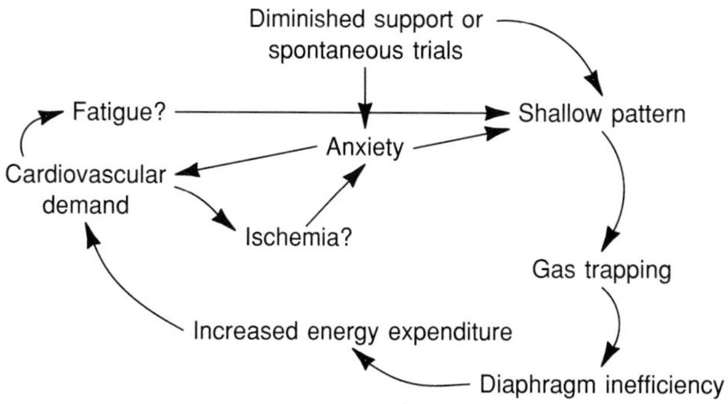

FIGURE 127-3 The cycle of cardiopulmonary instability that often arises during attempts to "wean." As mechanical support is diminished or the patient is placed on spontaneous ventilation, increased cardiovascular demands are made by exercising respiratory muscles. Anxiety often compounds this demand, and sympathetic drive may result in tachycardia, dysrhythmias, hypertension, or otherwise precipitate myocardial ischemia. The rapid breathing pattern typical of these patients coupled to severe airflow obstruction may result in gas trapping, diaphragm inefficiency, and further increases in energy expenditure. To the extent that cardiovascular reserves are limited (e.g., valvular heart disease, cardiomyopathy, ischemic heart disease), the result may be cardiovascular deterioration signalled by tachycardia, ischemia, or other manifestations. Alternatively, hypoperfusion could theoretically contribute to respiratory muscle dysfunction or fatigue.

Thus, when the NIF is some 2 to 3 times greater than the pressure cost of tidal volume delivery, we predict a high success for spontaneous breathing via a T-piece or CPAP system. Before that balance between strength and load is attained, a number of methods of exercising the patient may be utilized. Of course, very brief trials of spontaneous ventilation may still be tried, but this can initiate a cycle of patient apprehension, hyperventilation, and cardiac instability (see Fig. 127-3) that is uncomfortable to the patient and establishes a fear of physician-directed discontinuation of mechanical support. Alternative approaches utilize an SIMV circuit, with decreasing the number of breaths as a strategy to gradually increase patient effort. In our experience this carries a disadvantage, particularly in the patients most difficult to wean: an irregular breathing pattern, with patient breaths at a much lower tidal volume than is attained with machine breaths. Some patients exhibit a "ledge" at some machine rate below which agitation and the appearance of exhaustion quickly emerge. A useful alternative is to maintain a fixed low tidal volume (e.g., 5 to 7 mL/kg) with an A/C mode and then gradually decrease the sensitivity at which the patient triggers the ventilator, increasing patient effort in accord with what would be predictable on the basis of measurement of muscle strength (e.g., sensitivity during periods of exercise set at one-third of the NIF). This method of exercising the patient attains a more constant ventilatory pattern, but does carry the theoretical disadvantage of "front-loading" respiratory effort so that the patient must make a relatively large inspiratory effort prior to initiating gas flow. For this reason we do not advocate setting the trigger in excess of 6 to 7 cmH_2O, even in the relatively strong patient, since larger initial inspiratory efforts are likely to result in discomfort. Another alternative strategy calls for PS as a means of exercising the patient, with the level of support adjusted to attain a reasonable spontaneous tidal volume (e.g., 300 to 500 mL) and respiratory rate (under 30 breaths per min). The PS level can then be gradually decreased as deemed necessary to increase patient effort. A convenient measure of success during this period is to track the tidal volume and respiratory rate, since patient fatigue and inadequate levels of pressure support almost invariably are signaled by gradually increasing respiratory rates and shallow breaths. This method of "weaning" may become our standard, although clinical trials to date have not documented a clear benefit from this ventilator mode[43,47] (see Chap. 9).

In many ways the specific modes used to exercise the patient are irrelevant, as long as the patient is kept comfortable and adequately ventilated and the exercise can be graded so as to strengthen, and not fatigue, the patient. Indeed, it is useful to be familiar with a number of different "modes," since the patient's preference can then dictate which one is used in a particular circumstance. During the period of exercise it is crucial that the patient be rested in the evening, ideally with normal periods of sleep, and that exercise be restricted to defined periods during the day that are gradually increased in length. The improvements in lung mechanics and strength are documented by daily bedside measuments of airway pressures and NIF, with therapy titrated according to these measurements. This is also an excellent strategy to involve the patient in the process of discontinuing mechanical ventilation, since there are often components of frustration, fear, and depression related to dependence on this life-support system. The patient can be informed of the daily progress, the activity planned for the day, and the methodical approach to abnormalities that have been identified. In this fashion a participation is fostered that challenges the patient but is not overwhelming, and that facilitates the patient's earliest possible return to spontaneous breathing.

CASE PRESENTATION

A 56-year-old alcoholic man with a long history of tobacco use was involved in a home fire caused by his smoking in bed. He was brought to the emergency room, unconscious, with 35 to 40 percent second- and third-degree burns of the chest, abdominal wall, and left upper extremity. There were perioral facial burns, singed nasal hairs, and carbonaceous sputum. Direct inspection of the airway revealed marked thermal injury of the upper airway with significant edema. He was promptly intubated. Carbon monoxide poisoning and a structural central nervous system lesion were excluded, and he was moved to the ICU. An initial alcohol level of 280 mg/dL was noted.

His initial exam was remarkable for a pulse of 124 per min and a blood pressure of 110/80 mmHg. There was no complete eschar restricting chest excursion. The lungs revealed diffuse wheezing during bag ventilation. The extremities were cold and nailbed return poor. Bagging was notable for significant resistance. The patient was connected to the ventilator with an F_{IO_2} of 1.0, rate of 20, tidal volume of 700 mL, with an A/C mode. The patient seemed to be making struggling efforts; diazepam, 10 mg twice, and then pancuronium, 8 mg, were given intravenously. Respiratory efforts ceased and the patient received controlled ventilation. Almost immediately the heart rate rose to 160 and the blood pressure fell to 80/60. When the patient was briefly disconnected from the ventilator at end expiration there was a rush of air, and the blood pressure began to rise. The patient was slowly bagged with 100% oxygen while 3 L of crystalloid were rapidly infused and the maintenance fluids increased beyond the initial Parkland formula prediction. At this point the patient had a blood pressure of 120/80 mmHg and a pulse of 118.

Mechanical ventilation was reinstituted with a tidal volume of 550 mL, respiratory rate of 22, F_{IO_2} of 1.0, and inspiratory flow of 40 L/min. With these settings, the peak airway pressure was 60 cmH_2O; the plateau or end-inspiratory pressure 35 cmH_2O; and the PEEPi, measured at end expiration, 12 cmH_2O. The initial blood gas analysis revealed a Pa_{O_2} of 195 mmHg, Pa_{CO_2} of 44 mmHg, and pH of 7.30. Inhaled and intravenous bronchodilators were started. With an increase in the inspiratory flow to 60 L/min, peak airway pressure rose by 5 cmH_2O, but PEEPi fell to 8 cmH_2O. The F_{IO_2} was decreased to .50, following arterial saturation with pulse oximetry.

Over the next 24 h peak airway pressures rose to 80 cmH_2O with PEEPi of 20 cmH_2O. The Pa_{CO_2} remained at 40 to 45 mmHg. Sedation and muscle relaxation were maintained. With reduction of the tidal volume to 450 mL peak airway pressure fell to 70 cmH_2O, with PEEPi of 12 to 15 cmH_2O. Attempts to increase minute ventilation by increasing the rate further increased PEEPi. With the reduced tidal volume and rate of 18 the Pa_{CO_2} was 64 mmHg, with a pH of 7.24. The patient was maintained at this level of mechanical support, and bronchodilator therapy continued. Gradually, over the next 72 h, peak airway pressure and PEEPi levels fell, with Pa_{CO_2} falling as well.

By the fifth hospital day peak airway pressure had fallen to 45 cmH_2O with a plateau pressure of 35 cmH_2O and PEEPi of 5 cmH_2O, ascribed to underlying chronic airflow obstruction and the patient's recent inhalation injury. The chest radiograph revealed diffuse bilateral alveolar infiltrates; F_{IO_2} was gradually increased over the day to .80 to maintain an arterial hemoglobin saturation of 90%. Broad-spectrum antibiotics were started and a central venous hyperalimentation catheter with questionable purulence was discontinued. PEEP was added to the ventilator circuit in 5-cmH_2O increments. Up to 15 cmH_2O, the peak airway pressure rose by less than the incremental addition of PEEP; at 20 cmH_2O PEEP, the airway pressure rose by more than the PEEP added, and the blood pressure fell. With 15 cmH_2O PEEP, the F_{IO_2} was decreased to .60 with maintenance of arterial hemoglobin saturation above 90%.

A right heart catheterization revealed a pulmonary capillary wedge pressure of 14 mmHg and a cardiac output of 9.5 L/min. With fluid restriction and diuretic administration the wedge pressure fell to 5 mmHg with adequate cardiac output as judged by vital signs, urine output, and absence of a lactic acidosis. Over 2 to 3 days the alveolar infiltrates on chest radiograph cleared, and gas exchange improved markedly. PEEP was decreased over this period to 5 cmH_2O. At this point a left lower lobe collapse was noted radiologically; the patient's tidal volumes were increased to 600 mL, and sighs (8 per min at twice the tidal volume) were added. Reexpansion of the lobe was noted by exam and follow-up chest radiograph.

Over the next day, sedation was held and the patient became more responsive. A grand mal seizure was noted, and the patient was loaded with dilantin, and then phenobarbital, while the electroencephalogram was followed. A history was obtained, from an outside hospital, of an old seizure disorder.

By the fifteenth day the patient had undergone several surgical debridements of burn and two split-thickness graft attempts, as well as a tracheostomy. With therapeutic levels of his antiepileptic drugs he was responsive, followed simple commands, and was able to express his discomfort from his injury and the titration of his analgesics. When taken off the ventilator for suctioning he would maintain his minute ventilation of 14 L/min with a tidal volume of 350 mL and respiratory rate of 40, but was unable to sustain this for more than a few minutes. With the ventilator set at a tidal volume of 450 mL, the peak airway pressure was 32 cmH_2O, plateau pressure 16 cmH_2O, and the NIF 20 cmH_2O. It was discovered that bronchodilator therapy had been inadvertently stopped, and this was restarted. A careful review of his nutritional status indicated progressive hypoalbuminemia over the hospitalization, with a magnesium level of 0.8 mg/dL and a phosphate level of 1.2 mg/dL.

The patient was placed on a pressure support system during the days, with 25 cmH_2O supplied at the airway opening. With this he maintained a spontaneous breathing rate of 28 to 34. There was no progression of his breathing rate over the course of the day. In the evenings he was returned to full mechanical support with an A/C mode, and was given adequate sedation for sleep.

With further bronchodilator therapy the patient's peak airway pressures fell to 23 cmH_2O and the plateau pressure to 16 cmH_2O with a tidal volume of 450 mL. With correction of his electrolyte levels the NIF rose to 38 cmH_2O. With adjustment of his nutritional support to maximize lipid intake at the same calorie load, his minute ventilation diminished to 10 L/min. Over this 3- to 4-day interval his PS was decreased to 10 cmH_2O; with this he maintained a tidal volume of 300 to 350 mL and a rate of 25 to 30 breaths per min. At this point the patient was given a trial of spontaneous breathing with CPAP of 5 cmH_2O, selected to assist with likely underlying airflow obstruction. He tolerated this without difficulty and was placed on supplemental oxygen by tracheostomy; this was maintained throughout the remainder of his ICU course.

CASE DISCUSSION

This patient is typical of patients with complex critical illness, requiring frequent modification of the details of mechanical ventilation both to achieve adequate support and to liberate the patient most expeditiously from the machine. The initial lung mechanical abnormalities were dominated by severe airflow obstruction arising from the thermal injury to the airway. As with many such patients, even before mechanical ventilation could be undertaken, vigorous volume resuscitation was necessary to stabilize venous return in the face of high intrathoracic pressures arising from PEEPi and positive-pressure ventilation.

After stabilizing the circulation, the patient was sedated and muscle-relaxed to diminish carbon dioxide production. Initially, low tidal volume and high flow rate achieved adequate ventilation and acceptable peak airway pressures and gas trapping (as gauged by PEEPi). As airflow obstruction worsened over the first 24 h, a prudent decision was made to accept a degree of hypoventilation and hypercapnea, rather than to attempt to increase minute ventilation with the attendant risk of barotrauma.

As airflow obstruction improved with time and bronchodilators, the patient next developed low-pressure pulmonary edema, likely related to his inhalation injury or subsequent sepsis. This resulted in a large intrapulmonary shunt. Unlike the gas exchange abnormality associated with airway disease, large increases in the F_{IO_2} became necessary to achieve arterial hemoglobin saturation. At this point PEEP was added to the ventilator circuit, using bedside compliance to titrate to a level that then permitted reduction of F_{IO_2} to a nontoxic level. Low-tidal-volume ventilation was maintained to reduce the risk of barotrauma, minimize the impact of PEEP on venous return, and, conceivably, limit lung injury caused by large swings in volume and pressure. Finally, this phase of the patient's course involved manipulation of the circulation in pursuit of the lowest pulmonary vascular pressures associated with an adequate cardiac output, to shorten the duration of support with PEEP.

After recovery from acute lung injury, the patient received continued support while a number of surgical and medical issues were addressed. Accordingly, a tracheostomy was performed. By the time his general condition permitted consideration of discontinuation of mechanical ventilation, he was weak with abnormal lung mechanics. Fortunately, some component of his weakness was attributable to electrolyte abnormalities, and some component of his high airway resistance to bronchospasm—both of which conditions were readily reversible. His nutritional support during this time was modified to be adequate but to minimize carbon dioxide production, thus reducing his minute ventilation requirement. During this period he was exercised by day and rested at night. Eventually, when relatively simple bedside parameters predicted a high likelihood of success with spontaneous ventilation, he was liberated from mechanical ventilation and eventually discharged from the critical care unit.

References

1. Hall JB, Wood LDH: Liberation of the patient from mechanical ventilation. JAMA 257:1621, 1987.
2. Aubier M, Trippenbach T, Roussos C: Respiratory muscle fatigue during cardiogenic shock. J Appl Physiol 51:499, 1981.
3. Viires N, Sillie G, Aubier A, et al: Regional blood flow distribution in dogs during induced hypotension and low cardiac output: Spontaneous breathing versus artificial ventilation. J Clin Invest 72:935, 1983.
4. Summer WR, Curry P, Haponik EF, et al: Continuous mechanical turning of intensive care unit patients shortens length of stay in some diagnostic-related groups. J Int Care 4:45, 1989.
5. Marini JJ, Capps JS, Culver BH: The inspiratory work of breathing during assisted mechanical ventilation. Chest 87:612, 1985.
6. Marini JJ, Rodriguez RM, Lamb VJ: The inspiratory workload of patient-initiated mechanical ventilation. Am Rev Respir Dis 134:902, 1986.
7. MacIntyre NR: Respiratory function during pressure support ventilation. Chest 89:677, 1986.
8. MacIntyre NR, Leatherman NE: Ventilatory muscle loads and the frequency-tidal volume pattern during inspiratory pressure associated (pressure-supported) ventilation. Am Rev Respir Dis 141:327, 1990.
9. Kacmarek RM: The role of pressure support ventilation in reducing imposed work of breathing. Respir Care 33:99, 1988.
10. Hall JB, Wood LDH: Management of the critically ill asthmatic patient. Med Clin North Am 74(3):779, 1990.
11. Rodriguez-Roisin R, Ballester E, Roca J, et al: Mechanisms of hypoxemia in patients with status asthmaticus requiring mechanical ventilation. Am Rev Respir Dis 139:732, 1989.
12. Tuxen DV, Lane S: The effects of ventilatory pattern on hyperinflation, airway pressures, and circulation in mechanical ventilation of patients with severe airflow obstruction. Am Rev Respir Dis 136:872, 1987.
13. Tuxen DV: Detrimental effects of positive end-expiratory pressure during controlled mechanical ventilation of patients with severe airflow obstruction. Am Rev Respir Dis 140:5, 1989.
14. Schmidt GA, Hall JB: Acute on chronic respiratory failure. JAMA 261:3444, 1989.
15. Pepe PE, Marini JJ: Occult positive end-expiratory pressure in mechanically ventilated patients with airflow obstruction. Am Rev Respir Dis 126:166, 1982.
16. Braun NMT, Faulkner J, Hughes RL, et al: When should respiratory muscles be exercised? Chest 84:76, 1983.
17. Marini JJ: Should PEEP be used in airflow obstruction? Am Rev Respir Dis 140(1):1, 1989.
18. Petrof BJ, Legare M, Goldberg P, et al: Continuous positive airway pressure reduces work of breathing and dyspnea during weaning from mechanical ventilation in severe chronic obstructive pulmonary disease. Am Rev Respir Dis 141:281, 1990.
19. Fleury B, Murciano D, Talamo C, et al: Work of breathing in patients with chronic obstructive pulmonary disease in acute respiratory failure. Am Rev Respir Dis 131:822, 1985.
20. Marini JJ: Strategies to minimize breathing effort during mechanical ventilation. Crit Care Clin 6:635, 1990.
21. Dantzker RM: Gas exchange in the adult respiratory distress syndrome. Clin Chest Med 3:57, 1982.
22. Corbridge TC, Wood LDH, Crawford GP, et al: Adverse effects of large tidal volume and low PEEP in canine acid aspiration. Am Rev Respir Dis 142:311, 1990.
23. Malo J, Ali J, Wood LDH: How does positive end expiratory pressure reduce intrapulmonary shunt in canine pulmonary edema? J Appl Physiol 57:1002, 1984.
24. Suter PM, Fairley B, Isenberg M: Optimum end-expiratory airway pressure in patients with acute pulmonary failure. N Engl J Med 292:284, 1975.
25. Wood LDH, Prewitt RM: Cardiovascular management in acute hypoxemic respiratory failure. Am J Cardiol 47:963, 1981.
26. Humphrey H, Hall J, Sznajder JI, et al: Improved survival following pulmonary capillary wedge pressure reduction in patients with ARDS. Chest 97:1176, 1990.
27. Tharratt RS, Allen RP, Albertson TE: Pressure-controlled inverse ratio ventilation in severe adult respiratory failure. Chest 94:755, 1988.
28. Kacmarek RM, Hess D: Pressure-controlled inverse-ratio ventilation: Panacea or auto-PEEP? Respir Care 35:945, 1990.
29. Breen P, Ali J, Wood LDH: High frequency ventilation in lung edema: Effects of gas exchange and perfusion. J Appl Physiol 56:187, 1984.
30. Sznajder JI, Becker CJ, Crawford GP, et al: Combination of constant flow and continuous positive pressure ventilation in canine pulmonary edema. J Appl Physiol 67:817, 1989.
31. Mink SN, Light RB, Cooligan T, et al: The effect of PEEP on gas exchange and pulmonary perfusion in canine lobar pneumonia. J Appl Physiol 50:517, 1981.
32. Marini JJ, Smith TC, Lamb VJ: External work output and force generation during synchronized intermittent mechanical ventilation. Effect of machine assistance on breathing effort. Am Rev Respir Dis 138:1169, 1988.
33. Truwit JD, Marini JJ: Evaluation of thoracic mechanics in the ventilated patient. Part 2: Applied mechanics. J Crit Care 3(3):199, 1988.
34. Wright PW, Marini JJ, Bernard GR: In vitro versus in vivo comparison of endotracheal tube airflow resistance. Am Rev Respir Dis 140(1):10, 1989.
35. Haluszka J, Chartrand DA, Grassino AE, Milic-Emili J: Intrinsic PEEP and arterial P_{CO_2} in stable patients with chronic obstructive pulmonary disease. Am Rev Respir Dis 141:1194, 1990.
36. Marini JJ, Smith TC, Lamb VJ: Estimation of inspiratory muscle strength in mechanically ventilated patients: The measurement of maximal inspiratory pressure. J Crit Care 1(1):32, 1986.
37. Multz AS, Aldrich TK, Prezant DJ, et al: Maximal inspiratory pressure is not a reliable test of inspiratory muscle strength in mechanically ventilated patients. Am Rev Respir Dis 142:529, 1990.

38. Marini JJ: Monitoring during mechanical ventilation. Clin Chest Med 9:73, 1988.
39. LeMaire F, Teboul JL, Cinotti L, et al: Acute left ventricular dysfunction during unsuccessful weaning from mechanical ventilation. Anesthesiology 69:171, 1988.
40. Dhingra S, Solven F, Wilson A, et al: Hypomagnesemia and respiratory muscle power. Am Rev Respir Dis 129:497, 1984.
41. Fiaccadori E, Coffrini E, Ronda N, et al: Hypophosphatemia in the course of chronic obstructive pulmonary disease: Prevalence, mechanisms, and relationships with skeletal muscle phosphorus content. Chest 97:857, 1990.
42. Whittaker JS, Ryan CF, Buckley PA, et al: The effects of refeeding on peripheral and respiratory muscle function in malnourished chronic obstructive pulmonary disease patients. Am Rev Respir Dis 142:283, 1990.
43. Kreit JW, Capper MW, Pomerleau CM, et al: Work of breathing during pressure support ventilation is not less than the work of breathing during assisted mechanical ventilation. Am Rev Respir Dis 137:64, 1988.
44. Roussos C, Macklem PT: Diaphragmatic fatigue in man. J Appl Physiol 43:189, 1977.
45. Shikora SA, Bristrian BR, Borlase BC, et al: Work of breathing: Reliable predictor of weaning and extubation. Crit Care Med 18:157, 1990.
46. Montgomery AB, Holle RHO, Neagley SR, et al: Prediction of successful ventilator weaning using airway occlusion pressure and hypercapnic challenge. Chest 4:496, 1987.
47. Brochard L, Harf A, Lorino H, Lemaire F: Inspiratory pressure support prevents diaphragmatic fatigue during weaning from mechanical ventilation. Am Rev Respir Dis 139:513, 1989.

Chapter 128
ACUTE HYPOXEMIC RESPIRATORY FAILURE

JESSE B. HALL
LAWRENCE D.H. WOOD

KEY POINTS

- *Acute hypoxemic respiratory failure (AHRF) is characterized by severe hypoxemia that is relatively refractory to oxygen therapy; it results from processes that cause alveolar collapse or filling.*
- *Failure to visualize an obvious alveolar abnormality on chest radiograph in a patient whose blood-gas analyses suggest AHRF should cause consideration of the accuracy of the data [e.g., effective fraction inspired oxygen (F_{IO_2}) and true Pa_{O_2}] and the possibility of other types of right-to-left shunting (e.g., intracardiac, pulmonary arteriovenous malformation).*
- *Initial therapy for all patients includes supplemental oxygen in the highest concentration available, understanding that delivery by high flow mask and rebreathing devices achieves a maximal F_{IO_2} of approximately 0.6 to 0.7 under most clinical conditions; failure to achieve full arterial saturation confirms a large shunt fraction.*
- *The vast majority of patients with cardiogenic pulmonary edema (CPE) respond to standard measures to reduce pre- and afterload and to give inotropic support; during the hours that such pharmacologic therapies are effected, supplemental oxygen with or without continuous positive airway pressure (CPAP) by mask are usually adequate to achieve adequate oxygen delivery.*
- *Indications for elective intubation in patients with CPE include hypotension precluding the use of vasoactive drugs, complex and persistent arrhythmias, and failure to respond to therapy over the course of the first few hours.*
- *In contrast to patients with CPE, patients with the adult respiratory distress syndrome (ARDS) typically require early, elective intubation since the duration of AHRF is usually greater; exceptions to this generalization are postictal pulmonary edema, heroin-associated pulmonary edema, air embolization, and AHRF associated with tocolysis, all of which tend to have a more benign course.*
- *The acute phase of ARDS is characterized by an exudative lung lesion from pulmonary capillary leak; while interventions directed at inflammatory, cytokine, and other pathways of lung injury might be imagined, at the present time no specific pharmacologic therapy has been confirmed to be of benefit and the management of these patients is supportive while predisposing conditions are identified and corrected.*
- *Ventilator management of patients with exudative phase ARDS should begin with an F_{IO_2} of 1.0, tidal volume 6 to 7 mL/kg, and respiratory rate 20 to 28; during initial stabilization on the ventilator sedation and, often, muscle relaxation are advisable to minimize oxygen consumption ($\dot{V}_{O_2}$) and airway pressures.*
- *Subsequent goals of supportive therapy include the least positive end-expiratory pressure (PEEP) achieving 90% saturation of an adequate hemoglobin (14 g/dL) on a nontoxic F_{IO_2} (≤ 0.60)*
- *While controversial, circulatory management directed at reduction of the pulmonary capillary wedge pressure (Ppw) to the least level consistent with an adequate cardiac output and O_2 delivery ($\dot{Q}_{O_2}$) may reduce edemagenesis and thus the duration of potentially dangerous supportive therapy.*
- *Tissue hypoxia and lactic acidosis are ameliorated by combining measures to increase $\dot{Q}_{O_2}$ (cardiac output, O_2 saturation, hemoglobin) with measures to reduce $\dot{V}_{O_2}$ (ventilation, antipyretics, antibiotics); potential O_2 extraction defects are best prevented by early treatment of sepsis.*
- *Monitoring and manipulating the circulation in these patients must take into account the fact that altered perfusion may significantly impact on arterial saturation via the effects of shunted mixed venous blood, and vasoactive drugs may have varying arteriolar, venous, and pulmonary arterial effects on preload, afterload, and pulmonary shunt fraction; given these complexities, right heart catheterization may be useful.*
- *Late or proliferative phase ARDS is signaled by a large dead space fraction, high airway pressures, pulmonary hypertension and a 'honeycomb' appearance radiologically; edema may be minimal and hypovolemia poorly tolerated because of adverse effects on dead space and venous return.*
- *In focal lung disease producing AHRF such as lobar pneumonia or contusion, PEEP therapy may not significantly reduce and can in fact increase intrapulmonary shunt; accordingly it should be used cautiously with frequent confirmation of benefit.*
- *Focal lung diseases confer increased permeability on apparently noninvolved lung vessels, so circulating volume should be maintained at the lowest level allowing adequate cardiac output; other approaches to AHRF with focal lung disease include patient positioning to minimize shunt and split lung ventilation.*

Severe hypoxemia commonly prompts admission to the ICU or complicates the course of patients admitted for other reasons. When not readily corrected by supplemental oxygen, this gas exchange failure is termed *acute hypoxemic respiratory failure* (AHRF). Most typically, it is caused by diffuse lung lesions such as pulmonary edema or focal inflammatory lesions such as bacterial lobar pneumonia (Table 128-1). This chapter reviews the pathophysiology, clinical presentation, and treatment of these frequent causes of critical illness.

Acute severe refractory hypoxemia is lethal. That the antibiotic era has not reduced the substantial early mortality of bacterial pneumonia underlines the need for aggressive supportive therapy.[1] Subsequent description of the adult respiratory distress syndrome (ARDS) stimulated an ongo-

TABLE 128-1 Causes of Acute Hypoxemic Respiratory Failure

Homogenous Lung Lesions (Producing Pulmonary Edema)
Cardiogenic or hydrostatic edema
Left ventricular failure
Acute ischemia
Mitral regurgitation
Mitral stenosis
Ball-valve thrombus
Volume overload, particularly with coexisting renal and cardiac disease
Permeability or low pressure edema (ARDS)
Most common
Sepsis and sepsis syndrome
Acid aspiration
Multiple transfusions for hypovolemic shock
Less common
Near-drowning
Pancreatitis
Air or fat emboli
Cardiopulmonary bypass
Pneumonia
Drug reaction or overdose
Leukoagglutination
Inhalation injury
Infusion of biologics (e.g., interleukin-2)
Edema of unclear or "mixed" etiology
Reexpansion
Neurogenic
Postictal
Tocolysis-associated
Focal Lung Lesions
Lobar pneumonia
Lung contusion
Lobar atelectasis (acutely)

ing search for prevention and specific treatment of acute lung injury. Yet, as for pneumonia, definitive therapy—if and when it becomes available—is unlikely to improve outcome unless the patient is stabilized from the cascade of airspace flooding, intrapulmonary shunt, respiratory muscle fatigue, cardiovascular instability, and tissue hypoxia initiated by diffuse alveolar damage and pulmonary vascular leak.[2] Cardiogenic pulmonary edema (CPE) complicates left ventricular dysfunction, and the consequent hypoxemia and acidosis need urgent correction as part of the treatment of ischemic heart disease and congestive heart failure. Management of the patient with trauma is sometimes complicated by pulmonary contusion necessitating different volume resuscitation and ventilator therapy from other airspace-filling diseases. These four different manifestations of AHRF often present with such suddenness and severity that only early aggressive application of an informed understanding of cardiopulmonary pathophysiology can stabilize the patient to provide a window for recovery from the primary disease.

The diagnosis and management of these underlying diseases are discussed in more detail elsewhere in this book (see Chaps. 54, 63, 102, and 115), as are the common sequelae of AHRF such as multisystem organ failure (MSOF) and the proliferative phase of ARDS (see Chaps. 53 and 54). The goal of this chapter is to harness principles of pathophysiology described in Chaps. 1 and 2 to an effective approach to stabilizing the patient with AHRF by managing three interrelated problems: **1.** the reduction and clearance of airspace liquid without reducing the cardiac output; **2.** the informed manipulation of the ventilator to reduce intrapulmonary shunt and hypoxemia without reducing venous return or aggravating the acute lung injury through barotrauma or oxygen toxicity; and **3.** the correction of inadequate oxygen delivery and tissue hypoxia in the patient with increased oxygen consumption and potential defects in tissue oxygen extraction, all without increasing alveolar flooding. Our approach encourages aggressive implementation of effective therapy to achieve acceptable end points, followed immediately by rapid, titrated diminution of each therapy to the least amount maintaining the end point. We hypothesize that such aggressive supportive therapy minimizes the adverse effects of both hypoxia and therapy, thereby shortening the duration and complications of critical care.

Pathophysiology

The feature common to all lung diseases producing AHRF is collapse or filling of alveoli causing intrapulmonary shunt and lung mechanical abnormalities (see Chap. 1) (Fig. 128-1). It is useful conceptually and didactically to consider these processes as either homogeneous (e.g., pulmonary edema) or heterogeneous (e.g., lobar pneumonia or collapse). This is done with an understanding that much recent work has pointed to marked regional differences in lesions such as ARDS, heretofore considered to be prototypically homogeneous in their distribution.[3,4]

HOMOGENEOUS AHRF—PULMONARY EDEMA

Lung liquid flux is determined by the conductance of the pulmonary microcirculation (Kf) and the accompanying driving pressure (see Chap. 2 and Fig. 128-2.[5] Under normal conditions, a positive hydrostatic pressure gradient Pmv − Pis in Fig. 128-2) tends to move liquid from the circulation to the interstitial space; this is opposed by the oncotic pressure gradient ($\pi mv - \pi is$, Fig. 128-2) favoring movement of liquid back into the vascular space. Normally the vascular-lung interface maintains the oncotic gradient by virtue of its selective permeability to oncotic factors (primarily proteins), indicated by the coefficient of reflection (σ in Fig. 128-2), which ranges in value from 0.6 to 0.7. In uninjured lung, a small net pressure gradient results in movement of a transudate from the vessels into the interstitial space which collects in lung lymphatics and returns to the circulation; liquid does not collect to any appreciable extent in the alveoli.

CARDIOGENIC OR HIGH PRESSURE PULMONARY EDEMA. Elevation of the microvascular pressures of the lung is associated with an increased driving pressure to lung liquid flux. If pressure increases sufficiently to cause liquid flux to

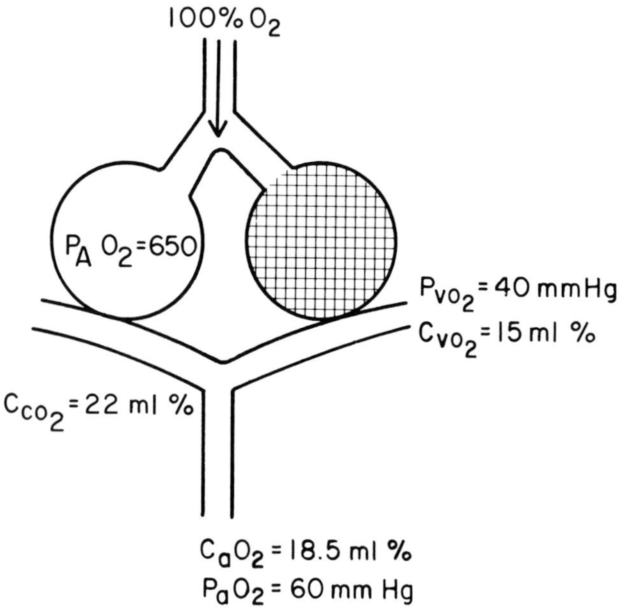

FIGURE 128-1 A cartoon of a two compartment model of lung perfusion and ventilation demonstrating the basis for gas exchange failure in AHRF. When large portions of the lung are nonventilated due to alveolar collapse or flooding (hatched area), blood flow to these units with a mixed venous P_{O_2} of 40 mmHg and content of 15 vol %, is effectively "shunted" through the lungs without resaturation occurring. Thus despite a high concentration of supplemental oxygen (100% in this example) and a high $P_{A_{O_2}}$ in ventilated units, these blood flows mix in accord with their contents. In this example of a 50 percent shunt, the result is systemic arterial hypoxemia with a Pa_{O_2} of 60 mmHg.

exceed lymphatic and other clearance mechanisms, liquid accumulates with eventual alveolar flooding. This can occur despite normal lung function (as indicated by a normal Kf and σ) and normal plasma oncotic pressure. Of course any degree of lung 'leak' (vide infra) or cause of a hypooncotic state (e.g., hypoalbuminemia) will result in increased lung liquid flux at a given microvascular pressure.[6] High microvascular pressures most commonly result from elevation of left ventricular end-diastolic pressure (LVEDP) associated with left ventricular failure or excess circulating volume, less commonly from mitral orifice obstruction (e.g., mitral stenosis or ball-valve obstruction) with associated left atrial pressure elevation, occasionally from mitral valve incompetence with transmission of ventricular pressures to the lung circulation during systole, and very rarely from pulmonary venoocclusive disease.

A number of conditions can result in ventricular dysfunction and elevated LVEDP. As shown in Fig. 128-3, the diastolic pressure-volume curve of the ventricle is shifted upward and to the left acutely by ischemia and chronically by myocardial hypertrophy as in long-standing hypertension. Infiltrative diseases such as amyloidosis or sarcoidosis may produce a similar shift, as does fibrosis related to injury or aging. Hypoxia, acidosis, tachycardia, acute increases in afterload, and interstitial edema (as in the vascular leak associated with sepsis) have been described to have direct or indirect effects that similarly decrease ventricular compliance.

Many of the same processes that cause diastolic ventricular dysfunction (e.g., ischemia) also result in systolic dysfunction (see Fig. 128-3), as represented by a rightward and downward displacement on the ventricular end-systolic pressure-volume relationship (see discussion of Figs. 2-2 through 2-6 in Chap. 2). In the setting of systolic dysfunction, any steady state cardiac output will occur at a higher ventricular filling pressure and predispose to pulmonary edema. Thus one "cost" of maintenance of adequate perfusion in the face of systolic dysfunction as in congestive cardiomyopathy is elevation of LVEDP. In some clinical circumstances this optimal ventricular filling pressure may be as high as 20 to 30 mmHg or higher, much above the nor-

FIGURE 128-2 The Starling equation for edema flow in the lungs (see text for discussion). Hydrostatic edema most typically occurs in conditions in which the pulmonary microvascular pressure (Pmv) is high because of elevations in LVEDP secondary to cardiac dysfunction.

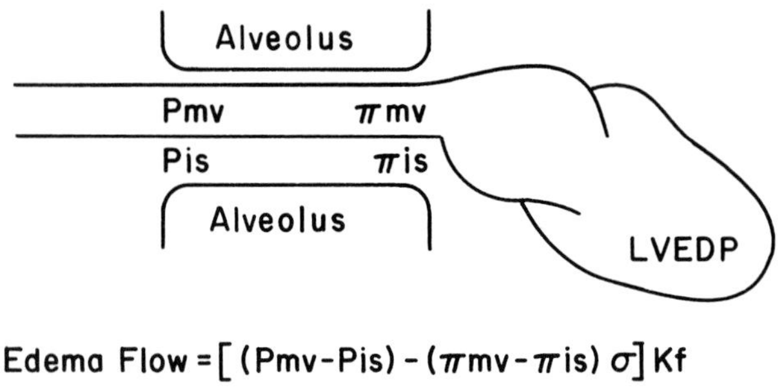

FIGURE 128-3 A ventricular pressure-volume curve demonstrating diastolic and systolic dysfunction (see text for discussion).

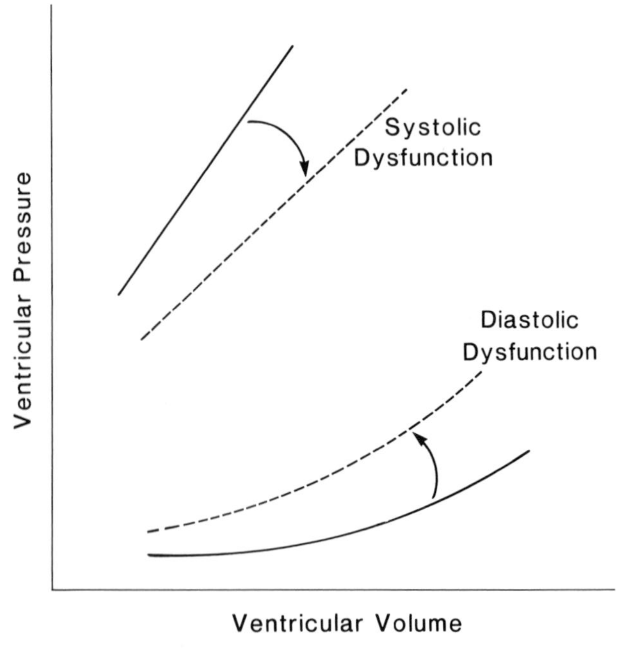

mal range of 3 to 8 mmHg. Small increments in filling pressure may overcome mechanisms of edema clearance and cause clinically apparent lung flooding.

Excessive fluid administration may significantly contribute to edemagenesis. With entirely normal cardiovascular and renal function, this is not likely to occur, since mechanisms of volume excretion are highly efficient. However, in the setting of critical illness, often with multiple factors contributing to impaired ventricular function or impaired renal water excretion, volume "overload" may occur. This may occur even without exogenous fluid administration, as when a vasoactive drug or the Trendelenburg position results in translocation of intravascular volume from the peripheral circulation to the central compartment.

A number of factors tend to limit the rate of lung flooding from high pressure pulmonary edema.[5] As water enters the interstitial space, the pressure in this compartment rises, thus narrowing the hydrostatic pressure gradient (Pmv − Pis) driving edemagenesis. Also, as lung liquid flux increases under conditions of high pressure edema, the small oncotic pressure of the lung interstitium is further reduced by washout of proteins. This widens the oncotic pressure gradient opposing fluid egress from the vasculature, and lung lymph flow increases many fold to remove the excess edema. When these defenses are overwhelmed, CPE tracks through tissue planes to cause interstitial perihilar edema; eventually, the alveolar tight junctions are disrupted and edema floods alveolar spaces.

LOW PRESSURE PULMONARY EDEMA. Low pressure pulmonary edema, also termed pulmonary capillary leak or ARDS, results from injury to the interface of the lung microcirculation with the interstitium and alveolar space.[7] Injury may be sustained from direct lung insults (e.g., aspiration, inhalation, or infectious agents) or indirectly by systemic processes (e.g., sepsis, traumatic shock with large volume blood product resuscitation). Regardless of initiating event, the result is a "leak" of fluid and protein into the interstitium (and eventually alveolar spaces) despite normal microvascular hydrostatic and oncotic pressures. As shown in Fig. 128-2, this is equivalent to an increase in Kf and a reduction of r toward zero.

Much experimental evidence suggests that the leukocyte is central to the mechanisms resulting in acute lung injury and ARDS. Direct lung insult or systemic events such as sepsis appear to cause activation and chemotaxis of neutrophils and macrophages. At least in models of sepsis, these events are followed by release of a number of mediators including tumor necrosis factor, prostaglandins, proteases, oxygen radicals, platelet activating factor, leukotrienes, and interleukins. These concatenating cellular and molecular pathways appear capable of resulting in endothelial cell injury, protein exudation, and interstitial and alveolar edema formation. In the lung this causes surfactant inactivation and pulmonary edema, a condition ultimately recognized as ARDS. In systemic insults such as sepsis these same events may cause hemodynamic and circulatory abnormalities and eventually multiorgan dysfunction. Pathways independent of the leukocyte may also play prominent roles in certain clinical circumstances. For example, endotoxin itself appears capable of direct injury to the endothelial cell, possibly initiating events in the microcirculation of the lung and elsewhere that result in a "leak." Certainly patients with profound neutropenia are not immune to acute lung injury, and ARDS complicating sepsis in these patients is a fairly common clinical problem.[8]

It is useful to distinguish between the early phases of acute lung injury and events occurring subsequently.[9] Pathologically, the early picture is of flooding of the lung interstitium and alveoli with proteinaceous fluid and minimal evidence of cellular injury, at least at a light microscopic level. Ultrastructural evidence of cell injury can be obtained by electron microscopy, with changes of endothelial cell swelling, widening of intercellular junctions, increased numbers of pinocytotic vesicles, and disruption and denudation of the basement membrane prominent. Some inflammatory cell infiltration of the lung interstitium may be seen (particularly in ARDS complicating sepsis or trauma), but it is often a subtle finding.[9] This early phase of diffuse alveolar damage (DAD) has been termed *exudative,* and is a period of time during which pulmonary edema and its effects are most pronounced, and when manipulations to affect the rate of edemagenesis are most likely to have impact (vide infra). Over the ensuing days hyaline membrane formation in the alveolar spaces is prominent, attributed to precipitation of serum proteins. Inflammatory cells become more numerous within the lung interstitium. As the process of DAD progresses, there is extensive necrosis of type I alveolar epithelial cells, which likely contribute cellular debris to the increasingly prominent hyaline membranes.

The latter phase of DAD is dominated by disordered healing. This can occur as early as 7 to 10 days after initial injury and may progress in a short period of time, resulting in extensive pulmonary fibrosis (Fig. 128-4). This has been termed the *proliferative* phase of DAD and appears to involve abnormal collagen deposition. Type II alveolar cells proliferate along alveolar septae, and within the alveolar wall fibroblasts and myofibroblasts become more prominent. Lung flooding may be minimal at this point, and the clinical picture is often dominated by large dead space fraction and high minute ventilation requirements, progressive pulmonary hypertension, slightly improved intrapulmonary shunt which is less responsive to PEEP, further reduction in lung compliance, and a tendency toward creation of zone 1 conditions of the lung if the patient develops hypovolemia (see Chap. 52). It is not clear what signals and controls this abnormal healing of the lung, and how healing might be modified to beneficially affect outcome.

A number of differences between low and high pressure pulmonary edema should be highlighted. For a given amount of lung water, alveolar flooding is greater with low pressure pulmonary edema, likely related to the lung injury that promotes water movement from the interstitial to the alveolar space.[10] In addition, active transport processes may be important in clearance of fluid from the alveolar space, and these transport mechanisms may be disrupted by acute lung injury.[11] Also, some of the mechanisms limiting edemagenesis in high pressure pulmonary edema (vide

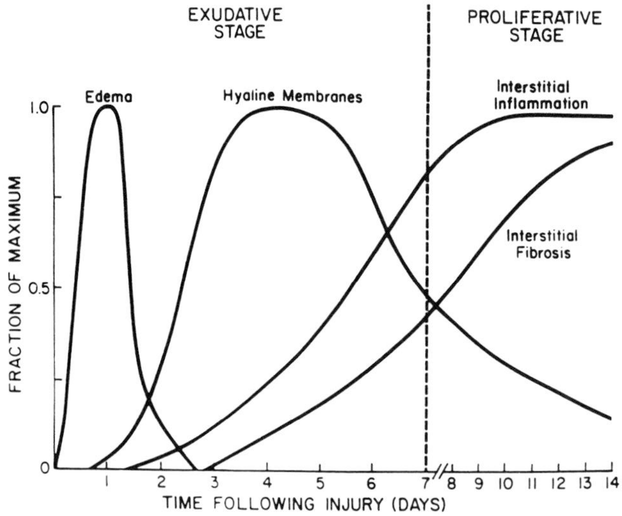

FIGURE 128-4 A schematic representation of the time course of evolution of ARDS. During the early or exudative phase the lesion is characterized by a pulmonary capillary leak with edema and then shortly thereafter hyaline membrane formation. Within as short a period of time as 7 to 10 days a proliferative phase may appear, with marked interstitial inflammation, fibrosis, and disordered healing (see text for discussion). (Reproduced with permission from Katzenstein AA, Askin FB: *Surgical Pathology of Non-neoplastic Lung Disease.* Philadelphia, Saunders, 1982.)

supra) may not be operative in low pressure pulmonary edema. Specifically, there is no "washout" of the interstitial proteins in ARDS and thus no tendency for a widened oncotic pressure gradient to oppose the hydrostatic pressures driving liquid flux; furthermore, the interstitial back pressure to edemagenesis (Pis) may be less evident due to the primary disruption of the alveolar barrier.[10]

PULMONARY EDEMA OF UNCLEAR ETIOLOGY. Some forms of pulmonary edema, although well-described clinically, remain obscure as to their etiology, at least in terms of basic Starling mechanism(s) (see Table 128-1). Neurogenic pulmonary edema, most commonly seen following catastrophic central nervous system (CNS) injury, has been ascribed to both high and low pressure mechanisms.[12] Reexpansion pulmonary edema, relatively common unilaterally after inflation of a collapsed lung by tube thoracostomy, has been held by many to result from a sudden decrease in lung interstitial pressures and thus from a widened hydrostatic pressure gradient. Some evidence in animal models, however, has suggested that reperfusion following reexpansion may result in lung injury analogous to reperfusion injury following organ transplantation, with a pulmonary capillary leak.[13] Pulmonary edema complicating tocolytic therapy is the most common form of lung flooding encountered during pregnancy, and the mechanisms remain obscure (see Chap. 88).

NONHOMOGENEOUS AHRF

The prototype of nonhomogeneous AHRF is acute lobar bacterial pneumonia. With this lung infection, shunt fractions may reach 40 percent of total cardiac output, despite consolidation involving only a single lobe and thus 20 percent of normal perfusion. One explanation for this large shunt fraction is the failure of alveolar hypoxic vasoconstriction to reduce pulmonary arterial flow to infected and consolidated lung segments, with this response to inflammation often resulting in normal or even increased blood flow.[14] The absence of a reduction in pulmonary blood flow may be mediated by local elaboration of prostaglandins, since inhibitors of these metabolic pathways allow the expected reduction in flow in animal models. Another contribution to the large shunt fractions encountered in pneumonia is the consumption of oxygen by the aerobically active leukocytes and bacteria within the consolidated lobe, causing the venous effluent from the infected region of the lung to have even a lower oxygen saturation than mixed venous blood.[14] Because PEEP is ineffective or aggravates the hypoxemia, it is worth testing postural effects (consolidated lobe uppermost) or unilateral PEEP[15] when shunt is severe. Yet shunt is not the only cause of hypoxemia in pneumonia, because adjacent lung regions become hypoventilated due to their mechanical interaction with the consolidated lobe. Consequently, about half of the hypoxia during air breathing is due to low ventilation perfusion ratios ($\dot{V}/\dot{Q}$), and that is very responsive to oxygen therapy.[14]

Another focal lung lesion that can result in significant hypoxemia is lung contusion. These lesions invariably emerge within hours after blunt chest trauma and are increased by fluid resuscitation and PEEP;[16] they result from direct mechanical injury to the lung and its blood supply. The central region of the contused lung often manifests significant hemorrhage and interruption of the pulmonary arterial circulation, so intrapulmonary shunt is minimal. Yet in the peripheral regions of the contusion and in adjacent segments and lobes mechanically interdependent with the poorly ventilated contusion, hypoventilation leads to low $\dot{V}/\dot{Q}$ and hypoxemia which is responsive to oxygen therapy. Accordingly, measures to improve ventilation (nerve blocks, analgesics, chest physiotherapy with deep breathing) and oxygen by facemask often correct the hypoxemia, and are preferred to positive-pressure ventilation with PEEP, which tends to increase the injury without ameliorating the hypoxemia. Undoubtedly, similar effects occur in the subsegmental inhomogeneity of ARDS as well, yet the major effects are shunt and its responsiveness to PEEP.

CONSEQUENCES OF ALVEOLAR FILLING OR COLLAPSE

GAS EXCHANGE. As demonstrated in Fig. 128-1, the consequence of alveolar flooding and collapse is intrapulmonary shunt as mixed venous blood traverses nonventilated airspaces (see discussion of Fig. 1-8 in Chap. 1).[17] Despite high concentrations of supplemental oxygen, arterial blood may remain unsaturated if shunt fractions are above 30 percent (Fig. 128-5). Nonetheless, even small increases in arterial oxygen tension may result in relatively large increases in arterial oxygen content, given the steep slope of the oxyhemoglobin dissociation curve in the range of Pa_{O_2} from 25

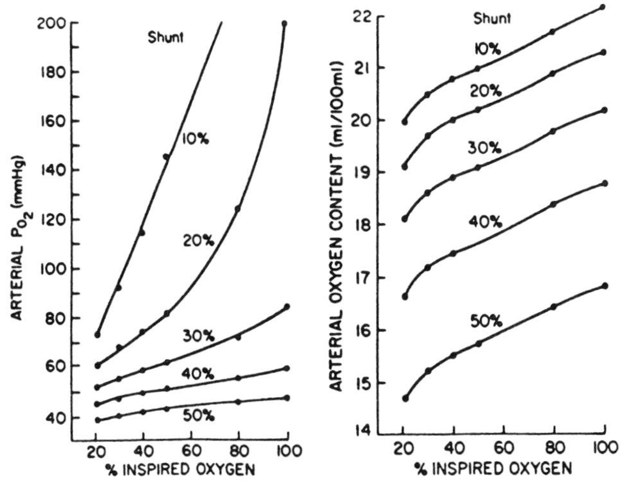

FIGURE 128-5 Demonstration of the effect of intrapulmonary shunt on gas exchange and oxygen delivery. On the graph on the left, Pa_{O_2} is plotted against FI_{O_2} for varying shunt fractions. Note that as shunt fraction rises above 30 percent, there is only a very small increase in arterial Pa_{O_2} despite increasing inspired oxygen to 100%. Nonetheless, as shown in the panel on the right, even these small changes in arterial Pa_{O_2} are associated with relatively large increases in arterial oxygen content, since these values are on the steep portion of the oxyhemoglobin dissociation curve. (Reproduced with permission from Reference 17.)

to 65 mmHg (see Fig. 128-5). In addition, maneuvers such as PEEP may be used to recruit alveoli and decrease intrapulmonary shunt (vide infra), and raising $\dot{Q}_{O_2}$ increases Pa_{O_2} for a given large shunt by raising the O_2 saturation of the mixed venous blood ($S\bar{v}_{O_2}$), which perfuses the flooded region (see Chap. 11). Invariably, the minute ventilation required to maintain eucapnea is increased due in part to increased physiologic dead space in the overventilated nonflooded airspaces; often this is aggravated by large tidal volumes and PEEP.[17]

LUNG MECHANICS. To a first approximation, the lung manifesting pulmonary edema or pneumonic consolidation behaves as a two compartment structure, with a population of alveoli exhibiting near normal compliance characteristics and another recruitable only by the application of increased transpulmonary pressures. This is consistent with the notion that fluid-filled or collapsed alveoli do not participate in ventilation until increased pressures are applied, which results in a degree of alveolar recruitment. In this sense, lung volume is decreased only because airspaces flood at about one-eighth their volume when air filled, (see discussion of Fig. 1-9 in Chap. 1); accordingly, a small volume of pulmonary edema floods eight times that volume of airspace,[18] as indicated by the large reduction in measured functional residual capacity (FRC). As assessed at the bedside in the mechanically ventilated patient, respiratory system static compliance is markedly reduced, often to the range of 20 to 40 mL/cmH_2O or less, in part because FRC is reduced and in part because flooded airspaces restrict the inflation of adjacent interdependent aerated lung segments. The consequence of this mechanical abnormality for the spontaneously breathing patient is an increased elastic contribution to the work of breathing; the consequence for mechanical ventilatory support is a higher elastic pressure imposed by the ventilator. In both cases, the aerated lung units are much overdistended and subject to barotrauma unless the patient or physician reduces the tidal volume; in general, spontaneously breathing patients reduce their tidal volume (to 5 to 7 mL/kg) much more than do their physicians who often select much higher tidal volumes on the ventilator.

In cardiogenic pulmonary edema[19] and the exudative phase of ARDS,[18] many collapsed and flooded alveoli can be recruited with the application of PEEP. Preventing alveolar and airway pressure from falling to atmospheric by application of a retard valve on the ventilator or providing a positive pressure by mask throughout the respiratory cycle exploits the hysteresis of the inflation and deflation limbs of each breath. Over the course of five to eight breaths the increased end-expired pressure increases end-inspired volume to achieve alveolar recruitment by expansion of collapsed units and translocation of fluid from flooded units to the interstitial space; then PEEP prevents the derecruitment of these units at end expiration (Fig. 128-6). The result is increased respiratory system compliance due to increased FRC and an improvement in gas exchange due to oxygenation of perfused recruited airspaces. Such recruitment with improvement in lung mechanics and gas exchange does not occur to the same extent in lobar pneumonia, probably because viscid alveolar pus does not flow into the lung interstitium,[15] or in advanced proliferative phase ARDS because edema contributes less to shunt while alveolar obliteration with fibrosis unresponsive to PEEP contributes more.[9]

Airway resistance is another lung mechanical feature that could conceivably be altered in patients with AHRF. CPE typically produces a narrowing of airway caliber, attributed to both airway edema and reversible bronchospasm or "cardiac asthma" (see Chap. 130). Airway resistance has been demonstrated to be increased in patients with ARDS,[20] although these measurements have not been corrected for aerated lung volume. Conceivably airway secretions, edema, or even bronchospasm induced by mediators released during lung injury could contribute to actual reductions in airway size. Although these phenomena have not been clearly demonstrated there may be a role for bronchodilator therapy in these patients; it will not likely substantially alter course nor other features of their management.[20] It is also important to appreciate that during mechanical ventilation of patients with acute respiratory failure the endotracheal tube itself as well as the various exhalation and PEEP valves used may introduce significant increases in resistence to the respiratory circuit.[21]

OXYGEN DELIVERY. Normal tissue function depends on adequate oxygen delivery ($\dot{Q}_{O_2}$) relative to consumption ($\dot{V}_{O_2}$) (see Chap. 1). A number of conditions may result in increased $\dot{V}_{O_2}$ in patients with AHRF, including the increased work of breathing, fever accompanying pneumonia or sepsis-induced ARDS, and the hypermetabolism associated with ARDS and its precursors (see Fig. 1-5 in Chap. 1). Unfortunately, inherent to AHRF is a reduction in $\dot{Q}_{O_2}$.

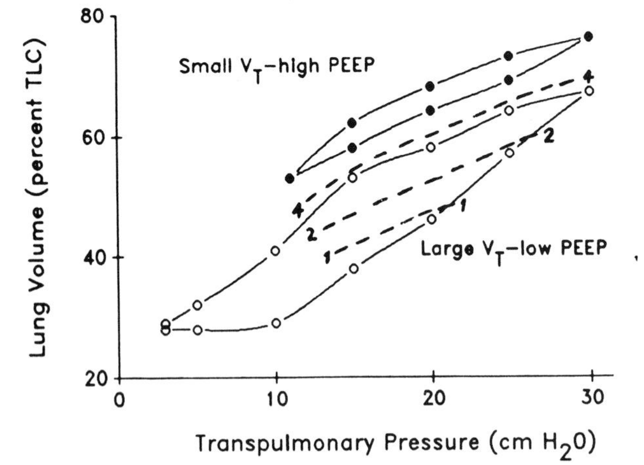

FIGURE 128-6 Comparison of pulmonary pressure-volume relationships during canine acid aspiration pneumonitis between two groups: open circles denote large tidal volume (VT)-low PEEP (3 cmH_2O); closed circles denote small VT-high PEEP (13 cmH_2O). Note that increasing PEEP by 10 cmH_2O caused a large increase in end-expired lung volume such that VT was halved to maintain similar end-inspired lung volume and transpulmonary pressure. This ventilatory pattern reduced the edema by 50 percent compared to the large VT-low PEEP pattern.

The interrupted lines illustrate how a patient with a large VT-low PEEP ventilatory pattern moves through the pulmonary P-V hysteresis with each breath after the VT is reduced and PEEP is increased. The increase in end-expired volume when PEEP is applied during breath 1 (see interrupted lines connecting the end-inspired and end-expired volumes denoted #1) occurs because less volume is expired than was inspired; accordingly, the next breath expands the lung to a greater end-inspired volume (denoted #2), and end-expired volume (see #2) increases further, presumably because part of the inspirate is retained in previously flooded airspaces which were recruited when alveolar liquid was displaced into the interstitium. Subsequent breaths (see #4) continue this process through about eight breaths, when alveolar recruitment is complete indicated by the closed circles; this large increase in end-expired volume at the same end-expired pressure occurs within the P-V hysteresis of the edematous lungs to reduce shunt and to increase thoracic volume and so pleural pressure more than predicted from the low lung compliance before PEEP was increased (for further discussion, see Figs. 1-9 and 1-13 in Chap. 1). (Reproduced and adapted from Corbridge TC, Wood LDH, Crawford GP, et al: Am Rev Respir Dis 142:311, 1990, with permission.)

This most obviously occurs as a result of hypoxemia with associated arterial desaturation, but may be further compounded by complicating anemia or hypoperfusion (e.g., left ventricular dysfunction accompanying CPE, PEEP reducing cardiac output in the treatment of ARDS). Because $\dot{V}_{O_2}$ is three times normal in Fig. 1-5, $\dot{Q}_{O_2}$ must be increased similarly to maintain aerobic metabolisms when the O_2 extraction limit is normal; if any or all of arterial desaturation, anemia, or reduced cardiac output conspire to reduce $\dot{Q}_{O_2}$ below the extraction limit, $\dot{V}_{O_2}$ decreases so anaerobic metabolism, lactic acidosis, and organ failure ensue.

In addition to the balance between $\dot{Q}_{O_2}$ and $\dot{V}_{O_2}$ being potentially adversely affected by diminished delivery and increased demand, in ARDS the possibility of a systemic oxygen extraction defect has been suggested (see discussion of Fig. 1-3 and 1-4 in Chap. 1). Specifically, a number of clinical investigators have suggested that in patients with ARDS and sepsis, interventions increasing oxygen delivery by a variety of mechanisms are associated with an increase in oxygen uptake over an abnormally wide range of deliveries. Not all human studies have been consistent in this finding, however, and some have suggested the purported correlation may be the result of measurement artifact. Nonetheless, as therapies are titrated to individual patients, often with the potential for opposite effects on oxygenation and perfusion, monitoring of the adequacy of oxygen delivery is advisable although difficult (see Chap. 56 and 57).

Clinical Presentation

If coincident CNS depression is not present and the patient has not progressed to a moribund state or respiratory arrest, the bedside appearance of the various forms of AHRF are remarkably similar and are characterized by marked tachypnea (respiratory rate > 30) and dyspnea. Physical examination reveals diffuse crackles in the case of pulmonary edema and focal findings of consolidation in the case of lobar pneumonia. It is not unusual to encounter a patient with pneumonia early during its evolution with marked dyspnea and minimal physical findings and radiologic abnormalities that over ensuing hours become more pronounced as intravenous fluids are administered; in our experience this is particularly true of pneumonia complicating diabetic ketoacidosis or other conditions accompanied by dehydration, as if low pulmonary vascular pressures reduce inflammatory edema in involved and apparently uninvolved lung regions.[22,23] Cardiogenic pulmonary edema may be accompanied by evidence of airflow obstruction, including wheezing, and on occasion it may be extremely difficult to determine whether the primary process is asthma, COPD, or CPE (see Chaps. 129 and 130). The presence of crackles, a radiologic appearance of high pressure edema (vide infra), and hypoxemia refractory to oxygen therapy all suggest pulmonary edema as a primary process. Cough and purulent sputum are hallmarks of infectious processes, while fulminant pulmonary edema often results in copious airway secretions producing rhonchous sounds and abundant expectoration. As early as the publication of Osler's *Textbook of Medicine* it was recognized that the character of the airway secretions in noncardiogenic edema differed from those of cardiogenic causes, being frothy and having the appearance of plasma (vide infra).

Not infrequently the clinician will be assisted, or potentially confused, by rapidly accumulated data regarding gas exchange. Initial room air arterial blood-gas analysis or pulse oximetry in the distressed patient with AHRF typically reveals Pa_{O_2} of 30 to 50 mmHg or saturation $< 85\%$. If supplemental oxygen by mask or cannula achieves $> 95\%$

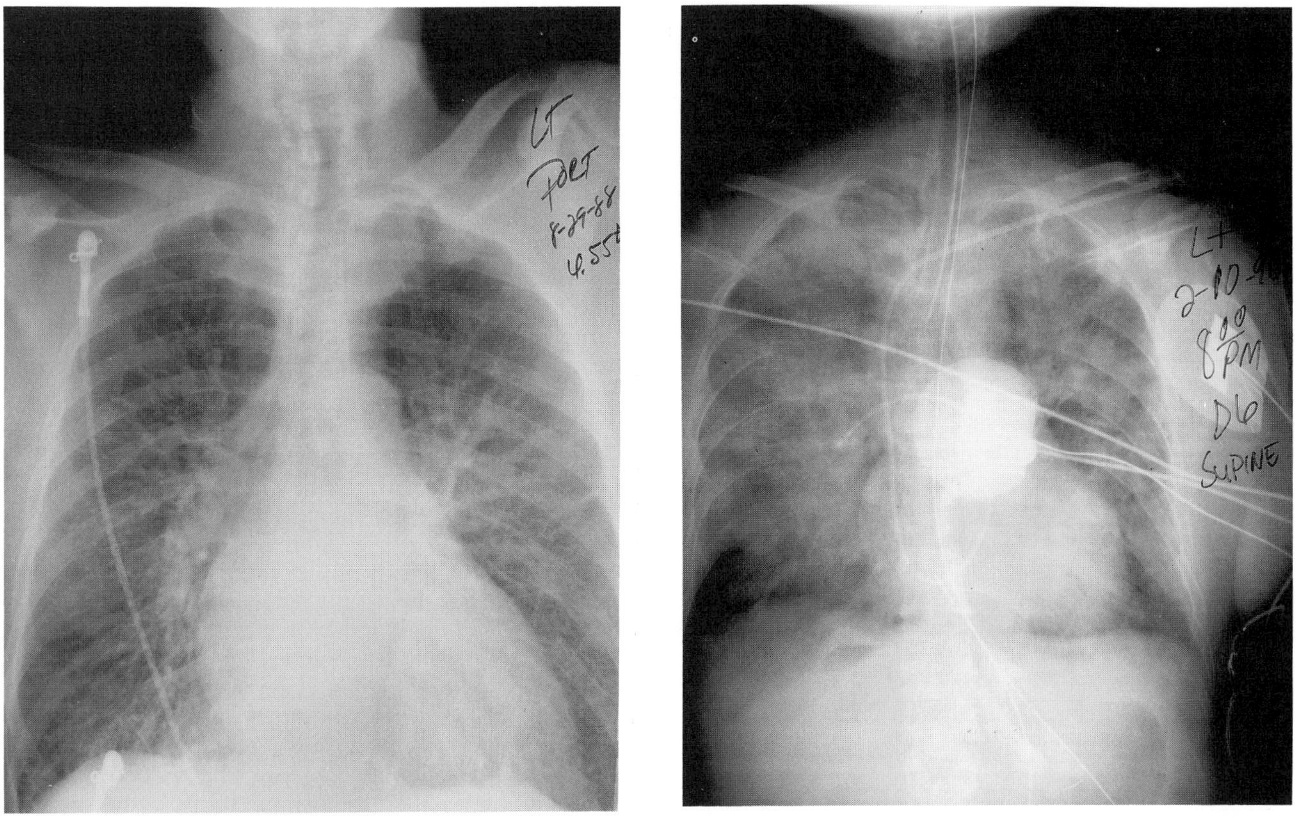

a

b

FIGURE 128-7 Radiologic examples of hydrostatic (cardiogenic) (*a*) and permeability (ARDS) pulmonary edema (*b*). Fig. 128-7*a* is remarkable for a large cardiac silhouette, a hilar "bat's wing" appearance, and Kerley B lines, all characteristic of CPE. Fig. 128-7*b* is remarkable for infiltrates extending to the lung periphery and a very dense appearance of the edema, characteristics of ARDS. Unfortunately, these signs do not have a very high accuracy in determining the etiology of pulmonary edema, as discussed in the text.

saturation of arterial hemoglobin, alternative explanations for respiratory distress should be considered, including airway disease, pulmonary embolus, or severe metabolic acidosis (see discussion of Fig. 11-1 in Chap. 11). Failure to achieve > 95% saturation of arterial blood with supplemental oxygen is consistent with AHRF and a large intrapulmonary shunt, and the specific alveolar filling process should be obvious by physical examination and chest radiograph. In the rare instance that the chest radiograph is entirely clear of alveolar infiltrates one should consider that the blood-gas data are incorrect or there is a right-to-left shunt at another site (e.g., pulmonary arteriovenous malformation or intracardiac shunt).

DETERMINING THE ETIOLOGY OF PULMONARY EDEMA

Inhomogeneous lung infiltrates are often easily identified as pneumonia or lung contusion, and the existence of pulmonary edema is often clear by examination of the distressed patient. Yet the specific etiology of pulmonary edema is often obscure. A number of clinical and laboratory data should be collated to inform the clinical judgment of distinguishing between hydrostatic and permeability edema.

CLINICAL SETTING. The most useful information derives from the setting in which the pulmonary edema develops. CPE is most often accompanied by systolic left ventricular or valvular dysfunction and the abnormal heart sounds and murmurs associated with each should be sought. Electrocardiographic (ECG) evidence of prior or ongoing ischemic injury suggests an obvious cause for CPE. Review of volume administration will often supply information suggesting the explanation for pulmonary edema in patients with left ventricular or renal dysfunction. ARDS too arises in typical settings (see Table 128-1). In most large series, sepsis, blood product resuscitation following trauma, and acid aspiration account for the majority of AHRF secondary to pulmonary capillary leak. Less common causes include pancreatitis, near-drowning, leukoagglutination reactions, lung infections with viral agents or pneumocystis, fat embolism syndrome, or drug toxicities.

CHEST RADIOGRAPH. A number of studies have assessed the utility of the chest radiograph in distinguishing hydrostatic from increased permeability edema.[24] Unfortunately the accuracy of this simple and widely available test varies significantly in these reports and there is not general agreement as to the most useful criteria to be applied. Some of the criteria that have been suggested to support a diagnosis of hydrostatic edema include increased heart size, increased width of the vascular pedicle, vascular redistribution toward upper lobes, septal lines, and a centrifugal pattern of spread with perhilar "bat's wing" distribution of the edema (Fig. 128-7). The lack of these findings and patchy peripheral infiltrates that extend to the lateral lung margins suggest ARDS. All of these signs overlap, however, and in the best of hands this test is unlikely to yield better than a 60 to 80 percent accuracy of diagnosis. Accordingly, they are best used in conjunction with clinical context and examination of the alveolar liquid to increase the accuracy of determination of edema etiology.

EDEMA FLUID ANALYSIS. If intubation is required, collection of endotracheal tube suckings for protein analysis should be routine. CPE is transudative in nature, with a protein content (E) < 50 percent of that of the patient's plasma (P). By contrast, the protein content of edema fluid in ARDS is close to that of plasma, usually 70 to 90 percent of the plasma concentration.[11,25] In our experience this simple test is extremely useful and generally underutilized. Subsequent analysis is consistent with the active clearance of crystalloid from alveolar liquid across the healed alveolar membrane, such that E/P increases as patients recover; by contrast, failure to concentrate alveolar protein signals persistent leak and a poorer prognosis.[11]

ECHOCARDIOGRAPHY. Echocardiography is increasingly applied to provide noninvasive information regarding cardiovascular function (see Chaps. 21 and 22). Findings supporting CPE include left ventricular dilation, regional or global wall motion abnormalities, or substantial mitral regurgitation on Doppler imaging. Conversely, a small, well-contracting ventricle imaged echocardiographically in a patient with pulmonary edema suggests pulmonary vascular leak (the exudative phase of ARDS) but intercurrent resolution of the high pulmonary vascular pressures predisposing to CPE must be ruled out.

INVASIVE HEMODYNAMIC MONITORING. Right heart catheterization is most often performed in patients with pulmonary edema to contribute to the evaluation of its etiology and to guide subsequent cardiovascular management. Much has been written concerning the wisdom of such invasive monitoring of patients. It has been suggested that this technology itself contributes to a poor patient outcome, given the large number of well-recognized complications (see Chaps. 25 and 54). One recent study has determined that physician understanding and facility with the information generated is remarkably poor.[26] We take as a given that the safe performance of the procedure and a full understanding of the interpretation of the information generated is a prerequisite for the use of such technology, and much of this text is devoted to such knowledge (see Chap. 25). We also recommend that invasive monitoring not be performed as routine or be dictated by preconditions, but rather that the clinician formulate specific questions regarding ventricular function, the adequacy of volume resuscitation, the degree of intrapulmonary shunt, and the adequacy of perfusion and oxygen delivery.[27] All other sources of information should then be exhausted in pursuit of the answers to these questions. If central issues remain unresolved, and both diagnosis of etiology of edema and subsequent therapy will be best guided by invasive monitoring, we advocate the use of right heart catheterization.

The specific pulmonary capillary wedge pressure (Ppw) that one selects as a determinant of "high pressure" versus "low pressure" pulmonary edema is necessarily arbitrary under clinical conditions, since degrees of lung injury, hypoalbuminemia, volume overload, and ventricular dysfunction may all promote lung flooding. In the mechanically ventilated patient with normal lung function and serum oncotic pressure, CPE is typically associated with a Ppw of 25 to 35 mmHg or higher, and ARDS with a Ppw of 0 to 18 mmHg.

DEFINING AND SCORING ARDS

Interestingly, there is not an infallible and widely accepted definition of ARDS. We find useful the following criteria (Table 128-2): **1.** a clinical presentation consisting of dyspnea and tachypnea; **2.** a clinical setting of either direct lung insult (e.g., acid aspiration, viral pneumonia, near-drowning) or a systemic process known to be associated with acute lung injury (e.g., sepsis, trauma with massive blood product resuscitation); **3.** three or four quadrant alveolar consolidation on chest radiograph; **4.** diminished respiratory system compliance (typically < 40 mL/cmH_2O measured in those patients requiring mechanical ventilation); **5.** impaired gas exchange with severe hypoxemia ($Pa_{O_2}/FI_{O_2} < 150$ or requirement of PEEP > 5 cmH_2O to maintain $Pa_{O_2} > 60$ mmHg on $FI_{O_2} > 0.5$); and **6.** when measured, a Ppw < 16mmHg. Since patients present with varying degrees of acute lung injury, a number of investigators[28] have found useful a scoring system that incorporates many of these features (Table 128-3).

Treatment of AHRF

Much of the attention and energy of the critical care physician will be directed at supportive therapy of patients with AHRF, with the goal of maintaining adequate oxygen delivery while processes such as pulmonary edema and focal lung infection are treated. This must be accomplished with an eye toward minimizing the complications of this potentially dangerous supportive therapy. It cannot be overemphasized that along with support of the patient a simultaneous search for and treatment of the underlying cause of the lung failure must be conducted, because supportive therapy alone will likely ultimately result in mounting complications and irreversible organ failures. Thus, it is essential to identify and treat myocardial ischemia or valvular incompetence as causes of CPE, or sepsis as a cause of ARDS, or pneumonia as a cause of focal disease. This is obvious on the face of it, but we often encounter situations in which the details of supportive care and rapidly changing clinical circumstances distract even good clinicians from

TABLE 128-2 Criteria for Diagnosis of ARDS

Clinical presentation
  Tachypnea and dyspnea
  Crackles on auscultation
Clinical setting
  Direct lung insult (e.g., aspiration) or systemic process with potential for lung injury (e.g., sepsis)
Radiologic appearance
  Three or four quadrant alveolar flooding
Lung mechanics
  Diminished compliance (<40 mL/cmH_2O)
Gas exchange
  Severe hypoxemia refractory to oxygen therapy ($Pa_{O_2}/FI_{O_2} < 150$)
Normal pulmonary vascular pressures
  PW < 16 mmHg

TABLE 128-3 Scoring System for ARDS

Chest roentgenogram score	
No alveolar consolidation	0
1 quadrant consolidation	1
2 quadrant consolidation	2
3 quadrant consolidation	3
4 quadrant consolidation	4
Hypoxemia score	
$Pa_{O_2}/FI_{O_2} \geq 300$	0
Pa_{O_2}/FI_{O_2} 225–299	1
Pa_{O_2}/FI_{O_2} 175–224	2
Pa_{O_2}/FI_{O_2} 100–174	3
$Pa_{O_2}/FI_{O_2} \leq 100$	4
Compliance (when ventilated) (mL/cmH_2O)	
≥80	0
60–79	1
40–59	2
20–39	3
≤19	4
PEEP required (when ventilated) (cmH_2O)	
≤5	0
6–8	1
9–11	2
12–14	3
≥15	4
Final value is obtained by dividing the aggregate sum by the number of components used	
Score:	
No injury	0
Mild to moderate injury	0.1–2.5
Severe injury (ARDS)	> 2.5

Modified and reproduced with permission from Reference 28.

these pursuits. Details of the diagnosis and management of these problems are discussed elsewhere in this book (see Chaps. 63, 74, 98, 102, 115, 116, 122, and 136).

MANAGING CARDIOGENIC PULMONARY EDEMA

As noted above, many features of the history, physical examination, and early laboratory tests will indicate the etiology of pulmonary edema to be cardiogenic so management of CPE overlaps considerably with the management of left ventricular systolic and diastolic dysfunction discussed in Chap. 115. Initial arterial blood-gas analysis typically reveals marked hypoxemia which, like other causes of AHRF, is only minimally responsive to oxygen therapy. For reasons that are not clear but may relate to intrapulmonary shunting of blood with high mixed venous P_{CO_2}, as many as a third of these patients will exhibit modest elevations of Pa_{CO_2}, despite obvious increased drive to breathe and prior to receiving narcotics (vide infra).[29] Although there is typically only a minimal increase in Pa_{O_2} with oxygen therapy, most patients rapidly respond to pharmacologic interventions and do not require mechanical ventilatory support.

PHARMACOLOGIC THERAPY. The primary goal of pharmacologic therapy is to reduce the left atrial and pulmonary vascular pressures responsible for CPE (Table 128-4). This is effected by reducing the central blood volume and so left ventricular preload; because the heart in CPE often exhibits poor systolic function, positive inotropic agents and afterload reduction also reduce edema while maintaining adequate cardiac output at reduced preload. Relieving edema improves oxygenation and reduces work of breathing. Secondary important goals are relief of hypoxemia and anxiety with its attendant sympathetic discharge (increasing blood

TABLE 128-4 Therapy of Cardiogenic Pulmonary Edema

Correction of Hypoxemia

Supplemental oxygen by mask or cannula
Consider CPAP by mask
Mechanical ventilation for unstable patients

Preload Reduction

Upright position
Morphine sulfate (2–5 mg IVP)
Furosemide (20–40 mg IVP)
Alternative diuretic regimens
  Bumetanide
  Metolazone and furosemide
  Low dose dopamine (1–4 μg/kg/min)
Topical or sublingual nitrates
If coexistent ischemia is evident, use IV nitroglycerin
Consider phlebotomy or rotating tourniquets to temporize when renal function is poor
Renal dialysis/ultrafiltration emergently if diuresis cannot be achieved

Afterload Reduction

Treatment of anxiety to lower systemic blood pressure (e.g., morphine sulfate)
Specific antihypertensive therapy
  Nifedipine (10–20 mg PO or SL)
  Sodium nitroprusside for accelerated hypertension
Intraaortic balloon pump (IABP) for refractory ventricular failure

Inotropic Support

Dobutamine, 5–10 μg/kg/min

Note: The majority of patients will improve with correction of hypoxemia and the initial therapies listed for reduction of preload and afterload. The more extensive and invasive interventions listed are required when ischemia, severe ventricular dysfunction, or renal failure complicate CPE.

pressure and oxygen consumption) and management of cardiac rhythm disturbances to improve cardiac output.

Therapy should begin with oxygen by nasal cannula or mask, titrated against oximetry or arterial blood-gas measurements. Patients invariably prefer the upright position, which should be facilitated if the blood pressure allows; this positioning should be maintained even after intubation and positive-pressure ventilation. A tight-fitting CPAP mask can be beneficial for the spontaneously breathing patient (vide infra). Morphine sulfate, 2 to 4 mg intravenously as an initial dose and followed by 2- to 4-mg doses each 5 to 10 min should be given, titrated against the patient's level of anxiety, level of consciousness, and angina, if any. In addition to its anxiolytic effect, which also tends to reduce hypertension related to excessive sympathetic tone, morphine decreases tone in the venous capacitance vessels, thus reducing preload via peripheral pooling of the intravascular volume.

Further preload reduction can be accomplished with furosemide. This agent has an immediate effect on preload by its venodilating action and a later effect resulting from diuresis;[30] it may also have pulmonary vascular effects which reduce intrapulmonary shunt directly.[31] An initial dose of 20 to 40 mg given intravenously is appropriate, although substantially larger doses may be required in patients with diminished renal function. The initial dose may be doubled if a response is not noted within 30 to 90 min. Alternative regimes to achieve diuresis include bumetanide (initial dose 1 to 2 mg intravenously) or the combination of furosemide and metolazone (initial dose 2.5 to 10 mg orally), particularly if the glomerular filtration rate is reduced. Alternative rapid preload reduction is effected by rotating tourniquets or phlebotomy, and can be used in conjunction with the venous dilating effects of nitroglycerin therapy, particularly if renal function is extremely compromised and there will be a substantial delay in instituting hemodialysis or ultrafiltration (see Chap. 155). When renal function is acceptable, longer term diuresis may be enhanced by intravenous administration of dopamine at a dose of 1 to 4 μg/kg/min (see Chap. 125). Continuous ECG monitoring should by started immediately and brady- or tachyarrhythmias treated as described elsewhere (see Chap. 120). Special considerations for the setting of pulmonary edema focus on the excess preload and diastolic wall tension produced by bradycardia, so oxygen, atropine, isoproterenol, and transvenous pacing should be implemented early.

Patients whose blood pressure does not fall to a normal range with morphine sulfate may have a component of accelerated or malignant hypertension contributing to ventricular decompensation (see Chap. 123). More aggressive control of blood pressure will then be necessary. For acute management of mild elevations of blood pressure a calcium channel blocker such as nifedipine may be used, given as 10 or 20 mg sublingually or by a "bite and swallow." More substantial elevations of blood pressure in the setting of pulmonary edema are best treated with sodium nitroprusside, started at a dose of 10 μg/min total dose and then doubled every 3 to 5 min until blood pressure is reduced to the range of 140 to 160/90 to 100 mmHg (see Table 115-3 in Chap. 115).

This relatively simple approach will result in rapid, dramatic improvement in many patients with mild and uncomplicated pulmonary edema (see Table 128-4). Indeed, such patients are often substantially improved by this approach initiated in the emergency department, with minimal symptoms on ICU admission. Subsequent management is directed at identification of the predisposing causes of ventricular dysfunction, and serial enzyme and ECG studies should be performed in most patients to exclude myocardial infarction. Subsequent echocardiographic assessment is also useful. Topical or oral nitrates can also be used in these relatively stable patients.

Clear evidence of ongoing ischemia as indicated by continued anginal chest pain or ischemic ECG changes should be treated more aggressively (see Chap. 116). Intravenous nitroglycerin is useful in this setting because it reduces preload by its effects on the venous circulation, can have a favorable effect on the distribution of myocardial blood flow, and is a mild afterload reducing agent. It should be started at 10 μg/min *total* dose and then doubled every 3 to 5 min, titrated until pain is resolved or blood pressure begins to fall. Patients who fail to achieve pain control with nitroglycerin should be considered for IABP assistance. Other details concerning management of acute ischemia are given in Chap. 116. All patients with transmural infarction or unstable angina should be considered for anticoagulation, thrombolytic therapy, or surgical intervention as described elsewhere (see Chap. 116). In these instances of severe ischemic injury or risk, mechanical ventilatory support will likely be required and should be instituted electively (vide infra).

Acute mitral regurgitation is suggested by the associated systolic murmur, a small cardiac silhouette with cardiogenic edema, a setting consistent with endocarditis, or a large v wave noted at the time of right heart catheterization (see Chap. 25). If systolic function is relatively well preserved, administration of inotropic agents may worsen the regurgitant fraction and is generally contraindicated. Therapy should begin with a readily titratable afterload reducing agent such as nitroprusside, started at 10 μg/min *total* dose and then doubled every 3 to 5 min. It is extremely useful to perform right heart catheterization in these patients to titrate both preload and afterload appropriately. Echocardiography and left heart catheterization are useful to determine the need for and timing of surgical repair.

Patients with significant systolic dysfunction will be identified by hypotension or evidence of hypoperfusion such as oliguria despite diuretic use or persistent lactic acidosis. These patients will benefit from inotropic drug support and we usually favor dobutamine at a dose of 5 to 15 μg/kg/min, titrated against measured cardiac output and clinical parameters of perfusion. After stabilization over the first few days in the ICU these patients often benefit from long-term management with afterload reducing agents such as the angiotension-converting enzyme inhibitors (see Chap. 125).

VENTILATORY SUPPORT. The majority of patients will respond sufficiently rapidly to avoid mechanical ventilatory support. If improvement is noted but the patient remains in significant respiratory distress with hypoxemia, one alternative is to institute CPAP by mask,[32] which can significantly improve gas exchange. Such patients require close monitoring by experienced staff since the mask must be tight-fitting to provide CPAP and loss of a seal can have immediate adverse effects on arterial hemoglobin saturation. In addition, gastric dilation with vomiting can have disastrous consequences.

Patients who fail to improve, present with hypotension, or develop significant hypotension during the course of therapy should be considered for elective intubation and mechanical ventilation (Table 128-5). In addition, severe ischemia, uncontrollable arrhythmias, and a need for angiographic studies or surgical intervention will often require controlled ventilation. At the time of intubation and immediately thereafter the patient should be heavily sedated; morphine sulfate can be used if blood pressure is adequate or a short-acting benzodiazepine of hypotension is present.

The institution of mechanical ventilation often has a beneficial cardiovascular effect since the work of breathing is reduced, oxygen consumption is diminished, perfusion requirements of the respiratory muscles may decrease, and positive-pressure ventilation may act to reduce the afterload on the dysfunctional left ventricle.[33] Initial ventilator settings should include an F_{IO_2} of 1.0, tidal volume of 6 to 8 mL/kg, and respiratory rate of 25. The patient may initiate breaths in an assist-control (A/C) or synchronized intermittent mandatory ventilation (SIMV) mode with the sensitivity set at a minimal level of -2 cmH_2O. PEEP may then be titrated against arterial saturation to permit a reduction in the F_{IO_2} to 0.6 or less; it is helpful to recall that PEEP has fewer adverse effects on venous return when the circulatory volume is increased as in CPE, and PEEP tends to enhance pump function in the damaged left ventricle by reducing preload and afterload.[34]

The ongoing requirement for ventilatory support will in most instances be dictated by correction of the underlying ventricular dysfunction and valvular or ischemic disease, if any. If new complications do not arise and cardiovascular function is stabilized, the patient may be returned to spontaneous breathing modes when preload is reduced and gas exchange improves, signaled by a diminishing requirement for PEEP (see Chap. 127).

TABLE 128-5 Indications for Intubation and Mechanical Ventilation in Cardiogenic Pulmonary Edema

- Hypotension, even of modest degree
- Clinical evidence of nonresolving ischemia
- Left ventricular failure refractory to medical support
- Coexisting lung disease
- Complex arrhythmias
- When angiography or surgery are required for ischemic or valvular heart disease

TREATMENT OF ARDS

As stated above, the predisposing conditions producing diffuse lung injury and pulmonary capillary leak must be identified and individually treated to ensure patient recovery (see Table 128-1). In addition, certain forms of pulmonary edema, while perhaps related to increased permeability, generally have a self-limited and benign course. These include tocolytic-associated pulmonary edema,[35] postictal pulmonary edema,[36] heroin-associated edema, and pulmonary edema associated with air emboli (see Chap. 118). Patients with these conditions will often respond to supplemental oxygen and diuresis; even when mechanical ventilation is required it is usually for a brief period of time, and the more extensive monitoring and circulatory manipulations described below are not typically indicated.

SPECIFIC PHARMACOLOGIC THERAPY. Given the incomplete understanding of the complex cellular and molecular events that precipitate and then perpetuate acute lung injury, it has been tempting to consider pharmacologic interventions to interrupt these pathways.[37] Many agents have been tried anecdotally, but recent controlled trials provide informed guidance concerning the absence of effective specific prevention and treatment.

Corticosteroids. One intervention that has been anecdotally held to be beneficial is corticosteroid therapy, presumably acting to limit neutrophil-mediated injury. When evaluated prospectively in patients with sepsis syndrome as their predisposition to lung injury, high dose (30 mg/kg every 6 h for a day) methylprednisolone did not prevent the development of ARDS nor reduce the mortality compared to an identical placebo-treated control group.[38] In addition, in another prospective randomized trial of steroids begun after ARDS was well established, no beneficial effect on gas exchange or lung mechanics could be demonstrated, and outcome was not improved.[39] In this investigation acute lung injury appeared related to a number of underlying conditions, including sepsis, aspiration, and pancreatitis.

Accordingly, we do not believe that corticosteroids are indicated in any instance of established ARDS in the exudative phase. Conceivably these agents could be of use to beneficially affect the disordered healing of proliferative phase disease, but this remains to be proven (vide infra). It is unlikely that "prophylactic" steroids have any role in most patients with conditions predisposing to ARDS, but it is worth considering that not all subgroups have been nor are likely to be exhaustively studied and some still advocate the early use of high dose methylprednisolone for witnessed aspiration or early after long bone fracture to prevent fat embolization syndrome (see Chap. 118).

Prostaglandin Administration or Inhibition. A number of basic animal investigations and clinical studies have suggested a role for prostaglandins as mediators of acute lung injury[40] and interventions have been performed involving both prostaglandin administration as well as inhibition of synthesis with nonsteroidal anti-inflammatory drugs (NSAIDs). Prostaglandin E_1 (PGE_1) has been thought to have potential salutary effects for patients with ARDS, given its ability to inhibit platelet aggregation and neutrophil chemotaxis as well as its other anti-inflammatory actions. It is also a pulmonary arterial vasodilator, and it has been hypothesized that primary treatment of the moderate pulmonary hypertension that often develops after acute lung injury is beneficial. In one investigation of PGE_1 in surgical patients with acute respiratory failure, an improvement in gas exchange was noted as well as a trend toward improvement in long-term survival.[41] These promising results were not supported by a more recent investigation of PGE_1 infusion for treatment of ARDS associated with both medical and surgical predispositions.[42] In this study the trend toward increased survival was present in the placebo-treated group, and many complications were noted in the treatment group, including hypotension, diarrhea, and fever. In addition, follow-up studies have failed to confirm any significant improvement in gas exchange following PGE_1 administration.[43] At the present time PGE_1 infusion cannot be considered routine nor proven therapy for ARDS.

Interestingly, inhibition of prostaglandin synthesis has also been considered to be of possible benefit in sepsis and ARDS. NSAIDs, inhibitors of cyclooxygenase and hence thromboxane A_2 and prostacyclin production, have been studied because of their ability to diminish platelet and neutrophil aggregation and generation of oxygen radicals. Limited human studies suggest benefit from use of ibuprofen in patients with sepsis,[44] but large series demonstrating benefit in terms of acute lung injury are lacking. Indomethacin reduced shunt in canine oleic acid edema, but this was due to reduced cardiac output without any reduction in edema.[45] At the present time NSAID use should be considered investigational.

Surfactant. In both animal models of acute lung injury and in bronchoalveolar lavage (BAL) fluid from patients with ARDS, decreased levels of or abnormal ratios of components of surfactant have been described.[38,46] BAL fluid from patients with ARDS also has diminished surface tension-reducing properties, consistent with low levels of surfactant or presence of inhibitor(s) of its action. Accordingly, surfactant replacement has been considered a potential therapy for this disorder.

Clinical data supporting the use of surfactant are most compelling in studies involving patients with the neonatal respiratory distress syndrome, a condition characterized by surfactant deficiency.[47] Early treatment of premature infants was associated with lesser PEEP requirements, less barotrauma, improved gas exchange and respiratory system compliance, reduced incidence of bronchopulmonary dysplasia, and improved survival in some but not all studies.[48] Although this therapy is becoming more widely used in neonates, there have only been limited trials in ARDS.[49] Until more completely investigated in adults, this therapy cannot be advocated for general use.

Pentoxifylline. Pentoxifylline is a phosphodiesterase inhibitor whose actions include inhibition of neutrophil chemotaxis and activation. It has also been demonstrated to inhibit cytokine release by macrophages. These properties have been thought to be of potential benefit in ARDS. In animal models this agent has been demonstrated to protect against endotixin-induced lung injury, perhaps by reducing neutrophil tropism to the lung and the subsequent inflammatory events.[50] Clinical evidence of benefit has not been demonstrated and this agent should be considered investigational.

SUPPORTIVE THERAPY. This review suggests that a 'magic bullet' to alter the course of cellular and molecular events following acute lung insult is desirable but as yet not available. In the future, these and newer agents, perhaps in combination and including antibiologics such as prophylactic antitumor necrosis factor antibodies in populations at risk,[51] may find application. At present, outside of clinical research trials, therapy is directed at supportive care and treatment of associated conditions; this includes ventilator management to reduce shunt and cardiovascular management to reduce edema, both accomplished while maintaining oxygen delivery or reducing oxygen consumption.

Respiratory Therapy. When the patient with ARDS presents to the ICU, therapy should begin simultaneously with evaluation. Supplemental oxygen should be provided by high flow or rebreather mask, although it should be recognized that such approaches in dyspneic and tachypneic patients rarely achieve a tracheal $F_{I_{O_2}}$ much above 0.60 (see Chap. 11). A large intrapulmonary shunt will be suggested by a minimal increase in Pa_{O_2} (to < 100 mmHg). Nonetheless, even small increases in Pa_{O_2} in the patient with arterial desaturation result in proportionally large increases in oxygen delivery (vide supra), so maximal oxygen therapy by mask should be implemented until endotracheal intubation is effected; interim CPAP by mask in alert, well-monitored patients usually improves saturation further.

In virtually all patients elective intubation should be performed early, to permit application of PEEP and to avert progression to fatigue. Possible exceptions are noted above. If hypoperfusion is present, as in the patient with hypotension, cardiovascular instability, or the hyperdynamic circulation of sepsis, sedation and muscle relaxation should be instituted immediately. Other patients with extreme hypoxemia should also have oxygen consumption lowered by this means to rest the respiratory muscles and allow cooling of the febrile patient without shivering (vide infra), at least for the first few hours of stabilization on the ventilator.

Initial ventilator settings are selected to provide adequate oxygenation and ventilation, with a minimal risk of barotrauma. This is best accomplished with an $F_{I_{O_2}}$ of 1.0, tidal volume of 6 to 8 mL/kg, and respiratory rate of 25. With muscle relaxation the ventilation is controlled; patients deemed stable to initiate breaths can be managed with A/C or SIMV with minimal sensitivity (-2 cmH_2O). The goal of low tidal volume use is to maintain airway pressures < 45 cmH_2O, which can usually be achieved with the strategy described despite marked reductions in lung compliance. Such low tidal volume ventilation is appropriate to the reduced FRC in edematous lungs and has been shown to be safe in a diverse population of patients.[52] This may avoid lung injury and capillary leak associated with larger tidal volumes and larger pressure excursions,[53] and facilitates the use of larger levels of PEEP to reduce shunt without excessive end-inspiratory pressures.

Intermittent positive-pressure ventilation (IPPV) with high concentrations of oxygen will achieve an acceptable Pa_{O_2} ($\geq$50 mmHg) and O_2 saturation ($Sa_{O_2} \geq 90\%$) in the majority of patients; unfortunately, ongoing administration of such high concentrations of oxygen causes further lung damage. This certainly seems to be the case in animal models and in normal human lung (see Chap. 58), although it is difficult to distinguish the sequelae of acute lung injury from the complications of the therapy it requires. On the other hand, one consequence of greater hypoxemia with Sa_{O_2} approaching 75% is global myocardial hypoxia with anaerobic metabolism and acute dilated cardiomyopathy, which progresses rapidly to bradycardic cardiac arrest. Accordingly it seems prudent immediately on stabilization of the patient on the ventilator to utilize PEEP to recruit alveoli, diminish intrapulmonary shunt, and decrease oxygen requirement (vide supra). We advocate titration of PEEP therapy to achieve an F_{IO_2} of $\leq$ 60. Since alveolar recruitment is associated with both improvement in respiratory system compliance and gas exchange, the former can be used at the bedside to follow the improvement in lung function (see Chap. 127). PEEP should be added in increments of 3 to 5 cmH_2O while following lung compliance ($C = V_T/(P_{plat} - PEEP)$). During such a PEEP "trial" alveolar recruitment and lung mechanical changes tend to be complete and stable after five to eight breaths, and thus the improvement in lung function can be rather rapidly determined, as opposed to the hours of assessment that might occur if many serial blood-gas determinations are performed, during which time clinical condition can change for a host of different reasons.

It is extremely useful to follow arterial saturation noninvasively with pulse oximetry at this time. When further increments of PEEP do not alter lung compliance or actually cause it to fall, it is likely that lung hyperexpansion is occurring without significant alveolar recruitment. This is often a point at which PEEP will have adverse consequences on venous return (see discussion of Fig. 2-16 in Chap. 2) and hypotension and tachycardia may be observed. Of course, this adverse cardiovascular effect of positive-pressure ventilation and PEEP may be encountered at any point following its institution, particularly if the patient is hypovolemic or receives drugs (e.g., morphine sulfate, muscle relaxants) which impair the reflex alterations in venous pressure (Pms) that permit constancy of venous return in the face of rising right atrial pressure. Furthermore, PEEP may actually increase resistance to venous return (RVR) such that cardiac output is reduced by PEEP even when Pms increases just as much as Pra;[55] accordingly, PEEP-induced hypotension needs to be treated early with expansion of the circulating volume and/or vasoactive drugs. There is no evidence that PEEP has any "prophylactic" role in preventing patients with no or minimal lung injury from progressing to ARDS. Early titration of PEEP therapy is often associated with an apparent improvement in the chest radiograph. This should be viewed as a result of increases in lung volume and not a decrease in lung water and does not suggest a change in the underlying pulmonary capillary leak.

Not uncommonly, the patient with ARDS presents with such severe alveolar flooding and hypoxemia that more rapid correction with PEEP seems prudent. Then immediate implementation of 15 cmH_2O PEEP (provided the tidal volume is 5 to 7 mL/kg) will improve oxygen saturation if it does not reduce blood pressure to an unacceptable level. Then PEEP can be titrated up or down from that level after reducing F_{IO_2} until Sa_{O_2} falls to about 90%; of course, a falling blood pressure with PEEP increment mandates lower PEEP until the circulatory volume is increased or vasoactive drugs are added to maintain venous return at the higher PEEP. This aggressive utilization of PEEP, guided by oximetry and blood pressure, can allow the experienced intensivist to arrive at a PEEP providing adequate Sa_{O_2} without hypotension within 10 min of intubating and ventilating the relaxed patient! Sometimes, PEEP of 20 cmH_2O does not achieve 90% saturation even on 100% O_2; then it is advisable to reduce the tidal volume as tolerated by arterial pH and have chest tubes available at the bedside as PEEP is increased further to achieve appropriate end points.[56]

In our experience this approach is useful in many, but not all, patients to define a range of PEEP that permits rapid titration of F_{IO_2} to 0.60 or less. We would not necessarily advocate a level of PEEP that achieves the highest lung compliance or the lowest intrapulmonary shunt, however. Rather, the goals are an adequate saturation (>90%) of an adequate hemoglobin (in these patients, 14 g/dL or more), all on a nontoxic F_{IO_2}. The least level of PEEP that achieves these goals will result in the fewest complications related to elevated airway and intrathoracic pressures and should be sought. Since PEEP does not reduce lung water but rather redistributes it from the alveoli to the peribronchovascular space, discontinuation of PEEP is associated with rapid alveolar flooding and deterioration in oxygenation. Thus, even during the course of suctioning, patients with ARDS in the exudative phase may develop arterial desaturation with adverse consequences. Accordingly, specimens should be collected early in the course of management for protein determination (vide supra), Gram stain, culture, or other purposes as necessary. During the first few days and thereafter, nursing and respiratory therapy staff should be instructed to keep airway disconnections to a minimum, or to use an in-line suctioning system that maintains sterility and positive pressure, usually via the suctioning catheter residing in a sterile sheath and entering the endotracheal tube via a tight sealing diaphragm. These suctioning systems are generally effective for lesser levels of PEEP (<15 cmH_2O) but often leak if higher levels are attempted; such failure to maintain a seal, of course, defeats efforts at maintaining higher airway pressures. These instructions for maintenance of PEEP must often be explicit, for the airway and ventilator tubing often fill with copious amounts of alveolar liquid in these patients, sometimes prompting frequent disconnections to clear the fluid, which actually promotes alveolar and so bronchial flooding, which is quite different from the bronchorrhea requiring repeated bedside suctioning in COPD or other airflow obstruction leading to ventilator therapy.

Circulatory Management of ARDS. The routine supportive therapy outlined above is widely applied to patients with ARDS. Unfortunately, many have noted that mortality for this disease process remains high and unacceptable.[2,57,58] While it might be argued that this high mortality relates to increasing severity of disease or only the most severely ill patients reported in most series,[57] it is still compelling to consider interventions to improve outcome.

If edemagenesis could be diminished early after the lung injury, the duration of potentially dangerous ventilator, PEEP, and oxygen therapy could be reduced and outcome conceivably improved. In this regard it is interesting that most patients with ARDS do not die during the early phase of disease as a consequence of severe hypoxemia, but rather over days to weeks, frequently with evidence of hypermetabolism, nosocomial infection, and MSOF (see Chaps. 53 and 54).[58] Much animal and some clinical investigation has evaluated strategies to achieve reductions in lung water. When leak is well established, attempts to increase serum oncotic pressure are not successful because lung vascular permeability to protein is so increased.[59] However, modest (5 mmHg) reduction of the Ppw, by analogy to the treatment of hydrostatic edema, reduced edema accumulation by 50 percent in 4 h in canine oleic acid lung injury.[59] Even greater reductions in extravascular lung liquid (EVLL) and gravimetric edema were produced by reducing Ppw 1 h after hydrochloric acid aspiration[60–62] and after kerosene aspiration.[63,64] Data from six studies of the treatment of canine aspiration pneumonitis are summarized in Fig. 128-8 to illustrate the effects of these cardiovascular therapies on edema *(upper panel),* cardiac output *(lower panel)* and shunt ($\dot{Q}$VA/$\dot{Q}$T on F_{IO_2} = 0.6, *middle panel*). Reduction in the Ppw from 12 mmHg (control) to 8 or 5 mmHg by either plasmapheresis[60,61,63] or infusion of nitroprusside[62] 1 h after lung injury results in decreased lung water and improvement in intrapulmonary shunt; yet similar reduction of Ppw by hemofiltration did not reduce edema, presumably because that intervention aggravates lung injury. Of course, reducing Ppw reduces cardiac output as illustrated by the fall from 7 L/min to 3 L/min in Fig. 128-8, *lower panel.* Note, however, that cardiac output was maintained at the baseline value when vasoactive drugs (nitroprusside, dopamine) accompanied the reduced Ppw. Note further that when hematocrit is maintained or increased as Ppw is reduced (as with plasmapheresis), $\dot{Q}_{O_2}$ can be increased at reduced Ppw.[60] Accordingly, it is quite possible in most patients with ARDS to reduce circulating volume while maintaining $\dot{Q}_{O_2}$ in order to minimize edemagenesis.[65]

While reduction of preload is virtually always successful in CPE with salutary effect on lung function and minimal if any adverse consequences on ventricular function, the possibility for diminishing cardiac output is quite real when ventricular diastolic function and preload are more nearly normal. Thus, the goals of this approach in the patient with

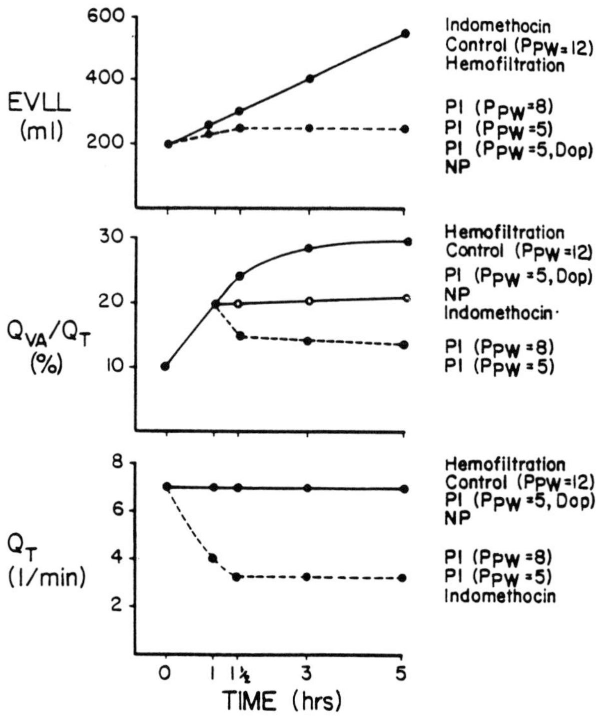

FIGURE 128-8 Schematic diagram illustrating the effects of reducing Ppw 1 h after hydrochloric acid or kerosene aspiration at time 0 h (abscissa) on extravascular lung liquid (EVLL by thermal dilution, upper ordinate), shunt ($\dot{Q}$VA/$\dot{Q}$T, middle ordinate), and cardiac output ($\dot{Q}$T, lower ordinate). The data are compiled from six studies by the same group with similar experimental protocols (see References 45, 60–64). *Upper panel.* Edema increases linearly with time after injury in the control group (Ppw = 12 continuous line), but reduction of Ppw to 8 or 5 mmHg at 1 h by plasmapheresis (Pl) or sodium nitroprusside (NP) attenuates or stops the edema accumulation (interrupted line), such that EVLL is less than half that in the control group by 5 h; all EVLL values were confirmed by gravimetric edema measures in the lungs excised at 5 h. Note that hemofiltration to Ppw = 5 mmHg did not reduce edema, and indomethacin had no effect on edemagenesis when Ppw was kept the same as the control group. *Middle panel.* Shunt increased in a curvilinear manner to about 30 percent as EVLL increased with time in the control group (continuous line through closed circles); when Ppw was reduced by plasmapheresis, $\dot{Q}$VA/$\dot{Q}$T stopped increasing and actually fell to about 15 percent due in part to reduced edema. Note that dopamine and NP also reduced $\dot{Q}$VA/$\dot{Q}$T when they reduced edema (continuous line through open circles), but that $\dot{Q}$VA/$\dot{Q}$T is greater in these groups than in plasmapheresis alone (interrupted line) because the vasoactive drugs increased $\dot{Q}$T; similarly indomethacin reduced $\dot{Q}$VA/$\dot{Q}$T compared to the control group despite similar edema because cardiac output decreased (see lower panel). *Lower panel.* $\dot{Q}$T did not change with time when Ppw was maintained in the control group; when Ppw was reduced by plasmapheresis, $\dot{Q}$T was maintained equal to the control group by dopamine and NP (continuous line). Plasmapheresis reduced $\dot{Q}$T by reducing Ppw (interrupted line), but reduced O_2 delivery less by increasing the hematocrit. Indomethacin reduced $\dot{Q}$T as the same Ppw suggesting decreased ventricular function; consequently, $\dot{Q}$VA/$\dot{Q}$T decreased with no change in edema.

ARDS are the least Ppw consistent with an adequate cardiac output. The question of the adequacy of cardiac output and hence oxygen delivery is further complicated in patients with sepsis and ARDS because of the potential defect in peripheral tissues in oxygen extraction (vide supra). Yet this uncertainty exists at any cardiac output, so we encourage use of careful hemodynamic evaluation while circulating volume and Ppw are reduced to the least value providing adequate $\dot{Q}_{O_2}$; when it is feasible, we measure $\dot{V}_{O_2}$ and excess lactate to detect anaerobic metabolism (see Chap. 57). Since even small reductions in preload significantly reduce cardiac output (See Fig. 128-8, *lower panel*), and the determination of adequate perfusion is difficult, undertaking this approach requires close monitoring of tissue function and hemodynamics. Since the adequacy of a given measured cardiac output or calculated oxygen delivery would be difficult to relate to patient needs, clinical end points of global organ system function are usually better parameters to follow. Accordingly, during any contemplated intervention, adequate nail bed perfusion, urine output, mental status, blood pressure, and absence of lactic acidosis are used to gauge the limits of preload reduction. The methods available to reduce preload include volume restriction (often difficult given the requirements of nutrition, antibiosis, and other drug administration in these patients), diuresis (or nitrates as venous dilators), phlebotomy and red blood cell reinfusion to maintain circulating hematocrit, or plasmapheresis. Diuresis with potent loop diuretics carries the disadvantage of confounding the use of urine volumes or urine electrolytes as indicators of the adequacy of renal perfusion.

As illustrated in the lower panel of Fig. 128-8, perfusion was augmented at a lower Ppw by the use of vasoactive drugs that confer inotropic (dopamine, dobutamine) or afterload reducing (nitroprusside) augmentation of cardiac output. Note that dopamine increased shunt *(middle panel)* at the same value of edema, probably by increasing pulmonary blood flow;[60] in the same way, indomethacin infusion, which did not reduce edema *(upper panel)*, reduces shunt by reducing cardiac output.[45] Sodium nitroprusside would be a natural choice as an agent which could both reduce preload and afterload; but it also increased shunt *(middle panel).* When studied in patients with ARDS, nitroprusside increased intrapulmonary shunt, likely secondary to its vasodilating effects on the pulmonary circulation with reversal of hypoxic vasoconstriction.[65,66] Dobutamine increases cardiac output at normal or reduced values of Ppw and also increases shunt. We interpret these studies to indicate $\dot{Q}_{O_2}$ can be maintained at reduced Ppw when circulatory volume is reduced, hematocrit is increased, and vasoactive drugs are titrated; the increase in shunt with these drugs is rarely a limit to this therapy because the increased $S\bar{v}_{O_2}$ maintains Sa_{O_2} in AHRF.[66]

While these circulatory manipulations are effective in reducing lung water and intrapulmonary shunt yet maintaining or improving oxygen delivery in acute animal models, extrapolation to clinical application must be done with appropriate skepticism. One clinical study has reported that extravascular lung water measured by single-pass multiple tracer technique does not correlate with the level of intrapulmonary shunt or survival in patients with ARDS.[67] Of course, this correlation does not address the specific question of whether reduction in lung water in a given patient could be accomplished safely and would have a salutary effect on outcome. Several retrospective or noninterventional studies have reported data showing a correlation between survival and net diuresis or reduction in Ppw.[68–70] Because a prospective randomized trial of this therapy has not been conducted, the circulatory management of these patients has been described as a therapeutic dilemma.[71] On the one hand judicious volume reduction may improve lung function. In the extreme, however, hypoperfusion and other organ failure could occur. Volume "loading" the patient could transiently increase cardiac output and hence oxygen delivery, but would likely worsen lung edema and escalate and extend treatment intensity and duration.

Our own experience is that reduction of Ppw can be safely accomplished in patients with ARDS,[70] and indeed focuses the clinician's attention on precisely the parameters of organ function that should be followed in all critically ill patients (e.g., mental status, urine output and concentration, circulatory adequacy, metabolic evidence of anaerobic metabolism). Reducing Ppw is in part accomplished by meticulous attention to limit all extraneous fluid administration. Active interventions can be individualized to a given patient but most often involve diuresis, with the caution that this may confound interpretation of renal function. In selected patients, particularly those with manifest systolic dysfunction, dobutamine may be used to maintain perfusion at a reduced Ppw. If volume administration must be increased in response to excessive reduction in preload, consideration should be first given to increasing circulating hemoglobin. While such an approach is both safe and successful anecdotally, it clearly requires confirmation by an appropriate clinical trial. In the interim, it seems reasonable use of current critical care capabilities to seek end points of therapy, and never should be misinterpreted as trading reduced pulmonary edema for a hypoperfusion state. Hence, we emphasize seeking the lowest pulmonary vascular pressures compatible with an *adequate* cardiac output and $\dot{Q}_{O_2}$.

Monitoring the Patient with ARDS. Changes in intrapulmonary shunt, oxygen consumption, or perfusion are frequent and relatively sudden in these patients, and therefore arterial saturation and hence oxygen delivery are volatile. Accordingly, careful monitoring for hypoxemia and the adequacy of oxygen delivery are advisable. If there is not gross hypoperfusion, continuous pulse oximetry is reliable and should be considered in all patients. Alternatively, frequent sampling of arterial blood-gases is advisable throughout the first day of management, as well as with major interventions or changes in clinical appearance of the patient.

The debate over use of invasive monitoring in these patients has been mentioned. If there is no question to be answered and therapy will likely not be altered by the data collected, pro forma right heart catheterization is of course not warranted.[27] We would offer a number of observations. Circulatory disturbances are frequent in these patients; on occasion, a patient with "clear-cut" ARDS will prove to have significant left ventricular dysfunction and hydrostatic edema. Of course, this determination may also be made by tests such as analysis of edema fluid or echocardiography (vide supra). Hemodynamic monitoring may be useful in patients with sepsis as an antecedent to ARDS. Many of these patients are hypovolemic, likely related to intravascular volume lost through their diffuse capillary leak and sequestration of circulating volume in the venous capacitance vessels. Volume resuscitation is appropriate to the extent that hypovolemia is the cause of hypoperfusion superimposed on their hypoxemia, but excessive volume administration carries the risk of worsening pulmonary edema. Measurements of Ppw and cardiac output may help avoid excessive fluid administration. Although these same patients tend to a hyperdynamic circulation following fluid resuscitation, varying degrees of ventricular dysfunction may exist and support with inotrope infusions can be titrated with invasive measurements. Treatment of these patients with positive-pressure ventilation, PEEP, and vasoactive drugs also carries the possibility of complex effects on intrapulmonary shunt, cardiac output, and $S\bar{v}_{O_2}$, which are difficult to discern simply from the vital signs and arterial blood-gas determinations; invasive monitoring is particularly useful in this setting. Specific interventions may be considered to reduce edema in these patients, and titration of such interventions is aided by invasive measurement. Finally, we note that the greatest uncertainty exists early in the course of management, so a low threshold for instituting early invasive measurements should be accompanied by an aggressive withdrawal as soon as the questions are answered.

INNOVATIVE SUPPORTIVE INTERVENTIONS REQUIRING FURTHER CLINICAL STUDY. *High Frequency Ventilation.* Since pressure or volume excursions during mechanical support of lung disease characterized by markedly diminished compliance may themselves contribute to lung injury and leak,[53,72] several alternative modes of mechanical ventilation for AHRF have been proposed; each aims to maximize the benefits of PEEP to reduce shunt, while minimizing the tidal volume excursions required to effect adequate alveolar ventilation. A number of high frequency ventilation strategies have been demonstrated to achieve ventilation and oxygenation in animal models. High frequency oscillatory ventilation (HFOV) reduces shunt in edematous lung regions in proportion to the end-expiratory alveolar pressure, which is underestimated by airway opening pressure.[73] The widest clinical application has been of high frequency jet ventilation (HFJV). A number of crossover and prospective randomized trials comparing HFJV to conventional ventilation have been reported.[74–76] Although this ventilatory mode does appear to be safe in the hands of investigators reporting these results, it did not confer benefit in terms of incidence of barotrauma, gas exchange, or outcome. A number of investigators have also noted that HFJV does not provide adequate CO_2 elimination in patients with high minute ventilation requirements or markedly reduced compliance.[74]

Constant flow ventilation (CFV) relies less on bulk flow and completely on intrapulmonary momentum exchange to effect alveolar ventilation,[77] but requires careful placement of the inflow gas jets to bypass the bottleneck of facilitated diffusion in the proximal airways.[78] A recent canine study demonstrated that a small tidal volume (3 to 4 mL/kg) in series with CFV effected eucapnia and reduced shunt at lower alveolar pressures in a canine model of AHRF.[79] Accordingly, these alternative ventilatory strategies cannot be considered at the present time to confer significant benefit over conventional ventilation, although further investigation of their utility is warranted. Of course, a judicious trial of any of these modes (HFOV, HFJV, CFV) by intensivists familiar with their unusual mechanics and adverse effects is warranted in unique circumstances when conventional therapy has been pushed unsuccessfully to its limit; in this regard, it is sobering to recall that no prospective trial has been conducted to establish the benefit of PEEP on morbidity and mortality, yet its benefit on arterial oxygenation in AHRF can be repeatedly and reversibly demonstrated.

Inverse ratio ventilation (IRV). Described elsewhere in the text (see Chap. 9), IRV involves prolongation of inspiratory time so that the inspiratory: expiratory time ratio (I:E) exceeds 1, as opposed to the usual ratios of 1:2 or 1:3 used during conventional ventilation. The purported benefits of this ventilatory strategy are more optimal distribution of ventilation and alveolar recruitment at lower airway inflating pressures.[80,81] A number of studies have indicated that intrapulmonary shunt can be reduced substantially with IRV and some authors have suggested it be used as a "salvage" strategy for patients who cannot be adequately treated with conventional ventilation and PEEP.[82,83] However, when the mechanism of alveolar recruitment and shunt reduction has been most carefully examined,[84] it appears that IRV results in auto- or intrinsic PEEP (see Chap. 9) as a result of incomplete alveolar emptying and gas trapping at the end of the shortened expiratory period. Thus it seems that IRV and PEEP set on the ventilator may result in nearly the same lung inflation and mean alveolar pressure for an equivalent degree of alveolar recruitment, suggesting little benefit to be derived from this strategy. Nonetheless, there may be patients who benefit from this alternative approach, and it warrants a comparison with PEEP and conventional therapy in the difficult patient; then, a check on auto-PEEP and end-inspiratory pressure should be included with evaluation of cardiac output, shunt, $\dot{Q}_{O_2}$, and Pa_{CO_2}. It should be noted that IRV is extremely uncomfortable for the patient with AHRF and virtually mandates complete sedation and muscle relaxation.

Patient Positioning. Side-to-side positioning of the patient is well described to improve gas exchange in the patient with asymmetric alveolar filling disease (vide infra). Similar reduction of intrapulmonary shunt and improved oxygenation has been described in patients with ARDS shifted to a prone position.[85,86] Computed tomography imaging of the chest has demonstrated that acute lung injury (ARDS) in supine ICU patients often has a heterogenous distribution, with more edema in dependent lung regions. In an interesting canine model of acute lung injury created in two groups of animals, one supine and the other prone, flipping animals in either group subsequent to the development of pulmonary edema improved oxygenation. These observations are consistent with positional changes in ARDS patients exploiting the gravitational distribution of blood flow to reduce shunt. We reserve this strategy for patients who cannot be adequately managed in the supine position.

Extracorporeal Membrane Oxygenation (ECMO). The details of this technology are described elsewhere (see Chap. 29). The hypothesis supporting such invasive management of patients is the provision of adequate oxygenation by an extracorporeal device, permitting a degree of lung "rest" during the period of injury and until organ recovery is well established. That is, ventilation and barotrauma may be reduced in the hope of diminishing lung injury, while FI_{O_2} may be reduced to reduce oxygen toxicity; in some circumstances of venoarterial ECMO, the lung bypass can also reduce pulmonary flow and vascular pressures to reduce edema.[63] The earliest large multicenter trial of this therapy, using venoarterial ECMO, was reported in 1979.[87] In this study, patients with advanced ARDS requiring toxic concentrations of oxygen were enrolled, and survival was not improved with ECMO. After this report, interest waned in the use of this technology in ARDS. Over the next decade, however, increased survival was demonstrated in neonates with respiratory distress syndrome and recent studies have suggested that it may be beneficial in this form of respiratory failure (see Chaps. 29 and 186). Concommitant with these reports from neonatal ICUs, a number of European and American investigators have returned to various ECMO strategies. Most popular is use of venovenous bypass to achieve extracorporeal carbon dioxide removal ($ECCO_2R$) with only a fraction of oxygenation provided by the extracorporeal circuit; further blood oxygenation is achieved by apneic ventilation in the paralyzed patient by continuous flow provided by a cannula placed in the trachea, along with low frequency positive-pressure ventilation.[88,89] Interestingly, reported survival is improved from earlier reports of ECMO in ARDS but clear differences in survival between this approach and conventional ventilator strategies have not been demonstrated. Final results of the single large American study are not yet available. At present this therapy is best considered experimental and should be restricted to large centers with both experience in and resources for this intensive therapy.

MANAGEMENT DURING RECOVERY FROM THE EXUDATIVE PHASE OF ARDS. Rapid recovery from ARDS, generally within 2 to 3 days, is encountered and is likely determined by resolution of the predisposing cause and arguably by appropriate cardiovascular interventions. Such recovery is heralded by diminished shunt, increased lung compliance, and diminishing oxygen requirements. When FI_{O_2} can be reduced to 0.40 to 0.50, consideration can be given to cautious reduction in PEEP. On occasion, however, even small decrements in PEEP will be associated with sudden arterial desaturation, perhaps related to alveolar flooding or collapse related to surfactant deficiency or dysfunction. When this occurs, PEEP levels often must be increased above the former level for alveolar recruitment. Accordingly, we recommend small decrements (2 to 3 cmH_2O) of PEEP, with several hours of observation between adjustments.

When the patient has achieved an FI_{O_2} of .40 and PEEP $<$ 10, evaluation for spontaneous ventilation can be undertaken. If CNS depression, muscle weakness, or new lung insults have not occurred during the course of acute illness, rapid progression to CPAP is appropriate, with prompt extubation (see Chap. 127). In anticipation of these events, sedation and muscle relaxation should be discontinued as soon as resolution of edema becomes clear.

MANAGEMENT OF THE PATIENT IN PROLIFERATIVE PHASE ARDS. Unfortunately many patients with ARDS will progress over the first week of mechanical ventilation to disordered healing and severe lung fibrosis. This is usually characterized by increasing airway pressures, diminished lung compliance, a "honeycomb" appearance on the chest radiograph, progressive pulmonary hypertension, and extremely high minute ventilation requirements ($>$20 L/min). Barotrauma is a prominent feature of their course and multiple organ failures often accrue. A number of observations regarding their supportive therapy should be made. Increased vascular permeability at this point in the course may be minimal, and strategies to reduce preload and edema are fraught with complications. Indeed, in view of the high alveolar pressures, attempts to reduce the Ppw may result in increased dead space and hypoperfusion (see Chap. 52). Thus, the circulatory management seeking the lowest Ppw providing adequate cardiac output and $\dot{Q}_{O_2}$ should not be pushed; instead, liberalization of fluid intake to provide a circulating volume in excess of that just adequate is a better strategy in this later phase of ARDS.

Interventions to directly influence the course of lung fibrosis are not well established, but anecdotally high doses of corticosteroids have been noted to confer benefit, similar perhaps to more chronic forms of lung fibrosis.[90] Nosocomial pneumonia is remarkably common during this period of time and is likely the major source of late sepsis in patients with ARDS.[91] The infecting organism is most often a gram-negative enteric or *Pseudomonas.* In view of the abnormal chest radiograph and gas exchange, multiple causes of fever and leukocytosis, and high incidence of colonization of the airway, diagnosis is difficult and maybe aided by various techniques to obtain protected specimens.[91]

If improvement is not marked by 10 to 14 days but recovery is still possible tracheostomy is reasonable for patient comfort and ongoing ventilator management. Nutritional support is crucial and should be instituted if recovery is not likely to be complete within the first day of management. Subsequent management of these patients is often protracted and difficult, with constant attention to the details of various organ failures and complications that inevitably arise over time.

PULMONARY SEQUELAE OF ARDS. Although there are a limited number of long-term follow-up studies of patients with ARDS, it appears that the range of outcomes is rather wide: patients may recover with minimal or no abnormality by routine lung function testing shortly after acute lung insult, or substantial impairment may persist for a year or longer, if not permanently.[92] In most studies, at 1 year approximately one-fourth of patients show no impairment, one-fourth moderate impairment, one-half mild impairment, and a very small fraction severe impairment. Exertional dyspnea is the most commonly reported symptom, although cough and wheezing are common as well. A reduced single-breath carbon monoxide diffusing capacity is the most common pulmonary function abnormality. Spirometry and lung volumes when abnormal tend to reveal mixed restrictive-obstructive abnormalities. The difficulty in determining which patients will manifest such problems and prognosticating for those who do suggest that at the time the patient is ready for discharge from the hospital, complete lung functions should be obtained. Those patients with substantial abnormalities should be referred for appropriate follow-up.

MANAGEMENT OF FOCAL LESIONS PRODUCING AHRF

LOBAR PNEUMONIA. Inflammatory pneumonias, even involving only a fraction of the lung volume, can produce significant lung shunt because of the increase in pulmonary blood flow and aerobic metabolism of the consolidated region.[14] Accordingly, supplemental oxygen often has only a modest effect in resolving the associated hypoxemia, but it may correct arterial desaturation due to hypoventilation of lung regions mechanically interdependent with the pneumonic consolidation. Accordingly, many otherwise healthy patients will stabilize with supplemental oxygen and appropriate antibosis until inflammation subsides over the first days of therapy.

Patients with concurrent problems (e.g., old age, debilitated state, sepsis) or those with extreme hypoxemia will require mechanical ventilatory support, in part to stabilize the cardiovascular collapse associated with pyrexia and excess work of breathing. Indications are similar to other forms of AHRF and include tachypnea (respiratory rate $>$ 35) and inability to achieve adequate arterial saturation. Once intubation has been performed, careful sampling of airway secretions for Gram stain and culture should be performed.

The guidelines for ventilator management are similar to those for patients with ARDS. However, PEEP therapy should be added cautiously, and with pulse oximetry in place. This is particularly so in these patients with focal disease, since PEEP may not recruit the consolidated lung but rather hyperinflate normal lung and at high levels cause an increase in intrapulmonary shunt.[93] Nonetheless, a trial of PEEP is warranted in most patients since varying degrees of lung edema may be present in regions distant from the radiologically apparent pneumonia.

If the patient cannot be adequately oxygenated with PEEP, consideration should be given to positioning with "the good lung down."[94] This maneuver can favor blood flow to normally ventilated lung regions and improve gas exchange. In those patients with substantial airway secretions, this carries the risk of soiling the normal lung.

Interventions to decrease blood flow to the infected lobe could conceivably improve gas exchange, and inhibition of prostaglandin synthesis with indomethacin has been demonstrated to reduce lung shunt in a canine model of pneumonia.[95] There is little experience with such approaches in human beings, however, and other effects of such agents may make their use inadvisable.

As for other patients with AHRF and severe hypoxemia, every attempt should be made to reduce oxygen consumption. In patients with pneumonia, sedation and muscle relaxation with controlled ventilation, correction of hyperthermia, and avoidance of shivering are all simple measures that can achieve this goal.

LUNG CONTUSION. Blunt chest trauma, particularly when sufficient to cause rib fracture, often results in contusion of the underlying lung. As discussed above, the contusion essentially stops blood flow to the consolidated hemorrhagic region probably by mechanical distortion or obliteration of the vessels. As a result the shunt in pulmonary contusion is very small but the hypoxia can be quite profound due to mechanical interdependence of the contused regions with the surrounding lung leading to large numbers of low $\dot{V}_A/\dot{Q}$ units there.[16] This is important to oxygen therapy, for hypoxemic patients with large lung contusions often become well oxygenated with modest amounts of supplemental oxygen by nasal prongs or mask in clinical circumstances where the associated pain or other injuries might lead the prudent physician to believe that intubation and stabilization on a ventilator is imperative for the presumed shunt lung disease. The frequent concurrence of flail chest with lung contusion impacts little on the already small shunt, but adds to the hypoventilation of associated regions having very low $\dot{V}_A/\dot{Q}$, leading to severe hypoxemia. Yet measures which enhance ventilation like pain control and mechanical stabilization of the flail segment often allow simple oxygen supplementation to correct the hypoxemia[96] and spare the patient intubation and positive-pressure ventilation.[97] This has a special advantage in lung contusion where positive-pressure ventilation especially with PEEP is associated with an increase in the underlying lung contusion.[98]

CASE PRESENTATION

A 32 year-old woman was admitted to the emergency room for fever, shortness of breath, and diminishing mental status over several hours duration. The patient had a long history of inflammatory bowel disease with several small bowel resections for obstruction resulting in a short bowel syndrome and malabsorption. She was managed with home parenteral nutrition administered through a tunneled left subclavian catheter. She had reported some tenderness over the catheter site to her family a day earlier. Today she noted a fever and rigor in the morning. By early afternoon she had become slightly short of breath with walking and later in the day was somewhat inappropriate in her responses to the family. She was then brought to the hospital.

On evaluation the patient was lethargic but responded to voice and could follow very simple commands. The temperature was 40.0°C (104°F) orally, pulse 135 and bounding, blood pressure 95/25, and respiratory rate 30. Skin examination was remarkable for several hemorrhagic vesicles in the axillae and one area of painless rounded induration with a central necrotic eschar suggesting ecthyma gangrenosum. In addition, there was induration, tenderness, and erythema along the subcutaneous track of the catheter. The cardiopulmonary examination was remarkable only for a hyperdynamic circulation and the abdomen was benign. No meningeal signs and no focal neurologic abnormalities were present.

The initial laboratory data included an arterial blood-gas determination on room air revealing a Pa_{O_2} of 80 mmHg, Pa_{CO_2} of 14 mmHg, and pH of 7.19. The glucose, creatinine, and BUN were normal and the arterial lactate level was 24 mg/dL. The hematocrit was 49 percent and white blood cell count 19,500 with 82 polys, 14 bands, and 4 lymphs. The peripheral smear suggested a microangiopathic hemolytic process and the platelet count was 85,000. The prothrombin and partial thromboplastin times were normal. The chest radiograph revealed a questionable interstitial infiltrate diffusely and a left subclavian catheter in good position. Urinalysis was unremarkable.

A 16 gauge peripheral intravenous line was started and blood cultures were obtained through the catheter and at peripheral sites. Urine cultures were obtained as well. Pulse oximetry was started. Loading doses of tobramycin and ceftazidime were given. While antibiotics were being administered, the blood pressure fell to 70/0 and the patient was slightly more tachypneic and less responsive. Elective intubation was performed and the blood pressure rose to 85 systolic after a liter of 0.9 N saline (NS) solution was given.

Surgical consultation was obtained in the emergency room and when pus could be expressed from around the catheter insertion site the subcutaneous tunnel was opened and irrigated, and the catheter was removed. By gross inspection infection appeared to involve the subcutaneous path of the catheter but not extend extensively into surrounding tissues nor extend fully to the venous insertion site. Gram stain of the pus within the tunnel revealed many white blood cells and gram-negative bacteria.

In view of the strong evidence of gram-negative septicemia including *Pseudomonas* species, the initial antibiotics were continued. While surgical evaluation was being conducted, the patient exhibited repeated episodes of hypotension and an additional 4 L 0.9 NS solution was given, resulting in modest increases in the blood pressure. Pulse oximetry revealed desaturation and the F_{IO_2} was increased to 100%. The patient was transferred to the ICU.

On arrival, benzodiazepines were given for sedation but the patient continued to make substantial respiratory efforts, and muscle relaxation was instituted with vecuronium (given as a loading dose of 0.1 mg/kg and then a maintenance infusion of 0.07 mg/kg/h). Sedation was continued. A cooling blanket was applied. The endotracheal tube now yielded abundant frothy sputum; sent for lab analysis, these airway suckings revealed a protein content of 75 percent of the serum value. The patient was placed on the ventilator at a tidal volume of 6 mL/kg and rate of 28 with an F_{IO_2} of 1.0. The peak airway pressure was 40 cmH_2O and the plateau pressure, determined with an inspiratory hold maneuver, 35 cmH_2O. The blood pressure was now 98/35 and the heart rate 118. An arterial blood-gas sample revealed a Pa_{O_2} of 45 mmHg, Pa_{CO_2} of 25 mmHg and pH of 7.33. A repeat chest film indicated good position of the endotracheal tube and diffuse alveolar infiltrates (Fig. 128-9).

PEEP was added to the ventilator circuit in 5 cmH_2O increments while monitoring Sa_{O_2} with a pulse oximeter, airway pressures, and vital signs (Table 128-6). A right heart catheter was placed and revealed a right atrial pressure of 8 mmHg, right ventricular pressure of 35/8 mmHg, pulmonary artery pressure of 32/16 mmHg, and Ppw of 14 mmHg. The cardiac output determined by thermal dilution was 9.0 L/min. With titration of PEEP the Pa_{O_2} rose to 85 mmHg, and F_{IO_2} was decreased to 70%, when Sa_{O_2} fell to 90% (Pa_{O_2} = 59 mmHg). The Pa_{CO_2} was now 23 mmHg and pH 7.37. A simultaneous mixed venous blood specimen revealed a P_{O_2} of 45 mmHg with a calculated intrapulmonary shunt fraction ($\dot{Q}s/\dot{Q}_T$) of 37 percent. Whenever the patient was disconnected from the ventilator, desaturation rapidly ensued and staff were instructed to not disconnect the circuit for purposes of suctioning.

The urine output in the first hour in the ICU was 45 mL. Antibiotics were maximally concentrated and fluids given at a keep open rate only. Intravenous furosemide was given at a dose of 40 mg, which resulted in a urine output of 600 mL over 3 h. Each hour during the early management urine output, vital signs, physical examination, hemodynamics, and arterial and mixed venous blood-gases were assessed by the clinicians at the bed-

TABLE 128-6 Titration of PEEP Therapy

PEEP Level	Pplat	Crs	Sa_{O_2}(%)	BP
0	35	12	88	98/35
5	39	12	90	98/30
10	40	14	94	96/35
15	42	16	96	94/35
20	52	13	93	85/35
17.5	43	16.5	98	94/35

PEEP, positive end expiratory pressure (cmH_2O); Pplat, plateau proximal airway pressure (cmH_2O; Crs, compliance of the respiratory system (mL/cmH_2O); Sa_{O_2}, arterial oxygen saturation; BP, blood pressure in mmHg.

TABLE 128-7 Hemodynamic Management of a Patient with ARDS

Hours after Admission	0	6	9	12	24	48
F_{IO_2}	0.70	0.70	0.70	0.60	0.50	0.40
PEEP (cmH_2O)	17.5	17.5	17.5	15	15	5
Ppw (mmHg)	14	10	6	5	4	5
$\dot{Q}_T$ (L/min)	9.0		7.0	9.5	8.0	7.0
Pa_{O_2} (mmHg)	59	54	51	60	69	79
$P\bar{v}_{O_2}$ (mmHg)	45		36	43	40	39
$\dot{Q}_S/\dot{Q}_T$	37		35		22	17
BUN:creatinine	14				20	
Dobutamine (μg/kg/min)		7.5	7.5	5.0		

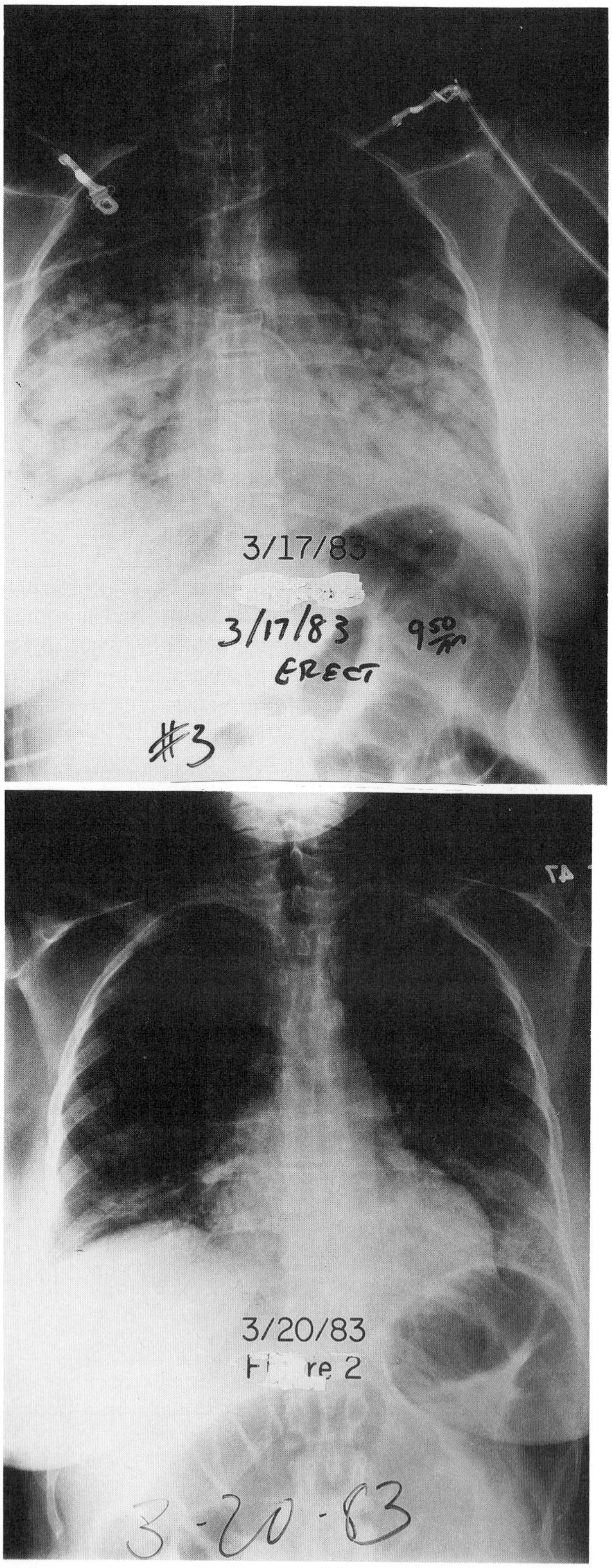

a

b

FIGURE 128-9 Chest radiographs shortly after intubation and right heart catheterization of this patient with ARDS (*a*), and 60 to 72 h following the management described in the text and after extubation (*b*).

side (Table 128-7). Serum creatinine and BUN were measured every 6 h.

Furosemide was given every 4 h at a dose of 40 mg in the first 24 h. After two doses, the Ppw fell to 10 mmHg, and after three doses the measured Ppw was 6 mmHg. At this point the heart rate rose to 130, the blood pressure fell to 80/45, and the measured cardiac output was 7.0 L/min with a $P\bar{v}_{O_2}$ of 36 mmHg (see Table 128-7). Dobutamine was started at a dose of 5 μg/kg/min and titrated to 7.5 μg/kg/min. The systolic blood pressure rose mimimally to 88 mmHg but the measured cardiac output rose to 9.5 L/min and $P\bar{v}_{O_2}$ to 43 mmHg.

Over the next 24 h the Ppw was maintained at 2 to 5 mmHg while the cardiac output, fluid balance, acid-base state, and gas exchange were closely followed (see Table 128-7). After a net diuresis of 4.5 L the ratio of BUN/creatinine rose from the initial value of 14 to 20. With the same tidal volume and rate Pa_{CO_2} rose gradually to 35 mmHg. These data were interpreted as indicating the limits of volume reduction and fluid administration was liberalized to maintain matched input and output.

Over hours 24 to 48 in the ICU gas exchange markedly improved (see Table 128-7). Blood cultures returned positive for *Pseudomonas* sensitive to the antibiotics selected. Ventilator support was gradually diminished in accord with the patient's improving status. Muscle relaxation was withheld on the first day sufficiently long to confirm neurologic function and then entirely held after 36 h. After 48 h the patient was able to communicate and was informed that she would be triggering the ventilator and over the next day assuming more of the work of breathing. From hours 48 to 72 the patient was managed with an A/C mode and trigger sensitivity of -2 cmH_2O. On the morning of the fourth ICU day the chest film had cleared dramatically (see Fig. 128-9) and the patient was placed on CPAP of 5 cmH_2O after demonstrating a negative inspiratory force (NIF) of -60 cmH_2O and spontaneous tidal volume of 400 mL with a respiratory rate of 26. She was extubated after a 30-min trial and managed with supplemental oxygen by mask. The following day she was transferred to the ward to receive a complete course of antibiotics and to await placement of a new catheter. Plans were initiated to obtain complete pulmonary function tests before discharge.

CASE DISCUSSION

This woman's acute illness occurred in a setting and with signs and symptoms making certain an initial diagnosis of gram-negative sepsis. Early on appropriate antibiotics were given, the likely infectious focus identified, and consideration given to any necessary surgical intervention. As is often the case in these patients, volume resuscitation was deemed necessary for the hypotension encountered early on. As is also often the case, this volume resuscitation was quickly followed by the development of AHRF. Indeed, early gas exchange abnormalities were present with the very first arterial blood-gas sample, which revealed an abnormal Pa_{O_2} given the patient's age and hyperventilation.

Arguably the initial volume resuscitation of this patient was excessive, but this judgment is difficult to make at the bedside with the information available by clinical assessment in the absence of measured hemodynamics. Elective intubation was warranted on the basis of this patient's shock alone (see Chap. 127) and certainly crucial in the management of the ARDS that quickly complicated her sepsis. Since sepsis is such a common predisposition to ARDS, careful monitoring of gas exchange (as with pulse oximetry in this case) should always be carried out during fluid resuscitation. Collection of edema fluid shortly after intubation confirmed a high protein content consistent with the exudative phase of pulmonary capillary leak.

Given the identification of the predisposing cause for ARDS in this case and its appropriate treatment, attention was then directed to the supportive management of the patient. Initial ventilator management included a high $F_{I_{O_2}}$ (confirming a large intrapulmonary shunt) with low tidal volumes and high rates to minimize high airway pressures. PEEP was then added while following lung mechanics and pulse oximetry as described in the preceding chapter. An optimal PEEP level of 17.5 cmH_2O was identified which maximized lung compliance. Had gas exchange been excellent at this level a strategy of "least" PEEP to achieve an arterial saturation of 90% with an $F_{I_{O_2}} \leq 0.60$ would have been reasonable; given the severity of shunt lung disease in this patient, even relatively high levels of PEEP required continued use of an $F_{I_{O_2}}$ as high as 0.70. Efforts were also directed at reducing tissue oxygen requirements during the early phase of AHRF, achieved by muscle relaxation to reduce the work of the respiratory muscles and to avoid shivering related to the patient's underlying infection, and by control of the patient's hyperthermia.

This approach to early supportive care has broad consensus among critical care physicians; unfortunately, morbidity and mortality for patients managed in this fashion remains unacceptably high. Also, within the present armamentarium of pharmacologic agents with potential to modify the course of acute lung injury, therapies of proven benefit have not yet been identified. Our own approach, supported by experimental data and clinical experience as described in this chapter, is to consider the possibility of minimizing edemagenesis in such patients by active management of the patient's circulation. Accordingly, this patient underwent right heart catheterization, which confirmed the clinical suspicion of a high flow shock state with improved acidosis following fluid resuscitation but diffuse lung flooding despite "normal" pulmonary vascular pressures as indicated by a Ppw of 14 mmHg. Cautious volume reduction was then carried out with fluid restriction and frequent doses of furosemide. The adequacy of the cardiac output was determined by bedside physical examination, measured cardiac output, the parameters of renal function such as the BUN:creatinine ratio, and the degree of acidosis that could be ascribed to hypoperfusion. Unfortunately, the requirement for muscle relaxation made serial neurologic examinations difficult, but in pursuit of some assessment of CNS function sedation and paralysis were periodically held. The choice of powerful diuretics to reduce intravascular volume in this patient precluded the use of urine electrolytes as sensitive markers for the adequacy of renal perfusion, although the utility of such a test in the face of sepsis might be compromised.

When net diuresis had been achieved, the Ppw fell (see Table 128-7) and at 9 h of therapy a degree of hypovolemia causing a lower cardiac output occurred. A response to this could have been further volume administration, although in the face of a continued pulmonary capillary leak this could result in further lung edema. Instead, cardiac output was augmented by dobutamine infusion, reasonable in view of a component of ventricular dysfunction in many cases of sepsis. Measured cardiac output rose with this intervention and the patient was then maintained at this intravascular volume. An elevation of BUN:creatinine and increasing Pa_{CO_2} at the same minute ventilation [likely indicating an increase in West zone I conditions of the lung (see Chap. 127)] suggested the limits of hypovolemia had been achieved.

Pulmonary vascular pressures were maintained at a low level and the predisposing infection was treated over the next 24 to 28 h associated with marked improvement in gas exchange and a deescalation of supportive care as $F_{I_{O_2}}$ and PEEP were decreased. Since the course of the patient's acute illness had been relatively short and intercurrent problems minimal, she was promptly encouraged to return to spontaneous ventilation and withdrawn from mechanical support when her gas exchange could be supported with supplemental oxygen supplied by mask alone.

References

1. Austrian R, Gold J: Pneumococcal bacteremia with especial reference to bacteremic pneumococcal pneumonia. Ann Intern Med 60:759, 1964.
2. Matthay MM: The adult respiratory distress syndrome: Definition and prognosis. Clin Chest Med 11:575, 1990.

3. Maunder RJ, Shuman WP, McHugh JW, et al: Preservation of normal lung regions in the adult respiratory distress syndrome. JAMA 255:2463, 1986.
4. Gattinoni L, Pesenti A, Bombino M: Relationships between lung computed tomographic density, gas exchange and PEEP in acute respiratory failure. Anesthesiology 69:824, 1988.
5. Crandall ED, moderator: Recent Developments in Pulmonary Edema (an edited summary of an interdepartmental conference arranged by the Department of Medicine of the UCLA School of Medicine, Los Angeles, California). Ann Intern Med 99:808, 1983.
6. Liez PL, Jacobson E, Shubin H, Weil MH: Pulmonary edema related to changes in colloid osmotic and pulmonary artery wedge pressure in patients after acute myocardial infarction. Circulation 51:350, 1975.
7. Rinaldo JE, Christman JW: Mechanisms and mediators of the adult respiratory distress syndrome. Clin Chest Med 11(4):621–632, 1990.
8. Ogibene FP, Martin SE, Parker MM, et al: Adult respiratory distress syndrome in patients with severe neutropenia, N Engl J Med 315(9):547, 1986.
9. Tomashefski JF: Pulmonary pathology of the adult respiratory distress syndrome. Clin Chest Med 11(4):593, 1990.
10. Montaver JSG, Tsang J, Evans KG, et al: Alveolar epithelial damage: A critical difference between high pressure and oleic acid induced low pressure edema. J Clin Invest 77:1786, 1986.
11. Matthay MA, Wiener-Kronish JP: Intact epithelial barrier function is critical for the resolution of alveolar edema in humans. Am Rev Respir Dis 142:1250, 1990.
12. Matthay MA (ed): Symposium on pulmonary edema. Clin Chest Med 6:229, 1985.
13. Pavlin J, Cheney FW Jr: Unilateral pulmonary edema in rabbits after re-expansion of collapsed lung. J Appl Physiol 46:31, 1979.
14. Light RB, Mink S, Wood LDH: Pathophysiology of gas exchange and pulmonary perfusion in pneumococcal lobar pneumonia in dogs. J Appl Physiol 50:524, 1981.
15. Light RB, Mink SN, Wood LDH: The effect of unilateral PEEP on gas exchange and pulmonary perfusion in canine lobar pneumonia. Anesthesiology 55:251, 1981.
16. Oppenheimer L, Craven KD, Forkert L, Wood LDH: Pathophysiology of pulmonary contusion in dogs. J Appl Physiol 47(4):718, 1979.
17. Dantzker RM: Gas exchange in the adult respiratory distress syndrome. Clin Chest Med 3:57–67, 1982.
18. Malo J, Ali J, Wood LDH: How does positive end-expiratory pressure reduce intrapulmonary shunt in canine pulmonary edema? J Appl Physiol 57(4):1002, 1984.
19. Pare PD, Warriner E, Baile M, Hogg JC: Redistribution of pulmonary extravascular water with positive end-expiratory pressure in canine pulmonary edema. Am Rev Respir Dis 127:590, 1983.
20. Wright PE, Bernard GR: The role of airflow resistance in patients with the adult respiratory distress syndrome. Am Rev Respir Dis 139:1169, 1989.
21. Marini JJ, Kirk W, Culver BH: Flow resistance of the exhalation valves and PEEP devices used in mechanical ventilation. Am Rev Respir Dis 131:850, 1985.
22. Cooligan T, Light RB, Wood LDH: Mink SN: Plasma volume expansion in canine pneumococcal pneumonia. Am Rev Respir Dis 126:86, 1982.
23. Kaplan JD, Calandrino FS, Schuster DP: A positron emission tomographic comparison of pulmonary vascular permeability during the adult respiratory distress syndrome and pneumonia. Am Rev Respir Dis, 143:150, 1991.
24. Aberle DR, Brown K: Radiologic considerations in the adult respiratory distress syndrome. Clin Chest Med 11(4):737, 1990.
25. Fein A, Grossman RF, Jones JG, et al: The value of edema fluid protein measurement in patients with pulmonary edema. Am J Med 67:32, 1979.
26. Iberti TJ, Fischer EP, Leibowitz AB, et al: A multicenter study of physicians' knowledge of the pulmonary artery catheter. JAMA 264:2928, 1990.
27. Chatterjee K, Parmley WW, Ganz W et al: Hemodynamic studies: Their uses and limitations. Am J Cardiol 64:30, 1989.
28. Murray JF, Matthay MA, Luce J, et al: An expanded definition of the adult respiratory distress syndrome. Am Rev Respir Dis 138:720, 1988.
29. Aberman A, Fulop M: The metabolic and respiratory acidosis of acute pulmonary edema. Ann Intern Med 76:173, 1972.
30. Dikshit K, Vyden JK, Forrester JS, Chatterjee K, et al: Renal and extra-renal hemodynamic effects of furosemide in congestive heart failure after acute myocardial infarction. N Engl J Med 288:1087, 1973.
31. Ali J, Wood LDH: Pulmonary vascular effects of furosemide on gas exchange in pulmonary edema. J Appl Physiol 57:160, 1984.
32. Väisänen IT, Räsänen J: Continuous positive airway pressure and supplemental oxygen in the treatment of cardiogenic pulmonary edema. Chest 92(3):481, 1987.
33. Permutt S, Wise RA, Sylvester JT: Interaction between the circulatory and ventilatory pumps, in Lenfant C (ed): *Lung Biology in Health and Disease. Vol 29—The Thorax,* part B. [Roussos C, Macklem PT (eds)]. New York, Marcel Dekker, 1985, pp 701–735.
34. Scharf SM, Bianco JA, Tow DD, Brown R: The effects of large negative intrathoracic pressure on left ventricular function in patients with coronary artery disease. Circulation 63:871, 1981.
35. Pisani RJ, Rosenow EC: Pulmonary edema associated with tocolytic therapy. Ann Intern Med 110(9):714, 1989.
36. Teplinsky K, Hall JB: Postictal pulmonary edema: Report of a case. Arch Intern Med 146:801, 1986.
37. Said SI, Foda HD: Pharmacologic modulation of lung injury. Am Rev Respir Dis 139:1553, 1989.
38. Luce JM, Montgomery B, Marks JD, et al: Ineffectiveness of high-dose methylprednisolone in preventing parenchymal lung injury and improving mortality in patients with septic shock. Am Rev Respir Dis 138:62, 1988.
39. Bernard GR, Luce JM, Sprung CL, et al: High-dose corticosteroids in patients with the adult respiratory distress syndrome. N Engl J Med 317:1565, 1987.
40. Goldstein G, Luce J: Pharmacologic treatment of the adult respiratory distress syndrome, in Wiedemann HP, Matthay MA, Matthay RA (eds): Clin Chest Med 11(4):773, 1990.
41. Holcroft JW, Vassar MJ, Weber CJ: Prostaglandin E_1 and survival in patients with the adult respiratory distress syndrome. Ann Surg 203:371, 1986.
42. Bone RC, Slotman G, Maunder R, et al: Randomized double-blind, multicenter study of prostaglandin E_1 in patients with the adult respiratory distress syndrome. Chest 96:114, 1989.
43. Melot C, Lejeune P, Leeman M, et al: Prostaglandin E_1 in the adult respiratory distress syndrome. Am Rev Respir Dis 139:106, 1989.
44. Bernard GR, Reines HD, Metz CA, et al: Effects of a short course of ibuprofen in patients with severe sepsis. Abstract. Am Rev Respir Dis 137:A138, 1988.
45. Mayers I, Breen PH, Gottlieb S, et al: The effects of indomethacin on edema and gas exchange in canine acid aspiration. Respir Physiol 69:149, 1987.

46. Hallman M, Spragg R, Harrell JH, et al: Evidence of lung surfactant abnormality in respiratory failure. J Clin Invest 70:673, 1982.
47. Jobe A, Ikegami M: Surfactant for the treatment of respiratory distress syndrome. Am Rev Respir Dis 136:1256, 1987.
48. Horbar JD, Soll RF, Sutherland JM, et al: A multicenter, randomized, placebo-controlled trial of surfactant therapy for respiratory distress syndrome. N Engl J Med 320:959, 1989.
49. Enhorning G: Surfactant replacement in adult respiratory distress syndrome. Am Rev Respir Dis 140:281, 1989.
50. Welsh CH, Lien D, Worthon GS, et al: Pentoxifylline decreases endotoxin-induced pulmonary neutrophil sequestration and extravascular protein accumulation in the dog. Am Rev Respir Dis 138:1106, 1988.
51. Tracey KJ, Lowry SF, Cerami A: Cachetin/TNF in septic shock and septic adult respiratory distress syndrome. Am Rev Respir Dis 138:1377, 1988.
52. Lee PC, Helsmoortel CM, Cohn SM, et al: Are low tidal volumes safe? Chest 97:425, 1990.
53. Corbridge TC, Wood LDH, Crawford GP, et al: Adverse effects of large tidal volume and low PEEP in canine acid aspiration. Am Rev Respir Dis 142:311, 1990.
54. Walley KR, Becker CJ, Hogan RA, et al: Progressive hypoxemia limits left ventricular oxygen consumption and contractility. Circ Res 63:849, 1988.
55. Fessler HE, Brower RG, Wise RA, Permutt S: Effects of positive end-expiratory pressure on the gradient for venous return. Am Rev Respir Dis 143:19, 1991.
56. Kirby RR, Downs JB, Civetta JM, et al: High level positive end expiratory pressure (PEEP) in acute respiratory insufficiency. Chest 67:156, 1975.
57. Rinaldo JE: Prognosis of the adult respiratory distress syndrome: Inappropriate pessimism? Chest 90:470, 1986.
58. Hyers TM, Fowler AA: Adult respiratory distress syndrome: Causes, morbidity and mortality. Fed Proc 45:25, 1986.
59. Prewitt RM, McCarthy J, Wood LDH: Treatment of acute low pressure edema in dogs: Relative effects of hydrostatic and oncotic pressure, nitroprusside, and positive end expiratory pressure. J Clin Invest 67:409, 1981.
60. Long GR, Breen PH, Mayers I, Wood LDH: Treatment of canine aspiration pneumonitis: Fluid volume reduction vs. fluid volume expansion. J Appl Physiol 65:1736, 1988.
61. Sznajder JI, Zucker AR, Wood LDH, Long GR: Effects of plasmapheresis and hemofiltration on acid aspiration pulmonary edema. Am Rev Respir Dis 134:222, 1986.
62. Gottlieb SS, Wood LDH, Hansen DE, Long R: The effect of nitroprusside on pulmonary edema, oxygen exchange, and blood flow in hydrochloric acid aspiration. Anesthesiology 67(2):47, 1987.
63. Zucker AR, Becker CJ, Berger S, et al: Pathophysiology of treatment of canine kerosene pulmonary injury: The effects of plasmapheresis and positive end-expiratory pressure on canine kerosene pulmonary injury. J Crit Care 4:184, 1989.
64. Zucker A, Wood LDH, Curet-Scott M, et al: Partial lung bypass reduces kerosene lung injury in dogs. J Crit Care, 1991. (In press)
65. Wood LDH, Prewitt RM: Cardiovascular management in acute hypoxemic respiratory failure. Am J Cardiol 47:963, 1981.
66. Oppenheimer L, Wood LDH, Prewitt RM: Acute effects of nitroprusside in patients with hypoxemic respiratory failure. Surg Forum 32:306, 1981.
67. Brigham KL, Kariman K, Harris TR, et al: Correlation of oxygenation with vascular permeability-surface area but not with lung water in humans with acute respiratory failure and pulmonary edema. J Clin Invest 72:339, 1983.
68. Eisenberg PR, Hansrough JR, Anderson D, Schuster DP: A prospective study of lung water measurements during patient management in an intensive care unit. Am Rev Respir Dis 136:662, 1987.
69. Simons RS, Berdine GG, Seidenfeld JJ, et al: Fluid balance and the adult respiratory distress syndrome. Am Rev Respir Dis 135:924, 1987.
70. Humphrey H, Hall J, Sznajder I, et al: Improved survival in ARDS patients associated with a reduction in pulmonary capillary wedge pressure. Chest 97:1176, 1990.
71. Hyers TM: ARDS: The therapeutic dilemma. Chest 97(5):1025, 1990.
72. Petersen GW, Horst B: Incidence of pulmonary barotrauma in a medical ICU. Crit Care Med 11(2):67, 1983.
73. Breen P, Ali J, Wood LDH: High frequency ventilation in lung edema: Effects on gas exchange and perfusion. J Appl Physiol 56(1):187, 1984.
74. MacIntyre NR, Follett JV, Dietz JL, et al: Jet ventilation at 100 breaths per minute in adult respiratory failure. Am Rev Respir Dis 134:897, 1986.
75. Borg UR, Stoklosa JC, Siegel JH, et al: Prospective evaluation of combined high-frequency ventilation in post-traumatic patients with adult respiratory distress syndrome refractory to optimized conventional ventilatory management. Crit Care Med 17:1129, 1989.
76. Carlon GC, Howland WS, Groeger JS, et al: Role of high-frequency jet ventilation in the management of respiratory failure. Crit Care Med 12:777, 1984.
77. Schumacker PT, Sznajder I, Nahum A, Wood LDH: Ventilation-perfusion inequality during constant flow ventilation. J Appl Physiol 62(3):1255, 1987.
78. Breen PH, Sznajder JI, Morrison P, et al: Constant flow ventilation in anesthetized patients: efficacy and safety. Anesth Analg 65:1161, 1986.
79. Sznajder JI, Becker CJ, Crawford G, Wood LDH: Combination of constant flow and continuous positive pressure ventilation in canine pulmonary edema. J Appl Physiol 67(2):817, 1989.
80. Abraham E, Yoshihara G: Cardiorespiratory effects of pressure controlled inverse ratio ventilation in severe respiratory failure. Chest 96:1356, 1989.
81. Gurevitch MJ, Van Dyke J, Young ES, et al: Improved oxygenation and lower peak airway pressure in severe adult respiratory distress syndrome: Treatment with inverse ratio ventilation. Chest 89:211, 1986.
82. Ravizza AF, Carugo D, Cerchiari EL, et al: Inversed ratio and conventional ventilations: Comparison of the respiratory effects. Abstract. Anesthesiology 59:A523, 1983.
83. Tharratt RS, Allen RP, Albertson TE: Pressure controlled inverse ratio ventilation in severe adult respiratory failure. Chest 94:755, 1988.
84. Cole AGH, Weller SF, Sykes MK: Inverse ratio ventilation compared with PEEP in adult respiratory failure. Intensive Care Med 10:227, 1984.
85. Piehl M, Brown R: Use of extreme position changes in acute respiratory failure. Crit Care Med 4:13, 1976.
86. Langer M, Mascheroni D, Marcolin R, et al: The prone position in ARDS patients. Chest 94:103, 1988.
87. Zapol WM, Snider MT, Hill JD. et al: Extracorporeal membrane oxygenation in severe acute respiratory failure. JAMA 242:2193, 1979.
88. Morris AH, Wallace CJ, Clemmer TP, et al: Extracorporeal CO_2 removal therapy for adult respiratory distress syndrome patients. Respir Care 35:224, 1990.

89. Gattinoni L, Pesenti A, Mascheroni D, et al: Low frequency positive-pressure ventilation with extracorporeal CO_2 removal in severe acute respiratory failure. JAMA 256:881, 1986.
90. Hooper RG, Kearl RA: Established ARDS treated with a sustained course of adrenocortical steroids. Chest 97:138, 1990.
91. Meduri GU: Ventilator-associated pneumonia in patients with respiratory failure: A diagnostic approach. Chest 97(5):1208, 1990.
92. Elliott CG: Pulmonary sequelae in survivors of the adult respiratory distress syndrome, in Wiedemann HP, Matthay MA, Matthay RA (eds): Clin Chest Med 11(4):789, 1990.
93. Mink SN, Light RB, Cooligan T, Wood LDH: The effect of PEEP on gas exchange and pulmonary perfusion in canine lobar pneumonia. J Appl Physiol 50:517, 1981.
94. Remolina C, Khan AU, Santiago TV, Edelman NH: Positional hypoxemia in unilateral lung disease. N Engl J Med 304:523, 1981.
95. Light RB: Indomethocin and acetylsalicylic acid reduce intrapulmonary shunt in experimental pneumococcal pneumonia. Am Rev Respir Dis 134:520, 1986.
96. Mackersie RC, Shackford SR, Hoyt DP: Continuous epidural fentanyl analgesia: Ventilatory function improvement with routine use in treatment of blunt chest injury. J Trauma 27:1207, 1987.
97. Barone JE, Pizzi WF, Nealon TF: Indications for intubation in blunt chest trauma. J Trauma 26:334, 1986.
98. Shorr RM, Crittenden M, Indeck M: Lung thoracic trauma: Analysis of 515 patients. Ann Surg 206:200, 1987.

Chapter 129
ACUTE ON CHRONIC RESPIRATORY FAILURE

GREGORY A. SCHMIDT
JESSE B. HALL

KEY POINTS

- *Severe chronic obstructive pulmonary disease (COPD) is usually clinically evident, but occasionally manifests as cryptic respiratory failure or postoperative ventilator dependence.*
- *Acute on chronic respiratory failure (ACRF) can occur when relatively minor, although often multiple, insults cause acute deterioration in a patient with advanced COPD.*
- *The wide variety of causes of ACRF may be compartmentalized into causes of incremental load, diminished neuromuscular competence, or depressed drive, superimposed on a limited ventilatory reserve.*
- *Intrinsic positive end-expiratory pressure (PEEPi) is a central contributor to the excess work of breathing in patients with ACRF.*
- *The most important therapeutic interventions are oxygen, bronchodilators, corticosteroids, and nutritional support.*
- *The decision to intubate a patient with ACRF requires clinical judgment and a bedside presence. Hypotension and severe alkalemia commonly complicate the immediate peri-intubation course, but are usually avoidable.*
- *Ventilator settings should mimic the patient's breathing pattern, with a relatively rapid rate (e.g., 20/min) and small tidal volume (V_T) (e.g., 450 to 550 mL).*
- *Prevention of complications such as gastrointestinal hemorrhage, venous thrombosis, and nosocomial infection is a crucial component of the care plan.*
- *The key to getting the patient off the ventilator is to increase neuromuscular competence while reducing respiratory system load.*

In the past 25 years mortality from COPD has risen dramatically. This trend is most apparent in men, is clearly related to cigarette smoking, and cannot be accounted for by changing diagnostic practices.[1] Admissions to ICUs for exacerbations of COPD account for a substantial portion of bed-days since these patients often require prolonged ventilatory support. In surgical ICUs COPD is an important problem as well, since it is one of the more common reasons for a prolonged postoperative recovery. An approach to this disease is an essential component of the intensivist's armamentarium.

Healthy adults expend very little effort to support the work of breathing, and blood flow to the respiratory muscles is but a small fraction of cardiac output. Normal individuals can tolerate substantial increments in respiratory workload or decrements in neuromuscular competence without a deterioration in ventilatory function. In contrast, patients with COPD spend their days perched on the precipice of respiratory failure. Minor insults to the respiratory system can tip a precarious balance, precipitating respiratory failure. This acute deterioration superimposed on stable disease is termed *acute on chronic respiratory failure* (ACRF).

Patients may present to the ICU with worsening dyspnea, deteriorating mental status, or respiratory arrest. Especially when there is a preexisting diagnosis of lung disease, the diagnosis of ACRF can be made easily. However, it is important to remember that not all patients with severe COPD will carry that label. In many patients with respiratory distress, congestive heart failure is considered first; making a correct diagnosis of ACRF requires a high index of suspicion. On occasion the disease is even more occult, e.g., in the postoperative patient who fails extubation, then is noted to have hyperinflation on the chest radiograph. Since optimal therapy depends on accurate diagnosis, underlying COPD should be considered within the differential diagnosis in most patients with dyspnea or inability to sustain unassisted ventilation.

Despite severe underlying pulmonary impairment, the prognosis for patients with ACRF is not uniformly poor. In an older study, 1 year mortality ranged from 26 percent if mechanical ventilation was not required to more than 50 percent when ventilation became necessary.[2] It is certain that long-term survival for patients with severe COPD has been improved by interventions such as long-term oxygen therapy (see Chap. 11) and likely that outcome for acute episodes of deterioration has improved as well. Many patients will return to an acceptable quality of life and even go back to work. Predictors of survival from acute bouts of respiratory failure include premorbid functional status, base-line dyspnea, and serum albumin level,[3] but these indicators are not refined enough to allow accurate prognostication in an individual patient. Ideally, patients followed in the clinic with known, severe COPD will be encouraged to discuss their wishes regarding intensive care with their physicians before acute deterioration. Unfortunately, this is only occasionally accomplished. It is our approach to fully support patients with COPD who believe their quality of life is acceptable, especially since the majority will be successfully liberated from the ventilator. On the other hand, when mechanical ventilation seems excessive in the patient's or physician's judgment, comfort measures alone may be appropriate.

Pathophysiology

Much of the pathophysiology of respiratory failure is detailed in Chap. 1. However, several points crucial to an understanding of the patient with ACRF will be presented here. The fundamental approach taken in this chapter is that the primary determinant of ACRF is inspiratory muscle fatigue (see Chap. 133). A functional definition of muscle

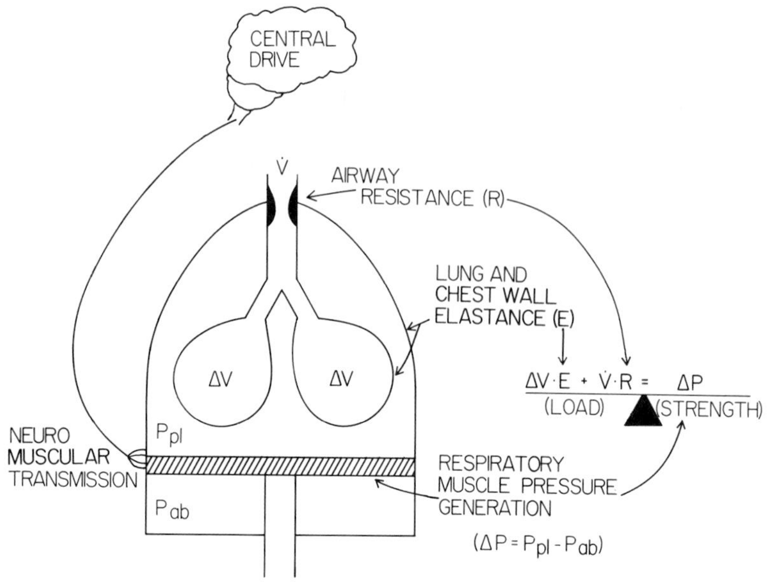

FIGURE 129-1 A drawing of the key elements of the respiratory system. Drive to breathe derives from CNS regulators of respiratory pattern. Neural afferents are the path for signals causing respiratory muscle contraction. Diaphragm contraction generates a pleural pressure (Ppl) and is opposed by any increased abdominal pressure (Pab). The Ppl generated must overcome the resistive (R) and elastic (E) forces acting on the respiratory system in producing a given minute ventilation ($\dot{V}$). (Reprinted from Reference 36, with permission.)

fatigue is the failure to develop the amount of tension generated before fatigue, no matter what the degree of stimulation. Skeletal muscles fatigue when their rate of energy consumption exceeds the energy supplied by blood flow for a sustained period of time.[4] Fatigue of respiratory muscles in normal persons has been demonstrated when the tension developed with each breath exceeded 40 percent of their maximal tension.[5] Once fatigue is established, the respiratory muscles become unable to sustain the mechanical load imposed on the system, and ventilatory failure ensues. Although controversy exists over the relative contributions of "central" versus "peripheral" mechanisms of fatigue, and the precise means of assessing fatigue in human respiratory failure remain elusive, this approach provides a useful conceptual framework for the treatment of patients with ACRF (see Chap. 133). This concept is developed in Fig. 129-1. The central nervous system (CNS) drives the inspiratory muscles via the spinal cord and phrenic and intercostal nerves. Inspiratory muscle contraction lowers pleural pressure (Ppl), thereby inflating the lungs. The pressure generated by the inspiratory muscles (neuromuscular competence) must be sufficient to overcome the elastance of the lungs and chest wall (elastic load), as well as the flow resistance of the airways (resistive load). Ventilation is sustained only as long as the inspiratory muscles are able to maintain adequate pressure generation.

In patients with COPD, the respiratory system load is chronically elevated due to abnormal airway resistance and increased elastance. The increment in airway resistance is accounted for by bronchospasm, airway inflammation, and physical obstruction by mucus and scarring. The most significant contributor to the elastic load is dynamic hyperinflation. The airflow obstruction and decreased elastic recoil typical of advanced COPD lead to prolongation of expiration. When the rate of lung emptying is slowed, expiration cannot be completed before the ensuing inspiration. Rather than reaching equilibrium at functional residual capacity (FRC) at the end of each breath, the respiratory system empties incompletely. Expiration terminates at this higher, dynamically determined FRC. At end expiration, there remains a positive elastic recoil pressure, called PEEPi, which opposes the inspiratory muscles on the subsequent breath. The phenomenon of PEEPi is easily demonstrated when a patient with COPD is mechanically ventilated, but it is present during spontaneous breathing as well.[6,7] The impact of PEEPi on the work of breathing is illustrated in Fig. 129-2.

At the same time that the respiratory system load is elevated, the inspiratory muscles are poorly able to tolerate it. The hyperexpansion of COPD forces the inspiratory muscles to operate on a disadvantageous portion of their force-length relationship. Moreover, these patients often suffer from chronic protein-calorie malnutrition, a condition which does not spare the respiratory muscles. Therefore, even when patients with severe COPD are compensated, the increased load and diminished neuromuscular competence are precariously balanced. Only minor additional decrements in strength or increments in load are sufficient to precipitate inspiratory muscle fatigue and respiratory failure.

ADDITIONAL CAUSES OF DECREASED NEUROMUSCULAR COMPETENCE (Fig. 129-3)

DEPRESSED DRIVE. In the usual patient who is dyspneic, tachypneic, diaphoretic, and using accessory muscles of respiration, impairment of drive is clearly not the cause of ACRF. When drive has been assessed in this setting, it is greatly elevated.[8] Nevertheless, in some patients new CNS insults or drug effects contribute to respiratory failure. Even small doses of sedatives or narcotics may cause respiratory failure; a careful history is essential to exclude this possibility. Occult hypothyroidism is not rare in the el-

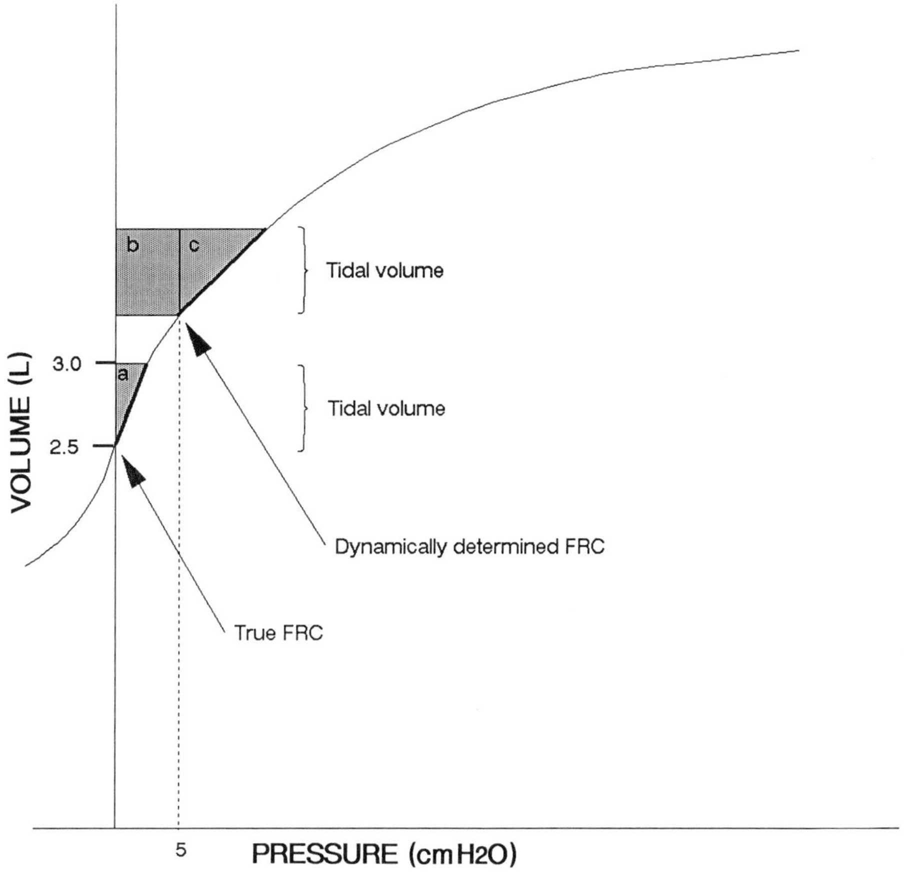

FIGURE 129-2 The effects of PEEPi on work of breathing. A volume-pressure curve for the respiratory system is shown. Under normal conditions, alveolar pressure is atmospheric at end expiration (shown as True FRC). As transpulmonary pressure is generated by the respiratory muscles, there is a V_T change (here from 2.5 to 3.0 L, a V_T of 0.5 L). The pressure-volume product or the external work is shown by shaded area a. With gas trapping due to airflow obstruction, FRC can become dynamically determined. In this example the end-expiratory pressure (PEEPi) is 5 cmH_2O, which raises the end-expired lung volume. Now for the same V_T generation the respiratory muscles must overcome the positive alveolar pressure (PEEPi) before flow occurs, and the work of breathing is increased accordingly (b + c). In addition, the V_T change can occur on a flatter portion of the volume-pressure curve, resulting in yet another increment in elastic load. The addition of continuous positive airway pressure (CPAP) in an amount to counterbalance the PEEPi has the ability to reduce the work of breathing from b + c to c only.

derly, particularly in women. Thyroid function testing should be part of the routine screening of patients with ACRF.

It has been proposed that central depression of drive contributes to the terminal stages of respiratory failure, irrespective of precipitant. According to this hypothesis, overworked respiratory muscles generate inhibitory signals which feed back to the CNS to reduce drive, thereby protecting the muscles from fatigue.[9,10] The relevance of this mechanism to respiratory failure remains to be demonstrated. Regardless of the contribution of central mechanisms to fatigue, the approach of restoring a more favorable balance between energy supply and expenditure remains the same.

FAILED NEUROMUSCULAR TRANSMISSION. To effect adequate ventilation, the CNS must transmit drive to the working muscles via the spinal cord and peripheral nerves. Thus, causes of neuromuscular failure such as spinal cord lesions, primary neurologic diseases, and neuromuscular blocking drugs may produce ACRF. One of the more common causes, especially in surgical patients, is phrenic nerve injury. This occult lesion may be induced by direct trauma to the nerve or more indirectly by cold cardioplegia during open heart surgery. A little known action of aminoglycosides is to act as mild neuromuscular blockers. Although this is unimportant in the great majority of patients, those with already impaired neuromuscular transmission, such as patients with myasthenia gravis, may experience a further loss of strength.

MUSCLE WEAKNESS. The most important causes of decreased neuromuscular competence fall into the category of muscle weakness. Especially prominent are electrolyte disturbances such as hypokalemia and hypophosphatemia. Hypophosphatemia may be exacerbated by many of the

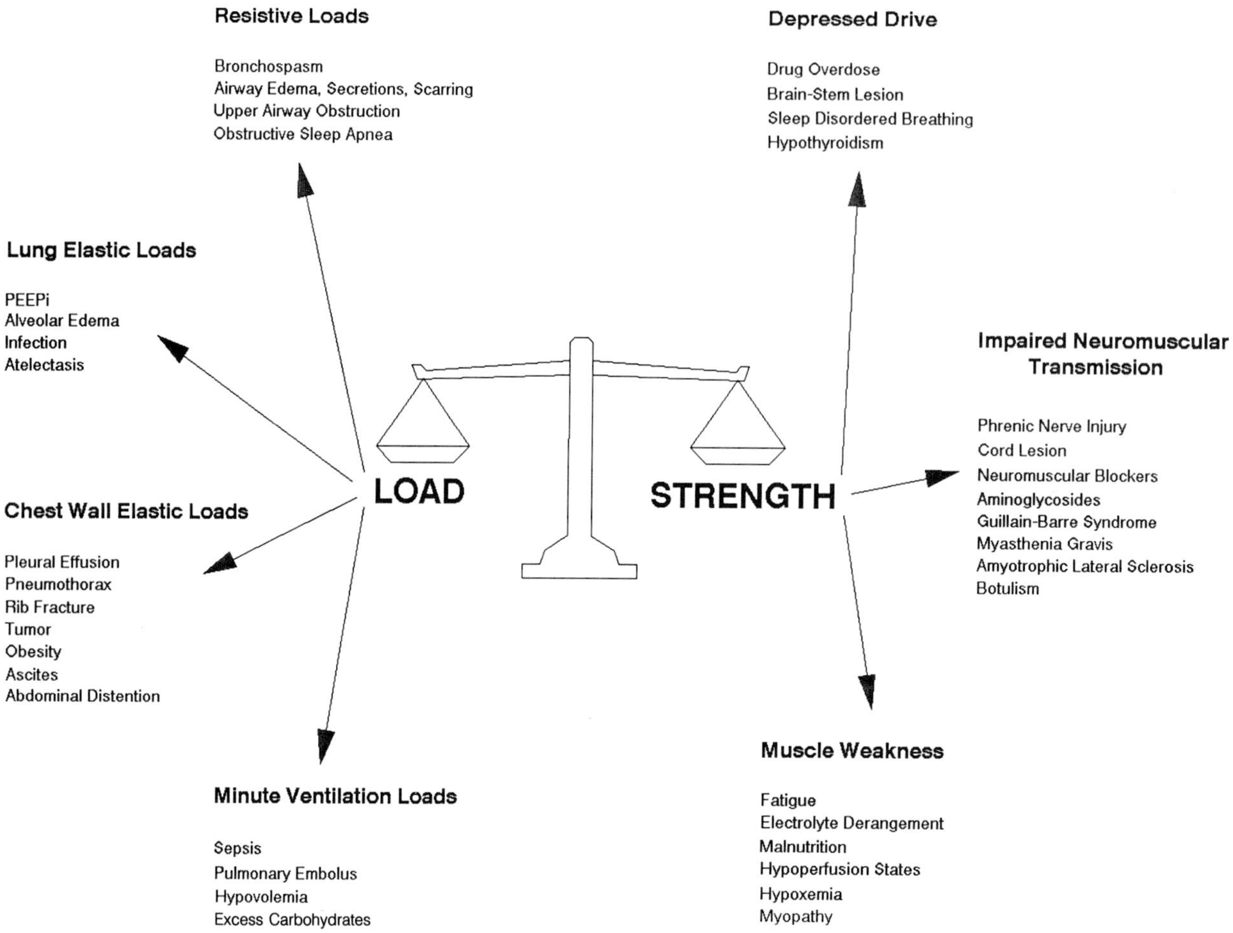

FIGURE 129-3 The balance between load upon and strength of the respiratory system determines progression to and resolution of ACRF.

drugs used to treat COPD, such as methylxanthines, β agonists, corticosteriods, and diuretics, accounting for its striking prevalence (about 20 percent in these patients).[11]

Muscle fatigue is the reversible loss of ability to develop force and is itself a cause of muscle weakness. The metabolic basis for such weakness may relate to inadequate supply of nutrients, excess generation of intracellular products such as lactate, or depletion of muscle glycogen. Evidence to support the importance of blood supply in the genesis of fatigue comes from studies of respiratory failure in animals with cardiogenic or septic shock.[12,13] In these animal models, fatigue is hastened by circulatory insufficiency. Hypoperfusion states, hypoxemia, and severe anemia have the potential to contribute to muscle fatigue and thereby to respiratory failure.

ADDITIONAL CAUSES OF INCREASED LOAD (see Fig. 129-3)

INCREASED RESISTIVE LOAD. One of the most common causes of ACRF, and the most amenable to pharmacologic intervention, is bronchospasm. The disease course in most patients with COPD includes an asthmatic component. Exacerbations of bronchospasm increase resistive workload, precipitating ACRF. Superimposed heart failure may also cause increased airway resistance, mimicking asthma ("cardiac asthma"). Upper airway obstruction is much less common, but since these patients frequently have a history of prior intubation, tracheal stenosis should be considered. Finally sleep apnea, which commonly coexists with COPD, may need to be excluded. Especially once the patient is intubated, clues to this underlying cause of dynamic upper airway obstruction (e.g., snoring) may be impossible to discern. In the proper setting (obese, hypersomnolent patient), this possibility should be vigorously pursued.

INCREASED LUNG ELASTIC LOAD. Contributors to lung stiffness include pulmonary edema (cardiogenic and noncardiogenic), pneumonia, interstitial inflammation, tumor, and atelectasis. As noted above, at the same time that bronchospasm causes increased flow resistance, it simultaneously worsens elastic load by augmenting PEEPi.

INCREASED CHEST WALL ELASTIC LOAD. The chest wall includes the thorax, diaphragm, and abdomen. Therefore, obesity, rib fracture, pneumothorax, pleural effusion, ascites, and abdominal distention contribute to the work of breathing. These factors are particularly relevant in the postoperative setting.

MINUTE VENTILATION LOADS. Dividing the work of breathing into resistive and static components is a useful way of analyzing the effort of each breath. However, even if the work of each breath remains constant, an increase in respiratory rate increases the load. Increased minute ventilation ($\dot{V}_E$) requirements can be divided into those due to excess carbon dioxide production ($\dot{V}_{CO_2}$) and those from worsened dead space. The first category includes excessive carbohydrate feeding, fever, and hypermetabolism because of injury or infection. New dead space may be caused by pulmonary embolism, hypovolemia, or shallower breathing (which raises the dead space fraction, V_D/V_T).

MULTIFACTORIAL RESPIRATORY FAILURE

To analyze respiratory failure in a way which facilitates management, it is important to dissect the very complex real-life patient into simple components of deranged neuromuscular competence and load. However, the patient with ACRF due to isolated rib fracture or hypokalemia is uncommon. More often, numerous contributors to both decreased strength and increased load are implicated. For example, a patient admitted with pneumonia and worsening bronchospasm may additionally have hypophosphatemia, heart failure, and malnutrition. Aspiration at the time of intubation, abdominal distention related to attempts to enterally feed, and overzealous parenteral nutrition with carbohydrates complete the picture of multifactorial ACRF. Although such a patient may seem overwhelmingly complex, a systematic approach to each component of respiratory failure leads logically to a plan for treatment.

Approach to the Patient

The patient with ACRF presents a challenge to the physician at each of three phases of management: before intubation, following institution of mechanical ventilation, and at the point of liberation from the ventilator.

PHASE 1, BEFORE INTUBATION

The goals of management in the patient not yet intubated are to forestall mechanical ventilation when this is possible and recognize progressive respiratory failure when it is not.

Avoiding mechanical ventilation nearly always depends on discerning the cause of ACRF and reversing it. Thus, the first step is to review each of the potential causes enumerated in Fig. 129-3 in light of the clinical presentation. On occasion, impending respiratory failure can be averted by a specific intervention targeted to one precipitant, such as rib fracture (intercostal nerve block) or pulmonary edema (diuresis, afterload reduction). More often several contributors are identified, such as worsened bronchospasm, electrolyte derangement, and infection, and treatment must be broad based. The treatments of many of these precipitants are discussed throughout this text; here, the use of oxygen, pharmacotherapy, and continuous positive airway pressure (CPAP) will be discussed.

OXYGEN. One of the most pervasive myths surrounding the treatment of ACRF is that these patients rely on hypoxic drive to breathe. Physicians are often hesitant to supply oxygen, fearing that patients will stop breathing, necessitating intubation. Since these patients are typically hypoxemic on presentation (P_{O_2} usually about 30 to 40 mmHg), failure to supply adequate oxygen is a potentially devastating treatment error. Unrelieved hypoxemia in the face of acidemia, fatiguing respiratory muscles, and an often failing right ventricle, risks arrhythmia, myocardial infarction, cerebral injury, renal failure, and respiratory arrest.

In several studies performed over the past decade, patients with COPD have been convincingly shown to nearly maintain $\dot{V}_E$ despite treatment with even 100% oxygen,[14,15] and to augment their drive in response to hypercapnia.[16] When oxygen is given, the P_{CO_2} typically rises, but this is attributed largely to worsened matching of ventilation and perfusion ($\dot{V}/\dot{Q}$) and the Haldane effect, not to hypoventilation. In one series, patients with ACRF had a mean initial P_{O_2} of 38, and P_{CO_2} of 65.[4] They were then placed on 100% oxygen, raising the mean P_{O_2} to 225, while the mean P_{CO_2} plateaued at 88. $\dot{V}_E$ fell by a small amount and drive remained supranormal.

High concentrations of inspired oxygen are not usually necessary in ACRF, unless pneumonia or pulmonary edema is present, since hypoxemia is largely due to $\dot{V}/\dot{Q}$ mismatching, not shunt. Nevertheless, we believe that the risks of oxygen therapy have been greatly overstated,[17] often leading physicians to withhold a potentially lifesaving therapy. The goal of oxygen therapy is to maintain 90% saturation of an adequate circulating hemoglobin. This can usually be attained with a facemask at 30 to 35% or nasal cannula at 3 to 5 L/min. A rise in P_{CO_2} is likely, but this in itself is of little importance. Patients may progress to respiratory failure *despite* oxygen therapy, but not because of it. For this reason, careful serial assessments by the ICU team of physician-nurse-respiratory therapist are essential.

PHARMACOTHERAPY. Bronchodilators are an essential part of the early management of these patients (Table 129-1). While much of the airflow obstruction of COPD is irreversible, most patients will have some reversible component.[18,19] Combined therapy with β agonists, ipratropium, aminophylline, and corticosteroids is usually used, and each of these is discussed below. Respiratory stimulants would be predicted not to work in this setting, since drive is already supranormal. Indeed, doxapram and similar drugs have now fallen out of favor since their toxicity is substantial and their efficacy minimal.[20] We believe there is no role for these drugs.

β Agonists. Inhaled, β_2-selective agents (albuterol, bitolterol, terbutaline, metaproterenol) should be given by me-

TABLE 129-1 Bronchodilator Therapy in ACRF

β Agonists
Albuterol or metaproterenol by MDI (Three puffs every 30–60 min)
or
Albuterol or metaproterenol by nebulizer (0.5 mL albuterol or 0.3 mL metaproterenol in 2.5 mL normal saline solution)
Ipratropium
Three puffs every 6 h by MDI
Consider high doses (100–600 μg every 6 h) in the intubated patient
Aminophylline
Loading dose is 5 mg/kg
Maintenance dose is approximately 0.5 mg/kg/h
Must be titrated against serum levels
Corticosteroids
Methylprednisolone, 0.5–2 mg/kg every 6 h
Assess ongoing need after 72 h

tered-dose inhaler (MDI), unless patient distress makes this impractical. Administration may be facilitated by the use of a chamber device. Higher doses than usual can be given, such as three puffs every 30 to 60 min, although there is no clear benefit from frequent doses. A handheld nebulizer (0.5 mL albuterol or 0.3 mL metaproterenol mixed with 2.5 mL saline solution) may be useful in patients who cannot use an MDI reliably, but otherwise this route confers no additional efficacy. Parenteral agents (e.g., epinephrine 0.3 mL subcutaneously), and their concomitant toxicity, can nearly always be avoided.

Ipratropium. The anticholinergic agent, ipratropium bromide, is as effective as metaproterenol in the treatment of ACRF,[21] and may even be better in stable COPD. An additional advantage of this drug is that, compared to metaproterenol, its use is associated with a small rise in Pa_{O_2}, rather than the small decline usually seen with β agonists. The addition of ipratropium to a regimen containing inhaled β agonists has not been shown to yield incremental benefit in patients with status asthmaticus or COPD.[22] Nevertheless, the only arguments against its use are cost and convenience. Until there is more solid evidence that the combination of ipratropium and β agonists is no better than either agent alone, we advise the use of both drugs. The usual dose of ipratropium in ACRF is three puffs every 30 to 60 min. Recently, much higher doses (400 to 600 μg) have been administered but the value of this in ACRF has not been established.[23]

Aminophylline. Aminophylline is a mildly effective bronchodilator in patients with COPD. In combination with β agonists, a synergistic effect has been noted.[24] It is therefore indicated in the treatment of ACRF. In addition to its actions as a bronchodilator, aminophylline has salutary effects on the diaphragm in experimental settings. These include inotropy and resistance to fatigue,[25] although the clinical relevance of these findings is yet to be demonstrated. The toxicity of these drugs is substantial, including arrhythmogenesis and CNS effects. Daily serum levels are necessary for safe use, especially in light of the significant interactions with other drugs. Aminophylline is initiated as a loading dose of 5 mg/kg infused over 30 min, then continued as an intravenous infusion at a rate of 0.5 mg/kg/h. In patients who are already taking an oral methylxanthine, intravenous loading and maintenance dosing should be guided by serum levels. Given the mild efficacy of the drug and the substantial toxicity, it is difficult to justify empirical partial loading doses. The serum level should be reassessed daily since aminophylline interacts with many other drugs given to critically ill patients.

Corticosteroids. Patients with ACRF given methylprednisolone, 0.5 mg/kg every 6 h in addition to standard bronchodilators show greater improvement in spirometric values than patients who are not.[26] This benefit is demonstrable at least as early as 12 h, and in some studies of patients with asthma, possibly after 1 h. Higher doses may also be of benefit in patients with asthma, but this has not been evaluated in ACRF. Therefore, any patient with ACRF should be given methylprednisolone, 0.5 to 2 mg/kg every 6 h. The benefit of corticosteroids beyond the first few days is not known. Since these drugs have important detrimental effects on metabolic and immune function, their continued use should be reevaluated after the first 72 h.

Antibiotics. Bronchitis is a common precipitant of ACRF. Nevertheless, the efficacy of antibiotics is controversial. Since benefit has been demonstrated in one study,[27] we give an inexpensive, broad-spectrum antibiotic (e.g., amplicillin, doxycycline, cotrimoxazole) empirically.

CONTINUOUS POSITIVE AIRWAY PRESSURE. As discussed above, a substantial component of the increased work of breathing in ACRF is related to PEEPi. The patient must generate sufficient force to overcome the remaining recoil pressure (equal to PEEPi) before his efforts result in any inspiratory flow. Therefore, the use of CPAP by facemask, in an amount up to the degree of PEEPi, should be capable of reducing the work of breathing in spontaneously breathing patients with impending respiratory failure (see Fig. 129-2). In intubated patients with ACRF, CPAP has been demonstrated to reduce the work of breathing by nearly 50 percent.[28] Additionally, all patients in this series subjectively felt less dyspneic. This approach will likely be limited by patient cooperation since it requires a tight-fitting mask over the face. In addition, potential dangers include barotrauma, hemodynamic compromise, and the risk of gastric insufflation and vomiting into the mask. Clearly this approach needs further investigation.

ARRHYTHMIAS. Arrhythmias are common in the setting of respiratory failure. Fortunately, they are typically more of a nuisance than a serious problem. Nevertheless, they can serve to distract the physician from more important issues, may limit the doses of bronchodilating drugs, and sometimes are significant in and of themselves. The most common rhythms are sinus tachycardia, atrial fibrillation, atrial flutter, multifocal atrial tachycardia, and ventricular premature beats. It can be difficult to judge the contributions of hypoxemia, cor pulmonale, metabolic derangements, underlying coronary artery disease, and drug toxicity. Treatment should focus on rectifying the underlying respiratory failure, since this usually has a beneficial impact on arrhythmias.[29] Hypoxemia and electrolyte abnormalities should be corrected as a first priority. Monitoring should be initiated, and if arrhythmias continue despite correction of apparent exacerbating factors, myocardial ischemia should be excluded. Atrial fibrillation can be controlled with a calcium channel blocker or digoxin. β-Blockers should generally be avoided for fear of worsening lung function, although short-acting, selective drugs have occasionally been used with success. Multifocal atrial tachycardia often responds to verapamil, sometimes with restoration of sinus rhythm.[30]

RECOGNIZING IMPENDING RESPIRATORY FAILURE. Despite aggressive attempts to find and reverse the causes of ACRF, some patients will progress nonetheless to frank respiratory failure. The decision to intubate requires clinical judgment and should be assessed by a physician present at the bedside (Table 129-2). Assessment of respiratory failure based solely on results of arterial blood-gas studies is fraught with error. We have taken care of a small number of patients in whom the P_{CO_2} rose to >150 mmHg while the patients were alert and conversant, and mechanical ventilation did not become necessary. On the other hand, many patients with ACRF will progress to respiratory arrest long before progressive hypercapnia is clearly documented. Respiratory arrest may be complicated by aspiration or cardiovascular instability, compromising future efforts to return the patient to spontaneous breathing. The goal at this stage of management is to intubate the patient *electively* once mechanical ventilation becomes unavoidable.

Useful bedside parameters of impending respiratory arrest include respiratory rate, mentation, pattern of breathing, and the patient's own assessment. The patient may be able to tell the physician whether he is improving or not; his degree of dyspnea over time is a useful guide to likelihood of success without intubation. Most patients with ACRF will be tachypneic, reflecting their excessive drive. A rate which remains above 35 to 40, or a rising rate despite therapy, is predictive of respiratory failure. Deterioration of mentation commonly precedes respiratory arrest. Patients become confused, less conversant, then poorly rousable. The pattern of respiratory muscle use may add further information. Thoracoabdominal paradox, or inward movement of a lax abdominal wall during inspiration (rather than the usual outward motion), may be a sign of diaphragmatic fatigue. Evaluation for this sign requires experience since most patients with ACRF are actively using their abdominal expiratory muscles. Thus, what appears to be inward movement of the abdomen can be simply the relaxing of expiratory muscles, rather than diaphragmatic paralysis.

TABLE 129-2 Assessment of the Need for Intubation in ACRF

1. This judgment must be made by the physician at the bedside.
2. Consider as ominous:
   Respiratory rates >36
   Use of all accessory muscles
   Thoracoabdominal paradox
   Even minor mental status changes
   Patient's subjective sense of exhaustion
3. Arterial blood-gas studies are of limited use in making this judgment and simply confirm clinical assessment.

Better methods of assessing ventilatory reserve are needed. As the role of respiratory muscle fatigue in ACRF is clarified, and as methods for assessing fatigue in spontaneously breathing patients are developed, our ability to intubate patients expeditiously, but not excessively, may improve.

In a small number of patients with ACRF, face mask ventilation has been described as an alternative to endotracheal intubation.[31,32] A tight-fitting mask allows substantial ventilatory assistance, yet provides for brief periods off of the ventilator during which patients can speak, inhale nebulized medications, expectorate, and swallow liquids. This form of ventilatory assistance has been used for prolonged periods (up to 8 d) and has been shown to relieve symptoms, reduce respiratory rate, improve gas exchange, and lessen the amplitude of the diaphragmatic electromyogram as well as the transdiaphragmatic pressure.[32] In 13 patients with ACRF who were judged to require, or be likely to require, intubation, only 1 patient treated with mask ventilation subsequently required endotracheal intubation.[32] In contrast, 11 of 13 matched historical controls required intubation. Similarly, those treated with the mask system had a more transient need for mechanical assistance and a shorter ICU stay. Complications of the mask have been minor and few; local skin breakdown has been attributed to the tight-fitting mask. Aspiration of gastric contents has not been noted in these patients; however, impaired mentation should contraindicate the use of mask ventilation. We are optimistic that this method may provide a safe, minimally invasive technique for managing the patient with ACRF.

PHASE 2, FOLLOWING INTUBATION

This phase consists of the immediate peri-intubation management and the first few days of mechanical ventilation. In many respects, treatment begun in the preintubation phase is continued, but several additional concerns become relevant. Care consists of stabilizing the patient on the ventilator, ensuring rest of the patient and respiratory muscles, improving neuromuscular competence, reducing load, and giving prophylaxis against complications. Optimal treatment at this time is likely to facilitate eventual liberation from mechanical ventilation.

PERI-INTUBATION RISKS. There are two common pitfalls in the postintubation period: life-threatening alkalosis and hypotension. These are both related to overzealous ventilation and can be avoided by considering the patient's own ventilatory pattern preceding intubation. Most patients with ACRF have a $\dot{V}_E$ of only about 10 L/min (sometimes much lower as respiratory failure evolves), and breathe at V_Ts of about 300 mL. Physicians commonly choose ventilator settings with higher V_Ts and correspondingly lower

V_D/V_T fractions. In addition, $\dot{V}_E$ levels >10 L/min are often used, particularly during hand-bag ventilation. Finally, as the work of breathing is assumed by the ventilator, $\dot{V}_{CO_2}$ drops by 20 percent or more. All of these factors join to dramatically lower the patient's P_{CO_2} once assisted ventilation begins. Since preexisting compensatory metabolic alkalosis is the rule, life-threatening alkalemia (pH > 7.7) can easily be achieved. This scenario can be avoided by simply aiming for a more reasonable $\dot{V}_E$, approximating the patient's own pattern of breathing. Our own practice is to select a V_T of 8 mL/kg and rate of about 20/min on an assist-control (A/C) mode of ventilation. There is no need to attempt to normalize pH, a maneuver which merely serves to waste the bicarbonate that has been so vigorously conserved during the evolution of respiratory failure.

Hypotension is a consequence of escalating PEEPi following intubation. The degree of dynamic hyperinflation is proportional to $\dot{V}_E$. PEEPi has the same deleterious consequences on venous return as extrinsic PEEP, and can cause serious hypoperfusion. Again, the key to avoiding this pitfall is to prevent excessive ventilation. When hypotension occurs, the circulation can usually be promptly restored by simply ceasing ventilation for 30 s, then instituting ventilation along with measures to reduce PEEPi.

ENSURING REST AND RECOVERY. Following intubation, most patients are exhausted and will sleep for the first day. Little or no sedation is typically necessary. The respiratory muscles will require 48 to 72 h of rest before substantial recovery, so that resumption of breathing efforts before that is counterproductive and likely to lead to recurrence of respiratory muscle fatigue.[33] We continue to encourage rest by maintaining ventilation, adding sedation when necessary. Rest can be achieved using any mode of ventilation, as long as settings are chosen which minimize patient effort. It is important to emphasize that having the patient connected to a ventilator is no guarantee that the patient is relieved of the work of breathing. Even when the ventilator is set at a very sensitive trigger, the presence of PEEPi causes the patient to make a substantial inspiratory effort to get a breath, even on A/C mode. For example, with a triggered sensitivity of -1 cmH_2O and PEEPi of 10 cmH_2O, the patient must lower his airway pressure by 11 cmH_2O to trigger a breath. It is incumbent on the physician to ensure that the patient is, in fact, rested. When this is achieved, respiratory muscle strength usually improves demonstrably over the first few days.

IMPROVING NEUROMUSCULAR COMPETENCE. Each of the factors discussed in phase 1 (and in Fig. 129-3) which contribute to depressed neuromuscular competence should be reviewed daily in the ventilated patient. In this phase, the signal importance of nutrition must be recognized. Malnutrition is a common partner of advanced COPD and contributes to respiratory muscle dysfunction as well as immune depression. In a randomized trial of standard feeding versus supplementation (1000 kcal above usual), malnourished inpatients with COPD were shown to develop greater respiratory muscle endurance and strength in only 16 days when given extra calories.[34] Excessive refeeding should be avoided, however, since unnecessarily high levels of carbon dioxide production ($\dot{V}_{CO_2}$) may result. On occasion, detailed nutritional information including indirect calorimetry may be helpful to guide nutritional management (see Chap. 91 and 94). When calorie requirements have been assessed, it is usually advisable to supply a large fraction (50 percent or more) of total calories in the form of lipids, to minimize the respiratory quotient and hence $\dot{V}_{CO_2}$. Especially with refeeding, hypophosphatemia commonly develops while the patient is in the ICU, and serum phosphate content should be assessed on a daily basis.

Once the respiratory muscles are rested, a program of exercise should be initiated. The goal is to encourage muscle power, tone, and coordination by allowing the patient to assume nonfatiguing respirations. This can be achieved using any ventilator mode, e.g., progressively lowering the triggered sensitivity on A/C, reducing the backup rate on intermittent mandatory ventilation (IMV), or lowering the inspiratory pressure on pressure support. After a period of work, the patient is returned to full rest to facilitate sleep at night. As strength improves, the amount of exercise can be increased in step, until full spontaneous breathing can be sustained.

DECREASING LOAD. Efforts to decrease load should continue. Once the patient is ventilated, it becomes possible to apportion the load into resistive and elastic components (see Chap. 14). These determinations may provide insight into the precipitants of respiratory failure and serve to guide therapy. For example, if the resistive load and PEEPi are minimal, but the elastic load is excessive, there is little to be gained from more aggressive bronchodilators. Rather, the source of the elastic load (lung, chest wall, abdomen—see Fig. 129-3) should be determined and corrected.

It is important to continue treatment with bronchodilators. Both ipratropium and β agonists can be successfully delivered from MDIs, using an adaptor into the ventilator circuit.[35] The usual number of puffs should be doubled to compensate for the reduced delivery of drug to the patient. Drug delivery may be facilitated by inserting an inspiratory pause coincident with the dose of medication. Prolonged use of any ventilator setting that decreases expiratory time, however, carries the risk of increasing PEEPi.

Other contributors to increased load, such as congestive heart failure, pulmonary embolization, or respiratory infection may be easier to discern once the patient is mechanically ventilated and should be sought during this phase. Congestive heart failure can usually be excluded by the physical examination and chest radiograph. Only occasionally is the additional information from pulmonary artery catheterization necessary. Pulmonary embolism (PE) is much more difficult to exclude. The incidence of PE as a precipitant of ACRF is unknown. The reported frequency of deep venous thrombosis ranges from 9 to 45 percent,[4] and pulmonary emboli are probably an order of magnitude less common. Nevertheless, PE is commonly found at autopsy. As a treatable condition, it is worth finding, but currently available methods make diagnosis difficult. Perfusion lung scanning is always abnormal, and the addition of lung scanning almost never solves the diagnostic dilemma (see Chap. 118). Noninvasive leg studies have been challenged in this setting as well. Recently, capnography has been suggested as a method for excluding PE in patients with ACRF.[36]

PROPHYLAXIS. The prevention of complications is an essential component of the management plan. As for most other bedridden, critically ill patients, subcutaneous heparin and antacids or sucralfate should be routine. Because some evidence indicates that acid neutralization in the stomach is a risk factor for pulmonary infection, many physicians choose sucralfate. One of the greatest risks to the mechanically ventilated patient is the development of nosocomial pneumonia. Establishing a diagnosis of pneumonia is problematic since clinical criteria are neither sensitive nor specific. Bronchoscopy with protected brush sampling and quantitative cultures may be useful in this respect, but whether the information gained will beneficially affect outcome is unknown.[37] Prophylaxis against pneumonia using nonabsorbable antibiotics is under active investigation, but cannot be considered routine.

PHASE 3, LIBERATION FROM THE VENTILATOR

The fundamental principle which guides management in this phase is that successful liberation from the ventilator requires that the premorbid, compensated relationship between neuromuscular competence and load must be reestablished. Therefore, a strategy for successfully discontinuing mechanical ventilation emphasizes increasing the strength and decreasing the load. Therapy may be highly focused, such as repleting inorganic phosphate or relieving a pneumothorax. More often, a broad assault on many potential precipitants, namely bronchospasm, infection, electrolyte derangement, and fatigue, is used. In either case, when load has been reduced and neuromuscular competence promoted, the patient will be able to breathe free of assistance. On the other hand, if a compensated balance of strength and load cannot be restored, attempts at spontaneous breathing will be futile. A corollary principle is that the specifics of ventilator management, such as the mode chosen or the device used, are largely irrelevant details.[38] Only the patient's improving physiology determines the ability to maintain ventilation. This issue is more fully elaborated in Chap. 127.

The progress of the patient can be easily followed by measuring respiratory parameters (negative inspiratory force [NIF], peak pressure [Ppk], static pressure [Pst], PEEPi—see Chap. 14) on a daily basis. The impact of therapeutic maneuvers can be assessed in this way as well. Finally, these parameters provide clues to the ability of the patient to sustain independent ventilation. For example, while PEEPi remains at 10 cmH_2O, there is little point in trying to make the patient breathe. Indeed, in such a circumstance efforts should be directed at attempting to reduce the work of breathing.[39] On the other hand, when PEEPi has resolved and strength is adequate (usually when the NIF $> 3 \times$ Pst), mechanical ventilation is no longer necessary.

When discontinuation of mechanical ventilation is imminent, it is useful to anticipate the respiratory pattern which the patient will soon assume. We have been impressed that patients ventilated at supraphysiologic V_Ts such as 800 to 1000 mL, experience respiratory distress and agitation when resuming their usual pattern of 30 breaths/min at a V_T of 300 mL. By choosing a pattern of mechanical ventilation which more closely approximates spontaneous respiration (e.g., A/C mode, V_T 450 mL, rate 18), the transition from the ventilator is smoothed.

Following extubation, careful serial assessments are in order. Deterioration in the hours just following extubation suggests upper airway edema. In the uncomplicated patient, the respiratory rate falls slightly through the first day, most often into the mid twenties to low thirties. Efforts must continue, to build strength and reduce load, to protect the gains that have already been made. Once the patient is stable off of the ventilator, a prompt transfer to the more benign setting of the general ward should be encouraged.

CASE PRESENTATION

A 72-year-old woman with COPD was admitted to an outside hospital with worsening dyspnea. There was a 70 pack-year history of cigarette smoking, and recent spirometric values obtained in the outpatient clinic were notable for a forced vital capacity (FVC) of 1.5 L and forced expiratory volume in 1 s (FEV_1) of 0.7 L. She was taking a theophylline preparation and albuterol. Four days before admission, the woman complained of worsening of her usual cough, but denied fever. Two days previously she confined herself to bed for worsening dyspnea. On the day of admission she was found confused and cyanotic by her family and transported to an emergency room. There was no history of heart disease or venous thrombosis.

On examination, the blood pressure was 160/90, the heart rate 105 and irregularly irregular, the respiratory rate 36, and the temperature 37°C (98.6°F). She was lethargic but in obvious respiratory distress, diaphoretic, and using accessory muscles of respiration. There were diminished breath sounds in all lung fields, with wheezes diffusely and a markedly prolonged expiratory phase. The heart sounds were distant and no extra sounds were appreciated. The abdomen was soft and nontender. An initial arterial blood-gas determination obtained on room air revealed a P_{O_2} of 36 mmHg, P_{CO_2} of 67, and pH of 7.29. Oxygen at 0.5 L/min by nasal cannula was begun, nebulized albuterol was administered, and an intravenous infusion of aminophylline started at 35 mg/h. A chest radiograph showed hyperinflated lungs, without infiltrates, effusion, or cardiomegaly. A repeat blood-gas determination, with the patient now on 0.5 L oxygen, showed a P_{O_2} 43, P_{CO_2} 66, pH 7.29. The oxygen was increased to 1 L/min and the patient admitted to the ICU. As she was being moved into bed, she became agitated and her distress intensified. She failed to improve with another albuterol treatment and was then intubated. She was placed on IMV at a rate of 20, VT 900 mL and sedated. A subsequent blood-gas sample on 60% oxygen was P_{O_2} 220, P_{CO_2} 30, pH 7.60. The rate was reduced to 16, and subsequently to 12. Treatment with a third generation cephalosporin was begun.

Over the ensuing 2 weeks, numerous attempts to discontinue ventilation were made, but each time the IMV rate was reduced from 8 to 6, the patient became tachypneic and hypertensive. A pulmonary artery catheter was placed, revealing a cardiac output of 4.1 L/min and pulmonary capillary wedge pressure of 18. When the family was told to plan for long-term ventilation in a chronic care hospital, they requested transport to our institution.

On arrival the patient was comfortable on an IMV of 8, VT 900 mL, fraction inspired oxygen (F_{IO_2}) 30%, with a P_{O_2} 95, P_{CO_2} 40, pH 7.38. Settings were changed to A/C, VT 450 mL, rate 18, at which time the patient was found to have 10 cm PEEPi. Her NIF was −18 cmH_2O, Ppk 36 cmH_2O, and Pst 26 cmH_2O. The pulmonary artery catheter was withdrawn and enteral feeding instituted at 2600 cal/day. Albuterol and aminophylline were continued, ipratropium was added, and methylprednisolone was given at 60 mg every 6 h. Sucralfate and subcutaneous heparin were begun, and the cephalosporin discontinued. Intravenous phosphate was given to correct hypophosphatemia, and calcium, magnesium, potassium, and theophylline levels were checked on a daily basis. An exercise program, consisting of turning the triggered sensitivity to −4 cmH_2O during the daytime only, was tolerated well. On the third day, the NIF had increased to 28 cmH_2O, the PEEPi was only 4 cmH_2O, the Ppk 30 cmH_2O, and the Pst 22 cmH_2O. After 1 week, PEEPi decreased to 2 cmH_2O and the patient was able to sit in a chair for several hours. After a 6 h trial of CPAP, she was extubated and successfully transferred to the ward. Prior to discharge, pneumococcal and influenza vaccines were administered.

CASE DISCUSSION

This patient's early course demonstrates some of the common errors in the management of ACRF. First, in the setting of severe hypoxemia, it is crucial to give adequate amounts of oxygen. Here it was meted out sparingly; a better approach would have been to give 40% oxygen by facemask, assuring adequate saturation of hemoglobin using pulse oximetry. Although no adverse effects of aminophylline loading were apparent, this drug has substantial toxicity. Its use should be guided by drug levels and empirical boluses avoided. A typical error at the time of intubation was the selection of ventilatory parameters which grossly overestimated the required $\dot{V}_E$, especially since CO_2 production falls following institution of mechanical ventilation. Severe alkalemia resulted, although this too was tolerated. Initial ventilator dependence was due to unrecognized (and therefore untreated) weakness, in the face of unresolved bronchospasm (indicated by PEEPi). When the patient was ventilated at an IMV rate of 8 ($\dot{V}_E$ 7 L), she was being fully ventilated. On reduction to IMV rate of 6, she was suddenly presented with a ventilatory challenge. Since her strength was poor and her load excessive, she was unable to sustain ventilation and became agitated. While lowering the rate from 8 to 6 seemed a small change to her physicians, it was the difference between full ventilation and respiratory failure. Pulmonary artery catheterization is sometimes necessary to exclude heart failure as a contributor to ACRF, but in this case seemed more motivated by frustration with the lack of progress by the patient. There was no suggestion of heart failure on examination or chest radiograph. While nosocomial pneumonia occurs in 25 to 35 percent of these patients, there is no evidence that broad-spectrum antibiotics can prevent infection. Oral ampicillin, doxycycline, or cotrimoxazole would have been less expensive alternatives.

On transfer, a more physiologic choice of ventilator settings was used. Contributors to impaired neuromuscular competence were sought, leading to correction of malnutrition, starvation, and hypophosphatemia. Similarly, factors adding to respiratory system load were defined (persistent bronchospasm) and additional bronchodilators added. Measures were instituted to reduce the likelihood of gastrointestinal hemorrhage, catheter-associated sepsis, and deep venous thrombosis, and the patient was mobilized. Once reversible factors were identified and corrected and the respiratory muscles exercised, only a brief additional period of mechanical ventilation was necessary. Like most patients with ACRF, a return to successful spontaneous breathing was possible.

References

1. Speizer FE: The rise in chronic obstructive pulmonary disease mortality: Overview and summary. Am Rev Respir Dis 140, (suppl):S106, 1989.
2. Sukumalchantra Y, Dinakara P, Williams MH: Prognosis of patients with chronic obstructive pulmonary disease after hospitalization for acute ventilatory failure: A three year follow-up study. Am Rev Respir Dis 93:215, 1966.
3. Menzies R, Gibbons W, Goldberg P: Determinants of weaning and survival among patients with COPD who require mechanical ventilation for acute respiratory failure. Chest 95:398, 1989.
4. Derenne JP, Fleury B, Pariente R: Acute respiratory failure of chronic obstructive pulmonary disease. Am Rev Respir Dis 138:1006, 1988.
5. Roussos CS, Macklem PT: Diaphragmatic fatigue in man. J Appl Physiol 43:189, 1977.
6. Fleury B, Murciano D, Talamo C, et al: Work of breathing in patients with chronic obstructive pulmonary disease in acute respiratory failure. Am Rev Respir Dis 131:822, 1985.
7. Haluszka J, Chartrand DA, Grassino AE, et al: Intrinsic PEEP and arterial P_{CO_2} in stable patients with chronic obstructive pulmonary disease. Am Rev Respir Dis 141:1194, 1990.
8. Aubier M, Murciano D, Fournier M, et al: Central respiratory drive in acute respiratory failure of patients with chronic obstructive pulmonary disease. Am Rev Respir Dis 122:191, 1980.
9. Respiratory Muscle Fatigue Workshop Group. NHLBI Workshop Summary: Respiratory muscle fatigue. Am Rev Respir Dis 142:474, 1990.

10. Yanos J, Keamy MF III, Leisk L, et al: The mechanism of respiratory arrest in inspiratory loading and hypoxemia. Am Rev Respir Dis 141:933, 1990.
11. Fiaccadori E, Coffrini E, Ronda N, et al: Hypophosphatemia in course of chronic obstructive pulmonary disease: Prevalence, mechanisms, and relationships with skeletal muscle phosphorus content. Chest 97:857, 1990.
12. Hussain SNA, Simkus G, Roussos C:Respiratory muscle fatigue: A cause of ventilatory failure in septic shock. J Appl Physiol 58:2033, 1985.
13. Aubier M, Trippenbach T, Roussos C:Respiratory muscle fatigue during cardiogenic shock. J Appl Physiol 51:499, 1981.
14. Aubier M, Murciano D, Fournier M, et al: Effects of the administration of O_2 on ventilation and blood gases in patients with chronic obstructive pulmonary disease during acute respiratory failure. Am Rev Respir Dis 122:747, 1980.
15. Sassoon CSH, Hassell KT, Mahutte CK: Hyperoxic-induced hypercapnia in stable chronic obstructive pulmonary disease. Am Rev Respir Dis 135:907, 1987.
16. Erbland ML, Ebert RV, Snow SL: Interaction of hypoxia and hypercapnia on respiratory drive in patients with COPD. Chest 97:1289, 1990.
17. Schmidt GA, Hall JB: Oxygen therapy and hypoxic drive to breathe: Is there danger in the patient with COPD? Intensive & Criti Care Dig 8:124, 1989.
18. Anthonisen NR, Wright EC, IPPB Trial Group: Bronchodilator response in chronic obstructive pulmonary disease. Am Rev Respir Dis 133:814, 1986.
19. Gross NJ: COPD: A disease of reversible airflow obstruction. Am Rev Respir Dis 133:725, 1986.
20. Moser KM, Luchsinger PC, Adamson JS, et al: Respiratory stimulation with intravenous doxapram in respiratory failure. N Engl J Med 288:427, 1973.
21. Karpel JP, Pesin J, Greenberg D, et al: A comparison of the effects of ipratropium bromide and metaproterenol sulfate in acute exacerbations of COPD. Chest 98:835, 1990.
22. Patrick DM, Dales RE, Stark RM, et al: Severe exacerbations of COPD and asthma: Incremental benefit of adding ipratropium to usual therapy. Chest 98:295, 1990.
23. Gross NJ, Petty TL, Friedman M, et al: Dose response to ipratropium as a nebulized solution in patients with chronic obstructive pulmonary disease. A three-center study. Am Rev Respir Dis 139:1188, 1989.
24. Jenne JW: Theophylline as a bronchodilator in COPD and its combination with inhaled beta-adrenergic drugs. Chest 92:75, 1987.
25. Murciano D, Aubier M, Lecocguic Y, et al: Effects of theophylline on diaphragmatic strength and fatigue in patients with chronic obstructive pulmonary disease. N Engl J Med 311:349, 1984.
26. Albert RK, Martin TR, Lewis SW: Controlled clinical trial of methylprednisolone in patients with chronic bronchitis and acute respiratory insufficiency. Ann Intern Med 92:753, 1980.
27. Anthonisen NR, Manfreda J, Warren CPW, et al: Antibiotic therapy in exacerbations of chronic obstructive pulmonary disease. Ann Intern Med 106:196,1987.
28. Petrof BJ, Legare M, Goldberg P, et al: Continuous positive airway pressure reduces work of breathing and dyspnea during weaning from mechanical ventilation in severe chronic obstructive pulmonary disease. Am Rev Respir Dis 141:281, 1990.
29. Incalzi RA, Pistelli R, Fuso L, et al: Cardiac arrhythmias and left ventricular function in respiratory failure from chronic obstructive pulmonary disease. Chest 97:1092, 1990.
30. Salerno DM, Anderson B, Sharkey PJ, et al: Intravenous verapamil for treatment of multifocal atrial tachycardia with and without calcium pretreatment. Ann Intern Med 107:623, 1987.
31. Meduri GU, Conoscenti CC, Menashe P, et al: Noninvasive face mask ventilation in patients with acute respiratory failure. Chest 95:865, 1989.
32. Brochard L, Isabey D, Piquet J, et al: Reversal of acute exacerbations of chronic obstructive lung disease by inspiratory assistance with a face mask. N Engl J Med 323:1523, 1990.
33. Braun NMT, Faulkner J, Hughes RL, et al: When should respiratory muscles be exercised? Chest 84:76, 1983.
34. Whittaker JS, Ryan CF, Buckley PA, et al: The effects of refeeding on peripheral and respiratory muscle function in malnourished chronic obstructive pulmonary disease patients. Am Rev Respir Dis 142:283, 1990.
35. Fernandez A, Lazaro A, Garcia A, et al: Bronchodilators in patients with chronic obstructive pulmonary disease on mechanical ventilation. Am Rev Respir Dis 141:164, 1990.
36. Chopin C, Fesard P, Mangalaboyi J, et al: Use of capnography in diagnosis of pulmonary embolism during acute respiratory failure of chronic obstructive pulmonary disease. Crit Care Med 18:353, 1990.
37. Meduri GU: Ventilator-associated pneumonia in patients with respiratory failure. A diagnostic approach. Chest 97:1208, 1990.
38. Schmidt GA, Hall JB: Acute on chronic respiratory failure: Assessment and management of patients with COPD in the emergent setting. JAMA 261:3444, 1989.
39. Marini J: Strategies to minimize breathing effort during mechanical ventilation. Crit Care Clin 6:635, 1990.

Chapter 130
STATUS ASTHMATICUS

JESSE B. HALL
LAWRENCE D.H. WOOD

KEY POINTS

- *Status asthmaticus is defined as asthma that is severe at its onset or progresses rapidly despite standard therapy; without successful management it may result in ventilatory failure and death.*
- *Bronchospasm, mucus plugging, and airway inflammation result in extreme increases in airways resistance.*
- *The consequences of airflow obstruction include ventilation-perfusion mismatch with hypoxemia; dynamic hyperinflation, and intrinsic positive end-expiratory pressure (PEEPi); pulsus paradoxus and conceivably circulatory inadequacy; increased work of breathing; and a potential for respiratory muscle fatigue.*
- *Signs and symptoms suggesting severe asthma include airflow obstruction despite maximal therapy, dyspnea precluding sleep or speech, accessory muscle use, pulsus paradoxus >18 mmHg, and a rising partial pressure of carbon dioxide (P_{CO_2}) with unresolving dyspnea.*
- *Status asthmaticus must be distinguished from other causes of dyspnea and wheezing including congestive heart failure, chronic obstructive pulmonary disease (COPD), upper airway obstruction or foreign body, or less severe asthma complicated by barotrauma, pneumonia, or pulmonary embolism.*
- *The key pharmacologic interventions for status asthmaticus include high doses of β agonists and corticosteroids; ipratropium and theophylline have adjunctive roles.*
- *Once intubation and positive-pressure ventilation (PPV) have become necessary, diminished venous return and hypotension are common because of high intrathoracic pressures; this problem is best treated with aggressive volume resuscitation and reduction of PEEPi.*
- *Most patients with status asthmaticus requiring mechanical ventilation will benefit from sedation and muscle relaxation early in their course to reduce carbon dioxide production and minimize PEEPi.*
- *Mechanical ventilatory support in status asthmaticus is optimal with low tidal volumes and high inspiratory flow rates titrated to minimize PEEPi (<15 cmH_2O) and peak airway pressures (<55 cmH_2O) with eucapnea.*
- *If eucapnea cannot be achieved within the limits of acceptable peak airway pressure and PEEPi, intentional controlled hypoventilation should be considered, with bicarbonate infusion to correct pH <7.20.*

Asthma is defined as a condition of airway hyperreactivity and reversible airflow obstruction that results in intermittent symptoms that include wheezing, dyspnea, and cough.[1] While the vast majority of patients with this relatively common pulmonary disease are managed in the ambulatory care setting, any patient with asthma has the potential to develop status asthmaticus. This is a type of asthmatic attack that is severe at the onset or progresses rapidly despite routine therapy and may result in ventilatory failure and death. In managing these patients, one must make a prompt initial assessment, apply clear-cut triage guidelines, titrate therapy to an often rapidly changing course, monitor carefully for deterioration, and institute mechanical support should ventilatory failure become imminent.

Pathophysiology

Airflow obstruction in asthma arises from smooth-muscle–mediated bronchoconstriction and airway inflammation. While a subset of asthmatic patients with very rapid onset and progression of symptoms has been described,[2] suggesting a predominant role for increased bronchomotor tone in these individuals, most patients with status asthmaticus have symptoms over several days, consistent with significant airway inflammation and edema. Mucus plugging of both large and small airways is a striking finding at postmortem in patients who have died of status asthmaticus.[3] These plugs consist of mucus, sloughed epithelial cells, eosinophils, and the fibrin and other serum components that leak readily through the denuded airway epithelium.[3]

ABNORMALITIES OF GAS EXCHANGE

Airway obstruction results in a maldistribution of alveolar ventilation relative to perfusion with consequent hypoxemia. As would be predicted by this mechanism of hypoxemia, correction of hypoxemia is achieved with modest amounts of supplemental oxygen. Even in those patients requiring mechanical ventilatory support, adequate arterial oxygen saturation can usually be achieved with an F_{IO_2} of 0.3 to 0.5, since true intrapulmonary shunt is trivial (see Chap. 1).[4] During acute treatment with bronchodilators hypoxemia may actually worsen;[5] this has been attributed to worsening of ventilation-perfusion matching as a result of the preferential effects of β-agonist bronchodilators on the less obstructed airways. Resolution of hypoxemia does not parallel spirometric improvement until late in the course of recovery;[6] this is explained by relief of bronchospasm in large airways, with improvement in peak expiratory flow rate (PEFR) and forced expiratory volume in 1 s (FEV_1), while small airway bronchoconstriction resulting in gas exchange abnormality persists until late in the course. Dead space increases substantially in asthma, presumably due to hypoperfusion of regions of hyperinflated lung.[4,6] Despite this increase in dead space, the majority of patients with asthma present with a low P_{CO_2}. In fact, it has been suggested that a normal P_{CO_2} signals early ventilatory failure, a point to be discussed further below.

LUNG MECHANICAL ABNORMALITIES

The severe airway obstruction in status asthmaticus raises airway resistance, so that the normal inspiratory transpulmonary pressure of 5 to 7 cmH_2O during quiet tidal breathing increases to 50 cmH_2O or more. Expiration becomes active during status asthmaticus, with large positive pressures generated during active expiratory muscle contraction being quite ineffective in increasing expiratory flow because of effort independence of forced expiration. Despite maximal efforts, FEV_1 is markedly reduced (to 10 to 20 percent of normal) and PEFR is less than 100 L/min in severe asthma.[6,7] At low lung volumes in normal individuals such expiratory efforts result in dynamic airway collapse. In status asthmaticus, expiratory times are prolonged and alveolar emptying is not complete at the end of expiration. Thus alveolar pressure in status asthmaticus does not reach atmospheric pressure. This condition is termed intrinsic or occult positive-end expiratory pressure (PEEPi).[8] Indeed, measurement of PEEPi determines the degree of dynamic hyperinflation in these patients (vide infra). Static gas trapping may also occur behind truly occluded airways.[9]

CIRCULATORY EFFECTS OF SEVERE AIRWAY OBSTRUCTION

Circulatory abnormalities during status asthmaticus are due in large part to the pressure excursions associated with breathing against obstructed airways. During expiration, increases in intrathoracic pressure diminish blood return to the right heart (see Chap. 2). Filling of the right heart greatly increases as intrathoracic pressure falls during the large inspiratory effort made against obstructed airways. During inspiration, right ventricular volume may increase sufficiently to shift the interventricular septum toward the left ventricle, compromising the volume of this chamber and resulting in incomplete filling. Large negative intrathoracic pressures also affect right and left ventricular systolic performance by increasing afterload. The net effects of these cyclical events are a stroke volume and arterial systolic pressure that varies with respiration, a phenomenon termed *pulsus paradoxus*. During quiet tidal breathing without airway obstruction, the pulsus, measured as the maximal drop in systolic blood pressure during inspiration, is typically less than 10 mmHg. During severe asthma the pulsus is greater than 15 mmHg, unless the patient has ceased making sufficient efforts to cause large intrathoracic pressure swings. Indeed, the degree of pulsus paradoxus can be used to track the course of status asthmaticus and its treatment.[9]

PROGRESSION TO VENTILATORY FAILURE

Status asthmaticus may result in respiratory muscle fatigue and ventilatory failure, even in a young and otherwise healthy individual. The work of breathing is greatly increased, with effort required throughout inspiration and expiration. Dynamic hyperinflation results in the diaphragm being placed in a mechanically disadvantaged position as a force generator. In addition, the PEEPi associated with dynamic gas trapping represents a positive alveolar pressure that must be overcome during inspiration before a pressure gradient driving gas flow is established from mouth to alveolus. These mechanical loads are imposed upon the respiratory muscles at a time when circulatory abnormalities, as described above, may result in hypoperfusion. A number of investigations have demonstrated lactic acidosis during status asthmaticus, likely due to increased muscle lactate production, the action of catecholamines used during treatment, and perhaps, diminished clearance related to perfusion abnormalities.[10,11] The presence of lactic acidosis may predict an increased risk of progression to ventilatory failure.[10]

Clinical Presentation and Differential Diagnosis

A history (see Table 130-1) will often be difficult to obtain from a patient with acute airflow limitation, since speech is often monosyllabic. The clinician should attempt to discern the length of prehospital symptoms, since a prolonged course suggests a substantial component of airway inflammation and a likelihood that response will be slow. Loss of sleep is useful to determine. Prior use of medications is essential information, particularly use of theophylline preparations, since prior use will help determine the appropriate loading dose. Discerning the patient's subjective sense of the severity of the attack is useful as well.

Clinical signs of severe asthma include tachycardia, tachypnea, hyperinflation, wheeze, accessory muscle use, pulsus paradoxus, and diaphoresis (Table 130-1). The absence of wheezing does not exclude a diagnosis of asthma, and in the period immediately preceding respiratory arrest the chest may be completely silent.

"All that wheezes is not asthma" is an appropriate clinical saw to consider at least once during patient evaluation.[12] In most cases, history and physical examination will help identify conditions that can be confused for or may

TABLE 130-1 Indicators of Severe Asthma

Long duration of symptoms
Progression despite optimal outpatient therapy
Dyspnea precluding sleep
Dyspnea precluding speech
Accessory muscle use
Tachycardia >120 beats/min
Respiratory rate >35 breaths/min
Pulsus paradoxus >15 mmHg
FEV_1 <1 L/min
PEFR <120 L/min
Rising or elevated Pa_{CO_2}

complicate status asthmaticus (Table 130-2). The absence of a prior history of asthma in an adult should alert the physician to other diagnoses. Cardiac asthma refers to the airway hyperreactivity that has been described in patients with congestive heart failure.[13] The presence of heart failure is usually evident by examination, but the distinction between airway obstruction and left ventricular dysfunction can be difficult, particularly in the elderly. Interestingly, bronchodilators may partially reverse the airflow obstruction associated with left ventricular failure.[14] The presence of a foreign body must be considered in all children with dyspnea and wheezing, and upper airway obstruction related to prior intubation may be occasionally encountered in adults. Physiologic demonstration of upper airway obstruction can be accomplished with flow-volume loops, but this is usually not feasible in the dyspneic, wheezing patient. The obstruction can also be demonstrated by direct inspection or radiologic imaging, although many of these patients are not stable enough to leave an observation unit for radiology and cannot tolerate bronchoscopy. In these circumstances they require stabilization as described elsewhere in this text (see Chap. 134). The most useful clues to upper airway obstruction in this setting are localized wheeze, inspiratory stridor localized over the trachea, or unilateral hyperinflation noted on chest radiograph.[15]

In large series of patients with pulmonary embolus, wheezing is not a reported sign, though it has been described anecdotally.[12] Airway obstruction would not be expected to be significant in pulmonary embolus, if it occurs at all, unless it were a preexisting abnormality. We feel it is particularly useful to measure PEFR or FEV_1 in patients with severe dyspnea seemingly out of proportion to other evidence of airflow obstruction. If airflow obstruction is not severe by these objective parameters, other diagnoses should be considered. As regards the diagnosis of pulmonary embolus, it is likely that ventilation-perfusion scanning is not reliable in the presence of airflow obstruction, and other diagnostic approaches will be required (see Chap. 118). Barotrauma is common in status asthmaticus, and both pneumomediastinum and pneumothorax correlate with progression to ventilatory failure. Chest pain, acute deterioration, tracheal deviation, subcutaneous emphysema, asymmetric breath sounds, and a mediastinal "crunch" on auscultation are all symptoms and signs that should prompt a search for barotrauma with chest radiography. Pneumonia complicating asthma is suggested by fever, purulent sputum, localizing signs on examination, and hypoxemia that does not correct with modest amounts of supplemental oxygen.

TABLE 130-2 Differential Diagnosis of Severe Dyspnea with Wheezing

Status asthmaticus
Upper airway obstruction
Foreign body
Left ventricular failure or ischemia
COPD
Asthma complicated by pulmonary embolus, pneumonia, or barotrauma

Assessment of Severity of Illness

The key junctures in decision making in the managment of severe asthma are **1.** does the patient need admission to the hospital? **2.** does the patient need admission to a critical care unit? and **3.** does the patient need intubation and mechanical ventilation? Although a number of different "scores" based on physical findings and spirometric measurements have been proposed, this decision making remains something of an art. It is best informed, however, by a number of simple determinations (Table 130-1). Asthma that worsens over days despite aggressive outpatient pharmacologic therapy (particularly if high does of corticosteroids have been given) is likely to respond slowly. Extreme interruption of sleep for two or more evenings is likely to predispose to exhaustion. Dyspnea precluding speech or permitting only monosyllabic responses, heart rate greater than 120, respiratory rate greater than 35, accessory muscle use, diaphoresis, pulsus paradoxus greater than 20 mmHg, PEFR less than 120 L/min, and FEV_1 less than 50 percent of predicted all indicate severe asthma. While the spirometric measurements are desirable and objective, the most severely ill patients usually cannot even perform the maneuver. If patients with these signs and symptoms do not respond to therapy within 1 h, admission to the hospital is advisable, although many facilities utilize a short-term, close-observation unit for stable patients with asthma. If the patient exhibits these signs of severe asthma on presentation but dramatically reverses and prior therapy was not optimal, discharge with close follow-up is acceptable. If the patient clearly improves in the first hour though not completely, admission to the regular ward is appropriate. *If improvement is not uniform across the signs and symptoms described, or if any deterioration is noted, the patient is best cared for in the intensive care unit.*

Once admission has been determined, the patient should have an arterial blood gas and chest radiograph, unless these tests have been obtained earlier for specific indications. A chest radiograph should be obtained immediately in all patients complaining of chest pain, and even in patients without chest pain unsuspected barotrauma may be identified.[7] Patients over the age of 40 should have an electrocardiogram obtained, although the clinician should be aware that a number of acute changes often accompany asthma, inluding sinus tachycardia, right axis deviation, clockwise rotation, and signs of right ventricular hypertrophy. Electrocardiographic changes caused by asthma resolve within hours of response to therapy. Other useful tests include serum electrolytes and glucose, sputum analysis (including staining for eosinophils if the diagnosis of asthma has been called into question), and a complete blood count.

Initial arterial blood gases should be interpreted with caution. If a compensated respiratory acidosis is discovered, chronic ventilatory failure is suggested. Although a rising P_{CO_2} in a patient with progressive signs of worsening asthma and respiratory muscle fatigue should be interpreted to herald respiratory arrest, at least one series has now reported adult asthmatics with initial hypercapnea who did not require mechanical ventilation and who had outcomes not different than patients presenting with hypo- or normocapnea.[16] Thus, the initial P_{CO_2} in patients with severe asthma must be interpreted in light of the other parameters given in Table 130-1 to determine the need for mechanical ventilatory support.

All patients requiring admission should have a large bore intravenous catheter established. This will be useful for administration of bronchodilators and is crucial should emergent airway management become necessary.

Therapy

PHARMACOLOGIC INTERVENTIONS

Patients sufficiently ill to be admitted to the hospital should be placed on enough supplemental humidified oxygen to achieve full arterial saturation. Resolution of hypoxemia improves oxygen delivery to the respiratory muscles, relieves any component of hypoxic-mediated pulmonary hypertension, and protects against a paradoxical worsening of gas exchange with bronchodilator therapy, and oxygen itself has been described to have bronchodilating properties.[12]

The mainstay of pharmacologic intervention is treatment with β agonists, which should be started on presentation (see Table 130-3). The preferred route of administration is by inhalation to minimize side effects. Terbutaline sulfate, metaproterenol sulfate, and albuterol are roughly similar in efficacy, duration of action, and incidence of undesirable side effects of tremor and cardiac arrhythmias. Metered-dose inhalers (MDI) are effective in mild to moderate asthma and can be used in intubated, mechanically ventilated patients.[17] However, most spontaneously breathing patients with status asthmaticus benefit from nebulized solutions given by nursing or respiratory therapy staff. Inhalation should be repeated every 20 min until there is a response or undesirable side effects occur. If intubation and mechanical ventilation becomes necessary, β agonists may be given continuously by inhalation. Prior use of inhaled β agonists should not preclude their use in the emergency room or ICU.[18] Some patients with severe asthma will not tolerate inhalation treatments. This judgment is difficult to make and is best accomplished by an experienced clinician or respiratory therapist. If the patient does not appear to tolerate or benefit from inhalation therapy, subcutaneous terbutaline sulfate or epinephrine can be administered every 20 min for the first hour. Known cardiac disease or age greater than 50 years are relative contraindications to parenteral use of these agents.[19] While β agonists have been used intravenously with success in pediatric patients with severe asthma, reports of fatal myocardial ischemia following their use in adults should preclude their use.[12]

Since most patients with status asthmaticus have a significant component of airway inflammation, corticosteroids should be started in all patients requiring admission to a hospital. Most clinical investigations have indicated that higher doses of intravenous corticosteroids result in an earlier but not greater improvement in PEFR or FEV_1.[12] Since patients with status asthmaticus admitted to the ICU are at risk for progression to ventilatory failure during the first hours to days of management, we believe use of higher doses of corticosteroids are warranted, and therefore recommend 250 mg of methylprednisolone or its equivalent every 6 h. There is no role during acute exacerbations for inhaled steroids, and they should not be given, even if the patient is on a maintenance regimen. It is possible that higher doses of these agents would benefit selected patients, but data are lacking to illuminate this point. Patients responding to initial therapy can quickly be tapered over 24 to 48 h to an oral maintenance dose.[20]

TABLE 130-3 Bronchodilator Therapy for Status Asthmaticus

Inhaled β agonists titrated to undesirable effects, (e.g., albuterol 5 mg by nebulization *q* 20 min)
If inhaled β agonists are not tolerated, consider parenteral epinephrine or terbutaline
High-dose corticosteroids for the first 24–48 h (e.g., methylprednisolone 250 mg IV *q* 6 h)
Theophylline titrated to a serum level of approximately 15 μg/mL
Ipratropium bromide may be of benefit in some patients (e.g., 100—200 μg by inhalation alternating with β-agonist administration)

Other agents must be considered auxiliary in the management of status asthmaticus, but multimodality therapy is preferred by most clinicians. Ipratropium bromide is an anticholinergic agent available for inhalation treatment that in some studies augments the bronchodilating action of β agonists in asthma.[21] If patients do not respond adequately to inhaled or parenteral β agonists, ipratropium may be added in alternating doses (see Table 130-3). Theophylline too may be used to potentiate other pharmacologic agents in status asthmaticus.[12] Theophylline should be administered intravenously to achieve a serum level of 10 to 15 μg/mL. If no drug has been taken prior to admission, a loading dose of 5 to 6 mg/kg is appropriate in the adult. If the patient has used a theophylline preparation prior to admission, a maintenance infusion should be started and serum levels determined (see Chap. 131). Maintenance infusions are generally in the range of 0.5 (mg/kg/h); old age, liver disease, and congestive heart failure usually impair clearance and result in lower infusion requirements. A number of drugs typically used in the critical care environment (cimetidine, erythromycin) interfere with metabolism, and careful titration of dose against serum level is necessary.

ASSESSMENT OF NEED FOR MECHANICAL VENTILATION

Some patients will present to the physician in respiratory arrest, and others may deteriorate prior to full assessment. Others may progress despite the therapy outlined above. In this latter group, the signs requiring intubation and ventilatory support are given in Table 130-4. Altered mental status

TABLE 130-4 Indications for Intubation

Respiratory rates >40 breaths/min
Climbing pulsus paradoxus
Falling pulsus paradoxus in the exhausted patient
Altered sensorium
Inability to speak
Patient's subjective sense of exhaustion
Complicating barotrauma
Unresolving lactic acidosis
Diaphoresis in the recumbent position
Silent chest despite respiratory effort
Elevation of Pa_{CO_2} with progressive signs and symptoms

is frequently seen in the patient immediately prior to respiratory arrest, although the manifestations are sometimes subtle and include distraction, slow response, and a slight inappropriateness.[12] We interpret these to be signs of exhaustion rather than specific metabolic encephalopathy. Marked diaphoresis and assumption of a recumbent position despite continued worsening of airflow obstruction have been described to herald respiratory arrest. Absence of breath sounds, a rising P_{CO_2}, and an increasing pulsus paradoxus (or a rapid fall in pulsus in a patient with failing respiratory muscles) have a similar ominous portent.

AIRWAY CONTROL

Presence of the signs described above mandates elective intubation, rather than awaiting respiratory arrest with its attendant instability. The decision to intubate should be made prospectively, with control of cardiopulmonary status as described below. Since manipulation of the airway may worsen bronchospasm and induce laryngospasm in these patients, and mask ventilation may be difficult, the procedure should be performed by the most experienced individual available.

Pretreatment with atropine and topical anesthesia minimizes the risk of worsened airflow obstruction. Sedation should be achieved with small doses of a short-acting benzodiazepine, such as midazolam, given as 1 to 2 mg intravenous boluses until the patient allows inspection of the airway. Morphine should be avoided because of deleterious effects on venous return (vide infra), possible induction of vomiting, and the potential for histamine release which could theoretically worsen bronchospasm. If the patient will permit passage of the endotracheal tube with sedation alone, this is preferred. An 8-mm or larger endotracheal tube is recommended since mobilization of mucus plugs often occurs during mechanical ventilation. If muscle relaxation is required, an agent that does not result in histamine release, such as vecuronium at a dose of 0.1 mg/kg should be used. This agent would have an expected duration of action of 20 to 40 min, during which PPV is essential.

ACHIEVING CIRCULATORY STABILITY

Following intubation and PPV with either a bag or mechanical ventilator, hypotension and hypoperfusion are relatively common. This is almost invariably due to diminished venous return (see Chap. 2). The large intrathoracic pressures associated with inspiration during PPV, and the dynamic hyperinflation with creation of PEEPi, result in increases in right atrial pressure. In addition, sedation and muscle relaxation cause mean systemic pressure to fall. These patients also often have a modest degree of hypovolemia due to poor intake during the dyspneic period preceding admission. These factors act to cause diminished venous return and hence cardiac output, signaled by tachycardia; a narrow pulse pressure; and hypotension. This pathophysiology can be confirmed by slowly bagging (4 to 6 breaths per minute) on 100% oxygen for approximately 1 min. The prolonged expiratory time will decrease PEEPi and usually result in a rise in blood pressure in the hypotensive patient. If this occurs, fluid boluses of 0.5 to 1.0 L normal saline should be given every 10 to 20 min until an adequate circulation is restored. Understanding this characteristic of management of the severely airway obstructed patient is important, since inappropriate exploration of other causes of hypotension is fraught with difficulties and distracts the clinician from addressing the immediate requirements of mechanical ventilation.

MANAGEMENT OF THE PATIENT ON A VENTILATOR

Management of these patients with mechanical ventilation is particularly challenging, since airway pressures are typically high and interventions to achieve normocapnea often result in more dynamic hyperinflation and greater risk of barotrauma. The goals of therapy are to achieve adequate alveolar ventilation, low levels of PEEPi, minimal circulatory compromise, and low risk of barotrauma. Often, innovative approaches are required.

Initial ventilator mode is irrelevant since the patient should be fully sedated and muscle relaxed. This will minimize airway pressures, allow determination of PEEPi, and lower CO_2 production.[12,22] Sedation can be achieved with short-acting benzodiazepines, ketamine, or droperidol.[12,23,24] Muscle relaxation should be accomplished with an agent that does not cause histamine release such as vecuronium. Even fully sedated and relaxed, many patients will still exhibit high airway pressures and difficulty in achieving adequate alveolar ventilation. Many combinations of tidal volume (VT), respiratory rate (RR), and inspiratory flow rate ($\dot{V}$I), have been suggested. When carefully studied,[22] patients with status asthmaticus mechanically ventilated to eucapnea have very remarkable dynamic hyperinflation, with end-inspired lung volume (VEI) as much as 3 to 4 L above apneic functional residual capacity (FRC) (see Fig. 130-1). This hyperinflation is associated with increased alveolar, central venous, and esophageal pressures as well as systemic hypotension. If one explores various combinations of tidal volume and respiratory rate while maintaining a constant minute ventilation (see Fig. 130-1*b*), one notes that at higher rates and lower tidal volumes, peak (Ppk) and end-inspired plateau (Pplat) pressures fall because of the lower VEI, while there is a small increase in

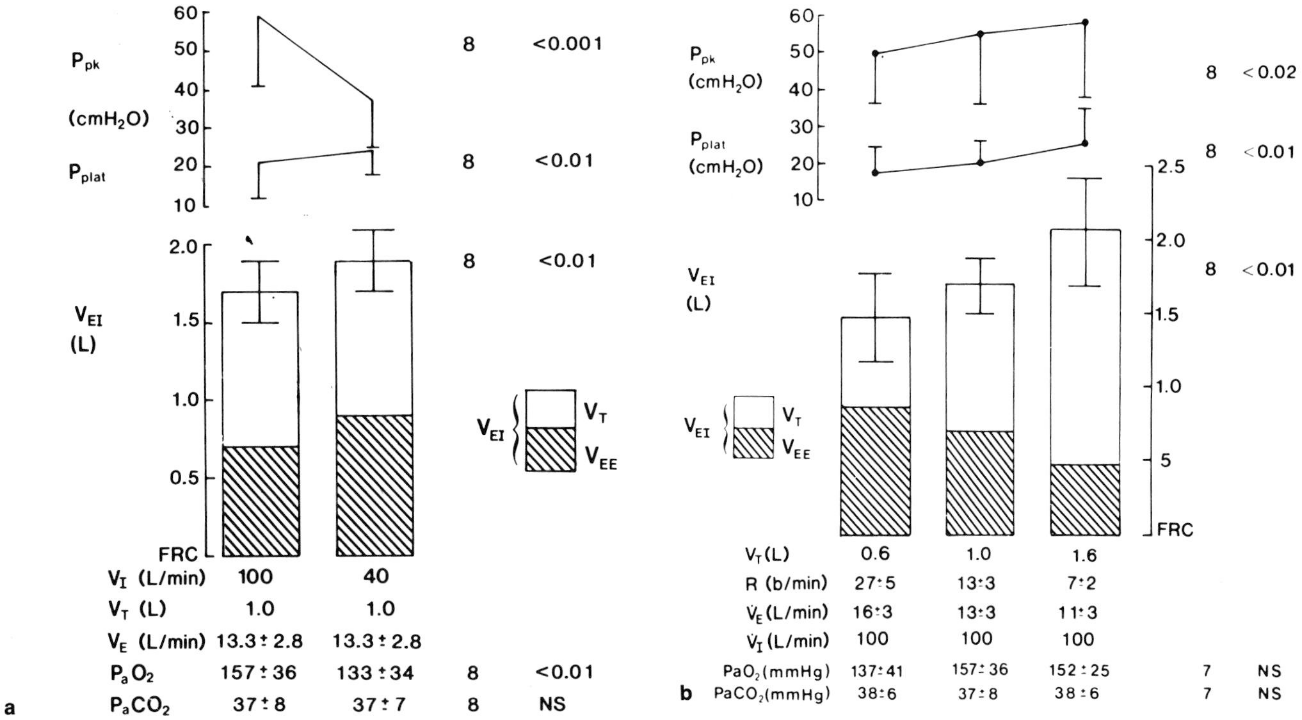

FIGURE 130-1 Effects of various ventilator settings on airway pressures and dynamic hyperinflation during normocapnic ventilation of eight muscle-relaxed asthmatic patients. VEE = lung volume at end expiration, VEI = lung volume at end inspiration, Ppk = peak airway pressure, Pplat = end-inspiratory plateau pressure, V̇I = minute ventilation, V̇I = inspiratory flow. (*a*) Note that as inspiratory flow is decreased from 100 to 40 L/min at the same minute ventilation, peak airway pressures fall but hyperinflation due to dynamic gas trapping increases significantly. (*b*) Dynamic hyperinflation can be reduced at low respiratory rates with high tidal volumes, but this results in Ppk and Pplat increasing. (Reproduced with permission from Tuxon and Lane.[22])

end-expired volume (VEE), due to slightly greater air trapping caused by the reduced time for expiration (TE). Figure 130-1*a* demonstrates that varying V̇I from 40 to 100 L/min while maintaining tidal volume and respiratory rate constant reduces VEE, VEI, and Pplat by allowing greater TE. These improvements in dynamic hyperinflation are at the cost of a Ppk that increases from 40 to 60 cmH_2O.

These data support an approach to mechanical ventilation in the patient with status asthmaticus using small tidal volumes and high inspiratory flow to minimize dynamic hyperinflation, thus minimizing risk of adverse circulatory consequences and barotrauma related to overdistension of alveolar structures. Peak pressures will be increased by higher V̇I, but in asthma these higher airway pressures are encountered largely by the robust proximal airways, while dissipation of pressure along the proximal airways protects against alveolar barotrauma. After the patient has been intubated and the circulation stabilized, mechanical ventilation should be initiated with a tidal volume of 8 to 10 mL/kg and respiratory rate of 12 to 15, with inspiratory flows of 60 L/min. With the patient sedated and muscles relaxed, PEEPi should be measured (see Fig. 130-2). This is most easily done by occlusion of the expiratory limb of the ventilator, which results in the proximal airway pressure gradually rising to a peak level as alveolar emptying is completed during the prolonged expiratory phase. Many ventilators facilitate this determination with an end-expiratory hold switch. This measurement helps determine the degree of dynamic hyperinflation but, of course, does not determine the amount of gas trapped beyond completely occluded airways.

The goals of ventilator therapy are an acceptable peak airway pressure (<55 cmH_2O), least intrinsic PEEP (<15 cmH_2O), eucapnea, and a stable circulation. In some patients this can be accomplished with sedation, muscle relaxation, and the initial ventilator settings suggested above. Unfortunately, in many patients airway pressures will be unacceptably high, as will PEEPi and P_{CO_2}. If this results despite full muscle relaxation, tidal volume can be varied in 100 mL increments with corresponding changes in RR and V̇I to attempt to optimize Ppk, PEEPi, and P_{CO_2}.

CONTROLLED HYPOVENTILATION AND OTHER MANEUVERS

While many patients can have Ppk titrated to 50 to 60 cmH_2O and PEEPi to 10 to 15 cmH_2O with the approach described above, in some this will be in association with a P_{CO_2} of 70 to 90 mmHg. Further attempts to decrease P_{CO_2} are met by worsened hyperinflation. Several series have now described managing such patients with controlled hypoventilation—accepting the high P_{CO_2}.[25,26] If the associ-

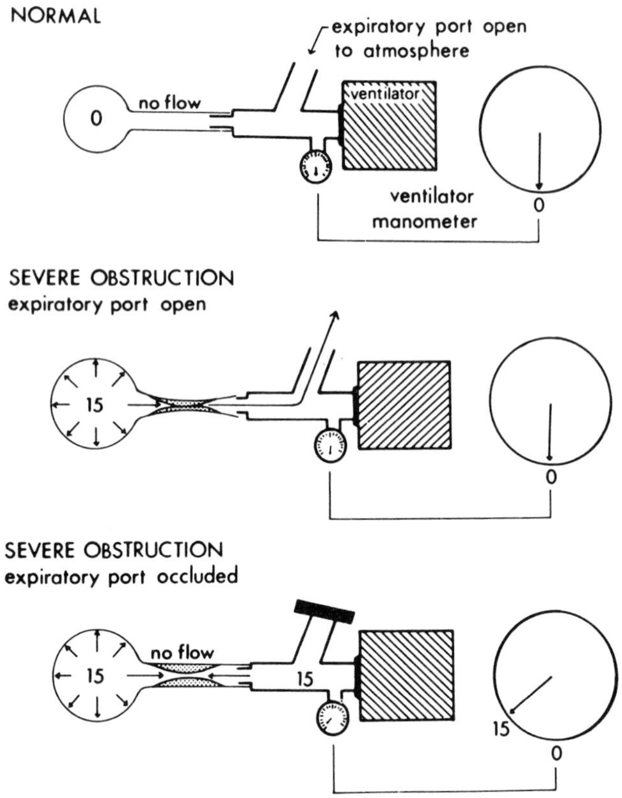

FIGURE 130-2 Measurement of PEEPi in mechanically ventilated patients. (*a*) Under normal conditions alveolar pressure is atmospheric at the end of passive exhalation. (*b*) With severe airflow obstruction, alveolar pressure may not equilibrate with atmospheric pressure at end expiration (i.e., there is positive PEEPi). However, this will not be reflected by pressure measurement at the airway opening if the expiratory limb of the ventilator is open, allowing pressure downstream from the site of the obstruction to approach atmospheric. (*c*) When the expiratory limb is occluded at end expiration in the muscle-relaxed patient, alveolar emptying is complete and proximal airway pressure rises as gas is discharged to the central airways. The rise in proximal airway pressures gives PEEPi. (Reproduced with permission from Pepe and Marini.[8])

ated acute respiratory acidosis is prohibitive (pH < 7.2), bicarbonate is infused to achieve a serum pH of approximately 7.25. While a strategy of bicarbonate infusion to correct pH has been called into question in other acid-base disturbances (see Chap. 158), the success of this approach in published series and our own hands suggest it is appropriate. Of course, it is possible many patients would tolerate a period of several days of acute respiratory acidosis until the status asthmaticus resolved or renal compensation occurred.

Other approaches to therapy have been suggested. A largely anecdotal literature suggests that general anesthesia may be used to reverse status asthmaticus,[12] and halothane and enflurane are the agents most frequently used. While a number of the inhalational anesthetics unquestionably have significant bronchodilating properties, the facts that bronchospasm can return following treatment with an inhalational agent, that the patient may manifest circulatory instability during this intervention, and, most importantly, that virtually all patients can be successfully managed with the ventilator strategies described above, suggest inhalational anesthesia should be used rarely, if at all. While some authors have suggested a role for bronchoscopy in status asthmaticus,[11,27] we believe the potential for barotrauma or exacerbation of bronchospasm should preclude its routine use. While PEEP may have some use during efforts to discontinue mechanical ventilation in patients with COPD (see Chap. 127), it should not be used during ventilation of patients with status asthmaticus since it can result in dangerous increases in lung volumes and airway pressures with resulting hypoperfusion and hypotension, as described above.[28,29] High-frequency ventilation does not offer any benefit in these patients and can result in further undesirable hyperinflation.[30] One interesting report has described improvement in seven ventilated asthmatics treated with a helium-oxygen gas mixture.[31] While this intervention is well described in the treatment of upper airway obstruction, it is surprising that benefit was seen in asthmatics, since resistance to airflow is much less dependent on gas density beyond the lobar bronchi. Since this therapy has only been described in a limited number of patients and since gas mixing of helium and oxygen requires some modification of standard ICU ventilators and gas delivery systems, its use must be considered experimental at the present time.

LIBERATION FROM MECHANICAL VENTILATION

During sedation and muscle relaxation, the paralyzing agent should be discontinued briefly every several hours to prevent accumulation. As airway pressures fall, sedatives, muscle relaxants, and bicarbonate infusions can be reduced to prepare the patient for a brief period of spontaneous ventilation and then extubation. While some patients with very labile asthma may respond to therapy within hours, more typically the patient will require 24 to 48 h of aggressive bronchodilator therapy until airway pressures and PEEPi fall. Once this begins, improvement is often rapid, with resolution of all dynamic hyperinflation over a period of 12 h not unusual. Patients with mucus plugging will often mobilize copious amounts of tenacious secretions that can even appear to be casts of the airway during this recovery phase, and careful attention to the possibility of occlusion of the endotracheal tube, particularly if a small-diameter tube has been used, is mandatory.

If pneumonia, central nervous system injury, or muscle weakness have not complicated the patient's course, progression to spontaneous ventilation and extubation should be prompt once airflow obstruction responds to therapy. Several anecdotal reports have noted significant myopathy complicating severe asthma.[32,33] High creatinine kinase levels on admission may be a marker for this problem. Various aspects of care of these patients could contribute to muscle injury or weakness, including high-dose corticosteroids, paralytic agents, and the disuse associated with mechanical ventilation during muscle relaxation. Assessment of respiratory muscle strength should be routine in these patients and is best accomplished by determination of negative inspiratory pressure (See Chap. 127).

If the patient has adequate muscle strength and no signs of ventilatory failure (vide supra) emerge during the brief period of spontaneous breathing, extubation should be performed since the endotracheal tube itself may perpetuate bronchospasm in these patients. Following extubation the patient should continue to receive vigorous bronchodilator and chest physiotherapy in the ICU until at least the next day. During this period and following discharge from the ICU, a careful program of education should be implemented to help the patient identify signs of worsening asthma, to optimize drug regimen, and to clarify the response to worsening airflow obstruction following discharge to obviate future episodes of life-threatening asthma.

CASE PRESENTATION

A 28-year-old woman was admitted to the emergency room with shortness of breath and wheezing. She had asthma since the age of 10 and required emergency room visits or admission to the hospital many times each year. She had never been intubated. She moved to this city 5 months ago and had not yet established contact with a physician. She had been using an inhaler, a long-acting theophylline preparation, and prednisone at a dose of 30 mg/day. She had baseline shortness of breath making it difficult for her to climb two flights of stairs. For the past 4 days she had been too ill to attend work, and for two evenings sleep was constantly interrupted by dyspnea. There had been no chest pain, fever, or productive cough.

In the emergency room, the patient was sitting bolt upright and answered questions in monosyllables or with a nod of the head. Her pulse was 150 and regular, respirations 40 and very labored, with use of all accessory muscles. Her blood pressure was 140/85 with 25 mmHg pulsus paradoxus and she was afebrile. There was no diaphoresis or rib retractions. The lung examination revealed diffuse inspiratory and expiratory wheezing with poor air movement. There was no tracheal deviation, subcutaneous emphysema, or mediastinal crunch. Brief cardiovascular and neurologic exams were within normal limits.

Oxygen was supplied by nasal cannula with 4 L/min flow. An attempt at PEFR determination was unsuccessful because the patient was unable to perform the maneuver. Albuterol, 5 mg by nebulization, was given immediately as a 16 gauge intravenous catheter was placed. Following placement of the catheter, 250 mg of Solu-Medrol was given and theophylline started at 40 mg/h by infusion pump. Since the patient was unable to tolerate the inhalation therapy, epinephrine 0.4 mg of 1:1000 strength was given subcutaneously every 20 min for three doses.

Because the patient improved minimally, a bed was arranged in the ICU. The patient was transported to this unit but in the course of transport did not receive further medications for 30 min. On arrival in the ICU her respiratory rate was 50, pulse 150, and she was now diaphoretic and slow to respond to questions. The chest was silent and the pulsus paradoxus was 15 mmHg, but her respiratory efforts seemed less forceful. While equipment was being gathered for intubation, she assumed a recumbent position. After 2 mg of intravenous midazolam, she was orally intubated with a 8-mm endotracheal tube without difficulty.

After the airway was secured, 2 mg of midazolam and 7 mg of vecuronium were given. The patient was difficult to bag, and during the first several minutes of bagging her heart rate climbed to 175, pulse pressure narrowed to 120/105, and then systolic blood pressure fell to 80 mmHg. When the patient was bagged slowly (2 breaths per minute) with 100% oxygen, the blood pressure rose and the heart rate fell. After two 1-L fluid boluses, each given over 10 min, the circulation stabilized.

After a stable blood pressure was achieved, the patient was placed on the mechanical ventilator with 100% oxygen, a tidal volume of 600 mL, RR of 15, and inspiratory flow rate of 60 L/min. With these settings, the peak airway pressure was 65 cmH_2O, intrinsic PEEP was 20 cmH_2O, and an arterial blood gas revealed a P_{O_2} of 300, P_{CO_2} of 68, and pH of 7.15. A chest radiograph revealed no evidence of barotrauma, marked hyperinflation, and good endotracheal tube position. The admitting electrolytes were normal except for a bicarbonate of 17, with an anion gap of 23 and arterial lactate level of 5.8 mg/dL. The creatine kinase level was elevated to 1300 U/mL, and the theophylline level was therapeutic at 15 μg/mL.

With several combinations of tidal volume, rate, and inspiratory flow, the optimal settings were a tidal volume of 475 mL, rate 18, and inspiratory flow of 70 L/min, giving a peak airway pressure of 57 cmH_2O, and PEEPi of 12 cmH_2O; minor increases in V_T or rate raised PEEPi above 15 cmH_2O. On these settings and a Fi_{O_2} of 0.4, the next arterial blood gas gave a P_{O_2} of 95, P_{CO_2} of 68, and pH of 7.18. A bicarbonate infusion was begun and titrated to give a pH of 7.25.

Over the next 24 h sedation was continued and muscle relaxant held every 4 h until muscle contraction was evident and then restarted. The patient received albuterol, 5 mg every 2 h by MDI connected by simple adapter to the ventilator tubing. Solu-Medrol, 250 mg every 6 h, was given by intravenous infusion, and ipratropium, 500 μg, was given by inhalation every 6 h. After 12 h of treatment, a large number of mucus plugs were suctioned from the airway, and after 30 h the peak airway pressures and PEEPi were noted to fall. At this same time P_{CO_2} began to fall on the same minute ventilation and the bicarbonate drip was discontinued. Several hours later all sedation and muscle relaxants were held, and after 52 h of mechanical ventilation the patient was able to sit up and breathe spontaneously, although her breaths were shallow and the measured negative inspiratory pressure was slightly low at 50 cmH_2O. Since her spontaneous breathing pattern was at a rate of 32 with no increase in P_{CO_2}, the patient was extubated.

During the next 24 h the patient was kept in the ICU. Bronchodilator and chest physiotherapy were continued and she demonstrated increasing stability as the frequency of treatments was reduced. She was then transferred to the ward where ongoing plans for outpatient management were made.

CASE DISCUSSION

Many features of the management of status asthmaticus are represented by this case. While some patients may present with relatively brief duration of symptoms, most, as in this case, will present on a number of medications with worsening symptoms over days. The severity of this attack was suggested by the relatively long duration of symptoms, the lack of sleep for two evenings, monosyllabic speech, pulse of 150, respirations of 40, and pulsus paradoxus of 25 mmHg. As if often the case, the patient could not perform a spirometric or peak flow maneuver.

Initial therapy was appropriately aggressive. Oxygen was administered, intravenous access established, and inhaled β agonists given. Since the inhaled agents were poorly tolerated, parenteral epinephrine was instituted promptly. High doses of corticosteroids were given, in anticipation of benefit over course of the next 24 h. Since the patient had been taking a long-acting theophylline preparation at home, a maintenance infusion was started and titrated against serum levels. It should be mentioned, however, that some clinicians would opt against the use of theophylline in this setting since it is a weak bronchodilator with a narrow therapeutic window and subjects the patient to many potential drug interactions and side effects.[34]

Since the patient failed to improve promptly, it was clear that admission to a critical care unit was necessary. Unfortunately, parenteral β-agonist therapy (or conceivably another attempt at inhalation therapy) was interrupted in the course of transporting the patient. Such patients may deteriorate with even brief interruptions in therapy. Close observation is essential, and arguably this patient's intubation occurred later than was ideal. Fortunately, cardiopulmonary arrest was averted.

Once PPV was instituted, sedation and muscle relaxation were effected. While this is appropriate, these medications in conjunction with the high intrathoracic pressures resulting from PPV caused hypoperfusion. This could be readily demonstrated by diminishing ventilation briefly and observing the rise in blood pressure and heart rate. Fluid resuscitation promptly restored a stable circulation, essential before proceeding to management of the patient on the ventilator.

Initial ventilator settings included relatively small tidal volumes and high inspiratory flow rates. Even with these, peak airway pressure and intrinsic PEEP were excessive and ventilation was inadequate. Fine adjustment of tidal volume, respiratory rate, and peak flow settings could achieve an acceptable airway pressure (peak <55 to 60 cmH_2O) and degree of hyperinflation (PEEPi <15 cmH_2O), but only at the cost of inadequate ventilation (P_{CO_2} = 68). Accordingly, the patient was hypoventilated with sedation and muscle relaxation continued. Bicarbonate infusion was used to maintain a pH of approximately 7.25.

Aggressive bronchodilator therapy continued with the patient on the ventilator, and airway resistance began to fall over 24 to 48 h, as is typical. Some improvement was no doubt related to clearing mucus plugs, a desirable goal but on occasion a threat to endotracheal tube patency. Once airflow obstruction resolved significantly, sedation and muscle relaxants were held. Since no evidence of muscle weakness or other complications were present, the patient was quickly converted to spontaneous breathing, and when she demonstrated stable and adequate ventilation, extubation was performed. Management continued in the ICU for the next day, to assure continued response and to establish a treatment plan to avert similar crises in the future.

References

1. American Thoracic Society: Standards for the diagnosis and care of patients with chronic obstructive pulmonary disease (COPD) and asthma. Am Rev Respir Dis 136:225, 1987.
2. Arnald AG, Lane DJ, Zapata E: The speed of onset and severity of acute severe asthma. Br J Dis Chest 76:157, 1982.
3. Hogg JC: The pathology of asthma. Clin Chest Med 5:567, 1984.
4. Rodriguez-Roisin R, Ballester E, Roca J, et al.: Mechanisms of hypoxemia in patient with status asthmaticus requiring mechanical ventilation. Am Rev Respir Dis 139:732, 1989.
5. Douglas JG, Rafferty P, Fergusson RJ: Nebulised salbutamol without oxygen in severe acute asthma: How effective and how safe? Thorax 40:180, 1985.
6. Roca J, Ramis L, Rodriguez-Roisin R, et al.: Serial relationships between ventilation perfusion inequality and spirometry in acute severe asthma requiring hospitalization. Am Rev Respir Dis 137:1055, 1988.
7. Rebuck AS, Read J: Assessment and management of severe asthma. Am J Med 51:788, 1971.
8. Pepe PE, Marini JP: Occult positive end-expiration pressure in mechanically ventilated patients with airflow obstruction. Am Rev Respir Dis 126:166, 1982.
9. Knowles GK, Clark TJH: Pulsus paradoxus as a valuable sign indicating severity of asthma. Lancet II:1356, 1973.
10. Appel D, Rubenstein R, Shrager K, et al.: Lactic acidosis in severe asthma. Am J Med 75:580, 1983.
11. Jederlinic PJ, Irwin RS: Status asthmaticus. J Int Care Med 4:166, 1989.
12. Hall JB, Wood LDH: Management of the critically ill asthmatic patient. Med Clin N Am 74(3):779, 1990.
13. Fishman AP: Cardiac asthma—a fresh look at an old wheeze. N Engl J Med 320:1346, 1989.
14. Cabanes LR, Weber SN, Matran R, et al.: Bronchial hyperresponsiveness to methacholine in patients with impaired left ventricular function. N Engl J Med 320:1317, 1989.
15. Baughman RP, Loudon RC: Stridor: differentiation from wheezing or upper airway noise. Am Rev Respir Dis 139:1407, 1989.

16. Mountain RD, Sahn SA: Clinical features and outcome in patients with acute asthma presenting with hypercapnia. Am Rev Respir Dis 138:535, 1988.
17. Fuller HD, Dolovich MB, Posmituck G, et al.: Pressurized aerosol versus jet aerosol delivery to mechanically ventilated patients. Am Rev Respir Dis 141:440, 1990.
18. Rossing TH, Fanta H, McFadden ER: Effect of outpatient treatment of asthma with beta agonists on the response to sympathomimetics in an emergency room. Am J Med 75:781, 1983.
19. Cydulka R, Davidson R, Grammer L, et al.: The use of epinephrine in the treatment of older adult asthmatics. Ann Emerg Med 17:322, 1988.
20. Ratto D, Alfonso C, Sipsey J, et al.: Are intravenous corticosteroids required in status asthmaticus? JAMA 260:527, 1988.
21. Rebuck As, Chapman KR, Abboud P: Nebulized anticholinergic and sympathomimetic treatment of asthma and chronic airways disease in the emergency room. Am J Med 82:59, 1987.
22. Tuxen DV, Lane S: The effects of ventilatory pattern on hyperinflation, airway pressures, and circulation in mechanical ventilation of patients with severe air-flow obstruction. Am Rev Respir Dis 136:872, 1987.
23. Strube PJ, Hallam PL: Ketamine by continuous infusion in status asthmaticus. Anaesthesia 41:1017, 1986.
24. Prezant DJ, Aldrich TK: Intravenous droperidol for the treatment of status asthmaticus. Crit Care Med 16:96, 1988.
25. Menitove SM, Goldring RM: Combined ventilator and bicarbonate strategy in the management of status asthmaticus. Am J Med 74:898, 1983.
26. Darioli R, Perret C: Mechanical controlled hypoventilation in status asthmaticus. Am Rev Respir Dis 129:385, 1984.
27. Fitzgerald JM, Hargreave FE: The assessment and management of acute life-threatening asthma. Chest 95:888, 1989.
28. Marini JP: Should PEEP be used in airflow obstruction? Am Rev Respir Dis 140:1, 1989.
29. Tuxen DV: Detrimental effects of positive end-expiratory pressure during controlled mechanical ventilation of patients with severe airflow obstruction. Am Rev Respir Dis 140:5, 1989.
30. Solway J, Rossing TH, Saari AF, et al.: Expiratory flow limitation and dynamic pulmonary hyperinflation during high frequency ventilation. J Appl Physiol 60:2071, 1986.
31. Gluck EH, Onorato DJ, Castriotta R: Helium-oxygen mixtures in intubated patients with status asthmaticus and respiratory acidosis. Chest 98:693, 1990.
32. Williams TJ, O'Hehir RE, Czarny D, et al.: Acute myopathy in severe asthma treated with intravenously administered corticosteroids. Am Rev Respir Dis 137:460, 1988.
33. Brun-Buisson C, Gherardi R. Hydrocortisone and pancuronium bromide: acute myopathy during status asthmaticus. Crit Care Med 16:731, 1988.
34. Newhouse MT: Is theophylline obsolete? Chest 98:1, 1990.

Chapter 131

BRONCHODILATORS

GARRETT FOULKE
TIMOTHY ALBERTSON

KEY POINTS

- *Inhaled β agonists are first-line bronchodilator therapy. Careful monitoring for cardiac toxicity and vasodilation is necessary since these drugs are often used at higher doses than recommended.*
- *On occasion, airflow obstruction is so severe that delivery of drug by inhalation is impossible; parenteral β agonists are useful in this circumstance.*
- *Inhaled anticholinergic agents are finding increasing application as adjuncts to β agonists in severe airflow obstruction.*
- *For both intubated, mechanically ventilated patients and more stable patients outside of the ICU, metered-dose inhalers (MDIs) may be used, although nebulized aerosol delivery is best for the most severe airflow obstruction.*
- *Knowledge of pharmacokinetics and monitoring of serum levels are vital to the safe use of theophylline.*
- *Theophylline exhibits many drug interactions with other agents used in critically ill patients, and dosing adjustment is often required.*
- *The intensivist should be familiar with inhaled and intravenous general anesthetic agents as therapy for severe bronchospasm and recognize that most support for this therapy is anecdotal.*
- *The pharmacologic properties of adjunctive agents (muscle relaxants, sedatives, etc.) can interact with bronchospastic disease.*

Bronchodilator drugs are extensively used in the critical care setting for both acute therapy of life-threatening airflow obstruction and ongoing treatment of chronic disease. This extensive use makes knowledge of the pharmacology, toxicity, and potential drug interactions of the commonly used bronchodilator drugs crucial for the intensivist. This chapter will review the pharmacologic features pertinent to the critical care setting.

β-Adrenergic Receptor Agonists

Inhalation of β_2-selective agents is widely considered to be the first-line therapy for acute bronchospasm in the critically ill patient (Table 131-1). There has been a relatively long experience with the parenteral administration of several of these agents (epinephrine, terbutaline). Used parenterally, bronchodilation is prompt, but side effects of sinus tachycardia, ventricular and supraventricular arrhythmias, hypotension, and potential for myocardial ischemia often limit dose, particularly in the older patient with multisystem disease. Accordingly, use of these drugs in North America and Europe has shifted in the past decade to inhalation as the preferred route of administration, with the rationales that reduced systemic doses and increased delivery to the active site are achieved with this method. These considerations may be extremely important in the critically ill patient receiving myriad medications with multiple drug interactions and toxicities possible. Several observations should be made in this regard. First, the most severe airway obstruction is now treated with near continuous inhalation of β agonists, both to spare patients intubation if they are still capable of spontaneous breathing and to minimize the duration of mechanical ventilation if ventilatory failure has supervened. Such use, justifiable in view of the severity of airway disease, may result in serious systemic side effects, and the patient must be monitored with this possibility in mind. In addition, subcutaneous administration may be necessary when profound bronchospasm prevents adequate drug delivery by aerosol. This judgment is one that can only be made at the bedside and relies on observation by the experienced physician, nurse, and respiratory therapist.

The subcutaneous route is associated with decreased β_2 specificity and thus tachycardia. Increased myocardial oxygen demand due to α- and β_1-adrenergic effects of subcutaneous epinephrine have long been a concern. Some studies suggest, however, that there is no difference in incidence of side effects between subcutaneous administration of epinephrine and terbutaline regardless of patient age.[1,2] Isoproterenol has been used intravenously for profound bronchospasm largely in the pediatric age group. The dose is approximately 10 percent of what is used for life-threatening bradyarrhythmias.[3] Even at this dose the drug has dangerous cardiac stimulation potential and should not be used in adults. Intravenous salbutamol appears to have a safer profile and a growing experience in Europe, but currently is not available in the United States.[3] Direct endotracheal instillation of salbutamol has been reported to be efficacious in a resuscitation setting,[4] but this and other β agonists are routinely administered by either nebulized aerosol or by direct use of an MDI.

PHARMACOLOGY

All β-adrenergic agonists are chemical modifications of phenylethylamine. As indicated in Table 131-1, the available agents are classified as catecholamines, resorcinols, and saligenins. The structural modifications in the agents result in differences in duration of action and β_2-receptor specificity. The enzymes catechol-O-methyltransferase (found in liver and kidney) and monoamine oxidase (presynaptic neurons) metabolize all catecholamines, limiting their duration of action. The noncatecholamine β_2 agonists are resistant to enzymatic degradation and therefore have a longer duration of action.

Binding of β-receptor agonists to cell membrane receptors produces an increase in intracellular smooth muscle cyclic adenosine monophosphate (AMP) and lowered intra-

TABLE 131-1 Aerosol/Parenteral Bronchodilators

Drug	Route	Adult Dose (Pediatric)	Duration (hr)	Type
β-adrenergics				
Catecholamines				
Epinephrine	sq	0.3–0.5 mL, 1:1000 (0.01 mL/kg)	1–2	$\alpha = \beta_1 = \beta_2$
Isoproterenol	aerosol	0.5 mL, 0.5% soln (0.01 mL/kg)	1–2	$\beta_1 = \beta_2$
	IV	0.1–1.2 μg/kg/min[b]	—	$\beta_1 = \beta_2$
Isoetharine		0.3–0.5 mL, 1% soln (0.02 mL/kg)	2–3	$\beta_2 \geq \beta_1$
Resorcinols				
Metaproterenol	aerosol	0.3 mL, 5% soln (0.01 mL/kg)	3–5	$\beta_2 > \beta_1$
Terbutaline	sq	0.25 mL, 1% soln (0.01 mL/kg)	4–6	$\beta_2 \geq \beta_1$
	aerosol[a]	0.1 mL, 1% soln (0.03 mL/kg)	4–6	$\beta_2 \gg \beta_1$
Fenoterol	aerosol	0.5 mL, 0.5% soln (0.01 mL/kg)	4–6	$\beta_2 \gg \beta_1$
Saligenin				
Salbutamol	aerosol	0.5 mL, 0.5% soln (0.01 mL/kg)	4–6	$\beta_2 \gg \beta_1$
Anticholinergics				
Ipratropium bromide	MDI only	2 puffs (36 μg)	4–6	Quarternary ammonium
Glycopyrrolate	aerosol[a]	0.8–2.0 mg	5–8	Quarternary ammonium
Atropine sulfate	aerosol[a]	1.75 mg (0.025–0.075 mg/kg)	3–5 3–5	Tertiary ammonium

MDI, metered-dose inhaler; sq, subcutaneous injection.
[a]Not FDA approved.
[b]Generally in children only.

cellular ionized calcium concentrations. This is thought to promote smooth muscle relaxation and bronchodilation. Additional effects include increased mucociliary transport and inhibition of histamine and slow reacting substance of anaphylaxis (SRS-A) release from mast cells. β-Adrenergic receptor agonists also may inhibit the release of acetylcholine from postganglionic cholinergic nerves in the airway.

Epinephrine is administered subcutaneously and has α-, β_1-, and β_2-adrenergic activity. Isoproterenol is a potent but infrequently used aerosol agent because of its significant β_1 activity. The remainder of the readily available agents (see Table 131-1) have moderate β_2-receptor specificity. The clinical differences between agents in the critical care setting are minimal. In general, catecholamine agonist activity peaks at 5 to 15 min with duration from 1 to 3 h. The noncatecholamine agents show onset of action at 5 to 15 min, peak effects at 1 to 2 h and a duration of action from 3 to 6 h. These data bear little relevance to dosing schedules in the critically ill bronchospastic patient. Here drug should be administered by inhalation if possible, parenterally if this is not effective. If inhalation therapy is chosen, treatments should be repeated at frequent intervals (every 10 to 30 min) until a response is noted or side effects are limiting. On occasion, continuous therapy may be desirable.[5]

UNWANTED EFFECTS/DRUG INTERACTIONS

Adverse effects associated with β-adrenergic receptor agonists include tremor, nervousness, insomnia, palpitations, and tachycardia. Tachycardia occurs both as a direct result of β_1 stimulation and as a reflex due to β_2-mediated peripheral vasodilation. Tremor occurs as a result of peripheral β stimulation. It is tolerated in many patients but may limit use in some. Since tremor and therapeutic effect both result from β stimulation, there is no counteractive therapy. Cardiac stimulation and vasodilation may increase myocardial oxygen demand or aggravate cardiac arrhythmias. Additionally, hypokalemia is induced by β stimulation. Stimulatory effects on skeletal muscle and an insulin-induced uptake of potassium have both been postulated.[6] β-Adrenergic agents have been used to treat hyperkalemic dialysis patients.[7] It appears that clinically important tachyphylaxis to the bronchodilator effects does not develop.[8]

The most frequent drug interaction seen with β agonists occurs when several β agonists are used simultaneously, with emergence of the side effects already mentioned. The combined use of aminophylline and β agonists may increase the incidence of (primarily supraventricular) cardiac arrhythmias, but these are well tolerated and the risk of more dangerous ventricular arrhythmias seems negligible.[9,10]

Methylxanthines

Theophylline is the only agent in this group in clinical use. It is typically selected as a second-line bronchodilator, or given with β agonists in patients with severe airflow obstruction. Problems with the clinical use of theophylline are related to a narrow therapeutic window and to individual variation in clearance.

PHARMACOLOGY

Theophylline's principle action(s) in the treatment of airway disease remain(s) elusive. It is a very weak phosphodiesterase inhibitor. It has activity as an adenosine-receptor antagonist but a similar compound, enprofylline, has greater bronchodilator potency without any adenosine antagonist properties. Other proposed mechanisms of action include increased binding of cyclic AMP and inhibition of intracellular calcium release. By one or more of these mechanisms, theophylline causes relaxation of bronchial smooth muscle. Theophylline also augments diaphragmatic contractility.[11] There has been considerable debate as to the absolute amount and clinical relevance (most data are from in vitro systems) of this phenomenon. One research group has provided evidence for slightly improved diaphragmatic function in patients with both chronic disease[12] and acute respiratory failure.[13] Theophylline's benefit in acute disease probably results from a combination of bronchodilator and diaphragmatic effects. Theophylline may also reduce mucosal edema and have anti-inflammatory actions. The critically ill patient can be affected in additional ways since theophylline is also reported to be a weakly positive myocardial inotrope, stimulate catecholamine release, cause mild diuresis, inhibit white cell function, cause dilation of most arteries and veins, stimulate gastric acid secretion, and decrease cerebral blood flow.[14]

Oral theophylline in an ambulatory patient results in peak serum levels at 1 to 2 h (4 h for slow release preparations). The timing and duration of drug absorption (especially with slow release preparations) in the critically ill should be considered unpredictable. This is particularly true following overdosage. The volume of distribution as well as the clearance rates for theophylline can fluctuate in a critically ill patient. Theophylline is hepatically metabolized and excreted by the kidneys. The half-life in healthy adults ranges from 7 to 9 h. This is reduced in smokers to 4 h and increased to 12 h or more in patients with liver disease or any condition which decreases liver blood flow (e.g., congestive heart failure). In addition, a number of drugs are known to alter theophylline clearance (Table 131-2). Theophylline infusion dosage, therefore, involves the use of rough guidelines (based on lean body weight) with subsequent reliance on serum theophylline levels to establish the necessary infusion rate. An admission theophylline level should be obtained and administration begun based on guidelines noted in Table 131-3. Subsequent adjustments are made based on serum levels (Table 131-4). If steady-state serum levels are low, further loading doses are given based on an estimate that 1 mg/kg of theophylline will produce a 2 mg/L rise in serum level.

There is evidence in asthmatic patients that increasing the theophylline level from low therapeutic (10 mg/L) to

TABLE 131-2 Theophylline Drug Interactions

Drug/Group	Potential Interaction(s)	Alterations
Cimetidine	Theo. Cl decreased 25–40%	Monitor level, may need dose reduction
Erythromycin (and other macrolide antibiotics)	Theo. Cl decreased ~25%	Monitor level, may need 25% dose reduction or change in antibiotic
Ciprofloxacin (and other fluroquinolones)	Theo. Cl decreased ≤30%	Monitor level
Allopurinol	Theo. Cl decreased ~25% if ≥600 mg/day	Monitor level, may need 25% dose reduction
Oral contraceptives/ estrogens	Theo. Cl decrease ≤30%	Monitor level
Propranolol	Theo. Cl decreased 20–40%	β Blocker contraindicated in bronchospactic disease
Troleandomycin	Theo. Cl decreased 40–60%	Reduce Theo. (50% minimum), monitor level, better–avoid troleandomycin
Isoproterenol (IV)	Theo. Cl **increased** ≤40%	Monitor level, may need increased dosage
Phenobarbitol	Theo. Cl **increased** 10–60% after ≥30 days	Monitor level, may need dose increase
Rifampin	Theo. Cl **increased** ≤25%	Monitor level
Phenytoin	Theo. Cl **increased** ~75% after ≥10 days	Monitor level, may need increase
	Phenytoin absorption may decrease	Monitor level, better–avoid phenytoin/Theo. combination
Lithium	Lithium Cl may increase	Monitor levels of both drugs

Theo. Cl, theophylline clearance.

TABLE 131-3 Intravenous Theophylline Guidelines

Loading Dose

No previous theophylline: 6 mg/kg of aminophylline (lean body weight) infused over 30 min.

If already on theophylline, reduce theophylline dose based on serum level (Cs mg/L):

Vol. of distribution (Vd) = 0.5 L/kg × Wt (kg)

Loading dose = Vd × desired changed in serum level (mg/L)
= Vd (Cs desired − Cs known)

For 50-kg patient with Cs of 8 mg/L and desired Cs of 18 mg/L:

Loading dose $= 0.5_{L/kg} \times 50_{Kg} \times (18_{mg/L} - 8_{m\mu g/L}) = 250$ mg
= 312.5 mg aminophylline
(80% theophylline)

If the level is unknown then the loading dose (if any can only be estimated based on dose interval (presumed to approximate half-life) and intake. If a q8h preparation was last taken 8 h ago, then a "half loading dose" (3 mg/kg) could be given (if 16 h ago, 4.5 mg/kg, etc.) A predose level should be drawn.

Initial Maintenance Dose

Group	Infusion Rate (mg/kg/h)
Adults	0.5
Smokers (60% Cl increase)	0.8
Liver disease (50% Cl decrease)	0.4
Severe COPD (cor pulmonale etc.)	0.4
Congestive failure (60% Cl decrease)	0.2
Viral illness (probable hepatic dysfunction)	0.4
Children	0.9–1.2

Subsequent adjustment as per Table 131-4.

TABLE 131-4 Aminophylline Maintenance Adjustments

After 24 h (presumed >4 half-lives and therefore steady state) adjustments based on steady-state serum level (Cs mg/L) and:

Clearance (C_L) = Dose/Cs

Maintenance Dose mg/h = Cl × desired Cs

If patient receiving 24 mg/h × 24 h and level is now 8 mg/L with desired level of 18 mg/L, then:

$$CL = \frac{24 \text{ mg/h}}{8 \text{ mg/L}} = 3 \text{ L/h}$$

Maintenance Dose = 3 L/h × 18 mg/L = 54 mg/h aminophylline

Prior to 24 h, adjustments can be made by two methods.

1. Give loading dose, obtain level, wait 2–4 h, obtain second level, determine half-live ($T_{1/2}$) via semi-log plot or computer calculation, determine clearance via:
   $CL = .693 \times Vd^a/T_{1/2}$
   Maintenance dose = as above (additional loading dose may be needed)[a]
2. Give loading dose, obtain level (to ensure loading adequate), begin maintenance, repeat level at 4–6 h, make estimated adjustments (e.g., if level falls by 20%/h, increase rate by 20%/h).
   Note: This process must ultimately be abandoned ×24 h to document steady-state level adequacy.

[a]See Table 131-3.

high therapeutic (near 20 mg/L) can add an additional 10 percent benefit (as measured by spirometric values).[15] In the critically ill, this benefit may warrant efforts to maximize theophylline level. A similar benefit has not been documented in acute on chronic respiratory failure. Approximate "target" levels for theophylline might therefore be set at 12 to 15 mg/L for chronic obstructive pulmonary disease (COPD), 14 to 16 mg/L for responding asthma, and 18 to 20 mg/L for unresponsive status asthmaticus.

UNWANTED EFFECTS/DRUG INTERACTIONS

Theophylline can produce nausea, vomiting, headache, diarrhea, and insomnia. Of greater concern are hyperglycemia, seizures, and cardiac arrhythmias, usually from excessive dosing. Theophylline-induced seizures are difficult to treat and have a mortality rate as high as 50 percent.[16] This is compounded by the fact that many patients do not manifest symptoms before the seizures. Seizures may be refractory to therapy but are treated conventionally (see Chap. 142). Serum theophylline monitoring is the only reliable means of preventing serious theophylline toxicity.[17] The incidence of serious theophylline side effects should be near zero below 15 mg/L, uncommon below 20 mg/L and 75 percent at >25 mg/L.[18] Levels up to 40 mg/L generally warrant discontinuation of the drug (with administration of activated charcoal for acute ingestions) and supportive care. Charcoal hemoperfusion should be considered above 40 mg/L with severe symptoms (seizures, ventricular arrhythmias) and above 60 mg/L even in the absence of symptoms.

Principle cardiac complications are tachycardia and exacerbation of supraventricular arrhythmias. Theophylline can produce multifocal atrial tachycardia.[19] Cardiac arrhythmias may be precipitated by infusion of the drug through a central venous catheter. Therapeutic drug levels should not produce ventricular arrhythmias but higher levels have been reported to do so. Ventricular arrhythmias are reported to respond promptly to lidocaine.[17] Profound hypotension and cardiovascular collapse can occur with rapid infusion of the drug.

Allergic reactions, such as urticaria, angioedema, bronchospasm, and pruritis have been reported with aminophylline. This is felt to be due to the ethylenediamine added to aminophylline to increase water solubility. Intravenous theophylline (rather than aminophylline) is now frequently used from premixed solution bags. It is best if dosages are based on mg of aminophylline (2 mg aminophylline = 1.6 mg theophylline) since all standard guidelines (as in Table 131-3) are in this form.

Theophylline has well-known drug interaction potential with many commonly used drugs.[17] Pertinent drug interactions with theophylline in the critical care setting are summarized in Table 131-2. The effect on lithium is a variable indirect effect, presumably due to diuretic effects of theophylline. There are also reports that calcium channel blocking agents may diminish theophylline's ability to enhance diaphragmatic contractility.[20] Limited reports suggest that thiabendizole may decrease theophylline clearance by 50 percent and carbamazepine may increase it by up to 100 percent. Accurate assessment of the carbamazepine data is hampered by the concomitant administration of phenobarbitol to many patients. Influenza vaccine is also reported to decrease clearance but this is a highly variable phenomenon.

NEW AGENTS

Enprofylline is a theophylline-like compound which does not have adenosine antagonist properties. There are few, if any, central nervous system (CNS) side effects from this drug. Clearance is not affected by hepatic metabolism since it is eliminated unchanged in the urine.[21] Since the drug does have potent bronchodilator properties, it is hoped that clinical studies will ultimately show it to be an effective alternative to theophylline.

Anticholinergic Agents

Anticholinergic agents are effectively used in the critical care setting as bronchodilators. Atropine sulfate has been used in an unapproved nebulized form by intensivists and emergency room physicians for many years. The compound glycopyrrolate is increasingly used in the same fashion. The approved aerosol drug ipratropium bromide is thus far available only in MDI, but can be readily administered to critically ill patients, including those requiring intubation.[22] The precise role of ipratropium in asthma and COPD—adjunct to β agonists, alternative to β agonists, etc.—remains to be defined. Nonetheless, it is likely that ipratropium and similar agents will find increasing use in severe airflow obstruction.

PHARMACOLOGY

All compounds in this group are antimuscarinic and block cholinergic (vagal) innervation to produce predominately large airway bronchodilation. Atropine sulfate, when given in a dose of 0.025 to 0.075 mg/kg has an onset of action at 15 to 30 min. Peak effect is seen at 30 min or more and duration of effect is between 3 and 5 h. Since this drug is a tertiary ammonium compound and is readily absorbed, the systemic side effects of tachycardia, drying of secretions, urinary retention, and CNS toxicity are all encountered. The quaternary ammonium compounds ipratropium and glycopyrrolate are both relatively free of this problem since they are charged and not systemically absorbed. Glycopyrrolate can be administered by inhalation (not approved by the Food and Drug Administration) of the injectable form. Dosage in an adult should start at 0.8 mg and can be increased to up to 2 mg. It has an onset and peak effect similar to atropine sulfate. The drug has a duration of action of up to 8 h after inhalation therapy.[23] The potential reduction in mucocilliary clearance with these agents does not appear to be a clinical problem.

NEW AGENTS

Another quaternary ammonium anticholinergic compound, oxitropium bromide, is undergoing extensive testing. It appears to have properties similar to the other agents in this class.[24] The muscarinic receptor is slowly being characterized into multiple subsets. It is hoped that in the future, agents which are specific for an airway smooth muscle receptor (perhaps M3) will be perfected.[25]

Other Bronchodilator Agents

General anesthetics can be used for unremitting bronchospasm. The reported experience with these agents is largely anecdotal. The most extensive experience is with halothane. This drug has bronchodilator properties that are effected through multiple mechanisms including direct bronchial smooth muscle relaxation. Pertinent side effects include arrhythmias and hypotension when used for status asthmaticus.[26] Additionally, myocardial depression and significant cerebral vasodilation must be anticipated. There is the potential that the hypoxemia of severe bronchospastic disease may increase myocardial toxicity. Because of these concerns, isoflurane has been advocated, again with only anecdotal support. The use of enflurane has also been reported but this agent failed in a patient who subsequently responded to halothane.[27] The uninitiated should not underestimate the difficulty of preserving cardiopulmonary function in the patient with status asthmaticus treated with inhaled anesthetics, and accordingly we suggest they be considered only when all other measures, including specific ventilator management, has failed (see Chap. 130).

Intravenous anesthesia can be achieved with ketamine. The drug produces bronchodilation, increased heart rate, and increased blood pressure without altering respiration. It has been effectively used in the asthmatic patient.[28,29] Because of these properties, the drug is gaining popularity for use in emergent intubation of asthmatic patients. Principle pharmacologic concerns are the CNS disturbances and hallucinations occurring during awakening. Thus, ketamine is relatively contraindicated in patients with possible cardiac ischemia, hypertension, and preeclampsia. Droperidol, an intravenous anesthetic agent, has also been reported to be of benefit for sedation in patients with status asthmaticus requiring mechanical ventilation.[30]

Intravenous magnesium sulfate has been reported to be an effective bronchodilator.[31] Of particular interest is the fact that patients who responded poorly to β agonist were treated effectively with magnesium sulfate.[32] An intravenous infusion of 1.2 g over 20 min. is recommended in adults. The mechanism of action is unknown but may be related to intracellular calcium flux. Skin flushing and a sensation of cutaneous warmth may be encountered. Pharmacologic concerns include the sedation and depressed neuromotor function that is seen with magnesium administration.

Currently available calcium channel blockers do have some effect on airway resistance, but these effects are mild and there has been little clinical benefit demonstrable.[33] Research continues into application of calcium antagonists and leukotriene antagonists. Several neuropeptides have been implicated in nonadrenergic, noncholinergic mechanisms of airway control and agents may become available which exploit these pathways.[34]

Other Pharmacologic Issues

Steroids and other anti-inflammatory therapies are central in treating airway disease, since most patients with airflow obstruction have a significant element of airway inflammation which causes airway edema and may potentiate bronchospasm.[35] It is assumed that virtually all patients with airflow obstruction which causes ventilatory failure will require treatment with corticosteroids (see Chaps. 129 and 130). Whether patients whose airflow obstruction is a relatively minor feature of other critical illness require corticosteroids and in what form is a decision that must be individualized.

Sedation and paralysis often are necessary once mechanical ventilation is instituted for status asthmaticus. Opiates, both naturally occurring and synthetic, are frequently used for sedation purposes. Most opiates cause histamine release with a potential for worsened bronchospasm. It is not clear that this action of the opiates is clinically relevant, but even small effects would be of concern in a patient requiring mechanical ventilation for airway disease. Accordingly, in most patients benzodiazepine sedation may be preferred. The same principle holds for paralytic agents. Depolarizing agents such as succinylcholine cause considerably more histamine release than nondepolarizing agents. Therefore, use of a nondepolarizing agent such as vecuronium may be in order.

Most β agonist and anticholinergic therapies depend on adequate aerosol delivery. The maximal effective delivery possible from any aerosol system is 13 percent (for an MDI). This is reduced to approximately 5 percent for most nebulizer systems used on critically ill patients.[36] There is a further reduction in the intubated mechanically ventilated patient where a mean of 2.9 percent deposition is achieved.[37] This reduced delivery requires larger doses to be administered to most severely affected patients.

CASE PRESENTATION

A 24-year-old white male asthmatic was admitted with 3 days of increasing wheezing and shortness of breath. The patient complained of moderate nausea but no vomiting or other gastrointestinal complaints. He denied chest pain, fever, sputum production, or other acute complaints. The past medical history included a smoking history for the past 6 years and asthma since childhood. He was being treated for peptic ulcer disease. His private physician placed him on erythromycin for "bronchitis" 10 days previously. Medications included a slow release theophylline preparation, metaproterenol inhaler, inhaled steroid preparation, cimetidine 300 mg every 6 h and erythromycin 500 mg four times a day.

Physical examination was pertinent for moderate respiratory distress with evidence of intercostal retractions. Vital signs were blood pressure 176/92, pulse 126, respirations 36, and temperature 37.2°C (99°F). No jugular venous distention or peripheral edema was present. Chest examination revealed limited airflow with diffuse wheezing. Bowel sounds were active. The patient received a metaproterenol nebulized aerosol treatment twice in his first hour in the emergency department (0.3 mL of a 5% solution by nebulized aerosol). He was given 125 mg methylprednisolone intravenously. An IV of normal saline at 125 mL/h was established and theophylline was withheld.

Pertinent laboratory values included a white cell count of 11,500/cm^3, a hematocrit of 42, a theophylline level of 27 μg/mL, and an arterial blood-gas sample that revealed P_{O_2} 62 mmHg, P_{CO_2} 48 mmHg, pH 7.31 on 40% inspired oxygen. Because of increasing respiratory distress, the patient was intubated. Anesthesia for intubation was intravenous ketamine after which midazolam was given for sedation.

Following this he appeared to be worse and was given another metaproterenol aerosol treatment. There was no improvement and he was given 0.8 mg glycopyrrolate as a nebulized aerosol and nebulized metaproterenol was repeated. The patient was transferred to the ICU and metaproterenol aerosol treatments every 4 h, glycopyrrolate aerosol treatments every 6 h, and 125 mg methylprednisolone IV every 6 h were instituted. Serial theophylline levels were obtained. A repeat theophylline level at 4 h was 22 μg/mL. Repeat levels remained at 22 μg/mL throughout the night. The patient was continued on intravenous cimetidine 50 mg/h because of the presence of guaiac-positive gastric aspirate and stool. The following morning the theophylline level was 20 μg/mL and an infusion at 0.4 mg/kg/h was begun. A daily repeat level was ordered. By the second day metaproterenol could be administered through the ventilator tubing with a simple adapter and an MDI; the respiratory therapy staff judged this to be equally effective to nebulization treatments, and this seemed confirmed by measurements of airway pressure on the ventilator.

After 2 days, the patient was improved and extubated. Plans were made to transfer him to oral agents over the next 2 days and to be discharged on oral theophylline, metaproterenol inhaler, and 80 mg prednisone daily on a tapering dose. The patient was instructed to return in 2 days for a checkup and a repeat theophylline level.

CASE DISCUSSION

This patient required intubation and mechanical ventilation after 1 h of emergency room management with an inhaled β-adrenergic agent. Arguably, inhalation treatments should have been more frequent, at a higher dose, or parenteral administration of epinephrine or terbutaline should have been attempted. When intubation was performed, ketamine and a benzodiazepine were selected for anesthesia and sedation on the theoretical basis of preventing histamine release and worsened bronchospasm.

The patient's elevated theophylline level was perhaps due to the interaction of theophylline with the H_2 blocker and antibiotic he had been placed on earlier. Since he was taking a time-release preparation, it was advisable to withhold intravenous aminophylline until his level began to fall. An infusion started at this time was at a rate lower than normal for a healthy adult because of the concomitant cimetidine and erythromycin administration. It was then titrated against measured serum level.

A quarternary ammonium anticholinergic agent was added to the β-adrenergic therapy and both continued by inhalation at frequent intervals. In the case of the metaproterenol, this could be achieved with an MDI, even during mechanical ventilation. The patient was gradually converted to an outpatient regimen, including high dose corticosteroids.

References

1. Cydulka R, Davison R, Grammer L, et al: The use of epinephrine in the treatment of older adult asthmatics. Ann Emerg Med 17:322, 1988.
2. Spiteri I, Millar A, Pavia D, Clarke S: Subcutaneous adrenaline versus terbutaline in the treatment of acute severe asthma. Thorax 43:19, 1988.
3. Bohn D, Kalloghlian A, Jenkins J, et al: Intravenous salbutamol in the treatment of status asthmaticus in children. Crit Care Med 12:892, 1984.
4. Verbeek P, Gareau A, Rubes C: Treatment of asthma-related respiratory arrest with endotracheal albuterol (salbutamol). Ann Emerg Med 17:358, 1988.
5. Moler F, Hurwitz M, Custer J: Improvement in clinical asthma score and Pa_{CO_2} in children with severe asthma treated with continuously nebulized terbutaline. J Allergy Clin Immunol 81:1101, 1988.
6. Vincent H, Boomsma F, Veld A, et al: Effects of selective and nonselective β-agonists on plasma potassium and norepineprine. J Cardiovasc Pharmacol 6:7, 1984.
7. Allon M, Dunlay R, Copkney C: Nebulized albuterol for acute hyperkalemia in patients on hemodialysis. Ann Intern Med 110:426, 1989.
8. Lipworth B, Struthers A, McDevitt D: Tachyphylaxis to systemic but not to airway responses during prolonged therapy with high dose inhaled salbutamol in asthmatics. Am Rev Respir Dis 140:586, 1989.
9. Eidelman D, Sami M, McGregor M, Cosio M: Combination of theophylline and salbutamol for arrhythmias in severe COPD. Chest 91:808, 1987.
10. Laaban J, Iung B, Chauvet J, et al: Cardiac arrhythmias during the combined use of intravenous aminophylline and terbutaline in status asthmaticus. Chest 94:496, 1988.
11. Aubier M, DeTroyer A, Sampson M, et al: Aminophylline improves diaphragmatic contractility. N Engl J Med 305:249, 1981.
12. Murciano D, Aubier M, Lecocguic Y, Pariente R: Effects of theophylline on diaphragmatic strength and fatigue in patients with chronic obstructive pulmonary disease. N Engl J Med 311:349, 1984.
13. Vire N, Aubier M, Murciano D, et al: Effects of aminophylline on diaphragmatic fatigue during acute respiratory failure. Am Rev Respir Dis 129:396, 1984.
14. Bowton D, Alford P, McLees B, et al: The effect of aminophylline on cerebral blood flow in patients with chronic obstructive pulmonary disease. Chest 91:874, 1987.
15. Vozeh S, Kewitz G, Perruchoud A, et al: Theophylline serum concentration and therapeutic effect in severe acute bronchial obstruction: The optimal use of intravenously administered aminophylline. Am Rev Respir Dis 125:181, 1982.
16. Zwilich CW, Sutton FD, Neff TA, et al: Theophylline-induced seizures in adults: Correlation with serum concentrations. Ann Intern Med 82:784, 1975.
17. Hendeles L, Weinberger M: Theophylline a "state of the art" review. Pharmacotherapy 3:2, 1983.
18. Jacobs M, Senior R, Kessler G: Clinical experience with theophylline: Relationships between dosage, serum concentration and toxicity. JAMA 235:1983, 1976.
19. Levine J, Michael J, Guarnieri T: Multifocal atrial tachycardia: A toxic effect of theophylline. Lancet 1:12, 1985.
20. Kolbeck RC, Speir WA: Diltiazem, verapamil, and nifedipine inhibit theophylline-enhanced diaphragmatic contractility. Am Rev Respir Dis 139:139, 1989.
21. Chung K, Barnes P: Respiratory and allergic disease. I. Br Med J 296:29, 1988.
22. Fernandez A, Lazaro A, Garcia A, et al: Bronchodilators in patients with chronic obstructive pulmonary disease on mechanical ventilation. Am Rev Respir Dis 141:164, 1990.
23. Ziment I, Au J: Anticholinergic agents. Clin Chest Med 7:355, 1986.
24. Frith P, Jenner B, Dangerfield R, et al: Oxitropium bromide dose-response and time-response study of a new anticholinergic bronchodilator drug. Chest 89:249, 1986.
25. Gross N, Barnes P: A short tour around the muscarinic receptor. Am Rev Respir Dis 138:765, 1988.
26. Rosseel P, Lauwers LF, Baute L: Halothane treatment in life-threatening asthma. Intensive Care Med 11:241, 1985.
27. Echeverria M, Gelb A, Wexler H, et al: Enflurane and halothane in status asthmaticus. Chest 89:152, 1986.
28. Corssen G, Gutierrez J, Reeves JG, et al: Ketamine in the anesthetic management of asthmatic patients. Anesth Analg 51:588, 1972.
29. L'Hommedieu CS, Arens JJ: The use of ketamine for the emergency intubation of patients with status asthmaticus. Ann Emerg Med 16:568, 1987.
30. Prezant D, Aldrich T: Intravenous droperidol for the treatment of status asthmaticus. Crit Care Med 16:96, 1988.
31. Okayama H, Aikawa T, Okayama M, et al: Bronchodilating effect of intravenous magnesium sulfate in bronchial asthma. JAMA 257:1076, 1987.
32. Skobeloff E, Spivey W, McNamara R, Greenspon L: Intravenous magnesium sulfate for the treatment of acute asthma in the emergency department. JAMA 262:1210, 1989.
33. Molho M, Gruzman C, Katz I, et al: Nifedipine in Astha. Dose-related effect on resting bronchial tone. Chest 91:667, 1987.
34. Barnes P: Neural control of human airways in health and disease. Am Rev Respir Dis 134:1289, 1986.
35. Barnes P: A new approach to the treatment of asthma. N Engl J Med 321:1517, 1989.
36. Newhouse MT, Dolovich MB: Current concepts. Control of asthma by aerosols. N Engl J Med 315:870, 1986.
37. MacIntyre N, Silver R, Miller C, et al: Aerosol delivery in intubated, mechanically ventilated patients. Crit Care Med 13:81, 1985.

Chapter 132

RESTRICTIVE LIMITATION TO BREATHING: MANAGEMENT OF PATIENTS WITH THORACIC CAGE DEFORMITY AND PULMONARY FIBROSIS

THOMAS CORBRIDGE
LAWRENCE D.H. WOOD

KEY POINTS

Kyphoscoliosis

- *Scoliotic curves greater than 100° are associated with dyspnea; curves greater than 120° are associated with alveolar hypoventilation and cor pulmonale.*
- *Patients with severe deformity in acute respiratory failure for the first time have a good prognosis with median survival of 9 years. Common precipitants include pneumonia, congestive heart failure, and upper respiratory tract infection, although precipitating factors are often minor and may remain obscure.*
- *Low tidal volumes and high respiratory rates minimize the risk of barotrauma during mechanical ventilation; antiatelectasis measures are necessary.*
- *Nocturnal hypoxemia is common in patients with kyphoscoliosis and may contribute to cardiovascular deterioration; routine polysomnography is recommended.*
- *Strategies for management of patients with chronic ventilatory failure include daytime intermittent positive-pressure ventilation (IPPV), nocturnal nasal continuous positive airway pressure (CPAP) and nasal IPPV, and nocturnal ventilation through a tracheostomy; corrective surgery is not recommended for most adult patients.*

Pulmonary Fibrosis

- *Acute deterioration often results from bacterial pneumonia, and chronic deterioration often represents disease progression.*
- *Pulmonary hypertension and cor pulmonale are common in patients with end-stage fibrosis.*
- *Low tidal volumes and high respiratory rates during mechanical ventilation minimize pneumothorax, high ratio of volume of dead space to tidal volume (V_D/V_T), and low cardiac output.*
- *Corticosteroids are the mainstay of medical management of many disorders leading to pulmonary fibrosis. Treatment typically requires high doses for prolonged periods of time and should not be started without a firm tissue diagnosis. Patients who deteriorate while taking steroids are candidates for cytotoxic therapy.*
- *Heart-lung and single-lung transplantation has been successful in patients with end-stage fibrosis who have failed medical therapy.*

Both thoracic cage deformity and pulmonary fibrosis result in a restrictive limitation to breathing. Although both disorders are relatively rare in the context of pulmonary intensive care, the potential problems they create can lead to long and complicated intensive care unit (ICU) admissions. In this chapter, we describe the chronic derangements in cardiopulmonary function associated with these disorders and how they affect management during acute, reversible decompensations. A primary goal of this chapter is to offer strategies for cardiovacular management and mechanical ventilation of these patients that minimizes the risk of ventilator-induced complications and maximizes the chance for early, successful extubation.

Patients with Thoracic Deformity

Kyphoscoliosis is the prototypical cause of severe thoracic deformity. It is defined as a combination of scoliosis (defined as a lateral deformity of the spine) and kyphosis (a posterior deformity of the spine) and is far more common than either kyphosis or scoliosis alone. As many as 200,000 people with severe kyphoscoliosis are at risk of developing respiratory failure at some time in their lives.[1] Most cases are idiopathic. Others result from congenital defects, poliomyelitis, thoracoplasty, syringomyelia, and tuberculosis.

Clinical symptoms and pathophysiologic consequences of kyphoscoliosis generally correlate with the degree of spinal curvature.[1,2] Severe deformity, however, is not incompatible with a long and relatively asymptomatic life,[3] and some patients with moderate deformity progress quickly to ventilatory failure and cor pulmonale. The reason for this variability is not clear, though in some patients sleep-disordered breathing contributes to an accelerated course.[4,5] The combination of a moderate kyphotic deformity and a moderate scoliotic deformity is functionally equivalent to a severe deformity of either alone,[2] yet the scoliotic deformity is worse. In patients with kyphoscoliosis, a scoliotic curve less than 70° (see Fig. 132-1) rarely results in cardiopulmonary sequelae, whereas angles greater than 70° place the patient at risk of developing respiratory failure.[1] Those reaching this angle earlier in life are at greater risk of eventual respiratory failure because spinal curvature increases with age by an average of 15° in 20 years from an initial angle of 70°.[6,7] Angles greater than 100° are associated with dyspnea, and angles of 120° or more may result in alveolar hypoventilation and cor pulmonale.[1] Patients with severe deformity typically take rapid and shallow breaths.

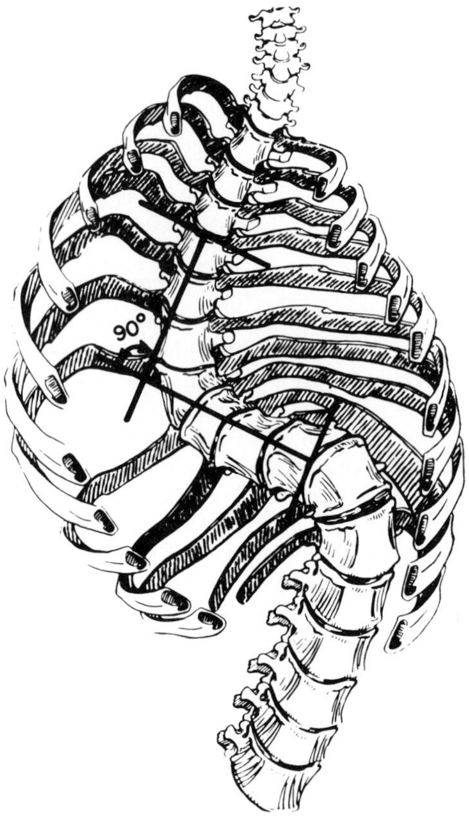

FIGURE 132-1 Determination of the scoliotic angle. The scoliotic deformity consists of a primary initiating curve and a secondary compensatory curve. The scoliotic angle is determined by the intersection of lines estimating the position of the upper and lower components of the primary curve. (Reprinted from Reference 9, with permission.)

Auscultation of the chest may reveal crackles or coarse wheezes reflecting atelectatic and deformed lungs; and cardiac examination may provide evidence for pulmonary hypertension such as a loud P_2, right ventricular heave, and jugular venous distension.[2]

PATHOPHYSIOLOGY

RESPIRATORY MECHANICS

In patients with scoliosis, pulmonary function tests typically show reduced total lung capacity (TLC) and vital capacity (VC) because inspiratory capacity (IC = TLC − FRC) is reduced (see Fig. 132-2). Functional residual capacity (FRC) is also reduced. Occasionally residual volume (RV) is low; but if so, it is decreased to a lesser extent than FRC. Expiratory reserve volume (ERV = FRC − RV) is also low. Patients with fibrothorax or thoracoplasty may show similar abnormalities.[1] By contrast, obesity mainly reduces FRC so as to reduce ERV without much change in RV, VC, or TLC; and in patients with ankylosing spondylitis, ERV and IC excursions are restricted around a normal FRC, such that RV increases and TLC decreases to reduce VC, a pattern similar to that of neuromuscular diseases of the chest wall.

In each of these disorders, it is the deformed chest wall that limits the excursion of the respiratory system; the lungs and respiratory muscles are affected secondarily and to a lesser degree. Whereas in health TLC is largely determined by the pressure-volume (P-V) curve of the lung, in scoliosis the P-V curve of the noncompliant chest wall dominates, lowering TLC and FRC while RV is relatively spared (see Fig. 132-3). Note that the P-V curve is shifted downward and to the right, requiring patients to generate large respiratory muscle efforts to take in small amounts of air. Normal lung compliance and respiratory muscle strength are assumed in Fig. 132-3, though reductions in both contribute to low lung volumes in many patients with scoliosis. Lung compliance falls from previous infection, atelectasis, or abnormalities in alveolar surface tension, and can be improved with IPPV. Intermittent positive-pressure ventilation can increase lung compliance by 70 percent for up to 3 h even when FRC does not increase, suggesting that inflation with IPPV lowers surface tension by altering the surfactant lining layer.[8] Inspiratory muscle dysfunction may result from operating at a mechanical disadvantage (created by the deformed thorax) or from respiratory muscle fatigue, and when kyphoscoliosis is a manifestation of neuromuscular disease, inspiratory muscles may be affected directly by the neuromuscular disease.

GAS EXCHANGE

Significant arterial hypoxemia is usually absent in patients with kyphoscoliosis until the late development of hypercapnia.[1] However, nocturnal hypercapnia and hypoxemia may occur early, particularly during rapid eye movement (REM) sleep, and may contribute to the cardiovascular deterioration in some patients.[4,5] Alveolar-arterial gradients $[(A - a)P_{O_2}]$, even in late stages, are usually no more than 25 mmHg.[1] This modest increase in $(A - a)P_{O_2}$ results primarily from ventilation-perfusion ratio ($\dot{V}/\dot{Q}$) inequality caused by atelectasis or underventilation of one hemithorax. Altered $\dot{V}/\dot{Q}$ ratios also contribute to the low diffusing capacity commonly found in these patients, as does the reduction in the vascular bed available for diffusion that occurs when portions of lung fail to grow in the distorted chest.

Alveolar hypoventilation results, in part, from an increase in V_D/V_T. This ratio of dead space to tidal volume is increased because V_T is reduced in hypercapneic patients, while anatomic and alveolar dead space are usually normal.[1] Minute ventilation is generally normal, but it is maintained by higher respiratory rates. The use of small V_T minimizes the work of breathing[9] and is also a sign of inspiratory muscle dysfunction.[10] As inspiratory muscle strength falls, the arterial partial pressure of carbon dioxide (Pa_{CO_2}) rises.[10] Progressive hypercapnia may in turn lead to further weakness.[11]

The ventilatory response to high concentrations of inspired CO_2 appears to be normal in eucapneic patients with severe kyphoscoliosis. However, in hypercapneic patients, the response is blunted either from buffering of the signal by elevated cerebral spinal fluid (CSF) bicarbonate or from a derangement in the central drive to breathe.[9]

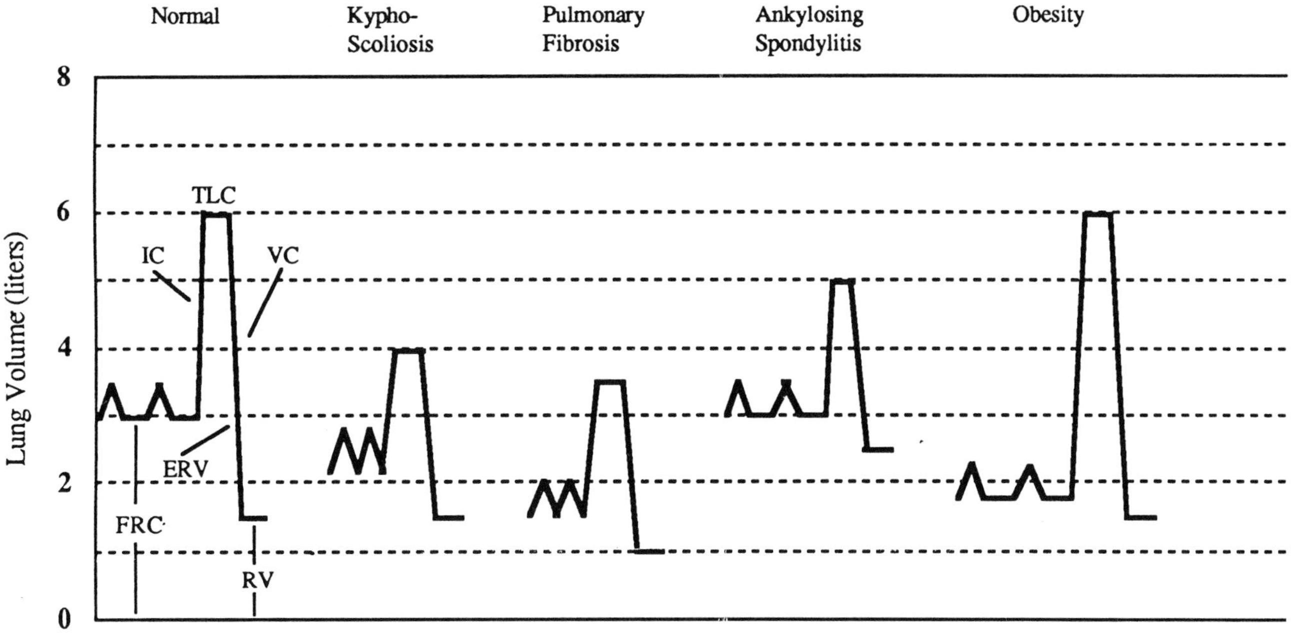

FIGURE 132-2 Schematic drawing of the abnormalities of lung volumes in common restrictive diseases. By contrast with normal subdivisions (left panel) of plethysmographic gas volumes (TLC, FRC, RV) and spirometric volumes (IC, VC, ERV), kyphoscoliosis and pulmonary fibrosis reduce VC and TLC by restricting IC, with lesser reductions in FRC (panels 2,3); anklyosing spondylitis (like neuromuscular diseases of the chest wall) limits IC and ERV excursions around a normal FRC, so TLC is reduced and RV is increased causing a large decrease in VC (panel 4); and obesity greatly reduces FRC to eliminate ERV without much change in TLC or RV, so VC is normal and IC is increased (panel 5).

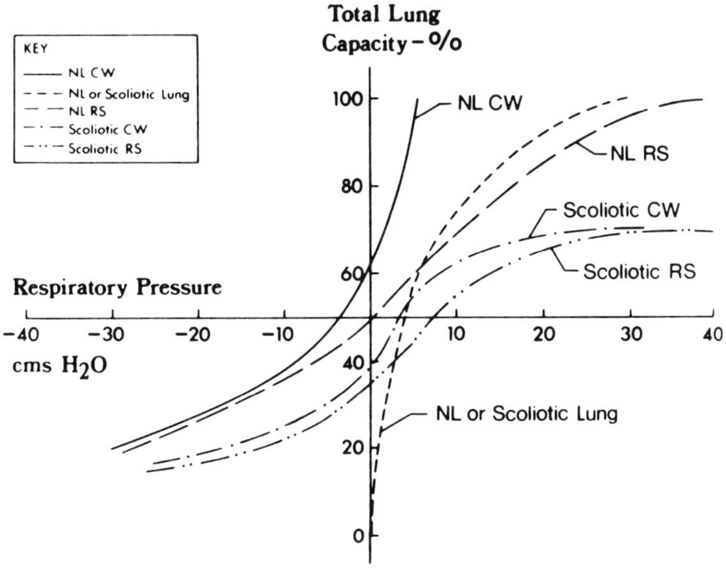

FIGURE 132-3 Pressure-volume curves of the chest wall, lung, and respiratory system in scoliosis.[1] The P-V curve is shifted downward and to the right requiring patients to generate large transpulmonary pressures to take in small amounts of air. NL = normal lung; RS = respiratory system; CW = chest wall.

PULMONARY CIRCULATION

A further consequence of severe kyphoscoliosis is pulmonary hypertension and cor pulmonale. Left untreated, patients with cor pulmonale typically die within 1 year.[2] Initially, pulmonary hypertension may occur only with exercise, but as the angle of spinal curvature increases, it occurs at rest as well. Pulmonary hypertension is usually the consequence of increased pulmonary vascular resistance (PVR) from either hypoxic pulmonary vasoconstriction or anatomic abnormalities and not from elevated left atrial pressure.[1] Thus, an increased gradient between the pulmonary artery diastolic pressure and the pulmonary capillary wedge pressure usually exists. Early use of supplemental oxygen in hypoxic patients, correction of reversible causes of hypercapnia, and the diagnosis and successful treatment of sleep-disordered breathing may lower pulmonary artery pressure in many patients and delay the onset of right ventricular failure.[12] Despite correction of these reversible causes, many patients are left with irreversible pulmonary hypertension associated with proliferation of the media in smaller, precapillary pulmonary vessels.[2] Normal blood flow through vessels narrowed by low lung volumes, the vascular effects of chronic hypoxia and hypercapnia, failure of portions of blood vessels to grow in compressed areas during childhood, or kinking of larger vessels as they travel through deformed lung are all potential causes of irreversible pulmonary hypertension.[1] Of course, in each patient with kyphoscoliosis and pulmonary hypertension, other treatable causes must be excluded such as pulmonary embolus, left ventricular failure, or intracardiac shunt, especially in patients with lesser angles of curvature.[13]

ACUTE CARDIOPULMONARY FAILURE

OUTCOME

Acute respiratory failure (ARF) in patients with severe thoracic deformity is most often precipitated by pneumonia, upper respiratory tract infection, and congestive heart failure.[14] Triggers may be minor and frequently remain obscure. In 20 patients with mean deformity of 113° admitted with ARF for the first time, admission blood gases showed severe arterial hypoxemia (Pa_{O_2} of 35 ± 7 mmHg), acute on chronic hypercapnia (Pa_{CO_2} of 63 ± 9 mmHg), and mild arterial acidemia (pH of 7.34 ± 0.08).[14] Cor pulmonale was present in 60 percent of patients. Of these 20 patients, 7 (35 percent) required intubation and mechanical ventilation, while the other 13 (65 percent) were managed successfully without mechanical ventilation. There were no statistical differences in admission blood gases, cause of respiratory failure, age, or degree of spinal curvature between patients who required mechanical ventilation and those who did not. Outcome was surprisingly good. All patients survived the initial episode of ARF and subsequently experienced 2.4 episodes of ARF each during the follow-up period (median of 6 years). Median survival after the first episode of ARF was 9 years. On discharge, mean Pa_{O_2} was 63 mmHg and mean Pa_{CO_2} was 55 mmHg. This study demonstrates the importance and success of early and aggressive therapy.

DETECTING REVERSIBLE FEATURES

Though the history obtained for a patient with ARF may be limited by dyspnea, the physician should seek information regarding duration and character of symptoms. The history takes on added importance in these patients since the physical exam is often difficult and confusing. For instance, areas of atelectasis may mimic the auscultatory findings of pneumonia, and crackles resulting from preexisting lung disease or atelectasis coupled with jugular venous distension from pulmonary hypertension may mimic left ventricular failure. Though airflow obstruction is not a common cause of ARF in these patients, clues to its presence should be sought. Cough remains a useful sign since it is unusual in the absence of other lung pathology; and unless there is associated neuromuscular weakness or obtundation, the cough is usually effective enough to clear secretions.[1] Remember that relatively minor insults such as viral upper respiratory tract infection are enough to precipitate ARF because of limited respiratory muscle function reserve and increased work of breathing.

OXYGEN THERAPY

The foremost goal in these patients is the early correction of arterial hypoxemia with supplemental oxygen. This is best accomplished using a pulse oximeter while increasing the fraction of inspired oxygen until arterial saturation approaches 100 percent. If this cannot be accomplished quickly without an endotracheal tube, we encourage early intubation and mechanical ventilation. Hypoxemia, in addition to its many adverse effects, causes pulmonary vasoconstriction and may precipitate right ventricular failure in these patients in whom pulmonary hypertension is common. Hypoxemia results not only from lung disease but also from perfusing lung units having very low $\dot{V}/\dot{Q}$ with a low mixed venous $P_{O_2}(Pv_{O_2})$, a frequent finding in patients with pulmonary hypertension and low cardiac output. Increasing venous saturation by raising cardiac output or hemoglobin, or by decreasing oxygen consumption, will in turn increase arterial saturation.

CARDIOVASCULAR MANAGEMENT

Evaluation of shock in patients with kyphoscoliosis is similar to that described elsewhere in this text (see Chaps. 114 and 117). When sepsis causes shock, patients with kyphoscoliosis and pulmonary hypertension may not mount the usual hyperdynamic response. Hypotensive patients not responding to an initial volume challenge, such as 500 mL of normal saline in 10 min, should have a pulmonary artery catheter inserted and bedside echocardiography for further directed therapy. In general, mechanical ventilation is indicated for all patients in shock, in part to decrease blood flow to the diaphragm, which can be as high as 20 percent of the cardiac output in patients with hypoperfused states and hyperventilation. Mechanical ventilation, sedation, and muscle relaxation decrease oxygen consumption (and thus oxygen requirement) and lactic acid generation.

When right ventricular failure causes shock, a vicious cycle can ensue. Conceivably, as the right ventricle fails, cardiac output and systemic blood pressure fall, limiting perfusion to the right ventricle from the aortic root. Right ventricular end-diastolic volume increases and shifts the interventricular septum to the left (often well visualized with echocardiography), thereby decreasing left ventricular compliance and further reducing cardiac output and blood pressure. Ensuring an adequate circulating volume, adding dobutamine, and correcting alveolar and mixed venous hypoxia to reduce pulmonary vasoconstriction are the first goals of therapy. Increasing systemic blood pressure and thus perfusion pressure of the right ventricle with norepinephrine may be helpful in some patients.[15] We recommend that noninvasive leg studies be performed in all patients with cor pulmonale to exclude deep venous thrombosis and, to ensure preventive therapy of venous thrombosis, that intermittent pneumatic compression stockings be used or low-dose heparin (5000 U given subcutaneously every 8 to 12 h) be given.

VENTILATOR MANAGEMENT OF THE PATIENT WITH RESTRICTIVE CHEST WALL DISEASE

Intubation is indicated for refractory hypoxemia, progressive ventilatory failure, shock, or a deteriorating mental status. Intubation can be difficult because of curvature of the cervical spine and distortion of the trachea. Furthermore, patients with kyphoscoliosis are at a higher risk of early desaturation during intubation because their smaller lungs contain less oxygen. Early assessment of anatomic abnormalities of the upper airway facilitate use of adjuncts such as fiber-optic bronchoscopy for intubation (see Chap. 5). Intubation should be considered early and planned carefully when less invasive therapies fail. Rarely, IPPV may stave off intubation in the patient able to cooperate with treatments, but this usually is not an option in acute situations. Negative-pressure ventilators are similarly not feasible in most acute situations because they require patients to lie flat and coordinate their breaths with the ventilator, and they are difficult to apply to patients with distorted chests. These devices have, however, averted mechanical ventilation in some patients.[14] During the peri-intubation period, a fraction of inspired oxygen (F_{IO_2}) of 1.0 is desirable, though it should be decreased as soon as possible to no greater than 0.6 once the patient is stable on the ventilator. Decreasing O_2 consumption with sedatives and muscle relaxants, providing positive end-expiratory pressure (PEEP), and increasing $P_{V_{O_2}}$ are strategies that allow for nontoxic F_{IO_2} in most patients. Positional changes, such as placing the patient in the decubitus position, may also improve oxygenation in patients with asymmetric chest walls.

Ventilatory failure results from a variety of causes of inspiratory muscle weakness including malnutrition, electrolyte abnormalities, sepsis, hypoxemia, or hypercapnia; or from any condition which increases the load on the respiratory system such as airflow obstruction, pulmonary edema, or pneumonia. Patients with chronic hypercapnia who require mechanical ventilation should be ventilated to a Pa_{CO_2} similar to their baseline value to achieve a normal pH. Ventilation to a normal Pa_{CO_2} results in bicarbonate wasting which, in turn, causes an acute fall in pH when patients start to breathe spontaneously, and hypercapnia invariably develops. Acute acidemia is poorly tolerated and may thwart attempts at discontinuing mechanical ventilation.

Respiratory muscle fatigue is best treated with 72 h of complete rest on the ventilator, with early nutritional supplementation and correction of metabolic irregularities. To achieve adequate rest, patients must be made comfortable on the ventilator; if they are not, work of breathing will remain high despite ventilator settings which apparently supply most of the minute ventilation. A ventilator mode should be selected that minimizes discoordinate breathing. Trigger sensitivity should be low (-1 or -2 cmH_2O), and adequate sedation should be given. We use theophylline titrated to a serum level of 10 μg/mL to increase respiratory muscle strength, help clear secretions, and treat bronchospasm. In patients with significant bronchospasm, we add inhaled bronchodilators and systemic steroids.

We use small tidal volumes (6 to 7 mL/kg) and high respiratory rates (20 to 30 breaths per minute) when ventilating patients with severe chest wall restriction to minimize the hemodynamic effects of positive-pressure ventilation and the risk of barotrauma. Since the chest wall is stiff in these patients, high alveolar pressures increase pleural pressure more than in diseases characterized by stiff lungs. High pleural pressures decrease venous return to the right atrium and result in a fall in cardiac output. Furthermore, high alveolar pressures increase the risk of pneumothorax, pneumomediastinum, and interstitial emphysema. Should pneumothorax occur, chest tube insertion is complicated by the distorted chest wall. In general, we aim to reduce peak airway pressures to less than 40 cmH_2O by using the least tidal volume needed to achieve correction of respiratory acidemia; of course, this goal is aided by accepting values of Pa_{CO_2} closer to 60 than 40 mmHg in the acute phase of stabilizing the patient on the ventilator. The use of small tidal volumes demands added attention to the prevention of atelectasis, especially in these patients prone to alveolar collapse. To this end, both PEEP and sighs are effective. We start with 5 cmH_2O PEEP and increase only if atelectasis is apparent or if 90 percent saturation of the arterial blood cannot be achieved with a F_{IO_2} of 0.6.

The approach to liberation from mechanical ventilation is similar to that described in Chap. 127. We favor the early determination of respiratory muscle strength as assessed by the maximum negative inspiratory force (NIF) measured at FRC, and of the load on the respiratory system as determined by the resistive and static pressures generated by a tidal volume similar to the patient's spontaneous breath (often about 300 mL). The goal is then to increase strength with many interventions including nutrition, rest, and theophylline while decreasing load by other interventions including bronchodilators, antibiotics, or diuresis. When extubation is near at hand, we find that ventilation with tidal volumes that mimic the patient's spontaneous tidal volume allow for smoother transition to spontaneous breathing. Although most patients in ARF for the first time are successfully extubated, some require prolonged ventilatory support. In these patients two other strategies may be helpful. First, in the patient who is able to breathe spontaneously on CPAP or a T-piece for several hours, consider negative-pressure ventilation. In spite of problems with fit and comfort, the addition of a cuirass may allow for prolonged periods off positive-pressure ventilation and eventual extubation. Second, by decreasing dead space, tracheostomy may allow for discontinuation of positive-pressure ventilation in the borderline patient. Tracheostomy is not without complications, however, and may be technically difficult in patients with severe cervical spine curvature and a distorted trachea. Each of these approaches needs to be considered as a transition to or part of chronic management.

CHRONIC MANAGEMENT

Plans for chronic management are best started in the ICU to optimize care on the general medical ward and at home. A primary consideration is whether home oxygen therapy is indicated. Evaluation should include arterial blood gas analysis at rest on room air and on exertion to a level likely to be achieved by the patient at home. Derangements in breathing pattern and oxygen desaturation during sleep should be excluded with polysomnography once the patient is stable. A broad spectrum of abnormalities, including central and obstructive sleep apnea, have been identified which contribute to chronic hypoxemia, cor pulmonale, and early death. Chronic respiratory failure was reversed in seven patients with severe kyphoscoliosis using noninvasive, nocturnal ventilatory support in the form of nasal CPAP or nasal IPPV.[16] Patients received nasal IPPV only when nasal CPAP did not prevent nocturnal hypoventilation. After 3 months of therapy, patients showed significant improvements in Pa_{O_2}, Pa_{CO_2}, respiratory muscle strength, and sleep patterns. Other useful strategies include daytime IPPV (25 cmH_2O for 5 min, 4 to 6 times daily),[8,17] negative-pressure ventilation, and nighttime mechanical ventilation through a permanent tracheostomy.[12] Ventilatory muscle training may also be of benefit by increasing the maximum inspiratory muscle strength. We favor early assessment of right ventricular function and pulmonary artery pressure with echocardiography. The presence of pulmonary hypertension gives added importance to oxygen therapy and mandates exclusion of other treatable causes such as pulmonary embolus. To this end, we encourage noninvasive leg studies in all patients with kyphoscoliosis and pulmonary hypertension. Though orthopedic surgery probably stabilizes the spine and prevents further deformity in some patients, it plays a limited role in the adult patient with severe kyphoscoliosis and alveolar hypoventilation. Finally, yearly influenza vaccination and one-time pneumococcal vaccination is indicated for all patients with thoracic deformity, and all efforts should be made to ensure cessation of smoking.

Patients with Pulmonary Fibrosis

CLINICAL PERSPECTIVES OF CRITICAL ILLNESS

The term *pulmonary fibrosis* refers to a condition of the lung in which normal air spaces and blood vessels are replaced predominantly by extensive fibrosis. Gas exchanging units are thickened, deformed, and dysfunctional, and the lungs are small and stiff. This term usually refers to patients without ongoing, prefibrotic inflammation, though this distinction is tricky since areas of fibrosis may lie adjacent to areas of inflammation. Therefore, fibrosis is generally used when referring to patients in whom therapeutic options are limited because at present no treatment exists to reverse fibrosis, and immunosuppressive agents are ineffective at this late stage. Nevertheless, new hope is found in the repeated success obtained with single lung and heart-lung transplantation for end-stage pulmonary fibrosis. The success of transplantation warrants renewed interest in the care of the patient with pulmonary fibrosis when acute decompensations arise, since some patients may eventually qualify for transplantation.

The etiologies of pulmonary fibrosis are legion (see Table 132-1), including acute and chronic insults of known and unknown etiologies. The pathogenesis of pulmonary fibrosis is beyond the scope of this chapter. Our focus is to identify potentially reversible features of the injury, which in part depends on the nature and severity of the initial insult, whether the insult persists, and whether the insult establishes an ongoing inflammatory response.[18–20]

SYMPTOMS AND SIGNS

Patients with end-stage pulmonary fibrosis are invariably dyspneic. Initially, dyspnea may be present only during exercise, but as the disease progresses it occurs at rest as well, bringing about a sedentary existence. Dyspneic patients typically breathe with small tidal volumes and fast respiratory rates at a higher minute ventilation.[21] Dyspnea is frequently associated with a nonproductive, annoying cough. If the cough is productive, alternate diagnoses such as bronchitis, pneumonia, or bronchiectasis should be considered. Constitutional symptoms include fatigue, malaise, weight loss, and commonly, arthralgias; symptoms associated with sleep-disordered breathing may also occur.

Auscultation of the chest frequently reveals dry, velcro-type crackles at the bases in patients with lower lobe fibrosis; cardiac examination may provide evidence for pulmonary hypertension such as a loud P_2, right ventricular heave, right-sided S_3, and jugular venous distension. Hepatomegaly and bilateral pedal edema also suggest right ventricular failure. Clubbing of the fingers and toes occurs commonly in patients with idiopathic pulmonary fibrosis and asbestosis, though it is occasionally seen in patients with other diseases. Other manifestations of hypertrophic osteoarthropathy are rare.

LABORATORY ABNORMALITIES

Resting hypoxemia and mild respiratory alkalosis are common as patients progress to end-stage fibrosis. Interest-

TABLE 132-1 Etiologies of Pulmonary Fibrosis

Acute (hours to days)	Chronic (weeks to years)
Oxygen toxicity	Idiopathic pulmonary fibrosis
Adult respiratory distress syndrome	Collagen vascular disease
Hypersensitivity pneumonitis	Hypersensitivity pneumonitis
Aspiration	Asbestosis
Drug-induced pneumonitis	Silicosis
Infection	Berylliosis
Inhalation injury	Coal dust disease (progressive massive fibrosis)
	Sarcoidosis
	Lymphangioleiomyomatosis
	Tuberous sclerosis
	Histiocytosis X
	Drug-induced pneumonitis
	Chronic aspiration
	Cystic fibrosis
	Talcosis
	Wegener's granulomatosis
	Bronchiolitis obliterans organizing pneumonia
	Goodpasture's syndrome
	Radiation pneumonitis
	Idiopathic pulmonary hemosiderosis
	Mitral stenosis
	Allergic bronchopulmonary aspergillosis
	Infection

ingly, hypoxemia may be worse when the patient is in the upright (rather than the supine) position or during sleep. Rarely, it results in polycythemia.[22] Other laboratory abnormalities, depending on the cause of fibrosis, include elevation in sedimentation rate, cryoglobulins, serum immunoglobulins, antinuclear antibodies, and rheumatoid factor.

The radiographic distribution of infiltrates is often characteristic of the underlying disorder, though there are numerous exceptions. Upper lobe predominant lesions include sarcoidosis, tuberculosis, fungal infection, silicosis, allergic bronchopulmonary aspergillosis, histiocytosis X, ankylosing spondylitis, berylliosis, cystic fibrosis, and hypersensitivity pneumonitis. Mid- and lower-lung field predominance is seen in idiopathic pulmonary fibrosis, collagen vascular diseases, asbestosis, chronic aspiration, talcosis, lymphangitic carcinoma, chronic pulmonary congestion, and lymphangioleiomyomatosis. Hilar adenopathy is associated with sarcoidosis, tuberculosis, histoplasmosis, malignancy, berylliosis, silicosis (classically with "eggshell" calcifications), coal worker's pneumoconiosis, and rarely, with hypersensitivity pneumonitis or adverse reactions to phenytoin or methotrexate. Pleural effusion suggests lymphangioleiomyomatosis, collagen vascular disease, mitral stenosis, asbestosis, or drug-induced lung disease. "Honeycombing" refers to cystic spaces within areas of fibrosis of 0.5 to 1.0 cm in diameter with white borders 2 to 3 mm thick.[23] It is a nonspecific finding in end-stage fibrosis; however, when present early or distributed evenly, honeycombing is suggestive of histiocytosis X, lymphangioleiomyomatosis, or tuberous sclerosis. These conditions also cause normal or increased lung volumes despite diffuse infiltrates and are more likely to cause pneumothorax.

PATHOPHYSIOLOGY

RESPIRATORY MECHANICS

In patients with end-stage pulmonary fibrosis, pulmonary function tests typically show reduced TLC, VC, and IC (see Fig. 132-2). FRC and RV are also reduced, though usually to a lesser extent than TLC or VC. Occasionally, RV is normal when there is early airway closure or decreased elastic recoil pressure at low lung volumes.[19] Forced expiratory volume at 1 s (FEV_1) is reduced, either in proportion to the FVC to maintain a normal FEV_1/FVC ratio, or less than the FVC to increase the FEV_1/FVC ratio; in this instance, high expiratory flow rates relative to volume reflect an increase in elastic recoil pressure. Airway resistance is usually normal, though significant reversible and irreversible obstructive defects do occur.

Since chest wall compliance and respiratory muscles are usually normal in patients with pulmonary fibrosis,[24] lung volumes are most affected by changes in the pressure-volume relationship of the noncompliant lung (see Fig. 132-4).[24] The P-V curve is shifted downward and to the right, such that increased elastic recoil of the lung limits TLC despite a very large maximum transpulmonary pressure. This lung stiffness requires patients to generate prohibitively large negative pleural pressures to achieve even moderate tidal volumes.

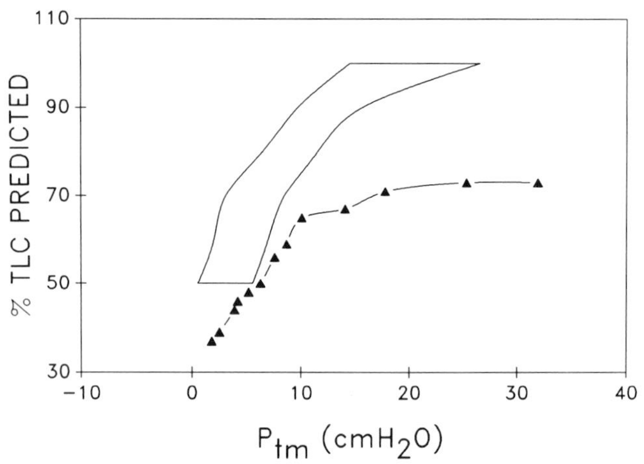

FIGURE 132-4 Pressure-volume curve of the lung in a 48-year-old man with sarcoidosis. The P-V curve is shifted downward and to the right of the normal range such that increased elastic recoil of the lung limits TLC despite a very large maximum transpulmonary pressure. This requires patients to generate prohibitively large negative pleural pressures to get in minimal amounts of air.

GAS EXCHANGE

Exercise-induced hypoxemia and a low DLCO are hallmarks of early disease, occurring even before the onset of symptoms or changes in the radiograph.[19] With time, arterial hypoxemia and a widened $(A - a)P_{O_2}$ are found at rest. In 20 percent of patients arterial hypoxemia is worse when they are in the upright position and is improved on recumbency.[22] This pattern is also seen in patients with intrapulmonary arteriovenous malformations and is opposite of the normal response. Arterial saturation also falls in many patients during REM sleep when arterial saturations can drop briefly below those found during maximal exercise.[25] Sleep-related desaturation is due to the exaggerated effects of normal nocturnal hypoventilation and $\dot{V}/\dot{Q}$ variance in those patients having awake hypoxemia, or to abnormal alveolar hypoventilation from respiratory muscle dysfunction or obstructive sleep apnea.

Early investigators thought the hypoxemia of pulmonary fibrosis was secondary to a thickened, fibrotic interstitium resulting in an anatomic barrier to diffusion of oxygen, a so-called alveolar-capillary block. This theory fell into disfavor when eight patients with varying types of interstitial lung disease were studied with the multiple inert gas elimination technique.[26] In these patients, $\dot{V}/\dot{Q}$ inequality was the principal defect, while diffusion limitation contributed to none of the $(A - a)P_{O_2}$ at rest and only 19 percent of the $(A - a)P_{O_2}$ during exercise. In a subsequent study, however, evidence for diffusion limitation at rest has been reported in patients with idiopathic pulmonary fibrosis (IPF). In fifteen patients with IPF studied by the multiple inert gas elimination technique, 19 percent of $(A - a)P_{O_2}$ at rest and 40 percent of $(A - a)P_{O_2}$ during exercise was attributed to diffusion limitation.[27] The $\dot{V}/\dot{Q}$ inequality was still the principal defect, contributing to 81 percent of the $(A - a)P_{O_2}$ at rest; yet during exercise $\dot{V}/\dot{Q}$ inequality did not increase. It was the combination of low $P\bar{v}_{O_2}$ from an inadequate cardiac output, increased diffusion limitation, and high $\dot{V}/\dot{Q}$ variance that accounted for the characteristic widening of $(A - a)P_{O_2}$ during exercise in these patients. Intrapulmonary shunt was small, averaging 2 percent of cardiac output at rest and 3 percent during exercise.

The V_D/V_T ratio is frequently greater than 0.4 (normal <0.3) in patients with end-stage fibrosis.[28] That is, half of the total ventilation is wasted in nonfunctional regions requiring greater minute ventilation to maintain a normal Pa_{CO_2}. In fact, mild respiratory alkalosis is common, perhaps the result of greater afferent stimuli from the fibrotic lung.[21] High V_D/V_T reflects not only an increase in the volume of alveolar dead space but also a decrease in tidal volume in most patients. Smaller tidal volumes may represent an adaptive response to minimize work of breathing which can be as high as 5 to 6 times normal.[29]

PULMONARY CIRCULATION

Pulmonary hypertension and cor pulmonale are common in patients with end-stage fibrosis, correlating with a DLCO less than 45 percent predicted and a VC less than 50 percent predicted.[30] Pulmonary hypertension occurs when blood vessels are destroyed by inflammation and progressive fibrosis, and when hypoxemia results in pulmonary vasoconstriction. Although supplemental oxygen may alleviate hypoxic pulmonary vasoconstriction, pulmonary hypertension resulting from destroyed and distorted vasculature may be irreversible unless there is a large inflammatory component to the injury. Pulmonary hypertension has been associated with redistribution of pulmonary blood flow to the upper lobes,[22] a pattern which has been seen to normalize in some patients treated with corticosteroids.[28] Since pulmonary vascular resistance is typically high, the gradient between the pulmonary artery diastolic pressure and the pulmonary capillary wedge pressure is usually wide. Occasionally, pulmonary hypertension reflects an increase in left atrial pressure when there is left ventricular failure, mitral valve disease, or ventricular interdependence. Since polycythemia and high blood flows are unusual in patients with pulmonary fibrosis, they rarely contribute to elevations in pulmonary artery pressure.

ACUTE CARDIOPULMONARY FAILURE

OUTCOME

Intensive management including mechanical ventilation is indicated for many patients with pulmonary fibrosis when acute decompensations occur, though mortality is high. Included are patients in whom a firm diagnosis has not been made or appropriate therapy has not been started; previously stable patients in whom an acute, reversible insult has occurred; and patients for whom transplantation is a consideration. This contrasts with patients who gradually develop end-stage fibrosis and cardiopulmonary failure despite appropriate therapy. In these patients, a prospective discussion and decision not to initiate resuscitative efforts should precede the anticipated terminal decompensation.

DETECTING REVERSIBLE FEATURES

The differential diagnosis of clinical deteriorations in patients with pulmonary fibrosis is quite broad (see Table 132-2). Acute deteriorations suggest pneumonia, pulmonary embolus, heart failure, or pneumothorax. Pneumonia most often results from community-acquired bacteria.[30] Fortunately, at least in patients with IPF, opportunistic infection is rare despite the widespread use of immunosuppressive agents.[30] There is, however, an increased incidence of pulmonary tuberculosis in patients with chronic interstitial lung disease,[31] particularly in patients with silicosis. Worsening pulmonary hypertension with right ventricular failure also causes acute decompensations. Precipitants include hypoxic pulmonary vasoconstriction and acute pulmonary embolus. Cardiogenic pulmonary edema is another cause of clinical deterioration and may be difficult to establish without echocardiography or hemodynamic measurements. Basilar crackles can reflect fibrosis or edema, jugular venous distension may be due to right ventricular failure alone, and a third heart sound may be right-sided instead of left-sided. Pneumothorax (especially in patients with end-stage, honeycombed lungs and in patients with histiocytosis X, lymphangioleiomyomatosis, and tuberous sclerosis) also results in sudden deteriorations. Because the lungs are stiff, reexpansion can be difficult, frequently requiring high levels of negative pressure for prolonged periods of time, and occasionally, thoracotomy with pleurodesis.

If deterioration occurs over a period of weeks to months, progressive fibrosis, bronchogenic carcinoma, steroid myopathy, cor pulmonale, and left ventricular failure should lead the list of diagnostic possibilities. Open lung biopsy is strongly recommended to evaluate the possibility of progressive disease, especially in patients in whom a diagnosis has not been made or in patients with a rapidly deteriorating course. The hope is that a specific diagnosis can be made and that there will be enough of an active inflammatory process to anticipate a response with immunosuppressive therapy. We have a low threshold for open lung biopsy and for initiating corticosteroid therapy; yet we strongly discourage the blind use of steroids because of the many complications associated with their use, including respiratory muscle weakness. Treatment with corticosteroids often requires high doses for prolonged periods of time, and patients may not manifest a favorable response for weeks to months. Patients who are rapidly deteriorating are candidates for both corticosteroids and cytotoxic agents (such as cyclophosphamide). When further benefit from steroid therapy appears questionable, they should be tapered slowly. Premature or rapid withdrawal of corticosteroids has been associated with rapid deterioration and death in some patients.[30] Although higher-dose corticosteroids appear to be better than lower dose in general, high-dose pulse therapy (methylprednisolone, 2 g) has not proved to be better than conventional doses of oral prednisone.[32] High-dose pulse cyclophosphamide, which is useful in other disorders, is as yet untested in patients with pulmonary fibrosis.

TABLE 132-2 Causes of Deterioration in Patients with Pulmonary Fibrosis

Acute	Chronic
Pneumonia	Progressive fibrosis
Pulmonary embolism	Steroid myopathy
Left ventricular failure	Bronchogenic carcinoma
Acute cor pulmonale	Chronic cor pulmonale
Aspiration	Fungal, mycobacterial pneumonia
Bronchospasm	Drug-induced pneumonitis
Pneumothorax	Chronic aspiration
	Left ventricular failure
	Poor conditioning

Bronchogenic carcinoma also causes subacute deterioration. Patients with pulmonary fibrosis are at greater risk of developing carcinomas within areas of fibrosis. The diagnosis of scar carcinoma is usually made successfully with transbronchial biopsy or bronchoalveolar lavage and portends a dismal prognosis. Other causes of clinical decompensation include drug toxicity, alveolar hemorrhage, airflow obstruction, and progression of underlying disease.

OXYGEN THERAPY

During the initial evaluation, the early identification and correction of arterial hypoxemia is vital. This is best checked by pulse oximetry while delivering supplemental oxygen until 90 percent arterial saturation is achieved. It is not unusual for patients with fibrosis to require higher flow rates than patients with COPD or asthma. If adequate oxygenation cannot be achieved quickly, intubation and mechanical ventilation are indicated. Hypoxemia, in addition to many other adverse effects, worsens pulmonary hypertension through hypoxic pulmonary vasoconstriction and may precipitate right ventricular failure in these patients who may have preexisting pulmonary hypertension. Hypoxemia results not only from abnormalities of the lung but also from perfusing lung units having very low $\dot{V}/\dot{Q}$ with a low $P_{\bar{v}O_2}$, a frequent finding in patients with pulmonary hypertension and low cardiac output. Increasing venous saturation by raising hemoglobin or cardiac output, or by decreasing oxygen consumption, will in turn increase arterial saturation.

CARDIOVASCULAR MANAGEMENT

Evaluation of shock in patients with pulmonary fibrosis is similar to that described in Chaps. 114 and 117. Hypotension with cool and clammy extremities and a narrow pulse pressure suggests an inadequate cardiac output from hypovolemia, left ventricular failure, cor pulmonale, pericardial effusion, or valvular heart disease; hypotension with a warm and bounding circulation and a wide pulse pressure suggests sepsis. Essential features of the special diagnostic and management approaches to cardiovascular dysfunction in patients with pulmonary fibrosis are identical with those described for patients with chest wall restriction.

VENTILATOR MANAGEMENT OF THE PATIENT WITH PULMONARY FIBROSIS

When mechanical ventilation is needed for refractory hypoxemia or shock, a strategy that minimizes risks of lung injury and circulatory compromise is desirable. When the usual practice of delivering tidal volumes of 10 to 12 mL/kg is followed or high levels of PEEP are used, patients with small fibrotic lungs generate high alveolar pressures. Recall that the shape of the P-V curve of the fibrotic lung which predicts high transpulmonary pressures will be generated when small tidal volumes are delivered. Additionally, variations in local compliance and airways resistance result in greater expansion of more compliant areas and areas supplied by low-resistance pathways.

The adverse consequences of overexpansion in these patients are many. Pneumothorax and bronchopleural fistula are more likely to occur in the presence of fibrotic, honeycombed lungs. Treatment may be difficult since large negative pressures are often required to reexpand the noncompliant lung. Prolonged chest tube drainage may be necessary. High alveolar pressures also compress alveolar vessels, diverting blood flow from ventilated units and increasing dead space. Increasing V_D/V_T from 0.4 to 0.6 requires an increase in minute ventilation of 50 percent to maintain a constant Pa_{CO_2}.[33] Increasing minute ventilation in mechanically ventilated patients by increasing respiratory rate or tidal volume, however, increases alveolar pressure and V_D/V_T further. A vicious cycle can ensue if minute ventilation is continually increased in a conventional, yet misguided, attempt to lower Pa_{CO_2}. Higher alveolar and pleural pressures increase right atrial pressure and so decrease venous return to the right atrium to reduce cardiac output, Pv_{O_2}, and blood pressure. PEEP and hypovolemia are frequent contributors to this unfortunate and not uncommon scenario. Additionally, diversion of blood flow by high alveolar pressures increases flow to nonventilated units, as in pneumonic consolidation, resulting in greater intrapulmonary shunt. Finally, large tidal volumes deplete surfactant,[34] which increases surface tension and lowers perimicrovascular pressure to aggravate pulmonary edema. Both surfactant depletion and pulmonary edema are diminished by increasing end-expiratory lung volume with PEEP and decreasing tidal volume excursion.[34]

To avoid excessive tidal volume excursions and high airway pressures we use small tidal volumes (6 to 7 mL/kg) and fast respiratory rates (25 to 30 breaths per minute) when ventilating patients with pulmonary fibrosis with the goal of maintaining peak airway pressures below 40 cmH_2O. Because of the positive correlation between minute ventilation and airway pressure, we choose the least minute ventilation necessary to maintain baseline Pa_{CO_2}, which in these patients is generally between 35 and 40 mmHg. For a given Pa_{CO_2}, minute ventilation is reduced further by decreasing CO_2 production; to this end, treating fever and agitation and avoiding excessive caloric and carbohydrate intake helps. Repleting intravascular volume and avoiding excessive PEEP also allows for a reduction in minute volume by decreasing V_D/V_T. A strategy of purposeful hypoventilation further lowers airway pressures in patients in whom high pressures persist.

We use the least PEEP necessary to provide 90 percent arterial saturation with an F_{IO_2} no greater than 0.6. Though F_{IO_2} of 1.0 is desirable in the peri-intubation period, it should be decreased as quickly as possible (to no greater than 0.6) to avoid oxygen toxicity. The use of sedatives and muscle relaxants to decrease oxygen consumption, providing PEEP, and increasing Pv_{O_2} allow for nontoxic F_{IO_2} in most cases. Occasionally, positional changes such as placing a patient in the decubitus or upright position improves oxygenation. PEEP also helps prevent atelectasis, which is of greater concern when tidal volumes are small. A minimum of 5 cmH_2O PEEP is generally needed for this purpose, though occasionally higher levels are needed to reexpand collapsed areas or to keep them open.

The approach to liberation from mechanical ventilation is similar to that discussed elsewhere.[35] We encourage the early determination of respiratory muscle strength as measured by the NIF (especially in patients on high-dose steroids) and of the load on the respiratory system as determined by the resistive and static pressures generated by a tidal volume similar to the patient's spontaneous breath (often about 300 mL). Lung compliance is then increased as much as possible by treating pulmonary edema, atelectasis, or pneumonia; airflow obstruction is treated when present with inhaled bronchodilators, steroids, and theophylline. Respiratory muscle strength is improved with correction of sepsis, shock, anemia, acidosis, electrolyte abnormalities, and with institution of theophylline, nutrition, and a nonfatiguing, graded program of respiratory muscle exercise. When extubation is near at hand, we find the use of small tidal volumes makes for an easier transition to spontaneous breathing, since patients consistently breathe with small volumes and high rates when extubated.

CHRONIC MANAGEMENT

Goals of chronic management include **1.** removal of ongoing insults to the lung such as drug-induced lung injury or hypersensitivity pneumonitis, **2.** treatment of inflammation in hope of preventing further fibrosis, **3.** treatment of associated complications such as hypoxemia and exercise intolerance, and **4.** evaluation for transplantation. Immunosuppressive therapy is the mainstay of medical management. High-dose corticosteroids are effective in many disorders that result in end-stage fibrosis (see Table 132-3). In IPF, corticosteroid therapy (prednisone 1 to 1.5 mg/(kg · day) results in objective improvement in about 20 percent of patients after several weeks of therapy, while over 50 percent report subjective improvement.[36] Patients in whom high-dose steroids are contraindicated (e.g., diabetes mellitus) or who deteriorate markedly while on steroids are candidates for cyclophosphamide, which induces objective and subjective responses in some patients after 3 to 6 months of therapy.[37] Cyclophosphamide is first-line therapy in patients with Wegener's granulomatosis in whom objective im-

TABLE 132-3 Corticosteroid Responsive Disorders

Hypersensitivity pneumonitis (extrinsic allergic alveolitis)
Idiopathic pulmonary fibrosis
Drug-induced pneumonitis
Acute lupus pneumonitis
Acute radiation pneumonitis
Polymyositis
Allergic bronchopulmonary aspergillosis
Bronchiolitis obliterans organizing pneumonia
Idiopathic pulmonary hemosiderosis
Goodpasture's syndrome
Wegener's granulomatosis (concurrent with cyclophosphamide)
Löffler's syndrome
Eosinophilic pneumonitis
Silo filler's disease
Berylliosis
Sarcoidosis
Histiocytosis X*

*Controversial.

provement can be seen as early as 1 week; complete remissions occur in most patients. Azathioprine has also been used with limited success in patients with IPF.

In patients who have already developed end-stage fibrosis, immunosuppressive agents are consistently ineffective because of the lack of an active inflammatory process. For these patients new hope is found in the repeated success obtained with heart-lung and single lung transplantation. Heart-lung transplantation is reserved for patients with irreversible pulmonary hypertension and right ventricular failure (see Chap. 79). In patients with adequate right ventricular function, defined by the Toronto Lung Transplant Group as a right ventricular ejection fraction of at least 20 percent, single lung transplantation is currently performed in patients up to 60 years of age.[38,39] Corticosteroids, which adversely affect healing of the bronchial anastamosis, are ideally stopped several weeks prior to transplantation. This may be difficult since steroid withdrawal can result in significant clinical deterioration, even in patients on low doses. Recently, however, some patients on low-dose steroids have had successful transplants. Postoperatively, patients have shown significant improvements in VC, FEV_1, Pa_{O_2}, and DLCO, and have returned to an active life-style. Postoperative immunosuppression includes prednisone, cyclosporine, and azathioprine (see Chap. 78).

All patients should be evaluated for home oxygen therapy. Evaluation should include arterial blood gas analysis on room air at rest and during exercise. We favor the early use of supplemental oxygen in hypoxemic patients, though there is little evidence for improved survival from long-term oxygen therapy. Oxygen therapy frequently improves exercise tolerance and may allow patients to exercise on a daily basis. Though sleep studies are not universally recommended in the routine management of patients with pulmonary fibrosis,[40] we maintain a low threshold for performing them, especially in patients with pulmonary hypertension. In some patients with restrictive ventilatory failure and sleep-disordered breathing, noninvasive nighttime ventilation with nasal IPPV improves daytime function and arterial blood gases.[41]

We favor early assessment of right ventricular function and pulmonary artery pressure with echocardiography and find serial exams invaluable in detecting persistent or progressive right ventricular dysfunction. The presence of pulmonary hypertension gives added importance to the evaluation for oxygen therapy and mandates exclusion of other treatable causes such as pulmonary embolus. To this end, we encourage noninvasive leg studies in all patients with pulmonary hypertension.

Other therapeutic considerations include treatment of bronchospasm with inhaled bronchodilators and theophylline, suppression of cough (though difficult) with codeine, and morphine for terminal dyspnea. Yearly influenza vaccination and one-time pneumococcal vaccination is strongly encouraged, and all efforts should be made to ensure patients never smoke.

CASE PRESENTATIONS

Case One (Kyphoscoliosis)

A 53-year-old woman with congenital kyphoscoliosis (scoliotic angle of curvature 110°) was admitted to the ICU with dyspnea, cough, and fever. She was in her usual state of health until 1 day prior to admission when she complained of feeling "tired" and "warm." On the day of admission the patient awoke coughing, severely short of breath, and confused.

Six months prior to admission spirometry showed a VC of 50 percent predicted without evidence for airflow obstruction; arterial blood gases on room air were Pa_{O_2} of 65 mmHg, Pa_{CO_2} of 53 mmHg, and pH of 7.39; and the patient reported dyspnea on exertion and intermittent leg swelling. There was no history of acute respiratory failure.

In the emergency room the patient appeared cyanotic. She was alert though minimally cooperative. Her temperature was 38.7°C, pulse was 120, respirations were 27, and blood pressure was 90/65 mmHg. There was obvious thoracic deformity. Bibasilar crackles were heard. Auscultation of the heart revealed sinus tachycardia and a loud P_2. The abdomen was normal, and there was mild pitting edema of both lower extremities.

Arterial blood gases on room air were Pa_{O_2} of 40 mmHg, Pa_{CO_2} of 67 mmHg, and pH of 7.30. The hematocrit was 48 percent, the white blood cell count was 18,000, with 75 percent neutrophils and 16 percent bands. The sodium was 145 mmol/L, the potassium 4.4 mmol/L, the chloride 105 mmol/L, and the carbon dioxide 32 mmol/L. The blood urea nitrogen was 20 mmol/L and the creatinine was 1.5 mg/dL. A chest x-ray revealed severe thoracic deformity and a possible right lower lobe infiltrate. An electrocardiogram showed sinus tachycardia with nonspecific ST and T wave abnormalities and right axis deviation.

Supplemental oxygen (FI_{O_2} = 1.0) was supplied by face mask without significant improvement in arterial saturation as measured by pulse oximetry. The patient was subsequently intubated without difficulty. Postintubation the blood pressure fell to 80/60 and the pulse increased to 135. The patient was given a 500-mL bolus of normal saline over 10 min, and the blood pressure increased to 105/70. Initial ventilator settings were F_{IO_2} of 1.0, tidal volume of 400 mL (7 mL/kg), respiratory rate of 20, and PEEP of 0 cmH_2O. Full arterial saturation and eucapnia were achieved, and the F_{IO_2} was decreased to 0.6 without a fall in arterial saturation. Respiratory rate was then decreased to 15 to allow Pa_{CO_2} to climb to the patient's baseline level of 50 mmHg. Peak airway pressure was 35 cmH_2O on these settings, with a minimal resistive pressure drop.

Gram stain of endotracheal suckings revealed multiple polymorphonuclear leukocytes with intracellular gram-positive dipplococci. Penicillin was given intravenously after blood and sputum cultures were obtained. The patient was placed on heparin (5000 U subcutaneously every 12 h).

The patient improved after 36 h of mechanical ventilation and antibiotics and was successfully extubated after a short trial of spontaneous breathing. She was transferred to the general medical floor 1 day later. Prior to discharge home, she had an echocardiogram which revealed mild right ventricular hypertrophy and pulmonary hypertension. Noninvasive leg studies showed no evidence for deep vein thrombosis. Arterial blood gases on room air were Pa_{O_2} of 65 mmHg, Pa_{CO_2} of 50 mmHg, and pH of 7.38, and the patient did not desaturate on walking down the hall. The patient was scheduled for an outpatient sleep study to rule out nocturnal desaturation.

Discussion

Severe kyphoscoliotic deformity, as demonstrated in this patient, is often associated with chronic alveolar hypoventilation and mild right ventricular failure. Acute respiratory failure is most often precipitated by pneumonia, congestive heart failure, and upper respiratory tract infection, though triggers may be minor and may remain obscure. Outcome is surprisingly good for the first episode of ARF with median survival of 9 years. A primary goal in these patients is the correction of arterial hypoxemia. If this cannot be done quickly without an endotracheal tube, early intubation is indicated. Intubation can be difficult because of curvature of the spine and distortion of the trachea and may require adjuncts such as fiber-optic bronchoscopy. When mechanical ventilation is required, we use small tidal volumes and high respiratory rates to minimize the hemodynamic effects of positive-pressure ventilation and the risk of pneumothorax. In this patient with pneumococcal pneumonia, initiating mechanical ventilation (even with a small tidal volume) was associated with a drop in systolic blood pressure of 10 mmHg. This occurs when high pleural pressures generated during positive-pressure ventilation decrease venous return to the right atrium and reduce cardiac output, a situation aggravated by an inadequate circulating volume. For this reason, we minimize airways pressures generated during mechanical ventilation by avoiding PEEP and high minute volume in the peri-intubation period and give a volume challenge to the hypotensive patient. Once the patient is stabilized on the ventilator, F_{IO_2} is decreased to no greater than 0.6 as long as full arterial saturation is maintained, and patients are ventilated with the least minute volume achieving a Pa_{CO_2} similar to their baseline. Ventilation to a normal Pa_{CO_2} results in bicarbonate wasting and respiratory acidemia when patients start to breathe spontaneously. Once this patient was successfully extubated, echocardiography was performed to evaluate the right ventricle and noninvasive leg studies were performed to exclude deep vein thrombosis as a cause of pulmonary hypertension. The patient was evaluated for home oxygen therapy and scheduled for a sleep study. A broad spectrum of abnormalities have been identified in these patients during sleep that contribute to chronic hypoxemia and cor pulmonale. Correction of these abnormalities with interventions such as CPAP has reversed chronic respiratory failure in some patients.

Case Two (Pulmonary Fibrosis)

A 69-year-old man with IPF required intubation and mechanical ventilation for pneumococcal pneumonia. He was transferred from another hospital for management of progressive hypoxemia and hypercapnia.

He was in his usual state of health until 1 day prior to admission when he complained of dyspnea. He was admitted to another hospital severely short of breath, intubated, and mechanically ventilated. The diagnosis of pneumococcal pneumonia was made by sputum gram stain (and was later confirmed by positive blood cultures) and appropriate antibiotics were started. Despite improvement in the chest x-ray and decrease in white blood cell count, arterial blood gases worsened over the ensuing 3 days when he was transferred for further management.

One year prior to admission, IPF was diagnosed in this patient by open lung biopsy. The patient was started on high-dose corticosteroids without objective or subjective improvement. Steroid therapy was stopped after 4 months, at which time the patient refused further care. Pulmonary function tests performed 8 months prior to admission showed a VC of 50 percent predicted with high FEV_1/FVC and a DLCO of 40 percent; arterial blood gases on room air were Pa_{O_2} of 60 mmHg, Pa_{CO_2} of 36 mmHg, and pH of 7.40.

On transfer, the patient was intubated, agitated, and uncooperative. The temperature was 37.9°C, the pulse was 130, the spontaneous respirations were 35, and the blood pressure was 90/65 mmHg. Bibasilar velcro-type crackles were present, and there was consolidation in right midthorax anteriorly. Auscultation of the heart revealed sinus tachycardia and a loud P_2. The abdomen was normal, and there was mild pitting edema of both lower extremities.

Ventilator settings were F_{IO_2} of 0.8, tidal volume of 850 mL (12 mL/kg), respiratory rate of 25, and PEEP of 10 cmH_2O. Peak airway pressures were 65 cmH_2O, with a

5-cmH_2O resistive pressure drop. Arterial blood gases were Pa_{O_2} of 45 mmHg, Pa_{CO_2} of 67 mmHg, and pH of 7.23. The hematocrit was 34 percent, the white blood cell count was 12,000, with 70 percent neutrophils and 10 percent bands. The sodium was 137 mmol/L, the potassium 4.4 mmol/L, the chloride 100 mmol/L, and the carbon dioxide 15 mmol/L. The blood urea nitrogen was 40 mmol/L and the creatinine was 2.5 mg/dL. A chest x-ray revealed small lungs with bibasilar fibrosis and an infiltrate in the right middle lobe. An electrocardiogram showed sinus tachycardia with nonspecific ST and T wave abnormalities.

The patient was sedated and paralyzed while the ventilator settings were changed to $F_{I_{O_2}}$ of 1.0, tidal volume of 8 mL/kg, respiratory rate of 20, PEEP of 10 cmH_2O. Arterial blood gases obtained 15 min later were Pa_{O_2} of 65 mmHg, Pa_{CO_2} of 45 mmHg, and pH of 7.36. $F_{I_{O_2}}$ was decreased to 0.6, PEEP was decreased to 5 cmH_2O, and tidal volume was lowered to 7 mL/kg, with a further increase in Pa_{O_2} and decrease in Pa_{CO_2}. Peak airway pressure on these settings was 35 cmH_2O. Blood pressure increased to 120/80, and the pulse fell to 110.

The patient rested on the ventilator for 48 h and was then successfully extubated after a 2-h trial of spontaneous breathing. He was discharged home 1 week later on oxygen at 2 L/min delivered by nasal cannula to keep his arterial saturation greater than 90 percent.

Discussion

When patients with stiff lungs require mechanical ventilation, the usual practice of delivering tidal volumes of 10 to 12 mL/kg or using high levels of PEEP generates dangerously high alveolar pressures. This diverts blood flow from ventilated units and increases V_D/V_T. Increases in V_D/V_T require minute ventilation to increase to maintain a constant Pa_{CO_2}, but increasing minute ventilation in mechanically ventilated patients increases alveolar pressure and V_D/V_T further. This creates a vicious cycle if minute ventilation is continually increased in a conventional, yet misguided, attempt to lower Pa_{CO_2}. Additionally, high alveolar pressures and pleural pressures increase right atrial pressure and so decrease venous return to the right atrium to reduce cardiac output, $P\bar{v}_{O_2}$, and blood pressure; and perfusing lung units with low V/Q with a low $P\bar{v}_{O_2}$ contributes to arterial hypoxemia. PEEP and hypovolemia are frequent contributors to this common, ill-fated scenario. Additionally, diversion of blood flow by high alveolar pressures increases flow to nonventilated units, as in this patient with pneumonic consolidation, resulting in greater intrapulmonary shunt. In this case, by lowering minute ventilation and PEEP, Pa_{CO_2} fell because dead space fell, and Pa_{O_2} increased because $P\bar{v}_{O_2}$ increased. Avoiding excessive airway pressures also protects against pneumothorax, which can be difficult to treat in these patients because large negative pressures are often required to reexpand the stiff lungs. The use of small tidal volumes also mimicked the patient's own tidal volume and allowed for a smoother transition to spontaneous breathing.

References

1. Bergofsky EH: Respiratory failure in disorders of the thoracic cage. Am Rev Respir Dis 119:643, 1979.
2. Bergofsky EH, Turino GM, Fishman AP: Cardiorespiratory failure in kyphoscoliosis. Medicine 38:263, 1959.
3. Rom WN, Miller A: Unexpected longevity in patients with severe kyphoscoliosis. Thorax 33:106, 1978.
4. Mezon BL, West P, Israels J, et al.: Sleep breathing abnormalities in kyphoscoliosis. Am Rev Respir Dis 122:617, 1980.
5. Guilleminault C, Kurland G, Winkle R, et al.: Severe kyphoscoliosis, breathing, and sleep. Chest 79:626, 1982.
6. Caro CG, DuBois AB: Pulmonary function in kyphoscoliosis. Thorax 16:282, 1961.
7. Collins DK, Ponseti IV: Long term follow-up of patients with idiopathic kyphoscoliosis not treated surgically. J Bone Joint Surg 51A:425, 1969.
8. Sinha R, Bergofsky EH: Prolonged alteration of lung mechanics in kyphoscoliosis by positive pressure hyperinflation. Am Rev Respir Dis 106:47, 1972.
9. Grippi MA, Fishman AP: Respiratory failure in structural and neuromuscular disorders involving the chest bellows, in Fishman AP (ed): *Pulmonary Diseases and Disorders,* 2d ed. New York, McGraw-Hill, Inc, 1988, chap. 149, p 2299.
10. Lisboa C, Moreno R, Fava M, et al.: Inspiratory muscle function in patients with severe kyphoscoliosis. Am Rev Respir Dis 132:48, 1985.
11. Keamy MF, III, Yanos J, Davis K, et al.: Canine diaphragm contractility is depressed by respiratory but not lactic acidosis. Am Rev Resp Dis 137:386, 1988 (abstract).
12. Hoeppner VH, Cockcroft DW, Dosman JA, et al.: Nighttime ventilation improves respiratory failure in secondary kyphoscoliosis. Am Rev Resp Dis 129:240, 1984.
13. Simonds AK, Carroll N, Branthwaite MA: Kyphoscoliosis as a cause of cardio-respiratory failure—pitfalls of diagnosis. Respir Med 83:149, 1989.
14. Libby DM, Briscoe WA, Boyce B, et al.: Acute respiratory failure in scoliosis and kyphosis. Prolonged survival and treatment. Am J Med 73:532, 1982.
15. Molloy WD, Lee KY, Girling L, et al.: Treatment of shock in a canine model of pulmonary embolism. Am Rev Resp Dis 130:870, 1984.
16. Ellis ER, Grunstein RR, Chan S, et al.: Noninvasive ventilatory support during sleep improves respiratory failure in kyphoscoliosis. Chest 94:811, 1988.
17. Simmonds AK, Parker RA, Branthwaite MA: The effect of intermittent positive-pressure hyperinflation in restrictive chest wall disease. Respiration 55:136, 1989.
18. Henson P: Mechanisms of cellular injury in interstitial lung disease. Chest 79(suppl):108S, 1986.
19. Kern JA, Fishman AP: End-stage fibrotic lung disease: treatment and prognosis, in Fishman AP (ed): *Pulmonary Diseases and Disorders,* 2d ed. New York, McGraw-Hill, Inc, 1988, chap. 144, pp 2237–2250.
20. Turner-Warwick M: Widespread pulmonary fibrosis, in Fishman AP (ed): *Pulmonary Diseases and Disorders,* 2d ed. New York, McGraw-Hill, Inc, 1988, chap. 50, pp 755–771.
21. Lourenco RV, Turino GM, Davidson LAG, et al.: The regulation of ventilation in diffuse pulmonary fibrosis. Am J Med 38:199, 1965.
22. Crystal RG, Fulmer JD, Roberts WC, et al.: Idiopathic pulmonary fibrosis: clinical, histologic, radiographic, scintigraphic, cytologic and biochemical aspects. Ann Intern Med 85:769, 1976.

23. Fraser RG, Pare JAP, Pare PD, et al. (eds): *Diagnosis of Diseases of the Chest*, 3d ed, glossary. Philadelphia, PA, Saunders, 1990, p xxi.
24. de Troyer A, Yernault JC: Inspiratory muscle force in normal subjects and patients with interstitial lung disease. Thorax 35:92, 1980.
25. Bye PTP, Issa F, Berthon-Jones M, et al.: Studies on oxygenation during sleep on patients with interstitial lung disease. Am Rev Respir Dis 129:27, 1984.
26. Wagner PD, Dantzker DR, Dueck R, et al.: Distribution of ventilation-perfusion ratios in patients with interstitial lung disease. Chest 69(suppl):256, 1976.
27. Agusti AGN, Roca J, Gea J, et al.: Mechanisms of gas exchange impairment in idiopathic pulmonary fibrosis. Am Rev Respir Dis 143:219, 1991.
28. McCarthy D, Cherniak RM: Regional ventilation-perfusion and hypoxia in cryptogenic fibrosing alveolitis. Am Rev Respir Dis 107:200, 1973.
29. West JR, Alexander JK: Studies on respiratory mechanics and the work of breathing in pulmonary fibrosis. Am J Med 27:529, 1959.
30. Panos RJ, Mortenson RL, Niccoli SA, et al.: Clinical deterioration in patients with idiopathic pulmonary fibrosis: causes and assessment. Am J Med 88:396, 1990.
31. Sachor Y, Schindler D, Siegal A, et al.: Increased incidence of pulmonary tuberculosis in patients with chronic interstitial lung disease. Thorax 44:151, 1989.
32. Keogh BA, Bernardo J, Hunninhake GW, et al.: Effect of intermittent high dose parenteral corticosteroids on the alveolitis of idiopathic pulmonary fibrosis. Am Rev Respir Dis 127:18, 1983.
33. Snyder JV, Froese A. Respirator lung, in Snyder JV, Pinsky MR (eds): *Oxygen Transport in the Critically Ill*, chap. 24. Chicago, IL, Year Book Medical Publishers, 1987, pp 358–373.
34. Corbridge TC, Wood LDH, Crawford GP, et al.: Adverse effects of large tidal volume and low PEEP in canine acid aspiration. Am Rev Respir Dis 141:311, 1990.
35. Hall JB, Wood LDH: Liberation of the patient from mechanical ventilation. JAMA 257:1621, 1987.
36. Turner-Warwick M, Burrows B, Johnson A: Cryptogenic fibrosing alveolitis: response to corticosteroid treatment and its effects on survival. Thorax 35:593, 1980.
37. Brown CH, Turner-Warwick M: The treatment of cryptogenic fibrosing alveolitis with immunosuppressant drugs. Q J Med 40:289, 1971.
38. The Toronto Lung Transplant Group. Experience with Single-Lung Transplantation for pulmonary fibrosis. JAMA 259:2258, 1988.
39. Grossman, RF, Frost A, Zamel N, et al.: Toronto Lung Transplant Group. Results of single-lung transplantation for bilateral pulmonary fibrosis. N Engl J Med 322:727, 1990.
40. Midgren B, Hansson L, Eriksson L, et al.: Oxygen desaturation during sleep and exercise in patients with interstitial lung disease. Thorax 42:353, 1987.
41. Goldstein RS, Avendano MA, De Rosie J, et al.: Intermittent positive-pressure ventilation via a nasal mask in patients with restrictive ventilatory failure. Chest 97(suppl):80S, 1990.

Chapter 133

RESPIRATORY MUSCLE FATIGUE AND VENTILATORY FAILURE

CHARIS ROUSSOS

KEY POINTS

- *Respiratory muscles fatigue when their work load exceeds the energy delivered; inspiratory fatigue occurs earlier when the load is a larger fraction of the muscle's maximal inspiratory force.*
- *The critical force causing respiratory muscle fatigue is affected by the duration of contraction each minute (pressure-time index), the velocity of contraction (VT/TI), and by the operational length (lung volume) and state of training of the muscle.*
- *Glycogen depletion, lactic acid accumulation, inability to utilize blood-borne energy sources, and decrease in the rate of adenosine triphosphate (ATP) hydrolysis explain the reduced contractile force generated by the fatigued diaphragm; secondary reductions in central nervous system (CNS) drive or neuromuscular coupling (or both) likely aggravate the hypoventilation which accompanies respiratory muscle fatigue.*
- *Tachypnea, abdominal paradox, and respiratory alternans are physical signs of respiratory muscle fatigue observed in normal subjects during loaded breathing, in patients during unsuccessful weaning, and in clinical conditions leading to ventilatory failure.*
- *Prevention and treatment of respiratory muscle fatigue is best approached by correcting the many factors which reduce muscle tone, power, and coordination and which increase the respiratory load.*

The respiratory system consists of two parts: the lung (the gas-exchanging organ) and the ventilatory pump that ventilates the lung. Failure of the lung leads mainly to hypoxemia. Failure of the pump leads mainly to alveolar hypoventilation, which in turn leads to hypercapnia (Fig. 133-1). The failure of the pump theoretically may occur at any site from the CNS to the contractile machinery. For practical purposes there are three major causes of pump failure.

1. The output of the CNS may primarily be inadequate (e.g., after barbiturate intoxication) or the pattern of breathing is not optimal (e.g., during an unsuccessful weaning period with the patient breathing with small tidal volume [V_T] resulting in an increase in V_D/V_T).
2. There may be a mechanical defect such as flail chest, nerve damage, or kyphoscoliosis.
3. The muscles may fail as force generator, i.e., the muscles become fatigued.

The failure may occur when patients breathe against excessive inspiratory load and the energy demand exceeds the energy supply. However, under these conditions one may intuitively envisage two additional possibilities: either feedback loops that reduce or modify the output of the CNS are activated, or the CNS itself, due to sustained effort, reduces or alters its output. It follows that respiratory muscle fatigue is a complex phenomenon that involves changes in the muscle as well as the nervous system.[1,2]

Respiratory muscle fatigue may be compared to a car (the muscles) and its driver (the CNS), which fail to achieve a required speed. If the demand for chemical energy (gasoline) exceeds the supply because of blocked fuel line or the car runs out of gas, this is analogous to fatigue within the respiratory muscles. If the driver slows down, it may be due to two mechanisms: because he perceives a fault in the engine (analogous to adaptation of the CNS as a result of the feedback loop) or because he has become tired and sleepy (analogous to fatigue of the CNS).

An important concept of respiratory muscle fatigue is that it occurs after a period of work, in contrast to weakness, which does not follow some sort of exercise. Furthermore, fatigue occurs when there is an imbalance between energy demand and supply. Thus, fatigue may occur not only at very high work loads but even with the very modest work of breathing, i.e., almost during quiet breathing if the blood supply to the muscle is severely reduced, as in shock.

Pathophysiology of Respiratory Muscle Fatigue

Fatigue is the loss of force consequent to muscular exercise, particularly during submaximal intermittent contraction.

FIGURE 133-1 The respiratory system is depicted as consisting of two parts: the lung, the gas-exchanging organ, the failure of which is manifested by hypoxemia, and the pump that ventilates the lung, consisting of the chest wall, the respiratory muscles, the respiratory centers that control them, and the nerves. Failure of the pump due to central depression, mechanical defect, or fatigue is manifested mainly by hypercapnia. (From Reference 2, with permission.)

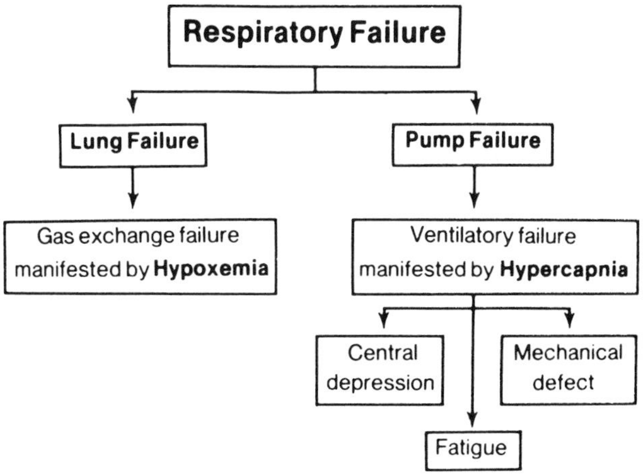

However, much evidence suggests that the physiologic events underlying fatigue commence very early, well before the loss of force. The site and mechanism of fatigue have remained a subject of controversy over the last century, and naturally this controversy has not left the respiratory system unaffected. It is interesting, however, that the consensus to be deduced from the following pages was outlined elegantly in the first experiments regarding respiratory muscle fatigue conducted by Davis, Haldane, and Priestly.[3] These investigators concluded that both the CNS and the muscles may be responsible for fatigue.

Since the generation of a voluntary contraction involves the whole pathway from the brain to the contractile machinery, the various potential sites of failure can be divided into three broad categories: those within the individual muscle fibers; those concerned with neural transmission from CNS to muscle; and those which lie within the CNS.

MUSCLE CONTRACTILE FAILURE

Skeletal muscle, including the diaphragm, is analogous to an engine. It converts chemical energy to heat and work. Thus, when the energy supply cannot meet the energy demand, fatigue ensues. Slow muscle, which has a high oxidative potential, is less susceptible to developing fatigue than fast muscle.[4] Extending these observations to the respiratory muscles, Farkas and Roussos submitted hamsters to daily treadmill exercise and demonstrated that a hamster's diaphragm becomes more resistant to fatigue after increasing its oxidative capability by developing lung emphysema (using elastase).[5]

The substances directly involved in the transformation of chemical energy into mechanical work in skeletal muscle are ATP, adenosine diphosphate (ADP), orthophosphate (Pi), hydrogen ions (H^+), magnesium ions (Mg^{2+}), and phosphocreatine (Pc). Using nuclear magnetic resonance (NMR), Dawson and colleagues[6] showed that Pc breaks down progressively, and creatine, ADP, and H^+ levels rise while ATP, the direct source of energy, is reduced by only 25 percent. The latter finding is consistent with the results obtained in normal subjects performing dynamic exercise until exhaustion.[7] Why, then does muscle fail?

To answer this, we must consider changes in chemistry that take place in muscle fiber: ATP is hydrolyzed to ADP, Pi, and H^+. Thus,

$$\text{MgATP} + H_2O \longrightarrow \text{MgADP} + \text{Pi} + H^+ \qquad (133\text{-}1)$$

As the muscles fatigue, the concentration of all products increases considerably, and therefore, this reaction is slowed. This observation leads to the hypothesis that the decline of muscle force is not due to depletion of ATP but to the reduced rate of ATP breakdown resulting from product accumulation. Similar experiments with NMR in the diaphragm have not been done as yet.

The increase in energy demands in excited muscles is provided mainly by the combustion of fat, blood glucose, and glycogen of the working muscles. The association of glycogen depletion with fatigue of the skeletal muscles and the diaphragm is well-established.[8] However, why glycogen depletion coincides with fatigue is not clear. Perhaps there is a rate-limiting step in utilizing the blood-borne fuels for which glycogen is used. Thus, fatigue will occur when glycogen is depleted.

Historically, lactic acid accumulation has received great attention as the culprit of fatigue in the skeletal muscles. Similarly, blood lactate elevation has also been found in subjects breathing through high inspiratory loads to exhaustion,[9] but there is no direct evidence that the lactic acid produced by the respiratory muscles is the culprit in diaphragmatic fatigue. In addition, animals with low cardiac output (pericardiac tamponade) or *Escherichia coli* endotoxic shock develop substantially less lactic acidosis if they are ventilated rather than breathing spontaneously. In these experiments, diaphragmatic lactic acid concentration is greater in the spontaneously breathing animals, which also develop diaphragmatic fatigue, than in the ventilated ones.[8] The effect of lactic acid on force generation is believed to be mediated by lowering pH. At low pH, Ca^{2+} is sequestered in the sarcoplasmic reticulum,[10] and a larger amount of Ca^{2+} is needed to produce a given tension. In addition, hydrogen ions exert a direct negative effect on the contractile process itself.[11]

To summarize, glycogen depletion, lactic acid accumulation, inability to utilize blood-borne substances, and decrease in the rate of ATP hydrolysis are merged to explain loss of force, but the exact interplay of all these factors is not yet identified either in skeletal muscle or in the diaphragm.

NEUROMUSCULAR TRANSMISSION FAILURE

When a nerve muscle preparation is stimulated continuously, failure of propagation between nerve and muscle can easily be demonstrated. This failure may occur presynaptically at nerve terminal branches, postsynaptically from a decrease of end-plate excitability, or from depletion of human muscles in vivo.[12] However, experiments during maximum voluntary contraction, with one exception,[13] do not support neuromuscular transmission failure.

For the diaphragm, evidence that neuromuscular transmission and cell membrane excitation are adequate has been found in experiments in dogs in cardiogenic and septic shock.[8,14] As the diaphragm became fatigued, the relationship of integrated phrenic nerve activity (Ephr) and diaphragmatic electromyographic (EMG) activity remained unaltered; i.e., when the diaphragm started failing as a force generator and greater stimulation was needed for an increment of transdiaphragmatic pressure, the relationship of Ephr and EMG was similar to that observed during the control period and to the earlier stage of the fatigue. However, these experiments may not be specific in testing this question; e.g., changes in the action potential through the run may have compensated for discrepancies between Ephr and EMG. Teleologically, transmission block could be beneficial in some instances. As suggested by Nassar-Gentina and coworkers,[15] the muscle is protected against excessive depletion of its ATP store which would ultimately lead to rigor mortis. Support for this hypothesis may be deduced from experiments by Lüttgaw, in which single muscle fibers were stimulated.[16] He demonstrated that the reduction in action potential amplitude (action potential fatigue) was minimized when contraction was inhibited by hypertonic solution and was abolished completely in noncontracting fibers poisoned with cyanide or iodoacetate; i.e., action potential was closely related to muscle fiber contraction. These experiments, therefore, suggest a close relationship between metabolism and fatigue of the neuromuscular junction. Neuromuscular transmission failure in man during diaphragmatic fatigue is not clearly understood. However, if high frequency fatigue is due to failure of the neuromuscular junction, it may be inferred that such a failure can exist in the diaphragm of man. It has been clearly shown that normal subjects breathing against inspiratory loads develop high frequency fatigue,[17] which may reflect neuromuscular junction failure.

FATIGUE OF THE CENTRAL NERVOUS SYSTEM

During short maximal contraction central fatigue does not, in some studies, appear to play a role,[18] since maximal nerve stimulation fails to increase the failing force. In contrast, during fatigue of intermittent submaximal contraction of the diaphragm, reduced CNS motor drive appears to be a factor.[1,19] Undoubtedly, the experimental protocol is complex, and the difference between the two muscle groups is intriguing. However, such findings are of particular importance in understanding the pathophysiology of ventilatory failure and need further testing.

Central fatigue must not be confused with progressive decrease in the firing rate during maximum contraction, during which superimposed supramaximal electric tetanic stimulation does not increase muscle force. Several investigators have clearly shown that the central firing rate decreases during fatiguing muscle contraction.[18] Experimentally, the gradual loss of force following prolonged maximum voluntary contraction can be accurately mimicked with electrical stimulation if the stimulation frequency can be accurately reduced, whereas, if high stimulation frequencies are maintained too long, force loss is more rapid. Thus, it was proposed that the decrease in firing frequency is an adaptive mechanism to the alteration of muscle contractile characteristics.[18]

It is well-established that fatigue is characterized not only by loss of force but also by slowing of the muscle contractile speed. In addition, it is known that for any muscle or motor unit the minimum excitation frequency required to generate force and tetanic fusion is proportional to its contractile speed. Thus, if during fatigue the degree of contractile slowing matches the decline in motor neuron firing rate, the latter does not result in any additional reduction in muscle force. Such an adaptation would be rather beneficial; it would avoid the failure of electrical propagation associated with high frequency fatigue as well as the complete depletion of vital chemicals within the muscle cell which might otherwise occur if high firing rates were maintained. An interesting question, of course, is how such an adaptation is brought about. In this context Hannerz and Grimby have presented evidence that motor neurons receive a tonic inhibitory drive from peripheral sources and that during a maximum voluntary contraction the motor neuron discharge rate increases if muscle afferents are partially blocked.[7]

In the diaphragm, during fatigue, muscle relaxation is prolonged,[20] but we have no information about alteration in firing rate. However, we have shown that afferent information via large (types I and II) and small (types III and IV) fibers affects the central respiratory controller's discharge in *terms* of firing rate, firing time, and frequency of breathing;[21] the latter is observed in states of diaphragmatic fatigue in both animals and human beings.[8,14,22] It is tempting, therefore, to hypothesize that as the contractile properties and the diaphragmatic chemistry change during fatigue, afferents via the phrenic nerve may affect the output of respiratory centers in terms of firing rate or timing (frequency of breathing, duty cycle).

SUMMARY

The diaphragm fails as a force generator whenever demand exceeds energy supply, during high resistive breathing, and/or during hypoxemia.[8,14,19] As fatigue ensues, contractile slowing increases[20] and central discharge firing decreases, either as fatigue of the CNS[19,23] or adaptation to the altered chemistry or contractile characteristics of the muscles, which may prevent their self-destruction by excessive activation. Extending and enlarging this to the respiratory system, we hypothesize that as the diaphragm contracts intermittently, the central controllers may modify the duration of contraction (Ti) and total duration of breathing cycle (TT). Such a strategy may optimize diaphragmatic function but at the cost, in some instances, of alveolar hypoventilation and CO_2 retention. This interaction, if it exists, is postulated to be mediated by the large and small phrenic afferents.

Determinants of Critical Task (Pressure, Work)

The *threshold of fatigue* is that level of exercise which cannot be sustained indefinitely. This level, therefore, can be expressed as a percentage of the maximum performance. Such a relationship during isometric contraction determines the critical force above which fatigue ensues; for intermittent contraction, this approach was adopted by Roussos and colleagues in their original work on fatigue of the respiratory muscles.[1,24] The model used in this approach was "the muscle as an engine," i.e., fatigue develops when the mean rate of energy demand ($\dot{U}d$) exceeds the mean rate of energy supply ($\dot{U}s$).

$$\dot{U}d > \dot{U}s \qquad (133\text{-}2)$$

$$\dot{W}/E > \dot{U}s \qquad (133\text{-}3)$$

or

$$\dot{W} > \dot{U}sE \qquad (133\text{-}4)$$

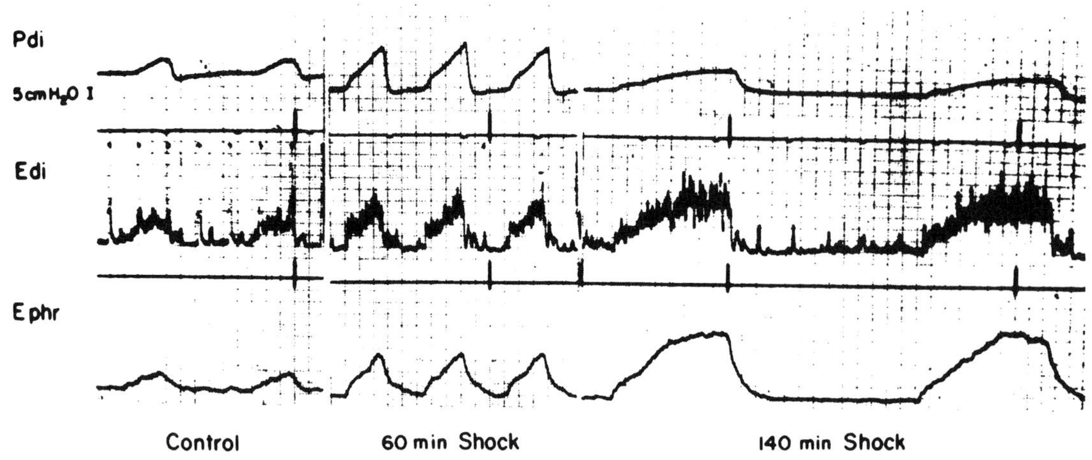

FIGURE 133-2 Tracings from a dog in cardiogenic shock shows typical evolution of transdiaphragmatic pressure (Pdi), integrated electrical activity of the diaphragm (Edi), and integrated electrical activity of the phrenic nerve (Ephr). The left panel represents a control. The middle panel shows a reading made 60 min after the onset of cardiogenic shock. The right panel shows a reading made 140 min after onset of cardiogenic shock and just before the death from respiratory arrest. While Edi and Ephr continue to increase, Pdi decreases (fatigue). The decrease in size of electrocardiographic artifact on the Edi tracing is a result of injection of saline into pericardium. (From Reference 8, with permission.)

where $\dot{W}$ = mean muscle power and E = efficiency. Clearly, when $\dot{U}sE > \dot{W}$, the muscle can continue to work indefinitely, but when $\dot{U}sE < \dot{W}$, there will be a finite endurance time. Thus, an increase in muscle power or a decrease in either efficiency or energy supplies should predispose to fatigue. In a system with volume displacement, as with the respiratory system, if the pressure generated by the inspiratory muscle assumes a square wave form, the term $\dot{W}$ in the inequality Eq. (133-3) becomes:

$$\dot{W} = P \cdot Vt \cdot f = P \cdot V_T \cdot 1/T_T \qquad (133\text{-}5)$$

where P = pressure, V_T = tidal volume, f = frequency of breathing, and T_T = total duration of the breathing cycle. Multiplying numerator and denominator by inspiratory time (T_I), Eq. (133-5) becomes:

$$\dot{W} = P \cdot V_T/T_I \cdot T_I/T_T \qquad (133\text{-}6)$$

where V_T/T_I=mean inspiratory flow and T_I/T_T the ratio of inspiratory time:total duration of breathing cycle (duty cycle). Substituting Eq. (133-6) into inequality Eq. (133-3) yields:

$$P \cdot V_T/T_I \cdot T_I/T_T > \dot{U}sE \qquad (133\text{-}7)$$

Clearly then, the power of the respiratory muscles can be greater than, equal to, or smaller than the available energy as a variety of combinations of P, V_T/T_I, and T_I/T_T. Thus, Roussos and his colleague[25] found that the critical pressure for the diaphragm is 40 percent of the maximum diaphragmatic pressure and for all the inspiratory muscles, 50 to 70 percent of this maximum, for a V_T/T_I of 0.6 to 0.9 L/s and T_I/T_T of 0.3 to 0.5. However, in keeping with predictions of inequality Eq. (133-7), Bellemare and Grassino[26] found that the critical transdiaphragmatic pressure decreases as the T_I/T_T increases at a constant V_T/T_I. They found that when the product of Pdi/Pdi_{max} and T_I/T_T exceeds 0.15, there was a finite endurance time.

One would predict that, if $\dot{U}sE$ decreases (either decreasing the energy supply or efficiency or both), the critical values of pressure or the combination of pressure, flow, and duty cycle will change. For example, reduction in $\dot{U}s$ by reducing cardiac output in dogs results readily in diaphragmatic fatigue[8,14] (Fig. 133-2). Similarly, altering the efficiency, as might occur in resistive breathing compared to unobstructed hyperventiltion, may substantially alter critical pressure or power.[25] Similar arguments may account for the smaller critical Pdi, if the diaphragm operates at shorter lengths during acute hyperinflation, when a given force requires much greater excitation.[25,27] Conversely, by increasing the oxidative capacity of the muscles, critical pressure is also increased[5] by improving the aerobic performance of the muscles.

In summary, there is clear evidence that there is a critical force which, if exceeded, results in fatigue. This critical force, however, is largely affected by other factors, e.g., the total duration of contraction per minute (pressure-time index), velocity of contraction, operational length, energy supply, efficiency of the muscles, and state of muscle training.

Respiratory Muscle Fatigue and Ventilatory Failure in Clinical Conditions

Ventilatory failure resulting in CO_2 retention implies alveolar hypoventilation for a given CO_2 production ($\dot{V}_{CO_2}$). The respiratory equation relates the arterial carbon dioxide tension (Pa_{CO_2}) to alveolar ventilation ($\dot{V}_A$)

$$Pa_{CO_2} = K\frac{\dot{V}_{CO_2}}{\dot{V}_A}, \qquad (133\text{-}8)$$

where K denotes the constant of proportionality. Since $\dot{V}_A = \dot{V}_E - \dot{V}_D$, where $\dot{V}_E$ denotes minute ventilation and $\dot{V}_D$ dead space ventilation, the respiratory equation may be expressed as follows:

$$Pa_{CO_2} = K\frac{\dot{V}_{CO_2}}{\dot{V}_E(1 - \dot{V}_D/\dot{V}_E)} = K\frac{\dot{V}_{CO_2}}{\dot{V}_E(1 - fV_D/fV_T)}$$
$$= K\frac{\dot{V}_{CO_2}}{\dot{V}_E(1 - V_D/V_T)} = K\frac{\dot{V}_{CO_2}}{V_T \cdot f(1 - V_D/V_T)} \qquad (133\text{-}9)$$

This new form of respiratory equation clarifies the factors that lead to the rise of CO_2, i.e., when the ratio of dead space volume to tidal volume (V_D/V_T) increases at constant $\dot{V}_E$ and $\dot{V}_{CO_2}$ or when $\dot{V}_E$ decreases at constant V_D/V_T and $\dot{V}_{CO_2}$, or both. An important point that may be deduced from this equation also is that, at constant $\dot{V}_E$, P_{CO_2} may rise by increasing the frequency, with a concurrent fall in V_T and hence increases in V_D/V_T. The $\dot{V}_E$ in the above equation may further be separated to its two components, namely flow and duty cycle:

$$\dot{V}_E = V_T \cdot f = V_T \cdot \frac{1}{T_T} = \frac{V_T}{T_I} = \frac{T_I}{T_T}, \qquad (133\text{-}10)$$

Thus, a reduction in mean inspiratory flow (V_T/T_I), duty cycle (T_I/T_T) or both will cause retention of carbon dioxide. In these equations it becomes apparent that Pa_{CO_2} may rise due either to inability of the muscles to generate pressure and thus, in turn, inspiratory flow (V_T/T_I) or to alterations in the pattern of breathing (f, T_I/T_T), or even to reduced neural output. These last two mechanisms, as may be deduced from the review in the section on the site of fatigue, might be due to an adaptation via a feedback mechanism or to fatigue, although this hypothesis remains to be proved.

FATIGUE DURING LOADED BREATHING

When a normal subject or patient breathes against a load that might lead to fatigue, there are distinct periods from the point of view of breathing pattern and ability to maintain the required task. Figure 133-3 depicts some of these changes as a normal person breathes against a fatiguing load, during which he/she attempts to maintain a constant mouth pressure. At the beginning, the timing of breathing and the mouth pressure remain constant. We call this period the *stage of infinite possibilities,* i.e., the subject has no indication that the task is of limited duration and, hence, the run might be from very short to very long. The last period, mainly the terminal four to five breaths, which we call the *stage of exhaustion,* is when the subject can no longer sustain the breathing task and gives up the effort. Between these two periods is a third period, which we call the *stage of alternative strategies.* We believe that during this period, whenever the breathing task eventually leads to exhaustion, i.e., when the task is above the critical level, the subject uses all possible strategies to maintain the target pressure or work to preserve ventilation. These notions are depicted in Fig. 133-3. One can see that, although mouth pressure remains constant, the pleural, or gastric, and transdiaphragmatic pressure vary almost in an alternative fashion. We interpret these changes as the result of recruitment and derecruitment between the diaphragm and intercostal/accessory muscles. We also explain this alternation as a strategy of partial resting of one group of muscles while the other group is doing most of the work. Frequency of breathing also increases. This strategy might also be advantageous to the inspiratory muscles because their shortening is limited and therefore their length and geometry remain at an optimal condition.

FATIGUE DURING WEANING

The three stages of breathing have also been observed in patients who cannot be weaned from the respirator.[22]

FIGURE 133-3 Recorded measurements of an experimental run at 75 percent of maximum mouth pressure (Pm_{max}). Except for transdiaphragmatic pressures (Pdi), all pressures were measured relative to atmospheric pressure. Swings in mouth pressure and esophageal pressure remained constant throughout the run, those in gastric pressure (Pga) and Pdi varied. (From Reference 24, with permission.)

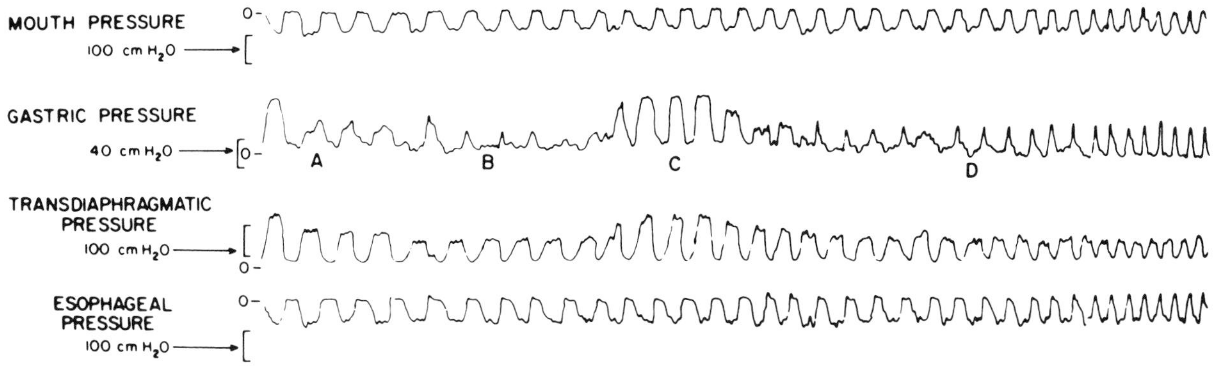

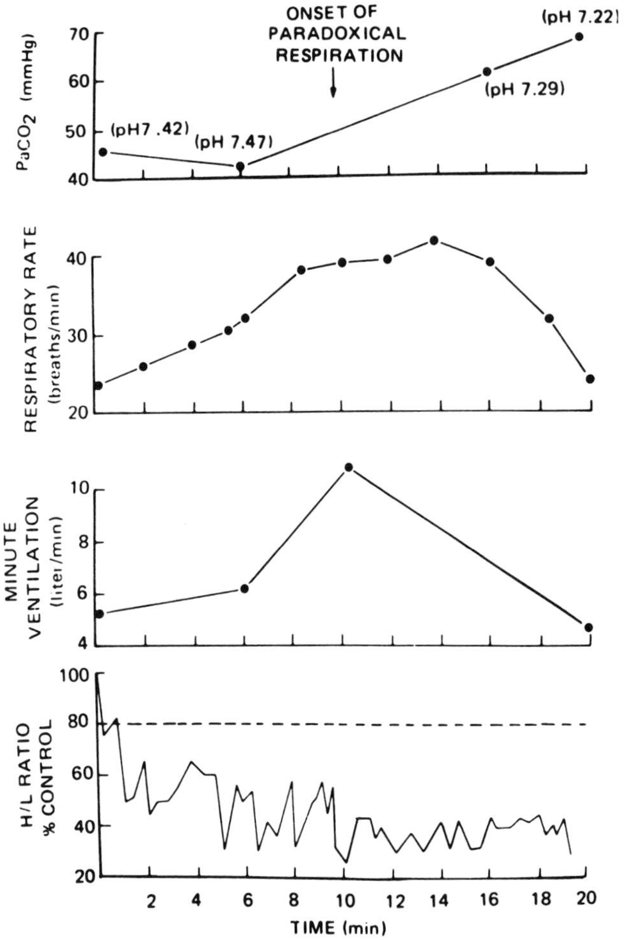

FIGURE 133-4 Sequence of changes in Pa_{CO_2}, respiratory rate, $\dot{V}_E$, and high:low (H:L) ratio of the diaphragm in a patient during a 20-min attempt at discontinuation of mechanical assistance. The initial change was the fall in H:L ratio (indicating fatigue), followed by a progressive increase in respiratory rate. The Pa_{CO_2} fell initially, and the patient became alkalemic. Paradoxical abdominal displacements were not noted until after there had been a substantial increase in respiratory rate and $\dot{V}_E$. Hypercapnia and respiratory acidosis did not develop until after abdominal paradox and alteration between rib cage and abdominal breaths were noted. Just before artificial ventilation was reinstituted, there was a sharp fall in respiratory frequency and $\dot{V}_E$ (from Reference 22).

These patients had also demonstrated respiratory muscle fatigue, as detected by EMG measurements. Figure 133-4 shows that very early there is an increase in frequency of breathing (tachypnea), while the muscles can still generate adequate ventilation. Bradypnea follows and invariably coincides with a decrease of inspiratory muscle pressure. Finally, if artificial ventilation is not instituted, central apnea ensues. In the same patients we have also observed paradoxical chest wall respiration resulting from either inward motion of the abdominal wall or "alternating breathing." During this type of breathing, patients breathe in an alternative fashion with the diaphragm and intercostal and accessory muscles. These observations are diagrammatically

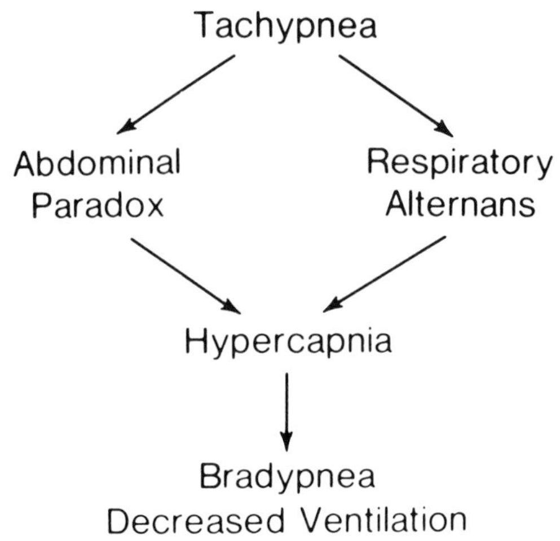

FIGURE 133-5 Schematic representation of the clinical signs of respiratory muscle fatigue, in sequence from top to bottom.

shown in Fig. 133-5. The clinician can observe all these changes by simple inspection and/or by palpation of the chest wall.

FATIGUE AS CAUSE OF RESPIRATORY FAILURE

Respiratory muscle fatigue is recognized in a number of clinical conditions, whereas in other conditions it is very likely that patients hypoventilate due to fatigue. From clinical experience hypercapnia occurs either acutely, as in shock, or chronically as in chronic obstructive pulmonary disease (COPD). It follows that, if fatigue plays a role in the CO_2 retention, fatigue may occur either acutely or chronically. Table 133-1 depicts these situations. Fatigue and, in turn, hypercapnia of acute onset are usually due to a combination of increased opposing forces of lung, a reduction of muscle strength, a decrease in efficiency, and a reduction of energy supplied to the inspiratory muscles. Prevention and management of respiratory muscle fatigue and the ensuing ventilatory failure has been approached as the mirror image of the cause; reducing load and increasing tone, power, and coordination.[28]

Patients with chronic hypercapnia develop CO_2 retention, usually insidiously. They may have to breathe against increased loads imposed either by the lung (as in COPD), the chest wall (as in kyphoscoliosis, extreme obesity, neuromuscular disorders), or both. We do not know the mechanism by which these patients insidiously develop CO_2 retention. However, we can hypothesize that as the disease progresses, the critical level of power output is exceeded to maintain normal $\dot{V}_A$. Thus, it is possible that the muscles become chronically fatigued, or alternatively, the central controllers may set a lower level of ventilation, which reduces the power output below the critical value. Our hypothesis is consistent with the findings of Sorli and colleagues.[13] They showed that in COPD patients with CO_2 retention, the T_I was decreased with a concomittent reduction in V_T while V_T/T_I, T_I/T_T, and central drive were not different from those in patients with COPD who did not

TABLE 133-1 Fatigue and Hypercapnia in Clinical Conditions

Hypercapnia of Acute Onset
Lung diseases
Asthma
Acute on chronic respiratory failure
Chest wall diseases
Prematurity
Atrophy secondary to artificial ventilation
Neuromuscular disorders
Lung and chest wall disease
Cardiogenic shock
Noncardiogenic pulmonary edema
Respiratory distress syndrome of infants
Hypercapnia of Insidious Onset
Lung diseases
Bronchitis
Emphysema
Bronchiectasis
Chest wall diseases
Kyphoscoliosis
Thoracoplasty
Pleural thickening
Extreme obesity
Neuromuscular disorders
Lung and chest wall diseases
Scleroderma
Polymyositis
Systemic lupus erythematosus

retain carbon dioxide. In addition, the CO_2 retainers had a lower forced expiratory volume at 1s (FEV_1) higher effective impedance, higher weight, and higher functional residual capacity (FRC) and FRC/TLC (total lung capacity) compared to non-CO_2 retainers. Thus, it is reasonable to speculate that the CO_2 retainers are better off by terminating T_I early, avoiding substantial deviation from the optimal muscle length and perhaps substantial geometric alteration of the diaphragm and intercostal muscles, than by taking a large V_T (long T_I). The price to pay, of course, is a reduction in V_T resulting in an increase in V_D/V_T, which in turn, as the respiratory equation predicts, will raise Pa_{CO_2}.

How is this reduction in T_I brought about? Is it due to afferent stimuli arising from the chest wall, stretch or irritant of J-receptors, or the result of a change in the rhythmicity of the respiratory centers due to chronic hypercapnia and hypoxia? To approach this question, we studied COPD patients with ($P_{CO_2} > 45$ mmHg) and without ($P_{CO_2} <$ 45 mmHg) CO_2 retention.[29] We found that patients with CO_2 retention developed a peak tidal Pdi of about 25 to 30 percent of Pdi_{max}, while the peak tidal Pdi in patients without CO_2 retention was less due to their smaller V_T and higher frequency, while T_I/T_T was not different. Using the results from normal subjects in which the critical pleural pressure (i.e., the pressure developed per inspiration, when exceeded, results in fatigue) at FRC plus one-half inspiratory capacity (IC) is 25 to 30 percent of the maximum, we may place the CO_2 retainers above or in the critical zone of fatigue, while the non-CO_2 retainers remain in the nonfatiguing zone (Fig. 133-6). Thus, it is tempting to speculate either that the CO_2 retainers are in a chronic state of fatigue or that the CNS sets a pattern of breathing in an attempt to avoid exhaustion.

The aforementioned notions clearly require a strong interaction between the muscles and CNS. The interrelationship between respiratory muscle energy expenditure and its central control was first suggested by Otis,[30] who concluded that for given $\dot{V}_A$ and mechanical properties of the system there is an optimal frequency at which minimal work is performed. Similarly, Mead pointed out that the optimal frequency during spontaneous breathing is more closely associated with the minimum average force.[31] By the same token, we propose that fatigue is not just a failure of physiologic function, but rather a protective mechanism for survival when the thorax is under excessive stress. Therefore, a regulatory mechanism must exist within the CNS to coordinate the motor neuron discharge to the

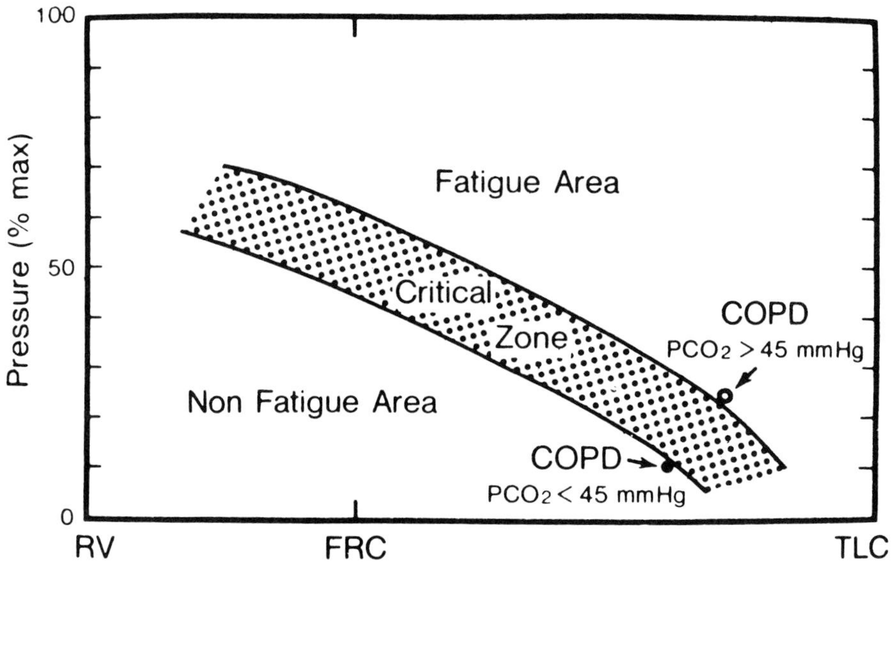

FIGURE 133-6 Pressure-volume diagram. Critical zone is constructed from data in normal subjects; at normal FRC the critical pressure above which fatigue occurs is 40 to 60 percent of maximum pleural or transdiaphragmatic pressure, while at FRC + one-half IC this critical pressure is 25 to 30 percent of the maximum. Note that patients with CO_2 retention are placed in the fatigue area, whereas normocapnic patients are placed in the nonfatigue area.

changes in the contractile speed of the motor unit they supply or alteration in the muscle chemistry.

It is almost certain that information travels via vagi affecting the CNS. The significance in this regard of chest wall or respiratory muscle afferents has recently generated interest among investigators. During loaded breathing in some recent studies, the effects of respiratory muscle afferents in the switch-off mechanism of the respiratory controllers have been clearly demonstrated.[21,23] Furthermore, we have shown the differential effect of large and small fibers of the phrenic nerve on the phrenic discharge.[21] Thus, it seems likely that respiratory muscle afferents have an important role in choosing the frequency or duty cycle of breathing. Our experiments in cardiogenic and septic shock under severe respiratory muscle stress or insult are consistent with such an operation.[8,14]

An alternative hypothesis is that, when fatigue ensues, the CNS alters either its firing output or its rhythmicity, which may be called *central fatigue*. The work of Bellemare and his colleagues supports the fact that a central component of diaphragmatic fatigue exists.[23] However, whether such a central fatigue is due to primary central failure and not to an adaptation of the CNS, as we speculate above, needs further investigation.

CASE PRESENTATION

A 65-year-old man presented to the clinic with cyanosis and marked dyspnea, was admitted directly to the ICU, and placed on high flow oxygen by facemask. A history could not be obtained. On examination the patient was cyanotic, in obvious respiratory distress, using all accessory muscles, and demonstrating paradoxical movement of the abdomen on inspiration. The blood pressure was 85/60, the heart rate 115, respirations 44, and the temperature 39°C (102.2°F). He withdrew from pain but was lethargic and unable to answer questions. There was no meningismus. On lung examination there were bronchial breath sounds over the right base posteriorly, along with diffuse expiratory wheezes. The patient was urgently intubated and mechanically ventilated. An arterial blood-gas sample drawn just prior to intubation revealed a P_{O_2} of 48 mmHg, P_{CO_2} of 34 mmHg, and pH of 7.24. A chest x-ray showed adequate placement of the endotracheal tube and confirmed the clinical impression of lobar pneumonia.

Thirty minutes following the institution of mechanical ventilation (assist-control, rate 28, V_T 550 mL, PEEP 5 cmH_2O, F_{IO_2} 0.6) repeat arterial blood-gas determination showed P_{O_2} 120 mmHg, P_{CO_2} 35 mmHg, and pH 7.30. The blood pressure had risen to 100/65 with a heart rate of 110. Gram stain of the first specimen retrieved after intubation revealed sheets of polymorphonuclear leukocytes with large numbers of gram-positive lancet-shaped diplococci. Broad-spectrum antimicrobials (cefotaxime, gentamicin, erythromycin) were instituted pending culture results. Parenteral nutrition was begun since an ileus precluded the enteral route.

On the third hospital day, the blood pressure was 120/70, the heart rate 100, the temperature was 37.4°C (99.5°F), and the patient was awake and able to follow commands. Sputum and blood cultures revealed *Streptococcus pneumoniae,* and the antibiotic regimen was changed to penicillin alone. On assist-control at a rate of 20, V_T 550 mL, and F_{IO_2} 0.4, the P_{O_2} was 85 mmHg, the P_{CO_2} 40 mmHg, and the pH 7.40; peak pressure was 28 cmH_2O and static pressure was 16 cmH_2O. Maximum negative inspiratory force (NIF) was −34 cmH_2O, and vital capacity (VC) was 700 mL. A brief trial of spontaneous ventilation was attempted, but after 60 min, the respiratory rate rose to 40, the patient became diaphoretic, and paradoxical respirations were again noted. Full mechanical ventilation was resumed. It had been learned that the patient was a long-time cigarette smoker who was being treated for COPD with bronchodilators and diuretics. Bronchodilators were instituted and additional contributors to respiratory failure were sought. Hypophosphatemia and hypomagenesemia were discovered and corrected.

On the following day, the patient remained afebrile and was alert. NIF was −60 cmH_2O and peak and pause pressure were 21 and 13 cmH_2O, respectively. He was able to breathe spontaneously with no apparent discomfort. After 6 h on a T piece, the respiratory rate was 24 and unlabored, and the patient was extubated. Continued attention to measures to reduce the respiratory load (bronchodilators, penicillin, antipyretics) and to maintain the strength (phosphate and magnesium repletion, nutrition) were assured, and the patient was moved to the ward.

CASE DISCUSSION

This case demonstrates the management of a patient with community-acquired pneumonia superimposed on COPD, focussing on the role of the respiratory muscles. The paradoxical abdominal movement on inspiration most likely represented diaphragmatic fatigue, and early treatment by intubation and ventilation presumably prevented the next stage of apnea. At no point in the ICU course was respiratory muscle fatigue established to be present, since this would have required exclusion of CNS or neuromuscular junction dysfunction by demonstration of reversible respiratory muscle weakness during supramaximal stimulation of the phrenic nerves.[19] Nevertheless, it is likely that respiratory muscle fatigue in the broad sense (contractile, neuromuscular or CNS failure) contributed to both the early impending respiratory failure, as well as the later failure to sustain spontaneous breathing on the third day.

Immediately after admission, several factors potentially contributed to respiratory muscle fatigue, including hypoxemia, hypoperfusion, and acidemia (each of which limits substrate delivery to working muscles), as well as pneumonia, COPD, and hyperpyrexia (all of which contribute to respiratory muscle load). These led to the clinical manifestations of encephalopathy, recruitment of accessory muscles, and thoracoabdominal paradox. Respiratory arrest was probably imminent at the time of intubation. By intervening to provide ventilatory support and to rest the fatigued muscles, the cardiac output was redirected to the heart, brain, and viscera, following which the cardiovascular status stabilized and the lactic acidosis was ameliorated.

On the third hospital day, respiratory failure recrudesced when spontaneous breathing was attempted before an acceptable balance of respiratory system strength (NIF, VC) and load (peak and static pressures) had been restored (see Table 1-2 in Chap. 1, and Chap. 127). Uncorrected electrolyte abnormalities and untreated bronchospasm conspired to overtax the respiratory muscles, leading once again to manifestations of respiratory muscle fatigue. However, attention to increasing the strength and decreasing the load, while maintaining nutrition and ensuring rest, led to successful liberation from the ventilator by the next day.

References

1. Roussos C, Macklem PT: Diaphragmatic fatigue in man. J Appl Physiol 43:189, 1977.
2. Roussos C, Macklem PT: The respiratory muscles: Medical progress. N Engl J Med 307:786, 1982.
3. Davies HW, Haldane JS, Priestly JG: The response to respiratory resistance. J Physiol (Lond) 53:60, 1919.
4. Edgerton, VR, Gaslow GE, Rassmusen SA, Spector SA: Is resistance of a muscle to fatigue controlled by its motor neurons? Nature 258:589, 1980.
5. Farkas G, Roussos C: Histochemical and biochemical correlates of ventilatory muscle fatigue in emphysematous hamsters. J Clin Invest 74:1214, 1984.
6. Dawson MJ, Gardian DG, Wilkie DR: Muscular fatigue investigated by phosphorous nuclear magnetic resonance. Nature 274:861, 1978.
7. Hannerz J, Grimby L: The afferent influence on the voluntary firing rate of individual motor units in man. Muscle Nerve 2:414, 1979.
8. Aubier M, Trippenbach T, Roussos C: Respiratory muscle fatigue during cardiogenic shock. J Appl Physiol 51:449, 1981.
9. Jammes Y, Bye PTP, Pardy RL, Roussos C: Vagal feedback with expiratory threshold load under extracorporeal circulation. J Appl Physiol 55:316, 1983.
10. Naess Y, Storm-Mathisen A: Fatigue of sustained tetanic contractions. Acta Physiol Scand 34:351, 1955.
11. Fabiato A, Fabiato F: Effects of pH on the myofilaments and the sarcoplasmic reticulum of skinned cells from cardiac and skeletal muscles. J Physiol (Lond) 276:233, 1978.
12. Jardin J, Farkas G, Prefaut C, et al: The failing inspiratory muscles under normoxic and hypoxic conditions. Am Rev Respir Dis 124:274, 1981.
13. Sorli J, Grassino A, Lorange G, Milic-Emili J: Control of breathing in patients with chronic obstructive lung disease. Clin Sci Mol Med 54:295, 1978.
14. Hussain S, Simkus G, Roussos C: Respiratory muscle fatigue, a cause of ventilatory failure in septic shock. J Appl Physiol 58:2033, 1985.
15. Nassar-Gentina V, Passonneau JV, Vergara JL, Rapoport SI: Metabolic correlates of fatigue and of recovery from fatigue in single frog muscle fibers. J Gen Physiol 72:539, 1975.
16. Lüttgaw HC: The effect of metabolic inhibitors on the fatigue of the action potential in single muscle fibers. J Physiol (Lond) 178:45, 1965.
17. Aubier M, Farkas G, De Troyer A, et al: Detection of diaphragmatic fatigue in man by phrenic stimulation. J Appl Physiol 50:538, 1981.
18. Bigland-Ritchie B, Johansson R, Lippold OCHJ, Woods JJ: Contractile speed and EMG changes during fatigue of sustained maximal voluntary contractions. J Neurophysiol 50:313, 1983.
19. Yanos J, Keamy MF III, Leisk L, et al: The mechanisms of respiratory arrest in inspiratory loading and hypoxemia. Am Rev Respir Dis 141:933, 1990.
20. Esau SA, Bellemare F, Grassino A, et al: Changes in relaxation rate with diaphragmatic fatigue in humans. J Appl Physiol 54:1353, 1983.
21. Jammes Y, Buchler B, Delpierre S, et al: Phrenic afferents and their role in inspiratory control. J Appl Physiol 60:854, 1986.
22. Cohen C, Zagelbaum G, Gross D, et al: Clinical manifestations of inspiratory muscle fatigue. Am J Med 73:308, 1982.
23. Bellemare F, Bigland-Ritchie B: Central components of diaphragmatic fatigue assessed from bilateral phrenic nerve stimulation. J Appl Physiol 62:1307, 1987.
24. Roussos C, Fixley M, Gross D, Macklem PT: Fatigue of inspirtory muscles and their synergistic behavior. J Appl Physiol 46:879, 1979.
25. Roussos C, Aubier M: Neural drive and electromechanical alterations in the fatiguing diaphragm, in Porter J, Whelan J (eds): *Human Muscle Fatigue: Physiological Mechanisms.* Ciba Foundation Symposium No. 82. London, Pitman Medical, 1981, pp 213–233.
26. Bellemare F, Grassino A: Effect of pressure and timing of contraction on human diaphragm fatigue. J Appl Physiol 53:1190, 1982.
27. Farkas G, Roussos C: Acute diaphragmatic shortening: In vitro mechanics and fatigue. Am Rev Respir Dis 130:434, 1984.
28. Hall JB, Wood, LDH: Liberation of the patient from mechanical ventilation. JAMA 257:1621, 1987.
29. Roussos C: The failing ventilatory pump. Lung 160:59, 1982.
30. Otis AB: The work of breathing. Physiol Rev 34:449, 1954.
31. Mead J: Control of respiratory frequency. J Appl Physiol 15:325, 1960.

Acknowledgment

This chapter was reprinted with permission from the *Aspen Lung Conference Supplement: Chronic Respiratory Failure* published in *Chest* 97:89S–96S, 1990. The editors are grateful to the author and the publisher for allowing us to add key points and an illustrative case, to reduce the number of references cited, and to make other minor revisions in this chapter in accord with the format of the book.

Chapter 134

UPPER AIRWAY OBSTRUCTION

E.G. KING
G.J. SHEEHAN
T.J. MCDONNELL

KEY POINTS

- *Upper airway obstruction (UAO) is one of the most serious life-threatening emergencies faced by critical care physicians.*
- *Definitive diagnosis and reestablishment of an effective airway are urgent considerations when UAO is apparent.*
- *Patients at rest can be surprisingly asymptomatic despite severe narrowing of the upper airway.*
- *Sudden deterioration of UAO patients is unpredictable.*
- *Direct visualization by bronchoscopy is the most effective way to establish a diagnosis and frequently also provides the best way to correct UAO.*
- *Other diagnostic aides include airway tomography or computed tomography (CT) and flow-volume loops.*
- *The use of heliox (a helium-oxygen gas mixture) in patients with severe UAO should not lead the clinician to a false sense of security; it should be used to provide temporary support pending definitive diagnosis and management.*
- *Mechanical obstruction cannot be significantly improved by pharmacologic manipulations.*
- *Critical care physicians must be competent in the full range of airway access techniques, including bronchoscopy and tracheotomy.*
- *Remember: All that wheezes is not asthma.*

UAO is one of the most serious life-threatening emergencies faced by critical care physicians.[1,2] The obstruction may be *functional* or *anatomic*, acute or chronic. For purposes of this chapter, "upper airway" is defined as encompassing the airway *from mouth and nares to primary carina.* A large number of conditions may be responsible for acute upper airway compromise (Table 134-1), but all require prompt diagnosis followed immediately by definitive restoration of airflow. This chapter will outline techniques of upper airway assessment and methods of airway restoration applicable to most causes of obstruction, and then will review some of the conditions encountered in critical care practice. From a practical critical care viewpoint, most UAO is related to the posterior oropharynx and larynx.

TABLE 134-1 Causes of Upper Airway Obstruction (UAO)

Traumatic
Facial injury (mandibular and maxillary fractures)
Acute laryngeal injury
Laryngeal stenosis
Airway burn
Hemorrhage
Infections
Ludwig's angina
Retropharyngeal abscess
Epiglottitis
Laryngitis
Diphtheria
Acute tonsillitis (quinsy)
Endotracheal tube trauma
Foreign Bodies
Tumors
Laryngeal tumors
Laryngeal papillomas
Intrinsic or extrinsic tumors causing tracheal narrowing
Laryngospasm
Angioedema
Angioedema of allergic origin
Hereditary angioedema
Vocal cord paralysis
UAO of obesity or pachylaryngopathy

Clinical Features

Signs and symptoms of UAO include marked respiratory distress; aphonia or dysphonia; the hand-to-the-throat "choking sign"; cyanosis; inspiratory stridor or crowing; suprasternal and intercostal indrawing; facial swelling and prominence of neck veins; absent air movement with no air entry into the chest on auscultation; and tachycardia. Thoracoabdominal paradox is often prominent. As asphyxiation progresses, bradycardia, hypotension, and death occur.

UAO is occasionally misdiagnosed as asthma. It can be associated with exercise-related shortness of breath and a variety of obstructive airway sounds. In contrast to asthma, however, the obstructive noises are intensified on inspiration and are usually localizable to the upper airway. Some patients with UAO will develop their problems at a time far removed from the occurrence of the underlying cause. Tracheal stenosis after tracheostomy, or subglottic laryngeal stenosis due to prolonged endotracheal intubation, may become apparent only after a considerable period of time has elapsed. A high index of suspicion must be maintained if there is a history—no matter how remote—of intubation, laryngeal injury, tracheostomy, or thyroid surgery.

Assessment and Diagnosis of UAO

The techniques chosen for assessment will depend on the urgency of the situation. Often, correction or bypassing of the acute obstruction can be coupled with the process of assessment. The rigid bronchoscope may be used both to directly examine a tracheal stenosis and to secure the airway by carefully insinuating the bronchoscope through the stenotic segment. Fiberoptic and rigid bronchoscopy, tracheotomy, interpretation of airway tomograms or CT images (Fig. 134-1),[3] and analysis of flow-volume loops (Fig. 134-2)[4] are basic requirements in the effective diagnosis and

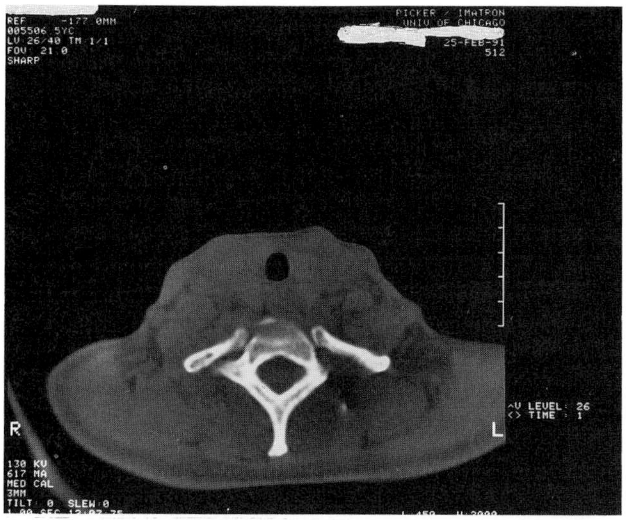

a

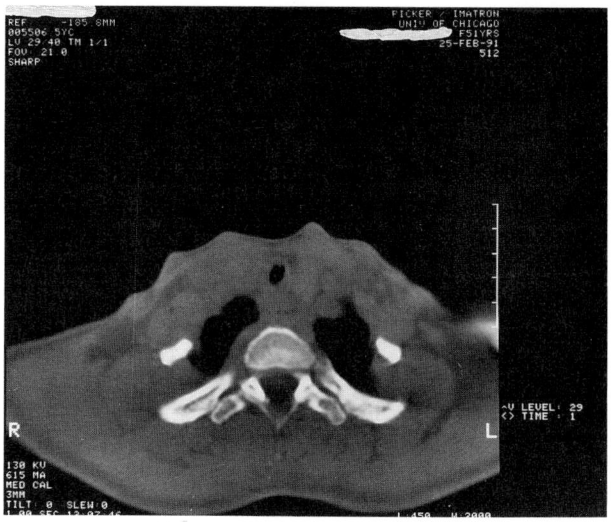

b

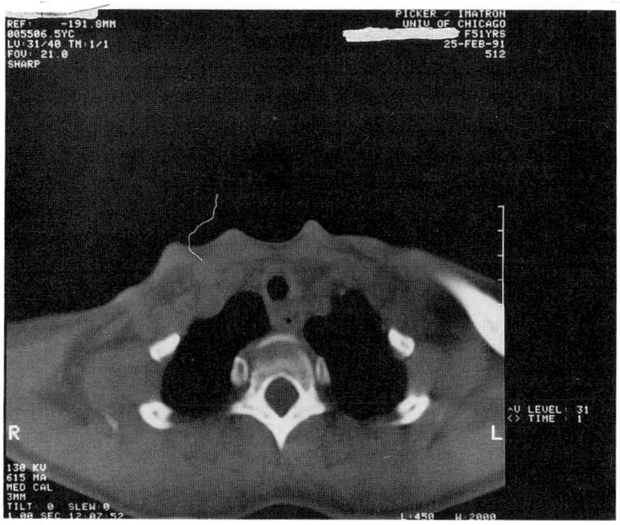

c

FIGURE 134-1 The utility of computerized tomography (CT) in defining anatomy in upper airway obstruction is demonstrated. This patient presented 4 months after an extended period of intubation with progressive dyspnea on exertion. Pulmonary function testing suggested fixed airway obstruction by flow-volume curve (see Fig. 134-2). The routine chest radiograph was unremarkable. These CT cuts visualize the trachea. Panel *a* indicates minimal narrowing, with maximal narrowing noted in panel *b* at the level of T1 (airway diameter measured as 7 mm). Panel *c* reveals an enlarging lumen below the area of stenosis. At surgery the diagnosis of postintubation tracheal stenosis was confirmed.

management of upper airway problems. More complex techniques, such as ultrasonography or high-frequency oscillation, can be used to measure oropharyngeal cavity size and conductance.

The most important diagnostic tools after a quick history taking and physical examination are the laryngoscope and the fiberoptic or rigid bronchoscope. These allow direct visualization of the oronasopharynx and larynx along with rapid translaryngeal intubation to secure patency of the airway. Lateral soft tissue x-ray views of the neck, tomograms, and oropharyngeal/cervical CT are occasionally useful in assessing the extent of airway obstruction, though they are seldom of value in cases of acute obstruction. Tracheal stenosis and airway compromise due to goiter, thyroid malignancy, vascular arches, and mediastinal or paratracheal tumors may require radiologic or radionuclide imaging techniques for complete assessment and consideration of proper management. Similarly, the extent of tracheal tumors, such as cystadenocarcinoma, may best be determined by radiologic methods. Flow-volume loops provide indices of UAO severity and may give a clue as to the site of airway compromise. While performance of these loops is of interest and provides a basis for ongoing assessment and comparison, they are seldom helpful in initial management and do not dictate therapy.

It is useful to separate patients with potential UAO into those with marked resting or progressive symptoms (i.e., the true emergency cases) and those with a somewhat more indolent or stable course who have features of airway obstruction with forced respiratory maneuvers or exercise. The latter, stable, group can undergo a full range of studies, albeit with watchful supervision. The former group, however, are potential disasters that require urgent diagnosis and management. It is to be emphasized that *since airway resistance varies inversely with the fourth power of the radius at the point of airway compromise, small advances in the underlying disease are likely to dramatically worsen the respiratory resistive load.* A number of events can produce rapid progression to asphyxiation; one such is manipulation of the upper airway by an inexperienced clinician who is not ready or able to establish an airway. In patients who are dyspneic at rest or are suffering rapid progression in airway obstruction, it is

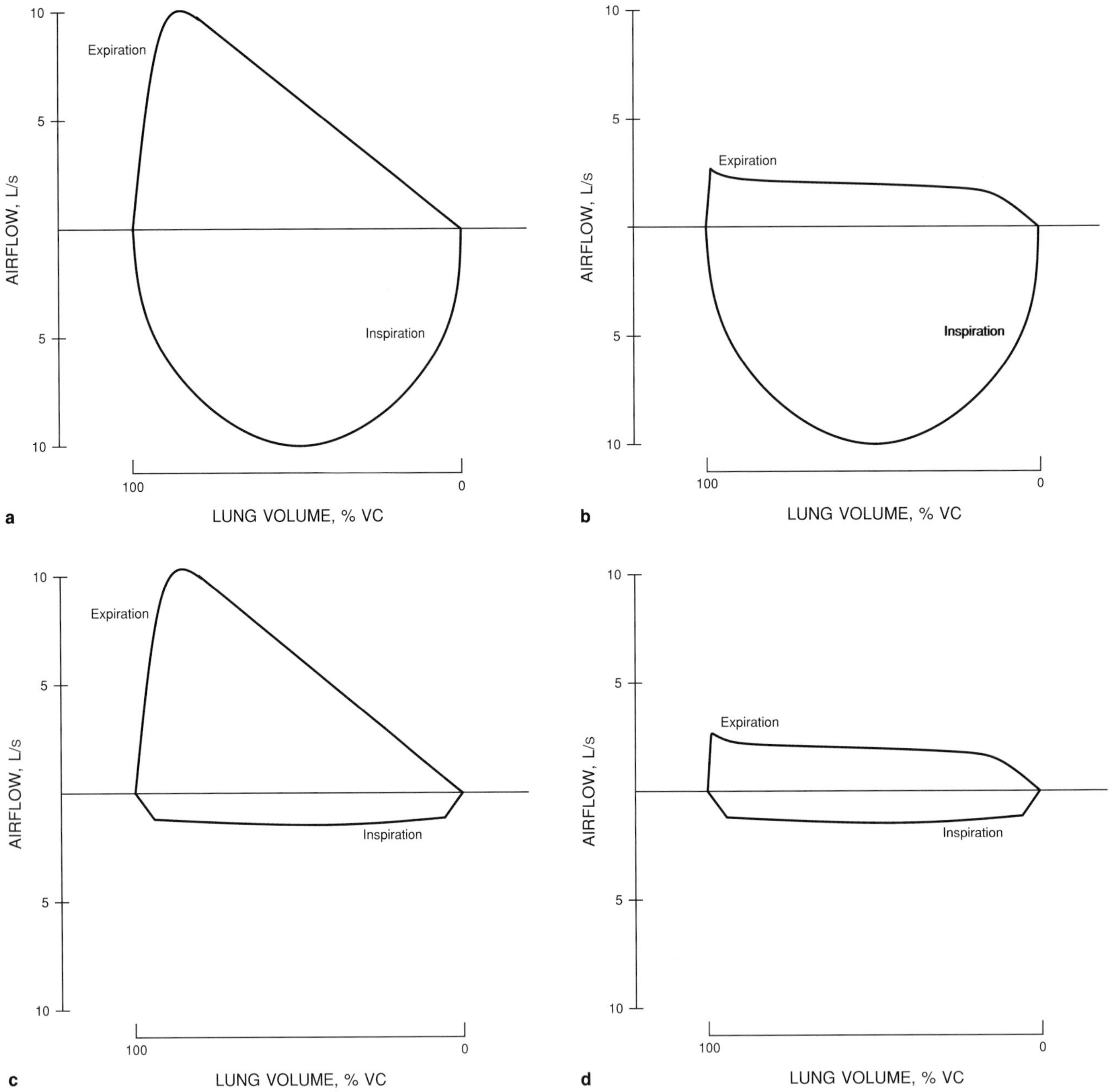

FIGURE 134-2 Simultaneous flow-volume curves performed during a maximal inspiration from residual volume to total lung capacity and then forced expiration back to residual volume. Figure 134-2*a* indicates the normal contour of the inspiratory and expiratory curves. With variable intrathoracic obstruction (e.g., tracheomalacia within the thorax), obstruction is marked during expiration with marked truncation of the expiratory curve (*b*). With variable extrathoracic obstruction (e.g., collapse of tracheal cartilage in the neck following trauma), obstruction is most marked during inspiration (*c*). Finally, with fixed obstructions (e.g., tracheal stenosis), both the inspiratory and expiratory curves are markedly truncated (*d*).

essential that the critical care physician be competent in the full range of techniques for gaining airway access, including rigid open bronchoscopy and tracheotomy.

Management Strategies Applicable to All Forms of Upper Airway Obstruction

Securing and maintaining a patent airway is of paramount importance in the resuscitation of asphyxiating patients. Measures required may include the use of pharyngeal airways, endotracheal intubation (either transnasally or orally), tracheotomy, endoscopy with an open bronchoscope, intubation over a fiberoptic bronchoscope, the use of helium-oxygen mixtures,[5,6] and various drugs, inhaled and systemic—such as epinephrine, norepinephrine, β-mimetics, antihistamines, steroids, and antibiotics.

Heliox, a helium-oxygen gas mixture, is effective in reducing the work of breathing by decreasing the resistive load by a decrease in the density-dependent pressure drop across the airway obstruction. In order to be effective, the heliox:oxygen ratio must be at least 70:30. When it is necessary to add high flows of supplemental oxygen in hypoxemic patients, gas density rises and the efficacy of heliox is lost. It is important to emphasize that although work of breathing may be diminished and dyspnea alleviated to some degree with heliox in a patient with a mechanically obstructed airway, it still leaves the mechanical obstruction in place. Heliox must be viewed as a temporizing measure only. Similar comments can be made about the pharmacologic approaches to managing airway obstruction: The use of airway-active drugs must not be allowed to lull the attending physician into a false sense of security when a serious underlying mechanical obstruction is present. If heliox is used in patients with pure UAO and no lung disease, then a fixed 21% oxygen mixture can be used. Unfortunately, most patients with UAO also have lung disease with varying degrees of hypoxemia. In these cases, we apply 21% heliox by mask, with supplemental oxygen by nasal cannula titrated against pulse oximeter readings. This avoids time-consuming adjustments of blenders used to achieve various helium-oxygen mixtures.

Other therapeutic options include CO_2 or neodymium:YAG laser clearing of laryngeal or endotracheal lesions, acute dilatation, the use of small endotracheal tubes when establishing a translaryngeal airway, and the temporary use of a jet catheter by cricothyroid membrane puncture while getting ready to progress to a more definitive procedure. It goes without saying that upper airway obstruction due to collapse of oropharyngeal structures in an unconscious or paralyzed patient can be easily managed by the jaw thrust maneuver.

The precise management strategy obviously depends on the diagnosis; every effort must be directed toward achieving this.

Selected Causes of UAO

FACIAL TRAUMA[7]

Motor vehicle trauma is often associated with facial injury that includes mandibular and maxillary fractures leading to upper airway compromise, particularly when accompanied by unconsciousness. Early establishment of an airway is the foremost resuscitative priority in this setting, but care should be taken to stabilize and protect the cervical spine during airway or endotracheal tube insertion. Where spinal stability is in doubt, intubation over a fiberoptic bronchoscope is favored by many authors. Hemorrhage and mucus commonly contribute to airway compromise under these circumstances and must be cleared through vigorous suctioning. Rarely, ethmoidal artery laceration may produce catastrophic ongoing hemorrhage requiring isolation and ligature; but this procedure can be done after the airway has been secured.

ACUTE LARYNGEAL INJURY

Laryngeal fractures are almost always due to motor vehicle trauma (e.g., laryngeal smash on the steering wheel), "clothesline"-type injuries, or martial arts "play." The clinical features are those of airway obstruction, dysphonia, loss of laryngeal prominence, and subcutaneous cervical emphysema. The fractures are associated with extensive submucosal edema and hemorrhage that may partially or completely obstruct the airway. Initial attempts to intubate the asphyxiating patient are frustrated by obstruction to tube passage at the laryngeal level. This demands urgent tracheotomy or even cricothyrotomy. Early bronchoscopic recognition of the problem is desirable, with control of the airway and appropriate stenting of the larynx in order to preserve not only airway patency but also as much function as possible. Unfortunately, functional results after severe laryngeal injury are frequently not ideal even with early diagnosis, airway control, and proper stenting. Common sequelae include voice change, laryngeal stenosis, and predisposition to aspiration.

LARYNGEAL STENOSIS

Laryngeal stenosis may develop after direct trauma, prolonged intubation, radiation, or relapsing polychondritis; or after laryngeal surgery or laser resections. Surprisingly, patients may not be symptomatic until the airway reaches a 3-mm diameter. Typical sites of obstruction are at the level of the cricoid and at the cords. Cricoid injury with resultant stenosis (subglottic stenosis) is a disaster, because corrective surgical techniques meet with variable and unpredictable success.

It is not uncommon for a patient in an intensive care unit (ICU), when first extubated, to exhibit alarming features of UAO. The typical pattern is that of relatively easy breathing for anywhere from 15 min to 2 or 3 h, followed by the gradual progression of dyspnea, inspiratory stridor, and increased work of breathing. These patients are commonly managed in a semireclining position and given heliox in a 70:30 mixture, which can be used to drive a nebulization system of racemic epinephrine. Other strategies include parenteral and inhaled steroid administration, and the use of aerosolized atropine sulfate or ipratropium bromide. Again, it must be emphasized that *these are all temporizing measures of dubious value.* Patients must be followed very carefully until the acute swelling and inflammation associated with the endotracheal tube has subsided. These patients should remain in the ICU under careful observation and should not be sent to the ward until it is apparent that upper airway obstruction has resolved or greatly improved. Patients with these problems should be followed with a fiberoptic bronchoscopic examination and flow-volume loop prior to hospital discharge. They should also be warned that if they ever again develop respiratory symptoms of obstruction, reexamination of the airway is advisable. In patients who are acutely deteriorating and whose work of breathing is leading to progressive ventilatory dyscoordination, reintubation with serious consideration of subsequent tracheotomy should be undertaken.

AIRWAY BURN[8]

Exposure to inhaled hot particulate material from fires, or to superheated or hot expanding steam or gas, may produce upper airway "scald"—superheated gas burns with severe swelling and inflammatory response. This reaction may involve the airway from nasooral cavities to mainstem bronchi, although the brunt of the injury is borne by the laryngeal structures. With head and neck burns or fires in enclosed spaces, burn injury to the upper airway must always be considered and, if suspected, confirmed by fiberoptic bronchoscopy. Rather trivial-appearing redness seen immediately after an airway burn may progress to a grotesquely swollen and obstructed oropharynx and/or larynx. This is partly related to the fluid resuscitation required in burn therapy. Prophylactic intubation has now become standard practice (see Chap. 68).

HEMORRHAGE[9]

Acute upper airway obstruction may occur in association with bleeding into perilaryngeal or cervical tissues. These bleeding episodes are generally related to anticoagulant therapy (usually Coumadin),[9] or to hereditary coagulation disorders (usually severe factor VIII deficiency). Correction of the bleeding may require administration of vitamin K, fresh frozen plasma, cryoprecipitate, platelets, or specific factor concentrates. Relief of airway obstruction should be regarded as an emergency, since bleeding may be accompanied by a rapid progression from airway patency to obstruction and cardiorespiratory arrest.

INFECTION WITH MIXED ANAEROBES OF ORAL OR ODONTOGENIC ORIGIN

Odontogenic infection arising from apical tooth spaces can spread to submandibular and cervical spaces and produce UAO. *Ludwig's angina,* an indurative cellulitis involving both the sublingual and submandibular spaces, usually has a dental origin. Treatment frequently requires the establishment of an airway. It is a polymicrobial anaerobic infection. Antimicrobial agents should be directed against oral anaerobes. Penicillin in high doses is usually sufficient, but the addition of metronidazole or substitution with clindamycin provides coverage for *Bacteroides* species. Surgical drainage of the involved spaces may be required.

Similar infection can occur in the lateral pharyngeal space. This space is shaped like an inverted cone with its apex at the hyoid bone and its base at the skull. Infection can arise secondary to pharyngitis, parotitis, otitis, and mastoiditis, as well as to odontogenic infection. In addition to mouth anaerobes, *Staphylococcus aureus* and *Streptococcus pyogenes* can also be involved. Trismus, swelling below the angle of the mandible, and medial displacement of the lateral pharyngeal wall are prominent when the anterior compartment of the lateral pharyngeal space is infected. When infection is confined to the posterior compartment, septicemia may be the only feature, with few local signs. CT of the neck is useful in delineating these infections and in defining their extent prior to surgical drainage.

Retropharyngeal space infection can cause asphyxiation by obstruction or, more commonly, by spontaneous rupture of pus or erosion of a blood vessel and subsequent hemorrhage. Such infection either is mixed anaerobic odontogenic or originates from suppurative lymphadenitis (usually *Streptococcus pyogenes*). Dysphagia, altered quality of the voice, and nuchal rigidity are seen. Bulging of the posterior pharyngeal wall may be seen. In addition to appropriate antibiotics, surgical drainage is indicated (see Chap. 105).

ACUTE EPIGLOTTITIS[10]

Most of our information on adult epiglottitis has come from case reports and small series. Nevertheless, it is now clear that epiglottitis is not rare in adults. Historical accounts strongly suggest that George Washington died of this condition. In a retrospective review, 42 cases were identified in the Edmonton Hospitals over a 10-year period. Similarly, MayoSmith et al[10] reported 56 cases over an 8-year period in the state of Rhode Island, an incidence of 10 cases per million per year. It is clear from these studies that adult epiglottitis differs from the childhood disease in a number of respects. In children, *Hemophilus influenzae* type B accounts for most cases. Bacteremia is usual and susceptability is related to absence of antibodies to a capsular antigen. In contrast, in adults only a minority of cases are related to *H. influenzae.* In the Rhode Island series, 6 of 25 (24 percent) blood cultures taken were positive (all with *H. influenzae*). Ninety-seven percent of adults have been shown to have anticapsular antibodies. Epiglottitis and bacteremia due to *H. influenzae* may arise only in persons whose immunity has waned or failed to develop. The bacteriologic etiology of the remainder of adult cases is uncertain, since cultures of the pharynx or the epiglottis surface may not reflect submucosal infection. Routine cultures usually identify *Streptococcus pyogenes* and some other aerobic pathogens from mucosal surfaces. Furthermore, it is clear from case reports that *Streptococcus pyogenes, Streptococcus pneumoniae,* and *Staph. aureus* may be important causes of adult epiglottitis. *Pasteurella multocida* has been described, as has *Candida albicans,* in immunocompromised hosts. Mixed anaerobic infection involving other spaces in the neck may also present as epiglottitis. The role of viruses, mycoplasmas, and *Chlamydia* species has not been properly investigated.

The clinical syndrome is characterized by rapid onset of dysphagia, sore throat, drooling, fever, shortness of breath, and muffled voice. Hoarseness is rare, since the vocal cords are not involved. Many patients assume a characteristic forward-leaning posture. Other conditions that on occasion mimic epiglottitis include peritonsillar abscess, croup, and diphtheria. Epiglottitis should perhaps be termed *supraglottitis,* since all of the tissues above the true cords are inflammed. Swelling of the epiglottis and aryepiglottic folds, with complete obliteration of the vallecular and pyriform sinuses, is typical. A diagnosis can be made by direct inspection of the epiglottis during indirect laryngoscopy, or by direct laryngoscopy during intubation. An unfounded folklore suggests that examination of the oropharynx is dangerous, but we recommend it as the best and quickest way to make the diagnosis. Lateral x-rays of the neck may reveal swollen supraglottic tissues, but should not be done in a patient in whom the diagnosis is strongly suspected; not only is time thus wasted, but fatalities have arisen in the radiology department. Successful resuscitation is rarely achieved once spontaneous obstruction has developed with cardiorespiratory arrest. We believe that the current pediatric practice of prophylactic intubation in all cases of epiglottitis should be extended to adults. The Rhode Island experience showed a 7 percent mortality rate, which is unacceptably higher than the 1 percent mortality rate currently reported in most pediatric series. There are no clinical features that allow prediction of imminent airway obstruction.

Once the diagnosis is made or strongly suspected, the operating room should be readied for intubation under inhalational anesthesia, and for possible emergency tracheotomy. With the surgeon ready, inhalational anesthesia with an oxygen-enflurane or oxygen-halothane mixture is given while the patient is still sitting. The supraglottic structures are frequently so swollen that the cords are obscured and the normal anatomy is not apparent; the bronchoscope must be aimed at the bubbles in the laryngeal aditus. Flexible bronchoscopy has the advantage that the patient may be supported in the sitting position while the airway is secured. Fixation of the tube by careful taping prevents death from dislodgement.

H. influenzae resistance to ampicillin ranges from 10 to 50 percent. Chloramphenicol resistance is rare, as is resistance to the second- and third-generation cephalosporins. Cefuroxime has the advantage of being active against *Staph. aureus* and the other possible bacterial causes. It is also active against most oral anaerobes, except *Bacteroides fragilis.* There is no role for steroids, racemic epinephrine, or helium-oxygen mixtures in the management of epiglottitis.

The endotracheal tube is left in place with the patient breathing spontaneously (T-piece, 1 to 3 cmH_2O continuous positive airway pressure [CPAP] or low-pressure support) until the inflammation and swelling of the upper airway and epiglottis are observed to subside and the patient is able to breathe around the tube. As a general rule, the intubation time is only 2 to 3 days, at which point the tube is removed and the patient carefully observed for recurrent UAO.

DIPHTHERIA

Diphtheria is now rare in the developed world. Small epidemics continue to appear, especially among the poor and elderly, due to inadequate or waning immunization. Even full immunization does not guarantee protection, since it is completely effective in only 75 percent of persons. Clinical diphtheria develops over a few days. Multiple sites in the upper respiratory tract may be involved, or it may be confined to the nares, pharynx, larynx, or trachea. The membrane initially appears white and glossy, but then deteriorates into a dirty-gray color. Local toxin production often produces striking submandibular and neck swelling, mimicking Ludwig's angina. The diagnosis may not become apparent until myocarditis or cranial neuropathies develop, or the reports of pharyngeal cultures become available. Prophylactic intubation or tracheostomy is indicated in many such patients. Penicillin or erythromycin should be administered along with diphtheria antitoxin.

OTHER INFECTIONS THAT MAY CAUSE UAO

Acute tonsillitis or pharyngitis due to *Staph. pyogenes* rarely progresses to airway obstruction. When it does, the cause of obstruction is usually abscess formation within the tonsillar or peritonsillar space (quinsy). Infectious mononucleosis uncommonly produces airway obstruction due to massive tonsillar enlargement. Systemic corticosteroids produce a rapid resolution of swollen tonsillar tissue, so intubation is rarely necessary.

FOREIGN BODIES

The lodgement of foreign bodies in the upper airway, with consequent UAO and asphyxiation, continues to receive public attention (the "cafe coronary").[11] Controversy exists over the application of the pulsive squeeze (the "Heimlich maneuver"), positioning, and back pounding. Whenever possible, the object should be grasped under direct vision by fingers or forceps. Failing that or pulsive dislodgement, it may be necessary to perform an urgent cricothyroidotomy to achieve an airway. Massive aspiration requires intubation, vigorous suctioning, and endoscopic piecemeal removal of food fragments. Great effort must be directed toward removing organic particulate material—such as peanuts, or meat or vegetable pieces—since their continued presence in more distal airways frequently causes pneumonia.

LARYNGEAL TUMORS

Laryngeal tumors (usually of the squamous cell type) usually are slow-growing; persons who have them usually present with hoarseness. An occasional patient, however, presents with acute or rapidly progressive airway obstruction. Only rarely are cordal swellings associated with significant airway obstruction. Diagnosis depends on direct inspection and biopsy where appropriate.

LARYNGEAL PAPILLOMAS[12]

Laryngeal papillomas are only rarely associated with acute UAO. They are caused by a DNA virus, are believed to be infectious, and may involve the airway from false cords to distal bronchi—although most commonly the polypi are in the larynx and upper trachea. Management is by CO_2 laser resection, interferon injection, or, more recently, argon-dye laser ablation after hematoporphyrin tissue sensitization. Securing the airway is seldom a problem with an open bronchoscope.

LARYNGOSPASM

The larynx is a complex device with a number of muscle groups and articulating cartilages that interact in intricate patterns during phonation, swallowing, and breathing maneuvers. This process occasionally becomes disordered, producing partial or complete closure of the upper airway—either at the level of the true cords or at the aryepiglottic folds, posterior commissure, or false cords, or both. The spasm may be precipitated by a variety of laryngeal stimuli, including blood, mucus, water, temperature extremes, and direct contact (e.g., during intubation without sufficient topical anesthesia). Visceral reflex and central emotional factors may also play a role. In regard to the latter, the syndrome of "hysterical respiratory distress," first described by Osler,[13] has been rediscovered by several authors and is now well described.[14,15] Although uncommon, these cases are striking in that respiratory distress is severe, there is no apparent anatomic abnormality present, and intubation may be difficult without resorting to paralysis. It is said that these patients can be identified and "cured" by commanding nasal breathing in the "sniffing position"; but in a number of cases that the authors have seen, laryngospasm was so severe that cyanosis and bradycardia dictated endotracheal intubation. Other patients, less seriously compromised, may well respond to reassurance and sedation alone.

ANGIONEUROTIC LARYNGEAL EDEMA

Angioneurotic edema (AE) is characterized by recurrent episodes of local swelling involving the face, the larynx, and the skin of the extremities. Commonly associated gastrointestinal disturbances include colicky pain, nausea, and vomiting. Laryngeal AE may be either allergic or nonallergic in origin; in the latter case it may be either hereditary or nonhereditary.

AE OF ALLERGIC ORIGIN

The usual offending allergens are foods, drugs, and inhaled substances. Bee stings, poison ivy, and poison oak, involving the head and neck or the tongue, are also occasionally associated with airway obstruction. In addition to avoiding the precipitating allergen, management consists of the immediate administration of parenteral epinephrine and antihistamines (see Chap. 89). Only rarely is intubation or other heroic airway access required.

HEREDITARY AE[16]

This is a potentially life-threatening condition caused by a deficiency of C1 esterase inhibitor. Precipitating events are often obscure; they may include trivial trauma, emotional stress, and upset. The condition is autosomal-dominant, with variable penetrance. Treatment of an acute episode may require urgent intubation or tracheostomy. With premonitory symptoms, there may be time to administer intravenous C1 esterase inhibitor. Patients who experience frequent attacks should keep this material at home. Long-term prophylaxis may also be achieved, in some patients, through regular use of ϵ-aminocaproic acid or danazol, both of which stimulate C1 esterase inhibitor production.

"PACHYLARYNGOPATHY," OBESITY

A small group of patients, most with associated sleep-disordered breathing, get into great difficulty with UAO when they are asleep, sedated, unconscious, or under anesthesia. In the latter circumstance it is not uncommon for intubation with a standard MacIntosh curved or straight-blade laryngoscope to be difficult, necessitating intubation over a fiberoptic bronchoscope. "Pachylaryngopathy" refers to marked lymphoid hyperplasia in the tonsillar, adenoidal, and lingual regions that may extend to involve the aryepiglottic folds and false cords of the larynx, and the pyriform fossae and valleculae. These patients are usually obese, with a small oropharyngeal cavity.

THE TRACHEA

Obstruction involving the trachea may be due to trauma or surgery-related injury, tumors (both intra- and extraluminal, including lymphomas), chondromalacia, foreign bodies, the thyroid, and vascular anomalies. Although the onset of airway compromise is usually gradual, some patients remain asymptomatic despite 2- to 3-mm diameter airways until complete blockage results from mucus, bleeding, or inflammation with swelling.

PULMONARY EDEMA ASSOCIATED WITH UAO[17,18]

Classic pulmonary edema has been noted to occur with severe partial UAO from many causes, including epidermolysis bullosa, esophageal achalasia and diverticulum, epiglottic cysts, necrotizing tracheobronchitis, laryngeal rheumatoid arthritis, inflammatory uvular edema, relapsing polychrondritis, stroke with bilateral vocal cord paralysis, acromegaly, vallecular cysts, etc. Generally, these conditions are associated with a more gradual onset of airway obstruction, and a systematic workup can be pursued. The pulmonary edema is thought to be due to the left ventricular afterload imposed by very negative pleural pressure, large negative interstitial pressure excursions and increased venous return; it generally subsides quickly with restoration of a patent airway. Occasionally, relief of UAO may be associated with the development of pulmonary edema.[17]

CASE PRESENTATION

Mrs. O.L., 62 years old, presented at the emergency room (ER) severely short of breath, with indrawing, cyanosis, and a rapid pulse. She was febrile (38.8°C) and had a 3-day history of respiratory tract infection, with a sharp unproductive cough, muscle aches and pains, and progressive respiratory distress. In the ER she was noted to have a pulsus paradoxus of 25 mmHg and a hyperinflated chest, and could speak only one or two words at a time. Wheezes were present in both lung fields on auscultation. Given inhaled albuterol, intravenous methylprednisolone, subcutaneous epinephrine, and oxygen by mask, she seemed to improve. After 5 h she was admitted to a general medical ward. Although she could not lie flat and was still very dyspneic, there was substantial improvement. She was started on intravenous ampicillin.

The patient had been quite well most of her life, aside from troublesome rheumatoid arthritis involving both hands. She had been involved in a car accident some 14 months previously and had been in an ICU for 18 days. During much of this time she had been mechanically ventilated with an endotracheal tube for multiple rib fractures. She also had a pneumothorax requiring tube drainage and had undergone internal fixation of humeral and femoral fractures. During the intervening 14 months, she had been inactive but generally well, despite several respiratory tract infections, each of which required antibiotics and bronchodilators to resolve.

Pulmonary function studies had been ordered as a routine by the admitting house officer; when these were performed the following morning, they demonstrated the classic features of severe variable inspiratory impairment with a "step." At the conclusion of the respiratory maneuvers associated with the pulmonary function studies, the patient suddenly became very dyspneic and was placed on salbutamol by nebulization, the system being driven by 70:30 heliox with supplemental oxygen at 10 L/min flow. She seemed to improve with this and was transported to the radiology department for quick three-cut tomograms of the trachea. These demonstrated narrowing of the tracheal lumen to an estimated 1- to 2-mm diameter about one-third of the way down the trachea. The stenotic segment spanned approximately 2.5 cm. In the radiology department the patient became so severely dyspneic that she struggled with her attendants and resisted efforts to keep the heliox and supplemental oxygen mask in place. She was given 8 mg of diazepam IV and seemed to settle down. The operating room was readied for a tracheotomy. While the patient was still in the radiology department an attempt was made to examine the airway with a fiberoptic bronchoscope, with the aim of inserting an endotracheal tube over the bronchoscope. During this maneuver the upper ostium of the stenosis was visualized, but it proved impossible to insert the endotracheal tube over the fiberoptic bronchoscope. This was abandoned after two tries because the patient became obtunded, cyanotic, with distended neck veins, and clearly moribund.

At this point the ICU team arrived and, using a 5-mm pediatric Storz bronchoscope with a bag-ventilating sidearm system, easily slipped the bronchoscope through the stenotic segment and reestablished the airway. The patient gratefully took a huge gasp of air, opened her eyes, and coughed a large amount of bloody mucus out through the bronchoscope!

After these harrowing events the patient underwent an uneventful resection of the stenotic tracheal segment, with primary end-to-end anastomosis. The patient ultimately was discharged and went home. Follow-up fiberoptic bronchoscopy showed a circumferential ring stenosis at the anastomotic site, but a good 5- to 6-cm lumen.

CASE DISCUSSION

The case of Mrs. O.L. clearly illustrates a number of the problems associated with UAO. Emergency room and medical house staff can be forgiven for a misdiagnosis of reactive airways disease in association with a respiratory tract infection; since the patient was in respiratory distress with indrawing, was not moving much air, and was febrile with bilateral rhonchi. They were not aware of the significant antecedant history. Furthermore, she apparently improved with oxygenation and bronchodilator therapy. It is of interest that the diagnosis of UAO was serendipitous, in that someone ordered pulmonary function studies (not normally useful during an acute attack of respiratory distress) that demonstrated the classic step pattern, on the inspiratory limb of the flow-volume loop, of extrathoracic UAO. The patient was then sent to have quick midchest tomograms to ascertain the extent and severity of the obstructive lesion. The frequency of patients with respiratory compromise coming to grief in pulmonary function laboratories and radiology departments is well known; it was surprisingly good luck that this patient did not close off her airway and die during the diagnostic maneuvers. The likelihood of successful resuscitation in an airway-obstructed patient with a bradycardic-asystolic cardiopulmonary arrest in a radiology department is rather remote, even with heroic intervention.

The use of heliox, particularly with high-flow oxygen augmentation, provided attending doctors with a false sense of security and was like "whistling past the graveyard." As none of those involved with the case had an appreciation for the rapidity of deterioration that can occur under these circumstances, they were not aware that UAO patients are often only one glob of mucus away from sudden death. Again, the patient and the operator were lucky that attempts to deal with the stenosis by fiberoptic bronchoscopic intubation did not produce a catastrophe by increasing mucosal edema or provoking bleeding. As it was, the patient seriously deteriorated after these maneuvers and was clearly asphyxiating. The case demonstrates the importance of critical care personnel's being comfortable with the job of establishing an effective airway by a full range of techniques, including stiff bronchoscopy and tracheotomy.

It is of interest that this woman's near-death was associated with an endotracheal tube cuff–related injury that had occurred so much earlier that none of those initially involved with the case, including the patient's husband, made the connection. It was the fortuitous, albeit misguided, flow-volume loop that prompted the correct diagnosis. Mrs. O.L.'s case also illustrates that patients with 2- to 3-mm airways get along surprisingly well at rest and become symptomatic only with exercise or with respiratory tract infections that produce mucosal engorgement. Finally, this case underscores the importance of critical care physicians' being acutely aware of the potential for rapid and unpredictable deterioration in UAO. Active intervention must occur at the mere suggestion that a life may be in danger from asphyxia.

References

1. Dailey RH: Acute upper airway obstruction. Emerg Med Clin North Am 1:261, 1983.
2. Jacobson S: Upper airway obstruction. Emerg Med Clin North Am 7:205, 1989.
3. Marcuso AA, Hanafee WN: Computerized tomography of the injured larynx. Radiology 133:139, 1979.
4. Miller RD: Obstructing lesions of the larynx and trachea: Clinical and pathophysiological aspects, in Fishman AP: *Pulmonary Diseases and Disorders,* 2d ed. New York, McGraw-Hill, 1988, pp 1173–1187.
5. Skrinskas GJ, Hyland RH, Hutcheon MA: Using Helium-oxygen mixtures in the management of acute upper airway obstruction. Can Med Assoc J 128:555, 1983.
6. Boorstein JM, Boorstein SM, Humphries GN, et al: Using helium-oxygen mixtures in the emergency management of acute upper airway obstruction. Ann Emerg Med 18:688, 1989.
7. Gruss JS (ed): Facial trauma, in McMurty RY, McLellan BA (eds): *Management of Blunt Trauma.* Baltimore, Williams and Wilkins, 1990, pp 359–441.
8. Haponik EF, Meyers DA, Munster AM, et al: Acute upper airway injury in burn patients: Serial changes of flow-volume curves and nasopharyngoscopy. Am Rev Respir Dis 135:360, 1987.
9. Rosenbaum L, Thurman P, Krantz SB: Upper airway obstruction as a complication of oral anticoagulation: Report of three cases. Arch Intern Med 139: 1151, 1979.
10. MayoSmith MF, Hirsch PJ, Wodzniski SF, et al: Acute epiglottitis in adults: An eight year experience in the state of Rhode Island. N Engl J Med 314:1133, 1986.
11. Mittleman RE, Wetli CV: The fatal cafe coronary. Foreign-body airway obstruction. JAMA 247:1285, 1982.
12. Abramson AL, Waner M, Brandsma J: The clinical treatment of laryngeal papillomas with hematoporphyrin therapy. Arch Otolaryngol Head Neck Surg 114:795, 1988.
13. Osler W: Hysteria, in Osler W (ed): *The Principles and Practice of Medicine.* New York, Appleton, 1902, pp 1111–1112.
14. Ramirez JR, Leon I, Rivera LM: Episodic laryngeal dyskinesia: Clinical and psychiatric characterization. Chest 90:16, 1986.
15. Synder HS, Weiss E: Hysterical stridor: A benign cause of upper airway obstruction. Ann Emerg Med 18:991, 1989.
16. Davis AE: C. inhibitor and hereditary angioneurotic edema. Ann Rev Immunol 6:595, 1988.
17. Galvis GA: Pulmonary edema complicating relief of upper airway obstruction. Am J Emerg Med 5:294, 1987.
18. Willms D, Shure D: Pulmonary edema due to upper airway obstruction in adults. Chest 94:1090, 1988.

Chapter 135 CARDIOPULMONARY FAILURE ASSOCIATED WITH SLEEP-DISORDERED BREATHING

MARK WYLAM
JESSE B. HALL

KEY POINTS

- *Sleep-disordered breathing (SDB) may present as cardiopulmonary failure.*
- *SDB represents a reversible form of pulmonary hypertension.*
- *In patients with SDB general anesthesia may lead to upper airway obstruction after extubation and may worsen central alveolar hypoventilation.*
- *Congestive heart failure may coexist and exacerbate SDB.*
- *Postoperative loads on the respiratory system may precipitate florid manifestations of previously unrecognized SDB.*
- *Within the differential diagnosis of acute on chronic respiratory failure are chronic obstructive pulmonary disease (COPD) and SDB, which often coexist.*

Breathing irregularities during sleep are extremely common and are increasingly recognized as producing clinical syndromes characterized by central nervous system (CNS) and cardiopulmonary dysfunction. These syndromes are most often identified in ambulatory patients, but they may complicate or first emerge during critical illness. We call to the reader's attention the need to consider sleep-disordered breathing (SDB) as a cause of or contributor to postoperative respiratory failure, hypercapnic respiratory failure with deterioration during oxygen therapy, and cor pulmonale.

Pathophysiology and Classification

Sleep is characterized by striking changes in the control of breathing as compared to the waking state. There is a greater reliance on metabolic regulation of breathing with generation of periodic breathing patterns.[1] Hypopneas and brief apneas are common. In health, these alterations in breathing do not result in significant hypercapnia nor arterial oxygen desaturation. Under many pathologic conditions, hypoventilation and hypoxemia may become extreme, with acute and chronic consequences for diverse organ systems.[2]

SLEEP APNEA SYNDROMES

Apnea during sleep may be classified as *central*, resulting from cessation of neural output from brain stem regulatory centers to the respiratory muscles, or as *obstructive*, resulting from closure of the upper airway, usually at the level of the base of the tongue (Figure 135-1). Many patients exhibit a mixed pattern, with both central and obstructive episodes. In mixed apnea, obstruction is felt to be a dominant underlying mechanism, and when obstruction is relieved (vide infra), both obstructive and central apneas resolve. The vast majority of patients with SDB have obstructive sleep apnea (OSA) and are obese.

The pathogenesis of the classic obstructive apnea is well formulated. A final common pathway of upper airway occlusion occurs, precipitating apnea, and repeats itself perhaps hundreds of times per night. Though some patients may have altered upper airway anatomy to promote obstruction, such as micrognathia, tonsillar hypertrophy, redundant soft tissue, or nasal obstruction, the majority have no specific abnormality. After the onset of sleep, negative oropharyngeal pressure during inspiration must be over-

FIGURE 135-1 A cartoon demonstrating obstruction of the upper airway in sleep apnea. Low intrathoracic pressures (Pes) will not be transmitted to the hypopharynx if the upper airway is patent (nonocclusive condition). If upper airway resistance is increased, pharyngeal pressures (Pph) may approach Pes favoring occlusion. In patients with obstructive sleep apnea, the increased compliance of the upper airway results in closure even at small negative pressures. (Reprinted with permission from Block AJ, Faulkner JA, Hughes RL, et al: Factors influencing upper airway closure. Chest 86:117, 1984).

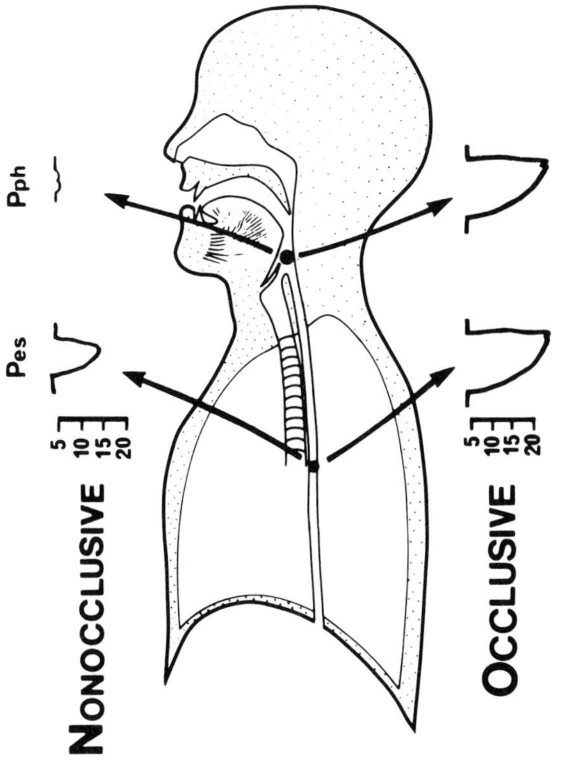

TABLE 135-1 Sleep-Disordered Breathing

Sleep apnea
Obstructive
Central
Mixed
Periodic breathing (including Cheyne-Stokes respiration)
Desaturation in lung and neuromuscular disease

come by upper airway musculature to prevent dynamic airway collapse. In OSA, upper airway collapse is facilitated by a reduction in tone of upper airway musculature, high pharyngeal compliance, and high upstream resistance to airflow.[3–5] These factors combine to produce a Starling resistor which produces airway closure when the critical closure gradient is exceeded. The critical closure pressure approximates -15 cmH_2O in subjects who never snore, -5 cmH_2O in patients who habitually snore, and -3 cmH_20 in patients with OSA. The precise mechanisms by which obesity produces airway obstruction during sleep remain to be elucidated but likely include narrowing of the upper airway, diminished compliance of pharyngeal tissues, increased respiratory elastic load, and direct effects upon brain stem regulatory centers.[7,8]

Central apneas are usually found in concert with obstructive apneas as a consequence of the exaggerated periodic breathing pattern that occurs with severe sleep fragmentation. However, primary central apnea may occur in diseases with anatomic damage to respiratory neurons. Among these are bulbar poliomyelitis, encephalitis, brain stem neoplasm, brain stem infarction, spinal cord surgery, and cervical cordotomy. A classification of SDB is given in Table 135-1.

CHEYNE-STOKES BREATHING PATTERNS

Cheyne-Stokes respiration represents a periodic crescendo-decrescendo alteration in tidal volume. Normal individuals exhibit this marked periodic breathing pattern during sleep at high altitude. This breathing instability is attributable to the hypoxemia associated with high altitude and is correctable with oxygen therapy. With uncorrected hypoxemia, Cheyne-Stokes breathing patterns (Fig. 135-2), are seen, with hypoventilation during and hypercapnia following the apneic phase. Severe congestive heart failure and bilateral frontal lobe neurologic disease may cause these patterns in the waking state under normoxic conditions. Sleep tends to worsen any degree of Cheyne-Stokes breathing and associated hypoxemia.[9]

NOCTURNAL DESATURATION IN LUNG AND NEUROMUSCULAR DISEASE

Nocturnal arterial oxygen desaturation is relatively common in patients with COPD, neuromuscular weakness, and severe restrictive lung disease. In the case of lung disease, this may result in part from base-line hypoxemia, with the patient positioned on the relatively "steep" portion of the oxyhemoglobin saturation curve. Small changes in $P_{A_{O_2}}$ associated with hypopneas or irregular breathing may result in significant desaturation. In the case of neuromuscular disease, brain stem involvement or weakness of upper airway muscles may predispose to central or obstructive apnea, respectively. Finally, for any degree of associated sleep apnea, patients with diminished pulmonary reserve may manifest greater gas exchange abnormalities.[10]

FIGURE 135-2 Instability and periodicity of breathing pattern induced by administration of hypoxic gas mixture to a normal subject during sleep. Beginning in Panel A, the onset of hypoxia in a normal subject is shown on the bottom line and is reflected by the fall in partial pressure of expired oxygen ($P_{ET}O_2$) and arterial oxygen saturation (SaO_2). The tidal volume (Vt) and breathing frequency vary progressively over the 11 minutes of hypoxia, over Panels A and B. When normoxia is restored (Panel B), periodic breathing eventually resolves. (Reprinted with permission from Berssenbrugge A, Dempsey JA, Iber C, et al: J Physiol (London) 343:507, 1983.)

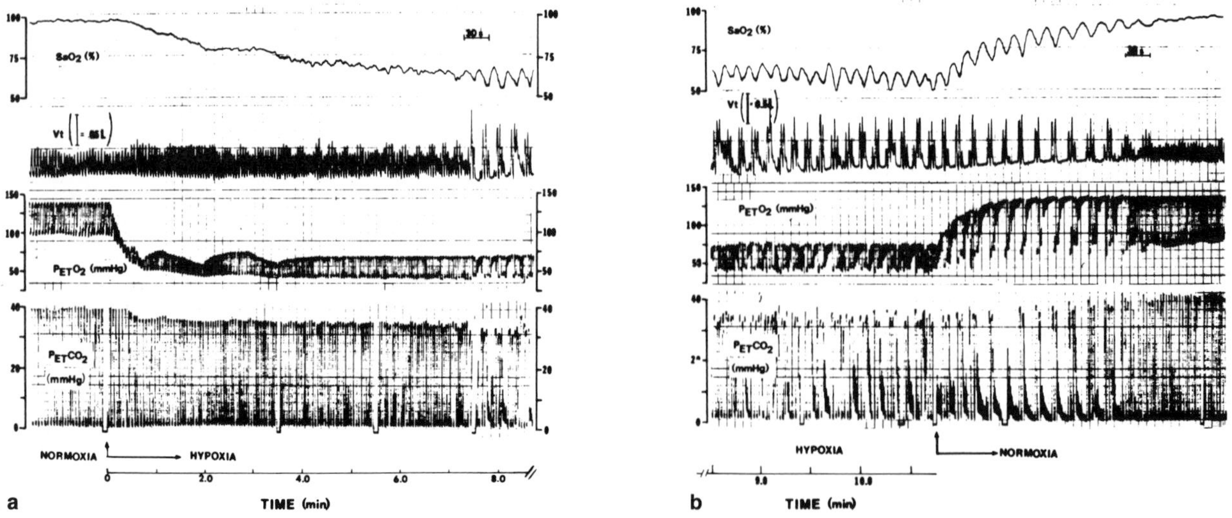

Consequences of Sleep-Disordered Breathing

Hypoventilation related to hypopneic or apneic episodes results in respiratory acidosis and hypoxemia. Hypoxemia may be exacerbated by ventilation ($\dot{V}/\dot{Q}$) perfusion mismatch in obese patients or those with underlying lung disease. Acutely, these metabolic disturbances may result in a multitude of organ system dysfunctions, with myocardial failure, ischemia, and arrhythmias of greatest concern.[11] Clinically, some patients progress to hypercapnia during the waking state (primary or obesity-related hypoventilation syndrome), marked hypersomnolence and stupor, and both right and left heart failure.

In fact, most of the adverse consequences of SDB appear to result from chronic and possibly the cumulative effects of recurrent hypoxemia. Hypoxia is a potent stimulus to awakening. Typically, patients do not regain full consciousness but rather partially arouse, with normal sleep architecture disturbed by literally hundreds of hypoxic episodes in severe sleep apnea. Interrupted sleep results in daytime hypersomnolence and appears to accumulate over time to result in personality changes, loss of job, and deterioration of family relationships. In the most severe cases, it produces an organic brain syndrome that may eventuate in stupor and coma.

Intermittent hypoxemia and respiratory acidosis cause pulmonary arterial vasoconstriction, potentially leading to pulmonary hypertension and cor pulmonale. It is likely that pulmonary hypertension and right heart failure related to sleep apnea occur mostly, if not exclusively, in patients with underlying lung or pulmonary vascular disease.[12–14] Nonetheless, severe OSA is a well-documented correctable cause of pulmonary hypertension and should be considered in the differential diagnosis of these disorders.

Autonomic discharge during and following episodes of OSA typically produces tachycardia and systemic hypertension. Some evidence suggests that sleep apnea produces sustained hypertension during the waking state as well.[15] In addition, significant inspiratory efforts against an obstructed upper airway can result in large negative pleural pressures, which increase left ventricular afterload.[16] An unusual but dramatic consequence of this increased afterload is pulmonary edema.[17] The combination of increased myocardial work and diminished oxygen supply related to nocturnal hypoxia could acutely precipitate ischemic injury or, over time, adversely affect left ventricular function. Finally, cor pulmonale associated with sleep apnea could result in left ventricular diastolic dysfunction on the basis of ventricular interdependence.

TABLE 135-2 Clinical Presentation of Sleep-Disordered Breathing

Symptoms	Signs
Disrupted sleep	Obesity
Snoring	Snoring
Hypersomnolence	Cardiac arrhythmias
Loss of intellectual abilities	
Morning headache	Pulmonary hypertension
Personality changes	Cor pulmonale
Stupor and coma	
Enuresis	Systemic hypertension
Impotence	Edema

Clinical Presentation

The symptoms and signs of SDB are given in Table 135-2. Patients with SDB may present because of underlying cardiopulmonary disease or with altered mental status and right heart failure related to their SDB. Obesity is almost invariably present in patients with obstructive and central sleep apnea. Excessive weight in these patients may be dramatic and fit the clinical description of the 'Pickwickian' syndrome (hypersomnolence, hypercapnia, erythrocytosis, and morbid obesity, defined as body weight >100 percent of ideal weight). It is important to note that many patients with clinically significant OSA have only a modest weight gain above their ideal weight. Frequently, a patient's recent 20 to 40-lb increase converts prominent snoring to more florid sleep apnea.

Since many of the signs and symptoms of SDB occur during sleep and with progressive disease, the patient's intellectual function and recognition of problems is impaired; collateral history from a sleeping mate is crucial. This is particularly true when this diagnosis is considered in the critically ill.

Precipitating Conditions

Although many patients exhibit an insidious and progressive clinical course, a number of conditions may accelerate signs and symptoms (Table 135-3). Acute upper airway infection, renal failure with generalized edema, and congestive heart failure can all result in narrowing of the airway, compounding the degree of obstruction.[18,19] Alcohol and sedative use dramatically worsen underlying OSA, with as little as several ounces of alcohol at bedtime converting snoring to complete obstruction with arterial oxygen desaturation. In the critical care unit, sedation from anesthetic or

TABLE 135-3 Factors Associated with Worsening Sleep Disordered Breathing

Acquired upper airway injury
Edema
Alcohol and sedative use
Hypothyroidism
Hypoxia
Normoxia

other agents can similarly precipitate florid OSA.[20] Hypothyroidism has been associated with both central and OSA and must be excluded in every patient with these disorders.[21] Hypoxemia associated with lung disease will worsen any component of pulmonary hypertension resulting from sleep apnea. Interestingly, correction of hypoxemia with oxygen therapy may cause a transient decline in level of consciousness as marked sleep deprivation perpetuated by intermittent hypoxemia is relieved and facilitates deep sleep for several days (vide infra).

Presentation of Sleep-Disordered Breathing in Critical Illness

While the usual presenting symptoms of SDB prompting evaluation of ambulatory patients is snoring or hypersomnolence, other scenarios are more likely in the ICU. SDB may first present as a complication of anesthesia or surgery, as the primary disease process precipitating acute on chronic respiratory failure, or it may lead to difficulty liberating patients from mechanical ventilation.

SLEEP-DISORDERED BREATHING IN POSTOPERATIVE RESPIRATORY FAILURE

A patient with undetected signs and symptoms of SDB may first manifest apnea after general anesthesia. It is not uncommon for postoperative obese patients to develop upper airway obstruction and apnea postextubation.[22] A semiawake patient with SDB may arouse suspicion when loud sonorous respiratory efforts are heard by recovery room personnel as the patient terminates apneic events. General anesthesia, like alcohol in the outpatient setting, selectively depresses upper airway muscle activity and promotes airway obstruction in susceptible patients. Oral-pharyngeal surgery with attendant laryngeal edema may likewise produce an incremental increase in upper airway narrowing, precipitating obstructive apnea. In addition, inhalational anesthetics can combine to blunt central respiratory center response to carbon dioxide, as well as to hypoxemia and acidosis.[23] These patients may exhibit depressed cognitive function, appearing "slow to wake up," with appreciable hypoventilation and hypercapnia. Closer examination with detection of elevated serum bicarbonate, polycythemia, and history from others may identify unsuspected signs of SDB.

Postoperatively, conditions such as atelectasis, respiratory muscle splinting, sedative/analgesics, and volume overload may lead to mild desaturation and be well tolerated in healthy patients. However, similar degrees of desaturation in patients with SDB may precipitate significant hypoxemia with attendant complications as they hypoventilate during rapid eye movement (REM) sleep. Specific attention to desaturation during sleep in these patients is best carried out by pulse oximetry.

SLEEP-DISORDERED BREATHING IN ACUTE ON CHRONIC RESPIRATORY FAILURE

The inclusion of SDB in the differential diagnosis of severe cardiopulmonary failure is not widely appreciated. SDB in patients with COPD is a frequent and clinically significant problem leading to severe oxygen desaturation, cardiac arrhythmias, and cor pulmonale. These patients may present in emergency settings with either the neurobehavioral manifestations of SDB "coma," or the cardiopulmonary manifestations of acute on chronic respiratory failure. Dyspnea may be diminished or absent secondary to CNS depression as a result of sleep fragmentation, chronic CNS hypoxia, or acute hypercapnia. The degree of hypersomnolence and stupor may approach coma and may mimic pharmacologic, metabolic, or infectious causes of coma. Secondary pulmonary hypoxic vasoconstriction is present and leads to right heart failure and venous hypertension. Results from several studies indicate that right-sided cardiac hemodynamics fail to improve in patients with apnea and lung disease in whom the apnea is not corrected.

It is interesting to note that patients with hypercapnia related to COPD do not have reduced drive to breathe as measured by P0.1 (the negative airway occlusion pressure 0.1 s after initiation of inspiration which is proportional to respiratory drive).[24] Also, existing evidence does not indicate that drive to breathe is affected detrimentally by oxygen therapy.[25,26] However, patients with COPD and a component of SDB may have reduced drive to breathe and may raise their PCO_2 during supplemental oxygen therapy to a point requiring mechanical support. We speculate that this is due to the induction of deep sleep by correction of the hypoxia that had resulted in long-term sleep interruption and deprivation. Therefore, when airflow obstruction is not severe enough to explain severe hypoventilation or the patient develops "CO_2 narcosis" with O_2 therapy, consider associated SDB. Such patients exhibit marked obesity and snoring.

Recognizing decompensated SDB, as distinct from acute on chronic respiratory failure due to advanced COPD, is essential, since specific therapy directed at the underlying sleep disorder can significantly reverse their multiple organ failures.

SLEEP-DISORDERED BREATHING IN "FAILURE TO WEAN"

Frequently, during treatment of decompensated obstructive apnea requiring an artificial airway and mechanical ventilation, underlying central alveolar hypoventilation may evolve. As a result, despite adequate resolution of airway obstruction or alveolar edema, restoration of sleep architecture and resolution of central apnea may lag behind other respiratory parameters.

Mechanical overventilation may decrease the renal compensation for chronic respiratory acidosis. This may frustrate attempts to decrease ventilatory support when central hypoventilation and respiratory acidosis recur during efforts to wean from mechanical ventilation. Also, since ac-

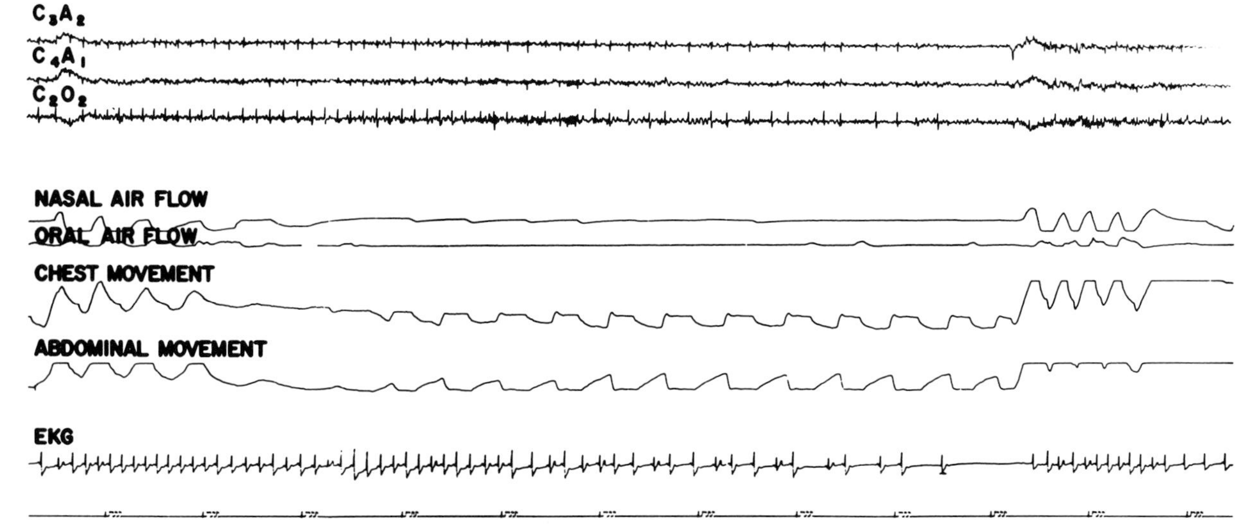

FIGURE 135-3 Polysomnographic tracing revealing obstructive apneas. Simultaneously recorded are the EEG (top three lines), air flow at the nose and mouth, chestwall-abdominal movement, and EKG. Note that airflow ceases (flattened lines) despite continued muscle activity, indicating airway obstruction. In central apnea muscle activity and airflow cease simultaneously. This apneic episode caused arterial saturation to fall from 90 to 62%, associated with a bradycardia as indicated on the EKG. The bottom line gives 5-second time intervals. (Reprinted with permission from Reference 2.)

quired pulmonary hypertension may cause right heart limitation of cardiac output, attention to central volume status and cardiopulmonary interactions is important. Finally, postextubation airway edema may result in sufficient SDB following extubation to give the appearance of hypercapnic respiratory failure. When patients who retain carbon dioxide following extubation do not manifest respiratory distress, the possibility of SDB should be considered.

Diagnosis

In all patients less ill or in those who have been stabilized, a good sleep history will give the most important clinical guide to the presence or absence of OSA. However, a positive diagnosis requires a polysomnogram (Fig. 135-3). This study will make the diagnosis, distinguish among the various forms of sleep apnea, assess the severity of the disease, and frequently, determine effective therapy. Formalized scoring of the entire polysomnographic record is recommended. Quantitative data should include information regarding sleep stages, types of respiratory patterns and their relationship to sleep stage and posture, arterial oxygen saturation, and cardiac rate and rhythm. Several indices have been used to describe the severity of illness: frequency of apnea, apnea duration, number of desaturations >4 percent, average desaturation per episode, and percentage of time below 90, 80, 70, and 60% saturation. These data are readily available by computer analysis.[27] Equally important, the effects of oxygen and nasal continuous positive airway pressure (CPAP) therapy can be evaluated using these parameters. Ideally, the sleep study is done in the ICU unit after extubation for seriously ill patients and includes response to therapy such as nasal CPAP.

Management

Not all patients with SDB will require diagnostic polysomnography prior to therapeutic intervention. Patients with hypercapnic respiratory failure, cor pulmonale, obtundation, and end-organ failure require prompt attention. Because compromised upper airway patency is frequent in these patients with advanced SDB, establishing an airway with endotracheal intubation is of paramount importance and can frequently be accomplished without sedation. A controlled airway minimizes the risk of aspiration and eliminates obstructive physiology immediately. Though the obstructive component of sleep apnea is relieved immediately, central apneas may increase for several days before waning[28] and hence, controlled ventilation is usually required. Frequently, patients with "end-stage" SDB will sleep for several days, with remarkable return of level of consciousness and cognitive function. Oxygen supplementation necessary to prevent desaturation during remaining apneas or to meet requirements of underlying lung disease relieves attendant hypoxic pulmonary vasoconstriction, improves right heart function and cardiac output, and contributes to a spontaneous diuresis. Oxygen administration alone is insufficient treatment for patients with critical levels of neurologic depression secondary to severe sleep fragmentation. Acutely, oxygen administration results in prolonged apneas, resulting in acute respiratory acidosis, despite the fact that chronic oxygen use may in fact reduce apneas.[29]

In patients less ill, there are a number of approaches to the treatment of SDB. However, foremost is the treatment of associated conditions which may hasten the resolution of SDB. Withdrawal of respiratory depressants and sedatives, treatment of underlying hypothyroidism, resolution of cor pulmonale with oxygen therapy, and reduction of airway edema associated with nephrotic syndrome and congestive heart failure are all to be undertaken simultaneously during therapy directed at upper airway obstruction and apnea. Prophylaxis for deep venous thrombosis and gastrointestinal hemorrhage are necessary due to their high incidence in these patients. A beneficial but difficult long-term goal is weight reduction.

Nasal CPAP is effective in the long-term treatment of OSA.[30] Patients generally accept nasal CPAP therapy fairly, well, though 5 percent do not tolerate it for reasons that include feelings of suffocation, nasal irritation, ear pain, and conjunctivitis. Surgical procedures, including uvulopalatopharyngoplasty, have been proposed to eliminate the site of upper airway obstruction. However, there is yet no sure way of identifying those patients with apneas who will improve with surgery. Tracheostomy is uniformly effective but is reserved for patients intolerant of nasal CPAP, since postoperative problems including stomal infection, speech interference, social acceptance, chronic cough, positional pain, and irritation are common.[31]

For the patient in the recovery room or ICU postoperatively with acute worsening of subclinical sleep apnea secondary to anesthetics, a temporizing measure is placement of an endotracheal tube nasally into the back of the pharynx without intubating the trachea. This prevents lower airway and laryngeal trauma but creates an effective channel to relieve obstruction. Soft compliant rubber nasopharyngeal catheters are ineffective since they collapse easily with negative pressure.The mechanism of action of this nasopharyngeal tube is probably to provide the sole conduit for airflow and not to serve as an airway stint, since apnea returns during temporary plugging of the tube.[32]

For the other groups of patients with chronic respiratory disease (COPD, cystic fibrosis, restrictive lung disease), neuromuscular disorders, and Cheyne-Stokes respirations, the clinician should maintain an awareness that these disorders frequently worsen with sleep, especially during critical illness.[33] The repercussions on gas exchange are more severe when baseline daytime hypoxemia exists. Continuous monitoring with pulse oximetry during critical illness will discern episodes of desaturation missed by intermittent arterial blood-gas sampling. Therapy directed at the underlying condition, along with supplemental oxygen and cardiac rhythm monitoring is usually sufficient.

CASE PRESENTATION

R.H., a 48 year-old man presented to the emergency room with shortness of breath and altered mental status. According to the family, the patient had noted dyspnea on exertion for several years, with intermittent choking sensations at night. During a recent clinic visit he was told he had "an enlarged heart" and hypertension, and he was begun on a diuretic and digoxin. He had made several emergency room visits in the past several months and was told he had "bronchitis and emphysema" and was started on inhaled bronchodilators. He had smoked one pack of cigarettes a day for 20 years. He had been moderately obese all his adult life, and in the past 6 months had gained an additional 40 lb. He was now 275 lb and 5 ft 7 in. tall.

On examination he was an obese gentleman who initially was stuporous but answered simple questions after being shaken. He was afebrile with a pulse of 110 and regular, blood pressure of 170/110, and respirations 18 and notable for stertorous sounds punctuated by silence as he dozed. His neck was stout, and no specific upper airway abnormality could be discerned. Lung examination revealed scattered expiratory wheezing. The heart sounds were rather indistinct but there was marked elevation of the jugular venous waveform and peripheral edema. The neurologic examination was nonfocal.

The initial laboratory data included an arterial blood-gas determination on room air with a P_{O_2} of 50 mmHg, P_{CO_2} of 65 mmHg, and pH of 7.33. The hematocrit was 49 with a normal white blood cell count and differential. The chest radiograph revealed clear lung fields and cardiomegaly. The creatinine was 2.6 mg/dL with a BUN of 65 mg/dL.

Oxygen was applied by nasal cannula at 4 L/min. A bronchodilator treatment by respiratory therapy was requested. The therapist arrived within 5 min, but the patient seemed more deeply obtunded. Sternal rub was necessary to elicit a response, and the patient pushed away examiners and would not answer questions. No respiratory distress was noted at any time. Endotracheal intubation was performed without difficulty or sedation. The patient remained stuporous following the procedure. He was moved to the ICU.

The patient remained minimally responsive for the next 48 h. Mechanical ventilation was instituted because the patient had episodes of apnea with desaturation noted by pulse oximetry. A brain computed tomography (CT) scan and toxicology screen of the urine were unrevealing. Further discussion with the family revealed a history of prominent snoring and gradual decline in cognitive function. An echocardiogram revealed right ventricular hypertrophy and dilation with paradoxical movement of the intraventricular septum. Estimated pulmonary artery pressure was 70/30. Bedside assessment of lung mechanics did not reveal intrinsic positive end-expiratory pressure (PEEP) or significant inspiratory resistance. Thyroid functions were within normal limits.

Over the first 2 days in the ICU the patient exhibited a marked diuresis without drug therapy. His BUN and creatinine levels fell. On the third day the patient awoke and responded normally to questions. The family observed he was "brighter than he had been for weeks." On the fourth ICU evening the patient was extubated and polysomnography was performed in the ICU. Within minutes of falling asleep, obstructive and central apneas were noted, with approximately 30 apneas/h noted, with a maximum duration of 38 sec. There was frequent arterial desaturation, to a nadir of 58%. Institution of nasal CPAP titrated to 13 cmH_2O resolved all obstruction, although central apneas persisted with desaturation. Supplemental oxygen added to the CPAP system eliminated all episodes of desaturation.

The patient was transferred to the ward and then home, with CPAP and oxygen to be used each evening. Marked improvement in neurologic function continued to improve over several weeks. He continued to diurese during the first week out of the ICU and then began a program of weight loss. When seen in follow-up 3 months later, a repeat echocardiogram revealed a smaller right ventricular diameter, normal septal movement, and an estimated pulmonary artery pressure of 45/20 mmHg.

CASE DISCUSSION

This patient presented with combined cardiorespiratory failure. In this obese male, the history of intermittent choking sensations at night (termination of OSA), prominent snoring, and gradual decline in cognitive function, combined with a primary symptom of dyspnea on exertion (from underlying pulmonary hypertension), suggested SDB. His systemic hypertension was probably multifactorial, but is nevertheless found in 50 percent of patients with SDB. Symptomatic airflow obstruction posed an additional risk factor for sleep-associated desaturation and his development of sustained pulmonary hypertension. The recent weight gain was temporally related to the advancing symptom complex. The laboratory findings of compensated respiratory acidosis and polycythemia are frequent markers of chronic alveolar hypoventilation. The moderate renal failure and CNS dysfunction are common end-organ failures in SDB.

The hypoventilatory response to supplemental oxygen with deterioration of mental status suggested an impaired drive to breathe not typical for most COPD patients. Removal of oxygen supplementation at that time, in an "attempt to increase ventilatory responsiveness" would have led to life-threatening hypoxemia. The correct therapy of relieving airway obstruction and applying supplemental oxygen was lifesaving.

The gradual neurologic improvement occurred during restoration of normal sleep architecture. Since metabolic, toxic, and CNS disorders can lead to a decreased drive to breathe, these disorders were appropriately excluded. The echocardiogram confirmed right ventricular dilation with pulmonary hypertension and compromised left ventricular function secondary to paradoxical septal motion. The spontaneous diuresis underscores the improvement in cardiac output after relief of hypoxic pulmonary vasoconstriction. Diuretic therapy is frequently unwarranted and poses the potential problem of decreased venous return, equating to decreased cardiac output, especially in patients receiving positive-pressure ventilation. The lack of intrinsic PEEP or dynamic inspiratory resistance suggested that airway obstruction was a relatively minor contributor to alveolar hypoventilation, compared to the SDB.

Coincident with mental status improvement, the patient's drive to breathe normalized, allowing for extubation. The ICU polysomnogram confirmed the diagnosis and demonstrated nasal CPAP to be effective therapy. Central apneas resolved with time, although temporary supplemental oxygen was necessary. The reduction in pulmonary artery pressures remind us to include SDB in the differential diagnosis of all cases of unexplained pulmonary hypertension.

References

1. Orem JM: Central neural interactions between sleep and breathing, in Sanders NA, Sullivan CE (eds): *Sleep and Breathing.* New York, Dekker, 1984 pp 91–136.
2. Hall JB: The cardiopulmonary failure of sleep-disordered breathing. JAMA 255(7):930, 1986.
3. Onal E, Lopata M: Periodic breathing and the pathogenesis of occlusive sleep apnea. Am Rev Respir Dis 126:676, 1982.
4. Rajagopal KR, Abbrecht PH, Tellis CJ: Control of breathing in obstructive sleep apnea. Chest 85(2):174, 1984.
5. Hudgel DW, Chapman KR, Faulks C, Hendricks C: Changes in inspiratory muscle electrical activity and upper airway resistance during periodic breathing induced by hypoxia during sleep. Am Rev Respir Dis 135:899, 1987.
6. Issa FG, Sullivan CE: Upper airway closing pressures in obstructive sleep apnea. J Appl Physiol 57:520, 1984.
7. Ray CS, Sue DY, Bray G, et al: Effects of obesity on respiratory function. Am Rev Respir Dis 128:501, 1983.
8. Burki NK, Baker RW: Ventilatory regulation in eucapnic morbid obesity. Am Rev Respir Dis 129:538, 1984.
9. Tobin MJ, Snyder JV: Cheyne-Stokes respiration revisited: Controversies and implications. Crit Care Med 12(10):882, 1984.
10. Fletcher EC, Costarangos C, Miller T: The rate of fall of arterial oxyhemoglobin saturation in obstructive sleep apnea. Chest 96(4):717, 1989.
11. Guilleminault C, Connolly SJ, Winkle RA: Cardiac arrhythmia and conduction disturbances during sleep in 400 patients with sleep apnea syndrome. Am J Cardiol. 52:490, 1983.
12. Bradley TD, Rutherford R, Grossman RF, et al: Role of daytime hypoxemia in the pathogenesis of right heart failure in the obstructive sleep apnea syndrome. Am Rev Respir Dis 131:835, 1985.
13. Fletcher EC, Schaff JW, Miller J, Fletcher JG: Long-term cardiopulmonary sequelae in patients with sleep apnea and chronic lung disease. Am Rev Respir Dis 135:525, 1987.
14. Weitzenblum E, Krieger J, Apprill M, et al: Daytime pulmonary hypertension in patients with obstructive sleep apnea syndrome. Am Rev Respir Dis 138:345, 1988.
15. Fletcher EC, DeBehnke RD, Lovoi MS, et al: Undiagnosed sleep apnea in patients with essential hypertension. Ann Intern Med; 102:190, 1985.
16. Tolle FA, Judy WV, Yu PL, Markand ON: Reduced stroke volume related to pleural pressure in obstructive sleep apnea. J Appl Physiol: Respirat Environ Exercise Physiol 55(6):1718, 1983.
17. Chaudhary BA, Nadimi M, Chaudhary TK, Speir WA: Pulmonary edema due to obstructive sleep apnea. South Med J 77(4):499, 1984.
18. Herlihy JP, Whitlock WL, Dietrich RA, Shaw T: Sleep apnea syndrome after irradiation of the neck. Arch Otolaryngol Head Neck Surg 115(12):1467, 1989.
19. Fein AM, Niederman MS, Imbriano L, Rosen H: Reversal of sleep apnea in uremia by dialysis Arch Intern Med 147(7):1355, 1987.

20. Dolly FR, Block AJ: Effect of flurazepam on sleep-disordered breathing and nocturnal oxygen desaturation in asymptomatic subjects. Am J Med 73:239, 1982.
21. Orr WC, Males JL, Imes NK: Myxedema and obstructive sleep apnea. Am J Med 70:1061, 1981.
22. Keamy MF, Cadieux RJ, Kofke WA, Kales A: The occurrence of obstructive sleep apnea in a recovery room patient. Anesthesiology 66(2):232, 1987.
23. Knill RL, Gelb AW: Peripheral chemoreceptors during anesthesia. Are the watch dogs sleeping? Anesthesiology 57:151, 1982.
24. Aubier M, Murciano D, Fournier M, et al: Effects of the administration of O_2 on ventilation and blood gases in patients with chronic obstructive pulmonary disease during acute respiratory failure. Am Rev Respir Dis 122:747, 1980.
25. Aubier M, Murciano D, Fournier M, et al: Central respiratory drive in acute respiratory failure of patients with chronic obstructive pulmonary disease. Am Rev Respir Dis 122:191, 1980.
26. Sassoon CSH, Hassell KT, Mahutte CK: Hyperoxic-induced hypercapnia in stable chronic obstructive pulmonary disease. Am Rev Respir Dis 135:907, 1987.
27. Medical Section of the American Lung Association. Indications and standards for cardiopulmonary sleep studies. Am Rev Respir Dis 138:591, 1988.
28. Guilleminault C, Cummiskey J: Progressive improvement of apnea index and ventilatory response to CO_2 after tracheostomy in obstructive sleep apnea syndrome. Am Rev Respir Dis 126:14, 1982.
29. Martin RJ, Sander MH, Gray BA, Pennock BE: Acute and long-term ventilatory effects of oxygen administration in adult sleep apnea syndrome. Am Rev Respir Dis 125:175, 1982.
30. Remmers JE, Sterling JA, Thorarinsson B, Kuna ST: Nasal airway positive airway pressure in patients with occlusive sleep apnea. Am Rev Respir Dis 130:1152, 1984.
31. Dayal VS, Brais F: Tracheotomy in long-term management of sleep apnea. J Otolaryngol 10:273, 1981.
32. Nahmias JS, Karetzky MS: Treatment of the obstructive sleep apnea syndrome using a nasopharyngeal tube. Chest 94:1142, 1988.
33. Krieger J, Weitzenblum, Racineux JL: Chronic respiratory disease and sleep in adults. Bull Eur Physiopathol Respir 23:479, 1987.

Chapter 136

ASPIRATION SYNDROMES

AARON R. ZUCKER
JACOB IASHA SZNAJDER

KEY POINTS

- *Aspirations must be excluded as the cause of respiratory distress or hypoventilation of obscure etiology.*
- *Aspiration syndromes are largely preventable with attention to the minimization of risks.*
- *Solid materials cause hypoxemia from large-airways obstruction; smaller objects cause bronchospasm, atelectasis, hemoptysis, bronchiectasis, and chronic infections.*
- *Liquid aspirations cause pulmonary capillary leak and acute hypoxemic respiratory failure, even in the absence of bacterial superinfection and pneumonia.*
- *Corticosteroids and other specific therapies for the capillary leak are ineffective; antibiotics should be used for specific indications.*
- *Edema is reduced by lowering pulmonary capillary hydrostatic pressures to the least value compatible with adequate cardiac output.*
- *Shunt and hypoxemia are reduced with the least positive end-expiratory pressure (PEEP) necessary to maintain oxygen saturation above 90 percent of a sufficient circulating hematocrit (i.e., a hematocrit of 35) while administering a nontoxic* F_{IO_2} *(<0.6).*
- *Barotrauma is minimized by ventilation with the least tidal volume preventing untoward respiratory acidosis (*$Pa_{CO_2} <$ *50 mmHg; pH > 7.30).*

The first description of clinical findings in women thought to have aspirated stomach contents during labor is often credited to Mendelson.[1] He reasoned that these women suffered from the effects of gastric acid on the tracheobronchial tree. Subsequent research showed that the pulmonary injury was largely dependent on pH, volume, and distribution of aspirates. Significant pulmonary dysfunction also resulted from aspiration of other nonacidic substances, particulate matter, and heavily infected gastrointestinal contents. These diseases are categorized as "aspiration syndromes" and are discussed separately under general headings of solid aspirations, liquid aspirations, and aspirations of infected materials. Their prevention and management is a daily concern for the intensivist, since etiologic studies have implicated them in approximately 40 percent of cases of the adult respiratory distress syndrome (ARDS).[2]

Risk of Aspiration

The body has a complex, efficient protective mechanism that minimizes the risk of aspiration of noxious substances while breathing, speaking, and swallowing. During breathing, the epiglottis remains in a resting position, allowing unobstructed air flow in either direction through the open vocal cords. During swallowing, entry of foreign substances and saliva into the nasopharynx is prevented as the soft palate moves upward and posteriorly. Simultaneously, the epiglottis descends to seal the glottis as the vocal cords adduct, thus protecting the lower respiratory tract from the oncoming bolus. The constrictor muscles of the pharynx then propel the substance past the glottis into the esophagus, where secondary peristaltic waves both push it through the lower esophageal sphincter into the stomach, and prevent its reflux toward the pharynx. Reflux is further minimized by the high resting tension of the lower esophageal sphincter (approximately 25 to 30 mmHg). These mechanisms act in concert to minimize entry of foreign materials into the respiratory tract. However, small amounts of gastric contents may asymptomatically reflux into the upper airways in normal people during sleep.

These protective mechanisms are efficient enough to prevent even the products of repetitive vomiting or gastroesophageal reflux from harming the airways. Clinically significant aspiration syndromes occur only when these defenses are overwhelmed for any of a variety of reasons (Table 136-1). In a pregnant woman, effects of the growing uterus can compound hormonally induced decreases in gastric motility and lower esophageal sphincter tone, thereby predisposing the woman to reflux. Patients with weakness of the musculature involved in airway protection may be alert but unable to muster the usual defenses against aspiration. Head trauma, coma, drug toxicities, central nervous system (CNS) infections, and seizures combine with vomiting and depressed reflexes to make aspiration a serious threat. Patients undergoing resuscitation and emergency intubation, especially those with a full stomach, may be difficult to intubate and may have a propensity to vomit and aspirate during the procedure. Patients requiring intubation after head and neck trauma run the added risk of aspirating blood. Surgical patients are at increased risk, especially if an operative procedure is emergently necessary before the stomach has been emptied. Patients fed through nasogastric or transpyloric tubes have decreased airway protection at both glottic and lower esophageal sphincter levels.

Prevention of Aspiration Syndromes

Some simple maneuvers can reduce the likelihood of aspiration in high-risk patients. For example, unconscious patients can be placed in a head-down lateral position, while patients with gastroesophageal reflux or swallowing disorders can be maintained at 30° head elevation.[3] Though clinical studies of multiple risk factors in adults have failed

TABLE 136-1 Conditions Predisposing to Aspiration Syndromes

Depressed central nervous system reflexes
Hypoxemia; hypercarbia
Coma
Head trauma
Drug overdoses and ethanol toxicity
Anesthesia and sedative drugs
Seizures
Metabolic encephalopathies
Nervous system infections
Sepsis
Dementia
Structural lesions of the central nervous system
Abnormal pharyngeal function
Guillain-Barré syndrome
Trauma to the neck and pharynx
Surgery of the neck and pharynx
Myasthenia gravis
Multiple sclerosis
Cranial nerve dysfunction
Amyotrophic lateral sclerosis
Botulism
Muscular dystrophy
Dermatomyositis
Nasogastric tubes, with or without feeding
Gastrointestinal bleeding
Miscellaneous disorders
Emergency and routine airway manipulations
Pregnancy
Intestinal obstruction
Gastroesophageal reflux
Scleroderma
Esophageal diverticula
Achalasia
Upper endoscopy
Vomiting
Near-drowning

to document a clear association between aspiration and depressed levels of consciousness or constant supine positioning, these recommendations are favored for such high-risk patients.[4] One must keep in mind that such manipulations cannot entirely prevent aspiration.

While many of the conditions in Table 136-1 cannot be modified by the physician, decreased consciousness and other reversible risks can be diagnosed and treated. Rapid treatment of seizures, as well as emptying the stomach prior to nonemergency surgery, will reduce the chance of vomiting and subsequent gastric aspiration. Should vomiting occur, anticipation of respiratory failure in deteriorating patients allows for well-planned, safe intubations that can be facilitated by sedation and/or muscle relaxation and the availability of large-bore suction catheters. Blood gas analysis revealing frank respiratory failure mandates prompt administration of supplemental oxygen and evaluation for the need for tracheal intubation. When emergency intubation is needed, Sellick's maneuver reduces, but does not eliminate, the chances of aspiration. Likewise, establishing an artificial airway does not preclude the risk of aspiration. In patients with endotracheal tubes or tracheostomies, the incidence of dye-detectable aspirations is as high as 80 percent.[5] Since many such patients have recurrent or progressive pulmonary disease, recurrent aspiration is the presumed cause. Although the mechanism by which either tube type adversely affects airway protection is obscure, the advent of thin-walled, high-volume, low-pressure cuffs is associated with decreased frequency of aspirations. When these cuffs are inflated to approximately 25 mmHg, the risk of aspiration is substantially reduced, but the cuffs still allow adequate capillary flow to the tracheal mucosa.[6,7]

In patients with stomach distension, the risk of aspiration due to stomach enlargement must be weighed against that due to nasogastric tube placement, since these tubes interfere with normal lower esophageal sphincter function. Stomach distension is usually the more pressing problem. Thus, patients with intestinal obstructions, gastrointestinal bleeding, or positive-pressure ventilation should have a nasogastric tube placed for decompression. Since the magnitude of lung damage from aspiration is significantly related to acidity, the common practice of administering antacids to increase gastric pH in order to prevent gastrointestinal ulceration might also reduce aspiration pneumonitis. However, there is no proof that this practice reduces morbidity or mortality in patients who aspirate stomach contents; in fact, it may increase the incidence of nosocomial pneumonia (see Aspiration of Infected Materials, below). Furthermore, particulate antacids have been shown to cause lung injury. While antacids increase the pH of previously secreted gastric juices, their benefit may be outweighed by the addition of liquid volume to the stomach contents already present. Histamine-2 antagonist drugs were developed to reduce peptic ulcer formation caused by gastric acidity, but their effect of reducing gastric liquid volume was invoked as a preoperative mechanism for reducing aspirations. Ranitidine is increasingly being used in intensive care units (ICUs) and operating rooms for prevention of both ulcers and aspiration.[8] Metoclopramide increases gastric motility and emptying and lowers esophageal pressure, thereby reducing the risk of regurgitation and aspiration. Theoretically, adding this drug to a histamine-2 antagonist combines their beneficial effects.[9]

Another common reason for stomach distension in ICU patients is over-aggressive nasogastric feedings. Frequently, methylene blue dye is put into the feedings of patients at risk for aspiration; if dye is later found in the airways, feeding practices are altered. Patients with chronically depressed CNS function often have repeated aspiration episodes, which may cause recurrent bronchospasm and lung damage. This is especially relevant to the pediatric population, where aspirations are a problem in children with cerebral palsy or other reasons for discoordinated swallowing. Although simple gastrostomy may suffice for adequate caloric intake, a significant percentage of these patients still aspirate. When long-term feeding problems are expected in spite of medical therapy, surgical interventions such as gastrostomy/enterostomy, often combined with an antireflux procedure (e.g., Nissen fundoplication), can be beneficial.[3]

Pathophysiology and Management of Aspiration Syndromes

ASPIRATION OF SOLIDS

Aspirated solid materials can be immediately life-threatening if they are large enough to obstruct the major airways. If awake, the victim may exhibit severe respiratory distress and cyanosis. Fatal hypoxemia can ensue unless the obstruction is promptly relieved. The Heimlich maneuver and other such methods can be used to forcefully dislodge the obstructing material by acutely raising intrathoracic pressure. Foreign body aspiration must also be suspected in patients with both depressed sensorium and either severe respiratory distress or hypoventilation. Initially, the pharynx should be assessed for the presence of foreign matter by inspection and oropharyngeal suctioning; an effort to obtain as much history as possible about the predisposing factors should also be made.

Prolonged inspiration accompanied by stridor may be heard if a partial upper airway obstruction is present; additional expiratory stridor and prolongation signify a greater functional extrathoracic obstruction. Smaller solid items, such as peanuts and other foodstuffs, children's toys, or teeth dislodged by trauma or during intubation attempts, may migrate to lower airways and cause coughing, chest pain, and varying degrees of hypoxemia, depending on the caliber of the airway they occlude. While examining a patient, one may hear localized or generalized wheezing both from airway turbulence caused by the object and from reflex bronchospasm. Alternatively, one may appreciate areas of diminished breath sounds due to atelectasis behind an obstructing foreign body. Chest x-rays may be useful for following the course of an aspiration and will reveal radiopaque foreign bodies or partial obstructive lesions. If evidence points to an object, or several objects, obstructing one or more large bronchi, bronchoscopy with either a rigid or flexible bronchoscope should be performed. The choice of apparatus depends on the size of the item(s) to be removed. This is important, because if the object is not promptly coughed up or actively removed, atelectasis distal to the obstruction may occur. In addition, some foreign materials provoke a chronic inflammatory reaction even after they are removed; this may progress to a localized pneumonitis and bronchiectasis.

ASPIRATION OF LIQUIDS

ASPIRATION OF STOMACH CONTENTS

After Mendelson's initial clinical description of the results of aspiration of stomach contents in pregnant women, animal research elucidated the mechanism of lung injury. The acidity of the aspirated liquid was shown to be important; as the pH of fluids instilled into the lungs fell below a critical value of 2.5, increasing damage to the respiratory epithelium occurred. Little further injury occurred when pH fell below 1.5.[10] However, the extent of lung injury is not solely dependent on pH, since even aspiration of gastric juice buffered to pH 5.9 provokes significant pulmonary inflammation and dysfunction if particulate matter is suspended in the fluid.[11] This may be followed by chronic bronchiolitis, pneumonitis, bronchiectasis, and granuloma formation.

Gastric acid itself causes acute pulmonary dysfunction in several ways. Even after small aspirations, immediate vagally mediated bronchospasm frequently occurs in both animal models and patients. After larger aspirations, dye added to the aspirate appears on the pleural surface within seconds as a result of chemically induced injury of the alveolar epithelium and endothelium.[12] Atelectasis is apparent within minutes, yet microscopic lesions and edema formation usually are not severe for 1 h or longer after injury in experimental animals. Within several hours, acid aspirations present as extensive permeability pulmonary edema, with severe hypoxemia due to shunt.[13] In addition to the direct membrane damage and pulmonary capillary leak caused by the acid, some investigators believe that the earliest hypoxemia is partially due to large areas of atelectasis resulting from dysfunction of pulmonary surfactant. This may result from actual destruction of surfactant by acid, and from surfactant inactivation by plasma and membrane proteins in the edema fluid.[14]

After gastric aspiration, patients may be minimally symptomatic and show little abnormality on chest x-ray. On the other hand, they may be severely distressed, with rapidly progressive hypoxemia and pulmonary infiltrates. The nature, volume, and distribution of the aspirate, along with the patient's hydration status, will determine the early course of disease. For severely ill patients, our approach combines early support with mechanical ventilation with attempts to minimize edema formation. We try to limit edema formation because laboratory and clinical evidence suggests that doing so decreases shunt and lung stiffness as well as the subsequent duration of ventilator, oxygen, and ICU therapies, which have their own complications (see Innovative Approaches to Aspiration Lung Injury, below).

Differential Diagnosis

Aspiration may occur as an isolated event or in the setting of a patient otherwise at risk for development of ARDS. Regardless, the final common pathway of increased pulmonary capillary permeability will result in pulmonary edema formation and hypoxemia from shunt. Careful observation and attention to recent medical history are helpful in separating aspiration pneumonitis from high-pressure pulmonary edema. Acute myocardial dysfunction and intravascular fluid overload must be excluded, since these entities require different approaches to care. While these latter conditions may be easy to discern clinically in individual cases, more objective assessment of hemodynamic parameters with a Swan-Ganz catheter may be necessary.

Oxygen Therapy and Mechanical Ventilation

Supplemental oxygen should be administered to patients with respiratory distress after a witnessed or suspected aspiration. Initially, respiratory distress and work of breathing may be mild, and blood gas analysis may show that increasing the inspired oxygen by face mask is all that is needed to maintain 90% saturation (Pa_{O_2} approximately 60 mmHg). If the patient remains alert and nonfatigued, and Pa_{O_2} stays above 60 mmHg while breathing oxygen-enriched air, intubation and mechanical ventilation may be avoided. While patients may initially satisfy these flexible criteria, they frequently worsen as edema forms and shunt increases. Shunt diseases are not responsive to simple oxygen therapy, so intubation and application of PEEP are necessary.

PEEP does not reduce alveolar edema, but redistributes it to the interstitial space, where it interferes less with gas exchange and lung mechanics.[15] We advocate using the "least PEEP" necessary to maintain hemoglobin saturation at or above 90%, while delivering relatively nontoxic concentrations of oxygen (i.e., below 60%). We also attempt to use the lowest tidal volume providing adequate carbon dioxide elimination (usually below 10 mL/kg), to reduce both adverse effects on cardiac output and the chances of pulmonary barotrauma. In normal rats and sheep, ventilation with high volumes and pressures directly increases lung permeability, resulting in frank edema after 30 min; dogs ventilated for 4 h after acid aspiration with high tidal volumes have 60 percent more edema than those ventilated with small tidal volumes.[16] After many aspiration injuries, relatively normal alveoli coexist with fluid-filled ones. If mechanical ventilation with "normal" ventilator tidal volumes (10 to 15 mL/kg) is instituted, preferential overdistension of the normal, more compliant alveoli may result in augmentation of the original lung injury, or in pneumothorax.

Cardiovascular Management of Severe Aspiration

Detailed discussions of the microcirculatory forces promoting edema formation appear in Chaps. 2 and 28. Following acid aspiration, protein-rich edema forms as the coefficient of vascular permeability (K_f) increases and the protein reflection coefficient (σ) decreases. Several studies have produced equivocal answers to the question whether steroids might reduce the lung injury following acid aspiration. We do not use steroids even in these circumstances, because of their potential for inducing fluid and electrolyte disorders and infection and the lack of evidence for improved outcome in similar lung injuries.[17] Since no other specific therapies exist to normalize either K_f or σ, only changes in the hydrostatic pressure gradient from capillary to interstitium (Pmv − Pis) affect edema formation. After aspiration of hydrochloric acid in dogs, edema decreases by 50 percent when pulmonary capillary hydrostatic pressures are reduced by 5 mmHg for 4 h[13,18]; there are associated reductions in shunt, hypoxemia, and lung stiffness. These canine studies provide compelling evidence that pulmonary vascular leak is reduced by lowering pulmonary vascular pressures after acute lung injury, and several reports support this approach in human beings.[19,20]

We approach fluid management by seeking the lowest pulmonary capillary wedge pressure (Ppw) consistent with an adequate cardiac output of a well-saturated red cell mass. We define "adequate cardiac output" as that at which there is no systemic metabolic acidosis, and clinical assessment of peripheral circulation (mentation, urinary output, capillary refill) is satisfactory. We maintain the hemoglobin level between 12 and 15 g/dL and use PEEP as described above. When lung leak is severe and a patient is unstable, Swan-Ganz catheterization adds objective support to the clinical examination and therapeutic decisions. There is no absolute value of Ppw that is acceptable; in some patients with left ventricular dysfunction, adequate cardiac output requires a Ppw of 20 mmHg, whereas most patients with aspiration pneumonitis have adequate cardiac output at a Ppw of less than 8 mmHg. Still others have sufficient cardiac function when the Ppw is lowered toward zero.[19,20] Accordingly, adjustments of circulating volume and Ppw must be titrated against changes in clinical examination of cardiac output in each patient.

Increments in PEEP raise the measured Ppw by increasing the pleural pressure surrounding the heart. Normally, pleural pressure increases by approximately 50 percent of applied PEEP; in situations of reduced lung compliance this may decrease slightly.[21] Therefore, the measured Ppw overestimates the transmural cardiac filling pressure by these amounts. In practice, these effects of PEEP on Ppw measurements are small, and they have no impact at all on the strategy of seeking the lowest Ppw compatible with adequate cardiac output on each level of PEEP. Yet worsening hypoxemia can require increased PEEP, which often reduces venous return and cardiac output. In such situations, inotropic support may be helpful to maintain adequate cardiovascular status while minimizing fluid administration. Patients with stiff lungs have an increased proportion of cardiac output to the laboring respiratory muscles, which increases minute oxygen consumption.[22] Sedation and neuromuscular paralysis are often helpful in minimizing these abnormalities, and allow redirection of blood flow and oxygen to other vital tissues. We advocate muscle relaxation and controlled mechanical ventilation in the early phases of severe pulmonary capillary leak states when difficulty is encountered in establishing adequate oxygenation and ventilation. After the patient has been stabilized, we discontinue paralysis and mechanically ventilate with either the synchronized intermittent mandatory mode or the assist control mode.

ASPIRATION OF OTHER LIQUIDS

In the initial investigations of the effects of acidic fluids on the lungs, small amounts of normal saline solution (pH 5.9) were also studied and did not cause lesions. When large amounts of neutral liquids are aspirated into the alveoli, however, serious pulmonary dysfunction ensues. Clinically, this occurs after near-drowning episodes, although a significant proportion of submerged victims do not aspirate large quantities of water. When water is aspirated into the terminal airways, displacement of air from the alveolar space causes pulmonary shunting and hypoxemia. In addition, surfactant may be washed out and/or inactivated, further contributing to hypoxemia by promoting air space collapse due to increased alveolar surface tension. This collapse causes the interstitial pressure surrounding pulmonary capillaries (Pis) to become more negative, increasing the hydrostatic driving pressure (Pmv − Pis) for edema formation.[23] Although the mechanism of this edema formation differs from the capillary leak state after acid injury, the end result is basically the same: flooded alveoli causing stiff, poorly functioning lungs. Near-drowning victims may also have additional lung injury caused by aspiration of stomach contents.

Blood may reach the terminal airways after head and neck trauma or surgery; pulmonary hemorrhage; disseminated intravascular coagulation; or any cause of hematemesis. The severity of the resulting hypoxemia and respiratory distress due to intrapulmonary shunting is primarily related to the amount of aspirated blood. Although the patient may be severely ill initially, the blood is typically cleared from the lungs in several days with only supportive care.

Hydrocarbon aspiration accounts for almost 20 percent of reported accidental intoxications in children under 5 years of age. Hydrocarbons with high vapor pressures (mineral seal oil, kerosene) spread throughout the tracheobronchial tree more readily, but any of them can cause severe alveolar injury, either during the initial aspiration or after regurgitation of the liquid or its vapor from the stomach. In the past, patients aspirating hydrocarbons often were given emetics or underwent gastric lavage and suction to remove any hydrocarbon from the stomach. However, with the realization that gastrointestinal absorption plays no role in the systemic toxicity after such events,[24] these interventions are no longer recommended unless it is known that another life-threatening toxin has also been ingested (organophosphate insecticides, etc.). Hydrocarbons cause pulmonary capillary leak by dissolving membrane-structural lipid molecules and/or directly inactivating surfactant. As with acid aspirations, the results are alveolar edema, stiff lungs, and intrapulmonary shunting.[25] In a canine model of hydrocarbon aspiration in which 0.25 mL of kerosene was instilled into each mainstem bronchus, plasmapheresis was used to reduce Ppw from 10 to 5 mmHg for 5 h post-injury. Edema formation was reduced significantly from control values, with an associated reduction in shunt and improved lung compliance—results similar to those seen after such interventions in hydrochloric acid aspiration injury. An integrated approach to the treatment of hydrocarbon aspiration as a model of permeability pulmonary edema will be presented at the end of this chapter.

ASPIRATION OF INFECTED MATERIALS

Many toxic substances initially provoke a severe, acute inflammatory reaction with infiltrates on x-ray, and fever. Yet infection rarely plays a significant role in the first few days after aspiration. Normally, the acidity of stomach contents minimizes the bacterial load entering the airways during an aspiration episode. In fact, most gastric aspirations are not followed by bacterial infections or superinfection; but when these consequences do occur (20 to 30 percent of cases), they are associated with a significant increase in morbidity and mortality. In patients aspirating outside the hospital, bacteria entering the lower respiratory tract are likely to represent those normally found in the oral cavity—i.e., a mixture of aerobes (*Staphylococcus aureus, Streptococcus pneumoniae,* etc.) and anaerobes (*Fusobacterium nucleatum, Peptostreptococcus, Bacteroides fragilis,* etc.). Patients who have been in the hospital, especially those with debilitating chronic diseases, endotracheal tubes, and oral disease (dental abscesses, etc.), are frequently heavily colonized with gram-negative organisms in the oropharynx or apparatus. In one large clinical study, patients with community-acquired secondary infection were more likely to have purely anaerobic isolates, while those with hospital-acquired disease frequently had mixed infections.[26]

This alteration of flora is also favored by the almost routine use, in many ICUs, of antacids and histamine antagonists (cimetidine, ranitidine) for gastric ulcer prevention. While having a salutary effect on the gastric mucosa, the increase in pH promotes the growth of bacteria, especially gram-negative species such as *Pseudomonas aeruginosa* and *Escherichia coli*. This has been correlated, in clinical studies, with an increase in nosocomial pneumonias after aspiration episodes.[27] To avoid this problem, clinicians have begun administering sucralfate instead of histamine antagonists. This compound acts as an adherent barrier to protect the gastric mucosa from the effects of acid and pepsin.

Empiric antibiotic therapy is indicated after aspiration of fecal material in patients with paralytic or obstructive ileus. In such circumstances, broad-spectrum antibiotic coverage should be instituted (e.g., clindamycin and an aminoglycoside). In other situations, some physicians assess the likelihood of specific pathogens (normal mouth anaerobes in healthy patients, enteric gram-negative bacteria in chronically ill patients, etc.), select antibiotics empirically (penicillin G in the former case, a third-generation cephalosporin plus an aminoglycoside in the latter), and observe for improvement. However, others feel that empiric therapy is unwarranted after most aspirations, since it may promote the emergence of resistant bacterial strains. An alternative strategy is to attempt isolation of the responsible organisms(s) while beginning therapy. Routine tracheal aspirate specimens may be helpful if they reveal pure growth of a pathogen, but contamination with oropharyngeal flora frequently occurs. To minimize specimen contamination, some authors advocate obtaining specimens of lower respiratory flora with a protected specimen brush catheter, either by blindly passing this through an endotracheal tube[28] or by using bronchoscopic guidance.[29] Selective antibiotic treatment can then be instituted in individual patients based on culture results.

Innovative Approaches to Aspiration Lung Injury

Even with the best of care, the capillary leak state following aspiration lung injury has a high mortality rate. This has led to investigations of other methods of treatment, including extracorporeal membrane oxygenation (ECMO), alternative modes of mechanical ventilation, surfactant replacement therapy, and biochemical interventions to reduce purported mediators of continuing lung injury.

The use of ECMO apparatus as a temporary artificial lung is being reevaluated as a method of patient support that might minimize barotrauma, improve oxygenation, and reduce morbidity and mortality. This technique is discussed in detail in Chap. 29. ECMO has been effective in treating neonates with refractory hypoxemia from such diseases as meconium aspiration, persistent fetal circulation syndrome, and hyaline membrane disease. These successes have regenerated interest in its utility for adult diseases, despite disappointing clinical experience more than a decade ago.[30] While some recent success has been reported,[31] the data have yet to be reproduced, so further studies will be important in determining the potential future use of ECMO.

Other alternative modes of mechanical ventilation have been evaluated, such as high-frequency ventilation, jet ventilation, high-frequency oscillation, and constant-flow ventilation. These share the common problem that pressure measured at the endotracheal tube underestimates alveolar pressures; this underestimation is due to momentum transfer and Bernoulli effect (see Chap. 127). At this time, each mode remains an experimental tool with little evidence of clinical utility. There are abundant reasons to anticipate complications, not the least of which is the distraction from effective therapy caused by a noisy ventilator without the usual alarms.

Exogenous surfactant has been successfully used to treat premature babies with hyaline membrane disease of the newborn, wherein absence of surfactant development is the primary cause of alveolar collapse and hypoxemia. Since secondary surfactant deficiency and dysfunction occur after many acute lung injuries,[32] the effects of surfactant replacement in animals and patients with increased pulmonary capillary permeability are being evaluated.[33,34] We recently studied the effects of exogenous bovine surfactant (100 mg of phospholipid per kg) on the course of edema formation in euvolemic dogs undergoing hydrochloric acid aspiration. One hour after injury, animals received either 45 mL of surfactant or an equal volume of saline placebo into each mainstem bronchus. After 5 h, gravimetric edema in excised lungs from the surfactant group was reduced by 50 percent compared to control dogs, accompanied by a significant reduction in shunt. These results suggest that surfactant replacement may be beneficial in the acute stages of aspiration pneumonitis; further studies and clinical trials are ongoing.

Other proposed therapies are being evaluated for the treatment of aspiration lung injury at the cellular and subcellular levels in animal models.[35] When neutrophils are activated during pulmonary injury, they may adhere to the lung capillaries and release membrane oxidants, such as oxygen free radical species. These can augment the original lung damage. Pentoxifylline is a chemical that reduces neutrophil adhesion to the pulmonary capillaries; to the extent that these cells amplify lung injury after the initial event, pentoxifylline therapy may be beneficial. Systemic administration of *N*-acetylcysteine increases levels of the antioxidant glutathione, which also might mitigate against the injury amplification caused by activated neutrophils and their oxidant products. Direct antioxidant therapies with DMSO and other oxygen radical–scavenging agents are also under study.

CASE PRESENTATION

A previously healthy 18-month-old female (body weight 10 kg) suddenly began coughing and vomiting. Nearby, an empty bottle which had contained kerosene for fueling a room heater, was found. The child appeared well for a short time, but on arrival at a local emergency room she was tachypneic and agitated. Supplemental oxygen by face mask was immediately administered, and the patient's distress decreased somewhat. An arterial blood gas determination revealed a pH of 7.14, Pa_{O_2} 48 mmHg, and Pa_{CO_2} 90 mmHg. Orotracheal intubation was attempted without sedation or neuromuscular paralysis; during this procedure the patient vomited twice. After intubation, hand-bagging with 100% oxygen was performed; an observer noted that this was difficult to perform in spite of certainty that the tube was correctly placed. A repeat blood gas analysis showed a pH of 7.18, Pa_{O_2} 58 mmHg, and Pa_{CO_2} 74 mmHg. Before transfer to a tertiary care facility, gastric lavage was performed, and activated charcoal was administered by nasogastric tube.

FIGURE 136-1 Photographic reproduction of the initial portable anterior-posterior chest x-ray, showing four-quadrant air space filling with air bronchograms and a heart that is not obviously enlarged. This severe pulmonary edema caused arterial desaturation (82%) on $F_{I_{O_2}}$ = 1.0 and PEEP = 8 cmH_2O.

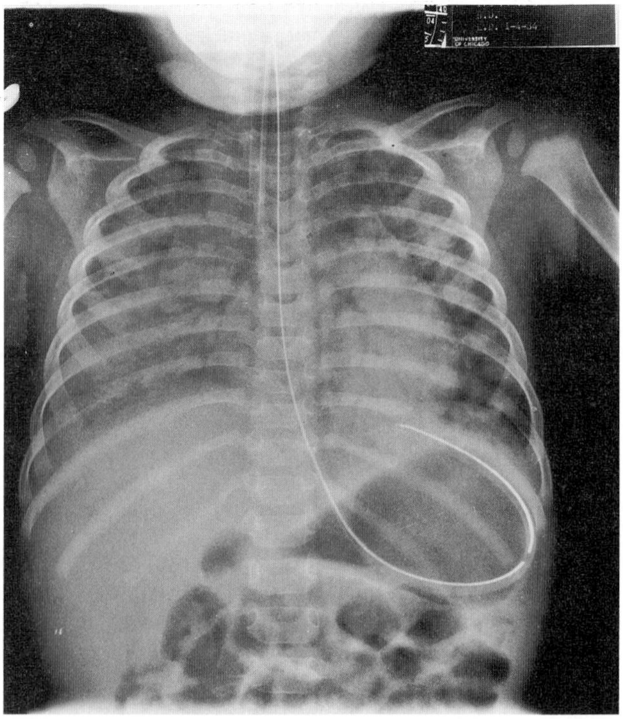

After transfer the patient remained severely distressed, with respiratory rate of 80 breaths per min, heart rate of 200 beats per min, and blood pressure of 94/40. Physical examination was otherwise unremarkable, except for diffuse rales and wheezes throughout both lung fields. She received mechanical ventilation with a volume ventilator with inspired oxygen fraction (F_{IO_2}) of 1.0, delivered tidal volume of 10 mL/kg, a ventilation rate of 50 breaths per min, and 8 cmH_2O PEEP. She struggled and did not allow effective ventilation to be performed. Therefore, intravenous midazolam and pancuronium bromide were administered. A chest x-ray showed widespread alveolar and interstitial infiltrates (Fig. 136-1). The next blood gas analysis showed pH 7.10, Pa_{O_2} 50 mmHg, Pa_{CO_2} 48 mmHg, and base deficit 14 meq/L. A pulse oximeter revealed 82% saturation. PEEP was increased stepwise to 14 cmH_2O until saturation exceeded 90%. Shortly thereafter, however, arterial blood pressure fell to 70/34 mmHg, and the peripheral circulation was clinically diminished. A dobutamine infusion was begun at 10 μg/kg per min, and a Swan-Ganz catheter was placed. The next systemic arterial blood gas revealed pH 7.22, Pa_{O_2} 28 mmHg, Pa_{CO_2} 48 mmHg, and base deficit 12 meq/L; the oximeter read 62% saturation. Simultaneous mixed venous results were pH 7.18, Pa_{O_2} 13 mmHg, Pa_{CO_2} 60 mmHg, and base deficit 18 meq/L. Cardiac index (CI) was 2.5 L/min per m^2, mean systemic arterial blood pressure was 50 mmHg, Ppw was 14 mmHg, and mean pulmonary artery pressure was 36 mmHg. The patient's hematocrit was 28, and calculated pulmonary shunt fraction was 80%.

The dobutamine infusion was increased to 20 μg/kg per min, with improvement in saturation (70%) and cardiac index (4.0 L/min per m^2). The patient received 10 mL/kg of packed red blood cells, which increased Ppw to 16 mmHg, associated with CI of 4.5 L/min per m^2; arterial blood gas analysis showed a Pa_{O_2} of 64 mmHg at an F_{IO_2} of 1.0. Static compliance of the respiratory system (C_{RS}) was 2.0 mL/cmH_2O, and peak inspiratory pressure was 68 cmH_2O. The PEEP was further increased, in increments of 2 cmH_2O, to 20; this time no hemodynamic compromise occurred. Systemic Pa_{O_2} rose to 120 mmHg, associated with an increase in C_{RS} to 3.6 mL/cmH_2O as peak airway pressure decreased to 54 cmH_2O. Cautious diuresis with furosemide (1 mg/kg per dose) was begun, while intravenous fluids were administered at a rate calculated at 75 percent of routine maintenance. Approximately 8 h later, pulmonary shunt fraction was 30%, hematocrit was 44, and CI was 4.8 L/min per m^2, while Ppw was 10 mmHg. Over the next 8 h this regimen was continued, and a net negative fluid balance of 250 mL was accomplished (Fig. 136-2). During that time, F_{IO_2} was slowly decreased to 0.6. Systemic saturation remained above 90%. As blood gases and clinical examination improved, PEEP was decreased from 20 to 12 cmH_2O by 24 h post-admission. During the next few days, total parenteral nutrition was instituted at the same restricted fluid rate, and pharmacologic diuresis was stopped. By 6 days, PEEP had been reduced to 5 cmH_2O at F_{IO_2} of 0.45.

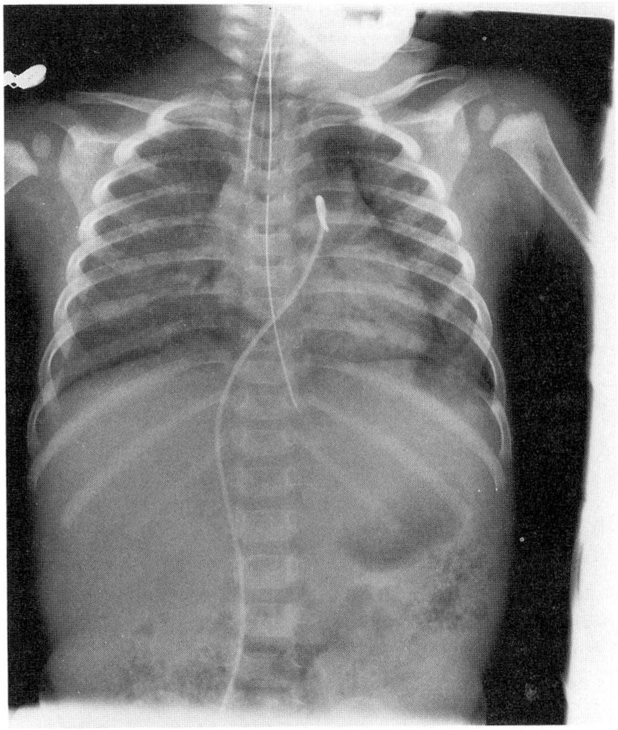

FIGURE 136-2 Chest x-ray taken about 24 h later than Fig. 136-1. A Swan-Ganz catheter is positioned in the pulmonary artery to measure Ppw = 10 mmHg and CI = 4.8 L/min per m^2 on PEEP = 20 cmH_2O. The air space filling is reduced; arterial saturation is 92% on F_{IO_2} = 0.6.

The patient breathed spontaneously at 50 breaths per min, with a tidal volume of 3 to 4 mL/kg. Peak airway pressure with ventilator breaths of 10 mL/kg was 32 cmH_2O; C_{RS} was 4.0. The baby was successfully extubated 7 days after admission.

CASE DISCUSSION

The management of this case underscores our approach to the treatment of permeability pulmonary edema due to aspiration of kerosene by an infant. These principles apply equally to many adult patients who develop ARDS after aspiration of various liquids. Following aspiration of a hydrocarbon and gastric contents, the patient was tachypneic, hypercapneic, acidotic, and hypoxic in spite of intubation and administration of supplemental oxygen, and in accordance with the extensive alveolar edema. Her agitation and work of breathing were so great that adequate mechanical ventilation was confounded, so she received an intravenous sedative and neuromuscular blocker. Even then, her systemic Pa_{O_2} was extremely low while receiving 100% oxygen and 8 cmH_2O PEEP, signifying severe intrapulmonary shunting. We began to increase PEEP in increments of 2 cmH_2O in the pursuit of the lowest value compatible with 90% arterial oxygen saturation. When 14 cmH_2O PEEP was reached, saturation was acceptable, but arterial blood pressure and peripheral pulses were diminished, because PEEP raised pleural and right atrial pressure to reduce venous return and cardiac output.

We resisted the initial temptation to administer intravenous fluids to increase cardiac preload and output, since the subsequent increase in pulmonary capillary hydrostatic pressure would have caused further edema formation and the need for greater ventilatory support. Instead, we administered intravenous dobutamine, which increased cardiac ouput at the same filling pressures. A Swan-Ganz catheter was placed so that objective data could be obtained to support decisions concerning fluid and inotropic interventions. The initial physiologic measurements and blood gas analysis showed low cardiac output with inadequate systemic oxygen delivery. While some improvement occurred after increasing the inotropic infusion, systemic oxygen saturation was still only 70%.

At that time, the Ppw was 14 mmHg, while PEEP was 14 cmH_2O, so the transmural Ppw was less than 14 mmHg—a value that was not too high in the face of a low cardiac output. Accordingly, we initiated a volume challenge with packed red blood cells to increase cardiac ouput and oxygen-carrying capacity significantly. The Ppw was then 16 mmHg, and the patient was then able to tolerate further increases of PEEP to 20 cmH_2O; arterial Pa_{O_2} rose to 120 mmHg and hemodynamic status stabilized. Approximately 8 h after the initial resuscitation, slow diuresis with furosemide was begun; a 250-mL net fluid loss occurred in the next 16 h. Still, the child remained hemodynamically stable, although Ppw was only 10 mmHg. During the next few days PEEP and oxygen were slowly decreased, and parenteral nutrition was begun. As the patient's needs for mechanical ventilation decreased, neuromuscular paralysis was stopped. With mild sedation the patient cooperated with respiratory support; she was successfully extubated a week after the initial insults.

References

1. Mendelson CL: The aspiration of stomach contents into the lungs during obstetrical anesthesia. J Obstet Gynecol 52:191, 1946.
2. Fowler AA, Hamman RF, Good JT, et al: Adult respiratory distress syndrome: Risk with common predispositions. Ann Intern Med 98:593, 1983.
3. Hogan WJ, Dodds WJ: Gastroesophageal reflux disease (reflux esophagitis), in Sleisenger MH, Fordtran JS (eds): *Gastrointestinal Disease: Pathophysiology, Diagnosis, and Management.* Philadelphia, WB Saunders, 1989, p 594.
4. Bone DK, Davis LJ, Zuidema GD, Cameron JL: Aspiration pneumonia. Ann Thorac Surg 18:30, 1974.
5. Cameron JL, Reynolds J, Zuidema GD: Aspiration in patients with tracheostomies. Surg Gynecol Obstet 136:68, 1973.
6. Bernhard WN, Cottrell JE, Sivakumaran C, et al: Adjustment of intracuff pressure to prevent aspiration. Anesthesiology 50:363, 1979.
7. Nordin U: The trachea and cuff induced tracheal injury. Acta Otolaryngol 345 Suppl: 1977.
8. Colman RD, Frank M, Loughnan BA, et al: Use of i.m. ranitidine for the prophylaxis of aspiration pneumonitis in obstetrics. Br J Anaesth 61:720, 1988.
9. Manchikanti L, Marrero TC, Roush JR: Preanesthetic cimetidine and metoclopramide for acid aspiration prophylaxis in elective surgery. Anesthesiology 61:48, 1984.
10. Wynne JW, Modell JH: Respiratory aspiration of stomach contents. Ann Intern Med 87:466, 1977.
11. Wynne JW, Ramphal R, Hood CI: Tracheal mucosal damage after aspiration: A scanning electron microscope study. Am Rev Respir Dis 124:728, 1981.
12. Hamelberg W, Bosomworth PP: Aspiration pneumonitis: Experimental studies and clinical observations. Anesth Analg 43:669, 1964.
13. Sznajder JI, Zucker AR, Wood LDH, Long GR: The effects of plasmapheresis and hemofiltration on canine acid aspiration pulmonary edema. Am Rev Respir Dis 134:222, 1986.
14. Holm BA, Notter R, Finkelstein J: Surface property changes from interactions of albumin with natural lung surfactant and extracted lung lipids. Chem Phys Lipids 38:287, 1985.
15. Malo J, Ali J, Wood LDH: How does positive end-expiratory pressure reduce intrapulmonary shunt in canine pulmonary edema? J Appl Physiol 57:1002, 1984.
16. Corbridge T, Wood LDH, Crawford G, et al: Adverse effects of large tidal volume and low PEEP in canine acid aspiration. Am Rev Respir Dis, 141:311, 1990.
17. Bernard G, Luce J, Sprung C, et al: High-dose corticosteroids in patients with the adult respiratory distress syndrome. N Engl J Med 317:1565, 1987.
18. Long GR, Breen PH, Mayers I, Wood LDH: Treatment of canine aspiration pneumonitis: Fluid reduction versus fluid expansion. J Appl Physiol 65:1736, 1988.
19. Eisenberg PR, Hansbrough JR: Anderson D, Schuster DP: A prospective study of lung water measurements during patient management in an intensive care unit. Am Rev Respir Dis 136:662, 1987.
20. Humphrey H, Hall J, Sznajder JI, et al: Improved survival following pulmonary capillary wedge pressure reduction in patients with ARDS. Chest 97:1176, 1990.
21. Jardin F, Genevray B, Brun-Ney D, Bourdarias JP: Influence of lung and chest wall compliances on transmission of airway pressures to the pleural space in critically ill patients. Chest 88:653, 1985.
22. Viires N, Sillye G, Aubier A, et al: Regional blood flow distribution in dogs during induced hypotension and low cardiac output. J Clin Invest 72:935, 1983.
23. Nieman GF, Bredenberg CE: High surface tension pulmonary edema induced by detergent aerosol. J Appl Physiol 58:129, 1985.
24. Dice WH, Ward G, Kelley J: Pulmonary toxicity following gastrointestinal ingestion of kerosene. Ann Emerg Med 11:138, 1982.
25. Zucker AR, Sznajder JI, Becker CJ, et al: The pathophysiology and treatment of canine kerosene pulmonary injury: Effects of plasmapheresis and positive end-expiratory pressure. J Crit Care 4:184, 1989.
26. Bartlett JG, Gorbach SL, Finegold SM: The bacteriology of aspiration pneumonia. Am J Med 56:202, 1974.
27. Garvey B, McCambley J, Tuxen B: Effects of gastric alkalinization on bacterial colonization in critically ill patients. Crit Care Med 17:211, 1989.
28. Zucker AR, Pollack M, Katz R: Blind use of the double-lumen plugged catheter for diagnosis of respiratory tract infections in critically ill children. Crit Care Med 12:867, 1984.

29. Wimberly N, Faling L, Bartlett J: A fiberoptic bronchoscopy technique to obtain lower uncontaminated respiratory secretions for bacterial culture. Am Rev Respir Dis 119:337, 1979.
30. Zapol WM, Snider MT, Hill JD, et al: Extracorporeal membrane oxygenation in severe acute respiratory failure, JAMA 242:2193, 1979.
31. Gattinoni L, Pesenti A, Mascheroni D, et al: Low-frequency positive-pressure ventilation with extracorporeal CO_2 removal in severe acute respiratory failure. JAMA 256:881, 1986.
32. Hallman M, Maasilta P, Sipila I, Tahvanainen J: Composition and function of pulmonary surfactant in adult respiratory distress syndrome. Eur Respir J 2:104, 1989.
33. Harris JD, Jackson F, Moxley MA, Longmore WJ: Effect of exogenous surfactant instillation on experimental lung injury. J Appl Physiol 66:1846, 1989.
34. Lachmann B: Animal models and clinical pilot studies of surfactant replacement in adult respiratory distress syndrome. Eur Respir J 2:98, 1989.
35. Said S, Foda HD: Pharmacologic modulation of lung injury. Am Rev Respir Dis 139:1553, 1989.

Chapter 137
LUNG HEMORRHAGE AND HEMOPTYSIS

RICHARD K. ALBERT

KEY POINTS

- *Ensure adequate oxygenation.*
- *Correct all coagulation abnormalities.*
- *Institute appropriate volume replacement and red blood cell (RBC) transfusion.*
- *Decide if surgery or other urgent intervention is indicated.*
- *Be prepared to position the patient in a posture that facilitates removal of secretions and limits the likelihood of aspiration.*

Hemoptysis means coughing up of blood. This manifestation has many causes (Table 137-1). It can range in severity from production of a small amount of blood-tinged sputum to massive bleeding (generally considered production of more than 300 to 600 mL in 12 to 24 h). The latter can cause death by asphyxiation or by intravascular volume depletion.

When the chest x-ray shows a diffuse, fine reticular pattern, patients with hemoptysis (sparse or massive) are generally classified as having a pulmonary hemorrhage syndrome (Table 137-1).

Determining that expectorated blood is coming from the lungs is generally a simple undertaking. However, the possibility that "hemoptysis" might be originating from the nasopharynx (being inhaled and then expectorated) or from the stomach (dark blood with an acidic pH, frequently mixed with food particles) should not be overlooked. Blood originating from the lungs is generally bright-red, has an alkaline pH, contains alveolar macrophages, and is frequently mixed with frothy or purulent sputum.

Stabilization and Initial Evaluation and Therapy

As with any acutely ill patient admitted to the intensive care unit (ICU), initial efforts should be directed at assuring airway patency and stabilizing the vital signs. The most common cause of death in patients with hemoptysis is asphyxia: the volume of blood being produced cannot be cleared, and the blood is aspirated diffusely.[1,2] Clearance of massive bleeding may be facilitated by placing the patient in the Trendelenburg position. Alternately, if the site of bleeding is known, placing the bleeding lung in the dependent position may help protect the other lung. Adequate oxygenation should be assured; and, depending on the

TABLE 137-1 Causes of Hemoptysis and Pulmonary Hemorrhage

Hemoptysis
- *Infections*
  - Bronchitis
  - Bacterial mycobacterial pneumonia
  - Mycetoma (*Aspergillus, Candida*)
  - Lung abscess
  - Bronchiectasis
- *Tumors* (suspect in patients >40 years old)
  - Carcinoma
  - Bronchial adenoma
- *Cardiovascular*
  - Mitral stenosis
  - Pulmonary infarction
  - Arteriovenous malformation
- *Trauma*
- *Drug- and toxin-induced*
  - Anticoagulants
  - D-penicillamine (few cases, Wilson's disease treated for 2–3 years)
  - Trimellitic anhydride (exposure in the manufacture of plastics, paint, and epoxy resins)
- *Other*
  - Sarcoidosis
    - Endobronchial granulomas
    - Mycetomatous colonization of cysts
  - Blood dyscrasia
    - TTP
    - Hemophilia
    - Leukemia
    - Thrombocytopenia from other causes
  - Ankylosing spondylitis
    - Traction bronchiectasis
    - Spontaneous pneumothorax
    - Mycetoma
  - Broncholithiasis

Pulmonary hemorrhage
- *Pulmonary-renal syndromes*
  - Anti–basement membrane antibody–induced (Goodpasture's syndrome)
  - Presumed immune complex–induced
    - Associated with systemic vasculitis
      - Cryoglobulinemia
      - Polyarteritis
      - Wegener's granulomatosis
      - Lymphomatoid granulomatosis
      - Churg-Strauss syndrome
      - Hypersensitivity angiitis
      - Behçet's syndrome
      - Henoch-Schönlein purpura
      - Necrotizing vasculitis
    - Associated with connective tissue disease
      - Systemic lupus erythematosus
      - Rheumatoid arthritis
      - Progressive systemic sclerosis
      - Mixed connective tissue disease
    - Idiopathic (alveolar hemorrhage + glomerulonephritis without immune complex deposition and without systemic vasculitis)
- Hemosiderosis

degree of bleeding, volume resuscitation and transfusion may be needed.

In extreme circumstances intubation of the mainstem bronchus going to the nonbleeding lung may protect the good lung and tamponade the lung that is bleeding (see Chap. 10).

Peripheral blood should be sent for a platelet count; fibrinogen determination; and thrombin time, prothrombin time, and partial thromboplastin time (Table 137-2). In some patients a bleeding time might be helpful. Any abnormalities should be corrected with the appropriate therapy (see Chap. 146).

A low platelet count may be partially corrected by transfusing platelets. In general, every unit transfused increases the platelet count by 10,000 per mm^3. Counts of approximately 50,000 per mm^3 should be the goal, as spontaneous bleeding rarely occurs with platelet counts higher than this.

TABLE 137-2 Interpretation of Studies Done to Evaluate Patients for Bleeding Disorders

Platelet count low, fibrinogen low
Disseminated intravascular coagulation (DIC)
Other forms of consumption
Platelet count low, fibrinogen normal
Platelet consumption
Idiopathic thrombocytopenic purpura (ITP)
Vasculitis
Hemolytic-uremic syndrome
Hypersplenism
Medication-induced
Decreased production
Aplastic bone marrow
Medications
Neoplasia
Acquired immunodeficiency syndrome (AIDS)
Platelet count normal, fibrinogen low
Primary fibrinolysis
Afibrinogenemia
Platelet count normal, fibrinogen normal, thrombin time long
Heparin
Presence of fibrin degradation products
Platelet count normal, fibrinogen normal, thrombin time normal
Partial thromboplastin time normal, prothrombin time long
Factor VII deficiency
Liver disease
Early warfarin effect
Partial thromboplastin time long, prothrombin time long
Factor V deficiency
Factor X deficiency
Prothrombin deficiency
Warfarin effect
Liver disease
Vitamin K deficiency
Circulating anticoagulants (e.g., systemic lupus erythematosus)
Partial thromboplastin time long, prothrombin time normal
Factor VIII deficiency
Factor IX deficiency
Factor XI deficiency
Circulating anticoagulants (e.g., lupus)

Immune platelet destruction may be treated with intravenous gamma globulin prior to platelet transfusions. If platelet dysfunction is the result of an interaction with a medica tion, the problem will improve within 24 h of stopping the offending agent. The platelet dysfunction associated with uremia may be treated with dialysis or by administration of cryoprecipitate or DDAVP (desamino-D-arginine-vasopressin).[3] Cryoprecipitate and DDAVP are also useful in treating patients with von Willebrand's disease and hemophilia A. Coagulation factor deficiencies are treated with vitamin K or, for a more rapid effect, large volumes of fresh frozen plasma.

Most experienced clinicians suggest administering small doses of codeine or morphine to blunt the cough reflex and slow the rate of bleeding. This recommendation must be tempered by concerns for the possibility that central depressants could increase the risk of aspiration.

In addition to obtaining a urinalysis, a blood urea nitrogen (BUN) level, a serum creatinine level, and a careful occupational history in patients with diffuse alveolar hemorrhage, the physician should also have blood sent for testing for antiglomerular basement antibodies (Goodpasture's syndrome), antineutrophil cytoplasmic antibody (Wegener's granulomatosis),[4] antinuclear antibodies (ANA), rheumatoid factor, complement, and circulating immune complexes (systemic lupus erythematosus or other vasculitis), and cryoglobulin (cryoglobulinemia). Determining if the alveolar macrophages contain hemosiderin may be helpful. The disorders causing immune complex–related pulmonary hemorrhage and hematuria can generally be differentiated by clinical evaluation and serologic testing. However, biopsy of the lung or kidney is needed to establish the diagnosis when vasculitis is the cause.[5]

Determining When Surgery or Bronchial Artery Embolization Should Be Considered

Most patients with hemoptysis have a sufficiently slow rate of bleeding that an elective evaluation can be undertaken. In some instances (e.g., trauma) emergent surgical intervention is clearly indicated. In others, especially in cases with rapid rates of bleeding, the decision is more difficult.

Most clinicians believe that patients with massive hemoptysis should be considered for immediate surgery. This opinion is based on the results of several studies that have addressed the question. Unfortunately, no definitive guidelines are available, because the definition of "massive hemoptysis" has varied (200 to 900 mL blood loss in 4 to 24 h), the number of causes of hemoptysis is large (over 100 different conditions reported—see Table 137-1) and, as yet, no study has used a prospective design with patients being randomized to surgical versus nonsurgical intervention. It is difficult to extrapolate from the data in these series to any single patient.

A widely cited nonrandomized study of patients who produced more than 600 mL of blood in 16 h reported an 81 percent survival rate in the group operated on, and a 22 percent survival rate in the group not receiving surgery because of "physician or patient procrastination."[6] Unfortunately, the number of patients not treated with surgery was small (n = 9), and many of these had lung abscesses (which other authors suggest are a particularly ominous cause of hemoptysis). Accordingly, it may not be appropriate to apply these results to other patients with hemoptysis.

What is clear, from both the literature and clinical practice, is that some patients abruptly die from hemoptysis, and that for these patients surgical intervention may be lifesaving. Given the relative inability to select those at risk of dying, a "conservative" approach might be to consider performing surgery on most, if not all, patients producing more than 200 to 300 mL of blood in 24 h. However, prior to surgery, two issues should be considered.

DETERMINING WHETHER THE PATIENT'S PULMONARY RESERVE IS SUFFICIENT TO TOLERATE SURGERY

Many patients have hemoptysis in the setting of diffuse lung disease (e.g., bronchiectasis attributable to cystic fibrosis or diffuse scarring from old tuberculosis; or lung cancer in a COPD patient with inadequate pulmonary function to tolerate resection). For these patients surgery is precluded and bronchial arteriography and possible embolization should be considered. Recent series suggest that (1) the frequency with which this technique is able to stop acute hemoptysis is high; (2) the rate at which hemoptysis recurs in the subsequent 1 to 3 years is low; and (3) complications are rare.[7] Accordingly, bronchial arterial embolization is the treatment of choice for persons with substantial, life-threatening hemoptysis who cannot tolerate parenchymal resection. From the same data it could also be argued that bronchial embolization might be considered the treatment of choice for all patients with massive hemoptysis, regardless of their pulmonary function. Unfortunately, in many instances the vascular anatomy precludes doing the procedure, either because a specific feeding vessel (or vessels) cannot be found, or because of concern about the possibility of interrupting blood flow to the spine.

DETERMINING WHETHER THE CAUSE OF THE HEMOPTYSIS IS AMENABLE TO SURGICAL CORRECTION

Localized bronchiectasis can be removed surgically, as can lung abscesses, many tumors (both benign and malignant), pulmonary infarctions, and one (or a few) arteriovenous malformations. Mycetomas are thought rarely to require surgery. Surgical intervention should not be considered as therapy for any of the systemic diseases associated with hemoptysis.

There is no convincing evidence that the prognosis of patients with idiopathic pulmonary hemorrhage can be improved by any form of therapy. Goodpasture's syndrome has been treated with corticosteroids with anecdotal success, but this therapeutic intervention is not generally accepted as being helpful. Bilateral nephrectomy followed by plasmapheresis, immunosuppression, and ultimately kidney transplantation (or chronic dialysis) appears to be the most beneficial therapeutic approach.[8]

When Bronchoscopy Should Be Performed

Bronchoscopy allows the site of bleeding to be determined in most patients with hemoptysis. The procedure is also extremely effective in determining some specific causes of bleeding—namely, bronchogenic carcinoma, bronchial adenomas, mycetomas, and bronchitis.

For most patients bronchoscopy should be carried out without waiting for the hemoptysis to stop. Although clinical outcome may not be affected by the timing of the procedure, the ability to determine the site of bleeding is markedly improved when the procedure is done early.[9] This information can be critically important should surgical or other urgent therapeutic interventions be needed. Two retrospective studies have suggested that bronchoscopy has a very low yield (and therefore can be deferred) in patients younger than 40 who are nonsmokers, have been bleeding for less than 1 week, and have normal chest x-rays.[9,10]

Fiberoptic bronchoscopy under local anesthesia allows optimal visualization of the endobronchial anatomy. In addition, endobronchial and/or transbronchial biopsies and aspirations, and bronchial brushings and washings, can be obtained, and endobronchial epinephrine or iced–saline solution lavage can be administered as therapeutic interventions. However, the suction channel of most fiberoptic bronchoscopes is only 7 mm in diameter; this results in a limited ability to remove large volumes of blood rapidly. Accordingly, when the rate of bleeding is brisk, straight bronchoscopy is the procedure of choice, despite that it allows inspection of only the more central airways. An additional benefit of straight bronchoscopy is that any of various occluding devices (Fogarty balloon catheter, Gelfoam, gauze, double-lumen endotracheal tube) can be inserted in an attempt to tamponade the bleeding or to protect the uninvolved lung (see Chap. 10).

Bronchoscopy is of only limited help in patients with pulmonary hemorrhage; its main value is that it can exclude other explanations for the bleeding. Few, if any, of the conditions associated with pulmonary hemorrhage require—or can be diagnosed with certainty by means of—a transbronchial biopsy.

Other Diagnostic Approaches

In many instances a specific cause for hemoptysis cannot be determined after fiberoptic or straight bronchoscopy. Other diagnostic procedures are available, such as bronchography, computed tomography (CT), pulmonary arteriography, and red blood cell scanning; however, these are only rarely indicated. Patients with hemoptysis, a normal chest x-ray (or at least a roentgenogram that shows no focal abnormality), and a normal bronchoscopy generally have an excellent prognosis. A retrospective series reported that, in patients meeting these criteria, (1) the hemoptysis resolved prior to discharge in more than 50 percent, and within 6 months in 90 percent; and (2) the hemoptysis recurred in fewer than 5 percent.[2] Only 1 patient of the 67 studied developed bronchogenic carcinoma, and this occurred nearly 2 years after the initial episode. Subsequent development or diagnosis of a bronchogenic carcinoma is extremely rare. On the basis of this data, patients meeting these criteria generally do not require additional evaluation or particularly careful follow-up. Rather, most should simply be instructed to return for an additional evaluation if the symptom recurs.

Obtaining arterial blood gases with the patient breathing 100% O_2 while upright, supine, and in Trendelenburg position, and at total lung capacity (TLC) and functional residual capacity (FRC), may allow the diagnosis of an arteriovenous malformations to be confirmed.[11] In stable patients with diffuse lung lesions *without* hemoptysis, the single-breath diffusing capacity can confirm the clinical suspicion of excess lung blood, to narrow the diagnostic possibilities.[12]

CASE PRESENTATION

A 39-year-old black male with a 25-year history of sarcoidosis and a 7-year history of chronic renal failure requiring dialysis came to the emergency room complaining of hemoptysis. While being evaluated he coughed up a sufficient quantity of blood to fill a kidney basin; he was admitted directly to the ICU. The patient denied symptoms of acute bronchitis and suggested that his bleeding seemed to be coming from the right lower lung area. He was tachypneic and tachycardiac, and his blood pressure was 110/60 without postural changes. Pulmonary examination was within normal limits, with the exception of diffuse rhonchi. His chest x-ray showed small lung volumes, diffuse fibrosis, no apparent cavities, and no infiltrates.

A large-bore intravenous catheter was inserted, and he was given O_2 (4 L/min via nasal prongs), codeine sulfate (30 mg orally), and desmopressin (DDAVP) (0.3 μg/kg in 50 mL normal saline, intravenously, over 30 min); and, because of a hematocrit of 14, 2 U of packed red blood cells were transfused. Peripheral blood was sent for a prothrombin time, a platelet count, and a partial thromboplastin time. These were normal.

Pulmonary function tests obtained 2 years earlier demonstrated a total lung capacity of 40 percent predicted and a DLCO of 32 percent predicted. These values were thought to preclude surgical intervention.

Although it was recommended that the patient undergo straight bronchoscopy, logistic considerations required that the procedure be done with a fiberoptic bronchoscope. At that time no bleeding was evident, but a few small thrombi were apparent around the orifice of the superior segment of the right lower lobe. Bronchial arteriography demonstrated an abnormal vascular pattern in this area, consistent with bronchiectasis. Embolization of two bronchial arteries feeding these abnormal vessels was performed.

The patient had no further bleeding for the remainder of his 5-day hospitalization or during the subsequent 30-day follow-up.

CASE DISCUSSION

This patient had massive hemoptysis from bronchiectasis associated with diffuse fibrotic lung disease. Because the platelet dysfunction associated with chronic renal failure might have contributed to his problem, he was treated with desmopressin. The question of surgical versus nonsurgical intervention became moot when old pulmonary function tests documented insufficient pulmonary reserve to tolerate parenchymal resection. While bronchoscopy did not yield a cause for his hemoptysis, it did suggest a site of origin. Directed bronchial arterial embolization effectively treated the problem.

References

1. Conlan AA, Hurwitz SS, Kriege L, et al: Massive hemoptysis. Review of 123 cases. J Thorac Cardiovasc Surg 85:120, 1983.
2. Adelman M, Haponik EF, Bleeker ER, Britt EJ: Cryptogenichemoptysis. Clinical features, bronchoscopic findings, and natural history in 67 patients. Ann Intern Med 102:829, 1985.
3. Mannuccio P, Remuzzi G, Pusineri F, et al: Deamino-8-D-arginine vasopressin shortens the bleeding time in uremia. N Engl J Med 308:8, 1983.
4. Nolle B, Specks U, Ludemann J, et al: Anticytoplasmic autoantibodies: The immunodiagnostic value in Wegener's Granulomatosis. Ann Intern Med 111:28, 1989.
5. Leatherman JW, Sibley RK, Davies SF: Diffuse intra-pulmonary hemorrhage and glomerulonephritis unrelated to antiglomerular basement membrane antibody. Am J Med 72:401, 1982.
6. Crocco JA, Rooney JJ, Fankushen DS, et al: Massive hemoptysis. Arch Intern Med 121:495, 1968.
7. Stoll JF, Bettmann MA: Bronchial artery embolization to control hemoptysis: A review. Cardiovasc Intervent Radiology. 11:263, 1988.
8. Briggs WA, Johnson JP, Teichman S, et al: Antiglomerular basement membrane antibody-mediated glomerulonephritis and Goodpasture's syndrome. Med 58:348, 1979.
9. Gong H Jr, Salvatierra C: Clinical efficacy of early and delayed bronchoscopy in patients with hemoptysis. Am Rev Respir Dis 124:221, 1981.
10. Weaver LJ, Solliday N, Cugell DW: Selection of patients with hemoptysis for fiberoptic bronchoscopy. Chest 76:7, 1979.
11. Terry P: Pulmonary arteriovenous malformation. N Engl J Med 308:1197, 1983.
12. Addleman M, Logan AS, Grossman RF: Monitoring intrapulmonary hemorrhage in Goodpasture's syndrome. Chest 87:119, 1985.

Chapter 138

PLEURAL DISEASE

EUGENE F. GEPPERT

KEY POINTS

- *In critically ill patients, pleural effusion may become evident not by symptoms but by signs of altered gas exchange or worsened compliance of the respiratory system.*
- *Most pleural effusions will necessitate thoracentesis for analysis of the fluid that allows its classification as either a transudate or exudate.*
- *Bedside ultrasound is extremely helpful in choosing a site for diagnostic thoracentesis.*
- *Some clues for the diagnosis do not come from thoracentesis. Consider pulmonary embolus, abdominal and pelvic diseases, and connective tissue diseases when ordering diagnostic tests.*
- *Closed or open pleural biopsy should be done when tuberculosis or metastatic cancer of the pleura need to be diagnosed.*
- *Empyema and intrapleural hemorrhage are emergencies that require rapid diagnosis and therapy with surgical drainage or thoracotomy.*
- *Pleural effusion associated with esophageal rupture has low pH (<6) and very high amylase; rapid surgical repair and drainage can be lifesaving.*

Presentation of Pleural Effusion

SIGNS AND SYMPTOMS

In the critically ill patient, the most prominent "signs" of pleural effusion may be those of impaired gas exchange or decreased compliance of the respiratory system. Although many pleural effusions are small and do not cause any signs or symptoms, conscious patients in the ICU who develop new pleural effusion may complain of dyspnea, cough, and chest pain. Even a small pleural effusion can cause dyspnea, especially if it compounds another condition that causes dyspnea such as anemia, heart disease, or parenchymal lung disease. The rapidity of onset of chest pain with pleural effusion should not be taken to indicate a disease with a known rapid onset such as acute pulmonary embolus; even rather subacute illnesses such as tuberculous pleurisy may cause the sudden onset of pleuritic chest pain. Physical examination typically reveals dullness to percussion over the effusion and egophony (E to A change) on auscultation near the upper level of the border between dull and resonant areas. Critically ill patients who are breathing without the aid of mechanical ventilation may attempt to splint the portion of the hemithorax where the pleuritic pain is perceived. This low tidal volume breathing pattern ("splinting") may in turn lead to atelectasis and hypoxemia.

RADIOLOGIC AND ULTRASOUND DETECTION

In the critically ill patient, pleural fluid is usually detected by portable chest radiogram, which is often done with the patient supine. In this posture, the pleural fluid layers behind the lungs in the posterior chest may be difficult to appreciate, appearing as a gray veil that uniformly covers the lung field. Even in chest radiograms that are exposed with the patient in a more upright posture, a pleural fluid collection may stay in the space immediately under the lung (subpleural effusion) and in this way may simulate an elevated or paralyzed diaphragm. The best method for discovering pleural effusions and evaluating their size in critically ill patients is to expose a portable chest radiogram with the patient in the lateral decubitus position, or to use ultrasonography which can detect even a small collection of pleural fluid (see Chap. 19). Computed tomography (CT) scanning of the chest is a sensitive way to detect small amounts of pleural fluid, but the study is rarely performed in critically ill patients with this purpose in mind. Portable chest radiographs exposed with the patient in the lateral decubitus position have the advantage of being reasonably easy to perform and are readily available; they can also detect small amounts of fluid.

A special problem encountered in critically ill patients is the hemithorax that is completely opacified on a chest radiograph (Fig. 138-1). Is the entire lung collapsed or does a massive pleural effusion overlie and displace the lung? There are some radiologic signs that can help in this differentiation. In a hemithorax in which the lung is completely collapsed, the interspaces between the ribs tend to be closer together than in the opposite hemithorax and the diaphragm is elevated as a consequence of volume loss. Many times, however, the distinction between these two entities cannot be made short of thoracentesis carried out to definitively answer the question. If the x-ray changes are caused by a massive pleural effusion, pleural fluid will be readily aspirated by the thoracentesis needle; if the changes are caused by lung collapse, no fluid will be obtainable. The intensivist faced with this dilemma should not hesitate to perform thoracentesis since the risk of pneumothorax is nil in a collapsed lung and very unlikely to occur in passing a needle into a massive pleural effusion.

Physiologic Effects

MECHANICAL EFFECTS

The mechanical effects of pleural effusion on the respiratory system include both restriction of lung volumes and outward expansion of the chest cage.[1,2] The compliance of the lung is not altered, but there is a decrease in chest wall compliance.[3] When pleural fluid is removed from the pleural space, an improvement in vital capacity is seen, but it is much smaller than the amount of fluid removed; this is because only a small portion of the fluid inside the thoracic cage is accommodated by an inward movement of the lung. The larger portion of the fluid is accommodated by an outward movement of the thoracic cage.[2] Because inspiratory muscles are allowed to operate more effectively, patients

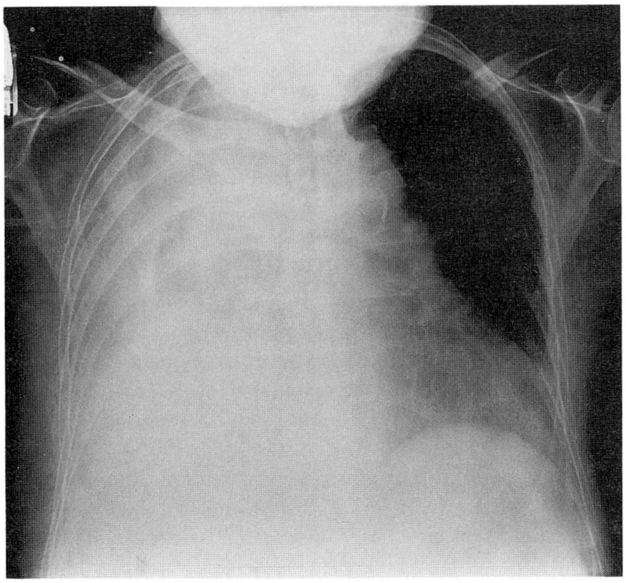

a

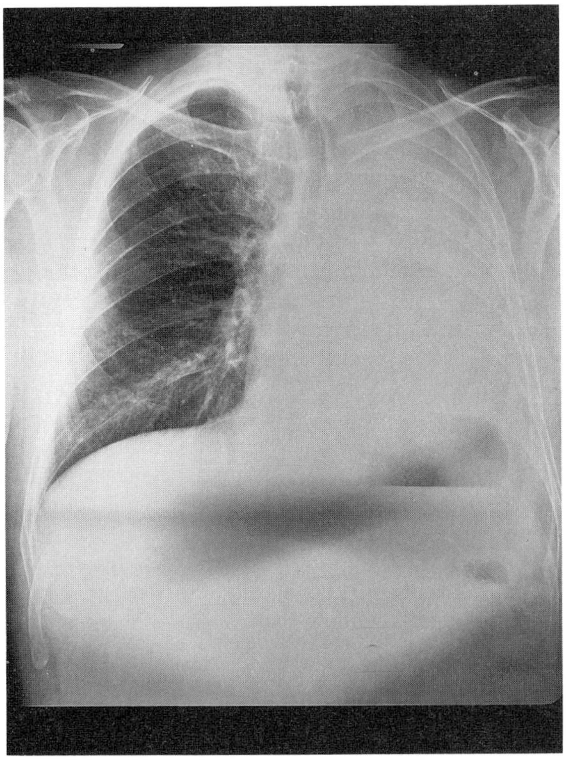

b

FIGURE 138-1 ***a.*** **Opacified right hemithorax due to pleural effusion. This is suggested by the lack of volume loss in the right side of the chest, suggestion of fluid tracking up the lateral wall, and air-containing lung seen in the perihilar region.** ***b.*** **Opacified left hemithorax due to complete lung collapse. This is suggested by mediastinal and tracheal shift.**

consistently experience relief of dyspnea when pleural fluid is removed.[1,2] The concurrent reduction in pleural pressure may facilitate venous return and so increase cardiac output.

GAS EXCHANGE EFFECTS

Pleural effusion causes a small increase in the $(\text{A}-\text{a})_{O_2}$ and in the physiologic pulmonary shunt. The result of these differences is a small decrease in Pa_{O_2} that improves after thoracentesis.[1] Also, when large effusions are removed from the pleural space, lung reexpansion may be associated with unilateral pulmonary edema, with a deterioration in gas exchange that lasts until this "reexpansion pulmonary edema" resolves.

Evaluation

CLASSIFICATION BASED ON THORACENTESIS

The vast majority of undiagnosed pleural effusions in critically ill patients should be diagnosed with thoracentesis (see Chap. 15). There may be times when clinical judgment can replace thoracentesis. An example of this might include a small pleural effusion accompanying pneumococcal pneumonia in which the diagnosis is proven decisively by positive blood culture and a convincing sputum Gram stain. Another example of an effusion that might not require thoracentesis is a small right-sided pleural effusion in an afebrile elderly patient with decompensated congestive heart failure. The pleural effusions associated with adult respiratory distress syndrome (ARDS) do not mandate diagnostic thoracentesis if they are very small and the patient does not have a fever. Small pleural effusions in postoperative patients during the first several days are common and need not be tapped. Even in these examples, thoracentesis is reasonable in the midst of a complex set of clinical problems. The presence of a pleural effusion in a patient with an undiagnosed fever requires thoracentesis as soon as possible, certainly on the same day that it is discovered. This is because the effusion might possibly be an empyema, and an evolving empyema can proceed within a matter of hours to convert the pleural space from its normal unilocular configuration to a honeycomb of multiloculated spaces, each of which represents a separate abscess in evolution. A sense of prudent hurry about performing thoracentesis in febrile, critically ill patients should increase the chance of early diagnosis of empyema, allow early institution of surgical drainage through tube thoracostomy or rib resection, and lessen the possibility of death due to sepsis syndrome.[4]

Large pleural effusions may be entered with a needle during thoracentesis with little difficulty and no need for ultrasonography. Small effusions or loculated fluid are best tapped with the help of pleural ultrasonography to localize the site and depth of the fluid; this technique may also help avoid puncture of nearby abdominal viscera. Failure to obtain pleural fluid during thoracentesis could mean that the fluid was not accessible in the site chosen. If the thoracentesis was done without ultrasound guidance, then another attempt should be made on the same day with the help of ultrasound.[5]

When thoracentesis does not result in a clear diagnosis, the intensivist should consider doing a closed pleural biopsy.[6] Pleural biopsy is most useful in diagnosing pleural tuberculosis, pleural coccidioidomycosis, and pleural cancer. The risks of closed pleural biopsy are similar to those of thoracentesis: pneumothorax and bleeding. In many cases, the need to document the presence of pleural tuberculosis to justify the toxicity of antituberculosis chemotherapy makes pleural biopsy a worthwhile risk in the critically ill patient. If the patient is judged unable to tolerate a pneumothorax, it is best to perform an open pleural biopsy in the operating room for diagnosis.

PLEURAL FLUID ANALYSIS

Pleural fluid collected at thoracentesis in critically ill patients should be analyzed in approximately the same manner as in patients outside the ICU. Pleural fluid from critically ill patients should be sent for analysis of pH and P_{CO_2}, total protein, lactate dehydrogenase (LDH), amylase, glucose, white blood cell (WBC) count and differential, red blood cell (RBC) count, cytologic studies, aerobic cultures, anaerobic cultures, culture for mycobacteria and fungi, and if appropriate, hematocrit and a wet preparation of spun sediment or a KOH preparation (to look for fungal forms). Pleural fluid protein and LDH values are used to categorize the pleural effusion as either a transudate or an exudate. A pleural fluid is an exudate if it satisfies at least one of the following criteria: **1.** the pleural fluid protein is 50 percent (or greater) of the total serum protein; **2.** the pleural fluid LDH is 60 percent (or greater) of the serum LDH; or **3.** the pleural fluid LDH is greater than two-thirds of the upper limit of normal serum LDH in the laboratory.[7] A pleural effusion whose analysis meets none of these three criteria is a transudate. Fortunately, the differential diagnosis of transudate is small. The most common causes of transudative pleural effusion include congestive heart failure, nephrotic syndrome, and cirrhosis; less commonly, acute pulmonary embolus or malignant pleural implants may cause a transudative pleural effusion.

The differential diagnosis of exudative pleural effusion is large and may require further diagnostic tests dictated by the clinical situation. If a special type of problem is suspected, it may require special studies. Bloody pleural fluid should have a hematocrit determination and the result should be compared to the patient's circulating hematocrit. The closer the hematocrit of the pleural fluid is to the hematocrit of the peripheral blood, the more likely that one is dealing with a hemothorax. In acute dissection of the thoracic aorta, for example, the two hematocrits will correspond closely. In traumatic thoracentesis or in malignant bloody pleural effusions, the pleural fluid hematocrit will usually be much lower than the peripheral blood value. If uncertainty remains after diagnostic thoracentesis as to whether a hemothorax is present or not, the best course of action is often to place a tube thoracostomy. The hematocrit of the bloody drainage can then be measured every 12 to 24 h to see if it is changing in a way that clarifies the situation. When it becomes clear that one is dealing with hemothorax, the decision can be made as to whether to perform thoracotomy.

If it is suspected that hyperalimentation fluid has infused into the pleural space through a perforated catheter or enteral feedings have infused into the pleural space through a perforation of the esophagus by the feeding tube, a glucose determination may give a rapid diagnosis since the concentration of glucose will be unphysiologically elevated in the fluid. In cases where infection is in the differential diagnosis, a sample of pleural fluid should be spun in a centrifuge and examined under a cover slip since amebae and fungi such as blastomycosis can be diagnosed much more quickly by this technique than by waiting for cultures. If the fluid appears milky and chylothorax is suspected, a determination of the presence of chylomicrons is diagnostic. It is a wise policy to draw an extra tube of heparinized pleural fluid and to save it in a refrigerator in case other analyses are desired later. For example, it is not routine to order a creatinine on pleural fluid; however, if a critically ill patient with pleural effusion is discovered to have ureteral obstruction after the thoracentesis has been performed, the entity of urinothorax may enter the differential diagnosis, and the intensivist will need to analyze a pleural fluid:urine creatinine ratio (normal <1.0), since elevation of this ratio strongly supports the diagnosis of urinothorax.[8]

FACTORS TO CONSIDER UNRELATED TO THORACENTESIS

At the same time that thoracentesis is being done, the intensivist should consider whether there is any clinical evidence for acute pulmonary embolism, congestive heart failure, abdominal disease, or connective tissue disease as the cause of the effusion. Each of these possibilities requires other evaluation in addition to thoracentesis.

The clinical prior probability of acute pulmonary embolus includes such elements as the presence of risk factors, plus a listing of the symptoms, signs, and laboratory values most commonly present in acute pulmonary embolus, such as dyspnea, chest pain, hemoptysis, tachycardia, tachypnea, electrocardiographic (ECG) changes, an acute widening of the $(A-a)_{O_2}$, and the presence of a new pleural effusion on chest radiogram, sometimes together with an elevated hemidiaphragm and platelike atelectasis. Further evidence relating to the possibility of acute pulmonary embolus can be collected in the ICU by performing Doppler, duplex scanning, or other noninvasive tests of the leg veins at the patient's bedside. These tests are performed to look for evidence of deep venous thrombosis of the leg veins, since this is a very important risk factor for acute pulmonary embolus and a disease process that in itself requires the patient to have either anticoagulation or the placement of an inferior vena cava umbrella. In many hospitals, a perfusion scan of the lungs can be done at the bedside in the ICU; perfusion scans are most useful when they are completely normal and in this way effectively rule out the possibility of acute pulmonary embolus. When the perfusion scan is read as showing a high probability of pulmonary embolus and there is no contraindication to anticoagulation of the patient, the intensivist may judge from the total clinical picture that the diagnosis of acute pulmonary embolus is correct and proceed with treatment. When the perfusion scan is not normal and not read as having a high probability of pulmonary embolus, further diagnostic efforts are needed, usually pulmonary angiography. In some cases, the critically ill patient with acute pulmonary embolus may have pleural effusion as the only evidence of the presence of this disease, since other signs, symptoms, and ECG evidence may be very hard to interpret in the critically ill patient (see Chap. 118).

The evaluation of the critically ill patient for the presence of congestive heart failure should include, in addition to the chest radiogram and the physical examination, an echocardiogram for the evaluation of ventricular function. In particular, Kerley B lines are searched for on the chest film and an S_3 third heart sound is sought on physical examination of the heart. In cases in which the diagnosis of congestive heart failure is in doubt, two courses of action may be helpful. If the patient has no hypotension or evidence of hypoperfusion, a trial of diuresis with furosemide may resolve the pleural effusion. In the unstable patient, right heart catheterization and measurement of pulmonary capillary wedge pressure can help determine the likelihood of a cardiogenic source of the effusion.

When there are clinical signs and symptoms of abdominal or pelvic disease, it is worthwhile to transport the critically ill patient with a pleural effusion to the radiology department for CT scanning of the abdomen and pelvis. Abdominal and renal ultrasound is also helpful in many cases. If ascitic fluid is present, paracentesis should be performed.

Connective tissue disease may present clinically for the first time in the ICU (see Case Presentation below). In the majority of cases of pleural effusion that remain undiagnosed after thoracentesis, it is worthwhile to perform serologic tests for the presence of connective tissue disease.

Types of Pleural Effusion

TRANSUDATES

When the pleural fluid of the critically ill patient is a transudate, differential diagnosis is limited. The most common causes include intravascular volume overload with congestive heart failure, severe hypoalbuminemia from nutritional or other factors, nephrotic syndrome, and hepatic cirrhosis (Table 138-1). Rarely, other diseases such as acute pulmonary embolus may cause a transudative pleural effusion.

TABLE 138-1 Common Causes of Transudates

Congestive heart failure
Cirrhosis of the liver
Nephrotic syndrome
Severe hypoalbuminemia of any cause

TABLE 138-2 Causes of Exudative Pleural Effusion in Critically Ill Patients

Venous thromboembolism
ARDS
Pulmonary embolus from intravascular catheter
Superior vena cava obstruction
Congestive heart failure (rare)
Empyema or complicated parapneumonic effusion
Simple parapneumonic effusion
Exudative ascites from abdominal or pelvic disease
Malignancy in the pleura or mediastinal lymph nodes
Tuberculous pleurisy
Amebiasis
Fungal disease
Acute exacerbation of systemic lupus erythematosus
Postoperative pleural effusion after thoracic surgery
Postoperative pleural effusion after abdominal or pelvic surgery
Postpartum state
Pancreatitis
Myxedema

EXUDATES

The differential diagnosis of exudative effusions in the critically ill patient is very large indeed. Some of the causes of exudative pleural effusion are listed in Table 138-2.

In the search for a diagnosis of a pleural exudate, it is best to send samples routinely for the following tests: protein determination, LDH, pH and P_{CO_2}, glucose, aerobic and anaerobic culture, acid fast and fungal stains, acid fast and fungal cultures, cytology, serologies for connective tissue disease (antinuclear antibody, etc.), WBC count, differential of WBCs, RBC count, and amylase determination. In selected cases it may be reasonable to add other determinations such as cryptococcal antigen determination or hematocrit.

COMPLICATED PLEURAL EFFUSION AND EMPYEMA

The concept of empyema and its treatment has undergone change in the recent past. If empyema is defined as a pleural effusion in which the cultures are positive for organisms, then this concept would not be broad enough to cover all of the clinical situations in which tube thoracostomy is required for satisfactory resolution of a parapneumonic pleural effusion (i.e., a pleural effusion associated with pneumonia). To clarify the concept, the notion of a complicated pleural effusion has been put forward as an alternative. A *complicated parapneumonic effusion* is present when the pH of the fluid is <7.10 and it is associated with a glucose of <40 mg/dL and a LDH value of >1000 U/L.[9] If this definition of complicated pleural effusion is accepted, an *empyema* can be simply defined as the presence of frank pus in the pleural space. Empyema or complicated pleural effusion is an emergency of the pleural space and all critically ill patients who have empyema or complicated pleural effusion should undergo placement of a chest tube to achieve surgical drainage. For patients who are suspected of having multiple loculations of pus, early thoracotomy with surgical drainage (rib resection) may be the best procedure since it is so reliable.[10] If surgical drainage cannot be performed for any reason on a critically ill patient, recent experience with the noncritically ill suggests that "medical" therapy with intravenous antimicrobial drugs may sometimes be successful.[11] In patients who have placement of a chest tube for empyema, radiographic dye should be injected through the chest tube to determine the size and configuration of the empyema cavity ("empyemogram").[12] An empyemogram allows the surgeon to determine whether or not the pus-filled space has been adequately drained. If there is an undrained site, another chest tube should be placed in it. In critically ill patients, the surgeon must decide between tube thoracostomy and thoracotomy. Frequently, critically ill patients are too sick to undergo the long anesthesia times and the major incision necessary for ideal surgical drainage. In these cases, tube thoracostomy placed by a surgeon or a drainage catheter placed by a radiologist are usually better choices. The placement of a tube thoracostomy into a critically ill patient who is breathing on a mechanical ventilator is best done without using a trochar for placement of the tube into the pleural space. It is preferable to first make the incision in the intercostal space, then use a Kelly clamp to introduce the tube into the pleural space. This maneuver helps to avoid possible impalement of the lung, which is more likely to happen when a trochar is used.

CHYLOTHORAX

Chylothorax is the presence of chyle (of small intestinal origin, transported through the lymphatics) in the pleural space. Chylous pleural effusion should be suspected when milky-appearing material is removed at thoracentesis. It should be differentiated from pseudochylous effusion. A chylothorax contains chylomicrons, high levels of triglyceride, and a predominance of lymphocytes, whereas a pseudochylous effusion contains cholesterol crystals, smaller amounts of triglycerides but no chylomicrons. A pseudochylous effusion is usually a chronic pleural effusion, often more than 5 years old, that looks milky to the naked eye because it contains cholesterol crystals and other lipids that result from the disintegration of cells and cell membranes over time.

Chylothorax may be discovered in the critically ill patient in various settings. Attempts to place intravenous catheters in the left internal jugular or subclavian veins can result in laceration of the thoracic duct. In the postoperative patient who has just had thoracic surgery, intraoperative laceration of a major chyle vessel is the likely cause. In patients with lymphoma, chylothorax is a complication of the lymphoma itself. Chylothorax also happens with no apparent cause.

When a chylothorax is discovered, conservative management with repeated thoracenteses or placement of a tube thoracostomy is in order to determine whether the rent in the vessel will close spontaneously, without the need for another thoracotomy.[12] In patients with lymphoma, specific antilymphoma therapy such as radiotherapy may allow the chylothorax to regress. In critically ill patients, a major consequence of chylothorax is nutritional, since most of the lipids ingested by the patient collect in the pleural space and are unavailable to metabolizing tissues. Also, immune function may be impaired in repeated drainage of the chylothorax because substantial numbers of lymphocytes are removed with the chyle. Chylothorax often requires that alternative methods of nutrition such as intravenous alimentation be instituted. When conservative measures fail, operative ligation of the thoracic duct below the leaking site is one option; another is surgical obliteration of the pleural space.[14]

HEMOTHORAX

Pleural hemorrhage can occur spontaneously in patients who are being treated with heparin or warfarin, in patients with polyarteritis nodosa, in patients who have suffered thoracic trauma, in postoperative patients, in patients with ruptured thoracic aortic aneurysm, and in patients whose chests have been punctured with needles (placement of central venous catheters, transthoracic needle aspiration, thoracentesis or pleural biopsy).

When blood is removed from the pleural space at thoracentesis, it may or may not undergo clotting if it is drawn into an unheparinized syringe. If the blood does not clot, it is very likely to be a hemothorax that has been present for many hours or days and it may contain little or no fibrinogen. If the blood clots, it may be a new hemothorax with a high fibrinogen content, or the blood may be completely fresh and result from the trauma of the thoracentesis itself. These observations stem from the natural history of hemorrhage into the pleural cavity. When blood first enters the pleural space, it undergoes clotting as a result of activation of fibrinogen by the pleural surface; thereafter the clot gradually undergoes fibrinolysis, leaving behind the reliquified blood that is depleted of fibrinogen. In summary, when nonclotting blood is withdrawn from the pleural space, this indicates that the blood was not the result of the trauma of the procedure itself but represents instead the result of pathologic bleeding of many hours' to days' duration.

If the pleural effusion is discovered to be bloody with a high hematocrit, the intensivist has a special problem since the ongoing rate of bleeding now becomes the most important variable to assess. The only reliable way to determine the rate of intrapleural hemorrhage is to insert a thoracostomy tube and measure the hourly rate of blood loss. Rapid bleeding is defined as a rate of bleeding that causes hypotension in the patient even after insertion of a thoracostomy tube has drained the pleural space.[15] Bleeding of >200 mL/h is also considered to be rapid bleeding even if the patient's blood pressure can be maintained by the infusion of blood products.[16] Rapid bleeding requires emergency thoracotomy with identification of the bleeding site and electrocautery of the torn vessel. Very slow rates of intrapleural hemorrhage may be treated with blood transfusion and observation. Both the thoracostomy tube and the chest radiograph should be watched closely because intrapleural clotting can obstruct the drainage tube, and the intensivist may therefore fail to appreciate the true bleeding rate.

Hemothorax in the context of sudden onset of severe chest pain should raise the possibility of aortic dissection; if the bleeding site in the aortic wall is small, the patient may survive long enough for a thoracentesis to be performed in the ICU. However, priority should be given to surgical intervention and to efforts to make a specific diagnosis if time allows, with an echocardiogram or CT scan or magnetic resonance imaging or aortogram. When hemothorax is the result of trauma or surgery, thoracotomy is often lifesaving. When hemothorax results from heparin or warfarin therapy in a patient with acute pulmonary embolus, the anticoagulants should be stopped and reversed and a vena cava umbrella should be inserted to protect the patient from repeat pulmonary embolus.

BLOODY PLEURAL EFFUSION

Pleural effusions that are bloody in gross appearance but that do not have a hematocrit comparable to circulating blood do not represent an emergency in themselves. Most of these effusions are caused by pleural metastases. When the cause of hemorrhagic pleural effusion is an acute pulmonary embolus, the hemorrhagic pleural effusion is not a contraindication to heparin therapy. Pleural tuberculosis and pleural effusion associated with pancreatitis are also often bloody.

ESOPHAGEAL DISEASES AND PLEURAL EFFUSION

Critically ill patients who are bleeding from esophageal varices are often treated by endoscopic esophageal variceal sclerotherapy in which the varices are injected with sodium morrhuate.[17–19] The sclerosing agent is thought to exude from the varix into the esophageal wall and from there it may leak into the mediastinum, since the esophagus is not covered by a serosal membrane. Mediastinal and pleural effusions form immediately after esophageal sclerotherapy in a large percentage of these patients, with many of them also having a fever in association with this process. In most cases, this reaction is self-limited and does not mandate diagnostic thoracentesis. Fever prolonged beyond 48 h together with progressive enlargement of the pleural effusions on chest radiograph, however, should be investigated with thoracentesis.

Critically ill patients who are vomiting with great forcefulness may suffer a through-and-through rupture of the esophageal wall, with spillage of bacteria and esophageal contents into the mediastinum and pleura. This complication is also seen in patient's who undergo esophageal instrumentation.[20,21] In most patients, rupture of the esophagus causes dyspnea, fever, and toxicity. Analysis of pleural fluid classically shows a very low pH (<6) and elevated amylase (of salivary origin). Patients with esophageal rupture should be treated with immediate thoracotomy to repair the esophagus and drain all infected spaces in the mediastinum and pleura.

Treatment of Pleural Effusions

The treatment of pleural effusion in the critically ill patient is dictated by the specific diagnosis; nevertheless, several generalizations are true for the treatment of pleural disease in general.

PLEURITIC PAIN

Most forms of pleuritic chest pain can be relieved with nonsteroidal anti-inflammatory drugs.[22] These are effective when given by rectal suppository or by intramuscular injection to patients who cannot take medication by mouth. Nonsteroidal anti-inflammatory drugs are usually more effective than narcotics in relieving pleuritic pain. An alternative to control of severe pleuritic chest pain in the critically ill patient is the performance of local nerve blocks by an anesthesiologist. These techniques include intercostal nerve block, epidural narcotic administration, and instillation of local anesthetic into the pleural space. The relief of pain through these methods can play an important role in the care of the patient not only in reducing suffering but also in enabling the patient to cough and take deep breaths, thus combating the tendency to develop pneumonia.

DYSPNEA AND THERAPEUTIC THORACENTESIS

The dyspnea of pleural effusion is often relieved by therapeutic thoracentesis. No matter what its cause, a very large pleural effusion causes dyspnea and may to a small extent impair ventilation in a critically ill patient, especially when that patient is breathing spontaneously. By performing a therapeutic thoracentesis, the intensivist can alleviate the patient's distress and improve lung volumes and arterial oxygen tension.[1] The relief of dyspnea following therapeutic thoracentesis results from a decrease in the size of the thoracic cage, which allows the inspiratory muscles to operate more effectively;[2] increased cardiac output may also correct respiratory muscle dysfunction to avoid intubation and ventilation of the hypoventilating patient.

TUBE THORACOSTOMY

Therapeutic thoracentesis is a good means of removing pleural fluid for relief of dyspnea when the rate of accumulation of pleural fluid is low and when the pleural effusion is small or moderate in size. Very large pleural effusions and those that recur rapidly are best drained with placement of a tube thoracostomy. A thoracostomy tube is also the best treatment for infections and ongoing hemorrhage into the pleural space.

A special difficulty in treatment of pleural effusion with a thoracostomy tube is encountered in the patient who has a massive pleural effusion associated with massive ascites. Patients with the combined abnormality often sit upright and are continuously dyspneic. The special dilemma in this instance is that thoracentesis is only transiently effective in lowering the volume of pleural fluid, since the ascites replaces whatever has been drawn out in a very short interval of time. The placement of a tube thoracostomy in a patient with combined pleural effusion and ascites is usually not a good choice since it effectively drains both the thoracic and abdominal compartments at such a fast rate that it may result in acute intravascular volume depletion and worsened hypoproteinemia from the net protein lost in the removed fluid. It is usually best, therefore, to manage the dyspnea of combined pleural effusion and ascites by positioning the patient for maximum comfort and by avoiding drainage of the serosal spaces.

SURGICAL INTERVENTIONS

Other surgical interventions that are available in the treatment of pleural effusion include chemical pleurodesis (tetracycline),[23] surgical pleurodesis (thoracotomy), and the surgical placement of a pleuroperitoneal shunt.[24] In *chemical pleurodesis,* the pleural space is first drained with a thoracostomy tube. Following full expansion of the underlying lung, a low pH solution of tetracycline (20 mg/mL) is introduced into the pleural space to cause inflammation, followed by adherence of the parietal and visceral pleura to each other, thereby obliterating the pleural space. Although often effective, chemical pleurodesis is occasionally accompanied by extremely severe chest pain that is often not controlled either by lidocaine mixed in with the tetracycline or by administering narcotics. *Surgical pleurodesis* involves a thoracotomy followed by stripping of parietal pleura to remove the potential space that previously existed between the two layers. After surgical pleurodesis, the visceral pleura is adherent to the chest wall. Some critically ill patients in our institution have done well following surgical pleurodesis performed through a small thoracotomy wound just below the axilla. *Pleuroperitoneal shunt* is an internal drainage procedure in which fluid drains through a modified Denver shunt into the peritoneal cavity. It has been used for draining large, recurrent pleural effusions from a wide variety of causes, including malignant pleural effusion.

CASE PRESENTATION

Mrs. M.M., a 69-year-old black woman, was admitted with a chief complaint of dyspnea and pleuritic chest pain. She was a nonsmoker with a history of a positive intermediate strength purified protein derivative (PPD) skin test (not treated with isoniazid chemoprophylaxis), and she had multiple medical problems that included chronic anemia, diabetes mellitus, peripheral vascular disease in her legs, and a recent left-sided hip fracture treated with open reduction and internal fixation. The hip surgery had been performed 1 month prior to admission and the patient had been recovering well at home. One week prior to admission she noted diffuse weakness and shortness of breath. Three days prior to admission she felt the abrupt onset of left-sided pleuritic chest pain and her degree of dyspnea increased. The patient sought help at the emergency room and was admitted. Medications on admission included only insulin. Her past medical history included resectional surgery for squamous cell carcinoma of the mouth (she was a chronic user of snuff) and chronic renal insufficiency with a serum creatinine level of 1.5 to 2.0 mg/dL.

Physical examination revealed a thin black woman in distress, holding her left anterior hemithorax. Her blood pressure was 140/70, pulse was 80, respiratory rate 20 and her oral temperature was 37.1°C (98.9°F). Chest examination showed dullness to percussion and decreased breath sounds at both lung bases. Heart examination showed a jugular venous pressure of 5 cm while she was sitting at a 45° angle; there was a left-sided S_4, fourth heart sound, a 2/6 systolic ejection murmur at the left lower sternal border and trace bilateral calf edema. Extremities revealed a well-healed hip wound and numerous toe amputations.

The chest radiograph showed bilateral moderate-sized pleural effusions. The ECG had normal sinus rhythm with no abnormalities. The WBC count was 10,300 with 68 neutrophils, 1 band, and 31 lymphs. Electrolytes were normal, BUN 29, and serum creatinine 2.3 mg/dL. Arterial blood-gas determinations drawn while the patient breathed room air were pH 7.48, P_{CO_2} 30 mmHg and P_{O_2} 51 mmHg. An echocardiogram showed a moderate pericardial effusion with no atrial or ventricular collapse. Since the pleural effusions were moderately large with no radiologic indications of loculation, ultrasound was not performed prior to thoracentesis. A thoracentesis was done on the left hemithorax without any difficulty; the fluid was clear and straw colored, and was an exudate with a protein of 3.7 g/dL, LDH of 273 U (normal 56 to 194), pH of 7.32, glucose 173, amylase 30, WBC count of 22,400/μL with 92 neutrophils, 4 lymphs, 2 macrophages, and 1 eosinophil; RBC count was 200/μL. Gram and AFB stains showed no organisms and cytology was negative. A Doppler examination of the leg veins was normal.

Concern over the patient's general instability (hypoxemia, high WBC count indicating possible new onset of sepsis) led to the decision to move her to the ICU unit on hospital day 1. Her cardiac monitor showed occasional bradycardia with rates as low as 25. She required intermittent intravenous injections of atropine for control of the bradycardia. She then had a psychotic episode manifested by hallucinations and agitation. A lumbar puncture was done which showed a protein of 65 mg/dL, glucose of 63 mg/dL with a concomitant serum glucose of 110 mg/dL, a WBC count of 13 with 85% lymphocytes, 13% mononuclear cells, and 2% plasma cells, a RBC count of 2, and no organisms were seen on Gram stain. Repeat thoracentesis continued to show an exudate and the differential diagnosis included prominently pleural tuberculosis, pulmonary embolus, viral pleuropericarditis, connective tissue disease manifesting as pleural effusion, abdominal disease, and idiopathic pleural effusion. Although pulmonary embolus was considered in the differential diagnosis in light of the patient's recent hip surgery and her low P_{O_2}, the absence of clot in the leg veins on noninvasive testing meant that the patient was unlikely to have another large pulmonary embolus immediately, thus allowing the investigations to proceed without the need to treat her with anticoagulants. Viral pleuropericarditis was possible since there was fluid in both the pericardial and pleural spaces. Viral cultures could be done, but the results would not be available immediately. There were no symptoms, signs, or laboratory findings to indicate abdominal disease.

The possibility of pleural tuberculosis led her physicians to perform a closed pleural biopsy using an Abrams needle in the ICU. Multiple pieces of parietal pleura were obtained and histopathology showed a marked pleuritis with no granulomas. On hospital day 3 the patient became thrombocytopenic with a platelet count of 52,000; serologies for connective tissue disease had been completed: antinuclear antibody was positive at 1:1600. An assay for double-stranded DNA was negative. Measures of complement were all reduced and an antinuclear antibody assay done on pleural fluid was positive at >1:1600. The pleural biopsy together with the pleural fluid analysis were considered to have made tuberculosis an unlikely cause of the effusion, and a diagnosis of late-onset systemic lupus erythematosus (SLE) was made. She was moved out of the ICU and started on glucocorticoid in the form of prednisone. Her condition slowly improved over several weeks. Isoniazid and rifampin were administered as a precaution for several weeks until pleural fluid and tissue cultures were reported as negative; at that point isoniazid was continued as chemoprophylaxis because of the patient's positive PPD skin test, together with her risk factors for reactivation: diabetes and immunosuppressive therapy.

CASE DISCUSSION

The presentation and course of this patient's illness illustrates features of late-onset SLE.[25] Pleuritis and pericarditis are the most common manifestations, whereas lymphadenopathy, Raynaud's phenomenon, alopecia, and skin rash are less common. The case also exemplifies a typical application of thoracentesis and pleural biopsy in the ICU setting. Since tuberculosis is a disease that activates in the presence of chronic debilitating illnesses, it is common to consider it in the differential diagnosis of critically ill patients with multisystem disease. When pleural tuberculosis is being considered, effective microbiologic diagnosis requires culture of both pleural fluid and pleural tissue, together with sputum, since the number of infecting organisms is low and the diagnosis is very difficult to make with pleural fluid alone. In this case, the use of thoracentesis and pleural biopsy allowed the physician to turn his diagnostic attention away from tuberculosis and to emphasize the treatment of the more likely cause of the pleural effusion, SLE. The possibility of acute pulmonary embolus was not investigated with a bedside perfusion scan in the ICU, but the leg veins were examined with the Doppler technique to see whether there was imminent risk of pulmonary embolus from the large veins of the legs. There was no particular clinical reason to suspect abdominal or pelvic disease and so CT scanning of these areas was not given priority. The pleural biopsy was given high priority and done when the patient had not yet developed thrombocytopenia; a few days later, the patient's platelet count had dropped and the risk of intrapleural hemorrhage from the procedure would have been higher. By providing evidence that the patient did not have active pleural tuberculosis, her physician felt comfortable in giving her the drug prednisone, which resulted in her rapid improvement and transfer out of the ICU.

References

1. Brown NE, Zamel N, Aberman A: Changes in pulmonary mechanics and gas exchange following thoracocentesis. Chest 74:540, 1978.
2. Estenne M, Yernault JC, De Troyer A. Mechanism of relief of dyspnea after thoracocentesis in patients with large pleural effusions. Am J Med 74:813, 1983.
3. Wright GW: Tuberculosis and pneumonia, in Fenn WO and Rahn H (eds.): *Handbook of Physiology*. Washington, DC, American Physiological Society, 1965, p 1617.
4. Lemmer JH, Botham MJ, Orringer MB: Modern management of adult thoracic empyema. J Thorac Cardiovasc Surg 90:849, 1985.
5. Rosenberg ER: Ultrasound in the assessment of pleural densities. Chest 84:283, 1983.
6. Sokolowski JH Jr, Burgher LW, Jones FL, et al: Guidelines for thoracentesis and needle biopsy of the pleura. Am Rev Respir Dis 140:257, 1989.
7. Light RW: *Pleural Diseases*. Philadelphia, Lea & Febiger, 1983, p 36.
8. Stark DD, Shanes JG, Baron RL, Koch DD: Biochemical features of urinothorax. Arch Intern Med 142:1509, 1982.
9. Sahn SA. The pleura. Am Rev Respir Dis 138:184, 1988.
10. Ferguson MK: The healing hand. Chest 97:4, 1990.
11. Berger HA, Morganroth ML: Immediate drainage is not required for all patients with complicated parapneumonic effusions. Chest 97:731, 1990.
12. Orringer MB: Thoracic empyema—Back to basics. Chest 93:901, 1988.
13. Light RW: *Pleural Diseases*. Philadelphia, Lea & Febiger, 1983, pp 213–215.
14. Strausser JL, Flye MW: Management of nontraumatic chylothorax. Ann Thorac Surg 31:520, 1980.
15. Weil PH, Margolis IB: Systemic approach to traumatic hemothorax. Am J Surg 142:692, 1981.
16. Light RW: *Pleural Diseases*. Philadelphia, Lea & Febiger, 1983, p 206.
17. Mauro MA, Jaques PJ, Swantkowski TM, et al: CT after uncomplicated esophageal sclerotherapy. AJR 147:57, 1986.
18. Bacon BR, Bailey-Newton RS, Connors AF: Pleural effusions after endoscopic variceal sclerotherapy. Gastroenterology 88:1910, 1985.
19. Saks BJ, Kilby AE, Dietrich PA, Coffin LH, Krawitt EL: Pleural and mediastinal changes following endoscopic injection sclerotherapy of esophageal varices. Radiology 149:639, 1983.
20. Bellman MH, Rajaratnam HN: Perforation of the oesophagus with amylase rich pleural effusion. Brit J Dis Chest 68:197, 1974.
21. Patton AS, Lawson DW, Shannon JM, et al: Reevaluation of the Boerhaave syndrome: A review of fourteen cases. Am J Surg 137:560, 1979.

22. Sacks PV, Kanarek D: Treatment of acute pleuritic pain: Comparison between indomethacin and a placebo. Am Rev Respir Dis 108:666, 1973.
23. Sahn SA: Malignant pleural effusions. Clin Chest Med 6:113, 1985.
24. Brofman JD, Hall JB, Scott W, Little AG: Yellow nails, lymphedema and pleural effusion: Treatment of chronic pleural effusion with pleuroperitoneal shunting. Chest 97:743, 1990.
25. Baker SB, Rovira JR, Campion EW, Mills JA: Late onset systemic lupus erythematosus. Am J Med 66:727, 1979.

Chapter 139

LIFE-THREATENING COMPLICATIONS OF CYSTIC FIBROSIS IN ADULTS

EUGENE F. GEPPERT

KEY POINTS

- *Infection of the bronchi with mucoid* Pseudomonas aeruginosa *plays an important role in the stepwise destruction of the lungs in patients with cystic fibrosis. Therapy during any critical illness emphasizes treating this and other infecting pathogens.*
- *Bronchiectatic cysts, interstitial cysts, and emphysematous bullae may lead to life-threatening pneumothorax.*
- *A minority of patients develop hepatic cirrhosis with portal hypertension and esophageal varices that may cause life-threatening upper gastrointestinal hemorrhage.*
- *Critically ill adults with cystic fibrosis do not tolerate the fasting state well and whenever possible should receive enteral feedings together with supplemental pancreatic enzymes.*
- *Adults with cystic fibrosis require larger doses of antimicrobial drugs than do other patients due to increased volume of distribution and to increased clearance of the drugs.*
- *Chest physiotherapy adds measurably to the pulmonary function of very ill patients with cystic fibrosis and should be performed in the critically ill four times a day.*
- *Endotracheal intubation and mechanical ventilation are ineffective in treating patients with end-stage cystic fibrosis who have acute ventilatory failure. Their use results in a very prolonged stay in the intensive care unit (ICU) followed by a fatal outcome. Use this form of therapy only as a bridge to overcome a temporary illness in patients with adequate baseline pulmonary function.*
- *Critically ill adults with cystic fibrosis are prone to develop the distal intestinal obstruction syndrome (partial small-bowel obstruction with right lower quadrant mass and pain). The intensivist should try to prevent this by giving the patient at least a small amount of supplemental pancreatic enzyme each day, even if the patient is not eating food.*

Cystic fibrosis is a systemic disease caused by an abnormal gene that is characterized biochemically by abnormalities in fluid and electrolyte transport in exocrine epithelial cells.[1] Clinically, cystic fibrosis is most noted for the secondary effects on organ systems of this abnormality: exocrine insufficiency in the pancreas, progressive bronchiectasis, and attacks of partial obstruction of the distal intestine. The disease runs a highly variable course and is often very severe during childhood. Statistics from the Cystic Fibrosis Foundation with its national registry of patients now show that many patients with cystic fibrosis are living into adulthood, and more than 50 percent of patients can now expect to survive to age 25. Many factors have contributed to this enhanced survival, but antimicrobial drugs have been extremely important since they help to combat the organisms such as *Pseudomonas aeruginosa* that infect the lungs of these patients and progressively injure the pulmonary bronchioles.

For many patients with cystic fibrosis adulthood is the period of life when the first critical illness appears. The current goal of treatment in adults with cystic fibrosis is to delay the crisis period for as long as possible. When the disease has progressed to the crisis point, it usually makes itself manifest as acute respiratory failure superimposed on chronic respiratory failure, as hemoptysis, or sometimes as hepatic failure with gastrointestinal hemorrhage.

Pathophysiology of Cystic Fibrosis

The precise nature of the genetic defect in cystic fibrosis is unknown, but current research efforts are producing a wealth of new information about the disease. In 1989, the gene responsible for cystic fibrosis was identified on the long arm of chromosome 7 and its deoxyribonucleic acid (DNA) was sequenced.[2] The gene codes for a protein of 1480 amino acids. Whatever may be the exact nature of the protein that is abnormal in cystic fibrosis, its defective function probably results directly in the biochemical derangements that have been documented in cystic fibrosis: excessive salt in sweat but a deficiency of salt and water in the bronchial, genitourinary, and gastrointestinal mucus. These biochemical abnormalities are present in utero. Even before birth, the abnormal gastrointestinal secretions may cause ileus that can be seen with uterine ultrasonography. At birth, the lungs are structurally normal, but over time, the secondary consequences of abnormal bronchial mucus result in the development of progressive bronchiectasis and widespread bronchiolitis obliterans.[3] Bronchiectasis and bronchiolitis obliterans are probably caused by more than just the water deficiency of bronchial mucus. The infection of bronchial mucus with large numbers of bacteria also plays an important pathogenetic role in the stepwise destruction of the lungs. The reasons why the airways of patients with cystic fibrosis are so readily infected with bacteria such as *Staphylococcus aureus* and *P. aeruginosa* are completely unknown. Nevertheless, the presence of these organisms is thought to play a major role in the ongoing cycle of lung destruction by releasing bacterial elastases and initiating other changes that result in tissue destruction.[4] Microcolonies and dense concentrations of *P. aeruginosa* can often be found at the location of destructive changes,[3] and it has been shown that intensive treatment with anti-*Pseudomonas* antimicrobial drugs can improve spirometric function.[5] The functional result of the pathologic changes in the lung is chronic airways obstruction. It results from unstable large central bronchi, narrowed peripheral bronchi, and widespread plugging of bronchial lumens with abnormally viscid mucus.[6] A late change in the disease is that the bronchial arteries become hypertrophic in response to the widespread bronchiectasis, richly supplying intraluminal and periluminal granulation tissue. It is this system of hypertrophied arteries that is responsible for the hemoptysis that is seen so frequently. In an advanced stage of lung disease, the lungs of patients with cystic fibrosis contain bronchiectatic cysts, interstitial cysts, and emphysematous bullae, all of which may rupture into the pleural space and cause pneumothorax.[7] Eventually cystic fibrosis lung disease reaches the stage of arterial hypoxemia and respiratory insufficiency that terminates with cor pulmonale. About 90 percent of patients with cystic fibrosis succumb with acute respiratory failure.[8] A small minority of patients with cystic fibrosis develop cirrhosis of the liver and may have esophageal varices. Strictures of the common bile duct are more common and usually become manifest as abdominal pain.[9] Most patients with cystic fibrosis have pancreatic exocrine insufficiency that requires them to supplement all meals and meal replacement formulas with pancreatic enzyme capsules.

General Care of the Cystic Fibrosis Patient during Critical Illness

NUTRITION

Critically ill patients with cystic fibrosis are usually anorectic and will lose a large amount of weight quickly unless immediate measures are taken to provide their daily caloric needs. In adult patients we prefer the enteral approach, either through use of a soft nasoenteral tube or through a gastrostomy or jejunostomy. The patients should be given meal replacement formulas supplemented by pancreatic enzymes to achieve a total caloric intake similar to that of other critically ill patients (see Chap. 92). Whenever possible, the daily caloric needs of a critically ill adult with cystic fibrosis should be measured by calorimetry. It is important to add vitamin E to the daily regimen at a dose of 100 to 200 units and to measure the serum levels of other fat-soluble vitamins to determine whether these should be given in increased amounts.

Critically ill adults with cystic fibrosis are prone to develop distal intestinal obstruction syndrome, and the intensivist should be vigilant for signs of right lower quadrant pain and partial bowel obstruction. Even when the patient is not being fed for some reason, small doses of pancreatic enzymes should be given in order to help prevent the onset of ileal obstruction. Also, some adult patients with cystic fibrosis will have lost islet tissue in the pancreas and may either be frankly diabetic or develop hyperosmolar coma when challenged with intravenous hyperalimentation. Much is still unknown about the optimal nutritional support of the critically ill adult with cystic fibrosis.

ANTIMICROBIAL THERAPY

Because almost every adult patient with cystic fibrosis who is critically ill has chronic bronchial infection with *P. aeruginosa,* supportive care requires intravenous antimicrobial therapy. An important principle to remember is that patients with cystic fibrosis need substantially larger doses of both the aminoglycosides and the penicillins, since the drugs have both increased clearance and increased volume of distribution.[10] Some guidelines for initial dosing are given in Table 139-1.

Whenever possible, serum levels should be measured and adjusted to achieve desirable peak and trough levels for each drug. If the patient was hospitalized previously, the antimicrobial dosages that achieved good serum levels on a previous occasion may be used as the starting doses. Two drugs should be used against *P. aeruginosa,* and penicillins should not be given simultaneously with the aminoglycosides, since there is evidence that the penicillins may inactivate the aminoglycosides in vivo.[11] If a sputum cul-

TABLE 139-1 Antimicrobial Agents and Doses for Critically Ill Adults with Cystic Fibrosis

Organism	Agent	Adult Dose(mg/kg/day IV)*	Doses Per Day
S. aureus	Oxacillin	150–200	4
P. aeruginosa	Gentamicin	8–20	3
P. aeruginosa	Tobramycin	8–20	3
P. aeruginosa	Amikacin	15–30	2–3
P. aeruginosa	Netilmicin	6–12	2–3
P. aeruginosa	Carbenicillin	250–500	4–6
P. aeruginosa	Ticarcillin	250–500	4–6
P. aeruginosa	Piperacillin	250–450	4–6
P. aeruginosa	Mezlocillin	250–450	4–6
P. aeruginosa	Azlocillin	250–450	4–6
P. aeruginosa	Ticar/Clavulanate	250–450	4–6
P. aeruginosa	Imipenem/cilastatin	4g/day IV	3–4
P. aeruginosa-cepacia	Ceftazidime	4–6g/day IV	3

*Except as noted.
SOURCE: Modified from Boat[13] with permission.

ture shows other pathogens, such as *S. aureus*, antimicrobial coverage should be expanded accordingly.

The goal of antimicrobial therapy in the critically ill adult with cystic fibrosis is to dramatically decrease the numbers of bacteria infecting the tracheobronchial tree. The benefits realized from this approach include better pulmonary function, decreased cough and sputum volume, better appetite, and a better sense of well being. Organisms are never totally eradicated, and the time period necessary to realize benefit is 2 weeks in most patients, with critically ill patients often requiring even more treatment.

PHYSICAL THERAPY

Chest physiotherapy contributes substantially to the respiratory care of adults with cystic fibrosis. Except in the circumstance of acute life-threatening hemoptysis, we advocate the use of chest physiotherapy by hand percussion for 3 min in each position four times a day.

Acute Ventilatory Failure

GENERAL CONSIDERATIONS

Most patients with cystic fibrosis eventually succumb to their disease through gradually worsening lung disease with cor pulmonale and acute ventilatory failure. Whenever possible, the patient's physician should try to talk to the patient who is worsening so that the patient's own desires can be taken into account at the moment when acute ventilatory failure supervenes. If the adult patient wishes to choose a conservative approach without endotracheal intubation and mechanical ventilation, the patient's desires should be legally recorded according to the requirements of the patient's local government. In Illinois, for example, the patient should fill out and sign a Power of Attorney for Health Care document, which designates another person who is legally empowered to make important decisions for the patient in the event the patient cannot do so himself. In counseling the patient, the physician should point out that endotracheal intubation and mechanical ventilation most often has had a bad outcome in adult patients with cystic fibrosis, and it is best reserved for those patients in whom it provides a "bridge" to recovery from a complication other than acute ventilatory failure (e.g., hemoptysis). For the adult patient with end-stage cystic fibrosis lung disease, the use of endotracheal intubation and mechanical ventilation as a means of dealing with acute ventilatory failure usually results in a prolonged stay in the ICU while struggling for a long period of time to be liberated from the mechanical ventilator and suffering multiple complications.[12,13] The amount of suffering involved is considerable, and the patient should only be subjected to this with full advance knowledge of what is involved and the probable outcome. Very often, the patient's personal physician will have prepared the patient and the patient's family for the terminal phase of the illness, and the physician's decision together with the intensivist will be not to offer mechanical ventilation as an option for dealing with the terminal stage of the disease.

CLINICAL PROGRESSION FROM CHRONIC COMPENSATED VENTILATORY INSUFFICIENCY TO ACUTE VENTILATORY FAILURE

Some clinical signs tend to predict the impending onset of acute ventilatory failure. Adult patients who are entering the final phase of their illness often show a failure to improve their FEV_1 following a 2-week course of intravenous antimicrobial therapy. They very often show a stepwise increase in their baseline arterial PCO_2. The echocardiogram often shows right ventricular dilation and interference with motion of the cardiac septum. The clinical signs of impending acute ventilatory failure are variable. Some patients develop increasing dyspnea at rest and struggle to breathe until exhaustion. Other patients, also exhausted, retain carbon dioxide progressively and lose consciousness. Agonal breathing may reveal itself by the use of head-bobbing movements during breathing and decreasing excursion of the chest wall.

Patients who are showing signs of cor pulmonale can now be considered for lung transplantation. There are many factors to be taken into consideration in making a decision about performing lung transplantation on an adult with cystic fibrosis, and at the present time the majority of patients with end-stage disease are not choosing to undergo the operation. As technical improvements advance the success of lung transplantation, more and more patients are likely to seek this form of therapy.

VENTILATOR MANAGEMENT OF PATIENTS WITH CYSTIC FIBROSIS

Very little has been written about the ventilator management of adult patients with cystic fibrosis, perhaps because most experts agree that it should be avoided as much as possible. If an adult patient with cystic fibrosis does undergo endotracheal intubation with mechanical ventilation, however, a few guidelines are in order. A tracheostomy should be performed unless it is clear that the patient will only be intubated for less than 2 weeks. The performance of a tracheostomy allows the patient more comfort in that the patient may be able to eat and talk with the tracheostomy in place. A nasal endotracheal tube will be prone to cause difficulty, since 50 percent of adult patients with cystic fibrosis have nasal polyps and they are susceptible to bacterial sinusitis. An oral endotracheal tube is clearly more uncomfortable for an awake patient than is a tracheostomy. We begin mechanical ventilation with the assist-control mode and a tidal volume of about 10 mL/kg. We also try to ensure excellent humidification of the inspired gas and practice frequent suctioning with the use of saline washes for bronchial toilet. Patients who struggle against the ventilator should be paralyzed and sedated for the first few days of mechanical ventilation if they cannot be made comfortable with manipulation of the ventilator. Because of the high risk of pneumothorax, we try to maintain peak airway pressures of less than 40 mmHg. The trigger sensitivity of the ventilator should be kept low (-1 or -2 cmH_2O). We employ the same criteria used in patients with chronic obstructive pulmonary disease (COPD) to predict when an adult with cystic fibrosis is ready to be liberated from the mechanical ventilator (see Chap. 127 and 129). Patients who are in acute ventilatory failure should get a program of nutrition that supplies them with the full complement of calories they metabolize, and they should be treated with bronchodilators such as theophylline (to achieve a serum level of about 10 to 15 mg/L) and long-acting β-adrenergic agonists. We avoid using steroid drugs except in adult patients with cystic fibrosis who are known to also have the complication of allergic bronchopulmonary aspergillosis. It is very important to suppress fever in these patients because oxygen delivery to their tissues is already marginal at best, and nothing should be done that promotes increased oxygen need by the tissues. We do not routinely perform fiberoptic bronchoscopy in adult patients with cystic fibrosis who are being mechanically ventilated unless there is some specific indication (lung collapse, hemoptysis, etc.).

MANAGEMENT OF ACUTE VENTILATORY FAILURE WITHOUT MECHANICAL VENTILATION

The usual method of managing adult patients with cystic fibrosis who go into acute ventilatory failure is conservative. This means that the patient is admitted to the hospital for a program of care that includes chest physiotherapy, intravenous antimicrobial drugs against infecting organisms present in the patient's sputum, oxygen therapy by nasal prongs or mask, supplemental nutrition, and measures to assure patient comfort. Usually this program can be carried out without using the ICU. In some patients who are severely dyspneic, we have found patient-controlled analgesia with morphine to be a useful and effective means of controlling the patient's overwhelming sense of shortness of breath. Of course, morphine is used with the knowledge that it will depress respiration, but there are instances where the relief of the patient's suffering takes precedence over this consideration.

MANAGEMENT OF COR PULMONALE

The management of cor pulmonale in adults with cystic fibrosis is not different from management of cor pulmonale resulting from most other lung diseases (see Chap. 115). The emphasis should be placed on treating the underlying lung disease with intravenous antimicrobials and treating alveolar hypoxia with supplemental oxygen.

Hemoptysis

A minor amount of hemoptysis (several tablespoons) is a frequent occurrence in adult patients with cystic fibrosis and in itself has no important clinical meaning. Major hemoptysis, however, defined as >300 mL of blood expectorated within 24 h, is a life-threatening complication of cystic fibrosis.

Hemoptysis in adult patients with cystic fibrosis is caused by bleeding in either bronchial arteries or in other nonbronchial systemic collateral arteries that provide the blood supply to a region of bronchiectatic lung. The bleeding sites are in areas of exuberant granulation tissue growth in bronchiectatic bronchi. The bronchial source of the blood supply means that there is a systemic head of blood pressure behind any weak point or rupture in these vessels, and for this reason the bleeding can be dramatic and even exsanguinating.

Patients who come to the emergency room with gross hemoptysis should be admitted to the ICU for observation. Mild narcotics such as codeine should be given to suppress cough and thereby hold down the risk of exacerbating the hemorrhage. Vitamin K should be administered and blood clotting function should be measured (prothrombin time, activated partial thromboplastin time, platelet count). No drugs should be administered that inhibit platelet function, such as aspirin. Blood should be prepared in the blood bank for transfusion. The patient should be treated with all the general support given to most hospitalized patients with cystic fibrosis: hydration and nutrition should be provided, and intravenous antimicrobials should be administered as would be given for a non-life-threatening exacerbation. While the patient is actively bleeding, inhaled bronchodilators and chest physiotherapy should be withheld since they often provoke coughing and increased bleeding.

After the patient has been stabilized in the ICU, bedside fiberoptic bronchoscopy should be performed to ascertain which lobe or segment is bleeding.[14] In some cases, the intensivist may prefer doing the fiberoptic bronchoscopy in the operating room under general anesthesia. After bronchoscopy, the patient should be taken to the angiography suite for selective bronchial arteriography. Since bronchial arteriography is usually very time consuming, physicians and nurses from the intensive care team will often need to be present in the angiography suite to maintain care of the patient during the procedure. The angiographer first localizes the bronchial artery that is bleeding by recognizing a blush of dye at the distal end of the injected artery (see Fig. 139-1). After identifying any spinal cord collaterals that may be present, so as to avoid them, the angiographer injects small particulate material (Gelfoam or Ivalon), and very often the hemoptysis stops immediately. If the hemoptysis does not stop after this embolization procedure, the difficult decision looms over whether or not to take the patient to the operating room for an emergency lobectomy. Ideally, pulmonary function tests will be available from the recent past to help guide the thoracic surgeon in assessing the risk of operation. Patients who have an FEV_1 of 1.6 L or better are the most reasonable candidates for emergency thoracotomy.[14] In the absence of an option of emergency resectional surgery, the available options are all poor ones. Consideration can be given to intubating the patient and placing him in bed with the bleeding lobe in a dependent position while

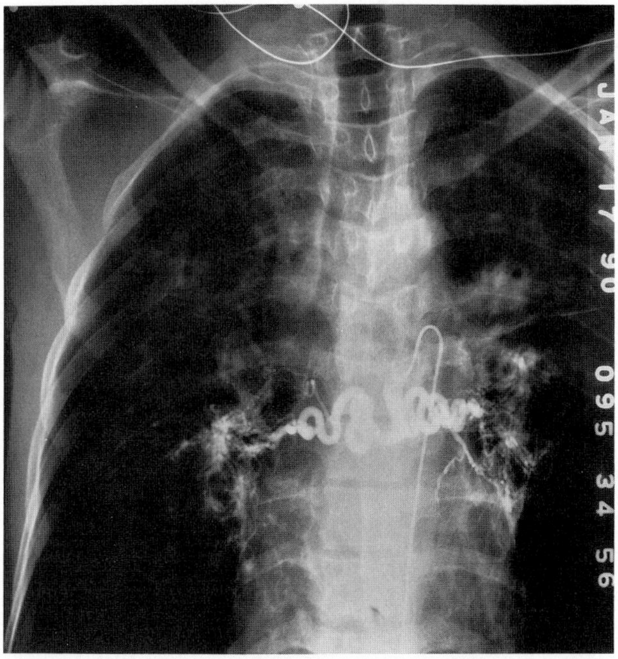

FIGURE 139-1 A bronchial angiogram done on an adult with cystic fibrosis and gross hemoptysis. Shown are the extremely enlarged and tortuous bronchial arteries that originate in the thoracic aorta and provide the blood supply to the site of bleeding (patch of white), which is a bed of granulation tissue in an area of severe bronchiectasis.

carrying on with transfusion and giving supplement oxygen. Many of these patients will go on to die. The recommended sequence of steps in the care of the adult cystic fibrosis patient with hemoptysis is lised in Table 139-2.

Pneumothorax

Spontaneous pneumothorax is very common in adults with cystic fibrosis and may require management in the ICU. The first time the patient has a pneumothorax, if it is a small one (10 percent), it may be watched in the hospital without intervention. When the pneumothorax is recurrent or when it is large enough to worsen the patient's dyspnea, exercise tolerance, or gas exchange, the pneumothorax should be treated.

TABLE 139-2 Sequence of Steps in Treatment of Hemoptysis in Adults with Cystic Fibrosis

Admission to ICU, conservative measures: reversal of clotting abnormalities with vitamin K or fresh frozen plasma, suppression of cough with codeine, nothing by mouth (except pills) while decisions are being made about definitive treatment, institution of intravenous antimicrobial therapy.
Fiberoptic bronchoscopy to localize bleeding site.
Selective bronchial arteriography with embolization.
If all else fails, consider thoracotomy with lobectomy.

TABLE 139-3 Sequence of Steps in Treatment of Pneumothorax in Adults with Cystic Fibrosis

Admission to ICU for medical stabilization and oxygen.
Temporary relief of pneumothorax by tube thoracostomy or modified Heimlich valve.
After preparation for surgery with chest physiotherapy, antimicrobials, and increased nutrition, take to operating room for transapical partial pleurectomy.

Our approach is to admit the patient with a large pneumothorax to the ICU for the definitive steps in therapy. The patient should be given supplemental oxygen to breathe and should be kept fasting except for oral medications while decisions are made concerning the possible need for surgical therapy. This means that the patient's nutritional needs should initially be handled by intravenous hyperalimentation. If the patient is highly prone to develop the distal intestinal obstruction syndrome (meconium ileus equivalent), it may be advisable to give the patient one or two enzyme capsules per day by mouth to help prevent this complication. Once the patient is stabilized in the ICU, a thoracic surgeon should place a chest tube or other device (modified Heimlich valve) to relieve the pneumothorax. For most patients, especially those with very poor pulmonary function or those who have recurrent pneumothorax, placement of a tube thoracostomy is not definitive therapy. Rather, we prefer to treat the problem with a thoracotomy done with an incision high in the axilla with the goal of performing an apical pleural stripping in order to fuse the lung to the chest wall and prevent future recurrences of pneumothorax. At thoracotomy, the thoracic surgeon can also oversew any blebs that may be actively leaking air and causing the pneumothorax. This partial pleurectomy is very well tolerated by most patients since the major accessory muscles of respiration are not injured during the surgery. We have found that most patients can be extubated promptly after surgery without going into acute ventilatory failure. We do not favor the use of chemical pleurodesis with sclerosing agents such as tetracycline because this procedure can be painful and has a high rate of failure. Talc pleurodesis is available at some centers and may be useful in selected cases where thoracotomy is not an option.[15] All of these procedures remove the option of a later lung transplant, but at the present time there are many more adult patients with cystic fibrosis who have life-threatening pneumothorax than there are opportunities to undergo lung transplantation. The recommended sequence of steps in the care of an adult with cystic fibrosis who has a large pneumothorax is listed in Table 139-3.

Critical Illness and Gastrointestinal Manifestations of Cystic Fibrosis

DISTAL INTESTINAL OBSTRUCTION SYNDROME

Adult patients with cystic fibrosis often suffer from partial or complete obstruction of the small bowel at the level of the distal ileum. The cause of this condition is intraluminal collection of abnormally viscid mucofeculant material in the terminal ileum and right colon.[16] Critically ill patients in the ICU are particularly prone to develop distal intestinal obstruction syndrome, perhaps because of interruption of their usual regimen of dietary intake, supplemental oral pancreatic enzyme therapy, and effects of dehydration due to critical illness. For this reason the intensivist should be vigilant for signs of right lower quadrant pain, often with a palpable fecal mass in that location. Differential diagnosis is complicated by the possibility of small-bowel obstruction from adhesions of previous surgery and by the possibility of intussusception. If complete small-bowel obstruction is seen with failure to pass feces or flatus, the patient should be treated as any other patient with small-bowel obstruction. If the obstruction is only partial, the patient will continue to pass flatus but will experience severe right lower quadrant pain and possibly vomiting. In the past, these patients have been treated by taking them to the department of radiology for a gastrografin enema, and this treatment is highly effective. Since it is often very difficult to transport patients from the ICU to radiology, another approach should be tried. The patient should be given a large volume (approx 4 to 6 L) of balanced intestinal lavage solution (Golytely), either orally or through a nasogastric tube, at a slow rate (500 mL/h, as tolerated). Before beginning therapy, it is best to administer 5 to 10 mg of metoclopramide to reduce nausea and vomiting.[16] This continuous lavage of the distal intestine from above can be very effective in relieving the patient's pain as the obstruction is washed away.

CIRRHOSIS WITH PORTAL HYPERTENSION AND ESOPHAGEAL VARICES

A small minority of adults with cystic fibrosis develop cirrhosis with portal hypertension and esophageal varices. These patients may be admitted to ICUs with acute upper gastrointestinal hemorrhage. They are most often treated with sclerotherapy, and selected cases may benefit from surgery (portal-systemic shunting with splenorenal anastomoses[17]). Often, these patients are treated in the same way as other patients with this condition (see Chaps. 163 and 164).

CASE PRESENTATION

JN was a 29-year-old white male with cystic fibrosis diagnosed in childhood who was admitted directly to the ICU from the emergency room with a chief complaint of gross hemoptysis.

As an infant, JN had failure to thrive and steatorrhea. A sweat test performed at age 2 made the diagnosis of cystic fibrosis. He was treated throughout childhood with supplemental pancreatic enzymes with meals and had a normal growth and development. During his teen years he neglected to return to his physician for follow-up. Three years prior to admission he was admitted to his local hospital for small-bowel obstruction, which remitted after 3 days with no surgery. Also in that year he had elective surgery for the removal of multiple bilateral nasal polyps. Two years prior to admission, JN returned to the medical care system when he sought the help of an adult pulmonary specialist. At that time he was employed as a parts specialist in an automobile supply store. His chief complaint was easy fatigueability, low body weight, and chronic productive cough. On initial evaluation he was 5 ft 9 in. tall with a weight of 125 lb. He appeared to be a very thin, pale white man in no acute distress. His chest exam revealed loud wheezes throughout together with early inspiratory crackles. He had 4+ clubbing of all fingernails.

His pulmonary function tests revealed a low total lung capacity (TLC) at 5.4 L, 76 percent predicted. His FEV_1 was 1.4 (33 percent), and his forced vital capacity was 2.4 (46 percent) with no improvement after inhalation of bronchodilator. His D_LCO was normal. Initial arterial blood gases showed a pH of 7.4, P_{CO_2} of 40 mmHg, and P_{O_2} of 74 mmHg on room air. His chest film showed diffuse bronchiectasis with the most severe changes in both upper lobes. Sputum culture grew out two species of mucoid *P. aeruginosa.*

He was started on a daily program at home of chest physiotherapy, rotating oral antimicrobial drugs, meal replacement dietary supplements, and inhaled bronchodilators. He did generally well and returned every 6 weeks for clinic visits.

Six months prior to admission he came to clinic complaining of increased cough and sputum together with expectoration of $\frac{1}{2}$ cup of blood. He was admitted to the hospital and started on intravenous ceftazidime and gentamicin, to which his organisms were sensitive. He was also given codeine, 30 mg every 6 h, for excessive cough. He underwent immediate fiberoptic bronchoscopy, which showed a stream of blood coming from the anterior segment of the right upper lobe. Bronchial arteriography was then performed, and the patient's bronchial arteries were found to be profoundly hypertrophic and tortuous; a blush was seen in the branch to the right upper lobe (Fig. 139-1). This was embolized and the bleeding stopped immediately. Following this the patient completed a 2-week course of intravenous antimicrobials and was discharged. Two weeks later he returned to work.

One month prior to admission, the patient related during a clinic visit that on two recent occasions he had coughed up 50 mL of bright red blood. He was advised to stay home from work, and he was placed on oral codeine and a new antimicrobial regimen. On the day of admission he coughed up several cups of bright red blood and came immediately to the emergency room, where he was admitted to the ICU. During the first hospital day he was started on intravenous gentamicin and ceftazidime, his cough was suppressed with codeine, and he was stabilized. A bedside fiberoptic bronchoscopy in the ICU showed that he was once again bleeding from the right upper lobe. While waiting to be taken to the angiography suite, the patient got out of his ICU bed, walked to his toilet, had massive hemoptysis, and fell to the floor in a state of respiratory arrest. Immediate cardiopulmonary resuscitation and endotracheal intubation were carried out. The patient was transfused (posthemoptysis hematocrit was 13) and taken to the angiography suite where repeat bronchial arteriography showed that the previously embolized region now contained a large arteriovenous fistula that was bleeding. Although some of the arterial branches feeding it were reembolized, other branches from more remote arteries could not be embolized. The patient's physician decided that the best approach to treatment would be immediate right upper lobectomy. He was taken by the thoracic surgeons to the operating room where it was necessary to resect both the right upper and middle lobes due to the presence of large collateral bronchial arteries. The patient tolerated the thoracotomy and the immediate postoperative period well. He fully regained consciousness and after stabilization his P_{CO_2} was 48 mmHg. After several weeks he was extubated, but on the second day after extubation he became exhausted from his heavy work of breathing and needed reintubation. One week later he underwent elective tracheostomy without difficulty. Following this he spent 8 weeks in the ICU where the therapeutic plan emphasized nutritional supplements, periods of rest at night followed by periods of spontaneous breathing or pressure-assisted breathing as tolerated. Unfortunately, the patient was never able to tolerate progressively longer periods of spontaneous breathing due to precipitous exhaustion. His P_{CO_2} progressively rose on the ventilator to the high 60's. During his terminal week he used patient-controlled analgesia to administer small doses of morphine to himself to control his worsening dyspnea. He died of progressive hypotension while still on the mechanical ventilator.

CASE DISCUSSION

In this case, the decision to intubate and mechanically ventilate the patient was made in the setting of an unexpected respiratory arrest brought on by exsanguinating hemoptysis. The hope was to provide him with a bridge to further survival after the cause of the hemoptysis was treated. The patient's recent measurement of FEV_1 (1.4 L) would ordinarily not have led to acute ventilatory failure. This FEV_1 is, however, less than the value of 1.6 L that one author considers a minimum value for successful thoracotomy in cystic fibrosis patients with hemoptysis.[14] In the end, the surgery was definitive in stopping the hemoptysis but the patient could not sustain his own ventilation after recovering from the acute effects of his bilobectomy. It seems very likely that his life was prolonged for 6 months by the benefit he achieved from his first bronchial artery embolization.

At the end of his life, the patient's physiologic state could be described as showing a number of severe derangements. His need for high minute ventilation refected the large amounts of alveolar dead space that resulted from the progression of his lung disease. He had cor pulmonale as judged by bedside echocardiography, and he was in a state of acute ventilatory failure superimposed on his chronic respiratory insufficiency, which had been moderate prior to surgery and became critically compromised after thoracotomy. He did not gain weight in spite of nutritional supplements. The humane care of the patient during the dying process consisted of setting the ventilator to control the patient's air hunger, providing for frequent visits from his family, and allowing the patient to use small doses of morphine to take away his dyspnea.

References

1. Quinton PM: Cystic fibrosis: A disease in electrolyte transport. FASEB J 4:2709, 1990.
2. Riordan JR, Rommens JM, Kerem B, Alon N, Rozmahel R, Grzelczak Z, Zielenski J, Lok s, Plavsic N, Chou J, Drumm ML, Iannuzzi MC, Collins FS, Tsui L: Identification of the cystic fibrosis gene: Cloning and characterization of complementary DNA. Science 245:1066, 1989.
3. Baltimore RS, Christie CDC, Walker Smith GJ: Immunohistopathologic localization of *Pseudomonas aeruginosa* in lungs from patients with cystic fibrosis. Am Rev Respir Dis 140:1650, 1989.
4. Fick RB: Pathogenesis of the pseudomonas lung lesion in cystic fibrosis. Chest 96:158, 1989.
5. Regelmann WE, Elliott GR, Warwick WJ, Clawson CC. Reduction of sputum *Pseudomonas aeruginosa* density by antibiotics improves lung function in cystic fibrosis more than do bronchodilators and chest physiotherapy alone. Am Rev Respir Dis 141:914, 1990.
6. Zach MS: Lung disease in cystic fibrosis: An updated concept. Pediatr Pulmonol 8:188, 1990.
7. Tomashefski JF, Bruce M, Stern RC, Dearborn DG, Dahms B: Pulmonary air cysts in cystic fibrosis: Relation of pathologic features to radiologic findings and history of pneumothorax. Human Pathol 16:253, 1985.
8. Fick RB, Stillwell PC: Controversies in the management of pulmonary disease due to cystic fibrosis. Chest 95:1319, 1989.
9. Gaskin KJ, Waters DLM, Howman-Giles R, De Silva M, Earl JW, Martin HCO, Kan AE, Brown JM, Dorney SFA: Liver disease and common-bile-duct stenosis in cystic fibrosis. N Engl J Med 318:340, 1988.
10. Bosso JA, Townsend PL, Herbst JJ, Matsen JM: Pharmacokinetics and dosage requirements of netilmicin in cystic fibrosis. Antimicrob Agents Chemother 28:829, 1985.
11. Konishi H, Goto M, Nakamoto Y, et al: Tobramycin inactivation by carbenicillin, ticarcillin and piperacillin. Antimicrob Agents Chemother 23:653, 1983.
12. Davis PB, di Sant'Agnese PA: Assisted ventilation for patients with cystic fibrosis. JAMA 239:1851, 1978.
13. Boat TF: Cystic fibrosis, in Murray JF and Nadel JA (eds): *Textbook of Respiratory Medicine.* Philadelphia, WB Saunders Company, 1988, p 1126–1152.
14. Trento A, Estner SM, Griffith BP, Hardesty RL: Massive hemoptysis in patients with cystic fibrosis: Three case reports and a protocol for clinical management. Ann Thor Surg 39:254, 1985.
15. Spector ML, Stern RC: Pneumothorax in cystic fibrosis: A 26-year exerience. Ann Thorac Surg 47:204, 1989.
16. Cleghorn GJ, Stringer DA, Forstner GG, Durie PR: Treatment of distal intestinal obstruction syndrome in cystic fibrosis with a balanced intestinal lavage solution. Lancet 7:8, 1986.
17. Stern RC, Stevens DP, Boat TF, Doershuk CF, Izant RJ, Matthews LW: Symptomatic hepatic disease in cystic fibrosis: Incidence, course, and outcome of portal systemic shunting. Gastroenterology 70:645, 1976.

SECTION K

NEUROPSYCHIATRIC DISORDERS IN THE CRITICALLY ILL

Chapter 140

DELIRIUM, PSYCHOTIC DISORDERS, AND ANXIETY

MICHAEL G. WISE
CLARK D. TERRELL

KEY POINTS

- *Delirium and anxiety occur frequently in critically ill patients; psychotic disorders are relatively rare.*
- *An acute change in a critically ill patient's behavior or mental status is delirium until proven otherwise.*
- *Delirium requires immediate evaluation and treatment.*
- *Bedside testing of cognitive function, which can be done rapidly, is an essential part of differentiating between psychiatric disorders.*
- *Agitation may be seen in delirium, psychosis, or anxiety.*
- *Anxiety may occur secondary to drugs (e.g., alcohol withdrawal, aminophylline), medical illness (acute congestive heart failure), or as an adjustment to a rapid deterioration in health.*
- *A medically ill patient who is psychotic is delirious until proven otherwise.*

Overview

This chapter tells how to recognize, evaluate, manage, and treat a patient who becomes acutely confused or agitated. In critically ill patients, all psychiatric diagnoses must be considered carefully because mental status changes are almost always secondary to underlying physiologic problems.

The critically ill patient who develops acute agitation, confusion, or psychosis presents a medical emergency. A good diagnostic rule in such patients is that any acute change in a patient's mental status is delirium until proven otherwise. Delirium is common, especially in critically ill patients. Any change in a patient's behavior, mood, psychomotor activity (agitation or apathy), or cognitive function can signal the onset of delirium. Without rapid diagnosis and treatment, the prognosis for recovery may be poor.

Agitation in the critically ill patient may reflect anxiety or psychosis, rather than delirium. Anxiety may be a reaction to the patient's illness and the stress of the hospitalization. It may also be a manifestation of the illness itself, an effect of medication, or the result of a preexisting psychiatric disorder. Understanding the etiology of a patient's anxiety permits the clinician to initiate treatment. This includes reversing anxiogenic conditions when possible, using supportive interventions, and ordering antianxiety medications. Any patient, with or without a known psychiatric disorder, can become anxious or worried when faced with a life-threatening illness.

Patients with preexisting psychiatric disorders may develop anxiety or psychosis in reaction to serious medical illness. Psychosis may be a symptom of a variety of conditions, including delirium, depression, and schizophrenia. The syndromes described are not mutually exclusive; delirium must first be considered even in a critically ill patient with a known psychotic disorder (e.g., schizophrenia) or other psychiatric condition (e.g., dementia, depression, or an anxiety disorder). This chapter attempts to provide useful guidelines to the diagnosis, evaluation, and treatment of delirium, psychotic disorders, and anxiety.

Delirium

Delirium as a diagnostic term has many synonyms (Table 140-1)[1]. One of the most descriptive of these is acute brain failure. Just as the heart, kidney, or liver can fail acutely, so can the brain. The patient manifests this change in physiologic status by a variety of acute mental status changes such as confusion, agitation, lethargy, anger, and anxiety.

Because delirium is extremely common, potentially lethal, and often overlooked, it must be considered immediately in the critically ill patient who has mental status changes.[2] Approximately 10 percent of all patients admitted to acute medical and surgical services develop delirium during their hospitalization; for medically ill patients aged 70 years or more, the incidence may increase to 50 percent. About 10 percent of hospitalized medical and surgical patients are delirious at any given time.[3]

TABLE 140-1 Synonyms for Delirium

Acute brain failure	Encephalopathy
Acute brain syndrome	Exogenous psychosis
Acute brain syndrome with psychosis	ICU psychosis
	Metabolic encephalopathy
Acute confusional state	Oneiric state
Acute organic psychosis	Organic brain syndrome
Acute organic reaction	Reversible cognitive dysfunction
Acute reversible psychosis	Toxic confusional state
Cerebral insufficiency	Toxic encephalopathy

Early recognition of delirium may permit critical care physicians to rapidly reverse causative physiologic factors and improve prognosis. From the days of Hippocrates, the rapid development of agitation and confusion has been recognized as a poor prognostic sign in the gravely ill. The mortality rate associated with delirium is significant. Of hospitalized patients who become delirious, 20 to 30 percent die during that hospitalization or soon after discharge.[4] In a recent follow-up study of 198 hospitalized patients who developed delirium, 34 percent died during the year following diagnosis. Most of these died within the first 90 days. Patients with delirium which followed an operative procedure had a lower mortality (17 percent) than patients with a delirium unrelated to any operative procedure (42 percent).[5]

No comprehensive studies have examined the morbidity associated with delirium. Delirious patients are at risk for self-harm as a result of dangerous behaviors, such as pulling out intravenous lines, nasogastric and nasopharyngeal tubes, arterial lines, and on one occasion known to the authors, an intra-aortic balloon pump. Patients who develop delirium have prolonged hospitalizations.[6] In addition, it is not uncommon for a delirious patient to become paranoid and misinterpret the intentions of the critical care staff; paranoid delirious patients may strike and injure hospital personnel. Although many patients with delirium have a full recovery, some develop chronic organic brain syndromes and permanent disability. Delirious patients may progress to stupor, coma, seizures, or death.

Patients are not at equal risk to develop delirium. Seven groups of patients are at increased risk (Table 140-2). Patients over 60 years of age have a high potential for acute brain failure.[7] As high as 67 percent of adult postcardiotomy patients develop delirium.[8] Third-degree burns place the patient at greater risk,[9] with delirium occurring in almost all patients with greater than 40 percent total body surface area burned.[10] Preexisting brain damage creates an increased risk of delirium.[11,12] Although few studies exist, the general consensus is that delirium is frequently encountered in hospitalized children.[13] In addition, patients with drug dependence, especially on alcohol, benzodiazepines, or barbiturates, often become delirious during acute drug withdrawal. Patients with the human immunodeficiency virus (HIV) spectrum of disorders are yet another group at increased risk.

When faced with a patient who is confused and perhaps agitated, the first question must be, "Is the patient delirious?" *The clinician should not attribute the change in mental status to an "ICU psychosis."* The brain's response to a physiologic insult, whether metabolic, anoxic, toxic, or infectious, is delirium.[14] Thus delirium should be considered as dire a medical emergency as acute renal failure or cardiac ischemia. Recognition of the clinical features of delirium is clearly essential for the critical care physician. The clinical features of delirium are summarized in Table 140-3. Three sources of information are useful in looking for these features. These include the patient, the medical record, and the patient's family. Review the medical chart, particularly the nurses' notes, for descriptions of behavioral or mood changes. Prodromal symptoms include restlessness, irritability, tearfulness, anxiety, or problems with sleep (odd cycles, insomnia, or hypersomnia). Family members are sometimes aware of early changes in the patient. A brief inquiry to the family will usually reveal their concerns. A thorough examination of the patient, including a mental status examination, is the key to confirming the diagnosis. An important clinical characteristic that differentiates delirium from dementia or psychotic disorders is the rapidly fluctuating (waxing and waning) course of delirium.[15] Within one-half hour, a delirious patient may transform from an alert, clear-thinking, and coherent person to a confused, disoriented person with disorganized thought processes. Given the rapid shift in the patient's mental status, it is not difficult to understand how different physicians who observe a delirious patient at varying points in time may form widely divergent clinical impressions.

The delirious patient's ability to maintain attention and sustain memory for recent events, such as the time of day, date, and situation, is impaired. Although many patients with delirium are hyperactive and agitated, others may be lethargic and apathetic. Some patients who have delirium will alternate between states of agitation and hypoactivity (i.e., mixed delirium). Unfortunately, the quietly confused, lethargic patient is often incorrectly diagnosed as depressed.[7] If a physician mistakes delirium for depression and prescribes an antidepressant medication, the delirium will worsen.

Emotional disturbances develop frequently in delirious patients. The range of emotional responses seen may include anxiety, anger, panic, fear, sadness, apathy, and (rarely) euphoria. These emotional responses may change rapidly. The patient's personality, physiologic dysfunction, the environment, and the disorganized thoughts and misperceptions all likely contribute to the emotional responses seen with delirium.[10]

TABLE 140-2 Patients at High Risk to Develop Delirium

Children
Drug-dependent
Elderly (age 60 or older)
HIV-spectrum disorders
Postcardiotomy
Preexisting brain damage
Severe burn injury

TABLE 140-3 Clinical Features of Delirium

Prodrome	Disorganized thinking and speech
Rapid fluctuations in mental status	Altered perceptions
Decreased attention span	Neurologic abnormalities
Diminished memory for recent events	Dysgraphia
Disorientation	Constructional apraxia
Agitation or lethargy	Dysnomic aphasia
Emotional disturbances	Motor abnormalities
Sleep-wake disturbances	EEG slowing

Patient ______________
Examiner ______________
Date ______________

"MINI-MENTAL STATE"

Maximum score	Score	
		Orientation
5	( )	What is the (year)(season)(date)(day)(month)?
5	( )	Where are we? (state) (country) (town) (hospital)(floor).
		Registration
3	( )	Name 3 objects: 1 second to say each. Then ask the patient all 3 after you have said them. Give 1 point for each correct answer. Then repeat them until he learns all 3. Count trials and record. Trials ______________
		Attention and Calculation
5	( )	Serial 7's. 1 point for each correct. Stop after 5 answers. Alternatively spell "world" backwards.
		Recall
3	( )	Ask for the 3 objects repeated above. Give 1 point for each correct.
		Language
9	( )	Name a pencil, and watch (2 points) Repeat the following "No ifs, ands or buts." (1 point) Follow a 3-stage command: "Take a paper in your right hand, fold it in half, and put it on the floor" (3 points) Read and obey the following: **Close your eyes (1 point)** Write a sentence (1 point) Copy design (1 point) Total score ASSESS level of consciousness along a continuum ______________ Alert Drowsy Stupor Coma

INSTRUCTIONS FOR ADMINISTRATION OF MINI-MENTAL STATE EXAMINATION

Orientation

(1) Ask for the date. Then ask specifically for parts omitted, e.g., "Can you also tell me what season it is?" One point for each correct.

(2) Ask in turn "Can you tell me the name of this hospital?" (town, country, etc.). One point for each correct.

Registration

Ask the patient if you may test his memory. Then say the names of 3 unrelated objects, clearly and slowly, about one second for each. After you have said all 3, ask him to repeat them. This first repetition determines his score (0–3) but keep saying them until he can repeat all 3, up to 6 trials. If he does not eventually learn all 3, recall cannot be meaningfully tested.

Attention and calculation

Ask the patient to begin with 100 and count backwards by 7. Stop after 5 subtractions (93, 86, 79, 72, 65). Score the total number of correct answers.

If the patient cannot or will not perform this task, ask him to spell the word "world" backwards. The score is the number of letters in correct order. E.g., dlrow = 5, dlorw = 3.

Recall

Ask the patient if he can recall the 3 words you previously asked him to remember. Score 0–3.

Language

Naming: Show the patient a wrist watch and ask him what it is. Repeat for pencil. Score 0–2.

Repetition: Ask the patient to repeat the sentence after you. Allow only one trial. Score 0 or 1.

3-Stage command: Give the patient a piece of plain blank paper and repeat the command. Score 1 point for each part correctly executed.

Reading: On a blank piece of paper print the sentence "Close your eyes," in letters large enough for the patient to see clearly. Ask him to read it and do what it says. Score 1 point only if he actually closes his eyes.

Writing: Give the patient a blank piece of paper and ask him to write a sentence for you. Do not dictate a sentence, it is to be written spontaneously. It must contain a subject and verb and be sensible. Correct grammar and punctuation are not necessary.

Copying: On a clean piece of paper, draw intersecting pentagons, each side about 1 in., and ask him to copy it exactly as it is. All 10 angles must be present and 2 must intersect to score 1 point. Tremor and rotation are ignored.

Estimate the patient's level of sensorium along a continuum, from alert on the left to coma on the right.

FIGURE 140-1 Mini-mental state examination. ***Source:*** **Reproduction from Folstein MF, Folstein SE, McHugh PR: Mini-mental state: A practical method for grading the cognitive state of patients for the clinician. J Psychiatr Res 12:189, 1975. Reprinted with permission.**

The sleep-wake cycles of patients with delirium are often reversed; increased sleep may occur during the day with reports from the night shift that patients are hyperactive, agitated, and confused. Thinking is generally disorganized and fragmented. The disjointed thought patterns and defective reasoning of delirious patients are reflected in their speech. Speech becomes increasingly incoherent as the severity of the delirium increases.[16] In severe delirium, speech becomes chaotic and patients may ramble from one subject to another. Perceptions may be altered in delirium, most often with illusions or overt hallucinations or both. Patients may misperceive the movement of a curtain to be someone about to attack them or the sound of a dropped chart as a gunshot. Tactile illusions may occur; for example, the movement of intravenous tubing against the skin may be interpreted as a snake crawling on the arm. Paranoid delusions occur frequently and cause patients to be fearful and, at times, aggressive.

Numerous neuropsychiatric signs are present. Dysgraphia (impaired writing), which is easily tested for by asking the patient to write, is a highly sensitive indicator for delirium. In one study, 34 of 35 acutely confused patients had impaired writing.[17] Nearly all delirious patients will also have constructional apraxia (difficulty drawing). A few patients may exhibit dysnomic aphasia (problems naming items). Dysfunction of the motor system such as tremor, asterixis, myoclonus, or symmetric reflex and muscle tone alterations may be detected in a delirious patient. A patient with a delirium of toxic-metabolic etiology may have a tremor that is absent at rest but apparent with movement. Myoclonus and asterixis occur in many toxic and metabolic conditions and are not restricted to hepatic encephalopathy.[18]

The electroencephalogram (EEG) reflects the global cerebral dysfunction found in delirium; EEG changes virtually always accompany delirium.[19] Slowing of the EEG is seen in lethargic, anergic, and hypoactive patients. Although slowing is most commonly seen, low voltage fast activity may be seen on the EEG of hyperactive, agitated patients (as in delirium tremens).[20] The EEG slowing is relative to a patient's normal background activity. For example, if a patient's base-line activity is 12 Hz, slowing of the background to 8 Hz may occur during metabolic encephalopathy. Since 8 Hz falls within the "normal" range, without a base-line study the EEG might be read as normal, although significant slowing is actually present. Although it is cumbersome to perform in critically ill patients and problematic to do in agitated patients, the EEG is a useful test to diagnose delirium if doubt exists.

Once delirium is suspected, one should administer a bedside examination of the patient's cognitive function. The mini-mental state examination (MMSE, Fig. 140-1) offers a reasonable, although not too sensitive, screening evaluation of cognitive function.[21] The MMSE takes only a few minutes to administer and tests the patient's concentration, orientation, attention, memory function, ability to

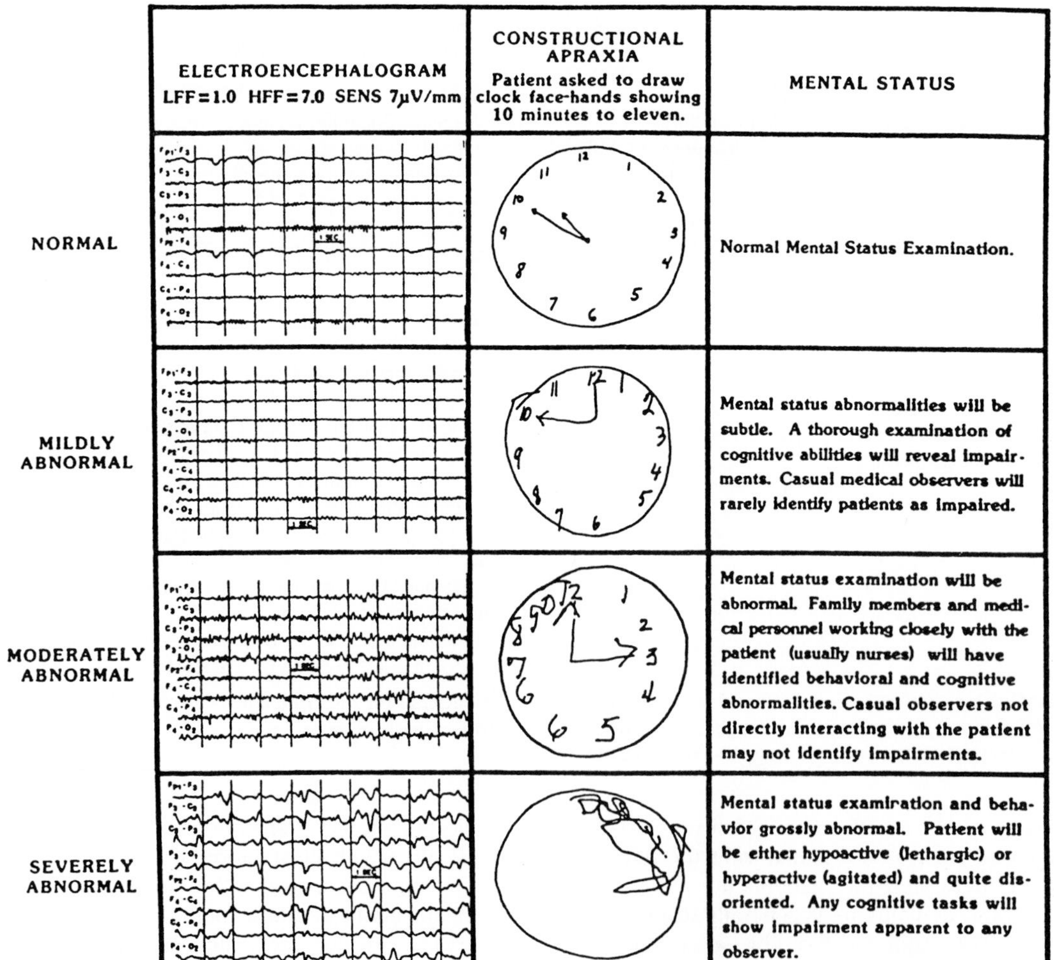

FIGURE 140-2 Comparison of EEG, constructional apraxia, and mental status. *Source:* Reprinted from Wise MG: Delirium, in Hales RE, Yudofsky, SSC (eds): *The American Psychiatric Press Textbook of Neuropsychiatry*. Washington, DC, American Psychiatric Press, 1987. Copyright 1987 by The American Psychiatric Press, Inc. Reprinted by permission.

write, ability to speak, and constructional praxis. A score of 20 or below (of a total score of 30) is suggestive of cognitive impairment (delirium, dementia, or delirium superimposed on dementia).

Further bedside testing of the patient's ability to reason and process information is often diagnostically helpful. For example, ask the patient to sequentially perform the following:

1. Place your right hand on your left elbow.
2. Place your right hand on your right ear.
3. Place your right hand on your right elbow.

The patient with delirium usually slowly performs the first two tasks, although sometimes making errors, and may look to the examiner for reassurance. A confused patient will either attempt the third task or will repeat the first two tasks (perseveration), despite repeated instructions to "place your right hand on your right elbow." The patient does not understand that the third task is impossible. The patient *without* delirium will quickly perform the first two instructions; when asked to perform the last directive, an unimpaired patient may laugh or smile, stating "I can't do that—it's impossible!"

It is easy to test for dysgraphia (impaired writing). Simply ask the patient to write a sentence or sign his or her name. Dysnomia (difficulty naming objects) can be tested by asking the patient to name items available at the bedside. Virtually anyone with delirium will have constructional apraxia (difficulty drawing objects). This can be demonstrated by asking the patient to draw the face of a clock, with the hands at a predetermined time (e.g., 10:50, as in Fig. 140-2.)[1] The ability to draw a clock is a highly sensitive test for delirium, correlating well with the degree of cognitive impairment and the degree of slowing seen on the EEG.

Besides delirium, other diagnoses to consider when evaluating a patient are dementia, psychosis, or depression. The clinical courses of these disorders differ. Dementia has a slowly progressive course, whereas delirium typically occurs acutely. Also, a patient with dementia is usually alert and has a relatively stable clinical picture, in contrast to the rapidly fluctuating course of the delirious patient. Patients with dementia have a lowered threshold for delirium; it is not unusual for a patient to have both disorders. When these disorders coexist, treating the delirium will improve the patient's behavior and reduce the degree of confusion.

When marked confusion, altered behavior, perceptual disturbances (hallucinations), and delusional thinking are seen in a patient, the clinician must differentiate delirium from a psychotic disorder, such as schizophrenia. The patient with schizophrenia will not exhibit the cognitive deficits seen in delirium (i.e., the MMSE score should be >20). A patient with a psychotic disorder is typically oriented, and delusions, if present, are well-developed and longstanding.[22] This is in contrast to the disorientation and the loosely knit, vague, and rapidly changing delusions of the delirious patient. Hallucinations are most commonly visual when they occur in delirium; they are most commonly auditory in psychotic disorders. The patient's prior history is helpful in the differential diagnosis. Because new onset

TABLE 140-4 Neuropsychiatric Evaluation of the Delirious Patient

MENTAL STATUS
Interview (assess level of consciousness, psychomotor activity, appearance, affect, mood, intellect, thought processes)
Performance tests (memory, concentration, reasoning, motor and constructional praxis)
PHYSICAL STATUS
Neurologic exam (reflexes, limb strength, cranial nerves, gait, meningeal signs, Babinski)
Vital signs (review past and present)
Medical chart (review diagnoses, labs [including VDRL], behavior changes)
Medication log (correlate abnormal behavior with medication changes)
LABORATORY EXAMINATION—BASIC
Blood chemistries (electrolytes, glucose, calcium, albumin, ammonia, magnesium, phosphorus, liver and thyroid function tests)
Blood count (hematocrit, MCV, WBC and differential, sedimentation rate)
Drug levels (toxic screen, medication blood levels)
Arterial blood gases
Urinalysis
Chest x-ray
FURTHER LABORATORY EXAMINATION—BASED ON CLINICAL JUDGMENT
Electroencephalogram
CT or MRI scan
Additional blood chemistries (heavy metals, thiamine and folate levels, LE prep, ANA, urinary porphobilinogen)
Lumbar puncture

SOURCE: Reprinted from Wise MG: Delirium, in Hales RE, Yudofsky, SC (eds): *The American Psychiatric Press Textbook of Neuropsychiatry.* Washington, DC, American Psychiatric Press, 1987. Copyright 1987 by The American Psychiatric Press, Inc. Reprinted by permission.

psychotic disorders are exceedingly rare in the elderly, delirium is always considered in an elderly patient who exhibits bizarre behavior.

Delirium with apathy and lethargy may mimic depression. Sleep disturbance, increased or decreased activity, impaired concentration, and altered appetite are common to both depressed and delirious patients. To complicate the differential diagnosis further, a patient with depression occasionally will also have a psychosis. Another patient who can appear delirious is a manic patient who has a bipolar disorder. Mania is characterized by sleep disturbance, increased activity, impaired concentration, and not uncommonly, psychotic symptoms. The clinician can differentiate depression and mania from delirium by past history and by looking for the episodic waxing and waning, disorganization, disorientation, EEG slowing, or other cognitive dysfunctions characteristic of delirium yet usually absent in mania and depression.

The search for an etiology of a patient's delirium can be a difficult task. An elderly, delirious patient often has multisystem organ disease and numerous medications prescribed. Each potential contributor to the delirium must be evaluated and abnormalities corrected, when possible. The following provides a systematic approach to the evaluation of delirium.

The evaluation of a delirious patient includes a physical examination, an abbreviated neurologic examination, records review, laboratory evaluation, and other tests and procedures (Table 140-4). Basic laboratory tests are obtained in the workup of a delirious patient, and, based on clinical judgment, additional procedures may be indicated (e.g., magnetic resonance imaging [MRI] scan, lumbar puncture).

TABLE 140-5 Drugs That Can Cause Delirium

Analgesics	*Anticonvulsants*	*Drug Withdrawal*
meperidine	phenobarbital	alcohol
opiates	phenytoin	barbiturates
pentazocine	valproic acid	benzodiazepines
salicylates	*Anti-inflammatory Drugs*	*Sedative-hypnotics*
Antibiotics	ACTH	barbiturates
acyclovir	corticosteroids	benzodiazepines
aminoglycosides	ibuprofen	glutethimide
amphotericin B	indomethacin	*Sympathomimetics*
cephalexin	naproxen	aminophylline
cephalosporins	phenylbutazone	amphetamines
chloramphenicol	steroids	cocaine
chloroquine	*Antineoplastic Drugs*	ephedrine
ethambutol	aminoglutethimide	epinephrine
gentamicin	asparaginase	phenylephrine
interferon	DTIC	phenylpropanolamine
isoniazid	5-fluorouracil	theophylline
rifampin	methotrexate (high dose)	
sulfonamides	tamoxifen	*Miscellaneous Drugs*
tetracycline	vinblastine	baclofen
ticarcillin	vincristine	bromides
vancomycin	*Antiparkinson Drugs*	chlorpropamide
Anticholinergic Drugs	amantadine	cimetidine
antihistamines	bromocriptine	disulfiram
(chlorpheniramine)	carbidopa	ergotamines
antispasmodics	levodopa	lithium
atropine/homatropine	*Antituberculosis Drugs*	metrizamide
belladonna alkaloids	isoniazid	metronidazole
benztropine	rifampin	phenelzine
biperidin	*Cardiac Drugs*	podophylline
diphenhydramine	β-blockers	(by absorption)
phenothiazines	(propranolol)	procarbazine
(especially thioridazine)	captopril	propylthiouracil
promethazine	clonidine	quinacrine
scopolamine	digitalis	ranitidine
tricyclic antidepressants	disopyramide	timolol ophthalmic
(especially amitriptyline)	lidocaine	
trihexyphenidyl	mexiletine	
	methyldopa	
	quinidine	
	procainamide	
	tocainide	

TABLE 140-6 Emergent Items in the Differential Diagnosis of Delirium (WHHHHIMP)

Diagnoses	Clinical Questions
Wernicke's encephalopathy/ withdrawal	ataxia? ophthalmoplegia? alcohol/drug history?, ↑ ↑ MCV?, ↑ SYMPATHETIC ACTIVITY (e.g., ↑ pulse, ↑ BP, sweating)? hyperreflexia?
Hypertensive encephalopathy	↑ ↑ ↑ BP?, papilledema?
Hypoglycemia	history of insulin-dependent diabetes mellitus?, ↓ ↓ glucose?
Hypoperfusions of CNS	↓ BP?, ↓ ↓ cardiac output (e.g., myocardial infarct, arrhythmia, cardiac failure)?, ↓ hematocrit?
Hypoxemia	arterial blood gases (↓ P_{O_2}?), history of pulmonary disease?
Intracranial bleed	history of unconsciousness?, focal neurologic signs?
Meningitis/encephalitis	meningeal signs?, ↑ WBC?, ↑ temp?, viral prodrome?
Poisons/medications	Should toxic screen be ordered? Signs of toxicity (e.g., pupillary abnormality, nystagmus, ataxia)? Is the patient on a drug that may cause delirium?

SOURCE: Reprinted from Wise MG: Delirium, in Hales RE, Yudofsky SC (eds): *The American Psychiatric Press Textbook of Neuropsychiatry*. Washington, DC, American Psychiatric Press, 1987. Copyright 1987 by The American Psychiatric Press, Inc. Reprinted by permission.

TABLE 140-7 I Watch Death

Infections	Encephalitis, meningitis, syphilis, sepsis
Withdrawal	Alcohol, barbiturates, benzodiazepines
Acute metabolic	Acidosis, alkalosis, electrolyte disturbance, hepatic or renal failure
Trauma	Heat stroke, postoperative state, severe burns
CNS pathology	Abscesses, hemorrhage, seizures, stroke, tumor, vasculitis, normal-pressure hydrocephalus
Hypoxia	Anemia, hypotension, carbon monoxide poisoning, cardiac/pulmonary failure
Deficiencies	B_{12}, niacin, thiamine
Endocrinopathies	Hyper/hypoadrenocorticalism, hyper/hypoglycemia
Acute vascular	Hypertensive encephalopathy, shock
Toxins/drugs	Medications, pesticides, solvents
Heavy metals	Lead, manganese, mercury

SOURCE: Reprinted from Wise MG: Delirium, in Hales RE, Yudofsky SC (eds): *The American Psychiatric Press Textbook of Neuropsychiatry*. Washington, DC, American Psychiatric Press, 1987. Copyright 1987 by The American Psychiatric Press, Inc. Reprinted by permission.

Medications are a common cause of delirium (Table 140-5). A review of the medication records and a complete drug history are essential. The clinician should check the nurses' medication records because drugs that are ordered are not always given as prescribed. Withdrawal from drugs such as alcohol, barbiturates, and benzodiazepines may create delirium. Correlation of behavioral changes with initiation, discontinuation, or dose alteration of a medication often helps clarify the etiology.

The physician must first consider etiologies for delirium that can rapidly cause irreversible injury or death. The mnemonic WHHHHIMP can help the clinician recall these emergent items (Table 140-6).

After these conditions have been investigated, a more comprehensive list of diagnoses may be considered. The mnemonic I WATCH DEATH (Table 140-7) summarizes many of the insults that may contribute to delirium. The intentionally melodramatic mnemonic serves as a reminder of the substantial morbidity and mortality that result from undertreatment of acute brain failure.

The primary objective in the treatment of a delirious patient is to identify and treat reversible causes. For example, if an ataxic, alcoholic patient with ophthalmoplegia develops a confusional state, immediate treatment with thiamine is indicated. Frequently, multiple potential causes of delirium are identified. The clinician must correct as many of these abnormalities as possible.

Whether or not an etiology is found, pharmacologic interventions are often necessary to control the agitated behavior and confusion of the delirious patient. Many medications which have been used in critical care settings, such as morphine, diazepam, and similar drugs, carry significant risks. The dangers of sedation, decreased respiratory drive, hypotension, and worsening cognitive function warrant that extensive use of these agents be avoided in the treatment of a delirious, agitated patient. There are exceptions: benzodiazepines are recommended for treating delirium secondary to withdrawal from benzodiazepines or alcohol, and benzodiazepines in low doses can be used to augment the calming effect of haloperidol in acutely agitated patients (as described later in this chapter). Pharmacologic management of a patient with delirium requires close supervision by the physician and nursing staff; prn orders are not advised. Nonessential medications should be discontinued, especially medications found on Table 140-5.

Haloperidol is a highly potent antipsychotic medication which effectively reduces agitation and psychotic thought and sedates without further dulling awareness. It has virtually no anticholinergic or hypotensive actions. Haloperidol can be given parenterally; for over 20 years in North America it has been used intravenously to manage delirium. Although the Food and Drug Administration (FDA) has not approved the intravenous use of haloperidol, local hospital pharmacy committees have approved haloperidol for intravenous use as an innovative treatment.[23] Large doses of intravenous haloperidol have been used in seriously ill patients without harmful side effects.[24,25] In one study which looked at the effects on respiration of haloperidol, chlorpromazine, and diazepam in patients with chronic airway obstruction, only haloperidol did not depress respiration.[26] In our clinical experience, high doses of haloperidol (up to 100 mg intravenous bolus) have been given to critically ill, delirious patients without evidence of respiratory depression. The clinical incidence of extrapyramidal symptoms (EPS) with intravenous haloperidol in the critically ill population is extremely low; *orally* administered high potency neuroleptics more commonly cause EPS. The risk of tardive dyskinesia is negligible with intravenous haloperidol used at the doses listed and for the brief time recommended.

Recommended guidelines for administration of intravenous haloperidol to an agitated patient are provided in Table 140-8. The lower dosage schedule is appropriate for the elderly patient. The calming action of haloperidol is not immediately seen. The dose is repeated every 20 to 30 min until the patient is relaxed or sedated. Once a tranquil state is achieved, a repeat dose is given if agitation returns.

TABLE 140-8 Suggested Guidelines for Haloperidol Use in Acute Agitation

Level of Agitation	*Starting Dose*
Mild	0.5–2.0 mg
Moderate	2.0–5.0 mg
Severe	5.0–10.0 mg

1. Clear intravenous IV line with normal saline.
2. For elderly, use starting doses in the low range.
3. Allow 20 to 30 min between doses.
4. For continued agitation, double previous dose.
5. After 3 doses, give 0.5–1.0 mg lorazepam IV concurrently, or alternate lorazepam with haloperidol every 30 min.
6. Once patient is calm, add the total mg of haloperidol given and administer this total dose over the next 24 h.
7. Assuming the patient remains calm, reduce dose 50% every 24 h.
8. Oral dosage is twice the IV dose.

SOURCE: Reprinted from Wise MG, Rundell JR: *Concise Guide to Consultation Psychiatry*. Washington, DC, American Psychiatric Press, 1988. Copyright 1988 by The American Psychiatric Press, Inc. Reprinted by permission.

Treatment with haloperidol should continue for 3 to 5 days to prevent recurrence of the delirium, tapering the total daily dose by no more than 50 percent every 24 h. In patients who do not respond to haloperidol alone, intravenous lorazepam (in doses from 0.5 to 2.0 mg) may be given for a synergistic calming effect.[27]

Droperidol is a butyrophenone similar to haloperidol. Although droperidol is an antipsychotic medication, it is probably better known as a preanesthetic agent and as an antiemetic. Droperidol is approved for intravenous use by the FDA; as an antipsychotic, it is as potent as haloperidol. When compared to haloperidol, however, droperidol produces greater sedation and has a slightly higher potential for hypotension.[28]

Lower potency antipsychotic medications, such as chlorpromazine and thioridazine, often cause hypotension and have significant anticholinergic side effects. For these reasons, it is best to avoid the low potency antipsychotic drugs in the critically ill delirious patient.

Additional supportive measures are indicated in the management of delirium. The patient requires close medical attention and constant observation. Careful monitoring of fluid balance, oxygenation, and nutrition permits early detection of medical deterioration. The staff should watch for dangerous behavior, such as crawling out of bed or pulling out central venous or arterial catheters.

Insomnia and reversal of the sleep-wake cycle are problems often encountered in delirious patients. Certain interventions are helpful in restoration of sleep and include avoiding unnecessary awakenings at night, maintaining lighting to simulate day and night, and minimizing daytime naps. When haloperidol, droperidol, or lorazepam are used in treatment, give a large portion of the dose at bedtime. If other medications are used, use short-acting compounds such as triazolam, alprazolam, or chloral hydrate. Avoiding unnecessary awakening of the patient at night helps restore the normal sleep-wake cycle.

If the patient is accustomed to a hearing aid or eyeglasses, use of these devices in the hospital may improve orientation. It is best to avoid the common practice of placing confused patients near each other; this makes reorientation more difficult and can increase the agitation and confusion of both patients.

Environmental interventions and family involvement are sometimes helpful. Family members often become distraught and frightened when witnessing delirium in a loved one; it is beneficial for the family to understand the patient's condition. In addition, the informed family may be able to help care for the patient. A calm, understanding relative or friend can stay with the paranoid delirious patient, offer reassurance, help prevent mishaps, and reduce the burden on the nursing staff. The family and nursing staff should be encouraged to frequently orient the patient to the date and surroundings. It may be helpful to place a clock, calendar, and familiar items in the room where they are easily seen by the patient. During evening hours, a nightlight may decrease misperceptions and confusion. If available, a room with a window may help orient a delirious patient to diurnal cues.[29]

After a delirium has resolved, it is therapeutic to help the patient and family understand the bizarre experience.[30] Family members and the patient typically do not understand what caused the confusional state; they are often reluctant to discuss their concerns and fears with anyone. Patients may fear they will reexperience the confusion and wonder if they will become permanently impaired or "crazy."

Psychotic Disorders

Psychosis is characterized by impairment in the ability to interpret reality and is usually associated with dysfunctional behavior and communication. Hallucinations and delusions are frequently seen in psychosis, reflecting abnormal thought. Although psychosis is a hallmark of certain illnesses, like schizophrenia and delusional disorders, it may be seen in several other conditions. Failure to understand this may lead less experienced clinicians to diagnose any patient with a psychotic symptom as having schizophrenia. From the preceding discussion, it should be apparent that psychotic thought, including delusions, misperceptions, and hallucinations, is usually seen in delirium. Similarly, psychotic symptoms are sometimes present in patients with mood disorders (major depression or a manic episode). Delusional thinking is frequently encountered in patients with dementia. For example, it is not uncommon for demented individuals to think that someone is stealing their money or household belongings. Intoxication with certain illicit drugs, such as lysergic acid diethylamide or phencyclidine (LSD, PCP), is also associated with psychotic symptoms.

In the evaluation of an acutely agitated patient, differentiating delirium from a psychotic disorder is an important part of diagnosis. The delusions present in chronic psychotic disorders are deeply integrated into the patient's perception of the world; these delusions are elaborately organized and highly resistant to change. The delusional thought seen in a delirious patient is usually fragmented, poorly developed, and changes rapidly. If hallucinations are present, the type of hallucination can be relevant, recalling that auditory hallucinations are most typical in psychotic disorders. The delirious patient will have definite cognitive deficits, such as dysgraphia, constructional apraxia, and EEG abnormalities, which are not present in psychotic disorders. The past psychiatric history will also identify the patient with a chronic psychotic illness, such as schizophrenia or a delusional disorder. In any elderly patient, the new onset of confusion and psychotic symptoms should be considered delirium until proven otherwise. Schizophrenia rarely presents de novo in the elderly.[31]

When a medically ill patient known to have a chronic psychotic disorder becomes acutely agitated and exhibits bizarre behavior, delirium must still be ruled out. Delirium is a medical emergency requiring urgent evaluation and treatment. If mental status examination reveals no cognitive deficit in such patients, it may be assumed the patient is experiencing an acute psychotic decompensation. If the patient's past psychiatric history is known, treatment usually involves prescribing an antipsychotic medication to which the patient previously responded. In emergency situations, or when prior treatment is unknown, the guidelines for dosing haloperidol in delirium (Table 140-8) may be followed. If oral dosing is preferred, the oral dose is twice the parenteral dose. With oral dosing, the chances of developing extrapyramidal symptoms (EPS) are greatly increased. Whereas laryngospasm is the most dangerous form of EPS (occurring rarely), muscle rigidity, torticollis, and oculogyric crisis (rolling of the eyes upward) are more commonly seen. In acute EPS reactions, 25 to 50 mg diphenhydramine (Benadryl) may be administered intravenously or intramuscularly.[32] Psychiatric consultation is generally indicated to assist in the evaluation and treatment of a medically ill patient with a psychotic disorder.

Anxiety

Anxiety is a physiologic and psychologic response to many conditions. By itself, anxiety is a symptom and not a specific disorder. Patients with both delirium and psychotic disorders often exhibit anxiety. In medically ill patients, anxiety may be a response to serious illness and hospitalization; it may also be a manifestation of the illness itself or a response to medications. Anxiety disorders, such as generalized anxiety disorder or panic disorder, are found in 5 to 20 percent of general medical inpatients.[33]

The physical signs and symptoms of anxiety can mimic or aggravate medical disorders (Table 140-9). Cardiovascular symptoms are most frequently encountered. When evaluating anxiety, it is helpful to consider several broad diagnostic categories. These include anxiety as a part of a medical illness, anxiety as a drug reaction, anxiety as an acute reaction to a life-threatening illness, and the presence of an anxiety disorder.

Certain medical conditions are frequently associated with anxiety symptoms: hyperthyroidism, akathisia, hypoglycemia, pulmonary edema, and congestive heart failure are examples (Table 140-10). Anxiety may result from a withdrawal syndrome, most notably from alcohol, benzodiaze-

TABLE 140-9 Somatic and Autonomic Manifestations of Anxiety

Anorexia	Headache	Sexual dysfunction
Chest pain	Hot or cold flashes	Shakiness
Choking sensation	Hyperventilation	Shortness of breath
Diarrhea	Jumpiness	Smothering sensation
Diaphoresis	Light-headedness	Stomach pain
Dizziness	Lump in throat	Sweating
Dry mouth	Muscle aches	Tachycardia
Dyspnea	Muscle tension	Trembling
Easy startle response	Nausea	Unsteady feeling
Faintness	Pallor	Urinary frequency
Fatigability	Palpitations	Vertigo
Fidgetiness	Paresthesias	Vomiting
Flushing	Restlessness	

pines, barbiturates, and opiates. Many medications can cause symptoms of anxiety; a few examples of anxiogenic medications include theophyllines, thyroid supplements, and sympathomimetics and stimulants (e.g., phenylephrine, epinephrine, amphetamines, and caffeine). A patient's past history will identify whether anxiety symptoms predate the onset of medical illness. Many patients with preexisting anxiety disorders already receive treatment. Pharmacologic treatment that predates the critical illness should be continued during hospitalization, unless medically contraindicated.

Because anxiety is associated with increased sympathetic nervous system activity, it is a particularly undesirable symptom in patients with recent cardiac injury or cardiac arrhythmias. Therefore, it is important that patients admitted to a coronary care unit receive medication to reduce anxiety.[34] One study showed that only two-thirds of patients in a coronary care unit actually received benzodiazepines which were ordered.[35] Many patients in such circumstances are undertreated, due to clinicians' excessive fear of sedation, fear of drug dependence, or failure of the staff to recognize anxiety.

TABLE 140-10 Medical Causes of Anxiety

Cardiovascular Conditions	*Drugs*
Angina pectoris	Alcohol withdrawal
Arrhythmia	Amphetamine
Congestive heart failure	Aminophylline
Hypovolemia	Anticholinergics
Intra-aortic balloon pump	Antihypertensives:
Myocardial infarction	reserpine, hydralazine
Syncope	Antituberculosis agents:
Valvular disease, especially	isoniazid, cycloserine
mitral valve prolapse	Barbiturate withdrawal
Endocrine Conditions	Benzodiazepine withdrawal
Hyperadrenalism	Caffeine
Hypocalcemia	Cocaine
Hyperthyroidism	Digitalis (toxicity)
Hypothyroidism	Dopamine
Immunologic Conditions	Ephedrine
Anaphylaxis	Epinephrine
Systemic lupus	Levodopa
erythematosus	Lidocaine
Metabolic Conditions	Methylphenidate
Anemia	Monosodium glutamate
Hypoglycemia	Neuroleptics (akathisia)
Hyponatremia	Nonsteroidal anti-
Hyperkalemia	inflammatory agents
Hyperthermia	Nicotinic acid
Porphyria	Phenylephrine
Neurologic Conditions	Phenylpropanolamine
Akathisia	Procarbazine
Encephalopathy	Pseudoephedrine
Essential tremor	Salicylates
Postconcussion syndrome	Steroids
Restless legs syndrome	Theophylline
Seizure disorder, especially	Thyroid preparations
temporal focus	*Respiratory Conditions*
Vertigo	Asthma
Peptic ulcer disease	Chronic obstructive
Secreting Tumors	pulmonary disease
Carcinoid	Pneumonia
Insulinoma	Pneumothorax
Pheochromocytoma	Pulmonary edema
	Pulmonary embolus
	Respirator dependence

SOURCE: Adapted from Geringer ES, Stern TA: Anxiety and depression in the medically ill, in Wise MG (ed): *Problems in Critical Care Medicine*. Philadelphia, Lippincott, 1988.

Benzodiazepines are the drugs of choice for treating anxiety in critically ill patients. Benzodiazepines are categorized according to their speed of onset, duration of action, sedation properties, and route of metabolism (Table 140-11). The onset of action correlates well with the lipid solubility of the benzodiazepine.[32] For example, diazepam is highly lipophilic and has a very rapid onset of action. Duration of action, which is determined by the benzodiazepine's half-life and physiologic metabolites, is also an important factor to consider. Lorazepam and oxazepam are metabolized by direct conjugation in the liver, resulting in shorter elimination half-lives than the other benzodiazepines, which undergo hepatic oxidation. In patients with severe liver disease, the use of lorazepam or oxazepam carries a lower potential for side effects.[36] In critically ill patients, the route of drug administration is important as well. Diazepam and lorazepam are available for intravenous use. Although both of these drugs may be administered intramuscularly as well, lorazepam is reported to have more reliable absorption by the intramuscular route.

Antianxiety medication is indicated when a patient has significant anxiety. Patients with a past history of substance abuse remain at higher risk for future substance abuse. However, patients without a history of drug abuse are at very low, if any, risk for abuse of benzodiazepines.

Buspirone is a new, nonbenzodiazepine antianxiety medication which does not impair cognitive function, does not cause sedation, and is not habit forming. However, the onset of action of buspirone is delayed for 1 to 2 weeks, reducing its usefulness in the treatment of acute anxiety. Nonetheless, it may be helpful for treating the chronically anxious, medically ill patient. Buspirone is initially dosed at 5 mg orally twice a day, with a recommended daily maximum dose of 60 mg.

Many critically ill patients experience anxiety because there are unknown aspects to their illness. Often the fear of dying is foremost in their thoughts. It is helpful to address this fear when talking with patients. Frequently patients will openly state that they believe they are dying. If death seems an unlikely outcome, explanations about the nature of the illness and expected recovery are generally reassuring. If death is an expected outcome, one may ask, "What frightens you most about dying?" Terminally ill patients may fear having severe pain as they die; in this case, offer reassurance that they will be kept comfortable and free of severe pain to the extent this is possible. Patients may have concerns of a religious nature which are best handled through a consultation visit from a chaplain.

When critically ill patients directly ask whether or not they are dying, a truthful answer is best. Patients usually suspect that they are dying when such a question is posed.

TABLE 140-11 Benzodiazepines: Profile for Use

	Equivalent Oral Doses (mg)	Onset of Action	Active Metabolite	Half-life (h)[a]	Degree of Sedation
Midazolam (Versed)	[b]	Fast	Yes	2–5	+++
Diazepam (Valium)	5.0	Fast	Yes	20–70	+++
Clorazepate (Tranxene)	7.5	Fast	Yes	[c]	++
Flurazepam (Dalmane)	15.0	Fast	Yes	[c]	+++
Triazolam (Halcion)	0.25	Intermediate	No	1.5–5	++
Lorazepam (Ativan)[d]	1.0	Intermediate	No	10–20	+++
Alprazolam (Xanax)	0.5	Intermediate	Yes	12–15	+
Halazepam (Paxipam)	20.0	Intermediate	Yes	12–15	++
Chlordiazepoxide (Librium)	10.0	Intermediate	Yes	5–30	++
Oxazepam (Serax)[d]	15.0	Slow	No	5–15	+
Temazepam (Restoril)	15.0	Slow	No	9–12	++
Clonazepam (Klonopin)	0.5	Slow	No	18–50	++
Prazepam (Centrax)	10.0	Slow	Yes	[c]	+

[a]Half-life of parent compound only.
[b]Available only in parenteral form in US.
[c]Prodrugs—metabolites are the active agents and have long half-lives (30–200 h).
[d]Direct hepatic glucuronide conjugation.

A quick, falsely reassuring reply, "Oh, you'll be feeling better soon," is generally irritating and impairs meaningful communication. Sometimes patients ask for reassurance and comfort when they are anxious about dying. Usually they will ask a nurse for this type of support.

To calm severely ill patients who becomes anxious, it is helpful to spend a few quiet moments at the bedside. Learn from the patients what the illness means to them and what are the fears. Give reasonable reassurance without offering false hope. Most patients benefit from being told accurate information about their illness and prognosis; however, this must be done in a gentle and caring manner.

Psychiatric consultation will be helpful in the management of patients with severe anxiety who have not responded to supportive care or antianxiety medication. When faced with a patient who has an anxiety disorder or whose personality fosters anxiety and prevents effective communication and interaction, a psychiatric consultant can provide assistance.

CASE PRESENTATION

I. R., a 61-year-old, retired office manager with a history of chronic obstructive pulmonary disease (COPD), congestive heart failure, and adult-onset diabetes mellitus, presented to the emergency department with acute respiratory distress. In the face of progressive respiratory decompensation, she was intubated and admitted to the medical intensive care unit (MICU). On admission she was alert, oriented, and although she appeared quite anxious, she was cooperative with the MICU staff. Mrs. R.'s daughter provided a list of the patient's medications: digoxin 0.125 mg po every day, theophylline 200 mg po every 12 h, and tolbutamide 500 mg po twice daily.

Mrs. R. was extubated 20 h following admission to the MICU. Her physician ordered digoxin 0.125 mg po daily, tolbutamide 500 mg po twice daily, increased theophylline to 300 mg po every 12 h, and added prednisone 60 mg po every day and albuterol 2.5 mg in 3 ml normal saline every 2 h. Her cardiac status remained stable, and her respiratory status slowly improved over the next 24 h. During day 3 in the MICU, the nursing staff noted that Mrs. R. was often drowsy and appeared preoccupied. She left her food tray untouched and ate only with strong, constant encouragement. At times she was tearful; when questioned, she said she was afraid of dying. Although she was not openly uncooperative, the patient was without energy or motivation, lying quietly in her bed.

Convinced that Mrs. R. was clinically depressed, her physician prescribed amitriptyline 50 mg po at bedtime. The next morning on rounds, the patient was somnolent and difficult to arouse. Later in the day, Mrs. R. was found trying to urinate in one of the drawers of her bedside table. When a male attendant attempted to help her back to her bed, the patient became agitated, screaming "Keep away from me!" She ran out of the room, tearing intravenous lines from her arms and cardiac monitoring leads from her chest. She fell to the floor outside her room. As she was helped from the floor to her bed, she cried and pled, "Please don't hurt me, have mercy on me!" Her physician requested psychiatric consultation, stating, "I have a patient who must be schizophrenic. She was fine until just now, when she became psychotic and crazy."

Mrs. R. was returned to her MICU bed, with no fractures detected. On mental status examination, the psychiatrist found the patient moderately agitated, dishevelled, and paranoid. She believed the hospital staff were trying to harm her. She was disoriented to time and place; she stated the year was 1945 and did not know where she was. She had no recollection of her illness or the events of the past 4 days. Reacting to a slight movement of the curtain at her bedside, she turned suddenly and stated, "Something just ran under my bed." On MMSE, she scored 18 of 30, with deficits in orientation, recent memory, calculation, attention, following a three-stage command, writing, and constructional ability. Her attempt to draw the face of a clock showed marked constructional apraxia. On physical examination, Mrs. R. was tachycardic (112 beats/min), tachypneic (24 respirations/min), hypertensive (185/108), and had an oral temperature of 37.5°C (99.5°F). Chest auscultation revealed no acute changes. A neurologic examination was remarkable for asterixis.

Mrs. R.'s husband and daughter reported that the patient had no prior psychiatric history. Two days ago they noticed that Mrs. R. "seemed different—not quite herself. She wouldn't talk to us and didn't seem to recognize us. She was sleepy and confused much of the day." Review of the nurses' notes in the chart revealed the patient had been awake most of the evening shift for the past two nights.

The medication record showed that the patient's theophylline dose was increased on admission, with a blood level of 14 μg/mL on the day following the dosage change. Her digoxin dose, amitriptyline dose, and her prednisone dose had remained constant. Review of the laboratory studies revealed a full workup on admission, with frequent arterial blood-gas determinations, which documented respiratory acidosis on admission, with progressive improvement to her base line.

CASE DISCUSSION

The patient had a delirium. In this case, delirium was manifest by a fluctuating course (with alternating lethargy and agitation), cognitive impairment, visual illusions, disorientation, memory dysfunction, dysgraphia, constructional apraxia, and delusional thoughts. With no prior history of psychiatric illness and the clinical picture described, a first schizophrenic psychotic episode at age sixty-six was ruled out. Unfortunately Mrs. R. was initially diagnosed with depression, and amitriptyline was ordered for her. The added burden of amitriptyline's strong anticholinergic effects most likely exacerbated the patient's condition.

Further evaluations were requested by the psychiatrist to include a theophylline level, digoxin level, blood chemistries, blood count, urinalysis, ECG, chest x-ray, and EEG (see Table 140-4). These tests revealed a digoxin level 2.3 mμg/mL (0.8 to 2.0 mμg/mL therapeutic range), theophylline level 31 μg/ml (10 to 20 μg/mL therapeutic range), white blood cell (WBC) count 9600 (8900 on admission), hematocrit 29 percent (unchanged from admission), and urinalysis with 15 to 20 WBC/ high power field (hpf). A urine specimen was sent for culture and sensitivity. Serum glucose was 48 mg/dL (decreased from 86 mg/dL on admission). Her VDRL was nonreactive. A blood-gas determination, with the patient on 2 L O_2 by nasal canula, revealed Pa_{O_2} 60 mmHg, P_{CO_2} 55 mmHg, pH 7.36, and HCO_3^- 30 meq/L. Her chest x-ray was without acute changes. An EEG documented diffuse slow background activity.

In this case, multiple possible causes of delirium were identified:

1. Medication effects
   a. Anticholinergic effects of amitriptyline
   b. Toxicity (theophylline and digoxin levels are above therapeutic ranges)
   c. CNS effects of steroids (prednisone)
2. Hypoglycemia
3. Infection (WBC in urine sample)
4. Hypoxemia

The two physicians agreed that the most immediate concern was to treat or reverse the pathologic conditions identified. Amitriptyline was discontinued to reduce anticholinergic effects. The next doses of theophylline and digoxin were held, with plans to adjust the dosages of each to reduce further toxicity, monitoring with serum drug levels. Although prednisone may be contributing to Mrs. R.'s delirium, it was currently an essential medication for treatment of her respiratory distress. Therefore, prednisone was continued at the current dose, with a plan to taper the dose as rapidly as possible.

Hypoglycemia was treated with an intravenous dextrose solution and by discontinuing tolbutamide. The patient's serum glucose level was more closely monitored. Her occult urinary tract infection was treated with trimethoprim-sulfamethoxazole, after clarifying she had no known allergies to these drugs. Culture of her urine revealed *Escherichia coli,* susceptible to trimethoprim-sulfamethoxazole. A workup to search for an etiology for her anemia was initiated. With 2 L of O_2 by nasal cannula, the patient maintained marginally adequate oxygenation. To effectively progress with treatment of her respiratory illness and to prevent hypoxemia, Mrs. R. had to cooperate with wearing her nasal cannula and with obtaining further blood-gas samples.

Intravenous haloperidol was administered to control the patient's agitation. She was calmer, better oriented, and less paranoid after three doses of 5 mg haloperidol were given intravenously at 30-min intervals. Supportive measures were initiated, providing close supervision to prevent dangerous behavior and to monitor her medical condition. Unnecessary awakenings were avoided at night to assist in restoration of her sleep-wake cycle. Mrs. R.'s eyeglasses were brought from home for her to wear. Her husband and daughter, reassured that Mrs. R. would most likely soon return to "her old self," offered to stay with her, to help with orientation and observation. The next day, 5 mg intravenous haloperidol was prescribed every 8 h. The patient's delirium resolved within 24 h after management and treatment are initiated. The dose of haloperidol was decreased by 5 mg daily.

References

1. Lipowski ZJ: Organic brain syndromes: A reformulation. Comp Psychiatry 19:309, 1978.
2. Wise MG: Delirium, in Hales RE, Yudofsky SC (eds): *The American Psychiatric Textbook of Neuropsychiatry*. Washington, DC, American Psychiatric Press, 1987, pp 89–105.
3. Lipowski ZJ: Delirium (acute confusional states). JAMA 258:1789, 1987.
4. Lipowski ZJ: Delirium in the elderly patient. N Engl J Med 329:578, 1989.
5. Wise MG: Unpublished data
6. Thomas RI, Cameron DJ, Fahs MC: A prospective study of delirium and prolonged hospital stay. Arch Gen Psychiatry 45:937, 1988.
7. Lipowski ZJ: Delirium, clouding of consciousness and confusion. J Nerv Mental Dis 145:227, 1967.
8. Dubin WR, Field NL, Gartfriend DR: Postcardiotomy delirium: A critical review. J Thoracic Cardiovasc Surg 77:586, 1979.
9. Andreasen NJC, Noyer R, Hartford C, et al: Management of emotional reactions in seriously burned adults. N Engl J Med 286:65, 1972.
10. Lipowski ZJ: *Delirium (Acute Brain Failure in Man)*. Springfield, IL, Charles C Thomas, 1980.
11. Layne OL, Yudofsky SC: Postoperative psychosis in cardiotomy patients: The role of organic and psychiatric factors. N Engl J Med 284:518, 1971.
12. Epstein LJ, Simon A: Organic brain syndrome in the elderly. Geriatrics 22:145, 1967.
13. Prugh DG, Wagonfeld S, Metcalf D, et al: A clinical study of delirium in children and adolescents. Psychosom Med 42(suppl):177, 1980.
14. Engel GL, Romano J: Delirium, a syndrome of cerebral insufficiency. J Chronic Dis 9:260, 1959.
15. Wells CE, Duncan GW: *Neurology for Psychiatrists*. Philadelphia, FA Davis, 1980.
16. Cummings JL: Acute confusional states, in Cummings JL (ed): *Clinical Neuropsychiatry*. New York, Grune & Stratton, 1985, pp 68–74.
17. Chedru F, Geschwind N: Writing disturbances in acute confusional states. Neuropsychologia 10:343, 1972.
18. Adams RD, Victor M: *Principles of Neurology*. New York, McGraw-Hill, 1989.
19. Pro JD, Wells CE: The use of the electroencephalogram in the diagnosis of delirium. Dis Nerv Sys 38:804, 1977.
20. Kennard MA, Bueding E, Wortis WB: Some biochemical and electroencephalographic changes in delirium tremens. Q J Studies on Alcohol 6:4, 1945.
21. Folstein MF, Folstein SE, McHugh PR: "Mini-mental state": A practical method for grading the cognitive state of patients for the clinician. J Psychiatr Res 12: 189, 1975.
22. American Psychiatric Association: *Diagnostic and Statistical Manual of Mental Disorders*. 3d ed, revised. Washington, DC, American Psychiatric Association, 1987.
23. Wise MG, Cassem NJ: Behavioral disturbances in the ICU, in Civetta JM, Taylor RW, Kirby RR (eds): *Critical Care*. Philadelphia, JB Lippincott, 1988, pp 1595–1604.
24. Tesar GE, Murray GB, Cassem NH: Use of high-dose intravenous haloperidol in the treatment of agitated cardiac patients. J Clin Psychopharmacol 5:344, 1985.
25. Sos J, Cassem NH: Managing postoperative agitation. Drug Ther 10(3):103, 1980.
26. Tandon MK: Effect on respiration of diazepam, chlopromazine and haloperidol in patients with chronic airways obstruction. Aust NZ J Med 6:561, 1976.
27. Adams F: Neuropsychiatric evaluation and treatment of delirium in the critically ill cancer patient. Cancer Bull 36:156, 1984.
28. Cassem NH, Hackett TP: The Setting of Intensive Care, in Cassem NH, Hackett TP (eds): *Massachussetts General Hospital Handbook of General Hospital Psychiatry*. 2d ed. Littleton, MA, PSG Publishing Company, 1987, pp 353–379.
29. Wilson LM: Intensive care delirium. Arch Intern Med 130:225, 1972.
30. Mackensie TB, Popkin MK: Stress response syndrome occurring after delirium. Am J Psychiatry 137:1433, 1980.
31. Babigian HM: Schizophrenia: Epidemiology, in Kaplan HI, Sadock JB (eds): *Comprehensive Textbook of Psychiatry*. 4th ed. Baltimore, Williams & Wilkins, 1985, pp 643–650.
32. Bernstein JG: *Handbook of Drug Therapy in Psychiatry*. 2d ed. Littleton, MA, PSG Publishing Company, 1988.
33. Strain JJ, Liebowitz MR, Klein DF: Anxiety and panic attacks in the medically ill. Psych Clin North Am 4:333, 1981.
34. Cassem NH, Hackett TP: Psychiatric consultation in a coronary care unit. Ann Intern Med 75:9, 1971.
35. Stern TA, Caplan RA, Cassem NH: Use of benzodiazepines in a cornary care unit. Psychosomatics 28:19, 1987.
36. Wise MG, Rundell JR: *Concise Guide to Consultation Psychiatry*. Washington, DC, American Psychiatric Press, 1988.

Chapter 141
CEREBROVASCULAR DISEASE

WILLIAM J. POWERS
DANIEL F. HANLEY, JR.

KEY POINTS

- *Non-arteriosclerotic causes of stroke, especially cerebral emboli of cardiac origin, occur commonly in patients admitted to intensive care units (ICUs) and should be carefully sought by appropriate diagnostic tests.*
- *The efficacy of anticoagulation in patients with acute cerebral ischemia or infarction of any cause has not been conclusively demonstrated. Any possible benefit must be weighed against the risk of iatrogenic hemorrhage.*
- *In patients with acute cerebrovascular disease, reduction of systemic blood pressure carries a significant risk of producing further neurologic deterioration.*
- *Emergency neurosurgical interventions should be strongly considered in patients with cerebellar infarction or hemorrhage and consequent brainstem compression.*
- *Lumbar puncture is the most sensitive test for detection of subarachnoid hemorrhage; CT or MRI may miss the diagnosis in 10 to 20 percent of cases.*
- *Early surgical clipping of ruptured aneurysms removes the risk of rebleeding and facilitates the effective management of delayed vasospasm and hydrocephalus.*

Etiology

Cerebrovascular diseases can be divided into three categories: cerebral ischemia and infarction, intracerebral hemorrhage, and subarachnoid hemorrhage.

Cerebral ischemia and infarction are caused by processes that impair cerebral perfusion. Global hypoperfusion due to systemic hypotension or increased intracranial pressure may produce infarction in the distal territories or border zones of the major cerebral arteries, producing characteristic symptoms of proximal arm and leg weakness, amnesia, or cortical blindness. Local arterial stenosis in combination with systemic hypotension rarely causes a focal brain infarction. Atherosclerosis is the most common cause of local arterial disease producing cerebral ischemia and infarction; it causes such disease primarily by serving as a nidus for thrombus formation with subsequent distal embolization. While emboli arising from the heart cause approximately 30 percent of all cerebral infarcts in a general population, they assume more importance in the ICUs. Atrial fibrillation, infective endocarditis, nonbacterial thrombotic endocarditis, and ventricular mural thrombus secondary to acute myocardial infarction or cardiomyopathy all are common causes of cerebral infarction in patients admitted to ICU. Rarer causes of cerebral infarction must also be considered in this setting; these include dissections of the carotid or vertebral artery after head or neck trauma, intracranial arterial or venous thrombosis secondary to meningeal or parameningeal infections, and paradoxic emboli.[1,2,3]

Hemorrhages into the basal ganglia and cerebellum, which most often occur in middle-aged patients with longstanding hypertension, are the most common type of intracerebral hemorrhage. Arteriovenous malformations must be considered, especially in younger patients. Amyloid angiopathy becomes increasingly important in patients in the seventh, eighth, and ninth decades. These hemorrhages usually occur in the subcortical hemispheric white matter. Rarer causes of intracerebral hemorrhage occurring in patients with other systemic diseases include thrombocytopenia, hemophilia, and disseminated intravascular coagulation. Intracranial aneurysms may rupture into the brain as well as the subarachnoid space, producing a predominantly intracerebral hematoma.

Spontaneous subarachnoid hemorrhage is almost always due to ruptured intracranial aneurysms, although arteriovenous malformations may ocassionally manifest themselves in this manner.

Clinical and Laboratory Diagnosis

The initial diagnostic evaluation of the patient serves (1) to determine whether neurologic symptoms are due to cerebrovascular disease or are caused by some other condition, such as encephalitis, a mass lesion, multiple sclerosis, epilepsy, or hypoglycemia; and (2) to distinguish among different types of cerebrovascular disease that require different treatments. The clinical history and examination remain the cornerstone of this process. Cerebrovascular disease produces the sudden onset of focal brain dysfunction. The primary exception to this is pure subarachnoid hemorrhage with symptoms restricted to the sudden onset of severe headache, with or without loss of consciousness. Focal brain dysfunctions may not always include an obvious hemiparesis. Isolated neurologic deficits, such as neglect, agnosia, aphasia, cortical blindness, and amnesia, may be the only manifestations of brain infarction or hemorrhage. Multiple small brain infarcts may mimic a metabolic or toxic encephalopathy with depressed consciousness and minimal or no focal neurologic deficits. The initial neurologic examination provides information about the location of the brain dysfunction and provides a baseline for monitoring the subsequent clinical course. A thorough medical evaluation is necessary to detect systemic diseases that may be the cause of the cerebrovascular problem. Careful examination of the heart is imperative to detect conditions that might predispose to embolization.

The primary role of diagnostic tests is to determine etiology. Differentiation between infarction and hemorrhage may be critical. X-ray computed tomography (CT) is the diagnostic test of choice for patients with acute cerebrovascular disease. It is rapid and can be easiy performed on acutely ill patients. Acute intracerebral hemorrhage is easily identified by noncontrast CT scan. Intravenous contrast administration increases sensitivity for detecting diseases that may mimic stroke, such as tumor, subdural hematoma, and abscess. Cerebral infarction may not be demonstrated by CT for several days; if small enough, it may never be apparent. Demonstration of cerebral infarction is rarely necessary, since the diagnosis can be made reliably by the clinical presentation and a negative CT scan to exclude hemorrhage and other conditions. Magnetic resonance imaging (MRI) is more sensitive than CT for lesion detection, especially in the early period following ischemic infarction and for lesions in the cerebellum and brain stem. However, it is more cumbersome to perform in acutely ill patients on life support systems, because of the requirement for longer imaging times and non-ferromagnetic support and monitoring devices. While MRI has no advantage over CT in the demonstration of acute hemorrhage, it does have superior sensitivity for detecting subacute or chronic hemorrhage.

In the patient who is awake and alert with acute focal brain dysfunction, the distinction between cerebral infarction and cerebral hemorrhage often has no bearing on immediate therapeutic decisions, and CT may be safely postponed. If the patient has signs or symptoms suggesting an intracranial mass lesion, however, emergency CT is critically important to determine the need for neurosurgical intervention.

Lumbar puncture with cerebrospinal fluid (CSF) examination is an extremely important test in the evaluation of the patient with cerebrovascular disease. It is essential to rule out meningitis with secondary stroke caused by thrombosis of arteries or cortical veins. Cerebrospinal fluid pleocytosis is common following septic embolism from infective endocarditis and can serve as a valuable clue to its presence. Lumbar puncture is the most sensitive test for detection of subarachnoid hemorrhage; CT or MRI may miss this diagnosis in 10 to 20 percent of cases. In the majority of patients, cerebral edema or mass lesion can be excluded by careful history and neurologic examination. Lumbar puncture can then be performed safely at the bedside without a prior brain-imaging study.

Differentiation of cerebral infarction due to atherosclerotic cerebrovascular disease from that caused by cardiac emboli may be important therapeutically (see Treatment, Cardiac Emboli, below). For patients over the age of 50 who present to the hospital with a cerebral infarction and who have no clinical or electrocardiographic evidence of heart disease, there is little diagnostic yield from cardiac monitoring or echocardiography. However, in younger patients or those hospitalized in an ICU with underlying systemic or cardiac disease, these tests can be of value to detect a cardiac lesion or arrythmia (especially atrial fibrillation) that may predispose to cerebral embolism.[1] Because of the high incidence of asymptomatic atherosclerosis and the inconsistent relationship between the degree of atherosclerotic disease and consequent brain infarction, examination of the extracranial carotid or vertebral arteries by Doppler or ultrasound studies has little value in differentiating cardioembolic from atherosclerotic causes of brain infarction. Cerebral arteriography can provide high-resolution images of both extracranial and intracranial vessels, which may be useful in identification of non-atherosclerotic cerebrovascular diseases, such as dissection, vasculitis, and venous thrombosis. Cerebral arteriography plays a more important role in the patient with subarachnoid hemorrhage by confirming the existence of an aneurysm and providing the necessary information to plan a surgical approach. In selected patients with intracerebral hemorrhage, arteriography may demonstrate vascular malformations or aneurysms. This is particularly true when the location of the hemorrhage and the patient profile are not typical for hypertensive hemorrhage or amyloid angiopathy.

Transcranial Doppler studies detect increases in flow velocity in the majority of patients with arteriographic vasospasm following subarachnoid hemorrhage. Vasospasm occurring in vessels other than those examined may not be detected. An increase in flow velocity due to luxury perfusion, hemodilution, or other mechanisms may be falsely interpreted as vasospasm. The value of cerebral blood flow measurements in the diagnosis and treatment of patients with cerebrovascular disease remains to be demonstrated. The diagnosis of cerebral infarction can be made reliably by means of the clinical picture and a CT scan. It is rarely, if ever, necessary to demonstrate a defect on a cerebral blood flow study. Cerebral blood flow measurement, as an adjunct in deciding either the appropriate therapeutic intervention in patients with cerebral infarction or the timing of surgery with patients with subarachnoid hemorrhage, has not been demonstrated to result in improved outcome.

Treatment

ATHEROTHROMBOTIC INFARCTION

No clinical evidence or pathophysiologic reason supports routine restriction of patients with acute brain infarction to bed. Prolonged bed rest carries increased risk of iliofemoral venous thrombosis, pulmonary embolism, and pneumonia. Patients should be out of bed and walking as soon as possible after a stroke. Occasionally, orthostatic hypotension with worsening of neurologic deficits will occur; in these cases a more gradual program of ambulation should be instituted. In hemiplegic patients, subcutaneous heparin should be administered to prevent iliofemoral venous thrombosis. Intermittently pumping antithrombotic stockings may provide added benefit. At the time of hospital admission, some patients may have mild intravascular volume depletion. In addition to normal maintenance requirements, careful fluid supplementation may be required. The composition of the intravenous fluid (normal saline solution, one-half normal saline solution, or 5% glucose) makes no difference as long as serum electrolyte and glucose concentrations remain normal. Care must be taken to avoid hypoosmolarity, which can exacerbate brain edema. This may be easier to accomplish if normal saline solution is used. Systemic arterial hypertension is common following acute stroke; in most cases, blood pressure returns to baseline levels without treatment in a few days. Appropriate treatment remains controversial. During the period following acute cerebral infarction, the normal mechanism of cerebral autoregulation of blood flow in response to changes in perfusion pressure is impaired. Any reduction in systemic blood pressure is likely to cause a decrease in cerebral blood flow, causing further damage in marginally perfused areas adjacent to the infarct. There are no known hazards to the brain from this spontaneous transient elevation in systemic blood pressure. When systemic hypertension is causing organ damage elsewhere (e.g., myocardial ischemia or dissecting aortic aneurysm), careful and judicious lowering of the blood pressure, with constant monitoring of neurologic status, is indicated. When undertaking antihypertensive therapy, it should be emphasized that *there is no level to which blood pressure can be reduced that does not carry the risk of further neurologic deterioration.* The use of supplemental inspired oxygen is rational only if the arterial oxygen content of the blood is decreased. No special diet is necessary for patients with acute stroke. It is important to remember that dysphagia occurs commonly, even with unilateral hemispheric lesions. Prior to instituting oral feeding, each patient's ability to swallow should be carefully checked. Incontinence also is common following acute stroke. Careful attention must be given to the prevention of decubitus ulcers in bedridden patients.

No therapeutic intervention has been shown to be of value in reducing brain damage due to acute cerebral infarction. Of vasodilators, hemodilution, calcium channel blockers, prostacyclin, and pentoxifylline, not one has been demonstrated to be of benefit in clinical trials.[4] Preliminary trials with streptokinase and tissue plasminogen activator in acute stroke are currently under way. Some experts advocate emergency carotid endarterectomy in selected patients with acute ischemic stroke. Since this operation has high rates of morbidity and mortality in this setting and prevailing evidence suggests that most hemispheric infarctions are due to distal embolization, no improvement in outcome is to be anticipated. Cerebral edema is the major cause of early mortality following cerebral infarction. No effective treatment is available. Corticosteroids and glycerol have not provided consistent improvements in morbidity or mortality. Mannitol and hyperventilation can temporarily reduce intracranial pressure, but have no long-term benefit. They may be of value to the patient with brain stem compression from edematous cerebellar infarct in whom craniotomy and removal of the edematous tissue is planned. This is the only situation in which surgical intervention for the treatment of cerebral edema following brain infarction is likely to provide benefit.

Recent studies have demonstrated no benefit from anticoagulation with heparin in patients with transient ischemic attack or partial stable stroke.[5,6,7] Although several controlled trials have demonstrated a benefit of long-term oral anticoagulation in patients whose initial presentation was progressing stroke, more recent evidence from uncontrolled trials of heparin in acute progressing stroke have demonstrated that further progression usually occurs in spite of early anticoagulation.[8,9] This issue is unresolved.[6] Aspirin and ticlopidine have been demonstrated to be modestly effective in the long-term prevention of recurrent stroke, but there are no data regarding their value during the acute period.

CARDIAC EMBOLI

The general care of the patient with cardioembolic brain infarction—as well as the choice of intravenous fluids, the control of blood pressure, and the lack of effective medical therapy for reducing brain damage or treating cerebral edema—are the same as for atherothrombotic infarction. Although not rigorously proven by controlled trials, there is evidence that early anticoagulation may be of value in preventing recurrent infarction from cardiac emboli, particularly in patients with acute myocardial infarction and atrial fibrillation.[6,10] The results of long-term anticoagulation in patients with cardiomyopathy, left ventricular aneurysms, and rheumatic valvular disease suggest that acute anticoagulation may be beneficial in these patients as well. The decision to institute anticoagulation with heparin after cardioembolic cerebral infarction, however, must take into account the small but real risk of producing hemorrhage into the infarct, resulting in neurologic deterioration. This risk appears to be greatest in hypertensive patients with large infarctions who are given anticoagulation within the first few days. Since recurrence occurs within 2 weeks in only 3 to 12 percent of patients, many experts recommend postponing the institution of heparin therapy for several days in all patients, and for as much as 1 week in those at higher risk of hemorrhagic transformation.[10]

OTHER CAUSES OF CEREBRAL INFARCTION

In general, the principles of general care—and the lack of effective treatment for edema and neuronal salvage—are applicable. Specific causes may require specific definitive therapy, such as exchange transfusions for cerebral infarction due to sickle cell anemia. Anticoagulation does not appear to be effective for patients with emboli due to nonbacterial thrombotic endocarditis. Cerebral venous thrombosis can present a particularly difficult situation. While there is some evidence that anticoagulation may be of value in improving the outcome, patients who present with large or hemorrhagic infarctions probably should not be given anticoagulation, because of the danger of brain hemorrhage.

INTRACEREBRAL HEMORRHAGE

The care of patients with primary intracerebral hemorrhage requires the same attention to the principles of general care, early ambulation, and intravenous fluids as that of patients with cerebral infarction. Systemic blood pressure is often elevated acutely, sometimes to very high levels. As with cerebral infarction, autoregulation is impaired, and reduction in systemic blood pressure may critically reduce blood flow to the ischemic region surrounding the hemorrhage. If the intracranial hemorrhage is large enough to increase intracranial pressure, cerebral perfusion pressure will be reduced, making the rationale for lowering systemic blood pressure even more problematic. In patients with increased intracranial pressure, the use of systemic antihypertensive agents may cause intracranial vasodilation, with further increases in intracranial pressure. The dangers of reducing systemic blood pressure in this situation are obvious. The benefits are unclear. Rebleeding occurs rarely; its relationship to early arterial hypertension is unknown.

No specific medical therapy has been shown to be of value in patients with acute intracerebral hemorrhage. Corticosteroids do not reduce morbidity and mortality due to edema. Mannitol and hyperventilation can be used effectively to reduce intracranial pressure temporarily if a definitive surgical intervention is planned. The primary goal of surgery is to alleviate the effects of the hematoma acting as an intracranial mass lesion, not to reverse the effects of local tissue destruction; thus surgery has no role in treating small hemorrhages. The value of surgery is best proven for cerebellar hemorrhages resulting in brain stem compression; here, surgical evacuation can be lifesaving. Ideally, however, surgical intervention should be undertaken before brain stem damage occurs. Prospectively determined criteria for the necessity and the timing of cerebellar hematoma evacuation are not available. Many patients with cerebellar hematomas do well without surgical intervention, or simply with ventricular drainage for hydrocephalus. Patients with large, deep hematomas arising from the basal ganglia do not benefit from surgical intervention. Those with more superficial hematomas and signs of increased intracranial pressure may show improvement after surgical evacuation. In the absence of clinical signs due to mass effect, however, such operations are not indicated.

Intracerebral hematomas due to arteriovenous malformations or ruptured aneurysms require special consideration and careful angiographic studies prior to any surgical approach. In patients with intracerebral hematomas due to bleeding diatheses (e.g., thrombocytopenia, hemophilia, or disseminated intravascular coagulation) the underlying problem should be corrected, if possible.

SUBARACHNOID HEMORRHAGE DUE TO RUPTURED INTRACRANIAL ANEURYSM

Following rupture of an intracranial aneurysm, three events commonly occur that can cause further brain damage; these are rebleeding, delayed ischemia (clinically known as *vasospasm*), and hydrocephalus. While little can be done to ameliorate the effects of initial hemorrhage, improved results in aneurysm treatment over the past decade strongly suggest that emergent clipping of ruptured intracranial aneurysms, coupled with acute ventricular drainage for hydrocephalus and prophylactic treatment for vasospasm, is associated with improved outcome.[11] However, the intensivist would be well advised to recognize that delayed surgery may still be appropriate for some patients when the care-providing team is not well practiced in urgent interventions for subarachnoid hemorrhage. The remainder of this section will discuss critical care management of subarachnoid hemorrhage patients on an urgent or emergent basis, recognizing that some controversy persists about this issue of surgical timing.

PREOPERATIVE CARE

Cerebral angiography should be performed emergently. After identification of an aneurysm, the assessment of operative risk factors—including Hunt-Hess clinical grade (Table 141-1), surgical accessibility of the lesion, presence of a mass effect caused by a hematoma, and/or presence of severe vasospasm—is necessary to determine the optimal timing of surgery. The most practiced teams are now operating on most patients in grades I to III in the first 24 to 48 h after presentation. Preoperative prophylactic medical therapy includes anticonvulsants and calcium channel blockers. Recent controlled studies suggest that calcium channel blockers administered prophylactically to aneurysm patients reduce the morbidity of vasospasm by about 50 percent.[12–14] The use of these medications is associated with transient mild lowering of the blood pressure and with impaired vascular responsiveness to vasoconstrictors.

No overall benefit has been demonstrated for antifibrinolytic therapy or for medical management of blood pressure. Antifibrinolytic drugs appear to be associated with increased incidences of both vasospasm and delayed hydrocephalus. Additional preoperative measures include bed rest, sedation, and limiting of activities to avoid cough and Valsalva maneuvers (as rupture appears to be temporarily related to these activities). Stool softeners can be particularly helpful.

POSTOPERATIVE CARE

For most ruptured aneurysms, definitive clipping can be accomplished; this removes the threat of rebleeding. The focus of postoperative care then becomes prevention and treatment of delayed vasospasm and hydrocephalus. Prophylactic use of calcium channel blockers should be continued. A second type of therapy for vasospasm is hypervolemic/hypertensive therapy. Prophylactic augmentation of circulating blood volume and event-predicated augmenta-

TABLE 141-1 Hunt-Hess Classification of Patients with Intracranial Aneurysms, According to Surgical Risk

Category	Criteria
Grade I	Asymptomatic, or minimal headache and slight nuchal rigidity
Grade II	Moderate-to-severe headache, nuchal rigidity; no neurologic deficit other than cranial nerve palsy
Grade III	Drowsiness, confusion, or mild focal deficit
Grade IV	Stupor, moderate-to-severe hemiparesis; possibly, early decerebrate rigidity and vegetative disturbances
Grade V	Deep coma, decerebrate rigidity, moribund appearance

SOURCE: Hunt WE, Hess RM.[15]

tion of both circulating blood volume and mean arterial pressure are associated with about 10 percent incidence of postoperative morbidity related to vasospasm.[16–18] This represents a 50 percent reduction, approximately, from the vasospasm-related morbidity of previous decades.

Hypervolemic/hypertensive therapy is delivered by intravenous administration of saline solution and colloid (such as blood or plasma extract) to achieve pulmonary capillary wedge pressures in the range of 15 to 18 mmHg.[19] Cardiotonic and pressor agents that minimize arrythmia production are used. A useful combination is dopamine and phenylephrine. A practical goal is doubling of cardiac output while maintaining heart rate less than 100 beats per minute. When this type of therapy is applied, frequent reversal of severe neurologic deficits is noted. Reversal usually occurs in 1 to 6 h, but may occur slowly over 24 to 36 h. Support for as long as 10 to 14 days may be required in order to prevent relapse of neurologic dysfunction. Concurrent problems that can exacerbate cerebral ischemia due to vasospasm include volume depletion secondary to diabetes insipidus (rare) or cerebral salt wasting (common); blood loss secondary to phlebotomy; and reduced cerebral perfusion pressure secondary to obstructive hydrocephalus. Complications of hypervolemic/hypertensive therapy include angina pectoris and congestive heart failure. The latter seems to occur more frequently when this therapy is administered concurrently with calcium channel blockers; for this reason many practitioners advocate discontinuing calcium channel blockers, or decreasing the dose of the administered blocker, if hypertensive/hypervolemic therapy is to be rendered concurrently.

Obstructive hydrocephalus is the third process that must be prevented or managed to produce the optimal result for each subarachnoid hemorrhage victim.[20] Frequent use of neuroimaging tests, such as CT and MRI, is helpful to define the development of hydrocephalus. Massive intraventricular bleeding frequently leads to aqueductal obstruction and the hyperacute presentation of obstructive hydrocephalus as coma. In this situation, temporary relief of the obstruction by placing an external ventricular drain is the treatment of choice. Management of these drains requires extreme diligence if meningitis is to be avoided. In the patient with unclipped aneurysm, drain placement and/or subsequent overdrainage may be associated with aneurysmal rupture. For patients with mildly dilated ventricles due to communicating hydrocephalus, and little or no alteration of mental state, lumbar puncture may prove to be the best monitoring modality, since it can be performed intermittently and is only rarely associated with infection. For persons with surgically clipped aneurysms who have impaired mental state and clear elevation of intracranial pressure, continuous monitoring and drainage of either ventricular or lumbar CSF should be performed.

Fever is a nearly universal accompaniment of subarachnoid hemorrhage and is usually treated symptomatically with antipyretic and anti-inflammatory drugs. The value of these drugs has been difficult to define. Since fever elevates cerebral metabolism, the control of fever in patients with impaired cerebral perfusion may be important to minimize ischemic damage. The value of anti-inflammatory drugs in subarachnoid hemorrhage is currently under investigation. The new discipline of interventional neuroradiology has been involved in the treatment of aneurysmal subarachnoid hemorrhage. Catheter-directed obliteration of the aneurysm sac has been performed, but remains an experimental procedure of undefined risks and unknown value in these patients. Balloon angioplasty for vasospasm is also a new treatment modality that is not currently in common practice. Recent case reports strongly suggest that this approach will be of value in patients who do not respond to conventional therapy for vasospasm, particularly if applied prior to development of irreversible brain infarction.

CASE PRESENTATION

Patient X is a 55-year-old man who presented with a history of a nocturnal seizure and coma. The patient's illness began acutely on the evening of admission, when, while having sexual intercourse with his wife, he complained of severe headache. The complaint was immediately followed by jerking of his arms and legs, posturing in an extensor position. This lasted for 5 to 10 min and was followed by a more prolonged period of unresponsiveness. He was transported to the nearest hospital, where examination revealed an unresponsive man with bilateral extensor posturing to painful stimuli. The pupillary light reflexes, corneal reflexes, and vestibuloocular reflex were intact. A CT scan demonstrated a 5-mm layer of blood in the interhemispheric fissure and basal cisterns. Substantial quantities of dense blood were noted in both lateral ventricles, and significant ventricular dilatation was present. A working diagnosis of acute subarachnoid hemorrhage and obstructive hydrocephalus was made, and the patient was transferred to the neurocritical care area. Upon admission to the ICU the patient's condition was unchanged from that seen at presentation. A ventricular catheter was inserted and bloody CSF drained. Initial monitoring revealed an intracranial pressure of 30 mmHg. The patient's CSF was allowed to drain to a level of 15 mmHg. Gradually, over the next 4 h, intracranial pressure came under control and remained at 15 mmHg. The patient regained consciousness within 24 h of ventricular drainage and underwent selective cerebral angiography, which demonstrated an anterior communicating artery aneurysm.

On the second day post-hemorrhage, the patient was arousable and oriented to person, place, and time. However, he was unaware of the events leading to his hospitalization. On limited neurologic examination, 4+/5 strength was easily demonstrable in all limbs; no cranial nerve palsies were evident. The patient preferred to close his eyes, but he was easily arousable to verbal commands. Both the patient and his wife gave consent to surgical clipping, which was performed 3 days after his presentation. A secure clip placement was achieved without intraoperative rupture.

On the first postoperative day, the patient was arousable but more lethargic, requiring touch, and occasionally pain, to awaken. No cranial nerve deficits or motor impairment were noted. Intracranial pressure remained between 10 and 15 mmHg. However, 150 mL of bloody CSF drainage was required to control intracranial pressure.

On the second postoperative day (fifth day post-hemorrhage) the patient was easily arousable, followed all commands, and occasionally participated in activities of daily living. Gradual improvement was seen through the sixth postoperative day. That evening he became less alert, however, and one of three observers noted new onset of the right pronator drift. Over the night, intermittent periods of high urine output occurred, with urine specific gravities of 1.004. CT scan at this time demonstrated significant residual interhemispheric and basilar cistern blood. No infarction or lucency was noted in the hemispheres. Ventricular size was reduced as compared to that seen at admission. A subsequent angiogram showed significant narrowing of both anterior communicating arteries and the proximal portion of the left middle cerebral artery. A clinical diagnosis of vasospasm was made; the patient was treated with rapid volume expansion using 250 mL/h of normal saline solution and boluses of plasma extract to increase the pulmonary capillary wedge pressure to 15 mmHg. A single dose of 5 U of Pitressin (vasopressin) was administered subcutaneously, with rapid reduction in urine output and an increase in urine specific gravity to 1.012. Over the subsequent 12 h the patient became alert, with return of symmetric motor function to all extremities. No further episodes of diabetes insipidus occurred. Intravenous volume therapy was continued for 6 days at a rate of 8 L of normal saline solution per day. During this period, two attempts to decrease the total volume administered were associated with a decline in mean arterial pressure from 125 to 110 mmHg and a fall in pulmonary capillary wedge pressure from 15 to 8 mmHg. These circulatory changes were accompanied by increased somnolence and were reversed by boluses of plasma extract.

Ventricular drainage was discontinued on the tenth postoperative day. Follow-up CT demonstrated resolution of subarachnoid space blood and diminished ventricular size consistent with resolved obstructive hydrocephalus. On the thirteenth postoperative day the patient had a normal neurologic examination, without augmented circulatory support, at a mean arterial pressure of 105 mmHg and a pulmonary capillary wedge pressure of 5 mmHg. After 24 h of further neurologic and circulatory monitoring, the arterial line and Swan-Ganz catheters were removed. The patient made an uneventful recovery from his surgery and was able to return to work after 3 months of convalescence.

CASE DISCUSSION

A number of essential points regarding the diagnosis and management of cerebrovascular disease in the critically ill are demonstrated by this case. The sudden catastrophic neurologic event, with headache and seizures as early manifestations, strongly suggested subarachnoid hemorrhage (SAH), which was confirmed by CT imaging. It is important to note that CT or MRI scanning may miss SAH in 10 to 20 percent of cases, particularly if anatomic derangements are less dramatic than in this case.

The early CT scan also identified one of the complications of SAH—obstructive hydrocephalus, which was treated with a ventricular drain, with improvement. Early cerebral angiography, increasingly advocated to plan surgical approach, was performed, and identified a ruptured aneurysm—the cause of SAH in the vast majority of cases.

The patient underwent early surgical clipping of the aneurysm. The rationale for early surgical intervention is discussed in detail in this chapter. Intracranial pressure (ICP) was followed carefully in the postoperative period; drainage of CSF was necessary to maintain an appropriate ICP. The postoperative period was also complicated by transient diabetes insipidus, a not-unusual problem following neurosurgical intervention. Finally, meticulous neurologic examination postoperatively identified a new abnormality on the sixth and seventh post-operative days, which prompted a repeat CT scan. When further bleeding and ventricular obstruction were excluded, a repeat angiogram revealed arterial narrowing, suggesting post-hemorrhage/postoperative vasospasm. The patient was treated with volume expansion therapy. With the need to expand volume within the limits of cardiopulmonary reserve, and in the face of complicating diabetes insipidus, invasive hemodynamic monitoring and titration of fluids to an optimal pulmonary capillary wedge pressure were particularly helpful interventions.

References

1. Hachinski V, Norris JW: *The Acute Stroke.* Philadelphia, FA Davis, 1985.
2. Levine SR: Acute cerebral ischemia in a critical care unit. Arch Intern Med 149:90, 1989.
3. Powers WJ: Stroke, in Pearlman AL, Collins RC (eds): *Neurobiology of Disease.* New York, Oxford University Press, 1990, pp 339–355.
4. Grotta J: Current medical and surgical therapy for cerebrovascular disease. N Engl J Med 317:1505, 1987.
5. Biller J, Bruno A, Adams HP Jr, et al: A randomized trial of aspirin or heparin in hospitalized patients with recent transient ischemic attacks—a pilot study. Stroke 20:441, 1989.
6. Scheinberg P: Controversies in the management of cerebrovascular disease. Neurology 38:1609, 1988.
7. Duke RJ, Bloch RF, Turpie AGG, et al: Intravenous heparin for the prevention of stroke progression in acute partial stable stroke: A randomized controlled trial. Ann Intern Med 105:825, 1986.
8. Haley EC Jr, Kassell NF, Torner JC: Failure of heparin to prevent progression in progressing ischemic infarction. Stroke 19:10, 1988.
9. Jonas S: Anticoagulant therapy in cerebrovascular disease: Review and meta-analysis. Stroke 19:1043, 1988.
10. Cerebral Embolism Task Force: Cardiogenic brain embolism. Arch Neurol 46:727, 1989.

11. Weir B: *Aneurysms Affecting the Nervous System*. Baltimore, Williams and Wilkins, 1987.
12. Pickard JD, Murray GD, Illingworth R, et al: Effect of oral nimodipine on cerebral infarction and outcome after subarachnoid hemorrhage: British aneurysm nimodipine trial. Br Med J 298:636, 1989.
13. Philippon J, Grob R, Dagreou F, et al: Prevention of vasospasm in subarachnoid hemorrhage. A controlled study with nimodipine. Acta Neurochirurgica 82:110, 1986.
14. Petruk KC, West M, Mohr G, et al: Nimodipine treatment in poor grade aneurysm patients. J Neurosurg 68:505, 1988.
15. Hunt WE, Hess RM: Surgical risk as related to time of intervention in the repair of intracranial aneurysms. J Neurosurg 28:14, 1968.
16. Awad IA, Carter LP, Spetzler RF, et al: Clinical vasospasm after subarachnoid hemorrhage: Response to hypervolemic hemodilution and arterial hypertension. Stroke 18(2):365, 1987.
17. Kassell NF, Peerless SJ, Durward QJ, et al: Treatment of ischemic deficits from vasospasm with intravascular volume expansion and induced arterial hypertension. Neurosurgery 11(3):337, 1982.
18. Solomon RA, Fink ME, Lennihan L: Early aneurysm surgery and prophylactic hypervolemic hypertensive therapy for the treatment of aneurysmal subarachnoid hemorrhage. Neurosurgery 23(6):699, 1988.
19. Hanley DF, Borel C: Hypervolemic hypertensive therapy for subarachnoid hemorrhage–induced vasospasm, in Long DM (ed.): *Current Therapy in Neurologic Surgery*, vol 2. Philadelphia, BC Decker, 1989, pp 169–172.
20. Yasargil MG, Yonekawa Y, Zumstein B, Stahl HJ: Hydrocephalus following spontaneous subarachnoid hemorrhage. J Neurosurg 39:255, 1973.

Chapter 142

STATUS EPILEPTICUS AND SERIAL SEIZURES

ILO E. LEPPIK

KEY POINTS

- *Status epilepticus or serial seizures must be recognized and treated promptly.*
- *Acute confusional states or aphasia may be forms of nonconvulsive status epilepticus.*
- *Prompt and appropriate treatment prevents brain damage and death.*
- *Morbidity and mortality from properly treated status epilepticus arise from the underlying process which precipitated the seizures.*
- *Two groups of persons present as status: Group 1 patients have no acute central nervous system (CNS) disorder but have epilepsy which has gone out of control; group 2 patients have acute CNS disease, such as intracerebral hemorrhage, infection, or tumor.*
- *Group 1 patients respond quickly to therapy and have low mortality; group 2 patients may need more than one medicine and have a high mortality rate due to the underlying disorder.*
- *Diazepam has a short brain half-life, and by itself is insufficient treatment for status epilepticus.*
- *Time is of the essence. If a person continues to have seizures after loading doses of phenytoin and phenobarbital, pentobarbital coma should be used.*

Presentation and Diagnosis

Status epilepticus (SE) requires prompt recognition and treatment to prevent brain damage and death. The classical form of status epilepticus, "a condition characterized by an epileptic seizure which is so frequently repeated or so prolonged as to create a fixed and lasting condition," is at the extreme end of a spectrum of seizure frequencies. It has been estimated that 50,000 to 60,000 persons in the United States will have at least one episode of convulsive SE in a given year.[1] The reported causes of SE vary from study to study, reflecting referral practices of the institutions performing the investigations. It is useful to classify patients with SE into two groups based on the etiology of seizures and the prognosis. Group 1 includes patients with a history of epilepsy who have an acute exacerbation of seizures, usually because of withdrawal of antiepileptic medication.[2] In some areas, alcohol or drug abuse involving phencyclidine (PCP, "angel dust"), cocaine (crack), or other street drugs may be frequent causes of SE or serial seizures (SS). Hypoglycemia, hypocalcemia, and other metabolic conditions may present as SE or SS. Unusual causes include baclofen withdrawal or secondary hyperparathyroidism. Group 1 patients usually respond well to treatment with first-line drugs and often do not require intensive care after hospitalization. Group 2 consists of patients with an acute neurologic insult such as head injury, rapidly growing brain tumor, or anoxic encephalopathy, and they usually need intensive care.

Other than the cumulative changes caused by seizures in close succession, there is little to distinguish a generalized tonic-clonic (GTC) or partial seizure occurring as part of SE from a seizure observed as a single, isolated event. After one seizure is over and the patient is still postictal, it cannot be predicted if the patient will recover completely or have another seizure. One should be prepared to vigorously treat subsequent seizures, especially if the patient is not recovering consciousness within 15 min of the last convulsion. A large number of patients presenting to a critical care facility do not meet the formal definition of SE but present with SS. These should be treated as vigorously as SE.

Any type of epileptic seizure can develop into SE (Table 142-1). The syndrome usually associated with the term SE in adults is "convulsive" SE. This consists of seizures manifested by tonic and clonic motor activity lasting 1 to 2 min followed by a postictal state of lethargy, stupor, or coma for 15 to 30 min before the next seizure. This form is most often seen in adults. Seizures may be generalized at onset or may generalize from partial seizures (Table 142-1). In children, the convulsions often last longer or are continuous for 10 to 20 min.[3] Serial seizures consist of individual seizures with recovery between each seizure; our approach is to treat anyone who has had three or more convulsions in less than 24 h as vigorously as if they had classical SE.

Nonconvulsive SE consists of more subtle seizures (Table 142-1). The differential diagnosis of an acute confusional state should always include absence (petit mal) SE and complex partial SE. Frequent or continuous absence seizures are characterized by clouding of consciousness and a confusional state.[4] Rapid blinking of the eyes, unfocused

TABLE 142-1 Types of Seizures which Can Manifest as Status Epilepticus

Convulsive	Nonconvulsive
GENERALIZED SEIZURES	
Tonic-clonic (grand mal)	Absence (petit mal)
PARTIAL SEIZURES	
Partial seizures (simple or complex) generalizing to tonic-clonic seizures	Simple partial seizures (no change in consciousness) Somatomotor (Kojevnikov's) Aphasic Complex partial seizures (altered consciousness) Confusional state

gaze, and subtle myoclonic activity may be present. While most common in children and adolescents, absence SE has occasionally been reported in adults and has been mistaken for a psychiatric disorder.

Simple partial seizures are characterized by stereotypical motor behavior or sensory phenomena, with no alteration in consciousness or awareness. The most representative of this is repetitive clonic activity of the mouth and face or of the hand or fingers. Aphasic SE is characterized by loss of speech, which may last a few hours to several days in an otherwise alert patient. Although rare, this syndrome must be considered in patients presenting with dysphasia or aphasia who appear to have had a stroke but do not have structural damage to the CNS.[5] Complex partial SE may present with clinical behavior that cycles from a "twilight" state with partial responsiveness and semipurposeful automatisms to total unresponsiveness, speech arrest, and stereotypical automatisms.[6] If not recognized and left untreated, it may persist for days.

In addition to epileptic seizures there are many nonepileptic behaviors which may confound diagnosis and treatment. Some of these are physiologic phenomena such as decorticate posturing, spinal seizures, spasticity, or tetany. Intermittent decorticate posturing can sometimes mimic tonic-clonic activity in a person with altered consciousness, yet treatment with benzodiazepines or barbiturates may further depress the level of consciousness or respiration. Ocular findings such as pinpoint pupils, large unreactive pupils, or unilateral pupillary dilation may be useful clues, indicating intracranial pathology, because following seizures, pupillary function returns to normal. Some persons with psychiatric conditions may present with repetitive motor behavior suggesting tonic-clonic seizures. Out-of-phase limb movements (right arm flexed while left is extended during tonic-clonic activity) and pelvic thrusting may be present and are often characteristic of nonepileptic seizures.

Because epileptic seizures are paroxysmal behaviors associated with abnormal electric discharges within the brain, an electroencephalogram (EEG) is necessary for establishing the correct diagnosis. A person in a confusional state due to absence seizures will have a generalized epileptiform discharge on the EEG, often the classic three per second spike and wave pattern. A person with aphasic SE will have a focal epileptiform discharge in the dominant (usually) left temporal region, and a person with complex partial SE with automatisms will have a focal or widespread epileptiform discharge. The EEG pattern of nonepileptic behavior may be generalized slowing in a person with decerebrate posturing, or be normal (except for movement artifact) in persons with tetany or psychogenic seizures.

Morbidity and Mortality

Morbidity and mortality from SE are related to three factors: damage to the CNS caused by the acute insult which precipitated the seizures; systemic stress from repeated GTC convulsions; and injury from repetitive electric discharges within the CNS.

While it is difficult to obtain precise mortality figures for convulsive SE, rates as high as 50 percent were reported in literature prior to 1960.[1] More recent figures for acute mortality have been in the 8 to 12 percent range. Currently, with appropriate therapy, mortality is related to the etiology of the SE. In appropriately treated patients, death results from the condition which precipitates SE, rather than from the repeated seizures themselves. In one series, 10 percent of patients with acute onset of seizures or SE died within 1 month.[2] They were all group 2 patients, and death was attributable to the underlying illness. No deaths from seizures or their treatment occurred.

The systemic consequences of repeated GTC seizures affect the cardiovascular, respiratory, and renal systems. The cardiovascular system is particularly stressed because of the excessive demands placed upon it by repeated tonic contractions of the skeletal muscle system. Tachycardia is common; however, bradycardia may occur from vagal tone modulated by CNS activity. Cardiac arrhythmias may result from hyperkalemia. Drugs used to treat status may compound these problems, because barbiturates are myocardial depressants, and phenytoin (PHT) PHT and its solvent, propylene glycol, may cause arrhythmias and hypotension.

A single GTC seizure is usually followed by great respiratory effort stimulated by acidemia and hypercarbia, but following a series of seizures, respiratory failure may occur. Respiratory drive may also be depressed by the disorder precipitating SE, as well as the barbiturates and benzodiazepines used to treat the patient. Noncardiogenic edema occasionally complicates seizures and can lead to acute hypoxemic respiratory failure. Finally, aspiration of gastric contents is an ever-present risk in any obtunded patient. For these reasons, an early assessment of the need for airway protection and endotracheal intubation is indicated in patients with SE. Some will need mechanical ventilation as well.

Rhabdomyolysis leads to myoglobinuria and may rarely cause renal failure. Metabolic-biochemical complications include metabolic acidosis, hypoxemia, azotemia, hyperkalemia, hypoglycemia, and hyponatremia. Lactic acidosis is the rule in convulsive SE. Following the control of muscular activity, the acidosis should resolve promptly. The blood lactate concentration should fall by half, 1 h after seizures stop. Persistent acidosis despite control of seizures should raise the possibility of an additional, occult stimulus for lactate production such as sepsis or hypovolemic hypoperfusion. Massive activation of both sympathetic and parasympathetic systems leads to severe autonomic nervous system disturbances including hyperpyrexia, excessive sweating, and salivary and tracheobronchial hypersecretion. There are also endocrine abnormalities including marked elevations in plasma prolactin, glucagon, growth hormone, and corticotropin.[7] Pleocytosis may occur in the cerebrospinal fluid (CSF) but is typically of insufficient magnitude to be confused with bacterial meningitis.[8] In the setting of alcohol withdrawal seizures however, pleocytosis may be more marked and include significant numbers of neutrophils. In such a patient, it is most prudent to institute empiric antibiotics for meningitis, pending the results of microbiologic investigation.

Blocking the systemic manifestations of convulsive SE and correcting the metabolic effects of hypoxia and hypoglycemia is not sufficient to prevent CNS damage, because prolonged electrical activity in the brain can cause irreversible neuronal damage.[9] There appears to be a 30- to 60-min period during which these changes are still reversible, but after 60 min, neuronal death is evident.[9] Prolonged, if not permanent, deficits of memory have been reported after complex partial seizures, and widespread neuronal necrosis has been seen following epilepsia partialis continua.[5] The developing brain is particularly vulnerable to seizure activity. Permanent damage may occur in the neonatal rat brain under conditions which do not affect a mature brain.[10]

Management of Status Epilepticus in the Adult

The first few minutes should be spent in bedside assessment. This begins with a judgment regarding the need for endotracheal intubation (airway). Secondly, whether the patient is breathing spontaneously or being mechanically ventilated, the adequacy of ventilation and oxygenation is determined from arterial blood gases and the pattern of respiration (breathing). Then, clues to hypovolemia or the cardiovascular complications of SE should be sought and treated (circulation). The patient should be examined for clues which might indicate a cause for this particular episode of SE. Many persons with epilepsy have Med Alert bracelets. Evidence of a recent head injury may suggest the presence of an intracerebral hematoma. Historical details surrounding the onset of SE should be obtained. This can often be provided by paramedical personnel or friends or relatives accompanying the individual.

Any person with SE or SS should be admitted for observation and treatment of the precipitating condition and any complications. Even if seizures are quickly brought under control and the patient appears alert, after SE or SS, most persons experience disorientation, confusion, fatigue, and other symptoms. SE may be the initial manifestation of epilepsy[1] and an EEG and structural studies [magnetic resonance imaging (MRI) or computed tomography (CT)] should be obtained. These tests should be performed as an emergency procedure on any person who continues to have seizures after loading doses of the first drug have been administered. In most patients without a clear precipitant of SE, and in any patient who remains febrile after seizures have ceased, a lumbar puncture (after MRI or CT) should be obtained to exclude bacterial or viral meningitis or encephalitis. When the suspicion of meningitis is high, empiric antibiotics should be given until intracranial mass lesions can be excluded (see Chap. 103). Because CSF pleocytosis may be present after SS or SE, antibiotic treatment may not be necessary unless there are clinical signs of meningitis (nuchal rigidity) or evidence of bacterial infection, such as bacteria on stain or positive cultures. Intravenous fluids should be pushed to maintain adequate urine output, especially if testing indicates the presence of myoglobinuria.

In the treatment of SE, time is of the essence. Every facility should have a predetermined protocol which includes a time frame (Table 142-2). It is easy to be distracted by other needs, and often attention is directed away from a patient with SE after seizures seem to have been stopped. The most important task in treating SE or SS is to prevent additional seizures.

DRUG TREATMENT (See Fig. 142-1)

The ideal drug for the treatment of SE should enter the brain rapidly, have an immediate onset of anticonvulsant activity, should not significantly depress consciousness or respiratory function, should have a long half-life so that the therapeutic concentrations are maintained for hours, and should effectively block both the somatic manifestations of seizures and the neuronal discharges. Recent studies of drug distribution to the brain have altered prior recommendations. Diazepam given by itself is no longer the treatment of choice because the recurrence of seizures with diazepam alone is greater than if a longer-acting drug is used.[2] In general, loading doses of long-acting antiepileptic medication should be started as soon as intravenous access is available; short-acting agents should be used only when needed to stop an active seizure.

TABLE 142-2 Treatment Protocol with Time Frame of Intervention

Time Frame, min	Treatment Protocol
0–5	Assess cardiorespiratory function, obtain history, and perform neurologic and physical examination. Take blood for antiepileptic drug levels, glucose, blood urea nitrogen, electrolytes, metabolic screen, and drug screen. Insert oral airway and administer oxygen only if needed.
6–9	Start intravenous infusion with saline solution. Administer 25 g of glucose and thiamine.
10–30	Begin infusion of PHT, 20 mg/kg, at a rate no faster than 50 mg/min. This may take 20–40 min. Monitor ECG and blood pressure. Lorazepam, 4 or 8 mg, or diazepam, 10 to 20 mg, may be given if convulsions occur while PHT is being infused.
31–60	If seizures persist, give phenobarbital, 10 mg/kg given at 100 mg/min intravenously.
60	If seizures persist, barbiturate coma or general anesthesia with agents with which the facility is familiar should be started.

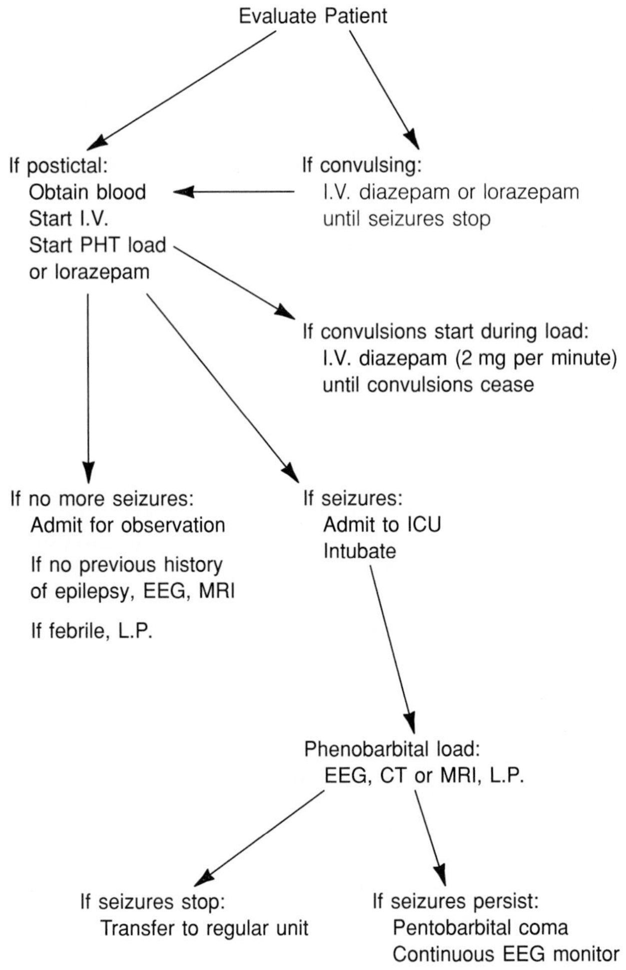

FIGURE 142-1 Diagnostic and treatment flow chart for status epilepticus.

Because of the need to obtain reliable and rapid blood concentrations of drugs, the intravenous route must be used except in unusual circumstances, such as inability to establish intravenous access quickly in infants. Under these conditions, rectal or intramuscular diazepam may be the only option.

PHENYTOIN

The main advantages of PHT are its effectiveness in controlling convulsions, relatively long half-life, and lack of significant CNS depression. Disadvantages are its cardiovascular toxicity if given too rapidly, the time required for giving the full loading dose, and its relative ineffectiveness in suppressing focal epileptic activity. PHT is effective in suppressing experimental seizures as soon as adequate brain concentrations are attained, which, in rats, requires only a few minutes.[11] The currently available parenteral form of PHT was developed in the 1950s for intramuscular use and contains propylene glycol and ethanol. Propylene glycol itself is cardiotoxic. The parenteral PHT preparation may be diluted to 5 mg/mL or less in normal saline solution.[12] This permits steady administration by infusion equipment. Injection of undiluted PHT by hand can be dangerous because of erratic administration, resulting in transiently high concentrations which may cause hypotension or cardiac arrhythmias. Blood pressure and electrocardiogram (ECG) should be monitored during PHT infusion. If seizures do not respond to PHT infusion, there is a very high probability that a significant acute CNS insult has occurred. Following intravenous PHT, with or without diazepam, 89 of 99 (90 percent) group 1 patients in one series had their seizures controlled. The remaining 10 patients had only isolated seizures. In contrast, 21 of 37 (57 percent) group 2 patients remained in SE or had additional seizures.[2] Many persons in group 1 are recovering consciousness during PHT administration, while group 2 patients remain comatose or stuporous. PHT infusion may thus aid in diagnosis, while using a CNS depressant such as phenobarbital or one of the benzodiazepines may make it difficult to assess the level of consciousness. The target PHT concentration is 25 to 30 μg/mL.

The volume of distribution of PHT in adults is approximately 0.75 L/kg.[2] This means that a loading dose of 20 mg/kg will result in concentrations of approximately 26 μg/mL at the end of infusion if the level was zero prior to the load. Doses less than 18 or 20 mg/kg are not sufficient to attain these high levels. The half-life of PHT after doses of 20 mg/kg is in excess of 36 h. Thus, after one PHT load, levels will be high for 24 h. If seizures continue after a loading dose of PHT, other agents should be used because administration of more PHT will result in levels above 30 μg/mL. High PHT levels are associated with severe ataxia and slurring of speech and may paradoxically precipitate more seizures. A phenytoin prodrug has been recently tested in volunteers. This preparation has the advantages of being water soluble, causing less venous sclerosis than the current PHT preparation, and being rapidly converted to PHT in humans.[13]

BENZODIAZEPINES

Diazepam (Valium) became popular in the mid-1960s following a few case reports of its success in treating SE. Its advantage is rapid onset of activity due to quick distribution to the brain. Disadvantages are its tendency to depress respiration and consciousness, and its short CNS half-life, limiting its effectiveness to less than $\frac{1}{2}$ h.[14] Diazepam should be used in conjunction with, or be followed by, PHT loading. In adults, doses of 5 to 10 mg may be needed. Use of larger doses may lead to respiratory and CNS depression. Although concentrations of 0.2 to 0.8 μg/mL have been suggested, specific target levels have not been established. Rather, the drug should be given until seizures stop. Use of a diazepam drip for the treatment of SE was recommended a few years ago. It has fallen out of favor because of the pharmacokinetics of diazepam. Although it attains high brain levels quickly, it is rapidly redistributed to bulk storage sites such as adipose tissue, which comprise a much larger fraction of body mass. Diazepam has a long elimination half-life of 20 to 30 h. Thus, if a diazepam drip of 10 to 15 mg/h is used for 12 to 24 h, body stores of 120 to 360 mg may accumulate and lead to persistent sedation.

Lorazepam has recently been advocated for the treatment of SE because of its longer CNS action. In the first large, double-blind, randomized study of benzodiazepines in SE, 4 mg lorazepam was compared with 10 mg diazepam and found to be equivalent in terms of effectiveness and number of side effects.[15] A study comparing PHT with lorazepam is in progress, and its results should permit assessment of the future role of lorazepam in SE.[16] Target concentrations for it have not yet been established, although 0.2 to 0.4 μg/mL may be considered adequate. Clonazepam has been used successfully in Europe, but a parenteral form is not available in the United States.

BARBITURATES
Phenobarbital (PB) has the advantage of having a very long half-life, can be administered more rapidly than PHT, and is effective in generalized and partial seizures. Disadvantages are depression of consciousness and respiration. The depression of respiration may be more profound in a patient initially treated with diazepam. Its volume of distribution is approximately 1 L/kg, meaning that 1 mg/kg should give approximately 1 μg/mL serum level of concentration. A dose of 10 mg/kg is often used and can be followed by an additional 10 mg/kg if needed. These will give levels of 10 to 20 μg/mL, the target levels for patients with SE. Higher levels are often encountered in persons being treated chronically with barbiturates for epilepsy, because they have developed tolerance. Acute levels of 20 μg/mL are quite sedating.

PARALDEHYDE
Paraldehyde has been used intermittently for treatment of SE but has not been well studied. It has been given intramuscularly, rectally, or intravenously.[17] Unfortunately, supplies of parenteral paraldehyde are becoming limited in the United States because of manufacturers' concern of cost of litigation.

OTHER DRUGS
Lidocaine, as a 50 to 100 mg push intravenously, followed by a 1 to 2 mg/min infusion has been used for SE, but because of the propensity for high doses to cause seizures, and its variable brain distribution during SE, its use must be discouraged.[18]

Valproic acid (VPA) has been given rectally for the treatment of SE. A major disadvantage is its relative slowness in absorption compared to drugs that are given intravenously. An intravenous VPA preparation may soon become available; its effectiveness in SE will need to be assessed and target levels need to be established.

Carbamazepine (CBZ) is not available in a parenteral form. Rectally administered CBZ suspension takes too long to reach peak concentration to be of value in treating SE.

PENTOBARBITAL COMA PROTOCOL
Pentobarbital coma has been successfully utilized in SE refractory to diazepam, PHT, and other drugs.[19] Its use should be carefully monitored by EEG recording. Doses should be tailored to maintain a flat or burst suppression pattern on the EEG. A loading dose of 6 to 8 mg/kg or more given over 1 h while monitoring the EEG is usually effective, followed by maintenance doses of 1 to 2 mg/(kg · h). Pentobarbital coma may be required for many days. Once coma with pentobarbital has been initiated, the EEG should be monitored often. If possible, an EEG machine with four or more channels should be available at the bedside. Scalp electrodes should be placed according to the International 10-20 system, and at least two channels of bipolar recording obtained from each hemisphere. The EEG can be recorded for 2 to 4 min every few hours to ascertain that flat or burst suppression conditions are established. An attempt to lighten coma can be made on a daily basis by decreasing the pentobarbital administration rate while observing the EEG. If epileptiform activity reappears, the rate can be increased. Pentobarbital must be tapered; rapid discontinuation may result in exacerbation of seizures. When only a small amount of pentobarbital is needed, lorazepam in 2 to 4 mg boluses every 6 to 8 h may be substituted.

In the past, general anesthesia was used instead of pentobarbital coma, and some centers unfamiliar with the procedure may still use inhalation therapy. However, prolonged use of inhalation anesthesia may lead to pulmonary complications, and it has not been as effective in our experience.

OTHER CONSIDERATIONS

In some situations, the underlying cause of SE may have implications for management. For example, in a patient with seizures due to tricyclic antidepressant overdose, hypotension may be a cardinal feature. In these instances, use of PHT needs to be monitored closely, since it may worsen hypotension. Further, since barbiturates may depress myocardial contractility, use of this drug may be associated with worsened hypotension.

Status Epilepticus in the Pediatric Population

Diagnosis of seizures in the neonate may be difficult because signs are subtle. These may include sucking, random eye movements, stretching, yawning, bicycling, and apnea. These seizures are unlike the events seen in older persons because of the lack of myelin and dendritic connections. Nevertheless, these seizures are often associated with serious CNS disturbances. A standard loading dose of 20 to 25 mg/kg of phenobarbital has been found to be effective and necessary to attain sufficient concentrations.[20] If ineffective, it may be followed by a PHT dose of 20 mg/kg. Diazepam, 0.3 to 0.5 mg/kg, or lorazepam, 0.1 mg/kg, intravenously are often effective. Paraldehyde, 0.3 to 0.4 mg/kg per rectum, may be used if this drug is available.

CASE PRESENTATION
A 23-year-old woman who had just graduated from college developed fever and headache during the third week of July. She did not seek medical attention at the

onset, but her headache became increasingly severe. An examination by her family physician was unremarkable. One day after the examination, she became lethargic and had a generalized tonic-clonic seizure. She was taken to the emergency room, where she was noted to be lethargic but with no focal neurologic deficits. She was admitted for evaluation and had her second tonic-clonic seizure approximately 4 h after her first. Diazepam, 5 mg, was given intravenously after the second seizure, and she became more lethargic. A third seizure occurred about 1 h after the second. A neurologist was consulted, and loading with phenytoin, 20 mg/kg at 50 mg/min, was started. A CT scan, performed for persistent lethargy, revealed no abnormality. Results of a lumbar puncture were compatible with viral encephalitis (total white blood cell count of 364, 90 percent lymphocytes). After her fourth generalized tonic-clonic seizure, she was intubated and a loading dose of phenobarbital 20 mg/kg was given.

An EEG showed almost constant spike and wave discharges, so pentobarbital coma with a load of 20 mg/kg followed by 3 mg/(kg · h) was given to induce burst suppression pattern on the EEG. She was given daily maintenance dosages of phenytoin and phenobarbital. For 2 weeks, every attempt at discontinuing pentobarbital coma was unsuccessful as determined by reappearance of spike-wave discharges on the EEG.

Eventually, the epileptogenic activity abated, pentobarbital coma was discontinued, and intermittent injections of 4 to 6 mg of lorazepam were successful. She slowly became more responsive, and 2 weeks after pentobarbital coma, she was discharged. Although there was some initial improvement during the first 6 months after discharge, she has moderate impairment of intellectual functioning and a seizure disorder, controlled by phenytoin and carbamazepine.

CASE DISCUSSION

Diazepam is often used as the initial drug after a first or second seizure. However, its effectiveness is short, and it may not prevent further seizures. After controlling the initial seizures, longer-acting antiepileptic medications such as PHT must be administered. If PHT fails to control seizures, the probability of a serious acute CNS lesion is high. Intubation must be initiated because the next line of drugs (phenobarbital, pentobarbital) severely depresses respiration. Morbidity and mortality of persons whose seizures are not controlled by PHT is high because of the nature of the CNS insult. An MRI or CT scan must be done immediately to determine the cause of SS or SE refractory to PHT. Likely causes include brain tumor, subarachnoid hemorrhage, stroke, meningitis, encephalitis, anoxic brain injury, and abscess. If structural studies are negative, a lumbar puncture must be performed to rule out meningitis.

Discontinuation of pentobarbital coma was tried on a daily basis by decreasing the rate of infusion while the EEG was monitored, but each attempt to reduce the rate below 2 mg/(kg · h) was accompanied by recurrence of epileptiform activity. Finally, the rate was decreased to 2 mg/(kg · h) and eventually to 1 mg/(kg · h) with control of epileptiform activity. At this point, maintenance of burst suppression was no longer necessary and some background activity could be seen on the EEG. When epileptiform activity of less than one burst per 10 min could be attained with 1 mg/(kg · h) of pentobarbital, lorazepam was substituted. Prolonged pentobarbital coma may be associated with hepatic failure, so pentobarbital coma must be tapered or discontinued if the liver enzyme concentrations become twice normal or greater.

References

1. Hauser A: Status epilepticus: epidemiologic considerations. Neurology 40:9, 1990.
2. Cranford RE, Leppik IE, Patrick B, et al.: Intravenous phenytoin in acute treatment of seizures. Neurology 29:1476, 1979.
3. Acardi J, Chevrie JJ: Convulsive status epilepticus in infants and children: a study of 239 cases. Epilepsia 11:187, 1970.
4. Porter RJ, Penry JK: Petit mal status. Adv Neurol 34:61, 1983.
5. Hamilton N, Matthews T: Aphasia, the sole manifestation of status epilepticus. Neurology 29:745, 1979.
6. Treiman DM, Delgado-Escueta AV: Complex partial status epilepticus. Adv Neurol 34:69, 1983.
7. Meldrum BS, Horton RW, Bloom RS, et al.: Endocrine factors and glucose metabolism during prolonged seizures in baboon. Epilepsia 20:527, 1979.
8. Schmidley JW, Simon RP: Postictal pleocytosis. Ann Neurol 9:81, 1981.
9. Meldrum B: Physiological changes during prolonged seizures and epileptic brain damage. Neuropadiatrie 9:203, 1978.
10. Wasterlain CG, Duffy TE: Status epilepticus in immature rats. Arch Neurol 33:821, 1976.
11. Leppik IE, Sherwin AL: Intravenous phenytoin and phenobarbital anticonvulsant action, brain content and plasma binding in rats. Epilepsia 20:201, 1979.
12. Cloyd JC, Bosch DE, Sawchuk RJ: Concentration-time profile of phenytoin after admixture with small volumes of intravenous fluids. Am J Hosp Pharm 34:313, 1978.
13. Leppik IE, Boucher BA, Wilder BJ, et al.: Pharmacokinetics and safety of a phenytoin prodrug given IV or IM in patients. Neurology 40:456, 1990.
14. Celesia GG, Booker HE, Sato S: Brain and serum concentrations of diazepam in experimental epilepsy. Epilepsia 15:417, 1974.
15. Leppik IE, Derivan AT, Homan RW, et al.: Double-blind study of lorazepam and diazepam in status epilepticus. JAMA 249:1452, 1983.
16. Treiman DM, DeGiorgio CM, Ben-Menachem E, et al.: Lorazepam versus phenytoin in the treatment of generalized convulsive status epilepticus: report of an ongoing study. Neurology 35(suppl 1):284, 1985.
17. Curless RG, Holzman BH, Ramsay RE: Paraldehyde therapy in childhood status epilepticus. Arch Neurol 40:477, 1983.
18. Simon RP, Benowitz NL, Culala S: Motor paralysis increases brain uptake of lidocaine during status epilepticus. Neurology 34:384, 1984.
19. Van Ness PC: Pentobarbital and EEG burst suppression in treatment of status epilepticus refractory to benzodiazepines and phenytoin. Epilepsia 31:61, 1990.
20. Lockman LA: Phenobarbital dosage for neonatal seizures. Adv Neurol 34:505, 1983.

Chapter 143

NEUROMUSCULAR DISEASES LEADING TO RESPIRATORY FAILURE

JOHN M. LUCE

KEY POINTS

- *Neuromuscular diseases may cause respiratory muscle weakness that leads to hypercapneic respiratory failure.*
- *The severity of respiratory failure is too often quantitated late by systemic arterial blood gas analysis; respiratory failure should be anticipated, and should be prevented by elective intubation indicated by declining respiratory muscle strength.*
- *The severity of respiratory muscle weakness may be quantitated by measure of maximum inspiratory and expiratory pressures at the mouth, vital capacity on spirometry, or transdiaphragmatic pressure.*
- *Specific diagnosis of the neuromuscular disease is facilitated by understanding of the forms of neuromuscular dysfunction variously involving upper motor neurons, lower motor neurons, peripheral nerves, the myoneural junction, and the muscles themselves.*
- *Treatment usually involves the administration of agents for specific neuromuscular diseases and precipitating factors; supplemental oxygen; mechanical ventilation; nursing care; and emotional support.*

A wide variety of neuromuscular diseases cause weakness or paralysis that may involve the respiratory muscles and lead to hypercapneic respiratory failure. This chapter focuses on how such failure comes about and what specific disorders may be responsible for it. The chapter begins with a review of normal neuromuscular function, neuromuscular dysfunction in specific diseases associated with respiratory failure, and the general management of patients with such disorders who receive intensive care. The chapter concludes with an illustrative case presentation.

Normal Neuromuscular Function

Normal neuromuscular function requires the integrated activity of several components. The first of these components is the upper motor neuron, which conveys impulses from the motor area of the cerebrum to lower motor neurons in the brain stem and spinal cord by way of the corticobulbar and corticospinal tracts. The lower motor neuron consists of a cell body in the anterior gray substance of the spinal cord or brain stem and its axon, which passes through the nerve root and peripheral nerve to the myoneural junction. These junctions are made up of the terminal membranes of the lower motor neurons, the postjunctional membranes of muscles, and the subneural cleft between them. The nerve axons synthesize acetylcholine (ACh) from acetic acid and choline and store it within vesicles in the distal axon. When the neurons are stimulated, they release ACh into the cleft. Receptors on the postjunctional membrane, which is also called the motor end-plate, accept ACh and open channels for the passage of calcium and sodium ions, which depolarize the muscle. Depolarization, in turn, triggers contraction of muscle myofibrils. The ACh is then broken down into acetic acid and choline by an enzyme, anticholinesterase, in the subneural cleft. These products are then taken up by the axons for resynthesis of ACh; the postjunctional membrane becomes repolarized, owing to ion flux; and the muscle returns to its former condition.[1]

The muscles of respiration comprise three groups: the diaphragm, the intercostal and accessory muscles, and the muscles of the abdomen.[2] The diaphragm is innervated by the lower motor neurons of the phrenic nerve, which originate at the C3–C5 spinal cord level. It is inserted in the lateral ribs; its fibers are normally directed upward, parallel to the rib cage. When the diaphragm contracts during a vital capacity (VC) maneuver, it pushes down on the abdominal viscera, displaces the abdominal wall outward, and increases abdominal pressure (Pab). At the same time, the diaphragm lifts the rib cage upward, causing an outward displacement because of its rib articulation, and generates a negative pleural pressure (Ppl) that inflates the lungs. The amount of respiratory work performed by the diaphragm and the normally lesser contribution of other inspiratory muscles during inspiration are reflected in the pressure gradient across the diaphragm, Pdi, which is the difference between Pab and Ppl. These values can be obtained by simultaneously recording pressure in gastric and esophageal balloons. The maximum inspiratory pressure (PI_{max}), measured at the mouth after exhaling completely to residual volume (RV) and then inspiring forcefully, reflects the power of the diaphragm and other inspiratory muscles.[3]

The intercostal muscles include the internal and external intercostals, whose fibers run in an anterior-posterior direction. The intercostals are innervated by lower motor neurons from the T1–T12 levels. Accessory muscles include the scalenes (innvervated by C4–C8), the sternocleidomastoids (cranial nerve XI, C2–C3) and the trapezoids (XI, C2–C4). The external intercostals, the parasternal internal intercostals, and the accessory muscles serve primarily an inspiratory function and are responsible for increasing the anterior-posterior diameter of the thorax. The scalenes, sternocleidomastoids, and trapezoids are recruited at high levels of inspiratory activity, at which point other back muscles that support the thorax also become involved. The lateral internal intercostals are used to exhale forcefully.

The abdominal respiratory muscles include the rectus and transverse abdominis and the external and internal obliques. These muscles are innervated at the T7–L1 levels. They are generally regarded as expiratory muscles, al-

TABLE 143-1 Disorders of Neuromuscular Function

Level	Examples	Clinical Characteristics	Cerebrospinal Fluid	Nerve Conduction	Electromyography
Upper motor neurons	Hemiplegia Quadriplegia	Weakness Spasticity Hyperreflexia Many have sensory and autonomic changes	Normal	Normal	Normal
Lower motor neurons	Paralytic poliomyelitis Amyotrophic lateral sclerosis	Weakness Atrophy Flaccidity Hyporeflexia Fasciculations Bulbar involvement No sensory changes	Little or no inflammation	Normal	Denervation potentials
Peripheral neurons	Guillain Barré syndrome Diphtheria	Weakness Flaccidity Hyporeflexia Bulbar involvement Sensory and autonomic changes	Increased protein	Reduced	Denervation potentials late in course
Myoneural junction	Myasthenia gravis Botulism Eaton-Lambert syndrome Organophosphate poisoning Tick paralysis	Fluctuating weakness Fatigability Normal reflexes Bulbar involvement (esp. eyes) No sensory changes May have autonomic changes May respond to cholinergic agents	Normal	Normal	Changes in muscle action potential during repetitive stimulation
Muscles	Muscular dystrophies Polymyositis Trichinosis Endocrinologic disease	Weakness Normal reflexes No sensory or autonomic changes May have pain	Normal	Normal	Small motor units

though they enhance the mechanical advantage of the diaphragm. The abdominal muscles are not used during quiet exhalation to functional residual capacity (FRC), which is accomplished through passive recoil of the lungs. However, they are called upon during forceful exhalation that allows lung deflation to RV. The maximum expiratory pressure (PE_{max}), measured at the mouth after a complete inspiration to total lung capacity (TLC) and then a forceful exhalation, reflects the power of the abdominal muscles and other expiratory muscles.

In addition to these acknowledged respiratory muscles, several other muscles also play vital roles in the breathing process. These include the muscles of the mouth (innervated by cranial nerve X), uvula and palate (cranial nerve XI), tongue (cranial nerves IX and XII), and larynx (C1). All these muscles are essential in keeping the upper airway open; they also subserve swallowing and speech.

Neuromuscular Dysfunction

DISORDERS OF UPPER MOTOR NEURONS

Neuromuscular dysfunction can involve any or all of the components of normal neuromuscular function described above (Table 143-1). Damage to the upper motor neurons extending from the motor cortex to synapse with lower motor neurons in the brain stem or spinal cord characteristically causes unilateral weakness. Lesions above the corticospinal tract decussation in the medulla produce contralateral weakness or paralysis, whereas those below the medulla produce ipsilateral weakness below the level of involvement if only one side of the spinal cord is damaged; most spinal cord lesions cause bilateral weakness, because of the close proximity of the tracts. Accompanying the weakness of upper motor neuron disease may be an increase in muscle tone, called *spasticity;* an increase in reflex activity; and the presence of the extensor plantar response (Babinski sign). Upper motor neuron lesions may also be accompanied by sensory and autonomic changes, depending on the level of involvement. Peripheral nerve conduction is normal in patients with upper motor neuron lesions, and muscle denervation potentials are not seen in the electromyogram (EMG).

As might be anticipated from the foregoing, cerebral infarction involving the motor cortex causes weakness of the contralateral upper and lower extremities that is known clinically as *hemiplegia.* Such hemiplegia is associated with sensory changes if the infarction involves the neighboring sensory cortex. Physical examination has suggested that hemiplegic patients exhibit decreased chest wall motion on the side of their extremity weakness. Their chest radiographs may also show elevation of the hemidiaphragm on the affected side. This is in keeping with reduced activity during voluntary inspirations in both the parasternal intercostal muscles and the hemidiaphragm on EMG.[4] In some cases the reduction of hemidiaphragmatic activity may be sufficient to limit regional lung ventilation and cause hypoxemia, especially when the patient lies in a lateral position.[5] However, hemiplegia is likely to compromise overall ventilation only when it coexists with other cardiopulmonary diseases.[6]

Quadriplegia resulting from acute cervical spinal cord trauma, spinal artery infarction, or cord compression by tumor is a much more serious process. Servere damage at or above cord segments C3 to C5 involves the phrenic nerves and causes partial or complete bilateral hemidiaphragmatic paralysis. Because the hemidiaphragms cannot contract effectively, the lower rib cage does not expand laterally during inspiration. In addition, intercostal muscle paralysis caudad to the lesion limits lateral extension of the middle and upper rib cage. Sternocleidomastoid, scalene, and trapezoid activity persists in high spinal cord injuries, but contraction of these muscles causes an increase primarily in the anterior-posterior dimensions of the upper rib cage and pulls the hemidiaphragms toward the head. Abdominal paradox, in which the abdominal wall is sucked in by the negative Pab as the hemidiaphragms ascend, is a sign of hemidiaphragmatic dysfunction in patients who inspire only with their accessory muscles.[7]

As a result of their profound respiratory muscle dysfunction, high-cervical quadriplegics are unable to generate an adequate VC during inspiration; therefore they manifest a high Pa_{CO_2} and a low Pa_{O_2}. The hypoxemia of these patients results both from hypoventilation and from microatelectasis; the latter occurs because of retained secretions, and because the inward recoil of the lungs is no longer affected by the outward recoil of the chest wall.[8] Hypercapnea and hypoxemia frequently worsen when the patient breathes spontaneously in the supine position and the abdominal contents force the hemidiaphragms cephalad. Alveolar hypoventilation is even more pronounced during sleep, a phenomenon that has been ascribed to diminished CO_2 responsiveness but more likely results from inhibition of intercostal and accessory muscle activity.

Quadriplegic patients with lesions in the lower cervical spinal cord, whose phrenic nerve nuclei are completely or partially intact, can contract their hemidiaphragms to a greater or lesser extent. Nevertheless, they lack the intercostal muscle activity necessary to stabilize the rib cage so that the hemidiaphragms can function properly. Hemidiaphragmatic contraction therefore results in paradoxical inward motion of the upper and middle rib cage during inspiration, until the chest wall stiffens due to spasticity or fibrosis of muscles—as it eventually does in most patients with chronic neuromuscular disease.[9] Furthermore, because these patients lack abdominal muscle tone, their hemidiaphragms cannot contract from the steeply domed position in which their fiber length-tension relationship is optimized. Thus, their VC and TLC are diminished. This diminution is most pronounced when such a patient sits up and the hemidiaphragms are not supported by the abdominal contents; it is minimized when the patient is supine.

The other major problem in patients with cervical spinal cord lesions at any level is that they cannot exhale forcefully to RV. This is primarily because they have lost the use of their abdominal and other expiratory muscles. At the same time, they cannot inhale to TLC, because of inspiratory muscle dysfunction. The combination of expiratory and inspiratory weakness prevents them from coughing and clearing secretions. Recent studies have demonstrated that some quadriplegics use the clavicular portion of their pectoralis major muscles to reduce RV toward normal, and have suggested that the patients might cough more effectively by training these muscles.[10] Nevertheless, many patients do not use their muscles in this fashion and therefore are at high risk for respiratory tract infections, including pneumonia.

DISORDERS OF LOWER MOTOR NEURONS

Lower motor neuron dysfunction is characterized by weakness, loss of deep tendon reflexes, and denervation atrophy of muscles whose motor neurons are destroyed. Diseases of the anterior horn cells also cause fasciculations, in which irritability of the motor neurons leads to sporadic discharges of the muscle fibers under their control. Sensory involvement does not occur, and the motor damage tends to be diffuse. In contrast, motor nerve root lesions that result, say, from herniated discs cause a myotomic distribution of weakness; because these lesions are not selective for anterior roots, they usually are accompanied by pain and sensory loss. Denervation potentials, including fasciculations and fibrillations, are seen in the EMGs of patients with lower motor neuron disorders. Nerve conduction velocities are normal, however, until the axonal loss is severe.

Paralytic poliomyelitis was once the most widespread lower motor neuron disease in the developed world; it remains a common disorder in underdeveloped nations where preventive vaccines are scarce. Poliomyelitis is an acute febrile illness that may produce signs of meningeal irritation and flaccid paralysis. The term *poliomyelitis* refers to inflammation of the gray matter of the spinal cord. The disease is caused by a ribonucleic acid virus that spreads from person to person via fecal-oral transmission and infects motor neurons in the spinal cord and brain stem. Paralysis, if it occurs, may develop within hours of acute infection, or may take an indolent course. Muscle weakness usually is asymmetric, may be widely distributed, and tends to involve the lower extremities and lower trunk.

Patients with paralytic poliomyelitis that is confined to the lower cervical spinal cord may exhibit the same respiratory muscle dysfunction as do patients with low cervical cord trauma, in that their diaphragmatic function remains intact. On the other hand, patients with upper cord and brain stem lesions usually lose diaphragmatic function. Bulbar poliomyelitis also may cause paralysis of the muscles involved in swallowing and speech, although the ocular motor nerves usually are spared. Weakness of the laryngeal muscles may precipitate upper airway obstruction, and aspiration may occur if the gag reflex is lost. In addition, patients may exhibit wide swings in blood pressure, pulse, and respiratory rate because of damage to the cardiovascular and respiratory control centers in the brain stem.

The diagnosis of paralytic poliomyelitis is based on clinical presentation, cerebrospinal fluid (CSF) findings of mild pleocytosis and minimal protein elevation, and the demonstration of denervation potentials on EMG. Therapy is supportive during the acute illness and, when necessary, thereafter. The prognosis for overall survival has exceeded 90 percent, except in older patients and those with the bulbar form of the disease. Most patients also recover some, if not all, motor function, although recovery is unlikely in areas of total paralysis. In some patients the reinnervation of denervated muscle may be followed, years later, by a syndrome of denervation, nerve weakness, and atrophy that is called *postpoliomyelitis motor neuron disease.*[11]

Amyotrophic lateral sclerosis (ALS) has succeeded paralytic poliomyelitis as the most common lower motor neuron disorder in advanced countries, although it is still uncommon. The disease usually occurs sporadically among older adults, but familial and Western Pacific forms are also known. ALS is classified as a disorder of lower motor neurons because it damages the anterior horn cells of the spinal cord and brain stem. Nevertheless, the disease also may affect upper motor neurons. Despite extensive investigations, the etiology of ALS is unknown.[12]

The clinical course of ALS varies; patients most often present with progressive muscle weakness and wasting that often involves the distal muscles initially. Although the extraocular muscles are spared in ALS, bulbar involvement may lead to impairment of the gag reflex; lingual atrophy and fasciculations; and laryngeal dysfuncation. Signs of upper motor neuron involvement, such as spasticity and hyperreflexia, may occur at any time, but generally exist if lower motor neuron damage has been present for over 1 year. The coexistence of upper and lower motor signs should strongly suggest the diagnosis. Electromyography will reveal changes of muscle denervation with normal motor nerve velocities until the axonal dropout is sufficiently severe to cause mild slowing. The CSF is normal in patients with ALS.

Specific therapy is not available for ALS, and the prognosis is generally poor. Indeed, more than 50 percent of patients die from complications such as aspiration and pneumonia within 3 years of diagnosis. Serial pulmonary function testing in such patients reveals a progressive decrease in VC and an increase in RV. These changes reflect widespread weakness of inspiratory and expiratory muscles, associated with severe hypercapnia and hypoxemia that can be corrected only by mechanical ventilatory support. Nevertheless, some patients with ALS stabilize after years of illness; hence prognosis must be individualized.[13]

DISORDERS OF PERIPHERAL NERVES

Damage to the peripheral nervous system results in a variable combination of muscle weakness, sensory change, autonomic dysfunction, and reflex loss. Such damage may involve either single nerves (mononeuropathy), multiple nerves (mononeuropathy multiplex), or a diffuse pattern (polyneuropathy), and may occur within the nerve plexus, trunks, or branches. Because the longest nerves are particularly vulnerable, the weakness associated with polyneuropathy tends to be greatest distally in the hands and feet and to ascend proximally as nerve damage progresses. The EMG characteristically shows slowing of the transmission of impulses and denervation if the axons are involved.

The polyneuropathy most often encountered in critical care practice, *acute postinfectious polyneuropathy,* is better known as the *Guillain-Barré syndrome.* It is characterized by a widespread, patchy, inflammatory demyelination of the peripheral and autonomic nervous systems that is thought to result from a hypersensitivity reaction. There is virtually no inflammation in the central nervous system. Many patients with Guillain-Barré syndrome recall on antecedent upper respiratory infection or gastrointestinal illness within 1 month of onset. Other purported predisposing factors include surgery, pregnancy, malignancy, and acute seroconversion to the human immunodeficiency virus.[14]

Guillain-Barré syndrome is a worldwide illness that occurs at all times of year and afflicts young and middle-aged adults. Characteristic features include progressive, usually symmetric, weakness that often includes facial and bulbar paresis and external ophthalmoplegia. This is accompanied by areflexia; mild sensory changes, such as distal paresthesias; and autonomic abnormalities, such as tachycardia, arrhythmias, and postural hypotension. These clinical manifestations generally are complete within 2 to 4 weeks. Although occasionally normal early in the illness, motor nerve conduction becomes abnormal over time on the EMG. The CSF protein level also is usually normal during the first few days of illness, but steadily rises, and remains elevated for several months—even after recovery has commenced.

Not all patients with Guillain-Barré syndrome develop respiratory failure, but all should be followed closely lest such failure occur. Daily bedside evaluation of VC and respiratory muscle strength aims to follow the muscle weakness objectively, so patients with decreasing respiratory reserve should be moved to the intensive care unit (ICU) before hypercapnea supervenes. Such patients should be electively intubated and ventilated when signs of respiratory distress are present and before the Pa_{CO_2} becomes elevated or the VC falls below 10 mL/kg. The care of patients who require mechanical ventilation or therapy for autonomic dysfunction will be discussed later in this chapter. In terms of specific therapy, corticosteroids are of no proven value in treating Guillain-Barré syndrome; plasmapheresis reduces hospital stays and the time spent on the ventilator if it is given to patients who do not improve or who worsen within the first 7 days.[15] Most patients survive the Guillain-Barré syndrome if they are adequately supported during the acute phase of their illness.[16] Recovery usually begins within 2 to 4 weeks after progression ceases, although some patients recover more quickly and others remain paralyzed for 1 year or longer. Although most patients eventually recover complete motor function, approximately 15 percent remain significantly handicapped by weakness.

DISORDERS OF THE MYONEURAL JUNCTION

Disorders of the myoneural junction are caused by abnormalities of ACh release or reception. They are therefore characterized by fluctuating weakness and fatigability that is particularly striking in certain muscle groups: the extraocular muscles, the eyelid levators, and other muscles of the head and neck. Because these disorders by definition involve the myoneural junction, they are not associated with sensory loss, altered reflexes, profound muscle atrophy, or the EMG findings of upper or lower motor neuron disease. Instead, the EMG reveals changes in muscle action potential during repetitive stimulation that often can be altered by drugs affecting ACh activity.

Myasthenia gravis is the prototypical myoneural junction disorder. Probably an immunologic disease, it results from circulating antibodies directed against ACh receptors in the myoneural junction. In addition to these humoral aspects, cell-mediated immunity, involving sensitized lymphocytes, and the thymus gland also are involved. The result is that potential interactions between ACh and receptor molecules are reduced, leading to low-amplitude motor end-plate potentials that may fail to trigger strong muscle contractions. This, in turn, causes weakness and fatigability superficially resembling those seen in poisoning by botulinum toxin.[17]

Myasthenia occurs in all decades of life, with the incidence peaking in the third decade. The most common presenting symptom is weakness of the eye muscles, manifested by diplopia or ptosis. Dysarthria and dysphagia also are common, as is proximal weakness of the upper and lower extremities. Selective respiratory muscle involvement is unusual; sensory and reflex changes imply the presence of another disorder. Myasthenia can be diagnosed on clinical grounds and by giving short-acting acetylcholinesterase-inhibiting agents that increase the interaction between ACh and its receptors. Thus, transiently increased strength should be achieved within seconds following the intravenous injection of edrophonium (Tensilon). Antibodies to the ACh receptor can also be detected in 90 percent of patients with unequivocal generalized myasthenia gravis.[18] A rapid decline in muscle action potentials on repetitive stimulation is seen on the EMG.

Myasthenia is treated on a chronic basis with relatively long-acting anticholinesterase agents, such as pyridostigmine (Mestinon), at a dosage that improves muscle weakness with a minimum of cholinergic side effects.[19] Plasmapheresis, which presumably removes antireceptor antibodies, may improve motor function for longer periods. Thymectomy leads to complete remission or substantial improvement in about 85 percent of myasthenia patients. Corticosteroids and other immunosuppressive agents are routinely given to patients with generalized disease.[20] Patients treated with these measures and provided with supportive care during exacerbations generally enjoy a good prognosis.[21] Such exacerbations may involve the need for mechanical ventilation; they occur in approximately 10 percent of patients. They usually are precipitated by infection, surgical stress, or the administration of aminoglycosides, neuromuscular blocking agents, or cholinergic agents.

Botulism is another disorder of the myoneural junction that may be encountered in critical care practice. This disease is not immunologic but is caused by a sporulating, gram-positive anaerobic bacterium, *Clostridium botulinum.* Ubiquitous in nature, this organism produces potent neurotoxins, designated A through G, that bind irreversibly to the presynaptic terminal and inhibit ACh release. Botulism occurs in three forms: food-borne botulism, in which preformed toxin is ingested in nonacidic home-canned or factory-canned vegetables or meat; infant botulism, in which the organism and its spores are ingested in honey or other foods, or from the environment; and wound botulism, in which *C. botulinum* and its spores contaminate traumatic or surgical wounds.[22,23]

Neuromuscular symptoms follow exposure to *C. botulinum* neurotoxin within 2 to 24 h. The bulbar musculature is affected first, with resultant diplopia and dysphagia. Ptosis, extraocular muscle weakness, and diminution of the gag reflex also are common. Because the neurotoxin also involves the autonomic nervous system, gastrointestinal symptoms such as nausea, vomiting and ileus also may occur, and the pupils may be dilated. Mentation remains normal, and there is no fever. Patients usually develop a symmetric descending weakness or paralysis of the skeletal muscles, including those used for respiration. Severe respiratory muscle involvement is paralleled by decreases in VC and TLC and an increase in RV, reflected in hypercapnia, hypoxemia, and the need for mechanical ventilation.

Botulism may be verified by the detection of the neurotoxin in serum, stool, or contaminated food. Some patients exhibit improvement in muscle strength following the administration of edrophonium, which may prompt confusion of this disease with myasthenia gravis. However, diagnosis is most readily confirmed by EMG, which shows small evoked muscle action potentials that increase in amplitude after repetitive stimulation. This pattern is dissimilar to that seen in myasthenia; it most closely resembles EMG findings in the Eaton-Lambert syndrome, a myasthenic variant described for the most part in patients with neoplasm.

Specific therapy for botulism involves elimination of unabsorbed neurotoxin from the gut by means of enemas and gastric lavage; administration of trivalent antitoxin (against neurotoxins A, B, and E) to neutralize circulating neurotoxin in the serum; administration of high-dose penicillin (3 million U intravenously every 4 h) to kill *C. botulinum* organisms, if present; and surgical debridement of offending wounds. Guanidine hydrochloride, which enhances ACh release and has been used in patients with Eaton-Lambert syndrome, also may be considered. Only about one-third of patients with botulism have respiratory failure severe enough to require mechanical ventilation, although aspiration is common in the disorder. Few patients die if treated properly, and even the extremely weak can usually be weaned from mechanical ventilation within months. Nevertheless, many patients report easy fatigability and exertional dyspnea years after recovery. When studied, some manifest diminished respiratory muscle strength, but a lack of cardiovascular fitness also may contribute to their fatigue.[24]

DISORDERS OF MUSCLES

The final components of neuromuscular function are the muscles themselves. Disorders of muscle are called myopathies. They may be genetic (e.g., the various muscular dystrophies), inflammatory (e.g., polymyositis), metabolic (e.g., glycogen storage diseases, such as acid maltase deficiency), or endocrinologic (e.g., hypo- and hyperthyroidism). Myopathic processes commonly involve the shoulder and pelvic girdles in a symmetric fashion. Sensory loss does not occur with the myopathies; reflex changes are minimal; muscle wasting is uncommon; and pseudohypertrophy may occur early in the course of certain dystrophies. Pain may be prominent, as may an increase in the serum concentration of creatine phosphokinase (CPK) and other muscle enzymes. Nerve conduction studies are normal. A predominance of small motor units is seen on EMG.

Muscular dystrophies are a subgroup of myopathies with three characteristics: hereditary transmission, progressive weakness, and biopsy evidence of muscle degeneration without evidence of stored material or structural abnormality. None of the muscular dystrophies is common; the Duchenne type is perhaps the best known. This dystrophy is associated with an X-chromosomal deficiency of the protein dystrophin that produces progressive proximal weakness starting in childhood.[25] This is paralleled by expiratory muscle weakness that limits cough, and later by inspiratory weakness that reduces RV and TLC.[26]

Patients with Duchenne dystrophy generally maintain near-normal arterial blood gas values while awake, until their disease is far advanced. However, hypercapnia and hypoxemia may be due primarily to reduced innervation of the intercostal and accessory muscles during rapid eye movement (REM) sleep.[27] Eventually patients become unable to walk and develop muscle contractures and kyphoscoliosis, as is true in other neuromuscular disorders. These thoracic cage abnormalities then combine with respiratory muscle weakness to cause severe respiratory failure. Respiratory tract infections become progressively more frequent, and most patients die in the third decade.

Duchenne dystrophy is generally not difficult to diagnose clinically. The trait is transmitted as a sex-linked recessive; once a patient is known, affected siblings can be identified in the neonatal period, because their CPK levels are always markedly elevated. One-third of cases, however, arise as spontaneous mutations. There is no specific treatment beyond the possible use of corticosteroids, which increase muscle strength but do not reduce wheelchair requirements.[28] Physical therapy, splints, braces, and corrective orthopedic surgery also have been recommended. Infections should be treated, and acute mechanical ventilation may be called for. The question whether to provide chronic ventilatory support for patients with advanced illness raises great ethical difficulties.

Management in the Intensive Care Unit (ICU)

Not all patients with neuromuscular disease require intensive care or elect to receive it. Nevertheless, significant numbers are admitted to the ICU, and an unfortunate few spend their last days of life there. The general management of such patients may be divided into five overlapping areas: the diagnosis and treatment of the specific neuromuscular disease, if possible; the diagnosis of precipitating factors prompting admission; the evaluation of the need for respiratory support; the provision of such support on an acute basis; and the consideration of chronic support when required.

DIAGNOSIS OF SPECIFIC NEUROMUSCULAR DISEASE

Neuromuscular disease will have been previously diagnosed in some patients who receive intensive care. Others will lack a diagnosis and may have to be supported before a diagnosis is made. Once weakness or paralysis is appreciated, most neuromuscular diseases causing these symptoms can be differentiated by means of physical examination; CSF analysis; provocative tests, such as the administration of cholinergic drugs; nerve conduction studies and EMG; and, occasionally, muscle biopsy. Once a diagnosis is made, specific therapy can be applied.

PRECIPITATING FACTORS

Although some patients with neuromuscular disease need intensive care solely because of progressive respiratory muscle dysfunction, admission is usually prompted by precipitating factors. The identification of such factors is essential, because they may be more amenable to therapy than the neuromuscular disease itself. Upper airway obstruction and aspiration should be suspected in patients with bulbar involvement, whereas microatelectasis and lower respiratory tract infections are common among all patients with generalized weakness. Pulmonary hypertension and right-sided heart failure should be anticipated in chronically hypoxemic patients, including those whose muscle weakness is compounded by kyphoscoliosis. Intercurrent illnesses, such as urinary tract sepsis, pulmonary embolism, or ischemic heart disease, also may occur, as may cholinergic crises in patients with myasthenia gravis.

EVALUATION OF THE NEED FOR RESPIRATORY SUPPORT

The need for respiratory support should be assessed in patients with neuromuscular diseases as early as possible. The finding of severe hypoxemia, hypercapnia, and acidemia on arterial blood gas analysis is perhaps the most compelling indication for such support; but by the time blood gas abnormalities occur, respiratory failure is already profound. Although it cannot be diagnosed solely on physical

TABLE 143-2 Respiratory Compromise Due to Neuromuscular Diseases Causing Weakness

Finding	Compromise
Maximum pressures	
Maximum expiratory pressure <40 cmH_2O	Inability to cough and clear secretions
Maximum inspiratory pressure <−20 cmH_2O	Inability to ventilate adequately
Vital capacity	
<30 mL/kg	Inability to cough adequately
<20 mL/kg	Inability to sigh or prevent atelectasis
<10 mL/kg	Inability to ventilate adequately
Bulbar weakness or paralysis	Inability to protect airway and avoid aspiration
Arterial blood gases	
Hypercapnia	Inability to ventilate adequately
Hypoxemia	Inability to oxygenate adequately

examination, respiratory failure is suggested by a rapid, shallow breathing pattern and by the presence of abdominal paradox.[29] Patients with neuromuscular disease should be observed during sleep for signs of upper rib cage paradox and upper airway obstruction. Respiratory muscle dysfunction may be documented by having a patient exhale forcefully or cough.

Determination of PI_{max} and PE_{max} is the most sensitive way to quantitate respiratory muscle weakness.[3] These pressures should be measured while breathing with maximum effort against mouthpiece systems that are occluded at RV and TLC, respectively. Observed pressures, either from a patient's baseline state or from therapeutic trials, may then be compared against published predicted values. In one study, PE_{max} was found to be less than 80 percent of predicted value in 87 percent of patients with generalized neuromuscular disease, and less than 50 percent in 66 percent. By contrast, PI_{max} exceeded 80 percent of predicted value in 83 percent of patients.[30] The PE_{max} averages approximately 100 cmH_2O in normal adults, whereas a pressure of less than 40 cmH_2O precludes effective coughing (Table 143-1). The average PI_{max} is −70 cmH_2O; a normal $PaCO_2$ cannot be maintained if the pressure is less (in the sense of absolute magnitude) than −20 cmH_2O.[31]

In lieu of determining maximum pressures, VC may be measured by spirometry, and RV and TLC by more sophisticated pulmonary function testing. Again, observed volumes may be compared with published predicted values. The VC averages approximately 50 mL/kg in normal adults; impaired secretion clearance occurs at a VC of less than 30 mL/kg, and ventilatory failure occurs at a VC of around 10 mL/kg[31] (Table 143-2). Spirometry and pulmonary function tests may also be performed before and after therapeutic interventions; or in various postures, to help determine in which position patients will breathe most effectively.

Further quantitation of respiratory muscle strength can be obtained by measuring Pdi during quiet breathing, and maximum Pdi (Pdi_{max}) on forced inspiration. Pdi increases from 0 to approximately 5 cmH_2O during a quiet inspiration in normal persons, whereas Pdi_{max} should exceed 25 cmH_2O.[32] Normal persons should also be able to sustain a Pdi of some 40 percent of Pdi_{max} over extended periods. Inability to generate normal pressures on a single breath, or over time, correlates with respiratory muscle weakness or fatigue, as does a concurrent shift in the power spectrum on diaphragmatic EMG.[33] Power spectrum analysis is a relatively sophisticated technique, however; neither it nor Pdi measurement are routinely available at most centers.

PROVIDING RESPIRATORY SUPPORT

Hypoxemic respiratory failure in patients with neuromuscular disease usually can be treated adequately with supplemental oxygen delivered through nasal prongs or a face mask, coupled with frequent positioning and periodic hyperinflations, or the delivery of positive end-expiratory pressure (PEEP) via face mask, to improve atelectasis. However, intubation and mechanical ventilation are usually called for if lung volumes and muscle strength have declined to the levels mentioned above; these measures are always necessary if hypercapnia is acute and severe. Patients with rapidly reversible muscle weakness or paralysis should be intubated by the translaryngeal route in most instances, but tracheostomy is indicated for any patient who requires intubation for more than a few weeks. A tracheostomy facilitates the suctioning of airway secretions and allows speech through special tubes that direct air exhaled through the larynx. It also provides access to the airway during weaning from mechanical ventilation.

No particular kind of mechanical ventilation has been demonstrated to be superior in patients with neuromuscular disease, although intermittent positive-pressure ventilation is preferred over intermittent negative-pressure ventilation in the developed world today. The relative merits of various modes of positive-pressure ventilation also are open to debate. Nevertheless, assist-control and intermittent mechanical (mandatory) ventilation can be used only for patients who can generate substantial respiratory efforts, so most patients with severe weakness or paralysis are ventilated, at least initially, in the controlled mode. Atelectasis can be prevented or treated in such patients with frequent sighs or moderate-to-high tidal volumes.

An ongoing debate exists regarding whether patients of all sorts should undergo respiratory muscle exercise or be rested while they receive mechanical ventilation. Although some patients might benefit from nonfatiguing exercise, this approach seems unreasonable in patients with neuromuscular disease. With such patients a more prudent course is to wait until muscle strength returns, either because of therapy or because of time, and then consider weaning. Weaning should be attempted only when patients demonstrate sufficient maximum pressure and lung volumes and have a minute ventilation of less than 10 L. Patient-initiated weaning modes, such as pressure support, should be used only when patients can initiate breaths and comfortably assume more work of breathing.

Patients with neuromuscular disease and concurrent lower airway obstruction due to asthma should be treated with aerosolized β-adrenergic agonists, systemic corticosteroids, and other drugs as indicated. Theophylline may also be used for this purpose; it has also been purported to improve the contractility of the diaphragm and other respiratory muscles.[34] Nevertheless, it is not clear that theophylline in therapeutic doses actually increases diaphragmatic contractility. Furthermore, no one has demonstrated that theophylline can reduce the ventilator dependence or facilitate the ventilator weaning of patients with neuromuscular disease or other disorders. If theophylline is administered empirically to such patients in hope of strengthening the respiratory muscles, drug levels should be followed closely to reduce the toxicity.

Patients with neuromuscular disorders require scrupulous nursing care to avoid nerve compression (especially involving the ulnar and peroneal nerves) and bedsores. Patients should be turned frequently and may benefit from insulating pads or kinetic beds. Footboards and wrist splints should be provided; physical therapy may prevent disuse (but not denervation) atrophy and improve patient morale. Nutrition should also be provided by the enteral route whenever possible, although aspiration must be avoided. Oral feedings may be used for tracheostomized patients who can swallow. On the other hand, nasointestinal feedings are desirable for patients who cannot swallow but are likely to regain neuromuscular function, whereas feeding jejunostomies may be more appropriate for those who are permanently weak or paralyzed. Low-dose subcutaneous heparin or pneumatic leg compression devices are indicated to prevent deep venous thrombosis and pulmonary embolism.

Autonomic dysfunction in patients with Guillain-Barré syndrome and other neuromuscular diseases may take the form of either over- or underactivity of the sympathetic nervous system. Hypertension, diaphoresis, and tachycardia may be treated with α- or β-adrenergic antagonists; short-acting, titratable agents are helpful in preventing overswings of pulse and pressure. The hypotension that accompanies cervical spinal cord injury and other conditions may be treated with intravenous fluids or short-acting α-adrenergic agonists, whereas bradycardia is treated with atropine. Patients with profound vagal tone in whom bradycardia occasionally progresses to asystole may be candidates for ventricular pacing.

Finally, patients receiving mechanical respiratory assistance on an acute basis also require emotional support. These patients frequently regress on a psychologic basis—some times because of central nervous system involvement by their disease, but more commonly because of their complete dependence on the people caring for them. Most such patients, and their families, need frequent reminders that their needs will be met by nurses, physicians, respiratory therapists, and other health professionals. If their neuromuscular function is amenable to time or treatment, they should also be told that their recovery can be expected, in months if not in days.

CONSIDERATION OF CHRONIC SUPPORT

There remains the difficult question what to tell patients who are not expected to recover neuromuscular function because of the type and severity of their disease. Current ethical standards suggest that such patients, or their surrogates, should be informed of their prognosis and offered respiratory support on a chronic basis if it is available. Some patients who accept chronic support and whose phrenic nuclei are damaged, but whose nerves and hemidiaphragms are intact, may be candidates for electrophrenic ventilation, in which the nerves are repetitively stimulated in the lower neck or upper thorax.[35] Others who maintain near-normal arterial blood gas measurements only while awake may be ventilated during sleep with rocking beds, chest cuirasses, and other intermittent negative-pressure devices; or by intermittent positive pressure delivered through the mouth or a tracheostomy.[36,37] Unfortunately, however, most patients with severe chronic neuromuscular disease must receive negative- or positive-pressure ventilation around the clock. Chronic home ventilation of this sort is effective, although it requires attendant care and is expensive. Furthermore, some patients refuse such treatment. It is ethically permissible to withhold or withdraw life support from these patients if they, or their surrogates, so desire.

CASE PRESENTATION

Mrs. A.Q., a 69-year-old Hispanic woman, was admitted to San Francisco General Hospital through its emergency room on December 6, 1989 with a history of orthopnea and fatigue. She had been treated previously for paroxysmal atrial fibrillation, hypertension, and ischemic heart disease, and was receiving digoxin, 0.25 mg PO qd; isosorbide, 20 mg PO qid; and enalapril, 5 mg PO bid. Two weeks prior to admission, the patient had fallen and bruised her right buttock. Three days prior to admission, she had been seen in a nearby emergency room for dyspnea and fatigue; the emergency room physician at that time could obtain little history from Mrs. A.Q., who spoke only Spanish. He noted cardiomegaly on her chest radiograph and left ventricular enlargement on her ECG. Her arterial blood gas values on room air were: pH 7.38, Pa_{CO_2} 49 mmHg, Pa_{O_2} 66 mmHg. She was assumed to have congestive heart failure and was sent home to take furosemide, 40 mg PO bid.

In the emergency room at San Francisco General Hospital, 3 days later, Mrs. A.Q. told a Spanish-speaking physician that she felt more fatigued than short of breath. Her fatigue was minimal in the morning but worsened as the day progressed. She also had difficulty swallowing;

her tongue felt swollen, and she could not sleep lying flat because her tongue fell back in her throat. She appeared to be in no distress, but her speech was somewhat slurred. Her vital signs were: pulse 122 and irregularly irregular, blood pressure 142/97 mmHg, temperature 37.4°C, respiratory rate 36. Her weight was 56 kg. She had a left-sided ptosis. Bibasilar rales were present on examination of the chest, but no extra heart sounds were heard. A 1-cm decubitus ulcer was noted on her right buttock. She seemed weak in all extremities and had intact sensation and reflexes, but she could not cooperate fully on neurologic examination.

Laboratory values in the emergency room were: Na^+ 132 meq/L, K^+ 4.3 meq/L, Cl^- 97 meq/L, HCO_3^- 33 meq/L, BUN 28 mg/dL, creatinine 1.1 mg/dL. Chest radiograph revealed cardiomegaly, small lung volumes, and discoid atelectasis at the bases. ECG revealed left ventricular enlargement and atrial fibrillation at a rate of 101 per minute. Arterial blood gas values obtained while breathing 2 L of oxygen were: pH 7.37, Pa_{CO_2} 52 mmHg, Pa_{O_2} 94 mmHg. Spirometry revealed a forced vital capacity (VC) of 800 mL and an expiratory volume, in 1 s, of 750 mL. Blood was sent for phosphate and thyroid function tests, which were subsequently reported as normal. The patient was admitted to the ICU for observation with diagnoses of muscle weakness and unexplained hypoventilation.

In the ICU, Mrs. A.Q. was given supplemental oxygen, monitored with frequent bedside spirometry, treated for her decubitus ulcer, and seen by a neurologist. The neurologist confirmed the left-sided ptosis and dysarthria and also detected bilateral nystagmus on external gaze. Mrs. A.Q. had intact reflexes and sensation, but she had diffuse muscle weakness involving the face as well as the extremities. She could not rise from a seated position and could not raise her hands over her head. She was given 2 mg of edrophonium (Tensilon) intravenously, with no response. After additional doses of 2 mg and then 5 mg, she was able to raise her hands, and her VC increased to 1350 mL. A tentative diagnosis of myasthenia gravis was made; blood was sent for acetylcholine receptor antibody levels, which subsequently proved to be elevated. Thereafter the patient was given pyridostigmine (Mestinon), 60 mg PO q 4 h; the dose ultimately was increased to 80 mg PO qid. She remained intermittently dysarthric and dysphagic, but maintained her VC above 1000 mL. She was instructed to use an incentive spirometer frequently. A CT scan of the chest revealed a mediastinal mass; the patient was scheduled for thymectomy.

On the day before surgery, Mrs. A.Q.'s VC was 1275 mL. PI_{max} and PE_{max}, measured at the mouth, were −60 mmHg and 52 mmHg, respectively. Mrs. A.Q. received plasmapheresis in the ICU. She underwent an uneventful thymectomy after intubation without the use of succinylcholine on December 12, 1989. She was returned to the ICU later that day, intubated and receiving mechanical ventilation, with an epidural catheter in place to allow for analgesic administration. Weaning from mechanical ventilation was considered the following morning; but Mrs. A.Q.'s VC was 750 mL, her PI_{max} was −28 mmHg, and her PE_{max} was 18 mmHg. She was continued on her medications and ventilated in the assist-control mode for 2 days. At this point, she was started on intravenous methylprednisolone, 60 mg qid.

Two days later, Mrs. A.Q. developed thick secretions attributed to bibasilar *Escherichia coli* pneumonia, which was treated successfully without the use of aminoglycosides. She subsequently underwent a second plasmapheresis. Her VC improved to 1300 mL, and her PI_{max} and PE_{max} rose to −52 mmHg and 48 mmHg, respectively; she was weaned from mechanical ventilation and extubated on December 25, 1989. She was discharged from the ICU, with a normal Pa_{CO_2} and Pa_{O_2}, 2 days later. Mrs. A.Q. left San Francisco General Hospital, on oral pyridostigmine and prednisone, on January 7, 1990.

CASE DISCUSSION

This case highlights the occasional difficulty of diagnosing respiratory failure due to neuromuscular disease, especially in patients who, by virtue of age or underlying poor health, may have other medical problems. Spirometry was essential in documenting Mrs. A.Q.'s respiratory muscle weakness, although tests of respiratory muscle strength also would have been useful. Myasthenia gravis was tentatively diagnosed in the patient on account of her response to edrophonium; this diagnosis was confirmed by the presence of acetylcholine receptor antibodies. Mrs. A.Q. received therapy appropriate to her condition, which was exacerbated by the stress of surgery and pneumonia. Her improvement with treatment was paralleled by increased lung volumes and muscle strength.

References

1. Ali HH, Savarase JJ: Monitoring of neuromuscular function. Anesthesiology 45:216, 1976.
2. Derrenne JPH, Macklem PT, Roussos CH: The respiratory muscles: Mechanics, control, and pathophysiology, parts I, II, and III. Am Rev Respir Dis 118:119, 118:373, 118:581, 1978.
3. Black LF, Hyatt RE: Maximal static respiratory pressures in generalized neuromuscular disease. Am Rev Respir Dis 103:641, 1971.
4. De Troyer A, De Beyl DZ, Thirion M: Function of the respiratory muscles in acute hemiplegia. Am Rev Respir Dis 123:631, 1981.
5. Ridyard JB, Stewart RM: Regional lung function in unilateral diaphragmatic paralysis. Thorax 31:438, 1976.
6. Lisboa C, Paré PD, Pertuzé J, et al: Inspiratory muscle function in unilateral diaphragmatic paralysis. Am Rev Respir Dis 134:488, 1986.
7. Luce JM: Medical management of spinal cord injury. Crit Care Med 13:126, 1985.
8. Schmidt-Nowara WW, Altman AR: Atelectasis and neuromuscular respiratory failure. Chest 85:792, 1984.
9. Estenne M, Heilporn A, Delhez L, et al: Chest wall stiffness in patients with chronic respiratory muscle weakness. Am Rev Respir Dis 128:1002, 1983.

10. Estenne M, Knoop C, Vanvaerenbergh J, et al: The effect of pectoralis muscle training in tetraplegic subjects. Am Rev Respir Dis 139:1218, 1989.
11. Cashman NR, Maselli R, Wollmann RL, et al: Late denervation in patients with antecedent paralytic poliomyelitis. N Engl J Med 317:7, 1987.
12. Tandan R, Bradley WG: Amyotrophic lateral sclerosis, part 1: Clinical features, pathology, and ethical issues in management. Ann Neurol 18:271, 1985.
13. Kreitzer SM, Saunders NA, Tyler HR, Ingram RH: Respiratory muscle function in amyotrophic lateral sclerosis. Am Rev Respir Dis 117:437, 1978.
14. Asbury AK, Arnason BG, Adams RD: The inflammatory lesion in idiopathic polyneuritis. Medicine 48:173, 1969.
15. Hughes RAC, Newsom-Davis JM, Perkin GD, Pierce JM: Controlled trial of prednisolone in acute polyneuropathy. Lancet 2:750, 1978.
16. Gracey DR, McMichan JC, Divertie MB, Howard FM: Respiratory failure in Guillain-Barré syndrome. Mayo Clin Proc 57:742, 1982.
17. Drachman DB: Myasthenia gravis, parts 1 and 2. N Engl J Med 298:136, 298:186, 1978.
18. Lindstrom JM, Seybold ME, Lennon VA, et al: Antibody to acetylcholine receptor in myasthenia gravis. Neurology 26:1054, 1976.
19. Mier-Jedrzejowicz AK, Brophy C, Green M: Respiratory muscle function in myasthenia gravis. Am Rev Respir Dis 138:867, 1988.
20. Dau PC, Lindstrom JM, Cassel CK, et al: Plasmapheresis and immunosuppressive drug therapy in myasthenia gravis. N Engl J Med 297:1134, 1977.
21. Gracey DR, Divertie MB, Howard FM: Mechanical ventilation for respiratory failure in myasthenia gravis. Mayo Clin Proc 58:597, 1983.
22. Merson MH, Dowell VR: Epidemiological, clinical and laboratory aspects of wound botulism. N Engl J Med 289:1005, 1973.
23. Hughes JM, Blumenthal JR, Merson MH, et al: Clinical features of types A and B food-borne botulism. Ann Intern Med 95:442, 1981.
24. Wilcox P, Andolfatto G, Fairbarn MS, Pardy RL: Long-term follow-up of symptoms, pulmonary function, respiratory muscle strength, and exercise performance after botulism. Am Rev Respir Dis 139:157, 1989.
25. Hoffman EP, Fischbeck KH, Brown RH, et al: Characterization of dystrophy in muscle-biopsy specimens from patients with Duchenne's or Becker's muscular dystrophy. N Engl J Med 318:1363, 1988.
26. Smith PEM, Calverley PMA, Edwards RHT, et al: Practical problems in the respiratory care of patients with muscular dystrophy. N Engl J Med 316:1197, 1987.
27. Smith PEM, Edwards RHT, Calverley PMA: Ventilation and breathing pattern during sleep in Duchenne muscular dystrophy. Chest 96:1346, 1989.
28. Mendell JR, Moxley RT, Griggs RC, et al: Randomized, double-blind six-month trial of prednisone in Duchenne's muscular dystrophy. N Engl J Med 320:1592, 1989.
29. Cohen CA, Zagelbaum G, Gross D, et al: Clinical manifestations of inspiratory muscle fatigue. Am J Med 73:308, 1982.
30. Griggs RC, Donohoe KM, Utell MJ, et al: Evaluation of pulmonary function in neuromuscular disease. Arch Neurol 38:9, 1981.
31. O'Donohue WJ, Baker JP, Bell GM, et al: Respiratory failure in neuromuscular disease. JAMA 235:733, 1976.
32. Newsom Davis J, Golman M, Loh L, Casson M: Diaphragm function and alveolar hypoventilation. J Med 177:87, 1976.
33. Roussos CS, Macklem PT: Diaphragmatic fatigue in man. J Appl Physiol 43:189, 1977.
34. Aubier M, De Troyer A, Sampson M, et al: Aminophylline improves diaphragmatic contractility. N Engl J Med 305:249, 1981.
35. Weese-Mayer DE, Morrow AS, Brouillette RT, et al: Diaphragm pacing in infants and children. Am Rev Respir Dis 139:974, 1989.
36. Goldstein RS, Molotiu N, Skrastins R, et al: Reversal of sleep-induced hypoventilation and chronic respiratory failure by nocturnal negative pressure ventilation in patients with restrictive ventilatory impairment. Am Rev Respir Dis 135:1049, 1987.
37. Bach JR, Alba AS, Bohatiuk G, et al: Mouth intermittent positive pressure ventilation in the management of postpolio respiratory insufficiency. Chest 91:859, 1987.

Chapter 144

COMA, PERSISTENT VEGETATIVE STATE, AND BRAIN DEATH

MATTHEW E. FINK

KEY POINTS

- *The neuroanatomy of coma can be divided into three major categories: diffuse brain dysfunction, primary brain stem disorders, and secondary brain stem compression from supratentorial mass lesions.*
- *Most cases of coma are due to metabolic disorders or exogenous drug intoxication.*
- *Patient evaluation must follow an orderly sequence, beginning with vital signs, general physical examination, and neurologic examination.*
- *The most important single sign distinguishing toxic-metabolic coma from primary brain disease is the presence of pupillary light responses.*
- *The neurologic examination of the patient in coma is brief and focuses on (1) level of consciousness, (2) pupils, (3) eye movements, (4) motor responses, and (5) respiratory pattern.*
- *Early computed tomography (CT) scanning of the brain is the most valuable test to diagnose structural causes of coma.*
- *Hypoxic-ischemic encephalopathy after cardiopulmonary arrest or shock states may be treatable by aggressive measures to increase cerebral blood flow after resuscitation.*
- Persistent vegetative state *describes a patient who fails to awaken from coma after 4 weeks.*
- *The Uniform Determination of Death Act states that "an individual who has sustained either (1) irreversible cessation of circulatory and respiratory functions, or (2) irreversible cessation of all functions of the entire brain, including the brain stem, is dead."*
- *The determination of death by brain criteria is based on clinical examination and, in most cases, does not require confirmatory tests. However, the cause of coma must be known, and the cause must be sufficient to explain the coma.*

Coma and Survival in Critical Care Units

The extreme severity of illness in critical care units makes them a focal point for the diagnosis and treatment of patients with critical organ failure. Coma is the clinical manifestation of severe, acute brain failure and has a major impact on the protocols and outcomes of treatment in the intensive care unit (ICU). Hypoxic-ischemic encephalopathy, a common cause of coma in hospitalized patients, often results in death or permanent neurologic impairment, even though stable cardiovascular function is restored by modern resuscitative techniques. Earlier studies have described the outcome of coma in a general hospital population, but little information is available regarding the prevalence, causes, and outcome of coma complicating the clinical course of patients in critical care units.[1,2]

To determine the significance of coma on the overall survival of patients in the six critical care units at Columbia-Presbyterian Medical Center, we prospectively screened every patient in our ICUs over a 10-month period to identify patients in coma. In our 1400-bed hospital with 70 critical care beds, we found 233 patients over the age of 10 who had prolonged unconsciousness (greater than 6 h) from either primary neurologic disorders (85) or secondary to systemic illnesses (144). We were able to follow 196 patients for 2 weeks to determine mortality, persistent coma, or awakening. Table 144-1 lists the frequency of diagnoses for all patients.

At the end of 2 weeks, 61 percent of the entire group of comatose patients were dead or in persistent coma, a condition likely to result in delayed death or persistent vegetative state. The largest group of patients had hypoxic/ischemic coma secondary to cardiopulmonary arrest or profound hypotension and had the worst prognosis, with 74 percent dead or still in coma. The best outcome, not surprisingly, was in the group with drug intoxication, with 21 percent having a poor outcome at 2 weeks. The severity of coma at time of diagnosis, using the Glasgow Coma Scale (Table

TABLE 144-1 Causes of Coma in 233 ICU Patients

Primary neurologic	
Intracerebral hemorrhage	20
Brain infarction	18
Brain trauma	12
Meningitis	11
Subarachnoid hemorrhage	11
Brain tumor	4
Intraventricular hemorrhage	3
Status epilepticus	3
Hydrocephalus	2
Brain abscess	1
	85
Secondary systemic	
Hypoxic/ischemic	52
Metabolic	48
Systemic infection	17
Drug intoxication	8
Anesthesia (narcotics)	7
Cardiac failure	5
Myocardial infarction	3
Blood dyscrasia	2
Systemic malignancy	2
	144
Unknown cause	4

TABLE 144-2 Glasgow Coma Scale

I. Best motor response	
Obeys	6
Localizes	5
Withdraws	4
Abnormal flexion	3
Extensor response	2
No response	1
II. Verbal response	
Oriented	5
Confused conversation	4
Inappropriate words	3
Incomprehensible sounds	2
No response	1
III. Eye opening	
Spontaneous	4
To speech	3
To pain	2
No response	1
Total score = Score I + II + III	

SOURCE: Adapted with permission from Lancet 2:81, 1974.

144-2), correlated weakly with outcome; the cause of coma had a more profound impact on prognosis.

The significance of these statistics is obvious. Overall mortality in ICUs is 8 to 15 percent. The presence of coma complicating the clinical course of a patient dramatically increases the risk of death or persistent vegetative state, whether due to primary neurologic disease or secondary to other systemic illnesses. We have not yet made a major impact in intensive care for the acutely damaged brain, and this limitation has a profound effect on the success of all critical care treatment.

Coma: Definitions, Anatomy, and Physiology

Coma is a state of "unarousable psychologic unresponsiveness in which the subject lies with eyes closed."[2] Upon casual inspection, the person appears asleep, but there is no understandable response to any internal or external stimulus. The severity of coma is subjectively measured by comparing the intensity of an external stimulus and the complexity and purposefulness of the response. Clinical descriptions should include these elements, and most coma scales adhere to this guideline (see Table 144-2).[3] Coma is the opposite of consciousness; in between these extremes are various states of depressed consciousness such as *obtundation* and *stupor*. To avoid confusion in various interpretations of these terms, it is preferable to describe the patient's level of consciousness in terms of a stimulus-response model.

There are other clinical syndromes that are often confused with coma and should be defined. *Hypersomnia* refers to a condition of excess drowsiness and excessive sleep. It may occur in the setting of narcolepsy, hypothalamic disorders, sleep disorders, or psychiatric illness. *Akinetic mutism* is a condition with silent, alert, and awake appearance, regular sleep-wake cycles, but no evidence of response to the environment, mental activities, or spontaneous movements. A variety of pathologic lesions have been described in this clinical condition. The *locked-in syndrome* is a state of total paralysis of all somatic musculature, with preserved consciousness, preventing the patient from showing a response even though full consciousness and most sensory modalities (vision, hearing, touch) are preserved.[4] Ventral pontine infarction is the most common cause for this syndrome. Such patients usually have preserved vertical eye movements, and communication is possible. Total neuromuscular paralysis can also cause locked-in syndrome.

The *persistent vegetative state* is a chronic condition that sometimes emerges after severe brain injury, usually hypoxic-ischemic damage, where the patient regains eye opening and sleep-wake cycles but has no recognizable signs of cognitive function.[5] Brain stem functions are intact, including breathing, and with attention to nursing care, the state can be maintained for months or years.[6]

Coma and specific focal signs of neurologic damage may occur together or independently. The neuroanatomy of consciousness is not linked to any specific motor, sensory, or cognitive function. Therefore, patients in coma can be divided into two major clinical categories, coma with or coma without focal neurologic signs. This simple division is often the best way to identify primary neurologic disease as the cause for coma.

Because coma is a sleeplike state, it is not surprising to find that the neuroanatomy of coma is closely related to brain stem structures that regulate daily cycles of wakefulness and sleep: the ascending reticular activating system (ARAS). Moruzzi and Magoun identified this structure in animals as lying within the center of the brain stem, extending from the midbrain into the hypothalamus and thalamus.[7,8] They further demonstrated that electrical stimulation of this region in a sleeping animal produced arousal, and ablation caused coma. The ARAS is in a pivotal location where all ascending sensory stimuli travel en route to the thalamus and secondarily to widespread areas of the cerebral cortex. Consciousness is due to arousal effects induced by the ARAS on the cerebral cortex, and most states of coma result from depression or destruction of the reticular formation.

In clinical situations, direct damage to the midbrain or pontine reticular formation, from infarction, hemorrhage, trauma, abscess, or neoplasm, can cause coma. In addition, secondary compression of the midbrain from supratentorial mass lesions can cause coma (transtentorial herniation). And last, massive damage to both cerebral hemispheres can cause coma. Drug intoxication and severe metabolic derangements cause coma by interfering with neuronal function throughout the brain. Such functional causes of coma are, theoretically, reversible, by correcting the underlying metabolic derangement or removing the offending drug.

Examination of the Patient with Depressed Consciousness

Acute depression in level of consciousness is a critical, life-threatening emergency that requires rapid diagnosis and treatment. A rigorous and systematic evaluation should be undertaken in an attempt to answer the following questions:

1. Is there systemic illness causing brain failure?
2. Is there evidence of diffuse or focal brain injury?
3. Is the patient improving or deteriorating?

The most important and most often neglected part of the evaluation is examination for systemic illness. In our experience, hospitalized patients who develop acute depression in consciousness are far more likely to have sepsis, acid-base and electrolyte disorders, hepatic, renal, or cardiac failure, rather than cerebral infarction or hemorrhage. Therefore, careful physical examination is performed with attention to vital signs before neurologic examination is done. Check for airway patency, observe spontaneous breathing patterns, and carefully auscultate the lungs and heart. Core body temperature is an important clue to drug overdose (hypothermia) or infection (hyperthermia). Emergency laboratory studies are obtained to identify the major metabolic derangements that can cause coma (Table 144-3). Emergency measures are taken to ensure vital functions even if the diagnosis is obscure (Table 144-4).

TABLE 144-3 Emergency Laboratory Tests for Metabolic Coma

1. Venous blood: hemoglobin, white blood count, platelets, glucose, electrolytes, calcium, blood urea nitrogen, creatinine, osmolality, coagulation studies, liver function tests, muscle enzymes, thyroid and adrenal functions, toxicology screen, blood cultures.
2. Arterial blood: pH, P_{CO_2}, P_{O_2}, carboxyhemoglobin, ammonia
3. Urine: toxicology, microscopic examination
4. Gastric aspirate: toxicology
5. Cerebrospinal fluid: cell count and gram stain, protein, glucose, culture, counterimmunoelectrophoresis, viral and fungal antigens, and antibody titers

TABLE 144-4 Emergency Treatment for Coma

1. Protect airway and provide oxygen
2. Evaluate for trauma and stabilize spine
3. Support and maintain circulation
4. Administer glucose, thiamine, and naloxone
5. Treat intracranial hypertension
6. Stop epileptic seizures
7. Treat infections
8. Treat hyperthermia
9. Correct electrolyte and acid-base disorders
10. Give specific antidote for identified toxins

The neurologic examination of the patient in coma is limited. Experience has demonstrated that five physiologic variables give most of the important information about the underlying cause of coma: (1) response to external stimulation, (2) motor responses, (3) size and reactivity of pupils, (4) eye movements and ocular reflexes, and (5) pattern of breathing.[2,9]

RESPONSE TO EXTERNAL STIMULATION

Attempts should be made to elicit a behavioral response by verbal command alone. If no response is obtained from shouting or shaking the patient, then noxious stimulation can be applied by digital pressure to the supraorbital nerves or nail-bed pressure to the fingers and/or toes. The examiner should record the type of stimulus and nature of the response for purposes of serial examinations. Purposeful attempts by the patient to remove the offending stimulus indicates preservation of brain stem function and intact connections to the appropriate cerebral hemisphere. Eye opening, either spontaneous or in response to stimulation, indicates preserved function of the *reticular activating system* in the upper brain stem and hypothalamus.

The Glasgow Coma Scale (Table 144-2) was developed to evaluate patients with head trauma and is reliable and reproducible in trauma patients.[3,10] Its application in nontraumatic conditions is less reliable, but it is still the most widely used clinical scale to evaluate the level of consciousness.[11] The scale is a simple and reproducible tool to compare examinations of different examiners at different times.

Frequent examination at regular intervals is the best way to document improving or worsening neurologic function.

MOTOR RESPONSES

Absence of any motor response, with flaccidity and areflexia, indicates severe brain stem damage and is found in terminal coma or severe sedative drug ingestion.

Decorticate, or flexor, posturing of the arms indicates bilateral cerebral hemisphere damage or toxic/metabolic depression of brain function. Decerebrate, or extensor, posturing of the arms indicates destructive lesions of the midbrain and upper pons but can also be present in severe metabolic insults, such as hepatic encephalopathy and anoxic-ischemic encephalopathy.

Withdrawal from pain and localizing responses indicate purposeful behavior. Ability to follow verbal commands is the best response.

Focal, unilateral cerebral hemisphere lesions will produce asymmetrical limb movements.

PUPILLARY RESPONSES

The size, equality, and light reactivity of the pupils should be noted.

Small, reactive pupils may be due to metabolic brain disease or increased intracranial pressure with hypothalamic dysfunction. Very small pupils (pinpoint) that react to naloxone are characteristic of narcotic overdose. Small pupils occur in pontine hemorrhage or infarction.

Bilateral, widely dilated, fixed pupils are due to sympathetic overactivity from an endogenous cause (seizures or severe anoxia/ischemia) or exogenous catecholamines (dopamine or norepinephrine). Atropinelike drugs may cause dilated and fixed pupils.

Midposition and fixed pupils imply both sympathetic and parasympathetic failure at the level of the midbrain. Such pupils are seen in brain death.

A unilateral dilated pupil, unresponsive to a bright light, usually means damage to the ipsilateral IIIrd nerve from transtentorial herniation. In the setting of head trauma, this implies an ipsilateral epidural, subdural, or intracerebral hematoma. In nontraumatic conditions, it usually occurs with large cerebral infarcts, spontaneous intracerebral hematoma, or supratentorial brain tumors.

EYE MOVEMENTS

Deeply comatose patients usually have no spontaneous eye movements.[12] Spontaneous roving, horizontal, and conjugate eye movements indicate that the brain stem is intact but do not require that the frontal or occipital cerebral cortex be functioning. Conjugate lateral deviation of the eyes suggests the presence of either a massive hemispheric lesion (eyes look toward the lesion) or a pontine lesion (the eyes look away from the lesion). Dysconjugate eyes are seen in all types of coma.

When cortical influences are depressed with intact brain stem function, the eyes will deviate conjugately to the side opposite the direction of passive head rotation, like a doll's head (doll's eyes reflex). This occurs in normal sleep, coma, or persistent vegetative state and implies intact connections between afferent sensory nerves in the neck, the vestibular nuclei in the medulla, and the nuclei of the third and sixth cranial nerves and their connections in the brain stem (medial longitudinal fasciculus). Unilateral brain stem lesions eliminate the response to the side of the lesion.

If the doll's eyes reflex is absent, the ice water caloric response is elicited by irrigating the external auditory canal with 30 mL of ice water. With the comatose patient supine and the head elevated 30°, the eyes will deviate conjugately and tonically to the side of the cold water. In an awake, intact patient, there will be deviation to the side of the cold water and rapid nystagmus away from the cold water. Structural brain stem disease eliminates the caloric response, as does inner ear disease, deep drug coma, and anticonvulsant drug overdose.

PATTERN OF BREATHING

Patients with acute, isolated brain injury uncomplicated by other critical medical illnesses may have characteristic breathing patterns (Fig. 144-1) that aid in neurologic diagnosis. However, these patterns are not reliable in patients with multiple organ system failures who are receiving mechanical ventilation. Nevertheless, a discussion is warranted.

Cheyne-Stokes respiration (Fig. 144-1a) is a periodic breathing pattern in which periods of hyperpnea regularly alternate with apnea in a smooth crescendo-decrescendo pattern. This neurogenic respiratory alteration occurs with frontal lobe damage, unilateral or bilateral, or secondary to cardiac or respiratory failure. It is the result of the loss of frontal lobe controls over respiratory patterns with excessive dependence on blood P_{CO_2} to trigger brain stem respiratory centers. Post-hyperventilation apnea often accompanies a Cheyne-Stokes pattern.

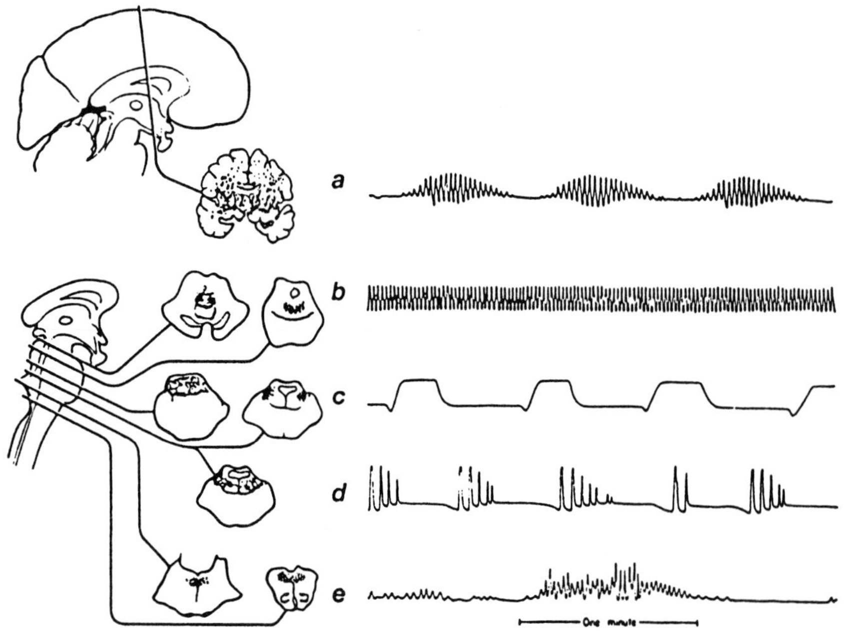

FIGURE 144-1 Abnormal respiratory patterns in coma. See text for explanation. (With permission from Plum F and Posner JB: *The Diagnosis of Stupor and Coma,* 3d ed. F.A. Davis, Philadelphia, 1980, 34.)

Central neurogenic hyperventilation (Fig. 144-1b) is sustained, rapid, deep hyperpnea that often occurs in patients with upper brain stem damage. It can only be diagnosed with arterial blood gas measurements, since hyperventilation will also occur secondary to hypoxemia and acidemia. Metabolic disorders, especially the early stages of hepatic coma, cause central neurogenic hyperventilation.

Apneustic breathing (Fig. 144-1c) is a prolonged inspiratory gasp. It is rarely observed but has been described in association with discrete lesions of the mid-to-lower pons. Most patients with this respiratory pattern require early intubation and mechanical ventilation.

Ataxic and irregular periodic breathing (Fig. 144-1d,1e) occur with medullary damage and are not compatible with sustained life. These are often terminal states.

Spontaneous yawning may occur in comatose patients. Apparently, neural networks for this complex respiratory response are integrated in the lower brain stem.

Differential Diagnosis of Coma

Metabolic causes and *toxic ingestions* account for the largest number of patients with depressed consciousness (Table 144-5).[13] The single most important sign distinguishing metabolic from structural coma is the presence of the pupillary light response.[12] In metabolic coma, confusion and stupor commonly precede symmetrical motor signs. Asterixis, myoclonus, tremor, and seizures are common. Central hyperventilation occurs frequently.

Supratentorial mass lesions causing compression or displacement of the upper brain stem (Table 144-6) usually present with focal neurologic signs that are asymmetrical. Neurologic dysfunction usually progresses in a rostral-caudal fashion, and the examination usually points to one anatomic area of the brain stem at a given point in time.

Subtentorial masses or destructive lesions causing coma (Table 144-6) usually have a history of brain stem dysfunction or sudden onset of coma. Brain stem signs always precede or accompany the onset of coma and always include abnormalities of eye movements. Cranial nerve palsies are usually present. Irregular respiratory patterns are common and usually appear at the onset of coma.

TABLE 144-5 Metabolic Causes of Coma

1. Hypoxia: decreased P_{O_2}, anemia, cyanide poisoning, carbon monoxide poisoning, methemoglobinemia
2. Ischemia: cardiac arrest, shock, blood hyperviscosity, cerebral arterial spasm after subarachnoid hemorrhage, disseminated intravascular coagulation, systemic lupus, multifocal embolism, hypertensive encephalopathy, arteritis
3. Hypoglycemia
4. Cofactor deficiency: thiamine, niacin, pyridoxine, vitamin B_{12}, folate
5. Infections: meningitis, encephalitis, postinfectious demyelinating encephalomyelitis, brain abscess
6. Hepatic or renal failure
7. Systemic diseases: septicemia, paraneoplastic syndromes, hypothyroidism, porphyria
8. Exogenous toxins and drugs: benzodiazepines, opiate analgesics, barbiturates, anticonvulsants, salicylates, ethanol, tricyclic antidepressants, anticholinergics, phenothiazines, amphetamines, cocaine, lithium, monoamine oxidase inhibitors, antihistamines, lysergic acid diethylamide (LSD), paraldehyde, methanol, ethylene glycol, cimetidine, heavy metals, organic phosphates, penicillins
9. Fluid and electrolyte disorders: hypo- and hypernatremia, hypo- and hyperosmolality, acid-base disorders, extreme values of calcium, magnesium, phosphorus
10. Hypothermia and heat stroke

TABLE 144-6 Focal Neurologic Lesions Causing Coma

Supratentorial lesions (compress the midbrain)
- Cerebral hemorrhage
- Large cerebral infarction
- Subdural hematoma
- Epidural hematoma
- Brain tumor
- Brain abscess

Posterior fossa lesions
- Brain stem infarction
- Cerebellar or brain stem hemorrhage
- Cerebellar or brain stem tumor
- Cerebellar abscess

Diagnostic Procedures in Evaluating the Comatose Patient

Keeping in mind the above differential diagnosis for states of coma, the sequence of diagnostic studies becomes clear. Rapid identification of metabolic or toxic causes of coma is determined by laboratory testing of blood, urine, gastric aspirate, and cerebrospinal fluid (CSF) (see Tables 144-3 and 144-5).

Intracranial mass lesions can be rapidly identified by computed tomography (CT) scanning. Although magnetic resonance imaging (MRI) is more sensitive than CT at identifying small brain lesions, CT is highly reliable at identifying supratentorial masses and acute intracranial hemorrhage of diverse cause. CT is the test of choice in acute trauma because it provides detailed images of bony structures of the skull base.[14] In addition, CT can be performed easily and rapidly in critically ill, intubated, and artificially ventilated patients. Full cardiac, respiratory, and hemodynamic monitoring may continue during CT scanning, a feat currently difficult with MRI. Identification of specific intracranial lesions (tumor, hematoma, hydrocephalus) should lead to rapid diagnosis and treatment by the appropriate neurologic consultant.

In cases of acute subarachnoid or intracerebral hemorrhage, early angiography may be indicated for rapid diagnosis of aneurysm or vascular malformations.[15] However, this procedure will always follow CT scanning.

Lumbar puncture and CSF examination is essential in the diagnosis of meningitis and encephalitis.[16] However, unless acute bacterial meningitis is strongly suspected, CT scanning should precede lumbar puncture to diagnose possible intracranial mass lesions, hydrocephalus, or brain edema. If it is essential to obtain CSF in states associated with intracranial masses and intracranial hypertension, ventriculostomy may be performed safely and provides an excellent tool for subsequent monitoring and treatment of intracranial hypertension.

Electroencephalography (EEG) is useful in the diagnosis of metabolic encephalopathies, although it is nonspecific in regard to cause (i.e., uremia versus hepatic failure).[17–19] A rare patient in coma from nonconvulsive status epilepticus will be identified by EEG. The primary use for EEG is as a confirmatory test for brain death when clinical criteria are inadequate.[20] Evoked-potential studies (visual, auditory, and somatosensory) have been used extensively in the hope they would provide information about prognosis in comatose patients with acute brain damage.[18,21] In general, they are no more useful than the clinical examination, except for somatosensory evoked-potential response (SSER). SSERs are resistant to sedative drug intoxication and may be present in drug overdose states that cause an "isoelectric" EEG. The persistence of cortical SSERs in comatose patients with head trauma predicts potential recovery in about one-third of patients; the absence of SSER predicts poor outcome in the vast majority.[22]

Selected Causes of Coma

Head trauma, drug intoxications, metabolic derangements, and *cerebrovascular diseases,* all important causes of coma in the ICU, are reviewed in other chapters.

Hypoxic-ischemic encephalopathy is the most common and most devastating cause of coma in most critical care units. The term is a pathologic diagnosis that refers to the effects of various degrees of global brain ischemia, sometimes complicated by hypoxemia. Cardiac arrest is the most common cause of global brain ischemia.[11,23–25] Each year, there are 200,000 attempts at cardiac resuscitation, and only 70,000 are successful. Of the early survivors, 30 percent leave the hospital, but only 10 percent resume their former lifestyle because of permanent neurologic deficits. Other important causes of global brain ischemia include severe hypotension, cardiac failure, strangulation, cardiopulmonary bypass, status epilepticus, diffuse cerebral atherosclerosis, increased intracranial pressure, cerebral arterial spasm, closed head trauma, and hyperviscosity.

The degree of neuronal injury in this condition depends on the degree of mismatch between metabolic demand and delivery of substrate (oxygen and glucose) to the brain.[26] For example, the brain can tolerate 45 min of total circulatory arrest with complete recovery if hypothermia to 18°C. is induced. Conversely, a brain with metabolic activity that is eightfold above normal during status epilepticus will sustain neuronal damage after 2 h, even with perfect maintenance of arterial oxygenation, glucose, and blood pressure.

The neurologic syndromes that follow cardiac arrest and resuscitation are diverse and depend on the duration of ischemia [time from arrest to cardiopulmonary resuscitation (CPR)], adequacy of CPR, underlying cardiovascular disease, degree of arterial atherosclerosis, and adequacy of postresuscitation cerebral perfusion. Patients in coma less than 12 h after resuscitation usually make an excellent recovery. Those in coma more than 12 h have permanent neurologic deficits due to focal or multifocal infarcts of the cerebral cortex in arterial border zones. They may be left with permanent amnesia, dementia, bibrachial or quadriparesis, cortical blindness, seizures, myoclonus, and ataxia.[27,28] If the coma persists for 1 week, recovery is rare, and most patients remain in a persistent vegetative state due to laminar necrosis of the cerebral cortex with preservation of brain stem function.[29,30]

Early in the course of hypoxic-ischemic encephalopathy, specific neurologic signs can predict outcome with a high degree of reliability. In a study of 210 patients, the absence of pupillary responses on the first day after CPR predicted poor outcome.[31] None of 52 patients recovered and only 3 regained consciousness. No patient who lacked corneal reflexes after the first day ever regained consciousness. After 3 days, a lack of purposeful motor responses predicted poor outcome in all patients (persistent vegetative state or severe disability). Certain early signs were associated with good recovery. At 1 day, the following signs were associated with at least a 50 percent chance of regaining independent function: verbal responses of any type, purposeful eye movements or motor responses, normal ocular reflexes, and response to verbal commands.

The cause of hypoxic-ischemic encephalopathy is not a simple response to circulatory arrest. Evidence has accumulated that the brain can tolerate a longer period of ischemia than previously thought if certain conditions are met. After a 10-min period of global brain ischemia, if the circulation is adequately restored, there is marked hyperemia, subsequently followed by a delayed, progressive fall in cerebral blood flow, to levels considerably below prearrest values.[32] In some cases, cerebral metabolism remains high in the face of low blood flow, a situation that worsens the effects of the initial ischemia. There is experimental evidence suggesting that if cerebral blood flow can be maintained at a hyperemic level, brain recovery can occur.[33] It appears that some of the damage is due to a lack of adequate reperfusion after resuscitation, the *no-reflow* phenomenon. The mechanisms of delayed hypoperfusion and no reflow are poorly understood but may be due to diffuse arterial spasm, calcium influx, vasoconstrictor prostaglandins, and intravascular coagulation. In addition, other biochemical changes are initiated after ischemia which can cause delayed neuronal injury: elevation of intracellular calcium, release of neurotoxic excitatory amino acids (glutamate and aspartate), reoxygenation injury from superoxide formation, and brain lactic acidosis.[34,35]

The pathophysiology of cerebral blood flow and metabolism following CPR is complex and points to several windows of opportunity, where the devastating effects of global brain ischemia may be ameliorated. Calcium channel blockers such as nimodipine, nicardipine, and lidoflazine are being investigated, experimentally and clinically, to determine if they can prevent neuronal damage following global brain ischemia and improve cerebral perfusion after resuscitation.[33] Excitatory amino acid antagonists (MK-801) may be effective at preventing delayed neuronal injury after ischemia.[36] Free radical scavengers and drugs which specifically treat brain acidosis are being developed.

Treatment of Coma

Treatment must be instituted immediately, even when the diagnosis is uncertain, to prevent further brain damage secondary to complications. Oxygenation must be assured, and airway protection is essential. All patients in coma should have a cuffed endotracheal tube placed quickly; the need for mechanical ventilation is determined by the degree of spontaneous breathing and the need for therapeutic hyperventilation. Trauma patients with suspected cervical spine injuries may need emergency tracheostomy to avoid extension of the neck during endotracheal tube placement. Subsequent ventilator adjustments are determined by arterial blood gases.

Arterial blood pressure must be maintained. Hypotension results in secondary brain ischemia. Intravascular volume replacement with blood or isotonic solutions often requires hemodynamic monitoring. The goals are to attain normal intravascular volume with normal central venous pressure, pulmonary artery wedge pressure, mean arterial pressure, and normal blood osmolality. Excessive volume replacement can aggravate intracranial hypertension, especially if hypotonic solutions are administered and serum osmolality falls. Inadequate intravascular volume will cause a fall in cardiac output and worsen brain ischemia. Inotropic and vasopressor drugs are administered as needed.

As part of the initial management of all patients with coma, glucose should be given (50 mL of 50% glucose) as soon as blood is sent to the laboratory. Although there is a theoretical risk of hyperglycemia causing brain lactic acidosis during ischemia, the risk of damage from hypoglycemic coma is much greater and requires emergency treatment. Thiamine, 100 mg intramuscular or intravenous, is administered with the glucose.

Seizures, regardless of cause, must be stopped. The treatment of recurrent seizures is described in Chap. 142.

Intracranial hypertension, if present, should be treated aggressively using intracranial pressure monitoring as a guideline for treatment.[14,37] Details of intracranial pressure monitoring and treatment are described in Chap. 34.

Systemic infections, especially gram-negative sepsis, can cause stupor or coma on a toxic basis and must be promptly treated. Severe acid-base disorders, while rarely responsible by themselves for coma, can worsen the overall situation by causing secondary cardiovascular and respiratory failure. Rapid correction of severe acidosis or alkalosis is essential.

Hyperthermia can accompany a variety of pathological states, either infectious or secondary to hypothalamic or brain stem damage. A 1°C elevation of body temperature will increase tissue metabolic demand by 3 percent. Therefore, hyperthermia can itself exacerbate the harmful effects of ischemia, hypoxia, or hypoglycemia. Hyperthermia should be aggressively treated; mild hypothermia exerts a protective effect on the brain.

Specific antidotes may be effective in coma secondary to drug intoxication. Details of treatment for drug overdose are described in other chapters.

Other than general measures, as outlined above, treatment depends on accurate diagnosis of cause and specific directed treatment, i.e., surgical evacuation of subdural hematoma.

Prognosis and the Persistent Vegetative State (PVS)

Prospective studies in the 1970s of patients with nontraumatic coma provide the best available information regarding prognosis in patients with PVS after hypoxic-ischemic encephalopathy.[1,29,31] Every year in the United States there are 2000 new patients with PVS after head trauma, but the long-term outcome of these patients is unknown.[38]

In the first few days after onset of coma, it is impossible to predict the likelihood of PVS. The absence of pupillary responses and corneal reflexes after the first day of coma predicts a poor outcome in 99 percent of patients but does not tell us which patients will die and which will survive in a vegetative state. It takes at least 2 weeks to determine, with a high degree of certainty, which patients will remain vegetative. In the Levy study of 24 patients who remained vegetative after 2 weeks and survived to 1 month, only 5 were alive at the end of 1 year, 3 permanently vegetative and 2 with overwhelming neurologic and mental impairments.

Hopefully, in the future, noninvasive cerebral blood flow and metabolic studies will allow us to predict with certainty, early on, which patients will have permanent, irreversible brain damage that will result in a PVS.[30] When we attain that capability, families of patients and physicians will be in a better position to make intelligent decisions about continuation or termination of medical treatments for critically ill patients in coma.[39,40]

Declaration of Death Using Neurologic Criteria

In recent years, the success rate of organ transplantation has increased dramatically and transplantation has become standard therapy for patients with end-stage kidney, heart, and liver disease. Unfortunately, thousands of critically ill patients will not receive needed organs due to a lack of understanding of the concepts and criteria for the declaration of death. We are wasting a rare and precious resource because health professionals, as well as the public, have been misinformed about definitions and procedures necessary to declare death in the setting of massive, irreversible brain damage.[41]

Although specific protocols for the determination of death vary slightly from institution to institution, guidelines in the United States were firmly established by the President's Commission in 1981 and have been uniformly accepted by the American Medical Association, American Academy of Neurology, and American Bar Association.[42]

The Uniform Determination of Death Act states that "an individual who has sustained either (1) irreversible cessation of circulatory and respiratory functions, or (2) irreversible cessation of all functions of the entire brain, including the brain stem, is dead. A determination of death must be made in accordance with accepted medical standards."

In 1987, the state of New York adopted the above statement as the legal definition of death. At the present time, 41 states have similar statutes, and an additional 6 states have high court judicial rulings permitting death determination by neurologic criteria.[43,44]

However, confusion still surrounds (1) the definition of death and (2) the criteria for determining death in a patient who has stable cardiovascular function but irreversible cessation of brain function. Part of this confusion arises from the continued use of the ambiguous term *brain death*, implying that there is more than one type of death. If health professionals are confused about this concept, it is no surprise that the public remains uncertain about the terminology.

The medical and legal definitions of death are clear: brain death and cardiac death are the same. Dissenting opinions from the strict religious orthodoxy of Roman Catholicism and Orthodox Judaism persist, however, due to individual interpretations and applications of religious beliefs and laws. It is unlikely that there will ever be a unanimously accepted definition of death due to diverse religious and ethical opinions. However, as a practical matter, religious objections to determination of death by brain criteria have little impact on overall organ donation efforts.

In the diagnosis of death by neurologic criteria, a correct neurologic diagnosis is essential. The President's Commission clearly states that the determination of death by neurologic criteria is a clinical diagnosis, with preconditions and confirmatory tests. The core of the clinical diagnosis is to establish unresponsiveness and brain stem areflexia. The preconditions are that (1) the cause of coma be known and (2) the cause be adequate to explain the coma.[45,46] Careful attention to these preconditions will alert the intensivist to special circumstances that require reevaluation and confirmatory tests. In the press for organ procurement, the cautious physician may be perceived as delaying the transplant process to ensure that the diagnosis of death is unequivocal.

The Commission's recommendations grew out of studies at Harvard Medical School in the 1960s, and extensive collaborative studies sponsored by the NINCDS in the years 1971–1972.[47,48] These clinical studies were performed before the availability of CT imaging, making the *cause of coma* and anatomic extent of brain damage uncertain in many cases. Therefore, the use of routine EEG became a standard part of many determination-of-death protocols. With the ability to directly visualize the extent of brain damage in comatose patients by CT, the determination of irreversibility became more precise. To this day, however, there continues to be uneccessary reliance on confirmatory laboratory tests rather than the use of objective clinical criteria.

In New York and most other states in the United States and many countries around the world, clinical criteria are sufficient to diagnose brain death. Confirmatory tests such as EEG and cerebral blood flow studies are reserved for situations where there is uncertainty regarding cause and reversibility of coma.

Determination of Death by Neurologic Criteria

The quoted material in this section is from the President's Commission.[42]

"A. An individual with irreversible cessation of all functions of the entire brain, including the brain stem, is dead."

The *functions* of the brain that are relevant are those that can be evaluated by clinical examination. It is important that the physician who examines a patient to make a determination of death is experienced in neurologic examinations and understands the significance of the findings.

"1. Cessation is recognized when evaluation discloses findings of a and b:

a. Cerebral functions are absent, and . . ."

The patient must be in deep coma and unresponsive to all external stimuli, including pain, bright light, or loud noises. Spinal reflexes and motor responses are permitted. Spontaneous movements other than of spinal origin and epileptic seizures must be absent. Certain neurologic disorders can result in total muscular paralysis with preserved consciousness and cognition (locked-in syndrome from discrete brain stem infarction or neuromuscular paralysis). In these circumstances, EEG or cerebral blood flow studies may be necessary to determine the integrity of the cerebral hemispheres.

"b. . . . brain stem functions are absent."

Pupils must be unreactive to stimulation with a bright light. Size is not important, and pupils may be small, midposition, or large. The pupillary light reflex may be altered by mydriatic agents, and drugs such as glutethimide, scopolamine, dopamine, norepinephrine, opiates, cocaine, amphetamine, atropine, and neuromuscular blocking agents. The presence of ocular trauma or previous eye surgery (cataracts) can alter the light reflex.

Ocular movements must be absent to passive head turning and to irrigation of patent ear canals with 30 mL of iced water with the head elevated 30°. Aural trauma, labyrinthine disease, sedatives, anticholinergic drugs, anticonvulsants, aminoglycoside antibiotics, and tricyclic antidepressants may alter this response.

Corneal reflexes are variable. When present, they are meaningful, but their absence does not necessarily mean irreversible damage to the brain stem.

Oropharyngeal reflexes ("gag" reflexes) are usually not testable in near-dead patients due to the presence of endotracheal tubes and other oral hardware. Bronchial reflexes can be assessed by passing a suction catheter into the trachea.

Apnea testing is a critical part of brain stem assessment and determines irreversible damage to the medulla.[49,50] Great variability is reported in the performance of this test, but there are minimum requirements. The patient must have a normal blood pressure and is ventilated with 100 percent oxygen for 10 min prior to testing. This assures adequate oxygen reserves to prevent hypoxemia during apnea. A maximum stimulus for breathing is attained when P_{CO_2} is greater than 60 torr. This level is attained in 10 to 15 min of apnea depending on the level of P_{CO_2} at the beginning of the test. Oxygen lines and tubes from the patient to the mechanical ventilator remain connected throughout the test. If adequate oxygenation is maintained, the test is easily performed without complication. Arterial blood gases will confirm the appropriate level of P_{CO_2}, and direct observation of respiratory movements by the physician will determine brain stem function. If the patient is not adequately oxygenated, the blood pressure will fall, cardiac arrhythmias will develop, and spinal cord hypoxia will result in spontaneous myoclonic spinal movements.

Decerebrate and decorticate posturings require intact brain stem structures at and below the level of the vestibular nuclei (pontomedullary junction) and are inconsistent with the diagnosis of death.

"2. Irreversibility is recognized when evaluation discloses findings of a and b and c:

a. The cause of coma is established and is sufficient to account for the loss of brain function."

With the advent of CT scanning, precise neurologic diagnosis became a routine matter. The combination of clinical history, neurologic examination, and cranial CT, in most cases, will identify the cause of coma and can precisely localize the extent of damage to the cerebral hemispheres and brain stem. Uncertainty exists in conditions that cause diffuse damage to the brain, such as cerebral hypoxia, ischemia, uremia, hepatic failure, meningitis, encephalitis, and drug intoxication. Appropriate testing will provide a correct diagnosis but may preclude the determination of death. Drug screening is an essential part of every examination, since drug intoxication may contribute to the clinical problem, if not the primary cause of coma.

In rare situations, the precise cause of coma cannot be immediately determined. In such cases, prolonged observation, EEG, and cerebral blood flow studies may be necessary for diagnosis. Such cases are often due to an unidentified drug, and much caution should be taken before declaring death.

"b. The possibility of recovery of any brain functions is excluded."

The most important reversible conditions are sedative drug intoxications, hypothermia, neuromuscular paralysis (primary or drug induced), and severe hypotension. By systematic evaluation, these conditions can be identified and corrected. If drug intoxication is diagnosed, prognosis is uncertain until the drug is metabolized or removed. Drug-induced coma may result in an electrically silent EEG; auditory and SSERs are usually preserved. Core temperature must be above 35°C to determine irreversible coma. Gradual warming can be attained with standard "warming blankets." Severe neuromuscular paralysis can be identified at the bedside with a peripheral nerve stimulator. Severe hypotension must be corrected before applying the criteria for determination of death.

"c. The cessation of all brain functions persists for an appropriate period of observation and/or trial of therapy."

In the absence of drug intoxication, hypothermia, young age, or hypotension and a precise diagnosis of structural damage to the brain fully accounting for the total absence of brain function, a period of 12 h of observation is sufficient to make a declaration of death.

Following global brain ischemia/hypoxia, a period of 24 h is sufficient time for initial treatment and observation before a diagnosis of death is made.

In clinical situations where there is doubt regarding the cause of coma, all available diagnostic studies should be utilized to make a definitive diagnosis. If this is still not possible, confirmatory tests such as EEG and cerebral blood flow studies should be used for evidence of death of the entire brain.

Confirmatory Tests for the Diagnosis of Death

ELECTROENCEPHALOGRAPHY

The "isoelectric" EEG was first associated with loss of brain function in 1959 and subsequently became important as part of the Harvard criteria for brain death in 1968.[47] The Harvard criteria recommended two separate EEG recordings, 24 h apart, both showing an absence of EEG activity. However, the authors were aware of the difficulties of requiring a technologically advanced test in all hospitals. They therefore stated that "in situations where . . . electroencephalographic monitoring is not available, the absence of cerebral function has to be determined by purely clinical signs."

In 1972, the United States Collaborative Study of Cerebral Death applied the Harvard criteria to a prospective cohort of 503 patients in deep apneic coma.[48] The Harvard criteria were much too restrictive, and the Collaborative Study found that unresponsivity, apnea, brain stem areflexia, and a single isoelectric EEG had 100 percent accuracy in predicting somatic death. The Collaborative Study also confirmed a critical fact: patients who recover from apneic coma with an isoelectric EEG have unrecognized sedative drug intoxication. Occasional patients with isolated loss of brain stem function due to infarction or hemorrhage have persistent EEG activity, as do those afflicted with total neuromuscular paralysis.

The influence of the Harvard criteria and the Collaborative NINDS Study are evident in the continued requirements for EEG confirmation of death in protocols in many hospitals throughout the United States. However, the President's Commission in 1971 recognized that the EEG is optional when the clinical diagnosis is uncertain, and the majority of states in the United States have adopted the Uniform Determination of Death Act and the recommendations of the President's Commission.[43,45]

If the cause of coma is clearly established from anatomic imaging studies of the brain and clinical criteria are met that all brain functions are absent, EEG confirmation is not necessary.[51] If there is doubt regarding diagnosis, then all available tests should be performed, and a declaration of death may not be made. Apneic coma and an isoelectric EEG in the face of normal brain imaging studies are strongly suggestive of sedative drug intoxication, and appropriate toxicology studies must be performed.

CEREBRAL BLOOD FLOW STUDIES

1. *Four-vessel cerebral angiography* may be performed in clinically dead patients who have an uncertain diagnosis.[45] Complete absence of cerebral circulation is an absolute confirmation of brain death. The major use of the technique is for rapid diagnosis of death in patients whose clinical examination is obscured by hypothermia or drug intoxication. The need for organ donation will usually prompt this examination; the alternative is to wait until complicating factors are corrected.

2. *Radioisotope brain scanning* can accurately document absent brain blood flow in the cerebral hemispheres but not in the vertebrobasilar circulation.[52] Some institutions have portable units that can be brought to the bedside in the ICU. Because this technique does not image the posterior circulation, the clinical diagnosis of brain stem areflexia becomes even more important. In situations of suspected or known drug intoxication, isotope brain scanning is not helpful, since it will not answer the question of whether brainstem areflexia is due to drug effect or irreversible damage.

3. *Transcranial Doppler sonography* is a noninvasive bedside technique that can measure, in a qualitative fashion, blood flow in the proximal portions of the middle cerebral arteries. An ultrasonic probe is placed over the temporal bones, and direction and velocity of flow can be measured. A number of investigators have shown that absence or reversal of diastolic flow in the middle cerebral arteries can be demonstrated in most patients who meet the traditional criteria for brain death.[53] About 10 percent of patients cannot be insonated because of excessive skull thickness. This technique is roughly equivalent to isotope brain scanning, since it only provides information about the anterior circulation.

4. *Xenon-enhanced CT* is a noninvasive technique for accurately measuring brain blood flow in all arterial territories. It has been used in young children and infants with great reliability to confirm the clinical criteria of death.[54] In children, especially, it overcomes many of the problems associated with EEG and cerebral angiography. Unfortunately, the technique is only available in a few large referral centers.

Special Considerations in Young Children and Infants

The criteria for determination of death outlined by the President's Commission in 1981 urged caution in applying the criteria to children under 5 years of age. It is generally assumed that the young brain has a greater capacity for recovery after acute insults; therefore, special modifications were recommended by the Task Force for the Determination of Brain Death in Children, published in 1987.[55]

The clinical and laboratory criteria are identical to those applied to older children and adults, i.e., apneic coma with brain stem areflexia. The modifications apply to the periods of observation recommended before determining irreversibility of coma.

1. Premature infants and term newborns: Newborns, premature or term, are difficult to evaluate after perinatal insults, and no specific criteria are recommended. It is suggested that a waiting period of 7 days after the acute insult be established before the extent and reversibility of brain injury is determined by clinical and laboratory investigations.
2. Seven days to 2 months: Two clinical examinations and EEGs separated by 48 h.
3. Two months to 1 year: Two examinations and EEGs separated by 24 h. A repeat examination and EEG may be omitted if a radionuclide angiogram demonstrates absence of the cerebral circulation.
4. Over 1 year: The criteria are the same as for older children and adults. When an irreversible cause exists, laboratory testing is not required.

CASE PRESENTATION

A 61-year-old man awoke in the morning with vertigo, nausea, vomiting, dysarthria, and ataxia. By the time he arrived at the hospital emergency room, he had a mild occipital headache, but the vertigo and nausea had resolved.

Past medical history was notable for atherosclerotic coronary artery disease. Nine years prior to the current admission, he underwent coronary artery bypass surgery for severe exertional angina pectoris and three-vessel coronary artery disease. He also had hypertension, hypercholesterolemia, and intermittent atrial fibrillation. Medications at the time of hospital admission were verapamil 120 mg daily, atenolol 25 mg daily, aspirin 325 mg daily, and lovastatin 20 mg daily.

Examination on admission was notable for blood pressure 190/100 and pulse 90 with irregularly irregular cardiac rhythm. Carotid pulses were brisk without bruits. Lungs were clear and cardiac auscultation revealed normal heart sounds without gallops or murmurs. The abdomen was soft with normal bowel sounds, and peripheral arterial pulses were normal. He was awake, alert, and attentive, fully oriented, and able to describe recent and past events with great accuracy. The only abnormalities on neurologic examination were mild dysarthria, horizontal nystagmus to the right and left, rotary nystagmus on up gaze, gait ataxia, and intention tremor of the right arm and leg.

Complete blood count and chemistry screen were normal. ECG showed atrial fibrillation with a ventricular rate of 95. Computerized tomography of the brain showed lucencies in both cerebellar hemispheres, compatible with bilateral cerebellar infarctions, most likely due to cardiogenic embolism related to atrial fibrillation.

The patient was admitted to the neurologic ICU for monitoring of neurologic signs and was started on intravenous heparin to prevent recurrent embolism. Ten hours after hospital admission, he suddenly became unresponsive to verbal stimuli with stridorous breathing. He was intubated and hyperventilated to maintain P_{CO_2} at 30 to 35 torr. Pupils were 2 mm, irregular in shape but reactive to light. There were no movements of the eyes to head turning or ice water caloric testing. Corneal reflexes were absent. Painful stimulation initiated extensor posturing of all four limbs. Heparin was discontinued even though coagulation studies were all at "control" values. Mannitol and dexamethasone were administered intravenously.

An emergency CT scan revealed a large hematoma in the right cerebellum, causing compression of the brain stem and obstruction of the IVth ventricle with acute hydrocephalus. Immediate neurosurgical consultation was obtained, and the patient underwent surgical evacuation of the hematoma and placement of an external ventricular drain.

On the second hospital day, he remained deeply comatose, without any response to pain, no reflex eye movements, and trace corneal reflexes but had small, equal pupils that remained reactive to light.

On the third hospital day, he awakened. He opened his eyes to voice and could protrude his tongue to verbal command. He was able to blink and move his eyes in all directions of gaze. Pupils remained at 2.5 mm and reacted briskly to light. Facial grimacing was appropriate. He was able to lift his right arm and leg in a purposeful fashion on verbal command.

Late on the third hospital day, he suddenly deteriorated and again became comatose with loss of all brain stem functions except pupillary responses. A repeat CT scan showed edema and residual hemorrhage in the cerebellum, with dilated lateral ventricles. Mannitol was given intravenously and a new ventricular drain was placed.

Over the next 5 days, there was minimal improvement. He did not respond to voice or visual threat. Painful stimulation elicited extensor posturing of all four limbs. Pupils remained reactive to light, and corneal reflexes were present. There were trace eye movements with the doll's head maneuver. Blood pressure control became extremely difficult due to abrupt extreme fluctuations from frank hypotension to severe hypertension.

On the eighth hospital day, the patient's wife requested a do-not resuscitate (DNR) order since the prognosis for recovery was poor. However, all aggressive treatment measures were continued.

On the ninth hospital day, the patient was awake. He opened his eyes to command, nodded his head yes/no appropriately, wiggled the toes of both feet, and was able to lift his right leg off the bed on request. The DNR order was canceled.

On the tenth day, he developed a fever to 103°F. Although all cultures were negative, ventriculitis was strongly suspected, and he was treated with vancomycin and ceftazidime. From the tenth until the fifteenth hospital day, he remained in deep coma, unresponsive to all external stimuli. Brain stem reflexes remained intact as documented by normal pupillary responses, corneal reflexes, and eye movement reflexes.

On the fifteenth hospital day, he awakened and was able to follow commands, blink, move his eyes, nod his head, and withdraw his limbs in a purposeful fashion.

On the eighteenth day, he was weaned from the ventilator and was medically stable.

On the ninteenth hospital day he suffered a major upper gastrointestinal hemorrhage accompanied by aspiration, severe hypoxemia, and shock. He remained pressor dependent for 48 h and required mechanical ventilation.

On the twenty-first hospital day, he was medically stable but deeply comatose and still required mechanical ventilation. There were no responses to any external stimuli, including pain. Continuous myoclonic movements of the face were noted and successfully treated with intravenous diazepam. Pupillary responses, reflex eye movements, and corneal reflexes persisted. The DNR orders were written again at the request of the family. No further neurologic improvement occurred over the next several days.

On the twenty-fourth hospital day, bradycardia and hypotension developed and were not treated. The patient died.

CASE DISCUSSION

This patient's hospital course was characterized by a complex series of both primary neurologic injury and medical complications. The interaction of these various factors ultimately determined the outcome.

On admission to the hospital, the problem was straightforward. The patient had a typical syndrome of cerebellar infarction in the setting of atrial fibrillation and cardiogenic embolism. The embolic events occurred while he was taking aspirin, and anticoagulation with heparin was clearly indicated in this setting. However, it is recognized that there is a small but definite risk of hemorrhagic transformation of large brain infarcts, and careful monitoring in the ICU was appropriate.

The abrupt onset of coma with respiratory compromise is characteristic of primary brain stem injury, and early loss of brain stem reflexes was consistent with that diagnosis. The preservation of pupillary responses indicated a small but definite chance for reversibility and recovery. The differential diagnosis at this point included cerebellar hemorrhagic infarction with brain stem compression, brain stem infarction from basilar artery occlusion, and acute hydrocephalus due to cerebellar edema. CT scanning was mandatory as an emergency diagnostic procedure. Mannitol and dexamethasone would have little effect on brain stem compression from a cerebellar hematoma because of the small volume of the posterior fossa. Surgical decompression was the only possible treatment option.

For the first 24 h after surgery, his neurologic examination indicated a severe degree of brain injury with loss of all brain stem reflexes except for pupillary responses. However, standard rating scales such as the Glasgow Coma Scale would not be helpful in predicting prognosis. The Glasgow Coma Scale does not include pupillary responses, and the patient would score the lowest possible value. The Levy criteria would indicate less than a 5 percent chance of good recovery. Yet the ability to recover from brain stem injury is astonishing and, with our current limitations in knowledge, difficult to predict. This uncertainty was demonstrated by the dramatic recovery on the third day, only to be followed by another abrupt deterioration within hours due to cerebellar edema and recurrent hydrocephalus from ventricular drain obstruction.

In spite of aggressive treatment, little improvement occurred. The labile blood pressure was indicative of changes in brain stem compression. Increasing compression causes brain stem ischemia, resulting in a compensatory rise in blood pressure to maintain brain stem perfusion (Cushing response). If the hypertensive peaks are treated too aggressively, it could precipitate brain stem infarction. In addition, sudden resolution of the Cushing response will cause a fall in blood pressure. If long-acting antihypertensive medications have been administered, dangerous hypotension can ensue. The management of these patients requires minute-to-minute adjustment of short-acting intravenous agents that can be rapidly discontinued.

An appropriate DNR order was written after 1 week passed without evidence of awakening from coma. This does not imply cessation of treatment and only addresses how medical and nursing personnel will respond to a cardiac arrest. All aggressive measures are continued. However, it is recognized that if a cardiac arrest occurs in the setting of severe brain injury causing prolonged coma, the additional damage from hypoxia and ischemia makes the situation irreversible.

On the eighth day, the patient again improved, again demonstrating the uncertainties in predicting neurologic recovery. His subsequent deterioration from the tenth to the fifteenth day was related to severe infection, probably verticulitis. His neurologic examination reflected a superimposed *metabolic encephalopathy* with normal brain stem functions but deep coma. Successful treatment of the infection resulted in reawakening on the fifteenth day.

He continued to improve until the nineteenth day when gastrointestinal bleeding, aspiration, hypoxemia and hypotension caused major hypoxic-ischemic cerebral injury superimposed on the primary brain stem pathology. This was manifested by profound and persistent coma with multifocal myoclonus in the setting of preserved brain stem function. After medical stabilization, his neurologic state was the same. After 3 days, the chance of good neurologic recovery was virtually nil, the probability of PVS high, and DNR orders were written. Cardiac death occurred on the twenty-fourth day. Determination of brain death was not necessary.

Although it is impossible to be certain, based on his neurologic examination on the fifteenth day, if no further medical complications had developed, the patient had better than a 50 percent chance of making a good neurologic recovery based on the Levy studies.

References

1. Levy DE, Bates D, Caronna JJ, et al: Prognosis in nontraumatic coma. Ann Intern Med 94:293, 1981.
2. Plum F, Posner JB: *The Diagnosis of Stupor and Coma,* 3rd ed. Philadelphia, F.A. Davis, 1980.
3. Longstreth WT, Jr, Diehr P, Inui TS: Prediction of awakening after out-of-hospital cardiac arrest. New Engl J Med 308:1378, 1983.
4. Hawkes CH: "Locked-in syndrome": Report of seven cases. Br Med J 4:379, 1974.
5. Jennett WB, Plum F: The persistent vegetative state: A syndrome in search of a name. Lancet 1:734, 1972.
6. Higashi K, Hatano M, Abiko S, et al: Five-year follow-up study of patients with persistent vegetative state. J Neurol Neurosurg Psychiatr 44:552, 1981.
7. Moruzzi G: The sleep-waking cycle. Rev Physiol 64:1, 1972.
8. Magoun HW: *The Waking Brain,* 2nd ed. Springfield, IL, Charles C. Thomas, 1963.
9. Fisher CM: The neurological examination of the comatose patient. Acta Neurol Scand 45(Suppl 36):1, 1969.
10. Pal J: The value of the Glasgow Coma Scale and Injury Severity Score in predicting outcome in multiple trauma patients with head injury. J Trauma 29:746, 1989.
11. Mullie A, Buylaert W, Michem N, et al: Predictive value of Glasgow Coma Score for awakening after out-of-hospital cardiac arrest. Cerebral Resuscitation Study Group of the Belgian Society for Intensive Care. Lancet 1:137, 1988.
12. Fisher CM: Some neuro-ophthalmological observations. J Neurol Neurosurg Psychiatr 30:383, 1967.
13. Ashton CH, Teoh R, Davies DM: Drug-induced stupor and coma: Some physical signs and their pharmacological basis. Adverse Drug React Acute Poisoning Rev 8:1, 1989.
14. Fink ME: Emergency management of the head-injured patient. Emerg Med Clin North Am 5:783, 1987.
15. Solomon RA, Fink ME: Current strategies for the management of aneurysmal subarachnoid hemorrhage. Arch Neurol 44:769, 1987.
16. Fishman RA: *Cerebrospinal Fluid in Diseases of the Nervous System.* Philadelphia, W.B. Saunders, 1980.
17. Austin, EJ, Wilkus RJ, Longstreth WT: Etiology and prognosis of alpha coma. Neurology 38:773, 1988.

18. Ganes T, Lundar T: EEG and evoked potentials in comatose patients with severe brain damage. Electroencephalogr Clin Neurophysiol 69:6, 1988.
19. Tasker RC, Boyd S, Harden A, et al: Monitoring in non-traumatic coma. Part II: Electroencephalography. Arch Dis Child 63:895, 1988.
20. Chatrian GE: Electrophysiologic evaluation of brain death: A critical appraisal, in Aminoff MJ (ed): *Electrodiagnosis in Clinical Neurology*, 2nd ed. New York, Churchill Livingstone, 1986, pp 669–736.
21. Cascino GD: Neurophysiological monitoring in the intensive care unit. J Intensive Care Med 3:215, 1988.
22. Ahmed I: Use of somatosensory evoked responses in the prediction of outcome from coma. Clin Electroencephalogr 19:78, 1988.
23. Bertini G, Margheri M, Giglioli C, et al: Prognostic significance of early clinical manifestations in postanoxic coma: A retrospective study of 58 patients resuscitated after prehospital cardiac arrest. Crit Care Med 17:627, 1989.
24. Brain Resuscitation Clinical Trial I Study Group: Randomized clinical study of thiopental loading in comatose survivors of cardiac arrest. N Engl J Med 314:397, 1986.
25. Earnest MP, Yarness PR, Merrill SL, et al: Long-term survival and neurologic status after resuscitation from out-of-hospital cardiac arrest. Neurology 30:1298, 1980.
26. Siesjo BK: Cerebral circulation and metabolism. J Neurosurg 60:883, 1984.
27. Caronna JJ, Finklestein S: Neurological syndromes after cardiac arrest. Stroke 9:517, 1978.
28. Krumholz A, Stern BJ, Weiss HD: Outcome from coma after cardiopulmonary resuscitation: Relation to seizures and myoclonus. Neurology 38:401, 1988.
29. Dougherty JH, Rawlinson, DG, Levy DE, et al: Hypoxic-ischemic brain injury and the vegetative state: Clinical and neuropathologic correlation. Neurology 31:991, 1981.
30. Levy DE, Sidtis JJ, Rottenberg DA, et al: Differences in cerebral blood flow and glucose utilization in vegetative versus locked-in patients. Ann Neurol 22:673, 1987.
31. Levy DE, Caronna JJ, Singer BH, et al: Predicting outcome from hypoxic-ischemic coma. JAMA 253:1420, 1985.
32. Beckstead JE, Tweed WA, Lee J, et al: Cerebral blood flow and metabolism in man following cardiac arrest. Stroke 9:569, 1978.
33. Safar P: Resuscitation from clinical death: Pathophysiologic limits and therapeutic potentials. Crit Care Med 16:923, 1988.
34. Krause GS, White BC, Aust SD, et al: Brain cell death following ischemia and reperfusion: A proposed biochemical sequence. Crit Care Med 16:714, 1988.
35. Rothman SM, Olney JW: Glutamate and the pathophysiology of hypoxic-ischemic brain damage. Ann Neurol 19:105, 1986.
36. Kochhar A, Zivin JA, Lyden PD, et al: Glutamate antagonist therapy reduces neurologic deficits produced by focal central nervous system ischemia. Arch Neurol 45:148, 1988.
37. Tasker RC, Matthew J, Helms P, et al: Monitoring in non-traumatic coma. Part I: Invasive intracranial measurements. Arch Dis Child 63:888, 1988.
38. Interagency Head Injury Task Force Report. National Institute of Neurological Disorders and Stroke, Department of Health and Human Services, Bethesda, MD, 1989.
39. American Academy of Neurology: Position of the American Academy of Neurology on certain aspects of the care and management of the persistent vegetative state patient. Neurology 38:125, 1989.
40. Munsat TL, Stuart WH, Cranford RE: Guidelines of the vegetative state: Commentary on the American Academy of Neurology statement. Neurology 38:123, 1989.
41. Bernat JL: Ethical issues in brain death and multiorgan transplantation. Neurol Clin 7:715, 1989.
42. Report of the Medical Consultants on the Diagnosis of Death to the President's Commission for the Study of Ethical Problems in Medicine and Biomedical and Behavioral Research: Guidelines for the determination of death. JAMA 246:2184, 1981.
43. Powner DJ: The diagnosis of brain death in the adult patient. J Intensive Care Med 2:181, 1987.
44. Walker AE: *Cerebral Death,* 3rd ed. Baltimore-Munich, Urban & Schwarzenberg, 1985
45. Black PM: Brain death. N Engl J Med 299:338, 393, 1978.
46. Black PM: Brain death in the intensive care unit. J Intensive Care Med 2:177, 1987.
47. Beecher HK: A definition of irreversible coma: Report of the ad hoc committee of the Harvard Medical School to examine the definition of brain death. JAMA 205:337, 1968.
48. NINCDS Collaborative Study: An appraisal of the criteria of cerebral death: A summary statement. JAMA 237:982, 1977.
49. Earnest MP, Beresford HR, McIntyre HB: Testing for apnea in suspected brain death: Methods used by 129 clinicians. Neurology 36:542, 1986.
50. Ropper AH, Kennedy SK, Russell L: Apnea testing in the diagnosis of brain death. J Neurosurg 55:942, 1981.
51. Grigg MM, Kelly MA, Celesia GG, et al: Electroencephalographic activity after brain death. Arch Neurol 44:948, 1987.
52. Goodman JM, Heck LL, Moore BD: Confirmation of brain death with portable isotope angiography: A review of 204 consecutive cases. Neurosurgery 16:492, 1985.
53. Petty GW, Mohr JP, Pedley TA, et al: The role of transcranial Doppler in confirming brain death: Sensitivity, specificity, and suggestions for performance and interpretation. Neurology 40:300, 1990.
54. Ashwal S, Schneider S, Thompson J: Xenon computed tomography measuring cerebral blood flow in the determination of brain death in children. Ann Neurol 25:539, 1989.
55. Task Force for the Determination of Brain Death in Children: Guidelines for the determination of brain death in children. Neurology 37:1077, 1987.

SECTION L

HEMATOLOGIC AND ONCOLOGIC DISORDERS IN THE CRITICALLY ILL

Chapter 145

ANEMIA, LEUKOPENIA, AND ELEVATED BLOOD COUNTS

R. BRIAN MITCHELL
PHILIP C. HOFFMAN

KEY POINTS

- *Assessment of the physiology and the morphology in each case of anemia or leukopenia will narrow the differential diagnosis.*
- *Anemia is due to hemorrhage until proven otherwise.*
- *A given degree of anemia affects each patient differently, depending on age, cardiac function, vascular integrity, oxygenation, and other concomitant disease.*
- *Compensatory mechanisms for anemia include increased cardiac output ($\dot{Q}_T$) and increased oxygen extraction.*
- *In patients with questionably adequate oxygen transport, blood transfusion to a hematocrit of 40 percent provides aerobic metabolism at lower $\dot{Q}_T$ and oxyhemoglobin saturation than during anemia.*

Approach to the Patient with Severe Anemia or Leukopenia

Patients with primary hematologic disorders are rarely admitted to an ICU because of their underlying disease, but frequently for complications of the disease or its treatment. On the other hand, hematologic disorders commonly develop in ICU patients. Anemia or leukopenia, of any cause, can range from mild to severe. Frequently, multiple etiologies are discovered. Clues to the underlying pathophysiology are found by examination of the patient, examination of the blood smear, and simple ancillary tests such as a reticulocyte count and a direct antiglobulin test. Classification based on cellular morphology will further limit the differential diagnosis (Table 145-1). Immediate decisions regarding transfusion or other therapy must be based on the underlying diagnosis and the patient's ability to tolerate anemia.

An isolated cytopenia suggests different diagnostic possibilities than does a trilineage abnormality. Examination of the blood smear may reveal both quantitative and qualitative abnormalities. White blood cell (WBC) effects may include neutropenia, lymphopenia, leukocytosis, increased early forms (myelocytes, promyelocytes, blasts), dysplastic changes (hypogranularity, chromatin abnormalities), or the presence of malignant cells (e.g., hairy cell leukemia, lymphoma). The many red blood cell (RBC) abnormalities (Table 145-2) are not entirely specific but are important to recognize when present. Reticulocytosis, polychromasia, basophilic stippling, or the presence of circulating nucleated RBCs indicates a component of blood loss or hemolysis. Platelet abnormalities include quantitative changes or the presence of giant platelets (>7 μm) or megakaryocyte fragments. If thrombocytopenia is detected by a machine count, platelet clumping must be excluded by performing a manual platelet estimation using the blood smear.

BONE MARROW EXAMINATION

As with any test, bone marrow examination should be performed when the findings will alter management of the patient. Bone marrow examination may not be required to discover the etiology of a pure anemia, but it may be necessary to decipher the effects of therapy or concomitant disease. Often the history, physical examination, complete blood count and differential, and peripheral blood morphology limit the differential diagnosis to two or three possibilities which can be confirmed by bone marrow examination. In cases of severe trilineage deficiencies, the marrow must be inspected for overall cellularity, the presence of dysplastic changes, and blast count to differentiate between

TABLE 145-2 Morphologic RBC Abnormalities

Morphologic Abnormality	Associated Diseases
Target cells	Liver disease Hemoglobinopathies-thalassemia, hemoglobin C
Spherocytes	Immunohemolytic anemia Hereditary spherocytosis
Schistocytes	Microangiopathic hemolytic anemia
Sickle or fusiform cells	Hemoglobinopathies
Spur cells or acanthocytes	Liver disease
Howell-Jolly bodies	Splenectomy
Heinz bodies (special stain)	G6PD or other enzyme deficiencies
Macroovalocytes	Folate or B_{12} deficiency
Bizarre cells (poikilocytosis)	Iron deficiency
Teardrop cells	Extramedullary hemopoiesis Marrow replacement Iron deficiency Myelodysplasia
Rouleaux	Hypergammaglobulinemia

TABLE 145-1 Pathophysiologic and Morphologic Differential Diagnosis of Anemia

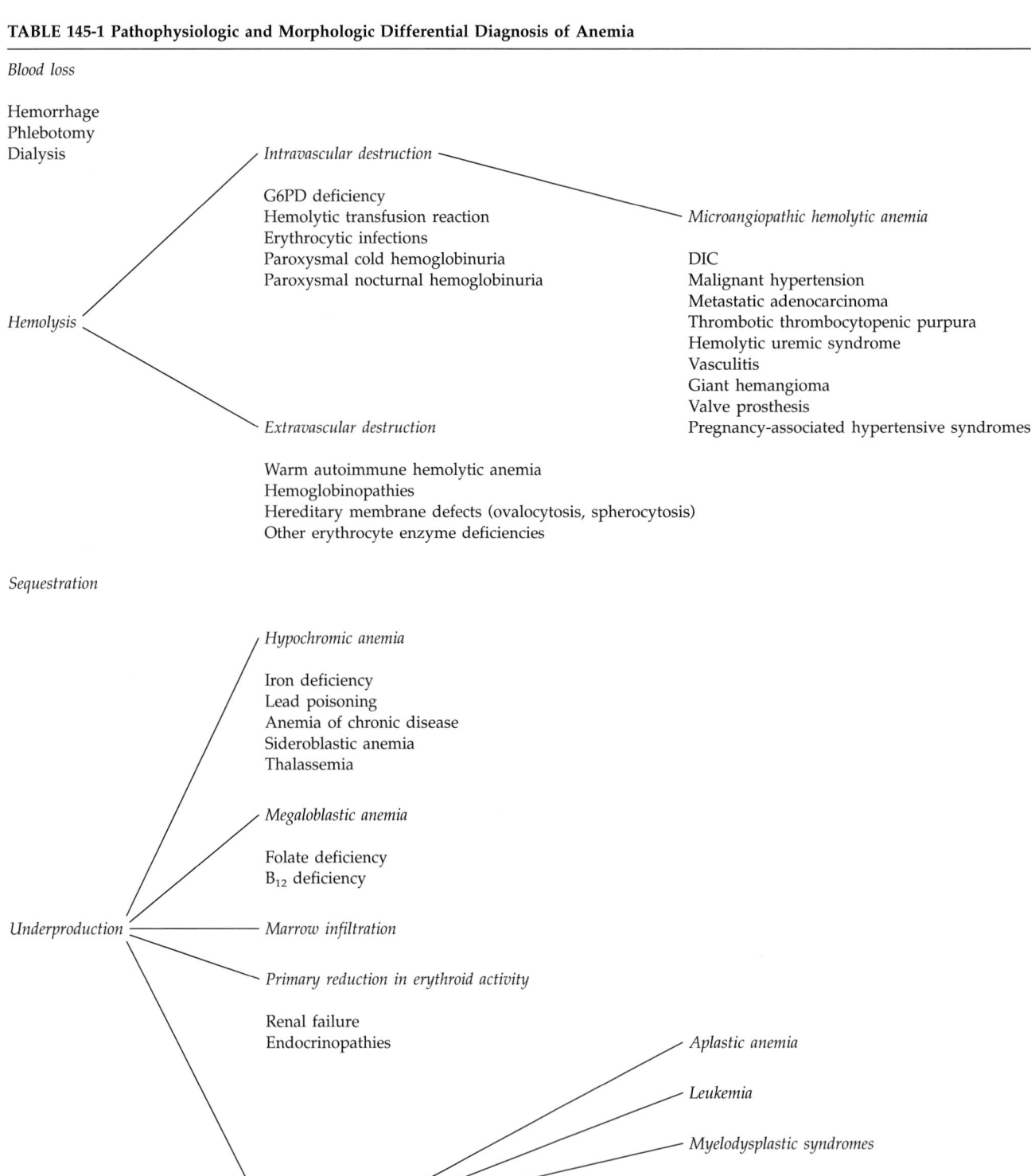

- *Blood loss*
  - Hemorrhage
  - Phlebotomy
  - Dialysis
- *Hemolysis*
  - *Intravascular destruction*
    - G6PD deficiency
    - Hemolytic transfusion reaction
    - Erythrocytic infections
    - Paroxysmal cold hemoglobinuria
    - Paroxysmal nocturnal hemoglobinuria
    - *Microangiopathic hemolytic anemia*
      - DIC
      - Malignant hypertension
      - Metastatic adenocarcinoma
      - Thrombotic thrombocytopenic purpura
      - Hemolytic uremic syndrome
      - Vasculitis
      - Giant hemangioma
      - Valve prosthesis
      - Pregnancy-associated hypertensive syndromes
  - *Extravascular destruction*
    - Warm autoimmune hemolytic anemia
    - Hemoglobinopathies
    - Hereditary membrane defects (ovalocytosis, spherocytosis)
    - Other erythrocyte enzyme deficiencies
- *Sequestration*
- *Underproduction*
  - *Hypochromic anemia*
    - Iron deficiency
    - Lead poisoning
    - Anemia of chronic disease
    - Sideroblastic anemia
    - Thalassemia
  - *Megaloblastic anemia*
    - Folate deficiency
    - B_{12} deficiency
  - *Marrow infiltration*
  - *Primary reduction in erythroid activity*
    - Renal failure
    - Endocrinopathies
  - *Stem cell disorders*
    - *Aplastic anemia*
    - *Leukemia*
    - *Myelodysplastic syndromes*
      - Refractory anemia
      - Refractory anemia with excess blasts
      - Chronic myelomonocytic leukemia
      - Refractory anemia with ringed sideroblasts
    - *Myeloproliferative disorders*
      - Chronic myelogenous leukemia
      - Polycythemia vera (treated)
      - Essential thrombocythemia
      - Myelofibrosis with myeloid metaplasia

the myelodysplastic syndromes, acute leukemia, aplastic anemia, or marrow replacement by tumor, fibrosis, or granuloma. Bone marrow examination may confirm overproduction of one or more cell lines in patients with cytopenias due to destruction or sequestration.

Indications and Contraindications to Transfusion

PHYSIOLOGIC CONSIDERATIONS

As with other body systems, a great deal of reserve is built into the oxygen delivery system. Overall oxygen delivery to the tissues depends on the hemoglobin concentration, the saturation of hemoglobin, and the $\dot{Q}_T$. Oxygen delivery to critical organs also depends on local blood flow. The severity of symptoms for a given degree of anemia reflects the adequacy of the patient's compensatory mechanisms. Mild anemia is asymptomatic except with exercise. Moderate anemia requires increased $\dot{Q}_T$ at rest to maintain adequate tissue oxygenation. In severe anemia, the limits of compensation are reached, and dyspnea at rest, heart failure, or altered mental status occur.

Compensatory mechanisms include increased $\dot{Q}_T$, peripheral vascular changes (vasoconstriction of noncritical vascular beds and vasodilatation in critical areas), increased oxygen extraction, and possibly changes in hemoglobin-oxygen affinity. $\dot{Q}_T$ determines overall blood flow, and local vascular tone governs individual organ perfusion. In normal human beings and animals, the cardiovascular system responds rapidly to anemia. In dogs, isovolemic hemodilution to a hematocrit of 20 percent is associated with a 70 percent increase in $\dot{Q}_T$ and no decline in tissue oxygenation.[1] The vasodilatory response has also been studied in dogs. Perfusion of the coronary artery with blood at a hematocrit of 10 percent and a constant perfusion pressure of 100 mmHg was adequately compensated by coronary artery dilatation, allowing increased blood flow.[2] This vasodilatory response to anemia was impaired at lower perfusion pressures, such that myocardial dysfunction occurred at a hematocrit of 17 percent. Because of the increased metabolic demands of acute illness, it is impossible to predict the effects of anemia on an individual patient, but these studies imply that systemic hypotension or local flow-limiting lesions, such as atherosclerotic plaques, will raise the limit of tolerable hemodilution. With anemia, strenuous exercise, increased metabolism, or poor perfusion, the tissues remove a higher percentage of oxygen from the blood. The limits of oxygen extraction for individual organs are reviewed fully in Chap. 57.

If anemia or hypoxia persist for several hours or days, increased levels of 2,3-diphosphoglycerate (2,3-DPG) within erythrocytes will raise the P50.[3] While the clinical relevance of the P50 to tissue oxygen utilization remains controversial, in one study, children with elevated RBC 2,3-DPG, and an associated elevation in P50, were asymptomatic, even during exercise, despite a mean hemoglobin concentration of 7.9 g/dL.[4] Children with an inadequate elevation in 2,3-DPG were markedly symptomatic at the same hemoglobin concentration. On the other hand, at normal oxygen tension, the P50 does not affect oxygen delivery, and the best evidence suggests that a left shift in the oxyhemoglobin dissociation curve does not impair oxygen extraction.[5] During hypoxia, such left shifts—from decreased 2,3-DPG, alkalosis, decreased P_{CO_2}, or hypothermia—increase oxygen delivery (increased O_2 saturation for a given low Pa_{O_2}) without impairing tissue extraction at the tissue level.[5] It should be noted that erythrocyte 2,3-DPG levels decline as length of storage increases, and 2,3-DPG levels require several days after transfusion to rise to normal levels.[4]

The work of attaining a given $\dot{Q}_T$ increases as the viscosity of the blood increases. Viscosity increases less than oxygen-carrying capacity as the hematocrit approaches 40 percent, such that in normovolemic states, peak oxygen delivery occurs at a hematocrit of 40 percent.[6] Because viscosity decreases with increased vessel diameter, peak oxygen delivery occurs at a higher hematocrit in hypervolemic states, assuming adequate vasodilatation and increases in $\dot{Q}_T$ occur. At the low shear rates present in the microvasculature, viscosity increases much more steeply as the hematocrit rises. Thus, the effects of viscosity on tissue oxygenation are difficult to predict. Although vascular stenoses may limit flow and impair oxygen delivery, this may be paradoxically worsened by increasing the hematocrit, and hence, the viscosity. Patients with normal vasculature can limit the increase in viscosity after blood transfusion by vasodilatation; patients with noncompliant vessels will be less able to accommodate a significant increase in hematocrit. With these caveats, it seems reasonable to return the low hematocrit to normal (40 percent) in critically ill patients vulnerable to tissue hypoxia. The potential complications of either raising $\dot{Q}_T$ (volume infusion, vasoactive drugs), or of raising oxygen saturation (positive end-expiratory pressure [PEEP], high fraction inspired oxygen [$F_{I_{O_2}}$]), are at least as great as the potential complications of increasing the hematocrit.

With an indwelling pulmonary artery (PA) catheter in place, it is possible to measure arterial and central venous P_{O_2}, P_{CO_2}, and pH, central venous (CVP) and pulmonary artery occlusion pressures, and $\dot{Q}_T$ output. When a normal P50 for the oxygen dissociation curve is assumed, small errors in venous oxygen saturation may be misleading, even when corrected for pH, temperature, and P_{CO_2}. $\dot{Q}_T$ and oxygen delivery can be determined before and after transfusion (keeping in mind the low 2,3-DPG of stored blood) to guide further therapy. A nomogram has been designed for this purpose, but its apparent complexity can distract the physician from relatively simple calculations of oxygen consumption and delivery.[7]

The lowest tolerable hematocrit depends on the patient's ability to compensate. An otherwise healthy patient, at rest, may easily tolerate a gradual fall in hematocrit to 20 percent. However, such a patient could be in grave danger if coronary artery disease were present or if acute infection were to develop. The margin of safety to provide each patient is not a measurable issue, but rather a clinical judgment. No matter how rigorously one calculates the physiologic parameters of oxygen delivery, the decision to transfuse must also be made on clinical grounds by comparing the estimated short-term and long-term risks of continued anemia versus those of blood transfusion.

IMMUNOLOGIC CONSIDERATIONS

In several hematologic disorders, transfusion should be avoided if possible. Patients with aplastic anemia who are candidates for bone marrow transplantation risk alloimmunization which could lead to graft rejection. Similarly, patients with aplastic anemia, acute leukemia, myelodysplasia, or other disorders which may necessitate long-term blood product support risk alloimmunization to either RBC antigens or human leukocyte antigens (HLAs), making future RBC transfusions difficult and platelet transfusions ineffective. Young patients without disease of other organs can usually tolerate a hematocrit well under 20 percent and a platelet count of 10,000 to 15,000/μL. On the other hand, patients with significant bleeding or who are at risk for central nervous system (CNS) hemorrhage should be given platelet transfusions. Patients with myelodysplasia are generally older, with abnormalities of other organ systems and may be at greater risk for bleeding or ischemia. Likewise, patients who, after receiving high dose chemotherapy, develop mucosal damage, prolonged pancytopenia, and dysfunction of other organ systems should receive liberal transfusions of RBCs and platelets. Leukocyte filters may minimize exposure to HLA antigens and inhibit alloimmunization to transfused platelets.[8] Patients who have undergone marrow ablative or similar high dose chemotherapy should receive irradiated blood products to prevent engraftment of immunocompetent cells and subsequent graft-versus-host disease (GVHD). Such patients who are seronegative for cytomegalovirus (CMV) should receive CMV-negative blood.

IRON OVERLOAD

Although an in-depth discussion of iron overload is beyond the scope of this text, its major, life-threatening manifestations are cardiac failure, arrhythmias, and complications of cirrhosis. The diagnosis of transfusional iron overload or idiopathic hemochromatosis requires demonstration of elevated serum iron content, transferrin saturation, and ferritin, and evidence for increased hepatic iron stores. Liver biopsy may be necessary. Focal periportal fibrosis, diabetes mellitus, and subclinical adrenal insufficiency occur in adults with pure transfusional iron overload after approximately 100 U RBCs (approximately 20 g iron).[9] Patients with thalassemia develop iron overload from overabsorption and from transfusion, and those patients who die of cardiac failure and arrhythmias usually have iron stores in excess of 40 g.[10]

Blood Loss

HEMORRHAGE

Hemorrhage must always be excluded during the initial evaluation of anemia and on a continuing basis in any case of persistent anemia. Gastrointestinal bleeding is a frequent reason for ICU admission, and it may complicate other serious illnesses. On occasion, "emergency released" type-specific blood must be given before the antibody screen is completed. The site of bleeding and the immediate risk of exsanguination can be estimated by evaluating orthostatic blood pressure and pulse, examining a stool sample and the nasogastric aspirate or emesis, and measuring the spun hematocrit. Patients with severe anemia, volume depletion, and active bleeding must be transfused immediately. It is always worthwhile to ask the patient about previous transfusion reactions, and it is imperative to obtain a sample for the blood bank before transfusion.

Any new fall in a patient's hematocrit should provoke a search for bleeding and for coagulopathy. Gastrointestinal bleeding is the most common site, but retroperitoneal, intrapleural, intramuscular, or mediastinal hemorrhage may result from invasive procedures such as central venous catheterization, cardiac catheterization, liver biopsy, paracentesis, etc.

PHLEBOTOMY

Phlebotomy may be a source of mild chronic blood loss in the ICU. A recent study[11] found that patients never admitted to the ICU lost a mean of 175 mL blood during an average hospital stay of 14 days; in contrast, ICU patients lost a mean of 760 mL during an average hospital stay. Patients with indwelling arterial catheters had the highest mean blood loss—over 70 mL daily while in the ICU, because an additional 3 mL blood was discarded with each phlebotomy. Compensation for a loss of 70 mL ($\approx$28 mL RBCs) daily requires manufacture of an additional 60,000 to 70,000 RBCs/μL/day—a two-fold increase in erythropoiesis. Hence, a normal person would develop a reticulocytosis to about 2.4 percent until iron deficiency occurred. Whole blood contains approximately 0.5 mg/mL of iron, and normal body iron stores range from 250 mg to 1000 mg. With a blood loss of 70 mL/day, iron deficiency could occur in 7 to 30 days. Patients with anemia from either hemolysis or underproduction, however, have already reached a steady state between erythrocyte production and destruction or senescence. These patients will be unable to increase erythropoiesis, and the hematocrit will fall approximately 0.5 percent daily. Two units of RBCs will be needed every 13 days to maintain a steady state.

Hemolysis

Erythrocyte destruction can be diagnosed by the findings of anemia, increased erythroid production (reticulocytosis, polychromasia, basophilic stippling, circulating nucleated RBCs, bone marrow erythroid hyperplasia), exclusion of hemorrhage, and evidence for increased RBC turnover (hemoglobinemia or hemoglobinuria, hyperbilirubinemia, increased serum lactate dehydrogenase [LDH] level, decreased haptoglobin). Extravascular erythrocyte destruction is more common, but acute intravascular hemolysis may be life-threatening.

Intravascular hemolysis causes hemoglobinemia which may be evident grossly or may be detected in the serum using a dipstick for urinary blood. (It must be remembered that hemolysis of the blood sample is a frequent sequela of hurried phlebotomy or improper technique). Hemoglobinuria may also be detected grossly or by dipstick testing of a fresh urine sample (myoglobinuria and hematuria must be excluded). Acute intravascular hemolysis may cause back pain, shock, anaphylaxis, chills, fever, adult respiratory distress syndrome, disseminated intravascular coagulation (DIC), and acute renal failure.

Many factors contribute to the development of renal failure in acute intravascular hemolysis, and the mechanism may vary with the cause of hemolysis. Acute tubular necrosis is the most common lesion, although in severe hemolytic transfusion reactions, renal cortical necrosis may occur. Both free hemoglobin and erythrocyte stroma have been implicated.[12,13] A recent study demonstrated that urine acidification dramatically increased the nephrotoxicity of hemoglobinuria, perhaps related to the conversion of hemoglobin to methemoglobin in acidic urine.[14] On the other hand, intravascular hemolysis does not invariably induce renal failure. In acute hemolytic transfusion reactions, nephrotoxicity is often related to the development of DIC.[15]

In addition to the disorders discussed below, ICU patients may suffer iatrogenic hemolysis. Intra-aortic balloon pumps, left ventricular assist devices, extracorporeal oxygenating devices, artificial heart valves, inadvertent rapid infusion of hypotonic solutions, and infusion of blood under pressure, especially via a small bore needle (smaller than 18 gauge), may cause hemolysis. *Blood should be infused with normal saline solution only*—never with other fluids or medications.

INTRAVASCULAR DESTRUCTION

GLUCOSE-6-PHOSPHATE DEHYDROGENASE DEFICIENCY (G6PD). Acute hemolytic anemia in a male who is of Mediterranean or African descent should raise the suspicion of G6PD deficiency. Because erythrocytes carry enormous relative quantities of oxygen, they are prone to oxidative damage, normally minimized by the free radical scavenger, glutathione. G6PD, the first enzyme of the hexosemonophosphate shunt, generates the reduced nicotinamide-adenine dinucleotide phosphate (NADPH) necessary for glutathione reductase to maintain adequate levels of reduced glutathione. Relatively few commonly used medications cause severe hemolytic anemia, particularly in patients with mild to moderate deficiency (Table 145-3).[16] Patients who suddenly develop renal or hepatic dysfunction may be more susceptible, because many other agents cause hemolysis at high concentration.

TABLE 145-3 Selected Causes of Hemolysis in G6PD Deficiency

Medications
Sulfonamides
Primaquine
Doxorubicin
Nitrofurantoin
Ingestions
Fava beans
Naphthalene (moth balls)
Infections (e.g, hepatitis)
Diabetic ketoacidosis

Of the several varieties of defective G6PD, some are clinically silent, while others cause life-long hemolytic anemia. Most individuals never experience severe hemolysis. Some persons of Mediterranean descent develop life-threatening hemolysis after eating fava beans. Acute infections, particularly hepatitis, and diabetic ketoacidosis have been associated with severe hemolysis.[17,18] Because the activity of G6PD—both normal and abnormal forms—decreases exponentially with time, younger RBCs are more resistant to oxidative damage. Thus, individuals exposed chronically to an oxidant drug may reach a steady state of hemolysis compensated by reticulocytosis. G6PD assays may be normal after an episode of acute hemolysis in which the older cells have been destroyed.

MICROANGIOPATHIC HEMOLYTIC ANEMIA (MAHA). A search for peripheral blood schistocytes should be performed in any case of hemolytic anemia. Table 145-1 lists the various causes of MAHA. In most cases, the anemia is mild. Transfusion is rarely required, and therapy is directed toward the underlying disorder. Most of these disorders are discussed elsewhere in this text. (See Chap. 147.)

TRANSFUSION REACTIONS. Hemolytic transfusion reactions are rare. The most severe transfusion reactions occur in cases of ABO mismatch because complement-fixing IgM isoantibodies are involved. With modern techniques, mismatches occur virtually only through clerical error, so double-checking is imperative both in the ICU and in the blood bank. On occasion, another RBC antibody (such as an Rh antibody) may cause a hemolytic transfusion reaction. This occurs most commonly when the initial antibody screen is negative, and the patient receives RBCs bearing an antigen to which he or she has been exposed previously. A delayed (anamnestic) reaction occurs—typically 7 to 14 days after the transfusion—and the only clues may be a fall in hematocrit, a rise in LDH and bilirubin, and the finding of an antibody not previously detected. Transfusion reactions are discussed in greater detail elsewhere in this text. (See Chap. 35.)

ERYTHROCYTIC INFECTIONS. Malaria, although rare in the United States, is the world's most common cause of hemolytic anemia, with a prevalence of roughly 300 million cases and an annual mortality of perhaps 1 million.[19] All four species of plasmodia infect RBCs, causing hemolysis as they proliferate intracellularly. Chromium 51 labeling of RBCs demonstrates shortened RBC survival and splenic accumulation, but anemia may also be related to dyshematopoiesis, drug-induced hemolysis, or marrow suppression related to malarial or concurrent bacterial infection.[20] In complicated falciparum malaria, capillary obstruction by the multitude of enlarged, infected erythrocytes leads to multisystem organ failure, including severe neurologic dysfunction and renal failure.

Babesiosis causes hemolytic anemia, fever, chills, and myalgias in patients living in temperate climates. Invasion of the erythrocyte by *Babesia microti* activates the alternative complement pathway, leaving infected RBCs coated with C3b, and resulting in intravascular hemolysis. The direct antiglobulin test is positive only with anticomplement. Without a spleen to filter and respond to blood-borne particulate antigens, asplenic patients are at particular risk for developing fatal babesiosis.[21]

EXTRAVASCULAR DESTRUCTION

SICKLE CELL DISEASE. Sickle cell disease is commonly encountered in the ICU because of the myriad complications (Table 145-4) spawned by a single amino acid substitution in the hemoglobin β chain. Sickling is a function of the hemoglobin S concentration and the deoxyhemoglobin: oxyhemoglobin ratio. Deoxyhemoglobin S forms polymers which induce a sickle or fusiform shape, reducing the pliability of the cell, and leading to capillary obstruction and shortened intravascular survival (hemolysis). In children, extravascular destruction occurs primarily in the spleen, until it is destroyed by repeated infarction, at which time the liver becomes the primary site of sickle cell destruction.

Patients with SS disease usually have moderate anemia with a hematocrit of 18 to 28 percent. In patients with SC disease, sickle/α-thalassemia, or sickle/β-thalassemia the hematocrit is typically 30 to 35 percent, and the disease is milder. Acute exacerbations of anemia may occur due to folate deficiency, splenic sequestration, or intercurrent infection. Parvovirus infection of erythroid precursors is responsible for many aplastic crises.[22] The diagnosis of parvovirus infection can be established by demonstrating IgM antibody to the virus, and by finding an apparent block in marrow erythropoiesis at the erythroblast stage, indicating destruction of later erythroid precursors.

To prevent or mitigate severe vasoocclusive complications, exchange transfusion or chronic transfusion therapy to maintain 50 percent hemoglobin A is necessary. Because of the risks of alloimmunization, hepatitis, and iron overload, this should be reserved for patients suffering from or at risk for organ-threatening or life-threatening complications.[23] For patients with such complications, partial exchange transfusion has the advantage of limiting the iron load of the transfusions, removing some of the patient's sickle hemoglobin, and avoiding hyperviscosity.[24] Patients with sickle cell disease should, if possible, receive relatively fresh blood from donors negative for sickle trait ("sickledex negative").

TABLE 145-4 Complications of Sickle Cell Disease

Hematologic	
	Chronic hemolytic anemia
	Aplastic crisis
	Megaloblastic crisis
	Iron overload
Infectious	
	Sepsis
	Pneumonia
	Meningitis
	Osteomyelitis
Pulmonary	
	Chest crisis
	Pulmonary infarction
	Pulmonary embolism
	Cor pulmonale
Abdominal disease	
	Liver crisis
	Symptomatic cholelithiasis
Cardiac	
	High output congestive heart failure
	Sudden death
Neurologic	
	Seizures
	Stroke
	Cerebral hemorrhage
Renal disease	
	Renal papillary necrosis
	Hematuria
	Isothsenuria
	Renal tubular acidosis
	Nephrotic syndrome
	Chronic renal failure
Miscellaneous	
	Painful crisis
	Osteonecrosis
	Priapism
	Leg ulcers
	Proliferative retinopathy

Patients with sickle cell disease may require ICU admission because of septic shock or complications of cardiopulmonary disease. Children, particularly, are prone to meningitis, sepsis, and pneumonia. All patients with sickle cell disease should be considered functionally asplenic and susceptible to encapsulated organisms. Streptococci, *Haemophilus influenza, Salmonella* species, enteric pathogens, and staphylococci are common pathogens.[25] Rarely, other bacteria which usually cause limited infection may cause catastrophic illness in sickle cell patients who lack a functioning spleen.

The cardiopulmonary complications of sickle cell disease are not well defined. Left ventricular dilatation may result from chronic volume overload, but overt left heart failure is rare. Hypertrophy and arrhythmias may occur in heavily transfused patients. It has been suggested that although increased preload and decreased afterload augment $\dot{Q}_T$, they may conceal left ventricular dysfunction.[26]

There are few large autopsy series of patients who die of sickle cell disease. One study found that acute chest syndrome, renal failure, and cerebrovascular accidents were the three leading causes of death in patients over age 20.[27] Acute chest crisis occurs in both children and adults with sickle cell disease; manifestations include chest pain, fever, pulmonary infiltrates, and hypoxia. Some series have found infection to be a common cause of acute chest syndrome in children, but others have found that, as in adults, documented infection is uncommon.[28-30] Sludging in the hypoxic environment of the small pulmonary arterioles (with or without pulmonary infarction) is the presumed cause of most cases of acute chest syndrome. Although one autopsy series found extensive pulmonary vascular abnormalities, including thrombi, marrow emboli, intimal narrowing and fibrosis, pleural fibrosis, and evidence of cor pulmonale,[31] no large series of sickle cell patients have undergone radionuclide studies or right heart catheterization to prove pulmonary vascular occlusion or pulmonary hypertension. Several case reports document chronic pulmonary disease with pulmonary hypertension and sudden death.[32]

Two autopsy studies found a high incidence of pulmonary thromboemboli in adults.[27,31] Although a recent report suggests that sickle cells may induce thrombus formation,[33] the incidence of pulmonary embolism and in situ thrombosis is not known, and the role of anticoagulation in sickle cell pulmonary disease is unclear. If suspected clinically, the diagnosis of pulmonary embolism should be pursued. There are reports of complications of intravenous contrast studies in sickle cell patients,[34] but there are also reports of patients who have tolerated intravenous contrast studies well.[35] There are no prospective studies of pulmonary angiography in sickle cell patients.

IMMUNOHEMOLYTIC ANEMIA. Immunohemolytic anemia may be mild, or patients may present with a hematocrit of <15 percent; these disorders often occur in elderly patients unable to tolerate severe anemia. Splenomegaly is often present, and lymphadenopathy is present in cases associated with lymphoma or infection. Jaundice occurs when hemolysis overwhelms the capacity of the liver to conjugate bilirubin.

Decisions regarding immediate transfusion should be made according to the clinical status of the patient as discussed above. ^{51}Cr-labeled donor RBCs survive as long as autologous RBCs, but RBC survival may be as short as 2 days. The diagnosis of immunohemolytic anemia is suggested by the findings of anemia, reticulocytosis, and spherocytosis; the presence of schistocytes implies a microangiopathic not an immunologic cause. Megaloblastic changes imply superimposed folate deficiency.

Autoimmune hemolytic anemia (AIHA) is most commonly due to warm-reactive, IgG antibodies. Underlying disorders include lymphoproliferative disorders (usually chronic lymphocytic leukemia), collagen-vascular disorders, immunodeficiency disorders (e.g., IgA deficiency), infection, thyroid disease, and gastrointestinal disease.[36] Approximately 5 to 20 percent of warm-reactive AIHA cases are drug-induced and therefore easily treated by removal of the offending agent. High dose penicillin, quinidine, and methyldopa are the drugs most commonly associated with AIHA.[37] As many as 20 to 50 percent of cases of warm-reactive AIHA are idiopathic.

Acute management of immunohemolytic anemias requires close cooperation with the blood bank. Laboratory studies may take days to complete, so the patient's transfusion requirement should be carefully evaluated. Transfusion is risky until concealed alloantibodies are excluded. Since the autoantibody is nearly always a panagglutinin, crossmatch-compatible blood is rarely available, and "least-incompatible" blood must be administered. If there is concern over the safety of transfusion (i.e., the laboratory investigations are not complete), blood should be given slowly, and in the smallest amount necessary to relieve symptoms.

Warm-reactive AIHA may respond, within several days, to intravenous IgG (0.4 g/kg intravenously over 4 to 6 h, daily for 3 to 5 days) or glucocorticoids (60 to 100 mg prednisone daily). Occasionally, splenectomy or cytotoxic therapy is indicated. Supplemental folate should always be given to patients with active hemolysis. Patients with cold-reactive autoantibodies generally do not respond to IgG, glucocorticoids, or splenectomy; warm blood should be infused.

Sequestration

Splenic sequestration (hypersplenism) may result from any cause of splenic enlargement—infectious (e.g., mononucleosis), immunologic (e.g., Felty's syndrome), mechanical (e.g., portal hypertension), or neoplastic (e.g., lymphoma). Anemia and thrombocytopenia are common findings; significant leukopenia is rarely due to splenic sequestration. Anemia may be caused by **1.** pooling of blood (dilutional anemia), **2.** lysis of RBCs after repeated journeys through the splenic cords, or **3.** active phagocytosis of antibody-coated erythrocytes or of structurally altered RBCs. Thrombocytopenia may be due to pooling or immunologic clearance. The normal spleen pools about 1 percent of the RBC mass and 30 percent of the platelet mass; in massive splenomegaly, as much as 50 percent of the RBC mass and 80 percent of the platelet mass may be sequestered within the spleen.[38] Examination of the peripheral blood may reveal spherocytes, giant platelets, and reticulocytosis. An enlarged spleen is not fully protected by the rib cage, and in many cases, architectural distortion renders it fragile and susceptible to minor trauma, especially if the enlargement has occurred rapidly or is due to infection.

Splenectomy may be beneficial if the underlying disorder cannot be treated rapidly or completely enough. Emergency splenectomy is rarely needed, except in cases of traumatic or spontaneous rupture, with intraabdominal hemorrhage. In patients with hematologic disorders, particularly if they have been recently treated, anemia may be due to some combination of marrow involvement, splenic sequestration, or toxicity of treatment. Thorough evaluation is necessary to avoid performing an unnecessary splenectomy.

Underproduction Anemia

The presence of anemia and a low reticulocyte count implies underproduction. At a hematocrit of 40 percent (4 to 5×10^6 RBCs/μL), there will be 50,000 to 60,000 reticulocytes/μL if RBC survival is normal (i.e., roughly 1 percent of the total RBCs/unit volume). Disorders such as iron deficiency and anemia of chronic disease are commonly encountered in the ICU, but are rarely the sole cause of severe anemia. Other disorders, such as pernicious anemia (B_{12} deficiency), are uncommonly encountered in the ICU, but may be associated with severe anemia. An in-depth discussion of all of the disorders listed in Table 145-1 is beyond the scope of this text, only a few pertinent comments will be made. Most underproduction anemias develop slowly, giving the cardiovascular system time to adjust. Thus, patients are typically normovolemic and may develop pulmonary edema if blood is infused too rapidly.

MEGALOBLASTIC ANEMIA

Folate deficiency may be seen in patients with alcoholism, malnutrition, hemolytic anemia, pregnancy, malignancy, or during acute severe illness.[39] Since acute starvation can rapidly lower the serum folate level, total body stores are more accurately assessed by measuring RBC folate levels. Any patient treated with folate for megaloblastic anemia, should be tested for B_{12} deficiency, in order not to camouflage the hematologic manifestations of B_{12} deficiency with folate administration, only to encounter the neurologic manifestations in the future. Patients with severe B_{12} deficiency may develop hypokalemia with the initiation of replacement therapy.

HYPOCHROMIC ANEMIAS

IRON DEFICIENCY ANEMIA. The presence of iron deficiency anemia indicates chronic gastrointestinal hemorrhage in men and postmenopausal women. Iron deficiency is difficult to diagnose in the setting of acute illness. Serum iron and transferrin levels often decrease in patients with acute or chronic illness. Ferritin, an acute phase reactant, may be elevated in acute and chronic illness.[40] If it is necessary to diagnose iron deficiency in an ICU patient, a bone marrow aspirate or particle section (not a biopsy, as decalcifying solutions may leach out iron) must be stained with Prussian blue.

MARROW INFILTRATION

Marrow infiltration by tumor, fibrosis, or granulomata may cause anemia, thrombocytopenia, or leukopenia. In some cases a myelophthisic (leukoerythroblastic) anemia may develop. Examination of the peripheral blood smear may reveal immature granulocytes, nucleated RBCs, and large platelets. Anisocytosis and poikilocytosis—particularly teardrop cells—may be present. Miliary tuberculosis is the most common benign cause of infiltrative myelopathy.[41] Other fungal or parasitic infections may cause a similar picture. Sarcoidosis may involve the bone marrow, but rarely causes a myelophthisic anemia.

PRIMARY REDUCTION IN ERYTHROID ACTIVITY

Because the kidney is the primary site of erythropoietin production, patients with chronic renal failure often become transfusion dependent and are thus exposed to the risks of infection and iron overload. With the availability of recombinant human erythropoietin, chronic transfusion therapy is no longer necessary in the majority of patients with renal failure. Recent studies have documented the effectiveness and safety of recombinant erythropoietin.[42] Side effects are minimal, although hypertension occurs in nearly one-third of patients. Because of the dramatic increase in erythropoiesis, iron deficiency is common, and iron supplementation should be prescribed for all patients except for those with iron overload. Seizures have occurred in patients receiving erythropoietin, occasionally associated with marked hypertension in the early phases of therapy. Moreover, the hematocrit can rise precipitously with erythropoietin therapy, causing hyperviscosity. However, it is not clear that the incidence of seizures in patients with chronic renal failure is increased because of erythropoietin therapy.[43] Antibody production to recombinant erythropoietin has not been documented, so any patient with chronic renal failure who is truly refractory to erythropoietin must be assumed to have a concomitant disorder (e.g., iron deficiency, myelodysplasia, gastrointestinal bleeding).

Primary bone marrow disorders resulting in severe underproduction anemia almost always involve the WBCs or platelets; these disorders are discussed below.

Leukopenia

Leukopenia, per se, is not a medical emergency, and even patients with severe leukopenia need not be hospitalized for their low WBC count alone. Neutropenia (absolute granulocyte count $<$500 to 1000/μL) *with fever,* however, *is* an emergency, and broad-spectrum antibiotics should be administered immediately after the appropriate cultures have been obtained. The risk of infection rises with the severity of neutropenia,[44] with a sharp increase in the risk of life-threatening gram-negative septicemia or fungal infections when the granulocyte count is $<$500/μL. Patients who have received chemotherapy that damages mucosal barriers are at even higher risk. Extra caution is required to prevent nosocomial infection in a seriously ill patient subjected to multiple invasive procedures. Handwashing, before and after each patient contact, and strict observance of sterile technique during invasive procedures are probably the most important precautions for neutropenic ICU patients.

Studies of granulocyte transfusion, both prophylactic and therapeutic are inconclusive. In a recent review,[45] the authors conclude that prophylactic granulocyte transfusions are unwarranted, and therapeutic transfusions should be reserved for patients who face prolonged neutropenia with a documented infection unresponsive to optimal antibiotics. Potential complications include pulmonary infiltrates with hypoxia (possibly exacerbated by concomitant amphotericin B administration), CMV infection, HLA alloimmunization, GVHD, and transfusion reactions.

Isolated leukopenia, without any qualitative or quantitative defects in the erythroid or platelet lines is uncommon, and is usually drug related (Table 145-5). In cases of toxic neutropenia, bone marrow examination may reveal an apparent block in differentiation, e.g., at the promyelocyte stage. If the patient has no other findings of acute leukemia, this is a good sign—indicating that the hemopoietic stem cells are unaffected and that circulating neutrophils should return several days after the offending agent is stopped. Other causes include cyclic neutropenia, mild congenital neutropenia (common in blacks), infection, or chemotherapy-induced neutropenia. Rare cases of autoimmune neutropenia may be idiopathic or may be associated with autoimmune diseases or lymphoproliferative disorders.

Leukopenia associated with qualitative abnormalities in the RBC line (anisocytosis, poikilocytosis, teardrop cells, nuclear budding, karyorrhexis) or with a trilineage cytopenia often represents a stem cell disorder. These disorders, namely, acute leukemia, myelodysplasia, aplastic anemia, and the myeloproliferative syndromes, can present similarly, so bone marrow examination is essential for correct diagnosis. Special studies, including chromosome analysis, cytochemistry, flow cytometry, or DNA analysis may be useful. In both acute leukemia and myelodysplasia there may be dysplastic circulating RBCs and granulocytes and occasional myeloblasts. Current therapy for myelodysplastic syndromes includes blood product support, aggressive treatment of infection, investigational hemopoietic growth factors, or chemotherapy as for acute leukemia.

TABLE 145-5 Drugs Implicated in Toxic Neutropenia

- Antibiotics
  - Chloramphenicol
  - Sulfonamides
  - β-Lactam antibiotics
  - Vancomycin
  - Antimalarial drugs
  - Antituberculous drugs
- Phenothiazines
- Tricyclic antidepressants
- Phenytoin
- Carbamazepine
- Anti-inflammatory agents
  - Phenylbutazone
  - Indomethacin
  - Gold
- Antithyroid drugs
- Antiarrhythmics
  - Quinidine
  - Procainamide
  - Lidocaine
  - Disopyramide
- Captopril
- Allopurinol
- Cimetidine
- Sulfonylureas
- Levamisole

Leukocytosis, Polycythemia, and Thrombocythemia

The finding of markedly elevated blood counts should raise concern about vascular occlusion or hemorrhage from vascular damage. However, many disorders are not associated with hyperviscosity or vascular occlusion, including leukemoid reactions, thrombocytosis associated with iron deficiency, secondary polycythemia (in the absence of hypovolemia), chronic myelogenous leukemia (CML), and chronic lymphocytic leukemia. Leukostasis occurs only in cases of acute leukemia as discussed in Chap. 148.

The myeloproliferative disorders (see Table 145-1) are clonal disorders in which cytopenias may occur because of overexpansion of another cell line. Anemia commonly occurs in CML and myelofibrosis and occasionally occurs in essential thrombocythemia (often from blood loss). In some cases, these disorders terminate in acute leukemia; nearly all patients with CML develop acute leukemia (blast crisis) within 5 years.

Patients with essential thrombocythemia and polycythemia vera have both quantitative and qualitative platelet abnormalities as demonstrated by platelet aggregometry and measurement of the bleeding time.[46] Bleeding or thrombosis are much more likely to occur than in cases of secondary thrombocytosis. Patients with severe hemorrhagic or thrombotic complications may improve dramatically with emergent plateletpheresis.[47]

In polycythemia vera, there is clonal overexpansion of all three lines. Whole blood viscosity increases rapidly above a hematocrit of 45 percent; although vasodilatation will ameliorate the effect of increased RBC mass in younger patients, older patients with less compliant vessels or with fixed obstruction to flow are more prone to vascular occlusion or bleeding. Signs and symptoms of hyperviscosity include headache, dizziness, visual disturbances, transient ischemic attacks, confusion, or stroke.

Patients with polycythemia vera are five times more likely than age-matched controls to suffer cerebral thrombosis.[48] Blood vessels in plethoric areas may rupture, leading to cerebral hemorrhage, gastrointestinal hemorrhage, and so on. Other thrombotic complications include deep venous thrombosis, pulmonary embolism, bowel ischemia and Budd-Chiari syndrome. Erythrocytosis is fairly easily controlled by removal of 250 to 500 ml every other day until the hematocrit is normal. Patients with acute symptoms of hyperviscosity should be given equivalent amounts of intravenous plasma, dextran, or saline solution to maintain hypervolemia. Phlebotomy alone may actually exacerbate thrombotic complications due to the compensatory increase in platelet count which accompanies blood loss and ultimately, iron deficiency.[49] Alkylating agents can be used to suppress excess proliferation of RBCs and platelets.

CASE PRESENTATION

A 69-year-old man was admitted to the ICU with unstable angina, fatigue, exertional dyspnea, and a hematocrit of 23 percent. Four weeks prior to admission he was referred to a hematologist with the diagnosis of nodular poorly differentiated lymphocytic lymphoma. At that time he had a WBC count of 5.5×10^9/L, a platelet count of 75×10^9/L, and a hematocrit of 31 percent. He was previously healthy, with no history of cardiac disease or angina. Examination revealed diffuse lymphadenopathy. The spleen was palpable 3 cm below the left costal margin in the midclavicular line. Bone marrow aspiration and biopsy revealed involvement of the marrow by lymphoma. Treatment was begun with cyclophosphamide, 100 mg/m^2/day by mouth, and interferon-α, 3,000,000 U/m^2 three times a week subcutaneously. Ten days prior to admission, the patient's WBC count was 3.4×10^9/L, the platelet count was 69×10^9/L, and the hematocrit was 29 percent.

At the time of admission to the ICU, the patient had no orthostatic changes in blood pressure or pulse, and examination of the stool was negative for occult blood. Intravenous nitroglycerin, an oral β blocker, and transfusion of 2 U packed RBCs were initiated. Myocardial infarction was ruled out and administration of cyclophosphamide and interferon was suspended. Although he developed no further chest pain, his hematocrit level rose to only 25 percent after transfusion. He was given another 3 U packed RBCs. On the third hospital day, the laboratory values were WBC count 3.1×10^9/L, platelet count 31×10^9/L, and hematocrit 28 percent. The patient remained asymptomatic without any evidence for gastrointestinal bleeding. The spleen was now palpable 6 cm below the left costal margin.

Cardiac catheterization was performed which revealed 90 percent stenosis of the left anterior descending coronary artery. Angioplasty was performed successfully, and the patient received another 2 U packed RBCs and 10 U single-donor platelets during the procedure. The following day the patient complained of left groin and left lower quadrant abdominal pain and a 4×6 cm hematoma was noted at the catheterization site. The hematocrit was 26 percent, and the platelet count was 17×10^9/L. Ten more units of single-donor platelets were given. On the following day the hematocrit was 22 percent, the reticulocyte count was 3.5 percent ($175{,}000 \times 10^9$/L), and the spleen was palpable 8 cm below the costal margin. Computed tomography of the abdomen did not demonstrate a retroperitoneal hematoma, although extensive retroperitoneal adenopathy and marked splenomegaly were noted.

The patient was transferred out of the ICU. One week later, after an additional 5 U packed RBCs, the following hematologic values were obtained: WBC count 4.6×10^9/L, platelet count 19×10^9/L, and hematocrit 29 percent. Bone marrow aspiration and biopsy revealed involvement by lymphoma, but also adequate megakaryocytes and erythroid hyperplasia. A splenectomy was performed with a blood loss of 500 mL. Three units of packed RBCs and 20 U single-donor platelets were given during and after surgery. Two weeks later the platelet count was 125×10^9/L and the hematocrit was 36 percent. Six weeks after surgery, cyclophosphamide and interferon were resumed without further complication.

CASE DISCUSSION

This case illustrates a severe anemia with multiple etiologies. This patient's anemia was a result of lymphomatous involvement of the bone marrow, splenic sequestration, and bone marrow suppression from chemotherapy. The clinicians involved were careful to exclude possible sources of bleeding, even though there were other evident explanations for the anemia. Splenectomy eliminated the problem of splenic pooling and destruction of erythrocytes and pooling of platelets, allowing the patient to resume treatment for his underlying disorder.

References

1. Mebmer K, Sunder-Plassmann L, Jesch F, et al: Oxygen supply to the tissues during limited normovolemic hemodilution. Res Exp Med 159:152, 1973.
2. Crystal GJ, Salem MR: Myocardial oxygen consumption and segmental shortening during selective coronary hemodilution in dogs. Anesth Analg 67:500, 1988.
3. Bunn HF, Jandl JH: Control of hemoglobin function within the red cell. N Engl J Med 282:1414, 1970.
4. Festa RS, Asakura T: The use of an oxygen dissociation curve analyzer in transfusion therapy. Transfusion 19:107, 1979.
5. Schumacker PT, Long GR, Wood LDH: Tissue oxygen extraction during hypovolemia: Role of hemoglobin P50. J Appl Physiol 62:1801, 1987.
6. Erslev AJ, Gabuzda TG: *Pathophysiology of Blood.* 3d ed. Philadelphia, Saunders, 1985, p 47.
7. Schneider AJ, Stockman JA, Oski FA: Transfusion nomogram: An application of physiology to clinical decisions regarding the use of blood. Crit Care Med 9:469, 1981.
8. Andreu G, Dewailly J, Leberre C, et al: Prevention of HLA immunization with leukocyte-poor packed red cells and platelet concentrates obtained by filtration. Blood 72:964, 1988.
9. Schafer AI, Cheron RG, Dluhy R, et al: Clinical consequences of acquired transfusional iron overload in adults. N Engl J Med 304:319, 1981.
10. Modell B: Advancers in the use of iron-chelating agents for the treatment of iron overload. Prog Hematol 11:267, 1979.
11. Smoller BR, Kruskall MS: Phlebotomy for diagnostic laboratory tests in adults: Pattern of use and effect on transfusion requirements. N Engl J Med 314:1233, 1986.
12. Schmidt PJ, Holland PV: Pathogenesis of the acute renal failure associated with incompatible transfusion. Lancet 1:1169, 1967.
13. Tam S, Wong JT: Impairment of renal function by stroma-free hemoglobin in rats. J Lab Clin Med 111:189, 1988.

14. Zager RA, Gamelin LM: Pathogenetic mechanisms in experimental hemoglobinuric acute renal failure. Am J Physiol 256(3 Pt 2):F446, 1989.
15. Goldfinger D: Acute hemolytic transfusion reactions—A fresh look at pathogenesis and considerations regarding therapy. Transfusion 17:85, 1977.
16. Beutler E: Glucose-6-phosphate dehydrogenase deficiency, in Williams WJ, Beutler E, Erslev AJ, Lichtman MA (eds): *Hematology*. 4th ed. New York, McGraw-Hill, 1990, p 591.
17. Salen G, Goldstein F, Haurani F, Wirts CW: Acute hemolytic anemia complicating viral hepatitis in patients with glucose-6-phosphate dehydrogenase deficiency. Ann Intern Med 65:1210, 1966.
18. Gellady AM, Greenwood RD: G-6-PD hemolytic anemia complicating diabetic ketoacidosis. J Pediatr 80:1037, 1972.
19. Jandl JH: *Blood: Textbook of Hematology*. Toronto, Little, Brown, 1987, p 319.
20. Pasvol G: The anaemia of malaria. Q J Med 58:217, 1986.
21. Rosner F, Zarrabi MH, Benach JL, Habicht GS: Babesiosis in splenectomized adults: Review of 22 reported cases. Am J Med 76:696, 1984.
22. Anderson LJ, Török TJ: Human parvovirus B19. N Engl J Med 321:536, 1989.
23. Greenwalt TJ, Zelenski KR: Transfusion support for haemoglobinopathies. Clin Haematol 13:151, 1984.
24. Charache S: Treatment of sickle cell anemia. Annu Rev Med 32:195, 1981.
25. Johnston RB: Increased susceptibility to infection in sickle cell disease: Review of its occurrence and possible causes. South Med J 67:1342, 1974.
26. Denenberg BS, Criner G, Jones R, Spann JF: Cardiac function in sickle cell anemia. Am J Cardiol 51:1674, 1983.
27. Thomas AN, Pattison C, Serjeant GR: Causes of death in sickle-cell disease in Jamaica. Brit Med J 285:633, 1982.
28. Barrett-Connor E: Acute pulmonary disease and sickle cell anemia. Am Rev Respir Dis 104:159, 1971.
29. Sprinkle RH, Cole T, Smith S, Buchanan GR: Acute chest syndrome in children with sickle cell disease: A retrospective analysis of 100 hospitalized cases. Am J Pediatr Hematol/Oncol 8:105, 1986.
30. Charache S, Scott JC, Charache P: "Acute chest syndrome" in adults with sickle cell anemia: Microbiology, treatment, and prevention. Arch Intern Med 139:67, 1979.
31. Oppenheimer EH, Esterly JR: Pulmonary changes in sickle cell disease. Am Rev Respir Dis 103:858, 1971.
32. Collins FS, Orringer EP: Pulmonary hypertension and cor pulmonale in the sickle hemoglobinopathies. Am J Med 73:814, 1982.
33. Chiu D, Lubin B, Roelofsen B, van Deenen LLM: Sickled erythrocytes accelerate clotting in vitro: An effect of abnormal membrane lipid asymmetry. Blood 58:398, 1981.
34. Rao AK, Thompson R, Durlacher L, James F: Angiographic contrast agent—Induced acute hemolysis in a patient with hemoglobin SC disease. Arch Intern Med 145:759, 1985.
35. Bashour TT, Lindsay J: Hemoglobin S-C disease presenting as acute pneumonitis with pulmonary angiographic findings in two patients. Am J Med 58:559, 1975.
36. Pirofsky B: Clinical aspects of autoimmune hemolytic anemia. Semin Hematol 13:251, 1976.
37. Jandl JH: *Blood: Textbook of Hematology*. Toronto, Little, Brown, 1987, p 306.
38. Jandl JH, Aster RH: Increased splenic pooling and the pathogenesis of hypersplenism. Am J Med Sci 253:383, 1967.
39. Davis RE: Clinical chemistry of folic acid. Adv Clin Chem 25:233, 1986.
40. Worwood: Ferritin in human tissues and serum. Clin Haematol 11:275, 1982.
41. Weick JK, et al: Leukoerythroblastosis: Diagnostic and prognostic significance. Mayo Clin Proc 49:110, 1974.
42. Eshbach JW, Abdulhadi MH, Browne JK, et al: Recombinant human erythropoietin in anemic patients with end-stage renal disease: Results of a phase III multicenter clinical trial. Ann Intern Med 111:992, 1989.
43. Eschbach JW, Adamson JW: Guidelines for recombinant human erythropoietin therapy. Am J Kidney Dis 2(suppl 1):2, 1989.
44. Bodey GP, Buckley M, Sathe YS, Freireich EJ: Quantitative relationships between circulating leukocytes and infection in patients with acute leukemia. Ann Intern Med 64:328, 1966.
45. Menitove JE, Abrams RA: Granulocyte transfusions in neutropenic patients. CRC Crit Rev Oncol 7:89, 1987.
46. Schafer AI: Bleeding and thrombosis in the myeloproliferative disorders. Blood 64:1, 1984.
47. Panilio AL, Reiss RF: Therapeutic plateletpheresis in thrombocythemia. Transfusion 19:147, 1979.
48. Chiefitz E, Thiede T: Complications and causes of death in polycythaemia vera. Acta Med Scand 172:513, 1962.
49. Berk PD, Goldberg JD, Donovan PD, et al: Therapeutic recommendations in polycythemia vera based on polycythemia vera study group protocols. Semin Hematol 23:132, 1986.

Chapter 146

BLEEDING DISORDERS

JOSEPH M. BARON
BEVERLY W. BARON

KEY POINTS

- *Assessment of the patient with a bleeding diathesis requires careful history-taking, bedside evaluation, and comprehensive base line coagulation testing.*
- *Uncomplicated vascular injury related to trauma or surgery is the first consideration before invoking a coagulopathy as the primary basis for bleeding.*
- *Consideration of coagulation abnormalities should include vascular disorders, platelet problems, impairment of the fibrin generation cascade, and excessive fibrinolytic activity.*
- *Disseminated intravascular coagulation (DIC) may present with either thrombotic or bleeding problems. Awareness of the possibility of the diagnosis and prompt appropriate laboratory confirmation may improve treatment selection and outcome.*
- *Invasive procedures in critically ill patients with coagulopathies need to be performed with special caution to prevent complications. Some guidelines are presented.*

Introduction to Bedside and Laboratory Diagnosis of Coagulopathies

Accurate diagnosis of the mechanism of a bleeding disorder is based on careful history-taking and bedside evaluation of the patient coupled with appropriate confirmatory laboratory testing.[1] Information obtainable from the patient or others about a preexisting congenital or acquired bleeding diathesis, medications being taken, and underlying disturbed organ function (e.g., hepatic or renal insufficiency) will facilitate the diagnostic process and provide the basis for empirical urgent therapy, if necessary, before laboratory testing can be completed.

Careful physical examination may clarify whether observed bleeding is strictly a *local* problem, i.e., limited to one site with the extent of bleeding not out of proportion to that expected from an observed injury or fixed lesion, or due to a *systemic* bleeding diathesis which should be suspected if multiple bleeding or bruising sites cannot be accounted for by the extent or intensity of known trauma. In some patients with a single mechanism of systemic coagulopathy, it may be possible to distinguish a vascular or platelet disorder characterized by *immediate bleeding* (prolonged continued bleeding after onset and dominant petechial/mucosal manifestations) from a fibrin generation (cascade) or fibrinolysis problem typified by *delayed bleeding* (rebleeding after initial hemostasis and prominent ecchymoses/deep muscle and joint hemorrhage). Complex coagulopathies such as DIC may have features of both categories. The presence of findings such as splenomegaly or telangiectases may also be helpful clues.

Several generalizations based on data from history and physical examination may help in directing work-up and treatment of bleeding problems. The *first* consideration in evaluating a bleeding patient before invoking a coagulopathy as a contributing cause is to exclude uncomplicated vascular injury (related to trauma or surgery) amenable to surgical hemostasis techniques. *Second,* brisk bleeding is almost never due to spontaneous hemorrhage due to a coagulopathy alone. *Third,* clinically significant bleeding often is the result of coexistence of trauma or a potential bleeding lesion (e.g., peptic ulcer) with presence of, or development of, a coagulopathy. *Fourth,* initial and follow-up laboratory screening of critically ill patients for the presence of a potential bleeding diathesis is important in predicting and preventing bleeding complications during interventions such as line placements and surgical procedures.

Systematic laboratory evaluation of the patient with a coagulopathy[2] is facilitated by considering the factors necessary for normal clot formation and degradation (Table 146-1). An appropriate screening laboratory survey for a hemostatic disorder in the critically ill patient would include a platelet count, review of peripheral smear for the presence of schistocytes and evaluation of platelet number and appearance, bleeding time (unless platelet count $<50{,}000/mm^3$), prothrombin time (PT), activated partial thromboplastin time (PTT), thrombin time, fibrin degradation products (FDPs), and D-dimer assay. These tests should be done simultaneously and not in sequential order in the critically ill patient.

The initial response to vessel injury with formation of the platelet plug depends on normal vascular and platelet function. Defects in these components are reflected in a prolonged *bleeding time.* Formation of the definitive fibrin clot requires proper functioning of the clotting factor cascade (Fig. 146-1). In vitro clotting times such as PT and PTT are useful, in combination, in detecting significant abnormalities in this pathway. The thrombin time depends on the final step of the cascade (fibrinogen conversion to fibrin) and, thereby, increases the sensitivity of detection of fibrinogen abnormalities and inhibitors acting at this level (e.g., heparin). Maintenance of the fibrin plug for a sufficient time to permit repair of vascular injury is necessary to prevent delayed or secondary bleeding. Excessive fibrinolysis leading to premature clot instability and lysis is detected by FDP/D-dimer testing. FDPs result from fibrinogenolysis and fibrinolysis, but D-dimer is a unique product of plas-

TABLE 146-1 Major Phases in Clot Formation, Maintenance of Its Integrity, and Eventual Dissolution

1. Blood vessels
2. Platelets
3. Fibrin generation cascade
4. Fibrin degradation

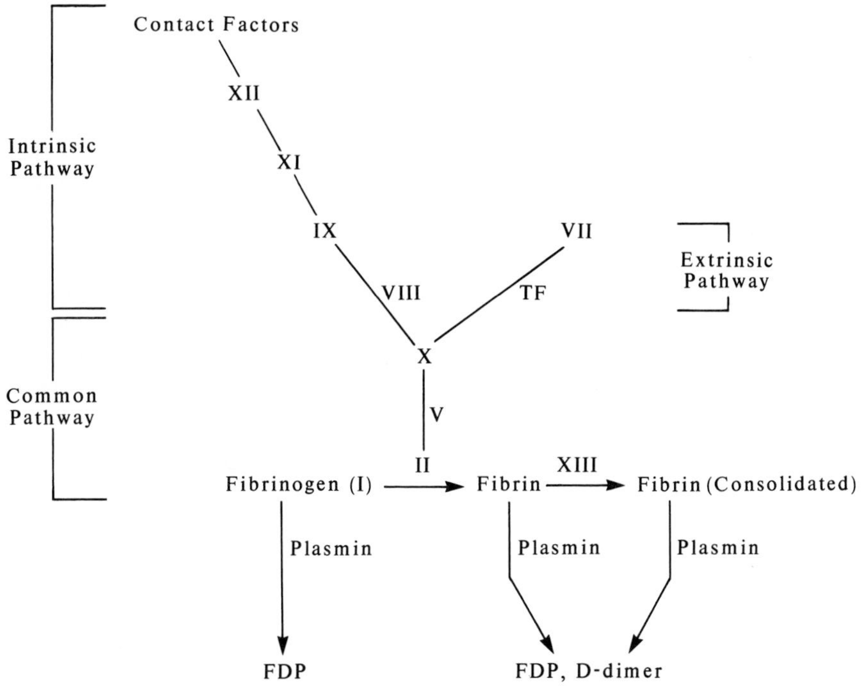

FIGURE 146-1 Fibrin generation cascade and fibrin degradation. TF, tissue factor; FDP, fibrin degradation products.

TABLE 146-2 Screening Coagulation Test Profiles in Selected Typical Fully Manifest Bleeding Disorders

Disorder	Platelet No.	Bleeding Time	PT	PTT	TT	FDP	D-dimer	Other
1. Vasculitis	N	I	N	N	N	N	N	Palpable purpura
2. Telangiectasia	N	N	N	N	N	N	N	Cutaneous and visceral lesions
3. Immune thrombocytopenia	D	I	N	N	N	N	N	Antiplatelet antibodies
4. Thrombotic thrombocytopenic purpura	D	I	N	N	N	N	N	Schistocytes, renal failure
5. Thrombocythemia	I	I or N	N	N	N	N	N	Large platelets
6. Thrombocytopathy	I, N, or D	I	N	N	N	N	N	Impaired platelet aggregation
7. Hypofibrinogenemia	N	N	I	I	I	N	N	Liver dysfunction
8. Hemophilia A	N	N	N	I	N	N	N	Low VIII:C
9. von Willebrand's disease	N	I	N	I	N	N	N	Low VIII:C, low ristocetin cofactor
10. Vitamin K deficiency	N	N	I	I	N	N	N	
11. Advanced liver disease	N or D	N or I	I	I	I	I	N	Elevated VIII:C, short euglobulin lysis time
12. Disseminated intravascular coagulation	D	I	I	I	I	I	I	Schistocytes, low fibrinogen and VIII:C, normal euglobulin lysis time
13. Heparin therapy	N	N	I	I	I	N	N	Low antithrombin III, positive circulating anticoagulant test
14. Warfarin therapy	N	N	I	I	N	N	N	Negative circulating anticoagulant test
15. Thrombolytic therapy	N	N	I	I	I	I	I	Low fibrinogen, short euglobulin lysis time

N, normal; I, increased; D, decreased; TT, thrombin time.

min degradation of fibrin. Thus, elevated D-dimer levels imply that clotting (fibrin formation) has taken place prior to plasmin activity. Screening profiles of a number of common coagulopathies are displayed in Table 146-2.

Vascular Disorders

VASCULITIS[3]

Patients with vasculitis due to a variety of etiologies (e.g., drugs, infections, neoplasms, systemic connective tissue diseases) may have increased risk of bleeding complications due to vascular fragility resulting from the inflammatory changes in vessel walls. Cutaneous rashes secondary to allergic drug reactions may have a significant vasculitic component. Vasculitis may be suspected by finding so-called palpable purpura—small hemorrhagic areas which are infiltrated and become palpable—in contrast to the typically flat purpura of thrombocytopenia.

Cutaneous vasculitis causes a prolonged bleeding time and may interfere clinically with the safety of even a small surgical incision through involved areas. A positive diagnosis of vasculitis may be made by a small punch biopsy of a purpuric lesion. Management consists of removing possible offending agents, treating underlying disorders (if possible), minimizing skin trauma, and use of anti-inflammatory agents such as corticosteroids, if not contraindicated by other clinical circumstances.

VASCULAR MALFORMATIONS

A variety of vascular malformations may bleed when traumatized or inadvertently entered at the time of closed-space biopsies. Hereditary hemorrhagic telangiectasia (Osler-Weber-Rendu disease) may be associated with cutaneous, mucosal, or deep visceral malformations. Usually there is no laboratory evidence of a coagulopathy. Family history (autosomal dominant inheritance) and careful inspection of cutaneous and mucosal sites for blanching "spiders" may help suggest the diagnosis. Unfortunately, rare patients have only unsuspected deep visceral malformations which may bleed. Occasional coexistence with von Willebrand's disease and hemophilia A has been noted.

Patients with congenital cavernous hemangiomas may have a coagulopathy related to consumption of platelets and clotting factors in stagnant vascular spaces (Kasabach Merritt syndrome).[4] There may be evident physical findings and laboratory features of DIC.

MICROCIRCULATORY OBSTRUCTION

Leukostasis secondary to very elevated myeloblast levels in acute nonlymphocytic leukemias may lead to small vessel obstruction and resulting purpura.[5] Brain, lung, and skin are particularly well recognized sites of clinical importance. Similar vasoocclusive sequelae may be seen in DIC, thrombotic thrombocytopenic purpura (TTP), and fat embolism after long bone fractures.

Platelet Disorders

THROMBOCYTOPENIAS (TABLE 146-3)

The platelet count is the result of the balance between production and removal rates of platelets from the circulation. Bone marrow normally has a six-to-eightfold reserve production capacity for the formed elements released into the blood which can help compensate for shortening of the normal platelet half-life. Although there is no simple readily available test corresponding to the reticulocyte count as an indicator of new red blood cell (RBC) production, the rate of platelet production can be estimated roughly from evaluation of Wright-stained peripheral blood smears for young (large, basophilic) platelets.

UNDERPRODUCTION STATES

HYPOPLASTIC MARROW. Lack of platelet production either as an isolated problem or as a contributing factor to thrombocytopenia is suspected by finding decreased overall cellularity or selective decrease in megakaryocyte number and size on bone marrow examination. A variety of suppressive factors may cause a generalized decrease in marrow mass or a selective decrease in megakaryocyte number. These include chemicals—either medicinal or environmental toxins; infectious agents—including bacteria, viruses, fungi, and mycobacteria; immune processes with either humoral or cellular mediated inhibition; radiation injury; and idiopathic hypoplastic or aplastic marrow. Marrow hypoplasia will be evident on examination of a bone core biopsy. Care should be taken not to sample marrow which is in the port of prior radiotherapy. Hypoplasia is expected in such an area and may be misleading if extrapolated to the status of the full marrow.

Ineffective Marrow

Ineffective marrow states are characterized by normal or increased cellularity but lack of release of precursors into the blood. An inappropriately low reticulocyte response to anemia is a convenient way to monitor marrow "effectiveness" in this circumstance. A common cause of ineffective marrow function is folate deficiency causing megaloblastic hematopoiesis. The finding of hypersegmented polymorphonuclear leukocytes, ovalomacrocytes, and lack of reticulocyte response in conjunction with thrombocytopenia should suggest this mechanism. Increased metabolic requirements, decreased folate intake in the diet, and therapy with certain chemotherapeutic agents predispose to folate deficiency. Ineffective marrow function is also a feature of various myelophthisic conditions in which marrow is replaced by such processes as tumor or granuloma or impaired functionally by metabolic disturbances such as azotemia or hypothyroidism. A variety of inflammatory conditions may cause increased or decreased platelet counts via mechanisms not clearly defined.

SHORTENED PLATELET SURVIVAL

The normal half-life of platelets in the blood (5 days) is usually shortened in patients who are ill. Fever, bleeding, and

TABLE 146-3 Thrombocytopenias in the Critically Ill

Mechanism	Selected Specific Causes
I. Underproduction of Platelets	
a. Bone marrow hypoplasia/aplasia	1. Drugs and chemicals (cytotoxic chemotherapy, ethanol, benzene, chloramphenicol, thiazides)
	2. Radiation therapy
	3. Infections (viral hepatitis, cytomegalovirus, tuberculosis)
b. Ineffective bone marrow	1. Myelophthisic (metastatic cancers, tuberculosis)
	2. Megaloblastic (folic acid, B_{12} deficiencies)
	3. Primary marrow diseases (leukemia, myeloma)
II. Shortened Platelet Survival	
a. Immune thrombocytopenia	1. Drugs (rifampicin, methicillin, sulfonamides, barbiturates, diphenylhydantoin, quinidine, α-methyldopa, thiazides, furosemide, gold salts, heparin, trimethoprimsulfamethoxazole
	2. Lymphomas
	3. Collagen vascular diseases (systemic lupus erythematosus)
	4. Viral infections (HIV-1)
b. Intravascular consumption	1. DIC
	2. TTP
	3. Cardiopulmonary bypass
	4. Hemodialysis
III. Sequestration	1. Hypersplenism (cirrhosis, lymphoma)
IV. Hemodilution	1. Massive transfusion

DIC, disseminated intravascular coagulation; TTP, thrombotic thrombocytopenic purpura; HIV-1, human immunodeficiency virus 1.

sepsis, in general, predispose to shortened platelet survival; some very specific circumstances include immune-mediated platelet removal by the reticuloendothelial system, hypersplenism, and consumptive coagulopathy. Otherwise uncomplicated shortened platelet life span is suspected by finding low circulating platelet count, normal or usually increased numbers of megakaryocytes on bone marrow examination, and presence of large, basophilic platelets on blood smear (indicative of effective marrow release of platelets).

Idiopathic Thrombocytopenic Purpura

Idiopathic (or autoimmune) thrombocytopenic purpura (ITP) is documented by finding antiplatelet antibodies in the patient's serum or on the patient's platelets. In instances where a drug is suspected as the cause, these studies done in the presence and absence of the candidate drug may help confirm the diagnosis. Since the testing may take some time, often an empirical decision is made to stop administration to the patient of one or more suspect drugs, when possible. Immune-mediated thrombocytopenia also may be associated with such conditions as collagen vascular disease, lymphomas, and viral infections.

The first step in therapy consists of discontinuation of any potential offending agents (e.g., quinidine, trimethoprim-sulfamethoxazole, diphenylhydantoin, thiazides). In addition, drugs which impair platelet function are contraindicated. It is often difficult to sort out a responsible drug in patients with complex medical conditions who are taking multiple medications, but in our experience a frequent offender in the ICU setting is intravenous furosemide given in repetitive doses. A switch to ethacrynic acid may be helpful sometimes. Corticosteroids may improve platelet survival by loosening of antibody attachment to platelets and decreasing reticuloendothelial clearance of the antibody-coated platelets. A longer term effect of corticosteroids is suppression of antibody production. Administration of platelets is usually of temporary benefit because their survival is shortened, presumably by mechanisms similar to those affecting the patient's platelets. Another intervention which may help improve platelet survival is infusion of intravenous γ-globulin, 0.4 to 1 g/kg/day for 3 to 5 days.[6] This product is thought to work by reticuloendothelial blockade and possibly also by reduction in amount of antiplatelet antibody available to attach to platelets due to presence of anti-idiotypic antibody in the preparation. In some patients receiving platelets, pretreatment with intravenous γ-globulin may help prolong survival of the platelets. Intravenous γ-globulin has few side effects. Benefit may not be seen for several days, and platelet rises which may be lifesaving and permit surgical procedures are temporary. Repeated doses may again be effective, but cost becomes an important consideration when selecting this as an ongoing treatment.

Splenectomy may be an effective treatment for ITP, but often the ICU patient is not a good candidate for the procedure, and therefore the emphasis is more on the medical interventions just outlined. Other agents such as azathioprine, vincristine, colchicine, danazol, and cyclophosphamide may be helpful adjuncts, but these are usually used in subacute and chronic management situations.

POSTTRANSFUSION PURPURA (PTP). Abrupt, often apparently unexplained, delayed appearance of severe thrombocytopenia may occur following blood transfusion in rare predisposed (usually $P1^{A1}$-negative) individuals. Shortened life span of both $P1^{A1}$-positive donor platelets (to which isoantibodies have been produced) as well as the patient's own platelets (mechanism unclear) is observed. In addition to the traditional treatment with whole blood or plasma exchange, recent favorable experience with infusions of intravenous γ-globulin (0.4 g/kg/day for 2 to 5 days) promises improved outlook for patients with this potentially serious problem.[7] The reader is referred to Chap. 35 for further discussion.

THROMBOTIC THROMBOCYTOPENIC PURPURA (see Chap. 147). In TTP[8] intravascular clumping of platelets accounts for secondary vasoocclusion and thrombocytopenia. The precise mechanism of initiation of the process is not understood, but triggers include infections, chemotherapeutic agents (especially mitomycin), and malignancies. The important diagnostic clues are schistocytes on blood smear, low platelet count usually with disproportionately low incidence of hemorrhagic symptoms, negative Coombs' test in the face of laboratory evidence of hemolysis, and (usually) normal coagulation studies. Evidence of vasoocclusion by platelet hyaline agglutinates may be seen in biopsies of organs such as skin, marrow, gingiva, and kidney. Treatment with corticosteroids, plasma infusion or exchange, and antiplatelet agents (e.g., dipyridamole and aspirin) usually results in significant improvement. Also, favorable responses to intravenous vincristine injections have been reported. Some patients may have a chronic relapsing course which may be suspected by detection of increased proportion of high molecular weight von Willebrand's factor (VWF) multimers in plasma obtained in intercritical periods (these are not present during an acute flare). Transfusion of platelets is to be avoided unless there is serious bleeding, because it has been noted to exacerbate the vasoocclusive process.

DISSEMINATED INTRAVASCULAR COAGULATION. A more extended discussion of DIC[9] appears later in this chapter. When thrombocytopenia is a manifestation of DIC, usually other aspects of the process are present, which permit recognition of the syndrome. Accompanying microangiopathic hemolysis, hypofibrinogenemia, elevated FDPs and D-dimer levels, and prolonged clotting times are cardinal features. In addition to low platelet counts in advanced DIC, qualitative platelet dysfunction due to thrombin-induced platelet storage pool depletion compounds the bleeding diathesis and may make platelet transfusions less effective.

HEPARIN-INDUCED THROMBOCYTOPENIA.[10] Bleeding is the most frequent complication of heparin therapy. However, an important, although fortunately rare, cause of thrombocytopenia is the immune mechanism related to heparin. This is of special interest in the ICU because of the almost ubiquitous exposure of patients to heparin if one considers its use in access and monitoring lines and the wide usage of 'heparin-bond' or 'heparin-coated' catheters.

It is common for patients to have a small drop in platelet count (usually within the normal range) within 1 to 2 days of initiating heparin therapy. This is felt to be secondary to some platelet aggregation caused by high molecular weight heparin species in the commercially available heparin. The dreaded immune-mediated thrombocytopenia (seen in less than 1 percent of heparin-treated patients) typically appears at about 5 to 7 days after first exposure, but an anamnestic response due to persistent antibody from previous sensitization to heparin may lead to thrombocytopenia earlier in some patients. The clinical picture may range from no symptoms to life-threatening thrombotic events which may be venous or arterial. Hemorrhage is less frequent despite quite severe thrombocytopenia in some individauls. Clinical suspicion of the syndrome should lead to discontinuation of all exposure of the patient to heparin (including locks, flushes of indwelling lines, and use of indwelling catheters that are heparin-coated). Laboratory confirmation of the presence of heparin-dependent antiplatelet antibodies may be helpful but is not always possible. The incidence of false-negative results even with the best testing methods often makes it necessary to make the decision about discontinuing heparin on clinical grounds.

It is important to emphasize that the severe antibody syndrome may occur with any type of heparin given via either intravenous or subcutaneous routes, and incidence is unrelated to dose administered. Management of the patient who still needs anticoagulation is difficult. It takes several days for the thrombocytopenia to improve after heparin discontinuation, and anticoagulation with warfarin cannot be accomplished immediately. Dextran and antiplatelet drugs such as dipyridamole and aspirin have been used with variable success in the "window period" between discontinuation of heparin and completion of warfarinization.[11] Some preliminary experimental results suggest the potent antiplatelet agent prostacyclin (PGI_2) as another alternative. Transfusion of platelets is usually contraindicated unless necessitated by hemorrhage. Some normal individuals have platelets which do not aggregate when incubated with the patient's plasma plus heparin. The platelets which do not aggregate might be expected to survive longer and not contribute to the vasoocclusive process. Theoretically, these might be safer to transfuse if platelets are needed or if the patient urgently requires a procedure (e.g., open heart surgery) in which heparin readministration is needed. A history of any adverse reaction to heparin in the past or necrotic changes at subcutaneous heparin injection sites should alert one to risk of serious vascular consequences on reexposure to the drug.

MECHANICAL SURFACE-RELATED THROMBOCYTOPENIA.[12] Variable lowering of platelet number is sometimes seen when platelets pass over or through foreign or distorted surfaces. Some such clinical situations include during cardiopulmonary bypass and the presence of intra-aortic balloon pumps or pulmonary artery catheters. For cardiopulmonary bypass, at least, platelet-related bleeding during or after bypass is much more likely to be secondary to impaired platelet function (vide infra) than severe depression of the platelet count.

SEQUESTRATION

HYPERSPLENISM. Thrombocytopenia with or without anemia and neutropenia may be a feature of hypersplenism.[13] This state of increased local sequestration, usually with shortened intrasplenic survival, frequently is accompanied by increased spleen size notable on physical examination or imaging study (bedside ultrasound is a safe, noninvasive method for assessing the spleen in ICU patients).

Hypersplenism may be a chronic stable condition antedating and then complicating a new problem (e.g., cirrhosis with splenomegaly prior to acute deterioration for another reason). Additionally, acute onset of hypersplenism with progressive splenic enlargement and sequestration may be a feature of such processes as splenic venous occlusion and sickle cell splenic sequestration crisis in children. It is unusual to encounter a platelet count $<30{,}000/\text{mm}^3$ in "compensated" hypersplenism associated with cirrhosis and portal hypertension accompanied by splenomegaly. Bone marrow evaluation is expected to reveal increased megakaryocyte number and overall hypercellularity. The peripheral smear should show decreased platelet numbers but some large basophilic platelets.

In situations of progressive splenomegaly with associated thrombocytopenia (and risk of splenic rupture), splenectomy may be the only available therapy. If the splenic enlargement is secondary to leukemic or lymphomatous involvement, radiation therapy may be of some benefit in shrinking the spleen, but the effect may be temporary, and there is the risk of paradoxical thrombocytopenia or neutropenia rather than count improvement.

THROMBOCYTOSIS/THROMBOCYTHEMIA

Elevated platelet counts are commonly seen in critically ill patients because inflammation, bleeding, surgery, hemolysis, severe injury, and neoplasia are among the major causes of reactive thrombocytosis. Usually, the count is elevated to levels $<1 \times 10^6/\text{mm}^3$, and no adverse effect is expected from such a secondary increase in qualitatively normal platelets.

In contrast, patients with elevated platelet counts secondary to myeloproliferative disorders[14] are at increased risk of bleeding or thrombotic sequelae, especially when the platelet count exceeds $1 \times 10^6/\text{mm}^3$. The diagnosis of an underlying myeloproliferative disorder may have been established prior to the patient's presentation with a complication, or it may be suspected from associated clinical features such as splenomegaly, abnormal platelet morphology on smear, and bone marrow examination revealing panmyelosis (increase in all cell lines) as well as qualitative abnormalities in megakaryocytes, which are also markedly increased in number.

If the patient is asymptomatic, a prolonged bleeding time may portend hemorrhagic problems. No definitive laboratory tests predict impending thrombotic complications in such patients, but it appears that the risk may be increased in older persons with fixed vascular disease. It is especially important to avoid splenectomy, either intentional or inadvertent, at the time of abdominal surgery for other reasons, because marked platelet elevations have been noted with some fatal vasoocclusive events following such an event.

Platelet levels may be quickly and effectively reduced in symptomatic thrombocythemic individuals by plateletpheresis. Chemotherapy with hydroxyurea or busulfan can be used to maintain normal platelet counts (usually seek to keep platelets $\leq 500{,}000/\text{mm}^3$). These drugs can also help prevent secondary rises in platelet count following surgical procedures and other factors which may precipitate reactive thrombocytosis.

THROMBOCYTOPATHY

Qualitative platelet abnormalities frequently are encountered in the ICU setting.[15] Often they contribute to other more serious bleeding diatheses, but may on occasion, present a significant problem in their own right. Exposure to external agents, such as ethanol, aspirin, and nonsteroidal anti-inflammatory drugs (NSAIDs) prior to admission is common. The resulting bleeding time prolongation varies in duration and severity. Once the offending agent has been removed, the bleeding problem can be overridden promptly by administration of exogenous normal platelets, if necessary, but usually passage of several days is sufficient for the patient's own production of platelets unexposed to the drug(s) to correct the prolonged bleeding time.

UREMIA

A more difficult problem is the thrombocytopathy associated with uremia. A variety of interventions may be helpful temporarily. Correction of the prolonged bleeding time may be needed prior to an intended surgical intervention (e.g., renal biopsy for diagnosis). The key step is appropriate dialysis; additional benefit sometimes is noted with administration of corticosteroids, infusions of cryoprecipitate[16] (usually 10 cryopacks every 12 h), intravenous DDAVP[17] (0.3 μg/kg), platelet transfusions, and conjugated estrogens.[18] Intravenous DDAVP, if effective in reducing the bleeding time, may be repeated at 6 to 12-h intervals, but tachyphylaxis is expected after 2 to 3 days of this therapy. It is also important to seek and correct other coexisting coagulopathies such as vitamin K deficiency.

MYELOPROLIFERATIVE DISORDERS

Patients with myeloproliferative disorders may have platelet dysfunction, especially when platelet counts are elevated. Usually, normalization of the platelet count results in return of bleeding time to normal, but individuals with long-standing polycythemia vera or myeloid metaplasia, for example, may still have abnormal bleeding, especially with surgical procedures, even when all counts have been normalized.

DRUGS

ASPIRIN. The classic drug inhibitor of platelet function is aspirin. It causes irreversible inhibition of cyclooxygenase, thereby leading to impaired prostaglandin metabolism. The net effect of aspirin is the result of inhibition of production of the platelet aggregant thromboxane A_2 versus decreased synthesis of prostacyclin—the potent endothelium-derived inhibitor of platelet aggregation. In most individuals on Western diets which contain limited amounts of the omega fatty acid precursors of prostacyclin synthesis, the net result is a prolonged bleeding time. When aspirin is discontinued, the exposed platelets remain impaired, but newly synthesized platelets with normal function soon begin to contribute to normalization of the bleeding time. Usually, the aspirin effect on bleeding time has dissipated significantly by 3 days after discontinuation.

NONSTEROIDAL ANTI-INFLAMMATORY DRUGS. NSAIDs cause reversible inhibition of cyclooxygenase and, therefore, a shorter time of bleeding risk than aspirin after discontinuation.

ANTIBIOTICS. Antibiotics of the penicillin family, epitomized by carbenicillin, may cause a complex coagulopathy. In addition to disturbance of intestinal flora synthesis of vitamin K, a thrombocytopathy characterized by prolonged bleeding time and interference with the conversion of fibrinogen to fibrin (resulting in prolongation of the thrombin time) is recognized. These phenomena usually are not of major clinical significance, but they may add to other coagulation defects and affect interpretation of coagulation laboratory evaluations. When bleeding from these mechanisms is serious, platelet transfusion after discontinuation of the drug should bypass the impaired function of platelets exposed to the drug.

DYSPROTEINEMIAS

Abnormal immunoglobulin concentrations, as seen in myeloma and Waldenstrom's macroglobulinemia, interfere with platelet function (causing prolonged bleeding times), presumably by physical "coating" of platelet surfaces, thus limiting access of clotting factors to the phospholipid surfaces provided by platelets which are needed to promote key reactions in the clotting cascade. In addition, prolongation of the thrombin time is often noted.

CARDIOPULMONARY BYPASS[12]

Acquired thrombocytopathy is regularly produced by platelet contact with membrane surfaces in bypass circuits. In some patients this may add to other mechanisms of increased bleeding risk (such as hypofibrinogenemia and inadequate heparin neutralization) after bypass. Transfusion of donor platelets (if clinically urgent) is expected to normalize the bleeding time once bypass is discontinued.

THROMBIN-INDUCED STORAGE POOL DEFECT (DIC)

Thrombocytopathy may contribute to the bleeding problems in DIC. During active DIC (e.g., in acute promyelocytic leukemia), an acquired platelet function defect with prolonged bleeding time may appear secondary to release of granule contents by excess thrombin. This is likely to be especially troublesome when patients are thrombocytopenic as well. Control of the DIC is the key to successful correction of this problem. Infusion of donor platelets is of benefit for only limited time periods, since these platelets are also exposed to excess thrombin while the DIC is active.

Fibrin Generation Disorders

SAMPLE COLLECTION AND INTERPRETATION

Accurate clotting time values, which form the basis for assessment of the integrity of the coagulation cascade, depend on collection of the correct quantity of blood relative to the amount of anticoagulant present in the sample tube; in addition, extraneous contamination by heparin must be avoided. It is important not to overfill collection tubes; rather, one should permit the vacuum to determine the correct amount of specimen per tube and then promptly invert to ensure adequate mixing with anticoagulants. Rapid delivery to the testing location decreases problems with cascade activation in the tube (which leads to prolonged clotting times). When drawing from heparinized lines, a double draw (discarding at least 10 ml initially and using the second aliquot) should prevent heparin contamination. Unexpectedly long PTT levels not corrected by a 1:1 mix with pooled normal plasma and corrected by incubation with heparin neutralizer powder (triethylaminoethyl cellulose) should indicate presence of heparin contamination.

Consideration of the results of PT and PTT in combination can help identify the site(s) of cascade deficiency (Table 146-4). Prolonged clotting times should be restudied after mixing patient's plasma with an equal volume of pooled normal plasma to differentiate between absence of factors in question and inhibition of their activity by circulating inhibitors. If the clotting time corrects on such 1:1 mix, a deficiency is present; if the clotting time of the mix remains prolonged, an inhibitor (such as heparin or an inhibitor directed against a specific clotting factor) is present.

ISOLATED FACTOR DEFICIENCIES

Isolated severe factor deficiencies may antedate and complicate the need for intensive care as in hemophilia A or B, or may be acquired as a consequence of the critical illness, e.g., hypofibrinogenemia secondary to DIC.

HYPOFIBRINOGENEMIA

Low functional fibrinogen levels in the ICU most commonly result from decreased hepatic synthesis or increased removal due to thrombin and plasmin action during DIC. Bleeding risk is increased by the anticoagulant effect of nonclottable fibrin split products in high titer. Spontaneous

TABLE 146-4 Use of Combined PT and PTT Results to Determine Site(s) of Fibrin Generation Cascade Defects

	PT–Normal	PT–Elevated
PTT–Normal	Result 1	Result 2
PTT–Elevated	Result 3	Result 4

Result 1: Normal screen of cascade (factor levels at least 30 to 35% of normal)
Result 2: Isolated low factor VII level—may be due to congenital deficiency or *early* liver disease, vitamin K deficiency or warfarin effect.
Result 3: Intrinsic pathway abnormality—low factor VIII, IX, XI or XII; typical pattern in hemophilia A and von Willebrand's disease
Result 4: Due to common pathway abnormality (factors I [Fibrinogen], II, V, X) and/or combined intrinsic and extrinsic pathway defects. Seen in *advanced* liver disease, vitamin K deficiency, full warfarin and heparin effects, and DIC.

clinical hemorrhage from hypofibrinogenemia is not expected above a concentration of 100 mg/dL in plasma and usually is not a serious risk until levels <50 mg/dL are reached. Fibrinogen may be replaced with fresh frozen plasma (FFP) or, more effectively, by cryoprecipitate; 1 cryopack is expected to raise the fibrinogen level approximately 4 mg/dL in a 70-kg patient. Although the plasma half-life of fibrinogen is approximately 4 days under normal circumstances, serial plasma fibrinogen level determinations will dictate frequency of infusions (as often as every 6 to 12 h especially in acutely ill patients with shortened fibrinogen half-life).

HEMOPHILIA A (FACTOR VIII DEFICIENCY)

Critical illness in a patient with hemophilia A requires careful correction of the preexisting coagulopathy, especially when complicated by such new problems as ITP, DIC, sepsis, and hepatic or renal dysfunction. Appearance of an inhibitor to factor VIII and development of a progressive pseudotumor may further increase the complexity of management. Preparation of the severe hemophiliac for surgery consists of checking to exclude an inhibitor and then replacing with factor VIII concentrate to achieve the desired percent correction (100 percent equals 1 U factor VIII/mL patient's plasma). For major surgery, a starting level at or above 100 percent is desirable. Additional doses are given intraoperatively. The doses are dictated by the amount of bleeding and stat factor VIII levels. The shortened half-life of factor VIII during bleeding leads to increased requirements for replacement (both higher doses and shorter intervals between doses). Sample calculation: a 70-kg patient with an hematocrit of 40 percent will have a blood volume of 4900 mL (70 mL/kg) and a plasma volume of 2940 mL (60 percent of his blood volume). If the starting factor VIII level is <1 percent, approximately 3000 U factor VIII concentrate will be needed to achieve correction to the 100 percent level. It is important to assess adequacy of correction by monitoring of factor VIII level before invasive procedures and to continue support for 10 to 14 days after a major surgical procedure or hemorrhage to prevent serious delayed bleeding. Maintenance postoperative factor VIII support usually is given every 8 to 12 h, with the goal that factor VIII plasma level nadirs not reach <40 to 50 percent before each dose.

Similar considerations apply to patients with hemophilia B (Christmas disease), except that replacement is with FFP or factor IX concentrate in severe deficiency states. A recombinant factor IX product is being tested.

FACTOR VII DEFICIENCY

This is a much less common inherited deficiency. It is a non-X-linked disorder with a variable severity, which may, in some patients, present as a severe hemophilia-like condition. Replacement with FFP or prothrombin complex is appropriate. The relatively short half-life of factor VII (4 to 7 h) may require dosing at 6 to 8 h intervals during major hemostatic challenges, but less frequent maintenance doses may be sufficient beyond the fourth day following some orthopedic procedures.[19]

Isolated factor VII deficiency is most often acquired due to vitamin K deficiency, early liver disease, and during initiation of warfarin anticoagulation. When factor VII deficiency cannot be corrected with vitamin K therapy, factor replacement with FFP or, when indicated, prothrombin complex can be accomplished. A recombinant factor VII product is being tested.

FACTOR XI DEFICIENCY

Factor XI deficiency is usually inherited, although in advanced liver disease factor XI deficiency may coexist with low levels of the other factors synthesized in liver parenchymal cells. FFP is the only replacement product.

FACTORS II, V, X

These deficiencies usually coexist with others, although isolated factor X deficiency with significant bleeding may be seen in amyloidosis. FFP replacement therapy is indicated, if needed, but may not readily correct an amyloid-associated factor X deficiency because of the rapid clearance of the factor, which attaches to the amyloid fibrils. Splenectomy may be helpful in such instances. FFP and prothrombin complex (for II and X) are the replacement products.

FACTOR XII

Factor XII deficiency causes a prolonged PTT, without clinically significant bleeding diathesis. Some have suggested that, paradoxically, patients severely deficient in XII may be hypercoagulable. It is important to identify this factor deficiency to avoid unnecessary correction of the PTT with FFP.

FACTOR XIII

Deficiency of factor XIII[20] is usually lifelong and may be associated with significant bleeding problems of the delayed type. In homozygotes there is a predilection for fatal intracranial bleeding; spontaneous abortion also has been noted. Rarely, acquired deficiency is seen in patients who develop an inhibitor while taking drugs such as isoniazid. The diagnosis cannot be made from the usual clotting or bleeding time tests. Rather, this deficiency must be suspected and assayed for directly. Clot dissolution in 5 *M* urea during overnight incubation indicates deficiency (<1 percent activity). The deficiency is readily corrected with FFP, cryoprecipitate, or a placental concentrate. More than 1 to 2 percent of the normal factor XIII level is adequate for hemostasis and intact clot stability. Prolonged half-life (8 days) permits long dosing intervals and easy prophylaxis when a hemostatic challenge is anticipated.

VON WILLEBRAND'S FACTOR[21]

Deficiency of VWF results in a bleeding disorder more akin to that associated with platelet dysfunction than to the hemophilias. Cardinal findings include prolonged bleeding time and moderately prolonged PTT with depression (usually mild) of factor VIII coagulant (VIII:C) level. Decreased ristocetin cofactor and von Willebrand's antigen levels are also found. The commonest variety (type I) is characterized by a defect in secretion of normal VWF from vascular endothelial cells. Less commonly, qualitative defects in multimeric structure (type II) or severe synthetic deficiency (recessively inherited type III) are seen. Type I patients may respond to infusion of DDAVP, a synthetic vasopressin analogue, with a rise in VWF and other released endothelial products some of which may have anticoagulant effects (such as prostacyclin [PGI_2] and tissue plasminogen activator). Usually, there is a net hemostatic benefit seen as an improved bleeding time over a several hour period. Repeat doses may be given, but tachyphylaxis after 2 to 3 days precludes effective long-term therapy with DDAVP.

The Duke bleeding time is considered by some[21] to be the best indicator of bleeding risk prior to procedures, although more extensive work-up, including functional (ristocetin cofactor, PTT, VIII:C) and antigenic (VIII-related antigen and multimer analysis) studies may be useful in characterizing the type and severity of defect. The usual goal of therapy is normalization of the bleeding time during active bleeding and before anticipated surgery or invasive procedures. A recent critical review of the bleeding time[22] raises questions as to the predictability of bleeding from the bleeding time result in individual cases. For severe deficiency and prolonged treatment, cryoprecipitate is indicated. DDAVP is contraindicated in type IIB and platelet type (or pseudo) von Willebrand's—two conditions in which platelet aggregation and thrombocytopenia may ensue.

INHIBITORS[23]

Coagulation factor inhibitors may create life-threatening situations, especially in otherwise critically ill patients. The potency of the inhibitor can be determined by titration of the effect of plasma dilutions on the result of mixing patient's plasma with pooled normal plasma (vide supra).

FACTOR VIII INHIBITORS

The most commonly encountered inhibitor is directed against factor VIII. This is seen most frequently in hemophiliac patients on supplementary factor replacement but can also occur sporadically in elderly individuals, postpartum, and in persons with an autoimmune diathesis or lymphoma.[24] Factor VIII inhibition usually is quantitated in Bethesda units; levels >10 u/mL indicate more potent inhibitors. For lesser titers, infusion of factor VIII concentrate often can override the inhibitor in the short term, although in some patients this will result in stimulation of a rising inhibitor titer. Other modes of therapy for high titer inhibitors include bypassing the factor VIII-dependent step with prothrombin complex concentrate, use of porcine factor VIII concentrates, and combined immunosuppressant programs which include cytotoxic agents, plasma processing over columns which remove IgG and immune complexes,[25] and high dose intravenous immunoglobulin.

Inhibitors found in nonhemophiliacs tend to be more responsive to simpler immunosuppressive treatments, e.g., azathioprine and prednisone. There is a significant risk of bleeding in these individuals when the inhibitor is not controlled. If an underlying tumor or autoimmune disorder is present, its management may help reduce the level of inhibitor. Surgical procedures in patients with inhibitors are obviously fraught with high risk, and meticulous hemostatic correction perioperatively is necessary. Correction needs to be maintained for at least 10 days after major procedures (as in uncomplicated hemophilia) to prevent delayed bleeding.

LUPUS ANTICOAGULANTS

The presence of the so-called *lupus anticoagulant*[26] is important to recognize, because, despite the usually associated prolonged PTT, it may imply a hypercoagulable state rather than a bleeding diathesis. This phospholipid inhibitor was first identified in patients with de novo systemic lupus erythematosus (SLE), but it is known to occur also in drug-induced SLE syndromes, in individuals with other autoimmune diseases, and in otherwise normal persons. The typical laboratory result is a long PTT with evidence of an inhibitor and interference with several of the coagulation factor assays. An abnormally steep rise in the PT with serial dilution of thromboplastin in vitro is a characteristic finding (tissue thromboplastin inhibition [TTI] test). This latter phenomenon may be mimicked by the presence of heparin and coumadin anticoagulation; therefore, it is preferable to perform the test, if possible, before anticoagulation is begun. Absorption of the patient's plasma with platelet phospholipid in vitro may remove the inhibitor and lead to normalization of the PTT and the TTI test, thus enhancing the specificity of diagnosis.

Most patients with the lupus anticoagulant do not have coagulation problems, but approximately 25 percent may have clinically important hypercoagulability. It is unclear whether empirical prophylactic long-term anticoagulation with warfarin is useful. Perioperative minidose heparinization is recommended to offset other hypercoagulable stimuli, which may be additive. If thrombotic problems—typically venous (deep venous thrombosis, pulmonary emboli) do occur, chronic anticoagulation with warfarin is recommended.

Reduction of potency of lupus anticoagulants may occur spontaneously, as a result of discontinuation of an offending drug (e.g., procainamide), or in response to immunosuppressive therapy (e.g., prednisone).

COMBINED FACTOR DEFICIENCY STATES

VITAMIN K DEFICIENCY.[27] The combination of poor dietary intake and antibiotic therapy so commonly seen in the ICU patient readily predisposes to vitamin K deficiency. Impaired absorption of fat-soluble vitamins, as in biliary obstruction, may contribute as well. Prolongation of the PT initially and then both PT and PTT is characteristic. Documentation of selected reduction of Factors II, IX, and X is rarely needed to make this diagnosis; usually the initial decline in VII in the absence of other explanations, such as liver disease or coumadin anticoagulation, is sufficient. Vitamin K supplementation therapy may be by oral, subcutaneous, intramuscular, or intravenous routes. The oral route is preferred, if possible, to avoid risk of hematoma or, rarely, anaphylaxis after intravenous dosing. Glucose-6-phosphate dehydrogenase (G6PD)-deficient individuals may experience hemolytic reactions from the oxidant effects of vitamin K preparations.

DYSFIBRINOGENEMIA

A qualitative abnormality of fibrinogen may or may not be associated with hypofibrinogenemia.[28] The diagnosis is made by finding disproportionately low functional fibrinogen relative to the antigenic fibrinogen level. In addition to the variety of inherited fibrinogen abnormalities associated with bleeding, clotting, and wound dehiscence problems which have been recognized, acquired decrease in fibrinogen function also is seen commonly in parenchymal liver disease.[29]

If it becomes clinically necessary to correct the hypofibrinogenemia, infusion of cryoprecipitate is the method of choice. A functional level of ≥100 mg/dL is the usual goal of therapy.

Fibrinolytic Disorders

DEFINITIONS AND LABORATORY TESTING METHODS

Clot strength and stability are the keys to prevention of rebleeding and consequent development of hemorrhagic infarction after initial hemostasis. Formation of covalent bonding of fibrin mediated by factor XIII is important for clot strength, and carefully regulated activity of the fibrinolytic system allows eventual clot degradation at a time when the vessel is strong enough to handle reestablished flow. The details of regulation of the fibrinolytic process, including its intensity and timing, are incompletely understood.

Fibrinolytic activity is mediated by plasmin, which is derived from the inactive plasma precursor plasminogen. Plasminogen can be activated by various endogenous kinases, including tissue plasminogen activator and urokinase, as well as by exogenous agents such as streptokinase. The activity of plasmin is regulated by a series of inhibitors, the most important of which is α_2-antiplasmin. The activity of the fibrinolytic system is assessed indirectly in vitro by measurement of concentrations of substrate (fibrinogen) and plasmin-generated breakdown products of fibrinogen and fibrin (FDPs, D-dimer). Lesser degrees of fibrinolysis may be detected by measuring plasmin-antiplasmin complexes.

PRIMARY FIBRINOLYSIS

It is helpful to distinguish so-called primary fibrinolysis, in which plasmin is generated from plasminogen by an activator in the plasma, from secondary fibrinolysis, in which plasmin is generated within a formed clot by activator which is also present. Primary fibrinolysis (fibrinogenolysis) is seen in states of tissue injury such as liver disease or therapeutic administration of activators, e.g., urokinase and streptokinase. Secondary fibrinolysis is the normal mechanism of clot degradation initiated by tissue plasminogen activator. The latter process is accelerated pathologically in DIC.

SECONDARY FIBRINOLYSIS

The in vitro tests of clot lysis, such as the euglobulin lysis time, are sensitive to generation of circulating plasmin and therefore are shortened in primary fibrinolysis but normal in secondary fibrinolytic states (e.g., DIC). Levels of fibrinogen and FDPs do not distinguish the two mechanisms. D-dimer is a unique degradation product of cross-linked fibrin not seen among the products of plasmin digestion of fibrinogen. As such, it is helpful in distinguishing fibrinogenolysis from fibrinolysis. This is especially helpful in evaluating states of increased clot formation such as DIC. However, it must be emphasized that elevated D-dimer levels do not indicate the mechanism of clot generation, e.g., during dissolution of a hematoma there may be high levels of D-dimer without the necessary implication that DIC was the basis for the original clot formation.

Complex Coagulopathies

ACUTE DISSEMINATED INTRAVASCULAR COAGULATION[9]

The most important complex coagulopathy in intensive care medicine is acute DIC. This is basically a state of increased propensity for clot formation triggered by a variety of stimuli related to such diverse underlying disorders as sepsis, tissue injury, and neoplasm. There may be clinical and laboratory evidence of hypercoagulability, but in acute cases, consumptive coagulopathy with hemorrhagic manifestations may predominate. The full-blown state is characterized by thrombocytopenia, prolonged clotting times, depressed circulating levels of cascade factors (especially factor VIII), and increased fibrinolysis manifested by high

FDP and D-dimer levels as well as hypofibrinogenemia. There may be associated hemolysis with evidence of microangiopathic changes on blood smear (schistocytes) in some patients. Organ dysfunction secondary to vasoocclusion or hemorrhage may be evident. DIC should be suspected when such a complex coagulopathy appears, especially if the clinical setting predisposes to it.

The key step in management is therapy of the condition (e.g., antibiotic treatment for infection) predisposing to the underlying hypercoagulable state. Transfusion of blood products, e.g., RBCs, platelets, FFP, and, if needed for correction of severe hypofibrinogenemia, cryoprecipitate, may protect the patient from hemorrhagic complications while the mechanism triggering the DIC is being eliminated. Although, in theory, blood product support may temporarily "feed the fire," often patients benefit from such treatment without requiring heparin therapy with its attendant potential complications.

In cases of purpura fulminans and massive thromboembolism, where the pace of the process is catastrophic, trial of heparin therapy is appropriate, along with blood product support, especially in patients who have potentially treatable underlying disorders which can be expected to respond in a relatively short time to appropriate specific therapy. Doses of heparin required are variable because of heparin resistance in DIC (due to low antithrombin III and elevated platelet factor 4 levels). The necessary dosages may vary from 5 to 10 U/kg/h by continuous intravenous infusion up to full therapeutic levels. The usual criteria used to determine whether heparin is helpful include clinical observation of lessened bleeding and rise in fibrinogen levels and platelet counts.

There are obvious risks to the use of heparin because of uncertainty as to the optimal dose and difficulty in clotting test interpretation created by the addition of an anticoagulant drug. Heparin therapy usually is not indicated for patients with bleeding in critical areas, e.g., intracranial locations. In addition, isolated antifibrinolytic therapy with agents such as ϵ-aminocaproic acid is *contraindicated* because of the risk of extensive thrombotic complications. For more chronic, low-grade DIC, subcutaneous heparin (e.g., 5000 U every 8 to 12 h) may be helpful in preventing clinical thrombotic complications.

Laboratory parameters for following DIC include: clotting times, platelet count, and fibrinogen level (assuming they are not simultaneously disturbed by an underlying process such as leukemia or liver failure). FDP levels are good markers for detection of fibrinolysis but tend to lag behind as indicators of improvement.

MASSIVE TRANSFUSION

Patients who have received one to two blood volumes replaced with stored RBCs are subject to development of a complex coagulopathy, the most important feature of which is thrombocytopenia due to both dilutional and consumptive mechanisms.[30] In addition, there may be impaired platelet function and lowered levels of plasma factor VIII and factor V. Successful management of this coagulopathy depends on recognizing the developing pattern and providing sufficient platelets and FFP to offset the effects of dilution (see Chap. 35). More serious disturbances of hemostasis appear if DIC as a consequence of the underlying shock and/or tissue injury becomes manifest (vide supra).

ANTIBIOTIC THERAPY

Use of multiple or broad-spectrum antibiotics predisposes to combined coagulation defects. Vitamin K deficiency is common. A mixture of impaired platelet function manifested by prolonged bleeding time and prolonged thrombin time has been observed with carbenicillin[31] and other related antibiotics.

LIVER DISEASE[32]

Because of the key role of the liver in clotting factor synthesis, coagulopathies are an important part of liver dysfunction. Not only are clotting times prolonged, but if there is associated hypersplenism, thrombocytopenia also may be present. In addition, primary fibrinolysis secondary to liver cell injury may add to a picture which may mimic DIC. It is not unusual to see DIC superimposed on liver failure causing a severe complex coagulopathy. When attempting to distinguish the coagulopathy of advanced liver failure from DIC, the pattern of fibrinolysis and factor VIII:C level may help. Primary fibrinolysis (short euglobulin lysis time) and elevated factor VIII:C levels are seen in liver disease; secondary type fibrinolysis (normal euglobulin lysis time) and low factor VIII:C levels (as well as elevated D-dimer) favor DIC.

Therapy for the coagulopathy of liver disease consists of replacement of clotting factors and correction of vitamin K deficiency. If volume considerations permit, FFP is used first. Often it is necessary to use prothrombin complex for adequate correction prior to invasive or surgical procedures. The risks of administration of this product include enhanced coagulation and, in some instances, DIC due to the presence of activated clotting factors in the concentrate. The cost and increased risk of transmission of viral agents from such pooled products are other considerations.

RENAL DISEASE

Uremic patients are likely to have a bleeding diathesis which most commonly is a thrombocytopathy characterized by prolonged bleeding time. The disease underlying the renal failure may also, of course, predispose to a coagulopathy (e.g., immune thrombocytopenia due to SLE, factor X deficiency secondary to amyloid, low antithrombin III and factor IX levels in nephrotic syndrome of various causes). The thrombocytopathy becomes especially important if surgical interventions such as renal biopsy are needed. One is usually able to obtain sufficient acute or subacute hemostasis by using one or more of the treatments discussed earlier, but chronic protection from bleeding is more difficult to achieve. Recent evidence suggests that hemostasis may be improved in uremia after treatment with recombinant human erythropoietin.[33]

DYSPROTEINEMIAS[34]

Patients with multiple myeloma or Waldenstrom's macroglobulinemia may have significant bleeding problems in addition to the thrombocytopenia which may accompany advanced disease or be a consequence of treatment. Both impaired platelet function (prolonged bleeding time) and prolonged thrombin time secondary to interference with fibrinogen conversion to fibrin may be seen. The mechanism of these effects is not fully understood but is thought to reflect physical effects of the paraproteins "coating" the platelets, thereby interfering with exposure of their needed phospholipid template for key cascade steps and possible steric hindrance of the process of fibrin formation. These adverse effects on coagulation tend to improve with a decline in paraprotein levels (by chemotherapy-induced decreased production or removal by plasmapheresis).

Coagulation Status: Guidelines for Invasive Procedures

GENERAL CONSIDERATIONS

Guideline 1: Perform procedures only when absolutely necessary in patients who have coagulopathies or can be expected to develop them as a result of their disease or its therapy.

Guideline 2: Make the intervention(s) as limited as possible and preferably perform procedures which can be done under direct vision. This facilitates assurance of primary hemostasis and easier follow-up for detection of delayed bleeding.

Guideline 3: Be certain that the preliminary coagulation status is fully delineated, so that potential bleeding risks can be anticipated accurately and the correct therapeutic agents can be available.

Guideline 4: If a preparatory treatment (e.g., infusion of factor VIII concentrate) or change in medication (e.g., discontinuation of an anticoagulant drug) is indicated, be certain to check that the expected beneficial effect has actually occurred before the procedure begins.

Guideline 5: Coordinate the timing of procedures for which supportive products are needed with the providers (e.g., blood bank or pharmacy) so that an adequate supply is available for the anticipated duration of support. Be liberal in estimating needs so that unexpected complications can be covered.

Guideline 6: Carefully follow the patient for both immediate and delayed bleeding to detect status changes early. Alert coworkers to the potential for bleeding and the appropriate therapy based on previous evaluation.

Guideline 7: Be alert to potential effects of changes in medical status (e.g., onset of sepsis) or newly added medications which may complicate the coagulation status of patients who have already been evaluated and treated appropriately for their initial coagulopathy. Be prepared to reassess the patient if there is decreasing response to initially appropriate therapy.

SPECIFIC COAGULOPATHIES

VASCULITIS

Patients with vasculitic rashes may have very long bleeding times which prohibit skin incision. Discontinuation of an offending drug and trial of corticosteroids may be useful. Platelets are not indicated unless thrombocytopenia or thrombocytopathy coexist.

THROMBOCYTOPENIA

Platelet counts for direct vision procedures such as limited biopsies or peripheral line insertions are usually adequate at 50,000 to 80,000/mm^3, depending on the extent of the intervention. For major surgical procedures, insertion of lines in large central vessels, or closed-space needle biopsies, initial levels at the 80,000 to 100,000/mm^3 range are preferred (assuming normal qualitative platelet function which may be assessed by the bleeding time). Lumbar punctures are usually performed safely at platelet counts $>$50,000/mm^3.

THROMBOCYTOPATHY

Thrombocytopathic bleeding can be very difficult to manage, especially if the environment into which new platelets are transfused is deleterious to their function. Thus, in uremia, for example, multiple transfusions of normal platelets may be ineffective. Other methods of therapy discussed in earlier sections of this chapter may be helpful in this situation. The bleeding time may not be corrected significantly in some patients. The predictive value of the skin incision bleeding time in individual patients has been questioned recently,[22] but it seems prudent to attempt to lower an elevated bleeding time, when possible, prior to invasive procedures.

Drug-induced thrombocytopathies may be easier to manage if the drug has a reasonably short half-life or reversible inhibitory effect on platelet function (e.g., NSAIDs). After the drug effect has dissipated following discontinuation, newly produced platelets by the patient's marrow and transfused normal platelets (if needed for an acute intervention) will correct the prolonged bleeding time.

THROMBOCYTHEMIA

Patients with myeloproliferative disorders and elevated platelet counts (normally in excess of 1×10^6/mm^3, but sometimes also in the 0.5×10^6 to 1×10^6/mm^3 range) often have excessive bleeding, either spontaneously or following trauma or surgery. It generally is advisable to lower the platelet count to the normal range, but despite this some patients will have considerable bleeding difficulties. The bleeding time may be a helpful predictor. It is wise to avoid or minimize procedures, when possible, in these individuals.

FIBRIN GENERATION CASCADE DEFECTS

Insist on at least normal PT and PTT levels, if achievable, for procedures in which excess bleeding seriously can compromise the outcome (e.g., intracranial neurosurgery) or when closed-space procedures are performed in which mechanical hemostasis is difficult to achieve or extent of bleeding may not be obvious until it is significant. More precise factor level correction than implied by normal clotting times is indicated for such procedures in patients with known factor deficiency states such as hemophilia A.

For direct vision procedures or line placements, there may be a greater tolerance of impaired clotting times. The clotting times should not exceed 1.2 to 1.3 times base line under these circumstances. In contrast to platelet-related problems, bleeding in patients with cascade deficiencies may be delayed in onset and, therefore, unexpected by uninformed medical and nursing staff.

FIBRINOLYTIC STATES

Hyperfibrinolytic states leading to short clot survival, hypofibrinogenemia, and elevated FDPs may be associated with serious bleeding during and after procedures. Intracranial bleeding, thrombotic events, and major surgical procedures are contraindications to initiation of fibrinolytic therapy, because of the risk of clot breakdown. Invasive procedures while the patient is in a fibrinolytic state are to be avoided if possible. If bleeding occurs during fibrinolytic therapy, the usual approach is to discontinue the drug, provide blood product support (including cryoprecipitate as a source of fibrinogen, if needed), and wait until the fibrinolytic state subsides.

ANTICOAGULANT EFFECTS

HEPARIN. The heparinized patient who needs a procedure usually can be managed by discontinuation of heparin approximately 6 h beforehand. In urgent circumstances, neutralization with protamine can hasten preparation.

WARFARIN. After discontinuation or tapering of warfarin therapy prior to an intended procedure, it may take two days or more for the PT to normalize. In emergent situations, use of FFP or prothrombin complex (if volume overload is a problem) can provide immediate correction by supply of the missing factors. Oral or intravenous vitamin K has onset of its effect after approximately 12 h. A state of subsequent warfarin resistance is likely to be established by its use in doses sufficient to correct the PT (e.g,. 25 mg daily for 3 days). Use of prothrombin complex may be associated with induction of a hypercoagulable state. It should be reserved, therefore, for urgent indications. During the period following tapering of warfarin, temporary heparinization with subsequent discontinuation of heparin 6 h before an invasive procedure will permit flexibility in planning of interventions.

CASE PRESENTATION

A previously healthy 57-year-old factory worker was admitted to the emergency room complaining of weakness, fever, and bilateral flank pain of 2 h duration. Although he had felt quite well 4 h before while eating dinner, he had had a single episode of gross hematuria and had noted some unexplained bruises on his legs 3 h before. Physical examination confirmed the presence of several purpuric areas on his legs without evidence of trauma, mild abdominal distention, epigastric tenderness, and a distended urinary bladder by percussion. Vital signs were: blood pressure, 100/60; pulse, 120/min; respiration, 20/min; and temperature, 39.4°C (103°F). He was alert but restless. Initial laboratory values revealed WBC 17,500/mm^3 with 20 percent bands; hemoglobin 9 g/dL; hematocrit 27 percent; platelets 200,000/mm^3; PT, 65; and PTT > 100 s. Schistocytes were seen on peripheral blood smear. Insertion of a Foley catheter yielded 300 mL of grossly bloody urine. A nasogastric tube returned 400 mL fresh and partially clotted blood. A detailed coagulation work-up was sent, RBCs and FFP transfusions were started, and empirical intravenous antibiotic therapy with ampicillin and gentamicin was started after cultures were obtained. Vital signs remained stable, and the patient was transferred to the ICU. Bleeding from intravenous puncture sites, nasogastric tube, and urinary tract continued, and new purpuric lesions appeared. Blood drawn into tubes without anticoagulant failed to clot. Supportive therapy with RBCs, fluids, and FFP continued, but the patient became first agitated then lethargic and was intubated.

Coagulation profile data;

1. PT and PTT—corrected to normal when patient's sample was mixed in equal volume with pooled normal plasma (no circulating inhibitor present)
2. FDP titer >2560 μg/mL (normal 10 to 20)
3. D-dimer 16 to 32 (normal < .5)
4. Repeat platelet count (after RBCs and FFP)—120,000/mm^3
5. Fibrinogen <15 mg/dL (normal 200 to 400 mg/dL)
6. Factor VIII:C 20 percent (normal 50 to 150 percent)
7. Factor V—50 percent
8. Liver function tests—bilirubin, albumin, alkaline phosphatase, SGPT—normal; SGOT and LDH moderately elevated.

When the fibrinogen level was obtained, 20 U cryoprecipitate was infused. Within 1 to 2 h spontaneous bleeding stopped; repeat fibrinogen of 80 mg/dL was obtained, and fever declined to 38.5°C (101.5°F). Another dose of cryoprecipitate (10 U) was given 6 h after the first. Over the course of the next 24 h, the coagulation picture improved. The patient was extubated 24 h after admission. Blood and urine cultures grew gram-negative bacteria. The patient continued to improve and was referred for urologic consultation.

CASE DISCUSSION

This dramatic case of DIC secondary to urosepsis and complicating bacteremia indicates the importance of supportive care until treatment of the underlying cause can become effective (in this case, bactericidal antibiotic therapy). The rapid onset and profound fibrinolytic parameters are more extreme than in most instances of DIC but serve to illustrate the potentially catastrophic consequences of this coagulopathy if not recognized and treated appropriately. The nature of the coagulopathy became evident when the detailed work-up was completed. In critically ill patients, it is wise to perform a comprehensive laboratory coagulation base-line work-up and then follow the key parameters serially during therapeutic interventions.

The high D-dimer level indicates that the very low fibrinogen level resulted from excess effect of both thrombin and plasmin (i.e., accelerated clot formation and degradation). If the patient had not sustained a rise in the fibrinogen level with cryoprecipitate, addition of heparin to the regimen at an initial dose rate of 5 to 10 U/kg intravenously hourly would have been considered in an effort to provide a temporary decrease in clot formation. ϵ-Aminocaproic acid was contraindicated in this clinical setting because resulting clot stabilization could have caused serious organ damage secondary to infarction.

References

1. Bowie EJW, Owen CA: The clinical and laboratory diagnosis of hemorrhagic disorders, in Ratnoff OD, Forbes CD (eds): *Disorders of Hemostasis.* Orlando, Grune & Stratton, 1984, p 43.
2. Thompson AR, Harker LA: *Manual of Hemostasis and Thrombosis,* 3d ed. Philadelphia, Davis, 1983, p 175 (Appendix A).
3. Winkelmann RK: Classification of vasculitis, in Wolff K, Winkelmann RK (eds): *Vasculitis.* London, Lloyd-Luke, 1980, p 1.
4. Kasabach HS, Merritt KK: Capillary hemangioma with extensive purpura: Report of a case. Am J Dis Child 259:1063, 1940.
5. McKee LC Jr, Collins RD: Intravascular leukocyte thrombi and aggregates as a cause of morbidity and mortality in leukemia. Medicine 53:463, 1974.
6. Bussel JB, Kimberly RP, Inman RD, et al: Intravenous gammaglobulin treatment of chronic idiopathic thrombocytopenic purpura. Blood 62:480, 1983.
7. Berney SJ, Metcalfe P, Wathen NC, Waters AH: Post-transfusion purpura responding to high dose intravenous IgG: Further observations on pathogenesis. Brit J Haematol 61:627, 1985.
8. Bukowski RM: Thrombotic thrombocytopenic purpura: A review. Prog Hemost Thromb 6:287, 1982.
9. Marder VJ, Martin SE, Francis CW, Colman RW: Consumptive thrombohemorrhagic disorders, in Colman RW, Hirsh J, Marder VJ, Salzman EW (eds): *Hemostasis and Thrombosis.* 2d ed. Philadelphia, Lippincott, 1987, p 975.
10. King DJ, Kelton JG: Heparin-associated thrombocytopenia. Ann Intern Med 100:535, 1984.
11. Kelton JG, Warkantin TE: Heparin-induced thrombocytopenia. Annu Rev Med 40:31, 1989.
12. Bick RL: Alterations of hemostasis during cardiopulmonary bypass: A comparison between membrane and bubble oxygenators. Am J Clin Pathol 73:300, 1980.
13. Harker LA, Finch CA: Thrombokinetics in man. J Clin Invest 48:963, 1969.
14. Hardisty RM, Wolf HH: Haemorrhagic thrombocythemia: A clinical and laboratory study. Br J Haematol 1:390, 1955.
15. Coller BS: Disorders of platelets, in Ratnoff OD, Forbes CD (eds): *Disorders of Hemostasis.* Orlando, Grune & Stratton, 1984, p 143.
16. Janson PA, Jubelier SJ, Weinstein MJ, Deykin D: Treatment of the bleeding tendency in uremia with cryoprecipitate. N Engl J Med 303:1318, 1980.
17. Mannucci PM, Remuzzi G, Pusineri F, et al: Deamino-8-D arginine vasopressin shortens the bleeding time in uremia. N Engl J Med 308:8, 1983.
18. Liu YK, Kosfeld RE, Marcum SG: Treatment of uraemic bleeding with conjugated estrogen. Lancet ii:887, 1984.
19. Kuzel T, Green D, Stulberg SD, Baron J: Arthropathy and surgery in congenital factor VII deficiency. Am J Med 84:771, 1988.
20. Lorand L, Losowsky MS, Miloszewski KJM: Human factor XIII: Fibrin-stabilizing factor. Prog Haemost Thromb 5:245, 1980.
21. Coller BS: von Willebrand's disease, in Ratnoff OD, Forbes CD (eds): *Disorders of Hemostasis.* Orlando, Grune & Stratton, 1984, p 241.
22. Rodgers RPC, Levin J: A critical reappraisal of the bleeding time. Semin Thromb Hemost 16:1, 1990.
23. Shapiro SS: Acquired inhibitors to the blood coagulation factors. Semin Thromb Hemost 1:336, 1975.
24. Green D, Lechner K: A survey of 215 non-hemophilic patients with inhibitors to factor VIII. Thromb Haemost 45:200, 1981.
25. Nilsson IM, Jonsson S, Sundqvist SB, et al: A procedure for removing high titer antibodies by extracorporeal protein-A-sepharose adsorption in hemophilia: Substitution therapy and surgery in a patient with hemophilia B and antibodies. Blood 58:38, 1981.
26. Shapiro SS, Thiagarajan P: Lupus anticoagulants. Prog Hemost Thromb 6:263, 1982.
27. Olson RE: Vitamin K, in Colman RW, Hirsh J, Marder VJ, Salzman EW (eds): *Hemostasis and Thrombosis.* 2d ed. Philadelphia, Lippincott, 1987, p 846.
28. Beck EA, Charache P, Jackson D: A new inherited coagulation disorder caused by an abnormal fibrinogen (fibrinogen "Baltimore"). Nature 208:143, 1965.
29. Francis JL, Armstrong DJ: Acquired dysfibrinogenemia in liver disease. J Clin Pathol 35:667, 1982.
30. Harrigan C, Lucas CE, Ledgerwood AM, Mammen ET: Primary hemostasis after massive transfusion for injury. Am Surg 48:393, 1982.
31. Shattil SJ, Bennett JS, McDonough M, Turnbull J: Carbenicillin and penicillin G inhibit platelet function in vitro by impairing the interaction of agonists with the platelet surface. J Clin Invest 65:329, 1980.
32. Joist JH: Hemostatic abnormalities in liver disease, in Colman RW, Hirsh J, Marder VJ, Salzman EW (eds): *Hemostasis and Thrombosis.* 2d ed. Philadelphia, Lippincott, 1987, p 861.
33. Moia M, Mannucci PM, Vizzotto L, et al: Improvement in the haemostatic defect of uraemia after treatment with recombinant human erythropoietin. Lancet 2:1227, 1987.
34. Furie B: Acquired coagulation disorders and dysproteinemias, in Colman RW, Hirsh J, Marder VJ, Salzman EW (eds): *Hemostasis and Thrombosis.* 2d ed. Philadelphia, Lippincott, 1987, p 841.

Chapter 147

THROMBOTIC THROMBOCYTOPENIC PURPURA AND THE APPROACH TO THROMBOTIC MICROANGIOPATHIES

LAWRENCE TIM GOODNOUGH

KEY POINTS

- *The thrombotic microangiopathies (TMA) include the spectrum of thrombotic thrombocytopenic purpura (TTP) and hemolytic-uremic syndromes (HUS), and related obstetric syndromes.*
- *The hallmarks of TMA are a microangiopathic hemolytic anemia (MAHA) and thrombocytopenia.*
- *TMA must be distinguished from other coagulopathies such as disseminated intravascular coagulation (DIC) or collagen vascular disease with vasculitis, since therapeutic approaches differ.*
- *The clinical presentation of TTP is characterized by a pentad of findings: MAHA, thrombocytopenia, neurologic abnormalities, renal dysfunction, and fever.*
- *Plasma exchange is the therapy of choice for TTP, with adjunctive therapies including plasma infusion, corticosteroids, splenectomy, and antiplatelet agents.*
- *TTP is a hematologic emergency and patients are at risk to develop tissue anoxia, lactic acidosis, renal failure, or catastrophic central nervous system (CNS) injury.*
- *Complications of plasma exchange which may be encountered in the critical care environment include bleeding at catheter sites, air embolus, citrate toxicity, and pulmonary edema.*

Clinical Presentation

Moschcowitz's original description of TTP in 1925 was based on a triad of findings: (microangiopathic hemolytic) anemia, thrombocytopenia, and neurologic symptoms. By 1966, 271 cases of TTP were reviewed and the features of fever and renal impairment were added to form a clinical pentad.[1] Subsequent series have confirmed that renal involvement is common, with proteinuria, hematuria, or azotemia seen in 80 percent of patients with TTP.[2] Indeed, the hemolytic-uremia syndromes (HUS, MAHA, thrombocytopenia, and renal failure) are now regarded as part of a spectrum of TMA which at one extreme consists of TTP with predominant neurologic findings and minimal renal abnormality, and at the other extreme consists of profound renal dysfunction with no or minimal CNS pathology.[3] These latter syndromes, falling within the rubric HUS, are more common in childhood, the postpartum period, and following use of chemotherapeutic agents (particularly mitomycin C). On occasion, the evolution of renal manifestations in TTP can become indistinguishable from HUS, at which point attempts at rigid distinction are generally unrewarding.

The age of onset of TTP ranges from infancy to the eighth decade, with a peak incidence in the third decade. Females are more frequently affected than males by a ratio of 3:2. Childhood HUS often presents with antecedent illness, typically gastroenteritis related to enterotoxin-producing strains of *Escherichia coli* or *Shigella*. TMA associated with pregnancy includes several syndromes with considerable overlap, making rigid prospective differentiation difficult.[4] Pregnancy-induced hypertension (PIH; eclampsia and preeclampsia) is often associated with subtle laboratory abnormalities consistent with a degree of underlying TMA; on occasion this becomes clinically significant. When *h*ypertension, *e*levated *l*iver enzymes, and *l*ow *p*latelets occur together as a *s*yndrome in pregnancy, the term HELLPS is applied. TTP may also be encountered in pregnancy; unlike thrombocytopenias associated with PIH, it may not improve rapidly with termination of the pregnancy and require further treatment. Thus, diagnosis of TTP in pregnancy is often made with this retrospective information. Finally, postpartum HUS is distinguished by its onset after delivery.

Recently, TTP syndromes have been described in patients receiving chemotherapeutic agents[5] and cyclosporine[6] following organ transplantation. These are particularly important observations, since these patient populations are growing, are likely to be encountered in the critical care environment, and are at risk for multiple diseases that may be associated with coagulopathy and cytopenia, making diagnosis challenging.

The symptoms of TTP vary according to the extent and severity of the thrombotic lesions. Neurologic findings can be nonspecific, including headache alone or minor changes in mental status. Often these seemingly minor manifestations of disease are found by careful history to precede more fulminant findings associated with anemia, thrombocytopenia, or renal failure, and these pieces of information become crucial in establishing a diagnosis. Neurologic findings may be more obvious, and include seizures, obtundation, and even coma. Fever is present in approximately two-thirds of cases.

Laboratory findings in TTP are often striking. Thrombocytopenia may be profound, with platelet counts <50,000/mm^3 frequently observed. Anemia is of a microangiopathic type, and the peripheral smear is usually remarkable for fragmented red blood cells (RBCs), polychromatophilia, nucleated RBCs, and markedly diminished platelets (Fig. 147-1; Plate 49). Intravascular hemolysis frequently causes elevation of total bilirubin (predominantly direct fraction) and lactate dehydrogenase (LDH). Urinalysis usually re-

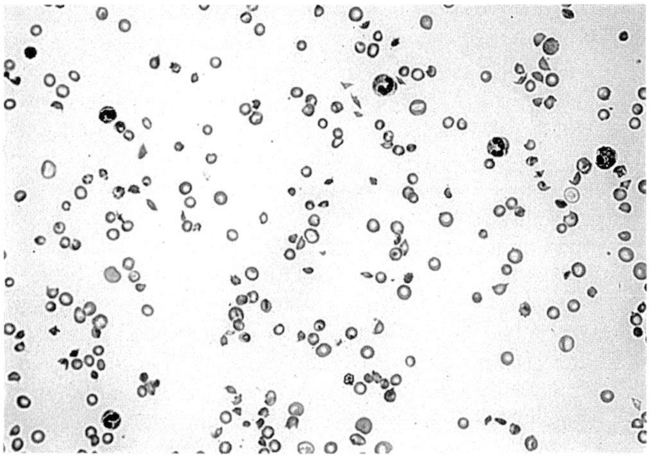

FIGURE 147-1 Admission (hospital day 1) peripheral blood smear (Wright-Giemsa stain) of patient B.B. showing characteristic RBC morphology of microangiopathic hemolytic anemia. Magnification ×350. (See Plate 49.)

veals proteinuria or hematuria; varying degrees of diminished glomerular filtration rate may be seen. Diagnosis of TTP by tissue biopsy has been advocated by some, but findings are often consistent with but not specific for TTP. Gingival biopsy, one of the more popular tests, lacks sensitivity and specificity.[7]

Pathophysiology

The earliest pathologic descriptions of TTP emphasized the presence of hyaline thrombi in the terminal arterioles and capillaries of the heart, liver, and kidneys. These hyaline deposits have subsequently been shown to consist largely of agglutinated platelets. A degree of associated fibrin deposition is felt to be a secondary phenomenon, since its presence is variable and patients with TTP do not routinely exhibit the coagulation abnormalities of DIC.

The pathogenesis of this diffuse microvascular thrombosis remains unclear. Presumably the initial event is inappropriate platelet adhesion, aggregation, and mediator release on endothelial surfaces. This results in vascular occlusion with the characteristic hyaline thrombi of platelets and fibrin. Plasma from some patients with TPP has been shown to lack a stimulatory factor for the release of prostaglandin (PGI_2) from vascular endothelial cells. Since PGI_2 is a potent natural inhibitor of platelet aggregation, its absence might explain this vascular lesion. In support of this hypothesis, vascular endothelial cells have been shown to have decreased PGI_2 production in the presence of TTP plasma compared to normal plasma. Since PGI_2 is an unstable compound, it has been suggested that normal plasma contains a compound which prolongs its activity. Conceivably, deficiency of this stabilizing factor leads to reduced levels of PGI_2 with consequent microvascular thrombosis.

A second hypothesis explaining the findings in TTP postulates the presence of a "toxic-agglutinin." It has been demonstrated that the plasma from some patients with TTP is capable of inducing aggregation of both normal and TTP platelets. Finally, an unusually large plasma factor VIII:von Willebrand factor has been identified in the plasma of patients with chronic relapsing TTP which disappears during periods of remission. Since this protein participates in platelet-endothelial cell adhesion, it may play a role in the pathogenesis of microvascular thrombosis in some patients. Of course, the spectrum of TTP and HUS syndromes may involve several of these pathophysiologic mechanisms, thus accounting for the variability in responses to plasma infusions and plasma exchanges.

Differential Diagnosis

The differential diagnosis of the thrombotic microangiopathies includes disease processes presenting with thrombocytopenia and MAHA (Table 147-1). Most commonly, the clinician must distinguish between TTP and the DIC syndromes, or distinguish TTP from a collagen vascular disease (CVD) such as systemic lupus erythematosus (SLE) with vasculitic activity (Table 147-2). DIC may be associated with many diseases (see Table 147-1) and results in

TABLE 147-1 Differential Diagnosis of Microangiopathic Hemolytic Anemia

DIC Syndromes
Purpura fulminans
Incompatible blood transfusion reaction
Sepsis
Amniotic fluid embolus
Dead fetus syndrome
Abruptio placentae
Massive tissue injury (trauma, burns)
Kasabach-Merritt syndrome (cavernous hemangioma)
SLE and Other Vasculitic Syndromes
Pregnancy-Associated Syndromes
PIH
HELLPS
HUS
Childhood-associated
Postpartum
Drug-induced (chemotherapy, cyclosporine, etc.)
TTP

TABLE 147-2 Laboratory Findings in Thrombotic Microangiopathies and Other Disorders

	TMA	DIC	SLE
RBC fragmentation	+++	+++	+
Thrombocytopenia	+++	+++	±
PT	Normal	Increased	Normal
PTT	Normal	Increased	Normal
Fibrinogen	Normal	Low	Normal
FDP	Low	High	Low
Complement levels	Normal	Normal	Low

widespread generation and deposition of intravascular fibrin in small blood vessels accompanied by a consumptive coagulopathy, with clotting factor activation as a primary process. This is to be distinguished from TTP, in which the primary process appears to be platelet aggregation at the vascular endothelial surface.

DISTINGUISHING THROMBOTIC THROMBOCYTOPENIC PURPURA AND DISSEMINATED INTRAVASCULAR COAGULATION

DIC may be initiated by either endothelial injury (intrinisic coagulation pathway) or release of tissue thromboplastin (extrinisic coagulation pathway). Either process can cause intravascular aggregation of platelets exposed to collagen and thrombin. The clinical manifestations of DIC arise from injury related to intravascular thrombosis or from bleeding that results from eventual depletion of clotting factors and platelets. Acute DIC syndromes usually present with bleeding and demonstrable hypo- or afibrinogenemia. In more chronic forms of DIC in which reticuloendothelial system clearance mechanisms, clotting factor production, and marrow cell production compensate for consumption, patients will present with thrombosis rather than hemorrhage. Typical thrombotic problems include deep vein or superficial thrombophlebitis, pulmonary embolus, cerebral vascular accidents, or nonbacterial (murantic) endocarditis.

DIC shares with TTP the features of MAHA and thrombocytopenia (see Table 147-2). In one series, the frequency of MAHA as judged by peripheral smear was 68 percent in patients with DIC. In the same series, thrombocytopenia (platelet count <150,000/mm^3) was seen in 96 percent of cases of DIC; however, significant thrombocytopenia (platelet count <50,000/mm^3) was much less common (57 percent).

A number of laboratory findings will help to distinguish TTP from DIC (see Table 147-2). As noted above, hypofibrinogenemia is typical of fulminant, consumptive DIC. In addition, as clotting factors are consumed, elevation of prothrombin time (PT) and partial thromboplastin time (PTT) is seen. Also, the systemic generation of fibrin can lead to activation of the fibrinolytic system, either by activation of plasminogen by tissue activators released from vascular endothelium or by Hageman factor-dependent activation. Fibrinolysis results in the appearance of fibrin degradation products (FDP) in the serum that can be measured. While no one of these laboratory tests can distinguish TTP from DIC, in the aggregate they are sufficiently powerful to permit specific diagnosis (see Table 147-2).

Finally, the clinical context will often help to determine if DIC is a viable explanation for the observed abnormalities. Most often, the disease or disorder that is the precipitant of DIC is obvious. Amniotic fluid embolus, retained products of conception, and abruptio placentae are obstetric complications often associated with DIC. Septicemia will be the substrate for DIC in many patients encountered in the ICU. The presentation of these patients may be fulminant, as in the Waterhouse-Friderichsen syndrome (shock, bleeding diathesis, and adrenal insufficiency in association with meningococcemia), or more indolent as in the complex postoperative patient with a "smoldering" intraabdominal source of infection. Trauma is a well-recognized cause of DIC and fibrinolysis resulting from the exposure of tissue thromboplastins and plasminogen activators to plasma.[8] In trauma patients, unexplained bleeding during or after a surgical procedure may be the first manifestation of DIC. In the setting of head injury, as many as 70 percent of patients may have clinical evidence of DIC.[9]

In summary, TTP can usually be distinguished readily from DIC by clinical context and a relatively simple set of laboratory parameters. This formulation is important to apply, since all of the 'defining' features of TTP—thrombocytopenia, MAHA, fever, neurologic dysfunction, and renal abnormality—are so common in the critically ill as to warrant a clear approach to this possible diagnosis.

APPROACH TO THE PREGNANT PATIENT

Hematologic aberrations associated with PIH (preeclampsia/eclampsia) include MAHA, thrombocytopenia, and alterations of the coagulation mechanism. Evidence of MAHA can be found in 2 to 15 percent of women with PIH, and thrombocytopenia has been reported in as many as 18 percent of patients. Thus, a subset of patients with PIH will have two of the cardinal hematologic abnormalities of TTP.[4] It has been suggested that PIH and TTP share pathophysiologic features, specifically aberration in prostaglandin metabolism at the platelet-endothelial cell interface. In this regard it is interesting that plasma exchange has been reported to be a successful therapy in PIH. A subset of patients with PIH and thrombocytopenia may have marked elevation of liver function tests (HELLPS). Right upper quadrant pain is often present and may mimic cholecystitis or peritonitis.

Postpartum HUS is characterized by predominant renal involvement; neurologic signs and fever are usually absent. It has been suggested that this syndrome is a clinical counterpart of the generalized Schwarzman reaction. It is hypothesized that bacterial endotoxins or vasoactive amines are discharged into the maternal circulation and either stimulate the coagulation cascade or initiate thrombosis by damage to the vascular endothelium.

As mentioned above, DIC syndromes accompany major complications of pregnancy. Usually these processes are associated with a catastrophic process such as amniotic fluid embolus or abruptio placentae. Less apparent and more indolent DIC may be encountered with retained products of conception.

Finally, TTP itself is encountered in pregnancy but is extremely rare, with fewer than 70 cases reported. It is likely that the majority of pregnant patients with thrombocytopenia and MAHA are best classified as PIH with hematologic abnormalities.[10] The key features distinguishing these patients from the group with HELLPS are the emergence of disease in late pregnancy, relatively mild hematologic irregularities, and prompt resolution of thrombocytopenia, MAHA, neurologic symptoms, and liver function abnormalities following delivery. HUS begins postpartum, with a predominance of renal dysfunction. DIC differs from TTP as described above (see Table 147-2). Finally, that small remaining group of patients whose clinical presentation is best described as TTP, are best treated in pregnancy with the usual treatments (vide infra), although the support for this is largely anecdotal.[10]

DISTINGUISHING THROMBOTIC THROMBOCYTOPENIC PURPURA FROM COLLAGEN VASCULAR DISEASE

An association between TTP and SLE has been reported. In one review, evidence of SLE was found in 7 of 64 cases initially diagnosed as TTP.[1] TTP has also been reported in association with other CVDs including rheumatoid arthritis, ankylosing spondylitis, and polyarteritis nodosa. On the other hand, vasculitis in association with SLE or other CVD may mimic TTP with findings of renal failure, fever, neurologic disturbance, thrombocytopenia, and MAHA. Serum complement levels are usually low in patients with vasculitis and normal in TTP (see Table 147-2). Antinuclear antibodies are positive in the great majority of patients with SLE. These CVD "screening tests" are useful in virtually all patients with a tentative diagnosis of TTP. If a diagnosis of a specific CVD can be made, therapy should be directed at this disorder, rather than the associated hematologic problems.

Therapy

TTP is a hematologic emergency. Patients will often need ICU admission because of profound anemia, shock, lactic acidosis, respiratory failure, or deteriorating neurologic function. Intubation and mechanical ventilation may be required because of ventilatory failure complicating CNS involvement or because of direct lung injury associated with pulmonary vascular involvement by TTP.[12]

PLASMA EXCHANGE

Once a diagnosis of TTP is made, plasma exchange is the therapy of choice. Since 1961, mortality for this disease has declined from over 90 percent to <50 percent, likely due to institution of plasma exchange. Prognosis in TTP is influenced by prompt recognition and treatment, so that emergency apheresis should be conducted in any patient with neurologic manifestations. Plasma exchange of 150 percent of plasma volume is instituted (3 to 4 L for normal-sized individuals) with single-donor plasma replacement. Two intravenous sites are required for the procedure through 17 gauge (draw line) and 18 gauge (return line) catheters. Alternatively, plasma exchange can be conducted through a double-lumen dialysis catheter. For initial catheter placement we prefer femoral vein placement, to avoid hemothorax or pneumothorax in a severely thrombocytopenic patient. Femoral catheters should be changed every 72 h. As the patient stabilizes and thrombocytopenia resolves, a subclavian line can be placed electively in the operating room if longer term access is necessary.

Complications of plasma exchange include bleeding, air embolus, hepatitis, citrate toxicity, and pulmonary edema. Bleeding is common not only because of thrombocytopenia but because anticoagulation is necessary to achieve adequate blood flow through extracorporeal lines. If heparin is used, this anticoagulation should be minimized. The risk of air embolus is reduced by experienced personnel. Machine safety devices include bubble traps and a bubble alarm that stops the machine when air is detected in the lines. Citrate toxicity can occur from the plasma citrate anticoagulant infused into the patient and is compounded by associated renal dysfunction. Citrate toxicity causes hypocalcemia and metabolic alkalosis, and presents as oral paresthesias, numbness or tingling in the extremities, or prolonged QT interval on the electrocardiogram. We prevent hypocalcemia by routinely administering 1 ampule calcium gluconate by constant infusion per liter of plasma exchanged. An additional one-half ampule may be administered if symptoms are experienced during the procedure. Periodic monitoring of ionized calcium levels is useful, as well. In all cases, the relative benefits and risks of the procedure should be discussed with the patient or guardians and informed consent obtained.

Plasma exchange should be performed daily until evidence indicates the disease is in remission. The patient should have normal mental status, renal function, and urinary sediment, and should be afebrile. The most sensitive indicator of response is a rising platelet count, which should normalize ($>150{,}000/mm^3$) before discontinuing plasma exchange. LDH is also a sensitive indicator of intravascular RBC turnover and can be used to monitor response to therapy. Sequential examination of RBC morphology on peripheral smear [Fig. 147-1 (Plate 49) and Plates 50 and 51] should be conducted, although improvement in cell fragmentation can lag behind clinical response (such as improving mental status) by several days. Bone marrow reticulocyte response may not be marked for 7 to 10 days. The patient should be given folate (1 mg or more daily) in this setting of poor dietary intake, plasma exchange, and increased marrow requirement.

The usual course of plasma exchange is 5 to 10 days. Patients can be moved from the ICU when mental status has normalized and hematocrit and platelet count are increasing. The shortest treatment requirement we have observed is 3 days. Late responses in occasional patients have occurred after 14 days of therapy. We continue plasma exchange for up to 3 weeks as long as the patient is stable or improving.

ADJUNCTIVE THERAPIES

In patients with incomplete clinical response, splenectomy should be considered. In a recent series of 12 patients with only a partial response to plasma exchange, 9 achieved complete remission after splenectomy with or without subsequent plasma exchange.[13] High dose steroid therapy has been advocated by some but without convincing evidence of benefit. Our current approach is to use steroids only in patients who do not respond to plasma exchange. Vincristine, presumably acting as an immunosuppressive, has also been reported to produce sustained remissions in a small series,[14] but we reserve use of this agent for exchange and steroid failures.

In view of the suspected pathogenetic mechanisms of TTP, antiplatelet agents seem a rational addition to treatment. However, clinical trials have not shown a convincing impact of these drugs, including intravenous prostacyclin. Aspirin is difficult to give to an obtunded or comatose patient, and we discourage nasogastric tube placement for this purpose because of risk of bleeding. Dipyridamole (Persantine) can be given intravenously. We add one baby aspirin (80 mg) daily and dipyridamole 200 mg twice daily when the patient is able to ingest oral medication, and continue them for at least several months. Larger series have shown that plasma exchange therapy coupled with antiplatelet agents results in complete remission in approximately two-thirds of patients.[15]

Plasma infusion therapy is useful in many patients, particularly those with chronic relapsing TTP. While plasma infusion (12 U every 24 h) can be used in patients with acute TTP, this therapy should not delay the institution of plasma exchange nor prevent the transfer of the patient to a fully equipped referral unit.

Platelet transfusion is contraindicated in TTP, based on clinical evidence that it leads to relapse.[16] If a diagnosis of TTP has been made, we do not recommend routine use of platelet support, even during invasive procedures. Heparin has been advocated for patients with HUS, but a randomized trial in pediatric patients failed to show benefit.[17] Supportive therapy often requires renal dialysis, and plasma exchange should be considered for patients with rapid disease progression.[11]

CASE PRESENTATION

B.B., a 20-year-old black woman, was admitted with thrombocytopenia and seizures. Eight days prior to admission she had undergone outpatient surgical excision and drainage of the left axilla for hydraadenitis suppurativa. A routine blood count that day revealed a platelet count of 14,000, a mildly elevated white blood cell (WBC) count, and a normal hematocrit (Table 147-3). A previous blood count 4 weeks prior to admission was normal. While undergoing evaluation in the emergency room the patient suffered a generalized seizure and was admitted. Previous history was noncontributory. Physical examination revealed a lethargic, disoriented patient. Temperature was 38.7°C (101.7°F), pulse was 114, and respiratory rate was 28. Blood pressure (supine) was 94/50. No focal neurologic signs were present. Laboratory evaluation revealed a hematocrit of 20.8 percent, a WBC of 24,200 and a platelet count of 4,000/mm^3. Peripheral blood smear (see Fig. 147-1) showed striking RBC fragmentation consistent with an MAHA, along with nucleated RBCs and polychromatophilic RBCs indicating increased bone marrow production. Platelets were absent. The remaining laboratory evaluation included a PT of 14.0 s (normal <12.4 s), a PTT of 24 s (normal <30 s), an LDH level of 2481, fibrinogen value of 225 mg/dL, and a creatinine content of 1.1 mg/dL. Urinalysis revealed 3+ protein, 4+ blood with occasional RBCs on microscopic evaluation, and occasional hyaline casts. Total bilirubin content was 1.7 mg/dL with direct (conjugated) bilirubin level of 0.3 mg/dL.

For the initial 18 h the patient was felt to have DIC

TABLE 147-3

CLINICAL COURSE

Day	−31	−8	0	1 (Admission)	2	3	4	5	6	7	8	10	13	15	20	25
Hematocrit (%)	43	40		20.8	14.2	29.0	27.7	29.3	32.7							
Platelet count (×1000/mm)	216	14		4	64	20	24	39	77		105	34	53	78	55	25
PT (s)				14.0	13.8	12.9		12.1								
PTT (s)				24	26	20		22								
Fibrinogen (mg/dL)				225		253										
LDH				2481		1241	828									
Plasma exchange (3 L)					*	*	*	*	*	*	*	***	*			
Platelets (U)				******												
RBCs (U)				*****										*		
γ-Globulin (5 days)														*		
Prednisone 1 mg/kg/day														*		
Splenectomy															*	
Vincristine																*

based on her left axillary infection, leukocytosis, and abnormal PT. She was given 6 U platelets which resulted in a platelet count increment of 64,000/mm^3. She was transferred to the medical ICU. Consultation with hematology was then obtained, whereupon a diagnosis of TTP was made and therapeutic plasma exchange recommended. The patient underwent daily plasma exchange for 7 days with rapid improvement in mental status, increase in platelet count to 105,000/mm^3, decrease in LDH level to 485, and improvement in peripheral RBC morphology after two exchanges (see Plate 50) and five exchanges (see Plate 51). Laboratory work-up for SLE was negative. The patient was begun on antiplatelet therapy (aspirin 80 mg daily and dipyridamole [Persantine] 200 mg twice daily). After 10 treatments, plasma exchange was discontinued because of reactions to plasma which included urticaria and wheezing despite diphenhydramine therapy. The patient's platelet count declined to 38,000/mm^3. Prednisone therapy (1 mg/kg/day) and high dose intravenous γ-globulin therapy (0.4 g/kg/day for 5 days) were begun, resulting in a transient rise in platelet count to 100,000/mm^3. When the platelet count declined to 55,000/mm^3, the patient underwent splenectomy. Postoperatively the platelet count continued to decline to 25,000/mm^3. Vincristine, 2 mg intravenously, was given on hospital day 23. Thereafter the platelet count increased to 405,000/mm^3, and the patient was discharged on hospital day 30.

CASE DISCUSSION

As often occurs, the initial diagnosis considered in this patient with TTP was DIC secondary to infection. Although thrombocytopenia, MAHA as indicated by peripheral smear, and elevation of the PT were consistent with this, a number of observations should direct the clinician to the appropriate diagnosis. First, the platelet count was profoundly depressed. Secondly, while infection was present earlier, it appeared to have been adequately treated and was responding. Thirdly, neurologic abnormality was substantial, with seizures noted on admission. It should be noted, however, that many patients with TTP will have more subtle neurologic findings or symptoms, and often only a careful history will identify a headache or other seemingly minor complaint that is a key to diagnosis. Finally, the fibrinogen level of 225 mg/dL argued against substantial fibrinolysis, a typical finding in DIC. Significantly, although TTP was an early working diagnosis guiding therapeutic interventions, continued diagnostic evaluations to exclude CVD, primarily SLE, were performed.

Prompt diagnosis permitted early institution of plasma exchange, as discussed in the chapter. Early observation and treatment in the ICU were appropriate, given the complications of therapy and general instability of this patient population. Response to therapy was prompt (see Table 147-3), and indicated by improving mental status, rising platelet count, decrease in LDH level, and improvement in peripheral smear [see Fig. 147-1 (Plate 49) and Plates 50 and 51]. The sequence of these events is typical for the patient achieving remission with plasma exchange. Antiplatelet agents were added to her regimen when she had improved to a point that they could be administered orally.

When plasma exchange alone failed to achieve a sustained remission and complications of therapy were encountered, adjunctive measures were taken, including intravenous γ-globulin, prednisone, splenectomy, and vincristine. Following a hospital course of a month, most of which was possible in the regular ward setting, the patient was discharged to be followed long-term as an outpatient.

References

1. Amorosi EL, Ultmann J: Thrombotic thrombocytopenic purpura: Report of 16 cases and review of the literature. Medicine 45:139, 1966.
2. Ridolfi RL, Bell WR. Thrombotic thrombocytopenic purpura: Report of 25 cases and a review of the literature. Medicine 60:413, 1981.
3. Byrnes JJ, Moake JL: Thrombotic thrombocytopenic purpura and the haemolytic-uraemic syndrome: Evolving concepts of pathogenesis and therapy. Clin Haematol 15:413, 1986.
4. Weiner CP: Thrombotic microangiopathy in pregnancy and the postpartum period. Semin Hematol 24:119, 1987.
5. Murgo AJ: Thrombotic microangiopathy in the cancer patient including those induced by chemotherapeutic agents. Semin Hematol 214:161, 1987.
6. Smith RE, Berg DD: Coagulation defects in cyclosporine A-treated allogeneic bone marrow transplant patients. Am J Hematol 28:137, 1988.
7. Goodman A, Ramos R, Petrelli M, Hirsch SA, et al: Gingival biopsy in thrombotic thrombocytopenic purpura. Ann Intern Med 89:501, 1987.
8. Kapsch DN, Metzler M, Harrington M, et al: Fibrinolytic response to trauma. Surgery 95:473, 1984.
9. Miner MED, Kaufman HM, Graham SH, et al: Disseminated intravascular coagulation fibrinolytic syndrome following head injury in children: Frequency and prognostic implications. J Pediatr 100:687, 1982.
10. Vandekerchhove F, Noens L, Colardyn F, et al: Thrombotic thrombocytopenic purpura mimicking toxemia of pregnancy. Am J Obstet Gynecol 150:320, 1984.
11. Spencer CD, Crane FM, Kumar JR, Alving BM: Treatment of postpartum hemolytic uremic syndrome with plasma exchange. JAMA 247:2808, 1982.
12. Bone RC, Henry JE, Petterson J, Amare M: Respiratory dysfunction in thrombotic thrombocytopenic purpura. Am J Med 65:262, 1978.
13. Schneider PA, Rauner AA, Linker CA, et al: The role of splenectomy in multimodality treatment of thrombotic thrombocytopenic purpura. Ann Surg 202:318, 1985.
14. Schreeder MT, Prchal JT: Successful treatment of thrombotic thrombocytopenic purpura by vincristine. Am J Hematol 14:75, 1983.
15. Myers TJ: Treatment of thrombotic thrombocytopenic purpura with combined exchange plasmapheresis and antiplatelet drugs. Semin Thromb Hemost 7:37, 1981.
16. Gordon LI, Dwaan HC, Rossi EC: Deleterious effects of platelet transfusions and recovery thrombocytosis in patients with thrombotic microangiopathy. Sem Hematol 24:194, 1987.
17. Vitaco M, Avalos JJ, Giantantonio CA: Heparin therapy in the hemolytic-uremic syndrome. J Pediatr 83:271, 1973.

Chapter 148

ACUTE LEUKEMIA

RICHARD A. LARSON

KEY POINTS

- *Many patients, especially children and younger adults, can be cured of acute leukemia with the use of intensive chemotherapy and skillful supportive care.*
- *The prognosis for ICU management depends on the specific type of leukemia, its stage, prior therapy, and underlying chronic medical problems.*
- *Infection and bleeding are due to the severe pancytopenia caused either by the leukemia itself or its myelosuppressive treatment; these problems resolve as the normal marrow recovers.*
- *The success of chemotherapy for acute leukemia depends not only on the drug susceptibility of an individual patient's particular leukemia but also on the ability of that patient to survive the toxicity of treatment.*
- *Blood transfusions should be used to maintain a hematocrit >30 percent and a platelet count >20,000/μL.*
- *Hyperleukocytosis with malignant myeloblasts must be treated as a medical emergency with leukapheresis and chemotherapy.*
- *Central nervous system (CNS) leukemia can be successfully treated with radiotherapy, intrathecal chemotherapy, and high dose systemic chemotherapy.*
- *Tumor cell lysis, aminoglycosides, disseminated intravascular coagulation (DIC), elevated lysozyme, hyperuricemia, and direct infiltration by leukemia cells can lead to renal failure which is reversible with proper care.*
- *Necrotizing enterocolitis requires aggressive medical management with blood transfusions, antibiotics, nasogastric suction, bowel rest, and maintenance of normal serum proteins and electrolytes.*
- *Hyperuricemia is proportional to the leukemia tumor burden and responds to effective chemotherapy together with fluids, bicarbonate and allopurinol.*

Acute leukemia is a malignant proliferation of bone marrow or lymphoid cells that is uniformly fatal when left untreated. However, with the use of intensive chemotherapy and skillful supportive care, many patients, particularly children and younger adults, may be cured of this devastating disease. Not uncommonly, the use of the medical ICU is necessary during the treatment of acute leukemia, either to manage the complications of the disease itself or the complications of intensive cytotoxic therapy. Such newly diagnosed patients deserve maximum aggressive supportive care in the medical ICU because most of the acute complications of leukemia resolve as a complete remission is achieved. The successful treatment of patients with acute leukemia requires a multidisciplinary approach with close collaboration between intensive care physicians, hematologists, infectious disease specialists, and the blood bank. Twenty-four-hour physician coverage is necessary to respond to emergencies that could otherwise lead to rapid deterioration of a patient in the midst of treatment. Although major challenges remain to be overcome, the majority of young and middle-aged adults can today be successfully treated for acute leukemia.

Appropriate decision making requires an understanding of the pathophysiology and clinical history of the leukemic disorders. The likelihood of a successful outcome from intensive care management depends in part on the specific type of leukemia and its stage. That is, the prognosis depends on whether the patient is newly diagnosed and not yet treated or is in an advanced stage following multiple relapses. Knowledge of prior therapy aids in the evaluation of subsequent complications, especially with regard to opportunistic infections or organ dysfunction. Since the best opportunity to cure acute leukemia requires appropriate diagnosis and optimal initial treatment and supportive care, it is highly desirable that newly diagnosed patients be referred to regional oncology centers where appropriate expertise and resources are readily available. This chapter will briefly review the treatment strategy for acute leukemia and then focus on the serious metabolic, circulatory, and infiltrative complications that most often require ICU care. The far more common bleeding and infectious complications and direct drug toxicities have been dealt with elsewhere (see Chaps. 35, 55, 96, 98, 99, 145, 146, 149–151).

Differential Diagnosis

Leukemia and other cancers result from genetic mutations in somatic cells. When mutational damage alters normal growth regulatory mechanisms in a hemopoietic stem cell, a clone of neoplastic cells may proliferate, overwhelming the normal bone marrow through a selective growth advantage although not necessarily more rapid growth. Leukemia cells usually retain characteristics of their original cell lineage, allowing classification (Table 148-1).[1] However, because these are neoplastic cells, aberrant expression of proteins not usually manifested by normal cells within a particular hemopoietic lineage may be detected, yielding a "mixed cell" phenotype. The acute leukemias include acute myeloid (nonlymphocytic) leukemia (AML: myeloblastic, myelomonocytic, monoblastic, erythroblastic, and megakaryocytic) and acute lymphoblastic leukemia (ALL) as well as the blastic transformations of chronic myelogeneous leukemia (CML) and the myelodysplastic syndromes (MDS). Therapy-related AML occurs in patients treated with chemotherapy or radiotherapy for an earlier cancer or other disease.

Acute leukemia almost always causes marked abnormalities in the peripheral blood counts. Anemia may be mild, moderate, or severe, and the red blood cells may be mildly macrocytic. Most patients will have moderate to severe

TABLE 148-1 French-American-British (FAB) Classification of Acute Leukemias

FAB Subtype	Type
	Acute Lymphoblastic Leukemia (ALL)
L1	Small cells; homogeneous
L2	Large cells; heterogeneous
L3	Large cells; homogeneous (Burkitt type)
	Acute Myeloid/Nonlymphoblastic Leukemia (AML/ANLL)
M1	Acute myeloblastic leukemia without maturation (AML)
M2	Acute myeloblastic leukemia with maturation (AML)
M3	Acute promyelocytic leukemia—hypergranular (APL)
M3V	Acute promyelocytic leukemia—microgranular (APL)
M4	Acute myelomonocytic leukemia (AMMoL)
M4Eo	Acute myelomonocytic leukemia with abnormal eosinophils (AMMoL-M4Eo)
M5a	Acute monoblastic leukemia—poorly differentiated (AMoL)
M5b	Acute monocytic leukemia—well-differentiated (AMoL)
M6	Erythroleukemia (EL)
M7	Acute megakaryoblastic leukemia (AMegaL)
	Chronic Myelogenous Leukemia (CML)
	Lymphoid blast phase
	Myeloid blast phase
	Therapy-related Acute Myeloid Leukemia (t-AML)
	Primary Myelodysplastic Syndrome (MDS)
	Refractory anemia with excess blasts in transformation (RAEB-T)

thrombocytopenia. Although an elevated white blood cell count and readily recognizable circulating blast cells are frequently present, not all patients have leukocytosis. Some patients actually present with leukopenia, and malignant cells may not be observed in the peripheral blood. A careful review of a blood smear often demonstrates dysplasia in one or more cell lines. In elderly patients, AML frequently evolves from a MDS; mature granulocytes are often hypocellular with poorly condensed nuclear chromatin, and platelets may be large in size but lacking normal granulation. An overt or a subclinical preleukemic phase may have been present for several months. The presence of greater than 30 percent blast cells in the marrow is the somewhat arbitrary dividing line between acute leukemia and the "preleukemic" MDS.

The diagnosis and subclassification of acute leukemia rest on the interpretation of an adequate bone marrow sample. A marrow aspiration specimen together with a bone marrow needle core biopsy from the posterior iliac crest provide important information. Auer rods are often observed in malignant myeloblasts. Cytochemical reactivity detects myeloperoxidase or nonspecific esterase activity in myeloid leukemias, whereas such activity is absent in lymphoid leukemias. Immunophenotypic analysis using flow cytometry or immunohistochemical techniques detects cell surface antigens which corroborate the diagnosis. Cytogenetic analysis of bone marrow specimens provides important diagnostic and prognostic information.[2] Metaphase cells are karyotyped after direct preparation or short-term (24 to 48 h) unstimulated cultures. Characteristic recurring chromosomal abnormalities include the gain of extra chromosomes, the loss of certain chromosomes, and structural rearrangements such as translocations, deletions, insertions, and inversions. Several distinct subtypes of acute leukemia can now be defined according to their characteristic morphologic, cytochemical, immunophenotypic, and cytogenetic features.[3,4] These disorders have a more predictable clinical course than less well-defined leukemias.

Management

The optimal chemotherapy for patients with acute leukemia has not yet been determined.[5,6] Recent clinical trials have identified different risk groups which are more or less likely to respond to standard chemotherapy programs. Treatment is given in two or three phases: remission induction and consolidation with or without maintenance. The goal of *remission induction chemotherapy* is to induce a complete remission. Any lesser response does not improve survival. The term *complete remission* is defined by the absence of detectable leukemia in the bone marrow and blood, the regeneration of normal marrow elements, and the return to normal levels of all three blood cell lines for at least a month. This reflects a reduction in the tumor cell mass by >3 logs (i.e., >99.9 percent). However, as many as 10^8 malignant cells may still survive at this point. If no postremission therapy were given, most patients with acute leukemia would relapse within 2 to 4 months. Thus, *consolidation chemotherapy* (sometimes called *intensification therapy*) is directed at destroying any clonogenic leukemia cells that remain undetected following initial treatment. Consolidation therapy uses several monthly cycles (commonly one to eight) of myelosuppressive chemotherapy, each sufficiently intensive to produce bone marrow hypoplasia and peripheral blood pancytopenia. Various strategies using allogeneic bone marrow transplantation or high dose chemotherapy followed by reinfusion of autologous marrow collected earlier during remission are being tested as postremission consolidation treatments. Low dose outpatient maintenance chemotherapy that does not lower the blood counts has not been proven to increase the fraction of patients with AML who are cured, although 18 to 24 months of prolonged maintenance treatment seems useful for patients with ALL.

Patients who suffer a relapse of acute leukemia after completion of all therapy can usually achieve a second remission with reinstitution of the original induction chemotherapy regimen. However, patients who relapse in the midst of initial treatment or while receiving maintenance therapy are less likely to achieve a second remission and rarely have long survival. Second and subsequent periods of remission are usually progressively shorter. The risks and costs of marrow transplantation are easily justified for patients who have had a relapse of leukemia because otherwise disease-free survival is generally (but not always) short. Patients who are less than forty years old and have a human leukocyte antigen (HLA)-identical sibling are good candidates for allogeneic transplantation. It may be possible to extend the upper age limit with the use of T cell depletion from the donor marrow to diminish the incidence and severity of graft-versus-host disease (GVHD). The use of marrow from a matched but unrelated donor is also feasible.

The success of chemotherapy for acute leukemia depends not only on the drug susceptibility of an individual patient's particular leukemia but also on the ability of that patient to survive the rigors of treatment. Significant advances have been made in the supportive care of patients undergoing intensive cytotoxic therapy. Prevention and early treatment of infection have been foremost. Prior to treatment, all patients should have a thorough dental evaluation to identify and eliminate potential oral sources for infections. Patients are placed in protective isolation within single rooms; in this way, these immunocompromised patients are protected from common infectious agents within the hospital environment. Laminar airflow rooms are not necessary for successful treatment, but patients are generally restricted from eating fresh fruits and vegetables to decrease their enteric bacterial flora. Strict attention to thorough handwashing by all medical and nursing personnel and visitors is necessary.

Patients with leukemia are severely immunocompromised both by their disease and by their treatment. Because chemotherapy damages mucosal barriers, these patients are prone to infection by endogenous organisms. Most common are gram-negative enteric bacteria, gram-positive cocci, and fungi such as Candida and Aspergillus species. Patients with ALL also are susceptible to pneumocystis, mycobacterial, and viral infections. Prophylactic use of oral antibiotics such as norfloxacin or trimethoprim-sulfamethoxazole can decrease the incidence and severity of infections in granulocytopenic patients, but these have not been widely used in part because of concerns that drug resistance will emerge.

Standard practice dictates that broad-spectrum antibiotic therapy must be initiated promptly and empirically in a granulocytopenic patient at the time of the first fever greater than 38.5°C (101.5°F). Blood, urine, and sputum cultures must be obtained, but the source of infection is rarely identified, in part, because there is little inflammatory response in the tissues. The first priority must be to prevent septic shock. Ceftazidime as a single agent or the combination of a semisynthetic penicillin plus an aminoglycoside is widely used, but the choice of regimen partly depends on renal function and history of allergies. Should initial cultures reveal a pathogen, antibiotic therapy should be adjusted for maximum bactericidal activity based on susceptibility testing in vitro. In general, however, broad-spectrum treatment continues until the chemotherapy is completed and the granulocyte count recovers to near normal. These concepts are discussed fully in Chaps. 96 and 99.

Patients with acute leukemia are characterized by bone marrow failure, either due to replacement by leukemia cells or to chemotherapy-induced hypoplasia. In either case, patients depend on blood transfusions to supply the formed elements in the blood to maintain the blood volume, carry oxygen, and protect against bleeding. Red blood cell transfusions are given to maintain a hematocrit of approximately 30 percent. A higher hematocrit should be maintained in hypoalbuminemic patients to keep the blood volume expanded and tissues perfused. Bleeding is a common problem, and the risk rises as the platelet count decreases (see Chap. 146). Platelets should be transfused prophylactically to maintain a platelet count $>20,000/\mu L$ to decrease the risk of spontaneous hemorrhage such as a stroke or gastrointestinal bleeding. No salicylates or other drugs which interfere with platelet function should be given nor should intramuscular injections be given to a thrombocytopenic patient. The use of single-donor platelets collected by apheresis will decrease the rate of alloimmunization in leukemia patients (see Chap. 35). Patients who become alloimmunized may require HLA-matched platelets or antibody crossmatched platelets to achieve adequate posttransfusion platelet counts. Techniques to remove leukocytes by filtration or centrifugation from red cell or platelet transfusion units may slow the rate of alloimmunization.

Granulocyte transfusions are rarely necessary for patients receiving chemotherapy for acute leukemia. The indications for their use are generally limited to severely granulocytopenic patients who remain febrile and bacteremic despite receiving antibiotics which have bactericidal activity against the particular organism in vitro. In this situation, the phagocytic activity of exogenous granulocytes can be lifesaving. One or two leukapheresis products are transfused daily for 4 to 7 days. Complications include respiratory distress from leukoagglutination, transmission of cytomegalovirus (CMV), and rapid alloimmunization. Pulmonary infiltrates may worsen as granulocytes migrate into infected lung tissues.

Soft Silastic right atrial catheters (e.g., double-lumen Hickman or Groshong) which tunnel under the skin and enter the innominate vein are widely used. They allow direct access to a large vein for infusion of chemotherapy, antibiotics, and blood transfusions, and also allow painless blood sampling for laboratory monitoring. Parenteral hyperalimentation can be administered easily through these catheters if necessary. Although a boon to both patient and physician, such chronic indwelling lines are not without hazard. They must be placed in a sterile fashion by a skilled surgeon, especially in a thrombocytopenic patient. A vigorous skin preparation preoperatively reduces the likelihood of a staphylococcal or corynebacterial subcutaneous tunnel infection or bacteremia. Although most gram-negative bacteremias can be treated successfully in a granulocytopenic patient by antibiotics alone without removing the catheter, gram-positive infections or candidal infections of the tunnel or vein may require catheter removal.

Hyperleukocytosis

A small proportion of patients with leukemia have an extraordinary elevation of circulating leukocytes. Hyperleukocytosis (>100,000 blast cells/μL) is a true medical emergency, but the risks of circulatory complications begin to rise above about 50,000/μL. These patients present special problems because of the rheologic effects of leukemia blast cells in the circulation of the lung, brain, and other organs, and the metabolic consequences when massive numbers of leukemia cells are destroyed simultaneously by cytotoxic drugs (see Chap. 151). Although in some cases the blood viscosity is markedly increased because of the elevated leukocrit, in most cases, the whole blood viscosity will not be increased above normal because hyperleukocytosis is most frequently associated with severe anemia.[7] Red blood cell transfusions can precipitate a hyperviscosity syndrome in a patient with hyperleukocytosis and should be delayed if possible until the white blood cell count falls. Nevertheless, viscosity may be high in the microcirculation. The high oxygen consumption and invasiveness of leukemia cells may interact with slow flow through the capillaries to lead to hypoxemia and vascular damage.

The contribution of blood cells to the viscosity of blood is a function of the deformability of individual cells and their fractional volume. Immature leukocytes are much larger and less deformable than erythrocytes. Leukemic myeloblasts are considerably larger than lymphoblasts, which are in turn larger than leukemic lymphocytes. Thus, the incidence of significant leukostasis is most common in CML in the blast phase, followed by AML, then ALL. In contrast, it is rare in patients with chronic lymphocytic leukemia (CLL) despite white cell counts as high as 500,000/μL. Similarly, well-hydrated patients with CML in the chronic phase can tolerate total white blood cell counts of 200,000/μL without difficulty, because only a small fraction are blasts or promyelocytes and the majority are mature granulocytes.

Leukostasis and hypoxia in the capillary beds can induce respiratory distress, cardiac arrhythmias, and CNS symptoms leading to coma. Death follows rapidly unless the circulation can be restored. Emergency measures include leukapheresis to remove a large mass of tumor cells directly from the bloodstream.[8] A single efficient leukapheresis can decrease the leukocyte count by approximately 50 percent within 2 to 3 h. A centrifuge technique rather than a filtration method should be used since blast cells do not adhere to glass wool filters. Prompt use of antimetabolite drugs such as oral hydroxyurea or intravenous cytarabine can rapidly reduce cell proliferation and transiently decrease the blast count. A single dose of cranial irradiation (200 to 400 cGy) can ameliorate CNS symptoms due to leukostasis. Diffuse pulmonary infiltrates and respiratory distress may also respond to thoracic irradiation. Once the circulation through the capillaries has been restored, systemic chemotherapy should be initiated rapidly.[9] Prophylactic platelet transfusions must be given to prevent bleeding as the circulation is restored to hypoxic tissues. The invasiveness of leukemic myeloblasts may lead to injury and disruption of vascular endothelium. Lysis of these cells in situ releases proteolytic enzymes causing further tissue damage and bleeding.

Tachypnea and pulmonary infiltrates in a patient with hyperleukocytosis can mimic pulmonary infection. Care must be taken to rule out "pseudohypoxemia" which results from the in vitro consumption of oxygen within an arterial blood-gas sample by blast cells in transit to the laboratory.[10] Such blood specimens should be rapidly transported on ice. Rarely, marked thrombocytosis can produce a similar artifact in addition to pseudohyperkalemia.

Tissue Infiltration

Leukemia is, from its genesis in the marrow, spleen, or thymus, a systemic disease. Malignant cells circulate through the bloodstream and lymphatics and can infiltrate the parenchyma of any tissue. ALL cells migrate preferentially to lymphoid organs such as lymph nodes, spleen, and liver, causing organomegaly. When malignant myeloblasts form a solid tumor, a granulocytic sarcoma or chloroma results. The term *chloroma* (green cancer) describes the greenish color which results from the myeloperoxidase reaction when a granulocytic sarcoma is exposed to air. Granulocytic sarcomas occur most often in patients with CML in blast phase or with AMoLs and most commonly involve bone and subperiosteum, lymph nodes, skin, soft tissues, and the gastrointestinal tract.[11] They most frequently cause pain but may also cause neuropathy or intestinal obstruction from their mass effect. They are quite responsive to local irradiation (1000 to 2000 cGy), but since they are a localized manifestation of a disseminated disease, systemic chemotherapy must also be used. Local therapy is often not necessary, because granulocytic sarcomas often shrink and disappear within a few days after chemotherapy begins.

CNS infiltration by leukemia cells is more common in ALL than AML and is more common in children than adults. Among patients with myeloid leukemia, the incidence of CNS involvement is greatest in children and in those with monoblastic leukemias or high circulating blast counts. Among the lymphoblastic leukemias, the risk is greatest in patients with the T cell or B cell immunophenotypes.[12] When the vascular leptomeninges surrounding the brain and spinal cord are infiltrated by malignant cells, leukemia cells can often (but not always) be found in the cerebrospinal fluid (CSF) by lumbar puncture. Cranial neuropathy and spinal radiculopathy result from impingement upon these nerves as they traverse narrow bony foramina by an expanding mass of leukemia cells. In contrast, a few malignant cells in the CSF at diagnosis are probably not significant since they often disappear during the initial induction chemotherapy treatment without specific attention to the CNS.

The most frequent symptoms in patients with overt CNS leukemia are those caused by increased intracranial pressure: vomiting, headache, papilledema, and lethargy. Diplopia results from oculomotor nerve palsy, especially the abducens. Facial nerve palsies are also common. Spinal radiculopathy and the cauda equina syndrome occur more commonly in adults than in children. Mass lesions within the brain substance itself or within the spinal cord are not common, and seizures are rarely present. Meningismus is also uncommon, and its presence suggests infection or subarachnoid hemorrhage.

The diagnosis is established by finding leukemia cells in the CSF. Usually, the CSF pressure is elevated in symptomatic patients, the glucose concentration is low, and the protein concentration is moderately elevated. Computed tomography (CT) scans may demonstrate thickening of the membranes around the base of the brain or the spinal nerves. Because spinal subarachnoid hemorrhage or focal hematomas can follow lumbar puncture in thrombocytopenic patients, transfusion of platelets to $>20{,}000/\mu L$ should be administered and any coagulopathy corrected first.

CNS leukemia is usually rapidly responsive to irradiation or intrathecal chemotherapy. Standard treatment for symptoms is 2400 cGy to the whole brain in 12 fractions. The spinal column is rarely irradiated except in patients with symptomatic radiculopathy because of the resulting damage to the underlying bone marrow. Dexamethasone (16 mg/day) can alleviate symptoms of increased intracranial pressure. The cord is best treated with preservative-free methotrexate (12mg/m^2 to a maximum dose of 15 mg) injected intrathecally every 3 days for at least six doses. Once the CSF is clear of malignant cells, intrathecal therapy should be administered once a month for the following year. Methotrexate can cause an inflammatory arachnoiditis with fever and nuchal rigidity. For this reason, hydrocortisone (50 mg) is often coadministered with the methotrexate. Alternative drugs for intrathecal use are cytarabine (50 mg) or less commonly thio-TEPA. Slow diffusion of methotrexate out of the CSF into the systemic circulation can cause myelosuppression and gastrointestinal toxicity. This can be lessened by giving leucovorin 24 to 36 h after each dose. Administration of intrathecal chemotherapy via lumbar puncture has the disadvantage of not treating the ventricles at all and the top surface of the brain only poorly. For this reason, an Ommaya reservoir is often placed in symptomatic patients who require chronic CNS therapy to allow an intraventricular (and easier) route of administration.

Clinical trials have suggested that the CNS is a sanctuary site for leukemia cells and is poorly treated by many intravenously administered drugs. Patients can have an isolated CNS relapse despite remaining in an apparent bone marrow remission. Since this can occur in as many as one-third of patients with ALL, all patients with lymphoblastic leukemia generally receive some prophylactic treatment of the CNS as part of their initial treatment program. Alternatives include high doses of cytarabine or methotrexate, two drugs which cross the blood-brain barrier and reach cytotoxic concentrations in the CSF even when administered intravenously.

Although uncommon, various paraneoplastic syndromes occur in patients with leukemia, such as Guillain-Barré polyneuritis and progressive multifocal leukencephalopathy. It is not known to what extent the leukemia itself or its treatment with chemotherapy or irradiation is responsible for these disorders. High doses of cytarabine (≥ 2 g/m^2 for 6 to 12 doses) can cause irreversible cerebellar ataxia, especially in elderly patients or those with renal failure.

Marked leukemic infiltration of the liver and spleen is infrequent in AML and occurs principally in patients with ALL or CML in the blast phase. Signs and symptoms may mimic an acute hepatitis with jaundice, tender hepatomegaly, and elevated serum transaminase levels. This problem usually resolves with effective chemotherapy, but the choice of initial chemotherapy may be compromised because many useful drugs are cleared through the liver. A biliary ultrasound examination should be performed to rule out bile duct obstruction. The spleen is rarely massively enlarged although it may be palpable at diagnosis due to leukemic infiltration. Vascular infarction can occur, causing painful subcapsular hematomas. A rub with respiratory variation will sometimes be heard over the left upper quadrant. Rarely, such an infarcted spleen ruptures, causing shock and signs of intraperitoneal hemorrhage. This is a surgical emergency. Splenic rupture can also occur during chemotherapy as the tumor cell mass is receding, but this is extremely rare.

Infiltration of the kidneys is more common in ALL than in AML. These patients present with oliguric acute renal failure. Renal ultrasound examination demonstrates homogeneous enlargement of both kidneys but no ureteral obstruction. Alternatively, enlarged retroperitoneal lymph nodes can cause ureteral obstruction and renal failure without intrinsic renal disease. These signs resolve during the course of effective chemotherapy, but the inability to excrete the breakdown products of tumor cell lysis can precipitate hyperkalemia and hyperuricemia with their resultant metabolic complications. One or two doses of radiation therapy (200 to 400 cGy) to include just the kidneys (or the ureters as necessary) can reestablish renal excretory function prior to the use of systemic chemotherapy and thus alleviate the risk of tumor lysis syndrome.

Typhlitis is a necrotizing enterocolitis particularly of the terminal ileum, appendix, cecum, and right colon which occurs in granulocytopenic patients.[13,14] Although most often seen in young patients who have recently received intensive chemotherapy, typhlitis can occur in any granulocytopenic patient, such as those with aplastic anemia or with acute leukemia not yet treated. Symptoms and signs are similar to those of inflammatory bowel disease: nausea, vomiting, abdominal pain and tenderness, profuse watery or bloody diarrhea, and fever. The intestinal mucosa is ulcerated, allowing invasion of enteric organisms into and through the bowel wall. Ileus and bowel dilatation result. Plasma proteins and electrolytes are lost into the bowel lumen as occurs with toxic megacolon. Bowel perforation and peritonitis may follow. Jaundice and hepatitis are common, probably because of bacterial seeding through the portal vein. Most patients are best managed with aggressive medical treatment: broad-spectrum antibiotics, transfusion of red blood cells, platelets, and fresh frozen plasma, maintenance of normal serum electrolytes (especially potassium), and bowel rest with nasogastric suction. Narcotic analgesics and paralytic agents such as Lomotil should be avoided because they increase the risk of ileus. Granulocyte transfusions in this setting can prove lifesaving in severely neutropenic patients. With appropriate treatment of the transmural gastrointestinal infection and the recovery of granulocytes, this problem usually resolves without sequelae. Patients with clear evidence of bowel perforation require surgery with ileal diversion or bowel resection. Peritoneal lavage can establish the correct diagnosis if blood or feculent material are recovered. Although the perioperative mortality is high in such cases, the likelihood of a granulocytopenic patient surviving a disseminated peritonitis is small. Radiographic evidence of air within the bowel wall (*pneumatosis intestinalis*) does not in itself require surgery, nor should a granulocytopenic patient who is otherwise doing well necessarily undergo laparotomy for intraperitoneal free air. Antibiotic-associated pseudomembranous colitis (*Clostridium difficile*), radiation enteritis, and GVHD are other causes of abdominal pain and bloody diarrhea in leukemia patients.

Hyperuricemia

Uric acid is the product of nucleic acid catabolism and is increased in diseases where cell turnover rates are high. The total body pool of uric acid is consistently elevated in patients with acute leukemia and occasionally, acute gouty arthritis may be the presenting symptom. Uric acid is largely excreted by the kidneys by both glomerular filtration and tubular excretion. Uric acid nephropathy in leukemia may be present at diagnosis, or it may occur as a complication of therapy.[15] Normal individuals secrete 300 to 500 mg uric acid in the urine daily. The rate of excretion may increase more than 50-fold in patients with acute leukemia. Hyperuricemia may be exacerbated and uricosuria increased as a result of successful cytolytic therapy as well as by drugs such as thiazide diuretics, probenecid, or aspirin.

In acid urine, uric acid quickly supersaturates and precipitates. Uric acid has a dissociation constant of 5.4. At pH 7.0 and above, over 99 percent of urates are in the ionized form and thus water soluble. At pH 4.5, on the other hand, 80 percent of urate is in the form of poorly soluble uric acid, and the combined uric acid–urate solubility falls below 8 mg/dL. In leukemia patients, therefore, the production of organic acids together with decreased urine formation from dehydration due to anorexia or fever frequently leads to precipitation of urates within the renal tubules and collecting system. Direct infiltration of leukemia cells into the kidneys also appears to enhance the local accumulation of uric acid. Leukemia patients with prior renal disease are more prone to develop uric acid nephropathy. Hyperphosphatemia due to tumor cell lysis can cause calcium deposition in the calyces and tubules.

Intratubular precipitation of urates leading to obstruction of urine flow is the more critical cause of nephropathy rather than renal cell injury per se. Effective management of hyperuricemia and hyperuricosuria in leukemia patients is based on reducing the production of uric acid and at the same time promoting the solubility of uric acid in the urine. An adequate urine flow (100 mL/h) should be established by oral or intravenous hydration. The blood volume must be expanded and acidosis corrected. Acetazolamide, a carbonic anhydrase inhibitor, can be given together with sodium bicarbonate to alkalinize the urine. Allopurinol (300 mg/day) will effectively inhibit the conversion of xanthine and hypoxanthine to uric acid. Allopurinol treatment with alkalinization of the urine markedly decreases the risk of uric acid nephropathy in nearly all cases of leukemia.[16] Once the tumor cell mass has been reduced, these measures can be safely discontinued. Allopurinol causes an allergic dermatitis in approximately 10 percent of patients, but this usually occurs only after more than a week of treatment, allowing time for leukemia cytoreduction. Fever and the Stevens-Johnson's syndrome may follow the systemic rash if allopurinol is continued.

Lysozymuria and Renal Tubular Dysfunction

Lysozyme is a small protein (molecular weight 14,000) with an unusually high isoelectric point (pH 11) that has a remarkable capacity to lyse cell walls of certain bacteria. It is also known as muramidase. Lysozyme is present in high concentrations in granulocytes and monocytes and also tissue macrophages. Patients with monocytic and myelomonocytic leukemia excrete large quantities of lysozyme in the urine.[17] Lysozymuria is also present in chronic inflammatory disorders such as sarcoidosis and tuberculosis. The small molecular weight of the protein permits its filtration through the glomerulus and subsequent tubular resorption. Lysozyme, however, is toxic to renal tubule cells and causes tubular dysfunction. Marked hypokalemia has generally accompanied lysozymuria in patients with monoblastic and myelomonocytic leukemias. These problems resolve with effective treatment of the leukemia.

Disseminated Intravascular Coagulation

Laboratory evidence of DIC is almost always present at diagnosis in patients with APL, but it can accompany any leukemia or infection where there is rapid cell lysis or tissue destruction. The pathophysiology is still controversial, but the coagulation cascade appears to be initiated by the release of intracellular thromboplastic material.[18] The syndrome is characterized by the consumption of plasma coagulation proteins and platelets, resulting in a prolonged prothrombin time (PT), thrombin time, and partial thromboplastin time (PTT) together with a decrease in fibrinogen levels and an elevation in fibrin degradation products (FDP). Oozing from venipuncture sites is common. Fibrin thrombi are usually present in the renal glomeruli leading to moderate renal insufficiency. Trauma to circulating red blood cells from fibrin strands causes schistocytes which are apparent on the blood smear. The DIC in patients with leukemia reaches its maximum intensity shortly after chemotherapy begins as the destruction of leukemia cells results in the release of procoagulant-rich granules. The DIC wanes as the tumor burden declines.

Management of DIC is always directed at correcting the underlying tissue destruction whether due to leukemia, infection, burn or crush injury, or obstetric complication. In the meantime, the consumption of coagulation proteins by fibrin formation and its associated secondary fibrinolysis can be rapidly brought under control using heparin. A continuous intravenous infusion of heparin at 5 U/kg/h is well tolerated even in thrombocytopenic patients and allows fresh frozen plasma or cryoprecipitate to be transfused safely without concern about adding substrate for renewed intravascular coagulation. Cryoprecipitate infusions should be used to maintain the fibrinogen concentration at >100 mg/dL. Several doses of vitamin K (10 mg/day) should be given. If the liver is functioning normally, the vitamin K-dependent factors II, V, VII, IX, and antithrombin III (AT-III) will be rapidly repleted, thereby avoiding the need for transfusion of large volumes of fresh frozen plasma. If after 24 h of heparin therapy the fibrinogen has not stabilized and the FDP levels have not decreased, the heparin infusion should be increased to 10 U/kg/h; a higher dose of heparin is rarely necessary. Lack of response to heparin may indicate a deficiency of the heparin cofactor AT-III, which can be repleted by transfusion of fresh frozen plasma. The optimal approach to DIC in leukemia remains to be determined, and it may be possible to manage the coagulopathy of APL with intensive chemotherapy and blood product support without the routine use of heparin.[19]

Lactic Acidosis

Significant elevations of blood lactate or pyruvate concentrations in patients with leukemia result from an increase in the rate of lactic acid production or a decrease in the rate of pyruvic acid utilization or both. Whether clinical acidosis results depends in part on other metabolic and respiratory factors which influence acid-base balance. Blood lactate elevations occur more commonly in patients with acute leukemia than in any other neoplastic disorder.[20] Lactic acidosis may also be secondary to inadequate oxygenation of the tissues due to hyperleukocytosis, septic shock, pulmonary edema, or severe anemia. The development of lactic acidosis despite apparently adequate oxygen supply to the tissues can sometimes reflect disseminated fungal infection with small vessel occlusion or extensive liver necrosis. Lactic acidosis associated with massive leukemia is seen most commonly in patients with ALL, and especially B cell ALL. Experiments in vitro suggest that although malignant leukocytes exhibit little lactic acid production under aerobic conditions, they can have considerable anaerobic lactic acid production. It has been estimated that a rapidly growing mass of leukemia cells crowded into organs where the cells may be poorly oxygenated and therefore dependent on anaerobic glycolysis for energy could produce as much as 300 to 600 m*M* lactic acid per h. Any interference with hepatic blood supply or hepatic metabolism can diminish the body's ability to handle this acid load, resulting in clinical acidosis.

The successful treatment of lactic acidosis in patients with acute leukemia depends on the institution of effective antileukemia therapy. Removal of lactic acid by hemodialysis or peritoneal dialysis may also be useful.

CASE PRESENTATION

A 22-year-old man presented to his family physician with a 1-week history of gum bleeding and epistaxis and fever to 38°C (100.4°F). His physical examination was remarkable for pallor and multiple ecchymoses and petechiae. Retinal hemorrhages were present as well as fresh blood in the nares and the mouth. There was no lymphadenopathy, and the spleen was not palpable.

The complete blood count showed a hemoglobin of 10.0 g/dL, a hematocrit of 30 percent, and a platelet count of 12,000/μL. The white blood cell count was 1200/μL; the differential was remarkable for only rare polymorphonuclear granulocytes, and the remainder of the cells were mature lymphocytes. The peripheral blood smear was remarkable for pancytopenia and the presence of schistocytes. The coagulation profile revealed a PT of 16 s and a PTT of 60 s. The fibrin split products were positive at >80 but <160 μg/mL. The fibrinogen concentration was 90 mg/dL. The blood chemistry was remarkable for a creatinine level of 2.2 mg/dL, uric acid value of 9.5 mg/dL, and a lactic dehydrogenase (LDH) level of 450 IU/ml. The chest x-ray was normal. The patient was immediately admitted to a comprehensive medical center with a diagnosis of aplastic anemia or acute leukemia and possible infection with DIC.

The patient was evaluated by a hematologic oncologist on admission to the hospital. Blood and urine cultures were obtained, and intravenous antibiotic therapy was begun with ceftazidime. A bone marrow examination was performed with aspiration and biopsy. A bone marrow sample was sent for cytogenetic analysis which later revealed the presence of t(15;17) in 80 percent of the metaphase cells. The aspirate smears and a bone core biopsy specimen revealed a massive infiltration by malignant granulated blast cells with bilobed nuclei and multiple Auer rods; the diagnosis was acute promyelocytic leukemia (APL). Allopurinol and intravenous hydration were initiated. Platelets and red blood cells were transfused. A double-lumen Hickman catheter was placed in the innominate vein, and chemotherapy was initiated with intravenous cytarabine and daunorubicin. The patient continued to ooze from venipuncture sites and a repeat fibrinogen level was 50 mg/dL. Heparin was begun at

5 U/kg/h by continuous intravenous infusion. Cryoprecipitate was then infused to maintain the fibrinogen concentration at >100 mg/dL. Three daily doses of vitamin K were also given. The following day, the fibrin split products were still >320 μg/mL, so the heparin infusion was increased to 10 U/kg/h. Two units of fresh frozen plasma were transfused to supply adequate AT-III, the vitamin K-dependent cofactor required for heparin inhibition of thrombin. All spontaneous bleeding soon stopped. Four days into chemotherapy, the fibrinogen level began to rise without further cryoprecipitate transfusions and the fibrin split products began to decline. Gradually, the serum creatinine concentration also returned to normal as the fibrin thrombi in the renal glomeruli lyzed, and the schistocytes disappeared from the peripheral blood smear. His fever resolved, but antibiotics were continued despite negative initial cultures because of the marked granulocytopenia. The chemotherapy treatment ended on day 7, and the bone marrow examination showed that the cellularity had declined from 100 percent to approximately 60 percent. Without further treatment, the bone marrow cellularity declined to <5 percent 1 week later and then began to regenerate with normal-appearing marrow cells.

The patient was doing quite well until suddenly on day 14, when his temperature increased to 40°C (104°F), and he became tachypneic. Antibiotics were changed empirically to mezlocillin and tobramycin. A chest radiograph demonstrated a midlung infiltrate, and blood cultures grew *Pseudomonas aeruginosa.* Because of hypotension and respiratory distress, the patient required fluid resuscitation and intubation, but there was a prompt response to antibiotics over 72 h, and he was easily extubated. The patient had profuse diarrhea and required continuous KCl infusions to maintain a serum potassium level of >4 meq/L. He developed crampy abdominal pain and bloody diarrhea. The diarrhea stool was positive for pseudomonas and for *C. difficile* toxin. Lomotil was inadvertently given, following which an ileus developed. The bowel began to dilate with evidence of pneumatosis coli on abdominal radiographs. An experienced oncology surgeon was consulted, who agreed with aggressive medical management rather than surgical exploration. The patient was placed on bowel rest with nasogastric suction. No narcotics were allowed. The serum potassium level was maintained at >4.5 meq/L, and the serum albumin was repleted using fresh frozen plasma. Blood transfusions were used to maintain the hematocrit >30 percent and the platelet count >20,000/μL. Intravenous metronidazole was added to the antibiotic regimen. Over several days, the abdominal distention and ileus resolved.

Twenty-eight days after initiating chemotherapy, the patient's blood count returned to normal, and all evidence of his pseudomonas sepsis with pneumonia and necrotizing enterocolitis resolved. The renal function returned to normal, and there was no further evidence of DIC. A bone marrow examination at this time revealed a normal bone marrow with no evidence of residual disease, and it was felt that the patient was in complete remission. This patient subsequently received three additional courses of intensive consolidation chemotherapy for his APL without complication; there has been no evidence of recurrent disease over the past 6 years.

CASE DISCUSSION

This case dramatically illustrates the benefits of appropriately aggressive intensive care in a patient with leukemia. In view of the complexity of supportive management in many patients with leukemia, referral to an oncology center should be routine. In this case, initial empiric antibiotic therapy with ceftazidime was chosen, rather than using an aminoglycoside, because of the concurrent renal insufficiency. DIC was apparent at the time of diagnosis, a common finding in patients with APL. Heparin at 5 U/kg/h was given by continuous intravenous infusion to treat the DIC which almost always worsens in APL when tumor cell lysis begins. When the DIC failed to resolve, it was appropriate to increase the heparin infusion to 10 U/kg/h, then to add fresh frozen plasma when the lack of response to heparin suggested the possibility of AT-III deficiency.

When the patient first deteriorated, intensive care, even including mechanical ventilation and aggressive support of the circulation, was instituted since the likelihood of response to chemotherapy was high. His ICU course included several typical life-threatening, yet reversible, complications of leukemia (or its treatment). Many of these are unavoidable and should be anticipated as part of the supportive management of leukemia. Lomotil should not have been given and may have contributed to the development of ileus. Chemotherapy can denude the gut epithelium allowing enteric flora to penetrate the mucosal barrier and even seed the portal blood. The transmural infection, gastrointestinal bleeding, and loss of plasma proteins and electrolytes into the gut lumen require vigorous management similar to that used for toxic megacolon in a patient with severe inflammatory bowel disease. With each such reversible complication it is important to keep in mind that an excellent outcome remains possible. Oncologists, surgeons, and intensivists with substantial experience in the support of patients with leukemia are invaluable when caring for critically ill patients with this disease.

References

1. Bennett JM, Catovsky D, Daniel MT, et al: Proposed revised criteria for the classification of acute myeloid leukemia: A report of the French-American-British Cooperative Group. Ann Intern Med 103:626, 1985.
2. Samuels BL, Larson RA, Le Beau MM, et al: Specific chromosomal abnormalities in acute nonlymphocytic leukemia correlate with drug susceptibility in vivo. Leukemia 2:79, 1988.
3. Koeffler HP: Syndromes of acute nonlymphocytic leukemia. Ann Intern Med 107:748, 1987.
4. Bitter MA, Le Beau MM, Rowley JD, et al: Associations be-

tween morphology, karyotype, and clinical features in myeloid leukemias. Human Pathol 18:211, 1987.
5. Wolff SN, Herzig RH, Fay JW, et al: High-dose cytarabine and daunorubicin as consolidation therapy for acute myeloid leukemia in first remission: Long-term follow-up and results. J Clin Oncol 7:1260, 1989.
6. Champlin R, Gale RP: Acute lymphoblastic leukemia: Recent advances in biology and therapy. Blood 73:2051, 1989.
7. Lichtman MA, Rowe JM: Hyperleukocytic leukemias: Rheological, clinical, and therapeutic considerations. Blood 60:279, 1982.
8. Cuttner J, Holland JF, Norton L, et al: Therapeutic leukapheresis for hyperleukocytosis in acute myelocytic leukemia. Med Pediatr Oncol 11:76, 1983.
9. Dutcher JP, Schiffer CA, Wiernik PH: Hyperleukocytosis in adult acute nonlymphocytic leukemia: Impact on remission rate and duration, and survival. J Clin Oncol 5:1364, 1987.
10. Hess CE, Nichols AB, Hunt WB, et al: Pseudohypoxemia secondary to leukemia and thrombocytosis. N Engl J Med 301:361, 1979.
11. Neiman RS, Barcos M, Berard C, et al: Granulocytic sarcoma: A clinocopathologic study of 61 biopsied cases. Cancer 48:1426, 1981.
12. Kantarjian HM, Walters RS, Smith TL, et al: Identification of risk groups for development of central nervous system leukemia in adults with acute lymphocytic leukemia. Blood 72:1784, 1988.
13. Starnes HF Jr, Moore FD Jr, Mentzer S, et al: Abdominal pain in neutropenic cancer patients. Cancer 57:616, 1986.
14. Shamberger RC, Weinstein HJ, Delorey MJ, et al: The medical and surgical management of typhlitis in children with acute nonlymphocytic (myelogenous) leukemia. Cancer 57:603, 1986.
15. Kanswar YS, Manaligod JR: Leukemic urate nephropathy. Arch Pathol 99:467, 1975.
16. Vogler WR, Bain JA, Huguley CM Jr, et al: Metabolic and therapeutic effects of allopurinol in patients with leukemia and gout. Am J Med 40:548, 1966.
17. Muggia FM, Heinemann HO, Farhangi M, et al: Lysozymuria and renal tubular dysfunction in monocytic and myelomonocytic leukemia. Am J Med 47:351, 1969.
18. Bauer KA, Rosenberg RD: Thrombin generation in acute promyelocytic leukemia. Blood 64:791, 1984.
19. Goldberg MA, Ginsburg D, Mayer RJ, et al: Is heparin administration necessary during induction chemotherapy for patients with acute promyelocytic leukemia? Blood 69:187, 1987.
20. Field M, Block JB, Levin R, et al: Significance of blood lactate elevations among patients with acute leukemias and other neoplastic proliferative disorders. Am J Med 40:528, 1966.

Chapter 149 THE ONCOLOGIC EMERGENCIES

WILLIAM J. GRADISHAR
PHILIP C. HOFFMAN

KEY POINTS

- *Patients with malignancy are subject to life-threatening complications of the primary disease, its treatment, or coexisting medical diseases.*
- *Complications are frequently worth treating since they are often associated with a higher acute morbidity and mortality than the malignancy.*
- *In premorbid or terminal patients restraint must be exercised in the diagnosis and treatment of oncologic complications.*
- *A high index of suspicion must be maintained to recognize oncologic complications since they often share features similar to other common medical illnesses.*
- *Frequent examinations of critically ill patients are necessary since such patients (intubated, bed-bound, hypotensive) are often unable to verbalize changes in their condition.*

Patients with an underlying malignancy can develop a number of different medical complications that arise by anatomic distortion and functional impairment by tumor or by metabolic and endocrine abnormalities that are frequently associated with the presence of a particular cancer. Since these acute complications can frequently cause more immediate morbidity and mortality than the underlying malignancy, they are appropriately referred to as oncologic emergencies. Clinicians must exercise sound clinical judgment when approaching a patient with one of the oncologic emergencies. In end-stage patients with an underlying malignancy, it is often more humane to leave the oncologic complication (e.g., hypercalcemia, spinal cord compression [SCC]) untreated rather than subject a patient to numerous diagnostic tests and therapeutic maneuvers that will not prolong or improve the patient's remaining life.

Patients with an underlying malignancy often have comorbid medical illnesses that can mask an acute complication of the cancer. Furthermore, the treatment of the malignancy with chemotherapy, radiation, or biologic response modifiers may cause these acute complications to develop. To recognize these disorders it is important to develop a differential diagnosis for common signs and symptoms that occur in critically ill cancer patients (Table 149-1). A high index of suspicion for these complications must always be complemented by frequent and thorough clinical assessments of the patient.

TABLE 149-1 Differential Diagnosis for Common Signs and Symptoms in Cancer Patients

Sign/Symptom	Differential Diagnosis
Nausea and vomiting	Hypercalcemia
	Renal failure
	Brain metastases or brain herniation
	Leptomeningeal carcinomatosis
	Liver metastases
Abnormal mental status	Hypercalcemia
	Hyponatremia
	Renal failure
	Sepsis
	Leptomeningeal carcinomatosis
	Brain metastases or brain herniation
Hemodynamic instability	Pulmonary embolism
	Pericardial tamponade
	Pericardial constriction
	Brain herniation
	Superior vena cava syndrome
Renal failure	Hypercalcemia
	Tumor lysis syndrome; hyperuricemia
	Obstruction
	Paraneoplastic changes
	Glomerulonephritis

Thoracic Syndromes

SUPERIOR VENA CAVA SYNDROME

The superior vena cava (SVC) syndrome is an oncologic problem that typically occurs in 3 to 8 percent of patients with carcinoma of the lung or lymphoma.[1,2] To understand the clinical manifestations of the syndrome, an appreciation of the regional anatomy is necessary (Fig. 149-1). Venous blood returning from the head and neck, upper extremities, and upper thorax reaches the right heart via the SVC. The SVC is situated in the right anterior superior mediastinum, adjacent to the right posterolateral aspect of the proximal ascending aorta and the anterior surface of the right pulmonary artery. It lies adjacent to the right mainstem bronchus and is encircled by mediastinal and paratracheal lymph nodes. Three mechanisms, alone or in combination, may account for the development of SVC syndrome. **1.** The SVC is susceptible to external compression by tumor because of the compliance of the vessel wall as well as the low intravenous pressure. **2.** Tumor may directly invade the vessel wall resulting in deformity of the SVC lumen. **3.** External compression by tumor may precipitate the formation of thrombosis within the SVC lumen causing a complete or partial obstruction. The syndrome tends to develop insidiously, resulting in progressive worsening of signs and symptoms over time.

Benign diseases (e.g., syphilitic aneurysm of the aorta, histoplasmosis, thyroid goiter, etc.) accounted for the majority of cases of SVC syndrome until relatively recently. Now the vast majority of cases (>90 percent) are caused by malignancy.[3] In a review of several large series of patients with SVC syndrome, 52 to 81 percent of cases were caused

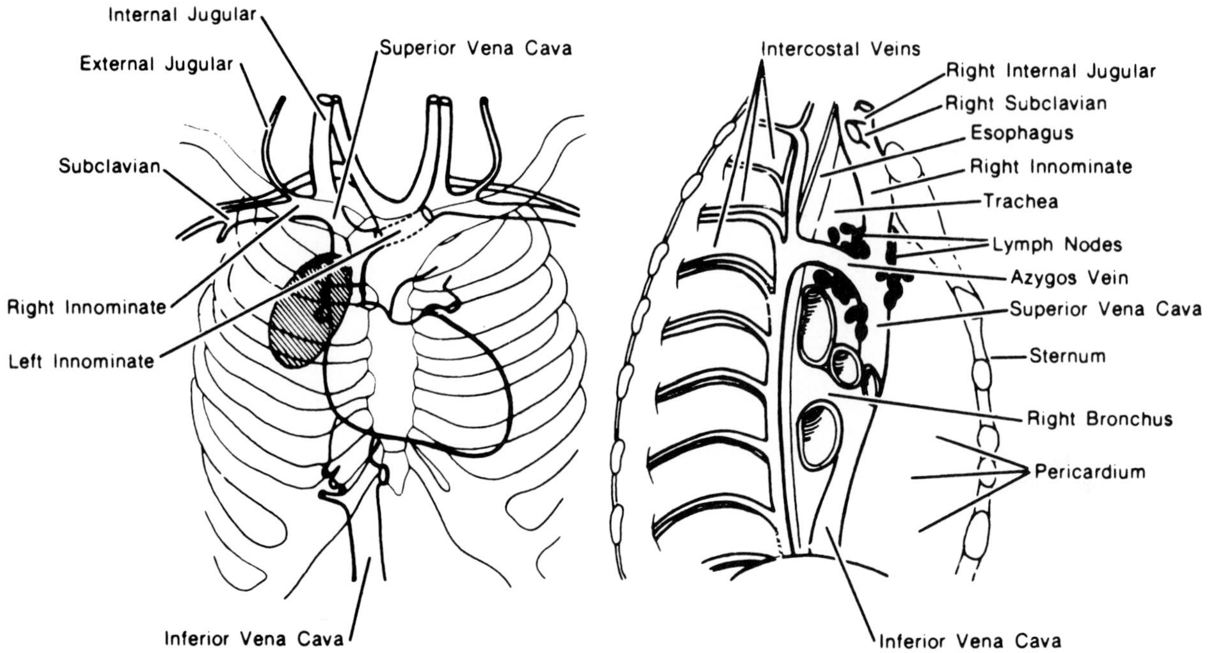

FIGURE 149-1 Frontal *(left)* and lateral *(right)* sections of the thorax depicting the anatomic structures adjacent to the SVC. The shaded area indicates the most common site of obstruction in SVC syndrome.

by lung cancer. The most common histologic subtype is anaplastic small cell cancer (41 percent) followed by squamous cell (27 percent), adenocarcinoma (14 percent), and large cell carcinoma (13 percent). The majority of the lung cancers, particularly small cell carcinomas, are centrally located near the right hilum.

The second most common malignancy causing the SVC syndrome and accounting for 2 to 15 percent of all cases is malignant lymphoma. The histologic subtypes of non-Hodgkin's lymphoma most commonly identified include diffuse large cell lymphoma (often with sclerosis) and lymphoblastic lymphoma. Hodgkin's disease rarely causes SVC syndrome. A minority of cases of SVC syndrome are caused by tumors metastatic to the mediastinum (e.g., breast) or by primary mediastinal tumors (e.g., germ cell tumors, thymomas).

Central vein catheters are commonly used in patients for hemodynamic monitoring, hyperalimentation, cardiac pacing, and the administration of chemotherapy and blood products. SVC syndrome caused by thrombus formation around these catheters is diagnosed with increasing frequency and must be considered in the appropriate setting.

The diagnosis of SVC syndrome is made on the basis of a constellation of symptoms and signs.[1,2] The most common presenting symptom is dyspnea. As a result of increased venous pressure, patients often complain of headache, dizziness, blurry vision, and a sensation of fullness in the head. Less commonly patients will complain of dysphagia, dysphonia, cough, and chest pain.

The characteristic physical findings develop as a result of partial or complete obstruction of the SVC. Venous distention of the neck and chest wall (50 to 90 percent), facial edema (50 percent), upper extremity edema (10 to 15 percent), cyanosis (15 to 20 percent), and facial plethora (20 percent) are common physical findings.

Usually the diagnosis of SVC syndrome is suspected entirely on the basis of signs and symptoms. Occasionally the SVC obstruction may be partial, making the clinical manifestations subtle, especially early in the clinical course. Additional diagnostic tests are obtained with the intention of characterizing the exact location and the cause of the obstruction (i.e., histology).

Chest x-rays will be abnormal in the majority of patients. The abnormalities include a widened superior mediastinum, a right hilar or mediastinal mass (usually anterior), and pleural effusions. Although the location of the abnormality is not conclusive, right-sided hilar masses are consistent with lung carcinoma, and anterior mediastinal masses suggest lymphoma.

A computed tomography (CT) scan with venous contrast material has recently been advocated as a noninvasive method of delineating the site and extent of SVC obstruction.[4] Information regarding the extent of collateral circulation as well as other structures involved with tumor may also be determined. Furthermore, if a pathologic diagnosis cannot be made from a more accessible site, a CT scan provides information useful when considering a percutaneous biopsy. Finally, the CT scan serves as a guide for planning the radiation ports used in treating some patients.

Radionuclide venography and contrast venography are methods of demonstrating the degree of patency and flow patterns within the SVC.[1] These methods also give insight into the degree of involvement of vena cava tributaries and the extent of collateral venous pathways. The images obtained with radionuclide venography are not as well defined as with contrast venography.

Definitive and supportive therapy for SVC syndrome should not be delayed in patients without a tissue diagnosis who are clinically deteriorating. In all patients the least invasive and most expedient method of obtaining a tissue diagnosis should be pursued. The positive yield from a number of diagnostic procedures was recently compiled (Table 149-2).[1,2] Sputum cytology will establish a diagnosis, usually lung carcinoma, in half the cases. Thoracentesis of a pleural effusion, if present, has a high positive yield (73 percent). Bone marrow biopsies will establish a diagnosis of malignancy, usually small cell carcinoma or lymphoma, in 25 percent of patients. Because lung carcinoma is the most common cause of the SVC syndrome, bronchoscopy has approximately a 50 percent diagnostic yield. Palpable supraclavicular lymph nodes have a high diagnostic yield if accessible for biopsy. Mediastinoscopy and thoracotomy can be considered when other approaches have failed to yield a diagnosis; however, the time involved in arranging for the procedure and the associated morbidity may result in further clinical deterioration of the patient. Long delays in obtaining unnecessary diagnostic tests can prove detrimental to the patient's outcome and add little useful information. In rare patients, a therapeutic intervention must take place before a tissue diagnosis is obtained. In a hemodynamically unstable patient, the time necessary to arrange a tissue biopsy (e.g., bronchoscopy, mediastinoscopy, etc.) may be detrimental to the patient's outcome. Therapy must begin empirically in such patients.

The goals of therapy, when treating SVC syndrome, are not only to palliate the associated signs and symptoms, but also to cure patients if they have a chemosensitive or radiosensitive malignancy.

Supportive measures that bring temporary relief of symptoms include the administration of supplemental oxygen, elevation of the head and chest of the patient, and the administration of oral or intravenous dexamethasone (4 mg every 6 h). Diuretics given intravenously may result in symptomatic relief in some patients, but their use cannot be advocated routinely.

In patients with small cell carcinoma of the lung, combination chemotherapy has been determined to be more effective (73 to 100 percent) than radiation therapy alone (40 to 65 percent) in achieving symptomatic relief of symptoms related to the SVC syndrome. The clinical manifestations of SVC syndrome usually resolve within 7 to 10 days after the initiation of therapy. Furthermore, the use of chemotherapy may eliminate the need to radiate a large lung field with its attendant complications. Finally, since chemotherapy is the mainstay of treatment for small cell carcinoma, this approach permits the early institution of systemic therapy.

TABLE 149-2 Diagnostic Yield of Various Tests in SVC Syndrome

Test	% Positive
Thoracotomy	98
Mediastinoscopy	77
Thoracentesis	73
Lymph node biopsy	67
Bronchoscopy	51
Sputum cytology	49
Bone marrow biopsy	23

The treatment of choice for patients with SVC syndrome caused by non-Hodgkin's lymphoma depends on the histology. Patients with aggressive lymphomas (e.g., diffuse histiocytic, lymphoblastic lymphoma) often achieve complete remission with the use of combination chemotherapy. Studies comparing radiation therapy versus chemotherapy versus combined chemoradiotherapy have shown comparable results. Relief of symptoms usually occurs within 2 weeks of starting therapy.

For patients without a tissue diagnosis or in patients with a diagnosis other than lymphoma or small cell cancer (e.g., non-small cell lung cancer, breast cancer), the primary modality of therapy is radiation therapy. When total radiation doses ranging between 4000 to 6000 cGy are administered, 90 percent of patients achieve symptomatic relief. Some radiotherapists advocate the use of high initial daily fractions of radiation therapy (e.g., 400 cGy $\times$ 3 to 4) followed by conventional fractions of radiation therapy (180 to 200 cGy/day) until the total dose is administered. Relief of symptoms seems to occur earlier in patients receiving high daily doses of radiotherapy, although survival may not be prolonged.

For patients with SVC syndrome secondary to thrombus formation around a central vein catheter, the use of tissue plasminogen activator, urokinase, or streptokinase has been advocated as a means of clot lysis.[5] In most situations the ideal approach is to remove the catheter while administering heparin to reduce peripheral embolization.

The overall prognosis of patients with SVC syndrome is directly related to the stage of the underlying disease. Patients with a malignancy of limited stage that responds to chemotherapy or radiation therapy (or both) have a good prognosis, whereas those with extensive disease that is unresponsive to therapy do poorly.

PERICARDIAL DISEASE

Although any part of the heart can be involved with malignancy, it is pericardial involvement that most commonly results in overt clinical manifestations. There are a variety of disorders in the differential diagnosis of a patient with an underlying malignancy who presents with signs and symptoms suggesting a cardiac or pulmonary disease. Included in the differential are chemotherapy-related ventricular dysfunction, radiation-induced pericardial disease, radiation-induced coronary artery disease, malignant pericardial or pleural effusion, pericardial infection, and right ventricular dysfunction due to pulmonary embolism or coexistent chronic obstructive pulmonary disease. Since many of the signs and symptoms of these disorders overlap, great care must be taken to determine the precise etiology of the clinical manifestation as treatment can vary greatly. Treatment of the underlying malignancy, especially with the use of radiation therapy, can also result in clinical syndromes primarily affecting the pericardium.

Primary malignancies of the heart are exceedingly rare, but the pericardium is a relatively frequent site of metastases. Autopsy series report that pericardial seeding with tumor occurs in 1 to 20 percent of patients with an underlying malignancy. The vast majority of these patients have clinically silent pericardial disease.[6,7]

The most common malignancies affecting the pericardium are lung carcinoma (squamous, small cell, adenocarcinoma) and breast carcinoma which each account for over 30 percent of cases in most series. These two cancers account for the largest fraction of cases in large part because of the high prevalence of the two diseases and because of their proximity to the pericardium. Other malignancies that commonly involve the pericardium include lymphoma, leukemia (lymphocytic more than nonlymphocytic), and melanoma. Much less commonly, ovarian carcinoma and gastrointestinal carcinoma have been reported to involve the pericardium.

Although pericardial metastases are diagnosed or suspected in a minority of patients (7 to 30 percent) antemortem, the clinical syndromes that can develop as a result of this complication are often immediately life-threatening unless recognition and intervention occur promptly. The clinical syndromes associated with malignant pericardial involvement are pericardial effusion, pericardial tamponade, and constrictive pericarditis. The differential diagnosis of these syndromes must be appreciated to recognize nonmalignant diseases that can mimic malignant pericardial disease and as a result drastically alter management.

Tumors that involve structures lying immediately adjacent to the heart (e.g., esophageal or lung carcinoma) can directly invade the pericardium. More commonly, seeding of the pericardium tends to occur via lymphangitic spread. Malignancy will commonly invade the lymph nodes that drain the mediastinum, and through retrograde spread, tumor cells course through the subepicardial and epicardial lymph vessels eventually infiltrating the pericardium. Less commonly, pericardial metastases can occur through hematogenous spread of tumor. In any patient with an underlying malignancy who develops hemodynamic instability, pericardial disease must be considered as a cause.

Large pericardial effusions may develop slowly and not cause symptoms; however, the enlarging pericardial sac may place pressure on adjacent anatomic structures resulting in cough, dysphagia, or hoarseness.

The symptoms that accompany evolving cardiac tamponade develop as a result of the changes in the circulation. As a result of an elevated venous pressure, patients commonly complain of a sensation of fullness in the head and neck. Similarly, elevated venous pressure in the inferior vena cava will cause hepatic and visceral congestion, sometimes resulting in complaints of nausea and vague abdominal pains. Patients will complain of dyspnea as a result of diminished cardiac output. In cases where tamponade develops quickly, patients will appear acutely ill with signs of shock including diaphoresis, hypotension, tachycardia, and altered mental status.

The diagnosis of cardiac tamponade is dependent on a high index of suspicion in patients with malignancy and circulatory failure.[8] Equally important is an ability to correctly recognize and interpret physical findings and hemodynamic data. Patients with cardiac tamponade usually have tachycardia, an elevated jugular venous pressure, a pulsus paradoxus, and a narrow arterial pulse pressure. A paradoxical pulse is defined as an *inspiratory* decline of systolic pressure exceeding 10 mmHg. Examination of a right atrial waveform will typically reveal the absence of the atrial y descent and a prominent x descent indicating that venous influx is impaired during diastole and that atrial filling will occur only during systole.

Occasionally the signs of cardiac tamponade are confused with congestive heart failure.[9] Both conditions cause dyspnea, elevated jugular venous pressure, and an enlarged cardiac silhouette on chest x-ray. However, pulsus paradoxus is almost always present in tamponade, but almost uniformly absent in heart failure. Pulmonary congestion and gallop rhythms characteristic of heart failure are almost never seen in tamponade.

Pulsus paradoxus by itself is not diagnostic of tamponade because it can occur in several other conditions, among them obstructive lung disease, constrictive pericarditis, pulmonary embolism, right ventricular infarction, restrictive cardiomyopathy, and shock. There are also conditions under which pulsus paradoxus may *not* be observed in patients with cardiac tamponade including severe left ventricular dysfunction, severe hypotension, atrial septal defect, aortic incompetence, hypovolemia, and positive-pressure breathing.[9]

Findings on chest radiographs are nonspecific. Severe tamponade can develop with a normal-sized cardiac silhouette particularly if the pericardial fluid accumulates rapidly. An enlarged cardiac silhouette without radiographic signs of pulmonary congestion should suggest the presence of tamponade rather than congestive heart failure.

The electrocardiogram (ECG) findings in tamponade are nonspecific. Sinus tachycardia and nonspecific ST segment changes are common. The ECG changes characteristic of acute pericarditis (ST segment elevation) may occur. Electrical alternans may develop, characterized by phasic alteration of the amplitude of the R wave (Fig. 149-2). Two-dimensional echocardiography is the most specific and sensitive noninvasive modality for documenting the presence of a pericardial effusion as small as 20 mL. Certain echocardiographic features support the diagnosis of cardiac tamponade: **1.** right ventricular compression, **2.** diastolic indentation of the right atrium and right ventricle, and **3.** enlargement of the inferior vena cava or lack of respiratory variation in the presence of normal systolic left ventricular and right ventricular function.[7] In some cases, these signs may not be present. As a result, Swan-Ganz catheterization may be necessary to determine the functional signifi-

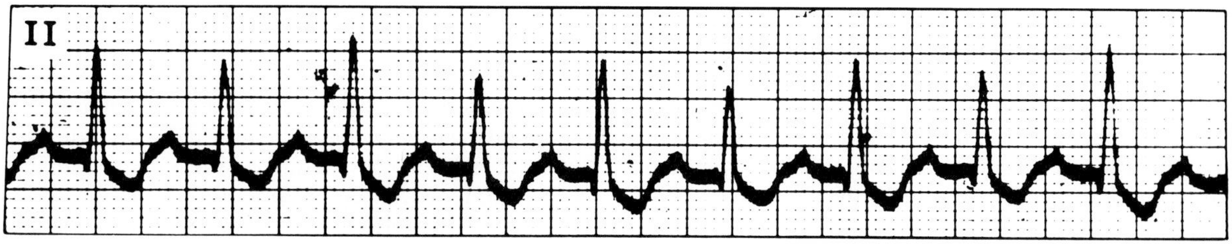

FIGURE 149-2 ECG depicting electrical alternans with variation in the amplitude of the QRS complex from beat to beat.

cance of a pericardial effusion. In cardiac tamponade, the right atrial, right ventricular, and pulmonary capillary wedge pressures are elevated and equal (see Chap. 121).

In constrictive pericarditis, a thickened, fibrotic pericardium limits the filling of all four heart chambers. Renal compensatory mechanisms increase salt and water retention and eventually cause ascites and edema. Signs and symptoms of left heart failure eventually develop manifested by dyspnea, cough, and orthopnea. A variety of nonmalignant etiologies can cause constrictive pericarditis. In cancer patients, the syndrome typically develops following radiation therapy to the mediastinum. In most series, patients with underlying lung carcinoma, breast carcinoma, and Hodgkin's disease account for the majority of cases. Constrictive pericarditis can develop 6 to 30 months following radiation therapy.

The symptoms associated with constrictive pericarditis typically develop insidiously over a period of months to years. Increasing abdominal girth and peripheral edema along with progressive exertional dyspnea are common complaints. As the disease progresses, symptoms suggestive of cardiac cachexia develop (e.g., weakness, dyspnea at rest, palpitations, etc.).

Patients generally have a normal or low blood pressure. Elevated venous pressure is demonstrated by jugular venous distention with a rapid *y* descent and rapid rebound. In contrast to cardiac tamponade, an inspiratory increase in jugular venous distention, Kussmaul's sign, occurs in constrictive pericarditis. The heart sounds are often distant. Hepatomegaly, pulmonary edema, and ascites are late clinical features of the syndrome.

Chest radiographs show an enlarged cardiac silhouette in only slightly more than 50 percent of cases. Occasionally intrapericardial calcifications are present; however, the absence of calcifications does not exclude constrictive pericarditis. ECG findings are nonspecific. Atrial fibrillation is observed in long-standing cases due to elevated atrial pressure.

M-mode and two-dimensional echocardiography can demonstrate pericardial thickening, but most findings are nonspecific. More recently, Doppler echocardiography has demonstrated that altered patterns of left ventricular filling can distinguish normal individuals from those with constrictive pericarditis.[7] Patients with constrictive pericarditis typically have a rapid deceleration of filling velocity and a shortened filling period.

In constrictive pericarditis, cardiac catheterization will demonstrate equilibration of diastolic pressures in all four chambers. The ventricular pressure tracing will demonstrate the characteristic dip- and plateau or "square-root sign" (Fig. 149-3). The early diastolic dip of ventricular pressure indicates abnormally rapid ventricular filling in constrictive pericarditis. The pulmonary artery pressure is slightly elevated, and the cardiac index is usually decreased. Angiography is able to demonstrate a thickened pericardium in most patients with constrictive pericarditis, and more recently CT has been shown to effectively distinguish between restrictive myocardial disease and constrictive pericarditis by the presence of a thickened pericardium.

The management of patients with large, symptomatic pericardial effusions or frank cardiac tamponade is directed toward reducing intrapericardial pressure by removing pericardial fluid.[8] The manner in which this is accomplished largely depends on the patient's hemodynamic stability. In

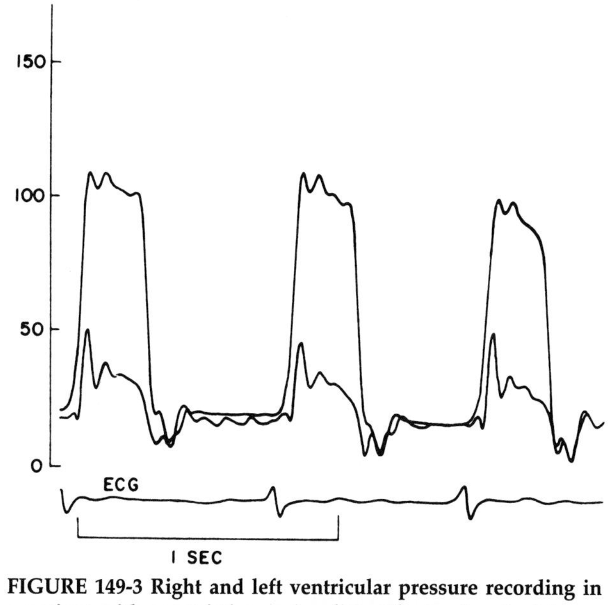

FIGURE 149-3 Right and left ventricular pressure recording in a patient with constrictive pericarditis. The tracing depicts equilibration of right and left ventricular diastolic pressures and the characteristic "square-root" sign of the diastolic wave form.

cases where the clinical status of the patient is rapidly deteriorating, pericardiocentesis must be performed immediately. The "blind" approach to aspirating pericardial fluid can be complicated by arrhythmias, sudden death, and laceration of coronary arteries. In a more controlled situation, echocardiography or CT scanning can guide the aspiration needle to the location likely to yield the most fluid with fewest potential complications.

Removal of pericardial fluid should occur slowly because pulmonary edema may be precipitated by suddenly decompressing the right heart which will in turn increase its output. The left heart may not be able to accommodate the sudden increase in venous return, resulting in overload of the left ventricle and the development of pulmonary edema.

Once fluid has been aspirated it should be analyzed for cytologic evidence of malignancy. Fluid should also be sent for culture to rule out common bacterial infections as well as opportunistic infections. Analysis of malignant effusions may reveal serous, serosanguineous, or hemorrhagic fluid; therefore, the gross appearance of the fluid is not helpful. The fluid usually has the characteristics of an exudate with high specific gravity, protein, and cell count; however, with the exception of malignant cells being present, no other feature distinguishes a malignant effusion from other causes.

For recurring or thick pericardial effusions, drainage of the fluid can be facilitated by pericardiostomy via a subxiphoid approach in the pericardial sac and inserting tubes that allow both irrigation and drainage of the fluid. This procedure can often be accomplished under local anesthesia. It also allows for the instillation of sclerosing agents (e.g., tetracycline) that will potentially obliterate the pericardial space and prevent the reaccumulation of fluid.[10]

Occasional patients, who otherwise may have a relatively long life expectancy (e.g., those with breast cancer), may develop recurring pericardial effusions that do not respond to conservative measures. In these cases a total or partial pericardiectomy can be considered. In patients with constrictive pericarditis due to tumor encasement or radiation fibrosis, pericardiectomy is the treatment of choice. Occasionally patients present with effusive-constrictive pericarditis which has features more like those of cardiac tamponade than those of chronic constrictive pericarditis. Effusive-constrictive pericarditis most frequently is radiation induced. A surgical approach that allows for removal of as much of the pericardium as possible is favored. In patients who are already debilitated and compromised because of their underlying malignancy and its treatment, undertaking a major surgical procedure carries with it significant morbidity and operative mortality. In patients with a very poor prognosis aside from this complication, supportive care is indicated.

Neurologic Syndromes

SPINAL CORD COMPRESSION

The recognition of SCC in patients with malignancy depends on a high index of suspicion and persistent clinical vigilance. Arriving at the diagnosis in patients who are cared for in the ICU can be even more of a challenge because patients are bed-bound, often sedated and intubated, and therefore unable to report pain or weakness. Not uncommonly, these patients are afflicted with more than one medical problem. As a result, a variety of overlapping signs and symptoms can be present. To have any chance of reversing the neurologic deficits that occur as a result of SCC (i.e., paralysis), the diagnosis must be made in a very timely fashion. Therefore, any suspicion of the diagnosis must be aggressively pursued with the appropriate evaluation.[11,12]

Clinical evidence of SCC occurs in approximately 5 percent of patients with malignancy. The syndrome can occur in any tumor that has the ability to metastasize, but certain tumors more commonly cause this syndrome than others. Lung cancer accounts for approximately 15 percent of cases, while myeloma, prostate cancer, melanoma, lymphoma, unknown primaries, and breast cancer each account for 9 to 12 percent of total cases. As a rule, patients usually have widespread disease at the time of diagnosis. However, SCC can be the presenting manifestation of cancer in some patients. On the other hand, there can be a latency period of many years between the initial diagnosis of cancer and the onset of symptoms related to a SCC (e.g., breast cancer).

SCC can occur as a result of several mechanisms. The most common mechanism causing SCC (85 percent of cases) is direct extension of a vertebral body metastasis to the epidural space. Solid tumors most commonly cause SCC through this mechanism. Approximately 10 percent of cases are caused by invasion of the intervertebral space by lymphoma-laden lymph nodes arising in the retroperitoneal space. Less commonly, the vascular supply to the spinal cord can be compromised by tumor compression of the spinal arteries supplying the cord. If the structural integrity of a vertebral body is compromised as a result of direct bone invasion (e.g., myeloma, breast and lung carcinoma), collapse of the vertebral body can occur, resulting in SCC.

No matter what mechanism accounts for the SCC, motor, sensory, and autonomic function below the level of the cord compression are affected. The clinical manifestations that result depend on the level at which the cord compression occurs (cervical–10 percent, thoracic–70 percent, lumbosacral–20 percent). Not uncommonly, more than one level (vertebral body) is involved by tumor.

The signs and symptoms of SCC in a bed-bound, intubated patient are more difficult to assess than in an alert, ambulatory patient. Pain localized to the spine or the paravertebral area is present in more than 90 percent of patients. The pain can be localized and present for weeks to months before neurologic deficits develop. The pain can be exacerbated by movement, straining, coughing, etc. Nerve root pain or radicular pain is characterized as a sharp pain radiating down both arms in cervical cord compression, or as a "bandlike" constriction around the chest in thoracic cord compression. Patients may complain of weakness in the extremities as well as loss of pain and temperature sensation below the level of the lesion. Patients unable to express themselves (due to sedation, altered mental status, or intubation) may not be able to offer these clues to the diagnosis. As autonomic fibers become affected, bowel function is altered (e.g., fecal incontinence or constipation) as is bladder control (urinary urgency-early; overflow incontinence-late). Patients in the ICU commonly have bladder catheters in place to monitor urinary output making this symptom of little value in this setting. Similarly, due to inactivity, pain medication, and tube feedings, bowel function would not be expected to be normal; therefore, this clue may be difficult to detect in patients with multiple medical problems.

Because patients often are unable to describe symptoms that would suggest the diagnosis, a high index of suspicion and thorough neurologic examinations are mandatory in high-risk patients. Frequent examinations must be done including a careful motor examination to detect any evidence of weakness. Sensory examinations with special attention to pain (e.g., pin prick) must be completed to detect hypesthesia. Deep tendon reflexes, Babinski reflexes, and sphincter tone must be evaluated regularly.

If a suspicion of SCC exists based on the neurologic examination, steps must be taken immediately to definitively diagnose and treat the problem. Consultation from medical oncology, radiation therapy, and neurosurgery must be included in management discussions. The approach to an individual patient is obviously tempered by the constraints of other ongoing medical problems. Radiologic studies may be difficult to obtain because the patient must be stable enough to leave the ICU to obtain an x-ray, CT scan, myelogram, or magnetic resonance imaging (MRI) scan. Therapeutic interventions must begin *immediately* in any patient with rapidly evolving neurologic signs, even before the diagnosis is confirmed radiologically.[12] Dexamethasone, 10 mg intravenously immediately, followed by 4 mg every 6 h, should start as soon as SCC is suspected. The decrease in edema surrounding the spinal cord that occurs as a result of steroid administration will often result in temporary improvement of back pain and neurologic deficits. The steroids should be continued until definitive therapy (surgery or radiation) is completed, at which point the steroids should be tapered.

Radiologic studies of the spine will demonstrate abnormalities of the vertebral bodies (e.g., destruction, collapse, loss of pedicles) in two-thirds of patients with back pain. These abnormalities will correctly predict the presence or absence of epidural metastases in over 80 percent of patients, but myelography with or without CT or MRI is necessary to confirm the diagnosis.[13] The myelogram, after instilling water-soluble contrast (metrizamide) into the cerebrospinal fluid (CSF), delineates the upper and lower limits of the lesion(s) allowing for treatment planning. A CT scan is obtained in many centers following routine myelography to better visualize the spinal processes. Similarly, the MRI scan is under extensive evaluation because it is noninvasive and has the ability to clearly distinguish between extradural and intradural lesions.[14]

Surgery or radiation therapy or both remain the primary modalities for the treatment of SCC. As a general rule, ***the degree of neurologic improvement following a therapeutic intervention depends on the degree and duration of neurologic impairment at diagnosis.*** Patients who are ambulatory at diagnosis have a 65 to 80 percent chance of being ambulatory following radiation therapy alone or decompressive laminectomy followed by radiation therapy. Patients who are paraparetic at presentation have approximately a 50 percent chance of being ambulatory following either treatment. Finally, patients who are paraplegic at diagnosis have less than a 10 percent chance of significant neurologic recovery, and the morbidity associated with either treatment approach is not acceptable in such patients.

A decompressive laminectomy is done in situations where the diagnosis of cancer has not been confirmed, the vertebral column is unstable, bone is impinging on the cord, the tumor is known to be particularly radioresistant, or the area has been previously irradiated. Surgery is accompanied by an operative mortality rate of 7 to 10 percent. Radiation therapy should follow surgery except in situations where the tumor is radioresistant (e.g., sarcoma) or normal tissue will not tolerate additional radiotherapy. Radiation therapy can be given alone in situations where the tumor is very radiosensitive (e.g. lymphoma, myeloma) and the spinal column is stable. Radiation doses of 3000 to 4000 rads are generally administered over 2 to 4 weeks.

CEREBRAL HERNIATION SYNDROME

Cerebral herniation syndromes are medical emergencies that can be caused by primary brain neoplasms or metastases to the brain from distant primary tumors. The most common cancers that metastasize to the brain are lung (15 to 30 percent), breast (15 to 25 percent), kidney (5 to 10 percent), and melanoma (autopsy series suggest that 75 percent of cutaneous melanomas metastasize to the brain).[15]

The clinical manifestations of herniation syndromes occur because the brain is confined within a fixed space. The cranial cavity is divided into compartments by the dura (Fig. 149-4). The falx cerebri separates the supratentorial space into the right and left hemispheres. The tentorium separates the occipital lobes from the cerebellum. Mass lesions in brain parenchymal tissue increase intracranial volume and induce the formation of surrounding edema. Because the intracranial contents are divided into compartments, there is a tendency for a pressure increase in one compartment to be equilibrated throughout the entire intracranial space by shifting brain tissue from one compartment to another. The specific location of the mass lesion will determine the particular herniation syndrome that occurs. In general, the three most important herniation syndromes are temporal lobe-tentorial, transtentorial, and cerebellar-foramen magnum.[16,17]

In the temporal lobe-tentorial herniation syndrome, the presence of a mass lesion in a temporal lobe causes an increase in the intracranial pressure (ICP) of that compartment. As a result, the medial portion of the temporal lobe, the uncus, is pushed through the tentorial opening where the midbrain is located. The midbrain and subthalamus are

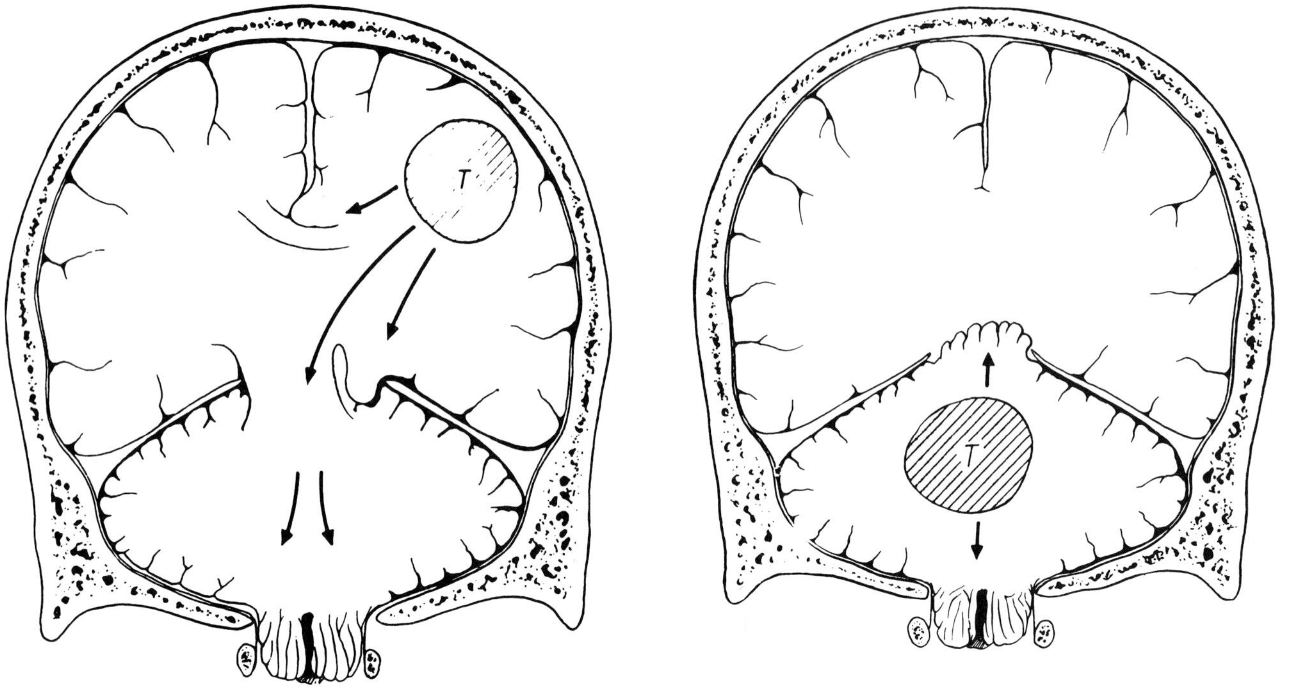

a *b*

FIGURE 149-4 ***a.*** **Schematic indicating brain tissue displacement that accompanies a parietal lobe tumor.** ***b.*** **Schematic indicating brain tissue displacement that accompanies a tumor in the posterior cranial fossa.**

then pushed to the opposite side. The shift in structures places pressure on the surrounding vasculature and cranial nerves resulting in the clinical manifestations that are observed. The oculomotor nerve (III) normally abuts the underside of the temporal lobe; however, the shift of anatomic structures compresses the nerve. As a result, ptosis and pupillary dilation occur due to compression of parasympathetic fibers that travel in the lateral part of III. Paralysis of the superior, inferior, and medial rectus muscles innervated by III along with intact innervation of the lateral rectus muscle (VI) results in the eye turning outward. Due to the compression of the third cranial nerve and shift of the midbrain, the oculocephalic response (doll's eyes) should be absent since this maneuver tests the integrity of the midbrain and pons. Similarly, caloric testing should be abnormal in comatose patients with an uncal herniation since brain stem function is compromised due to compression and a shift from its normal position. Hemiparesis usually occurs on the side contralateral to the mass lesion. Typically, third nerve paralysis occurs prior to disturbances of consciousness. Depending on the tempo of the herniation, however, patients can present in a stuporous state or be frankly comatose. As the syndrome progresses, Cheyne-Stokes respirations develop, evolve into weak irregular breathing, and ultimately lead to respiratory arrest. The motor signs can eventually evolve into decerebrate or decorticate posturing.

Central or transtentorial syndromes occur when the brain herniates through the tentorium compressing the diencephalon and lower brain stem. This syndrome is classically characterized by a steady progression of signs and symptoms as more brain tissue is affected in retrocaudal progression. Initially, patients have an impaired level of consciousness and often present in stupor. Respirations are irregular or follow a Cheyne-Stokes pattern. Babinski reflexes are present bilaterally, and the pupils are small and reactive. As the patient becomes more obtunded, decorticate posturing may develop and responses to noxious stimuli become absent. Pupils will become fixed in midposition. Testing with both caloric and oculocephalic responses may be abnormal at this point as midbrain function is compromised. Decorticate or decerebrate posturing will be prominent features of the physical examination. In the final stage of the syndrome, the patient is completely unresponsive with shallow respirations, fixed pupils, and flaccid paralysis.

The cerebellar-foramen magnum herniation syndrome occurs due to the downward displacement of inferior parts of the cerebellar hemispheres through the foramen magnum. The cerebellar tissue displaced may be from one cerebellar hemisphere or both. The mass lesion that causes cerebellar herniation can be located in the cerebellum, though centrally placed frontal tumors can also cause cerebellar herniation. The lethal outcome that ultimately occurs is the result of compression of the medulla, which results in respiratory arrest. Clinically, the signs that characterize the syndrome include loss of consciousness, tonic extension and arching of the neck and back, bradycardia or tachycardia, and loss of deep tendon reflexes.

Herniation syndromes must be considered in any patient with an underlying malignancy who rapidly develops a constellation of neurologic deficits. Once the diagnosis is suspected, therapeutic maneuvers must be instituted immediately, even before a confirmatory CT scan of the brain is obtained. Furthermore, a lumbar puncture should not be performed in any patient suspected of having an evolving herniation, since the sudden release of CSF and ICP may bring a herniation to completion.

The management of a patient with an evolving herniation must be undertaken in the ICU. Acute medical management is a stabilizing maneuver until definitive radiation therapy or surgery can be initiated. ICP depends on body temperature, systemic blood pressure, and intrathoracic venous resistance.[18] In patients who have had neurologic damage, autoregulation of cerebral blood flow is lost or impaired. As a result, changes in systemic blood pressure can have an exaggerated and detrimental effect on brain tissue. Similarly, cerebral blood flow increases in parallel with body temperature resulting in increases in ICP. Increases in intrathoracic venous resistance also result in increases in ICP. Maneuvers such as tracheal suctioning or positive end-expiratory pressure can therefore cause increases in ICP, resulting in worsening of the neurologic impairment. Management of patients often requires manipulation of body temperature, venous pressure, or determinants of cerebral blood flow.

Patients are typically intubated and ventilated.[19,20] *Hyperventilating* comatose patients to a P_{CO_2} of 25 to 30 mmHg will reduce cerebral blood flow and decrease ICP. *Dexamethasone* (100 mg intravenously, then 25 mg four times daily) can reduce the edema surrounding a mass lesion and as a result decrease the symptoms and signs associated with an expanding lesion. *Osmotic agents* such as mannitol (100 g intravenously in a 20% solution; then 25 g intravenously as needed) reduce ICP by increasing the flow of fluid from brain tissue to the intravascular space through use of an osmotic gradient (see Chap. 4). Following these manipulations the patient should be evaluated for radiation therapy and surgical decompression.

LEPTOMENINGEAL CARCINOMATOSIS

Leptomeningeal carcinomatosis refers to the widespread dissemination of tumor cells throughout the leptomeninges and ventricles. Certain lymphomas, leukemias, and solid tumors (Table 149-3) have a high propensity for spread to the meninges.[21,22] Meningeal involvement has been reported in 33 percent of adult patients with acute lymphoblastic leukemia, 20 percent of patients with acute myelogenous leukemia, and in 1 percent of patients with chronic lymphocytic leukemia. Lymphomatous involvement of the meninges occurs commonly with certain subtypes of non-Hodgkin's lymphoma, especially those with high-grade histology. Meningeal involvement will occur in up to 30 percent of patients with diffuse histiocytic lymphoma. Autopsy series have reported meningeal involvement in up to 75 percent of patients with Burkitt's lymphoma. The low-grade, nodular lymphomas have a relatively low incidence of clinically overt meningeal involvement.

The solid tumors that most commonly involve the meninges include breast cancer, gastric cancer, melanoma, and lung cancer.[22] Autopsy studies have suggested meningeal involvement with tumor in up to 5 percent of breast cancer cases and 28 percent of small cell lung cancer cases. In the

TABLE 149-3 Tumors Associated with Leptomeningeal Carcinomatosis

Acute lymphocytic leukemia
Acute nonlymphocytic leukemia
Diffuse histocytic lymphoma (large cell)
Burkitt's lymphoma
Breast carcinoma
Lung carcinoma
(Adenocarcinoma > oat cell > squamous)
Malignant melanoma
Adenocarcinoma of unknown primary
Gastrointestinal cancer

majority of cases where leptomeningeal carcinomatosis has been described, particularly with lymphomas and solid tumors, the disease is widespread when the clinical manifestations of central nervous system (CNS) involvement become apparent.

The signs and symptoms of leptomeningeal carcinomatosis are often vague and nonspecific, adding to the challenge of diagnosing this entity in the intensive care setting. Furthermore, tumor seeding of the meninges can occur anywhere along the neuroaxis, resulting in a variety of unrelated symptoms and signs. Vague, unrelenting headaches are the most common symptom. Personality changes, altered levels of consciousness, memory loss, hallucinations, confusion, and dementia have all been described. Signs suggesting meningeal irritation (e.g., nuchal rigidity, neck pain, pain with straight leg raising) are commonly observed. Radicular nerve root involvement is suggested by weakness of the extremities, bladder incontinence, and paresthesias. Cranial nerve involvement is common, especially III and VI, resulting in oculomotor palsies and decreased visual acuity. Not uncommonly, deep tendon reflexes are diminished and diffuse sensory abnormalities are present.

The diagnosis of leptomeningeal carcinomatosis is made by examination of the CSF obtained from a lumbar puncture *(A lumbar puncture should not be performed when signs suggestive of an expanding mass lesion are present.)* The definitive diagnosis of leptomeningeal carcinomatosis is made by detecting tumor cells in the CSF, and multiple fluid samples may be necessary before the diagnosis is made. Usually 7 to 10 mL CSF is obtained with each lumbar puncture, and techniques such as cytocentrifugation and Millipore filtering will often increase the detection of tumor cells. Other findings suggesting, but not confirming, the diagnosis are an elevated CSF pressure, a decreased CSF glucose concentration, an elevated CSF protein concentration, and a monocytic pleocytosis. Other tumor markers, such as β_2-microglobulin and β-glucuronidase, are nonspecific and investigational. Patients with lymphoma or leukemia who present with cranial nerve palsies in the absence of mass lesions or hemorrhage should be assumed to have meningeal involvement.

CT and MRI scans may be of benefit in situations where repeated examinations of CSF fail to detect tumor cells. In this situation, especially in a patient with diffuse neurologic manifestations, a CT or MRI scan may detect tumor implants along with the neuroaxis that explain the clinical findings.

The treatment of leptomeningeal carcinomatosis usually involves intrathecally administered chemotherapy or radiation therapy or both.[23] Administering chemotherapy systemically is largely ineffective due to the blood-brain barrier which prevents the most effective chemotherapy from achieving adequate CSF concentrations. Methotrexate, thio-TEPA, and cytosine arabinoside are the drugs most commonly administered intrathecally. The drugs can be instilled directly into the CSF by lumbar puncture or through an Ommaya reservoir, a device surgically implanted into a lateral ventricle. Using a small scalp vein needle, the reservoir can be accessed percutaneously to sample CSF or to administer chemotherapy. The toxicities that can occur with the use of intrathecal chemotherapy include aseptic meningitis, encephalitis, and rarely brain necrosis. The dose of drug administered intrathecally rarely causes significant systemic symptoms such as myelosuppression or nausea and vomiting.

Radiation therapy can be used as an adjunct to intrathecal chemotherapy or as a primary means of treating carcinomatous meningitis. Radiation ports should not encompass the entire neuroaxis since significant myelosuppression can occur. Rather, radiation is directed to specific areas of known or presumed tumor implants, such as to the posterior fossa in cases with cranial neuropathies.

Treatment of leptomeningeal carcinomatosis can result in significant palliation.[21] Forty to 50 percent of patients can be expected to improve or remain stable with appropriate treatment, However, the long-term prognosis for these patients remains dismal due to the widespread extent of disease.

Metabolic Syndromes

HYPERCALCEMIA

One of the most common metabolic complications of cancer is hypercalcemia. Although hyperparathyroidism is a more common cause of hypercalcemia, patients with an underlying malignancy account for the majority of cases of hypercalcemia in hospitalized patients. Because of the myriad of physiologic functions of calcium, abrupt variations in calcium homeostasis can have a greater immediate threat to a patient's life than the underlying malignancy. Approximately 5 to 10 percent of hospitalized patients with a malignancy will develop a complicating hypercalcemia.[24] Patients cared for in the ICU often have several medical problems that can mask the signs and symptoms of hypercalcemia; therefore, one must maintain a high index of suspicion for this disorder, since failure to recognize it can have fatal consequences.

At least four mechanisms account for the hypercalcemia associated with malignancy.[25,26] Breast cancer, and less commonly Hodgkin's disease, non-Hodgkin's lymphomas, pancreatic carcinoma, and non-small cell lung cancer cause hypercalcemia by a mechanism directly related to *bone metastases.* Tumor cells may be able to directly resorb bone or a tumor cell product (e.g., prostaglandins) may stimulate surrounding osteoclasts to resorb bone. Between 30 and 50 percent of breast cancer patients will develop hypercalcemia at some point during their clinical course, usually when the disease is widespread.

Secondly, 50 percent of patients with multiple myeloma and less commonly patients with T cell and Burkitt's lymphoma, will develop hypercalcemia due to the production of cytokines (previously known as osteoclast activating factor) by malignant plasma cells. Cytokines include lymphotoxin, and possibly tumor necrosis factor and interleukin-1. These molecules are potent stimulators of osteoclast activity.

Thirdly, certain tumors secrete a parathyroid hormone (PTH)-like peptide that mediates the hypercalcemic state.[25,27] The tumors most commonly associated with this syndrome include squamous cell carcinomas (head and neck, lung, and esophagus), renal carcinoma, transitional cell bladder carcinoma, and ovarian carcinomas. The peptide, although not identical to PTH, has structural similarities. It appears to enhance osteoclastic bone resorption and to enhance renal tubular calcium reabsorption.

Finally, elevated levels of 1,25-dihydroxycholecalciferol (vitamin D_3) have been detected in some cases of Hodgkin's and non-Hodgkin's lymphoma. This substance enhances osteoclastic bone resorption and increases gastrointestinal calcium absorption.

The symptoms of hypercalcemia are nonspecific and can be similar to those caused by the underlying disease or its treatment. Further complicating the recognition of hypercalcemia, particularly in the intensive care setting, are concurrent medical problems, the use of sedative medications, and the frequent need for mechanical ventilatory support. Moreover, the immobility in an ICU exacerbates hypercalcemia. The signs and symptoms of hypercalcemia are outlined in Table 149-4. The clinical manifestations of hypercalcemia depend on both the degree of hypercalcemia and the time period over which the hypercalcemic state develops. Patients with long-standing hypercalcemia may have few symptoms, whereas a mild elevation that occurs over a short period can have overt clinical manifestations. Generalized fatigue, lethargy, polyuria, nausea, vomiting, and

TABLE 149-4 Symptoms and Signs of Hypercalcemia

Symptoms	Signs
Weight loss	Hyporeflexia
Anorexia	Confusion, psychosis
Pruritus	Seizure
Polydipsia	Obtundation, coma
Fatigue	Ileus
Lethargy	Renal insufficiency
Muscle weakness	Bradycardia
Nausea, vomiting	Prolonged PR interval
Constipation	Shortened QT interval
Polyuria	Atrial, ventricular arrhythmias

constipation are the most common presenting complaints. Poor oral intake and excessive urine output can compromise volume status, worsening the hypercalcemic state. Patients can present in an obtunded or comatose state if the calcium concentration is markedly elevated (14 mg/dL or higher) or if the elevation occurs quickly.

Although there are many causes of hypercalcemia, primary hyperparathyroidism and the hypercalcemia of malignancy account for the majority of cases. To distinguish the two, it is important to rely on the clinical history and well chosen laboratory tests. Hypercalcemia that develops quickly in a patient with a malignancy supports a diagnosis of malignancy-associated hypercalcemia. A patient who has chronic symptoms, asymptomatic hypercalcemia, and no known malignancy is more likely to have primary hyperparathyroidism or some other cause of hypercalcemia. A low or normal serum immunoreactive PTH level will usually exclude the diagnosis of primary hyperparathyroidism.

The management of patients with malignancy-associated hypercalcemia is often made difficult by complications related to the underlying malignancy or its treatment. Furthermore, many patients who develop hypercalcemia have widespread disease and are refractory to therapy. The goal of therapy is to decrease calcium resorption from bone, increase renal excretion of calcium, and treat the underlying malignancy.[27] The latter maneuver is often not possible to initiate in the ICU because of other medical problems (e.g., respiratory failure, sepsis, pancytopenia, etc.) and because the complications related to hypercalcemia require an immediate reduction in the serum calcium concentration which may not be achieved with chemotherapy alone.

Patients with malignancy-associated hypercalcemia are almost always intravascularly volume depleted. This is due to both the fluid losses associated with vomiting and to the obligate water loss associated with calciuresis (a calcium-induced nephrogenic diabetes insipidus). Infusions of isotonic saline solution will replete the intravascular volume, thereby decreasing resorption of calcium in the proximal convoluted tubule of the kidney. Furthermore, calcium excretion will be promoted by the exchange of calcium for sodium in the distal tubule of the kidney.

The actual rate of fluid administration is dictated by the patient's cardiac, pulmonary, and renal function. Patients with impaired cardiac function, pulmonary disease, or renal insufficiency may not tolerate large or rapid boluses of fluid. Normal saline infusion rates of 250 to 500 mL/h can be initiated along with careful and frequent clinical assessments of cardiopulmonary status and urine output. With aggressive hydration over 24 to 48 h (4 to 10 L/day) approximately 25 to 30 percent of patients will achieve an improvement in serum calcium concentration. During this period, potassium (10 meq/L infused saline) and magnesium losses resulting from the saline infusion must be replaced.

Although loop diuretics (e.g., furosemide) are commonly used along with saline infusions to enhance calciuresis, no controlled clinical studies have been reported which demonstrate an added benefit over saline infusions alone. The use of diuretics can prevent the hypernatremia and pulmonary edema caused by aggressive saline infusions, but they must be used cautiously due to their ability to cause hypokalemia, hypomagnesemia, and hypovolemia.

Since the major cause of hypercalcemia is enhanced osteoclastic activity, therapy should be directed at reducing bone turnover. Mithramycin is a cytotoxic antibiotic that directly kills osteoclasts, resulting in decreased bone resorption. Mithramycin is usually administered as a bolus infusion in a dose of 25 μg/kg or as an infusion over 2 to 4 h. The hypocalcemic effect is usually seen after *24 to 48 h*. The dose can be repeated every 3 to 4 days, but the toxicity of the drug is increased with multiple doses. Caution must be exercised when using mithramycin in patients with hepatic or kidney dysfunction. Thrombocytopenia is a common side effect. A prolonged prothrombin time can develop as well as minor elevations in tests of liver and kidney function.

Calcitonin is useful for rapid reduction of calcium levels but the peak hypocalcemic effect occurs at 48 h and decreases thereafter despite repeat doses. In pharmacologic doses, calcitonin inhibits bone resorption and enhances calciuresis. Although various schedules exist, for markedly elevated levels of calcium, calcitonin should be administered intramuscularly at a dose of 8 IU/kg every 6 h. The hypocalcemic effect of calcitonin can be observed within 2 to 3 h of administration. There is no associated toxicity with the use of calcitonin. Some investigators have suggested that steroids enhance the effect of calcitonin, but this observation has largely been anecdotal and seen in malignancies expected to respond to the antitumor effect of prednisone (e.g., myeloma, lymphoma, leukemia, breast cancer).

Diphosphonates are a class of compounds chemically related to pyrophosphate. Diphosphonates have an affinity for hydroxyapatite in areas of increased bone turnover such as a metastatic site. Once in these areas diphosphonates are taken up by osteoclasts and inhibit bone resorbing activity.[28] Etidronate (Didronel) is commercially available and is administered intravenously, 7.5 mg/kg/day in 500 mL of normal saline solution over 3 h for 5 to 7 consecutive days. The hypocalcemic effect of etidronate is usually seen within 3 to 5 days. The drug can then be continued orally at an average dose of 20 mg/kg body weight/day for 30 days. Etidronate has been free of significant toxicity.

Inorganic phosphate compounds have been used successfully in the past to treat malignancy-associated hypercalcemia, but the use of intravenous phosphates in emergency situations has largely been abandoned due to toxicity. The rationale for using phosphate compounds is to increase the serum phosphate concentration, which inhibits calcium resorption from bone and reduces urinary calcium excretion. However, phosphate shifts calcium from the blood to other tissues. When the product of [calcium] $\times$ [phosphorus] exceeds 58, precipitation of calcium salts can occur. Because of severe hypocalcemia, renal failure, hypotension, and extraskeletal calcification that can occur with the parenteral use of phosphate, this drug has largely been abandoned in the acute, symptomatic setting.

Glucocorticoids have been used to treat malignancy-

TABLE 149-5 Stepwise Treatment of Hypercalcemia

1. Normal saline infusion	250–500 mL/h (4–10 L/day)	1. Replace K^+, Mg^{2+} losses 2. Observe cardiopulmonary status 3. Consider diuretics to enhance calciuresis
2. Mithramycin	25 μg/kg (bolus infusion or IV over 2–4 h)	1. Repeat dose every 3–4 days 2. Increased toxicity with multiple doses
3. Calcitonin	8 IU/kg IM or SC every 6–12 h	
4. Diphosphonates (i.e., etidronate) disodium	7.5 mg/kg/day in 250–500 mL of normal saline infused over 2–3 h for 3 days	
5. Inorganic phosphates	Not recommended	
6. Prednisone or hydrocortisone	20–40 mg PO daily 100–150 mg IV every 12 h	

associated hypercalcemia. Patients with tumors that respond to the cytolytic action of glucocorticoids (e.g., myeloma, leukemia, lymphoma) are the same patients who will respond to the hypocalcemic effect of corticosteroids. There are also occasional patients with breast cancer who develop a "flare" of their disease when treated with hormones (e.g., tamoxifen or stilbestrol) and develop hypercalcemia. Corticosteroids can sometimes control the hypercalcemia in this setting. The usual dose is prednisone, 20 to 40 mg orally daily, or hydrocortisone, 100 to 150 mg intravenously every 12 h (Table 149-5).

THE SYNDROME OF INAPPROPRIATE ANTIDIURETIC HORMONE SECRETION (SIADH)

Diagnosis of SIADH is made by excluding other causes of hyponatremia. In critically ill patients the cause of hyponatremia may be multifactorial. A more complete discussion of the diagnosis and treatment of hyponatremia is outlined elsewhere (see Chap. 156). Other disorders where water metabolism is impaired must be excluded before considering a diagnosis of SIADH.[29] There should be no clinical or laboratory evidence supporting a diagnosis of hypovolemia, edema-forming disorders, adrenal insufficiency, renal insufficiency, or hypothyroidism. In SIADH, antidiuretic hormone (ADH) release may result from the ectopic production of the hormone by tumor tissue, drugs that mimic ADH activity, or conditions that stimulate the release of ADH from the posterior pituitary (Table 149-6).

The ectopic synthesis and release of ADH should be considered as a cause of hyponatremia in patients with an underlying malignancy who have no other causes of altered water metabolism of SIADH (see Table 149-6). Small cell carcinoma of the lung is the most common histologic type of cancer associated with clinically evident SIADH. Up to 10 percent of patients with small cell lung cancer develop hyponatremia caused by SIADH. Several other tumors (see Table 149-6) have been associated with clinically significant SIADH, although much less commonly. On the other hand, subclinical SIADH has been reported to occur in as many as 40 percent of patients with colon cancer and lung cancer.

If all other potential causes of hyponatremia can be excluded in a patient with an underlying malignancy, then the ectopic production of SIADH by tumor tissue should be investigated. *(Parenchymal brain metastases or leptomeningeal carcinomatosis from any cancer can cause SIADH.)* ADH levels can be checked by radioimmuno-assay, though this test is not widely available. Simpler laboratory tests can support the diagnosis. The laboratory features characteristic of SIADH are:

1. Normal renal, adrenal, and thyroid function
2. Normal volume status
3. Urinary sodium excretion in excess of 20 meq/L
4. A urine osmolality inappropriately high (>500 mO/kg) for the low serum osmolality (≤280 mO/kg)

Pathologically, hypoosmolar, hyponatremic states are characterized by intracellular swelling. The clinical manifestations (Table 149-7) of the fluid shifts include increased neuromuscular excitability, seizures, muscle fasciculations, and coma. Permanent neurologic damage or death can occur as a result of prolonged, severe hyponatremia (<120 meq/L). The clinical manifestations of SIADH depend on the degree of hyponatremia and hypoosmality as well as the pace at which they developed.

In patients in whom SIADH is caused by ectopic tumor production of ADH, the ideal therapy is to treat the tumor. However, therapies directed toward eliminating the tumor with chemotherapy, radiation therapy, or surgical intervention may result in an unacceptable delay before the

TABLE 149-6 Disorders Associated with SIADH

Carcinomas	Pulmonary Disorders	CNS	Drugs
Small cell lung cancer	Viral, bacterial pneumonias	Meningitis, encephalitis	Morphine
Bronchial carcinoids	Abscess	Primary or metastatic tumors	Nicotine
Prostate	Tuberculosis	Abscess	Cyclophosphamide
Adrenal		Head trauma—skull fractures	Vincristine
Head and neck		Subdural hematoma	Alcohol
Duodenal, colorectal		Subarachnoid hemorrhage	Chlorpropamide
Pancreas		Pain	
Esophagus		Cerebritis	
Hodgkin's and non-Hodgkin's lymphoma			

TABLE 149-7 Clinical Manifestations of Hyponatremia

Symptoms	Signs
Headache	Personality changes
Lethargy, apathy	Muscle fasciculations
Confusion	Hyperreflexia, asterixis
Nausea, vomiting	Weakness
Muscle cramps	Delirium, seizures
	Coma

hyponatremia is corrected. The initial therapeutic measure in patients with *severe, symptomatic* hyponatremia (<120 meq/L) must be directed toward increasing the serum sodium concentration to 120 to 125 meq/L.[30] Severe, symptomatic hyponatremia should be treated with 3% saline solution and a loop diuretic (e.g., furosemide).

Once the serum sodium concentration improves and the clinical manifestations of hyponatremia resolve, antineoplastic therapy can be initiated. However, cyclophosphamide and vincristine, which are common antineoplastic drugs, especially in the treatment of small cell lung cancer, can cause a drug-induced SIADH by directly stimulating pituitary secretion of ADH.

Less severe cases of hyponatremia can be treated with demeclocycline or lithium carbonate, agents which block the action of ADH at the level of the renal tubule. More recently, the administration of oral urea (10 to 60 g/day) has been used to induce an osmotic diuresis resulting in increased free water excretion.[31]

LACTIC ACIDOSIS

Lactic acidosis is an acid-base disorder that occasionally occurs in patients with underlying malignancies. In those patients where it does occur the underlying cancer is usually a leukemia or a rapidly growing lymphoma (undifferentiated and Burkitt's lymphomas) or rarely a solid tumor.[32] Lactic acidosis tends to occur in cancer patients especially when there is significant liver involvement leading to impaired lactate metabolism.

Lactic acidosis is suspected when an anion gap metabolic acidosis is present without an associated history of toxic ingestions, renal failure, or alcoholism. The other laboratory values should not suggest significant azotemia or ketosis.

The treatment of lactic acidosis is controversial. If possible, the cause of the hyperlactatemia must be treated (e.g., intravenous fluids, antibiotics, and vasoactive drugs in the case of septic shock). The administration of sodium bicarbonate in patients with lactic acidosis is theoretically sound, but clinical trials have shown that alkali administration may be deleterious to patient outcome[33] (see Chap. 158). Other therapies for lactic acidosis (e.g., hemodialysis, sodium dichloroacetate) remain investigational. The principal modality of therapy is chemotherapy, and lactic acidosis is one of the few indications for emergency chemotherapy.

TUMOR LYSIS SYNDROME

Tumor lysis syndrome occurs following treatment of certain malignancies that are exquisitely sensitive to the effects of chemotherapy, hormonal therapy, or biologic therapy. Malignancies that commonly cause lactic acidosis (e.g., Burkitt's lymphoma, leukemias, rarely solid tumors) also lead to the tumor lysis syndrome. Metabolic abnormalities that characterize tumor lysis syndrome typically appear from hours to days following administration of systemic chemotherapy. However, the syndrome has also been described following the administration of tamoxifen for metastatic breast cancer, α-interferon for a T cell lymphoma, and spontaneously in rare cases.[34,35] Hyperuricemia, hyperkalemia, hyperphosphatemia, and hypocalcemia occur as a result of the rapid and massive killing of tumor cells which release their intracellular contents into the bloodstream. Patients who are at risk of developing tumor lysis syndrome must be recognized prior to initiating treatment so that measures can be taken to prevent severe metabolic abnormalities from developing.

The most life-threatening complications that can develop in the tumor lysis syndrome are cardiac arrhythmias due to hypocalcemia or hyperkalemia and renal failure due to hyperuricemia. Hypocalcemia develops as a result of hyperphosphatemia when phosphate is released from dying tumor cells. Calcium phosphate salts form when the product of calcium and phosphate concentrations exceed their solubility product. Precipitation of calcium phosphate salts in the renal tubules may result in azotemia or acute renal failure. Similarly, hyperphosphatemia that develops in the setting of underlying renal insufficiency may cause rapid progression to renal failure. The hypocalcemia that develops secondary to hyperphosphatemia can precipitate cardiac arrhythmias, tetany, and seizures. Hyperuricemia and hyperuricosuria develop as a result of increased uric acid production arising from the breakdown of DNA and RNA contained in tumor cells. A more extensive discussion of hyperkalemia, hyperphosphatemia, and hypocalcemia can be found elsewhere (see Chaps. 153 and 156).

A general framework for the management of patients who develop severe tumor lysis syndrome centers on correcting the severe metabolic abnormalities.[36]

1. Patients must be aggressively hydrated with half-normal saline solution to ensure a urine output of at least 100 to 200 mL/h. Diuretics may be needed to increase urine output in patients with azotemia.
2. Allopurinol, 300 to 600 mg orally daily, should begin 12 h prior to initiating chemotherapy.
3. Alkalinization of the urine (pH 7 to 7.5) promotes uricosuria. The addition of sodium bicarbonate to intravenous solution (50 meq/L) will produce an alkaline urine pH. Once the serum uric acid concentration is normal, however, alkalinization of the urine should be discontinued since calcium phosphate salt formation is promoted at a high pH, which may aggravate the symptoms of hypocalcemia.
4. Hemodialysis should be initiated early for patients with worsening renal function, congestive heart failure, serum potassium >6 meq/L, serum creatinine >10 mg/dL, serum phosphorus $\geq$10 mg/dL, or serum uric acid $\geq$10 mg/dL.

UROLOGIC EMERGENCIES

Patients with an underlying malignancy are at risk of developing a number of unique urologic complications.[37] These complications must be distinguished from any of the more common disorders affecting the kidneys, ureters, and bladder that have been extensively discussed (see Chaps. 107 and 153). Three urologic disorders related to an underlying malignancy or its treatment are chemotherapy and radiation-induced hematuria, obstructive uropathy, and uric acid nephropathy.

Hematuria can develop in cancer patients from causes that affect the general population; however, even urinary tract infections or renal calculi can represent life-threatening problems in a debilitated and immunocompromised cancer patient. The clinical manifestations, evaluation, and treatment of the common causes of hematuria are similar to patients without a malignancy. Generally, hematuria caused by an infection will resolve once appropriate antibiotics are administered, but infections that are resistant to treatment may originate proximal to a site of extrinsic or intrinsic obstruction. Hematuria caused by renal calculi will be accompanied by colicky pain and will resolve after the stone is passed.

More serious hematuria due to hemorrhagic cystitis can develop in patients treated with high-dose cyclophosphamide (Cytoxan). This complication has been reported to occur in 10 to 70 percent of patients, with the higher incidence occurring in patients undergoing allogeneic bone marrow transplantation with a preparative regimen containing high dose cyclophosphamide.[38] Hemorrhagic cystitis has also been reported in patients receiving long-term cyclophosphamide in a lower dose. Therefore, both the dose as well as the cumulative exposure to the drug are important.

The urothelium of the bladder wall is damaged by a metabolic breakdown product of cyclophosphamide, acrolein, which is excreted in the urine and concentrated in the bladder. In patients who are volume depleted, the urine is concentrated, exposing the urothelium to high concentrations of acrolein, thereby precipitating hemorrhagic cystitis. Prophylactic measures that reduce the exposure of the bladder mucosa to acrolein include aggressive intravenous hydration, frequent emptying of the bladder, and the administration of 2-mercaptoethane sulfonate (Mesna) which acts as an acrolein scavenger. Generally, the onset of bleeding occurs during or shortly following the administration of high dose cyclophosphamide, although bleeding occurring months following the administration of cyclophosphamide has been reported.

Examination of the bladder mucosa in patients with radiation or chemotherapy-induced hemorrhagic cystitis will reveal diffuse mucosal and submucosal edema. There will be multiple areas of punctate hemorrhage, and depending on the severity, there may be areas of ulceration and necrosis that extend through the bladder wall.

The management of patients who develop hemorrhagic cystitis begins by immediately discontinuing the cyclophosphamide and volume repleting the patient. Local measures to control bleeding should be undertaken in consultation with the urology service. Several investigators have successfully used formalin directly instilled into the bladder to control hemorrhagic bleeding. Initially, the bladder is completely irrigated to remove blood clots. It is then visually inspected by cystoscopy to determine the severity of the mucosal damage and to fulgurate any exposed bleeding vessels. A 1% to 4% formalin solution is then instilled into the bladder and allowed to coat the mucosa for a short time. The bladder is then irrigated for up to 24 hours.[39] Patients who continue to bleed despite conservative therapeutic measures may require surgery (e.g., cystectomy, urinary diversion, or ligation of the hypogastric arteries).

Patients with an underlying malignancy who develop progressive azotemia or acute renal failure must be evaluated to rule out a *urinary tract obstruction*. The differential diagnosis and the approach to a patient with renal failure is discussed extensively in Chap. 153. The discussion that follows will focus on the malignant and treatment-related causes of upper and lower urinary tract obstruction.

The signs and symptoms of urinary obstruction depend on the anatomic site of the obstruction as well as whether it is a unilateral or bilateral obstruction. Upper urinary tract obstructions occur above the level of the bladder. A pathologic process that affects the drainage of one kidney (unilateral obstruction) may cause complete or partial obstruction on the affected side. As a result, the patient may be completely asymptomatic while progressive hydronephrosis may develop along with progressive deterioration of kidney function on that side. If the opposite kidney and ureter are normal, there may be no decrease in urine output or increase in serum creatinine content. A pathologic process in the upper urinary tract that simultaneously affects the drainage of both the left and right kidneys may cause progressive renal insufficiency or acute renal failure. Malignant causes of upper urinary tract obstructions include tumors that involve the retroperitoneum (e.g., Hodgkin's disease, non-Hodgkin's lymphoma, sarcoma, and germ cell carcinoma). Bladder carcinomas or other pelvic carcinomas may compress one or both ureters at their point of entry into the bladder. A treatment-related cause of upper urinary tract obstruction is retroperitoneal fibrosis caused by long-term busulfan therapy or by radiation therapy directed to the retroperitoneum.

Evaluation of suspected upper urinary tract obstruction is initiated with ultrasonography which will demonstrate unilateral or bilateral hydronephrosis. The level of obstruction may not be clearly delineated; however, since nephrotoxic contrast dyes are to be avoided if possible, a CT scan without contrast, as opposed to an intravenous pyelogram, is helpful in determining the level and extent of the obstruction.

The immediate goal of a therapeutic intervention is to preserve renal function with as little morbidity as possible. Percutaneous nephrostomy tubes (unilateral or bilateral) can be placed by a urologist or radiologist under local anesthesia. As long as the obstruction has not been present for a prolonged period, renal function in the affected kidney(s) will normalize following placement of percutaneous nephrostomy tubes. For long-term management of an upper urinary tract obstruction, ureteral stents can be placed by retrograde ureteral catheterization which will dilate the lumen of the ureter. For patients who are not candidates for these procedures and who have a good short-term prognosis, surgically diverting the urinary tract should be considered. The obstruction may eventually resolve following treatment of the malignancy if it is chemosensitive or radiosensitive.

Lower urinary tract obstruction commonly presents with progressive renal insufficiency along with the signs and symptoms of bladder outlet obstruction. Prostate carcinoma may compress the intravesical urethra, or an enlarging tumor (rectal, cervical, ovarian, etc) may encroach on the bladder outlet thus causing obstruction. Previous radiation therapy may also result in urethral stricture causing bladder obstruction.

Physical examination may reveal a distended bladder. Rectal or pelvic examination may reveal a pelvic mass. Urethral catheterization, if feasible, may demonstrate a full bladder characteristic of a bladder outlet obstruction. An empty bladder in the setting of anuria suggests an obstruction at a level above the bladder or another cause of acute renal failure (see Chap. 153). Diagnostic tests using radiocontrast dye should be avoided since nephrotoxic dyes may further compromise renal function. A CT scan can determine the size and extent of the pelvic tumor. Cystoscopy can detect the level of bladder outlet obstruction, as well as the extent of bladder wall involvement.

Therapy is directed toward relieving the obstruction. If a urethral catheter cannot be placed, then a suprapubic cystostomy can be created. A percutaneous catheter is then inserted for drainage. In patients who cannot undergo urethral catheterization or suprapubic cystostomy, because of the extent of tumor involvement or a fibrotic bladder wall, consideration can be given to surgically diverting the urinary tract (e.g., ileal conduit) or increasing the capacity of the bladder (e.g., dilation or surgical augmentation). Obstruction caused by a urethral stricture may be relieved by dilation of the urethra. If the underlying tumor is sensitive to hormones (e.g., prostate cancer), chemotherapy, or radiation therapy, tumor regression may occur resulting in relief of the obstruction.

In all cases of urinary obstruction, the aggressiveness of the therapeutic intervention must be tempered by the prognosis of the patient. Procedures that carry a high morbidity and mortality must be avoided. Similarly, care must be taken to correct electrolyte imbalances and to treat urinary tract infections which add to the morbidity associated with this complication.

Acute hyperuricemic nephropathy can occur following the treatment of chronic myeloproliferative disorders, acute or chronic myelocytic leukemia, multiple myeloma, acute lymphoblastic leukemia, and lymphoma. These disorders are characterized by normal to increased urinary uric acid secretion in untreated patients; when effective cytotoxic chemotherapy or radiation therapy is administered, massive tumor lysis can occur. As a result, tumor cells release large amounts of nucleoprotein which is metabolized to uric acid, raising the serum uric acid concentration to high levels. The large load of uric acid that is filtered by the kidney exceeds the kidney's capacity to excrete uric acid. As a result uric acid crystals precipitate in the renal medulla, distal tubules, collecting ducts, and renal pyramids. Renal failure commonly occurs when uric acid levels exceed 20 mg/dL. Prophylactic measures to prevent uric acid nephropathy routinely include vigorous hydration, alkalinization of the urine, and the administration of allopurinol.

When acute renal failure develops in patients with a hematologic malignancy, acute hyperuricemic nephropathy must be considered. The diagnosis can be confirmed by a markedly elevated serum uric acid concentration and an ultrasound study that discloses no signs of obstruction. A urinalysis will reveal an acid pH and uric acid crystals.

The treatment of this disorder is directed toward clearing uric acid stones from the urinary tract (kidney medulla, pelvis, ureters). This may be accomplished by ureteral and medullary lavage, via nephrotomy or direct ureteral cannulation. In some patients an open surgical procedure may be necessary to remove uric acid stones. For patients who develop anuric acute renal failure, dialysis may be necessary to support the patient until kidney function returns. A more aggressive approach (i.e., dialysis) for the treatment of acute hyperuricemic nephropathy can be advocated because the underlying malignancies which typically cause it often allow a prolonged survival, and the complication reflects the effectiveness of the therapy.

CASE PRESENTATION

A 72-year-old man with a history of adenocarcinoma of the lung was admitted to the hospital complaining of new-onset shortness of breath and a cough productive of white sputum. Three months earlier he was noted to have a 3-cm nodule in the left upper lung. A needle biopsy of the lesion confirmed a diagnosis of cancer. The patient refused surgery but agreed to a course of radiotherapy. A chest x-ray obtained following the completion of radiotherapy revealed a slight decrease in the size of the lesion. Physical examination on admission to the hospital revealed a pulsus paradoxus, increased jugular venous pressure, bilateral basal pulmonary rales, and hepatomegaly. An ECG showed electrical alternans, and a chest x-ray revealed an enlarged cardiac silhouette with a 2.5-cm nodule in the left upper lung. The systolic blood pressure varied between 80 and 100 mm Hg in both arms with a resting heart rate of 120/min.

Through a subxiphoid pericardiostomy 720 mL serous fluid containing malignant glandular cells was removed. The hemodynamic status of the patient improved immediately; however, the fluid reaccumulated rapidly over the following 48 h. A pericardiectomy was performed and an additional 1200 mL fluid was removed. At the time of surgery the lung nodule was removed, which revealed a poorly differentiated adenocarcinoma. The resected pericardium showed chronic inflammation and sheets of malignant cells within the pericardial tissue. The patient received a course of radiotherapy to the mediastinum. At the completion of the treatment the patient felt well, but the lung cancer eventually recurred, and the patient died despite receiving several courses of chemotherapy.

CASE DISCUSSION

This case illustrates one of the most dramatic oncologic complications, cardiac tamponade. The optimal treatment of this patient would have been to surgically remove the tumor nodule at diagnosis. Although radiation therapy can be curative in small peripheral lung tumors, a recurrence in the pericardium is not surprising since the tumor drains directly into the lymphatics of the mediastinum.

A pericardiostomy was performed in this patient because of his relatively stable condition. In patients who become hemodynamically unstable very quickly, a pericardiocentesis is indicated. The rapid reaccumulation of malignant pericardial fluid in this patient resulted in the surgical "stripping" of the pericardium. A pericardectomy effectively removes the space in which fluid can accumulate and potentially cause hemodynamic compromise. Although the therapeutic intervention was aggressive in this patient, he was able to live for several more months without the debilitating symptoms associated with malignant pericardial disease.

References

1. Nieto A, Doty D: Superior vena cava obstruction: Clinical syndrome, etiology, and treatment. Curr Prob Cancer 10:442, 1986.
2. Ahmann, F: A reassessment of the clinical implications of the superior vena cava syndrome. J Clin Oncol 2:961, 1984.
3. Lochridge SK, Knibbe WP, Doty DB: Obstruction of the superior vena cava. Surgery 85:14, 1979.
4. Schwartz EE, Goodman LR, Haskin ME: Role of CT scanning in the superior vena cava syndrome. Am J Clin Oncol 9:71, 1986.
5. Capek P, Cope C: Percutaneous treatment of superior vena cava syndrome. AJR 152:183, 1989.
6. Thurber DL, Edwards JE, Achor RW: Secondary malignant tumors of the pericardium. Circulation 26:228, 1962.
7. Shabetai R: Progress in cardiac tamponade and constrictive pericarditis. Prog Cardiol 14:87, 1986.
8. Theologides A: Neoplastic cardiac tamponade. Semin Oncol 5:181, 1978.
9. Fowler N: Cardiac tamponade in medical patients: The rarity of Beck's triad. Prog Cardiol 14:35, 1986.
10. Shepard F, Ginsberg J, Evans W: Tetracycline sclerosis in the management of cardiac tamponade secondary to malignant pericardial effusion. J Clin Oncol 3:1678, 1985.
11. Bruckman J, Bloomer W: Management of spinal cord compression. Semin Oncol 5:135, 1978.
12. Portenoy R, Lipton R, Foley K: Back pain in the cancer patient: An algorithm for evaluation and management. Neurology 37:134, 1987.
13. Rodichok LD, Ruckdeschel JC, Harper GR, et al: Early detection and treatment of spinal epidural metastasis: The role of myelography. Ann Neurol 20:696, 1986.
14. Smoker WRK, Godersky JC, Knutzon RK, et al: The role of MR imaging in evaluating metastatic spinal disease. AJNR 8:901, 1987.
15. Posner J, Chernick N: Intracranial metastases from systemic cancer. Adv Neurol 19:575, 1980.
16. Adams, R, Victor M: *Principles of Neurology*. 3d ed. New York, McGraw-Hill, 1985, pp 478–479.
17. Plum F, Posner JB: The Diagnosis of stupor and coma. *Contemporary Neurology Series*. 3d ed, vol 19. Philadelphia, Davis, 1980.
18. Howland WS, Carlon GC: *Critical Care of the Cancer Patient*. Chicago, Year Book Medical Publishers, pp 25–28.
19. Heffner JE, Sahn SA: Controlled hyperventilation in patients with intracranial hypertension. Application and management. Arch Intern Med 143:765, 1983.
20. Cairncross JG: Neurological emergencies in cancer patients. Prog Clin Biol Res 132D:319, 1983.
21. Bleyer W, Byrne T: Leptomeningeal cancer in leukemia and solid tumors: Curr Prob Cancer 12:183, 1988.
22. Sorenson S, Eagan R, Scott M: Meningeal carcinomatosis in patients with primary breast or lung cancer. Mayo Clin Proc 59:91, 1984.
23. Wasserstrom W, Glass J, Posner J: Diagnosis and treatment of leptomeningeal metastases from solid tumors: Experience with 90 patients. Cancer 49:759, 1982.
24. Fisken RA, Heath DA, Somers S, et al: Hypercalcemia in hospital patients: Clinical and diagnostic aspects. Lancet 1:202, 1981.
25. Mundy G. Ibbotsan K, D'Sooza S, et al: The hypercalcemia of

cancer: Clinical implications and pathogenic mechanisms. N Engl J Med 310:1718, 1984.
26. Silverman P, Distelhorst CW: Metabolic emergencies in clinical oncology. Semin Oncol 16:504, 1989.
27. Burtis W, Wu T, Insogna K, Stewart A: Humoral hypercalcemia of malignancy. Ann Intern Med 108:454, 1988.
28. Caufield R: Rationale for diphosphonate therapy in hypercalcemia of malignancy. Am J Med 82(suppl 2A):1, 1987.
29. Robinson AG: Disorders of antidiuretic hormone secretion. Clin Endocrinol Metab 14:55, 1985.
30. Narins RG: Therapy of hyponatremia: Does haste make waste? N Engl J Med 314:1573, 1986.
31. Decaux G, Brimioulle S, Genette F, Mockel J: Treatment of the syndrome of inappropriate secretion of antidiuretic hormone by urea. Am J Med 69:99, 1980.
32. Kreisberg RA: Pathogenesis and management of lactic acidosis. Annu Rev Med 35:181, 1984.
33. Stacpoole PW: Lactic acidosis: The case against bicarbonate therapy. Ann Intern Med 105:276, 1986.
34. Tsokos G, Balow J, Spiegel R, et al: Renal and metabolic complications of undifferentiated and lymphoblastic lymphoma. Medicine 60:218, 1981.
35. Boccia R, Longo D, Licher M, et al: Multiple recurrences of acute tumor lysis syndrome in an indolent non-Hodgkin's lymphoma. Cancer 56:2295, 1985.
36. Cohen LF, Balow JE, Magrath IT, et al: Acute tumor lysis syndrome: A review of 37 patients with Burkitt's lymphoma. Am J Med 68:486, 1980.
37. Fair W: Urologic emergencies, in DeVita VT Jr, Hellman S, Rosenberg SA (eds): *Cancer: Principles and Practice of Oncology*. 2d ed. Philadelphia, Lippincott, 1989, pp 2016–2028.
38. De Fronzo R, Braine H, Colvin O, et al: Cyclophosphamide in the kidney. Cancer 33:483, 1974.
39. Spiro L, Hecht H, Horowitz A, et al: Formalin treatment for massive bladder hemorrhage. Urology 2:699, 1983.

Chapter 150

BONE MARROW TRANSPLANTATION AND GRAFT-VERSUS-HOST DISEASE

STEPHEN W. CRAWFORD
KEITH M. SULLIVAN

KEY POINTS

- *Principles and approaches to critical care of bone marrow transplant (BMT) recipients are similar to those for other immunosuppressed hosts.*
- *Specific complications tend to occur within well-defined time periods.*
- *The primary distinguishing features of BMT recipients are the high prevalence of graft rejection, graft-versus-host (GVH) reactions and chemoradiotherapy-related toxicities.*
- *Acute graft-versus-host disease (GVHD) represents a major problem to allogeneic marrow transplantation.*
- *Hepatic veno-occlusive disease (VOD) is the most common lethal chemoradiotherapy-related toxicity after marrow transplantation.*
- *Diffuse pneumonia after marrow transplantation occurs in over 40 percent of cases; cytomegalovirus (CMV) is the most common infectious cause.*
- *Noninfectious (idiopathic) pneumonias remain a major cause for mortality and have no proven effective treatment.*

Bone Marrow Transplantation (BMT)

Transplantation of human bone marrow has become the primary therapy for several malignant and nonmalignant diseases. BMT serves as a "salvage" therapy for restoring marrow function after marrow-ablating doses of chemoradiotherapy to eradicate malignant cells in leukemias, myelodysplastic syndromes, multiple myeloma, malignant lymphomas, and assorted solid tumors, such as breast carcinoma and neuroblastoma. BMT can also be used to replace dysfunctional hemopoietic or lymphoreticular precursors and correct congenital or acquired deficiencies, such as aplastic anemia, thalassemia, and congenital immune deficiency syndromes.[1]

Antigenic differences between the marrow donor and recipient may result in graft rejection or, since the marrow graft contains immunocompetent lymphocytes, initiate GVH reactions. Antigenic determinants that mediate tissue graft rejection responses are primarily the human leukocyte antigens (HLA). These are coded for by genes of the major histocompatibility complex (MHC) located on chromosome 6.

Donor marrow may be obtained from several sources. Autologous marrow from the patient can be used for malignant disease treatment if it is free of malignancy and harvested before chemoradiotherapy conditioning. It may be cryopreserved for an extended period prior to reinfusion. Alternatively, syngeneic marrow from an identical twin is also ideal for transplant because it is genetically indistinguishable from that of the recipient.

In many cases, BMT is undertaken with allogeneic (phenotypically similar) marrow. Ideally, HLA-identical siblings serve as allogeneic donors to minimize antigenic disparity. Siblings have a 25 percent chance of having HLA identity. Allogeneic BMT also may be performed using partially HLA-matched donor marrow. International tissue typing banks may identify unrelated volunteer donors with HLA identity.

IMMUNOLOGIC ALTERATIONS

Intensive chemoradiotherapy conditioning regimens produce predictable alterations in host defenses related to granulocytopenia and ablation of humoral and cell-mediated immunity.[2] Circulating granulocytes generally recover within the first 3 weeks after marrow infusion. Normal numbers of lymphocytes are seen within a month after BMT, but antibody production is often delayed for 3 or more months. Host immunoglobulins may circulate for 3 months. At 1 year serum levels of IgM and IgG are usually normal, but serum and secretory IgA levels remain low for a longer period. T-dependent antigen production, response to vaccination, and skin reactivity to antigens may be delayed for months to a year. Alveolar macrophages of host origin persist for weeks to months before being replaced by donor cells (Fig. 150-1).

Patients with chronic GVHD have persistently decreased cell-mediated immunity and antigen-specific antibody responses.[3] These alterations occur due to the GVHD and are independent of immunosuppressive treatment.

Complications of Marrow Transplantation

Although conceptually a straight-forward procedure, the utility of BMT is limited by a relatively high morbidity and mortality primarily related to relapse of malignancy, conditioning-related toxicities, infection, and donor-recipient antigenic disparity (leading to graft rejection or GVHD) (Table 150-1): these BMT-related complications have been extensively reviewed elsewhere.[4] Specific complications tend to occur within well-defined periods of immunologic alteration after intensive conditioning regimens.[5] Knowledge of these periods makes diagnostic decisions in the marrow recipient easier than in many other immunosuppressed hosts. About 40 percent of marrow recipients at major transplantation units require intensive hemodynamic

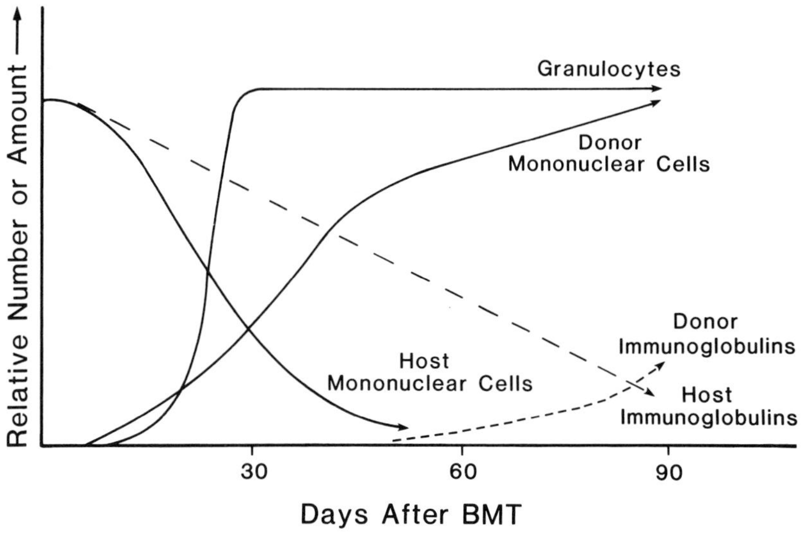

FIGURE 150-1 Alterations in host defenses after marrow transplantation.

monitoring or critical care procedures such as hemodialysis or mechanical ventilation. In this section, the incidence and presentation of complications of concern to the critical care provider will be discussed. With the exception of the immunologic aspects, complications of BMT are similar to those of intensive antineoplastic therapy. Significant differences will be stressed.

COMPLICATIONS OF CYTOREDUCTIVE CHEMOTHERAPY

Infections are very common after BMT. Bacteremia or serious bacterial infection is noted in up to 50 percent of marrow recipients. *Aspergillus* species infections and *Candida* colonization and infection have also become major clinical problems.[6] The risks for bacterial and fungal infections are mainly related to the uniform use of central venous access lines (e.g., Hickman catheters), prolonged neutropenia, and immunosuppression to prevent GVHD.

TABLE 150-1 Complications after Marrow Transplantation

- Rejection of marrow graft
- Relapse of malignancy
- Conditioning-related toxicity
  - Hepatic VOD
  - Oral mucositis
  - Idiopathic pneumonia
  - Leukoencephalopathy
  - Neuropathy
  - Myopericarditis
  - Hepatitis
- Infection
  - Venous access line infection
  - Bacteremia/fungemia
  - Pneumonia
    - Viral
    - Fungal
    - Bacterial
    - *P. carinii*
- GVHD
  - Acute
  - Chronic
- Idiopathic pneumonia
- Obliterative bronchiolitis

Gastrointestinal manifestations of conditioning-related toxicities are the rule. Desquamation of the oropharyngeal and gastrointestinal mucosa (mucositis) secondary to high dose radiotherapy and antimetabolites generally occurs within the first 3 weeks of transplantation. The mucositis and opiate analgesics administered to temper the pain increase the risk of pulmonary aspiration and mandate intravenous alimentation.

Although relatively uncommon, congestive cardiomyopathies and pleuropericarditis syndromes associated with cyclophosphamide and anthracycline-containing preparative regimens are occasionally seen. Central nervous system (CNS) complications may also be seen with specific drug treatments. Both Guillian-Barré syndrome and peripheral neuropathies have been described after cytosine arabinoside treatment. Toxicity due to cyclosporine may cause altered sensorium and coma. Cancer therapy complications such as cyclophosphamide-induced hemorrhagic cystitis, tumor lysis syndromes and chemotherapy-related neurologic and pulmonary reactions also may be observed.

RELAPSE AND REJECTION

Relapse of primary malignancy and rejection of the donor marrow are fatal complications. Fortunately, immunologically mediated graft rejection is relatively uncommon (<1 percent) in recipients of HLA-identical marrow prepared with total body irradiation (TBI). It occurs more frequently with increasing degree of HLA disparity, as well as in previously transfused patients with aplastic anemia not prepared with TBI. Recurrence of malignancy after transplant occurs in approximately 20 percent of patients transplanted in early stage leukemia (i.e., first remission or chronic phase) and in 50 to 70 percent of patients transplanted in advanced leukemia (relapse or blast crisis).[7] Most relapses occur with host type cells and signal ineffective antineoplastic treatment. Extramedullary conditioning-related toxicities limit the intensity of the cytoreductive regimens that can be used. Second transplantation following repeat preparative conditioning may be successful, but mortality remains high due to prolonged pancytopenia.

GRAFT-VERSUS-HOST DISEASE (GVHD)

This clinicopathologic syndrome is an immunologic reaction of donor lymphocytes to "foreign" antigens present on the surface of host cells. Transplantation (HLA) antigens are important, as are "minor" antigens not detected by current typing techniques. Overall, acute GVHD occurs in 20 to 50 percent of allografts and in up to 80 percent of recipients of HLA nonidentical grafts.[7] GVHD is categorized as acute or chronic according to time of presentation, organ involvement, and histology.

ACUTE GVHD

Incidence

Acute GVHD occurs within the first 3 months after BMT. The reactions are seen in 20 to 50 percent of HLA-identical marrow recipients. The incidence increases with patient age and degree of HLA disparity with the donor.

Manifestations

The histologic hallmark of acute GVHD is lymphocytic infiltration of the epidermis and gastrointestinal tract. The clinical syndrome is composed of dermatitis, enteritis, and hepatitis. The severity of GVHD is commonly determined by a grading system (Table 150-2). The grade depends on the stage of GVHD within the skin, liver, and gut (Table 150-3). Fever, diffuse macular dermatitis (often leading to bullae and desquamation), cramping abdominal pain, watery to bloody diarrhea, and jaundice with cholestasis and hepatocellular necrosis may be seen. The most dramatic presentation, in the absence of prophylactic immunosuppression, occurs as early as 7 days after BMT. This hyperacute GVHD is accompanied by exfoliative dermatitis, shock, and hyperpyrexia. Mortality increases with increasing severity of acute GVHD and often is related to associated infectious complications.

TABLE 150-2 Grading of GVHD

Grade	Degree of Organ Involvement
1	+ to ++ skin rash; no gut involvement; no liver involvement; no decrease in clinical performance
2	+ to +++ skin rash; + gut involvement or + liver involvement (or both); mild decrease in clinical performance
3	++ to +++ skin rash; ++ to +++ gut involvement or ++ to +++ liver involvement (or both); marked decrease in clinical performance
4	Similar to grade 3 but with ++ to ++++ organ involvement and extreme decrease in clinical performance

Immunology

The principle effector cells responsible for GVHD appear to be immunocompetent donor cytotoxic T lymphocytes. These differentiate and proliferate in response to host histocompatibility antigens. It is likely that lymphokine production from sensitized lymphocytes recruits additional effector mononuclear cells to participate in the alloimmune response.

Although histocompatibility matching is an important first step in trying to reduce the severity of acute GVHD, this alone is ineffective in preventing GVHD. Almost all recipients of unmodified allogeneic marrow develop GVHD if not given posttransplant immunosuppression. Methotrexate and cyclosporine appear to be equally effective in decreasing the incidence of acute GVHD. Their combined use is superior to either agent alone. Attempts at removing donor T lymphocytes from the marrow inoculum have been effective in lessening GVHD, but advantages are offset by increasing rates of graft rejection and recurrent leukemia.

CHRONIC GVHD

Incidence

Chronic GVHD is seen in 20 to 50 percent of allografts. It develops more than 3 months after BMT, usually following prior acute GVHD. Twenty to thirty percent of chronic GVHD develops de novo, without prior acute GVHD.

Manifestations

Chronic GVHD mainly involves skin, mucosal membranes, and liver. Pigmentation and sclerosis of the skin, lichenoid oral plaques, esophagitis, polyserositis, and oral and ophthalmic sicca syndrome resemble collagen vascular disorders. Elevated alkaline phosphatase and transaminase levels occur in 90 percent of cases. Chronic wasting due to anorexia is common in untreated patients. Chronic pulmonary diseases are seen in 10 to 20 percent and are divided between diffuse interstitial pneumonias and obliterative bronchiolitis.

Mortality from chronic GVHD is related to type of onset and extent of disease. Mortality is lower in disease limited to skin and liver only and with a de novo onset (in the absence of prior acute GVHD). Death is usually caused by infection.

Immunology

Minor histocompatibility antigen differences and deficient thymic function may play a role in the immunopathogenesis of chronic GVHD. These patients have an increase in nonspecific suppressor lymphocyte function and lack the specific suppression of cytotoxic reactivity to host alloantigens. Cytokine mediators may propagate autoimmune-like tissue injury.

Chronic immunodeficiency remains as long as the dis-

TABLE 150-3 Staging of Acute GVHD

Stage	Skin	Liver	Gut
+	Maculopapular rash <25% body surface	Bilirubin 2–3 mg/dL	Diarrhea 500–1000 mL/day
++	Maculopapular rash 25–50% body surface	Bilirubin 3–6 mg/dL	Diarrhea 1000–1500 mL/day
+++	Generalized erythroderma	Bilirubin 6–15 mg/dL	Diarrhea >1500 mL/day
++++	Desquamation and bullae	Bilirubin >15 mg/dL	Pain or ileus

ease is active and places these patients at risk for opportunistic infection. Immunoglobulin deficiencies are common and likely responsible for the increased incidence of fatal infections with *Streptococcus pneumoniae*.

HEPATIC VENO-OCCLUSIVE DISEASE (VOD)

Liver disease is a common and complex problem after BMT. The most serious complication is hepatic VOD (Table 150-4).

Incidence

Incidence of hepatic VOD ranges from <2 percent among patients transplanted for nonmalignant conditions without TBI conditioning to 20 to 60 percent for those with malignancy conditioned with chemotherapy and TBI.[8] Higher rates are seen with increasing age of marrow recipients and prior hepatitis. The mortality rate of hepatic VOD is approximately 30 percent. There is no known effective treatment.

TABLE 150-4 Gastrointestinal Disease after Marrow Transplantation

		DAYS AFTER TRANSPLANTATION		
	Pretransplant	Day 0–20	Day 20–100	Beyond Day 100
Liver disease	Viral hepatitis, leukemia, drug effect, tuberculosis	VOD, bacteremia, drug effect, fungal infection, parenteral nutrition, early GVHD	Acute GVHD, viral hepatitis, persistent VOD, fungal infection, drug effect, EBV lymphoma	Chronic GVHD, viral hepatitis (chronic), drug effect, infection (mycobacteria)
Ascites	—	VOD, peritonitis	Persistent VOD, acute GVHD, peritonitis, hepatic vein obstruction, pericarditis, pancreatitis	Chronic hepatitis (virus, chronic GVHD)
Diarrhea	Fungal infection, parasites, drug effect	Conditioning therapy, drug effect, infection, early GVHD	Acute GVHD, infection, drug effect	Persistent acute GVHD, infection, bacterial overgrowth (chronic GVHD)
Nausea/ vomiting	Bacteremia, liver disease, drug effect	Conditioning therapy, drug effect, infection, early GVHD	Infection (herpes virus), acute GVHD, drug effect	Drug effect, chronic GVHD
Esophageal symptoms	Infection, reflux esophagitis	Esophagitis (fungal, bacterial)	Esophagitis (viral), reflux esophagitis	Chronic GVHD, reflux esophagitis
Intestinal bleeding	Peptic ulcer	Esophagitis (infections), "stress ulcers," Mallory-Weiss tears	Esophagitis (infections), "stress ulcers," GVHD, viral ulcers (mostly CMV), EBV lymphoma	Persistent acute GVHD
Abdominal pain	—	VOD, conditioning therapy enteritis	Acute GVHD, infection, drug effect (ileus), liver abscess, cholecystitis, peritonitis, pancreatitis, cystitis, herpes zoster	Persistent acute GVHD, infection

EBV, Epstein-Barr virus; GVHD, graft-versus-host disease; VOD, veno-occlusive disease. Adapted from reference 8.

Presentation

Hepatic VOD is distinguished from other liver diseases in part by the timing of presentation. Occurring within 2 weeks of BMT, it appears earlier than hepatic manifestations of acute GVHD. Typically seen are progressive weight gain with peripheral edema, a peaking of hepatic enzymes within 2 weeks, jaundice, ascites, and painful hepatomegaly. Metabolic encephalopathy and coma may ensue. Renal failure consistent with the hepatorenal syndrome occurs in many patients and complicates treatment.

Pathogenesis

The pathologic lesion is terminal hepatic venule occlusion and hemorrhage. Subendothelial thickening with edema and deposition of fibrin and clotting factors are later replaced by cellular debris and fibrotic reaction involving terminal venules and sinusoids. Hepatocellular injury around the terminal venule is prominent.

Endothelial cell damage from high dose chemoradiotherapy is a likely inciting event. Deposition of coagulants and microthrombosis probably lead to venular obstruction. Resulting passive congestion and ischemia cause necrosis of surrounding hepatocytes. Toxicities of antimetabolic drugs and viral hepatitis may impair cellular metabolic repair mechanisms and contribute to hepatic injury.

PNEUMONIA

Incidence and Pathogenesis

Pneumonia develops in 40 to 60 percent of marrow recipients and remains a major cause of morbidity and mortality.[9] Both infectious and noninfectious etiologies are seen, and the prevalence of these vary with time after BMT (Table 150-5).

Infectious Pneumonia

Approximately half of pneumonias are due to infection. The true incidence of bacterial bronchopneumonia is unknown but ranges from 2 percent (documented by open lung biopsy) to over 25 percent (noted at autopsy).[10] The frequency of invasive fungal disease due to *Aspergillus* and *Candida* species is increasing. *Aspergillus* infection most often involves lung and is seen in 10 to 15 percent of BMT. Invasive *Candida* infection is also prevalent in BMT patients, and autopsy data suggest that 50 percent of cases have pulmonary involvement.[10]

Sixty percent of diffuse pneumonias are due to CMV.[11] For the period between 30 and 150 days after BMT this rate increases to 80 percent.[12] These occur primarily among recipients with previous infection documented by positive pretransplant serology. Other herpes group viruses, such as herpes simplex virus (HSV) and varicella zoster virus (VZV), are less commonly seen because of the prophylactic administration of acyclovir. Likewise, *Pneumocystis carinii* is rare after a pretransplant course of trimethoprim-sulfamethoxazole prophylaxis.

TABLE 150-5 Incidence of Common Etiologies for Pulmonary Infiltrates after BMT

Complications within 100 Days	Approx. Incidence (%)
Pulmonary edema syndromes	0–50
Infectious pneumonia	30–40
Bacterial	2–30
Fungal	10–20
Viral	20–30
Protozoal	<5
Idiopathic pneumonia	10–20
Pulmonary VOD	rare
Complications after 100 Days	
Bacterial bronchopneumonia	20–30
Idiopathic pneumonia	10–20
Viral pneumonia	0–10
Obliterative bronchiolitis[a]	10–20

[a]Obstructive airflow among marrow recipients with chronic GVHD

Noninfectious Causes of Pulmonary Infiltrates

In 20 to 30 percent of patients with suspected pneumonia after BMT no infection is demonstrated. The causes of noninfectious pulmonary disease after BMT include pulmonary hemorrhage, edema, adult respiratory distress syndrome (ARDS), and idiopathic interstitial pneumonia. Less common are thromboemboli and leukemic infiltrate.

Presentations

The etiologies and severity of lung diseases seen vary with the time after BMT. Focal or patchy infiltrates in the first 30 days after BMT frequently represent bacterial or fungal infection during this period of granulocytopenia. Bacteria are an unusual cause for diffuse infiltrates. Focal radiographic lesions with masslike appearances that develop or persist despite antibiotics are pulmonary fungal infections in the majority of cases.[13] Occasionally, *Legionella* and rarely *Nocardia* species are identified within localized lesions.

Within the first 30 days, diffuse infiltrates rarely are infectious. Pulmonary edema related to excess intravascular volume administration, cardiotoxic chemotherapy, or ARDS from chemoradiotherapy injury or sepsis, in addition to pulmonary hemorrhage due to thrombocytopenia (<20,000/mm^3) cause the majority of diffuse infiltrates. These patients frequently suffer from multiorgan disease from conditioning-related toxicities or grade 2 to 4 (moderate to severe) acute GVHD. Thus, pancytopenia, hepatic and renal failure, desquamative skin lesions, and mucositis complicate both evaluation and management. Within 30 days, diffuse infiltrates often are acute in onset and progress rapidly to respiratory failure.

Beyond 30 days, viral pneumonias, especially CMV, predominate as causes for diffuse pulmonary infiltrates. Onset may vary from insidious to rapid progression from tachypnea to hypoxia with respiratory failure. Unfortunately, similar presentations are seen with idiopathic interstitial pneumonia or *Pneumocystis* pneumonia. There is little to clinically distinguish these etiologies. The severity of illness and rapidity of onset after 30 days is usually less than at earlier times. However, progression to profound respiratory failure often follows.

Late after BMT (>100 days), diffuse pulmonary disease is most often insidious in onset. These late pneumonias occur predominantly among allogeneic marrow recipients with chronic GVHD.[14] Viral pneumonias (CMV and VZV) are seen but become less common after day 100. *Pneumocystis* infection occasionally presents in patients with chronic GVHD and inadequate trimethoprim-sulfamethoxazole prophylaxis. Idiopathic pneumonias, possibly due to late radiation or cyclophosphamide-induced pulmonary damage, are clinically identical in presentation to other diffuse pneumonias.

OBLITERATIVE BRONCHIOLITIS

Incidence

Recently it has been recognized that 10 percent of allogeneic marrow recipients develop chronic airflow obstruction. This is most notable among long-term survivors with chronic GVHD and has been demonstrated histologically to represent an obliterative bronchiolitis pattern.[15] It is unclear whether airflow obstruction seen within 100 days of BMT is similar in histology or possibly related to airway infection. This early presentation is often associated with acute GVHD. The relationship between airflow obstruction and GVHD has led to speculation that bronchial epithelial cell expression of class II histocompatibility antigen triggers cytotoxic lymphocyte response.

Manifestations

The diagnosis depends on demonstration of airflow obstruction by pulmonary function testing. Some recipients are asymptomatic when this is detected. Typical manifestations are insidious progression of dyspnea on exertion and cough.[16] There may be few physical findings, and the chest radiograph may be normal. Rarely, the onset is acute and profound wheezing is noted, particularly when symptoms are seen early after BMT.

Although often progressive and resulting in death because of respiratory failure, the rapidity of onset and rate of progression predict the outcome.[16] Control of chronic GVHD with increased immunosuppression may achieve stabilization of the airway disease.

Diagnosis and Management of BMT Complications

PRINCIPLES OF CARE

INFECTION CONTROL. Infection is a major cause of morbidity and mortality among severely immunosuppressed marrow graft recipients. Efforts to decrease the incidence of infections have a significant impact on development of disease and death. The types of infections addressed include bacterial, fungal, viral, and parasitic.

Infection control begins prior to BMT. Experience suggests that the outcome of patients given intensive chemoradiotherapy during active fungal infection is poor. Efforts should be made to diagnose and treat potential pulmonary, hepatic, or renal foci of infection prior to consideration of BMT.

Prophylactic daily administration of oral trimethoprim-sulfamethoxazole for the 2 weeks prior to BMT and twice weekly after adequate granulocyte engraftment has virtually eliminated the occurrence of *Pneumocystis* pneumonia. Patients with sulfa allergies who cannot undergo desensitization may be considered for intravenous or aerosolized pentamidine. Long-term intravenous pentamidine is limited in cumulative dose by potential hepatic toxicity; we have seen failures of aerosolized and intravenous pentamidine prophylaxis in this population.

Placement of marrow recipients in protective environments with filtered laminar airflow (LAF) for the duration of neutropenia decreases infection in all patients but reduces mortality only among patients transplanted for aplastic anemia. The reasons for the lack of survival advantage for malignancy patients are not clear but may be related to TBI-associated nausea and vomiting which reduce the success of total gut decontamination. In most cases, LAF is combined with decontamination of the gastrointestinal tract with oral nonabsorbable antibiotics. Efforts are underway to identify antibiotic combinations that will eliminate aerobic pathogens without eradicating anaerobic flora that prevent candidal overgrowth. An unexpected benefit noted with LAF use was a decrease in incidence of acute GVHD in patients with aplastic anemia not receiving TBI. This finding has led to speculation that bacterial antigens may contribute to stimulation of donor cytotoxic lymphocytes by host alloantigens.

Prophylactic measures have decreased the incidence of herpesvirus infections. Pretransplant serologic testing identifies previously infected recipients who are at risk for reactivation infection with CMV and HSV. Transmission of CMV infection can be avoided by providing the recipient with blood products from CMV seronegative donors.[17] Similarly, the rate of HSV reactivation after BMT can be suppressed by prophylactic acyclovir after BMT. Surprisingly, this also decreases the incidence of CMV infection by about a third even though acyclovir has little in vitro activity against CMV. Studies are in progress to evaluate other agents, such as immunoglobulins and ganciclovir, as prophylaxis.

GVHD PROPHYLAXIS. Prevention of GVHD is of paramount importance. Clearly morbidity and mortality increase with increasing grades of GVHD. GVHD causes direct organ damage and may lead to fatal hepatic failure, gastrointestinal bleeding, or diffuse exfoliative dermatitis. In addition, it increases the incidence of other potentially fatal complications such as CMV enteritis, pneumonia, and bacterial and fungal infection. Virtually all allograft recipients who do not receive in vivo immunosuppressive prophylaxis develop acute GVHD. As noted above, prophylaxis with a combination of methotrexate and cyclosporine decreases the incidence of acute GVHD to about 25 percent.

TOTAL PARENTERAL NUTRITION (TPN). Provision of adequate nutrition during the periods of inadequate oral intake is an important part of the supportive care of the BMT patient. Most transplant units provide TPN through large bore indwelling venous access catheters if severe mucositis, nausea, vomiting, or respiratory failure preclude oral alimentation. Few studies clearly demonstrate that TPN decreases the rate of infectious complications or speeds engraftment and hematologic recovery. However, there is evidence that overall mortality is lower among marrow recipients who receive TPN.

SEPSIS SYNDROME

Hypotension and fever are common in marrow recipients, especially during the period of neutropenia. Whereas the basic approach to these situations is similar to that described elsewhere for other neutropenic hosts (see Chapter 99), the marrow transplant recipient poses several distinct problems.

Bacteremia is noted in at least 50 percent of marrow recipients. As in other hospitalized patients, gram-negative enteric organisms are common. However, gram-positive cocci and yeast are also seen with increasing regularity. Among these, coagulase-negative staphylococci and *Candida* species predominate. These prevalences influence antibiotic choices and frequently prompt the empiric addition of antistaphylococcal agents and amphotericin.

Systemic viral infections are seen with higher frequency after BMT than after conventional chemotherapy. Herpesviruses, and CMV in particular, almost uniformly reactivate after allogeneic BMT in previously infected patients developing acute GVHD and may present with a septic appearance. CMV viremia has been associated with high cardiac output and low systemic vascular resistance (SVR) suggestive of the sepsis syndrome. It is unclear whether this response is due to viremia or concomitant processes often associated with CMV infection, such as GVHD.

The primary diagnostic dilemma posed by sepsis syndrome is differentiation of true bacterial or fungal sepsis from acute GVHD. The cardiovascular responses to systemic cytotoxic lymphocyte activation in acute GVHD may be indistinguishable from that of endotoxemia. As with endotoxemia, acute GVHD may be associated with high levels of circulating tumor necrosis factor (TNF) and other vasoactive cytokines. In our experience, profoundly decreased SVR and relative hypotension are seen with the acute onset of GVHD. In patients with uncompromised myocardial function, stroke volume increases and cardiac output may exceed three times normal. These patients have fever, diffuse cutaneous hyperemia, and bounding peripheral and precordial pulses. Diffuse pulmonary infiltrates, azotemia, and altered sensorium may follow in severely ill patients.

GVHD increases the risk of infection and subsequent sepsis, and the two conditions often coexist. Allogeneic marrow recipients with clinical sepsis should therefore be presumed to have infection. Empiric antibiotic coverage should be started and modified on the basis of culture results and locally endemic infection and resistance patterns. The assessment of potential GVHD should be made on clinical grounds and biopsy of appropriate tissues. Often the pattern of dermatitis may strongly suggest acute GVHD and biopsy may confirm suspicions.

Confounding the evaluation and treatment of sepsis syndrome in the marrow recipient is the frequent finding of relative intravascular volume expansion. As many as 50 percent of BMT recipients develop pulmonary edema within the first weeks after BMT. This is generally attributable to excessive administration of crystalloid fluids. In addition to exogenous fluid administration, intravascular volume is often replete due to fluid and sodium retention from hepatic VOD. Thus, brisk volume replacement often is not necessary in these patients to maintain arterial blood pressure when SVR declines. However, blood loss, often from occult gastrointestinal sources, may complicate the volume management of the marrow recipient with sepsis.

One critical determinant of survival in such situations appears to be cardiac function. Inability to respond with an increased cardiac output is associated with high mortality. The clinical assessment of intravascular volume necessary to provide adequate left ventricular filling is extremely difficult in these rapidly changing patients. Given the potential complexities of diagnosis and management, central hemodynamic monitoring with a flow-directed pulmonary artery catheter often is useful. With appropriate precautions, percutaneous introduction of the pulmonary artery catheter via the internal jugular or femoral vein can be performed safely in most cases. Such monitoring allows support of arterial pressure with vasoactive drugs while avoiding excessive volume administration. We provide positive inotropic support for those patients with inadequate stroke volume despite "normal" pulmonary artery occlusion pressures.

GVHD

Diagnosis and management of acute GVHD is crucial to success in allogeneic BMT. These aspects of care often involve the critical care physician in collaboration with the oncologist. Acute GVHD most frequently occurs during the initial hospitalization for BMT. Such patients are at risk of death as a result of multisystem involvement of the GVHD and frequently require intensive care management. In addition to the acute illness associated with the onset of acute GVHD, risks of potentially fatal bacterial or fungal infection are also present.

In contrast to acute GVHD, chronic GVHD primarily presents a limitation to long-term survival. The major life-threatening problems relate to infectious complications of prolonged deficits in antigen-specific antibody production, increased nonspecific suppressor lymphocyte activity, and phagocytic dysfunction. Thus, acute disseminated bacterial infections and opportunistic pulmonary infections pose the greatest threats. These occur primarily in the ambulatory care setting and only later involve the critical care physician.

ACUTE GVHD

Since acute GVHD is a clinicopathologic syndrome, the presentation may only suggest the diagnosis. Dermatitis, jaundice, and enteritis may be caused by various insults such as chemoradiotherapy, disseminated infection, or drug toxicity. Histologic confirmation of the diagnosis is made by biopsy (often repeated) of affected organs. Skin is the most often involved and biopsied; however, liver and gastrointestinal tract are also amenable to this approach. Thus, invasive procedures are usually necessary to confirm the diagnosis of acute GVHD in the presence of skin, liver, or gastrointestinal tract disease. Occasionally, fever may be the major manifestation and biopsy of other organs too risky. In this case, "blind" biopsy of skin becomes necessary for diagnosis.

However, verification of the diagnosis does not eliminate concomitant causes of similar features, such as infection. Repeated blood cultures should be prompted by persistent fever. Nausea and vomiting should be evaluated by endoscopy to exclude viral, bacterial, or fungal infection, and diarrheal stool should be examined and stained for bacterial pathogens. Vigilant search for other etiologies should continue. Exfoliative dermatitis should be biopsied to exclude toxic epidermal necrolysis due to drug sensitivity. Liver and endoscopic gastrointestinal tract biopsies may be necessary to exclude infectious complications.

Treatment of established acute GVHD is often difficult. Current strategies use increased immunosuppression with corticosteroids (methylprednisolone, 2 mg/kg/day), antithymocyte globulin (ATG), and continued methotrexate and cyclosporine.[18] The survival rates for steroid-resistant GVHD are poor, and death is most often due to infection. The administration of monoclonal antibodies directed against T lymphocytes shows promise as a method of "turning-off" the disease.

Supportive care of the marrow recipient with acute GVHD assumes great importance because of the difficulties posed by treatment and the threat of fatal infectious complications. Continued surveillance for viral, bacterial, or fungal infection is mandatory. A chest x-ray is obtained at least weekly and abnormalities aggressively evaluated. Prophylactic broad-spectrum antibiotics should be continued for the duration of neutropenia or in the presence of fever and immunosuppressive therapy.

Adequate nutrition is vital but often poses problems in the presence of severe enteric GVHD. Malabsorption is common and return to oral feeding often delayed. TPN may be required for prolonged periods. Cramping and diarrhea may necessitate parenteral opiate analgesics, even at the risk of ileus.

Depression of marrow function and systemic viral infection are sometimes manifestations of severe acute GVHD. Thrombocytopenia due to decreased platelet production may be compounded by rapid turnover because of fever and bleeding. Support of hemostasis usually requires repeated transfusions of platelets. Vitamin K should be given when the prothrombin time is elevated, but may fail to correct the problem in the presence of hepatic failure, requiring the administration of plasma to correct the hemostatic defect. Bleeding from the gastrointestinal tract is common and may be severe. A thorough evaluation for the site(s) of severe or persistent bleeding is recommended. Often diffuse intestinal hemorrhage because of ulceration from GVHD is found at endoscopy. However, focal bleeding from infectious ulcers or peptic disease may be identified. Angiography or nuclear medicine studies may be useful, and surgical correction of localized bleeding may be successful.

HEPATIC FAILURE

DIFFERENTIAL DIAGNOSIS. Liver disease is increasingly common after BMT. The etiologies are varied and interactions complex (see Table 150-4). Hepatic VOD and GVHD account for the majority of cases and in part can be differentiated on the basis of time of presentation and biochemical patterns.[19] However, drug toxicities (cyclosporine, antibiotics, and antimetabolites) and infections, especially viral (hepatitis B, hepatitis C, CMV, HSV, and Epstein-Barr) and bacterial or fungal, may also cause liver disease. Renal impairment prevents the normal excretion of conjugated bilirubin and continued hemolysis contributes to jaundice beyond that expected for the degree of liver disease.

Levels of hepatic transaminases rise and peak within 2 weeks of transplant in hepatic VOD. Fluid retention and jaundice develop early in the course and may be severe. Hepatic VOD must be distinguished from passive hepatic congestion from right heart failure, pancreatitis, hepatic vein thrombosis, invasive fungal disease, and septicemia with peritonitis.

Liver disease due to GVHD tends to occur after day 20 and in the presence of clinical disease in other organs. Elevations in alkaline phosphatase may peak at twenty times normal levels, much higher than seen in hepatic VOD.

Imaging modalities such as computed tomography (CT) and ultrasonography are useful in defining liver density, focal lesions, collateral circulation, and presence of ascites. Percutaneous liver biopsy carries risks of hemorrhage in thrombocytopenic patients but may be critical in defining pathology and providing culture material in difficult cases. Transjugular approaches to the hepatic vein for liver biopsy may prove to be safer. Occasionally, paracentesis is required to exclude fungal or bacterial infection and to relieve pressure in cases with respiratory embarrassment.

MANAGEMENT. Therapy does not appear to alter the natural history of VOD of the liver. Supportive measures may be ineffective in preventing progressive hepatic failure. Restriction of fluid and sodium intake along with judicious use of loop diuretics may avoid extracellular fluid accumulation. However, ascites and edema often develop prior to overt jaundice and suggest that active sodium retention due to renal disturbance is important. A major cause of mortality is the development of the hepatorenal syndrome. Care must be exercised to avoid compromising renal perfusion while trying to decrease ascites. We advocate efforts to maintain intravascular volume with replacement of blood products to ensure renal perfusion. However, hemodialysis may be necessary. Renal failure in these settings is often multifactorial. The administration of multiple nephrotoxic drugs appears to play a part. We have witnessed a decrease in the incidence of renal failure requiring hemodialysis with diminished use of aminoglycoside antibiotics and improved monitoring of cyclosporine levels.

Surgical shunting procedures to decompress the portal circulation are risky and of unproven benefit in this setting. Management of ascites with peritoneovenous shunt likewise poses great risks. Potential treatments to limit venule obstruction by microthrombosis may include prophylactic anticoagulation or thrombolytic therapy. This theoretical approach is certainly not without risk in the setting of prolonged thrombocytopenia.

Liver disease caused by GVHD requires intensive therapy for the GVHD, as discussed above. Specific interventions do not appear beneficial. Hepatic encephalopathy is approached as it is with any chronic liver disease (see Chap. 164). Modifications in dietary protein intake and clearing of the gastrointestinal tract with lactulose should be instituted.

PNEUMONIA

DIAGNOSTIC APPROACH. The clinical presentations of pulmonary disease after BMT have been reviewed in this chapter and in recent literature.[9] The diagnostic approach to pulmonary disease after BMT differs from other categories of immunosuppressed hosts due to the difference in prevalence of specific etiologies.

In the 30 days following BMT, diffuse pulmonary infiltrates often do not require invasive diagnostic evaluation because of the low prevalence of infectious causes noted.[20] A thorough clinical evaluation and empiric treatment with broad-spectrum antibiotics is recommended. Empiric diuresis and sodium restriction frequently improves the clinical status of the patient. Occasionally, pulmonary artery wedge measurement (or cardiac echocardiography) is necessary to exclude pulmonary edema and guide therapy. Correction of bleeding disorders, including adequate platelet support, may help prevent further pulmonary hemorrhage. If clinical deterioration ensues, fiberoptic bronchoscopy with bronchoalveolar lavage (BAL) is recommended to exclude treatable pulmonary infection.

After 30 days, unless pulmonary edema is strongly suspected as the cause of diffuse pulmonary infiltrates, we proceed to fiberoptic bronchoscopy with BAL. These specimens are processed with rapid detection techniques for viral pathogens, especially CMV. The techniques include direct fluorescent monoclonal antibody stains and centrifugation culture (shell vial) for CMV.[21,22] High sensitivity for the detection of virus in as little as 16 h has been noted for these tests. In addition to bacterial, fungal, and cytologic stains, a quantitative bacterial culture is performed.

Experience has shown that in the marrow transplant recipient, open lung biopsy for the evaluation of diffuse infiltrates is unlikely to reveal pathogens not detectable by BAL. For this reason, we have curtailed our use of this modality. Thoracotomy is reserved for marrow recipients with nondiagnostic BAL (sometimes repeated) who have high risk of undiagnosed infection, such as *Pneumocystis*, if prophylaxis was not received.

Focal pulmonary lesions are aggressively evaluated since there is a high probability of bacterial or fungal infection. CT scanning of the chest often reveals a masslike appearance of the lesion with a zone of attenuation highly suggestive of invasive pulmonary fungal infection. Additional lesions, not appreciated on plain chest radiograph, may also be seen. This often alters the approach to diagnosis.

The diagnostic approach to localized lesions in part depends on the radiographic appearance and location(s). Areas of bronchopneumonia can usually be approached with fiberoptic bronchoscopy and BAL. Protected microbiologic brushings increase the diagnostic yield. Peripheral lesions may be amenable to percutaneous needle aspiration biopsy for diagnosis; the diagnostic yield for masslike lesions is about 67 percent but the negative predictive value only 50 percent.[13] Thus, a nondiagnostic evaluation should prompt repeat of the procedures or progression to more definitive measures. The most definitive study appears to be biopsy at thoracotomy. Complete surgical resection of pulmonary fungal infection may be both diagnostic and curative in selected patients.

TREATMENT

BACTERIAL. Fever in the marrow recipient should be presumed to represent bacterial infection, and empiric antibiotics should be given after appropriate cultures are obtained. In this regard, management is identical to other immunosuppressed or neutropenic hosts (see Chap. 99). Marrow recipients have a high prevalence of coagulase-negative staphylococcal infections, yet it is unclear how often these cause pneumonia. Late after BMT, chronic GVHD increases the prevalence of systemic pneumococcal infections and mandates prophylactic penicillin or trimethoprim-sulfamethoxazole for the duration of active disease.

VIRAL. CMV pneumonia previously was fatal in over 85 percent of affected marrow recipients. Multiple experimental treatment modalities were unsuccessful in altering outcome. Recently, several centers have reported favorable responses to combination therapy with ganciclovir and high-titer anti-CMV immunoglobulin.[23–25] Various treatment regimens have been used successfully, usually initially involving administration of ganciclovir 2.5 mg/kg q 8h for at least 2 weeks together with CMV immune globulin 400–500 mg/kg three to five times weekly for between 2 and 3 weeks. In some series, continued therapy with lower dose ganciclovir and CMV immune globulin for a period of several weeks after successful therapy has been suggested to avoid early relapse.

Treatment of other herpes group viruses is with intravenous acyclovir at doses of 500 mg/m^2 every 8 h for at least 7 days. Except for CMV, HSV, and VZV, the efficacy of therapy for other viral respiratory infections in this setting remains unproven; however we do currently use and recommend aerosolized ribavirin as treatment for respiratory syncytial virus (RSV) and parainfluenza pneumonias.

FUNGAL. Invasive pulmonary infections with filamentous fungi such as *Aspergillus* species carry an extremely high mortality, especially early in the transplant procedure or in the presence of GVHD. This is due to prolonged neutropenia and the frequent administration of corticosteroids to treat GVHD. Similar problems exist for infections with *Mucor, Rhizopus, Pseudallescheria* and others. Treatment is with intravenous amphotericin B at doses of 1.0 mg/kg/day until resolution of infection. Most often, survival requires recovery of an adequate neutrophil count and discontinuation of corticosteroids. Surgical resection of infected lung has been used with success in patients with localized infection. This approach is warranted in cases with impending hemorrhage due to large blood vessel invasion by the fungus or those in whom prolonged periods of neutropenia or continued use of corticosteroids are likely.

Candida species infections are common and rarely seen without evidence of oropharyngeal or gastrointestinal tract colonization. Disseminated microabscesses complicate these infections and may be difficult to detect premortem. Therapy is similar to other immunosuppressed populations.

OTHER INFECTIONS. Management of *P. carinii, Legionella* species, *Nocardia,* and other unusual infections among marrow transplant recipients does not differ substantially from that used elsewhere. Few data exist to suggest that outcome of these infections after BMT is different from other patient populations. Survival is more closely related to the underlying immune deficiencies, GVHD, or conditioning-related toxicities.

IDIOPATHIC PNEUMONIA. No proven treatment exists for diffuse idiopathic pneumonia after BMT. When the syndrome presents early in the transplant course, a biopsy of the lung most often reveals the histologic pattern of diffuse alveolar damage. We believe that these patients behave identically to others with ARDS. Supportive management, including assisted mechanical ventilation, is appropriate. However, the overall mortality rate in patients requiring mechanical ventilatory support approaches 95 percent by 6 months after insult.[26] Treatment of ARDS-like conditions after BMT with corticosteroids has not been evaluated in clinical trials and carries the risk of increasing the incidence of infection.

Idiopathic interstitial pneumonia, usually appearing somewhat later in the course, displays histopathology of mononuclear interstitial infiltrates and may be an immunologically mediated process. No data exist to support the empiric use of corticosteroids in these conditions. Nevertheless, we have seen successful outcomes with this approach. We advocate managing idiopathic interstitial pneumonia, especially more than 100 days after BMT, in the same manner as idiopathic pulmonary fibrosis in the nontransplant population. In the presence of active GVHD, increased immunosuppression to control that condition is also advised.

AIRFLOW OBSTRUCTION. Obstructive airflow in the presence of chronic GVHD is managed primarily by addressing the GVHD with increased immunosuppression. This approach has been noted to halt the progression of pulmonary disease in some cases. In addition, we recommend aerosolized bronchodilator treatment for symptomatic patients. Early and aggressive antibiotic treatment for any potential lower respiratory infection should be initiated. Prophylactic trimethoprim-sulfamethoxazole is encouraged. Most patients with chronic GVHD and airflow obstruction have hypogammaglobulinemia. A pathogenic role of this deficit in recurrent sinopulmonary infection contributing to the airflow obstruction has been proposed. We recommend the routine intravenous replacement of immunoglobulin for those with low class or subclass levels.

Similar management is recommended for airflow obstruction that develops early in the BMT course. Evaluation for possible airway infection by viruses (such as RSV) or fungus should be undertaken in rapidly developing obstruction, especially in the presence of acute GVHD.

CASE PRESENTATION

Allogeneic marrow transplantation from a sibling donor with a single HLA disparity (at the B locus) was undertaken as treatment for a 23-year-old man with acute nonlymphocytic leukemia in relapse. Prior to transplantation, he was clinically well without evidence of hepatic, renal, or respiratory disease. Preparation for transplantation included administration of oral doses of trimethoprim-sulfamethoxazole for 2 weeks as prophylaxis against *P. carinii* pneumonia. Cytoreductive and marrow-conditioning preparation included cyclophosphamide (total dose of 120 mg/kg) and TBI (total dose of 13.2 Gy in 11 fractions). Serologic testing revealed the presence of CMV antibodies but no evidence of HSV exposure. Posttransplant immunosuppression was used with methotrexate (15 mg/m^2 on day 1; 10 mg/m^2 on days 3, 6, and 11) and cyclosporine (1.5 mg/kg every 12 h intravenously, then 6.25 mg/kg every 12 h orally) as GVHD prophylaxis.

By day 10 after transplantation, the patient was febrile to 38.6°C (101.8°F), tachypneic to 30 breaths/min, and had gained 7 kg in body weight (from 69 to 76 kg). He complained of severe oral pain, dysphagia, right upper quadrant abdominal fullness, and dyspnea with minimal exertion. On physical examination, there was diffuse cutaneous erythema, severe oral mucositis which bled easily, bilateral inspiratory crackles in the lung bases, tender hepatomegaly and 2 + pedal edema. The remainder of the examination, including cardiac auscultation, was within normal limits. Specifically, no cardiac murmur or friction rub was noted. Blood pressure was normal without pulsus paradoxus.

Additional medications at this time included broad-spectrum antibiotics (mezlocillin, ceftizoxime and vancomycin) and morphine sulfate for control of oral pain.

Laboratory evaluation revealed multiple abnormalities. Absolute neutropenia persisted. Hemoglobin was 11 g/dL and daily platelet counts ranged from 10,000 to 20,000/mm^3 despite frequent transfusions. Serum bilirubin concentration had risen to 7 mg/dL with minimal elevations in hepatic transaminases and alkaline phosphatase. Mild hyponatremia (Na, 130 mg/dL) was present. The blood urea nitrogen (BUN) value was 45 mg/dL and the serum creatinine was unchanged from base line. Serum albumin was 2.2 g/dL. Chest x-ray revealed cardiomegaly and diffuse alveolar infiltrates. Posterior costophrenic angle blunting was considered to be consistent with small bilateral pleural effusions. Electrocardiogram was normal except for a sinus tachycardia. Arterial blood-gas values were pH, 7.50; Pa_{O_2}, 58 mmHg; Pa_{CO_2}, 30 mmHg.

The clinical diagnoses of hepatic VOD and pulmonary edema were made. Supplemental oxygen was administered by nasal cannula. An echocardiogram excluded pericardial effusion, and the ventricular chambers were normal in dimension. Diuresis was then initiated with repeated doses of furosemide and a constant infusion of dopamine (1 to 2 μg/kg/min). Urine output was achieved that exceeded fluid intake by approximately 1 L/day. Intravascular volume was maintained with the transfusion of blood products and albumin solutions. Additional sodium chloride was removed from all intravenous fluids, including TPN. The hemoglobin was kept at 13 to 14 g/dL and serum albumin levels above 2.5 g/dL. Appropriate cultures were obtained and were unrevealing. Amphotericin (0.5 mg/kg/day) was empirically administered in view of the persistent fever and neutropenia despite broad-spectrum antibiotics.

A coagulation screen was performed, and no coagulation defects were revealed. Platelet transfusions were given daily to maintain platelet counts above 30,000/mm^3. Mouth care was meticulously provided to minimize oral bleeding. In addition, morphine sulfate infusions were adjusted to provide adequate analgesia without impairing sensorium.

Respiratory symptoms improved over the next 24 h, and the chest x-ray revealed improvement in the extent of the infiltrates and size of the cardiac silhouette. Oxygenation also improved. However, the serum creatinine increased from 1.1 to 1.6 mg/dL and the bilirubin remained unchanged. Because of concern about impending renal failure associated with hepatic VOD and pulmonary edema, a flow-directed pulmonary artery catheter was placed via the right internal jugular vein. The following central hemodynamic values were obtained: pulmonary artery wedge pressure, 10 mmHg; cardiac index, 5.6 L/min/m^2. Mean arterial blood pressure was 75 mmHg.

These hemodynamic data confirmed that cardiac output was adequate with an acceptable pulmonary artery wedge pressure and a decreased SVR. The use of potentially nephrotoxic drugs was reconsidered. Vancomycin and amphotericin were discontinued (on the basis of negative cultures) and the dose of cyclosporine reduced.

Fluid management continued unchanged over the next few days with gradual improvement in respiratory and hepatic function. The pulmonary artery catheter was discontinued after 48 h. Total body weight returned to base line, and renal function remained stable without further increase in the creatinine level. The oral mucositis reached its zenith on day 12 and displayed gradual resolution over the next week as marrow engraftment ensued and circulating granulocytes returned.

Persistent diffuse erythematous skin rash prompted a punch biopsy of the skin on day 20. Acute GVHD was confirmed and methylprednisolone (2 mg/kg/day) was begun. Despite reinstitution of *P. carinii* pneumonia prophylaxis, control of GVHD and tapering of the corticosteroids, dry cough and dyspnea developed on day 60 after transplant. Chest x-ray displayed diffuse infiltrates. Bronchoscopy with BAL was performed. Microbiologic stains, cultures, and cytologic examinations were unrevealing. Centrifugation cultures and immunofluorescent monoclonal antibody staining for CMV were positive within 16 h of lavage. Respiratory symptoms and roentgenographic abnormalities responded to treatment with ganciclovir and high-titer CMV-specific immunoglobulin over 14 days.

CASE DISCUSSION

This case illustrates common clinical problems associated with "high-risk" marrow transplantation. Factors that placed this marrow recipient at high risk of complications were his age (over 21 years), hematologic malignancy in relapse, HLA disparity with the marrow donor, and seropositivity for CMV. Typical complications involving the liver, lungs, and kidneys ensued. Although the causes of such complications are myriad, the clinical presentations made clinical assessment and management relatively straightforward.

Jaundice within the first 2 weeks after transplantation is more commonly related to VOD than hepatic GVHD. The associated findings of rapid weight gain secondary to fluid retention and the lack of marked elevation of the hepatic transaminases and alkaline phosphatase are typical of hepatic VOD. Treatment is unsatisfactory; however, judicious diuresis is attempted while efforts are made to maintain renal perfusion by ensuring adequate intravascular volume and osmotic pressure. As illustrated by this case, invasive hemodynamic monitoring with a pulmonary artery catheter is occasionally useful in assessing cardiac output (and by inference, renal perfusion) in relationship to intravascular filling pressures.

Diffuse pulmonary infiltrates occur in up to 40 percent of marrow transplant recipients. CMV is the most common infectious etiology, and this patient was at risk as a result of previous exposure (evident by seropositivity). However, pulmonary edema syndromes are also common, especially within the first 2 weeks after transplant, and CMV pneumonia rarely occurs within the first 30 days. There were ample signs of total body volume excess (increased weight, pedal edema, cardiomegaly, and pleural effusions). Pulmonary edema was therefore the most likely diagnosis at initial presentation of respiratory disease. Pleuropericarditis was excluded by echocardiography. Pulmonary hemorrhage could not be excluded and may have contributed to the radiographic presentation since it is frequently associated with profound thrombocytopenia (<20,000/mm^3). BAL might have confirmed this suspicion; however, management would not have been altered. Infectious causes for diffuse infiltrates within this time period are uncommon, especially after pretransplant *P. carinii* pneumonia prophylaxis. Thus, bronchoscopy would have been unlikely to have altered therapy and was not used. Had the patient not responded to initial management, bronchoscopy with BAL would have been performed. When infiltrates occurred on day 60 after transplant, CMV pneumonia was the most likely diagnosis. BAL was quickly performed to confirm the diagnosis and initiate therapy, which fortunately proved successful.

References

1. Thomas ED, Storb R, Clift RA, et al: Bone-marrow transplantation. N Engl J Med 292:832, 895, 1975.
2. Lum LG. A review: The kinetics of immunologic recovery after human marrow transplantation. Blood 69:369, 1987.
3. Witherspoon RP, Matthews D, Storb R, et al: Recovery of in vivo cellular immunity after human marrow grafting: Influence of time postgrafting and acute graft-versus-host disease. Transplantation 37:145, 1984.
4. Press OW, Schaller RT, Thomas ED: Bone marrow transplant complications, in Toledo-Pereyra LH (ed): *Complications of Organ Transplantation*. Chap. 22. New York, Marcel Dekker, 1987, pp. 399–424.
5. Clark JG, Crawford SW: Diagnostic approaches to pulmonary complications of marrow transplantation. Chest 91:477, 1987.
6. Meyers JD: Infection in bone marrow transplant recipients. Am J Med 81 (suppl 1A):27, 1986.
7. Sullivan KM, Storb R: Bone marrow transplantation and graft-versus-host disease, in Brent L, Sells R (eds): *Bailliere's Clinical Immunology and Allergy*. London, Bailliere Tindall Ltd, 1989, 91–118.
8. McDonald GB, Shulman HM, Wolford JL, et al: Liver disease after human marrow transplantation. Sem Liver Dis 7:210, 1987.
9. Krowka MJ, Rosenow EC, Hoagland HC: Pulmonary complications of bone marrow transplantation. Chest 87:237, 1985.
10. Hackman RC: Lower respiratory tract, in Sale GE, Shulman HM (eds): *The Pathology of Bone Marrow Transplantation*. Chap. 9. New York, Masson Inc, 1984, pp. 156–170.
11. Meyers JD, Flournoy N, Thomas ED: Nonbacterial pneumonia after allogeneic marrow transplantation: A review of ten years' experience. Rev Infect Dis 4:1119, 1982.
12. Crawford SW, Hackman RC, Clark JG: Open lung biopsy diagnosis of diffuse pulmonary infiltrates after marrow transplantation. Chest 94:949, 1988.
13. Crawford SW, Hackman RC, Clark JG: Biopsy diagnosis and clinical outcome of focal pulmonary lesions after marrow transplantation. Transplantation 48:266, 1989.
14. Wingard JR, Santos GW, Saral R: Late-onset interstitial pneumonia following allogeneic bone marrow transplantation. Transplantation 39:21, 1985.
15. Chan CK, Hyland RH, Hutcheon MA, et al: Small-airways disease in recipients of allogeneic bone marrow transplants. Medicine 66:327, 1987.
16. Clark JG, Crawford SW, Madtes DK, et al: Obstructive lung disease after allogeneic marrow transplantation: Clinical presentation and course. Ann Intern Med 111:368, 1989.
17. Bowden RA, Sayers M, Flournoy N, et al: Cytomegalovirus immune globulin and seronegative blood products to prevent primary cytomegalovirus infection after marrow transplantation. N Engl J Med 314: 1006, 1986.
18. Sullivan KM: Acute and chronic graft-versus-host disease in man. Int J Cell Clon 4(S1):42, 1986.
19. McDonald GB, Shulman HM, Sullivan KM, et al: Intestinal and hepatic complications of human marrow transplantation. Gastroenterology 90:460, 770, 1986.
20. Crawford SW, Hackman RC, Clark JG: Open lung biopsy diagnosis of diffuse pulmonary infiltrates after marrow transplantation. Chest 94:949, 1988.
21. Crawford SW, Bowden RA, Hackman RC, et al: Rapid detection of cytomegalovirus pulmonary infection by bronchoalveolar lavage and centrifugation culture. Ann Intern Med 108:180, 1988.
22. Emanuel D. Peppard J, Stover D, et al: Rapid immunodiagnosis of cytomegalovirus pneumonia by bronchoalveolar lavage using human and murine monoclonal antibodies. Ann Intern Med 104:476, 1986.
23. Emanuel D, Cunningham I, Jules-Elysee K, et al: Cytomegalovirus pneumonia after bone marrow transplantation successfully treated with the combination of ganciclovir and high-dose intravenous immune globulin. Ann Intern Med 109:777, 1988.
24. Reed EC, Bowden RA, Dandliker PS, et al: Treatment of cytomegalovirus pneumonia with ganciclovir and intravenous cytomegalovirus immunoglobulin in patients with bone marrow transplants. Ann Intern Med 109:783, 1988.
25. Schmidt GM, Kovacs A, Zaia JA, et al: Ganciclovir/immunoglobulin combination therapy for the treatment of human cytomegalovirus-associated interstitial pneumonia in bone marrow allograft recipients. Transplantation 46:905, 1988.
26. Crawford SW, Schwartz DA, Petersen FB, et al: Mechanical ventilation after marrow transplantation: Risk factors and clinical outcome. Am Rev Respir Dis 137:682, 1988.

Chapter 151

TOXICITIES OF CHEMOTHERAPY

GINI FLEMING
NICHOLAS J. VOGELZANG

KEY POINTS

- *Drug toxicity is most often a diagnosis of exclusion.*
- *Dose, schedule, and drug combinations are key parameters used to determine the likelihood of drug toxicity.*
- *Not all toxicities are known, and drug regimens are constantly modified.*
- *Therapy is supportive for most chemotherapy-related toxicity.*
- *Pelvic and spinal radiation will potentiate the myelosuppressive effects of chemotherapeutic agents.*
- *Bleomycin is a frequent drug-related cause of interstitial lung disease, with a sporadic incidence of toxicity below doses of 450 mg and a rising incidence above this dose.*
- *The majority of cardiac events in cancer patients is related to preexisting heart disease or direct invasion of the heart; nonetheless, drug toxicity must often be considered, particularly when anthracyclines have been administered.*
- *One to 10 percent of patients receiving >550 mg/m² of doxorubicin will develop a chronic cardiomyopathy.*
- *Vincristine is unique among chemotherapeutic agents in that its dose-limiting toxicity is neurologic.*
- *In high dose regimens, cytosine arabinoside and methotrexate may produce dramatic central nervous system (CNS) syndromes.*
- *Renal injury is often dose limiting in the use of cisplatin.*
- *Magnesium wasting in cisplatin-related renal injury may be profound and accompanied by hypocalcemia and hypokalemia.*
- *Mesna is helpful in limiting the hemorrhagic cystitis associated with cyclophosphamide.*
- *Venoocclusive disease (VOD) is a major hepatic toxicity of regimens used in bone marrow transplantation.*
- *Biologic agents increasingly used in the treatment of cancer have a wide range of actions involving virtually all organ systems.*

As more intensive anticancer regimens are being used to achieve cure, an increasing number of oncology patients are admitted to ICUs for complications of treatment. Several general principles about drug-induced toxicity should be kept in mind.

Drug toxicity is often a diagnosis of exclusion. The toxic reaction to an antineoplastic drug or drugs is frequently clinically and even pathologically nonspecific. Other causes should always be considered. Infection, tumor effect, and toxicity from other drugs such as antiemetics or antibiotics are frequently elements of the differential diagnosis.

Dose, schedule, and combination make a difference. Most antineoplastic drugs are given in combination, and drugs and radiation are often combined. The toxicities of a given combination may be more severe than the effects of the individual agents would suggest. Moreover, a different drug schedule, e.g. a 5-day continuous infusion rather than a single bolus dose, may have a very different spectrum of side effects. Until recently, the dose-limiting toxicity of most agents has been myelosuppression, but the recent successes of autologous marrow reinfusion for rescue after very high dose drug regimens have exposed a plethora of new toxicities.

Not all toxicities are known. New drugs and new combinations of drugs are constantly being tried and may be widely used before all toxicities are well-characterized. Moreover, the diagnosis of drug reactions that are sporadic rather than dose related is often difficult, particularly in cancer patients who have many symptoms regardless of treatment. Much of the literature consists of case reports. The tables in this chapter list the most common or notorious toxicities and are not intended to be complete.

Treatment is supportive. The importance of a diagnosis of treatment-related toxicity is generally that the offending agent can be stopped and useless remedies or diagnostic procedures can be withheld. Only rarely is specific therapy indicated.

Myelosuppression[1,2]

Complications of myelosuppression, including infections and bleeding, account for most therapy-related ICU admissions in cancer patients. Management of these problems is discussed elsewhere. Granulocytes (circulating half-life 6 h) are usually affected earliest and most severely, followed by platelets (half-life 5 to 7 days), with red blood cells (RBCs) (half-life 120 days) being relatively spared unless the patient has received high doses or multiple courses of chemotherapy. Bleeding and other causes of anemia must be considered before a very low hemoglobin is attributed to antineoplastic chemotherapy alone. There is variation in which cell lines are most suppressed; the nitrosoureas and mitomycin C, for example, typically produce a late, severe, thrombocytopenia. For most drugs the nadir of the granulocyte count is 7 to 14 days after administration of a single dose, with recovery by 21 to 28 days. Some agents produce a more delayed pattern (Table 151-1). Patients who have received pelvic or spinal radiation or who have had multiple courses of chemotherapy will suffer more severe and prolonged myelosuppression. The critically ill cancer patient may also have a multitude of other causes for cytopenias, but if doubt exists as to the cause of abnormal blood counts, a bone marrow biopsy should be obtained. This can safely be performed on even the sickest patients and is an invaluable aid in excluding many possible diagnoses, particularly marrow infiltration by tumor.

TABLE 151-1 Granulocytopenia Induced by Antineoplastic Drugs

Drug	Nadir (days)	Recovery (days)
Most agents	7–14	21–28
Busulfan	21–28	42–56
Melphalan	21	28–40
Mitomycin C	21–28	40–55
Nitrosoureas (BCNU,CCNU, methyl-CCNU)	21–28	35–60

Mucositis[2,3]

Like the cells in the bone marrow, cells of the gastrointestinal tract, from mouth to rectum, proliferate rapidly and are therefore particularly susceptible to damage by antineoplastic drugs. Toxicity ranges from mild mouth sores to severe bloody diarrhea with a measurable mortality (Table 151-2). Breakdown of the mucosal barrier also contributes to morbidity and mortality by providing a portal for the entry of infectious agents, particularly in a neutropenic patient. High dose chemotherapy regimens with or without radiation frequently cause severe mucositis. Several essentials should be kept in mind.

TREATMENT

Candida and herpes viruses commonly cause or worsen stomatitis and esophagitis. *Clostridium difficile* should always be considered in hospitalized patients with diarrhea, particularly those on antibiotics, even if they have also received diarrhea-producing anticancer therapy. Since high dose metoclopramide is frequently used as an antiemetic it should be appreciated that it too can cause diarrhea.

Patients' mouth should be kept scrupulously clean using soft swabs and saline or peroxide rinses. Various antiseptic mixtures have been recommended to prevent superinfection; we suggest chlorhexidene gluconate 0.12%.

The discomfort caused by stomatitis may be severe. If topical anesthetics do not control it, systemic narcotics should be administered in ample doses. Diarrhea and stomatitis often severely compromise enteral feeding. Intravenous alimentation should be considered early.

TABLE 151-2 Antineoplastic Drugs which Cause Mucositis

Drug	Effects
Bleomycin	Stomatitis
Cytosine arabinoside	Stomatitis, diarrhea; can be quite severe with high doses
Doxorubicin	Ulcerative stomatitis; enhanced by radiation
High dose etoposide (VP-16)	Oropharyngeal mucositis is dose-limiting extramedullary toxicity
5-Fluorouracil	Stomatitis, anal sores, diarrhea (may be bloody); continuous infusion or combination with leucovorin may (rarely) produce fatal diarrhea
High dose melphalan	Esophagitis, stomatitis, diarrhea, and colitis
High dose mitoxantrone	Structurally related to the anthracyclines, similar but less intense stomatitis
Methotrexate	Stomatitis; severity enhanced by high dose therapy or concomitant radiation
High dose Thio-TEPA	Mucositis, diarrhea

Pulmonary Toxicity[4,5]

A large number of antineoplastic drugs can cause pulmonary symptoms (Table 151-3). Syndromes reported include acute pleuritic chest pain, hypersensitivity lung disease, and noncardiogenic pulmonary edema,[6,7] but the vast majority of cases fall into the pneumonitis/fibrosis category described below. It is classically associated with the three Bs: busulfan, bleomycin, and BCNU (carmustine) and is, for many agents, sporadic rather than dose related. Methotrexate lung toxicity is symptomatically similar but is believed to be a form of hypersensitivity reaction.[8,9]

CLINICAL PRESENTATION

The onset may be after prolonged continuous treatment, which is typical for busulfan, after only a few cycles of therapy, as is frequently reported with the m-BACOD (methotrexate, bleomycin, doxorubicin, cyclophosphamide, vincristine, dexamethasone) regimen,[10] or even years after therapy has ended, as can be seen with BCNU. Signs and symptoms are nonspecific and range from mild to life-threatening. Patients invariably present with dyspnea. A dry cough, fatigue, fever, and end-expiratory rales are common but not universal features. The symptoms typically appear gradually over several weeks, but acute presentations are not unusual. The patient ill enough to arrive in the ICU will generally by hypoxic with diffuse pulmonary infiltrates on chest x-ray and the full spectrum of possible causes for this presentation, including infection (much more common than drug toxicity in most series), radiation, cardiogenic edema, pulmonary embolus, hemorrhage, leukoagglutinin reaction, and progressive tumor, must be considered.

HISTOPATHOLOGY

The histopathology closely resembles that of idiopathic diffuse interstitial pulmonary fibrosis. There is endothelial cell swelling, necrosis of type I pneumocytes and atypical proliferation of type II pneumocytes, with generalized fibrosis in end-stage disease. The character of the inflammatory infiltrate, when one is present, is variable; eosinophilia suggests a hypersensitivity reaction which may be particularly responsive to corticosteroids. Studies with bronchoalveolar lavage report certain predominant cell populations to be associated with specific drugs, but the clinical usefulness of this technique has yet to be established.[11,12]

TABLE 151-3 Antineoplastic Drugs with Pulmonary Toxicity

Agent	Type of Toxicity	Incidence, %	Comments
Bleomycin	Pneumonitis/fibrosis	2–40	Chest x-ray may be atypical
	Hypersensitivity pneumonitis	Rare	Eosinophilia may be seen on lung biopsy; steroids felt to be useful
	Acute chest pain	Rare	Substernal pressure or pleuritic; self-limited over 4–72 h
Busulfan	Pneumonitis/fibrosis	4	Insidious onset after prolonged therapy; poor prognosis
Carmustine (BCNU)	Pneumonitis/fibrosis	20–30	Toxicity dose-related; common in pretransplant regimens; may appear years after therapy has ended
Cyclophosphamide	Pneumonitis/fibrosis	< 1	May potentiate toxicity of bleomycin, BCNU
High-dose cytosine arabinoside	Noncardiogenic pulmonary edema	4–20	Care is supportive; prognosis variable
Methotrexate	Hypersensitivity pneumonitis	8	Prognosis good; dramatic response to corticosteroids reported
	Acute pleuritic pain	Rare	May be associated with pleural effusion or friction rub; subsides over 3–5 days
	Noncardiogenic pulmonary edema	Rare	Few reports, most with intrathecal injection
Mitomycin C	Pneumonitis/fibrosis	3–12	
Procarbazine	Acute hypersensitivity Rare pneumonitis		Onset within hours after drug dose; recovery rapid

DIAGNOSTIC TESTING

The chest x-ray will generally be normal or reveal a basilar or diffuse reticulonodular pattern, but an atypical chest x-ray should not rule out a diagnosis of drug toxicity. Bleomycin is particularly notorious for occasionally producing a nodular appearance which may mimic recurrent tumor, while methotrexate may be associated with a pleural effusion or hilar adenopathy. Pulmonary function tests reveal a reduced diffusing capacity for carbon monoxide (DLCO) and, sometimes, a restrictive ventilatory defect. Gallium scans are often reported to be positive in early bleomycin toxicity, but are certainly not positive in all cases of the pneumonitis/fibrosis syndrome. Since the histologic findings are not specific, even a lung biopsy may not absolutely establish the diagnosis of drug-induced toxicity, although it is usually helpful. Whether and when to take which acutely ill cancer patient with hypoxia and diffuse pulmonary infiltrates for an open lung biopsy remain controversial.[13,14] The decision should be individualized based on the patient's disease, clinical status, and previous therapy.

TREATMENT

Treatment is supportive. The precipitating agent should be discontinued. While there are no good data establishing the efficacy of corticosteroid therapy, there are many anecdotal reports of its usefulness, and it is often given a trial.[15] The syndrome may be reversible, particularly in mild cases, or it may be progressive even in the absence of further exposure to the drug.

BLEOMYCIN[4]

Bleomycin is a particularly frequent and well-studied cause of pneumonitis. Lung sensitivity to bleomycin may result from concentration of the drug in pulmonary tissue or the lung's relative deficiency of the hydrolase enzyme that detoxifies bleomycin. Most large series report a 1 to 2 percent incidence of fatal bleomycin toxicity with a variety of doses and regimens. Toxicity is sporadic rather than dose related below a threshold of 450 to 500 mg. Above this threshold the incidence rises dramatically.

Attempts have been made to predict and prevent pulmonary toxicity by following serial DLCOs. Stopping therapy in patients with a significant decrease in DLCO is strongly recommended, but this practice has not been shown to alter the incidence of fatal toxicity and a recently normal DLCO should not preclude consideration of drug toxicity. Age over 70, prior or concomitant radiation to the lungs, and concomitant treatment with cyclophosphamide, which by itself causes pulmonary damage only rarely, are reported to potentiate bleomycin lung toxicity. Less well-documented risk factors include renal dysfunction, prior administration of other pulmonary toxic agents, and administration of the drug by intravenous bolus rather than by continuous infusion. Preexisting lung disease has not been shown to be a risk factor.

The dangers of oxygen therapy in bleomycin-treated patients are a source of some controversy in the scant literature on the subject (see Chap. 58). There is a theoretical attractiveness to the concept since bleomycin may exert its toxic effects on the lung through the generation of reactive oxygen species which it does produce in vitro when incubated with iron in the presence of oxygen. Moreover, hypoxia diminishes the pneumonitis produced by bleomycin in animals whereas the acute administration of oxygen potentiates it. However, animal data do not show any increased lung damage when the hyperoxic exposure is delayed 3 or more weeks after drug administration. Data in human beings is extremely sparse. An early report noted the deaths of five consecutive testicular cancer patients ages 21 to 54 who developed severe postoperative respiratory distress 6 to 12 months after receiving fairly high doses (135 to 595 mg) of bleomycin. All patients had significantly reduced preoperative DLCOs (50 to 60 percent of predicted). Intraoperative inspired oxygen concentration (F_{IO_2}) ranged from 35 to 42%. The authors then limited their next 12 patients, who were comparable in age, bleomycin dosage, time from treatment to surgery, operation performed, and preoperative DLCO, to intra- and postoperative F_{IO_2} of 22 to 26% and had no significant pulmonary morbidity.[16] Moreover, they subsequently operated on over 700 bleomycin-treated patients, limiting F_{IO_2} to <30%, and had no episodes of postoperative pulmonary failure.[17] Numerous other reports of otherwise unexplained perioperative respiratory failure in bleomycin-treated patients given over 30% F_{IO_2} have appeared. Most authors therefore recommend limiting intra- and perioperative F_{IO_2} to <30%, although this advice has been disputed on the basis of some small retrospective series.[18] In the absence of better data, and despite the fact that no reports of pulmonary damage in bleomycin-treated patients from oxygen therapy *not* related to surgery exist, it is probably wise to use supplemental oxygen in these patients only when necessary, particularly if the patient has had documented bleomycin pneumonitis or has had very recent administration of the drug.

Cardiovascular Toxicity[19,20]

The vast majority of cardiac events in cancer patients is related to preexisting heart disease or tumorous involvement of the myocardium or pericardium, not to anticancer drugs, most of which produce cardiac damage rarely and sporadically, if ever (Table 151-4). Anthracyclines are the exception. Doxorubicin and daunorubicin have very similar effects on the heart; doxorubicin is much more commonly used and its cardiac effects have been better studied.

TABLE 151-4 Antineoplastic Drugs with Cardiac Toxicity

Drug	Effect	Incidence, %	Comments
Amsacrine	Acute QT prolongation, atrial and ventricular arrhythmias	1	Investigational agent mechanistically similar to anthracyclines; some deaths reported during infusion
	Cardiomyopathy	< 1	May develop in days or weeks after treatment; risk increased by prior anthracycline therapy
Anthracyclines	Acute ECG changes	Common	Almost always benign and reversible
	Acute myocarditis/pericarditis syndrome	Rare	
	Chronic cardiomyopathy	1–2	
High dose cyclophosphamide	Acute hemorrhagic cardiac necrosis	10–30	
5-Fluorouracil	Angina/myocardial infarction	Rare	Usually within hours of drug dose; asymptomatic ECG changes more common
Mitoxantrone	Cardiomyopathy	?	Structurally related to anthracyclines, incidence of cardiomyopathy probably somewhat less, risk dose-related
Vinca alkaloids	Angina/myocardial infarction	Rare	Scattered case reports

ELECTROCARDIOGRAPHIC CHANGES AND ARRHYTHMIAS

Cisplatin and other drugs may, of course, produce secondary effects through alterations in plasma potassium, calcium, and magnesium levels. Direct effects appear to be caused mainly by the anthracyclines and the investigational agent amsacrine (m-AMSA). Electrocardiographic (ECG) changes occur in up to 40 percent of patients during doxorubicin infusion. The most frequently noted effects are nonspecific ST-T wave changes, but premature atrial and ventricular contractions, sinus tachycardia, and decreased QRS voltage are also common; almost every conceivable type of arrhythmia has been reported. While sudden death presumed due to acute anthracycline-induced arrhythmia has been reported, it is extremely rare; cardiac monitoring during drug infusion is not warranted. The ECG changes are, with the possible exception of the decreased QRS voltage, transient. They are not a reason to discontinue therapy and are not associated with the subsequent development of heart failure.

MYOCARDIAL ISCHEMIA AND INFARCTION[21]

These are very rarely the result of anticancer drugs. Radiation therapy to the heart may result in accelerated atherogenesis, but this becomes symptomatic only years after treatment. The vinca alkaloids have been reported to precipitate myocardial infarction in a few instances, sometimes when given with bleomycin, which is known to cause Raynaud's syndrome and other vasospastic symptoms. Up to 4 percent of patients treated with 5-fluorouracil (5-FU) have been reported to suffer anginal symptoms, and a greater number have transient asymptomatic ECG changes suggestive of ischemia;[22] prolonged infusions appear to cause more problems. Myocardial infarction may occur. The mechanism is unknown, but agents such as nitrates and calcium channel blockers which reverse vasospasm may be helpful.

CARDIOMYOPATHY AND PERICARDITIS

The anthracyclines and high dose cyclophosphamide may produce fatal cardiomyopathies.

ANTHRACYCLINES.[23,24,25] The myocarditis-pericarditis syndrome describes an acute drop in ejection fraction seen in the hours to weeks after drug administration. This is sometimes associated with a pericardial effusion and may result in the precipitous death of the patient from severe congestive failure. Fortunately, it is exceedingly rare.

A chronic cardiomyopathy, on the other hand, develops in from 1 to 10 percent of patients receiving 550 mg/m^2 of doxorubicin, depending on how vigorously it is sought. The symptoms are nonspecific; patients develop tachycardia, dyspnea, cardiomegaly, and peripheral and pulmonary edema. Pathologic changes are similar to those seen in cardiomyopathy of other causes. Grossly the heart is pale and dilated; electron microscopy shows myofibrillar loss and sarcoplasmic dilatation with coalescence into cytoplasmic vacuoles.

Total dose is the single most important risk factor for developing doxorubicin-related cardiomyopathy, though extremes in age and prior cardiac irradiation may increase susceptibility. There is no cutoff point below which failure does not occur, but the slope of the curve increases at 550 mg/m^2. Symptoms usually appear around 30 to 60 days after what appears to have been the precipitating dose of doxorubicin, but may also first be noted a year or more after the end of treatment. Classically, the onset of failure was held to be abrupt, the damage irreversible and the mortality extremely high. More recent series, in which ejection fractions have been regularly monitored, suggest that many cases are mild or moderate and respond well to conventional therapy. Moreover, in some patients, even some with failure severe enough initially to require vasopressors, there may be a gradual return of the ejection fraction to normal.

There is no specific therapy for anthracycline-induced cardiotoxicity once it has occurred; care is supportive. Further drug administration is absolutely contraindicated. Perhaps, if the promise of new cardioprotective agents such as ICRF-187 is borne out, this common complication of a useful drug will become a problem of the past.

CYCLOPHOSPHAMIDE.[26] The major nonhematologic dose-limiting toxicity of cyclophosphamide is a severe hemorrhagic myopericarditis which is usually seen only at doses higher than 1.55 g/m^2, typically used in marrow-ablative regimens. In its most virulent form, cyclophosphamide-induced cardiotoxicity appears within 48 h after the last drug dose. Patients rapidly die of cardiogenic shock. More typically, edema, tachycardia and tachypnea develop 7 to 10 days after therapy, usually preceded by a decrease in QRS amplitude on the ECG. Not all patients, however, who have a decrease in QRS amplitude will develop symptoms. A hemorrhagic or serosanguinous pericardial effusion develops frequently, with possible signs of tamponade. Pericardiocentesis often does not produce any clinical improvement, possibly because of the severity of the underlying myocardial damage, and some centers no longer perform the procedure in this situation.

Hearts in patients dying of cyclophosphamide cardiomyopathy are increased in weight with thickened walls, dilated ventricles, and, in the worst cases, patchy transmural hemorrhages. Microscopically there is endothelial damage resulting from vasculitis with microthrombi in small vessels, interstitial edema, and fibrin deposition prominent in the myocardium.

ECG findings include a markedly increased thickness of the septum and posterior wall, probably caused by interstitial edema and hemorrhage. Ventricular dilatation is not prominent, and reduced fractional shortening may not distinguish between symptomatic and asymptomatic patients.

Treatment is supportive. If patients survive the acute phase complete recovery can be expected, and there may be no residual evidence of cardiac damage even at autopsy.

TABLE 151-5 Antineoplastic Drugs with Neurologic Toxicity

Drug	Incidence, %	Comments
Acute Encephalopathy		
L-Asparaginase	25–50	Ranges from drowsiness to stupor; usual onset day after start of therapy; generally resolves rapidly when therapy over
High dose busulfan	15	Acute obtundation, seizures; prophylactic anticonvulsants often used
High dose carmustine (BCNU)	10	Severe acute or chronic encephalomyelopathy; time of onset variable; not reversible; encephalopathy also seen with intracarotid therapy
Cisplatin		With intracarotid therapy only
High dose cytosine arabinoside	10–20	Ranges from disorientation to coma; usual onset 5–7 days after start of therapy; prognosis variable
Hexamethyl-melamine	Variable	Toxicity ranges from depression to hallucinations; usually reversible when drug withdrawn
Ifosfamide	5–30	Frequency greater with higher doses; ranges from mild somnolence to coma; onset hours after infusion, recovery usually within days
High dose methotrexate	2–15	Usual onset 1 week postdrug; most common presentation strokelike syndrome; usually reversible
Mitotane	40	Lethargy, somnolence, dizziness, vertigo
Procarbazine	10	Usually mild drowsiness or depression, rarely stupor or manic psychosis
High dose Thio-TEPA	Dose-dependent	Somnolence, seizures, coma; dose-limiting extramedullary toxicity
Vincristine/ vinblastine	Rare	SIADH
Acute Cerebellar Syndrome		
High dose cytosine arabinoside	10–20	Ranges from mild dysarthria to disabling ataxia; onset 5–7 days after start of therapy; prognosis variable
5-Fluorouracil	<1	Usually seen with large bolus doses; reversible in 1–6 weeks
Acute Paraplegia		
Intrathecal: Cytosine arabinoside Methotrexate Thio-TEPA	Rare	These are the only drugs normally given intrathecally; all cause acute reversible arachnoiditis fairly commonly, paralysis exceedingly rarely; paralysis may or may not be reversible
Other Neuropathies		
Cisplatin	Dose-dependent	Ototoxicity; distal sensory neuropathy which may be severe enough to cause disabling ataxia
Etoposide	Anecdotal	Mild distal paresthesias; tendon reflex depression; may be synergistic with vincristine
Hexamethyl-melamine	Variable	Peripheral paresthesias and weakness; usually reversible when therapy discontinued
Procarbazine	10–20	Decreased tendon reflexes, mild distal paresthesias; usually reversible when therapy discontinued
Vinca alkaloids	See text	Symmetrical areflexia and distal paresthesias; symmetrical motor weakness starting with dorsiflexors, jaw pain cranial nerve palsies, paralytic ileus

Neurotoxicity[27,28]

Only rarely will the neurologic toxicity (Table 151-5) of an anticancer drug be severe enough to be the primary reason for admission to the ICU. Neurologic problems are common in cancer patients, but most of these are produced by local effects of tumor, like brain or epidural metastases. The antiemetic premedications given to patients often include combinations of high doses of corticosteroids, metoclopramide, and benzodiazepines, all of which can cause dramatic neurologic changes that must be considered when symptoms developing acutely after therapy are being evaluated.

VINCA ALKALOIDS

Vincristine is unique among antineoplastic agents in that its dose-limiting toxicity is neurologic. Vinblastine causes similar side effects, but the frequency and intensity are lower. Fortunately neither drug crosses the blood-brain barrier well, and except for cases of syndrome of inappropriate antidiuretic hormone (SIADH), which these agents can produce, massive overdose, or accidental intrathecal injection (which is reported to be uniformly fatal despite a variety of heroic measures), causes for CNS symptoms should be sought elsewhere.

PERIPHERAL NEUROPATHY. The most common toxic manifestation of vincristine is a symmetric mixed sensorimotor neuropathy which may, in severe cases, progress to quadriparesis. It is dose related and gradual in onset. Peripheral nerve conduction velocities are characteristically normal despite severe clinical deficits. Mononeuropathies have been reported only very rarely. Another cause for them should be assumed. Paresthesias and motor weakness may or may not gradually improve. No treatment is known to heal vinca-related neuropathies.

Transient severe muscle pain or "Velban myalgias," sometimes requiring opiates for relief, are seen most often in children. This phenomenon is not well understood. A characteristic severe jaw pain that can begin within hours of a first dose of vincristine may represent trigeminal nerve toxicity. This resolves spontaneously within days and usually does not recur with subsequent doses.

CRANIAL NERVE PALSIES. One or another cranial nerve palsy including vocal cord paralysis, dysphagia, optic atrophy (rare), ptosis, ophthalmoplegias or facial nerve paralysis may be seen in up to 10 percent of vincristine-treated patients. Unlike the peripheral nerve findings, cranial neuropathies may be so abrupt in onset as to mimic a brain stem stroke. They tend to be bilateral and are usually reversible with discontinuation of the drug.

AUTONOMIC NEUROPATHY. Autonomic symptoms including ileus, bladder atony, impotence, and orthostatic hypotension may occur even in patients with no sign of peripheral nerve toxicity. Severe paralytic ileus presenting as an acute abdomen is not rare and can occur acutely or following long-term vincristine or vinblastine administration. It is usually reversible over the course of several days. Nasogastric tube drainage is the only standard therapy; metoclopramide has been reported to be helpful and may be tried if there is no suspicion of mechanical obstruction.

L-ASPARAGINASE

Twenty-five to 50 percent of patients receiving this drug on a wide variety of dosing schedules will have some evidence of cerebral dysfunction, adults more commonly than children. Toxicity ranges from mild depression and drowsiness to confusion, stupor, and coma. Evidence of encephalopathy often occurs on the first day after administration of asparaginase and usually clears rapidly after the end of therapy. The syndrome resembles hepatic encephalopathy and may or may not be associated with high ammonia levels. The electroencephalogram (EEG) in most cases shows a diffuse slowing that returns to normal when the drug is stopped. The cause of the encephalopathy remains unknown. L-Asparaginase itself does not cause focal neurologic abnormalities, but thrombotic and hemorrhagic cerebrovascular accidents due to asparaginase-induced clotting abnormalities have been reported.

CYTOSINE ARABINOSIDE (ARA-C)[29,30]

Given at conventional doses of 100 to 200 mg/m^2 by continuous infusion, Ara-C is not neurotoxic. However, it is increasingly being used in much higher doses (e.g., 2 to 3 g/m^2 given twice daily), usually for the treatment of acute nonlymphocytic leukemia. The sustained cerebrospinal fluid drug levels achieved with these regimens have been implicated in the 10 to 20 incidence of cerebellar and cerebral toxicity observed. Larger cumulative doses and age over 55 are associated with more frequent and more irreversible neurologic damage.

The cerebellar changes are more common and usually more severe than the cerebral ones. The onset of symptoms is usually 5 to 7 days after the start of Ara-C therapy (within 24 h of the final dose on a typical schedule). Mild cerebellar findings may include intention tremor, dysarthria, and horizontal nystagmus; in severe cases limb and truncal ataxia may render the patient completely unable to walk or even eat unaided. Cerebral symptoms range from mild somnolence to disorientation, memory loss and coma. Seizures have been reported. EEGs show diffuse slowing; findings on lumbar puncture and computed tomography (CT) are normal. Toxicity may abate over a few days to weeks, or it may be irreversible. Rarely, it is fatal. Supportive care and withdrawal of Ara-C are the only therapies. Postmortem examinations reveal severe loss of Purkinje cells and cerebellar gliosis. Interestingly, intrathecal Ara-C has not been associated with cerebellar toxicity, though it may cause a rare paralysis similar to that described below with methtrexate.

METHOTREXATE[31,32]

Like Ara-C, methotrexate used in conventional doses is not neurotoxic. When it is used in very high doses (1 to 7 g/m^2) cytotoxic levels are achieved in the cerebrospinal fluid (CSF), and a 2 to 15% incidence of transient, varied CNS syndromes has been reported. The time of onset ranges from several hours to several weeks after treatment with a mean of about a week. Signs develop abruptly and often resemble a stroke with, for example, hemiplegia and a speech disorder. Neurologic findings may fluctuate; focal or generalized seizures are common. Electrolytes and radiologic studies are normal, EEGs show a variety of abnormalities, and examination of the CSF may or may not reveal an elevated protein level. The mechanism of these neurologic reactions is unknown and care is only supportive. Patients recover completely over several days and symptoms may or may not recur with subsequent courses. In general, the CSF methotrexate level will not be elevated at the time of toxicity; the relationship to prior high or prolonged levels is not clear.

Intrathecal methotrexate can also cause neurologic damage. The most common symptom is an acute arachnoiditis which resolves over 12 to 72 h without sequelae. Rarely, the presentation may be severe enough to mimic bacterial meningitis. Very rarely an acute reaction which may include paralysis, cranial nerve palsies, or seizures is seen. Examination of the CSF may show increased pressure, high protein concentrations, and a reactive pleocytosis. Recovery is often, but not always, complete. A necrotizing leukoencephalopathy sometimes occurs after the combination of cranial radiation and intrathecal methotrexate, but this is a delayed effect which usually begins insidiously months after treatment.

Renal and Urinary Toxicity[33]

Cisplatin is the only antineoplastic drug used frequently in current oncologic practice that causes renal failure. Hyperuricemic nephropathy with or without a full blown tumor lysis syndrome may occur following rapid cell lysis in sensitive cancers with large tumor volumes; it is not the effect of any particular drug and is discussed elsewhere. Cyclophosphamide and ifosfamide can cause a hemorrhagic cystitis which is difficult to manage and is occasionally fatal. Table 151-6 lists the common renal abnormalities caused by antineoplastic drugs.

CISPLATIN[34,35]

Renal injury characterized pathologically by focal necrosis of the distal tubules and collecting ducts is a dose-limiting toxicity of cisplatin. Acute renal failure can occur. Vigorous pretreatment hydration with saline solution minimizes but does not eliminate the damage; all patients will have some decline in glomerular filtration rate with sufficient dosage. Aminoglycoside therapy and preexisting renal dysfunction are believed to increase the incidence. The creatinine level begins to rise a few days after therapy, peaks at 3 to 14 days and then, usually, declines towards pretreatment levels. Toxicity is cumulative; multiple courses and higher doses produce more severe and less reversible damage.

Cisplatin also causes a variety of electrolyte disorders. Renal magnesium wasting, not necessarily associated with azotemia, is seen in half the patients receiving cisplatin and may persist for years. Though serum magnesium levels are often strikingly low, and symptomatic muscular irritability has been reported, most patients are asymptomatic. Of particular concern in the ICU are the hypocalcemia and hypokalemia that frequently accompany the magnesium wasting, and which may be refractory to treatment if serum magnesium levels are not first corrected. Oral magnesium therapy is of uncertain benefit; intravenous or intramuscular doses should be administered. Renal salt wasting resulting in hyponatremia and symptomatic orthostatic hypotension has also been reported.

METHOTREXATE

High doses of methotrexate (>50 mg/kg) are potentially quite toxic and are normally given in the hospital with careful hydration and urine alkalinization to promote drug excretion. Plasma methotrexate levels are measured after drug administration, and leucovorin rescue is continued until the drug concentration has fallen to a safe level. Despite these precautions, an acute azotemia believed to result from the precipitation of methotrexate crystals in the distal nephron can be seen. Methotrexate-induced renal failure is usually, although not always, reversible over the 2 to 3 weeks following drug withdrawal. However, because the kidney is the primary route of excretion for methotrexate, dangerously high drug levels will persist for some time. This can produce other morbidity, particularly cytopenias and mucositis. A similar situation occurs when methotrexate has inadvertently been given to a patient with a third space fluid reservoir, such as a pleural effusion or ascites, from which the drug is only gradually released. Methotrexate cannot be cleared effectively by peritoneal or hemodialysis, so continued administration of leucovorin until plasma levels fall below $5 \times 10^{-8} M$ is necessary.

CYCLOPHOSPHAMIDE[36,37]

Urologic complications, including bladder fibrosis, bladder cancer, and hemorrhagic cystitis, are among the most troublesome side effects of cyclophosphamide.

Susceptibility to hemorrhagic cystitis is somewhat idiosyncratic, and symptoms can occur after a few small doses, but the incidence is much higher with prolonged or high

TABLE 151-6 Antineoplastic Drugs Producing Renal and Electrolyte Abnormalities

Agent	Toxicity	Comments
Cisplatin	Magnesium, calcium, potassium wasting; renal insufficiency	See text
Cyclophosphamide	Impaired free water excretion	Transient; seen with doses >50 mg/kg
High dose methotrexate	Acute renal failure	Usually reversible
Mithramycin	Azotemia or renal failure with tubular necrosis	Unusual at lower doses used for hypercalcemia
Mitomycin C	Renal failure with microangiopathic hemolytic anemia	Common with cumulative dose >60 mg
Nitrosoureas (BCNU, CCNU, methyl-CCNU)	Progressive renal failure appearing after large cumulative doses	Decrease in renal size may be noted, effect may be years after therapy
Streptozotocin	Renal failure, proximal renal tubular acidosis, nephrotic syndrome	Transient proteinuria earliest manifestation

dose therapy. Ifosfamide, an analogue of cyclophosphamide, is even more likely to produce urothelial toxicity.

PREVENTION. Local bladder irritation from acrolein, one of the metabolites of cyclophosphamide, is believed to cause the damage. Sodium 2-mercaptoethane sulfonate (Mesna) can help prevent it by providing free sulfhydryl groups which neutralize the acrolein in the urine. Mesna is not useful in treating established cystitis. Adequate prehydration with frequent voiding to decrease the length of time the acrolein is in contact with the bladder is also an important measure, particularly with high single doses of cyclophosphamide. Unfortunately, these same high doses produce inappropriate water retention with hyponatremia and elevated urinary sodium levels, an effect thought to result from potentiation of the effects of vasopressin on the kidney. Hypotonic solutions should not be used to hydrate patients on high dose cyclophosphamide therapy. Furosemide may help prevent the electrolyte abnormalities, which are usually seen starting 8 h and ending 24 h after the drug dose.

CLINICAL PRESENTATION. The acute form of hemorrhagic cystitis appears within the first few days after drug treatment. Symptoms range from minimal hematuria with mild dysuria, urgency and frequency, to massive hemorrhage requiring transfusion. The thrombocytopenia seen with high doses of cyclophosphamide aggravates the blood loss. The bleeding is usually self-limited and will stop after a median duration of a month, even in severe cases, if the patient can be supported that long.

TREATMENT. Mild episodes do not require treatment other than cessation of drug therapy. In serious cases vigorous hydration to promote urine flow, maintenance of adequate platelet counts (>50,000/mm^3), and rapid constant bladder irrigation through a large bore catheter are indicated. The catheter must be carefully kept free of obstructing clots which can cause renal obstruction with severe pain.

If these initial measures fail to control bleeding, instillation of a variety of agents into the bladder should be considered. *Alum* is an astringent which acts by precipitating superficial proteins on the bladder surface. Irrigation with a 1 to 2% solution produces minimal local toxicity and little or systemic absorption, although some authors suggest that aluminum levels be monitored in patients with renal failure. Disadvantages of this therapy are that the alum may clog the catheter and may provide only partial or transient amelioration of bleeding. Intravesical instillation of certain *prostaglandin analogues* such as 0.2% carboprostamethamine is a new and promising treatment that has been reported to result in complete and lasting resolution of hemorrhage with no significant side effects. Experience with these agents is limited, however. *Formalin* treatment has been used for many years. It produces significant pain, and must be given with the patient under anesthesia. Too weak a concentration may be ineffective and too strong a concentration can produce significant side effects, such as hydronephrosis and bladder contracture. More extreme measures, such as urinary diversion, can be taken if all else fails; exact management will depend on local urologic expertise.

Hepatotoxicity[38–40]

Although a large number of cytoxic agents can damage the liver in a variety of ways, few of them regularly do so

TABLE 151-7 Cytotoxic Agents with Hepatic Toxicity

Drug	Frequency	Comments
L-Asparaginase	Common	Fatty metamorphosis; decreased synthetic function; reversible
Azathioprine	Uncommon	Cholestasis/necrosis; hyper-bilirubinemia; variable prognosis
High dose cytosine arabinoside	Common	Elevated bilirubin and transaminases; reversible
Floxuridine (FUDR)	Common	Biliary sclerosis with hepatic intra-arterial infusion
Methotrexate	Common	Cirrhosis, fibrosis, fatty metamorphosis; laboratory data may be normal; seen with prolonged daily therapy; variable prognosis
High dose methotrexate	Common	Elevated transaminase levels, usually reversible in weeks
6-Mercaptopurine	Common	Cholestasis or necrosis; usually reversible
Mithramycin	Common	Necrosis; rarely seen with lower doses used for hypercalcemia
Nitrosoureas (BCNU, CCNU)	Occasional	Generally mild and reversible
Vincristine	Rare	May produce severe damage when combined with radiation to the liver

rhagic necrosis in tumors has prompted widespread phase I investigation.

Fever, chills, nausea and anorexia are universally seen with TNF administration. These symptoms are not dose dependent. Bolus doses cause hypertension during the infusion. This hypertension is followed by a dose-related drop in blood pressure which reaches a nadir 2 to 6 h after the start of infusion and returns to pretreatment levels within 24 h. The hypotension has been reported to be relatively resistant to dopamine and steroids. It becomes less marked with repeated daily doses. Peripheral cyanosis (without hypoxemia), dyspnea, and chest tightness can all be seen with a bolus infusion; myocardial infarction has been reported. However, the dose-limiting toxicity of repeated daily bolus dosage is hepatotoxicity. The dose-limiting toxicity of a 5-day continuous infusion, on the other hand, is thrombocytopenia. Interestingly, accelerated cachexia has not been noted, although elevated triglyceride levels are seen during prolonged infusions.

CASE PRESENTATION

A 66-year-old woman whose past history was significant only for mild hypertension and a 30 pack year smoking history presented to the oncology clinic with diffuse adenopathy. A diagnosis of stage IV large cell lymphoma was made, and she was started on the m-BACOD regimen:

Methotrexate 200 mg/m2 IV day 8 and 15
Leucovorin 10 mg PO every 6 h for 8 doses starting 24 h after each dose of methotrexate
Bleomycin 4 U/m^2 day 1
Doxorubicin 45 mg/m^2 day 1
Cyclophosphamide 600 mg/m^2 IV day 1
Vincristine 1 mg/m^2 PO days 1–5
Repeat every 21 days

Multiple dose reductions of cyclophosphamide and doxorubicin were required for cytopenias. However, the patient responded well to treatment with rapid disappearance of her adenopathy. After the third cycle an asymptomatic interstitial infiltrate was noted on her chest x-ray. Repeat PFTs were obtained.

	Pretreatment	Repeat
Pa_{O_2} (room air)	72	58
Pa_{CO_2}	42	40
pH	7.41	7.41
RV	2.82	2.14
TLC	5.71	4.96
FRC	3.3	2.74
DLCO	16.5	N/A

Bleomycin pulmonary toxicity was suspected. Day 1 of the fourth cycle was administered without the bleomycin. One week later the patient presented to clinic appearing acutely ill and mildly dyspneic. She had a temperature of 38.8°C (102°F), a systolic blood pressure of 70, and bibasilar inspiratory crackles. The remainder of her physical examination was unremarkable. She was admitted to the ICU.

Her WBC count was 2.0 with 56 polymorphonuclear cells and 40 bands. Blood-gas determinations on a 2 L nasal cannula showed P_{O_2} 89, P_{CO_2} 39, and pH 7.42. Her chemistry panel was within normal limits. A chest x-ray was unchanged from the one obtained the previous week.

Her blood pressure responded to fluids and remained normal thereafter. On the assumption that her WBC were decreasing she was started on mezlocillin, vancomycin, and tobramycin.

Contrary to expectations, the patient's neutrophil count did not decrease but returned to normal over the next few days. However, she remained febrile and gradually became severely dyspneic. Trimethoprim-sulfa was added to her drug regimen. Four days after admission her P_{O_2} obtained on a 50% face mask was 71, P_{CO_2} 38, pH 7.42. Blood, urine, and sputum cultures were negative. A chest x-ray showed somewhat increased infiltrates. A gallium scan (which had not revealed any pulmonary abnormalities in the staging work up) showed intense uptake in both lungs. All pressure readings taken with a pulmonary artery catheter were within normal limits.

On the fifth ICU day she was taken for an open lung biopsy which revealed mild septal fibrosis with no evidence of cytomegalovirus, fungi, pneumocystis, or tumor. Cultures were negative. An attempt at extubation after the biopsy produced marked hypoxemia and hypotension; the patient was reintubated. Trimethoprim-sulfa was discontinued, and the patient was placed on methylprednisolone 250 mg daily for presumed bleomycin pneumonitis.

Her temperature did not rise above 38°C (102°F) thereafter and her oxygenation gradually improved. Six days later she was successfully extubated. She was transferred from the ICU, and the steroids were rapidly tapered with no recurrence of her symptoms. At discharge the patient had a room air blood-gas valve with a P_{O_2} of 63, P_{CO_2} of 38, and pH of 7.48; she was not dyspneic with normal exertion. She refused all further chemotherapy and remains without evidence of lymphoma 2 years later.

CASE DISCUSSION

The case illustrates many of the features of a sporadic drug toxicity of any type, and some features particular to pulmonary toxicity in the cancer patient. First, the diagnosis was not at all obvious initially. Hypotension and fever with mild dyspnea in a lymphoma patient could have many etiologies. This patient had never had pulmonary irradiation, her disease was responding well to therapy, and she had no evidence of cardiac failure on examination or central venous pressure readings, so infection and drug toxicity were uppermost in the clinicians' minds. Early bleomycin toxicity had already been suspected because of a decline in pulmonary function. However, recently normal tests would not by any means have excluded bleomycin pneumonitis, and the recent decline did not rule out infection as the cause for this patient's acute illness.

Second, even the open lung biopsy did not make a definitive diagnosis of bleomycin pneumonitis; it only excluded several other diagnoses. Since drug toxicity is often a diagnosis of exclusion, the clinician must maintain a high index of suspicion based on a knowledge of what antineoplastic drugs a patient has received and what toxicities are likely. If the diagnosis is not suspected, it will be missed. Acute reactions to very low cumulative doses of bleomycin are not unusual in the setting of this particular drug combination. In this case this fact helped guide the thinking of the team.

Third, the patient was started on low doses of oxygen at the time of ICU admission. While the risk for exacerbating bleomycin lung damage should always be kept in mind, the prudent policy is to give oxygen if it seems needed, using as low an F_{IO_2} as possible while maintaining adequate oxygenation.

Finally, open lung biopsy was performed when the patient's condition continued to deteriorate despite withdrawal of bleomycin and institution of broad-spectrum antibiotic coverage. The need for and timing of open lung biopsy must be determined individually for each case. Since no specific therapy for bleomycin pneumonitis is available, and the likely infections could be treated for a few days with minimal morbidity, a wait-and-see approach was reasonable for this woman. Open lung biopsy probably contributed to the respiratory failure she experienced but it allowed the team to discontinue unnecessary antibiotics and allayed fears that some pulmonary infection was being missed.

High dose corticosteroids were started after the biopsy. It is impossible to know what role they played in this patient's recovery, but it is interesting to note that her illness began 2 days after she stopped dexamethasone. It has been reported[56] that patients with Hodgkin's disease may have activation of occult radiation injury to the lung a day or two after stopping the high dose steroids in the MOPP (meclorethamine, vincristine, procarbazine, prednisone) protocol. Something similar may occur with bleomycin lung injury.

In summary, a review of the chemotherapeutic history, a knowledge of what toxic effects are likely and a realization that multiple explanations are possible for most situations should guide any evaluation of the acutely ill cancer patient. A diagnosis of drug toxicity is made by excluding other etiologies. Supportive care is usually the appropriate treatment.

References

1. Hoagland HC: Hematologic complications of cancer chemotherapy. Semin Oncol 9:95, 1982.
2. See-Lasley K, Ignoffo RJ: *Manual of Oncology Therapeutics.* St. Louis, Mosby, 1981, p. 249.
3. Mitchell EP, Schein PS: Gastrointestinal toxicity of chemotherapeutic agents. Semin Oncol 9:52, 1982.
4. Cooper JAD, White DA, Matthay RA: Drug-induced pulmonary disease. Part I: Cytotoxic drugs. Am Rev Respir Dis 133:321, 1986.
5. Ginsberg SJ, Coomis RL: The pulmonary toxicity of antineoplastic agents. Semin Oncol 9:34, 1982.
6. Andersson BS, Cogan BM, Keating MJ, et al: Subacute pulmonary failure complicating therapy with high-dose Ara-C in acute leukemia. Cancer 56:2181, 1985.
7. Haupt HM, Hutchins GM, Moore GW: Ara-C lung: Noncardiogenic pulmonary edema complicating cytosine arabinoside therapy of leukemia. Am J Med 70:256, 1981.
8. Sostman HD, Matthay RA, Putman CE, et al: Methotrexate-induced pneumonitis. Medicine 55:371, 1976.
9. Carson CW, Cannon GW, Egger MJ, et al: Pulmonary disease during the treatment of rheumatoid arthritis with low dose pulse methotrexate. Semin Arth Rheum 16:186, 1987.
10. Bauer KA, Skarin AT, Balikan JP, et al: Pulmonary complications associated with combination chemotherapy programs containing bleomycin. Am J Med 74:557, 1983.
11. White DA, Rankin JA, Stover DE, et al: Methotrexate pneumonitis: Bronchoalveolar lavage findings suggest an immunologic disorder. Am Rev Respir Dis 139:18, 1989.
12. White DA, Kris MG, Stover DE: Bronchoalveolar lavage populations in bleomycin-induced pulmonary toxicity. Thorax 42:551, 1987.
13. Cheson BD, Samlowski WE, Tang TT, Spruance SL: Value of open-lung biopsy in 87 immunocompromised patients with pulmonary infiltrates. Cancer 55:453, 1985.
14. Potter D. Pass HI, Brower S, et al: Prospective randomized study of open lung biopsy versus empirical antibiotic therapy for acute pneumonitis in nonneutropenic cancer patients. Ann Thorac Surg 40:422, 1985.
15 White DA, Stover DE: Severe bleomycin-induced pneumonitis: Clinical features and response to corticosteroids. Chest 86:723, 1984.
16. Goldiner PL, Carlon GC, Cvitkovic E, et al: Factors influencing postoperative morbidity and mortality in patients treated with bleomycin. Br Med J 1:1664, 1978.
17. Hulbert JC, Grossman JE, Cummings KB: Risk factors of anesthesia and surgery in bleomycin-treated patients. J Urol 130:163, 1983.
18. LaMantia KR, Glick JH, Marshall BE: Supplemental oxygen does not cause respiratory failure in bleomycin-treated surgical patients. Anesthesiology 60:65, 1984.
19. Von Hoff DD, Rozencweig M, Piccart M: The cardiotoxicity of anticancer agents. Semin Oncol 9:23, 1982.
20. Hallahan DE, Vogelzang NJ, Borow KM, et al: Cardiac metastases from soft-tissue sarcomas. J Clin Oncol 4:1662, 1986.
21. Doll DC, Ringenberg QS, Yarbro JW: Vascular toxicity associated with antineoplastic agents. J Clin Oncol 4:1405, 1986.
22. Rezkalla S, Kloner RA, Ensley J, et al: Continuous ambulatory ECG monitoring during fluorouracil therapy: A prospective study. J. Clin Oncol 7:509, 1989.
23. Schwartz RG, McKenzie WB, Alexander J, et al: Congestive heart failure and left ventricular dysfunction complicating doxorubicin therapy. Am J Med 82:1109, 1987.
24. Haq MM, Legha SS, Choski J, et al: Doxorubicin-induced congestive heart failure in adults. Cancer 46:1109, 1980.
25. Saini J, Rich MW, Lyss AP: Reversibility of severe left ventricular dysfunction due to doxorubicin cardiotoxicity: Report of three cases. Ann Intern Med 106:814, 1987.
26. Steinherz LJ, Steinherz PG: Cyclophosphamide cardiotoxicity. Cancer Bull 37:231, 1985.
27. Weiss HD, Walker MD, Wiernik PH: Neurotoxicity of commonly used antineoplastic agents. N Engl J Med 291:75, 1974.

28. Kaplan RS, Wiernik PH: Neurotoxicity of antineoplastic drugs. Semin Oncol 9:103, 1982.
29. Lazarus HM, Herzig RH, Herzig GP, et al: Central nervous system toxicity of high-dose systemic cytosine arabinoside. Cancer 48:2577, 1981.
30. Gottlieb D, Bradstock K, Koutts J, et al: The neurotoxicity of high-dose cytosine arabinoside is age-related. Cancer 60:1439, 1987.
31. Jaffe N, Takaue Y, Anzai T, Robertson R: Transient neurologic disturbances induced by high-dose methotrexate treatment. Cancer 56:1356, 1985.
32. Ackland SP, Schilsky RL: High-dose methotrexate: A critical reappraisal. J. Clin Oncol 5:2017, 1987.
33. Schilsky RL: Renal and metabolic toxicities of cancer chemotherapy. Semin Oncol 9:75, 1982.
34. Blachley JA, Hill JB: Renal and electrolyte disturbances associated with cisplatin. Ann Intern Med 95:628, 1981.
35. Hutchison FN, Perez EA, Gandara DR, Renal salt wasting in patients treated with cisplatin. Ann Intern Med 108:21, 1988.
36. Levine LA, Richie JP: Urological complications of cyclophosphamide. J Urol 141:1063, 1989.
37. Zalupski M, Baker LH: Ifosfamide. J Natl Cancer Inst 80:556, 1988.
38. Perry MC: Hepatotoxicity of chemotherapeutic agents. Semin Oncol 9:65, 1982.
39. Zimmerman HJ: Hepatotoxic effects of oncotherapeutic agents, in Popper H, Schaffner F(eds): *Progress in Liver Diseases,* Volume VIII. New York, Grune & Stratton, 1986, p. 621.
40. Woolley PV III: Hepatic and pancreatic damage produced by cytotoxic drugs. Cancer Treat Rev 19:117, 1983.
41. Rollins BJ: Hepatic venoocclusive disease. Am J Med 81:297, 1986.
42. Shulman HM, McDonald GB, Matthews D, et al: An analysis of hepatic venocclusive disease and centrilobular hepatic degeneration following bone marrow transplantation. Gastroenterology 79:1178, 1980.
43. Dulley FL, Kaunfer EJ, Appelbaum FR, et al: Venocclusive disease of the liver after chemoradiotherapy and autologous bone marrow transplantation. Transplantation 43:870, 1987.
44. Jones RJ, Lee KSK, Beschorner WE, et al: Venoocclusive disease of the liver following bone marrow transplantation. Transplantation 44:778, 1987.
45. Quesada JR, Talpaz M, Rios A, et al: Clinical toxicity of interferons in cancer patients: A review. J Clin Oncol 4:234, 1986.
46. Deyton LR, Walker RE, Kovacs JA, et al: Reversible cardiac dysfunction associated with interferon alpha therapy in AIDS patients with Kaposi's sarcoma. N Engl J Med 321:1246, 1989.
47. Rohatiner AZS, Prior P, Burton A, et al: Central nervous system toxicity of interferon. Prog Exp Tumor Res 29:197, 1985.
48. Lotze Mt, Matory YL. Rayner AA, et al: Clinical effects and toxicity of interleukin-2 in patients with cancer. Cancer 58:2764, 1986.
49. Gaynor ER, Vitek L, Sticklin L, et al: The hemodynamic effects of treatment with interleukin-2 and lymphokine-activated killer cells. Ann Intern Med 109:933, 1988.
50. Nora R, Abrams JS, Tait, NS, et al: Myocardial toxic effects during recombinant interleukin-2 therapy. J Natl Cancer Int 81:59, 1989.
51. Snydman DR, Sullivan B, Gill M, et al: Nosocomial sepsis associated with interleukin-2. Ann Intern Med 112:102, 1990.
52. Sherman ML, Spriggs DR, Arthur KA, et al: Recombinant human tumor necrosis factor administered as a five-day continuous infusion in cancer patients: Phase I. Toxicity and effects on lipid metabolism. J Clin Oncol 6:344, 1988.
53. Creaven PJ, Brenner DE, Cowens JW, et al: A Phase I clinical trial of recombinant human tumor necrosis factor given daily for five days. Cancer Chemother Pharmacol 23:186, 1989.
54. Creaven PJ, Plager JE, Dupere S, et al: Phase I clinical trial of recombinant human tumor necrosis factor. Cancer Chemother Pharmacol 20:137, 1987.
55. Kuei JH, Tashkin DP, Figlin RA: Pulmonary toxicity of recombinant human tumor necrosis factor. Chest 96:334, 1989.
56. Castellino RA, Glatstein E, Turbow MM, et al: Latent radiation injury of lungs or heart activated by steroid withdrawal. Ann Intern Med 80:593, 1974.

Chapter 152
COMPLICATIONS OF RADIATION THERAPY

DAVID G. BRACHMAN
RALPH R. WEICHSELBAUM

KEY POINTS

- *The clinical expression of radiation damage varies widely from organ to organ and may be delayed by weeks, months, or years.*
- *It is important to consider the possibility of adverse effects of radiation in any patient who has received radiotherapy.*
- *The affected organ may be a tissue that is within the radiation portal but is not necessarily the original site of disease.*
- *Complications of radiation may be modified by prior, concurrent, or subsequent chemotherapy.*
- *Life-threatening complications are seen, including radiation pneumonitis, acute and chronic pericardial disease, and endocrine hypofunction.*

In order to understand and deal with the consequences of any particular medical treatment, a basic understanding of the therapy itself is needed. Few specialties are as poorly understood by the nonpractitioner as radiation therapy. It has been estimated that 60 percent of all cancer patients receive radiotherapy at some point in their clinical course. Because of either the underlying illness or the treatment received, some cancer patients are likely to be found in an intensive care setting. Therefore, a conceptual understanding of radiotherapy is essential for effective management of these patients. A basic (and necessarily oversimplified) discussion of the physical, biological, and clinical aspects of radiation therapy will be presented, to be followed by a clinical case from our institution, along with pertinent points on diagnosis and management.

Radiation Biology

The therapeutic agent employed in radiation therapy is *ionizing radiation;* its principal lethal effect appears to be the induction of double-strand DNA breaks. The radiation itself can be either electromagnetic or particulate. The most commonly used clinically of the former are photons (x-rays and gamma rays); of the latter, electrons. Although the *physical* characteristics of the various types of radiation differ, their ultimate effects on tissue do not. Photons and electrons can interact directly with DNA or may instead interact first with intracellular water to produce free radicals. Free radicals are highly reactive chemically and are the proximate cause of most DNA damage with these types of radiation. The probability of a tumor or normal tissue sustaining damage depends on many factors, including the total dose of radiation and certain microenvironmental features—including the concentration of cellular oxygen and the presence of intracellular sulfhydryl groups. The organ expression of cellular damage, once it has been sustained, is even more variable. Normal tissues can maintain functional integrity through the processes of repopulation by undamaged stem cells or recruitment from outside the treatment area. Furthermore, as the vast majority of radiation effects are expressed at the time of cell division, the time to clinical expression of radiation damage varies widely from organ to organ, according to the cell turnover time characteristics of the irradiated tissue.

The extent and timing of cell renewal needed to maintain the functional integrity of a tissue forms the basis for the differential diagnosis of the various clinical syndromes seen following radiation therapy. Tissues such as gastrointestinal mucosa, bone marrow, and skin require continued cellular proliferation for proper function. Acute damage to these tissues is usually manifested during a course of fractionated radiotherapy. These reactions may be heightened by, and may present somewhat earlier with, the use of concomitant chemotherapy; but they are still characteristic for the organ involved (see Table 152-1). Those tissues, such as muscle and nerve, whose continued functional activity does not require regular cell renewal are often termed "resistant" to radiation, in distinction to the "sensitive" tissues noted above. These terms are misleading, however, because late effects usually limit the dose of radiation that is deliverable to a specific organ. Stem cell drop-out and small-vessel damage appear to be the final common pathways with respect to most late-occurring radiation effects. These effects typically take at least several months to occur, and may continue to be first manifested for many years post-therapy. In the above examples, the presumed ultimate cause of the observed effects is the same—i.e., the disruption of DNA by ionizing radiation.

Organ volume treated, total dose, fraction (dosage increment) size, and overall treatment time determine tissue response. External beam irradiation, with few exceptions, is delivered over a prescribed period of time in discrete increments (fractions) to a usually predetermined total dose. This dose is prescribed in grays (Gy) (1 Gy = 100 rads). As an example, in head and neck cancer patients treated with curative intent the total dose is often between 65 and 70 Gy given in fractions of 1.8 to 2 Gy/day, 5 days per week. At 2 Gy/day, this would require a total treatment duration of 7 weeks to reach 70 Gy. Commonly practiced radiotherapy treatment regimens—in terms of overall treatment time, total dose, and daily fraction size—have evolved in order to balance tumor control with short- and long-term treatment sequelae. The relationship between the dose delivered and the likelihood of tumor control, versus a normal-tissue complication, can be represented by a pair of sigmoidal curves, with probability on the vertical axis and total dose on the horizontal axis (Fig. 152-1). The degree of horizontal separation of the curves gives an idea of the therapeutic index—i.e., the likelihood of cure for a given level of toxicity at a certain dose. In addition to the total dose, local con-

TABLE 152-1 Selected Post–Radiotherapy Organ Syndromes and Their Management

Organ	Time to Onset after Start of Radiotherapy*	Syndrome	Fractionated Dose Range Needed to Produce Syndrome†	Clinical Signs and Symptoms	Etiology	Rx	Comment
Lung	Acute	Airway obstruction	≥2 Gy	Dyspnea, stridor, cough, hemoptysis, localized wheezing	Edema of endobronchial lesion(s)	Steroids (high-dose); bronchoscopic YAG laser, endoscopic stent, further radiotherapy (external beam or endobronchial ^{192}Ir) all potentially useful	Bronchoscopy or high-speed CT most useful in diagnosis
	Early	ARDS	Unclear, but probably >40 Gy to large volume	Progressive hypoxemia, not corrected with increasing FI_{O_2}; decreased compliance, etc.; diffuse pulmonary infiltrates, not limited to RT port	Capillary leak (?) type II pneumocyte loss	See Chap. 128	True incidence unknown, but appears rare; need to exclude other causes; histologic changes seen both in and out of RT field
	Intermediate	Pneumonitis	≥18 Gy (whole lung) ≥35 Gy (limited volume)	Cough, dyspnea, low-grade fever, occ. hemoptysis; linear/diffuse infiltrates corresponding to RT field; effusion uncommon	Type II pneumocyte loss with decreased surfactant production; ? hypersensitivity reaction	Supportive; steroids without proven role, but may be useful in severe cases; if instituted, prolonged use may be necessary to avoid flare upon withdrawal	Usually 6–12 weeks after completion of Rx and resolves in 4–8 weeks; worse with concurrent/recent use of actinomycin D, bleomycin, cyclophosphamide, methotrexate, and doxorubicin; variable progression to fibrosis

TABLE 152-1 Selected Post–Radiotherapy Organ Syndromes and Their Management (Continued)

Organ	Time to Onset after Start of Radiotherapy*	Syndrome	Fractionated Dose Range Needed to Produce Syndrome†	Clinical Signs and Symptoms	Etiology	Rx	Comment
	Chronic	Fibrosis	As for pneumonitis	Ranges from asymptomatic to ventilatory insufficiency; chest x-ray shows linear stranding from hilum, volume loss, pleural thickening	Progressive alveolar fibrosis within RT field	Supportive; avoid further insults	Chest x-ray changes stabilize at 6 months to 1 year
Liver	Early	Hepatitis	≥30 Gy, whole liver	Moderate elevation in AST, ALT; occ. jaundice; rare decrease in synthetic function	Sinusoidal congestion	Supportive; avoid hepatotoxins	Usually asymptomatic; recovery is the rule
	Intermediate	Hepatic insufficiency	>35 Gy, whole liver	Jaundice, ascites, decreased synthetic function, encephalopathy	Venous fibrosis	Supportive	Rare; avoided by partial sparing during treatment
Kidney	Intermediate/late	Nephrosclerosis	>20 Gy bilateral whole kidneys	Hypertension, edema; decreased GFR; epithelial casts, hyaline casts, microscopic hematuria	Small-vessel sclerosis	Supportive	Rare
Hemopoietic	Acute/early	Decreased counts	Highly volume-dependent; i.e., with total body radiation (TBI) ≥6 Gy; mantle radiotherapy ≥20 Gy; pelvic RT ≥40 Gy	Sensitivity; Lymphocytes ≫ Granulocytes > Platelets > RBC	Lymphocytes undergo "interphase death"; remaining elements experience variable degrees of maturation arrest	Supportive; recovery (full/partial) occurs along the timeframe of a particular element's half-life	Generally, precipitous drops are not due to radiation except for lymphocytes in TBI or total nodal RT; little effect is seen (either short or long term) when not irradiating either axial

							skeleton or spleen; marrow recovery in previously irradiated regions can occur over 4–8 weeks by either regeneration (lower doses) or repopulation (less than 40 Gy); greater than 40 Gy usually results in localized marrow fibrosis with compensatory hyperplasia in unirradiated areas
Heart	Acute	Pacemaker failure	≥5 Gy	Any manifestation of pacer failure from subtle alterations in sensitivity to complete pulse generator failure	Direct effect of radiation on CMOS (complementary metaloxide semiconductor) chips; bipolar-type chips probably less sensitive	Supportive; evaluation of patients native rhythm prior to treatment and continuous monitoring during the time the beam is on is recommended.	Avoid direct irradiation of pacer whenever possible; spontaneous recovery of pacer function can occur within minutes to hours but is inconsistent
	Acute/early	Acute pericarditis	≥40 Gy to large volume	Usual signs and symptoms of acute pericarditis	Direct cellular injury with inflammatory response	NSAIA/steroids; pericardial drainage if clinically indicated	Rule out malignant etiology
	Intermediate/late	Constrictive pericarditis	≥40 Gy to large volume	Usual signs and symptoms of constrictive pericarditis; 50% incidence of effusion	Pericardial fibrosis	Pericardiectomy	Hodgkin's disease, breast cancer most common reasons for RT; rule out malignant etiology

TABLE 152-1 Selected Post–Radiotherapy Organ Syndromes and Their Management (Continued)

Organ	Time to Onset after Start of Radiotherapy*	Syndrome	Fractionated Dose Range Needed to Produce Syndrome†	Clinical Signs and Symptoms	Etiology	Rx	Comment
	Late	Premature atherosclerosis	≥35 Gy (?)	"Premature" CAD	Intimal injury	Optimize on individual basis	Hodgkin's disease best studied; incidence probably ~10%.
Brain	Early/ intermediate	Hypersomnolence	≥35 Gy	Nonfocal except for excessive sleeping (up to 20+ h/day); EEG shows diffuse slowing; CSF mild pleocytosis, with moderate elevation of protein	Transient, widespread demyelination	Supportive; full recovery in 3–6 weeks usually seen; avoid further insults	Rare; usually limited to setting of RT and IV/IT methotrexate for pediatric leukemia
	Intermediate/ late	Radionecrosis	>54 Gy (whole brain) >60 Gy (limited volume)	Often mimics symptoms of recurrent tumor; patient may have decreased intellectual capacities, focal motor findings, 6th nerve palsy, papilledema. LP findings as with hypersomnolence syndrome; CT/ MRI nonspecific, often variable mass effect with low intensity center (tumor vs. necrosis); EEG shows high voltage, slow wave (c/w a destructive lesion)	Ischemic necrosis and/or stem cell depletion of myelin-producing oligodendroglial cells	Surgical therapy is both diagnostic and therapeutic, is often life saving, and can result in dramatic improvement; steroids can be of temporary benefit if significant edema is present	Positron emission tomography appears capable of accurately differentiating recurrent tumor (increased glucose utilization) from necrosis (decreased glucose utilization); worse with BCNU, other chemoagents

Hypothalamic-pituitary axis	Late	Hypofunction	≥45 Gy	Can be occult or overt; adrenal, thyroid, and gonadal function appear equally susceptible	Probable microvascular sclerosis	Replacement therapy as needed	Up to 66% incidence in patients receiving RT after incomplete removal of pituitary adenoma; 50% in similar patients without surgery
Thyroid	Late	Hypofunction	≥35 Gy	Varies with severity	Probable microvascular sclerosis	Replacement therapy	Increasing incidence with increased dose and increased time from irradiation; at 18 months, clinical hypothyroidism <5% incidence at 40 Gy but 20% at 60 Gy; occult hypothyroidism approximately double the overt incidence
Stomach	Intermediate/late	Ulceration	≥45 Gy	As expected	Single or multiple ulcers; exact pathophysiology unclear	Standard therapy	Low incidence (<3%)
Intestine	Intermediate/late	Obstruction	≥45 Gy	Subacute onset common	Small-vessel ischemia	Varies with clinical picture	Incidence <3% but more likely with previous surgery, history of GI disease, or concurrent chemotherapy

*All time periods are approximate. "Acute" refers to the time period during treatment; "Early" is from completion of treatment to 6 weeks after completion; "Intermediate" is from 6 weeks to 6 months; "Late" is more than 6 months after completion.

†Doses in grays (Gy); 1 Gy = 100 rads. *Unless otherwise stated, doses are literature minimums needed to produce syndrome at 5 percent occurrence level.*

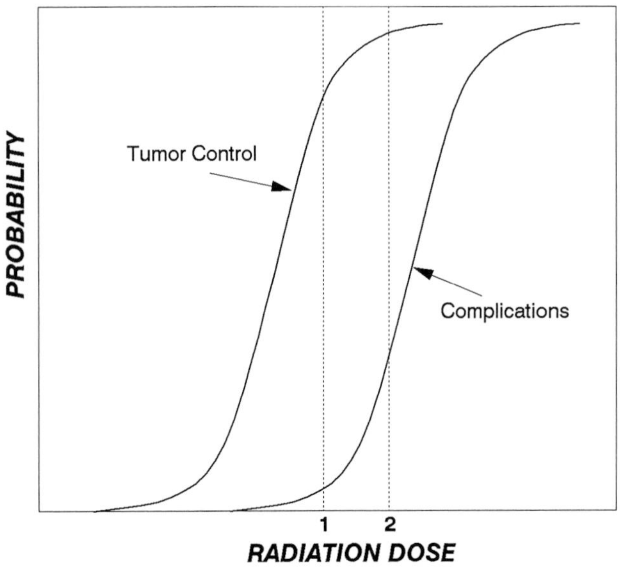

FIGURE 152-1 Graphic representation of therapeutic index. 1. Dose for tumor contour with minimum complications. 2. Maximum tumor dose with significant complications.

trol of a tumor is influenced by the overall treatment time involved and the fraction size. When the other parameters are kept constant, longer overall treatment times *or* lower doses *or* smaller daily fraction sizes may result in decreased tumor control. In certain circumstances where cure is not possible and the goal of treatment is palliative, it may be advantageous to shorten the overall time of treatment—e.g., when treating for pain or airway obstruction, or in other, similar, clinical situations. The dose per fraction is often increased in these instances; this larger daily dose—along with the accompanying decrease in overall treatment time—can result in equivalent tumor control rates with lower total doses. The increased daily fraction size may result in a higher likelihood of late sequelae in a patient in whom long-term survival is achieved. These same relationships apply to normal tissue damage, but an additional factor—*volume*—needs to be considered. The greater the volume of a particular normal tissue included in a radiotherapy field, the greater the deleterious effect for a given total dose. This relationship is often expressed as

$$\text{biological effect} \propto \frac{\text{dose} \times \text{volume}}{\text{time}} \qquad (152\text{-}1)$$

where "time" refers to the overall course of therapy (e.g., days or weeks). This relationship holds best for organs that are relatively homogenous in terms of function, such as lungs, liver, and kidneys. Generally speaking, one rarely irradiates an entire uninvolved organ, except when **1.** the anticipated dose is below the minimum tolerance level, or **2.** the involved organ is one of a pair, of which the second is known to have adequate function (i.e., one of two kidneys, one of two eyes) and is out of the beam path.

Clinical Assessment of Radiation-Induced Complications

In order to recognize the various possible radiation-induced complications, the physician encountering the patient must first be aware of the possibility of their occurrence. Radiation can be used as either a local, a regional, or a systemic mode of therapy. Examples of these uses include a very restricted *local* field for a pituitary adenoma; *regional* therapy, which, for a pyriform sinus cancer, e.g., would likely involve treatment to the primary site as well as the cervical and supraclavicular lymph nodes up to the entry point of the jugular vein at the base of the skull, the jugular foramen; and *systemic* therapy, which, e.g., would take the form of total body radiation prior to bone marrow transplantation. Thus, the affected organ may be a tissue within the radiation portal and not the original site of disease. For example, the close proximity of the pituitary gland to the nasopharynx mandates its partial inclusion within the treatment field for nasopharyngeal carcinoma, a commonly cured malignancy. If one is unaware of this, the diagnosis of secondary adrenal insufficiency as the cause of hypotension unresponsive to vasoactive drugs is unlikely to be considered highly in one's algorithm for a patient with a remote history of this malignancy. Likewise, little diagnostic energy should be spent on a finding that is clearly not related to previous radiotherapy. An example of this situation would be listing radiation pneumonitis among the etiologic possibilities of a right middle lobe infiltrate in a patient who had received radiation for head and neck cancer, where only the pulmonary apices are included in the radiation field (as they lie immediately beneath the supraclavicular lymph nodes).

CASE PRESENTATION

P.M., a 31-year-old white female, was transferred from an outside hospital for management of respiratory distress.

She had been well until 6 months before admission, when a chest x-ray taken because of a dry cough, fever, and weight loss had disclosed a large mediastinal mass with possible lingular extention. Matted left supraclavicular lymph nodes had been present on physical examination, and a gallium scan had shown uptake in the mediastinum, left hilum, lingula, and left supraclavicular nodes. Pathology from the left supraclavicular site had disclosed Hodgkin's disease, of the nodular sclerosis subtype. Neither bone marrow aspiration nor bipedal lymphangiogram had disclosed evidence of additional disease; the patient had been staged as II B. Combined modality therapy with three cycles of MOPP (mechlorethamine, vincristine, procarbazine, and prednisone), followed by mantle radiotherapy and three additional cycles of MOPP, had been prescribed at an outside hospital. After completion of the initial three cycles of chemotherapy, mantle radiotherapy had been undertaken to a midplane dose of 40 Gy in increments of 1.8 Gy per frac-

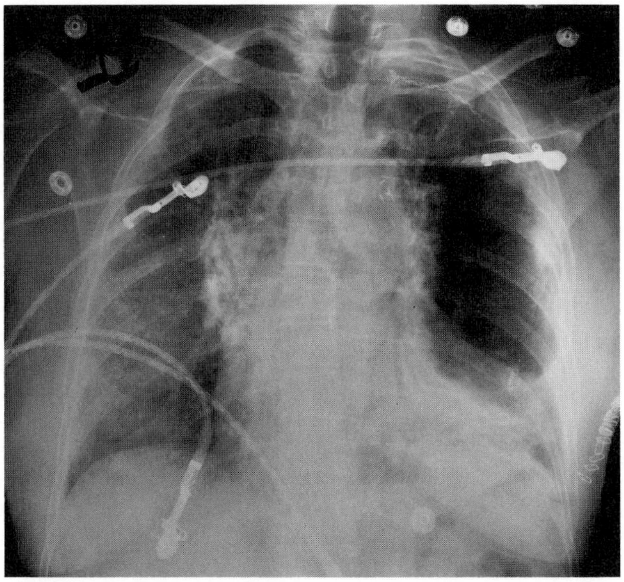

a

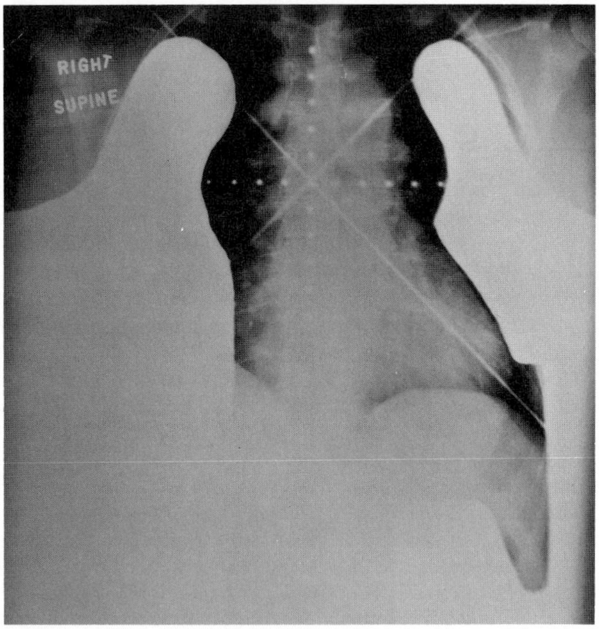

b

FIGURE 152-2 *a.* **Chest x-ray upon transfer, showing retrocardiac and bilateral hilar infiltrates. Patient is S/P open lung biopsy.** *b.* **Pre-radiotherapy planning x-ray ("simulation film") for patient's mantle field. The radiotherapy beam transits all structures** *not* **shielded by custom blocks. Note the very close concordance with subsequent infiltrates. (The uppermost portion of the field, not included in the photograph, includes the node-bearing regions up to the base of the skull.)**

tion; because of the possible lingular extension, no cardiac blocking had been used until completion of 30 Gy. Radiotherapy had been completed without difficulty, but shortly after the fifth cycle of chemotherapy (3 months after completion of RT) the patient had developed a nonproductive cough, dyspnea, and fever to 38.4°C, and had been empirically started on erythromycin. Four days later her symptoms had worsened, necessitating admission to the hospital. The white cell count then had been 2000, with 20 percent bands. Treatment had included second- and third-generation cephalosporins, erythromycin, trimethoprim-sulfamethoxazole, and acyclovir, but dyspnea and hypoxemia had progressed. A chest x-ray at that time reportedly had shown perihilar infiltrates; the differential diagnosis had included opportunistic infections, drug reaction, radiation pneumonitis, and progressive Hodgkin's disease. Serologic studies for fungal and viral infections had been negative, and bronchoscopy with biopsy had failed to reveal an infecting organism. Impending respiratory failure on the fifteenth hospital day had led to open-lung biopsy, empiric therapy with methylprednisolone, and transfer to this institution.

Physical examination on admission to our hospital revealed a thin woman in respiratory distress on 60% oxygen, speaking in short phrases. The respiratory rate was 34. Room air P_{O_2} was 35 mmHg, which corrected to 60 mmHg on a 60% oxygen mask. The admission chest x-ray (Fig. 152-2*a*) disclosed volume loss on the left with left lung base and bilateral hilar air space infiltrates. These findings corresponded well to the radiation port (Fig. 152-2*b*) and were consistent with radiation pneumonitis. Review of the open lung biopsy showed changes typical of that diagnosis and, furthermore, failed to show evidence of infection or tumor.

The patient was given supportive therapy, prednisone was given at a dose of 40 mg daily, and there was gradual improvement over 2 weeks. Pulmonary functions at discharge showed severe restriction (FVC 1.08, FEV_1.96) with resting hypoxemia (P_{O_2} 55 mmHg on room air); the patient was discharged on home oxygen and steroids, to be tapered slowly as symptoms allowed.

CASE DISCUSSION

In this patient the diagnosis of radiation pneumonitis is strongly supported by the radiographic localization of infiltrates to the radiation portal, as well as by the symptomatic clinical presentation at about 12 weeks after completion of radiotherapy and the typical histopathologic findings. These features, along with a lack of other demonstrable etiologies despite an extensive work-up, make pneumonitis the likely cause of her severe respiratory difficulties.

The earliest (and clinically silent) effect of pulmonary radiation seems to be upon the type II pneumocytes, with hyperplasia and early release of surfactant. After a latent period of 1 to 3 months, accumulated unrepaired genetic damage leads to a loss of reproductive capacity by both vascular endothelium stem cells and type II pneumocytes. The resultant depletion of endothelial lining cells and lowered surfactant production produce a situation in which capillary leak and increased surface tension both contribute to air space loss.

Chemotherapy before, during, and—to a lesser degree—subsequent to radiation may augment the pulmonary effects of treatment and lower the threshold for symptomatic radiation pneumonitis. Actinomycin D, bleomycin, cyclophosphamide, methotrexate, and doxorubicin are the agents most commonly associated with increased risk of pulmonary damage. Other drugs implicated as lowering the threshold of susceptibility to pneumonitis include medroxyprogesterone acetate (Megace), and propoxyphene-acetaminophen (Darvocet). The occurrence of steroid withdrawal–induced onset of radiation pneumonitis is a well-documented, but poorly understood, phenomenon. It tends to occur when drugs of this class are administered either during or shortly after a course of radiotherapy and withdrawn within the usual latent period seen for onset of radiation pneumonitis—i.e., 1 to 3 months after completion of radiotherapy. This situation can arise (as it did in our patient) when steroids are used in chemotherapy combinations or for coexisting but unrelated conditions, such as chronic obstructive pulmonary disease (COPD) or autoimmune disease. Similarly, too rapid a withdrawal of these agents after their institution for treatment of pneumonitis may also lead to a recurrence of the presenting symptoms. Treatment is the same in all instances; reinstitution of steroids at the lowest level possible to ameliorate the patient's symptoms after other possible etiologies have been ruled out. A recent study[1] of 590 patients with Hodgkin's disease who received mantle radiotherapy found an overall incidence of 6 percent for symptomatic radiation pneumonitis. Mantle radiotherapy alone was associated with a 3 percent occurrence, whereas the rate for radiation plus initial chemotherapy was 11 percent. Sixteen of twenty-six patients (44 percent) were treated with steroids, three were treated with antibiotics, sixteen recovered without further treatment, and one fatality was seen. The treatment of acute pneumonitis is largely supportive, the primary goals being symptomatic relief and prevention of additional pulmonary insults. There is no clinical evidence that the use of steroids in either the latent or the symptomatic state prevents or lessens the development of subsequent pulmonary fibrosis. Moderate doses (40 to 60 mg prednisone per day, or equivalent) are usually employed; once this treatment is instituted, the use of steroids may need to be continued for a prolonged period to avoid a withdrawal "flare."

The other significant finding encountered in this patient was not evident from either her physical, physiologic, or routine biochemical evaluations. As can be seen from Fig. 152-2, the thyroid gland is included in the "mantle" treatment field because of its close physical proximity to cervical chain nodes. The incidence of clinical hypothyroidism after this form of treatment is not clearly known; biochemical hypothyroidism has been estimated to occur in anywhere from 21 to 78 percent of cases.[2,3]

The incidence appears to rise with increasing time from treatment,[2] younger age at time of treatment, and increasing doses received.[3] Most cases are subclinical, but patients may fail to respond appropriately to dynamic testing with thyroid releasing hormone; this indicates a lack of ability to increase output under physiologic stress. Alteration of endocrine function after radiotherapy is not unique to Hodgkin's disease. Primary hypothyroidism has been reported following radiation for head and neck cancer,[4] and secondary hypothyroidism and adrenal insufficiency from pituitary failure have been seen after treatment for head and neck cancer,[5] pituitary adenoma, or medulloblastoma.[6,7] The diagnosis of primary hypothyroidism is often difficult in the ICU setting, as is discussed in further detail in Chap. 161. In this patient the T_4, free thyroid index, T_3, and rT_3 were all low; the TSH was high-normal. The decision was made, on the basis of both the biochemical findings and the a priori likelihood of hypothyroidism, to undertake thyroid replacement. After the drawing of a serum cortisol level, the patient was started on levothyroxine, 0.1 mg/day.

References

1. Tarbell NS, Thompson L, Mauch P: Thoracic irradiation in Hodgkin's disease: Disease control and long-term complications. Int J Radiat Oncol Biol Phys 18:275, 1990.
2. Mauch P, Tarbell N, Weinstein H, et al: Stage IA and IIA supradiaphragmatic Hodgkin's disease: Prognostic factors in surgically staged patients treated with mantle and paraaortic irradiation. J Clin Oncol 6:1576, 1988.
3. Constine LS, Donaldson SS, Link MP: Pediatric Hodgkin's disease: Pulmonary, cardiac, and thyroid function following combined modality therapy. Int J Radiat Oncol Biol Phys 16:679, 1989.
4. Posner MR, Weichselbaum RR, Fitzgerald TJ, et al: Treatment complications after sequential combination chemotherapy and radiotherapy with or without surgery in previously untreated squamous cell carcinoma of the head and neck. Int J Radiat Oncol Biol Phys 11:1887, 1985.
5. Perry-Keene DA, Connelly JF, Young RA, et al: Hypothalamic hypopituitarism following external radiotherapy for tumors distant from the adenohypophysis. Clin Endocrinol 5:373, 1976.
6. Snyder PJ, Fowble BF, Schatz NJ, et al: Hypopituitarism following radiation therapy for pituitary adenomas. Am J Med 81:457, 1986.
7. Pasqualini T, Diez B, Domene H: Long-term endocrine sequelae after surgery, radiotherapy and chemotherapy in children with medulloblastoma. Cancer 59:801, 1987.

SECTION M

RENAL AND METABOLIC DISORDERS IN THE CRITICALLY ILL

Chapter 153

ACUTE RENAL FAILURE

DAVID M. GILLUM
STEPHEN BRENNAN

KEY POINTS

- *Acute glomerulonephritis and vasculitides are the most common causes of acute renal failure (ARF) developing outside the hospital, whereas prerenal azotemia and acute tubular necrosis (ATN) account for the overwhelming majority of hospital-acquired cases.*
- *ARF is present in at least 10 to 30 percent of patients admitted to an ICU and is associated with a mortality rate of about 50 percent despite advances in supportive care and technology.*
- *The most important diagnostic classification to be made in the evaluation of patients with ARF is based on the site of the renal lesion (pre-, intra-, or postrenal).*
- *Since there are few specific therapies available in patients with established ATN, the major clinical focus is on prevention of ARF by identification of subjects at highest risk.*
- *All aspects of treatment of ATN, including dialysis, are basically supportive. The nondialytic measures of greatest importance are maintenance of nutritional, volume, and electrolyte homeostasis.*
- *Prophylactic dialysis is indicated when the blood urea nitrogen (BUN) value exceeds 100 mg/dL or the creatinine level is >9 mg/dL. Emergent dialysis is indicated in the management of ARF when pulmonary edema, hyperkalemia, refractory acidosis, or symptomatic uremia develops.*

Acute renal failure (ARF) can be defined as an abrupt decrease of clearance of nitrogenous waste by the kidneys resulting from a variety of processes. Such a process is initially manifest by rising plasma levels of BUN and creatinine and a variable decrease in urine output. This definition of ARF includes the designations of prerenal, renal, and postrenal causes. Postrenal causes of ARF include any process resulting in obstruction to urine flow; renal causes result from parenchymal insults (e.g., ischemia, nephrotoxins) to the kidneys. Prerenal causes of ARF are processes [such as volume depletion or congestive heart failure (CHF)] which result in hypoperfusion of otherwise intact kidneys. Prerenal azotemia is readily reversible following correction of the underlying disorder.

When considering causes of ARF (Table 153-1), it is useful to distinguish between hospital-acquired and nonhospital-acquired etiologies. Acute glomerulonephritis and vasculitic syndromes are much more common in the nonhospital-acquired ARF, while prerenal azotemia is the most common form of hospital-acquired ARF, accounting for 40 to 60 percent of cases,[1] with volume depletion, hypotension, and heart failure being the usual contributors. The condition of prerenal azotemia is a predisposing factor for the development of ATN from other insults (such as nephrotoxins, ischemia), and, therefore, must be vigorously sought and treated in the patient at risk. Postrenal causes of ARF are discovered in 1 to 15 percent of hospitalized azotemic patients,[1] with the largest number occurring in the elderly. Because postrenal causes are often reversible, it is imperative that these are recognized by the physician. Complete recovery of kidney function may ensue after relief of uncomplicated obstruction of up to 10 to 14 days' duration. Obstruction to urine flow is only partially responsible for the reduced glomerular filtration rate (GFR), however. It has been demonstrated that renal vasoconstriction occurs in response to ureteral obstruction, and this response is mediated by thromboxanes. Although most obstructive causes of kidney failure are extrarenal, it is diagnostically useful to consider intrarenal causes of obstruction resulting from occlusion of tubules by precipitation of crystals (e.g., uric acid, methotrexate, calcium oxalate, acyclovir) or protein (multiple myeloma). These forms of ARF often respond to therapy which promotes diuresis and high tubular fluid flow rates.

When prerenal and postrenal causes of azotemia have been excluded in the patient with ARF, then the diagnostic effort is focused on the renal parenchyma. One framework for delineating the cause of intrinsic ARF is to consider those processes which affect blood vessels, glomeruli, or tubules and interstitium. Pathologic processes confined to small renal vessels which may cause ARF include hemolytic uremic syndrome, scleroderma, malignant hypertension, and vasculitis. Occlusion of the main renal arteries by emboli, thrombi, or mechanical causes may also result in ARF. Acute inflammation of glomeruli (glomerulonephritis) or the tubulointerstitial compartment (acute interstitial nephritis) may also result in a syndrome of ARF. Of patients developing ARF, glomerular and interstitial diseases comprise 1 to 10 percent, but the most common cause of intrinsic acute renal failure is ATN.[1] In the critical care setting, ATN accounts for the overwhelming majority of cases of intrinsic ARF.

The principal factors predisposing to ATN are renal ischemia resulting from prolonged prerenal azotemia, nephrotoxins, and pigmenturia. Settings in which ATN may be commonly observed include emergent or elective repair of abdominal aortic aneurysms, major trauma, other postsurgical states, and gram-negative bacterial sepsis. ARF has been reported in 2 to 5 percent of patients admitted to general medical-surgical hospitals, but in patients admitted to

TABLE 153-1 Causes of Acute Renal Failure

Prerenal
- Volume Depletion
  - Gastrointestinal fluid loss, excessive diuresis, salt wasting nephropathy
- Volume Redistribution
  - Peripheral vasodilation (sepsis, antihypertensives), peritonitis, burns, pancreatitis, hypoalbuminemia (nephrotic syndrome, hepatic disease)
- Reduced Cardiac Output
  - Pericardial tamponade, complications of myocardial infarction, acute or chronic valvular disease, cardiomyopathies, arrhythmias

Renal
- Ischemia
  - Trauma, surgery, sepsis, pigment nephropathy (hemolysis, rhabdomyolysis), cardiac or aortic hemorrhage
- Nephrotoxic
  - Radiocontrast, antibiotics (aminoglycosides, amphotericin) nonsteroidal anti-inflammatory drugs, carbon tetrachloride, ethylene glycol, heavy metals (lead, mercury, arsenic, cadmium, uranium), pesticides, fungicides, cyclosporine
- Disorders of Glomeruli and Blood Vessels
  - Poststreptococcal glomerulonephritis, infective endocarditis, systemic lupus erythematosus, malignant hypertension, thrombotic microangiopathies (hemolytic uremic syndrome, thrombotic thrombocytopenic purpura, postpartum renal failure), Goodpasture's syndrome, polyarteritis nodosa, Wegener's granulomatosis; Henoch-Schönlein purpura, idiopathic rapidly progressive glomerulonephritis, renal artery embolism, renal artery dissection, bilateral renal vein thrombosis
- Interstitial Nephritis
  - Drug-induced
    - Semisynthetic penicillin analogues (e.g., methicillin, ampicillin, nafcillin), cephalosporins, rifampin, ciprofloxacin, cotrimoxazole, sulfonamides, thiazides, furosemide, allopurinol, phenytoin, tetracyclines, warfarin, phenindione
  - Associated with infection
    - Streptococcal, staphylococcal, leptospirosis, infectious mononucleosis, diphtheria, brucellosis, Legionaire's disease, toxoplasmosis.

Postrenal
- Malignancy
  - Lymphoma, renal adenocarcinoma, bladder/ureteral carcinoma, gynecologic cancers, prostate cancer, other pelvic tumors, metastatic disease
- Inflammatory Processes
  - Tuberculosis, inflammatory bowel disease, retroperitoneal abscess, postradiation therapy
- Vascular Diseases
  - Aortic aneurysm, renal artery aneurysm
- Papillary Necrosis
  - Diabetes mellitus, sickle hemoglobinopathy, analgesic abuse, prostaglandin inhibition, hepatic cirrhosis
- Intratubular
  - Uric acid, calcium phosphate, Bence-Jones proteins, methotrexate, acyclovir, sulfonamide antibiotics
- Miscellaneous
  - Nephrolithiasis, ureteral ligation, retrograde pyelography with ureteral edema, neurogenic bladder, neuropathic ureteral dysfunctions, obstructed urinary catheter

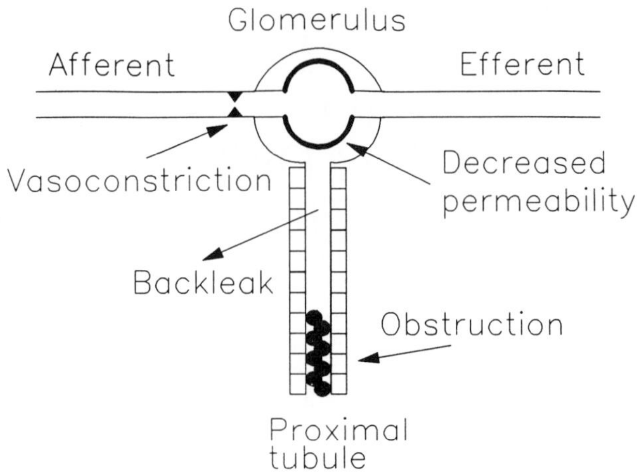

FIGURE 153-1 Pathogenesis of acute renal failure. Glomerular filtration can be depressed by vasoconstriction of the afferent arteriole, decreased permeability of the glomerular filtration surface, or obstruction of the tubular lumen by cellular debris, casts, or crystals. Filtration becomes ineffective when tubular backleak permits reasorption of normally excreted solutes. These factors are present in varying degree depending on the etiology of the renal failure.

ICUs, the incidence increases to 10 to 30 percent. Despite advances in dialysis technology and the great strides in critical care, the mortality rate for ARF remains high (20 to 80 percent), and development of ARF in hospitalized patients increases mortality sixfold.[2,3]

Basic research during the past decade has illuminated the physiologic factors[4] resulting in the loss of glomerular filtration in ATN (Fig. 153-1). The three leading pathogenetic theories to explain loss of filtration are hemodynamic, tubular backleak, or tubular obstruction. Investigators of a potential hemodynamic basis have focused on persistent afferent arteriolar constriction[5], loss of glomerular permeability, and efferent arteriolar dilation. Renal vasoconstriction is most prominent in the initiation phase of ATN although it may be evident in the maintenance phases as well. Nevertheless, when vasodilators are infused raising renal blood flow (RBF), GFR does not increase in parallel fashion suggesting other factors are of more importance in the maintenance of ATN.

Backleak of tubular fluid across denuded basement membranes and injured proximal tubule cells has been demonstrated in several experimental models of ARF,[6] and a recent study measuring dextran clearances in human ischemic ARF suggested a tubular backleak mechanism.[7] Intratubular obstruction arising from occlusion by cellular debris plays a definite role in the pathogenesis of experimental ARF[8,9] and likely contributes to human ARF along with tubule backleak and vascular factors.

Studies of cellular injury in ARF have examined the respective roles of increases in cellular calcium and the generation of toxic O_2 metabolites.[4] Elevation of free Ca^{++} in the cytosol exerts many detrimental effects including depletion of cellular adenosine triphosphate (ATP) stores and activation of phospholipases with a secondary increase in cytosolic free fatty acids. In view of these detrimental effects, investigators have argued that elevated cytosolic Ca^{++} is the primary mediator of cell injury with ischemia.[10] At present, there is no consensus regarding the role of Ca^{++} as the primary mediator of cell injury. However, while it remains uncertain whether an increase in cytosolic Ca^{++} alone accounts for significant cell damage during the ischemic period, it is likely that during the reperfusion period Ca^{++} may be of greater importance.[11]

Oxygen-free radicals are highly toxic metabolites which have been implicated in diverse pathophysiologic conditions including toxic chemical injury, radiation therapy, chemotherapy, acute glomerulonephritis as well as ischemia and reperfusion injury to kidney and other organs.[12] The toxic O_2 metabolites include superoxide (O_2^-), hydrogen peroxide (H_2O_2) and the hydroxylradical ($OH\cdot$) which is the most toxic of the oxygen-free radical species. Scavenging systems which protect the eukaryotic cell against oxygen-free radicals include superoxide dismutases which convert superoxide to hydrogen peroxide, catalase which catalyzes the detoxification of H_2O_2, and glutathione which reduces H_2O_2. The accumulation of oxygen-free radicals during ischemia results from the xanthine oxidase reaction. Stores of hypoxanthine are greatly augmented during ischemia, and the action of xanthine oxidase on the excess substrate likely results in the accumulation of oxygen-free radicals. While tissue protection from oxygen-free radical damage is evident in experimental circumstances following infusion of free radical scavengers and allopurinol, the subcellular site of damage due to these species is poorly defined. Phospholipases (A, B, and C) may also be activated during ischemia contributing further to tissue injury.

The mechanism of aminoglycoside-induced renal injury is not well understood. Aminoglycosides are tubule toxins and the earliest morphologic changes consist of vacuolization of proximal tubules, loss of brush border, and the presence of myeloid bodies within proximal tubule cells. Clinical evidence also attests to the tubular toxicity of aminoglycosides; maximum urine osmolality falls and renal wasting of Mg^{++} and K^+ ensues. The relationship between this tubule damage and reduced GFR remains unclear, although in experimental models using high doses of aminoglycosides, tubule obstruction and backleak can be demonstrated. In experimental models of aminoglycoside nephrotoxicity, relatively small doses decrease glomerular permeability while larger doses cause renal vasoconstriction. The relevance of these hemodynamic changes to human aminoglycoside nephrotoxicity is not known.

Myohemoglobinuric ARF resulting from intravascular hemolysis or rhabdomyolysis is characterized in animal models by an early, prominent reduction of RBF which can be reversed by volume expansion. Obstructing pigmented casts are a salient histologic feature of tubules in myohemoglobinuric ARF; however, the functional significance of these casts remains uncertain. Tubule obstruction is probably more important in the initiation phase of ARF, and tubule backleak seems to account for a small fraction of the reduced GFR.

Approach to Diagnosis of Acute Renal Failure

The diagnostic approach to ARF involves assignment of the cause to prerenal, renal, or postrenal categories, with further refinement of the diagnosis based on additional laboratory testing.[13]

HISTORY AND PHYSICAL EXAMINATION IN ACUTE RENAL FAILURE

Any decrease in effective perfusion of the kidneys can result in the syndrome of prerenal ARF. This may be the result of an absolute decrease in the extracellular fluid (ECF) volume, redistribution of ECF from vascular to interstitial locations (*third-spacing*), or impaired delivery of blood to the kidneys such as can occur in patients with renal arterial stenosis, vasculitis, or depressed cardiac function. Third-space losses should be suspected in the presence of severe burns, pancreatitis, peritonitis, or recent abdominal surgery. Absolute decreases in the ECF volume are most common in the setting of gastrointestinal fluid losses or in patients receiving excessive doses of diuretics.

Decreases in weight, if known, can provide some information about the degree of ECF loss. However, weight changes are subject to misinterpretation if the nature of fluid loss is not taken into account (Fig. 153-2). The ability of pure water loss (which is spread out across the total body water) to cause volume depletion is only one-third as great as an equivalent loss of isotonic fluid (all of which must come from the smaller ECF compartment). Thus, the im-

FIGURE 153-2 Effect of fluid loss on body water distribution. Because water is in osmotic equilibrium across biologic membranes, loss of 3 L solute free water will be spread across the total body water resulting in a small decrease (0.3 L) in plasma volume. A similar loss of isotonic fluid, which does not obligate osmotic water movement, leads to a much greater decrease (1.0 L) in plasma volume. This is based on assumption of 45 L total body water, two-thirds of which is intracellular. Of the extracellular fluid, about one-third is plasma and the remainder extravascular (interstitium).

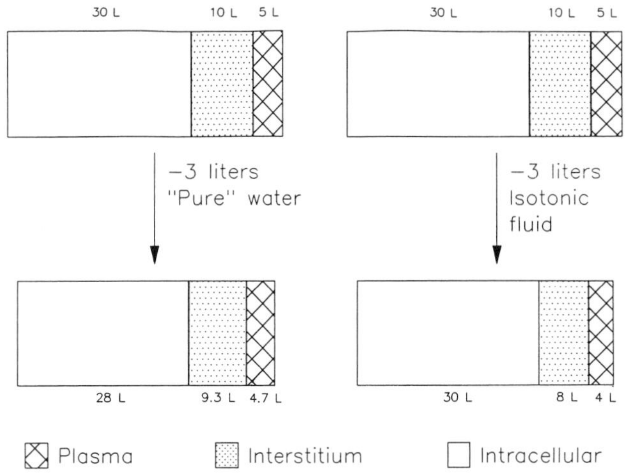

portance of changes in weight cannot be assessed without knowledge of the serum sodium concentration.

The cardinal signs of ECF volume depletion are changes in hemodynamic parameters and in the skin. An orthostatic increase in pulse of 15 beats/min or decrease in diastolic blood pressure of 10 mmHg can detect losses of 5 percent of the ECF volume. Skin changes which accompany volume depletion include cool, mottled extremities, dry mucous membranes and axillae, and skin tenting (particularly over the forehead and sternum, where age-related changes in skin elasticity are not as pronounced as elsewhere).

Obstruction of the urinary tract must be considered in every patient with an acute deterioration of renal function. The symptoms of acute urinary tract obstruction (severe flank pain, hematuria, changes in urine flow) are often mistaken for urinary tract infection. Of more importance from a historical standpoint is the identification of preexisting conditions which predispose to urinary obstruction. Some of these are listed in Table 153-1. Physical findings suggestive of obstruction include palpably enlarged kidneys, pelvic or abdominal masses, bladder enlargement, prostatic hypertrophy, aneurysmal dilation of the aorta, and signs of inflammatory bowel disease.

Intrinsic ARF can be the final result of many diverse renal insults. While space limitations do not permit a thorough review of all aspects of the history and physical examination in intrinsic ARF, some points deserve comment. ARF due to therapeutic or recreational drugs (e.g., cocaine-induced rhabdomyolysis) is so common that a detailed drug history is mandatory.[14] The presence of a skin rash should suggest the possibility of a systemic vasculitis with renal involvement or acute tubulointerstitial nephritis (TIN). Palpable purpura due to leukocytoclastic vasculitis is characteristic of Henoch-Schönlein purpura. One of the pulmonary-renal syndromes should be considered if prominent thoracic complaints accompany ARF. These include, among others, Goodpasture's syndrome, Wegener's granulomatosis, systemic lupus erythematosus (SLE), and Churg-Strauss syndrome.

TABLE 153-2 Urine Flow Rates in the Diagnosis of Acute Renal Failure

Anuria (<100 mL/day)
Complete urinary tract obstruction
Bilateral renal arterial or venous occlusion
Bilateral cortical necrosis
Overwhelming ATN
Severe acute glomerulonephritis
Oliguria (100–500 mL/day)
Prerenal azotemia
Intrinsic ARF
Tubular necrosis
Interstitial nephritis
Glomerulonephritis
Partial/intermittent obstruction
Polyuria/Nonoliguria (>500 mL/day)
Tubular necrosis
Interstitial nephritis
Partial/intermittent obstruction

DIAGNOSTIC TESTS IN ACUTE RENAL FAILURE

The majority of cases of ARF can be diagnosed by history and physical examination. However, in a significant minority, the cause remains obscure after initial evaluation and further evaluation is necessary.

Daily urine flow must be measured in patients in whom the etiology of ARF is obscure. Bladder catheterization is both diagnostic and therapeutic in patients with obstruction at the level of the bladder neck or urethra. Urine production is classified as anuria (urine output <100 mL/day), oliguria (urine output <500 mL/day), or nonoliguria (urine output >500 mL/day). Causes of ARF associated with various urine flow patterns are listed in Table 153-2. Prerenal ARF with polyuria may very rarely be seen if excessive urine losses are the cause of the prerenal state. This occurs in adrenal or mineralocorticoid deficiency states and excessive diuresis. Although occasional polyuric patients with urinary indices suggestive of prerenal ARF have been described,[15] it is believed that the majority of them in fact have polyuric ATN rather than prerenal ARF. The continued use of an indwelling bladder catheter after the cause of ARF has been determined is frequently unnecessary and merely increases the risk of nosocomial urinary tract infection. This is particularly true in the oligoanuric patient. Intermittent bladder catheterization once or twice daily can provide useful information with a lower risk of urosepsis. An external condom-type catheter does not provide sufficient information to replace the Foley catheter in persons with ARF. Because it is also associated with an increased risk of urinary infection, it cannot be recommended in this setting.

Urinalysis is also useful in patients with ARF. The urinary specific gravity tends to be >1.020 in patients with prerenal failure. On the other hand, patients with intrinsic or postrenal ARF are generally isosthenuric with urine specific gravity approximately 1.010. Substantial proteinuria (3+ or more) strongly suggests the possibility of intrinsic glomerular injury. Urine pH is generally more acidic in prerenal azotemia than in the other forms. Glycosuria in the absence of hyperglycemia strongly suggests proximal tubular injury. A positive reaction for blood in the urine is consistent with acute glomerular or tubular injury, urinary tract infection, or nephrolithiasis. If blood is present on dipstick but not microscopically, a pigment nephropathy (hemoglobinuria or myoglobinuria) should be considered. The urine sediment is usually unremarkable in prerenal and postrenal azotemia, except for occasional hyaline casts. In postrenal ARF due to stones, blood and crystals can be seen. Intrinsic ARF is often associated with a characteristic (or even diagnostic) urine sediment. A careful microscopic examination can frequently distinguish between glomerulonephritis, ATN, and TIN. In particular, detection of large numbers of eosinophils in the urine strongly suggests the diagnosis of drug-induced TIN. Hansel's stain of the urine is more sensitive than Wright's stain for the detection of urinary eosinophils.[16] The Hansel method correctly identified 10 of 11 patients with TIN, as opposed to only 2 of 11 correctly classified using Wright's stain. False-positive results with the Hansel technique are most commonly caused by rapidly progressive glomerulonephritis or acute prostatitis.

Several measurements of urine composition have been suggested as ways to differentiate between prerenal azotemia and intrinsic ARF in the oliguric patient.[17] Urine electrolytes are most useful in this regard, especially the fractional excretion of sodium (FE_{Na}), calculated as:

$$FE_{Na} = (U_{Na} \times P_{Cr})/(P_{Na} \times U_{Cr}) \qquad (153\text{-}1)$$

where U_{Na} and P_{Na} are urine and plasma sodium concentrations and U_{Cr} and P_{Cr} are urine and plasma creatinine concentrations. Values of $FE_{Na} < 0.01$ (1 percent) in oliguric patients suggest avid tubular sodium reclamation and prerenal azotemia with functioning renal tubules, whereas values >0.03 (3 percent) suggest tubular injury. The FE_{Na} is less useful in patients who are not oliguric.[18] Contrary to common belief, however, it may be useful in diuretic-treated patients. Although an elevated value may be a result of ATN or the effects of the diuretic, a low level in the face of diuretic therapy strongly suggests volume depletion and prerenal ARF. Some causes of ARF presenting with a low FE_{Na} are listed in Table 153-3. Other urinary diagnostic indices do not show any clearcut superiority over FE_{Na} in distinguishing prerenal azotemia from ATN; however, they are independently useful in the assessment of tubular function. A low U_{Na} (<10 meq/L) as an isolated measurement is often used as evidence of a prerenal state. However, this measurement depends exquisitely on the state of water balance in addition to sodium balance. It cannot be said that it is any easier to use than FE_{Na}, since an independent evaluation of water balance must be made to interpret it. Therefore, it is not recommended as an isolated measurement in the routine evaluation of ARF.

Injury to the nephron and urinary tract is accompanied by release of cellular enzymes into the urine. At this time, enzymuria is a nonspecific finding and adds little diagnostic information. Detection of renal tubular antigen in the urine may be a rapid, simple test for the diagnosis of intrinsic ARF, but it is not yet widely available. Urine uric acid: creatinine ratios > 1:1 are consistent with acute urate nephropathy.[19]

TABLE 153-3 Causes of Acute Renal Failure with Low FE_{Na}

Prerenal azotemia
Nonoliguric ATN
Acute glomerulonephritis
Acute obstruction (early)
Acute TIN
Contrast nephropathy
Nontraumatic rhabdomyolysis
Uric acid nephropathy

Several radiographic studies are useful in the evaluation of patients with ARF. Plain films of the abdomen can assess kidney size, detect >90 percent of renal stones, and detect skeletal abnormalities of secondary hyperparathyroidism which imply chronic renal insufficiency rather than ARF. In our view, the potential hazards of intravenous pyelography make this test of little benefit in the work-up of ARF. Renal ultrasound is a sensitive and specific method for detecting hydronephrosis. It is probably indicated in nearly every patient with ARF unless obstruction can be proven more quickly in another manner (e.g., by bladder catheterization in a patient with symptoms of bladder neck obstruction) or if some diagnosis other than obstruction is made with certainty early in the evaluation. If clinical suspicion of obstruction persists despite a "negative" ultrasound, retrograde pyelography is the definitive diagnostic maneuver. Computed axial tomography (CT) of the kidneys does not have any advantages over ultrasound and retrograde pyelography in the detection of obstruction, but may help clarify its cause. Radionuclide scans of the kidneys may be useful in the evaluation of patients with suspected vascular accidents of the kidneys.

The great majority of the time, volume status can be ascertained by history and physical examination alone. Occasionally, one is presented with a patient in whom the ECF volume status cannot be determined with certainty on clinical grounds, particularly subjects with significant third-space losses. A typical example would be a patient with sepsis, hypotension, noncardiogenic pulmonary edema, anasarca, and oliguria. In this case, the clinician is often faced with the contradictory choice of using either diuretics or intravenous fluids. It is obviously inappropriate to treat a patient as if volume overload and hypovolemia were present simultaneously; in this setting, invasive hemodynamic monitoring with a pulmonary artery catheter can be an invaluable diagnostic adjunct.

Clinical Syndromes of Acute Renal Failure

PRERENAL AZOTEMIA

The major symptoms and signs related to ECF volume depletion have been discussed in the previous section. It is important to emphasize that edema and prerenal azotemia can coexist in states such as CHF, cirrhosis, and severe hypoalbuminemia. Treatment of patients with prerenal azotemia in the face of massive peripheral edema is often a frustrating experience for both physician and patient. Causes of prerenal ARF are listed in Table 153-1.

In addition to a low FE_{Na}, common laboratory features of prerenal ARF are a BUN:creatinine ratio >20, polycythemia, mild hypercalcemia, hyperuricemia, and increases in plasma albumin and cholesterol levels. Metabolic acidosis may be present in patients with diarrhea or grossly impaired tissue perfusion (lactic acidosis); on the other hand, metabolic alkalosis is more common in patients with prerenal azotemia due to diuretic treatment or prolonged emesis. Hyponatremia is frequently present due to nonosmotic stimulation of antidiuretic hormone (ADH) release. When prerenal azotemia is suspected in the setting of adult respiratory distress syndrome or CHF, measurement of central pressures with a Swan-Ganz catheter can be invaluable. A diagnostic fluid challenge (500 to 1000 mL of intravenous isotonic saline solution over 30 min) is frequently helpful. There is no point in giving smaller fluid boluses or over a longer period of time; the rapid extravascular redistribution of crystalloid solutions markedly decreases the diagnostic sensitivity of more prolonged infusions.

Treatment of prerenal ARF is aimed at rapidly correcting the "effective arterial volume" to normal. Ongoing gastrointestinal or renal fluid losses should be halted. When there is an absolute decrease in ECF volume, expansion is best accomplished with intravenous isotonic saline solution or transfusions of appropriate blood products. In CHF, efforts to correct hemodynamic abnormalities should take precedence. In general, it is helpful to consider that peripheral edema is usually a cosmetic problem which can be tolerated if cardiac and pulmonary functions are adequate. Intravenous isotonic saline solution should be considered in patients whose renal function worsens with diuretic therapy. In the ICU, a common problem is the severely hypoalbuminemic patient with gross anasarca. One frequent approach to this type of patient is the concomitant use of various combinations of albumin (to increase oncotic pressure and mobilize interstitial fluid) plus furosemide (to accelerate renal sodium excretion) plus dopamine (to increase urine output). Under most circumstances this is unnecessary and may be harmful. If, as is usually the case, the patient has a low effective blood volume, the mobilization of interstitial edema will be short-lived due to the brief half-life of intravenously administered albumin. As edema reaccumulates, the vascular volume will become further contracted because of the imposed diuresis. Therefore, this course should not be undertaken unless cardiac filling pressures are already elevated or the edema is so severe it poses an independent threat to the patient's health.

OBSTRUCTIVE RENAL DISEASE

Urinary tract obstruction is found at autopsy in about 3.8 percent of the population (see Table 153-1). Between the ages of 20 and 60 years, women predominate due to pregnancy and gynecologic malignancies, whereas obstruction due to prostatism is the most common cause in men over age 60.[20] Intrarenal obstruction can occur from crystal or protein deposition within the nephron. In addition to structural causes of obstruction, neuromuscular abnormalities may result in a neurogenic bladder and a functional state of obstruction. Retroperitoneal fibrosis can be associated with urinary tract obstruction in the absence of hydronephrosis.

Some of the clinical and laboratory features of obstructive nephropathy have already been discussed. Additional findings include an elevated plasma BUN:creatinine ratio, impaired urinary concentration and dilution, hyperkalemia, and defective urine acidification. Hypertension is unusual. The two most important diagnostic tests when obstruction is suspected are bladder catheterization and renal ultrasonography. In rare cases when obstruction is still suspected despite an apparently normal sonogram, retrograde pyelography is indicated. Examples would be ARF in a patient with a completely normal urinalysis and subjects with a history of recurrent nephrolithiasis.

The degree and rate of return of renal function following relief of obstruction depend on the severity and duration of the initial lesion. Thus, early treatment is of paramount importance. The presence of infection in an obstructed kidney is a urologic emergency requiring immediate relief. The urinary tract can be drained with an indwelling Foley catheter, internal ureteral stents, or by percutaneous nephrostomy. Once the patient's condition has stabilized, specific therapy directed toward the underlying cause of the obstruction can be undertaken.

INTRINSIC ACUTE RENAL FAILURE

Postischemic/Septic Acute Renal Failure

The usual clinical settings in which postischemic ARF develops are the perioperative patient and following massive trauma. In most of these patients several factors act synergistically to produce renal insufficiency, including circulating myoglobin or hemoglobin, concurrent use of antibiotics, volume depletion, hypotension, use of radiographic contrast, and use of vasopressors. Therefore, in actual practice it is often impossible to ascribe the azotemia to a single cause. However, this is frequently unnecessary, since management of established ATN due to ischemia or sepsis is largely independent of the actual inciting agent(s).

The clinical features of ATN are variable. Normal urine output or mild oliguria may be seen early in the course, which can then progress to severe oligoanuria. Too often, clinicians tend to prescribe inadequate fluid early and excessive fluid late in the evolution of ATN. It is important to keep in mind that oliguria is a symptom rather than a disease; it is inappropriate to continue pushing IV fluids in established oliguric states simply to try to improve urine flow unless true volume depletion is present. The characteristic "muddy brown" urine sediment loaded with coarse granular and cellular casts, hematuria, cellular debris, and tubular epithelial cells is usually seen and practically diagnostic. The FE_{Na} is usually >3 percent, particularly in oliguric states. Ultrasound of the kidneys is generally unremarkable except for a slight increase in size due to parenchymal edema. Renal flow scan may suggest vascular disease; absence of flow is an ominous prognostic sign.

Nephrotoxic Acute Renal Failure

Countless diagnostic, therapeutic, endogenous, and industrial compounds are associated with intrinsic ARF. Herein are considered those toxic nephropathies associated with radiocontrast agents, aminoglycosides, cancer chemotherapy, and nonsteroidal anti-inflammatory drugs (NSAIDs).

AMINOGLYCOSIDES. Neomycin is occasionally used as a surgical irrigant or orally in preparation for bowel surgery,

TABLE 153-4 Risk Factors for Aminoglycoside Nephrotoxicity

Preexisting renal disease
Advanced age
Volume depletion
Obstructive jaundice
Severe infection
Drug interactions
Cephalosporins
Vancomycin
Prostaglandin inhibitors

and acute azotemia can still be ascribed to this drug, particularly in patients with preexisting renal impairment. Gentamicin is less toxic than neomycin but more toxic than tobramycin, amikacin, or netilmicin.[21] Perhaps the most sensitive marker of aminoglycoside toxicity is a steady increase in plasma trough drug levels on a constant dose. The serum creatinine level usually increases after 7 to 10 days of therapy, but urine output is generally well preserved except in severe cases. Occasionally ARF becomes apparent after the drug has been discontinued. A concentrating defect is an early sign of tubule injury and the patient may report polyuria. Enzymuria is not necessarily predictive of significant nephrotoxicity. The treatment of aminoglycoside nephrotoxicity is prophylactic and supportive. Given the growing number of antibiotics with broad gram-negative coverage, by identification of patients at high risk (Table 153-4) it is often possible to avoid aminoglycosides altogether and thus prevent the problem. Even the most careful monitoring of drug levels does not entirely prevent nephrotoxicity, especially if coexistent liver disease is present,[22] but its incidence and severity are diminished. Spontaneous recovery of renal function may be delayed for days or weeks after the drug is discontinued.

RADIOCONTRAST NEPHROPATHY. The clinical course of contrast nephropathy is characterized by an osmotic diuresis beginning within 30 min of contrast administration.[23] A rapid increase in serum creatinine concentration develops within 24 to 48 h after the contrast study; urine output is frequently well preserved but oliguria may be seen. The FE_{Na} is unexpectedly low (<1 percent) in many of these patients. The incidence of contrast nephropathy is <5 percent overall but greater risk is present in some patients (Table 153-5). The major therapeutic emphasis in contrast-induced ARF is on prevention.[24] ECF volume should be expanded prior to contrast administration in subjects in high-risk groups. Some clinicians use combinations of saline, mannitol, and bicarbonate, but our experience suggests that the particular regimen used is less important than awareness of the problem. Prophylactic dialysis to expedite contrast removal has not been beneficial.

TABLE 153-5 Risk Factors for Radiocontrast Nephrotoxicity

Preexisting renal failure
Diabetes mellitus
Volume depletion
Previous contrast nephropathy
Multiple contrast procedures
High contrast dose (>2 mL/kg)
Congestive heart failure
Elderly patient
Gout/hyperuricemia

CANCER CHEMOTHERAPY. In any patient with cancer and ARF, the primary diagnostic consideration is urinary tract obstruction. Once this possibility has been excluded other diagnoses must be considered, including drug effects (Table 153-6). The most common offending chemotherapeutic agents are cisdiamminedichloroplatinum (cis-DDP, cisplatin), the nitrosoureas, and methotrexate. Cisplatin causes dose-dependent ATN 4 to 10 days after the drug is administered. Renal magnesium wasting also occurs. The incidence of renal dysfunction due to nitrosoureas is a function of the cumulative drug dose. ARF and Fanconi's syndrome are the toxic effects of streptozotocin at cumulative doses above about 4 g/m^2. Nephrotoxicity is frequently seen where methotrexate is used in very high doses, usually accompanied by citrovorum rescue. Renal injury is usually the result of intratubular precipitation of methotrexate, particularly in acidic urine. Awareness of the potential nephrotoxicity of chemotherapeutic agents combined with appropriate prophylactic measures has greatly decreased the incidence of ARF due to these compounds.

NONSTEROIDAL ANTI-INFLAMMATORY DRUGS: Several different syndromes of ARF have been associated with NSAIDs. The most common is prerenal ARF due to decreased activity of vasodilatory prostaglandins, especially PGE_2 and PGI_2 (prostacyclin). This is particularly likely to occur in states of functional volume depletion, such as CHF, cirrhosis, and hypovolemia, in which the prostanoids may be critical in the maintenance of normal RBF. Some of

TABLE 153-6 Causes of Renal Dysfunction in Malignancy

Obstruction
Ureteral
Retroperitoneal lymphatic involvement
Primary ureteral tumor
Bladder neck
Primary bladder tumor
Prostate
Intrarenal
Intratubular crystallization
Light-chain proteins
Renal Parenchymal Invasion
Renal cell carcinoma
Metastases to kidneys
Tumor infiltration (leukemias/lymphomas)
Drug Effects
Cisplatin
Nitrosoureas
Methotrexate
Mithramycin
Mitomycin
Radiation Nephritis

the NSAIDs, particularly phenacetin, are associated with papillary necrosis and obstructive uropathy. The NSAIDs can also cause an allergic-type TIN which is unique because of the presence of nephrotic range proteinuria.

Acute Tubulointerstitial Nephritis

Inflammatory lesions of the renal interstitium and tubules occur in many clinical scenarios. The most common cause is an allergic-type reaction to drugs, but renal or systemic infections and neoplastic diseases can also lead to this complication. The most common offending drugs are antibiotics, NSAIDs, anticonvulsants, and diuretics. The so-called classic triad of TIN (fever, skin rash, eosinophilia) occurs in a minority of patients; however, an empirical diagnosis of TIN should be questioned in the absence of all three signs.[25] Tubular dysfunction (Fanconi's syndrome, distal renal tubular acidosis, hyperkalemia) occurs in the majority of patients. Substantial proteinuria is rare except in cases of NSAID-induced TIN. TIN may be idiopathic, presumably on an autoimmune basis, and occasionally coexists with anterior uveitis.

When urinary eosinophils exceed 5 percent of total urinary leukocytes, the diagnosis of TIN is highly likely. Gallium scans of the kidney are strongly positive in TIN but false-positive results occur in the setting of the nephrotic syndrome. The usual treatment is withdrawal of the offending drug and general supportive care. Steroids may hasten recovery from TIN but do not improve the generally good prognosis for this disorder.

Glomerulonephritis and Vasculitis

Glomerulonephritis is a generic term which encompasses a broad variety of entities whose final result is inflammation of the glomerulus. Postinfectious glomerulonephritis is the model for the syndromes of acute disease. Many bacterial, viral, fungal, and parasitic infections can cause postinfectious glomerulonephritis. ARF is more common in acute glomerulonephritis associated with visceral abscess formation or a recent streptococcal infection than in the face of other infections. Hematuria, edema, proteinuria, and hypertension are the rule, but typical nephrosis is unusual.

The common feature of vasculitis is inflammation and necrosis of blood vessels throughout the body. In patients with vasculitis, some degree of clinical and pathologic renal involvement is practically universal, although serious renal pathology is uncommon and ARF is rare. When it does occur, ARF is usually attributable to renal ischemia or crescentic rapidly progressive glomerulonephritis. Vasculitis in which renal disease is more prominent include polyarteritis nodosa, leukocytoclastic vasculitis, mixed cryoglobulinemia, Henoch-Schönlein purpura, and Wegener's granulomatosis.[26]

In cases of postinfectious glomerulonephritis, eradication of the infection is usually associated with resolution of ARF. Steroids and occasionally cytotoxic drugs are frequently useful in the treatment of vasculitis, SLE, Goodpasture's syndrome, and Wegener's granulomatosis. Aggressive immunosuppressive therapy is usually to no avail if oliguria or anuria has occurred. Adjunctive plasmapheresis is very useful in anti-glomerular basement membrane (GBM) disease.[27]

Thrombotic Microangiopathies

Hemolytic-uremic syndrome (HUS) and the closely related entity thrombotic thrombocytopenic purpura (TTP) are characterized by renal involvement early in their course. Renal disease tends to be more fulminant in HUS than in TTP. Nearly 100 percent of patients with HUS have ARF at some point in their course (which is severe in at least 60 percent) as compared to a total incidence of renal failure of even mild severity in TTP which is <50 percent. Clinical features of these disorders are more thoroughly discussed in Chap 147.

In the syndrome of disseminated intravascular coagulation, the pathologic picture is cortical necrosis. This can be prevented in some experimental models by the infusion of the angiotensin antagonist saralasin. Some authors consider malignant hypertension to be a form of microangiopathic nephropathy.[26] Acute deterioration in renal function is common if not universal in malignant hypertension. Renal failure is due to glomerular microthrombus formation and subsequent fibrinoid necrosis.

Tumor Lysis Syndromes

If large numbers of malignant cells suddenly die, as in spontaneous necrosis or successful chemotherapy of large tumors, ARF can occur. This is most commonly noted in patients with germ cell tumors or hematologic malignancies because of their rapid turnover. The tumor lysis syndrome is a nephropathy due to the toxic effects of intracellular constituents. The most common pathogenetic mechanism involved is acute urate nephropathy. When serum uric acid levels exceed about 20 mg/dL, the risk of ARF is high. The urinary ratio of uric acid:creatinine is >1. Synergistic factors in the development of the acute nephropathy include volume depletion and acidosis. The usual pathophysiology of urate nephropathy is intratubular deposition of urate crystals causing intrarenal obstruction. Less commonly, ureteral obstruction may be seen. Once oliguria occurs, diuretics are seldom useful in restoring urine flow.[28] Hemodialysis usually results in prompt improvement of renal function. Peritoneal dialysis is not recommended because urate clearances by this modality are 10- to 20-fold less than with hemodialysis. If dialysis does not result in diuresis within a week, ureteral catheterization should be performed to exclude ureteral obstruction. Allopurinol and alkaline diuresis are effective measures when instituted prophylactically, but do not reverse established urate nephropathy.[28]

Severe hyperphosphatemia (levels >20 mg/dL) can be associated with tumor lysis and subsequent ARF.[29] The pathogenesis of the renal dysfunction can be either intratubular crystallization of phosphate or metastatic calcification in the renal parenchyma. It is important to make the distinction between this entity and urate nephropathy, because urinary alkalinization will worsen phosphate crystallization. The treatment of this condition is aimed at reducing phosphate levels by diuresis. There may be a theoretical advantage in the use of agents such as mannitol which act in the proximal tubule, the major site of renal phosphate reabsorption.

Hepatobiliary Disease and Acute Renal Failure

ARF frequently occurs in the setting of severe liver disease. Prerenal azotemia can be a consequence of ascitic redistribution of the ECF (or its excessive treatment with diuretics), gastrointestinal fluid losses (vomiting, diarrhea, hemorrhage), or cardiac dysfunction (alcoholic cardiomyopathy). If a coagulopathy is present, blood clots in the collecting system can cause obstructive uropathy. Cirrhosis may predispose to the occurrence of papillary necrosis. Intrinsic ARF in subjects with liver disease is classified into disorders which simultaneously injure liver and kidney, and those in which the renal disease is a consequence of the hepatic process (Table 153-7). The kidney is generally much more sensitive to the effects of potential nephrotoxic agents if jaundice is present. A relatively specific glomerular lesion called cirrhotic glomerulosclerosis has been identified and is usually asymptomatic; however, it probably predisposes to ARF of other causes. The most serious of coexistent hepatic and renal diseases is the hepatorenal syndrome (HRS).

TABLE 153-7 Coexistent Renal and Liver Failure

- **Simultaneous Liver and Renal Injury**
  - Cardiovascular collapse/shock
  - Drugs and toxins
    - Chlorinated solvents
    - Heavy metals (arsenic, chromium, copper)
    - Antibiotics
      - Isoniazid
      - Rifampin
      - Tetracyclines
      - Sulfonamides
    - Acetaminophen
    - Mushroom poisoning *(Amanita phalloides)*
  - Infections
    - Viral hepatitis
    - Bacterial sepsis
  - Miscellaneous
    - Reye's syndrome
    - Acute fatty liver
    - SLE
    - Polyarteritis nodosa
- **Sequential Liver and Renal Injury**
  - Prerenal azotemia
    - Ascites
    - Alcoholic cardiomyopathy
    - Emesis
    - Excessive diuresis
  - Intrinsic ARF
    - Cirrhotic glomerulosclerosis
    - ATN
    - Hepatorenal syndrome
  - Obstructive nephropathy
    - Blood clots in collecting system
    - Papillary necrosis

HRS is difficult to distinguish from prerenal ARF in the setting of advanced liver failure; indeed, many authorities consider the two conditions to be part of a single spectrum. Perhaps the best operational definition of HRS is severe prerenal azotemia that does not respond to volume repletion. The principal functional abnormalities which have been described are renal vasospasm in the setting of peripheral vascular resistance which is abnormally low.[30] There is no "typical" structural lesion of HRS.[31] Oliguria and a low FE_{Na} are frequent if not universal findings; the diagnosis of HRS should be considered untenable in their absence.

The therapy of HRS has been very disappointing. A trial of empirical volume expansion with colloid solutions, with an end point of clear-cut increases in ascites and peripheral edema, can be used diagnostically to differentiate prerenal ARF from HRS. Attempts to modify low systemic vascular resistance have been unsuccessful in reversing this condition, as have attempts at selectively increasing renal perfusion.[32] Paracentesis, ascitic reinfusion, and use of peritoneovenous shunts have not produced substantial improvements in patient survival in the few available controlled studies.[33] Attempts to redistribute ascitic fluid into the vascular tree and then excrete it with various combinations of albumin, furosemide, and dopamine have not improved long-term results.[33] Hemodialysis and related modalities have not been shown to improve survival and cannot generally be recommended except in two general settings. If there is any doubt about whether the patient may have potentially reversible ATN (such as by demonstration of a $FE_{Na} > 1$ percent), or if the patient is a candidate for hepatic transplantation, all supportive measures including dialysis should be considered.

Pregnancy and Acute Renal Failure

The incidence of ARF complicating pregnancy has been decreasing for the past 25 years. This is attributable to improvements in prenatal care and obstetric science and fewer complications related to septic abortions. The timing of ARF in pregnancy has a bimodal distribution.[34] The early peak, which occurs during the first 20 weeks of gestation, is due to septic abortions, while the later peak (at 36 to 40 weeks) is secondary to preeclampsia and bleeding complications.

Preeclampsia and eclampsia are accompanied by decreases in GFR of 20 to 25 percent which are seldom clinically significant. However, in a small proportion of pregnant women, the renal dysfunction progresses to severe ARF. Women with preeclampsia are at increased risk for the development of cortical necrosis. Cortical necrosis can also occur as a complication of placental abruption (often with concealed blood loss) or prolonged intrauterine death. Although severe irreversible renal failure may be seen, partial recovery of renal function due to "patchy" cortical necrosis is more common.[35] The diagnosis of complete cortical necrosis should be established by renal biopsy or arteriography to exclude patchy cortical necrosis and ATN, from either of which a degree of functional recovery is to be expected.

Coexistent ARF and fulminant hepatic failure have been described in gravid subjects. In women with acute fatty liver of pregnancy, ARF is present in over half. Although the mortality rate for both mother and fetus in this condition has been reported to be at least 70 percent, the prognosis may be improving because of increased recognition of less severe cases. The recently described syndrome known by the acronym HELLP (hemolysis, elevated liver enzymes, low platelets) is a variant of unusually severe preeclampsia. The great majority of these patients have evidence of hepatic dysfunction and sinusoidal congestion which may culminate in liver rupture. The mean creatinine clearance in these women is about 55 mL/min (less than half normal), while 10 percent have severe ARF with creatinine clearance <20 mL/min.

The rare but well-defined clinical entity of idiopathic postpartum ARF[36] is characterized by the onset of ARF in the peripartum period following a previously normal pregnancy and childbirth. The serum creatinine level rises rapidly within a few days to several weeks following parturition. There is often an associated consumptive coagulopathy. Other common clinical features include malignant hypertension, lethargy, seizures, and a dilated cardiomyopathy. The pathophysiology of this disorder is unknown. The outcome is poor; most patients have severe chronic renal failure, require dialysis, or die.

Acute Renal Failure in Renal Transplantation

The approach to the transplant patient with ARF is no different from that in any other patient, with the exception that several unique entities must be considered. It is simplest to consider these in relation to the time since transplantation occurred. Within the first few hours or days after surgery, technical problems are the first consideration. In addition to hypovolemia and ATN, these include vascular thrombosis, ureteral stenosis, urinary leaks, and obstructive fluid collections such as hematomas or lymphoceles. Hyperacute rejection, though often apparent at the time of surgery, may not be recognized for several hours or days. Thorough diagnostic evaluation is mandatory, including renal ultrasound, confirmatory tissue typing (particularly the direct crossmatch), and occasionally angiography or transplant biopsy. Surgical intervention is often required in addition to the usual supportive measures.

During the period beginning approximately a week after surgery and continuing for the next several months, drug effects, acute rejection, and infectious processes are of particular concern. It is during this time that antirejection drug dosages are at their highest levels, and as a result, complications related to these drugs are most frequent. The immunosuppressive drug cyclosporine is a frequent cause of dose-dependent acute nephrotoxicity, and levels should be monitored closely. Therapeutic cyclosporine levels in whole blood are between 50 and 150 μg/mL. The clinical diagnosis of acute rejection is often difficult to make, frequently requiring histologic confirmation or empirical, antirejection therapy. Although an acute rejection episode occurs in the majority of renal transplant recipients within the first year following engraftment, it is increasingly uncommon thereafter. Thus, a diagnosis of acute rejection several years after transplantation is less likely as long as the patient complies with therapy.

One of the most frequent and severe infections compromising renal function in transplant recipients is cytomegalovirus (CMV), which can cause dysfunction in many organ systems, including the central nervous system (CNS), lungs, liver, and kidneys. CMV is often suspected clinically on the basis of fever, multisystem organ involvement (including ARF), and progressive leukopenia. It is more common in patients who have received intensive immunosuppression for severe or recurrent rejection episodes.

Late causes of ARF in transplant recipients include recurrence of the patient's original renal disease, de novo transplant glomerulopathy, infections, transplant artery stenosis, and urologic problems such as stricture or rejection of the ureter. In addition to renal ultrasound, transplant biopsy is often useful in defining the cause of ARF late in the course of a kidney transplant.

Prevention of Acute Renal Failure

Frequently, ARF develops in hospitalized patients in whom it is predictable and can be prevented or ameliorated. To intervene effectively, it is important to identify the patients at risk (Table 153-8). There is an additive interaction among the risk factors. Unfortunately, most attempts to modify the course of ARF are probably too late if tubular damage has already begun.[37]

PHARMACOLOGIC INTERVENTION

Diuretics

The evidence in the literature is by no means convincing that diuretics have a beneficial effect on the course of ARF. However, theoretical arguments as well as some clinical and experimental evidence suggest that diuretics are not entirely without benefit.[38,39] In particular, mannitol and loop diuretics can behave as vasodilators under some conditions and thus may be useful if vasospasm is prominent. Furosemide can diminish renal oxygen demand and may thus protect at least some nephron segments during ischemia. If the decrease in GFR seen in clinical renal failure is at least partly due to intratubular obstruction, high flow rates

TABLE 153-8 Risk Factors for the Development of Acute Renal Failure

Preexistent chronic renal failure
Volume depletion
Diabetes mellitus
Elderly patients
Postoperative patients
CHF
Urinary tract infection
Prior history of ARF

induced by diuretics may prevent nephron obstruction.

Mannitol may be effective in the prevention of ARF if administered before the occurrence of the renal insult. It is much less effective when given substantially after the fact. Its beneficial effects cannot be explained entirely by changes it induces in RBF. It is most useful in those situations in which a known renal insult is about to take place (e.g., radiocontrast administration or renal arterial surgery). Despite its greater diuretic potency, furosemide is less effective than mannitol in ARF prevention. The differences between furosemide and mannitol may be due to a greater degree of volume depletion in the furosemide group. In ischemic ARF, the loop diuretic was able to decrease renal injury if given before ischemia occurred.

Clinical studies have shown modest benefits of diuretics in human ARF. In groups of patients with established ARF, the need for dialysis may be slightly reduced, but there is little improvement in speed of recovery, and mortality is not affected by diuretics.[39] Urine output tends to increase, which may simplify fluid management. However, the repeated use of intravenous diuretics simply to preserve urine flow does not enhance recovery of renal function and cannot be recommended. It is our practice to administer a large one-time dose of furosemide (200 to 400 mg by slow intravenous infusion) once ARF has become established. If urine output does not increase, no further diuretics are indicated.

Calcium Antagonists

It has been suggested that calcium channel blockers may prevent or mitigate renal failure[40] by favorably affecting renal hemodynamics and inhibiting cellular calcium uptake. When given both before and after experimental renal ischemia induced by norepinephrine or renal artery occlusion, verapamil and diltiazem substantially improve GFR compared to placebo. Fewer data are available in clinical ischemic ATN. The studies which have been done are largely in the setting of cadaveric renal transplantation. In these studies, the incidence of delayed graft function (analogous to ischemic ATN) is decreased in patients receiving treatment with diltiazem, but long-term outcome is unchanged. Whether these agents can diminish the need for acute dialysis or lessen mortality in other forms of ARF remains to be seen.

Dopamine

Dopamine in relatively low doses (<5 μg/kg/min) is used in the treatment of ARF of many etiologies. It is clear that some patients will convert from an oliguric to a nonoliguric state when treated with dopamine. However, it has not been shown that most of the usual end points of ARF (mortality, length of hospitalization or ICU stay, need for dialysis) can be materially improved. It may be that so-called renal dose dopamine only hastens recognition of those patients whose prognosis is inherently good. However, even though dopamine alone has not been shown to improve outcome from ARF, there is a reasonable expectation that it may be of benefit when used in combination with other agents. The combination of dopamine and furosemide is more effective than either agent alone in raising urine output in oliguric states.[41] This is presumably on the basis of increased blood flow due to dopamine which allows better delivery of furosemide to its active site.

Several other agents have been used in attempts to modify the course of experimental ARF. These include atrial natriuretic hormone, ATP-$MgCl_2$, amino acids and small oligopeptides (e.g., glutathione), and thyroxine. It is of interest that ATP-$MgCl_2$ can exert its protective effects even if given after renal injury has taken place. Clinical data using these compounds are scanty or nonexistent.

Nondialytic Therapy of Acute Renal Failure

When a diagnosis of intrinsic ARF has been firmly established and potentially reversible causes have been excluded or treated, the patient is then monitored for early detection of complications. Conservative measures consist of hospital observation with attention to blood pressure, volume status, neurologic function, and evidence of hemorrhagic or infectious complications. Electrolytes (Na^+, K^+, Cl^-, CO_2, Ca^{++}, PO_4), BUN, and creatinine should be monitored daily, although the hyperkalemic patient will require more frequent monitoring.

Fluid intake should be adjusted to replace urine and insensible losses, while Na^+ and K^+ are allowed in amounts to replace urine and gastrointestinal losses. Obviously, fluid and electrolyte restriction will be more severe in the oliguric patient. A small, daily reduction in weight is expected in the patient with ARF, but weight loss >1 kg/daily indicates severe catabolism or volume loss. On the other hand, it should be emphasized that maintenance of weight or weight gain indicates volume expansion.

The guiding principle of nutritional management in the nondialyzed case of ARF is slowing the accumulation of nitrogen waste products and avoiding severe electrolyte perturbations. If the oral route can be used, the patient should receive a daily diet with 40 g high-quality protein to meet a minimum daily requirement of 0.6 g/kg. When dialysis becomes necessary, protein intake must be increased to provide 1.0 to 1.5 g/kg/day. Calories can be provided in the form of simple carbohydrates such as jelly and sugar. Caloric requirements increase in proportion to the severity of the underlying illness, and intake of 3000 kcal/day or more may be necessary to blunt catabolism. Should the patient be incapable of eating due to anorexia or other reasons, a small, soft feeding tube may be inserted into the stomach and tube feeding administered by constant infusion or intermittent bolus. In general, tube feedings with lower K^+ and Na^+ concentrations are chosen. For the patient who cannot tolerate enteral feeding, total parenteral nutrition (TPN) becomes necessary. Because of the volume of fluid required for TPN, earlier institution of dialysis and ultrafiltration is often necessary.

The management of various electrolyte abnormalities often associated with ARF is described in greater detail in Chap. 156 and will only be touched upon here. Administration of excessive amounts of free water is the most common cause of hyponatremia in patients with ARF. Less important causes of hyponatremia in this setting include water production from carbohydrate metabolism and water release from injured tissue. Judicious fluid management will prevent any untoward complications from hyponatremia. Hyperkalemia is the most grave of the electrolyte perturbations which may complicate ARF. The clinical consequences of hyperkalemia are largely confined to the cardiovascular and neuromuscular systems. The earliest hyperkalemic effects are manifest in the ECG. ECG changes are uniformly present above a K^+ of 8 meq/L; below 7 meq/L changes may not be evident. The treatment of hyperkalemia is summarized in Table 153-9.

Disturbances of divalent ion metabolism are common in ARF. Hyperphosphatemia is an almost universal accompaniment of oliguric ARF. Control of hyperphosphatemia in the acute setting is achieved by oral administration of aluminum hydroxide gels. Short-term administration of aluminum-containing compounds to patients with renal failure does not result in aluminum intoxication. However, concurrent administration of oral citrate compounds must be avoided, because citrate enhances gut absorption of aluminum and accelerates the development of aluminum intoxication.

Hypocalcemia is an expected complication of ARF, but is generally of no clinical significance and does not require intervention. Severe depression of serum Ca^{++} may complicate rhabdomyolysis-induced ARF, however. Nevertheless, calcium salts are contraindicated except as part of the treatment of life-threatening hyperkalemia or if hypocalcemic tetany develops. Hypercalcemia may be observed when rhabdomyolysis-induced ARF enters the diuretic phase, and Ca^{++} deposited in damaged muscle is released. It is usually self-limited.

Uric acid levels may rise by 1 to 2 mg/dL/day in cases of ARF not due to rhabdomyolysis, but rarely does the level exceed 15 mg/dL. This plateau is thought to result from enhanced metabolism of uric acid by gut bacteria. Extreme elevations in uric acid levels have been observed in cases of exertional rhabdomyolysis and following treatment of some lymphomas.

Metabolic acidosis occurs commonly in ARF, and in cases of trauma or sepsis the fall in plasma bicarbonate may exceed 15 meq/24 h. In the catabolic patient with ARF, acid is released from metabolism of sulfur- and phosphorus-containing compounds, all of which contribute to a rise in the anion gap. Acidosis may be treated with sodium bicarbonate; however, the additional volume is hazardous in the patient with compromised renal function. Uncontrollable acidosis may mandate dialysis therapy.

Metabolic alkalosis may complicate ARF in the patient with nasogastric suction, but is a less frequent acid-base disturbance in these patients. Although nasogastric suction-induced metabolic alkalosis normally responds to saline supplementation, this maneuver is ineffective in ARF and carries the hazard of potential volume overload. Severe metabolic alkalosis in ARF may require dialysis using a reduced concentration of bicarbonate or acetate in the bath. Alternatively, 0.1 *N* HCl may be administered by slow intravenous infusion. Development of metabolic alkalosis in the patient on nasogastric suction may be prevented or attenuated by use of histamine H_2 blockers such as cimetidine.

Infection continues to be a leading cause of death in the patient with ARF, and pneumonia, urinary tract infection, and wound infection are most common. Infection has been the cause of death in up to 70 percent of cases of ARF and has contributed to 50 percent of deaths occurring during the diuretic phase.[42] In several large series of ARF, the incidence of septicemia exceeds 50 percent, and intraabdominal sepsis is known to be a particularly important determinant of survival. In the septic patient without an obvious source, intraabdominal sepsis must be vigorously excluded. Imaging procedures of value for detecting an abdominal source include CT scanning and ultrasound, with CT scan the better of the two. The severity of infection in ARF is undiminished despite the advent of new antibiotics and other advances in general medical care. Prophylactic antibiotics are not recommended for the patient with ARF and may be harmful.

Prior to the use of antacids and histamine H_2 blockers (cimetidine, ranitidine) to prevent gastric stress ulceration in ARF, gastrointestinal hemorrhage was the second lead-

TABLE 153-9 Therapy of Hyperkalemia

Drug	Dose	Onset	Duration	Mechanism
Ca gluconate	10–20 mL IV	1–5 min	0.5 h	Membrane antagonist
$NaHCO_3$	1–2 ampules (44–88 meq) IV	30 min	1–4 h	Cellular shift
Glucose + insulin	500 mL $D_{10}W$ with 10 U reg insulin IV	30 min	1–4 h	Cellular shift
Polystyrene sulfonate (Kayexalate)	30–50 g with sorbitol PO, or as retention enema	1–2 h	4–6 h	Increased excretion

ing cause of death. Now, many centers report a dramatic decline in gastrointestinal hemorrhage.[43] Recent advances in the therapy of uremic bleeding include use of deamino-8-1-arginine vasopressin (DDAVP), cryoprecipitate, and conjugated estrogens.[44] These drugs are most useful in patients with clinically significant bleeding episodes who lack evidence of any other (nonuremic) coagulopathy. DDAVP is typically infused over 30 min in a dose of 0.3 μg/kg body weight and is effective within minutes.[45] Unfortunately, because of the short duration of action of this compound (1 to 4 h) frequent dosing may be required. The use of cryoglobulin infusions (10 U intravenously over 15 min) may also serve as a temporary expedient in patients with uremic bleeding. Conjugated estrogens (0.6 mg/kg intravenously daily for 5 days) have a very delayed onset of action (3 to 5 days) but the duration of the therapeutic effect can be as long as 14 days.[46]

In the absence of other strong indications, it is recommended that prophylactic dialysis be initiated when the BUN value exceeds 100 mg/dL or the serum creatinine level exceeds 9 mg/dL. This recommendation is based on a recent prospective evaluation of the role of intensive dialysis in the management of ARF.[47] It is important to recognize, however, that in patients with reduced muscle mass (e.g., the elderly), serum creatinine clearance may be lower than expected for a given degree of renal dysfunction. In these settings dialysis is initiated at creatinine levels significantly < 9 mg/dL.

The most common indications for urgent dialysis include volume overload and pulmonary edema, pericarditis, refractory hyperkalemia, uncontrollable acidosis and CNS manifestations of uremia including encephalopathy and seizures.

CASE PRESENTATION

A 72-year-old black female with a 30-year history of essential hypertension and noninsulin-dependent diabetes mellitus presented to the emergency room complaining of the abrupt onset of severe colicky periumbilical abdominal pain. She denied previous episodes of abdominal pain, and thought she had been in relatively good health. The initial evaluation was nonspecific, and she was placed in an observation unit. Laboratory evaluation revealed the following: serum sodium 142 meq/L, potassium 4.8 meq/L, chloride 102 meq/L, carbon dioxide content 24 meq/L, creatinine 0.9 mg/dL, BUN 18 mg/dL, and glucose 188 mg/dL. Urinalysis was unremarkable and serum amylase was normal. A supine abdominal x-ray demonstrated modest dilation of several loops of small bowel. Four hours later the intensity of the abdominal pain had increased, her temperature had risen to 38.2°C (101.8°F), and tachycardia had supervened. Repeat abdominal x-rays revealed progressive dilation of the small bowel loops with the additional finding of irregular thickening of the bowel wall. Mesenteric angiography was performed, demonstrating significant occlusive disease involving the origins of the celiac axis, superior and inferior mesenteric arteries, and an acute occlusion with bowel infarction in the territory of the superior mesenteric artery. Broad-spectrum antibiotics and pressor support were initiated, and the patient was taken to surgery for resection of necrotic bowel and revascularization of the compromised segments. Pressor support was required throughout the surgery. Postoperatively in the ICU the patient was noted to be oliguric. Laboratory evaluation at that time revealed a serum sodium of 136, potassium 5.7, chloride 94, carbon dioxide 17, BUN 47, creatinine 1.9. Urinalysis demonstrated occasional dark granular casts and an FE_{Na} of 3.6 percent. A diagnosis of ATN was made. Furosemide, 1 mg/kg, was administered IV, followed by a second dose of 5 mg/kg after 1 h when there was no response to the initial dose. Oliguria persisted, and no additional furosemide was administered. Dopamine was continued at 10 μg/kg/min for blood pressure support. TPN was begun, and broad-spectrum antibiotics continued. Over the next 3 days daily urine output remained <200 mL, and the serum creatinine and BUN rose progressively to levels of 5.6 mg/dL and 114 mg/dL, respectively. Progressive volume overload resulting from TPN, medications, and blood products necessitated ultrafiltration of 4 L on day 2, and regular hemodialysis was initiated on day 3 via a double-lumen subclavian catheter. The patient remained dialysis dependent for 16 days; dialysis and/or ultrafiltration were required 4 to 5 days each week. On day 13 the urine output had increased to 550 mL, and by day 17 urine output had increased to over 2 L/24 h. By day 16 the serum creatinine level plateaued and began falling spontaneously the next day. Over the next 6 days the serum creatinine level fell to a base line of 1.7 mg/dL.

CASE DISCUSSION

This case study illustrates a typical course of oliguric ATN. The etiology was multifactorial and included gram-negative septicemia, radiocontrast nephrotoxicity, and renal ischemia during surgical revascularization of the small bowel. Supporting evidence for the diagnosis included the FE_{Na} of 3.6 percent, pigmented urinary casts, absence of obstructive uropathy, and an appropriate clinical setting. The patient was markedly catabolic, explaining the rapid rise of the BUN level and institution of hemodialysis on day 3. Ultrafiltration was performed a day earlier because of progressive volume overload in the setting of oliguria. Over the next 2 weeks the patient remained oliguric and dialysis dependent. The therapeutic objective of dialysis was to maintain the predialysis BUN value <100 mg/dL and to avoid other complications of ARF such as volume overload and hyperkalemia. PN was continued until the patient had an adequate oral intake. Her recovery from ATN was heralded by the increasing urine output, followed by stabilization, and ultimately spontaneous decrease, in the serum creatinine to near normal levels.

References

1. Hou SH, Bushinsky DA, Wish JB, et al: Hospital-acquired renal insufficiency: A prospective study. Am J Med 74:243, 1983.
2. Kennedy AC, Burton JA, Lukes RG, et al: Factors affecting the prognosis in acute renal failure. Q J Med 42:73, 1973.
3. Thibault GE, Mulley AG, Barnett OG, et al: Medical intensive care: Indications, interventions and outcomes. N Engl J Med 302:938, 1980.
4. Bonventre JV, Leaf A, Malis CD: Nature of the cellular insult in acute renal failure, in Brenner BM, Lazarus JM (eds): *Acute Renal Failure.* 2d ed., New York, Churchill Livingstone, 1988, p 3.
5. Brezis M, Rosen S, Silva P, Epstein FH: Renal ischemia: A new perspective. Kidney Int 26:375, 1984.
6. Donohoe FJ, Venkatachalam MA, Bernard DB, Levinsky NG: Tubular leakage and obstruction after renal ischemia: Structure-function correlations. Kidney Int 13:208, 1978.
7. Myers BD, Chui F, Hilberman M, Michaels AS: Transtubular leakage of glomerular filtrate in human acute renal failure. Am J Physiol 237:F319, 1978.
8. Venkatachalam MA, Bernard DB, Donohoe JF, Levinsky NG: Ischemic damage and repair in the rat proximal tubule: Differences among the S_1, S_2, and S_3 segments. Kidney Int 14:31, 1978.
9. Patel R, McKenzie JK, McQueen EG: Tamm-Horsfall urinary mucoprotein and tubular obstruction by casts in acute renal failure: Lancet 1:457, 1964.
10. Schanne FAX, Kane AB, Young EE, Farber JC: Calcium dependence of toxic cell death: A final common pathway. Science 206:700, 1977.
11. Malis CD, Bonventre JV: Mechanism of calcium potentiation of oxygen free radical injury to renal mitochondria. A model for post-ischemic and toxic mitochondrial damage. J Biol Chem 261:14201, 1986.
12. Slater TF: Free-radical mechanisms in tissue injury. Biochem J 222:1, 1984.
13. Rudnick MR, Bastl CA, Elfinbein IB, et al: The differential diagnosis of acute renal failure, in Brenner BM, Lazarus JM (eds): *Acute Renal Failure.* 2d ed., New York, Churchill Livingstone, 1988, p 177.
14. Koffler A, Friedler RM, Massry SG: Acute renal failure due to non-traumatic rhabdomyolysis. Ann Intern Med 85:23, 1976.
15. Miller PD, Krebs RA, Neal BJ, McIntyre DO: Polyuric prerenal failure. Ann Intern Med 140:907, 1980.
16. Nolan CR, Anger MS, Kelleher SP: Eosinophiluria—A new method of detection and definition of the clinical spectrum. N Engl J Med 315:1516, 1986.
17. Miller TR, Anderson RJ, Linas SL, et al: Urinary diagnostic indices in acute renal failure. A prospective study. Ann Intern Med 89:47, 1978.
18. Pru C, Kjellstrand CM: The FE_{Na} test is of no prognostic value in acute renal failure. Nephron 36:20, 1984.
19. Kelton J, Kelley WH, Holmes EW: A rapid method for the diagnosis of acute uric acid nephropathy. Arch Intern Med 138:612, 1978.
20. Bell ET: *Renal Diseases.* Philadelphia, Lea & Febiger, 1946. pp 113–139.
21. Meyers RD: Risk factors and comparisons of clinical nephrotoxicity of aminoglycosides. Am J Med 80 (suppl B):119, 1986.
22. Desai TK, Tsang TK: Aminoglycoside nephrotoxicity in obstructive jaundice. Am J Med 85:47, 1988.
23. D'Elia JA, Gleason RE, Alday M, et al: Nephrotoxicity from angiographic contrast material. A prospective study. Am J Med 72:719, 1982.
24. Parfrey PS, Griffiths SM, Barrett BJ, et al: Contrast material-induced renal failure in patients with diabetes mellitus, renal insufficiency, or both. N Engl J Med 320:143, 1989.
25. Linton AL, Clark WF, Driedger AA, et al: Acute interstitial nephritis due to drugs. Review of the literature with a report of nine cases. Ann Intern Med 93:735, 1980.
26. Salant DJ, Adler S, Bernard DB, Stilmant MM: Acute renal failure associated with renal vascular disease, vasculitis, glomerulonephritis, and nephrotic syndrome, in Brenner BM, Lazarus JM (eds): *Acute Renal Failure.* 2d ed. New York, Churchill Livingstone, 1988, p 371.
27. Thysell H, Bygren P, Bengtsson V, et al: Immunosuppression and the additive effect of plasma exchange in the treatment of rapidly progressive glomerulonephritis. Acta Med Scand 212:107, 1982.
28. Robinson RR, Yarger WE: Acute uric acid nephropathy. Editorial. Arch Intern Med 137:839, 1977.
29. Kaplan BS, Hebert D, Morrell RE: Acute renal failure induced by hyperphosphatemia in acute lymphoblastic leukemia. Can Med Assoc J 124:429, 1981.
30. Epstein M, Schneider N, Befeler B: Relationship between systemic and intrarenal hemodynamics in cirrhosis. J Lab Clin Med 89:1175, 1977.
31. Papper S: Hepatorenal syndrome. Contrib Nephrol 23:55, 1980.
32. Cohn JN, Tristani FE, Khatri M: Renal vasodilator therapy in the hepatorenal syndrome. Med Ann DC 39:1, 1970.
33. Levenson DJ, Skorecki KL, Newell GC, Narins RG: Acute renal failure associated with hepatobiliary disease, in Brenner BM, Lazarus JM (eds): *Acute Renal Failure.* 2d ed. New York, Churchill Livingstone, 1988, p 535.
34. Chugh KS, Singhal PC, Shamra BK, et al: Acute renal failure of obstetric origin. Obstet Gynecol 48:642, 1976.
35. Kleinknecht D, Grunfeld JP, Gomez PC, et al: Diagnostic procedures and long-term prognosis in bilateral renal cortical necrosis. Kidney Int 4:390, 1973.
36. Ferris TF: Postpartum renal insufficiency. Kidney Int 14:383, 1978.
37. Schusterman N, Strom BL, Murray TG, et al: Risk factors and outcome of hospital-acquired acute renal failure. Am J Med 83:65, 1987.
38. Levinsky NG, Bernard DB: Mannitol and loop diuretics in acute renal failure, in Brenner BM, Lazarus JM (eds): *Acute Renal Failure.* 2d ed. New York, Churchill Livingstone, 1988, p 841.
39. Cantarovich F, Galli C, Benedetti L, et al: High dose frusemide in established acute renal failure. Br Med J 4:449, 1973.
40. Russell JD, Churchill DN: Calcium antagonists and acute renal failure. Am J Med 87:306, 1989.
41. Lindner A: Synergism of dopamine and furosemide in diuretic resistant, oliguric acute renal failure. Nephron 33:121, 1983.
42. Montgomerie JZ, Kalmanson GM, Guze LB: Renal failure and infection. Medicine 47:1, 1968.
43. Remuzzi G: Bleeding in renal failure. Lancet 1:1205, 1988.
44. Bridges KR: Hemorrhagic complications associated with renal failure. J Crit Illness 4:17, 1989.
45. Mannucci PM, Remuzzi G, Pusineri F, et al: Deamino-8-D-arginine vasopressin shortens the bleeding time in uremia. N Engl J Med 308:8, 1983.
46. Janson PA, Kosfeld R, Marcum S: Treatment of uremic bleeding with conjugated oestrogen. Lancet 2:887, 1984.
47. Gillum DM, Dixon BS, Yanover MJ, et al: The role of intensive dialysis in acute renal failure. Clin Nephrol 25:249, 1986.

Chapter 154
RHABDOMYOLYSIS AND MYOGLOBINURIA

THEODORE H. LEWIS JR
JESSE B. HALL

KEY POINTS

- *Muscle injury, with ensuing metabolic and renal disturbances, is common in many settings of critical illness, particularly drug abuse, trauma, and seizures.*
- *Clinical evidence of injury includes myalgias and muscle swelling, but often the condition is clinically silent.*
- *Abnormal urine or serum laboratory tests are often the initial clue to the diagnosis.*
- *The diagnosis of rhabdomyolysis should prompt a search for an ischemic tissue bed, infection, and potential myotoxins.*
- *Patients with rhabdomyolysis are often massively volume depleted.*
- *Metabolic disturbances include hyperuricemia, hyperphosphatemia, and hyperkalemia; the latter may be life-threatening and require early dialysis.*
- *Hypocalcemia may occur; it is usually clinically insignificant and should only be treated in the setting of severe hyperkalemia or ventricular dysfunction.*
- *The renal failure of rhabdomyolysis is characterized by a rapid rise in serum creatinine (>1 mg/dL/day).*
- *Aggressive volume administration may prevent the development of renal failure; the benefits of urine alkalinization, mannitol, and diuretics remain controversial.*

Rhabdomyolysis is a condition caused by skeletal muscle injury and release of muscle cell contents into the circulation.[1,2] It may result in myoglobinuria, the filtration of myoglobin into the urine, and is often associated with acute renal failure (ARF). Rhabdomyolysis may complicate many different disease states. In some, such as crush injury, muscle injury is obvious; in others, such as drug overdose, it may never be apparent. Rhabdomyolysis may occur in the setting of an altered mental status, and even in the conscious patient may occur with minimal symptoms or physical findings. Therefore, diagnosis requires a high level of suspicion and appropriate sensitivity to abnormal laboratory values.

In addition to complicating many critical illnesses, rhabdomyolysis may require intensive care because of its life-threatening complications. Hypovolemia may be profound. Hyperkalemia may require electrocardiographic (ECG) monitoring and emergent dialysis. Thus, rhabdomyolysis and myoglobinuria pose a challenge to physicians in many specialties and subspecialties and to the intensivist in particular.

Etiologies

MECHANISMS OF CELLULAR INJURY

Many insults can precipitate rhabdomyolysis and myoglobinuria. Disruption of the muscle cell membrane may result from a direct mechanical or toxic insult to the membrane or an inability to maintain ionic gradients across the membrane. Knochel postulated in a hypophosphatemic model of acute muscle injury that decreased intracellular phosphate leads to decreased activity of the sodium-potassium adenosine triphosphatase (Na,K ATPase), allowing the movement of sodium and calcium into the cell.[2,3] Increased intracellular calcium was then postulated to activate phospholipases and endopeptidases, causing cell lysis. Such a mechanism may also explain muscle injury in energy-deficient states such as ischemia or extreme exertion.

DISORDERS ASSOCIATED WITH RHABDOMYOLYSIS

Although a formulation of events at the sarcolemma may improve understanding of the pathophysiology of muscle injury, it does not at present have an impact on management or help form a differential diagnosis of the cause of acute muscle injury. Table 154-1 lists some of the precipi-

TABLE 154-1 Conditions Associated with Rhabdomyolysis

Energy Imbalances	*Drug Related*
Ischemia	Illicit drugs
Crush injury	Alcohol
Vascular occlusion	Heroin
Compartment syndrome	Phencyclidine
Trauma	Cocaine
Exertional	Amphetamines
Untrained athletic activity	Prescription drugs
Status asthmaticus	Lipid-lowering agents
Delerium tremens	Anesthetics
Seizures, myoclonic activity	Succinylcholine
Neuroleptic malignant syndrome	Aminocaproic acid
Congenital enzyme deficiencies	Terbutaline
Glycolytic pathway defects	Aminophylline
Carnitine-palmityltransferase	Diuretics
Temperature related	
Heat stroke	
Malignant hyperthermia	
Electrolyte Abnormalities	*Infections*
Hypokalemia	Viral
Hypophosphatemia	Coxsackie
Hyperosmolar states	Echo
Hyperglycemia (both DKA and NKC)[a]	Influenza
Hypernatremia	Measles
	Bacterial
	Clostridium
	Staphylococcus
	Legionella
	Typhoid
	Tularemia

[a]DKA, diabetic ketoacidosis; NKC, nonketotic hyperosmolar coma

tants of rhabdomyolysis, categorized by the mechanism of muscle injury. It is immediately apparent that several of these conditions, such as ischemia, severe metabolic derangements, and seizures, are common to many disease states seen in the ICU. Similarly many infections are associated with the development of rhabdomyolysis. A detailed discussion of all the causes of rhabdomyolysis listed in Table 154-1 exceeds the spatial limits of this text, but several warrant special mention.

TRAUMA. Crush injury was the first entity in which the association between muscle injury and ARF was made.[4] In addition to direct pressure injury to the muscle, blood flow is reduced by mechanical forces and possibly vasospasm. Consequent tissue hypoxia probably contributes to the injury as well. When the external pressure is removed from the muscle, blood flow is restored. If significant muscle damage has occurred, the complications of rhabdomyolysis begin. Such injury commonly occurs in settings of building collapse or burying. It may also occur from the weight of a patient's body resting on an extremity or portion of the trunk for an extended period of time, as seen in coma or prolonged general anesthesia.

ALCOHOL. In Gabow's series of 87 cases of rhabdomyolysis, alcohol was the sole precipitant noted in approximately 20 percent and was identified as a potential cause in two-thirds of the cases.[1] Alcohol appears to have a direct myotoxic effect, which may result from an inhibition of calcium uptake by the sarcoplasmic reticulum, change in sarcolemmal fluidity, or inhibition of the Na,K ATPase.[5] The effects of alcohol may be potentiated by hypokalemia and hypophosphatemia, two metabolic derangements that may themselves precipitate rhabdomyolysis and occur frequently in the alcoholic population. Rhabdomyolysis may also occur secondary to alcohol withdrawal seizures or prolonged compression during periods of unconsciousness from alcohol intoxication.

OTHER DRUG ABUSE. Heroin and phencyclidine (PCP, angel dust) have previously been the street drugs most commonly associated with the development of rhabdomyolysis, but this complication is increasingly seen in cocaine (crack, coke) abusers.[6] In heroin abuse, immobility leading to compression is thought to play a significant causative role. A direct toxic effect is also likely as rhabdomyolysis associated with heroin abuse has been linked to myocardial cell damage.[7] Furthermore, rhabdomyolysis is reported in patients treated with methadone who have not experienced periods of unconsciousness.[8] Phencyclidine may cause rhabdomyolysis by isometric muscle contraction (such as contraction against restraints), seizures, or compression and resultant crush injury secondary to loss of pain perception. In a series of 1000 patients with phencyclidine intoxication, 22 cases of rhabdomyolysis were noted.[9] Seizures, compression, and severe muscle contraction may also be important causes of rhabdomyolysis in cocaine intoxication. Other possible mechanisms include hyperthermia and ischemia secondary to vasoconstriction. The incidence of cocaine-associated rhabdomyolysis is not yet defined, but is probably increasing with the growing use of the drug. Finally, rhabdomyolysis has been reported in patients abusing amphetamines.[10]

Clinical Presentation and Evaluation

The clinical presentation of rhabdomyolysis is variable (Table 154-2). In the awake, cooperative patient symptoms may include cramping pain in the involved muscle group(s), frequently the calves and lower back; progressive weakness; and discoloration of the urine. However, these complaints may be absent, even in the alert patient. In Gabow's series, 50 percent of patients with reliable histories complained of muscle pain.[1]

Physical examination may be notable for fever or volume depletion. The muscles involved may demonstrate swelling, tenderness, and a firm or doughy consistency. Hemorrhagic discoloration of overlying skin is sometimes noted. Once again, these findings are not universal and in Gabow's series only 5 percent of patients had objective findings of muscle injury on presentation.[1]

Gross examination of the urine may suggest the diagnosis of rhabdomyolysis and myoglobinuria. Circulating myoglobin is not highly protein bound and is readily filtered at the glomerulus. Thus, release of myoglobin in large amounts during muscle injury results in its filtration into the urine. Myoglobin visibly colors water at 50 mg/L, but in urine is not visible until its concentration exceeds 100 mg/L. Since the serum concentration of myoglobin rarely exceeds 25 mg/L, even after muscle injury, discoloration of the serum is very unusual in rhabdomyolysis and should suggest hemolysis.[2,11]

The laboratory values found in patients with rhabdomyolysis and myoglobinuria reflect acute muscle cell lysis, as well as the primary insult or its complications. Disruption of cell membranes allows the release of potassium, phosphate, proteins, and purines: hyperkalemia, hyperphosphatemia, and hyperuricemia may be prominent abnormalities. However, in Gabow's series only 7 percent of patients demonstrated hyperkalemia.[1] The hallmark of muscle damage is elevation of creatine kinase (CK) concentration, which is present in all patients with rhabdomyolysis. CK content is usually elevated to such a degree that the diagnosis of myocardial infarction or cerebral vascular accident is excluded. CK isoenzyme analysis is useful if there is concern over myocardial damage, but may also be misleading since up to 7 percent of muscle CK may be of the MB isoform. Serum analysis for myoglobin is also diagnostic but requires special techniques such as gel electrophoresis,

TABLE 154-2 Clinical Presentation of Rhabdomyolysis

Symptoms (Often absent)	Signs (Often absent or minimal)
Muscle pain	Muscle swelling
Weakness	Doughy consistency to muscle
Parethesias	Paralysis
Abnormal urine	Anesthesia

radioimmunoassay, or enzyme-linked immunosorbent assay (ELISA). Aldolase, lactate dehydrogenase (LDH) and glutamic oxaloacetic transaminase (SGOT) levels are also frequently elevated, but only aldolase is specific for muscle injury. Calcium deposition in the damaged muscle may cause hypocalcemia. Release of creatine from muscle and its spontaneous hydration to creatinine results in elevation of creatinine. Creatinine and blood urea nitrogen (BUN) levels may also be elevated by prerenal azotemia or ARF. Disseminated intravascular coagulation (DIC), as indicated by thrombocytopenia, prolongation of the prothrombin (PT) and partial thromboplastin times (PTT), and elevation of fibrin degradation products, is frequently seen.

The presence of myoglobin in the urine establishes the diagnosis of rhabdomyolysis and myoglobinuria. However, myoglobinuria is not always detected. It may be detected by reaction with orthotoluidene (urine dipstick) at concentrations as low as 0.15 mg/L to 0.62 mg/L, but orthotoluidene also reacts with the globin fragment of hemoglobin.[2,11] Therefore, in the presence of red blood cells or hemolysis its specificity is limited. However, in the absence of significant hematuria its presence should suggest rhabdomyolysis or hemolysis. Radioimmunoassay is more sensitive and specific than dipstick; immunodiffusion, immunoelectrophoresis, and hemagglutination are more specific, but all are more expensive.[2] In one series of patients who had rhabdomyolysis, without hematuria, 74 percent were noted to have orthotoluidine-positive urine.[1]

Complications

The complications of rhabdomyolysis arise from the local effects of muscle cell lysis and the systemic effects of the substances released (Table 154-3). When sarcolemmal integrity is compromised there are several consequences: ionic gradients across the cell membrane are lost, resulting in an influx of sodium, calcium, and extracellular fluid into the cell; and an efflux of intracellular components such as potassium, phosphate, and sulfate-containing anions into the extracellular and intravascular spaces. These electrolyte and solute shifts may cause significant acute biochemical and hemodynamic abnormalities in the hours to days following muscle injury.

TABLE 154-3 Complications of Rhabdomyolysis

Acute	Late
Systemic	Hypercalcemia
Volume depletion	
Biochemical abnormalities	
Hyperkalemia	
Hyperuricemia	
Hyperphosphatemia	
Hypocalcemia	
Metabolic acidosis	
DIC	
Renal failure	
Local	
Compartment syndrome	

HYPOVOLEMIA

The influx of fluid into the damaged muscle may cause hypovolemia to the point of shock. Volume requirements in the initial period after muscle injury can exceed 10 L/day. Indices of volume status such as urine output, urine sodium concentration, and BUN:creatinine ratio may all be misleading in rhabdomyolysis. Invasive hemodynamic monitoring may be necessary to better assess volume status.

ELECTROLYTE DISTURBANCES

The release of large amounts of potassium can cause life-threatening hyperkalemia. This complication usually occurs in the setting of oliguric acute renal failure and requires frequent measurement of serum potassium levels. Theoretically the hyperkalemia associated with rhabdomyolysis is less responsive to traditional therapy that relies on shifting potassium intracellularly, such as the infusion of insulin and glucose, because potassium transport mechanisms are likely impaired in injured muscle and transported potassium may immediately leak from the intracellular compartment.

The large amounts of organic phosphate released may lead to hyperphosphatemia. Hyperphosphatemia may worsen hypocalcemia by decreasing the production of 1,25-dihydroxycholecalciferol.[12] In the presence of normal calcium levels the calcium-phosphate product may increase sufficiently to cause metastatic calcification.

The release of purines from damaged muscle and subsequent hepatic conversion to uric acid can cause hyperuricemia. High concentrations of uric acid, particularly in the setting of hypovolemia with low urine flow and pH, may cause sludging of urate crystals in the renal tubules. The role of urate nephropathy in the pathogenesis of ARF in rhabdomyolysis is not clear, but it may contribute to some degree.

Sulfur-containing proteins in muscle can be released in large amounts during injury. Hydrogen and sulfate loads may overwhelm renal excretory mechanisms, resulting in an anion gap acidosis, which may be severe.[13] Other causes of acidosis that may occur in the setting of rhabdomyolysis include lactic acidosis from ischemia and the acidosis of uremia.

HYPOCALCEMIA AND HYPERCALCEMIA

Shifts in serum calcium concentrations frequently complicate rhabdomyolysis. Hypocalcemia may be noted acutely, although it rarely causes symptoms or hemodynamic effects. The etiology of the hypocalcemia is multifactorial. Deposition of calcium in the damaged muscle has been demonstrated in both experimental models pathologically and clinically by nuclear medicine techniques.[14] This is probably the major mechanism responsible for acute hypocalcemia.[15] In addition, levels of 1,25-dihydroxycholecalciferol are reduced acutely in rhabdomyolysis.[12] This reduction may reflect the effects of hyperphosphatemia and uremia. Decreased responsiveness of bone to increased levels of parathyroid hormone probably also accounts for some of the decrease in serum calcium.

Whereas hypocalcemia may be noted acutely in rhabdomyolysis and during oliguric myoglobinuric renal failure, hypercalcemia may complicate the diuretic phase of resolution of renal failure. This hypercalcemia is felt to be secondary to mobilization of calcium previously deposited in injured muscle. It is augmented by elevation of 1,25-dihydroxycholecalciferol, which is likely produced in increased quantities by the recovering kidneys. Hypercalcemia may occur at any point during the recovery phase of ARF, from days to weeks after the initial insult.[16]

ACUTE RENAL FAILURE

Perhaps the most significant complication of rhabdomyolysis is acute renal failure (ARF), seen in approximately 30 percent of patients.[1,17] Early studies by Bywater using infusions of muscle extracts suggested that myoglobin was nephrotoxic.[18] Morphologically, plugging of the renal tubules with precipitated material was seen. Subsequent investigators have questioned the role of myoglobin.[19] In the absence of aciduria myoglobin may not be nephrotoxic. Myoglobin is converted to ferrihemate at a pH <5.6, and ferrihemate has been shown to be toxic to renal tubules, as well as to precipitate in them.[20] In addition to tubular obstruction by myoglobin, or other muscle constituents, other mechanisms may be important in the development of renal failure. Injection of glycerol in rats, a model of myoglobinuric renal failure, causes a dramatic reduction in renal blood flow, which correlates morphologically with both afferent and efferent arteriolar vasoconstriction.[21] Injection of muscle extracts in rabbits causes glomerular microthrombi.[19] Recently several authors have demonstrated a potential role for oxygen-free radicals in the renal injury seen in glycerol-induced myoglobinuria, as well as in hemoglobinuria. Pretreatment with dimethylthiourea, a free radical scavenger, protects against azotemia in glycerol-induced renal dysfunction.[22] Similarly, deferoxamine appears to protect against renal injury in a glycerol-injected rat model. This finding suggests that iron, perhaps derived from the heme groups of myoglobin, may be the source of free radical generation.[21,23] Finally, it is of note that chronic saline loading and alkalinization of the urine protect against the development of renal failure in many experimental models.

The clinical characteristics of the ARF associated with myoglobinuria have been described in several series. One retrospectively examined 88 cases of nontraumatic rhabdomyolysis.[1] Azotemia was present on admission in 25 percent of cases. Twenty-seven percent of this subset were thought to be volume depleted and azotemia resolved with fluid administration. The remainder developed renal failure. In addition, 20 percent of those cases that were not azotemic on admission developed renal failure, resulting in a 33 percent incidence for all cases. A comparable incidence of 43 percent was noted in a second series of patients with ARF complicating rhabdomyolysis.[17] Oliguria ranged in incidence from 38 to 73 percent in these two series. Another study of renal failure in nontraumatic rhabdomyolysis noted oliguria in 88 percent of cases reported.[1,24] The laboratory values, as described above, are typical of ARF of any etiology, except that hyperkalemia and hyperphosphatemia tend to occur early, and serum creatinine concentration tends to be higher than expected for a given level of azotemia, perhaps because of the release of previously formed creatine from damaged muscle.[17] The duration of oliguria varied from 3 to 38 days.[17,23] Dialysis was required in 46 percent of patients who developed ARF in one series[17] and 78 percent in another.[24]

Attempts to predict those patients at greatest risk for the development of ARF have relied on retrospective analysis of clinical series. Discriminant analysis of the previously noted series concluded that the likelihood of renal failure was best predicted by the serum potassium, phosphate, and albumin levels at presentation.[1] There was no correlation with the level of CK and the development of renal failure. A subsequent retrospective study suggested the probability of renal failure was low in patients whose CK level was <6000 IU.[25] Elevated potassium and phosphate concentrations and dehydration on admission were also predictive of renal failure.

COAGULOPATHY

Disseminated intravascular coagulation may complicate rhabdomyolysis. It probably results from the activation of the clotting cascade by components released from the damaged muscle. In rabbits injection of muscle extracts causes prolongation of the PT and PTT, hypofibrinogenemia, and thrombocytopenia.[19] Histologic evidence of thrombosis is also noted. Overt clinical bleeding or thrombosis rarely complicates DIC associated with rhabdomyolysis. It should be noted that cocaine ingestion and hyperthermia may be complicated by fulminant hepatic failure, and careful evaluation to distinguish between DIC and liver failure should be undertaken, where appropriate.

LOCAL COMPLICATIONS

In addition to these systemic complications, local complications may occur as well. Injured muscle often becomes edematous. In muscle groups confined by fascial planes, swelling may cause a rise in the pressure within the compartment leading to reduced blood flow with ischemia and further muscle and nerve damage. This further muscle damage is manifest as the "second wave phenomenon," the persistent elevation or rebound elevation in CK levels at 48 to 72 h after the initial muscle injury. Failure of the CK levels to decrease by approximately 50 percent every 48 h should raise suspicion of further ischemic muscle damage.

SURVIVAL

Survival in nontraumatic rhabdomyolysis with or without ARF is excellent. In the large series of cases of rhabdomyolysis with and without renal failure, the overall survival rate was 90 percent; survival in those patients who developed ARF was 80 percent.[1] It was not noted whether survivors or nonsurvivors suffered traumatic or nontraumatic rhabdomyolysis. In those series of cases of ARF complicating rhabdomyolysis, survival ranged from 95 to 100 percent.[24,17]

Therapy

The therapy of rhabdomyolysis should be directed at two objectives. The first is the treatment of any reversible cause of muscle damage. Examples are an infection or carbon monoxide poisoning. This obvious tenet is often overlooked.

The second objective is the management and prevention of complications. Because hypovolemia is often present in patients with rhabdomyolysis, aggressive volume resuscitation should be instituted. Two to three liters of saline per hour are often required during the initial management, and 300 to 500 mL/h once hemodynamic stability has been achieved. Failure to provide adequate volume replacement is probably the most frequent error made in the management of rhabdomyolysis. In the oliguric patient with evidence of myoglobinuric renal failure, assessment of volume status may require central venous or pulmonary artery pressure monitoring.

Electrolyte abnormalities in the acute stages of rhabdomyolysis often will require therapy. In particular, hyperkalemia requires frequent serial determinations, ECG monitoring, and treatment if levels should exceed 6 meq/L or cause rhythm or conduction system disturbances. Conventional therapy with insulin and glucose infusions, β-adrenergic agents, and sodium bicarbonate may be ineffective because of loss of sarcolemmal integrity, and therefore early use of exchange resins or dialysis may be necessary. If hyperuricemia is severe, uric acid levels greater than 20 mg/dL, consideration should be given to treatment with allopurinol. Hyperphosphatemia should be treated with phosphate binders. Therapy with calcium infusion may worsen the deposition of calcium in injured muscle and lead to higher levels of hypercalcemia in the diuretic phase of recovery from ARF. For these reasons calcium administration should only be used for the therapy of severe hyperkalemia or if ventricular dysfunction has resulted in hypoperfusion.

Therapy aimed at preventing the onset of acute myoglobinuric renal failure is controversial. It is clear from many animal studies that low urine volumes and aciduria potentiate the renal insult seen in muscle injury. In a recent study of rats infused with myoglobin, the effects on renal function of urine pH with and without solute loading were examined. Renal injury appeared to depend on urine pH, and no injury occurred at a urine pH of 8.0. Dilution of urine with nonresorbable salt protected renal function at low urine pH. The investigator concluded that bicarbonate administration protects against renal injury in myoglobinuria by both its alkalinizing effect and a solute diuretic effect.[26]

Animal studies support vigorous fluid administration to maximize urine flow and alkalinization. Two clinical studies have used such therapy. The first study retrospectively examined the course of patients given an infusion of mannitol and sodium bicarbonate.[27] Twenty patients were found to have received such therapy. All were oliguric and 19 were azotemic. Nine of these patients demonstrated improved urine flow and resolution of azotemia. Eleven patients (55 percent) progressed to ARF, in comparison with a 72 percent incidence in a similar group of patients.[1] In the second study, 20 victims trapped in a collapsed building were treated with aggressive volume resuscitation in the field.[28] On arrival at the hospital 7 patients were found to have myoglobinuria. These patients all received alkaline diuresis with sodium bicarbonate and mannitol (after adequate volume replacement). None of the 7 patients developed ARF.

These studies suggest that alkaline diuresis is effective in preventing ARF in patients with myoglobinuria. However, there was no control group in either study. High urine flows may increase urine pH without requiring bicarbonate administration. Might bicarbonate administration be detrimental? Metabolic alkalosis could theoretically worsen the hypocalcemia seen in rhabdomyolysis. In one of the two clinical studies acetazolamide was administered to prevent the development of such a metabolic alkalosis.[28] Based on the available animal and clinical data, it is clear that increased urine volume is beneficial in attempts to prevent ARF in patients with myoglobinuria. Alkalinization of the urine probably adds to the beneficial effect of high urine flow, but whether its effect is clinically relevant and worth the potential risk remains to be studied.

Similarly the role of mannitol has not been studied in a controlled fashion. Osmotic diuresis is protective in animal models. Both clinical studies noted administered mannitol as part of the fluid resuscitation protocol.[27,28] Mannitol administration may reduce renal tubular oxygen consumption by reducing sodium resorption.[29] This reduction in oxygen consumption might, in turn, reduce renal ischemic damage. Caution should be used in administering mannitol because an osmotic diuresis without adequate volume replacement might worsen hypovolemia.

In summary, treatment to prevent the development of ARF in rhabdomyolysis is controversial. At our institution patients who are at risk for rhabdomyolysis and myoglobinuric renal failure are closely monitored for evidence of hypovolemia or electrolyte disturbances and serum CK values are followed. If myoglobin is present in the urine or if the serum CK level exceeds 5000 IU, then normal saline infusion is instituted with a goal to achieve a urine flow in excess of 200 mL/h. (This may require rates of intravenous volume administration in the range of 500 mL/h.) If the urine pH is <6, then sodium bicarbonate is administered as well, although this therapy is not uniformly supported among our ICU staff. The serum pH is followed closely and if it exceeds 7.45 then the bicarbonate infusion is discontinued or acetazolamide is administered. If a successful diuresis is not achieved with vigorous volume administration, then central venous pressure monitoring is used to ensure adequate volume resuscitation. If the patient is no longer hypovolemic, mannitol is added at a dose of 25 g every 6 h. These measures are continued until myoglobinuria has resolved, unless volume overload limits intravenous fluid or serum osmolarity limits mannitol administration. If there is no response in urine output to these measures, then furosemide is administered at a dose of 40 mg intravenously and increased to 200 mg intravenously or until a diuresis occurs.

Local therapy is extremely important in rhabdomyolysis of either traumatic or nontraumatic origin. Close attention should be paid to the decline of serum CK levels. If the level does not fall by 50 percent over 48 h, a careful search should be made for evidence of increased tissue pressures in the involved muscle groups. If such evidence is found, then close attention should be focused on neurovascular function in effected limbs. Some authors recommend monitoring compartmental pressures, whereas others feel physical examination is adequate.[30,31] If circulatory compromise, compartmental pressures in excess of 40 mmHg, or compartmental pressures within 30 mmHg of the diastolic blood pressure is noted, fasciotomy should be performed. In the absence of compartment syndrome, debridement of necrotic muscle with intact skin overlying is contraindicated given the risk of infection in the open wound.[31] This contrasts with situations where the skin has been broken, such as a compound crush injury where wide debridement of the necrotic muscle is indicated.[31]

CASE PRESENTATION

L.T. is a 34-year-old intravenous drug abuser who presented with disorientation and left flank pain.

The day prior to admission the patient was found by a family member striking his head against the wall. He was confused and complaining of left flank pain. He was brought to the emergency room where 0.3 mg naloxone was given. His mental status improved and he gave a history of "speed balling" heroin and cocaine. He continued to complain of left flank pain. He was held overnight for observation.

Oliguria was noted, which prompted bladder catheterization. Cola-colored urine was obtained. Urine dipstick revealed 4+ blood, 3+ protein. Microscopic urinalysis revealed occasional RBCs and occasional WBCs. The serum CK value was 15,330 IU. The patient was admitted to the ICU.

Past medical history was of note only for drug abuse.

Physical examination revealed a well-developed black male in moderate distress secondary to back pain. Vital signs demonstrated a pulse of 120, blood pressure of 120/80 with orthostatic changes, respiratory rate of 20, and temperature of 36.2°C (97.3°F). The chest was clear. There was no jugular venous pulsation at 30°. The cardiac examination was normal, including intact pulses in all extremities. There was tenderness to palpation over the left flank. Rectal examination revealed guaiac-positive stool. Extremities were warm, and the skin was not tense. The neurologic examination was of note for loss of pinprick over the painful flank area.

Initial laboratory results in the ICU yielded a hemoglobin of 12.7 g/dL, a WBC count of 24,000/μL, platelet count of 142,000/μL, PT 20.9 s (control 12.0 s), PTT 42.9 s (control 26.0 s), fibrinogen 92 mg/dL; sodium 137 meq/L, potassium 3.7 meq/L, chloride 102 meq/L, bicarbonate 19 meq/L, BUN 26 mg/dL, creatinine 2.9 mg/dL; calcium 7.0 mg/dL, phosphate 4.9 mg/dL, uric acid 19.4 mg/dL; CK was 48,989 IU, lactate dehydrogenase was 8276, AST was 3026, ALT was 1626, total bilirubin was 3.1 mg/dL. Urinalysis revealed dark brown colored urine, pH 5, 3+ blood, 4+ protein, and 5 to 10 RBCs per high-power field.

A diagnosis of rhabdomyolysis was made. The patient was treated with intravenous fluids at a rate of 300 mL/h. The intravenous fluid administered was 0.45 sodium chloride with one ampule of sodium bicarbonate added to each liter. This therapy resulted in a urine output that averaged 200 mL/h.

The rest of the hospital course (Table 154-4) was remarkable for early hypocalcemia, late hypercalcemia, and the eventual need for dialysis for azotemia. The patient was discharged with modest elevation of the serum creatinine concentration.

CASE DISCUSSION

This patient had many possible causes of rhabdomyolysis, including heroin, cocaine, and possibly a period of coma. The symptoms of muscle injury were obscured by his obtundation. Once narcotic effects were treated with an antagonist, he did note severe pain in the flank, a characteristic symptom of rhabdomyolysis. He had no physical findings of muscle injury except for anesthesia over the involved muscle group.

The patient's laboratory evaluation was also characteristic of rhabdomyolysis. Initial electrolytes included a normal potassium value and an anion gap acidosis, initial BUN and creatinine values were elevated, with a low BUN:creatinine ratio. Hypocalcemia was present, as was hyperphosphatemia and hyperuricemia. The CK content was markedly elevated, with a lesser elevation of the LDH. Thrombocytopenia and elevation of the PT and PTT time suggested DIC. The urinalysis grossly suggested rhabdomyolysis by its cola color. This was supported by the orthotoluidene positivity with minimal hematuria; however, hemolysis may also have contributed to this finding.

The initial management with aggressive volume resuscitation was aimed at increasing urine output to greater than 200 mL/h. Bicarbonate was added to alkalinize the urine, with the understanding that the benefit of this therapy is controversial. Indeed the patient developed a metabolic alkalosis during the bicarbonate infusion. Therapy with allopurinol was considered but was not given; the level of elevation of the uric acid was not felt to justify its use. Despite volume resuscitation with alkaline fluids, the patient developed nonoliguric renal failure. The renal failure was remarkable for a rapid rise in creatinine level and persistently low BUN:creatinine ratio. After 7 days of progressive increase of the BUN and creatinine values, dialysis was initiated and continued through day 14 when the serum creatinine level began to normalize. This time course is typical of patients with nontraumatic rhabdomyolysis. Finally, it is of note that the patient was hypocalcemic, but because there were no symptoms, no signs of hyperkalemia, and no ventricular dysfunction, treatment was withheld. Late hypercalcemia developed, nonetheless, but was asymptomatic and resolved quickly.

TABLE 154-4 Clinical and Laboratory Course of Case

Hospital Day	1a	1b	2a	2b	3	5	9	14(DC)	30
Clinical	Severe flank pain			Asymptomatic					
Treatment	IV fluids (NaCl and HCO_3) 200 mL/h			Diuretics		Dialysis			
Chemistries									
K	3.7	3.5	3.6	3.2	5.0	4.3	4.2	5.2	4.5
BUN	26	31	36	40	46	115	122	86	15
Creatinine	2.9	3.5	4.8	6.0	6.5	8.2	12.7	8.9	2.0
Ca	7.0	6.8	6.0	5.8	5.1	8.2	8.7	9.6	12.5
PO_4	4.9	5.3	5.3	4.8	4.5	6.3	5.4	7.6	3.7
Urinalysis	19.4	18.1	19.6	17.8	16.8	11.4	10.6	8.8	4.4
CK × (10^3)	48.9	55.5	51.7	47.0	32.6	26.6	2.2	0.4	0.2
LDH × (10^3)	15.7	21.0	24.0	14.8	9.3	2.0	1.0	0.4	0.1

References

1. Gabow P, Kaehny W, Kelleher S: The spectrum of rhabdomyolysis. Medicine 61:141, 1982.
2. Knochel J: Rhabdomyolysis and myoglobinuria. Ann Rev Med 33:435, 1982.
3. Knochel J, et al: Hypophosphatemia and rhabdomyolysis. J Clin Invest 62:1240, 1978.
4. Bywaters E, Beall D: Crush injuries with impairment of renal function. Br Med J 4185, 1941.
5. Haller R, Knochel J: Skeletal muscle disease in alcoholism. Med Clin North Am 68:91, 1984.
6. Roth D, Alarcon F, Fernandez J, et al: Acute rhabdomyolysis associated with cocaine intoxication. N Engl J Med 319:673, 1988.
7. Schwartzfarb L, Singh G, Marcus D: Heroin-associated rhabdomyolysis with cardiac involvement. Arch Intern Med 137:1255, 1977.
8. Koppel C: Clinical features, pathogenesis, and management of drug induced rhabdomyolysis. Medical Toxicol Adverse Drug Experience 4:108, 1989.
9. McCarron M, Schulbe B, Thompson G, et al: Acute phencyclidine intoxication: Clinical patterns, complications, and treatment. Ann Emerg Med 10:290, 1981.
10. Kendrick W, Hull A, Knochel J: Rhabdomyolysis and shock after intravenous amphetamine administration. Ann Intern Med 86:381, 1977.
11. Hamilton R, Hopkins M, Shihabi Z: Case conference: Myoglobinuria, hemoglobinuria, and acute renal failure. Clin Chem 35:1713, 1989.
12. Llach F, Felsenfeld A, Haussler M: The pathophysiology of altered calcium metabolism in rhabdomyolysis-induced acute renal failure. N Engl J Med 305:117, 1981.
13. McCarron D, Elliot W, Rose J, Bennett W, et al: Severe mixed metabolic acidosis secondary to rhabdomyolysis. Am J Med 67:905, 1979.
14. Frymoyer P, et al: Technetium Tc99m medronate bone scanning in rhabdomyolysis. Arch Intern Med 145:1991, 1985.
15. Akmal M, et al: Hypocalcemia and hypercalcemia in patients with rhabdomyolysis with and without acute renal failure. J Clin Endocrinol Metab 63:137, 1986.
16. Feinstein E, et al: Delayed hypercalcemia with acute renal failure with nontraumatic rhabdomyolysis. Arch Intern Med 141:753, 1981.
17. Grossman R, et al: Nontraumatic rhabdomyolysis and acute renal failure. N Engl J Med 291:807, 1974.
18. Bywaters E, Stead J: The production of renal failure following injection of solutions containing myohemoglobin. Q J Exp Physiol 33:53, 1944.
19. Blachar Y, Fong J, Chadarévian JP, et al: Muscle extract infusion in rabbits: A new experimental model of the crush syndrome. Circ Res 49:114, 1981.
20. Braun S, Weiss F, Keller A, et al: Evaluation of the renal toxicity of heme proteins and their derivatives: A role in the genesis of acute tubule necrosis. J Exp Med 131:443, 1970.
21. Ayer G, Grandchamp A, Wyler T, Truneger B, et al: Intrarenal hemodynamics in glycerol-induced myohemoglobinuric acute renal failure in the rat. Circ Res 29:128, 1971.
22. Shah S, Walker P: Evidence suggesting a role for hydroxyl radical in glycerol-induced acute renal failure. Am J Physiol 255:F438, 1988.
23. Paller M: Hemoglobin- and myoglobin-induced acute renal failure in rats: Role of iron in nephrotoxicity. Am J Physiol 255:F539, 1988.
24. Koffler A, Friedler R, Massry S: Acute renal failure due to nontraumatic habdomyolysis. Ann Intern Med 85:23, 1976.
25. Ward M: Factors predictive of acute renal failure in rhabdomyolysis. Arch Intern Med 148:1553, 1985.
26. Zager R: Studies of mechanisms and protective maneuvers in myoglobinuric acute renal injury. Lab Invest 60:619, 1989.
27. Eneas J, Schoenfeld P, Humphreys M: The effect of infusion of mannitol-sodium bicarbonate on the clinical course of myoglobinuria. Arch Intern Med 139:801, 1979.
28. Ron D, Tattelman V, Michealson M, et al: Prevention of acute renal failure in traumatic rhabdomyolysis. Arch Intern Med 144:277, 1984.
29. Knochel J: Rhabdomyolysis and myoglobinuria. Sem Nephrol 1:75, 1981.
30. Reis N, Michaelson M: Crush injury to the lower limbs: Treatment of the local injury. J Bone Joint Surg 68:414, 1986.
31. Whitesides T, Haney T, Morimoto K, Harada H, et al: Tissue pressure measurements as a determinant for the need of fasciotomy. Clin Orthop 113:43, 1975.

Chapter 155

DIALYSIS IN THE CRITICAL CARE PATIENT

ELEANOR D. LEDERER
DAVID M. GILLUM

KEY POINTS

- *The major indications for dialysis are volume overload, hyperkalemia, and uremia. Dialysis may also be useful for intractable volume overload secondary to heart failure or nephrotic syndrome, for facilitation of nutritional support, or for treatment of drug intoxication.*
- *There are many forms of dialytic therapy that can be tailored to the clinical situation. Ultrafiltration can be accomplished by continuous arteriovenous hemofiltration (CAVH), intermittent ultrafiltration via a single vascular catheter, or peritoneal dialysis. Dialysis can be accomplished via CAVH with concomitant flow-through of dialysate, intermittent hemodialysis, or peritoneal dialysis.*
- *Slow continuous ultrafiltration has the advantage of being hemodynamically less stressful than other modalities while being capable of removing massive volumes safely. However, vascular access, tendency to thrombosis, and patient immobilization are notable disadvantages of this technique.*
- *Intermittent hemodialysis is the most efficient form of dialysis; this makes it the preferable modality in most acutely ill, severely catabolic critical care patients. Difficulties of vascular access and hemodynamic stresses are the major drawbacks.*
- *Peritoneal dialysis is technically easier to perform, does not require specialized personnel, and is hemodynamically nonstressful. On the other hand, it may not be efficient enough to clear uremic toxins adequately in severely catabolic patients, and it is not possible in patients who have had recent abdominal surgery or multiple adhesions.*

Indications for Dialysis

The maintenance of normal fluid and electrolyte status is the result of complex interactions between the kidneys, heart, liver, and endocrine system. Failure of any of these organ systems can result in fluid and/or electrolyte abnormalities; however, in the absence of frank renal failure, most such abnormalities can be managed conservatively. Dialysis is indicated most frequently therefore, when acute or chronic renal failure complicates the clinical situation (see Table 155-1).

TABLE 155-1 Indications for Dialysis

Volume overload
Severe hypertension
Pulmonary edema
Electrolyte imbalance
Hyperkalemia
Profound acidosis/alkalosis
Hypercalcemia
Hypermagnesemia
Hyper- or hyponatremia
Uremic symptoms
Altered mental status or seizures
Anorexia, nausea, vomiting
Pericarditis
Bleeding
Drug intoxication
Salicylates
Methanol
Ethylene glycol

FLUID OVERLOAD

Fluid overload is one of the most common indications for dialysis or ultrafiltration in the ICU patient. The complications of volume overload that are amenable to fluid withdrawal include hypertension, pulmonary edema with hypoxemia, and congestive heart failure. Particularly in the renal failure patient, volume overload can result in severe hypertension and can be resolved easily with simple fluid removal, thus diminishing, or completely eliminating, the need for pharmacotherapy. Pulmonary edema of the cardiogenic or noncardiogenic variety may respond more or less to fluid removal, especially if the underlying condition has been complicated by the development of renal insufficiency or severe congestive heart failure. End-stage cardiac failure frequently renders the patient relatively refractory to diuretics, even if they are given in combination and parenterally. Moreover, continuous high-dose diuretic therapy may result in a number of other side effects, such as electrolyte abnormalities, prerenal azotemia, interstitial nephritis, and deafness.[1] Under these circumstances, simple ultrafiltration can be accomplished with a minimum of metabolic and hemodynamic consequences. Even if the individual can maintain a relatively stable volume and electrolyte status in the nonstressed state, his or her nutritional needs may necessitate administration of large volume loads that exceed excretory capabilities. Ultrafiltration, alone or combined with dialysis, can markedly facilitate nutritional management.

ELECTROLYTE IMBALANCES

Electrolyte imbalances are another indication for dialysis. Hyperkalemia, the most common electrolyte indication for acute dialysis, can be managed medically most of the time (see Chap. 156). However, when hyperkalemia is complicated by renal failure or a severely catabolic condition, such as rhabdomyolysis, sepsis, or other tissue necrosis, its management is markedly facilitated by dialysis. But the decision to institute dialysis does not obviate the use of more conservative management techniques, either before dialysis access can be achieved or between dialysis procedures. Occasionally, profound and refractory acidosis may be an indication for dialysis. Less commonly, severe symptomatic hyponatremia, hypernatremia, hypercalcemia, hypermagnesemia, and severe alkalosis, especially in the individual with renal insufficiency, may all be considered indications for dialysis.

UREMIA

In the absence of severe electrolyte perturbations and volume overload, the most common indication for urgent dialysis is central nervous system (CNS) dysfunction. Early CNS manifestations of uremia include diminished concentration; insomnia; and drowsiness advancing to stupor, coma, or seizures as uremia worsens. Asterixis or clonus may presage generalized seizure activity in the uremic patient. Other uremic complications that may respond to dialysis include nausea, vomiting, and anorexia.[2,3] Gastrointestinal bleeding due to stress ulceration has been a leading cause of morbidity and mortality in acute renal failure (ARF); however, early use of histamine H_2–receptor blockers (cimetidine, ranitidine) or other antacid therapy has greatly diminished this problem. Abnormalities of platelet function are responsible for the bleeding tendency in uremic patients. This complication, manifested clinically as a prolongation of the bleeding time with normal prothrombin and partial thromboplastin times, usually improves with dialysis. Therefore, a bleeding tendency in a uremic patient mandates dialysis therapy.[4] Therapy with DDAVP, conjugated estrogens, or cryoprecipitate may also be useful in the management of uremic bleeding (see Chap. 153). A not-uncommon cardiovascular complication of ARF is uremic pericarditis, the incidence of which has declined with earlier institution of dialysis therapy. Pericarditis is frequently correlated with the severity of uremia and level of blood urea nitrogen (BUN), although cases have been reported at BUN concentrations lower than 100 mg/dL.[5] Nonuremic causes of pericarditis must be excluded, even as therapy is begun for presumed uremic pericarditis.

DRUG INTOXICATION

In general, hemodialysis can be useful in the treatment of intoxication if the clearance of the agent is significantly increased over the endogenous clearance rate (see Chap. 168). Agents that are highly protein-bound or have a large volume of distribution are unsuitable for removal by hemodialysis. Hemodialysis is most commonly applied to the treatment of salicylate intoxication; other intoxications that may be improved by hemodialysis include those with methanol, ethylene glycol, bromide, chloral hydrate, isopropyl alcohol, and lithium.

Following a massive overdose of salicylates, the plasma half-life may increase from 2.4 to 19 h. This increase is accompanied by a reduction in plasma protein binding. Clinical manifestations of salicylate intoxication may include acid-base disturbances (respiratory alkalosis followed by profound metabolic acidosis), tinnitus, gastrointestinal hemorrhage, bleeding diathesis, and CNS alterations (see Chap. 177). Very few patients with salicylate intoxication require dialysis, but it may be life-saving in the setting of massive overdosage with plasma salicylate levels exceeding 80 mg/dL. Salicylate clearance during hemodialysis exceeds 100 mL/min, and plasma half-life is reduced to 4 h.[6] Charcoal hemoperfusion has also been successfully applied to the treatment of severe salicylate intoxication.

MULTIPLE METABOLIC DERANGEMENTS

Occasionally a patient with a potentially reversible condition requiring an aggressive therapeutic intervention, such as surgery for an intraabdominal abscess, may present with multiple electrolyte abnormalities with or without acute renal failure. Since severe hyperkalemia, acidosis, or hypocalcemia greatly increases surgical risk, stabilization of the patient with dialysis prior to surgery may be indicated to optimize survival. Likewise, the patient with an aggressive tumor and a large cell kill after chemotherapy may develop tumor lysis syndrome with concomitant renal failure, hyperkalemia, hyperphosphatemia, hyperuricemia, and hypocalcemia. The tumor may respond to chemotherapy; however, during this massive cell lysis, dialysis may be needed to avert a potentially lethal metabolic complication.

Choice of Extracorporeal Therapy

Many alternatives for dialytic therapy are available and can be adapted to the patient's needs (see Table 155-2). The choice of dialysis procedure depends on several factors: the specific goals of therapy for the particular patient, the clinical condition of the patient, the expertise of the physician, and the available technical support. Table 155-3 lists the advantages and disadvantages of each procedure. Often, in a given case, many of the options are feasible; in that circumstance the choice of procedure would be based on the physician's and/or the patient's choice.

ULTRAFILTRATION ALONE

Massive volume overload in a patient who is unresponsive to diuretics often mandates some form of ultrafiltration therapy. This circumstance is not uncommonly encountered in cardiovascular surgery patients (e.g., those undergoing aneurysm repair) who receive massive volume resuscitation during surgery. If adequate diuresis is impossible because of unfavorable postoperative systemic and renal hemodynamics or acute renal failure, then ultrafiltration may be required. Other postsurgical states or trauma, when complicated by acute renal failure and massive volume overload, may also require intervention with an ultrafiltra-

TABLE 155-2 Blood Purification and Ultrafiltration Procedures

Procedure	Type of Kidney/ Filtration Device	Description
Hemodialysis	Hollow-fiber, parallel-plate dialyzer	Diffusive removal of solutes
Intermittent ultrafiltration	Hollow-fiber, parallel-plate dialyzer	Convective fluid removal
Slow continuous ultrafiltration (SCUF)	High-flux (Hemofilter) membrane Amicon Diafilter 10, 20 or 30 Hospal Biospal	Continuous convective fluid removal
Continuous arteriovenous hemofiltration (CAVH)	High-flux membrane Amicon Diafilter 10, 20 or 30 Hospal Biospal	Continuous slow convective solute/fluid removal with replacement by substitution fluid
Hemodiafiltration	High-flux membrane Amicon Diafilter 10, 20 or 30 Hospal Biospal	Combination of CAVH with diffusive solute removal
Continuous arteriovenous hemofiltration dialysis (CAVHD)	Hollow-fiber, parallel-plate dialyzer	Continuous diffusive removal of solutes

TABLE 155-3 Relative Advantages and Disadvantages of Different Dialysis Procedures

Technique	Advantages	Disadvantages
Ultrafiltration (simple)	Rapid fluid removal for emergent state	Requires vascular access Requires trained personnel
CAVH (and related modalities)	Large-volume continuous fluid removal Hourly adjustable rate of fluid removal No requirement for trained personnel	Inefficient dialysis Need for full anticoagulation Tendency toward thrombosis Large-bore vascular access Patient immobilization
Hemodialysis	Easy access Efficient removal of fluid and solutes for emergent situation	Requires vascular access Requires trained personnel Multiple potential complications in unstable patient (e.g., bleeding, hypotension, arrhythmias, hypoxemia)
Peritoneal dialysis	Gentle removal of fluid and solute Easy access, at bedside if necessary No requirement for trained personnel Hemodynamically nonstressful	Less efficient Possibility of peritonitis Limited utility in patients with abdominal surgeries or other processes

tion procedure. In a critically ill patient with acute renal failure, periodic ultrafiltration may be required to accommodate aggressive parenteral nutrition. Medical conditions in which ultrafiltration may find application include the nephrotic syndrome with massive proteinuria and anasarca, as well as intractable congestive heart failure[7,8] and ARDS in the setting of oliguria.

LARGE-VOLUME ULTRAFILTRATION

Choice of an ultrafiltration procedure will depend on the patient's cardiovascular stability and the urgency of the need for volume removal. Life-threatening pulmonary edema requires immediate intervention and removal of large volumes of plasma; peritoneal dialysis, with its slower rates of ultrafiltration, is generally or often not suitable in this circumstance. For the patient without hemodynamic compromise, intermittent large-volume ultrafiltration is indicated. In a typical ultrafiltration session up to 6 L of fluid may be removed over 1 to 3 h, depending on the hemodynamic response. This procedure requires all of the extracorporeal equipment and personnel used in hemodialysis. In the face of poor cardiac function, circulatory collapse, and sepsis, large-volume ultrafiltration may worsen hypotension and may be poorly tolerated. A slower rate of ultrafiltration in these patients will often permit the necessary volume removal without further hemodynamic compromise. If not, then alternative modes of volume removal, such as hemofiltration or peritoneal dialysis, must be entertained.

SLOW CONTINUOUS ULTRAFILTRATION (SCUF)

Slow continuous ultrafiltration has proven to be of great value in the above circumstances.[9] Access to the circulation is most commonly achieved with large-bore catheters (No. 8 French) in a femoral artery and vein. The arterial catheter is then connected to the inlet port of the high-flux membrane filtration device, while the venous catheter is attached to the outlet. Blood flow through the device is entirely dependent on the patient's arteriovenous pressure gradient, as well as on the type of vascular access and the resistance properties of the needle or catheter making the arterial connection. Blood flow through these filtration devices is low, rarely exceeding 50 to 80 mL/min even at relatively higher systemic blood pressure (compared to the average blood flows of 250 to 300 mL/min in the artificial kidney used for intermittent hemodialysis or ultrafiltration). The rate of ultrafiltration is determined by the oncotic pressure exerted by plasma proteins and the hydraulic pressure across the membrane. Typically, the net filtration pressure in a SCUF device is only 50 to 60 mmHg, resulting in a filtration rate of 8 to 12 mL/min. The advantage of SCUF is that it results in a low but constant rate of ultrafiltration, allowing large amounts of fluid removal even in a relatively unstable patient. In a 24-h period, up to 17 L of fluid may be removed. Disadvantages are the requirement for systemic anticoagulation to prevent clotting of the filtration device, and the risk of arterial thrombosis at the site of catheter placement. For anticoagulation the filter is primed with 2000 IU heparin, and a constant infusion is begun at 10 IU/kg per h. For the patient in whom systemic heparinization is contraindicated, alternative modes of anticoagulation are possible. If the patient already has a bleeding diathesis (e.g., disseminated intravascular coagulation or hepatic failure), no exogenous anticoagulation may be needed, especially if blood pressure is adequate and the flow through the device is under low resistance. Even under these circumstances, however, the flow is so low that clotting frequently occurs. If the patient's problem is bleeding, then regional anticoagulation can be accomplished by infusing heparin into the outlet line and reversing the effects with a constant protamine infusion into the return line.[10,11] This method, though effective, requires very frequent monitoring of coagulation parameters and is quite cumbersome. Very low-dose systemic heparinization is probably equally effective, and is much easier. If systemic heparin is contraindicated because of heparin-associated thrombocytopenia, then regional citrate anticoagulation can be employed, in which sodium citrate is infused into the outlet line and calcium chloride is infused into the return line to reverse the anticoagulant effects.[12,13] Not only is this method cumbersome, but it can also lead to both sodium and citrate intoxication, resulting in severe hypernatremia and alkalosis, since there is incomplete removal of the sodium or citrate by the filter.[14,15] This form of anticoagulation should be used only with extreme caution, and only by experienced personnel.

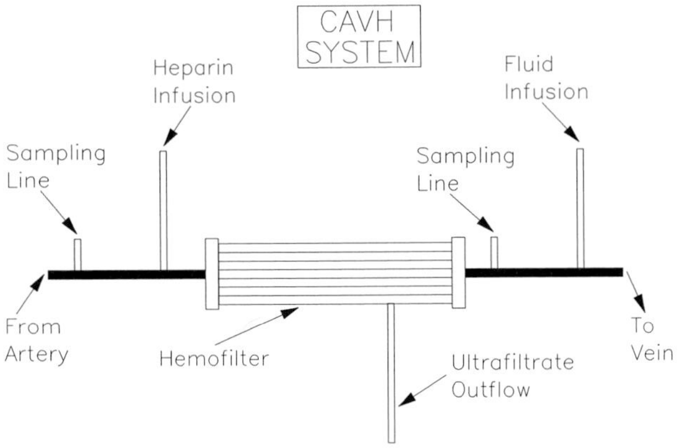

FIGURE 155-1 Schematic diagram of a typical continuous arteriovenous hemofiltration (CAVH) system.

CONTINUOUS ARTERIOVENOUS HEMOFILTRATION (CAVH)

The procedure from which SCUF is an outgrowth is continuous arteriovenous hemofiltration.[16,17] In principle CAVH is similar to SCUF, in that the same filtration device is used, and access to the circulation is gained through the femoral vessels (Fig. 155-1). CAVH differs from SCUF in that once euvolemia is achieved, the ultrafiltrate is replaced, on an hourly basis, with a substitution. Fluid removed during CAVH has an electrolyte composition identical to that of plasma, and although there is no commercially available substitution fluid for CAVH in the United States, many centers have used Ringer's solution ($[Na^+]$ = 130 meq/L, $[K^+]$ = 4 meq/L, $[Ca^{2+}]$ = 3 meq/L, $[Cl^-]$ = 109 meq/L, and [lactate] = 28 meq/L). Replacement of 15 L or less of ultrafiltrate in a 24-h period may not keep the BUN level below 100 mg/dL in the critically ill patient with acute renal failure. Modifications to CAVH that may overcome this problem include use of the pre-dilution mode, in which the substitution fluid is infused into the arterial line (entering the filtration device) instead of into the venous line, as is commonly practiced. Pre-dilution increases the rate of ultrafiltration by decreasing oncotic pressure inside the filter, and may diminish the problem of clotting in the filter.

Another means by which solute clearance may be increased is the incorporation of diffusive transport with the convective solute removal of CAVH. This technique has been named *continuous arteriovenous hemodiafiltration*, and is

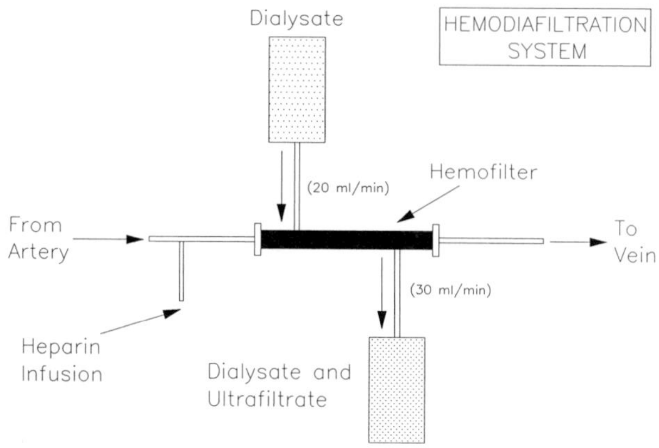

FIGURE 155-2 Schematic diagram of a typical continuous arteriovenous hemodiafiltration system.

accomplished by circulation of dialysate through the filter[18] (see Fig. 155-2). This can be done by gravity, or with an infusion pump, at a rate of up to 20 mL/min. Another technique, known as *continuous arteriovenous hemofiltration dialysis (CAVHD),* has been described, in which a standard artificial kidney is used in the circuit and solute clearance is achieved by diffusive transport.[19] The rate of ultrafiltration is low, however, precluding the use of this technique in patients with marked volume overload. The complications of CAVH and the other continuous renal replacement procedures are those related to anticoagulation and vascular complications at the site of cannulation. Frequent clotting of the filter may be a problem, especially with lower blood flows and hypotension. The vascular complications of principal concern are arterial thrombosis, aneurysm and fistula formation, and dissection. Furthermore, the patient must remain in bed for a long time.

HEMODIALYSIS

Hemodialysis is the most commonly used form of renal dialytic therapy, both in acute and in chronic situations. In some clinical conditions hemodialysis and peritoneal dialysis may be considered of equal efficacy, and, thus, the choice may become a simple matter of the physician's preference. Some clinical situations, however, may make hemodialysis preferable to peritoneal dialysis. Severely catabolic patients may overwhelm the clearance capabilities of peritoneal dialysis. Examples include acute rhabdomyolysis, sepsis complicating acute renal failure, and multiorgan failure syndromes. In these situations, daily hemodialysis may be necessary to control azotemia, uremia, or any of the multiple electrolyte abnormalities that can occur with acute renal failure—especially hyperkalemia. Additionally, patients who have undergone recent abdominal surgery, such as cholecystectomy or aneurysm repair; patients who have suffered an acute abdominal process, such as bowel rupture; and patients with a history of multiple intraabdominal procedures, may have extensive adhesions and are poor candidates for peritoneal dialysis. Therefore, hemodialysis offers them a better form of therapy.

Access to the intravascular space is a necessity and can be accomplished via one of several techniques. For the single dialysis procedure, large-bore catheters can be placed in a femoral artery and vein and removed at the end of dialysis. This technique has some advantages: the catheters are placed percutaneously at the bedside and are removed at the end of the procedure, thus lessening the chances of infection. However, for patients who need dialysis on a more long-term basis, this approach is impractical. Several temporary dialysis catheters are now available for short-term dialysis patients. These catheters are all large-bore and are inserted preferably into the subclavian or femoral vein, but occasionally into the jugular vein. The catheters can be single- or double-lumen; most are double-lumen with parallel intake and outflow paths. Many can be placed at the bedside, whereas others have to be placed in the operating room. These catheters have the advantages that they are relatively easy to place as minor surgical procedures and can be used immediately. On the other hand, the placement and use of these catheters is associated with a number of complications, both immediate and late[20–23] (see Chap. 24). Possible immediate complications include puncture of a major vascular structure with exsanguination, hemothorax, pneumothorax, and pericardial rupture and tamponade with catheters placed in the subclavian or internal jugular vein. Possible late complications include infection, subclavian vein thrombosis, and stenosis. Another form of temporary access is the Schribner shunt. This access device consists of two lengths of tubing placed within an artery and the adjacent vein, extending beyond the skin and linked into a loop by a connecting piece such that the two ends can be pulled apart and attached to dialysis tubing. The placement of such an access requires reasonably intact vasculature and some degree of technical expertise. These accesses function well but do have the disadvantages of destruction of the used vasculature, infection, and ischemia of distal tissue. While it is virtually impossible to predict how long a patient will require dialysis, the number of dialysis procedures generally corresponds to the overall severity of the patient's condition, the severity of the initial renal damage, and the likelihood of ongoing repetitive renal insults.[24] However, most episodes of acute renal failure resolve within 1 month, and only a small percentage of courses extend beyond 2 months. Because 4 to 8 weeks is well within the useful life span of a single venous catheter, and because these catheters are so easy to place, single-catheter access devices have become more popular and prevalent. If it is known from the outset that the likelihood of chronic renal failure is overwhelming—e.g., in the case of nephrectomy of all or most functioning renal tissue, or severe vascular compromise—then one may elect both to place a temporary central venous access and to create, simultaneously, a permanent vascular access (not in the same arm). Thus one can use the temporary access while awaiting maturation of the permanent access. If it is not possible to place the permanent access immediately, one should take care to avoid vascular punctures in the arm designated for the permanent access.

With hemodialysis, clearance is accomplished via diffusion and convection. The technique involves pumping blood from a large-caliber blood vessel into a filtration device composed of a biocompatible semipermeable material, then returning the blood to the vasculature. On the opposite side of the membrane is dialysate solution, the composition of which can be adjusted to achieve desired alterations in plasma composition. Generally, the sodium level is around 135 meq/L and the chloride level 100 to 110 meq/L. Levels of potassium and bicarbonate (or acetate, as a bicarbonate equivalent) can be varied according to the needs of the patient. The calcium level is generally high, at 3.0 to 3.5 meq/L ionized fraction, but can also be altered to accommodate a specific clinical situation. The magnesium level is 1 to 1.5 meq/L.

Dialysate may be single-pass—i.e., the dialysate flows through the system once and is then discarded—or regenerative. Single-pass dialysis is used in chronic dialysis units and most acute dialysis units. If a source of water and a mechanism for water purification, such as a portable deionizing unit, are available, then portable single-pass dialysis is possible in the critical care unit. An acceptable alternative to single-pass dialysis is the use of a cartridge system such as the REDY Sorbsystem, in which the dialysate is a single 5- or 6-L pool that is continuously "regenerated" via passage through a cartridge containing a series of filtration and absorption materials.[25] In most circumstances either source of dialysate is acceptable. Regenerative systems, however, have a few shortcomings. First, very high BUN concentrations may overwhelm the cartridge's filtration capacity, resulting in ammonia accumulation. Second, since the 5- or 6-L dialysate pool equilibrates against the total body water pool, it may be difficult to alter sodium, chloride, and bicarbonate concentrations unless the bath is changed frequently during the procedure.

The efficiency with which a substance is cleared from the blood is a function of a number of factors: blood flow rate, dialysate flow rate, surface area of the filter, characteristics of the membrane, pressure across the membrane, and the size and charge of the specific substance. The blood flow rates range between 150 and 350 mL/min, depending on the type and site of vascular access. Increasing blood flow tends to increase clearance. While 300 to 350 mL/min is usually easily accomplished with a permanent access, single-catheter temporary devices may not permit such high flow. Thus the blood flow rate can be a limiting factor in efficiency of dialysis. Dialysate flow rates are generally 500 mL/min. Little increase in clearance results from dialysate flow rates in excess of 500 mL/min. Dialysis membranes are manufactured by several firms; the ultrafiltration coefficient and the clearance properties of each membrane are published by its manufacturer. A higher ultrafiltration coefficient increases efficiency of fluid removal. For usual dialysis, the membranes are all very similar in these characteristics. The membranes used for SCUF, on the other hand, have a much higher ultrafiltration coefficient in order to accomplish such massive volume loss at minimum blood flows and pressure differentials. Within a given manufacturer's line, a higher model number indicates a greater surface area and, thus, greater ultrafiltration and clearance per unit time. On the whole, small particles, such as urea, tend to be cleared more efficiently than larger molecules, such as creatinine. Likewise, for the same size, charged particles move less readily than neutral ones.

Generally, during a single dialysis procedure the expected drop in BUN concentration should be greater than 60 percent. Increased clearance can be accomplished by increasing the blood flow rate, applying pressure at the venous return line to increase ultrafiltration, using a larger filter, or increasing dialysis time. If the urea concentration remains elevated despite apparently adequate dialysis sessions (4 to 5 h), one should examine the dialysis record to confirm adequate blood flow (300 mL/min or more) for the entire dialysis period and calculate the percentage of recirculation of blood within the vascular access. The *percentage of recirculation* is the percentage of blood entering the arterial outflow line that is derived from newly dialyzed blood being returned to the body via the venous return line. Up to 10 percent recirculation is considered tolerable within an established fistula or graft; higher values (up to 15 or 20 percent) are seen with single-needle devices. Recirculation is calculated as follows:

$$\frac{P - A}{P - V} \times 100 = \% \text{ recirculation} \qquad (155\text{-}1)$$

where P, A, and V are the concentrations of urea in a peripheral artery or vein, the arterial outflow line, and the venous return line, respectively. Higher-than-usual recirculation suggests a malfunctioning access. Persistent elevations of the BUN level despite adequate flow rates, acceptable recirculation percentage, and a greater than 60 percent decrease in BUN per dialysis treatment must be the result of enhanced urea generation. Increased rates of urea production occur with excessive protein loads (e.g., in parenteral nutrition), gastrointestinal bleeding, or severely catabolic states, such as sepsis or multiorgan failure. Efforts to decrease the BUN level, then, should be directed at decreasing nonessential protein sources (such as gastrointestinal blood) and further intensifying dialysis efforts.

COMPLICATIONS

The complications of the hemodialysis procedure may preclude its application to some patients.[26] Hypotension is the most common, occurring in over 70 percent of the patients with acute renal failure in a recent survey of our experience. The possible causes of hypotension are several, including allergic reaction to the dialysis membrane, volume depletion, pericardial effusion, peripheral vasodilation, dialysis-associated hypoxemia, acute bleeding, and hypocalcemia. Thus patients with very poor cardiac function, autonomic neuropathy, sepsis, or underlying pulmonary disease may be at high risk for this complication. Generally, dialysis-associated hypotension is easily managed with fluid repletion, the use of a small-sized dialysis filter, or low-dose vasopressors. If fluid removal is a necessity, ultrafiltration alone, followed by hemodialysis, is sometimes better tolerated from a hemodynamic standpoint.[27] Additionally, there may be some benefit in prophylactically increasing inspired oxygen concentration prior to dialysis and planning transfusions of blood products while dialysis is in progress. Severe and repeated hypotensive events on hemodialysis suggest that an alternative dialytic modality may be indicated, and should prompt evaluation for pericardial effusion. Also, since acetate has been associated with myocardial depression and peripheral vasodilation, a dialysate containing bicarbonate, rather than acetate, is preferable.[28]

Two other potentially life-threatening complications of hemodialysis are cardiac arrhythmias and hypoxemia. Cardiac arrhythmias may be secondary to acute electrolyte abnormalities, such as hypokalemia caused by dialysis against a very low-potassium bath; hypoxemia secondary to dialysis-induced hypoventilation and complement activation is aggravated when cardiac output is reduced during dialysis. Patients with underlying cardiac arrhythmias (or cardiac failure) and patients on digoxin should be dialyzed against a bath of relatively normal potassium concentration, with close attention also to maintenance of a relatively normal pH. Hypoxemia occurring on dialysis results from at least two different mechanisms.[29–32] Removal of carbon dioxide by dialysis results in hypoventilation and a decreased minute ventilation, thus causing hypoxemia. Additionally, contact of the patient's blood with the dialysis membrane results in activation of complement, causing sequestration of leukocytes in the pulmonary vasculature and leading to ventilation/perfusion ($\dot{V}/\dot{Q}$) mismatch and subsequent hypoxemia. In a patient with relatively normal pulmonary function and arterial blood gases, the small decrement in P_{O_2} is of little clinical significance. However, in a patient with substantial underlying pulmonary disease even this small change may result in significant desaturation. Thus supplemental oxygen or pulse oximetry is recommended for these patients.

Besides hypoxemia, complications related to the dialysis membrane itself include leukopenia and the so-called first-use syndrome.[33–35] Leukopenia, a result of complement activation and leukocyte sequestration, occurs within the first hour of dialysis and generally resolves by the end of the procedure. It is important to recognize that this complication occurs, and to avoid obtaining white blood cell counts after dialysis is initiated. *First-use syndrome* is a cluster of symptoms that occurs in some patients experiencing dialysis with a certain type of dialysis membrane for the first time. Symptoms generally start about 30 min after the initiation of dialysis and may include chest pain, abdominal cramps, shortness of breath, and back pain. On examination the patient may have wheezes and flushing of the upper chest and neck. These symptoms can be treated conservatively, and dialysis continued. Very rarely a patient will experience a true anaphylactic reaction to a kidney membrane, particularly those containing cuprophane.[36] Many patients may experience other relatively nonspecific, but fairly common, symptoms, such as nausea, vomiting, and muscle cramps. If the patient is extremely azotemic and is dialyzed very aggressively, then he or she may suffer from symptoms of fatigue, washout, and, under most unusual circumstances, dialysis disequilibrium. Dialysis disequilibrium is characterized by altered sensorium and headache, and even by seizures in extreme cases; it can be prevented by more conservative early dialysis.

Technical errors can also lead to potentially severe complications, such as air embolism or acute hemolysis secondary to the use of improperly prepared, or contaminated, dialysate. The use of heparin for anticoagulation may be complicated by bleeding or thrombocytopenia. The two alternatives to heparin that may be more suitable in the critical care setting are sodium citrate and frequent saline flushes.

ALTERNATE FORMS OF DIALYSIS

Other forms of dialysis requiring vascular access include high-flux hemodialysis, hemodiafiltration, and charcoal hemoperfusion. The first two have been used only rarely in the acute setting. High-flux dialysis requires the use of an exceedingly porous membrane with high clearances of higher-molecular-weight molecules. Control of volume loss is accomplished through built-in hydrostatic pressure controls. Thus the machinery is somewhat more expensive, but its use can result in lower dialysis times and better clearances of some of the substances thought to contribute to the uremic syndrome, such as β_2-microglobulin. The usefulness of this technique in the acute setting is unknown. Hemodiafiltration involves removal of large volumes of plasma ultrafiltrate during an intermittent hemodialysis session with concomitant replacement by crystalloid solutions. Again, experience in application of this technique in the acute setting is lacking. Charcoal hemoperfusion has been used in two major clinical settings: acute poisoning and hepatic failure. This technique involves exposing blood to a filter containing activated charcoal particles, which absorb a wide variety of known and unknown substances. Hemoperfusion is more effective in removing highly lipophilic or protein-bound substances than regular hemodialysis. Thus salicylates and barbiturates are removed more effectively by hemoperfusion than by hemodialysis; however, the percentage of poisonings that require intervention of this nature is quite limited.[37] Charcoal hemoperfusion has been attempted for removal of a large number of different chemicals, but there are few comparative studies or sizable trials. Decision-making on the use of this technique in the treatment of poisoning relies heavily on clinical judgment. The same is true for the use of this technique in fulminant hepatic failure. Anecdotal reports document its usefulness on a temporary basis in the treatment of acute hepatic coma, but there is no evidence of any impact on mortality in any large clinical trials. The major complications of this modality are thrombocytopenia and hypocalcemia.

PERITONEAL DIALYSIS

Because of less efficient clearance of small solutes, peritoneal dialysis is not the procedure of first choice for the catabolic patient with acute renal failure. Nevertheless, in circumstances where hemodialysis cannot be safely performed (hypotension, cardiogenic shock, acute myocardial infarction), peritoneal dialysis may be indicated. Further, peritoneal dialysis is more easily performed than hemodialysis in small children, and is an alternative mode of therapy when blood access cannot be obtained. Conditions that may contraindicate peritoneal dialysis, or make it difficult, include postoperative or traumatized abdomen and disorders associated with reduced peritoneal clearance, such as shock, disseminated intravascular coagulation, peritoneal fibrosis, intraabdominal adhesions, and vascular disease of the peritoneum (e.g., scleroderma, malignant hypertension).

The principal advantages of peritoneal dialysis include ease of setup and fewer complications related to less abrupt changes in solute concentration. Access to the peritoneal cavity is achieved with an acute or chronic catheter. Acute catheters are rigid and are placed percutaneously by direct puncture a few centimeters below the umbilicus, in a midline position. We prefer the chronic catheter (e.g., Tenckhoff), which is placed under sterile conditions in an operating room.

Several techniques of peritoneal dialysis are usable in the critical care setting. For intermittent peritoneal dialysis (IPD), 2 L of peritoneal dialysate is instilled over 10 min, is permitted to dwell 30 min, and then is drained over the next 20 min, for a cycle time of 1 h. This may be done manually, but requires close nursing attention and is complicated by higher rates of peritonitis. The exchange volume may be adjusted from 1 to 3 L, according to the patient's abdominal capacity and underlying pulmonary compromise. With manual techniques it is difficult to maintain a dialysate exchange rate greater than 2 L/h. Automated techniques using cyclers permit an increase in dialysate flow; a standard protocol may use an exchange cycle with 5- to 10-min infusion time, 5- to 15-min dwell time, and 10- to 20-min drain time, resulting in a dialysate flow of up to 4 L/h. Such a protocol results in a urea clearance of 20 to 25 mL/min and a creatinine clearance of 12 to 20 mL/min. More rapid cycling (greater than 4 L/h) may increase urea clearance toward a maximum of 30 mL/min, but is likely to be poorly tolerated. Once control of uremia has been achieved with continuous 24-h IPD, it may be possible to switch to a regimen of nightly peritoneal dialysis [known as *continuous cyclic peritoneal dialysis* (CCPD) if a cycler is employed]. With such a regimen dialysis is performed for 10 to 12 h each night, with a 2 L/h exchange rate.

An approach that may improve the efficiency of intermittent peritoneal dialysis regimens is known as *tidal peritoneal dialysis*. With this technique a constant volume of dialysate remains in the peritoneal cavity, and a tidal volume is circulated rapidly. The advantage of this technique is that dialysate is always present in the peritoneal cavity and large volumes of dialysate flow are possible. The disadvantage of the technique is the requirement and expense of large volumes of fluid, as well as the need for a reciprocating pump device. It is claimed that the best clearances of urea and creatinine are obtained with a residual and tidal volume of 1.5 L. At present this method is not practical for use in the ICU setting. Other ways to increase the efficiency of peritoneal dialysis include the use of intraperitoneal or systemic vasodilators. Nitroprusside administered by the intraperitoneal route may double the clearance of solutes with larger molecular weights, but clearances of smaller solutes are augmented by less than 20 percent. Only rarely does nitroprusside have a role in peritoneal dialysis for the patient with acute renal failure.

SOLUTIONS FOR PERITONEAL DIALYSIS

Commercially available solutions for peritoneal dialysis (Dianeal, Travenol) have the following composition: [Na^+] 132 meq/L, [Cl^-] 96 meq/L, [Ca^{2+}] 3.5 meq/L, [Mg^{2+}] 0.5 meq/L, [lactate] 40 meq/L. Potassium may be added up to a concentration of 4.0 meq/L, depending on the patient's serum K^+ level. Glucose concentration is varied according to the need for ultrafiltration; 1.5% Dianeal has a D-glucose concentration of 1.5 g/dL, 2.5% contains 2.5 g/dL, and 4.25% has 4.25 g/dL. The osmolalities of these solutions are 346, 396, and 485 mOsm per kg H_2O, respectively. Rates of ultrafiltration with the 4.25% solution may approach 700 mL/h, and even with the 1.5% solution a modest ultrafiltration of 100 to 200 mL per 2-L exchange may be observed.

EFFICIENCY OF PERITONEAL DIALYSIS

Clearance of small solutes by peritoneal dialysis is less than 20 percent of the rate attained with hemodialysis. Because of this, peritoneal dialysis may be unsuitable for the catabolic patient with ARF. Rates of potassium removal on peritoneal dialysis are generally less than 12 meq/H, whereas hourly sodium polystyrene sulfonate (Kayexalate) enemas (30 g) may remove up to 30 meq/h.[38] Metabolic acidosis is corrected by peritoneal dialysis, albeit more slowly than with hemodialysis. Ultrafiltration rates are also less than those seen with hemodialysis, but with 4.25% solutions they may approach 700 mL/h. Clearance of high-molecular-weight solutes (MW approximately 5000) is comparable to that seen with hemodialysis.

RESULTS AND COMPLICATIONS OF PERITONEAL DIALYSIS

While no formal controlled comparison has been made of peritoneal dialysis versus hemodialysis in the management of ARF, reported mortality rates are similar.[39] Complications of peritoneal dialysis include mechanical events, such as fluid leakage around the catheter, inadequate drainage, and edema of the scrotum and abdominal wall. Infectious complications include peritonitis, as well as infections at the exit site or in the catheter tunnel. Peritonitis is diagnosed by the appearance of cloudy drainage fluid and the presence of a WBC count greater than 100 cells per mm^3, predominantly polymorphonuclear leukocytes. Treatment consists of parenteral or intraperitoneal antibiotics. If there is no response to an appropriate antibiotic in proper dosage after 24 to 36 h, consideration should be given to removing the catheter. Tunnel abscess or catheter biofilms, if present, may preclude recovery from peritonitis. Pulmonary complications directly related to peritoneal dialysis include basal atelectasis and the occasional pleural effusion (sometimes massive). Pleural effusion may arise because of a diaphragmatic hernia (congenital or acquired) and may respond to dialysis in a more upright position.

Metabolic complications of peritoneal dialysis include hyperglycemia, postdialysis hypoglycemia, hypernatremia, and protein loss. Hyperglycemia most commonly accompanies the frequent use of 4.25% solutions. If necessary, insulin can be administered by the intraperitoneal route or parenterally. More intensive insulin therapy is required in diabetic patients; it is estimated that during hourly exchanges of peritoneal dialysis fluid, one-half of the administered glucose may be absorbed. Hypernatremia is an unusual complication, but can occur in the setting of frequent monitoring of the serum electrolyte concentrations. It is recommended that electrolyte and glucose measurements be performed within the first four hours of peritoneal dialysis, and rechecked as indicated, generally at least daily.

CASE PRESENTATION—1

A 50-year-old woman with hepatic failure secondary to chronic active hepatitis undergoes orthotopic liver transplant. During surgery she has several hypotensive episodes and receives over 50 U of blood products and 10 L of crystalloid. Urine output during the 8 h surgery is 650 mL. Postoperatively her systolic blood pressure hovers around 80 mmHg on dopamine, 12 μg/kg per min. Her weight is 25 kg in excess of her preoperative condition; she has pulmonary edema as well as diffuse peripheral edema. Urine output is less than 10 mL/h, despite high-dose parenteral furosemide. Because of persistent bleeding, the surgery team wish to administer coagulation products, but are concerned about volume status. The BUN and creatinine levels are 25 and 0.9 mg/dL, respectively. The serum potassium level is 4.8 meq/L.

CASE DISCUSSION—1

The ideal form of dialytic therapy for this woman would be slow continuous ultrafiltration. The major goal of therapy in this case is removal of fluid. Her recent abdominal surgery precludes peritoneal dialysis. Her serum chemistries do not indicate an urgent need for dialysis. Hemodynamically she appears somewhat unstable so intermittent hemodialysis or ultrafiltration may precipitate worse hypotension. SCUF offers the ability to remove large volumes continuously, thus allowing continued administration of blood products as needed. With her coagulopathy, there is risk associated with catheter insertion, but this would be true for any form of access.

CASE PRESENTATION—2

A 25-year-old construction worker sustains a massive crush injury on the job. He is admitted to the ICU in acute oliguric renal failure secondary to rhabdomyolysis. Blood pressure is 160/90, pulse 120. On examination he has bilateral rales, myoedema, and an ileus. Laboratory analysis shows a BUN level of 40 mg/dL, creatinine 5.4 mg/dL, and potassium 6.3 meq/L. Despite insulin/bicarbonate infusions and sodium polystyrene sulfonate enemas his potassium level rises to 7.8 meq/L. Urine output does not increase in response to high-dose furosemide and chlorothiazide combined.

CASE DISCUSSION—2

The only feasible means of dialyzing this man is acute hemodialysis. The primary goal of therapy is control of acute hyperkalemia. Since he is oliguric, volume overload will become a problem soon as well. With his healthy muscle mass, this man is severely catabolic, and the rate of potassium release would exceed the capacity of peritoneal dialysis or CAVHD. At the bedside, an acute hemodialysis catheter could be placed and dialysis against a dialysate bath containing no potassium could be initiated within 1 h. Dialysis may be required even more often than daily, if dictated by the electrolytes.

CASE PRESENTATION—3

A 68-year-old diabetic man with severe congestive heart failure secondary to ischemic heart disease is admitted with progressive peripheral edema and shortness of breath. Physical examination reveals a dyspneic man with a blood pressure of 85/50 and massive anasarca. High-dose parenteral diuretics result in the development of hyponatremia, hypokalemia, and azotemia. He complains of nausea, anorexia, worsening muscular weakness, and excessive sleepiness.

CASE DISCUSSION—3

In this case, aggressive treatment of the hypoperfusion state should be the primary goal of therapy. In addition, peritoneal dialysis would be an excellent choice of dialytic therapy. The primary goal of dialytic therapy here is volume removal. Ultrafiltration via a vascular access may be hazardous in this patient with severe heart failure and hypotension. Likewise, being diabetic, he may have autonomic neuropathy and be unable to vasoconstrict peripherally in response to rapid fluid removal. CAVH would necessitate bed rest and systemic anticoagulation—both unnecessary and undesirable complications to add to his condition. Peritoneal dialysis offers slow, continuous, hemodynamically nonstressful fluid removal with little risk of hypotension or bleeding. Additionally, it would correct his electrolyte abnormalities as well as his azotomia.

References

1. Suki WN, Stinebaugh BJ, Frommer JP, et al: Physiology of diuretic action, in Seldin DW, Giebisch G (eds): *The Kidney: Physiology and Pathophysiology*. New York, Raven Press, 1985, pp 2144–2154.
2. Merrill JP, Hampers CL: Uremia. N Engl J Med 285:953, 1970.
3. Giovannetti S, Berlyne GM: An outline of the uremic syndrome. Nephron 14:119, 1975.
4. Shattil SJ, Bennett JS: Platelets and their membranes in hemostasis: Physiology and pathophysiology. Ann Intern Med 94:108, 1981.
5. Oriieke J, Le Pailleur C, Zingraff J, et al: Uremic cardiomyopathy and pericarditis. Adv Nephrol 9:33, 1980.

6. Schreiner GE, Maher JF, Argy WP Jr, et al: Extracorporeal and peritoneal dialysis of drugs, in Brodie BB, Gillette JR (eds): *Concepts in Biochemical Pharmacology,* Handbook of Experimental Pharmacology, vol 28. Berlin, Springer-Verlag, 1971, p 403.
7. DiLeo M, Pacitti A, Bergerone S, et al: Ultrafiltration in the treatment of refractory congestive heart failure. Clin Cardiol 11:449, 1988.
8. Shilo S, Slotki IN, Iaina A: Improved renal function following acute peritoneal dialysis in patients with intractable congestive heart failure. Isr J Med Sci 23:821, 1987.
9. Kramer P, Wigger W, Rieger J, et al: Arteriovenous hemofiltration: A new and simple method for treatment of overhydrated patients resistant to diuretics. Klin Wochenschr 55:1121, 1977.
10. Swartz RD, Port FK: Preventing hemorrhage in high risk hemodialysis: Regional versus low-dose heparin. Kidney Int 16:513, 1979.
11. Shapiro WB, Faubert PF, Poruch JG, et al: Low-dose heparin in routine hemodialysis monitored by activated partial thromboplastin time. Artif Organs 3:73, 1979.
12. Ashouri OS: Regional sodium citrate anticoagulation in patients with active bleeding undergoing hemodialysis. Uremia Invest 9:45, 1985–1986.
13. Lohr JW, Slusher S, Diederich DA: Regional citrate anticoagulation for hemodialysis following cardiovascular surgery. Am J Nephrol 8:368, 1988.
14. Silverstein FJ, Oster JR, Perez GO, et al: Metabolic alkalosis induced by regional citrate hemodialysis. ASAIO-Trans 35:22, 1989.
15. Suki WN, Boneulos RD, Yocom S, et al: Citrate for regional anticoagulation. Effects on blood P_{O_2}, ammonia and aluminum. ASAIO-Trans 34:524, 1988.
16. Kramer P, Kaufhold C, Grove HJ, et al: Management of anuric intensive-care patients with arteriovenous hemofiltration. Int J Artif Organs 3:255, 1980.
17. Golper JA: Continuous arteriovenous hemofiltration in acute renal failure. Am J Kidney Dis 6:373, 1985.
18. Rong C, Brendolan S, Bragantini L, et al: Arteriovenous hemodiafiltration: A combined therapy for acute renal failure in the hypercatabolic patients, in La Greca G, Fabris A, Ronco C: *CAVH.* Milan, Wichtig Editore, 1986, p 171.
19. Geronemus R, Schneider N: Continuous arteriovenous hemodialysis: A new modality for treatment of acute renal failure: Trans Am Soc Artif Intern Organs, 30:610, 1984.
20. Moss AH, McLaughlin MM, Lempert KD, et al: Use of a silicone catheter with a Dacron cuff for dialysis short term vascular access. Am J Kidney Dis 12:492, 1988.
21. Donnelly PK, Hoenich NA, Lennard TW, et al: Surgical management of long-term central venous access in uraemic patients. Nephrol Dial Transplant 3:57, 1988.
22. Schwab SJ, Butler GL, McCann RL, et al: Prospective evaluation of a Dacron cuffed hemodialysis catheter for prolonged use. Am J Kidney Dis 11:166, 1988.
23. Tilney NL, Kirkman RL, Whittemon AD, et al: Vascular access for dialysis and cancer chemotherapy. Adv Surg 19:221, 1986.
24. Myers BD, Moran SM: Hemodynamically mediated acute renal failure. N Engl J Med 314:97, 1986.
25. Drukker W, Van Doorn AWJ: Dialysate regeneration, in Maher JF (ed): *Replacement of Renal Function by Dialysis.* Kluwer Academie Dordrecht Holland, 1989, pp 421–426.
26. Lazarus JM: Complications in hemodialysis: An overview. Kidney Int 18:783, 1980.
27. Ing TS, Chen WT, Daugirdas JT, et al: Isolated ultrafiltration and new techniques of ultrafiltration during dialysis. Kidney Int 18:S77, 1980.
28. Velez RL, Woodard TD, Henrich WL: Acetate and bicarbonate hemodialysis in patients with and without autonomic dysfunction. Kidney Int 26:59, 1984.
29. Cardoso M, Vinay P, Vinet B, et al: Hypoxemia during hemodialysis: A critical review of the facts. Am J Kid Dis 11:281, 1988.
30. Eiser A, Jayamanni D, Kohsing C, et al: Contrasting alterations in pulmonary gas exchange during acetate and bicarbonate hemodialysis. Am J Nephrol 2:123, 1982.
31. Garella S, Chang BS: Hemodialysis-Associated hypoxemia. Am J Nephrol 4:273, 1984.
32. Oh MS, Uribarri J, DelMonte ML, et al: A mechanism of hypoxemia during hemodialysis. Am J Nephrol 5:366, 1985.
33. Hakim RM, Breillatt J, Lazarus JM, et al: Complement activation and hypersensitivity reactions to dialysis membranes. N Engl J Med 311:878, 1984.
34. Arnaout MA, Hakim RM, Todd RF, et al: Increased expression of an adhesion-promoting surface glycoprotein with granulocytopenia of hemodialysis. N Engl J Med 312:457, 1985.
35. Ogden DA: New dialyzer syndrome. N Engl J Med 302:1262, 1980.
36. Daugirdas JT, Ing TS, Roxe DM, et al: Severe anaphylactoid reaction to cuprammonium cellulose hemodialyzers. Arch Intern Med 145:489, 1985.
37. Lorch JA, Gaulle S: Hemoperfusion to treat intoxications. Ann Intern Med 91:301, 1979.
38. Brown SJ, Ahearn DJ, Nolph KD: Potassium removal with peritoneal dialysis. Kidney Int 4:67, 1973.
39. Tirmat J, Zucchini A: Peritoneal dialysis in acute renal failure, in Trevino-Becerra A, Boen JS (eds): *Today's Art of Peritoneal Dialysis,* Contributions to Nephrology, vol 17. Basel, S. Karger, 1979, p 33.

Chapter 156

SEVERE ELECTROLYTE DISTURBANCES

STEPHEN BRENNAN
ELEANOR D. LEDERER

KEY POINTS

- *One should always measure plasma osmolality before beginning treatment for hyponatremia or hypernatremia.*
- *Treatment of symptomatic hyponatremia should often be begun before its cause has been determined.*
- *Because of a large intracellular pool, disorders of the serum potassium level are frequently caused by altered distribution of the cation between intra- and extracellular sites.*
- *Hyperkalemia of any severity should be treated emergently if typical ECG changes are present.*
- *Hypocalcemia does not require urgent treatment unless it is symptomatic.*
- *Hypomagnesemia frequently accompanies hypokalemia and hypocalcemia; it may be necessary to correct the magnesium deficit before the potassium and calcium level will return to normal.*
- *Symptomatic phosphorus depletion can be present with a normal serum phosphorus level; treatment should begin if a high index of suspicion is present.*
- *Severe hyperphosphatemia occurs almost exclusively in the setting of significant renal failure or severe cell lysis.*

Abnormalities of Body Fluid Tonicity

The osmolality of all body fluids is usually maintained within a narrow range (285 to 295 mOsm/kg). Because water is in equilibrium across cell membranes, any change in the ratio between total body solutes and water will result in an abnormal plasma tonicity. Disorders of plasma osmolality (Posm) are usually diagnosed because of abnormalities in the plasma sodium level. Hyponatremia usually is associated with hypotonic plasma, and hypernatremia is associated with hyperosmolality. In order to diagnose and treat disorders of plasma tonicity effectively, an understanding of the normal mechanisms that defend the Posm is essential.[1] These are summarized in Fig. 156-1.

Production of dilute urine requires adequate delivery of solute and water to the so-called diluting segment of the nephron (the cortical thick limb of Henle's loop), which then reabsorbs NaCl and KCl but not water. This renders the tubular fluid hypotonic with respect to plasma. In the absence of antidiuretic hormone (ADH), the water permeability of the more distal nephron segments is normally very low, preventing further water reabsorption. Urinary

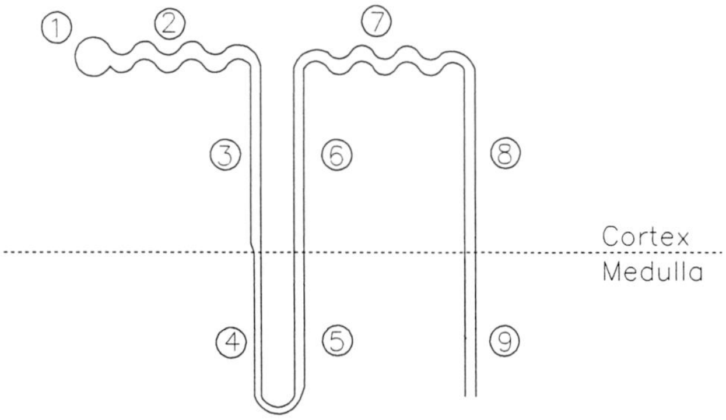

FIGURE 156-1 Regulation of renal water excretion. Normal water balance depends on normal filtration of water and solutes (1) and intact reabsorptive function of the proximal convoluted tubule (2) and the proximal straight tubule (3). The thin descending limb (4) allows water extraction so that high solute concentrations are presented to the thick ascending limb for reabsorption. In the concentrating segment of the nephron (medullary thick limb of Henle's loop) (5), active solute reabsorption results in the creation of a hypertonic medullary interstitium. In the diluting segment (cortical thick limb of Henle's loop) (6), continuing solute reabsorption results in the production of tubular fluid, which is hypotonic with respect to plasma. This process reaches its maximum in the distal convoluted tubule (7). In the absence of ADH the remainder of the nephron is essentially water-impermeable. In the presence of ADH, over 80 percent of tubular water is reabsorbed in the cortical collecting tubule (8), and most of the remainder is reabsorbed as the urine achieves its highest osmolality while traversing the medullary region (9) in the medullary and papillary collecting ducts.

concentration requires, in addition, the intact function of the concentrating segment (the medullary thick limb of Henle's loop), which generates medullary hypertonicity, and of the vasa recta, which maintain this osmolar gradient. The water permeability of the distal nephron increases in the presence of ADH, allowing water to diffuse from the tubular lumen into the renal interstitium for return to the plasma. ADH levels are regulated mainly by the plasma osmolality, but other factors[2] that stimulate ADH release are hypovolemia, pain, nausea, and some drugs (especially narcotic analgesics).

Changes in Posm are of clinical importance because of secondary effects on cell volume and composition.[3,4] Since water can freely pass cell membranes, hypotonicity causes cell swelling, while the converse occurs with hypertonicity. Cell volume regulation occurs in somatic cells following changes in Posm. Restoration of cell volume occurs by active increases or decreases in intracellular solute levels. This process begins within a few hours in the brain and is virtually complete within 2 to 3 days. These adaptive responses are of paramount importance when considering the clinical syndromes of hyper- and hypoosmolality.

HYPOTONICITY/HYPONATREMIA

Hyponatremia is of clinical importance only if it is associated with hypotonicity. Although hyponatremia is usually

TABLE 156-1 Causes of Pseudohyponatremia

Plasma osmolality normal	
	Hyperlipidemia
	Hyperproteinemia
Plasma osmolality elevated	
	Hyperglycemia
	Mannitol infusion
	Radiographic contrast agents (diatrizoate sodium)
	Glycerol administration

associated with a low osmolality as well, normal plasma osmolality or even hypertonicity may be seen.[1,5] Those conditions in which the plasma Na level is low despite normal or elevated Posm are referred to collectively as *pseudohyponatremia* and are listed in Table 156-1. Their existence underscores the importance of measuring Posm directly, before treatment of hyponatremia is begun. In this chapter we will use the term *hyponatremia* to mean a true state of hypotonicity in which the Posm has been proven to be low. The symptoms of hyponatremia depend on its duration and the rapidity with which it develops. We thus consider the problem from the standpoint of whether hypotonicity is acute or chronic.

Acute hyponatremia is defined as a hypotonic state that develops within 24 h, before regulation of cell volume has occurred. There are only a few clinical settings in which it usually occurs. In postoperative patients, nonosmotic stimuli for the release of ADH (pain, narcotics, nausea) can result in hyponatremia,[6] particularly with the administration of hypotonic fluids perioperatively. This is particularly true in the patient undergoing transurethral resection of the prostate, in whom electrolyte-free solutions are required for irrigation of the operative field.[7] Patients with psychiatric disorders are also at risk for the development of acute hyponatremia,[8] because the neurochemistry of the psychotic state itself causes increases in ADH levels. The effects of psychotropic medications on stimulating ADH release may be a factor in a small minority of patients. Although most patients with psychogenic polydipsia never develop acute or severe hyponatremia, a substantial fraction of cases of severe symptomatic hyponatremia occurs in this population. The therapeutic use of oxytocin (which possesses ADH activity) in salt-free water can cause serious hyponatremia.[9] If high doses of oxytocin are used, the increased rate of drug delivery is accompanied by increased free water administration as well. This can even be seen occasionally in normal labor and delivery. Finally, diuretic medications (particularly thiazides) can lead to hyponatremia,[10] which has been shown to develop within 24 to 48 h in some patients. The mechanism by which this occurs is thought to be nonosmotic (volume depletion) stimulation of ADH release, coupled with stimulation of thirst and diluting segment dysfunction.

Chronic hyponatremia is a pathophysiologic state that is fundamentally different from acute hyponatremia, although no less critical.[11] The most common etiologies for chronic hyponatremia are diuretic use, edema-forming states, and the syndrome of inappropriate ADH secretion (SIADH). Diuretic-induced hyponatremia is caused by chronic stimulation of ADH secretion due to volume depletion, combined with inhibition of the function of the diluting segment (particularly with thiazide diuretics). The edema-forming states (heart failure, cirrhosis, and the nephrotic syndrome) are characterized by gross expansion of the extracellular fluid (ECF). However, the kidneys behave as if they were hypoperfused: the glomerular filtration rate (GFR) is diminished, proximal tubule reabsorption of salt and water are enhanced, and urinary excretion of Na is very low. ADH secretion is supranormal. *SIADH* is defined as hyponatremia that occurs in the absence of any known physiologic stimulus for ADH release (especially volume depletion), and excretion of urine that is not maximally dilute (normal subjects given a water load can achieve a urinary osmolality of <100 mOsm/kg). Usually SIADH is a complication of pulmonary or CNS diseases, or is a paraneoplastic syndrome. Causes are listed in Table 156-2.

As acute hypotonicity develops, the neurons swell within the rigid cranial vault. Perhaps because of hormonally mediated differences in water permeability of the brain,[12] females seem to be particularly susceptible to symptomatic hyponatremia. The early symptoms are nonspecific, including agitation, nausea, delirium, and weakness, ultimately progressing to seizures and hypotension. Later, herniation may occur. However, Arieff[13] has shown

TABLE 156-2 Causes of the Syndrome of Inappropriate ADH Secretion (SIADH)

Malignancies	
	Pharyngeal
	Genitourinary (bladder, ureter, prostate)
	Lymphoma
	Pancreas
Pulmonary disorders	
	Bronchogenic carcinoma
	Mesothelioma
	Pneumonia
	Pneumothorax
	Positive-pressure ventilation
	Asthma
CNS diseases	
	Infections (encephalitis, meningitis, abscess)
	Trauma
	Brain tumors
	Intracranial hemorrhage
	Acute psychosis
	Multiple sclerosis
Drugs	
	Chlorpropamide
	Carbamazepine
	Antidepressants (?)
	Clofibrate
	Antineoplastic drugs (vincristine, cyclophosphamide)
	Narcotic analgesics
	Nonsteroidal anti-inflammatory drugs
	Isoproterenol
	Nicotine

that devastating hyponatremia can occur very abruptly in previously healthy young women. The nonspecific nature of the symptoms often leads to a substantial delay before the correct diagnosis is entertained and ultimately treated. On occasion, the first symptom of acute hyponatremia is respiratory arrest. Because of the efficiency of the adaptive processes, chronic hyponatremia is usually asymptomatic. Since the brain's water content is nearly normal, cerebral edema generally does not occur. Any symptoms that develop are the consequences of alterations in cell solute content and of changes in transmembrane ion gradients that require a more severe decrement in plasma Na. The clinical complaints include weakness, lethargy, nausea, and, ultimately, seizures and coma when the limits of adaptive cell volume regulation have been breached.

The diagnostic evaluation in cases of suspected acute hyponatremia is relatively straightforward. The most important tests are the osmolality and electrolyte composition of urine and plasma. Unfortunately, the osmolality measurements alone do not discriminate between those solutes that are "effective" osmoles (i.e., not freely permeable across cell membranes) and the "ineffective" osmoles, of which urea is quantitatively the most important. It is sometimes useful to compute a corrected value of Posm (^{c}Posm) using the formula

$$^{c}\text{Posm} = \text{Posm (measured)} - (\text{BUN in mg/dL})/2.8 \quad (156\text{-}1)$$

The normal range is 280 to 290 mOsm/kg. An analogous calculation can also be applied to obtain the corrected urine osmolality (Uosm). The corrected Uosm is usually elevated; however, it may be surprisingly low in the edema-forming states, because of avid Na reclamation (a reflection of the functional state of volume depletion).[14] The documentation of a low Uosm in the face of serum hypoosmolality is virtually diagnostic of "pure" water intoxication. If SIADH is suspected, the Uosm should be less than maximally dilute (in fact, it is usually more concentrated than the plasma); there should be no evidence for the existence of an edema-forming condition; and tests of thyroid, renal, and adrenal function must all be normal.

Standard texts usually attempt to classify hyponatremia on the basis of a volume model (i.e., division into volume-contracted, euvolemic, and volume-overloaded groups). Although this has some benefits from a diagnostic standpoint, we believe that it tends to deemphasize important aspects of pathophysiology and treatment. We offer an alternative scheme for classification of hyponatremia, based on three principles. First, and most important: Is the patient symptomatic? If not, diagnostic evaluation can proceed at a more composed pace. Second: Is the hyponatremia acute, or chronic? The treatments for these entities may be very different particularly if they are very severe. Third: Is the ADH level high (in either a relative or an absolute sense), and, if so, why? The vast majority of patients with hyponatremia have some elevation of ADH levels, the reason for which forms the basis for subsequent evaluation. These principles are summarized in Fig. 156-2.

When one considers the situations in which acute hyponatremia occurs, it becomes apparent that prevention is often possible. This can best be accomplished by the administration of isotonic fluids whenever possible, particularly to postoperative patients. If hyponatremia is asymptomatic, appropriate treatment consists of fluid restriction and withdrawal of any offending medications. If it is symptomatic, acute hyponatremia represents a medical emergency demanding prompt therapy. Once symptoms occur, the prognosis becomes much worse.[11] It is our practice to administer normal saline solution intravenously to correct any volume depletion; this is followed rapidly by hypertonic saline solution given in a dose sufficient to render the patient asymptomatic and seizure-free. Furosemide should be employed if volume overload is present. Loop-acting diuretics are most useful in those states characterized by a urine osmolality greater than that of plasma. Urine and plasma electrolytes and osmolality must be measured frequently, and urine losses of Na should be replaced by parenteral infusion—particularly if ECF volume contraction is also present. The following guidelines must be observed to minimize the complications of therapy[15]: First, the serum Na level must not be allowed to increase by more than 20 to 25 meq/L during the first 48 h of therapy under any circumstances, regardless of its initial value. [In fact, marked clinical improvement is usually seen with rather modest increases in the serum Na level (10 to 15 meq/L) during treatment, after which more gradual correction can be used.] Second, complete correction to normal is not desirable, and hypernatremia occurring during the course of therapy is to be absolutely avoided. We set an arbitrary upper limit of 130 meq/L for the maximum level of serum Na during the initial correction phase. By following these guidelines, the majority of patients will become asymptomatic with an acceptably low risk of developing neurologic complications, especially the rare condition known as central pontine myelinolysis (CPM).

The rate of correction of hyponatremia affects morbidity and mortality. Patients undergoing a rapid increase in the serum Na level (20 meq/L over 6 to 8 h) suffer only a 10 percent mortality, compared to patients undergoing slow correction (20 meq/L over 36 to 48 h), in whom the mortality is 50 percent. Some investigators have proposed a link between rapid correction and CPM.[16,17] However, careful review of reported cases of CPM associated with treatment of hyponatremia suggests that the overwhelming majority of patients had excessive correction (more than 25 meq/L in the first 48 h), or had a final serum Na level higher than 130 meq/L. Thus, although a vigorous controversy exists in the literature, we believe that if the above guidelines are followed rapid correction offers the best hope for a good outcome.[18]

Practical guidelines for the use of hypertonic saline solution are fairly straightforward. First, the target value for final serum Na level is chosen as either an increase in the serum sodium of 20 to 25 meq/L or an absolute value of 130 meq/L, whichever is lower. The amount of NaCl required to achieve this target is then calculated as

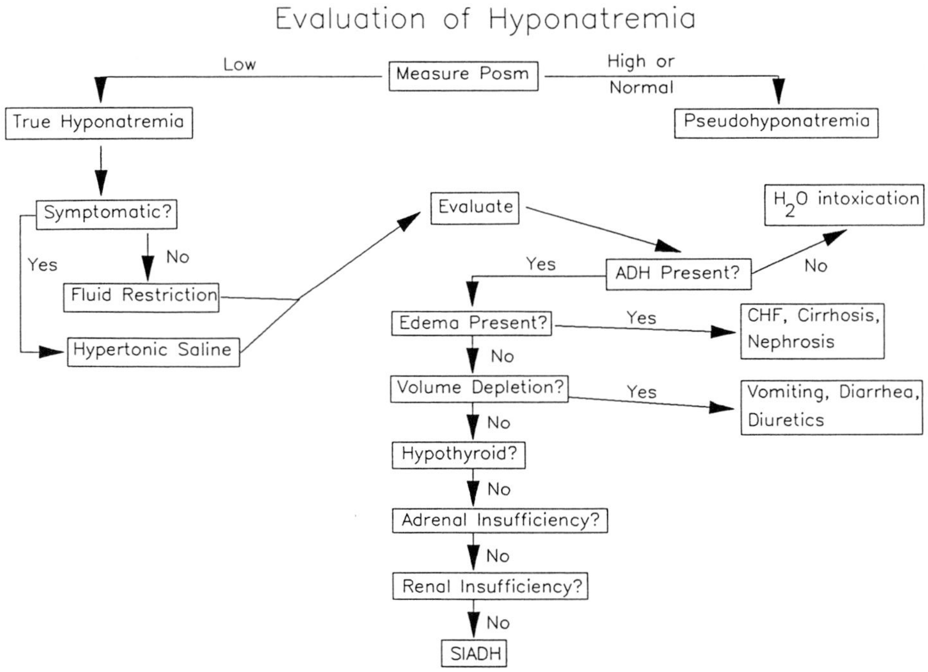

FIGURE 156-2 Evaluation of patients with hyponatremia. Hypoosmolality must be verified by the presence of a low serum osmolality. Once true hyponatremia has been confirmed, treatment with 3% saline solution should be started in symptomatic cases. The first step in evaluation is demonstration of the presence or absence of ADH activity (i.e., high or low urinary osmolality). Once water intoxication has been excluded, appropriate causes of high ADH activity are sought. In their absence—and if thyroid, adrenal, and renal function are normal—a diagnosis of SIADH is made.

$$\text{meq NaCl} = (0.6) \times (\text{weight in kg}) \times (\text{target Na} - \text{plasma Na}) \quad (156\text{-}2)$$

Since 3% NaCl solution is 513 mM, the volume of hypertonic saline solution needed to administer the calculated amount of Na is

$$3\%\ \text{NaCl (mL)} = (1000) \times (\text{meq NaCl})/513 \quad (156\text{-}3)$$

This solution should be infused at a rate calculated to increase the serum Na level by 1 to 1.5 meq/L per h. It should be noted, however, that the actual rate of correction is often significantly slower than that predicted by the above formulas, chiefly because of ongoing renal Na and water losses. Therefore, the importance of frequent surveillance of plasma and urine chemistries cannot be overemphasized.

HYPERTONICITY/HYPERNATREMIA

Hypernatremia is always associated with hypertonicity.[19] Thus, "pseudohypernatremia" does not exist, although hypertonicity may be present even if the plasma Na level is normal or low. Acute hypernatremia is uncommon and has relatively few causes; these include water deprivation, administration of a large solute load, and osmotic diuretics. Assuming a daily requirement of 1.5 L of water daily in an afebrile person at rest, it can be shown that the serum Na level will increase by about 5 meq/L per day if fluid ingestion is nil. These changes will be more dramatic if the person is physically active or febrile, or has impaired urinary concentrating ability. This is most often a problem at the extremes of age, when the patient cannot express thirst or obtain water independently and may have impaired water conservation. It is unusual for water intake to cease entirely; therefore, the hypernatremia that develops mainly because of inadequate intake usually occurs slowly, allowing cell volume regulation to occur. On the other hand, patients exposed to large solute loads may be unable to adapt rapidly enough, and acute symptomatic hypertonicity can result. In the ICU setting this is usually due to the administration of extremely concentrated fluids—especially $NaHCO_3$ administered during cardiac resuscitation. The most common cause of hyperosmolality due to endogenous solute accumulation is diabetic hyperosmolar nonketotic coma. In this entity, severe hyperosmolality can occur with a normal, or even a low, plasma Na level. Hyperosmolar coma is described in more detail in Chap. 159. The use of osmotic diuretics, such as mannitol, can cause hypernatremia by accelerating the loss of water in comparison to salt; in addition, the drug itself is osmotically active and will cause hypertonicity out of proportion to the degree of hypernatremia. This fact underscores the importance of determining the Posm during an evaluation for suspected hyperosmolality.

Chronic hypernatremia is much more common than the acute form. Their pathophysiology is often similar, a combination of inadequate water ingestion and excessive water losses. In addition to the syndromes described above, a few other entities can cause chronic hypertonicity.[20,21] Diabetes insipidus is caused by deficiency of ADH or resistance to its action on the nephron. Significant hypernatremia seldom develops unless access to water is impaired. Conn's syndrome and Cushing's syndrome may rarely be associated with significant hyperosmolality, particularly if drug treatment includes diuretics that accelerate water losses. Several mini-epidemics of neonatal hypernatremia have been reported as resulting from improper preparation of infant feeding formulas[22]; in these instances large solute burdens were administered to those least well equipped to deal with them.

The symptoms of hypernatremia are nonspecific. They depend on both the severity of the hypertonicity and the rapidity with which it develops. CNS signs predominate, including altered mental status, nausea, seizures, nystagmus, and central hyperventilation. If neuronal shrinkage occurs rapidly, physical separation of the brain from the meninges can occur. This can become clinically apparent as intracranial hemorrhage.[23] Extracranial findings include myoclonus of the limbs, metabolic acidosis, and hyperglycemia due to peripheral resistance to insulin.[24] This latter finding has important therapeutic implications, to be discussed below. ECF volume depletion is to be expected in most cases. If euvolemia or volume overload is present, excessive solute ingestion should be strongly suspected.

The diagnostic evaluation of all patients with suspected hypertonicity includes measurement of urine and plasma electrolyte levels and osmolality. Of course, the Posm should be corrected for the contribution of the ineffective osmole urea. Most other diagnostic testing, including water deprivation tests and hormonal determinations, can be deferred until the patient's clinical condition has stabilized. Continued measurements of plasma and urine chemistries are essential during therapy in order to modify treatment as necessary.

The treatment of hypernatremia is two-pronged. The first step is to halt ongoing water losses and correct volume depletion with normal saline solution, or blood products if indicated. This is combined with replacement of the established water deficit. Because of the insulin resistance that is characteristic of hyperosmolar states, we believe that the typical solution used (5% dextrose in water) is relatively contraindicated. This fluid can actually worsen hypertonicity by providing an additional effective osmole that will be only gradually metabolized to CO_2 and eliminated.[19] The first choice of fluid should be tap water or distilled water given orally or via nasogastric tube. In patients with paralytic ileus or gastric retention, parenteral solutions of 0.45% NaCl can be infused without substantial risk of hemolysis. If adequate correction does not occur with this fluid, dextrose-containing solutions may be employed. Close monitoring of the serum glucose level is mandatory. With careful observation of trends in the urine and plasma chemistries, appropriate adjustments in fluid administration can be made promptly. When salt poisoning is present, the excretion of Na is accelerated by the use of furosemide. This drug also causes a water diuresis, however; increases in water administration may therefore become necessary. Dialysis is occasionally indicated for rapid removal of salt in patients with coexistent pulmonary edema.

The rate at which correction should proceed is being actively investigated. In acute hypernatremia, we believe that rapid correction is advisable. However, the active treatment should stop when either **1.** the patient is asymptomatic, or **2.** the serum Na level has fallen by 20 to 25 meq/L, or **3.** the serum Na level has fallen to 148 meq/L. In chronic hypernatremia, similar guidelines apply. Neuronal cell uptake of solutes (amino acids and other unidentified "idiogenic osmoles") is the adaptive process that prevents brain cell shrinkage during chronic hypernatremia. These substances do not exit the cell instantly during correction of hypernatremia, and may be responsible for the cerebral edema and seizures that sometimes complicate overzealous treatment of chronic (but not acute) hypertonic states.[25] These so-called rehydration seizures are almost certainly completely analogous to seizures that complicate acute hyponatremia. It has been shown that the incidence of rehydration seizures in children is decreased when rehydration is accomplished by the oral route.[26]

When feasible, the patient should be allowed to correct the hypertonic state by ad lib ingestion of tap water. Alert patients with hypernatremia invariably drink enough water to self-correct hypernatremia safely and effectively, unless a thirst disorder or gastrointestinal problem is present. When oral ingestion is not possible, nasogastric or parenteral water administration is necessary. The desired final Na concentration (Na_f) is either 148 meq/L or a decrease from the initial sodium concentration (Na_i) of 20 to 25 meq/L, whichever is higher. The amount of water needed to induce this change is calculated as

$$\text{water (L)} = (0.6) \times (\text{weight in kg}) \times [(Na_i)/(Na_f) - 1] \qquad (156\text{-}4)$$

This volume can be administered at a rate predicted to decrease the plasma sodium by 1 to 1.5 meq/L per h. It must be borne in mind that 0.45% NaCl is completely equivalent to an equal mixture of normal saline solution and free water; therefore, if 0.45% saline solution is chosen, only half the infused volume is effective in replacing the water deficit (the other half being equivalent to normal saline solution). As with hyponatremia, the actual rate of correction often lags behind that predicted, because of ongoing water losses and simultaneous administration of salt for coexistent ECF volume depletion.

Symptomatic hypernatremia is associated with major mortality and morbidity. In the elderly, the overall mortality is over 40 percent, with another 40 percent being left with significant neurologic deterioration.[20] Mortality is probably comparable in children, although long-term neurologic sequelae may be less frequent than in adults.[11] Surprisingly, nosocomial hypernatremia is associated with mortality rates at least as high as, if not higher than, hypernatremia developing outside the hospital.

Abnormalities of the Serum Potassium Concentration

The marked disparity between the intracellular and extracellular concentration of K is the major determinant of the transmembrane potential difference of the cell.[27] Relatively minor deviations from normal can produce potentially life-threatening complications in excitable tissues such as skeletal muscle, smooth muscle, cardiac muscle, the cardiac conduction system, and the nervous system. The vast majority of the body stores of K are intracellular. What is measured in the serum is only a tiny fraction of the body content; thus, extrapolating total body content of K from an isolated serum measurement is a gross estimation at best. Additionally, small changes in the intracellular concentration of K have few consequences; on the contrary, relatively slight changes in the extracellular concentration can have profound effects.[28,29]

The normal daily intake of K is around 100 meq. The kidney excretes 90 percent of the daily load; the gastrointestinal tract excretes the remainder. Several factors can influence renal K secretion, the most important being the presence or absence of aldosterone.[30,31] Aldosterone stimulates Na reabsorption, thus creating a favorable gradient for K secretion into the distal tubular lumen. Increased mineralocorticoid activity will enhance K excretion, while aldosterone deficiency or resistance will inhibit this process.

While the kidney is primarily responsible for the maintenance of the day-to-day K balance, the minute-to-minute regulation of serum K concentration is a function of a different set of factors[32,33] (Table 156-3). Several hormones play a crucial role in this setting. Insulin favors K entry into cells, while glucagon stimulates K exit. β-Adrenergic stimulation causes K entry while α-adrenergic stimulation causes the opposite.[34] There is also some evidence that aldosterone may stimulate K entry into skeletal muscle cells. Alkalemia may stimulate K uptake into cells, while the opposite may occur with acidemia. The degree of K shift with acid-base disturbances is highly variable, depending on whether the disturbance is metabolic or respiratory, on the underlying medical conditions, and on the type of insult. Finally, hyperosmolality alone may stimulate K exit from cells into the extracellular space. This can occur in patients given contrast media or hypertonic saline solution, or in diabetic patients with spontaneous or iatrogenic hyperglycemia.

TABLE 156-3 Potassium Distribution

Factors stimulating entry into cells
Hormonal
Insulin
β-Adrenergics
Aldosterone (?)
Physical
Alkalemia
Factors stimulating exit from cells
Hormonal
Glucagon
α-Adrenergics
β Blockade
Physical
Acidemia
Hyperosmolality

HYPOKALEMIA

Hypokalemia is defined as a serum K concentration of less than 3.5 meq/L. The etiologies fall into the following categories: decreased intake, increased output, and a shift from the extracellular to the intracellular space (Table 156-4). Hypokalemia based on poor intake is uncommon but may occur in alcoholics, elderly individuals on a very poor diet (tea and toast diet), and those hospitalized and unable to eat for prolonged periods. Despite an inadequate K intake the kidney continues to excrete a small but obligatory amount of K. If poor intake is suspected, 24-h urinary K losses of less than 20 meq/day would be confirmatory. A random urine sample that contains less than 20 meq/L of K suggests dietary K deficiency or extrarenal K losses. Hypokalemia based on increased output, through either the urinary or the gastrointestinal tract, is more common. Gastrointestinal losses may be direct (through diarrhea), in which case the urine K excretion should be very low. The metabolic alkalosis and volume depletion accompanying vomiting will cause renal K wasting leading to urine K concentrations in excess of 20 meq/L. Other causes of renal K wasting include excess mineralocorticoid activity, the use of diuretics, osmotic diuresis, the presence of a non-reabsorbable anion in the distal tubule (such as bicarbonate or carbenicillin), a high urine flow rate, and alkalosis. A few drugs, such as cisplatin and amphotericin B, may cause renal K wasting secondary to direct tubular effects.[35–37] In all of these clinical settings, the spot urinary K concentration exceeds 20 meq/L and the daily K secretion exceeds 40 meq/day. In somewhat less common conditions, hypokalemia results

TABLE 156-4 Etiologies of Hypokalemia

Decreased intake
Unusual diet (e.g., tea and toast)
Parenteral fluids deficient in K^+
Increased excretion
Renal
Increased mineralocorticoid effect
Primary hyperaldosteronism
Secondary hyperaldosteronism
Volume depletion
Vomiting
Cirrhosis
Congestive heart failure
Mineralocorticoid administration
Osmotic diuresis
Tubular defects
Hypomagnesemia
Gastrointestinal
Diarrhea
Intracellular Shift
Hormonal
Insulin
β-Adrenergics
Aldosterone
Physical
Alkalemia
Miscellaneous
Hypokalemic periodic paralysis
Thyrotoxic periodic paralysis

from the sudden shift of K from the extracellular to the intracellular space. Some examples include glucose and insulin infusion, β-adrenergic agonists, bicarbonate infusion,[38] hypokalemic periodic paralysis, and thyrotoxic periodic paralysis. In these situations the spot urine K concentration is low, indicating no evidence of renal potassium wasting.

The clinical manifestations of hypokalemia are protean. The most life-threatening involve the cardiac conduction system and the neuromuscular system. Hypokalemia characteristically produces flattening of the T wave, with the appearance of U waves on ECG; potentiates digitalis toxicity (particularly the supraventricular arrhythmias); and provokes atrial and ventricular arrhythmias, alone or in the setting of acute myocardial infarction.[39,40] From a neuromuscular standpoint, the most apparent complication of hypokalemia is flaccid paralysis of the skeletal muscle and lack of tone in the smooth muscle. Clinically this may produce profound muscle weakness resulting in respiratory failure, ileus, and rhabdomyolysis secondary to the inability of the vasculature of the skeletal muscle to respond to metabolic demands. Hypokalemia may also produce both insulin resistance and depression of insulin release, leading to clinically significant glucose intolerance. From a renal standpoint, K depletion results in an impairment of urinary concentrating ability; it may also impair magnesium reabsorption.

If a treatable cause of K wasting can be found, the offending agent or condition should be treated and supplemental K given. For mild, minimally symptomatic hypokalemia, oral potassium supplements are generally satisfactory. Administration of 40 to 80 meq/day, given in divided doses, is generally adequate for initial therapy. In the patient with ongoing losses and normal renal function, it is useful to measure K concentration in the fluids being lost, calculating the total 24-h loss, and then administer that amount plus 40 meq extra. For the patient with impaired excretory ability (as in renal failure) it is safer to give a smaller amount (20 to 25 meq) initially, then recheck the serum K concentration before giving further doses. The alkalemic patient (as from vomiting) should receive KCl (K-Ciel or K-Lyte Cl); the acidemic patient would benefit from potassium bicarbonate or its equivalent (e.g., potassium citrate). For severe hypokalemia (K^+ below 2.0 or life-threatening symptoms) intravenous K should be administered. An initial rate of 10 meq/h is safely tolerated by most patients. After 40 meq is given, the serum K^+ level should be remeasured before further doses are given. Particular care must be taken in the patient with impaired renal function or impaired cellular uptake mechanisms (e.g., patients on β blockers), and more frequent checks of the K level are imperative. This can be frequently accomplished with relative ease in the ICU setting itself.[41] Sudden hyperkalemia can result in acute cardiac standstill even in patients with normal renal and cardiac function. For life-threatening hypokalemia, intravenous K may be given at a rate of 40 meq/h, but only with continuous monitoring.[42]

TABLE 156-5 Etiologies of Hyperkalemia

Increased intake (usually coupled with decreased excretion)
Unusual diet (low Na^+, K^+ supplement, salt substitute)
Excessive parenteral administration
Decreased excretion
Renal failure
Decreased mineralocorticoid effect
Addison's disease
Type IV renal tubular acidosis
Urinary obstruction
Drugs
ACE inhibitors
K^+ sparing diuretics
Nonsteroidal anti-inflammatory drugs
Extracellular shift
Hormonal
Glucagon
β Blockade
α-Adrenergics
Insulin deficiency
Physical
Acidemia
Hyperosmolality (radiocontrast, mannitol)
Miscellaneous
Hyperkalemic periodic paralysis
Digoxin toxicity

HYPERKALEMIA

Hyperkalemia is defined as a serum K level higher than 5.0 meq/L. An isolated elevated K value, particularly in the absence of any risk factors or clinical manifestations, should prompt a repeat K level as well as exclusion of spurious hyperkalemia secondary to in vitro hemolysis of red cells or thrombocytosis. True hyperkalemia may result from excessive intake, decreased output, and shift of K from the intracellular to the extracellular space (Table 156-5). Excessive intake alone as a cause of hyperkalemia is extraordinarily unusual. More commonly, excessive K intake occurs in the setting of a limited capacity to excrete a K load. The use of salt substitutes that contain K—or a low-Na high-K diet—in the presence of renal insufficiency or mineralocorticoid deficiency may produce hyperkalemia.[43,44] Certain drugs also impair K excretion.[45–47] On occasion the impairment of renal K secretion may be extremely subtle. In these patients with decreased renal K clearance, lethal hyperkalemia may occur quickly once mechanisms of extrarenal K disposal are saturated. The suspicion of renal excretory impairment can be confirmed by measurement of a spot urine K concentration of less than 20 meq/L in the face of hyperkalemia.

Less commonly, hyperkalemia is a result of a massive shift of K from the intracellular to the extracellular space. This may occur with massive cell lysis; with any of several hormonal alterations; with acidosis; or with acute hypertonicity. Severe digitalis intoxication may be accompanied by hyperkalemia due to impaired K uptake. In these clinical conditions, the spot urine K concentration will be clearly in excess of 40 meq/L, suggesting no abnormalities in the renal excretory process.

The consequences of hyperkalemia are confined primarily to the cardiac conduction and neuromuscular systems. Every clinician should recognize the ECG manifestations of hyperkalemia, since this complication is swiftly fatal. Mild degrees of hyperkalemia—5.5 to 6.0 meq/L—produce peaking of the T waves. As the degree of hyperkalemia worsens, the PR interval lengthens, the P waves disappear, and the QRS interval widens. The final event is cardiac standstill. Occasionally hyperkalemia may present as severe bradyarrhythmias and varying degrees of AV block. From a neuromuscular standpoint the manifestations of hyperkalemia are quite similar to those of hypokalemia, including flaccid paralysis of skeletal and smooth muscle.

Treatment of hyperkalemia depends on both the severity and the cause. For mild hyperkalemia, a thorough search for the cause of hyperkalemia, with close observation, is appropriate. Offending agents may be discontinued. Diets (especially salt substitutes in patients admitted to the emergency room or ICU from home), drugs (potassium salts of penicillin), and intravenous infusions (parenteral nutrition) should be reviewed. Renal excretion of K can be maximized by the administration of furosemide or another loop-acting diuretic. An exchange resin such as sodium polystyrene sulfonate (Kayexalate) can be administered orally or rectally in small doses. On the other hand, severe hyperkalemia is a true medical emergency. Therapy should be directed at minimizing cardiac toxicity, enhancing K movement into the cells, and removing K from the body. Calcium, by altering the threshold for spontaneous firing, can directly protect the heart from the deleterious effects of hyperkalemia on the conduction system. Generally, calcium gluconate 10%, 10 mL, given intravenously, acts instantaneously and lasts for 20 to 30 min. Simultaneous maneuvers to enhance K entry into cells should be initiated, including 10% glucose with 10 U/L regular insulin intravenously at a rate of 250 to 500 mL/h. The practice of sodium bicarbonate administration has recently been questioned, since there is some evidence that the associated hypertonicity may mitigate its hypokalemic effects. Another therapeutic maneuver described recently is inhalation of the β agonist albuterol, which was recently shown to decrease the serum K level in a small group of asymptomatic patients with chronic renal failure and mild hyperkalemia.[48,49] The use of this agent is still somewhat experimental. There should also be attempts made to eliminate K from the body. Furosemide, or another loop diuretic, given intravenously will markedly increase renal K excretion. In the emergent situation, exchange resins should be given only per rectum, for two reasons. In case of cardiorespiratory arrest, the patient may aspirate orally administered sodium polystyrene sulfonate; also, the site of action of the exchange resin is the colon. It is best administered via a rectal tube with an inflatable balloon for 30-min retention, in a dose of 50 to 100 g in 100 mL 70% sorbitol. Finally, where appropriate, dialysis may be initiated. This option should be considered in patients with life-threatening levels of hyperkalemia and the inability to stimulate K excretion by any route, at least for the short term (e.g., in severe acute renal failure or advanced chronic renal failure).

Abnormalities of the Serum Calcium Level

Most of the Ca in the human body is bound by the bony structures of the skeletal system, apparently fixed, yet constantly in dynamic equilibrium with extracellular fluid to maintain normal serum Ca concentration or to buffer acid loads.[50] The majority of extraskeletal Ca is found in the extracellular space in a concentration of approximately 10 mg/dL (2.5 mmol/L). Serum Ca exists in three forms: free ionized; bound to serum proteins (primarily albumin); and complexed to negatively charged compounds. From a clinical standpoint, however, it is the free ionized Ca concentration that exerts physiologic effects.

The maintenance of a normal serum Ca concentration depends on the interaction of the Ca regulatory hormones parathyroid hormone (PTH) and vitamin D on three organs: the kidney, the small intestine, and the skeleton.[50] Under physiologic conditions, these two hormones maintain normal body Ca balance as well as serum Ca concentration by enhancing intestinal Ca absorption and modifying release from, or uptake into, skeletal stores. Daily Ca intake ranges between 500 and 1000 mg, but absorption varies considerably. There is an obligate daily loss of 100 to 200 mg Ca via the gastrointestinal tract, even in the absence of Ca ingestion. Intestinal Ca absorption is enhanced by elevated PTH and vitamin D activity, and is depressed by decreased PTH or vitamin D; steroids; achlorhydria; malabsorption syndromes; and renal insufficiency. Renal Ca excretion is increased by calcitonin, the absence of PTH, and natriuresis. The loop-acting diuretics enhance Ca excretion, while the thiazide diuretics actually enhance renal Ca absorption. Other factors that increase Ca reabsorption by the kidney include PTH, vitamin D, ECF volume depletion, and insulin.

PTH secretion occurs almost exclusively in response to hypocalcemia. In addition to its direct stimulatory effect on renal Ca reabsorption, PTH releases Ca from bone to help restore a normal plasma concentration. PTH also stimulates 1-α hydroxylation of 25-OH-cholecalciferol to form active vitamin D, which enhances Ca absorption from the intestine. Formation of vitamin D, the other primary Ca-regulating hormone, is enhanced by hypocalcemia, hypophosphatemia, and elevated parathyroid hormone levels, and is inhibited in the presence of renal failure, hyperphosphatemia, hypercalcemia, and acidosis. Vitamin D stimulates Ca reabsorption from the intestine and kidney. Markedly elevated levels of vitamin D may result in Ca release from the bone. Calcitonin is a weak hypocalcemic hormone, inhibiting release of Ca from bone and enhancing Ca loss in the urine.

HYPOCALCEMIA

Hypocalcemia is a relatively uncommon clinical condition (see Table 156-6), but up to 70 percent of patients in critical care units may show hypocalcemia if tested routinely. It carries a poor prognosis.[51–53] Low total serum Ca levels with normal ionized Ca concentrations are seen in hypoalbuminemic states, such as nephrotic syndrome. Since the ionized fraction is physiologically most important, the low measured total Ca concentration in this clinical setting is of no clinical significance. One can correct for the degree of hypoalbuminemia by:

$$\text{Corrected Ca} = \text{measured Ca} + 0.8 \times (4 - \text{plasma albumin})$$

While convenient at the bedside, this method has been shown to result in erroneous estimates of the ionized Ca level when compared to measurements made by ion-specific electrode.[54,55] True hypocalcemia generally is seen with either a deficit of PTH effect, sequestration of Ca, or vitamin D deficiency. Most commonly, hypoparathyroidism is due to end organ resistance, such as severe hypomagnesemia or vitamin D deficiency, or is postsurgical. Primary hypoparathyroidism is rare. Ca sequestration may occur in the setting of acute pancreatitis[56] or rhabdomyolysis, or with the infusion of a Ca-chelating substance, such as phosphate, oxalate, or citrate—e.g., in the rapid administration of blood.[57] Additionally, acute alkalemia, such as with rapid administration of parenteral bicarbonate or with hyperventilation, can produce clinical hypocalcemia with a normal serum Ca concentration secondary to an increase in the complexed fraction and a resultant decrease in the ionized fraction. Vitamin D deficiency occurs with renal failure; in patients with excessive urinary losses due to nephrotic syndrome; with enhanced hepatic metabolism, which has been noted in patients using phenytoin; and, occasionally, as a congenital deficiency.

The signs and symptoms of hypocalcemia are related primarily to the excitable tissues. Tetany is the major clinical sign, and in mild degrees can be elicited by testing for Trousseau's or Chvostek's sign.[58] Additionally, hypocalcemia can be associated with a prolonged QT interval on ECG and can result in ventricular arrhythmias. Hypocalcemia may also cause depression of myocardial output, and may be at least partially responsible for the low-output state associated with severe septic shock.[59] Myocardial depression is most pronounced in patients with underlying cardiac disease, but occasionally presents in individuals with otherwise normal cardiac function. Hypocalcemia may also provoke bronchospasm, laryngospasm, and respiratory failure.[60]

TABLE 156-6 Causes of Hypocalcemia

Total Ca low, ionized Ca normal
Hypoalbuminemia
Total Ca low, ionized Ca low
Hypoparathyroidism
Primary deficit in production
End organ resistance
Renal failure
Hypomagnesemia
Sequestration
Pancreatitis
Rhabdomyolysis
Infusion of phosphate, oxalate, citrate
Total Ca normal, ionized Ca low
Acute alkalemia

The treatment of hypocalcemia depends on its severity. The serum magnesium level should be checked and significant deviations from the normal range corrected. Ionized Ca should also be determined to ascertain whether or not true hypocalcemia exists. In mild cases, simple oral Ca supplementation is sufficient. The typical initial dose is 2 to 4 g daily in four divided doses. Calcium carbonate (Os-cal, Tums) is usually satisfactory, except in patients with achlorhydria (pernicious anemia, therapy with H_2 blockers), for whom calcium citrate is preferred.[61] In symptomatic cases, parenteral Ca may be necessary, particularly with the presence of tetany or cardiac arrhythmias. Generally 100 to 200 mg of elemental Ca given intravenously, followed by a slow infusion of 0.5 to 2.0 mg/kg per h with frequent determinations of total and ionized Ca, is desirable. Ca administration to the asymptomatic patient should be done very cautiously and should be avoided in rhabdomyolysis (see Chap. 154), since exogenous Ca will worsen cell necrosis and result in severe rebound hypercalcemia.

HYPERCALCEMIA

Hypercalcemia is a relatively common ion disorder (see Table 156-7).[62] In a hospitalized patient, hypercalcemia generally results from malignancy[63] or hyperparathyroidism.[64] Other etiologies that are less common but must be considered include hyperthyroidism, Addison's disease, viral infections,[65] vitamin D intoxication,[66] vitamin A intoxication,[67] immobilization, and long-term parenteral nutrition.[68] Additionally, granulomatous illnesses,[69–73] such as sarcoidosis, tuberculosis, and fungal diseases, may also be accompanied by hypercalcemia, generally via enhanced production of vitamin D. Once the diagnosis of true hypercalcemia has been confirmed—i.e., by an elevated ionized Ca concentration—laboratory evaluation and therapy should begin simultaneously.[74] The hypercalcemia associated with malignancy is frequently acute, associated with profound symptoms such as altered mental status and dehydration, and not accompanied by either nephrolithiasis or nephrocalcinosis.[75] On the other hand, the hypercalcemia of hyperparathyroidism is more frequently asymptomatic or mildly symptomatic and may be associated either with classic parathyroid bone disease or with renal stones. Calcification of soft tissues, such as the vasculature and kidneys, is also more commonly seen in hyperparathyroidism. Although hypophosphatemia points toward a diagnosis of hyperparathyroidism, this laboratory value may be normal in hyperparathyroidism. It lacks specificity, and may be present in malignancy as well. The finding of an inappropriately elevated PTH level in the face of hypercalcemia confirms the diagnosis of hyperparathyroidism. If the PTH level is normal or low, then further workup is war-

TABLE 156-7 Causes of Hypercalcemia

Malignancy
Bony metastases (e.g., prostate)
PTH-like substance (e.g., squamous cell of esophagus)
Lymphokine production (e.g., multiple myeloma)
Prostaglandin-mediated (e.g., breast) (?)
Hyperparathyroidism
Vitamin D excess
Excessive ingestion
Granulomatous diseases (e.g., tuberculosis, sarcoidosis)
Lymphoma (rare)
Miscellaneous
Hyperthyroidism
Vitamin A intoxication
Aluminum intoxication
Immobilization
Paget's disease
Long-term parenteral nutrition

ranted, including serum protein electrophoresis, vitamin D level, and thyroid hormone.

The treatment of hypercalcemia depends on the severity of the symptoms. Mild hypercalcemia (below 12 mg/dL) can be managed conservatively by restriction of Ca intake, observation, and treatment of the underlying disorder. Volume depletion should be corrected if present, and vitamin D, calcium supplements, and thiazide diuretics discontinued. Generally these simple measures will adequately control Ca concentration until the cause can be discovered and treated more specifically.

Severe hypercalcemia is associated with a number of potentially life-threatening complications, often requiring emergency treatment before diagnostic evaluation can be completed. Altered mental status and muscle weakness are prominent complaints. Prominent manifestations of muscular weakness include adynamic ileus, nausea, vomiting, and severe constipation. The renal effects of hypercalcemia include decreased GFR, a decrease in urinary concentrating ability, and—if the hypercalcemia is severe and prolonged—nephrocalcinosis. Thus such patients who have both altered mental status, with nausea and vomiting, and an inability to concentrate the urine may present profoundly volume-depleted, to the point of hypovolemic shock. The cardiac effects of hypercalcemia include shortening of the QT interval and cardiac arrhythmias, especially supraventricular arrhythmias. Since most patients with severe hypercalcemia are volume-depleted, parenteral saline solution should be given. Patients with relatively well-preserved cardiac and renal function may tolerate up to 1 L/h, especially if coupled with high-dose (100 to 200 mg every 2 h) furosemide.[76] However, older patients with impaired cardiac, renal, or pulmonary function require more cautious volume replenishment, often with the aid of a central venous pressure monitor. Simple volume replenishment may decrease the Ca concentration to a far safer level without the need to resort to more dangerous agents. The addition of furosemide also enhances Ca excretion through the kidney, both because of its calciuretic properties (which may be manifest only at high doses[76]) and by increasing the amount of saline solution that can be given before volume overload supervenes. Furosemide is contraindicated in hypercalcemic patients with coexistent volume depletion and should be initiated only after volume status is clearly corrected. The diuresis that ensues can be massive—up to 500 mL/h urine output. Frequent monitoring of electrolytes—especially potassium, magnesium, and phosphate—is a necessary adjunctive measure. Other useful therapeutic agents for refractory hypercalcemia include calcitonin and mithramycin.[75] (See Chap. 149.)

Abnormalities of the Magnesium Level

Mg is second only to potassium as the most abundant cation in the intracellular space, yet abnormalities of the Mg level are commonly overlooked.[77–79] Like potassium, therefore, the serum concentration of Mg is at best only an approximation of total body Mg content.[54,80] The total body stores of this cation are distributed approximately 50 percent in the skeleton and the rest in soft tissue, particularly liver and skeletal muscle. A diet of normal composition provides a more than adequate amount of Mg, which is absorbed primarily in the small intestine. The kidney filters Mg readily and, under normal conditions, reabsorbs more than 80 percent of the filtered load. Under conditions of either Mg depletion or hypomagnesemia, Mg disappears from the urine. On the other hand, Mg loading suppresses Mg reabsorption so effectively that the kidney can excrete virtually the entire filtered load if necessary. Gastrointestinal absorption of Mg depends on normal small bowel function and, in contrast to calcium, does not depend on vitamin D.

HYPOMAGNESEMIA

Since the normal diet generally contains enough Mg to prevent negative Mg balance, hypomagnesemia rarely occurs on a dietary basis alone.[81] A potential clinical condition would be the very poor diet of neglected elderly persons, or a magnesium-free parenteral nutritional regimen. Thus, common etiologies of clinical hypomagnesemia can be divided into two major categories: excessive losses, and shifts into the intracellular space. Of the two, excessive loss is by far the more common. Mg wasting can occur either through the gastrointestinal tract or through the kidneys. Gastrointestinal loss of Mg can be seen with diarrhea, malabsorption syndromes of many types, vomiting, and biliary fistulas. Urinary loss of Mg is generally seen either with marked diuresis or with renal tubular dysfunctions, such as some forms of renal tubular acidosis. A few drugs commonly result in Mg wasting—most prominently, cisplatin,[82] cyclosporin, loop diuretics, amphotericin B,[83] and the aminoglycosides.[84] Shifting of Mg from the extracellular to intracellular space may occur in the setting of an acute myocardial infarction,[85] as well as in an alcoholic who presents in alcohol withdrawal after a binge. The serum Mg level may be normal on admission and then fall promptly on administration of a glucose-containing solution. A similar situation may be seen in the patient receiving total parenteral nutrition.[86] In both of these conditions, there is generally some degree of total body Mg depletion as reflected in the avid uptake of Mg into the tissues upon provision of glucose.

Determination of the cause of hypomagnesemia, once it has been discovered, depends heavily on a careful history taking.[87] Since dietary deficiency alone is so unusual, the primary differential is between gastrointestinal and urinary losses. If the source of loss is in doubt, measurement of the urinary Mg level will give the answer. In the face of true hypomagnesemia, the urine should be virtually free of the cation.

The consequences of hypomagnesemia are primarily related to the nervous and neuromuscular systems.[81,88,89] In severe cases, altered mental status, hyperreflexia, and even tetany can be seen and can mimic hypocalcemia.[90] In fact the two abnormalities, hypocalcemia and hypomagnesemia, may coexist (e.g., in malabsorption syndromes). If they coexist and are sufficiently severe, it may not be possible to correct either abnormality without correcting the other concomitantly.[90–93] The neuromuscular manifestations of Mg deficiency include hypotension, hypoventilation, dysphagia, dysphonia, and pseudoasthma.[94] Hypomagnesemia is also associated with ventricular arrhythmias,[95] congestive heart failure,[96,97] and an increased thrombotic tendency. Hypomagnesemia is commonly accompanied by hypokalemia or hypophosphatemia.[35–37]

Mild hypomagnesemia can be managed with oral Mg salts, bearing in mind that many of them have laxative effects if used in large doses.[98] Maalox (30 mL qid), milk of magnesia (5 mL qid), or MgO (250 to 500 mg qid) are all useful. For severe hypomagnesemia (Mg level less than 1.0 mg/dL, or associated with tetany or seizures) parenteral administration is warranted. In patients with normal renal function, $MgSO_4$ can be given intravenously at a rate of 50 meq over 4 to 6 h. Rapid administration can cause hypotension, vasodilation with facial flushing, and renal wasting of as much as 50 percent of the dose. Serum levels should be measured every 4 to 6 h to prevent overdosage.

HYPERMAGNESEMIA

Hypermagnesemia is virtually unknown except in persons with acute or chronic renal failure, because of the efficiency with which the kidney can excrete Mg. Therefore, the finding of hypermagnesemia should prompt a check of renal function if none has already been performed. Elevations of the serum Mg level are fairly common in women receiving active treatment of preeclampsia, because of the universal presence of some degree of depression in the GFR and routine therapeutic use of $MgSO_4$. Mild degrees of hypermagnesemia, even up to levels of 5 or 6 mg/dL, are generally well tolerated. However, Mg concentrations greater than 6 mg/dL are generally associated with symptoms related to the central nervous system and the neuromuscular system. Altered mental status, lethargy, depressed deep tendon reflexes, and flaccid paralysis are the major hallmarks of severe hypermagnesemia. Since hypermagnesemia can result in respiratory depression,[99] swift intervention for symptomatic hypermagnesemia is mandated. Initially any Mg-containing substances should be withdrawn. Calcium, 10 to 20 meq, can immediately reverse the clinical signs. If the patient has normal renal function, loop-acting diuretics can hasten Mg excretion. Patients with renal failure may require dialysis.

Disorders of Phosphorus Homeostasis

Total body P stores are approximately 10 g/kg body weight, mostly in the form of phosphate (PO_4). Less than 1 percent of the body P is present in the ECF; 85 percent is in bone, and the remainder is intracellular. As with potassium, the intracellular localization of P can make it difficult to assess the state of P balance on the basis of serum measurements. Furthermore, transcellular shifts in its distribution make it possible to observe either hypo- or hyperphosphatemia in patients with normal body stores. Most Americans ingest about 1400 mg P daily, of which about 500 mg is excreted in the stool. Minimal fecal excretion of PO_4 is about 150 to 250 mg/day. The remainder is eliminated by the kidneys. Phosphate deprivation tends to decrease excretion of PO_4, whereas parathyroid hormone (PTH) increases its excretion.[100]

HYPOPHOSPHATEMIA

Hypophosphatemia may occur as a result of either cellular redistribution or PO_4 depletion. The principal factors leading to PO_4 redistribution are respiratory alkalosis and administration of nutrients such as glucose and fructose.[101] In the ICU, the latter phenomenon is most frequently seen during initiation of enteral or parenteral hyperalimentation. This transient decrease in PO_4, although occasionally quite profound, is of no clinical significance unless there is a coexistent total body P deficiency.[102] Unfortunately, there is no convenient laboratory study that can reliably distinguish transient cellular redistribution from true PO_4 depletion. In patients who have a history or physical findings of malnutrition or burns, or are recovering from catabolic states (e.g., sepsis or surgery), PO_4 depletion is usually present.

True PO_4 depletion can occur by either inadequate ingestion or excessive losses of P. Almost any diet that is otherwise nutritionally sound contains sufficient PO_4 to avoid hypophosphatemia. Conversely, however, if malnutrition is present, PO_4 depletion is more likely. Most causes of significant hypophosphatemia are due to PO_4 wasting in the gastrointestinal tract or the urine. Vitamin D deficiency can impair PO_4 absorption in the gut. Intestinal diseases can lead to malabsorption of both PO_4 and vitamin D.[100] Ions that can bind phosphorus (Al, Mg, Ca, Fe) can produce striking negative PO_4 balance by inhibiting uptake of dietary P and forming insoluble complexes with PO_4 secreted into the intestinal lumen.[103]

Renal losses of P are more common than gastrointestinal losses, however. Both metabolic acidosis and alkalosis are associated with significant phosphaturia.[104,105] Respiratory acidosis causes phosphaturia, but also an increase in the serum PO_4 level. Respiratory alkalosis causes hypophosphatemia in the face of intense renal PO_4 conservation. Diuretics, such as acetazolamide, that inhibit sodium reabsorption in the proximal tubule also elicit phosphaturia. PO_4 wasting is an integral part of Fanconi's syndrome, which is generalized dysfunction of proximal tubular reabsorption. Excessive PO_4 losses are common following recovery from acute renal failure due to tubular necrosis or obstructive nephropathy. After renal transplantation, small numbers of patients have marked phosphaturia despite otherwise normal renal function; the reason for this is unclear.[106] Significant hyperglycemia is also associated with PO_4 wasting, presumably because of the concomitant osmotic diuresis.

The acute manifestations of PO_4 deficiency are due to depletion of energy stores such as adenosine triphosphate (ATP) and 2,3-diphosphoglycerate. Findings of CNS dysfunction include lethargy, altered mental status, and ataxia.[107] Neurologic findings may be focal. In addition, muscular weakness, myalgias, and even rhabdomyolysis can occur in severe hypophosphatemia. Cardiac damage, expressed as a refractory dilated cardiomyopathy that responds only to PO_4 repletion, has been described. Hemolytic anemia can be found in cases of very severe hypophosphatemia. A reversible defect in phagocytosis and killing of bacteria by granulocytes is also attributed to ATP deficiency. Thrombocytopenia can also occur in severe PO_4 depletion. Major renal effects include marked hypercalciuria and hypermagnesiuria, and occasionally bicarbonaturia and glycosuria.

The diagnosis of hypophosphatemia is based on a serum PO_4 level of less than 2.5 mg/dL. Unfortunately, it is much more difficult to assess the true state of P balance. Measurements of urinary PO_4 excretion can be helpful. In a hypophosphatemic patient, a low random urine PO_4 level (below 15 mg/dL) suggests either acute respiratory alkalosis or appropriate renal P retention in the face of extrarenal losses. A high random urine PO_4 level (above 75 mg/dL) is more consistent with renal P losses' causing the problem. However, it is generally much more important, in an individual case, to consider if any aspects of the clinical history suggest a potential cause of PO_4 wasting—such as malnutrition or sudden improvements in nutritional state, hyperglycemia, diarrhea, or diuretic treatment.

Hypophosphatemia can be treated by supplementation with oral or intravenous P salts. In mild asymptomatic cases (serum PO_4 1.5 to 2.5 mg/dL), the halting of P losses, combined with an adequate diet, should be sufficient to correct the problem. When additional agents are required, we prefer the use of balanced sodium and potassium salts of PO_4 (Neutra-Phos-K) in a dose of 250 mg every 8 h for 5 to 7 days. Patients with severe symptomatic hypophosphatemia (serum PO_4 level below 1.0 mg/dL) require more aggressive therapy. We use intravenous sodium phosphate ($Na_2HPO_4 \cdot 7H_2O$) or potassium phosphate (K_2HPO_4) at a rate of 2 mg phosphorus per kg body weight every 6 h, until the serum PO_4 level exceeds 2.0 mg/dL; then we complete replenishment with oral preparations if possible. In any patient being treated for hypophosphatemia, meticulous attention must be paid to serum chemistries, particularly calcium, PO_4, and magnesium. In an effort to prevent hypophosphatemia, we believe that any nutrition given to a patient whose PO_4 level is below 5 mg/dL should contain at least 500 mg P daily.

HYPERPHOSPHATEMIA

Hyperphosphatemia can occur because of release of P from intracellular sites, inadequate excretion, or excessive ingestion. Life-threatening hyperphosphatemia is much less common than similarly severe hypophosphatemia, and when it does occur is usually the result of liberation of intracellular stores.[100] The most common scenarios are of lysis of red blood cells, skeletal muscle, or tumor cells. A normal serum PO_4 level in a patient with rhabdomyolysis suggests prior severe PO_4 depletion that may have been etiologically important.

Since the bulk of dietary P is ultimately excreted by the kidneys, renal insufficiency causes hyperphosphatemia. Serum PO_4 levels may be over 10 mg/dL in patients with chronic renal failure, but seldom exceed 8 mg/dL in acute renal failure unless the cause of the renal dysfunction is related to cellular lysis. Renal clearance of PO_4 can be depressed in patients with hyperthyroidism and in those receiving diphosphonates for the treatment of hypercalcemia. Hyperphosphatemia due to increased intake is unusual, but can be seen in patients receiving PO_4-containing laxatives or enemas, or as a complication of therapy with intravenous P for PO_4 depletion.

The major clinical presentations of hyperphosphatemia are hypocalcemia due to the formation of biologically inactive Ca-PO_4 complexes; increased susceptibility to acute renal failure, both directly and synergistically with other nephrotoxins; and, on a more chronic basis, ectopic (or "metastatic") deposition of Ca-PO_4 crystals in the soft tissues.

Hyperphosphatemia is classified as mild-to-moderate (with values between 5 and 8 mg/dL) or severe (serum PO_4 level above 10 mg/dL). If renal P excretion is normal (above 500 mg P per day), either tissue redistribution or excessive ingestion must be present. The usual blood chemistry pattern associated with cell lysis (elevated potassium and urate levels, depressed sodium and calcium levels) can be helpful in making the diagnosis. A thorough diet and medication history will frequently uncover an unsuspected source of exogenous PO_4 ingestion.

The first line of therapy in hyperphosphatemia is the use of enteric PO_4 binders. Calcium, magnesium, or aluminum salts, in doses of 30 mL or more every 6 h, can induce negative balance of more than 250 mg of P daily if a patient is taking nothing else by mouth. If renal function is adequate, phosphaturia can be induced by volume expansion or the use of carbonic anhydrase inhibitors, such as acetazolamide. Alkaline diuresis may be useful, but its benefits must be weighed against the risks of decreased P solubility in alkaline urine and a possible decline in ionized calcium levels secondary to the induction of systemic alkalemia. In patients with marked compromise in renal function and severe hyperphosphatemia, dialysis is the treatment of choice.

CASE STUDIES

Case Presentation

A 79-year-old man was admitted to the hospital because of lethargy and dysarthria. His past history was remarkable for significant coronary artery disease treated with a triple aortocoronary bypass 6 years prior to admission. After the bypass he was treated with quinidine gluconate for frequent ventricular premature beats. He was otherwise in good health until 36 h prior to admission, when he was seen in an emergency room because of urinary retention. He was noted to have an enlarged prostate gland; a bladder catheter was passed with difficulty and the patient was discharged with instructions to follow up with a urologist of his choosing. No laboratory analyses were performed at that time.

He did well until 24 h later (12 h prior to admission), when a family member was unable to arouse him from a nap; paramedics then brought him to the emergency room. At that time he was found to have a blood pressure of 168/96 without orthostatic changes; pulse 84; respiratory rate 16; and no fever. His weight was 64 kg. General physical examination findings were normal except for frequent premature beats and a grade 3/6 systolic cardiac murmur best heard at the left upper sternal border. Neurologic examination revealed an elderly lethargic man who was responsive to his name. He was disoriented as to person, place, and time. Although he did not follow commands well, there did not appear to be asymmetry of his motor strength, sensation, cranial nerves, or deep tendon reflexes.

Laboratory studies revealed a serum sodium of 112 meq/L, potassium 3.6 meq/L, chloride 77 meq/L, bicarbonate 23 meq/L, BUN 18 mg/dL, creatinine 1.3 mg/dL, glucose 91 mg/dL, and uric acid 4.2 mg/dl. The remainder of his admitting blood chemistries were normal. His CBC was within normal limits. Urinalysis was remarkable for a specific gravity of 1.027, trace blood, 4 to 6 RBCs per hpf, and 0 to 2 WBCs per hpf. Chest x-ray revealed changes consistent with prior median sternotomy but was otherwise normal. The ECG showed 10 PVCs per min and nonspecific ST-T wave changes. A CT brain scan was "normal for age." A lumbar puncture was attempted but was unsuccessful.

The patient was admitted to the neurologic ICU for further observation and management. Repeat serum sodium was 111 meq/L 4 h after the initial assessment. Plasma osmolarity at that time was 241 mOsm/kg. Urine chemistries revealed osmolarity 597, sodium 54, potassium 66, and creatinine 118. Because of the patient's CNS findings, active treatment with 3% saline solution was begun. The total infusion volume was calculated, from Equations 156-2 and 156-3, as

$$\text{3\% saline (mL)} = [(64) \times (0.6) \times (130 - 111) \times 1000]/513 = 1422 \text{ mL}$$

This fluid was given over 19 h (1 meq/L per h) at a rate of 75 mL/h. Within 12 h the patient was fully alert and cooperative. Repeat plasma sodium after 18 h was 123 meq/L. Over the next 48 h, while the patient was on a fluid restriction of 1200 mL per 24 h, the sodium gradually increased to 137 meq/L. During this interval there was no evidence of pulmonary congestion, peripheral edema, or ascites. Renal function remained normal. Tests of thyroid and adrenal function were normal. During a trial of ad lib water intake, plasma sodium decreased to 128 meq/L within 24 h. Because the patient had difficulty complying with his fluid restriction, demeclocycline 300 mg bid was added to his regimen. Following correction of his hyponatremia, the patient underwent an uneventful transurethral resection of the prostate and was discharged to his home. When he was seen as an outpatient 3 weeks later, his serum sodium level was 136 meq/L.

Case Discussion

This patient presented with a typical case of severe symptomatic hyponatremia. As is frequently seen, treatment was delayed several hours while other possible causes of altered mental status were investigated. Once treatment was begun, the patient had a dramatic clinical response. Despite attempts to raise his serum sodium at a rate of 1 meq/L per h, the actual rate achieved was only 0.7 meq/L per h, because of ongoing losses of electrolytes in the urine. Once his condition had stabilized, investigation of the cause of his hyponatremia was undertaken. Since he had no evidence of volume depletion, edema-forming disorder, or renal insufficiency, and his thyroid and adrenal function were normal, a diagnosis of idiopathic SIADH was made. Treatment with fluid restriction and demeclocycline resulted in normalization of his serum sodium level. The role of the probable lower urinary tract obstruction in the pathogenesis of his hyponatremia is a matter of speculation.

Case Presentation

A 34-year-old man presented to the emergency room after collapsing while attempting to complete a 10-mile run in 100° (F) weather. He had noticed some nausea and diarrhea during the week prior to admission, but these symptoms had abated by 1 to 2 days prior to the race. He was complaining of weakness, nausea, and diffuse myalgias. His past medical history was unremarkable. He had recently begun to train extensively with weight lifting and daily running, but generally trained in a much cooler environment.

Physical examination showed a young man in moderate distress. Vital signs were: blood pressure 92/64 supine, 84/50 sitting; heart rate 116 supine, 140 sitting; respiratory rate 24; temperature 100°F. His peripheral pulses were thready. Extensive swelling and tenderness were noted over many muscle groups. Cardiac examination was normal except for tachycardia. The lungs were clear, the abdominal examination was unremarkable, and neurologic examination was nonfocal.

Laboratory studies revealed a hemoglobin of 15.8 gm/dL, hematocrit 50.1, platelets 122,000 per mm^3, white blood cells 21,900 per mm^3 with 92 percent neutrophils and 8 percent lymphocytes. Serum Na was 152 meq/L, K 7.1 meq/L, Cl 118 meq/L, HCO_3 24 meq/L, BUN 22 mg/dL, creatinine 2.8 mg/dL, Ca 8.2 mg/dL, PO_4 5.8 mg/dL, albumin 4.7 g/dL, uric acid 19.6 mg/dL. The serum ALT was 1005 IU/L, AST 2211 IU/L, LDH 1955 IU/L, CPK 104,200 IU/L. Urinalysis revealed a specific gravity of 1.026, pH 5.0, large blood, 2 + protein, 0 to 1 RBC per hpf, 2 to 3 pigmented casts per lpf. Chest x-ray showed some prominence of the pulmonary vasculature but was otherwise normal. The ECG was remarkable for sinus tachycardia, borderline prolongation of the QRS interval, and peaking of T waves in the precordium.

The patient was admitted to the medical ICU with a diagnosis of acute exertional rhabdomyolysis. He received a fluid bolus of 1 L of D_5NS over 30 min, followed by D_5NS with 25 g/L mannitol at 250 mL/h. Urine output increased from 10 mL/h on admission to 90 mL/h after 8 h of fluid resuscitation, at which time the IV fluids were decreased to 100 mL/h. Vital signs at that time were blood pressure 122/76, heart rate 96. The patient was given a single dose of 1 g $CaCl_2$ IV and Kayexalate retention enemas every 4 h as treatment of his hyperkalemia; there followed prompt resolution of the ECG abnormalities. Oral administration of a gel of aluminum hydroxide $[Al(OH)_3]$ (Amphojel) was begun in a dose of 30 mL every 4 h. Serial lab values were:

Time	Na	K	Cl	HCO_3	BUN	Cr	Ca	PO_4	CPK
4 h	152	7.6	100	24	35	3.2	7.4	7.2	175,600
12 h	154	7.0	110	21	28	3.0	6.8	7.8	204,200
24 h	150	5.9	112	18	28	2.6	6.5	7.2	211,900

Case Discussion

This case demonstrates some of the classic electrolyte features of acute rhabdomyolysis. Muscle necrosis results in release of K, creatinine, PO_4, uric acid, LDH, and AST into the extracellular fluid. Thus creatinine increases out of proportion to BUN; and K, PO_4, and uric acid increase out of proportion to the degree of renal failure. Ca levels decrease secondary to sequestration in damaged muscle, hyperphosphatemia, and diminished renal production of active vitamin D_3. One typical finding not seen in this case is hyponatremia due to dilution of the ECF by the Na-poor intracellular fluid. It was not present here because of excessive hypotonic fluid losses (perspiration) prior to admission.

The therapy consists of aggressive volume replacement with maintenance of a good urine output to enhance excretion of K, PO_4, uric acid, and free myoglobin, and to minimize the potential nephrotoxic effects of uric acid and myoglobin. Hyperkalemia is treated with Kayexalate enemas and Ca; glucose and insulin are likely to be only minimally effective in facilitating K entry into damaged skeletal muscle. If necessary, hyperphosphatemia can be treated with early use of enteral PO_4 binders. Hypocalcemia may become severe, but generally is asymptomatic and should not be corrected unless symptoms develop (note that in this case parenteral Ca was used as a treatment for hyperkalemia, not for hypocalcemia). Administration of Ca in this clinical setting carries the risk of Ca-P deposition and severe rebound hypercalcemia. If renal function in this patient had continued to deteriorate, or if hyperkalemia had been uncontrollable, dialysis would have been necessary.

References

1. Berl T, Anderson RJ, McDonald KM, Schrier RW: Clinical disorders of water metabolism. Kidney Int 10:117, 1976.
2. Schrier RW, Berl T, Anderson RJ: Osmotic and nonosmotic control of vasopressin release. Am J Physiol 236:F321, 1979.
3. Fishman RA: Cell volume, pumps, and neurologic function: Brain's adaptation to osmotic stress. Res Publ Assoc Nerv Ment Dis 53:159, 1974.
4. Siebens AW: Cellular volume control, in Seldin DW, Giebisch G (eds): *The Kidney: Physiology and Pathophysiology*. New York, Raven Press, 1985, p 91.
5. Covey CM, Arieff AI: Disorders of sodium and water metabolism and their effects on the central nervous system, in Brenner BM, Stein JH (eds): *Contemporary Issues in Nephrology*, Vol I: *Sodium and Water Homeostasis*. New York, Churchill Livingstone, 1978, p 212.
6. Chung HM, Kluge R, Schrier RW, Anderson RJ; Postoperative hyponatremia: A prospective study. Arch Intern Med 146:333, 1986.
7. Sunderrajan S, Bauer JH, Vopat RL, et al: Post-transurethral resection hyponatremic syndrome: Case report and review of the literature. Am J Kidney Dis 4:80, 1984.
8. Raskind M, Barnes RF: Water metabolism in psychiatric disorders. Semin Nephrol 4:316, 1984.
9. Morgan DB, Kirwan NA, Hancock KW, et al: Water intoxication and oxytocin infusion. Br J Obstet Gynecol 84:6, 1972.
10. Friedman E, Shadel M, Halkin H, Farfer Z: Thiazide induced hyponatremia. Ann Intern Med 110:24, 1989.
11. Brennan S, Ayus JC: Treatment of hypoosmolar and hyperosmolar states, in Suki WN, Massry SG (eds): *Therapy of Renal Diseases and Related Disorders*, 2d ed. Boston, Kluwer, 1991, p 1.
12. Fraser CL, Kucharczyk J, Arieff AI, et al: Sex differences result in increased morbidity from hyponatremia in female rats. Am J Physiol 256:R880, 1989.
13. Arieff AI: Hyponatremia, convulsions, respiratory arrest, and permanent brain damage after elective surgery in healthy women. N Engl J Med 314:1529, 1986.
14. Rose BD: New approach to disturbances in the plasma sodium concentration. Am J Med 81:1033, 1986.
15. Brennan S, Ayus JC: Central pontine myelinolysis and electrolyte disorders, in Riggs R, Arieff AI (eds): *Neurologic Manifestations of Systemic Disorders*. Boston, Little Brown, 1991 (in press).

16. Sterns RH: Severe symptomatic hyponatremia: Treatment and outcome. Ann Intern Med 107:656, 1987.
17. Kleinschmidt-DeMasters BK, Norenberg MD: Rapid correction of hyponatremia causes demyelination: Relation to central pontine myelinolysis. Science 211:1068, 1981.
18. Ayus JC, Krothapalli RK, Arieff AI: Treatment of symptomatic hyponatremia and its relation to brain damage. N Engl J Med 317:1190, 1987.
19. Brennan S, Ayus JC: Acute versus chronic hypernatremia: How fast to correct ECF volume? J Crit Illness 5:330, 1990.
20. Snyder NA, Feigal DW, Arieff AI: Hypernatremia in elderly patients. Ann Intern Med 107:309, 1987.
21. Perkins RM, Levin DL: Common fluid and electrolyte problems in the pediatric intensive care unit. Pediatr Clin North Am 27:567, 1980.
22. Finberg L, Kiley J, Luttrell CN: Mass accidental salt poisoning in infancy. JAMA 184:187, 1963.
23. Simmons MA, Adcock EW, Bard H, Battaglia FC: Hypernatremia and intracranial hemorrhage in neonates. N Engl J Med 291:6, 1974.
24. Nitzan M, Zelmanovsky S: Glucose intolerance in hypernatremic rats. Diabetes 17:579, 1968.
25. Hogan GR, Dodge PR, Gill SR, et al: Pathogenesis of seizures occurring during restoration of plasma tonicity to normal in animals previously chronically hypernatremic. Pediatrics 43:54, 1969.
26. Blum D, Brasseur D, Kahn A, Brachet E: Safe oral rehydration of hypertonic dehydration. J Pediatr Gastroenterol Nutr 5:232, 1986.
27. Kassirer JP, Wish JB: Disorder of potassium metabolism, in Suki WN, Massry SG (eds): *Therapy of Renal Diseases and Related Disorders.* Boston, Martinus Nijhoff, 1984, p 63.
28. Weisberg LS, Szerlip HM, Cox M: Disorders of potassium homeostasis in critically ill patients. Crit Care Clin 3:835, 1987.
29. Huerta BJ, Lemberg L: Potassium imbalance in the coronary care unit. Heart Lung 14:193, 1985.
30. Wright FS, Giebisch G: Regulation of potassium excretion, in Seldin DW, Giebisch G (eds): *The Kidney: Physiology and Pathophysiology.* New York, Raven Press, 1985, p 1223.
31. Field MJ, Giebisch GJ: Hormonal control of renal potassium excretion. Kidney Int 27:379, 1985.
32. Bia MJ, DeFronzo RA: Extrarenal potassium homeostasis. Am J Physiol 240:F257, 1981.
33. Brown RS: Extrarenal potassium homeostasis. Kidney Int 30:116, 1986.
34. Williams ME, Gervino EV, Rosa RM, et al: Catecholamine modulation of rapid potassium shifts during exercise. N Engl J Med 312:823, 1985.
35. Rodriguez R, Solanki DL, Whang R: Refractory potassium repletion to cisplatin-induced magnesium depletion. Arch Intern Med 349:2592, 1989.
36. Whang R, Flink EB, Dyckner T, et al: Magnesium depletion as a cause of refractory potassium depletion. Arch Intern Med 145:1686, 1985.
37. Whang R, Oei TO, Aikawa JK, et al: Predictors of clinical hypomagnesemia, hypokalemia, hypophosphatemia, hyponatremia, and hypocalcemia. Arch Intern Med 144:1794, 1984.
38. Salerno DM: Postresuscitation hypokalemia in a patient with a normal prearrest serum potassium level. Ann Intern Med 108:836, 1988.
39. Kafka H, Langevin L, Armstrong PW: Serum magnesium and potassium in acute myocardial infarction: Influence on ventricular arrhythmias. Arch Intern Med 147:465, 1987.
40. Lipworth BJ, McDevitt DG, Struthers AD: Prior treatment with diuretic augments the hypokalemia and electrocardiographic effects of inhaled albuterol. Am J Med 86:653, 1989.
41. Willats SM, Myerson K: Electrolyte measurement by clinicians. Intensive Care Med 13:411, 1987.
42. Kruse JA, Carlson RW: Rapid correction of hypokalemia using concentrated intravenous potassium chloride infusions. Arch Intern Med 150:613, 1990.
43. Findling JW, Waters VO, Raff H: The dissociation of renin and aldosterone during critical illness. J Clin Endocrinol Metab 64:592, 1987.
44. Kalin MF, Poutsky L, Seres DS, Zumoff B: Hyporeninemic hypoaldosteronism associated with acquired immune deficiency syndrome. Am J Med 82:1035, 1987.
45. Rimmer JM, Horn JF, Gunnar J: Hyperkalemia as a complication of drug therapy. Arch Intern Med 147:867, 1987.
46. Ponce SP, Jennings AE, Madias NE, Harrington JT: Drug-induced hyperkalemia. Medicine 64:357, 1985.
47. Lachaal M, Venuto RC: Nephrotoxicity and hyperkalemia in patients with acquired immunodeficiency syndrome treated with pentamidine. Am J Med 87:260, 1989.
48. Blumberg A, Weidmann P, Shaw S, Gnadinger M: Effect of various therapeutic approaches on plasma potassium and major regulating factors in terminal renal failure. Am J Med 85:507, 1988.
49. Montoliu J, Lens XM, Revert L: Potassium-lowering effect of albuterol for hyperkalemia in renal failure. Arch Intern Med 147:713, 1987.
50. Agus ZS, Goldfarb S: Renal regulation of calcium balance, in Seldin DW, Giebisch G (eds): *The Kidney: Physiology and Pathophysiology.* New York, Raven Press, 1985, p 1323.
51. Desai TK, Carlson RW, Geheb MA: Prevalence and clinical implications of hypocalcemia in acutely ill patients in a medical intensive care unit setting. Am J Med 84:209, 1988.
52. Zaloga GP, Chernow B: Hypocalcemia in critical illness. JAMA 256:1924, 1986.
53. Zaloga GP, Rainey TG: Hypocalcemia in the critically ill: When to suspect and what to do. J Crit Illness 1:12, 1986.
54. Zaloga GP, Wilkins R, Tourville J, et al: A simple method for determining physiologically active calcium and magnesium concentrations in critically ill patients. Crit Care Med 15:813, 1987.
55. Thode J, Juul-Jrgensen B, Bhatia HM, et al: Ionized calcium, total calcium and albumin corrected calcium in the serum in 1213 patients with suspected calcium metabolic diseases: A prospective multicenter study. Ugeskr-Laeger 151:2423, 1989 (Danish).
56. Stewart AF, Longo W, Kreutter D, et al: Hypocalcemia associated with calcium-soap formation in a patient with a pancreatic fistula. N Engl J Med 315:496, 1986.
57. Rutledge R, Sheldon GF, Collins ML: Massive transfusion. Crit Care Clin 2:791, 1986.
58. Riggs JE: Neurologic manifestations of fluid and electrolyte disturbances. Neurol Clinics 7:509, 1989.
59. Levine SN, Rheanes CN: Hypocalcemic heart failure. Am J Med 78:1033, 1985.
60. Brussel T, Matthay MA, Chernow B: Pulmonary manifestations of endocrine and metabolic disorders. Clinics Chest Med 10:645, 1989.
61. Recher RR: Calcium absorption and achlorhydria. N Engl J Med 313:70, 1985.
62. Forster J, Querusio L, Burchard KW, Garen DS: Hypercalcemia in critically ill surgical patients. Ann Surg 202:512, 1985.
63. Burtis WJ, Wu TL, Insogna KL, Stewart AF: Humoral hypercalcemia of malignancy. Ann Intern Med 108:454, 1988.

64. Fitzpatrick LA, Bilezikian JP: Acute primary hyperparathyroidism. Am J Med 82:275, 1987.
65. Zaloga GP, Chernow B, Eil C: Hypercalcemia and disseminated cytomegalovirus infection in the acquired immunodeficiency syndrome. Ann Intern Med 102:331, 1985.
66. Audron M, Kumar R: The physiology and pathophysiology of vitamin D. Mayo Clin Proc 60:851, 1985.
67. Gleghorn EE, Eisenberg LD, Hach S, et al: Observations of vitamin A toxicity in three patients with renal failure receiving parenteral alimentation. Am J Clin Nutr 44:107, 1986.
68. Shike M, Harrison JE, Sturtridge WC, et al: Metabolic bone disease in patients receiving long term total parenteral nutrition. Ann Intern Med 92:343, 1980.
69. Barbour GL, Coburn JW, Slatopolsky E, et al: Hypercalcemia in an anephric patient with sarcoidosis: Evidence for extrarenal generation of 1,25-dihydroxy vitamin D. N Engl J Med 305:440, 1981.
70. Murray JJ, Heim CR: Hypercalcemia in disseminated histoplasmosis. Am J Med 78:881, 1985.
71. Gkonos PJ, London R, Hindler ED: Hypercalcemia and elevated 1,25-dihydroxyvitamin D levels in a patient with end stage renal disease and active TB. N Engl J Med 311:1683, 1984.
72. Kantarjian HM, Saad MF, Esley EH, et al: Hypercalcemia in disseminated candidiasis. Am J Med 74:721, 1983.
73. Parker MS, Dokoh S, Woolfinden JM, Buchsbaum HW: Hypercalcemia in coccidioidomycosis. Am J Med 76:341, 1984.
74. Boyd JC, Ladenson JH: Value of laboratory tests in the differential diagnosis of hypercalcemia. Am J Med 77:863, 1984.
75. Mundy GR, Yates JP: Recent advances in pathophysiology and treatment of hypercalcemia of malignancy. Am J Kidney Dis 14:2, 1989.
76. Suki WN, Yium JJ, Von Minden M, et al: Acute treatment of hypercalcemia with furosemide. N Engl J Med 283:836, 1970.
77. Quamme GA, Dirks JH: Magnesium: Cellular and renal exchanges, in Seldin DW, Giebisch G (eds): *The Kidney: Physiology and Pathophysiology*. New York, Raven Press, 1985, p 1269.
78. Whang R, Ryder KW: Frequency of hypomagnesemia and hypermagnesemia. Requested vs. routine. JAMA 263:3063, 1990.
79. Ryzen E: Magnesium homeostasis in critically ill patients. Magnesium 8:201, 1989.
80. Reimhart RA: Magnesium metabolism: A review with special reference to the relationship between intracellular content and serum levels. Arch Intern Med 148:2415, 1988.
81. Whang R: Magnesium depletion: Pathogenesis, prevalence, and clinical implications. Am J Med 82(3A):24, 1986.
82. Buckley JE, Clark VL, Meyer TJ, Pearlman NW: Hypomagnesemia after cisplatin combination chemotherapy. Arch Intern Med 144:2347, 1984.
83. Barton CH, Pahl M, Vaziri ND, Cesario T: Renal magnesium wasting therapy associated with amphotericin B therapy. Am J Med 77:471, 1984.
84. Kes P, Reiner Z: Symptomatic hypomagnesemia associated with gentamicin therapy. Magnesium and Trace Metals 9:54, 1990.
85. Rasmussen HS, Aurup P, Hajberg S, et al: Magnesium and acute myocardial infarction: Transient hypomagnesemia not induced by renal magnesium loss in patients with acute myocardial infarction. Arch Intern Med 146:872, 1986.
86. Chernow B, Bamberger S, Stoiko M, et al: Hypomagnesemia in patients in postoperative intensive care. Chest 95:391, 1987.
87. Baldwin TE, Chernow B: When to suspect hypomagnesemia in critically ill patients. J Crit Illness 2:60, 1987.
88. Flink EB: Clinical manifestations of acute magnesium deficiency in man, in *Magnesium in Health and Disease*. Spectrum Publications, 1980, p 865.
89. Durlach J: Clinical aspects of chronic magnesium deficiency, in *Magnesium in Health and Disease*. Spectrum Publications, 1980, p 883.
90. Levine BS, Coburn JW: Magnesium, the mimic/antagonist of calcium. N Engl J Med 310:1253, 1984.
91. Kelnar CJH, Taor WS, Reynolds DJ, et al: Hypomagnesemic hypocalcemia with hypokalemia caused by treatment with high dose gentamicin. Arch Dis Child 53:817, 1978.
92. Wheeler PG, Smith T, Golindano C, et al: Potassium and magnesium depletion in patients with cirrhosis on maintenance diuretic regimens. Gut 18:683, 1977.
93. Ryzen E, Rude RK: Low intracellular magnesium in patients with acute pancreatitis and hypocalcemia. West J Med 152:145, 1990.
94. Fiaccadori E, DelCanale S, Coffrini E, et al: Muscle and serum magnesium in pulmonary intensive care unit patients. Crit Care Med 16:751, 1988.
95. Njinimbam G, Ryder KW, Glick MR, et al: Identification of hypomagnesemia and hypokalemia in patients receiving digoxin. Clin Chem 365:575, 1990.
96. Gottlieb SS: Importance of magnesium in congestive heart failure. Am J Cardiol 63:39G, 1989.
97. Kurnik BR, Marshall J, Katz SM: Hypomagnesemia-induced cardiomyopathy. Magnesium 7:49, 1988.
98. Oster JR, Epstein M: Management of magnesium depletion. Am J Nephrol 8:349, 1988.
99. Fassler CA, Rodriguez M, Babisch DB, et al: Magnesium toxicity as a cause of hypotension and hypoventilation: Occurrence in patients with normal renal function. Arch Intern Med 145:1604, 1985.
100. Lau K: Phosphate disorders, in Kokko JP, Tannen RL (eds): *Fluids and Electrolytes*. Philadelphia, Saunders, 1986, p 398.
101. Sheldon GF, Brzyb S: Phosphate depletion and repletion: Relation to parenteral nutrition and oxygen transport. Ann Surg 182:683, 1975.
102. Knochel JP: The pathophysiology and clinical characteristics of severe hypophosphatemia. Arch Intern Med 137:203, 1977.
103. Shields HS: Rapid fall of serum phosphorus secondary to antacid therapy. Gastroenterology 75:1137, 1978.
104. Mostellar ME, Tuttle EP: Effects of alkalosis on plasma concentration and urinary excretion of inorganic phosphate in man. J Clin Invest 43:138, 1964.
105. Kempson SA: Effects of metabolic acidosis on renal brush border membrane adaptation to a low phosphorus diet. Kidney Int 22:225, 1982.
106. Rosenbaum RW, Hruska KA, Korkor A, et al: Decreased phosphate reabsorption after renal transplantation: Evidence for a mechanism independent of calcium and parathyroid hormone. Kidney Int 19:568, 1981.
107. Lotz M, Zisman E, Bartter FC: Evidence for a phosphorus depletion syndrome in man. N Engl J Med 278:409, 1968.

Chapter 157
DIABETES INSIPIDUS

JESSE HALL
GARY ROBERTSON

KEY POINTS

- *Polyuria (urine volume over 30 mL/kg per day) is common in critically ill patients and must be interpreted in light of large fluid losses and loads.*
- *In assessing polyuria, the clinician must first exclude solute diuresis.*
- *If water diuresis is identified (hypotonic polyuria), a distinction must be made between excessive water administration (secondary diabetes insipidus) and a disorder of vasopressin secretion or action (primary diabetes insipidus).*
- *If the plasma sodium level is high (above 145 meq/L), primary diabetes insipidus is strongly suggested, and DDAVP should be given to distinguish neurogenic from nephrogenic forms.*
- *If the plasma sodium level is low (below 145 meq/L), water deprivation testing with frequent serial determination of urine and plasma osmolality will often determine the cause of the observed polyuria.*
- *All but the most unstable patients can undergo water deprivation, since plasma osmolality will increase and maximally stimulate functional vasopressin secretion mechanisms well before hypovolemia results in hypoperfusion.*
- *Whenever patients are given replacement therapy for diabetes insipidus, frequent determinations of plasma sodium and osmolality should be made to avoid water intoxication.*

In the critically ill patient, urinary output is carefully measured and closely followed as a guide to the adequacy of the circulation. When urinary output is greater than anticipated, the clinician must determine whether water intake or administration has been excessive, and the observed excretion appropriate, or whether a pathologic process has caused inappropriate urinary fluid loss. To make this distinction one must be familiar with both the physiologic and the pathophysiologic mechanisms of water balance.[1,2]

Normal Physiology

OSMOTIC CONTROL OF WATER BALANCE

Plasma osmolality is tightly regulated by mechanisms that control thirst and the secretion of antidiuretic hormone (ADH, also called arginine *vasopressin*). Both thirst and secretion of vasopressin are mediated by osmotically sensitive neurons located in the anterior hypothalamus. Vasopressin is synthesized by neurosecretory cells in the hypothalamus, transported intracellularly, and stored in neurosecretory granules in cell axons that terminate in the posterior pituitary. When released into the circulation, vasopressin affects water balance by promoting water reabsorbtion in the renal collecting ducts, thus reducing free water clearance.

Below a threshold level of about 280 mOsm/kg, thirst is absent and plasma vasopressin levels decrease to undetectable levels (see Fig. 157-1). Under these conditions, urine becomes maximally dilute and urine volume increases. With normal renal function such water diuresis will protect against a further fall in plasma osmolality despite a water intake amounting to many liters per day. At the upper threshold for plasma osmolality, estimated to be 295 to 300 mOsm/kg, plasma vasopressin rises to levels sufficient to effect maximal antidiuresis and stimulate thirst (see Fig. 157-1). Renal water loss is minimal; if water intake is achieved, dehydration will be prevented even when water losses are high. Thus the drinking of water and renal water clearance are counterpoised actions, linked by hypothalamic control, that serve to maintain water balance by regulating plasma osmolality between the respective thresholds for vasopressin release and thirst.[3]

NONOSMOTIC INFLUENCES ON WATER BALANCE

While thirst and vasopressin secretion are predominantly osmoregulated, there are other influences that may be significant in the critically ill.[2,3] Marked hypovolemia promotes hormone release, probably via stimuli arising from vascular sensors of the pressure-volume state. Small-to-moderate reductions in blood volume (5 to 15 percent) are much less effective than comparable changes in osmolality in stimulating hormone release (see Fig. 157-2). Thus water deprivation will maximally stimulate vasopressin secretion, via osmotic mechanisms, prior to the development of hypovolemia sufficient to result in hypoperfusion and hypotension. Several other influences may be significant in critically ill patients: Positive-pressure ventilation results in antidiuresis; negative-pressure ventilation causes water diuresis, which can be abolished by administration of vasopressin. Also, nausea and/or vomiting of any cause can result in 100- to 1000-fold elevations of serum vasopressin above baseline. Patients with protracted nausea or vomiting may develop water intoxication while receiving intravenous fluids, particularly if large hypotonic volumes are administered.

Pathophysiology

Polyuria is defined as urinary output in excess of 30 mL/kg per day. In a critically ill patient such urine volumes require interpretation in light of frequent large fluid losses (wound drainage, nasogastric suction and diarrhea, burns, etc.) and large administered volumes (multiple drug infusions, hyperalimentation, blood products, etc.).

When water intake is sufficient to reduce plasma osmolality, then vasopressin secretion ceases and hypotonic polyuria (urine osmolality less than 300 mOsm/kg and urine specific gravity less than 1.010) occurs. This is termed *secondary diabetes insipidus.* While critically ill patients rarely

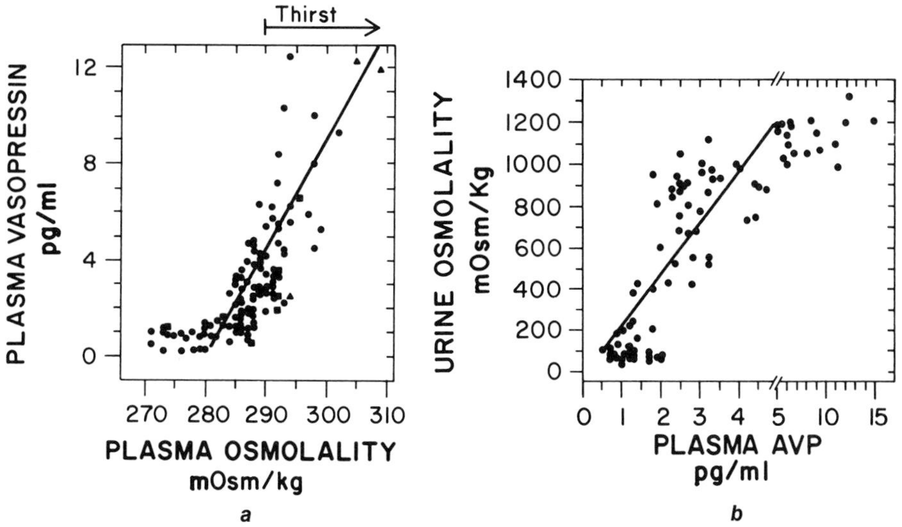

FIGURE 157-1 Plasma vasopressin levels are shown in relation to plasma and urine osmolality. Plasma vasopressin levels rise progressively as plasma osmolality increases above a threshold of approximately 280 mOsm/kg (*a*), associated with a progressive rise in urine osmolality to a plateau of approximately 1200 mOsm/kg (*b*). Thirst is stimulated at a plasma osmolality threshold of approximately 290 to 295 mOsm/kg. See text for explanation. [Reproduced, with permission, from Robertson GL et al: Osmotic control of vasopressin function, in Andreoli TE, Grantham JJ, Rector FC (eds): *Disturbances in Body Fluid Osmolality*. Bethesda, MD, American Physiological Society, 1977.]

take fluids ad libitum, intravenous water administration may become excessive, particularly when orders are written for fluids to "match," or exceed by a specific amount, the urine volume.

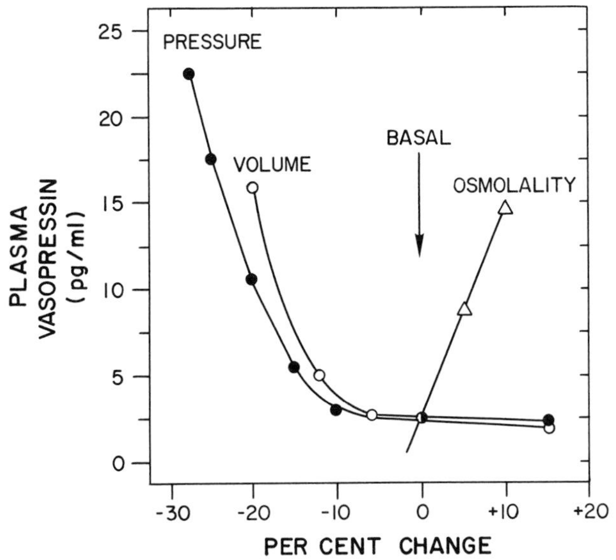

FIGURE 157-2 Effects of percent change in serum osmolality, blood volume, and arterial pressure on plasma vasopressin levels. Note that vasopressin levels are much more responsive to small changes in osmolality than to equivalent percent changes in pressure or volume. (Reproduced, with permission, from Robertson GL, Berl T.[1])

Alternatively, an increased urinary output may be an indicator of a disturbance of water balance. Polyuria may result from solute diuresis (as in uncontrolled diabetes mellitus, or following administration of mannitol or contrast media). Under these conditions urine solute excretion is high (over 1 mOsm/min) and urine osmolality approaches isotonicity. Hypotonic polyuria, on the other hand, signifies primary diabetes insipidus, arising from inadequate vasopressin secretion (*central*, or *neurogenic*, diabetes insipidus), resistance to the action of vasopressin at a renal tubular level (*nephrogenic* diabetes insipidus) or, as recently described in pregnancy, resistance to hormone action arising partly from degradation of vasopressin by vasopressinase, which is produced in large amounts by the placenta.[4]

Causes of Diabetes Insipidus

NEUROGENIC DIABETES INSIPIDUS

Given the frequencies with which central nervous system and renal injuries occur during critical illness, it is not surprising that diabetes insipidus is one of the more commonly encountered endocrinopathic complications (see Table 157-1). Neurogenic diabetes insipidus is seen after massive brain injuries of many types (trauma, infection, poisoning, post-anoxia). Some authors have suggested that it may be a marker for poor prognosis.[5] Given the facts that it occurs in only a minority of patients meeting clinical criteria for brain death, that it can reverse despite neurologic deterioration,

TABLE 157-1 Causes of Diabetes Insipidus

Vasopressin deficiency (neurogenic diabetes insipidus)
Acquired
Closed and open head trauma*
Postoperative*
Meningoencephalitis*
Vascular injury*
Post-anoxic/ischemic injury*
Granulomatous disease (sarcoid, histiocytosis)
Tumor
Familial
Vasopressin insensitivity (nephrogenic diabetes insipidus)
Acquired
Pyelonephritis*
Postobstructive*
Sickle cell disease and trait
Polycystic kidney disease
Amyloidosis
Metabolic disturbances (hypokalemia, hypercalcemia)*
Granulomatous disease
Pharmacologic causes*
Multiple myeloma
Familial
Excessive water intake (secondary diabetes insipidus)
Resetting of thirst osmostat
Neurosarcoid
Meningitis
Head trauma
Multiple sclerosis
Psychogenic polydipsia
Excessive IV fluid administration*

*Denotes entities commonly encountered in critical care environment.

and that it can be seen after minor injuries with no substantial neurologic dysfunction, it is unlikely to be a particularly useful prognostic indicator.[3] Interestingly, vasopressin administered to patients with brain death may be useful in preventing cardiac arrest and thus help to preserve organ function for ultimate harvest and transplantation.[6]

Trauma is a relatively uncommon cause of diabetes insipidus in the general population, but is an extremely important one in surgical intensive care. In closed head injury, diabetes insipidus is usually seen only after trauma sufficient to cause skull fracture or cranial nerve injury. It typically manifests 1 to 14 days following injury, although patients with minor injury and delayed onset have been described.[3,7–9]

Pituitary and suprasellar surgical procedures often result in postoperative abnormalities in water balance. The reported incidence of diabetes insipidus ranges from as low as 2 percent to as high as 81 percent.[3] This wide range is attributable to differences in surgical procedure, patient population, and, most significant, the sensitivity of tests used to identify vasopressin insufficiency.[3] Post-neurosurgical diabetes insipidus usually follows one of three patterns[3,10]: Onset may be abrupt, within several days of surgical intervention, and resolve within the first week. For some patients with abrupt onset, however, the disorder is not transient, and abnormalities of hormone secretion persist indefinitely. Finally, some patients exhibit a "triple response." In such cases, after early onset of diabetes insipidus there is a period of remission, with normalization or even excessive hormone release (*syndrome of inappropriate antidiuretic hormone secretion*, or *SIADH*), followed by a return of vasopressin insufficiency. The period of SIADH has been ascribed to unregulated hormone release from damaged and degenerating neurons.

Tissue hypoxia is a final common pathway for hypothalamic and hypophyseal injury. Disorders of vasopressin secretion have been reported and must be considered after diverse processes, including cardiopulmonary arrest, hypoxemia, obstetric hemorrhagic shock, gastrointestinal hemorrhage with shock, and carbon monoxide poisoning.[3,11–12]

NEPHROGENIC DIABETES INSIPIDUS

Many drugs, intrinsic renal diseases, and metabolic disturbances (see Table 157-1) can cause acquired nephrogenic diabetes insipidus in the critically ill patient.[3,13] While urine concentration mechanisms are perturbed in most forms of renal dysfunction, the associated reduction in glomerular filtration rate blunts the degree of polyuria. A number of disorders have disparate effects on renal tubular concentration function and thus may be notable for the observed urinary outputs that they cause. These disorders include amyloidosis, obstructive nephropathy, and multiple myeloma with light chain nephropathy.

The action of vasopressin may be impaired by a number of drugs, including lithium, methoxyflurane, and amphotericin.[13] In addition, hypercalcemia and hypokalemia impair renal concentrating mechanisms. While these electrolyte disturbances produce only modest polyuria in and of themselves, it is important to correct such abnormalities before embarking on an assessment of polyuria.

Approach to Diagnosis

The usual entry point for evaluation of a patient is the observation of polyuria. The plasma osmolality and sodium level are usually within, or near, normal ranges. However, if free water clearance is abnormal and water intake and/or administration is insufficient, dehydration may be significant and hypernatremia extreme (over 160 meq/L). If a lucid, hypernatremic, dehydrated patient does not manifest thirst, damage to hypothalamic osmoreceptors may be inferred.

Once polyuria is observed, the first task is to exclude solute diuresis (see Table 157-2). In this circumstance the urine is usually isotonic or slightly hypertonic relative to plasma, and total solute excretion exceeds 20 mOsm/kg per day. Glycosuria is readily identified. Careful review of drug administration and recent radiologic procedures should identify mannitol- or contrast-induced diuresis. Urea diuresis should be considered in highly catabolic (e.g., burn, septic, or postoperative) patients receiving high protein loads. Diuretics must be discontinued 12 to 24 h prior to

TABLE 157-2 Causes of Solute Diuresis

Sodium diuresis
Diuretics
Salt-wasting renal disease
Dopamine
Glycosuria
Urea diuresis
Contrast dye
Mannitol
Glycerol

assessment of polyuria, because of their prolonged action. In this regard, dopamine, often infused at low "dopaminergic" rates (1 to 4 μg/kg per min), must be considered as a natriuretic agent[14] and should be discontinued prior to attempts to elucidate the cause of polyuria.

If solute diuresis is absent, the polyuria is due to a water diuresis—otherwise known as diabetes insipidus. In this condition the urine is hypotonic to plasma, and the solute excretion rate [urinary output (L) × urine osmolality (mOsm/kg)] is normal (under 20 mOsm/kg per day). The most likely cause of hypotonic polyuria in modern intensive care is excessive water administration and/or use of potent loop diuretics, so-called secondary diabetes insipidus. Usually, when these etiologies are recognized after careful review of fluid and drug administration, formal assessment of water balance is not necessary, and free water restriction or discontinuation of loop diuretics (as appropriate) resolves the observed polyuria. In some cases the etiology of polyuria remains unclear despite review of these data, and a more detailed algorithm should be used in diagnosis (see Fig. 157-3).

If free water administration is excessive, vasopressin levels are nil and diuresis is maximal. Accordingly, the plasma osmolality and sodium level tend toward the lower limits of their normal ranges (usually around 280 mOsm/kg and 135 meq/L, respectively). Water deprivation causes plasma osmolality and sodium concentration to rise; vasopressin release promotes urine concentration and antidiuresis. In hypotonic polyuria arising from a severe deficiency of vasopressin secretion or action, plasma osmolality and sodium concentration rise, but urinary concentration does not occur. Thus the hypernatremia and hyperosmolality are progressive. Under these conditions, assessing the urinary response to exogenous vasopressin should distinguish between hormone insufficiency and renal resistance to hormone effect.

Unfortunately this simple paradigm may be easier to describe than to apply.[3] Because of great variability in the osmolal set point for thirst and vasopressin secretion in normal subjects, the plasma osmolality and sodium concentration are imperfect discriminators of primary diabetes insipidus from secondary diabetes insipidus. Moreover, in patients with neurogenic and nephrogenic diabetes insipidus the deficiency of hormone secretion or action is often incomplete; thus, during fluid deprivation such patients can exhibit varying degrees of renal concentration that are difficult to distinguish from those seen in patients whose polyuria is due to excessive water intake and/or administration. Also, hypotonic polyuria from any cause may "wash out" the renal medullary concentration gradient, resulting in a blunting of maximum concentrating capacity that may be mistaken for nephrogenic diabetes insipidus.

Despite these confounding factors, an approach using the plasma sodium concentration is useful[3] (Fig. 157-3). When an ion-selective electrode is used to make this measurement, the sodium concentration in plasma water is determined. Flame photometry (an older, and now less often used, technique) measures the sodium concentration in total volume; thus conditions that displace significant amounts of plasma water (e.g., excessive hyperlipidemia or hyperproteinemia) may result in artifactually low sodium concentrations—a result termed *pseudohyponatremia.*

The first task in diagnosis is to exclude solute diuresis. This is usually simple, requiring a review of the patient's history and allowing 24 h following diuretic, mannitol, or radiocontrast administration for diuresis to resolve. If necessary, determination of low urine osmolality (under 300 mOsm/L) in a spot determination, or normal solute excretion (500 to 1500 mOsm/day) in a 24-h collection, will confirm water diuresis.

Patients in whom solute diuresis has been excluded and in whom polyuria of unclear cause persists are divided into those with normal (under 145 meq/L) and those with high (over 145 meq/L) plasma sodium level.[3] In the latter group excessive intake of water is unlikely and the physician may proceed directly to administration of hormone to distinguish between neurogenic and nephrogenic diabetes insipidus. This is best done with a therapeutic trial of the vasopressin analogue desamino-D-arginine-8-vasopressin (DDAVP, also called *desmopressin*), administered parenterally at a dose of 1 μg subcutaneously. If urine osmolality increases to more than 150 percent of the baseline value, neurogenic diabetes insipidus is confirmed and replacement therapy is instituted. If urine osmolality fails to increase by this amount, attention should be directed to potential causes of nephrogenic diabetes insipidus (see Table 157-1).

Patients with plasma sodium levels below 145 meq/L should be considered for fluid deprivation testing. Fluid restriction should be continued until the plasma osmolality or sodium level exceed 295 mOsm/kg or 145 meq/L, respectively. This degree of dehydration can be achieved with no more than a 3 to 4 percent loss of total body water (1 to 2 L), of which only a fraction (0.5 L or less) is from the intravascular compartment. This implies that all but the most unstable patients should be able to undergo sufficient fluid deprivation to test vasopressin release and action. Also, it is not necessary to institute invasive monitoring of patients for this purpose alone. Since the venous circulation has a high compliance and volume, this small decrement in volume during water deprivation is unlikely to alter pressure beyond the limits of error of this measurement. In our experience, clinicians following the central venous pressure minute-to-minute during such testing often overreact to small decrements and terminate water deprivation in the

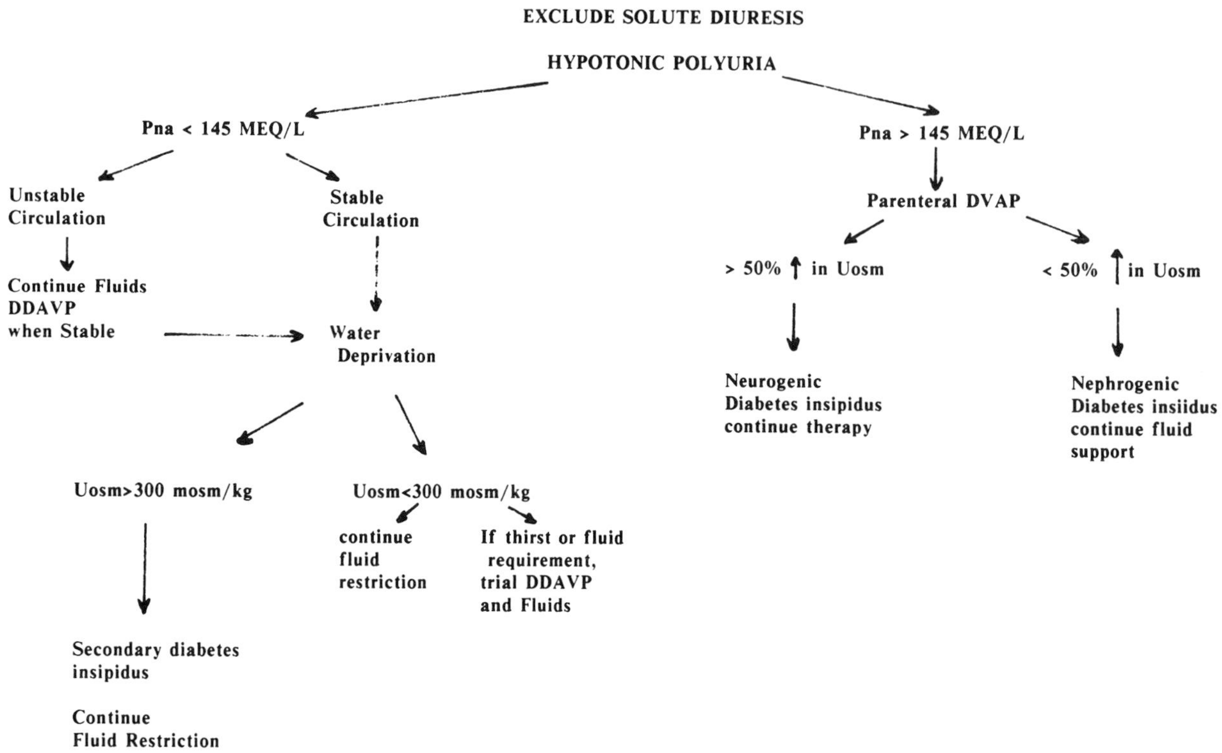

FIGURE 157-3 An algorithm for the evaluation and treatment of polyuria in critically ill patients. P_{Na} = plasma sodium; Uosm = urine osmolality. All patients considered to have complete or partial primary diabetes insipidus should be referred for full evaluation following resolution of their critical illness. (Reproduced, with permission, from Hall JB, Robertson GL.[3])

absence of other indications of adverse hypovolemia.[3] Much more important is the careful measurement of hour-to-hour fluid intake and output, and serial measurement of the plasma sodium level with matched urine osmolality.

If intravenous medications cannot be withheld in a critical case, attempts should be made to concentrate them maximally and to reduce fluids to 1 to 2 L/day. Nonessential fluids can then be withheld, and urine output, osmolality, and plasma sodium followed serially.

If the plasma sodium level rises to the high-normal range in the face of a urine osmolality below 300 mOsm/L, excessive water intake is excluded as a cause, and DDAVP can be given to distinguish between neurogenic and nephrogenic diabetes insipidus.[3] If the plasma sodium level and osmolality increase significantly and urine osmolality rises above 300 mOsm/L, secondary diabetes insipidus is suggested, though similar results often occur with partial neurogenic or nephrogenic diabetes insipidus; hence, the result is nondiagnostic. In ambulatory patients a measurement of plasma vasopressin levels is often used at this juncture to distinguish various forms of diabetes insipidus.[15] This approach is not practical in the critical care setting, since the delay for obtaining and interpreting measurements is often unacceptable. Accordingly, a different approach is warranted. If the fluid deprivation is well tolerated then a trial of reduced fluid intake should continue, on the suspicion that the observed polyuria is a result of excessive water administration. However, if the patient develops thirst or manifestations of hypovolemia prior to resolution of the polyuria, DDAVP therapy *with close monitoring of water balance* may be undertaken until formal testing can be conducted safely.[3]

If a patient requires vasoactive drugs to support circulatory function or manifests hypoperfusion (low measured cardiac output, wide arteriovenous oxygen content difference, lactic acidosis, arterial hypotension), then fluid deprivation is not advisable. Of course, polyuria is extremely unusual in these circumstances. If polyuria is present, volume administration should be continued as deemed necessary according to the usual endpoints of preload adequacy. DDAVP can be administered as well, to determine if polyuria abates, but *fluid balance must be monitored very closely to guard against water intoxication.*

Treatment

If excessive water administration is confirmed as a cause of polyuria, fluid administration should be reduced while clinical assessment of intravascular volume status and measurement of the plasma sodium level continue on a frequent basis.

Treatments for neurogenic and nephrogenic diabetes insipidus differ according to several factors.[16–21] Critically ill patients with neurogenic diabetes insipidus usually need initial hormone replacement to restore normal water bal-

TABLE 157-3 Replacement Therapy for Diabetes Insipidus

Agent	Dose	Route	Duration
Desmopressin (DDAVP)	1–2 μg	SC	12–24 h
	5–20 μg	Intranasal	12–24 h
Aqueous vasopressin	5–10 U	SC, IM	4–6 h
Vasopressin tannate (in oil)	2.5–50 U	IM	24–72 h

ance. Several vasopressin preparations are available; their dosages, routes, and durations of action are summarized in Table 157-3. DDAVP is a preferred agent, since it can be administered parenterally or intranasally, or placed directly on the buccal mucosa. It has a long duration of action (8 to 16 h), facilitating once- or twice-daily dosing, and lacks the vasoconstrictor and intestinal motility effects of high doses of vasopressin. Thus it avoids the side effect of abdominal pain that may result from inadvertent administration of excessive doses of the hormone. This problem is not rare, since Pitressin, a common injectable vasopressin preparation, is supplied in a very concentrated form and requires careful dilution prior to administration.[3]

Complications associated with the use of DDAVP seem rare, but experience with this agent in critically ill patients is somewhat limited. A noteworthy report tells of venous thromboembolism in a patient receiving DDAVP for diabetes insipidus.[22] Causality may exist in this case, since high doses of DDAVP increase plasma concentrations of coagulation factor VIII procoagulant activity, von Willebrand factor, and ristocetin cofactor activity. The drug has been used to reduce the incidence of bleeding in uremia, hemophilia, and von Willebrand's disease. It remains to be determined if this agent will place critically ill patients at higher risk for thromboembolic disease.

Critically ill patients with impaired thirst and ability to communicate will be dependent on the physician's assessment of osmolality and hydration during hormone replacement. Urinary output, urine osmolality, and the plasma sodium level should be followed daily, or more frequently if they are highly variable. If hypernatremia is initially extreme (over 160 meq/L), correction should proceed over 36 to 72 h, with plasma osmolality decreasing at approximately 1 mOsm/kg per h. This tempo is recommended to avoid cerebral edema.

Regardless of the initial sodium concentration, a risk of water intoxication exists while the physician is administering hormone and fluids. This is particularly true in cases of transient diabetes insipidus, most often described in the neurosurgical patient population. We recommend that patients with trauma and postoperative syndromes have replacement therapy withheld after 3 to 5 days, and then be reassessed. Patients with a triphasic course may require fluid restriction for a period of time, and ultimately may manifest vasopressin deficiency again.

Patients with nephrogenic diabetes insipidus should be carefully screened for drugs associated with this disorder. During critical illness, fluids should be titrated against urinary output and the plasma sodium level.

Finally, all patients receiving a diagnosis of primary diabetes insipidus during critical illness should be referred for complete assessment of pituitary function upon recovery. Long-term diagnostic and therapeutic strategies are best planned at the time of discharge from the ICU.

CASE PRESENTATION

A 36-year-old man was trapped in a home fire and sustained a 27 percent second- and third-degree burn of the back and legs. To escape, he jumped 2 stories onto an asphalt pad, sustaining a broken femur, chest contusions, and skull fracture with associated epidural hematoma. After resuscitation and diagnostic brain CT scan in the emergency room he was immediately taken to the operating room for hematoma evacuation and placement of an intracranial pressure (ICP) monitor. He received an initial dose of mannitol on presentation to the emergency room, and arrived in the burn ICU with mannitol infusion and hyperventilation by mechanical ventilation in place.

Serial measurements of plasma sodium and plasma osmolality are given in Table 157-4. The urine volumes and IV fluids administered each day are summarized as well. The patient's weight on admission to the ICU was 80 kg. During the first hospital day the patient was heavily sedated with intermittent muscle relaxation to facilitate supportive therapy. From day 2 to day 3 neurologic recovery was apparent, with spontaneous movement of the extremities and continued improvement over the remaining course. For the first 4 days mannitol was titrated to maintain ICP below 20 to 25 mmHg. By day 4, hyperventilation and mannitol infusion were gradually tapered, with continued neurologic improvement; the patient was extubated on ICU day 5.

By day 5, urinary output had risen to 4.8 L/day. This was initially ascribed to possible solute diuresis. Following discontinuation of mannitol urinary output continued to increase, to 8 to 9 L/day (see Table 157-4). At this point urine osmolality was measured, and hypotonic polyuria (250 mOsm/kg) was confirmed.

A review of fluid history did not clarify the cause of this polyuria, since the daily intravenous input was generally consistent with that typically given in comparable burn cases. The patient was not able to communicate regarding thirst. On day 9 the plasma sodium level was 143 meq/L and the plasma osmolality 290 mOsm/kg. The next morning all intravenous fluids other than hyperalimentation were held. Over the course of 5 hours, urinary output remained high (400 mL/h) and plasma sodium and osmolality rose to 155 meq/L and 305 mOsm/kg, respectively, with urine osmolality changing little (250 to 275 mOsm/kg). DDAVP, 1 μg subcutaneously, was given; urinary output fell, with a rise in urine osmolality to 600 mOsm/kg.

The patient was kept on DDAVP for 4 days. Plasma sodium fell as low as 129 meq/L at one point (Table 157-4) and responded to adjustment of free water intake. When DDAVP was withheld, after 7 days, plasma osmolality and sodium rose, with recurrence of polyuria. The patient was again started on DDAVP.

TABLE 157-4 Daily Summary of Clinical Data from Case Presentation

Day	1	2	3	4	5	6	7	8	9	10	11	12	13	14	15	16	17	18
Urinary Output (L)	1.2	1.8	2.0	3.0	4.8	7.8	8.0	9.0	8.0	5.0	2.5	1.5	1.5	1.8	1.0	1.8	4.8	2.5
IV fluids (L)																		
0.5 NS	3	2	1	1	1	1	1	1	—	0.1	0.5	—	—	—	—	—	—	—
D5LR	7	5	3	2.5	3.5	4.0	5.5	5.0	0.2	2.5	2.5	2	2.4	2.4	2.4	2.4	2.4	2.4
Hyper-alimentation	—	3.5	3.5	3.5	3.5	3.5	3.5	3.5	3.5	3.5	3.5	3.5	3.5	3.5	3.5	3.5	3.5	3.5
Mannitol dosage (g)	140	110	100	80	45	20	—	—	—	—	—	—	—	—	—	—	—	—
Plasma sodium (meq/L)	139	149	153	151	146	144	143	143	155	139	134	129	134	137	134	140	145	140
Plasma osmolality (mOsm/kg)	295	300	310	315	300	296	—	290	305	280	270	260	270	275	280	285	290	280
Urine osmolality (mOsm/kg)	—	—	—	—	—	—	—	250	275	600	—	—	—	—	—	—	—	—
DDAVP dosage (μg)	—	—	—	—	—	—	—	—	1	1	1	1	—	1	1	—	—	1

After 3 weeks the patient was discharged from the ICU to a rehabilitation center. DDAVP was continued, with frequent assessment of plasma sodium, until complete endocrinologic evaluation was undertaken.

CASE DISCUSSION

A number of features of diabetes insipidus in the critically ill are represented here. Early interpretation of polyuria was confounded by many factors, including large amounts of administered fluids (as a requirement of burn management), mannitol infusion, and early hyperalimentation (conceivably contributing to solute diuresis). The persistence of the polyuria beyond the period of mannitol infusion confirmed that it was hypotonic.

While a component of this patient's polyuria could be ascribed to a mild solute diuresis (total solute excretion = 9.0 L/day × 250 mOsm/kg = 2250 mOsm/day, which is more than 20 mOsm per kg body weight per day), which perhaps was attributable to hyperalimentation, the prominent hypotonic polyuria appropriately focused attention on the possibility of primary or secondary diabetes insipidus.

Since a review of volume history did not clarify the cause of polyuria, the general algorithm described in this chapter was applied. With a high-normal plasma sodium level, fluid restriction was instituted; urine and plasma parameters were followed. As is often the case with critically ill patients, some ongoing fluid administration (in this case, hyperalimentation) was necessary. Despite the severity of his illness, the patient tolerated sufficient water deprivation for hyperosmolality and hypernatremia to emerge. As we have mentioned, this almost invariably occurs before significant volume depletion takes place.

Administration of DDAVP confirmed neurogenic diabetes insipidus—the most likely problem in this case of closed head trauma. Despite careful monitoring of the plasma sodium level and osmolality, a degree of hyponatremia developed, as is often the case with closed head trauma. In view of this difficulty in management and of the fact that diabetes insipidus may be transient after neurologic insult, replacement therapy was discontinued after 1 week. The patient promptly demonstrated return of polyuria, and DDAVP was again administered on a daily basis, with no further need for formal water deprivation. Ultimately the patient underwent full endocrinologic assessment, which we recommend in all such cases.

References

1. Robertson GL, Berl T: Water metabolism, in Brenner BM, Rector FC (eds): *The Kidney*. Philadelphia, WB Saunders, 1986, pp 386–433.
2. Robertson GL: Posterior pituitary, in Felig P, Baxter JD, Broadus AE, et al (eds): *Endocrinology and Metabolism*. New York, McGraw-Hill, 1987, pp 338–385.
3. Hall JB, Robertson GL: Diabetes insipidus, in *Endocrine Emergencies*, Problems in Critical Care. Philadelphia, JB Lippincott (in press).
4. Durr JA, Hoggard JG, Hunt JM, et al: Diabetes insipidus in pregnancy associated with abnormally high circulating vasopressinase activity. N Engl J Med 316:1070, 1987.
5. Keren G, Barzilay Z, Schreiber M, et al: Diabetes insipidus indicating a dying brain. J Crit Care Med 10(11):798, 1982.
6. Yoshioka T, Sugimoto H, Uenishi M, et al: Prolonged hemodynamic maintenance by the combined administration of vasopressin and epinephrine in brain death: A clinical study. Neurosurg 18(5):565, 1986.
7. Notman DD, Mortek MA, Moses AM: Permanent diabetes insipidus following head trauma: Observations in ten patients and an approach to diagnosis. J Trauma 20:599, 1980.
8. Kern KB, Meislin HW: Diabetes insipidus: Occurrence after minor head trauma. J Trauma 24(1):69, 1984.
9. Hadani M, Findler G, Shaked I, Sahar A: Unusual delayed onset of diabetes insipidus following closed head trauma. J Neurosurg (63)456, 1985.
10. Verbalis JG, Robinson AG, Moses AM: Postoperative and posttraumatic diabetes insipidus, in Czernichow P, Robinson AG (eds): *Diabetes Insipidus in Man*, Frontiers of Hormone Research, vol 13. Basel and London, S Karger, 1985, pp 2470–265.
11. Glauser FL: Diabetes insipidus in hypoxemic encephalopathy. JAMA 235:932, 1976.
12. Halebian P, Yurt R, Petito C, Shires GT: Diabetes insipidus after carbon monoxide poisoning and smoke inhalation. J Trauma 25(7):662, 1985.
13. Singer I, Forrest JN Jr: Drug-induced states of nephrogenic diabetes insipidus. Kidney Int 10:82, 1976.
14. McDonald RH, Goldbert LI, McNay JL, et al: Effects of dopamine in man: Augmentation of sodium excretion, glomerular filtration rate, and renal plasma flow. J Clin Invest 43:1116, 1964.
15. Robertson GL: Diagnosis of diabetes insipidus, in Czernichow AP, Robinson A (eds): *Diabetes Inspidus in Man*, Frontiers of Hormone Research, vol 13. Basel and London, S Karger, 1985, p 127.
16. Robinson AG: dDAVP in the treatment of central diabetes insipidus. N Engl J Med 294:507, 1976.
17. Cobb WE, Spare S, Reichlin S: Neurogenic diabetes insipidus: Management with dDAVP (1-desamino-8-D-arginine-vasopressin). Ann Intern Med 11:183, 1978.
18. Shucart WA, Jackson I: Management of diabetes insipidus in neurosurgical patients. J Neurosurg 44:65, 1976.
19. Chanson P, Jedynak CP, Dabrowski G, et al: Ultralow doses of vasopressin in the management of diabetes insipidus. J Crit Care Med 15(1):44, 1987.
20. Cunnah D, Ross G, Besser GM: Management of cranial diabetes insipidus with oral desmopressin (DDAVP). Clin Endocrin 24:253, 1986.
21. Grossman A, Fabbri A, Goldberg PL, Besser GM: Two new modes of desmopressin (DDAVP) administration. Br Med J ii:12, 1980.
22. Albert SG, Salvato-Lechner V, Joist HJ: Venous thromboembolism and transient thrombocytopenia in a patient with diabetes insipidus treated with desmopressin acetate (DDAVP). Thromb Research 50(5):695, 1988.

Chapter 158

ACID-BASE DISORDERS

V. THEODORE BARNETT
GREGORY A. SCHMIDT

KEY POINTS

- *Acid-base disorders are common in the ICU, and mixed disorders are often seen. These can be identified by the use of a few simple diagnostic steps.*
- *Acidemia has deleterious effects on the myocardium, the vasculature, the central nervous system, and diaphragmatic function.*
- *Alkalemia can lead to decreased cerebral blood flow, tetany, and refractory arrhythmias.*
- *The anion gap and the osmolal gap are useful in the diagnosis of metabolic acidosis.*
- *Lactic acidosis occurs from a large number of causes, but most commonly represents tissue hypoxia.*
- *The use of bicarbonate in the treatment of organic acidosis is controversial and is not recommended.*
- *Most metabolic alkaloses are preventable with attention to fluid and electrolyte status. Severe or symptomatic metabolic alkalosis can be treated with infusion of 0.1 N HCl.*
- *Respiratory acidosis represents ventilatory failure and should be treated accordingly.*
- *Respiratory alkalosis is very common and often is benign, but requires determination of cause (e.g., early sepsis or pulmonary embolism).*

Disturbances of acid-base equilibrium occur in a wide variety of critical illnesses and are among the most commonly encountered disorders in the ICU. In addition to reflecting the seriousness of the underlying disease, these disorders have their own morbidity and mortality.

The maintenance of acid-base homeostasis is discussed in Chap. 3. In this chapter we will deal with the clinical effects of alterations in hydrogen ion concentration and with the disorders of acid-base balance encountered in the ICU. Particular emphasis is placed on the physiologic effects of acidemia and on lactic acidosis and its treatment.

A blood pH less than normal is called *acidemia;* the underlying process causing acidemia is called *acidosis.* Similarly, *alkalemia* and *alkalosis* refer to the pH and the underlying process, respectively. While an acidosis and an alkalosis may coexist, there can be only one resulting pH. Therefore, acidemia and alkalemia are mutually exclusive conditions.

The approach to acid-base derangements should emphasize a search for the cause, rather than an immediate attempt to normalize the pH. Many disorders are mild and do not require treatment. Further, treatment may be more detrimental than the acid-base disorder itself. More important is a full consideration of the possible underlying pathologic states. This may facilitate a directed intervention that will benefit the patient more than normalization of the pH would. This chapter will conclude with a full discussion of the diagnostic approach to acid-base disturbances.

Physiologic Effects

ACIDEMIA

The effects of acidemia are rarely encountered in patients without a coexisting disease that modifies and obscures physiologic changes. Experiments utilizing acute acid-base changes in humans are often unreliable, because of the artificiality of methods used to induce acid-base changes and the short time courses of many experiments. Conclusions drawn from basic science investigations of acidemia are compromised by lack of uniformity of experimental conditions (temperatures, species, time course, etc.) and questionable applicability to the clinical arena. With these caveats in mind, we have summarized the physiologic consequences of respiratory and metabolic acidemia (see also Chap. 3).

CARDIOVASCULAR EFFECTS

In isolated cardiac muscle and mammalian hearts, cardiac contractility begins to decrease with small changes from normal pH and continues to fall as pH is lowered. Depression of the slow inward calcium current by intracellular hydrogen ions appears to be the primary cause of this decrement in inotropy; increased extracellular calcium can counter the effect. Both metabolic and respiratory acidemia cause a similar degree of myocardial depression, but the effect of respiratory acidemia occurs more promptly—presumably because of the rapid entry of CO_2 into the cardiac cell.

Metabolic acidemia decreases the threshold for ventricular fibrillation in animals. The effect of respiratory acidemia is less clear, with at most a slight decrease in the fibrillation threshold. Clinically no increase in arrhythmias is seen in patients with respiratory failure and hypercapnia, except that attributable to hypoxia.[1] Once fibrillation is established, acidemia has no effect on the success of conversion to sinus rhythm.[2]

In isolated vessels acidemia causes vasodilation, although at very low pH (below 7.15) vascular resistance begins to rise toward the control level. The response to acidemia in patients or intact animals is even more complex. Acidemia causes stimulation of the sympathetic-adrenal axis. In severe acidemia this effect is countered by a depressed responsiveness of adrenergic receptors to circulating catecholamines. The net effect on ventricular performance, heart rhythm, and vascular tone depends on the relative effects of these competing influences. For example, mild acidemia causes increased cardiac output, a response that can be prevented by β-adrenergic blockade. Severe acidemia typically causes a decrease in cardiac output and vasodilation despite sympathetic stimulation. However, since intracellular hydrogen ion concentration depends on the mechanism of, and rate of change of, blood pH, there is no arterial pH at which myocardial depression will reliably occur.

NEUROMUSCULAR EFFECTS

Acute respiratory acidemia causes marked increases in cerebral blood flow. In human beings, acute elevation of P_{CO_2} to more than 60 mmHg causes confusion and headache. When P_{CO_2} exceeds 70 mmHg, loss of consciousness and seizures can occur. This is likely due to an abrupt lowering of intracellular pH rather than to any effect of CO_2 per se. In fact, chronic increases in CO_2, as seen in chronic obstructive pulmonary disease, are typically well tolerated even when the P_{CO_2} is as high as 150 mmHg. The encephalopathy of acute-on-chronic respiratory failure is poorly understood, but may include elements of intracellular acidosis, hypoxia, and endogenous neuropeptide secretion. Thus the term "CO_2 narcosis," which implies a direct effect of CO_2, is a misnomer.

Acute hypercapnia causes depression of diaphragmatic contractility and a decrease in endurance time.[3] This effect may contribute to the downward spiral of respiratory failure in patients with acute CO_2 retention. Whether chronic respiratory acidosis impairs diaphragmatic function has not been determined. The effect of metabolic acidemia on the respiratory muscles is less clear, but probably also consists of depression of contractility.

EFFECTS ON ELECTROLYTE LEVELS

Acute infusion of hydrochloric acid causes an increase in the serum potassium concentration. However, administration of organic acids, such as lactic acid and ketoacids, does not raise the potassium level, and may even lower it.[4] The hyperkalemia commonly observed in both lactic acidosis and ketoacidosis is due to factors other than the pH change.[5] Acute respiratory acidemia causes no change, or a slight increment, in the serum potassium level. Both respiratory and metabolic acidemia cause increased extracellular phosphate concentrations. Clinically, lactic acidosis and ketoacidosis are associated with hyperphosphatemia.[6]

ALKALEMIA

CARDIOVASCULAR EFFECTS

Alkalemia appears to increase myocardial contractility, at least to a pH of 7.7. At higher pH, in vitro studies generally show a decline in contractility. There is little effect on the threshold for ventricular fibrillation,[7] but some animals exhibit spontaneous ventricular fibrillation at pH levels above 7.8.[8] There are reports of alkalemic patients with atrial and ventricular arrhythmias that were refractory to treatment until the alkalemia was corrected.[9]

The effect of alkalemia on the vasculature in vitro is to cause vasodilation, which is maximal at pH 7.65. At higher levels of pH, vasoconstriction occurs, with a return to baseline vascular tone by pH 7.8.[10] Clinically, hyperventilation causes a decrease in systemic vascular resistance. However, alkalemia can also cause coronary artery spasm with ECG evidence of ischemia. In fact, respiratory alkalosis can be used as a provocative stimulus in the diagnosis of vasospastic angina.[11]

NEUROMUSCULAR EFFECTS

Acute respiratory alkalemia causes a decrease in cerebral blood flow, which falls to 70 percent of control at a P_{CO_2} of 30 mmHg. The maximal decrease, to 50 percent of basal flow, occurs at a P_{CO_2} of 20 mmHg. This effect lasts only 6 h.[12] Acute hyperventilation can produce confusion, myoclonus, asterixis, and loss of consciousness. Both respiratory and metabolic alkalemia can lead to seizures. The effects of alkalemia on skeletal muscle, including the diaphragm, are poorly understood; respiratory muscle contractility may be slightly increased.

EFFECTS ON ELECTROLYTE LEVELS

Acute hypocapnea causes a slight reduction in the serum levels of sodium, potassium, and phosphorus.[13] Alkalemia causes a small rise in the lactate concentration (on the order of 1 to 2 mmol/L), because of the hydrogen ion modulation of phosphofructokinase activity and consequent increased glycolysis.[14] Ionized calcium levels fall .03 to .09 mmol/L for each rise in pH of 0.1 unit. The paresthesias, carpal-pedal spasm, and tetany seen with acute hyperventilation, however, are due to direct effects of hydrogen ion concentration on neurons.[15]

PULMONARY EFFECTS

In patients with respiratory failure and increased pulmonary shunt, alkalemia can cause a decrease in P_{O_2}. This is due to a deterioration in ventilation/perfusion relationships.[16]

EFFECTS ON OXYGEN DELIVERY

Alkalemia causes an increase in hemoglobin's affinity for oxygen. However, there are also an increase in the concentration of 2,3-diphosphoglycerate in red blood cells and a change in red cell morphology, which oppose this effect.[17] The clinical effect of alkalemia-induced changes in oxygen delivery is minimal. Only in patients with tissue hypoxia are the small, acute changes potentially relevant.

Metabolic Acidosis

PATHOPHYSIOLOGY

Metabolic acidosis is characterized by a primary decrease in HCO_3 (bicarbonate) concentration and a compensatory decrease in the CO_2 concentration. Metabolic acidosis occurs from either loss of HCO_3 or addition of H^+. Bicarbonate loss generally occurs through the kidneys or the bowel. The body produces 50 to 100 meq of H^+ per day from normal metabolism. An increase in this fixed acid production, or a decrease in the renal ability to excrete the acid load, will produce a metabolic acidosis. Acidosis from decreased renal excretion generally is slow to develop. In contrast, acidosis from increased acid production—as in lactic acidosis or ketoacidosis—can exceed maximal renal excretion and cause a rapidly developing, and severe, acidosis.

APPROACH TO DIAGNOSIS

The etiologies of metabolic acidosis are divided into those that cause an increase in the anion gap and those associated with a normal anion gap. The *anion gap* is the difference between measured cations and measured anions; it is defined as $[Na^+] - [Cl^-] - [HCO_3^-]$, with a normal value of 8 to 14 meq/L. A normal-anion-gap acidosis occurs when chloride replaces the bicarbonate lost in buffering H^+. An increase in the anion gap in metabolic acidosis occurs when the anion replacing the bicarbonate is not one that is routinely measured. Anions always equal cations, but if the anion is not chloride then the anion gap calculated from routine chemistries will increase.

Normal-anion-gap acidosis occurs from the loss of bicarbonate, through the kidneys or through the gut, or from the addition of an acid with chloride as the accompanying anion. The most common cause of normal-gap metabolic acidosis in the ICU is diarrhea; in the absence of diarrhea a renal tubular acidosis is likely. The causes of renal tubular acidosis encountered in the ICU are listed in Table 158-1 and are discussed in depth in Chap. 3. The other causes of normal-anion-gap acidosis are usually obvious from the surgical history and medication list. The etiologies of normal-anion-gap metabolic acidosis are listed in Table 158-2.

The etiologies of increased-anion-gap metabolic acidosis are given in Table 158-3. The most important increased-anion-gap acidosis in intensive care medicine is lactic acidosis, which is discussed separately below.

KETOACIDOSIS

Ketoacidosis occurs when there is an increase in free fatty acid production and a preferential shunting of fatty acids in the liver to the formation of ketones. This occurs in states of

TABLE 158-1 Etiologies of Renal Tubular Acidosis (RTA) in the ICU

Proximal RTA
- Primary renal disease
  - Nephrotic syndrome
- Systemic diseases
  - Amyloidosis
  - Multiple myeloma
  - Systemic lupus erythematosus (SLE)
- Drugs and toxins
  - Heavy metal toxicity
  - Carbonic anhydrase inhibitors

Type I Distal RTA
- Primary renal disease
  - Obstructive uropathy
  - Renal transplant rejection
  - Nephrocalcinosis
  - Pyelonephritis
- Systemic diseases
  - Cirrhosis
  - Multiple myeloma
  - Sickle cell disease
  - Amyloidosis
  - SLE
- Drugs and toxins
  - Amphotericin
  - Lithium
  - Analgesic abuse

Type IV Distal RTA
- Primary renal disease
  - Obstructive uropathy
  - Hyporeninemia
- Systemic diseases
  - Diabetes mellitus
  - Addison's disease
  - Sickle cell disease
- Drugs and toxins
  - Spironolactone
  - Triamterene
  - Amiloride

TABLE 158-2 Etiologies of Normal-Anion-Gap Metabolic Acidosis

Gastrointestinal Loss of Bicarbonate
- Diarrhea
- Urinary diversion
- Small bowel, pancreatic, or bile drainage (fistulas, surgical drains)
- Cholestyramine

Renal Loss of Bicarbonate (or Bicarbonate Equivalent)
- Renal tubular acidosis
- Recovery phase of DKA
- Renal insufficiency

Acidifying Substances
- HCl
- NH_4Cl
- Arginine HCl
- Lysine HCl
- $CaCl_2$ or $MgCl_2$ (oral)
- Sulfur

TABLE 158-3 Etiologies of Increased-Anion-Gap Metabolic Acidosis

Etiology	Anion
Ketoacidosis	Acetoacetate, β-hydroxybutyrate
Diabetic	
Alcoholic	
Starvation	
Lactic acidosis	Lactate
Uremia	Phosphates, sulfates, organic anions
Toxins	
Ethylene glycol	Glycolate, lactate
Methanol	Formate, lactate
Salicylate	Salicylate, lactate, organic anions
Paraldehyde	Unknown

low insulin and increased glucagon. Diabetic ketoacidosis is a common reason for ICU admission and is easily diagnosed from glucose and ketone measurement. Alcoholic ketoacidosis (AKA) generally occurs after binge drinking in alcoholics who have no food intake and repeated vomiting. It is characterized by a normal or slightly elevated serum glucose level with increased ketones. Because of the altered redox state of the liver, much of the ketones in AKA occur in the form of β-hydroxybutyrate, which is not measured by the Ketostix or Acetest. Specific enzymatic testing is necessary to detect β-hydroxybutyrate; unfortunately, this test is not available at many hospitals. Starvation ketoacidosis is usually a mild and self-limited acidosis. During a 1-month fast, pH stabilizes at an average of 7.35 and the fall in bicarbonate is rarely greater than 5 meq/L. Ketoacidosis is discussed in detail in Chap. 159.

TOXINS

Toxin ingestion is an uncommon but important cause of increased-anion-gap acidosis. Any patient who presents with an anion-gap acidosis that is not explained by tests for ketones and lactate should be suspected of having ingested a toxin. However, it should also be remembered that lactic acidosis can occur with toxin ingestion and that an increased lactate level does not rule out an acidosis from toxins. Often the laboratory diagnosis of toxin ingestion is slow; thus the diagnosis must be suspected, and clinical clues sought, prior to laboratory confirmation. Specific tests must be ordered, since methanol and ethylene glycol are not included in a routine toxicology screen. Salicylate intoxication is the most common of these ingestions and often presents with a mixed respiratory alkalosis and metabolic acidosis, which can be an important diagnostic clue. The pH in salicylate-intoxicated adults is typically normal or alkaline.

Methanol and ethylene glycol are two toxins that, when ingested, can cause a severe increased-anion-gap metabolic acidosis—among other clinical manifestations. The toxic effects of both drugs, including the metabolic acidosis, are mediated by metabolites—glycolate in the case of ethylene glycol, and formaldehyde and formate in the case of methanol. The osmolal gap, which is the difference between measured osmolality and that calculated from the formula $Osm = 2[Na^+] + [glucose]/18 + [BUN]/2.8 + [ethanol]/4.6$, is increased above its normal value of less than 10 mosmol/L when there are unmeasured osmotically active particles present. It is usually, although not invariably, increased in methanol and ethylene glycol poisoning. In addition, the retinal sheen seen with methanol poisoning and the characteristic urinary oxalate crystals seen with methylene glycol poisoning can be important diagnostic clues. A detailed discussion of these ingestions is presented in Chap. 170.

The identification of the anion associated with an increased-anion-gap acidosis in the ICU is not as precise as it might seem from the relatively short list of possibilities. In some cases of acidosis, either no anion is found or the rise in anions accounts for only a fraction of the rise in the anion gap; the identity of the offending anion, or anions, in these circumstances has not been determined.[18]

TREATMENT

In general, all medications or administered substances contributing to an acidosis should be removed, if possible. However, a mild acidosis secondary to a necessary treatment (e.g., hyperalimentation) can be tolerated. In normal-anion-gap acidosis characterized by ongoing loss of bicarbonate, bicarbonate therapy is indicated in amounts equal to losses.

Bicarbonate therapy has not been found to be efficacious in the treatment of diabetic ketoacidosis. Several trials, including a small prospective study in patients with severe ketoacidosis (pH 6.90 to 7.14), showed no difference in the rate of bicarbonate increase, or pH increase, with bicarbonate therapy.[19] In addition, bicarbonate therapy can result in rebound alkalemia as ketones are metabolized and bicarbonate regenerated. In most cases alcoholic ketoacidosis responds rapidly to glucose infusion, and neither bicarbonate nor insulin therapy is needed. Starvation ketoacidosis is easily treated with nutritional support.

Salicylate overdose is treated with alkaline diuresis and, if severe, with hemodialysis. Methanol and ethylene glycol poisoning, if severe and accompanied by a metabolic acidosis, should be treated by ethanol infusion, which competitively inhibits metabolism to toxic products via alcohol dehydrogenase; and, if the acidosis remains significant, by hemodialysis. The ethanol infusion should maintain a blood ethanol level above 100 mg/dL.

LACTIC ACIDOSIS

DEFINITION AND SIGNIFICANCE

Lactic acidosis is the most common and most important acidosis encountered in the ICU. The acidemia has physiologic significance and, perhaps more important, serves as a marker for a diverse group of serious underlying conditions. In addition, the presence, magnitude, and course of the acidosis have important prognostic implications.

Many patients in the ICU have small elevations in lactate level, usually in the range of 2 to 5 mmol/L, that are due to a variety of stimuli, including sympathetic activation. Mild increases in the serum lactate level may indicate early tissue hypoxia, but also may reflect the hypermetabolic state accompanying many critical illnesses. The definition of lactic acidosis is arbitrary; it is commonly defined as a lactate level greater than 5 mmol/L with an arterial pH less than 7.35.[20]

Increasing lactate levels correlate well with increasing mortality in patients with cardiogenic shock. In other types of shock the correlation is not as good, and there is considerable overlap in lactate levels between survivors and nonsurvivors. This lack of correlation is due, in part, to the influence on lactate levels of such factors as nutritional status and liver disease. However, the trend in lactate levels in a given patient can be helpful in gauging the effect of therapy and assessing prognosis.

ETIOLOGIES

The etiologies of lactic acidosis are numerous and are listed in Table 158-4. Most cases of lactic acidosis encountered in the ICU occur secondarily to a handful of processes; shock, either septic, cardiogenic, or hypovolemic, is the most common cause. Hypoxia, seizures, regional ischemia (i.e., mesenteric or in an extremity), and toxin exposure account for a majority of the remaining cases. A few examples will be discussed further, to give insight into the various mechanisms causing lactic acidosis.

TABLE 158-4 Etiologies of Lactic Acidosis

Increased Oxygen Consumption
Strenuous exercise
Grand mal seizure
Neuroleptic malignant syndrome
Severe asthma
Pheochromocytoma
Decreased Oxygen Delivery
Decreased cardiac output
Hypovolemia
Cardiogenic shock (including pericardial and pulmonary vascular disease)
Decreased arterial oxygen content
Profound anemia
Severe hypoxemia
Regional ischemia (mesentery or extremity)
Microcirculatory disturbances
Sepsis
Alterations in Cellular Metabolism
Diabetes mellitus
Thiamine deficiency
Severe alkalemia
Hypoglycemia
Malignancy
Toxins and Drugs
Carbon monoxide
Ethanol, methanol
Biguanides
Ethylene glycol, propylene glycol
Salicylates
Isoniazid
Streptozocin
Cyanide, nitroprusside
Papaverine
Acetaminophen
Nalidixic acid
Ritodrine
Terbutaline
Fructose, sorbitol, xylitol
Epinephrine, norepinephrine
Congenital
Glucose-6-phosphatase deficiency
Fructose-1,6-diphosphatase deficiency
Pyruvate carboxylase deficiency
Pyruvate-dehydrogenase (PDH) deficiency
Oxidative phosphorylation defects
Decreased Lactate Clearance
Fulminant hepatic failure
D-Lactate

Sepsis

Sepsis is a common cause of lactic acidosis in the ICU. Several mechanisms act to produce increased lactate. Some cases of sepsis exhibit frankly diminished oxygen delivery and inadequate tissue oxygenation. In other cases a hyperdynamic circulation exists, with a delivery of oxygen far exceeding usual requirements. There is evidence that occult tissue hypoxia exists in this state. This condition is called *pathological supply dependency of oxygen utilization,* since increased oxygen delivery (even when it is supranormal) increases oxygen consumption. This is discussed further in Chap. 57. In addition, sepsis is a hypermetabolic state with increased substrate flux, leading to increased circulating levels of many metabolic compounds, including alanine, lactate and pyruvate.

Seizures

Grand mal seizures cause tremendous muscle energy usage and glycogen breakdown, with much of the glucose converted to lactate. The lactic acidosis associated with seizures is illustrative of the handling of an acute lactate load. Immediately following a seizure, a lactic acidosis is present, with a lactate level often greater than 10 mmol/L and a pH below 7.20. In 1 h, lactate levels fall to half their post-seizure levels and pH normalizes.[21]

Malignancy

Lactic acidosis has been reported in a variety of malignancies, most commonly in leukemia and lymphoma. The excess lactate is apparently produced by the malignancy through enhanced glycolysis without the cellular control mechanisms that normally link glycolysis with oxidative phosphorylation. Extensive liver metastases are commonly found in lactic acidosis associated with solid tumors; diminished hepatic lactate extraction is contributory in many cases, although hepatic metastases are not required for lactic acidosis to occur. It is important to remember, however, that most cases of lactic acidosis in patients with malignancy are due to shock and sepsis.

Hepatic Failure

The liver is the major lactate-metabolizing organ. With severe hepatic disease, lactate clearance is decreased. Because of the excess capacity for lactate metabolism that is normally available, stable patients with chronic liver disease do not manifest a rise in serum lactate even with severe hepatic dysfunction. However, the capacity to clear a lactate load is diminished, and any condition that increases lactate production will cause an exaggerated rise and delayed fall in blood lactate levels.

EFFECTS OF LACTATE

Lactate has physiologic effects independent of changes in hydrogen ion concentration. Human neutrophils and fat cells in vitro show a decrease in β-adrenergic responsiveness with acidosis; this is exaggerated by increased lactate levels.[22,23] Animal experiments have shown direct lactate effects on the myocardium. These include inhibition of glyceraldehyde-3-phosphate dehydrogenase (and, thus, a decreased rate of glycolysis) and mitochondrial swelling (which decreases the ability to couple oxidative phosphorylation). Further, lactate decreases the slow inward calcium current, causing a negative inotropic effect even at a pH of 7.4.[24,25] It remains to be seen whether these in-vitro results will be confirmed in clinical situations.

TREATMENT

The treatment of lactic acidosis is primarily the treatment of the disease causing the metabolic derangements. Without successful treatment of the process precipitating lactic acidosis, survival is unlikely. Therapies aimed at ameliorating the lactic acidosis itself are attempts to prevent further deterioration until the primary process can be controlled.

Bicarbonate

Bicarbonate has long been the standard therapy for lactic acidosis, but its effects have only recently come to be studied in any systematic way. Data concerning the physiologic effects of bicarbonate use are limited to anecdotes from patients with lactic acidosis, experimental models of lactic acidosis in animals, and a single human study. The recent data have called into question the traditional arguments for bicarbonate use, and a controversy has arisen over whether bicarbonate use in patients with lactic acidosis is warranted.

The results of bicarbonate therapy have been reported in several patients with lactic acidosis secondary to malignancy, both with and without liver metastases. In these patients therapy with bicarbonate causes increased lactate production. There is often a near-stoichiometric relationship between bicarbonate administered and lactate produced.[26] Animal studies have also shown an increase in lactate levels after bicarbonate administration.

Administration of bicarbonate causes an increase in CO_2 production, because of the metabolism of bicarbonate to H_2O and CO_2. Ventilation must be increased if a rise in P_{CO_2} after bicarbonate administration is to be avoided. However, many patients with severe lactic acidosis are at near-maximal ventilation and cannot achieve a significant increase in ventilation. In patients in whom ventilation can be increased who are mechanically ventilated, an increase in minute ventilation can be used to lower the P_{CO_2} and raise the pH without the administration of bicarbonate.

Increased P_{CO_2} after bicarbonate administration translates into decreased intracellular pH (pHi), since CO_2 equilibrates across cell membranes more rapidly than bicarbonate. Indeed, several animal studies have demonstrated a fall in pHi in the liver and in muscle following bicarbonate administration.[27]

The value of bicarbonate in improving hemodynamic derangements in critically ill patients with lactic acidosis has also been brought into question. A prospective controlled study in patients with lactic acidosis, comparing bicarbonate with hypertonic saline solution as a therapeutic agent, found bicarbonate to be no more effective than saline solution in increasing cardiac output and not effective in increasing mean arterial pressure. Bicarbonate also increased P_{CO_2} and decreased the ionized calcium level, possibly mitigating the cardiovascular effects of the increased pH seen with bicarbonate.[28] Studies in animal models of lactic acidosis demonstrate that bicarbonate is not superior to saline solution in improving mean arterial pressure or cardiac output, and may lower cardiac output. In addition to the above, bolus injection of bicarbonate into animals causes a decrease in blood pressure—an effect due to the hyperosmolality of the solution. The effectiveness of bicarbonate in these studies did not depend on the severity of the acidemia. Bicarbonate was no more effective at a pH of 6.9 to 7.0 than at higher pH levels.[27]

In animal models of lactic acidosis—including the hypoxic and hemorrhagic types, and lactic acidosis induced by phenformin administration and pancreatectomy—the mortality rate of animals treated with bicarbonate is no different from that of animals treated with normal saline solution (89 to 100 percent).[27] In the same models of lactic acidosis, dichloroacetate (DCA) therapy is associated with a mortality rate of 22 to 33 percent.

Carbicarb

Carbicarb is a combination of 0.33 *M* sodium carbonate (Na_2CO_3) and 0.33 *M* sodium bicarbonate ($NaHCO_3$) that has been developed as an alkalinizing agent. Carbicarb was formulated to cause a smaller increase in P_{CO_2} than bicarbonate (an effect that has been demonstrated in laboratory animals). It effectively increases arterial pH. Further, it provides buffering equal to that obtained with bicarbonate, with a lower sodium load and a lower—although still high—osmolality.[29] Trials of Carbicarb in human beings are currently underway; it use, therefore, must be considered experimental.

Dichloroacetate (DCA)

DCA lowers blood lactate, glucose, and triglyceride levels in human beings. It increases the activity of the pyruvate-dehydrogenase complex (PDH) by inhibiting the protein-kinase–mediated inactivation of PDH.[30] PDH is the rate-limiting enzyme that converts pyruvate into acetyl-CoA and thereby controls entry of pyruvate into the tricarboxylic acid (TCA) cycle. Inhibition of PDH increases the flow of pyruvate, and thus lactate, into the TCA cycle. The effect of DCA occurs mainly in skeletal muscle, where the pyruvate dehydrogenase complex is most abundant.

In animal models of lactic acidosis, DCA causes an increase in bicarbonate levels, arterial pH, and intracellular pH in both liver and muscle. This is accomplished by a decrease in lactate production from the gut and an increase in the hepatic extraction of lactate. Mortality at 4 h was 19 percent in DCA-treated animals, and 79 percent in those treated with bicarbonate.[27]

Two uncontrolled trials of DCA therapy in human beings have been conducted.[30,31] DCA therapy in patients who were resistant to therapy with bicarbonate caused significant reductions in lactate levels and increases in bicarbonate levels and arterial pH. In addition, 10 of 13 patients studied had an increase in systolic blood pressure, and cardiac output increased by 21 percent in the 4 patients in whom it was measured. However, all but 1 of the patients died of their underlying disease. In an open prospective trial, 26 of 29 patients responded to DCA therapy, response being defined as a decrease in lactate levels of 20 percent or more within 6 h. Among responders there was a 74 percent decrease in arterial lactate concentration, a 47 percent increase in bicarbonate, and normalization of pH. Mean survival time of responders was 60 h, compared with 26 h among nonresponders. No adverse affects are seen with acute administration of DCA. The results to date are promising, but a determination of the clinical place of DCA awaits the results of a controlled, prospective, randomized, multicenter trial of DCA therapy in lactic acidosis. Such a study is currently under way.

Dialysis

Both hemodialysis and peritoneal dialysis have been used in the treatment of lactic acidosis.[32] Either bicarbonate or acetate, which is converted to bicarbonate, is used as the buffer. Dialysis does not correct acidemia by removing hydrogen ions; its utility lies in its ability to prevent volume overload during the administration of large amounts of bicarbonate. The use of bicarbonate with dialysis is complicated by the same potential for adverse effects as with intravenous bicarbonate. Dialysis has the advantage of removing lactate, which, as described above, may have direct negative effects on the myocardium and cellular metabolism.

Recommendations

The decision whether to use bicarbonate is a difficult one. It is the choice between a long-standing but unproven therapy with potential deleterious effects, and reliance on data from experimental animal models with limited confirmatory human data; neither is an entirely satisfactory choice. Until additional controlled, randomized, double-blind trials of bicarbonate therapy are conducted, the debate will most likely continue. Because of the lack of data supporting bicarbonate use in human beings and the arguments reviewed above, we do not recommend the use of bicarbonate in lactic acidosis, *regardless of the pH.*

As with any therapy with potential deleterious effects, if bicarbonate therapy is attempted, close monitoring of its effects on a patient's hemodynamics, P_{CO_2}, pH, and clinical condition is necessary to determine response and detect any adverse effects. Further, if bicarbonate is used, it should be administered slowly, and preferably in an isotonic mixture.

Metabolic Alkalosis

PATHOPHYSIOLOGY

Metabolic alkalosis is characterized by a primary increase in the bicarbonate concentration and a compensatory increase in the P_{CO_2}. The normal kidney can excrete bicarbonate loads up to 10 meq/kg per day. Therefore, for a metabolic alkalosis to persist there must be both a process that elevates serum bicarbonate concentration and a stimulus for renal bicarbonate reabsorption.[33] The process that elevates bicarbonate is usually acid loss from the stomach or from the kidney. The stimulus for reabsorption generally is either hypovolemia with a chloride deficit; hypokalemia; or an increase in mineralocorticoid activity. In metabolic alkalosis associated with volume and chloride deficit, the renal tubules have a strong sodium avidity. When chloride deficit is present, bicarbonate is reabsorbed with sodium. The metabolic alkalosis will persist until the chloride deficit is replaced.[7] Hypokalemia increases tubular bicarbonate reabsorption and may cause vasoconstriction of the afferent renal arteriole, with reduced glomerular filtration. Mineralocorticoid excess causes increased bicarbonate by way of increased secretion of hydrogen ions in the cortical collecting tubule.

APPROACH TO DIAGNOSIS

The major causes of metabolic alkalosis in the ICU—vomiting, nasogastric suction, diuretics, corticosteroids, and overventilation of patients with chronically increased bicarbonate levels—are obvious (when present) from a patient's history and medication list. A careful search of all substances given to the patient is needed to disclose administration of compounds, such as citrate with blood products, and acetate in TPN, that can raise the bicarbonate level. If the etiology is not clear, a trial of volume and chloride replacement, as well as correction of hypokalemia, can be attempted. If this does not effect an improvement in the alkalosis, a search for increased mineralocorticoids may be warranted. The etiologies of metabolic alkalosis are listed in Table 158-5.

TREATMENT

Most cases of metabolic alkalosis encountered in the ICU are predictable and preventable. Replacement of diuretic-induced potassium losses with KCl, minimization of nasogastric suction, use of H_2 blockers with required prolonged nasogastric suction, and avoidance of rapid decreases in P_{CO_2} in patients with chronic obstructive pulmonary disease (COPD) will prevent the occurrence of metabolic alkalosis in many cases. Once a metabolic alkalosis is established, removal of the precipitating factors and correction of electrolyte deficits generally suffice to restore acid-base balance.

In patients who require continued diuresis but exhibit rising bicarbonate levels, acetazolamide can be used to reduce the bicarbonate level. Potassium replacement is mandatory when acetazolamide is used in patients with metabolic alkalosis. Patients in whom more severe volume overload is combined with metabolic alkalosis can be treated with a combination of continuous arteriovenous hemodialysis, which will remove bicarbonate in proportion to its concentration in plasma, and fluid replacement with a lesser volume of bicarbonate-free NaCl.

In rare cases more rapid correction may be indicated. The

TABLE 158-5 Etiologies of Metabolic Alkalosis

Chloride-Responsive
- Renal H^+ loss
  - Diuretic therapy
  - Posthypercapnia
  - Penicillin therapy
- Gastrointestinal H^+ losses
  - Vomiting
  - Nasogastric suction
  - Villous adenoma
  - Congenital chloridorrhea
  - Watery diarrhea hypokalemia achlorhydria syndrome (VIPoma/pancreatic cholera)
- Alkali administration
  - Bicarbonate
  - Citrate in blood products
  - Acetate in TPN
  - Nonabsorbable alkali (MgOH, AlOH) and exchange resins

Chloride-Resistant
- Increased mineralocorticoid activity
  - Primary aldosteronism
  - Cushing's syndrome
  - Drugs with mineralocorticoid activity
- Profound hypokalemia
- Refeeding
- Bartter's syndrome
- Parathyroid disease
- Hypercalcemia

pH level at which treatment is instituted is arbitrary. A pH of 7.6 is often used, because it is thought that the risks of serious adverse effects increase dramatically above this level, although the supporting evidence is minimal. Treatment is clearly indicated if adverse effects of alkalemia occur (such as arrhythmias and CNS depression), regardless of the degree of alkalemia.

Several methods of rapid correction have been used in the past, including arginine hydrochloride, ammonium chloride, and hydrochloric acid. Arginine hydrochloride and ammonium chloride have recently been shown to potentially increase intracellular pH.[34] This paradoxical increase in intracellular pH might exacerbate the effects of alkalemia. In addition, arginine hydrochloride causes hyperkalemia independent of pH change, and neither arginine hydrochloride nor ammonium chloride should be used in patients with liver disease. These treatments should be abandoned.

Hydrochloric acid in concentrations of 0.1 to 0.2 *N* (100 to 200 meq/L) can be used safely for the correction of metabolic alkalosis.[35] It should be infused into a central vein, and arterial pH should be monitored every hour. The initial infusion rate ranges from 20 to 50 meq/h, according to the severity of alkalemia and its effects. Normalization of the pH is not necessary. In patients who require fluid restriction, concentrations of hydrychloric acid up to 1 *N* have been used safely. However, concerns have been raised about catheter deterioration with concentrated solutions.[36] If central venous access is not attainable then hydrochloric acid can be infused safely into a peripheral vein, if it is mixed with an amino acid solution and infused with fat emulsion.[37]

Treatment of alkalosis secondary to mineralocorticoid excess is aimed at identifying and removing the source of mineralocorticoid. If removal of the source is not possible, the combination of sodium restriction, potassium supplements, and spironolactone or amiloride should prove successful at controlling the alkalosis.

Respiratory Acidosis

PATHOPHYSIOLOGY

Respiratory acidosis is characterized by a primary increase in the arterial P_{CO_2} and a compensatory increase in the bicarbonate concentration. Tissue buffers can raise the bicarbonate level only 4 to 5 meq/L in acute respiratory acidosis, so severe acidemia can ensue. Chronic respiratory acidosis is further buffered by increased renal reabsorption of bicarbonate, so acidemia is consequently less severe, even with marked hypercapnea.

Respiratory acidosis represents ventilatory failure. The pathophysiology, etiology, and treatment of ventilatory failure are discussed fully in Chap. 127. A basic approach to the patient with respiratory acidosis is presented here. Respiratory acidosis occurs when alveolar ventilation is decreased relative to CO_2 production. Decreased alveolar ventilation arises from a decrease in minute ventilation, or from an increase in dead space without a compensatory rise in minute ventilation. A rise in CO_2 production will not produce hypercapnea unless ventilation does not increase appropriately. This can be the case in patients at near-maximal ventilation, or with fixed mechanical ventilation.

APPROACH TO DIAGNOSIS

The etiologies of respiratory acidosis can be classified according to which part of the respiratory system is affected. Thus hypercapnea can result from abnormalities in the neural control of respiration, in the chest wall and respiratory muscles, or in the lung and upper airway. Pulmonary disease is the most common cause of respiratory acidosis in the ICU. Drugs that depress respiratory drive should always be sought in a patient presenting with ventilatory failure, particularly if no pulmonary disease is present. The disorders of respiratory muscles and sleep apnea are less common diseases, but ones for which a high index of suspicion is necessary to make the diagnosis. The etiologies of respiratory acidosis are listed in Table 158-6.

TREATMENT

Treatment for respiratory acidosis is aimed at reversing the disorders that led to decreased alveolar ventilation. Ideally, the specific pathophysiology causing the hypercapnea can be reversed. However, treatment is aimed at improving all of the factors that may lead to respiratory acidosis. This includes increasing minute ventilation, decreasing dead

TABLE 158-6 Etiologies of Respiratory Acidosis

Inhibition of Respiratory Control
- Drugs (narcotics, sedatives, anesthetics)
- Sleep apnea
- CNS lesions
- Myxedema

Disorders of the Chest Wall
- Kyphoscoliosis
- Morbid obesity
- Burns

Neuromuscular Disease
- Myasthenia gravis
- Amyotrophic lateral sclerosis
- Guillain-Barré syndrome
- Poliomyelitis
- Botulism
- Severe hypokalemia
- Severe hypophosphatemia
- Multiple sclerosis
- Periodic paralysis
- Spinal cord injury
- Myopathy

Upper Airway Obstruction
- Foreign body
- Laryngospasm
- Obstructive sleep apnea
- Tracheal stenosis

Disorders of the Lung
- COPD
- Asthma
- Severe pneumonia
- Pulmonary edema
- Pneumothorax
- ARDS

space, and decreasing CO_2 production. Some diseases are amenable to rapid correction of hypercapnea with treatment of the underlying disorder (e.g., narcotic overdose); however, intubation and mechanical ventilation are often necessary to increase alveolar ventilation, decrease P_{CO_2}, and improve the acidemia. An alternate approach combines controlled hypoventilation with a bicarbonate infusion to prevent severe acidemia. Several small uncontrolled studies of persons with severe asthma show good results with this method, but no controlled trials have been conducted (see Chap. 130). Respiratory acidosis associated with neurologic injury is of special importance, since acidemia can increase cerebral blood flow and intracranial pressure and thus may require aggressive correction.

Respiratory Alkalosis

PATHOPHYSIOLOGY

Respiratory alkalosis is characterized by a primary reduction in the arterial P_{CO_2}. A secondary two-phase reduction in the bicarbonate concentration occurs, with a small acute decrease due to tissue buffers and a larger chronic decrement due to a decrease in renal titratable acid excretion and an increase in renal bicarbonate excretion. Respiratory alkalosis occurs when alveolar ventilation is increased relative to CO_2 production.

TABLE 158-7 Etiologies of Respiratory Alkalosis

Hypoxia
- High altitude
- Pulmonary disease
- Decreased $F_{I_{O_2}}$
- Profound anemia

CNS Disturbances
- Anxiety and pain
- Voluntary hyperventilation
- CNS disease (CVA, tumor, infection, trauma)
- Fever
- Sepsis and endotoxin
- Drugs (salicylates, catecholamines, progesterone)
- Hyperthyroidism
- Liver disease
- Pregnancy

Pulmonary Disorders
- Pneumonia
- Pulmonary embolism
- Restrictive lung disease
- Pulmonary edema
- Bronchospasm
- Pleural effusion
- Pneumothorax

Mechanical Ventilation

APPROACH TO DIAGNOSIS

Respiratory alkalosis is a very common abnormality in the ICU. Hyperventilation is a nonspecific response to a variety of stimuli, ranging from the benign to the life-threatening. The challenge is to distinguish those respiratory alkaloses that are manifestations of serious disease. This requires a thorough clinical review, with particular emphasis on signs of sepsis and pulmonary or CNS disease.

The causes of respiratory alkalosis can be grouped according to where the stimulus for increased ventilation occurs. Virtually any disorder affecting the lungs can cause stimulation of pulmonary parenchymal receptors and hyperventilation. Hypoxia, sensed by carotid body chemoreceptors, stimulates the respiratory center. The respiratory center can also be directly stimulated by a number of toxins, hormones, and primary CNS processes. Inappropriate mechanical ventilation is an important and correctable cause of respiratory alkalosis in the ICU. The etiologies of respiratory alkalosis are listed in Table 158-7.

TREATMENT

The primary treatment of respiratory alkalosis is treatment of the underlying cause of hyperventilation. The alkalemia itself generally does not require treatment. In cases where a severe alkalemia is present—generally, when a respiratory alkalosis is superimposed on a metabolic alkalosis—sedation may be necessary. In sepsis, where a significant portion of cardiac output can go to the respiratory muscles, intubation and muscle relaxation are often required to control hyperventilation and redirect blood flow.

Approach to Acid-Base Disturbances

Diagnosing disorders of acid-base homeostasis in the ICU can be challenging. Many critically ill patients have combinations of disorders. In addition, many patients admitted to the ICU have preexisting disturbances—such as respiratory acidosis in patients with COPD, and metabolic alkalosis in patients on diuretics—that must be taken into account when one is judging subsequent changes.

Several steps must be taken to diagnose acid-base disturbances. Required laboratory information includes the pH, the P_{CO_2}, the bicarbonate level, and electrolyte levels. The first step is to determine whether an acidemia or an alkalemia is present—i.e., whether the pH is below 7.36 or above 7.44. In mixed disorders the pH may be in the normal range. In these cases, alterations in the bicarbonate level, the P_{CO_2}, and the anion gap are the markers for acid-base disturbances and should be routinely assessed in all patients.

Next, the source of the primary disturbance is determined to be of metabolic or respiratory origin. With an acidemia, a P_{CO_2} above 44 mmHg identifies a respiratory acidosis, and a bicarbonate level below 20 meq/L signifies a metabolic acidosis. In an alkalemia, a P_{CO_2} below 36 mmHg signifies a respiratory alkalosis, and a bicarbonate level above 28 meq/L signifies a metabolic alkalosis.

The third step is to determine whether appropriate compensation for the primary disturbance has occurred. Metabolic disturbances are accompanied by predictable and consistent respiratory compensation; respiratory disturbances are accompanied by a two-step change in bicarbonate concentration that is somewhat less consistent. An acute change is due to tissue buffers, and a more chronic change is due to renal compensatory changes. The expected degree of change in the bicarbonate level thus depends on the duration of the primary disturbance. The expected compensations for both respiratory and metabolic disturbances are listed in Table 158-8. If a predicted response is not present, then an additional acid-base disturbance is present or the compensation is not yet complete. (It may take 12 to 24 h for respiratory compensation to become complete, and several days for metabolic compensation.) For example, in a chronic metabolic acidosis with a bicarbonate level of 16 meq/L, the predicted P_{CO_2} is 30 to 34 mmHg. If the actual P_{CO_2} is 38 mmHg, a respiratory acidosis is also present.

The final step is to check the anion gap. The anion gap—the difference between measured anions and measured cations—is defined under Metabolic Acidosis, above. The better part of unmeasured anion is accounted for by plasma proteins, primarily albumin. The remainder consists of phosphate, sulfates, lactate, and other organic anions. An increased anion gap does not always signify a metabolic acidosis. The anion gap increases in alkalemia, because of an increase in the net anionic charge on plasma proteins.[38] Dehydration will also increase the anion gap, because of an increased protein concentration. However, if the anion gap is greater than 20 meq/L, a metabolic acidosis should be suspected and investigated. Seventy percent of patients with an anion gap greater than 20 meq/L will have an identifiable organic anion, as will virtually all of those with an anion gap greater than 30 meq/L.[39]

These steps should allow recognition and classification of most acid-base disorders. As discussed above, proper classification of disorders requires a knowledge of baseline acid-base status from which to measure deviations. Diagnosis of the cause of the acid-base derangements identified depends, of course, on the individual patient and the clinical situation.

TABLE 158-8 Appropriate Compensation in Simple Acid-Base Disorders

Metabolic acidosis
$P_{CO_2} = (1.5 \times HCO_3^-) + 8 \pm 2$
Metabolic alkalosis
$P_{CO_2} = (0.7 \times HCO_3^-) + 21 \pm 1.5$*
Respiratory acidosis
Acute: $HCO_3^- = [(P_{CO_2} - 40)/10] + 24$
Chronic: $HCO_3^- = [(P_{CO_2} - 40)/3] + 24$
Respiratory alkalosis
Acute: $HCO_3^- = [(40 - P_{CO_2})/5] + 24$
Chronic: $HCO_3^- = [(40 - P_{CO_2})/2] + 24$

*For a bicarbonate (HCO_3^-) level greater than 40 the formula to be used is: $P_{CO_2} = (.75 \times HCO_3^-) + 19 \pm 7.5$

CASE PRESENTATION

A 63-year-old woman with a history of congestive heart failure presented to the emergency room with a chief complaint of increasing shortness of breath over the preceding 2 days. She also complained of a fever to 102°F and a cough productive of thick yellow sputum. She had no history of respiratory illness and was a nonsmoker. Her past medical history was remarkable only for hypertension and congestive heart failure treated with furosemide, 20 mg/day, and digoxin, 0.25 mg/day. She was on no other medication.

Physical examination showed a dyspneic woman in mild distress. Vital signs were: blood pressure 140/84, heart rate 100, respiratory rate 30, and temperature 39°C. Her heart had a regular rate and rhythm with no murmur or gallop. Lung examination revealed right-sided basilar crackles. There was no accessory muscle use. The remainder of the examination was unremarkable.

Initial laboratory values included a white blood cell count of 14×10^3 cells per mm^3, with 18 percent band forms and a hemoglobin of 13.4 g/dL. Electrolytes were: sodium 139 meq/L, potassium 3.4 meq/L, chloride 98 meq/L, and bicarbonate of 29 meq/L. Arterial blood gas analysis on room air was pH 7.59, P_{CO_2} 31 mmHg, and P_{O_2} 51 mmHg. Chest x-ray showed a lobar infiltrate in the right lower lobe. Sputum examination showed gram-positive diplococci and many white blood cells.

The patient was admitted to a medical floor and begun on penicillin, 1 million U every 6 h, and placed on 3 L/min of oxygen by nasal cannula. Twelve hours after admission she complained of increased shortness of breath. On examination she was breathing at 42 breaths per min and using accessory muscles. Blood pressure was 110/64 and heart rate was 120. Her lung examination showed diffuse crackles and her heart showed no gallop or murmur. Arterial blood gas analysis revealed a pH of 7.40, a P_{CO_2} of 48 mmHg, and a P_{O_2} of 44 mmHg. The patient was intubated, transferred to the ICU, and begun on mechanical ventilation in an assist-control mode, with a rate of 16, a tidal volume of 600 mL, an FI_{O_2} of 1, and 5 cmH_2O PEEP. Chest x-ray showed good position of the endotracheal tube and a diffuse pulmonary infiltrate. Her antibiotics were changed to ampicillin, gentamicin, and erythromycin.

Two hours after the patient's arrival in the ICU her blood pressure fell to 86/40. Normal saline infusion was increased to 500 mL/h. Arterial blood gas analysis showed a pH of 7.24, a P_{CO_2} of 38 mmHg, and a P_{O_2} of 86 mmHg. Serum bicarbonate was 16 meq/L, the anion gap was 23, and an arterial lactate level was 8 mmol/L. The ECG showed left ventricular hypertrophy with nonspecific T-wave changes and was unchanged from the admission ECG.

Because of the patient's history of congestive heart failure and onset of hypotension, a pulmonary artery catheter was inserted. The pressures were: RA 10, RV 38/8, PA 34/18, and Ppw 14 mmHg. Cardiac output by thermodilution was 4.7 L/min. The arteriovenous oxygen content difference was 2.3 mL O_2/dL. A bedside echocardiogram showed mild-to-moderate global hypokinesis with no regional wall motion abnormalities. She was begun on dobutamine at 5 μg/kg per min; her blood pressure increased to 98/54.

By the next morning her arterial blood gas showed a pH of 7.34, a P_{CO_2} of 38 mmHg, and a P_{O_2} of 72 mmHg on 50% O_2. Her serum bicarbonate was 20; her blood pressure was 122/74 and her heart rate 100. The dobutamine was discontinued. She was restarted on furosemide, 40 mg/day IV, and begun on total parenteral nutrition (TPN) for nutritional support.

Two days later her blood cultures returned with *Streptococcus pneumoniae,* and her antibiotics were changed to penicillin, 1 million U every 6 h. Her oxygenation continued to improve, but she became increasingly alkalemic, with an arterial pH of 7.55, a P_{CO_2} of 44 mmHg, and a bicarbonate level of 38 meq/L.

Her furosemide was discontinued, acetazolamide begun, and enalapril added for afterload reduction. Her alkalemia, however, continued to worsen over the next 48 h; her arterial pH rose to 7.60, with a P_{CO_2} of 46 mmHg and a bicarbonate level of 44 meq/L.

A careful search of all medications and substances administered revealed that the patient's parenteral nutrition solution contained 70 meq of acetate per L. The TPN was discontinued, and she was begun on enteral nutrition. She was also treated with oral KCl and mild liberalization of her sodium intake. Over the next several days her alkalosis resolved, with bicarbonate decreasing to 26 meq/L and arterial pH to 7.42. She was extubated without difficulty, and the remainder of her hospital stay was uneventful.

CASE DISCUSSION

This patient had a complex series of acid-base disturbances. The initial presentation was of a severe alkalemia. The P_{CO_2} was decreased, indicating a respiratory alkalosis. But the bicarbonate level was at the upper end of normal, not appropriately decreased; this denoted a metabolic alkalosis. Combined with the patient's history, this can be seen to have been a chronic metabolic alkalosis secondary to diuretics, and an acute respiratory alkalosis secondary to pneumonia. Next the patient developed ventilatory failure. Arterial blood gas analysis revealed a normal pH but a P_{CO_2} of 48 mmHg, reflecting a respiratory acidosis. This was balanced by the chronic increase in the bicarbonate level. As sepsis progressed, the patient developed an acidemia with a decreased bicarbonate level and an increased anion gap, consistent with lactic acidosis. The compensatory P_{CO_2} expected (in mmHg) is calculated from the formula $P_{CO_2} = (1.5 \times HCO_3) + 8 \pm 2$, where HCO_3 is the bicarbonate level in meq/L; this gives an expected value of 30 to 34 mmHg when the bicarbonate level is 16 meq/L. This compensation was not present, since the patient's P_{CO_2} was 38 mmHg. Therefore, either a respiratory acidosis was also present or the compensation had not yet had time for completion. The lactic acidosis resolved with treatment of the patient's infection. Her final acid-base disorder was a severe alkalemia of metabolic origin, with a bicarbonate level rising to 44 meq/L. Appropriate respiratory compensation for a severe metabolic alkalosis shows a wide range of variation. The expected P_{CO_2} for a bicarbonate of 44 meq/L is 44.5 to 62.5 mmHg. Since the observed value of 46 mmHg fell within this range, no second disturbance was present. The metabolic alkalosis was initially thought to be secondary to diuretics, but eventually was found to be due to administration of acetate in the TPN solution. In a normal fluid and electrolyte state, the bicarbonate produced from the acetate would have been excreted in the urine. However, with intravascular volume depletion, the kidneys are sodium-avid; in the face of hypochloremia, sodium bicarbonate is reabsorbed, perpetuating the alkalosis.

This case illustrates several important points in the diagnosis and treatment of acid-base disorders. **1**. preexisting diseases are common and may exacerbate or mitigate the degree of pH change; **2**. acid-base equilibrium in the ICU is a dynamic system, and multiple disorders may occur simultaneously or sequentially; **3**. most acid-base disorders resolve with treatment of the underlying disorder and do not require treatment of the pH itself; and **4.** unexplained disorders should prompt a thorough search of all administered substances.

References

1. Sideris DA, Katsadorus DP, Valianos G, Assioura A: Type of cardiac dysrhythmias in respiratory failure. Am Heart J 89:32, 1975.
2. Harrington JT, Cohen JJ: Metabolic acidosis, in Cohen JJ, Kassirer JP (eds): *Acid-Base.* Boston, Little, Brown and Co, 1982, p 121.
3. Juan G, Calverley P, Talamo C, et al: Effect of carbon dioxide on diaphragmatic function in human beings. N Engl J Med 310:874, 1984.
4. Oster JR, Perez GO, Vaamonde CA: Relationship between blood pH and potassium and phosphorus during metabolic acidosis. Am J Phys 235:F345, 1978.
5. Fulop M: Serum potassium in lactic acidosis and ketoacidosis. N Engl J Med 300:1087, 1979.
6. Oster JR, Alpert HC, Vaamonde CA: Effect of acid-base status on plasma phosphorus response to lactate. Can J Phys Pharm 62:939, 1984.
7. Rimmer JM, Gennari FJ: Metabolic alkalosis. J Intensiv Care Med 2:137, 1987.
8. Streisand RL, Gourin A, Stuckey JH: Respiratory and metabolic alkalosis and myocardial contractility. J Thorac Cardiovasc Surg 62:431, 1971.
9. Ayres SM, Grace WJ: Inappropriate ventilation and hypoxemia as causes of cardiac arrhythmias. Am J Med 46:495, 1969.
10. Carrier O, Cowsert M, Hancock J, Guyton AC: Effect of hydrogen ion changes on vascular resistance in isolated artery segments. Am J Phys 207:169, 1964.
11. Ardissino D, De Servi S, Falcone C, et al: Role of hypocapnic alkalosis in hyperventilation-induced coronary artery spasm in variant angina. Am J Cardiol 59:707, 1987.
12. Raichle ME, Posner JB, Plum F: Cerebral blood flow during and after hyperventilation. Arch Neurol 23:394, 1970.
13. Arbus GS, Herbert LA, Levesque PR, et al: Characterization and clinical application of the "significance band" for acute respiratory alkalosis. N Engl J Med 280:117, 1969.
14. Relman AS: Metabolic consequences of acid-base disorders. Kidney Int 1:347, 1972.
15. Somjen GG, Allen BW, Balestrino M, Aitken PG: Pathophysiology of pH and Ca^{++} in bloodstream and brain. Can J Phys Pharm 65:1078, 1987.
16. Brimioulle S, Kahn RJ: Effects of metabolic alkalosis on pulmonary gas exchange. Am Rev Respir Dis 141:1185, 1990.
17. Bellingham AJ, Detter JC, Lenfant C: Regulatory mechanisms of hemoglobin oxygen affinity in acidosis and alkalosis. J Clin Invest 50:700, 1971.
18. Rackow EC, Mecher C, Astiz ME, et al: Unmeasured anion during severe sepsis with metabolic acidosis. Circ Shock 30:107, 1990.
19. Morris LR, Murphy MB, Kitabchi AE: Bicarbonate therapy in severe diabetic ketoacidosis. Ann Intern Med 105:836, 1986.
20. Luft D, Deichsel G, Schmulling R, et al: Definition of clinically relevant lactic acidosis in patients with internal diseases. Am J Clin Pathol 80:484, 1983.
21. Orringer CE, Eustace JC, Wunsch CD, Gardner LB: Natural history of lactic acidosis after grand-mal seizures. A model for the study of an anion-gap acidosis not associated with hyperkalemia. N Engl J Med 297:796, 1977.
22. Davies AO: Rapid desensitization and uncoupling of human β-adrenergic receptors in an in vitro model of lactic acidosis. J Clin Endocrinol Metab 59:398, 1984.
23. DePergola G, Cignarelli M, Nardelli G, et al: Influence of lactate on isoproterenol-induced lipolysis and β-adrenoreceptors distribution in human fat cells. Horm Metab Res 21:210, 1989.
24. Mochizuki S, Kobayashi K, Neely JR: Effects of L-lactate on glyceraldehyde-3-P dehydrogenase in heart muscle. Rec Adv Stud Card Struc Metab 12:175, 1978.
25. Jurkowitz M, Scott KM, Altschuld RA, et al: Ion transport by heart mitochondria. Arch Biochem Biophys 165:98, 1974.
26. Fraley DS, Adler S, Bruns FJ, Zett B: Stimulation of lactate production by administration of bicarbonate in a patient with a solid neoplasm and lactic acidosis. J Engl J Med 303:1100, 1980.
27. Graf H, Arieff AI: The use of bicarbonate in the therapy of organic acidosis. Intensiv Care Med 12:285, 1986.
28. Cooper DJ, Walley KR, Wiggs BR, Russell JA: Bicarbonate does not improve hemodynamics in critically ill patients who have lactic acidosis. A prospective controlled clinical study. Ann Intern Med 112:492, 1990.
29. Sun JH, Filley GF, Hord K, et al: Carbicarb: An effective substitute for $NaHCO_3$ for the treatment of acidosis. Surgery 102:835, 1987.
30. Stacpoole PW, Harman EM, Curry SH, et al: Treatment of lactic acidosis with dichloroacetate. N Engl J Med 309:390, 1983.
31. Stacpoole PW, Lorenz AC, Thomas RG, Harman EM: Dichloroacetate in the treatment of lactic acidosis. Ann Intern Med 108:58, 1988.
32. Vaziri NB, Ness R, Wellikson L, et al: Bicarbonate-buffered peritoneal dialysis. An effective adjunct in the treatment of lactic acidosis. Am J Med 67:392, 1979.
33. Sabatini S, Kurtzman NA: The maintenance of metabolic alkalosis: Factors which decrease bicarbonate excretion. Kidney Int 25:357, 1984.
34. Rothe KF, Fluchter StH, Schorer R: Studies on therapy of metabolic alkalosis during experimental uremia. Urol Int 41:161, 1986.
35. Martin WJ, Matzke GR: Treating severe metabolic alkalosis. Clin Pharmacol 1:42, 1982.
36. Kopel RF, Durbin CG: Pulmonary artery catheter deterioration during hydrochloric acid infusion for the treatment of metabolic alkalosis. Crit Care Med 17:688, 1989.
37. Knutsen OH: New method for administration of hydrochloric acid in metabolic alkalosis. Lancet i:953, 1983.
38. Madias NE, Ayus JC, Adrogue HJ: Increased anion gap in metabolic alkalosis. The role of plasma-protein equivalency. N Engl J Med 300:1421, 1979.
39. Gabow PA, Kaehny WD, Fennessey PV, et al: Diagnostic importance of an increased serum anion gap. N Engl J Med 303:854, 1980.

Chapter 159

DIABETIC KETOACIDOSIS, HYPERGLYCEMIC HYPEROSMOLAR NONKETOTIC COMA, AND HYPOGLYCEMIA

JOHN B. BUSE
KENNETH S. POLONSKY

KEY POINTS

- *Diabetic ketoacidosis (DKA), hyperglycemic hyperosmolar nonketotic coma (HHNC), and hypoglycemia are life-threatening disorders of glucose metabolism.*
- *Altered glucose metabolism should be considered in the differential diagnosis of all patients with mental status changes, neurologic deficits, and severe illness.*
- *Therapy of DKA and HHNC requires replacement of deficits of fluids, electrolytes, and insulin.*
- *Mixed anion gap acidosis and hyperosmolarity are often encountered in the same patient.*
- *Continuous insulin therapy is essential in DKA.*
- *In DKA and HHNC, careful physical examination and laboratory follow-up with a flow sheet allow for prevention of the disastrous consequences of aggressive therapy—cerebral edema, pulmonary edema, hypoglycemia, hypokalemia, and hyperchloremic metabolic acidosis.*
- *A search for the underlying cause of metabolic decompensation is required.*
- *Therapy of hypoglycemia requires immediate establishment and maintenance of modest hyperglycemia (glucose concentration above 100 mg/dL).*

Diabetes mellitus and its major life-threatening complications—DKA, HHNC, and hypoglycemia—may precipitate or complicate critical illness. This chapter will focus on the management of DKA, since it has been more exhaustively studied and since the management principles of its therapy are applicable to HHNC. A brief review of the physiology and therapy of hypoglycemia will follow. These conditions have been the subject of other reviews, which are referenced for additional reading.[1–9]

Pathophysiology of Diabetic Emergencies

Currently, the majority of patients with diabetes can be classified as having either type I (previously known as *juvenile onset, ketosis-prone, insulin-dependent,* or *brittle*) diabetes or type II (previously, *adult onset, nonketosis-prone, non-insulin–dependent,* or *obesity-related*) diabetes.

Type I diabetes results from the autoimmune destruction of the insulin-secreting beta cells in the pancreas, with consequent insulin deficiency. Most persons with type I diabetes present in childhood or early adulthood, though well-documented cases have also been described in the geriatric population. Hyperglycemia is usually not present until approximately 90 percent of insulin secretory capacity is lost. In times of stress (either physiologic or emotional), however, insulin requirements increase and often precipitate metabolic decompensation because of inadequate insulin secretory reserve. Patients with insulin deficiency require insulin therapy for survival. The half-life of insulin in the circulation is 7 min, and therapy for insulin deficiency requires continuous delivery of insulin to the circulation by infusion or by diffusion of insulin from depot injections.

The pathoplysiology of type II diabetes is less well understood. At presentation, persons with type II diabetes usually have normal or high insulin levels and an insulin action that is impaired—so-called insulin resistance. Today insulin resistance can be overcome only by **1.** increasing circulating insulin concentrations, with insulin (often at high doses) or oral hypoglycemic agents; **2.** calorie restriction; **3.** exercise; or **4.** therapy directed at its reversible causes: obesity; hyperglycemia; sepsis; uremia; catecholamine, glucocorticoid, growth hormone, or thyroxine excess; and antibodies to insulin or its receptor. Most persons with type II diabetes present in middle age and are overweight and sedentary. However, there is a not-uncommon familial adolescent form of the disorder termed *maturity onset diabetes of youth,* or *MODY.*

DKA is the life-threatening metabolic consequence of insulin deficiency. Insulin deficiency, in concert with excess secretion of glucagon (primarily), catecholamines, glucocorticoids, and growth hormone, produces hyperglycemia by stimulating glycogenolysis and gluconeogenesis and impairing glucose disposal. As has been elegantly demonstrated by Foster and McGarry,[10] this hormonal milieu also results in lipolysis and unrestrained fatty acid oxidation, producing acetone, beta-hydroxybutyrate, and acetoacetate—and, thereby, ketoacidosis.

HHNC is the most severe presentation of a syndrome in which insulin resistance and relative insulin deficiency produce hyperglycemia. The glucose remains largely in the extracellular space and osmotically shifts water from the intracellular compartment. Glucose, water, and salts are filtered at the glomerulus; because of a limit in renal tubular reabsorptive capacity for glucose of approximately 200 mg/min, an osmotic diuresis occurs with water lost in excess of salts. A vicious circle of cellular dehydration and diuresis is produced, which can only be compensated by adequate fluid intake. With inadequate fluid intake, hyperosmolarity and hypovolemia develop, further increasing insulin resistance and hyperglycemia.

Patients rarely fit purely insulin-deficient or insulin-resistant physiology, particularly when in extremis. Patients with type I diabetes who are not well controlled or who are under stress are insulin-resistant. Patients with poorly controlled type II diabetes may become insulin-deficient through a process of beta cell exhaustion. In fact, when careful studies of insulin levels, secretory dynamics, and tissue sensitivity are performed, there is considerable overlap between patients with DKA and patients with HHNC. One of the keys to the management of these patients is recognizing the contributions of insulin deficiency and resistance and optimizing their individual therapies.

DKA, HHNC, and Differential Diagnosis

Early in their course patients with uncontrolled diabetes present with nonspecific complaints. If the disease follows an indolent course over months to years (more common of type II than of type I diabetes), patients can present with profound wasting, cachexia, and prostration similar in degree to patients with long-standing malignancy or chronic infection. With significant physical or emotional stress, sudden metabolic decompensation can occur. The cases of DKA and HHNC that are missed usually occur in patients with new-onset diabetes. All patients with nonspecific complaints should be questioned about more specific symptoms of diabetes. Polyuria (or at least nocturia) and weight loss are almost always present, though often not reported by the patient. Any patient with severe illness (acute or chronic) or neurologic changes should have his or her glucose and electrolyte levels measured.

HISTORY AND PHYSICAL EXAMINATION

DKA and HHNC are easily recognized, when considered (Table 159-1). In DKA, metabolic decompensation develops over a period of hours to a few days. Patients with severe DKA classically present with lethargy and a characteristic hyperventilation pattern with deep slow breaths (Kussmaul respirations) associated with the fruity odor of acetone. They often complain of nausea and vomiting; abdominal pain is somewhat less frequent. The abdominal pain can be quite severe and may be associated with distension, ileus, and tenderness without rebound, but usually resolves relatively quickly with therapy unless there is underlying abdominal pathology. Most patients are normotensive, tachycardic, and tachypneic, with signs of mild-to-moderate volume depletion. Hypothermia has been described in DKA, and patients with underlying infection may not manifest fever. Cerebral edema does occur.

Patients with HHNC are usually stuporous, with obvious profound dehydration, and often demonstrate focal neurologic deficits such as Babinski reflexes, asymmetric reflexes, cranial nerve findings, paresis, fasciculations, and aphasia. The syndrome evolves over days to weeks with a progressive decrease in fluid intake and mental status; usually there is no prior history of diabetes. These patients are hypotensive and exhibit normal-to-depressed ventilation. Hypothermia again is common, while cerebral edema is rare.

LABORATORY TESTS AND DIFFERENTIAL DIAGNOSIS

Once DKA or HHNC is considered, the diagnosis can be made quickly with routine laboratory tests. DKA and HHNC need to be differentiated from each other and from the other causes of ketosis and metabolic acidosis. This is often quite difficult; in fact, these disorders often coexist. Table 159-2 and the following discussion are provided to help make that distinction. Blood and urine glucose and ketone levels can be obtained in minutes using glucose oxidase–impregnated strips and the nitroprusside reaction, respectively.

The sine qua non of HHNC is hyperosmolarity. The osmolarity can be measured by freezing point depression, or can be estimated using the following formula:

$$\text{Osmolarity (mOsm/L)} = 2 \times \text{sodium} + \text{glucose}/18 + \text{BUN}/2.8 + \text{ethanol}/4.6 \qquad (159\text{-}1)$$

where glucose, BUN, and ethanol are in mg/dL.

In HHNC, the osmolarity is generally greater than 350 mOsm/L and can exceed 400 mOsm/L. The serum sodium and potassium levels can be high, normal, or low, and do not reflect total body levels, which are uniformly depleted. The glucose concentration will usually be greater

TABLE 159-1 Signs and Symptoms of Glucose Metabolism Disorders

UNCONTROLLED DIABETES			
Polyuria	Nocturia	Thirst	Polydipsia
Polyphagia	Weight loss	Blurred Vision	Dizziness
Vaginitis	Skin infection	Fatigue	Malaise
DIABETIC KETOACIDOSIS			
Dyspnea	Nausea	Vomiting	Abdominal pain
Normotension	Tachycardia	Tachypnea	Abdominal tenderness
Hypo/hyperthermia	Lethargy to coma	Fruity breath	Orthostasis
Cerebral edema			
HYPERGLYCEMIC HYPEROSMOLAR NONKETOTIC COMA			
Dehydration	Stupor to coma	Shallow respiration	Hypotension to shock
Hypo/hyperthermia	Focal neurologic signs or seizures		

TABLE 159-2 Distinguishing HHNC, DKA, and Other Metabolic Acidoses

	HHNC	DKA	Lactate	Starvation	Uremia	Rhabdo-myolysis	Ethanol	Methanol	Ethylene Glycol	Salicylate
Glucose	++++	+++	0	0	0	0	−,+	0	0	0,−,+
Ketones	0,+	++++	0	+	0	0	+++	0	0	0,++
pH	0,−	−−−−	−−−−	−	−−	−−−−	−−−	−−−	−−−	−−−
Anion Gap	0,+	++++	++++	+	+	+	+++	++	++	++
Osmolarity	++++	++	0	0	+	++	+	++	++	+

0 denotes normal levels; + denotes increased levels; − denotes decreased levels; scale from mild (+,−) to extreme (++++,−−−−).

than 600 mg/dL, with levels over 1,000 mg/dL quite common. In pure HHNC, there is usually no significant metabolic acidosis or anion gap. However, severe anion gap metabolic acidosis of uncertain etiology has been reported in HHNC.[11]

The sine qua non of DKA is ketoacidosis. As mentioned earlier, there are two ketoacids produced in DKA—beta-hydroxybutyrate and acetoacetate—as well as the neutral ketone acetone. The nitroprusside reaction commonly used to detect ketone bodies detects aceotoacetate much better than acetone and does not react with beta-hydroxybutyrate at all. Particularly in severe DKA, beta-hydroxybutyrate is the predominant ketone, and it is possible, though unusual, to have a negative serum nitroprusside reaction in the face of severe ketosis. The urine beta-hyroxybutyrate level can be measured at many centers, and commercially, but this service usually is not readily available. Fortunately, there is a readily available index for unmeasured anions in the blood—namely, the "anion gap" (normally less than 14 meq/L):

$$\text{anion gap} = \text{sodium} - (\text{chloride} + \text{bicarbonate}) \quad (159\text{-}2)$$

Most persons with DKA present with an anion gap greater than 20 meq/L, and some with an anion gap greater than 40 meq/L. However, some patients have a hyperchloremic metabolic acidosis without a significant anion gap.[12] Patients with DKA almost invariably have large amounts of ketones in their urine. The serum glucose level in DKA is usually about 500 mg/dL. However, an entity known as *euglycemic DKA* has been described, particularly in the presence of decreased oral intake or pregnancy, where the serum glucose level is normal or near normal but the patient requires insulin therapy for the clearance of ketoacidosis.[13] The arterial pH is commonly less than 7.3 and can be as low as 6.5. There is partial respiratory compensation with hypocarbia. Patients are often mildly hyperosmolar, though osmolalities greater than 330 mOsm/kg are unusual without mental status changes.

Not all patients with hyperglycemia and an anion gap metabolic acidosis will have DKA. Lactic acidosis is the most common cause of metabolic acidosis in hospitalized patients and can be seen in uncomplicated diabetes, as well as in DKA and HHNC. Lactic acidosis usually occurs in the setting of decreased tissue oxygen delivery resulting in the nonoxidative metabolism of glucose to lactic acid. Lactic acidosis complicates other primary metabolic acidoses as a consequence of dehydration or shock. Thus, assessing its relative contribution can be difficult. The presentation is identical to that seen in DKA. In pure lactic acidosis, the serum glucose and ketone levels should be normal and the serum lactate concentration should be greater than 5 mM. The therapy of lactic acidosis is directed at the underlying cause and at optimizing tissue perfusion.[14]

Starvation ketosis results from inadequate carbohydrate availability resulting in physiologically appropriate lipolysis and ketone production to provide fuel substrates for muscle. The blood glucose level usually is normal. Though the urine can have large amounts of ketones, the blood rarely does. Usually the arterial pH will be normal and the anion gap will be, at most, mildly elevated.

Alcoholic ketoacidosis is a more severe form of starvation ketosis wherein the appropriate ketogenic response to poor carbohydrate intake is increased through as-yet poorly defined effects of alcohol on the liver. Classically, these patients are longstanding alcoholics for whom ethanol has been the main caloric source for days to weeks. The ketoacidosis manifests itself when, for whatever reason, alcohol and caloric intake decreases. In isolated alcoholic ketoacidosis, the metabolic acidosis is usually mild-to-moderate in severity. The anion gap is elevated. Serum and urine ketones are always present. However, alcoholic ketoacidosis produces an even higher ratio of beta-hydroxybutyrate to acetoacetate than DKA, and negative or weakly positive serum nitroprusside reactions are common. Respiratory alkalosis associated with delirium tremens, agitation, or pulmonary processes often normalizes the pH, but should be evident with careful analysis of acid-base status. Usually the patient is normoglycemic or hypoglycemic; sometimes mild hyperglycemia is present. Patients who are significantly hyperglycemic should be treated as if they had DKA. The therapy of alcoholic ketoacidosis consists of thiamine, carbohydrates, fluids, and electrolytes, with special attention to the more severe consequences of alcohol toxicity, alcohol withdrawal, and chronic malnutrition. In more severely ill patients where alcoholic ketoacidosis is considered a possibility, there is usually other underlying illness, such as pancreatitis, gastronintestinal bleeding, hepatic encephalopathy, delerium tremens, or infection complicated by concomitant lactic acidosis.[15]

Uremic acidosis is characterized by very large elevations in the blood urea nitrogen (BUN) level (often above

200 mg/dL) and creatinine level (above 10 mg/dL) with normoglycemia. The pH and anion gap are usually only mildly abnormal. The treatment is supportive, with careful attention to fluid and electrolytes until dialysis can be performed. Rhabdomyolysis is a cause of renal failure where the anion gap can be significantly elevated and acidosis can be severe. There should be marked elevation of CPK and myoglobin levels. It should be noted that mild rhabdomyolysis is not uncommon in DKA, but the presence of hyperglycemia and ketonemia leaves no doubt as to the primary etiology of the acidosis.[16]

Toxic ingestions can be differentiated from DKA by history and laboratory investigation. Salicylate intoxication can produce an anion gap metabolic acidosis, usually with a respiratory alkalosis. The plasma glucose level is normal or low and the osmolality normal, and salicylates are detected in the urine or blood. Salicylate uncouples oxidative phosphorylation; consequently, ketonemia and lactic acidosis develop. It should be noted that salicylates can cause a false-positive glucose determination when using the cupric sulfate method and a false-negative result when using the glucose oxidase reaction. Methanol and ethylene glycol also produce an anion gap metabolic acidosis without hyperglycemia or ketones, but need to be kept in mind, primarily because they produce an increase in the measured serum osmolality but not in the calculated serum osmolality—an "osmolar gap." Their serum levels can also be measured. Isopropyl alcohol does not cause a metabolic acidosis but needs to be remembered because it is metabolized to acetone, which can produce a positive reaction in the nitroprusside reaction commonly used for the detection of ketoacids. Therapy of these intoxications is discussed elsewhere.[17–19] Rare cases of anion gap acidoses have been reported with other ingestions, including toluene, iron, hydrogen sulfide, nalidixic acid, papaverine, paraldehyde, strychnine, isoniazid, and outdated tetracycline.

It should be remembered that patients often present with combinations of the above conditions. As already noted, DKA not uncommonly appears with hyperosmolarity and coma. HHNC can have mild-to-moderate ketonemia and acidosis. Alcoholic ketoacidosis can contribute to either DKA or HHNC; and lactic acidosis is common in severe DKA and HHNC. We believe that any patient with hyperglycemia above 250 mg/dL and an anion gap metabolic acidosis should be treated by the general principles outlined below, with special consideration for possible other contributing metabolic acidoses (see Chaps. 158, 170).

Therapy

The optimum management of DKA and HHNC has been the object of considerable controversy over the past half century. Only recently have prospective studies of various therapeutic approaches been performed. The guidelines we propose rely heavily on prospective studies of DKA by Kitabchi and coworkers[1] and are readily applicable to HHNC. The general approach (Table 159-3) is to **1.** provide necessary fluids to restore the circulation, **2.** treat insulin deficiency with continuous insulin, **3.** treat electrolyte disturbances, **4.** follow the patient closely and carefully, and **5.** search for underlying causes of metabolic decompensation.

TABLE 159-3 Treatment of Severe Disorders of Glucose Metabolism

Diabetic ketoacidosis
- Fluids (usual deficit 5–10 L)
  - If hypotensive: 1 L 0.90% NaCl in first hour
  - If normotensive: 1 L 0.45% NaCl in first hour
  - In subsequent hours:
    - match urine output with 0.45% NaC1
    - if hypotensive, 200–1000 mL/h 0.9% NaCl (consider pulmonary artery catheter and colloid solutions)
    - otherwise calculate free water deficit and replace 50% over 12 h with 5% dextrose in water
    - after glucose reaches 250–300 mg/dL, add dextrose to IV fluids (~100 g per 24 h)
- Insulin
  - 10-U IV bolus
  - 0.1 U/kg/h IV or IM
  - Check glucose hourly and adjust drip to decrease glucose 10% per h to a level of 250 mg/dL
- Potassium (usual deficit 200–1000 meq)
  - Establish that the patient is not oliguric
  - ECG monitoring for hyperkalemia and hypokalemia
  - If hyperkalemic, follow hourly
  - If normokalemic, 10–20 meq/h
  - If hypokalemic, 20–40 meq/h
  - Half as chloride and half as phosphate salts
- Bicarbonate
  - None if pH >7.1
  - Consider $NaHCO_3$ 1 meq/kg IV for pH <6.9
  - For pH 6.9–7.1, consider for hyperkalemia or shock
  - In general avoid >50 meq/h
- Search for underlying cause
- Monitor
  - ECG
  - Vital signs
  - Hourly glucose and electrolytes
  - Every 2–4 h: calcium, magnesium, phosphate
  - Every 6–24 h: BUN, creatinine, ketones

Hyperglycemic hyperosmolar nonketotic coma (HHNC)
- HHNC should be treated like DKA, though patients will generally require more fluids and less insulin.

FLUIDS

Volume contraction is one of the hallmarks of DKA and HHNC. It can contribute to acidosis via lactic acid production as well as decreased renal clearance of organic and inorganic acids. It contributes to hyperglycemia by decreasing renal clearance of glucose. If decreased tissue perfusion is significant, it causes insulin resistance by decreasing insulin delivery to the sites of insulin-mediated glucose disposal—namely, muscle and adipose tissue—as well as through stimulation of catecholamine and glucocorticoid secretion. Fluid deficits on the order of 5 to 10 L are common in DKA and HHNC. It should be remembered that the urine produced during the osmotic diuresis of hyperglycemia is approximately half-normal with respect to sodium content. Therefore, water deficits are in excess of sodium deficits. Historically, large quantities of isotonic IV fluids have been rapidly administered to patients in DKA or HHNC. We tend to be more cautious; for patients with a history of congestive heart failure, chronic or acute renal failure, severe hypotension, or significant pulmonary disease, we give early and frequent consideration to the use of invasive hemodynamic montoring.

When there is physical evidence of dehydration—i.e., hypotension, decreased skin turgor, or dry mucous membranes—we generally administer 1 L of normal saline solution over the first hour and 200 to 500 mL/h in subsequent hours, until hypotension resolves and an adequate circulation is maintained. If hypotension is severe, with clinical evidence of hypoperfusion, and does not respond to crystalloid, then therapy with colloid is considered, often in combination with invasive hemodynamic monitoring. If there is no hypotension and no concern of renal failure, we administer 1 L of half-normal saline solution over the first hour.

During that first hour, the laboratory data usually returns; it can be quite helpful in planning further therapy. Despite the excess of water losses over sodium, the measured sodium level is usually low, because of osmotic effects of glucose. These osmotic effects can be corrected using a simple formula:

$$\text{corrected sodium concentration} = \text{measured sodium} + 0.016\,(\text{glucose} - 100). \quad (159\text{-}3)$$

Severe hypertriglyceridemia, which is common in severe diabetes, can cause a false decrease in the serum sodium concentration by approximately 1.0 mEq/L at a serum lipid concentration of 4.6 g/L.[20] An estimated water deficit can be calculated using the corrected sodium:

$$\text{water deficit in liters} = 0.6\,(\text{weight in kg})\,[(\text{corrected sodium}/140) - 1]. \quad (159\text{-}4)$$

Using these formulas, a 70-kg patient with a measured sodium level of 140 meq/L and a glucose level of 1000 mg/dL would have a calculated water deficit of 4.3 L. If the patient is normotensive after the first liter of fluids, we replace urinary losses with one-half normal saline solution and additionally provide approximately one-half the water deficit as 5% dextrose over the first 12 to 24 h (using the example above the amount would be 2 L), and the remainder over the subsequent 24 h. The plan for fluid therapy should be continuously reevaluated in light of the clinical and laboratory response of the patient. Once the serum glucose level reaches 250 to 300 mg/dL, fluids should contain 5% dextrose, and therapy should be aimed at maintaining the serum glucose in that range for 24 h to allow slow equilibration of osmotically active substances across cell membranes. At least 100 g of dextrose per 24 h (at least 80 mL/h of 5% dextrose if the patient is NPO) must be given to prevent ketogenesis. In late pregnancy approximately 100 percent more carbohydrate may be needed, so 10% dextrose should be used.

The primary goal of fluid therapy is to maintain adequate circulation, and the secondary one is to maintain brisk diuresis. Beyond that, pulmonary edema, hyperchloremic metabolic acidosis, and a rapid fall in the serum osmolality should be avoided by frequent monitoring of the patient, the glucose level, and the electrolyte levels. It has been demonstrated that fluid administration and subsequent continued osmotic diuresis is responsible for a large portion of the initial decline in glucose during therapy. In general, persons with HHNC present with more profound dehydration and require more IV fluids than persons with DKA.

INSULIN

Insulin is the mainstay of therapy of DKA, which is essentially an insulin-deficient state. In the past, high doses of insulin (upwards of 50 U/h) were favored. In more recent studies, low-dose insulin therapy (0.1 U/kg/h) has been shown to be equally effective in producing a decrease in serum glucose and affecting clearance of ketones. Furthermore, low-dose therapy results in a dramatic reduction in the major morbidity of intensive insulin therapy—i.e., hypoglycemia and hypokalemia.

Studies have also shown that IV insulin is significantly more effective than IM or SC insulin in lowering ketone body concentration over the first 2 h of therapy. The SC route is inappropriate for critically ill patients, because of the possibility of tissue hypoperfusion and the slower kinetics of absorption. Numerous studies attest to the efficacy of IM therapy in severe DKA. In cases where there is insufficient nursing monitoring or IV access to allow for safe IV administration, IM therapy is the route of choice. It is important that a needle of adequate length—at least 1.5 in. for adults—be used.

Lastly, it has been shown that a 10 U IV priming dose of insulin, when one is starting a patient on insulin therapy, significantly improves the glycemic response to the first hour of therapy. The rationale is to fully saturate insulin receptors before beginning continuous therapy and to avoid the lag time necessary to achieve steady-state insulin levels. When mixing insulin in normal saline solution, it does not seem to be necessary to add albumin to prevent insulin absorption onto the infusion set. However, the IV tubing should be flushed with the insulin infusate prior to use.

In those rare instances where the glucose level does not decrease at least 10 percent, or 50 mg/dL in 1 h, the insulin infusion rate should be increased and a second bolus of IV insulin administered. As the glucose level decreases, it is usually necessary to decrease the rate of infusion. After the glucose level reaches approximately 250 md/dL, it is prudent to decrease the insulin infusion rate and administer dextrose as described under Fluids, above. It is a common mistake to discontinue IV insulin in response to a falling glucose level. Insulin must be continued until ketones are cleared from the circulation, usually 12 to 24 h after hyperglycemia is controlled. With resolution of ketosis, the rate of infusion approaches the physiologic range of 0.3 to 0.5 U/kg/per day.

When the decision is made to feed the patient, the patient should be switched from IV or IM therapy to SC therapy. SC insulin should be administered before a meal and the insulin drip discontinued approximately 30 min later. The glucose level should be checked in 2 h and at least every 4 h subsequently, until a relatively stable insulin regimen is determined. A fair proportion of patients with HHNC do not require therapy for their diabetes after hospitalization, and most do not require insulin.

POTASSIUM

Potassium losses during the development of DKA and HHNC are usually quite high (3 to 10 meq/kg) and are mediated by shifts to the extracellular space secondary to acidosis and protein catabolism compounded by hyperaldosteronism and osmotic diuresis. Most persons with DKA or HHNC have normal or even high serum potassium levels, at presentation, but the initial therapy with fluids and insulin will cause the serum potassium level to fall. Our approach has been to monitor the ECG for signs of hyperkalemia (peaked T-wave, QRS widening) initially, and to administer potassium if these signs are absent and the serum potassium level is less than 5.5 meq/L. If the patient is oliguric, we do not administer potassium unless the serum concentration is less than 4 meq/L or if there are ECG signs of hypokalemia (U wave)—and even then, only with extreme caution. With therapy of DKA, the potassium level always falls, usually reaching a nadir after several hours. We usually replace potassium at 10 to 20 meq/h, one-half as potassium chloride and one-half as potassium phosphate, and monitor serum levels at least every 2 h initially, as well as following ECG morphology. Some patients with DKA who have had protracted courses with vomiting present with hypokalemia and acidosis; they may require 20 to 40 meq/h by central line to avoid further decreases in the serum potassium concentration.

PHOSPHATE

Like potassium, phosphate is depleted in patients with DKA and HHNC. Though patients usually present with an elevated serum phosphate level, the serum level declines with therapy. Though no well-documented clinical significance of this finding has been determined, and no benefit of phosphate administration has been demonstrated, most authorities recommend phosphate therapy as above, and monitoring for its possible complications—hypocalcemia and hypomagnesemia.

BICARBONATE

The serum bicarbonate level is always low in DKA, but no true deficit is present, because the ketoacid and lactate anions are metabolized to bicarbonate during therapy. The use of bicarbonate in the therapy of DKA is highly controversial; no benefit of bicarbonate therapy has been demonstrated in clinical trials. In fact, in two trials hypokalemia was more common in bicarbonate-treated patients. There are theoretical considerations against the use of bicarbonate; namely, cellular levels of 2,3-diphosphoglycerate are depleted in DKA, causing a leftward shift in the oxyhemoglobin dissociation curve and thus impairing tissue oxygen extraction. Acidemia has the opposite effect; therefore, reversing acidosis acutely might decrease tissue oxygen extraction. Additionally, there is in vitro data to suggest that pH is a regulator of cellular lactate metabolism and that correction of acidosis could increase lactate production. Most important, bicarbonate administration acutely elevates P_{CO_2}, which may lower intracellular pH. We do not administer bicarbonate routinely, but we understand that other authors advocate its use. We think that such use should be restricted to (1) patients with severe acidosis (pH below 6.9), (2) cases of hemodynamic instability where the pH is less than 7.1 and (3) cases of hyperkalemia with ECG findings. When bicarbonate is used, it should be used sparingly as a temporizing measure while definitive therapy with insulin and fluids are under way. Approximately 1 meq/kg of bicarbonate is administered as a rapid infusion over 10 to 15 min, with further therapy based on repeat ABG every 30 to 120 min. Potassium therapy should be considered prior to treatment with bicarbonate, since transient hypokalemia is a not-uncommon complication of the administration of alkali (see Chaps. 3, 158).

MONITORING

It is possible to manage many cases of mild DKA without ICU admission, depending on staff availability. We routinely admit patients with DKA to the ICU if they have a pH below 7.3. If mental status is compromised then prophylactic intubation is considered, and nasogastric suctioning is always performed, because of frequent ileus and danger of aspiration. If the patient cannot void at will, bladder catheterization is necessary to adequately follow urine output. ECG monitoring is continuous, with hourly documentation of QRS intervals as well as T-wave morphology. Initially, serum glucose, electrolytes, BUN, creatinine, calcium, magnesium, phosphate, ketone, lactate, CPK, and liver function tests are obtained, as well as urinalysis, ECG, upright chest x-ray, complete blood count (CBC), and ABG. If there is any concern about possible toxic ingestions, toxicology screening is also performed. Subsequently, glucose and electrolyte levels are measured at least hourly; calcium, magnesium, and phosphate every 2 h; and BUN, creatinine, and ketones every 6 to 24 h. The urine ketone concentration is a more sensitive indicator of ongoing or recurrent hepatic ketogenesis. It is often not necessary to routinely monitor arterial blood gases, since bicarbonate and the anion gap are relatively good indices of the response to therapy. Monitoring venous pH has also been shown to adequately reflect acidemia and response to therapy. Usually, frequent blood work is necessary only for the first 12 h or so. In severely ill patients with obvious underlying disease, the course is often more protracted; when venous access is a problem, early consideration should be given to placement of an arterial line. A flow sheet tabulating these findings, as well as mental status, vital signs, insulin dose, fluid and electrolytes administered, and urine output allows easy analysis of response to therapy. Once the acidosis begins to resolve and the response to therapy becomes predictable, it is reasonable to curtail laboratory use. If cardiovascular status is unclear or troublesome, invasive hemodynamic monitoring is an appropriate guide for fluid therapy. The goal should be to rapidly achieve hemodynamic stability and to fully correct DKA in 12 to 36 h.

THE SEARCH FOR UNDERLYING CAUSES

After stabilizing the patient, a careful history taking and physical examination and a diagnostic strategy should be aimed at determining the precipitating event. In our practice, the most common cause of DKA is noncompliance with insulin therapy; this is usually easily treated. The second most common cause is infection, with urinary tract infection, pelvic inflammatory disease, and pneumonia predominating. It is often difficult to determine initially if the patient is infected. Fever can be absent in a significant proportion of patients with diabetic emergencies. The white blood count (WBC) is not uncommonly elevated to the range of 20,000 or higher, even in the absence of infection.[21] We therefore perform cultures on most patients with DKA or HHNC, and if there is a significant concern about infection we cover them empirically and broadly with antibiotics pending microbiologic findings. Special consideration of ruling out meningitis should be made in any patient with altered mental status. In this regard, our approach has been to perform lumbar punctures on all patients with meningismus and on patients for whom we cannot convince ourselves that the history documents clearly the progression of mental status changes in phase with, but temporally lagging behind, the metabolic insult. If our index of suspicion is lower, we often gear our antibiotic therapy to cover bacterial meningitis and perform a lumbar puncture if the mental status does not improve quickly with therapy. The cerebrospinal fluid (CSF) glucose level is not particularly useful in determining if the fluid is infected, but a CSF glucose level of less than 100 mg/dL is unusual when the serum glucose level is greater than 250 mg/dL.[22] The relative frequency of sinus infection (particularly mucormycosis), foot infection, bacterial arthritis, cholecystitis, cellulitis, and necrotizing fasciitis should be considered. Pneumonia can be difficult to diagnose in patients with dehydration, since the alveolar edema fluid, which shows up as an infiltrate on chest x-ray, often is not present but develops along with progressive hypoxia during hydration. To avoid this occurrence, we are particularly judicious with fluid administration in patients we suspect of having pneumonia. Pancreatitis and pregnancy are common precipitants and need to be specially considered while assessing the abdominal pain, which is almost ubiquitous at presentation. Abdominal guarding and tenderness associated with vomiting is common. Rebound is present only rarely. These symptoms and findings usually resolve quickly with therapy in the absence of intraabdominal pathology. The serum amylase level is often elevated without pathologic significance, but a high lipase level is usually more specific.[23] Acute myocardial infarction and stroke, as well as thromboembolic phenomena, are frequent precipitants and complications of DKA.

Precipitating factors are similar in HHNC, but they are found more commonly and are often more severe. Common associated illnesses are chronic renal insufficiency, pneumonia, gastrointestinal hemorrhage, sepsis (particularly with gram-negative organisms), myocardial infarction, pulmonary embolism, and intracranial events. Burns, hyperalimentation, dialysis, heatstroke, thyrotoxicosis, acromegaly, pancreatitis and a variety of drugs (mostly diuretics, steroids, and β blockers) have also been associated.

The more insulin-resistant the patient seems to be, the more likely one is to find a precipitating cause. If a precipitating cause is found, treatment is essential if adequate metabolic control is to be achieved.

COMPLICATIONS AND PROGNOSIS

At the close of the twentieth century it should be possible to successfully treat almost all cases of DKA. The most troublesome complication is cerebral edema. It is particularly common in children and can be fatal. In most series specific causes cannot be assigned, though aggressive hydration, particularly with hypotonic fluids, may contribute.[24] In 50 percent of patients who subsequently have a respiratory arrest, there are premonitory symptoms; despite early intervention, only half of such patients avoid severe or fatal brain damage. Cerebral edema is much less common in HHNC but may be associated with decreases in plasma glucose below 250 mg/dL during the first day of therapy.[25] Other complications of life-threatening severity that have been reported include the adult respiratory distress syndrome (ARDS) and bronchial mucous plugging.[26–28]

The most common complication of HHNC is death. Female gender, lack of prior knowledge of diabetes, and acute infections are risk factors for the development of HHNC. Despite aggressive therapy, mortality is in the range of 20 to 50 percent in most recent case series. Prognosis is inversely related to serum osmolality, BUN level, and sodium level, though large differences in values are not apparent between survivors and nonsurvivors.[29] The mortality seems to be in large part a function of the underlying illness and the duration of illness prior to appropriate medical therapy. Though complete recovery of neurologic function in survivors is the rule, persistent coma is not infrequent. Arterial and venous thromboembolic events are quite common. Standard prophylactic low-dose heparin is certainly a reasonable precaution for patients with HHNC, but currently no indication exists for full anticoagulation.

Hypoglycemia

Though not a complication of diabetes per se, severe hypoglycemia is a not-uncommon complication of its therapy. It may also be a major complication of critical illness—

particularly hepatic failure, drug overdose, and sepsis. The serum glucose concentration is very strictly regulated in normal persons, between approximately 60 and 140 mg/dL. The differential diagnosis of hypoglycemia can be divided into fasting and postprandial forms (Table 159-4). Fasting hypoglycemia can result from endocrine disorders, hepatic dysfunction, antibodies to insulin or the insulin receptor, or substrate deficiency. The major endocrine causes are excess insulin or insulin-like growth factor secretion, and growth hormone or cortisol deficiency. Insulin hypersecretion can be from an insulinoma or can come from normal islet tissue because of pharmacologic stimulation. Certain malignancies, particularly sarcomas, hepatomas, and tumors of the biliary tract, can cause elevated free insulin-like growth factors and can present with hypoglycemia, often in the presence of cachexia. Any cause of severe hepatic dysfunction—toxins, viruses, congestive heart failure, or shock—as well as enzymatic defects causing decreased gluconeogenesis or glycogen storage diseases, can cause hypoglycemia. Hypoglycemia can occur with fasting in alcoholism, pregnancy, or uremia due to substrate unavailability, but otherwise occurs only with end-stage protein calorie malnutrition. Postprandial hypoglycemia can be caused by rapid gastric emptying due to postsurgical changes, or it can be idiopathic in etiology. It has been associated with early type II diabetes. Drugs that can cause hypoglycemia include alcohol, insulin, sulfonylureas, salicylates, β blockers, pentamidine, some antiarrhythmic agents, akee fruit, and the rat poison Vacor.

TABLE 159-4 Causes of Hypoglycemia

Fasting hypoglycemia
Hypersecretion of insulin or increased insulin-like growth factors
- Insulinoma
- Nesidioblastosis
- Certain carcinomas (sarcoma, hepatoma, others)

Hyposecretion of counterregulatory hormones
- Growth hormone deficiency
- Cortisol deficiency

Hepatic failure
- Toxic, (esp. alcohol)
- Infectious
- Congestive
- Shock
- Inborn errors of metabolism

Starvation
- Uremia
- Pregnancy
- Severe protein calorie malnutrition

Autoimmune disorder (antibodies to insulin or insulin receptors)

Postprandial
- Idiopathic
- Alimentary
- Early Type II diabetes mellitus

Factitious or drug-related
- Insulin
- Sulfonylureas and other sulfa compounds
- Salicylates
- β blockers
- Pentamidine
- Antiarrhythmic agents
- Glucose consumption in test tube by leukocytes

The symptoms of hypoglycemia initially result from sympathoadrenal responses and consist of palpitations, anxiety, tremulousness, sweating, and hunger. If hypoglycemia progresses, neuroglycopenic symptoms develop. These include headache, nightmares, fatigue, confusion, bizarre behavior, hallucinations, seizures, coma, and focal neurologic deficits. The absolute glucose concentration at which these symptoms develop is highly variable; in part it depends on the rate of fall in glucose concentration. In critically ill patients, symptoms may be obscured by concurrent problems until profound hypoglycemia, with seizures or coma, evolves.

Patients who present with signs and symptoms compatible with hypoglycemia should have blood glucose measured, and glucose administered—by mouth if conscious, or intravenously otherwise. The disappearance of symptoms over a period of minutes suggests that hypoglycemia is the likely etiology. IV administration of 50 mL of 50% dextrose will awaken more than 80 percent of hypoglycemic patients destined for neurologic recovery.

Patients with hypoglycemia should be fully evaluated to determine etiology. A complete history, physical examination, and routine laboratory tests will result in a likely diagnosis in the majority of cases. The various studies that can be used in less obvious cases should be considered only with the help of a specialist and are beyond the scope of this review. Glucose tolerance testing is usually nondiagnostic, except in rare cases of postprandial hypoglycemia. A 72-h fast will produce a diagnosis in the vast majority of patients with fasting hypoglycemia. At a minimum, glucose, insulin, C peptide, proinsulin, and urine and serum drug screens should be obtained in both the normal and the hypoglycemic state.

TREATMENT

The most critical step in the therapy of hypoglycemia is recognizing the cause, and thereby determining the likely duration and severity, of hypoglycemia. If a patient took his or her insulin, forgot to eat breakfast, and subsequently lost consciousness, an ampule of 50% dextrose in the field

TABLE 159-5 Treatment of Hypoglycemia

Consider the diagnosis
Determine capillary glucose concentration
Confirm with serum glucose and insulin
Oral calories if conscious
Reassess; if glucose < 100 mg/dL, *then* administer 50 mL 50% dextrose
Reassess; if glucose <100 mg/dL, *then* infusion of 10% dextrose to maintain glucose >100 mg/dL
Reassess; if glucose <100 mg/dL, *then* infusion of 10% glucose +100 mg/L hydrocortisone + 1 mg glucagon
Reassess; if glucose <100 mg/dL, *then* add infusion of diazoxide

and breakfast would almost certainly be curative. However, if a patient made a suicide gesture after drinking a quart of liquor by taking long-acting oral hypoglycemic agents, aspirin, and β blockers, then the hypoglycemia is likely to be severe and long-lasting and will require intensive therapy for days. Similarly, patients with hepatic failure will require continuous therapy with hypertonic glucose once hypoglycemia develops, until hepatic function returns.

The goal of therapy is to establish and maintain modest hyperglycemia immediately and to monitor intensively using hand-held blood glucose monitors. Seltzer[9] has described a protocol for use in severe hypoglycemia: in the presence of documented hypoglycemia, whether or not the patient responds to 50 mL of 50% dextrose, a continuous infusion of 10% glucose at a rate sufficient to keep the blood glucose level above 100 mg/dL should be started. If more than 200 mL/h is necessary to maintain hyperglycemia, then 100 mg of hydrocortisone and 1 mg of glucagon are added to each liter of 10% dextrose for as long as necessary. Intravenous diazoxide can also be considered to decrease insulin secretion. If the patient awakens, a high-carbohydrate diet should be initiated. Progressive hyperglycemia is the signal that therapy can be tapered. With early aggressive therapy, usually coma is reversed and focal deficits resolve over time.

CASE PRESENTATION

A 57-year-old white male was brought to the emergency room by family members because of progressive weakness, weight loss, fever, productive cough, nausea, and vomiting. When he arrived, he told the physician in attendance that in the previous 6 months he had lost approximately 30 lb. Because of a long history of cigarette smoking (2 packs a day for the past 40 years) and the death of his father, at age 60, of lung cancer, the patient believed he had lung cancer. He had become quite despondent and had begun to neglect himself, eating poorly and consuming approximately a fifth of whiskey a day. He denied losing consciousness. In the day before presentation, he developed fevers and chills, a cough productive of moderate amounts of purulent sputum, and some shortness of breath. Nausea and vomiting, without abdominal pain, had developed. He claimed to have had a normal physical exam and screening laboratory tests approximately 18 months earlier. His latest chest x-ray was 10 years old and was reportedly normal.

On physical exam he was an ill-appearing, oriented, moderately cachectic man with a temperature of 38.5°C and deep, though nonlabored, respirations at a rate of 20. He was orthostatic, with a blood pressure and pulse of 140/90 and 112 supine, which changed, while sitting, to 100/70 and 132. The rest of his exam was remarkable for dry mucous membranes, signs of consolidation in the right upper lobe, and mild epigastric tenderness. A CBC, electrolytes, BUN, creatinine, amylase, and arterial blood gases were drawn; IV saline was started at 250 mL/h; and 2 L per minute oxygen, by nasal cannula, was administered. A chest x-ray revealed that the right upper lobe was consolidated, with some collapse; abdominal radiographs were unrevealing. The emergency room physician informed the resident on call that he was admitting a moderately ill, dehydrated patient with pneumonia, which was possibly postobstructive secondary to lung cancer. Blood and sputum cultures were obtained and the patient was treated for possible anaerobic or aerobic pneumonia.

Approximately 1 h later, the resident arrived to admit the patient. The laboratory tests showed a hemoglobin of 17 and a white count of 16,000 with a left shift. The serum sodium was 136, chloride 102, potassium 5.0, bicarbonate 13, BUN 40, and creatinine 2.0. The amylase was elevated twofold. The resident noted a urinal containing 300 mL of clear urine next to the patient's gurney; this struck him as odd in light of the patient's reported dehydration. On questioning, the patient also described polyuria and nocturia as well as blurred vision for the past few months. He denied ingesting aspirin, methanol, or ethylene glycol. The physician noted that the patient was somewhat confused and disoriented and that his respiration, at a rate of 24, interfered with his speech. The patient's breath had a slightly fruity odor. The blood pressure was 110/70 with a pulse of 124. Otherwise the physical exam was unchanged, except for more severe epigastric tenderness and guarding without rebound. Bowel sounds were absent. The patient was mildly tremulous and diffusely hyperreflexic. Fundoscopy was normal and the neck was supple. The resident made a diagnosis of ketoacidosis of either diabetic or alcoholic etiology and performed three tests immediately: a finger stick blood glucose determination read "high" on two separate readings; urinalysis showed +++ ketones and ++++ glucose; a nitroprusside test for serum ketones was also floridly positive. A diagnosis of diabetic ketoacidosis was confirmed. Blood samples were sent for repeat serum electrolytes, glucose, calcium, magnesium, phosphate, ketones, osmolality, arterial blood gases, and lactate. Though the resident felt that the amylase was nonspecifically elevated, with the abdominal findings on exam, he also sent a serum lipase. Because of mental status changes, vomiting, and more severe abdominal pain, a nasogastric tube was placed and drained 1 L of viscous fluid without blood or bile. There was some relief of the abdominal tenderness.

The resident ordered (1) 1 L of 0.9% sodium chloride administered IV over 1 h; (2) thiamine, 10 mg IV; (3) 10 U of regular human insulin, to be administered IM with a 1.5-inch needle into the deltoid muscle; and (4) 10 U of regular human insulin IV. An ECG was completely normal and, in particular, showed no evidence of hyperkalemia. Before the therapy could be administered the patient had a generalized seizure. Though the history clearly revealed that the patient's mental status changes had progressed in an expected fashion and that the seizure was probably due to metabolic causes or alcohol withdrawal, there was sufficient concern about both intracranial bleeding (in an alcoholic) and metastases (in a patient with a potential lung cancer and meningitis) that a CT scan and lumbar puncture were performed after adjusting his antibiotics for improved central nervous system (CNS) penetration and gram-negative coverage. They were both unrevealing. The CSF glucose level was 400 mg/dL.

One-half hour later, the repeat laboratory results revealed the following: serum sodium 137, chloride 100, potassium 5.4, bicarbonate 8, glucose 596, osmolality 315, and a positive acetone at a dilution of 1:8; arterial blood pH 7.13, P_{O_2} 70, P_{CO_2} 20; magnesium was low, at 1.0 meq/L. Calcium, lipase, phosphate, and lactate were within normal limits. The patient was transferred to the ICU. On arriving there, the patient's blood pressure was 110/74 with a pulse of 120. Repeat serum glucose and electrolytes were sent. Though the relative contributions of alcoholic ketoacidosis and DKA were unknown, the resident decided to treat the patient as if he had DKA and alcoholism. One hundred units of regular human insulin were mixed in a 250-mL bag of 0.9% sodium chloride, and the tubing was flushed before starting the insulin drip at 0.1 U/kg per h (6 U/h). The corrected sodium was calculated to be 145, and the free water deficit was calculated to be 1 L. IV magnesium was administered. Consideration was given to administration of anticonvulsants and benzodiazepines, because of the seizure and the possibility of early delirium tremens. None was given. No arterial line was placed, because the patient had good venous access. Urine output was approximately 300 mL/h; maintenance fluids, of half-normal saline containing 30 meq/L potassium chloride and 30 meq/L potassium phosphate, at 350 ml/h were ordered. Because of continued hypotension, normal saline (500 mL) over the next hour was also ordered. Physical examination failed to reveal other sources of infection. Sputum Gram stain was not diagnostic. Nasal cannula oxygen was increased to 4 L/min. Acetaminophen was administered, and a flow sheet was started.

One-half hour later, the laboratory tests were essentially unchanged, including a glucose of 592 despite 1 h of insulin therapy and hydration. The insulin drip was increased to 0.2 U/kg per h (12 U/h) and an additional 10 U were administered as an IV bolus. An hour later the patient seemed somewhat improved. His abdominal discomfort had largely resolved. The blood pressure was 120/76 with a pulse of 112. The IV fluids were decreased to 200 mL/h. Repeat serum electrolytes, glucose, and blood gases were obtained: sodium 137, chloride 102, potassium 4.4, bicarbonate 12, glucose 522, pH 7.29, P_{O_2} 90, P_{CO_2} 22. For the next 2 h, chemistries were obtained hourly and revealed a continued improvement with the serum glucose decreasing approximately 50 mg/dL per h. No more blood gases were obtained, as the serum bicarbonate and anion gap were slowly returning toward normal. Once the serum glucose was below 400, finger stick glucose monitoring was continued hourly and serum electrolytes and glucose were obtained every 2 h; calcium, magnesium, phosphorus, osmolality, and acetone every 6 h; and BUN and creatinine daily. Four hours after the patient was admitted to the ICU the serum glucose decreased 100 mg/dL to 355, and the insulin drip was decreased to 1.5 U/kg per h.

Seven hours after admission to the ICU, the glucose reached 270 mg/dL. The patient was still orthostatic, though his resting pulse had decreased to 92 and his respiratory rate to 18. Serum ketones were still positive at 1:4 dilution. The sodium was 138, potassium 4.0, chloride 103, and bicarbonate 19, with an anion gap of 16. His urine output was 200 mL/h and his IV fluid was changed to half-normal saline with 5% dextrose and 20 meq/L of both potassium phosphate and potassium chloride, at a rate of 250 mL/h. The normal saline was discontinued. The insulin drip was decreased to 0.1 U/kg/h.

Twenty-four hours after admission, the patient was much improved, his vital signs were normal, and his serum glucose was 220. His serum ketones were negative. He was tolerating clear liquids. The resident ordered a 2800-calorie ADA diet. The IV fluids were discontinued and the insulin drip was substituted, with two doses per day of mixed regular and long-acting human insulin. The patient's meal tray was delayed in coming up from the cafeteria; the nurse on duty held his insulin dose, and 2 h later his blood glucose was 390 and he had trace acetone in his serum. He recovered quickly from this setback with an additional dose of intramuscular insulin and was transferred to the floor. His sputum and blood cultures grew pneumococci. His antibiotics were changed to IV penicillin. He received education on home glucose monitoring, insulin administration, diet, and diabetes self-care before hospital discharge, on the fourth hospital day, on oral antibiotics and a split-mixed insulin regimen. One month later his chest x-ray was normal and he was gaining weight and feeling well, though he still required insulin therapy.

CASE DISCUSSION

This case illustrates almost all the key points in the therapy of diabetic emergencies. First, initially the diagnosis was missed, largely because it was not considered in an older patient with no antecedent history of diabetes; appropriate questions were not asked of the patient. Second, other potential contributing factors in the pathophysiology of acidosis were considered and ruled out, though a mild hyperosmolar state was detected and treated. Third, careful physical exam and laboratory follow-up allowed for adjustments in therapy aimed at ensuring an adequate circulation while producing a slow, steady decline in glucose and acidemia. Fourth, investigation led to the diagnosis of the underlying cause and its appropriate treatment. Special consideration was given to meningitis and abdominal pathology as etiologies, because of mental status changes and abdominal tenderness; they were ruled out. Fifth, this patient's DKA relapsed when his insulin drip was stopped, because his subcutaneous insulin dose was held for misguided reasons. Insulin therapy must be continuous in DKA, as insulin deficiency is the pathophysiology and intravenous insulin has a half-life of just minutes. This patient did well at least in part because he presented relatively early in the course of his illness and the precipitating cause was relatively easy to treat. He did not suffer any ill effects from his therapy, and in particular did not develop a hyperchloremic metabolic acidosis, pulmonary edema, cerebral edema, hypoglycemia, or hypokalemia.

References

1. Kitabchi AE: Low-dose insulin therapy in diabetic ketoacidosis: Fact or fiction? Diabetes Metab Rev 5:337, 1989.
2. Krane EJ: Diabetic ketoacidosis. Pediatr Clin North Am 34:935, 1987.
3. Brumfield CG, Huddleston JF: The management of diabetic ketoacidosis in pregnancy. Clin Obstet Gynecol 27:50, 1984.
4. Marshall SM, Alberti KGMM: Hyperosmolar non-ketotic diabetic coma, in Alberti KGMM, Krall LP (ed): *The Diabetes Annual*, 4th ed. Elsevier, 1988, p 235.
5. Pope DW, Dansky D: Hyperosmolar hyperglycemic nonketotic coma. Emerg Med Clin North Am 7:849, 1989.
6. Shafrir E, Bergman M, Felig P: The endocrine pancreas: Diabetes mellitus, in Felig P, Baxter JD, Broadus AE, Frohman LA (eds): *Endocrinology and Metabolism*. New York, McGraw-Hill, 1987, pp 1043–1178.
7. Field JB: Hypoglycemia. Endocrinology and Metabolism Clinics of North America 18:27, 1989.
8. Sherwin RS, Felig P: Hypoglycemia, in Felig P, Baxter JD, Broadus AE, Froliman LA (eds): *Endocrinology and Metabolism*. New York, McGraw-Hill, 1987, pp 1179-1202.
9. Seltzer HS: Drug-induced hypoglycemia. Endocrinol Metab Clin North Am 18:163, 1989.
10. Foster DW, McGarry JD: The metabolic derangements and treatment of diabetic ketoacidosis. N Engl J Med 309:159, 1983.
11. Arieff AI, Carroll HJ: Nonketotic hyperosmolar coma with hyperglycemia: Clinical features, pathophysiology, renal function, acid-base balance, plasma-cerebrospinal fluid equilibria and the effects of therapy in 37 cases. Medicine 51:73, 1972.
12. Adrogué HJ, Wilson H, Boyd AE III, et al: Plasma acid-base patterns in diabetic ketoacidosis. N Engl J Med 307:1603, 1982.
13. Munro JF, Campbell IW, McCuish AC, Duncan LJP: Euglycaemic diabetic ketoacidosis. Br Med J 2:578, 1973.
14. Madias NE: Lactic acidosis. Kidney International 29:752, 1986.
15. Fulop M: Alcoholism, ketoacidosis, and lactic acidosis. Diabetes Metab Rev 5:365, 1989.
16. Möller-Petersen J, Andersen PT, Hjörne N, Ditzel J: Nontraumatic rhabdomyolysis during diabetic ketoacidosis. Diabetologia 29:229, 1986.
17. Brenner BE, Simon RR: Management of salicylate intoxication. Drugs 24:335, 1982.
18. Turk J, Morrell L, Avioli LV (eds): Ethylene glycol intoxication. Arch Intern Med 146:1601, 1986.
19. Rich J, Scheife RT, Katz N, Caplan LR: Isopropyl alcohol intoxication. Arch Neurol 47:322, 1990.
20. Weisberg LS: Pseudohyponatremia: A reappraisal. Am J Med 86:315, 1989.
21. Burris AS: Leukemoid reaction associated with severe diabetic ketoacidosis. South Med J 79:647, 1986.
22. Powers WJ: Cerebrospinal fluid to serum glucose ratios in diabetes mellitus and meningitis. Am J Med 71:217, 1981.
23. Campbell IW, Duncan LJP, Innes JA, et al: Abdominal pain in diabetic metabolic decompensation. JAMA 233:166, 1975.
24. Rosenbloom AL: Intracerebral crises during treatment of diabetic ketoacidosis. Diabetes Care 13:22, 1990.
25. Arieff AI: Cerebral edema complicating nonketotic hyperosmolar coma. Miner Electrolyte Metab 12:383, 1986.
26. Brun-Buisson CJL, Bonnet F, Bergeret S, et al: Recurrent high-permeability pulmonary edema associated with diabetic ketoacidosis. Crit Care Med 13:55, 1985.
27. Brandstetter RD, Tamarin FM, Washington D, et al: Occult mucous airway obstruction in diabetic ketoacidosis. Chest 91:575, 1987.
28. Hansen LA, Prakash UBS, Colby TV: Pulmonary complications in diabetes mellitus. Mayo Clin Proc 64:791, 1989.
29. Wachtel TJ, Silliman RA, Lamberton P: Predisposing factors for the diabetic hyperosmolar state. Arch Intern Med 147:499, 1987.

Chapter 160

ADRENOCORTICAL INSUFFICIENCY IN THE INTENSIVE CARE UNIT

STEVEN KOENIG
GREGORY A. SCHMIDT

KEY POINTS

- *The cardiovascular consequences of adrenocortical insufficiency include hypotension and death.*
- *The five most important causes of adrenocortical insufficiency in the intensive care unit (ICU) are recent or ongoing glucocorticoid administration, autoimmune adrenalitis, tuberculosis, adrenal hemorrhage, and drugs.*
- *Clues to the diagnosis include hyperpigmentation, absence of axillary or pubic hair in a female, hyperkalemia, hyponatremia, hypoglycemia in the presence of hypotension, eosinophilia, unexplained hypotension unresponsive to aggressive fluid and vasoactive drug therapy, and past or family history of autoimmune disease.*
- *Since the presenting signs, symptoms, and laboratory abnormalities of adrenocortical insufficiency may be nonspecific, a high index of suspicion is required to make the diagnosis.*
- *A random cortisol level and rapid adrenocorticotropic hormone (ACTH) stimulation test should be performed whenever there is suspicion of adrenocortical insufficiency.*
- *When the diagnosis is possible and the patient is hemodynamically unstable, empiric treatment with dexamethasone sodium phosphate, 4 mg intravenously along with glucose-containing saline solution, should precede diagnostic tests.*
- *Hydrocortisone sodium succinate, 100 mg every 6 to 8 h IV, has sufficient glucocorticoid and mineralocorticoid activity for any level of stress or surgery. It is the standard of treatment for adrenocortical insufficiency.*
- *The diagnosis of adrenocortical insufficiency should prompt a search for the underlying cause.*

Adrenocortical insufficiency is an uncommon diagnosis in the ICU. It is nevertheless important, since it is easily treated once the diagnosis is made but can be lethal if missed. In addition, since critical illness is often the precipitant of overt adrenocortical insufficiency, the intensivist may have the first—and the only—chance to make the diagnosis. Because the presenting symptoms, signs, and laboratory abnormalities of adrenocortical insufficiency may be nonspecific, a high index of suspicion is required to make the diagnosis. Broad application of random serum cortisol levels and the rapid adrenocorticotropic hormone (ACTH) stimulation test allows exclusion of adrenocortical insufficiency in the majority of critically ill patients in whom the diagnosis is considered.

Adrenocortical Physiology

For practical purposes, glucocorticoid synthesis is regulated by three mechanisms: a negative feedback loop involving cortisol or synthetic cortisol-like steroids, a diurnal rhythm, and stress.

Glucocorticoid production by the adrenal cortex is regulated primarily by the hypothalmus and pituitary gland. Corticotropin releasing factor (CRF), produced by the hypothalmus and perhaps other regions in the central nervous system, regulates the synthesis of ACTH by the pituitary. ACTH, in turn, acts on the adrenal cortex to stimulate production of cortisol. When the circulating level of cortisol (or synthetic cortisol-like steroids) becomes supraphysiologic, CRF and ACTH synthesis is suppressed and the adrenal gland ceases its secretory activity until the cortisol concentration returns to normal. Conversely, when cortisol levels are subnormal, CRF and ACTH secretion increase, stimulating the adrenal gland to produce cortisol until levels return to normal.

Normal persons with regular sleeping habits have a diurnal ACTH-cortisol secretory pattern. In addition, cortisol is secreted in a series of bursts rather than in a steady, continuous manner. These phenomena need to be taken into account when one is interpreting single values of plasma cortisol; they contribute to the lack of sensitivity of random cortisol levels in the diagnosis of adrenal diseases.

The "stress response" is characterized by continuous ACTH secretion despite hypercortisolemia. Regardless of the time of day or concentration of plasma cortisol, stress overrides other regulatory mechanisms and increases cortisol secretion by the adrenal cortex. Other things being equal, the greater the stress, the greater the elevation of cortisol. Two- to fivefold increases in plasma cortisol are associated with septic shock, severe trauma, and surgical procedures. Acute respiratory failure causes a 50 to 100 percent rise in cortisol levels.

While glucocorticoids have diverse physiologic effects, the most important during critical illness are those related to the cardiovascular system. Glucocorticoids help maintain vascular tone and cardiac contractility. Their presence is important to the physiologic effects of catecholamines on vascular smooth muscle. The clinical correlate of these points is that the hypotension of adrenocortical insufficiency may be poorly responsive to treatment with fluids and vasoactive drugs alone.

The normal daily output of cortisol by the adrenal gland is 20 to 30 mg. Twenty milligrams of hydrocortisone in the morning (8 A.M.) and 10 mg in the evening (4 to 6 P.M.) or its equivalent (Table 160-1) reproduces the daily output, as well as the diurnal rhythm, of cortisol secretion by the normal adrenal gland. When under maximal physiologic stress, the normal adrenal gland secretes approximately 10 to 12 times the normal daily output of glucocorticoid. The

TABLE 160-1 Glucocorticoid and Mineralocorticoid Preparations

	Relative Glucocorticoid Potency	Relative Mineralocorticoid Potency	Equivalent Glucocorticoid Dose
Hydrocortisone (Cortef, Solu-Cortef)	1.0	1.0	100 mg PO,IV
Prednisone (Deltasone, Meticorten)	4.0	0.7	25 mg PO
Methylprednisolone (Medrol, Solu-Medrol)	5.0	0.5	20 mg PO,IV
Dexamethasone (Decadron, Hexadrol)	25.0	2.0	4 mg PO,IV
Fludrocortisone (Florinef)	10.0	400	—*

*The usual mineralocorticoid replacement dose has no significant glucocorticoid activity.

clinical correlate is that 300 mg of hydrocortisone or its equivalent is considered a "stress dose" of glucocorticoid.

The renin-angiotensin system is the major regulator of aldosterone secretion. Perfusion pressure to the kidney, also known as "effective blood volume," is the most potent modulator of this system. Other potent stimulators of renin synthesis include hyponatremia, hypokalemia, prostaglandins, vasodilators such as nitroprusside, and activation of the sympathetic nervous system (probably through β receptors). Potassium also modifies aldosterone secretion independently of its effect on renin; hyperkalemia inhibits renin production but enhances aldosterone synthesis. Although ACTH regulates mineralocorticoid secretion, it is of minor importance compared to the renin-angiotensin system and serum potassium concentration.

Mineralocorticoids are important for normal salt and water homeostasis. Their absence leads to loss of salt in the urine and impaired excretion of potassium. Although rarely life-threatening, the hyperkalemia, hyponatremia, hemoconcentration, and hypovolemia that result from mineralocorticoid deficiency provide important clinical clues to the diagnosis of primary adrenocortical insufficiency. Because ACTH is not a potent regulator of aldosterone production, secondary adrenocortical insufficiency is not associated with hyperkalemia. If hyponatremia and volume depletion are present, they are not as pronounced as in patients with primary adrenocortical hypofunction.

Causes of Adrenocortical Insufficiency

Adrenocortical insufficiency is classified as primary (Addison's disease) when it results from direct involvement of the adrenal gland and as secondary when it results from deficient ACTH production by the pituicytes or from CRF deficiency. The most common cause of adrenocortical hypofunction—that arising from glucocorticoid therapy—is an example of secondary adrenocortical insufficiency.

PRIMARY ADRENOCORTICAL INSUFFICIENCY (Table 160-2)

AUTOIMMUNE DISEASE

The most common cause of primary adrenocortical insufficiency is autoimmune adrenalitis, which is responsible for approximately 80 percent of cases.[1] Associated autoimmune disorders, such as hypoparathyroidism, hypogonadism, hypo- and hyperthyroidism, diabetes mellitus, pernicious anemia, chronic active hepatitis, celiac disease, vitiligo, and alopecia are present in 40 to 70 percent of cases and may provide a clue to the diagnosis.[2] Autoimmune adrenalitis often occurs in young white females; it has a mean duration of symptoms, before diagnosis, of approximately 3 years.

TUBERCULOSIS

Mycobacterium tuberculosis is the second most common cause of primary adrenocortical insufficiency, accounting for fewer than 20 percent of cases.[1] Although active tuberculosis is present at other sites in 97 percent of cases, adrenocortical insufficiency has become manifest years after the initial presentation of disease.[3] The most common areas of extra-adrenal involvement are the lungs, the genitourinary tract, and the gastrointestinal system.[2] Both sexes are equally involved; the mean duration of symptoms prior to diagnosis is 6 to 9 months.

FUNGAL DISEASE

Adrenal involvement by fungal disease can similarly result in adrenocortical insufficiency. As with tuberculosis, disease is usually present elsewhere. Of the fungi, *Histoplasma capsulatum* is the most common, adrenal involvement occurring primarily with the disseminated form of the disease.[4] In one study, more than 50 percent of patients with disseminated histoplasmosis had adrenocortical insufficiency, and it was the most common cause of death.[4] Adrenal involvement may be seen during the active phase of dissemination or may evolve years later, after the disease has become "inactive."[2]

MALIGNANCY

Autopsy studies have demonstrated a 27 to 40 percent incidence of metastases to the adrenals in patients dying with malignancy.[5] Yet metastatic carcinoma accounts for fewer than 1 percent of cases of Addison's disease.[1] This discrepancy probably results from the fact that 90 percent of the adrenal cortex must be destroyed before hypofunction results, and from the underdiagnosis of adrenocortical insufficiency in malignancy.[6] Underdiagnosis can be attributed at least in part to the similarity of the symptoms of adrenocortical insufficiency and those of malignancy. The four most common tumors to involve the adrenals are lung cancer, breast cancer, melanoma, and lymphoma.[5] Adrenal insufficiency typically occurs in the setting of widespread disease, but is rarely the initial manifestation of malignancy.

HEMORRHAGE

Although uncommon, adrenal hemorrhage is a very important cause of adrenocortical insufficiency in the ICU. Adrenal hemorrhage associated with fulminant sepsis was initially described with *Neisseria meningitidis* (Waterhouse Friderichsen syndrome). However, infections with pneumococcus, *Haemophilus influenzae* type b, or DF-2 can also cause this syndrome. In patients with meningococcal meningitis, the presence of petechiae correlates with adrenocortical dysfunction. We consider all critically ill patients with meningococcal infection to have adrenocortical insufficiency, and treat them empirically with corticosteroids pending the results of diagnostic tests.

Additional conditions that predispose to adrenal hemorrhage are trauma to the abdomen or thorax, recent surgery, severe medical illness, history of thromboembolism, coagulopathy, and anticoagulant therapy.[7] In these settings, the sudden onset of abdominal, back, flank, or chest pain (86 percent of cases), anorexia, nausea, or vomiting (47 percent), confusion or disorientation (42 percent), fever (66 percent), orthostatic hypotension (48 percent), abdominal rigidity or rebound (22 percent), or a sudden fall in hematocrit, should immediately raise the possibility of adrenal hemorrhage.[7] The typical laboratory abnormalities of Addison's disease may not be present; this should not deter one from considering the diagnosis.

TABLE 160-2 Etiology of Primary Adrenocortical Insufficiency[1,2,7,21]

- Autoimmune (idiopathic) (80%)
- Mycobacterium tuberculosis (<20%)
- Miscellaneous (<1%)
  - Hemorrhage (sepsis, anticoagulants, coagulopathy, history of thromboembolic disease, post-surgery, trauma, "difficult" pregnancy, burns, leukemia, metastatic carcinoma, pancreatitis, vasculitis, postadrenal venography)
  - AIDS (fungi, mycobacteria, CMV, Kaposi's sarcoma)
  - Fungal infection (histoplasmosis, coccidioidomycosis, paracoccidioidomycosis, *Cryptococcus*, blastomycosis, candidiasis, torulopsis)
  - Metastatic carcinoma
  - Lymphoma
  - Drugs (rifampin, ketoconazole, aminoglutethimide, metyrapone, trilostane, etomidate, cyproterone acetate, o p' DDD)
  - Bilateral adrenalectomy
  - Irradiation
  - Sarcoidosis
  - Amyloidosis
  - Hemochromatosis
  - Congenital conditions

DRUGS

Drugs constitute a rare, but important, cause of Addison's disease (Table 160-2). Of particular interest to the intensivist are ketoconazole and rifampin. Ketoconazole decreases glucocorticoid production and is an antagonist at the glucocorticoid receptor. Rifampin increases the catabolism of glucocorticoids. Administration of either of these drugs, by worsening an adrenal reserve already decreased by fungal or tuberculous adrenalitis, can cause acute adrenocortical insufficiency.

ACQUIRED IMMUNODEFICIENCY SYNDROME (AIDS)

Patients with AIDS are at risk of developing adrenocortical insufficiency by several mechanisms. Fungi, mycobacteria, cytomegalovirus, and Kaposi's sarcoma may involve the adrenal glands in up to 50 percent of patients.[8] Although one autopsy series reported that no patient had more than 70 percent destruction of the adrenal gland, there are documented cases of adrenal insufficiency in patients with AIDS.[9] As patients with AIDS survive longer, it is likely that clinically important adrenocortical insufficiency will occur more frequently.[10]

SECONDARY ADRENOCORTICAL INSUFFICIENCY (Table 160-3)

Secondary adrenocortical hypofunction occurs because of diminished secretion of ACTH by the pituitary gland. This ACTH deficiency can result from chronic glucocorticoid therapy, intrinsic pathology of the pituitary corticotrophs, or absence of CRF. With the exception of chronic glucocorticoid therapy, secondary adrenocortical insufficiency is much less common than primary adrenal disease.

Most patients entering an ICU with secondary adrenocortical insufficiency are receiving glucocorticoids or have been on them in the prior year. Both the pituitary gland and the adrenal glands are suppressed by chronic glucocorticoid therapy. The degree of suppression varies according to the glucocorticoid preparation, the dose, the timing of the dose, and the duration of therapy. Controversy exists regarding the concentration and duration of steroid therapy necessary to cause clinically important inhibition of the hypothalamic-pituitary-adrenal axis. Prednisone at 25 mg bid for 2 days, 12.5 mg/day for 6 months, and 5 mg/day for 5 years causes suppression of adrenal responsiveness.[11,12]

TABLE 160-3 Etiology of Secondary Adrenocortical Insufficiency[21,22]

Glucocorticoid therapy
Tumors (pituitary adenoma, craniopharyngioma, meningioma, glioma, hamartoma, pinealoma, metastatic carcinoma [breast, lung, GI], lymphoma, leukemia)
Vascular
  Pituitary apoplexy (almost always related to primary pituitary tumor)
  Sheehan's syndrome (postpartum)
  Intracranial aneurysm
  Cavernous sinus thrombosis
  Diabetes mellitus
  Vasculitis
  Sickle cell disease and trait
  Arteriosclerosis
  Eclampsia
Pituitary surgery
Irradiation (to nasopharynx, sella turcica)
Head trauma
Infection (tuberculosis, fungal disease, syphilis, malaria, brucellosis, nocardiosis, actinomycosis, abscess, viruses)
Autoimmune disorders
Sarcoidosis
Histiocytosis X
Hemochromatosis
Lipid storage diseases
Isolated ACTH deficiency
Congenital conditions

Yet in other studies, prednisone in doses below 40 mg/day given in the morning for 5 to 7 days did not result in significant adrenal suppression.[13] Moreover, even when inhibition of the hypothalamic-pituitary-adrenal axis is demonstrated, it is unclear how this biochemical suppression translates into clinically relevant adrenocortical insufficiency. A reasonable guideline is to consider all patients who have been on 40 mg/day of prednisone, or its equivalent, for a period greater than 2 to 3 weeks as adrenally compromised, especially if they have become cushingoid. (In this setting, adrenocortical insufficiency can occur in response to stress as long as 1 year after steroids have been discontinued.[14]) All such patients should have their adrenal function evaluated and be considered for interim coverage with "stress doses" of steroids.

Clinical Features of Adrenocortical Insufficiency

Three groups of patients may require management of adrenocortical insufficiency in the ICU. The first includes patients known to have adrenocortical insufficiency or presumed to have iatrogenic adrenocortical hypofunction on the basis of prior glucocorticoid therapy. Diagnosis and treatment are straightforward once the history is obtained. More challenging are patients with previously undiagnosed chronic adrenocortical insufficiency who present in hypoadrenal crisis; in this situation a high index of suspicion and a thorough understanding of the signs, symptoms and laboratory abnormalities of chronic adrenocortical insufficiency are essential for considering and making the diagnosis. Finally, patients who enter the ICU with normal adrenal function may develop acute adrenal hemorrhage secondary to therapy or their acute illness. Knowledge of the presenting signs and symptoms of adrenal hemorrhage, as well as of the settings in which it occurs, is critical to establishing the diagnosis.

SYMPTOMS AND SIGNS

A patient with acute adrenocortical insufficiency has many of the symptoms, signs, and laboratory abnormalities of chronic adrenocortical insufficiency (Table 160-4), but they are of much greater severity in the acute case. Weakness and apathy are extreme, often with confusion. Anorexia, nausea, and vomiting are severe, and contribute to intravascular volume depletion. Abdominal pain is frequent and can mimic acute abdomen. Except for adrenal hemorrhage, however, localizing signs are usually absent, though there may be tenderness and pain on deep palpation. Hyperpigmentation of skin and mucous membranes is a helpful clue when present but will not be seen in secondary adrenocortical insufficiency or in acute adrenocortical destruction. Fever is common, even without underlying infection.

LABORATORY FINDINGS

In patients with acute decompensation of a chronic hypoadrenal state, the laboratory findings associated with chronic adrenocortical insufficiency (Table 160-5) are usually more pronounced and occur more frequently. However, the laboratory abnormalities associated with acute and chronic Addison's disease are not invariably present. Moreover, in secondary adrenocortical insufficiency, hyperkalemia is not a feature, since mineralocorticoid production remains unaffected. Therefore, the absence of the classic laboratory findings of adrenocortical insufficiency cannot be used to exclude the diagnosis. Although most of the laboratory abnormalities of hypoadrenal crisis are nonspecific, hypoglycemia in a hypotensive patient should immediately raise the possibility of this diagnosis. One

TABLE 160-4 Clinical Features of Chronic Primary Adrenocortical Insufficiency[21,23]

Condition	% of Cases
Weakness and fatigue	100
Weight Loss	100
Anorexia	100
Hyperpigmentation	92
Hypotension	88
Gastrointestinal symptoms	56
Salt craving	19
Postural symptoms	12
Muscle and joint pains	4

TABLE 160-5 Laboratory Features of Chronic Primary Adrenocortical Insufficiency[23]

Hyponatremia	88%
Hyperkalemia	64%
Prerenal azotemia	NA*
Hypoglycemia	NA*
Hypercalcemia	6%
Anemia	NA*
Eosinophilia	NA*
Lymphocytosis	NA*

*NA denotes no data available

would expect "stress hormones" like catecholamines and cortisol to cause hyperglycemia.

WHEN TO CONSIDER THE DIAGNOSIS (Table 160-6)

This uncommon diagnosis demands a high index of suspicion, since its manifestations are frequently nonspecific. It is better to "oversuspect" adrenocortical insufficiency in critically ill patients than to wait for a "classic" patient with all the signs, symptoms, and laboratory abnormalities. The diagnostic tests are easily performed (see below), and the side effects of a short course of "stress" steroids are minimal. On the other hand, the consequences of a missed diagnosis are grave.

Diagnosis

SCREENING TESTS (Fig. 160-1)

The two screening tests useful for detecting adrenocortical insufficiency in the ICU are random cortisol levels and the rapid ACTH stimulation test.

SERUM CORTISOL

A random cortisol level greater than 20 μg/dL makes the diagnosis of adrenocortical insufficiency very unlikely.[2] On the other hand, in the setting of shock, a cortisol level less than 20 μg/dL is highly suggestive of hypoadrenalism and should prompt a rapid ACTH stimulation test.[15]

TABLE 160-6 When to Consider the Diagnosis of Adrenocortical Insufficiency

History of treatment with glucocorticoids (within the past year)
Hypotension (systolic BP <110 mmHg) with a chronic history of weight loss and weakness
Hypotension with a history or evidence of tuberculosis, malignancy, AIDS, polyendocrine deficiency, vitiligo, or coagulopathy
Hyperkalemia and hyponatremia, especially in the absence of chronic renal failure
Hypotension with hypoglycemia or eosinophilia
Hypotension with hyperpigmentation
Hypotension with the absence of axillary or pubic hair in a female
Unexplained hypotension unresponsive to aggressive fluids and vasoactive drugs

RAPID ACTH STIMULATION TEST

This "dynamic" test of adrenocortical function measures the response of the adrenal gland to stimulation by exogenous ACTH. It can be performed at any time of day. After the drawing of samples for basal levels of cortisol, aldosterone, and ACTH, 250 μg of synthetic ACTH (cosyntropin) is administered intravenously. Repeat samples for cortisol and aldosterone are then drawn 30 and 60 min later. "Normal" response varies, depending on the laboratory and the criteria used. A recent review proposed that a peak cortisol level greater than 20 μg/dL is a sufficient single criterion for normal adrenal function. Use of the cortisol increment as a criterion for normalcy increased neither the sensitivity nor the specificity of the test.[16]

Following withdrawal of glucocorticoids, the pituitary gland recovers first, followed by the adrenal cortex. Therefore, except in very early ACTH deficiency, a normal response to a rapid ACTH stimulation test not only indicates an intact adrenal cortex, but also implies a normal hypothalamic-pituitary-adrenal axis as well.[14,17] A blunted or flat cortisol response can be due to primary or secondary adrenocortical insufficiency.

The rapid ACTH stimulation test is only a screening procedure. A clearly normal response eliminates the possibility of primary adrenocortical insufficiency and makes the diagnosis of secondary hypoadrenalism unlikely. However, because rare patients with secondary adrenocortical insufficiency show a normal response, and because there are occasional false-positives, the test results should be verified when the patient's condition stabilizes.[18] The "gold standard" is the standard ACTH stimulation test. Other investigations to test the integrity of the hypothalamic-pituitary-adrenal axis include the metyrapone test, CRF stimulation test, and insulin-hypoglycemia test.

Management (Fig. 160-1)

The pace of therapy depends on the degree of suspicion of adrenocortical insufficiency and the acuteness of the patient's illness.

PREEXISTING OR PRESUMED ADRENOCORTICAL INSUFFICIENCY

Patients who are known to have adrenocortical insufficiency or who have a history of glucocorticoid treatment in the past year should be given "stress doses" of corticosteroids during severe intercurrent illness and during surgical procedures. The use of hydrocortisone sodium succinate, 100 mg intravenously every 6 to 8 h, effectively eliminates the possibility of adrenocortical insufficiency. Hydrocortisone should be promptly tapered to maintenance levels once the acute illness has resolved.

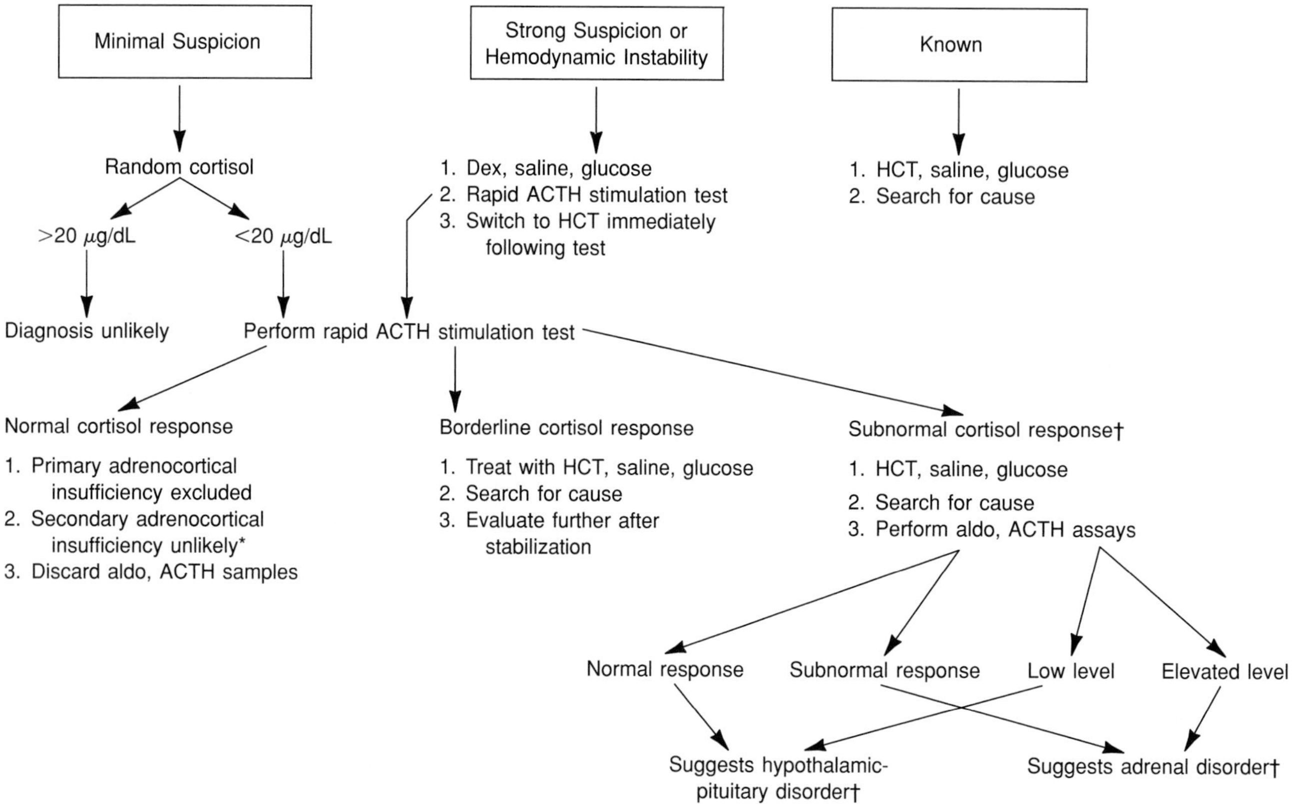

FIGURE 160-1 Flow diagram for the diagnosis and management of adrenocortical insufficiency. *Dex* denotes dexamethasone sodium phosphate, 4 mg IV; *ACTH*, adrenocorticotropic hormone; *HCT*, hydrocortisone sodium succinate, 100 mg q 6–8 h IV; *Aldo*, aldosterone. (*If secondary adrenocortical insufficiency still is entertained seriously, treat as borderline cortisol response. † Verify after stabilization.)

THE HEMODYNAMICALLY STABLE PATIENT

Measurement of plasma cortisol and a rapid ACTH stimulation test should precede initiation of "stress doses" of steroids. Hypovolemia should be treated with glucose-containing saline solution using the usual clinical guidelines. If the diagnosis is confirmed, hydrocortisone sodium succinate, 100 mg intravenously every 6 to 8 h, should be instituted.

THE HEMODYNAMICALLY UNSTABLE PATIENT

Acute adrenal insufficiency is life-threatening and requires prompt and aggressive therapy to effect an optimal outcome. Dexamethasone sodium phosphate, 4 mg, should be given intravenously immediately. Dexamethasone is preferred as the initial glucocorticoid replacement because, unlike hydrocortisone, it does not interfere with the assay for cortisol, and thus will not preclude performance of the rapid ACTH stimulation test. Although dexamethasone possesses no mineralocorticoid activity, vigorous hydration with saline solution will allow the patient to tolerate this lack easily for the 1 h required to perform the rapid ACTH stimulation test. Once the diagnostic tests are concluded, hydrocortisone should be substituted promptly for dexamethasone, since it has sufficient mineralocorticoid activity so as not to require concomitant mineralocorticoid replacement. Intramuscular preparations of glucocorticoids should be avoided, because of the uncertainty of adequate absorption in hypoperfused states. Vigorous hydration with normal saline solution and glucose should also be initiated. In general, persons with acute adrenocortical insufficiency have a deficit of approximately 20 percent of their extra cellular fluid volume and should receive at least 3 L of glucose-containing saline solution. The rapidity of infusion depends on the patient's hemodynamic status and the presence of underlying cardiovascular disease. The patient's fluid, electrolyte, and glucose status should be carefully monitored during resuscitation. A central venous or pulmonary artery catheter may be helpful in guiding fluid therapy. The precipitating cause of the adrenal decompensation, especially infection, should be sought. Prophylactic antibiotics are not indicated.

In patients with coexistent hypothyroidism, either from hypopituitarism or from autoimmune thyroiditis, glucocorticoid replacement should begin prior to thyroid hormone replacement. Administration of thyroid hormone increases the metabolism of glucocorticoids. Thus, treatment with thyroid hormone before glucocorticoids might worsen the hypoadrenal state, perhaps precipitating a crisis.

ETIOLOGIC DIAGNOSIS OF ADRENOCORTICAL INSUFFICIENCY

Since the cause of adrenocortical insufficiency has implications for management, a thorough search for the etiology should be undertaken once the diagnosis is made. To screen for the possibility of tuberculosis, a purified protein derivative (PPD), chest x-ray, abdominal x-ray (adrenal calcification is found in 30 to 50 percent of cases), and urinalysis should be checked. An abnormal prothrombin time, partial thromboplastin time, or platelet count may reveal an unsuspected coagulopathy, increasing the likelihood of adrenal hemorrhage. Antiadrenal antibodies are found in approximately 70 percent of patients with autoimmune adrenalitis—a very specific finding, since they are noted in fewer than 0.1 percent of normal control subjects and in fewer than 1.5 percent of persons in other disease groups.[19] A computed tomography (CT)-scan of the adrenals can be very helpful in determining the etiology of Addison's disease. Although the density and contours of the glands can yield useful information, the two most useful parameters are size and the presence of calcification (adrenal calcification is detected in 53 percent of cases of tuberculosis but in 0 percent of cases of autoimmune adrenalitis).[20] A CT scan of the head will detect sellar and suprasellar masses. If the diagnosis of autoimmune adrenalitis is made, other autoimmune endocrine diseases should be sought.

CASE PRESENTATION

A 56-year-old black man presented with a 2-day history of severe shortness of breath. His past medical history was unremarkable, although his wife reported a 6-month history of fatigue, generalized weakness, and a 15-lb weight loss. Two days prior to admission, the patient complained of abrupt onset of shortness of breath, a cough productive of blood-flecked green sputum, pleuritic chest pain, fever to 103° F, and a single rigor. (On admission he also noted severe abdominal pain, anorexia, nausea, and vomiting.) When the shortness of breath progressed to dyspnea at rest, his wife finally persuaded him to seek medical attention.

On examination the patient was a thin, cachectic, very dark-skinned black man, lethargic and using accessory muscles of respiration. Blood pressure was 85/65 mmHg, falling to 70 mmHg palpable when seated. The pulse was 125 beats per min (bpm) and regular, the respirations 36 and moderately labored, and the temperature 38° C. Chest exam revealed bronchial breath sounds at the left base. Cardiac exam was normal. Examination of the abdomen revealed slightly decreased bowel sounds and diffuse tenderness on deep palpation, but no rebound. The patient was confused, but the neurologic exam was nonfocal. Laboratory data included: white blood cell count 14,600 per mm^3 with 23 percent band forms, 10 percent eosinophils; hemoglobin 9.7 g/dL, hematocrit 29.9; sodium 129 meq/L, potassium 4.9 meq/L, urea nitrogen 45 mg/dL, creatinine 1.7 mg/dL, glucose 55 mg/dL. Results of urinalysis and abdominal x-ray were normal. Gram stain of the sputum showed sheets of polymorphonuclear leukocytes with intracellular gram-positive diplococci. Chest x-ray revealed left lower lobe consolidation. Room air arterial blood gas analysis demonstrated pH 7.42, P_{O_2} 55, P_{CO_2} 23. Lumbar puncture was normal.

The initial impression was pneumococcal pneumonia and dehydration with a presumed underlying malignancy. Treatment included O_2, isotonic saline solution with glucose, and intravenous penicillin. Hypotension persisted despite 3 L of fluid. Pulmonary artery catheterization revealed a pulmonary artery wedge pressure of 18 cmH_2O and a cardiac output of 4.3 L/min. After addition of dopamine as high as 15 μg/kg per min, the blood pressure remained 80/60. The combination of hyponatremia, hypoglycemia, eosinophilia, and hypotension unresponsive to fluids and pressors in a patient with an underlying chronic illness raised the suspicion of coexistent adrenocortical insufficiency. A cortisol level was sent. Hypotension persisted until the following morning. The cortisol level was found to be 9 μg/dL. A rapid ACTH stimulation test yielded a maximum cortisol response of 11 μg/dL, confirming the diagnosis of adrenocortical insufficiency. The patient was then begun on hydrocortisone, 100 mg intravenously every 8 h. Hypotension dramatically resolved over 2 h. The patient was discharged from the ICU the following day with a resolving pneumonia, normal blood pressure, and a good appetite.

CASE DISCUSSION

This is a classic presentation of a patient with chronic compensated adrenocortical insufficiency who developed an intercurrent pneumonia. This stress precipitated acute adrenocortical insufficiency, with typical manifestations of hypotension unresponsive to volume and vasoactive drugs; gastrointestinal signs and symptoms; confusion; hyperpigmentation; hyponatremia; hypoglycemia; azotemia; and eosinophilia. Usually, the most likely explanation for such a patient's hypotension is septic shock, which may also respond poorly to fluids and drugs. However, the history of chronic illness obtained from the patient's wife, combined with the admitting laboratory data—particularly the eosinophilia and hypoglycemia—provide such strong evidence for adrenocortical insufficiency that the diagnosis is almost inescapable. Given the severity of illness, simply sending a random cortisol level was inappropriate. Presumptive treatment with dexamethasone sodium phosphate, 4 mg intravenously, should have been begun immediately. A rapid ACTH stimulation test should then have been performed to confirm the clinical suspicion. Finally, while the most likely etiology of this patient's adrenocortical insufficiency is autoimmune adrenalitis, he should be referred for confirmation of adrenocortical insufficiency and investigation of its cause.

References

1. Irvine WJ, Barnes EW: Adrenocortical insufficiency. Clin Endocrinol Metab 1:549, 1972.
2. Kannan CR. Addison's disease, in *The Adrenal Gland*. New York, Plenum Medical Book Co, 1988, pp 31–96.
3. Guttman PH: Addison's disease. A statistical analysis of 566 cases and a study of the pathology. Arch Pathol 10:742, 1930.
4. Sarosi GA, Voth DW, Dahl BA, et al: Disseminated histoplasmosis: Results of long-term follow-up. A Center for Disease Control cooperative mycoses study. Ann Intern Med 75:511, 1971.
5. Redman BG, Pazdur R, Zingas AP, Loredo R: Prospective evaluation of adrenal insufficiency in patients with adrenal metastasis. Cancer 60:103, 1987.
6. Rosenthal FD, Davies MA, Burden AC: Malignant disease presenting as Addison's disease. Br Med J 1:1591,1978.
7. Rao RH, Vagnucci AH, Amico JA: Bilateral massive adrenal hemorrhage: Early recognition and treatment. Ann Intern Med 110:227, 1989.
8. Knowlton AI. Adrenal insufficiency in the intensive care setting. J Intensive Care Med 4:35, 1989.
9. Glascow BJ, Steinsapir KD, Anders K, Layfield LJ: Adrenal pathology in the acquired immune deficiency syndrome. Am J Clin Pathol 84:594, 1985.
10. Dluhy RG: The growing spectrum of HIV-related endocrine abnormalities (editorial). J Clin Endocrinol Metab 70:563, 1990.
11. Kehlet H, Binder C: Adrenocortical function and clinical course during and after surgery in unsupplemented glucocorticoid-treated patients. Br J Anaesth 45:1043, 1973.
12. Streck WF, Lockwood DH: Pituitary adrenal recovery following short term suppression with corticosteroids Am J Med 66:910, 1979.
13. Christy NP, Wallace EZ, Jailer JW: Comparative effects of prednisone and of cortisone in suppressing the response of the adrenal cortex to exogenous adrenocorticotropin. J Clin Endocrinol Metab 16:1059, 1956.
14. Graber AL, Ney RL, Nicholson WE, et al: Natural history of pituitary-adrenal recovery following long-term suppression with corticosteroids. J Clin Endocrinol 25:11, 1956.
15. Mattingly D, Tyler C: Plasma 11-hydroxycorticoid levels in surgical stress. Proc R Soc Med 58:1010, 1965.
16. May ME, Carey RM: Rapid adrenocorticotropic hormone test in practice: Retrospective review. Am J Med 79:679, 1985.
17. Kehlet H, Lindholm J, Bjerre P: Value of the 30 min ACTH-test in assessing hypothalamic-pituitary-adrenocortical function after pituitary surgery in Cushing's disease. Clin Endocrin 20:349, 1984.
18. Cunningham SK, Moore A, McKenna TJ: Normal cortisol response to corticotropin in patients with secondary adrenal failure. Arch Intern Med 143:2276, 1983.
19. Nerup J: Addison's disease—a review of some clinical, pathological and immunological features Dan Med Bull 21:201, 1974.
20. Doppman JL, Gill JR, Nienhuis AW, et al: CT findings in Addison's disease. J Comput Assist Tomogr 6:757, 1982.
21. Baxter JD, Tyrrell JB: The adrenal cortex, in Felig P, Baxter JD, Broadus AE, Frohman LA (eds): *Endocrinology and Metabolism,* 2d ed. New York, McGraw-Hill, 1987, pp 511–650.
22. Kannan CR: Hypopituitarism, in *The Pituitary Gland*. New York, Plenum Medical Book Co, 1988, pp 423–441.
23. Nerup J: Addison's disease—clinical studies. A report of 108 cases. Acta Endocrinol 76:127, 1974.

Chapter 161

HYPOTHYROIDISM, NONTHYROIDAL ILLNESS, AND MYXEDEMA COMA

ROY E. WEISS
SAMUEL REFETOFF

KEY POINTS

- *Only primary hypothyroidism can be of sufficient clinical severity as to require immediate hormone replacement.*
- *Virtually all patients admitted to an ICU have low serum triiodothyronine (T_3) and 30 to 50 percent have low thyroxine (T_4) with normal or low serum thyrotropin (TSH).*
- *Patients with a $T_4 < 3.0$ µg/dL despite normal T_4-binding proteins have a 68 to 84 percent mortality rate.*
- *T_3 is the logical choice for critically ill patients requiring thyroid hormone replacement.*
- *Early intubation and mechanical ventilation are crucial for successful treatment of myxedema coma.*
- *Management of myxedema coma should include administration of glucocorticoids while the adrenal status is being assessed.*
- *Hypothyroidism reduces the metabolism of almost all drugs, and the doses need careful adjustment to prevent drug toxicity.*

Hypothyroidism is a state of tissue deprivation of thyroid hormone. This is manifested by general reduction of the metabolic rate accompanied by specific symptoms and signs. Usually hypothyroidism is caused by a decreased supply of thyroid hormone due to: **1.** failure of the gland to synthesize and secrete thyroid hormone; **2.** failure of the pituitary to secrete TSH; or **3.** hypothalamic disease resulting in thyrotropin-releasing hormone (TRH) deficiency.

Perhaps the most controversial, if not challenging aspect of thyroidology for the intensivist, is how to interpret thyroid function tests in critically ill patients, and when the tests are abnormal, what to do. Clinically important hypothyroidism in its most severe form usually is seen in patients with primary hypothyroidism and occurs over several weeks culminating in myxedema coma. Equally challenging are the thyroid function abnormalities seen in patients with concurrent severe illness and the assessment of the thyroid hormone status at the tissue level.

Evaluation of Thyroid Function in Patients with Severe Nonthyroidal Illness

DEFINITION OF NONTHYROIDAL ILLNESS

Virtually all critically ill patients have reduced serum levels of T_3 and approximately 30 to 50 percent have also low T_4 concentration both associated with normal or low serum TSH values.[1] This phenomenon has been termed the *low T_3 syndrome, Nonthyroidal illness* (NTI) or the *euthyroid sick syndrome.* Each of these descriptive terms assumes *a priori* that such patients are euthyroid despite reduced thyroid hormone levels. The condition is not limited to acute illness. Patients with chronic hepatic or renal failure, calorie deprivation, and a variety of other illness present similar thyroid hormone profiles.[2] Serum T_3 as well as the T_4 concentrations are also decreased following nonthyroid surgical procedures.[3] In patients with a T_4 value <3.0 µg/dL, the mortality rate is 68 to 84 percent,[4] indicating that abnormal to low TSH in the face of a low T_4 concentration is a marker for mortality in the critically ill population. To understand this phenomenon and develop a rational basis for treatment, it is useful to review the thyroid physiology with emphasis on processes occurring in NTI.

THYROID HORMONE PHYSIOLOGY IN CRITICAL ILLNESS

Ninety percent of hormone secreted by the thyroid gland is T_4 while the remainder is T_3. Thyroid hormone is metabolized in peripheral tissues by stepwise monodeiodination until the molecule is completely stripped of iodine. This process uses specific enzymes, *deiodinases.* The deiodination of T_4 can take one of 2 pathways—removal of the iodine from the outer phenolic ring (5′ position) resulting in 3, 3′,5-triiodothyronine (T_3) or removal of the iodine from the inner phenolic ring (5 position) yielding 3,3′,5′-triiodothyronine (reverse T_3 or rT_3). T_3 is the active form of the hormone while rT_3 has no biologic activity. The same enzyme that removes iodine from the 5′ position of the T_4 molecule also is responsible for deiodination of the 5′ iodine from rT_3. Therefore, reduction in the 5′-deiodinase activity, invariably associated with severe illness and malnutrition, not only reduces the serum T_3 level but also increases that of rT_3.

The nature of perturbations of the hypothalamic-pituitary-thyroid axis in critically ill patients is less well understood. The basal TSH values in serum can be normal or low, but the response of TSH to TRH is usually attenuated.[2] Stress and malnutrition may be partly responsible. More importantly, drugs commonly administered to ICU patients have inhibitory effects on the hypothalamic and pituitary function. Dopamine is one such drug which inhibits TSH even when infused at "renal" doses.[5,6] Critically ill patients who will eventually recover from their illness have as a rule less impairment of the TSH response to TRH.

TABLE 161-1 Interpretation of Thyroid Function Tests

Diagnosis	T_4	T_3	TSH	rT_3
Primary hypothyroidism	dec	dec/N	inc	dec/N
Central hypothyroidism	dec	dec	N	???
NTI	dec/N	dec	N/dec	N/inc

N, normal

INTERPRETATION OF THYROID FUNCTION STUDIES (TABLE 161-1)

Many critically ill patients have thyroid hormone and TSH levels measured at some point during the course of hospitalization. Low concentrations of thyroid hormone without an appropriate increase in serum TSH level would under normal conditions raise the suspicion of pituitary (secondary) or hypothalamic (tertiary) hypothyroidism, but in a critically ill patient, the diagnosis of primary hypothyroidism with inadequate pituitary response needs consideration. A modest elevation of serum TSH level without an increase in rT_3 concentration is a strong indication of primary hypothyroidism. With the exception of renal failure, a decreased rT_3 level raises the possibility of hypothyroidism and should prompt a search for the etiology. While these diagnoses are being investigated, thyroid hormone replacement and glucocorticoid treatment are indicated. Since results of rT_3 measurement are often not readily obtained, this test is useful in retrospect for ruling out primary endocrine dysfunction and adds little to the decision of initial management of patients. Since only primary hypothyroidism is usually of such severity as to require emergency treatment, its recognition depends on some degree of TSH elevation, prior history of thyroid disease, and physical findings compatible with hypothyroidism.

TO TREAT OR NOT TO TREAT

Should patients with low serum levels of thyroid hormone in the face of catastrophic NTI receive hormonal replacement? In a randomized prospective study to determine the effect of T_4 treatment in NTI, 11 patients admitted to an ICU with reduced thyroid hormone levels were treated with intravenous T_4 and 12 patients not given the hormone served as controls.[7] The study indicated an earlier mortality in the treated group, although the number of survivors was not significantly different between both groups. It was concluded that T_4 therapy was not beneficial, and inhibition of TSH secretion by the administration of T_4 may be detrimental to the recovery of thyroid function. Yet many physicians find it difficult to withhold treatment in a dying patient with virtually undetectable thyroid hormone levels.

Data on the benefit of thyroid hormone treatment are not only limited but the seriousness of the intercurrent illness is such that it is unlikely that an answer will be forthcoming considering the difficulty in interpreting the effect of thyroid hormone replacement in individuals receiving multiple drugs. Thus, the argument centers not only on the question whether such patients are truly hypothyroid, thus the term *euthyroid sick,* but whether this temporary hypothyroidism may not, in fact, be beneficial. Inhibition of the type I 5′-deiodinase is the principal mechanism reducing the supply of biologically active thyroid hormone, T_3 to peripheral tissues of the severely ill. Experimental work in a rat model indicates that this peripheral tissue hypothyroidism is maintained by preventing compensatory TSH increase through the local generation of normal T_3 levels in the pituitary gland which utilizes a different form of 5′-deiodinase.[8,9] This type II enzyme is actually more active in severe illness. Teleologists argue that it is not by accident that this mechanism of reduced delivery of thyroid hormone to peripheral tissues has been put in place and thus, reduced metabolic activity may be beneficial in the face of the increased catabolism characteristic of severe illness. The question is, does the physician or nature know best? At our institution there is no uniform consensus on this subject. Table 161-2 may serve as a bedside guide to the intensivist to select patients for thyroid hormone treatment.

WHAT TO TREAT WITH

If the decision is made to treat a sick patient who has reduced thyroid hormone levels, the logical choice is T_3. Administration of T_4 does not change significantly the serum T_3 concentration—it only increases the level of the biologically inactive rT_3.[5] The problem with T_3 treatment is its theoretical cardiac "toxicity." Another difficulty with the use of T_3 is its availability in only oral form. However, intravenous T_3 can be obtained from the medical director of Smith Kline and French Corp., Philadelphia, PA, generally within 24 h for use in myxedema coma. A solution of T_3 for intravenous use can also be prepared by the hospital pharmacist by dissolving L-T_3 in 0.1 *N* NaOH followed by a 10-fold dilution in normal saline containing 2 percent albumin to a final concentration of 25 μg T_3/mL. The solution is sterilized by a single passage through a 0.22 μm Millipore filter and stored, for no longer than 1 week, at 4°C, protected from light.

TABLE 161-2 Indications for Thyroid Hormone Treatment in Patients with Severe NTI

History of thyroid disease
History of radioactive iodine treatment
Hyporeflexia
Hypothermia
Macroglossia
Goiter
Increased serum TSH concentrations
Increased serum creatine phosphokinase (CPK)
Hypercholesterolemia
Unexplained pleural or pericardial effusions

Myxedema Coma

DIAGNOSIS

Myxedema coma is caused by marked and prolonged depletion of thyroid hormone. The cardinal features of myxedema coma are: **1.** defective thermoregulation to the point of hypothermia; **2.** altered mental status to the point of coma; and **3.** identifiable precipitating event. The condition is a medical emergency since it is potentially fatal in approximately one-half of cases.[10] Typically, this rare entity occurs in elderly women with long-standing hypothyroidism who develop an intercurrent illness and lapse into coma, or less severely hypothyroid persons exposed to cold or given tranquilizers, narcotics, or sedatives sufficient to push them to the brink of myxedema coma. Table 161-3 lists events likely to precipitate myxedema coma. The usual features of severe hypothyroidism (myxedema) include dry, coarse skin, scaly elbows and knees, yellowness in the skin without scleral icterus, coarse hair, thinning of the lateral aspect of eyebrows, macroglossia and hoarseness, obtundation, delayed deep tendon reflexes, and hypothermia. When these signs are backed by a markedly reduced serum T_4 level and an elevated TSH concentration, the diagnosis is obvious. However, as is the case in thyrotoxic crisis, initiation of treatment should not be delayed until the results of the thyroid functions studies become available. Furthermore, because of intercurrent illness, TSH values may not be elevated in proportion to the severity of hypothyroidism. A high index of suspicion in a patient presenting as described above should prompt immediate treatment after a blood sample is taken for laboratory confirmation of the diagnosis.

PULMONARY AND CARDIOVASCULAR COMPLICATIONS

Alveolar hypoventilation is known to occur in myxedema.[11] It is thus not surprising that patients with underlying lung pathology experience worsening of their symptoms. It has been demonstrated that the hypoxic ventilatory drive is depressed in patients with myxedema and that it responds to hormone replacement.[12] The hypercapnic ventilatory response is also significantly depressed but does not change with replacement of thyroid hormone. Therefore, a reduced central nervous system drive to breathe and decreased respiratory muscle activity are the main reasons for respiratory depression in myxedema coma. Secondary aspiration pneumonia, laryngeal obstruction, and reduced surfactant contribute to lung dysfunction. It should be emphasized that failure of early aggressive management of impaired respiration (i.e., intubation) is a common error in the management of these patients.

TABLE 161-3 Common Precipitating Factors of Myxedema Coma

Exposure to cold
Infection
Surgery
Strokes
Occult gastrointestinal bleeding
Trauma
Drug overdose
Sedatives
Tranquilizers
Narcotics
Anesthetics
Congestive heart failure

TABLE 161-4 Laboratory Findings in Myxedema Coma

Hypoglycemia
Hyponatremia
Hyperkalemia
Hypercortisolemia
Anemia
Leukocytosis with a left shift
Serum creatinine >2.0 mg/dL
Increased P_{CO_2} in arterial blood
Decreased P_{O_2} in arterial blood

The cardiovascular complications in myxedema coma are caused by the combination of hypothyroid cardiomyopathy, hypothermia, and hypoxia. Pericardial effusion is almost a universal finding which less often can lead to tamponade. It is best demonstrated by echocardiography. In patients with long-standing hypothyroidism, hypercholesterolemia may accelerate the progress of atherosclerosis leading to ischemic heart disease. The reader is referred to the discussion of hypothermia and its cardiovascular complications (see Chap. 72).

The intercurrent illness and decreased food intake caused by the mental obtundation of myxedema may reduce the serum levels of cholesterol and TSH, diminishing their value as indicators of the severity of the myxedema. Patients presenting with a more profound hypothermia have a poor prognosis. The laboratory findings in patients with myxedema coma are listed in Table 161-4.

TREATMENT

THYROID HORMONE. Although severe hypothyroidism, especially in the elderly, should be treated cautiously with gradual increments of small doses of thyroid hormone, myxedema coma makes an exception to this rule. The immediate threat to life takes precedence to the risks of rapid hormone replacement. The theoretical advantage of treating critically ill patients with T_3 as opposed to T_4 has been discussed above. In hypothyroid patients without major intercurrent illness, T_4 therapy alone may be sufficient to increase the serum T_3 level to normal in 2 to 3 days. This is unlikely to occur in ICU patients with multiorgan system failure. The principle of hormonal treatment is to rapidly replenish the extrathyroidal pool of thyroid hormone, consisting mainly bound to serum proteins, and to provide the tissues with the daily requirement of the biologically active hormone. Replenishment is best achieved by the immediate administration of T_4, a hormone with considerably longer half-life (7 days) and higher affinity for serum proteins.[11–13] The active form of the hormone, T_3, can then be provided, which becomes readily available to tissues with lesser risk of accumulating in excessive amounts (half-life approximately 1 day).

Several investigators have estimated that the average extrathyroid T_4 pool is approximately 800 μg/1.73 m^2.[13–16] Based on this estimate and the normal turnover rate of T_4, its daily requirement is on the average 80 μg, possibly 50 μg in hypothyroidism due to reduced rate of hormone degradation. Intensivists using only T_4 for treatment should give initially 500 μg L-T_4 followed by 50 to 100 μg daily. The serum T_4 concentration should be in the normal range within 24 to 48 h. Daily electrocardiographic monitoring for ischemic changes and continuous monitoring of rhythm are essential.

We prefer the regimen of both T_4 and T_3 treatment. Following the intravenous loading dose of T_4, 25 μg T_3 should be given every 6 h through a nasogastric tube until improvement is noted and provided the diagnosis has been confirmed by laboratory tests. The dose is then reduced to maintenance level but changed to T_4 only after recovery from intercurrent illness.

USE OF STEROIDS. The metabolism of all drugs and compounds is markedly reduced in patients with myxedema coma. Hence, the absolute requirement for steroids is, if anything, reduced. However, because of the 5 to 10 percent incidence of associated primary hypoadrenalism, glucocorticoids should be given until evidence for intact adrenal function is secured by the cortisol measurement on a blood sample obtained on admission. The usual dose of hydrocortisone is 50 mg every 6 h. The steroid dose can then be tapered rapidly after confirmation of a normal pituitary adrenal axis. Alternatively, the initial dose can be 2 mg dexamethasone and a 1-h ACTH (Cosyntropin) stimulation test can be done on the spot to assess adrenocortical function.[16]

SUPPORTIVE CARE. Early intubation and mechanical ventilation are believed to be the hallmarks for the successful treatment of myxedema coma. To observe how the patient may do without intubation has no rationale. Severe hemodynamic collapse in the presence of a large pericardial effusion may necessitate immediate pericardiocentesis. Because hypothyroidism can cause an elevation of serum CPK, obtaining a base-line value is helpful in the follow-up, particularly if a myocardial infarction is later suspected. Moderate elevations of blood urea nitrogen (BUN) and creatinine values are not uncommon and are not necessarily indicative of chronic renal failure.

Hypothermia is treated with blankets, letting internal heat generation slowly warm the body.[10] External warming runs the risk of shock by producing peripheral vasodilation in a patient with already reduced cardiac output. Measurement of right heart pressure is useful to guide therapy. Patients with myxedema are rarely volume overloaded, and the use of diuretics runs the risk of further reducing the cardiac output. Hyponatremia is best treated by water restriction because total body sodium is increased due to its storage in glycosaminoglycan, forming the myxedematous accumulation which becomes mobilized with thyroid hormone treatment. Antiulcer prophylaxis is recommended. More importantly, it should be remembered that hypothyroidism reduces the metabolism of all drugs, and their dosage needs careful adjustment to prevent drug toxicity. Diligent investigation into the precipitating causes should include blood, urine, sputum cultures, and empiric treatment with antibiotics.

The presence of anemia should be investigated and corrected by blood transfusion to increase the oxygen-carrying capacity. Use of α-adrenergic agents should be avoided because patients are already vasoconstricted.

EFFICACY OF TREATMENT

Assuming that an accurate diagnosis has been made and proper therapeutic measures have been carried out, how is progress and efficacy of treatment followed? The physician is committed to treat the patient for several days and as long as the serum TSH concentration remains elevated. Reduction of the TSH level provides the earliest evidence for response to thyroid hormone therapy. Irreversible damage to the respiratory centers has been observed with failure of spontaneous respiration despite full repletion of thyroid hormone. There are no useful laboratory measurements helpful in assessing the peripheral tissue responses to thyroid hormone in the critical care setting. The ultimate gauge of successful treatment is complete clinical recovery.

Goiter and Acute Airway Obstruction

Large goiters, 150 g or more, can cause some degree of tracheal obstruction. In a series of 2908 goiters, only 58 (2.0 percent) presented with tracheal obstruction. Tracheal compression obstructing up to 75 percent of the tracheal lumen often remains asymptomatic.[17] Although dyspnea on exertion has been attributed to goiter, the symptoms are often only nocturnal, manifesting as stridor or when more severe, sleep apnea. This can be confirmed by x-ray views of the trachea at rest and during reverse Valsalva and by sleep studies.[18]

Growth of the goiter would have to be extensive to cause direct tracheal compression. In Reidel's struma, there is tracheal cartilage destruction by fibrous invasion, which can also cause bilateral vocal cord paralysis. Several case reports have been published describing the acute presentation of tracheal obstruction associated with goiter.[19,20] Management of these patients is somewhat difficult because emergency tracheostomy may be difficult to perform due to interference by the thyroid gland. The use of small endotracheal tubes and immediate subtotal thyroidectomy should reduce the need for tracheostomy. It should be noted that subtotal thyroidectomy may not be successful in the presence of tracheomalacia which may require prosthetic supports.[21] In some instances, a simple division of the thyroid isthmus may be sufficient to relieve the symptoms.

CASE PRESENTATIONS

Case 1

An 82-year-old man with a history of emphysema, enlarged prostate, abdominal aortic aneurysm, and alleged hypothyroidism underwent transuretheral resection of the prostate. On postoperative day 2 he developed dyspnea, abdominal pain, and severe hypotension. Abdominal computed tomography (CT) scan revealed leakage from the aortic aneurysm. Surgical repair of the aneurysm was complicated by intraoperative myocardial infarction (MI). Over the ensuing 50 days the patient had two episodes of pneumonia, acute tubular necrosis requiring hemodialysis, and lower gastrointestinal bleeding. On postoperative day 6 it was realized that the patient had not been receiving his replacement T_4 dose of 50 μg/day, which was then restarted. Because attempts to liberate him from the ventilator were unsuccessful, a tracheostomy was performed on day 22. Thyroid function tests on day 55 revealed a T_4 of 1.1 μg/dL (normal 5.0 to 12.0), and free T_4 index (FT_4I) of 1.4 (normal 6.0 to 10.5), and a TSH of 62 mU/L (normal 0.5 to 4.0). Several days later the TSH level was found to have increased to 74 mU/L at which point the endocrine service was consulted. It was recommended to give 400 μg T_4 as an intravenous bolus followed by 100 μg T_4 daily, and 25 μg T_3 every 6 h via nasogastric tube. On day 61 the patient seemed more alert, did not require mechanical ventilation, and was successfully extubated. Within 4 days, serum TSH concentration had dropped to 12.6 mU/L and the FT_4I had increased to 4.6. T_3 treatment was then discontinued, but the patient continued to receive T_4. By day 72 the TSH level had increased to 27 mU/L, and T_3 therapy was reinstated, which led to a prompt drop in the TSH concentration to 7.8 mU/L. The patient remained extubated and on day 77 was transferred from the ICU to a regular hospital room. The results of thyroid function tests are depicted in Fig. 161-1.

Discussion

This case illustrates primary hypothyroidism (most likely autoimmune as the patient had high antithyroid antibody titers). The elevated TSH despite illness and drug treatment supports the presence of primary hypothyroidism. The ability to extubate the patient shortly after initiation of hormonal therapy attests to its efficacy. Even though the patient received several weeks of T_4 therapy, the T_3 values remained low. The increase in rT_3 illustrates the shunting of T_4 to the inactive metabolite rT_3 in severe NTI. When T_3 was given in conjunction with T_4 the TSH level rapidly decreased, and the patient showed clinical improvement. Although many of this patient's initial complications were unrelated to the myxedema, attention to detail regarding prompt and appropriate continuation of medications including thyroid hormone may have averted the necessity for mechanical ventilation. Administration of T_3 in the immediate post-MI period

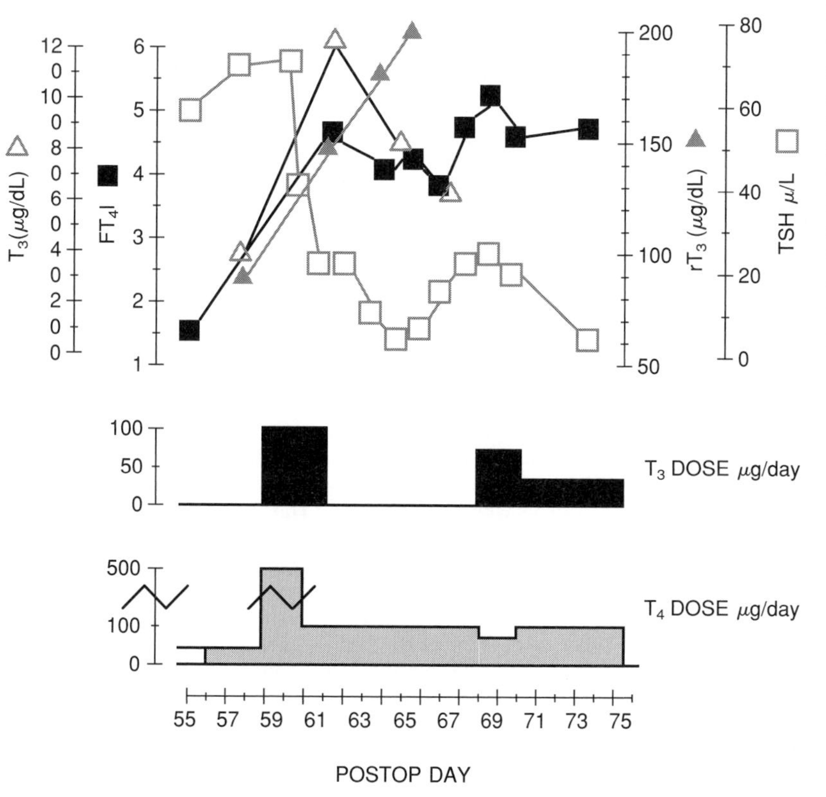

FIGURE 161-1 A diagrammatic representation of Case 1 discussed in this chapter. An 82-year-old man with alleged hypothyroidism underwent surgical repair of an abdominal aortic aneurysm and subsequently had a perioperative myocardial infarction. Difficulty in liberating the patient from the ventilator prompted thyroid evaluation. Results of these tests showed the patient to be significantly hypothyroid. The response of the various thyroid parameters to T_3 and T_4 treatment are illustrated. Improvement of the clinical condition best correlated to the T_3 treatment. A further discussion is in the text.

should be done with caution for fear of inducing further ischemia by increasing myocardial oxygen demand; however, careful monitoring of T_3 levels and electrocardiograms as in this patient did not detect any adverse side effects.

Case 2

The endocrine service was asked to consult regarding a 79-year-old woman 2 weeks after repair of an abdominal aortic aneurysm. She had no history of thyroid disease, and T_4 values were normal on routine examination 1 month earlier. The patient's postoperative course was somewhat stormy with episodes of intra-abdominal bleeding requiring brief treatment with dopamine for maintenance of blood pressure and surgical reexploration. Thyroid function studies revealed an FT_4I of 2.8 (normal 6 to 10.5) and a TSH of 0.9 mU/L (normal 0.4 to 4.0). The surgical team had instituted treatment with intravenous T_4 200 μg/day for the previous 2 weeks. The recommendation of the endocrine consultant was to obtain serum T_3 and rT_3 levels, to discontinue treatment with T_4, and recheck thyroid function studies when the patient recovered. Serum T_3 level was < 10 mμg/dL (normal 90 to 185) and rT_3 250 mμg/dL (normal 14.5 to 30). The markedly high rT_3 indicates that the T_4 given was primarily converted by the very ill patient to rT_3.

Discussion

These data confirm the futility of T_4 treatment under these circumstances because of the inability of the patient to generate the active form of the hormone.

Case 3

An 83-year-old woman was brought to the emergency room because of abdominal discomfort and distention accompanied by diarrhea for 3 days. She had a history of chronic constipation and laxative use. She was seen at another hospital a week earlier for a renal ailment and was given trimethoprim-sulfamethoxazole. Her past history was significant for a "goiter" treated surgically 40 years earlier. Although presumably on thyroid replacement therapy, her recent compliance was uncertain. Other medications included diclofenac (Voltaren) and oxybutynin chloride for chronic urinary incontinence.

The patient was lethargic on admission with a rectal temperature of 35.2°C (95.5°F), blood pressure of 118/60 mmHg, regular pulse at 53/min, and a respiratory rate of 30/min. Her skin was dry. She had a transverse neck scar with no thyroid tissue palpable. Bibasilar rales extended two-thirds up the lung fields. Cardiac examination results were unremarkable. Her abdomen was distended and tympanitic with hypoactive bowel sounds. Though lethargic, she was arousable. Deep tendon reflexes showed delayed relaxation.

Laboratory values were: sodium, 138; potassium, 8.0; chloride, 109; and bicarbonate 23 meq/L; blood urea nitrogen of 65 and creatinine of 3.8 mg/dL. Blood sugar level was 53 mg/dL. The blood cell count revealed a hemoglobin of 10 g/dL with 12,700 WBC/mm^3 (31 percent segmented, 60 percent band forms). Arterial blood-gas values on room air showed a pH of 7.4, a P_{O_2} of 49 mmHg (85 percent saturated), and P_{CO_2} of 31 mmHg. Chest radiograph demonstrated left lower lobe retrocardiac infiltrate and probable right middle lobe infiltrate. Heart size was unremarkable. Abdominal radiograph showed a dilated large colon 9.5 cm wide with multiple air-fluid levels.

On admission to the ICU the patient was intubated. A right heart catheter was placed, which revealed a cardiac output of 1.0 L/min and a pulmonary capillary wedge pressure of 5 mmHg. She was given intravenous fluids, dobutamine, antibiotics, hydrocortisone, and L-T_4. The diagnosis of hypothyroidism was subsequently confirmed by laboratory tests showing no detectable T_4 and a TSH concentration of >50 mU/L. The serum cortisol level before institution of treatment was 32 mg/dL. She continued to improve and was off pressors and ventilatory support by the third hospital day. By day 6, she had good bowel function and was able to eat. She was discharged on thyroid hormone replacement therapy on day 14.

Discussion

This case illustrates the typical presentation and laboratory findings of myxedema precoma. This elderly patient, who had a history of goiter, presented with a surgical scar on her neck and a history of not taking T_4. There is little question that this patient was hypothyroid, based on this history and on physical examination. Initial assessment resulted in the prompt initiation of specific therapy with intravenous T_4. This case differs from Case 1 in that in the absence of severe NTI, T_3 therapy is not necessary and that T_4 alone is effective in correcting the hypothyroidism. Intubation and mechanical ventilation ensured proper tissue oxygenation and were appropriately started early in the course of treatment. Antibiotics given for aspiration pneumonia may have masked the hypothermia and the precipitating event. Aggressive treatment averted the progression to frank myxedema coma. Treatment with glucocorticoids proved retrospectively not to be necessary, but there is no evidence their inclusion was detrimental.

References

1. Kaptein EM, Weiner JM, Robinson WJ, et al: Relationship of altered thyroid hormone indices to survival in nonthyroidal illnesses. Clin Endocrinol (Oxf) 125:565, 1982.
2. Wartofsky L, Burman KD: Alterations in thyroid function in patients with systemic illness: The "euthyroid sick syndrome." Endocr Rev 3:164, 1982.
3. Burr WA, Black EG, Griffiths RS, et al: Serum triiodothyronine and reverse triiodothyronine concentrations after surgical operation. Lancet 2:1277, 1975.
4. Baue AE, Gunther B, Hartl W, et al: Altered hormonal activity in severely ill patients after injury or sepsis. Arch Surg 119:1125, 1984.
5. Delatlia D: Dopamine and TSH secretion in man. Lancet II:760, 1977.
6. Scanlon MF, Weightman DR, Shale DJ, et al: Dopamine is a

physiological regulator of thyrotrophin (TSH) secretion in normal man. Clin Endocrinol (Oxf) 10:4, 1979.
7. Brent GA, Hershman JM: Thyroxine therapy in patients with severe nonthyroidal illnesses and low serum thyroxine concentration. J Clin. Endocrinol Metab 62:1, 1986.
8. Lim VS, Henriquez C, Seo H, et al: Thyroid function in a uremic rat model: Evidence suggesting tissue hypothyroidism. J Clin Invest 66:946, 1980.
9. Lim VS, Passo C, Murata Y, et al: Reduced triiodothyronine content in liver but not pituitary of the uremic rat model: Demonstration of changes compatible with thyroid hormone deficiency in liver only. Endocrinology 114:280, 1980.
10. Blum M: Myxedema coma. Am J Med 264:432, 1972.
11. Wilson WR, Bedell GN: The pulmonary abnormalities in myxedema. J Clin Invest 39:42, 1960.
12. Zwillich CW, Pierson DJ, Hofeldt FD, et al: Ventilatory control in myxedema and hypothyroidism. N Engl J Med 292:662, 1975.
13. Holvey DM, Goodner CJ, Nicoloff JT, et al: Treatment of myxedema coma with intravenous thyroxine. Arch Intern Med 113:89, 1964.
14. Ingbar SG, Freinkel N: Simultaneous estimation of rates of thyroxine degradation and thyroid hormone synthesis. J Clin Invest 34:808, 1955.
15. Sterling K, Chodos RB: Radiothyroxine turnover studies in myxedema, thyrotoxicosis and hypermetabolism without endocrine disease. J Clin Invest 35:806, 1956.
16. Nicoloff JT: Thyroid storm and myxedema coma. Med Clin North Am 69:1005, 1985.
17. Melliere D, Saada F, Etienne G, et al: Goiter with severe respiratory compromise: Evaluation and treatment. Surgery 103:367, 1988.
18. Karbowitz SR, Edelman LB, Nath S, et al: Spectrum of advanced upper airway obstruction due to goiters. Chest 87:18, 1985.
19. Tseng KH, Felicetta JV, Rydstedt LL, et al: Acute airway obstruction due to a benign cervical goiter. Otolaryngol Head Neck Surg 97:72, 1987.
20. Torres A, Arroyo J, Kastanos N, et al: Acute respiratory failure and tracheal obstruction in patients with intrathoracic goiter. Crit Care Med 11:265, 1983.
21. Geelhoed GW: Tracheomalacia from compressing goiter: Management after thyroidectomy. Surgery 104:1100, 1988.

Chapter 162

THYROTOXICOSIS

ROY E. WEISS
SAMUEL REFETOFF

KEY POINTS

- *Autonomous hypersecretion and exogenous overdose of thyroid hormone are the most common causes of severe thyrotoxicosis.*
- *Hyperpyrexia and altered mental status are the hallmarks of thyroid storm.*
- *Medical treatment usually normalizes circulating thyroid hormone levels in 2 to 3 weeks, except under circumstances of iodine overload, in which case hyperthyroxinemia may persist for months.*
- *Blockade of hormonal secretion is best accomplished by the addition of stable iodine to an antithyroid drug regimen.*
- *β Blockers prevent thyroid storm in the thyrotoxic patient undergoing surgery, and they may ameliorate cardiovascular dysfunction in thyroid storm, but their side effects often confound therapy in the elderly, patients with asthma, and patients with cardiomyopathy.*
- *After gastric aspiration and lavage, only symptomatic and supportive treatment is needed in cases of levothyroxine overdose.*
- *Neonatal thyrotoxicosis can be life-threatening; it is usually caused by transplacental transfer of thyroid-stimulating antibodies. It is transient and requires only short-term treatment.*

Thyrotoxicosis occurs when the supply of thyroid hormone exceeds the amount needed for normal tissue function. The source of thyroid hormone may be **1.** excessive synthesis and secretion of hormone from the thyroid gland stimulated by abnormal thyroid-stimulating substances or by thyrotropin (also called thyroid-stimulating hormone, or TSH), **2.** autonomous hypersecretion or abnormal release of preformed hormone, or **3.** an exogenous or ectopic source of hormone.[1] Manifestations can be mild or severe, depending on the degree of hormone excess and its duration as well as on the presence of intercurrent illness. Aspects related to thyrotoxicosis in the severely ill patient will be the focus of this chapter.

A few basic facts of thyroid physiology are important for understanding the therapeutic approach to thyroid disorders: Iodine is actively transported into the thyroid gland, where it is organified and covalently bound to tyrosine. The iodinated tyrosines are coupled to form mainly thyroxine (T_4) and some triiodothyronine (T_3), both within the thyroglobulin molecule. It is in the form of thyroglobulin that the hormone is stored in the colloid of the thyroid follicles. Under the stimulation of TSH or an abnormal stimulator, thyroglobulin is digested by proteolysis, and the liberated hormone—predominantly T_4—is secreted into the circulation. In blood, T_4 is transported bound to specific serum proteins. In virtually all peripheral tissues, T_4, derived from blood, is converted into the active hormone, T_3, by removal of a single iodine atom from the 5′ position in the outer phenolic ring of the molecule. This reaction is mediated by a tissue specific 5′-deiodinase. Removal of iodine from the inner phenolic ring yields an inactive form of the hormone, reverse T_3 (rT_3). Intracellular T_3 binds to nuclear receptors, through which it exerts its effects.

Diagnosis in the ICU

Thyrotoxicosis may be manifested by adverse changes in every organ system. Pyrexia, tachycardia, congestive heart failure, oxyhemoglobin desaturation, and hypertension are the hallmarks of thyrotoxic crisis. There may also be involvement of the central nervous system, ranging from tremulousness to seizures and coma, or involvement of the respiratory system with tachypnea and respiratory muscle fatigue. Goiter and exophthalmos may be absent as frequently as they are present. Unfortunately, at the time of presentation in the ICU, most patients with these characteristics may have only modest elevations of thyroid hormone concentration in serum (see Chap. 161). Failure to recognize these symptoms as manifestations of thyrotoxicosis might result in nonspecific treatment with ensuing morbidity, and even mortality. On the other hand, not to treat pyrexia as a sign of sepsis, or tachycardia as a sign of ischemia or hypoxia, could be equally devastating. "Stat." laboratory measurement of thyroid hormones is not always available to provide firm laboratory support to the diagnosis and specific treatment. A 2-h radioiodine uptake test could conceivably be done at the bedside using a portable gamma counter probe, but probably is not practical. Therefore, the preliminary diagnosis of thyrotoxicosis is usually based on a careful history taking and physical examination. Useful findings are **1.** previous diagnosis and treatment of thyrotoxicosis, **2.** presence of exophthalmos, **3.** goiter, **4.** history of thyroid hormone ingestion, **5.** evidence of previous thyroid surgery, including an anterior neck surgical scar, and **6.** recent use of iodine-containing radiologic contrast agents. Such information only supports the suspicion that the suggestive physical signs may be related to thyrotoxicosis.

Physiologic Consequences and Cardiovascular Complications

Thyroid hormone exerts its tissue effect directly by interaction with specific nuclear receptors, and indirectly through activation of the sympathoadrenal system. Each of these actions causes unique effects on various tissues. The physiologic basis of the sympathomimetic effect of thyroid hormone is unknown. Table 162-1 summarizes the cardiopulmonary complications of thyrotoxicosis.

TABLE 162-1 Cardiopulmonary Complications of Thyrotoxicosis

Increased metabolic demand with increased O_2 consumption and CO_2 production
Respiratory muscle weakness
Increased work of breathing
Hyperdynamic circulation
Potential for high-output heart failure
Potential for myocardial ischemia
Arrhythmias

Perhaps the most detrimental effect of thyrotoxicosis, and clearly evident in the more severe state of thyroid storm (see below), is pyrexia. Increased body temperature may be secondary to the increased basal metabolic rate or actual resetting of hypothalamic thermoregulation. Pyrexia further increases cardiovascular stress; therefore, reduction of body temperature is an important goal of therapy.

Neurologic complications of severe thyrotoxicosis span the neuromuscular disorders of myopathy (in over 50 percent of all hyperthyroid patients; classified as "severe" in 4 percent),[2] exophthalmic ophthalmoplegia, aggravation of myasthenia gravis, and thyrotoxic periodic paralysis (primarily in Asian men). With the exception of the irritability and tremulousness, the delirium, stupor, coma, and convulsions may be related to the direct action of thyroid hormone on the brain.[3] Thyroid hormone can affect the concentrations and distributions of various neurotransmitters.[4] Hematologic manifestations of thyrotoxicosis[5] are rarely life-threatening. It is useful for the intensivist to be aware that hyperthyroidism can cause slight anemia. Anemia may be secondary to hemodilution because of increased blood volume, but true reduction of red blood cell mass may be caused by reduced iron absorption and vitamin B_{12} deficiency associated with autoimmune reduction of gastric acidity and intrinsic factor. Minimal thrombocytopenia, with rare instances of idiopathic thrombocytopenic purpura, has been reported.[6] Moderate eosinophilia may occur, which has been attributed to relative or absolute hypoadrenalism. There may be a variable relative and absolute lymphocytosis associated with hyperthyroidism. These manifestations may cloud the picture of a critically ill patient who may have other hematologic perturbations for different reasons.

Hypercalcemia is the most common life-threatening electrolyte abnormality seen in thyrotoxicosis.[5] Severe hypercalcemia (11.8 to 19.2 mg/dL) has been reported in several patients with thyrotoxicosis.[7]

The most notable effect of thyrotoxicosis on the gastrointestinal system is hypermotility with malabsorption.[8] The myopathy of hyperthyroidism may cause weakness of the striated muscles of the pharynx and, perhaps, the smooth muscle of the esophagus. Such patients could have dysphagia, then could aspirate and develop pneumonia.[9] Patients with hyperthyroidism appear to have a higher incidence of gastritis.[10] This is consistent with the hypergastrinemia seen in thyrotoxic patients.[11] Treatment with H_2 blockers is indicated.

Rarely, fulminant hepatic necrosis or less severe hepatic injury may occur. Although thyroid hormone has no direct toxic effect on the liver, the change in cardiac output, with diminished oxygen supply to the liver, can result in hepatic failure. In patients receiving propylthiouracil (PTU), drug toxicity is more likely the cause of fulminant hepatic necrosis.[12] Any thyrotoxic patient who presents with jaundice or other signs of hepatic injury should have a thorough evaluation for possible alternative causes of liver damage.

Thyroid Storm

Thyroid storm, or *thyrotoxic crisis,* is a life-threatening, though rare, complication of severe thyrotoxicosis. The diagnosis is clinical, bearing no direct relation to the absolute levels of thyroid hormones in serum. The cardinal features of thyroid storm are marked tachycardia, hypertension, and widened pulse pressure; hyperpyrexia (usually greater than 38.5°C); and altered mental status. In extreme cases, cardiovascular collapse and shock may be seen. Some investigators contend that abnormal mentation is the most important diagnostic component of thyroid storm.[13] Of course, these clinical features can occur with a multitude of illnesses in the absence of thyrotoxicosis. A blood sample for the measurement of T_4, free T_4 or the free T_4 index (FT_4I), and TSH, by a sensitive method, should immediately be obtained in all individuals suspected of having this disorder. Empiric treatment should then begin. It is prudent to obtain a blood sample for cortisol determination before administration of "stress doses" of steroids, in order to decide later whether long-term therapy is necessary. Laboratory findings in thyroid storm are listed in Table 162-2.

PRECIPITATING FACTORS

Patients who develop thyroid storm usually have poorly controlled thyrotoxicosis; often there is an identifiable precipitating factor (see Table 162-3).[13,14] In many cases it is difficult to determine whether the intercurrent illness is the cause or the consequence of the thyroid storm.

TREATMENT

The treatment of thyroid storm should take a four-pronged approach to prevent irreversible cardiovascular collapse—

TABLE 162-2 Laboratory Findings in Thyroid Storm

Elevated T_4 and free T_4 (FT_4I)
Elevated T_3
Hyperglycemia
Leukocytosis with left shift
Anemia
Hypercalcemia
Hypokalemia
Abnormal liver function tests
Hypercortisolemia

TABLE 162-3 Factors Precipitating Thyroid Storm

Surgery
Infection
Acute psychiatric illness
Congestive heart failure
Diabetic ketoacidosis
Pulmonary embolism
Bowel infarction
Parturition
Trauma
Vigorous palpation of thyroid gland
Withdrawal of antithyroid medication
Radioactive iodide therapy
Iodine-containing contrast agents
"Health food" preparation containing seaweed or kelp

namely, **1.** therapy aimed to reduce the serum thyroid hormone levels, **2.** therapy to reduce the action of the thyroid hormones on peripheral tissues, **3.** therapy to prevent cardiovascular decompensation and to maintain normal homeostasis, and **4.** treatment of the precipitating event(s).

THERAPY AIMED TO REDUCE THYROID HORMONE LEVELS

An antithyroid drug, either PTU or methimazole (MMI), is given to prevent further synthesis of thyroid hormone. These drugs are not available in parenteral form; they can only be given orally or by nasogastric tube. There may arise an occasion when PTU or MMI cannot be given even by nasogastric tube—as, for example, in patients with infarcted bowel. PTU offers a slight advantage over MMI in that, in addition to its inhibitory effect on hormone synthesis, it decreases the conversion of T_4 to T_3 in peripheral tissue. PTU should be given in a dose of 200 to 250 mg every 6 h, or MMI in a dose of 25 mg every 6 h. Some authors recommend an initial loading dose of 600 to 1000 mg PTU, but this has not been proved to be advantageous. MMI tablets may be crushed and placed in an aqueous solution and administered rectally (40 mg every 6 h); PTU is not water-soluble, and so cannot be prepared in this manner. The onset of action of PTU is immediate, in its blocking the synthesis of thyroid hormone; but it may take several weeks to normalize the serum levels, because of stored hormone. In severe thyrotoxicosis with decreased glandular content of hormone, significant decline in serum levels may be observed in a matter of a few days. We usually repeat thyroid function tests every other day while the patient is acutely ill, to help guide management.

Blockade of hormonal secretion is usually best accomplished by the addition of stable iodine to the antithyroid drug regimen. Iodine can be administered as Lugol's solution or a saturated solution of potassium iodide (ssKI) given 2 drops every 12 h, or by intravenous drip as sodium iodide (0.5 mg every 12 h). It is important to avoid using iodine without antithyroid drug blockade, as new hormone synthesis may occur and result in delayed release of hormone. There have been several cases where the use of iodine alone resulted in the precipitation of thyroid storm. Administration of antithyroid drugs 1 h before iodine is sufficient to establish blockade of hormone synthesis. A combination of antithyroid drugs and ssKI should decrease the serum T_3 level to the normal range in 1 to 5 days; however, the metabolic response may lag behind by 2 to 3 days.[15] Corticosteroids and propranolol, which also decrease the peripheral conversion of T_4 to T_3, can be used to further reduce serum T_3 concentration (see Tables 162-4 and 162-5).

In the event that antithyroid drugs cannot be used because of previous history of reactions, such as agranulocytosis or hepatotoxicity, iodine and oral cholecystographic agents may have to be used alone—the latter in the form of ipodate or iopanoate (iopanoic acid). These agents are strong inhibitors of the 5′ deiodination; thus they decrease serum T_3 and increase T_3.[16] They also bind to the thyroid hormone receptor, but it is unclear whether this results in competitive inhibition of T_3 action.[17] These agents have a high iodine content (approximately 60 percent by weight) and thus also act by releasing iodine in the course of their degradation. As in the case of iodine treatment, their administration without antithyroid drugs requires careful monitoring of the clinical status. Iopanoic acid (Telepaque) may be given in amounts of 1 to 3 g daily. We have found that 3 g/day often causes diarrhea; this can be prevented by giving 0.5 g 3 times per day, with no reduction of the drug's therapeutic efficacy. Alternatively, sodium ipodate (Oragrafin) may be used at 0.5 mg/day, which can reduce serum T_3 by 62 percent in 1 day.[18]

For the rare case of hypersensitivity to antithyroid drugs *and* a history of anaphylaxis to iodine-containing contrast media, lithium carbonate and perchlorate are alternative drugs. Lithium carbonate can be given in doses of 300 mg every 6 h, with subsequent adjustments to maintain a serum lithium level of 0.7 to 1.4 meq/L. Caution should be exercised in patients over 60 years of age. This drug acts by blocking iodide uptake and hormone release by the thyroid gland. Perchlorate competes with iodide uptake by the thyroid gland, ultimately reducing the production of T_4. Its serious side effects, including aplastic anemia and nephrotic syndrome, limit its use.

Successful reduction of thyroid hormone concentrations in serum has been reported using plasma exchange in 3 patients (2 of whom were pregnant).[19] Filtration through a resin bed that removes T_3 and T_4 has not yet been used clinically.[20] Intravenous administration of thyroxine-binding globulin has been shown experimentally to decrease thyroid hormone transfer from blood to tissues.[21]

PREVENTION OF DECOMPENSATION

Reduction of the body temperature decreases the demands on the cardiovascular system. This can be achieved by cooling and by pharmacologic blockade of the thermoregulatory centers. Use of a cooling blanket and ice packs alone will induce shivering; treatment with chlorpromazine, 25 to 50 mg, and meperidine, 25 to 50 mg, IV every 4 to 6 h will decrease the severe shivering and limit further generation of heat.[13]

Patients in thyroid storm lose excessive amounts of fluid, because of **1.** increased insensible water loss associated

TABLE 162-4 Mechanisms of Action of Antithyroid Drugs

	PTU	MMI	$LiCO_3$	$KClO_4$	ssKI	IOP	β Blockers	GLUCO	Cholestyramine	TBG
Reduction of serum hormone levels										
Block thyroidal I^- uptake			++	+++						
Block T_4 synthesis	+++	+++				+				
Block T_4 release			+ +	+	+++	+				
Block T_4-to-T_3 conversion	++					+++	+	+		
Decrease intestinal absorption of hormone									+	
Reduction of action on peripheral tissues										
Increase T_4 binding to serum protein										+++
Block thyroid hormone receptor						+				
Block sympathomimetic activity							+++	+		

+ = minor effect; ++ = moderate effect; +++=strong and principal effect; PTU = propylthiouracil; MMI = methimazole; $LiCO_3$ = lithium carbonate; $KClO_4$ = potassium perchlorate; ssKI = saturated solution of potassium iodide; IOP = iopanoic acid; GLUCO = glucocorticoids; TBG = thyroxine-binding globulin.

TABLE 162-5 Drugs Used in the Treatment of Thyrotoxicosis

Drug	Dose	How Supplied	Adverse Effects
Propylthiouracil (PTU)	200–250 mg q 6 h PO	50-mg TAB	Rash, agranulocytosis, hepatic toxicity
Methimazole (MMI)	25 mg q 6 h PO	5- and 50-mg TAB	Rash, agranulocytosis, hepatic toxicity
Lithium carbonate	300 mg q 6 h PO	150-, 300-, and 600-mg TAB	Nausea, vomiting, arrhythmias, pseudotumor cerebri
Lugol's solution	2 drops q 12 h PO	8 mg iodine/drop	Hypersensitivity
ssKI	1 drop q 12 h PO	50 mg iodide/drop	Hypersensitivity
Iopanoic acid	0.5 g tid PO	0.5-g TAB	Abdominal cramps, diarrhea, hypersensitivity, nephrotoxicity
Perchlorate	1.0 g qd	0.5-g TAB (66.7% organically bound)	Aplastic anemia
Propranolol	40 mg q 6 h PO 1 mg SLOW IVP	10-, 20-, 40-, 60-, and 80-mg TABS; 1-mg/mL vials	Asthma, heart block
Hydrocortisone	100 mg IVPB q 8 H	100-mg vials	Immunosuppression

with hyperthermia and tachypnea, **2.** decreased antidiuretic hormone, and **3.** vomiting and diarrhea associated with increased intestinal motility. Thus, patients may present with either high- or low-output failure and fluid management may necessitate right heart catheterization to determine filling pressures and guide management. Solutions containing crystalloid for volume replacement, and dextrose to replenish hepatic glycogen stores and minimize the breakdown of body protein, are used. Treatment with high doses of propranolol, as will be discussed below, can further necessitate the use of 5 to 10% dextrose solutions. Multivitamins are often administered to replenish the B-complex vitamins.

Treatment of congestive heart failure is usually supportive. While reduction of the high body temperature should be attempted before specific treatment is instituted, the judicious use of inotropic agents and diuretics should also be considered. Since patients are often volume-depleted, diuretics should be used carefully, and always with meticulous monitoring of intravascular volume. Impending shock should be treated with rapid correction of volume and inotropic agents, as indicated. Atrial fibrillation is a known complication of thyrotoxicosis. Control of ventricular response can be attained with β blockers, but conversion to sinus rhythm can be achieved only after the patient is made euthyroid.

Since relative hypoadrenalism is thought to occur in thyroid storm because of accelerated metabolism of glucocorticoids, it is prudent to give 300 mg of hydrocortisone IV, followed by 100 mg every 8 h to provide adequate stress levels. Additionally, glucocorticoids can be beneficial for their effect in reducing the conversion of T_4 to T_3 in peripheral tissue. Use of parenteral H_2 blockers is indicated to reduce the likelihood of ulcer formation. In thyrotoxicosis there is rapid clearance of drugs. Therefore, doses of digitalis, insulin, and antibiotics need to be increased to be effective. Two exceptions are adrenergic drugs and anticoagulants.[22] Furthermore, it is necessary to remember to reduce drug doses with improvement of the thyrotoxicosis.

REDUCTION OF THYROID HORMONE ACTION ON BODY TISSUES

The effects of thyroid hormone can be reduced by **1.** decreasing its conversion to the active form, T_3; **2.** counteracting its sympathomimetic effects; **3.** displacing it from its receptor; and **4.** reducing its transport to tissues.

The oral cholecystographic agents, as discussed above, may act in part by displacement of T_3 from its site of action at the receptor in cell nuclei. Other analogues of thyroid hormone with reduced thyromimetic activity, which nevertheless compete with thyroid hormone at its site of action, deserve theoretical consideration.[23] The activity of 5′-deiodinase is regulated by the concentration of T_4, as well as by catecholamines and other factors. PTU, glucocorticoids, propranolol, oral cholecystographic agents, and amiodarone also reduce the activity of this enzyme and thus decrease the generation of T_3, resulting in reduction of serum T_3 concentration. Severe acute or chronic nonthyroidal illness also suppresses T_3 generation in peripheral tissues.

β Blockers, useful in the preparation of thyrotoxic patients for surgery, should be used with caution in thyroid storm. Whereas surgical stress is clearly related to increased catecholamines, and thyroid storm can be prevented by the use of propranolol, it is unclear whether thyroid storm induced by other mechanisms is equally responsive to β blockers. However, when there is evidence of increased adrenergic activity short of thyroid storm (i.e., no evidence of hyperpyrexia, nor of mental status changes), 1 mg of propranolol can be administered by slow IV push every 5 min until an effect on pulse rate is seen. Usually a total daily dose of 300 to 400 mg oral propranolol is required to achieve effective β blockade in the severely thyrotoxic patient. It appears that younger patients are more prone to hyperadrenergic states with more labile courses, and do better with the β blockers.[13] This is in contradistinction to elderly patients, who may present with "apathetic" thyrotoxicosis without elevation in body temperature and without severe tachycardia. These elderly patients more often experience cardiotoxic effects in response to β blockers. Therefore, β blockers should be used with caution in thyroid storm and in severe thyrotoxicosis, except in the elderly, in asthmatics, and in patients with evidence of dilated cardiomyopathy. When surgery is indicated in such patients, careful titration of the adverse adrenergic cardiovascular effects (tachycardia, large pulse pressure) can be implemented with shorter duration β blockers (esmolol), preceded by maximal bronchodilator therapy in asthmatic patients or right heart catheterization in the elderly and in patients with prior heart failure.

TREATMENT OF PRECIPITATING EVENTS

Without an antecedent history of surgery, any patient with thyroid storm should be suspected of being septic until proven otherwise. Blood, urine, and other body secretions (i.e., ascitic or pleural fluid and sputum) should be Gram-stained and cultured. Empiric use of broad-spectrum antibiotics is recommended.

In a seriously ill patient in whom an infection or other precipitating cause, such as diabetic ketoacidosis, cannot be identified, pulmonary thromboembolism[24,25] or bowel infarction should be considered.

THYROID STORM IN PREGNANCY

The approach to treatment of thyroid storm in pregnant patients is similar to that outlined above. Thyroid storm is clearly a life-threatening condition for the mother. The basic approach to prevent decompensation is aggressive fluid replacement, along with treatment of the precipitating event and antithyroid therapy. β Blockers may have deleterious effects on the fetus at all stages of fetal development; therefore, their use must be weighed against maternal safety. While administration of iodide often results in the development of massive fetal goiter, PTU can be given to the toxic pregnant patient with only a small likelihood of adverse effects on the fetus.

Anesthesia and Surgery: Risks and Management in Thyrotoxic Patients

The Swiss surgeon Emil Theodor Kocher (1841–1917) was not only the first to operate on hyperthyroid patients; he was also among the first to recognize that thyroidectomy carried a high rate of mortality in "unprepared" thyrotoxic patients. The stress of any form of surgery or anesthesia alone could push a mildly decompensated thyrotoxic patient into a thyroid crisis, a life-threatening condition (see above). Therefore, it is important to control thyrotoxicosis prior to surgery. Ideally the FT_4I should be below the upper limit of normal. Unfortunately, even in the presence of a rapid turnover rate, thyroxine has a half-life of at least 72 h, and frequently it takes more than 1 week to achieve a normal FT_4I—an unacceptable wait, especially when the need for surgery is urgent. In such instances the preoperative therapeutic goal is to prevent the occurrence of thyroid storm. Blocking the effect of thyroid hormone on the sympathetic nervous system, particularly on the heart, is an alternative (if not an ideal) approach to therapy.[26] An arbitrary goal of maintaining a heart rate below 90 beats per min may not always be achieved in patients who have a pulse rate of 210 beats per min at the outset. In fact, there are no strict criteria for the response to therapy prior to surgery. Propranolol is the most widely used drug[27–29]; although other parenteral preparations are now available, there is no clear evidence of advantages of one over another. Propranolol, however, has the added effect of decreasing the conversion of T_4 to T_3 in peripheral tissues. This effect may not be shared by other β blockers, such as atenolol.[30] By and large, β blockers have little effect on the serum concentration of T_4 or on the metabolic status of the patient. The use of an antithyroid drug (PTU or MMI) and iodide, combined, provides the most rapid means of reduction of thyroid hormone in serum; these agents block its synthesis and its release, respectively. Although the results of determinations of serum thyroid hormone concentrations may not be available on a STAT basis, it is important to obtain a blood sample before initiating treatment.

We would like to discuss three scenarios for the preoperative treatment of thyrotoxic patients. First, consider an ICU patient who is in a septic condition with severe cholecystitis. The presence of thyrotoxicosis has been confirmed by an FT_4I of 21 (normal range 6 to 10.5) and a TSH level below 0.1 mU/L (normal range 0.4 to 4.0 mU/L). A cholecystectomy is planned as the definitive treatment, to take place in approximately 1 week. In this instance the physician has time to institute therapy aimed at reduction of the thyroid hormone concentration and to follow serum hormone levels as guides of therapeutic response. Initiation of PTU, 200 mg every 8 h orally or via nasogastric tube, followed by 1 or 2 drops of ssKI twice daily, is the suggested method for treatment of this patient's thyrotoxicosis. The reason for starting PTU before iodide is to prevent flooding the gland with iodide, which has been shown to produce, on occasion, a later exacerbation of thyrotoxicosis. A full discussion of these drugs appears under Thyroid Storm, above, and in Table 162-4. Thyroid function tests should be obtained every 2 days.

Second, consider a 65-year-old woman admitted for semi-emergent aortic valvuloplasty for severe aortic stenosis due to rheumatic carditis. She has been noted to be thyrotoxic; recent thyroid function tests revealed an FT_4I of 19 and a TSH of less than 0.1 mU/L. The valvuloplasty has been scheduled for tomorrow morning. While antithyroid drugs and ssKI should be given at the onset, in this case there is little chance for this treatment to reduce the thyroid hormone levels in 24 h. Propranolol can provide a rapid and effective preparation for surgery.[27] An initial dose of 40 mg every 6 h is appropriate, to be followed by increments of 20 mg every 6 h, depending on the response as judged by the heart rate. Although the usual dose is approximately 40 mg every 6 h, doses of up to 320 mg/day may be required. Symptoms of tachycardia, anxiety, and sweating should be relieved within 12 h. Intraoperative propranolol may be administered for tachycardia as needed. Propranolol should be resumed within 4 to 6 h following surgery and maintained for 48 h. If the patient is unable to take oral medication perioperatively, then propranolol can be administered as a 1.0- to 2.0-mg slow IV bolus. On postoperative day 3 the dose of propranolol can be halved; it can be halved again on day 4, and discontinued completely on day 5, 6, or 7, depending on the symptoms and the response to antithyroid drug therapy. Propranolol is not indicated in patients with bronchial asthma, advanced grades of heart block, or unstable insulin-dependent diabetes; nor in those patients taking quinidine or psychotropic drugs that augment adrenergic activity. Although β blockers are generally contraindicated in congestive heart failure, when administered with caution they are useful in correcting the high-output failure of thyrotoxicosis. Three cases have been reported in which thyroid storm followed surgery prepared only with propranolol.[31,32]

Third, consider a 25-year-old 38-week primigravida who must undergo emergent cesarean section for fetal distress. The patient is known to have active Graves' disease. She has not been compliant in taking the prescribed PTU, and is febrile, tachycardiac, and hallucinating. Appropriate preparation for this patient prior to general anesthesia and emergency cesarean section would be intravenous propranolol, 1.0 to 2.0 mg as a slow IV bolus. Then 10 to 15 mg propranolol can be added to 500 mL 5% dextrose and infused while the patient's and fetus's heart rates are monitored. Continuation of the propranolol after surgery would be indicated, as discussed above. The use of atropine to control bronchial secretions during surgery should be avoided in thyrotoxic patients, because of possible exacerbation of the sympathomimetic activity. There are reports of the use of plasma exchange in severe thyrotoxicosis of pregnancy.[18]

Levothyroxine Overdose

Levothyroxine ($L\text{-}T_4$) is commonly dispensed and, in the United States, accounted for 1.4 percent of all prescriptions written in 1986 (approximately 12 million prescriptions).[33] This wide availability leads to frequent overdoses, with reports of 2000 to 5000 acute toxic exposures annually in this country.[33,34] Despite the high frequency of overdosage, with documented blood levels of T_4 up to 16 times normal, there has been no reported mortality from $L\text{-}T_4$ ingestion.[35] Clearly, patients do become symptomatic, with tachycardia, nervousness, diarrhea, and even seizures; but these symptoms are generally self-limited.

The most commonly used thyroid preparation today is synthetic $L\text{-}T_4$, which has practically no T_3, in contrast to the thyroid preparations of 20 years ago (which consisted of thyroid gland extracts containing considerable amounts of T_3). Therefore, ingestion of a large quantity of $L\text{-}T_4$ does not cause immediate toxic effects. Symptoms occur after a significant amount of T_4 has been converted to T_3, usually about 24 h after ingestion. After gastrointestinal decontamination, by induction of vomiting with syrup of ipecac and gastric lavage using charcoal, only symptomatic and supportive treatment is indicated. Recommendations by Lehrner and Weir,[36] based on experience with two cases and review of the literature, are aggressive treatment with **1.** gastrointestinal decontamination; **2.** cholestyramine, to increase fecal elimination of the hormone; **3.** prednisone and propylthiouracil; and **4.** propranolol. Recently, Gorman et al[35] recommended only gastrointestinal decontamination and propranolol if the patient is markedly symptomatic. They suggest home gastrointestinal decontamination when 0.5 mg $L\text{-}T_4$ has been ingested, and determination of serum T_4 with ingestions on the order of 2.0 to 4.0 mg. Elderly patients and persons with underlying cardiac disease warrant hospitalization for observation if the serum T_4 level is high or the patient is symptomatic. The use of other medical therapy should await the onset of symptoms.

Neonatal Thyrotoxicosis

Neonatal thyrotoxicosis is a rare emergency that is treatable, but nevertheless is associated with a 12 to 16 percent rate of mortality.[37,38] A neonate presents signs of thyrotoxicosis within the first 24 h of life or later if the mother was on thyroid-suppressive therapy. Physical findings are goiter, tachypnea, tachycardia, cardiomegaly, hyperkinesis, restlessness, diarrhea, and poor weight gain. Flushing, periorbital edema, and exophthalmos may also be present.

Most infants with neonatal thyrotoxicosis are born to mothers with hyperthyroidism. Neonatal thyrotoxicosis can also occur with no documented maternal thyroid disease, and even in the presence of maternal hypothyroidism. In most cases this disease is caused by transplacental transfer of thyroid-stimulating immunoglobulin.[39] In others, where such a substance cannot be demonstrated in the mother's serum, there may be de novo formation of thyroid-stimulating immunoglobulins in the fetus due to neonatal Graves' disease.

Treatment of neonatal thyrotoxicosis is short-term until the placentally transferred immunoglobulins have disappeared. PTU is given at doses of 5 to 10 mg/kg per day in 3 divided daily doses. Iodide solutions (10% potassium iodide, 76.6 mg/mL) may be given in a dose of 1 drop, or about 4 mg, every 8 h. High-output congestive heart failure and other sympathomimetic effects can be treated with propranolol, 2 mg/kg per day in 2 or 3 divided doses. Caution should be exercised in the use of propranolol, since severe bradycardia and hypoglycemia may result.[40]

Iodide-induced Thyrotoxicosis (Iod-Basedow)

Iodide, in the form of dietary supplements or medication (e.g., antitussive agents, amiodorone, or contrast agents), can induce thyrotoxicosis, especially in patients who are relatively iodide-deficient. Treatment requires special considerations, since antithyroid drugs alone are slow to act (because of a flooded iodine pool). To deplete the gland of iodine, perchlorate must be added to the therapeutic regimen—particularly in amiodarone-induced thyrotoxicosis.[41] Naturally, iodide treatment is not indicated.

CASE PRESENTATION

A 52-year-old black female with a history of rheumatoid arthritis, occlusive coronary artery disease, and mild renal insufficiency for 2 years was admitted for cardiac catheterization because of angina pectoris of 6 months' duration. History and physical findings were suggestive of hyperthyroidism; review of the patient's thyroid function studies obtained 14 months prior to admission revealed a T_4 of 16 μg/dL (normal value, 5.0 to 12.0) an FT_4I of 19.2 (normal value, 6.0 to 10.5), and an undetectable (under 0.1 mU/L) TSH (normal value, 0.5 to 4.0). Creatinine at that time was 2.1 mg/dL, thought to be secondary to hypertensive renal disease with an associated type IV renal tubular acidosis. Results of tests covering the entire course of this patient's illness are shown in Fig. 162-1. On the day of admission the patient had an FT_4I of 14.4, a TSH under 0.01 mU/L, and a T_3 of 233 ng/dL (normal value, 90 to 185). Medications included ibuprofen and oral nitroglycerin. Because exacerbation of her underlying coronary artery disease by thyrotoxicosis was considered to be the reason for anginal symptoms, she was started on PTU, 150 mg tid, and was discharged from the hospital without the cardiac catheterization having been performed. She was readmitted 13 days later because of diarrhea and pruritic rash over extremities and trunk. Three days earlier, she had discontinued the PTU. Her FT_4I was 20.4, TSH under 0.1 mU/L, and—because the white blood cell count was normal (9.9×10^3 cells per mm^3)—PTU treatment was reinstituted. Twenty-four hours later it was noted that the rash had worsened; within 72 h the patient developed fever and confusion associated with a reduction of the white blood cell count to 1.4×10^3 cells per mm^3 (associated with 1 percent band forms, 13 percent neutrophils, 39 percent lymphocytes, 30 percent monocytes, and 17 percent eosinophils). Serum creatinine was 2.5 mg/dL. The patient was started on iopanoic acid and ssKI. Within 1 week the FT_4I decreased to 14.5, and, as expected, the rT_3 increased to 182 ng/dL, with marked improvement and complete recovery of mental function. One month later, in a follow-up clinic visit, the FT_4I was normal, at 8.2, with maintenance of suppressed T_3 at 79 ng/dL, but the creatinine was noted to be 4.9 mg/dL. Under hospital supervision the iopanoic acid was discontinued and propranolol was added to the ssKI. On day 6 the patient underwent a subtotal thyroidectomy. The pathologic findings were consistent with Graves' disease. The patient had an uneventful postoperative recovery, but required thyroid hormone replacement because of postoperative hypothyroidism (TSH 18.6 mU/L 1 month after surgery).

CASE DISCUSSION

This case illustrates a number of aspects presented in this chapter. On the second hospital admission (period B, Fig. 162-1) the patient fulfilled the criteria for thyroid storm (hyperpyrexia and altered mental status). The complicating event that followed was PTU-induced leukopenia and a rash. Iopanoic acid and ssKI were given as an alternative treatment of thyroid storm, along with adjunctive therapy. Note the marked increase in rT_3 as a consequence of the inhibitory effect of iopanoic acid on 5′-deiodinase and the reduction of serum T_4 by the ssKI-induced blockade of T_4 release from the thyroid gland. The decrease in renal function associated with the use of iopanoic acid has also been reported (manufacturer's package insert). It was particularly severe in this patient, probably because of the already-compromised renal function. This new development necessitated yet another change in the approach to therapy. Since radioiodide could not be used, because of suppressed thyroidal uptake by the treatment with stable iodine, the only viable therapeutic alternative was surgical thyroidectomy.

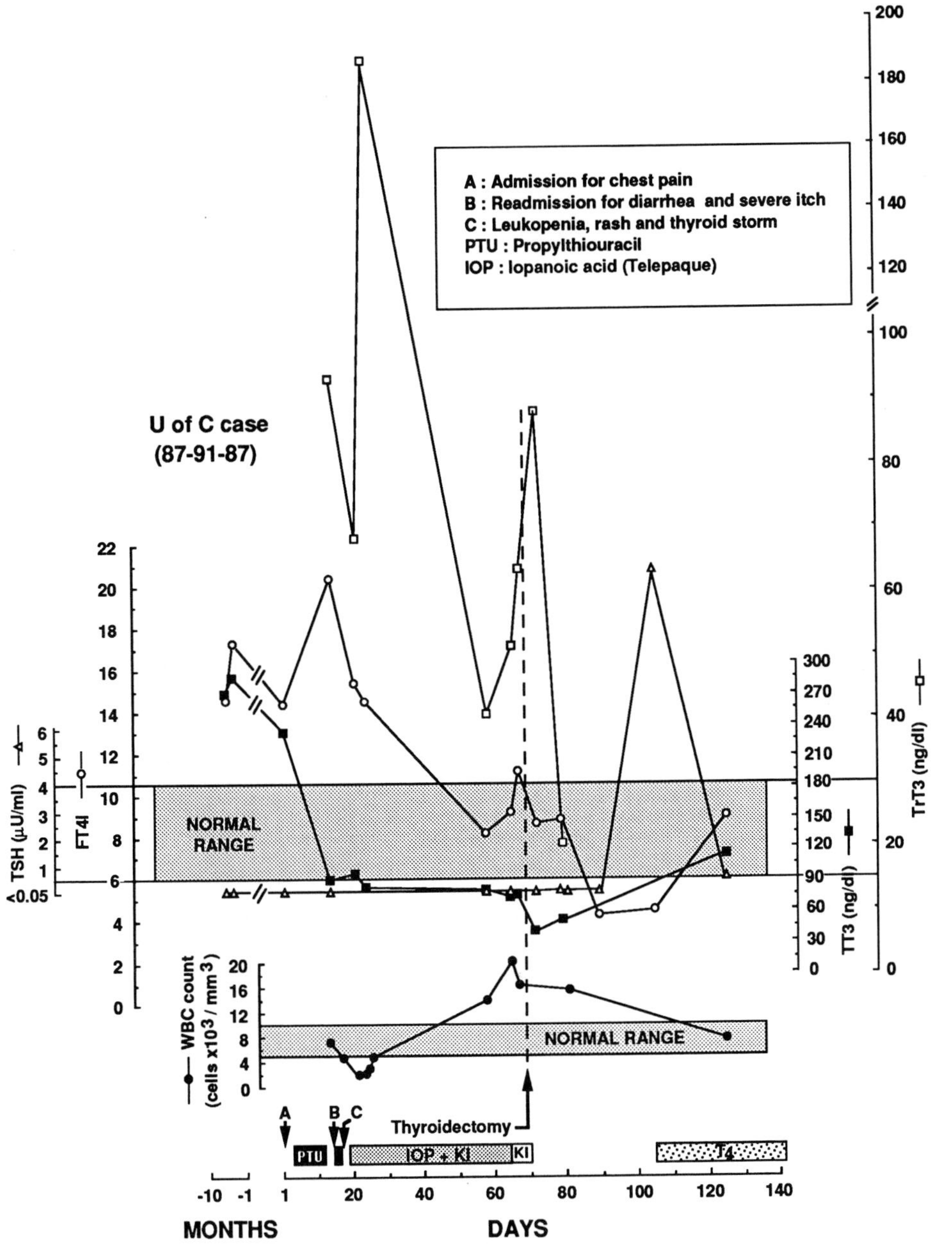

FIGURE 162-1 Diagrammatic representation of the course of illness in a 52-year-old female who presented with thyrotoxicosis. In brief, the patient initially presented with chest pain; the diagnosis of thyrotoxicosis was made, and the patient treated with PTU. Improvement of thyroid function and disappearance of the chest pain were noted. She was admitted several days later for diarrhea, fever, leukopenia, and a rash, which was diagnosed as PTU toxicity; she subsequently developed thyroid storm with hyperpyrexia and altered level of consciousness, and was treated with ssKI and iopanoic acid. Her thyroid function again improved on this regimen, but she was noted to have worsening renal function. The iopanoic acid was discontinued and the patient was admitted for a third time for surgical thyroidectomy, which resulted in permanent hypothyroidism. For further details, refer to text.

Preparation for surgery consisted of continuing the ssKI and addition of propranolol. The postoperative course was unremarkable, except for the inability of the residual gland to maintain euthyroidism. Lifelong need for L-T_4 replacement is anticipated.

References

1. Ingbar SH: Classification of the causes of thyrotoxicosis, in Ingbar SH, Braverman LE (eds): *The Thyroid*. Philadelphia, JB Lippincott, 1986, p 809.
2. Kudrjavcev T: Neurologic complications of thyroid dysfunction. Adv Neurol 19:619, 1978.
3. Vaccari A: Effects of dysthyroidism on central monoaminergic neurotransmission (review). Monogr Neural Sci 9:78, 1983.
4. Adams RD, DeLong GR: The neuromuscular system and brain, in Ingbar SH, Braverman LE (eds): *The Thyroid*. Philadelphia, JB Lippincott, 1986, p 885.
5. Katz Al, Emmanouel DS, Lindheimer MD: Thyroid hormone and the kidney. Nephron 15:223, 1975.
6. Herbert V: The blood, in Ingbar SH, Braverman LE (eds): *The Thyroid*. Philadelphia, JB Lippincott, 1986, p 878.
7. Parfitt AM, Dent LE: Hyperthyroidism and hypercalcemia. Q J Med 39:171, 1970.
8. Sellin JH, Vassilopoulou-Sellin R, Lester R: The gastrointestinal tract and liver, in Ingbar SH, Braverman LE (eds): *The Thyroid*. Philadelphia, JB Lippincott, 1986, p 871.
9. Sack TL, Sleisenger MH: Effects of systemic and extraintestinal disease on the gut, in Sleisenger MH, Fordtran JS (eds): *Gastrointestinal Disease*. Philadelphia, WB Saunders, 1989, p 488.

10. Siurala M, Lamberg BA: Stomach in thyrotoxicosis. Acta Med Scand 165:181, 1952.
11. Sagara K, Shimada T, Fujiyama S, Sato T: Serum gastrin levels in thyroid dysfunction. Gastroenterol Jpn 18:79, 1983.
12. Hanson JS: Propylthiouracil and hepatitis. Two cases and a review of the literature. Arch Intern Med 144:994, 1984.
13. Nicoloff JT: Thyroid storm and myxedema coma. Med Clin North Am 69:1005, 1985.
14. Wartofsky L: Thyrotoxic storm, in Ingbar SH, Braverman LE (eds): *The Thyroid*. Philadelphia, JB Lippincott, 1986, p 974.
15. Wartofsky L, Ransil BJ, Ingbar SH: Inhibition by iodine of the release of thyroxine from the thyroid glands of patients with thyrotoxicosis. J Clin Invest 49:78, 1970.
16. Wu S-Y, Chopra IJ, Solomon DH, Johnson DE: The effect of repeated administration of ipodate (Oragrafin) in hyperthyroidism. J Clin Endocrinol Metab 47:1358, 1978.
17. DeGroot LJ, Rue PA: Roentgenographic contrast agents inhibit triiodothyronine binding to nuclear receptors in vitro. J Clin Endocrinol Metab 49:538, 1979.
18. Shen DC, Wu SY, Chopra IJ, et al: Long term treatment of Graves' hyperthyroidism with sodium ipodate. J Clin Endocrinol Metab 61:723, 1985.
19. Derksen RHWM, van de Wiel A, Poortman J, et al: Plasma exchange in the treatment of severe thyrotoxicosis in pregnancy (case reports). Eur J Obstet Gynecol Reprod Biol 18:139, 1984.
20. Burman KD, Yeager HC, Briggs WA, et al: Resin hemoperfusion: A method of removing circulating thyroid hormones. J Clin Endocrinol Metab 42:70, 1976.
21. Wahl R, Schmidberger H, Fessler E, et al: Effects of human thyroxine-binding globulin and prealbumin on the reverse flow of thyroid hormones from extravascular space into the bloodstream in rabbits. Endocrinology 124:1428, 1989.
22. Kellett HA, Sawers JS, Boulton FE, et al: Problems of anticoagulation with warfarin in hyperthyroidism. Q J Med 58:43, 1986.
23. Jorgensen ES: Stereochemistry of thyroxine and analogues. Mayo Clin Proc 39:560, 1964.
24. Giddings NB, Surks MI: Cerebral embolism in atrial fibrillation complicating hyperthyroidism. JAMA 240:2567, 1978.
25. Parker, JL, Lawson PH: Death from thyrotoxicosis. Lancet 2:894, 1973.
26. Toft AD, Irvine WJ, Sinclair I, et al: Thyroid function after surgical treatment of thyrotoxicosis. N Engl J Med 298:643, 1978.
27. Lee TC, Coffey RJ, Currier BM, et al: Propranolol and thyroidectomy in the treatment of thyrotoxicosis. Ann Surg 195:766, 1982.
28. Haddad JF, Tibblin S: Preoperative treatment of thyrotoxicosis in developing countries: A comparative study of carbimazole and propranolol. Ann R Coll Surg Engl 70:357, 1988.
29. Crooks JF, Forrest AL, Hamilton WF, Gunn A: Propranolol in the surgical treatment of hyperthyroidism, including severely thyrotoxic patients. Br J Surg 68:865, 1981.
30. How ASM, Khir AN, Bewsher PD: The effect of atenolol on serum thyroid hormones in hyperthyroid patients. Clin Endocrinol 13:299, 1980.
31. Eriksson M, Rubenfeld S, Garber A, Kohler P: Propranolol does not prevent thyroid storm. N Engl J Med 296:263, 1977.
32. Jamison M: Postop thyrotoxic crisis in a patient prepared for thyroidectomy with propranolol. Br J Clin Pract 33:82, 1979.
33. 1986 Annual Report of the American Association of Poison Control Centers National Data Collection System. Am J Emerg Med 5:405, 1987.
34. Kulig K, Golightly LK, Rumack BH: Levothyroxine overdose associated with seizures in a young child. JAMA 254:2109, 1985.
35. Gorman GL, Chamberlain JM, Rose SR, Oderda GM: Massive levothyroxine overdose: High anxiety—low toxicity. Pediatrics 82:666, 1988.
36. Lehrner LM, Weir MR: Acute ingestion of thyroid hormone. Pediatrics 73:313, 1984.
37. Hollingsworth DR, Mabry CC: Congenital Graves' disease, in Fisher DA, Burrow GN (eds): *Perinatal Thyroid Physiology and Disease*. New York, Raven Press, 1975, p 163.
38. Samuel S, Pildes RS, et al: Neonatal hyperthyroiditis in an infant born to a euthyroid mother. Am J Dis Child 121:440, 1971.
39. Singer J: Neonatal thyrotoxicosis. J Pediatr 91:749, 1977.
40. Gardner LI: Is propranolol alone really beneficial in neonatal thyrotoxicosis? Am J Dis Child 134:819, 1980.
41. Martino E, Aghini-Lombardi F, Mariotti S, et al: Treatment of amiodarone-associated thyrotoxicosis by simultaneous administration of potassium perchlorate and methimazole. J Endocrinol Invest 9:201, 1986.

SECTION N

GASTROINTESTINAL DISORDERS IN THE CRITICALLY ILL

Chapter 163

GASTROINTESTINAL HEMORRHAGE

IRA M. HANAN

KEY POINTS

- *Aggressive blood and volume replacement and airway protection are paramount in the management of the acutely bleeding patient.*
- *Diagnostic evaluation should take place only after adequate hemodynamic stabilization.*
- *Medical therapy is largely supportive.*
- *Early team approach, involving medical and surgical personnel, should be used.*
- *Pharmacologic therapy may be of limited value for continued bleeding, heightening the importance of endoscopic, angiographic, and surgical therapies.*

Gastrointestinal bleeding accounts for 2 percent of all medical and surgical hospital admissions in the United States.[1] Despite greater diagnostic capabilities afforded by gastrointestinal endoscopy and angiography, as well as improved drug therapy for peptic ulcer disease, mortality from gastrointestinal bleeding remains approximately 10 percent. Fifteen percent of patients require surgical intervention. The constant 10 percent mortality rate may reflect a changing patient population. Patients who would have died from exsanguination survive because of improved transfusion capabilities, while high-risk patients with various medical conditions, such as cancer, live longer to the point that they may develop gastrointestinal bleeding. Such patients are less likely to survive a bleed when it occurs. These factors may confound our ability to prove that early recognition of adverse risk factors limits morbidity and ultimately reduces mortality. Identifying the patient at risk of recurrent or ongoing bleeding may result in earlier surgical intervention and reduced surgical mortality.

Clinical Considerations

The identification of high-risk patients is important to plan appropriate diagnostic evaluation and therapeutic management of the bleeding patient. The rate at which bleeding occurs will determine the symptoms and signs. Additionally, regardless of the etiology or location of bleeding, the rate generally will determine the outcome.

The American Society of Gastrointestinal Endoscopy's (ASGE) 1981 study of upper gastrointestinal bleeding highlighted risk factors in patients with upper gastrointestinal bleeding.[2] Although a study in lower gastrointestinal bleeding has not been undertaken, the risk factors would likely be the same.

Age is an important determinant of outcome from gastrointestinal bleeding. Mortality for patients older than sixty is 30 percent higher than for patients sixty years or less (13.4 vs 8.7 percent). Morbidity is also higher in the older patient. The general medical history of an individual patient is important in assessing risk. Various concomitant diseases add further risk to the bleeding patient. Congestive heart failure and arrhythmias appear to be associated with increased mortality, while angina and hypertension do not. Concomitant central nervous system (CNS) disease, including acute and chronic encephalopathies or cerebral vascular accidents, may significantly increase the mortality from gastrointestinal bleeding. Not surprisingly, the presence of coexisting liver disease, even in patients with nonvariceal bleeding, heightens mortality. The ASGE study also highlights concomitant neoplastic, pulmonary, or renal disease, factors likely to significantly increase mortality, even in patients not requiring surgery.

Patients presenting to the hospital with a gastrointestinal bleed fare better than patients who bleed while hospitalized. Patients who have onset of bleeding in the hospital have a mortality rate of >30 percent. This likely reflects the high mortality associated with stress-related bleeding, which is more apt to account for gastrointestinal bleeding which presents during hospitalization.

The manner in which a patient bleeds may reflect the rate of bleeding and thus the outcome. For upper gastrointestinal bleeding, the presence of black stool, as opposed to brown stool, does not carry a higher mortality, morbidity, or need for surgery. However, patients passing red stool with an upper gastrointestinal bleed do have a poorer outcome. Likewise, the color of the nasogastric aspirate is important, with red blood predicting a higher mortality, morbidity, and need for surgery than coffee-ground color or clear aspirate. When combined, the stool color and nasogastric aspirate color can be important predictors of outcome. Patients with brown stool and a clear nasogastric aspirate have a favorable 8 percent mortality, compared with a 30 percent mortality rate in those with red blood in the stool and nasogastric aspirate. The underlying pathology accounting for bleeding, although not initially evident in most cases, can be predictive of eventual outcome. It is well recognized that one-third of patients presenting with esophageal variceal hemorrhage will die during the initial

TABLE 163-1 Initial Management for Severe Gastrointestinal Bleeding

1. Maintain two large bore IV catheters.
2. Resuscitate with crystalline fluid to restore blood pressure.
3. Delay endoscopy until patient is adequately resuscitated.
4. Transfuse packed red cells early to maintain hematocrit >30%.
5. Use platelet, fresh frozen plasma transfusions as needed to correct thrombocytopenia or coagulopathy.
6. CVP or Ppw monitoring may be helpful if bleeding from varices is suspected. A CVP <10 mmHg helps prevent recurrent variceal bleeding.
7. Nasogastric tube should be inserted if patient has hematemesis.
8. Use peripheral vasopressin nitroglycerin patch therapy in young cirrhotics with suspected variceal bleeding.
9. Obtain surgical consultation.

hospitalization.[3] On the contrary, a Mallory-Weiss tear of the gastroesophageal junction is associated with a low mortality rate, <5 percent.[2]

Regardless of the etiology and site of gastrointestinal bleeding, the initial management is similar (Table 163-1). When profound hemorrhage results in shock, orthostatic hypotension, or tachycardia, prompt blood and volume replacement are essential. Two large bore intravenous catheters should be maintained at all times. Initial volume replacement with crystalloid (normal saline or Ringer's solution) should be administered promptly. Although often not essential, central venous pressure (CVP) monitoring is useful in patients with suspected or known portal hypertension. This subgroup of patients should have CVP monitoring whenever possible to avoid fluid overload which may result in a further rise of portal pressure, thereby precipitating an additional bleeding episode. In the instance of left-sided heart failure, monitoring of pulmonary artery wedge pressure (Ppw) may be necessary after the patient is stabilized.

Prompt replacement of blood with packed red cells must follow crystalline replacement as soon as possible. While volume restoration with crystalloid will normalize blood pressure, the oxygen-carrying capacity will remain low, possibly resulting in myocardial or intestinal ischemia. In most instances, there is sufficient time to allow typing and crossmatching of red cells. Yet, if exsanguination is occurring, the transfusion of non-crossmatched type specific blood may be necessary (see Chap. 35).

The quantity of packed red blood cells to be transfused is variable, yet the goal of transfusion should be to keep the hematocrit above 30 percent. This will provide sufficient tissue oxygenation in the face of bleeding. Transfusion of platelets or fresh frozen plasma should be administered promptly if thrombocytopenia or coagulopathy accompany the bleeding episode. Attempts to raise the platelet count above 60,000 and lower the prothrombin time to within 2 s of control are desirable. The initial management of the bleeding patient should include nasogastric suctioning if hematemesis is occurring. The primary function of a nasogastric tube is to prevent aspiration by maintaining gastric decompression. The use of nasogastric lavage for diagnostic purposes, i.e., the documentation of an upper gastrointestinal bleeding source, is not necessary in most instances. The patient presenting with rectal bleeding and orthostasis or hypotension should have esophagogastroduodenoscopy (EGD) performed as the first diagnostic procedure regardless of the presenting features (see Chap. 33).

Surgical consultation should be sought early in the course of management. Collaboration with the surgical team allows coordinated planning, permitting appropriate timing of surgical intervention, if needed.

Upper Gastrointestinal Bleeding

DIAGNOSTIC EVALUATION OF UPPER GASTROINTESTINAL BLEEDING

Most patients who bleed from a source proximal to the ligament of Treitz will present with melena. Nearly 60 percent of bleeding episodes include melena as a feature, while red blood per rectum accompanies 17 percent of upper gastrointestinal bleeding.[2] More than half the episodes of upper gastrointestinal bleeding will be accompanied by a history of hematemesis, most often with red blood rather than coffee-ground material.[2]

Most patients do not have other significant symptoms. The majority of patients with upper gastrointestinal bleeding do not have abdominal pain, even when peptic ulcer disease is present. Absence of epigastric pain is particularly noted in the elderly when bleeding complicates peptic ulcer disease.

After stabilization, the diagnostic evaluation of the bleeding patient can begin. When an upper gastrointestinal bleeding source is suspected, or can easily be excluded in appropriate instances, EGD should be performed (see Chap. 33). EGD will provide diagnostic accuracy of >85 percent in patients with an upper gastrointestinal source of bleeding. Failure to identify the bleeding site generally is attributable to excessive hemorrhage or clot obscuring the field of vision.

When EGD fails to identify adequately the site of bleeding, two options exist. General support measures, including blood and volume replacement, nasogastric aspiration, among others, are continued, and EGD is repeated 6 to 12 h later if bleeding appears to have slowed. This may be evident by hemodynamic stabilization, ease of maintaining the hematocrit, or clearing the nasogastric aspirate. The second attempt by the endoscopist will identify the cause of bleeding in 70 percent of patients in whom the initial procedure did not.[4] Alternatively, if massive bleeding confronts the endoscopist, angiography may be used promptly, especially if surgical intervention is apparent.

The angiographic diagnosis of acute arterial hemorrhage is based on visualization of extravasated contrast material into the gastrointestinal tract. Therefore, it necessitates active bleeding at the time the study is performed. The bleeding must be of sufficient briskness, 0.5 to 1.0 mL/min to be demonstrable. When used correctly, angiography may demonstrate a bleeding site in 75 percent of patients with a brisk upper gastrointestinal bleed.[5] The majority of bleeding episodes, 85 percent, originate from a branch of the left gastric artery; the right gastric and short gastric arteries comprise 5 percent each.[6]

For variceal hemorrhage, the angiographic diagnosis is indirect, relying on visualization of varices during the venous phase of selective mesenteric angiography and the exclusion of an arterial bleeding site.[7] Obviously, confusion could exist in the cirrhotic patient in whom angiography is performed when bleeding has slowed. Varices may be present, yet may not account for the active hemorrhage, resulting in an angiographic study revealing only varices.

Radionuclide studies occasionally aid in detecting the site of acute gastrointestinal bleeding. Technetium 99m-labeled red blood cells and technetium 99m-labeled sulfur colloid both may be used to detect acute gastrointestinal bleeding with rates of bleeding <0.5 mL/min. It is important for the clinician to understand differences between these two techniques, because the method used in a particular bleeding scan may affect the sensitivity of the examination. Technetium 99m-labeled sulfur colloid disappears within minutes after injection, thereby requiring active bleeding during the time of immediate injection. Technetium 99m-labeled red blood cells remain in the blood pool for days, allowing repeated imaging for 1 to 2 days following injection. This difference has made the technetium 99m-labeled red blood cell technique the preferred one when attempting to determine gastrointestinal bleeding. When used in selected patients, the sensitivity may be >90 percent, with very high specificity.[8] However, caution regarding reproducibility of such results is warranted, because patient selection may influence the outcome of such studies. Furthermore, radionuclide studies suggest only an anatomic region from which bleeding may occur and do not offer an etiologic source. A positive result should prompt a repeat endoscopy or, if emergency surgery is planned, angiography to localize precisely the bleeding site, allowing the surgeon to limit a resection.

THERAPY

ACUTE VARICEAL HEMORRHAGE

The mainstay of therapy for acute variceal hemorrhage is supportive by maintaining hemodynamic parameters and preventing complications such as aspiration and ischemic injury to vital organs. Despite various pharmacologic and endoscopic interventions, the mortality rate from acute variceal hemorrhage is 30 percent. Controversy remains whether pharmacologic agents and sclerotherapy influence short-term survival of the bleeding patient (Fig. 163-1).

Vasopressin

Vasopressin, a potent vasoconstrictor, is widely used in the treatment of variceal hemorrhage. The theoretical beneficial effect is due to vasoconstriction of the splanchnic circulation, resulting in diminished portal blood flow and decreased portal venous pressure. Since 1956, when it was first used to control variceal hemorrhage, vasopressin has become standard therapy. However, the evidence supporting the benefit of vasopressin is largely anecdotal. Few well-controlled trials assessing vasopressin's ability to halt variceal bleeding and improve mortality have been undertaken. When compared with placebo, vasopressin has not improved mortality,[9] although it may transiently control bleeding.[10]

The presumption of efficacy of vasopressin in the control of variceal hemorrhage results from studies showing suc-

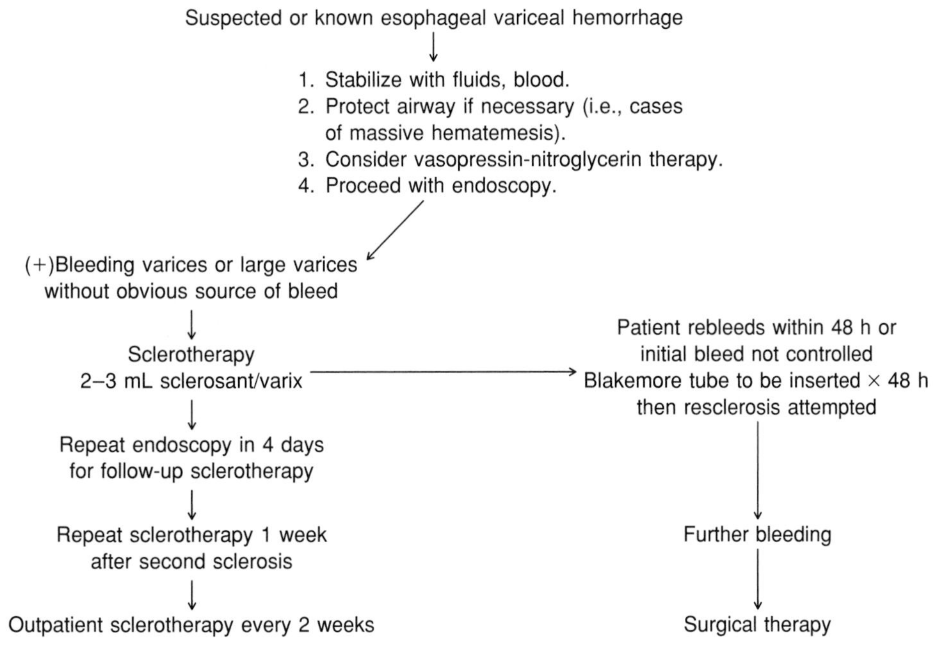

FIGURE 163-1 Evaluation and therapy of variceal hemorrhage.

cessful cessation of bleeding by intraarterial infusions of vasopressin. Noncontrolled trials suggest selective infusion of vasopressin into the superior mesenteric artery has controlled hemorrhage in more than half the patients treated, yet comparison with placebo is lacking.[11,12] Some authors have suggested equal benefit of both intravenous and intraarterial vasopressin, recommending the former due to the ease of administration.

Despite the controversy regarding its benefit, vasopressin remains widely used. An initial bolus of 20 U should be administered via peripheral intravenous access. Thereafter, infusion of 0.4 to 0.6 U/min should be continued. The higher dose should be used for the patient without known cardiac or peripheral vascular disease. This dose should be continued for at least 24 h, at which time tapering can begin if bleeding has been controlled. Tapering should proceed slowly over the next 24 h. Infusion through a central line may result in high concentrations reaching the cardiac vasculature, potentially resulting in vasoconstriction. For any given patient, the physician must assess the potential benefit of vasopressin weighed against the potential risks encountered in its use. As a vasoconstrictor, vasopressin's action is not limited to the splanchnic circulation. This accounts for multiple adverse systemic hemodynamic effects and particularly for a high rate of cardiovascular complications.

The minor complications encountered with intravenous vasopressin include abdominal pain, nausea, vomiting, pallor, transient hypertension, and sinus and junctional arrhythmias, including profound sinus bradycardia.[9] Major complications, including left-sided heart failure, pulmonary edema,[13] myocardial infarction, intracerebral hemorrhage,[9] and scrotal and abdominal skin necrosis[14] have been reported. Although intraarterial infusion reduces the systemic complications attributable to vasopressin, local complications may occur, including bleeding from or thrombosis of the femoral artery, thrombosis of the superior mesenteric artery, and mesenteric ischemia.

The younger patient, without suspected peripheral or cardiac vascular disease, generally can tolerate intravenous vasopressin infusion. The physician must keep in mind the lack of conclusive evidence that vasopressin controls bleeding when managing the elderly patient who is more likely to develop cardiovascular complications.

The concurrent use of transdermal or sublingual nitroglycerin with vasopressin has received attention. Nitroglycerin reverses the undesirable hemodynamic response to vasopressin while potentiating vasopressin's reduction of portal venous pressure.[15] Trials comparing vasopressin alone versus vasopressin and nitroglycerin for the control of variceal hemorrhage have not shown any improvement in mortality, although major complications attributable to vasopressin are reduced when nitroglycerin is used.[16,17] Currently, the concomitant use of transdermal nitroglycerin with vasopressin is advisable.

Alternate Pharmacotherapy

Long-acting analogues of somatostatin have been used to control variceal hemorrhage. Pharmacologic doses of somatostatin produce selective splanchnic vasoconstriction, thereby reducing portal pressure and blood flow.[18] Unlike vasopressin, these potentially beneficial effects of somatostatin are not associated with systemic hemodynamic effects. Several uncontrolled studies have shown that somatostatin infusion can control bleeding from esophageal varices.[19,20] However, further controlled trials assessing the effectiveness of somatostatin in the management of variceal hemorrhage are necessary.

The chronic prophylactic use of β-blocker therapy to prevent recurrent variceal hemorrhage in cirrhotics has been advocated by some.[21] Its benefit in nonalcoholic cirrhotic patients is disputed.[22] β-Blocker therapy is never indicated in the acute management of variceal bleeding. Although intravenous β-blocker drugs may acutely reduce portal venous pressure, their effects on heart rate are undesirable in the acutely bleeding patient.

Sclerotherapy

First described in 1939 to control variceal hemorrhage, endoscopic variceal sclerotherapy (EVS) has become a first-line therapy to control acute variceal hemorrhage, as well as to prevent rebleeding. EVS is indicated at the time of diagnostic endoscopy when active bleeding from a visible varix is seen, or when large nonbleeding esophageal varices are present without other obvious etiologies to account for recent hemorrhage. In the former situation, EVS can control bleeding in 95 percent of patients[23] when performed by an experienced endoscopist. Rebleeding, however, represents a formidable problem in patients receiving EVS. Controlled studies note rebleeding rates within 48 h to range from 20 percent to 74 percent.[23,24] The timing of EVS may have an impact on the outcome of a variceal hemorrhage. Rebleeding rates, complications, and death from exsanguination may be greater when EVS is delayed until after initial control of bleeding with vasopressin and tamponade tube.[24] Blood transfusion requirements are reduced in patients receiving immediate EVS.[25] Since it appears to be more effective in controlling acute hemorrhage, with a lower complication rate than with the use of a tamponade tube, EVS should be attempted prior to the use of such tubes. When compared to portacaval shunt, EVS is less costly and equally effective in controlling variceal hemorrhage in severe cirrhotics. Neither therapy has an advantage in lowering mortality.[26]

If EVS is successful in controlling active hemorrhage, it must be continued until obliteration of varices is complete. This generally requires months of treatment, which can effectively be accomplished on an outpatient basis.[27] Following the initial therapy, EVS should be repeated approximately 4 days after the first session, presuming ulceration of the distal esophagus is not profound. In such an instance, further EVS may need to be delayed a week. Two or three EVS treatments should be scheduled over a 10-day period while the patient is hospitalized. Thereafter, therapy should be continued every 1 to 3 weeks, depending on individual ulceration rate and patient acceptance. Sclerotherapy should only be performed twice within the initial 3 days, because more frequent therapy may result in esophageal necrosis. Therefore, any patient who has recurrent bleeding after two sessions of sclerotherapy within the first 3 days should be considered a sclerotherapy failure. The more frequently EVS can be performed, the sooner varices will be obliterated. Complete obliteration of varices is necessary to prevent future variceal hemorrhage. When complete obliteration is accomplished, long-term rebleeding rates are lower and survival improved.[28]

It is essential that the endoscopist exclude other sources of gastrointestinal hemorrhage, ensuring that the esophageal varices account for the bleeding episode. The presence of large esophageal varices, which have never bled, does not warrant prophylactic therapy, because the complication rate outweighs benefit.[29]

Sclerotherapy is not advisable for large bleeding gastric or duodenal varices. Although anecdotal reports exist,[30] the rebleeding and mortality rates are high,[31] likely due to the extremely high pressure in such varices.

Tamponade Tubes

Balloon tamponade of esophageal varices generally is reserved for hemorrhage which fails to stop after therapy with vasopressin and sclerotherapy. The Sengstaken-Blakemore (S-B) tube is most frequently used. Its double-balloon system allows for compression of gastric and esophageal varices, as opposed to the less frequently used Linton tube, which tamponades only gastric varices. Additionally, both tubes have a large bore lumen for gastric lavage and suction. The S-B tube is indicated for active variceal hemorrhage sufficient to cause hemodynamic instability or lead to aspiration. It has no role as prophylaxis against recurrence once bleeding has ceased. Because aspiration may complicate the insertion of an S-B tube, endotracheal intubation for airway protection generally is advised. The S-B tube can be passed either nasally or orally to full insertion. After inflation of approximately 30 mL air into the gastric balloon, radiographic confirmation of the gastric balloon's position in the stomach should be made. Thereafter, the gastric balloon can safely be inflated to its maximal capacity. Maximal inflation of a gastric balloon inadvertently located in the esophagus can result in esophageal perforation. Following insufflation of the gastric balloon, it is preferable to insufflate the esophageal balloon to 35 mmHg, a pressure exceeding the intravariceal pressure, although some inflate the esophageal balloon only if tamponade of the cardiofundic region by the gastric balloon fails to control hemorrhage. Traction is necessary to maintain proper positioning of the apparatus. Compression of varices for 48 h is recommended. Prolonged use of the S-B tube is limited by local ischemia produced by compression of the esophageal wall. A nasogastric tube inserted above the esophageal balloon prevents aspiration of oropharyngeal secretions which pool above the inflated apparatus. Alternatively, a tamponade tube with an esophageal suction channel can be used. Following deflation of the balloons, the S-B tube should be left in place for an additional 24 h so that it can easily be reinflated should bleeding recur. If rebleeding does not occur during this time, the S-B tube can be removed. If rebleeding occurs immediately on deflation, it should be reinflated but only until definitive therapy, such as a shunt procedure, can be performed. Aspiration and esophageal perforation comprise the major complications of tamponade tube use, resulting in a 3 percent mortality rate.

Balloon tamponade can control hemorrhage in more than 90 percent of cases, yet the effects are often temporary with an early rebleeding rate as high as 25 percent.[32] Therefore, balloon tamponade should be considered to control ongoing bleeding, allowing stabilization of the patient until definitive therapy, either repeated sclerotherapy or surgical therapy, can be performed.

TABLE 163-2 Indications for Surgical Therapy for Variceal Hemorrhage

Child's class A or B patient in whom vital signs can not be stabilized despite medical management
Patients who bleed continuously for >48 h despite sclerotherapy and tamponade tube
Patients who present with third acute variceal hemorrhage despite previous variceal sclerotherapy
Patients presenting with acute variceal hemorrhage after noncompliance with planned sclerotherapy

Surgical Therapy

Unremitting or recurrent variceal hemorrhage may require surgical intervention to relieve portal hypertension or to resect varices (Table 163-2). Patients who continue to bleed for more than 48 h have a higher mortality. Surgical therapy should be considered if the patient falls into Child's class A or B once vasopressin, sclerotherapy, and a tamponade tube fail to control bleeding. Immediate and long-term mortality after portosystemic shunting is higher in patients with more advanced cirrhosis. When performed emergently as a last resort for active variceal hemorrhage, mortality for portosystemic shunting approaches 50 percent[33] and is even higher in a Child's class C patient. Some suggest that earlier surgical intervention in such patients may lower mortality to <20 percent.[34,35] Patients who present with a third variceal hemorrhage, despite sclerotherapy during two previous hospitalizations, should be deemed sclerotherapy failures and considered for surgical therapy. This includes patients noncompliant with outpatient sclerotherapy. Using sclerotherapy as a primary therapy, while reserving surgery for "rescue," yields good results.[36]

The most commonly used surgical therapy for bleeding varices is the portosystemic shunt. Designed to direct blood from the high pressure portal system into the low pressure systemic venous system, portosystemic shunts are effective in lowering portal venous pressure, resulting in cessation of bleeding. However, experience has shown that elective portosystemic shunts for recurrent bleeding have failed to improve survival of cirrhotic patients, although rebleeding rates are diminished. Shunted patients die from progressive liver failure, exacerbated by diminished portal blood flow.

Various techniques allow portosystemic shunting of blood, including mesocaval, portocaval, and splenorenal shunting procedures. In the setting of acute variceal hemorrhage, the mesocaval shunt generally is preferred due to the relative ease by which the surgeon anastomoses the superior mesenteric vein to the inferior vena cava using a graft.

Recently, other surgical approaches have been used for control of variceal hemorrhage. Esophageal and gastric devascularization with esophageal transection may be preferred by a surgeon experienced in performing this procedure. The necessary combined thoracic and abdominal approach limits its use in severely ill cirrhotic patients.

Variceal hemorrhage may occur in noncirrhotic patients. Esophageal varices may result from extrahepatic portal venous obstruction. Generally, such patients are better operative candidates than cirrhotic patients and carry a lower mortality rate. When large gastric varices accompanied by small or absent esophageal varices are identified, splenic or portal vein thrombosis should be considered as the cause, rather than cirrhosis. Splenic and portal vein thrombosis may occur in the setting of acute pancreatitis, pancreatic cancer, abdominal trauma, and hypercoagulable states. It is imperative to identify this subgroup of patients with variceal hemorrhage, because splenectomy rather than a portosystemic shunt is definitive therapy for recurrent bleeding. Evaluation with a celiac angiogram should be undertaken.

NONVARICEAL HEMORRHAGE

The prognosis for nonvariceal upper gastrointestinal bleeding is better than for variceal hemorrhage in part because of the self-limited nature of most upper gastrointestinal bleeding. Those lesions which continue to bleed account for the 10 percent mortality rate from gastrointestinal bleeding (Fig. 163-2).

Mallory-Weiss Tear

Mallory-Weiss tear generally is a self-limited form of bleeding, rarely requiring more than supportive intervention. Mortality is half that of other forms of nonvariceal hemorrhage.[2] In the rare instance of continued bleeding from a Mallory-Weiss tear, endoscopic therapy by either electrocoagulation or injection therapy should be attempted prior to surgical oversewing of the lesion. Surgery should be considered if more than 10 U packed cells is required to maintain the hematocrit.

Peptic Ulcer Disease

Most upper gastrointestinal bleeding occurs as a complication of peptic ulcer disease. Although H_2-receptor antagonists, antacids, and sucralfate are effective healers of peptic ulcers, they have little effect on stopping ulcer-related bleeding or lowering the rate of rebleeding. Numerous trials have failed to show benefit of cimetidine or ranitidine, when compared to placebo, in the management of acute bleeding from ulcers.[37] Similarly, high dose antacid therapy

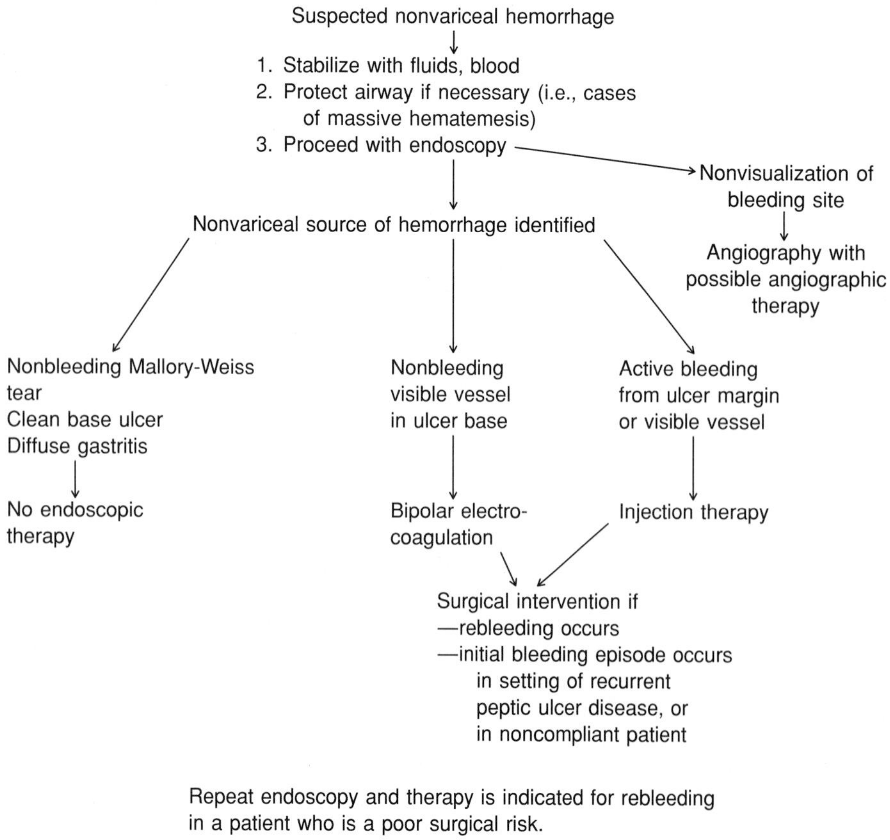

FIGURE 163-2 Evaluation and therapy of nonvariceal hemorrhage.

does not control bleeding or prevent recurrent hemorrhage.[37] Combined antacid and H_2-receptor antagonist therapy may lower rebleeding rates,[37] although additional trials are necessary.

Endoscopic therapy, using either bipolar electrocoagulation or injection therapy (see Chap. 33), is indicated when active bleeding in the form of oozing or pulsating hemorrhage, or nonbleeding visible vessels, is seen at the time of endoscopy (see Plates 26 and 27). Blinded, sham-controlled studies suggest rebleeding rates, transfusion requirements, and length of hospitalization are reduced when bipolar coagulation is used to control hemorrhage in this setting.[38] Injection therapy appears to provide permanent hemostasis from active bleeding.[39] However, controlled studies assessing its effectiveness are needed.

Angiographic therapy for acute upper gastrointestinal hemorrhage is generally reserved for the high-risk operative patient or for the control of bleeding in the unstable patient awaiting surgery. The angiographer may use two approaches to control acute upper gastrointestinal bleeding—the intraarterial infusion of vasoconstrictive drugs and embolization (see Chap. 20). Although systemic vasopressin, via peripheral venous access, does not effectively control nonvariceal hemorrhage,[37] therapeutic efficacy of intraarterial vasopressin infusion has been shown.[40] Often the effects of intraarterial infusion may be permanent, sparing surgical intervention, in a poor operative candidate.

Embolization therapy uses various substances, most frequently Gelfoam, to selectively embolize the bleeding vessel. Necrosis of the stomach, duodenum, gallbladder, liver, or spleen may follow embolization therapy. Because the duodenum derives its blood supply from the celiac axis and superior mesenteric artery, spontaneous infarction is rare. The patient with advanced atherosclerotic vascular disease, or in whom previous gastric surgery entailed ligation of collateral vessels, is at greater risk of infarction due to compromised collateral circulation.[41] In view of the higher morbidity associated with embolization therapy, it should be used only after vasopressin fails to control bleeding.

Surgical intervention for bleeding peptic ulcers should be considered in two situations. First, surgery is used to control life-threatening hemorrhage which has failed to respond to medical management and endoscopic means. In fact, in the low operative risk patient, effectively stabilized to allow surgery, angiographic therapy should not even be attempted. Second, surgery should be considered in the patient in whom medical management has failed to heal or prevent recurrence of peptic ulceration, particularly if there have been previous complications attributed to peptic ulcer disease, e.g., previous bleeding. The patient who has recurrent hemorrhage due to noncompliance with maintenance antiulcer therapy should be considered for elective surgical therapy once bleeding has stopped. The ICU personnel are vital to the outcome of surgery for bleeding ulcers. Morbidity and mortality are greatly reduced when the surgeon operates electively in the nonbleeding patient. Likewise, the prompt correction of volume and blood loss, prevention of aspiration, and correction of the coagulation profile prepare the patient with continued bleeding, thereby allowing a safer operation.

The surgical procedure performed depends on the location of the ulcer, as well as the stability of the patient. The patient with active hemorrhage, undergoing an emergent operation, will have the bleeding point of the ulcer oversewn, along with truncal vagotomy and pyloroplasty. Vagotomy and antrectomy may be considered if the patient has been adequately stabilized. However, when performed as an emergency procedure for hemorrhage, gastric resection carried a 46 percent mortality rate in one series, compared with 8 percent for vagotomy and pyloroplasty.[42] Selective vagotomy with either pyloroplasty or antrectomy, an option in the elective situation, is not advisable in the unstable patient.

Gastric ulcer bleeding is treated with the same approach as a bleeding duodenal ulcer, except that resection is recommended if the situation allows. Partial gastrectomy carries a slightly lower mortality in the setting of gastric ulcer bleeding than when performed for a bleeding duodenal ulcer.[43] Resection for actively bleeding gastric carcinoma is recommended only when performed electively, because it is a prolonged procedure which might be unsuitable for an unstable patient.

Morbidity approaches 30 percent after surgical therapy for bleeding ulcers. Postoperative wound infection is the major complication.

Gastritis

Acute hemorrhagic gastritis, commonly seen in alcoholic patients, or in the setting of physiologic stress (stress-related mucosal damage [SRMD]), accounts for nearly 25 percent of upper gastrointestinal bleeding.[2] It is the most common cause of gastric bleeding in series from municipal hospitals where alcoholism is prevalent. Most patients will stop bleeding spontaneously. Nonsurgical therapy including acid suppression and angiographic therapy should be instituted to avoid surgery. Surgical therapy, consisting of total gastrectomy, should be avoided due to its high mortality rate.[44]

Acute Lower Gastrointestinal Bleeding

Acute lower gastrointestinal bleeding is defined as bleeding from below the ligament of Treitz. On occasion, patients with hematochezia actually may be bleeding briskly from a location above the ligament of Treitz, rather than a lower gastrointestinal source. Therefore, upper gastrointestinal endoscopy should be the first diagnostic procedure performed in the patient with hematochezia if bleeding is brisk enough to require intensive care management.

Most patients who experience severe lower gastrointestinal bleeding are elderly, the average age being 65, and have concomitant medical problems including cardiac and respiratory disease.[45] Therefore, prompt resuscitative measures are indicated in these patients.

The color of the blood passed should not be used to predict the site of bleeding, because right-sided colonic and small bowel bleeding may be brisk enough to result in bright red bleeding, as may a left-sided colonic diverticulum. A cecal bleeding site may produce melena rather than maroon or bright red bleeding, although this is uncommon.

Lower gastrointestinal bleeding significant enough to produce orthostasis or tachycardia is generally from a vascular source rather than a mass, such as polyp or carcinoma. Most frequently, diverticulosis or angiodysplasia is the source of such vascular bleeding in the elderly. Angiodysplasia may be congenital, causing bleeding in the young patient. More frequently, it is an acquired lesion, most commonly located in the right colon, cecum, or distal small bowel. Nonvascular lower gastrointestinal bleeding may arise from small bowel or colonic ulcerations (as may occur in inflammatory bowel disease), yet hemodynamic instability is rare. Unless the patient has a previous known history, bowel ulcers should rarely be considered in the differential diagnosis. Massive bleeding in younger patients suggests a bleeding Meckel's diverticulum, which can be diagnosed with a Meckel's scan.

DIAGNOSTIC EVALUATION

Controversies exist regarding the diagnostic evaluation of the patient with lower gastrointestinal bleeding. Keeping in mind the likely differential diagnosis for various age groups, as well as the presence of ongoing bleeding, should help direct appropriate evaluation.

ANGIOGRAPHY

Unfortunately, angiography requires active bleeding at a rate of at least 1 mL/min to allow detection. Bleeding must be from a vascular origin, such as an artery within a diverticulum or from angiodysplasia. Such bleeding generally is intermittent, likely accounting for some reports that angiography is not sensitive for detecting lower gastrointestinal bleeding. Therefore, prompt examination is essential when active bleeding is suspected by ongoing hypotension, orthostasis, or tachycardia. When instituted promptly in patients with massive lower gastrointestinal bleeding, superior and inferior mesenteric angiography may localize bleeding in over 70 percent of patients.[45] Localization permits the use of angiographic therapy or may limit surgical resection (see Chap. 20).

COLONOSCOPY

The use of emergency colonoscopy during severe bleeding largely has been avoided because it generally is nondiagnostic and impractical. Visualization of the colonic mucosa is impaired in the unprepared bleeding patient. Regional localization of bleeding, when the precise site is not seen, may help limit surgical resection. However, retrograde flow of blood throughout long segments of colon, and even into the terminal ileum, may falsely indicate the region of bleeding. Despite the conventional avoidance of clearing preparations in the bleeding patient, some argue in favor of their use, allowing complete emergent colonoscopy, yielding a diagnosis in nearly 75 percent of patients.[46] However, most endoscopists urge conservative support until bleeding has subsided or stopped before preparing the patient and proceeding with colonoscopy.

Flexible sigmoidoscopy is of limited value in the bleeding patient and should generally be avoided in favor of complete colonoscopy.

RADIONUCLIDE SCANS

Radionuclide bleeding scans are frequently used to localize bleeding sites in patients with lower gastrointestinal bleeding. Although the sensitivity may be greater than for angiography, its specificity may impair accurate diagnosis. Caution should be exercised against surgical intervention based on the results of a bleeding scan alone. Rather, the scan should redirect one's attention to specific sites of the gastrointestinal tract when pursuing repeat angiography or endoscopy.

THERAPY

Supportive therapy remains the mainstay for patients with lower gastrointestinal bleeding, since most episodes stop spontaneously. However, the rebleeding rate remains high, particularly in patients who undergo blind hemicolectomy for severe bleeding.[47] Although surgical resection of the bleeding area is required in most patients with massive bleeding, nonsurgical therapy may allow nonemergent surgery or even spare surgery in the high-risk patient.

ANGIOGRAPHIC THERAPY

Following identification of a bleeding site by angiography, selective intraarterial infusion of vasopressin may halt bleeding in the majority of patients. However, rebleeding occurs in nearly half of those who are initially controlled.[45] The operative mortality rate is lowered when angiographic therapy is initiated to stabilize the actively bleeding patient.[45] Its use should be encouraged if an experienced angiographer is available. The complications of intraarterial vasopressin therapy for lower gastrointestinal bleeding are similar to those for upper gastrointestinal hemorrhage.

ENDOSCOPIC THERAPY

Endoscopic therapy exists for lower gastrointestinal bleeding, although its use is a fraction of that for upper gastrointestinal bleeding. Lesions amenable to endoscopic therapy (as many as 30 percent in one series)[46] include angiodysplasia and bleeding from polypectomy sites. Endoscopic coagulation should be attempted by an experienced endoscopist since it may prevent the need for surgical intervention. Even endoscopically guided infusion of epinephrine into a bleeding diverticulum has been reported,[48] but generally is not feasible.

SURGERY

Surgical resection of the bleeding segment of bowel is indicated if severe bleeding is not controlled or is recurrent. Although timing of surgical intervention is not always clear, many consider it necessary if the transfusion requirement exceeds 6 to 8 U packed cells over a 24-h period. Despite aggressive diagnostic evaluation, the site of ongoing bleeding may not be ascertained. The medical and surgical teams are then faced with the dilemma of a blind resection. In the elderly patient, often this will entail a subtotal colectomy from the cecum to proximal rectum, with an ileoproctostomy. This generally will ensure resection of the unidentified bleeding site. Yet, when performed emergently, the mortality rate may be 40 percent.[49] The future prospect of debilitating diarrhea in the elderly patient makes this approach unattractive unless life-threatening bleeding continues. Some surgeons may opt for a blinded, left-sided colectomy, based on the high prevalence of left-sided diverticulosis in the elderly population. Such an approach may carry a risk of rebleeding which approaches 33 percent.[47]

The surgeon should be alerted that angiodysplasia may be confined to the small bowel, particularly in the distal terminal ileum.[50] Resection of the distal 30 to 60 cm of the terminal ileum should be considered if a right hemicolectomy for suspected angiodysplasia is undertaken. Intraoperative small bowel endoscopy, allowing examination of the distal terminal ileum, should be considered in the setting of cecal angiodysplasia when surgery is performed. Angiography demonstrating cecal angiodysplasia may fail to identify a similar small bowel lesion.

Surgical resection of an identified Meckel's diverticulum is definitive therapy for bleeding in the young patient. The diagnosis is often made by a ^{99m}Tc pertechnetate scan, which has a sensitivity of 75 percent.[51]

Bleeding of Unknown Origin

Occasionally, a patient with significant acute gastrointestinal bleeding will undergo extensive evaluation without a source of bleeding identified. Despite endoscopic and radiologic evaluation, the etiology of bleeding may not be apparent. Occult sources of acute bleeding include angiodysplasia, located in various areas of the gastrointestinal tract, as well as hemobilia.

Angiodysplasia of the upper gastrointestinal tract may produce clinically significant hemorrhage, but may not be identified easily by endoscopy or angiography. These lesions may be small, vascular lesions mistaken for traumatic injury from a nongastric tube or endoscope. They may be single or multiple, located in the stomach or postbulbar duodenum. Gastric angiodysplasia may account for significant bleeding in patients with chronic renal failure.[52] Careful, meticulous inspection of the gastric and duodenal mucosa is paramount in the patient with hematemesis without an identifiable lesion. The cecum may also harbor angiodysplasia missed at the time colonoscopy is performed. However, such lesions likely will be identified by angiography, even if not actively bleeding. Small bowel angiodysplasia may account for obscure bleeding. Intraoperative endoscopy may identify such lesions. An endoscopist and surgeon, experienced in performing intraoperative endoscopy, should consider the inspection of the entire small bowel prior to blind colectomy in the patient with bleeding of unknown origin.

Hemobilia is bleeding from either the liver and bile ducts or from the pancreas through the ampulla of Vater and is a rare cause of gastrointestinal bleeding. Hepatic hemobilia usually results from blunt or sharp trauma to the liver. A hepatic artery aneurysm, which erodes into the right hepatic or common bile duct, produces melena and occasionally right upper quadrant abdominal pain. Jaundice is infrequently present. Pancreatic hemobilia is even less common. Pancreatitis, with resultant pseudoaneurysm formation of the splenic artery, is generally present in such cases. Acquired splenic artery aneurysms may erode into the pancreas, resulting in hemobilia without pancreatitis.

Hemobilia should be suspected when melena occurs in conjunction with jaundice or after blunt trauma or acute pancreatitis. Following a negative forward-viewing diagnostic endoscopy, the endoscopist should examine the duodenal papilla using a side-viewing duodenoscope. Active bleeding or a clot emanating from the papilla may be seen. Alternatively, angiography may reveal active bleeding or associated aneurysms from the hepatic or splenic artery. Angiographic therapy may provide temporary control of hemobilia,[53] but definitive surgery generally is needed.

Aortoenteric fistula is a rare development following abdominal vascular surgery with the placement of a synthetic graft. The fistula generally arises from the proximal anastomosis of the graft, communicating with the fourth portion of the duodenum. Graft infection generally is present, and likely plays a role in the pathogenesis of the fistula.[54] Bleeding from aortoenteric fistula generally is intermittent, yet with episodes of massive bleeding. The evaluation of suspected aortoduodenal fistula includes endoscopy or angiography. The endoscopist must examine the fourth portion of the duodenum, where bleeding or the graft itself may be seen. If endoscopy fails to identify a fistula, angiography should be performed if clinical suspicion is high. Surgical correction of the fistula, including removal of the graft, is necessary to prevent potential exsanguination.

Stress-Related Mucosal Damage (Stress Ulcers)

SRMD, commonly referred to as stress ulcers, is the result of multiple major system failure in the critically ill patient. SRMD, often resulting in severe gastric hemorrhage, poses an additional threat to these patients. The mortality rate is >30 percent, partly owing to the difficulty of controlling such bleeding, as well as to the underlying disease. As in most chronic peptic ulcers, SRMD is not the result of hypersecretion of acid and pepsin. Rather, weakening of the gastric mucosal resistance, created by local ischemia, is the likely inciting event. Acid and pepsin secretion are normal or low in most critically ill patients. Only in patients exhibiting Cushing's ulcers, related to CNS trauma or infection, is acid secretion increased.

Bleeding from SRMD may be *overt*, resulting in hypotension, tachycardia, and requiring blood transfusion, or *occult*, detectable only by gastroccult testing of the gastric

TABLE 163-3 Comparison of Measures for Stress Ulcer Prophylaxis

	Antacids	H_2-Receptor Antagonists	Sucralfate
Drug/pharmacy costs	Low	High	Low
Nursing "cost"	High	Low	Low
Preferred dosage schedule	Hourly	Continuous	Every 4 h
Potential disadvantages	Diarrhea Hypermagnesemia Nosocomial pneumonia	Mental confusion Drug-drug interactions Nosocomial pneumonia	?

contents. Although occult bleeding may occur frequently in the critically ill patient, it is of little clinical significance because few of these patients progress to overt bleeding. Clinically significant bleeding from SRMD occurs in 5 to 20 percent of patients in the ICU.[55] Attempts have been made to assess the relative importance of the underlying disease.[56,57] Patients at risk include those with burns on more than 50 percent of their body, sepsis, respiratory failure or prolonged ventilator support, fulminant hepatic failure, prolonged hypotension, or renal failure. Although some authors suggest a correlation between the number of risk factors noted in a particular patient and the risk of bleeding,[56] others warn that some risk factors, including sepsis, shock, and the need for prolonged mechanical ventilation, may be more significant than others.[58]

Endoscopically, SRMD may appear as multiple erosions or submucosal hemorrhage when mild. Multiple acute gastric ulcerations, generally found on the lesser curvature or fundus of the gastric body, are more often associated with overt hemorrhage. Bleeding usually manifests as oozing of blood from the margins of these multiple lesions. However, hemorrhage from a major artery may occur, with the typical endoscopic appearance of an ulcer with a visible vessel.

THERAPY

The mainstay of therapy for SRMD is supportive, while the intensivists attempt to reverse the underlying stress factors. However, the same skepticism should be raised regarding actual benefits of H_2-receptor antagonists and antacids, as discussed in regard to nonstress ulcer bleeding. The ability to reverse stress factors is the major determinant of outcome. Endoscopic and angiographic therapies should be attempted, but their role in this setting is not well established. The presence of multiple lesions, often over a large area of mucosa, may render endoscopic and angiographic therapy useless in many cases.

Surgery should largely be avoided, because a near total gastrectomy is required in most instances, and mortality exceeds 50 percent. Only in instances in which massive hemorrhage continues, despite nonsurgical therapy in a viable patient with treatable medical problems, should gastrectomy be undertaken.

PROPHYLAXIS

Since hemorrhage from SRMD is difficult to treat, yet carries a high mortality, much attention has been given to prophylactic therapy (Table 163-3). Despite the finding of SRMD in the setting of low or normal acid secretion, prophylaxis has been directed toward measures to neutralize acid or suppress its secretion. Antacid titration, using 30 to 60 mL of a potent antacid delivered hourly through a nasogastric tube, may significantly reduce the occurrence of stress-related hemorrhage. Overt bleeding is more likely to occur in high-risk patients if the gastric pH falls below 3.5. The low nursing compliance rate and the development of diarrhea in these patients, limit its practicality and therefore its benefit. Acid suppression by the use of intravenous H_2-receptor antagonists may be useful to prevent hemorrhage, although the benefits remain controversial. Early studies used intermittent cimetidine rather than continuous infusion therapy. The former method allowed frequent falls of the gastric pH below 3.5, possibly explaining its ineffectiveness in some trials. Continuous infusion therapy (following a bolus) is recommended because it maintains the gastric pH above 3.5, theoretically providing greater protection. Clinical trials assessing its benefit are forthcoming. Omeprazole, a potent inhibitor of the H^+/K^+ chief cell pump, produces complete achlorhydria. Whether such an agent, capable of total acid suppression, will further reduce the occurrence of stress-related hemorrhage is not known, but of great interest.

Sucralfate, a basic aluminum salt of sucrose octasulfate, is an effective ulcer-healing drug. It neither neutralizes acid nor suppresses acid production. Sucralfate increases mucosal blood flow, mucus secretion, and local prostaglandin production. These physiologic effects bolster mucosal resistance against acid and pepsin, allowing ulcer healing. Sucralfate recently has been used to prevent stress ulceration. It appears to be as effective as high dose antacids or cimetidine for the prevention of stress ulceration.[59,60]

Because sucralfate does not raise gastric pH, colonization of gastric juice by gram-negative bacteria is not as great as when antacids or H_2-receptor antagonists are used.[61] This may explain why patients requiring mechanical ventilation develop nosocomial pneumonia more frequently when treated with antacids or cimetidine than when sucralfate is used for prophylaxis.[62] Therefore, sucralfate may be preferred, because it is as effective as acid neutralization and suppression, and it is safer.

Despite aggressive prophylaxis, hemorrhage in the critically ill patient may develop. Combination drug therapy, using antacids, H_2-receptor antagonists, and sucralfate may be warranted in the most critically stressed patients.

CASE PRESENTATION

D.H., a 61-year-old white man with a history of alcoholic cirrhosis, peptic ulcer disease, and squamous cell carcinoma of the mouth presented to the emergency room complaining of "vomiting blood." The hematemesis, consisting of bright red blood and clots, was accompanied by the passage of bright red blood per rectum. He complained of light-headedness, but denied syncope. There was no history of abdominal pain.

The patient's past medical history included years of alcohol abuse with resultant cirrhosis, complicated by a documented variceal hemorrhage. Sclerotherapy had been instituted 2 years previously with good results. A gastric ulcer had been documented several years previously. The patient continued maintenance antiulcer therapy with ranitidine 150 mg at bedtime. Two years earlier, a squamous cell carcinoma of the floor of the mouth, with metastasis to the mediastinum, was discovered. Chemotherapy, using bleomycin, methotrexate with leucovorin, and cisplatin had been used. Later, radiation therapy was required.

On presentation to the emergency room, the patient appeared alert, but pale. His systolic blood pressure measured 60 mmHg, with a pulse of 108, in the supine position. The skin had multiple spider angiomata on the chest and face. The lungs were clear. Heart tones were normal. The abdomen was nondistended; shifting dullness was absent. Mild right upper quadrant tenderness was noted. The liver edge was 3 cm below the right costal margin. Splenomegaly was absent. The rectal vault contained bright red blood.

Following placement of two large bore intravenous lines, including a subclavian catheter, normal saline was administered until packed red blood cells were available. The systolic blood pressure rose to 100 mgHg within 30 min. The patient was promptly admitted to the ICU.

The initial hematocrit was 22.4 percent with a hemoglobin of 7.7 g/dL. The platelet count was 95,000. The coagulation profile and electrolytes were within normal limits, while the serum BUN value was 23 with a serum creatinine level of 1.2 g/dL. The ECG recorded after fluid resuscitation was normal as was the chest x-ray.

Following ICU admission, the patient received 3 U packed red cells over 4 h, resulting in a rise of the hematocrit only to 25 percent. Oxygen per nasal cannula at 2 L/min was administered. The blood pressure was maintained at 100 to 110 systolic, with an average pulse of 90. The patient had no further hematemesis, although he continued to pass melena. Urgent surgical consultation was requested.

Shortly after stabilization of the blood pressure and pulse rate, and after transfusion of 3 U packed cells, EGD was performed. Following the use of topical cetacaine spray to anesthetize the hypopharynx, 4 mg midazolam was administered intravenously for conscious sedation. Endoscopy revealed a 3-cm ulcer on the posterior wall of the duodenal bulb. A 3-mm visible vessel within the ulcer was noted. The vessel was not actively bleeding. No other lesions were present. Esophageal and gastric varices were absent. Following complete inspection of the upper gastrointestinal tract, the visible vessel was treated by electrocoagulation. While oozing was noted during therapy, it had completely resolved by the completion of the procedure. The surgical service was notified of the endoscopic findings. Surgical therapy was recommended in view of active peptic ulceration despite maintenance therapy. Elective surgery was planned for the third following day.

The patient remained in the ICU for only 24 h. Following EGD, the nasogastric tube was not replaced, because there was no active bleeding. Following additional transfusion of 2 Units blood, his hematocrit rose to 30 percent. He had no melena or hematemesis for the next 24 h. The patient was transferred from the ICU.

Twelve hours later, the patient vomited clots of blood and passed bright red blood per rectum. His systolic blood pressure dropped to 80 mmHg, and his pulse rose to 130 beats/min. He was promptly transferred back to the ICU. Endotracheal intubation was necessary to maintain airway control in the setting of massive hematemesis. Following fluid resuscitation and transfusion of 3 U packed red blood cells, the blood pressure and pulse returned to normal. The hematocrit was maintained at 30 percent. In view of the history of chronic peptic ulcer disease and recurrent bleeding within 48 h, surgery was recommended. A vagotomy and antrectomy, with resection of the duodenal ulcer, was performed without complication. The postoperative course was uncomplicated. The patient was discharged 9 days after surgery.

CASE DISCUSSION

This case illustrates important diagnostic and therapeutic points to recall when managing the bleeding patient. The patient's history of cirrhosis and earlier variceal hemorrhage did not predict recurrent bleeding from varices. Cirrhotic patients with portal hypertension will frequently bleed from nonvariceal sources. The finding of a visible vessel accurately predicted the recurrence of bleeding within the next 48 h. Such a finding mandates immediate surgical consultation if it has not already been sought. Adequate intravenous access must be maintained despite the initial cessation of bleeding. The outcome from the second bleeding episode may have been undesirable if prompt resuscitation could not be initiated due to the lack of adequate intravenous access. Fortunately, in this instance the massive rebleeding episode was recognized promptly by the ward staff. The less intensive observation of the noncritical care setting may result in late recognition of bleeding.

On rebleeding, the patient was not treated with antacid therapy because it does not affect the course of active bleeding. Vasopressin does not affect bleeding from nonvariceal sources. Fortunately, the patient responded quickly to resuscitation, allowing surgery to proceed. Had he remained unstable, angiographic therapy to control bleeding would have been used to stabilize him before he went to surgery. This patient bled from a gastric ulcer, despite a prophylactic antiulcer regimen. This feature made the decision regarding surgical intervention easy. However, once elective surgery is planned for the bleeding patient, it should be performed as soon as possible, avoiding the potential for rebleeding and resultant instability.

References

1. Levy M: Aspirin use in patients with major upper gastrointestinal bleeding and peptic-ulcer disease. N Engl J Med 290:1158, 1974.
2. Silverstein FE, Gilbert DA, Tedesco FJ, et al: The national ASGE survey on upper gastrointestinal bleeding: II. Clinical prognostic factors. Gastrointest Endosc 27:80, 1981.
3. Graham DY, Smith JL: The course of patients after variceal hemorrhage. Gastroenterology 80:800, 1981.
4. Dagradi AE, Arguello JF, Weingarten ZG: Failure of endoscopy to establish a source for upper gastrointestinal bleeding. Am J Gastroenterol 72:395, 1979.
5. Irving JD, Northfield TC: Emergency arteriography in acute gastrointestinal bleeding. Br Med J 1:929, 1976.
6. Kelemouridis V, Athanasoulis CA, Waltman AC: Gastric bleeding sites: An angiographic study. Radiology 149:643, 1983.
7. Keller FS, Rosch J: Value of angiography in diagnosis and therapy of acute upper gastrointestinal hemorrhage. Dig Dis Sci 26(July suppl):78, 1981.
8. Eckstein MR, Athanasoulis CA: Gastrointestinal bleeding: An angiographic perspective. Surg Clin North Am 64:37, 1984.
9. Fogel MR, Knauer CM, Andres LL, et al: Continuous intravenous vasopressin in active upper gastrointestinal bleeding. Ann Intern Med 96:565, 1982.
10. Merigan TC Jr, Plotkin GR, Davidson CS: Effect of intravenously administered posterior pituitary extract on hemorrhage from bleeding esophageal varices: A controlled evaluation. N Engl J Med 266:134, 1961.
11. Johnson WC, Widrich WC, Ansell JE, et al: Control of bleeding varices by vasopressin: A prospective randomized study. Ann Surg 186:369, 1977.
12. Chojkier M, Groszmann RJ, Atterbury CE, et al: A controlled comparison of continuous intraarterial and intraveneous infusions of vasopressin in hemorrhage from esophageal varices. Gastroenterology 77:540, 1979.
13. Kravetz D, Bosch J, Teres J, et al: Comparison of intraveneous somatostatin and vasopressin infusions in treatment of acute variceal hemorrhage. Hepatology 4:442, 1984.
14. Gogel HK, Sherman RW, Becker LE: Scrotal and abdominal skin necrosis complicating intraveneous vasopressin therapy for bleeding esophageal varices. Dig Dis Sci 30:460, 1985.
15. Groszmann RJ, Kravetz D, Bosch J, et al: Nitroglycerin improves the hemodynamic response to vasopressin in portal hypertension. Hepatology 2:757, 1982.
16. Tsai Y-T, Lay C-S, Lai K-H, et al: Controlled trial of vasopressin plus nitroglycerin vs. vasopressin alone in the treatment of bleeding esophageal varices. Hepatology 6:406, 1986.
17. Gimson AES, Westaby D, Hegarty J, et al: A randomized trail of vasopressin and vasopressin plus nitroglycerin in the control of acute variceal hemorrhage. Hepatology 6:410, 1986.
18. Bosch J, Kravetz D, Rodes J: Effects of somatostatin on hepatic and systemic hemodynamics in patients with cirrhosis of the liver: Comparison with vasopressin. Gastroenterology 80:518, 1981.
19. Thulin L, Tyden G, Samnegard H, et al: Treatment of bleeding oesophageal varices with somatostatin. Acta Chir Scand 145:395, 1979.
20. Jenkins SA, Baxter JN, Corbett W, et al: A prospective randomized controlled clinical trial comparing somatostatin and vasopressin in controlling acute variceal haemorrhage. Br Med J 290:275, 1985.
21. Lebrec D, Poynard T, Hillon P, et al: Propranolol for prevention of recurrent gastrointestinal bleeding in patients with cirrhosis: A controlled study. N Engl J Med 305:1371, 1981.
22. Burroughs AK, Jenkins WJ, Sherlock S, et al: Controlled trial of propranolol for the prevention of recurrent variceal hemorrhage in patients with cirrhosis. N Engl J Med 309:1539, 1983.
23. Paquet KJ, Feussner H: Endoscopic sclerosis and esophageal balloon tamponade in acute hemorrhage from esophagogastric varices: A prospective controlled randomized trial. Hepatology 5:580, 1985.
24. Prindiville T, Trudeau W: A comparison of immediate versus delayed endoscopic injection sclerosis of bleeding esophageal varices. Gastrointest Endosc 32:385, 1986.
25. Larson AW, Cohen H, Zweiban B, et al: Acute esophageal variceal sclerotherapy: Results of a prospective randomized controlled trial. JAMA 255:497, 1986.
26. Cello JP, Grendell JH, Crass RA: Endoscopic sclerotherapy versus portacaval shunt in patients with severe cirrhosis and variceal hemorrhage. N Engl J Med 311: 1589, 1984.
27. Korula J: Outpatient esophageal variceal sclerotherapy: Safe and cost-effective: A prospective study. Gastrointest Endosc 32:1, 1986.
28. Westaby D, MacDougall BRD, Williams R: Improved survival following injection sclerotherapy for esophageal varices: Final analysis of a controlled trial. Hepatology 5:827, 1985.
29. Santangelo WC, Dueno MI, Estes BL, et al: Prophylactic sclerotherapy of large esophageal varices. N Engl J Med 318:814, 1988.
30. Kirkpatrick JR, Shoenut JP, Micflikier AB: Successful injection sclerotherapy for bleeding duodenal varix in intrahepatic portal obstruction. Gastrointest Endosc 31:259, 1985.
31. Trudeau W, Prindiville T: Endoscopic injection sclerosis in bleeding gastric varices. Gastrointest Endosc 32:264, 1986.
32. Hunt PS, Korman MG, Hansky J, et al: An 8-year prospective experience with balloon tamponade in emergency control of bleeding espohageal varices. Dig Dis Sci 27:413, 1982.
33. Prandi D, Rueff B, Roche-Sicot J, et al: Life-threatening hemorrhage of the digestive tract in cirrhotic patients: An assessment of the postoperative mortality after emergency portacaval shunt. Am J Surg 131:204, 1976.
34. Villeneuve J-P, Pomier-Layrargues G, Duguay L, et al: Emergency portacaval shunt for variceal hemorrhage: A prospective study. Ann Surg 206:48, 1987.
35. Orloff MJ, Bell RH Jr: Long-term survival after emergency portacaval shunting for bleeding varices in patients with alcoholic cirrhosis. Am J Surg 151:176, 1986.
36. Henderson MJ, Kutner MH, Millikan WJ, et al: Endoscopic variceal sclerosis compared with distal splenorenal shunt to prevent recurrent variceal bleeding in cirrhosis: A prospective, randomized trial. Ann Intern Med 112:262, 1990.
37. Zuckerman G, Welch R, Douglas A, et al: Controlled trial of medical therapy for active upper gastrointestinal bleeding and prevention of rebleeding. Am J Med 76:361, 1984.

38. Laine L: Multipolar electrocoagulation in the treatment of active upper gastrointestinal tract hemorrhage: A prospective controlled trial. N Engl J Med 316:1613, 1987.
39. Hirao M, Masuda K, Noda K, et al: Endoscopic local injection of hypertonic saline-epinephrine solution to arrest hemorrhage from the upper gastrointestinal tract. Gastrointest Endosc 31:313, 1985.
40. Athanasoulis CA: Angiographic methods for the control of gastric hemorrhage. Am J Dig Dis 21:174, 1976.
41. Shapiro, N, Brandt L, Sprayregan S, et al: Duodenal infarction after therapeutic Gelfoam embolization of a bleeding duodenal ulcer. Gastroenterology 80:176, 1981.
42. McArdle CS, Tilney NL: Surgery for peptic ulcer disease: Operative complications and immediate morbidity. J R Coll Surg Edinb 21:285, 1976.
43. Foster JH, Hickok DF, Dunphy JE: Factors influencing mortality following emergency operation for massive upper gastrointestinal hemorrhage. Surg Gynecol Obstet 117:257, 1963.
44. Hubert JP, Kiernan PD, Welch JS, et al: The surgical management of bleeding stress ulcers. Ann Surg 191:672, 1980.
45. Browder W, Cerise EJ, Litwin MS: Impact of emergency angiography in massive lower gastrointestinal bleeding. Ann Surg 204:530, 1986.
46. Jensen DM, Machicado GA: Diagnosis and treatment of severe hematochezia: The role of urgent colonoscopy after purge. Gastroenterology: 95:1569, 1988.
47. McQuire HH, Haynes BW: Massive hemorrhage from diverticulosis of the colon. Ann Surg 175:847, 1972.
48. Ballardini G, del Poggio P: Therapeutic use of colonoscopy in active diverticular bleeding. Letter. Gastrointest Endosc 31:290, 1985.
49. Potter GD, Sellin JH: Lower gastrointestinal bleeding. Gastroenterol Clin North Am 17:341, 1988.
50. Duray PH, Marcal JM, Jr, LiVolsi VA, et al: Small intestinal angiodysplasia in the elderly. J Clin Gastroenterol 6:311, 1984.
51. Berquist TH, Nolan NG, Stephen DH, et al: Specificity of ^{99m}Tc pertechnetate in scintigraphy diagnosis of Meckel's diverticulum: Review of 100 cases. J Nucl Med 17:465, 1976.
52. Clouse RE, Costigan DJ, Mills BA, et al: Angiodysplasia as a cause of upper gastrointestinal bleeding. Arch Intern Med 145:458, 1985.
53. Fagan EA, Allison DJ, Chadwick VS, et al: Treatment of haemobilia by selective embolisation. Gut 21:541, 1980.
54. Busuttil RW, Rees W, Baker JD, et al: Pathogenesis of aortoduodenal fistula: Experimental and clinical correlates. Surgery 85:1, 1979.
55. Shuman RB, Schuster DP, Zuckerman GR: Prophylactic therapy for stress ulcer bleeding: A reappraisal. Ann Intern Med 106:562, 1987.
56. Zinner MJ, Zuidema GD, Smith PL, et al: The prevention of upper gastrointestinal tract bleeding in patients in an intensive care unit. Surg Gynecol Obstet 153:214, 1981.
57. Knaus WA, Draper EA, Wagner DP, et al: Apache II: A severity of disease classification system. Crit Care Med 13:818, 1985.
58. Zuckerman GR, Cort D, Shuman RB: Stress ulcer syndrome. Intensive Care Med 3:21, 1988.
59. Tryba M, Zevounou F, Torok M, et al: Prevention of acute stress bleeding with sucralfate, antacids, or cimetidine: A controlled study with pirenzepine as a basic medication. Am J Med 79 (suppl 2C):55, 1985.
60. Borrero E, Bank S, Margolis I, et al: Comparison of antacid and sucralfate in the prevention of gastrointestinal bleeding in patients who are critically ill. Am J Med 79(suppl 2C):62, 1985.
61. Driks, MR, Craven DE, Celli BR, et al: Nosocomial pneumonia in intubated patients given sucralfate as compared with antacids or histamine type 2 blockers. N Engl J Med 317:1367, 1987.
62. Craven DE, Kunches LM, Kilinsky V, et al: Risk factors for pneumonia and fatality in patients receiving continuous mechanical ventilation. Am Rev Respir Dis 133:792, 1986.

Chapter 164

ACUTE AND CHRONIC HEPATIC DISEASE

THEODORE H. LEWIS JR
GREGORY A. SCHMIDT

KEY POINTS

- *Fulminant hepatic failure (FHF) is defined as the onset of hepatic encephalopathy (HE) within 8 weeks of the onset of liver-related symptoms.*
- *Common complications in patients with FHF or with cirrhosis include encephalopathy, infection, bleeding, and renal failure.*
- *In addition, FHF may be complicated by cerebral edema, cardiovascular instability, and hypoglycemia.*
- *Supportive management of FHF consists of* **1.** *airway protection,* **2.** *treatment of HE with lactulose or nonabsorbable antibiotics,* **3.** *monitoring clinical signs of increased intracranial pressure,* **4.** *aggressive treatment of bleeding with blood product transfusions,* **5.** *treatment of hypotension with volume resuscitation and empirical therapy for sepsis, and* **6.** *avoidance of hypoglycemia.*
- *Orthotopic liver transplantation (OLT) is the definitive therapy for FHF. It should be considered early for patients with poor prognosis lesions such as hepatitis B or non-A, non-B hepatitis.*
- *Additional complications of cirrhosis include spontaneous bacterial peritonitis, variceal hemorrhage, and hypoxemia.*
- *The mainstay of therapy for variceal hemorrhage is sclerotherapy; pharmacotherapy is a minimally effective temporizing measure.*
- *In all patients with severe liver disease, prevention of infection and pulmonary aspiration deserve emphasis.*

Patients admitted to the ICU with severe liver disease comprise two main groups: those with fulminant hepatic failure (FHF) and those having cirrhosis. Such patients have a very high risk of dying. Moreover, death is often due to a complication during hospitalization, rather than to the initial precipitant of admission. These complications and their therapies require close monitoring and aggressive supportive care, which are best delivered in the ICU. The cooperation of the gastroenterologist, intensivist, and transplant surgeon is of paramount importance to delivery of "state of the art" care.

Although there are several important differences in the presentation, complications, and management of these two groups, there are also many issues in common. Attention to infection surveillance, airway protection, coagulation, nutrition, and the adverse effects of drugs is essential to maximizing the chances for recovery in both groups, and in this chapter, these topics are covered first. Reversible neuropsychiatric dysfunction associated with acute or chronic liver disease, termed hepatic encephalopathy (HE), is then reviewed. Subsequently, particular concerns in the management of patients with FHF and cirrhosis are discussed.

General Supportive Measures

INFECTION SURVEILLANCE

Infection is extremely common in both acute and chronic liver failure. In a prospective study of infection in patients with FHF, at least one infection developed in 80 percent of the patients studied.[1] Pneumonia and urinary tract infection were the most common; bacteremia was documented in 26 percent. *Staphylococcus aureus* was the organism most frequently isolated from the tracheobronchial tree, gram-negative rods from the urinary tract, and *Staphylococcus epidermidis* from the blood. Clinical manifestations varied greatly, and over 25 percent of patients with bacteriologic evidence of infection failed to demonstrate an increase in temperature or white blood cell count. In 20 percent of patients who died, death was directly attributable to infection.

Many types of bacterial infection [e.g., spontaneous bacterial peritonitis (vide infra), pneumonia, endocarditis] are seen with increased frequency in patients with cirrhosis, especially in those with cirrhosis attributed to alcohol. In one series of 187 alcoholic cirrhotics, 46 percent had a bacterial infection on admission or developed one during hospitalization.[2] Infection is the proximate cause of death in up to one-fourth of cirrhotics.

Several potential contributors to the risk of infection have been identified. Patients often have significantly impaired consciousness, blunting their ability to protect against aspiration. Invasive catheters, which violate surface defenses, are frequently used. Furthermore, patients with FHF have been shown to have reduced polymorphonuclear (PMN) leukocyte function, perhaps secondary to circulating inhibitors of chemotaxis. Opsonization is also defective; reduced levels of complement and fibronectin are believed to be responsible. In those with cirrhosis, extensive portosystemic collaterals allow bacteria to bypass the hepatic reticuloendothelial system (RES). Finally, impaired phagocytosis of RES cells and defective opsonization have also been identified in cirrhotics.

In patients with hepatic failure, hyperpyrexia or elevated white blood cell count should prompt a careful evaluation for pneumonia, urinary tract infection, and infected catheter sites. In addition, because clinical indicators of infection may be absent, empirical broad-spectrum antimicrobial therapy is appropriate in any hemodynamically unstable patient.

AIRWAY PROTECTION

Patients with liver disease are at substantial risk of unpredictable airway compromise. Aspiration may be precipitated by gastrointestinal hemorrhage, infection, drug effect, worsening of HE, or iatrogenic intervention (endoscopy, placement of esophageal tamponade balloon). The superimposition of severe pneumonitis or nosocomial pneumonia on hepatic failure is frequently lethal. All too often the need to secure the airway is only recognized after a catastrophe ensues. Airway assessment must be an ongoing part of daily care. It is our practice to intubate when we believe the risk of aspiration is more than trivial, preferring to subject our patient to a well-planned, early intubation rather than chance an urgent procedure performed too late. In those with cerebral edema, measures must be taken to avoid a further increase in intracranial pressure (ICP) related to airway manipulation (vide infra).

COAGULOPATHY

Some derangement of coagulation is nearly universal in patients with severe liver disease. Coagulopathy may, in part, underlie the admission to the ICU (e.g., variceal hemorrhage) or complicate the delivery of intensive care (e.g., risk of invasive procedures). The tendency towards bleeding is usually related to deficiency of hepatic coagulation factors, but in some patients thrombocytopenia, disseminated intravascular coagulation, or fibrinolysis may contribute (see Chap. 146). Appropriate therapy depends on the major contributor to coagulopathy, but in the usual circumstance of variceal bleeding includes transfusion of fresh frozen plasma. Vitamin K (10 mg subcutaneously for 3 days) should be given to all patients with chronic liver disease since deficiency of this fat-soluble vitamin may supervene due to cholestasis or malnutrition. In FHF, replacement of clotting factors has not been shown to prevent clinically significant bleeding, and some authors discourage their prophylactic use.[3] However, fresh frozen plasma and platelets should be transfused prior to any surgical or invasive procedure.

Efforts to reduce bleeding risks cannot be overemphasized. H_2 antagonists or antacids should be used to raise the gastric pH above 5, which reduces the incidence of gastrointestinal hemorrhage and transfusion requirements.[4] The decision to insert central venous or arterial catheters should be carefully considered and the procedure performed by experienced personnel. Endotracheal tubes should be placed through the mouth because of the risk of life-threatening epistaxis following nasotracheal intubation.

NUTRITION

Malnutrition characterizes the patient with severe liver disease. Even in acute hepatic failure, anorexia often limits dietary intake before admission to the ICU. Those with chronic liver disease are particularly likely to be cachectic and to have specific deficiencies of micronutrients. Institution of full nutritional support should be an early priority. The presence of HE is not a contraindication to the provision of nutrition (vide infra and see Chap. 93). Patients with liver disease, especially those with FHF, have a propensity to hypoglycemia. High concentration glucose infusion is sometimes necessary to maintain blood glucose levels, with total daily glucose needs occasionally exceeding 1000 g. Finally, these patients must receive thiamine and folic acid because preexisting dietary inadequacy is the rule.

DRUG METABOLISM

Drug administration in patients with acute or chronic hepatic failure may be complicated by reduced protein binding as well as impaired hepatic degradation (or activation). Further, the common occurrence of renal failure in these critically ill patients mandates regular assays of drug levels when these are available and attention to adverse drug effects (see Chap. 169).

Hepatic Encephalopathy

Liver disease is frequently complicated by a syndrome of neurologic and psychiatric dysfunction, called hepatic or portosystemic encephalopathy. HE in chronic liver disease differs from the encephalopathy of FHF in clinical manifestations, response to therapy, prognosis, and possibly in pathogenesis. In patients with cirrhosis, HE is usually reversible, especially if a precipitant can be found. In contrast, the HE of FHF responds poorly, if at all, to standard treatment measures.

PATHOPHYSIOLOGY

The pathophysiology of HE is not known. However, in the past decade, much has been learned about potential mechanisms. It is generally believed that HE consists of profound neural depression mediated through an endogenous inhibitory neurotransmitter complex. The leading candidate is the γ-aminobutyric acid A ($GABA_A$)-benzodiazepine receptor system, the principle inhibitory neurotransmitter system in mammals.[5] It is postulated that gut-derived GABA circulates in increased amounts or that endogenous (or possibly diet-derived) benzodiazepines are present, leading to activation at the GABA-benzodiazepine receptor. In one report, plasma GABA levels correlated with the stage of encephalopathy in patients with acute hepatic failure, but not those with cirrhosis, suggesting a difference in pathogenesis in these two groups of patients.[6] Urine and plasma benzodiazepine activities correlate with the severity of encephalopathy in a group of patients with alcoholic cirrhosis who had not taken benzodiazepine medications.[7] The benzodiazepine antagonist, flumazenil, has induced variable but distinct improvements in mentation and electroencephalographic (EEG) findings in cirrhotics,[8] providing further support for the GABA-benzodiazepine hypothesis, although negative results have been published as well. In rats with experimentally induced FHF, flumazenil improves behavioral abnormalities and visual evoked responses.[9] These data suggest that increased GABA, increased effect of GABA, or a benzodiazepine-like substance is probably important in the pathogenesis of HE. It seems likely that current investigations will solve some of the puzzle of HE, possibly leading to new therapies.

TABLE 164-1 Clinical Stages of Acute Hepatic Encephalopathy

Stage	Mental State	Tremor	Electroencephalographic Changes
Stage I, prodrome (often diagnosed in retrospect)	Euphoria: occasionally depression; fluctuant, mild confusion; slowness of mentation and affect; untidiness; slurred speech; disorder in sleep rhythm	Slight	Usually lacking
Stage II, impending coma	Accentuation of stage I: drowsiness; inappropriate behavior; inability to maintain sphincter control	Present (easily elicited)	Abnormal: generalized slowing
Stage III, stupor	Patient sleeps most of the time but is rousable; speech is incoherent; confusion is marked	Usually present (if patient can cooperate)	Always abnormal
Stage IV, coma	Patient may (stage IVA) or may not (stage IVB) respond to painful stimuli	Usually lacking	Always abnormal

From Reference 3 with permission.

CLINICAL MANIFESTATIONS

Neuropsychiatric abnormalities range from subtle findings on psychometric testing to deep coma. In patients with cirrhosis, depressive signs usually predominate, without the antecedent agitation often seen in acute HE. Reversal of the sleep cycle may be an early finding. Obtundation and coma present grave risks to airway protection and therefore receive the greatest attention. However, more subtle changes in personality, behavior, or intellect may provide clues to impending HE, allowing early therapy. It is important to remember that severe liver impairment is not always apparent from the history, examination, or laboratory tests. Therefore, any critically ill patient with unexplained encephalopathy should be evaluated for the possibility of occult liver disease.

To facilitate communication between physicians and allow correlation between groups of patients, the severity of encephalopathy has been stratified (Table 164-1). Early, or stage I, encephalopathy is often diagnosed retrospectively. It is characterized by subtle personality changes and reduced cognitive function. A fine tremor may be present. Stage II encephalopathy is manifest by drowsiness, lethargy, or more overt changes in personality. Asterixis is often present, although this finding is also seen in uremia, anoxia, and salicylate poisoning. Ataxia and dysarthria may also be noted. Stage III encephalopathy is marked by delirium, disorientation, and somnolence; seizures may occur. Hyperreflexia and Babinski's sign can often be elicited. Deep coma characterizes stage IV encephalopathy. Decerebrate posturing and brisk oculocephalic reflexes may be seen. In FHF, rapid progression from stage I to stage IV is common.

DIAGNOSIS

There is no single test on which to base a diagnosis of HE. In the setting of cirrhosis, progressive obtundation following a known precipitant of HE (Table 164-2) strongly suggests the diagnosis. However, HE can be mimicked by nearly any of the causes of encephalopathy and coma. Several conditions deserve special mention. Patients with liver disease are particularly susceptible to sedative and narcotic medications. Because specific therapy may be available (e.g., naloxone), drug effects must not be overlooked. Ethanol and other drugs of abuse may cause coma as well, so that screening for these substances is often a part of the diagnostic evaluation. Other causes of impaired mentation related to underlying hepatic disease include hypoglycemia, subdural hematoma, meningitis, subclinical status epilepticus, hypoxemia, and Wernicke's encephalopathy. Therefore, arterial blood-gas analysis, serum chemistries, neurodiagnostic imaging, lumbar puncture, and an EEG may be necessary before a diagnosis can be made confidently.

The arterial ammonia level may provide helpful information. Although this test does not correlate well with the presence or degree of encephalopathy, when elevated it can provide support for the diagnosis. There are characteristic EEG findings of paroxysmal triphasic waves, but these

TABLE 164-2 Precipitants of Hepatic Encephalopathy

Gastrointestinal hemorrhage
Spontaneous bacterial peritonitis
Systemic infection
Drugs (especially benzodiazepines and barbiturates)
Acute deterioration in liver function (e.g., hepatitis, hepatotoxin)
Dietary protein load
Alkalosis
Diuretic therapy, especially with hypokalemia
Diarrhea or dehydration
Constipation
Azotemia

are neither sensitive nor specific. Visual evoked responses may be more useful. Even after a full investigation it may not be possible to make a diagnosis of HE with certainty. In this situation a trial of therapy for HE may be both diagnostic and therapeutic.

THERAPY

Treatment of HE is based on the removal of precipitants and a reduction in colon-derived nitrogenous substances. Oral protein should be eliminated, and all oral intake stopped to reduce the risk of aspiration. Blood in the gastrointestinal tract should be removed by nasogastric suction and enemas. Nonabsorbable disaccharides (lactulose, lactitol) are effective when given by nasogastric tube (30 to 45 mL hourly, adjusted downward to induce three loose stools per day) or rectally (300 mL in saline solution as a retention enema for 30 to 60 min every 6 h). Neomycin is an alternative, given as 2 g every 8 h via a nasogastric tube. The effects of lactulose and neomycin are additive in some patients.

Nutrition is important in these critically ill patients and can be given without contributing to HE. In cirrhosis, impaired hepatic catabolism of aromatic amino acids raises their plasma amino acid level, possibly contributing to HE by generating false neurotransmitters in the brain. One of the rationales for branched-chain amino acid solutions (BCAA) is that they may compete with aromatic amino acids for entry into the central nervous system. In fact, in some trials, BCAAs have increased the likelihood of awakening from HE. While this area remains controversial (see Chap. 93), a recent meta-analysis of published trials suggests that BCAAs lead to a significant improvement in the degree of HE and possibly to an improvement in survival.[10]

Despite aggressive treatment of HE the potential for deterioration must be appreciated. Serial examinations are essential, with attention to the patient's ability to guard the airway.

Fulminant Hepatic Failure

Fulminant hepatic failure is defined as the development of HE within 8 weeks of the initial presentation of liver-related symptoms. Thus, FHF is typically a complication of acute liver disease such as viral or drug-induced hepatitis. FHF may also be the initial presentation of a previously compensated chronic liver disease such as Wilson's disease or chronic active hepatitis. In addition to HE, FHF may affect coagulation, cardiovascular stability, and renal function, and may predispose to life-threatening infection.

Previously, despite aggressive supportive care, FHF resulted in a very high mortality. However in the last 5 years the application of OLT to FHF has resulted in a dramatic improvement in survival among select patient groups. The advent of this new, effective therapy demands that patients with FHF be considered for OLT and transferred to a transplant center when possible. (see Chap. 80).

ETIOLOGIES

Fulminant hepatic failure may occur in the setting of hepatocellular necrosis or microvesicular steatosis. Hepatocellular necrosis is the pathologic change noted in viral or drug-induced hepatitis, while microvesicular steatosis is seen in fatty liver of pregnancy, tetracycline toxicity, or Reye's syndrome. The toxins implicated in FHF include drugs, both prescribed and illicit, chemicals, and peptide toxins produced by fungi. Commonly identified etiologies in our institution include hepatitis B, drug reaction, and non-A, non-B hepatitis; however, often no etiology can be determined[11] (Table 164-3).

Viral hepatitis is the most common cause of FHF worldwide, accounting for 50 to 70 percent of cases.[12] Hepatitis B is the most common viral cause of FHF, and is responsible for 25 to 75 percent of cases. Coinfection with hepatitis D appears to increase the incidence of FHF. In two series of patients presenting with FHF who had anti-HBc IgM (acute fulminant hepatitis B), coinfection with hepatitis D was demonstrated in 30 percent.[13] Newly acquired infection

TABLE 164-3 Principal Causes of Fulminant Hepatic Failure

Infections
Viral hepatitis
Type A
Type B
Type D
Non-A, non-B
Yellow fever
Miscellaneous viral infections
Coxiella burnettii infection
Poisons, Chemicals, and Drugs
Amanita phalloides
Acetaminophen
Tetracycline
Phosphorus
Halothane and certain other, chiefly halogenated, hydrocarbons
Ethanol
Isoniazid
Methyldopa
Monoamine oxidase inhibitors
Sodium valproate
Pirprofen
Ischemia and Hypoxia
Hepatic vascular occlusion
Acute circulatory failure
Heat stroke
Gram-negative bacteremia with shock
Congestive cardiac failure
Pericardial tamponade
Miscellaneous Metabolic Anomalies
Acute fatty liver of pregnancy
Reye's syndrome
Jejunoileal bypass
Wilson's disease
Galactosemia
Hereditary fructose intolerance
Hereditary tyrosinemia

From Reference 3 with permission.

with hepatitis D may also cause FHF in the setting of chronic infection with hepatitis B. Hepatitis A is an unusual cause of FHF, accounting for 1 to 6 percent of viral-related cases. Finally, many patients with FHF due to non-A, non-B hepatitis, or with "no cause identified" may prove to have hepatitis C.

CLINICAL PRESENTATION

The clinical presentation of FHF is variable and, in part, depends on the etiology of the liver disease. The predominant symptoms relate to the development of HE. Typical physical findings are fetor hepaticus and signs of HE such as asterixis, confusion, or obtundation. Jaundice is common when the hepatic injury has been established but is not uniformly present. Patients with hepatic necrosis sometimes develop fever. Tachycardia and hypotension may be due to FHF alone or to superimposed gastrointestinal hemorrhage or sepsis.

Laboratory abnormalities may vary with the etiology of hepatic injury. Patients with extensive hepatic necrosis commonly demonstrate dramatic elevations of serum aminotransferase levels. However, in patients with microvesicular steatosis these may be only modestly elevated. An abnormal prothrombin time indicates hepatocellular damage and loss of synthetic function. Elevation of the serum ammonia level is common. Although these laboratory abnormalities are useful in the assessment and management of the patient with liver disease, it is the presence of HE, not any particular test result, which distinguishes FHF from severe hepatitis.

COMPLICATIONS

CEREBRAL EDEMA

Cerebral edema complicates as many as 50 to 80 percent of cases of FHF in autopsy and clinical series.[14,15] Cerebral edema may precipitate uncal or cerebellar herniation. In some series cerebral edema is the leading cause of death in patients with FHF.[16]

PATHOGENESIS. Whether cerebral edema is a distinct complication of FHF or part of the spectrum of HE is not known. Cerebral edema may occur because of disordered cellular processes which result in swelling of glial cells (cytotoxic edema), because of increase transit of fluid across the blood-brain barrier (vasogenic edema), or because of excess extracellular fluid (interstitial edema). All of these mechanisms may be active in the cerebral edema associated with FHF. Serum from human beings or animals with acute hepatic failure depresses the activity of animal neural membrane Na^+, K^+-ATPase.[17,18] Such depressed activity might cause loss of osmotic gradients and cell swelling. Substances which do not normally cross the blood-brain barrier, such as insulin and L-glucose, are found in the brains of rats with FHF, demonstrating abnormal transport and, therefore, a component of vasogenic edema.[19]

Whatever its pathogenesis, cerebral edema ultimately causes morbidity and mortality by increasing ICP. An increase in ICP adds ischemic injury to the initial cerebral insult. Additional factors that may exacerbate cerebral edema or reduce cerebral perfusion pressure are often present in FHF. Volume overload or a hypooncotic state may worsen cerebral edema. Hypotension, as a complication of FHF, gastrointestinal hemorrhage, or sepsis, may reduce the cerebral perfusion pressure. Finally, sepsis and hypoglycemia may each independently contribute to cerebral injury.

CLINICAL MANIFESTATIONS. Cerebral edema is usually present only in those patients with significant HE (stage III or IV). The earliest sign of increased ICP is heightened muscle tone, but this finding is often subtle. As ICP rises above 30 mmHg, abnormal pupillary reflexes are common.[18] Decorticate and decerebrate posturing are seen as the ICP continues to rise. Opisthotonus may also be seen at very high levels of ICP. Hypertension with bradycardia (Cushing's reflex) may occur as a preterminal event.

The diagnosis of increased ICP may be apparent on physical examination; however, on many occasions ICP is increased without significant physical findings. Computed tomography (CT) may demonstrate obliteration of sulci and narrowing of cerebral ventricles. Invasive ICP monitoring (see Chap. 34) may be used to better monitor patients at high risk for increased ICP or to tailor strategies to reduce ICP.

MANAGEMENT. The management of cerebral edema in patients with FHF is challenging. Because it is difficult to diagnose early, some transplant centers advocate early invasive ICP monitoring in patients with FHF and stage III or IV encephalopathy. Others have suggested that ICP monitoring adds little to clinical examination, but these authors performed careful neurologic examinations every 5 min.[20]

Efforts to prevent the development of cerebral edema have proven ineffective. Prophylactic dexamethasone administration and hyperventilation failed to reduce the incidence of increased ICP or to improve survival.[15,20] Fluid restriction and blood pressure control are probably important, but have not been studied in detail. Most centers recommend nursing the patient in a "head upright position"; however, in a recent study, head elevation did not prevent increases in ICP.[21] Maneuvers in which the head is turned or flexed may decrease venous return from the head and increase ICP. These maneuvers, such as assessment of oculocephalic reflexes, should be avoided. Patients at risk for elevated ICP (stage III and IV encephalopathy) should usually be intubated (vide supra) because of the risk of aspiration. However, airway manipulation dramatically raises ICP. Therefore, intubation should be performed electively, with appropriate premedication, and by the most experienced personnel available. Mask hyperventilation should be used in an effort to reduce the ICP prior to the intubation. Short-acting barbiturates are probably the anesthetic agents of choice because of their effects on ICP. In addition, intravenous lidocaine (100 mg IVP) may be added for its airway and general anesthetic effects.

Two forms of therapy have been effective in reducing ICP: hyperventilation[22] and osmotic diuretics. The effect of hyperventilation is transient because cerebrovascular and renal compensation for the acute hypocapnia occur. In addition, since hyperventilation works by reducing cerebral blood flow, it has the potential to worsen rather than improve cerebral blood flow. The ICP response to osmotic diuretics is longer lasting. Mannitol (1 g/kg) reduces ICP or arrests the rise in patients with FHF.[23] Mannitol may be given as necessary (while monitoring the ICP) as long as serum osmolarity does not exceed 320 mO. Mannitol and hyperventilation should be titrated to an ICP < 30 mmHg or a cerebral perfusion pressure > 40 mmHg.

CIRCULATORY IMPAIRMENT

Hypotension is extremely common in patients with FHF. Although hemorrhage and infection contribute, in 60 percent of instances of hypotension, no explanation is found.[24] Hemodynamic evaluation of normotensive patients with FHF reveals a baseline increased cardiac output and reduced peripheral resistance. During periods of hypotension cardiac output decreases, but peripheral resistance falls to an even greater degree. Because associated bradycardia is seen in some patients, centrally mediated vasodilation has been postulated. Another potential explanation is the vasodilating effects of endotoxin, which has been shown to be present in increased amounts in patients with FHF.

In addition to disordered tone of the resistance vessels, evidence suggests that impaired microvascular regulation exists in FHF. An analysis of oxygen transport and extraction in 32 patients with FHF revealed that in those patients who died of liver failure there was a low extraction ratio (oxygen consumed divided by oxygen delivered) despite apparently reduced tissue perfusion (increased venous lactate) implying impaired oxygen utilization.[25] The apparent dependence of oxygen consumption on oxygen delivery further supports this concept.[26] The etiology of such microvascular dysfunction remains unclear. Circulating endotoxin, increased levels of vasoactive intestinal peptide, and substance P[27] have been proposed as potential mechanisms.

METABOLIC, RENAL, AND PULMONARY DERANGEMENTS

Extensive hepatocellular necrosis depletes hepatic glycogen stores and impairs hepatic gluconeogenesis. This combination results in significant hypoglycemia in many patients with FHF. Dextrose requirements may be unusually high. Commonly, 10% dextrose solutions are needed and as much as 2000 g has been given to maintain an acceptable plasma glucose level. Impaired hepatic metabolism of lactate may result in severe lactic acidosis. Sodium bicarbonate is probably not indicated, since in animal models of lactic acidosis due to hepatic failure, bicarbonate appears to increase lactate production (see Chap. 158).

Renal failure complicates 30 to 70 percent of cases of FHF. Renal failure may be due to acute tubular necrosis (ATN) or be functional in nature, with the latter predominating[28] (vide infra, Cirrhosis).

Arterial hypoxemia may be due to pulmonary vascular abnormalities or pulmonary edema. Pulmonary edema occurs in >30 percent of cases and often is associated with low intravascular pressures. A common mechanism underlying the pulmonary edema and cerebral edema of FHF has been proposed.[27]

PROGNOSIS

The prognosis in FHF may depend on the etiology of the hepatic damage. In several large series <10 percent to as many as 50 percent of patients survived.[29] Survival is more likely with acetaminophen overdose (53 percent) and hepatitis A (67 percent). Patients with hepatitis B, non-A, non-B hepatitis, and drug-induced injury (other than acetaminophen) are less likely to recover. Furthermore, in a retrospective multivariate analysis of prognostic variables in FHF, the authors suggested that etiology was the most important predictor of outcome.[30] However, in a pooled analysis of several other studies, a difference in survival between viral hepatitis (all types) and toxic injury could not be demonstrated.[31] Although etiology is important in determining prognosis, it is not the sole factor.

Survival correlates with the severity of liver injury. A markedly elevated prothrombin time and metabolic acidosis are associated with decreased survival in patients with acetaminophen-induced FHF.[30] The degree of HE also parallels survival.[32] In addition to these static variables, progression of HE over time and inability to correct the coagulopathy with the administration of vitamin K and clotting factors also indicate a poorer outcome. Such prognostic criteria may be important in determining which patients should be considered for OLT. Those lacking poor prognostic criteria might be spared a difficult surgical procedure and lifelong immunosuppressive therapy. Patients predicted to do poorly might undergo transplantation earlier, preempting the life-threatening complications of FHF.[30]

SPECIFIC THERAPIES

The substantial mortality of patients with FHF despite an aggressive supportive approach has sparked interest in artificial hepatic support and transplantation.

ARTIFICIAL HEPATIC SUPPORT

The rationale for artificial hepatic support presumes a group of patients whose liver dysfunction is so severe that survival is not possible, but whose liver might regenerate if the patient could be kept alive long enough.[33] In the past, cross-perfusion with primate livers, cross-circulation with normal donors, and exchange transfusion (including whole blood washout) have been attempted. Current interest has focused on hemoperfusion through columns of activated charcoal. In animals with FHF, charcoal hemoperfusion improves survival.[34] In one clinical trial, early institution of charcoal hemoperfusion benefitted patients with FHF and stage III encephalopathy when compared with treatment of historical controls.[35] However a recent, randomized controlled study in patients with stage IV encephalopathy demonstrated no difference in survival between treatment and control groups. Furthermore, survival rates of both groups were dramatically higher than those in the previous study. The authors concluded that the intensive management of complications rather than charcoal hemoperfusion improved survival, especially in patients with better "intrinsic survival" (i.e., those with acetaminophen intoxication or hepatitis A).[29] Although artificial hepatic support does not currently offer an additional benefit to aggressive supportive care, it remains an area of active research.

HEPATIC TRANSPLANTATION

The development of OLT has dramatically changed the management of FHF. Several series have demonstrated improved survival in patients who were transplanted in stage III or IV encephalopathy when compared with historic controls or patients who were not transplanted because of lack of organ availability.[11] Currently OLT is indicated in those patients with a poor prognosis, such as hepatic injury due to non-A, non-B hepatitis or Wilson's disease, and advanced encephalopathy. The difficult decisions arise in those patients who have a relatively good prognosis lesion such as acetaminophen toxicity and significant encephalopathy, or those with a poor prognosis lesion but only mild to moderate encephalopathy.

Chronic Liver Disease

Patients admitted to the ICU with complications of chronic liver disease usually have cirrhosis, but may also have chronic active hepatitis, hepatic vein thrombosis (Budd-Chiari syndrome), or nodular regenerative hyperplasia. Although HE is common, it is usually not the overriding complication as in FHF, since the HE of cirrhosis is more amenable to treatment and is not complicated by cerebral edema. Rather, the ICU course is dominated by variceal hemorrhage, spontaneous bacterial peritonitis (SBP), and the hepatorenal syndrome (HRS).

VARICEAL HEMORRHAGE

Bleeding from varices is a common complication of cirrhosis and a frequent cause of death. However, patients suspected of variceal hemorrhage are bleeding from other sites (e.g., portal hypertensive gastropathy, peptic ulcer disease, Mallory-Weiss tear) in about 30 percent of cases, making early definitive diagnosis with esophagogastroduodenoscopy essential.[36] Acute variceal hemorrhage is due to rupture of a dilated submucosal vein, usually just above the gastroesophageal junction. In about 15 percent of patients, bleeding is from a gastric varix, a point which has implications for management (vide infra). Prominent gastric varices in the absence of esophageal varices suggest splenic vein thrombosis, a condition which can be cured by splenectomy.

It is common for bleeding to cease spontaneously, making assessment of therapeutic interventions difficult. In one series of variceal bleeding, 85 patients underwent endoscopy within 4 h of active bleeding, before any definitive therapy was begun: only 25 percent were still bleeding.[37] For this reason, evaluation of therapeutic efficacy must be based on carefully designed prospective randomized trials rather than uncontrolled observations. Despite the frequency of spontaneous cessation of hemorrhage, rebleeding is the rule if definitive therapy is not undertaken. Therefore, some intervention is essential even when bleeding stops. New treatment options are evolving, and controlled, comparative trials of existing approaches have often yielded conflicting results. Therefore, the best therapy for acute variceal bleeding is not agreed on. Rather, treatment strategies depend on local expertise, individual interpretations of the literature, and personal preference. The approach given here is an attempt to synthesize a wide diversity of opinion.

SUPPORTIVE MANAGEMENT

The first goal is hemodynamic resuscitation. The approach to hemorrhagic shock is developed in Chap. 114, but several points are worth noting here. At least two large bore peripheral intravenous catheters should be maintained at all times, even if the patient appears to have stabilized. Intravascular volume should be repleted using crystalloid initially, adding packed red blood cells and fresh frozen plasma as needed. It is crucial that this stabilization be accomplished before the patient is subjected to endoscopy; otherwise this procedure may precipitate hemodynamic collapse and death. While adequate volume resuscitation is essential, hypervolemia raises portal pressure and the likelihood of continued hemorrhage. Therefore, in patients with severe hemorrhage, management may be aided by a central venous catheter, or if heart or lung disease is present, a pulmonary artery catheter. A central venous pressure of 10 cmH_2O and a pulmonary capillary wedge pressure of 12 to 16 cmH_2O are reasonable target pressures although these have not been validated in clinical trials. Coagulopathy should be reversed, if possible. Several units of blood should be kept in the blood bank until the patient has clearly stabilized and definitive therapy has been provided.

The second major goal in the first minutes of stabilization in the ICU is to assess the need for endotracheal intubation. Hematemesis, hemodynamic instability, HE, instrumentation near the airway (nasogastric tube, esophageal tamponade tube, endoscope), and drug therapies all contribute to a risk of massive blood aspiration or subsequent aspiration pneumonia. This airway assessment must be repeated and ongoing throughout the ICU course, so that intubation can be performed prophylactically, not belatedly. Clear indications for intubation include massive hematemesis, hemodynamic instability, and lethargy from HE. In addition, nearly all patients in whom esophageal tamponade tubes are placed should first be intubated. Diagnostic endoscopy

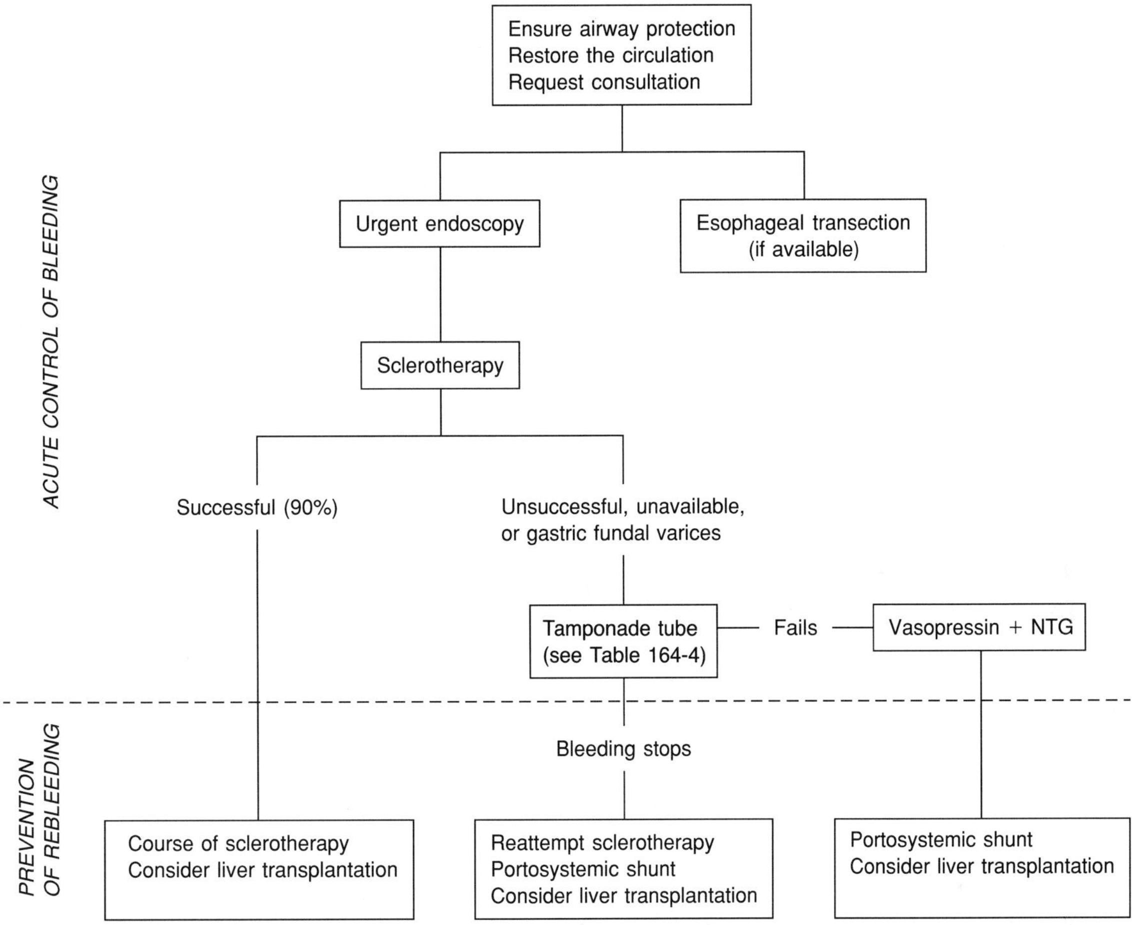

FIGURE 164-1 An approach to acute variceal hemorrhage is outlined. NTG, nitroglycerine (see text).

is an additional indication, particularly if bleeding is active, mental status is abnormal, or sedation is necessary.

Once acute resuscitation and airway control are established, attention can turn to control of bleeding (Fig. 164-1). It is useful to separately consider the acute control of bleeding and the subacute prevention of rebleeding, although these therapies overlap to some degree. As early as possible, consultation from a general surgeon, a hepatologist, and sometimes from a liver transplant surgeon should be obtained, even if bleeding seems minor.

ACUTE CONTROL OF BLEEDING

SCLEROTHERAPY. Urgent therapeutic endoscopy deserves the highest priority. Although sclerotherapy is technically more challenging during active hemorrhage, it can almost always be successfully accomplished by an experienced endoscopist. The technical aspects of sclerotherapy are discussed in Chap. 33. Acute control of bleeding is achieved in about 90 percent of patients. Transfusion requirements are reduced by sclerotherapy; however, survival, which is more related to hepatic function, is not improved. Gastric varices, which are the source of bleeding in up to 20 percent of cirrhotics, can be treated with sclerotherapy if they are on the lesser curvature or within a hiatus hernia. However, gastric fundal varices should generally be treated with a portosystemic shunt (PSS).

BALLOON TAMPONADE. Control of bleeding can be achieved in about 85 percent of patients with variceal tamponade tubes. The two most commonly used devices are the single gastric balloon Linton-Nachlas (L-N) tube and the gastric plus esophageal balloon Sengstaken-Blakemore (S-B) tube. In a comparative trial, bleeding control was equivalent (L-N 83 percent, S-B 90 percent).[38] We prefer the S-B tube, but begin by inflating only the gastric balloon (Table 164-4). This alone will cause cessation of bleeding in close to two-thirds of patients. If bleeding continues, the esophageal balloon is inflated as well.

Significant complications attend the use of these tubes. Aspiration is common, especially when the esophageal part of the S-B tube is inflated. Esophageal perforation, asphyxia, and nosocomial pneumonia are also seen. Since these devices are used only sporadically in most ICUs, placement should be guided by an established protocol and is best supervised by an experienced clinician. Acute rebleeding occurs when the balloon is deflated in about half

TABLE 164-4 Use of the Sengstaken-Blakemore Tube

1. Assess the need for airway intubation. **With rare exceptions (e.g., alert, cooperative, hemodynamically stable patient), an endotracheal tube (ETT) should be placed first.** The sedation typically mandated by the tube itself is often an indication for airway protection in itself.
2. This three-lumen tube consists of a distal (gastric) balloon, an esophageal balloon, and a distal suction/lavage port. Before placement, the integrity of both balloons must be ensured. The gastric (distal) balloon is a "volume" balloon which is filled with 250 mL air. The esophageal balloon is a "pressure" balloon and should be tested at 40 mmHg using a mercury manometer and a three-way stopcock.
3. Deflate the balloons, lubricate the device, and insert it through the mouth and into the stomach. A cooperative patient may be able to assist passage by swallowing. Placement in the stomach should be confirmed by injecting air through the distal lumen while listening for a rush of air over the stomach.
4. The gastric balloon should be partially inflated (100 mL) and a chest radiograph obtained to confirm adequate placement in the stomach. Then the balloon is fully inflated (total volume 250 mL). The tube is gently snugged against the gastroesophageal junction and affixed to an external device to maintain traction, a maneuver which will usually stop bleeding. **A conventional suction tube should be placed through the mouth, into the esophagus, to remove pooled secretions which will collect above the balloon.**
5. A repeat chest radiograph should be obtained to confirm proper placement of the gastric balloon against the gastroesophageal junction.
6. If bleeding continues, the esophageal balloon should be inflated to 25 to 40 mmHg, using the least pressure which maintains hemostasis. Some advocate deflating the esophageal balloon for 30 min each 12 h to reduce the likelihood of esophageal mucosal necrosis. The gastric balloon should never be deflated while the tube is in place.
7. Plans should be made for more definitive therapy to control bleeding.
8. In an emergency, the tube can be removed after cutting across all three lumens.

the patients so that this approach should be considered only as a bridge to one of the more definitive therapies.

PHARMACOTHERAPY. Intravenous vasopressin has long been used in variceal hemorrhage. However, its efficacy has never been shown,[39] and complications are frequent. Thus, its wide application is explained more by the triumph of optimism over experience than by rigorously established utility. In a meta-analysis of controlled trials of vasopressin, control of initial bleeding was achieved in 52 percent, rebleeding occurred in 45 percent, complications were frequent, and survival was not affected.[40] Typically, vasopressin is given at 40 U/h until bleeding stops, following which it is reduced to 20 U/h, then continued for 24 h or longer. Doses up to 90 U/h have been given, although complications are dose related. Common adverse effects include cardiac ischemia, myocardial infarction, bradycardia, hyponatremia, abdominal cramping, and hypertension.

In an attempt to reduce the toxicity of vasopressin, combination therapy with various vasodilators has been tried. Vasopressin has been combined with nitroglycerin (NTG), nitroprusside, isoproterenol, and isosorbide dinitrate, hoping to counter the detrimental systemic vasoconstriction which underlies most complications. The most useful combination appears to be with NTG, which can be given sublingually, intravenously, or transdermally. The addition of NTG further reduces portal pressure, while ameliorating systemic vasoconstriction.[41] Regimens which have been advocated include intravenous NTG titrated to lower the systolic blood pressure to 100 mmHg, using 40 to 400 μg/min,[42] or 0.4 mg given sublingually every 30 to 60 min. In a hemodynamically unstable patient, NTG should only be given intravenously in case it must be abruptly discontinued.

Alternative pharmacologic therapies have included triglycyl-lysine vasopressin and somatostatin. Experience with each of these remains somewhat limited, but both may have advantages over vasopressin. Triglycyl-lysine vasopressin is given as a 2-mg bolus every 4 h and is gradually metabolized to vasopressin. It has been shown to be superior to placebo in the control of bleeding while most side effects are minimal.[43] Somatostatin, 4.2 μg/min, has been compared with vasopressin and found to be more efficacious and safer, although mortality was unaffected and this drug is very expensive.[44] Propranolol has no role in the acutely bleeding patient and remains of controversial utility for chronic prevention of rebleeding.

In summary, standard pharmacotherapy is of little efficacy for the control of bleeding and often causes serious complications. It should be used only when sclerotherapy is unavailable or has failed and not at all in patients with coronary artery disease. Moreover, it should only be relied on as a temporizing measure until more effective therapy can be applied. Concomitant NTG should be given to reduce complications. The roles of triglycyl-lysine vasopressin and somatostatin remain to be determined.

PREVENTION OF REBLEEDING

After acute bleeding ceases spontaneously or is controlled by sclerotherapy, balloon tamponade, or pharmacotherapy, rebleeding is very common and often lethal. Therefore, definitive therapy must be instituted to preserve the gains of initial stabilization. At this point it is also useful to reassess the need for airway protection, plan for nutrition, administer cathartics to reduce the likelihood of HE, and begin surveillance for nosocomial infection. Further therapy for variceal bleeding includes liver transplantation, continued sclerotherapy, esophageal transection, and PSS. As noted above, β blockers have been advocated beginning 24 h after cessation of hemorrhage, but their use remains investigational.

LIVER TRANSPLANTATION. This therapy is discussed fully in Chap. 80. Transplantation is the ideal approach for candidates who have advanced or symptomatic liver disease. Not only is bleeding prevented, but the underlying disease is addressed as well. Since rebleeding may compromise the success of transplantation, candidates should be transplanted as soon as a donor liver is available. In patients who are considered transplant candidates, PSS operations should be avoided because they will complicate or even prevent future transplantation.

CONTINUED SCLEROTHERAPY. For the majority of patients who will not be acutely transplanted, chronic sclerotherapy is the treatment of choice. This approach has the advantages of maintaining portal perfusion and hepatic function, and probably reduces the incidence of HE.[45] Nevertheless, rebleeding occurs in about one-third of patients with prolonged follow-up.

ESOPHAGEAL TRANSECTION. This approach requires laparotomy during which a stapling device is inserted through a gastrotomy incision, and the esophagus is transected. It has not been widely applied but may be as effective as sclerotherapy for initial control of bleeding. It can also be used in patients who have failed sclerotherapy, especially those who are transplant candidates.[46] However, rebleeding after 6 months is common.

PORTOSYSTEMIC SHUNTING. Possibly the most controversy in the management of variceal bleeding surrounds the application of PSS. It has been advocated as the procedure of choice in high-risk patients by some and considered a last resort by others. In general, PSS is used in patients who are not transplant candidates and who have failed sclerotherapy. For all types of PSS, operative mortality is very high. Moreover, long-term survival is uncommon because most patients have severe hepatic insufficiency, and this is exacerbated by PSS. Therefore, before deciding to shunt any patient, an assessment of prognosis should be made.

Although PSS is usually effective in preventing further hemorrhage, it accelerates the deterioration in hepatic function. Therefore, HE is common and prolonged survival is unusual. The two most common surgical procedures are the portocaval shunt and the interposition mesocaval shunt. The advantage of the former is that early mortality is lower, while the second is preferred if future transplantation is an option (since the graft can simply be ligated at the time of transplant). A third approach, the distal splenorenal shunt, was devised to preserve portal flow with the hope of maintaining hepatocyte function. Despite encouraging initial results, several trials have failed to show a benefit in terms of HE for this more complex operation.

Since acute sclerotherapy is effective in the majority of patients with variceal hemorrhage, and less costly and invasive than portocaval shunting, it will remain the procedure of choice in most patients. However, the small number of cirrhotics who fail initial sclerotherapy, but are not transplant candidates, may benefit from PSS. For patients with gastric fundal varices, PSS is the treatment of choice.

SPONTANEOUS BACTERIAL PERITONITIS

Spontaneous bacterial peritonitis is an infection of preexisting cirrhotic ascites, without an apparent perforated viscus. Approximately 10 percent of hospitalized cirrhotics will have or develop SBP. This infection is associated with a substantial risk of in-hospital death (>50 percent) as well as 1 year mortality (62 percent[47]). However, most of those who die succumb to another complication of end-stage liver disease, rather than to SBP. Because SBP is a marker for a poor long-term prognosis, affected patients should be evaluated for possible liver transplantation.

The portal of entry of bacteria to the ascitic fluid is thought to be the bloodstream in the majority of cases. Alternative hypotheses that may account for abdominal seeding in some patients include infected abdominal lymph, intestinal transmural migration of bacteria, and spread from continguous sites of infection. Gastrointestinal endoscopy and radiologic procedures, liver biopsy, and intravenous catheters may be sources of bacteremia in some patients. Paracentesis only rarely results in perforation of bowel and cannot be implicated in the great majority of patients.

Most infecting organisms are gram-negative aerobic bacilli (69 percent), with *Escherichia coli* leading the list (47 percent), followed by streptococci (26 percent), and *Klebsiella* species (11 percent). SBP is uncommonly polymicrobial (8 percent).

CLINICAL MANIFESTATIONS

At the time of diagnosis, some patients are totally asymptomatic, while others have fulminant sepsis. Common findings include fever, abdominal pain or tenderness, increasing ascites, encephalopathy, and leukocytosis. These signs in a cirrhotic should always prompt diagnostic paracentesis because early treatment of SBP is crucial for optimal outcome. Since SBP is often very subtle, paracentesis should also be performed in cirrhotics with deteriorating renal function, hypothermia, new-onset diarrhea, or unexplained encephalopathy.

DIAGNOSIS

Numerous criteria have been proposed as a basis for the diagnosis, but each relies on an analysis of the ascitic fluid. These include a fluid PMN leukocyte count $>250/\text{mm}^3$, pH < 7.35, arterial pH to ascitic fluid pH gradient (A − AF pH) > 0.1, and fluid lactate concentration >25 mg/dL.[48] The most sensitive indicator is a PMN count $>250/\text{mm}^3$ (sensitivity 94 percent); therefore this serves as an indication for beginning treatment. Less sensitive parameters are A − AF pH > 0.1 and ascitic fluid pH < 7.31; however either of these results virtually ensures the diagnosis of SBP (specificity 99 percent).[48] Positive ascitic fluid cultures confirm the diagnosis, but these are negative in some patients. The yield has been increased by direct inoculation of fluid into blood culture bottles at the bedside.[49] Blood cultures are frequently positive as well and should be performed whenever the diagnosis of SBP is considered.

When a patient with ascites is found to have peritonitis, it is important to consider the possibility of an underlying abdominal infection (secondary peritonitis). Although most cirrhotics with peritonitis will have SBP, these patients are not immune to appendicitis, cholecystitis, and diverticulitis. It is impossible to distinguish SBP from secondary peritonitis based on the physical examination. Factors which may indicate underlying perforation of a viscus include polymicrobial ascitic infection, lack of response to antibiotics, a rising ascitic fluid PMN count, free intraabdominal air, glucose level <50 mg/dL, fluid lactate dehydrogenase level >225 mU/mL, or total protein concentration >1 g/dL.[50]

TREATMENT
Treatment with antibiotics should begin in any patient with an ascitic fluid PMN count >250/mm^3. A Gram stain of the fluid may provide a guide to antibiotic selection in some patients, especially if a polymicrobial flora is demonstrated (mandating anaerobic coverage). The preferred empirical regimen is cefotaxime, 2 g intravenously every 6 h, since this drug is at least as effective as ampicillin plus an aminoglycoside, yet is less nephrotoxic.[51] Subsequently, the regimen should be adjusted based on results of ascitic fluid or blood cultures and should continue for 10 to 14 days. If all cultures are negative, SBP is not excluded. If the initial ascitic fluid PMN count is >500/mm^3, SBP is highly likely despite negative cultures, and empirical therapy should continue. If cultures are negative, the clinical suspicion of SBP is low, and the initial ascitic fluid PMN count is <500/mm^3, antibiotics can be discontinued.[48] If the patient is unimproved in 48 h, paracentesis should be repeated to assess the effectiveness of therapy.

HEPATORENAL SYNDROME

The HRS is functional renal failure complicating severe hepatic disease, usually in patients with tense ascites. Although the kidneys are structurally and histologically normal, HRS is nearly always irreversible. Successful hepatic transplantation can restore normal renal function; far less commonly, the syndrome spontaneously remits. Often, it is the final, lethal complication of cirrhosis. It may be precipitated by critical illness (hypotension, sepsis, variceal hemorrhage) or medical interventions (paracentesis, diuresis, prostaglandin inhibitors), prompting admission to the ICU.

PATHOPHYSIOLOGY
The pathogenesis of HRS is not known with certainty, but its likelihood parallels the severity of the hepatic failure. The most attractive hypothesis to explain the syndrome, the "peripheral arterial vasodilation hypothesis," was proposed in 1988.[52] In this model, the fundamental defect is the extreme peripheral vasodilation characteristic of severe liver disease. This results in marked "arterial underfilling," a term distinct from hypovolemia (see Chap. 3). As a consequence, plasma renin, aldosterone, antidiuretic hormone, and norepinephrine levels rise, causing intense renal vasoconstriction. Renal vasoconstriction causes sodium and water retention (adding to ascites and edema), culminating in functional renal failure. Renal vasodilator prostaglandins are synthesized in an attempt to maintain renal perfusion, a response which delays the evolution of renal failure. This mechanism explains the marked sensitivity of decompensated cirrhotics to prostaglandin inhibitors.

DIAGNOSIS
The diagnosis is typically considered when azotemia or oliguria is noted, usually in the setting of tense ascites, and typically following one of the precipitants identified above. The differential diagnosis includes most of the causes of acute renal failure (see Chap. 153), but hypovolemic prerenal azotemia and ATN deserve mention. It is crucial to exclude hypovolemia, because this can mimic HRS in all respects. If hypovolemia cannot be confidently ruled out on clinical grounds, it may be necessary to place a pulmonary artery catheter. An alternative is to give a rapid fluid challenge (500 to 1000 mL), observing the response. Because hypovolemia is easily reversible, while HRS is lethal, it is hard to overemphasize the importance of ensuring adequate intravascular volume. ATN is less likely to masquerade as HRS, but it, too, may be reversible. Precipitants such as aminoglycosides, radiographic dye, and hemorrhagic hypotension should be sought. In HRS the urinalysis is benign, resembling that seen in prerenal azotemia. Urine electrolyte analysis can be especially useful; in prerenal azotemia, the urinary sodium concentration is low and the urine:plasma creatinine ratio is elevated. In ATN, the urine sodium content is usually, but not invariably, higher than 20 meq/L, while the urine:plasma creatinine ratio is <20. Renal tubular casts may be identified in a fresh urine specimen of the patient with ATN. In all instances of renal failure, prostaglandin inhibitors must be avoided or discontinued.

TREATMENT
This syndrome has been largely refractory to therapy short of hepatic transplantation. Rarely, patients have responded spontaneously or to portocaval shunting or peritoneal-venous drainage. Dialysis can treat uremia and its complications but does not reverse HRS. Therefore, when the diagnosis of HRS is certain, dialysis should only be instituted as a bridge to more definitive therapy (transplantation). Other potential treatments such as the use of vasoactive drugs or diuretics are generally ineffective.

HYPOXEMIA

Severe hypoxemia is an uncommon complication of severe chronic liver disease. The pathophysiology was the subject of speculation for many years, but has recently been delineated with the use of the multiple inert gas elimination technique (MIGET). Whie some patients have demonstrable right-to-left shunting, in most patients hypoxemia is attributable to ventilation perfusion ($\dot{V}/\dot{Q}$) mismatching.[53,54] Some patients with cirrhosis do not manifest hypoxemia, despite significant $\dot{V}/\dot{Q}$ mismatching, because they compensate with increased cardiac output and hyperventilation. This may bear on the cirrhotic who becomes critically ill since, as oxygen consumption rises or cardiac output becomes limited, the gas exchange defect may become manifest.[55] Hypoxemia may temporarily respond to increasing the inspired oxygen fraction; however, the only long-term solution is restoration of hepatic function. While severe hypoxemia has generally been considered a contraindication to hepatic transplantation, the $\dot{V}/\dot{Q}$ abnormality, as well as intrapulmonary shunt, is reversible, and we have successfully transplanted one patient with a resting room air P_{O_2} of 43 mmHg.

CASE PRESENTATION

A 55-year-old white woman in previous good health was admitted from another hospital with the diagnosis of FHF.

The patient was in her usual state of health until approximately 2 weeks prior to admission when she and her husband consumed several wild mushrooms, which they had picked themselves. The following morning the patient developed nausea, vomiting, abdominal pain, severe headache, and diffuse myalgias. She was seen by a physician who felt she was suffering from a viral gastroenteritis. Her symptoms persisted.

She was then admitted to another institution. Her physical examination was of note only for dehydration. Admitting laboratory data revealed a metabolic acidosis and hypoglycemia, serum ALT was 5110 U/L, serum AST was 4950 U/L, LDH was 5170 U/L, alkaline phosphatase was 181 U/L, total bilirubin was 3.1 mg/dL and PT was >50 s. Progressive lethargy and confusion developed. The history of mushroom ingestion was obtained from the husband and a presumptive diagnosis of *Amanita* intoxication was made. She was transfered for evaluation for OLT.

On transfer the patient was obtunded. Her physical examination was notable for jaundice, stable vital signs, and a liver span of 8 cm. She did not respond to painful stimuli; examination of the cranial nerves revealed intact pupillary and cold caloric reflexes with diminished gag reflex; muscle tone was increased diffusely. Laboratory data revealed a hemoglobin level of 15.5 g/dL, a WBC count of 5.0×10^3/mL, and a platlet count of 124×10^3/mL; PT was >100 s, PTT was 64 s, fibrinogen was 55 mg/dL; total bilirubin was 9.8 mg/dL, ALT was 1670 U/L, AST was 1806 U/L, LDH was 1200 U/L, the alkaline phosphatase was 164 U/L and γ-glutamyl transferase was 84 U/L. An arterial ammonia level was 348 μg/dL and arterial lactate was 5.5 meq/L.

Because of stage IV encephalopathy the patient was electively intubated after mask hyperventilation and administration of thiamylal (200 mg) and intravenous lidocaine (100 mg). An emergent CT scan of the brain revealed obliteration of the sulci and loss of the white-gray matter border, consistent with cerebral edema and increased ICP. Therapy for HE with lactulose was initiated via nasogastric tube. Hyperventilation was used to achieve a Pa_{CO_2} of 25 mmHg. Oxygenation was well maintained (Pa_{O_2} of 110 mmHg on an $F_{I_{O_2}}$ of 30%) with 3 cmH_2O positive end-expiratory pressure. Mannitol (0.5 g/kg) was administered by rapid bolus infusion and repeated as necessary according to clinical parameters of increased ICP (muscle rigidity, decorticate posturing, pupillary responses) and serum osmolarity. Mild hypotension (90/40) prompted the insertion of a pulmonary artery catheter to better assess volume status: it revealed a pulmonary capillary wedge pressure of 3 mmHg with a cardiac output of 9 L/min. Because of adequate urine output, high mixed venous oxygen saturation (82%) and stable metabolic acidosis, no effort was made to increase filling pressures or cardiac output. Penicillin was administered to prevent further hepatic uptake of *Amanita* toxins. Silibinin was not given because of the long delay following exposure. The patient received 10% dextrose and saline solution at 125 mL/h (300 g/day glucose). Blood glucose was monitored frequently, and serial neurologic examinations were performed. The patient was placed on the United Network for Organ Sharing stat listing.

Aggressive support was continued with no change in the patient's mental status or coagulopathy. On hospital day 4, OLT was performed. The procedure was relatively uncomplicated and the next day the patient was following commands appropriately. Her postoperative course was complicated by infection and pulmonary edema, but she eventually left the hospital for rehabilitation.

CASE DISCUSSION

Fulminant hepatic failure following ingestion of *Amanita* species of mushrooms is uncommon in the United States, but frequently reported in Europe. Early diagnosis allows therapy with silibinin and penicillin, which may reduce the hepatic injury (see Chap. 181). Unfortunately, in this instance the hepatic injury was well established when the diagnosis was made.

The rapid progression of HE seen in this case is typical of the course followed by patients with FHF. The failure of encephalopathy to respond to conventional therapy is also common. Early management should be focused on airway protection and exclusion of alternative causes of encephalopathy. Because stage IV encephalopathy is often associated with increased ICP, intubation was performed under the most controlled circumstances possible: the patient was mask hyperventilated, and anesthesia with a short-acting barbiturate and lidocaine was used. Hypoglycemia and electrolyte imbalance were excluded. A CT scan of the head was performed to exclude a structural cause for encephalopathy. While no focal structural lesion was seen, changes consistent with cerebral edema and increased ICP were noted.

Because of the CT and physical examination findings consistent with early increased ICP, hyperventilation and mannitol infusion were initiated. In our institution ICP monitoring is not available to patients with FHF, so therapy must be titrated against physical examination findings alone. While currently available studies suggest that invasive ICP monitoring adds little to the survival of patients with FHF, the titration of therapy for increased ICP is difficult without it.

The remainder of care in the medical ICU was focused on maintaining normal renal function and reducing the likelihood of infection or other complications. The insertion of a pulmonary artery catheter to monitor fluid status might be viewed as aggressive, but volume shifts related to therapy with mannitol as well as those associated with FHF alone might lead to hypovolemia and increase the likelihood of renal failure. The hypotension noted was typical of that associated with FHF as the cardiac output was high with a low peripheral resistance, suggesting disordered vascular regulation. The patient did not demonstrate significant hypoxemia and no radiographic evidence of pulmonary edema was seen. Hypoxemia in FHF is typically due to pulmonary edema or pneumonia, whereas severe ventilation perfusion abnormalities and some right-to-left shunt characterize the hypoxemia noted in cirrhosis. Fresh frozen plasma was infused prior to catheter insertion, but no other attempt was made to correct the coagulopathy. Ranitidine was infused to prevent stress ulceration.

Finally, because of the extremely poor prognosis of a patient with toxin-related FHF presenting with stage IV encephalopathy and PT $>$100 s, the decision was made early in the hospital course to perform OLT as soon as an organ was available. Her operative course was of note for minimal blood requirements, a testimony to the ability of massive plasma replacement at the time of surgery to correct the coagulopathy as well as the continued improvement in surgical technique. Our patient, like many in reported series, had dramatic improvement in mental status immediately following OLT.

References

1. Rolando N. Harvey F, Brahm J, et al: Prospective study of bacterial infection in acute liver failure: An analysis of fifty patients. Hepatology 11:49, 1990.
2. Rimola A, Bory F, Planas R: Infecciones bacterianas agudas en la cirrhosis hepatica. Gastroenterol Hepatol 4:453, 1981.
3. Jones EA, Schafer DF: Fulminant hepatic failure, in Zakim D, Boyer T (eds): *Hepatology: A Textbook of Liver Disease.* Philadelphia, Saunders, 1990.
4. MacDougall BR, Williams R: H_2-receptor antagonists in the prevention of acute upper gastrointestinal hemorrhage in fulminant hepatic failure: A controlled trial. Gastroenterology 74:464, 1978.
5. Jones EA, Skolnick P, Gammal SH, et al: The gamma-aminobutyric acid A ($GABA_A$) receptor complex and hepatic encephalopathy. Ann Intern Med 110:532, 1989.
6. Levy LJ, Losowsky MS: Plasma gamma aminobutyric acid concentrations provide evidence of different mechanisms in the pathogenesis of hepatic encephalopathy in acute and chronic liver disease. Hepatogastroenterology 36:494, 1989.
7. Mullen KD, Szauter KM, Kaminsky-Russ K: "Endogenous" benzodiazepine activity in body fluids of patients with hepatic encephalopathy. Lancet ii:81, 1990.
8. Bansky G, Meier PJ, Riederer E, et al: Effects of the benzodiazepine receptor antagonist flumazenil in hepatic encephalopathy in humans. Gastroenterology 97:744, 1989.
9. Gammal SH, Basile AS, Geller D, et al: Reversal of the behavioral and electrophysiological abnormalities of an animal model of hepatic encephalopathy by benzodiazepine receptor ligands. Hepatology 11:371, 1990.
10. Naylor CD, O'Rourke K, Detsky AS, et al: Parenteral nutrition with branched-chain amino acids in hepatic encephalopathy: A meta-analysis. Gastroenterology 97:1033, 1989.
11. Emond J, Aran P, Whitington P, et al: Liver transplantation in the management of fulminant hepatic failure. Gastroenterology 96:1583, 1989.
12. Bansky G, Meier PJ, Riederer E, et al: Effects of the benzodiazepine receptor antagonist flumazenil in hepatic encephalopathy. Lancet ii:81, 1990.
13. Govindarajan S, Chin KP, Redecker AG, et al: Fulminant B viral hepatitis: Role of delta agent. Gastroenterology 86:1417, 1984.
14. Ware AJ, D'Agostino AN, Combes B: Cerebral edema; a major complication of massive hepatic necrosis. Gastroenterology 61:877, 1971.
15. Canalese J, Gimson A, Davis C, et al: Controlled trial of dexamethasone and mannitol for the cerebral oedema of fulminant hepatic failure. Gut 23:625, 1982.
16. Silk DBA, Hanid MA, Trewby PN, et al: Treatment of fulminant hepatic failure by polyacrylonitrile membrane haemodialysis. Lancet ii:1, 1977.
17. Seda HW, Hughes RD, Gove CD, Williams R: Inhibition of rat brain Na^+, K^+-ATPase activity by serum from patients with fulminant hepatic failure. Hepatology 4:74, 1984.
18. Ede RJ, Gove CD, Willaism R: Reduced Na^+, K^+-dependent ATPase activity during acute hepatic failure in the rat: A possible cause of encephalopathy and cerebral oedema. Clin Sci 66:62, 1984.
19. Zaki AEO, Ede RJ, Davis M, Williams R: Experimental studies of blood brain barrier permeability in acute hepatic failure. Hepatology 4:359, 1984.
20. Ede RJ, Gimson AE, Bihari D, Williams R: Controlled hyperventilation in the prevention of cerebral oedema in fulminant hepatic failure. J Hepatol 2:43, 1986.
21. Davenport A, Will E, Davison A: Effect of posture on intracranial pressure and cerebral perfusion pressure in patients with fulminant hepatic and renal failure after acetaminophen self-poisoning. Crit Care Med 18:286, 1990.
22. Ede RJ, Williams R: Hepatic encephalopathy and cerebral edema, in Williams R (ed): Semin Liver Dis 6:107, 1986.
23. Hanid MA, Davies M, Mellon PJ, et al: Clinical monitoring of intracranial pressure in fulminant hepatic failure. Gut 21:866, 1980.
24. Trewby PN, Williams R: Pathophysiology of hypotension in patients with fulminant hepatic failure. Gut 18:1021, 1977.
25. Bihari D, Gimson A, Waterson M, Williams R: Tissue hypoxia during fulminant hepatic failure. Crit Care Med 13:1034, 1985.
26. Gimson A, Bihari D, Wilson C, et al: Delivery dependent oxygen consumption in acute liver failure. Clin Sci Mol Med 66:12, 1984.
27. Bihari D, Gimson A, Williams R: Cardiovascular, pulmonary and renal complications of fulminant hepatic failure, in Williams R (ed): Semin Liver Dis 6:119, 1986.
28. Ring-Larsen H, Palazzo U: Renal failure in fulminant hepatic failure and terminal cirrhosis: A comparison between incidence, types and prognosis. Gut 22:585, 1981.
29. O'Grady JG, Gimson AE, O'Brien CJ, et al: Controlled trials of charcoal hemoperfusion and prognostic factors in fulminant hepatic failure. Gastroenterology 94:1186, 1988.
30. O'Grady JG, Alexander GJ, Hayllar K, Williams R: Early indicators of prognosis in fulminant hepatic failure. Gastroenterology 97:439, 1989.
31. Tygstrup N, Ranek L: Assessment of prognosis in fulminant hepatic failure, in Williams R (ed): Semin Liver Dis 6:159, 1986.

32. Trey C, Lipworth L, Davidson CS: Parameters influencing survival in the first 318 patients reported to the Fulminant Hepatic Failure Surveillance Study. Gastroenterology 58:306, 1970.
33. Tygstrup N, Andreasen PB, Ranek L: Liver failure and quantitative liver function, in Williams R, Murray-Lyon IM (eds): *Artificial Liver Support.* Turnbridge Wells, England, Pitman Medical, 1975, p 286.
34. Chang TMS, Lister C, Chirito E, et al: Effects of hemoperfusion rate and time of initiation of ACAC charcoal hemoperfusion on the survival of fulminant hepatic failure rats. Trans Am Soc Artif Intern Organs 24:243, 1978.
35. Gimson AE, Braude S, Mellon PJ, et al: Earlier charcoal haemoperfusion in fulminant hepatic failure. Lancet 2:681, 1982.
36. Terblanche J: Has sclerotherapy altered the management of patients with variceal bleeding? Am J Surg 160:37, 1990.
37. Mitchell KJ, Macdougall BRD, Silk DBA, et al: A prospective reappraisal of emergency endoscopy in patients with portal hypertension. Scand J Gastroenterol 17:965, 1982.
38. Teres J, Cecilia A, Bordas JM, et al: Esophageal tamponade for bleeding varices: Controlled trial between the Sengstaken-Blakemore tube and the Linton-Nachlas tube. Gastroenterology 75:566, 1978.
39. Sherlock S: Vasopressin and vasopressin analogues in liver disease. J Hepatol 5:232, 1987.
40. Grace ND: Variceal hemorrhage: Pharmacologic approach, in McDermott WV, Bothe A (eds): *Surgery of the Liver.* Boston, Blackwell Scientific Publications, 1988, pp 303–314.
41. Grace ND: A hepatologist's view of variceal bleeding. Am J Surg 160:26, 1990.
42. Teres J, Planas R, Panes J, et al: Vasopressin/nitroglycerin infusion vs. esophageal tamponade in the treatment of acute variceal bleeding: A randomized controlled trial. Hepatology 11:964, 1990.
43. Soderlund C, Magnusson I, Torngren S, et al: Terlipressin (triglycyl-lysine vasopressin) controls acute bleeding oesophageal varices. Scand J Gastroenterol 25:622, 1990.
44. Saari A, Klvilaakso E, Inberg M, et al: Comparison of somatostatin and vasopressin in bleeding esophageal varices. Am J Gastroenterol 85:804, 1990.
45. Rikkers LF: Definitive therapy for variceal bleeding: A personal view. Am J Surg 160:80, 1990.
46. Terblanche J, Burroughs AK, Hobbs KEF: Controversies in the management of bleeding esophageal varices. N Engl J Med 320:1393, 1989.
47. Tito L, Rimola A, Gines P, et al: Recurrence of spontaneous bacterial peritonitis in cirrhosis: Frequency and predictive factors. Hepatology 8:27, 1988.
48. Wilcox CM, Dismukes WE: Spontaneous bacterial peritonitis: A review of pathogenesis, diagnosis, and treatment. Medicine (Baltimore) 66:447, 1987.
49. Runyon BA, Umland ET, Merlin T: Inoculation of blood culture bottles with ascitic fluid: Improved detection of spontaneous bacterial peritonitis. Arch Intern Med 147:73, 1987.
50. Runyon BA, Hoefs JC: Spontaneous vs secondary bacterial peritonitis: Differentiation by response of ascitic fluid neutrophil count to antimicrobial therapy. Arch Intern Med 146:1563, 1986.
51. Felisart J, Rimola A, Arroyo V, et al: Cefotaxime is more effective than ampicillin-tobramycin in cirrhotics with severe infections. Hepatology 5:457, 1985.
52. Schrier RW, Arroyo V, Bernardi M, et al: Peripheral arterial vasodilation hypothesis: A proposal for the initiation of renal sodium and water retention in cirrhosis. Hepatology 8:1151, 1988.
53. Rodriguez-Roisin R, Roca J, Agusti A, et al: Gas exchange and pulmonary vascular reactivity in patients with liver cirrhosis. Am Rev Respir Dis 135:1085, 1987.
54. Melot C, Naeije R, Dechamps P, et al: Pulmonary and extrapulmonary contributors to hypoxemia in liver cirrhosis. Am Rev Respir Dis 139:632, 1989.
55. Agusti AG, Roca J, Rodriguez-Roisin R, et al: Pulmonary hemodynamics and gas exchange during exercise in liver cirrhosis. Am Rev Respir Dis 139:485, 1989.

Chapter 165

ACUTE PANCREATITIS IN THE CRITICALLY ILL

BRYCE R. TAYLOR

KEY POINTS

- *Etiology of acute pancreatitis in the ICU setting is multifactorial, and patients with hypoperfusion injury from various causes are most at risk.*
- *Serial computed tomography (CT) scanning is most useful in confirming the diagnosis and in following the inflammatory process.*
- *The likelihood of multisystem failure is high, and preventive measures must be instituted early.*
- *Initial treatment is supportive, with aggressive fluid and electrolyte replacement and close monitoring of hemodynamic, pulmonary, and renal status.*
- *Surgical intervention is indicated for deteriorating patients with a surgically correctable lesion and in patients with complications of the disease such as major hemorrhage, abscess, or symptomatic pseudocyst.*
- *Close supervision by an experienced abdominal surgeon is important for assessing the indications for surgical exploration.*

Acute pancreatitis can be a frustrating disease to diagnose and treat. Causes are myriad and poorly understood, pathologic variation is great, diagnosis is often difficult, and treatment in most cases is nonspecific and supportive only. Pancreatitis usually presents as a self-limiting disease from which the patient recovers without complication or intervention. In its most severe form (approximately 10 percent of cases), it is a potentially lethal disease complicated by multisystem failure and sepsis, often requiring sophisticated intensive care and judiciously timed surgical debridement, carrying a mortality rate of up to 30 to 40 percent.[1,2] Most intensivists are therefore well familiar with the patient who presents with acute necrotizing pancreatitis and who may occupy a bed for many months, often ultimately dying of septic complications.

The subject of this chapter is the increasingly recognized entity of acute pancreatitis in the patient who is already critically ill from other causes. Discussion will focus on the associated diseases reported to date, the pathogenesis of this unusual form, its recognition, and finally its management.

Etiology

Many causes of acute pancreatitis have been recognized, the most common being alcohol and gallstones. Table 165-1 lists the reported diverse causes of acute pancreatitis under various headings.

Whatever the initiating cause, the pathogenetic mechanism common to all forms of acute pancreatitis seems to be an intense inflammatory response caused by the release of activated pancreatic enzymes, with resultant tissue destruction, fluid and electrolyte loss, hypotension, renal and pulmonary complications, late septic complications, and in 20 to 40 percent of severe cases, multisystem organ failure (MSOF) and death.[3]

The list of illnesses in the critically ill patient that may precede the development of pancreatitis in the ICU is a growing one and appears in Table 165-2. Why are these seemingly disparate groups of patients at risk to develop this apparently unrelated and possibly lethal condition? The answer is not known and may be multifactorial.

After cardiopulmonary bypass, important factors may be microembolism and venous thrombosis,[4,5] a low postoperative flow state, prolonged bypass,[6] intraoperative or postoperative bleeding, hypothermia,[7] and the use of both nar-

TABLE 165-1 Acute Pancreatitis—Etiologic Factors

Metabolic	Obstructive/Mechanical	Infections	Idiopathic	Hypoperfusion
Alcohol	Gallstones	Mumps	Familial	Vascular
Hypercalcemia	Afferent loop obstruction	Coxsackie		PAN[c] and other collagen disorders
Drugs	Duodenal obstruction	*Mycoplasma*		Embolic
Hyperlipidemia	Periampullary tumors	Ascariasis[a]		Low flow states
	Duodenal ulcer	Clonorchiasis[a]		
	Pancreas divisum			
	Trauma			
	Blunt			
	Penetrating			
	Postoperative			
	After ERCP[b]			

[a]May cause pancreatitis by an obstructive mechanism.
[b]Endoscopic retrograde cholangiopancreatography
[c]Polyarteritis nodosa

TABLE 165-2 Pre-existing Conditions/Procedures

1. Cardiopulmonary bypass
2. Cardiac transplantation
3. Abdominal aortic aneurysm repair
4. Renal transplantation
5. Liver transplantation
6. Shock from any cause
7. Major upper abdominal surgery

cotics and vasopressors.[8] After cardiac transplantation, the pancreatitis frequently reported may be related to the effect of heparin on platelet aggregation[9] and the administration of cyclosporin A[10] and prednisone,[11] in addition to the factors suggested for cardiopulmonary bypass. Abdominal aortic aneurysm repair, especially after acute rupture, may produce hypotension, microemboli, and vasoconstriction, with prolonged hypoperfusion of the pancreas.[12]

Postrenal transplant pancreatitis may be related to hypercalcemia,[13] specific operative factors, or to immunosuppression as for cardiac transplantation. The reasons for severe pancreatitis after liver transplantation may include direct dissection in some cases, blood loss and hypovolemia, or obstruction to pancreatic venous outflow during prolonged venous bypass. One group has suggested that a hepatitis B infectious factor may be involved.[14]

Review of these possible mechanisms for pancreatitis developing in the critically ill patient seems to confirm hypoperfusion injury as a major pathogenetic mechanism. In fact, one group suggested that *any* patient in shock from a variety of causes (oligemic, cardiogenic, or septic) is at risk to develop pancreatitis.[15] The actual mechanism of this injury causing release of activated enzymes and an inflammatory response is not known.

Hypoperfusion may play an important role in the conversion of a less severe self-limiting pancreatitis into the more lethal necrotizing form, even when the more common etiologic factors such as alcohol and gallstones are major contributors in the noncritical care setting.[16]

Many major upper abdominal procedures have been reported to be complicated by pancreatitis, usually from direct dissection or injury of the gland at surgery (see Table 165-2). However, since any patient subjected to a period of hypotension intraoperatively is a candidate for hyperamylasemia or pancreatitis or both, these cases previously thought to have a mechanical cause only may well be multifactorial.

Diagnosis

Whatever the cause of the new disease in the ICU patient, the physician must diagnose the condition early, attempt to assess the severity of the process, institute appropriate aggressive supportive management, and use judgment to decide the timing and selection of surgical intervention, if necessary. Most patients may improve even if the disease is virtually ignored; those few whose pancreas becomes necrotic and infected need aggressive and timely surgery to avoid MSOF and death.

Clinical signs and symptoms are notoriously variable in patients with pancreatitis[12] and even more difficult to evaluate in the critically ill. The patient may complain of abdominal pain, nausea, and vomiting; often the patient will demonstrate nonspecific features, such as elevated temperature, leukocytosis, or in more severe cases, unexplained hemodynamic instability and increased fluid requirements without major clinical findings. Serum amylase,[17–19] random urinary amylase, and the amylase : creatinine clearance ratio may be useful[20,21] but not reliable in all patients. Serum lipase[22] may be more reliable and specific than serum amylase but has not gained wide acceptance. Isoamylase determinations,[23] serum elastase, phospholipase A_2, and trypsin have been suggested but have not been practically useful.[24,25]

In addition to clinical evaluation and frequently unreliable biochemical tests, morphologic assessment of the retroperitoneum is necessary. Patients presenting initially with suspected pancreatitis usually undergo routine abdominal and chest films which rule out other significant catastrophes such as perforation and mechanical intestinal obstruction. These films may also suggest pancreatitis by demonstrating pleural effusions, localized jejunal or colonic ileus, outline of a widened duodenal C loop, pancreatic calcification, associated radiopaque gallstones, or obliteration of psoas shadows and free intraperitoneal fluid. However, convenience, positioning, and the inconclusive nature of these findings have led to reliance on other radiologic tests, namely ultrasound and CT scan.

ULTRASOUND

Ultrasonography is the modality of choice in patients with edematous pancreatitis who rapidly respond to conservative therapy, in suspected biliary pancreatitis with a mild clinical course, and in follow-up of a retroperitoneal collection or phlegmon for resolution or development of a pseudocyst.[26] It has also been suggested that Doppler ultrasound may be valuable in detecting pseudoaneurysms >1 cm. However, paralytic ileus and obesity together severely hamper the ultrasonographer's ability to evaluate the retroperitoneum.

High resolution real-time scanners now examine in detail the pancreatic gland, its peripancreatic compartments, and the associated biliary tract, with the patient in the semierect, sitting, and supine positions. These maneuvers unfortunately may be difficult in a critically ill patient.

The abnormalities detected on ultrasound may be variable. The gland itself may be diffusely enlarged and hypoechoic or have a normal appearance, depending on a number of factors such as timing of the study, presence of underlying chronic disease, and the degree of intrapancreatic fat or hemorrhage. Ductal diameter is similarly variable and may be increased, normal, or decreased. The ultrasonographer is just as interested in the peripancreatic retroperitoneal spaces, looking for evidence of acute fluid collections in the lesser sac, phlegmon, and hemorrhage. It is also possible to detect displacement of the gastrointestinal tract and the presence of intraperitoneal fluid. Fluid collections in the lesser sac usually regress as the clinical picture improves. Those that do not and are surrounded by a dense pseudocapsule may be legitimately termed *chronic pseudocysts* and be treated usually by some sort of radiologic or surgical intervention.

Critical in the assessment of the retroperitoneum is the detection of scattered pancreatic necrosis and the involvement of peripancreatic tissues with fat necrosis, hemorrhage, and ultimately abscess formation; unfortunately, ultrasonography is limited in its ability to define these subtle changes in tissue density.[26]

CT SCAN

CT scanning is the most useful tool in assessing the retroperitoneum morphologically, especially in complicated cases. The procedure in the acutely ill patient may be somewhat inconvenient and cumbersome because of endotracheal intubation, multiple lines, and hemodynamic instability, but these problems are not insurmountable.

A mildly inflamed pancreas may show slight diffuse enlargement with irregular borders and patchy densities. Peripancreatic fat may increase in density as it necroses. The more severe forms of pancreatitis are accompanied by an increase in peripancreatic inflammatory exudate and intrapancreatic fluid collections. Often the pancreas is markedly enlarged, with irregular fluid collections in the retroperitoneum and poor enhancement in scattered areas within the gland. Unlike ultrasonography, CT is an excellent method to identify high density fluid collections in the transverse mesocolon, small bowel mesentery, and pararenal and perirenal spaces.[27]

The critical value of CT is in the recognition and follow-up of significant complications. Pancreatic abscess consists of pancreatic necrosis which becomes infected and liquefied; it presents on CT as ill-defined or poorly encapsulated fluid collections of different densities with air bubbles being recognized in about 20 percent of cases. Pseudoaneurysms may also be detected by CT, and with enhancement, may be highlighted.

SEVERITY OF DISEASE

The intensivist must identify not only the presence of the new condition, but also its severity, and the likelihood of progression to necrosis and complications. Ranson's criteria[28] have been used to indicate severity and prognosis in the patient who presents with pancreatitis (Table 165-3), but are clearly difficult to evaluate in the critically ill patient who develops pancreatitis as a secondary disease. These indicators are directed toward the systemic effects of the disease, and in the patient under consideration, a number of Ranson's criteria may already be present before the onset of the pancreatitis.

Numerous blood tests have been suggested as indicators of severity (areas of necrosis within the gland), e.g., cyclic adenosine monophosphate, albumin, methemalbumin,[29] ribonuclease,[30] C-reactive protein,[31] and fibrinogen.[24] Another group has reported that the volume and color of peritoneal aspirate at diagnosis is useful.[32] None of these tests has been as accurate, however, as clinical assessment of the patient and serial CT scans of the abdomen, especially in the ICU setting.[33,34] The development of abdominal pain, tenderness, fever, leukocytosis, hemodynamic instability, and CT changes within 1 to 2 weeks of the presumed onset of the pancreatitis provides the best assessment of the severe complications of the disease.

In the patient who is deteriorating or is persistently septic, and whose CT scan demonstrates features typical of pancreatic necrosis listed above, percutaneous aspiration of the retroperitoneum with microscopic examination and cultures can be valuable[35–37] and is frequently used in our unit to direct further management.

TABLE 165-3 Early Objective Prognostic Signs Used to Estimate the Risk of Death or Major Complications from Acute Pancreatitis

At Admission or Diagnosis	During Initial 48 h
Age >55	Hematocrit fall >10 percentage points
White cell count >16,000/mmm^3	BUN rise >5 mg/100 mL
Blood glucose >200 mg/100 mL	Serum calcium level below 8 mg/100 mL
Serum LDH >350 IU/L	Arterial O_2 <60 mmHg
SGOT >250 U/dL	Base deficit >4 meq/L
	Estimated fluid sequestration >6 L

SOURCE: From Ranson JHC, Rifkind KM, Turner JW: Prognostic signs and nonoperative peritoneal lavage in acute pancreatitis. Surg Gynecol Obstet 143:209, 1976. Reproduced by permission.

Treatment

After the patient has been stabilized systemically and the disease has been identified to be severe, attention is initially turned to the possible etiologic factors listed in Table 165-1. An ICU patient may develop pancreatitis related to causes other than the described hypoperfusion injury—drugs, gallstones, or other obstructive/mechanical factors may be critical. (Very frequently, as is the case with gallstone pancreatitis, the disease will be short, self-limiting, and may be treated in selected cases with immediate or delayed endoscopic or surgical intervention as the case demands. The most common scenario is for a quick resolution of the acute inflammation, with recommendation of surgery in the same admission if the gallbladder remains in situ or endoscopic sphincterotomy and gallstone removal if the gallbladder was removed previously. In the critically ill person, however, this intervention, unless indicated early by persistent jaundice and acute pancreatitis should be delayed until after resolution of the primary illness.)

However, we will assume that the disease in the ICU patient has been initiated by a hypoperfusion injury to the gland and that no immediate "corrective" intervention is appropriate.

Principles of treatment include careful monitoring, correction of the metabolic and hemodynamic effects of the inflammatory process, respiratory and renal support, nutrition, control of pancreatic enzyme secretion and its sequelae, and prevention and treatment of the local complications of necrotizing pancreatitis.

Ongoing evaluation and management of this patient from the outset must be a collaborative effort between the intensivist and an abdominal surgeon experienced in the medical and surgical measures which may become necessary. The decision-making with regard to surgery is based to some extent on hard data which can be measured, such as biochemistry and x-rays, but also on clinical experience and intuition.

MONITORING

The critically ill patient who develops pancreatitis is likely already hemodynamically monitored in the ICU setting, with close evaluation of heart rate, arterial blood pressure, hourly urine output, and central venous pressure. Since patients with severe pancreatitis may well have major fluid derangement, renal failure, sepsis, and especially pulmonary complications, Swan-Ganz lines are usually necessary to measure and monitor left atrial filling pressures, cardiac indices, systemic vascular resistance, and the oxygen-derived variables (delivery, uptake, and utilization).

Frequent determinations of blood counts, blood urea nitrogen (BUN), blood sugar, electrolytes, creatinine, calcium, magnesium, and arterial blood-gas levels are useful in detecting deteriorating pulmonary or renal status, the adequacy of treatment, and the evolution of septic complications. In a patient who is slow to respond, serial ultrasounds and CT scans are critical in the ongoing evaluation of the retroperitoneum.

METABOLIC AND HEMODYNAMIC EFFECTS

The need for volume replacement in the patient with severe pancreatitis cannot be overemphasized. This patient, in effect, has a massive retroperitoneal burn, with ongoing third space losses in the retroperitoneum, peritoneal cavity, and bowel lumen. Requirements may vary from small amounts to 8 to 10 L isotonic fluid in the first 24-h period. In the ICU, especially if the patient has a preexisting brittle cardiovascular status, fluid replacement and its effects may have to be followed closely; however, a postcardiopulmonary bypass or cardiac transplantation patient developing pancreatitis still requires adequate salt and fluid replacement. Those patients, who with appropriate massive fluid administration develop hemodynamic instability, may require inotropic and even temporary pressor support. The frequency of this circumstance has led some to postulate a myocardial depressant factor (MDF) as being an important pathogenetic mechanism.[38]

Because hemorrhage can occur as a complication of the retroperitoneal proteolytic enzyme extravasation, blood administration may be necessary; for those who develop hypoalbuminemia related to significant protein loss, plasma or albumin or both can be given.

It should be stressed that the reason why one patient progresses to pancreatic necrosis while another patient has a benign self-limiting course, remains a mystery; however, in the usual case of pancreatitis and especially in the ICU with a critically ill patient, this deterioration may well be enhanced by hypotension and hypoperfusion related to inadequate attention to volume replacement.

Metabolic acidosis, hyperglycemia, hypocalcemia, and hypomagnesemia must be recognized and treated. However, early fluid management and stabilization are usually sufficient to correct the acidosis. Correction of the other biochemical abnormalities should be done with caution, since some measurements such as the serum calcium level may be spuriously lowered by the hypoalbuminemic state. (Determination of serum ionized calcium is a more accurate reflection of "true" calcium levels.)

RESPIRATORY AND RENAL SUPPORT

Many mechanisms are implicated in the development of typical adult respiratory distress syndrome (ARDS) in this setting. After major heart or transplantation surgery, the patient's pulmonary function may already be compromised by anesthetics, opiates, and pain related to the procedure. In addition, elevation of diaphragms, pleural effusions, abdominal pain leading to further splinting and atelectasis, and overaggressive fluid replacement may contribute to the respiratory failure. The most important factors may occur in the lung itself, with increased capillary permeability related to serotonin release, breakdown of surfactant by the enzyme phospholipase A released by the necrosing pancreas, or the activation of the complement cascade with elaboration of vasoactive prostaglandins and leukotrienes. Whatever the mechanisms, aggressive ventilatory support is often required and should be anticipated. If the patient is previously ill and develops respiratory insufficiency with the acute pancreatitis or requires multiple operations for its complications, ventilatory support may be prolonged for many weeks. Tracheostomy may become necessary for adequate tracheobronchial toilet or occasionally for protracted ventilation.

No specific renal injuries have been recognized in the patient with acute pancreatitis, apart from the secondary effects of volume loss and hypotension. However, as reviewed previously, many of the ICU-related pancreatitis patients may have a hypoperfusion injury as a cause; therefore, renal injury may be anticipated in many. Aggressive support with fluid, judicious use of diuretics when adequate fluid has been replaced, and hemodialysis in selected cases of acute tubular necrosis (ATN) are all used.

One group examining the incidence of pancreatitis in patients undergoing abdominal aortic aneurysm repair found that there was a high correlation of pancreatic injury with ischemic injury to the kidney[15] (ATN), suggesting similar etiologies and the necessity for monitoring closely the renal function.

NUTRITION

Nutritional support for the seriously ill patient is critical, even though no specific benefit to the patient with an inflamed pancreas has been proven. Most of the conditions listed in Table 165-2 occur in patients at risk for developing pancreatitis; yet, these patients entered the ICU with an expectation of returning to normal feeding within days. The recognition of pancreatitis, however, should carry with it the realization that a prolonged stay is possible. All too often, the intensivist withholds total parenteral nutrition (TPN) until the course of the disease is declared, only to find that after 2 weeks, the patient is not improving significantly and now has been starved unnecessarily.

The patient who develops pancreatitis in this setting should be regarded with suspicion and TPN instituted early. On the other hand, long-term TPN in a sick, possibly septic patient has its own frequent complications, among which are line sepsis and opportunistic infections.

CONTROL OF PANCREATIC ENZYME SECRETION

Many therapeutic steps have been taken to minimize pancreatic enzyme secretion or limit its effects. Studies to examine the possible benefits in acute pancreatitis of nasogastric suction,[39] anticholinergics,[40] H_2 blockers,[41] somatostatin,[42] calcitonin,[43] and glucagon[44] have not supported the routine use of these agents.

Similarly, the effects of the proteolytic enzyme inhibitor Trasylol,[45,46] the antitrypsin agent EACA (ϵ-aminocaproic acid)[47] and a phospholipase A inhibitor[48] have not been convincing. Nasogastric suction is still used routinely, especially in the obtunded patient, to decompress paralytic ileus, control vomiting, perhaps decrease stimulation of the pancreas, and prevent aspiration.

The numerous modalities used and tested in the treatment of the severe form of this disease attest to the failure of most to alter the course of the inflammatory process. The mainstay of initial treatment is resuscitation with fluid and electrolytes, combined with respiratory and nutritional support, as well as attention to the primary disease state in the case of the critically ill patient. Patients who die from necrotizing pancreatitis, however, do not usually die in the early resuscitation phase, or even in the first 2 weeks, owing to excellent intensive care.

The next step is to evaluate and follow the pathologic process in the retroperitoneum, at the same time as all supportive measures are continued.

LOCAL COMPLICATIONS OF NECROTIZING PANCREATITIS

At the outset, the clinician must be aware of the pathologic conditions that secondarily occur as a result of acute pancreatitis.

The complications of necrotizing pancreatitis are pancreatic necrosis, pancreatic abscess, and pseudocyst formation.[49]

Aggressive early hemodynamic stabilization is probably the only rational way to prevent further hypoperfusion injury to the pancreas and the development of these complications.

Institution of peritoneal dialysis via the percutaneous or minilaparotomy route accelerates early improvement in some patients, but does not appear to offer any statistical benefit in decreasing development of complications and death.[50]

The patients who develop retroperitoneal necrosis (fat or pancreatic) are at high risk for morbidity and mortality. Those who do not will usually survive with appropriate supportive measures only.

PANCREATIC AND PERIPANCREATIC NECROSIS

Pancreatic necrosis consists of patchy devitalization of the pancreatic gland developing within a few days or up to weeks after the onset of the inflammatory process. The patient will usually have abdominal pain, persistent fever (possibly low grade) and leukocytosis. CT scanning with vascular enhancement may demonstrate local or diffuse areas of nonenhancement. Needle aspiration at this stage will show no growth or culture, if necrosis is present without infection.

The treatment of this entity is controversial. It is difficult to predict how many patients with pancreatic necrosis (without infection) will go on to spontaneous resolution if simply supported and how many will develop sepsis, clearly requiring debridement. Undoubtedly, some patients *do* resolve and would clearly not benefit from laparotomy. Every pancreatic surgeon has had the experience of extensively debriding sterile retroperitoneal necrosis, subjecting the patient to perhaps many future debridements (which now, of course, involve tissue which *is* infected), and wondering whether the noninfected condition at the outset might have resolved spontaneously. In addition, many "sequestrectomies" performed for pancreatic necrosis are likely excisions of necrotic fat only, rather than necrotic gland. The differentiation between these two pathologic entities, in terms of their morbidity and mortality, has not been reported. A retroperitoneum with a well-perfused pancreas surrounded by necrotic fat may have a different outlook than if the gland itself is compromised. Therefore, removal of uninfected necrotic fat only might be a fruitless exercise.

There has been a suggestion that only 40 percent of patients with pancreatic and peripancreatic necrosis become infected.[51] Because of that, and the aforementioned fear that surgery in the sterile situation may actually cause more harm than good, we tend to avoid major debridement unless sepsis is confirmed. Therefore, if the patient remains stable hemodynamically, has only low-grade fever and leukocytosis, CT findings that do not suggest extensive glandular necrosis and infection, and a sterile percutaneous retroperitoneal sample, we continue with supportive management without intervention. However, the patient may ultimately require intervention even without gross septic parameters simply because of a prolonged "smoldering" course showing no clinical improvement.

The role of antibiotics in the patient with pancreatic necrosis or sepsis is similarly controversial.[52,53] All would agree that these patients require antibiotics, but most would admit that their use in pancreatic necrosis (with or without sepsis) is for systemic rather than local treatment or prophylaxis. Patients with sterile necrosis usually receive broad-spectrum antibiotics for systemic protection while the intensivist monitors the retroperitoneum, and those with infected necrosis must be actively treated to prevent or manage bacteremia with no delusion that the established retroperitoneal sepsis will improve without debridement or drainage. Consequently, antibiotics are administered if there is evidence of pancreatic necrosis with or without infection.

INFECTED NECROSIS AND PANCREATIC ABSCESS

Some patients with pancreatic and peripancreatic necrosis develop spontaneous infection of the necrotic tissue, presumably because of direct contamination by bacteria from the transverse colon. Although some authors do not distinguish between infected necrosis and pancreatic abscess, others differentiate them on the basis of suitability for drainage percutaneously, i.e., infected pancreatic necrosis requires extensive surgical debridement and possibly pancreatic resection because of solid necrotic areas, whereas a pancreatic abscess may require just percutaneous drainage if liquefaction has taken place, leaving little solid necrotic tissue remaining.

There is no question that sepsis in the retroperitoneum requires intervention to avoid almost certain death. This has significant implications in the patient who is critically ill from a primary illness.

The diagnosis of retroperitoneal sepsis, whether infected pancreatic necrosis or pancreatic abscess, is made by recognition of a deteriorating clinical course which may be more precipitous than with pancreatic necrosis, more pronounced fever and leukocytosis, typical CT findings, and a positive percutaneous aspirate. When the patient is maintained on broad-spectrum antibiotics (with perhaps decreased immunosuppression in the transplant patient), preparations are made for surgical debridement. Although some cases may be amenable to percutaneous drainage only, in our experience, the majority require laparotomy.

Principles of Surgical Debridement

The conventional indications for surgery in acute pancreatitis include diagnosis, failure of early medical management, unresolving gallstone pancreatitis, and pancreatic sepsis. In the critical care setting, the diagnosis should always be made; aggressive supportive care has virtually eliminated the need for early operation; as stated before, a persistent gallstone pancreatitis may be treated effectively by early endoscopic sphincterotomy. Therefore, the main indication for surgery in the critically ill patient with pancreatitis is the late development of necrosis or sepsis.

Recommended methods of surgical debridement vary considerably and are beyond the scope of this chapter, but principles of the different approaches are similar; the critical step is the selection of the appropriate patient for debridement followed by the quick execution of that surgery with excellent anesthesia and postoperative intensive care.

Surgery should consist of wide debridement of all devitalized peripancreatic fat and pancreatic tissue followed by adequate dependent drainage, which is generous enough to allow drainage of thick, purulent, often particulate material.[54,55] Since multiple operations for repeated abdominal toilet are often required, some surgeons have advocated open packing of the abdomen to facilitate the repeated procedures.[56]

Our own preference is a radical excision of all necrotic and infected material followed by generous dependent sump drainage and closure of the abdomen. Extensive infection and necrosis may be better treated with open packing if repeated laparotomy is anticipated. Intubation of the gastrointestinal tract (cholecystostomy, gastrostomy, and jejunostomy were enthusiastically advocated in the past[57]) is to be avoided in this septic setting. Temporary packing of the retroperitoneum may occasionally be necessary to control venous oozing from the bed of the necrotic tissue.

The extent of pancreatic resection varies, depending on the degree of necrosis of the gland itself. Although some surgeons have recommended major pancreatic resection routinely,[58,59] we debride the gland itself only if necessary; only necrotic portions are removed, and major anatomic dissections are avoided if possible in these often unstable patients.

PANCREATIC PSEUDOCYST

With more frequent use of ultrasound and CT in the early stages of pancreatitis, recognition of fluid collections in and around the lesser sac has become the rule rather than the exception. Most collections probably consist of inflammatory exudate, and in fact, most resolve as the pancreatitis settles. The persistence of a lesser sac fluid collection (or fluid in a variety of areas such as the peritoneal cavity, the retroperitoneum, or even mediastinum) implies a communication with a ruptured pancreatic duct system. The collection that develops thick fibrous walls consisting of the surrounding stomach, colon, and mesentery, can be properly termed a *chronic pseudocyst*. Diagnosis of such a condition does not mandate immediate treatment, unless the pseudocyst grows quickly, becomes infected, bleeds, or ruptures into the peritoneal cavity or adjacent bowel. In an already sick patient, a quickly enlarging or infected pseudocyst is best treated with percutaneous decompression, whereas immediate surgery is required for bleeding or free rupture. Spontaneous rupture into the intestinal tract, a rare occurrence, can be treated expectantly in this setting if the patient is otherwise stable. The uncomplicated pseudocyst which is stable in size, and at least 6 weeks old (to allow the walls to "mature" enough to accept sutures) is conventionally drained internally at laparotomy; in the intensive care situation, percutaneous drainage can be done safely to avoid the dreaded complications, but must be used with full knowledge that recurrence is frequent.

Acute pancreatitis is usually a benign self-limiting disease which spontaneously resolves with conventional supportive measures. Necrotizing pancreatitis is a potentially lethal disease, killing patients by causing major hemodynamic derangements early and septic complications late. Although a number of pathogenetic mechanisms have been postulated, the pancreatitis which develops in the critically ill patient may be related in major part to a hypoperfusion injury to the gland.

The intensivist must have a high index of suspicion, must diagnose the disease and evaluate its severity early, and institute aggressive management and monitoring to both resuscitate the patient and evaluate the pathologic process in the retroperitoneum. Surgical intervention is not necessary in most cases, but development of life-threatening complications, such as infected pancreatic necrosis, requires timely and radical surgery.

CASE PRESENTATION

A.L., a 52-year-old man, had end-stage chronic liver disease related to cryptogenic cirrhosis and underwent orthotopic liver transplantation. He had no known history of pancreatitis and was hepatitis B negative. The transplant procedure was uneventful with no periods of hypotension or major blood loss (6 U replacement), using a venous bypass of 90 min duration.

The patient was transferred to the ward from the surgical ICU on day 5. He was treated early in the postoperative period with standard immunosuppression consisting of Minnesota antilymphoblast globulin (MALG) and Solu-Medrol with replacement of the MALG at day 7 by

FIGURE 165-1 CT scan of percutaneous drainage of a sterile lesser sac collection. L, liver; S, stomach; C, colon; SP, spleen; P, phlegmon of pancreas; PDC, percutaneous drainage catheter in lesser sac collection.

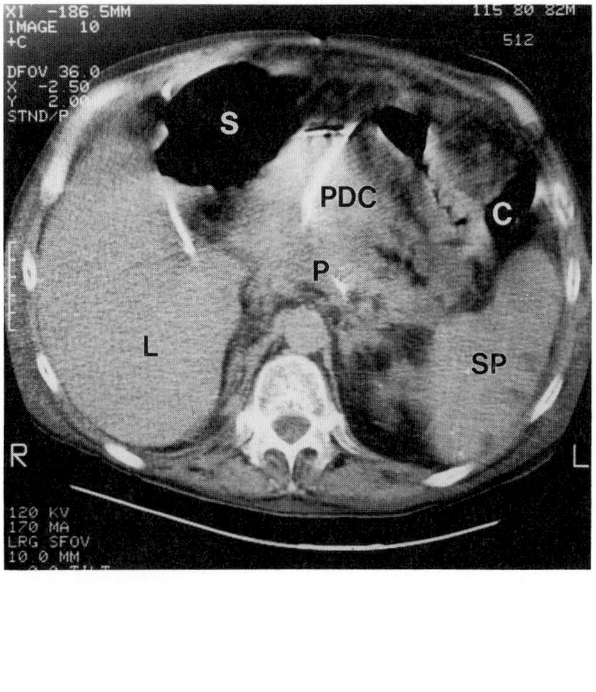

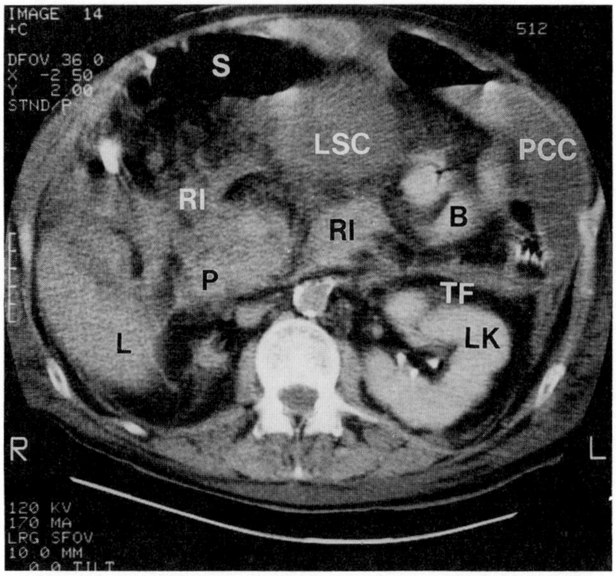

FIGURE 165-2 CT scan of massive inflammation in retroperitoneum with necrotizing pancreatitis. L, liver; S, stomach; LSC, lesser sac collection; PCC, paracolic collection; B, bowel; TF, thickened fascia; LK, left kidney; RI, retroperitoneal inflammation; P, phlegmon in head of pancreas.

cyclosporin. Nephrotoxicity prompted a switch from cyclosporin to Imuran on day 9.

On day 10 the patient had diffuse abdominal pain and tenderness, a serum amylase level of 700 IU (upper limit of normal 200 IU), and an ultrasound study which showed diffuse mild enlargement of the pancreas. He was given supportive treatment including TPN.

On day 17, continuing with mild abdominal pain and tenderness, he became hemodynamically unstable with respiratory distress and was readmitted to the ICU. A diagnosis of sepsis and ARDS was made. He was treated with high dose broad-spectrum antibiotics, ventilation, fluid support, and a slight decrease in immunosuppression. A CT scan and ultrasound suggested ongoing pancreatitis with an enlarged edematous gland and retroperitoneal fluid collections, despite a now normal serum amylase concentration.

On day 26, a liver biopsy suggested acute rejection, which was treated with recycling of the steroid regimen (starting with 200 mg Solu-Medrol on the first day with later tapering).

On day 31 abdominal CT scan revealed an upper abdominal collection which, on percutaneous drainage, proved to be sterile, with an amylase level of 27,500 IU (Fig. 165-1).

On day 34, a course of amphotericin B was begun because of positive yeast cultures from both urine and bile. The patient improved initially. On day 43, he developed respiratory distress once more, and a CT scan showed massive retroperitoneal inflammation with an edematous pancreas without evidence of air bubbles (Fig. 165-2). Percutaneous aspiration retrieved mixed gram-negative bacteria on Gram stain and culture. Laparotomy the following day consisted of a wide debridement of massive infected fat necrosis in the back of the abdomen. Large amounts of purulent foul-smelling particulate matter (which grew a variety of gram-negative bacteria on culture) were removed although the gland itself appeared grossly viable. The abdomen was irrigated and packed open and subjected to frequent relaparotomy and packing change over the ensuing 4 weeks. The patient required further surgery for splenic artery bleeding related to the sepsis and long-term packing.

The liver and renal function remained stable, and the ARDS gradually resolved. He experienced a number of other unrelated complications, but was ultimately discharged after a total of 4 months in hospital, in good health, with good liver function, and on a full diet. He remains well 9 months after surgery.

CASE DISCUSSION

This case illustrates the difficulties presented by a critically ill patient who develops necrotizing pancreatitis. The patient had had an uncomplicated liver transplant procedure and had been treated with Solu-Medrol, cyclosporin, and Imuran, all of which have been implicated in pancreatitis. At the outset, the abdominal signs and symptoms were difficult to assess, and serum amylase content had been mildly elevated but had decreased to normal levels by the time severe pancreatitis had become evident. The pancreatitis initially was mild, but repeated episodes of clinical deterioration and serial changes on CT and ultrasound led to the diagnosis of a pseudocyst and ultimately infected pancreatic necrosis. In this case, the pathologic condition consisted of massive infected retroperitoneal fat necrosis. Diagnosis and treatment were further complicated by recycling of steroids for rejection, nosocomial infections, and a very brittle pulmonary status as the patient went in and out of sepsis. The clinical course would suggest that the patient had developed mild pancreatitis at first, but because of a number of additional factors which may have compromised perfusion to the pancreas, a necrotizing form evolved.

Ultimate success in this case was achieved by recognition of the disease and aggressive debridement of necrotic infected retroperitoneal tissue amidst heroic efforts by the intensivists to provide respiratory, hemodynamic, antimicrobial, and nutritional support.

References

1. Peterson LM, Brooks JR: Lethal pancreatitis, a diagnostic dilemma. Am J Surg 137:491, 1979.
2. Trapnell J: The natural history and management of acute pancreatitis. Clin Gastroenterol 1:147, 1972.
3. Keynes M: Heretical thoughts on the pathogenesis of acute pancreatitis. Gut 29:1413, 1988.
4. Colon R, Frazier OH, Kahan BD: Complications in cardiac transplant patients requiring general surgery. Surgery 103:32, 1988.
5. Feiner H: Pancreatitis after cardiac surgery: A morphologic study. Am J Surg 131:684, 1976.
6. Moneta GL, Misbach GA, Ivey TD: Hypoperfusion as a possible factor in the development of gastrointestinal complications after cardiac surgery. Am J Surg 149(5):648, 1985.
7. Mikhailidis DP, Hutton RA, Jeremy JY, Dandona P: Hypothermia and pancreatitis. J Clin Pathol 36:483, 1983.
8. Rose DM, Ranson JHC, Cunningham JN, Spencer FC: Patterns of severe pancreatic injury following cardiopulmonary bypass. Ann Surg 199:168, 1984.
9. Greenbaum RA, Barradas MA, Mikhailidis DP, et al: Effect of heparin and contrast medium on platelet function during routine cardiac catheterization. Cardiovasc Res 21:878, 1987.
10. Grace AA, Barradas MA, Mikhailidis P, et al: Cyclosporine A enchances platelet aggregation. Kidney Int 32:889, 1987.
11. Dandona P, Junglee D, Katrak A, et al: Increased serum pancreatic enzymes after treatment with methylprednisolone: Possible evidence of subclinical pancreatitis. Br Med J 291:24, 1985.
12. Victor DW, Rayburn JL, McCready RA, Hyde GL: Pancreatitis following aneurysmectomy. J Ky Med Assoc 86(6):285, 1988.
13. Frick TW, Fryd DS, Sutherland DER, et al: Hypercalcemia associated with pancreatitis and hyperamylasemia in renal transplant recipients. Am J Surg 154:487, 1987.
14. Alexander JA, Demetrius AJ, Gavaler JS, et al: Pancreatitis following liver transplantation. Transplantation 45(6):1062, 1988.
15. Warshaw AL, O'Hara.PJ: Susceptibility of the pancreas to ischemic injury in shock. Ann Surg 188:197, 1978.
16. Popper HL, Necheles H, Russell KC: Transition of pancreatic edema to pancreatic necrosis. Surg Gynecol Obstet 87:79, 1948.
17. Read G, Braganza JM, Howat HT. Pancreatitis: A retrospective study. Gut 17:945, 1976.
18. Janowitz HD, Dreiling DA: The plasma amylase: Source, regulation and diagnostic significance. Am J Med 27:924, 1959.
19. Salt WB, Schenker S: Amylase: Its clinical significance: A review of the literature. Medicine 55:269, 1976.
20. Warshaw AL, Fuller AF: Specificity of increased renal clearance of amylase in the diagnosis of acute pancreatitis. N Engl J Med 292:325, 1975.
21. Leckie PA, Ferreira P, Debas HT: Assessment of the amylase-creatinine clearance ratio in postoperative patients. Ann Surg 192:195, 1980.
22. Lifton LJ, Slickers KA, Pragay DA, Katz LA: Pancreatitis and lipase: A reevaluation with a five minute turbidimetric lipase determination. JAMA 229:47, 1974.
23. O'Donnell MD, FitzGerald O, McGeeney KF: Differential serum amylase determination by the use of an inhibitor, and design of a routine procedure. Clin Chem 23:560, 1977.
24. Bery AR, Taylor TV, Davies GC: Diagnostic tests and prognostic indicators in acute pancreatitis. J R Coll Surg Edinb 27:345, 1982.
25. Delcourt A: Controversies in the biological diagnosis of acute pancreatitis, in Hollender LF (ed): *Controversies in Acute Pancreatitis.* New York, Springer-Verlag, 1982, pp 38–44.
26. Jeffrey RB: Sonography in acute pancreatitis. Radiol Clin North Am 27(1):5, 1989.
27. Balthazar EJ: CT diagnosis and staging of acute pancreatitis. Radiol Clin North Am 27(1):19, 1989.
28. Ranson JHC, Rifkind KM, Turner JW. Prognostic signs and nonoperative peritoneal lavage in acute pancreatitis. Surg Gynecol Obstet 143:209, 1976.
29. Kelly TR, Klein RL, Porquez JM, Homer GM: Methemalbumin in acute pancreatitis: An experimental and clinical appraisal. Ann Surg 175:15, 1972.

30. Warshaw AL, Lee KH: Serum ribonuclease elevations and pancreatic necrosis in acute pancreatitis. Surgery 86:227, 1979.
31. Buchler M, Malfertheimer P, Schoetensack C: Sensitivity of antiproteases, complement factors and C-reactive protein in detecting pancreatic necrosis. Int J Pancreatol 1:227, 1986.
32. McMahon MJ, Pickford IR, Playforth MJ: Early prediction of severity of acute pancreatitis using peritoneal lavage. Acta Chir Scand 146:171, 1980.
33. Balthazar EJ, Ranson JHC, Naidich DP: Acute pancreatitis: Prognostic value of CT. Radiology 156:767, 1985.
34. Kivisarri L, Somer K, Standertskjold-Nord-Enstam CG: Early detection of acute fulminant pancreatitis by contrast enchanced computed tomography. Scand J Gastroenterol 15:633, 1980.
35. Gerzof S, Banks P, Spechler S: Role of guided percutaneous aspiration in early diagnosis of pancreatic sepsis. Dig Dis Sci 29: 950, 1984.
36. Hill MC, Dach JL, Barkin J: Role of percutaneous aspiration in diagnosis of pancreatic abscess. AJR 141:1035, 1983.
37. Karlson KB, Martin EC, Fanuchen EI: Percutaneous drainage of pancreatic pseudocysts and abscesses. Radiology 142:619, 1982.
38. Lefer AM, Spath JA Jr: Pancreatic hypoperfusion and the production of a myocardial depressant factor. Ann Surg 179:868, 1974.
39. Levant JA, Secrist DLM, Resin H: Nasogastric suction in the treatment of alcoholic pancreatitis: A controlled study. JAMA 229:51, 1974.
40. Switz DM, Vlahcevic ZR, Farrar JT: The effect of anticholinergic and/or nasogastric suction on the outcome of acute alcoholic pancreatitis: A controlled trial. Gastroenterology 68:974, 1975.
41. Meshkinpour H, Molinari MD, Gardner L: Cimetidine in the treatment of acute alcoholic pancreatitis: A randomized double-blind study. Gastroenterology 77:687, 1979.
42. Usadel KH, Leuschner U, Uberla KK: Treatment of acute pancreatitis with somatostatin: A multicenter double-blind trial. N Engl J Med 303:999, 1980.
43. Goebell H, Ammann R, Herfarth CH: A double-blind trial of synthetic salmon calcitonin in the treatment of acute pancreatitis. Scand J Gastroenterol 14:881, 1979.
44. Olazabal A, Fuller R: Failure of glucagon in the treatment of alcoholic pancreatitis. Gastroenterology 74:489, 1978.
45. Trapnell JE, Rigby CC, Talbot CH: A controlled trial of Trasylol in the treatment of acute pancreatitis. Br J Surg 61:177, 1974.
46. Skyring A, Singer A, Tornya P. Treatment of acute pancreatitis with Trasylol: A report of a controlled clinical trial. Br Med J 2:627, 1965.
47. Konttinen YP: Epsilon-aminocaproic acid in the treatment of acute pancreatitis. Scand J Gastroenterol 6:715, 1971.
48. Tykka HT, Vaittinen EJ, Mahlberg KL: A randomized double-blind study using $CaNa_2$ EDTA, a phospholipase A_2 inhibitor in the management of human acute pancreatitis. Scand J Gastroenterol 20:5, 1985.
49. Frey CF, Bradley EL, Beger HG: Progress in acute pancreatitis. Surg Gynecol Obstet 167(4):282, 1988.
50. Ranson JHC, Spencer FC: The role of peritoneal lavage in severe acute pancreatitis. Ann Surg 187:565, 1978.
51. Berger HG, Krauzberger W, Bittner R: Results of surgical treatment of necrotizing pancreatitis. World J Surg 9:972, 1985.
52. Howes R, Zuidema GD, Cameron JL: Evaluation of prophylatic antibiotics in acute pancreatitis. J Surg Res 18:197, 1975.
53. Finch WT, Sawyers JL, Schenker SA: A prospective study to determine the efficacy of antibiotics in acute pancreatitis. Ann Surg 183:667, 1976.
54. White TT, Heimbach DM: Sequestrectomy and hyperalimentation in the treatment of hemorrhagic pancreatitis. Am J Surg 132:270, 1976.
55. Crist DW, Cameron JL: The current management of acute pancreatitis. *Advances in Surgery*. Vol. 20. Chicago, Year Book Medical Publishers, 1987, pp 69–124.
56. Davidson ED, Bradley EL III: "Marsupialization" in the treatment of pancreatic abscess. Surgery 89:252, 1981.
57. Lawson DW, Daggett WM, Civetta JM: Surgical treatment of acute necrotizing pancreatitis. Ann Surg 172:605, 1970.
58. Watts GT: Total pancreatectomy for fulminant pancreatitis. Lancet 2:384, 1963.
59. Norton L, Eiseman B: Near total pancreatectomy for hemorrhagic pancreatitis. Am J Surg 127:191, 1974.

Chapter 166
TOXIC MEGACOLON

RICHARD K. REZNICK

KEY POINTS

- *Toxic megacolon is usually a complication of ulcerative colitis.*
- *Toxic megacolon has a 10 to 25 percent medical-surgical mortality rate.*
- *Clinical features include an extremely ill patient with massive colonic dilatation.*
- *Complications and mortality are linked to colonic perforation.*
- *Combined medical-surgical care is essential.*
- *Medical treatment includes resuscitation, steroids, and frequent examinations.*
- *Surgical intervention is indicated if dramatic improvement is not seen within 12 to 24 h.*
- *Surgical treatment is most often an emergency subtotal colectomy.*

Toxic megacolon, or toxic dilatation of the colon, is perhaps the most dreaded and certainly the most lethal complication of colitis. Successful treatment of toxic megacolon requires constant vigilance, expert resuscitative management, combined medical-surgical expertise, and thoughtful judgment.

In the vast majority of cases, toxic megacolon is a complication of ulcerative colitis but can afflict patients with granulomatous colitis (Crohn's colitis), infective colitis, pseudomembranous enterocolitis, and ischemic colitis. Although it can occur at any age, it is most often a disease of young patients, and up to 70 percent of those afflicted are under the age of thirty. In a large proportion of patients with toxic megacolon, it is the initial presentation of the disease process. This results in the presentation to the critical care physician of an often young, previously healthy patient, who is overwhelmingly ill, with a 10 to 25 percent chance of dying. The challenge is formidable but must be met because early recognition of the disease process, aggressive medical treatment, thorough resuscitation, and appropriately timed surgery can make the difference between survival and death.

The incidence of toxic megacolon in patients with ulcerative colitis ranges from 1.6 to 21.4 percent depending on the series reported. The more frequently cited figures are in the lower ranges, and one can generally expect that a moderate-sized general hospital will encounter two to five patients per year. The term, toxic megacolon, was first used by Marshak in 1950.[1] However, case reports dating back to 1930 describe several patients with typical features of toxic megacolon—a young acutely ill patient with ulcerative colitis who presents to the emergency department with bloody diarrhea, dehydration, abdominal distention, signs of peritoneal irritation, and radiologic evidence of profound and dangerous dilatation of the colon. As the name implies, patients with toxic megacolon are usually extremely ill. Typically, they have a high fever, severe fluid and electrolyte abnormalities, metabolic alkalosis, and confusion. Swift recognition of the problem is paramount, and resuscitation must be immediate.

Etiology and Pathogenesis

Toxic megacolon is a disease complex with the principal feature being dilatation of the colon. Indeed, it is colonic perforation that is responsible for the major complications of this disease. Ulcerative colitis is a disease of the mucosa and submucosa. It does not generally afflict the muscle layers or serosa of the colon. Toxic megacolon is the singular exception to this "rule." Why a mucosal disease suddenly and dramatically becomes transmural and the colon dilated to dangerous proportions is the subject of much of the efforts aimed at explaining the pathogenesis of toxic megacolon. Two theories prevail. Neither theory, however, has overwhelming acceptance in part because there are no pathognomonic histologic findings in toxic megacolon. The first theory is simply that the inflammatory process extends beyond the submucosa and into the muscularis propria of the colon. This is substantiated by the finding of granulation tissue replacement of colonic wall muscle and areas of muscle necrosis in pathology specimens. What might trigger this extension of the inflammatory process is only speculative. The second theory invokes destruction of the myenteric plexus leading to intestinal paralysis and subsequent dilatation. However, although sometimes seen, neural damage is an inconsistent finding in toxic megacolon specimens leading to doubt about its pathogenic significance. It has also been proposed that the metabolic disturbances frequently seen in toxic megacolon, such as hypokalemia, hypocalcemia, hypomagnesemia, hypophosphatemia, and metabolic alkalosis may play a part in the pathogenesis of this disorder.

Approximately 50 percent of the time, the development of toxic megacolon is preceded by some event or therapy which has been implicated in the pathogenesis of this disorder (Table 166-1). Most notable is the concern that a barium enema done on a patient with active ulcerative colitis may be the precipitating event leading to toxic megacolon.

TABLE 166-1 Factors That May Precipitate Toxic Megacolon

Barium enema
Opiates
Anticholinergics
Antidiarrheal agents
Electrolyte imbalance
? Pregnancy

Whether it is the preparation for the barium enema or the barium enema itself, several authors have cautioned that frequently a temporal association is noted between the diagnostic procedure and the disease. One explanation for this association has to do with the fact that in the past, barium frequently contained tannic acid. The astringent properties of tannic acid can stimulate colonic contraction and make the barium adhere to the colonic wall, conditions which might theoretically predispose to the development of colonic dilatation.[2] Despite controversy regarding this issue, it is considered inappropriate to do a barium enema in a patient with acute fulminating colitis or any degree of colonic dilatation.

Opiates and anticholinergic drugs have also been implicated as precipitating factors in the development of toxic megacolon. Both of these compounds have a profound inhibitory effect on colonic motility which may induce or exacerbate colonic dilatation. These agents are, therefore, contraindicated in acute ulcerative colitis.

Lastly, pregnancy has been thought to be a possible factor in precipitating toxic megacolon. Although it is generally agreed that pregnancy, in and of itself, does not affect the course of ulcerative colitis, many reported series of toxic megacolon include a substantial number of pregnant patients.

Disease Processes

INFLAMMATORY BOWEL DISEASES

The most common disease process that can be complicated by the development of toxic megacolon is ulcerative colitis (Table 166-2). In one large series, it accounted for 70 percent of documented cases.[3] Frequently, toxic megacolon is the initial presentation of the patient's illness. It occurs more frequently in patients with pancolitis and is rare when colitis is limited to the distal sigmoid and rectum (proctosigmoiditis). It has been reported that toxic megacolon is more likely to be seen in patients with frequent exacerbations and remissions of ulcerative colitis than in the patients whose disease is chronically active. It has been suggested that aggressive treatment of acute attacks of ulcerative colitis may reduce the possibility of toxic megacolon. Although not as common as in ulcerative colitis, toxic megacolon can complicate granulomatous (Crohn's) colitis. The characteristics of the toxic megacolon in Crohn's colitis and ulcerative colitis are similar, and treatment is essentially the same.

TABLE 166-2 Disease Processes That Can Be Complicated by Toxic Megacolon

Ulcerative colitis
Crohn's colitis
Amebic colitis
Salmonellosis
Cholera
Pseudomembranous colitis
Ischemic colitis
Behçet's syndrome
Methotrexate therapy

INFECTIOUS DISORDERS

Although unusual in North America, toxic megacolon can be a complication of infectious colitis. Most notable are salmonellosis, amebiasis, and cholera. This possibility underscores the importance of a good history because patients with infectious toxic megacolon, particularly salmonellosis, have a recent travel history and a short-lived illness, and frequently the accompanying diarrhea is nonbloody. All patients in whom toxic megacolon is suspected to be due to ulcerative colitis should have stool and blood cultures done and if rectal ulceration is prominent on proctosigmoidoscopy, the ulcers should be swabbed. In most cases of amebiasis, this will be diagnostic by the finding of trophozoites. If amebic colitis is suspected, indirect hemagglutination tests should be performed. Although infectious etiologies are unusual, it is critical to exclude them because treatment of these disorders is usually specific and medical. The exception to this is amebic colitis where early failure of medical management is an indication for surgical intervention.

OTHER DISEASES

Rarely, toxic megacolon develops in patients with a variety of other disorders. Principal among these is pseudomembranous colitis. This disorder, which results from an overgrowth of *Clostridium difficile* secondary to antibiotic administration, can be recognized on proctosigmoidoscopy by its characteristic dirty grayish yellow pseudomembranes. Of course, *C. difficile* culture or toxin identification confirms the diagnosis. Isolated case reports have described the development of toxic megacolon as a complication of ischemic colitis, Behçet's syndrome, and methotrexate therapy.

Diagnosis

The three features necessary to make a diagnosis of toxic megacolon are colitis, colonic dilatation, and a toxic-appearing patient (Table 166-3). Often the presentation is dramatic, and patients arrive in the emergency department critically ill and in obvious need of acute resuscitation. A history of inflammatory bowel disease is helpful but by no means necessary for the diagnosis, because toxic megacolon may be the first presentation of the disease. Patients present with complaints of an acute illness, including fever, diarrhea, and abdominal pain. Of note, the frequency of bowel movements may decrease just prior to the onset of toxic megacolon. On examination, the strikingly ill patient usually is dehydrated and tachycardic, often hypotensive, and may be confused. Abdominal examination reveals tenderness and distention. Signs of peritoneal irritation may be present and alert the examiner to the possibility of perforation. The abdominal distention appreciated clinically is

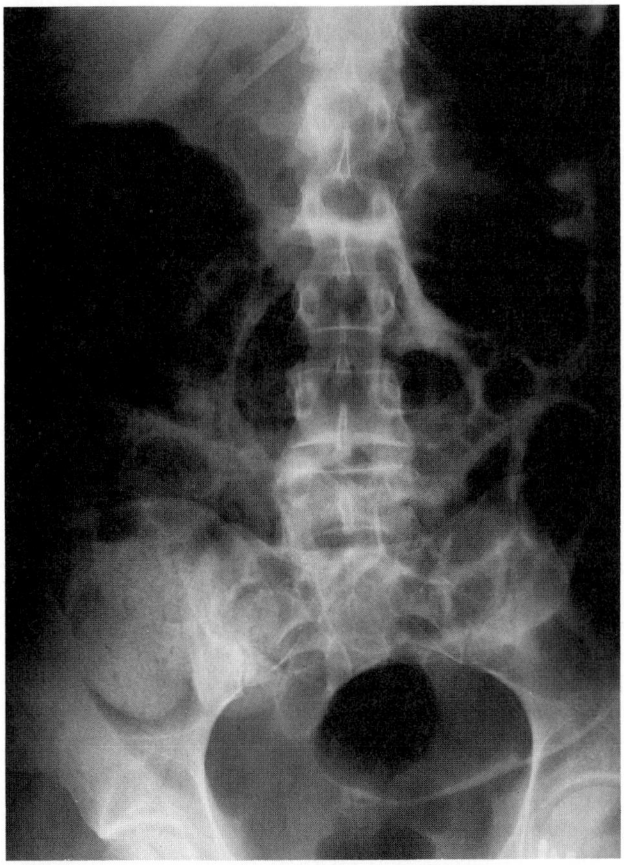

FIGURE 166-1 Abdominal radiograph shows massive colonic dilatation, most prominent in the transverse colon and free intraperitoneal air. These findings are consistent with a diagnosis of toxic megacolon complicated by colonic perforation.

often trivial when compared with the degree of colonic dilatation seen on plain film of the abdomen. All patients should have three views of the abdomen and an upright chest x-ray, the latter looking for free air under the diaphragm. The characteristic finding on abdominal views is marked colonic dilatation, particularly of the transverse colon. The reason that the transverse colon is most prominently dilated is not that disease is more active in that segment but rather due to gravity and colonic anatomy. The degree of transverse colon dilatation necessary to label the process toxic megacolon has been variably reported to range from 6 to 9 cm. In addition to being dilated, the involved colon has other abnormalities appreciable on a plain abdominal film[4] (Fig. 166-1). These include edema or loss of the normal haustral pattern, a nodular contour of the bowel wall, and an illusion of bowel wall thickening resulting from a combination of serosal edema and congested mucosa. Indeed, quite the contrary, the bowel wall in cases of toxic megacolon is most often perilously thin. There may be a striking appearance of round projections into the air column, a result of pseudopolyp formation. On occasion, air in the bowel wall may be seen on lateral projections, making it advantageous to order both left and right lateral decubitus films (four views of the abdomen).

TABLE 166-3 Diagnostic Features of Toxic Megacolon

Acute illness including fever, diarrhea, and abdominal pain
Patient appears severely ill
Dehydration
Abdominal distention
Signs of peritoneal irritation
Marked colonic dilatation on plain abdominal radiograph

Work-up of a patient with suspected toxic megacolon should include routine hematology and biochemistry and arterial blood-gas determinations. Typical findings include anemia, leukocytosis, hypocalcemia, hypomagnesemia, hypoalbuminemia, and metabolic alkalosis. In patients with this disorder, a gentle and careful proctosigmoidoscopic examination using a rigid scope should be carried out. Minimal insufflation of air should be used. The purpose of the examination is to confirm the suspicion of active colitis, to obtain stool cultures or swabs from mucosal ulceration, and to identify specific forms of colitis such as pseudomembranous colitis. Just as important as what investigations should be done, are what should not be done. Both barium enema and total colonoscopy are contraindicated in the patient with suspected toxic megacolon. Abdominal ultrasound and computed tomography (CT) are generally not helpful.

Management

Patients with toxic megacolon should be managed in an ICU (Table 166-4). These individuals are critically ill, often need invasive monitoring, and require intensive observation once the diagnosis is established. Resuscitative measures are the initial priority. All patients should have large bore intravenous lines, a Foley catheter, and a measure of filling pressure in the form of a central venous pressure (CVP) line or a Swan-Ganz catheter. Patients should be crossmatched for at least 4 units blood in consideration of the possibility of massive hemorrhage and the need for urgent surgical intervention. Correction of fluid and electrolyte abnormalities is the principal consideration in the initial hours of management. Patients should not be fed orally, should have nasogastric or long tube gastrointestinal decompression, and be considered for total parenteral nutrition (TPN).

TABLE 166-4 Management of Toxic Megacolon

Combined medical-surgical team in an ICU
Resuscitation
Emergency operation for certain or imminent perforation
Corticosteroids
Broad-spectrum antibiotics
Frequent clinical and radiologic assessment
Urgent surgical intervention if dramatic improvement fails to occur within 12–24 h

At the outset, patients with toxic megacolon must be cared for by a combined medical-surgical team. It is inappropriate to deny such a patient the benefit of the expertise of both the gastroenterologist and the abdominal surgeon. Together with the intensivist, a plan of management can be established that will optimize the chance of a successful outcome.

Morbidity and mortality of the disorder are very much linked to the presence or absence of colonic perforation. In a collective review of 497 cases, the overall mortality rate for toxic megacolon with perforation was 56.6 percent in contrast to an 8.7 percent mortality rate in patients without perforation.[5] Therefore, the primary aim of therapy is urgent treatment directed at reducing dilatation of the thin-walled inflamed colon.

Opinion varies widely as to whether medical or surgical therapy should predominate in this disorder. Some authors view medical therapy as a necessary preparation for early surgical treatment in all cases. Others view surgical intervention as having a role only in the event of failure of prolonged medical therapy. A middle-of-the-road approach predominates. Most authors agree that aggressive medical therapy should be tried for a limited time with urgent surgical intervention for those patients who fail to show quick and dramatic improvement. Clearly, patients presenting with signs indicating that perforation has already occurred, such as diffuse peritonitis or free air under the diaphragm, need resuscitation followed by emergency surgery. Other indications for emergency surgery include unequivocal features of septic shock, imminent rupture of the transverse colon (12 cm or greater), and the presence of at least three of the following: temperature >103°F (39.4°C), tachycardia >150, positive blood cultures, and partial loss of consciousness.

MEDICAL MANAGEMENT

Medical management of toxic megacolon has three components—resuscitative, therapeutic, and observational. As mentioned, all patients need urgent fluid and electrolyte replacement and ongoing monitoring. Therapeutic maneuvers aimed at reducing the acuity of the disease process have been largely the administration of steroids or ACTH. As with other conditions treated in the critical care environment, the use of steroids has its proponents and adversaries. Although there is no convincing proof of the efficacy of steroids, their use in chronic ulcerative colitis, acute fulminating colitis, and toxic megacolon has become so engraved that withholding steroids at this time is likely unacceptable. This being the case, the critical care physician using steroids in patients with toxic megacolon must be aware that high dose steroids may mask clinical signs and have been theorized to increase the risk of colonic perforation. Perhaps the greatest "risk" of using steroids is physicians' dependence on them to cure the disease process and subsequent reduced vigilance. Many patients with toxic megacolon have been on steroids chronically as treatment for ulcerative colitis, and in these patients there is no question that intravenous steroid administration is essential. The average dosing regimen is 100 mg hydrocortisone given every 6 h. Some authors prefer to use ACTH, and doses range from 40 to 180 U/24 h.

The use of antibiotics as part of the medical management of toxic megacolon is controversial but most authors suggest using wide-spectrum gram-negative and antianaerobic coverage.

Recently, the concept of rolling has been introduced into the medical management.[6] A group from Mount Sinai Hospital in New York reported 19 patients treated by steroids, long intestinal tube, and rolling the patient into the prone position for 10 to 15 min every 2 to 3 h. The concept of rolling is based on the observation that patients are routinely nursed in the supine position with the head up, which leads to the accumulation of air in the transverse colon because it is the most anterior and superior colonic segment. Rolling the patient theoretically redistributes this gas throughout the colon, thus lessening the chance that critical dilatation will result in perforation. Of the 19 patients treated, all had successful diminution of colonic diameter. However, 2 of the 19 patients died.

Whatever the mode of medical management used, frequent clinical and radiologic examination is mandatory. The patient should have an abdominal examination every 3 to 4 h and radiologic examination every 12 to 24 h. One should put limits on how long a trial of medical therapy is to be given prior to surgical intervention. Parameters for measurement of success should include: **1.** return of active bowel sounds; **2.** a decrease by at least 2 cm of colonic dilatation; **3.** a measurable decrease of abdominal girth; **4.** disappearance of abdominal pain; **5.** normal temperature and pulse; and **6.** a return to normal white blood cell count.[4] If the patient fails to manifest the majority of these parameters of improvement, then surgical treatment is warranted. The most important parameter is improvement in the patient's "toxic" appearance. If after 48 to 72 h of medical treatment, the patient still looks profoundly ill, an operation is mandatory.

The success of medical therapy is variable. In Binder's review of 497 patients, 28.9 percent were managed successfully medically, with an overall "medical mortality" rate of 30.3 percent. Of patients dying under medical management, 32.6 percent had perforations.[5] More recent articles offer encouragement for a trial of medical therapy. Katzka, Katz, and Morris report medical success in 17 of 29 cases of toxic megacolon with no mortality.[8] The report from Mount Sinai using the rolling technique reported a high success rate. Others, however, have argued that initial success with medical therapy may not be all that significant because most patients who have suffered one attack of toxic megacolon will ultimately need surgical intervention. A group from the Mayo Clinic reported on the fate of 38 patients treated medically with success.[9] Eleven of 38 eventually had a second attack of toxic megacolon, 15 eventually had urgent colectomy, and 60 percent overall had a long-term unsatisfactory result. The authors state that their results have "strengthened our opinion that medical management should be regarded almost exclusively as a preparation for imminent surgery." This view is perhaps best substantiated by the statistics from the group from Université de Montréal.[3] They treated 59 patients with toxic megacolon with initial medical therapy. There were 6 initial successes with no mortality, 36 failures requiring urgent surgical intervention with a 6 percent mortality rate, and 14 patients who initially had successful medical treatment but in whom toxic megacolon recurred necessitating surgical treatment, on average, 11 days after presentation. Of these 14 patients, 3 died. The overall success rate of medical therapy was only 10 percent. The authors' bias is that a very intensive and short trial of medical therapy is warranted, particularly in patients who have toxic megacolon as their initial presentation, and particularly if Crohn's colitis is the suspected etiology. If the patient is not *dramatically* better in 12 to 24 h, surgical intervention is necessary.

SURGICAL MANAGEMENT

Regardless of the surgical option exercised, operations for toxic megacolon are challenging and demanding. Collective reported mortality is 20 percent, although several groups have had better results. These operations are difficult because of the massive colonic distention, the thin-walled nature of the colon, and the frequent findings of gross or sealed-off perforations. Three operations are currently in use for toxic megacolon: subtotal colectomy and ileostomy, total proctocolectomy and ileostomy, and the Turnbull-Weakley blow-hole operation. The most frequently used procedure is a subtotal colectomy and ileostomy. This removes all of the diseased colon but leaves the rectum as a closed-off segment (Hartmann procedure) or as a mucous fistula. The rationale for this procedure is that it removes most of the disease process, treats the acute emergency of dangerous colonic distention, and maintains future options of restoration of intestinal continuity in the forms of ileorectal anastomosis or mucosal proctectomy and ileal pouch-anal anastomosis. On occasion, the rectum may be the source of active hemorrhage or severely active disease necessitating synchronous rectal excision. As restorative procedures are becoming more common and desirable in patients with ulcerative colitis, total proctocolectomy should be limited to the aforementioned circumstances, and every effort made to save the rectum. Predicated on the concept that trying to mobilize a thin-walled inflamed colon is hazardous, Turnbull and colleagues have advocated the blow-hole operation which does not involve any resection.[10] This operation consists of a loop ileostomy, transverse colon colostomy, and when the sigmoid colon is very dilated, a sigmoid colostomy as well. They claim that this is preferable to conventional extirpative procedures because mobilization of the colon can result in exposing and interrupting sealed-off perforations. After the acute attack has subsided, patients require a second procedure to extirpate the diseased colon. Their results are impressive—only 1 of 42 treated patients died. Despite this, few groups have reported experience with this technique, perhaps because of the diminished appeal of leaving an actively inflamed, thin-walled colon in situ.

CASE PRESENTATION

D.M., a 35-year-old man, presented to the emergency department with a 2-week history of increasing abdominal pain, bloody diarrhea, and anorexia. He was brought in by his friend who discovered that he was slightly confused and very weak. Two weeks before presentation, he had been a healthy man with no previous medical illness. On questioning, it became apparent that he had several episodes of vomiting, crampy abdominal pain, frequent bloody diarrhea until 24 h prior to admission when the diarrhea decreased, and he developed a fever. He attributed his symptoms to a bad "flu." On examination he appeared ill. His temperature was 103°F (39.4°C), pulse 130, and blood pressure 120/70 dropping to 95 systolic on sitting. He appeared dehydrated, lethargic, and confused. Positive findings were limited to the abdomen, which was distended and tympanitic. Abdominal tenderness was limited, and there was no rigidity, rebound, or guarding. Bowel sounds were diminished. Rectal examination revealed blood-tinged stool. An upright chest x-ray and three views of the abdomen revealed no free air under the diaphragm, minimal small bowel gas, and a grossly distended colon with the transverse colon measuring 9.5 cm in diameter. A gentle sigmoidoscopy was performed by the surgical team, and it revealed diffuse erythema, ulceration, and mucosal friability consistent with a diagnosis of ulcerative colitis. Stool cultures for bacteria and ova and parasites were sent. Routine hematology and biochemistry revealed: hemoglobin, 95 g/L; white blood cell count, 19.0 × 109/L; potassium, 3.3 mmol/L; sodium, 129 mmol/L; and urea, 15.9 mmol/L.

Based on the history and physical examination, a presumptive diagnosis of ulcerative colitis with toxic megacolon was made. He was seen jointly by the surgical team and gastroenterology service and admitted to the ICU. He was kept NPO, and instrumented with a nasogastric tube, Foley catheter, CVP line, and two large bore intravenous lines. The CVP measured 2 cm H_2O. Fluid resuscitation was initiated with 2 L normal saline solution in the first 2 h followed by normal saline solution delivered at 500 mL/h for the next 8 h. He was transfused with 3 U packed red blood cells. He was started on intravenous hydrocortisone, 100 mg every 6 h and 2 g cefoxitin every 6 h. He was examined by the combined medical-surgical team every 4 h and had repeat plain films of the abdomen every 12 h.

The patient quickly and dramatically improved by all measurable parameters. Most importantly, he became lucid and looked less ill. His tachycardia diminished, and his blood pressure became normal. The transverse colon diameter 24 h after admission was 7.0 cm. Abdominal examination revealed less distention and no signs of peritoneal irritation. Within 48 h after admission, the patient was transferred to the medical floor. Subsequent investigations revealed pancolitis consistent with a diagnosis of ulcerative colitis.

The patient continued to improve and was eventually discharged on oral prednisone, 20 mg/day. He was well until 4 weeks after discharge when he once again presented to the emergency department extremely ill. Clinical examination revealed a recurrence of toxic megacolon with a transverse colon diameter of 10.0 cm. After appropriate resuscitation, he was taken urgently to the operating room where a subtotal colectomy was performed.

The patient's postoperative course was stormy, complicated in part by the development, 10 days after operation, of a left subphrenic abscess treated successfully by percutaneous drainage. The patient gradually recovered and is now being considered for an ileal pouch-anal anastomosis procedure.

CASE DISCUSSION

The features of this case illustration are typical. The patient developed toxic megacolon as the first manifestation of his disease process. On arrival in the emergency department the patient was seriously ill. The approach adopted in his management was intensive medical management with a view to obviating the need for urgent surgical intervention. The mainstay of medical management was fluid resuscitation, steroids, antibiotics, and close observation by a joint medical-surgical team. The patient improved and was subsequently treated medically. This is a debatable point. Some would advocate that he should have undergone semiemergent operation as soon as he improved. This philosophy is based on the substantial possibility of developing further problems, which he indeed did. A second episode of toxic megacolon carries with it again a substantial risk of dying, somewhere between 10 and 25 percent. When he presented with this second episode, there was no debate. Surgery was prompt but nonetheless, complicated by a potentially life-threatening problem, a subphrenic abscess. This development likely resulted from the "unroofing" of a sealed-off perforation during the mobilization of the colon. This possibility has led some surgeons to use the blow-hole operation instead of resection. In this case, the surgical team opted to perform a subtotal colectomy instead of a total proctocolectomy. This has resulted in the possibility of performing, at a later date, a restorative procedure, thus avoiding the need for a permanent ileostomy in this patient.

References

1. Marshak RH, Lester LJ, Freedman AI: Megacolon, a complication of ulcerative colitis. Gastroenterology 16:768, 1950.
2. Ondyniaec NA, Judd ES, Sauer WG: Toxic megacolon, significant improvement in surgical management. Arch Surg 94:638, 1967.
3. Heppell J, Farkough E, Dube S, et al: Toxic megacolon: Analysis of 70 cases. Dis Colon Rectum 29:789, 1986.
4. Halpert RD: Toxic dilatation of the colon. Radiologic Clin North Am 25:147, 1987.
5. Binder SC, Patterson JF, Glotzer DJ: Toxic megacolon in ulcerative colitis. Gastroenterology 66:904, 1974.
6. Present DH, Wolfson D, Gelernt IM, et al: Medical decompression of toxic megacolon by "rolling." J Clin Gastroenterol 10:485, 1988.
7. Soyer MT, Aldrete JS: Surgical treatment for toxic megacolon and proposal for a program of therapy. Am J Surg 140:421, 1980.
8. Katzka I, Katz S, Morris E: Management of toxic megacolon: The significance of early recognition in medical management. J Clin Gastroenterol 1:307, 1979.
9. Grant CS, Dozois RR: Toxic megacolon: Ultimate fate of patients after successful medical management. Am J Surg 147:106, 1984.
10. Turnbull RP, Hawk WA, Weakley FL: Surgical treatment of toxic megacolon: Ileostomy and colostomy to prepare patients for colectomy. Am J Surg 122:325, 1971.

Chapter 167

MESENTERIC ISCHEMIA

ELIZABETH T. CLARK
BRUCE L. GEWERTZ

KEY POINTS

- *Mesenteric ischemia may result from acute arterial emboli, thrombotic events, primary vasoconstriction ("nonocclusive" ischemia), or venous thrombosis.*
- *Acute mesenteric embolic or thrombotic events classically present with severe abdominal pain out of proportion to the findings on physical examination. If peritoneal signs are elicited, it is likely that intestinal infarction has already occurred.*
- *Barium studies are contraindicated and interfere with the essential diagnostic study—arteriography.*
- *In cases of nonocclusive ischemia, intraarterial infusion of papaverine into the superior mesenteric artery (SMA) may be considered the primary mode of therapy.*
- *All patients with suspected embolic or thrombotic occlusions should undergo urgent laparotomy.*
- *If there is any question of viability at the resected margins, exteriorization with cutaneous enterostomies or a "second-look" laparotomy at 24 h should be performed.*

Mesenteric ischemia encompasses a wide variety of disorders ranging from chronic intestinal angina to catastrophic mesenteric infarction. The continued high mortality of these syndromes reflects the difficulties in accurately identifying patients at risk and the lack of reliable noninvasive diagnostic tests. Furthermore, the problems associated with the recognition of acute intestinal ischemia are even more confounding when ischemia is a secondary process, superimposed on another life-threatening illness. This discussion will focus on the pathophysiology of acute mesenteric ischemia and address current diagnostic and therapeutic options.

Anatomy and Regulation of the Mesenteric Circulation

The mesenteric circulation receives approximately 10 to 15 percent of the cardiac output. Resting intestinal blood flow ranges from 50 to 70 mL/min/100 g tissue.[1] Approximately 70 percent of the intestinal blood flow is directed to the mucosal and submucosal layers, whereas 30 percent supplies the muscularis and serosal layers. Blood flow increases approximately 25 to 30 percent with food ingestion because of the increased metabolic needs of mucosal transport and peristalsis.[2]

Three vessels provide the primary arterial supply to the splanchnic bed: the *celiac artery*, supplying the foregut, liver, and spleen; the *superior mesenteric artery* (SMA), supplying the intestine from the duodenal-jejunal junction to the midtransverse colon; and the *inferior mesenteric artery*, supplying the midtransverse colon to the rectum.

Importantly, extensive, but highly variable collaterals are present in this system. Collateral flow between the celiac and superior mesenteric distribution occurs primarily through branches of the gastroduodental artery including the superior and inferior pancreaticoduodenal arteries. Numerous collaterals exist between the superior and inferior mesenteric circulations, the most prominent of which is the marginal artery of Drummond connecting the middle colic and left colic arteries. Sigmoidal-hemorrhoidal vessels from the internal iliac vessels also anastomose with branches of the left colic artery. Extensive submucosal vascular plexi provide additional communications. Because of this collateral network, it is generally true that at least two of the three major vessels must be occluded before chronic ischemic symptoms develop. However, acute occlusion of a single vessel may result in severe vascular compromise depending on the underlying atherosclerotic disease and the degree of collateral involvement.

Neural, humoral, and intrinsic mechanisms all contribute to the regulation of the mesenteric circulation. The principal *neural input* is via the sympathetic nervous system. Electric stimulation of sympathetic nerves results in frequency-dependent increases in mesenteric vascular resistance reflecting constriction of large and medium-sized arterioles. Mesenteric venous capacitance is also regulated by the sympathetic nervous system. In some experiments, total splanchnic blood volume is decreased by more than 50 percent following direct stimulation of sympathetic nerves.[3]

A large number of circulating vasoconstrictors participate in *humoral regulation* of the intestinal circulation.[4] Although epinephrine and norepinephrine are involved, vasopressin and angiotensin are the most potent blood-borne substances. These agents are responsible for sustaining the posthemorrhagic mesenteric vasoconstriction initiated by sympathetic nerves. Exogenous vasoactive compounds have differential effects on the intestinal vasculature, many of which are dose dependent. For example, low doses of epinephrine, norepinephrine, dopamine, and acetylcholine result in vasodilation, whereas high doses cause vasoconstriction. Histamine is thought to cause vasodilation secondary to H_1-receptor stimulation, whereas glucagon causes vasodilation by relaxation of precapillary sphincters.

Intrinsic control mechanisms are reflected in the ability of the intestine to locally regulate blood flow and metabolism independent of neural input and circulating vasoactive agents. Local mechanisms are often characterized as either myogenic or metabolic in nature.[5] *Metabolic control* is initiated when oxygen demand transiently exceeds oxygen delivery. Local vasodilators such as hydrogen ions and adenosine are released locally and blood flow increases to maintain aerobic metabolism. Postprandial intestinal hyperemia is a classic example of metabolic flow regulation.[6] *Myogenic control* arises from a tendency of vascular smooth muscle to maintain a constant wall tension despite variations in perfusion pressure. Since wall tension equals pressure times radius, this is accomplished by modifying the contractile force of the circular-oriented smooth muscle cells thereby changing the effective radius of the lumen. Hence, when perfusion pressure decreases, vessels dilate (or increase radius) and when perfusion pressure increases, vessels constrict (or decrease radius).[7] These adjustments serve to maintain or "autoregulate" blood flow at near normal levels regardless of arterial pressure.

Despite the theoretical differences in metabolic and myogenic hypotheses of local blood flow regulation, it is difficult to delineate which is predominant in a given setting. Often, the directional response to a specific perturbation is the same regardless of mechanism. For example, abrupt reductions in perfusion pressure will elicit both myogenic vasodilation (to maintain tangential wall tension) and metabolic vasodilation (to correct tissue hypoxia).[8]

Pathophysiology

Mesenteric ischemia may result from acute arterial emboli, thrombotic events, primary vasoconstriction ("nonocclusive" ischemia) or venous thrombosis. The reported incidence of each mechanism varies widely, reflecting the differing patient populations of each large clinical series.

Embolism is one of the most frequently encountered causes of acute ischemia, accounting for roughly one-third of all mesenteric vascular catastrophes.[9] Most emboli occur in association with cardiac arrhythmias (especially atrial tachyarrhythmias) or myocardial infarctions. The SMA is the site of most embolic occlusions due to its oblique origin from the abdominal aorta. As many as 5 percent of all peripheral emboli lodge in this vessel. Occlusion typically occurs distal to the origin of the artery; only 15 percent of emboli remain impacted at the ostium of the SMA while approximately 50 percent migrate to the level of the middle colic artery.[10]

Acute thrombosis of an already compromised vessel lumen occurs in another one-third of cases. Such preexisting atherosclerotic lesions are often associated with prodromal symptoms. In fact, over 50 percent of patients who die due to SMA thrombosis have a history of postprandial abdominal pain.[10,11] In situ thrombosis typically occurs at the origin of the SMA, resulting in severe ischemia from the proximal jejunum to the midtransverse colon. In some patients with advanced atherosclerotic disease, extensive collateralization may predate the acute occlusion providing an extended "grace period" before infarction occurs or moderating the eventual ischemic insult.

Nonocclusive mesenteric ischemia, which comprises most of the remaining cases of mesenteric ischemia, involves the SMA distribution almost exclusively. The mechanism is multifactorial but usually involves moderate to severe mesenteric atherosclerosis, marginal cardiac reserve, and administration of vasoactive agents, especially digitalis preparations.[12] The onset is often predated by an acute decrease in cardiac function with reductions in mesenteric perfusion pressure. Paradoxical splanchnic vasoconstriction then ensues with microvascular collapse, formation of microthrombi, and capillary sludging. If there is associated systemic hypotension, catecholamines may further the vasoconstrictive process. Since the majority of patients suffering from nonocclusive mesenteric ischemia have histories of digitalis use, the effects of this drug on the mesenteric vasculature have been closely studied.[13] Digitalis compounds have been shown to induce contraction of arterial and venous smooth muscle in vitro and in vivo and to accentuate the myogenic vasoconstriction of arterioles in response to acute venous hypertension.[14–16]

Venous thrombosis, a final and relatively uncommon cause for mesenteric vascular compromise, may begin *peripherally* in the small veins of the mesenteric arcade or *centrally* in the major trunks of the portal system.[17,18] Venous occlusion is accompanied by substantial splanchnic fluid sequestration and hemorrhagic intestinal infarction. Like arterial thrombosis, venous thrombosis is most common in the superior mesenteric vessels.

Risk Factors

Multiple risk factors have been identified for acute mesenteric ischemia. These include age over 50 years, severe valvular atherosclerotic heart disease, congestive heart failure, cardiac arrhythmias, and recent myocardial infarction. Hypovolemia or hypotension, especially that associated with trauma, burns, pancreatitis, or gastrointestinal hemorrhage are commonly associated with both nonocclusive mesenteric ischemia and in situ thrombosis.

Over 40 percent of patients suffering from mesenteric venous thrombosis have a history of deep venous thrombosis of the extremities.[18] Hypercoagulable states such as polycythemia, thrombocytosis, antithrombin III deficiency, and malignancy increase the risk for mesenteric venous thrombosis. Unopposed estrogen stimulation, as seen with oral contraceptive use, pregnancy, or chemotherapy for prostate cancer, also increases risk.[10]

Clinical Presentation

Acute mesenteric emboli or *thrombotic* events classically present with severe abdominal pain out of proportion to the findings on physical examination. The pain is usually steady, severe, and localized in the mid abdomen. If peritoneal signs are elicited, it is likely that intestinal infarction has already occurred.

Embolism should be suspected if the onset of symptoms is acute and cardiac arrhythmias are documented. In contrast, in situ arterial thrombosis may mimic small bowel obstruction, presenting with a more gradual onset of symptoms including abdominal distension and emesis. A history of postprandial pain and weight loss may be elicited. "Intestinal angina" typically occurs 15 to 60 min after eating and is more closely related with the volume of food consumed rather than any specific type of food. The wasting mimics that associated with visceral malignancy and is indicative of decreased food intake ("food fear") not malabsorption.[10]

Nonocclusive mesenteric ischemia is also accompanied by periumbilical pain but occasionally occurs in the absence of such complaints. Clinical signs may be limited to shock, acidosis, hemoconcentration, and sepsis of unknown etiology. Mesenteric venous thrombosis generally presents with constant, diffuse abdominal pain, although symptoms may be intermittent at first. Roughly half these patients complain of distention and nausea with low-grade fever (39°C, 102.2°F). The two types of venous occlusion are reflected in the clinical presentations. Peripheral thrombosis has an insidious course over 1 to 2 weeks, whereas occlusion of a major venous trunk (e.g., portal vein or superior mesenteric vein) is associated with a sudden onset of symptoms.[17] Serosanguinous ascites may be present, and hypovolemia is a common clinical sign due to the substantial fluid sequestration that occurs.

The clinician's single greatest tool for the successful diagnosis of a mesenteric vascular event is a high index of suspicion in patients with multiple risk factors. Early diagnosis and institution of therapeutic measures prior to bowel infarction is essential to decrease mortality. If diagnosis occurs within 24 h, 60 percent of patients survive; survival decreases to <30 percent if more than 24 h pass between onset and diagnosis.[19,20] Although many laboratory abnormalities occur with mesenteric ischemia and infarction, most are nonspecific and thus not diagnostic.[21] These include hemoconcentration, leukocytosis with a significant "left shift," metabolic acidosis, hyperamylasemia, and hyperphosphatemia. Aspartate aminotransferase, lactic dehydrogenase, and creatine phosphokinase levels are commonly elevated but not until 6 to 12 h after infarction occurs. Precordial echocardiography and Holter monitoring are often "normal" subsequent to well-documented embolic events.

Abdominal plain x-ray is useful in excluding other causes of abdominal pain such as mechanical small bowel obstruction, perforation of a hollow viscus, or appendicitis with fecalith. As many as 70 percent of patients with mesenteric ischemia show at least one of the following signs on abdominal film: ileus, ascites, small bowel dilation, thickening of valvulae conniventes, and separation of small bowel loops. On occasion, a "gas-less" abdomen is seen due to prominent fluid accumulation within the lumen. A grave radiographic finding is the presence of intramural or portal air indicative of infarction and colonization with gas-forming organisms.

Colonscopy may be useful in the diagnosis of subacute colonic ischemia but is often misleading early in the course of the disease and is of no value in detecting small bowel ischemia. Its principal application is detection of sigmoid ischemia after vascular reconstructive procedures involving the abdominal aorta.

Barium studies are usually contraindicated but, if performed, may show evidence of small bowel dilation and focal mucosal hemorrhage ("thumbprinting"). The considerable disadvantage of intraluminal contrast studies is the potential for interference with the essential diagnostic study—arteriography. In fact, problems with all diagnostic tests except arteriography are the lack of specificity and reliability.

Successful arteriography mandates prior hemodynamic stabilization of the patient because hypotension alone may cause significant splanchnic vasoconstriction and preclude an adequate study. Any vasoactive drugs with splanchnic vasoconstrictive properties should be terminated, if possible. Both anterior-posterior (AP) and lateral views of the aorta are required. The AP view best demonstrates collateral vessels while lateral aortography better visualizes the origins of major visceral arteries that overlie the aorta in the AP plane.

Arteriographic signs can generally differentiate embolic from thrombotic occlusions. Emboli usually lodge just proximal or distal to the origin of the middle colic artery whereas thrombotic occlusions of preexistent stenotic lesions more often occur at the SMA origin and are associated with both generalized atherosclerosis of the aorta and the presence of extensive collaterals. Mesenteric venous thrombosis is characterized by general slowing of arterial blood flow (up to 20 s) in conjunction with nonopacification of the corresponding mesenteric or portal veins. The process is usually segmental in nature and thus is distinct from nonocclusive arterial ischemia which is more diffuse and shows normal venous filling. Nonocclusive ischemia characteristically shows narrowing and irregularity of major branches of the SMA which has been termed the "string of sausages" sign.

Therapy

When the diagnosis of mesenteric ischemia is considered, every effort should be made to discontinue or greatly reduce the administration of vasoactive drugs with significant α-adrenergic (vasoconstrictive) effects. In cases of nonocclusive ischemia, intraarterial infusion of papaverine into the SMA may be considered the primary mode of therapy. In fact, use of intraarterial papaverine is appropriate in the postoperative period even in patients suffering acute embolic or thrombotic occlusions.[10,20] The drug has been shown to increase intestinal blood flow to marginally perfused tissue and may significantly improve bowel salvage. Papaverine should be administered as a constant infusion at a rate of 30 to 60 mg/h for at least 24 to 48 h. Operation may be avoided in patients with nonocclusive ischemia if the diagnosis is clear on arteriography and abdominal signs and symptoms totally resolve with papaverine infusion.

In contrast, all patients with suspected embolic or thrombotic occlusions should undergo urgent laparotomy. Fluid resuscitation and administration of both heparin and antibiotics are indicated prior to surgery. Often, an embolus can be directly extracted from a transverse arteriotomy in the SMA at the base of the mesentery.[19] If adequate inflow is obtained following the passage of an embolectomy catheter, no additional arterial reconstruction may be required. If thrombosis of an atherosclerotic lesion is suspected, or if

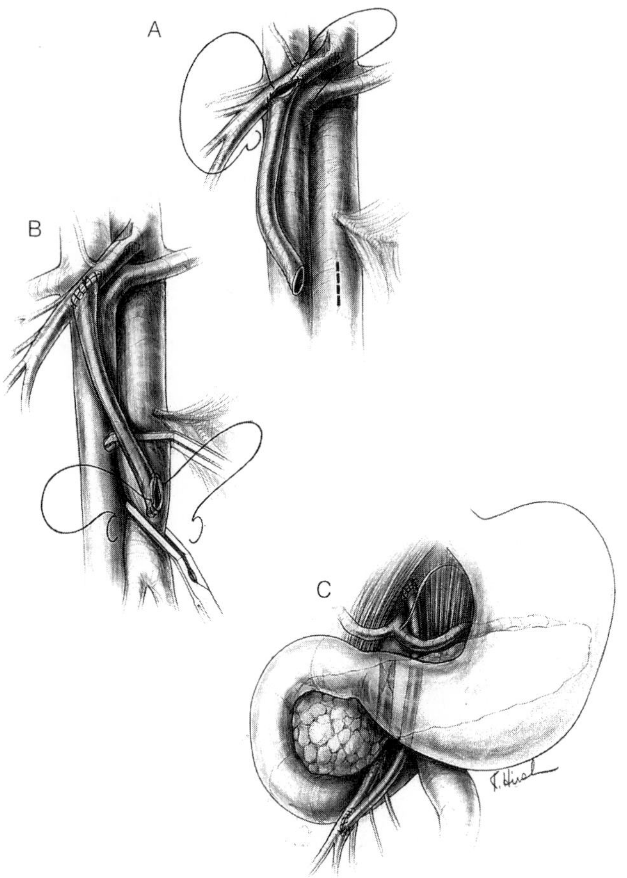

FIGURE 167-1 Illustration of operative technique for two forms of bypass of the SMA. *A* and *B* illustrate construction of a bypass graft in a retrograde fashion. The distal anastomosis is performed first to the SMA (*A*). The graft is tailored in length and anastomosed proximally to the infrarenal aorta (*B*). Antegrade bypass (*C*) originates in the supraceliac aorta with a distal anastomosis approximately 10 cm from the origin of the SMA.

complete extraction of the embolic material is not possible, some form of aortomesenteric bypass should be considered.[22] This can be constructed in an antegrade fashion with a graft originating in the suprarenal aorta or in a retrograde fashion with a graft from the infrarenal aorta (Fig. 167-1). The principal difficulty of the latter procedure is orientation of the vein or prosthetic graft to avoid kinking or compression by the mesentery. The operative approach to venous thrombosis involves resection of infarcted bowel. Venous thrombectomy can be considered in the larger more proximal veins, although the likelihood of recurrent thrombosis is relatively high.

Intraoperative determination of intestinal viability may be performed using a variety of techniques. Clinical judgments are based on the return of normal bowel color, mesenteric arterial pulsations, and visible peristalsis. In experienced hands, these assessments are fairly accurate, but on occasion may be too conservative (resulting in unnecessary bowel resection) or, worse yet, too optimistic (leaving ischemic or infarcted bowel in place). Hence, other more objective methods for determining viability have been developed.[23] These include detection of pulsatile mural blood flow by intraoperative Doppler ultrasound or fluorescein injection and inspection with a Wood's light.[24]

Once intestinal viability is determined and resection completed, a decision must be made regarding restoration of intestinal continuity. If there is any question of viability at the resected margins, exteriorization with cutaneous enterostomies may prevent a "second-look" laparotomy at 24 h. It should be cautioned that the decision for repeat laparotomy should be based on the findings at the time of the initial operation and must not be affected by apparent clinical improvement in the immediate perioperative period.

Careful attention to fluid management in the perioperative period is essential. Antibiotic coverage with broad-

FIGURE 167-2 Aortogram demonstrates acute occlusion of the SMA (arrow) associated with probable chronic occlusion of the celiac axis.

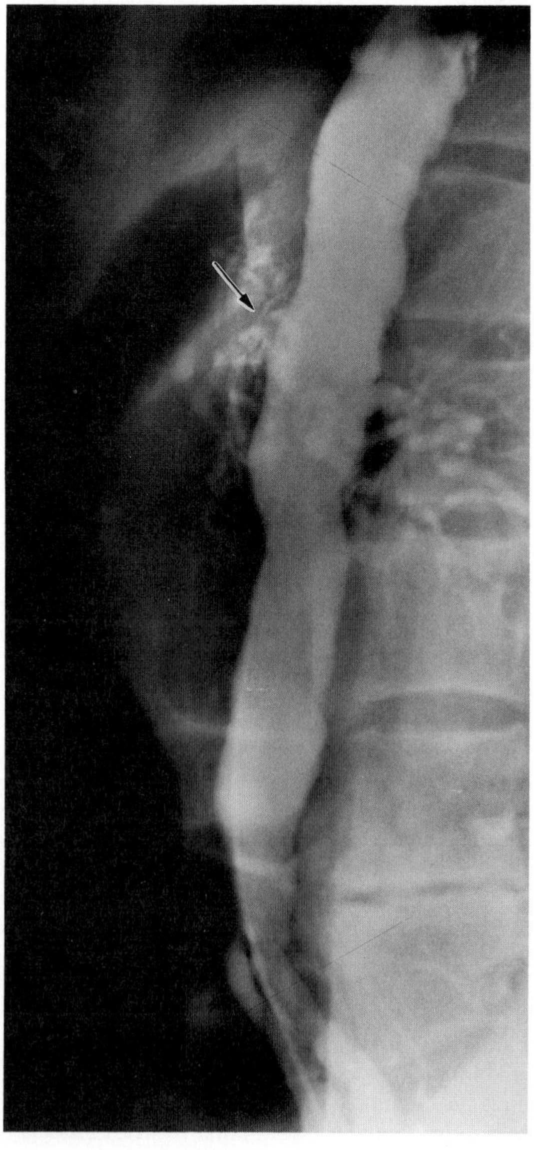

spectrum agents should be continued for at least 5 days. Unless specific contraindications are apparent, heparin anticoagulation followed by at least 3 months of warfarin therapy is appropriate. If a vascular reconstruction has been performed, postoperative arteriography is prudent prior to discharge to document graft patency and orientation.

CASE PRESENTATIONS

Case 1. A 75-year-old white man with a history of coronary artery disease, congestive heart failure, and hypertension presented to the emergency room with signs and symptoms of acute calculous cholecystitis. At operation, the diagnosis was confirmed and the gallbladder removed. His postoperative course was complicated by an episode of reversible myocardial ischemia and systemic hypotension 12 h after surgery, which responded to fluid resuscitation. Six hours following this episode he began complaining of diffuse abdominal pain, nausea, and distention despite a functioning nasogastric tube. On questioning, the patient related a history of abdominal pain following meals that had resulted in a 10-lb weight loss over the 6 months prior to this admission. The diagnosis of mesenteric ischemia was considered, and the patient underwent arteriography.

Arteriography demonstrated generalized infrarenal aortic atherosclerosis. There was a sharp termination of contrast just distal to the origin of the SMA (Fig. 167-2). A presumptive diagnosis of SMA thrombosis was made. After fluid resuscitation and placement of a pulmonary artery catheter, the patient was taken to the operating room. On exploration, he was found to have acute SMA thrombosis with resultant infarction of 60 cm of small bowel from the proximal jejunum to mid ileum. Thrombectomy of the SMA at the base of the mesentery was performed, and revascularization was accomplished with a saphenous vein bypass graft from the infrarenal aorta to the distal SMA. The ischemic intestine was resected, and a primary anastomosis was performed. The patient had an uneventful postoperative recovery, and an angiogram was obtained prior to discharge (Fig. 167-3).

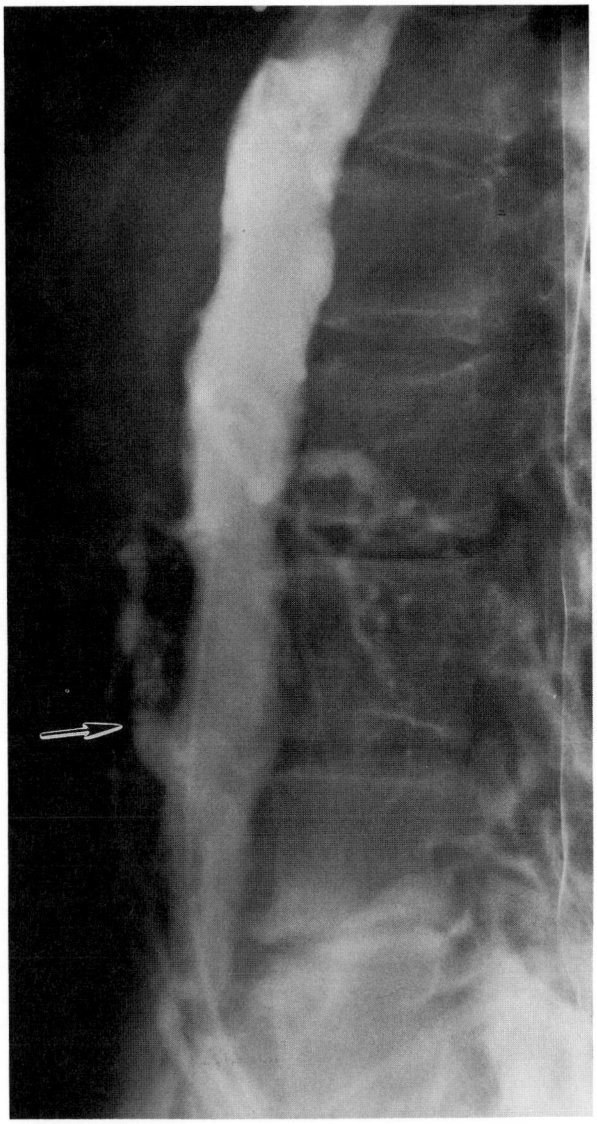

FIGURE 167-3 Arteriogram obtained following vein graft bypass (arrow) from infrarenal aorta to SMA. Note filling of distal portion of artery.

Discussion

This patient demonstrates the classic history of mesenteric arterial thrombosis. In this particular case, it occurred as a secondary phenomena to another acute illness and was associated with relative dehydration, hypotension, and marginal cardiac output. The history of intestinal angina and weight loss is common in patients experiencing acute thrombosis of atherosclerotic lesions.

The salutory outcome in this case was a direct reflection of the early arteriographic diagnosis and exploratory laparotomy. Adequate mesenteric revascularization is absolutely necessary. In the operating room, resection of marginal intestinal segments should be performed last, after revascularization is complete. In this case, no "second-look" operation was deemed necessary.

Case 2. A 58-year-old black man with a history of congestive heart failure treated with digitalis, presented to his physician complaining of crampy, left lower quadrant pain. A barium enema was performed. Diverticuli were demonstrated and the presumptive diagnosis of diverticulitis was made. He was hospitalized and treated with bowel rest, intravenous antibiotics, and fluids.

Twenty-four hours after admission, the patient became slightly hypotensive (90/60) and complained of more severe periumbilical pain. Dopamine infusions were initiated. The patient's blood pressure increased to 110/70, and an arteriogram was performed.

The study revealed multiple areas of narrowing of the major SMA branches (Fig. 167-4). Papaverine infusion was begun at 40 mg/h, and vasoconstriction improved substantially. After 24 h, the arteriographic study was repeated, and an essentially normal vascular pattern was visualized. Papaverine was discontinued; the patient recovered without incident.

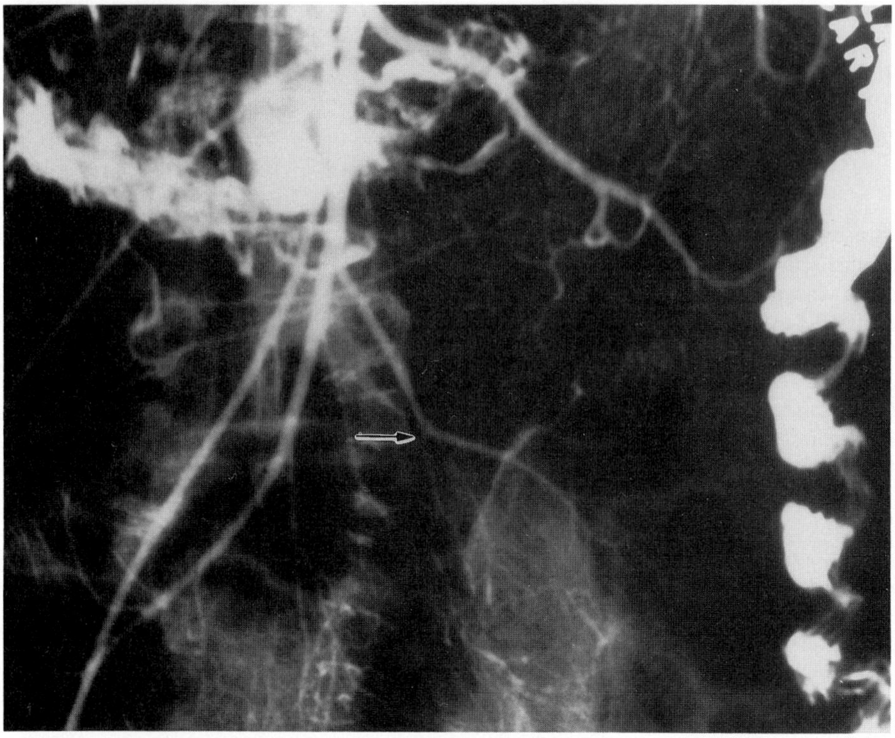

FIGURE 167-4 Selective arteriogram demonstrates diffuse spasm of branches of the SMA. Vessels are irregular and small with "cuffing" or constriction at branching points (arrow). No mucosal blush is seen.

Discussion
Unfortunately, this patient with signs and symptoms compatible with diverticulitis was initially misdiagnosed. The actual pathology of nonocclusive mesenteric ischemia became evident only 24 h after admission when more severe periumbilical pain ensued. The arteriographic findings are classic for nonocclusive ischemia. Fortunately, his response to papaverine infusion was excellent, and abdominal pain resolved. Should the patient have demonstrated persistent abdominal pain, free air in the abdomen on x-ray, leukocytosis, or new Hematest-positive stools, exploration would have been required.

Case 3. A 62-year-old white man with a long-standing history of polycythemia rubra vera presented to the emergency room with severe abdominal pain that awoke him from sleep approximately 3 h earlier. He complained of nausea but no emesis. Ascites was present, and the patient's mild hypotension (100/70) responded to fluid resuscitation. In view of his hematologic history, a diagnosis of acute venous thrombosis was thought likely, and an angiogram and computed tomography (CT) scan were obtained.

Arterial filling was delayed on angiography, and there was no opacification of the SMA. Thrombus was identified in the superior mesenteric vein on CT scan (Fig. 167-5). The patient's symptoms persisted, and an emergency laparotomy was carried out. Superior mesenteric venous thrombosis was confirmed, and 40 cm of discolored, ischemic, and dilated ileum was resected. A primary anastomosis was carried out although the determination was made to reexplore the patient in 24 h to assess the progression of disease. No attempt was made to thrombectomize the superior mesenteric vein.

The next day, repeat laparotomy was performed and the abdominal contents were inspected. The previously marginally perfused bowel was viable. He was treated with heparin followed by warfarin and recovered without complications.

FIGURE 167-5 Infused CT scan demonstrates thrombus in superior mesenteric vein (arrow). Diagnosis can be confirmed by lack of filling of vein on delayed phase of mesenteric arteriogram or duplex scanning of abdomen.

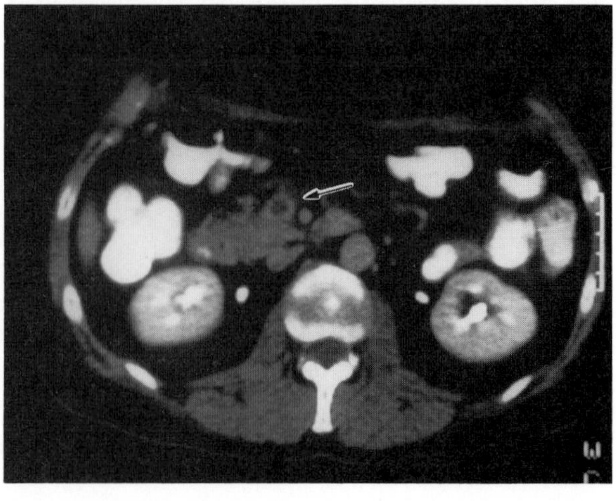

Discussion

Mesenteric venous thrombosis is an unusual diagnosis which is difficult to make in the absence of a significant hematologic history. In this specific case, the association with polycythemia was recognized, and aggressive diagnostic maneuvers were carried out. Although slowing of arterial flow and absent visualization of the major mesenteric veins is diagnostic, often CT scans are more specific in demonstrating the extent of the venous thrombosis. With improved noninvasive tests including duplex imaging, it is likely that earlier diagnosis will be possible.

In general, thrombectomy of mesenteric veins is unsuccessful. Operative therapy is generally limited to resection of ischemic gut rather than any venous reconstructive procedure. Anticoagulation in the perioperative period has significant risks, but unfortunately is essential to the appropriate management of patients suffering venous thrombotic disorders.

References

1. Parks DA, Jacobson ED: Physiology of the splanchnic circulation. Arch Intern Med 145:1278, 1985.
2. Granger DN, Richardson PDI, Kvietys PR, et al: Intestinal blood flow. Gastroenterology 78:837, 1980.
3. Brooksby GA, Donald DE: Dynamic changes in splanchnic blood flow and volume in dogs during activation of sympathetic nerves. Circ Res 29:227, 1971.
4. McNeill JR, Wilcox WC, Pang CCY: Vasopressin and angiotensin: Reciprocal mechanisms controlling mesenteric conductance. Am J Physiol 232:H260, 1977.
5. Granger HJ, Norris CP: Intrinsic regulation of intestinal oxygenation in the anesthetized dog. Am J Physiol (Heart Circ Physiol 7) 238:H836, 1980.
6. Valleau JD, Granger DN, Taylor AE: Effect of solute-coupled volume absorption on oxygen consumption in cat ileum. Am J Physiol 236(2):E198, 1979 or Am J Physiol:Endocrinol Metab Gastrointest Physiol 5(2):E198, 1979.
7. Shepherd AP: Myogenic responses of intestinal resistance and exchange vessels. Am J Physiol 233:H547, 1977.
8. Norris CP, Barnes GE, Smith EE, Granger HJ: Autoregulation of superior mesenteric flow in fasted and fed dogs. Am J Physiol 237(2):H174-H177, 1979 or Am J Physiol:Heart Circ Physiol 6(2):H174, 1979.
9. Sachs SM, Morton JH, Schwartz SI: Acute mesenteric ischemia. Surgery 92:646, 1982.
10. Boley SJ, Brandt LJ, Veith FJ: Ischemic disorders of the intestines. Curr Probl Surg 15:46, 1978.
11. Mikkelsen WP: Intestinal angina. Am J Surg 94:262, 1957.
12. Gazes PC, Holmes CR, Moseley V, Pratt-Thomas HR: Acute hemorrhage and necrosis of the intestines associated with digitalization. Circulation 23:358, 1961.
13. Ferrer MI, Bradley SE, Wheeler HO, et al: The effect of digoxin in the splanchnic circulation in ventricular failure. Circulation 32:524, 1965.
14. Mason DT, Braunwald E, Karsh RB, Bullock FA: Studies on digitalis. Effects of ouabain on forearm vascular resistance and venous tone in normal subjects and in patients in heart failure. J Clin Invest 43:532, 1964.
15. Mikkelsen E, Andersson KE, Pedersen OL: Effects of digoxin on isolated human mesenteric vessels. Acta Pharmacol Toxicol 45:25, 1979.
16. Kim EH, Gewertz BL: Chronic digitalis administration alters mesenteric vascular reactivity. J Vas Surg 5(2):382, 1987.
17. Grendell JH, Ockner RK: Mesenteric venous thrombosis. Gastroenterology 82:358, 1982.
18. Naitove A, Weismann RE: Primary mesenteric venous thrombosis. Ann Surg 161:516, 1965.
19. Boley SJ, Feinstein FR, Sammartano R, et al: New concepts in the management of emboli of the superior mesenteric artery. Surg Gynecol Obstet 153:561, 1981.
20. Boley SJ, Sprayegan S, Siegelman SS, et al: Initial results from an aggressive roentgenological and surgical approach to acute mesenteric ischemia. Surgery 82(6)848, 1977.
21. Jamieson WG, Marchuk S, Rowsom J, Durand D: The early diagnosis of massive acute intestinal ischemia. Br J Surg 69(suppl):S52, 1982.
22. Ottinger LW: The surgical management of acute occlusion of the superior mesenteric artery. Ann Surg 188:721, 1978.
23. Bulkley GB, Zuidema GD, Hamilton SR, et al: Intraoperative determination of small intestinal viability following ischemic injury. Ann Surg 193:628, 1981.
24. Galandiuk S, Fazio VW, Petras RE: Fluorescein endoscopy: A technique for noninvasive assessment of intestinal ischemia. Dis Colon Rectum 31:848, 1988.

SECTION O

OVERDOSE AND POISONING

Chapter 168

GENERAL MANAGEMENT OF POISONING

URI TAITELMAN
MATTHEW J. ELLENHORN

KEY POINTS

- *All comatose patients should receive dextrose, thiamine, and naloxone.*
- *Flumazenil, a benzodiazepine antagonist, may be of both diagnostic and therapeutic value in drug overdoses.*
- *Arterial blood gases; serum glucose, electrolytes, and osmolality; blood urea nitrogen; and hematocrit are useful early laboratory tests in severe poisonings.*
- *Gut decontamination by inducing emesis should not be undertaken if there is a diminished gag; any reduction in level of consciousness; a history of ingestion of strychnine, camphor, or small quantities of hydrocarbons; or in children under the age of 6 months.*
- *Activated charcoal is recommended for most ingestions but cannot be given repeatedly if an ileus develops.*
- *The emergency department and intensive care unit should post the drugs actually screened by the available toxicology lab to inform clinicians of the limitations of this test.*
- *An osmolal gap of greater than 10 mOsm/L suggests ingestion of ethanol, methanol, ethylene glycol, or isopropanol.*
- *Co-oximetry is useful to confirm carbon monoxide poisoning or methemoglobinemia.*
- *All poisonings and drug overdoses should be considered for specific antidotes or means to enhance elimination.*
- *The emergent management of corrosive ingestion is aggressive washout with any available diluent; emesis, gastric lavage, and activated charcoal administration are contraindicated.*
- *Corrosive ingestions require early evaluation for perforation which requires prompt surgical intervention.*

Principles which guide the physician in the treatment of any life-threatening disease apply to acute poisoning. Criteria for admission to the intensive care unit (ICU) include failure of vital functions or a prediction that vital functions may deteriorate. In many institutions, the ICU is the area designated for continuous monitoring because a prompt response to life threats is available.

First Assessment

Evaluation and support of vital functions are the initial mandatory steps in the first assessment, and only after their completion should the issue of poisoning be dealt with. A rapid assessment of respiratory, circulatory, and central nervous system (CNS) function must be performed.

Respiratory system assessment includes respiratory rates; presence or absence of labored breathing with retractions and use of accessory muscles; presence or absence of paradoxical, alternate, or asynchronous breathing; and most importantly, maintenance of upper airway patency. Diminished gag, sonorous breathing, stridor, resolution of airway obstruction by jaw thrust maneuver, and an obviously retrolapsed tongue all point to the need for an artificial airway. Measurement of vital capacity can be used to assess muscle strength in poisonings which affect respiratory muscle function but is difficult or impossible if there is any significant depression in level of consciousness. Circulatory system assessment includes palpation of central and peripheral pulses, capillary refilling time, blood pressure measurement, heart auscultation, and electrocardiographic recording. Assessment of the CNS must distinguish between two types of coma. "Quiet" coma is characterized by suppression of reflexes and muscular tone, bradypnea, and frequently, hypothermia. Hyperactive coma is characterized by agitation and increased muscular activity. In severe hyperactive coma convulsions, hyperthermia, and fluctuation of blood pressure are seen.

This rapid assessment should determine if the patient needs supplemental oxygen, bronchodilators, intubation, mechanical ventilation, a peripheral or central venous line for fluid resuscitation, and drug administration to correct acute circulatory failure. A defibrillator, temporary pacemaker, or in severe cases, cannulation for circulatory bypass may be indicated.

Anoxic and ischemic brain damage are major determinants of morbidity and mortality in acute poisoning, and their prevention is the first priority. Early suppression of convulsions is mandatory; in most cases benzodiazepines, phenytoin, and when necessary, barbiturates are used (see Chap. 142).

If the body temperature exceeds 40.0°C (from any unknown cause), internal and external cooling is initiated, and consideration can be given to treatment with intravenous dantrolene (1 to 5 mg/kg up to 10 mg/kg). Even if the suspicion of drug or toxin ingestion is strong, all febrile patients should be considered for lumbar puncture to exclude meningitis. The decision regarding dantrolene administration is influenced by the rate of temperature rise, by the peak temperature, and by the presence of muscular rigidity. Irreversible tissue injury can occur at central temperatures above 41°C, and core temperature is usually 0.5

to 1°C above rectal temperature. Contraindications to dantrolene administration include evidence of hepatic failure or advanced liver disease.

The comatose patient should receive an intravenous administration of hypertonic dextrose (50 mL of 50% dextrose in water to an adult, 1 mL/kg diluted 1:1 with water to a child), thiamine (100 mg intravenously or intramuscularly), and naloxone (at least 2 mg to an adult, 0.03 mg/kg to a child). Flumazenil (2.5 mg intravenously by slow infusion, then 0.1 mg/min as required up to 5 mg), a benzodiazepine antagonist, is currently in use in Europe and carries investigational drug status in the United States. It is of use diagnostically to determine if benzodiazepine overdose is present, but it may not shorten the duration of hospitalization or improve outcome. In addition, it may "unmask" undesirable effects of co-ingested substances, such as seizures (see Chap. 172).

Arterial blood gases, serum glucose, sodium, potassium, osmolality, blood urea nitrogen, and hematocrit determination should be included in the first assessment of severe poisoning. Initial history, physical examination, and laboratory data will determine the need in the first hours for serum ethanol, acetaminophen, and other drug levels as well as toxicologic screening of urine, blood, gastric aspirate, or other body fluids.

Decontamination: Prevention of Further Absorption

After a first assessment and completion of all necessary emergency interventions, treatment of the poisoned patient will include an attempt to confirm the diagnosis but, more importantly, prevention of further absorption. The exact identity of the toxic agent is often not evident at this stage, but the route of exposure is frequently known. Therefore, prevention of further absorption must immediately be instituted. If exposure has been by ingestion, emptying of the stomach and decontamination of the gut should be considered. Contraindications to stomach emptying include ingestion of corrosive agents, ingestion of small amounts (less than 1 mL/kg) of petroleum distillates, ingestion of sharp objects, a hemorrhagic diathesis, or serious damage to the stomach. Emesis should not be induced if there is loss of the gag reflex, existing or impending unconsciousness or convulsions, a history of strychnine or camphor ingestion, or severe heart disease or in a child under the age of 6 months. The emptying of the stomach after ingestion of fluids is effective if performed very early. An estimate of the volume of one swallow in children is 5 mL.[1] Emptying time of ingested fluid is rapid and proportional to the square root of the ingested volume. For solids such as tablets, emptying of the stomach may be effective many hours after ingestion since a conglomerate may form which remains for a considerable period in the stomach.

Emptying of the stomach can be achieved by emesis or lavage. Emesis should be induced only in a fully conscious patient with normal gag reflexes. Syrup of ipecac has been used for induction of emesis at a dose of 15 to 20 mL for children and 30 to 50 mL for adolescents and adults. Clear fluids (up to 240 to 480 mL) should be ingested immediately after the syrup of ipecac since emptying of a full stomach appears to be more effective than that of a partially empty one. Syrup of ipecac is of limited therapeutic benefit unless administered soon after overdose. In addition, its administration may make the diagnosis of poisoning more difficult to confirm because the vomiting, lethargy, and diarrhea that are induced are features which often mimic those of overdose. Even in conscious patients, syrup of ipecac may lead to aspiration pneumonitis. Emesis usually occurs 15 to 20 min after administration of ipecac but may be delayed up to 30 min. The initial dosage may be repeated if vomiting has not occurred after 30 min, although the patient should first be reevaluated for evidence of diminished gag reflex or level of consciousness.

If the patient is unconscious, gastric aspiration and lavage (after intubation for protection of the airway) should be used to empty the stomach. The patient is placed in the left-side head-down position and a large-bore orogastric tube (32–40F in adults; 16–26F in children) sufficiently large to aspirate tablets and fragments should be introduced into the stomach. The contents are then aspirated and kept for analysis, and following this, repeated lavage with 300 to 500 mL of warm saline is performed until the return is clear. Complications associated with gastric lavage include epistaxis, pulmonary aspiration, aspiration pneumonia, an inability to retrieve lavage fluid, bradycardia, premature ventricular contractions, and hypochloremic alkalosis. Contraindications have been discussed above.

Emptying of the stomach should be followed by administration of activated charcoal through the orogastric tube. Activated charcoal is a substance which has the property of adsorbing a number of different drugs and chemicals. Adsorption is more effective for larger and nonionized molecules. Mild poisoning in the early stage can be treated with single administration of 1 g/kg of activated charcoal by drinking or via gastric tube. Repeated activated charcoal administration is indicated in cases of massive ingestion and in cases where significant enterohepatic recirculation of the ingested compound or of its metabolites may be present. Doses currently used are 0.5 to 1 g/kg every 4 h. Since charcoal may delay bowel transit and even cause impaction, sorbitol 1 g/kg may be added to one or two doses of activated charcoal. Sorbitol does not significantly modify the total adsorption capacity of activated charcoal. Precautions for repeated activated charcoal administration include prevention of aspiration and monitoring of fluid and electrolyte balance. Adverse effects associated with charcoal use include abdominal cramps, nausea, vomiting, diarrhea, and aspiration pneumonitis. There are no known contraindications to the use of charcoal, although patients should be monitored for the development of ileus, a common complication of many drug ingestions. Such bowel immotility often limits the ability to give multiple doses of charcoal. Since it adsorbs and inactivates ipecac, it is best to administer charcoal after emesis. If the ingestant is known to be adsorbed by charcoal, charcoal should be administered

TABLE 168-1 Composition of Polyethylene Glycol Electrolyte Lavage Solution

Constituent	g/L
Polyethylene glycol 3350	60.0
Sodium chloride	1.46
Potassium chloride	0.75
Sodium bicarbonate	1.68
Sodium sulfate	5.68
Water	To 1 L

through the lavage tube followed by lavage. Compounds poorly adsorbed by charcoal include the alcohols (ethanol, methanol, etc.), aliphatic hydrocarbons, alkalis, boric acid, caustic acids, cyanide, heavy metals, and lithium.

Cathartics (sorbitol, magnesium sulfate, sodium sulfate) may be added to the initial charcoal administration to aid in the passage of the charcoal. When used together with each dose of a multiple-dose activated charcoal regimen, they may induce excess loss of fluid and electrolytes. If cathartics are used, careful monitoring of fluids and electrolytes, especially in children, is indicated. Repeat cathartics should not be administered if bowel sounds are absent. Multiple doses of magnesium-containing cathartics may lead to hypermagnesemia. Though the use of cathartics in the treatment of poisoning is widespread, benefit has not been substantiated by controlled clinical trials.

Whole bowel irrigation (WBI) has been employed for gut decontamination and is usually performed after emptying of the stomach by lavage or emesis. Equilibrated solutions of polyethylene glycol and electrolytes in water are used for WBI (Table 168-1).[2] WBI may be useful in the early treatment of ingestion of potentially lethal substances and after ingestion of very large amounts of toxic substances (iron tablets, mixed drug ingestions, and even heroin plastic packs).[2,3]

The rate of solution administration for WBI is 1.6 to 2 L/h for adults and 0.5 L/h for children.[2] WBI is completed when the effluent is clear without solid particles. Activated charcoal can be used before or after but not during WBI. A contraindication to WBI is paralytic or mechanical ileus. An advantage of the use of WBI is mechanical cleaning of the entire gut with no fluid or electrolyte imbalance.

Skin absorption can be the portal of entry for serious poisoning. Removal of the clothes and washing of the skin and mucous membranes with tap water is recommended for decontamination in most cases of skin exposure. If the skin is intact, mild alkaline soap can be used. If chemical or thermal burns are present, 0.9% sodium chloride in water (saline solution) is preferable. In a few cases specific ointment should be applied, e.g., 10% calcium gluconate ointment for hydrofluoric acid skin burns. Decontamination of the eyes is usually performed by washing with water or saline for 20 min with open eyelids. Contact lenses should be removed. Any ocular exposure with symptoms requires an ophthalmologic examination.

Confirmation of Diagnosis

Diagnosis is evident in many cases: (a) on the basis of a detailed history of the exposure, (b) by the existence of a container or an original package, (c) from the clinical signs and symptoms after physical examination, and (d) following laboratory analysis. After examining the patient, a consultation with a poison information center may be indicated to complete information on the pharmacologic and toxicologic properties of the causative agent. It is useful for the emergency department and ICU to post telephone numbers for the regional poison information service and to list the drugs that are routinely screened when urine, blood, or other samples are sent for toxicologic analysis. It is important to remember that for intentional poisoning history is often unreliable, and polypharmaceutical ingestion is common.

Laboratory Analysis

Many routine laboratory analyses are helpful in the diagnosis and evaluation of the severity of a poisoning. Poisons associated with hyperosmolality and an osmolar gap are, for example, ethanol, methanol, ethylene glycol, and isopropanol. Examples of poisonings causing a metabolic acidosis are presented in Table 168-2. A co-oximeter can assist in confirmation of the diagnosis of carbon monoxide poisoning or methemoglobinemia. Even when the identity of a poison appears evident after initial examination, it is recommended that confirmation be obtained where possible by quantitative or qualitative analysis. Waiting for such confirmation, in most cases, should not delay immediate

TABLE 168-2 Some Causes of Metabolic Acidosis

Ingredient	Type of Acid	Anion Gap
Cyanide	Lactic	High
Carbon monoxide	Lactic	High
Toluene (glue sniffing)	Renal tubular acidosis	Normal
Fluoroacetate (rodenticide)	Lactic	High
Methanol	Formic + lactic	High
Ethylene glycol	Glycolic + formic +oxalic	High
Paraldehyde	Acetic	High
Salicylate	Salicylic + lactic + organic	High
Uncoupling agent: pentachlorophenol dinitrophenol	Lactic	High
Phenformin	Lactic	High

NOTE: Many poisonings induce a high anion gap metabolic acidosis due to lactic acidosis. Lactic acidosis results from (a) perfusion failure (cardiac failure, volume loss, or peripheral vasodilation resulting from drug ingestion); (b) convulsions seen following overdose with tricyclic antidepressants, aminophylline and theophylline, isoniazid, organophosphates, organochlorine insecticides; and (c) direct block of aerobic metabolism.

institution of treatment of the poisoned patient. The physician should indicate to the analytic laboratory a suspected ingredient or group of ingredients which could be causative agents under consideration. Many ingredients can be identified by one of the following methods available in many hospitals:

1. Urine thin-layer chromatography (TLC)
2. Spectrophotometry
3. Gas chromatography (GC)
4. Flame photometry
5. Serum radioimmunoassay (RIA)
6. Enzyme multiple immunoassay technique (EMIT)

Specialized laboratories also utilize the following:

7. Gas chromatography with mass spectrometry (GC-MS)
8. High-pressure liquid chromatography (HPLC)
9. Atomic absorption photometry for electrolytes and metals
10. Flameless atomic absorption photometry for metals

Early in management, urine (50 to 100 mL), gastric contents, and blood (in hermetically sealed tubes) should be obtained and retained. Before specimens are sent to the analytic laboratory a direct communication between the physician and the laboratory analyst can improve mutual understanding.

If a poison is suspected to be the cause of coma, most laboratories can perform a coma screen analysis (usually of the urine) which includes the most common drugs responsible for coma: benzodiazepines, barbiturates, phenothiazines, tricyclic antidepressants, antihistamines, tranquilizers, hypnotics, and natural and synthetic opiates. After initial rapid identification by TLC of the urine, blood levels can be determined for most drugs. The clinician should be aware of the substances searched for in any "screening" test and should never assume that all poisonings have been excluded by any given screen.

Complete Assessment

Complete assessment includes a detailed medical history of the patient, detailed physical examination and laboratory analysis of renal and liver functions, a complete blood count, prothrombin time and partial thromboplastin time, and when necessary, calcium, phosphorus, magnesium, and creatine kinase.

Problem of Delayed Toxicity

After a complete physical examination of an asymptomatic patient, the physician should always consider the possibility of delayed toxicity. In such poisonings, symptoms may appear hours or days after exposure. Treatment is effective only if applied early. Some of the most common and most dangerous of such poisonings are described in detail in this section and follow ingestion of methanol, ethylene glycol, paraquat, acetaminophen, and mushrooms. Other poisonings may exhibit a symptom-free interval after the first symptoms appear, following which severe delayed symptoms occur. Typical examples of this group include carbon monoxide, oxides of nitrogen, phosgene, and methyl bromide inhalation and ingestion of fluoroacetate or colchicine. Cyclic antidepressant and monoamine oxidase inhibitor poisonings often develop catastrophic hemodynamic instability within hours following an admission evaluation revealing minimal physical signs of abnormality (see Chap. 173). Minor abnormalities (e.g., sinus tachycardia) may presage a severe clinical course. Such patients may require monitoring for at least 24 h.

Use of Antagonists and Antidotes

Antagonists and antidotes can be divided into two categories: those which should be readily available for immediate use in the emergency room and in the ICU (Table 168-3) and those which should be available in the central pharmacy for use within hours (Table 168-4).

Factors involved when considering use of antagonists and antidotes include severity of poisoning and efficacy and side effects of the therapy. For example, the use of fragment antibodies to treat digitalis poisoning is based mainly on clinical judgment (life-threatening arrhythmias, age, hyperkalemia) and not solely on the blood levels of digoxin. Use of a drug such as physostigmine for tricyclic antidepressant overdose may provoke more problems (bronchospasm, seizures) than it solves. In most cases, antagonists and antidotes are only a part of the therapy. For example, diazoxide may be used together with glucose administration in sulfonylurea-induced hypoglycemias; glucagon may be used with β agonists in treating overdose with β blockers; and antidotes such as sodium nitrite or hydroxocobalamin may accompany use of high concentrations of inspired oxygen in treating cyanide poisoning.

Enhancement of Elimination

Solute diuresis is recommended to increase elimination of substances usually excreted by the kidney with partial reabsorption by renal tubules. In cases of poisoning by lithium carbonate and bromide salts, this method enhances elimination. It is also a recommended treatment for mild renal failure caused by lithium poisoning. In severe lithium poisoning, however, hemodialysis should be utilized.

Alkaline diuresis enhances the elimination of long-acting barbiturates, salicylates, and chlorophenoxy herbicide compounds.[4] The preferred alkalinizing agent is sodium bicarbonate. The doses are titrated according to the acid-base status of the patient. The urine pH must be continuously monitored to be kept at a pH of 7.5 to 8. The desired urine volume is 2 to 4 mL/kg/h. This method is well tolerated by previously healthy young patients but is tolerated less (and usually necessitates intravascular monitoring) in patients

TABLE 168-3 Medications and Antidotes To Be Readily Available in the Emergency Room and ICU

Ingredient	Major Indication	Mode of Use
Deferoxamine	Iron	IV, intramuscular oral[a]
Potassium permanganate 1:10,000 in water	White phosphorus	Oral[a]
Potassium permanganate 1:5000 in water	White phosphorus	Dermal
Prussian blue (potassium hexacyanoferrate)	Thallium	Oral
Calcium gluconate 10%	Fluorides, oxalates	IV, Oral[a] intra arterial
Ethanol 10%	Methanol, ethylene glycol	Oral, IV
4 methylpyrrazole (4 MP)[b]	Methanol, ethylene glycol	IV
Sodium nitrite	Cyanide	IV
Amyl nitrite pearls	Cyanide	Inhalation
Sodium thiosulfate 25%	Cyanide	IV
Dicobalt edetate 1.5% (Kelocyanor[b])	Cyanide	IV
Hydroxocobalamin	Cyanide	IV
N-acetylcysteine	Acetaminophen	Oral, IV
Starch powder	Iodine	Oral[a]
Obidoxime[b] or Pralidoxime	Organophosphate insecticides	IV
Naloxone	Synthetic and natural opiates	IV
Flumazenil[b]	Benzodiazepines	IV
Digoxin immune FAB	Digoxin and other digitalis preparations	IV
Glucagon	Beta blockers	IV
Procyclidine (Kemadrin)	Dystonic reaction	IV
Biperiden hydrochloride (Akineton)	Dystonic reaction	IV
Diphenhydramine (Benadryl)	Dystonic reaction	IV
Sodium dantrolene (Dantrium)	Malignant hyperthermia, neuroleptic malignant syndrome	IV
Physostigmine	Central anticholinergic syndrome	IV
Diazoxide	Sulfanyl urea overdose	IV, oral
Vitamin B6 (pyridoxine phosphate)	Isoniazid	IV
Methylene blue	Methemoglobinemia	IV
Tetrahydrofolic acid (leucovorin)	Methanol, antifolics:methotrexate, trimethoprim, pyrimethamine	Intramuscular, IV
Vitamin K	Anticoagulant rodenticides	IV

[a] Used for gastrointestinal lavage or decontamination
[b] Not available in the United States

with renal, heart, and lung insufficiency. Alkaline diuresis should be considered to protect against myoglobinuric renal failure when convulsions or prolonged muscle compression during coma complicate drug overdose.

The efficacy of drug or toxin elimination by *hemodialysis* depends on the concentration of unbound water-soluble substance in the extracellular fluid compartment and is inversely proportional to the molecular weight (MW) (effective for substances with a molecular weight less than 500 daltons). It is more effective for products not strongly bound to plasma proteins. Thus, hemodialysis is the method of choice for severe methanol and ethylene glycol poisoning. The clearance of methanol (MW 32) is proportional to the blood flow through the hemodialyzer. The advantages of hemodialysis include rapid correction of acid-base and electrolyte disturbances. Complications of hemodialysis include hypotension, electrolyte and osmolar imbalance (signaled by muscle cramps, confusion, coma, or

TABLE 168-4 Medications and Antidotes To Be Available in the Pharmacy

Ingredient	Major Indication	Mode of Use
Antisera: venomous snakes, scorpions, spiders	Snake bites, scorpion stings, spider bites	IV
Botulism, antitoxin	Botulism	IV
Cholestyramine	Halogenated hydrocarbon insecticides	Oral
Dimercaptosuccinate (DMSA)[a]	Heavy metals	Oral, IV
Dimercaptopropansulfonate (DMPS)	Heavy metals	Oral, IV
Penicillamine	Heavy metals	Oral
Calcium disodium ethylenediamine tetraacetate (EDTA)	Heavy metals	IV
Diethylenetriamine pentaacetic acid (DPTA)[a]	Heavy metals	Intramuscular
Triethylene tetramine (trientine)	Copper	Oral
British Anti Lewisite (BAL) (dimercaprol)	Lewisite (arsenic mustard)	Subcutaneous, intramuscular
Colchicine immune FAB	Colchicine overdose	IV
Paradimethylaminophenol (4-DMAP)	Cyanide	IV

[a]Not available in the United States.

convulsions), hypoxemia, spontaneous bleeding, and mechanical complications (e.g., air embolism, blood leak).

Hemodialysis should be considered when the poison is known to be removed effectively by this route and the following conditions pertain: acute renal failure; severe intoxication with hypotension, apnea, or hypothermia unresponsive to supportive care; clinical deterioration and complications in spite of maximal supportive care; prolonged coma; chronic obstructive pulmonary disease (COPD) progressing during coma; lethal drug levels (by history or after gut decontamination); toxic metabolite potential (methanol, ethylene glycol); or after a poison with delayed toxicity.

Hemodialysis can be employed before blood levels are known following methanol or ethylene glycol poisoning. It may be effective after blood levels are known and the clinical condition permits in cases of salicylate, isopropanol, and lithium poisoning. In all cases, its use must be justified by the following:

1. The dialysis clearance of the substance is known to be significant.
2. The poisoning is severe with significant morbidity and/or mortality.
3. Hemodialysis has been proven to reduce morbidity and/or mortality in poisoning by the considered substance.

Extracorporeal hemocomplexation with hemodialysis is a technique in which blood is exposed to a chelating agent before entering the dialyzer. The chelating agent with its chelated metal is then dialyzed. This technique may be effective in severe organic mercurial poisonings.[5]

Charcoal and resin hemoperfusion are effective methods for removal of toxins from the blood. Clearance does not depend on water solubility. Removal persists at low plasma concentrations and is effective even when protein binding is significant (but not complete). However, normal constituents of blood are absorbed during the procedure, and thrombocytopenia, leukopenia, loss of clotting factors, and decreased glucose and calcium may occur. This technique requires heparinization. Hemoperfusion is contraindicated where there is inadequate supportive care to maintain the patient, in the presence of shock, and when anticoagulation cannot be tolerated. It is of use as an ancillary measure in nonbarbiturate sedative-hypnotic poisoning (ethchlorvynol, glutethimide, meprobamate, methaqualone) and following theophylline and disopyramide overdose, among others. It is useful in some cases of salicylate poisoning in which control of severe electrolyte and acid-base imbalance is necessary. The use of this technique should be justified by the following:

1. Significant clearance of the substance by the procedure (Table 168-5).

TABLE 168-5 Compounds Effectively Removed by Hemoperfusion

Barbiturates	Meprobamate
Carbamazepine	Methaqualone
Chloral hydrate	Methotrexate
Ethchlorvynol	Phenytoin
Glutethimide	Theophylline

2. Severe poisoning with significant morbidity or mortality.
3. Proof that the procedure has reduced morbidity or mortality.

Hemodialysis and hemoperfusion are ineffective for removal of substances with a high apparent volume of distribution (over 1 L/kg body weight). They are invasive procedures necessitating anticoagulation. Their use should therefore be justified by high blood levels of a substance with high clearance causing severe manifestations.

Corrosive Ingestion

Most corrosive agents are either strong acids or strong alkalies (Table 168-6). The severity of the damage depends on strength, concentration, amount, and viscosity of the corrosive agent. Strong acids and alkalies are fully dissociated and induce extreme pH changes in one molar concentration (one molar HCl in water has a pH of 0; one molar sodium or potassium hydroxide in water produces a pH close to 14.

Concentration is a very important factor. For example, vinegar is a 5% solution of acetic acid and is not corrosive; however, a 50% solution of the same substance is corrosive and will cause more damage than diluted hydrochloric acid, although the pH of dilute hydrochloric acid is below 1 and that of 50% acetic acid is above 2. Concentrated corrosive solutions usually have a high viscosity and cause severe damage to the esophagus and stomach. Solid corrosives usually cause more damage to the proximal portion of the esophagus.

Ingestion of strong acid causes severe pain. In adults, it is always intentional. Acids cause coagulation of proteins, and therefore, ingestion of liquid acid results in a layer of coagulated protein on the esophagus. The only exception is ingestion of hydrofluoric acid, which causes liquefaction necrosis. Most of the damage is restricted to the distal stomach where the liquid acid accumulates. In massive strong acid ingestion, the stomach, esophagus, and proximal small bowel are usually damaged.

Strong alkali has the capability of dissolving protein and fats and therefore causes a liquifaction necrosis of tissues. If a strong alkali is ingested, pain may be delayed. Ingestion of corrosive alkali may occur accidentally. Most of the damage is usually in the esophagus.

There are three phases in the evolution of tissue damage by corrosive agents: (a) an acute inflammatory stage which is maximal in 24 to 48 h followed by sloughing of necrotic tissue leaving ulcers or perforations, (b) formation of granulation tissue which is maximal in 3 to 4 days, and (c) formation of collagen scar tissue which replaces granulation tissue and may lead to fibrotic stenosis or deformation.

TABLE 168-6 Corrosive Ingestion

	Pathophysiology	Site of Maximal Damage
Strong acid	Coagulation necrosis	Gastric outlet
Strong alkali	Liquifaction necrosis	Midesophagus

The emergency treatment of corrosive ingestion is dilution and washout with fluids. The time element of dilution is more important than the choice of the fluid. If water is readily available, it should be used, although milk mixed with egg white may be a better choice when available since it dilutes and buffers as well. Fluid washout is effective if delivered immediately after ingestion (less than 2 min) and of questionable value after 30 min. Emesis, gastric lavage, and activated charcoal administration are contraindicated after corrosive ingestion. Neutralization of the corrosives by weak acids or weak alkalies is also contraindicated because of the generation of an exothermic reaction with resultant tissue damage and possible gas emission.

Most patients arrive at a hospital more than 30 min after ingestion with at least three of the following symptoms:

1. visible burns and inflammation of the mouth and oropharyngeal mucosa,
2. retrosternal and abdominal pain,
3. vomiting or frank hematemesis,
4. sialorrhea, and
5. dysphagia or inability to swallow.

In many cases, vital signs are abnormal. These patients should be evaluated for upper airway obstruction due to inflammation or edema and hypovolemic shock due to extensive burns of the gastrointestinal tract and necessitating fluid resuscitation.

Once a patient is stabilized, a chest x-ray including the upper abdomen (preferably in the erect position) should be performed for detection of pneumomediastinum, pneumothorax, or pleural effusion due to esophageal perforation and pneumoperitoneum due to gastric or small bowel perforation.

Severe hematemesis and radiographic signs of visceral perforation or signs of an acute abdomen are considered indications for immediate surgery. In all other cases, the need for surgical intervention is guided by early endoscopy performed by an experienced endoscopist, preferably during the first 48 h. After this time, there may be a significant incidence of perforation during the procedure. Radiographic visualization of the esophagus is a possible alternative to endoscopy. If perforation is suspected, water-soluble contrast material should be used instead of barium. If surgery is not performed after an initial assessment, follow-up in the ICU must be focused on early recognition of perforation of the esophagus or intraabdominal viscera and on acute bleeding.

Influence of Genetic Susceptibility and Enzyme Deficiency on Acute Poisoning

Genetic and enzymatic deficiencies may predispose to severe reactions during acute poisoning. For example, there is a relation between acute methemoglobinemia and hemolysis and the presence of a glucose-6-phosphate dehydrogenase (G6PD) deficiency, the most common cause of drug-induced hemolysis.[6] G6PD deficiency is the most common genetic disorder in human beings; it is estimated that about 300 million people all over the world are G6PD deficient.[7] The deficiency appears with a high frequency in certain ethnic groups; the transmission is X chromosome linked. There are several varieties of G6PD abnormality, and within each variety several degrees of severity can be found.[8] Some of the agents known to cause hemolytic anemia and hemolysis in G6PD-deficient individuals are listed in Table 168-7.

Many ingredients known to cause hemolysis in G6PD deficiency are also known to cause methemoglobinemia. They include direct oxidants of hemoglobin, such as nitrites and chlorates, and cyclic methemoglobin-inducing agents such as aminobenzenes (anilines), aminophenols, and quinones. Cyclic methemoglobin-inducing chemicals may cause massive methemoglobinemia in G6PD-deficient patients even after exposure to small amounts. The evaluation of a patient suspected to be poisoned by one of these substances includes a determination of a possible G6PD deficiency.

G6PD deficiency not only increases the incidence or severity of methemoglobinemia and hemolysis following exposure to many chemicals but also limits the use of methylene blue, an effective antidote for the methemoglobinemia of normal erythrocytes. The normal erythrocyte contains several enzymatic systems which reduce methemoglobin to hemoglobin. These systems depend on both aerobic and anaerobic glycolysis. Aerobic glycolysis in the erythrocyte depends on the activity of G6PD (Fig. 168-1).

Acute methemoglobinemia with levels above 40% of normal hemoglobin is a medical emergency. If the patient is not G6PD deficient, methylene blue 1 to 3 mg/kg in dextrose solution is the treatment of choice. Methylene blue reduces methemoglobin by using NADPH as a substrate. Since NADPH can be formed in the erythrocyte only by aerobic glycolysis (shunt of pentose phosphate), methylene blue is an ineffective and potentially hazardous therapy in severely G6PD-deficient patients. In such cases, other modes of therapy (transfusion or exchange transfusion) should be considered.

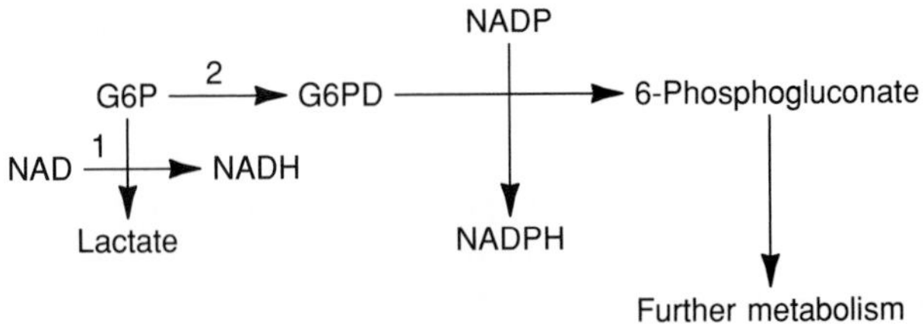

FIGURE 168-1 (1) During anaerobic glycolysis NAD is reduced to NADH. NADH dehydrogenase reduces methemoglobin to hemoglobin. (2) During aerobic glycolysis (requiring G6PD) NADPH is formed from NADP. NADPH is required to restore reduced glutathione which protects the erythrocyte membrane and also reduces methemoglobin to hemoglobin. NADPH is required for reduction of methemoglobin to hemoglobin by methylene blue.

The diagnosis of methemoglobinemia is a clinical diagnosis. Above a methemoglobin level of 15%, a grey cyanosis appears on mucous membranes and skin; above 30%, tachycardia and tachypnea occur. The diagnosis is confirmed by the chocolate brown color of blood (venous or arterial). Arterial blood analysis by co-oximeter (or another spectrophotometric method) demonstrates an increased methemoglobin concentration and decreased oxyhemoglobin saturation together with normal levels of measured arterial P_{O_2}.

Psychiatric Liaison

Psychiatric consultation should be obtained for any patient who has a substantiated history of intentional overdose. Nonpsychiatric physicians are also valuable in assessing

TABLE 168-7 Compounds Causing Hemolytic Anemia and/or Methemoglobinemia in G6PD Deficiency

Acetanilid	Isoniazid	Quinidine
Acetophenetidin	Menadiol	Quinocide
Acetylphenylhydrazine	Methylene blue	Salazopyrin
Aminopyrine	Nalidixic acid	Salazosulfapyridine
Aminoquinoline	Naphthalene	Salicylazosulfapyridine
Antipyrine	Niridazole	Sulfacetamide
Benzocaine	Nitrofurazone	Sulfafurazole
Chlorates	Pamaquin	Sulfamethazole
Chloroquine	Paraaminosalicylate	Sulfanilamide
Diaminodiphenylsulfone	Paracetamol	Sulfapyridine
Diazoxide	Pentaquine	Sulfasalazine
Dimercaprol	Phenacetin	Sulfisoxazole
Dipyrone	Phenazopyridine	Sulfonamides
Fava beans	Phenylhydrazine	Thiazolesulfone
Furadantin	Prilocaine	Toluidine blue
Furaltadone	Primaquine	Trinitrotoluene
Furazolidone	Probenecid	
Glafenine	Propylphenazone	

suicidal risk. After initial treatment has stabilized the patient, one-to-one staffing and frequent checks of status are indicated. Any possibly harmful objects such as glass, belt, shoelaces, and mirrors should be removed or made inaccessible. Prior to discharge a plan should be formulated based on the assumption of an adequate living environment and a compact with the patient to follow a posthospital treatment plan. This should include next-day follow-up with the physician or psychiatrist, an agreement by the patient to call either an emergency department or local suicide prevention center (give telephone number to the patient) if a suicidal urge becomes overwhelming, and an arrangement with family members to closely observe the patient and to remove all possible means to suicide, such as pills, weapons, razors, and knives.

CASE PRESENTATION

A 24-year-old obtunded woman is brought to the emergency room by paramedics for possible drug overdose. They were called to her apartment by a neighbor, who found her sitting on the front porch of the house, crying, lethargic, and claiming to have taken "all the pills in the bathroom." On arrival the paramedics find her lethargic but answering simple questions. They bring a number of empty bottles from the counter of the bathroom, which include acetaminophen with codeine, aspirin, oxazepam, and amitriptyline. The paramedics note that during the 10-min trip to the hospital she has become appreciably less alert.

On examination the patient is obtunded, barely responsive to voice, with a heart rate of 115, blood pressure of 110/65, respirations 10 and shallow, and she is afebrile. Her neck is supple and there is no abnormality on examination of the head, ears, nose, or throat. The lungs are clear and the cardiovascular examination unremarkable. The abdomen is benign. The neurologic examination is without focal abnormality, but the patient has a nearly absent gag and by the end of the examination responds only to deep pain.

Emergent intubation is performed with cricoid pressure to avoid aspiration. An intravenous catheter is placed, and immediately after collecting a blood sample the patient is given 50 mL of 50% glucose, 2 mg of naloxone, and 100 mg of thiamine, without response. An electrocardiogram reveals a sinus tachycardia with a prolonged QT interval. The arterial blood gas immediately after intubation on an F_{IO_2} of 0.4 reveals a Pa_{O_2} of 210, Pa_{CO_2} of 32, and pH of 7.47. The glucose, BUN, and serum electrolytes are normal and there is no osmolar gap.

Following intubation a large-bore orogastric tube is placed and the stomach is lavaged. No pill fragments are seen. Following vigorous lavage, the patient receives activated charcoal at a dose of 1 g/kg. Sorbitol 1 g/kg is added after the initial dose of charcoal. The patient is moved to the ICU for ongoing care and mechanical ventilation is instituted. A sample of blood and urine is sent for toxicologic screening.

Five hours after admission, an estimated six or more hours after drug ingestion, acetaminophen and salicylate levels are sent. There are no detectable salicylates, but acetaminophen is present but below a level requiring antidote therapy, as indicated by the Rumack-Matthew nomogram. The general toxicology screen indicates the presence of acetaminophen, codeine, oxazepam and metabolites, and amitriptyline.

Attempts to repeat doses of activated charcoal and cathartics are unsuccessful because of development of an ileus. Within 12 h the patient's level of consciousness is improved, and 30 h following intubation she is responsive, following simple commands, and breathing spontaneously without difficulty. She is extubated and monitored in the ICU over the next day, during which time her sinus tachycardia and prolonged QT interval resolve. Psychiatric liaison begins at the time she is extubated and continues when she leaves the ICU for a monitored telemetry bed for a full 24 h following normalization of the electrocardiogram. Long-term psychiatric follow-up on an outpatient basis is then established.

CASE DISCUSSION

This case is typical of many drug overdoses in that ingestion was polypharmaceutical, specific antidote therapy was appropriately considered but not appropriate based upon the documented drugs involved, and the patient improved with routine supportive care.

On presentation, the patient's rapidly deteriorating level of consciousness warranted therapy with dextrose, thiamine, and naloxone. Of the drugs ultimately documented by toxicology screen, only codeine would be expected to be reversed by naloxone. It is not surprising in this polypharmaceutical ingestion that a dramatic response to naloxone was not seen. It is interesting to speculate that the benzodiazepine antagonist, flumazenil, may have been of use in this patient.

Induction of emesis would have been a grave error in this patient, given her diminished level of consciousness, poor gag response, and generally rapid decline in neurologic function. Intubation and ventilatory support was appropriately begun early and electively. Following intubation and protection of the airway, gastric decontamination could be performed with a large-bore tube. Following this activated charcoal was administered but subsequent dosing was not possible due to development of an ileus.

The initial laboratory screen included a screen for abnormalities of glucose metabolism, electrolytes, renal function, acid-base status, or gas exchange. No abnormalities hinting at specific poisonings were identified. In addition, there was no osmolar gap to suggest ingestion of significant quantities of the alcohols (see Chap. 170). Six hours after admission, a long enough period of time to allow serum levels to rise but within a window of opportunity to treat, salicylate and acetaminophen levels were determined but did not indicate a need for measures to enhance secretion or initiate antidote therapy (see Chaps. 177, 178).

The history and laboratory testing confirmed ingestion

of a cyclic antidepressant, a likely contributor to her coma and cause of her sinus tachycardia and widened QT interval. Had acidosis occurred, a more aggressive approach to alkalinization would be warranted (see Chap. 173). Without acidosis, seizures, or more severe cardiac arrhythmias, care is supportive. The component of cyclic antidepressant overdose in this case was a likely explanation for her somewhat delayed toxicity and the need for prolonged monitoring. Finally, as the patient was stabilized and supportive therapy could be gradually withdrawn, psychiatric liaison was established to provide ongoing counseling and an appropriate discharge plan with follow-up.

References

1. Jones DV, Work CE: Volume of a swallow. Am J Dis Child 102:173, 1961.
2. Tenenbein M: WBI as a gastrointestinal decontamination procedure after acute poisoning. Med Toxicol 3:77, 1988.
3. Tenenbein M: WBI in iron poisoning. J Pediatr 1:142, 1987.
4. Flanagan RJ, Meredith TJ, Ruprah M, Onyon LJ, Liddle A: Alkaline diuresis for acute poisoning with chlorophenoxy herbicides and ioxynil. Lancet 1:454, 1990.
5. Taitelman U, Kostucki W, Yannai S: Efficiency of extracorporeal complexation with cysteine in methylmercury poisoning. Vet Human Toxicol Suppl:168, 1982.
6. Luzzato L: Inherited haemolytic states: Glucose-6-phosphate dehydrogenase deficiency. Clin Haematol 4:83, 1975.
7. Piomelli S: Chemical toxicity of red cells. Environ Health Perspectiv 39:65, 1981.
8. WHO Scientific Group: Standardization of procedures for the study of G6PD. WHO Tech Rep Ser 366: Geneva, 1967.

Chapter 169

PHARMACOKINETICS AND IATROGENIC DRUG TOXICITY IN THE INTENSIVE CARE UNIT

T.E. ALBERTSON
G.E. FOULKE
S. THARRATT
R. ALLEN

KEY POINTS

- *Rational therapeutic dosing is determined by being familiar with the basic concepts of pharmacokinetics.*
- *Frequently reviewed and accurately maintained medication flow sheets with scheduled stop orders and appropriate serum drug level monitoring can reduce adverse drug actions and untoward drug-to-drug interactions.*
- *Drug interactions can occur at any of the stages of drug absorption, action, distribution, biotransformation, or elimination.*
- *Computerized programs of drug interactions and the careful review of the medication list by the health care team can reduce adverse drug interactions.*
- *Adverse drug actions or complications can affect every organ system.*
- *The intensive care unit (ICU) clinician must always consider drug-induced causes of new onset organ system compromise.*
- *Differentiating between a drug-induced complication, a new medical problem, and an extension of a current disease process can be difficult.*

The critical care unit is a challenging and complicated arena for the practice of rational drug therapy. Adverse drug reactions and drug interactions contribute significantly to morbidity and mortality in the critically ill patient. Adverse drug effects represent one of the largest sources of iatrogenic complications occurring in hospitalized patients. The estimated incidence is between 20 and 40 percent in patients receiving more than 10 pharmaceutical agents.[1–4] The median number of concomitant drugs administered to hospitalized medical service patients has been estimated to be between 6 and 13 with many patients receiving 20 or more drugs.[1,4,5] A basic working understanding of pharmacokinetics as well as a knowledge of important drug interactions and adverse actions is useful to the critical care clinician.

Pharmacokinetics

A detailed discussion of pharmacokinetics is beyond the scope of this chapter. However, a brief review of some of the most important concepts, assumptions, and formulas involved is provided for use by the practicing intensivist. The reader is referred to several textbooks for a more complete review and discussion of this important aspect of clinical pharmacology.[3,5–8]

The critical care physician must be aware of a large number of factors which may influence the absorption, distribution, and elimination of drugs. The bioavailability (F) of a compound is the fraction of a presented dose which eventually becomes systemically absorbed. In the gastrointestinal tract absorption is affected by solubility, the presence of material that can chelate or complex with the compound, and the relative concentrations of the compound in the gastrointestinal tract versus other body fluids. In addition, critically ill patients add other important variables to bioavailability. Reductions in blood flow to the gastrointestinal tract and alterations in intestinal hydrogen ion concentrations (with change of a compound's ionization) can limit the rate of drug absorption. Altered motility ranging from delayed gastric emptying to the absence of peristalsis can significantly alter delivery of drug to sites of absorption. The intravenous route is therefore preferred in the critically ill patient, but this does not guarantee complete bioavailability. Drugs can precipitate in the intravenous tubing and bags (from contact with other compounds or electrolytes), chemically degrade before injection (e.g., secondary to light or chemical reactions), or precipitate in the vein itself.

The desired effect of a drug, be it killing bacteria or altering arterial blood pressure, is usually dependent on delivery of a critical threshold amount of compound. A graduated effect may occur with increasing drug concentration. Limiting toxicity usually results from excessive stimulation of the same target organ or receptor or by reaching the critical threshold for a different organ or receptor with resultant toxic response. Drug elimination is simultaneous with absorption, distribution, and drug effect. It occurs from metabolism (i.e., the liver and, to a small degree, the kidney), excretion (i.e., primarily the kidney with a small contribution from the lungs, skin, and gastrointestinal tract), and extracorporeal devices (e.g., dialysis and hemoperfusion).

The majority of clinically important therapeutic agents follow first-order or linear elimination kinetics. This implies that a constant percentage of drug is removed per unit of time. Thus, as the concentration or rate of drug presented to the eliminating organ increases, the absolute amount of drug that is removed increases. The time it takes to reduce the serum concentration by half (i.e., serum half-life or $T_{1/2}$) remains constant no matter what the initial concentration of drug presented to the organ(s) of drug elimination. This is in contrast to zero-order or saturable elimination kinetics where the absolute amount of drug eliminated tends to be fixed per unit time. The percentage of eliminated drug then varies with the concentration of drug presented to the organ(s) of elimination. Thus, the serum $T_{1/2}$ for saturable or

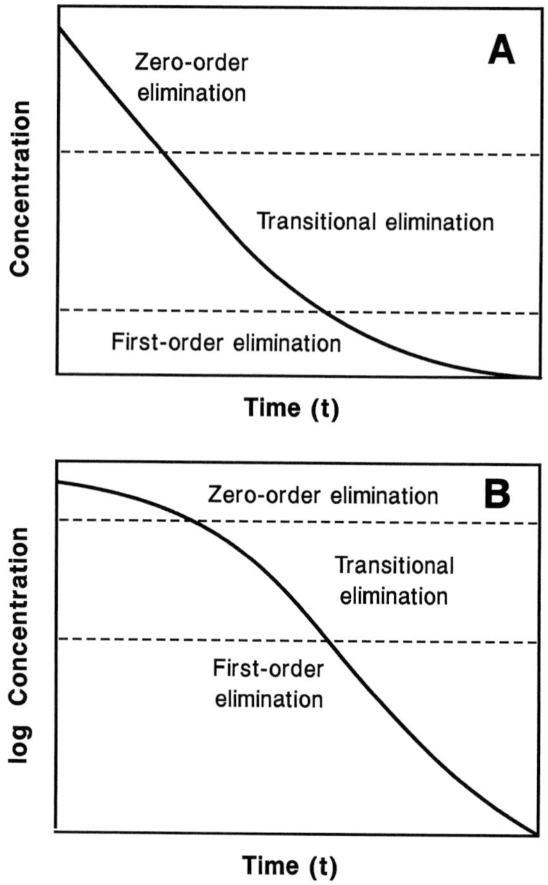

FIGURE 169-1 Linear plot (A) and semilogarithmic plot (B) of the plasma concentration versus time course of a drug displaying zero-order elimination kinetics at high levels that transitions into first-order elimination kinetics. The elimination drug half-life ($T_{1/2}$) is determined from the linear plot.

zero-order elimination kinetics increases with increasing concentrations of the drug. A given drug may show both zero- and first-order elimination functions. If the first-order elimination process becomes saturated at very high drug concentrations, a zero-order elimination process will predominate, followed by a transitional or hybrid phase of elimination, and, finally, first-order kinetics (Fig. 169-1).

Total body clearance (Cl) of a drug is the theoretical amount of blood, serum, or plasma from which all drug is cleared per unit time. When a drug level is constant or has reached equilibrium, the rate of elimination and the rate of administration (R_A) are equal:

$$R_A = \frac{\text{absorbed drug}}{\text{dose interval}} = \frac{F \times \text{dose}}{T}$$

where T = dosing interval and F = fraction available or bioavailability.

$$\text{Cl} = \frac{R_A}{\text{steady-state serum concentration}} = \frac{F \times \text{dose}}{C_{ss} \times T}$$

where C_{ss} = concentration at steady-state. The apparent volume of distribution (V_d) is a proportionality constant that has no direct physiologic meaning and does not refer to a real volume. It does, however, reflect the degree to which the drug concentrates in the blood or serum compartment versus other body compartments. Drugs that are highly lipid soluble, for example, will have large volumes of distribution (e.g., partitioned in brain or fat) with most of the drug remaining outside of the compartment sampled (blood). Highly water soluble compounds remain in the extracellular fluid compartment that includes the blood and thus have small volumes of distribution. Significant alterations in the apparent volume of distribution can occur with fluid status changes, starvation, obesity, and other metabolic conditions. The volume of distribution is related to the initial or time zero drug concentration (C_0) (see Fig. 169-2).

$$\text{Volume of distribution} = V_d = \frac{\text{IV dose}}{C_0} = \frac{F \times \text{dose}}{C_0}$$

Thus if the volume of distribution (V_d) of a drug that follows first-order elimination kinetics is known, a loading dose can be determined for a given desired serum concentration:

$$\text{Loading dose} = \frac{V_d \times \text{desired serum concentration}}{F} = V_d \times C_d, \quad \text{if IV dose } (F = 1.0)$$

where C_d = desired concentration.

Further, if the patient has a known present drug concentration (C_p) and a higher new concentration is desired (C_d), the same formula is used to determine the "reloading" dose:

$$\text{Dose} = \frac{V_d \times (C_d - C_p)}{F} = V_d \times (C_d - C_p) \quad \text{if IV dose } (F = 1.0)$$

Meticulous care in confirming consistent units of measure must be followed when using these formulas. For example, the literature will often report the volume of distribution of a compound in liters per kilogram (usually lean body weight). It is necessary then to multiply the known V_d by the patient's weight to determine the individual V_d. Similarly, drug concentration units must be consistent throughout the formula.

Additional useful pharmacokinetic relationships include formulas that relate the elimination rate constant (K_e) to the $T_{1/2}$. The K_e is determined by calculating the slope of the terminal (beta) phase of a first-order elimination plot of the

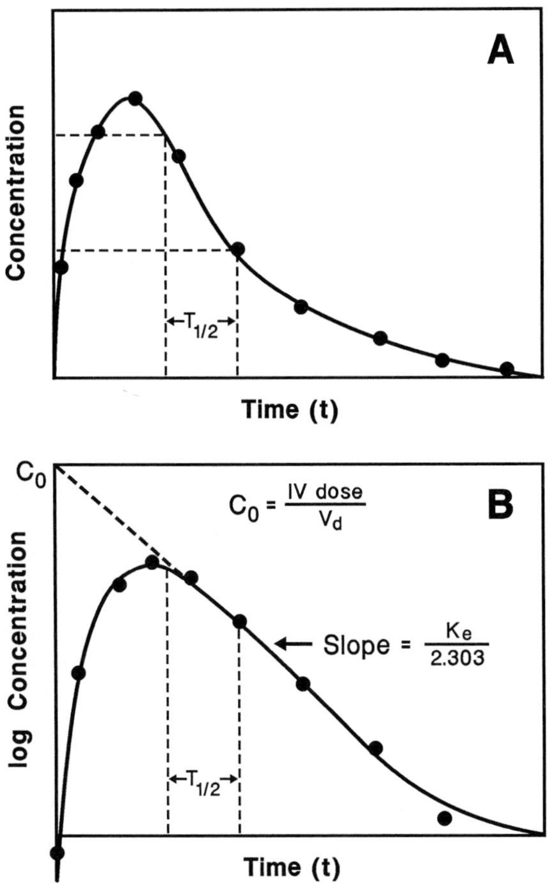

FIGURE 169-2 Linear plot (A) and semilogarithmic plot (B) of the plasma concentrations versus time course of a drug. The C_0 represents the calculated time zero concentration used to determine the volume of distribution (V_d) of a drug in an individual. The elimination constant (K_e) is a function of the slope of the semilogarithmic elimination curve.

logarithm of the concentration of drug versus time (Fig. 169-2).

$$T_{1/2} = \frac{0.693}{K_e}$$

$$K_e = \frac{0.693}{T_{1/2}}$$

Further, K_e relates to total body clearance Cl by the formula:

$$\mathrm{Cl} = K_e V_d$$

but as noted above, $K_e = 0.693/T_{1/2}$, so,

$$\mathrm{Cl} = \frac{0.693 V_d}{T_{1/2}}$$

Thus, if the half-life of a drug is short, the total elimination of the drug will tend to be fast. It should be emphasized that K_e and $T_{1/2}$ depend on clearance and V_d, not vice versa. Total body clearance and V_d are measured, whereas K_e and $T_{1/2}$ are derived variables.

A drug will accumulate if dosage and dosing intervals are held constant and the total drug load exceeds total body elimination per given time. A steady-state concentration C_{ss} is achieved when there is equilibrium between the amount of drug administered and amount eliminated by total body clearance. It generally takes four to five half-life intervals to reach steady-state concentrations when repeated doses are given. An initial accurate loading dose will significantly reduce the time needed to reach steady-state concentrations (Fig. 169-3). Clearance determinations may be used to calculate maintenance doses:

$$\text{Maintenance dose} = \frac{\mathrm{Cl} \times C_{ss} \times T}{F}$$

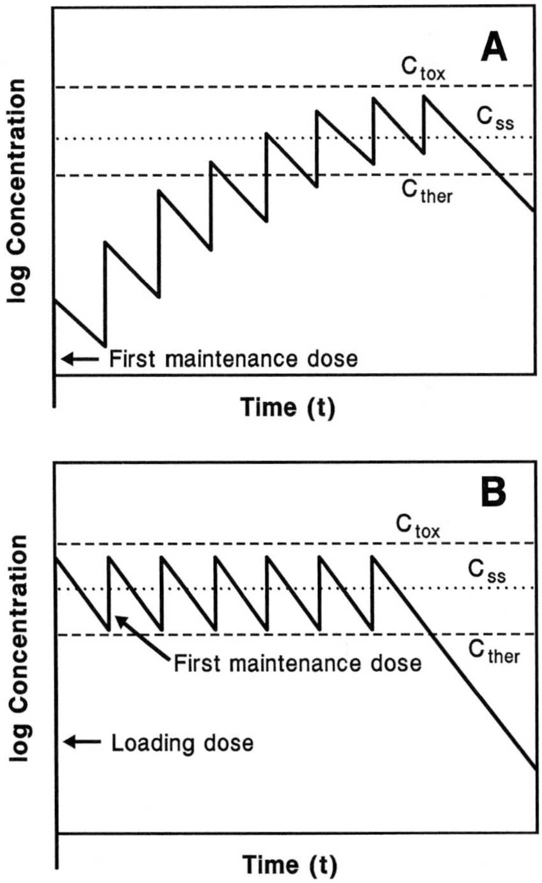

FIGURE 169-3 The semilogarithmic plot of the plasma concentrations versus time course of a drug with (A) no loading dose and (B) a loading dose followed by several maintenance doses. Without a loading dose approximately five to six dosing intervals are needed to reach steady-state plasma concentrations (C_{ss}). The dosing regimen is based on the drug elimination ($T_{1/2}$) and drug absorption characteristics, distribution rate constants, minimal therapeutic plasma concentrations (C_{ther}), and minimal toxic-plasma concentrations (C_{tox}).

and

$$\text{IV maintenance dose} = \frac{0.693 V_d C_{ss} T}{T_{1/2}}$$

or

$$\frac{\text{IV maintenance dose}}{T} = \frac{0.693 V_d C_{ss}}{T_{1/2}}$$

Thus the $T_{1/2}$ influences the interval at which a drug should be administered (T). This dosing interval is usually equal to or shorter than the $T_{1/2}$ for intermittent dosing. With constant infusion dosing, the interval approaches 0 (essentially $T = 1$ per minute) and the serum concentration fluctuations are minimal.

The window of dosing error for a given compound is governed by the relative margin of safety between toxic serum concentrations and therapeutic threshold concentrations (Fig. 169-3). Constant infusion dosing offers the best way to minimize serum level fluctuations. Another measure of this margin of dosing safety is the therapeutic index (TI):

$$\text{TI} = \frac{\text{TD}_{50}}{\text{ED}_{50}}$$

where TD_{50} is the drug dose that is toxic to 50 percent of the exposed population and ED_{50} is the drug dose that is effective in 50 percent of the exposed population. Obviously the known TI of a compound gives the clinician an approximation of the relative degree of safety of a compound. For the critically ill patient, monitoring of serum concentrations of compounds with narrow margins of safety should be utilized whenever possible. Although both peak and trough levels of a compound may be associated with toxicity, trough levels tend to be most useful especially in following aminoglycoside-induced nephrotoxicity.[3,5]

Drug Interactions and Adverse Actions

INDIVIDUAL VARIABILITY

The variability in clinical response to pharmaceutical agents is multifactorial. Pharmacogenetics, age, fluid status, disease states, nutritional condition, sex, body habitus, previous drug exposures, hemodynamic status, and concomitant drug administration all can affect toxicity and efficacy.

Genetic differences in drug biotransformation may be significant. Drug oxidation is an important biotransformation process and appears to be controlled by a polygenic inheritance pattern. In twin and family studies, more of the variability in biotransformation of drugs such as oral anticoagulants, tricyclic antidepressants, phenytoin, and phenylbutazone can be attributed to genetic rather than exogenous factors.[9] Hepatic acetylation of drugs such as hydralazine, procainamide, and isoniazid varies between individuals and appears to be genetically controlled. Patients with a low activity of hepatic *N*-acetyl transferase metabolize isoniazid with a half-life of approximately 100 h. Genetically "rapid" acetylators have a half-life of approximately 40 h. Slow acetylators are predisposed to hydralazine-induced lupus erythematosus and isoniazid-induced neuropathies. Isoniazid-induced hepatic injury is more common in the rapid acetylators. Approximately one-half of white and black Americans have the homozygous recessive trait of slow acetylation, whereas rapid acetylators predominate among Japanese and Eskimos.

Plasma cholinesterase enzymes represent another important genetic biotransformation variance. This enzyme and its variants appear to be controlled by at least four allelic autosomal genes. In the United States 1 in 2500 individuals is homozygous for a protein, with consequently diminished hydrolysis of succinylcholine in the plasma. Marked prolongation of succinylcholine-induced paralysis may result.

The geriatric population is at increased risk for adverse drug actions in the ICU setting.[4,10–12] Older individuals have a greater incidence of multiple illnesses and, therefore, receive more medications. Baseline reductions in kidney, liver, cardiac, and other organ function occur with age. These important factors, along with changes in body fat and a 10 to 15 percent reduction in total body water, can result in significant pharmacokinetic alterations in the elderly. Increased sensitivity to central nervous system active drugs may be related to alterations in specific brain receptors or overall pharmacokinetic changes in the elderly. Mental status changes in the elderly ICU patient may be related to a number of nondrug causes,[13] but the presence of drugs such as lidocaine, an H_2-receptor blocker, a benzodiazepine agonist, or a phenothiazine agent on the patient's medication list will often explain an otherwise puzzling change in mental status.

At the other end of the age spectrum, the pharmacokinetics of pediatric patients proves to be a challenging and poorly studied problem. Neonatal alterations in absorption, plasma protein binding, and metabolism require special vigilance and expertise in dosing therapeutic agents. Any drug dosing formula in pediatric patients offers only an estimate. Some clinicians have advocated (with few prospective studies) that doses in this age group may be better predicted by the surface area of the body rather than by unit of weight.

An important variable in determining individual patient pharmacokinetics is concomitant disease. Table 169-1 offers examples of disease states which alter the clearance of various compounds. Generally, these alterations increase the possibility of drug-induced toxicity. However, biotransformation may also lead to formation of an active drug (e.g., prodrug compound) or more active metabolite. Simply placing a patient on mechanical ventilation can significantly reduce lidocaine clearance and increase half-life without altering the V_d.[14] Alterations in body habitus, including cachectic and morbid obesity states can change the regional binding characteristics of various drugs. When dosing markedly obese or volume overloaded patients, conservative dose estimates should initially be made utilizing the ideal or lean body weight rather than the measured weight. Frequent adjustments in dosing schedules will often re-

TABLE 169-1 Disease States that Affect Drug Levels

Disease State	Mechanism	Drug Level	Example
Heart failure	Decreased metabolic clearance	Increased	Lidocaine Theophylline Cimetidine Procainamide Ranitidine
	Decreased renal clearance	Increased	Digoxin
	Decreased oral absorption	Decreased	Furosemide
Liver failure	Decreased metabolic clearance	Increased	Lidocaine Theophylline Diazepam Ethanol Cyclosporine Pentazocine
	Increased bioavailability after oral dose (decreased "first pass" effect)	Increased	Propranolol
Renal failure	Decreased clearance	Increased	Aminoglycosides Cephalosporins Cimetidine Digoxin Penicillin Lorazepam Ranitidine

SOURCE: Modified from reference 13.

quire utilization of the principles of pharmacokinetics previously outlined after appropriate measurement of drug blood levels.

Drug Interactions

Adverse drug interactions contribute significantly to additional morbidity and mortality in critically ill patients. Minimizing the incidence and severity of this problem requires a high index of suspicion, familiarity with the major drug interactions of frequently prescribed agents, and scrupulous record-keeping to avoid preventable occurrences. Meticulous patient record-keeping and open communication between physicians, pharmacists, and nurses are particularly important in the ICU to help reduce this problem. Frequent review of accurately maintained and easily accessible medication flow sheets by each member of the therapeutic health care team will prevent superfluous drugs as well as known drug incompatibilities and interactions. Automatic stop orders for certain high-risk or important agents forces the clinician to review the appropriateness of and need for continuing a medication. Regular monitoring of serum drug levels or physiologic parameters [e.g., clotting times for patients on warfarin (Coumadin), heart rate of patients receiving propranolol] can further reduce the incidence of adverse drug interactions. Determination and use of pharmacokinetic variables, often with the help of a clinical pharmacologist, clinical pharmacist, or pharmacokinetic consultative service will add clarity to the large cast of potential drug interactions in an individual patient. Several reference books and computerized programs catalog the multitude of known drug interactions.[8,15–20] More recently, hospital pharmacies have been able to acquire drug interaction programs which run simultaneously with programs designed to store, order, bill, and record patients' medications while they are in the hospital. These programs have the ability to highlight known drug interactions in the patient's medication list for the pharmacist, nurse, or physician.

Table 169-2 offers a summary of major processes and mechanisms of potential drug interactions in the ICU. Avoidance of drugs with known interactions is not always possible nor in the patient's best interest. Knowledge about drug interactions will allow the clinician to alter dosing or switch medications depending on the relative risks and costs.[21,22] It should be noted that most drug interaction studies report on small numbers of non-critically ill patients or volunteers. Knowledge of potential drug interactions should prompt a higher level of vigilance, but it does not necessarily mean that interacting drugs have to be abandoned.

ABSORPTION

Interaction between drugs at the level of absorption is common. Table 169-3 offers various possible mechanisms. Even antacids and enteral feeding mixtures must be considered to potentially influence drug absorption. Recently phenytoin absorption was found to vary with enteral feeding type. Protein hydrolysate-based feedings allowed less phenytoin absorption than a similar amount of protein in a meat-based product, and both allowed less absorption than

TABLE 169-2 Frequent Types of Drug Interactions in an Intensive Care Unit

General Process	Specific Process	Mechanism	Example A/B (Drug A Affects Drug B)
Absorption	Prevention of absorption	Formation of complexes/chelation	Antacids/digoxin Antacids/warfarin Antacids/phenothiazines Antacids/tetracycline Antacids/propranolol Enteral feeding/phenytoin
	Reduced absorption	Alteration of gastric pH and ratio of drug ionization or dissociation	Antacids/cimetidine Antacids/ranitidine H_2 blockers/ketoconazole
	Decreased peak absorption	Decreased gastric motility	Opiates/acetaminophen
	Increased peak absorption	Increasing gastric motility	Metoclopramide/acetaminophen
Distribution	Plasma binding alteration	Displacement at plasma binding sites of one drug by another, leading to increased free or unbound drug levels	Lidocaine/succinylcholine Phenylbutazone/warfarin Phenytoin/warfarin Phenytoin/salicylates Phenytoin/valproic acid Salicylates/valproic acid Valproic acid/diazepam
	Alteration of distribution	Displacement of tissue binding and reduction of volume of distribution	Quinine/digoxin Spironolactone/digoxin
Metabolism	Increased metabolism	Induction of metabolic enzymes	Barbiturates/warfarin Barbiturates/digitoxin Barbiturates/phenytoin Barbiturates/cortisol Barbiturates/theophylline Chronic ethanol/pentobarbital Chronic ethanol/phenytoin Carbamazepine/warfarin Carbamazepine/phenytoin Phenytoin/quinidine Rifampin/mexiletine
	Decreased metabolism	Inhibition of xanthine oxidases	Allopurinol/azathioprine Chloramphenicol/phenobarbital Chloramphenicol/tolbutamide
	Decreased metabolism	Enzyme inhibition or reduction of hepatic blood flow	Cimetidine/theophylline Cimetidine/warfarin Cimetidine/diazepam Ciprofloxacin/theophylline Diltiazem/cyclosporine Erythromycin/carbamazepine Erythromycin/theophylline Acute ethanol/pentobarbital Acute ethanol/phenytoin Metoprolol/lidocaine Metronidazole/warfarin Nicardipine/cyclosporine Propranolol/lidocaine Propranolol/theophylline Propoxyphene/doxepin Propoxyphene/phenytoin Ranitidine/theophylline Sulthiame/carbamazepine Thiabendazole/theophylline Thioridazine/phenytoin Verapamil/cyclosporin
Excretion	Increased excretion; prevention of reabsorption	Acidification of urine, ion trapping of organic bases	Ammonium chloride/amantadine Ammonium chloride/amiloride Ammonium chloride/cimetidine

TABLE 169-2 Frequent Types of Drug Interactions in an Intensive Care Unit (Continued)

General Process	Specific Process	Mechanism	Example A/B (Drug A Affects Drug B)
		Alkalinization of urine, ion trapping of organic acids	Bicarbonate/salicylates Bicarbonate/captopril Bicarbonate/cephalosporins Bicarbonate/furosemide Bicarbonate/heparin
	Decreased excretion	Decreased glomerular filtration rate	Furosemide/gentamicin
		Renal clearance mechanisms	Thiazides/lithium Probenecid/methotrexate Probenecid/penicillin Salicylates/methotrexate Cimetidine/procainamide Ranitidine/procainamide Quinidine/digoxin Amiodarone/digoxin
Pharmacodynamics	Drug synergism	Cellular potentiation of action (nonspecific)	Acute ethanol/barbiturates Aminoglycosides/pancuronium Barbiturates/benzodiazepines Dextran/heparin Verapamil/propranolol
		Agonism of the same receptor	Morphine/meperidine Diazepam/clonazepam
	Drug antagonism	Cellular antagonism of action (nonspecific)	Vitamin K/warfarin Thiazide diuretics/tolbutamide Cortisol/tolbutamide
		Antagonism of receptor and synapse	Flumazenil/benzodiazepines Naloxone/morphine Physostigmine/atropine Propranolol/norepinephrine
	Physicochemical complexing	Neutralization or chelation	Deferoxamine/iron Protamine/heparin

SOURCE: Modified from reference 13.

control (no enteral feeding).[23] Drug incompatibilities in intravenous parenteral nutrition fluids can also present drug interaction or absorption problems. Precipitation or chemical alteration may occur prior to parenteral dosing. Knowledge of in vitro drug incompatibilities is therefore essential.

Intramuscular and subcutaneous absorption in the critically ill patient may be decreased and erratic because of alterations in muscle and skin blood flow. For these reasons, as well as the potential for necrosis and infection with repeated injections, these routes of administration are not widely used in the ICU except for certain drugs (e.g., heparin).

DISTRIBUTION

Drug distribution may be altered when another agent displaces the drug from tissue or plasma binding sites. The potential for toxicity is based on the therapeutic index and is related to free drug levels of displaced drug. Important variables in determining the potential for displacement include the relative amount of the drug in the plasma or tissue, the relative affinity of the drugs for the various protein receptors, and the V_d of the displaced drug. The greater the concentration and receptor affinity of the displacing drug, the greater the displacement (Table 169-4). The smaller the V_d of the displaced drug, the more free drug is available in the plasma for pharmacologic effect. Finally, the clearance and elimination rate and elimination kinetics will determine if toxicity will result from drug displacement. Because first-order elimination is based to a great extent on the amount of free plasma drug available for biotransformation, displacement interactions are usually transient. They occur during the time when displaced free drug levels are increased to maximum and before first-order elimination has resulted in a new steady-state concentration. This new steady-state free drug concentration occurs with a reduced total drug level (total drug = free drug + bound drug) because the reduction in bound drug exceeds the slight increase in free drug. Since most therapeutic blood monitoring utilizes total drug level measurements, the clinician may be unaware of the new increased steady-state free drug level (free serum drug levels are slowly becoming clinically available using dialysis techniques).

TABLE 169-3 Potential Mechanisms of Drug Absorption Interaction in the ICU

1. Changes in physical properties of gastrointestinal tract contents
   - Volume, composition, viscosity, and osmotic pressure
2. Physicochemical interactions in the gastrointestinal tract
   - Formation of complexes or chelation
3. Changes in mucosal permeability and active transport
   - For example, neomycin and colchicine have toxic effects on intestinal mucosa and cause malabsorption syndrome and reduction in digoxin, iron, folate, and vitamin B_{12} absorption
4. Changes in gastrointestinal tract blood flow
   - Drugs can modify splanchnic blood flow
5. Changes in first-pass metabolism
   - Presystemic drug metabolism by liver, intestinal mucosa, and gut bacteria
   - Changes in fraction reaching the systemic circulation
6. Changes in pH of gastrointestinal tract fluids
   - Usually affect rate, not extent of absorption
7. Changes in gastric emptying
   - Drugs poorly absorbed from stomach; therefore, gastric emptying may be rate limitor
   - Usually affect rate, not total extent of absorption
8. Changes in gastrointestinal tract motility
   - May affect both rate and extent of absorption
   - Increasing motility generally causes increased rate of absorption
   - Increasing motility with special slow-release formulations may decrease rate and extent of absorption
   - Slowing motility generally causes decreased rate of absorption
   - Slowing motility with special slow-release formulations may increase rate and extent of absorption

SOURCE: Modified from reference 24.

TABLE 169-4 Examples of Drugs with High Plasma- and Protein-Binding Affinities

1. Digitoxin
2. Dihydroxycoumarin (Dicumarol)
3. Warfarin
4. Diazoxide
5. Phenytoin
6. Clofibrate
7. Valproic acid
8. Hydralazine
9. Quinidine
10. Sulfonamides
11. Tolbutamide
12. Salicylates
13. Nonsteroidal anti-inflammatory agents

TABLE 169-5 Examples of Agents in the ICU with Active Metabolites

Agent	Active Metabolite
Adriamycin (doxorubicin)	Adriamycinol
Allopurinol	Alloxantin, oxipurinol
Amitriptyline	Nortriptyline
Amphetamine	Parahydroxyamphetamine
Carbamazepine	Carbamazepine 10–11 epoxide
Cephalothin	Desacetylcephalothin
Chlordiazepoxide	*N*-desmethylchlordiazepoxide, *N*-desmethyldiazepam, demoxepam, oxazepam
Chlorpromazine	7-Hydroxychlorpromazine
Clonazepam	7-Aminoclonazepam
Codeine	Morphine, norcodeine
Cortisone	Cortisol
Diazepam	*N*-Desmethyldiazepam, oxazepam, *N*-methyloxazepam
Digitoxin	Digoxin
Disopyramide	*N*-Desisopropyldisopyramide
Doxepin	Desmethyldoxepin
Flurazepam	*N*-Desalkylflurazepam, flurazepam *N*-1-ethanol
Imipramine	Desipramine
Lidocaine	Monoethylglycinexylidide, glycinexylidide
Meperidine	Normeperidine
Nitroprusside	Thiocyanate
Prednisone	Prednisolone
Primidone	Phenobarbitol, phenylethylmalonamide
Procainamide	*N*-Acetylprocainamide
Propranolol	4-Hydroxy propranolol
Quinidine	2-Hydroxy quinidine
Spironolactone	Canrenone, canrenoate
Thioridazine	Mesoridazine

SOURCE: Adapted from reference 6.

METABOLISM

Metabolism or biotransformation of compounds generally results in progressively more polar, water-soluble products with each step. Many metabolites are pharmacologically active (Table 169-5). Initial biotransformations tend to be nonsynthetic reactions including oxidation, reduction, and hydrolysis. Alcohol and aldehyde dehydrogenase (nonmicrosomal enzymes found in the liver), monoamine and diamine oxidase, and a large number of esterases and amidases are important in initial biotransformation. Quantitatively, the cytochrome P-450 microsomal enzyme system is most important for initial metabolic conversion. It contains monooxygenases or mixed-function oxidases located in the cellular smooth endoplasmic reticulum of many tissues, although liver enzymes are responsible for most drug metabolism. These enzymes undergo induction (the ability of a substrate to enhance the activity of an enzyme). Common inducers of the cytochrome P-450 enzyme system include androgens, barbiturates, carbamazepine, chloral hydrate, chlordiazepoxide, corticosteroids, imipramine, phenytoin, and tolbutamide. Enzyme induction may result in increased rate of elimination of other drugs. The process of enzyme induction is relatively slow, taking days to weeks to manifest. Cigarette smoking has been shown to be an excellent inducer of the isoenzymes responsible for theophylline metabolism. Similarly, competition of two drugs for the same metabolizing enzyme system could result in a decrease in elimination of the first drug if the second drug has a higher affinity for the saturable enzyme sites.

Later phases of drug biotransformation include energy requiring synthetic reactions resulting usually in conjugation. Conjugation with glucuronic acid is the most prominent pathway to inactivate a drug. Conjugations with glutathione, glycine, or sulfate, as well as acetylation and methylation, are additional important late-phase biotransformations. Another mechanism for decreased drug clearance is reduction of blood flow to the biotransforming organ. The β-adrenergic blocking agents propranolol, nadolol, and metoprolol have been demonstrated to decrease lidocaine clearance by up to 20 to 50 percent via alterations in liver blood flow. Improvement of blood flow to an organ important in drug biotransformation (improvement of a disease state) can increase elimination rate. Drug interactions during biotransformation represent one of the largest and most important categories of adverse drug interactions.

EXCRETION

Drug or metabolite excretion occurs primarily in the kidney. Compounds in the blood can be passively filtered, actively secreted, and/or reabsorbed (active and passive). All three aspects of renal handling of compounds can potentially lead to drug interactions.

Drugs which result in intravascular volume depletion can reduce renal perfusion and therefore reduce glomerular filtration rate (GFR). This in turn can limit passive renal filtration of a second agent and, thus, its renal clearance or elimination. Furosemide, a potent diuretic, can by this mechanism reduce the elimination of other drugs such as gentamicin.

Active secretion of drugs in the proximal tubule (and to an extent in the distal tubule) may be by specific mechanisms (one for organic acids and one for organic bases). Competition for the organic acid transport system by several endogenous and exogenous organic acid compounds (e.g., penicillins, nonsteroidal anti-inflammatory agents, methotrexate, sulfonamides, and cephalosporins) can lead to important drug interactions. An example of this is the drug interaction of quinidine and digoxin.[25] This is a complicated drug interaction which can result in a doubling of serum digoxin concentrations with the addition of quinidine. It occurs as a result of both alteration in muscle and tissue binding of digoxin (altering the V_d of digoxin) and, more importantly, by a competition between quinidine and digoxin for renal excretion. This competition results in a reduction in digoxin elimination.

The reabsorption of secreted or filtered compounds occurs in the distal tubule or collecting duct. It is a function of drug concentration, urinary flow, and the pH of the urine. Alterations in distal urine pH can cause ion trapping of certain weak acids or bases and reduce passive reabsorption (passive movement of ionized compounds across membranes is poor).

Lithium is reabsorbed with sodium in the kidney by the same renal mechanism. In cases of volume depletion from chronic diuretic use, renal increases in sodium and lithium reabsorption occur leading to potentially toxic lithium levels.

PHARMACODYNAMICS

Drug interactions that occur at a cellular, physiologic, or physicochemical level in vivo fall under the category of pharmacodynamic interactions. These interactions can be at the same cellular receptor site (e.g., the benzodiazepine receptor antagonist flumazenil reversing or blocking the benzodiazepine receptor agonist diazepam). Additionally, drugs can antagonize or augment the action of other drugs by nonspecific physiologic or cellular mechanisms that do not involve single receptor sites. For example, an oral hypoglycemic drug such as tolbutamide may have its glucose lowering effect reversed by simultaneous exposure to a drug that causes hyperglycemia such as the thiazide diuretics. In vivo chelation of a drug by another drug is a type of pharmacodynamic interaction which usually neutralizes the action of both drugs. An example of therapeutic importance for the ICU would be the neutralization of aminoglycoside antibiotics by the semisynthetic penicillins. Finally, a drug can alter the environment of the body. One drug can alter serum electrolytes and allow toxicity of a second drug to be expressed. An example of this type of drug interaction includes diuretics or amphotericin B causing a depletion of total body potassium which, in turn, makes digoxin toxicity more probable.

AVOIDING DRUG INTERACTIONS

Significant effort should be made to prevent toxicity from drug interactions. Periodic evaluation of symptoms, signs, and laboratory measures is necessary. Scrupulous medication records with frequent review by the health care team to identify known potential drug interactions helps prevent drug interaction toxicity. Attempts must be made to individualize drug therapy using the least number and most appropriate medications. Frequent reevaluation of medication dosing must reflect the rapidly changing patient condition. Finally, the clinician must maintain a high degree of suspicion in order to detect and minimize toxic drug interactions in the ICU.

Adverse Drug Reaction

Every organ system can potentially be adversely affected by drug exposures. Drug-induced illness represents a major cause of iatrogenic complications in the hospitalized patient.[4,11] Certain patient populations are uniquely vulnerable to adverse drug effects. The elderly patient has a two to three times higher incidence of adverse drug reactions than young adults.[26] Cognitive impairment in the elderly is due to an adverse drug reaction 13.7 percent of the time when six or more drugs are simultaneously prescribed.[10] Even the inert ingredients of pharmaceutical formulations have been associated with significant adverse effects.[27,28] In view of this situation, the ICU clinician is often faced with

TABLE 169-6 Types and Mechanisms of Drug Fever

Type of Drug Fever	Mechanism	Drug
Administration related	Local phlebitis	Vancomycin
		Diazepam
	Unknown	Amphotericin B
		Bleomycin
	Sterile abscess	Paraldehyde
		Pentazocine
Pharmacologic actions		
Herxheimer's reaction	Endotoxin release	Antibiotics
Cancer chemotherapy	Tumor necrosis	Antineoplastics
Altered thermo-regulation	Direct CNS effect	Cocaine
		Phenothiazines
	Decreased heat loss	Atropine
	Increased metabolism	Thyroxine
Idiosyncratic		
Malignant hyperthermia	Unknown	Anesthetics
Glucose-6-phosphate dehydrogenase deficiency	Hemolysis	Quinidine
		Sulfonamides
Hypersensitivity	Immunologic	Penicillins
		Sulfonamides
		Streptomycin
		Vancomycin
		Tetracyclines
		Isoniazid
		Phenytoin
		Barbiturates
		Iodides
		Methyldopa
		Hydralazine
		Procainamide
		Quinidine
		Ibuprofen

SOURCE: Adapted from reference 13.

the question of whether a patient's poor clinical course is related to the underlying medical condition, a new undiscovered medical problem, or an adverse drug response. The clinician may simultaneously remove or change multiple drugs that a patient may be receiving. When an adverse effect disappears after removal of a drug from a patient, then a probable relationship appears to exist. Improvement in medical condition or another previously removed drug with a long $T_{1/2}$ may in fact account for this improvement. Rechallenging the patient with the suspicious agent would confirm that a particular drug is or is not the causative agent. Most ICU clinicians are unwilling to reexpose the patient to an adverse experience; therefore, it is difficult to prove a drug relationship for an individual patient. Retrospective adverse drug reaction studies are limited in number and generally only categorize potential drug reactions as probable, definite, or possible.

DRUG FEVER

The ICU patient frequently develops fever without an obvious source. After a thorough physical examination and culturing to detect infectious causes, the clinician should consider drug-induced fevers. Fever can occur simultaneously with systemic and cutaneous features of an adverse drug reaction, but it is thought to be relatively rare as the primary or sole manifestation of a drug reaction.[29] Early diagnosis of drug fevers will limit morbidity and may reduce ICU mortality.

Table 169-6 outlines five pathophysiologic categories for drug-related fevers: **1.** drug administration, **2.** altered thermoregulation, **3.** pharmacologic actions of the drug, **4.** idiosyncratic or heritable patient conditions, and **5.** hypersensitivity reactions. Table 169-7 provides a summary of the causes of 148 new and previously reported drug-induced fevers.[30] Antibiotics, cardiovascular drugs, and central acting agents were the largest categories of drugs causing fever.

The hypersensitivity-type reaction in which the patient may develop a rash, urticaria, serum sickness, and fever is an important drug reaction. The actual incidence is unknown,[30] and the diagnosis is often made by exclusion. Neither the magnitude of the fever nor the pattern (e.g., continuous, remittent, intermittent, or hectic) is helpful in making the diagnosis. Elevated temperatures from hypersensitivity drug-induced fevers may appear from 7 to 10

TABLE 169-7 Agents Responsible for Drug-Induced Fevers

Drug Class	Agent	Drug Class, %	Agent, %
Cardiovascular agents		25.7	
	α-Methyldopa		10.8
	Quinidine		8.8
	Procainamide		4.0
	Hydralazine		0.7
	Nifedipine		0.7
	Oxprenolol		0.7
Antimicrobials		31.1	
	Penicillin G		6.1
	Ampicillin		1.4
	Methicillin		4.1
	Cloxacillin		1.4
	Cephalothin		4.7
	Cepharin		0.7
	Cefamandol		0.7
	Tetracycline		1.4
	Lincomycin		0.7
	Sulfonamide		1.4
	Sulfatrimethoprim		0.7
	Streptomycin		0.7
	Nitrofurantoin		1.4
	Vancomycin		0.7
	Colistin		0.7
	Isoniazid		3.4
	Para-aminosalicylic acid		0.7
	Mebendazole		0.7
Antineoplastics		8.1	
	Bleomycin		2.0
	Daunorubicin		0.7
	Procarbazine		0.7
	Cytarabine		0.7
	Streptozocin		1.4
	6-Mercaptopurine		0.7
	L-Asparaginase		0.7
	Chlorambucil		0.7
	Hydroxyurea		0.7
Central nervous system agents		20.2	
	Phenytoin		7.4
	Carbamazepine		2.0
	Chlorpromazine		0.7
	Nomifensine		1.4
	Haloperidol		0.7
	Triamterene		0.7
	Benztropine		0.7
	Thioridazine		1.4
	Trifluoperazine		0.7
	Amphetamine		1.4
	Lysergic acid		3.3
Anti-inflammatory agents		2.1	
	Ibuprofen		0.7
	Tolmetin		0.7
	Aspirin		0.7
Miscellaneous agents		12.8	
	Iodide		4.0
	Cimetidine		1.4
	Levamisole		0.7
	Metoclopramide		0.7
	Clofibrate		0.7
	Allopurinol		0.7
	Folate		0.7
	Prostaglandin E_2		1.4
	Ritodrine		0.7
	Interferon		1.4
	Propylthiouracil		0.7

SOURCE: Adapted from reference 30. Represents 148 agents.

days postexposure but can occur within hours if there has been prior exposure. Patients with hypersensitivity drug-induced fever have been noted to have fevers as high as 40°C and yet generally appear well.[29] This finding may be an important clue to the presence of a drug-related fever. Resolution of the fever would be expected upon withdrawal of the agent, but a rechallenge would be necessary to confirm that the fever was in fact drug-induced.

DRUG WITHDRAWAL REACTIONS

The classic sedative, depressant, or opiate withdrawal syndrome has been seen by most ICU clinicians and has recently been reviewed in detail.[31]

To manifest a classical withdrawal syndrome to a sedative, depressant, or opiate, both tolerance and dependence must have developed. Hypermetabolism and "sympathetic overdrive" appear early with sedative depressant withdrawal as the patient progresses to a syndrome characterized by fever, hypertension, mental confusion, seizures, and cardiac arrhythmias. The clinician is often faced with diagnostic confusion when these manifestations occur at the same time as another critical illness. Diagnosis is made under such circumstances by review of historical data, elimination of other causes, and response to treatment.

Therapeutic withdrawal or detoxification of a narcotic-, sedative-, or hypnotic-habituated patient is performed by first establishing the patient's daily need for a short-acting similar compound. A long-acting related compound (which allows a smooth daily withdrawal) is then substituted. This is rarely done in the ICU setting unless an iatrogenic component exists. For example, a long-term ventilator-dependent ICU patient may become addicted to opiates. As the pulmonary function improves and ventilator dependence is reduced, it would be reasonable to begin a controlled slow withdrawal of opiates. Substitution of benzodiazepines (often in large doses) for preexisting ethanol or short-acting barbiturate addiction may be necessary. Withdrawal reactions from nicotine, opiates, and ethanol have been recently treated with clonidine, a centrally acting α_2-adrenergic agonist.

Important other clinical drug withdrawal syndromes exist (Table 169-8). The ICU clinician must be aware of these major syndromes. Sudden withdrawal of β-adrenoceptor antagonists can precipitate coronary artery ischemia. Abrupt withdrawal of exogenous steroids can result in Addisonian crisis or a dramatic exacerbation of the underlying disease for which steroids were prescribed. Withdrawal of antihypertensive agents such as clonidine can precipitate a life-threatening hypertensive crisis. Before altering long-standing drug regimens and risking withdrawal syndromes, the intensivist must consider the risk/benefit ratio of these actions in the critically ill patient.

TABLE 169-8 Drugs Associated with Clinical Withdrawal Syndrome

Cardiovascular agents
Centrally acting agents
Clonidine
Methyldopa
Guanabenz
Timenidine
β-Adrenoceptor antagonists
Calcium channel blocking agents
Adrenergic neuron blockers
Guanethidine
Bethanidine
Other antihypertensive agents
Reserpine
Diuretics
Saralasin
Nitroprusside
Corticosteroids
Parenteral
Inhaled (high dose)
Topical (high dose)
Central nervous system active agents
Neuroleptics
Lithium
Antidepressants
Hypnotics and sedatives
Barbiturates
Benzodiazepines
Ethanol
Anticonvulsants
Opioid analgesics

SOURCE: Adapted from reference 31.

MENTAL CONFUSION AND SEIZURES

In the ICU, mental confusion is a common problem. The multiple factors that contribute to an altered mental status in an ICU patient have recently been reviewed.[12] These include sensory-perceptual derangements brought on by an ICU, abnormal electrolytes, the underlying disease process, and multiple drug exposures while in the ICU.[32] Drugs that have been reported to alter mood and increase mental confusion include high doses of or withdrawal from corticosteroids, cimetidine, theophylline, barbiturates, benzodiazepines, digoxin, antidepressants (e.g., tricyclic antidepressants), anticholinergics, antihistamines, penicillins, lidocaine, quinidine, opiates, and phenothiazines (including antiemetics).

Table 169-9 offers a listing of important drug-induced or drug-promoted seizures. If acute alcohol withdrawal is excluded, the incidence of drug-induced convulsions is low and is estimated to be about 0.8 percent in hospitalized patients or a total of 1.7 percent of all seizures in hospitalized patients.[33]

ANAPHYLACTIC OR ANAPHYLACTOID REACTIONS

Anaphylaxis has been associated with exposure to many drugs in the ICU (Table 169-10). The symptom complex that makes up anaphylaxis is a continuum that may include urticaria, profound hypotension, upper airway obstruction (stridor), bronchospasm, and even cardiac arrest. Immuno-

TABLE 169-9 Drugs Reported to Cause Convulsions

Amphetamine	Imipenem-cilastatin
Anticholinesterase agents	Isoniazid
Antihistamines	Lead chelation
Antidepressants (tricyclic)	Local anesthetics (Lidocaine, procaine, bupivacaine)
Antipsychotics (phenothiazines)	Methylxanthines
Baclofen	Metronidazole
β-Blockers	Nalidixic acid
Chlorambucil	Narcotic analgesics
Cocaine	Penicillins
Cycloserine	Phenobarbital
Cyclosporine	Phenytoin
Ergonovine	Pitressin (secondary to water intoxication)
Folic acid	Prednisone (hypocalcemia)
General anesthetics (ketamine, enflurane, halothane)	Radiocontrast agents
Hyperbaric oxygen	Salicylates
Hypoglycemic agents	Sympathomimetics
Hypoosmolar parenteral solutions	Vitamin K oxides

SOURCE: Modified from references 13 and 33.

TABLE 169-10 Anaphylaxis or Anaphylactoid-Inducing Substances in the ICU

Adrenocorticotropic hormone	Nonsteroidal anti-inflammatory agents
Aminopyrine	Opiates
Amphotericin B	Penicillin
Cephalosporins	Plasmanate
Ciprofloxacin	Polymyxin
Demethylchlortetracycline	Protamine sulfate
Dextran	Radiocontrast agents
Ethambutol	Semisynthetic penicillins
Gamma globulin	Snake antivenom
Hydroxyethyl starch	Sulfonamides
Insulin	Tetanus antitoxin
Ketamine	Thyroid-stimulating hormone
Local anesthetics	Vancomycin
Muscle blockers	
Nitrofurantoin	

SOURCE: Modified from reference 13.

logic IgE-mediated responses (e.g., penicillin) have been discovered to be the pathophysiologic mechanisms of anaphylaxis. Penicillin is the most common drug to cause allergic reactions with an allergy incidence of 10 percent of the population. Approximately 10 percent of the patients with penicillin allergy have the potential for anaphylaxis.

A similar type of reaction is called the anaphylactoid reaction which is not IgE mediated. One mechanism for these reactions is the direct release of histamine from mast cells by morphine. Alternatively, a drug may activate complement leading to anaphylatoxins which can release mediators from mast cells and basophils. Examples of drugs causing this response would include aspirin and radiocontrast media. Anaphylactoid reactions have been reported to occur in 0.5 to 2.0 percent of patients exposed to radiocontrast agents.[34] Treatment for both anaphylaxis and anaphylactoid reactions has centered around immediate administration of epinephrine, intravascular volume expansion, oxygen, and the use of other vasopressors to maintain oxygen delivery. Antihistamines, aminophylline, and steroids play an important ancillary role but may be very useful as prophylactic measures in patients likely to experience contrast-related reactions.

CARDIOVASCULAR REACTIONS

Most agents active against cardiovascular disease are themselves capable of producing cardiovascular system toxicity, either an idiosyncratic or dose-dependent side effect. Obviously careful monitoring of serum levels of antiarrhythmic agents such as procainamide, quinidine, mexiletine, and disopyramide guides therapeutic use and helps to reduce toxicity. Despite such monitoring these agents have the ability to aggravate arrhythmias without obvious clinical predictive indicators. This finding has led both to the belief that the ICU patient must be carefully monitored when a new antiarrhythmic agent is started and to the more widespread use of electrophysiologic testing.

Drug-induced arrhythmias, both supraventricular (e.g., induced by theophylline) and ventricular (e.g., induced by tricyclic antidepressants, theophylline, or β-adrenergic receptor agonists) are not limited to specific cardiovascular therapeutic agents. Agents which change the internal electrolyte environment such as diuretics can indirectly predispose patients to cardiac arrhythmias. Certain agents which alter the corrected Q-T (Q-T_c) interval, such as procainamide, tricyclic antidepressants, and phenothiazine antipsychotic agents have been correlated with a highly lethal torsades de pointes phenomenon. This polymorphic ventricular tachyarrhythmia usually resolves when the offending agent has been metabolized. Treatment with isoproterenol, overdrive pacing, and intravenous magnesium has been used with some success.

Hypotension caused by drug exposure is a common cardiovascular adverse effect. Rapid infusion of many agents including H_2 blockers, phenytoin, and sedative-hypnotics can result in hypotension. Drug-induced hypertensive episodes are more rare and usually short-lived. Acute increases in blood pressure are common with the infusion of irritating substances such as amphotericin B, while more sustained hypertension has been noted with chronic high-dose corticosteroid use.

RESPIRATORY REACTIONS

Modification of the respiratory system by drug exposure falls into five major categories: **1.** depression of alveolar ventilation mediated by central nervous system depression, **2.** alveolar hypo- or hyperventilation induced by systemic and central nervous system alteration in pH, **3.** bronchospasm, **4.** neuromuscular blockade, and **5.** parenchymal lung disease. Comprehensive reviews of drug-induced pulmonary disease are available.[35,36]

Narcotics, barbiturates, phenothiazines, benzodiazepines, and other central nervous system acting depressants can induce alveolar hypoventilation. Specific pharmacologic antagonists (e.g., naloxone for opiates and flumazenil for benzodiazepines) are available for some ventilatory depressants and may provide a useful diagnostic challenge for the hypoventilating ICU patient.

Both depolarizing and nondepolarizing neuromuscular blocking agents are clinically useful in the ICU and obviously cause alveolar hypoventilation. This effect can be enhanced or mimicked by the simultaneous use of aminoglycoside antibiotics, particularly in patients with neuromuscular disease or if the patient has a genetic deficiency of serum cholinesterase (which metabolizes depolarizing agents such as succinylcholine).

Drug-induced bronchospasm occurs with β-adrenergic blockers, carbamate acetylcholinesterase inhibitors (e.g., neostigmine or physostigmine), or, rarely, from opiate narcotics (probably by histamine release from mast cells in some patients). Acetazolamide, the carbonic anhydrase inhibitor used both in the treatment of glaucoma and as an anticonvulsant agent, can be clinically used to stimulate alveolar ventilation by altering systemic pH (increasing renal bicarbonate loss causing a metabolic acidosis). Acetate is frequently added to total parenteral nutrition solutions as a way to provide bicarbonate. If excessive amounts are given, a metabolic alkalosis develops which can cause alveolar hypoventilation.

Table 169-11 offers a summary of various drugs that can cause parenchymal lung injury. Hypersensitivity lung disease is brought on by many of these same drugs[35,36] and may include manifestations of pulmonary edema, pulmonary hemorrhage, and pulmonary vasculitis.[37,38]

TABLE 169-11 Drug-Induced Pulmonary Parenchymal Injury

Cytotoxic Drugs	Noncytotoxic Drugs
Antibiotics	Antibacterial agents
Bleomycin	Nitrofurantoin
Mitomycin	Amphotericin B
Neocarzinostatin	Other antibiotics
Alkylating agents	Analgesics
Busulfan	Acetylsalicylic acid (aspirin)
Cyclophosphamide	Opiates
Chlorambucil	Heroin
Melphalan	Propoxyphene
Nitrosoureas	Methadone
Carmustine (BCNU)	Sedatives
Semustine (methyl CCNU)	Ethchlorvynol
Lomustine (CCNU)	Chlordiazepoxide
Chlorozotocin	Anticonvulsants
Antimetabolites	Phenytoin
Methotrexate	Carbamazepine
Azathioprine	Diuretics
Mercaptopurine	Hydrochlorothiazide
Cytosine arabinoside	Major tranquilizers
Miscellaneous	Haloperidol
Procarbazine	Fluphenazine
VM-26	Antiarrhythmics
Vinblastine	Amiodarone
Vindesine	Lidocaine
	Tocainide
	Miscellaneous
	Gold salts
	Penicillamine
	Colchicine
	Propranolol

SOURCE: Adapted from references 35 to 38.

HEMATOLOGIC REACTIONS

In the ICU patient, hematologic abnormalities are common either as a primary effect of the disease process, as a secondary bone marrow suppression from malnutrition, or from the nonspecific systemic stress of a severe illness. Drug-induced hematologic disorders including pancytopenia, hemolytic anemia, thrombocytopenia, and granulocytopenia are well described.[39–41]

Hemolytic anemias are rare in ICU patients. Agents which have been associated with hemolytic anemia include alpha-methyldopa, penicillins, cephalosporins, sulfonamides, quinidine, procainamide, isoniazid, chlorpromazine, and insulin. Idiosyncratic hypoplastic or aplastic anemia which is often irreversible has been noted after exposure to chloramphenicol, gold salts, trimethadione, the hydantoins, the H_2 blockers, the sulfonylurea hypoglycemics, captopril, and the sulfonamides.

Both thrombocytopenia and agranulocytopenia are difficult and common problems in the ICU. Tables 169-12 and 169-13 offer summaries of drugs associated with or proven to cause these conditions. The incidence of heparin-induced thrombocytopenia is thought to be 5 to 10 percent.[40] Existing data do not define the relative incidence of most drug-induced hematologic abnormalities in the ICU patient. In the outpatient setting, where concomitant disease processes are easier to control, studies suggest a rate of one episode of drug-induced blood disorders per 100,000 person-years.[39]

DERMATOLOGIC REACTIONS

When local chemical skin injury from extravasation of drugs or intravenous solutions is included, drug-induced dermatologic reactions are a common problem in the ICU. Local infiltration with an α-adrenergic blocker such as phentolamine may limit the extent of local tissue necrosis after extravasation of vasoconstricting catecholamines such as dopamine or norepinephrine.

Drug-induced skin reactions including macular-papular morbilliform exanthems, urticaria, or fixed drug eruptions have been commonly reported with trimethoprim-sulfamethoxazole, ampicillin, penicillins, blood products, sulfonamides, and erythromycin. Of concern to the intensivist are the three major types of drug-induced skin diseases with the potential for life-threatening complications. These include erythema multiforme (Stevens-Johnson syndrome), toxic epidermal necrolysis, and exfoliative erythroderma. Drug-related erythema multiforme is usually a self-limited,

TABLE 169-12 Drug-Induced Thrombocytopenia

Analgesics and anesthetics	Paramethadione
Acetaminophen	Primidone
Aminopyrine	Trimethadione
Aspirin and sodium salicylate	Valproate sodium
Chloroquine	Cardiovascular agents
Codeine	Chlorothiazides
Indomethacin	Diazoxide
Lidocaine	Digitoxin, digoxin, and digitalis
Meperidine	Ethacrynic acid
Phenacetin	Furosemide
Phenylbutazone	Iopanoic acid (Telepaque)
Antiarrhythmics	Mercurial diuretics
Amrinone	Methyldopa
Hydantoin	Nitroglycerin
Lidocaine	Reserpine
Quinidine	Spironolactone
Antibiotics	Miscellaneous agents
Amphotericin B	Allopurinol
Cephalosporin	Bismuth ethanol
Chloramphenicol	Chlorpheniramine
Chloroquine	Chlorpropamide
Erythromycin	Cimetidine
Hydroxychloroquine	Colchicine
Isoniazid	Disulfiram
Novobiocin	Ergotamine
Organic arsenicals	Gold salts
p-Aminosalicylic acid	Interferon
Penicillin derivatives	Intralipid
Primaquine	Potassium iodide
Pyrimethamine	Prednisone
Quinacrine	Propylthiouracil
Quinine	Quinine
Rifampin	Tetraethylammonium
Streptomycin	Tolbutamide
Sulfamethoxazole	Sedatives and central agents
Sulfisoxazole	Alcohol
Tetracycline	Barbiturates
Anticoagulants	Chloral hydrate
Heparin	Chlordiazepoxide
Anticonvulsants	Chlorpromazine
Acetazolamide	Desipramine
Barbiturates	Dextroamphetamine sulfates
Carbamazepine	Ethchlorvynol
Diazepam	Meprobamate
Ethosuximide	Prochlorperazine
Hydantoin	Promethazine

SOURCE: Modified from reference 13, 18, and 39.

acute, inflammatory cutaneous or mucocutaneous disease that is manifested by typical target-shaped lesions and diagnostic histopathologic findings. Penicillins, sulfonamides, salicylates, phenytoin, barbiturates, codeine, thiazide diuretics, furosemide, cimetidine, clindamycin, and ethosuximide are well-documented causes of erythema multiforme. Toxic epidermal necrolysis may be a maximal expression of the Stevens-Johnson syndrome. Diffuse blistering with large areas of skin sloughing, hypovolemic shock, pulmonary edema, and renal failure define the syndrome of toxic epidermal necrolysis. Antibiotics, salicylates, barbiturates, and narcotics have been associated with exfoliative erythroderma. This erythema is associated with induration of the skin and continuous desquamation and scaling involving almost all skin surfaces.

GASTROINTESTINAL TRACT REACTIONS

Changes in gastrointestinal tract motility including diarrhea and obstipation are common in the ICU. Anticholinergic agents, opiates, and aluminum-containing antacids are frequently associated with drug-induced constipation. Magnesium-containing antacids, quinidine, theophylline, and colchicine frequently cause diarrhea. A particularly aggressive diarrhea associated with other systemic symptoms is caused by *Clostridium difficile*. The pseudomembranous colitis syndrome is caused by an overgrowth of enteric *C. difficile* and release of toxins into the stool. It is frequently the consequence of broad-spectrum antibiotic exposure, but other drugs and conditions may contribute to it. The eradication of this toxin-producing organism requires enteral or systemic vancomycin or metronidazole. The condition has been reported to be a nosocomial hazard in the ICU.[42]

Stress-induced gastritis with bleeding may be potentiated by drugs such as heparin, aspirin, glucocorticoids, theophylline, and nonsteroidal anti-inflammatory agents. Prophylactic measures for stress gastritis including H_2 blockers, antacids, and sucralfate may modify the incidence of this problem.

As the primary organ for drug biotransformation, the liver is heavily exposed to compounds. Commonly used drugs can result in adverse effects mimicking almost all patterns of liver disease including hypersensitivity reaction, direct hepatocyte toxicity, deposition of microvesicular fat, fibrosis, and cholestasis.[43–45] Table 169-14 outlines some major types and examples of drug-induced liver disease.

RENAL REACTIONS

Drug-induced or drug-augmented nephropathy remains a major cause of increased morbidity and contributes to overall mortality of the critically ill patient. The aminoglycoside antibiotics and radiographic contrast materials are the leading causes of acute nephrotoxic renal failure in the ICU patient. Risk factors for the development of acute nephrotoxic renal failure include advanced age, sex (greater for females than males), prior renal disease, intravascular volume depletion, hypokalemia, and simultaneous use of other nephrotoxic agents. Table 169-15 offers a summary of mechanisms and examples of drug-induced nephropathies.

METABOLIC REACTIONS

Significant electrolyte abnormalities including potassium and sodium wasting are commonly seen with the use of potent loop diuretics and drugs such as amphotericin B. Serious hyperkalemia can be seen with the use of high doses of aldosterone-blocking diuretics such as spironolactone and triamterene. In addition, hyperkalemia in the ICU patient can be the result of exposure to exogenous potas-

TABLE 169-13 Drug-Induced Agranulocytosis

Analgesic/anti-inflammatory	Antimicrobials	Mepazine
drugs	Aminosalicylic acid	Methylpromazine
Amidopyrine	Amodiaquine	Perazine
(aminopyrine)	Ampicillin	Prochlorperazine
Antipyrine (phenezone)	Carbenicillin	Pramazine
Aspirin	Cephalexin	Thioridazine
Benoxaprofen	Cephalothin	Trimeprazine
Colchicine	Cephradine	Antithyroid drugs
Fenoprofen	Chloramphenicol	Carbimazole
Gold salts	Clindamycin	Methimazole
Ibuprofen	Cloxacillin	Methylthiouracil
Indomethacin	Co-trimoxazole	Propylthiouracil
Naproxen	Dapsone	Thiouracil
Oxyphenbutazone	Doxycycline	Diuretics
Paracetamol	Flucytosine	Acetazolamide
(acetaminophen)	Gentamicin	Bumetanide
Phenylbutazone	Griseofulvin	Chlorthalidone
Zomepirac	Hydroxychloroquine	Chlorothiazide
Antiarrhythmic drugs	Isoniazid	Ethacrynic acid
Aprindine	Lincomycin	Hydrochlorothiazide
Disopyramide	Methicillin	Mercurials
Procainamide	Metronidazole	Methozolamide
Propafenone	Mezlocillin	Other drugs
Propranolol	Nafcillin	Allopurinol
Quinidine	Nitrofurantoin	Brompheniramine
Tocainide	Novobiocin	Chlordiazepoxide
Anticonvulsants	Oxacillin	Cimetidine
Carbamazepine	Oxophenarsine	Diazepam
Ethosuximide	Penicillin	Ethanol
Mephenytoin	Pyrimethamine	Levamisole
Phenytoin	Quinine	Levodopa
Primidone	Rifampicin (rifampin)	Mebendazole
Sodium valproate	Ristocetin	Meprobamate
Trimethadione	Streptomycin	Methydroline
Antidepressants	Sulfadiazine	Metiamide
Amoxipine	Sulfamethoxypyridazine	Penicillamine
Clomipramine	Sulfapyridine	Phenindione
Desipramine	Sulfasalazine	Promethazine
Imipramine	(salicylazosulphapyridine)	Ranitidine
Maprotiline	Sulfathiazole	Thenalidine
Antihypertensives	Thiacetazone	Ticlopidine
Captopril	Ticarcillin	Tolbutamide
Diazoxide	Antipsychotics	
Hydralazine	Chlorpromazine	
Methyldopa	Clozapine	
Nifedipine	Fluphenazine	
Propranolol		

SOURCE: Adapted from reference 41.

sium chloride supplements, potassium drug salts (e.g., potassium penicillin), and transfusion of stored blood.

Phenformin, acetazolamide, salicylates, and drug preservatives and diluents (e.g., benzylalcohol and propylene glycol) all can cause metabolic acidosis in a patient exposed to high doses. High-dose glucocorticoids expectedly can cause hyperglycemia. In addition, antihypertensive agents such as diazoxide, thiazide diuretics, and β blockers have been associated with glucose intolerance.[46] Medication-related metabolic and electrolyte complications are particularly common when adverse effects of total parenteral nutrition are included.

CASE PRESENTATION

A 56-year-old 68-kg man presented with evidence of an acute anterior myocardial infarction. He was treated in the emergency room with thrombolytics and developed profound ventricular ectopy and improvement in his electrocardiogram changes. In the ICU, he was given 100 mg of lidocaine intravenously followed by an addi-

TABLE 169-14 Examples of Acute Drug-Induced Liver Diseases

Histopathologic Findings	Agents
Acute hepatocellular necrosis	
Centrilobular	Acetaminophen Halothane
Diffuse spotty necrosis	Isoniazid α-Methyldopa
Microvesicular steatosis	Tetracycline Valproic acid
Cholestasis	
Cannulicular blind-bile plugs	C-17 Alkylsteroids Estrogens
Exudative microscopic cholangitis	Chlorpromazine Erythromycin Estolate
Mixed pattern	
Atypical hepatitis	Phenytoin
Granulomatous hepatitis (hypersensitivity)	Quinidine Allopurinol
Vascular	
Veno-occlusive disease	Irradiation Cytotoxic drugs
Sinusoidal dilatation	Azathioprine Sex hormones
Hepatic vein obstruction	Sex hormones
Portal vein obstruction	Sex hormones

SOURCE: Adapted from references 43 to 45.

tional dose of 50 mg of lidocaine within 5 min with control of his ventricular ectopy. A peak lidocaine level (C_0) drawn within minutes of the second dose resulted in a blood level of 2 mg/L. It was calculated that his volume of distribution (V_d) was 75 L (1.1 L/kg). He was immediately started on a constant intravenous infusion of 2.5 mg/min of lidocaine. A steady-state blood level (C_{ss}) drawn 6 h later was 3 mg/L. Attempts to reduce his lidocaine dose over the next few days resulted in recurrence of his malignant ventricular ectopy. He was started on propranolol 40 mg orally every 6 h for return of his hypertension and postmyocardial infarction protection. After 24 h, the patient was noted to be confused and had a witnessed grand mal seizure. A blood lidocaine level was drawn and the infusion was stopped. This second level (C_{ss}) was found to be 10 mg/L. His mental status improved after lidocaine withdrawal without return of his ventricular ectopy. He was discharged 1 week later on aspirin and propranolol.

CASE DISCUSSION

This case demonstrates a number of important applications of pharmacokinetic principles in the intensive care setting. The established loading dose of 150 mg of lidocaine resulted in a low peak therapeutic blood level in this "average" 70-kg man. The calculated V_d in this patient was determined using the previously given formulas:

$$V_d = \frac{\text{IV dose}}{C_0} = \frac{150\text{ mg}}{2\text{ mg/L}} = 75\text{ L}$$

or

$$\frac{75\text{ L}}{68\text{ kg}} = 1.1\text{ L/kg}$$

From the C_{ss} determined on lidocaine, 2.5 mg/min, the clearance (Cl) and half-life ($T_{1/2}$) of lidocaine can be determined.

$$\text{Cl} = \frac{F \times \text{dose}}{C_{ss} \times T}$$

where F equals the bioavailability and T equals the dosing intervals.

$$\text{Cl} = \frac{1}{C_{ss}} \times \frac{\text{dose}}{T} = \frac{1 \times 2.5\text{ mg/min}}{3\text{ mg/L}} = 0.83\text{ L/min}$$

or

$$\frac{0.83\text{ L/min}}{68\text{ kg}} = 0.0122\text{(L/min)/kg}$$

Also,

$$\text{Cl} = \frac{0.693 V_d}{T_{1/2}}$$

$$T_{1/2} = \frac{0.693 \times V_d}{\text{Cl}} = \frac{0.693 \times 1.1\text{ L/kg}}{0.0122\text{(L/min)/kg}}$$

$$= 62.5\text{ min}$$

The addition of propranolol to this patient's therapeutic regimen resulted in a drug interaction with lidocaine. The reduction of clearance of lidocaine is thought to be in part due to the reduction in hepatic blood flow from propranolol. In this patient, the resulting reduction in lidocaine clearance produced a new C_{ss} of 10 mg/L of lidocaine. This lead to the adverse effect of altered mental status and seizure. The new $T_{1/2}$ can be determined:

$$\frac{\text{IV maintenance dose}}{T} = \frac{0.693 \times V_d \times C_{ss}}{T_{1/2}}$$

$$2.5\text{ mg/min} = \frac{0.693 \times 1.1\text{ L/kg} \times 68\text{ kg} \times 10\text{ mg/L}}{T_{1/2}}$$

$$T_{1/2} = 207.3\text{ min}$$

The new maintenance dose on propranolol needed to give a C_{ss} of 3 mg/L is calculated:

$$\frac{\text{IV maintenance dose}}{T} = \frac{0.693 \times 1.1\text{ L/kg} \times 68\text{ kg} \times 3\text{ mg/L}}{207.3\text{ min}}$$

$$\text{New maintenance dose} = 0.75\text{ mg/min}$$

TABLE 169-15 Drug-Induced Nephropathies

Location	Process	Drugs
Glomerulus	Glomerulonephritis	D-Penicillamine
		Gold
	Hypersensitivity	Phenytoin
		Sulfonamides
Proximal renal tubules	Fanconi's syndrome	Outdated tetracycline
	Acute renal tubular necrosis	Aminoglycosides
		Methoxyflurane
		Indomethacin
		Ibuprofen
		Radiocontrast agents
Distal tubules	Renal tubular acidosis	Amphotericin B
		Acetazolamide
Interstitium	Interstitial nephritis	Methicillin
		Rifampin
		Phenindione
		Allopurinol
		Ibuprofen
		Indomethacin
		Thiazides
		Furosemide
Collecting duct	Diabetes insipidus	Lithium
		Methoxyflurane
		Demethylchlortetracycline
Renal blood flow	Anaphylaxis	Penicillin
		Sulfonamides
		Radiocontrast agents
	Vasodilation	Nitroprusside
		Nitroglycerin

SOURCE: Modified from reference 13.

References

1. Smith J, Seidl L, Cluff L: Studies on the epidemiology of adverse drug reactions. Ann Intern Med 65:629, 1986.
2. Trunet P, Le Gall JR, Lhoste F, et al.: The role of iatrogenic disease in admissions to intensive care units. JAMA 244:2617, 1980.
3. Spector R: *The Scientific Basis of Clinical Pharmacology.* Boston, Little, Brown and Company, 1986.
4. Steel K, Gertman P, Crescenzi C, et al.: Iatrogenic illness on a general medical service at a university hospital. N Engl J Med 304:638, 1981.
5. Gilman A, Goodman L, Rall T, et al.: *Goodman and Gilman's The Pharmacological Basis of Therapeutics,* 7th ed. New York, Macmillan Publishing Co, 1985.
6. Gerson B: *Essentials of Therapeutic Drug Monitoring.* New York, Igaku-Shoin Medical Publishers, Inc, 1983.
7. Gibaldi M, Perier D: *Pharmacokinetics.* New York, Marcel Dekker, Inc, 1975.
8. Endrenyi L: Pharmacokinetics, in Kalent H, Roschlau W (eds): *Principles of Medical Pharmacology,* Chap 5. Philadelphia, Decker, Inc, 1989, pp 49–59.
9. AMA Division of Drugs, *AMA Drug Evaluations,* Chicago, American Medical Association, 1983.
10. Larson E, Kukull W, Buchner D, et al.: Adverse drug reactions associated with global cognitive impairment in elderly persons. Ann Intern Med 107:169, 1987.
11. Jahnigen D, Hannon C, Laxson L, et al.: Iatrogenic disease in hospitalized elderly veterans. J Am Geriatr Soc 30:387, 1982.
12. Easton C, Mackenzie F: Sensory-perceptual alterations: delirium in the intensive care unit. Heart Lung 17:229, 1988.
13. Prasad P, Albertson T, Turner J: Adverse drug reactions and interactions in neurosurgical patients, in Youmans (ed): *Neurological Surgery, Vol II.* Philadelphia, WB Saunders Comp, 1990.
14. Richard C, Berdeaux A, Delion F, et al.: Effects of mechanical ventilation on hepatic drug pharmacokinetics. Chest 90:837, 1986.
15. Lerman F, Weibert RT: *Drug Interaction Index.* Oradell, Medical Economics Company, Inc, 1982.
16. Pitlick W: *Antiepileptic Drug Interactions.* New York, Demos Publications, 1989.
17. Hansten P: *Drug Interactions.* Philadelphia, Lea and Febiger, 1985.
18. Chernow B: *The Pharmacologic Approach to the Critically Ill Patient.* Baltimore, Williams and Wilkins, 1988.
19. Rudd C, Wikman J, Lamb P: Drug interactions in critical care, in Lamb P, Bryan-Brown C (eds): *Complications in Critical Care Medicine.* Chicago, Year Book Medical, 1988.
20. Hosan R: *Drug Information Advisor.* Baltimore, Williams & Wilkins Electronic Media, 1986.
21. Tamai I, Strome S, Marshall C, et al.: Analysis of drug interactions among nursing home residents. Am J Hosp Pharm 46:1567, 1989.
22. Naranio C, Busto U: Adverse drug reactions, in Kalant H, Roshlau W (eds): *Principles of Medical Pharmacology.* Philadelphia, Decker, Inc, 1989, pp 658–665.
23. Guidry J, Eastwood T, Curry S: Phenytoin absorption in volunteers receiving selected enteral feedings. West J Med 150:659, 1989.
24. Neuvon P: Drug absorption interactions, in Prescott L, Nimmo W (eds): *Drug Absorption.* New York, ADIS Press, 1979, pp 228–232.

25. Bigger J, Leahey E: Quinidine and digoxin, an important interaction. Drugs 24:229, 1982.
26. Montamat S, Cusack B, Vestal R: Management of drug therapy in the elderly. N Engl J Med 321:303, 1989.
27. Golightly L, Smolinske S, Bennett M, et al.: Pharmaceutical excipients adverse effects associated with "inactive" ingredients in drug products (Part I). Med Toxicol 3:128, 1988.
28. Golightly L, Smolinske S, Bennett M, et al.: Pharmaceutical excipients adverse effects associated with "inactive" ingredients in drug products (Part II). Med Toxicol 3:209, 1988.
29. Kumar K, Reuler J: Drug fever. West J Med 144:753, 1966.
30. Mackowiak P, LeMaistre C: Drug fever: a critical appraisal of conventional concepts. Ann Intern Med 106:728, 1987.
31. George C, Robertson D: Clinical consequences of abrupt drug withdrawal. Med Toxicol 2:367, 1987.
32. Hollister L: Drug-induced psychiatric disorders and their management. Med Toxicol 1:428, 1986.
33. Messing R, Closson R, Simon R: Drug-induced seizures: a 10-year experience. Neurology 34:1582, 1984.
34. Greenberger P, Halwig J, Patterson R, Wallemark C: Emergency administration of radio contrast media in high-risk patients. J Allergy Clin Immunol 77:630, 1986.
35. Cooper J, White D, Matthay R: Drug-induced pulmonary disease. Part 1. Cytotoxic drugs. Am Rev Respir Dis 133:321, 1986.
36. Cooper J, White D, Matthay R: Drug-induced pulmonary disease. Part 2. Noncytotoxic drugs. Am Rev Respir Dis 133:488, 1986.
37. Kumar K, Holden W: Drug-induced pulmonary vascular disease-mechanisms and clinical patterns. West J Med 145:343, 1986.
38. Gauthier-Rahman S, Akoun G, Milleron B, et al.: Leukocyte migration inhibition in propranolol-induced pneumonitis. Chest 97:238, 1990.
39. Danielson D, Douglas S, Herzog P, et al.: Drug-induced blood disorders. JAMA 252:3257, 1984.
40. Bell W: Diagnosing and managing heparin associated thrombocytopenia. J Crit Illness 2:11, 1987.
41. Heimpel H: Drug-induced agranulocytosis. Med Toxicol 3:449, 1988.
42. Foulke G, Silva J: Clostridium difficile in the intensive care unit: management problems and prevention issues. Crit Care Med 17:822, 1989.
43. Kaplowitz N, Aw T, Simon F, et al.: Drug-induced hepatotoxicity. Ann Intern Med 104:826, 1986.
44. Zimmerman H, Lewis J: Drug-induced cholestasis. Med Toxicol 2:112, 1987.
45. Sherlock S: The spectrum of hepatotoxicity due to drugs. Lancet 2:440, 1986.
46. Houston M: Adverse effects of antihypertensive drug therapy on glucose intolerance. Cardiol Clin 4:117, 1986.

Chapter 170

THE ALCOHOLS

MATTHEW J. ELLENHORN

KEY POINTS

- *Chronic alcohol abuse causes adverse effects in all organ systems; these often complicate the diagnosis and management of critical illness in the alcoholic patient.*
- *Acute ethanol intoxication may cause coma, hypoventilation, hypothermia, and hypotension when blood levels exceed 300 mg/dL; ventilatory support, rewarming, volume expansion, and hemodialysis may be indicated.*
- *Convulsions in alcoholic patients are of four types, requiring an adjusted diagnostic and management approach.*
- *Acute ethanol withdrawal in alcoholic patients causes five distinct but overlapping syndromes, each requiring specific prevention or treatment; therapeutic benefit is shared from thiamine, multivitamins, glucose, volume, magnesium, haloperidol, benzodiazepines, and adrenergic blocking agents.*
- *Metabolic acidosis in the alcoholic patient is multifactorial, including ketoacidosis (starvation and alcoholic), lactic acidosis (seizures and liver dysfunction) and coingested toxins.*
- *Severe metabolic acidosis with osmolal gap indicates poisoning with methanol or ethylene glycol; early treatment with ethanol and hemodialysis is indicated and 4-methylpyrazole may be useful.*
- *Coingested toxins are common; isopropyl (rubbing) alcohol poisoning is detected by acetone odor and blood levels with osmolar gap without acidemia; severe intoxication is treated with respiratory support and dialysis.*

Alcohol poisoning[1] may result in extensive central nervous system (CNS), abdominal, or renal pathologic conditions and can lead to death. Aspects of alcohol toxicity of special interest to the critical care physician include **1.** the myriad problems encountered with ethyl alcohol abuse, **2.** seizures in the alcoholic patient, **3.** alcohol withdrawal syndromes, **4.** the severe metabolic acidosis and CNS depression observed with methanol and ethylene glycol, and **5.** the severe CNS depression seen with isopropyl alcohol poisoning.

The alcohols are a group of compounds largely metabolized by alcohol dehydrogenase in the liver (ethyl alcohol, methyl alcohol, ethylene glycol, isopropyl alcohol) to produce metabolites which can lead to a high anion gap and high osmolal gap metabolic acidosis (ethylene glycol, methyl alcohol), the production of unusual amounts of acetone (isopropyl alcohol), or, infrequently, ketoacidosis (ethyl alcohol) (Table 170-1). In acute excess, all produce serious and perhaps fatal CNS damage and varying degrees of severe abdominal symptoms (gastritis and pancreatitis). Chronic excess of ethyl alcohol, in fact, is protean[2,3] in its production of clinical disorders. The critical care physician will be required to treat effects of alcohol overdose such as hematemesis, hepatic failure, aspiration pneumonia, rhabdomyolysis, seizures, coma, hypoglycemia, severe metabolic acidosis, and withdrawal syndromes (Table 170-2).

Ethanol

Ethanol abuse[4] results in serious, often life-threatening clinical states following acute intoxication, during chronic use, and after withdrawal. It may lead to death following sudden arrhythmias, respiratory failure, or hypoglycemia. Mortality and morbidity from the regular use of alcohol rapidly increase with the daily consumption of three to five drinks and rises further after six drinks per day. In fact, more than 200,000 Americans die annually from alcohol-related disorders and alcohol dependency is observed in perhaps 5 to 10 percent of Americans. It is the most common single drug taken by patients. Alcohol determinations are the most frequently performed medicolegal test. In all

TABLE 170-1 Acute Toxicity of the Alcohols

	Ethanol	Methanol	Ethylene Glycol	Isopropanol
CNS depressant	+	+	+	+
Convulsion	+	+	+	+
Odor	+	−	−	+ (acetone)
Blood gases	respiratory acidosis ketoacidosis	severe metabolic acidosis	severe metabolic acidosis	mild metabolic acidosis
Anion gap	+	+++	+++	+
Osmolar gap	+	+	+	+
Oxalate crystaluria	−	−	++	−
Symptom onset	30 min	12–48 h	30 min–12 h	rapid
Lethal dose	5–8 g/kg	1–5 g/kg	1.5 g/kg	3–4 g/kg
Lethal blood level (mg/dL)	350–500	80	200	400
Special treatment	HD	ETOH; HD	ETOH; HCO_3, HD	HD; HCO_3

HD, hemodialysis

TABLE 170-2 Ethanol Toxicity in the Critical Care Setting

Suicides/Trauma	
	Traffic accidents
	Suicide attempts
	Cervical and cerebral trauma
	Subdural hematoma
Gastrointestinal	
	Acute and chronic recurrent pancreatitis
	Mallory-Weiss syndrome
	Hematemesis—ruptured esophageal varices
	Hepatic failure with encephalopathy
Respiratory	
	Aspiration pneumonia
	Atelectasis
	Pneumothorax
	Fractured ribs
Muscular	
	Rhabdomyolysis
	Myoglobinuria
Neurologic	
	Seizures
	Central pontine myelinosis
	Polyradiculoneuropathy
	Wernicke's encephalopathy
	Korsakoff's psychosis
	Pellagra encephalopathy
	Coma
Cardiovascular	
	Hypertension
	Subarachnoid hemorrhage
	Depressed left ventricular function
	Supraventricular arrhythmias
	Cardiomyopathy
Endocrine/Metabolic	
	Hypoglycemia, especially young children
	Acidosis, metabolic and respiratory
	Hypokalemia, hypomagnesemia
Ethanol Withdrawal Syndromes (see Table 170-3)	
Coingested Alcohols	
	Methanol, ethylene glycol, isopropyl alcohol

its manifestations, alcohol-related disorders make heavy demands on emergency and intensive care facilities throughout the world.

PHARMACOLOGY

Ethanol absorption occurs within 30 to 60 min. Delay in gastric emptying delays absorption. It distributes into total body water and penetrates the blood-brain barrier and placenta. The apparent volume of distribution is 0.6 L/kg in healthy adults, 0.7 L/kg in children.

Ethanol is metabolized mostly in the liver according to zero-order kinetics (i.e., elimination rate is concentration independent). The kidney and lungs excrete about 5 to 10 percent of an absorbed dose unchanged. The average adult metabolizes 7 to 10 g/h and reduces the ethanol level 15 to 20 mg/dL/h. The rate of reduction is increased in chronic alcoholics and children.

The liver cell metabolizes ethanol by the alcohol dehydrogenase pathway (major pathway), by a microsomal ethanol-oxidizing system (MEOS) and by a peroxidase-catalase system (minor pathway). Ethanol is converted to acetaldehyde by alcohol dehydrogenase; this is the rate-limiting step in its metabolism. The aldehyde is further metabolized by an acetaldehyde dehydrogenase. Finally, the acetate is converted to acetyl coenzyme, CO_2, and H_2O via the Krebs cycle.

PATHOPHYSIOLOGY AND CLINICAL MANIFESTATIONS

In the acutely intoxicated individual, ethanol acts as a CNS depressant.[5] Alteration of thought and mood occur before changes in vision (occipital lobe) and coordination (cerebellum). In nontolerant individuals, decrements in cognitive ability, motor coordination, and sensory perception may begin at blood ethanol concentrations as low as 50 mg/dL.

Profound metabolic changes include production of lactate, resulting in acidosis, elevation of serum uric acid content, accumulation of hepatic triglycerides, reduced gluconeogenesis, depressed protein synthesis, and reduction in active bone resorption and formation.

Psychopharmacologic agents (tricyclic antidepressants, propoxyphene, acetaminophen) are frequently coingested by alcoholics for treatment of anxiety and depression. Laboratory studies should include these drugs, if suspected. Alcoholics may complicate their often unreliable histories with simultaneous ingestions of other alcohols such as ethylene glycol, methanol, or isopropyl alcohol. The critical care physician must be alert for concomitant presence of complicating medical conditions (head trauma, intracranial bleeding, meningitis, pneumonia, alterations in electrolytes and blood glucose, external injuries, burns, and other overdoses from both prescription and over-the-counter drugs) when confronted with the often unruly and demanding alcoholic patient.

The blood alcohol level may not by itself reflect the seriousness of an alcohol intoxication. The intensivist should consider the above medical conditions including drug interactions and other disease factors when treating the alcoholic patient. A rough correlation of blood ethanol levels (mg/dL) with clinical status in nontolerant individuals suggests progressive deterioration from sobriety (<30), euphoria and excitement (30 to 250), confusion and stupor (180 to 400) to coma and death (>350).

TREATMENT OF ACUTE ETHANOL INTOXICATION

Acute alcohol ingestion in nontolerant patients usually responds to careful supportive care. Fifty percent dextrose (50 to 100 mL intravenously) is given to all obtunded patients after a blood glucose level is obtained. Comatose patients should be treated with initial attention to airway, breathing, and circulation, and should be given glucose, naloxone, and thiamine. Cervical immobilization should be considered and cervical x-rays obtained. The intensivist should look for cranial or other body trauma. Unless coma or coingestion of another drug delays absorption, gastric emptying is usually not necessary. Cathartics and charcoal probably are not useful in single ingestions. Fructose may lead to vomiting, abdominal pain, pruritus, lactic acidosis, and shock.

Hemodialysis can increase ethanol clearance, but supportive care is usually sufficient. Naloxone has not been shown conclusively to be useful in ethanol-induced coma. Analeptic agents should not be used.

The patient should be observed closely for respiratory depression. Nutritional deficiencies should be replaced as required with magnesium, thiamine, pyridoxine, and vitamins K and C. An underlying illness should be sought in the chronic alcoholic. The intensivist should watch for the development of withdrawal syndromes. Dehydration, electrolyte imbalance, and acid-base imbalances must be corrected.

Seizures in the Alcoholic Patient

Any patient arriving at the emergency department with seizures should be questioned about alcohol intake.[6] It is involved in up to 40 percent of adults with seizures admitted to a hospital and in about 15 percent of patients with status epilepticus.[7]

Seizures may be classified in an alcoholic population as follows:

1. Solitary, convulsive seizure in alcoholics. No prior epileptic convulsions, no other epileptogenic disease, no relation to withdrawal or massive intake of alcohol.
2. Convulsive seizure of alcoholics. Includes withdrawal seizures and seizures related to massive alcohol intake.
3. Seizures in alcoholics with potentially epileptogenic disease such as head injury, idiopathic epilepsy, cerebrovascular disease, and other drugs facilitating seizures.
4. Alcoholic epilepsy. Recurrent seizures in alcoholics; no history of epilepsy, potentially epileptogenic diseases, withdrawal, or massive intake of alcohol.

Seizures with alcohol use are dose dependent and may be causal, independent of alcohol withdrawal. Alcohol contributes to seizure frequency in the general epileptic population. This may be enhanced by sleep deprivation, enhanced photic sensitivity, and accelerated metabolism of antiepileptic drugs due to drinking alcohol.

Factors associated with alcohol withdrawal and considered most likely to precipitate seizures are hypoglycemia, hypomagnesemia, and respiratory alkalosis. Alcohol withdrawal also heightens photic sensitivity and can lead to television-induced seizures.

A history of seizures before age eighteen years or before the onset of heavy drinking is usually due to idiopathic epilepsy. Alcohol withdrawal seizures appear 6 to 48 h after either cessation or precipitous decline of alcohol intake. The true alcohol withdrawal seizure will be manifest prior to the onset of delirium tremens (DT). It is a generalized seizure and does not manifest an aura, a focal onset, or a significant period (e.g., more than 30 min) of postictal confusion, agitation, or aggression.[8] Persons who differ from this pattern (i.e., have an aura, begin the seizure with a focal presentation, have onset during DT, have an extended period of postictal confusion, suffer a second seizure) should be carefully evaluated for other conditions. Alcohol withdrawal may exacerbate partial (focal) seizures common with posttraumatic epilepsy. Partial seizures must be considered indicative of a mass lesion until proven otherwise. Seizures in a setting of alcohol consumption or withdrawal will usually not require long-term anticonvulsant therapy since the seizures are self-limited.

TREATMENT

Seizure treatment should include an intravenous line with 5% dextrose and saline solution established; 100 mg thiamine, 25 g dextrose, and 1.2 mg naloxone, are given intravenously to reverse Wernicke's syndrome, hypoglycemia, or narcotic ingestion; metabolic disorders, toxic ingestion, infection, and structural abnormality are ruled out by history, repeated physical examinations, laboratory data, and computed tomography (CT) scan, if required.

If an alcoholic develops status epilepticus (uncommon in alcohol withdrawal), an attempt is made to terminate the seizure in <60 min to prevent irreversible brain damage. Oral airway or an endotracheal tube is maintained and supplementary oxygen used. Two intravenous lines are started. After thiamine, dextrose, and naloxone are given, a loading dose of phenytoin (13 to 18 mg/kg) is started in one line with normal saline with a filter (0.22 or 0.45 μm) designed to remove phenytoin microcrystals which may form when it is mixed in solution. An intravenous infusion pump is recommended. The flow rate is kept at 40 to 50 mg/min, with caution in patients with preexisting heart disease. In a second line, diazepam is given at 2 to 4 mg/min, up to 20 mg. Diazepam has a short duration of action (20 to 30 min) and is given for immediate seizure control, with caution in the elderly who are more vulnerable to respiratory depression and hypotension; here, lorazepam may be useful (see Chap. 172). If seizures persist, a diazepam drip is begun, with 50 to 100 mg diazepam diluted in 500 ml 5% dextrose in water (D_5W) and run at 40 mL/h. If there is no response to phenytoin or diazepam, or if cardiac disease or phenytoin allergy preclude its use, intravenous phenobarbital is given at 25 to 50 mg/min after a loading dose of 7 to 20 mg/kg. Phenobarbital should not be administered together with an intravenous diazepam drip because of their potential incompatibilities in solution. By the time that phenobarbital is added, endotracheal intubation and mechanical ventilation are invariably helpful.

For the alcoholic in withdrawal with no present seizure but a past history of withdrawal seizures, phenytoin is added to the regimen for alcohol withdrawal (either an intravenous loading dose to those admitted or an oral loading dose of 19 to 20 mg/kg in two to three divided doses over 6 h with no more than 600 mg/dose to outpatients). For withdrawal seizures, the patient is maintained on phenytoin 300 mg/day for 5 days. The alcoholic who has already had a single or short burst of seizures and is alert may only need treatment for the alcohol withdrawal. Further seizures will be rare if adequately treated with a benzodiazepine. The patient should be observed for at least 6 h after the seizure before discharge. Possible causes of a decreased level of consciousness following seizures in the obtunded patient include postictal state, occult head trauma, unrecognized metabolic disorder, or poisoning. In alcohol withdrawal with no history of seizures, benzodiazepines are used (see Alcohol Withdrawal). Long-term anticonvulsant therapy is not indicated. For hypomagnesemia, 1 g magnesium sulfate (2 mL 50% solution, after a blood magnesium level is obtained) may be required four times daily for 1 to 2 days to replete magnesium stores.

Alcohol Withdrawal Syndromes

When large amounts of alcohol are consumed over a few days, or when smaller amounts of ethanol are ingested at frequent intervals and for prolonged periods, a state of physical dependence may be induced, which becomes most evident by the appearance of clinical abnormalities when the concentration of ethanol in the brain declines.[9,10] The onset of this syndrome usually occurs after a 5 to 10 year latency period, but in very heavy drinkers the onset may require only a few months. This state may follow not only cessation of drinking but simply a reduction in intake (Table 170-3).

The alcohol withdrawal syndrome derives from the effects of excess sympathetic activity and excessive release of norepinephrine in the brain and periphery (anxiety, arousal, agitation, tremor, sweating, tachycardia, hypertension, nausea, vomiting, sleeplessness, hyperreflexia, hyperthermia, and tinnitus). Other withdrawal symptoms such as seizures may be due to a central γ-aminobutyric acid deficiency. Dopaminergic excess may cause the hallucinations and delusions often seen in those suffering with alcohol withdrawal. Other symptoms (pruritus, loss of appetite, depression, paresthesia, weakness, and malaise) may represent changes in other transmitters yet to be evaluated.

ABSTINENCE SYNDROME AND DT

PATHOPHYSIOLOGY AND CLINICAL MANIFESTATIONS

The common withdrawal syndrome appears within 6 to 8 h after cessation of drinking and has a duration of approximately 72 h. It is characterized by a generalized tremor, a mild confusional state with agitation, sleep disturbances, startle reaction, autonomic hyperactivity (tachycardia, elevated blood pressure, diaphoresis, nausea, vomiting), hyperreflexia, hyperexcitability, craving for alcohol and other CNS depressants, headache, flushed facies, and conjunctival injection.

TABLE 170-3 Ethanol Withdrawal Syndrome Times of Onset after Cessation of Drinking

Common abstinence syndrome	6–8 h
Alcoholic hallucinations	24–36 h
Seizures (rum fits)	7–48 h (peak 24 h)
DTs	3–5 days (up to 14 days)
Alcoholic ketoacidosis (AKA)	24–72 h

Within 24 to 36 h after cessation of drinking, a perceptual disorder may appear, manifested by nightmares and visual or auditory illusions and hallucinations. Prior symptomatology which developed earlier may persist if left untreated. The patient can remain fully oriented.

Generalized tonic-clonic seizures (rum fits), generally multiple (two to six over 6 to 8 h with brief postictal episodes), may begin in a lesser number of subjects from 7 to 48 h after cessation of drinking with a peak incidence at 24 h. Loss of consciousness may not occur during the tonic-clonic movements. When patients present in this manner, without focal neurologic deficits or signs of acute head trauma, CT scanning is unlikely to indicate the presence of a treatable abnormality. If patients manifest focal seizures or signs, evidence of trauma, more than six seizures, seizures continuing longer than 6 h, or a prolonged postictal confusional state, further diagnostic evaluation is indicated.

In any case, patients having their first ethanol-related seizures should be hospitalized for diagnostic studies and observed for the occurrence of additional seizures or DT. More than 50 percent of such patients will have only one seizure. Seizures rarely develop after hallucinations but more than one-third of patients with withdrawal seizures will progress to DT. This stage of seizures is not indicative of epilepsy and does not require long-term anticonvulsive treatment. In fact, anticonvulsant drugs such as phenytoin are usually ineffective in preventing recurrences and may precipitate status epilepticus when patients simultaneously discontinue ethanol and anticonvulsants.[11] However, when withdrawal is accompanied by status epilepticus, prompt treatment is required.

Finally, the most delayed and most serious clinical manifestation of alcohol withdrawal is DT, a severe confusional state characterized by profound agitation, insomnia, hallucinations or delusions, tremor, and signs of autonomic hyperactivity which may include tachycardia, hyperthermia, hypertension, diaphoresis, vascular collapse, and death. Typically, it begins about 4 days after the reduction or cessation of ethanol intake and persists for 1 to 3 days. Seizures occur in approximately one-third of patients with DT and usually precede the onset of the DT. DT is associated with a 9 to 15 percent mortality rate, which may be higher among older patients and those with concurrent diseases, but can be reduced by appropriate treatment.

DT is a major impediment to the diagnosis and treatment of other critical illnesses. Concurrent illness such as infection (meningitis, pneumonia), metabolic disease, and trauma must be considered in the differential diagnosis. Detection of DT in an otherwise hemodynamically and metabolically unstable patient with respiratory depression may be difficult. A careful history of alcoholism and cessation of drinking, presence of signs of autonomic hyperactivity, and response to medication (see Treatment) may assist the intensivist in the management of this often intractable problem.

TREATMENT

Symptoms of the common withdrawal syndrome can be suppressed by the resumption of drinking or the administration of drugs such as barbiturates, phenothiazines, antihistamines, paraldehyde, or benzodiazepines. The benzodiazepines are preferred because they are safer and more effective. The long-acting benzodiazepines such as chlordiazepoxide may result in accumulation but also may help to smooth the waxing and waning of symptoms. Chlordiazepoxide (50 to 100 mg loading dose with repeat doses at 1 to 3 h) is useful. Up to 400 to 600 mg may be required in the first 24 to 48 h because of cross-tolerance. Because most of these patients are at risk for severe liver disease, a short-acting benzodiazepine such as oxazepam (half-life of 8 h) may be indicated in doses of 15 to 60 mg every 6 to 8 h. Chlordiazepoxide, though widely used, is not the ideal drug for management of the acute alcohol withdrawal syndrome. Because of its long half-life (up to 30 h), toxic effects of the drug may persist beyond the requirement for sedation, and patients often remain lethargic, ataxic, or confused for several days after the withdrawal state has resolved. A further disadvantage is its potential for respiratory decompensation, especially in patients with chronic pulmonary disease. Many alcoholics also suffer from obstructive pulmonary disease. Chlordiazepoxide is also a controlled drug, with potential for physical and psychologic dependence. It has its own withdrawal reactions.

Clorazepate dipotassium, 15 mg orally four times a day with rapid tapering by day 5, has been useful as a prophylactic against potential withdrawal seizures.[12] Intravenous phenobarbital[13] (260 mg initially followed by 130 mg every 30 min to an end point of light sedation) and calcium channel blockers[14] have shown early evidence of usefulness. Additional confirmatory studies are indicated, however. β-Adrenergic receptor antagonists such as atenolol (50 to 100 mg/day) may attenuate mild to moderate symptoms of alcohol withdrawal.[15]

Acute alcohol withdrawal may be primarily a central hyperadrenergic state. Withdrawal syndromes are known to correlate with increases in norepinephrine and 3-methoxy-4-hydroxyphenylglycol (MHPG) concentrations in the CNS.[16] Clonidine reduces both central and peripheral appearance of norepinephrine and MHPG concentrations.[17] The mechanism of action for clonidine in alcohol withdrawal appears to be mediated through stimulation of centrally located α_2-adrenergic receptors, resulting in a decrease in noradrenergic outflow from neurons located in the nucleus locus ceruleus.[18,19]

Clonidine, 0.2 mg four times on the first day, rapidly tapering to once on the fourth day, appeared effective in reducing heart rate, systolic blood pressure, and other adrenergically mediated signs and symptoms of acute alcohol withdrawal.[20] It may eventually supersede chlordiazepoxide as a drug of choice.

The DT patient is managed best in an ICU with continuous monitoring for any cardiac arrhythmias, and where fluid and electrolyte imbalances can be replenished with crystalline solutions. Fluid should be replaced with great care, because alcoholics may have an impaired ability to excrete water and a tendency to develop cerebral edema.[21] Magnesium supplementation will be needed to restore serum level deficiencies. The patient may require treatment for associated hyperthermia or hypothermia, hypoglycemia, pancreatitis, thiamine deficiency, alcoholic ketoacidosis, gastrointestinal bleeding, cerebral trauma, and any other disease underlying chronic alcoholism.

When sedation must be given quickly to the agitated patient with DT, one approach begins diazepam intravenously with a 10-mg loading dose followed by 5 mg every 5 to 10 min until the patient is calm.[22] Doses of 50 mg are often used for initial sedation; up to 215 mg has been given.[23] For severe agitation, 2 to 4 mg haloperidol intramuscularly may be useful. Then oxazepam is initiated at 30 mg every 6 h combined with clonidine at 0.2 mg every 6 h on the first day, both tapering to zero by day 4. The intensivist should watch carefully for any evidence of oversedation or hepatic encephalopathy, which are difficult to detect in these patients. A parenteral vitamin preparation containing thiamine and pyridoxine should be given daily for about 5 days to prevent the development of Wernicke's encephalopathy and Korsakoff's syndrome. Niacin should be added to prevent pellagra encephalopathy (vide infra).

The patient in DT may require restraints. As soon as feasible after admission skull films, CT scans of the head, and lumbar puncture should be obtained, as indicated. Steroids and ACTH should be avoided because they may mask infection and lead to sodium and electrolyte imbalance.

ALCOHOLIC KETOACIDOSIS

PATHOPHYSIOLOGY AND CLINICAL MANIFESTATIONS

Alcoholic ketoacidosis (AKA) follows withdrawal from alcohol and develops in chronic alcoholics with a recent history of heavy alcohol intake several days to several weeks prior to the episode.[24,25] Such patients have experienced vomiting and decreased food intake often due to gastritis, hepatitis, or pancreatitis or related to alcohol withdrawal, fatty liver infiltration, or aspiration pneumonia. They become volume depleted and usually have abruptly stopped or markedly decreased their alcohol intake 24 to 72 h before presentation. The patient becomes confused, drowsy, and occasionally comatose. Tachypnea is a common symptom, and the patient may present with breathlessness in a Kussmaul breathing pattern compensatory for the ketoacidosis. These patients often have no measurable blood alcohol levels when first seen in a health care facility. The blood glucose level is usually normal to slightly elevated. Most patients will respond to glucose-containing intravenous fluids without insulin. In some areas, AKA is the causative factor in up to 20 percent of patients presenting with ketoacidosis. Patients are usually conscious and able to give a good history.

The moderate to severe AKA is due to the formation of β-hydroxybutyrate (BOHB) and acetoacetate (AcAc). The BOHB usually predominates and therefore, testing with Ketostix and Acetest, which are most sensitive to AcAc, less so to acetone, and not at all to BOHB, may show only a weakly positive reaction when levels of BOHB are highest. The finding of ketonuria without glycosuria suggests the diagnosis. Serum lactate levels are only moderately elevated. Severe lactic acidosis would suggest another serious disorder such as hypoxemia or hypoperfusion.

Metabolic effects associated with AKA include hormonal changes (increased levels of cortisol, growth hormone, glucagon, free fatty acids, catecholamines, decreased levels of insulin and antidiuretic hormone) and effects secondary to any increase in the reduced nicotinamide-dinucleotide: nicotinamide-dinucleotide (NADH:NAD) ratio (increase in the BOHB:AcAc ratio and lactate production; decreased gluconeogenesis and citric acid cycle activity).

Electrolyte, glucose, and arterial blood-gas measurements are essential in making a diagnosis. The basic acid-base abnormality in AKA is an elevated anion gap metabolic acidosis. Hypokalemia and hypochloremia are often seen due to the bouts of prolonged vomiting. Serum potassium levels must be carefully monitored during treatment. The blood pH may vary from 6.96 to 7.61. A significant respiratory alkalosis may be seen as a compensatory response to the metabolic acidosis or from alcohol withdrawal or other associated illnesses. The protracted vomiting can lead to a primary metabolic alkalosis. The initial blood pH and bicarbonate levels are not good indicators of eventual outcome.

Serum ketone levels are markedly elevated. AcAc levels >2 meq/L (normal, <0.05) and BOHB levels over 10 meq/L (normal, <0.05) may be present. The BOHB:AcAc ratio (normally 1:1) rises to 5 to 10:1. When alcoholics with ketoacidosis are treated, the BOHB is oxidized to AcAc and later to acetone. Thus, the nitroprusside test may worsen when the patient is actually improving. It must be remembered that severe elevations of the anion gap (>30 meq/L) are found in ketoacidosis, hyperosmolar coma, lactic acidosis, and ingestion of ethylene glycol or methanol.

TREATMENT

Management of these patients requires correction of volume depletion and administration of glucose. The volume depletion is usually amenable to infusion of solutions of normal saline with dextrose. When the volume deficit is corrected (normal orthostatic blood pressure and pulse), 0.5 *N* saline with dextrose may be continued. Such intravenous therapy is continued until the serum bicarbonate level reaches 18 to 20 meq/L, signs of orthostasis have resolved, and oral fluids are well tolerated. Patients will respond to therapy within 12 h. Close monitoring (every 4 to 6 h) of serum potassium and phosphorus levels during treatment is important because hypokalemia and hypophosphatemia may ensue quickly. Potassium supplementation may be required. Sodium bicarbonate administration is usually not necessary except in severe cases of acidosis (pH <7.1). Insulin therapy is not required. Thiamine (50 to 100 mg) should be given to prevent development of the Wernicke-Korsakoff syndrome. Magnesium and multivitamins may be considered.

Wernicke's Encephalopathy and Korsakoff's Psychosis

PATHOPHYSIOLOGY AND CLINICAL PRESENTATION

Thiamine deficiency in alcoholics results from a combination of inadequate dietary intake, reduced gastrointestinal absorption, decreased hepatic storage, and impaired use of the vitamin.[26] A subset of thiamine-deficient alcoholics have Wernicke's encephalopathy, possibly due to an inherited or acquired abnormality of the thiamine-dependent enzyme, transketolase, which leads to a reduction in its affinity for thiamine. It only takes 18 days to become thiamine deficient on a thiamine-free diet,[27] and the Wernicke-Korsakoff syndrome has been precipitated in nonalcoholics receiving intravenous glucose therapy alone.[28,29]

Alcoholics account for most cases of Wernicke's encephalopathy in the United States, but patients with malnutrition due to hyperemesis gravidarum, starvation, thyrotoxicosis, gastric plication, bowel obstruction, renal dialysis, gastric malignancy, hyperparathyroidism, or acquired immunodeficiency syndrome are also at risk.[30]

Thiamine is a cofactor for transketolase, α-ketoglutarate dehydrogenase, pyruvate dehydrogenase, and branched-chain α-keto acid dehydrogenase. It may also have a function in axonal conduction and synaptic transmission.[31] A deficiency of thiamine can lead to decrease in use of glucose by the cerebrum. Sudden increases in glucose use by the brain accompany bursts of metabolic activity in vulnerable brain areas where structural brain lesions may develop.[32] This sudden increase in the use of glucose may indicate a shift from aerobic metabolism to rapid glycolysis, and such excitotoxicity may contribute to the pathogenesis of Wernicke's encephalopathy.[5]

Characteristic brain lesions of Wernicke's encephalopathy include symmetrical discoloration of structures surrounding the third ventricle, aqueduct, and fourth ventricle, with petechial hemorrhages in occasional acute cases and atrophy of the mamillary bodies in a majority of chronic cases. Subclinical cases can be diagnosed postmortem because of these distinctive findings. Autopsy studies have revealed a higher (0.8 to 2.8 percent) incidence of Wernicke's lesions in the general population than is predicted by clinical studies (0.04 to 0.13 percent).[33] This suggests that the classic clinical triad of encephalopathy, ophthalmoplegia, and ataxia is either not recognized or not invariably present.

In its classic form, Wernicke's encephalopathy is a neurologic disorder of acute onset, characterized by ocular abnormalities, ataxia, and a global confusional state.[34] However, the critical care physician may find patients with this syndrome who are comatose, hypothermic, or hypotensive.[35] In fact, only one of three patients will present with the classic clinical triad. Most are profoundly disoriented, indifferent, and inattentive. Some will have an agitated delirium following ethanol withdrawal.

Ocular signs are a hallmark of Wernicke's encephalopathy. Horizontal nystagmus is present in 85 percent of patients, bilateral paralysis of the lateral rectus muscles in 54 percent, and horizontal conjugate gaze palsies in about 45 percent.[35] Vertical nystagmus also may be present. Less often pupillary abnormalities (sluggishness to reaction and anisocoria), ptosis, retinal hemorrhages, and papilledema are observed.

The global confusional state described above may be the only clinical feature of Wernicke's encephalopathy. Gait ataxia occurs in about 90 percent of cases and probably results from a combination of polyneuropathy, cerebellar involvement, and vestibular paresis. Hypothermia may be due to involvement of the temperature regulating center and hypotension due to a defect in efferent sympathetic outflow and decreased peripheral resistance. Coma may be the only manifestation of Wernicke's encephalopathy.

Laboratory abnormalities reflect the chronic disease state of such patients and include anemia, leukocytosis, and liver function test results often seen in alcoholics. The lumbar puncture may reveal an elevated cerebrospinal fluid (CSF) protein in up to one-third of cases, a nonspecific finding in many CNS diseases. CT scanning may demonstrate some ventricular enlargement, but this is not specific for this condition. Serum transketolase activity assays the thiamine stores but may be difficult to perform and is not easily available in many laboratories. A depressed serum magnesium level may indicate depressed function of the transketolase function.

TREATMENT

Patients suspected of having Wernicke's encephalopathy should be treated immediately with 100 mg thiamine daily, infused slowly in 500 mL fluid for at least 5 days.[5] At the same time, deficiencies of other vitamins including niacin, minerals, and electrolytes, especially magnesium, should be corrected. Intravenous glucose should be given only in conjunction with thiamine since the glucose alone can precipitate Wernicke's encephalopathy in thiamine-deficient patients.[35] Fortification of alcoholic beverages with thiamine has been suggested.[36]

KORSAKOFF'S SYNDROME

With prompt use of thiamine, the ocular signs of Wernicke's encephalopathy improve within hours to days. Ataxia may improve within days to weeks. Nevertheless, most patients are left with horizontal nystagmus, some ataxia, and a disabling memory disturbance characterized by marked deficits in anterograde and retrograde memory, apathy, an intact sensorium, and otherwise normal intellectual abilities. Confabulation and decreased initiative are evident. About 25 percent of patients with this syndrome do not recover and require long-term care; only 20 percent recover during follow-up care. The memory disorder appears to correlate with areas of decreased sensitivity on the CT scans of the dorsomedial thalamus. Treatment is largely supportive. Long-term administration of fluvoxamine, a serotonic-uptake blocker, has improved word recall in some patients.[37]

ALCOHOLIC PELLAGRA ENCEPHALOPATHY

Recent studies indicate that some alcoholic patients who have received thaimine and pyridoxine but not niacin have developed a secondary pellagra consisting of confusion or an altered state of consciousness, oppositional hypertonus, and myoclonus.[38,39] Such findings may develop over a period of weeks or during hospitalization several days after admission and apparent recovery from Wernicke's encephalopathy. Treatment with niacin may result in dramatic improvement. Stimulation of metabolic pathways by pyridoxine and thiamine may increase the relative deficit of niacin.

Severe Metabolic Acidosis with Osmolar Gaps

Poisonings with methanol and ethylene glycol share many clinical similarities. First, they characteristically produce a high anion gap metabolic acidosis with rapid production of acid. Next, patients present as apparently drunk without the odor of alcohol (ethanol) or the presence of ethanol in the blood. Third, analysis of plasma electrolytes and osmolality aids in the diagnosis. The measured plasma osmolality (freezing point depression method) exceeds the calculated osmolality, resulting in an osmolal gap.

$$2\ Na^+ + BUN/2.8 + glucose/18 = 280 \text{ to } 300 \text{ mOsm normally} \quad (170\text{-}1)$$

Methanol and ethylene glycol uniquely produce both a severe metabolic acidosis and a discrepancy between measured and calculated serum osmolality (Table 170-4).

Both are treated by ethanol infusion and hemodialysis. Metabolic acidosis in an alcoholic patient may develop in association with other concomitant diseases. Intensivists must be alert to the proclivity of some alcoholics to drink anything resembling ethyl alcohol.

TABLE 170-4 Effect of Some Solutes on Serum Osmolality

For Each 1 mg/dL of:	Serum Osmolality Will Increase (mOsm/kg H_2O):
Methanol	0.34
Ethanol	0.22
Ethylene glycol	0.20
Acetone	0.18
Isopropyl alcohol	0.17

An Increase in Serum Osmolality of 1 mOsm/kg H_2O Caused by:	Corresponds to a Concentration of (mg/dL):
Methanol	2.6
Ethanol	4.3
Ethylene glycol	5.0
Acetone	5.5
Isopropyl alcohol	5.9

SOURCE: Kulig K, Duffy JP, Linden CH, et al: Toxic effects of methanol, ethylene glycol and isopropyl alcohol. *Top Emerg Med* 6:16, 1984. Used with permission.

TABLE 170-5 Clinical Summaries of Toxicity of Other Alcohols

Methanol
- Metabolic acidosis, severe with anion gap and osmolal gap
- Visual difficulties
- Abdominal pain, nausea and vomiting, pancreatitis
- Latent period of 12–14 h

Ethylene Glycol
- Ethanol-like intoxication with no odor
- CNS depression, coma
- Metabolic acidosis, severe: large osmolal and anion gap
- Onset within 1 to 12 h
- Calcium oxalate crystals in urine
- Hypocalcemia, possible

Isopropyl (Rubbing) Alcohol
- Deep coma of acute onset (30–60 min)
- Early decreased or absent deep tendon reflexes
- Pinpoint unreactive pupils (dilated in fatal cases)
- Hypothermia
- Respiratory depression
- Odor of acetone on breath and in vomitus
- Acetonuria without acidemia
- Hypotension
- Melena or hematemesis
- Sponging with rubbing alcohol history, no hyperpnea
- Acetonuria without prominent glycosuria or acidemia
- Osmolal gap

METHANOL

Methanol toxicity[40–42] frequently results from the consumption of methanol-contaminated whiskey and may be fatal. It is a colorless, volatile liquid with a specific gravity (0.81) similar to ethanol (0.79), and has a distinctive odor that may be masked by impurities added during the production process. Adults have survived ingestions of 500 to 600 mL but 30 mL generally is considered a minimal lethal dose. As little as 10 mL may cause blindness (Table 170-5).

PHARMACOLOGY

Methanol is absorbed from the gastrointestinal tract, with peak serum levels occurring within 30 to 90 min. Skin and lung absorption can be significant. It has an apparent volume of distribution of 0.6 to 0.7 L/kg. Concentrations in the vitreous humor and optic nerve are high. About 90 to 95 percent of methanol in human beings is metabolized in the liver by the enzyme alcohol dehydrogenase to formaldehyde, which is rapidly converted by aldehyde dehydrogenase to formic acid. A folate-dependent pathway oxidizes formic acid to carbon dioxide. Ethanol is metabolized preferentially by alcohol dehydrogenase. Methanol is oxidized ten times more slowly than ethanol and thus has a longer elimination half-life.

The serum half-life of methanol with mild toxic ingestions is 14 to 20 h and, following severe exposure, 24 to 30 h. Concurrent administration of ethanol increases the serum half-life to 30 to 35 h by its competitive inhibition of alcohol dehydrogenase.

PATHOPHYSIOLOGY AND CLINICAL PRESENTATION

Accumulation of formic acid produces the severe toxicity (blindness, metabolic acidosis) seen after methanol poisoning. Formic acid appears to correlate better with clinical toxicity than serum methanol levels and may account for a significant portion of the bicarbonate deficit in severe poisoning.[40]

Following methanol exposure, symptoms (CNS depression, coma, visual difficulties, gastrointestinal symptoms—vomiting, abdominal pain, pancreatitis) may begin after an interval of 40 min to 72 h.[41] Methanol produces CNS depressant effects similar to those of ethanol. Such symptoms may be delayed by concomitant alcohol ingestion. A profound metabolic acidosis requiring large amounts of bicarbonate occurs in severe methanol poisoning due to the rapid formation of formic acid. Methanol causes a significant osmolal gap (see Table 170-4).

Asymptomatic individuals generally have peak methanol levels below 20 mg/dL. CNS symptoms appear above 20 mg/dL, ocular symptoms above 100 mg/dL, and fatalities in the range of 150 to 200 mg/dL if the patient is untreated. The blood level of methanol alone is not a reliable prognostic indicator because toxicity results mainly from formic acid production.

Laboratory examinations following methanol exposure should include blood methanol and ethanol levels, serum electrolyte determination with calculation of anion and osmolal gaps, serum calcium level, complete blood count, serum blood urea nitrogen (BUN) and creatinine concentrations, urinalysis, serum osmolality, hepatic aminotransferase levels, serum amylase content (isoamylase analysis indicates that a substantial portion of the elevation may be caused by salivary-type amylase), and serum creatine kinase concentration.

TREATMENT

Airway, breathing, and circulation should be evaluated in all patients. For obtunded patients, naloxone, glucose, and thiamine are given. Respiratory status is monitored carefully. Blood should be drawn for arterial blood-gas determinations to screen for metabolic acidosis and hypoxemia. Ipecac or lavage is useful if the patient presents within 2 h of ingestion and may be useful up to 4 h after ingestion if coma or coingested drugs reduce gastrointestinal motility. Charcoal and cathartics are not effective. Forced diuresis is not useful. Hemodialysis can remove methanol (100 to 200 mL/min clearance) and formic acid, whereas hemoperfusion removes neither. Hemodialysis is considerably more effective than peritoneal dialysis. Indications for dialysis procedures include the following[1,42]:

1. A peak methanol level >50 mg/dL is recommended in the medical literature, but the exact level is debatable. Dialysis reduces the prolonged ICU time required for ethanol therapy at methanol levels >50 mg/dL.
2. Metabolic acidosis not immediately correctable with bicarbonate therapy. High formate levels (i.e., >20 mg/dL) suggest the need for hemodialysis.
3. Any visual impairment
4. Renal failure

Dialysis may be stopped when the methanol level falls below 25 mg/dL. Ethanol also is dialyzed so the maintenance ethanol blood levels must be increased during dialysis. Ethanol levels should be maintained between 100 and 150 mg/dL to completely inhibit toxic metabolite formation. Intravenous ethanol is used because it is more reliable than oral administration, although it may be irritating to the veins. An intravenous solution of 10% ethanol in D_5W is optimal. Ethanol infusion is continued until the methanol level falls below the range of 20 to 25 mg/dL. Ethanol prolongs the elimination half-life of methanol to 24 to 30 h; hence, several days may be required to reduce the methanol level below 25 mg/dL when hemodialysis is not used.

Indications for ethanol use include:

1. Peak blood methanol levels >20 mg/dL
2. A history of methanol ingestion of 0.4 mL/kg, or any symptomatic patient, pending confirmatory blood methanol levels.
3. Acidosis
4. Any patient considered for hemodialysis

In severe adult poisoning where medical care will be delayed for several hours, three to four 1-oz oral "shots" of whiskey should be given before or during transport to the hospital. Administration of folate provides increased cofactor for the oxidation of formic acid to carbon dioxide. Folic acid, 50 mg intravenously every 4 h for several days, has been recommended as a large but safe dose. The use of folate is especially important in alcoholics, who may be folate depleted. Folate efficacy in human beings, however, has not been proven. Leucovorin is the active form of folate and may be substituted for folic acid.

Although it is still an investigational drug in the United States, 4-methylpyrazole may be an effective adjunctive agent to decrease methanol toxicity by inhibiting alcohol dehydrogenase.[43] Administration of 20 mg/kg/day orally or intravenously adequately inhibits alcohol dehydrogenase for about 24 h. Further clinical studies are required before this investigational drug is generally available.

Supportive care should include correction of the metabolic acidosis with bicarbonate therapy; consideration of hypoglycemia, hypocalcemia, and myoglobinuria; blood analysis including a complete blood count, electrolytes, creatinine, calcium, BUN, amylase, hepatic aminotransferases, serum methanol and ethanol levels; and phenytoin or diazepam for controlling seizures.

If there is a latency period before treatment is begun exceeding 10 h and a blood formate level above 50 mg/dL, severe methanol poisoning can ensue, possibly leading to permanent sequelae (ocular damage, death).[44]

ETHYLENE GLYCOL

Ethylene glycol, often used as an alcohol substitute or ingested in a suicide attempt, is a colorless, odorless, sweet-tasting compound with wide commercial use as an antifreeze, coolant, preservative, and glycerine substitute. Ingestion may result in death. Its metabolites lead to CNS, cardiopulmonary, and renal dysfunction together with severe metabolic acidosis.[45,46] The approximate minimum lethal dose is about 1 to 1.5 mL/kg (~ 100 mL in an adult).

PHARMACOLOGY

Ethylene glycol is rapidly absorbed orally with peak blood levels at 1 to 4 h; it distributes evenly throughout body tissue, is filtered through the renal glomeruli, and is then passively resorbed. It is partially metabolized to oxalic acid; the liver oxidizes ethylene glycol primarily to glycoaldehyde, glycolate, and then glyoxylate. The plasma half-life of ethylene glycol is approximately 3 to 5 h. At ethanol levels of 100 to 200 mg/dL, the half-life of ethylene glycol is prolonged to 17 h because of the 100-times-greater affinity of ethanol for alcohol dehydrogenase.

PATHOPHYSIOLOGY

Ethylene glycol ingestion results in a CNS depression similar to that caused by ethanol and methanol. Cranial nerve dysfunctions (bilateral facial paralysis, hearing loss) may occur between 6 and 13 days after ingestion.[47,48] It also produces toxic metabolites. The accumulation of glycolic acid leads to metabolic acidosis, an anion gap, and an osmolal gap (primarily from glycolic acid and some lactic acid formation).

Similar to ethanol and methanol, ethylene glycol produces severe gastrointestinal symptoms. Renal involvement (oliguria, flank pain, acute tubular necrosis) is prominent with ethylene glycol ingestion. Visual problems do not occur generally.

Urinary oxalate crystals (octahedral or tent-shaped dihydrate crystals and needle-like crystals, the monohydrate form) are frequently observed in ethylene glycol intoxication.

Hypocalcemia with QT prolongation and tetany may be due to the formation of the oxalate metabolite which rapidly precipitates as calcium oxalate mainly in the monohydrate form in various tissues such as brain, kidney, myocardium, and pancreas. This precipitation most probably leads to the characteristic lowering of the serum calcium and to arrhythmias, tetanic contractions, or even generalized seizures. A high anion gap metabolic acidosis with elevation of the osmolal gap is often observed. Glycolic acid and bicarbonate levels correlate with the clinical picture better than serum ethylene glycol levels, because the former two levels reflect the action of the toxic metabolities (see Table 170-5).

TREATMENT

Acidosis, fluid and electrolyte imbalance, and respiratory depression must be corrected. Emesis or lavage may be effective early after ingestion. Charcoal and cathartics probably are not effective.

Hemodialysis is superior to peritoneal dialysis. Dialysis can lead to a decrease in glycolic acid levels. Indications for early dialysis include deteriorating vital signs, metabolic acidosis not easily corrected, crystalluria, and serum ethylene glycol levels over 50 mg/dL. Dialysis should be to a serum ethylene glycol level of 10 mg/dL or less.

Ethanol therapy, by competitive inhibition of alcohol dehydrogenase, reduces the formation of toxic metabolites. A blood alcohol level of 100 mg/dL fully saturates human liver alcohol dehydrogenase. Indications for ethanol therapy include a strong suspicion of significant ethylene glycol ingestion pending determination of serum levels, peak serum ethylene glycol levels >20 mg/dL (with or without symptoms), and acidemia, regardless of ethylene glycol levels. The ethanol must be administered early after ingestion because the elimination half-life of ethylene glycol is 3 h at low concentrations. The dosage is the same as that for methanol poisoning and may be given intravenously or orally. For severe adult poisoning in which medical care will be delayed several hours, three to four 1-oz oral "shots" of 86-proof whiskey should be given before or during transport to the hospital. The intensivist should watch for hypoglycemia. Additional ethanol is used in the dialysate to replace the ethanol lost during the procedure.

Pyridoxine (100 mg four times daily for 2 days) may aid in promoting the metabolism of glyoxalate to glycine; thiamine (100 mg four times daily for 2 days) may facilitate the metabolism of glyoxalate from glycolic acid to a nontoxic metabolite, α-hydroxy-β-ketoadipate. Serum magnesium levels should be determined to guide magnesium replacement. 4-Methylpyrazole may be useful.[43] Supportive care should include the careful observation of electrolyte and fluid balance and monitoring of serum calcium and arterial pH levels. Intravenous bicarbonate can be used as required.

Isopropyl Alcohol

Isopropyl alcohol exhibits CNS depressant properties similar to those of ethanol, methanol, and ethylene glycol. The principal metabolite of isopropanol, acetone, is not associated with the renal, cardiac, retinal, or metabolic toxicity seen with the metabolites of ethylene glycol (glycolic acid) or methanol (formic acid). Isopropanol is second to ethanol as the most commonly ingested alcohol and is a common cause of drug overdosage. Toxicity results both from ingestion and from inhalation in poorly ventilated spaces, such as that which occurs in young children given isopropanol sponge baths.

Isopropyl alcohol is a clear, volatile liquid with a burning, bitter taste and an aromatic odor. It is used in industry as a solvent and disinfectant and in the home as a constituent of rubbing alcohol, skin and hair products, and antifreeze. It is twice as potent a CNS depressant as ethanol. The toxic dose is about 1 mL/kg of a 70% isopropanol solution (as commonly seen in rubbing alcohol), but as little as 0.5 mL/kg may cause symptoms. The lethal dose in an adult is roughly 240 mL (2 to 4 mL/kg). Adults have survived ingestions of a liter.

High concentrations cause nausea, headache, lightheadedness, and eventually, coma. More than three swallows of 70% isopropanol usually results in symptoms in children. Such ingestion requires medical observation.

PHARMACOLOGY

Most of an oral dose is absorbed within 30 min and complete absorption occurs within 2 h. Large overdoses can delay absorption. Skin absorption, although small, contributes to toxicity with prolonged contact, such as after an isopropanol sponge bath. About 20 to 50 percent of an absorbed dose is excreted unchanged.[49] Most isopropanol is oxidized to acetone with the aid of alcohol dehydrogenase. Acetone is eliminated slowly in the lung or kidney and is further metabolized to acetate formate and finally, CO_2.[50] Isopropanol metabolism follows concentration-dependent (first-order) kinetics. In intoxicated chronic alcoholics, isopropanol elimination exhibits first-order kinetics with a half-life of 2.5 to 3.2 h. The elimination half-life of the active metabolite, acetone, may be more prolonged. Small amounts of isopropanol are excreted into the stomach and saliva. Ketoacids are not produced in sufficient quantities to cause a severe metabolic acidosis.[51]

PATHOPHYSIOLOGY AND CLINICAL MANIFESTATIONS

Isopropanol is both a potent CNS depressant and, in large doses, a cardiovascular depressant. Acetone may potentiate and lengthen the duration of CNS symptoms. Conversion of acetone to acetic acid and formic acid may lead to a mild acidosis. The shift in the NAD:NADH ratio brought about by the action of alcohol dehydrogenase may cause decreased gluconeogenesis and hypoglycemia similar to ethanol.

Isopropanol intoxication occurs rapidly (30 to 60 min) and peaks in several hours. It presents similar to ethanol intoxication without an early elation phase. The duration of action is longer because of acetone formation, and the odor of acetone is more prominent. Severe poisoning presents early with deep coma, respiratory depression, and hypotension.

Initial dizziness, poor coordination, headache, and confusion may progress to stupor, coma, and loss of deep tendon reflexes in serious cases. Such serious CNS depression can persist for 24 h. Pupils may be miotic and accompanied by nystagmus. Gastric irritation occurs with abdominal pain and vomiting. Hematemesis can occur.

Hypotension with large overdoses may result from peripheral vasodilation but serious arrhythmias are not seen. Tachycardia is a common finding.

Acetone levels and ethanol tolerance must be considered when evaluating isopropanol blood levels. Blood isopropanol levels of 120 to 200 mg/dL have been associated with coma and death and have been considered lethal levels, but no close correlation has been found between blood isopropanol levels and physical findings in overdose.[1]

Isopropanol is an alcohol that produces an osmolal gap (see Table 170-4). Seriously toxic levels of 200 mg/dL can produce a 34-mOsm change in the osmolal gap. Because acetone produces similar changes in osmolality, acetone levels must be considered in correlating osmolality to blood isopropanol levels.

Screenings for electrolytes, BUN, creatinine, glucose, arterial blood-gas, serum acetone, hepatic aminotransferase concentrations, and complete blood counts are indicated in severe isopropanol ingestion with depressed mental status. High serum ketone levels with minimal acidosis are characteristic of isopropanol ingestion (see Table 170-5).

Acetone does not appear to be shunted into the formation of acetoacetic and β-hydroxybutyric acids. Blood and urine glucose is either normal or slightly elevated following isopropyl alcohol poisoning, further differentiating this condition from diabetic ketoacidosis. Normoglycemic ketoacidosis is rare but does occur.

Intoxication with isopropyl rubbing alcohol should be suspected in alcoholics with a positive nitroprusside reaction (Acetest) in the presence of a normal anion gap and a normal serum bicarbonate level.

TREATMENT

Careful cardiac and respiratory monitoring together with immediate intravenous access are required for the rapid-onset respiratory depression and hypotension produced by serious ingestions.

Isopropanol is rapidly absorbed and, therefore, the usefulness of emesis or lavage 2 h postingestion may be limited. Ipecac is most effective when given within 30 min postingestion. Activated charcoal and cathartics are not useful. Isopropanol overdoses may respond to either peritoneal dialysis or hemodialysis, especially if initiated early. Dialysis should be considered in patients whose hypotension is not easily corrected with fluids, those with evidence of deterioration of vital signs, patients in deep coma with or without complicating underlying disease, or those with high blood isopropanol levels (see Table 170-1). About 30 g isopropyl alcohol and 6 g acetone can be removed per hour with hemodialysis. This is approximately fifty times the rate of removal achieved by urinary excretion.

No antidotes are available.

Supportive care includes treatment of hypotension with fluids and observation for respiratory depression with arterial blood-gas and bedside assessment.

CASE PRESENTATION

A 22-year-old man, admitted to the hospital because of a question of drug ingestion, was reported to be a frequent abuser of illicit drugs including phencyclidine, lysergic acid, and methaqualone. He had no history of diabetes mellitus. Five days before admission he began to vomit repeatedly and complained of abdominal pain. Four days later he appeared improved but depressed. He ate very little. He was found asleep a few hours after his parents had left home and then became incoherent and violent. He vomited a colorless liquid.

Taken to the hospital, he admitted having ingested "something." Examination revealed tachycardia and dilated but reactive pupils. No needle marks were observed. The tongue appeared swollen. He became belligerent; restraints were applied and haloperidol was given. During the next few hours, unresponsiveness and Kussmaul respirations ensued and he was intubated. Urine (600 mL) was drained by an indwelling catheter. Naloxone hydrochloride was administered by vein. An ECG demonstrated a wandering atrial pacemaker. The blood pressure rose to 190/90 mmHg, and the heart rate fell to 55. A nasotracheal tube was passed, and dexamethasone and furosemide were administered by vein. Arterial blood-gas determination on an oxygen-enriched mixture disclosed Pa_{O_2} of 170 mmHg, Pa_{CO_2} of 41 mmHg, and pH of 7.00. Mannitol and several ampules of sodium bicarbonate were infused by vein. He developed right-sided jacksonian seizures. One can of antifreeze was found half-empty at his home.

The patient had been well except for a history of headaches and dizziness on fasting that was ascribed to hypoglycemia. He was not known to ingest alcohol, although his driver's license was revoked a month before admission on a charge of "driving while intoxicated."

Temperature was 36.7°C (97.8°F), the pulse 74, and the respirations 34. The blood pressure was 120/70 mmHg.

The patient was comatose, without spontaneous movement except for intermittent right-sided seizure activity. No lymphadenopathy or cutaneous evidence of sepsis was found, and no signs of trauma were seen; a nasotracheal tube was present in the right nostril. The neck was supple, and the carotid arteries were normal. Inspiratory rales were heard throughout both lungs, most prominently over the left upper lobe. The heart was not enlarged; a grade 2 systolic ejection murmur was heard along the upper left sternal border. The abdomen was normal. Rectal examination disclosed decreased sphincter tone but was otherwise negative. Neurologic examination showed a lack of response to noxious stimuli. The eyes were in midposition; a doll's-head maneuver and caloric stimuli yielded no response. The pupils were 7 mm in diameter and constricted <1 mm on exposure to light; the optic fundi appeared normal. The extremities were flaccid, and no tendon reflexes were elicited. During the examination, a seizure began with clonic movements of the right thumb that spread to the hand, arm, and right side of the face and then became generalized, lasting about 30 s.

The serum glucose level by Dexi-Stik was 250 mg/dL or greater. A ferric chloride test and tests on the urine and serum for ketones were negative. The urine gave a +++ test for protein and a + test for glucose; there were five white blood cells and innumerable red blood cells per high-power field; a few uric acid crystals were seen, without oxalate or hippurate crystals. The hematocrit was 50.6%; the white cell count was 36,200, with 75 percent neutrophils. A stool specimen gave a negative test for occult blood. The BUN was 18 mg/dL, the creatinine 3.3 mg/dL, the glucose 376 mg/dL, the calcium 8.1 mg/dL, the phosphorus 5.4 mg/dL, the bilirubin 0.3 mg/dL, the ammonia 4.3 μg, and the globulin 3.5 g/dL. The sodium was 152 meq/L, the potassium 4.8 meq/L, the chloride 91 meq/L, the carbon dioxide 3 meq/L, the lactate 6.7 meq/L, and the osmolality 432 mOsm/Kg. The serum aspartate aminotransferase (SGOT) was 29 U, the lactic dehydrogenase 271 U, the creatine phosphokinase 68 U, the amylase 14 U, and the alkaline phosphatase 32 IU/L. A specimen of arterial blood, drawn while the patient was breathing an oxygen-enriched mixture, showed that the Pa_{O_2} was 101 mmHg, the Pa_{CO_2} 32 mmHg, and the pH 6.93. An ECG demonstrated an idioventricular rhythm or junctional rhythm with aberrant conduction of 40/min; the complexes were wide and low, with flat T waves; no intrinsic atrial activity was observed, although there were occasional retrograde P waves. An x-ray film of the chest revealed ill-defined diffuse parenchymal opacities, with focal consolidation in the left upper lung field: an endotracheal tube was in an appropriate position, with its tip 5 cm above the carina; a central venous pressure line was coiled in the superior vena cava but terminated centrally; the heart appeared normal. A "toxic screening test" gave negative results for methanol, ethanol, ketones, salicylate, barbiturate, and other drugs. Microscopical examination of stained specimens of aspirated sputum disclosed a moderate number of neutrophils and gram-positive intracellular diplococci.

Ventilatory assistance was given, and 50% glucose and additional doses of naloxone hydrochloride were administered, without effect. After the rapid intravenous injection of 6 ampules of sodium bicarbonate, a specimen of arterial blood, drawn while the patient was breathing an oxygen-enriched mixture, revealed that the Pa_{O_2} was 77 mmHg, the Pa_{CO_2} 41 mmHg and the pH 6.87. Physostigmine was administered by vein; the pupils did not constrict, the heart rate fell to 38/min, and the patient became hypotensive. An infusion of isoproterenol resulted in an increased heart rate. He became anuric; an intravenous infusion of mannitol was ineffective. Dopamine was begun. Brief seizures recurred, and phenytoin sodium was given, without effect; pancuronium bromide was administered. Pyridoxine, thiamine, and 5% ethanol were administered by vein, together with 11 ampules of sodium bicarbonate. The patient was transferred to the ICU. The eyes were slightly abducted and immobile; the corneal reflexes were absent, but the retinas and optic disks appeared normal. The limbs were flaccid and areflexive; plantar stimulation evoked no response. A cisternal puncture yielded 5 mL slightly xanthochromic fluid, without gross blood; the initial pressure was 300 mmH_2O after 10 s off the respirator; microscopical examination revealed 124 white blood cells, of which 80 percent were neutrophils and 20 percent lymphocytes, and 24 red blood cells/mm^3; no microorganisms or crystals were observed; the glucose value was 258 mg/dL and the protein 1520 mg/dL.

Penicillin, nafcillin, and gentamicin were administered by vein, with 2000 mg methylprednisolone. Extracorporeal hemodialysis was initiated, with a bath of sodium bicarbonate solution. Nine more ampules of sodium bicarbonate were given, with calcium salts. Anuria persisted, and the hypotension became more severe. Large volumes of dopamine, isoproterenol and levarterenol bitartrate were administered, but the systolic pressure did not rise above 70 to 80 mmHg. The patient died 9 h after admission.[52]

CASE DISCUSSION

This young drug abuser had a sudden change in mentation, becoming incoherent and violent, and passed into coma in a few hours. He developed focal seizures, evidence of meningitis, hypertension followed by hypotension, cardiac arrhythmias, diffuse pulmonary involvement, and renal failure. A severe, progressive metabolic acidosis ensued resistant to large amounts of bicarbonate. There was a very high anion gap (58 meq/L). The degree of acidosis was out of proportion to the extent of the renal failure and was resistant to large amounts of bicarbonate. Starvation ketosis decreases the serum bicarbonate level only by a few milliequivalents. He was not a chronic alcoholic. This helps rule out alcoholic ketoacidosis. Lactic acidosis was not a significant factor (lactate in blood was far less than the anion gap of 58 meq/L). Salicylate toxicity is ruled out by the absence of salicylates in the blood and paraldehyde by absence of a typical odor and no history of ingestion.

Methanol and ethylene glycol both develop a high anion gap metabolic acidosis with rapid production of acid. In addition, the apparent drunkenness without the odor of alcohol on the breath or its presence in the blood is suggestive. The measured plasma osmolality exceeded the calculated osmolality by about 80 mOsm/kg water. Ethanol can produce this, though there was none measured. A history of drinking a half-can of antifreeze (about 50 mL?) was enough to cause death. Test of the serum for methanol was negative, and there were no retinal changes. The early CNS findings (appearing drunk, comatose, convulsions within 12 h, CSF findings of meningoencephalitis, presence of hypertension and leukocytosis, myopathy (increased serum creatine phosphokinases level), accelerated course, and mild hypocalcemia all point to ethylene glycol, even in the absence of oxalate crystals in the urine which are positive in about 50 percent of poisonings by this substrate.[53]

The toxicology screen, which was received after the patient's death, revealed the highly toxic ethylene glycol level of 200 mg/dL. At autopsy, the kidneys exhibited bifringent sheathlike crystals in the proximal and distal tubules. Calcium oxalate crystals were also found in the walls of many brain vessels, with patchy focal necrosis of the brain and a sterile meningitis. The lungs were edematous, probably due to the cardiopulmonary toxicity of ethylene glycol combined with the large amounts of fluid administered.

Patients are often admitted to hospitals which are not capable of performing analysis of ethylene glycol or its metabolites on a 24-h basis. Specific treatment with ethanol and hemodialysis is often delayed, with fatal consequences, because of delayed diagnosis. When specific analysis capabilities are not available or the diagnosis is not immediately apparent, calculation of the anion and osmolal gaps may permit earlier diagnosis and treatment. Repetitive urine microscopies may disclose the presence of the typical calcium oxalate monohydrate crystals.

In this case, the half-empty can of antifreeze, the high anion gap metabolic acidosis, the high osmolal gap, and the inadequacy of very large amounts of sodium bicarbonate to restore a normal blood pH may have suggested a possible diagnosis of ethylene glycol poisoning. Ethanol therapy (intravenous solution of 10% ethanol in D_5W) sufficient to maintain a blood ethanol level in the range of 100 to 150 mg/dL will inhibit toxic metabolite formation.

Hemodialysis can supplement the ethanol administration since it becomes, especially in the presence of compromised renal function, the major route for removal of ethylene glycol from the body and speeds removal of the toxic metabolite glycolic acid. Hemodialysis and ethanol should be continued until ethylene glycol is no longer detected in the plasma and acidosis is corrected. If blood enthylene glycol determinations are not available, hemodialysis should be continued for at least 8 h and rapidly repeated if acidosis reappears.

References

1. Ellenhorn MJ, Barceloux DG: *Medical Toxicology. Diagnosis and Treatment of Human Poisoning.* New York, Elsevier Scientific Publishing Company, 1988, pp 781–812.
2. Lovejoy FH Jr: Ethanol intoxication. Clin Toxicol Rev 4:1, 1981.
3. Lieber CS: Biochemical and molecular basis of alcohol-induced injury to liver and other tissues. N Engl J Med 319:1639, 1988.
4. American Academy of Pediatrics. Committee on Adolescents: Alcohol use and abuse, a pediatric concern. Pediatrics 79:450, 1987.
5. Charness ME, Simon RP, Greenberg DA: Ethanol and the nervous system. N Engl J Med 321:442, 1989.
6. Ng SKC, Hauser WA, Brust JCM, et al: Alcohol consumption and withdrawal in new-onset seizures. N Engl J Med 319:666, 1988.
7. Brennan FN, Lyttle JA: Alcohol and seizures: a review. J R Soc Med 80:571, 1987.
8. Anstadt GW: Alcohol withdrawal and seizures. J Occup Med 31:888, 1989.
9. Lerner WD, Fallon HJ: The alcohol withdrawal syndrome. N Engl J Med 313:951, 1985.
10. Mendelson JH: Biologic concomitants of alcoholism. N Engl J Med 283:24, 1970.
11. Aminoff MJ, Simon RP: Status epilepticus: Causes, clinical features and consequences in 98 patients. Am J Med 69:652, 1980.
12. Haddox VG, Bidder G, Waldron LE, et al: Clorazepate use may prevent alcohol withdrawal convulsions. West J Med 146:695, 1987.
13. Young GP, Rores C, Murphy C, et al: Intravenous phenobarbital for alcohol withdrawal and convulsions. Ann Emerg Med 16:847, 1987.
14. Koppi S, Eberhardt G, Haller R, et al: Calcium-channel-blocking agent in the treatment of acute alcohol withdrawal—Caroverine versus meprobamate in a randomized double-blind study. Neuropsychobiology 17:49, 1987.
15. Horwitz RI, Gottlieb LD, Kraus ML: The efficacy of atenolol in the outpatient management of the alcohol withdrawal syndrome. Arch Intern Med 149:1089, 1989.
16. Borg S, Kvande H, Sedvall G: Central norepinephrine metabolism during alcohol intoxication in addicts and healthy volunteers. Science 213:1135, 1981.
17. Martin PR, Ebert MH, Gordon EK, et al: Effectiveness of clonidine in central and peripheral catecholamine metabolism. Clin Pharmacol Ther 35:322, 1984.
18. Svensson TH, Bunney BS, Aghajanian GK: Inhibition of both noradrenergic and serotonergic neurons in brain by the alpha adrenergic agonist clonidine. Brain Res 92:291, 1975.
19. Linnoila M, Mefford I, Nutt D, et al: Alcohol withdrawal and noradrenergic function. Ann Intern Med 107:875, 1987.
20. Baumgartner GR, Rowen RC: Clonidine vs chlordiazepoxide in the management of acute alcohol withdrawal syndrome. Arch Intern Med 147:1223, 1987.
21. Mander AJ, Weppner GJ, Chick JD, et al: An NMR study of cerebral edema and its biological correlates during withdrawal from alcohol. Alcohol Alcohol 23:97, 1988.
22. Chick J: Delirium tremens. Try to spot it early. Br Med J 298:3, 1989.
23. Brown CG: The alochol withdrawal syndrome. West J Med 138:579, 1983.
24. Adams SL, Mathews JJ, Flaherty JJ: Alcoholic ketoacidosis. Ann Emerg Med 16:90, 1987.
25. Thompson CJ, Johnston DG, Baylis PH, et al: Alcoholic ketoacidosis: An underdiagnosed condition? Br Med J 292:463, 1986.
26. Thomson AD, Ryle PR, Shaw GK: Ethanol, thiamine and brain damage. Alcohol Alcohol 18:27, 1983.
27. Ziporin ZZ, Nunes WT, Powell RC, et al: Excretion of thiamine and its metabolites in the urine of young adult males receiving restricted intakes of the vitamin. J Nutrit 85:287, 1965.
28. Nadel AM, Burger PC: Wernicke's encephalopathy following prolonged intravenous therapy. JAMA 235:2403, 1976.
29. Watson AJS, Walker JF, Tomkin GH, et al: Acute Wernicke's encephalopathy precipitated by glucose loading. Irish J Med Sci 150:301, 1981.
30. Davtyan DG, Vinters HV: Wernicke's encephalopathy in AIDS patient treated with zidovudine. Lancet 1:919, 1987.
31. Iwata H: Possible role of thiamine in the nervous system. Trends Parmacol Sci 3:171, 1982.
32. Hakim AM, Pappius HM: Sequence of metabolic, clinical and histological events in experimental thiamine deficiency. Ann Neurol 13:365, 1983.

33. Harter C: The incidence of Wernicke's encephalopathy in Australia—A neuropathological study of 131 cases. J Neurol Neurosurg Psychiatr 46:593, 1983.
34. Reuler JB, Girard DE, Cooney TG: Wernicke's encephalopathy. N Engl J Med 312:1035, 1985.
35. Victor M, Adams RD, Collins GH: The Wernicke-Korsakoff syndrome and related neurologic disorders due to alcoholism and malnutrition. *Contemporary Neurology Series.* Vol 3. Philadelphia, FA Davis, 1989.
36. Centerwall BS, Criqui MH: Prevention of the Wernicke-Korsakoff Syndrome. A cost-benefit analysis. N Engl J Med 299:285, 1978.
37. Martin PR, Adinoff B, Eckhard MJ, et al: Effective pharmacotherapy of alcoholic amnestic disorder with fluvoxamine: Preliminary findings. Arch Gen Psychiatry 46:617, 1989.
38. Sedaru M, Hauser-Hauw C, La Plane D, et al: The clinical spectrum of alcoholic pellagra encephalopathy. Brain 111:829, 1988.
39. Noel S, Telerman-Toppet N: Ethanol and the nervous system. N Engl J Med 322:407, 1990.
40. McMartin K, Ambre JJ, Tephly TR: Methanol poisoning in human subjects. Role for formic acid accumulation in the metabolic acidosis. Am J Med 68:414, 1980.
41. Martensson E, Olofsson V, Heath A: Clinical and metabolic features of ethanol-methanol poisoning in chronic alcoholics. Lancet 1:327, 1988.
42. Osterloh JD, Pond SM, Grady S, et al: Serum formate concentrations in methanol intoxication as a criterion for hemodialysis. Ann Intern Med 104:200, 1986.
43. Baud FJ, Galliot M, Astier A, et al: Treatment of ethylene glycol poisoning with intravenous 4-methylpyrazole. N Engl J Med 319:97, 1988.
44. Mahieu P, Hassoun A, Lauwerys R.: Predictors of methanol intoxication with unfavourable outcome. Human Toxicol 8:135, 1989.
45. Saladino R: Ethylene glycol. Clin Toxical Rev 11:1, 1989.
46. Jacobsen D, Hewlett TP, Webb R, et al: Ethylene glycol intoxication: Evaluation of kinetics and crystalluria. Am J Med 84:145, 1988.
47. Palmer BF, Eigenbrodt EH, Henrich WL: Cranial nerve deficit: A clue to the diagnosis of ethylene glycol poisoning. Am J Med 87:91, 1989.
48. Mallya KB, Mendis T, Guberman A: Bilateral facial paralysis following ethylene glycol ingestion. Can J Neurol Sci 13:340, 1986.
49. Natowicz M, Donahue J, Gorman L, et al: Pharmacokinetic analysis of a case of isopropanol intoxication. Clin Chem 31:326, 1985.
50. Lacouture PG, Heldreth DD, Shannon M, et al: Characteristics and testing for acetonemia/acetonuria after isopropyl alcohol ingestion. Vet Hum Toxicol 29:486, 1987.
51. Gaudet MP, Fraser GL: Isopropanol ingestion: Case report with pharmacokinetic analysis. Am J Emerg Med 7:297, 1989.
52. Case 38-1979. Case records of the Massachusetts General Hospital. Levinsky NG, discussant. N Engl J Med 301:650, 1979.
53. Jacobsen D, McMartin KE: Methanol and ethylene glycol poisonings. Mechanism of toxicity, clinical course, diagnosis and treatment. Med Toxicol 1:309, 1986.

Chapter 171

BARBITURATES AND OTHER SEDATIVE-HYPNOTIC DRUGS

MATTHEW J. ELLENHORN

KEY POINTS

- *Severe poisoning is signaled by the ingested dose, blood levels, coma, and hypotension.*
- *There are no antidotes for these drugs; gut decontamination with lavage and possibly activated charcoal may lessen toxicity.*
- *Forced alkaline diuresis and hemodialysis aid elimination of phenobarbital only.*
- *Effective supportive therapy includes: intubation for airway protection, ventilation for respiratory depression, volume expansion for hypotension, and occasionally, the need for inotropic agents for myocardial depression.*
- *Prevent or treat early the complications of supportive care of prolonged coma: hypoglycemia, aspiration pneumonia, pulmonary edema, gastrointestinal hemorrhage, rhabdomyolysis, renal failure, sepsis, hypothermia, and venous thrombosis.*
- *Physical and psychologic dependence on these drugs develop when taken at three to ten times the sedative dose from 1 to 2 months; abstinence syndrome produces psychosis, seizures, and sympathetic hyperactivity and can be prevented or treated with graded withdrawal of the equivalent doses of phenobarbital.*

Sedative-hypnotics consist of a number of chemically different compounds, both barbiturate and nonbarbiturate. Overdose or self-poisoning with these products may lead to a serious and often life-threatening condition. Of the relatively small number of patients who may not survive, death has been reported to be directly related to respiratory complications in many cases.[1] The critical care physician will encounter patients with poisoning or overdose by sedative-hypnotics, or withdrawal effects usually following long-term high dose ingestion of these drugs. Fortunately, the frequency of poisonings with many of these products has decreased over the past 20 years because of a perceived safety and often misuse of benzodiazepines[2] (see Chap. 172). With only a few exceptions, the treatment of poisoning with sedative-hypnotic drugs requires support of the patient on a ventilator with adequate replacement of circulating volume for hypotension and careful attention to details of preventing complications until the coma resolves.

Barbiturates

Barbiturates have been used in medical practice since 1903. By the early 1970s, barbiturate overdose was a leading cause of drug-induced death. The overdose and abuse potential of barbiturate sedatives led to development of the safer and more effective benzodiazepines. Toxic exposure to benzodiazepines is four times more common than to barbiturates, resulting in a 50 percent reduction in barbiturate-induced deaths over the last 10 years and a reduction in mortality to < 2 percent of hospitalized barbiturate overdose cases.[3]

Barbiturates are available to treat anxiety, gastrointestinal upset, pain, and sleep disorders. Although long-acting barbiturates are effective anticonvulsant drugs, diazepam and phenytoin are more commonly administered anticonvulsants in the emergency department. Ultrashort-acting barbiturates (Table 171-1) used for induction of anesthesia are an effective measure for situations such as emergency intubation. Barbiturates tend to reduce intracranial pressure and cerebral oxygen consumption after cranial surgery, cerebral trauma, and cardiac arrest. However, cardiovascular side effects limit their usefulness.[3]

PHARMACOLOGY

The parent compound, barbituric acid, has no intrinsic central nervous system (CNS) depressant properties. Substituting an alkyl, alkenyl, or aryl group primarily at position 5 confers sedative properties to the basic compound. Barbiturate compounds are divided into four categories based on their elimination half-lives in animals: ultrashort-acting (anesthetics), short-acting (sedative-hypnotics), intermediate-acting (sedative-hypnotics), and long-acting (antiepileptics) (see Table 171-1). The observed clinical effect depends on absorption, redistribution from tissue stores, and the presence of active metabolites. Therefore, the duration of action does not always correlate well with the elimination half-life. The more lipid soluble the barbiturate, the more rapid its onset, the shorter its duration, and the greater the degree of hypnotic activity.

Barbiturates are capable of producing all levels of CNS depression—from mild sedation to hypnosis to deep coma to death. They are strong respiratory depressants: respiratory depression begins when about three times the usual therapeutic dose is exceeded, and severe toxicity may result from ten times the hypnotic dose. At these concentrations, respiratory centers become insensitive to carbon dioxide, and the control of respiration becomes solely dependent on hypoxic drive. With further increases in barbiturate concentration, the hypoxic drive to respiration will fail, leading to cessation of respiration.

Since hepatic enzyme induction, coingested drugs, and ethanol can influence outcome, fatal doses are difficult to predict. Table 171-2 lists the therapeutic, toxic, and lethal blood levels for most sedative-hypnotics. Lethal adult doses are: phenobarbital, 8 to 10 g; secobarbital, pentobarbital, 2 to 4 g; amobarbital, butabarbital, 2 to 3 g. However,

TABLE 171-1 Barbiturate Pharmacokinetic Data[3]

	$T_{1/2}$ (h)	V_D (L/kg)	Protein Binding (%)	pK_a	Duration of Action (h)
Ultrashort-Acting (Anesthetics)					
Methohexital	1–2	1.1	73	7.9	0.3
Thiopental	6–46	1.4–6.7	72–86	7.6	0.3
Short-Acting (Sedative-Hypnotics)					
Pentobarbital	20–30	0.5–1.0	65	7.9	3
Secobarbital	22–29	1.6–1.9	46–70	7.9	3
Intermediate-Acting (Sedative-Hypnotics)					
Amobarbital	15–40	0.9–1.4	59	7.9	3–6
Aprobarbital	14–34	0.6–0.7	55–70	8.1	3–6
Butabarbital	34–42			7.9	3–6
Long-Acting (Antiepileptics)					
Barbital	48	0.4–0.6	25	7.8	6–12
Mephobarbital	48–52	2.6	40–60	7.8	6–12
Metharbital				8.5	
Phenobarbital	48–144	0.5–0.6	50	7.2	6–12

survival has occurred in an adult who reportedly ingested 20 g of amobarbital.[4] Gut decontamination should be induced in all cases where suspected ingested dose exceeds 5 to 6 mg/kg. Barbiturates are well absorbed (primarily from the small intestine). The onset of action is much more rapid with the short-acting drugs. Alcohol also increases the rate of absorption, possibly by increasing blood flow through the gastric mucosa.

Lipid solubility of the barbiturates is the dominant factor in their distribution in the body. The highly lipid-soluble ultrashort-acting barbiturates distribute into the gray matter of the brain within 30 s. As lipid solubility decreases, cerebral uptake decreases. Barbiturates such as phenobarbital accumulate more slowly in the brain. The highest concentrations of barbiturate occur at the steady state in the liver and kidney. The apparent volume of distribution ranges from 0.6 to 2.6 L/kg. Barbiturates rapidly cross the placenta and equilibrate in fetal fluid. They are also found in breast milk.

TABLE 171-2 Sedative-Hypnotic Drug Blood Levels (mg/dL)

	Therapeutic	Toxic	Lethal
Barbiturates			
Short-acting	0.1–0.8	0.7–1.4	3–4
Intermediate-acting	0.1–0.5	1–3	3
Phenobarbital	ca. 1.0	4–6	8–15
Barbital	ca. 1.0	6–8	10–20
Chloral hydrate	1.0	10	25
Ethchlorvynol	0.5	2	15
Glutethimide	0.2	1–8	3–10
Meprobamate	1	8–12	20
Methaqualone	0.5	1–3	3
Methyprylon	1.0	3–6	10

Barbiturates are slowly metabolized chiefly by the microsomal enzymes of the liver. Phenobarbital and other barbiturates induce liver microsomal enzymes and may accelerate metabolism of other concomitantly administered drugs metabolized by these enzymes (e.g., anticoagulants, digoxin/digitoxin, quinidine, tricyclic antidepressants, phenothiazines, testosterone, corticosteroids, and vitamin D or K). Metabolites may be active. Metabolism is generally more rapid in children and reduced in infants and in the elderly. The barbiturates which are most highly lipid soluble (and usually highly protein bound) are reabsorbed by the renal tubules. Tubular resorption is decreased when barbiturate ionization is increased. Thus, urinary alkalinization augments renal excretion of phenobarbital having a p*K*a of 7.2, but not other short-acting barbiturates having a higher p*K*a (see Table 171-1). Liver dysfunction, renal failure, chronic use, and age can affect the half-life, which ranges from an average of 1 h (methohexital) to 86 h (phenobarbital).

PATHOPHYSIOLOGY AND CLINICAL MANIFESTATIONS

Barbiturates are CNS depressants. These effects are most likely mediated through the inhibition of γ-aminobutyric acid (GABA) synapses of the brain and involve the $GABA_A$-benzodiazepine receptor-chloride iontophore system (see Chap. 172). Noradrenergic activity may also be selectively depressed. Barbiturates abolish the central respiratory drive. Respiratory depression is the usual cause of death in patients without ventilator support. As barbiturate concentrations rise, skeletal, smooth, and cardiac muscle are suppressed, leading to depressed myocardial contractility, vasodilation, and hypotension. In the gastrointestinal tract, reduced motility results in ileus.

Clinical effects arise from the CNS and cardiovascular system depressions. Short-acting barbiturate overdoses produce symptoms within 15 to 30 min and peak effects at 2 to 4 h. Overdoses of long-acting barbiturates lead to toxic reactions at 1 to 2 h with peak effects at 6 to 18 h. Initial fatalities result from cardiorespiratory arrest. Short-acting barbiturates appear more potent than other barbiturates in producing early apnea. Later causes of death result from respiratory failure, pneumonia, and pulmonary and cerebral edema. The major causes of hospital mortality are pulmonary edema and aspiration pneumonia. Problems related to difficulties with endotracheal intubation can affect ultimate morbidity and mortality.[1]

Toxic effects following barbiturate overdosage may initially resemble ethanol inebriation with slurred speech, ataxia, lethargy, nystagmus, headache, paresthesias, vertigo, and confusion. Unless hypoxia or coingestions complicate the clinical picture,[3] five stages of coma generally correlate with the severity of toxicity.

- Stage 0 Stuporous but responsive to verbal command
- Stage 1 Responsive to painful but not verbal stimulus
- Stage 2 Unresponsive to all stimuli but reflexes; vital signs intact
- Stage 3 Unresponsive, areflexic, but stable vital signs
- Stage 4 Unresponsive, areflexic and unstable vital signs

Since suppression of deep tendon reflexes correlates poorly with the depth of medullary depression, abnormalities in vital signs may be a more reliable sign in differentiation of stages 3 and 4 coma. Pupils are constricted but reactive early in coma but later dilate. Respiratory depression occurs early in coma, with slow or shallow respirations progressing to compromise of tidal volume and minute ventilatory volume. Hypoglycemia may contribute to CNS depression.

A weak and rapid pulse, cyanosis, cool and clammy skin, decreased urine output, and confusion indicate shock. The low cardiac output and tissue hypoperfusion are due to the relative hypovolemia which results from inhibition of vascular smooth muscle. Despite depression of myocardial contractility by barbiturates, the low output and hypotension are frequently responsive to fluid challenges. As such, placement of pulmonary pressure catheters is limited to patients vulnerable to pulmonary edema who remain hypotensive after initial fluid challenge. Hypothermia commonly occurs, especially in those patients in stage 3 or 4 coma.

Bullous skin lesions can develop primarily over pressure points, but not necessarily over areas of maximum pressure. These lesions are tense bullae surrounded by areas of erythema and commonly involve the fingers, malleoli, and medial aspect of the knee. They always appear in patients previously comatose, usually within 24 h.[5] Bullae are not diagnostic of barbiturate intoxication, since coma due to poisoning by carbon monoxide, amitriptyline, methadone, and other sedative-hypnotics (meprobamate, glutethimide, nitrazepam) produce similar lesions.[6]

Slowed gastrointestinal activity may be associated with a nonocclusive intestinal infarction after a phenobarbital overdose. Synergistic CNS depression occurs with general anesthetics, aliphatic alcohols (e.g., ethanol), narcotic analgesics, and other sedative-hypnotic drugs.

Serum barbiturate levels (see Table 171-2) complement clinical judgment but are not required for management. They may not reflect the brain barbiturate levels. Clinical effects depend on tolerance, underlying disease, age-related metabolism, and coingested drugs. The ingested dose and plasma barbiturate level may be the best correlates to serious intoxication. Short-acting barbiturates are more toxic at a given level than long-acting barbiturates (e.g., mortality is 5 percent for short-acting barbiturate levels over 3 mg/dL and 3 percent for long-acting barbiturate levels over 8 mg/dL).[3]

Evaluation of a patient with moderate to severe overdose should include a complete blood count, serum electrolytes, glucose, creatinine, urine myoglobin, and chest x-ray. Arterial blood-gas levels and tidal volumes should be obtained when clinical evidence of hypocapnia or hypoxemia appears. Generally, the electroencephalogram (EEG) displays a predictable progression of changes depending on the depth of coma. In severe cases, the EEG may be isoelectric, without the presence of irreversible brain damage.

Other Sedative-Hypnotics

CHLORAL HYDRATE

The usual recommended adult sedative dose of chloral hydrate is 500 mg to 1 g taken 30 min before surgery or sleep. A dose of >2 g may produce toxic symptoms. Ingestion of over 5 to 10 g may be lethal, although fatalities have resulted from the ingestion of 3 g and survival has followed a 36-g ingestion. Chloral hydrate is an alcohol. Its major metabolite, trichloroethanol, appears in the blood stream soon after ingestion. The initial sedative action may derive from the parent compound but prolonged effects are probably due to the active metabolite. The therapeutic half-life of chloral hydrate is 4 to 5 min whereas that of trichloroethanol is 8 to 12 h. Most of the trichloroethanol undergoes glucuronide conjugation and is excreted by the kidneys. A smaller part of trichloroethanol is oxidized to trichloroacetic acid, an inactive metabolite which has a half-life of 60 to 70 h.

In overdose, chloral hydrate produces significant CNS depression, gastrointestinal irritation, hepatitis, and proteinuria. Chloral hydrate induces a decrease in myocardial contractility and shortening of the refractory period. This can lead to resistant cardiac arrhythmias, particularly ventricular fibrillation, ventricular tachycardia, and supraventricular tachycardia, which are the usual modes of death following an overdose.

Additional points of interest following chloral hydrate ingestion include a disulfiramlike reaction when it is ingested with alcohol. Symptoms include headache, flushing, tachycardia, and hypotension, a distinct pearlike odor, and the early development of lethargy and a deep coma within 1 to 2 h after ingestion. The pupils, constricted early, may later dilate. Chloral hydrate is radiopaque, an additional useful indicator for effectiveness of decontamination procedures.[7]

ETHCHLORVYNOL

Sedative doses for therapeutic use of ethchlorvynol range from 500 to 700 mg. Between 4 and 10 g may produce mild to moderately toxic symptoms, depending on coingested drugs. Fatalities have followed doses of 5 g alone or 2.5 g when ethanol is coingested. Survival has been reported following ingestions of 80 to 125 g when vigorous supportive care and dialysis were instituted. Following a therapeutic dose, the elimination half-life of ethchlorvynol is about 25 h, but after an overdose the half-life of this drug may extend to 100 h.

Significant factors to be considered following an overdose of ethchlorvynol include its tendency to induce a prolonged (up to 17 days) coma, hypotension with relative bradycardia, hypothermia, a pungent or sweet breath odor, marked respiratory depression, development of noncardiogenic acute pulmonary edema and chest pain, especially following intravenous drug abuse, and excess salivation similar to that found in the cholinergic crisis following an organophosphate intoxication. Bilateral pleural effusions may follow intravenous use of ethchlorvynol and may result from increased extravascular lung water without a contribution of systemic venous hypertension. Pulmonary capillary wedge, pulmonary artery, and systemic venous pressures fall or remain unchanged following ethchlorvynol intoxication.[8–10]

GLUTETHIMIDE

Glutethimide is usually prescribed as a sedative-hypnotic in a dose of 250 to 500 mg. Toxic effects begin at doses of approximately 3 g, and ingestion of 10 g may be lethal. However, survival has followed an ingestion of 45 g. Following therapeutic doses, the elimination half-life of glutethimide is approximately 10 to 12 h. In acutely intoxicated patients, the half-life may rise to between 40 and 100 h.

Three significant findings in addition to those observed with most sedative-hypnotic drugs may be associated with a glutethimide overdose. First, severe poisoning can be associated with deep coma which fluctuates and is prolonged. This cyclic pattern of coma may be due to intermittent absorption from the gastrointestinal tract resulting from a drug-induced ileus, and enterohepatic recirculation of the drug and its active metabolite, 4-hydroxy-glutethimide (4-HG). Following an overdose the metabolite may increase in the plasma while the concentration of the parent compound decreases.

After an acute toxic ingestion, anticholinergic signs and symptoms are often prominent with pupillary dilation, ileus, urinary retention, warm dry skin, and inhibition of salivary secretion. These findings may persist for many hours after the patient has regained consciousness. Although respiratory depression is usually not severe after a glutethimide overdose, pulmonary edema and a pneumonitis often preceded by thick bronchial secretions may supervene and require intensive pulmonary care. Sudden apnea may occur.

Glutethimide is known to be subject to drug abuse, especially in combination with codeine, alcohol, or other CNS depressants. Cerebral edema and convulsions may be associated with an acute toxic ingestion.[11–12]

MEPROBAMATE

The usual adult therapeutic dose of meprobamate is 600 to 1600 mg daily. Toxic effects may develop following ingestions of 2 to 5 g. Fatalities have followed an overdose with 12 g; however, survival has occurred after a 40-g ingestion. Shock, pulmonary edema, and death are more commonly seen after ingestions exceeding 40 g. The elimination half-life of meprobamate after therapeutic doses is approximately 8 to 12 h; following an overdose, it may rise to 25 to 27 h.

An unusual feature associated with acute ingestions of meprobamate is its propensity to form concretions in the stomach. This may result in varying and discontinuous absorption of the drug, leading to fluctuating levels of consciousness with coma lasting over 24 h. In some cases, an initial recovery to full consciousness may precede a relapse to coma with respiratory arrest. When this occurs, gastroscopy may be indicated.

Following high doses of meprobamate, hypotension may appear early in the development of coma due to the depression of cardiac contractility. This drop in blood pressure can occur without significant respiratory depression. Care must be exercised with use of fluids to avoid precipitating pulmonary edema.[13–15]

METHYPRYLON

The usual adult hypnotic dose of methyprylon is 200 to 400 mg. Doses of 800 mg produce toxic effects. Ingestions >3 g produce stupor or a semicoma without alterations in blood pressure or respiration. Doses >6 g lead to a deep prolonged coma frequently accompanied by marked depressions of blood pressure and respiration and abnormal liver function. Death may occur following an ingestion of 6 g. However, survival has followed a 30-g ingestion treated with only supportive care. The elimination half-life of methyprylon following a therapeutic dose is 3 to 6 h. After overdose, the half-life is significantly prolonged.

Methyprylon overdosage may be associated with CNS depressant effects similar to those of the barbiturates. During the recovery phase the acutely methyprylon-intoxicated patient may exhibit seizures, delirium, tachycardia, paradoxical excitement, or hyperthermia.[3,16]

METHAQUALONE

Methaqualone is no longer available in the United States but is available elsewhere. The adult hypnotic dose is 150 to 200 mg. Coma lasting 4 and 90 h after ingestion of 3 and 7.5 g, respectively, has occurred. The lethal adult dose is 8 to 20 g, although an adult survived with supportive care following an ingestion of 24 g. The elimination half-life of methaqualone following a therapeutic dose is 10 to 50 h. This is prolonged in overdose.

Some unique aspects of acute intoxication with methaqualone that differ markedly from the other barbiturate and nonbarbiturate sedative-hypnotics include a tendency to produce muscular hyperactivity sufficient to require succinylcholine and curare for control. Assisted ventilation may be required. Overdoses may lead to a selective depression of polysynaptic spinal reflexes resulting in increased muscle tone, clonus, and muscle twitches.

Toxic doses of methaqualone result in inhibition of the first and second phase of platelet aggregation, prolongation of the prothrombin and partial thromboplastin times, and decrease in factors V and VII, all of which can lead to conjunctival, retinal, and gastrointestinal hemorrhage, together with purpura and petechiae to the skin. Coma may last 2 to 4 days following an acute overdose.[17–18]

Treatment of Poisoning with Barbiturates and Other Sedative-Hypnotic Drugs

Most patients with overdoses of sedative-hypnotic drugs respond to careful supportive care and require no special measures. Blood levels confirm drug ingestion but rarely improve patient management, except perhaps in severe poisoning when lethal levels suggest the need for hemoperfusion. Because of tolerance, coingested drugs, large tissue stores, underlying medical disease, and active metabolites, clinical evaluation correlates better with outcome than with blood levels. The intensivist should always screen for ethanol and other sedative-hypnotics when the clinical picture does not correlate with barbiturate blood levels, because most CNS depressants have synergistic actions (i.e., general anesthetics, alcohols, narcotics, sedative-hypnotics).

STABILIZATION

Because respiratory arrest is the major cause of early death, the patency of the airway and the adequacy of ventilation must be assessed first. No effective antidotes are available. Respiratory and CNS stimulants increase complications and should be avoided. Supplemental oxygen, head tilt-chin lift, intubation, and assisted ventilation are usually helpful and should be initiated early and maintained until the sedation has subsided sufficiently to allow spontaneous ventilation. This is often signaled by the patient's desire to remove the endotracheal tube. Careful bedside anticipation of this possibility can allow a planned nontraumatic extubation. Be aware that respiratory arrest may occur suddenly (e.g., during lavage procedure) and that mental status may fluctuate, leading to respiratory arrest after initial lightening of coma (e.g., meprobamate). An intravenous line is established with Ringer's lactate and a fluid challenge up to 2 L is given to hypotensive patients. A Foley catheter allows determination of fluid balance. Reduced urine output usually results from hypovolemia; diuretics are, therefore, not appropriate. Cardiac arrhythmias are rare but have been reported. Glucose, naloxone, and thiamine should be administered to all patients with depressed mental status.

ENHANCING DRUG ELIMINATION

As a result of decreased gastrointestinal motility and delayed gastric emptying, gut decontamination may be useful in obtunded patients up to 6 to 8 h postingestion. Induction of emesis is dangerous for any patient likely to develop early CNS depression (e.g., short-acting barbiturates). Comatose patients are lavaged only after a cuffed endotracheal tube has been inserted and the patient placed in the left lateral, head down position. The initial gastric aspirate should be saved for drug analysis. Barbiturates are well absorbed by charcoal; ten times the ingested dose (or 1 g/kg body weight) should be given together with a cathartic (sorbitol, magnesium citrate). Repeat doses of activated charcoal alone can reduce the average serum half-time of intravenous and oral phenobarbital. However, there may be no significant reduction in the duration of coma even after patients have received activated charcoal in 70 mL of 70 percent sorbitol every 4 h. Persistent diarrhea following sorbitol use can cause electrolyte and fluid depletion. Serial charcoal remains an unproven adjunctive therapy for comatose patients.

Urinary alkalinization (sodium bicarbonate 1 to 2 meq/kg every 4 to 6 h) may increase phenobarbital excretion five to ten times. Forced alkaline diuresis requires a urine flow of 3 to 6 mL/kg/h and a urinary pH over 7.5. Excessive fluid loads may aggravate cerebral or pulmonary edema. Potassium supplementation may be necessary to accomplish alkalinization. Alkaline diuresis is ineffective for short- and intermediate-acting barbiturates. The use of alkaline diuresis requires adequate renal perfusion and cardiac function to be effective and, therefore, is not indicated in patients having unstable hemodynamics and hypotension. In such patients, the use of alkalinization without diuresis is preferable.

Hemodialysis is more effective for long-acting barbiturates. Resin hemoperfusion with XAD-4 efficiently removes lipid-soluble barbiturates. As with hemodialysis, this measure should be reserved for severely intoxicated patients (e.g., respiratory failure) who do not respond well to supportive care or those who have lethal barbiturate levels. Release of barbiturates from tissue stores may be accompanied by late clinical deterioration.

PREVENTION AND EARLY TREATMENT OF COMPLICATIONS

Patients who ingest long-acting barbiturates may be comatose for 2 to 3 days. Prevention and early detection of the complications of both coma and barbiturate overdose are the mainstays of treatment. Common preventable complications are hypoglycemia, aspiration pneumonia, gastrointestinal hemorrhage, rhabdomyolysis, renal failure, sepsis, hypothermia, venous thrombosis, and pulmonary edema. Severely intoxicated patients with significant depression of myocardial function, as manifested by hypotension unresponsive to fluid challenge, require hemodynamic measurements using catheters in the pulmonary and systemic arteries to diagnose the cause of hypoperfusion and to titrate fluid and inotropic drug therapy. Consider early use of hemoperfusion and hemodialysis to hasten phenobarbital elimination in such patients. Treat bullous lesions as second-degree burns with layered dressings to protect the bullae (e.g., nonadherent dressing next to the skin surrounded by coarse gauze and a wrapping layer).

Dependence and Withdrawal

Similar to all other sedative-hypnotic drugs, barbiturates produce physical dependence when taken in three to five times the sedative dose for 1 to 2 months. Abrupt withdrawal from prolonged barbiturate use results in anxiety, agitation, confusion, delusions, hallucinations, tremor, ataxia, and hyperreflexia. Seizures occur in up to 75 percent of patients withdrawing from high dose pentobarbital therapy, and morbidity results from both seizures and trauma secondary to impaired judgment. For short- to intermediate-acting barbiturates, nausea, vomiting, orthostatic hypotension, and agitation develop 12 to 16 h after cessation of barbiturate use and peak at 48 to 72 h, with seizures and delirium. Resolution occurs in 4 to 7 days.[6] Timing and grading of barbiturate withdrawal symptoms are similar to ethanol-induced delirium tremens.[19] Confusion, impaired memory, and disorientation are primary manifestations. Withdrawal seizures may occur prior to the onset of confusion and often are more severe than those seen in ethanolism. Visual hallucinations are common, whereas delusions and other types of hallucinations present less frequently. Symptoms subside 3 to 4 days after withdrawal and rarely persist over a week.

Any sedative-hypnotic, with the exception of the opiates, can be withdrawn with the use of phenobarbital or benzodiazepines because of cross-tolerance. The development of barbiturate withdrawal symptoms may require reinstituting the usual barbiturate dose with gradual reduction (10 percent every 3 days) until discontinued.[20] Phenobarbital has a wider margin of safety in the setting of barbiturate withdrawal than short-acting barbiturates. The stabilizing dose of phenobarbital can be calculated by knowing the equivalency of the sedative-hypnotic drug with 30 mg phenobarbital.[19] Phenobarbital in a stabilizing dose is given for 2 days in three to four divided doses based on the drug history (Wesson method). After stabilization, the phenobarbital dose is reduced by 30 mg/day. If minor withdrawal symptoms develop, 200 mg pentobarbital is administered intramuscularly, and the daily phenobarbital dose is decreased by 25 percent. If signs of phenobarbital toxicity appear, the daily dose is reduced by 50 percent, and withdrawal is continued. Coaddiction to opiates should be considered in difficult cases, because opiate withdrawal may be difficult to differentiate from sedative-hypnotic withdrawal.

CASE PRESENTATION

A 58-year-old woman with a prior psychiatric history but no major medical problems was admitted to a local hospital in grade 4 coma with suspicion of drug intoxication. The systolic blood pressure was 70 mmHg. She was intubated and treated with gastric lavage and charcoal administration. Intravenous naloxone, 0.4 mg, was given without effect. Intensive supportive therapy had no effect. She was transferred to the ICU 10 h after admission still in grade 4 coma. Her systolic pressure was 60 mmHg, pulse rate 65/min, and temperature 31°C (88°F). No tendon reflexes or pupillary responses were present. Laboratory data showed the hemoglobin to be 11.6 g/dL, sodium 128 mmol/L, potassium 2.9 mmol/L, chloride 91 mmol/L, and normal BUN and creatinine. Plasma meprobamate concentration was elevated. No benzodiazepines, salicylate, barbiturates, propoxyphene, acetaminophen, or ethanol were detected.

She was put on a respirator, rewarmed to 36°C (96.8°F), and given a dopamine infusion, increased to 10μg/kg/min with increase of systolic pressure to 80 mmHg and of heart rate to 90/min. A central venous pressure (CVP) catheter was introduced into the left internal jugular vein with an initial reading of 4 cmH_2O. A fluid challenge of 250 mL saline solution was administered over 15 min and raised the CVP to 6 cmH_2O and the systolic pressure to 100 mmHg. A lumbar puncture produced normal spinal fluid except for an elevated pressure (26 cmH_2O). She was treated with mannitol intravenously. Due to her critical condition, charcoal hemoperfusion was initiated 4 h after admission. Her pupils began to react to light. There was no other apparent change in her condition during hemoperfusion until after 3.6 h when she exhibited asystole. She was immediately resuscitated with external cardiopulmonary resuscitation, epinephrine, and DC shock. These efforts resulted in sinus rhythm after 20 min. One hour after termination of hemoperfusion, she suddenly deteriorated with cyanosis and no recordable blood pressure. The clinical diagnosis of left-sided tension pneumothorax was made, and she was treated with a chest tube. After 4 days, the chest tube and ventilator were no longer necessary, and her condition gradually improved. A complicating bronchopneumonia was treated with antibiotics, and she was discharged from the unit. After 9 days, mitral insufficiency was diagnosed by routine auscultation and phonocardiography. This was probably due to papillary muscle dysfunction following myocardial infarction. Her cardiac status was reasonably compensated by treatment with digoxin and diuretics.

CASE DISCUSSION

The signs and symptoms reported in this case are typical of severe meprobamate poisoning. Unfortunately, this patient suffered cardiac arrest several hours after the start of the hemoperfusion, initiated or complicated by an acute myocardial infarction. Treatment consisted of intensive supportive therapy mainly directed toward hypotension, hypothermia, and respiratory failure. The use of a vasoconstrictor to raise blood pressure in this hypovolemic patient is controversial. Her physicians were concerned that fluid administration would worsen presumed cerebral edema. In such a patient a pulmonary artery catheter might aid fluid management while intracranial pressure determination would provide endpoints for the titration of fluids.

Gastric lavage should be performed after the airway is secured and followed by activated charcoal in repeated doses, since they may reduce the elimination half-life of meprobamate. Hemoperfusion was implemented because this meprobamate intoxication was complicated by severe hypotension, hypothermia, and respiratory depression not responsive to supportive therapy. Hemoperfusion should be continued for 5 to 6 h unless marked clinical improvement allows earlier discontinuation. With a half-life of plasma meprobamate of 2 to 4 h during hemoperfusion, the drug level should then be reduced to about 25 percent of the initial level.[13] A second hemoperfusion might be indicated if bezoar formation causes rebound effect and relapse into complications. In such cases, gastroscopy with destruction of the drug mass and lavage of the resulting fragments may also be indicated.[14] As commonly occurs, the patient's recovery was slowed by a hospital-acquired pneumonia.

References

1. Jay SJ, Johanson WG Jr, Pierce AK: Respiratory complications of overdose with sedative drugs. Am Rev Respir Dis. 112:591, 1975.
2. Bertino JS Jr, Reed MD: Barbiturate and nonbarbiturate sedative hypnotic intoxication in children. Ped Clin North Am 33:703, 1986.
3. Ellenhorn MJ, Barceloux DG: *Medical Toxicology. Diagnosis and Treatment of Human Poisoning.* New York, Elsevier 1988, pp 576–580.
4. Terplan M, Unger AM: Survival following massive barbiturate ingestion. JAMA 198:322, 1966.
5. Parrish J, Arndt KA: Skin lesions in barbiturate poisoning. Lancet 2:764, 1970.
6. Gaudreault P: Barbiturates. Clin Toxicol Rev 3:1, 1981.
7. Graham SR, Day RO, Lee R, Fulde GWO: Overdose with chloral hydrate: A pharmacological and therapeutic review. Med J Aust 149:686, 1988.
8. Miller KS, Sahn SA: Bilateral exudative pleural effusions following intravenous ethchlorvynol administration. Chest 95:464, 1989.
9. Burton WN, Vender J, Shapiro BA: Adult respiratory distress syndrome after Placidyl abuse. Crit Care Med 8:48, 1980.
10. Teehan BP, Maher JF, Carey JJH, et al: Acute ethchlorvynol (Placidyl) intoxication. Ann Intern Med 72:875, 1970.
11. Wright N, Roscoe P: Acute glutethimide poisoning. Conservative management of 31 patients. JAMA 214:1704, 1970.
12. Greenblatt DJ, Allen MD, Harmatz SC, et al: Correlates of outcome following acute glutethimide overdosage. J Forensic Sci 24:76, 1979.
13. Jacobsen D, Wiik-Larsen E, Saltvedt E, Bredesen JE: Meprobamate kinetics during and after terminated hemoperfusion in acute intoxications. Clin Toxicol 25:317, 1987.
14. Schwartz HS: Acute meprobamate poisoning with gastrotomy and removal of a drug containing mass. N Engl J Med 195:1177, 1976.
15. Allen MD, Greenblatt DJ, Noel BJ: Meprobamate overdosage: A continuing problem. Clin Toxicol 11:501, 1977.
16. Pancorbo AS, Palagi PA, Piecoro JJ, et al: Hemodialysis in methyprylon overdose: Some pharmacokinetic considerations. JAMA 237:470, 1977.
17. Lawson AHH, Brown SS: Acute methaqualone (Mandrax) poisoning. Scot Med J 12:63, 1967.
18. Bailey DN: Methaqualone ingestion. Evaluation of present status. J Anal Toxicol 5:279, 1981.
19. Khantzian EJ, McKenna GJ: Acute toxic and withdrawal reactions associated with drug use and abuse. Ann Intern Med 90:361, 1979.
20. Smith DE, Wesson DR: A new method for treatment of barbiturate dependence. JAMA 213:294, 1970.

Chapter 172

THE BENZODIAZEPINES

MATTHEW J. ELLENHORN

KEY POINTS

- *Severe benzodiazepine (BZD) overdose is often combined with other poisons.*
- *When present, respiratory depression is treated with ventilatory support and hypotension with vascular volume expanders, until the drug wears off.*
- *Forced diuresis and hemodialysis are not helpful.*
- *Flumazenil is a BZD antagonist which reverses respiratory depression but may aggravate toxic effects of coingested drugs.*

The BZDs are among the world's most widely prescribed drugs. They have become popular because of their efficacy as anxiolytics, sedative-hypnotics, anticonvulsants, and muscle relaxants and because of their safety.[1] Few documented cases have been published attributing fatalities solely to BZD overdose. For the intensivist working in a critical care unit, contact with this group of drugs will largely be restricted to **1.** its use in the treatment of severe convulsions (status epilepticus); **2.** care of overdose, most often when the BZD has been ingested with another sedative-hypnotic, alcohol, or tricyclic antidepressant; **3.** patients who have severe withdrawal effects following the development of a BZD-dependent state; and **4.** its use as a sedative, particularly during management of unstable patients on the ventilator or during patient withdrawal from drugs of abuse, such as alcohol or cocaine. In the latter circumstances, large doses are often administered, and care must be taken to not have drug accumulation or dependence develop.

Pharmacology

The BZDs are generally well absorbed from the gastrointestinal tract. Following intramuscular administration of chlordiazepoxide hydrochloride or diazepam, absorption is slow and erratic. Absorption of lorazepam and midazolam hydrochloride by this route, however, appears to be rapid and complete (Table 172-1). Prazepam and flurazepam undergo first-pass metabolism in the liver. Plasma concentrations are low after oral use. In fact, plasma concentrations of the BZDs and their frequently active metabolites usually peak 1 to 3 h after ingestion. Blood levels are considerably varied between patients, and therapeutic plasma concentrations are difficult to define. Such levels confirm acute ingestions but do not guide clinical management.

TABLE 172-1 BZD Groups and Elimination Half-Life (h)

Ultrashort-Acting (<10 h)	
Midazolam (Versed)	2–5 h
Temazepam (Restoril)	10 h
Triazolam (Halcion)	1.7–3 h
Short-Acting (10–24 h)	
Alprazolam (Xanax)	11–14 h
Lorazepam (Ativan)	10–20 h
Oxazepam (Serax)	3–21 h
Long-Acting (>24 h)	
Chlordiazepoxide (Librium)	5–30 h
Chlorazepate (Tranxene)	36–200 h
Clonazepam (Clonopin)	10–50 h
Diazepam (Valium)	20–50 h
Flurazepam (Dalmane)	50–100 h
Prazepam (Centrex)	26–200 h

SOURCE: Adapted with permission from Ellenhorn MJ, Barceloux DG: *Medical Toxicology. Diagnosis and Treatment of Human Poisoning*. New York, Elsevier Science Publishing Co, 1988, p 581.

The BZDs are quickly and widely distributed into the tissues. For example, volumes of distribution (V_D) of diazepam are 0.95 to 2 L/kg, chlordiazepoxide 0.26 to 0.58 L/kg, triazolam 0.8 to 1.3 L/kg, and alprazolam 0.97 to 1.17 L/kg. This accounts for the fact that the duration of action of a single dose is much shorter than the long elimination half-life would tend to indicate. In fact, orally administered BZDs produce anxiolytic, skeletal muscle relaxant, and anticonvulsant effects after the first dose.

Based on differences in the elimination half-life, the BZDs are classified into long-, short-, and ultrashort-acting groups (see Table 172-1). These drugs are highly protein bound and highly lipid soluble, with parent drugs and metabolites crossing the placenta and being excreted in breast milk. There is a rapid uptake by the gray matter of the brain after absorption. Following an intravenous injection of diazepam, gray matter uptake occurs within 15 to 20 s, a factor which may be responsible for its rapid anticonvulsant effect.

Many BZD drugs are eliminated by metabolism in the liver. Biotransformation of BZD drugs by hepatic microsomal enzyme systems occurs, for example, initially by demethylation (diazepam) to active metabolites which can prolong the original drug effects. This step is prolonged in the elderly, in neonates, in patients with liver disease, and after concomitant use of drugs which inhibit the P-450 microsomal enzyme system. A second step, glucuronide conjugation, is not affected by these factors. Such conjugates are excreted in the urine. The elimination half-life may determine the ability of a BZD to accumulate but does not necessarily correlate with drug effect. Nonetheless, it is in the patients receiving accelerating or large doses for anxiety or withdrawal that accumulation with eventual prolonged action occurs—the physician must always explore the least dose achieving therapeutic goals. The duration of BZD effect is inversely correlated with the apparent V_D of the drug and not with its half-life.[2] In high dose abusers, the diazepam half-life ranges from 48 to 94 h.[3] The short-acting BZDs such as oxazepam and lorazepam are metabolized in the liver only by glucuronidation, have no active metabolites, and do not appear to be affected by liver disease. BZDs are not appreciably removed by hemodialysis. Many patients experience extensive sedative effects from the use of BZDs because of the effects of their underlying critical illness on liver function.

Pathophysiology

The clinical use of BZDs is based on a central nervous system (CNS) action mediated through central BZD receptor sites which modulate γ-aminobutyric acid (GABA)-activated transmission. The $GABA_A$-BZD receptor-chloride ionophore complex located on the subsynaptic membrane of the effector neuron is the principal inhibitor neurotransmitter of the human CNS. This receptor complex is activated (chloride channel open) by GABA agonists binding to $GABA_A$ receptors, or by barbiturates or BZD agonists interacting with their specific receptors in the presence of GABA.[4]

Activation of the GABA receptor increases neuronal membrane permeability to Cl^- by opening the Cl^- ionophore. When the Cl^- resting potential is more negative than the neuronal resting membrane potential, Cl^- will enter the neuron, resulting in hyperpolarization. In turn, this hyperpolarization depresses neuronal activity. This is the mechanism of GABA-ergic inhibitory neurotransmission. Such an increase in neurotransmission can alter cortical and subcortical function to the extent that consciousness and motor control are impaired.[5] The anxiolytic, sedative, and anticonvulsant properties of BZD-receptor agonists are mediated through this mechanism. The $GABA_A$ receptor is widely distributed in brain, mainly in cortical and limbic structures.[6] BZD acts mainly at the limbic system (anxiolytic effect), at the midbrain reticular formation (sedative-hypnotic effect), through prevention of generalization of epileptic activity (anticonvulsant effect), and centrally (muscle relaxant effect).[7]

Another class of BZD receptors, the peripheral BZD receptors, are present in a number of nonneuronal tissues. A substance similar to a BZD-receptor agonist may contribute to the pathogenesis of hepatic encephalopathy by functionally increasing GABA-mediated transmission.[8] Flumazenil, a BZD-receptor antagonist, may, in fact, have some ameliorative effects in hepatic encephalopathies.

Overdosage

Serious intoxications in adults following oral overdose with a BZD derivative alone is unusual.[9] The critical care physician will rarely see such cases. Such overdose usually results in somnolence, confusion, weakness, dizziness, diplopia, and dysarthria. Ataxia and coma may be seen in larger overdoses. Elderly patients and very young children appear to be more susceptible to the CNS depressant action of the BZDs. In these groups, death has been reported after overdose.[10]

Paradoxical delirium, aggressive behavior, respiratory depression, and hypotension are uncommon and can be controlled with and require general supportive care. Parenteral administration of a BZD may produce apnea, hypotension, bradycardia, or cardiac arrest, particularly in the elderly, in severely ill patients, and in patients with limited pulmonary reserve or unstable cardiovascular status and in instances where the drug is administered too rapidly intravenously.

Respiratory and cardiovascular depressant effects may result partially from the propylene glycol in a diazepam injection. Serious overdoses are more frequently reported following use of the short-acting (alprazolam, lorazepam, oxazepam) and ultrashort-acting (midazolam, temazepam, triazolam) derivatives.

When BZDs are ingested together with other CNS depressants (ethanol, sedative-hypnotics, antidepressants), severe life-threatening respiratory depression may ensue, requiring assisted ventilation and hemodynamic monitoring. The presence of coma following ingestion of a BZD in a patient unresponsive to a painful stimulus and marked by hypotension and severe respiratory depression should prompt a careful search (blood, urine, gastric contents) for coingested drugs, trauma, or an underlying medical disease.

Treatment of Overdose

Gastrointestinal decontamination (syrup of ipecac-induced emesis or lavage) is indicated in a recent substantial ingestion of a BZD, unless the patient is or is about to rapidly become obtunded, comatose, or convulsive. Such measures are most effective if begun within 30 min to 2 h after ingestion. These procedures are followed by activated charcoal (1 g/kg) and a saline cathartic administration. Multiple doses of activated charcoal (0.5 g/kg every 4 to 6 h) may be useful, but repeated doses of cathartics should be avoided. Cathartics should not be used if the patient has an ileus, a not uncommon complication of polypharmaceutical overdose. Vital signs are monitored regularly. Assisted ventilation should be provided for respiratory failure and hypotension treated with expansion of circulating volume. Forced diuresis and hemodialysis are not effective. Hemoperfusion has not been adequately studied in such cases.

Flumazenil, an investigational drug in the United States, may lead to more rapid awakening. Aminophylline may also be useful in reversing the sedative effects of diazepam, flurazepam, lorazepam, flunitrazepam, and midazolam.[11] Naloxone, physostigmine, and doxepram have been used with inconsistent results. Accordingly, it is problematic whether these drugs lead to a beneficial outcome in these patients.

FLUMAZENIL

Flumazenil (Ro 15-1788), marketed as Anexate by Roche overseas, is an investigational new drug in the United

States and has been shown to reverse the respiratory depressant and sedative effects of some BZDs.[12] Patients with coma due to BZD poisoning have in many cases responded to flumazenil with immediate awakening or at least considerable improvement in the stages of coma. In fact, some studies indicate that an absence of improvement in alertness after administration of 5 mg flumazenil rules out BZD in the origin of CNS depression.[13]

PHARMACOLOGY

Flumazenil is rapidly and well absorbed by both oral (600 mg) and intravenous (0.5 to 1.0 mg) routes. It is widely distributed in the tissues (V_D of 0.63 to 1.5 L/kg) and has a high hepatic clearance. There are three metabolites: *N*-desmethylflumazenil, *N*-desmethylflumazenil acid, and desmethylflumazenil acid. Each also is conjugated to a glucuronide. The activity of the metabolites has not been evaluated. It is cleared from the plasma at the rate of 520 to 1300 mL/min. The plasma half-life, 0.7 to 1.3 h, is clearly shorter than the half-life of most BZDs. Approximately 40 percent of flumazenil is protein bound and 50 to 60 percent circulates in the free state. It freely enters the CNS and <0.2 percent is excreted unchanged. Its duration of action after intravenous use is short (15 to 140 min). Flumazenil crosses the placenta.

Mechanism of Action

Flumazenil is the first BZD-receptor antagonist to be studied extensively throughout the world and marketed outside of the United States. In the United Kingdom, the intravenous injection is licensed for the termination of general anesthesia induced or maintained with BZDs, for the reversal of BZD sedation in short diagnostic or therapeutic procedures, and in intensive care. It was first thought to be a simple antagonist, but it may also stimulate BZD receptors and have non-BZD actions.

In BZD overdose, flumazenil does not appear to improve the generally satisfactory outcome; however, it may help to clarify the diagnosis when the contribution of the BZD to depressed consciousness is in doubt, and to avoid the need for ventilatory support when BZD contributes significantly to severe respiratory depression.[14]

Dose

The definitive dose of flumazenil as an antidote to BZD remains to be determined. In diazepam- or midazolam-induced coma, 25 μg/min after a 2.5-mg bolus seems to be sufficient to maintain arousal.[15] Alternatively, an initial dose of 200 μg is followed with further 100-μg increments at 60-s intervals until sedation is reversed, up to a maximum dose of 2 mg.[15] In severe poisoning with a long-acting BZD, continuous infusion may be useful to prevent relapse of the coma.

PROBLEMS

Undesirable effects which may be induced by flumazenil are summarized in Table 172-2. Although flumazenil has a pharmacologically fascinating role in BZD overdose, it is not clear whether the hospital stay of a BZD-overdosed patient is reduced by the use of this antidote. Even so, it may keep a few such patients out of the ICU, and the diagnosis established may reduce unnecessary procedures (computed tomography scans, lavage) in the treatment of a patient with coma of unknown etiology.[16] Patients with BZD poisoning (coma, high Pa_{CO2} levels) who suddenly become alert after flumazenil use may be predisposed to a "catecholamine rush" similar to that occasionally seen after naloxone use for opiate-induced CNS depression. This may lead to such undesirable effects as hypertension or cardiac arrhythmias. Furthermore, flumazenil can unmask convulsive properties of other drugs as illustrated in the following case presentation.[17]

TABLE 172-2 Flumazenil—Undesirable Effects

1. Unmasking effect of proconvulsant drug: can induce convulsions and ventricular tachycardia in a patient after multiple drug overdose with a tricyclic antidepressant and a BZD
2. Induction of convulsions in epileptics controlled by BZD
3. Incomplete reversal of BZD-induced respiratory depression (may still require tracheal intubation, ventilatory assistance)
4. Insufficient dose
5. Tachycardia and arrhythmia on sudden awakening after flumazenil given for BZD sedation (catecholamine rush); bradycardia
6. Production of withdrawal state in a patient dependent on BZD; may occur in a postoperative recovery room
7. Resedation because of short half-life of flumazenil and longer half-life of the BZD
8. May increase sympathetic effects on heart in a mixed overdose by removing the protective effect of BZD, leading, for example, to chloral hydrate-induced ventricular arrhythmias
9. May lead to status epilepticus in mixed overdoses
10. Increase in blood pressure in patient with preexisting hypertension
11. Flushing, sweating, agitation, nausea, vomiting, hypotension

CASE PRESENTATION

A 57-year-old woman was found unrousable in bed by her husband. She had been well apart from depression, for which she had been receiving lorazepam, 2 mg/day, and amitriptyline, 75 mg/day, but no empty bottles were found at home. On admission, she was deeply unconscious with no response to pain and absent tendon reflexes. Pupils were mid dilated and nonreacting. The extremities were cool, and systolic blood pressure was 55 mmHg. She was bradypneic with a poor tidal volume and a core temperature of 34.4°C (94°F). The cardiac monitor showed a nodal rhythm and frequent multifocal ventricular premature beats, ventricular couplets, triplets, and salvos of ventricular tachycardia. The patient was intubated. A large bore gastric tube was placed and gastric lavage performed. Warming measures were instituted. Respiratory depression was treated with ventilatory support and hypotension with vascular volume expanders. No vasoactive drugs were administered.

In view of the depth of the coma, probable hypoventilation, and history of presumptive BZD ingestion, a trial of flumazenil was undertaken. It was given intravenously, slowly to reduce the likelihood of unmasking the CNS stimulatory effects of the tricyclic antidepressant. Two 50-μg boluses were given, each in 30 s, 2 min apart, followed by 100 μg every 3 to 4 min to a total dose of 500 μg. Respiratory rate increased to 20/min accompanied by increased depth of respiration but with no change in consciousness level. Five minutes later she developed grand mal convulsions. These convulsions were followed 15 s later by ventricular tachycardia, with no blood pressure, which reverted to sinus rhythm, with DC cardioversion. The convulsions ceased spontaneously after 30 s but recurred within 2 min, again followed by sustained ventricular tachycardia. This pattern of events recurred, with a total of nine cardioversions being made. Convulsions were eventually terminated with intravenous diazepam and thiopentone. Supportive treatment was continued in the ICU, and the patient recovered over 48 h. A history of lorazepam and amitriptyline overdose was later obtained.

CASE DISCUSSION

Supportive care was adequate and effective in treating this patient for the coma, respiratory depression, hypothermia, and hypovolemic shock complicating her ingestion of lorazepam and amitryptyline. Despite the clinical suspicion of BZD overdose, aminophylline and vasoactive drugs were not considered necessary; in retrospect, their use might have precipitated the convulsions and arrhythmias she suffered after flumazenil.

This specific BZD antagonist was used to reverse the central sedative effect of lorazepam, in the hope of shortening the duration of ventilator management and coma. Although respiratory depression was ameliorated, flumazenil unmasked the epileptogenic effects of the coingested tricyclic antidepressant. The ensuing convulsions probably accentuated the cardiac sensitivity to amitryptyline by inducing acidosis and increased circulating catecholamines. In addition, there may have been a lessening by flumazenil of the expected lorazepam inhibition of sympathetic outflow.

References

1. Ellenhorn MJ, Barceloux DG: *Medical Toxicology. Diagnosis and Treatment of Human Poisoning.* New York, Elsevier Science Publishing Co, 1988, pp 580–586.
2. Greenblatt DJ, Shader RI, Abernethy DR: Current status of benzodiazepines. N Engl J Med 309:354, 1983.
3. Rhodes PJ, Rhodes RS: Elimination kinetics and symptomatology of diazepam withdrawal in abusers. Clin Toxicol 22:371, 1984.
4. Paul SM, Marangos PJ, Skolnick P: The benzodiazepine-GABA-chloride ionophore receptor complex: Common site of minor tranquilizer action. Biol Psychiat 16:213, 1981.
5. Jones EA, Gammal SH, Martin P: Hepatic encephalopathy: New light on an old problem. Q J Med New Series 69:851, 1988.
6. Mohler H, Richards JG: The benzodiazepine receptor: A pharmacological control element of brain function. Eur J Anaesthesiol suppl 2:15, 1988.
7. Amitai Y: Benzodiazepines. Clin Toxicol Rev 7:1, 1985.
8. Skolnick P: The γ-aminobutyric acid A (GABA) receptor complex and hepatic encephalopathy. Some recent advances. Ann Intern Med 110:532, 1989.
9. Greenblatt DJ, Allen MD, Noel BJ, Shader RI: Acute overdosage with benzodiazepine derivatives. Clin Pharmacol Ther 21:497, 1977.
10. Sunter JP, Bal TS, Cowan WK: Three cases of fatal triazolam poisoning. Br Med J 297:719, 1988.
11. Gallen JS: Aminophylline reversal of midazolam sedation. Anesth Analg 69:260, 1989.
12. Prischl F, Donner A, Grimm G, et al: Value of flumazenil in benzodiazepine self-poisoning. Med Toxicol 3:334, 1988.
13. Hofer P, Scollo-Lavizzari G: Benzodiazepine antagonist Ro 15-1788 in self-poisoning: Diagnostic and therapeutic use. Arch Intern Med 145:663, 1985.
14. Flumazenil—The first benzodiazepine antagonist. Drug Ther Bull 27:39, 1989.
15. Lheureux P, Askenasi R: Specific treatment of benzodiazepine overdose. Human Toxicol 7:165, 1988.
16. Burkhart K, Kulig K, Rumack BH: The diagnostic utility of flumazenil (a benzodiazepine antagonist) in coma of unknown etiology. Vet Hum Toxicol 31:376, 1989.
17. Marchant B, Wray R, Leach A, Nama M: Flumazenil causing convulsions and ventricular tachycardia. Br Med J 299:860, 1989.

Chapter 173 CYCLIC ANTIDEPRESSANT OVERDOSE

JESSE HALL
GREGORY A. SCHMIDT

KEY POINTS

- *Cyclic antidepressant overdose is a frequent cause for ICU admission.*
- *Any patient with anticholinergic, neurologic, or cardiac toxicity (including QRS duration >100 ms) requires monitoring.*
- *Neurologic deterioration can be abrupt and unpredictable.*
- *Ventricular arrhythmia, respiratory arrest, hypotension, and seizures are the most important causes of morbidity and mortality.*
- *Acidemia, which potentiates toxicity, must be prevented or aggressively treated.*
- *Therapeutic alkalemia using sodium bicarbonate or hyperventilation may be beneficial.*

Cyclic antidepressants are commonly involved in suicide attempts and accidental overdoses. These drugs, which are widely available in North America and Europe, lead to substantial morbidity and mortality. In most critical care physicians' experience only illicit drug overdose is a more frequent cause of ICU admission. Because cardiovascular and neurologic complications of these drugs are life-threatening, the physician must be particularly alert to their occurrence.

Clinical Pharmacology

The cyclic compounds used first in the treatment of depression were phenothiazine analogues which contained a three-ringed nucleus and were referred to as *tricyclic antidepressants* (TCAs). In the past decade many new agents have been introduced, including tetracyclics (e.g., maprotiline), monocyclics, bicyclics, dibenzoxazepines (e.g., amoxapine) and various structurally unique congeners (e.g., trazodone) (Table 173-1). Several authors have encouraged the use of the term *cyclic antidepressants* for this growing class of drugs, with attention to specific subclasses since toxicities may differ.[1,2] Although the manifestations of acute overdose of most of the TCAs and the tetracyclic drug maprotiline are similar, the structurally dissimilar agents amoxapine and trazodone may exhibit substantially less cardiac toxicity.[1,3] The actual risk associated with these newer agents will be better defined with more experience.

TABLE 173-1 Classes of Cyclic Antidepressants

Tricyclics	*Bicyclics*
Imipramine[a]	Viloxazine
Desipramine[a]	
Amitriptyline[a]	*Dibenzoxazepines*
Nortriptyline[a]	Amoxapine[a]
Trimipramine[a]	*Other*
Protriptyline[a]	Trazodone[a]
Doxepin[a]	Fluoxetine[a]
Butriptyline	Bupropion[a]
Clomipramine	
Dibenzepin	
Dothiepin	
Tetracyclics	
Maprotiline[a]	
Mianserin	

[a] Available in the United States

In therapeutic doses, the cyclic antidepressants are well absorbed from the gastrointestinal tract. With overdose, however, the anticholinergic effects can dramatically impair gut motility and delay absorption. Therefore, measures to evacuate the stomach and to bind gut stores are important aspects of management. The volume of distribution of these drugs is large because they are both very lipid soluble and highly protein bound. The fraction of free TCA in the serum is significantly affected by serum pH, which may explain why acidosis potentiates toxicity. Metabolism of TCAs takes place primarily in the liver so that drugs which interfere with hydroxylation (e.g., morphine, haldol) may impede clearance.[4] Renal excretion of these drugs is minimal.

The implications of the binding and clearance characteristics of these drugs are: **1.** body stores are large and clearance may be prolonged after toxic ingestion; **2.** forced diuresis, hemodialysis, and hemoperfusion are unlikely to substantially enhance clearance; and **3.** drugs or diseases which impair hepatic metabolism can lead to protracted toxicity.

The usual therapeutic dose of the TCAs is 2 to 4 mg/kg/day. Toxicity is increasingly prominent when more than 10 to 15 mg/kg/day is taken. Childhood fatalities have been seen with doses as low as 15 mg/kg so that even a few tablets may be lethal to an infant.[5] In an adult, more than 2 g is typically taken before life-threatening complications of ventilatory failure, arrhythmia, or seizure occur. Of course, details regarding precise dose, or even the drug taken, are rarely available or reliable during early management. Moreover, as with any toxic ingestion, the physician must consider and exclude the possibility of multiple intoxicants.

Manifestations of Acute Overdose

Even in therapeutic doses, the cyclic antidepressants may cause sedation, generalized anticholinergic effects, and orthostatic hypotension. "Quinidinelike" membrane effects

TABLE 173-2 Major Toxicities in Acute Overdose

CNS Abnormalities	*Hypotension and Hypoperfusion*
Hallucinations	
Seizures	*Cardiac Arrythmias*
Coma	Supraventricular tachycardias
Anticholinergic Crisis	Ventricular tachycardia
Mydriasis and blurred vision	Torsade de pointes
Urinary retention	Ventricular fibrillation
Dry mucous membranes	Advanced heart block
Constipation and ileus	Bradycardia and asystole
Sinus tachycardia	
Hyperthermia or hypothermia	
Confusion, agitation, hallucination	

can lead to cardiac arrhythmias. In acute overdose, the major toxicities can be viewed largely as amplifications of these side effects (Table 173-2).

CENTRAL NERVOUS SYSTEM (CNS) ABNORMALITIES

The most common manifestation of overdose is depression of the level of consciousness. In addition, agitation, confusion, extrapyramidal signs, and hallucinations have been described. Progression from lethargy to coma and even to ventilatory failure can be extraordinarily rapid, more so than in other drug ingestions.[6] This may be related to rapid absorption of large quantities of drug or to redistribution of drug into the CNS. This phenomenon has important implications for early management (vide infra). It is important to note that coma from uncomplicated TCA overdose tends to resolve rapidly, usually within 12 to 24 h.[7] Accordingly, protracted obtundation should prompt consideration of other causes, such as coingested drugs, anoxic encephalopathy related to shock, or occult trauma. Some of the newer non-TCAs (e.g., maprotiline) have longer half-lives which may prolong coma.

Seizures are relatively common in patients requiring hospitalization and are associated with increased mortality.[8] Generalized seizures may herald cardiopulmonary arrest.[9] It is possible that tonic-clonic seizure activity potentiates cardiac toxicity by producing a metabolic acidosis which increases free drug concentration. Generalized seizures, therefore, require immediate control and a heightened awareness of the potential for sudden arrhythmias.

ANTICHOLINERGIC CRISIS

Cyclic antidepressants vary in their degree of muscarinic-receptor blockade and hence in their anticholinergic action. Sinus tachycardia, the most common rhythm abnormality in these patients, is most often due to this drug effect. Blurred vision, urinary retention, and dry mucous membranes are relatively common findings. Anticholinergic effects on the gut are of particular importance. Diminished peristalsis and delayed gastric emptying make drug recovery from the gut possible. Also, the possibility of ileus requires constant vigilance when repeated doses of activated charcoal are given, since gastric overdistention may lead to aspiration.

HYPOTENSION AND HYPOPERFUSION

TCAs cause both central and peripheral α-receptor blockade. This is the likely cause of the postural hypotension occasionally noted with therapeutic use. In acute overdose, hypotension may be profound, causing hypoperfusion and lactic acidosis. Hypotension can be followed shortly by cardiac arrest.[10,11] Although the peripheral vascular effects of these drugs account for the hypotension in most cases, it has been speculated that ventricular dysfunction may also occur.[12]

CARDIAC ARRHYTHMIAS

Mortality in cyclic antidepressant overdose is most often related to severe hypotension or cardiac arrhythmia.[10] Mechanisms of arrhythmogenesis include: **1.** anticholinergic effects; **2.** blockade of norepinephrine uptake resulting in increased adrenergic tone; **3.** quinidinelike effects which lead to depressed His-Purkinje conduction and facilitate reentrant ventricular arrhythmias; and **4.** myocardial ischemia from hypotension.[13]

The cardiac arrhythmias seen include tachyarrhythmias as well as advanced heart block and asystole (see Table 173-2). Sinus tachycardia is a common antecedent to more unstable rhythms, but malignant ventricular arrhythmias can interrupt normal sinus rhythm. Although sinus tachycardia is a sensitive marker for the anticholinergic effects of these drugs, it may not predict other mechanisms of cardiac toxicity.

The electrocardiographic (ECG) manifestations of cyclic antidepressant overdose include sinus tachycardia, QRS prolongation, rightward axis or right bundle branch block, PR and QT interval prolongation, and ST-T wave abnormalities. Limb lead QRS prolongation of $>$100 ms identifies a subpopulation of patients at greater risk for both seizures and arrhythmias.[14]

Management

REQUIREMENTS FOR ADMISSION AND MONITORING

Since QRS prolongation predicts subsequent toxicity, its use has been advocated as the primary determinant of the need for admission and monitoring. In one series negligible toxicity was noted when the maximal QRS duration was $<$100 ms on an admission ECG.[14] In a subsequent study, however, significant numbers of patients who lacked QRS prolongation went on to have seizures or ventricular arrythmias.[15] Nonetheless, all large series of patients with cyclic antidepressant overdose have reported that anticholinergic, CNS, and cardiac toxicities appear within 6 h of ingestion, if at all.

Accordingly, the combination of clinical assessment supplemented by measurement of the QRS duration can safely determine the need for admission. In any suspected cyclic antidepressant overdose, prolongation of the maximal initial limb lead QRS duration beyond 100 ms mandates continuous ECG monitoring and observation for CNS or circulatory deterioration. If the initial QRS duration is <100 ms *and no anticholinergic manifestations or CNS abnormalities are present,* the patient can be observed in the emergency department for 6 h. If *no* such abnormalities develop, the likelihood of significant toxicity is very low and referral for psychiatric evaluation may be made. If any abnormalities develop during this period of observation, however, admission to the closely monitored environment of the ICU is warranted.

Most qualitative urine and blood screens will detect the majority of cyclic antidepressants or major metabolites, but the clinician is advised to determine the limitations of the particular tests used in each hospital. Quantitative serum levels of these drugs can also be readily performed, but only correlate roughly with toxicity and are therefore unlikely to affect management.

MODIFICATION OF GENERAL MANAGEMENT

Because life-threatening arrhythmias may occur without warning, intravenous access should be established early (Table 173-3). Patients with *depressed consciousness of any degree* require extremely close monitoring, because deterioration may be abrupt. Dextrose, naloxone hydrochloride, and thiamine should be given to address potentially correctable contributors to lethargy. Activated charcoal should be given to bind unabsorbed drug. It is unwise to administer syrup of ipecac to symptomatic patients, because seizures or rapid deterioration of consciousness may lead to aspiration.

If consciousness is depressed, careful monitoring of the adequacy of ventilation is required, with frequent determination of arterial P_{CO_2} and pH. *Any degree of respiratory acidosis* should be treated with prompt intubation and mechanical ventilation. Obtundation with compromise of airway protection is an additional indication for endotracheal intubation. Once intubation is accomplished, gastric lavage should be carried out with a large bore tube, followed by activated charcoal and a cathartic. Careful serial assessments of the anticholinergic effects on the gastrointestinal tract must also be made. Absence of bowel sounds, development of abdominal distention, or large gastric residuals should prompt discontinuation of charcoal and institution of gastric suction. If bowel peristalsis is present, repeat doses of charcoal can be given every 6 h.

Given the pharmacokinetics of these drugs, forced diuresis, hemodialysis, and peritoneal dialysis have no role in the management of overdose. Hemoperfusion has been demonstrated to hasten drug clearance but is not generally recommended.[16]

TABLE 173-3 General Management Principles

Early IV access and activated charcoal
Avoid ipecac syrup and type I antiarrhythmic drugs
Admit and monitor based on QRS duration, symptoms, and signs
Gastric lavage if airway is protected
Early intubation and mechanical ventilation
No role for diuresis or dialysis
Maintain serum pH 7.45–7.55

THERAPEUTIC ALKALEMIA

Acidemia is thought to potentiate cardiac and CNS toxicity by increasing the concentration of free drug in the serum. The two major acidemic threats to patients with TCA overdose are lactic acidosis following seizures and respiratory acidosis resulting from coma. Numerous anecdotal reports have suggested that evolution of acidemia causes a "vicious cycle" of hypoperfusion and seizures that leads to worsening acidosis followed by ventilatory failure and death.

Accordingly, it is strongly recommended that any degree of hypoventilation be promptly reversed with mechanical ventilation. Similarly, generalized seizures must be promptly controlled. In any patient with significant toxicity—hypotension, respiratory depression requiring ventilatory support, seizures, ventricular arrhythmias, or advanced heart block—serum pH should be maintained between 7.45 and 7.55. Either bicarbonate infusion[1] or hyperventilation[17] to achieve metabolic or respiratory alkalemia, respectively, appears effective. If a patient requires mechanical ventilation and serum pH can be maintained above 7.45 with hyperventilation to a P_{CO_2} of 25 to 30, no further manipulation of pH is suggested. If the patient does not require mechanical ventilation or if hyperventilation cannot achieve the suggested degree of alkalemia, bicarbonate should be infused (2 ampules sodium bicarbonate/L 5% dextrose solution).

PHYSOSTIGMINE

We do not advise the use of physostigmine in cyclic antidepressant overdose. Physostigmine salicylate blocks cholinesterase and has been used in a number of poisonings with anticholinergic agents (see Chap. 168). It rapidly reverses coma and extrapyramidal side effects in TCA overdose and has been recommended for both CNS and cardiac toxicity. However, improved mentation is usually transient. In addition, this agent has been associated with worsened seizures, bradycardia, vomiting, and asystole.

MANAGEMENT OF SPECIFIC COMPLICATIONS (TABLE 173-4)

HYPOTENSION: Development of arterial hypotension should prompt rapid determination of serum pH and alkalinization. In the mechanically ventilated patient, hyper-

TABLE 173-4 Treatment of Specific Complications

Hypotension Alkalinization Volume infusion Right heart catheterization in persistent hypotension *Seizures* Alkalinization Diazepam (0.15 mg/kg IV, repeat as necessary) Phenytoin (15 mg/kg IV, over 30 min)	*Arrhythmias (avoid class I agents)* QRS widening Alkalinization Phenytoin (15 mg/kg IV, over 30 min) Ventricular arrhythmias Alkalinization Lidocaine (or overdrive pacing) Bradyarrhythmias/asystole Isoproterenol (atropine usually ineffective) Pacemaker

ventilation can be achieved within minutes. Volume infusion should also be given, with repeated 500-mL boluses of crystalloid. If hypotension is not corrected with 2 or 3 L of fluid, particularly if other evidence of hypoperfusion exists, consideration should be given to right heart catheterization as a useful guide to resuscitation. Management should then follow the general principles of management of shock as outlined in Chap. 114. Since malignant ventricular arrhythmias are the leading cause of death in cyclic antidepressant overdose, it seems particularly wise to avoid vasoactive drugs and their arrhythmogenic potential.

SEIZURES: Prophylactic antiepileptics do not have a clear role in TCA overdose. Since generalized seizures may be followed by cardiac arrhythmias or ventilatory failure, a physician should be at the bedside prepared to treat these complications. Alkalinization should be initiated and, except in rare circumstances, an endotracheal tube placed. Diazepam, 0.15 mg/kg, should be given intravenously and repeated at 15- to 20-min intervals until seizures are controlled or to a total of 30 to 40 mg. Intubation and mechanical ventilation will be required as larger doses are given. Phenytoin should also be given at the onset of seizures (15 mg/kg given intravenously over 30 min). Serum levels should then be measured and additional doses given as necessary to achieve a serum level of 20 μg/mL. Seizures that fail to respond to this regimen should be treated as other forms of status epilepticus (see Chap. 142).

ARRHYTHMIAS: Sinus tachycardia does not require treatment. Class I antiarrhythmic drugs (procainamide, diisopyramide, and quinidine) are contraindicated because their membrane effects amplify antidepressant toxicity. QRS widening, ventricular arrhythmia, and bradyarrhythmias should all prompt alkalinization of the blood.

Benefit from "prophylactic" phenytoin for patients with QRS widening has been suggested in one study,[18] and we recommend its use. Ventricular tachycardia, ventricular fibrillation, symptomatic bradyarrythmias, and asystole should be managed routinely, with the caution that class I antiarrhythmics be avoided. In addition, atropine is unlikely to be effective in bradyarrhythmias and heart blocks, because the predominant drug effect is below the bundle of His. β-Blocking agents and bretylium have been reported to cause worsened hypotension. It is notable that patients may be successfully resuscitated from malignant arrhythmias after considerable time. One individual recovered fully after 5 h of cardiopulmonary resuscitation.[19]

CONTINUOUS ECG MONITORING

Although most deaths after toxic ingestion occur within the first 24 h, there have been numerous reports of late deaths following TCA ingestion.[2] The majority of these patients were discharged from the ICU though they still had manifestations of drug effect—tachycardia, QRS prolongation, and CNS depression. Therefore, we routinely monitor patients until they are fully awake, arrhythmia free, and with normal conduction for 24 h. In many patients this can be accomplished in a telemetry unit and may not require the full services of the ICU. At the earliest possible time, coordination of long-term care with psychiatric staff should be initiated.

CASE PRESENTATION

A recently separated 39-year-old woman was brought by her husband to the emergency room following a possible drug overdose. The husband thought his wife had been started on some medication for depression 6 months earlier. Several hours earlier he had received a call from his wife who seemed very upset. When he arrived at her apartment, she stated that she had been drinking alcohol and had just taken "all the pills in the bottle."

On admission to the emergency room the patient was tearful, unwilling to answer questions beyond yes or no, slightly slow in responding, and had slurred speech. The heart rate was 120 and regular, blood pressure 110/60, and respirations 14 and unlabored. The neurologic examination was otherwise unremarkable. Her mucous membranes were dry, and her pupils were slightly dilated. An 18 gauge intravenous catheter was placed and an infusion of 2 ampules sodium bicarbonate in 5% dextrose solution started. The husband was instructed to try to obtain information regarding her psychiatrist, prescriptions, and pharmacy, and a drug toxic screen was sent. ECG revealed a sinus tachycardia, QRS duration of 150 ms, and nonspecific ST-T wave changes.

An attempt was made to place a nasogastric tube, but the patient began thrashing and striking out at staff. She apologized following this and claimed to have taken a month's supply of Elavil (amitriptyline). She admitted to a prior suicide attempt during which she had received ipecac in the emergency room. Syrup of ipecac (30 mL) was administered.

Approximately 5 min later the patient became stuporous with myoclonic jerking of her legs. The patient had a generalized seizure while attempts were made to draw an arterial blood-gas sample. She then became apneic and during intubation vomited and apparently aspirated. Diazepam, 10 mg intravenously, was given and followed by 1 g phenytoin over 30 min. An arterial blood-gas determination 15 min after her seizure revealed a pH of 7.30, P_{O_2} of 150 mmHg, and P_{CO_2} of 38 mmHg.

The patient was transferred to the ICU. Immediately on arrival, and prior to being connected to the ventilator, pulseless ventricular tachycardia developed. She was treated with a 200-joule countershock, 1 ampule sodium bicarbonate, and lidocaine (100-mg bolus followed by 2 mg/min). Following restoration of sinus tachycardia, the systolic blood pressure was 70 mmHg. A 1-L fluid challenge was given and a second intravenous line started. A large bore orogastric tube was placed but no pill fragments could be lavaged. A charcoal slurry was administered.

The initial ventilator settings were a tidal volume of 600 mL, rate of 25, and fraction inspired oxygen (F_{IO_2}) of .50. An arterial blood-gas sample 30 min after initiating mechanical ventilation revealed a pH of 7.48, P_{O_2} of 225 mmHg, and P_{CO_2} of 22 mmHg. Despite fluid challenges totalling 3 L, hypotension persisted. Right heart catheterization revealed a pulmonary capillary wedge pressure of 16 and cardiac output of 8 L/min; the systolic blood pressure remained 80 mmHg. After evidence of an ileus developed, no further charcoal was given and the orogastric tube was placed on suction.

Lidocaine was tapered after 12 h of infusion and phenytoin titrated to a serum level of 20 μg/mL. Blood pressure gradually rose to 110/70. The patient regained consciousness within 18 h. She was extubated on the second hospital day but required oxygen therapy for a right lower lobe infiltrate (presumed to be aspiration pneumonitis). By the third ICU day her sensorium was entirely normal, but QRS prolongation persisted. The ECG was normal the following day. She was discharged to the psychiatric service on the fifth hospital day.

CASE DISCUSSION

Even before the patient admitted to taking amitriptyline, her history of depression and signs of anticholinergic poisoning led to a clinical suspicion of cyclic antidepressant overdose. Because neurologic manifestations were apparent initially, securing venous access and beginning sodium bicarbonate therapy were clearly indicated. Both the neurologic findings and the prolonged QRS duration on the ECG were evidence of serious intoxication. The potential for abrupt deterioration made administration of ipecac unnecessarily dangerous. In addition, the post-intubation pH of 7.30 should have mandated further efforts to alkalinize the blood, using more aggressive sodium bicarbonate therapy or hyperventilation. It is possible that acidemia, superimposed on TCA toxicity, led to her cardiac arrest.

Once she was stabilized in the ICU, persistent hypotension was unresponsive to fluids. This led appropriately to right heart catheterization to determine whether she was still hypovolemic. When her filling pressures were not found to be low, we accepted the high output hypotension as adequate perfusion of the heart and brain in this young woman.

She awoke within 24 h as is typical in most cyclic antidepressant overdoses. Nevertheless, persistent ECG abnormalities led to the need for prolonged observation in the ICU.

References

1. Ellenhorn M, Barceloux DG: Antidepressants in, *Medical Toxicology: Diagnosis and Treatment of Human Poisoning.* New York Elsevier Ellenhorn M, Barceloux DG (eds): pp. 402–415, 1988.
2. Frommer DA, Kulig KW, Marx JA, Rumack B: Tricyclic antidepressant overdose: A review. JAMA 257:521, 1987.
3. Lesar T, Kingston R, Dahms R, et al: Trazodone overdose. Ann Emerg Med 12:221, 1983.
4. Van Brunt N: The clinical utility of tricyclic antidepressant blood levels: A review of the literature. Ther Drug Monit 5:1, 1983.
5. Saraf KR, Klein AF, Gittelman-Klein R, et al: Imipramine dose effects in children. Psychopharmacologia 37:265, 1974.
6. Herson VC, Schmitt BD, Rumack BH: Magical thinking and imipramine poisoning in two school-aged children. JAMA 241:1926, 1979.
7. Thorstrand C: Clinical features in poisoning by tricyclic antidepressants with special reference to the ECG. Acta Med Scand 199:337, 1976.
8. Biggs JT, Spiker DG, Petit JM, Ziegler VE: Tricyclic antidepressant overdose: Incidence of symptoms. JAMA 238:135, 1977.
9. Crome P, Newman B: Fatal tricyclic anti-depressant poisoning. JR Soc Med 72:649, 1979.
10. Callaham M, Kassel D: Epidemiology of fatal tricyclic antidepressant ingestion: Implications for management. Ann Emerg Med 14:1, 1985.
11. Sedal L, Korman MG, Williams PO, et al: Overdosage of tricyclic antidepressants: A report of two deaths and a prospective study of 24 patients. Med J Aust 2:74, 1972.
12. Jefferson JW: A review of the cardiovascular effects and toxicity of tricyclic antidepressants. Psychosom Med 37:160, 1975.
13. Marshall JB, Forker AD: Cardiovascular effects of tricyclic antidepressant drugs: Therapeutic usage, overdose, and management of complications. Am J Cardiol 103:401, 1982.
14. Boehnert MT, Lovejoy FH: Value of the QRS duration versus the serum drug level in predicting seizures and ventricular arrhythmias after an acute overdose of tricyclic antidepressants. N Engl J Med 313:474, 1985.
15. Foulke GE, Albertson TE: QRS interval in tricyclic antidepressant overdosage: Inaccuracy as a toxicity indicator in emergency settings. Ann Emerg Med 16:160, 1987.
16. Lorch JA, Garella S: Hemoperfusion to treat intoxications. Ann Intern Med 91:301, 1979.
17. Bessen HA, Niemann JT, Haskell RJ, Rothstein RJ: Effect of respiratory alkalosis in tricyclic antidepressant overdose. West J Med 139:373, 1983.
18. Boehnert M, Lovejoy FH: The effect of phenytoin on cardiac conduction and ventricular arrhythmias in acute tricyclic antidepressant overdose. Abstract. Vet Hum Toxicol 28:297, 1985.
19. Orr DA, Bramble MG: Tricyclic antidepressant poisoning and prolonged external cardiac massage during asystole. Br Med J 283:1107, 1981.

Chapter 174

NARCOTICS

R. STEVEN THARRATT
TIMOTHY E. ALBERTSON

KEY POINTS

- *The triad of coma, respiratory depression, and miotic pupils suggests opioid intoxication.*
- *Respiratory depression is the major threat to life; careful attention to airway, breathing, and circulation minimizes adverse outcomes.*
- *Naloxone is the antidote of choice. Doses of 0.4 to 10 mg are given and titrated to patient response. Large doses may be required. Continuous infusion may be required for ingestions of opioids with long half-lives.*
- *A careful examination for coexistent medical conditions is required in all opioid intoxications.*
- *Consider and treat the second drug that often accompanies opioid intoxications.*
- *Noncardiogenic pulmonary edema and rhabdomyolysis may occur.*
- *Blood and urine assays may confirm the diagnosis but are not necessary for clinical management of most ingestions. Response to naloxone administration may confirm the diagnosis. Routine drug assays may not detect fentanyl and fentanyl analogue ingestions.*
- *Extracorporeal removal, forced diuresis, pH alteration, or partial antagonist antidotes have no role in the management of opioid intoxication.*
- *Acute withdrawal is unpleasant but not usually life-threatening in the adult.*

The term *narcotic* refers to any drug producing narcosis or sleep and is often used interchangeably with the term *opiate*. Opiates refer to natural compounds isolated or derived from the poppy plant, *Papaver somniferum*. *Opioids* define any compound that has pharmacologic activity at any of several specific receptors distributed throughout the central (CNS) and peripheral nervous systems and include synthetically derived compounds and the naturally occurring endogenous polypeptides of the endorphin and enkephalin families.[1] Clinical management of toxic exposures to these compounds is relatively straightforward and involves basic intensive care and the use of pharmacologic antagonists to opioid receptors.

Pharmacology

A brief review of opioid-receptor pharmacology is necessary to understand the signs and symptoms of opioid ingestion and management principles. Opioid receptors can be divided into at least four classes of which three are clinically significant in man.[2–4] Mu (μ) receptors are responsible for the majority of supraspinal analgesia produced by the opioids. Respiratory depression and miosis are also mediated by stimulation of these receptors. The euphoria responsible for the illicit abuse of these drugs is thought to be mediated by mu receptors. Kappa (κ) receptors mediate spinal analgesia, miosis, mild respiratory depression, and sedation. Sigma (σ) receptors mediate dysphoria and hallucinations and produce mild respiratory stimulation. All opioids have variable agonist and antagonist effects at these three receptors. The majority of clinically significant compounds are either agonists at all receptors (morphine and its congeners), mixed agonists and antagonists (pentazocine, nalorphine, and similar drugs), or pure antagonists at all receptors (naloxone and naltrexone) (Table 174-1).

Signs and Symptoms of Opioid Intoxication

Classic signs and symptoms of opioid intoxication reflect agonist effects at the various receptors and establish the opioid toxidrome.[3] The triad of decreased level of consciousness, constricted pupils, and respiratory depression strongly suggests opioid ingestion. Evidence of both old and recent intravenous injections ("tracks") or small skin ulcers ("skin popping") may be seen. Opioid users become adept at intravenous injection. As peripheral sites become sclerosed, they often use the central veins of the neck and groin. Pneumothorax or metallic needle fragments in the soft tissues of the neck may be seen on radiographs, reflecting these central venous injection attempts.

Bradycardia results from decreases in sympathetic and increases in parasympathetic tone. Peripheral vasodilation may decrease venous return with resultant hypotension. Hypoxemia secondary to respiratory depression may contribute to this hypotension. Seizures directly produced by the opioids are uncommon. When present, they suggest propoxyphene or meperidine intoxication. Anoxia produced by any of the opioids or the adulterant(s) used in illicit manufacture are more common causes of seizures.

Hypoxemia is usually secondary to hypoventilation. When an abnormal alveolar-arterial gradient (A − a gradient) is present, opioid-induced noncardiogenic pulmonary edema must be considered.

Management Guidelines

Table 174-2 summarizes the major principles of management of opioid intoxication. The clinician should be attentive to airway, breathing, and circulation. The majority of fatalities from opioid ingestion relate to respiratory failure with resulting hypoxemia or aspiration pneumonia or both. Muscle relaxation may produce airway obstruction from glossal obstruction. Hypotension is usually due to a combination of venous vasodilation and hypoxemia, and it often

TABLE 174-1 Opioid Receptors, Clinical Effects, Agonists, and Antagonists

	RECEPTOR		
	Mu (μ)	Kappa (κ)	Sigma (σ)
Clinical Effects	Supraspinal analgesia Respiratory Depression Sedation Miosis Euphoria	Spinal analgesia Respiratory Depression Sedation Miosis	Hallucinations Dysphoria Respiratory stimulation Delusions
Prototype Agonists	Morphine Codeine Fentanyl	Morphine Codeine Fentanyl Pentazocine Nalorphine	Morphine Codeine Fentanyl Pentazocine Nalorphine
Prototype Antagonists	Naloxone Naltrexone Pentazocine Nalorphine	Naloxone Naltrexone	Naloxone Naltrexone

responds to supplemental oxygen administration. If oxygen administration fails to improve hypotension, fluid resuscitation with crystalloid usually will correct hypotension. Vasoactive drugs are reserved for hypotension unresponsive to naloxone, oxygen, and fluids. Aggressive control of the airway with endotracheal intubation, mechanical ventilation, and supplemental oxygen is the cornerstone of management of severe opioid intoxications.

Naloxone (Narcan) is the specific antidote of choice. It has pure antagonist properties at all clinically important opioid receptors.[5] In critical overdoses with hemodynamic instability, 0.4 mg naloxone should be given initially and rapidly titrated to stabilization of the patient or a total dose of 10 mg. If the patient has not responded in any way to 10 mg naloxone, the intensivist should consider the possibilities of an incorrect diagnosis of opioid intoxication, mixed ingestions with CNS depressants other than opioids, head trauma, supervening hypoxemia, or coexisting medical conditions such as sepsis, hypoglycemia, or electrolyte imbalances. Patients with catastrophic CNS events such as pontine infarction or hemorrhage can present with coma, pinpoint pupils, and respiratory depression. These patients can usually be distinguished by computed tomographic scanning or magnetic resonance imaging of the brain. Partial response to the initial dose of naloxone suggests intoxication with "designer opioids" (fentanyl derivatives), mixed agonist-antagonist opioids, mixed ingestions with other CNS depressants in which the opioid was the principle component, or opioid intoxications with coexisting medical-surgical conditions. Additional naloxone should be administered and a careful history and physical examination performed to determine coexistent intoxications and conditions.

In less critical patients without hemodynamic instability, an initial naloxone dosage of 0.4 to 2.0 mg is titrated to effect, observing for increased respirations, improved level of consciousness, or belligerent behavior. Since sudden improvement in the level of consciousness may occur with naloxone usage, all patients should be restrained, if possible prior to administration, to ensure the safety of both staff and the patient. In opioid-tolerant patients, the use of naloxone may produce the acute abstinence syndrome (withdrawal). With the exception of sporadic case reports, this has been the predominant adverse effect seen with even massive administrations of naloxone. The withdrawal syn-

TABLE 174-2 Management Principles in Opioid Intoxications

1. Aggressive control of the airway with administration of supplemental oxygen and assisted ventilation as necessary
2. Naloxone is the antidote of choice.
   - Severe intoxications: 0.4–10 mg titrated to effect
   - Mild intoxications: 0.4–2 mg titrated to effect
   - Mixed agonist-antagonist opioids:
     - 2–10 mg titrated to effect
   - Fentanyl analogues: 10–20 mg titrated to effect
   - Continuous infusion: 0.4 mg/h titrated to effect

   The IV route is preferred; alternatives include intramuscular, subcutaneous, sublingual injection and endotrachael instillation.
3. Consider an incorrect diagnosis, mixed ingestions, coexistent hypoxemia-anoxia, electrolyte abnormalities, and cranial trauma in nonresponders to naloxone.
4. Consider and exclude coexistent medical conditions.
5. Consider and treat the second drug that often accompanies opioid intoxication.
6. Be prepared to treat noncardiogenic pulmonary edema and rhabdomyolysis.
7. Blood or urine drug assays may confirm the diagnosis but are not necessary for management. A negative assay does not exclude the diagnosis of opioid intoxication.
8. Extracorporeal removal techniques, pH alteration, and forced diuresis have no role in management of opioid intoxications.

drome, though unpleasant to the patient, is usually not life-threatening. The half-life of naloxone is approximately 60 min, whereas the half-lives of most opioid agonists are longer. Patients thus must be closely monitored for return of symptoms of opioid intoxication. Naloxone can be administered and titrated via continuous infusion[6] (e.g., 4 mg in 1000 mL intravenous fluid administered at 100 mL/h = 0.4 mg/h). Intravenous administration of naloxone is preferred because of rapid onset of action and predictable absorption. Some opioid-tolerant patients may present difficulties in establishing intravenous access. Alternative routes of administration include intramuscular, subcutaneous, sublingual injection, and endotracheal instillation. Intramuscular injection of naloxone results in a slower onset of action (15 min) and erratic absorption in hypotensive patients. Sublingual injection into the vascular plexus beneath the tongue results in good absorption, but administration may be difficult in the presence of trismus. Endotracheal instillation of naloxone appears to be effective;[7] however, it is not approved for administration by this route by the manufacturer or the Food and Drug Administration. Naloxone exerts its principal antagonist properties at mu receptors.[4,8] Since most clinically used agonist-antagonist opioids are antagonists at mu receptors and agonists at kappa and sigma, larger doses (5 to 10 mg) of naloxone may be required to reverse the respiratory depression seen with these drugs. Fentanyl derivatives may require extremely large (10 to 20 mg) amounts of naloxone because of their extreme potency relative to morphine.[9] Patient response to administration of naloxone is strong evidence of the presence of opioids even in the face of negative results on drug screening. There are no current clinical indications for the use of partial antagonists such as nalorphine or levallorphan. The risks of respiratory depression and agonist effects at kappa and sigma receptors outweigh any benefit.

A careful physical examination is important to identify coexistent medical conditions related to the life-style of an opioid addict. Hypoglycemia, trauma, infection, sepsis, hepatitis, and HIV infection are commonly seen in these patients and may contribute to the presentation of the patient and require immediate intervention.[10]

Gastric lavage and activated charcoal-cathartic may be useful after oral ingestion of opioids, especially if the opioid was combined with anticholinergics. Gastric decontamination is not required in parenteral or respiratory exposures to opioids. However, these patients often abuse multiple drugs, and gastrointestinal decontamination may be required for an orally ingested second drug.

The second drug that often accompanies opioid ingestion may present more danger to the patient than the opioid component. Acetaminophen, aspirin, and caffeine frequently are combined with codeine in analgesic formulations. Combining heroin with amphetamines or cocaine ("speed balling") is popular among some heroin abusers. These patients often present with both respiratory depression and evidence of sympathetic stimulation. Once the respiratory depression is reversed with naloxone, the catecholamine release mediated by naloxone may potentiate the hypertension induced by the stimulant amphetamine or cocaine. Management of this mixed ingestion involves reversal of the opioid component with naloxone followed by specific supportive treatment of the amphetamine-induced toxicity, if required. Pentazocine and tripelennamine ("t's and blues")[11] or glutethimide and codeine ("loads")[12] are sometimes abused by destitute heroin users seeking an inexpensive substitute for the euphoria produced by heroin. These patients present with signs and symptoms of opioid ingestion combined with anticholinergic (tripelennamine) or additional CNS depression (glutethimide). The opioid component is first reversed with naloxone; the second ingestion is managed supportively.

Street samples of heroin typically contain 2 to 6 percent of the opioid, with the remaining 98 to 94 percent consisting of various adulterants.[13] Though usually inert from a toxicologic standpoint, contaminants can occasionally produce life-threatening symptoms requiring specific treatment. Adulterants that mimic the physical or sensory properties of the opioid are often chosen. Quinine and strychnine have been used because their bitter taste resembles heroin, and additional stimulation is produced on injection. Seizures and cardiac arrhythmias may result and require specific therapy. Local anesthetics such as lidocaine and procaine are used for their numbing properties ("freeze"). Most commonly, these compounds are used to adulterate cocaine. Seizures can occur with overdoses of the local anesthetics. Sugars such as lactose, mannitol, and dextrose mimic the consistency of heroin. Toxic effects relate primarily to vascular sclerosis and pulmonary thromboembolism. Opioids that are smuggled into the country by couriers who swallow balloons or condoms filled with opioids ("body packers") may be contaminated with gram-negative enteric bacteria and produce septic shock when intravenously injected. Unfortunately, most opioid users cannot provide a detailed description of the adulterants in their last injection. Most clinical toxicology laboratories cannot determine the identity of the adulterants rapidly enough to provide clinically useful information. The history that the patient has obtained his drug supply from a new source may suggest toxic effects from adulterants or a different concentration of opioid. Management is usually supportive and directed by an understanding of the adulterants commonly present in opioids and currently in use in a particular geographic location.

Cotton fever refers to the fever and diffuse pulmonary infiltrates that develop within minutes of an intravenous injection of the water extract of the cotton used to filter a dose of heroin. Cotton fever requires only supportive therapy but must be distinguished from the fever and infiltrates of primary pulmonary or endocardial infection or sepsis.

Opioid-induced noncardiogenic pulmonary edema is most commonly seen following heroin overdose but has been reported after overdoses with most opioids.[14] The pulmonary edema is thought to be produced by altered permeability of the pulmonary capillaries that is mediated by the opioid. Physiologically a low Pa_{O_2}, low to normal Pa_{CO_2} (which may be masked by hypoventilation from respiratory depression), increased pulmonary shunt, and a low to normal pulmonary capillary occlusion pressure are seen. The hypoxemia, which may be severe, usually responds to supplemental oxygen and positive end-expiratory pressure (PEEP).

Rhabdomyolysis may occur secondary to immobility following overdose or possibly through a direct effect of the opioid.

Blood and urine assays can confirm the presence of opioids but are not usually necessary for management. The response of a patient to the opioid antagonist naxolone is virtually pathognomonic of opioid exposure. Laboratory screening for opioids is usually done by enzyme-linked immunosassays of urine for morphine and morphine metabolites. Naxolone does not cross-react in these assays. The fentanyl derivatives ("China white" and others) present special difficulties in analysis because they are not detected by the usual opioid assays.[15] Radioimmunoassays are available for detection of these compounds; however, because of the large number of fentanyl analogues, their presence in millimicrogram amounts in body fluids, and the separation steps required in analysis, they are not widely used outside of research or forensic settings.[16]

The Withdrawal (Abstinence) Syndrome

Opioid withdrawal is not usually life-threatening to the adult patient.[17] Opioid withdrawal can be tolerated without pharmacologic intervention, although it may be extremely unpleasant for the patient. Clonidine, an α_2 agonist, has been used in modulating the symptoms of opioid withdrawal as a component of a comprehensive drug detoxification program.[18] It is not usually used in the ICU because acute detoxification of an opioid-dependent patient is not usually attempted during an intercurrent illness that precipitates an ICU admission. Attempts at pharmacologic detoxification without attention to the psychosocial component of addiction are not likely to be successful.

The withdrawal syndrome in newborn infants is potentially life-threatening especially if unrecognized.[19] Irritability, tremors, high-pitched cry, and inconsolability are all signs of an opioid-dependent infant. Symptoms usually begin within 48 h of birth. Seizures represent the largest threat to life, although sudden infant death syndrome appears to be higher in opioid-dependent infants. Treatment of the infant requires gradual opioid detoxification, usually using tincture of opium, morphine, or paregoric.

In opioid-dependent adults, the fear of inducing acute abstinence symptoms should not deter the use of naloxone to treat signs of overdose. Staff should be prepared for a sudden increase in level of consciousness and possible violent reaction when treating an unconscious patient with naloxone. Opioids such as heroin are easily reversed by naloxone and rapid titration with small amounts of naloxone may prevent "overshooting" the opioid reversal and inducing acute withdrawal symptoms. Acute withdrawal symptoms should be managed supportively; narcotics should not be given after naloxone in patients who have overdosed on opioids in an attempt to control naloxone-induced withdrawal symptoms.

A long-acting oral opioid antagonist, naltrexone, is occasionally used in opioid detoxification. If an opioid is required in a patient receiving naltrexone (for a specific clinical situation such as severe pain or angina), a rapidly acting opioid should be used with caution. Large amounts may be required to overcome the naltrexone-induced antagonism with resulting severe respiratory depression.

Management of Opioid Dependence in the ICU

Opioids are widely used in intensive care for their analgesic, sedative, anesthetic, and to a lesser extent, antianxiety and vasomotor properties. The fear of inducing dependence should not hinder their use for clear indications. Less addicting compounds should be used when the patient's clinical condition permits. The time course for induction of opioid dependence varies greatly and depends on the particular opioid used, the dosing schedule, duration of use, and the underlying physical and psychologic condition of the patient. Opioid tolerance may be induced rapidly in the ICU, especially with continuous infusions of opioids. A high degree of suspicion must be maintained and the patient closely monitored for signs and symptoms of withdrawal (Table 174-3). These signs are nonspecific and may be confused with the patient's underlying condition. The treatment of a therapeutically induced opioid-dependent state depends on the underlying condition of the patient. Patients still requiring ongoing intensive care are maintained with dosages of opioids sufficient to prevent withdrawal. Once stable, a patient should have all opioids converted to a long-acting opioid such as methadone which is then withdrawn incrementally over 7 to 14 days. Supportive treatment of withdrawal symptoms may also be required during this period. The long-acting opioid should be administered on a time-contingent basis, not on a symptom-contingent basis. No other opioid should be administered during this time.

Specific Opioids

DIPHENOXYLATE HYDROCHLORIDE AND ATROPINE (LOMOTIL)

This fixed opiate-anticholinergic combination is widely used as an antidiarrheal agent. In children, this preparation is capable of producing significant toxicity that may bear no relation to the dose ingested.[20] Signs and symptoms of anticholinergic toxicity (tachycardia, mydriasis, dry flushed skin, confusion, and urinary retention) may be seen in addition to the classic respiratory depression and coma due to the opioid. Decreased gastrointestinal motility may prolong or delay absorption. Enterohepatic recycling may play a role in diphenoxylate elimination. Treatment includes naloxone; large doses over prolonged periods may require continuous infusion. Children presenting with ingestions of diphenoxylate should be monitored closely for 12 to 24 h

TABLE 174-3 Signs and Symptoms of Opioid Withdrawal

Symptoms	Signs
Agitation	Dilated pupils
Restlessness	Hypertension
Anorexia	Tachycardia
Irritability	Piloerection
Nausea	Lacrimation
Vomiting	Rhinorrhea
Abdominal and bone pain	Fever
Diarrhea	

because of this variable and occasionally delayed toxicity.

Gastrointestinal decontamination may be useful since intestinal motility is often impared. Multiple doses of activated charcoal may also absorb drug undergoing enterohepatic recirculation. Physostigmine should be reserved for life-threatening anticholinergic symptoms (uncontrollable tachycardia or severe hallucinations), because physostigmine may produce cholinergic crisis or cardiac arrest or both.

HEROIN (DIACETYLMORPHINE)

Heroin is a popular drug of abuse because of the intense euphoria ("rush") generated. Heroin abuse has been supplanted somewhat by illicit use of the synthetic fentanyl and meperidine derivatives. Heroin is rapidly metabolized to 6-monoacetylmorphine and then metabolized to morphine by the liver. Toxicity is primarily related to morphine. Rapid death, often with the needle still in the vein, has been reported. The exact mechanism(s) of rapid death is not clear. It may be related to anaphylactoid reaction to the opioid or other adulterants, toxic reaction to quinine (often used to dilute heroin), or massive underestimation of the purity of the opioid injected with resulting respiratory failure. A cheaper form of heroin, called tar heroin because of its resemblance to roofing tar, has been implicated in many rapid deaths. These deaths are probably related to the opioid concentration which may be forty times greater than other sources. Treatment of tar heroin overdose is the same as for other opioids.

HEROIN SUBSTITUTES ("LOADS")

Destitute heroin abusers searching for a rush similar to heroin have combined glutethimide and codeine.[12] Referred to as "loads," the synergistic CNS depression can be fatal. The codeine component will respond to naloxone; however, glutethimide ingestions may require intensive respiratory and cardiovascular support for prolonged periods of time.

FENTANYL AND FENTANYL ANALOGUES ("DESIGNER DRUGS")

Fentanyl was introduced to the United States as an anesthetic agent in 1968. By 1979 various minor and easily produced synthetic modifications of the fentanyl molecule resulted in compounds that produced clinical effects similar to other abused opioids, yet were technically legal to possess since the specific molecule did not yet appear on the lists of controlled drugs. Popularly referred to as "designer drugs," the term is also applied to meperidine derivatives as well as some hallucinogenic amphetamine compounds.[21–23] These opioid compounds display tremendous variation in potencies (3-methylfentanyl is 7000 times as potent as morphine). While clinically similar to other opioids, they are chemically distinct and do not cross-react with usual immunoassays.[21] Large doses of naloxone are often required to reverse the respiratory depression and coma seen in these patients. Fentanyl derivatives should be suspected in patients who present with clinical signs and symptoms consistent with opioid ingestions, who respond to large doses of naloxone, and who have no evidence of opioids in urine assays.

MEPERIDINE AND MEPERIDINE ANALOGUES

Meperidine is the prototype of the phenylpiperidine opioids. In addition to classic signs of opioid toxicity, meperidine can produce myoclonic jerks and seizures, especially in the presence of renal insufficiency. Seizures may result from accumulation of normeperidine, a renally excreted meperidine metabolite.[24] Seizures usually respond to discontinuance of meperidine. Naloxone will not reverse normeperidine-induced seizures, although it will reverse the respiratory depression and other opioid manifestations of meperidine. Persistent seizures can be treated with diazepam and phenytoin. Phenobarbital should be avoided because of the risk of additional CNS depression. Persistent seizures suggest a non-opioid etiology such as anoxia, sedative-hypnotic withdrawal, or an underlying organic cerebral disorder.

Synthetic congeners of meperidine include 1-methyl-4-phenyl-4-propionoxypiperidine (MPPP). A potential contaminant of the synthesis of MPPP is 1-methyl-4-phenyl-1,2,3,6-tetrahydropyridine (MPTP). This contaminant, when metabolized by monoamine oxidase B in the brain to 1-methyl-4-phenylpyridinium (MPP^+), selectively destroys the zona compacta of the substantia nigra resulting in a drug-induced parkinsonism.[25] Epidemics of MPTP-induced parkinsonism have been observed in geographic clusters resulting from distribution of contaminated MPPP.[26] Treatment of MPTP-induced parkinsonism is similar to idiopathic Parkinson's disease. The long-term prognosis is not known, but it does not appear to be reversible.

METHADONE

Methadone is a synthetic opioid widely used for opioid detoxification and maintenance therapy. Methadone is used for detoxification primarily because of the absence of significant euphoria and its long half-life. Treatment with naloxone may be required for 48 to 72 h in methadone intoxications because of a methadone half-life of 15 to 25 h. Infants addicted to methadone in utero may have evidence of ventilatory depression for as long as 31 days after birth.[27]

CAMPHORATED TINCTURE OF OPIUM (PAREGORIC)

This compound is most often used as an antidiarrheal agent and occasionally to control withdrawal symptoms in newborn infants of opioid-dependent mothers. It is a mixture of opium, anise oil, benzoic acid, camphor, alcohol, and glycerin. It is approximately equivalent pharmacologically to 40 percent morphine. Prior to legal controls on dispensing this compound, paregoric was orally abused despite its pungent taste. Intravenous administration can produce severe inflammatory reactions and thrombosis. The camphor in paregoric may result in seizures, especially in children.

PENTAZOCINE

A mixed agonist-antagonist, pentazocine has agonist properties at kappa and sigma receptors and antagonist properties at mu receptors. It was thought that this drug would result in less respiratory depression and potential for addiction. Unfortunately, this was not borne out in clinical experience. Hallucinations may occur even with therapeutic doses probably due to sigma-receptor agonism.[28] Naloxone may need to be given in higher dosages to antagonize respiratory depression produced by pentazocine. Pentazocine has been illicitly combined with an antihistamine, tripelennamine, to give a euphoria qualitatively similar to heroin. This combination is referred to as "Ts and blues" (the tripelennamine tablet is blue), "tops and bottoms," "Ts and Bs," or "Teddies and Betties." Patients mix pentazocine:tripelennamine in 2:1, 3:1 or 4:1 ratios, then dissolve it in water and inject the mixture parenterally.[11] Life-threatening complications relate to CNS stimulation produced by the antihistamine. More than 100 mg tripelennamine (2 tablets) or a 1:1 ratio of pentazocine: tripelennamine increases the risk of tonic-clonic seizures.[29] Parenteral abuse of this combination has become more difficult since pentazocine has been reformulated to contain 0.5 mg naloxone. This amount of naloxone has no effect orally, but is capable of inducing acute abstinence symptoms in opioid-dependent patients who abuse the drug parenterally. Acute hypertensive crisis have been reported following the use of this new formulation parenterally.

OTHER OPIOID AGONISTS/ANTAGONISTS (BUTORPHANOL, NALBUPHINE)

These compounds are similar to pentazocine in their opioid-receptor physiology and respond similarly to naloxone. Exposures to these drugs do not appear to produce severe respiratory depression, perhaps due to agonism at sigma receptors. Overdoses with these compounds have not been widely reported. Intoxications would be expected to respond to standard management techniques of opioid overdosage.

CASE PRESENTATION

An 18-year-old Hispanic man presented to the emergency department *in extremis*. He was unconscious with a blood pressure of 50/30 mmHg, heart rate 40/min, and respirations 4/min and agonal. He was endotracheally intubated and placed on 100 percent oxygen. Two large bore intravenous lines were started and fluid resuscitation begun with lactated Ringer's solution. Physical examination was significant for 3 mm nonreactive pupils and a distended rigid abdomen without bowel sounds. Family members reported that the patient had complained for 48 h of increasing abdominal discomfort; they denied any history of drug use. The patient was emergently taken to the operating room for a presumed intraabdominal catastrophe; total time in the emergency department was 15 min. Naloxone was not given. Exploratory laparotomy was completely normal; as the abdomen was being closed, severe hypoxemia developed that was refractory to 10 cmH_2O of PEEP. In the recovery room PEEP was further titrated to 20 cmH_2O with persistence of a large intrapulmonary shunt. Chest radiographs showed diffuse alveolar infiltrates. Right heart and pulmonary artery wedge pressures were normal. Over the next 72 h the patient's condition improved, allowing rapid reduction in ventilatory support. The urinary drug screen result was positive for morphine metabolites. After extubation, the patient was able to give the history that he had been attempting to self-detoxify from heroin addiction; his abdominal cramping had become too severe, and he had self-injected one and a half times his usual heroin dose to control his abdominal pain. On discharge the patient was referred to a methadone detoxification program.

CASE DISCUSSION

This patient presented with classic signs of opioid overdose. Symptoms of intraabdominal catastrophes are not common but do occur with heroin overdoses. Although emergent surgery was felt to be indicated by the patient's presenting signs and symptoms, a response to naloxone in the emergency department may have altered initial therapy. Perioperatively the patient manifested noncardiogenic pulmonary edema. His condition rapidly improved over 72 h. The diagnosis of acute opioid use was made by urinary drug screen. The morphine metabolites suggested heroin intoxication, because heroin is metabolized to morphine. This excluded narcotics (fentanyl) given during surgery. The results of the urine drug screen did not alter management. The history supplied by the patient confirmed the diagnosis. A high level of suspicion must be maintained for opioid intoxication in patients presenting with coma, pinpoint pupils, and respiratory depression. A trial of naloxone is safe and may be diagnostic in these patients.

References

1. Thompson JW: Opioid peptides. Br Med J 288:259, 1984.
2. Gilman AG, Goodman LS, Gilman A (eds): *The Pharmacological Basis of Therapeutics*. 6th ed. New York, Macmillan, 1980, p 494.
3. Ellenhorn MJ, Barceloux DG: *Medical Toxicology. Diagnosis and*

Treatment of Human Poisonings. New York, Elsevier, 1988, pp 687–751.
4. Martin WR: Pharmacology of opioids. Pharmacol Rev 35:283, 1984.
5. Goldfrank LR: The several uses of naloxone. Emerg Med 16:105, 1984.
6. Bradberry JC, Raebel MA: Continuous infusion of naloxone in the treatment of narcotic overdosage. Drug Intell Clin Pharmacol 15:945, 1981.
7. Tandberg D, Abercrombie D: Treatment of heroin overdosage with endotracheal naloxone. Ann Emerg Med 11:443, 1982.
8. Sawynok J, Pinsky C, LaBella FC: Minireview on the specificity of naloxone as an opiate antagonist. Life Sci 25:1621, 1979.
9. Henderson GL: Designer Drugs: The California Experience, in Klein M, Saoienza H, McClain H, Kahn I (eds): *Clandestinely Produced Drugs, Analogs and Precursors*. United States Department of Justice Drug Enforcement Administration, Washington, DC, 1989, p 7.
10. Sternbach G, Moran J, Eliastam M: Heroin addiction: Acute presentation of medical complication. Ann Emerg Med 9:161, 1980.
11. Poklis A, Case MES, Ridenour GC: Abuse of pentazocine/tripelennamine combination. T's and blues in the City of Saint Louis, Missouri. Medicine 80:21, 1983.
12. Sramek JJ, Klajawall A: "Loads." N Engl J Med 305:231, 1981.
13. O'Neal PJ, Baker PB, Gough TA: Illicitly imported heroin products. Some physical and chemical features indicative of their origin. J Forensic Sci 24:889, 1984.
14. Duberstein JL, Kaufman DM: A clinical study of an epidemic of heroin intoxication and heroin induced pulmonary edema. Am J Med 51:704, 1971.
15. Hammargran WR, Henderson GL: Analyzing normetabolites of the fentanyls by gas chromatography/electron capture detection. J Anal Toxicol 12:183, 1988.
16. Henderson GL, Harkey MR, Jones AD: Rapid screening of fentanyl (China White) powder samples by solid phase radioimmunoassay. J Anal Toxicol 14:172, 1990.
17. George CF, Robertson D: Clinical consequences of abrupt drug withdrawal. Med Toxicol 2:367, 1987.
18. Gossop M: Clonidine and the treatment of the opioid withdrawal syndrome. Drug Alcohol Depend 21:253, 1988.
19. Sweet AY: Narcotic withdrawal syndrome in the newborn. Pediatr Rev 3:285, 1982.
20. Curtis JA, Goel KM: Lomotil poisoning in children. Arch Dis Child 54:222, 1979.
21. Henderson GL: Designer drugs: Past history and future prospects. J Forensic Sci 33:569, 1988.
22. Soine WH: Clandestine drug synthesis. Med Res Rev. 6:41, 1986.
23. Buchanan JF, Brown CR: Designer drugs: A problem in clinical toxicology. Med Toxicol 3:1, 1988.
24. Goetting MG: Neurotoxicity of meperidine. Ann Emerg Med 14:1007, 1985.
25. Langston JW, Ballard PA: Parkinsonism induced by 1-methyl-4-phenyl-1,2,3,6-tetrahydropyridine (MPTP): Implications for treatment and the pathogenesis of Parkinson's disease. Canadian J Neurol Sci 1:160, 1984.
26. Ballard PA, Tetrud JW, Langston JW: Permanent parkinsonism due to 1-methyl-4-phenyl-1,2,3,6-tetrahydropyridine (MPTP), seven cases. Neurology 35:949, 1985.
27. Olsen GD, Lees MH: Ventilatory response to carbon dioxide of infants following chronic prenatal methadone exposure. J Pediatr 96:983, 1980.
28. De Nosaquo N: The hallucination effect of pentazocine. JAMA 210:502, 1969.
29. Lahmeyer H, Steingold RG: Medical and psychiatric complications of pentazocine and tripelennamine abuse. J Clin Psychiatry 41:275, 1980.

Chapter 175

INHALED TOXINS

URI TAITELMAN
GREGORY A. SCHMIDT

KEY POINTS

- *Inhaled toxins cause illness through anoxia, direct lung injury, and systemic effects.*
- *Most toxic inhalations occur in closed, confined spaces, but massive release of toxic gases can lead to critical illness even in the open, where meteorologic and topographic conditions are major determinants.*
- *Chlorine inhalation primarily causes alveolar damage.*
- *High concentrations of hydrogen sulfide (H_2S) cause loss of consciousness with apnea, rapidly followed by cardiac arrest.*
- *Smoke inhalation is a complex exposure with components of thermal injury, pulmonary irritants, carbon monoxide (CO), and often cyanide or other toxicities.*
- *Pulmonary dysfunction after smoke inhalation may be immediate or delayed.*
- *CO poisoning should be anticipated in all victims of smoke inhalation. Prompt oxygen therapy is the most crucial intervention.*
- *Comatose patients who are rescued from fires involving synthetic or natural fibers should be considered to have combined CO-cyanide poisoning until proven otherwise.*

The respiratory system is a major route for poisoning by inhalation. Toxins which may be inhaled include gases, vapors of volatile liquids, and aerosols. Aerosols consist of suspensions of solid particles or liquid droplets, and may contain dusts, fumes (in particular, metal oxides formed by combustion, sublimation, or condensation), and mists and fogs (formed from condensation of gases or from liquid uptake by hygroscopic particles).[1] This chapter focuses on the acute aspects of inhalation injury due to molecular chlorine, H_2S, smoke, and CO. Acute cyanide poisoning is discussed fully in Chap. 176. The chronic manifestations of inhaled toxins are beyond the scope of this chapter.

Toxicokinetics

When particles are inhaled, their penetration along the airways toward alveoli depends essentially on size (Table 175-1).[2] When gases or vapors are inhaled, several factors determine their deposition in the airways or their diffusion to the alveolar space. Water-soluble gases, such as hydrochloric acid, hydrofluoric acid, sulfuric acid, and ammonia, predominantly affect the large, medium, and small airways. Nevertheless, when inhaled in high concentrations or for a prolonged period, they affect alveoli as well. Nonionized and poorly water-soluble gases, such as molecular chlorine, nitrogen oxides, phosgene, and methyl bromide, have a significant effect on the alveoli. Transfer of these substances across the alveolar capillary membrane depends on the diffusion coefficient of each gas, the concentration gradient between the alveolar space and the pulmonary capillaries, water solubility, and the mechanism of uptake. Thus, CO diffuses very rapidly through the alveolar capillary membrane due to its high diffusibility and to its rapid uptake by erythrocytic hemoglobin. On the other hand, gases with relatively low water solubility, such as nitrous oxide, depend on a high alveolar partial pressure to maintain high plasma concentrations. Such gases are rapidly eliminated by the lung when the alveolar fraction falls. The tissue distribution of toxic gases depends on the partition coefficient and tissue uptake. Thus, aliphatic and cyclic halogenated hydrocarbons tend to accumulate in tissue due to their very high lipid solubility and are very slowly eliminated. For example, after significant inhalation, carbon tetrachloride can be detected in exhaled breath for several days.[3]

To evaluate the kinetics of inhaled toxins, knowledge of particle size, molecular weight and density, vapor pressure, water solubility, and diffusion and partition coefficients is helpful.

Pathophysiology

Although there are many individual inhaled toxins, most can be categorized into those which displace air causing anoxia (e.g., carbon dioxide), others which produce acute lung disease (e.g., chlorine, hydrochloric acid, toluene diisocyanate), and those which lead to systemic toxicity (e.g., CO, hydrogen cyanide, H_2S). Of course, in many cases, several concurrent mechanisms of toxicity are apparent. For example, accidents in sewage systems usually include exposure to H_2S and inhalation of an hypoxic gas mixture. Similarly, silo filler's disease is due to inhalation of an hypoxic gas mixture with superimposed pulmonary edema from oxides of nitrogen.

TOXINS PRODUCING ANOXIA

Inhalation of gas mixtures which contain a low concentration of oxygen leads to anoxia. In most instances, the gas is heavier than air, displacing it as the concentration rises. Typically, disease due to this mechanism is related to release of a gas into a confined, inadequately ventilated space. However, massive release of a heavy gas can lead to

TABLE 175-1 Particle Penetration along Airways

Average Particle Size	Area of Deposition	Mechanism
5–30 μ	Nasopharynx	Inertial impaction
1–5 μ	Trachea, major bronchi	Sedimentation
<1 μ	Alveoli	Diffusion

a critical reduction in oxygen concentration even in the open. The organs most sensitive to the resultant hypoxemia are the central nervous system (CNS) and the heart. The pathophysiology and pathology are identical to other anoxic heart and brain insults.

TOXINS CAUSING ACUTE LUNG INJURY

One mechanism of acute lung injury is severe irritation or corrosion of the airways caused by strong water-soluble acids or alkalies in gaseous or aerosol form (e.g., hydrochloric acid, hydrofluoric acid, sulfur dioxide, ammonia). Alternatively, acute airway spasm and inflammation can be caused by allergic mechanisms (e.g., toluene diisocyanate, hay and pollen dusts) or during acute cholinergic crisis (see Chap. 184). Acute pulmonary edema is frequently the result of nonionized, poorly water-soluble, highly lipid-soluble gases such as molecular chlorine or some oxides of nitrogen. These gases cause pulmonary edema, which may be separated from the initial exposure by a symptom-free interval.

Fumes of metals and polymers can induce disease through immunologic mechanisms. These syndromes, which often affect welders or manipulators of heated, synthetic polymers, are known as metal fume or plastic fume fever. Chills, fever, cough, and dyspnea are common symptoms, typically developing several hours after exposure. The chest x-ray may be normal or reveal peribronchiolar infiltrates.

TOXINS LEADING TO SYSTEMIC TOXICITY

Toxic gases may interfere with oxygen transport by blood or oxygen utilization by tissues (e.g., hydrogen cyanide, H_2S, CO). Examples of these different mechanisms are listed in Table 175-2. As a general rule, the effect of a nonallergic, toxic gas is directly proportional to the product of the inhaled gas concentration and the duration of exposure (Haber's law).[4]

Specific Toxic Inhalations

CHLORINE

Accidental exposure to molecular chlorine commonly occurs when the gas is released from pressurized containers. In addition, it may occur in the home when hypochlorite bleach is mixed with acids, generating molecular chlorine gas. The gas has an unpleasant odor, is an irritant at low concentrations (2 to 3 ppm), and therefore provides a strong warning. However, chlorine is more than two times heavier than air and thus accumulates in low places. Moreover, it has a vapor pressure of more than 1 atmosphere at 20°C (68°F) so that rupture of a container of pressurized liquid chlorine will rapidly fill even a large, enclosed space. Therefore, release of large amounts of chlorine is highly dangerous, despite the fact that its presence is easily detected.

Once inhaled, chlorine produces lung injury. The gas dissolves in the water-saturated atmosphere of the airways, releasing hydrochloric acid (HCl), leading to airway inflammation, injury, and bronchospasm. Chlorine also reaches the alveoli, then readily penetrates the alveolar lining cell membranes due to its high lipid solubility. Once inside cells, chlorine slowly reacts with intracellular water to form HCl (a strong acid) and hypochlorous acid (HOCl, a strong oxidant). HCl causes protein coagulation and HOCl oxidizes intracellular components, in particular the free sulfhydryl groups of proteins and enzymes. These reactions (which develop slowly) explain the appearance or aggravation of symptoms many hours after exposure.

Patients present with lacrimation, conjunctival irritation, dyspnea, cough, and nausea. It is usually possible on the initial examination to distinguish between minor exposure (necessitating no medical treatment and only brief observation) and moderate to severe exposure (necessitating admission). Dyspnea and chest x-ray abnormalities indicate a potential for deterioration. Bronchospasm is occasionally prominent. Patients with severe exposures may develop acute hypoxemic respiratory failure due to fulminant diffuse alveolar damage (see Chap. 128). Pneumomediastinum and pneumothorax have also been described after chlorine exposure.[5]

Treatment is generally supportive and should include decontamination of exposed skin and mucous membranes. Oxygen should be given routinely. Bronchodilators may relieve dyspnea and reduce cough. The use of corticosteroids is controversial. Anecdotal reports and theoretical predictions indicate that steroids may speed healing of the acute insult as well as reduce the incidence of long-term complications. Their efficacy has not been proved in prospective, randomized, double blind, large scale studies. Patients needing mechanical ventilation are prone to pulmonary infections, to bronchial mucosal sloughing, and to alveolar rupture causing pneumothorax. During mechanical ventilation, attempts should be made to minimize peak and mean airway pressures. Meticulous airway toilet may be necessary to ensure airway patency.

The prognosis and consequences of chlorine exposure are difficult to predict. Most patients will heal completely with simple treatment consisting of rapid termination of exposure, administration of humidified oxygen, and bronchodilators. Three types of long-term complications have been described, but their occurrence is unpredictable. The first is the reactive airway dysfunction syndrome.[6] This entity is characterized by hyperreactivity to any nonspecific irritation of the airways, leading to bronchospasm and airflow limitation, for many weeks following exposure. This syndrome usually resolves after several months. The second potential long-term consequence of chlorine exposure is bronchiolitis obliterans, a progressive disease in which airways become obstructed by hypertrophic intraluminal scarring. Finally, some patients develop interstitial pulmonary fibrosis.

TABLE 175-2 Examples of Mechanisms of Toxicity of Inhaled Substances

Toxin	IDLH (ppm)	Mechanism of Acute Toxicity	Site of Major, Direct Injury
Pulmonary Allergens			
Toluene diisocyanate	10	Allergic bronchoconstriction	Airways
Pollens		Allergic bronchoconstriction and infiltrates	Airways and interstitium
Metal and polymer fumes		Allergic reaction	Airways and interstitium
Systemic Toxins			
Arsine	4	Severe hemolysis due to inhibition of RBC catalase	Red blood cells
Phosphine	200	General protoplasmic poison and pulmonary irritant	CNS. Also, tissues with a high metabolic rate (liver, heart, kidneys)
Carbon tetrachloride	300	Free radical generation in the liver, hypersensitivity of the heart to catecholamines	Liver, heart
Asphyxiants			
Propane		Displacement of oxygen from inhaled gas mixture	Brain, heart
Sulfur hexafluoride		Displacement of oxygen from inhaled gas mixture	Brain, heart
Nitrous oxide		Displacement of oxygen from inhaled gas mixture, CNS depression	Brain, heart
Impaired Oxygen Utilization			
Hydrogen cyanide	50	Inhibition of aerobic metabolism	Brain, heart
H_2S	300	Inhibition of aerobic metabolism	Brain
CO	1500	Decreased oxygen transport, availability, and utilization	Red blood cell, brain, heart
Acute Lung Dysfunction			
Hydrofluoric acid	20	Strong acid causing inflammation and damage of airways	Large and small airways
Ammonia	500	Strong alkali causing inflammation and damage of airways	Large and small airways, alveoli
Ozone	10	Strong oxidant causing oxidative damage	Small airways, alveoli

IDLH, immediately dangerous to life and health as defined by NIOSH;[13] ppm, parts per million.

HYDROGEN SULFIDE

A major cause of poisoning in any confined space where organic matter decays, the gas is produced by complete bacterial reduction of sulfur to H_2S. H_2S is heavier than air and tends to accumulate in low places. At low concentrations it has a disagreeable odor of rotten eggs, but above 300 ppm paralysis of the olfactory system occurs and cancels its warning property. Exposure to a nonlethal concentration causes headache, nausea, conjunctivitis, and irritation, edema, and inflammation of airways. A single breath at a concentration above 1000 ppm will cause immediate loss of consciousness and apnea, rapidly followed by cardiac arrest. Accidents usually occur when a worker descends toward an increasing concentration of H_2S, then suddenly collapses.

H_2S is weak acid with a p*K*a of 8.4; therefore at the pH of body fluids, it exists mostly as a nonionized, freely diffusing gas. It inhibits cellular aerobic metabolism in the brain, probably by binding the iron of cytochrome aa_3 (and resembles cyanide poisoning in this respect). Decreased oxygen concentration in confined spaces is a frequent aggravating factor in H_2S poisoning, compounding the anoxic insult.

Because H_2S is oxidized by oxyhemoglobin to sulfate, prompt resuscitation with pure oxygen is the major determinant of survival and neurologic recovery. Methemoglobin reacts with sulfide bound to cytochrome oxidase, creating sulfmethemoglobin and restoring oxidative metabolism. Indeed, induction of methemoglobinemia has a protective and therapeutic effect in experimental animals. However, in human poisoning oxygen has been more effective than induced methemoglobinemia,[7] probably because oxygen itself reacts with sulfide. Experimentally, hyperbaric oxygen (HBO) is even more effective than normobaric oxygen,[8] and a beneficial effect has been anecdotally reported. However, the role of HBO, like that of induced methemoglobinemia, remains to be determined.

Smoke Inhalation

THE COMPONENTS OF SMOKE

Fire is defined as rapid oxidation with the production of heat and light. However, there are two exceptions to this definition: fire may be produced by thermonuclear reaction; and overheated electrical cables may produce flame and toxic smoke by nonoxidative pyrolysis of the insulator, usually a polymer. Two distinctive interrelated processes occur during fire—oxidation (complete or incomplete) and pyrolysis. Complete oxidation of carbon produces carbon dioxide, of hydrogen produces water, and of sulfur produces sulfur dioxide (a toxic gas). Nonoxidized and partially oxidized substances are always emitted by flames as well. For example, when carbon-containing fuels are consumed, important constituents of smoke include CO (partially oxidized carbon) and elemental carbon (nonoxidized particles). Pyrolysis is an effect of temperature; in part it consists of the gases released from melting and boiling of constituents of the fuel. In addition, heat causes breakdown of large molecules to smaller ones. This thermal decomposition generates many new compounds,[9] among which are highly reactive free radicals. In a fire, the products of both oxidation and pyrolysis react with each other, generating and releasing a huge number of new compounds. The nature of these molecules depends on the composition of burning material, on the amount of oxygen available, and on the temperature generated by the fire. Up to a temperature of 700°C (1484°F) breakdown of large molecules to smaller ones is the rule; above 800°C (1696°F) cyclic compounds and hydrogen cyanide result. The cyclic compounds have important carcinogenic and chronic toxic properties which are beyond the scope of this chapter. Thus, toxicologically, two types of toxic combustion products can be described: gases having a toxic effect mainly on the lung and gases with

TABLE 175-3 Combustion Products Causing Acute and Delayed Lung Injury

Typical Parent Compound Consumed by Fire	Toxin	IDLH (ppm)
Wood, oils	Formaldehyde	100
	Acetaldehyde	10,000
	Acrolein	5
PVC, halogenated hydrocarbons used as solvents and chemical intermediates	Chlorine	25
	Hydrochloric acid	100
	Phosgene	2
Teflon and similar fluorocarbons	Perfluoroisobutylene	<1
Sulfur-containing fuels, leather, and other organic compounds containing sulfur	Sulfur dioxide	100
Nitrocellulose and all other compounds containing NO moieties; oxides of nitrogen; N_2 and O_2 from air in very hot fires	Nitric oxide	50
	Nitrogen dioxide	100

IDLH, immediately dangerous to life and health as defined by NIOSH;[13] ppm, parts per million; PVC, polyvinyl chloride.

systemic toxicity. The most common simple molecular products of combustion are listed in Table 175-3.

PATHOPHYSIOLOGY

The pathophysiology of disease caused by smoke inhalation includes the effects of temperature of the inhaled smoke, hypoxia due to decreased oxygen concentration, gases causing respiratory dysfunction, and gases causing systemic poisoning. Inhalation of dry hot gas (above 150°C, 318°F) does not cause thermal injury but may cause severe laryngospasm leading to immediate death.[10] Inhalation of steam causes severe thermal damage to the airways since the amount of heat carried by steam is very high. Smoke containing solid heated particles may cause thermal damage to the major airways. When the particles consist of carbon, inhalation may cause both thermal and chemical damage because the particles adsorb other toxic chemical molecules. In most open fires, the smoke is a dry hot gas mixture. Nevertheless, the thermal consequences of smoke inhalation may dominate the clinical picture, as discussed more fully in Chap. 68.

The decreased oxygen concentration during fire in confined spaces (as oxygen is consumed by the fire) depends on the nature of the burning substances. Gasoline will self-extinguish when the ambient oxygen fraction falls to 15 percent, while other compounds (especially those containing oxygen in their molecular structure) may burn until the concentration of oxygen falls below 10 percent. The isolated effect of decreased oxygen concentration is shown in Table 175-4. When ambient oxygen falls by even a few percent it has an important potentiating effect on the toxicity of other gases, especially CO and hydrogen cyanide.

Short-chain aldehydes (formaldehyde, acetaldehyde, acrolein) are produced when wood or oils are burned. The most toxic is acrolein, which produces acute pulmonary edema in a few minutes at a concentration above 10 ppm. In fires where PVC (widely used for building, floor lining, and furniture) is consumed, molecular chlorine, hydrochloric acid, phosgene, and chlorine free radicals are produced. Molecular chlorine, discussed above, reaches the alveoli. Hydrochloric acid is highly water soluble and causes chemical burns and bronchoconstriction of the water-saturated airways. Phosgene is produced when oxygen, chlorine, and carbon react at a temperature above 250°C (530°F).

TABLE 175-4 Correlation Between Hypoxic Gas Inhalation and Symptoms at Sea Level (1 ATA)

Inhaled FI_{O_2}	Symptoms
20% or more	None; normal concentration in air
12–15%	Tachycardia; loss of muscular coordination for skilled movements
10–12%	Nausea and vomiting; faulty judgment; even mild exertion impossible
6–8%	Rapid collapse and unconsciousness
<6%	Death in 6–8 min

FI_{O_2}, fraction inspired oxygen; ATA, atmospheres absolute.

Phosgene causes acute respiratory failure at very low concentrations. Sulfur dioxide becomes sulfuric acid in the water-saturated airways leading to further airway injury. Oxides of nitrogen (NO, NO_2 N_2O_4) are produced especially when molecules containing nitro groups (such as nitrocellulose) are involved. Oxides of nitrogen produce small airway and alveolar damage. These gases produce immediate pulmonary dysfunction due to airway inflammation and to pulmonary edema and in severe instances can lead to death. However, symptoms may be delayed or progress for the first 24 to 36 h. In addition, there is a substantial risk of severe, delayed (2 to 3 weeks) bronchiolitis obliterans.

The effect of these gases is frequently progressive or delayed and not manifest on initial chest x-rays. In addition to physical examination and arterial blood gas analysis, evaluation should include flow-volume loops when possible, repeated fiber optic bronchoscopy, and xenon 133 washout scans in critically ill patients. In mechanically ventilated patients, lung compliance and airflow resistance should be serially evaluated, and secondary infection should be excluded.

CARBON MONOXIDE POISONING

As the most important and frequently encountered toxic gas in smoke, CO has no odor, taste, color, or irritating characteristics. It is produced by pyrolysis and oxidative decomposition during combustion and is a major contributor to death during and shortly after smoke inhalation. Malfunctioning of domestic equipment using cooking gas (a mixture of propane and butane) causes CO poisoning and hypoxemia (due to displacement of oxygen). CO poisoning is, therefore, a very frequent cause of acute poisoning in the home.

MECHANISM OF TOXICITY. The affinity of CO for ferrous ion of hemoglobin is 200 to 240 times higher than the affinity of oxygen for hemoglobin. The uptake of CO by the blood from the alveolar space is usually rapid and complete because CO diffuses well through the alveolar capillary membrane, and then combines with hemoglobin to form carboxyhemoglobin (HbCO). Several mechanisms of CO toxicity have been suggested. First, formation of HbCO decreases the oxygen-carrying capacity of the blood. However, this is clearly an incomplete explanation because anemia, which reduces oxygen delivery to an equivalent degree, is much more readily tolerated than CO poisoning. For example, a fall in the hemoglobin concentration to 7.5 g/dL (half of normal) is often asymptomatic. In contrast, an HbCO concentration of 50 percent can cause coma or collapse. A second potential contributor to the toxicity of CO is that HbCO shifts the oxyhemoglobin dissociation curve to the left, decreasing the off-loading of oxygen to the tissues. Third, CO reacts with myoglobin in working muscle to form carboxymyoglobin, thereby limiting oxygen uptake. This effect is very important in the heart where oxygen uptake is normally high, facilitated by the high myoglobin content of cardiac muscle. Fourth, enzymes of the mitochondrial electron-transfer chain (in particular cytochromes b and aa_3) are inhibited by CO to a degree which is inversely proportional to the availability of oxygen to mitochondria.[11] The significance of this in human CO poisoning has yet to be determined. Finally, CO binds and inhibits the activity of intracellular enzymes and pigments containing iron, in particular cytochrome P-450 and reduced nicotinamide-adenine dinucleotide phosphate (NADPH) reductase. To the extent that these final three mechanisms of toxicity are operative, they may provide a rationale for the utilization of hyperbaric oxygen therapy, even once blood HbCO falls to low levels.

MANIFESTATIONS OF TOXICITY. The severity of the poisoning depends on the minute ventilation, the concentration of CO, and the duration of exposure. Unfortunately, these features cannot be determined in most smoke inhalation situations. Breathing a gas mixture with a simultaneously decreased oxygen concentration potentiates the toxicity of CO. The main target organs of CO poisoning are the heart and brain. Even a healthy, young patient may develop electrocardiographic (ECG) manifestations resembling acute ischemia with typical ST and T changes. The sensitivity of the heart to CO increases significantly in the presence of coronary artery disease. Human volunteers demonstrate a significant decrease in the time and energy necessary to induce angina pectoris after a short exposure to low concentrations of CO.[12] One-third of smoke inhalation fatalities are attributable to CO-exacerbated coronary insufficiency.

The neurologic manifestations of acute CO poisoning include loss of consciousness in severe cases and neuropsychiatric dysfunction in milder cases. In addition to these two major syndromes, many cerebral and cerebellar syndromes have been described, including extrapyramidal findings related to the high sensitivity of the basal ganglia to CO, especially when hypoxia is superimposed.

EVALUATION OF THE PATIENT. All victims exposed to smoke must be suspected of having CO poisoning. Patients declaring loss of consciousness, those presenting with any motor or sensory deficit, and all patients with abnormal neurobehavioral tests are considered to have significant CO poisoning until proven otherwise. Pulsating temporal headaches and extreme generalized muscular weakness are the most common neurologic findings in CO poisoning. The presence of coma after smoke inhalation is nearly always an indicator of severe CO poisoning. ECG changes resembling acute ischemia are all but diagnostic when they occur in young patients with healthy hearts who are rescued from fire.

LABORATORY CONFIRMATION. A level of HbCO performed by cooximetry or other spectrophotometric method is available in most hospitals. Levels up to 10 percent are found in cigarette smokers and in automobile passengers following an hour of freeway driving. An HbCO concentration between 10 and 40 percent has only a weak correlation with the severity of the poisoning and particularly with the neurologic outcome. Therefore the HbCO level is a good diagnostic but a poor prognostic indicator. Arterial blood gases usually demonstrate a normal P_{O_2}, contrasting with low oxyhemoglobin saturation measured by cooximeter. Metabolic acidosis is present in severe CO poisoning. Pulse oximeters cannot be used to monitor arterial saturation in patients with smoke inhalation.

TREATMENT. The majority of CO poisoning victims arriving alive to the hospital will improve with administration of oxygen and appropriate supportive treatment. Many have complete resolution of their symptoms within 2 to 3 days; however, in up to 30 percent a secondary syndrome of CO poisoning will develop 7 days to 3 weeks after exposure. In many cases, the secondary syndrome leads to long-term neurologic sequelae, particularly involving higher cerebral functions.

Pure oxygen should be administered as soon as possible after rescue from fire or smoke. HBO significantly increases the elimination of CO from the body (Table 175-5). It also displaces CO effectively and more rapidly from the intracellular compartment and may improve mitochondrial function. However, its routine use is controversial. Opponents claim that its superiority over normobaric oxygen treatment has not been unequivocally proven and that it does not prevent the secondary syndrome of CO poisoning. Supporters claim that it does reduce the severity and the incidence of long-term neurologic sequela. The issue will remain controversial until a well-designed, large scale, randomized, prospective trial is available. Currently, any patient with a history of unconsciousness or positive neurologic findings, including neurobehavioral psychometric abnormalities, is a candidate for hyperbaric therapy, because this treatment is relatively brief and safe. Since the pathophysiology of the secondary syndrome and the mechanism of the beneficial effect of HBO therapy are not fully clarified, when HBO is thought to be indicated, the first session should be initiated as soon as possible.

COMBINED CO-CYANIDE POISONING

Hydrocyanic acid (HCN) is produced when natural and synthetic fibers (e.g., polyurethane, acrylonitrile, nylon, wool, and cotton) are consumed by fire. The combination of CO, HCN, and hypoxic gas mixtures is frequently fatal because the toxicities of these factors potentiate each other. However, with rapid and effective modern rescuing tech-

TABLE 175-5 Effect of Oxygen Therapy on the Carboxyhemoglobin Level

Therapy	Half-life of HbCO
Room Air	3–4 h
100% O_2	40 min
HBO	15 min

HBO indicates hyperbaric oxygen at 2.8 atmospheres absolute.

niques, many victims are now retrieved alive. A prominent clinical feature of CO-CN poisoning is severe lactic acidosis. However, any comatose patient rescued from such a fire should be treated as a combined CO-CN poisoning until proven otherwise. Treatment includes pure oxygen ventilation and intravenous sodium thiosulfate administration as soon as possible. Induction of methemoglobinemia in CO-CN poisoning is contraindicated during prehospital care.

CASE PRESENTATIONS

Case 1

A group of 30 adolescents, aged 11 to 14 years, was exercising in an indoor swimming pool. Twelve were swimming while 18 were waiting out of the water, when a malfunction of the chlorination system caused a sudden, brief release of chlorine gas from a pressurized container. The 18 who were outside of the water escaped immediately after being warned by the irritating smell. On arrival in the emergency room they complained of irritation of the throat and eyes, 10 of them also coughed, but none were dyspneic. They all improved and felt well after 4 h of observation. Before their discharge from the emergency room, they were all found to have a normal flow-volume loop.

The 12 swimmers presented with cough and hoarseness and had wheezing and dyspnea on examination. Three of them had vomited repeatedly before arriving at the emergency room. They were immediately treated with humidified oxygen (FI_{O_2} 50%) by face mask and with albuterol aerosol. Chest x-rays performed 3 h after the exposure demonstrated diffuse alveolar and interstitial infiltrates in 4 patients. One patient had a pneumomediastinum. Five hours after the exposure a flow-volume loop was performed in all patients, revealing evidence of small airway disease in 8. Corticosteroids were then added (60 mg prednisolone by mouth to 4 patients and 100 mg of methylprednisolone intravenously to those unable to swallow). The patients with normal chest x-rays and net improvement during observation were transferred to an intermediate care unit; 4 others were transferred to the ICU for monitoring. Twenty hours after the exposure, decreased breath sounds in the right lung were noted in the patient with pneumomediastinum; a chest tube was inserted and he improved immediately. Twenty-four hours after the exposure, progressive pulmonary edema developed in 2 patients in the ICU and in 2 others who were in the intermediate care unit. They were all electively intubated, ventilated, and treated with oxygen and positive end-expiratory pressure (PEEP). Corticosteroid therapy was continued. The next day 2 intubated patients improved significantly and were extubated after 16 h of mechanical ventilation. After 4 days, corticosteroids were stopped in all patients. On day 7, an additional patient was successfully extubated. He was subsequently followed for recurrent episodes of bronchospasm classified as reactive airway dysfunction syndrome. The last patient in the ICU needed mechanical ventilation for 2 weeks and eventually was found to have bronchiolitis obliterans.

Discussion

The adolescents who were out of the water were exposed to lower concentrations of chlorine because their heads were above the water surface where the heavy gas accumulated. They also had a shorter exposure because they immediately escaped. The swimmers had significantly higher exposures because their heads were near the water and especially because they were breathing heavily while swimming and to escape.

The decision to use corticosteroids was a difficult one, but for short-term use in previously healthy persons, the benefits may outweigh the risks. As is typical after chlorine inhalation, delayed pulmonary toxicity was seen. This is attributed to the time necessary for oxidant and free radical-induced cellular injury to become clinically apparent. For this reason, it is essential to observe patients for at least 24 h following substantial exposure to chlorine gas.

Case 2

Two sailors descended the stairway to the lower deck of a ship transporting loads of fish meal for agricultural use. The ship had passed through stormy weather before reaching port, and sea water had penetrated the shipholds. The sailors descended unprotected despite a heavy unpleasant odor, and the lead sailor suddenly collapsed. The second sailor tried to help, but dropped at the first sailor's side. This accident was observed by their mates and a rescue team was organized. Two unprotected rescuers, followed by a rescuer equipped with self-containing underwater breathing apparatus (SCUBA), descended. The unprotected rescuers collapsed at the same level where the first two sailors dropped, but the protected rescuer succeeded in lifting all victims up by rope. However, the first two victims were declared dead after prolonged cardiopulmonary resuscitation efforts. The two rescuers immediately responded to resuscitative efforts and mechanical ventilation with pure oxygen. One of them recovered full consciousness, the other remained comatose for 4 days and then regained only a part of his mental and motor functions. Analysis of air from the shiphold revealed the following gas concentrations: H_2S 2000 ppm (0.02%), oxygen 13 percent, CO_2 6 percent, other gases (excluding nitrogen) 2 percent.

Discussion

Features typical of H_2S poisoning included the sudden loss of consciousness, especially on descending into a closed space. The first two victims suffered a prolonged anoxic insult due to impairment of oxidative metabolism by the toxic gas, precluding survival. The rescuers had a lesser exposure, and responded to resuscitation with oxygen. In all cases, the injury was probably compounded by the low ambient oxygen concentration. The neurologic impairment of the second rescuer is typical of postanoxic encephalopathy.

References

1. Menzel DB, McClellan RO: Toxic responses of the respiratory system, in Klaassen CD, Amdur MO, Doull J (eds): *Casarett and Doull's Toxicology: The Basic Science of Poisons,* Macmillan, New York, 1980, pp 255–258.
2. Casarett LJ: The vital sacs: Alveolar clearance mechanisms in inhalation toxicology, in Hayes WJ, Jr. (ed), *Essays in Toxicology, Vol 3,* Academic Press, New York, 1972, pp 1–35.
3. Stewart RD, Boettner EA, Southworth RR, et al: Acute carbon tetrachloride intoxication. JAMA 183: 994, 1963.
4. Haber F: Fünf vorträge aus den jahren 1920–23. Springer Verlag, Berlin, 1924.
5. Gapany-Gapanavicius M, Yellin A, Almog S, et al: Pneumomediastinum: A complication of chlorine exposure from mixing household cleaning agents. JAMA 248:349, 1982.
6. Decker WJ: Chlorine poisoning at the swimming pool revisited: Anatomy of two minidisasters. Vet Hum Toxicol 30:584, 1988.
7. Ravizza AG, Carugo D, Cerchiari EL, et al: The treatment of hydrogen sulfide intoxication: Oxygen versus nitrites. Vet Hum Toxicol 24:241, 1982.
8. Bitterman N, Talmi Y, Lerman A, et al: The effect of hyperbaric oxygen on acute experimental sulfide poisoning in the rat. Toxicol Appl Pharmacol 84;325, 1986.
9. Woolley WD, Fardell PJ: Basic aspects of combustion toxicology. Fire Safety J 5:29, 1982.
10. Zapp JA: Fire, toxicity and plastics, in *Physiological and Toxicological Aspects of Combustion Products,* International Symposium 1974, National Academy of Sciences, Washington, DC, 1976, p 62.
11. Piantadosi CA, Sylvia AL, Jobsis-Vandervliet FF: Differences in brain cytochrome responses to carbon monoxide and cyanide in vivo. J Appl Physiol 62:1277, 1987.
12. Birky MM, Clarke FB: Inhalation of toxic products from fires. Bull NY Acad Med 57:997, 1981.
13. NIOSH Pocket Guide to Chemical Hazards. USA, National Institute for Occupational Safety and Health, Publication No. 85-114, 1985, p 14.

Chapter 176

ACUTE CYANIDE POISONING

URI TAITELMAN

KEY POINTS

- *Cyanide is a rapidly acting poison, especially when it is inhaled as hydrogen cyanide (HCN).*
- *The progression of symptoms may be delayed (up to 1 h) after ingestion of cyanide.*
- *Prompt resuscitation, particularly with intubation, mechanical ventilation, and administration of 100% oxygen, is the most important therapeutic intervention.*
- *Pure oxygen and intravenously administered sodium thiosulfate are safe and effective antidotes and should be given as soon as possible.*
- *Induction of methemoglobinemia and administration of dicobalt ethylenediaminetetraacetate (EDTA) are effective but potentially hazardous therapeutic options.*
- *Intravenous hydroxocobalamin is an effective and safe antidote but is not available yet in many countries.*

In 1704 Diesbach, a German colormaker, synthesized Prussian blue (ferric ferrocyanide). In 1782 hydrogen cyanide (HCN) was produced from Prussian blue by the Swedish chemist Scheele and named prussic acid. HCN gas is the most toxic and rapidly acting form of cyanide-containing poisons. Acute human intoxication with cyanides occurs mainly during manipulation of cyanides used in different chemical and industrial procedures, in particular during metal processing–steel hardening (case hardening), electroplating, metal cleaning, and recovery of gold and silver from ores. Cyanides are involved in the preparation of acrylonitrile, which is used to produce acrylic fibers, synthetic rubber, and plastics. HCN is also a common combustion product of natural and synthetic fiber polymers. Many plants contain cyanogenic glycosides that may cause acute or chronic cyanide poisoning. Cyanide poisoning may also occur during treatment of hospitalized patients with sodium nitroprusside.

Toxicokinetics

The toxicity of cyanide-liberating compounds is directly proportional to the amount and rate of HCN formation. HCN is a weak acid with a pK_a of 9.4 and a boiling point of 25°C. Therefore, at body temperature and the pH of body fluids, it is in the form of nonionized HCN gas that diffuses very rapidly through all body compartments. Cyanides have a volume of distribution 1.5 L/kg. This high volume is due to intracellular fixation of cyanide. For example, erythrocytes contain 100-fold more cyanide than plasma. Cyanide has a high affinity for the ferric (Fe^{3+}) iron of enzymes and pigments and in particular for the cytochrome aa_3 of the electron transfer chain of the mitochondrial membrane. Inhibition of cytochrome aa_3 and interruption of aerobic respiration is the major mechanism of cyanide toxicity.

ROUTE OF EXPOSURE

INHALATION

The effect of inhalation of HCN is immediate. Inhalation of 10 ppm is considered the permissible exposure limit since this concentration can be completely detoxified by humans; 45 to 54 ppm is tolerated for about 30 min without difficulty; 180 ppm is fatal after 10 min; above 280 ppm is immediately fatal.

INGESTION

The rapidity of HCN formation in the stomach after ingestion of cyanide-containing compounds depends on gastric pH and the stability of the cyanide-liberating molecule. Thus potassium (KCN) and sodium (NaCN) cyanide are very toxic if ingested on an empty stomach, since they liberate HCN rapidly at an acid pH; ingestion when the stomach is full of alkaline food or buffered fluids may lead to a slowly developing clinical syndrome (delayed up to 1 h). Silver (AgCN) and copper ($CuCN_2$) cyanide are less toxic since they generate HCN less rapidly. Ingestion of plants containing cyanogenic glycosides (see Chap. 181) usually causes slow development of symptoms because the liberation of cyanides depends on enzymatic action. Enzymes capable of releasing cyanide may be produced by the plant and coingested with the glycoside or may be present in the intestine. The activity of these enzymes is higher in the alkaline pH of the small bowel.

SKIN EXPOSURE

Alkaline salts of cyanides (KCN and NaCN) are skin and mucous membrane irritants and may cause burns if concentrated. However, skin contact with these salts usually does not cause systemic cyanide poisoning.[1] HCN can be absorbed through human skin, but acute poisoning due to percutaneous absorption is not common.

BIOTRANSFORMATION: NATURAL DETOXIFICATION

All mammals have several detoxification pathways for cyanides. The major route of biological cyanide detoxification in humans is by conversion to relatively nontoxic thiocyanate (SCN^-), which is rapidly excreted by normal kidneys. This conversion requires a source of sulfane sulfur—a divalent sulfur bonded to another sulfur. Several sulfur-containing compounds[2] participate in the sulfur pool essential for the formation of thiocyanate including thiosulfate, bisulfides, mercaptopyruvate, cysteine, glutathione, elemental sulfur, and serum albumin. All of these compounds are in an equilibrium due to the activity of several enzymes known as sulfur transferases: rhodanese, mercaptopyruvate sulfurtransferase, and thiosulfate reductase. Thiocyanate formation occurs both in intracellular and extracellular compartments. The most important enzyme for thiocyanate formation in the intracellular compartment is rhodanese, which forms thiocyanate from cyanide if sulfane sulfur atoms are available. Rhodanese is located mainly in the lipid layer of the mitochondria, thus being in proximity to cytochrome oxidases, the prime targets of cyanide toxicity. The liver and kidneys contain high intracellular concentrations of rhodanese, while the brain contains a relatively small amount. The liver is the most effective organ for detoxifying cyanide to thiocyanate. In the extracellular compartment, serum albumin has two remarkable properties related to cyanide detoxification: It is a sulfane sulfur carrier, bringing sulfur to the liver, thereby equilibrating the intracellular with extracellular sulfane sulfur pool, and it has sulfurtransferase activity, forming thiocyanate from cyanide.

Vitamin B_{12} exists in the body in three forms as methylcobalamin, hydroxocobalamin, and cyanocobalamin. Hydroxocobalamin, a natural chelating agent, is transformed to cyanocobalamin by chelation of cyanide ion. A small amount of cyanide is detoxified by binding to hydroxocobalamin in this way.

Less than 1 percent of a cyanide load is eliminated in the gas form by the lung.[3] Other routes of natural detoxification of cyanides include oxidation to cyanates, formation of cyanohydrine compounds, and complete oxidation to CO_2, but these contribute only minimally to cyanide detoxification.

Toxicodynamics

The major target organs of acute cyanide poisoning are the central nervous system (CNS) and the heart. At low concentration cyanides stimulate the CNS. The respiratory center is stimulated as well, which increases intake if the poisoning is by inhalation. At higher levels of cyanide exposure, unconsciousness occurs, frequently with convulsions and apnea. The effect on the heart is at first stimulation (at low levels), causing increased cardiac output. At higher levels arrhythmias are seen, especially complete atrioventricular block, extreme bradycardia, ventricular tachycardia, ventricular fibrillation, and asystole. In animal experiments, apnea always precedes life-threatening cardiac dysfunction.

Clinical Manifestations

The severity of clinical manifestations depends on the amount and rate of cyanide absorption. If exposure is by inhalation, absorption is immediate. Thus, a patient that is asymptomatic despite an inhalation exposure needs only a short period of observation and no antidotal therapy. Inhalation of moderate amounts of HCN, especially when there is coexposure to other toxic gases, may cause persistent severe manifestations and necessitate full treatment. Up to one-third of patients with smoke inhalation who are rescued from domestic fires (proven by high carboxyhemoglobin levels) also have high blood levels of cyanide.[4]

If exposure is by ingestion, symptoms develop slowly in many cases. Three successive phases can be observed: the excitement or stimulation phase, the depression phase, and the adynamic phase (Table 176-1). However, following massive ingestion, the first phase is very short or missing. The patient may rapidly develop coma, seizures, apnea, and circulatory collapse. Survival with few or no sequelae can be achieved in this case only if the patient is intubated and mechanically ventilated with oxygen before or immediately following apnea. Patients resuscitated in the third phase are typically left with severe neurologic sequelae typical of anoxic brain damage.

Diagnosis

A diagnosis of cyanide poisoning is typically made based upon the circumstances of exposure or the resulting clinical syndrome. For example, the diagnosis may be obvious following industrial or laboratory exposure to cyanides. It should also be considered in comatose smoke inhalation victims who may have combined carbon monoxide and cyanide poisoning. Most suicide attempts are by chemists who have access to cyanides.

The typical clinical syndrome is notable for the coexistence of rapidly developing coma, cardiac dysfunction, and severe lactic acidosis in the setting of a high mixed venous oxygen saturation. The funduscopic examination may reveal red retinal veins, correlating with the elevated venous oxyhemoglobin saturation. When such findings are present in a setting consistent with cyanide exposure, empiric therapy should be given pending confirmation of the diagnosis.

Whole blood cyanide levels should always be performed since they are valuable for confirmation of the diagnosis and for evaluation of the effects of treatment. Samples should be drawn according to the instructions of the labora-

TABLE 176-1 Manifestations of Progressive Acute Cyanide Poisoning by Ingestion

I. Excitement or stimulation phase	Anxiety, dyspnea, sensation of chest constriction, headache, hyperpnea, giddiness, confusion, hypertension, tachycardia
II. Depression phase	Auditory and visual disturbances, coma, fixed dilated pupils, convulsions, hypoventilation, apnea, hypotension, bradycardia, ventricular arrhythmias
III. Adynamic phase *(état de mort apparent)*	Deep coma, loss of muscular tone, loss of spontaneous activity and all reflexes, absence of blood pressure and pulse

TABLE 176-2 Treatment of Cyanide Poisoning

Widely agreed-upon strategies
Prompt cardiopulmonary resuscitation
Ventilation with 100% oxygen
Sodium thiosulfate, 25% solution, 150 mg/kg intravenously
Gastric decontamination
Additional therapies, not universally available or agreed upon
Hydroxocobalamin, 4 g intravenously
Induction of methemoglobinemia
Amylnitrite 0.2 mL perle, crushed and inhaled 30 s of each minute until sodium nitrite is given
Sodium nitrite, 10% solution, 5–10 mg/kg intravenously
Paradimethylaminophenol (4-DMAP), 1–3 mg/kg intravenously
Dicobalt EDTA, 300–600 mg intravenously

tory that will perform the analysis since cyanide is volatile, oxidizable, and unstable.

Treatment

Prompt cardiopulmonary resuscitation (CPR) is the major determinant of survival from acute cyanide poisoning (Table 176-2). Most patients who have survived acute poisoning were treated with prompt CPR and oxygen administration.[5] In addition, several antidotes are available. Oxygen and sodium thiosulfate are efficacious, and their use in cyanide poisoning is universally accepted. Cobalt derivatives, especially hydroxocobalamin, are useful in addition. Other therapeutic modalities, such as induction of methemoglobinemia, are more controversial. Since treatment of cyanide poisoning is complex yet prompt therapy is essential, medical centers should consider developing a standard protocol for dissemination to the medical staff.

OXYGEN

Oxygen has been demonstrated to be an effective antidote in experimental animal and human cyanide poisonings. Its mechanism of action has not been elucidated, but it may relate to a change in the affinity of cytochrome aa_3 for oxygen during cyanide poisoning. Oxygen is protective when given before the poisoning and therapeutic when given after the exposure.[6–10] It also potentiates the effect of other antidotes.[11] Therefore, ventilation with pure oxygen is a major therapeutic intervention in the treatment of cyanide poisoning. Hyperbaric oxygen is even more effective experimentally.[11–13] However, its use in human cases is rarely practical because of the time element. The ultimate fate of the patient with severe cyanide poisoning is usually determined within minutes.

SODIUM THIOSULFATE

Sodium thiosulfate is an effective and safe antidote. It acts as an excellent sulfur donor to rhodanese and other sulfane sulfur transferases. The average normal plasma concentration of healthy volunteers is around 1 mg/dL. Administration of radioactive thiosulfate causes an immediate increase in all components of the sulfane sulfur pool.[2] At a dose of 150 mg/kg administered intravenously, sodium thiosulfate has practically no toxicity. The volume of distribution is 150 mL/kg. The half-life of the distribution phase is 23 min and of the elimination phase 180 min. About 40 percent of an injected dose is eliminated within 3 h in the urine if renal function is normal. The major disadvantage of thiosulfate administration is its slow penetration to the intracellular compartment. Nevertheless, administration of 150 mg/kg increases the extracellular concentration of thiosulfate a hundred times, thus favoring intracellular penetration. The only relative contraindication to thiosulfate administration is renal failure. Thiocyanate is readily removed by hemodialysis.

HYDROXOCOBALAMIN

Hydroxocobalamin is a natural precursor form of vitamin B_{12} which becomes cyanocobalamin after complexing cyanide. The compound is safe, is rapid acting, does not liberate cobalt, and only rarely causes hypersensitivity.[14] Hydroxocobalamin is particularly useful during the immediate treatment of comatose smoke inhalation victims who have a high probability of cyanide poisoning. A disadvantage of hydroxocobalamin administration is that large doses are necessary since 1 mol of hydroxocobalamin chelates only 1 mol of cyanide. The compound is poorly soluble in water so that a volume of 80 mL has to be infused in order to administer the initial dose of 4 g. Preparation of the compound necessitates great expertise and there is only one supplier (Pharmacie Central des Hôpitaux, France).

OTHER COBALT DERIVATIVES

For many years it has been known that cobalt atoms bind cyanide to form a stable complex. Dicobalt ethylenediaminetetraacetate (EDTA)(Kelocyanor) is a very potent and rapid acting antidote for cyanide poisoning in the experimental setting, capable of reversing deep coma and apnea.[15] Its potency is partially due to liberation of free cobalt in the extracellular fluid and to penetration of the blood-brain barrier.[16] The initial dose of dicobalt EDTA is 300 to 600 mg for an adult, followed by glucose infusion. If given in excess, this antidote may cause cardiac arrhythmias and hypotension, probably due to chelation of calcium and magnesium by EDTA. Since cyanide decreases the toxicity of dicobalt EDTA, toxicity is more apparent in nonpoisoned individuals, resulting in severe nausea, vomiting, and hypotension. Severe allergic reactions are seen as well.[1,17] Thus titration of the drug is delicate; it should be used only by an experienced physician in very severe cases of cyanide poisoning (*état de mort apparent*) and only when the diagnosis is unequivocally established.

INDUCTION OF METHEMOGLOBINEMIA

Induction of methemoglobinemia is used in several countries. Cyanide has a very high affinity for the ferric iron of methemoglobin. Experimentally, conversion of 30% hemoglobin to methemoglobin effectively protects or treats cyanide poisoning.[11] In North America, sodium nitrite is administered intravenously at a dose of 5 to 10 mg/kg or amylnitrite is given by inhalation. In Germany, 4-DMAP is given intravenously at a dose of 1 to 3 mg/kg. Induction of methemoglobinemia potentiates the beneficial effects of oxygen and thiosulfate, so that the combination of the three is very effective.

There are several disadvantages to induction of methemoglobin for patients with cyanide poisoning. First, this method is contraindicated after smoke inhalation (the most frequent cause of acute human cyanide poisoning), because the reduction in oxygen-carrying capacity due to 30% methemoglobinemia, superimposed on coexisting carboxyhemoglobinemia, is potentially dangerous. Further, components of smoke may independently cause methemoglobinemia.[18] Second, induction of methemoglobinemia takes time (10 to 30 min).[19] Third, the dose-response relationship between administration of sodium nitrite or 4-DMAP is unpredictable. In many cases methemoglobin is not produced, while in others excess methemoglobin may seriously compromise the patient.[20,21] Theoretically the dose should be adjusted to the patient's hemoglobin level and to the total enzymatic reducing power of the erythrocytes at the time of the injection, factors that are impossible to evaluate in most emergency situations. Fourth, induction of methemoglobinemia in a glucose-6-phosphate dehydrogenase (G6PD) deficient patient may cause fatal methemoglobinemia or hemolysis. Finally, since the safe use of methemoglobin-inducing antidotes requires the ability to monitor the resulting methemoglobinemia and the availability of immediate treatment for excessive methemoglobinemia, its use at the site of accidental poisoning by nonphysician rescuers is controversial.

Decontamination

In acute cyanide poisoning by ingestion, the order of therapeutic interventions is **1.** prompt CPR as needed, **2.** 100% oxygen and intravenous antidotes, and **3.** gastric lavage and decontamination following initial therapy.

Several methods have been described in the literature for stomach decontamination after ingestion of cyanide salts. One aims to form a stable precipitate of ferrous ferrocyanide (Berlin white) by introducing two solutions into the stomach. Solution A consists of 16% ferrosulfate and 0.3% citric acid. Solution B is 6% sodium carbonate. Equal volumes of solutions A and B are mixed and immediately instilled into the stomach. This is followed by a washout of the stomach with 6% sodium carbonate or water.[22]

Alternative approaches include washing of the stomach with an oxidizing solution such as 1:10,000 potassium permanganate or 3% hydrogen peroxide; a solution of hydroxocobalamine; 600 mg of dicobalt EDTA as a 1.5% aqueous solution; or a solution of activated charcoal.[23] There are no data comparing the efficacy of these methods. The most readily available solution is activated charcoal.

CASE PRESENTATION

Emergency medical services were alerted by the wife of a 40-year-old chemist who was found unconscious in his study shortly after dinner. A bottle containing white powder and an empty glass were on the table. The man was lying on the floor, unresponsive, with evidence of emesis on his clothes. His pupils were dilated and unreactive to light. The blood pressure was 80/50 with a pulse of 40. Shortly afterward he developed grand mal seizures followed by apnea. He was immediately intubated and ventilated with pure oxygen. A femoral catheter was placed and infusion of saline and dopamine started. He was brought to the nearest hospital within 15 min.

In the emergency room the blood pressure was 70/50. A central venous line was inserted revealing a central venous pressure (CVP) of 24 cmH_2O. The electrocardiogram (ECG) showed a slow junctional rhythm at 40/min with frequent PVCs and severe ST depression in all leads. Gastric lavage was performed and the local poison information center was consulted. The anion gap was 30. Arterial blood and venous blood from the CVP line were sent for blood gas analysis. The arterial pH was 6.95, the P_{CO_2} 30, and the arterial P_{O_2} 300 mmHg, while the venous P_{O_2} was 85 mmHg. Arteriovenous oxygen content difference was 1 mL/dL.

Sodium thiosulfate, 150 mg/kg, was slowly infused immediately after samples for toxicologic analysis were drawn. Fifteen minutes after thiosulfate administration, the blood pressure rose to 110/70, the heart rate was 100/min, and normal sinus rhythm was present on the ECG monitor. Fifteen minutes later the patient recovered consciousness. Metabolic acidosis slowly resolved within the next hour. It was learned that the patient's family history was notable for G6PD deficiency. The chest roentgenogram confirmed right lower lobe aspiration pneumonitis. The patient was extubated 4 h after arriving in the emergency room and was hospitalized for further care of pneumonia and for psychiatric evaluation.

It was subsequently discovered that he had been depressed for the prior 2 weeks and took potassium cyanide from his laboratory. He mixed one teaspoon of the powder with water and swallowed it shortly after dinner. The whole blood cyanide level on admission was 5 mg/dL. The white powder was sent to a specialized analytical laboratory for cyanide analysis and revealed that it was a mixture of 50% potassium cyanide and 50% potassium cyanate. It was established that the original bottle was opened to air several times since it was purchased some years ago, explaining the oxidation of 50% of the contents.

CASE DISCUSSION

A suicide attempt performed by a chemist, rapidly followed by coma, convulsions, and circulatory failure, is highly suspicious for acute cyanide poisoning. However, rapidly developing coma and cardiac dysfunction should always prompt consideration of this toxicity even when the setting is less obvious. The development of lactic acidosis with an elevated venous oxygen saturation is highly suggestive of cyanide poisoning, and, in this case, is all but diagnostic. The favorable outcome in this chemist is attributable to the deterioration of the potassium cyanide in the bottle due to oxidation, the fact that the salt was ingested after a large meal (thus blunting gastric acidity and delaying release of HCN), and the prompt resuscitation. Had the patient been intubated, ventilated, and oxygenated more than a few minutes after apnea, the outcome might have been different.

In a young healthy person, severe CNS depression precedes cardiac arrest from cyanide poisoning, and cardiac recovery during treatment is faster than CNS recovery, as demonstrated in this case. It is probable that cardiac activity could have been restored even if resuscitation had been delayed, but severe neurologic sequelae of anoxic brain damage would have been likely. The only antidotes given to this patient were oxygen and thiosulfate. Sodium nitrite was not administered since the patient belonged to a family with known G6PD deficiency. Cobalt compounds, especially hydroxocobalamin, could have been given as well but were unavailable in this case.

References

1. McKiernan MJ: Emergency treatment of cyanide poisoning (letter). Lancet 2:86, 1980.
2. Westley J, Adler H, Westley L, Nishida C: The sulfurtransferases. Fund Appl Toxicol 3:377, 1983.
3. Sylvester DM, Hayton WL, Morgan RL, Way JL: Effects of thiosulfate on cyanide pharmacokinetics in dogs. Toxicol Appl Pharmacol 69:265, 1983.
4. Clark CJ, Campbell D, Reid WH: Blood carboxyhemoglobin and cyanide levels in fire survivors. Lancet 1:1332, 1981.
5. Bismuth C, Cantineau JP, Pontal P, Baud F, Garnier R, Poulos L: Intoxication cyanhydrine: Primauté du traitement symptomatique. Vingt-cinq observations. Presse Med 41:2493, 1984.
6. Way JL, Gibbon SL, Sheehy M: Cyanide intoxication: Protection with oxygen. Science 152:210, 1966.
7. Cope C: The importance of oxygen in the treatment of cyanide poisoning. JAMA 12:109, 1961.
8. Isom GE, Way JL: Effect of oxygen on cyanide intoxication. VI. Reactivation of cyanide-inhibited glucose metabolism. J Pharmacol Exper Therapeut 1:235, 1974.
9. Isom GE, Way JL: Effects of oxygen on the antagonism of cyanide intoxication—cytochrome oxidase, in vivo. Toxicol Appl Pharmacol 65:250, 1982.
10. Isom GE, Way JL: Effects of oxygen on the antagonism of cyanide intoxication—cytochrome oxidase, in vitro. Toxicol Appl Pharmacol 74:57, 1984.
11. Way JL, End E, Sheehy MH, et al: Effect of oxygen on cyanide intoxication. IV. Hyperbaric oxygen. Toxicol Appl Pharmacol 22:415, 1972.
12. Skene WG, Norman JN, Smith G: Effect of hyperbaric oxygen in cyanide poisoning. Protocols 3rd Int Conf Hyperbaric Med: 705, 1966.
13. Litovitz TL, Larkin RF, Myers RAM: Cyanide poisoning treated with hyperbaric oxygen. Am J Emerg Med 1:99, 1983.
14. Posner MA, Tobey RE, McElroy H: Hydroxocobalamin therapy of cyanide intoxication in Guinea pigs. Anesthesiology 2:157, 1976.
15. Paulet G, Chary R, Bocquet P, Fouilhoux M: Valeur comparée du nitrite de sodium et des chelates de cobalt dans le traitement de l'intoxication cyanohydrique chez l'animal (chien-lapin) non anesthésie. Arch Int Pharmacodyn 1–2:104, 1960.
16. Bartelhemer EW: Analyse der akuten kobaltvergiftung im tierversuch. Arch Exper Pathol Pharmacol 243:254, 1962.
17. Nagler J, Provoost RA, Parizel G: Hydrogen cyanide poisoning: Treatment with cobalt EDTA. J Occupat Med 6:414, 1978.
18. Hoffman RS, Sauter D: Methemoglobinemia resulting from smoke inhalation. Vet Human Toxicol 31:168, 1989.
19. Moore SJ, Norris JC, Walsh DA, Hume AS: Antidotal use of methemoglobin forming cyanide antagonists in concurrent carbon monoxide/cyanide intoxication. J Pharmacol Exper Therapeut 242:70, 1987.
20. Berlin CM: The treatment of cyanide poisoning in children. Pediatrics 46:793, 1970.
21. van Heijst AN, Douze JM, van Kesteren RG, et al: Therapeutic problems in cyanide poisoning. J Toxicol Clin Toxicol 25:383, 1987.
22. Marrs TC: Antidotal treatment of acute cyanide poisoning. Adverse drug reactions. Acute Poison Rev 4:179, 1988.
23. Lambert RJ, Kindler BL, Schaeffer DJ: The efficacy of superactivated charcoal in treating rats exposed to a lethal oral dose of potassium cyanide. Ann Emerg Med 17:595, 1988.

Chapter 177

SALICYLATES

BIANCA RAIKHLIN-EISENKRAFT
JESSE HALL

KEY POINTS

- *Chronic intoxication with salicylates may be subtle in presentation and can occur at relatively low serum salicylate levels.*
- *The standard nomogram predicting toxicity after single ingestions* cannot *be used for patients using salicylates chronically or having ingested enteric-coated preparations.*
- *Acidosis favors tissue penetration of salicylates.*
- *Most moderate to severe intoxications are characterized by respiratory alkalosis and metabolic acidosis, although the latter is often most prominent in children.*
- *Salicylate overdose may cause adult respiratory distress syndrome (ARDS).*
- *Alkalinization of urine enhances salicylate elimination.*
- *Hypokalemia must be treated aggressively to succeed in urinary alkalinization.*
- *Carbonic anhydrase inhibitors* should not *be used to alkalinize the urine.*
- *Seizures, refractory acidosis, and coma are indications for hemodialysis.*

The glycoside *salicin* was purified from the bark of the willow in 1827 by Leroux, but its antipyretic properties were known in England almost a hundred years earlier.[1] In the modern era, an extraordinarily large number of products containing acetylsalicylic acid (ASA) are sold over-the-counter. Although acute intoxications, particularly in children, have decreased in incidence in the past one to two decades, chronic toxicity remains a significant problem, often with a subtle presentation.[2–5] We review the pharmacology, pathophysiology, clinical presentation, and management of both acute and chronic intoxications.

Pharmacology

COMMON PREPARATIONS AND THERAPEUTIC USES

The most commonly used salicylates are aspirin (ASA), salicylic acid, and methylsalicylic acid. The stomach and blood rapidly hydrolyze ASA to salicylic acid and acetic acid. Methyl salicylate is present in topical salicylate preparations (Oil of Wintergreen, Ben Gay). It is a very infrequent cause of poisoning, but it is important to note that these preparations are extremely concentrated; 1 tsp Oil of Wintergreen contains approximately 7 g salicylate, roughly equivalent to 20 adult aspirin tablets.[2]

Aspirin is used for its analgesic and anti-inflammatory properties, as an antipyretic, and as an antiplatelet drug. Therapeutic benefits derive largely from the action of this class of drugs to inhibit prostaglandin biosynthesis. Platelet adhesiveness is impaired by ASA, while anti-inflammatory and most toxic effects appear to be mediated largely by salicylic acid.

Therapeutic adult dosage of aspirin is up to 650 mg every 4 h. If dosage is to be increased beyond this for management of chronic conditions such as rheumatoid arthritis, serum levels should be monitored. Pediatric dosage is 10 to 20 mg/kg every 6 h with no more than 60 mg/kg given in 24 h. Children's aspirin comes as an 80-mg tablet with containers in the United States limited to 36 tablets.

PHARMACOKINETICS

ASA is a weak acid with a p*Ka* of 3. As such, half an oral dose appears in the stomach in nonionized form and is rapidly absorbed. Peak therapeutic levels occur within 2 h. Enteric-coated preparations delay peak concentrations markedly. The standard nomogram for using serum level to predict toxicity cannot be applied to ingestions of these forms of aspirin. ASA is poorly soluble and often precipitates in the stomach, particularly in massive ingestions. This further confounds simple predictions of absorption. Finally, despite the relatively high intraluminal pH of the small bowel, ASA absorption at this site is substantial due to the large surface area.

Within the plasma compartment, 50 to 80 percent of salicylate is bound to albumin, whereas the remainder is present in active ionized form. States with diminished binding sites (hypoalbuminemia, presence of drugs competing for binding sites) result in greater amounts of free drug with the potential for tissue penetration and toxicity. Acidosis also enhances tissue penetration.[4] Thus, a number of conditions will markedly increase the volume of distribution of salicylates.

With small single doses, drug elimination is largely by conjugation in the liver. In this lower dose range the kinetics of drug elimination are first order (see Chap. 169), but with multiple or large single doses hepatic elimination pathways are saturated, renal excretion of unchanged drug becomes increasingly important, and drug elimination follows zero-order kinetics. Under these latter conditions, the plasma half-life of therapeutic doses (2 to 5 h) can increase tenfold.[6,7]

Two factors are of major importance clinically in maximizing renal excretion of salicylate. An alkaline urine greatly favors excretion by increasing the ionized form of the molecule in the urine which is less well reabsorbed. Similarly, avoidance of hypokalemia prevents preferential tubular excretion of hydrogen ion, acidification of urine, and diminished salicylate excretion. Of course, the metabolic acidosis of salicylate overdose diminishes renal excretion and is, in this regard, self-perpetuating.

Salicylates cross the placenta and are poorly metabolized by the fetus. Fetal demise attributable to ASA overdose has been reported.[8] Salicylates are generally contraindicated in pregnancy, particularly the third trimester, because of possible adverse consequences of prostaglandin synthesis inhibition.

Pathophysiology

ACID-BASE AND METABOLIC DISTURBANCES

Salicylate intoxication has two effects which can produce significant acid-base disturbances: increased alveolar ventilation and endogenous acid production.[9,10] The former results from either direct stimulation of brain stem centers or increased sensitivity to the usual metabolic signals controlling respiration. The latter has been attributed to uncoupling of oxidative phosphorylation and inhibitory effects on a number of Krebs cycle enzymes. Although the uncoupling of oxidative phosphorylation results in an increase in carbon dioxide production, this effect is "buried" in the more than compensatory concomittant increase in alveolar ventilation.

The metabolic acidosis seen in salicylate intoxication on rare occasions causes extreme acidemia but most typically blood pH is near normal.[11] Resistance to its development increases with age, and thus, acidosis tends to dominate the acid-base disturbance in infants, and "pure" forms of respiratory alkalosis are seen most often in the elderly. It is important to note that most patients exhibit a complex mixed acid-base disturbance. The respiratory alkalosis causes some appropriate excretion of base in compensation and independent increased acid production. A small fraction of the decrement in plasma bicarbonate is attributable to salicylic acid itself, but this is usually not significant. Lactate levels are usually modestly elevated, but severe lactic acidosis is rare unless shock supervenes. Ketoacidosis may play a small role in patients with protracted vomiting or nausea. The net result of this interplay of acid-base disturbances and compensations is usually respiratory alkalosis and metabolic acidosis, the latter accompanied by an elevated anion gap (mean anion gap approximately 20 in most patients with uncomplicated salicylate ingestion).[11]

Perturbations of glucose metabolism occur in salicylate overdose, and both hyperglycemia and hypoglycemia may be encountered.[12] Hyperglycemia is more common and has been ascribed to increased glucose-6-phosphatase activity and increase glycogenolysis. Interestingly, concurrent administration of glucose with salicylate in an animal model led to increased brain glucose concentrations and marked improvement in survival.[13] It is likely that serum glucose levels do not accurately reflect availability of this substrate in the central nervous system (CNS). Hypocalcemia with tetany has also been noted during salicylate overdose and may be exacerbated by bicarbonate therapy.

COAGULOPATHY

Even at very low doses ASA inhibits platelet adhesiveness, an action which is exploited therapeutically. At higher doses inhibition of factor VII synthesis is seen, indicated by an elevation of the prothrombin time (PT). Massive overdose can result in hepatic necrosis with typical associated coagulopathy.

PULMONARY CAPILLARY LEAK AND NEUROLOGIC MANIFESTATIONS

Low pressure pulmonary edema, or the adult respiratory distress syndrome (ARDS), is a well-described complication of salicylate overdose, as is cerebral edema.[14,15] It is unclear whether there are shared mechanisms of injury. It is likely that direct effects of salicylates, metabolic disturbances, and edema act in concert to produce the frequent and often dramatic neurologic manifestations of this overdose.

Clinical Presentation

Most guidelines for predicting severity of overdose have been generated from single ingestions in the pediatric population. Though this presentation is decreasing in incidence, chronic toxicity is still seen and is often unusual in its presentation. Furthermore, diagnosis is frequently delayed.

In general, acute ingestions of 150 to 300 mg/kg correlate to mild toxicity, 300 to 500 mg/kg to moderate toxicity, and >500 mg/kg to severe toxicity, with the potential for death (Table 177-1). Of course, in many circumstances the precise quantity of salicylates ingested will not be known to the physician. The Done nomogram may be used to predict severity of intoxication *for single ingestions* (Fig. 177-1).[2,16] We emphasize that this predictor is not to be used for chronic ingestions, when enteric preparations are involved, or if coexisting disease or ingestion will complicate outcome.[2,6] It is recommended that a level 6 h or longer after ingestions be used, to ensure that levels have reached their peak.

In chronic ingestions, toxicity may appear at much lower initial serum levels, related to greater tissue penetration and the possibility of levels continuing to rise over the first 24 h in hospital. Any serum level over 25 mg/dL in an adult with chronic ingestion and consistent findings should be considered to potentially indicate toxicity. Since salicylism may be rather cryptic in presentation, particularly in chronic ingestions in the elderly, it is recommended that this diagnosis be considered if obvious alternative explanations do not exist: **1.** for any mixed respiratory alkalosis and metabolic acidosis; **2.** in every patient with decreased level

TABLE 177-1 Toxicity Related to Ingested Dose and Serum Levels

Dose (mg/kg)	Level of Toxicity	Serum Level (mg/dL)
<150	None expected	<50
150–300	Mild to moderate	50–80
300–500	Severe	>80
>500	Potentially lethal	>160

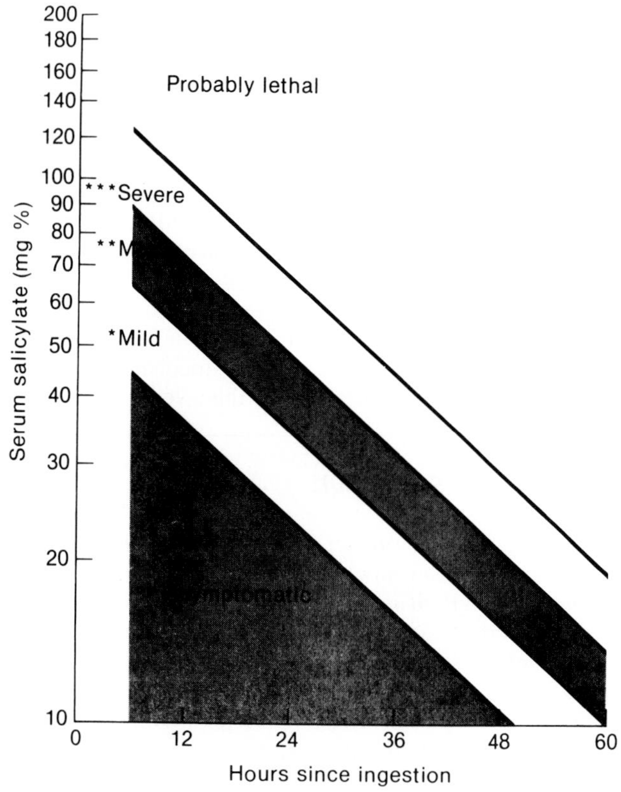

FIGURE 177-1 Nomogram relating serum salicylate level to general severity of intoxication. This nomogram should not be applied to chronic intoxication or ingestion of enteric-coated preparations. Note that the nomogram begins 6 h after ingestion to provide that serum levels have peaked. [Reprinted with permission from Done AK: Aspirin overdose: Incidence, diagnosis and management. Pediatrics 62(suppl):895, 1978.]

TABLE 177-2 Clinical Findings in 177 Patients Admitted to an ICU

Clinical Signs	%
Neurologic abnormalities (depressed consciousness)	61
Acid-base disturbances	50
Pulmonary complications	43
Hyperpyrexia	20
Circulatory disorders (hypotension)	14
ECG abnormalities	
Wide QRS, first- and second-degree atrioventricular block, ventricular arrhythmia	10
Coagulation disorders	38
Renal abnormalities (oliguria)	7

SOURCE: Modified and reprinted with permission from Thisted B, Krantz T, Strom J, Sorenson B: Acute salicylate self-poisoning in 177 patients treated in ICU. Acta Anaesth Scand 31:312, 1987.

TABLE 177-3 Clinical Features of Salicylate Intoxication

Mild to Moderate	Severe
Headache	Lethargy
Dizziness	Hallucinations
Tinnitus	Delirium
Deafness	Seizures
Hyperventilation	Coma
Nausea	Respiratory alkalosis
Vomiting	Gastrointestinal bleeding
Vasodilation	Hypotension
Tachycardia	Metabolic acidosis
	Pulmonary edema
	Cerebral edema
	Hypoglycemia
	Hyperpyrexia
	Renal and liver failure

of consciousness, particularly when accompanied by typical acid-base disturbances; and **3.** in every patient with respiratory distress due to low pressure pulmonary edema.

Neurologic signs tend to dominate the presentation (Table 177-2) and are a good gauge to the severity of the overdose (Table 177-3). Mild toxicity is characterized by tinnitus and lethargy. More severe intoxication or progression results in irritability or disorientation. The most severe intoxications are usually replete with findings, including hallucinations, seizures, and coma.

Gastrointestinal symptoms are prominent. Nausea and vomiting may reflect CNS disturbance or direct irritation of the upper tract. Minor bleeding from gastric erosion and ulceration is common but transfusion is rarely necessary, despite the associated coagulopathy. Gastric perforation has been reported with massive overdose.[17]

Hyperthermia is seen in as many as 20 percent of patients. ARDS is most likely in adults with chronic intoxication and is more frequent in patients with significant metabolic acidosis and marked CNS abnormalities. Acute renal and hepatic failure have been described, but are usually self-limited and reversible.

Management

DIAGNOSIS

We stress again that a high index of suspicion is necessary to make this diagnosis in obscure cases. Urine testing can be performed with ferric chloride or Phenistix, but these are qualitative and nonspecific tests. When clinical suspicion of salicylate intoxication exists, plasma levels should be measured.

LABORATORY TESTS AND MONITORING

Once a diagnosis of salicylate toxicity is made, laboratory tests including complete blood count with platelet count, electrolytes, blood urea nitrogen (BUN), creatinine, glucose, urinalysis including pH, and arterial blood-gas levels should be obtained. A repeat salicylate level after 2 to 3 h will help define those patients with rising levels and potential for worsening toxicity. For moderate to severe intoxications likely to be admitted to the ICU, a PT, serum calcium, chest radiograph, and liver function profile should be obtained. Since hypoxemia may develop early and rapidly in patients with pulmonary edema, monitoring with pulse oximetry is strongly advised. Serial neurologic examination as for all obtunded or comatose patients is essential and will help guide subsequent therapy.

SUPPORTIVE THERAPY

Emesis or gastric lavage may be useful up to 12 h after massive ingestions, presumably because large quantities of drug precipitate in the stomach. Because impaired level of consciousness is so frequent in these patients, the airway may need to be secured prior to attempts at evacuation (see Chap. 6). Activated charcoal binds salicylate and impairs absorption and should be given at a dose of 1.0 g/kg and repeated every 4 h for a total of three to four doses.[18] Development of an ileus in critically ill patients often makes this impossible. Cathartics such as magnesium sulfate may also enhance elimination.

All patients presenting with coma should have glucose and naloxone administered immediately (see Chap. 144). Since both hyperglycemia and hypoglycemia may complicate this intoxication, levels should be followed very frequently early in the course. Although naloxone does not appear to reverse the CNS effects of salicylates, polypharmaceutical ingestions are common, and since profound CNS depression is an indication for dialysis, other sources of altered mental status should be considered and treated.[19] The development of seizures should raise the possibility of a new electrolyte disturbance or hypoglycemia. Aside from correcting these metabolic abnormalities, seizures should be treated in the usual fashion (see Chap. 142).

Temperature in excess of 40°C (104°F) should be treated with passive cooling. Dehydration is common with severe intoxications, due to hyperthermia, nausea, vomiting, and possibly to a diffuse capillary leak. Fluid resuscitation should be vigorous and directed at achieving a urine output of 200 to 300 mL/h in the adult. Specific fluid recommendations are given below. During fluid resuscitation arterial oxygenation should be followed carefully and continuously with pulse oximetry. The presence of tachypnea (>40 breaths/min), diffuse crackles on examination, three or four quadrant airspace filling on the chest radiograph and requirement for high concentrations of inspired oxygen indicate well established ARDS. Supportive therapy is similar to other instances of low pressure pulmonary edema and includes early intubation, mechanical ventilation, positive end-expiratory pressure (PEEP), and circulatory manipulation (see Chap. 128).

If hypocalemia is associated with symptoms or electrocardiographic (ECG) changes, replacement therapy should be given intravenously with 10 mL calcium gluconate in the adult. An elevated PT can often be corrected with vitamin K therapy.

MANEUVERS TO ENHANCE ELIMINATION

Since metabolic acidosis promotes penetration of salicylate into tissues, pH correction should be undertaken immediately. It is usually possible to correct pH initially from 7.25 to 7.30 with boluses of bicarbonate (1 meq/kg each) while following serial arterial blood-gas levels. Since this bicarbonate preparation is extremely hypertonic and can induce hypernatremia, serum electrolytes should be followed very frequently. Other contributions to metabolic acidosis, such as lactic acidosis from hypoperfusion or from excessive respiratory muscle use, may complicate the acid-base changes typical of uncomplicated salicylism. Such critically ill patients require early intubation, muscle relaxation, mechanical ventilation, and correction of hypovolemia or ventricular dysfunction (see Chap. 127).

As noted above, alkalinization of the urine will markedly enhance renal excretion, the predominant route of drug clearance in massive overdose.[20–22] At a urine pH of 7.5, renal clearance of free salicylate begins to increase dramatically. This should be an initial goal of alkalinization therapy (Fig. 177-2). If possible, urine pH of 8.0 to 8.5 should be ultimately attained. We prefer adding 2 ampules bicarbonate to 1 L 5% dextrose solution and beginning the infusion rate at 200 to 300 mL/h, *after correcting initial blood pH to approximately 7.30 and treating any significant hypovolemia.* It is important that hypokalemia be rapidly corrected; without

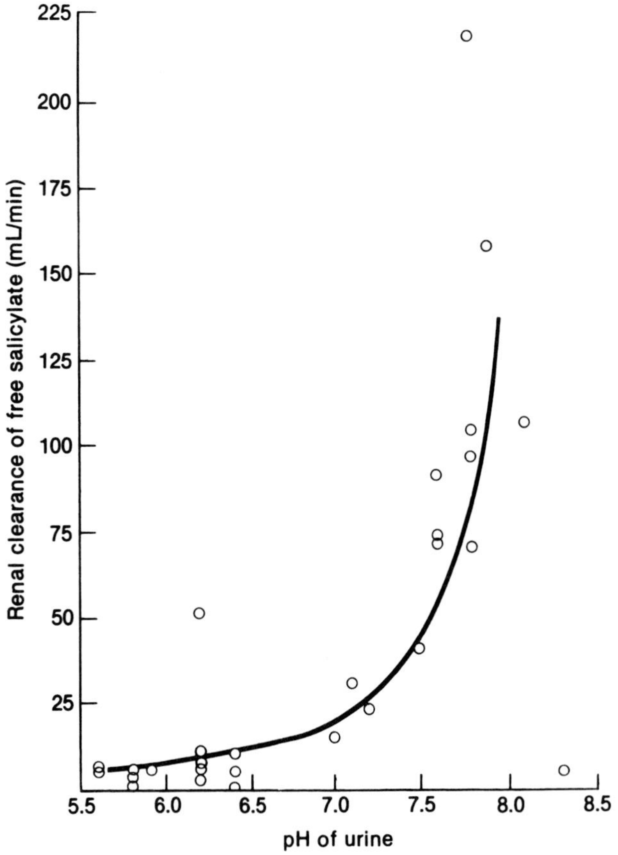

FIGURE 177-2 Relationship of renal clearance of salicylates to urinary pH. Note the marked increase in clearance as urine pH is taken above 7.5. (Reprinted with permission from J Pharmacol Exp Ther 87:253, 1946.)

this, alkalinization of the urine is impossible. KCl infusions of 20 to 30 meq/h may be necessary early on. If alkalinization of the urine continues to be difficult despite bicarbonate infusions over several hours, persistent or new hypokalemia should be considered and treated, if present, while bicarbonate infusion is continued at a higher rate. Hypocalcemia and pulmonary edema are always possible complications of this intervention.[23,24]

Drugs such as acetazolamide, which are used to alkalinize the urine under other circumstances, *should not* be used in salicylate overdose, because it is possible that a metabolic acidosis will be engendered prior to any benefit from enhanced elimination.[25]

Hemodialysis is an effective means of removing drug while simultaneously correcting fluid and electrolyte abnormalities.[26] This modality should be considered in single ingestions with levels above 120 mg/dL. It may be appropriate to dialyze chronic ingestions at lower levels (50 to 100 mg/dL) if complicating factors such as renal and cardiac failure make urine alkalinization difficult, if metabolic acidosis does not respond to standard measures, or if seizures and deep coma are present. Charcoal hemoperfusion is somewhat more effective in removing drug, but since most patients have profound electrolyte and acid-base disturbances that are equally pressing in terms of correction, dialysis is preferred. Peritoneal dialysis should not be performed.

CASE PRESENTATION

A 78-year-old patient was brought to the emergency department by his family. He lived alone and took unknown medications for hypertension, heart failure, and arthritis. His family last spoke to him a week previously and he seemed fine, although he complained of increased difficulty getting about. On this day they called him and he seemed to be confused so they visited his apartment. When they arrived, they found him lying on a couch, restless, not recognizing them and breathing rapidly.

On evaluation in the emergency room he was lethargic, lying curled on the gurney, responding to a loud voice and to pain, but not following any instructions. The pulse was 122 and regular, blood pressure 130/95 mmHg supine, respirations 35, and temperature 39.0°C (102.2°F) rectally. Orthostatic maneuvers caused the systolic blood pressure to drop 20 mmHg. Lung examination revealed bibasilar crackles. The cardiovascular examination was remarkable for no elevation of the jugular venous waveform, a displaced point of maximal impulse (PMI) and a third heart sound. No murmurs were heard. The patient had joint changes of severe osteoarthritis and was generally stiff. There was a question of nuchal rigidity but he was uncooperative. The rest of the physical examination was unremarkable, including a nonfocal neurologic examination within the limits of cooperation.

The initial laboratory data included an hematocrit of 36 percent, white blood cell count of 11,500, without remarkable differential, and platelet count of 110,000/mm^3. The sodium level was 138, potassium 2.9, chloride 101, and bicarbonate 16. An arterial blood-gas determination on room air revealed a P_{O_2} of 66, P_{CO_2} of 24, and pH of 7.46. The BUN was 45 mg/dL, creatinine 2.0 mg/dL, and glucose 196 mg/dL. Other screening chemistry results were within normal limits. An arterial ammonia level was normal. The urinalysis was unremarkable, but the urine was dipstick positive for ketones with a pH of 6.0. The PT was 2 s elevated and the partial thromboplastin time (PTT) was normal. A chest radiograph revealed questionable diffuse lower lobe hazy infiltrates.

The initial differential diagnosis was possible systemic or CNS infection, possible cerebrovascular event, and possible drug overdose. An intravenous line was started and normal saline solution was infused at 300 mL/h after a 500-mL bolus. A 20 meq KCl rider was also started. An immediate dose of ceftazidime was given after blood cultures were drawn, and because the patient would not cooperate with fundoscopic examination he was sent for computed tomogram (CT) of the brain. This required sedation and was normal. A lumbar puncture was performed; results were normal. A toxicology screen of the urine was obtained. The patient was admitted to the ICU.

Orthostatic blood pressure changes had resolved on admission to the ICU but the patient was more tachypneic. A repeat blood-gas determination on a 40% mask revealed a P_{O_2} of 49, P_{CO_2} of 29, and pH of 7.30. On a 100% rebreathing mask there was 90% arterial hemoglobin saturation by pulse oximetry but the patient exhibited declining mental status and continued tachypnea. An elective intubation was performed. A repeat chest radiograph revealed diffuse hazy infiltrates, and the patient was begun on mechanical ventilation, tidal volume 6 mL/kg, rate 30, and PEEP titrated to allow adequate arterial saturation on a 60% fraction inspired O_2 (F_{IO_2}).

Broad-spectrum antibiotics were continued. A repeat blood-gas sample revealed P_{O_2} of 68, P_{CO_2} of 31, and pH of 7.28. The patient had a grand mal seizure which responded to diazepam and dilantin. The urine toxicologic screen was returned 12 h after entry to the emergency department and was positive for salicylates. A serum level was therefore belatedly determined to be 75 mg/dL. Hemodialysis was begun.

With hemodialysis, hypokalemia and acidosis were rapidly corrected, and the patient was maintained in slight negative fluid balance. Lung edema gradually cleared over 24 to 48 h, and the serum salicylate levels fell to normal with several hemodialysis sessions. With return of normal CNS function within 72 h, the patient was extubated and discharged from the ICU.

CASE DISCUSSION

Many features of salicylate intoxication are represented by this case. Increasingly, physicians will likely encounter subtle presentations of chronic intoxication, particularly in the elderly. The diagnosis is rarely clear-cut; many other diagnoses must be considered and excluded. Unfortunately, as in this case, the confirmation of salicylate intoxication by measurement of serum levels is often delayed.

The picture of a mixed acid-base disturbance (respiratory alkalosis and metabolic acidosis) with CNS dysfunction should have prompted determination of serum salicylate level immediately on entry to the emergency department. As is often the case in adult overdoses, the respiratory alkalosis dominated the acid-base disturbance, at least early in the course. The salicylate level that was eventually measured—75 mg/dL—would not suggest severe intoxication in acute single ingestion overdose, but it should be stressed that significant toxicity occurs at much lower serum levels in chronic intoxication.

It is possible that early identification of salicylate intoxication might have avoided the protracted course in this case. Early selection of bicarbonate-containing fluids may have prevented development of a more severe acidosis favoring further tissue penetration and toxicity. It is important to stress that urine alkalinization would have been possible only with correction of hypokalemia, an electrolyte disturbance that drives continued acid excretion into the urine. Once metabolic acidosis has worsened, seizures have occurred, and ARDS has complicated fluid management, hemodialysis is clearly indicated to correct acid-base and fluid abnormalities and enhance drug elimination.

References

1. Flower RJ, Moncada S, Vane JR: The salicylates, in Goodman LS, Gilman A (eds): *The Pharmacological Basis of Therapeutics.* 7th ed. Macmillan, 1985, pp 680–690.
2. Ellenhorn MJ, Barceloux DG: Salicylates, in Ellenhorn MJ, Barceloux DG (eds): *Medical Toxicology, Diagnosis and Treatment of Human Poisoning,* Elsevier, 1988, pp 562–572.
3. Anderson RJ, Potts DE, Gabow PA, et al: Unrecognized adult salicylate intoxication. Ann Intern Med 85:745, 1976.
4. Gaudreault P, Temple AR, Lovejoy FH: The relative severity of acute versus chronic salicylate poisoning in children: A clinical comparison. Pediatrics 70:566, 1982.
5. Netter P, Faure G, Regent MC, et al: Salicylate kinetics in old age. Clin Pharmacol Ther 38:6, 1985.
6. Levy G: Clinical pharmacokinetics of salicylates: A reassessment. Br J Clin Pharmacol 10:285S, 1980.
7. Levy G, Tsuchiya T: Salicylate accumulation kinetics in man. N Engl J Med 287:430, 1972.
8. Rejent TA, Aik S: Fatal in utero salicylism. J Forensic Sci 30:942, 1985.
9. Millhorn DE, Eldridge FL, Waldrop TG: Effects of salicylate and 2,4-dinitrophenol on respiration and metabolism. J Appl Physiol 53:925, 1982.
10. Ring T, Andersen PT, Knudsen F, et al: Salicylate induced hyperventilation. Lancet 1:1450, 1985.
11. Gabow PA, Anderson RJ, Potts DE, et al: Acid-base disturbances in the salicylate intoxicated adult. Arch Intern Med 138:1481, 1978.
12. Arena FP, Dugowson C, Saudek CD: Salicylate induced hypoglycemia and ketoacidosis in a nondiabetic adult. Arch Intern Med 138:1153, 1978.
13. Thurston JH, Pollock PG, Warren SK, Jones EM: Reduced brain glucose with normal plasma glucose in salicylate poisoning. J Clin Invest 49:2139, 1970.
14. Heffner JE, Sahn SA: Salicylate induced pulmonary edema. Clinical features and prognosis. Ann Intern Med 95: 405, 1981.
15. Walters JS, Woodring JH, Stelling CB, et al: Salicylate induced pulmonary edema. Radiology 146:289, 1984.
16. Done AK: Salicylate intoxication. Significance of measurements of salicylate in blood in cases of acute ingestion. Pediatrics 26:800, 1960.
17. Robins JB, Turnbull JA, Robertson C: Gastric perforation after acute aspirin overdose. Hum Toxicol 4:527, 1985.
18. Hillman RJ, Prescott LF: Treatment of salicylate poisoning with repeat oral charcoal. Br Med J 291: 1472, 1985.
19. Leslie PJ, Dyson EH, Proudfoot AT: Opiate toxicity after self poisoning with aspirin and codeine. Brit Med J 292:96, 1986.
20. Prescott LF, Balali-Mood M, Critchley JAJH, et al: Diuresis or urinary alkalinization for salicylate poisoning? Br Med J 285:1383, 1982.
21. Prescott LF, Critchley JAJH, Proudfoot AT: Diuresis or urinary alkalinization for salicylate poisoning? Br Med J 286:147, 1983.
22. Vale JA, Buckley GM, Meredith TJ: Algorithm for modified alkaline diuresis in salicylate poisoning. Br Med J 290:155, 1985.
23. Fox GN: Hypocalcemia complicating bicarbonate therapy for salicylate poisoning. West J Med 141:108, 1984.
24. Zimmerman GA, Clemmer TP: Acute respiratory failure during therapy for salicylate intoxication. Ann Emerg Med 10:104, 1981.
25. Cowan RA, Hartnell GG, Lowdell CP, et al: Metabolic acidosis induced by carbonic anhydrase inhibitors and salicylates in patients with normal renal function. Br Med J 289:347, 1984.
26. Jacobsen D, Wiik-Larsen E, Bredersen JE: Hemodialysis or hemoperfusion in severe salicylate poisoning. Hum Toxicol 7:161, 1988.

Chapter 178

ACETAMINOPHEN POISONING

BARRY H. RUMACK
JEFFREY BRENT

KEY POINTS

- *Acetaminophen (APAP), when taken in overdose, may cause hepatotoxicity.*
- *The overdose itself may be clinically subtle until the hepatotoxicity is manifested in 1 to 3 days.*
- *All overdose patients should be screened for APAP.*
- *The antidote for APAP poisoning is N-acetylcysteine (NAC), which is completely effective if therapy is initiated within 8 h of the overdose. After that, its efficacy wanes, and it completely loses its protective effect if treatment is not initiated by 16 to 24 h.*

History

Acetaminophen (APAP) has been marketed since 1950 following the realization that it is a less nephrotoxic metabolite of the analgesic phenacetin. It is a safe and effective analgesic and antipyretic. However, in overdose, it may cause hepatic and, less frequently, renal toxicity.

The first report of APAP hepatotoxicity was in 1966,[1] following which there were published a variety of individual cases and series of APAP overdoses with consequent liver injury. Although APAP hepatotoxicity occurs only after the ingestion of very large amounts of the drug, its widespread use and availability make it the second most common cause of drug-induced hepatotoxicity, profoundly dwarfed in this regard by ethanol.

Pathophysiology of APAP Poisoning

The clinical course, pathologic observations, and rationale of therapy of APAP poisoning may be understood on the basis of its metabolism and the cellular effects of specific metabolites. Over 95 percent of an ingested dose of APAP is metabolized, primarily by the liver. All but approximately 5 percent of this is conjugated to form the sulfate or glucuronide derivative. Approximately equal amounts of both of these conjugates are produced, although children below the age of nine tend to predominantly generate the sulfate conjugate.[2] Acetaminophen itself and these two conjugates have no direct hepatotoxic effects. Less then 5 percent of a dose of APAP is oxidized via the hepatic P-450 mixed function oxidase system to N-acetyl-p-benzoquinonimine (NAPQI). As shown in Fig. 178-1, NAPQI has one of two potential fates. Being an electrophile it displays a predictable avidity toward cellular nucleophiles, the most prevalent ones being sulfhydryl groups. Of the available sulfhydryls, the two most significant are cysteine groups on

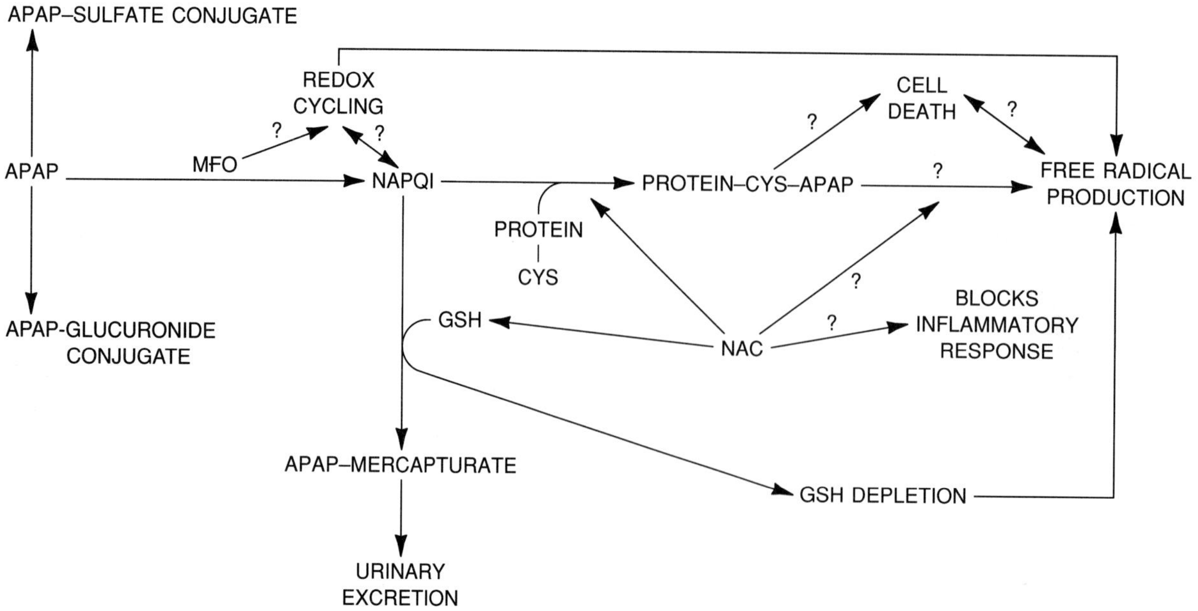

FIGURE 178-1 Mechanisms postulated for APAP hepatotoxicity and protection by NAC. [MFO: hepatic microsomal mixed function oxidase system. GSH: glutathione. CYS: cysteine] See text for details.

cellular proteins and soluble thiols, particularly glutathione. The formation of the adduct of NAPQI plus protein cysteine residues may adversely affect the function of hepatocellular enzymes and structural proteins and may thus be responsible for APAP-induced hepatotoxicity.

The glutathione conjugate is ultimately excreted in the form of the mercapturic acid, which has no known toxicity. Thus, glutathione is a protective molecule, detoxifying the microsomally generated APAP oxidation product.

A feature of APAP toxicity which distinguishes it from most other acute drug overdoses is the latency of its clinical effects. Although there may be mild gastrointestinal discomfort with perhaps some emesis at the time of an initial overdose, this may be sufficiently subtle that it may not be appreciated by the evaluating physician nor felt to be significant by the patient. Once APAP has been systemically absorbed, the metabolic events described above ensue. In an overdose, the ratio of conjugated to microsomally metabolized products appears to be similar to that seen after therapeutic dosing.[3] Thus, it appears that the kinetics of APAP metabolism are for all practical purposes nonsaturable. Although the amount of APAP metabolized via the microsomal mixed function oxidase pathway still amounts to approximately 5 percent of the total dose, the NAPQI thus formed may be sufficient to overcome hepatic glutathione stores. At such time that glutathione is depleted, NAPQI becomes free to react directly with cellular proteins. Studies in mice, which are an excellent model for human APAP toxicity, indicate that hepatic necrosis occurs following an APAP overdose when approximately 70 percent of glutathione stores are depleted.[4]

Although the modification of cellular proteins is most frequently theorized to be the cause of APAP toxicity, several alternative theories have been suggested. Free radical formation has been proposed as the mechanism of APAP toxicity. Although data suggest that free radicals may form during APAP poisoning, this is likely the result of glutathione depletion and not a primary cause of the toxicity.[5] Free radical-protecting agents have been shown to reduce lipid peroxidation following APAP toxicity but generally do not attenuate hepatic toxicity.[6] Although clearly more work needs to be done in this area before definitive conclusions can be made, present data indicate that free radical effects are not an essential step in the effect of APAP on hepatotoxicity. An APAP-induced immune reaction against the hepatocyte has also been proposed as a possible mechanism of the hepatotoxicity.[7]

APAP poisoning may also be associated with kidney damage. This renal toxicity may be either a component of a hepatorenal syndrome secondary to the hepatotoxic effect of APAP, or alternatively, may be due to a direct effect on the kidney. The kidney is capable of metabolizing APAP and thus may be vulnerable to damage caused by a metabolite.

No current data suggest that a hepatotoxic syndrome is associated with chronic APAP use with doses less than those required to cause acute poisoning. Although it is often stated that alcoholics have greater sensitivity to APAP poisoning, this has not been proven conclusively.

The Clinical Picture of APAP Toxicity

Acetaminophen toxicity may be viewed as a disease with a temporally related spectrum of presentations. Patients presenting early after an overdose often are asymptomatic or manifest mild to moderate abdominal discomfort with nausea and vomiting. Unfortunately, this is the time when treatment is most effective.[8] The exception to this clinical picture is the rare patient with an extremely high plasma APAP level, who may manifest early lethargy or coma.

Because of the subtlety of the typical early presentation of APAP poisoning, one must always have a high index of suspicion for this when dealing with any potential overdose. It is, therefore, advisable to screen for APAP in the evaluation of any overdose patient.

It is during the early period that circulating APAP levels are highest and, therefore, so is the synthesis of NAPQI. Initiation of NAC (Mucomyst) therapy during this early phase of NAPQI formation and consequent glutathione depletion is hepatoprotective.

The diagnosis of APAP poisoning is made by obtaining a plasma APAP level and interpreting its hepatotoxic potential by the Rumack-Matthew nomogram (Fig. 178-2), which relates level to time after ingestion.[9] A plasma APAP level above the lower nomogram line is an indication for NAC therapy. If the time of ingestion is unknown, the detection of any amount of APAP potentially above the nomogram line mandates that NAC therapy be initiated, at least until the time of ingestion can be determined accurately. Levels drawn 4 h postingestion are uninterpretable.

Untreated, APAP poisoning may progress to the stage of clinically manifest hepatotoxicity. Often, it is this picture of chemical hepatitis with right upper quadrant pain and tenderness, jaundice, and emesis that brings the patient to medical attention. By the time the hepatotoxicity is clinically evident there may be no circulating APAP, so the diagnosis is nonspecific based on the clinical picture, history, and an index of suspicion. At this time, laboratory studies reflect hepatocellular necrosis. Both alanine aminotransferase (ALT) and aspartate aminotransferase (AST) often rise to levels much higher than seen in alcoholic or viral hepatitis. It is not unusual for transaminase levels to peak at the 10,000 to 20,000 IU/mL range with similarly dramatic elevations in bilirubin and prothrombin time (PT). Liver biopsy during this time will show either a predominantly centrilobular pattern of toxicity or, in fulminant cases, total necrosis of the hepatic lobule. Recent animal studies have shown that as the hepatocyte breaks down, the NAPQI-cysteinyl adduct may be detected in the circulation by a sensitive immunoassay technique.[10] In addition, immunohistochemical studies of stained liver sections from mice can detect this adduct. However, this, technique remains experimental.

Many patients with significant APAP-related hepatotoxicity show transient alterations of their renal function. Other end-organs occasionally involved in severe APAP poisoning included the pancreas, in which pancreatitis has been reported, and the heart (myocarditis).

Most patients with APAP poisoning fully recover. Prog-

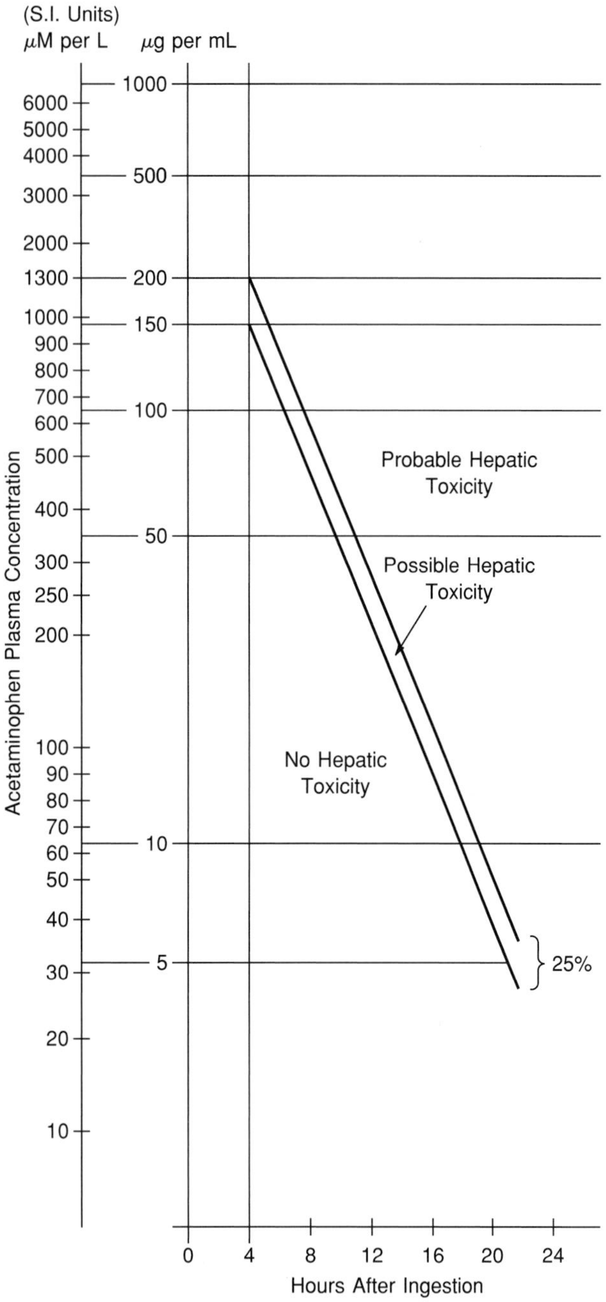

FIGURE 178-2 Rumack-Matthew nomogram for predicting APAP hepatotoxicity. (From Rumack BH: Pediatr Clin North Am 33:698, 1986. Used with permission.)

nostic factors suggesting a poor outcome include a bilirubin value >4 mg/dL and a PT ratio of >2.2.

Therapy of APAP Poisoning

Several sulfhydryl agents have been evaluated to determine the most efficacious antidote for APAP poisoning. Among the first agents tried were the chelators BAL (dimercaprol) and D-penicillamine. These were not effective and the latter agent actually enhanced APAP nephrotoxicity. Cysteamine had some degree of efficacy and was in fact used in Europe at one time, but suffered from the disadvantages of requiring intravenous administration and being very dysphoric when administered by this route. Intravenous cysteamine has also been associated with significant cardiovascular instability. Methionine, also in use for some time in Europe, can be administered orally without the side effects described for intravenous cysteamine, but appeared to worsen hepatic encephalopathy. Animal and human trials have shown that NAC is efficacious in attenuating APAP-induced hepatotoxicity, and this agent has become widely accepted as the drug of choice for the treatment of APAP overdoses.

There are a variety of theories regarding the exact therapeutic mechanism of NAC. NAC is metabolized to glutathione, and this may indeed be its primary mode of action. This theory explains why NAC is almost completely protective if administered within the first 8 h after APAP overdose,[8] during which time glutathione stores would be falling but perhaps not depleted. Animal data also suggest that free radicals may be induced during APAP poisoning.[5] NAC could be protective against free radical effects as well since glutathione may function as an endogenous free radical scavenger. There is also the suggestion that during the period of APAP hepatotoxicity polymorphonuclear cells infiltrate into the liver.[7] It has been argued that this is associated with immunologically mediated liver injury, and NAC has been suggested as a protective agent in this regard as well.

Three regimens for NAC administration are in current use (Table 178-1). The only approved treatment in the United States involves oral therapy with a loading dose of 140 mg/kg followed by 17 maintenance doses of 70 mg/kg at 4-h intervals. In Europe and Canada, NAC therapy is commonly administered by an intravenous protocol in which 300 mg/kg is infused over 20 h. A clinical regimen presently being studied involves 48 h of intravenous therapy administered as an initial 140 mg/kg loading dose followed by 70 mg/kg every 4 h. Although there has never been a strict comparison between these three treatments, it appears that for those patients with a delay in starting treatment, the 48-h intravenous protocol is superior.[11]

The administration of oral NAC is often challenging. Being a sulfhydryl reagent, it has both the taste and smell of rotten eggs and therefore is a potent emetic. The problem of vomiting oral NAC is compounded by the dyspepsia of an APAP overdose. NAC is supplied as a 20% solution. This should be diluted to a 5% solution by a 3:1 dilution in soda or fruit juice. If an oral dose is vomited within 1 h of administration, it may be beneficial to repeat it. Although it is reasonable to attempt oral therapy by having the patient drink the NAC solution, repeated emesis mandates a more aggressive approach. Once the 8-h postingestion period is passed, any delay in the effective administration of NAC results in a diminution of its efficacy.[8] Among the strategies that may be used to achieve satisfactory oral administration of NAC are administration in an ice cold solution through a

TABLE 178-1 Protocols for NAC Administration*

	Length (hours)	Administration	Loading Dose	Doses	FDA Approval
I	72	Oral	140 mg/kg	70 mg/kg every 4 h for 17 doses	Yes
II	20	Intravenous	150 mg/kg over 15 min	50 mg/kg over 4 h followed by 100 mg/kg over 16 h	No
III	20	Intravenous	300 mg/kg over 20 h		No

*From Brent J, Rumack BH: Acetaminophen poisoning, in Harwood-Nuss A/(ed): *Clinical Practice of Emergency Medicine,* Philadelphia, PA, Lippincott, 1991, p. 456. Used with permission.

straw in a covered container and antiemetics such as droperidol or metaclopramide. Failing these measures, NAC may be given as a slow drip through a nasogastric tube or, if this is unsuccessful, through a long tube inserted into the duodenum.

Because NAC is effective only if administered within approximately the first 20 h after overdose, it is unlikely to be of any benefit in the patient who presents with manifest hepatotoxicity. However, if elevated hepatic transaminases suggestive of an acetaminophen overdose and a significant amount of circulating APAP are noted, NAC therapy may be beneficial in an attempt to attenuate further hepatic damage from the unmetabolized drug.

Patients who present within the first several hours after APAP overdose, or who have taken APAP as part of a polydrug ingestion, should be treated with oral activated charcoal. In the context of a pure APAP overdose, where an effective antidote is available, it is probably sufficient to give a single dose of activated charcoal. However, if a polydrug ingestion is known or suspected, then multiple dose activated charcoal is more appropriate. Although activated charcoal adsorbs NAC, it does not appear to affect the absorption of this antidote to a clinically significant degree. Thus, the dose of oral NAC does not require adjustment for concomitant activated charcoal therapy. However, it is prudent to avoid the simultaneous administration of activated charcoal and NAC. Since both of these agents are administered typically on an every 4-h basis, they could be spaced in such a way as to be given 2 h apart from each other. Alternatively, gastric contents could be evacuated by suction prior to the administration of each oral NAC dose. Although oral NAC can be challenging to administer, it is the only route approved in the United States. In other countries, NAC is routinely given intravenously. The emesis induced by oral NAC is avoided by parental therapy. However, anaphylactoid reaction may occur with intravenous NAC.

Because of the data suggesting free radical generation and lipid peroxidation in the livers of animals treated with toxic amounts of APAP, the question of free radical-protecting modalities in the therapy of APAP overdose has been raised.[5] Although hepatocytes in cell culture and animals pretreated with free radical-protecting modalities are protected from APAP toxicity, no data suggest that a free radical-protecting agent is protective when administered after the dose of APAP. Thus, at this time no evidence supports the use of these agents in the treatment of APAP overdose. Further research is required to determine whether there is any potential role for this approach.

Animal studies show that pretreatment with cimetidine protects against APAP poisoning. Cimetidine is an inhibitor of microsomal APAP metabolism and therefore would be expected to prevent the generation of NAPQI. However, animal data suggest that this effect is most demonstrable only with pretreatment with very large doses (in the range of 1200 mg/kg). A recent prospective clinical trial comparing standard NAC therapy to NAC plus cimetidine (300 mg every 6 h failed to reveal any beneficial effects of this therapy.[12] At the present time, it is unknown whether higher doses of cimetidine may inhibit microsomal APAP metabolism and therefore provide an effective addition to treatment.

Acetaminophen is a small molecule with a low volume of distribution (1 L/kg) and low protein binding and should be removable by extracorporeal techniques. Indeed, a reduced half-life can be demonstrated following hemodialysis or hemoperfusion. However, it is unclear if a significant amount of drug is actually cleared by these procedures. In view of the specific antidote available for the treatment of APAP poisoning, extracorporeal drug removal techniques do not appear to play a significant role in the treatment of APAP poisoning. Patients who present late with severe hepatotoxicity should be treated with standard supportive care (see Chap. 168). They will not benefit from NAC therapy. If there is progressive worsening of transaminases, PT, encephalopathy, and hyperbilirubinemia then the possibility of fulminant hepatic necrosis should be considered. Liver transplantation is the only therapy effective for fulminant hepatic failure. An extremely small fraction of APAP-poisoned patients will progress to this degree of hepatotoxicity. Profoundly elevated hepatic transaminases, even to the 10,000 to 20,000 range, and significantly prolonged PTs, even beyond two times control, are by themselves not indications for transplantation in view of the resolution of the hepatotoxicity that can be expected in the majority of these patients. However, a progressively worsening PT and steeply rising bilirubin level at a time when the hepatic transaminase values are falling may indeed herald ensuing hepatic failure. Patients with this clinical picture may be treated most prudently in a facility capable of providing hepatic transplantation to ensure that appropriate preliminary steps are taken should this become a necessity.

CASE PRESENTATIONS

Case 1

A generally well 13-year-old girl overdosed on approximately 11 g APAP. She presented to a local hospital where an APAP level, drawn 7.5 h after admission, was 112 μg/mL. She was given an oral loading dose of 140 mg/kg Mucomyst, however, this induced vomiting shortly after she was given the drug. A nasogastric tube was inserted and intravenous droperidol was administered, yet she continued to have emesis following her Mucomyst doses. She was therefore transferred to a hospital where intravenous NAC was available through an experimental protocol, and she received a full course of therapy. There were no other coingestants, and her physical examination was always normal. Daily liver function tests were within normal limits except for an initial elevation of the PT to 2.5 s longer than control. However, this normalized without any vitamin K therapy. She was evaluated by a psychiatrist, and both she and her family were enrolled in psychiatric counseling. She was totally asymptomatic at the time of discharge.

Discussion

This is a fairly typical case of a potentially significant APAP poisoning treated with NAC. The difficulties encountered in the administration of oral NAC were not unusual; however, most patients will ultimately tolerate oral therapy. Although it is unknown how much hepatotoxicity may have been engendered by this overdose in the absence of therapy, it is likely that the extremely benign course in this patient was related to the timely NAC therapy.

Case 2

A 29-year-old man presented after 3 days of ingesting multiple 500-mg APAP tablets for a toothache. It was estimated that he ingested approximately 75 of these tablets over the prior 60 h. At the time of admission, he had a nondetectable APAP level. His PT was 16.2 s with control of 11.2 s, other liver function tests included an ALT of 1524 IU/mL, AST of 2176 IU/mL, and a total bilirubin of 7.9 mg/dL. He was not encephalopathic, had a normal BUN and creatinine, and had right upper quadrant tenderness with emesis. He had one episode of hematemesis although he was hemodynamically stable with a normal hematocrit. It should be noted that the patient did have history of peptic ulcer disease.

There are a variety of therapeutic issues related to this patient. The first and most obvious is: would NAC therapy be of any benefit at this point? It would be unlikely that this treatment would be helpful in view of the fact that the patient had no more circulating APAP to be metabolized and detoxified. This conceptual approach is somewhat supported by the fact that no data suggest that NAC is effective at this late stage after overdose. In view of the elevated PT with evidence of gastrointestinal bleeding, large bore intravenous access lines should be started and blood should be typed and screened for antibodies. Frequent hematocrits and vital sign monitoring is mandatory. Although one would normally not treat a mild elevation of the PT such as this, vitamin K therapy was indicated in view of the gastrointestinal bleeding. Should there be further evidence of bleeding, correction of the coagulapathy with fresh frozen plasma would be required. Over the next 24 h the patient's hepatic transaminases rose with the ALT peaking at 6930 IU/mL. Over the next several days, the transaminases returned to normal and the PT corrected without any additional vitamin K. There was no further gastrointestinal bleeding, and by the fifth hospital day the bilirubin was normal.

Discussion

This case is a fairly typical presentation of untreated APAP hepatotoxicity. Although many cases will ultimately clinically resolve, if there is involvement of a large amount of liver, there may be insufficient residual hepatocyte mass to regenerate or to support the patient's metabolic needs during the regeneration process. The patient will then progress to fulminant hepatic necrosis.

References

1. Davidson DGD, Eastham WN: Acute liver necrosis following overdose of paracetamol. Br Med J 2:497, 1966.
2. Jollow DG, Thorgeirsson SS, Potter WZ, et al: Acetaminophen-induced hepatic necrosis. VI. Metabolic disposition of toxic and nontoxic doses of acetaminophen. Pharmacology 12:251, 1974.
3. Davis M, Labadarios D, Williams RS: Metabolism of paracetamol after therapeutic and hepatotoxic doses in man. J Intern Med Res (suppl 4):40, 1976.
4. Mitchell JR, Jollow DJ, Potter WZ, et al: Acetaminophen-induced hepatic necrosis. IV. Protective role of glutathione. J Pharmacol Exp Ther 187:211, 1973.
5. Brent J, Rumack BH: The role of free radicals in toxic hepatic injury. II. Are free radicals the cause or the consequence of toxin-induced liver injury? J Toxicol Clin Toxicol. In press.
6. Tounes M, Siegers CP: The role of iron in the paracetamol- and $CC1_4$-induced lipid peroxidation and hepatotoxicity. Chem Biol Interact 55:322, 1985.
7. Mitchell JR: Acetaminophen toxicity. Editorial. N Engl J Med 314:1601, 1988.
8. Smilkstein MJ, Knapp GL, Kulig KW, et al: Efficacy of oral N-acetylcysteine in the treatment of acetaminophen overdose. N Engl J Med 319:1557, 1988.
9. Rumack BH, Matthew H: Acetaminophen poisoning and toxicity. Pediatrics 55:871, 1975.
10. Pumford NR, Hinson JA, Potter DW, et al: Immunochemical quantitation of 3-(Cystein-S-yl) acetaminophen adducts in serum and liver proteins of acetaminophen-treated mice. J Pharmocol Exp Ther 148:190, 1989.
11. Bronstein AC, Linden CH, Hall AH, et al: Intravenous N-acetylcysteine for acute acetaminophen poisoning. Vet Hum Toxicol 27:316, 1985.
12. Burkhart K, Janco N, Kulig K, et al: Cimetidine as adjunctive treatment for acetaminophen overdose. Vet Hum Toxicol 31:337, 1989.

Chapter 179

HALLUCINOGENS

R. STEVEN THARRATT
TIMOTHY E. ALBERTSON

KEY POINTS

- *Hallucinations may occur secondary to illicit drugs, therapeutically administered drugs, withdrawal syndromes, organic diseases, and psychiatric disorders.*
- *New-onset hallucinations in a patient over age 40 with no previous psychiatric history should prompt a search for an organic cause.*
- *Hallucinogens themselves rarely result in direct life-threatening conditions. Behavioral and environmental complications represent the largest threat to life.*
- *Most ingestions of hallucinogenic agents respond to supportive therapy and minimizing sensory input. Drug therapy may be necessary to control sympathomimetic "storm," anticholinergic crisis, or severe agitation.*
- *Monitor for rhabdomyolysis, intracranial bleeding, and status epilepticus.*
- *Phencyclidine (PCP)-intoxicated patients may become violent and difficult to control at any time. Nystagmus is commonly seen.*
- *Respiratory support may require sedation with benzodiazepines or haloperidol to allow the use of mechanical ventilation. Neuromuscular blockade may be necessary to safely deliver mechanical ventilation in severe cases of PCP intoxication.*
- *Gastric decontamination and activated charcoal are only occasionally helpful. Decontamination must be balanced against the sensory stimulation produced.*
- *Elimination enhancement, pH alteration, forced diuresis, and extracorporeal drug removal techniques play no role in management of hallucinogenic intoxications.*

Patients presenting with symptoms that include hallucinations represent a challenge to the intensivist because of the wide spectrum of compounds abused for this effect and the variety of medical and psychologic conditions that may produce hallucinations.

Hallucinations may be defined as gross distortions in perception. It is rarely necessary to know the specific identity of the hallucinogen since the management of toxicity resulting from these agents tends to be primarily supportive. Specific antidotes do not exist. The majority of hallucinogenic drug classification schemes focus on structural similarities of the compounds.[2–4] A more useful clinical scheme is to classify hallucinogens by their associated symptomology (Table 179-1).

TABLE 179-1 Classification of the Hallucinogenic Compounds

1. Hallucinogens with sympathomimetic effects
   - A. Phenylethylamine derivatives (hallucinogenic amphetamines)
   - B. Peyote and mescaline
   - C. Cocaine
   - D. Disassociative anesthetics (PCP and ketamine)
   - E. Indole alkylamines (magic mushrooms and tryptamine derivatives)
2. Hallucinogens with cholinergic effects
   - A. Anticholinergic plants (atropinelike compounds)
   - B. Muscimol and ibotenic containing mushrooms (group V)
3. LSD
4. Cannabinoids
5. Miscellaneous hallucinogens
   - A. Therapeutic drugs
   - B. Ethanol withdrawal
   - C. Hydrocarbons
   - D. Opioids

The major direct risks to the patient exposed to hallucinogens include associated effects on the central nervous (CNS) and cardiovascular systems. Complications indirectly associated with exposure to hallucinogens include gastric aspiration, respiratory insufficiency, rhabdomyolysis, and the trauma associated with failure of the patient to appropriately respond to the environment due to distortion of perception.

General Management Principles for Hallucinogenic Intoxication (Table 179-2)

Initial evaluation of the patient presenting with hallucinations attempts to determine if the hallucinations are due to a psychiatric or organic cause. Obtaining a history of previous psychiatric disorders, family history of psychiatric disorders, and a complete medication history is critical to this evaluation. All patients presenting with hallucinations should be presumed to have an organic etiology until proven otherwise. It is unusual to see the new onset of hallucinations or psychosis from a primary psychiatric cause in a patient older than age forty who has no previous history of a psychiatric disorder.

If the hallucinations are felt to be nonpsychiatric are they secondary to an underlying medical disorder or are they due to a toxicologic exposure? Many systemic diseases including electrolyte imbalances, ethanol withdrawal, and CNS infections may present with hallucinations and require specific management.

If a toxicologic etiology is suspected are the predominant symptoms best explained by sympathetic nervous system stimulation, cholinergic nervous system stimulation, disassociation from the environment, or none of these? This classifies the possible ingestant and guides supportive management. Table 179-3 contrasts the signs of sympatho-

TABLE 179-2 General Management of Hallucinogenic Intoxications

If hallucinogenic drugs are suspected, is the symptomology of the patient best explained by sympathetic or cholinergic stimulation?
In mild intoxications minimize sensory input. In severe intoxications aggressively control vital signs and agitation. Parenteral medications with short half-lives are preferred.
Aggressively control the airway and support ventilation in severe intoxications with respiratory depression.
Protect the patient from environmentally induced trauma. Protect the staff from a violent hallucinating patient.
Monitor for rhabdomyolysis, intracranial bleeding, and status epilepticus.
Forced diuresis, pH alteration, and extracorporeal removal techniques are not recommended.
Gastric decontamination is rarely helpful.

TABLE 179-3 Distinguishing Sympathomimetic and Anticholinergic Signs and Symptoms

Sympathomimetic	Anticholinergic
Diaphoresis	Dry Skin
	Absent bowel sounds
	Urinary retention
Tachycardia	Tachycardia
Hypertension	Hypertension
Pupillary dilatation	Pupillary dilatation
Hyperthermia	Hyperthermia
Flushed skin	Flushed skin
Hallucinations	Hallucinations

mimetic and anticholinergic toxicity; skin changes are a key distinguishing feature.

Aggressive control of sympathetic hyperactivity, including blood pressure, heart rate, and temperature, is often vital in the management of amphetamine-related hallucinogens. For critical life-threatening symptoms, preference should be given to parenteral formulations with short half-lives. Table 179-4 lists some suggested drugs and their dosages.

Hallucinogens themselves rarely result in direct life-threatening conditions. Death often results from trauma sustained because of altered perception of the environment, sympathomimetic stimulation, and cardiovascular collapse. Associated serious consequences include rhabdomyolysis secondary to isotonic muscle activity, electrolyte imbalance, and injuries resulting from forcible restraint. If mechanical restraints are required for patient and staff safety, strong consideration should be given to the use of benzodiazepines or haloperidol titrated to effect. Phenothiazines are less preferable due to potential adverse effects on hemodynamics and potential anticholinergic effects.[5]

The complications of rhabdomyolysis and seizures secondary to hallucinogenic drug ingestion do not require different management from that described in Chaps. 142 and 153.

Specific laboratory analyses of blood and urine for hallucinogens are not needed to successfully manage these intoxications, although they may have important forensic and legal implications. In general, urine assays will detect a wider array of hallucinogenic compounds and their metabolites than blood assays. Urine is preferred for analysis because most hallucinogens are rapidly metabolized, and urine metabolites are generally found in higher concentrations. Most commercially available enzyme-linked immunoassays (ELISA) use urine. Assays for lysergic acid dethylamide (LSD) and the hallucinogenic mushrooms are not routinely available.

Gastric decontamination is not generally indicated. A possible exception is recent ingestion of massive amounts of amphetamine-related hallucinogenic drugs. Generally these patients will present either with the clinical history of massive oral ingestion or with hemodynamic instability. The sensory stimulation of gastric emptying must be balanced against the small clinical benefit in minor oral ingestions of hallucinogenic compounds. The possibility of multiple drug ingestion must always be considered before deciding to forego gastric decontamination. Forced diuresis, alteration of pH, and extracorporeal drug removal have no role in the management of these ingestions.

Specific Hallucinogenic Agents

HALLUCINOGENS AFFECTING THE SYMPATHETIC NERVOUS SYSTEM

These drugs include the largest collection of chemicals capable of producing hallucinations and those most likely to cause the severe complications necessitating intervention by the intensivist. These chemicals can be further subdivided into: the phenylethylamine derivatives (hallucinogenic amphetamines), cocaine, the disassociative anesthetics, and the indole alkaloids that contain primarily tryptamine. The major complications of these compounds relate to an associated stimulation of the sympathetic nervous system with resultant life-threatening alterations in cardiovascular and CNS function.

HALLUCINOGENIC AMPHETAMINES

The prototype phenylethylamine backbone provides the starting point for the synthesis of a wide range of neurotransmitters. Norepinephrine, epinephrine, and ephedrine all share this backbone as do amphetamine and methamphetamine. The substitution of methoxyl groups on the phenyl ring leads to several synthetic hallucinogens.[6] Because these drugs are not found in nature, but rather are the product of illicit synthetic organic chemistry, these compounds are often mistakenly labeled as "designer drugs." This descriptive term is most commonly used for the chemically and pharmacologically unrelated narcotic fentanyl and meperidine analogues.

Since these compounds all share the phenylethylamine backbone, sympathomimetic side effects are often prominent. The chemical substitution on the phenyl ring blunts

TABLE 179-4 Useful Drugs in the Management of Hallucinogenic Intoxications

Symptom	Drug	Comments
Hypertension	Labetol 0.2–0.4 mg/kg, IV titrated every 10–15 min	Balanced α- and β-blocker
	Sodium nitroprusside 0.5 μg/kg/min IV	Protect from light
	Hydralazine 10–40 mg IV	
Supraventricular tachycardias	Labetol 0.2–0.4 mg/kg IV titrated every 10–15 min	
	Propranolol 0.5–2 mg IV	Caution with unoppossed α-adrenergic stimulation
	Esmolol loading dose 500 μg/kg/min Maintain dose 25–50 μg/kg/min	Requires continuous infusion with complex dosing regimen
	Verapamil 2.5–10 mg IV	Hypotension can occur
Agitation	Haloperidol 2–10 mg IM	
	Droperidol 2.5–10 mg IM or IV titrated	
	Chlorpromazine 25–50 mg IV or IM	Caution in anticholinergic and LSD intoxications
Anxiety	Diazepam 2–10 mg IV	Painful on IM injection
	Midazolam 1–4 mg IV	Watch for respiratory depression
Cholinergic crisis	Physostigmine 1–2 mg IV or IM	Can produce cardiac arrest; to be used *only* for life-threatening cholinergic phenomena

the sympathetic effect of most of the hallucinogenic amphetamines.[6] However, fatal sympathomimetic crises have occurred with dosages twice that originally recommended for 3,4-methylenedioxymethamphetamine (MDMA, Adam, ecstasy). Methylenedioxyamphetamine (MDA) represents the prototype of these compounds.[7]

The compound MDMA has been used as an adjunct to psychotherapy although it is now classified as a Schedule I controlled substance. MDMA developed popularity as a drug of abuse in the 1970s because of its subjective effect to enhance communication, self-esteem, and mood. It was used as a non-FDA (Food and Drug Administration) approved adjunct to psychotherapy by some therapists. Despite the notion that it has a wider margin of safety than MDA, animal data suggest similar toxic ranges for MDMA and MDA. The LD_{50} approximates 10 to 20 mg/kg in monkeys for both compounds.[7,8] Absorption is rapid from the gastrointestinal tract, and peak plasma levels are reached in 1 to 2 h. Volume of distribution is variable but large. This together with high protein binding (usually 15 to 40 percent) prevents the use of extracorporeal removal techniques (hemodialysis and hemoperfusion). Elimination is via hepatic modification and renal excretion.

Signs and symptoms of MDMA intoxication include restlessness, tachycardia, hypertension, diaphoresis, and confusion. Life-threatening complications include hypertensive crisis, supraventricular tachyarrhythmias, hyperthermia, seizures, intracerebral hemorrhage, and related trauma. Table 179-4 suggests pharmacologic intervention for these complications. The decision to pharmacologically control symptoms must be made on an individual basis and take into account age, underlying medical condition, and the risk to the patient if only supportive care is used. Propranolol has been used successfully in the management of these intoxications; however, it carries the potential risk of unopposed α-adrenergic stimulation with paradoxical hypertension. If propranolol is used, phentolamine may be required for α-adrenergic blockade.

Massive overdosages with the hallucinogenic amphetamines may result in a paradoxical catecholamine-depleted state. This may produce hypotension, relative bradycardia, and be refractory to the use of indirect pressors such as dopamine. Small titrated amounts of direct-acting catecholamines such as norepinephrine or phenylephrine may be required to maintain cardiovascular stability.

PEYOTE AND MESCALINE

A mixture of approximately 15 phenylethylamine and isoquinoline alkaloids, peyote is the dried crown of the cactus *Lophophoria williamsii*. Legally available for the religious rites of the Native American Church, it is illicitly distributed in the general population for its psychoactive properties. Symptoms of peyote toxicity include mild sympathetic stimulation and gastrointestinal distress. Hallucinations are similar to those in LSD intoxication. In contrast to the other phenylethylamine compounds, peyote in high doses has been associated with hypotension, bradycardia, and respiratory depression. Treatment is supportive.

COCAINE

Although abused primarily for its euphoric effects, cocaine also possesses poorly understood hallucinatory effects. Chronic abuse can produce a psychosis similar to that of chronic amphetamine abuse and paranoid schizophrenia.[3] Hallucinations may comprise part of this psychosis. In a series of 137 patients with cocaine ingestion seen in one emergency department, 37 percent presented with altered mental states that included hallucinations.[9] These hallucinations can affect any of the senses. Management of cocaine ingestion is supportive and similar to the management of the sympathomimetic amines.

DISASSOCIATIVE ANESTHETICS

Members of this class of hallucinogens (phencyclidine and ketamine) represent a unique class of anesthetics that result in a dissociation of the patient from the environment, profound analgesia, and moderate anesthesia while preserving spontaneous ventilation, laryngeal and pharyngeal reflexes.[10] PCP was removed from the pharmaceutical market in 1963 due to hallucinations, agitation, and muscle rigidity on emergence. Early oral abuse of PCP (PeaCe Pill) led to a negative reputation because of severe unpleasant reactions. The drug underwent a resurgence in popularity in localized areas of the United States (Los Angeles, New York) with the institution of PCP smoking. This route leads to better titration of the desired altered effects on the sensorium. Ketamine is available as an uncontrolled anesthetic drug and is widely used in veterinary medicine. It produces less vivid hallucinations and does not appear to be a widely abused street drug.

PCP is usually smoked and often is sprinkled on marijuana. It is well absorbed from both the pulmonary and gastrointestinal systems. Approximately 60 percent is inactivated by pyrolysis. The volume of distribution approximates 6 L/kg, and the plasma protein binding is 65 percent, preventing extracorporeal removal of the drug. The terminal half-life approximates 18 to 24 h. Excretion is via hepatic transformation and renal excretion.

PCP produces complex effects physically and psychologically. These effects appear somewhat independent of dose and highly dependent on route of administration, social setting, previous experience with the drug, and personality type.[11] PCP appears to affect several central neurotransmitters and their precursors, including tryptophan, tyrosine, dopamine, and acetylcholine.[12]

In low doses, mild stimulant effects may be seen. Moderate doses may produce muscle rigidity, hallucinations, and psychosis; high doses can produce coma, seizures, and brief periods of agitation. Profound violent behavior and insensitivity to pain can be seen at any time and with any amount ingested. PCP can mimic organic brain syndromes, psychosis, and affective syndromes.[11] A particular environmental disassociation mimics a catatonia. Nystagmus, first horizontal then vertical or rotary, can be seen even in low doses and may be helpful in making a clinical diagnosis.[13]

Life-threatening complications are primarily a result of dopaminergic storm. Hypertension may progress to intracerebral hemorrhage, and seizures may be difficult to control. Rhabdomyolysis results from direct toxicity of the drug or secondarily from mechanical restraints and the trauma induced during attempts to detain or restrain the victim. Treatment guidelines include minimizing sensory stimulation with patient monitoring being accomplished as noninvasively as possible. Gastric decontamination is usually of little clinical benefit and attempts at nasogastric or orogastric tube placement may cause extreme agitation and be counterproductive. Activated charcoal may be useful in binding ingested drug. Haloperidol or droperidol are the tranquilizers of choice. Extreme care must be exercised to protect the staff from sudden unprovoked violent outbursts. These patients can be profoundly insensate to pain and require five or more persons to restrain and control them.

Key to management of PCP ingestions is to distinguish the patient who will respond to supportive care alone from those who will require aggressive intensive care. Careful, continuous monitoring of the respiratory status of the patient will often distinguish these groups. At the first sign of impending respiratory insufficiency, aggressive control of the airway is mandatory. Endotrachael intubation may be difficult due to muscle rigidity and may require neuromuscular blockade.

Agitation may complicate the use of mechanical ventilation and require large amounts of sedation. If sedation alone is insufficient to deliver mechanical ventilation safely, then neuromuscular blockade with sedation is necessary. PCP appears to retain first-order kinetics even in massive overdoses.[14] Attempts to decrease sedation or mechanical ventilation can usually be made after one to two half-lives (36 to 48 h) and the response of the patient monitored. Careful monitoring of renal and electrolyte balance is required because a large percentage of these patients develop myoglobinuria and rhabdomyolysis.

PCP is a weak base which can be trapped in acidified urine, and this has been suggested as a possible means to enhance excretion.[11,13,15] However, the volume of distribution of PCP is large, the major (90 percent) route of excretion is hepatic, first-order elimination kinetics are retained even in massive overdoses, and the amount of drug recovered in acidified urine is a small fraction of the total drug cleared. The benefits of urinary acidification in severely intoxicated patients appear insufficient to justify the risk of aggravating myoglobinuria, renal failure, electrolyte imbalance, and instrumentation.[14,16] Extracorporeal removal is not effective. Urine assays for PCP metabolites are available and may be useful in confirming an ingestion but are not generally required for patient management.

INDOLE ALKYLAMINES

These compounds contain derivatives of tryptamine. Most commonly encountered are the psilocin and psilocybin containing mushrooms of the *Psilocybia, Gymnopilus,* and *Panelous* genera (so-called magic mushrooms). In addition to hallucinations, dysphoric reactions may occur and prompt presentation to the emergency department. Visual hallucinations have been reported in as many as 39 percent of ingestions.[17] Patients may also present with drowsiness. Sympathomimetic symptoms are seen in fewer than 50 percent of cases. Major complications after ingestion are rare although seizures have been reported. Trauma related to dysphoria represents the largest threat to the patient. Because of the short duration of symptoms (<12 h), ICU admission and specific therapy are rarely needed.

Ingestions of tryptamine, dimethyltryptamine (DMT), and bufitenine are less commonly seen. Fatalities with these compounds have not been reported; treatment is supportive.

HALLUCINOGENS AFFECTING THE CHOLINERGIC NERVOUS SYSTEM

The majority of these hallucinogens are found in plants and are either mistakenly consumed while foraging for edible plants or occasionally consumed specifically for their hallucinogenic potential. The plant family Solancace (potato) includes the *Datura* species jimsonweed, henbane, belladonna, and mandrake, all of which contain the anticholinergic alkaloids atropine, hyoscyamine, and scopolamine. Signs and symptoms reflect classic anticholinergic toxicity with pupillary dilation, tachycardia, dry flushed skin, dry mucous membranes, fever, and hallucinations. It is key to distinguish these intoxications from hallucinogens with sympathomimetic symptoms which will also include tachycardia, pupillary dilation, and agitation. Sympathomimetic ingestions, however, will not produce dry mucous membranes, urinary retention, and decreased gastrointestinal motility which are classic for anticholinergic toxicity (see Table 179-3). Severe hallucinations with agitation, seizures, or tachyarrhythmias unresponsive to supportive management may require use of the pharmacologic antagonist physostigmine. Physostigmine is a cholinergic agonist that can provoke bronchorrhea, bradyarrhythmias, and intractable cardiac arrest. Its use should be reserved for life-threatening intoxications. It may be repeated if symptoms recur. More than 2 to 5 mg is rarely required. Drugs with anticholinergic effects, such as phenothiazines, and haloperidol should be avoided in patients with significant anticholinergic signs; benzodiazepines may be used for agitation.

The ibotenic acid- and muscimol-containing mushrooms (group V)[18] of the *Amanita* species produce psychoactive symptoms via complex effects on γ-aminobutyrate (GABA) receptors. Clinical signs and symptoms are both cholinergic and anticholinergic. Fever, agitation, tachycardia, and dry mucous membranes are most commonly seen. Hallucinations usually involve alterations in visual perceptions rather than true visual hallucinations and are usually mild. Patients ingesting these mushrooms usually do not seek medical aid but may be brought to the emergency department by anxious parents or friends. These mushrooms are not hepatotoxic (although they are in the same family as the hepatotoxic *Amanita phalloides*). Specific therapy is not needed. Atropine and physostigmine may aggravate the symptoms and should not be used. Benzodiazepines may be used if anxiety is severe, although reassurance that symptoms last only 4 to 6 h is usually all that is needed.

LYSERGIC ACID DIETHYLAMIDE (LSD) AND LSD-LIKE COMPOUNDS

These compounds represent a wide variety of naturally occurring and synthetically substituted indole alkylamines whose primary effect is intense visual and to a lesser extent auditory hallucinations. Medical complications usually result from trauma related to the hallucinations.

A variety of plants in the morning glory (Convolvulaceae), and the Myristicaceae (nutmeg) families, as well as the fungus *Claviceps purpurea* (epidemic ergotism, Saint Anthony's fire) produce these compounds.[19]

LSD is the diethylamide derivative of the alkaloid. It is tasteless, odorless, and rapidly absorbed from both the gastrointestinal and nasal mucosa. The drug is effective in doses of 35 μg and has been distributed on sugar cubes, stamp backing ("panes"), and small pieces of gelatin ("dots"). Tolerance may develop rapidly. Metabolism appears to be via hydroxylation with an elimination half-life of approximately 3 h. LSD appears to exert its effects via modulation of central serotonin receptors.[20]

Signs and symptoms relate primarily to perceptional alterations and misrepresentation of sensory stimulation.[21] Insight usually remains intact and patients understand they are experiencing drug-induced hallucinations. Pupils may be dilated slightly; however, vital signs usually remain normal. Flashbacks, consisting of a repetition of previously experienced hallucinations months after ingestion, may occur but probably have been overrated in terms of clinical significance. Focal neurologic deficits have been reported with LSD use that may be mediated by vasospasm.

Since the majority of patients retain insight while under the influence of the drug, the mainstay of therapy has been to provide supportive reassurance in an environment that minimizes external sensory stimulation. This is referred to as "talking down" the patient. Diazepam intravenously or haloperidol intramuscularly can be useful if agitation is severe. Several reports of cardiovascular collapse suggest that phenothiazines such as chloropromazine should be avoided.[22] Careful monitoring of respiratory function is required if sedatives are administered. Gastric decontamination and activated charcoal are not usually necessary. Laboratory determination of LSD in body fluids is not widely available and is not necessary for treatment. There is no role for forced diuresis or extracorporeal dialysis due to the short half-life and absence of severe life-threatening reactions.

CANNABINOIDS

The plant parts of the Indian hemp plant *(Cannabis sativa)* contain over 61 monoterpenoid compounds collectively referred to as cannabinoids and abused primarily for their euphoric and hallucinogenic effects. The major psychomimetic compound is Δ^9-tetrahydrocannabinol (THC). This compound has also been investigated for treatment of glaucoma and is legally available as dronabinol for use as an antiemetic against chemotherapy-induced nausea. THC is rapidly absorbed from the respiratory and gastrointestinal mucosa. However, a large hepatic first-pass effect minimizes oral bioavailability. Peak plasma levels of THC are reached within 10 min of smoking and 45 min of oral ingestion. THC is widely distributed in fat and extensively metabolized by the liver with predominant excretion in the urine. Blood levels are not clinically helpful and assays of the urine can detect metabolites for confirmation of use. CNS effects rarely last more than 2 to 3 h. Marijuana produces mild alterations in mood, sensory perception, and coordination. High doses may produce lethargy. Mild elevations in vital signs are seen. Congestion of conjunctival blood vessels leading to reddened conjunctiva is a highly sensitive but not specific indicator of recent marijuana use. Few life-threatening symptoms have been documented with oral or inhaled marijuana use, although mild increases in heart rate and cardiac output have been reported. Trauma related to perceptual alterations are the most serious risks to life. Severe rhabdomyolysis, renal insufficiency, and cardiovascular collapse have been reported several hours after intravenous administration of marijuana extract.[23,24] Treatment of these marijuana-exposed patients is supportive. Specific therapy directed at inhalant exposures is not usually needed. Gastric decontamination and oral activated charcoal is occasionally useful in massive oral ingestions or recent oral ingestions in children. Intravenous exposures should be closely monitored with careful attention directed to intravascular fluid status, electrolyte balance, and renal function.

MISCELLANEOUS HALLUCINOGENS

A large number of pharmaceuticals used in ICUs have the propensity to produce hallucinations. Distinguishing these from illicitly obtained material is usually easy, although we have seen cases of patients abusing illicit drugs while hospitalized in the ICU. The determination of which one of several concurrently used pharmaceuticals is producing hallucinations presents much more of a challenge. Table 179-5 lists some of the more common drugs associated with hallucinations. Discontinuation of suspect drugs is often the only way to determine therapeutic drug-induced hallucinations. The management principles remain unchanged.

An extremely common cause of hallucinations in the ICU is ethanol withdrawal. Intoxicated patients often will emerge from sedation in the ICU 48 to 72 h after their last drink and enter ethanol withdrawal. Blood ethanol levels will be absent or low. A high index of suspicion will identify the majority of these patients. Therapy with benzodiazepines will control the majority of symptoms.

TABLE 179-5 Therapeutic Drugs Associated with Hallucinations

Antihistamines	*Anticolvulsants*	*Miscellaneous*
Cimetidine	Carbamazepine	Corticosteroids
Diphenhydramine		Metaprotereol
Chlorpheniramine	*Benzodiazepines*	Levodopa
Ranitidine	Clonazepam	Phenothiazines
	Lorazapam	Tricyclic anti-depressants
Antihypertensives		
Clonidine	*Cardioactive Drugs*	
Methyldopa	Digoxin	
	Disopyramide	
Anti-infectives	Quinidine	
Acyclovir	Procanamide	
Amantidine	Propranolol	
Cephalexin	Streptokinase	
Chloroquine		
Cycloserine	*Opioids*	
Dapsone	*Miscellaneous Drugs*	
Gentamicin	Baclofen	
Griseofulvin	Cyclobenzaprine	
Isoniazid	Bromocriptine	
Minocycline	Cyclosporin	
Nalidixic Acid	Disulfiram	
Pentamidine	Indomethacin	
Penicillin		
Vidarabine		

Some hydrocarbon solvents, particularly the aromatic hydrocarbons toluene, benzene, and xylene, have been abused for their euphoric effects. All hydrocarbons are CNS depressants and can produce hallucinations, seizures, and cardiac arrythymias. Treatment is supportive and symptoms terminate rapidly on removal from the environment.

Occasionally opioids, including the "designer opioids" are abused for their hallucinogenic potential. Treatment involves the use of naloxone and is more fully discussed in Chap. 173.

CASE PRESENTATION

A 16-year-old woman presented to the emergency department in a severe state of agitation pulling at her clothes and tearing at her hair. The patient was screaming "the bugs are attacking me." On questioning the patient stated she had been out "partying" with friends when the bugs attacked her. No friends were available for additional history. Vital signs on admission included blood pressure 170/100 mmHg, heart rate 150/min, respiration rate 30/min, and temperature 39.8°C (103.5°F). Pupils were 3 mm and bilaterally reactive; there was no nystagmus. The skin was flushed and moist. The remainder of the physical examination was normal. Telephone discussion with the patient's parents identified no prescription medication and no history of psychiatric disorders. The patient's parents commented that she had been "running around" with elements of the drug subculture.

Shortly after arrival the patient became violent and required forcible restraint. Blood pressure rose to 200/

110 mmHg, with a heart rate of 160/min. Intravenous access was obtained, and the patient was given 20 mg labetolol intravenously, a continuous blood pressure monitor was applied, and external cooling measures were begun. Haloperidol, 2 mg intramuscularly, was administered with some reduction in agitation. The patient was admitted to intensive care. Cultures of blood, urine, and cerebral spinal fluid were obtained. The urine drug screen was positive for amphetamine metabolites.

Over the next 6 h the patient required 60 mg labetolol and 4 mg haloperidol to control sympathetic hyperstimulation. Blood creatine phosphokinase concentration peaked at 4000 IU/dL, but myoglobinuria was not present. Within 12 h her mental status returned to normal, and she was able to relate the history that she ingested "speed" to get high with her friends. The remainder of her hospital course was unremarkable, and she was discharged 24 h after admission with a referral to a drug rehabilitation program.

CASE DISCUSSION

This young woman presented with hallucinations as a prominent symptom. There was no history of prescription drugs or previous psychiatric disorder. The circumstances of the patient's presentation strongly suggested illicit drug use. The patient's signs and symptoms, especially her blood pressure and heart rate, suggested sympathomimetic stimulation. The skin was moist and bowel sounds were present. This distinguished the patient's symptoms from anticholinergic toxicity. Shortly after arrival the patient's condition deteriorated and restraint was required. Haloperidol was chosen for sedation. The patient's sympathomimetic state required treatment. The blood pressure of 220/110, which appeared to be rising rapidly, prompted intervention. Labetolol was chosen because this drug will treat both hypertension and tachycardia in this setting. A search to rule out coexisting organic causes for her hallucinations was conducted, and the patient was closely monitored for the complications of rhabdomyolysis and intracranial hemorrhage. Her urine drug screen results confirmed the clinical diagnosis but did not affect therapy. In addition to treatment of her acute medical condition, interventions directed at the psychosocial pressures leading to illicit drug use were addressed prior to discharge.

References

1. Asaad G, Shapiro B. Hallucinations: Theoretical and clinical overview. Am J Psychiatry 143:1088, 1986.
2. Ellenhorn MJ, Barceloux DG: *Medical Toxicoloy. Diagnosis and Treatment of Human Poisoning*. New York, Elsevier, 1988.
3. Leikin JB, Krantz AJ, Zell-Kanter M, et al: Clinical features and management of intoxication due to hallucinogenic drugs. Med Toxicol Adverse Drug Exp 4:325, 1989.
4. West LJ: A clinical and theoretical overview of hallucinatory phenomena, in Siegal et al (eds): *Hallucinations: Behavior, Experience and Theory*. Los Angeles, Wiley, 1975, p 287.
5. Dubin WR, Weiss KJ, Dorn JM: Pharmacotherapy of psychiatric emergencies. J Clin Psychopharmacol 6:210, 1986.
6. Stone WH: Clandestine drug synthesis, in *Medicinal Research Reviews*. Los Angeles, Wiley, 1986, p 41.
7. Climko RP, Roehrich H, Sweeney DB, Al-Razi J: Ectasy: A review of MDMA and MDA. Intl J Psychiatry Med 16:359, 1986.
8. Davis WM, Hatoum HT, Waters IW: Toxicity of MDA considered for relevance to hazards of MDMA (ecstasy) abuse, Alc Drug Res 7:123, 1987.
9. Derlet RW, Albertson TE: Emergency department presentation of cocaine intoxication. Ann Emerg Med 18:182, 1986.
10. Phencyclidine: Pharmacologic and clinical review. Psych Med 2:189, 1984.
11. McCarron MM, Schulze BW, Thompson GA: Acute phencyclidine intoxication: Clinical patterns, complications and treatment. Ann Emerg Med 10:290, 1981.
12. Leonard BE, Tonge SR: Some effects of a hallucinogenic drug (phencyclidine) on neurohumoral substances. Life Sci 9:1141, 1970.
13. Barton CH, Sterling ML, Vaziri ND: Phencyclidine intoxication: Clinical experience in 27 cases confirmed by urine assay. Ann Emerg Med 10:243, 1981.
14. Jackson JE: Phencyclidine pharmacokinetics after a massive overdose. Ann Intern Med 111:613, 1989.
15. Aronow R, Done AK: Phencyclidine overdose: An emerging concept of management. JACEP 7:56, 1978.
16. Chiang W, Goldfrank L: The medical complications of drug abuse. Med J Aust 152:83, 1990.
17. Francis J, Murray VSG: Review of inquiries made to the NPIS concerning Psilocybe mushroom ingestion. Hum Toxicol 2:349, 1983.
18. Mitchell DH. Amanita mushroom poisoning. Annu Rev Med 31:51, 1980.
19. Shulgin AT: LSD. J Psychedelic Drugs 12:173, 1980.
20. Khun DM, White FJ, Appel JB: The discriminative stimulus properties of LSD: Mechanisms of action. Neuropharmacology 17:257, 1978.
21. Cohen S: Psychotomimetic agents. Annu Rev Pharmacol 7:301, 1967.
22. Solursh LP, Clement WR: Hallucinogenic drug abuse. Manifestations and management. CMA J 98:407, 1968.
23. Vaziri ND, Thomas R, Sterling M: Toxicity with intravenous injection of crude marijuana extract. Clin Toxicol 18:353, 1981.
24. Brandenberg D, Wernick R: Intravenous marijuana syndrome. West J Med 145:94, 1986.

Chapter 180
COCAINE

EDWARD A. PANACEK

KEY POINTS

- *Cocaine is currently the number one cause of drug-related emergency department visits in the urban United States and the second greatest cause of drug-related deaths.*
- *Cocaine toxicity should be suspected in any patient who presents with otherwise unexplained acute myocardial infarction, severe hypertension, new seizures, rhabdomyolysis, intracranial hemorrhage, or spontaneous pneumomediastinum.*
- *The major medical complications of cocaine abuse can be induced in young, otherwise healthy normal individuals without underlying medical problems.*
- *Cocaine-related fatalities are generally due to status epilepticus, ventricular dysrhythmia, myocardial infarction, or malignant hyperthermia.*
- *Cocaine-related fatalities often do not occur in close temporal relationship to the cocaine ingestion itself and may present up to 24 h later.*
- *The initial focus of pharmacologic therapy for both the hyperkinetic and hyperdynamic states is diazepam.*

By 1990, cocaine had become the recreational drug of choice in the United States as well as many other parts of the world. In the United States it is now the number one cause for drug-related emergency department visits in urban settings and is showing an increasing association with intensive care unit (ICU) admissions. Although the mechanisms of cocaine toxicity are not well understood, the drug can affect nearly every organ system. It is an important cause of fatalities and is currently the second most common cause of drug-related death. Physicians should maintain a high index of suspicion for the presence of cocaine use in appropriate patient populations and should be aware of the broad range of medical toxicity which can be associated with its use.[1]

Clinical Pharmacology

Cocaine is an ester type of anesthetic from the family of natural alkaloids. The drug derives its local anesthetic properties by interfering with neuronal sodium channels. Unlike other local anesthetics, it also impairs the presynaptic reuptake of catecholamines and upregulates postsynaptic receptors. This is the mechanism by which it acts as a vasoconstrictor. Cocaine also appears to have other, poorly understood actions within the central nervous system (CNS). It is this combination of pharmacologic effects which makes cocaine relatively unique.[2] Biochemically, cocaine bears only a passing resemblance to other substances to which it is most commonly compared, such as lidocaine, amphetamines, and phencyclidine (PCP). Cocaine hydrochloride is a white powder and is the formulation of all legal and, previously, most illicit cocaine. However, this form is poorly volatile; more recently it is being converted to the free (alkaloidal) base using simple extraction procedures. The resultant crystalline form is heat stable and can be smoked. When burnt, it often crackles, ergo the name "crack."[3]

An individual may administer cocaine by any one of a number of different routes. Smoking is the general practice, but intranasal and intravenous use continue to be popular. It is a common, but false, belief that orally ingested cocaine is inactivated in the acid environment of the stomach. Oral cocaine use is relatively equivalent to intranasal administration. Each achieves peak plasma concentrations in roughly 60 min, with effects lasting up to 2 h. Cocaine which is smoked or taken intravenously yields peak serum concentrations in 5 to 15 min and has a half-life of only 30 to 45 min.

The chemical name for the active substance in cocaine is methylbenzoylecgonine. It has a relatively large volume of distribution (2.1 L/kg) and is metabolized via hepatic and plasma esterases. There is genetic variability in the activity of these enzymes, which may explain the individual variability in physiologic response to cocaine use. Renally excreted metabolites (e.g., benzoylecgonine) can generally be detected in the urine for 2 to 3 days and longer in the setting of chronic use or underlying renal insufficiency.

As with all illicit street drugs, it is important to remember that these substances are absolutely unpredictable in terms of concentration or the presence of adulterants. Street cocaine, in particular, is notorious for being contaminated with or entirely replaced by various other drugs. Some of the more common and concerning adulterants are amphetamines, PCP, lysergic acid diethylamide (LSD), quinine, and heroin. A very unfortunate adulterant is strychnine, which can mimic the hyperexcitability effect of cocaine and goes by the street name "death hit."

Manifestations of Cocaine Toxicity

The medical complications associated with cocaine use range from single organ system involvement to death. Nearly every organ, and therefore every subspecialty of medicine, can be involved in its toxicity (Table 180-1). Most fatalities are associated with seizures, stroke, cardiac dysrhythmia, or acute myocardial infarction. Each of these conditions can be induced by cocaine in otherwise healthy normal individuals. A common misbelief is that severe toxicity associated with cocaine use must appear in close temporal association with the cocaine ingestion itself. Although about one-third of fatalities related to cocaine use occur within 1 h of the ingestion, another third will not occur until 6 to 24 h later.

An individual patient may present with a generalized picture of stimulant abuse or with focused toxicity of a specific organ system. It is important to note that a patient may

TABLE 180-1 Medical Complications of Cocaine Abuse

Cardiovascular: dysrhythmias, myocardial ischemia/infarction, myocarditis, cardiovascular collapse, hypertension, dilated cardiomyopathy, ruptured aorta, deep vein thrombosis
Central nervous system: agitation, anxiety, generalized seizures, vascular headaches, cerebral infarction, subarachnoid hemorrhage, psychosis, cerebral vasculitis
Pulmonary: alveolar hemorrhage, hemoptysis, acute pulmonary edema, black sputum bronchitis, hypersensitivity pneumonitis, barotrauma, bronchiolitis obliterans organizing pneumonia, (BOOP)
Gastrointestinal: bowel ischemia, body packer syndrome, hepatitis
Obstetric and Perinatal: spontaneous abortion, abruptio placentae, premature labor, neonatal cerebral infarction, neonatal seizures, neonatal myocardial infarction
Miscellaneous: rhabdomyolysis, hyperthermia, acute renal failure, effects of adulterants, infectious diseases (IV use)

develop fatal toxicity without the usual preceding progression of generalized symptoms. Certain organ system toxicities are particularly likely to prompt ICU admission.

CARDIOVASCULAR EFFECTS

The first reported cardiac manifestations of cocaine toxicity were atrial and ventricular dysrhythmias. These range from sinus tachycardia to ventricular fibrillation with sudden cardiac death and can be induced in otherwise healthy individuals. Electrophysiologic studies have failed to demonstrate a tendency toward dysrhythmia generation in the absence of cocaine use.[4]

The aspect of cocaine's toxicity which has engendered the most attention is myocardial infarction. By 1985, it had clearly been demonstrated that cocaine use could be associated with acute myocardial infarction in young healthy adults. Although it was known that cocaine could aggravate underlying coronary artery disease, it is now accepted that it can induce infarction in the absence of underlying coronary atherosclerosis.[5] Attempts to demonstrate vasospastic ischemia in these individuals, using ergonovine tests, have been unsuccessful. When catheterization is performed in the acute setting, the findings are generally those of thrombus superimposed on underlying normal coronary arteries. Further investigations have revealed that even low therapeutic doses of cocaine can increase myocardial oxygen demand and decrease coronary artery flow.[6] These effects seem to be most marked in normal, nonatherosclerotic coronary arteries and, in vivo, are blocked by the administration of phentolamine. However, the underlying mechanism by which cocaine induces infarction remains unclear. Postulated mechanisms include vasospasm, endothelial abnormalities, and induction of platelet aggregation.

Other cardiovascular effects of cocaine toxicity include myocarditis,[7] aortic rupture,[8] and cardiovascular collapse. In addition, a dilated cardiomyopathy which improves with the strict avoidance of further cocaine use has recently been described.[9] It appears to resemble the myocardial dysfunction of pheochromocytoma and chronic amphetamine abuse.

CENTRAL NERVOUS SYSTEM TOXICITY

With the recreational use of cocaine, one of the desired effects is obviously CNS stimulation. This occurs as a result of an increase in adrenergic neural transmission and a decrease in transmission along serontin-mediated pathways. Common side effects include hyperactivity, tremors, fasciculations, and headache.

Cocaine also causes both ischemic and hemorrhagic strokes.[10] More commonly, cocaine has been associated with subarachnoid hemorrhage.[11] When this was first recognized, it was usually in the setting of an underlying berry aneurysm or arteriovenous malformation. Therefore, it was postulated that cocaine caused severe hypertension, leading to rupture at a site of underlying vascular weakness. More recently, subarachnoid hemorrhage has been reported in the absence of demonstrable vascular malformations, prompting speculation that cocaine causes a form of vasculitis.[12]

The most common major CNS toxicity associated with cocaine use is generalized seizures.[13] Cocaine's capacity to induce seizures has been clearly demonstrated in animals. In some models the long-term, repeated administration of cocaine results in a progressive lowering of the seizure threshold. In some instances, seizures eventually occur spontaneously, in the absence of further cocaine administration.[14] Therefore, unlike most other drugs of abuse which demonstrate tolerance with long-term use, repeated administration of cocaine may result in increased sensitivity to its effects. Cocaine use is being found with increasing frequency in both adults and children who present with a new-onset seizure disorder.

Although the user of cocaine generally desires euphoria, the resultant effect may often be one of dysphoria, delirium, paranoia, or even psychosis. Auditory and visual hallucinations may occur as well as altered tactile sensation. Classically, the patient complains of ants crawling under his skin (formication) and may be driven to severe self-excoriation.

Cocaine has been demonstrated to have effects on the temperature-regulating areas of the hypothalamus. Hyperthermia may be a significant contributor to acute fatalities. This is generally seen in association with rhabdomyolysis (vide infra) but can be an isolated effect of cocaine abuse, particularly during the warmer summer months.

PULMONARY TOXICITY

The toxic effects on the lungs depend upon the route of administration.[15] Intravenous cocaine is mixed with a broad array of impurities, which are filtered by the pulmonary circulation. All forms of cocaine use, though, have been reported to cause noncardiogenic pulmonary edema. A capillary leak has been demonstrated in animal models of cocaine toxicity.

Patients who smoke cocaine often perform a deep, prolonged, and forceful Valsalva maneuver; subcutaneous emphysema, pneumomediastinum, and pneumothorax are all possible complications.[16] Pulmonary hemorrhage has been found in cocaine smokers as well. Usually this is an occult finding on biopsy or autopsy, but massive hemoptysis may be seen occasionally. BOOP has also been reported.[17] An entity called "crack lung," characterized by bronchospasm, fever, and transient pulmonary infiltrates, has also been described. Eosinophilia and elevated serum IgE levels lend support to the belief that this is a hypersensitivity reaction.

OTHER MAJOR TOXICITIES

Cocaine-induced rhabdomyolysis was first recognized in 1987.[18] It is usually seen in association with hyperpyrexia and hyperkinesis, although these findings are not universally present. The serum creatine phosphokinase (CPK) level can reach several hundred thousand, and the release of myoglobin can cause acute renal failure. The mechanism of cocaine-induced rhabdomyolysis is unclear but may be due to muscular overexertion, ischemia of skeletal muscles, or a direct toxic injury to the myocyte. Rhabdomyolysis caused by cocaine use is generally more severe and prolonged than that due to other etiologies. Urinalysis, or even gross examination of the urine, may provide a clue to the diagnosis. On occasion, this problem is overlooked until renal failure ensues.

Cocaine abuse during pregnancy has been associated with serious maternal and fetal complications. Unfortunately, the obstetric patient is not immune to the aforementioned toxicities, including acute myocardial infarction. In addition, cocaine use is associated with abruptio placentae, spontaneous abortion, and preterm labor. Cocaine has been shown to cause constriction of uterine vascular beds, with resultant placental ischemia. Finally, the drug crosses the placenta and has been implicated in myocardial and cerebral infarction in the fetus.[19]

Just as cocaine can cause ischemic infarcts in the coronary and cerebral circulations, it can also cause mesenteric ischemia and bowel infarction. Acute hepatitis has also been described in association with cocaine abuse, although the mechanism is not entirely understood.[20]

Diagnosis

Most cocaine-related fatalities occur outside the hospital; by the time these patients are seen in an emergency department, resuscitative efforts are usually not successful. The patient who arrives alive should generally survive the drug insult if he receives proper comprehensive and supportive care.[21] Given the current social climate, clinicians should have a very high index of suspicion for the involvement of cocaine in a broad array of medical conditions. Ulceration or perforation of the nasal septum can provide a helpful diagnostic clue to the presence of cocaine use. However, with an increasing tendency toward smoking rather than snorting cocaine, this finding is becoming less common.

Cocaine is very difficult to detect in blood because it undergoes very rapid metabolism. Drug screening methods are designed to detect cocaine metabolites in the urine. These metabolites can be detected within minutes after intravenous or inhalational use and will continue to be present for at least 2 days after a single administration. Frequent abuse of high doses of cocaine, or underlying renal insufficiency, may result in prolongation of a positive urine screen for up to 3 weeks. It is also anticipated that a hair analysis screening test will soon become generally available. Such a test would provide the capability to screen for remote cocaine use.

The differential diagnosis of the patient who presents with sympathetic stimulation includes other drug ingestions as well as non-drug-related medical illnesses. It may be very difficult to differentiate between amphetamine and cocaine abuse, although the clinical management is similar. PCP intoxication can also mimic cocaine effects (see Chap. 179). With PCP use, agitation is generally intermittent, the psychosis is more prolonged, the pupils are constricted rather than dilated, and there is usually a prominent bidirectional nystagmus. Psychiatric disorders and other systemic or environmental diseases must also be considered, especially thyrotoxicosis, hypertensive encephalopathy, heat stroke, neuroleptic malignant syndrome, malignant hyperthermia, CNS infection, and alcohol withdrawal.

Management

The basic supportive care of these patients should begin with consideration of airway, breathing, and circulatory stabilization (Table 180-2). The patient who presents with a change in mental status should receive 100 mL of 50% dextrose in water (or rapid bedside confirmation of adequate blood glucose) and naloxone hydrochloride 2 mg intravenously (particularly if coincident narcotic use is suspected). Appropriate toxicology screens should be initiated, although care should not be delayed pending the results. When the possibility of cocaine abuse is entertained, one must screen for occult complications. The possibility of sub-

TABLE 180-2 General Management Principles

Early intravenous access and electrocardiogram (ECG) monitoring.
Diazepam for agitation, seizures, or hyperadrenergic states.
Urine toxicology screen to confirm the diagnosis and exclude cointoxicants.
Laboratory screening to rule out myocardial infarction, rhabdomyolysis, and acute renal failure.
Avoid isolated use of beta blockers.
Rule out pneumomediastinum in patients with chest pain.
Consider head computed tomography (CT) scan to rule out subarachnoid hemorrhage.

arachnoid hemorrhage, acute myocardial infarction, and rhabdomyolysis must all be carefully considered.

There is no specific antidote to counteract the general toxicity or the multisystem complications of cocaine abuse. There is limited information available from animal studies to help guide therapeutic decisions, but there are no confirmatory human trials. The one agent which has most consistently shown protective and therapeutic benefits in the general management of these patients is diazepam.[22] It helps prevent hyperthermia, acidemia, agitation, and seizures, and it moderates the cardiovascular responses to cocaine. Diazepam should be considered the initial drug of choice unless there is a specific contraindication to its use. Further therapeutic recommendations are based on the specific end-organ toxicity (Table 180-3).

HYPERTENSION

A hyperadrenergic state with tachycardia and hypertension is commonly seen with cocaine toxicity. This will often respond to the use of diazepam alone. Previously, propranolol was used in this setting, but animal studies have shown increased mortality and morbidity associated with its use. There is a theoretical risk that beta blockade will allow an unopposed alpha effect, resulting in increased hypertension and coronary artery vasoconstriction. Most clinicians have had better results with intravenous labetalol, a combined alpha- and beta-adrenergic antagonist.[23] This is now the drug of choice when diazepam alone is not successful. If hypertension is severe, does not respond to labetalol, or is complicated by aortic dissection, addition of a vasodilator is indicated, as in other hypertensive emergencies. A very effective combination is that of nitroprusside and esmolol.

TABLE 180-3 Treatment of Specific Complications

Hypertension
Diazepam (0.05–0.15 mg/kg intravenously, repeated as needed)
Labetalol (0.25 mg/kg intravenously over 2 min, repeated every 10 min as needed, up to a total of 300 mg)
Nitroprusside and esmolol (by continuous infusion)
Myocardial infarction and ischemia
Nitrates, morphine
Avoid beta blockers used alone
Judicious use of thrombolytic therapy, after excluding severe hypertension and intracranial hemorrhage
Seizures
Serial assessment of the need to intubate or mechanically ventilate
Diazepam (0.15 mg/kg intravenously, repeated as needed)
Phenobarbital (10 mg/kg at 100 mg/min)
Midazolam by continuous infusion
Rhabdomyolysis
Saline hydration
Alkalinization of the urine
Mannitol (1 g/kg intravenously)
Hyperthermia
Rectal probe thermometer
External cooling
Consider dantrolene for severe, persistent cases

MYOCARDIAL INFARCTION

There are no available prospective clinical studies regarding the specific treatment of cocaine-induced myocardial ischemia. In general, these patients should be treated similarly to those who have the usual form of myocardial ischemia. Sublingual nitrates and morphine are used initially followed by a continuous infusion of nitroglycerine if pain continues. Although it is attractive to postulate that coronary vasospasm plays a prominent role, calcium channel blockers have not proven helpful.[22] Likewise, the use of beta-adrenergic antagonists raises concern regarding unopposed alpha-adrenergic vasoconstriction.[24] Coronary thrombosis has been demonstrated in these patients, and thrombolytic therapy has been used successfully. A note of caution, however, is that chronic ST-T elevations have been noted on the ECGs of long-term cocaine users. In addition, severe hypertension is common with cocaine abuse and is a relative contraindication to thrombolytic therapy. The blood pressure must be well controlled before thrombolysis can be considered. Any possibility of a subarachnoid hemorrhage must also be addressed before considering the use of these agents. Therefore, thrombolytic therapy should be used with caution, taking into account all historical and clinical factors.

CARDIAC DYSRHYTHMIAS

Most supraventricular tachydysrhythmias will respond to the measures outlined above. When significant ventricular dysrhythmias occur, lidocaine has been used with some success. Of concern is the fact that lidocaine exerts its antiarrhythmic properties by inhibiting fast sodium channels similar to the effect of cocaine. Therefore, it is possible that lidocaine could aggravate the toxicity of cocaine.[25] Our own practice is to aggressively treat the hyperadrenergic state; if significant dysrhythmias continue, bretylium is the antiarrhythmic of choice.

SEIZURES

The seizures seen with cocaine abuse are most often self-limited. Recurrent or prolonged seizures should be treated acutely with diazepam. Therapy for further prophylactic seizure control is less clear. There is some evidence that phenytoin may not be highly effective in preventing further cocaine-related seizures. Phenobarbital appears to be more effective in this setting. For particularly difficult to control seizures, we have had success with constant midazolam infusions. As in any patient with status epilepticus, careful consideration must be given to ensuring adequate oxygenation, ventilation, and blood glucose levels (see Chap. 142). Early consideration of elective intubation and mechanical ventilation is appropriate. Individuals without a previous seizure history should be evaluated with a CT scan, electroencephalogram (EEG), and screening laboratory tests.

ALTERED MENTAL STATUS

A change in mental status in the setting of drug abuse should always raise a broad list of clinical possibilities. In the setting of cocaine use, one must have a high index of suspicion for cerebral infarction or intracranial hemorrhage. Even in the absence of focal neurologic findings, we have a very low threshold for obtaining a head CT scan and performing a lumbar puncture. There are no specific therapeutic recommendations for cocaine-induced cerebral infarction or intracranial hemorrhage beyond the treatments usually employed. Severe psychosis, with or without agitation, will sometimes improve with diazepam alone. Haldol may be used, judiciously, when agitation persists.

PULMONARY COMPLICATIONS

Pneumomediastinum is generally a benign entity which resolves spontaneously and requires no specific treatment.[16] The only exception to this is when it is seen in the setting of bronchospastic disease; such patients need to be followed closely.

Noncardiogenic pulmonary edema should be approached as in any patient with acute respiratory distress syndrome (ARDS) (see Chap. 128). Treatment includes oxygen, mechanical ventilation with positive end-expiratory pressure (PEEP), and attempts to reduce the left ventricular filling pressure. The duration of illness is typically more brief than with other etiologies of ARDS, and early discontinuation of mechanical ventilation should be anticipated.

Bronchiolitis obliterans organizing pneumonia and "crack lung" (which appears to be a hypersensitivity reaction) generally respond to avoidance of further cocaine use. Occasionally glucocorticoids may be required.[17]

RHABDOMYOLYSIS AND HYPERTHERMIA

These complications can often be minimized through the early, aggressive use of diazepam. Serum creatine kinase levels should be determined in all cocaine abusers, particularly when subjective complaints of muscle tenderness or myalgias are present. Standard measures to treat rhabdomyolysis should be employed, including the maintenance of a high urine output, possibly with measures to alkalinize the urine (see Chap. 154). Consideration should also be given to the use of mannitol. The patient should be observed for development of a compartment syndrome, and renal function should be monitored.

Hyperthermia may be seen independently of rhabdomyolysis and should be treated aggressively when the temperature exceeds 41°C (106°F). The patient should receive external cooling since antipyretics are usually unsuccessful. Dantrolene sodium has been reported to be efficacious in this setting although there is a paucity of clinical experience (see Chap. 73).

CASE PRESENTATION

Paramedics were called to transport a 28-year-old man with agitation. While en route and again upon arrival at the emergency department, the patient was witnessed to have generalized seizures. The paramedics noted that the scene was suspicious for illicit drug use, although there was no history for any specific drug ingestion or intoxication.

Upon evaluation in the emergency department, the patient was agitated but moved purposefully only to noxious stimuli. Vital signs revealed a blood pressure of 210/140, heart rate 120 and regular, respiratory rate of 28, and a temperature of 38.9°C (102°F). The patient was diaphoretic and flushed. The chest examination revealed good air movement. The only evidence of trauma was a tongue laceration attributed to the patient's previous seizures. Pupils were 8 mm, equal, and weakly reactive to light. There was no evidence of nystagmus. The rest of the exam was unrevealing, without focal neurologic deficit or meningismus. An 18-gauge intravenous catheter was placed and 5% dextrose and water (D5W) begun at a keep open rate. The patient was put on a 50% O_2 ventimask and a monitor. General screening laboratory tests were obtained, and 50 mL of 50% dextrose in water and 100 mg thiamine were given intravenously. There was no change in the patient's condition, and he was then given naloxone 2 mL intravenously. There was still no improvement.

An ECG revealed sinus tachycardia with borderline voltage criteria for left ventricular hypertrophy. There were also 1 mm ST elevations in leads V3 to V6. A urinary catheter was placed and a urine toxic screen was sent. An attempt was made to place a nasogastric tube, but the patient became very agitated and suffered another generalized seizure. This was controlled with 10 mg of intravenous diazepam. The patient then was noted to have snoring respirations and a decreased gag response. He was orally intubated and mechanical ventilation begun. Initial ventilator settings included a tidal volume of 900 mL, rate of 18, and F_{IO_2} of 50%. An arterial blood gas revealed a pH of 7.32, P_{O_2} of 275, and P_{CO_2} of 22. Gastric lavage was performed using a large-bore tube. Aspiration revealed normal stomach contents without evidence of pills or pill fragments. After the lavage was cleared, the patient was given 50 g of activated charcoal in sorbitol through the nasogastric tube and admitted to the ICU.

Initial evaluation in the ICU revealed repeat vital signs of 200/130, pulse 126, and a temperature of 39.4°C (103°F). A cooling blanket was placed and a rectal probe inserted for constant monitoring of the patient's temperature. He was less agitated and had a withdrawal response to noxious stimuli in each extremity. Laboratory evaluation revealed a serum bicarbonate of 16 meq/L, calcium of 4.3 mg/dL, BUN of 32, and creatine of 1.8. The anion gap was 21. Urinalysis was positive on dip stick for blood, and a serum CPK was 232,000.

The patient was given labetalol by intermittent infusion and topical nitropaste, with good blood pressure control. Blood and urine cultures were obtained. Because of persistent mental obtundation, a head CT scan and lumbar puncture were performed (both normal). Mannitol was given and an alkaline diuresis induced because of massive rhabdomyolysis. Serum lactate level was 7 m*M*/L. The patient had no further dysrhythmias nor seizure activity, slowly regained consciousness over the subsequent 12 h, and was successfully extubated the next morning.

The ECG changes persisted, but acute myocardial infarction was ruled out by isoenzymes. Toxic screens were positive only for cocaine metabolites in the urine. Despite aggressive measures to treat rhabdomyolysis, the patient developed severe acute tubular necrosis (ATN) and required hemodialysis for 1 week. He was transferred from the ICU to the medical floor on the fourth hospital day and had a good recovery thereafter.

CASE DISCUSSION

Any patient with an acute change of mental status should prompt an initial focus on the airway, breathing, and circulation (ABCs) and be given dextrose and naloxone. The absence of a response to these measures, coupled with the patient's clinical presentation, raised the possibility of stimulant-related toxicity. The presence of miosis (rather than mydriasis) and the lack of nystagmus suggested intoxication with cocaine or amphetamine rather than PCP. Intracranial infection and focal cerebral lesions were thought unlikely but were appropriately excluded by further testing. It was important to obtain early control of the patient's agitation and seizures in order to avoid further complications. More early and aggressive use of benzodiazepines would have been appropriate rather than waiting for recurrent seizures.

Appropriate screening tests were performed to rule out coingestants and to detect rhabdomyolysis. Persistent ECG changes consistent with ischemia can sometimes be seen in chronic cocaine abusers; indeed, this patient was not found to have evidence of an acute myocardial infarction. Despite therapy directed at rhabdomyolysis, acute renal failure was not avoided. This patient's toxicity was typical for cocaine in that the seizures, severe hypertension, and acute tubular necrosis were transient and responded well to supportive measures.

References

1. Cregler LL, Mark H: Medical complications of cocaine abuse. N Engl J Med 317:1495, 1986.
2. Van Dyke C, Byck R: Cocaine. Sci Am 246:128, 1982.
3. Crack. Med Letter 28:8369, 1986.
4. Cregler LL, Mark H: Cardiovascular dangers of cocaine abuse. Am J Cardiol 57:1185, 1986.
5. Pasternack PF, Colvin SE, Baumann FG: Cocaine induced angina pectoris and myocardial infarction in patients younger than 40 years. Am J Cardiol 55:847, 1985.
6. Lange RA, Cigarroa RG, Yancy CW, et al: Cocaine-induced coronary artery vasoconstriction. N Engl J Med 321:1557, 1989.
7. Isner JM, Estes M, Thompson PD, et al: Acute cardiac events temporarily related to cocaine abuse. N Engl J Med 315:1438, 1986.
8. Barth CW, Bray M, Roberts WC: Rupture of the ascending aorta during cocaine intoxication. Am J Cardiol 57:496, 1986.
9. Chokshi SK, Moore R, Pondion NG, et al: Reversible cardiomyopathy associated with cocaine intoxication. Ann Intern Med 111:1039, 1989.
10. Seaman ME: Acute cocaine abuse associated with cerebral infarction. Ann Emerg Med 19:34, 1990.
11. Lichtenfeld PJ, Rubin DB, Feldman RS: Subarachnoid hemorrhage precipitated by cocaine snorting. Arch Neurol 411:223, 1984.
12. Kay BR, Fainstate M: Cerebral vasculitis associated with cocaine abuse. JAMA 258:2104, 1987.
13. Myers JA, Barnett MF: Generalized seizures and cocaine abuse. Neurology 344:1675, 1984.
14. Post RM, Kopanda RT: Cocaine, kindling, and psychosis. Am J Psych 133:627, 1976.
15. Itkonen J, Schnoll S, Glassroth J: Pulmonary dysfunction in "freebase" cocaine users. Arch Int Med 144:2195, 1984.
16. Shesser R, Davis C, Edelsten S: Pneumomediastinum and pneumothorax after inhaling alkaloidal cocaine. Ann Emerg Med 10:213, 1981.
17. Patal RC, Dutta D, Schonfeld SA: Free-base cocaine use associated with bronchiolitis obliterans organizing pneumonia. Ann Intern Med 107:186, 1987.
18. Merigian KS, Roberts JR: Cocaine intoxication: Hyperyrexia, rhabdomyolysis, and acute renal failure. Clin Toxicol 25:135, 1987.
19. Woods JR, Plessinger MA, Clark KE: Effect of cocaine on uterine blood flow and fetal oxygenation. JAMA 257:957, 1987.
20. Perinol LE, Warren GE, Levine JS: Cocaine induced hepatoxicity in humans. Gastroenterology 93:176, 1987.
21. Bessen HA: Treatment of cocaine toxicity. Ann Emerg Med 16:1922, 1987.
22. Derlet RW, Albertson TE: Agents that protect against cocaine induced death and seizures. Ann Emerg Med 18:446, 1989.
23. Dusenberry SJ, Hicks MJ, Mariani PJ: Labetalol treatment of cocaine toxicity. Ann Emerg Med 16:235, 1987.
24. Ramoska E, Sacchetti AD: Propranol-induced hypertension in treatment of cocaine intoxication. Ann Emerg Med 14:1112, 1985.
25. Derlet RW, Albertson TE: Potentiation of cocaine toxicity with lidocaine. Ann Emerg Med 19:464, 1990.

Chapter 181

PLANT POISONING

JEFFREY BRENT
BARRY H. RUMACK

KEY POINTS

- *There are a large variety of plant poisons in nature.*
- *There are few specific antidotes.*
- *Acute gastroenteritis is a feature of most plant poisonings. Organic brain syndromes are common.*
- *Supportive care and decontamination (gastrointestinal tract and others) are the mainstays of treatment.*
- *Identification of the plant is important for anticipating clinical events.*
- *In plant-related cardiac glycoside toxicity, antidigoxin Fab fragments may be of use.*
- *Mucosal irritation, renal failure, and hypocalcemia characterize plant-related oxalate toxicity.*
- *Life-threatening mushroom poisonings tend to have a delay of at least 6 h prior to the onset of symptoms. After that, hepatic, renal, or central nervous system complications may develop, depending on the type of mushroom ingested.*

Plant poisonings are an extremely heterogenous group of toxic syndromes. They typically occur as a result of direct ingestion or the use of plant parts in the preparation of derivative foods, commonly teas. Potentially toxic plant exposures rarely cause major illness. Only a very small proportion of them, which will be the focus of this chapter, require intensive care.

General Considerations in Plant Toxicology

The study of plant toxicology is hindered by the paucity of acutely ill patients. Prospective clinical trials are unheard of, and good clinical series are rare. Furthermore, there are an immense number of potential toxins in the plant kingdom, undoubtedly, many of them yet uncharacterized. Many of the cases in the literature predate the advent of modern intensive care medicine and, therefore, were more prone to a poor outcome. In addition, many of the clinical features of these patients were uncharacterized. Even today many of the case reports suffer from imprecise identification of the offending species. When ingestion of a toxic plant material is suspected, this can rarely be verified by identification of the toxin or quantitative blood levels.

There are a variety of phenomena which can occur following ingestion of plants unrelated to botanical toxins. A benign plant may be ingested and yet cause illness, because of the simultaneous ingestion of pesticides on the plant. Additionally, some plants are prone to produce an allergic response which may, at times, be difficult to distinguish from other kinds of toxic reactions.

Although there are a huge number of botanical toxins in nature, those causing a well-characterized clinical syndrome do so in remarkably similar ways. Acute gastroenteritis is an almost universal feature of plant toxin poisonings. In most cases, this will be the only manifestation. The second most common manifestation of plant poisoning, often seen along with, or following, the gastroenteritis, is an organic brain syndrome. This tends to be seen in the more severe cases and is usually characterized by some alteration in mental status manifested by delirium, coma, or seizures.

The treatment of plant poisoning is expectant and supportive. In very few cases are there specific antidotes which may be utilized. The major reason for identifying the particular plant material ingested is to know what to anticipate and what specific treatments may be useful.

General Management of Acute Plant Intoxication

Patients who have ingested poisonous plants should be treated by the steps given in Table 181-1. Initially, appropriate resuscitation should be performed and naloxone and glucose given as needed. Gastric lavage, with a large bore tube, should be performed if the patient presents immediately postingestion.

All patients who have ingested potentially poisonous plant material should receive activated charcoal, repeated approximately every 4 h until charcoal-laden stools are passed. Since most botanical toxins produce acute gastroenteritis, with diarrhea often a prominent component, it is wise to avoid using cathartics in conjunction with the charcoal therapy.

Attempts should be made to identify the plant. This may be done directly or by retrieving plant parts in gastric material. Regional poison control centers may be utilized in an attempt to locate local experts who can identify plants. Horticulturists, including hospital gardeners, can also be of help. Although supportive care is the mainstay of the treatment of plant intoxication, occasionally specific antidotes are available. Regional poison centers may provide advice regarding the specific management of the patient.

TABLE 181-1 General Principles of the Management of Plant Poisoning

1. Stabilize airway, breathing, and circulation as needed
2. Administer naloxone and dextrose for altered mentation
3. Gastrointestinal tract decontamination
   a. Lavage if early
   b. Activated charcoal
4. Identification of plant
5. Consultation with regional poison control center
6. Specific antidotes if available

TABLE 181-2 Plants Commonly Causing Specific Toxidromes

Anticholinergic Syndrome	
Deadly nightshade (*Atropa belladonna*)	
Angel's trumpet (*Datura suaveolens*)	
Jimson weed (*D. stramonium*)	
Matrimony vine (*Lycium halimifolium*)	
Henbane (*Hyoscyamus niger*)	
Cardiac Glycoside Syndrome	
Christmas rose (*Helleborus niger*)	
Lily of the Valley (*Convallaria majalis*)	
Foxglove (*Digitalis purpurea*)	
Common oleander (*Nerium oleander*)	
Yellow oleander (*Thevetia* sp.)	
Pyrrolizidine Alkaloid Syndrome	
Threadleaf (*Senecio longilobus*)	
Heliotrope (*Heliotropium europaeum*)	
Russian comfrey (*Symphytum xuplandicum*)	
Horsefoot (*Tussilage farfara*)	
Oxalate Syndrome	
Dumbcane (*Dieffenbachia* sp.)	
Elephant's ear (*Colocasia antiquorum*)	
Rhubarb (*Rheum* sp.)	
Jack-in-the-pulpit (*Arisaema atrorubens*)	
Skunk cabbage (*Symplocarpus foetidus*)	
Swiss cheese plant (*Monstera* sp.)	
Philodendron (*Philodendron* sp.)	
Caladium (*Caladium bicolor*)	
Solanine Alkaloid Syndrome	
Jerusalem cherry (*Solanum pseudo-capsicum*)	
Common potato (*S. tuberosum*)	
Eggplant (*S. melongena*)	
Woody nightshade (*S. dulcamara*)	
Horse nettle (*S. carolinense*)	
Common nightshade (*S. nigrum*)	
Tomato (*Lycopersicon esculentum*)	
Trumpet flower (*Solandra* sp.)	
Nicotine Syndrome	
Tobacco (*Nicotiana* sp.)	
Poison hemlock (*Conium maculatum*)	
Indian tobacco (*Lobelia inflata*)	
Cyanogenic Glycosides Syndrome	
Common fruit pits (Rosaceae family)	
Cherry laurel (*Prunus laurocerasus*)	
Cassava (*Manihot esculenta*)	
Bamboo (*Phylostachys aurea*)	
Elderberry (*Sambcucus* sp.)	
Bitter almonds (*Prunus dulcis*)	
Hydrangea (Saxifragaceae family)	
Lima beans (*Phaseolus lunatus*)	
Chokecherry (*Prunus virginiana*)	
Toxalbumin Syndrome	
Castor bean (*Ricinus communis*)	
Jequirity bean (*Abrus precatorius*)	
Sandbox tree (*Hura crepitans*)	
Bellyache bush (*Jatropha gossipifolia*)	
Black locust (*Robinia pseudoacacia*)	
Desert potato (*J. macrorhiza*)	
Colchicine Syndrome	
Autumn crocus (*Colchicum autuminate*)	
Glory lily (*Gloriosa superba*)	

TABLE 181-2 Plants Commonly Causing Specific Toxidromes (Continued)

Acute Gastroenteritis	
Holly berries (*Illex* sp.)	
Pokeweed (*Phytolaccia americana*)	
English ivy (*Hedera helix*)	
Aloe vera	
Multiple bulbs	

Specific Plant Syndromes

ANTICHOLINERGIC SYNDROME

Plants containing the tropane alkaloids, commonly atropine and scopolamine, are capable of giving rise to an anticholinergic syndrome (ACS). Plants containing these alkaloids are listed in Table 181-2. Among the most common plant causes of an ACS are *Datura stramonium* (jimson weed) and *Atropa belladonna* (deadly nightshade). The most frequent cause of intoxication by these plants is from teas. Anticholinergic plant poisoning is occasionally induced purposefully in an attempt to capture the hallucinogenic anticholinergic effects.

The toxicity of these alkaloids derives from their activity as a competitive antagonist at the cholinergic-muscarinic receptor. They cross the blood-brain barrier and thus cause central as well as peripheral effects. The clinical picture of an ACS is often described as "mad as a hatter, hot as a hare, dry as a bone, red as a beet, and blind as a bat." Another prominent clinical feature of the syndrome is tachycardia. Although this is usually sinus, a variety of supraventricular as well as ventricular dysrhythmias may occur. A striking feature of the ACS is the profound alteration in mentation including confusion, agitation, disorientation, hallucinations, and seizures. Physical examination will usually reveal mydriasis, absence of perspiration, and relatively parched mucous membranes on physical examination. Because of peripheral cutaneous dilation, these patients may appear flushed. Fever is common.

Patients with an ACS should be observed for cardiac dysrhythmias, hemodynamic instability, agitation, and seizures. Significant agitation is best treated with benzodiazepines, since neuroleptic agents have anticholinergic properties of their own.

Physostigmine is a potential antagonist for an ACS. The cholinergic stimulation associated with physostigmine may result in bradydysrhythmias, asystole, or seizures. Its use should be restricted to either patients with life-threatening ACS unresponsive to conservative therapies, or diagnostic dilemmas. The usual dose of physostigmine is 2 mg (0.5 mg for pediatric patients) intravenously over at least 2 min. A syringe containing atropine should be kept at the bedside in case bradydysrhythmias occur. Contraindications to physostigmine are asthma, peripheral vascular disease, bowel obstruction, urinary tract obstruction, or gangrene.

CARDIAC GLYCOSIDES

Plants from a large diversity of genera contain cardiac glycosides (Table 181-2). The specific chemical identity of these compounds may vary, depending on the nature of either of their two components: the steroid moiety (aglycone or genin) and the sugar.

The presentation of plant cardiac glycoside poisoning is similar to that described for medicinal glycosides. There is an initial period of gastrointestinal discomfort followed by multiple cardiac conduction abnormalities and hyperkalemia. The major source of variability of the clinical syndromes relates to the diversity of these glycosides found in nature. For example, the foxglove plant (*Digitalis purpurea*) contains predominantly digitoxin, which has a long half-life and causes a prolonged clinical syndrome. Alternatively, the European snapdragon (*Digitalis lanata*) contains mostly digoxin and causes a more abbreviated syndrome.

Because these glycosides have a variable degree of cross-reactivity, digoxin levels cannot be used as an absolute indication of body burden. Cardiac glycosides are known to bind to activated charcoal. Digitoxin is one of the few molecules for which a true enterohepatic circulation has been demonstrated, and therefore multiple doses of activated charcoal should be administered. Scrupulous management should be directed to potassium homeostasis.

There is some controversy about the efficacy of antidigoxin Fab fragments in the treatment of plant cardiac glycoside poisoning. There have been cases where this strategy has been used with apparent success.[1] Because of the cross-reactivity of antidigoxin antibodies with other cardiac glycosides, it may be theorized that Fab fragments would be efficacious. However, the exact amount of this material to be administered cannot be precisely calculated. In the case of plant glycosides, it is necessary to simply treat to the clinical endpoint of stability.

PYRROLIZIDINE ALKALOIDS

Pyrrolizidine alkaloid poisoning was first recognized in 1954 in Jamaica following which there have been multiple reports of hepatic veno-occlusive disease related to drinking herbal teas or eating contaminated cereals. These compounds represent a diverse but related group of substances. Common examples of plants containing these alkaloids are given in Table 181-2.

Consumption of these alkaloids causes endothelial edema of small and medium size hepatic veins and venules. This may result in sclerosis and occlusion. The congestion of hepatic sinusoids and central veins results in centrilobular hemorrhagic necrosis. The large hepatic veins are unaffected, distinguishing pyrrolizidine alkaloid hepatic veno-occlusive disease from the Budd-Chiari syndrome.

The presentation of pyrrolizidine alkaloid poisoning is typically one of right upper abdominal quadrant pain, nausea, vomiting, diarrhea, hepatomegaly, splenomegaly, ascites, jaundice, hypoglycemia, and extremely high elevations of hepatic transaminases. Because the syndrome occurs frequently in infants and children there may be some confusion between pyrrolizidine alkaloid poisoning and Reye's syndrome. Chronic ingestion, such as described in people consuming herbal teas, causes a progressive picture of hepatic veno-occlusive disease and cor pulmonale.

There is no specific antidote to pyrrolizidine alkaloid-induced disease. Treatment is supportive and directed to the management of coagulopathy, hypoglycemia, pulmonary hypertension, and encephalopathy. It is not known whether liver transplantation is beneficial.[2]

OXALATE SYNDROME

A diverse group of plants, including common house plants, contain oxalate (Table 181-2). Although the syndrome caused by oxalate ingestion is primarily one of mucosal irritation, severe systemic toxicity may occur. The plant that most commonly causes an oxalate syndrome is the *Dieffenbachia*. There have also been a number of cases of oxalate poisoning from the chronic ingestion of rhubarb leaves.

Oxalates can be found in the plant kingdom in either soluble or insoluble forms. Insoluble calcium oxalate crystals, known as rhaphides, are found in the *Dieffenbachia* and *Caladium* plants. Rhaphides tend to exist in the form of extremely sharp and irritating spicules. The major syndrome associated with calcium oxalate rhaphide-containing plants is severe mucosal irritation. This can be very dramatic, with significant oropharyngeal edema which may progress to airway compromise. Significant salivation may be associated with this.

Other plants contain oxalates in the form of soluble salts. Although not quite as irritating as rhaphides, these salts are more prone to systemic absorption and diffuse effects.

The systemic syndrome associated with oxalates is characterized by mucosal irritation, gastroenteritis, renal failure, and hypocalcemia. If the oxalates are ingested in the more soluble forms, such as occurs following rhubarb leaf ingestion, the initial oral irritant effects may be extremely subtle and symptoms may be delayed for 6 to 24 h. With significant acute soluble oxalate ingestion there will be symptoms of gastroenteritis including abdominal pain, hematemesis, and bloody diarrhea. Circulating oxalate combines with calcium to form insoluble calcium oxalate, resulting in hypocalcemia manifested by paresthesias, tetany, hyperreflexia, muscle twitches, seizures, and a prolonged Q-T interval. Oxalate is cleared by the kidney in the form of nephrotoxic crystals. Following chronic low levels of oxalate ingestion, such as occurs with dietary rhubarb leaf, renal failure may be the initial manifestation.

The initial management should be directed toward the airway in view of the potential for oropharyngeal edema. If there has been significant ingestion of oxalate, oral fluids, preferably milk, should be administered in an attempt at dilution. An electrocardiogram (ECG) and serum calcium should be obtained. Acute hemodynamic deterioration may be associated with either hypovolemia, gastrointestinal tract bleeding, or severe hypocalcemia. A microscopic urinalysis should always be performed looking for oxalates. With either presumed oxalate intoxication or the demonstration of oxalate crystals in the urine, intravenous fluids should be administered to maintain brisk urine output, and renal function should be followed.[3]

SOLANINE ALKALOIDS

Plants of the Solanaceae family (the nightshade or potato plants) contain parts that are toxic by virtue of the alkaloid solanine and closely related compounds (see Table 181-2). The great majority of these plants contain the solanine alkaloids in nontoxic amounts and in only certain, traditionally nonedible, parts of the plant.

These alkaloids contain a steroid-like aglycone covalently bonded to a sugar. Although the clinical syndromes caused by these plants are generally related to solanine, another closely related alkaloid with apparently a relatively unique syndrome is the cardioinhibitory solanocapsine.

Cases of severe solanine alkaloid poisoning are rare. Most cases derive from ingestion of either poisonous parts of the common potato plant or potatoes that, because of either improper handling or harvesting, contain an inordinate amount of solanine. This can occur when potatoes are harvested while still green, are improperly stored, or are traumatized.

Solanine alkaloids are poorly absorbed through the gastrointestinal tract, although their ingestion does cause mucous membrane irritation and a gastroenteritis picture, which may be severe. Gastric acid hydrolyzes solanine alkaloids to the component sugar and aglycone. The aglycones may be responsible for hypotension, an organic brain syndrome, headaches, and seizures. If the alkaloid solanocapsine is ingested, the predominant effect may be decreased cardiac output, severe hypotension, and bradydysrhythmias. Many of the solanine alkaloid–containing plants also contain atropine which may be responsible for a superimposed ACS. Symptoms of solanine alkaloid poisoning may be delayed for up to 24 h. Fever and a burning sensation of the mouth and oropharynx are frequently the initial sign and symptom of solanine alkaloid poisoning. In general the syndrome is limited because of the bitter taste of these alkaloids which tends to discourage significant ingestion.

Patients presenting with solanine alkaloid toxicity should be treated with supportive measures and gastrointestinal tract decontamination with activated charcoal. Among the problems that should be anticipated are an organic brain syndrome, seizures, hemodynamic instability from either gastrointestinal tract bleeding or inhibition of myocardial function, and an ACS.[4]

NICOTINE ALKALOID–CONTAINING PLANTS

The nicotine alkaloids are extremely potent. They are found in such common plants as the tobacco plant and poison hemlock (see Table 181-2). Nicotine alkaloids have resulted in poisoning when used as purgatives and enemas. Poison hemlock root has been confused with wild carrots and eaten. The leaves of the poison hemlock are likewise toxic and similar in appearance to parsley.

The pathophysiology of nicotine alkaloid poisoning is extremely complex. These alkaloids are readily absorbed through all mucous membranes as well as through the skin. Following ingestion, there tends to be rapid emesis through both a direct effect and stimulation of the medullary chemoreceptor trigger zone. The alkaloids are stimulatory to postsynaptic receptors between the pre- and postganglionic autonomic neurons, and motor end plates. They are also stimulating to the central nervous system. The stimulatory effect is somewhat counterbalanced by the potential prolonged depolarizing depression of postsynaptic receptors. Thus one may see, in any aspect of the nervous system, either stimulatory or depressive effects. Often there is initially stimulation followed by depression. These effects can be predominantly sympathomimetic or cholinergic. The patient can therefore present with either miosis, bradycardia and diaphoresis; or hypertension, tachycardia, and mydriasis. Death from nicotine alkaloid poisoning is often within an hour of ingestion.[5] This can occur after ingesting either the plants or the alkaloids in the form of cigarettes or nicotine-containing gum. The cause of death is usually depolarization blockade of the neuromuscular junction causing respiratory failure.

If there has been dermal exposure, for example to a nicotine alkaloid containing insecticide, thorough skin decontamination should occur. If there has been ingestion, activated charcoal should be given in a multidose fashion since there is some evidence that nicotine alkaloids are secreted into the stomach.[6] Respiratory status must be closely monitored. The treatment of clinically significant hemodynamic abnormalities should be with short-acting agents since there can be rapid transition between cholinergic and sympathomimetic states. Seizures should be anticipated.

CYANOGENIC PLANTS

Cyanide is one of the most potent and rapid acting poisons known. It is widely distributed in the plant world in the form of cyanogenic glycosides which are sugar compounds of cyanide. These glycosides may be hydrolyzed by either plant enzymes simultaneously ingested or endogenous enzymes to liberate hydrogen cyanide.

There are hundreds of varieties of plants from over 40 families that contain cyanogenic glycosides. Common examples are given in Table 181-2. The most common glycoside is amygdalin, which is found in a variety of pits including those of such common fruits as the plum, peach, apricot, bitter almond, cherry, pear, and apple. Amygdalin is the major glycoside in the product sold as Laetrile. Although amygdalin itself is nontoxic, these pits also contain a complex of enzymes known as emulsin in their coats. When the pits are chewed, emulsin is liberated and metabolizes the glycoside to free hydrogen cyanide.

Linamarin is another commonly occurring cyanogenic glycoside found in lima and cassava beans. Because the latter is a major dietary staple in tropical areas, particularly Nigeria, chronic cassava consumption has been associated with a form of chronic cyanide poisoning known as tropical or Nigerian ataxic neuropathy.[7]

The diagnosis of cyanide poisoning is based primarily on a high index of suspicion. If a patient presents with hypotension, seizures, an altered mental status, or a persistent metabolic acidosis in the setting of the potential ingestion of cyanogenic plants, this diagnosis should be strongly considered. The odor of bitter almonds is a further clue; however, this is of limited utility since it is not always present and cannot be detected by up to 40 percent of the population. Serious poisoning needs to be treated before cyanide levels are obtainable. If there is the suspicion of cyanide poisoning, the patient should be treated with activated charcoal and antidotes should be administered. At present in the United States the only approved antidote for cyanide poisoning is the Lilly cyanide antidote kit. Hydroxocobalamin is presently being evaluated in clinical trials in the United States. European data suggest that it is an effective antidote.[8] More details on the antidotes for cyanide poisoning can be obtained in Chap. 176.

TOXALBUMIN-CONTAINING PLANTS

Although a variety of plants (Table 181-2) contain a group of related toxins known as toxalbumins, virtually all the serious poisonings have been from the castor bean or jequirity bean. Most cases have resulted from accidental poisoning in children. Abrin, the active toxin in the jequirity bean, and ricin, which is found in the castor bean, are among the most potent natural toxins known when administered parenterally. Ingestion of these beans is usually not associated with toxicity because of the resistance of the intact bean to hydrolysis by gastrointestinal tract enzymes. However, if they are chewed, substantial toxicity may ensue. Most life-threatening cases have been from the ingestion of jequirity beans. In addition to the direct toxic effects that these proteins have on cells, they are also extremely antigenic and thus they cause a hypersensitivity reaction. Castor bean toxicity tends to be an acute, and sometimes quite severe, gastroenteritis. The jequirity bean also contains glycyrrhizin, which may cause hyperaldosteronism.

It is often stated that as little as one jequirity bean when chewed can be lethal to a child, although this is not well documented. However, there is little doubt that a single bean can cause severe gastroenteritis.[9] Toxalbumin ingestion has an acute caustic effect on the gastrointestinal tract. The resulting gastroenteritis can be persistent and severe. Occasional cases of toxalbumin poisoning cause a delayed syndrome of persistent gastroenteritis and encephalopathy characterized by stupor, seizures, and coma. Some cases have progressed to a multiple organ system failure picture with prominent pancreatitis, hepatotoxicity, hemolysis, and renal failure. In general the toxicity is more severe with abrin than with ricin. In addition, a primary irritant dermatitis has been described following dermal exposure to these substances. The management of patients with toxalbumin poisoning includes standard supportive care and activated charcoal. Severe hemorrhagic gastroenteritis should be anticipated. There are no specific antidotes.

COLCHICINE POISONING

Colchicine is an alkaloid present in members of the lily family (Table 181-2). In view of the large amount of plant that needs to be ingested, true botanical colchicine poisoning is quite unusual. The clinical syndrome engendered by colchicine poisoning involves an initial acute gastroenteritis, which may be severe and hemorrhagic. Other problems, which can be seen within days, are ascending motor paresis, bone marrow depression, rhabdomyolysis, renal failure, disseminated intravascular coagulation, and an adult respiratory distress syndrome, which is usually the cause of death. There may be an organic brain syndrome manifested by seizures and delirium. Atropine appears to be antidotal to the gastrointestinal effects of colchicine. Activated charcoal should be administered. Because many of these patients will develop an ileus, it may be impossible to administer multiple doses of charcoal. Rhabdomyolysis should be anticipated and attempts should be made to maintain brisk urine output. This may be challenging in view of the circulatory shock and possibility of renal failure from the direct nephrotoxic effects of the colchicine. Central venous or Swan-Ganz monitoring may be required.[10]

MISTLETOE TOXICITY

Mistletoe contains a variety of potentially toxic substances including β-phenylethylamine, tyramine, lectin, cardiotoxins, and mucosily irritating alkaloids. Cases of mistletoe toxicity have been reported following ingestion of the whole plant, mistletoe extract used as an abortifacient, and the berries. Severe toxicity is rare. Most cases are restricted to a gastroenteritis-like syndrome. It can also cause a toxic organic brain syndrome with hallucinations, delusions, seizures, and coma. Although the literature refers to cardiovascular collapse, bradydysrhythmia, and high grade of heart block, true cases are difficult to document. The treatment of mistletoe poisoning involves supportive care and activated charcoal.[11]

PODOPHYLLUM POISONING

Podophyllum is a resin consisting of multiple substances derived from the mandrake or mayapple plant. The major constituent is podophyllotoxin. Podophyllum poisoning occurs most commonly in the setting of either overzealous dermal application of medicinal solutions, ingestion of the topical compound, or overuse of podophyllum resin cathartics. Podophyllum plant poisoning is rare. The picture of podophyllum poisoning is one of multiple organ system involvement, causing significant gastroenteritis of which diarrhea is the most common feature, fever, an organic brain syndrome, and hypotension. There may also be delayed bone marrow depression and diffuse peripheral neuropathy of both efferent and afferent nerves. Treatment of podophyllum poisoning should involve scrupulous dermal decontamination if exposure has been topical, as well as gastrointestinal tract decontamination with activated charcoal. Patients presenting early following podophyllum ingestion should be observed since symptoms have been reported to occur as late as 13 h postingestion.[12] There is no specific antidote.

PENNYROYAL OIL

Pennyroyal oil is a volatile, or essential, oil derived from several herbs. It is widely used by herbalists as an abortifacient. Hepatotoxicity, renal failure, diffuse intravascular coagulation, seizures, and multiple organ system failure have been reported following pennyroyal oil ingestion.[13] Because pennyroyal oil–induced hepatic necrosis is associated with glutathione depletion, *N*-acetylcysteine (NAC) has been proposed as a treatment. Animal studies support this approach. There are a variety of therapeutic protocols in the use of NAC for acetaminophen poisoning. These are known to be safe and may thus be used in pennyroyal oil poisoning. They are reviewed in Chap. 178.

EUCALYPTUS OIL

Eucalyptus oil is another essential oil, the predominant component of which is eucalyptol. It is rapidly absorbed and causes gastrointestinal distress followed by seizures, pulmonary edema, and an organic brain syndrome. The seizures may occur up to 4 h postingestion. Treatment of ingestion involves activated charcoal, and expectant management of gastroenteritis, seizures, and adult respiratory distress syndrome.[14]

HALLUCINOGENIC PLANTS

There are multiple hallucinogenic plants known. However, the only ones known to cause significant enough toxicity to warrant intensive care management are those containing indolealkylamine derivatives, which are thus related to lysergic acid diethylamide (LSD). Plant materials containing these substances include the peyote cactus and morning-glory seeds. These cause a clinical picture similar to LSD intoxication; however, they are much less potent. The peyote cactus contains a variety of alkaloids of which mescaline is the most active. It is usually ingested in the form of dried cactus caps known as buttons, although a variety of other forms are available for either injection or ingestion. Ingestion of either peyote or a large number of morning-glory seeds causes an initial gastroenteritis and sympathomimetic syndrome followed by an organic brain syndrome characterized by visual hallucinations. In massive doses, these alkaloids have been known to cause respiratory depression. Severe emotional reactions including suicidal ideation and severe paranoia have been observed.[15]

Nutmeg, which is an extract of the fruit of the nutmeg tree, similarly can cause a clinical syndrome of hallucinations, gastroenteritis, tachycardia, flushing, agitation, and dry mouth. Hallucinations associated with ingestion of large amounts of nutmeg are primarily visual, similar to other hallucinogenic plant materials.

Treatment of hallucinogenic plant intoxication is supportive. Sedating medications may be needed. There is considerable discussion in the literature suggesting that neuroleptic tranquilizers such as haloperidol be avoided in view of the potential exacerbating effect of the anticholinergic properties of these agents. This, however, has not been observed clinically.

AKEE FRUIT POISONING

The unripened fruit of the akee tree (*Blighia sapida*) contains hepatotoxic compounds known as hypoglycins that are responsible for the Jamaican vomiting sickness, which bears a resemblance to Reye's syndrome. The clinical picture, which has been reported to have a high mortality in serious cases, involves severe hypoglycemia, organic brain syndrome characterized by seizures and central nervous system depression, acute fatty liver, and metabolic acidosis. There may be initial nausea and vomiting. The treatment involves standard supportive measures and activated charcoal. Patients should be observed for hypoglycemia, volume depletion, hepatic or renal failure, and seizures. Although the metabolic acidosis may be severe, there is no data addressing whether bicarbonate therapy is beneficial in this setting.[16]

TAXINE (YEW) POISONING

The genus *Taxus* comprises a variety of ornamental evergreen shrubs known as yews. These contain several alkaloids known as taxines. Significant human poisonings are rare. Those cases that do occur are usually restricted to a minor gastroenteritis. However, there have been cases reported of fatal yew intoxication. Several of these involved children who masticated yew seeds. The taxines produce both a negative inotropic and chronotropic effect on the heart; however, fatal cases have been reported to progress to fatal ventricular dysrhythmias. An organic brain syndrome with seizures has also been reported.[17] There is no specific antidote. Patients who become ill usually do so in 2 to 4 h. Patients presenting prior to that time period should be treated with observation, and gastrointestinal tract decontamination.

FAVA BEAN POISONING

The fava bean comes from the plant *Vicia fava*. Most people can ingest these beans without difficulty. However, individuals who are glucose-6-phosphate dehydrogenase deficient may develop a syndrome known as favism following either ingestion of the bean or inhalation of the pollen. This is characterized by initial gastrointestinal discomfort followed by the sudden onset of hemolytic anemia, which may progress to hemoglobinuria, jaundice, hepatosplenomegaly, and vascular collapse. In severe cases, the syndrome may take weeks to resolve. A hypersensitivity component has also been postulated as playing a role in favism.

The treatment involves hemodynamic support and monitoring for hemoglobinuria.[18]

WATER HEMLOCK POISONING

Water hemlock (*Cicuta* sp.) is an extremely toxic member of the carrot family. The plant grows in wet, swampy areas and contains the very potent cicutoxin. Poisonings have occurred by a variety of reasons including confusion with wild parsnips, carrots, and ginseng. The clinical syndrome induced by the cicutoxin is a muscarinic-cholinergic one, similar to that caused by organophosphate pesticides, followed by status epilepticus and, frequently, hypotension. A review of reported cases in this century reveals an overall mortality of 30 percent.[19] Severe rhabdomyolysis may occur. There is no specific antidote. Anticholinergic agents such as atropine do not appear to be helpful.[20]

RHODODENDRON POISONING

Rhododendrons, which include the azaleas, contain a variety of polyalcoholic diterpene resinoids. Rhododendron poisoning is extremely rare. Cases have been reported from the ingestion of honey, derived from bees using the nectar of these plants, and the ingestion of flowers or other parts of the plant. Symptoms usually begin within several hours of ingestion and include local irritation of oropharyngeal mucous membranes followed by acute gastroenteritis. Hypotension and bradycardia have been reported following significant ingestions. In addition, salivation, rhinorrhea, weakness, and an organic brain syndrome with coma and seizures may occur. Management of rhododendron poisoning should consist of administration of activated charcoal and general supportive care. There is controversy in the literature as to whether atropine is effective for the bradydysrhythmias associated with these toxins. Studies with experimental animals administered pure toxin have not shown a response to atropine. However, a clinical case report suggests atropine may have been of benefit in one case.[21] Hyperkalemia may occur.

DAPHNE POISONING

The shrub daphne contains a glycoside known as daphnin, as well as a resin which causes severe vesiculation. True cases of daphnin poisoning are very difficult to document in the modern literature. The older literature suggests that ingestion of any part of the shrub can result in intense burning and a vesiculation reaction, followed by severe gastroenteritis with hematochezia; an organic brain syndrome characterized by weakness, stupor, and coma; and renal failure with associated hematuria.[22]

GASTROENTERITIS SYNDROMES

Although abdominal pain, nausea, vomiting, and diarrhea are extremely common features of a great number of plant poisonings, there are some plants which commonly induce this syndrome as a primary manifestation of their toxicity. Common examples of this group of poisonous plants are given in Table 181-2. These plants contain a variety of gastrointestinal tract irritants. The ingestion of the gastroenteritis-producing plants should be treated with activated charcoal and appropriate fluid management.

MUSHROOM POISONING

Mushroom-induced toxic syndromes can be separated into eight groups as shown in Table 181-3. The principle of general management for plant poisonings outlined in Table 181-1 applies to mushrooms as well. The three life-threatening mushroom syndromes are those caused by the cyclopeptides, monomethylhydrazine, orelline, and orellanine. As seen in Table 181-3, each of these potentially extremely serious syndromes shares the characteristic of a delay of at least 6 h prior to the onset of symptoms. Cyclopeptide poisoning is generally caused by deadly amanitas. Specific management of poisoning by these mushrooms consists of prolonged multiple-dose activated charcoal therapy. There are some data which show that high-dose penicillin G therapy may be hepatoprotective. Fulminant amatoxin-induced hepatic failure has been treated with transplantation. Monomethylhydrazine poisoning is generally due to the inadvertent ingestion of false morel *Gyromitra esculenta*. Specific management of poisoning by this mushroom consists of the administration of methylene blue for clinically significant methemoglobinemia and the treatment of seizures with pyridoxine. A complete discussion of the clinical features and management of mushroom poisoning can be found in recent publications.[23]

CASE PRESENTATION

A 12-year-old male was noted to ingest some carrotlike plant material. Within approximately 30 min of the ingestion, he developed emesis and a staggering gait followed shortly by status epilepticus. He was brought to the hospital where he was intubated and intravenous lines were established. He was treated with naloxone, glucose, and diazepam. His seizures abated with multiple doses of diazepam and a loading dose of phenobarbital. He was lavaged with a large bore orogastric tube, and activated charcoal was instilled following the gastric emptying. His initial blood gas revealed a pH of 6.91; however, this quickly resolved with seizure control. He was continued on barbiturates and had no further seizures. The plant material was identified by a horticulturist as water hemlock.

The patient required 2 days of mechanical ventilation and becoming intermittently agitated, required sedation and muscle relaxation with pancuronium. Neurologic evaluation, done frequently between doses of these medications, revealed agitation but no further seizure activity. He developed significant rhabdomyolysis, but brisk urine output was maintained and he had no subsequent

TABLE 181-3 Summary of Common Mushroom-associated Syndromes

Syndrome	Clinical Course	Toxins	Typical Causative Mushrooms
Delayed gastroenteritis followed by hepatorenal syndrome	Stage I. 6–24 h after ingestion: onset of nausea, vomiting, profuse cholera-like diarrhea, abdominal pain, hematuria Stage II. 12–48 h after ingestion: apparent recovery. Hepatic enzymes are rising during this stage. Stage III. 24–72 h after ingestion: progressive hepatic and renal failure, coagulopathy, cardiomyopathy, encephalopathy, convulsions, coma, death	Cyclopeptides principally amatoxin	"Deadly amanitas" *Galerina* sp.
Anticholinergic syndrome	30 min to 2 h postingestion: delirium and hallucinations typically associated with anticholinergic findings.	Muscinol Ibotenic acid	*Amanita muscaria* *Amanita pantherina*
Delayed gastroenteritis with central nervous system abnormalities	6–24 h postingestion: nausea, vomiting, diarrhea, abdominal pain, muscle cramps, delirium, convulsions, coma. Hemolysis and methemoglobinemia may occur.	Monomethylhydrazine	*Gyromitra esculenta* ("false morel")
Cholinergic syndrome	30 min to 2 h postingestion: bradycardia, bronchorrhea, bronchospasm, salivation, perspiration, lacrimation, convulsions, coma	Muscarine	*Boletus* sp. *Clitocybe* sp. *Inocybe* sp. *Amanita* sp.
Disulfiram-like reaction with ethanol	30 min after drinking ethanol (may occur up to a week after eating coprine-containing mushrooms): flushing of skin of face and trunk, hypotension, tachycardia, chest pain, dyspnea, nausea, vomiting, extreme apprehension	Coprine	*Coprinus atramentarius*
Hallucinations	30 min to 3 h after ingestion: hallucinations, euphoria, drowsiness, compulsive behavior, agitation	Indoles Psilocybin Psilocin	*Psilocybe* sp.
Delayed gastritis and renal failure	Abdominal pain, anorexia, vomiting starting over 30 h postingestion followed by progressive renal failure 3–14 days later	Orelline Orellanine	*Cortinarius* sp.
General gastrointestinal tract irritants	30 min to 2 h after ingestion: nausea, vomiting, abdominal cramping, diarrhea. May recover without treatment	Unidentified, probably multiple	*Chlorophyllium molybidites* Backyard mushrooms ("little brown mushrooms") and many others

SOURCE: From reference 23 with permission.

deficit in renal function. He was extubated 2 days postingestion and had no central nervous system sequelae.

CASE DISCUSSION

This is a fairly typical case of cicutoxin poisoning following water hemlock ingestion. The steps described in Table 181-1 were expeditiously followed. Seizures were controlled by standard supportive measures, as was rhabdomyolysis. Like most serious plant poisonings, there was no specific antidote and the management was primarily gastrointestinal tract decontamination and supportive care. Identification of the plant was helpful in that it verified the cause of the clinical syndrome observed.

References

1. Shumaik GM, Wu AW, Ping AC: Oleander poisoning: Treatment with digoxin-specific Fab antibody fragments. Ann Emerg Med 17:732, 1988.
2. Kumana CR, Ng M, Lin HG, et al.: Hepatic veno-occlusive disease due to toxic alkaloids in herbal tea. Lancet 2:1360, 1983.
3. Drach G, Maloney WA: Toxicity of the common houseplant Dieffenbachia: Report of a case. JAMA 184:1047, 1963
4. McMillan M, Thompson JC: An outbreak of suspected solanine poisoning in school boys: An examination of criteria of solanine poisoning. Q J Med 190:227, 1979.
5. Battersby E, Cable J: Nicotine poisoning. N Z Med J 63:367, 1964.
6. McGuigan MA: Nicotine. Clin Toxicol Rev 4:1, 1982.

7. Freeman A: Chronic cyanide intoxication. Br Med J 282:1321, 1981.
8. Hall AH, Rumack BH: Hydroxocobalamin/sodium thiosulfate as cyanide antidote. J Emerg Med 5:115, 1987.
9. Hart M: Jequirity-bean poisoning. N Engl J Med 268:885, 1963.
10. Naidus RM, Roduien R, Mielke H: Colchicine toxicity. A multisystem disease. Arch Intern Med 137:394, 1977.
11. Hall AH, Spoerke DG, Rumack BH: Assessing mistletoe toxicity. Ann Emerg Med 15:1320, 1986.
12. Cassidy DE, Drewry J, Fanning JP: Podophyllum toxicity: A report of a fatal case and a review of the literature. J Toxicol Clin Toxicol 19:35, 1982.
13. Sullivan JB, Rumack BH, Thomas H, et al.: Pennyroyal oil poisoning and hepatotoxicity. JAMA 242:2873, 1979.
14. Courtemanche NJ, Li M, Peterson RG: Coma following acute ingestion of eucalyptus oil in a child. Vet Hum Toxicol 25:46 (suppl), 1983.
15. LaBarre W: Peyote and mescaline. J Psychedelic Drugs 11:33, 1979.
16. Tanaka K, Kean EA, Johnson B: Jamaican vomiting sickness: Biochemical investigation of two cases. N Engl J Med 295:461, 1976.
17. Thompson J: Poisoning by yew berry. Lancet 95:530, 1868.
18. Kattamis CA, et al: Favism, Clinical and biochemical data. J Med Genet 6:34, 1969.
19. Starreveld E, Hope CE: Cicutoxin poisoning (water hemlock). Neurology 25:730, 1975.
20. Nelson RB, North DS, Kaneriya M, et al.: The influence of biperiden, benztropine, physostigmine and diazepam on the convulsive effects of Cicuta douglasii. Proc West Pharmacol Soc 21:137, 1978.
21. Klein-Schwartz W, Litovitz T: Azalea toxicity. An overrated problem. Clin Toxicol 23:91, 1985.
22. Spoerke DG: Plants—Euphorbiace, in Rumack BH (ed): *Poisindex,* Denver, *Micromedex,* 1990.
23. Brent J, Rumack BH: Mushroom poisoning, in Haddad LM, Winchester JF (eds): *Clinical Management of Poisoning and Drug Overdoses, 2d ed.* Philadelphia, Saunders, 1990.

Chapter 182
ANIMAL POISONING

RICHARD C. DART
FINDLAY E. RUSSELL

KEY POINTS

- *Venoms are produced by various animals for purposes of prey capture and digestion, defense, and, perhaps, other activities.*
- *Venoms are complex substances, sometimes mixtures of proteins, lipids, mucopolysaccharides, etc., and usually have multiple sites of action. It is the toxicity of the* whole *mixture that causes the clinical presentation of poisoning in the patient.*
- *Venom poisoning is a dynamic process. Management of the patient may require immediate changes in therapeutics as new problems develop. Thus, continuous observation of the patient is fundamental.*
- *The administration of antivenin is necessary in many patients managed in the ICU. Close observation and the ability to treat immediate anaphylaxis are essential.*

There has been an increasing tendency to treat certain venomous animal injuries in the ICU following their preliminary evaluation and treatment in the emergency department. This has been particularly true for snake envenomations and for poisonings precipitated by the eating of tetraodonic and ciguateric fishes. Indeed, when an antivenin is needed, many medical facilities in the United States now administer the drug in the ICU. This reflects the progress in general medical care and the availability of specialized equipment and drugs in the ICU for treating complex entities such as venom poisoning.

The emergency department, however, remains the link in the care of the poisoned patient. The emergency physician is specifically trained in the recognition and emergent management of venom poisonings and anaphylactic reactions. It must be remembered that venom poisoning is a medical emergency requiring immediate attention and considerable judgment. It is particularly important to remember that no two cases of poisoning will be the same; a venom is a complex group of toxins, even within a single species. The problem of determining the severity of envenomation is difficult, and the importance of autopharmacologic reaction differences in patients makes venom poisoning a particularly difficult therapeutic problem. With these concepts in mind, this chapter focuses on the management of patients in critical care facilities, particularly those suffering from venom or fish poisonings encountered in the United States. When urgent information is required, the physician should contact a Regional Poison Control Center or the Arizona Poison and Drug Information Center [(602)626–6016], which operates the *Antivenin Index.*

Snakes

BIOLOGY AND VENOM

Approximately 375 of the more than 3500 species of snakes are considered dangerous to human beings. The venomous snakes can be divided into the **Elapidae**—the cobras, kraits, mambas, and coral snakes; **Hydrophiidae**—the true sea snakes; **Laticaudidae**—the sea kraits; **Viperidae**—the Old World vipers and adders; **Crotalidae**—the rattlesnakes, water moccasins, fer-de-lances copperheads of North America, and the bushmaster; and certain **Colubridae,** of which the clinically important are the boomslang and bird snake of Africa and the red-necked keelback of Asia.[1–5] Several other colubrids must be viewed with concern.[6] Antivenins are available for most of the medically important venomous snakes.[1,3,4]

In the United States, 21 of the approximately 120 species of snakes can be considered dangerous. It is estimated that 45,000 snakebite cases occur a year, of which 8000 are inflicted by venomous snakes. There are two families of venomous snakes indigenous to the United States—the Crotalidae and the Elapidae. The latter account for only 20 to 25 bites a year.[4]

Snake venoms are complex mixtures, containing chiefly proteins, many of which have enzymatic activity. Some of the more lethal proteins of snake venoms are small peptides. Other components are metalloproteins, glycoproteins, lipids, biogenic amines, free amino acids, and inorganic substances such as metals and electrolytes.[4,7] The primary function of a snake venom is to immobilize and, in most cases, kill the prey. It also facilitates the digestion of prey and serves as a defense against predators. Collectively, snake venoms have an effect on almost every organ system. However, in most crotalid envenomations the deleterious effects are seen in the hematologic, cardiovascular, respiratory and nervous systems. With rattlesnake venoms vascular resistance and permeability may be altered, red blood cell integrity and viscosity impaired, hypoperfusion induced, and neuromuscular transmission suppressed. Because there are multiple sites of action, one should not label or treat a poisoning as a "neurotoxin," "hemotoxin," or "cardiotoxin."[3]

CLINICAL PRESENTATION

A bite from any species of crotalid is capable of three clinically important manifestations. First, *local swelling* and *tissue changes* may occur, particularly when digits are involved (Fig. 182-1; Plate 46). Swelling is caused by injury to the small vessels and capillaries and results in transudation of blood components. Swelling may range from very mild to massive; if massive, it may compromise local perfusion or central blood volume. Edema in a particular area, such as the face or a muscle compartment, may threaten life or limb without the presence of apparent systemic effects. Secondly, venom components may cause *coagulopathies.* A coagulation anomaly resembling disseminated intravascular coagulation is a common laboratory finding. Although evi-

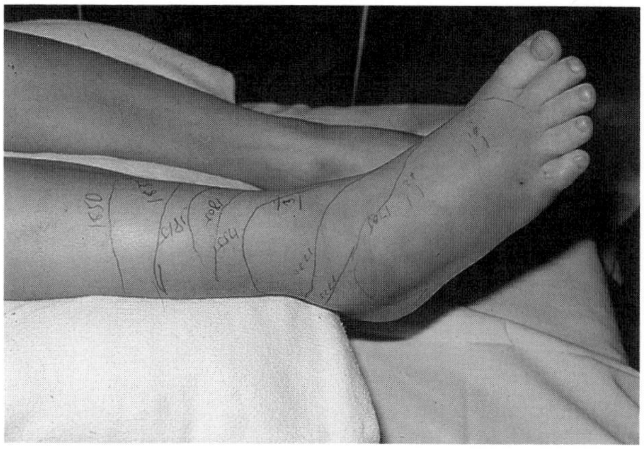

FIGURE 182-1 Local manifestations of *Crotalus atrox* Envenomation. This seven-year-old patient demonstrates two puncture wounds at the base of the little toe. A surrounding area of ecchymosis is evident. The lines represent serial markings of the advancing edge of swelling (using visual evaluation and palpation of induration). Circumferential measurements of the swelling were also followed at the sites marked #1, #2, and #3. Measurements were made every 15 to 30 min. (See Plate 46.)

dence of intravascular hemolysis on the peripheral blood smear is unusual, abnormal fibrinogen, prothrombin time (PT), activated partial thromboplastin time (PTT), or platelet counts are common. Thirdly, crotalid venom components may cause *systemic changes,* such as abnormal taste sensation, nausea and vomiting, or depressed levels of consciousness.

The severity of poisoning following a crotalid bite is variable. Approximately 25 percent of such bites are "dry," showing no evidence of venom injection. Crotalid bites are generally classified as *minimal, moderate,* or *severe,* depending on the degree of local and systemic injury, and on laboratory evidence[3,4] (Table 182-1). The critical care physician may be involved in the management of any grade of poisoning.

LOCAL INJURY

Evidence of local injury usually begins to develop within 30 min of envenomation, often sooner. Fang wounds associated with local pain and swelling are the most common early manifestations. However, cases in which severe swelling developed hours after a bite have been reported.[8] Thus, the patient should be closely observed for at least 6 h after a bite.

Various treatments for minimizing swelling have been proposed. Standard supportive measures include immobilization of the limb at heart level. Antivenin (Crotalidae) Polyvalent is the treatment of choice for limiting swelling and improving functional outcome.[4,9,10] Local debridement of clearly nonviable tissue may be necessary a few days after an envenomation, but it should be limited in nature since recovery of apparently compromised tissue often occurs.

TABLE 182-1 Grading of Crotalid Bite Severity on Admission (30 min–4 h)

The grading of a bite should be based on the physician's assessment of local injury, systemic signs and symptoms, and the results of laboratory tests. The grading of the bite should be determined by the most severe symptom or sign (e.g., a patient with no swelling but having a systolic blood pressure of 70 mmHg should be considered as severely envenomated).

Minimal Envenomation

Swelling, erythema, and ecchymosis limited to immediate area of the bite site.

Systemic signs and symptoms not present or minimal

Coagulation parameters all normal. No other significant laboratory abnormalities.

Moderate Envenomation

Swelling, erythema and ecchymosis present, may involve most of an extremity, and may be spreading slowly.

Systemic signs and symptoms present, but not life-threatening. These may include nausea, vomiting, oral paresthesias or unusual tastes, mild hypotension (SBP >80 mmHg), mild tachycardia, and tachypnea.

Coagulation parameters may be abnormal, but no clinically significant bleeding is present. Severe abnormalities of other laboratory tests are not present.

Severe Envenomation

Swelling and ecchymosis involve the entire extremity and are spreading rapidly.

Systemic signs and symptoms are markedly abnormal, including severe alteration of mental status, nausea and vomiting, hypotension (SBP <80 mmHg), severe tachycardia, tachypnea, or other respiratory compromise.

Coagulation parameters abnormal with serious bleeding present or threat of spontaneous bleeding, including PT unmeasurable, PTT unmeasurable, platelets <20,000/μL, or fibrinogen undetectable. Severe abnormalities of other laboratory values should also be considered severe envenomations.

COAGULOPATHY

Much debate has surrounded the significance of the coagulopathy following rattlesnake bites. Both blood component therapy and antivenin have been proposed as treatment. We recommend the use of antivenin with judicious addition of blood components when needed. Use of this approach permits reversal of clotting abnormalities, even in severe cases, while minimizing the patient's transfusion risks.

Minor alterations in coagulation parameters, if not associated with other significant clinical manifestations and if not progressive, do not require antivenin or blood component therapy. Serial determination of the PT, PTT, and platelet count should be performed to ensure that the coagulopathy is not worsening. Patients with moderately prolonged PT or PTT, depressed platelet counts, hypofibrinogenemia, or evidence of minimal bleeding (hematuria or minor gum bleeding) should be treated with antivenin alone. Severe abnormalities (e.g., unmeasurable PT, PTT, or fibrinogen, or platelet count <20,000/μL) should be treated with larger doses of antivenin. Administration of fresh frozen plasma or platelet concentrate should be considered when bleeding is profuse or involves critical areas or when the coagulopathy does not respond to antivenin therapy. However, these factors may be simply consumed without significantly altering the coagulopathy.[11]

SYSTEMIC MANIFESTATIONS

Systemic manifestations may be as benign as a metallic taste, sweating, perioral paresthesias, weakness, or anxiety. Although these manifestations require no specific treatment, they are regarded as indicators of the systemic spread of the venom and of impending deterioration.

The most important systemic effect of crotalid venom poisoning is hypotension. Hypotension may be mild or life-threatening and appears to be caused by intravascular volume depletion secondary to venom-induced increased vascular permeability. Loss of plasma often causes an initial hemoconcentration followed by hemodilution during volume resuscitation. Review of fatal snakebite cases strongly suggests that inadequate treatment of hypotension greatly contributes to mortality.[1,12,13]

MANAGEMENT

HYPOVOLEMIA

The initial management of hypotension should be rapid intravenous isotonic fluid infusion. Several liters may be required. In severe cases, colloid infusion may be more effective than crystalloid.[14] Antivenin should not be delayed because of requirements for fluid resuscitation.[3,15] Starting antivenin infusion in the emergency department often saves considerable time. If volume shifts are not easily assessed, central venous or pulmonary capillary wedge pressure monitoring may be needed. However, central line insertion may present risks because of coagulopathy. Central monitoring is generally limited to the most ill patients or to those with preexisting cardiopulmonary disease and should not delay antivenin administration.

ANTIVENIN ADMINISTRATION

The use of Antivenin (Crotalidae) Polyvalent, the only antivenin approved in the United States for treatment of crotalid bites, is recommended for envenomations that show evidence of poisoning and progression. Progression is defined as worsening of a patient's local injury, e.g., pain, ecchymosis and swelling; laboratory abnormalities, as evidenced by worsening hemoglobin, platelet count, clotting times or other tests; or systemic manifestations, as evidenced by unstable vital signs or abnormal mental status. In addition, antivenin is recommended for the treatment of any poisoning that appears to be life-threatening or to be developing a compartment syndrome. Antivenin should be used as soon as indicated, because its effectiveness declines as the time between envenomation and administration increases.[3,15] Unfortunately, many hospitals stock insufficient amounts of antivenin, even in endemic areas. Every hospital in endemic areas should stock at least 10 vials, an amount sufficient to initiate appropriate care of a severely envenomated patient.

Before administering the antivenin, an intradermal skin test should be performed using the material provided with each vial of antivenin. A positive test (wheal or erythema >10 mm in diameter appearing within 30 min) strongly suggests that the patient may develop an allergic reaction to antivenin infusion, whereas a negative result usually indicates that the patient will tolerate the infusion.[3,4,16] To prevent a delay while waiting for the skin test results, the initial dose of antivenin can be mixed. Since the antivenin takes about 30 min to go into solution, it will be ready when the skin test is interpreted.

The initial dose of antivenin should be: minimal findings and progression, 5 to 8 vials of antivenin; moderate findings and progression, 8 to 13 vials; severe envenomations, 13 to 20 vials. Patients in whom cardiovascular collapse appears imminent should receive an initial dose of 20 or more vials.

The instructions for the administration of antivenin included in the package insert are, for the most part, adequate. Several suggestions, however, should be considered. It may require 20 to 30 min to solubilize the lyophylized antivenin. Faster dissolution may occur if an isotonic solution is added to vials at room temperature.[17] Once mixed, the antivenin should be diluted in 250 to 500 mL crystalloid and slowly infused, about 50 mL/h for 10 min, until it is evident that anaphylaxis will not occur. If a reaction does not develop, the rate should be increased in a stepwise manner every few minutes until a rate of 250 to 500 mL/h is reached. Thus, once the decision to give antivenin is made, it still requires 45 to 60 min to achieve adequate antivenin infusion rates!

Most patients will show cessation or reversal of their findings during the first antivenin infusion, but some patients will require more antivenin if there is worsening local injury, failure to reverse laboratory findings, or worsening of systemic manifestations. Laboratory determinations are repeated every 4 h or after each course of antivenin therapy, whichever is more frequent. Unless the patient is hemodynamically unstable, the initial antivenin dose may be repeated in these patients. If the patient is unstable, the dose of antivenin should be at least 20 vials.

Antivenin reactions are a common problem.[3,18,19] These are classified as acute and delayed serum reactions. Early reactions are type I hypersensitivity reactions mediated by histamine. Delayed serum reactions (serum sickness) are type III hypersensitivity reactions. Early reactions occur in about 15 percent of patients during antivenin infusion. Under close observation and with appropriate pharmacologic intervention, acute reactions in patients requiring antivenin can nearly always be treated successfully, allowing the completion of antivenin infusion. Our procedure for handling antivenin reactions is shown in Table 182-2. Delayed reactions will usually occur after the patient has left the ICU. These are treated with antihistamines and corticosteroids.

Several other treatments, particularly large doses of ste-

TABLE 182-2 Management of Early Antivenin Reactions

1. Stop antivenin infusion immediately.
2. Re-evaluate the benefit: risk ratio of antivenin use in the patient. While further administration is safe with close observation and management, the possibility of death from anaphylaxis does exist. In general, further antivenin attempts are warranted for severe envenomations and many moderate envenomations. Most minimal cases do not require antivenin therapy.
2. In mild reactions, administer 50 mg diphenhydramine IV and epinephrine, 0.01 mg/kg of 1:1000 concentration, SC (total dose not to exceed 0.5 mg).
3. In moderate to severe reactions, administer 50 to 100 mg diphenhydramine IV, 300 mg cimetidine IV (or other H_2 blocker) and epinephrine, 0.3 mg of 1:1000, intramuscularly or infuse a 1:50,000 concentration of epinephrine slowly as needed up to several milliliters.
4. Antivenin may be cautiously restarted after symptoms have resolved. Before restarting the infusion, the antivenin should be further diluted (i.e., put vials in 500 to 1000 ml crystalloid) and infused very slowly. The rate may be slowly increased to infuse the antivenin over 2 h, if tolerated by the patient.
5. Patients with severe initial reactions (clear hypotension or airway compromise) should undergo further attempts at antivenin infusion only if their envenomation is life-threatening. The approach in step 4 is used with the addition of continuous epinephrine infusion.

TABLE 182-3 Management of Possible Compartment Syndrome after Crotalid Envenomation

1. Determine intracompartmental pressure.
2. If not elevated, continue standard management.
3. If signs of compartment syndrome are present and compartment pressure is >30 mmHg:
   a. Elevate limb.
   b. Administer mannitol 1 to 2 g/kg IV over 30 min.
   c. Administer *additional* Antivenin (Crotalidae) Polyvalent, 10 to 15 vials IV over 60 min.
   d. If elevated compartment pressure persists over 1 h, consider fasciotomy.

Notes: 1. Elevated compartment pressure is caused by the action of the venom on the tissues, and thus, the most effective treatment is to neutralize the venom, which in most cases will reduce the compartment pressure.
2. This protocol delivers a high osmotic load and should not be used when contraindicated. The protocol must be completed promptly so that, if ever needed, fasciotomy may be performed as early as possible.

roids, have been advocated for the treatment of crotalid envenomation. As in many other diseases, however, a beneficial effect has not been demonstrated. Thus, it is recommended that the mainstay of treatment remain antivenin and aggressive life support.

Recommended supportive care measures include immobilization of the limb in a functional position until swelling is receding and coagulation tests are normal. Then the bitten part, particularly the hand, should be used or physical therapy utilized to maintain range of movement and strength. If indicated, tetanus prophylaxis should be given. Antibiotics that will cover typical human skin flora are recommended only when infection is clinically evident. Blebs, bloody vesicles, or superficial necrosis can be debrided several days after the injury, and the area is then treated as a second-degree burn.

Compartment syndrome is an unusual but serious development. Diagnosis is often difficult in a leg that is already painful and swollen, since almost all bites by crotalids are subcutaneous. If compartment syndrome is suspected, compartment pressures should be measured. Although controversial, current evidence suggests surgery does not improve outcome and should be limited to refractory cases.[3,4,10,20] Our approach to potential compartment syndrome is shown in Table 182-3.

ELAPID AND EXOTIC SNAKEBITES IN THE UNITED STATES

The keeping of foreign snakes has become increasingly popular, leading to a rising frequency of *exotic snakebite*. The primary clinical management of exotic bites is similar to that of native species: recognition of hypotension and coagulation abnormalities and treatment with the appropriate antivenin. However, elapids and several foreign snakes also produce greater neuromuscular changes. These may lead to respiratory insufficiency, paralysis, and death, if untreated. Furthermore, because of their rare occurrence, it is often difficult for the ICU physician to evaluate the patient and to secure antivenin for treatment.

In coral snake bites, the general principles noted above for pit viper envenomation should be applied. Three vials of antivenin *(Micrurus fulvius)* should be given when a diagnosis of coral snake envenomation has been established. If symptoms develop, 3 to 5 additional vials may be given. Ventilatory support may be required, and the patient must be observed closely for respiratory muscle weakness or hypoventilation.[3] To assist in securing exotic antivenins for cases requiring antivenin treatment, the American Association of Zoos, Parks and Aquariums, and the American Association of Poison Control Centers have cooperated to produce the *Antivenin Index*. This listing records the antivenins kept by participating zoos in the United States. The *Antivenin Index* can be consulted by calling your regional poison control center or the Arizona Poison and Drug Information Center [(602)626–6016].

Arthropods

The phylum Arthropoda includes the spiders, scorpions, insects, ticks, kissing bugs, caterpillars, moths, centipedes, and millipedes, among others. Some arthropods sting (bees, scorpions, etc.), others bite (spiders, centipedes, kissing bugs, etc.), while still others discharge a toxic secretion (millipedes, caterpillars, etc.). Almost all of the 20,000 species of spiders are venomous, but luckily only a small number have fangs long and strong enough to penetrate the human skin. Several species of scorpions are a danger to man, and numerous species of bees, wasps, yellow jackets, and ants are of medical importance.[21]

The treatment of most arthropod bites and stings can be completed in the emergency department. However, severely ill patients, children, the elderly, and anyone with a debilitating disease who has been envenomated by the widow spiders (*Latrodectus* species), the brown or violin spiders (*Loxosceles* species), or displays any anaphylactic or serious sensitivity reaction should be followed in the ICU. This chapter will include the toxic effects of these venoms.

SPIDERS

WIDOW SPIDERS (*Latrodectus* Species)

The black widow spider found in the eastern United States is *L. mactans,* whereas in the West it is *L. hesperus.* Only females have fangs capable of penetrating human skin. Mature females range in body length from 10 to 18 mm and have a red hourglass or other red marking on the ventral abdomen. The venom causes nonspecific release of synaptic vesicles by allowing influx of Ca^{2+} ions. This particularly affects the neuromuscular junction, causing unrestrained muscle contraction and cramping.[22]

In most patients, there is an initial sharp, pinprick-like bite followed by a dull, numbing pain in the affected extremity and by pain and cramping in one or several large muscle masses. Muscle fasciculations and sweating may be observed. Pain in the low back, thighs, and abdomen is common, particularly in severe cases. The syndrome may mimic an acute abdomen.

There is usually little local tissue reaction at the bite site. Two very small puncture wounds may be found on close examination. These may be surrounded by a slightly blanched area and an erythematous blush, which in time becomes pallid. Minimal localized edema may be present. Unusual neuromuscular manifestations, including opisthotonus, mydriasis, salivation, and convulsions occur following the bites of some species. Mild to moderate hypertension is common, often developing about 2 to 4 h after the bite, and may require treatment. There may also be changes in the electrocardiogram, varying from simple ST segment depression and prolongation of the QT interval to complete heart block.[22]

Treatment of weakness and cramping may include calcium gluconate, methocarbamol, benzodiazepines, and/or narcotics. The critical care physician should monitor high-risk patients and treat those developing any life-threatening complications: respiratory insufficiency, hypertension and hypotension, and cardiac conduction abnormalities. Patients at the extremes of age and those with underlying pulmonary or cardiovascular disease are most prone to develop complications. These problems can be approached using standard advanced life support measures. The early use of antivenin should be considered in seriously ill patients. Antivenin *(L. mactans)* is often effective in reversing the *L. mactans* and *L. hesperus* poisonings. The patient's clinical response to antivenin may be variable because the venom used in producing the antibody in horses comes from a South American species. Although it is an equine product, like crotalid antivenin, it is less refined. Thus, the benefits of the antivenin must be weighed against the risks of anaphylaxis. The use of 1 to 2 vials, administered intravenously over 15 min, is recommended in patients with severe pain or muscle spasm unresponsive to standard treatment, and in the few patients who develop respiratory or cardiovascular compromise, especially those at the extremes of age.

VIOLIN SPIDERS (*Loxosceles* Species)

These spiders are variously known in North America as the fiddleback, brown, or brown recluse spiders. The violin on the dorsal cephalothorax is brown to black and distinct from the paler background. Both sexes are venomous. The bite of this spider may produce pain similar to an ant sting, but frequently patients recall no pain. Pruritus is often

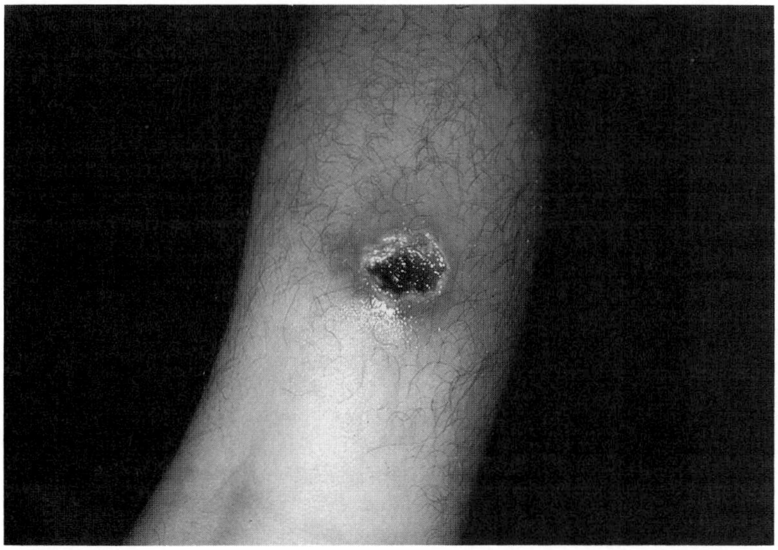

FIGURE 182-2 Necrotic arachnidism of the calf. This patient represents a typical presentation of presumed necrotic arachnidism. He presented to the emergency department on the third day after developing a systemic syndrome consisting primarily of weakness, malaise, and a feverish feeling in conjunction with the development of an enlarging leg lesion which later ulcerated. Systemic complications did not occur. Healing over the next 2 months resulted in a scarred area the size of the original lesion. Brown spiders as well as wolf spiders were found in the home. (See Plate 47.)

present. The bite site begins to redden and enlarge over the first several hours and may be surrounded by a blanched area. A small bleb or vesicle often forms at the site, subsequently rupturing and forming a pustule. Overall, the lesion may resemble a bull's eye (Fig. 182-2; Plate 47).

In some cases, systemic manifestations will develop, including fever, malaise, stomach cramps, nausea and vomiting, jaundice, splenomegaly, hemolysis, hematuria, hemoglobinuria, and thrombocytopenia. Fatal cases are rare and are usually preceded by intravascular hemolysis and its complications.[21]

No effective first-aid or Food and Drug Administration (FDA)-approved antivenin is available at the present time. The primary concerns are the elimination of other diagnoses and the prompt treatment of any complications. The most common serious complication is acute intravascular hemolysis, which may result in acute renal failure. Maintenance of adequate urine flow and alkalinization of the urine are usually effective in preventing renal failure.

SCORPIONS

In the United States members of the genera *Hadrurus, Vejovis,* and *Uroctonus* are capable of inflicting painful stings. The bark scorpion, *Centruroides exilicauda* (formerly *C. sculpturatus*), is the only native scorpion that causes severe illness. It inhabits Arizona, southern New Mexico, California, and Mexico.[23]

The management of children and adults stung by *C. exilicauda* must be considered separately. Adults develop severe local pain that radiates proximally. Minimal local swelling without ecchymosis may develop. Hypertension may develop but rarely requires treatment. Development of systemic findings rarely occurs. Children complain of pain, although it rarely appears to be severe. Some children are unaware of the sting. The area becomes sensitive to touch and merely pressing lightly over the injury (the "tap test") will elicit more severe pain. Children become restless and display abnormal and random head, neck, and body movements, as well as roving eye movements. Tachycardia may be evident within 45 min, and hypertension may be present 1 h after the sting, although it is not seen as early or as severely as it is in adults. Fasciculations may be seen over the face or large muscle masses, and the child may be weak. The respiratory distress from hypersalivation and respiratory weakness may proceed to respiratory arrest. Convulsions have been reported.[21,23,24]

The principles of care for the critically ill child are airway control and management of parasympathetic tone. Patients with a serious syndrome but without airway compromise may be treated with sedation or antivenin, if available, as described below. Intubation may be extremely difficult due to the jerky movements and the excessive secretions. Once airway control is established, one of several routes may be followed. Simple sedation with short- or long-acting benzodiazepines has been used effectively. Phenobarbital has been used, but its usefulness is limited by the fact that doses of >30 mg/kg are often needed to achieve sedation. Caution must be used with any type of sedation, because it may promote the development of respiratory failure. Nitroprusside is recommended for the rare development of hypertension severe enough to warrant treatment. Intravenous β-blockers may be of value. Propranolol has been useful in patients.[24] Labetolol is theoretically preferable due to its α- and β-receptor blockade. When available, the most effective drug for the treatment of *Centruroides* stings is *C. exilicauda* antivenin. However, this goat serum product is produced and distributed only within the state of Arizona. It should be used in severe poisonings only, using the same precautions recommended for any type of antivenin use.[21,23,24]

Fish Poisonings

With increased travel to the Caribbean and South Pacific, and the disruption of the biota, the number of fish and marine animal poisonings has increased at least tenfold during the past decade.[25–27] Although most of these poisonings can be treated in the office or emergency department, several, such as ciguatera and tetraodon poisoning, may require care in the ICU.

CIGUATERA FISH POISONING

Ciguatera fish poisoning is generally characterized by certain gastrointestinal and neurologic symptoms and signs. It may occur following the ingestion of tropical reef and semipelagic marine fishes such as the snappers, groupers, sea basses, barracudas, surgeonfish, and butterflyfish, as well as several gastropods. More than 100 species of fishes have now been implicated in ciguatera poisoning. Most of the toxic species are either carnivores or benthonic algal feeders. The principal toxin causing ciguatera fish poisoning is ciguatoxin. The toxin is thought to start in a dinoflagellate. The dinoflagellate is then eaten by small fish which are, in turn, eaten by larger fish, until a size edible by people is reached. Among the carnivorous species there appears to be a positive relationship between the amount of fish in the diet and the degree of toxicity. Larger ciguateric fishes tend to be more toxic than the smaller fish of the same species. In most cases the flesh is less toxic than are the viscera. The liver is usually the most toxic part of the fish.[27]

The majority of poisoned patients in the United States report having eaten offending fish in the Caribbean, although many cases have followed the consumption of toxic fish from a United States market. A smaller number of patients is seen in Hawaii, although by far the largest number of cases occur in the South Pacific.[26–28]

Ciguatera poisoning is complex, probably because it may involve several toxins, the most important being ciguatoxin and maitotoxin. The amounts of these and the lesser toxins and their distribution in fishes can account for the extremely variable clinical manifestations. Ciguatera poisoning might be divided into: those cases in which the neurologic findings predominate over the gastrointestinal, those in which the reverse is true, and those much rarer cases in which the manifestations are purely neurologic or gastrointestinal.[28]

In groups where neurologic findings predominate, there are paresthesias in the extremities and circumorally, feelings of electric shock, pain, or burning on contact with cold objects, some abdominal distress, nausea and occasionally vomiting, followed by weakness, headache, vertigo, chills, asthenia, pain in the large muscle masses and joints, feeling of looseness of the teeth, and ataxia. In mild cases there is no evidence of muscle weakness; reflexes are usually normal and there are no pathologic reflexes. The asthenia, weakness, and paresthesia may persist for months. In the most severe cases vertigo, weakness, paresis of the legs, dysmetria, nystagmus, prostration, bradycardia, coma, and sometimes death may occur.

In groups where gastrointestinal findings predominate, symptoms begin between 30 min and 12 h after ingestion. Nausea, repeated vomiting, abdominal and sometimes leg cramps develop; diarrhea, lassitude, weakness, and perioral paresthesia with tingling of the hands and feet often follow. Pruritus and diffuse body aches are common. The principal difference between the various forms of poisoning lies in the timing and severity of the major initial manifestations. Reversal of hot and cold sensations occurs in about 65 percent of all forms of ciguatera poisoning as a later development. All types of poisoning may result in serious arrhythmias. Fortunately, the fatality rate is <1 percent.[26–28]

Treatment, in addition to basic life-support measures, consists of gastric lavage, if carried out soon after the poisoning; calcium gluconate up to 1 g by drip as early as possible (and if not contraindicated), followed by atropine, 0.01 mg/kg by infusion for symptomatic bradycardia; dopamine, 5 to 20 μg/kg/min for hypotension; cyproheptadine for severe itching; and diazepam and diphenylhydantoin for convulsions.

Recently, amitryptiline and tocainide have been suggested as treatment, but current evidence is not convincing. Mannitol was tested in an uncontrolled study of 24 patients with acute ciguatera poisoning. The patients showed a marked lessening of neurologic and muscle dysfunction following injection of mannitol.[29] Gastrointestinal symptoms abated more slowly.

PUFFERFISH POISONING

Tetrodotoxication is caused by eating certain pufferfish, variously known as globefish, blowfish, balloonfish, swellfish, tambores, or fugu among others. It is also caused by other fishes, including ocean sunfish, porcupinefish, and triggerfish. Review of the literature shows approximately 125 fish species with tetrodotoxin (TTX). Between 1955 and 1975, more than 3000 individuals were reported to have been poisoned from eating puffers in Japan; 1537 (51 percent) died.[26,27] These authors verified the presence of TTX in the stomach contents and sera of eight patients who had died following manifestations of muscular weakness, paralysis, respiratory failure, and who had eaten puffers 13 h previously. During a sabbatical in Japan of one of us (FER), we learned that 37 people had committed suicide the year before by eating fugu.

Puffer poisoning is characterized by rapid onset (5 to 30 min) of weakness, nervousness, sweating, increased salivation, pallor, dizziness, nausea, and oropharyngeal paresthesia, often described as a tingling or pricking sensation. Vomiting is often repeated and violent. A weak pulse and tachycardia may develop early. The patient may complain of generalized numbness and a sensation of floating in air. Superficial and deep reflexes are usually decreased, and respiratory distress may be present. Dyspnea, cardiac arrhythmias, and generalized muscular weakness often follow, with paralysis, shock, and respiratory arrest developing in the more severe cases. Death may ensue in 6 to 24 h. Marked congestion and edema of the lungs and gastrointestinal tract have been observed at postmortem examination.[26,27]

The treatment of puffer poisoning has varied considerably. Oral bicarbonate of soda, emetics, laxatives, enemas, oxygen, intravenous fluids, posterior pituitary extracts, picrotoxin, physostigmine, atropine, caffeine, hexeton, coramine, cardiazole, lobeline pentylenetrazol, and stimulation of the phrenic nerve have been suggested. Currently, none of these can be recommended.

Treatment consists primarily of respiratory support. If the patient is treated soon after ingestion, decontamination of the gastrointestinal tract with gastric lavage and activated charcoal may be helpful. Otherwise, the patient is treated supportively with oxygen, intravenous fluids, nasogastric suction, and atropine for bradycardia.

PARALYTIC SHELLFISH POISONING (PSP)

PSP is caused by ingestion of filter-feeding organisms that have fed on unicellular organisms containing saxitoxin and other toxic compounds. Saxitoxin is not destroyed by typical food preparation techniques. The clinical syndrome consists of oral paresthesias starting minutes to hours after ingestion and rapidly spreading to other parts of the body. Other associated symptoms include light-headedness, incoordination, hyperreflexia, dysarthria, nausea, vomiting, and diarrhea, among others. Flaccid paralysis and respiratory insufficiency leading to death may occur in some cases. Treatment is supportive. Unless an anoxic insult has occurred, intubation and ventilation until the toxin effects wear off should suffice. If the ingestion is recent, gastric lavage and administration of activated charcoal may reduce the absorption of the toxin.

CASE PRESENTATION

A 36-year-old entomologist, walking in tall grass, suddenly developed pain in his left ankle. He found a spot of blood just above his shoe. About an hour later he came to the emergency department complaining of pain and swelling of the ankle.

On admission to the emergency department, the patient was in moderate pain and felt weak. The heart rate was 130 and regular, blood pressure 105/60, and respirations 18 and unlabored. The skin was dry. The physical examination was unremarkable except for the left leg. One puncture wound was evident, with a drop of dried blood at the opening. A 2.5-cm mildly ecchymotic area surrounded the puncture. The extremity displayed nonpitting swelling to the knee and was slightly warm and tender, but not discolored. No cords were palpable. Marked tenderness was found in the left inguinal area.

A diagnosis of crotalid envenomation was made. Two intravenous lines of normal saline at 200 mL/h, oxygen by nasal cannula, and heart monitoring were initiated. Specimens were sent for a blood count, PT, PTT, platelet count, fibrinogen, and urinalysis. Over the next 30 min the pain and swelling were noted to have advanced to just above the knee. It was decided to administer antivenin for an apparent moderate crotalid envenomation. A skin test was placed to determine horse serum sensitivity, using the material provided with the antivenin. While waiting for the skin test result, 10 vials of antivenin (Crotalidae) polyvalent were mixed according to the package insert (antivenin takes about 30 min to go into solution) and injected into a 500-mL bag of normal saline. During this procedure, the laboratory results returned showing: hemoglobin 19 g/dL, PT 42.4 s, PTT 95.6 s, platelets 110,000/mm^3, and fibrinogen 75 mg/dL. The skin test was negative at 30 min.

The antivenin infusion was started at 25 mL/h, with a physician at the bedside. This was increased to 50 and then 75 mL/h over the next 20 min. At this time the patient began sneezing. On closer examination, the patient was noted to have an urticarial rash. Auscultation of the chest showed scattered expiratory wheezes. The antivenin infusion was immediately discontinued. Epinephrine, 0.5 mL of 1:1000 solution, was administered subcutaneously, followed by 50 mg diphenhydramine and 300 mg cimetidine, given intravenously. The antivenin was further diluted from 500 to 1000 mL. After the urticarial reaction subsided, the infusion was restarted and the rate gradually increased until a rate of 250 mL/h was reached. The remainder of the antivenin was infused without difficulty.

After the antivenin infusion was completed, the physical examination and laboratory tests were repeated. No further swelling had developed, and the repeat laboratory test results were: hemoglobin 12.5 g/dL, PT 16.0 s, PTT 40.0 s, platelets 100,000/mm^3, and fibrinogen 100 mg/dL.

After this time the patient was reexamined every hour for 4 h to ensure that his condition was not worsening. Laboratory parameters were rechecked every 4 h. The laboratory tests had all returned to normal by the next afternoon. At that time the swelling had decreased by 50 percent, and the pain had completely resolved. The patient was cautioned concerning serum sickness and a follow-up appointment for 1 week was made.

CASE DISCUSSION

Even before the laboratory results were known, it was clear that this patient had suffered a pit viper envenomation. The combination of the presence of a puncture wound, ecchymosis, and rapidly developing pain and swelling in a locale known to be populated by pit vipers makes the diagnosis secure. Although unlikely, other possibilities include a large local reaction to a hymenoptera sting, deep venous thrombosis, cellulitis, or venous insufficiency.

The obvious progression of the swelling made it clear that antivenin was necessary. Therefore, the laboratory results did not need to be known before initiating treatment. Occasionally, patients will not develop dramatic swelling, but will develop a worsening coagulopathy or signs of systemic toxicity, including nausea, vomiting, confusion, and hypotension. These patients should also be treated with antivenin.

Periodic reevaluation of the patient is necessary to determine the necessity of further antivenin infusion. As in this patient (see also Fig. 182-1; Plate 46), worsening of local signs, systemic signs, or the coagulopathy after antivenin administration indicates the need for further antivenin infusion.

Early antivenin reactions during or just after antivenin infusion occur in about 20 percent of patients. These are treated as type I hypersensitivity reactions with epinephrine, diphenhydramine, and cimetidine. This approach will nearly always be successful in allowing completion of the antivenin infusion. The risk of death from an antivenin reaction is often overstated. When managing a probable rattlesnake bite, in particular, the risk of dying from appropriate antivenin infusion is much less than dying of the venom poisoning.

The administration of antivenin does not complete the care of an envenomated patient. Serial, careful clinical evaluations for the worsening of local or systemic manifestations, or the development of a compartment syndrome, must be performed. The initial treatment for a worsening clinical picture is more antivenin. Consultation with a physician experienced in the care of complicated snakebites may be helpful.

References

1. Dowling H, Minton SA Jr, Russell FE: *Poisonous Snakes of the World*. Washington, DC, US Government Printing Office, 1968.
2. Minton SA Jr, Minton MG: *Venomous Reptiles*. New York, Charles Scribner's Sons, 1969.
3. Russell FE: *Snake Venom Poisoning*. Great Neck, NY, Scholium International, 1983.
4. Russell FE, Dart RC: Toxic effects of animal toxins, in Doull J, Klassen CD, Amdur MO (eds): *Casarett and Doull's Toxicology: The Basic Science of Poisons*. 4th ed. New York, Macmillan Publishing, 1990. (In press)
5. Visser J, Chapman DS: *Snakes and Snakebite*. Cape Town, Purnell and Sons, 1978.
6. Minton SA Jr: A list of colubrid envenomations. Kentucky Herp 7:4, 1976.
7. Bieber AL: Metal and nonprotein constituents in snake venoms, in Lee C-Y (ed): *Snake Venoms*. New York, Springer-Verlag, 1979, pp 295–306.
8. Hurlbut KH, Dart RC, Spaite D, et al: Reliability of clinical pre-

sentation for predicting significant pit viper envenomation. Abstract. Ann Emerg Med 17:439, 1988.

9. Russell FE, Carlson RW, Wainschel J, et al: Snake venom poisoning in the United States: Experiences with 550 cases. JAMA 233:341, 1975.
10. Stewart RM, Page CP, Schwesinger WH, et al: Antivenin and fasciotomy/debridment in the treatment of the severe rattlesnake bite. Am J Surg 158:543, 1989.
11. LaGrange RG, Russell FE: Blood platelet studies in man and rabbits following *Crotalus* envenomation. Proc West Pharmacol Soc 13:99, 1970.
12. Hardy DL: Fatal rattlesnake envenomation in Arizona: 1969–1984. Clin Toxicol 24:1, 1986.
13. Russell FE, Buess FW, Strassberg J: Cardiovascular response to *Crotalus* venom. Toxicon 1:5, 1962.
14. Schaeffer RC Jr, Carlson RW, Puri VK, et al: The effects of colloidal and crystalloidal fluids on rattlesnake venom shock in the rat. J Pharmacol Exper Therap 206:687, 1978.
15. Russell FE, Ruzic N, Gonzalez H: Effectiveness of antivenin (Crotalidae) polyvalent following injection of *Crotalus* venom. Toxicon 11:461, 1973.
16. Spaite D, Dart RC, Hurlbut RM, McNally JT: Skin testing: Implications in the management of pit viper envenomation. Abstract. Ann Emerg Med 17:389, 1988.
17. Chalfin L, (ed): Tricks of the trade: Antivenin advice (Russell). Emerg Med, April 30, 1988, p 155.
18. Corrigan P, Russell FE, Wainschel J: Clinical reactions to antivenin, in Rosenberg P (ed): *Toxins: Animal, Plant and Microbial.* Oxford, Pergamon Press, 1978, pp 457–465.
19. Jurkovich GJ, Luterman A, McCullar K, et al: Complications of crotalidae antivenin therapy. J Trauma 28:1032, 1988.
20. Garfin SR, Castilonia RR, Mubarak SJ, et al: Rattlesnake bites and surgical decompression: Results using a laboratory model. Toxicon 22:177, 1984.
21. Russell, FE: Venomous bites and stings, in Berkow RB (ed): *Merck Manual.* Rahway, NJ, Merck & Co, 1987, pp 2565–2576.
22. Maretic Z, Lebez D: *Araneism.* Belgrade, Nolit Publishing, 1979, pp 60–73.
23. Rimza ME, Zimmerman DR, Bergeson DS: Scorpion envenomation. Pediatrics 66:298, 1980.
24. Rachesky IJ, Banner W, Dansky J: Treatments for *Centruroides exilicauda* envenomation. Am J Dis Child 138:1136, 1984.
25. Russell FE: Marine toxins and venomous and poisonous marine animals. *Adv Mar Biol* 3:255, 1965; see also *Marine Toxins and Venomous and Poisonous Marine Animals,* TFH Publishers, Neptune City, NJ, 1971.
26. Russell FE: Marine toxins and venomous and poisonous marine animals (invertebrates). Adv Mar Biol 21:59, 1984.
27. Halstead BW: *Poisonous and Venomous Marine Animals of the World.* Darwin Press, Princeton, NJ, 1988.
28. Russell FE: Ciguatera, in Toxin Rev, 1991. (In press)
29. Palafox NA, Jain AZ, Pinano TM, et al: Successful treatment of ciguatera fish poisoning with intravenous mannitol. JAMA 259:2740, 1988.

Chapter 183

PARAQUAT

URI TAITELMAN

KEY POINTS

- *Any amount of concentrated paraquat should be considered potentially lethal if ingested.*
- *Paraquat causes delayed toxicity; the patient may be asymptomatic many hours after ingestion and die days later from irreversible pulmonary fibrosis.*
- *There is a good correlation between the amount of ingested paraquat, plasma levels during the first 24 h, and outcome.*
- *Lung damage is the most prominent injury in severe paraquat poisoning.*
- *Lung toxicity may be potentiated by exposure to high concentrations of oxygen.*
- *Massive paraquat poisoning causes multiorgan failure.*

Paraquat (1,1′dimethyl-4,4′ bipyridilium dichloride) is an abbreviation of the term *paraquat*ernary-bipyridyl. This agent was first synthesized in 1932 by Michaelis and named by him methyl viologen because it could be readily reduced to a stable free radical having a violet or blue color, and was used as an oxidation-reduction indicator.[1] In 1955, its herbicidal properties were discovered, and it was marketed in 1962. Paraquat has since been used throughout the world as a contact herbicide due to its ability to disrupt chlorophyll photosynthesis. It is a basic water-soluble cation that is rapidly inactivated and degraded in soil. By 1966 the first descriptions of fatalities due to ingestion of paraquat were reported. In France, 60 fatal cases were reported in a single year.[2]

Toxicokinetics

Death may occur within 2 or 3 weeks of oral ingestion and is usually due to progressive pulmonary fibrosis preceded and aggravated by renal failure. Oral ingestion of as little as 10 mL of a 20% solution has proven fatal.[3] However, any amount of ingested, concentrated paraquat should be considered potentially lethal.

From 8 to 12 percent of ingested paraquat is absorbed by the gastrointestinal tract, mainly in the small bowel. Peak paraquat levels are achieved 3 to 7 h after ingestion.[4,5] It is then distributed (apparent volume of distribution 1.2 to 1.6 L/kg) mainly to three compartments: a central intravascular compartment, a tissue compartment consisting of highly vascularized and well-perfused tissues (kidney, liver, muscle), and a third compartment, the lung parenchyma. Paraquat is not metabolized in the body and is not significantly bound to plasma proteins. It is freely soluble in body water. Paraquat is excreted largely unchanged by the kidney, and clearance of paraquat closely parallels creatinine clearance. Paraquat is both passively filtered and actively excreted. Renal failure may markedly diminish clearance.

Toxicodynamics

Concentrated paraquat solutions are corrosive to the skin and mucous membranes. Erosions and ulcerations develop within hours if large amounts of concentrated formula are ingested and within 2 to 3 days if lesser amounts or concentrations are ingested. Nausea, vomiting, and abdominal pain are common symptoms in the first hours after ingestion. There is a good correlation between the amount ingested, plasma levels,[6] and outcome.

Three levels of systemic intoxication may be present following paraquat ingestion: **1.** *mild poisoning* (<20 mg paraquat ion/kg body weight)—all patients fully recover and suffer only minimal gastrointestinal symptoms; **2.** *moderate to severe poisoning* (20 to 40 mg paraquat ion/kg body weight)—death is usually delayed 2 to 3 weeks, with renal failure and pulmonary fibrosis usually the major causes of death; and **3.** *acute fulminant poisoning* (>40 mg paraquat ion/kg body weight)—multiorgan failure occurs early and death usually follows within a few days.[7] The multiorgan failure includes shock, renal failure, hypoxemic respiratory failure, and liver and pancreatic dysfunction. The majority of fatal cases following paraquat ingestion are characterized by progressive hypoxemic respiratory failure associated with pulmonary fibrosis.

Fatalities due to dermal exposure have been reported[8] and usually result from paraquat contact with preexisting skin lesions or repetitive and continuous dermal contact. A single accidental contact with healthy skin causes no systemic poisoning if the skin is rapidly washed.[9] Paraquat and, particularly, its homologue, diquat, are very corrosive and toxic to the eyes.

Inhalation of paraquat may be fatal though this route is considered less hazardous than oral ingestion because of the high dilution of paraquat used for spraying and the size of its droplets which limits its ability to reach very small airways and the alveoli.

Pathophysiology

At least three mechanisms contribute significantly to the pulmonary toxicity of paraquat. *Active uptake* of paraquat by pulmonary epithelium, and in particular type II alveolar epithelial cells, results in up to ten to twenty times greater concentration of paraquat in the lung than in the plasma. This active uptake is energy consuming and is increased when alveolar oxygen partial pressure increases. This active uptake is believed to be accomplished by a polyamine transport system.[10]

Generation of toxic species of oxygen results from the spontaneous reduction of paraquat to a paraquat radical in the presence of reduced nicotinamide-adenine dinucleotide phosphate (NADPH). Reduced paraquat radical causes a one-electron reduction to a dioxygen molecule, transforming molecular oxygen to a superoxide anion (Fig. 183-1). Thus, a redox recycling system including NADPH, paraquat, and molecular oxygen will cause superoxide anion formation as long as NADPH is available for re-forming paraquat radical from paraquat. If the amount of superoxide anion formed exceeds the rate of inactivation by superoxide dismutase (by transformation to hydrogen peroxide which is then enzymatically cleaved to water and molecular oxygen), accumulated superoxide anion will cause generation of hydroxyl free radicals (OH ·) which are very active and toxic oxygen free radicals (see Chap. 58). The generation of oxygen free radicals may lead to alterations of the lipid components of cells and cell membrane (lipid peroxidation) and may also affect water soluble components of the cell, in particular, enzyme and protein sulfhydryl groups.

Depletion of NADPH occurs since the coexistence of NADPH, paraquat, and molecular oxygen leads to conversion of NADPH to nicotinamide-adenine dinucleotide phosphate (NADP). NADPH is essential to the synthesis of surfactant by type II pulmonary epithelial cells and for the functioning of the glutathione peroxidase system, considered to be a major repair system after oxidative damage to the pulmonary cell. Thus, paraquat ingestion simultaneously results in free radical generation and inhibition of the cellular mechanisms repairing the damage caused by the oxygen free radicals (see Figure 183-1).

Two phases of histologic change in the lung parenchyma are observed after paraquat injury. The *inflammatory phase* usually begins a few days after exposure with proteinaceous pulmonary edema, hyaline membrane formation, and infiltration of the lung parenchyma by activated polymorphonuclear leukocytes, and by macrophages. A *proliferative phase* follows with proliferation of fibroblasts and abundant collagen formation, which can eventuate in progressive fatal pulmonary fibrosis. Neither the mechanisms by which the proliferative phase is generated nor the means to stop it is known.

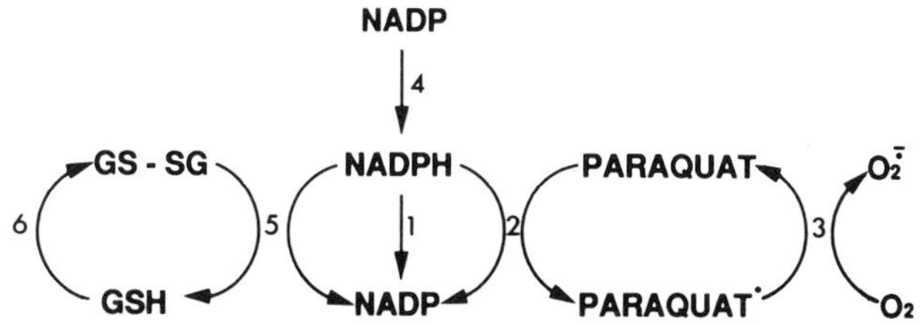

FIGURE 183-1 Mechanism of paraquat activity. NADPH is oxidized to NADP as paraquat is reduced to paraquat radical (steps 1 and 2). Paraquat radical reduces dioxygen to superoxide anion (O_2^-) (step 3). NADPH is re-formed from NADP during aerobic glycolysis (step 4). NADPH is indispensable to restore reduced glutathione (GSH) from oxidized glutathione (GS-SG) (step 5). GSH is converted to GS-SG during repair of cellular oxidative damage (step 6).

Clinical Presentation

The corrosive properties of paraquat often result in injury to exposed surfaces with symptoms of dysphagia, eye and skin pain, and substernal chest pain. Gastroenteritis is prominent in severe ingestions, and vomiting and diarrhea may result in dehydration.

Although these early symptoms follow from direct epithelial injury by paraquat, subsequent symptoms in progressive cases arise from the multiorgan failure occurring over days to weeks. Hypoxemic respiratory failure is often most prominent and presents with dyspnea and tachypnea.

Management

Since any amount of ingested concentrated paraquat should be considered potentially lethal, a useful intervention is decontamination and prevention of further absorption (Table 183-1). Delaying this in an asymptomatic patient may lead to a fatal outcome. Gastric lavage, followed by repeated administration of adsorbent, should be performed as soon as possible after ingestion, especially in an asymptomatic patient. Many adsorbents can adsorb paraquat including activated charcoal, Fuller's earth, bentonite, and kayexalate.[11] Cathartics (mannitol or sorbitol) may be added to the adsorbent solution. Once severe ulcerations of the pharynx and esophagus form, gastric lavage is impossible and may be hazardous because of possible perforation and aspiration. These complications may be fatal in and of themselves.

A plasma level of paraquat (accomplished by radioimmunoassay) should be obtained as soon as possible, because it is a most valuable diagnostic and prognostic test.[6] Evaluation of such levels is related to the time elapsed from the ingestion to the drawing of blood samples. Plasma levels equal to or above 2 mg/L at 4 h, 0.9 mg/L at 6 h, 0.3 mg/L at 10 h, 0.16 mg/L at 16 h, and 0.1 mg/L at 24 h may indicate a poor prognosis.[6] Other important factors determining prognosis include: **1.** the concentration of ingested formula (up to 70 percent mortality was reported after ingestion of 20% paraquat solutions compared to 10 percent mortality after ingestion of 5% solutions);[6] **2.** the amount ingested; and **3.** the condition of the stomach (if the stomach is full before ingestion, prognosis is generally better).

TABLE 183-1 Management of Paraquat Poisoning

Decontaminate gastrointestinal tract and skin.
Avoid gastric lavage if ulceration of pharynx and esophagus has occurred.
Determine plasma paraquat level for diagnostic and prognostic purposes.
Avoid excessive supplemental oxygen therapy.

Excessive oxygen supplementation should be avoided since it may potentiate paraquat toxicity. Positive end-expiratory pressure (PEEP) or continuous positive airway pressure (CPAP) with air should be tried before increasing the fraction of inspired oxygen (F_{IO_2}) in dyspneic and hypoxemic patients. Furthermore, supplemental oxygen, if used, should be maintained at the lowest possible levels.

Correction of dehydration resulting from the frequent vomiting and diarrhea is important because paraquat is excreted by the kidney, and functional renal failure due to hypovolemia may potentiate pulmonary and nephrotoxicity. Fluid repletion should be performed carefully to avoid water accumulation in the lungs. In this regard, pulmonary artery catheterization is often helpful. Solute diuresis does not protect the kidney from the toxic effects of paraquat. Close monitoring of renal function is essential for early detection of renal failure. This is usually a serious prognostic sign, since a decrease in renal function causes an increase of paraquat accumulation in the lung.[4] Renal failure from paraquat poisoning is usually reversible. Total parenteral nutrition (TPN) is necessary for patients unable to swallow.

The intensivist is frequently tempted to use a number of regimens that appear rational or have been cited anecdotally in the medical literature. It should be emphasized that none of the following treatments has been shown to reduce mortality in human cases of paraquat poisoning: *Hemodialysis,* and more particularly, *hemoperfusion* can effectively remove paraquat from the blood, but they do not reduce mortality in either animals[12] or human beings.[4] Hemodialysis should be restricted to the treatment of renal failure. *Antioxidants* (ascorbic acid, niacin, vitamin E, butylated hydroxytoluene) have all been found ineffective when studied.[13] *Corticosteroids* administered to stimulate endogenous superoxide dismutase production have failed to provide any benefit. *Desferoxamine* administered to chelate iron (a catalyst for hydroxyl radical formation) has not been evaluated yet in man. *Cyclophosphamide or radiation therapy* to decrease fibroblast proliferation and collagen formation in the lung have not been verified to reduce the incidence of lung fibrosis. *N-acetylcysteine, liposomal preparations of superoxide dismutase, and other free radical scavengers* have not yet been evaluated in man. Three *lung transplantations* have been performed in paraquat-poisoned patients. None of the patients survived. However, this was prior to the era of cyclosporine and before accumulation of information on paraquat kinetics in patients. Paraquat has biphasic pharmacokinetic characteristics. During the first phase (distribution and elimination phase), half-life is approximately 5 h; during the second phase (elimination phase), half-life increases to 84 h.[5] In cases of progressive pulmonary fibrosis and after complete recovery of renal function, lung transplantation should be considered.

CASE PRESENTATION

A soft drink bottle containing a mixture of 13% paraquat and 7% diquat was left unattended. Two mouthfuls were ingested by a 6-year-old girl. She was brought to the hospital 10 h later when her parents noticed that she had nausea and abdominal pain and questioned her and were told about the ingestion.

On admission, she was asymptomatic. Physical examination was essentially normal. Blood and urine samples were obtained. A solution of 900 mL 0.45% sodium chloride, 100 mL 20% mannitol, and 150 g Fuller's earth was prepared and instilled into the stomach by a nasogastric tube until a watery diarrhea containing Fuller's earth was observed. Hydration of the patient was accomplished with intravenous fluids. A qualitative dithionite test of the urine confirmed the presence of paraquat. The plasma paraquat level was 1.5 mg/L 11 h after ingestion. Charcoal hemoperfusion was performed for 3 h.

The following day the patient complained of a sore throat and was unable to swallow. Examination disclosed ulcerations of the pharynx and the base of the tongue. Chest x-rays and an arterial blood-gas analysis were normal. The serum creatinine level was 0.8 mg/dL on arrival and increased to 1.5 mg/dL by the second day. The plasma paraquat level was 0.2 mg/L on the second day. Another charcoal hemoperfusion was performed for 3 h. Peripheral parenteral nutrition was started and the urine volume monitored.

On the third day the serum creatinine level was 2.5 mg/dL, creatinine clearance 20 mL/min, and blood urea nitrogen (BUN) 40 mg/dL. The urine volume persisted at 1 mL/kg/h. On the fourth day the child became dyspneic. The Pa_{O_2} while she was breathing room air was 65 mmHg. A chest x-ray demonstrated diffuse bilateral interstitial and alveolar infiltrates. The BUN rose to 60 mg/dL, and the creatinine clearance decreased to 15 mL/min.

On the fifth day, the Pa_{O_2} dropped to 55 mmHg. With a CPAP mask (pressure 5 cmH_2O) the Pa_{O_2} was 65 mmHg on room air. The creatinine clearance remained unchanged. The BUN rose to 80 mg/dL, and the urine volume persisted as before. On the following day the child was again noted to be dyspneic and tachypneic. The Pa_{O_2} was 45 mmHg. A chest x-ray revealed a worsening diffuse lung injury. She was intubated and mechanically ventilated with F_{IO_2} of 0.25 and PEEP of 7 cmH_2O with adequate arterial hemoglobin saturation. On the following days renal function improved progressively. However, the pulmonary compliance decreased progressively and the F_{IO_2} had to be increased to maintain a Pa_{O_2} of 55 mmHg. The child died from refractory hypoxemic respiratory failure on the eighteenth day. A postmortem lung biopsy revealed massive pulmonary fibrosis.

CASE DISCUSSION

This patient ingested a concentrated paraquat solution. Medical treatment (gut decontamination) was begun more than 10 h after ingestion. Plasma paraquat was probably at its peak level a few hours prior to the gut decontamination. The two charcoal hemoperfusion sessions performed on the first 2 days did not likely influence the course of the disease. Thus, this therapy should not be used routinely. The most important prognostic indices were ingestion of concentrated formula, followed by plasma levels of paraquat above 0.3 mg/L at the tenth hour and the development of renal failure. The nonoliguric renal failure from paraquat poisoning was reversible, as is often the case. The lung was the main target organ. Refractory hypoxemic respiratory failure because of progressive irreversible pulmonary fibrosis caused death, as is usually the case in fatal ingestions. This occurred despite appropriate efforts to minimize oxygen toxicity, including tolerance of relatively low Pa_{O_2} before beginning any therapy, use of CPAP to improve gas exchange prior to use of supplemental oxygen, and use of the least supplemental oxygen when this additional therapy became necessary.

References

1. Smith P, Heath D: Paraquat. CRC Crit Rev Toxicol 4:411, 1976.
2. Bismuth C, Baud JF, Conso F, et al: *Toxicologie Clinique 4: Herbicides et protecteurs des bois*. Paris, Flammarion Medicine-Sciences, 1987, p 441.
3. Pond SM, Johnston SC, Schoof DD, et al: Repeated hemoperfusion and continuous arteriovenous hemofiltration in a paraquat poisoned patient. Clin Toxicol 25:305, 1987.
4. Bismuth C, Scherrmann JM, Garnier R, et al: Elimination of paraquat. Hum Toxicol 6:63, 1987.
5. Houze P, Baud FJ, Movy R, et al: Toxicokinetics of paraquat in humans. Hum Toxicol 9:5, 1990.
6. Proudfoot AT, Stewart MS, Levitt T, Widdop B: Paraquat poisoning: Significance of plasma-paraquat concentrations. Lancet 2:330, 1979.
7. Vale JA, Meredith TJ, Buckley BM: Paraquat poisoning: Clinical features and immediate general management. Hum Toxicol 6:41, 1987.
8. Wohlfahrt DJ: Fatal paraquat poisonings after skin absorption. Med J Aust 1:512, 1982.
9. Hofer E, Taitelman U: Exposure to paraquat through skin absorption: Clinical and laboratory observations of accidental splashing on healthy skin of agricultural workers. Hum Toxicol 8:483, 1989.
10. Smith LL: Mechanism of paraquat toxicity in lung and its relevance to treatment. Hum Toxicol 6:31, 1987.
11. Meredith TJ, Vale JA: Treatment of paraquat poisoning in man: Methods to prevent absorption. Hum Toxicol 6:49, 1987.
12. Hampson ECGM, Eyles DW, Pond SM: Effects of paraquat on canine bronchoalveolar lavage fluid. Toxicol App Pharmacol 98:206, 1989.
13. Bateman DN: Pharmacological treatments of paraquat poisoning. Hum Toxicol 6:57, 1987.

Chapter 184

ORGANOPHOSPHATE POISONING

URI TAITELMAN

KEY POINTS

- *Organophosphate (OP) insecticides inactivate acetylcholinesterase (AChE), leading to a severe cholinergic syndrome.*
- *Cholinergic manifestations including bronchoconstriction, bronchorrhea, salivation, lacrimation, perspiration, miosis, and bradycardia are common. However, sympathetic stimulation leading to tachycardia and hypertension also occurs.*
- *Muscle fasciculation, rare in other intoxications, suggests OP poisoning.*
- *Coma and seizures are frequent presenting symptoms of severe, acute OP poisoning.*
- *The leading cause of death is respiratory failure due to muscle weakness, depressed drive, bronchoconstriction, and bronchorrhea.*
- *Cardiac ventricular arrhythmias are common.*
- *Treatment includes resuscitation, decontamination, atropine, and reactivation of AChE with oximes.*
- *Red blood cell cholinesterase (ChE) levels are useful in diagnosing and managing OP poisoning.*

Organophosphate (OP) acetylcholinesterase (AChE) inhibitors are used throughout the world as insecticides. Acute human poisoning may occur during the manufacturing or handling of these products, which are readily and rapidly absorbed through the skin, lungs, and gastric and intestinal mucosa. They are particularly life-threatening if a large amount of a concentrated OP formulation is ingested. Subsequent toxicokinetics depend on liposolubility and enzymatic biotransformation. In massive overdose, redistribution from tissue stores may result in a prolonged or rebound clinical syndrome.[1]

Pharmacology

Tissue AChE has two active binding sites: an *anionic site* which binds the quaternary ammonium of choline, and an *esteratic site* which binds the acetyl moiety of acetylcholine (ACh) (Fig. 184-1). The structure of the OP AChE inhibitor molecules is described in Fig. 184-2. The major difference among OP insecticides is in the nature of the leaving moiety (which dissociates from the phosphate to enable binding to the esteratic site of AChE).

OPs complex with high affinity at the esteratic site of AChE, leading to phosphorylation and subsequent inhibition of AChE activity (see Fig. 184-2). Only phosphates di-

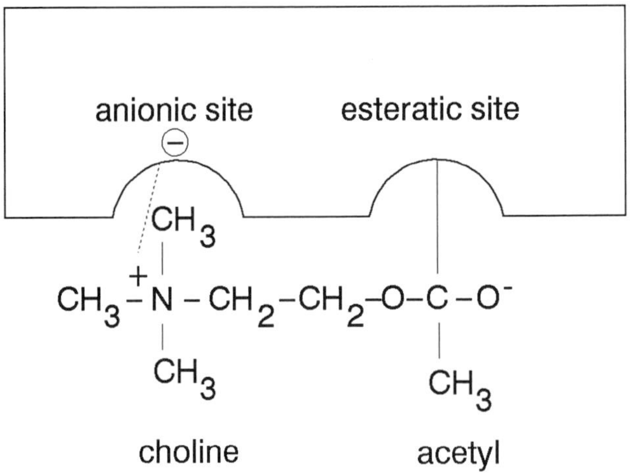

FIGURE 184-1 The enzyme AChE has two active binding sites, an anionic site which binds the choline moiety and an esteratic site which binds the acetyl moiety.

rectly act as AChE inhibitors; phosphorothioates must be activated to phosphates in the liver (substitution of sulfur by oxygen, Fig. 184-3). Phosphorothioates are more stable and more liposoluble than phosphates. Compounds possessing ethoxy radicals are more stable and liposoluble than those having methoxy radicals. A chlorinated, cyclic-leaving moiety increases the liposolubility of the compound.[1] The bond between the OP and AChE changes with time and becomes irreversible when one of the alkyl radicals is separated from the OP (see Fig. 184-2). This phenomenon of dealkylation is known as *aging*.

The time course of the aging phenomenon depends on the molecular structure of the OP. It is shorter for methoxy (CH_3O) as compared to ethoxy (C_2H_5O) radicals, and even shorter with isopropyl (i-C_3H_7O) radicals. The aging period of OP insecticides used in agriculture is estimated to be 24 to 48 h. Once aging has occurred, AChE is irreversibly and definitively inactivated. Oximes, which are of potential therapeutic value in OP poisoning, are reactivators of phosphorylated AChE. The oxime itself becomes phosphorylated and the adduct then dissociates, leaving a restored AChE (Fig. 184-4). However, oximes are inactive after aging has occurred.

In contrast to OP insecticides, most of which are much more toxic to insects than to mammals, several OP AChE inhibitors are particularly toxic to mammals. These compounds are synthesized and stored for use as potential chemical warfare agents. One of the most toxic of these compounds—soman—is characterized by an LD_{50} of 0.03 mg/kg and an aging period of 2 min. Only a few records of accidental human poisonings with such compounds have been described. Treatment of poisonings with these products is similar to that following acute OP insecticide exposure. Oxime therapy in the case of soman will, however, usually be of limited value.

OP compounds react with and are inactivated by many enzyme systems in mammals,[2] in particular by esterases such as arylesterases, aliesterases, and carboxylesterases.

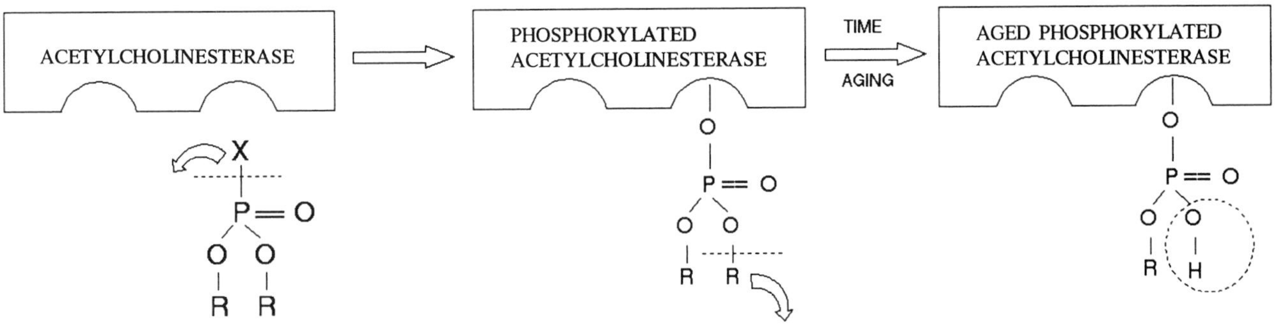

FIGURE 184-2 OP compounds consist of a phosphate group, a leaving moiety (X), and alkyl groups which are usually methyl, ethyl, or isopropyl groups. When the insecticide reacts with AChE, the leaving moiety is cleaved from the phosphate, which then binds to the esteratic site, and inactivates the enzyme. With time, this bond becomes irreversible as an R group separates from the OP in a phenomenon called *aging*.

In addition they are inactivated by hydrolases, transferases, and enzymes causing oxidative dearylation, oxidative *O*-dealkylation, and oxidative *N*-dealkylation.[2] For most OP insecticides, detoxification involves modification or hydrolysis of the leaving moiety or the alkyl radical. A few examples of such detoxification are shown in Fig. 184-5.

Pathophysiology

AChE is a large protein molecule present in cholinergic synapses. It hydrolyzes ACh to choline and acetate and has high affinity and activity for ACh hydrolysis (one molecule of AChE hydrolyzes 10^5 to 10^6 molecules of ACh/min). It is estimated that when ACh is discharged at the presynaptic site, only 15 percent reaches and activates the postsynaptic site. The remainder is hydrolyzed prior to reaching the postsynaptic receptors. Inhibition of more than 70 percent of tissue AChE is required before significant accumulation of ACh occurs in the synapses. The accumulation of ACh due to OP poisoning results clinically in the cholinergic syndrome.

The two types of ACh receptors are muscarinic and nicotinic. *Muscarinic receptors* are present at all synapses between the parasympathetic postganglionic fiber and the effector organ. These receptors can be activated by the alkaloid muscarine, hence their name. Atropine exhibits a high affinity for these muscarinic receptors and is a competitive inhibitor of ACh at these sites. Most of the receptors for ACh in the central nervous system (CNS) are muscarinic, but they are surrounded by the blood-brain barrier and constitute a distinct compartment.

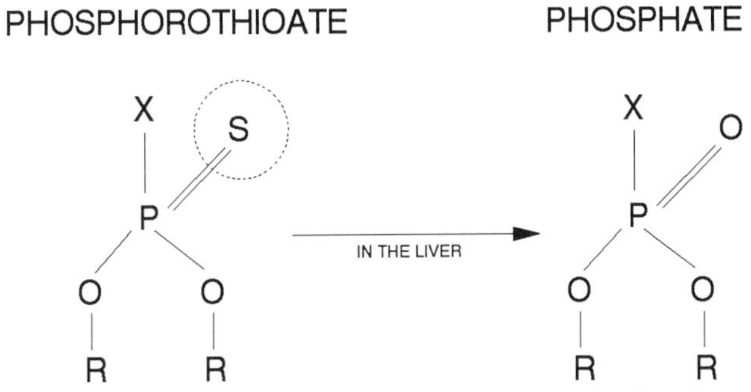

FIGURE 184-3 Phosphorothioates must be metabolized to the active phosphate by the liver.

Nicotinic receptors for ACh are present in all synapses between the pre- and postganglionic neurons of the sympathetic and parasympathetic autonomic systems. Their activation causes secretion of ACh by the parasympathetic postganglionic neurons and secretion of catecholamine by the sympathetic postganglionic neurons. Nicotinic receptors are also present at the junction of peripheral motor neurons and striated muscles.

Clinical Manifestations

ACUTE CHOLINERGIC SYNDROME

The acute cholinergic syndrome results from inhibition of AChE. Symptoms include three major types of clinical manifestations: a peripheral muscarinic syndrome, a nicotinic syndrome, and a CNS syndrome (Table 184-1.)

MUSCARINIC SYNDROME. The peripheral muscarinic syndrome is manifested by bronchorrhea and bronchoconstriction which may result in acute respiratory failure and death due to hypoxemia. All of the exocrine glands are activated, causing salivation, lacrimation, perspiration, and hypersecretion of gastric and intestinal fluid with diarrhea. Contraction of smooth muscles, including the gastric, intestinal, and urinary bladder musculature, may lead to vomiting, abdominal cramps and, in severe cases, involuntary urination and defecation. Bradycardia, miosis, and conjunctival hyperemia are also present.

NICOTINIC SYNDROME. The nicotinic syndrome is manifested by muscle fibrillations and fasciculations (especially of fine subcutaneous muscles such as pectoral, shoulder, and arm muscles), weakness, and decreased muscular strength. In severe cases, paralysis of striated muscles including the diaphragm and chest wall also occurs and leads

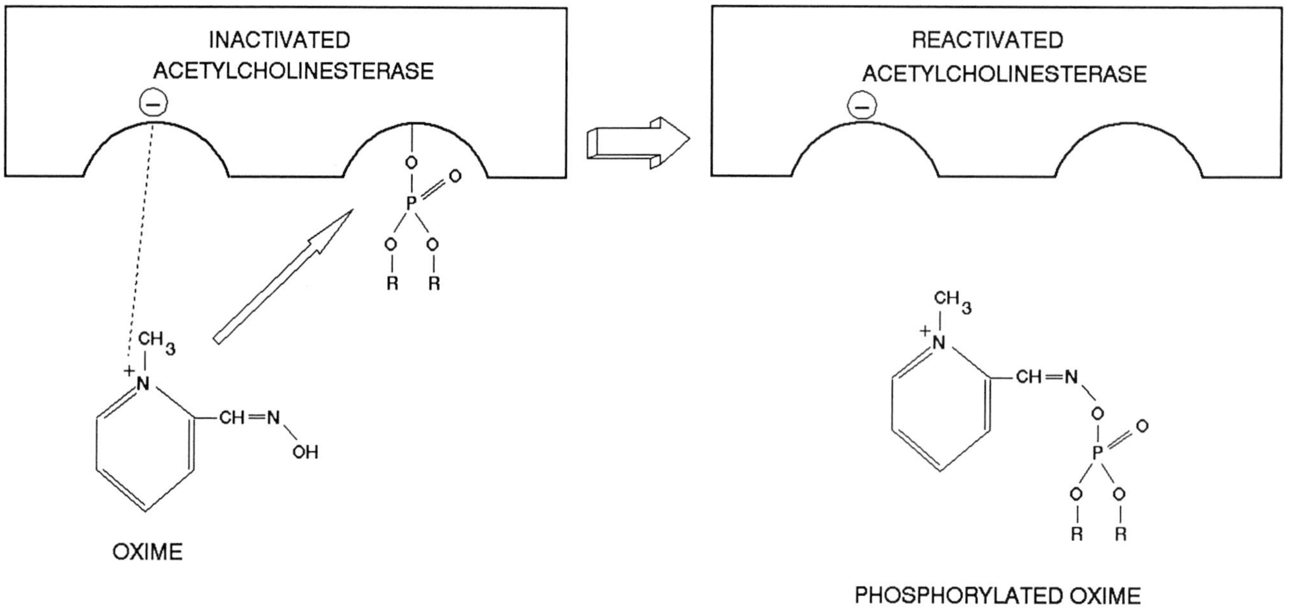

FIGURE 184-4 Oximes can reactivate AChE if given before aging occurs. The oxime reacts with the OP, forming a phosphorylated oxime, and restoring the esteratic site of the enzyme.

TABLE 184-1 Clinical Manifestations of OP Poisoning

Peripheral muscarinic signs	Bronchospasm, bronchorrhea, bradycardia Activation of exocrine glands: salivation, lacrimation, rhinorrhea, perspiration, diarrhea Contraction of smooth muscle: miosis, abdominal cramps, vomiting, involuntary defecation, and urination
Nicotinic signs	Fibrillations, fasciculations, muscular weakness (including diaphragm and chest wall muscles), tachycardia, hypertension, hyperglycemia
CNS signs	Coma, seizures, apnea, ataxia, slurred speech, drowsiness, confusion, tremor, restlessness, emotional lability, headache

to death due to hypoventilation. There may be stimulation of the sympathetic nervous system manifested by tachycardia, hyperglycemia, hypertension, and decreased gastrointestinal motility. Some effects of parasympathetic autonomic stimulation may be opposed by sympathetic stimulation, resulting in variable and unpredictable effects. Tachycardia is as frequent as bradycardia.

CNS SYNDROME. The CNS syndrome is manifested in mild and moderate cases by insomnia, irritability, and decreased mental performance. Severely affected patients demonstrate agitation, decreased consciousness, coma, convulsions, and variable and changing motor deficits. Depression of the respiratory control centers is a major cause of death. The CNS syndrome is most prominent following severe and massive OP poisoning. Clinical evaluation of the patient with acute OP poisoning should include a separate description of the muscarinic, nicotinic, and CNS syndromes.

NONCHOLINERGIC MANIFESTATIONS. Some of the toxic manifestations of OP poisoning are not correlated with the cholinergic syndrome and are not directly related to AChE inhibition. These include cardiac arrhythmias, peripheral neuropathy, and pulmonary toxicity. The pathophysiology of ventricular arrhythmias has not been fully elucidated. These arrhythmias may occur when the cholinergic syndrome is resolving. Delayed peripheral neuropathy is not due to AChE inhibition, but to the inhibition and aging of a neuronal target esterase. Direct toxicity of some of the OP compounds to the lung has been demonstrated.[4] However, aspiration of petroleum distillates, which are frequently used as solvents in OP preparations, can be an aggravating factor in the development of lung injury.

Diagnosis

Confirmation of diagnosis is based on the following:

1. Evidence of a cholinergic syndrome and, in particular, fasciculations, which are infrequently observed in other acute diseases
2. A detailed history of the exposure, including the existence of a container or an original package
3. A low measured level of ChE: in acute OP poisoning, the

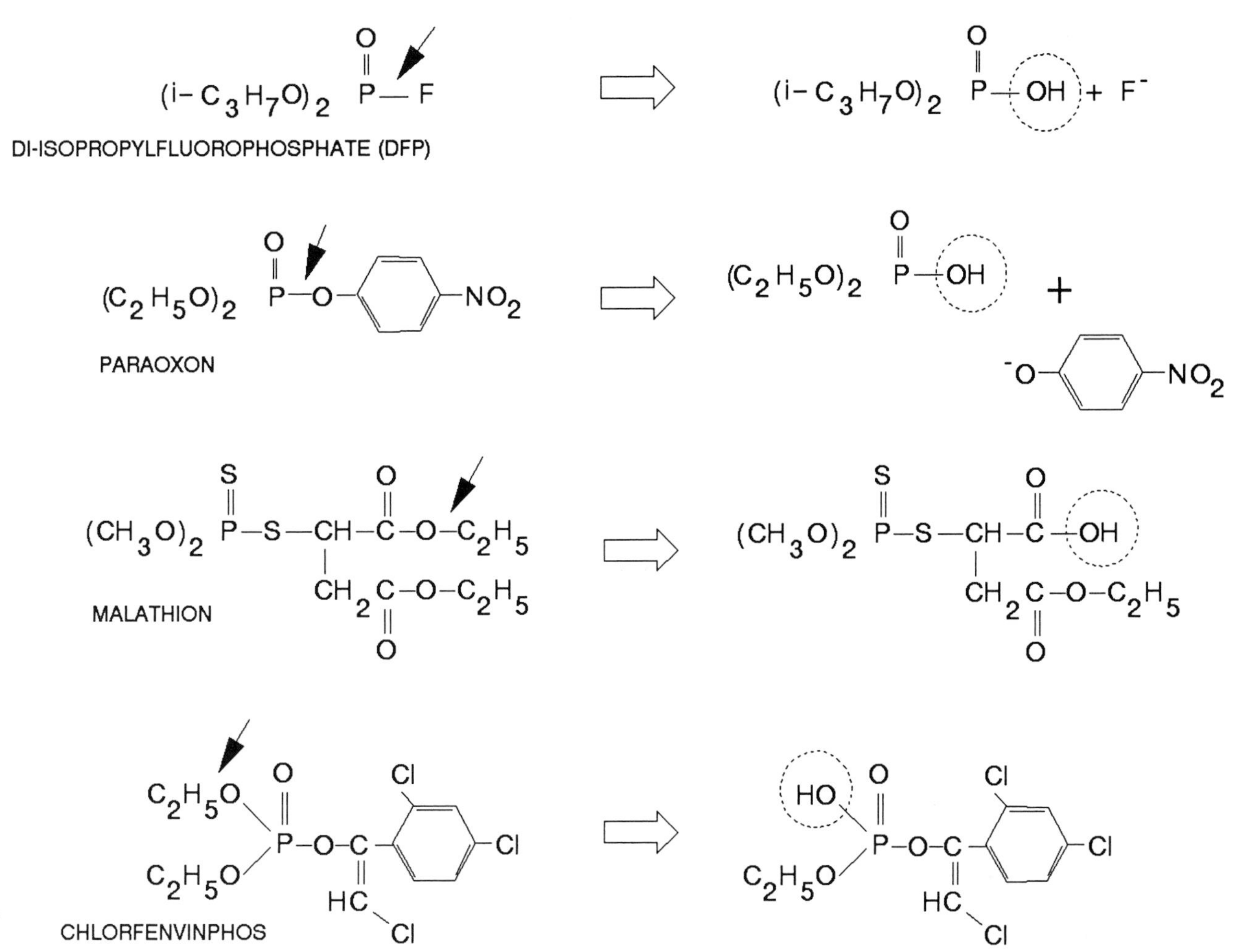

FIGURE 184-5 This figure illustrates the biotransformation of several OP insecticides. The compounds on the left are the active compounds which are detoxified to the inactive compounds on the right. An arrow marks the site of enzymatic detoxification. A broken circle highlights the change which makes the product inactive as a ChE inhibitor. Among the four OPs presented here, the di-isopropylfluorophosphate (DFP) is the most toxic. Its oral LD_{50} is 4 mg/kg. It is hydrolyzed by hydrolases to di-isopropylphosphate, which is not a ChE inhibitor. Paraoxon (active derivative of parathion) has an estimated LD_{50} of 10 mg/kg. The toxicity of paraoxon is modified by the presence or absence of paraoxanase reacting with the leaving moiety of paraoxon. Malathion has an oral LD_{50} of 1000 mg/kg due to its high affinity to carboxylesterase present in mammals. When carboxylesterases are blocked by pretreatment with triorthocresylphosphate (which blocks carboxylesterase but is not a ChE inhibitor), the LD_{50} of malathion becomes 10 mg/kg. Malathion is one of the most utilized insecticides in agriculture and in urban and rural insect control. Exposure to low doses of this compound leads to a relatively low risk of acute poisoning because of its effective detoxification. However, ingestion of large amounts of its concentrated formula is associated with a high morbidity and mortality.[3] Chlorfenvinphos has an LD_{50} of about 30 mg/kg and is inactivated by dealkylation.

ChE activity drops to below 30 percent of normal and is frequently close to 0 percent (vide infra). ChE levels should be determined in any patient with coma of an unknown origin who might have been exposed to OPs. Deep coma, with or without convulsions, is frequently the prominent presenting syndrome of severe acute OP poisoning.

A difficult diagnostic problem is the distinction between a cholinergic syndrome caused by OPs (which are long-acting AChE inhibitors) and one due to carbamate insecticides (short-acting AChE inhibitors). Carbamate poisonings exhibit a relatively moderate CNS syndrome, since most of the carbamates do not significantly penetrate the blood-brain barrier. When ChE levels are performed serially over hours, they will increase following carbamate poisoning due to the spontaneous decarbamylation of ChE. In contrast, the ChE activity will remain persistently depressed following OP poisoning. Some laboratories have the capability to measure red blood cell ChE activity before and after the in vitro addition of oximes. A significant increment in ChE activity indicates OP poisoning rather than carbamate poisoning. Oximes (reactivators) are an important part of OP poisoning treatment, but have no place in the treatment of carbamate poisoning. Therefore, specific diagnosis is clinically relevant.

Treatment

Prevention of death or anoxic brain damage from acute respiratory failure is the first priority in dealing with acute OP poisoning. In severe cases, endotracheal intubation, ventilation with an adequate fraction of inspired oxygen ($F_{I_{O_2}}$), and pharmacologic control of bronchospasm and bronchorrhea are the determinants of survival. Once the patient is stabilized, decontamination and specific therapy with atropine or oximes may be indicated.

DECONTAMINATION. OP compounds are hydrolyzed in an alkaline pH and are well adsorbed by activated charcoal. Therefore, following the initiation of atropine therapy (vide infra), all patients should undergo gastric lavage, followed by activated charcoal administration, removal of clothes, and washing of the skin with mild alkaline soap and water. The treating personnel should wear protective gloves and aprons.

ATROPINE. Bronchospasm, bronchorrhea, and bradycardia are treated by parenteral administration of atropine in doses of 1 to 2 mg intravenously for adults and doses of 0.03 to 0.05 mg/kg for children. After the first injection, atropine boluses may be repeated at intervals of 10 min or more until bronchorrhea and bronchospasm are controlled. Intravenous atropine may induce ventricular arrhythmias in the setting of hypoxemia. Thus, preoxygenation with 100% oxygen before each dose is recommended.[5] Several boluses are usually necessary in the initial phase of treatment, followed by increasing intervals between boluses. After the initial doses, atropine can be administered by continuous intravenous infusion titrated by the degree of bronchospasm, bronchorrhea, or bradycardia. This may be particularly useful if signs persist after the first few hours. The infusion should be initiated at a dose of 1 mg/h. When bronchorrhea and bronchospasm are controlled, the dose is reduced to 0.5 mg/h. If symptoms do not recur, the dose can again be halved to 0.25 mg/h, then finally stopped. The patient with normal lung auscultation and no bradycardia may need no atropine. Administration of atropine until full atropinization (maximal tolerance to atropine) is achieved is unnecessary and potentially harmful. The degree of perspiration and the size of pupils are unreliable guides for continued atropine administration in OP poisoning. Atropine has practically no effect on the nicotinic syndrome.

OXIMES. Oximes (reactivators of AChE) are a major treatment modality in OP poisoning. In most countries, either obidoxime or pralidoxime is available. Oximes are mild ChE inhibitors themselves, so two dosing regimes are used according to the clinical severity of the cholinergic syndrome. In mild cases (not requiring endotracheal intubation), 4 mg obidoxime/kg every 6 h, or 20 mg pralidoxime/kg every 6 h is recommended. An oxime bolus should be given slowly over 20 min by the intravenous route. In severe cases (necessitating endotracheal intubation), higher doses are recommended; 6 mg obidoxime/kg every 5 h or a continuous infusion titrated to achieve an obidoxime blood level of 4 to 8 mg/L. Pralidoxime should be given as a 1-g bolus over 20 min followed by continuous infusion rather than repeated boluses, to achieve serum levels of 10 to 15 mg/L. This may require an infusion of up to 500 mg/h.[6] Oxime levels should be checked at least once on the day that therapy is initiated and again each time the dose is modified. Obidoxime is more active but potentially more toxic than pralidoxime. High doses of obidoxime may lead to liver dysfunction. Therefore, monitoring of liver enzymes and bilirubin is mandatory when using obidoxime. The major disadvantage of oxime therapy is its low penetration through the blood-brain barrier. Although obidoxime penetrates the brain-blood barrier better than pralidoxime, propralidoxime (dihydropralidoxime), which is not a quarternary ammonium, penetrates ten times better than pralidoxime. It is transformed in situ to pralidoxime; unfortunately there is no clinical experience with this promising compound.

If blood levels of oximes are not available, the following estimation can be used for adults with normal liver and kidney functions. For obidoxime, the average plasma half-life is 80 to 90 min, volume of distribution 0.2 L/kg, and clearance 0.1 L/kg/h. Pralidoxime is filtered and actively excreted by the kidneys. Its clearance is slightly higher than the creatinine clearance. Its plasma half-life is about 60 min, and the volume of distribution is 0.6 to 0.8 L/kg. Oxime therapy should be started as soon as possible in every symptomatic patient and continued until full clinical recovery is achieved. Premature interruption in oxime administration is frequently associated with reappearance of symptoms. The duration of oxime therapy is necessarily longer in cases of massive ingestion of highly liposoluble OP compounds.

ANCILLARY THERAPY. Benzodiazepines (diazepam and lorazepam) are recommended for control of convulsions and agitation. Scopolamine has been used as a central anticholinergic drug, but we do not recommend its use because of the narrow toxic to therapeutic range. The role of standard bronchodilator therapy in OP poisoning is unknown. Aminophylline should probably not be given since hypoxemia and ventricular arrhythmias are common. Ipratropium bromide has been found to be useful in several case reports. There is no information regarding the use of β-agonists.

Laboratory Analysis and Monitoring

Pseudocholinesterase (butyryl ChE) is helpful for confirming the diagnosis, but has no value for clinical patient monitoring, because it may remain depressed many days following clinical improvement. Erythrocyte AChE exhibits a better correlation with the clinical syndrome and should be followed serially if possible. This test should be performed initially and after clinical improvement has begun. In severe, prolonged cases, it should be performed every 4 days. Some specialized laboratories can perform the detection of urine metabolites such as alkyl phosphates or the leaving moieties of the original compound. Oxime blood levels are also helpful for appropriate therapeutic drug monitoring.

Blood sugar levels should be monitored repeatedly. Hypoglycemia and hyperglycemia are frequently encountered.[7,8] Serum and urine myoglobin levels should be monitored especially during and after severe convulsions. Serum creatinine and creatinine clearance should be serially measured. Liver enzymes and bilirubin must be followed in cases treated by obidoxime. Pancreatitis has been described as a result of OP poisoning; serum amylase levels should be obtained daily.[9,10]

Evolution and Complications of Acute OP Poisoning

The major cause of death from OP poisoning is respiratory failure.[11,12] Aspiration pneumonitis is frequent and may become superinfected. Bacterial pneumonia is a frequent problem and a potential source of severe sepsis. The usual criteria for discontinuation of mechanical ventilation and for extubation should be modified in acute severe OP poisoning. Extubation should be performed only after spontaneous breathing through a T piece succeeds for several hours, and *never* after only a single measurement of adequate weaning parameters. Life-threatening cardiac arrhythmias are the second most common cause of death in treated OP poisonings. Whenever the QT interval exceeds half the RR interval, the ICU staff should be standing by to insert an emergency temporary pacemaker. If the hospital setting is such that emergency pacemaker insertion is logistically unfeasible, then a pacemaker should be inserted electively and prophylactically. Ventricular overdrive pacing is a recommended treatment for torsade de pointes in OP poisoning.[13] Renal dysfunction is usually manifested as acute, nonoliguric renal failure and occurs in about 13 percent of treated severe cases.[11] The pathophysiology is not known, but it is prudent to avoid hypovolemia and treat myoglobinuria. Liver dysfunction is frequent and has to be carefully monitored, especially in cases treated by obidoxime.[11]

The CNS manifestations often fluctuate. Peripheral motor deficits are frequently asymmetric and variable, and have no prognostic significance during the initial period. Regression psychosis is also a frequent complication occurring usually at the resolution of a severe cholinergic crisis. The syndrome is reversible within 4 to 6 weeks and necessitates involvement of a specialized psychiatric team.

Delayed peripheral neuropathy may occur, usually several weeks after the acute event. All patients should therefore be referred to a neurologist following discharge from the ICU. The diagnosis is based on clinical examination, electromyography, and nerve conduction studies. Neurotoxic esterase assay (performed by specialized laboratories) and sural nerve biopsy assist in making this diagnosis.

CASE PRESENTATION

Case 1

A 34-year-old farmer was brought to the emergency room after he collapsed during spray application of Mevinphos (phosdrin). He had been spraying each morning for the past 10 days and was working with a higher concentration of the compound than recommended by the manufacturer. On examination he was drowsy but arousable and had constricted pupils. The heart rate was 45/min. Bronchospasm and bronchorrhea were evident on auscultation. Pectoral fasciculations were noted. Muscular strength was decreased and he was perspiring heavily.

Humidified oxygen via a face mask was administered. An intravenous line was inserted and 2 mg atropine was administered. His clothes were removed and he was washed with mild alkaline soap and water. Blood samples were obtained and sent for analysis. Obidoxime, 4 mg/kg intravenously, was administered slowly. An electrocardiogram (ECG) showed slight QT prolongation, sinus bradycardia, and occasional premature atrial contractions. Plasma ChE (butyryl ChE) activity was 15 percent of normal with erythrocyte ChE activity also markedly reduced. The patient's condition improved rapidly. He received only four other doses of atropine, 1 mg at 1-h intervals, and three additional doses of obidoxime at 6-h intervals. The next day he was asymptomatic. Plasma ChE activity was still 20 percent of normal, but erythrocyte AChE activity was at the lower limits of normal.

The patient was discharged the next day with instructions to avoid any contact with OP or carbamate insecticides during the next month. He was referred to an occupational outpatient clinic.

Case 2

Emergency medical services were alerted by the family of a 62-year-old farmer who was found unconscious near a container of 50% malathion dissolved in kerosene. He was promptly intubated and manually ventilated with oxygen. After administration of 2 mg atropine intravenously, he was transferred to a local hospital.

Initial assessment revealed a strong odor from his mouth, sinus bradycardia at 50 beats/min, blood pressure of 100/60, wheezing and crackles in both lungs, decreased air entry to the right lower lung, constricted and unreactive pupils, and intense salivation, lacrimation, and perspiration. Neurologic examination revealed deep coma with slight response to pain, generalized decreased muscular strength, and fibrillations and fasciculations of the shoulder muscles and chest wall.

The patient was connected to a ventilator and given 50% oxygen. Two 1-mg boluses of atropine were given at 10-min intervals. The heart rate increased to 80 beats/min, and the bronchospasm and bronchorrhea decreased. A gastric tube was inserted and the stomach fluid was aspirated and sent to a specialized laboratory. Gastric lavage was performed and followed by 60 g activated charcoal. The skin and the hair were washed with mild alkaline soap and water. Blood samples were sent for toxicologic and routine analysis, and the patient was transferred to the ICU. The local Poison Information Center was consulted and, based on PoisIndex recommendations,[14] 1 g pralidoxime chloride was given as a bolus over 20 min. This was followed by a continuous infusion of 500 mg/h.

The first chest radiogram revealed typical findings of right lower lobe aspiration. The patient was mechanically ventilated with 50% oxygen and 5 cm positive end-expiratory pressure. During the first day he received seven boluses of atropine (1 mg) at progressively increasing intervals of 30 min to 3 h. Two other doses of 60 g activated charcoal were introduced into the stomach at 4-h intervals. A slight prolongation of the QT interval and rare premature atrial and ventricular contractions were noted. Provisions were made for emergency placement of a temporary pacemaker. The patient received four doses of diazepam (10 mg) for control of restlessness.

Results from the toxicology laboratory revealed the presence of malathion and petroleum distillate in the gastric aspirate. Pseudo ChE (butyryl ChE) activity was 0 percent and erythrocyte AChE activity was 5 percent of normal.

The next day mental status improved significantly; the patient oscillated between consciousness and drowsiness. The pralidoxime infusion was decreased to 100 mg/h.

On the third day the patient was again deeply comatose, with agitation and two episodes of grand mal seizures. Pralidoxime infusion was increased to 500 mg/h; diazepam and lorazepam were administered for control of convulsions and agitation. The same afternoon tachyarrhythmias were noted on the monitor. A 12-lead ECG confirmed atrial flutter with an atrial rate of 300/min and a ventricular rate of 150 beats/min. The blood pressure dropped from 140/85 to 105/80. Shortly thereafter, ventricular tachycardia developed and the blood pressure dropped still further. The patient was immediately cardioverted with 200 joules. After cardioversion, the QT interval was noted to be normal.

The patient remained comatose until the fifth day, when he progressively awakened. Pralidoxime infusion was stopped the next day. Although the patient was able to obey commands, he still needed mechanical ventilation because of muscular weakness and severe right lower and left upper lobe pneumonia.

On the ninth day of hospitalization he was disconnected from the ventilator and left with a T piece and supplemental oxygen for the next 24 h. Two weeks after ICU hospitalization, he was extubated and transferred to the intermediate care unit. He was discharged from the hospital 6 days later and referred to a neurologist for an ambulatory follow-up.

CASE DISCUSSION

These two cases illustrate the differences between acute poisoning due to occupational exposure, which is usually easily reversible if treated promptly, and massive ingestion of concentrated formula, resulting in severe and prolonged disease and necessitating prolonged ICU therapy. In the first case the patient appeared to progressively inhibit his ChE. He became symptomatic when 70 percent of his ChE was inhibited.

In the second case malathion was probably distributed to the tissues and progressively released during several days. This explains the reappearance of signs and deterioration when oxime therapy was prematurely decreased on the second day. In cases of massive ingestion, oxime therapy should be continued until full recovery and only then reduced. Since the ICU was prepared for emergency insertion of a temporary pacemaker had it been required, there was no need to place one prophylactically. When malignant arrhythmias later occurred, they were in the setting of a normal QT interval; thus, pacemaker placement was not indicated. Given the fluctuating nature of neurologic signs, the patient was left spontaneously breathing through the T piece for 24 h prior to extubation to avoid emergency reintubation.

References

1. Davies JE, Baquet A, Freed VH, et al: Human pesticide poisonings by a fat-soluble organophosphate insecticide. Arch Environ Health 30:608, 1975.
2. Dauterman WC: Biological and nonbiological modifications of organophosphorus compounds. WHO Bull 44:133, 1971.
3. Namba T, Greenfield M, Grob D: Malathion poisoning: A fatal case with cardiac manifestations. Arch Environ Health 21:533, 1970.
4. Durham Sk, Gijbels MJJ: Long-term morphologic and biochemical changes induced by O,O,S,-trimethyl phosphorothioates in the rat lung. Toxicol Appl Pharmacol 98:465, 1989.
5. Taitelman U, Adler M, Levy I: Treatment of massive poisoning by the organophosphate pesticide methidathion. Clin Toxicol 8:277, 1975.
6. Namba T, Nolte CT, Jackrel J, Grob D: Poisoning due to organophosphate insecticides: Acute and chronic manifestations. Am J Med 50:475, 1971.
7. Meller D, Fraser I, Kryger M: Hyperglycemia in anticholinesterase poisoning. Can Med Assoc 124:745, 1981.
8. Hruban Z, Schulman S, Warner NE, et al: Hypoglycemia resulting from insecticide poisoning. JAMA 184:590, 1963.
9. Moor PG, James OF: Acute pancreatitis induced by acute organophosphate poisoning? Postgrad Med J 57:660, 1981.
10. Dressler TD, Goodale RL, Arneson MA, Borner JW: Pancreatitis as a complication of anticholinesterase insecticide intoxication. Ann Surg 189:199, 1979.
11. Finkelstein Y, Kushnir A, Raikhlin-Eisenkraft B, Taitelman U: Antidotal therapy of severe acute organophosphate poisoning: A multi-hospital study. Neurotoxicol Teratol 11:593, 1989.
12. Bardin PG, Van Eeden SF, Joubert JR: Intensive care management of acute organophosphate poisoning: A 7 year experience in the Western Cape. S Afr Med J 9:593, 1987.
13. Ludomirsky A, Klein HO, Taitelman U, et al: QT prolongation and polymorphous (torsade de pointes) ventricular arrhythmias associated with organophosphorus insecticide poisoning. Am J Cardiol 49:1654, 1982.
14. Micromedex, Computerized Clin Info System, August, 1989.

PART IV

PERSPECTIVES ON CRITICAL CARE

EDITORS' INTRODUCTION

In planning a comprehensive review of adult critical care, we noted five important topics which were underemphasized. Although each topic is addressed in previous chapters of this book in the course of discussions of specific critical illnesses, it seemed appropriate to provide a comprehensive review of each of these recurring themes. Accordingly, we invited experts in these areas to contribute their perspective on how these topics impact on critical care.

Much has been and is being written concerning the diverse aspects of medical ethics in critical care. Indeed, our own university has a vigorous academic Center for Clinical Medical Ethics which is involved in research and development in our intensive care units and which staffs an active consultation service. We chose to invite this perspective from an actively practicing academic intensivist who has published extensively on this topic. Dr. Tom Raffin brings a refreshing clarity to the implementation of ethical principles in the daily practice of critical care. We anticipate that his viewpoints concerning defining and applying these principles are sufficiently honed by the clinical reality of critical care as to be most helpful to the practicing intensive care physician–nurse team.

Critical illness in children has so many differences from critical care in adults as to warrant a separate book for the pediatric intensivist. Yet there are similar principles, and many adult intensivists are invited to help care for critically ill children in their own or neighboring ICUs. In our experience, the exchange of critical care principles and practice between adult and pediatric intensivists is helpful and often leads to the innovative approaches which arise from interdisciplinary communication of all sorts. Accordingly, we invited Drs. O'Rourke and Crone—two pediatric intensivists with much experience interacting with their counterparts in adult critical care—to guide the reader concerning key similarities and differences in the principles and practice of pediatric critical care.

Our practice of critical care is based on nurse—physician teamwork, and we believe that all components of this book are relevant to all critical care team members. Nevertheless, unique features of the profession of critical care nursing warrant separate discussion, so that both physicians and nurses gain an informed view of the research advances, areas of special concern, and unique contributions of this discipline to the principles of critical care. Of course, entire books are devoted to critical care nursing, so we invited a prominent contributor to such books—Dr. Marguerite Kinney—to provide the reader with a summary of the contemporary issues. In turn, Dr. Kinney organized the invited experts in providing their perspectives.

Clinical investigation of critical illness is essential for the continued growth of effective critical care. Yet the practice of critical care is often so demanding that the intensivist's time is consumed with providing "state of the art" care. Accordingly, clinical investigation in the ICU requires an organized program parallel to and integrated with the practice of critical care. To assist in the important development of such programs, we invited two intensivists who have contributed significantly to clinical investigations of critical illness in North America and in Europe—Drs. John Murray and Roberto Rodriguez-Roisin—to share their perspective on the principles and disciplines required to initiate and sustain productive clinical investigation in the ICU.

Recent history reveals a synchronous development of the principles and practice of critical care throughout the world. Yet much of this book has a North American bias in the description of critical care. To help balance this view and to provide readers with a more informed understanding of critical care outside North America, we invited a European intensivist with unusual familiarity with intensive care practices throughout the world—Dr. Jean-Louis Vincent—to organize this international perspective. In turn, Dr. Vincent asked critical care colleagues from many nations to describe unique aspects of their critical care programs for comparison and contrast with those in North America.

Each of these perspectives is much more than a chapter in this book, for each addresses multiple topics, often by several authors expert in specific components of the topic. Some, like the pediatric and nursing perspectives, allow the reader to search our specific information concerning detailed approaches to commonly encountered problems. All provide an information base for reflection on aspects of critical care encountered daily.

Chapter 185

PERSPECTIVES ON CLINICAL MEDICAL ETHICS

THOMAS A. RAFFIN

Goals of Critical Care Medicine

Intensive care units have evolved over the past 70 years from postoperative recovery rooms and specialized care units devoted to patients with burns, trauma, war-related injuries, and polio.[1] A little more than 30 years ago, the potential of externally applied countershock to terminate ventricular fibrillation was described. Soon thereafter, mouth-to-mouth ventilation and closed-chest massage were reported, which gave rise to the widespread use of cardiopulmonary resuscitation (CPR). In the early 1960s, only 10 to 20 percent of American acute care hospitals had ICUs. However, by the late 1980s, 80 to 90 percent of the more than 6000 acute care hospitals had designated ICUs, and many large hospitals had numerous specialty critical care units including medical, surgical, cardiac, neurosurgical, cardiovascular surgical, trauma, and burn units.[1]

There are approximately 65,000 ICU beds in America's acute care hospitals, and the overall average daily charge for critical care ranges from $2000 to $8000/day. Using total daily charges, it is estimated critical care costs more than $50 billion/year. Since total health care expenditures in 1990 will be more than $600 billion (and are expected to climb to $1.5 trillion in the year 2000) critical care expenditures now account for almost 10 percent of all national health care expenditures.[2] The current gross national product (GNP) of the United States is close to $6 trillion, and total health care expenditures are more than 12 percent of the GNP. Therefore, the cost of intensive care accounts for almost 1 percent of the GNP.[1]

Along with the expanding numbers of ICU beds, cost, and remarkable growth in medical technology and treatment came inevitable dilemmas in ethical decision-making. In the mid to late 1970s, spurred on by the national publicity devoted to the 1976 Karen Ann Quinlan case in New Jersey, an intense national dialogue emerged over how to make ethical decisions when confronted by critically ill patients who were hopelessly ill.

Physicians, nurses, respiratory therapists, and other members of the ICU health care team have two major goals when caring for patients in ICUs. The first goal is to *save the salvageable.* This means a medical judgment must be made whether or not a patient is salvageable, and then, if the patient appears to be salvageable, the health care providers do all in their power to save the patient as long as this is consonant with the wishes of the patient. Fundamentally, the critical care team is following two age-old tenets of medicine: to restore health and to relieve suffering. These goals of medicine have been handed down through the ages from Hippocrates, Galen, Maimonides, clinicians, philosophers, and ethicists who have attempted to define the goals of medicine. What critical care practitioners do is stop a patient who is in the process of dying by placing the patient on life support such as mechanical ventilation, massive fluid resuscitation with inotropic support, dialysis, or total parenteral or nasogastric tube feeding. Once the patient is stable on life support and the illnesses and injuries have been treated, the critical care team waits for the patient to heal and regain strength. In effect, it is the *wisdom of the body* which dictates which organ systems will heal and which patients will survive. Critical care team members can only do so much. The rest is in the wise hands of nature.

The second major goal of critical care practitioners is to *help the dying have a peaceful and dignified death.* This is a vital goal since so many patients who are admitted into ICUs are admitted to die. This can easily be understood by reviewing mortality rates of specific subpopulations of patients admitted to ICUs (vide infra). Since many patients admitted to ICUs will die, it is important for critical care team members to understand death is both an enemy and a colleague. In other words, it is entirely appropriate and, in fact, a thoughtful and sensitive act to assist a hopelessly ill patient to die with peace and dignity. This should not be perceived as an onerous task to be avoided if possible or as a failure. It takes tremendous skill and sensitivity to work with patients, their families or surrogates, and other health care team members in orchestrating a sensitive and compassionate death. Close attention to the needs of family members who will be left behind can result in a more effective and shortened grieving process and a healthier return to functional life.

The overall death rate for all patients admitted to ICUs is approximately 15 to 20 percent.[3] However, this includes large numbers of patients in subpopulations with low mortality rates. For example, patients who have coronary artery bypass graft (CABG) surgery are admitted to ICUs for 2 to 3 days. Of the more than 300,000 patients in America who had CABG procedures in 1989, the mortality rate was approximately 4 to 6 percent, and the overall cost was $4 to $6 billion. Of the hundreds of thousands of Americans who took overdoses as suicide attempts, only 5 to 10 percent needed to be admitted to ICUs, and of this subpopulation, the overall mortality rate was approximately 5 to 6 percent.[3] These low mortality rates are also seen in other subpopulations of surgical patients who require intensive care such as following carotid endarterectomies and major vascular surgery. In estimating the overall mortality rates of patients in American ICUs, if one eliminates subpopulations of patients with low mortality rates, then a truer overall mortality rate would be 30 to 40 percent.

Since the mid 1970s, investigators have been publishing mortality statistics from individual ICUs.[3] For example, in 1984, Cullen and coworkers updated an earlier study published in 1976 on the outcome of critically ill patients in a surgical ICU.[4] The overall mortality rate was 69 percent as compared to a 73 percent mortality rate in 1976. One difference in the two studies is that, in 1984, it appeared the survivors' quality of life was significantly better. A study by LeGall and coworkers from France revealed 66 percent of patients were discharged from the ICU alive, but the survival rate fell to 50 percent at 6 months and was 49 percent at 1 year.[5]

An important international research effort during this time was the development of classification systems to standardize data concerning critically ill patients. One of the most well known classification systems was the APACHE (acute physiology assessment and chronic health evaluation) system developed by Knaus and coworkers.[6] The original APACHE study gave rise to the APACHE II severity of disease classification system for acutely ill patients.[7] This system uses a point score based on admission values of 12 routine physiologic measurements, age, and previous health status to provide a measure of severity of disease. Investigators discovered an increasing score was closely correlated with the subsequent risk of hospital death for 5815 admissions from 13 hospitals. In 1985, this group published a classic article analyzing the prognosis of ICU patients who have acute organ system failures.[8] Knaus and coworkers developed objective definitions for five organ system failures (cardiovascular, respiratory, renal, hematologic, and neurologic) and then monitored ICU admissions. The number and duration of organ system failures were linked to outcome at hospital discharge for each of 2719 ICU patients (48 percent) who developed them. Their data have been important in understanding the prognosis of critically ill patients in ICUs and providing accurate informed consent to both patients and families. Specifically, their data revealed for all medical and most surgical admissions a single organ system failure lasting more than a day resulted in a mortality rate approaching 40 percent. Among both medical and surgical patients, two organ system failures for more than a day increased death rates to 60 percent. Mortality for 99 patients with three or more organ system failures persisting after 3 days was 98 percent. Advanced chronologic age increased both the probability of developing organ system failure and the probability of death once organ system failure occurred. The APACHE II classification system has helped us understand prognosis in critical care units and has given rise to numerous studies and new research projects among which is the APACHE III project to gain a stronger and more effective data base.

Many subpopulations of critically ill patients in the ICU have death rates as high as 80 to 100 percent. Patients with the adult respiratory distress syndrome (ARDS) have death rates ranging from 65 to 100 percent.[3,9] The prognosis is significantly worse when ARDS is due to bacterial sepsis. Schuster and Marion performed a classic study on ICU outcome in patients with hematologic malignancies.[10] Seventy-seven patients who were admitted to a medical ICU over a 21-month period had their records reviewed. The overall hospital mortality rate was 80 percent. Sixteen patients (21 percent) were discharged from the ICU but died in the hospital. Only 4 of 52 patients who required mechanical ventilation left the hospital alive. Any patient on mechanical ventilation for longer than 5 days died.

A number of studies have identified the marked increase in mortality risk if critically ill patients develop renal failure.[3,8,11] Liver failure has also been shown to carry with it a high mortality rate in ICU patients.[3,12] In a classic study published in 1977, the decision-making autonomy of burn patients was maximized when it was clear from their presentation survival was unprecedented.[13] Imbus and Zawacki took the position that when burns are so severe, survival is unprecedented, and thus, an aggressive approach to decision-making should be invoked to preserve patient autonomy. While still lucid, and with sufficient information, the patient was asked whether or not he or she wished to choose between a full therapeutic regimen or ordinary care. There are clearly patients with severe burns who have, in essence, no chance to survive.

An axiomatic statement can be made about a critically ill patient who is admitted into an ICU: The longer a patient is in the ICU, the greater the chance for severe morbidity or death. This seems like a paradox since there is no safer place for a critically ill patient than an ICU. However, there is also no more dangerous a place. The leading cause of death for critically ill patients is infection, and the ICU, with its invasive procedures and resistant bacteria, is the worst place to become infected. In a 1985 study by Montgomery and colleagues, the causes of mortality in patients with ARDS were evaluated.[9] Forty-seven patients with ARDS had a 68 percent mortality rate. However, only 16 percent of these patients died due to unmanageable respiratory failure. Seventy-three percent of the patients died from sepsis and multisystem organ failure (MSOF). Clinicians who are not familiar with the discipline of critical care would find these data surprising since most would presume patients with respiratory failure on mechanical ventilation die because of difficulties in managing the respiratory failure. As the above study demonstrates, it is uncommon for patients in respiratory failure on mechanical ventilation to die because of difficulty in managing the patient's ventilation. The leading infections in critically ill patients in ICUs are sepsis, pneumonia, and other nosocomial infections such as catheter-related urinary tract infections.[14] For example, it is estimated patients with ARDS experience a 60 percent incidence of nosocomial pneumonia.[15] Nosocomial pneumonia with or without sepsis can lead to MSOF and a grim prognosis. Other key factors leading to death of critically ill patients in ICUs include cardiac arrest and arrhythmias, gastrointestinal bleeding, acute airway problems, abdominal catastrophes, pneumothorax, and pulmonary embolism.[16]

For patients and families, the ICU is a foreign, frightening, and bewildering place. In street clothes, nonhealth care professionals clearly feel out of place. Odd noises assault their ears: high-pitched regular beeps, buzzers, and alarms, and the deep, rhythmic swooshing sounds of machines that aid breathing. Intravenous bottles with tubes dangle from the ceiling like mysterious vines and remind family members of chilling science fiction movies like "Coma." Patients and family members feel completely out of control and as if they were once again children. They are surrounded by frighteningly ill patients who are the center of attention in a massive struggle between highly trained health care providers, remarkable new technology, and the power of nature. Given all the difficulties of critical care for patients and their families, what, indeed, are the survivors' preferences regarding intensive care? A 1988 study was performed investigating patients' and families' preferences for medical intensive care.[17] Patients were interviewed who were at least 55 years old and had been in an ICU during a 1 year period. Family members were interviewed if the patient had died. Of interest, 70 percent of patients and families were 100 percent willing to undergo intensive care again to achieve even a 1 month survival. Only 8 percent were completely unwilling to undergo intensive care to achieve any prolonged survival. Patient or family preferences were not well correlated with functional status or quality of life for 82 percent of the respondents. Age, severity of critical illness, length of stay, and charges for intensive care did not influence willingness to undergo intensive care. This is one of the few studies evaluating patient or family preferences for intensive care. A 1986 paper studied the preferences of homosexual men with AIDS for life-sustaining treatment and found many were willing to forego life-sustaining treatment if the prognosis were extremely poor.[18]

Many individuals who have never been admitted to an ICU are concerned and hesitant about being placed on life support in an effort to save their lives. Additionally, many health care professionals who work in ICUs understand that the struggle of some critically ill patients can be unrelenting torture with no hope for recovery. However, in agreement with the results from the above 1988 study, it seems clear that "substituted judgments" for incompetent patients concerning whether or not to provide or continue critical care must be made with objectivity and great thoughtfulness to ensure reflecting only the values of the patient.

Fundamental Principles of Biomedical Ethics

Biomedical ethics came of age in the 1980s. In 1976, the Karen Ann Quinlan case in New Jersey established that patients with, in essence, no chance to regain a reasonable quality of life could be withdrawn from extraordinary life support.[19] In 1983, the President's Commission for the Study of Ethical Problems in Medicine and Biomedical and Behavior Research published its extensive and groundbreaking report to the nation.[20] During this period, physicians, lawyers, scholars, ethicists, and ethics committees began to study biomedical ethics and the ethical dilemmas which confront medicine.[1,21–27] Because of the exponential growth in technology and the abilities of modern medicine, we are suddenly confronted with novel and highly complex ethical quandaries wherever we turn: the use of human fetal tissue, genetic alteration of nonhuman species, gene therapy in man, and newer approaches to in vitro fertilization. As we stand and pass judgment on these advances in medicine and science, we still remain in conflict over older and extremely complex ethical problems: relieving suffering with powerful analgesics in irreversibly impaired patients which might hasten their deaths, withdrawing food and water from patients in chronic, persistent vegetative states, use of animals in education and research, and the role of abortion.

TABLE 185-1 Four Fundamental Biomedical Ethical Principles

1. Beneficence
2. Nonmaleficence
3. Autonomy
4. Justice

To understand, critically analyze, and make thoughtful judgments about the biomedical ethical dilemmas which confront us in critical care medicine, it is important we are well grounded in the fundamental principles of biomedical ethics.

Ethics is a generic term for a variety of ways of investigating and attempting to define a moral life. Two major ethical theories, consequentialist and deontological, provide the basis for analyzing biomedical ethical issues.[24–27] The consequentialist ethical theory states actions are right or wrong according to their consequences rather than any intrinsic features they may have. One of the key consequentialist theories is utilitarianism whose origins are found in the writings of David Hume, Jeremy Bentham, and John Stuart Mill. Deontological ethical theory states that certain things are inherently right or wrong. Both ethical theories have strengths and weaknesses. In fact, there are major similarities between both theories and a careful analysis of ethical theory and moral reasoning has given rise to the development of four key biomedical ethical principles which can be used in analyzing a particular problem (Table 185-1).

BENEFICENCE

The first biomedical ethical principle is *beneficence* which means to do good or, in medicine, to restore health and relieve suffering. It is the primary duty of the physician to benefit the patient. Fundamentally, this means the health care provider attempts to preserve the patient's life. Preserving life and the appreciation of the sanctity of life has its roots in most religious traditions.

NONMALEFICENCE

The second fundamental ethical principle is *nonmaleficence* which means to do no harm (*primum non nocere*). This is an exceedingly important ethical principle and means a health care provider should not deliver a therapy if the odds are greater it might harm rather than benefit the patient. A good example of a violation of this ethical principle is when a health care practitioner provides a nonindicated therapy to a patient which results in morbidity or mortality. In the ICU, an example of this might be placing a nonindicated intravascular catheter which results in harm or injury. Such an act is in direct violation of the principle of nonmaleficence. Unfortunately, it is common for health care providers to violate this principle because of the great complexity and enormity of available diagnostic and therapeutic modalities. Another example of a violation of the principle of nonmaleficence would be when a patient asks a physician for an antibiotic to treat a viral cold. The physician knows the patient will not be benefitted by an antibiotic. Nevertheless, the physician succumbs to the patient's strong argument and prescribes a commonly used antibiotic. Unfortunately, 6 days later the patient has a violent hypersensitivity reaction to the antibiotic, becomes critically ill, and dies. This type of example which, thankfully, occurs rarely gives us insight into how easily any physician can violate the principle of nonmaleficence.

One of the most frightening violations of the principle of nonmaleficence occurs in the critical care unit. When health care practitioners are caring for patients on life support who have, in essence, no chance to regain a reasonable quality of life and who are simply languishing and suffering, we are violating the principle of nonmaleficence or first do no harm. The Hippocratic oath expresses a duty of nonmaleficence together with beneficence: "I will use treatment to help the sick according to my ability and judgment, but I will never use it to injure or wrong them."[26]

One possible violation of the ethical principle of nonmaleficence has been occurring in the United States since the early 1950s. This has been the practice by some health care providers of attempting to accumulate great wealth through the practice of medicine. We are commonly presented with unfortunate examples of corporations and individuals who have attempted to accumulate inappropriate levels of wealth and profit on the backs of their patients or society's ability to pay for health care. In the American system of health care, this has been a destructive force. Actions such as these clearly "wrong" our patients and society. Examples include inappropriate large profits by corporations producing medical supplies, equipment, and drugs; overutilization of diagnostic and therapeutic modalities including endoscopy and surgery; and charges which allow some health care professionals to have salaries significantly beyond many hundreds of thousands of dollars per year. Entrepreneurial spirit has made American commerce strong, but should our troubled health care system be undermined by lack of effective regulation?

AUTONOMY

The third fundamental ethical principle is *autonomy* which has only become central to the ethical practice of medicine over the past half century. Autonomy means respecting the individuality and personhood of others which allow them to be self-determining agents. Patients should not be treated as children in a paternalistic physician-patient relationship but as partners in adult-to-adult transactions. Patients are more than equal partners in arriving at decisions affecting their own lives and should be encouraged to assume the responsibilities of this partnership. Autonomy is a term derived from Greek and meant self-rule or self-governance in Greek city-states. Citizens made their own laws rather than having them imposed on them. In the Judeo-Christian tradition, great emphasis is placed on respect for other persons. A legally competent adult American who is not trying to commit suicide is in charge of his or her own health care. If a patient refuses treatment, the legal basis for this is the common law right of self-determination and a constitutionally derived right of privacy which is an interpreted right from our Constitution. This legal right of autonomy was recognized by the United States Supreme Court as long ago as 1891, when it stated:

> No right is held more sacred or is more carefully guarded by the common law than the right of every individual to the possession and control of his own person, free from all restraints or interference by others, unless by clear and unquestionable authority of law.[28]

It is paramount in the practice of modern medicine to provide informed consent to patients so they understand the risks and benefits of a diagnostic or therapeutic procedure, and therefore, through their autonomy, make a decision whether or not they want that diagnostic or therapeutic procedure. It is incumbent on the critical care practitioner to be honest and to make sure the communication has been truthful.[29] If an adult patient is not legally competent to receive informed consent, then a close relative or surrogate decision-maker should be involved in decision-making. This will be further discussed in the section on legal precedents. It is important to point out minors in America do not have autonomy under law to make health care decisions for themselves. Additionally, our courts believe they have more responsibility than parents in making key health care decisions for minors. For example, if a family discovers their child has acute leukemia and they want to take the child to be treated with unproven apricot pit (laetrile) therapy instead of standard-of-practice therapy for leukemia, the court will intercede and take the child away from the parents to ensure the child receives standard-of-practice care. Recent decisions concerning children with Christian Scientist parents reluctant to obtain standard-of-practice health care underscore this point. The bottom line for intensive care physicians is that, if a critically ill, definitely salvageable patient who is legally competent and not clearly trying to commit suicide elects not to be admitted to an ICU where mechanical ventilation or other life support could save the patient's life and return the patient to a reasonable quality of life, it is the right of the patient through his or her ethical and legal autonomy to decide not to receive indicated critical care treatment. As will be discussed further on, decision-making capacity lies in the hands of the patient, not in the hands of health care providers.

JUSTICE

The fourth fundamental ethical principle is *justice* which supports the fair allocation of medical resources. At the present time in America, we do not have just allocation of medical resources. Disadvantaged Americans suffer greater morbidity and mortality from major illnesses and die younger in most disease-specific categories than the middle class. Additionally, federal and state governments pass regulations and statutes which provide unjust care for the poor and disadvantaged. For example, to not allow the poor to receive transplantations or abortions while allowing the middle class these treatments is not consonant with a just system of health care.

These four fundamental ethical principles can be used to analyze complex biomedical ethical issues on a daily basis. A scholarly and time-consuming ethical analysis of justice might require studying egalitarian, libertarian, deontological, and utilitarian theories. However, for critical care practitioners, this extent of sophisticated analysis should serve as theoretical background and is not useful in day-to-day decision-making. Using the four fundamental ethical principles helps to place into perspective the ethical dilemmas which confront us and can lead to a more thoughtful and ethical practice of medicine. It is important to remember the four fundamental ethical principles are based on many complex and, at times, antagonistic ethical theories which have evolved through history.

The four ethical principles of beneficence, nonmaleficence, autonomy, and justice can interact in a dynamic and often antagonistic fashion when a specific biomedical issue is analyzed. Depending on one's point of view, an individual can use one or more of these principles to support an argument even though another person may use the same ethical principle to support a diametrically opposed position. One example of how these fundamental ethical principles can come into conflict can be appreciated in the current controversy concerning the management of human immunodeficiency virus (HIV) infections: preventing infections in persons unknowingly exposed to HIV conflicts with respecting the autonomy of infected persons and the confidentiality of their HIV test results.

Legal Precedents in Ethical Decision-Making

Many state courts and legislatures have handed down decisions which have helped build the legal framework in our nation's approach to biomedical ethical issues. It is important to remember that a court decision or legislative action in one particular state does not make precedent or law for any other state. Furthermore, just as individual concepts and insights into morality and ethics differ, so too do the arbitrary judgments of different state and federal courts and legislatures. There is no question that the family histories, life experiences, politics, and personal feelings of individual jurists and legislators play a role in forming their ultimate decisions. Thus, there is an important arbitrary component in judicial and legislative action, but taken as a whole of many sums, the ultimate evolution of decisions reflects society's morality.

The ground-breaking Karen Ann Quinlan case adjudicated in 1976 concerned a 22-year-old woman who became comatose after the probable ingestion of alcohol and tranquilizers.[19] She was maintained on mechanical ventilation, and although not brain dead, appeared to have a dismal prognosis. Her father arranged to have himself appointed legal guardian and, believing that Karen would never want to live under such circumstances, asked her physicians to remove her from the ventilator and allow her to die. The physicians refused, and the Quinlan case went to court.

The New Jersey Supreme Court examined "the reasonable possibility of return to cognitive and sapient life as distinguished from . . . biological vegetative existence."[19] The Quinlan court suggested a benefit exists when life-sustaining treatment contemplates "at very least, a remission of symptoms enabling a return toward a normal functioning, integrated existence." Additionally, the Quinlan court felt these ethical decisions should be made by the physician and family:

> . . . to treat a patient, must deal with medical tradition and past case histories. They must be guided by what they do know. The extent of their training, their experience, consultation with other physicians, must guide their decision-making processes in providing care to their patient. The nature, extent, and duration of care by societal standards is the responsibility of a physician. Mortality and conscience of our society places this responsibility in the hands of the physician. What justification is there to remove it from the control of the medical profession and place it in the hands of the courts?[19]

The New Jersey Supreme Court ruled that Karen had a constitutional "right to privacy" to be removed from the ventilator if the family, the physicians, and hospital ethics committee agreed. Furthermore, the court ruled that, in the absence of information from the patient herself, the physicians and the family had the right to make the decision to withdraw life support; the court clearly implied that, in such situations, the family's wishes could overrule the physician's concerns. In other words, "substituted judgment" could be made for the incompetent adult. As is often the case in patients who are in a chronic, persistent vegetative state, after the ventilator was removed, Karen was able to breath on her own and lived for 10 years with no cognitive function before she died.

In 1977, the Supreme Court of the State of Massachusetts decided in the *Saikewicz v. Superintendent of Belcher State School* case that, without information from the patient and his family, only the court—not the physician and family—has the right to make "substituted judgments" and thus decisions to withhold life support.[30] This decision caused great concern among health care professionals in the State of Massachusetts since they became frightened about making decisions concerning withholding and withdrawing life support without the assistance of the courts. In 1978, the Massachusetts Court of Appeals ruling in the *Dinnerstein* case decided that family and physician could make a thoughtful judgment concerning withholding life support without having to bring in the courts.[31] This judgment along with one or two other cases helped to support the role of physicians and families in making life and death decisions for patients in the State of Massachusetts.

In 1981, Clarence Herbert, a 55-year-old Californian, had a postoperative myocardial infarction which left him with severe brain damage. Two days after the heart attack, his family agreed with his physicians and asked he be withdrawn from life support, citing the patient's earlier comments he did not wish to be kept alive artificially. As with Karen Ann Quinlan, Mr. Herbert did not die after the ventilator was discontinued. Two days later, his family agreed routine life support should be stopped which included intravenous fluids and nutrition. Mr. Herbert died a week later. The two physicians who cared for Mr. Herbert were prosecuted for murder by the Los Angeles District Attorney in 1983 in *Barber v. Superior Court*.[32] The California Trial Court dismissed the charges. The court relied on the vital concept of proportionality as the criterion to be used in deciding whether to withdraw life support. The court stated, "Proportionate treatment is that which, in the view of the patient, has at least a reasonable chance of providing benefits to the patient which outweigh the burdens attendant to the treatment."[32] The Barber court relied on the Quinlan decision when attempting to define such terms as benefits and burdens. The Barber court felt nutrition and hydration were medical procedures and should be evaluated by health care providers:

> Medical procedures to provide nutrition and hydration are more similar to other medical procedures than to typical human ways of providing nutrition and hydration. Their benefits and burdens ought to be evaluated in the same manner as any other medical procedure.[32]

The Barber court also discussed who can appropriately decide for incompetent patients. When patients are incompetent, physicians must identify a surrogate to make a "substituted judgment" on the patient's behalf. The California court stated barring legislation to the contrary, it is legal to bypass formal conservatorship proceedings. The court reasoned the spouse and children are the most appropriate surrogates because they are in the best position to know the patient's feelings and desires regarding treatment, would be affected by the treatment decision, are concerned for the patient's comfort and welfare, and have expressed an interest in the patient through visits or inquiries to the patient's physician or hospital staff.

The right of competent adult patients with imminently fatal diseases to refuse treatment over the objection of physicians and hospitals was affirmed in a California case, *Bartling v. Superior Court*.[33] Mr. Bartling, who was legally competent, and his family desired to have him removed from a ventilator since his prognosis was so poor. The physicians and hospital refused, but eventually, the California Appeals Court ruled in favor of Mr. Bartling following his death. The Appeals Court stated:

> If the right of the patient to self-termination as to his own medical treatment is to have any meaning at all, it must be paramount to the interests of the patient's hospital and doctors. The right of a competent ill patient to refuse medical treatment is a constitutionally guaranteed right which must not be abridged.[33]

A 1986 decision in California established the right of a patient to refuse both nourishment and hydration in *Bouvia v. Superior Court*.[34] In this well-publicized case, an intelligent young quadriplegic woman with cerebral palsy demanded the hospital treating her halt all food and water so she could die because she was in constant pain, was totally dependent on others, and she found her quality of life unacceptable. The California State Court of Appeals, in April 1986, overturned a lower court's decision and held that state policy does not require that "all and every life must be preserved against the will of the sufferer." Thus, Bouvia was allowed to leave the hospital. At this writing, she remains alive.

In 1986, the Massachusetts case, *Brophy v. New England Sinai Hospital*, supported the withholding of nutrition and hydration from a patient in a chronic, persistent vegetative state.[35] The Massachusetts Court took this position because the evidence revealed the patient would never regain cognitive behavior, the ability to communicate, or the capability of interacting purposefully with his environment. The Massachusetts Supreme Judicial Court observed in the Brophy case:

> In certain, thankfully rare circumstances, the burden of maintaining the corporeal existence degrades the very humanity it was meant to serve. The law recognizes the individual's right to preserve his humanity even if to preserve his humanity to allow processes of a disease or affliction to bring about a death with dignity.[35]

In 1987, the New Jersey Supreme Court adjudicated more cases concerning withholding and withdrawing life support and held that a person's right to determine his or her own fate took precedence over even the state's interests.[36,37] The rulings are the first to specifically provide immunity from liability for relatives or friends found to have made decisions on behalf of a patient "in good faith."

In 1988, the State of California in the *Drabick* case ruled mentally incapacitated patients are entitled to have appropriate decisions made in their behalf by surrogate decisionmakers.[38] In this case, the family wanted nutrition and hydration withdrawn from Mr. Drabick who was in a chronic, persistent vegetative state. The court supported the Drabick family, and life support was withdrawn. In 1983, the report of the President's Commission urged adoption of the "proportionate treatment test" in situations where an individual did not make his wishes known in a legally acceptable writing or by some other reliable means such as a living will. In the 1983 *Barber v. Superior Court* decision, the court relied on a proportionate treatment analysis. The Drabick court also focused on the question of whether the benefits of the treatment outweigh the detriments. Specifically, it stated:

> Proportionate treatment is that which, in the view of the patient, has at least a reasonable chance of providing benefits to the patient, which benefits outweigh the burdens attendant to the treatment. Thus, even if a proposed course of treatment might be extremely painful or intrusive, it would still be proportionate treatment if the prognosis was for complete cure or

> significant improvement in the patient's condition. On the other hand, a treatment course which is only minimally painful or intrusive may nonetheless be considered disproportionate to the potential benefits if the prognosis is virtually hopeless for any significant condition.[38]

In the face of the progressive Drabick court decision in California in 1988, the state courts in New York and Missouri made it more difficult to withhold or withdraw life-sustaining treatment from incompetent patients.[39,40] In the New York case of Mary O'Connor, the court ruled treatment must be given unless there is unequivocal evidence the patient would have chosen to refuse it.[39] This rigid and strict decision set a standard of proof few patients are likely to satisfy. In the case of Nancy Cruzan, the Missouri court declared the state had an "unqualified" interest in prolonging life.[40] The Missouri court severely limited the right of families to make decisions on behalf of incompetent patients. It stated families cannot make the decision to have treatments stopped without "the most rigid of formalities." The court set the bright line of either a living will or clear and convincing evidence of a patient's refusal to be treated. However, the Missouri court went on to undermine the power of all advance directives (living wills): "It is definitionally impossible for a person to make an informed decision—either to consent or to refuse—under hypothetical circumstances."[40] Of importance, Missouri's living will law does not permit the refusal of artificial feedings. The court specifically determined that continued tube feedings were "not heroically invasive" because the "invasion took place when the gastrostomy tube was inserted."[40]

In June 1990, the Supreme Court of the United States made its landmark ruling on the Nancy Cruzan case which had been appealed from the State of Missouri.[40–43] This was the first case the Supreme Court of the United States ever ruled on concerning the biomedical ethical issue of withholding and withdrawing life support. The Supreme Court upheld the State of Missouri in its position a state can prohibit families from withdrawing life support from a legally incompetent loved one if there is not definite and convincing data which will support the fact the loved one wanted life support to be withheld or withdrawn. The Supreme Court voted 5 to 4 in upholding the Missouri law requiring clear and convincing evidence of an unconscious patient's wishes before sustenance is removed. At first glance, the decision might appear to have sweeping implications. However, it is actually a narrow ruling which upholds the rights of states to decide what type of evidence they require when allowing families and physicians to withhold or withdraw life support. For example, there are already many states which uphold or support the right of families and physicians to withhold or withdraw life support. Additionally, there are a number of states which have supported the withdrawing of nutrition and hydration from patients in a chronic, persistent vegetative state.[38] Chief Justice William Rehnquist of the Supreme Court wrote: ". . . There is no automatic assurance that the view of close family members will be necessarily the same as the patient's would have been had she been confronted with her situation while competent." Of great importance in the opinion written by Chief Justice Rehnquist, he implied that, if Nancy Cruzan had filled out a living will (which was legally available in the State of Missouri), then the Supreme Court might have honored such a signed statement by the patient. Therefore, the Cruzan decision both supported states rights to decide how to handle withholding and withdrawing life support and also upheld the importance of advance directives which could determine whether or not life support could be withheld or withdrawn from an incompetent patient. Chief Justice Rehnquist wrote, "For purposes of this case, we assume that the United States Constitution would grant a competent person a constitutionally protected right to refuse life saving hydration and nutrition."

There are certain to be future state and Supreme Court decisions concerning biomedical ethical issues germane to the practice of critical care medicine. Withholding and withdrawing life support is probably the most important biomedical ethical issue in intensive care, but there are many others which have an important impact on the care of critically ill patients.

Government Legislation and Regulations in Ethical Decision-Making

In the early 1980s, state legislatures began to pass living will legislation which would allow state citizens the right of dictating what type of health care they would receive if they became legally incompetent.[44] There are three types of living will or advanced directive documents passed by individual states. First, some states call them living wills. Second, some statutes are known as natural death act directives. Finally, many states are beginning to pass legislation to support legal durable powers of attorney for health care.[45] Generic living wills (not necessarily passed by a specific state legislature) are available from the Society for the Right to Die or Concern for Dying.[28] It is important to remember that if a living will has not been approved by a specific state legislature, then it is not legally binding. Thus, if you have a Durable Power of Attorney for Health Care from the State of California and become critically ill and lose your legal competence in the State of Missouri, the California living will document does not have validity in Missouri. However, living will documents are still of much value to families, loved ones, friends, and health care providers in determining what the patient would have wanted. More than 40 states have passed living will legislation.

Probably the most effective type of advance directive is a durable power of attorney for health care. The first durable power of attorney for health care was passed in the State of Pennsylvania in 1982. In 1984, the legislature of the State of California developed the California Durable Power of Attorney for Health Care which identifies a legally protected feature whereby people can indicate treatment preferences in various situations and designate an "attorney in fact" who is empowered to make medical decisions should a patient become unable to decide for him- or herself.[45]

In the same way a will is extremely important to American citizens because it guarantees the person's wishes concerning his or her estate are carried out after death, a living will is a document which all adult Americans should have to guarantee that their wishes are carried out concerning what health care should be delivered to them if they become legally incompetent. Extensive court precedent and legislative action support the view that life-sustaining treatment can be withheld if it can be determined the incompetent patient would not have wanted it.[1,20,21,32,38] It is not necessary for persons filling out a living will to list all the specific management approaches they would like taken if a specific illness or catastrophe befalls them. Living wills should be completed with generic statements such as: "If I have, in essence, no chance to regain a reasonable quality of life, please withhold and withdraw life support (including nutrition and hydration) from me so I can die with peace and dignity." There are some lawyers who encourage individuals to develop contingency plans in response to a wide variety of potential critical medical problems. Since every critically ill patient and medical circumstances are somewhat different, this type of laundry list approach is not of much value. Therefore, in the *Cruzan* case decided by the Supreme Court of the United States, "clear and convincing evidence" should be fulfilled by the above statement and not a hypothetical extensive list of management approaches.[40] In the 1988 *O'Connor* case in the State of New York, there is also a strong call for an unreasonable extent of documentation to identify what the patient would have wanted in a specific clinical situation. This might have been solved by a living will with a generic statement. Partially in response to the *O'Connor* case, the New York State legislature in June 1990 adopted a law letting the sick designate a proxy to make health care decisions for them when they no longer are able. The measure is similar to California's Durable Power of Attorney for Health Care.

Besides the growing availability of state court decisions and legislated living wills, the United States executive branch became involved in biomedical ethics by passing regulations concerning the withholding and withdrawing of life support from infants: the "Baby Doe" rule.[46] The "Baby Doe" rule which was specified in the 1985 Child Abuse and Neglect Prevention and Treatment Program attempted to regulate when it was appropriate to withhold and withdraw life support from infants. The "Baby Doe" rule came about due to a case in 1982 when a child with Down syndrome and esophageal atresia with a tracheoesophageal fistula did not have surgery because of the parents' refusal, and a juvenile court judge upheld the rights of the parents to make this decision. "Baby Doe" died several days later. President Reagan instructed the Secretary of Health and Human Services to notify health care providers of the applicability of regulations passed in 1973 to the treatment of handicapped patients (newborns). Following this, the Department of Health and Human Services developed the "Baby Doe" rule. After many court hearings, much publicity, and finally congressional debate, Congress passed the Child Abuse Amendments of 1984. Essentially, the "Baby Doe" rule states that life support can only be withheld or withdrawn if the baby is already dead or definitely going to die. For a neonatologist caring for hopelessly ill low-birth-weight infants in an ICU, these guidelines are not of significant assistance, and in fact can interfere with sound and sensitive decision-making. For example, if a neonate on a ventilator for 7 weeks is catastrophically impaired with the infant respiratory distress syndrome and profound cerebral damage from bleeding, and it has, in essence, no chance to regain a reasonable quality of life, the "Baby Doe" rule as passed in the Child Abuse Amendments of 1984 would not support the withdrawal of life support unless it could be proven the neonate was definitely going to die. Most experts from the fields of neonatology, pediatrics, and ethics believe it is appropriate to consider "quality of life" issues in deciding whether or not to withhold or withdraw life support from neonates. In fact, there is no question many parents and physicians are considering the infant's future potential "quality of life," and if it appears the infant has almost no chance to survive and if he survived, he would be catastrophically impaired, then decisions are being made to withdraw life support, and let infants such as these die. This unusual type of governmental regulation has not been repeated in other complex biomedical ethical settings, and it is hoped future directions in ethical decision-making not be encumbered by regulations emanating from the executive branch of the government. If anything, a well-intentioned government which attempts to practice medicine makes itself vulnerable to violation of the fundamental ethical principle of nonmaleficence—first do no harm.

TABLE 185-2 Four Key Practical Principles for Ethical Decision-Making in Critical Care Medicine

1. Establish the source of authority for decision-making
2. Achieve effective communication with patients and families
3. Early determination and ongoing review of patient desires
4. Recognition of patients' rights

Key Practical Principles in Ethical Decision-Making

There are four key practical principles which must be followed when considering withholding and withdrawing life support or other biomedical ethical issues dealing with patient care (Table 185-2). These four practical principles are: **1.** establish the source of authority for decision-making; **2.** achieve effective communication with patients and families; **3.** early determination and ongoing review of patient desires; and **4.** recognition of patients' rights.[1,21]

SOURCE OF AUTHORITY

The most important key practical principle in ethical decision-making in the ICU is the constant awareness of the true source of authority. Although physicians identify the options available to patients, all involved should recognize the actual authority over the patient never resides with the physician. Patients have the ethical and legal autonomy to decide what type of health care they will receive. If the patient is incompetent, then appropriately identified family or other surrogates (e.g., "attorney-in-fact" identified in a durable power of attorney for health care) have the right to decide what happens to them. Many of the ethical problems and controversies in critical care are a result of overt or covert violations of this principle. Physicians are, in effect, consultants engaged to evaluate their patient's problems, present reasonable options for diagnosis and management in straightforward and understandable language, and facilitate thoughtful decision-making. Except in emergencies, physicians should not proceed with diagnostic or therapeutic plans until those with the true authority have clearly decided.

EFFECTIVE COMMUNICATION

The second key practical principle in ethical decision-making in critical care medicine is the necessity of health care providers being able to communicate effectively with patients and families. Excellence in communication skills varies considerably among critical care providers from physicians through social workers. Especially in critical care situations, stress, fear, intimidation, and unfamiliarity with the setting can overwhelm even sophisticated patients and families. Critical care professionals are responsible not merely for attempting to communicate, but for ensuring that effective communication takes place. In essence, the solution to thorny problems involving withholding and withdrawing life support comes through effective communication with patients, families, and surrogates. There is no more important a skill to have in the intensive care setting.

Some physicians communicate better than others. When physicians are made aware of communication problems by patients, families, or members of the health care team, they should promptly enlist a proven facilitator—a social worker, chaplain, rabbi, ethicist, or psychotherapist, for example. There are several reasons why communication in the critical care setting is difficult for physicians. First, each case is stressful and emotionally wrenching, taking a major physical and psychologic toll on physicians. Second, the accumulation of many such cases exacts a high price from physicians in terms of emotional fatigue and distance, personal fear of death, guilt, insecurity, and anxiety. In fact, it is probable many critical care providers will "burn out" due to the remarkably high stress of their job. Third, effective communication in catastrophic situations requires time, a scarce commodity among physicians. With the demands of stress and time in such a work environment, it is understandable why physicians often have difficulty in nurturing their personal lives. It is important to again emphasize that outside facilitators can be extremely valuable on the health care team because they have the communication skills and the time to exercise them. Unfortunately, physicians and other critical care providers sometimes feel a loss of control when they involve facilitators to assist them in handling difficult cases often dealing with withholding and withdrawing life support. It should be a rule rather than an exception to bring in a facilitator at an early stage whenever it appears the ethical decision-making will be difficult.

A number of things can be done to optimize effective communication: **1.** Create an environment that fosters communication. Rushed or chaotic settings such as a hospital corridor hinder effective decision-making. **2.** Remember that stress often impairs the reasonability of patients, families, and health care providers. Keep communication simple until it is clear that more detail will be helpful rather than overwhelming. **3.** Encourage patients and families to ask questions and express their feelings. This helps to counteract the intimidation many people experience when dealing with health care providers and ICUs.

Remember to present information in the language and at the level of detail that best enables patients or surrogates to decide. It is not useful to speak honestly about a situation if you are distancing people with an esoteric medical vocabulary, unnecessary details, or an inappropriate emotional tone. Ask patients and families to summarize what has been said to check the accuracy of communication, provide a chance to correct misunderstandings, and assess their level of comprehension and reasoning. All critical care providers should make an effort to gain insight into and optimize their communication skills. Colleagues who act as observers can be most helpful in this endeavor.

An example of poor communication in a critical care setting would be when a physician tells a family their critically ill loved one is "stable" without much in the way of further explanation. Perhaps, a more truthful report to the family would be: "Your husband is as sick as any person could be, and the odds are overwhelming he will not survive. His status has not changed in the last 24 hours, and if he does not improve over the next several days, we might have to begin to discuss decreasing our level of critical care support."

Another example of poor communication is when a health care provider tells a family their critically ill sister has improved after 3 days whereas in fact her overall status still carries a dismal prognosis, and only one small relatively unimportant physiologic criteria has mildly improved. This type of inappropriate good news, although making the health care provider feel better, puts the patient's family and loved ones on an unrealistic roller coaster and inappropriately alters their expectations. Great care should be used in attempting to identify at all times what the true prognosis for any patient is before discussing daily, often unimportant, fluctuations in status.

QUALITY-OF-LIFE VALUES

The third key practical principle in ethical decision-making is the necessity for early determination and ongoing review of individual quality-of-life values. The ethics of life support require physicians to learn, whenever possible, the views of each patient or surrogate on the balance between quality and mere prolongation of life—this is the concept of proportionality which was discussed in the section on legal precedents. Critical care professionals should diligently avoid making assumptions in this area, especially with patients of different religious or ethnic backgrounds. The balance between the probable extension of life and the reduction in quality of life resulting from any treatment must be explicitly described and discussed with each patient. It is essential to be both truthful and sensitive when discussing the level of discomfort associated with any anticipated treatment.

When physicians were more paternalistic several decades ago as compared to being partners in health care exemplified by today's practice of critical care, they also painted an unduly optimistic picture. This was a significant error, and certainly is one now, since physicians who do this unintentionally appear untrustworthy at a time when the ability to trust one's physician is particularly critical. The same applies to families who want to withhold information from patients. In almost all cases, it is a physician's duty to be honest and straightforward with the patient for whom he cares concerning diagnosis, treatment options, and prognosis. Specific treatment options for probable complications should be explored as early as possible to avoid unnecessary guilt in surrogates who are forced to decide for incompetent patients. After permission from patients, family members should be included in anticipatory decision-making so they have no doubt about the patient's wishes. For example, having a patient agree with a do-not-resuscitate (DNR) order without informing the family might result in a situation where the patient becomes legally incompetent and the family refuses to follow the wishes of the patient even though the patient's wishes were stated in front of several critical care providers. What can result is a complex, highly emotional, and adversarial relationship between the patient's surrogates and the health care team.

As an illness progresses, patients commonly reassess the relative costs and benefits of treatments as they gain understanding into available therapies and prognosis. Thus, it is important to evaluate patients' insights into proportionality if the patient's status changes significantly. Such reassessment also requires active and careful exploration of the feelings of families because they might participate in decision-making or influence those of the patient.

Any medical intervention should be oriented toward the patient's goals as well as toward solving a clinical dilemma. In many cases, there is a critical point beyond which medical interventions may act less to prolong accessible life than to extend a miserable dying process.[1,20,21,25,47,48] Professionals cannot expect patients or families to take the lead in raising these questions.

PATIENTS' RIGHTS

The fourth key practical principle in ethical decision-making in critical care medicine is the recognition that patients have significant rights. Unbeknownst to most physicians, the American Hospital Association developed a code of patients' rights, and this code has been enacted into law in many states.[49] If critical care practitioners observe the spirit of these rights, then ethical decision-making will not be a major difficulty. Some of the most important of these patients' rights are: **1.** to receive considerate and respectful care; **2.** to receive information about the illness, the course of treatment, and the prospects for recovery in terms the patient can understand; **3.** to receive as much information about any proposed treatment or procedure as the patient may need to give informed consent or to refuse this course of treatment (except in emergencies, this information should include a description of the procedure or treatment, the medically important risks involved in this treatment, alternative courses of treatment or nontreatment and the risks involved in each, and the name of the person who will carry out the treatment or procedure); **4.** to participate actively in decisions regarding the medical care (to the extent permitted by law, this includes the right to refuse treatment); and **5.** to have patients' rights applied to the person who may have legal responsibility to make decisions about medical care on behalf of the patient.[21]

Brain Death and Organ Transplantation

The development of organ transplantation has been one of the most exciting and remarkable stories in modern scientific medicine. Transplantation of kidneys, hearts, and bone marrow is commonplace. Heart-lung, bilateral lung, and unilateral lung transplantation is now becoming established as an effective therapy for selected patients.[50] In the early days of the development of organ transplantation, the definition of death was redefined so physicians who removed organs from patients who were on life support were not accused of murder. In the early to mid 1960s there was no widely accepted definition of brain death. Courts and state legislatures felt the definition of death had to be decided by the expert testimony of physicians. The traditional definition of death was still intact which stated death was recognized by the cessation of function of both the heart and the lungs.

In 1968, the Ad Hoc Committee of the Harvard Medical School published their landmark report "To Define Irreversible Coma as a New Criterion for Death."[51] Death is now defined as the total and irreversible loss of brain function.[20] To identify brain death, one must demonstrate irreversible loss of cerebral hemispheric and brain stem function including ventilatory reflexes. If patients have been taking drugs which affect the central nervous system or are hypothermic, they cannot be declared brain dead until these conditions have been reversed. It is not mandatory to perform electroencephalography or cerebral blood flow studies in patients to confirm brain death. Family or surrogate approval is not required before brain death is determined because clinical diagnosis is a medical issue. However, it is mandatory family or surrogate approval be given before retrieval of organs for transplantation.

Uncommonly, families will not allow physicians to withdraw life support from their brain dead relatives. This usually occurs because of bewildering emotional turmoil caused by the catastrophic injury to their loved one. However, with honest and sensitive communication, most of these problems can be solved within 1 to 2 days.

Since one of the major limitations to widespread transplantation in the United States is scarcity of donor organs, it is extremely important to make sure health care providers discuss this issue with family members or surrogates of patients who are brain dead or near brain death and might be ideal organ donors. These issues must be discussed in a truthful and compassionate fashion. Recently, several states have adopted legislation which requires discussion of potential transplant donor status with the surrogates of patients who are brain dead. Some of this legislation identifies legal liability for health care providers who do not hold such discussions.

Withholding Basic Life Support

Providing basic life support such as food, water, and supplementary oxygen are difficult to forego in medical practice. Oftentimes, health care professionals provide these basics of care as a reflex, without fully considering if they are performing a truly caring act.

In critical illness, thoughtful clinicians need to replace such impulses with a careful decision-making process that takes into account several important points: **1.** Every medical intervention should serve what patients consider to be their best interests as determined in an active truthful dialogue with their families and their physicians. **2.** As in most cases involving the withholding or withdrawing of life support (or any major medical intervention), it is wise to include close family members in the decision-making process whenever possible. This will enlist the family on the side of the eventual treatment course, minimizing the possibility of emotional and adversarial conflicts at times of significant stress. **3.** Physicians should anticipate the likely medical course or courses and obtain clearly in advance the specific choices the patient wishes to make for each major situation. **4.** Once any medical intervention is begun in grave illness, withdrawing it to avoid an agonizing dying process requires a direct action that may result in a death. However necessary and humane such an action may be, those forced to make such decisions and those who carry them out are inevitably left with disturbing feelings. Additionally, the types of medications used need to be evaluated carefully. For example, patients who are terminally ill, suffering, and awaiting death, might be better served by not having infections treated with antibiotics or cerebral edema treated with steroids. It is horrible to observe comatose, hopelessly ill patients being pulled back needlessly from a painless death to live out an extra few days or weeks in pain and indignity. When this situation occurs, it is possibly due to some physicians, who are frustrated by underlying illnesses that defy medical intervention, attempting to gain a sense of control by treating conditions and not treating the patient. If family members or legal surrogates for the patient want every possible measure taken to keep the patient alive, professionals should comply with this request. If the desire to persist in treatment seems inappropriate to the critical care providers, a direct, logical challenge will often fail, whereas a sensitive and compassionate exploration of underlying feelings can result in more thoughtful ethical decision-making.[21]

Physicians need to clarify the purpose of placing intravenous lines. Unless a patient-oriented goal has been defined, it is not acceptable to begin intravenous therapy for hydration and nutrition. As in all forms of therapy, once an intravenous line is in place, it becomes harder to stop treating infections and chemical imbalances that might provide a humane death. The same reasoning applies to ordering laboratory tests or assessing vital signs. Once a treatment problem is identified, it becomes harder not to act especially because of the fear of plaintiff's attorneys and legal liability. Obviously, cautions similar to placing intravenous lines apply to the placement of feeding tubes, especially in patients in chronic, persistent vegetative states.

Withholding Advanced Life Support

The application of CPR raises many ethical issues. A patient in cardiac or pulmonary arrest presents professionals with a critical care emergency that requires a set of automatic responses if function is to be restored before severe organ damage or death occurs. Unless they are aware of the patient's previously expressed wishes about resuscitation, physicians must act first and evaluate later. No one is interested in paramedics on a routine basis delaying CPR while attempting to analyze the ethics of the situation.

A 1983 study of all the resuscitations at a major medical center in 1 year revealed only 14 percent of those who received CPR survived to leave the hospital.[52] Only 19 percent of all patients discussed the procedure with their physicians, and in only 32 percent of the cases was the family consulted about resuscitation, even though more than 95 percent of the physicians claimed to believe such consultations appropriate. In a 1986 study, 22 percent of patients and 86 percent of families were involved in decisions not to resuscitate.[53] The families identified the attending physician as a source of help with their decisions. Other useful factors included the presence of coma or brain death, indicating a hopeless prognosis; support and reassurance from physicians and nurses that the decision was appropriate; assurances from staff that care and comfort would be maintained; and previous conversations with the patient about CPR.

A 1989 study determined the success rate of CPR in 503 consecutive patients aged 70 and over in five Boston health care institutions.[54] Initially, 22 percent of the patients survived, but only 3.8 percent survived to hospital discharge. Only 2 of 244 patients with out-of-hospital cardiopulmonary arrest left the hospital alive. Only 17 of 259 patients with in-hospital arrest survived to discharge. Most of these survivors had ventricular arrhythmias and were resuscitated within minutes. The poorest outcomes were for patients with unwitnessed arrests, terminal arrhythmias such as asystole and electromechanical dissociation, and patients with CPR lasting more than 15 min.

The above studies underscore the ethical dilemma presented by CPR. Given the invasive and, at times, almost brutal nature of the procedure, it is hard to reconcile the small chance of a successful outcome with the loss of a more dignified death. This is especially so in the setting of chronic, severely debilitating, or terminal conditions. In attempting to minimize the occurrence of this type of dilemma, the critical care provider should take several important points into account: **1.** Since cardiopulmonary arrest is likely to occur during the hospitalization of an elderly, chronically ill or terminally ill person, there is little ethical justification for not discussing it in advance. This imperative also applies to similar patients who remain at home or in nursing homes. **2.** The code status of patients should be identified early and efficiently conveyed to patients, families, and all health care providers. **3.** Prominent signs in the front of medical charts or records are useful. **4.** Attending physicians must take the lead in bringing up this matter. If they neglect to do so, everyone pays a high price. Physicians who feel uneasy with such decision-making or who are not fully prepared to support it have an obligation to seek education or counselling to prepare them to perform this duty effectively. All critical care medicine training programs should devote a component of their educational program to this area. Where there is any doubt or a persistent lack of unanimity on the critical care team, it is often of significant help to enlist the aid of a facilitator to discuss the thoughts and feelings of each member of the team.

Some physicians have difficulty in asking patients about whether or not they want a DNR order written in the chart. The reasons for this have been described above and include stress, time limitations, and the emotional difficulty of having such a discussion with a patient—especially a long-term patient who might even be a friend. Another reason why some physicians do not regularly discuss potential DNR orders with their patients is because most severely ill patients when asked whether or not they want a DNR order elect not to have one written in the chart. The main reason for this is man's tenacity in holding on to life. A look down from the precipice into the jaws of death is frightening and something which we attempt to avoid at all costs even when death is near. However, physicians should not be dissuaded from asking patients about DNR orders. In fact, to make this type of discussion more productive, physicians should always ask two questions (Table 185-3). The first question is whether or not the patient wants a DNR order written on the order sheet in the medical chart. The second question in Table 185-3 should be asked if the patient does not want a DNR order. The majority of patients who will not agree to a DNR order will agree to this second proposal. If a patient does agree with this second question, then it should be documented in the medical chart in front of witnesses, and the family and legal surrogates should immediately be notified to make sure they are aware of the patient's plan. Thus, talking with patients about whether or not they want CPR is vitally important and, in almost all cases, will assist health care providers in understanding how to care for their patients.

TABLE 185-3 Two Questions to Ask Patients When Discussing DNR Orders

1. "Would you like us to write a DNR order in your medical chart? This means, if you have a cardiopulmonary arrest, you will not be resuscitated, and therefore, you will probably not survive."
2. To be asked if the patient wants CPR: "Let's presume you are successfully resuscitated and admitted to the ICU on life support. If the critical care team determines after 72 h of doing all in their power to save your life that you have, in essence, no chance to regain a reasonable quality of life, would you agree to let us withdraw life support and let you die with peace and dignity?"

In the late 1980s, biomedical ethicists began to define the obligations of the physician when care was medically futile. In 1988, Tomlinson and Brody stated, "The right of self-determination, as well as the patient's preferences, is irrelevant to the determination that resuscitation would be of no medical benefit. When this is the rationale for a DNR decision, the physician has no duty to ascertain the patient's preferences."[55] Although the physician should always make an effort to ascertain the patient's preferences to optimize sensitive and thoughtful communication, the underlying point is that, if a diagnostic or therapeutic management option is medically futile, the critical care team is not clearly obligated to pursue the option. Some hospitals in the United States have CPR policies which state CPR does not have to be administered if it is deemed to be medically futile by the physician(s) of record.

The key problem in all of this is: What is the definition of medical futility? Many believe three criteria need to be met to establish medical futility. First, the disease must be terminal. Second, the disease must be irreversible. Third, death must be imminent. However, the definition of imminent is not clear. Most health care providers, patients, jurists, and ethicists would agree that imminent could easily be defined as 24 to 48 h. However, does imminent death mean within 7 days, 2 weeks, or 2 months? Additionally, there have not been enough significant court cases to help us define medical futility. Therefore, to claim care is medically futile should not be used as an excuse not to effectively communicate with the patient or the patient's family or legal surrogates. Thoughtful decision-making comes through communication.

In 1989, Siegler and colleagues wrote an article concerning the illusion of futility in clinical practice.[56] The authors made the point a physician is under no obligation to offer, or even discuss, futile therapies. They identify how this is supported by moral reasoning in ancient and modern medical ethics, by public policy, and by case law. However, they quickly point out there are no strict criteria for defining futility. They emphasize the importance of health care providers following both clinical judgment and an explicit consideration of the patient's goals for therapy. Claims of medical futility should not be used to avoid difficult discussions with patients, their families, or surrogates.

In 1990, Schneiderman and colleagues attempted to find a practical way of identifying medical futility.[57] They proposed, ". . . When physicians conclude (either through personal experience, experiences shared with colleagues, or consideration of published empiric data) that, in the last 100 cases a medical treatment has been useless, they should regard that treatment as futile. If a treatment merely preserves permanent unconsciousness or cannot end dependence on intensive medical care, the treatment should be considered futile."[57] This is an interesting proposal and will be one of many which are eventually settled by state judicial decisions defining when physicians can determine a course of treatment is medically futile and withhold treatment. The issue of medical futility will prove to be one of the most important biomedical ethical issues in the 1990s.

Withdrawing Advanced Life Support

The decision to withdraw advanced life support can be one of the most difficult for critical care providers, family members, and surrogates.[1,21,58–60] Ideally, if such measures are carefully considered as outlined above, the guidelines for their withdrawal will have been well defined by patients, families, or surrogates. In reality, such clear definition is more the exception than the rule. The following are some suggestions for critical care providers when considering withdrawing advanced life support.

Carefully judge the likelihood of medical benefit using published data from studies such as APACHE II.[3]

Assess whether or not a patient is legally competent. A sound evaluation of mental status is vital to decision-making, and psychiatric consultation should be sought when the state of competence cannot be clearly identified.

Always attempt to seek unanimity among members of the critical care team. Problems arise when critical care team members feel excluded from the decision-making process. Because critical care nurses provide the great majority of the intensive care, they often have unique information about patients and families that is available only to those who spend long hours at the bedside.

Vigorously solicit the patient's judgment regarding withdrawal of life support. Although most persons on life support will be legally incompetent, a significant percentage will not be as was exemplified in the California court case of Mr. Bartling (vide supra).[33] Competent patients who request life support be stopped must be evaluated carefully. Such patients have a legal right to control their health care, and professionals who do not comply may be committing battery.

Do not rush decision-making with families. These are delicate processes which have their own timing and often are not worked out for many days. Facilitation by nonphysician experts, especially representatives of organized religion or social workers, is often invaluable. Calling in facilitators early as compared to later is a wise choice. The health care team should work with the family toward making a unanimous decision regarding the life support of incompetent patients.

It is extremely valuable to establish time-limited goals based on clinical judgment and information from published studies. After being advised that life support should be discontinued, families are often overwhelmed with confusion and guilt and may resist the advice. They can be helped in their decision-making if concrete, temporal milestones can be identified that herald improvement or failure. For example, the physician might say to the adult children of a man who had been on a ventilator with respiratory and renal failure for 2 weeks, "If we see no signs your father has improved over the next 72 h, then we believe you should consider withdrawing life support. We believe your father is suffering and has essentially no chance to regain a reasonable quality of life. To withdraw life support would allow him a more peaceful and dignified death."[21]

Time-limited goals for decision-making can be from several to many days. The most important thing is, if one simply attempts to make decisions on a day-by-day basis, it is extremely difficult to step back and gain a broad perspective in understanding the real prognosis. The interlude provided by time-limited goals is a period for families to let go of their unrealistic expectations and begin to accept the sad situation. Competent and sensitive facilitation of this process is extremely valuable. Sometimes, before patients and families can come to a thoughtful decision, they may need to express anger and mistrust generated by suboptimal communication with health care providers. Regularly, physicians must tolerate expressions of hostility without becoming defensive. Patient and family anger usually subsides once it is perceived critical care team members are truly understanding and supportive. Even if patients or families do not express anger, it is wise to attempt to facilitate patients and families in expressing it. Statements such as, "This may have turned out to be a lot more than you bargained for. It wouldn't surprise me if you are angry about it," can open the way to the expression and resolution of feelings.

An effective way of telling patients or families that you believe life support should be withdrawn is to say, "It is my best judgment, and that of the other physicians and nurses, that your relative has essentially no chance to regain a reasonable quality of life. I am saying this based on what I understand to be your relative's desires for quality of life. We believe life support should be withdrawn, which means your relative will probably die." There are two important components of this statement. First, the statement is realistically qualified in a way that implies a decision must be shared. Second, it makes clear that death is the probable result of the recommended course. Without this knowledge, there is no true informed consent, and potential emotional and legal liability looms.

It is not uncommon for grief-stricken or guilty family members to attempt to relieve their distress at the patient's expense by pressing for disproportionate treatment. A good example of this would be a son returning home to visit his critically ill mother on a ventilator who has, in essence, no chance to regain a reasonable quality of life. Because the son has not written or communicated with his mother for 10 years, he is overwhelmed by guilt. It is common in such a situation for the son to be totally against withdrawing life support. Such insistence usually dissolves once the underlying feelings are acknowledged and understood.

As a general principle, health care professionals should avoid involving themselves with cases which are inconsistent with their ethical principles. Resentment inevitably arising under such circumstances may compromise clinical judgment. If the critical care professional desires, the care of the patient can be transferred in an appropriate fashion to another professional. This should be an unusual event. If involvement with the patient cannot be avoided by the critical care professional, then frequent ventilation of feelings with understanding colleagues will make optimal care more likely.

If patients are legally incompetent and no documented written or oral communication about withdrawal of treatment exists, the problem is greater. This was true in the recent Supreme Court decision about Nancy Cruzan and the New York ruling on the *O'Connor* case.[39,40] However, it must be remembered, in these two cases, the key issue was withdrawing basic life support which is hydration and nutrition as compared to withdrawing advanced life support. Critical care providers must be knowledgeable about their own state's laws when attempting to care for incompetent patients with no written or oral communication about withdrawal of treatment. Overall, the most satisfactory resolution of such cases occurs when professionals and families painstakingly explore the quality of life values previously held by the patient. Once family members have agreed the patient would not have wanted to go on, consent to withdraw treatment usually follows. If no one knows the patient well enough to provide information about his or her quality of life values, professionals can establish an interdisciplinary group composed of physicians, nurses, families or friends, and two to three patient advocates (at least two of whom represent an organized religion, preferably that of the patient). This group identifies what it believes to be the most thoughtful "substituted judgment." Decisions should be made by family, friends, health care providers, and facilitators. Only rarely is legal assistance necessary.

Withdrawing Basic Life Support

The withdrawal of basic life support such as hydration or nutrition by intravenous lines or feeding tubes is legally controversial. This has been covered significantly in the section on legal precedents. Since it is now a state's rights issue as to whether or not it is legal to withdraw basic life support in patients who have not left clear instructions such as in a living will, all critical care providers should be familiar with their own state's laws. For example, to withdraw basic life support from a patient who did not leave "clear instructions" in the State of Missouri would be against the law.

The key to resolving ethical problems in this area lies in clarifying patient's interests. In the presence of truly informed consent and sensitive psychosocial management of decision-making, most painful ambiguities can be resolved. Communication, as always, is the key. The patient's wishes regarding withdrawal of treatment should be in writing. If possible, conflicts between the patient's wishes and those of the family should be mediated toward a consensus, although the patient's wishes must be controlling. Families need assurances that comfort and caring will be maintained, and critical care providers will not abandon the patient.

Euthanasia

There is a great deal of international debate and experimentation with euthanasia today.[1,25,61] From the practice of euthanasia in Holland, to anonymous reports of euthanasia in American medical journals, to citizens in states who are attempting to legalize euthanasia through referendums, we are confronted with controversy surrounding euthanasia on a daily basis. One of the key difficulties with discussing euthanasia is: What is its definition? A dictionary would state euthanasia is the act of putting to death without pain a person suffering from an incurable and painful disease or condition. Euthanasia is derived from the Greek, and its direct translation is "an easy death." However, how does withdrawing life support from a hopelessly ill patient differ from euthanasia?

Some individuals speak of passive euthanasia, where foregoing life support is a prime example. Active euthanasia would be the direct putting to death in a painless fashion of a person who is hopelessly ill and in pain. Because of the vagueness surrounding the definition of euthanasia, it is probably best to only use this term when describing the direct and active putting to death of a patient by a physician. An example of this would be a lethal injection. When using the term euthanasia, one should not be describing such acts as withholding or withdrawing life support and the provision of narcotic analgesics or hypnotics to relieve pain where, in some cases, hopelessly ill patients may overdose with such medications.

Currently, 85 to 90 percent of critical care professionals have stated they are withholding and withdrawing life-sustaining treatments from patients who are dying from terminal and irreversible diseases.[62] However, many leading physicians, philosophers, and biomedical ethicists including this author are opposed to physicians participating in active euthanasia in America. There is a long and impressive history of opposition to euthanasia in the practice of medicine. The Hippocratic oath declares opposition to the practice of euthanasia.[63,64] In 1988, the Council on Ethical and Judicial Affairs of the American Medical Association reaffirmed its opposition to euthanasia.[65] In 1988, the Journal of the American Medical Association published an anonymous first-person account of euthanasia.[66] This resulted in a strong call to have doctors not participate in euthanasia.[65,67]

Most critical care physicians are clearly opposed to participating in euthanasia. There are a number of strong criticisms against the practice of euthanasia. There is great concern euthanasia will expand from a practice which is desired by a legally competent patient to something which is used by surrogates of legally incompetent patients and eventually as an act which might be used to terminate life at an earlier stage of hopelessly ill patients who are in disadvantaged or vulnerable groups. Additionally, euthanasia is not consistent with the role of the physician as a healer who is committed to the sanctity of life. If an American citizen is intent on being euthanized, it is not necessary for a physician to be involved in the process.

Although at first glance it would seem likely euthanasia will not occur in America because of ample opposition, this is not clearly the case.[68,69] There are strong supporters of euthanasia, and there is an active program of euthanasia in the Netherlands.[70] The technique in Holland for performing euthanasia is to administer an hypnotic-like barbiturate which is then followed by a lethal injection of a paralytic agent. It is estimated 5000 to 10,000 Dutch are euthanized each year.[70]

Currently, two states in America are actively attempting to place bills legalizing euthanasia before the voters as referenda. In California, a bill entitled The California Humane and Dignified Death Act gathered only 130,000 of the necessary 450,000 signatures which would allow it to go to the voters in 1989. However, it is expected in the next 1 to 2 years enough signatures will be obtained.[71] It was reported in public opinion polls that up to 70 percent of California citizens favor the initiative, and many observers were surprised the initiative did not succeed. In 1990, the California legislation will again go through the referendum process and so, too, will a similar piece of legislation in the State of Washington. In Washington, only 150,000 signatures are needed, and there is a very active campaign to support this referendum. Although many citizens believe they should have the right to decide to end their lives when they have an incurable disease and are suffering, they do not have the right to demand physicians administer a lethal injection to provide them with their desired release.

If euthanasia referenda are passed by states, which appears quite likely over the next several years, physicians should not agree to administer lethal injections. If after fully considering the pros and cons of euthanasia, citizens still desire to have this option available, then they must identify other individuals to help them die, such as family members, friends, or counsellors.

AIDS and Ethics

The devastation from the HIV epidemic has only begun to be felt. The number of human beings who are now infected with HIV is in the millions, and the numbers continue to inexorably increase, especially in underdeveloped countries. The total of human loss, pain, and suffering is incomprehensible. The only other calamities to befall the earth of a similar magnitude include World War II and the black plague of the Middle Ages. It is estimated that by 1991 medical costs in America for new cases of AIDS alone will approach $6 billion.[72] For the critical care practitioner, a number of key ethical issues concern the care of patients with HIV. These ethical issues are: **1.** indications for life-sustaining treatment, **2.** confidentiality of HIV test results, **3.** the physician's obligation to care for seropositive patients, and **4.** the impact of the HIV epidemic on the allocation of medical resources.

Some patients with AIDS develop severe pulmonary infections, respiratory failure, and only have a chance to survive if placed on mechanical ventilation and other life support in ICUs. Since 1984, numerous studies have addressed the prognosis of AIDS patients with or without respiratory failure admitted to ICUs.[73] The studies in the mid 1980s revealed an in-hospital mortality rate for AIDS patients on mechanical ventilation of 86 to 100 percent. However, beginning in 1987, several studies were published which demonstrated a lower mortality rate for AIDS patients with respiratory failure admitted to ICUs and placed on mechanical ventilation.[73] These newer studies reveal an overall mortality rate of 50 to 60 percent. Of course, this is a mortality rate quite similar to many subpopulations of patients who are routinely admitted to ICUs for critical care. Certainly, caring for AIDS patients in respiratory failure on mechanical ventilators is not medically futile.

Competent patients have the right to refuse life-sustaining treatment and intensive care.[1,21,47,59,74] Even legally incompetent patients who have made clear what their wishes are have the right to refuse life-sustaining treatment. For patients with AIDS, especially if they do not have a legally recognized partner, the ability to fill out a durable power of attorney for health care and name their partner as an attorney-in-fact has been extremely valuable in preserving their decision-making capacity when they become legally incompetent. In a study by Steinbrook and colleagues in San Francisco of 118 homosexual men with AIDS, 45 percent indicated they would not want intubation or mechanical ventilation, despite an overly optimistic estimate of the outcome of intensive care.[18] In this study, three-fourths of the patients wanted to discuss life-sustaining treatment with their physicians, but only one-third had done so.

As one might expect, physicians who care for large numbers of AIDS patients are more aware of the poor prognosis after intensive care than those with less experience. Medical house staff at Bellevue Hospital and the University of California, San Francisco (each of whom had cared for more than 15 AIDS patients in the previous year) were able to accurately estimate the prognosis of AIDS patients requiring mechanical ventilation. On the other hand, residents at the University of Iowa and Providence Hospital, Oregon, who had seen one-fifth as many AIDS patients, significantly overestimated the prognosis of AIDS patients requiring intensive care. There was a high degree of correlation between the number of AIDS patients cared for, accuracy of outcome assessment, and tendency to initiate discussions with AIDS patients concerning life-sustaining treatment in intensive care.[75]

Confidentiality is an important ethical principle governing critical care providers and their obligations to their patients. Because of the importance of the ethical issue of confidentiality in the care of patients with HIV infection, confidentiality has been raised to the status of a major ethical principle somewhat like beneficence, nonmaleficence, autonomy, or justice. Some biomedical ethicists believe confidentiality is one of the key rules governing the professional-patient relationship.[26] Other key rules governing the professional-patient relationship include veracity, privacy, and fidelity. Everyone would agree that preserving the confidentiality of medical information protects a patient's privacy. It enables patients to seek care with confidence and discuss problems frankly with health care providers. If confidentiality is not maintained, patients with HIV infection will encounter stigma and discrimination.[76] Reports abound of HIV patients losing jobs, housing, health insurance, and being abandoned by family and friends. Unfortunately, due to the size and complexity of modern American medicine, breaches of confidentiality can be common. Therefore, some states have taken strong measures to maintain the confidentiality of HIV-positive individuals.

Health care professionals should do all in their power to encourage appropriate individuals to be tested for HIV in the hopes of decreasing transmission and instituting early therapy. If individuals discover they are seropositive, they have a moral duty to notify sexual or drug partners who are at risk for infection. In cases where seropositive patients refuse to notify other individuals whom they might have placed at great risk, physicians may have an ethical and legal duty to do so. In both California and New York, laws have been passed which allow physicians to notify sexual and intravenous drug-using contacts of seropositive persons about their risk without obtaining the approval of the original HIV-positive individual.

Therefore, a difficult balance exists between the confidentiality of the HIV-positive individual and the protection of third parties placed at risk after participating in certain practices with the HIV-positive person. Critical care providers and all other health care professionals must assist in decreasing the stigma of HIV infection. We need laws which will protect HIV-positive individuals against discrimination. This will facilitate more HIV testing and better public health control measures.

All health care providers, including critical care providers, are concerned about a random accident which would inoculate them with HIV. Since HIV is currently incurable and apparently in almost all cases, will result in death, this is certainly a realistic concern. Health care providers who perform invasive procedures or surgery and are in frequent contact with blood and bodily fluids are exposed to the greatest risk. Therefore, critical care providers are exposed to a significant risk but probably not as great a risk as an orthopedic or cardiovascular surgeon. There is growing concern among young physicians in training about the risk of being accidentally infected with HIV. This subject received a good deal of attention during the 1990 International AIDS Conference in San Francisco.

Leaders in clinical medicine and biomedical ethics believe a commitment to the profession of healing obligates physicians to care for HIV-positive patients even though it entails a risk.[77–79] The American Medical Association Council on Ethics and Judicial Affairs stated in 1988, "A physician may not ethically refuse to treat a patient whose condition is within the physician's current realm of competence solely because the patient is seropositive. If a physician is not able to provide the services required by persons with AIDS, he or she should make the appropriate referral to those physicians or facilities that are equipped to provide such services."[80] The American College of Physicians and the Society for Infectious Disease have stated there is an obligation to treat HIV-infected patients.[81]

Because of the enormity of the AIDS epidemic not only in America but throughout the world, it has a tremendous impact on the allocation of health care resources. By 1991, it is estimated there will be close to 300,000 patients with AIDS in the United States. Internationally, the reliability of estimated numbers of cases of HIV-infected and AIDS patients is poor. Obviously, the cost of AIDS is rising sharply, and it is projected that the total direct cost of AIDS will be 1.5 percent of total health expenditures in 1991. By 1991, it has been estimated that 12.4 percent of acute care beds in San Francisco and 8.1 percent in New York will be needed for persons with AIDS. This will have a significant impact on bed utilization in ICUs. The total cost for caring for AIDS patients is similar to the costs of other illnesses such as cancer or heart disease.[82]

Many persons with AIDS must be cared for in public hospitals because of their lack of medical insurance and financial resources. With the increasing demands for money to care for these patients and our current crisis atmosphere of health care financing, it is not clear who will provide the financial support needed to manage this enormous problem. In many large urban centers, ICUs and critical care providers find themselves with no available beds in their ICU because many beds are taken up by patients with AIDS. Since the mortality rate of AIDS patients admitted to ICUs and placed on mechanical ventilation approaches the mortality rates for patients with sepsis and organ system failure, ARDS, liver failure, and other common critical care problems, it is not reasonable or ethical to suggest access to ICU care should be restricted for patients with AIDS. If anything, the AIDS epidemic has forced physicians to become more conversant with biomedical ethics, the legality of withholding and withdrawing life support, and the necessity for assisting patients in making key health care decisions. Thus, critical care practitioners are challenged as are all other members of society to act ethically with sensitivity and compassion in caring for patients with HIV disease.

Ethics Consultations

When critical care practitioners are confronted by a thorny ethical dilemma in the ICU or a tense and possibly adversarial relationship with a legally incompetent patient's family or surrogate, then it is wise to call in a facilitator as soon as possible. A facilitator could be a representative from organized religion who is trained in the ethics and legalities in critical care medicine, a social worker, an ethicist, or a psychotherapist. Many hospitals have developed ethics committees, and it is expected that all accredited American hospitals will have ethics committees within the next few years. Ethics committees have approached the issue of ethics consultations in various ways. For example, some ethics committees have the whole committee become involved in an ethical case. Other committees identify a panel of potential consultants, any one of whom can become involved in a case.[1,21,25,83]

In 1988, La Puma and colleagues reported on the prospective evaluation of a newly established ethics consultation service in a university teaching hospital.[84] A physician-ethicist interviewed and examined patients, interviewed families, and others as needed and wrote a consultation note in the medical record. Fifty-one consultation requests were received from 45 physicians from July 1986 through June 1987. Thirty-three percent of the 51 patients were in the ICU, and 37 percent of the total number of patients were oriented at the time of consultation. Overall, 61 percent of the patients left the hospital alive. The requesting physician asked for assistance with decision-making concerning withholding and withdrawing life support in 49 percent of the cases. Questions concerning CPR were brought up in 37 percent of the cases, and legal issues were addressed in 31 percent. In 76 percent of the cases, assistance was asked with more than one issue. In 71 percent of the cases, the requesting physician stated the consultation was "very important" in assisting in-patient management. In 1985, a national conference on ethics consultation reported there was an average of nine formal requests for consultation per institution annually. The study by La Puma and colleagues from 1986 to 1987 reviewed 51 consultations. Thus, utilization of ethics consults appears to be increasing. The ethics consultation service helped health care team members in several ways: **1.** They facilitated patient-family participation in decision-making, **2.** The consultant reassured the physician that patients who were dying could be allowed to die without equating this with abandonment, **3.** The consultants helped physicians speak with patients and their families about quality of life and significant socioeconomic factors when the patient's wishes were unclear.

Brennan and colleagues reported in 1988 the results of the Optimum Care Committee of the Massachusetts General Hospital.[85] The Optimum Care Committee gave advice as do all ethical consults. Apparently, they only provided consultations on 73 cases from 1974 to 1987. However, from 1983 to 1986, their committee began to be more frequently consulted. At the Massachusetts General Hospital, only physicians could consult the Optimum Care Committee, and the nursing staff could not. This was unfortunate; nurses should always be allowed to consult the ethics committee because they provide a unique type of care, especially critical care nurses. The report by Brennan and colleagues is an example of an entire committee which functions in ethics consultations as compared to individual ethics consultants. There is room for many different models of ethics consultations. From our experience at Stanford University Medical Center, we prefer training and identifying skilled individual ethical consultants as compared to committee deliberations.

Health Care Rationing

Rationing has existed in health care and in the ICU over the past several decades.[86] Patient's income and geographic location of physicians and health care facilities have historically restricted the availability of medical services to many Americans, especially the disadvantaged. Additionally, reimbursement regulations imposed by third-party payers (now called "managed care") can also result in health care rationing. Isn't the fact that one in seven Americans currently has no health care insurance a form of rationing?

Because of the progressively more severe financial problems in our health care system, much more significant rationing will occur in the next several years. From 1947 to 1987, health care expenditures in America grew 2.5 percent per year faster than expenditures for other goods and services.[87] The percentage of the GNP for health care rose from under 5 percent during this time period to more than 12 percent at the present time. Health care prices rose more rapidly than other prices and the quantity of health care delivered grew faster than other quantities. The evolution of the American health care system had been characterized by a strong entrepreneurial nature, few cost controls, and a reliance on scientific progress and high technology to deliver the best possible care to all Americans without regard to cost.

There have been six major forces which have stimulated the growth and costs of our health care system so that now we spend more than $600 billion/year: technology, price of services, an aging population, defensive medicine, bureaucracy, and the contribution of third-party payments. Technology with new and advanced diagnostic and therapeutic procedures continues to inflate the cost of health care. It is probable many of our advances are not cost effective in terms of the overall health of our nation. Examples of new expensive technologies include erythropoietin, a hormone that stimulates the production of red blood cells. If this drug is provided to patients on chronic dialysis, the annual cost will approach three-quarters of a billion dollars.[88] If automatic implantable cardiac defibrillators were used in 20,000 potential candidates, the cost would be $1 billion. The estimated cost for AZT therapy in HIV patients is $5 billion annually. Newer low-osmolar radiopaque contrast agents which could eliminate 300 fatal reactions per year would increase the overall cost of radiopaque contrast media by $1 billion. The list of expensive new potential technologies goes on and on.

A second driving force which increases health care costs is the tendency for the price of services characterized by low-growth productivity to rise relative to the price of commodities. Many of the services provided in the hospital have not changed but have become more expensive. Our aging population is the third force causing increased health care costs. Almost 30 percent of all Medicare expenditures are devoted to the 6 percent of enrollees who are in the last years of life. The fourth force, defensive medicine to limit our legal liability, practiced by most physicians including critical care medicine physicians, is extremely expensive. In

America today, it is accepted that suing physicians and hospitals is a way of obtaining more funds to help in the care of a debilitated citizen. Additionally, malpractice suits are accepted as a legitimate business practice to generate enormous earnings both for plaintiffs and attorneys. The fifth force is the enormous bureaucracy involved in administering our complex health care system. Some estimates place the cost as high as 22 percent of total health care spending.[88] With the marked increase in health care insurance and the passage of Medicare and Medicaid legislation in 1965, there was an enormous infusion of funds into the health care system. This sixth force stimulated the extent and cost of the system and has been a major factor in the exponential growth of health care expenditures.

Comparisons are often made between the American health care system and those in the United Kingdom and Canada. Canada spends under 9 percent of their GNP for health care, and the United Kingdom spends under 7 percent even though they have universal insurance.[87] Per capita spending on health care, about one-third in Britain of that in the United States, entails a degree of rationing which is far beyond anything which is conceivable in America.[88] Essentially, physicians in the United Kingdom act as economic gate keepers, and services which are not available are simply not presented as options to patients unless they can afford private health care through a small, growing private system which is separate from the National Health Service program. In Canada, a set amount of funds is budgeted for health care expenditures, and physicians and hospitals simply cannot overspend their budget. Therefore, physicians in Canada also are confronted by a dilemma of not being able to provide certain advanced or state-of-the-art treatments to patients who cannot afford them through nongovernmental health care.

In the United States, there is great consternation over how to stabilize or decrease our health care costs since it is apparent we simply cannot afford our increasing fiscal commitment to health care. Increasing costs are destructive to private enterprise, to our competitiveness in international markets, and to the functioning of our government. The federal government has attempted to decrease health care costs by instituting competition and the diagnosis-related group (DRG) program to decrease costs. Recently, the legislature of the State of Oregon developed a plan to ration health care to the poor on the basis of what the citizens of Oregon felt were the most and least important types of health care delivered. For example, they have recommended that organ transplantation not be an option for Medicaid patients. This raises very significant ethical questions since middle class patients who have health insurance do have the option of becoming transplant candidates. Simply because an American is poor and must use governmental health care insurance, does this mean options for survival should be limited?

A definite technique of rationing health care has been the third-party's strategy of making it remarkably inconvenient for physicians and hospitals to obtain authorization and utilization review.[89] How to overcome this burgeoning negativistic bureaucracy is an important question. Ethically speaking, physicians and institutions should not try to subvert health care rationing through inconvenience by filling out forms in an untruthful fashion. It is better to be truthful and bring the problem to the attention of the American public and government.

Daniel Callahan, director of the Hastings Center for Bioethics, has played a major role in thinking about biomedical ethics in America. In 1987, he wrote a book recommending we ration health care, in part, based on the age of members of our society.[90] Callahan's position has engendered much negative reaction.[91] In 1990, Callahan proposed we limit medical progress since the cost of high technology with questionable significant benefit is stopping us from gaining affordable health care.[92]

Critical care providers are on the front lines of patient care rationing decisions because they must decide which patients are admitted or discharged from ICUs. In most acute care hospitals, there are either enough ICU beds to accommodate all critically ill patients or transfer of patients to ICUs in other hospitals is possible. However, more and more urban center hospital critical care providers are beginning to be forced to make triage decisions when ICU beds are limited because there are too many critically ill patients, and other hospital ICUs will not accept patients in transfer.

Triaging patients based on their ability to survive and function is an important component of American military or disaster medical care. Intermittently, triage has been used in modern American medicine such as during the early development of hemodialysis when equipment was limited. Interdisciplinary committees decided who would be dialyzed and who would die. If ICU beds are limited and critical care providers are asked to make triage decisions which will result in "earlier patient death," then it is vital several steps are taken:

First, triage decision policies should be developed by hospital and medical staff interdisciplinary committees. Second, day-to-day ICU triage decisions should be, at the least, reviewed by interdisciplinary committees (e.g., ethics committees). There will be times when these committees should be involved in the decision-making process. Critical care providers should not make triage decisions without carefully developed guidelines and rigorous review. Third, the American public should be made aware triage decisions are taking place. It is vital to keep the public informed and maintain the integrity of the American health care system. The public does not want to be surprised with the fact that critically ill Americans are being triaged from ICUs to an "earlier patient death."

There are many experts in health care who believe our system can be improved sufficiently to avoid systematic rationing or restriction of access through pricing. However, given the extent of our problems and the lack of accountable, courageous national leadership, it is doubtful the health care system will be significantly improved without anything less than a major overhaul. Unfortunately, until the crisis is so severe that fundamental changes must be made, we will be caught as critical care providers between a rock and a hard place. Patients, families, and surrogates will demand the best of care, plaintiffs' attorneys in courts will challenge us if we do not provide this care, and the federal government and insurance companies will make it difficult for us through bureaucracy, inconvenience, and restrictions to provide the care. The only way for critical care physicians to survive in this setting is to follow the four key biomedical ethical principles, to be truthtelling, and to inform our local communities, regions, and national government of the problems we must face and to work together to attempt to develop a national health care program. The critical care physician is not an economic gate keeper. Critical care physicians should deliver ethical, compassionate, and thoughtful care to patients within the constraints imposed by society.

References

1. Raffin TA, Shurkin J, Sinkler WS: *Intensive Care: Facing the Critical Choices.* New York, Freeman, 1988.
2. Ginzberg E: US health policy: Expectations and realities. JAMA 260:3647, 1988.
3. Raffin TA: ICU survival of patients with systemic illness. Am Rev Respir Dis 140:S28, 1989.
4. Cullen DJ, Keene R, Waternaux C, et al: Results, charges and benefits of intensive care for critically ill patients: Update 1983. Crit Care Med 12:102, 1984.
5. LeGall J, Brun-Buisson C, Trunet P, et al: Influence of age, previous health status and severity of acute illness on outcome from intensive care. Crit Care Med 10:575, 1982.
6. Knaus WA, Zimmerman JE, Wagner DP, et al: APACHE. Acute physiology and chronic health evaluation: A physiologically based classification system. Crit Care Med 9:591, 1980.
7. Knaus WA, Draper EA, Wagner DP, Zimmerman JE: APACHE II: A severity of disease classification system for acutely ill patients. Crit Care Med 6:685, 1985.
8. Knaus WA, Draper EA, Wagner DP, Zimmerman JE: Prognosis in acute organ-system failure. Ann Surg 202:685, 1985.
9. Montgomery AB, Stager MA, Carrico CJ, Hudson LD: Causes of mortality in patients with ARDS. Am Rev Respir Dis 132:485, 1985.
10. Schuster DP, Marion JM: Precedents for meaningful recovery during treatment in a medical intensive care unit: Outcome in patients with hematologic malignancy. Am J Med 75:402, 1983.
11. Fowler AA, Hammon RF, Zerbe GO, et al: Adult respiratory distress syndrome. Prognosis after onset. Am Rev Respir Dis 132:472, 1985.
12. Goldfarb G, Noel O, Poynard T, Rueff B: Efficiency of respiratory assistance in cirrhotic patients with liver failure. Intensive Care Med 9:271, 1983.
13. Imbus SH, Zawacki BE: Autonomy for burn patients when survival is unprecedented. N Engl J Med 297:308, 1977.
14. Pinilla JC, Ross DF, Martin T, Crump M: Study of the incidence of intravascular catheter infection in associated septicemia in critically ill patients. Crit Care Med 11:21, 1983.
15. Tobin MJ, Grenvik A: Nosocomial lung infection and its diagnosis. Am Rev Respir Med 12:191, 1984.
16. Girard K, Raffin TA: The chronically critically ill: To save or let die? Respir Care 30:339, 1985.
17. Danis M, Patrick DL, Sutherland LI, Green ML: Patients' and families' preferences for medical intensive care. JAMA 260:797, 1988.
18. Steinbrook R, Lo B, Moulton J, et al: Preferences of homosexual men with AIDS for life sustaining treatment. N Engl J Med 314:457, 1986.
19. In re Quinlan, 70 N.J. 10, 355 A.2d 647 (1976).
20. President's Commission for the Study of Ethical Problems in Medicine and Biomedical and Behavioral Research: Deciding to forego life-sustaining treatment. Washington, DC: US Government Printing Office, 1983.
21. Ruark JE, Raffin TA, and the Stanford University Medical Center Committee on Ethics: Initiating and withdrawing life support: Principles and practices in adult medicine. N Engl J Med 318:25, 1988.
22. Thomas JA, Hamm TE Jr, Perkins PL, Raffin TA, and the Stanford University Medical Center Committee on Ethics: Special Report: Animal Research at Stanford University: Principles, policies, and practices. N Engl J Med 318:1630, 1988.
23. Greely HT, Hamm T, Johnson R, Price CR, Weingarten R, Raffin TA, and the Stanford University Medical Center Committee on Ethics: The ethical use of human fetal tissue in medicine. N Engl J Med 320:1093, 1989.
24. Brody H: *Ethical Decisions in Medicine.* Boston, Little, Brown. 1976.
25. Young EWD: *Alpha and Omega: Ethics at the Frontiers of Life and Death.* Palo Alto, Addison Wesley, 1988.
26. Beauchamp TL, Childress JF: *Principles of Biomedical Ethics.* 3d ed. New York, Oxford University Press, 1983.
27. Johnson AR, Siegler M, Winslade WJ. *Clinical Ethics.* 2d ed. New York, Macmillan, 1986.
28. Society For The Right To Die: *The Physician and the Hopelessly Ill Patient.* New York, Society for the Right to Die, 1985.
29. Bok S: *Lying: Moral Choice in Public and Private Life.* New York, Pantheon, 1978.
30. Saikewicz v. Superintendent of Belcher State School, 373 Mass. 728, 370 N.E.2d 417 (1977).
31. In re Dinnerstein, 380 N.E.2d 134 (1978).
32. Barber v. Superior Court of Los Angeles, 147 Cal. App.3d 1006, 195 Cal.Rptr. 484 (1983).
33. Bartling v. Superior Court, 163 Cal.App.ed 196, 209 Cal.Rptr 220 (1984).
34. Bouvia v. Superior Court, 179 Cal.App.3d 1127, 225 Cal.Rptr.297 (1986).
35. Brophy v. New England Sinai Hospital, Inc., 390 Mass. 417; 497 N.E.2d 626 (1986).
36. In re Farrell, 108 N.J. 335, 529 A.2d 404 (N.J. 1987).
37. In re Jobes, 108 N.J. 394, 529 A.2d 434 (1987).
38. In re Drabick, 200 Cal.App.3d 185, 245 Cal.Rptr. 840 (Cal. Ct. App. 1988), reviewed denied (Cal., July 28, 1988), cert. denied, 109 S.Ct. 399 (1988).
39. In re O'Connor, 72 N.Y.2d 517, 531 N.E.2d 607, 534 N.Y.S.2d 886, (1988).
40. Cruzan v. Harmon, 760 S.W.2d 408 (1988).
41. Lo B, Rouse F, Dornbrand L: Family decision making on trial: Who decides for incompetent patients? N Engl J Med 322:1228, 1990.
42. Angell M: Prisoners of technology: The case of Nancy Cruzan. N Engl J Med 322:1226, 1990.
43. Snyder L: Life, death, and the American College of Physicians: The Cruzan case. Ann Intern Med 112:802, 1990.
44. Raffin TA: Value of the living will. Chest 90:444, 1986.
45. Gilfix M, Raffin TA: Withholding or withdrawing extraordinary life support: Optimizing rights and limiting liability. West J Med 141:387, 1984.
46. Stevenson DK, Ariagno RL, Kutner JS, et al: The 'Baby Doe' rule. JAMA 255:1909, 1986.
47. Luce JM, Raffin TA: Withholding and withdrawal of life support from critically ill patients. Chest 94:621, 1988.
48. Luce JM: Ethical principles in critical care. JAMA 263:696, 1990.
49. Title 22, Section 70707, California Administrative Code.

50. Stevens JH, Raffin TA, Baldwin JC: The current status of lung transplantation. Surg Gynecol Obstet 169:179, 1989.
51. Guidelines for Determination of Death: Report of the medical consultants on the diagnosis of death to the President's Commission for the Study of Ethical Problems in Medicine and Biomedical and Behavioral Research. JAMA 246:2184, 1981.
52. Bedell SE, Delbanco TL, Cook EF, Epstein FH: Survival after cardiopulmonary resuscitation in the hospital. N Engl J Med 309:569, 1983.
53. Bedell SE, Pelle D, Maher PL, Cleary PD: Do-not-resuscitate orders for critically ill patients in the hospital: How are they used and what is their impact? JAMA 256:233, 1986.
54. Murphy DJ, Murray AM, Robinson BE, Campion EW: Outcomes of cardiopulmonary resuscitation in the elderly. Ann Intern Med 111:199, 1989.
55. Tomlinson T, Brody H: Ethics and communication in do-not-resuscitate orders. N Engl J Med 318:43, 1988.
56. Lantos JD, Singer PA, Walker RM, et al: The illusion of futility in clinical practice. Am J Med 87:81, 1989.
57. Schneiderman LJ, Jecker NS, Johnsen AR: Medical futility: Its meaning and ethical implications. Ann Intern Med 112:949, 1990.
58. NIH Workshop Summary: Withholding and withdrawing mechanical ventilation. Am Rev Respir Dis 134:1327, 1986.
59. Hastings Center: Guidelines on the termination of life-sustaining treatment in the care of the dying: A report. Hastings Report, 1987.
60. Dracup K, Raffin TA: Withholding and withdrawing mechanical ventilation: Quality of life considerations. Am Rev Respir Dis 140:S44, 1989.
61. Singer PA, Siegler M: Euthanasia—A critique. N Engl J Med 322:1881, 1990.
62. The Society of Critical Care Medicine Ethics Task Force: Attitudes of critical care medicine professionals concerning foregoing life-sustaining treatments. Crit Care Med 17:589, 1989.
63. Angell M: Euthanasia. N Engl J Med 138:1000, 1988.
64. Wanzer SH, Federman DD, Adelstein SJ, et al: The physician's responsibility toward hopelessly ill patients: A second look. N Engl J Med 320:844, 1989.
65. The Council on Ethical and Judicial Affairs of the American Medical Association: *Euthanasia. Report: C (A-88). AMA Council Report.* Chicago: American Medical Association: 1988, p 1.
66. It's over, Debbie. JAMA 259:272, 1988.
67. Gaylin W, Kass LR, Pellegrino ED, Siegler M: 'Doctors must not kill.' JAMA 259:2139, 1988.
68. Risley RL: *A Humane and Dignified Death: A New Law Permitting Physician Aid-in-Dying.* Glendale, CA. Americans Against Human Suffering, 1987.
69. Humphry D, Wickett A: *The Right to Die: Understanding Euthanasia.* New York, Harper & Row, 1986.
70. de Wachter MAM: Active euthanasia in the Netherlands. JAMA 262:3316, 1989.
71. Parachini A: Mercy, murder, and morality: Perspectives on euthanasia; The California Humane and Dignified Death Initiative. Hastings Cent Rep 19(1)(Suppl):10, 1989.
72. Miller A: Can you afford to get sick? Newsweek January 30, 1988, p 44.
73. Wachter RM, Luce JM, Lo B, Raffin TA: Life-sustaining treatment for patients with the acquired immunodeficiency syndrome. Chest 95:647, 1989.
74. ACCP-SCCM Consensus Panel: Ethical and moral guidelines for the initiation, continuation, and withdrawal of intensive care. Chest 97:949, 1990.
75. Wachter RM, Cooke M, Hopewell PC, Luce JM: Attitudes of residents regarding intensive care for patients with the acquired immunodeficiency syndrome. Arch Intern Med 148:149, 1988.
76. Mangione CM, Lo B: Beyond fear: Resolving ethical dilemmas regarding HIV infection. Chest 95:1100, 1989.
77. Zuger A, Miles SH: Physicians, AIDS, and occupational risk: Historic traditions and ethical obligations. JAMA 258:1924, 1987.
78. Pellegrino ED: Altruism, self-interest, and medical ethics. JAMA 258:1939, 1987.
79. Lo B, Raffin TA, Cohen NH, et al: Ethical dilemmas about intensive care in patients with AIDS. Rev Infect Dis 9:1163, 1987.
80. AMA: Ethical issues involved in the growing AIDS crisis. JAMA 259:1360, 1988.
81. American College of Physicians Health and Public Policy Committee, Infectious Diseases Society of America: The acquired immunodeficiency syndrome (AIDS) and the infection with the human immunodeficiency virus (HIV). Ann Intern Med 108:460, 1988.
82. Bloom D, Carliner G: The economic impact of AIDS in the United States. Science 239:604, 1988.
83. Rosner F: Hospital medical ethics committees: A review of their development. JAMA 255:2693, 1988.
84. La Puma J, Stocking CB, Silverstein MD, et al: An ethics consultation service in a teaching hospital: Utilization and evaluation. JAMA 260:808, 1988.
85. Brennan TA: Ethics committees and decisions to limit care: The experience of the Massachusetts General Hospital. JAMA 260:803, 1988.
86. Relman AS: Is rationing inevitable? N Engl J Med 322:1809, 1990.
87. Fuchs VR: The health sector's share of the gross national product. Science 247:534, 1990.
88. Aaron H, Schwartz WB: Rationing health care: The choice before us. Science 247:418, 1990.
89. Grumet GW: Health care rationing through inconvenience: The third party's secret weapon. N Engl J Med 321:607, 1989.
90. Callahan D: *Setting Limits: Medical Goals in an Aging Society.* New York, Simon & Schuster, 1987.
91. Levinsky NG: Age as a criterion for rationing health care. N Engl J Med 322:1813, 1990.
92. Callahan D: Rationing medical progress: The way to affordable health care. N Engl J Med 322:1810, 1990.

Chapter 186

PEDIATRIC AND NEONATAL INTENSIVE CARE

P. PEARL O'ROURKE
ROBERT K. CRONE

Many adult intensivists are invited to participate or consult in the care of critically ill children. Often the communication between adult and pediatric intensivists reveals fresh approaches to the understanding and management of critical illness across all ages of patients. The *raison d'être* for a perspective on pediatric intensive care in a book of adult intensive care is to address issues unique to the critically ill child. Although the principles of intensive care are similar in the adult and child, the old adage, children are not small adults, is in part true. This chapter attempts to highlight aspects of pediatric critical care which differ from adult critical care. One challenge is that it is easy to gloss over important areas. A second is that in some areas of importance, we may be too narrow in stating our own diagnostic and therapeutic preferences when there is controversy within the field of pediatric critical care. We have been encouraged by our editors to be specific in our choices of therapy so that readers from the adult intensive care community may have clear guidelines.

Childhood includes the periods of active growth and maturation from prematurity through adulthood: this necessitates an understanding of developmental anatomy, physiology, pharmacology, and psychology. In addition, the fact that the child is physically smaller limits invasive therapy and monitoring. The basic pathophysiology of disease also differs. The adult's clinical status often primarily or secondarily reflects degenerative or self-inflicted diseases of use and abuse. For example, many admissions are precipitated or complicated by atherosclerosis, obesity, lung disease from smoking, hypertension or diabetes mellitus. As a result, the intensive care unit (ICU) admission of adults is often characterized by multisystem disease. In contrast, because children are relatively healthy with no appreciable baseline organ dysfunction, they more commonly suffer single-organ failure with fewer multisystem complications.

Special Differences of Pediatric from Adult Critical Care

TECHNOLOGICAL DIFFERENCES

There are a number of differences in philosophy of invasive monitoring in the pediatric versus the adult patient. Part of this philosophy is generated by the increased difficulty of invasive monitoring in the smaller pediatric patient, and part is generated by differences in pathophysiology of organ dysfunction.

Vascular cannulation for monitoring of intravascular pressures and blood gases is common in the ICU. Percutaneous arterial lines are routine in even the premature infant. The arteries are smaller, and line placement requires more skill and patience. Central venous pressure (CVP) is measured less frequently than in the adult ICU. As discussed in the cardiovascular section (vide infra), most pediatric patients can initially be treated and volume resuscitated using clinical assessment of volume status. In fact, a CVP catheterization is only considered if a reasonable volume replacement has not improved the clinical status of the patient. Then CVP lines are placed in the internal or external jugular, subclavian, or femoral vein.

Pulmonary artery (PA) catheters are also less commonly placed because of the infrequent need for measurement of pulmonary capillary wedge pressure (PWP) or cardiac output. The child rarely suffers isolated left ventricular failure; hence, a CVP value is usually adequate for volume assessment. But PA lines are useful for guiding therapy in cold septic shock, myocarditis, or myocardiopathy. The smallest quadriluminal catheter is 5 French, which has a distance of 15 cm between the distal PA port and the proximal CVP port. This distance obviously limits the applicability of this catheter in smaller children and infants. As a result, PA catheters are rarely used in children who weigh less than 15 kg. If PA monitoring is required in a small child, a separate catheter can be placed.

Routine monitoring of pulmonary function tests (PFT) can be difficult in the child because of the lack of patient cooperation. There are a number of approaches used which obviate the need for any cooperation. One example of this is the measurement of the crying vital capacity (VC). While a child is stimulated to cry, a tight-fitting mask is held over the mouth and nose and the exhaled volume is measured for each breath. The three largest breaths are then averaged for a VC.[1] In addition, PFTs in the endotracheally intubated child are unreliable because the air leak around uncuffed endotracheal tubes limits both pressure and volume measurements. Transcutaneous measurements of O_2 saturation, P_{O_2}, and P_{CO_2} are easily obtained in the child. End-tidal gas measurement has been difficult because these devices add dead space to the system, which can be a relatively large volume when compared to the small patient tidal volumes.[2]

SOCIAL ISSUES

Any critically ill patient must be considered as an individual as well as a member of a family or social group. The age spectrum of pediatric patients presents extreme situations. Virtually every pediatric patient is accompanied by a guardian who serves as the consenting party. The exception to this is the emancipated minor who, although not of majority age, is either married or financially independent. Despite children's dependence on a guardian, every effort should be made to help them understand and participate in their medical care. When appropriate, they should be asked for consent or assent. An adolescent can often be approached as an adult. Any healthy child over 4 years should be offered explanations and active participation appropriate to her age; obviously severely ill children of similar age are generally unable to participate.

Because the child is not the consenting individual, we go to the guardian(s) for guidance in situations of withdrawing or withholding medical support. The concept of a living will is obviated. Decisions to limit support for a child can be extremely difficult. They are often colored by the sentiment that "children should not die." In fact, physicians and nurses often suffer this same response. In addition, parents often cannot accept the fact that their child's condition is out of their control. Many parents blame themselves when they have been unable to protect their child from a critical illness. These feelings are best addressed by honest and precise discussions about the medical situation with the help of nursing, social service, and, if appropriate, clergy.

ASSESSING PATIENT COMFORT AND COOPERATION

Much of our care in the ICU setting requires patient compliance or at least a workable interface between patient and technology. In adults, the need for cooperation can usually be discussed and negotiated with the patient unless the clinical status is complicated by hypoxemia, encephalopathy, or other neurologic decompensation. In the pediatric intensive care unit (PICU) many patients are too young or too ill to understand and participate in their own care. All care is seen as an assault, and the separation from parents and familiar faces makes the environment hostile and the child's behavior counterproductive.

Another misconception is that "babies do not feel pain." While this was often used in defense of oxygen and muscle relaxant anesthesia, a number of elegant studies have shown elevated catecholamines in response to stimulation in these infants.[3] These studies have also demonstrated improved survival in the group receiving analgesia.

The child often cannot verbally express his discomfort or anxiety. An acute awareness of problems with parent separation, pain, and immobility must be anticipated. Beyond pharmacology, simple routine maneuvers that can help include parent attendance, sibling visiting, television, VCR tapes, head sets, and access to favorite toys.

In order to safely provide care and monitoring, pharmacologic cooperation and comfort are routinely induced. A titrated combination of narcotics and anxiolytics is the most common regimen. For analgesia, we usually administer morphine sulfate as a bolus (0.1 mg/kg) every 1 to 2 h or preferentially as an infusion (20 μg/(kg · h)) after an initial bolus. Diazepam (0.2 to 0.5 mg/kg every 4 to 6 h) or midazolam (0.05 to 0.2 mg/kg every 1 to 2 h) is added for anxiolysis. Short-term sedation is fairly easy to maintain, but long-term sedation is difficult and can produce a number of complications (dependence, tachyphylaxis, withdrawal). At this time there is no perfect method to guarantee chronic patient compliance.

TEMPERATURE CONTROL

Normothermia is maintained by thermoregulation which describes the patient's balance between heat production and heat loss. In the young child, and especially the premature infant, thermoregulation is often inadequate secondary to inappropriate heat loss. Small children have very large body surface areas, decreased insulation (less fat), and an inability to control their own environment; e.g., thermostat, blanket, and clothing decisions are made for them. Healthy children can increase their basal metabolic rate and nonshivering thermogenesis to maintain homeostasis for a short period, but this is not acceptable for the chronic situation or for the compromised infant. Because of baseline fragile thermoregulation, the infant is at high risk for developing hypothermia from exposure extremes. Any situation in which the child is wet increases this risk because heat loss is approximately 30 times as rapid in a wet environment. This describes the child at birth and the near-drowning victim. In both situations, it is imperative to dry the child immediately. The small child can also lose heat rapidly with low ambient temperature, such as in an operating room or even a hospital ward. In these settings, temperature control must be diligently monitored.

There are basic prevention as well as therapeutic approaches to hypothermia. Many of these modalities overlap. Ambient temperature should be increased whenever possible. This can be done with radiant warmers, isolettes, or warming lamps. The child should be dry, wrapped in blankets or clothes, and the head covered. Some commonsense maneuvers such as covering the cold radiologic plate with a towel or diaper can prevent conductive heat loss. If the child has clinical hypothermia (core temperature less than 35°C), more aggressive warming should be added to the above. This includes warm humidified air; warming blankets; nasogastric, colonic, or peritoneal lavage with warm saline; and in extreme cases cardiopulmonary bypass. The manifestations of hypothermia should be recognized. The critical organ systems affected are the brain and the heart. As the child cools to 30 to 32°C, there may be atrial arrhythmias: ventricular arrhythmias occur in the 27 to 30°C range and asystole at 18 to 20°C. Neurologically, the child loses consciousness at approximately 32°C, loses reflexes at 28°C, and becomes flaccid at 25°C. The child can, in fact, look dead secondary to hypothermia. The clinician should be aware of the clinical spectrum and be comfortable with diagosing hypothermia versus death. The child is dead if she is asystolic with a temperature greater than 30°C, or if despite aggressive rewarming attempts the child cannot be warmed to 30°C.

The very young child can also become hyperthermic if placed in too hot an environment. This is exaggerated in premature infants, because they do not sweat and, hence, may have inadequate evaporative losses for an extremely hot environment.

The Cardiovascular System

Circulatory well-being in infants and children is dependent on progression of structural and functional maturation. An understanding of this age-dependent process is essential to the diagnosis and treatment of circulatory failure in infants and children.

DEVELOPMENT OF THE CIRCULATION

Adult and fetal circulation differ in many ways.[4] Fetal circulation is distinguished by **1.** the placenta as the organ of respiration, **2.** high pulmonary vascular resistance, **3.** low systemic vascular resistance, and **4.** the fact that the fetal ventricles pump in parallel with a dominant right ventricle. In addition, the fetus exists in a remarkably hypoxic environment compensated for by a relatively high cardiac output and a hemoglobin with a high affinity for oxygen. The fetus compensates for the placement of the placenta in the systemic circulation by several shunts: the ductus arteriosus, ductus venosus, and the foramen ovale. When the fetus becomes an extrauterine being, a number of important changes occur to bring the circulation to an adult form:

1. With the first breath, the increase in oxygen saturation, as well as other potential neurohumoral mediators, relaxes the pulmonary vasospasm that existed in utero. Pulmonary blood flow then increases.
2. The placenta separates from the uterine wall, the placental blood vessels constrict, and systemic vascular resistance (SVR) and left ventricular afterload increase. As the pulmonary vascular resistance (PVR) decreases and SVR increases, left atrial pressures rise above the right, and the "flap valve" foramen ovale restricts left-to-right blood flow, causing functional closure of the foramen ovale.
3. The ductus arteriosus closes as the Pa_{O_2} increases. Other mediators such as the prostanoids and kinins, as well as changes in autonomic vascular tone, may also promote closure of the ductus arteriosus. It is usually functionally closed during the first 24 to 96 h of life, and anatomic obliteration follows during the next several weeks.
4. The ductus venosus passively closes with the removal of the placental circulation and readjustment in the portal pressure relative to inferior vena cava (IVC) pressure.
5. There is a further gradual decline in PVR due to a structural remodeling of the muscular layer of pulmonary blood vessels: During fetal life the central pulmonary vascular bed has a relatively thick muscle layer. After birth, this muscle coat thins and extends to the periphery of the lung, a process that takes months to years to complete.[5]

DEVELOPMENT OF AUTONOMIC CONTROL OF THE CIRCULATION

There is still considerable speculation regarding the functional integrity of autonomic circulatory control during fetal and perinatal development. It has been shown in several species that the fetal heart has a reduced store of catecholamines and an increased sensitivity to exogenously administered norepinephrine. The sympathetic nerves first develop in the atria and grow into the ventricles toward the apex at a variable and species-specific rate.[6]

In fetal lambs, resting α-adrenergic tone begins at approximately 0.6 of gestation and is nearly complete at birth, but resting β-adrenergic control does not begin until 0.8 gestation and is incompletely developed at birth. Adrenergic innervation of the human myocardium may be complete between 18 and 28 weeks gestation. However, low cardiac stores of norepinephrine, as well as an incomplete development of sympathetic nerves, have been demonstrated in humans after birth. Adrenergic responses are apparently present but diminished in the newborn human.

Development of cholinergic (vagal) control of the heart is also variable and species specific. In human newborn infants, the cholinergic system appears completely developed at birth and the heart is sensitive to vagal stimulation. This provides for a relative vagal predominance of neural cardiovascular control, making bradycardia a more likely response to any increase in autonomic tone.

The chemoreceptor and baroreceptor reflexes have important developmental implications in the infant and child; the baroreceptor reflex is present but is incompletely developed at term in the human. In preterm infants, postural changes elicit no change in heart rate, but some increase in peripheral vascular resistance, illustrating an incomplete and attenuated baroreceptor response.[7] The chemoreceptor response seems to be well developed in utero. Fetal bradycardia in response to hypoxia is thought to be mediated through the chemoreceptors and may be similar to the oxygen-conserving mechanisms of diving animals.

MYOCARDIAL METABOLISM

Adult cardiac muscle is almost exclusively dependent on oxygen for its metabolism. Its efficiency of oxygen extraction appears to be greater than other organs. Anaerobic metabolism is nearly nonexistent in adult cardiac muscle, so the heart is extremely sensitive to hypoxia or ischemia. Either of these conditions, however brief, will alter the energy supply and affect the mechanical response of the adult heart.

Because relative hypoxia is normal in utero, it is important to assess the metabolic characteristics of the fetal myocardium. Asphyxia for up to 30 min has no effect on the fetal electrocardiogram (ECG),[8] and the young heart endures hypoxia better than adult hearts.[9] This may be due to high concentrations of glycogen in the fetal myocardiac tissue. In addition, lactate is produced by the hypoxic fetal myocardium, suggesting that fetal myocardial tissue is capable of anaerobic glycolytic metabolism. Glucose injection prolongs survival of anoxic newborn lambs, whereas insulin injection reduces survival time. Newborn lambs reduce their oxygen consumption in the presence of hypoxia, whereas adult lambs do not.[10] In addition, fetal hemoglobin

TABLE 186-1 Age-Related Circulatory Variables

Heart Age	Systolic Rate, beats/min	Diastolic BP,* mmHg	Stroke BP, mmHg	Cardiac Volume, mL/beat	O_2 Index, L(min · m^2)	Hb Consumption, mL/(kg · min)	Concentration, g/dL	P_{50}, mmHg	Oxygen Unloaded, mL/100 mL at 95% Saturation
Term newborn	133 ± 18	80 ± 16	46 ± 16	4.5 ± 5.0	2.5 ± 0.6	6.0 ± 1.0	16.5 ± 1.5	18	1.8
6 months	120 ± 20	89 ± 29	60 ± 10	7.4 ± 2.0	2.0 ± 0.5	5.0 ± 0.9	11.5 ± 1.0	24	3.9
12 months	120 ± 20	96 ± 30	66 ± 25	11.5 ± 3.0	2.5 ± 0.6	5.2 ± 0.9	12.0 ± 75	30	4.7
2 years	105 ± 25	99 ± 25	64 ± 25	16.9 ± 4.5	3.1 ± 0.7	6.4 ± 1.2	12.5 ± 0.5	27	4.7
5 years	90 ± 10	94 ± 14	55 ± 9	27.8 ± 7.5	3.7 ± 0.9	6.0 ± 1.1	12.5 ± 0.5	29	4.7
12 years	70 ± 17	113 ± 18	59 ± 10	53.5 ± 14.5	4.3 ± 1.1	3.3 ± 0.6	13.5 ± 1.0	27.9	4.7
Adult	75 ± 5	—	—	85.5 ± 6.0	3.7 ± 0.3	3.4 ± 0.6	14.0 ± 1.0	27	4.9

*BP: blood pressure.

is more efficient than adult hemoglobin in relatively hypoxic environments. These mechanisms make the heart of the fetus and newborn relatively resistant to the destructive effects of hypoxia, provided that oxygenation and perfusion are reestablished within a reasonable period of time. Oxygen consumption increases precipitously after birth, presumably owing to thermogenesis. The full-term infant's oxygen consumption in a neutral thermal environment is approximately 5 mL/(kg · min) and increases to 7 mL/(kg · min) and 8 mL/(kg · min) at 10 days and 4 weeks, respectively. Thereafter, oxygen consumption and cardiac output decline gradually over the ensuing months.[11]

AGE-RELATED CIRCULATORY VARIABLES

Important circulatory variables are listed in Table 186-1, with normal values given from the newborn to the adult.

COMMON CARDIOVASCULAR DISEASE STATES

CONGENITAL HEART DISEASE

Although a complete discussion of congenital heart disease is not possible here, a variety of abnormalities that produce significant alterations in oxygenation, perfusion, and myocardial function after birth are worthy of attention.[12] The more common lesions include obstruction to systemic outflow (e.g., congenital aortic stenosis and coarctation of the aorta) and lesions that alter the adequacy of pulmonary blood flow (e.g., tricuspid or pulmonary atresia and tetralogy of Fallot). Many of these lesions are associated with other abnormalities that facilitate mixing or diversion of blood flow from one circuit to the other, in order to permit even marginal survival. Patent fetal conduits such as the ductus arteriosus or foramen ovale may exist in isolation or in association with other "shunt" lesions and, in some circumstances, rather than helping survival, may become a source of cardiac decompensation.

Newborns with significant congenital heart disease commonly present with either cyanosis or congestive heart failure (CHF). It is important to recognize that the degree of dysfunction changes during the first months of life since the neonatal circulation is dynamic and changing. The pulmonary vascular resistance decreases to adult levels by approximately 2 to 3 months of age. As this resistance falls, left-to-right shunts can increase and the symptoms of CHF become more apparent. In the newborn, the usual signs and symptoms of CHF include poor feeding, irritability, sweating, tachycardia, tachypnea, decreased peripheral pulses, poor cutaneous perfusion, and hepatomegaly. Cyanosis may indicate structural cardiac disease; however, respiratory disease, neurologic disease, pulmonary vascular disease (persistent pulmonary hypertension), and methemoglobinemia must also be considered.

Common cyanotic congenital heart lesions in the newborn include

- Tetralogy of Fallot
- Transposition of the great arteries
- Hypoplastic left heart syndrome
- Pulmonary atresia with intact ventricular septum
- Single ventricle
- Total anomalous pulmonary venous return
- Tricuspid atresia

Common congenital heart lesions presenting with CHF in the newborn include:

- Ventricular septal defect
- Patent ductus arteriosus
- Hypoplastic left heart syndrome
- Critical aortic stenosis
- Coarctation of the aorta

The diagnosis of congenital heart disease can be made on the basis of the physical examination, the ECG, chest radiograph, and the echocardiogram. Cardiac catheterization may be performed after initial stabilization and prior to either definitive or palliative cardiac surgery.

The initial medical treatment of congenital heart disease is aimed at relieving CHF, improving systemic perfusion, and maintaining pulmonary blood flow. In some situations (e.g., hypoplastic left heart syndrome, aortic stenosis, or atresia), the patency of the ductus arteriosus may be crucial to provide perfusion to the body. In these cases, prostaglandin E_1 (PGE_1) infusion has proved useful in maintaining the patency of the ductus arteriosus until definitive surgical correction can be performed.[13]

ACUTE CIRCULATORY FAILURE IN CHILDREN

Acute circulatory failure is defined as any clinical condition in which systemic blood flow is inadequate to meet the metabolic demands of the body. The clinical syndrome of shock includes the signs and symptoms of both an inadequate circulation and an attempt to compensate for circulatory failure.[14] The child has a remarkable ability to compensate for an inadequate circulation, with both endogenous catecholamine release as well as increased peripheral autonomic tone. The signs of compensation are often the earliest clinical clues that a child is in shock. Anxiety or irritability; cool, pale extremities; and an unexplained tachycardia are usually the earliest signs. Tachypnea, moderate metabolic acidosis, oliguria, and somnolence are signs of inadequate tissue perfusion, whereas obtundation, periodic breathing, or apnea are signs of impending cardiopulmonary arrest. The presence and severity of a metabolic acidosis correlates well with the degree of circulatory failure in children, making the arterial pH the single most important laboratory value in the evaluation of an inadequate circulation in infants and children. Blood pressure is not usually a good indicator of the adequacy of perfusion in children. The child's ability to constrict the peripheral circulation is so efficient that central blood pressure may be normal despite impending circulatory collapse. Circulatory failure can result from pump failure or from intravascular hypovolemia. Intravascular hypovolemia is a consequence of either true volume loss (blood, plasma, water) or an alteration in peripheral vascular resistance (see Table 186-2).

In children, the most common cause of circulatory failure is hypovolemia related to an excessive loss of volume.[15] This produces a decreased ventricular preload that decreases stroke volume and cardiac output. The most common causes of acute hypovolemia are **1.** blood loss (e.g., trauma, gastrointestinal tract bleeding), **2.** plasma loss (e.g., capillary leak syndrome associated with sepsis and acidosis, hypoproteinemia, burns, peritonitis), and **3.** water loss (e.g., vomiting and diarrhea, glycosuric diuresis in diabetic ketoacidosis).

Relative intravascular hypovolemia secondary to decreased peripheral vascular resistance and increased vascular capacitance also reduces cardiac output by decreased preload. Anaphylaxis and septic or endotoxic shock are two clinical examples of this condition. In addition, the ingestion of ganglionic blocking agents or of direct smooth muscle relaxants such as antihypertensive agents, major tranquilizers, and barbiturates not only decreases peripheral vascular resistance but can also produce toxic myocardial depression leading to circulatory failure at any age.

Cardiogenic shock is a relatively uncommon cause of circulatory failure in the pediatric patient when compared to the incidence in adults.[16] When it occurs in the neonate, the usual cause is congenital heart disease with outflow obstruction or systemic-to-pulmonary shunting, although viral or bacterial sepsis are also common causes. In any child, extrinsic inflow or outflow obstruction associated with tension pneumothorax, hemopericardium, or pneumopericardium, as well as pericardial effusion, must also be considered. Lastly, primary pump failure associated with viral, collagen-vascular, or infiltrative cardiomyopathies or with metabolic derangements such as hypoglycemia, sepsis, or uremia can produce circulatory failure that is refractory to treatment. Atrial or ventricular arrhythmias such as paroxysmal atrial tachycardia (PAT) or atrioventricular (AV) block can also precipitate circulatory failure in children (see Figure 186-1).[17]

Treatment

The etiology and functional physiology of shock can frequently be discerned from a history and physical examination. Specific therapy may differ in various clinical condi-

TABLE 186-2 Circulation Etiologies of Acute Circulatory Failure in Infants and Children

DECREASED INTRAVASCULAR VOLUME (90% INCIDENCE)		NORMAL INTRAVASCULAR VOLUME (10% INCIDENCE)
Loss of Volume (Vasoconstriction)	Loss of Resistance (Vasodilation)	Cardiogenic
1. Blood loss	1. Anaphylaxis	1. Pump failure
a. Trauma	a. Histamine SRS-A	a. Myocarditis
b. Gastrointestinal bleeding		b. Cardiomyopathy
2. Plasma loss	2. Sepsis	2. Inflow obstruction
a. Burns	a. Endotoxin	a. Pericarditis
b. Capillary leak syndrome		b. Tension pneumothorax
3. Water loss	3. Drug ingestion	3. Outflow obstruction
a. Gastroenteritis	a. Psychotropic agents	a. Pulmonary embolus
b. Diabetic ketoacidosis		b. Aortic stenosis
		c. Coarctation of the aorta
		4. Left-to-right shunts
		a. VSD
		b. AVMs
		5. Dysrhythmias

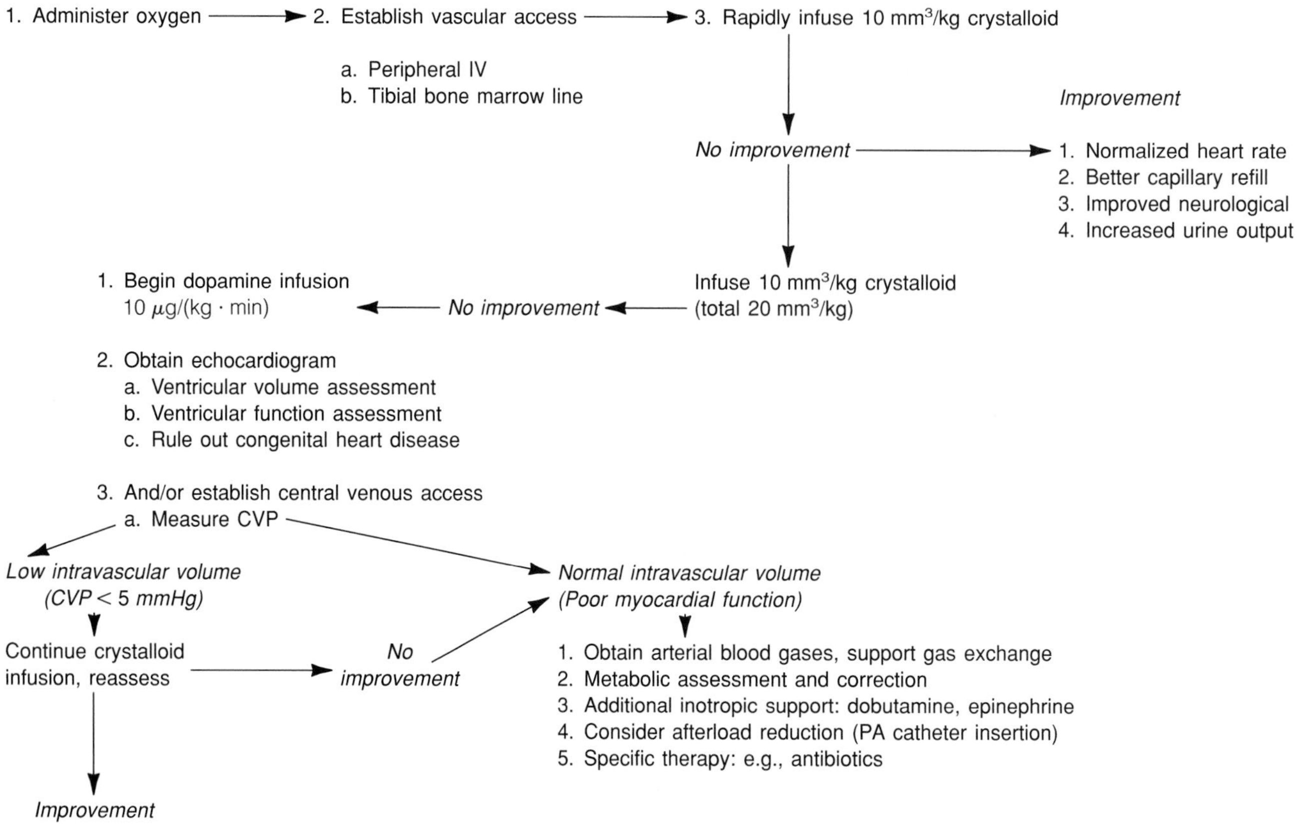

FIGURE 186-1 The child in shock.

tions, but immediate therapy should include assessment of the airway, administration of oxygen, and establishment of venous access. Occasionally, a peripheral venous site may be cannulated; quite commonly, however, peripheral cutaneous perfusion is too poor to allow this. In such instances, the external jugular or internal jugular vein may be cannulated, or a saphenous vein cutdown may be undertaken. In instances of cardiopulmonary arrest or profound circulatory collapse, the saphenous vein is ideal for cannulation by cutdown, because its anatomic position is nearly invariant and it is well out of the field of airway manipulation and external cardiac massage. More recently, intraosseous fluid administration has gained acceptance in many pediatric emergency facilities. Percutaneous placement of a stiff, short-beveled trocar needle into the anterior surface of the midshaft of the tibia has been shown to be an effective means for delivering fluid and noncaustic medication to the central circulation in infants and children. If possible, saphenous vein cannulation and lower extremity interosseous infusions should be avoided in the patient with abdominal trauma because the vena cava may be interrupted. In such instances, percutaneous internal jugular or subclavian venous cannulation may be the preferable approach. It should be attempted only by those familiar with the technique in infants and children, as these procedures carry high incidences of complications, including carotid arterial puncture, hemothorax, pneumothorax, and perforation of the superior vena cava or right atrium, when performed by unskilled personnel. Alternatively, antecubital vein cutdown is reasonably rapid and simple, but care must be taken to avoid injury to arterial and nervous structures in the antecubital fossa.

Specific therapy for circulatory failure is directed toward increasing cardiac output and normalizing peripheral organ perfusion. Because the determinants of cardiac output are heart rate and stroke volume, an increase in either may be beneficial. If tachycardia does not already exist, heart rate may be increased either by vagolysis or by cardiac β-stimulation (positive chronotrophy). The principal vagolytic agent is atropine (0.03 mg/kg), and the most commonly used positive chronotropic agents are isoproterenol or epinephrine. In children, a 30 to 50 percent increase in heart rate over control levels is well tolerated and will usually increase cardiac output substantially. Stroke volume is increased by **1.** increasing preload, **2.** decreasing afterload, or **3.** improving contractility.

Because most children in shock are hypovolemic, preload augmentation is the usual initial therapy (Figure 186-1). Once a venous cannula is established, the blood volume should be augmented with an infusion of blood, plasma, or crystalloid. The nature of the volume infusion depends primarily on availability and the characteristics of the losses. In a life-threatening situation, a balanced salt solution is probably the ideal infusate because it is immediately available and it can be very rapidly infused. The amount and rate of infusion depend on the clinical condition; however, a starting point is an infusion of 10 mL/kg of estimated body weight of lactated Ringer's solution over a few minutes. If there is no improvement in the patient's blood pressure or cutaneous perfusion, a second bolus of 10 mL/kg of body weight should be infused. If no improvement is observed after the second bolus of crystalloid, ongoing losses or a different cause should be suspected and further diagnosis pursued.

The first approach to further diagnoses is to accurately assess intravascular volume. This may be accomplished noninvasively through the use of echocardiography or invasively by the placement of a CVP catheter. Echocardiography has the advantage of being rapid and noninvasive, but it requires the immediate availability of sophisticated equipment and personnel skilled in interpreting pediatric echocardiograms. In addition, structural cardiac abnormalities can be ruled out simultaneously and myocardial function can be qualitatively assessed in real time.[18]

Central venous pressure monitoring is also effective and can be accomplished by cannulation of the internal jugular or subclavian vein. This procedure may take additional time to perform and is associated with complications that may be life threatening. Nevertheless, most infants and children who need ongoing assessment and cardiovascular support will require a CVP catheter.

Although a CVP value of 5 mmHg is a reasonable estimate for adequate intravascular volume, there is no single optimal CVP; only with careful incremental infusions of volume (10 mL/kg per bolus) can the effect on cardiac output be assessed. Several extracardiac factors, including lung compliance, the level of positive end-expiratory pressure (PEEP), peak inspiratory pressure (PIP), and increasing abdominal pressure, affect CVP or right ventricular filling pressure; thus, each patient's optimal CVP may differ considerably. Once a reasonable CVP has been obtained, if there is no improvement in blood pressure, cutaneous perfusion, or urine output, cardiogenic causes of circulatory failure must be considered.[19] Arterial blood gases, hematocrit, serum electrolytes, glucose, and calcium should be determined. Correction of acidosis, hypoxemia, or metabolic derangement is essential. Blood and other appropriate sites must be cultured and broad-spectrum parenteral antibiotic coverage begun if sepsis is a possibility.

Urine output can be an important indicator of the adequacy of the circulation. A urine output of greater than 1 mL/(kg · h) usually indicates an adequate renal blood flow and cardiac output. An output less than 0.5 mL/(kg · h) indicates circulatory failure, renal failure, or obstruction to urine flow.

Myocardial contractility can be improved by correcting existing metabolic derangements (hypoxia, acidosis, hypoglycemia) and by administering positive inotropic agents such as the sympathomimetic amines (β agonists), xanthines, and cardiac glycosides.[20] Ideally, before further cardiovascular support is initiated, a flow-directed thermodilution Swan-Ganz catheter should be placed. Right and left ventricular filling pressures, right atrial and pulmonary capillary wedge pressures, pulmonary artery pressure, and cardiac output can then be measured. From these data, pulmonary and systemic vascular resistances are calculated. A cardiac index of less than 2.5 L/(min · m^2) is indicative of circulatory failure and will require further therapy. Data collected will guide the therapeutic regimen, that is, to further increase inotropy, to augment intravascular volume, or to reduce vasomotor tone (afterload reduction).

However, in clinical pediatric practice, the PA catheter is less frequently used than when treating adult patients. In contrast to the adult with preexisting coronary artery disease, most conditions causing circulatory failure in children are associated with biventricular failure. In these cases, left ventricular filling pressures are reflected by the right atrial pressure. In most pediatric situations, the CVP is an adequate indicator of left- and right-sided filling pressures. The PA catheter in children is usually used for monitoring of PA pressure or for intermittent measurement of cardiac output by thermodilution technique.[21]

Afterload reduction may be indicated specifically when "pump failure" coexists with an elevated SVR. Under these circumstances, there may be an advantage to reducing afterload and ventricular work in order for the ventricle to pump more efficiently with an increase in stroke volume.[22] Afterload reduction may be effected with a direct vasodilator such as sodium nitroprusside, a β agonist (isoproterenol), or an α antagonist (phentolamine or tolazoline). Afterload reduction is frequently unpredictable, and the associated hypotension may reduce coronary perfusion to such a degree as to reduce cardiac efficiency rather than improve it. Vasodilators should be used with extreme caution, and vasoconstricting agents (phenylephrine or norepinephrine) should be available for immediate use. Afterload reduction is most safely employed with the use of a PA catheter in that endpoints of therapy, namely, an increased cardiac output and a decreased SVR, can be measured reliably and repeatedly.[23]

Pharmacologic vasoconstriction is used when hypotension results from an inappropriately low SVR such as in anaphylaxis and septic shock. The major complication of this therapy is that vasoconstricting agents produce an increase in the myocardial work and myocardial oxygen consumption, with the result that any primary myocardial decompensation may be worsened.

CARDIOVASCULAR PHARMACOLOGY IN CHILDREN

Pharmacologic support of the circulation includes positive inotropic and chronotropic agents, vasoconstrictors and vasodilators (afterload reduction), and antiarrhythmics. Most drugs currently used have not been adequately studied in children, so dosage recommendations and anticipated effects are extrapolated from studies in adults as well as from anecdotal clinical experience in children.[24]

Positive inotropic agents are often used in children to augment cardiac output in a variety of situations associated with circulatory failure. Most inotropic agents also affect heart rate and vasomotor tone. Tachycardia is often a deleterious side effect in the adult with limited myocardial oxygen reserve, whereas in the child an increase in heart rate is usually well tolerated and often beneficial.[14] Particularly in the neonate, whose ventricles are relatively noncompliant and in whom stroke volume is less variable, tachycardia is an important component of cardiac output augmentation. Because all agents that increase heart rate or contractility also increase myocardial oxygen consumption, it is imperative to ensure adequate arterial oxygenation and adequate supply of metabolic substrate during their administration. In addition, it is important to note that the cardiovascular response to the sympathomimetic amines is attenuated in the presence of acidosis; higher infusion rates of these drugs are required, which will need readjustment as acidosis improves.

EPINEPHRINE

Epinephrine has α-, β_1-, and β_2-adrenergic effects. It is used primarily in children with cardiac arrest or with profound myocardial depression and hypotension. As it is both a potent inotrope as well as vasoconstrictor, epinephrine supports the intravascular perfusion pressure. However, intense peripheral vasoconstriction can lead to renal, splanchnic, and cutaneous ischemia if epinephrine is continued for prolonged periods. After initial stabilization with epinephrine, support is usually continued with dopamine, dobutamine, or isoproterenol, which produce less peripheral vasoconstriction. Epinephrine is the drug of choice in severe circulatory failure or in cardiopulmonary arrest (vide infra).[25]

DOPAMINE

Dopamine is a sympathomimetic amine with α-, β-, δ-agonist properties. The properties of dopamine are extremely dose dependent.[26] In low doses, there is a δ effect with selective dilation of the splanchnic and renal vascular beds. In intermediate doses, it is a positive inotrope with little effect on heart rate or vasomotor tone; at high doses, it continues to have inotropic effects, but with the addition of an α effect on peripheral blood vessels. Specific doses in micrograms per kilogram differ between patients, but as a rule the young child requires higher doses than the adult to produce the same cardiovascular effect. In one recent study, an infusion of 15 μg/(kg · min) of dopamine was necessary to increase cardiac output above control in a group of infants following cardiac surgery.[27] This may reflect the decreased releasable stores of norepinephrine in the myocardium of immature ventricles. There are rare undesirable side effects of dopamine use in children, making it relatively safe and often the first agent chosen for inotropic support.

ISOPROTERENOL

Isoproterenol is a pure β agonist that produces positive inotropy, positive chronotropy, and a decrease in systemic vascular resistance secondary to dilation of the skeletal muscle vascular bed. If the patient has any degree of intravascular volume depletion, this vasodilation can cause a decrease in filling pressures, with resultant hypotension. The profound chronotropic effect of this drug limits its use in adults, but in children the increased heart rate is well tolerated and often beneficial.

DOBUTAMINE

Dobutamine is a direct-acting sympathomimetic amine that was initially purported to be similar to isoproterenol (positive inotropy and afterload reduction) but safer because of the lower incidence of tachycardia. With increasing experience, however, it appears that the vasomotor effects of dobutamine may vary with dosage in a manner similar to that seen with dopamine.[28] Dobutamine is often used in conjunction with dopamine to enhance myocardial contractibility without altering heart rate or systemic vascular resistance to the degree seen with isoproterenol.

NOREPINEPHRINE

Norepinephrine, an α- and β-adrenergic agonist, is the naturally occurring mediator of sympathetic activity whose effects are also dose dependent. Norepinephrine accounts for 80 to 90 percent of the circulating catecholamines in the newborn; by contrast, epinephrine is the major circulating catecholamine in the adult. Exogenously administered norepinephrine is only rarely used in the child and is reserved for situations in which cardiac function is near normal and extreme peripheral vasodilation has occurred. This may be seen in anaphylaxis, in septic shock, during spinal or epidural anesthesia, or with drugs that block the sympathetic nervous system. If myocardial dysfunction exists, the increase in afterload associated with peripheral vasoconstriction may not be tolerated without additional concurrent inotropic support.

AMRINONE

Amrinone is a relatively new xanthine derivative that is a nonglycoside, noncatecholamine cardiotonic agent. It has both positive inotropic effects as well as pulmonary and systemic vasodilator effects. While clinical experience with this drug in infants and children is still somewhat limited, it has been shown in clinical and laboratory studies to be a potent inotropic agent while directly decreasing right and left ventricular afterload. As is the case with the sympathomimetic amines, a higher infusion of amrinone on a weight basis is necessary to maintain a therapeutic effect when compared to similar infusions in adults.[29] One study suggests that in infants an initial bolus dose of 3 to 4.5 mg/kg in divided doses followed by an infusion of 10 μg/(kg · min) is necessary, whereas in neonates an infusion rate of 5 μg/(kg · min) is necessary. Although a potent inotropic agent, hypotension and thrombocytopenia may limit amrinone's usefulness as a first-line drug in infants and children.

DIGITALIS

Digitalis is the inotropic agent most commonly used for the chronic treatment of myocardial failure. In addition to its inotropic effects, it reduces sinoatrial (SA) node automaticity and AV conduction and is used for control of supraventricular tachycardias, including atrial fibrillation and flutter and AV nodal paroxysmal tachycardia. The main problem with digitalis use is toxicity. Because of the long half-life of digitalis and the unpredictability of digitalis toxicity in patients who demonstrate changing levels of serum potassium, ionized calcium, and pH, many clinicians avoid the initiation of digitalis in the unstable, acutely ill patient. More rapid acting and predictable inotropic drugs can be substituted.

CALCIUM

Calcium is another inotropic agent. When serum ionized calcium levels are low, the administration of calcium produces a positive inotropic effect; if ionized calcium levels are normal, however, the inotropic effect is much less marked. Low ionized calcium levels are most commonly documented in patients with septic shock, after massive volume replacement with citrated blood, and in neonates with relatively unstable calcium metabolism.[30] Calcium can also have a number of effects on the conduction system. In children with a normal ionized calcium, the rapid administration of calcium through a central venous catheter can cause severe bradycardia or asystole. This effect can be exaggerated in the presence of hypokalemia and digitalis; therefore, calcium should only be administered to such patients with great caution. There have also been reports of calcium precipitating malignant ventricular arrhythmias in adult patients with coronary artery disease; the relative absence of coronary artery disease in children minimizes this complication in the pediatric patient. The vasomotor effects of calcium are somewhat controversial, but most reports show an increase in SVR. Increased pulmonary resistance has also been documented.

BICARBONATE THERAPY

Acidosis profoundly depresses myocardial function and is a sensitive indicator of inadequate tissue perfusion. Although controversial, initial correction with 1 to 2 mEq/kg of sodium bicarbonate is recommended in children for a pH of less than 7.20 after establishment of adequate ventilation ($P_{CO_2} < 40$ mmHg). The circulatory system is refractory to sympathomimetic amines in the presence of severe acidosis; thus, inotropic agents, even in massive doses, are rendered ineffective unless acidosis is corrected.[31] After initial correction of the pH, the persistence or reappearance of metabolic acidosis suggests a return to an underperfused state and is cause for immediate alarm and therapeutic action. Sodium bicarbonate therapy can only be used as a stopgap measure to render the circulation amenable to pharmacologic support. Repeat infusions of sodium bicarbonate rapidly lead to hypernatremia and hyperosmolarity and cannot neutralize the ongoing lactic acidosis associated with inadequate tissue perfusion.

VASODILATORS

Vasodilators are used in children for four main purposes: to control systemic hypertension, to increase cardiac output by decreasing afterload, to control pulmonary hypertension, and to attempt to control cardiac shunting.[32] The use of vasodilators for control of systemic hypertension and for increasing cardiac output in children with CHF has been quite successful. On the other hand, treatment of pulmonary hypertension and cardiac shunting with vasodilators has shown mixed results. Responses of the pulmonary vasculature and of cardiac shunting to vasodilators seem to vary from patient to patient. The primary problem with these two uses is that all available vasodilators seem to work on the systemic circulation as well as on the pulmonary circulation. Systemic hypotension and increases in left-to-right shunting have resulted from attempts to treat pulmonary hypertension with vasodilators.

Sodium Nitroprusside

Sodium nitroprusside relaxes arteriolar and venous smooth muscle, producing a decrease in the afterload and possibly a decrease in the preload. The half-life is only minutes; as such, it is very safe to titrate infusions of this drug to a desired effect. Most common indications for its use are to control severe systemic hypertension, to precipitate an intraoperative episode of controlled hypotension in an attempt to decrease blood loss, and to increase cardiac output in children with low output syndrome (e.g., myocarditis, postcardiac surgery). Sodium nitroprusside can be used for days without problems. Potential difficulties include cyanide and thiocyanate poisoning. Cyanate is an intermediate metabolite of nitroprusside; thiocyanate is the final metabolite and is slowly cleared via renal extretion.[33] Thiocyanate toxicity is more common than cyanate toxicity. Thiocyanate levels of 10 mg/dL are associated with weakness, hypoxia, nausea, muscle spasms, and disorientation. The development of a metabolic acidosis is a sign of possible toxicity. Treatment involves discontinuing the administration of nitroprusside.

Nitroglycerine

Intravenous nitroglycerine is similar in effect to sodium nitroprusside, except that nitroglycerine has a relatively stronger vasodilating effect on the venous capacitance system than on the arterial bed. It has also been suggested as a pulmonary vasodilator, particularly in infants with pulmonary hypertension following cardiac surgery. There is very little reported experience of use of this drug in children.

Hydralazine

Hydralazine is routinely used to control systemic hypertension. It produces vascular smooth muscle relaxation in the arterial system much more than in the venous system.[34] There have also been some preliminary reports of hydralazine therapy for treatment of pulmonary hypertension.[35] A number of unpleasant effects of hydralazine therapy (i.e., headache, nausea, dizziness, sweating, tremors) have been described. The most important acute side effect is reflex tachycardia. A β antagonist (e.g., propranolol) is often used as adjunctive therapy to counteract this effect.

Tolazoline and Phentolamine[36]

Tolazoline and phentolamine are competitive α-adrenergic blockers that have been used in the treatment of pulmonary hypertension. The success of this therapy is not uniform, and these drugs are now rarely used. Serious side effects of these drugs include tachycardia, ventricular arrhythmias, systemic hypotension, and tissue edema.

Prostaglandin E_1

Although classified as a vasodilator, PGE_1 is a unique drug that has greatly improved the care of neonates with heart disease. PGE_1 acts directly on vascular smooth muscle, infused at a rate of 0.1 μg/(kg · min), it will maintain patency of the ductus arteriosus or even reopen the ductus in neonates up to 7 days of age and perhaps even older.[13] This response is dependent on factors such as age and the state of contraction of the ductus arteriosus. Side effects of apnea, hypotension from systemic vasodilation, or central nervous system (CNS) excitability should be anticipated. This drug is indispensable in patients with ductus-dependent cardiac lesions such as interrupted aortic arch, critical aortic stenosis, or hypoplastic left heart syndrome, where systemic flow is supplied by the ductus arteriosus. It is equally indispensable in pulmonary atresia and critical pulmonic stenosis, where pulmonary blood flow is supplied by the ductus arteriosus. It has also been used to treat pulmonary hypertension with varying degrees of success.

PRACTICAL USE OF INOTROPIC AGENTS IN INFANTS AND CHILDREN

There are a variety of approaches to pharmacologic support of the circulation in pediatric patients. We present one reasonably reliable and rational method for inotropic support. It is not uncommon that steps to support the circulation must begin before invasive hemodynamic monitoring can be accomplished in children. Dopamine is the first line of inotropic support in most circumstances (Table 186-3). Dopamine can be infused via a peripheral or central vein as well as through a tibial marrow needle. Care must be taken when infusing the drug through a peripheral vein, since it can cause local vasoconstriction and possible tissue necrosis if perfusion is extremely poor or if extravasation occurs. Infants and children are relatively resistant to dopamine and usually need higher infusion rates than adults. Five and even 10 μg(kg · min) is often a starting dose. Children rarely develop the α-vasoconstrictive effects of dopamine until an infusion rate of 20 μg/(kg · min) is reached. Arrhythmias are only rarely associated with dopamine use in children, and thus it is a relatively safe drug to initiate, even before intravascular status is fully evaluated and an etiology is established.

If an infusion rate of dopamine at 20 μg/(kg · min) is inadequate to restore the circulation (after appropriate volume resuscitation), dobutamine may be *added* to the dopamine infusion at 5 μg/(kg · min) (Table 186-3). This can be increased until 20 μg/(kg · min) of this agent is reached. Alternatively, if perfusion is extremely poor, or if cardiac arrest has occurred, epinephrine at an infusion rate of 0.1 μg/(kg · min) can be started. This infusion rate should be doubled every 5 to 10 min until perfusion is restored. Infusion rates up to 3 μg/(kg · min) are occasionally used in poorly perfused patients, but care must be taken since the α-vasoconstrictive effect of epinephrine can cause renal and cutaneous ischemia when infusion rates greater than 0.5 μg/(kg · min) are used for extended periods of time.

In addition to these inotropic agents, afterload reduction using sodium nitroprusside is occasionally useful. Patients with primary pump failure as seen in myocarditis, cardiomyopathy, and post-cardiac surgery, will often benefit from a reduction in afterload. This is most safely accomplished with the aid of a thermodilution PA catheter so that cardiac index can be measured and systemic vascular resistance can be calculated. Nitroprusside is usually begun at an infusion rate of 0.1 μg/(kg · min) and increased until cardiac index increases or systemic hypotension occurs. When initiating nitroprusside, volume infusion will be necessary to compensate for the increased vascular capacitance.

In addition to cardiac output measurement, repeated two-dimensional echocardiography is very useful in reassessing ventricular performance and end-diastolic filling volume on a real-time basis and is an important tool in guiding pharmacologic and fluid therapy in these patients.

ANTIARRHYTHMICS

The most common arrhythmia in pediatric patients is bradycardia caused by hypoxia. Therefore, any list of antiarrhythmic drugs must begin with oxygen.

PROPRANOLOL

Propranolol is a β antagonist used in children to control supraventricular tachycardias and as an adjunctive agent to

TABLE 186-3 Typical Dilutions and Infusion Rates of Inotropes

Dopamine and Dobutamine	5–25 μg/(kg · min)	Add 60 mg of agent to 100 mL of D_5W. Infuse at the child's body weight (in kg) in mL/h to equal 10 μg/(kg · min)
[(e.g., 15-kg child: 60 mg of dopamine in 100 mL of D_{10} W. Run at 15 mL/h to equal 10 μg/(kg · min)]		
Epinephrine	0.1–3 μg/(kg · min)	Add 1 mg of epinephrine to 100 mL D_5W and infuse at the child's body weight (in kg) in mL/h to equal 0.17 μg/(kg · min)
[e.g., 15-kg child: Add 1 mg of epinephrine to 100 mL of D_5W. Infuse at 15 mL/h to equal 0.17 μg/(kg · min).]		

control hypertension, cyanotic spells in patients with tetralogy of Fallot,[37] and hypertrophic obstructive cardiomyopathy. Because it is a β blocker, propranolol must be used with caution in patients with asthma and in patients with myocardial failure. It can also precipitate hypoglycemia, especially in small children.[38]

VERAPAMIL

Calcium channel blockers, exemplified by verapamil, are becoming the drug of choice in supraventricular tachycardias. In infants rapid intravenous doses of 0.125 to 0.25 mg/kg of verapamil have been shown to be quickly effective in terminating more than 90 percent of supraventricular tachycardias without obvious side effects.[39] Toxicities include severe bradycardia and hypotension, which can be reversed with isoproterenol.

OTHER ANTIARRHYTHMICS

Other drugs useful in controlling ventricular arrhythmias in children include lidocaine, 1 mg/kg, and procainamide, 3 to 6 mg/kg, over 5 min intravenously. Use of much larger doses of procainamide has been reported. Phenytoin has also been used, especially in cases of suspected digitalis toxicity, in an intravenous dose of 5 mg/kg over 5 min. Oral phenytoin has been used for chronic control of ventricular arrhythmias in children. For life-threatening refractory ventricular arrhythmias unresponsive to other drugs, bretylium given in a dose of 5 to 10 mg/kg intravenously over 10 min is recommended.[40] Adenosine has recently been released for the acute termination of supraventricular tachycardia in infants and children. The effective dose range is reported to range widely, from 37.5 to 350 μg/kg with a mean value of 131 μg/kg.

HYPERTENSIVE CRISES IN INFANTS AND CHILDREN

The acute onset of severe systemic arterial hypertension constitutes a medical emergency because of the potential for cardiovascular decompensation as well as the CNS complications of encephalopathy, seizures, or intracranial hemorrhage. In older children, the neurologic manifestations of hypertension are more likely to precede cardiovascular decompensation. By contrast, severe hypertension in the neonate often presents with the nonspecific cardiorespiratory symptoms of CHF. The causes of severe hypertension in children are listed in Table 186-4.

Treatment of acute severe hypertension requires careful and constant monitoring of arterial blood pressure and of respiratory and neurologic function. The most common pharmacologic agents used in the treatment of acute hypertensive crises are diazoxide, hydralazine, and sodium nitroprusside. Diazoxide is a potent vasodilator that reduces blood pressure rapidly after an intravenous bolus. Hypotension, tachycardia, and nausea and vomiting are common side effects. Its duration of action is brief and must be followed by other agents of longer duration.

TABLE 186-4 Causes of Severe Hypertension in Children

Renal
- Acute glomerulonephritis (e.g., poststreptococcal, Henoch-Schönlein)
- Hemolytic uremic syndrome
- Chronic glomerulonephritis (all types)
- Acute and chronic pyelonephritis
- Congenital malformations (dysplasia, hypoplasia, cystic diseases)
- Tumors (e.g., Wilms', leukemic infiltrate)
- Postrenal transplantation; also with rejection
- Oliguric renal failure
- Trauma
- Obstructive uropathy
- After genitourinary surgery
- Blood transfusions in children with azotemia

Cardiovascular
- Coarctation of the aorta
- Renal artery abnormalities (e.g., stenosis, thrombosis)
- Takayasu's disease

Endocrine
- Pheochromocytoma
- Neuroblastoma
- Adrenogenital disease
- Cushing's syndrome
- Hyperaldosteronism
- Hyperthyroidism
- Hyperparathyroidism

Iatrogenic
- Intravascular volume overload
- Sympathomimetic administration (e.g., epinephrine, ephedrine)
- Corticosteroid administration
- Rapid intravenous infusion of methyldopa

Miscellaneous
- Immobilization (e.g., fractures, burns, Guillain-Barré syndrome)
- Hypercalcemia (e.g., hypervitaminosis D, metastatic disease, sarcoidosis, some immobilized patients)
- Hypernatremia
- Stevens-Johnson syndrome
- Increased intracranial pressure (any cause)
- Dysautonomia
- Postresuscitation

The Respiratory System

Respiratory insufficiency or failure is a common diagnosis in the PICU. Because pathophysiology changes with the age of the child, an understanding of normal development and maturation is helpful.

DEVELOPMENT

The bronchial tree and accompanying arteries develop during the first 16 weeks of gestation. For the next 19 months the bronchi undergo distal arborization with growth of companion arteries. Thick-walled alveolar precursors or alveolar saccules are present at birth and capable of gas exchange. Postnatally these saccules thin, becoming true alveoli. The number of alveoli increases dramatically in the first 8 years of life from approximately 24 million at birth to 300 million by age eight. After this time, further lung growth is accomplished by an increase in the size of the alveoli.[41] This normal pattern of lung growth has attracted interest in terms of catch-up growth in young children who have either hypoplasia or lung injury. But obviously because the number of large airways is completed in utero the scope of postnatal growth is limited to arborization of small terminal airways and an increase in the number of alveoli.

Another important pattern of maturation is the development and extension of elastin. At birth there is little elastin in the lung and it is present only to the level of the terminal bronchioles. Over time elastin slowly extends to the alveolar surface reaching a maximum during late adolescence.[42] The decreased amount of elastin in combination with smaller and fewer alveoli results in decreased lung compliance in the child. This can be further compromised at birth secondary to thick-walled alveolar precursors and potential immaturity of the surfactant system as seen in hyaline membrane disease (HMD).

In contrast, the child's chest wall is more compliant because of flexible cartilagenous ribs, the boxlike configuration of the chest wall, and decreased intercostal and diaphragmatic muscle strength. The combination of decreased lung compliance and increased chest wall compliance can result in alveolar collapse and a decreased FRC. During health, the child uses several dynamic mechanisms to maintain adequate inflation and FRC. But when a child becomes ill a number of events (i.e., abdominal distension, immobility, sedation) can exacerbate the normal tendency toward collapse.

The child also has higher airway resistance secondary to smaller airway size. This is most problematic in the first 6 years of life before there is growth and significant increase in the caliber of the airways.[43] Because of this, any disease process associated with even minor airway edema or obstruction can be symptomatic in the young child.

There are also maturational differences in the control of breathing. Apnea is encountered in the neonate secondary to a number of stresses: hypothermia, sepsis, and, paradoxically, hypoxemia.[44]

Finally there are differences in oxygen transport. At birth the child has an elevated oxygen consumption of 6 to 8 mL/(kg · min) which decreases to 5 to 6 mL/(kg · min) by age 1 year. In the first year of life meeting this elevated oxygen demand is complicated by the presence of fetal hemoglobin (decreased P50) and a normally occurring physiologic anemia at age 3 to 4 months. To overcome these potential limitations, the infant has a relatively high minute ventilation and cardiac output.

ETIOLOGIES OF RESPIRATORY FAILURE IN CHILDREN

In the adult or child the causes of respiratory failure can be subdivided into three major categories: hypoventilation with normal lungs, intrinsic alveolar or interstitial disease, and airway obstruction. Specific causes of these vary with the age of the child. The neonate is often considered separately because of the problems of immaturity (HMD), abnormal development (congenital diaphragmatic hernia, Potter's syndrome which is bilateral renal agenesis with associated pulmonary hypoplasia), perinatal stresses (persistent fetal circulation), and infections (*Listeria*, group B *Streptococcus*) specific to neonates.

HYPOVENTILATION WITH NORMAL LUNGS

Hypoventilation with normal lungs produces a pattern of shallow tachypnea with resultant atelectasis and hypoxemia. The causes of hypoventilation include muscle weakness from neuromuscular disease, central hypoventilation, an unstable chest wall, and extrinsic compression of the lungs.

Central sleep apnea is a relatively common diagnosis in infants. It can present as hypoventilation or complete apnea during sleep (Ondine's curse). Although etiology is uncertain, immaturity or abnormality of the medullary chemoreceptors is invoked.[45] Therapy includes time and maturation, theophylline as a stimulant, and cardiorespiratory home monitoring. If there is complete sleep apnea, tracheostomy and mechanical ventilation during sleep are required. Obstructive sleep apnea can be caused by an anatomic mandibular hypoplasia, Pierre Robin syndrome, tonsillar hypertrophy, or dynamic obstruction (lax pharyngeal muscles). This can occur at any age. Symptoms include very loud snoring with episodes of total obstruction that cause arousal from sleep. As a result these patients are usually sleep deprived and constantly fatigued. The goal of therapy is to bypass the obstruction: often a tonsillectomy and adenoidectomy are done to maximize the existing airway. Some patients require tracheostomy.[46]

ALVEOLAR OR INTERSTITIAL DISEASE

Alveolar or interstitial disease is physiologically the same in the adult and child, with the understanding that bacterial pathogens differ. The neonate is susceptible to group B *Streptococcus, E. coli,* and *Listeria.* The preschool child is most commonly affected by *Hemophilus influenzae* and *S. pneumoniae.* Although it has not been adequately studied, it appears that adult respiratory distress syndrome (ARDS) is a less common diagnosis in the PICU versus adult ICU. ARDS has been reported in 1 to 3 percent of PICU admissions.[47] Similar to adults, the mortality is highest if sepsis or malignancy complicate the course.

AIRWAY OBSTRUCTION

Upper airway obstruction is more common in the child than the adult. Because the child's airway is smaller at baseline even a small amount of edema or intrinsic or extrinsic compression can have a fatal effect. Common upper airway diagnoses in the PICU include epiglottitis, laryngotracheobronchitis (LTB or croup), and aspiration of a foreign body. Epiglottitis is a bacterial (*H. influenzae*) infection of the supraglottic tissues. A true medical emergency, it is characterized by rapid progression of swelling which can produce a fatal airway obstruction. Initial treatment is to secure an artificial airway and to administer antibiotics (usually ampicillin and chloramphenicol). Airway management is best performed by endotracheal intubation in the operating room where if need be, rigid bronchoscopy or tracheostomy can be safely performed. LTB or croup is the most common cause of upper airway obstruction in the child aged 3 months to 3 years. It is a viral infection which causes circumferential subglottic edema. Treatment includes increased ambient oxygen, mist, and racemic epinephrine. Steroids although of unproven benefit are frequently administered.[48] In our opinion, steroid administration is appropriate pending adequate studies. Endotracheal intubation is only performed if the preceding therapies fail and the child suffers respiratory failure. On occasion, Heliox has been used; the main impediments include inadequate scavenging systems, a lowered inspired oxygen concentration, and general unfamiliarity with use of this gas mixture (see Chap. 11).[49]

Foreign-body aspiration can occur at any age, but peak incidence is 6 months to 3 years. In the child the subglottic area is the narrowest part of the airway. If a foreign body lodges in this area, it can be difficult to remove by either coughing or manual extrication. Treatment of foreign-body aspiration is tailored to the degree of the child's respiratory difficulty. Heimlich maneuvers, abdominal thrusts, and back slaps are all reserved for near complete upper airway obstruction with little or no air movement. Of note, Heimlich maneuvers are avoided in children less than 4 to 6 years of age because an enthusiastic Heimlich maneuver could potentially cause hepatic rupture. For less dramatic upper airway obstruction or lower airway mechanical obstruction, therapy includes laryngoscopy, bronchoscopy, postural drainage, bronchodilators, chest physiotherapy, or surgical removal.[50]

Obstruction of the lower airways is common in pediatrics because of the small native diameter of these airways. Common diagnoses include asthma (vide infra) and viral infections—particularly respiratory syncytial virus (RSV) bronchiolitis and anything that causes airway edema. These patients present with a heterogeneous disease of air trapping and atelectasis causing an increased work of breathing, hypoxemia, and CO_2 retention. Specific therapy includes increased ambient oxygen, pharmacologic bronchodilation, and, when necessary, mechanical ventilation. RSV infections deserve separate discussion. Virtually 90 percent of children are infected by 2 years of age with almost 5 percent requiring hospitalization for bronchiolitis or pneumonia and many of these needing mechanical ventilation. While morbidity is high, mortality is less than 1 percent and is primarily seen in children with pulmonary vascular hypertension.[51] Conventional respiratory support remains the mainstay of therapy. The role of ribaviran is controversial; clinical studies have not demonstrated a clear benefit and there are concerns regarding personnel exposure during its administration.[52]

STATUS ASTHMATICUS

Status asthmaticus is one of the most common admitting diagnoses in pediatric hospitals, and is a common reason for admission to the PICU. Diagnosis and evaluation is virtually the same as in the adult, with the exception that children can present with severe hypoxemia as their major symptom without any CO_2 retention. These children are concerning because they can progress to respiratory failure without showing progressive elevation in their Pa_{CO_2}.

The treatment of status asthmaticus includes oxygen, steroids, and pharmacologic bronchodilation with the goal of avoiding endotracheal intubation. Because children do not have coronary artery disease they can safely tolerate more aggressive drug therapy with β-adrenergic agonists and theophylline than their adult counterparts. Theophylline is given as a 6-mg/kg bolus followed by an infusion of 0.5 to 1 mg/(kg · h) with the goal of a serum level of 15 to 20 μg/mL. Infants require lower doses because of decreased hepatic drug clearance. Beta-adrenergic agents are given by aerosol or intravenously. The aerosol route has become more popular in the past few years. Routine doses are isoproterenol (0.5%) 0.01 mL/kg: albuterol (0.5%) 0.01 mL/kg, and metaproterenol (5%) 0.01 mL/kg. These doses are diluted with 2 mL normal saline. Constant aerosolization has also been used. Intravenous isoproterenol is favored by some: the starting dose is 0.1 μg/(kg · min), and this is doubled for effect with close monitoring of the heart rate and ECG.[53]

It is uncommon to intubate a pediatric asthmatic. This probably reflects the incredible amount of energy the child can put into breathing and the child's tolerance for large doses of drugs. Most clinicians will only intubate a child with asthma once the child demonstrates mental status changes from fatigue. It is impossible to define the need for intubation by any specific Pa_{CO_2}. In our PICU, the majority of intubated asthmatics are children who were intubated at referring hospitals before they received an adequate trial of drugs.

PRINCIPLES OF MANAGEMENT OF CHILDHOOD RESPIRATORY FAILURE

Treatment of respiratory failure includes the following general categories: **1.** optimal body position, **2.** increase of ambient oxygen, **3.** relief of an obstruction either by airway instrumentation or pharmacology, **4.** treatment of infection, **5.** correction of fluid overload, **6.** maximizing nonpulmonary organ system function, **7.** negative- or positive-pressure ventilation, and **8.** innovative approaches including surfactant therapy, high-frequency ventilation, and extracorporeal membrane oxygenation (ECMO).

CONVENTIONAL MANAGEMENT

The young child is often dependent on an adult for his assumed body position. It should be remembered that respiratory status is optimal in a semiupright position with the head in midline. Because the larynx is so anterior and superior in a child, excessive neck flexion can produce obstruction and hence should be avoided. In fact, during cardiopulmonary resuscitation (CPR) or other active airway manipulation, the child should be placed in the "sniffing" position by placing a small towel or diaper under the occiput. This can then be followed by routine jaw thrust. Increase of ambient oxygen can be accomplished in a number of unstressful ways: face masks, face tests, nasal prongs, croup tents, or just "blow-by." The frightened child will often not tolerate any apparatus around the face, particularly if it in any way obstructs his vision.

The gold standard for respiratory support is the use of positive-pressure mechanical support. This is performed almost exclusively via an endotracheal tube (ETT) or tracheostomy tube. The appropriate size by internal diameter can be estimated in children > 1 year of age with the following equation:

$$\frac{\text{Age} + 16}{4}$$

Once a tube is placed, there should be an audible leak at approximately 20 to 25 cm H_2O pressure. Placement of an oral-tracheal tube is easier, but a nasal-tracheal tube is generally more comfortable and better tolerated by the child. Uncuffed ETTs are used in children less than 8 years of age because the flexible tracheal cartilage and relative subglottic narrowing provide an excellent seal without a cuff. ETTs are being safely left in children for increasing periods of time (6 to 8 weeks) before progressing to a tracheostomy. Once the need for long-term airway support is obvious, an earlier tracheostomy is appropriate.

With the ETT in place, the child can be treated with continuous positive airway pressure (CPAP) or positive-pressure ventilation. CPAP can also be administered with nasal prongs or a face mask. Because neonates are obligate nose breathers, nasal CPAP can be effective. But in the older child, nasal CPAP is unreliable. Face mask CPAP is used in adults and children, with the limitation of cutaneous pressure sores and gastric distension. Positive-pressure ventilation can be delivered by a number of different modes of ventilators: volume preset, pressure preset, or time-flow preset. In children weighing under 10 kg, the time-flow preset is most commonly used. These ventilators have the advantage of rapid response time at rapid ventilator rates with continuous-flow intermittent mandatory ventilation (IMV). Time-flow ventilators are used because inaccurate volumes are delivered with volume ventilators in the small child. The delivered volume is unreliable because of the variable leak around the uncuffed ETT, and the relatively large gas compression volume lost in the expanding tubing of the ventilator in comparison to the relatively small tidal volume. Obviously discrepancies in delivered volume from a volume preset ventilator would be even larger if the patient were experiencing large swings in lung compliance or resistance. Therefore, for children less than 10 kg time-flow preset ventilators are preferred because these ventilators pressure-limit delivered tidal volumes. In children over 10 kg, volume preset ventilators are used.[54]

Sedation or analgesia is required in virtually any conscious or semiconscious child at the beginning of mechanical ventilation. The amount of sedation should be tailored to the specific situation with the goals of patient comfort to facilitate the patient breathing in phase with the ventilator. There is no perfect drug regimen for sedation, but common combinations include a narcotic and a benzodiazepine. If the child does require very elevated airway pressures or $F_{I_{O_2}}$, then muscle relaxants should be added.

Weaning a pediatric patient from mechanical ventilation is generally the same as in the adult. One problem is concomitant weaning of sedation, in that it is often difficult to pharmacologically maintain patient compliance without depressing respiratory drive. A second problem is inability to reliably measure lung function (vide supra). A final difference is the fact that many of the routine "adult weaning" ventilator modes are difficult to use in the smaller child. Conventional assisted ventilatory breaths are problematic because of the work required to trigger the machine as well as the poor machine response time to the child's normal tachypnea. Pressure support ventilation has proven beneficial in older children, but in infants the relative tachypnea and small tidal volumes make it difficult for the machine to deliver appropriate pressures.[55]

NEW METHODS OF SUPPORT

The administration of exogenous surfactant has slowly been gaining popularity since the first description of decreased surfactant in HMD.[56] Completed as well as ongoing studies are available testing the efficacy and safety of surfactant administration in the neonate. To date, the data are very encouraging for this group of patients. Prophylactic administration to premature neonates has become accepted therapy. Rescue or therapeutic administration to infants with respiratory distress or failure is of less proven benefit.[57] Application to the older child and adult needs further study but may well be limited by the dose requirement, cost, and presence of surfactant inhibitors.

Negative-pressure ventilators can be used for children with chronic respiratory insufficiency who may benefit from intermittent, usually night-time ventilation (e.g., patients with Duchenne's muscular dystrophy). The iron lung is usually used in the hospital setting, but the body cuirass and the raincoat negative-pressure ventilators are appropriate for home use. The advantage of negative-pressure support is that it obviates the need for airway instrumentation. The disadvantage is that the patient must have nearly normal lungs, a normal upper airway, and be able to handle her own pulmonary toilet. In the neonate, the use of negative-pressure ventilation is limited because of the difficulty maintaining a neck seal without compressing the airway.

High-frequency ventilation includes three major types of machines: the high-frequency positive-pressure ventilator (HFPPV), the high-frequency jet (HFJ) and the high-frequency oscillator (HFO). All use rapid rates but differ in technical design and execution of gas delivery.[58] Each of these ventilators has been used in neonatal and pediatric patients. The HFJ has been used in the adult and the pediatric population with reported success in patients who have significant air leaks from barotrauma. HFO experience has primarily been in neonates. Despite sporadic enthusiasm, it remains of unproven benefit. One multicenter HFO trial which received study design criticism, demonstrated no

TABLE 186-5 Normal Ages for Major Developmental Milestones

Age, months	Motor Function	Language	Adaptive Behavior
1–1½	Lifts head from prone position and turns from side to side	Cries	Smiles
4	Shows no head lag when pulled to sitting from supine position; tries to grasp large objects	Utters sounds of pleasure	Smiles, laughs aloud, and shows pleasure to familiar objects or persons
5	Grasps voluntarily with both hands; plays with toes	Makes primitive sounds (ah, goo)	Smiles at self in mirror
6	Grasps with one hand; rolls prone to supine; sits with support	Has increased range of sounds	Expresses displeasure and food preferences
8	Sits without support; transfers objects from hand to hand; rolls supine to prone	Combines syllables (baba, dada, mama)	Responds to "no"
10	Sits well; crawls; stands holding; finger–thumb apposition in picking up small objects		Waves bye-bye; plays patty-cake and peek-a-boo
12	Stands holding; walks with support	Says two or three words with meaning	Understands names of objects; shows interest in pictures
15	Walks alone	Utters several intelligible words	Requests by pointing; imitates
18	Walks up and down stairs holding; removes clothes	Says many intelligible words	Carries out simple commands
24	Walks up and down stairs by self; runs	Makes two- or three-word phrases	Engages in organized play; points to some parts of body

advantages of HFO over conventional treatment in a neonatal population.[59] Further studies are necessary before HFO gains acceptance as more than an experimental tool.

ECMO is presently accepted as therapy for neonates greater than 34 weeks gestation with severe reversible respiratory failure.[60] The National Neonatal ECMO Registry reports an 82 percent survival rate for more than 4000 infants who have met institutional criteria for 80 percent or greater predicted mortality.[61] The major morbidity of ECMO is neurologic. In short-term follow-up, 15 to 20 percent of the infants suffer some neurologic sequela, ranging from minor to severe.[62] Long-term follow-up studies are presently in progress. There is increasing interest to expand the ECMO population to include children and adults with respiratory failure and to patients of any age with cardiovascular failure. The experience with respiratory failure in older children is limited but growing. Preliminary reports of 140 patients show a 43 percent survival rate with ECMO in patients who had an 80 to 100 percent predicted mortality.[61] The problem with this group is the identification of patients who are sick enough to warrant exposure to the risks of ECMO, but who have not progressed to irreversible disease. ECMO for cardiovascular support has primarily been used in the perioperative period. The survival rate for this is also in the range of 40 percent.[61]

The Central Nervous System

Neurologic dysfunction as a primary or secondary disease is a common concern in the PICU. The most common diagnoses are seizures, head trauma, tumor, infection, hypoxic or metabolic encephalopathy, and hemorrhage. Assessment of CNS function in any of these diseases requires an understanding of normal motor and cognitive development. Most observers who are uncomfortable with children usually grossly under- or overestimate what a child should be able to do.

Motor function is dependent on gestational age more than postnatal age. This is important to remember when evaluating a child with a history of prematurity.[63] Cognitive development is first seen as adaptive interactive behavior (eye contact, smiling, etc.). In the first year of life there are a number of motor, language, and behavior milestones that can be used as measuring tools (Table 186-5).

Assessment in the clinical setting includes observation and examination. The Glasgow Coma Scale (GCS) is used to categorize patients with an abnormal neurologic status; for very young children the verbal responses have been altered (Table 186-6).[64] Laboratory assessment is the same as in the adult: examination of the spinal fluid, radiologic imaging [plain films, computed tomography (CT), magnetic resonance imaging (MRI)], electroencephalogram (EEG), and brain stem evoked potentials. Of note, neonatal encephalography is less than a well-developed science, and results may often be difficult to interpret. Intracranial pressure (ICP) monitoring can be done by ventriculostomy or subarachnoid screw. The subarachnoid screw can only be used in older children once the skull plate is thick enough to support the apparatus.

TABLE 186-6 Glasgow Coma Scale

Eye opening		
Spontaneous	4	
To voice	3	
To pain	2	
None	1	
Best verbal response (For older children and adult)		Best verbal response (For very young children)
Oriented	5	Appropriate words or social smile, fixes and follows
Confused	4	Cries but consolable
Inappropriate	3	Persistently irritable
Incomprehensible	2	Restless, agitated
None	1	None
Best motor response		
Obeys commands	6	
Localizes pain	5	
Withdraws globally	4	
Decorticate posturing	3	
Decerebrate posturing	2	
None	1	

HEAD TRAUMA

Head injury accounts for 75 percent of all trauma admissions and 70 percent of trauma deaths that occur within the first 48 h of hospitalization.[65] Injury from trauma is both primary (contusion, shearing, and penetrating), as well as secondary (anoxia, ischemia). Unfortunately in the child as in the adult, increased ICP is the final common pathway for most head trauma. Children with significant head injuries have fewer skull fractures than their adult counterparts, and the fractures that do occur in children tend to be more diastatic and, hence, more difficult to diagnose.

The treatment of head injury includes basic support of ventilation, oxygenation, and perfusion. The indications for ICP monitoring and potential therapy are controversial. One set of criteria for monitoring is **1.** the patient who requires neurosurgery, **2.** the patient who has a GCS less than 8, **3.** the child who requires prolonged paralysis for mechanical ventilation, or **4.** the child who is going to have general anesthesia for a non-CNS surgical procedure.[66] These criteria may be too conservative: There is reported experience of no increased ICP in children with GCS greater than 6, but an 81 percent incidence of increased ICP if the GCS was 3 to 4.[67]

When any child is evaluated with a closed head injury, it is imperative to consider child abuse (shaken baby) in the differential.

TUMORS

Brain tumors are a common pediatric diagnosis and explain a number of PICU admissions for acute neurologic deterioration. Because childhood brain tumors are frequently situated in the posterior fossa, these patients may present with signs and symptoms of increased ICP secondary to obstructive hydrocephalus.

REYE'S SYNDROME

Reye's syndrome must be mentioned because of its pediatric predominance. This is a syndrome of encephalopathy, malignant cerebral hypertension, and fatty degeneration of the liver and is commonly associated with a viral infection (post varicella or influenza). Reye's syndrome has also been related to the use of aspirin. Because of this association, aspirin use in children has been avoided since the late 1970s and the incidence of Reye's syndrome has dramatically decreased to the point that it has virtually disappeared from PICUs. Children with Reye's syndrome are staged by both clinical parameters (Lovejoy, stages I to V) and EEG characteristics (grades I to IV). Elevated morbidity and mortality are associated with a rapid progression from minor to severe disease and extremely elevated levels of ammonia (>700 mg/L) at diagnosis. The treatment includes routine medical support of hepatic failure and treatment of increased ICP. The indication for invasive ICP monitoring is not exact but should be considered for any patient with a Lovejoy scale of 2 or greater. Because Reye's syndrome is so rare, the reader is referred to references for further discussion.[68]

SEIZURES

Seizures are frequently encountered in the PICU. The known etiologies include head trauma, infection, metabolic abnormalities (hypocalcemia, hyponatremia) hypoxemia, hypoglycemia, brain tumor, and fever. Evaluation is essentially the same as for the adult: metabolic screen, examination of spinal fluid, radiographic imaging, and EEG examination. Initial supportive treatment controls the airway and provides adequate ventilation and oxygenation. The specific goal of therapy is to stop the seizure. Usual medications are diazepam 0.1 mg/kg intravenous or per rectum, phenobarbital 10 to 20 mg/kg loading dose, and phenytoin 10 to 20 mg/kg loading dose. Caution is required whenever diazepam and phenobarbital are used together; apnea requiring intubation and ventilation may result. In fact, the most common reason for placement of an endotracheal tube in a patient with seizures is for the treatment of iatrogenic apnea.[69]

INCREASED INTRACRANIAL PRESSURE

Increased intracranial pressure (ICP) is the final common pathway for a number of injuries. Although evaluation and treatment are similar in the child and the adult, there are a few issues specific to children. Changes in mental status can be more difficult to assess in the child because the alterations can be very subtle, yet the child's physical examination is enhanced by the presence of the fontanelle and open sutures. A young child who has a chronic increase in intracranial volume will have split sutures which can be easily assessed by palpating the head. The fontanelle also offers a window into the status of the intracranial volume. With either acute or chronic increases in volume, the fontanelle becomes full and then bulges. This can be difficult for the nonpediatrician to assess. Most children when lying flat or crying will have fullness of the fontanelle; but when they are calm and held in a sitting position, the fontanelle should flatten.

Treatment is no different in the child or the adult. Any inciting events should be reversed and treated with antibiotics, metabolic correction, and/or anticonvulsants. Basic resuscitation should always focus on cardiopulmonary status: adequate gas exchange and arterial perfusion must be supported. Any fever should be treated immediately. Specific therapy then begins. The head should be positioned in the midline at a slant of about 30°. Hyperosmolarity is achieved and maintained by decreasing the intake as well as causing a diuresis with mannitol (0.25 to 1.0 gm/kg per dose) or lasix. Glycerol is rarely used because of the limitations of the oral route. Endotracheal intubation and hyperventilation are usually used if the ICP is elevated. Prophylactic hyperventilation is not recommended because over hours cerebral blood flow will reequilibrate to lower levels of Pa_{CO_2} (see Chap. 4). Steroids are only used for the treatment of edema immediately around a tumor margin. The use of barbiturates is controversial. While barbiturates will decrease the ICP, they have never been proven to improve survival or neurologic outcome. Nembutal is usually administered: 3 to 30 mg/kg as an intravenous bolus followed by 1 to 2 mg/(kg · h), with the blood level goal of 20 to 40 mg/L. They are less commonly used now than 10 years ago; if barbiturates are used, intracranial monitoring should be in place.[70]

BRAIN DEATH

Brain death has been a particularly difficult diagnosis to agree upon in the pediatric population. There are a number of proposed criteria. The most conservative restrict the definition to children over 5 years of age; more liberal ones limit it to children over 1 week of age.[71,72] Each practitioner is cautioned to review and understand local definitions of brain death because each hospital and state may have specified guidelines.

Despite regional differences, there are a number of general approaches. The clinical examination is paramount. This must be an exam which carefully documents no neurologic function. This examination should include evaluation of motor responses, cranial nerves, and an apnea test (documenting no respiratory effort in the face of a Pa_{CO_2} above 45 mmHg).[73] The clinical examination should be repeated a number of times during an observation period spanning 6 to 72 h. Most clinicians will also have one to two other staff-level physicians evaluate the child and document their findings in the medical record. Laboratory evaluations are seen as adjuncts or confirmatory tests and are only used as needed. There seems to be an increased reliance on the laboratory assessment in the situations of organ donation or when there is a question of homocide.

Obviously the diagnosis of brain death requires that the physician make every attempt to ascertain the cause of the event. If the cause cannot be identified, then the diagnosis of brain death is more unsettling. The physician must also exclude any circumstances present that may mimic brain death, e.g., hypothermia or drug ingestion.

The Renal System

RENAL FAILURE

Acute renal failure (ARF) is an abrupt, often temporary loss of renal function following an insult that may or may not be evident on presentation in the acutely ill infant and child. Oliguria is the rule, polyuria the exception, and anuria uncommon. Urine volume and composition are altered, and fluid, electrolyte, and acid-base disorders are commonly associated. Therapy is directed at maintaining normal metabolic and fluid homeostasis, supporting nutrition, and exhibiting patience. The causes of ARF are prerenal, postrenal (obstructive), or intrinsic renal (see Table 186-7). Prerenal causes are related to the adequacy of renal blood flow. Reducing cardiac output or renal blood flow by any mechanism will reduce urine output and ultimately azotemia and ischemic renal damage. Measurement of the adequacy of the circulating blood volume by CVP and cardiac output, as well as assessment of renal blood flow with nuclear imaging techniques, are useful in differentiating prerenal from renal causes of azotemia.[74]

Postrenal obstruction to urine flow can occur anywhere within the collecting system. Chronic partial obstruction at the level of the bladder neck, ureterovesicle, or ureteropelvic junction is a common form of congenital malformation. Posterior urethral valves are a frequent cause of obstruction

TABLE 186-7 Common Causes of Renal Failure in Children

I. Renal hypoperfusion
  A. Decreased intravascular volume
    1. Dehydration
    2. Hemorrhage
    3. Capillary leak syndrome
  B. Cardiogenic
    1. Pump failure
    2. Obstruction to inflow or outflow of blood
    3. Dysrhythmias
  C. Renal vascular obstruction
    1. Renal vein thrombosis
    2. Aortic or renal artery obstruction
II. Obstructive uropathy
  A. Urethral obstruction
    1. Congenital urethral valves
    2. Meatal or urethral stenosis
    3. Foreign body
    4. Prostatic or perineal neoplasm
  B. Bladder outlet obstruction
  C. Bladder dysfunction
    1. Neurogenic bladder
    2. Pharmacologic
      a. Opiates
      b. Regional anesthetics
III. Intrinsic renal failure
  A. Renal disease
    1. Glomerulonephritis and nephropathies
    2. Interstitial nephritis
    3. Microangiopathic nephropathies
      a. Hemolytic uremic syndrome
  B. Congenital disorders of the kidney
    1. Polycystic kidney disease
    2. Renal hypoplasia and dysplasia or agenesis
    3. Congenital nephrosis
  C. Nephrotoxins
    1. Aminoglycosides
    2. Heavy metals
    3. Hemoglobin, myoglobinuria
    4. Cyclosporin
    5. Uric acid in tumor lysis syndrome
    6. Ethylene glycol, hydrocarbons

in males. All these malformations can be the cause of mechanical obstructive nephropathy and renal injury or renal failure. Signs of obstruction may be subtle and require radiologic, ultrasonic, or endoscopic evaluation. Recurrent urinary tract infections are frequently the clinical presentation of obstructive lesions in older children.

Intrinsic renal failure may be due to disorders of renal glomeruli, tubules, or blood vessels. Glomerular diseases include hemolytic uremic syndrome, postreptococcal glomerulonephritis, and Henoch-Schönlein purpura, as well as other glomerular inflammatory and immune complex diseases. Acute tubular injury is most commonly caused by hypoxia and ischemia; other causes are rhabdomyolysis, sepsis, hyperthermia, hemolysis, and a myriad of nephrotoxins, such as mercury, carbon tetrachloride, and ethylene glycol. Vascular disease, including arterial embolus and venous thrombosis as well as congenital malformations, can lead to acute renal failure.

HEMOLYTIC UREMIC SYNDROME

Hemolytic uremic syndrome (HUS) represents a group of symptoms, signs, and laboratory findings associated with ARF, microangiopathic hemolytic anemia, and thrombocytopenia (see Chap. 147).[75] This disease is found almost exclusively in infants and children, but it does share some of the clinical features of thrombotic thrombocytopenia purpura, a more serious disease seen in adults. In fact, in some instances, the most striking difference between these two entities is the age of onset of illness. Thus, the younger the age of onset, the more typical the illness of HUS and the better its prognosis.

Hematologic abnormalities include acute hemolysis and thrombocytopenia. The hemolysis is often severe, with hemoglobin concentrations falling as low as 4 to 5 g/dL. The peripheral blood smear reveals damaged erythrocytes suggestive of a microangiopathic process. Coombs' tests are negative. There is usually an elevated bilirubin, decreased haptoglobin, and reticulocytosis. The thrombocytopenia lasts 7 to 14 days and reflects peripheral platelet consumption. Platelet survival is reduced, and there is increased platelet uptake in the reticuloendothelial system. Abnormal platelet function with reduced levels of prostacycline have been reported in patients with HUS. Glomerular capillary endothelial injury is the most consistent renal finding in HUS. Glomerular and/or arterial injury may predominate, depending on the presence and extent of renal insufficiency (glomerular injury) and hemolysis and hypertension (arterial injury).

Although the cause is unknown, a number of viruses, including coxsackie virus, echo virus, and adenovirus, as well as *Salmonella* and *Shigella* infections have been frequently associated with individual patients or small epidemics of HUS. It has also occurred in two or more family members. This may be due to sharing a common environment or a common genetic predisposition. Recent data would suggest that the vast majority of cases of idiopathic HUS is associated with cytotoxin-producing microorganisms such as *Shigella dysenteriae* and certain *E. coli* (0157:H7 and others). These organisms produce cytotoxins that cause endothelial cell injury or death.[76]

The clinical course is characterized most commonly by an antecedent gastrointestinal tract illness that may include bloody diarrhea. Mildly affected patients exhibit anemia, thrombocytopenia, azotemia, decreased urine output, and an uncomplicated course. In severely affected patients, anuria is common, hypertension and seizures may occur, and the duration of the illness is protracted. A small number of children will exhibit progressive and permanent renal insufficiency, severe and recurrent hemolysis, thrombocytopenia, and neurologic impairment. Occasionally a child will present with an acute abdomen with severe colitis requiring surgical abdominal exploration.

Treatment is usually conservative, with careful management of intravascular volume, hemoglobin concentration, and fluid and electrolyte balance, and treatment of hypertension when necessary. Peritoneal- or hemodialysis has proved quite helpful in managing electrolyte and intravascular volume derangements as well as uremia in patients with severe HUS and anuria. Specific treatments with anticoagulants, prostaglandin inhibitors, fibrinolytic agents, and plasmapheresis have been proposed but have not been adequately studied to date. Although most patients recover renal function, permanent renal failure may ensue, necessitating chronic dialysis or renal transplantation. Treatment of acute renal failure includes the assessment and correction of any prerenal factors that may be impairing urine output. Central venous pressure measurement is quite helpful, and in children with cardiac dysfunction a PA catheter can be useful for measuring cardiac output. Nephrotoxic drugs should be avoided if possible or their dose modulated and serum levels of the drug closely monitored. Daily fluids should be restricted to replacing insensible losses, urine output, and any ongoing losses, using fluids that reflect the electrolyte content of the losses. Caloric support is essential, bearing in mind that a significant protein load will accelerate the degree of azotemia. Serum electrolyte concentrations and acid-base balance must be carefully monitored. Hypertension commonly accompanies many forms of ARF and should be controlled to avoid myocardial and CNS complications of acute hypertension.

Controversial areas of treatment include the use of dopamine at infusions of 2 to 5 μg(kg · min) to enhance urine output. Mannitol may reduce or prevent the oliguric phase of acute tubular necrosis if used early in a period of hypotension or ischemia, but it will elevate serum osmolarity if it is not excreted by the kidneys. Similarly, furosemide may prevent or reduce tubular injury but is nephrotoxic and ototoxic if high serum levels persist.

DIALYSIS

Peritoneal- or hemodialysis is reserved for children who exhibit oliguria or anuria with severe volume overload and CHF, for those whose electrolyte abnormalities are uncontrollable by other means, or for those in whom uremia is rapid and severe. Peritoneal dialysis used to be preferred over hemodialysis in the acute setting because vascular access in children often requires surgical intervention and because patients with multisystem organ disease and ARF are often hemodynamically unstable. More recently, improved techniques in vascular access and new catheter designs have allowed acute hemodialysis to gain in popularity in the pediatric ICU setting.[77]

The technique for peritoneal dialysis includes the placement of a soft catheter with multiple holes into the peritoneal cavity through an anterior abdominal wall incision. This can be performed in the ICU with the use of local anesthesia. Once the patency and placement of the catheter are confirmed, a commercially available dialysate solution is infused into the peritoneal cavity, where it equilibrates with the plasma and extracellular fluids, using the parietal and visceral surfaces as semipermeable dialysis membranes. The period of fluid instillation for equilibration can be varied, depending on the clinical conditions; it is referred to as the dwell time. The composition of the dialysis fluid tends to be similar to plasma, containing approximately 130 mEq/L of sodium, 100 mEq/L of chloride, 35 mEq/L of acetate or lactate as a buffer, 3.5 mEq/L of calcium, and 1.5 mEq/L of magnesium. The glucose concentration can be varied to be either isosmotic with 1.5% glucose or hyperosmotic with 4.25% glucose. The latter concentration allows for additional intravascular and extracellular fluid to equilibrate with the dialysate fluid so that this fluid as well as electrolytes can be removed when the peritoneal cavity is evacuated. Complications of peritoneal dialysis include respiratory compromise from increased abdominal pressure during dwell time; and intubation and mechanical ventilation are sometimes required in children with impaired respiratory function. Peritonitis from bacterial or fungal agents is another complication, because contamination of the dialysis catheter or dialysate can occur in a patient whose host defenses are not normal. Severe dehydration, including circulatory collapse and metabolic derangements, can occur if peritoneal dialysis is too rapidly or improperly performed.

The principles of hemodialysis are essentially the same as those of peritoneal dialysis, using the blood compartment to interface with a semipermeable membrane rather than the peritoneum. Some authors argue that hemodialysis is more efficient than peritoneal dialysis and, therefore, more appropriate for the acute setting. More recently, the technique of hemofiltration or ultrafiltration has gained popularity. This is another extracorporeal process in which uremic blood is cleansed by a technique based solely on the principle of convective solute transport. During this procedure, an ultrafiltrate of the plasma is created by hydrostatic pressure exerted across a highly permeable membrane. Simultaneously, the blood volume is replaced by a modified lactated Ringer's solution.

OUTCOME

The prognosis in ARF depends on the patient's age, underlying disease, and the extent of the precipitating insult. In general, children tend to have a better outcome than adults; in fact, they usually recover completely from a renal insult of hypoxia or ischemia within a short time, provided that other organ systems are not involved. In children in whom chronic renal failure develops, long-term outpatient peritoneal dialysis or chronic hemodialysis is necessary for survival unless a renal transplant can be performed.

The Endocrine System

ADRENAL ABNORMALITIES

Congenital adrenal hyperplasia is an autosomal recessive disease that results in a deficiency of one of the hydroxylase enzymes. Twenty-one hydroxylase deficiency is the most common. This disease is characterized by low levels of cortisone and aldosterone and buildup of intermediary metabolites. In the partial deficiency states, the children have simple virilization. In complete deficiency states, salt wasting with hyponatremia and hyperkalemia is present. The children usually present in the first weeks of life with vomiting, failure to thrive, and cardiovascular collapse, and the diagnosis can be confused with pyloric stenosis. Treatment is acute volume resuscitation and steroid replacement therapy: hydrocortisone acetate 1.5 to 2.0 mg/kg intravenous and desoxycorticosterone acetate 1 to 2 mg/day intramuscular. Patients with 11 or 17 hydroxylase deficiency do not have salt wasting but do become virilized and may have systemic hypertension.

DIABETIC KETOACIDOSIS

Diabetic ketoacidosis (DKA) describes the state of glucose and ketone overproduction and underutilization with resultant hyperglycemic ketoacidosis. Clinically the patients present with metabolic acidosis, compensatory hyperventilation, and severe dehydration secondary to the forced hyperglycemic diuresis. They can also present with neurologic changes ranging from altered mental status to brain death. The laboratory evaluation reveals hyperglycemia, hyperosmolarity, hyperlipidemia, low or normal serum sodium, and potassium depletion. The treatment is volume resuscitation (initially with a non-glucose-containing solution) and administration of insulin. Ten-mL/kg boluses of isotonic fluid are given to correct cardiovascular collapse. Once perfusion has been established, the remainder of the fluid deficit is corrected over 24 to 48 h. Glucose is added to the resuscitation fluid when the serum glucose falls below 200. In DKA, insulin is given as a continuous infusion of approximately 0.1 U/(kg · hr). The infusion is tailored to achieve a glucose drop of 50 per hour. The patient should be closely monitored for replacement of potassium as well as phosphate. Bicarbonate is not used in these patients for fear of precipitating a paradoxical CNS acidosis.

These patients should be watched in the PICU if there is major metabolic or cardiovascular derangement or if there is any evidence of CNS decompensation. The main CNS problem is increased intracranial pressure: the etiology of this is not understood. Possible explanations include rapid change in the glucose, osmolality, or pH.[78,79] When intracranial hypertension does occur, it can prove fatal despite aggressive therapy. The best approach is anticipatory and to treat early with mannitol and, if required, hyperventilation. The association of DKA and malignant intracranial hypertension is much more common in the pediatric age group.[80]

The Gastrointestinal System

Gastrointestinal problems in the PICU include organ dysfunction and organ failure from acquired disease as well as congenital anatomic malformations and dysfunction. In addition, delivery of adequate nutrition is perhaps the most critical concern in the care of the critically ill infant and child.

CONGENITAL MALFORMATIONS

Gross anatomic malformations are usually diagnosed during the first few days of life. Some are apparent on initial physical examination, such as omphalocele, gastroschisis, diaphragmatic hernia, and imperforate anus. Others present in the first few days of life as enteral feeding failures, such as intestinal atresia, microcolon, tracheoesophageal fistula, and meconium ileus. Other malformations present difficult diagnostic and therapeutic dilemmas after the neonatal period. Specific clinical problems are discussed below.

INTESTINAL MALROTATION AND MIDGUT VOLVULUS

Malrotation of the intestine is related to the incomplete rotation of the fetal midgut during migration into the abdominal cavity. This abnormal rotation can lead to either partial or complete duodenal obstruction by peritoneal (Ladd's) bands or, more importantly, to a volvulus of the midgut. The midgut (duodenum to transverse colon) and its vascular supply hang on a single pedicle; if this twists, vascular infarction of the entire midgut can result. Infants with omphalocele almost invariably have associated malrotation. Symptomatic infants usually present within the first 3 weeks of life with signs of high intestinal obstruction (bilious vomiting) or signs of an acute abdomen, intestinal perforation, and sepsis. Treatment is surgical reduction and fixation of the volvulus with resection of nonviable bowel. Postoperative respiratory support and total parenteral nutrition are often required in those infants who were severely compromised before surgery.

MECKEL'S DIVERTICULUM

Meckel's diverticulum represents a persistence of the omphalomesenteric or vitelline duct that clinically comes to attention as a cause of painless lower gastrointestinal tract bleeding. The site of bleeding is an ulceration in the bowel mucosa caused by secretion of gastric acid. Although these bleeds are usually self-limited, massive and life-threatening bleeds have been reported.[81] The diagnosis is often a diagnosis of exclusion and can be difficult to make. The technetium-pertechnetate isotope scan is helpful only if there is gastric mucosa in the diverticulum. Therapy is supportive, with particular attention to blood replacement. The definitive therapy is surgical resection.

HIRSCHSPRUNG'S DISEASE (CONGENITAL AGANGLIONIC MEGACOLON)

Hirschsprung's disease is characterized by absence of the parasympathetic ganglion cells in varying distal lengths of the rectum and colon. The lack of these ganglion cells produces a relatively narrowed segment of bowel: the normal proximal bowel becomes distended. The resultant clinical diseases can be relatively minor with abdominal distention and stool retention or as severe as toxic megacolon with peritonitis and perforation. Toxic megacolon usually presents in the younger child; reported mortality rates are as high as 75 percent.

The diagnosis of Hirschsprung's disease can sometimes be made on the basis of history and physical examination. Barium enema should reveal a narrowed segment with ballooning of the proximal bowel. The definitive diagnosis is made by rectal or colon biopsy looking for the presence or absence of ganglion cells. Treatment of toxic megacolon is both supportive, with meticulous volume reexpansion and antibiotic coverage, as well as definitive, with surgical decompression by creating a colostomy in the region of normal bowel. A number of diseases present after the neonatal period; these can be newly acquired diseases or progression of chronic congenital diseases. These are discussed as either hepatic or intestinal disease.

OTHER INTESTINAL DISORDERS

Intestinal disorders can produce bleeding, obstruction, or inflammation with secondary problems of malabsorption and bowel perforation. Gastrointestinal bleeds in children are caused by inflammatory diseases (gastritis), ulcers, varices, or vascular malformations. Although ulcer disease is an uncommon presenting complaint in the pediatric patient, the problem of stress ulcer or stress gastritis must be anticipated in any critically ill child. Prophylactic antacids or an H_2 receptor antagonist should be considered. Bowel obstruction can occur in the form of intussusception, twisting of the bowel around congenital or postsurgical bands, and twisting of the bowel on itself (volvulus). Intussusception is relatively common in the pediatric age group, usually occurring in the distal ileum.[82] Only in a few cases can a leading point be identified, such as a polyp or localized edema as seen in Henoch-Schönlein purpura. The treatment of intussusception can be either surgical, or, if there is no evidence of necrotic bowel, many lesions can be successfully decompressed with a carefully manipulated barium enema. Inflammatory bowel diseases include the familial diseases of Crohn's disease and regional enteritis. Infectious agents that must also be considered include *Salmonella, Shigella,* and *Yersinia*. These patients can present with diarrhea; evidence of malabsorption, especially with lactose intolerance; and bloody diarrhea. They can also present with a toxic acute abdomen.

NECROTIZING ENTEROCOLITIS

A specific disease that merits separate discussion is necrotizing enterocolitis, commonly referred to as NEC.[83] Necrotizing enterocolitis is a fulminant neonatal disease characterized by ulceration and necrosis of the small bowel and colon. It has been reported to occur in 2.4 per 1000 live births. The cause is unknown, but most hypotheses suggest bowel ischemia as the main precipitating factor. Umbilical artery catheters, perinatal asphyxia, respiratory distress syndrome (RDS), and persistent patent ductus arteriosus have all been implicated. The vast majority of children have had enteral feedings before clinical NEC develops; some investigators suggest that a specific preexisting bowel flora carries a risk of the disease. Feeding intolerance, abdominal distention, and bloody stools are the most common presenting signs. Intestinal obstruction, perforation, and sepsis may follow. Treatment consists of withholding enteral feedings, administering appropriate antibiotics, and surgical exploration if an acute abdomen with free air is evident. Total parenteral nutrition is often required for several weeks, and intestinal obstruction can occur weeks to months after a relatively benign course of NEC.[84]

HEPATIC FAILURE

Hepatic failure can occur with chronic or acute liver disease. The etiologies and clinical presentations differ: chronic liver failure can be caused by biliary atresia, inborn errors of metabolism (tyrosinosis, Wilson's disease, galactosemia, cystic fibrosis), or chronic inflammatory hepatitis. Children with chronic disease often present with the signs and symptoms of synthetic dysfunction (malnutrition, hypoalbuminemia, abnormal coagulation), degradation dysfunction (icterus and hyperammonemia), and portal hypertension (hypersplenism and varices). Acute liver failure is most commonly caused by infectious hepatitis, type A and type B. Toxic hepatic failure is a close second.[85]

The physical examination is important for the identification of the liver and spleen size, evidence of bleeding, edema, and other organ dysfunction. The laboratory evaluation should include a screen of the synthetic function [albumin, prothrombin time (PT), partial thromboplastin time (PTT)], degradation screen (bilirubin, ammonia), and values of all the liver enzymes. Hepatic ultrasound, radiographic contrast studies, and liver biopsy are indicated on an individual basis.

The life-threatening complications of liver failure include acute bleeding, cardiovascular compromise secondary to massive intravascular hypovolemia from fluid shifts, and intracranial hypertension from the toxic encephalopathy. Treatment is expectant and supportive. A 10% dextrose infusion is used to guarantee an adequate carbohydrate supply. Low-protein diets tend to minimize ammonia production. Coagulation is supported with the administration of vitamin K, fresh frozen plasma, and platelets as required. Plasmapheresis with fresh frozen plasma and platelets can be used to improve coagulation while maintaining normovolemia. Oral lactulose and neomycin enemas are given in an attempt to decrease the enterohepatic cycle of ammonia production and absorption. Cardiovascular and respiratory functions should be closely monitored and supported as required.

It is important to anticipate the complications of intracranial hypertension. Serum ammonia levels are often used to monitor or track the neurologic dysfunction, but it is important to remember that it is unknown whether ammonia is the primary CNS toxin or is just one of many chemical markers. There are a number of other specific and controversial therapies as well. Steroids have been proposed for some forms of inflammatory hepatitis. Exchange transfusions and plasmapheresis have been advocated to decrease the load of toxins. This therapy has had variable results, and to date there is no strong evidence that morbidity and mortality are changed with this intervention. Patients with certain forms of acute hepatic failure, including those of toxic as well as infectious etiologies, may be considered candidates for acute liver transplantation.[86]

EXTRAHEPATIC BILIARY ATRESIA

Extrahepatic biliary atresia occurs once in every 8000 to 10,000 live births. The atresia differs from patient to patient, involving variable degrees of obstruction or discontinuity of the biliary tree between the duodenum and the proximal branches of the hepatic ducts.[87] The treatment is surgical (jejunal Roux-en-Y anastomosis and portoenterostomy) and is tailored to the amount of extrahepatic bile duct architecture present. These procedures are most successful in patients operated on at an early age (before 6 to 9 months). Despite some success, there are many acute and chronic complications of this surgery, including hepatic failure, ascending cholangitis, and cirrhosis with portal hypertension and varices. Until recently, the treatment of these complications has been aggressive ICU medical therapy, but the development of liver transplantation technology offers a new hope.

LIVER TRANSPLANTS

The recent emergence of improved immunosuppressive drugs, especially cyclosporin A, has increased the interest in and success of liver transplantation. The perioperative and postoperative periods require a coordinated approach of many disciplines: surgery, gastroenterology, anesthesia, immunology, and ICU staff. Reports to date suggest that although these children are critically ill, they do not pose unique clinical problems.[88] Most of the clinical issues that arise can be anticipated. These children experience large blood losses and require massive replacement therapy in the operating room. Because of this, the intravascular volume status, renal status, and hematology and coagulation profiles must be closely monitored and basic liver failure therapy is indicated. The immunosuppression required for graft survival puts the patient at risk of infection, both with "normal" as well as opportunistic organisms. Surveillance cultures and early aggressive antibiotic therapy are indicated. Perhaps the only unanticipated complication has been systemic hypertension, which appears unrelated to elevated CVP or PWP. Many patients have required aggressive therapy to control blood pressure (e.g., hydralazine, diazoxide, captopril).[89]

NUTRITIONAL SUPPORT IN THE CRITICALLY ILL

Adequate nutritional support of the child with critical disease is of paramount importance, as it can decrease morbidity and mortality. It is essential to try to meet the caloric and mineral requirements of these patients. The nutritional requirements for healthy children have been well defined, but the requirements of critically ill children are less well understood: the measurements of oxygen consumptionand nitrogen balance are not easy bedside maneuvers.

Even when caloric needs can be ascertained, it can be difficult to deliver adequate amounts because of extenuating circumstances; such as bowel compromise, severe fluid restriction for either renal or CNS disease, and glucose intolerance. Therefore, all avenues of nutrition (enteral and parenteral) must be explored, and nutritional intervention must be implemented early, before a catabolic state ensues.

ENTERAL NUTRITIONAL SUPPORT

Use of the gastrointestinal tract for alimentation is usually the safest and most efficient approach as long as the gut is functionally intact. A variety of commercial formulas with variable sources and quantities of protein, fat, and carbohydrate are available. Protein requirements can be met by ysing whole protein, protein hydrolysates, or individual amino acids. Whole protein, which has the least osmotic effect, allows for greater nutrient density. However, it can only be used in children with normal pancreatic function and no allergy. Children with protein allergy, pancreatic deficiency, or severe intestinal mucosal disease may benefit from a protein hydrolysate. However, these formulas have a high osmolarity and there are relatively few commercially available. Free amino acid formulas are also available and are used in chemically defined diets restricted by specific requirements or intolerances.

The high caloric density of fat makes it an important component in nutritional support. Long-chain triglycerides (LCTs) yield approximately 9 kcal/g, whereas medium-chain triglycerides (MCTs) yield 8.3 kcal/g. Although of greater caloric density, LCTs are less readily absorbed. MCTs are hydrolyzed more rapidly and are converted almost exclusively into free fatty acids and glycerol. MCTs are absorbed even in the absence of lipase owing to their relative water solubility and emulsification properties. However, there are drawbacks. For example, MCTs may cause an osmotic diarrhea, and they contain no essential fatty acids, so linoleic acid must be added to the diet separately.

Secondary disaccharidase deficiency is a common carbohydrate absorption problem in the critically ill child. Lactase function is easily impaired by hypoxia and ischemia as well as by infection and malnutrition. In these situations, lactose should be avoided and replaced with sucrose or polycose, which have the least osmotic effect. Enteral feeds can be delivered orally, through a nasogastric tube or a gastrostomy tube. Children with endotracheal tubes in place can be safely fed through a nasogastric tube; the risk of aspiration is minimized by using continuous infusion of formula rather than bolus feeds and by placing the child in an upright semisitting position. Narcotic analgesics and muscle relaxants hinder enteral feeding; if possible, these groups of drugs should be avoided.

PARENTERAL ALIMENTATION

Parenteral nutrition is used in children who cannot tolerate enteral feedings. It is used as supportive therapy in the critically ill child with acute respiratory or gastrointestinal disease and as a primary treatment in children with chronic short bowel syndrome, Crohn's disease, and renal failure. When intravenous alimentation is considered, 10% dextrose in water ($D_{10}W$) is administered at 1 to 1.5 maintenance for 24 h. The patient is closely monitored for glucosuria, hyperglycemia, and edema. If glucose load is tolerated, a $D_{10}W$ solution with amino acids (parenteral nutrition, PN-10) can then be initiated. Administration of $D_{10}W$ with or without amino acids can be done safely

TABLE 186-8 Maintenance Fluid Rates in Pediatric Patients Parenteral Nutrition

Body Weight, kg	Regular Maintenance, mL/kg/day	Malnourished Maintenance, mL/kg/day
1st 10	100	80–90
2nd 10	50	40
>20	20	20

through either a central or a peripheral catheter. Any more concentrated formula will sclerose peripheral veins and therefore must be given through a centrally placed line. If a central line has been placed and the patient is tolerating the relatively high glucose loads of 1.5 maintenance with PN-10 or $D_{10}W$, one may switch to PN-20 and simultaneously decrease the fluid rate to maintenance, to permit accommodation to the higher glucose load. The PN-20 is then advanced over 2 days to the 1.5 maintenance rate. The patient should gain relatively little weight until 1.5 maintenance with PN-20 is achieved. In general, if a patient is malnourished (less than 0.80 weight for height), fluid rates must be adjusted downward to roughly 80 percent of those for children of the same weight. After 1 week of nutritional rehabilitation, regular maintenance fluids may be used (Table 186-8).

Often the physician has determined a different maintenance fluid rate for a particular patient on the basis of previous intake-output data. If this is the case, the patient should be started on $D_{10}W$ at the low side of the maintenance rate and advanced to the maximum tolerable rate. When switching to $D_{20}W$, the low rate is again used and the advance in rates is repeated. Initial fluid and electrolyte deficits and ongoing losses (e.g., diarrhea) should not be repleted with PN solutions. A separate intravenous solution and line should be used for these extra losses. It should be adjusted every 8 h to equal the patient's losses. If a patient has severe hypoalbuminemic or edematous malnutrition, or both, great care must be exercised in the management of fluid status. Edema, hypervolemia, and hypovolemia may develop rapidly in these patients.

LIPID IN CENTRAL INTRAVENOUS ALIMENTATION

With central intravenous alimentation lipid is necessary only to prevent essential fatty acid deficiency and should be given at 5 to 10 percent of the total calories. The following fluid rate permits rough determination of the lipid rate necessary to prevent essential fatty acid deficiency during central intravenous alimentation: 5 to 10 mL/kg for the first 10 kg, 2.5 to 5 mL/kg for the second 10 kg, and 1.25 to 2.5 mL/kg for weight above 20 kg. Lipids are usually introduced a number of days after PN has been started. There are multiple reasons for withholding lipid during the initiation of intravenous alimentation. First, the tolerance of lipid products is improved if the patient has been primed by a period of adequate caloric intake. Second, fatty acids may impair the patient's tolerance of the large dextrose load. When increasing dextrose administration, the simultaneous introduction of fat products may confuse the interpretation and treatment of glycosuria. Lipemia checks should be done whenever lipid is used.

LIPID IN PERIPHERAL INTRAVENOUS ALIMENTATION

With peripheral intravenous alimentation (10% concentration), the lipid product must constitute a major component of the caloric intake, as it is the only isosmolar product of sufficient caloric density to provide significant caloric intake by peripheral vein. Thus, once the patient on peripheral alimentation has reached a maximum rate of PN-10, intralipid may be added at a rate of 10 mL/(kg · day) and advanced by 10 mL/(kg · day) to a maximum of 40 mL/(kg · day). During the initial 15 min of the infusion on the first day, the rate should be 0.1 mL/min. If tolerated, the rate may be advanced to a maximum of 10 mL/kg every 4 h. If lipid infusions exceed this flow rate, fat overload may develop. Lipid clearance may be facilitated by administering lipid continuously over 24 h. Serum lipemia is monitored daily while the patient is on lipid. A hematocrit tube of blood taped to the wall or spun immediately is observed for gross lipemia (opaque serum), which is an indication to discontinue or decrease the lipid infusion. Visible lipemia (cloudy serum) is an indication for more frequent monitoring and/or modest decrease in lipid dose. After the patient has stabilized on the maximum lipid dose, the lipemia check is repeated every other day or twice weekly. Because total fluid volume imposed by 1.5 maintenance PN-10 plus 40 mL/kg of lipid is often prohibitive for malnourished patients, PN-10 rate may be decreased while lipid is increased. However, lipid calories must not exceed 60 percent of the total calories. Often persistent lipemia limits lipid administration to levels less than the maximum recommendation. For calculations, the caloric densities shown in Table 186-9 may be used. The recently approved higher-calorie 20% lipid formulation offers a distinct advantage over the 10% solution. It is used at essentially one-half the previously mentioned flow rates for standard 10% lipid. Maximum infusion rates are 20 mL/(kg · day) or 60 percent of total calories as fat.

TABLE 186-9 Calculated Caloric Density of Lipid Products Used in Pediatric Peripheral Alimentation

Lipid Product	Caloric Density
Amino acids	3.33 cal/g
Dextrose 10%	0.34 cal/mL
Dextrose 20%	0.68 cal/mL
PN-10	0.39 cal/mL
PN-20	0.73 cal/mL
Lipid 10%	1.1 cal/mL
Lipid 20%	2.0 cal/mL

PERIPHERAL VERSUS CENTRAL ALIMENTATION

Energy Considerations

Peripheral intravenous alimentation is a stopgap measure that rarely permits caloric intakes in excess of maintenance requirements. Therefore, there are few extra calories for growth and repletion. Moreover, intravenous sites must be changed at least every 48 to 72 h to prevent phlebitis. Thus, the patient is subjected to frequent painful episodes of intravenous placement when peripheral alimentation is used for extended periods. The time spent searching for intravenous sites further decreases the total caloric intake. Peripheral intravenous alimentation should therefore be limited to 2 weeks' duration. By contrast, central alimentation can provide caloric and nitrogen requirements for both growth and maintenance. However, there is an increased risk of infection associated with prolonged indwelling catheters.

Caloric requirements represent the energy intake necessary for maintenance, growth, and activity. When intake is less than the maintenance level, the patient is in negative energy balance and loses weight. At intakes greater than maintenance, a positive energy balance provides net energy for growth and activity. Even hospitalized children often increase spontaneous activity when positive energy balance is obtained. The energy necessary for maintenance may increase by 50 to 100 percent with severe stress (infection, trauma). The energy necessary for activity obviously varies considerably among infants. Whatever net energy is left after allowance for maintenance and activity is available for growth. The caloric cost of growth is at least 5 calories per gram of weight. Normal growth is approximately 25 to 30 g/day for the first 6 months of life, 10 to 15 g/day for the next 6 months, and roughly 7 to 10 g/day thereafter. Representative maintenance energy requirements for the nonstressed state are listed in Table 186-10. Using this data, intravenous alimentation can be adjusted to produce normal or moderate catch-up growth rates. Weight gain in the face of inadequate calorie intake (less than maintenance) inevitably results from edema formation. If the goal of nutritional therapy is merely supportive over 1 to 2 weeks, growth may not be necessary and peripheral alimentation may therefore be adequate. If significant catch-up growth or long-term support is required, the child's growth and activity requirements should be met.

TABLE 186-10 Maintenance Energy Requirements for Nonstressed Patients

Age	Maintenance Energy, kcal/g
<2 years	75–80
2–5 years	70–75
5–10 years	55–70
10–17 years	40–55
Adult	40

Monitoring of Children on Total Parenteral Nutrition

Careful assessment of intake, output, and body weight should be made on a daily basis. The site of alimentation, either peripheral or central, should be evaluated regularly for signs of obstruction, extravasation, or occlusion. Skin and mucous membranes should be evaluated regularly for evidence of trace metal deficiency. Liver size and function must be monitored: intrahepatic cholestasis, excessive fat and glycogen deposition, and elevated liver functions tests have been documented in patients on total parenteral nutrition (TPN). Other metabolic studies should include routine screening of electrolytes, glucose, blood urea nitrogen, and creatinine, as well as ammonia. A serum lipemia check should be done daily. Total protein, albumin, hemoglobin, and triglycerides should be checked regularly but less frequently.[90]

Outcome

A child's survival obviously depends on adequate nutritional intake. It has been shown that an infant with a nonfunctioning gastrointestinal tract can survive on TPN for a period of years, but this is clearly a stopgap measure. The risk of complications from central vein cannulation increases with time, and vascular access in the child becomes increasingly limited as sites are used. Attention to alimentation has improved outcome in the ICU. Although difficult to quantify, it is our impression that children with any critical illness benefit from improved nutritional intake with faster recovery and decreased morbidity.

The Hematologic System

Hematologic problems in the ICU include abnormalities of coagulation, immunity, and the red blood cell (RBC) mass. These abnormalities can be primary isolated defects, or they can be secondary to multiorgan system failure. The immune system is discussed in the section on infectious disease.

THE COAGULATION SYSTEM

Normal clotting includes an initial phase of platelet hemostatic plug formation and a second stage of fibrin production that occurs by either the intrinsic or extrinsic pathways. For both of these phases to occur, platelets, coagulation factors, and an intact blood vessel are essential. Neonates have a number of measurable coagulation abnormalities that rarely have clinical manifestations. Term infants and most preterm infants show normal platelet-vessel interaction, but platelet aggregation is transiently impaired. In addition, many coagulation factors are decreased in activity or concentration in the fetus and in the newborn. Of greatest importance are the vitamin K–dependent factors, namely, factors II, VII, IX, and X. These are low at birth and fall to even lower levels during the first week of life unless vitamin K is administered. Factors V and VIII are close to adult levels in all but the most premature infants. Although routine screening tests for coagulation activity are prolonged in infants, the newborn's blood clots more rapidly in vitro owing to a deficiency of naturally occurring protease inhibitors, principally antithrombin III.

DIAGNOSIS OF HEMOSTATIC DISORDERS

Coagulation disorders are diagnosed on the basis of history, physical examination, and laboratory data. It is important to elicit any history of easy bleeding, bruising, drug ingestion, associated illnesses, or a family history of bleeding. The patient should be closely examined for evidence of petechiae or bruises, bleeding gums, or hepatosplenomegaly. Any sites of bleeding or venipuncture should be observed for fresh clot or oozing. The laboratory evaluation of PTT, PT, thrombin time, platelet count, and bleeding time gives valuable information as to the nature of the hemostatic defect.

SPECIFIC COAGULATION DISORDERS

CONGENITAL DISORDERS OF COAGULATION

Hereditary deficiencies of most of the coagulation factors are described, but classic hemophilia (factor VIII) and Christmas disease (factor IX) account for the vast majority. Since the advent of modern factor replacement therapy, these disorders only rarely cause life-threatening hemorrhage requiring intensive care management.[91]

FACTOR VIII DEFICIENCY OR HEMOPHILIA A

Factor VIII deficiency or hemophilia A is transmitted by sex-linked recessive inheritance and occurs in 1 in 10,000 male infants. The severity of the clinical disease is determined by the amount of circulating factor; severe disease is associated with less than 1 percent of normal levels, moderately severe disease with 1 to 5 percent, and very mild disease with 5 to 30 percent of normal levels.[91] The most common sites of bleeding are the joint spaces such as the knees or ankles, but hemorrhage may also occur in the peritoneal cavity, gastrointestinal tract, muscle, skin, or CNS. Severe trauma or surgery can cause extensive bleeding. The diagnosis is made by demonstrating an elevated PTT and decreased levels of factor VIII. Treatment requires adminstration of factor VIII in the form of plasma or cryoprecipitate, which contains more concentrated factor VIII derived from multiple plasma donors. Many of these patients have become seropositive for human immunodeficiency virus because of their exposure to multiple blood donors.

VON WILLEBRAND'S DISEASE

Von Willebrand's disease occurs nearly as commonly as hemophilia A and is transmitted to both sexes by an autosomal dominant inheritance. It is characterized by abnormalities of the factor VIII molecule as well as by qualitative platelet dysfunction. Skin and mucous membrane bleeding, particularly nosebleeds and menorrhagia, are the most frequent clinical problems. The PTT and bleeding time are prolonged in this disorder, as are some tests of platelet function. Serious bleeding is treated by infusing factor VIII concentrate or fresh frozen plasma.[92]

HEREDITARY THROMBOCYTOPENIA

Hereditary thrombocytopenia is an uncommon congenital defect. Most cases are associated with the familial sex-linked immune deficiency diseases such as the Wiskott-Aldrich syndrome. Platelet transfusions are given to control clinical bleeding.

ACQUIRED DISORDERS OF COAGULATION

A variety of circumstances can impair the production of coagulation factors. The vitamin K–dependent factors are the most commonly affected. These factors are decreased in the presence of liver disease, warfarin (Coumadin) therapy, and malabsorption syndromes secondary to either bowel disease or altered bowel flora with chronic antibiotic therapy. In addition, untreated vitamin K deficiency in the neonatal period results in hemorrhagic disease of the newborn. In these disorders, the PT is prolonged, and specific assays will demonstrate low levels of factors II, VII, IX, and X. The administration of vitamin K usually reverses these deficiencies unless synthetic function of the liver is markedly compromised.

Acquired platelet abnormalities include problems of decreased production, increased destruction, and decreased function. Decreased production or hypoproliferative states include marrow diseases such as leukemia and aplastic anemia and, perhaps most commonly, as the side effect of chemotherapeutic agents. Increased destruction can be immune mediated (e.g., idiopathic thrombocytopenic purpura)[93] or from consumption (e.g., microangiopathic states, hemolytic uremic syndrome, or thrombotic thrombocytopenic purpura). Finally, platelet dysfunction has been demonstrated in the presence of uremia and chronic polycythemia seen with cyanotic heart disease.[94] Treatment of all the acquired thrombocytopenias includes supportive platelet transfusions and, if possible, correction of the underlying disorder. Therapeutic splenectomy has been used to increase platelet survival in some of the severe immune-mediated diseases.

Disseminated intravascular coagulation (DIC) is characterized as a consumptive coagulopathy with decreased platelets and fibrinogen, increased PT, PTT, and thrombin time and an elevation of fibrin degradation products. DIC complicates a number of nonspecific conditions including sepsis, anaphylaxis, shock, acidosis, massive tissue trauma, sickle cell disease, and certain malignancies, particularly acute myelogenous leukemia in childhood.[95] Purpura fulminans is a particularly severe type of DIC associated with ecchymosis and thrombosis of the skin, subcutaneous tissue, and distal extremities. This condition is seen with acute meningococcemia as well as with other bacterial, viral, and fungal septicemias. Purpura fulminans is associated with a high morbidity and mortality; the main morbidity is the ischemic loss of distal extremities.[96]

Treatment of DIC consists of removing the triggering event whenever and as soon as possible. General support of the vascular volume and oxygen transport is essential. When active bleeding is present, transfusion of platelets (0.2 U/kg) and fresh frozen plasma (10 mL/kg) every 4 to 6 h as a bolus or continuous infusion will replenish platelet and clotting factors as well as coagulation antagonists such as antithrombin-3 (AT-3). Heparin has been advocated by some; however, it has not been shown to improve outcome and may enhance clinical bleeding. Transfusion with factor concentrates may be helpful when fresh frozen plasma therapy is limited by intravascular hypervolemia. Occasionally, exchange transfusion with fresh whole blood, or plasma exchange or plasmapheresis with fresh frozen plasma and platelets, may be necessary to treat severe DIC effectively.

RED BLOOD CELL ABNORMALITIES

Abnormalities of the RBC include either a decrease in the RBC mass or the presence of abnormally functioning RBCs. The RBC mass is reduced by either decreased production or increased loss. Decreased production is associated with factor deficiencies (iron, folate, vitamin B_{12}), with bone marrow disease (aplastic anemia, leukemia), with chronic diseases (infection, neoplasm, renal disease), and rarely with a congenital deficiency of RBC precursors (Diamond Blackfan syndrome). RBC loss is either extracorporeal blood loss (hemorrhage) or red cell destruction (hemolysis). Hemolysis can be caused by intrinsic RBC abnormalities or by extrinsic factors. Intrinsic anomalies include membrane defects (spherocytosis, elliptocytosis), enzyme defects [glucose-6-phosphate dehydrogenase (G6PD) pyruvate kinase deficiencies], and hemoglobinopathies (hemoglobin S, C, D, E, and thalassemia). The extrinsic abnormalities can be immune mediated, infection and toxin mediated, or secondary to microangiopathic destruction.

Regardless of the cause of RBC mass decrease, the signs, symptoms, and therapy depend on the acuity and severity of the blood loss. The acute loss of massive amounts of blood (hemorrhage) can cause hypovolemic shock. Treatment is oxygen and emergency intravascular volume reexpansion and ultimately replacement of RBCs. In the absence of hypovolemia, acute and chronic RBC loss is tolerated until there is a critical loss of oxygen-carrying capacity, which results in high-output cardiac failure. Treatment of these severe anemias includes oxygen and replacement of the RBC mass done very cautiously and slowly in an attempt to avoid the complications of fluid overload. Partial exchange transfusions are sometimes necessary to deliver an adequate RBC load safely.

The main functional abnormality of the RBC is an inability to carry oxygen; sulfhemaglobinemia and methemoglobinemia are the most common of these abnormalities. Methemoglobinemia and sulfhemoglobinemia can be either congenital or acquired disorders that produce hemoglobin that cannot bind oxygen. The congenital forms are usually asymptomatic and require no therapy, but the acquired or toxic forms may be fatal. The treatment includes oxygen, intravenous administration of methylene blue, and occasionally exchange transfusion.

SICKLE CELL ANEMIA

In addition to RBC loss and abnormal oxygen binding, grossly deformed RBCs can cause vaso-occlusive disease. Sickle cell anemia is the best example of this pathophysiology. Sickle cell anemia is a hemoglobinopathy. The major ICU complication is vaso-occlusive disease that can present as a painful crisis; if the vaso-occlusion occurs in the cerebral vessels or in another vital organ supply, it can present as a stroke or infarction. Vaso-occlusive disease of the lung is referred to as acute chest syndrome and presents clinically as ARDS. Treatment is hydration, oxygen, and, when severe, exchange transfusion and mechanical ventilation. The other potentially fatal crisis of sickle cell disease is splenic sequestration, which occurs in infants and young children who have not undergone autosplenectomy. Splenic sequestration presents with severe anemia and hypovolemic shock. The treatment is aggressive supportive therapy with emergency surgical splenectomy. Other children with sickle cell disease have usually had a functional autosplenectomy from multiple splenic infarcts. These children are at risk of severe infection from encapsulated organisms. Routine pneumococcal vaccine is administered as a precaution.

COMPLICATIONS OF TRANSFUSION THERAPY

Although the administration of blood products can be lifesaving, a number of potential complications should be anticipated. Whenever massive transfusion therapy is employed, the risks of citrate toxicity, transfusion reactions, as well as leukocyte and platelet sensitization, must be kept in mind.[97] In addition, depending on the age and type of blood component being employed, electrolyte disturbances such as hypocalcemia, hyperkalemia, and hypernatremia can occur. Whenever in doubt, a sample of the infusate should be sent for electrolyte analysis, and patient serum values of electrolytes and ionized calcium should be followed during therapy. Transfusion-acquired infections, including hepatitis, cytomegalovirus, and acquired immunodeficiency syndrome (AIDS), are particularly important risks for the chronically transfused and immunocompromised infant and child.[98]

Finally, hemochromatosis complicates the care of those patients who require chronic transfusion therapy for the treatment of an RBC abnormality. Efforts to decrease this often lethal complication include aggressive iron chelation therapy and the selective transfusion of young RBCs in an attempt to increase the time interval between required transfusions.

Oncologic Problems

Neoplastic disease in the child usually involves the hematopoietic system, central and sympathetic nervous system, soft tissue, bone, or kidney. Although much of oncology has become an outpatient subspecialty, a number of clinical situations do require hospitalization and intensive care.

BLAST CRISIS IN LEUKEMIA

Children who present with an initial white blood cell (WBC) count of greater than 100,000 are at a high risk of two potentially lethal complications: leukostasis and metabolic crisis (tumor lysis syndrome).

LEUKOSTASIS

Leukostasis is a syndrome of vascular obstruction caused by the high viscosity of blood when there are elevated cell counts or by the WBCs themselves. This syndrome should be anticipated in acute lymphoblastic leukemia (ALL) patients with presenting WBC counts greater than 500,000 and in acute myelogenous leukemia (AML) patients with WBC counts greater than 200,000. The leukemic cell in AML is less deformable than the lymphoblast; therefore, in AML, a lower WBC count can cause the same syndrome.

The two major target organs for leukostasis are the brain and the lung; the pathophysiology is vascular plugging, causing infarct.[99] Presenting symptoms include tachypnea, respiratory distress, clouding of the mental status, and focal neurologic deficits.[100] In addition to supportive therapy, the goal is to decrease the circulating tumor load and thereby decrease the viscosity.[101] Leukapheresis and exchange transfusion will transiently lower the tumor mass.[101] Cranial radiation may reduce the CNS load, and chemotherapy will interrupt cell production and possibly destroy circulating cells. The initial chemotherapy is aimed at stopping cell production without a large amount of cell lysis; this gives the advantage of halting a continually growing tumor load without causing a huge metabolic crisis before adequate perfusion is reestablished.

TUMOR LYSIS SYNDROME

Tumor lysis syndrome is a metabolic crisis precipitated by acute lysis of a large tumor load. The main abnormalities that result are elevations in uric acid, potassium, and phosphate; the elevated phosphate results in hypocalcemia. The hyperkalemia and hypocalcemia can be life threatening; the increased uric acid causes ARF, which further exacerbates the other metabolic imbalances.

Specific therapy is anticipatory monitoring with alkalinization of the urine and diuresis. Before any chemotherapy is administered, the renal function should be assessed and allopurinol therapy begun. In most cases, this conservative approach of a forced diuresis and allopurinol is adequate, but occasionally dialysis must be used. Basic indications at our institution for the initiation of dialysis include:

- Potassium >6 mEq/L
- Uric acid >19 mg/L
- Creatinine >10 mg/L
- Phosphorus >10 mg/L or rapidly rising
- Volume overload
- Symptomatic hypocalcemia

If dialysis is necessary, it is usually only needed for a few days until tumor lysis is nearly complete.

RESPIRATORY DISTRESS AND MEDIASTINAL MASS

The child with a mediastinal mass and respiratory distress presents a difficult therapeutic and diagnostic dilemma.[102] These children often complain of cough, difficulty in breathing, and shortness of breath, and stridor may be present. They prefer to sit upright and cannot tolerate supine positioning. The chest radiograph usually shows a large mediastinal mass, often with obliteration or obscuring of the tracheal air column. These tumors can be malignant (87 percent Hodgkin's and non-Hodgkin's lymphoma) or benign, and the prognosis and therapy rely on an accurate diagnosis. The diagnosis is best made by tissue sampling prior to any therapy. But a problem results from the fact that tissue sampling of a mediastinal mass requires anesthesia and surgery; by necessity, the airway must be manipulated and instrumented.[103] The obstructed intrathoracic trachea presents a major anesthetic risk; it is often impossible to maintain such an airway with the patient supine, deeply anesthetized, or receiving muscle relaxants. The care of these patients clearly requires individualized and creative approaches. If the airway compromise is severe, blind tumor therapy at the expense of obscuring the tissue diagnosis must precede any diagnostic procedure. Mediastinal radiation and systemic steroids are the two modes of emergency therapy most commonly administered. Sometimes this diagnostic dilemma can be circumvented; peripheral nodes or masses can be biopsied under local anesthesia or, if the tumor mass is very large, some of the tumor may remain outside the radiation field. In summary, although diagnosis is the key to neoplastic disease, mediastinal mass is one situation in which the risk may far outweigh the benefit of tissue diagnosis.

FEVER AND NEUTROPENIA

The most common admission diagnosis for children with neoplastic disease is fever and neutropenia. The neutropenic immunocompromised state caused by chemotherapy is a high-risk period for life-threatening infections.

Infectious Disease

The neonate and older child should be considered separately for the problems of infectious disease. The neonate's immature immune system with decreased cell-mediated immunity and B cell immunoglobulin production places her at higher risk for infection. There is some compensatory protection from transplacental IgG transfer, but these levels decay over the first 2 to 3 months.[104]

Neonatal infections are divided into congenitally and postnatally acquired. The congenitally acquired are usually viral infections of the TORCH group (TO = toxoplasmosis, R = rubella, C = CMV, and H = type II herpes simplex).

These infections can cause an overwhelming systemic illness with cardiorespiratory collapse or, more frequently, an insidious disease with a combination of thrombocytopenia, hepatosplenomegaly, skin rashes, and neurologic abnormalities. Whenever considering acquired infectious disease in the neonate, it is important to remember that the neonate does not localize infection well. The findings of sepsis may be very subtle and include hypothermia or hyperthermia, periodic breathing or apnea, lethargy, or hypotonicity.

The postnatally acquired infections are commonly caused by group B *Streptococcus*, (GBS), *E. coli*, *Listeria monocytogenes*, and type II herpes. These organisms which are obtained as the child travels through the vaginal tract can cause overwhelming sepsis with multisystem failure. GBS in the first days of life causes cardiorespiratory collapse, but late GBS (over 2 weeks of age) causes a milder disease with meningitis as the predominant feature.[105] After the neonatal period, the child is susceptible to different organisms. In the first 4 years of life *H. influenzae* is the common pathogen, followed by *S. pneumoniae*.

MENINGITIS

In the United States, 15,000 infants and children develop bacterial meningitis each year, with the peak incidence at 6 to 9 months of age. Approximately 75 percent of the cases occur in patients under the age of 15 years. The mortality rate is estimated at 5 to 10 percent with morbidity as high as 25 to 40 percent.[106] Unfortunately, the introduction of new antibiotics has not improved the outcome for these children.

The neonatal bacterial pathogens are *E. coli* and GBS. In children 2 months to 4 years, *H. influenzae* is the predominant organism followed by *S. pneumoniae* and *Neisseria meningitidis;* and in children over 4 years, *S. pneumoniae* and *N. meningitidis* prevail. A number of these children require PICU admission for treatment and support of increased ICP or the systemic effects of sepsis. Any child with bacterial meningitis must be closely observed for the complications of DIC, SIADH, subdural fluid collections, and metastatic infection such as arthritis, pericarditis, and pneumonia. Therapy is directed at irradication of the bacterial agent and systemic support. Most children are kept at a moderate fluid limit, both for the fear of increased ICP, as well as the propensity to develop SIADH. Steroids are now suggested for the younger child with *H. influenzae* meningitis.[107] There is some evidence that giving steroids before or with the first dose of antibiotics may decrease the morbidity of hearing loss with this disease. The dose is 0.6 mg/(kg · day) of Solu-Medrol four times daily for 4 days.

SEPSIS

Septic shock in the child goes through the same phases as in the adult, with warm vasodilated septic shock followed by cold constricted septic shock. The child can actually tolerate cold septic shock better than the adult because of the relatively normal baseline cardiovascular system without coronary artery disease. The treatment is the same with cardiorespiratory support and irradication of the infection. The use of naloxone (Narcan) is controversial. The use of steroids is limited to replacement therapy for possible adrenal hemorrhage.

IMMUNE COMPROMISED DISEASES

There are a number of congenital immune deficiency diseases that should be considered as a diagnosis for any child who has frequent infections and failure to thrive in the first year of life.[108] AIDS is becoming increasingly common. Eighty percent of pediatric AIDS infections are perinatally acquired from a seropositive mother. Approximately one-third of pregnancies in seropositive mothers yields a seropositive infant.[109] These children may first present with an opportunistic infection or with wasting syndrome, chronic diarrhea, lymphadenopathy, parotitis, recurrent bacterial infections, lymphoid interstitial pneumonitis (LIP), or encephalopathy. Young pediatric patients (less than 6 months) with *Pneumocystis carinii* (PCP) infection have a different clinical disease than adults. In the young child, PCP infection is an acute usually fatal disease unlike the insidious onset of PCP infection in the older child and adult.[110] The criteria for a PICU admission for a pediatric AIDS patient must be reviewed at the institutional level.

Trauma

PRENATAL AND PERINATAL

Prenatal injuries are secondary to severe maternal trauma, the most common being blunt abdominal trauma and gunshot wounds. Fetal mortality is much higher for the fetus than the mother and is usually caused by ischemia rather than direct injury (see Chap. 88). Perinatal injuries occur at the time of birth or in the immediate postnatal period. Birth injuries are most common in the large-term infant, in breech presentations, and in precipitous premature births. Skull fractures, cephalohematomas, and subdural, subarachnoid, and intraventricular or intraparenchymal hemorrhages can occur and may be associated with the development of increased intracranial pressure and secondary neuronal damage. Neck trauma with resultant torticollis or even cord transection is also reported after difficult breech deliveries. Other less devastating nerve injuries, bone fractures, or abdominal injuries may also be encountered.

PEDIATRIC

Accidents and trauma are the leading cause of death in children between the ages of 1 and 19 years. In statistics from 1986: 47 percent of pediatric trauma deaths were related to motor vehicle accidents, 17.8 percent secondary to homocide, 9.6 percent from suicide, and 9.2 percent from drowning. Of note, 30 percent of the deaths directly resulted from head injury.[111] The types of body injuries differ from adults. Children are usually victim to blunt rather than penetrating trauma; as a result, solid organ injury is more common than a ruptured viscus, and, because of the child's small size with more organs crowded into a smaller space, blunt injuries are usually multiorgan. The flexibility of the skeletal system has three major effects: **1.** bony fractures are less common; **2.** spinal cord injuries are less common; and **3.** there can be significant damage to internal organs without an overlying bony fracture (e.g., lung contusion without rib fractures). When bone fractures do occur, it is important to evaluate their effect on the growth plate—any disruption could have severe ramifications for subsequent limb growth.

Evaluation of the pediatric trauma patient is similar to the adult. While vital signs are critical to monitor, it is important to recognize that an elevated heart rate with a normal blood pressure may be the only sign of hypovolemia in the child. Because there are more solid organ injuries, abdominal scans are more frequently indicated. The role of diagnostic peritoneal lavage (DPL) is somewhat selective in the child. Most agree that DPL is indicated in a child who **1.** is comatose, **2.** is about to undergo nonabdominal surgery, **3.** has unexplained cardiovascular decompensation (shock), **4.** has penetrating chest injury below the nipple line, or **5.** has worsening abdominal examination.[112]

Initial therapy is basic resuscitation. Particular attention is given to the adequacy of volume resuscitation and temperature control. After trauma, the child is at high risk for hypothermia. The large body surface area to body volume ratio renders them susceptible to massive heat loss. Indications for abdominal surgery are free air or massive uncontrollable hemorrhage. Because children very frequently and nonspecifically develop an ileus, a nasogastric tube for decompression should be considered. Once the child is stabilized, he should be sent to an institution that is comfortable in the care of critically ill children.

CHILD ABUSE

Child abuse must always be considered in any injured child. Although physical and emotional abuse to children has always been present, the term "battered child" was first introduced by Kempe et al. in 1962.[113] Child abuse must be considered whenever there is a discrepancy between the severity of the injury and the proposed history. It should also be part of the differential diagnosis for any of the following: subdural hemorrhages; retinal hemorrhages; perioral injuries; genital and perianal injuries; multiple scars or fractures of different ages; any long-bone fracture in a child less than 3 years of age; burns; human bites; and any evidence of injury suggesting ropes, belts, etc.[114]

Although abuse can be emotional as well as physical, in the PICU, physical abuse is of critical import. Whenever there is suspicion, the history should be meticulously recorded and any alterations of that history documented. The physical exam should include detailed diagrams and descriptions of all bruises: an attempt should be made to date them. Often photographs can be helpful. Laboratory evaluation should include skeletal survey, hematocrit, platelet count, PT, PTT, and if sexual abuse is suspected, throat and genital cultures. It is important that the PICU physician remain the medical physician and not the judge. Social services and trauma specialists should be consulted immediately.

DROWNING

Drowning and near-drowning should be mentioned in any section on pediatric trauma. In some states it is the most common accidental cause of death in children less than 5 years of age. Fresh water drowning is more common than salt water drowning, with private swimming pools being the most common site.[115] Victims of drowning and near-drowning events are subject to primary pulmonary injury from aspiration and the cascade of multisystem injury from hypoxemia and possibly cardiac arrest. Similar to any child after a cardiac arrest, the target organ of greatest concern is the brain. Most children who have morbidity or mortality after surviving the initial event and resuscitation suffer primary CNS damage. The treatment is the same as discussed for increased ICP.[116]

The prognosis for near drowning has been correlated with a number of patient and event characteristics: duration of submersion and the cardiopulmonary and neurologic status at the scene and on arrival in an emergency room.[117] Unfortunately, there are no universally accepted factors for prognostication. An important component of the PICU care of the near-drowning or drowning victim is an understanding of prevention. As stated above, private swimming pools are the most common site; many of these accidents could be avoided if fences were appropriately placed around pools.

INGESTION

Ingestions are a common admission diagnosis in the PICU with patients requiring evaluation and treatment of cardiovascular and CNS dysfunction. Fifty percent of ingestions are accidental with a mean age of 2 years: these usually involve drugs that are readily available in the home. The other 50 percent are suicide gestures with a mean age of 15 years.[118] The basic treatment is systemic support, identification, decontamination, and elimination of the drug and efforts to minimize the side effects. It is imperative to consult social services for all accidental ingestions for the purpose of investigating how the child got the drug. Remember that poisoning can be a form of child abuse or child neglect. It is also important to have a low index of suspicion for possible suicide gestures: although we classically think of the adolescent in this group, children as young as 6 or 7 years are capable of suicide

BURNS

The peak incidence of burns is between the ages of 1 and 5 years. In younger children, scald burns to the upper extremities, head, and neck are the most common.[119] Although most burns are cared for in a burn ICU, a basic understanding is needed in the PICU. Burns should be evaluated immediately for percent body surface area (BSA) and severity or depth. The percent BSA estimate can be made with the "rule of nines" in children over 15 years of age. Under that age, special pediatric charts should be used.

Initial therapy after resuscitation includes placement of a nasogastric tube and Foley catheter. An ETT is placed if there is any evidence of airway burn. The burns should be elevated and dressed in a sterile manner. There are a number of formulas for calculating volume resuscitation. It is important to be comfortable with whichever one you select. One example is the modified Brooke and Parkland formulas:[120]

- First 24 h: maintenance plus 4 ml/kg for each percent BSA burn, first half given in the first 8 h and second half given in the next 16 h
- Second 24 h: maintenance as D_5 $\frac{1}{2}$NS and anything needed for blood pressure support

The child should also be closely monitored for delivery of adequate calories and infectious complications. The psychologic trauma from a burn injury can be overwhelming. Family as well as patient support and therapy are imperative.

Cardiopulmonary Arrest

Cardiopulmonary arrests are less common in the child than in the adult, with the pediatric incidence of out-of-hospital cardiac arrests estimated to be 13 percent of the adult incidence.[121] The causes of arrest differ dramatically. Sixty percent of adults have cardiac arrest because of a primary cardiac problem, myocardial ischemia with pump failure, or an arrhythmia. This can be considered a "primary cardiac arrest." In this situation, the time of end-organ damage is limited to the time of arrest until reestablishment of an adequate circulation. The child has normal coronaries and, hence, will not suffer a primary cardiac event. Rather, the child's cardiac arrest will be secondary to hypoxemia, acidosis, hypovolemia, or a metabolic disturbance. In this situation, the cardiac arrest is "secondary," and the time for potential end-organ injury includes time prior to the arrest.[122]

Another difference is the nature of the terminal arrhythmia. Adults most commonly have an episode of ventricular irritability prior to asystole (usually ventricular fibrillation). The child is more likely to have sinus bradycardia progressing directly to asystole.[123] This is important in that countershock may be helpful for the adult but will do nothing for the child.

The best treatment of cardiac arrest is anticipatory and preventative. It is much more important to recognize impending cardiac or respiratory failure before an arrest occurs. Once an arrest occurs, treatment is similar as for an adult with a few differences. Airway has been discussed previously. Hand placement for cardiac compressions changes with the age of the child. In one-person CPR, five compressions for each breath are given for children less than 6 years of age. In older children, the adult ratio of 15 compressions to each breath is used. In two-person CPR, five compressions to each breath are given. The rate of compressions is 80 to 100 for infants, 60 to 80 for the school-age child, and 60 per minute for the adolescent.[124]

TABLE 186-11 Drugs Used in Cardiopulmonary Resuscitation

Drug	Dose	Route
Epinephrine	0.01 mg/kg (0.1 mL/kg)	IV, IO, IT*
Sodium bicarbonate	0.5–1.0 mEq/kg	IV, IO
Atropine	0.02 mg/kg	IV, IO, IT
Glucose	0.5–1.0 gm/kg	IV, IO
Calcium chloride	0.2–0.25 mL/kg (5.0–7.0 mg/kg elemental calcium/kg)	IV, IO
Lidocaine	1.0 mg/kg	IV, IO, IT
Bretylium	5.0 mg/kg	IV, IO

*IV = intravenous; IO = intraosseous; IT = intratracheal.

Vascular access is important. The endotracheal tube can be used for the administration of many medications (epinephrine, atropine, lidocaine) (see Table 186-11). Intravascular catheters can be placed in the same sites as in an adult, but placement may be more difficult because of the size of the patient. It is now taught that in any child in whom an intravenous cannot be established, an intraosseous line (IO) should be placed for resuscitation. This is placed in the anterior tibial plateau 2 to 3 cm below the tibial tuberosity. The IO can be used for the administration of medications, volume, and infusions of vasoactive drugs.[125]

There are a few caveats for pediatric CPR. One is hypothermia. The child's vulnerability to hypothermia has been discussed elsewhere, but in the code situation this is critical. If a child is asystolic and has a temperature of less than 30°C, she is cold. But if the child has a temperature of at least 30°C and asystolic despite aggressive resuscitative efforts, she is dead. Efforts to rewarm a child should include active and passive surface rewarming and active core rewarming including warmed intravenous fluids; nasogastric lavage, enemas, and peritoneal dialysis.

Sudden Infant Death Syndrome

Sudden infant death syndrome (SIDS) is a major cause of death and morbidity in infants under 1 year of age claiming 2 to 3 victims per 1000 live births with an incidence which peaks between 3 and 4 months of age. SIDS deaths are sudden and unexplained. The death itself appears to be "quiet" in that there is no evidence of struggle or arousal. Many cases are temporally related to upper respiratory tract infections, immunizations, or recent anesthesia and surgery; but these events have never proven to be causative. There are many proposed etiologies for SIDS; the most common include central hypoventilation with sleep, central and/or peripheral chemoreceptor abnormalities, upper airway obstruction, primary hypoxemia, and cardiac conduction abnormalities.

The PICU cares for a number of infants who have been resuscitated from SIDS. Some of these infants die after their resuscitation if there was a prolonged period of cardiopulmonary arrest. Infants will survive if they are fortuitously discovered early and quickly resuscitated. These infants are then labeled as "near-miss SIDS." Further evaluation, treatment, and monitoring of these infants is controversial. The basic evaluation tool is a sleep pneumogram with a positive test documenting apnea and/or prolonged episodes of periodic breathing. Adjuncts to the pneumogram recordings can include cardiac monitoring, oximetry, EEG, and even esophageal pH probes to rule out gastroesophageal reflux. Some clinicians feel that a pneumogram is unnecessary in that, regardless of the results, therapy for a near-miss SIDS would still be the same; the strength of the history is enough to drive therapy.[126]

The possible treatments for these infants are limited. Theophylline has been used as a respiratory stimulant. But the mainstay is to teach the parents CPR and send the child home on a cardiorespiratory monitor.[127] Extensive home support is needed for families involved in monitoring programs. This support includes physician availability, technical backup, and respite care. There are a number of parent groups as well as the National Foundation for Sudden Infant Death, which can provide some of these supportive services.

References

1. Chiswick ML, Milner RDG: Crying vital capacity. Arch Dis Child 51:22, 1976.
2. Shapiro BA, Cane RD: Blood gas monitoring: Yesterday, today, and tomorrow. Crit Care Med 17:573, 1989.
3. Anand KD, Hickey PR: Pain and its effects in the human neonate and fetus. N Engl J Med 317:1321, 1987.
4. Rudolph AM, Heymann MA: Circulatory changes with growth in the fetal lamb. Circ Res 26:298, 1970.
5. Hislop A, Reid L: Pulmonary arterial development during childhood: Branching patterns and structure. Thorax 28:129, 1973.
6. Friedman WF, Pool PE, Jacobowitz D, et al.: Sympathetic innervation of the developing rabbit heart: Biochemical and histochemical comparison of fetal, neonatal and adult myocardium. Circ Res 23:25, 1968.
7. Waldman S, Krauss AN, Auld PAM: Baroreceptors in preterm infants: Their relationship to maturity and disease. Dev Med Child Neurol 21:714, 1979.
8. Enhornung G, Westin B: Experimental studies of the human fetus in prolonged asphyxia. Acta Physiol Scand 31:359, 1954.
9. Mott JC: The ability of young animals to withstand total oxygen lack. Br Med Bull 17:1245, 1961.
10. Cross KW, Dawes GS, Mott JC: Anoxia, oxygen consumption and cardiac output in newborn lambs and adult sheep. J Physiol (Lond) 146:316, 1959.
11. Rudolph AM, Heymann MA: Fetal and neonatal circulation and respiration. Annu Rev Physiol 36:187, 1974.
12. Rudolph AM: The changes in the circulation after birth. Their importance in congenital heart disease. Circulation 41:343, 1970.
13. Freed MA, Heymann MA, Lewis AB, et al.: Prostaglandin E_1 in infants with ductus arteriosus–dependent congenital heart disease. Circulation 64:899, 1981.
14. Crone RK: Acute circulatory failure in children. Pediatr Clin North Am 27:575, 1980.
15. Perkins RM, Levin DL: Shock in the pediatric patient. J Pediatr 101:319, 1982.
16. Perkins RM, Levin DL: Shock, in Levin DL, Morriss FC (eds): *Essentials of Pediatric Intensive Care.* St. Louis, Quality Medical Publishing, 1990.
17. Wetzel RC, Rogers MC: Dysrhythmias and their management, in Rogers MC (ed): *Textbook of Pediatric Intensive Care.* Baltimore, William and Wilkins, 1987.
18. Silverman NH, Ports TA, Snider AR, et al.: Determination of left ventricular volume in children: Echocardiographic and angiographic comparisons. Circulation 62:548, 1980.
19. Green TP: Therapeutic approach to the failing heart. Pediatr Ann 14:304, 1985.
20. Witte MK, Hill JH, Blumer JL: Shock in the pediatric patient. Adv Pediatr 34:139, 1987.
21. Pollack MM, Fields AJ, Ruttmann UE: Sequential cardiopulmonary variables of infants and children in septic shock. Crit Care Med 12:554, 1984.
22. Applebaum A, Blackstone EH, Kouchoukos NT, et al.: Afterload reduction and cardiac output in infants early after intracardiac surgery. Am J Cardiol 39:445, 1977.
23. Dillon TR, Janos GG, Meyer RA, et al.: Vasodilator therapy for congestive heart failure. J Pediatr 96:623, 1980.
24. Zaritsky A, Chernow B: Use of catecholamines in pediatrics. J Pediatr 105:341, 1984.
25. Otto CW, Yakaitis RW, Blitt CD: Mechanism of action of epinephrine in resuscitation from asphyxial arrest. Crit Care Med 9:364, 1981.
26. Driscol AS, Gillette PC, McNamara DC: The use of dopamine in children. J Pediatr 92:309, 1978.
27. Outwater K, Lang P, Treves S, et al.: Hemodynamic effects of dopamine in infants following cardiac surgery. J Clin Anesth 2:253, 1990.
28. Perkin RM, Levin DL, Webb R, et al.: Dobutamine: A hemodynamic evaluation in children with shock. J Pediatr 100:977, 1982.
29. Lawless S, Burckart G, Diven W, et al.: Amrinone pharmacokinetics in neonates and infants. J Clin Pharmacol 28:283, 1988.
30. Tsang RC, Donovan EV, Steichen JJ: Calcium physiology and pathology in the neonate. Pediatr Clin North Am 23:611, 1976.
31. Orlowski JP: Cardiopulmonary resuscitation in children. Pediatr Clin North Am 27:495, 1980.
32. Beekman RH, Rocchini AP, Rosenthal A: Hemodynamic effects of nitroprusside in infant with a large ventricular septal defect. Circulation 64:553, 1981.
33. Davies DW, Greiss L, Steward DJ: Sodium nitroprusside in children: Observations on metabolism during normal and abnormal responses. Can Anaesth Soc J 22:553, 1975.
34. Brent B, Berger H, Mahler D, et al.: Acute effects of hydralazine on the pulmonary circulation and right ventricular function in chronic lung disease and pulmonary hypertension. Clin Res 30:4A, 1982.
35. Rubin LJ, Peter RH: Oral hydrolazine for primary pulmonary hypertension. N Engl J Med 302:69, 1980.

36. Heymann MA, Hoffman JIE: Persistent pulmonary hypertension syndromes in the newborn, in Weir EK, Reeves JT (eds): *Pulmonary Hypertension.* Mt. Kisko, NY, Futura, 1984.
37. Strand DG, Sell CG, Oates JA: Hypertrophic obstructive cardiomyopathy in an infant: Propranolol therapy for three years. N Engl J Med 285:243, 1971.
38. Zeligs MA, Lockhart CH: Perioperative hypoglycemia in a child treated with propranolol. Anesth Analg 62:1035, 1983.
39. Porter CJ, Gillette PC, Garson A, et al.: The effects of verapamil on supraventricular tachycardia in children. Am J Cardiol 48:487, 1981.
40. Kock-Weser J: Bretylium. N Engl J Med 300:473, 1979.
41. Hislop A, Reid L: Growth and development of the respiratory system, in Davis J, Dobbling J (eds): *Scientific Foundations of Pediatrics.* Philadelphia, W. B. Saunders, 1974.
42. Bryan AC, Mansell AL, Levison H: Development of the mechanical properties of the respiratory system, in Hodson WA (ed): *Development of the Lung.* New York, Marcel Dekker, 1977, p. 446.
43. Hogg J, William J, Richardson J, et al.: Age as a factor in the distribution of lower airway conductance in the pathologic anatomy of obstructive lung disease. N Engl J Med 283:1283, 1970.
44. Rigatto H, Brady J, de la Torre Verduzco R, et al.: Chemoreceptor reflexes in preterm infants. The effect on gestational age and postnatal age in ventilatory response to inhalation of 100% and 15% oxygen. Pediatrics 55:604, 1975.
45. American Academy of Pediatrics Task Force on Prolonged Apnea: Prolonged infantile apnea: 1985. Pediatrics 76:129, 1985.
46. Ariagno RL, Guilleminault C: Apnea during sleep in the pediatric patient. Clin Chest Med 6:679, 1985.
47. Lyrene RT, Truog WE: Adult respiratory distress syndrome in a pediatric intensive care unit: predisposing conditions, clinical course and outcome. Pediatrics 67:790, 1981.
48. Leipzig B, Oskin FA, Cummings CW, et al.: A prospective randomized study to determine the efficacy of steroids in treatment of croup. J. Pediatr 94:144, 1979.
49. Orr JB: Helium-oxygen mixture in the management of patients with airway obstruction. Ear Nose Throat J 67:868, 1988.
50. Cohen S: Foreign bodies in the airway: five year retrospective study with special reference to management. Ann Otol 89:437, 1980.
51. Outwater KM, Crone RK: Management of respiratory failure in infants with acute viral bronchiolitis. Am J Dis Child 138:1071, 1984.
52. Committee on Infectious Diseases: Ribavirin therapy of respiratory syncytial virus. Pediatrics 79:475, 1987.
53. Barnes PJ: A new approach to the treatment of asthma. N Engl J Med 321:1517, 1989.
54. Haddad D, Richards CC: Mechanical ventilation of infants: significance of compression volume and elimination of compression volume. Anesthesiology 29:365, 1968.
55. MacIntyre NR: Respiratory function during pressure support ventilation. Chest 89:677, 1986.
56. Avery ME, Mead J: Surface properties in relation to atelectasis and hyaline membrane disease. Am J Dis Child 97:517, 1959.
57. Kendig JW, Notter RH, Cox C, et al.: Surfactant replacement therapy at birth: final analysis of a clinical trial and comparisons with similar trials. Pediatrics 82:756, 1988.
58. O'Rourke PP, Crone RK: High frequency ventilation. JAMA 250:2845, 1983.
59. The HiFi Study Group: High-frequency oscillatory ventilation compared with conventional mechanical ventilation in the treatment of respiratory failure in preterm infants. N Engl J Med 320:88, 1989.
60. Bartlett RH, Toomasian J, Roloff D, et al.: Extracorporeal membrane oxygenation (ECMO) in neonatal respiratory failure: 100 cases. Ann Surg 204:236, 1986.
61. Extracorporeal Life Support Organization (ELSO): Neonatal ECMO Registry, September 1990.
62. Towne GH, Lott IT, Hicks DA, et al.: Long-term follow-up of infants and children treated with extracorporeal membrane oxygenation (ECMO): a preliminary report. J Pediatr Surg 20:410, 1985.
63. Amiel-Tison C: Neurologic examination of the maturity of newborn infants. Arch Dis Child 43:89, 1968.
64. American College of Surgeons Committee on Trauma: Advanced Trauma Life Support Instructor Manual, Chapter 10, Pediatric Trauma, 1989, p. 226.
65. Davis RJ, Dean JM, Boldberg AL, et al.: Head and spinal cord injury, in Rogers MC (ed): *Textbook of Pediatric Critical Care.* Baltimore, Williams and Wilkins, 1987, p. 649.
66. Bruce DA, Schut L, Bruno LA, et al.: Outcome following severe head injury in children. J Neurosurg 48:679, 1978.
67. Bruce DA, Raphaely RC, Goldberg AI, et al.: Pathophysiology, treatment and outcome following severe head injury in children. Childs Brain 5:174, 1979.
68. Rockoff MA, Pascucci RC: Reye's syndrome emergency. Med Clin North Am 1:87, 1983.
69. Shields WD: Status epilepticus. Pediatr Clin North Am 36:383, 1989.
70. Dean JM, Rogers MC, Traystman RJ: Pathophysiology and clinical management of the intracranial vault, in Rogers MC (ed): *Textbook of Pediatric Intensive Care.* Baltimore, Williams and Wilkins, 1987, p. 527.
71. Ad Hoc Committee on Brain Death, The Children's Hospital, Boston: Determination of brain death. J Pediatr 110:15, 1987.
72. Freeman JM, Terry PC: New brain death guidelines in children: further confusion. Pediatrics 81:301, 1988.
73. Outwater KM, Rockoff MA: Apnea testing to confirm brain death in children. Crit Care Med 12:357, 1984.
74. Ellis D, Gartner JC, Galvis AG: Acute renal failure in infants and children: Diagnosis, complications, and treatment. Crit Care Med 9:607, 1981.
75. Fong JSC, Dechadarevian JP, Kaplan BS: Hemolytic uremic syndrome: Current concepts and management. Pediatr Clin North Am 29:835, 1982.
76. Cleary TG: Cytotoxin producing *E. coli* and the hemolytic uremic syndrome. Pediatr Clin North Am 35:485, 1988.
77. Potter DE: Comparison of peritoneal dialysis and hemodialysis in children. Dial Transplant 7:800, 1978.
78. Krane EJ, Rockoff MA, Wallman JK, et al.: Subclinical brain swelling in children during treatment of diabetic ketoacidosis. N Engl J Med 312:1147, 1985.
79. Rogers B, Sills I, Cohen M, et al.: Diabetic ketoacidosis neurologic collapse during treatment followed by severe developmental morbidity. Clin Pediatr 29:451, 1990.
80. Rosenbloom AL, Riley WJ, Weber FT, et al.: Cerebral edema complicating diabetic ketoacidosis in childhood. J Pediatr 96:357, 1980.
81. Mackey WC, Dineen P: A fifty year experience with Meckel's diverticulum. Surg Gynecol Obstet 156:56, 1983.
82. Wayne ER, Campbell JB, Barrington JD, et al.: Management of 344 children with intussusception. Radiology 107:597, 1973.
83. Brown EG, Sweet AY: Neonatal necrotizing enterocolitis. Pediatr Clin North Am 29:1149, 1982.

84. Schwartz MZ, Richardson CJ, Hayden CK, et al.: Intestinal stenosis following successful medical management of necrotizing enterocolitis. J Pediatr Surg 15:890, 1980.
85. Rogers EL, Rogers MC: Fulminant hepatic failure and hepatic encephalopathy. Pediatr Clin North Am 27:701, 1980.
86. Paradis KJ, Freese DK, Sharp HL: A pediatric perspective on liver transplantation. Pediatr Clin North Am 35:409, 1988.
87. Weber TR, Grosfeld JL: Contemporary management of biliary atresia. Surg Clin North Am 61:1079, 1981.
88. Riegle CM, Thompson AE, Gartner JC: Intensive care unit course following pediatric hepatic transplantation. Crit Care Med 12:220A, 1984.
89. Cienfuegos JA, Dominguez RM, Tamelchoff LW, et al.: Surgical complications in the postoperative period of live transplants in children. Transplant Proc 16:1230, 1984.
90. Reimer SL, Michener WM, Steiger E: Nutritional support of the critically ill child. Pediatr Clin North Am 27:647, 1980.
91. Buchanan GR: Hemophilia. Pediatr Clin North Am 27:309, 1980.
92. Nilsson IM, Holmberg L: Von Willebrand's disease today. Clin Haematol 8:147, 1979.
93. McWilliams NB, Maurer HM: Acute idiopathic thrombocytopenia in children. Am J Hematol 7:87, 1979.
94. Maurer HM, McCue CM, Caul J, et al.: Impairment in platelet aggregation in congenital heart disease. Blood 40:207, 1972.
95. Preston FE: Disseminated intravascular coagulation. Br J Hosp Med 28:129, 1982.
96. Toews WH, Bass JW: Skin manifestations of meningococcal infection. An immediate indicator of prognosis. Am J Dis Child 127:173, 1974.
97. Phillips TF, Soulier BA, Wilson RF: Outcome of massive transfusion. Exceeding two blood volumes in trauma and emergency surgery. J Trauma 27:903, 1987.
98. Friedland GH, Klein RS: Transmission of the human immunodeficiency virus. N Engl J Med 317:1125, 1985.
99. Vernant JP, Brun B, Mannoni P: Respiratory distress of hyperleukocytic granulocytic leukemias. Cancer 44:264, 1979.
100. Dearth J, Salter M, Wilson E, et al.: Early deaths in acute leukemia in children. Med Pediatr Oncol 11:225, 1983.
101. Kamen BA, Summers CP, Pearson HA: Exchange transfusion as a treatment for hyperleukocytosis, anemia, and metabolic abnormalities in a patient with leukemia. J Pediatr 96:1045, 1980.
102. King RM, Telander RL, Smithson WA: Primary mediastinal tumors in children. J Pediatr Surg 17:512, 1982.
103. Halpern S, Chatten J, Meadows AT: Anterior mediastinal masses: Anesthetic hazards and other problems. J Pediatr 102:407, 1983.
104. Wilson CB: Immunologic basis for increased susceptibility of the neonate to infection. J Pediatr 108:1, 1986.
105. Baker CJ: Summary of the workshop on perinatal infections due to Group B streptococcus. J Infect Dis 136:137, 1977.
106. Kaplan SL, Fishman MA: Supportive therapy for bacterial meningitis. Pediatr Infect Dis 6:679, 1987.
107. Committee on Infectious Diseases: Dexamethasone therapy for bacterial meningitis in infants and children. Pediatrics 86:130, 1990.
108. Hughes WT, Tutenkeji H, Bartley DL: The immune compromised host. Pediatr Clin North Am 103:30, 1983.
109. Cooper ER, Pelton SI, LeMay M: Acquired immunodeficiency syndrome: A new population of children at risk. Pediatr Clin North Am 35:1365, 1988.
110. Bernstein LJ, Bye MR, Rubinstein A: Prognostic factors and life expectancy in children with acquired immunodeficiency syndrome and pneumocystis carinii pneumonia. Am J Dis Child 143:775, 1989.
111. Division of Injury Control, Center for Environmental Health and Injury Control. Center for Disease Control. Childhood injuries in the United States. Am J Dis Child 144:627, 1990.
112. Drew R, Perry JF Jr, Fischer RP: The expediency of peritoneal lavage for blunt trauma in children. Surg Gynecol Obstet 145:885, 1977.
113. Kempe CH, Silverman FN, Steele BF, et al.: The battered-child syndrome. JAMA 181:105, 1962.
114. Johnson CF: Inflicted injury versus accidental injury. Pediatr Clinic North Am 37:791, 1990.
115. Wintemute GJ: The causes, impact and preventability of childhood injuries in the United States: childhood drowning injuries in the United States. Am J Dis Child 144:663, 1990.
116. Orlowski JP: Drowning, near-drowning and ice water submersions. Pediatr Clin North Am 34:75, 1987.
117. Allman FD, Nelson WB, Pacentine GA, et al.: Outcome following cardiopulmonary resuscitation in severe pediatric near-drowning. Am J Dis Child 140:571, 1986.
118. Fazen LE, Lovejoy FH, Crone RK: Acute poisoning in a children's hospital: A 2 year experience. Pediatrics 77:144, 1986.
119. McLoughlin E, McGuire A: The causes, impact and preventability of childhood injuries in the United States. Childhood burn injuries in the United States. Am J Dis Child 144:677, 1990.
120. Carvajal HF: Controversies in fluid resuscitation, in Carvajal HG, Parks DH (eds): *Burns in Children: Pediatric Burn Management.* Chicago: Year Book Medical Publishers, Inc, 1988.
121. Eisenberg M, Bergner L, Hallstrom A: Epidemiology of cardiac arrest and resuscitation in children. Ann Emerg Med 12:672, 1983.
122. O'Rourke PP: Outcome of children who are apneic and pulseless in the emergency room. Crit Care Med 14:466, 1986.
123. Walsh CK, Krongrad E: Terminal cardiac electric activity in pediatric patients. Am J Cardiol 51:557, 1983.
124. American Heart Association: *Textbook of Advanced Pediatric Life Support.* Dallas: The Association, 1987.
125. Rosetti VA, Thompson BM, Miller J, et al.: Intraosseous infusion: An alternative route of pediatric intravascular access. Ann Emerg Med 14:885, 1985.
126. Shannon DC, Kelly DH: SIDS and near-SIDS (Part I). N Engl J Med 306:959, 1982.
127. Shannon DC, Kelly DH: SIDS and near-SIDS (Part II). N Engl J Med 306:1022, 1982.

Chapter 187

NURSING PERSPECTIVES ON CRITICAL CARE

MARGUERITE R. KINNEY

Long before critical care units were integrated into the structure of American hospitals, Florence Nightingale recognized the importance of placing the sickest soldiers closest to the nurse. While the armamentarium of the nurse in Nightingale's day was indeed meager, this proximity of nurse and patient did allow the nurse to "put the patient in the best condition for nature to act upon him"[1] (p. 75). In the 1960s, the experience in newly developed coronary care units (CCUs) demonstrated that nurses with specialized knowledge and skill working in close proximity to patients and having the sophisticated technology available could positively influence mortality rates. The eminent physician Paul Dudley White noted that the critical care nurse was much closer to the patient than was the physician and thus "should have much to say . . . for the edification of the doctor"[2] (p. 35). Indeed, in the early years of critical care in this country, nurse and physician collaboration and cooperation in patient management was an important ingredient in the critical care environment.

In recent years nursing has emerged as a discipline directed toward the diagnosis and treatment of human responses to actual or potential health problems. While the focus in medicine is diagnosis and treatment of disease and injury, critical care nursing is concerned specifically with human response to life-threatening illness. Considerable effort is being focused on an understanding on these human responses in the difficult environment of the CCU.

The American Association of Critical-Care Nurses describes the scope of critical care nursing as being defined by "the dynamic interaction of the critically ill patient, the critical care nurse, and the critical care environment"[3] (p. 18). In this chapter, selected phenomena of concern congruent with the scope of critical care nursing practice are presented. These examples illustrate the ongoing effort to describe, explain, and predict human responses to life-threatening illnesses and treatment and to prescribe appropriate nursing interventions. The phenomena selected for presentation are also of concern to physicians, and the work presented here may serve to edify them, not only about the phenomena themselves but also about the scientific contributions of nurse investigators. Almost 20 years ago, Dr. Tinsley R. Harrison wrote that science is needed in both medicine and nursing, although he thought the need was greater in medicine.[4] Perhaps a more contemporary view is that the need is great in both disciplines; the focus of the inquiry is, however, different.

Patient care can only be enhanced as both physicians and nurses employ the tools of science to gain a better understanding of the illness, the environment in which care is delivered, and the patient's response to that care. Collaboration and communication are essential in the generation and application of knowledge gained through scientific inquiry and based on the different but complementary perspectives of each discipline.

The phenomena selected for inclusion in this chapter represent biopsychosocial dimensions of critical illness and are important in the care of patients regardless of the subspecialty or setting. The topics addressed demonstrate a recognition of the interrelationship between body and mind and the reciprocal effects exerted by the one on the other. The presentations acknowledge the need to understand phenomena such as pain, dyspnea, and separation from family from the patient's perspective if caregivers are to make progress in the delivery of humane care to the critically ill. A clear direction for the discipline of nursing provides the opportunity for nurses to contribute to the body of knowledge needed by all who care for the critically ill. While a comprehensive discussion of the phenomena addressed by nursing is beyond the scope of this chapter, the phenomena selected draw attention to the concerns shared by nurses and physicians and point to the rewards to be reaped by collaboration and cooperation.

REFERENCES

1. Nightingale F: *Notes on Nursing*. London, Harrison & Sons, 1959.
2. White PD: Heart and lung: A journal primarily directed to the education of nurses but useful for everyone involved in the care of the cardiac patient. Heart Lung 1:34, 1972.
3. Disch J: Scope of practice defined. Focus on AACN 7:18, 1980.
4. Harrison, TR: A potential by-product of critical care. Heart Lung 1:337, 1972.

187A/Endotracheal Suctioning

MARA M. BAUN

Endotracheal suctioning is a common procedure performed in critical care. Depending on patient status and the amount of secretions present, the procedure may be performed as often as every 15 or 20 min. While the procedure has seemed benign, recent investigations have provided new data that demonstrate the potential for serious untoward side effects.

During endotracheal suction, when the suction catheter is passed down the endotracheal tube and negative pressure is applied, air flows from the atmosphere into the tracheobronchial tree and up the catheter into the suction apparatus. There is a fall in pressure from the atmosphere to the airway, and again from the airway to the suction apparatus. The pressure change from atmosphere to trachea is related to the resistance of the pathway from the atmosphere through the airway. If the resistance of the pathway from the catheter tip to the atmosphere is high, a great portion of the negative pressure developed by the apparatus will also be developed in the airway. A decrease in transpulmonary pressure, a reduction in lung volume, and the possibility of atelectasis result. If the suction catheter stimulates the cough reflex, the pressure gradient might be reversed. As soon as solid or liquid aspirate is drawn into the suction catheter, the pressure in the airway once again becomes atmospheric.[1]

When an equilibrium is reached during suctioning, air flows down the trachea at the same rate as it flows up through the catheter. The pressure drop across each of these paths equals the product of flow and path resistance. Thus, the ratio of the outside diameter of the suction catheter to the inside diameter of the endotracheal tube through which it is passed is an important factor in determining the relative resistances of the two pathways and, therefore, the tracheal pressure. Experiments using a mock lung have determined that if the suction catheter has an outside diameter of not more than half of the inside diameter of the airway, negative pressures in the lungs are avoided.[1]

Even subatmospheric airway pressures of brief duration, such as those produced by suctioning with a large suction catheter through a narrow endotracheal tube, can cause a decrease in compliance and shunting. The mechanism responsible for this decrease in compliance is probably the collapse of alveoli. If the capillary blood flow is maintained through the collapsed, and thus unventilated, areas of the lungs, venous admixture to arterialized blood will occur. If enough alveoli collapse but continue to be perfused, the venous admixture, or shunt, will assume such proportions that a measurable fall in arterial oxygen tension will result. Collapse of the alveoli can also cause a decrease in functional residual capacity.

Decreased arterial oxygen tension, which has been reported during and after endotracheal suction in a wide variety of subjects, has a number of mechanisms in addition to atelectasis: (1) dilution of the alveolar gas with air in instances where the inspired oxygen tension is greater than room air; (2) apnea in patients requiring constant artificial ventilation; and (3) atelectasis resulting from the development of intraairway negative pressures, with an accompanying increase in shunt and alveolar-to-arterial oxygen tension difference. It is possible that any or all three of these mechanisms may operate in any one patient.

Hyperinflation and hyperoxygenation prior to and after endotracheal suction are practices employed in some clinical settings. Numerous studies of lung hyperinflations of 100% oxygen prior to and after endotracheal suction have reported that arterial oxygen tensions or saturations have remained at or above baseline during the entire suction-hyperinflation sequence.[2–4] It should be noted that most of these studies reported the effects of preoxygenation on arterial blood gases only, used postoperative patients with largely normal lungs, and did not include measures of cardiovascular function.

Only two studies[5,6] have addressed the effectiveness of inspired oxygen concentrations of less than 100% but greater than maintenance levels. In both of these studies, mean arterial oxygen tensions or saturations remained above baseline during the entire procedure, but an 8 percent decrease in tension occurred after return to the ventilator.

Recently, several reports have addressed the use of the lung hyperinflations themselves as methods of pre- and postoxygenation. While oxygenation was adequate, lung hyperinflations delivered by a volume ventilator resulted in mean increases ranging from 9 to 15 mmHg in mean arterial pressure (MAP) over three lung hyperinflation and suctioning sequences.[7,8] When some type of anesthesia bag was used, increases in MAP were greater than with the ventilator. Based on these and current studies in progress, it is suggested that the use of lung hyperinflations as preventative measures with endotracheal suctioning needs to be reconsidered. Since progressive increases in MAP might be deleterious to some patients, it is suggested that the use of lung hyperinflations as preventive measures with endotracheal suctioning should be used only when there is a demonstrated need to hyperinflate the lungs.

The use of modified endotracheal tube adapters to minimize the arterial oxygen desaturation that accompanies endotracheal suction has been reported in a number of studies. In general, some of these have concluded that suctioning through adapters was the preferable method.[2,9–11] Comparative protocols in these studies included disconnecting the subject from the ventilator with no preoxygenation and "bagging" with 100% oxygen at various rates and for variable periods of time before, after, or before and after suctioning. It is difficult to draw conclusions from these studies, however, because in some cases the comparative protocols were not sufficient to prevent arterial oxygen desaturation. In addition, in most of the studies, arterial blood gases were the only variables reported. Also, no consideration was given to effects of the use of the adapter on the cardiovascular system.

Special consideration needs to be given to those patients requiring positive end-expiratory pressure (PEEP) therapy in order to maintain adequate oxygenation. It has been postulated that "breaking" PEEP in order to perform endotracheal suctioning (ETS) would of itself result in potentially serious decreases in arterial oxygenation. Only two studies, however, have addressed specifically the discontinuation of PEEP for suctioning. A 123 percent increase in shunt was reported[12] when adult respiratory failure patients were removed from the ventilator for suctioning, accompanied by a 43 percent decrease in arterial oxygen tension ($P_{A_{O_2}}$).

A number of studies have compared the effects of suctioning through an adapter while PEEP is maintained as opposed to breaking PEEP by removing the subject from the ventilator.[13–15] Results of these studies lead to several conclusions that support the need for further investigation of the use of modified endotracheal tube adapters. First, suctioning subjects on PEEP results in different and potentially more deleterious cardiorespiratory effects than suctioning subjects not on PEEP. Presumably, some of these effects result from the seriousness of the respiratory impairment, which necessitates the use of PEEP, and some from the consequences of even short-term discontinuation of this therapy in order to perform the suctioning. Second, the use of a closed system using an adapter has been reported as the preferred protocol in some studies, but it has had equivocal results in others when compared to conventional forms of suctioning. It is difficult to draw generalizations from the studies reported, however, since protocols have differed greatly. In addition, most of these studies have reported the effects of closed system suctioning on respiratory variables only and have not looked at the effects of both the discontinuation of PEEP and the use of closed system suctioning on the cardiovascular system. It is possible that although arterial oxygenation appears adequate in some of the protocols studied, deleterious cardiovascular effects may be occurring that would be hazardous to subjects with compromised cardiovascular systems.

Another group of patients who require careful ETS are those with increased intracranial pressure (ICP). All of the few studies of ETS in this subgroup of patients have demonstrated that ETS, regardless of the protocol used, will increase ICP. These increases are greatest in those with cerebral hypertension who are least able to tolerate further increased ICP.[16]

Although considerable research has been done on various aspects of the ETS procedure, there are still numerous unresolved questions. Based on existing data, the following recommendations can be made:

1. Suctioning mechanically ventilated subjects needs to be accompanied by some form of supplemental oxygenation.
2. Suction flow rate, the number of suction sequences, and the length of time suction is applied should be the minimum required to remove secretions.
3. The suction catheter used should have an external diameter sufficiently small to allow the retrograde flow through the endotracheal tube to minimize the fall in tracheal pressure.
4. Much future research is needed to address details of all aspects of the suction process and to determine ways to "customize" suctioning to a given patient.

REFERENCES

1. Rosen M, Hillard EK: The effects of negative pressure during tracheal suction. Curr Res Anesth Anaig 41(1):50, 1962.
2. Brown SE, Stansbury DW, Merrill EJ, Linden GS, Light RW: Prevention of suctioning-related arterial oxygenation desaturation. Chest 83:621, 1983.
3. Baun MM, Flones MI: Cumulative effects of three sequential endotracheal suctioning episodes in the dog model. Heart Lung 13(2):145, 1984.
4. Pierce JB, Piazza DE: Differences in postsuctioning arterial blood oxygen concentration values using two postoxygenation methods. Heart Lung 16(1):34, 1987.
5. Buchanan L, Baun MM: The effect of hyperinflation, inspiratory hold, and oxygenation on cardiopulmonary status during suctioning in a lung injured model. Heart Lung 15(2):127, 1986.
6. Rogge JA, Bunde L, Baun MM: Effectiveness of oxygen concentrations of less than 100% before and after endotracheal suction in patients with chronic obstructive pulmonary disease. Heart Lung 18(1):64, 1989.
7. Preusser B, Stone K, Gonyon D, Winningham M, Groch K, Karl J: Effects of two methods of preoxygenation on mean arterial pressure, cardiac output, peak airway pressure, and postsuctioning hypoxemia. Heart Lung 17(3):290, 1988.
8. Stone KS, Vorst EC, Lanham B, Zahn S: Effects of lung hyperinflation on mean arterial pressure and postsuctioning hypoxemia. Heart Lung 18(4):377, 1989.
9. Bodai BI: A means of suctioning without cardiopulmonary depression. Heart Lung 11(2):172, 1982.
10. Craig KC, Benson MS, Pierson DJ: Prevention of arterial oxygen desaturation during closed-airway endotracheal suction: Effect of ventilator mode. Respir Care 29(10):1013, 1984.
11. Jung RC, Newman J: Minimizing hypoxia during endotracheal airway care. Heart Lung 11(3):208, 1982.
12. Spitzer PW, Smith SJ: Transient interruptions of PEEP in routine patient care: The effect on arterial blood gases in patients with adult Respiratory Distress Syndrome. Am Rev Resp Dis 117(4):213, 1978.
13. St. Onge D, Kirilloff LH, Zullo TG: The effect of maintaining and removing positive end-expiratory pressure during endotracheal suctioning. Heart Lung 11(3):259, 1982.
14. Schumann L, Parsons GH: Tracheal suctioning and ventilator tubing changes in adult respiratory distress syndrome: Use of a positive end-expiratory pressure valve. Heart Lung 14(4):362, 1985.
15. Douglas S, Larson E: The effect of a positive end-expiratory pressure adapter on oxygenation during endotracheal suctioning. Heart Lung 14(4):396, 1985.
16. Rudy EB, Baun M, Stone K, Turner B: The relationship between endotracheal suctioning and changes in intracranial pressure: A review of the literature. Heart Lung 15(5):488, 1986.

187 B/Shivering

BARBARA J. HOLTZCLAW

Most people consider shivering a ubiquitous healthy warming response that occurs when they are chilled. The sequelae and metabolic cost of shivering are generally unappreciated even among physicians and nurses. Vigorous shivering involves aerobic muscle activity that increases metabolic rate in healthy adults three to five times the resting value. Oxygen consumption during severe shivering parallels that consumed while bicycle riding or shoveling snow.[1] Despite its heavy metabolic toll, the efficiency of shivering in raising body temperature has been estimated at only 11 percent.[2] Shivering actually contributes to heat loss by increasing circulation to cooler body areas and the skin. When this occurs, the protective shell of insulation provided by superficial vasoconstriction is lost. Heat is further dissipated by convection during muscle movement. While healthy individuals may compensate fairly well for the exertion of shivering, seriously ill patients may tolerate sequelae poorly. Patients in critical care settings are often at risk for shivering due to (1) inadvertent heat loss during surgery and anesthesia, (2) induced heat loss during central or surface cooling, (3) febrile chills during infection, (4) febrile reactions to drugs and blood products, and (5) compromised ability to maintain and conserve heat. Early recognition and action by critical care nurses and physicians may forestall the serious consequences of shivering in vulnerable patients.

THE PHENOMENON OF SHIVERING

Shivering, in this discussion, refers to a course of involuntary generalized skeletal muscle contractions that occurs in response to heat loss. Phasic bursts of muscle contractions tend to punctuate periods of relaxation during a course. Shivering as a thermoregulatory response is differentiated from transitory tremors or shudders of autonomic origin in (1) pattern of muscle involvement, (2) duration of activity, and (3) pathways of impulse transmission. Tension of the muscle spindle sets up feedback oscillation so that each efferent impulse results in numerous rebound fasciculations.[3] Thus, the extrapyramidal motor activity of shivering is facilitated by tension from autonomic sources.[4] In situations where both occur, clear distinctions between cold-induced shivering and tremor may be difficult to make.[5]

THERMOREGULATION AND SHIVERING

Compensatory thermoregulatory responses occur when core temperatures rise above or fall below the thermostatic set point. This range is from about 36.4 to 37.3°C (97.5 to 99.5°F). The hypothalamus coordinates thermal balance through a complex feedback system that includes (1) sensory inputs, (2) integration and/or comparison, and (3) physiologic and behavioral output effector mechanisms. Both heat loss *and* heat gain mechanisms should be considered in any discussions of thermoregulation, because aggressive attempts to therapeutically raise or lower body temperature usually trigger compensatory responses that oppose the desired effect. Sensed *heat loss* initiates (1) shivering via the gamma efferent motor system, (2) vasoconstriction via autonomic stimulus, (3) postural changes as muscles tense and extremities are drawn closer to the body, and (4) warmth-seeking behavioral activities. Sensed *heat gain* causes (1) sweating and vasodilation, (2) muscle flaccidity and relaxation, and (3) behaviors, such as shedding clothes, to lose heat. Each mechanism accomplishes heat loss or gain through radiation, conduction, convection, or evaporation. In adult human beings, shivering is the primary mechanism by which heat is generated. Vasomotor responses serve only to conserve and maintain heat.

Afferent input for the shivering response begins with stimulation of functionally specific heat loss sensors in the skin, spinal cord, and brain. Impulses are transmitted via the spinal tracts to the preoptic anterior hypothalamus for integration. The hypothalamic comparator senses discrepancies between the set point and the integrated stimuli. The body temperature reference point for shivering stimulus is not a fixed or absolute temperature but rather a *threshold* below which shivering starts. This threshold is strongly influenced by skin temperature and skin-to-core gradients.[6] Gradients between the hypothalamic thermostatic set point and the skin are widened by cooling the skin or by elevation of the set point by a pyrogen. Chilling the skin, for example, can elicit shivering without making any appreciable change in core temperature. When set point levels are raised by a pyrogen, less cooling of skin is necessary to stimulate shivering.

STAGES OF SHIVERING PROGRESSION

Shivering in human beings follows a cephalad-to-caudal pattern of progression beginning in the masseters with hard-to-detect tremors and extending to include extremities.[7] Electromyographic (EMG) studies of healthy subjects during surface cooling demonstrate that masseter tremor is followed by neck and chest muscle contractions, which precede generalized shaking. Clinical nursing observations verified this phenomenon in hypothermic patients.[8] This progression was noted by nurse researchers who delineated the following stages in studies of surface and centrally cooled hypothermic patients[9,10]:

- 0—no shivering activity
- 1—nonvisible masseter contractions
- 2—neck and chest fasciculations
- 3—abdominal contractions
- 4—generalized shaking including extremities and teeth chattering

Staging provides a clinically important means for caregivers to consistently communicate the extent and severity of shivering activity. Standard measurements also provide the means for evaluating the efficacy of interventions to prevent or alleviate shivering.

CONDITIONS LEADING TO SHIVERING

The most common cause of shivering in surgical critical care settings is intraoperative heat loss. *Inadvertent intraoperative heat loss* occurs during most surgical procedures due to cold room air, averaging 21°C (70°F) or less, skin and visceral exposure, and use of wound irrigants. During operative procedures, anesthesia and analgesia suppress shivering and vasoconstriction. Shivering is completely obliterated by neuromuscular blocking agents such as pancuronium, d-tubocurarine, and metocurine. Cardiovascular drugs, such as nitroglycerine or sodium nitroprusside, contribute to heat loss by dilating superficial vascular beds. *Induced hypothermia* in critical care patients may be associated with intentional intraoperative cooling during cardiac or neurologic surgery. During cardiopulmonary bypass, hypothermia is induced without shivering under protection of anesthesia and muscle relaxants. During postanesthesia rewarming, however, shivering may be vigorous and accompanied by increased metabolic expenditure. Cooling blankets are also used to induce hypothermia to prevent cerebral edema after brain trauma or to treat refractory fever. Surface cooling is induced when heat from the patient's skin is transferred to circulating coolant in coils of the hypothermia blanket by conduction. Vigorous shivering follows, until compensatory responses are overwhelmed by drastic heat loss and the patient becomes poikilothermic. *Impaired heat conservation* makes shivering a major problem for patients with burns, large denuded areas of skin, or conditions that require skin to be kept moist and exposed. Elderly, weak, and/or debilitated patients may lack muscle mass and vasomotor tone needed to conserve heat. Shivering draws on caloric and metabolic stores needed by these patients for maintenance and recovery. Anemic patients tolerate the oxygen expenditure of shivering poorly due to the already diminished oxygen-carrying capacity of their blood.

Febrile shivering plays a role in both the cause and the effect of fever, whether the causative pyrogen is a microorganism, a foreign protein, or a drug. The pyrogen upwardly displaces the hypothalamic set point, and the *chill phase* of fever represents compensatory responses to raise core temperature to the higher level. As core temperature rises to the new set point, a *plateau* is reached. As temperature exceeds the set point, heat loss mechanisms such as vasodilation and sweating are activated and *defervescence* takes place.[1,11] These phases tend to be cyclic, with alternating bouts of chills and fever persisting as long as the pyrogen is present. The exact chemical nature of endogenous pyrogen was unknown until recently, although prostaglandins and cyclic nucleotides were thought to play a major role. The final common pathway is now believed to be the formation of a potent *endogenous pyrogen*, which may be the same as or closely related to *interleukin-1*. Interleukin-1 is known to enhance mitogenesis of T-lymphocytes, induce antibody formation by B-lymphocytes,[12] and activate lymphocytic response to antigen or mitogen.[13] Thus the benefits and management of fever are currently being debated. There is no evidence that the chills and shivering play a role in these immune processes. Thus they continue to warrant treatment and concern. Febrile shivering induced by drugs, blood products, or other infusions may be exhausting to seriously ill or debilitated patients. Amphotericin B, for example, is notorious for producing body-wracking chills or rigors, accompanied by increases in blood pressure and heart rate. Some anemic patients experience dyspnea and a significant fall in arterial oxygen saturation during severe drug-induced shivering.

SHIVERING SEVERITY AND SEQUELA

Stages of progression are closely linked to shivering severity because each advancing stage recruits more muscle mass. As muscle activity increases, oxygen consumption and production of carbon dioxide and lactic acid increase. Even well-ventilated cardiac surgery patients, who shiver after hypothermic bypass, show significant increases in oxygen consumption and carbon dioxide production.[14] Metabolic byproducts contribute to the already low serum pH caused by the return of accumulations of fixed acids from previously unperfused vascular beds.

Circulatory responses during aerobic activity are proportional to oxygen use. As shivering increases and oxygen is consumed, cardiac wall tension, rate, and contractility increase. Rate pressure product [(RPP) systolic blood pressure times heart rate] provides a reliable index of myocardial oxygen consumption (MV_{O_2}). RPP is considered by some authorities to be a critical measure in defining response of the coronary circulation to myocardial oxygen demands during exercise.[15] Among cardiac patients, RPP levels ranging from 14,000 to 20,000 are frequently associated with angina.[16]

Vigorous shivering in postoperative cardiac surgery patients is accompanied by a fall in mixed venous oxygen saturation. As oxygen stores are consumed, the shivering muscle derives energy substrate from *anaerobic* pathways and thus incurs an "oxygen debt" that must be repaid. In hypothermic patients, this anaerobic debt is added to that incurred aerobically by body-warming processes. The heart is able to use a greater variety of substrates than skeletal muscle but relies predominantly on *aerobic* means of metabolism. During ischemia or hypoxemia, cellular anaerobic glycolysis is stimulated and myocardial glycogen is rapidly depleted. The high-energy phosphates produced by glycolysis can therefore be supplied for only a limited period. Continued myocardial blood flow is particularly important to wash away accumulated metabolic products and hydrogen ions. If allowed to accumulate, lactate and other metabolites depress activity of enzymes required for glycolytic pathways.[17]

In rewarming after hypothermia, a common complication of vigorous shivering and profound vasoconstriction is *overshoot*: a rise in core temperatures to above set point levels. Overshoot refers to the common tendency for regulatory mechanisms to rebound or overcompensate. In these cases, body temperatures may rise to febrile levels.

SHIVERING MANAGEMENT

SHIVERING PREVENTION IN GENERAL CARE

Prevention is the key element in management of shivering from inadvertent heat loss. Patients with diminished ability to maintain and conserve heat are at greatest risk: the elderly, the cachectic, those with extensive burns and exposed moist skin, and those receiving drugs that prevent peripheral vasoconstriction. Staff may be unaware when patients become hypothermic unless thermometers are accurate and capable of measuring temperatures below 30°C. Standard mercury-in-glass clinical thermometers are inadequate for monitoring hypothermic patients because they do not measure below 34.4°C (94°F). Also, some brands of glass thermometers tend to lose accuracy when left unused on storage shelves.[18] All caregivers should be conscious of the dynamics of heat exchange in patient care. Heat is removed rapidly from the skin by (1) conduction to cool surfaces or liquids; (2) evaporation of sweat, irrigants, or bath water; (3) convection from air currents from drafts or laminar flow systems; and (4) radiation to cooler objects without direct contact. Adequate covering, control of heat and humidity, and prevention of drafts are simple but profoundly influential steps in reducing shivering.

SHIVERING MANAGEMENT AFTER GENERAL SURGERY

Warmed humidified gases are effective measures in reducing postoperative shivering in mild inadvertent hypothermia.[19] Warming blankets, warmed intravenous fluids, and radiant lights have also been used for rewarming with success.[20] Intravenous narcotics, such as morphine sulfate and meperidine, are frequently given as a postoperative shivering suppressant.[21] Whether these drugs relieve shivering by central suppression, by blocking neuromuscular transmission, or by peripherally dilating cutaneous vasculature is not clear at this time.

SHIVERING MANAGEMENT AFTER CARDIAC BYPASS

The rewarming measures mentioned in the preceding paragraph are insufficient and in some instances inappropriate for rewarming the centrally cooled patient with induced moderate or deep hypothermia. These patients are profoundly cool, with deep zones of unperfused tissue. Although the blood is rewarmed by the bypass pump at the end of surgery, vasoconstricted zones in peripheral regions remain cool. Heat is lost from the blood to cooler regions, and by the time patients reach the recovery area, they become hypothermic. Shivering ensues as the effects of anesthesia and muscle relaxants diminish. There is growing cautiousness about the speed at which the rewarming process should take place after hypothermic cardiac bypass. Too rapid rewarming can tax the compromised cardiovascular system as metabolic rate and oxygen consumption increase with each degree gain in body temperature. Rapid rewarming also causes constricted vascular beds to open, emptying fixed acids and metabolites into the circulation. Methods that allow slow uniform rewarming of tissues are thought to be less likely to produce the steep temperature gradients that initiate shivering. Thus, drugs to promote vasodilation and narcotics to suppress shivering are often used in conjunction with warm humidified gases to allow slow passive rewarming. Neuromuscular blockade with agents such as metocurine iodide is used less commonly to prevent shivering during passive rewarming.[22] Even though this method requires a longer period of mechanical ventilation and slows the rewarming process, it has been found to improve hemodynamic and cardiorespiratory stability in hypothermic patients. Because paralysis induced by neuromuscular blocking agents does not affect wakefulness, perception of pain, or other sensations, nursing assessment for pain must be particularly astute. Nurses must be alert to signs of sympathetic nervous system activity, such as rapid heart rate, increased blood pressure, or adrenergic sweating, as these may be possible manifestations of pain.

SHIVERING MANAGEMENT DURING SURFACE COOLING

The electrically controlled hypothermia blanket, with circulating liquid coolant, effectively transfers heat from the febrile patient's body. In the unanesthetized patient, however, the drastic heat loss from the skin elicits vigorous shivering, an initial rise in metabolic rate, and considerable distress. Heat-generating mechanisms are unable to keep pace with heat lost to the blanket and core temperatures tend to slide rapidly in the direction of skin temperatures. A rapid fall in core temperature of 0.5°C or more within a 15-min period, known as "drift," contributes to shivering and vasomotor instability. Drift occurs less often when the rate of cooling is controlled to allow core temperatures to fall more gradually. The energy expenditure resulting from responses to surface cooling makes premedication with shivering suppressant or muscle relaxant drugs a prerequisite. When the hypothermia blanket was first introduced, chlorpromazine was used as a shivering suppressant. Such adverse effects as hypotension, tachycardia, and a tendency to core temperature drift made the drug undesirable for this purpose. Narcotics, such as meperidine, may be given intravenously to suppress shivering. Nonnarcotic analgesics such as acetaminophen and ibuprofen may help reduce shivering in some patients if given prior to cooling.

MANAGEMENT OF FEBRILE SHIVERING

The chills of fever are combined effects of pyrogen-induced shivering and vasoconstriction. As the pyrogen moves the thermostatic set point higher, neutral or cool temperatures evoke mechanisms to warm the body. Efforts to cool the febrile patient during the chill phase of fever will usually accomplish the opposite effect. Ice packs and cool sponge baths may cause such severe shivering and vasoconstriction that fever climbs higher. Even tepid sponge baths will stimulate shivering in a febrile patient because of the steep temperature gradient between the skin and the water. Evaporation causes further chilling and triggers compensatory efforts to generate and conserve heat. Responses of individuals with fever vary considerably with different environmental temperatures. Research indicates that pyrogen-induced fevers do not cause shivering when room temperatures are raised to 32°C, and no tendency was found for fever to be more severe under these conditions.[23] These findings offer a variety of possibilities for nursing interventions to reduce febrile shivering.

When febrile shivering is caused by pyrogenic drugs such as amphotericin B, chills and shivering occur as the set point rises higher than existing blood and skin temperatures. Intravenous meperidine and hydrocortisone are often prescribed to diminish febrile effects, but results are variable among patients. Aspirin, ibuprofen, and acetaminophen may also reduce febrile symptoms if patients can tolerate them, but their effectiveness in reducing shivering remains uncertain. Many patients receiving amphotericin

B, blood products, and other products with pyrogenic properties are immunosuppressed, anemic, and thrombocytopenic.[24] In these patients, use of prostaglandin inhibitors may be contraindicated because of their effects on blood clotting and their tendency to erode gastric mucosa.

CURRENT RESEARCH IN SHIVERING

POSTOPERATIVE SHIVERING AND HYPOTHERMIA

Much of the research in shivering has centered on hypothermic patients in the immediate postoperative period. These problems are of concern to both medicine and nursing. Thus collaborative research among surgeons, anesthesiologists, nurse anesthetists, and nurse researchers appears in the literature.[14,20] Studies of the incidence and intraoperative environmental influences on hypothermia have also helped to identify factors contributory to postoperative shivering. Sophisticated instruments for metabolic measurement enabled researchers to estimate the caloric and oxygen costs of shivering.[14] Measures to prevent intraoperative and postoperative hypothermia have been investigated and include (1) heated blankets, (2) reflective "survival" blankets, (3) heated humidified inspired gases, and (4) warming vests, caps, leggings, and plastic hoods to conserve heat during the surgical procedure.[19,20,25]

A CLINICAL PREDICTOR OF SHIVERING

In a study of 24 postoperative hypothermic cardiac surgery patients, a nurse researcher found that nonvisible masseter contractions of stage 1 shivering are referred to the mandible. These are palpable as a vibratory "hum" to the examiner's fingertips placed along the jaw line. This early prodromal sign was predictive of postoperative shivering and was verifiable by EMG recordings.[10] Stage 1 shivering caused no appreciable increases in oxygen consumption, carbon dioxide production, heart rate, or blood pressure. However, with onset of stage 2 shivering significant increases occurred in each of these variables. As duration and extent of shivering progression increased, so did each indicator of metabolic expenditure. Myocardial oxygen consumption above pre- or postshivering levels was consistent with demands of heavy aerobic exercise, and the RPP was indicative of diminished myocardial oxygenation. The presence of masseter contractions as a predictor of more vigorous shivering may provide a useful assessment tool for caregivers.[10,14]

CONTROL OF SHIVERING DURING SURFACE COOLING

Little clinical research has been reported on the problem of hypothermia-induced shivering during surface cooling. One notable exception is an investigation of a nonpharmacologic nursing measure to prevent shivering. Three layers of dry terry cloth toweling were applied to patients' extremities, from toes to knees and fingertips to elbows, prior to application of the hypothermia blanket. This intervention was based on evidence that the skin sensors lead thermoregulatory responses before core changes take place. Sensors on the hands and feet were believed to have dominant influence in total afferent heat loss impulses. Extremity wraps protected sensors against shivering stimulus, while heat was conducted to the cooling blanket from the less sensitive trunk. In both a pilot study ($n = 17$) and a larger investigation ($n = 35$), significantly fewer subjects with extremity wraps shivered than did controls.[9,26]

EFFECTS OF A NURSING MEASURE ON DRUG-INDUCED SHIVERING

Efficacy of a nursing intervention to control amphotericin B–induced febrile shivering was tested in 40 hospitalized adult patients with cancer. Three layers of terry cloth toweling were wrapped from toes to groin and fingertips to axillae to modify the rate of heat loss from skin. Studies of environmental influences on febrile responses gave support to the study. Use of the wraps was based on the same physiologic principles as was the wrapping intervention for surface cooling. Duration of shivering and amount of meperidine required for shivering suppression were compared between treatment and control groups. Total shivering duration was shorter and severity less in the treatment group than in the control group. Less meperidine was administered to the treatment group than to controls, although differences were not statistically significant.[27]

FUTURE DIRECTIONS

Many questions remain unanswered about the nature of shivering and its most effective management. Its specific neurophysiology, the precise location of hypothalamic centers, and the neurotransmitters involved in impulse transmission continue to be investigated. Major findings in any of these areas might have consequences for treatment or prevention of shivering. Biochemical discoveries show great promise in the pharmacologic management of febrile shivering. Drug-carrier technologies are being designed to encapsulate toxic drugs in liposomes, which may reduce such side effects as febrile shivering.

Other shivering-related research has lagged behind. While effects of shivering on healthy subjects have been studied for several decades, few studies of shivering effects in hospital settings are found before the early 1960s. Studies of interventions in shivering are even more recent, with many appearing within the last decade. Many studies involve too few subjects to be conclusive, so further replication is warranted. Many investigations should be extended to include other patient groups or situations. The influence of skin-to-core gradients on shivering remains relatively unexplored in patients who are centrally cooled. Clinical studies are needed to further investigate the influence of environment on febrile shivering using carefully controlled humidity and room temperature. Extension of the previously cited studies using extremity wraps to protect dominant skin sensors needs to be done with different populations and differing age groups. Strategies for alleviating shivering in the burned patient warrant investigation. Also notably absent are published studies of subjective perceptions and emotional responses related to postoperative shivering, although most patients readily recall distress from this phenomenon. No published clinical studies were found on the use of relaxation techniques, hypnosis, or psychic imaging to alleviate shivering.

Research, by its very nature, builds on the progress of previous work from diverse sources. In the study of shivering, many clues to clinical application lie dormant in the literature of the basic sciences. Advances in neurophysiology, pharmacology, and biochemistry may offer new directions for ongoing, independent, and collaborative research in this area by medicine and nursing.

REFERENCES

1. Brown AC, Brengelmann G: Energy metabolism, in Ruch TC, Patton HD (eds): *Physiology and Biophysics*. Philadelphia, WB Saunders, 1965, pp 1030–1049.
2. Horvath SM, Spurr GB, Hutt BK, Hamilton IH: The metabolic cost of shivering. J Appl Physiol 8:595, 1956.
3. Sato H: Fusimotor modulation by spinal and skin temperature changes and its significance in cold shivering. Ex Neurol 72:21, 1981.
4. Ingram WR: Central autonomic mechanisms, in Field J, Magoun HW, Hall VE (eds): *Neurophysiology*. Washington, DC, American Physiological Society, 1960, p 966.
5. Sessler DI, Israel D, Pozos RS, Pozos M, Rubinstein EH: Spontaneous post-anesthetic tremor does not resemble thermoregulatory shivering. Anesthesiology 68(6):843, 1988.
6. Strom G: Central nervous regulation of body temperature, in Field J, Magoun HW, Hall VE (eds): *Neurophysiology*. Washington, DC, American Physiological Society, 1960, p 1186.
7. Hemingway A: Shivering. Physiol Rev 43:415, 1963.
8. Hickey MC: Hypothermia. Am J Nurs 65(1):116, 1963.
9. Abbey JC, Andrews C, Avigliano K, Blossom R, Bunke B, Clark E, Engberg N, Healy P, Halliburton P, Peterson J: A pilot study: The control of shivering during hypothermia by a clinical nursing measure. J Neurosurg Nurs 5(2):78, 1973.
10. Holtzclaw BJ: Postoperative shivering following cardiac surgery: A review. Heart Lung 15(3):292, 1986.
11. Stitt JT: Neurophysiology of fever. Fed Proc 40:2835, 1981.
12. Kluger MJ, Kauffman CA: Biologic mechanisms of fever, in Murray HW (ed): *FUO: Fever of Undetermined Origin*. Mt Kisco, NY, Futura, 1983, pp 9–23.
13. Dinarello CA, Conti P, Mier JW: Effects of human interleukin-1 on natural killer cell activity: Is fever a host defense mechanism for tumor killing? Yale J Biol Med 59:96, 1986.
14. Holtzclaw BJ, Geer RT: Shivering after heart surgery: Assessment of metabolic effects. Anesthesiology 65(3A):A18, 1986.
15. Gobel FL, Nordstrom LA, Nelson RR, Jorgenson CR, Wang Y: The rate-pressure product as an index of myocardial oxygen consumption during exercise in patients with angina pectoris. Circulation 57:549, 1978.
16. Cokkinos PV, Voridis EM: Constancy of pressure-rate product in pacing induced angina pectoris. Br Heart J 38:39, 1976.
17. Ross J: Cardiac energetics and myocardial oxygen consumption, in West JB (ed): *Best and Taylor's Physiological Basis of Medical Practice*, 11th ed. Baltimore, Williams & Wilkins, 1985, p 246.
18. Abbey JC, Anderson AS, Close EL, Hertwig EP, Scott J, Sears R, Willen RM, Packer AG: How long is that thermometer accurate? Am J Nurs 78(8):1375, 1978.
19. Pflug AE, Aasheim GM, Goster C, Martin R: Prevention of post anaesthesia shivering. Can Anaesth Soc J 25:43, 1978.
20. Vaughan MS, Vaughan, RW, Cork RC: Radiation versus conduction for postop rewarming of adults. Anesthesiology 53:S195, 1980.
21. Pauca AL, Savage RT, Simpson S, Roy RC: Effect of Pethidine, fentanyl and morphine on post-operative shivering in man. Acta Anaesthesiol Scand 28:138, 1984.
22. Rodriguez JL, Weissman C, Damask MC, Askanazi J, Hyman AI, Kinney JM: Physiologic requirements during rewarming: Suppression of the shivering response. Crit Care Med 11(7):490, 1983.
23. Palmes ED, Park CR: The regulation of body temperature during fever. Arch Environ Hlth 11:749, 1965.
24. Rutledge DN, Holtzclaw BJ: Amphotericin B-induced shivering in cancer patients: A nursing approach. Heart Lung 17(4):432, 1988.
25. Radford P, Thurlow AC: Metallized plastic sheeting in the prevention of hypothermia during neurosurgery. Br J Anaesth 51:237, 1979.
26. Abbey JC, Close L: A study of control of shivering during hypothermia. *Commun Nurs Res* 12:2, 1979.
27. Holtzclaw BJ: Effects of extremity wraps to control drug-induced shivering: A pilot study. Nurs Res 39(5):280, 1990.

187C/Wound Healing

NANCY A. STOTTS

Repair of wounds, an essential part of care for the critically ill, focuses on restoration of tissue integrity without loss of function or production of disfigurement. Generally, wound healing in critical care patients is associated with surgery or trauma; however, it is also an integral part of recovery after medical conditions associated with tissue damage (e.g., myocardial infarction).

Nurses play a pivotal role in facilitating wound healing in the critical care unit. They provide ongoing assessment, local treatment, and systemic support for healing and collaborate with physicians, dietitians, and other members of the health care team in planning and providing care. Nursing care and nurses' ability to work with others facilitates repair and mitigates wound-related complications in the critical care unit.

Nurses have contributed to the scientific basis for care. Various models of wound healing are used by nurse researchers in exploring the field,[1–4] and there is beginning debate as to the value of various models for wound healing. Although there have been a few basic research studies conducted by nurses in the area of wound healing,[1,3] most work reported by nurses has been clinical research.

In this section, studies that have applicability for critical care and represent nursing contribution to the field of wound healing will be reviewed. Work completed by nurses on assessment of wound status will be described as well as research that focuses on interventions to support wound healing.

One of the major issues in wound management is the assessment of wound healing. Objective, quantitative, standardized measures of healing are sought. Instrumentation to quantify healing has improved, and increasing numbers of studies evaluate wound healing with objective measures such as digitized photography[1] and histological photography.[3]

An area that has received increased attention is the development of instruments to assess wound healing at the bedside.[2,5,6] Various approaches have been used, and there is appreciation of the need for a consistent and systematic approach to evaluate wound status that, when used over time, will provide data on the trajectory of healing. Before an instrument for use in clinical care is adopted widely, there is a need to establish its validity and reliability under a variety of conditions and with the diverse populations seen in the critical care unit.

Open wounds, those healing by secondary intention, are especially difficult to assess in the clinical area. The instruments used to measure the status of these wounds often address only one dimension of healing (e.g., size or color). One such instrument that measures wound volume in open wounds is the Kundin Wound Gauge.[7] It has established validity and reliability but is limited in that it measures only volume.

An important issue is how to make the link between assessment of wound status in open wounds and selection of the most appropriate treatment for the wound. A paradigm that uses color as the criterion for planning treatment was established by nurses in the Dutch Wound Care Consultant Society.[8] This approach, the three-color concept, suggests that treatment for an open wound is based primarily on the color of the wound surface (i.e., if the wound is red, it is kept moist and protected; if yellow, kept clean; if black, debrided). This paradigm has been introduced in the United States, but validity and reliability data on it have not yet been reported.

Studies examining the effects of various dressings have been of major interest. A multicenter study was conducted to test the performance and effects of two occlusive hydrocolloid dressings on the healing of noninfected partial thickness wounds.[9] Subjects ($n = 66$) were randomly assigned to the experimental treatment (Restore, Hollister, Inc., Libertyville, IL) or the control treatment (DuoDerm, ConvaTec, Inc., Princeton, NJ) and treated for a period of 28 days or until the wound healed. The experimental treatment performed better than the control treatment in terms of wearing time, conformity, flexibility, and containment of drainage. The percentage of wounds that healed entirely or partially also was greater with the experimental than with the control group dressing. The authors do, however, caution against applying these findings in clinical practice because of the small sample size and the fact that the convenience sampling methodology used does not ensure representativeness of the sample.

A similar study examined the performance of the same two hydrocolloid dressings.[10] The researchers studied the dressings' absorbance, wear time, flexibility, conformity, adhesive properties, and durability and the rate of healing in 50 subjects randomly assigned to the experimental treatment (Restore) or the control treatment (DuoDerm) group. The experimental dressing was superior in all dimensions studied. Subjects in the two groups were not different in age, weight, or other demographic variables. Findings from these two studies show there is a difference in the performance and rate of healing using these two hydrocolloids, and clinical practice can be directed by findings from these studies.

The effect of topical agents in promoting wound repair has been the focus for study by nurse researchers. The effects of varying concentrations of epidermal growth factor on the rate of keratinocyte migration, mitosis, and rate of differentiation of keratinocytes over the wound was studied in an animal model.[3] The rate at which the wound was reepithelialized was increased, and the cells covering the wound formed a triple rather than a single layer, indicating a positive preliminary effect on wound healing.

Moist dressings (sometimes called damp-to-damp or moist-to-moist or wet-to-dry) are a mainstay in the treatment of open wounds, and their effectiveness is the gold standard against which new products are evaluated. The effect of the temperature of moist dressings on the rate of healing of rabbit wounds has been examined.[4] Specifically, the effects of moist dressings of 39 to 40°C were compared with moist dressings applied at 26 to 28°C. There was no difference between the two treatments, an effect explained by the rapid rate at which the warmer dressings cooled and the cooler dressings warmed when in contact with the animal tissue.

Studies also have examined the effects of various dressing change techniques. The irritation and stripping effects of two adhesive tapes (Micropore and Transpore) on the superficial layers surrounding the midsternotomy incisions in postoperative coronary artery bypass patients were examined.[11] The study was undertaken because dressing changes with tape occur frequently in the surgical critical care patient and there is a high risk of denuding skin and thereby disrupting the patient's first line of defense against infection. The use of critically ill patients in the study is noteworthy because they are a vulnerable population with high potential for detrimental effects with any impingement upon their defenses. The investigators found that both tape types were safe, with the Micropore tape causing less irritation and stripping than the Transpore tape. Both tapes, however, increased skin stripping by postoperative day 3 as a result of daily dressing changes.

The safety of using clean gloves to provide wound care is a frequently asked question by today's hospital administrators with their emphasis on risk management and cost containment. A study of 13 critically ill burned patients assessed whether the risk of infection was increased when clean rather than sterile gloves were used on all noninvasive procedures including dressing change.[12] The difference in cost of sterile and clean gloves also was examined. Each patient had an individual box of clean gloves placed at the bedside and replaced weekly. Air analysis and contact culture found all boxes holding the clean unused gloves were contaminated; *Saccharomyces aureus* was the most frequently occurring organism. Of the 13 subjects, 11 had antibiotic-resistant strains of organisms present in the boxes, and 7 of these appeared after the strain was cultured in the corresponding patient. When nonsterile gloves were used for all procedures, an approximate 40% annual cost savings resulted in the burn unit. These data suggest that nonsterile gloves can be used safely in the care of the critically ill, but because they become contaminated with an individual patient's flora, use of a single box of gloves by more than one patient could result in cross transfer of organisms. In addition, considerable cost saving could be realized if clean gloves were used for all noninvasive procedures in the care of the critically ill, including dressing change.

Nurses frequently are responsible for changing dressings of patients, a procedure that is often considered stressful and painful. Based on knowledge that excessive stress is correlated with impaired healing, the use of relaxation and guided imagery were examined as interventions to reduce stress in surgical patients with cholecystectomy incisions healing by primary intention.[5] Spielberger's state anxiety scale and cortisol levels were used to measure stress. The tissue response to stress at the incision line was measured with a wound assessment inventory. State anxiety was less in the experimental group, while cortisol level and inflammatory response did not differ between groups until day 3 when the subscale on the wound assessment inventory showed less erythema at the incision line. These data suggest that the subjective experience of stress was less when imagery and relaxation were used. Lack of data in the field as to the usual or appropriate amount of inflammation at a surgical incision line suggests further work in the area must be performed before the data on the inflammatory response with this intervention can be used meaningfully in the clinical area to modify healing.

The effect of the stressor intermittent noise on the rate of wound healing was examined in albino rats.[1] Using a two-group experimental design, the experimental group of rats was exposed to noise (2 to 16 kHz for 15 min/h for 19.5 days); the control group was not exposed to noise. Rate of healing was measured with digitalized photographs taken every other day. Repeated-measure analysis of variance showed the experimental group had slower healing. Although it is premature to draw implications for practice from these data, the study does provide a model to use in exploring the effects of noise on healing in patients who are exposed to constant noise levels, such as those experienced by critical care patients. It also provides the basis for clinical studies in this area.

The effects of music on adult postoperative abdominal surgery patients' pain during wound packing also has been explored.[13] Using a crossover design, subjects were randomly assigned to the music or nonmusic control group. Pain was measured using the McGill Pain Questionnaire and the Pain Ladder, a nine-point vertical visual analogue scale. The group who received the music had statistically significant lower pain scores on both scales. There was no difference in the amount of analgesia received by the groups or in the effects of the music on pain when scheduled versus emergency surgery was considered.

Transcutaneous electrical stimulation (TENS), another therapy to reduce pain during the dressing change procedure, has been explored with incisional pain caused by cleaning and packing abdominal surgical wounds.[14] Subjects ($n = 75$) were randomly assigned to one of three groups: TENS, placebo-TENS, or no treatment. The treatment was administered during the routine dressing change 2 days after surgery. Pain was significantly less for the TENS treatment than for the other two groups. Drug administration did not contribute to the level of pain reported. Appreciation of the theoretical link of pain with increased catecholamine levels and decreased perfusion lays the foundation for study of the impact of this therapy on wound healing in the critical care population.

Seminal work has been completed that focuses on wound assessment and local wound care. Further attention is needed to address the effects of specific therapies in critical care on dimensions of wound healing. An area that has not been addressed but is important clinically is the effect of the patient's psychological status on healing (e.g., depression, hopelessness). Also, the effect of the manipulation of internal environment (e.g., nutritional status, perfusion, oxygenation) on wound healing is an area with great potential for nurses interested in wound healing in critical care. Future nursing research in wound healing in the critically ill must be approached zealously to establish a comprehensive scientific basis for practice.

REFERENCES

1. Wysocki AB: The effect of intermittent noise exposure on the rate of wound healing in albino rats. Unpublished dissertation. University of Texas at Austin, Austin, TX, 1986.
2. Cooper DM: Development and testing of an instrument to assess the visual characteristics of open, soft tissue wounds. Unpublished PhD dissertation. University of Pennsylvania, Philadelphia, PA, 1990.
3. Gill, BP, Atwood JR: Reciprocy and helicy used to relate mEFG and wound healing. Nurs Res 30:68, 1971.
4. Quinn AD: The effect of the temperature of a wet dressing on the rate of wound healing in rabbits. Unpublished master's thesis. University of California, San Francisco, CA, 1981.
5. Holden-Lund C: Effects of relaxation with guided imagery on surgical stress and wound healing. Res Nurs Hlth 11:235,1988.
6. Stotts N, Cooper D: Development of an instrument to assess wound status. Calif Nurs 80(7):10, 1984.
7. Kundin JI: A new way to size up a wound. Am J Nurs 89(2):206, 1989.
8. Willemsteijn B: Postoperative complications: Wound care. Second International Intensive Care Nursing Conference, Hague, Netherlands, 1986.
9. Myers RB, Moore K, Mulder GD, Pike RA, Kissil MT: Report of a multicenter clinical trial on the performance of two occlusive hydrocolloid dressings in the treatment of noninfected, partial-thickness wounds. JET 15(4):158, 1988.
10. Watts C, Shipes E: A study to compare the overall performance of two hydrocolloid dressings on partial thickness wounds. Ostomy/Wound Manag 21:28, 1988.
11. Weber BB, Speer M, Swartz D, Rupp S, O'Linn W, Stone KS:

Irritation and stripping effects of adhesive tape on skin layers of coronary artery bypass graft patients. Heart Lung 16(5):567, 1987.
12. Sadowski DA, Pohlman S, Maley MP, Warden GD: Use of non-sterile gloves for routine noninvasive procedures in thermally injured patients. JBCR 9(6):613, 1988.
13. Angus JE, Faux S: The effect of music on adult postoperative patients' pain during a nursing procedure, in SG Funk, EM Tournquist, MT Champagne, LA Copp, RA Wiese (eds): *Key Aspects of Recovery: Management of Pain, Fatigue, and Nausea*. New York, Springer Publishing Company, 1989, pp 166–172.
14. Hargreaves A, Lander J: Use of transcutaneous electrical nerve stimulation for postoperative pain. Nurs Res 38(3):159, 1989.

187 D/Dyspnea

VIRGINIA KOHLMAN-CARRIERI

Dyspnea, or breathlessness, is one of the most common symptoms of pulmonary disease, heart disease, and neuromuscular disorders affecting the respiratory muscles. This subjective sensation of labored, uncomfortable breathing is a sensory experience that is perceived, interpreted, and rated only by the patient himself.[1] Although the exact incidence and prevalence of dyspnea in critically ill patients is not known, it can be hypothesized to be great in the clinical states prevalent in critical care.

Dyspnea is most likely to occur in conditions that increase patients' awareness of respiratory muscle effort, heighten their awareness of increased respiratory drive, or increase the perception that breathing is uncomfortable in the absence of physiologic dysfunction.[2] Respiratory effort is the specific sensation most closely related to dyspnea.[3]

Research and subsequent knowledge related to the measurement, correlates, or management of dyspnea in the critically ill patient are meager and scattered. Measures, such as lung volumes, oxygen tension or saturation, respiratory muscle strength, and estimates of the work of breathing are significant reflections of pulmonary function; however, they do not measure dyspnea.[4–6] Recently, "patient comfort" has been measured in retrospective interviews following the testing of different modes of ventilation.[7] This outcome criterion may be related to dyspnea; however, the exact relationship of this sensation to breathlessness is unknown.

Nurse researchers have focused primarily on the beginning steps in the analysis of the concept of dyspnea. A conceptual model derived from a review of literature and clinical experience has been suggested to direct further study of the symptom. Nurse researchers have tested a variety of instruments to measure the sensation of dyspnea. Within descriptive or correlational studies, visual analog scales (VASs), the modified Borg scale, magnitude estimation, and qualitative interviews have been administered to subjects to capture several dimensions of the symptom. One investigator found that the vertically oriented VAS is more sensitive, produces higher scores, and is easier for subjects to use.[8] Another found a strong and significant correlation between the VAS and the modified Borg scale in ventilator-assisted patients.[9] A significant correlation has also been found between the American Thoracic Society (ATS) Grade of Breathlessness Scale and a VAS.[10] Recently magnitude estimation was reported to be a reliable measure of one dimension of dyspnea.[11] Beginning small correlational studies have provided some insight into the relationship of significant variables to the symptom of dyspnea. At the present time studies of therapies to modulate the symptom have not been conducted with critically ill patients.

A theoretical model for guiding the study of the phenomenon of dyspnea describes the symptom as being modulated by the patient's coping and self-care strategies and appropriate nursing and medical therapies.[12] Antecedents, or those factors that may affect the symptom, are categorized into personal, health status, and situational. Like pain, the sensation of breathlessness is thought to have both sensory and affective dimensions. Both normal subjects and patients with lung disease are capable of distinguishing between the magnitude of an intrinsic or external load placed on their breathing (sensory) and a level of discomfort created by that load (affective). This detection threshold has been shown to be influenced by emotional and environmental factors. As depicted in the model for nursing research, it has also been suggested that the tolerance for dyspnea, or the distress level, is affected by situational and contextual determinants, individual behavior, and personality characteristics.[13] No two individuals will react to breathlessness in the same way.

Although it is the impression of clinicians that critically ill patients at one time or another experience dyspnea, until very recently this empirical observation had not been tested. Because dyspnea is not usually measured in the intensive care unit (ICU), the frequency and intensity of the symptom is not documented, making it difficult to retrieve information related to the symptom. The fact that critically ill patients do experience dyspnea is supported by recent descriptive studies with small samples in which patients were asked to recall sensations felt during acute episodes of respiratory distress or to rate the intensity of the symptom while on a ventilator.

Four primary causes of weaning failure were identified by the patients: inadequate understanding of the weaning process, lack of confidence in their breathing pattern, and environmental and staff factors.[14] Mechanically controlled breaths and frequent interruptions by caregivers during the weaning process prevented patients from controlling their own breathing patterns and produced associated sensations of increased effort and dyspnea. Patients stated they were unable to use strategies they had developed to cope with chronic usual dyspnea. Close confinement in the intensive care environment precipitated feelings of claustrophobia, worsening the intensity of dyspnea. Lack of confidence in breathing ability often was associated with feelings of nervousness, anxiety, and fear, all emotions that have been shown to be related to increasing shortness of breath.

In another study designed to identify negative experiences related to mechanical ventilation,[15] patients reported 11 different negative experiences. Although shortness of breath was not an exact sensation by patients, the sensations of "it gagged me" and "I felt like my chest was going to burst" were the feelings described with suctioning, positive pressure ventilation, and extubation. These are sensations that can be presumed to be related to the sensation of uncomfortable breathing.

In a recent qualitative study, 96 subjects with chronic obstructive pulmonary disease (COPD) were asked to recall their feelings associated with the sensation of shortness of breath during hospitalization and to comment about the actions of nurses while they were short of breath.[16] The described feelings were categorized into themes of fear, helplessness, vitality, preoccupation, and legitimacy. According to these subjects, fear triggered by dyspnea contributed to the problem by making breathing more difficult. Shortness of breath precipitated fear and the mechanism seemed cyclic to most subjects; the more excited and frightened the subjects became, the more they became short of breath. Subjects described breathing as demanding effort and concentration. They were consumed by breathing, having a morbid drive to continue to breathe no matter what the circumstance.

Other nurse investigators have studied the relationship between dyspnea and physiologic or psychologic correlates. Five ventilator-assisted patients all experienced dyspnea in a descriptive study of the factors occurring before, during, and after dyspneic episodes in the ICU.[9] These patients with restrictive or obstructive pulmonary disease rated the intensity of their dyspnea on both a VAS of 0 to 100 mm and a modified Borg scale at 4-h intervals, concomitant with complaints of dyspnea. Concurrent physiologic and environmental variables were recorded by nurses 30 min before dyspnea was rated by the patient and following the actual measurement. There was a strong significant relationship ($r = 0.79$ to $r = 0.98$) between the two instruments, suggesting that both the VAS and the Borg scale are valid and reliable and can be used to measure dyspnea in the ventilated patient. A moderate, positive significant correlation was found between the number of environmental events and severity of dyspnea in these patients. Acute episodes of dyspnea tended to coincide with an increase in treatments, environmental events, and nursing activities. It is unknown whether the dyspnea triggered the increase in activities and events or, in fact, was a result of these variables. Minimal correlation was found between the physiologic variables and dyspnea; for example, arterial partial pressure of oxygen ($P_{A_{O_2}}$) did not correlate significantly with dyspnea. In one patient, static inspiratory pressure (SIP) correlated significantly with dyspnea intensity. SIP might be expected to be related to shortness of breath if the current proposed physiologic mechanisms for dyspnea are valid.[17] An additional finding of this study was that nurses' estimations of patient dyspnea were not necessarily corroborated by patients' ratings of dyspnea intensity. This discrepancy between the rating of a sensation by health professionals and patients has been shown with pain in acutely ill patients and suggests that it is important for clinicians to measure the patient's perception of dyspnea rather than relying on their own observations of respiratory distress or related physiologic and environmental parameters.

A study of clinical signs and emotional states during high, medium, and low dyspnea revealed that subjects used their accessory muscles of respiration significantly more during times of high dyspnea than during low dyspnea.[8] Anxiety was significantly higher during high or medium dyspnea when compared with low. Although respiratory rate and depth did increase from low to high dyspnea, these commonly used parameters were not significantly different during varying levels of dyspnea. Interestingly, airway obstruction as measured by peak expiratory flow rates (PEFRs) was not significantly different among dyspnea levels. This study confirmed previous findings that anxiety is related to dyspnea and suggested that accessory muscle use is one nursing observation that may indicate increasing dyspnea.

In a study of adult asthmatics, measurements were made during the initial visit to the emergency room when the patients were experiencing severe dyspnea and just prior to discharge during low dyspnea.[18] During times of high dyspnea, PEFRs and oxygen saturation were significantly lower, while heart rate, anxiety, depression, somatization, hostility, and feelings of panic, congestion, and fatigue were significantly higher than during times of low dyspnea. Subjects sighed, used accessory muscles, and wheezed more during times of high dyspnea when compared to low. There were no differences in respiratory rate, cough, irritability, worry, anger, or loneliness between times of high dyspnea when compared to low. This study contributed to the identification of correlates of dyspnea in the asthmatic patient that could be used to identify the patient who is short of breath and is unable to verbalize this sensation.

Within an interdisciplinary study, one nurse researcher studied the relationship between dyspnea and the pressure-time index (PTI) and an index of mechanical efficiency, the respiratory system gain (RSG).[19] The PTI is determined by dividing the average inspiratory esophageal pressure during a trial of spontaneous breathing by the maximum inspiratory pressure and multiplying this number by the inspiratory fraction of total cycle time. The RSG is the minute ventilation divided by the PTI. These investigators concluded that the PTI and the efficiency of converting pressure to air movement may be important determinants of dyspnea in the critically ill ventilated patient. These physiologic measures may be important correlates of dyspnea in the critically ill ventilated patient.

The relationship between dyspnea and specific nursing activities was studied with five mechanically ventilated patients.[20] These patients also had dyspnea with the intensity of the sensation on a 100 mm VAS ranging from 7 to 96; the group mean was 43. There were no significant changes in dyspnea associated with the activities of bathing, weighing, or repositioning. There was a significant decrease in dyspnea from pre- to post-ETS. No significant relationships were found between usual measures of cardiopulmonary function, such as respiratory rate, peak inspiratory pressure, or heart rate, and dyspnea. Although it has been suggested that abdominal paradox may be used as a sign of muscle fatigue and presumably dyspnea, this observation was not significantly related to dyspnea in these patients.

A study of the relationship between recruitment of specific respiratory muscles and the sensation of dyspnea revealed that recruitment of the diaphragm decreased during resistance breathing and increasing dyspnea; however, the EMG of the sternomastoid muscle increased.[21] Rib cage and accessory muscle recruitment was the predominant pattern of breathing related to dyspnea during the inspiratory resistance breathing. Asynchronous breathing, ranging from some lag between the rib cage and abdominal movement to complete paradoxical breathing, was significantly related to dyspnea. These findings suggest that dyspnea may be related to the recruitment of the accessory muscles rather than the recruitment of the diaphragm and that, in COPD patients, a shift in the work of breathing from rib cage and accessory muscles to the diaphragm, such as may happen in diaphragmatic breathing, may result in the reduction in dyspnea. In addition, asynchronous breathing may be an important correlate of dyspnea in the critically ill patient.

Future nursing research related to the symptom of dyspnea depends on the measurement of that sensation in the critically ill patient. Major emphasis must be placed on teaching nurses how to measure the symptom and on routine assessment with all patients who are alert and able to rate their dyspnea, even if this rating is a number on a scale of 0 to 10. Objective measurements of dyspnea should be included in initial nursing assessments as baseline data and in the progress notes of flow sheets in critical care units. This documentation would provide an opportunity for the surveillance of the pattern of dyspnea over time and the use of dyspnea as an outcome measure for the testing of alternative therapies. At this time, the lack of documentation of this symptom limits investigation of this important sensation in the critically ill patient.

Different instruments require testing with critically ill patients who may not be alert or oriented and may be viewing scales from different positions. Future research should explore the relationship between dyspnea and physiologic measurements that are obtainable by the nurse at the bedside in differing types of diseases. Clinical indicators of increased work of breathing, such as facial signs of distress, vital signs, breathing pattern, and paradoxical breathing, need to be related to the frequency of dyspnea.[22] In addition, there may be specific physiologic measures that correlate with dyspnea in a certain group of patients or disease group and not in others.

It is important to test theoretically proposed therapies to modulate dyspnea as nursing research related to this phenomenon progresses toward controlled clinical trials. Therapies such as pursed lip breathing, diaphragmatic breathing, relaxation, imagery, fans to the face, and "bagging" are just a few of the many strategies that may modulate the sensation of dyspnea in the critically ill patient.

REFERENCES

1. Widimsky J: Dyspnea. Cor VASA 21:128, 1979.
2. Stulbarg M: Treatment of dyspnea: A physiological approach, in *Clinical Challenge in Cardiopulmonary Medicine: A Continuing Education Series from the American College of Chest Physicians*, vol 7. American College of Chest Physicians, Park Ridge, IL, 1986, pp 1–6.
3. Fishbein D, Kearon C, Killian KJ: An approach to dyspnea in cancer patients. J Pain Symptom Manage 4:76, 1989.
4. Fiastro JF, Habib M, Shon B, Campbell S: Comparison of standard weaning parameters and the mechanical work of breathing in mechanically ventilated patients. Chest 94:232, 1988.
5. Marini J, Rodriguez M, Lamb V: Bedside estimation of the inspiratory work of breathing during mechanical ventilation. Chest 89:56, 1986.
6. Marini J, Capps J, Culver B: The inspiratory work of breathing in mechanical ventilation. Chest 87:612, 1985.
7. McIntyre NR: Respiratory function during pressure support ventilation. Chest 89:677, 1986.
8. Gift AG, Plaut SM, Jacox A: Psychologic and physiologic factors related to dyspnea in subjects with chronic obstructive pulmonary disease. Heart Lung 15:595, 1986.
9. Lush MT, Janson-Bjerklie S, Carrieri VK, Lovejoy N: Dyspnea in the ventilator-assisted patient. Heart Lung 17:528, 1988.
10. Janson-Bjerklie S, Carrieri VK, Hudes M: The sensation of pulmonary dyspnea. Nurs Res 35:154, 1986.
11. Nield MA, Kim MJ: The reliability of magnitude estimation for dyspnea measurement. AARD 139:A243, 1990.
12. Carrieri VK, Janson-Bjerklie S, Jacobs S: The sensation of dyspnea: A review. Heart Lung 13:436, 1984.
13. Cherniack NS, Altose MD: Mechanisms of dyspnea. Clin Chest Med 8:207, 1987.
14. Knebel AR: Patient perceptions of the weaning experience following prolonged mechanical ventilation. ARRD 139:A97, 1989.
15. Gries ML, Fernsler J: Patient perceptions of the mechanical ventilation experience. Focus Crit Care 15:52, 1988.
16. DeVito AJ: Dyspnea during acute hospitalizations for acute phase of illness as recalled by patients with COPD. Heart Lung 19:186, 1990.
17. Wasserman K, Casaburi R: Dyspnea: Physiological and pathophysiological mechanisms. Ann Rev Med 29:503, 1988.
18. Gift AG, Cahill CA: Psychophysiologic aspects of dyspnea in chronic obstructive pulmonary disease: A pilot study. Heart Lung 19:252, 1990.
19. Truwitt JD, Lamb VJ, Knebel AR, Marini JJ: Pressure-time index and mechanical efficiency correlate with dyspnea during ventilatory stress. ARRD 139:A321, 1989.
20. Ruma S: Dyspnea in the mechanically-ventilated patient. Master's Thesis. University of California, San Francisco, 1986.
21. Breslin E, Garoutte BC, Carrieri VK, Celli BR: Correlations between dyspnea, diaphragm, and sternomastoid recruitment during inspiratory resistance breathing in normal subjects. Chest 98:298, 1990.
22. Pardee N, Winterbauer R, Allen J: Bedside evaluation of respiratory distress. Chest 85:203, 1984.

187E/Pain

KATHLEEN A. PUNTILLO

Pain in critically ill patients arises from underlying disease or from the many invasive procedures conducted in this environment. Pain has sensory-discriminative, motivational-affective, and cognitive dimensions. The magnitude of the pain as well as its spatial and temporal characteristics encompass the sensory-discriminative dimensions of pain. Motivational-affective dimensions include the unpleasant emotions and aversive drives associated with pain perception. Aversive drives, in turn, initiate motor responses that are evidenced physiologically and behaviorally. Finally, cognitive processes, such as evaluation and meaning derivation, can influence and control the sensory-discriminative and motivational-affective dimensions of pain. Attention to all of these dimensions reveals more information about the full extent of an individual's pain.

Nursing research clearly implicates pain as a leading cause of critical care patient stress with potentially negative consequences.[1–3] Despite this, medical and nursing research effort in this area is somewhat limited. A number of possible reasons exist for this dearth of research: the difficulties of controlling confounding variables in this complex patient population; problems assessing pain in patients with communication barriers; or troubles isolating physiologic measures such as autonomic nervous system (ANS) response as valid indicators of pain versus another phenomenon such as stress.

Nevertheless, research on pain in the critically ill is of vital importance to health professionals and patients. The following is a presentation of the "state of the science" on nursing pain research in critically ill adults, including identification of areas that merit further study in the future.

PATIENT REPORTS OF PAIN DURING CRITICAL ILLNESS

To define the prevalence, severity, and etiology of pain, a study was undertaken in 24 ICU patients.[4] Patient interviews were conducted an average of 3 days after these patients had been transferred from the ICU. Almost two-thirds recalled their ICU pain intensity to be moderate to severe, and there were many sources of pain in this predominantly surgical population besides incisions. Intubated patients described difficulties in communicating pain and noted nonverbal behaviors (moving legs and feet up and down, grabbing at nurses) that were necessary to capture staff attention. Most recalled receiving analgesics for pain even when doses used were minimal. Few of these patients recalled the use of nonpharmacologic interventions for pain.

The various dimensions of the postoperative pain of coronary artery bypass graft (CABG) patients have also been studied.[5] Using the McGill Pain Questionnaire (MPQ), the investigator interviewed 44 patients on two different occasions: 3 to 6 days after surgery (time A) and 17 to 20 days after surgery (time B). Since all patients had been transferred from the ICU by time A, their early critical care pain was not emphasized. However, in addition to their descriptions about present pain, these patients volunteered information about their ICU stays. For example, many patients recalled chest tube removal pain as the most excruciating pain they had ever experienced, a finding that has been reported by others.[6] These patients described such other ICU experiences as loss of control, ventilator dependence, and the feeling of chest crunching with inspiration as "terrifying." Interestingly, the majority of those identifying the whole front chest as the source of their most intense pain had undergone internal mammary artery (IMA) grafting, a procedure previously noted for its pain intensity.[7]

Patient and staff interviews confirm that critically injured burn victims suffer pain that is intense, prolonged, and extremely challenging to endure and manage.[8] Patients chronicled how they learned about their pain's probable trajectory; the acceptable methods of expressing and controlling it; and how they relied on other patients as major support systems. Nurses devised ways to cope with the patient pain they often inflicted. It was observed that nurses assessed patient pain to be less intense than did patients themselves. Additionally, more experienced nurses used less pain medication than did those with less experience.

THE PAIN OF PATIENTS WITH MYOCARDIAL INFARCTION

A number of studies have focused on pain in myocardial infarction (MI). Patients with larger infarcts have reported more intense pain and consumed more analgesics while in the CCU than those with smaller infarcts.[9] In a group of Mexican males, the most significant predictor of pain intensity was the extent to which these men used nonverbal behaviors indicative of pain, such as restlessness, facial grimacing, and vocalizations. Physiologic measures, such as heart rate and systolic blood pressure, were not good predictors of intensity.[10] Patients in a CCU do not always report their pain to the staff. Seventy-four percent of patients in one study[11] admitted to having unreported pain while in a CCU. The most frequent reason given for not reporting pain was that the pain was not considered to be severe enough to warrant reporting. All but one patient remembered being told to report pain, but miscommunication about the importance of reporting pain still exists.

The efficacy of nursing assessments and interventions for relief of cardiac chest pain has also been investigated.[12] Surprisingly, 56 percent of the time, interventions observed did not result in pain relief, even when narcotics were administered. This high percentage of pain relief failure in patients with underlying myocardial insufficiency is disturbing indeed.

NONPHARMACOLOGIC INTERVENTIONS FOR CRITICAL CARE PAIN RELAXATION TECHNIQUES FOR CARDIAC SURGICAL PAIN

Progressive relaxation was taught preoperatively, and daily visits were made to one group of CABG and cardiac valve replacement patients; only daily visits were made to a second group; and only consent was obtained from a third group.[13] For nine postoperative days, including the patients' first days in the cardiac recovery unit, pain was measured by patient self-reports on a vertical VAS and indirectly by the number of pain medications administered. However, there were no statistically significant decreases in pain reports or the use of pain medications in the group using relaxation postoperatively.

Researchers designing similar critical care studies would benefit from knowing how to promote and verify use of the relaxation exercises during the immediate postoperative period. It would also be helpful to know the success of these patients in completing a VAS that, in noncritical care populations, has a failure rate of 7 to 11 percent.[14]

Two relaxation interventions were also used to decrease pain and its ANS responses caused by ambulation in post-CABG patients in a cardiac stepdown unit.[15] Only one technique, systemic relaxation, decreased the distress associated with the pain of ambulation, while neither relaxation intervention decreased diastolic blood pressure or pulse. While systolic blood pressure or respiratory rate did decrease significantly in at least one of the relaxation groups, this finding could not be attributed to pain reduction alone.

MUSIC THERAPY FOR ICU PATIENTS

Music therapy offered to 22 ICU patients has had a positive influence on pain reduction.[16] Specifically, pain scores measured on a VAS of 0 to 5 significantly decreased after 20 min of patient- or family-selected music. Patient diagnoses and pain etiologies—information that could provide guidance for further research and clinical practice—were not reported. However, since the use of music requires little patient or staff time or energy, particularly when compared with a relaxation intervention, its application to pain relief in critically ill patients is promising.

ANALGESICS AND CRITICAL CARE PAIN RELIEF

Analgesic administration has often been used as a measure (albeit indirect) of pain relief in critical care patients. In nursing research, analgesic administration has been used as an outcome measure of pain reduction due to use of relaxation techniques with CABG patients.[13] However, analgesic use did not differ among the experimental and control groups.

Analgesic prescription and administration practices as indicators of pain relief were reviewed through retrospective chart audits of 100 cardiac surgery adults and children (50 per group).[17] This review indicated that children were prescribed significantly less potent narcotics than adults during the first three postoperative days. In fact, 6 of the 50 children had no postoperative analgesics prescribed. During the first five postoperative days, children received less than 30 percent of all administered analgesics while adults received over 70 percent. Furthermore, by the fifth postoperative day, almost all analgesics were discontinued for children. These documented discrepancies in analgesic practices for adults and children deserve further nursing and medical attention, especially in light of current knowledge concerning pain perception in infants and children.

Analgesics are by far the primary methods of pain relief in critically ill patients. Therefore, it is surprising to note the almost complete absence of nursing research evaluating the effectiveness of various types and modes of analgesics used alone or in conjunction with nonpharmacologic interventions. Recently, however, the effectiveness of nurse-administered versus patient-controlled analgesia (PCA) during tubbing procedures in burn patients was compared.[18] These two methods of morphine analgesia administration were alternated during tubbing procedures for 2 days in 15 acutely injured burn patients.

PCA did not result in less intense pain for these patients; nor did the amount of administered analgesics differ between the two methods. In fact, some patients reported they did not want to be concerned with administering their own medications and preferred nurse administration. Apparently, self-control over this specific part of their care was not of particular concern to them.

Certainly, no conclusive results can be drawn from only one study of PCA in critical care. Yet, while PCA has achieved tremendous recent popularity, it is clearly not superior or desirable in all situations of critical care pain relief, as evidenced from the PCA study. However, considering the loss of control frequently inherent in an ICU environment, future research may document the benefits of PCA use in selected patient populations.

IMPLICATIONS FOR FUTURE RESEARCH

The number of studies addressing pain in critically ill patients is small, and the majority have been conducted within the past 3 years. Clearly, pain in critical care patients is a phenomenon of concern for nursing, and research is in its infancy. We have seen that nurse researchers have explored patient perceptions and descriptions of their pain and its intensity. Although nurses have been successful in measuring the intensity of pain, comprehensive assessment of the multiple dimensions of pain is rare. Knowledge gained about nurse assessment and treatment practices may provide a framework for future pain intervention studies. Yet, while nurse researchers have been interested in the effects of nonpharmacologic interventions, only one analgesia study has been reported. Thus far, neither relaxation interventions nor PCA have proved more effective than traditional pain relief practices. However, the success of music in lowering ICU patient pain level warrants its increased use as a pain-relieving modality.

Certainly, nurses have chosen to study patients with cardiac disease or surgery more than any other critical care group. Assessment and management practices for pain in critically ill trauma and intubated patients have, thus far, been neglected. Pain characteristics, trajectories, and management techniques in these patients need exploration.

Opioid tolerance that sometimes develops in long-term severely ill patients necessitates the use of alternative pharmacologic modalities. However, the efficacy of many newer drugs has not yet been determined through clinical research in critically ill patients. Nurses adept at assessment and knowledgeable about analgesic pharmacology can collaborate with their medical colleagues to make valuable contributions to these types of analgesia studies. These researchers might also document the value of PCA or epidural analgesia in influencing the affective as well as the sensory dimensions of patient's pain. Finally, nurses can propose methods to more effectively control ICU procedural pain, such as that experienced during chest tube removal, extensive dressing changes, or burn wound care. In fact, the critical care arena is a fertile field for nursing research of pain in these patients.

REFERENCES

1. Nastasy EL: Identifying environmental stressors for cardiac surgery patients in a surgical intensive care unit. Heart Lung 14:302, 1985.
2. Bouckoms AJ: Pain relief in the intensive care unit. J Int Care Med 3:32, 1988.
3. O'Gara PT: The hemodynamic consequences of pain and its management. J Int Care Med 3:3, 1988.
4. Puntillo KA: The pain experiences of intensive care unit patients. Heart Lung 19:526, 1990.
5. Heye ML: Patient pain perceptions and coping strategies used in early convalescence from coronary bypass surgery. PhD Dissertation. The University of Texas at Austin, 1989.
6. Paiement B, Boulanger M, Jones CW, Roy M: Intubation and other experiences in cardiac surgery: The consumer's views. Can Anaesth Soc J 26:173, 1979.
7. Jansen KJ, McFadden PM: Postoperative nursing management in patients undergoing myocardial revascularization with the internal mammary artery bypass. Heart Lung 15:48, 1986.
8. Fagerhaugh SH: Pain expression and control on a burn care unit. Nurs Outlook 22:645, 1974.
9. Hofgren K, Bondestam E, Gaston Joahansson F, Jern S, Herlitz J, Holmberg S: Initial pain course and delay to hospital admission in relation to myocardial infarct size. Heart Lung 17:274, 1988.
10. Douglas MK: Physiologic and behavioral responses to acute myocardial ischemic pain in Mexican male patients. DNSc Dissertation. University of California, San Francisco, 1989.
11. Schneider AC: Unreported chest pain in a coronary care unit. Focus Crit Care 14:21, 1987.
12. Bourbonnais FE, MacKay RC: The influence of nursing interventions on chest pain. Nurs Pap 13:38, 198.
13. Bafford DC: Progressive relaxation as a nursing intervention: A method of controlling pain of open-heart surgery patients, in Batey M (ed): *Communicating Nursing Research, Vol. 8, Nursing Research Priorities: Choice or Chance*. Boulder, CO, Western Interstate Commission for Higher Education, 1977, p 284.
14. Scott J, Huskisson EC: Vertical or horizontal visual analogue scales. Ann Rheum Dis 38:560, 1979.
15. Horowitz BF, Fitzpatrick JJ, Flaherty GG: Relaxation techniques for pain relief after open heart surgery. Dim Crit Care Nurs 3:364, 1984.
16. Stone S, Rusk F, Chambers A, Chafin S: The effects of music therapy on critically ill patients in the intensive care setting. Proceedings of the 16th Annual National Teaching Institute of the American Association of Critical-Care Nurses, Atlanta, GA, May 15–18, 1989, p 624, Am Assoc of Critical-Care Nurses, Newport Beach, CA, 1989.
17. Beyer JE, DeGood DE, Ashley LC, Russell GA: Patterns of postoperative analgesic use with adults and children following cardiac surgery. Pain 17:71, 1983.
18. Moyer MA: The use of patient-controlled analgesia for burn pain, in Funk S, Torquist E, Champagne M, Copp L, Wiese R (eds): *Key Aspects of Comfort*. New York, Springer, 1989, p 135.

187F/Pressure Ulcers

NANCY BERGSTROM

Pressure ulcers, defined as localized areas of tissue necrosis over bony prominences, are a costly, life-threatening problem that has been recognized by the Joint Commission for the Accreditation of Healthcare Organizations[1] as one of 13 indicators of quality of care. Other federal, state, and corporate bodies recognize the seriousness of the problem, and legislation and public policy are focusing on the problem. It is important to note that pressure ulcers remain one of the leading causes of death among patients with spinal cord injuries. Furthermore, pressure sores contribute to the increasing cost of health care with one 1984 estimate of the cost of healing a Stage IV ulcer placed at $30,000 to $40,000.[2] The cost is even higher for para- and quadriplegics who, once a sore develops, may be limited in future rehabilitation and employment options.

INCIDENCE, PREVALENCE, AND DESCRIPTION OF PRESSURE ULCERS

The incidence (number of new cases appearing during a specified period) of pressure ulcers reported among medical-surgical patients in hospital settings ranges from 2.7 percent[3] to 9 percent.[4] The prevalence (cross-sectional count of the number of cases at a specific point in time) ranges from 4 percent[5] to 14 percent.[6] The incidence is even higher among patients with spinal cord injuries (60 percent)[7] and fractured hips (82 percent).[8] One prospective study of 60 medical intensive care patients found that 40 percent developed pressure ulcers within 2 weeks of admission to the medical ICU, but only one of these became a deep ulcer (Stage IV).[9] The higher incidence of pressure ulcers in this study may be due to the classification of erythematous lesions as pressure ulcers or to the failure of other investigators to study patients for an adequate length of time.

Pressure ulcers are characterized in relation to stage, surface size, depth, location, and other descriptors reflecting infected versus healing tissue. The staging system recommended by the National Pressure Ulcer Advisory Panel (NPUAP)[10] is as follows:

- Stage I: Nonblanchable erythema of intact skin. The heralding of skin ulceration.
- Stage II: Partial thickness skin loss involving epidermis and/or dermis. The ulcer is superficial and presents clinically as an abrasion, blister, or shallow crater.
- Stage III: Full thickness skin loss involving damage or necrosis of subcutaneous tissue that may extend down to, but not through, underlying fascia. The ulcer presents clinically as a deep crater with or without undermining of adjacent tissue.
- Stage IV: Full thickness skin loss with extensive destruction, tissue necrosis, or damage to muscle, bone, or supporting structures (e.g., tendon and joint capsule).

There is some debate regarding the appropriateness of including Stage I pressure sores when calculating incidence and prevalence. The Consensus Panel included Stage I pressure ulcers in the recommended classification system, recognizing the importance of early identification and treatment of ulcers in the prevention and worsening of pressure sores.

A more precise measure of the area of an ulcer using stereophotography has been developed.[11] This highly sophisticated technique is more appropriate for monitoring advanced pressure ulcers undergoing treatment than it is for studies that screen for incidence and prevalence.

PREDICTING PRESSURE ULCER RISK

Pressure ulcers are the result of the amount and duration of pressure over bony prominences and the ability of tissue to tolerate pressure (see Fig. 187-1).[4] The critical determinants of pressure are activity, mobility, and sensory perception. In this schema, persons who are unconscious or cognitively compromised, sedated, immobilized, or paralyzed or who have peripheral neuropathy may be at risk for pressure sores.

Despite the best efforts of nurses to reduce pressure or limit exposure, pressure sores can develop if tissues are less able to tolerate pressure. Tissue tolerance refers to the ability of the tissue to withstand or tolerate pressure. Extrinsic factors compromising tissue tolerance include friction that abrades the skin and shearing that results in the tearing of blood vessels and underlying connective tissue from the epidermis. Shearing usually results in deep ulcers, but an area of dark tissue or even eschar may conceal the extent of the damage for a considerable period of time before sloughing begins. Additionally, moisture from any source including incontinence of urine or feces or moisture from perspiration or draining wounds can lead to maceration of the tissue. Intrinsic factors including nutritional status, age,

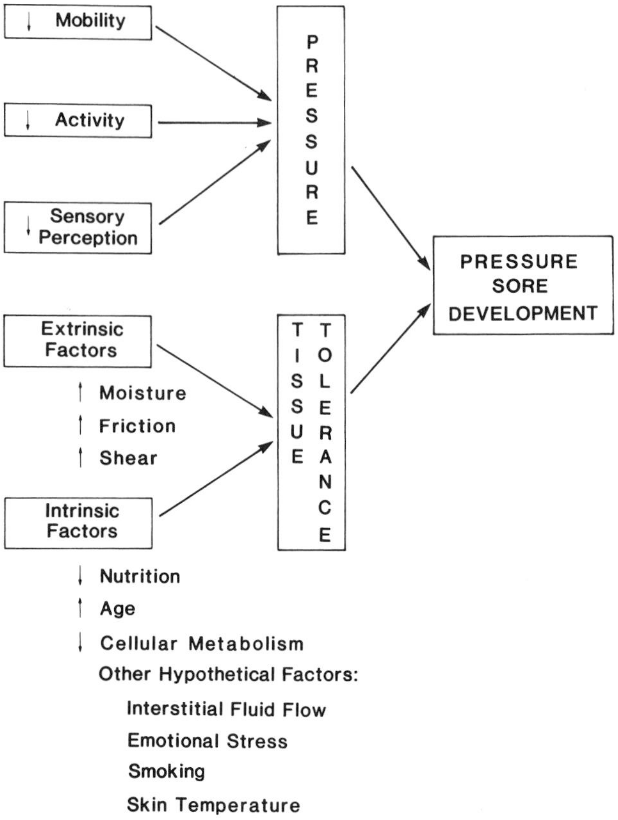

FIGURE 187-1 Conceptual framework of pressure and tissue tolerance for pressure.

blood pressure, body temperature, smoking history, hypoxia, and others may reduce tissue tolerance by altering the architecture of the skin, collagen, and supporting structures or the mechanisms supporting cellular maintenance (nutrition and oxygenation). Alterations in these extrinsic and intrinsic factors can reduce the amount and duration of pressure the tissue can withstand before developing lesions.

A number of instruments have been developed to predict risk for pressure sore development.[4,12,13] These instruments are alike in that they are composed of a series of subscales that rate specific risk factors; summing scores on the subscales provides an overall score indicating level of risk. The risk factors most consistently identified in these instruments include immobility, inactivity, fecal and urinary incontinence, altered level of consciousness, and nutrition. The Norton scale[12] and the Braden Scale for Predicting Pressure Risk[4] have been tested more systematically than the other instruments.

When these instruments are evaluated for high sensitivity and specificity denoting predictive validity and ease of use, clinically, the Braden Scale is somewhat superior (see Fig. 187-2). A summary of clinical tests of these tools provides details of the sensitivity, specificity, and predictive value of positive and negative tests (see Table 187-1).

The Norton scale[12] has highly variable sensitivity and specificity and has a tendency to overpredict. This tool was

Braden Scale

FOR PREDICTING PRESSURE SORE RISK

Patient's Name ______________________ Evaluator's Name ______________________ Date of Assessment

SENSORY PERCEPTION ability to respond meaning-fully to pressure-related discomfort	**1. Completely limited:** Unresponsive (does not moan, flinch, or grasp) to painful stimuli, due to diminished level of con-sciousness or sedation. OR limited ability to feel pain over most of body surface.	**2. Very Limited:** Responds only to painful stimuli. Cannot communicate discomfort except by moaning or restlessness. OR has a sensory impairment which limits the ability to feel pain or discomfort over 1/2 of body.	**3. Slightly Limited:** Responds to verbal com-mands, but cannot always communicate discomfort or need to be turned. OR has some sensory impairment which limits ability to feel pain or discomfort in 1 or 2 extremities.	**4. No Impairment:** Responds to verbal com-mands. Has no sensory deficit which would limit ability to feel or voice pain or discomfort.	
MOISTURE degree to which skin is exposed to moisture	**1. Constantly Moist:** Skin is kept moist almost constantly by perspiration, urine, etc. Dampness is detected every time patient is moved or turned.	**2. Very Moist:** Skin is often, but not always moist. Linen must be changed at least once a shift.	**3. Occasionally Moist:** Skin is occasionally moist, requiring an extra linen change approximately once a day.	**4. Rarely Moist:** Skin is usually dry, linen only requires changing at routine intervals.	
ACTIVITY degree of physical activity	**1. Bedfast:** Confined to bed	**2. Chairfast:** Ability to walk severely limited or non-existent. Cannot bear own weight and/or must be assisted into chair or wheel-chair.	**3. Walks Occasionally:** Walks occasionally during day, but for very short distances, with or without assistance. Spends majority of each shift in bed or chair.	**4. Walks Frequently:** walks outside the room at least twice a day and inside room at least once every 2 hours during waking hours.	
MOBILITY ability to change and control body position	**1. Completely Immobile:** Does not make even slight changes in body or extremity position without assistance.	**2. Very Limited:** Makes occasional slight changes in body or extremity position but unable to make frequent or significant changes independently.	**3. Slightly Limited:** Makes frequent though slight changes in body or extremity position independently.	**4. No Limitations:** Makes major and frequent changes in position without assistance.	
NUTRITION usual food intake pattern	**1. Very Poor:** Never eats a complete meal. Rarely eats more than 1/3 of any food offered. Eats 2 servings or less of protein (meat or dairy products) per day. Takes fluids poorly. Does not take a liquid dietary supplement. OR is NPO and/or maintained on clear liquids or IV's for more than 5 days.	**2. Probably Inadequate:** Rarely eats a complete meal and generally eats only about 1/2 of any food offered. Protein intake includes only 3 servings of meat or dairy products per day. Occasion-ally will take a dietary supplement. OR receives less than optimum amount of liquid diet or tube feeding.	**3. Adequate:** Eats over half of most meals. Eats a total of 4 servings of protein (meat, dairy products) each day. Occasionally will refuse a meal, but will usually take a supplement if offered. OR is on a tube feeding or TPN regimen which probably meets most of nutritional needs.	**4. Excellent:** Eats most of every meal. Never refuses a meal. Usually eats a total of 4 or more servings of meat and dairy products. Occasionally eats between meals. Does not require supplementation.	
FRICTION AND SHEAR	**1. Problem:** Requires moderate to maximum assistance in moving. Complete lifting without sliding against sheets is impossible. Frequently slides down in bed or chair, requiring frequent repositioning with maximum assistance. Spasticity, contractures or agitation leads to almost constant friction.	**2. Potential Problem:** Moves feebly or requires minimum assistance. During a move skin probably slides to some extent against sheets, chair, restraints, or other devices. Maintains relatively good position in chair or bed most of the time but occasion-ally slides down.	**3. No Apparent Problem:** Moves in bed and in chair independently and has sufficient muscle strength to lift up completely during move. Maintains good position in bed or chair at all times.		
				Total Score	

CON-63 (12/88)

FIGURE 187-2 Braden scale for the assessment of pressure sore risk.

TABLE 187-1. Sensitivity, Specificity, and Predictive Value of Positive and Negative Tests of Pressure Sore Prediction Tools*

Tool/Study	Sensitivity (%)	Specificity (%)	Predictive Value of Positive Test (%)	Predictive Value of Negative Test (%)
Norton/Norton et al.[12]	63	70	39	86
Norton modification/	100	49	31	100
Goldstone and Roberts[26]	76	58	50	81
Norton/Goldstone and Goldstone[27]	89	36	53	80
Norton modification/Warner and Hall[28]	65	89	15	96
Norton/Lincoln et al.[29]	0	94	0	85
Gosnell/Gosnell[13]	50	73	22	90
Braden/Bergstrom et al.[4]	100	90	44	100
Braden/Bergstrom/Demuth/Braden[9]	83	64	61	85
Braden/Hoenshell-Nelson/Miller (AICU)[15]	83	42	8	100
Braden/Hoenshell-Nelson/Miller (MICU)[15]	100	68	13	100

*NOTE: Caution must be used when comparing results from different studies because different definitions of pressure sores may be used, scores used in calculations may be determined at different points in time, different methods may be used to obtain scores, and other methodologic variables may influence the results and prevent comparison.

SOURCE: Taylor.[14]

developed specifically for use with elderly populations, and it is uncertain how it will perform with other age groups. The Braden Scale[4] has promising sensitivity and specificity and has been tested in critical care populations. One test of the Braden Scale rated 60 consecutively admitted AICU patients for risk on admission to the unit and subsequently assessed skin condition over a 2-week period.[9] Using a score of 16 to determine risk, the sensitivity was 83 percent and the specificity was 64 percent. Two major drawbacks in interpreting these results are (a) risk was only assessed upon admission and risk levels change as patient conditions change and (b) the investigator rated both risk and skin condition.

A subsequent study of 100 consecutively admitted patients in a Veterans' Administration (VA) Hospital yielded similar sensitivity.[15] Risk and skin condition, rated by different investigators who remained blind to findings, showed that a score of 16 was 83 percent sensitive and 41 percent specific. The disappointing specificity in this study, with a good deal of overprediction, might be attributed to the setting (VA) where mattress overlays and specialty beds, gel pads, and other pressure-relieving devices not charged to patients were readily available and did not require special prescriptions. The investigators were ICU staff who were especially sensitive to skin condition and had a responsibility for preventing pressure ulcers on the unit. The myocardial infarction subsample ($N = 40$) in the same study had somewhat better sensitivity and specificity.

Further tests of these instruments are required to determine the predictive validity with specific populations, to determine the frequency with which risk should be reassessed, and to evaluate the role of risk assessment in the prevention of pressure ulcers. Systematic studies for the purpose of refinement of these tools and for determining the generalizability to various settings and populations have been recommended by the NPUAP.[10]

OTHER RISK FACTORS

Pressure is the most important risk factor in the etiology of pressure ulcers, but other risk factors alter the ability of the skin to tolerate pressure as presented in the preceding conceptualization. Specifically, moisture from any source, friction and shearing force, age, nutrition, body temperature, hypotension, and perhaps hypoxia have been identified as factors reducing extrinsic or intrinsic tolerance. The NPUAP suggested that a better understanding of the etiology and natural history of pressure ulcers is needed, and nutrition was singled out as an area needing special attention in relation to the etiology, prevention, and treatment of pressure sores.

AGE

Age has been related to pressure ulcer development in a near linear relationship. The decrease in muscle mass and elastin that accompanies aging is hypothesized to allow a greater transfer of mechanical load from supporting structures to underlying tissue.[16]

NUTRITION

There is growing evidence to support the relationship between dietary intake, nutritional status, and the development of pressure ulcers. The dietary intake of calories, protein, vitamin C, and zinc have all been hypothetically related to risk. Only one prospective study of dietary intake in 200 newly admitted, elderly nursing home residents over a 3-month period has examined all these relationships, demonstrating that poor dietary intake of protein and calories was linked to pressure sore development and healing.[17]

The sequela to prolonged inadequate intake of calories and protein is kwashiorkor, marasmus, or mixed kwashiorkor-marasmus. Kwashiorkor, protein malnutrition, is diagnosed by visceral proteins such as serum albumin and by total lymphocyte count. Marasmus, calorie or energy malnutrition, is diagnosed by anthropometric measurements. Kwashiorkor-marasmus, a combination of both deficiencies, is diagnosed by deficiencies in markers of both visceral proteins and anthropometric measurements.

Serum albumin less than 3.5 mg/100 mL has been shown in several recent studies to be related to the development and presence of pressure ulcers.[17,18] An inverse relationship was demonstrated between stage of pressure sore and serum albumin levels in cross-sectional studies.[18,19] Poor dietary intake has been a more important indicator of risk in prospective studies.

A great deal remains to be learned about the role of nutrition in the development and healing of pressure ulcers, but the evidence to date supports nutritional assessment and dietary supplementation, particularly for the elderly and malnourished patients who are unable or unwilling to ingest adequate amounts of food for more than 2 or 3 days.

HYPOTENSION

Hypotension, defined as a diastolic blood pressure below 60 mmHg, has been associated with pressure ulcer development.[13,17] Hypothetically, the lowered blood pressure results in decreased peripheral perfusion. While dilation of a local tissue bed is a response to locally decreased blood flow, global hypotension will result in generalized vasoconstriction with poor skin flow.

SMOKING

Smoking has been linked to pressure ulcers in studies of spinal cord patients[19] and in a follow-up study of an aged cohort.[20] Smoking is known to cause vasoconstriction and to impair oxygen-carrying capacity; hence, these intrinsic factors may reduce the tolerance of tissue for decreased blood flow due to local pressure. The current use of cigarettes increases the odds of developing pressure sores threefold.[20]

TEMPERATURE

Core temperature, ambient temperature, and interface temperature all have the potential to influence pressure sore risk. Each degree increase in body temperature is hypothesized to increase the metabolic need by 10 percent. Persons with fever may be more susceptible to local tissue damage when the metabolic rate is increased and nutrients and oxygen delivered to tissues are decreased. On the other hand, an increase in ambient temperature and the temperature between the skin and certain fabrics or materials may lead to sweating and maceration of the skin. An increase in the temperature of the skin over bony prominences may also increase the risk of a pressure ulcer in this area. Evidence to support this relationship is just beginning to emerge.

INTERVENTIONS TO PREVENT PRESSURE ULCERS IN AT-RISK POPULATIONS

Clinical screening tools identify "at-risk" persons for the purpose of early intervention and pressure sore prevention. The prevention of pressure sores is the desired norm and can be accomplished by intervention strategies employed early in the course of illness, since many pressure ulcers have been documented to occur within 2 weeks of admission.[9,12,17]

PRESSURE RELIEF

Pressure is the first and foremost factor in the development of pressure sores; hence, methods to relieve pressure by moving the patient more often, helping the patient be aware of the need to move, if able, and reducing the pressure have all received a great deal of attention. Frequent turning regimens (usually every 2 h) are usually instituted as part of a care plan for at-risk subjects. When more frequent turning is necessary, a scheduled turning regimen may be supplemented with planned small shifts in body weight. The efficacy of this intervention has been described[12] and a protocol for implementation recommended.[21] While this intervention remains to be tested, protocols to provide small shifts in body weight may be a very promising adjunct to the turning regimen and deserve further evaluation. In the rehabilitative phase, patients are taught to shift their weight at intervals while sitting or lying down, and some devices have been introduced to remind them of time to turn.

Special mattresses, mattress overlays, and cushions are often used when frequent turning is difficult or is not possible as well as when patients are at greater levels of risk. These devices are classified as static (nonmoving) or dynamic (movement of air currents by electrical systems). The static systems include foam-, water-, gel-, and air-filled devices that are placed over the mattress or chair surface. These devices serve to provide for more even weight distribution but still require manual turning of patients. The dynamic support systems adjust weight distribution by alternating air currents and may be of two types: mattress overlays such as alternating current pads and air-fluidized beds. Numerous studies compare these pressure-relieving devices, but many have never been subjected to scientific review and are presented as unpublished reprints by product manufacturers.

Studies of pressure under bony prominences have shown that pressures under inflated surfaces were not always lower than pressures under static surfaces and that pads placed over the surface of the mattress for protection of incontinence do not increase or decrease pressure.[22–24] A comparison of conventional mattresses, a convoluted 2-in. foam, a Biogard flotation unit, and Soft-Care bed cushions showed that the mean of three pressure measurements was lowest over the sacrum and trochanter with Soft-Care and over the heel with Biogard.[22] These studies illustrate that the use of special mattresses or mattress overlays does not relieve the nurse of the need to turn the patient frequently and to systematically assess the skin for early signs of pressure.

In the case of the specialty bed, no statistically significant difference was found[17] between the mean of three pressure readings when subjects rested on Mediscus or Clinitron beds. These products are tested and compared frequently, but systematic studies are still needed to determine if these beds completely reduce the risk of pressure sores and the degree to which other complications such as phlebitis, renal calculi, and respiratory problems may be increased by lack of turning.

Studies considering the efficacy of one product over another have often used normal subjects or heterogenous patient populations; have not considered level of risk; have not controlled for covariates such as age, sex, race, weight, activity, mobility, etc.; and have tested the product at only one point in time (during the 1- to 2-h study). Studies are needed to evaluate clinical interventions. In order to be useful for clinical judgment these studies should (1) be prospective versus retrospective or cross-sectional; (2) include control or comparison groups; (3) test appropriate interventions for assessed levels of risk; (4) assess risk with reliable and valid risk predictor tools; (5) provide for documentation of standard care given to control groups and standard care given in addition to the intervention being tested; (6) evaluate skin condition and other clinical outcomes at specific intervals using trained data collectors rather than information from patient records; and (7) document useful information such as staffing patterns, nurse-patient ratios, and level of education of the caregiver.

NUTRITIONAL SUPPLEMENTATION

Nutrition is being recognized as an important variable in pressure sore risk and in other complications; hence, early nutritional support is essential for preventing complications. Interdisciplinary teams that provide for nutritional support are essential for critically ill patients.

THE TREATMENT OF PRESSURE ULCERS

The choice of treatment for ulcers depends on the stage, the presence or absence of infection or necrosis, and the location of the ulcer. Stage I and II ulcers can be readily treated and prevented from worsening through a combination of strategies aimed at relieving pressure, keeping the wound clean, preventing infection, and nourishing the patient. The enterostomal therapist (ET) has the most experience and training in the treatment of pressure ulcers and should be consulted for dealing with at-risk populations.

Over 2200 topical preparations have been recommended for treatment of ulcers.[25] A review of the myriad of products that has been applied to the skin is of interest from a historical perspective, but the current wisdom is that nothing should be applied to the ulcer that would not be appropriate to put into the eye. The specific recommendations for occlusive dressings and treatment of skin lesions are discussed in the section on wound healing. The major concern in the treatment of ulcers is to begin to treat the ulcer as soon as it is identified to prevent worsening and infection.[26–29]

REFERENCES

1. Joint Commission for the Accreditation of Healthcare Organizations: Critical indicators of quality of care. Chicago, 1987.
2. Curtin L: Wound management: Care and cost. Nurs Manag 15(2):22, 1984.
3. Gerson LW: The incidence of pressure sores in active treatment hospitals. Int J Nurs Stud 12:201, 1975.
4. Bergstrom N, Braden BJ, Laguzza A, Holman V: The Braden Scale for predicting pressure sore risk. Nurs Res 36:205, 1987.
5. Ek AC, Boman G: A descriptive study of pressure sores: The prevalence of pressure sores and the characteristics of patients. J Adv Nurs 7:51, 1982.
6. Langemo DK, Olson B, Hunter S, Burd C, Hansen D, Cathcart-Silberberg T: Incidence of pressure sores in acute care, rehabilitation, extended care, home health, and hospice in one locale. Decubitus 2(2):42, 1989.
7. Mawson AR, Biundo JJ, Neville P, Linares H, Winchester Y, Lopez A: Risk factors for early occurring pressure ulcers following spinal cord injury. Am J Phys Med Rehab 67(3):123, 1988.
8. Versluysen M: Pressure sores in elderly patients, the epidemiology related to hip operations. J Bone Joint Surg 67-B:10, 1985.
9. Bergstrom N, Demuth PJ, Braden BJ: A clinical trail of the Braden Scale for predicting pressure sore risk. Nurs Clin Am 22(2):417, 1987.
10. National Pressure Ulcer Advisory Panel, Pressure ulcers' prevalence, costs and risk assessment: Consensus Development Conference Statement. Decubitus 2(2):24, 1989.
11. Frantz R: The effect of TENS on healing of decubitus ulcers. *Proceedings of the Scientific Sessions, 30th Biennial Convention of Sigma Theta Tau International*. Indianapolis, Sigma Theta Tau, 1989, p 100.
12. Norton D, McLaren R, Exton-Smith AN: *An Investigation of Geriatric Nursing Problems in Hospitals*. London, National Corporation for the Care of Old People, 1962.
13. Gosnell DJ: An assessment tool to identify pressure sores. Nurs Res 22:55, 1973.
14. Taylor KJ: Assessment tools for the identification of patients at risk for the development of pressure sores: A review. J Enterostomal Ther 15(5):201, 1988.
15. Hoenshell-Nelson NA, Miller SM: The validity of the Braden Scale for predicting pressure sore risk in adult intensive care unit patients, Master's Thesis. University of Nebraska Medical Center, 1988.
16. Krouskop TA: A synthesis of the factors that contribute to pressure sore formation. Med Hypotheses 11:255, 1983.
17. Bergstrom N, Braden B: Nutrition/pressure sore link: Nutritional status during the development and resolution of pressure sores in the elderly, in Funk (ed): *Key Aspects of Recovery: Improving Mobility, Rest and Nutrition in Infants, Adults, and the Elderly*. Chapel Hill, NC, in press.
18. Pinchcofsky-Devin GD, Kaminski MV: Correlation of pressure sores and nutritional status. J Am Geriatr Soc 34(6):435, 1986.
19. Lamid S, ElGhatit AZ: Smoking, spasticity and pressure sores in spinal cord injured patients. Am J Phys Med 62(6):300, 1983.
20. Guralnik, JM, Harris TB, White LR, Cornoni-Huntley JC: Occurrence and predictors of pressure sores in the national health and nutrition examination survey follow-up. J Am Geriatr Soc 36(9):807, 1988.
21. Horsley JA, Crane J, Haller KB, Bingle JD: *Preventing Decubitus Ulcers*. New York, Grune & Stratton, 1981.
22. Maklebust J, Mondoux L, Sieggreen M: Pressure relief characteristics of various support surfaces used in prevention and treatment of pressure ulcers. J Enterostomal Ther 13(3):85, 1986.
23. Douglass HO, Jr, Holyoke ED, Goodwin PM, Priore RL: Skin pressure measurements on various mattress surfaces in cancer patients. Am J Phys Med 62(5):217, 1983.
24. Krouskop T, Williams R, Krebs M: The effectiveness of air flotation beds. *Care Science and Practice*, 1984.
25. Parish LC, Witkowski JA, Crissey JT: *The Decubitus Ulcer*. Chicago: Year Book Medical Publishers, 1983.
26. Goldstone LA, Roberts BV: A preliminary discriminant function analysis of elderly orthopaedic patients who will or will not contract a pressure sore. Int J Nurs Stud 17:17, 1980.
27. Goldstone LA, Goldstone J: The Norton score: an early warning of pressure sores? J Advanced Nursing 7:419, 1982.
28. Warner A, Hall DJ: Pressure sores: A policy for prevention. Nurs Times 82:59, 1986.
29. Lincoln R, Roberts R, Maddox A, et al: Use of the Norton Pressure Sore Risk Assessment Scoring System with elderly patients in acute care. J Enterostomal Ther 13:132, 1986.

187G/Weaning from Mechanical Ventilatory Support

JOHN M. CLOCHESY

Many critically ill patients require mechanical ventilatory support (MVS) which may last weeks to months or longer in debilitated patients. Successful weaning from MVS requires neuromuscular integrity, physiologic stability, and psychologic readiness. Figure 187-3 diagrams the general sequence used to wean patients from MVS. In the absence of neuromuscular integrity, traditional weaning modes are ineffective. In ventilator-dependent patients, physiologic stability requires adequate respiratory muscle mass, strength, and endurance and that metabolic demand not exceed capacity.

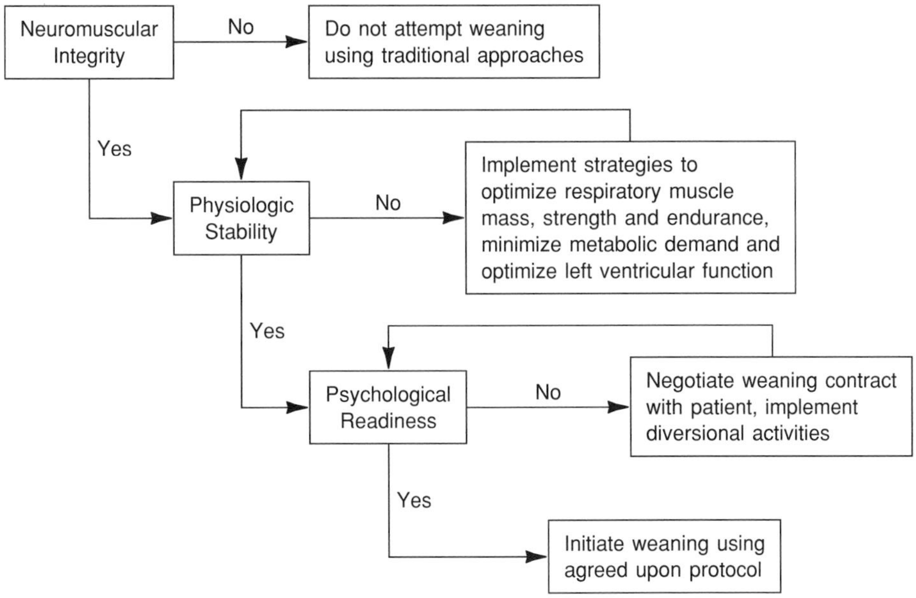

FIGURE 187-3 Weaning algorithm. (Copyright 1990 by John M. Clochesy. Used with permission.)

While the majority of patients successfully wean from MVS within 1 week, approximately 9 percent do not.[1] Weaning these patients requires special attention to physiologic stability and psychologic readiness. Psychologic readiness includes a willingness on behalf of the patient and a state of preparation that results in a particular stage of developmental maturity.[2] Table 187-2 lists the components of physiologic stability, clinical indicators, conditions necessitating nursing care,[3] and potential interventions used to promote physiologic stability. Three common modes of weaning from MVS include synchronized intermittent mandatory ventilation, assist-control ventilation with T-tube trials, and pressure support ventilation. Table 187-3 compares some uses and advantages of each, but it should be kept in mind that many approaches are successful (see Chap. 127.)

RESEARCH TO DATE

Research into weaning from MVS includes several descriptive, correlational, and experimental studies. Three themes emerge from the literature: predicting successful weaning from MVS, inspiratory muscle training, and the psychologic factors influencing weaning.

PREDICTING SUCCESS

Clinical criteria commonly used to predict successful weaning (Table 187-4) are not specific or sensitive.[4] Possibly more useful are the ventilator score (VS) and the adverse factor score (AFS).[5] Each of these scores is the sum of weighting of factors with potential to interfere with the weaning process. Investigators have found that if VS + AFS > 55, then progressive weaning is likely to be unsuccessful at that time. In a sample of 101 patients, the investigators, using all determinations for all patients, found that the sum of the two scores had a sensitivity of 93 percent and a specificity of 86 percent. The false-negative rate therefore is 7 percent, and the false-positive is 14 percent. A reorganization of the factors in the VS and AFS to fit within a framework of conditions necessitating nursing care (CNNC)[3] while maintaining the original weighting and scoring system has been proposed.[6] An individual patient's score within a CNNC identifies primary conditions requiring nursing intervention. Further development of this approach could lead to subscales that predict nursing care requirements and success in progressive weaning from MVS.

INSPIRATORY MUSCLE TRAINING

Inspiratory muscle training in patients with COPD resulted in a significant increase in inspiratory muscle strength following 1 month of training.[7] In a later double-blind study, patients with COPD significantly increased their maximal inspiratory pressure (MIP) and 12-min distance walk following training at 30 percent of their MIP for 2 months.[8] Inspiratory muscle training increases MIP in mechanically ventilated patients.[9] Further work is needed to identify the optimal resistive load and training protocol to increase respiratory muscle strength in mechanically ventilated patients.

PSYCHOLOGIC FACTORS

Many clinicians believe that psychologic stressors interfere with successful weaning from MVS. The effect on weaning of nursing contact, holding the patient's hand, and verbally interacting with 26 patients being weaned from MVS by the

TABLE 187-2. Components of Physiologic Stability, Clinical Indicators, Conditions Necessitating Nursing Care, and Potential Interventions

Physiologic Factors	Clinical Indicators	Conditions Necessitating Nursing Care	Potential Interventions
Respiratory muscle mass	Weight, serum albumin	Altered nutrition: less than body requirements	1. Initiate feeding protocol with adequate protein and energy sources. 2. Use a high-fat, low-carbohydrate diet to minimize the respiratory quotient.
Respiratory muscle strength and endurance	Maximal inspiratory pressure (MIP), vital capacity (VC), maximum voluntary ventilation (MVV)	Ineffective breathing pattern	1. Initiate formal exercise training program. 2. Allow adequate rest for diaphragmatic recovery between exercise sessions.
Metabolic demand	Oxygen consumption ($\dot{V}_{O_2}$)	Activity intolerance	1. Arrange environment to minimize energy expenditure
		Sleep pattern disturbance	2. Encourage strictly enforced periods of uninterrupted sleep and rest.
Left ventricular function	Ejection fraction (LVEF); heart rate (HR); blood pressure before, during, and after weaning	Altered cardiac output: decreased	1. Control fluid intake pattern. 2. Position patient with head of bed elevated. 3. Schedule and administer diuretics and afterload reducers so that peak effect coincides with weaning trial.

TABLE 187-3. Comparison of Common Modes of Weaning Patients from Mechanical Ventilatory Support

Weaning Mode	Use	Advantages
Synchronized intermittent mandatory ventilation (SIMV)	Weaning from MVS <72 h duration	Does not allow deconditioning of respiratory muscles
Assist-control ventilation with T-tube trials (T-tube)	Weaning from MVS >72 h duration	Allows muscles to rest/recover from fatigue
Pressure support ventilation (PSV)	Failure to wean with T-tube, patients with poor left ventricular function	Gradual decrease in positive intrathoracic pressure allows the body to adapt to decreased stroke volume and increased preload in patients with left ventricular failure.

TABLE 187-4. Criteria Commonly Used to Predict the Likelihood of Successful Weaning from Mechanical Ventilatory Support

Spontaneous ventilatory rate	<30 breaths/min
Minute ventilation	<10 L/min
Maximal inspiratory pressure	≥30 cmH_2O
Maximum voluntary ventilation	≥2 x baseline minute ventilation

T-tube method did not demonstrate any difference in patient outcome based on nursing contact.[10] Further research is needed to describe the nature of psychologic factors influencing weaning from MVS, including stressors and patients' perceptions of their own readiness.

THE WORK REMAINING

Several indicators of cardiovascular performance have been included in the adverse factor score.[5] Other investigators[11–13] describe differences in cardiac output, ventricular ejection fraction, central vascular pressures, and systemic vascular resistance between patients who successfully wean from MVS and those who do not. Further inquiry into the relationship of left ventricular function to successful weaning from MVS is warranted.

REFERENCES

1. Nett LM, Morganroth M, Petty TL: Weaning the unweanable. Am J Nurs 87:1181, 1987.
2. Simpson JA, Weiner ESC: *Oxford English Dictionary*. Oxford, Clarendon Press, 1989.
3. Fitzpatrick JJ, Kerr ME, Saba VK, Hoskins LM, Hurley ME, Mills WC, Rottkamp BC, Warren JJ, Capenito LJ: Translating nursing diagnosis into ICD code. Am J Nurs 89:493, 1989.
4. Shekleton ME, Balk RA, Szidon JP, Bone RC: Clinical indicators of the ability to sustain spontaneous ventilation, in *Proceedings of the Twelfth Annual Midwest Nursing Research Society Conference*. Indianapolis, Midwest Nursing Research Society, 1988, p 158.
5. Morganroth ML, Morganroth JL, Nett LM, Petty PL: Criteria for weaning from prolonged mechanical ventilation. Arch Intern Med 144:1012, 1984.
6. Dettenmeier PA: Using a numerical score to predict optimal weaning interval, in Boller J (ed): *Proceedings of the Sixteenth Annual National Teaching Institute of the American Association of Critical Care Nurses*. Newport Beach, CA, American Association of Critical-Care Nurses, 1989, pp 398–401.
7. Larson M, Kim MJ: Respiratory muscle training with the incentive spirometer resistive breathing device. Heart Lung 13:341, 1984.
8. Larson JL, Kim MJ, Sharp JT, Larson DA: Inspiratory muscle training with a pressure threshold breathing device in patients with chronic obstructive pulmonary disease. Am Rev Respir Dis 133:A100, 1986.
9. Aldrich TK, Karpel JP, Uhrlass, Sarapani MA, Eramo D, Ferranti R: Weaning from mechanical ventilation: Adjunctive use of inspiratory muscle resistive training. Crit Care Med 17:143, 1989.
10. Henneman EA: Effect of nursing contact on the stress response of patients being weaned from mechanical ventilation. Heart Lung 18:483, 1989.
11. Beach T, Millen E, Grenvik A: Hemodynamic response to discontinuance of mechanical ventilation. Crit Care Med 1:85, 1973.
12. Biondi JW, Hines RL, Matthay RA, Barash PG: Comparative right ventricular function during assist control, intermittent mandatory and spontaneous ventilation. Anesth Analg 65:S18, 1986.
13. Mathru M, Rao TLK, E1-Etr AA, Pifarre R. Hemodynamic response to changes in ventilatory patterns in patients with normal and poor left ventricular reserve. Crit Care Med 10:423, 1982.

187H/The Spouse and Family of the Critically Ill Adult

DEBRA K. MOSER
KATHLEEN DRACUP

Over the past few decades, both physicians and nurses have expressed the belief that the most effective health care requires the involvement of all members of a patient's family. As early as 1945 a physician wrote that "to say that patients have families is like saying that the diseased organ is part of the individual."[1] He went on to admonish physicians that effective medical care required viewing the patient within the context of the family and including family members in various aspects of treatment and evaluation. Nurses, also, have considered themselves oriented toward family care. For example, in the Social Policy Statement of the American Nurses' Association the family is identified as "the necessary unit of service."[2]

This commitment to the family as the unit of care rather than just the individual patient might be quite surprising to anyone who has spent time in an ICU. Here, every regulation is directed toward keeping the family at bay. In most critical care units, doors are closed and entrance is only permitted by telephoning or knocking to receive permission to enter. Visiting regulations severely restrict the amount of time families can spend with patients. A national survey[3] of critical care nurses conducted in 1985 demonstrated that 73 percent of respondents restricted the number of times family members could visit per day, with 22 percent setting that number at four visits in a 24-h period. The majority of respondents (84 percent) said that visits were limited by time, usually to 10 or 15 min. The number of visitors was also limited to two visitors by 87 percent of respondents. In 89 percent of units surveyed, the visitor must be a certain age to be allowed to enter, usually 12 or 14 years. These results are relatively unchanged from a survey conducted in 1980 about visiting policies in the ICUs and CCUs.[4]

The restrictions to the family's presence that exist in the unit, imposed at a time when patient and family most need mutual support and reassurance, reflect the conflict that exists among critical care nurses and intensivists about including the family in the critical care experience. On the one hand, the family can be viewed as a negative force. Members of the family may be highly anxious about the patient who has been hospitalized with a potentially disabling or life-threatening illness or injury, and this anxiety can be manifested in demanding, hostile behavior toward staff. Even if their behavior is "reasonable," the family needs staff time to receive information and ask questions. Time is often what the busy ICU nurse and physician feel they have least to give. Family members frequently report that their need for daily information from the physician is rarely met.[5] Nurses are not expected to spend time with family members nor are they accountable to document their assessment and interventions with family members in the hospital record. On the other hand, the family can be viewed as a positive force. They are a potential source of reassurance and support from the patient. Such support can be critical to the recovery of a patient who is experiencing a physiologic and psychologic crisis.

Investigations concerning family members of the critically ill have focused on four areas: (1) the physical and emotional responses of family members to the hospitalization of a loved one in an ICU; (2) the needs families experience related to that hospitalization and the degree to which those needs are met; (3) family-oriented interventions designed to meet these needs and reduce negative physical and emotional sequelae; and (4) the effect of family-patient interaction on patient physical and psychologic outcomes. A considerable body of literature exists in the first two areas, while the data supporting family-oriented interventions are quite sparse.

EFFECT OF CRITICAL ILLNESS ON PATIENT'S FAMILY

The vast majority of research on families' response to intensive care has been conducted on spouses of patients with cardiac disease. Although this fact limits our ability to generalize these findings to children, siblings, and other members of the adult patient's extended family, many similarities are assumed to exist. The same assumption can be made across diagnostic categories.

In interviewing the spouses of patients hospitalized in intensive care, researchers have consistently documented severe emotional distress, often continuing long after the initiating incident. This distress is manifested by anxiety, fear, depression, feelings of helplessness, sleep and appetite disturbances, and the inability to concentrate.[6–8] These disturbances are likely a reaction to a multitude of psychological stresses: sudden threat of loss of mate or threat of loss of health in the mate, fears of worrying or upsetting the patient, fears over the possibility of a radically altered future, family role changes, the burden of child and household care, and financial problems.

Surgery also produces distress and dysfunction in family members, with the experience often perceived as more stressful by the spouse than by the patient. Fear of loss of the patient, panic, and feelings of numbness that can interfere with decision making occur in families upon discovering that one of their members must have coronary artery surgery. Families of patients scheduled for coronary artery bypass surgery frequently report that waiting for the surgery to be performed is a major source of stress.[9] Other sources of stress include financial strain related to hospital costs, inability of the sick family member to function as usual, alterations in family relations and expectations, and feelings of helplessness and inability to comfort or assist the patient. Spouses are additionally stressed by feelings of isolation and a lack of support from other family members.

Rather than being able to derive support from health care professionals, many family members find that relations with nurses and physicians are further sources of stress. Some families struggle with frustration at lack of access to physicians caring for their family member, lack of preoperative instruction and information about expected immediate and long-term postoperative care, lack of staff concern for their fears, and depersonalization by staff.

NEEDS OF FAMILIES OF CRITICALLY ILL PATIENTS

Over the past decade, investigators have thoroughly described the needs of families of critically ill patients.[5,10–16] In general, these needs can be divided into six categories, although obvious overlap exists: (1) the need for relief of anxiety; (2) the need for information; (3) the need to be with the patient; (4) the need to be helpful to the patient; (5) the need for support and ventilation; and (6) personal needs.

NEED FOR RELIEF OF ANXIETY AND NEED FOR INFORMATION

Families frequently identify needs under the category of anxiety relief and needs for information as very important.[5,12–14,16] The need for hope, particularly, has been identified across several studies as important. Families strongly feel the need to know that their family member is receiving the best possible care and that staff members care about the patient. The need to know the patient's prognosis or expected outcome of the illness and specific facts concerning the patient's progress, such as proposed treatment and rationale for treatment, are important for relief of family member anxiety. Family members often are reluctant to leave the hospital for fear that their family member's condition will deteriorate. Thus, many families strongly feel the need to be called at home if the patient's condition changes and want to feel comfortable calling the unit to ask about the patient. They want honest answers in understandable terms. A frequent family frustration is inaccessibility of the patient's physician. One investigator[5] found that most family members wanted to talk to a physician at least once daily but that this need was met only 10 percent of the time.

NEED TO BE WITH PATIENT AND NEED TO HELP PATIENT

Family and patient needs have been traditionally ignored in the development of critical care unit hospital visiting policies. Restrictive visiting hours are a major source of stress to both families and patients. Families express a great need to be able to see the patient frequently, to remain with them, and to be able to visit whenever they want.[5,12,14,15] The more severely ill the patient is perceived to be, the greater the desire to visit frequently. Additionally, families want to help with the care of the patient.

NEED FOR SUPPORT AND VENTILATION

The need for support can partially be fulfilled by meeting informational and anxiety reduction needs. Families also need the staff to accept them, to reassure them that the patient is doing well (if that is the case) and that it is appropriate for them to leave the hospital for a while.[5,12,13] Possibly because families of critically ill patients see the role of the nurse as limited to patient care and exclusive of family concerns, family members do not consistently consider the need to ventilate their feelings as important.

PERSONAL NEEDS

Personal needs such as help with financial and family problems and easy access to food, bathrooms, and other conveniences are not deemed highly important by most families.[5,12,14] Again, this finding may be related to family member feelings that patient needs are foremost.

INTERVENTIONS FOR FAMILIES OF THE CRITICALLY ILL

Recognizing the importance of family-inclusive care, critical care nurses have implemented a number of interventions based upon the descriptive research summarized in the previous section. These interventions, many of which have appeared in the clinical literature, are aimed at reducing the adverse effects of a critical care hospitalization on the family. They are summarized in Table 187-5. Only a few of these interventions have been tested empirically.

TABLE 187-5. Interventions for Family Members of Critically Ill Patients.

1. Prepare families for first visit to unit.
2. Provide written orientation material that is both general (e.g., the American Association of Critical-Care Nurses booklet, "It's Critical That You Know: A Resource for Families of Critically Ill Patients") and specific to the unit.
3. Identify one family member who will communicate with the nursing staff about the patient.
4. Give unit phone number and set up schedule for phone calls to family members.
5. Provide unrestricted visiting.
6. Arrange physical structure of the unit so that a family member can remain with the patient.
7. Identify primary nurses on each shift.
8. Hold information meetings with the family each day, with both the physician and primary nurse in attendance.
9. Invite family member(s) to participate in the physical care of the patient as appropriate.

In one early experimental study, the use of a standardized care plan designed to meet the needs of spouses of critically ill CCU patients significantly increased the number of spouse needs that were met.[11] Components of the care plan included flexible visiting hours, calling the spouse at home twice a day to inform him or her of the patient's status, providing a consistent primary nurse on each shift, and 15-min conferences each shift between the spouse and primary nurse in which information was provided and the spouse was encouraged to ventilate his or her emotions. Generalizing from this study, care plans have been developed to meet the needs of families of hospitalized ICU patients.[28]

The effects of an ICU family support group on the family's appraisal of stress, social support, and hope was recently tested.[17] There were no significant differences on any of the outcome measures when families who participated in the support group were compared to a control group. Although the family members in the experimental group indicated that the group was beneficial in providing a forum to express feelings, gain information, and feel support, the lack of significant results suggests that a formalized support group intervention may not meet the special needs of this population. As noted by the investigators, the need for support occurs when a crisis is occurring,which is not necessarily the time when the support sessions can be held. Frequent informal discussions with nursing and medical staff may be more appropriate for the critical care setting.

Interventions based on the theoretical perspectives of family, stress, and social support have been proposed. For example, programs have been developed to meet the needs of families of medical ICU patients based on family crisis precepts. Elements of such programs include family assessment, concerted efforts at consistent information giving to meet the many informational needs identified by families, family crisis intervention program coordinators, daily phone calls to family members with a detailed report of the patient's condition, introductions to the staff and physicians caring for the patient, family-patient follow-through programs, and waiting room support. Additionally, routine family assessment coupled with the use of such nursing strategies as health teaching and information giving; the consistent use of an honest, empathetic, communication style; frequent explanations, in simple terms, of the critical care environment and equipment; individualized visiting hours; and allowing family participation in care have been promoted as important to caring for families in potential crisis. Multidisciplinary family conferences or discussion groups (whose members might include, in addition to the family members, a critical care nurse or clinical nurse specialist, physician, social worker, and psychologist) have been recommended to decrease stress in families and meet the needs for support.

EFFECT OF FAMILY-PATIENT INTERACTION

Failure to include the family in the patient's plan of care can have adverse consequences for the patient as well as the family. The family can be a powerful source of support for the patient, effectively mitigating some of the consequences of physiologic and psychologic stressors.

Investigators have demonstrated that interventions involving families need not be elaborate to be effective. In an early experimental study, one group of families was prepared for an initial CCU visit by means of a simple booklet offering answers to commonly asked questions.[18] Patient anxiety was significantly reduced after visits from prepared family members when compared to patients whose families were not prepared for the visit. Family instruction has also been demonstrated to reduce some of the manifestations of postcardiotomy psychosis.[19] Patients whose family members had received instruction concerning ICU equipment, routine postoperative care, and the patient's need for eye contact, frequent touch, and orientation had fewer manifestations of postcardiotomy psychosis than patients whose family members received no such instruction.

Naturally occurring family support has generally been associated with positive patient outcomes. In a recent study,[20] the effect of social support on recovery of patients from coronary artery bypass surgery was investigated. Support was measured as proportion of days visited (number of days visited divided by number of days hospitalized). Based on a median split of proportion of days visited, patients were divided into low- and high-support conditions. Unmarried patients (none of whom were visited more than twice the entire hospitalization) comprised a separate group. Married patients who received high support had significantly better outcomes, as measured by less need for pain medication, earlier discharge from the surgical ICU, and earlier discharge from the hospital than married patients receiving low support. Unmarried patients had better recovery than the married, low-support patients. Quality of the marital relationship did not significantly affect recovery. The results of this study provide strong evidence for the positive role that families can play in the recovery of the critically ill patient and have important implications for changing restrictive visiting policies.

Under the premise of providing time for the patient to rest and reducing patient stress, visiting policies in critical care areas are often highly restrictive.[21] However, the preponderance of evidence suggests not only that health care workers are responsible for most interruptions of rest[22] and that staff-patient interactions may be more stressful than family-patient interactions[23] but also that the intervention of allowing unrestricted visiting has a positive influence on patient recovery and family health.

IMPLICATIONS FOR RESEARCH AND PRACTICE

Researchers have adequately characterized the perceived needs of families of critically ill patients. Future research should concentrate on testing interventions designed to meet these needs in large controlled trials. Which types of interventions, singly or in combination, best meet the needs of families? Of the many possible ways to deliver information, which are most effective? What are the physical and psychologic outcomes in both patient and family members when family-centered interventions are employed? Are complex family programs necessary or is the consistent use of a well-designed family care plan sufficient to meet family needs?

Much of the research conducted in critically ill populations has concentrated on male cardiac patients. Thus, much family research is limited to findings in female spouses. Research in male spouses, in family members other than spouses, and in patients with diagnoses other than cardiac disease is indicated.

Although family-inclusive care for the critically ill is espoused by many, it is rarely seen in most critical care units. Two factors are important for implementation of critical care that routinely includes the family: (1) education of nurses and physicians and (2) development of systematic, structured, research-tested interventions for family-inclusive care.

A first step in the provision of family-inclusive care for the critically ill is the uniform education of nurses and physicians in the provision of family care. Many feel that they do not have the theoretical knowledge and psychosocial skills to effectively deal with families, and most feel that supporting families in need is emotionally exhausting.[24] Nurses often find family visits a source of stress.[21] Ultimately, the educational preparation of both physicians and nurses needs to provide those practitioners with a degree of comfort in dealing with families and a set of values that ascribes importance to meeting the needs of family members.

Nurses and physicians need to implement systematic, structured, research-tested interventions for family-inclusive care. Such care includes lifting restrictive visiting policies, providing frequent information sessions for the family, and including the family in daily discussions about treatment options. Structured family care involves the inclusion of the family in all preoperative, postoperative, and rehabilitation instruction that the patient receives. The growing number of intensivists and consultants makes frequent informational meetings for families essential.

It is important that the philosophy of every critical care unit reflect a family-centered approach. Families need to meet with physicians on a daily basis and should be told how this meeting will be accomplished. Nurses need to meet with family members outside the ICU and colleagues should expect to cover those nurses' patient care responsibilities during family conferences. Managers must hold their staff accountable for identifying family needs and implementing effective interventions. Ultimately, family-inclusive care requires the commitment and support of all the members of the critical care team.

REFERENCES

1. Richardson HB: *Patients Have Families*. NY, The Commonwealth Fund, 1945, p. 1.

2. American Nurses' Association: *Nursing: A Social Policy Statement*. Kansas, American Nurses' Association, 1980, p 5.
3. Stockdale LL, Hughes JP: Critical care unit visiting policies: A survey. Focus Crit Care 15:45, 1988.
4. Kirchhoff K: Visiting policies for patients with myocardial infarction: A national survey. Heart Lung 11:571, 1982.
5. Molter NC: Needs of relatives of critically ill patients: A descriptive study. Heart Lung 8:332, 1979.
6. Caplin MS, Sexton DL: Stresses experienced by spouses of patients in a coronary care unit with myocardial infarction. Focus Crit Care 15:31, 1988.
7. Mayou R, Foster A, Williamson B: The psychological and social effects of myocardial infarction on wives. Br Med J 1:699, 1978.
8. Bedworth JA, Molen MT: Psychological stress in spouses of patients with myocardial infarction. Heart Lung 11:450, 1982.
9. Gillis CL: Reducing family stress during and after coronary artery bypass surgery. Nurs Clin N Am 19:103, 1984.
10. Hampe SO: Needs of the grieving spouse in the hospital setting. Nurs Res 245:113, 1975.
11. Dracup KA, Breu CS: Using nursing research findings to meet the needs of grieving spouses. Nurs Res 27:212, 1978.
12. Daley L: The perceived immediate needs of families with relatives in the intensive care setting. Heart Lung 13:231, 1984.
13. Norris L, Grove S: Investigation of selected psychosocial needs of family members of critically ill adult patients. Heart Lung 15:194, 1986.
14. Leske J: Needs of relatives of critically ill patients: A follow-up. Heart Lung 15:189, 1986.
15. Stillwell SB: Importance of visiting needs as perceived by family members of patients in the intensive critical care unit. Heart Lung 13:238, 1984.
16. Freismuth C: Meeting the needs of families of critically ill patients: A comparison of visiting policies in the intensive care setting. Heart Lung 15:309, 1986.
17. Sabo KA, Kraay C, Rudy E, Abraham T, Bender M, Lewandowski W, Lombardo B, Turk M, Dawson D: ICU family support group sessions: Family members' perceived benefits. App Nurs Res 2:82, 1989.
18. Doerr BC, Jones JW: Effect of family preparation on the state anxiety level of the CCU patient. Nurs Res 28:315, 1979.
19. Chatham MA: The effect of family involvement on patients' manifestations of postcardiotomy psychosis. Heart Lung 7:995, 1978.
20. Kulik JA, Mahler HIM: Social support and recovery from surgery. Health Psych 8:221, 1989.
21. Woellner DS: Flexible visiting hours in the adult critical care unit. Focus Crit Care 15:66, 1988.
22. Walker BB: The postsurgery heart patient: Amount of uninterrupted time for sleep and rest during the first, second, and third postoperative days in a teaching hospital. Nurs Res 21:164, 1972.
23. Fuller BF, Foster GM: The effects of family/friend visits vs. staff interaction on stress/arousal of surgical intensive care patients. Heart Lung 11:457, 1982.
24. Hickey M, Lewandowski L: Critical care nurses' role with families: A descriptive study. Heart Lung 17:670, 1988.

187 I/The Elderly Patient

MARQUIS D. FOREMAN

Elderly patients admitted to the ICU present unique and complex challenges to medical and nursing intensivists. Typically, elderly patients are admitted to the ICU for acute exacerbations of chronic health conditions presenting as multi–organ system failure. These acute exacerbations of chronic health conditions, or acute-on-chronic organ failure, are made even more complex given the decline in physiologic reserve that accompanies aging, a decline more recently thought to be more a function of disease than of aging per se, but an omnipresent factor nonetheless.

Although elderly patients constitute approximately 46 percent of all patients admitted to ICUs,[1] great debate continues about the appropriateness of intensive therapy for the elderly. Opponents of such therapy argue that the elderly, as compared with younger patients, receive less benefit from such costly and highly technologic care. Opponents cite the higher rates of morbidity and mortality associated with intensive therapy for older patients, outcomes reputed to be a direct extension of age. It has been reported that elderly patients experience more iatrogenic complications; longer ICU and hospital stays; higher mortality while in the ICU, in the hospital, and in the immediate posthospital period; and generate greater hospital costs within the context of diminished productivity and contributions to society, diminished functional capacity, poorer quality of life, and the imminence of death.[2]

Conversely, advocates of intensive therapy for the elderly argue that when these findings of higher morbidity and mortality are examined by severity of illness, age is no longer important, i.e., that health status rather than age is more predictive of the outcomes of intensive therapy. Findings such as these clearly indicate that elderly as compared to younger patients derive equivalent benefit from intensive therapy, at equivalent costs and comparable long-term outcomes and rates of survival.[1] Nonetheless, the contradictions present in these opposing viewpoints make it impossible for a consensus to be reached relative to the appropriateness or range of intensive therapy for older adults, a stalemate that heightens the dilemmas and complexities in providing therapy to these patients.

Despite the apparent need to resolve this dilemma, intensive therapy for critically ill elders continues to be a poorly researched area of clinical practice. Although knowledge about the phenomena reviewed in this chapter, as well as much of that in this text, has relevance for elderly patients, this knowledge typically has not been generated with the elderly as a primary focus. Subjects used to gain knowledge about these phenomena have included elderly patients by virtue of the elderlys' being recipients of intensive therapy. However, these data have not been analyzed to reveal age-specific information. Yet there is rather universal agreement that many phenomena behave differently in elderly persons. As a result, the elderly have contributed to knowledge specific to certain phenomena, but the knowledge of these phenomena relative to the elderly is meager.

One exception to this situation is the study of delirium. The study of this phenomenon by nurses is reviewed with supportive literature (conducted by nonnurses and with non-ICU samples) cited as appropriate.

DELIRIUM

Delirium, also known as acute confusional states, ICU psychosis, or postcardiotomy delirium, is characterized as a transient, organic mental syndrome of diffuse cerebral dysfunction resulting in global cognitive impairment, i.e., simultaneous impairments of perception, memory, and thinking.[3] A common yet serious health problem, delirium is reported to afflict 24 to 80 percent of elderly hospitalized patients,[4] with case fatality rates of 25 to 33 percent.[5] Delirium often is the only symptom of physical illness in the elderly[6] and occurs more frequently and in more severe forms with critical illness.[7]

Development of delirium is associated with increased morbidity, increased intensity of nursing care, longer hospitalization, increased rates of nursing home placement upon discharge, and increased mortality, both during the critical illness and recuperative phases.[5,8] All of these factors contribute to the increased per-day hospital costs. Furthermore, it has been estimated that if the length of stay of each delirious elderly hospitalized patient could be reduced by just 1 day, the savings to Medicare would amount to $1 to $2 billion per year.[5]

Despite the obvious importance of this condition, 37 to 72 percent of patients who become delirious while hospitalized are never recognized by nurses or physicians as suffering from a delirium.[9] This underrecognition of delirium has been attributed to the myths and attitudes of health care professionals toward the aged, the variable clinical manifestations of delirium, and the lack of effective assessment and treatment protocols for this patient population.

RESEARCH INTO DELIRIUM

Research into the phenomenon of delirium conducted by nurse investigators falls into the categories of (1) detection and assessment, (2) variable clinical manifestations, (3) predictors, (4) etiologies, and (5) interventions. Each category of study is discussed separately; an extrapolation of these findings to clinical practice follows. Recommendations for research conclude this section.

DETECTION AND ASSESSMENT OF DELIRIUM

Because of the consequences of delirium, efforts to promptly and accurately detect its presence in the critically ill elderly patient are vital. However, the detection and assessment of delirium in this patient population is problematic at best, since problems arise from the characteristics of the phenomenon itself, the critical illness and intensive therapies, and the methods themselves.[10]

To facilitate the accurate and timely detection of delirium, the diagnostic value of the cognitive and behavioral features of delirium were examined.[11] These features were studied with 238 elderly medical patients, 47.5 percent of whom met the criteria for delirium.[3] Measures of attention and concentration were found to best discriminate delirious from nondelirious patients, with a diagnostic accuracy of 90 percent. Of additional relevance for critically ill elderly patients is the fact that these aspects can readily be assessed using nonverbal methods. Conversely, measures of disorientation and agitated behaviors, long considered classic manifestations of delirium, were nonspecific as they did not discriminate at all. Thus, delirium is detected more effectively by focusing on concentration and attention rather than orientation and psychomotor behavior.[11]

VARIABLE MANIFESTATIONS OF DELIRIUM

Anecdotally, it has been noted that the clinical manifestations of delirium vary between individuals and within an individual across time.[10] Yet, until recently, there has been no research to support these clinical anecdotes. Recently, three patterns of delirium based on predisposing factors and pathological processes have been identified.[12] Pattern I, labeled cognitive restricted, results from environmental challenges, i.e., an environment that is sensory depriving, overloading, and unfamiliar, characteristics typical of ICU environments. Additionally, it is also thought that pattern I may be a precursory state, since these individuals frequently progress to pattern II and/or pattern III.[12] Pattern II, or physiologic instability, has fluctuating symptomatology and arises from pathophysiologic states such as hypoxemia. Pattern III, or metabolic instability, is manifested by motor symptoms typically observed in encephalopathies and results from the toxic challenges of impaired hepatic or renal function or from the polypharmacy so often practiced with the elderly. These patterns of delirium not only are congruent with the variable and fluctuating nature of delirium but also can potentially facilitate more effective pattern-specific intervention.[12]

ETIOLOGY OF DELIRIUM

The etiology of delirium has been the most prevalent focus of nursing studies.[7,13–15] Although subjects have varied by age and illness, studies have consistently identified factors such as intraoperative hypotension, postoperative hypothermia, age, and physiologic alterations.

Extrapolating from this profile of delirium,[7] recommended parameters for nursing actions include maintaining or reestablishing normal physiologic status, creating an environment that promotes orientation, assisting in the accurate interpretation of information, and administering medications judiciously.

MANAGEMENT OF DELIRIUM

Nursing interventions traditionally have been rooted in the manipulation of interpersonal and environmental factors. These approaches have been aimed at the strange environment, altered sensory input, loss of control and independence, disruption in life pattern, immobility, pain, and disruption in elimination patterns.[16]

Testing various combinations of these approaches, interventions that provided orientation and clarification, corrected sensory deficit(s), and provided continuity of care were found to be the most effective in reducing delirium in the elderly postoperative patients.[16] However, since over 40 percent of the subjects in this study still manifested some degree of delirium, these interventions may be necessary but not sufficient components of an effective approach to reducing or preventing delirium.

Currently there is much work in progress to test various approaches for treating delirium. The underlying principle of these approaches is the belief that to be effective an intervention must be specific to the circumstances of the individual. Following the rubric of (1) eliminating or correcting the underlying cause and (2) providing supportive and symptomatic measures, individualized interventions for delirium are part of a cluster of interdisciplinary studies recently funded by the John A. Hartford Foundation.

APPLICATION OF THE FINDINGS TO PRACTICE

These nursing studies have included most aspects of delirium and were conducted with samples of adult patients of various ages and illnesses. Despite these differences, the findings are rather consistent. Additionally, integrating these findings creates a comprehensive protocol for the care of elderly patients at risk of becoming or who have become delirious. First, by virtue of the concomitants of aging and critical illness, these patients should be considered at high risk for this problem, and thus, surveillance efforts must be a routine part of their care. These surveillance efforts for delirium should occur in the initial period of hospitalization or early in the postoperative phase, since these are the times when a delirium is most likely to develop. Furthermore, efforts at detection should focus on the assessment of the patient's ability to concentrate and to attend to stimuli, an assessment best accomplished using a mental status questionnaire in combination with a behavioral rating scale.[17] Second, because the etiology is typically multifactorial and dynamic in nature, a pattern-specific[14] or algorithmic[18] approach is recommended to effectively identify the cause(s) and, subsequently, to intervene. Last, the parameters considered necessary to effectively intervene consist of (1) eliminating or correcting the underlying pathophysiologic condition and (2) providing symptomatic and supportive measures.

RECOMMENDATIONS FOR RESEARCH ABOUT DELIRIUM

Although consensus is developing about many of the clinical aspects of delirium, debate continues about the fundamental nature of the phenomenon. Some consider delirium to be a disturbance in consciousness, historically the position advocated by neurologists.[19] Others contend that delirium is a global impairment in cognition, concepts that are related but are vastly different.[3,7,14] Surprisingly, this is an aspect of the knowledge of delirium that has profound implications for the detection, assessment, and management of this clinical phenomenon, and yet it is an aspect of the study of delirium that continues to be avoided. Attention from the scientific community is warranted.

Clinically, much work remains. Specifically, interdisciplinary efforts are needed that focus on (1) obtaining definitive evidence linking specific pathologic conditions to the pathogenesis of delirium, (2) confirming the clinical and diagnostic features of delirium, (3) examining the phenomenon across multiple illnesses to determine whether or not certain features are specific to the delirium or the illness, (4) describing the evolution and resolution of the phenomenon, and (5) delineating effective protocols for the detection, prevention, and intervention of delirium.

Beyond a doubt, delirium is a complex dilemma for the afflicted critically ill elder, the patient's family, the involved nursing and medical intensivists, health care institutions, and society at large. However, delirium is not the only complicating factor in the intensive therapy for this patient population. Basic, applied clinical, ethical, and health policy research relative to the intensive therapy for the critically ill elderly patient population is vital. Answers to basic questions are required about the appropriateness of intensive therapy for elderly persons and rationing of life-sustaining technologies and services. It is essential that this research be methodologically sound, rigorous, and free of any bias, especially age bias. Additionally, research must be conducted to examine which factors commonly associated with aging interact to produce the less than desirable outcomes of intensive therapy so often attributed to the elderly. For example, is it the severity of illness, the multiple chronic health conditions, malnutrition, poor physiologic reserve, or some other factor(s) yet to be discovered? And although this work has relevance for patients other than the elderly, it is the latter for which it is of vital importance.

REFERENCES

1. Fedullo AJ, Swinburne AG: Relationship of patient age to cost and survival in a medical ICU. Crit Care Med 11:155, 1983.
2. Sage WM, Hurst CR, Silverman JF, Bortz WM: Intensive care for the elderly: Outcome of elective and nonelective admissions. J Am Geriatr Soc 35:312, 1987.
3. American Psychiatric Association (APA): *Diagnostic and Statistical* Manual of Mental Disorders, 3rd ed, rev. Washington, DC, APA, 1987.
4. Williams MA, Campbell EB, Raynor WW, Jr, Musholt MA, Mlynarczyk SM, Crane LF: Predictors of acute confusional states in hospitalized elderly patients. Res Nurs Health 8:31, 1985b.
5. Levkoff SE, Besdine RW, Wetle T: Acute confusional states (delirium) in the hospitalized elderly. Ann Rev Gerontol Geriatr 6:1, 1986.
6. Lipkowski, ZJ: Delirium in the elderly patient. N Engl J Med 321:264, 1989.
7. Foreman MD: Confusion in the hospitalized elderly: Incidence, onset, and associated factors. Res Nurs Health 12:21, 1989.
8. Williams MA, Ward SE, Campbell EB: Issues in studying con-

fusion in older patients. Paper presented at New Frontiers in Nursing Research, sponsored by the University of Alberta Faculty of Nursing, Edmonton, Alberta, Canada, 1986.
9. Palmateer LM, McCartney JR: Do nurses know when patients have cognitive deficits? J Gerontol Nurs 11:6, 1985.
10. Foreman MD: Acute confusional states in the hospitalized elderly: A research dilemma. Nurs Res 35:34, 1986.
11. Foreman MD: The cognitive and behavioral nature of acute confusional states. Scholarly Inq Nurs Prac 5(1):3, 1991.
12. Neelon VJ, Champagne MT, Moore KA: Acute confusion in hospitalized elders: Vertical and horizontal patterns of development—Implications for interventions. Paper presented at Elder Care: Today's Research, Tomorrow's Practice, sponsored by the Center for the Advancement of Nursing Practice, Beth Israel Hospital, Boston, MA, April 8, 1989.
13. Quinless FW, Cassese M, Atherton N: The effect of selected preoperative, intraoperative, and postoperative variables on the development of postcardiotomy psychosis in patients undergoing heart surgery. Heart Lung 14:334, 1985.
14. Roberts BL, Lincoln RE: Cognitive disturbance in hospitalized and institutionalized elders. Res Nurs Health 11:309, 1988.
15. Sadler PD: Incidence, degree, and duration of postcardiotomy delirium. Heart Lung 10:1084, 1981.
16. Williams MA, Campbell EB, Raynor WW, Jr, Mlynarczyk SM, Ward SE: Reducing acute confusional states in elderly patients with hip fractures. Res Nurs Health 8:329, 1985.
17. Foreman MD, Gillies DA, Wagner D: Impaired cognition in the critically ill elderly patient: Clinical implications. Crit Care Nurs Quart 12(1):61, 1989.
18. Foreman MD: Acute confusional states in the elderly: An algorithm. Dimens Crit Care Nurs 3:207, 1984.
19. Engel GL, Romano J: Delirium: A syndrome of cerebral insufficiency. J Chronic Dis 9:260, 1959.

Chapter 188

CLINICAL INVESTIGATION IN CRITICALLY ILL PATIENTS

JOHN F. MURRAY
ROBERTO RODRIGUEZ-ROISIN

Modern medical research is an enormous enterprise, that includes basic science in a variety of disciplines; experiments in thousands of different models of health and disease; epidemiologic analyses; clinical trials; and measurements and observations of patients and normal subjects. But the overall aim of this complex activity—the bottom line, in current parlance—is to improve the health and well-being of human beings. Clinical investigation in critically ill patients occupies only a tiny niche in the immense continuum of medical research, but its goals, although focused on a relatively small and highly selected group of patients, are incorporated in the overall objective:

> To provide new knowledge that leads to improvements in the diagnosis, treatment, and prevention of disorders that cause critical illness in human beings.

Note that there are two distinct, but interrelated, parts to this objective. Clinical investigation begins with the acquisition of new knowledge from the study of seriously ill patients, and then uses this knowledge to improve their condition. Clinical investigation of any variety often presents formidable difficulties; for reasons we will point out, clinical investigation of critical illness is probably the most demanding of all, because it centers on extremely sick patients. We are referring here, of course, to experiments that are carried out on patients while they are in intensive care units (ICUs)—research that involves diagnostic manipulations or therapeutic interventions that would not ordinarily be done, followed by assessment of the outcome of these innovations. This focus creates medical, ethical, and financial conflicts that are less intense, or simply absent, in other forms of medical research.

Because our interests and expertise lie mainly in the field of respiratory medicine, many of the examples we will cite come from this specialty and from our own experience. This orientation in no way discounts the importance of studies in other disciplines related to critical care medicine, and the general principles that we will discuss here apply to all specialties. With this caveat in mind, we would like to provide an example of how the results of clinical investigation of critical illness have advanced knowledge and improved care of patients in ICUs.

Nosocomial pneumonia is a common and devastating complication in patients with respiratory failure who are being mechanically ventilated.[1] For example, in a prospective study of 129 patients with adult respiratory distress syndrome (ARDS), among whom 108 episodes of various infections developed, pneumonia was the most common cause (68 percent) and the mortality rate in those in whom it occurred was 88 percent.[2] The diagnosis of pneumonia in patients with respiratory failure is difficult, because there are many causes of fever, leukocytosis, and radiographic infiltrations, and the high incidence of airway colonization leads to positive sputum cultures; thus the traditional hallmarks of bronchopulmonary infection are unreliable. An important advance in dealing with this problem was made in 1979 by Wemberly and coworkers,[3] who introduced the method of collecting specimens from the lower respiratory tract for quantitative bacterial culture through a telescoping plugged catheter (TPC) guided through a fiberoptic bronchoscope. Subsequently, Torres and coworkers,[4] in a study of 25 mechanically ventilated patients with suspected pneumonia, showed that a simpler and less expensive technique, using a Métras catheter, for blindly inserting the TPC into the airways gave as good results as directing the TPC visually through a fiberoptic bronchoscope. More recently, Torres and coworkers[5] compared the diagnostic value of quantitative cultures of specimens obtained by bronchoalveolar lavage and by TPC in 35 patients and showed that the two methods were equally valuable. Finally, the results of studies by Fagon and colleagues [6] also supported the use of TPC and quantitative cultures as a way of reducing both toxicity from unnecessary use of antimicrobial drugs and the overall cost of patient management. Collectively, these studies involved more than 200 seriously ill patients with respiratory failure, all of whom were bronchoscoped while being mechanically ventilated—which is not an easy thing to do. But that is not the end of the story; there remains doubt about the reliability of these methods for diagnosing pneumonia in patients who have been taking antimicrobial agents, and neither the sensitivity nor the specificity of the procedures is as high as one would like. Thus, many more such examinations, or different tests, need to be done in patients in ICUs to completely solve the problem.

How to do Clinical Research in Critically Ill Patients

In this section we will describe the basic principles involved in formulating, planning, and carrying out clinical investigation of critically ill patients. In the next, companion, section we will discuss the innumerable impediments to clinical investigation in an ICU that must be recognized and anticipated in order to be avoided. These two sections should not be regarded as a manual on "how to do" clinical research, which requires sophisticated training and experience. Moreover, the planning and logistic considerations must be tailored, as needed, to the particular needs of the

TABLE 188-1 Essential Steps in Clinical Research in Critically Ill Patients

Formulate an hypothesis
Prepare a protocol
Obtain Institutional Review Board (Committee on Human Research) approval
Obtain funding
Perform the study
Communicate the results

patient group that will be studied and the acute care facility in which the research will be performed. The essential steps in clinical study of seriously ill patients are shown in Table 188-1.

FORMULATE AN HYPOTHESIS

All research begins with an hypothesis, which can be thought of as a tentative supposition, made without assumption of its truth, that serves as a starting point for further investigation. An hypothesis, therefore, is an inference made from known facts or observed data in order to test its logical or empirical consequences. This definition implies that there are two steps in the formulation of an hypothesis: the first step is to assimilate a foundation of facts or data, and the second is to reason about what should naturally follow. In clinical medicine the hypothesis may be about basic mechanisms of disease, new methods of treatment, or other areas of uncertainty. Knowledge may be sought for its own sake, but clinical investigation nearly always is performed in an effort to answer a specific medical question—one that should be formulated as an hypothesis. On the basis of the particular hypothesis, experiments are then designed to test whether what *should* follow actually *does.* If it does not, the original hypothesis is invalid and a new one must be derived. Experimental evidence can only support, but never *prove,* an hypothesis. The results of additional experiments may finally disprove an hypothesis that, until then, has been supported by considerable evidence. An hypothesis becomes a "truth" when all the evidence in favor of it becomes incontrovertible.

We cannot overemphasize the importance of having an explicit hypothesis, because it is the hypothesis that defines what experiments need to be done. It is always wise, when one is writing a research protocol (usually the first step in a clinical investigation project) or preparing the results for publication (usually the last step), to enumerate the salient underlying facts and the reasoning from them that led to the specific hypothesis being tested.

PREPARE A PROTOCOL

After a brief introduction that states the hypothesis to be tested, the body of a research protocol is basically a "methods section" that describes in considerable detail exactly how the experiment(s) will be carried out from beginning to end. The essential elements of a research protocol for clinical investigation of critically ill patients are listed in Table 188-2. (The introduction and hypothesis have already been described.)

TABLE 188-2 Essential Elements of a Research Protocol

Introduction and hypothesis
Define patients
Inclusion criteria
Exclusion criteria
Number of subjects
Experimental group
Control group
End points
Outcome variables
Statistical analysis
Interventions
Clinically indicated
For purposes of study
Sequence of measurements
Variables
Frequency
Duration of study
Safeguards
Adverse reactions
Safety and monitoring
Significance
To patient
To others

DEFINE THE PATIENTS

A precise definition of the patients to be enrolled in the study is mandatory but is often neglected. The more general the enrollment criteria (i.e., the more heterogeneous the patient population), the greater the possibility of overlooking an effect (positive or negative) in one of the incorporated but undefined subgroups; this is especially true of research in critically ill patients, because the number of subjects in the entire study is usually small. Nothing better illustrates the problem created by the lack of a precise definition in clinical investigation than the legacy of inconclusive data surrounding that nebulous condition ARDS. It is likely that a crisper classification of patients into the various subgroups that make up ARDS would accelerate the acquisition of knowledge concerning its pathogenesis and treatment.[7]

It is always a good idea to list the specific inclusion and exclusion criteria and to refer to this list each time a patient is evaluated for possible enrollment in the study. These inclusion criteria must specify not only how the condition to be studied will be identified, but how its severity will be judged. There are several ways of assessing severity of illness; a useful and widely applied method is to use the Apache score, or some combination of its variables.[8] Enrollment must depend on the results of routine clinical examinations and laboratory tests that are already available at the time the patient is evaluated. Special studies cannot be done until the patient has been formally entered into the protocol, which requires signed consent (see Consent, under Obtain IRB Approval, below) and permission from the physician responsible for the care of the patient.

NUMBER OF SUBJECTS

In preparing the protocol, considerable thought must be given to the number of patients to be enrolled in the study, in both the experimental and the control group. The number depends on the hypothesis to be tested and on the magnitude of the anticipated difference(s) between the experimental and the control groups—which, of course is not known ahead of time and must be assumed on the basis of available data from preliminary studies. Tables are available in statistical texts that define how many patients need to be studied to achieve a certain *power*, which is the likelihood that if the assumed difference between groups were actually present it will be detected.[9] An inconclusive study that has a low power because of inadequate numbers of subjects loses much of its potential impact.

Once the number of subjects has been defined, the next step is to determine whether the patient resources in the institutional acute care units are sufficient to meet that particular need and during what period of time. For logistic purposes, it is wise to provide documentation, based on past experience, that the necessary number of patients will be available. (Such documentation is mandatory for purposes of obtaining funds from most granting agencies.) If sufficient patients are not available, the project should be abandoned or should be organized as a collaborative effort.

The discussion thus far has assumed that the study will include a control group. Without a suitable control population, the results of experimental studies are descriptive, not comparative; in other words, they describe only what happened under the conditions of the particular experiment. Such information may be useful in documenting pathogenic mechanisms or in creating a receptive environment for subsequent controlled trials. But the results of uncontrolled clinical investigation studies are rarely definitive and should not serve as a basis for widespread revisions of patient care. Matthay[10] cites several examples of "advances" in critical care medicine, based on reports of uncontrolled studies, that affected the practice of the specialty until, much later, the disappointing truth of their ineffectiveness emerged from controlled trials. The popularity of extracorporeal membrane oxygenation (ECMO) after its enthusiastic—but uncontrolled—introduction into clinical practice,[11] and its subsequent demise after a controlled trial was performed,[12] provides but one striking example of this phenomenon. We have the impression that this cycle is now being repeated with low-frequency ventilation with extracorporeal CO_2 removal.

When control subjects are included, the investigators should indicate how patients will be assigned to either the control or the experimental group. Usually this is done by random allocation.

END POINTS

It may seem obtuse to discuss end points, or outcome variables, near the beginning of a description of how to prepare a protocol; but the success of a research project depends on the relevance of what is being measured to the hypothesis being tested, as well as on the accuracy of measurement. So end points need to be considered early, because the data that must be obtained determine the interventions and the method of procedure.

Sufficient information, such as age, sex, and severity of illness indices, should be obtained to categorize the patients thoroughly and to compare the experimental and control groups. But the research question being asked is invariably answered by certain specific outcome variables that must be defined in advance to ensure that they are quantified in the best possible way. Many, many measurements can be made to define responses in critically ill patients, but the results of such a "fishing expedition" more often confuse than clarify, and the key variables may be ignored in the process.

A corollary of the need to specify the outcome variables that will be measured is to identify the statistical methods used to analyze them. Many clinical investigators cannot think beyond a t test, but that method is greatly misused, and many more powerful and precise statistical techniques are available.[13] It is always wise to consult a statistician while preparing the protocol, rather than (as is often the case) after the experiments have been performed.

INTERVENTIONS

One of the most difficult parts of planning clinical investigation in critically ill patients concerns the interventions that may need to be performed in order to obtain essential data. By definition, these patients are already desperately sick; it is always better, when possible, to simplify rather than complicate their care, and, above all, to avoid unnecessary procedures. Every intervention—*without exception*—has undesirable complications. This raises the important question whether any unnecessary procedure can be justified in a critical care setting. For example, is it ethically defensible to do an invasive procedure, such as catheterizing the pulmonary artery to record pressure and measure cardiac output, solely for purposes of an investigation? Pulmonary artery catheters are associated with appreciable complications.[14]

The way around this, of course, is to indicate that the presence of a pulmonary artery catheter *already inserted for clinical purposes* is one of the criteria for enrollment in the study. In this way the decision to do the catheterization, although it may restrict the number of patients available for the study, is made by the clinicians responsible for the patient and is not (or should not be) influenced by the needs of the experiment. However, this convenient solution is not applicable to some types of clinical investigation that include elective procedures with a small but finite risk, such as bronchoalveolar lavage to study patients with ARDS,[15] or bronchial biopsies in symptomatic asthmatics.[16] To keep matters straight, the protocol should specify which interventions will *have* been done for clinical purposes and which *will* be done for purposes of the study. Then the latter must be justified on the basis of a favorable balance between the potential risks of the procedure(s) and the likely benefits of the study.

SEQUENCE OF MEASUREMENTS

It is important to define ahead of time, and to indicate in the protocol, exactly which variables will be measured and when. This greatly facilitates analysis of the results, because all subjects in a given series will be studied similarly. The preparation of reporting forms that specify the variables to be measured and exact timing of measurements will greatly aid the team of investigators that performs the study, and will ensure uniformity of data collection. This section of the protocol should also indicate when the study will end. If it is open-ended, the criteria for termination (or continuation) should be enumerated.

SAFEGUARDS

The investigators must acknowledge that the well-being of the patients is their primary consideration, and the protocol should state how the patients' safety will be guaranteed. Obviously, if unanticipated clinical events occur, such as a fall in blood pressure or arterial P_{O_2} or a rise in temperature or P_{CO_2}—whether related to the study or not—the study should be terminated to permit additional diagnostic or therapeutic maneuvers. This decision can be made either by the attending physician or by the leader of the investigative team.

Most institutional review boards (IRBs, described in full below) require that any adverse reactions—any untoward effect conceivably related to the study—be reported to them promptly. Forms are often available for this purpose. Adverse reactions that involve new equipment must be reported to the equipment's manufacturer; and, in the United States, those that involve new drugs must be reported to the Food and Drug Administration (FDA).

As a further safeguard, it is customary for any study involving many patients who are enrolled in experimental and control groups over a long period of time to include a data safety and monitoring committee composed of scientists who are not directly involved with the investigation. This group of experts is particularly useful for assessing the progress of on-going studies in which the investigators are unaware (blinded) of the results, as in the recently concluded study of the use of high-frequency ventilation in newborn babies with infant respiratory distress syndrome.[17] A data safety and monitoring committee periodically reviews the latest results of the study in progress to determine whether it should continue. An investigation is terminated prematurely (i.e., before the anticipated number of subjects has been enrolled) if **1.** a clear statistical difference in results, either favorable or unfavorable, is found between the experimental and control groups, and it becomes unethical to continue, or **2.** continuation of recruitment would be unlikely to result in either a positive or a negative treatment effect.

SIGNIFICANCE

The written protocol concludes with a statement about the expected significance of the results. This section should not be a hypothetical promissory note, but a realistic appraisal of the importance of the knowledge to be gained from the study and of its likely effect on the care of patients with critical illness. In many instances the results of an experiment in a particular patient will not benefit that patient directly, but the aggregate results from several patients may improve the care of subsequent patients. The applicability of the results to enrolled and/or future patients should be indicated.

The description of the significance of the results is useful to members of IRBs and study sections, who must judge whether the anticipated knowledge to be gained from the study is sufficiently new and important to offset any of the study's possible adverse effects, and to justify funding. Suffice it to say, this section of the protocol should be persuasive and honest.

OBTAIN IRB APPROVAL

Because of the widespread belief, which was partly justified, that the extant system of unregulated research by physicians had led to excesses and had infringed on the rights of experimental subjects, the United States government in 1966 began to require prior review and approval of all federally funded research using human subjects. The mechanism by which this review is carried out is an IRB or a committee on human research (CHR), which have become an integral part of clinical investigation. Nowadays clinical research cannot be performed, virtually anywhere in the world, without first having been approved by the local IRB. Moreover, IRB approval is necessary before most granting agencies will consider a proposal for possible funding. The IRBs are composed of clinician-scientists from a wide variety of disciplines; nurses; and persons from the social and behavioral sciences, law, and theology. Usually at least one community member not affiliated with the institution serves on the IRB.

ACTIVITIES SUBJECT TO REVIEW

To clarify the distinction between innovative clinical practice, on the one hand, and clinical investigation, on the other, the Committee on Human Research of the University of California, San Francisco (UCSF) states:

> Thus, an established and accepted diagnostic or therapeutic procedure done for the benefit of the patient is not an experiment, and hence not within CHR jurisdiction to review, unless it is done as part of a comparison of standard practices. However, questions often arise about the necessity of submitting various innovations in diagnosis and therapy for CHR review. Previous DHEW [Department of Health, Education, and Welfare] guidelines stated that: "This policy is not concerned with the risks inherent in professional practice, as long as these do not exceed the bounds of established and accepted procedures, including innovative practices applied in the interests of individual patient, student or client." The Committee has interpreted this passage to mean that risks of any innovation applied to a patient for the *sole* purpose of aiding that individual are governed by the customary ethics of medicine (e.g., consultation with peers, obtaining informed consent from the patient or family), and do not require CHR review.

> On the other hand, when innovative diagnostic or therapeutic procedures are considered part of a study, they must be reviewed by the CHR in accordance with DHHS [Department of Health and Human Services] regulations. For example, a research study is by definition undertaken if, in addition to patient care, information is gathered for scientific purposes, i.e., with the intent of obtaining "generalizable knowledge," or if it is contemplated that innovative treatment on one patient will be repeated in the same or other patients in order to compare it to standard treatment.

CONSENT

One of the key elements in a research project involving human beings is to ensure that the individual subject gives free and informed consent to participate in the study. The Committee on Human Research of UCSF explicitly states, "Any person who is to be a subject of research, whether designed for his/her own direct benefit or for the advancement of scientific knowledge in general, must understand as completely as possible what is to be done and what the potential risks and benefits are. The person must give his/her consent freely, without pressure or inappropriate inducement." To ensure that free and informed consent is indeed obtained, the IRB reviews the recruitment and consent process, which obviously must be listed in the research proposal, and the consent form itself, which must be included with the protocol.

The requirement for free and informed consent is not easily satisfied in the ICU, because of the nature of the illnesses that cause people to be hospitalized there. By definition, ICU patients are nearly always extremely sick; they are often drugged, intubated, restrained, or otherwise rendered incapable of participating in the type of meaningful exchange that should precede enrollment in a clinical research project. This poses serious problems that are discussed below, under Impediments to Clinical Research in Critical Illness.

RISK-BENEFIT ASSESSMENT

The final step in the IRB approval process is an evaluation of the risks and benefits inherent in the study. The IRB must decide on the basis of the material submitted to it whether "The risks to the subject are so outweighed by the sum of the benefit to the subject and importance of the knowledge to be gained as to warrant a decision to allow the subject to accept [those] risks."[18] Such an assessment is a complex task. The risks may be physical, psychological and/or social; the benefits may pertain to the person, the group to which he or she belongs, and/or society. To assess the types and degrees of both risk and benefit, the IRB must rely heavily on information provided in the research protocol and consent form. Thus the study must be scientifically sound, and the nature and likelihood of all risks and benefits must be fully delineated in the protocol. There is no justification for placing any patient at risk, however minimal, if the design of the study and method of procedure are inadequate and no benefit will accrue from the investigation.

OBTAIN FUNDING

"Obtain funding" for clinical research in critically ill patients is more easily said than done, and during the past few years has become steadily more difficult. The reasons for this are complex, but include the facts that clinical research is widely seen as far from the cutting edge of modern medical science; that research expenses for clinical personnel and patient studies are extremely high; and that results are slow to be realized. Nevertheless, because the costs of the research cannot be passed on to third-party carriers or to the hospital, separate funds must be obtained to cover at least those costs that are related to the research itself (i.e., those interventions performed solely for purposes of the study). In California, third-party carriers generally do not pay for most experimental treatments nor for any research activities in the care of patients; therefore, physicians and hospitals are unlikely to receive any reimbursement except through granting agencies.

When applying for research funds, it is perfectly legitimate, and in some places obligatory, to include itemized requests for salaries of personnel, equipment, supplies, and hospitalization costs. But everything must be justified on the basis of the actual time that the investigative team will spend in the study; and this, in turn, depends on the number of experiments to be performed. Considerable clinical research support, of which only a small fraction supports studies in critically ill patients, is provided by the U.S. National Institutes of Health through their Special Centers of Research (SCOR) and contract (RFP) programs. But as everyone who has sought them realizes, these are highly competitive awards. Moreover, at least as judged by the authorship of articles in top-notch medical journals that report the results of clinical investigation, contributions by American scientists to this important activity are declining—a decrease that may be linked to a slowed growth of funding from the National Institutes of Health for clinical research.[19] This is occurring at a time when increasing numbers of non-American scientists are conducting studies that have a quite different basis of funding; research activities and costs are often integrated within the implementation and reimbursement structures providing critical care within each institution, and supplemented for special costs of investigation by grants from industrial and pharmaceutical firms.

Professional organizations contribute somewhat to clinical research, but more and more support seems to come from pharmaceutical companies and equipment manufacturers. These corporations underwrite much high-quality and useful research, but generally in fields in which they have commercial or proprietary interests. Clearly, one of the problems that need to be addressed by the leaders in critical care medicine and their professional organizations is how to fund unrestricted (i.e., non-drug or non-machine-oriented) clinical investigation in the future.

PERFORM THE STUDY

When one has progressed this far, actually carrying out the study is almost anticlimactic, and in some ways is the easiest part. But it is also the part that requires consummate attention to detail and thoughtful consideration of the logistic constraints of clinical investigation in an ICU. An elaborate or complex research project often begins with a few preliminary "pilot" studies. These enable the investigator to test the protocol under actual experimental conditions, after which it can be modified, if needed; any substantial changes will require reapproval by the IRB. Some of the problems that pertain to how the study is performed, such as the recruitment of patients, ethical aspects, selection of personnel, technical difficulties, and publication delays, are discussed under Impediments to Clinical Research in Critical Illness, below.

COMMUNICATE THE RESULTS

When Dr. Julius H. Comroe, Jr., was Director of the Cardiovascular Research Institute of the University of California, San Francisco (1958–1973), he made a point of telling each new trainee that a research project was not finished until the results were published. This is still true. Science progresses by building on already established facts; this means that the methods, raw data, and calculations of new experiments must be made available for other scientists to review and reflect on. Abstracts, oral presentations, and posters are useful means of scientific communication, but lack the "clout" of an original article published in a rigorously edited, peer-reviewed journal. Such a publication should be the goal of all serious investigators, and the senior member of the research team has the responsibility for ensuring that the report is not only written but finally published. Part of the education of young physician-scientists is to learn communication skills; the results of a research project provide the customary material on which to base a seminar or to write a paper. But there are inherent in this system some built-in delays to publication, which we will discuss next.

Impediments to Clinical Research of Critical Illness

We have said or implied several times, thus far, that clinical investigation of critically ill patients is not easy. In this section we discuss the reasons why this is so, and will suggest some ways to avoid the most common problems.

RECRUITMENT OF PATIENTS

All clinical research, by definition, involves patients in one way or another. In a study of highly selected patients it is particularly important that all eligible candidates be identified and enrolled, if possible, in the investigation. This presents special problems when the patients are in ICUs.

IDENTIFICATION

The first responsibility of the investigators is to set up a system that allows prompt identification of every patient who is a candidate for enrollment. Suitable patients are seldom easy to find and overlooking even a single one is a serious setback. The most effective way of recruitment, in our experience, is to have a member of the investigative team—usually a research fellow—survey the acute care units once or twice a day, every day, to find potential patients. Because many studies intend to examine patients with early or new-onset disorders, the recruitment system often needs to operate 24 hours a day; this stipulation nearly always requires the participation of the ICU nurses or house staff, who usually are very busy and are not committed to the project. In fact, nurses and house staff may believe that it is a nuisance for them to cooperate—and, possibly, that it is not in the patients' best interest to participate in the investigation. To ensure their assistance, the ICU staff need to be thoroughly briefed about the objectives, methods, and importance of the investigation. In particular, staff members must be reassured that their role will be only to notify a study physician that a prospective candidate is in the unit, and that *someone else* will evaluate the patient, obtain the consent, and collect the data. It is unreasonable—and unworkable—to expect nurses and house staff, who are already stressed, to take on extra work voluntarily, and they cannot be made to do it. We have also found that some sort of tangible inducement to the groups involved (e.g., house staff) helps to secure their participation; "finder's fees" have rightly been declared unethical.[20]

Once a patient has been identified as an eligible candidate, the investigator must ensure that all of the entry criteria and none of the exclusion criteria are present at the time the study actually begins, which may be a few hours later, or even the next day. For instance, a steady-state condition (defined as ± 5 percent at maximum in heart rate, respiratory frequency, tidal volume, and end-tidal P_{O_2} and P_{CO_2}), a mandatory methodological criterion for any investigation in pulmonary gas exchange, may come and go. Changes in a patient's status from suitable for enrollment to unsuitable are particularly apt to occur when patients are seen in the middle of the night or on weekends—times when the necessary human and technical resources for the investigation are difficult to mobilize. If studies of acute illness are planned, personnel must be available around the clock. In one of our studies in Barcelona on the patterns of ventilation-perfusion distributions in acute asthma,[21] the principal research fellow was on call 24 hours a day, 7 days a week, to evaluate potential patients, enroll them into the study when possible, and then perform the first series of measurements, which were obtained as soon as regular breathing could be maintained through a unidirectional valve for at least 10 to 15 min. The success of this investigation depended entirely on the availability of a person who was able not only to do the evaluation and obtain the consent, but then to carry out the initial tests, *regardless* of when the patient was admitted to the hospital.

CONSENT

Permission to perform studies on seriously ill patients is a delicate matter that has been addressed by most IRBs. At UCSF, for example, "the informed consent concept is extended to those studies in which subjects are not able to give personal consent for themselves. Here the consent document is addressed to those who have been designated responsible for the subject's well-being (e.g., parents for children). The Committee's concern is to verify that the consent process and documents are likely to assist these persons to make an informed decision which is in the best interests of the subject." But problems often arise when patients are too sick (e.g., shock), have certain illnesses (e.g., meningitis), or are receiving drugs (e.g., benzodiazepines or morphine) that affect consciousness and reason, and therefore cannot give informed consent. These kinds of patients are commonly encountered in ICUs.

In one of our studies, in San Francisco, of the effectiveness of methylprednisolone in septic shock,[22] we attempted to obtain informed consent from patients eligible for enrollment in the study when the patients were able to make informed decisions themselves. However, this was rarely possible because of the abnormal mental status commonly associated with hypotension and presumed sepsis. In cases where a close relative was identified and was available, that person was asked to act on behalf of the patient. However, this too was seldom possible, because of the acute nature of many patients' deterioration and the unavailability of suitable relatives in many instances. When neither patients nor their relatives could provide informed consent, the patients' attending physician and house staff were consulted for approval, and other physicians, familiar with the patients' condition but neither directly caring for them nor personally involved in the study, determined whether the patients could be enrolled. This consent process had been approved by the Committee on Human Research of UCSF and was contingent, at all times, on the satisfaction of four criteria: (1) that the study offered significant potential benefit and only minimal risk to patients in the study; (2) that the waiver or alteration of a research subject's informed consent would not adversely affect his or her welfare; (3) that the research could not practicably be carried out without the waiver or alteration; and (4) that whenever possible, the patients were to be provided with additional pertinent information upon participation in the study. Other IRBs have developed their own methods of waiving the usual procedure for obtaining informed consent from seriously ill patients who may be candidates for clinical research.

ETHICS

The basic ethical principles that govern human investigation are detailed in the Nuremberg Code of 1947 and the World Medical Association Declaration of Helsinki, revised in 1975.[23] These statements emphasize that participation in clinical investigation must be voluntary and stress that the interests of the subject must predominate over those of science and society. These irreducible principles serve as the fundamental guidelines for the evaluation process and the actions taken by IRBs (see above), and apply throughout the world, regardless of regional customs and requirements.[24] However, as was pointed out in a recent debate on the ethics of international collaborative research, investigators need to respect local sensitivities and to accommodate community traditions in obtaining consent and informing subjects about the risks and benefits of clinical investigation.[25]

The reason why the subject of ethics is addressed here, under Impediments to Clinical Research, is not that the principles themselves present a problem, but that they may present the investigator with a conflict of interest that needs to be recognized and dealt with. A potential conflict is inherent in the fact that the physician who acquires the informed consent is nearly always a member of the investigative team and, as such, stands to profit directly—and personally—from the patient's participation in the study. Investigators may benefit in several different ways from enrolling a subject: by obtaining results that lead to funds for further research, by gaining enhanced professional stature and promotion, and by satisfying the intellectual curiosity and emotional investment that led to a commitment to the project in the first place. Of course, these are the fuels that drive clinical research toward new and useful knowledge, and without this impetus critical care will not improve. Thus, when the research requires seriously ill patients to suffer discomfort, indignity, or danger beyond that necessary for ordinary clinical care, the investigators' goals may conflict with the patients' best interests. The way to avoid this, of course, is to have someone obtain the consent who does not stand to gain if the patient participates in the study; but this is not always possible. The next best solution is to be sure that whoever does interview the patient for possible enrollment is sensitive to the patient's needs and aware of the delicacy of the situation.

Another conflict between the patient's best interests and the researcher's desires may occur during the course of the study itself. For example, the principal aim of an investigation done by one of us[26] was to determine the mechanisms of abnormal pulmonary gas exchange in a series of critically ill patients with status asthmaticus who were selected because they were so sick that they required intubation and mechanical ventilation. To obtain an estimate of the most abnormal gas exchange conditions, according to the original protocol that had been approved, it was planned to perform the initial measurements as soon as possible after ventilatory support was begun. We soon learned, however, that desperately ill asthmatic patients are in a particularly unstable and precarious condition at the very time at which we wanted to make our measurements. Because patient welfare is paramount and would have been compromised by our interventions, we deferred our studies until it was perfectly safe to continue. Investigators must recognize that a conflict may arise between what they would like to do and what can safely and prudently be done, and must *always* give way to the patient's needs when this occurs.

PERSONNEL

There are two categories of personnel concerned with clinical research of critically ill patients: medical and technical. Both contribute importantly to the success or failure of the investigation.

MEDICAL

It is widely acknowledged that the clinical benefits of being hospitalized in an ICU derive largely from the skilled and devoted attention provided by the nursing staff. Accordingly, these key people must welcome clinical investigation, which they may perceive as an intrusion, into their units if the research is to have the maximum likelihood of success. To create a receptive environment, the principal investigator—and preferably, also, the medical staff who will be directly involved in the collection of data at the bedside—should meet with the nursing staff before the study begins. At this meeting, the investigators should explain the objectives of the study, the reasons for carrying it out, and the methods that will be used; the respective roles of the nurses, attending physicians, and researchers should be clearly established, all questions answered, and all concerns dispelled.

TECHNICAL

The considerations that apply to the selection of personnel for investigation in the ICU should follow the general principle of "the less the better." People occupy precious space around the bedside, and sometimes, perversely, tend to stay put in emergencies and may be harder to displace than machines. So only indispensable personnel should be in the ICU during the study. Others can wait outside the unit, or in their laboratories, for specimens or records to be delivered for analysis or examination. And, as has been implied throughout, the one or two members of the research team who are at the bedside should be knowledgeable about clinical investigation in critically ill patients, and should be prepared and able to respond quickly and appropriately to any emergency. Personnel in training must know ahead of time how to react if things go wrong. Obviously, nurses and physicians who have already had some ICU experience are the most desirable persons to perform clinical research of seriously ill patients.

TECHNICAL CONSIDERATIONS

Much of today's medical research involves the use of complicated "high-tech" instruments, and clinical investigation in the ICU is no exception. However, the ever-increasing sophistication of equipment sometimes creates problems in the study of critically ill patients.

EQUIPMENT

Careful consideration must be given to the choice of equipment to be used at the bedside. ICUs are already crowded, and access to the bedside is frequently limited by ventilators, pumps, drainage systems, traction devices, and other medical and surgical paraphernalia. The last thing a nurse wants to see rolled into the unit is another piece of hardware that further compromises his or her ability to care for the patient. A huge, bulky gamma camera detector, for example, when positioned over the thorax to record radioactivity in the lungs or heart, prevents turning the patient, makes suctioning extremely difficult, and creates an impossible situation during a cardiorespiratory arrest or other emergency. Space constraints are particularly bad in units that are subdivided into a series of small rooms with separate doors; under these circumstances, adding a large piece of equipment may actually block the door, or one side of the room, and severely restrict access to the patient.

When equipment is brought to the bedside, it should stay there for as short a time as possible. This requires not only tight scheduling of the personnel who will use the equipment, but the performance in advance, outside the unit, of as much setting-up and calibrating as possible.

OPERATION

There may also be problems with the operation or performance of the equipment. Murphy's Law—that if something can go wrong, it will—seems to have particular application in the ICU. The investigators need to check continuously to ensure that all the parts and pieces involved in the experimental procedure are working properly. All sorts of unexpected problems with the equipment can occur at any time without warning, either while data are being collected during the experiment or during the subsequent analysis and processing of specimens. To avoid operational failures it is advisable, first, to calibrate all the instruments as many times as possible, particularly those that are prone to technical lapses; second, to verify that the control (baseline) measurements are within the expected range; and third, to collect the data without problems. If there are doubts, mistakes, or difficulties, it is always better to stop the experiment temporarily and try to correct them. When everything is working properly again the experiment can continue, provided that the schedule of data collection has not been irrevocably altered and that it still appears worthwhile to go ahead. As a general rule, it is not advisable to use equipment that is not under the direct supervision (maintenance, operation, and quality control) of the investigators and their technical team. It goes without saying that the technicians must be well trained in the methods used and must be confident about their roles in the experiment. An experienced team of medical and technical personnel is indispensable for this kind of research.

ANALYSIS

Many physiologic variables, such as blood pressure, heart rate, temperature, and ventilator settings, are measured and recorded at the bedside. But many other measurements—e.g., of P_{O_2}, P_{CO_2}, pH, biochemical and hematologic variables, and radioactivity—are made in laboratories that may be some distance from the ICU in which the patients are being studied. This poses logistic problems that need to be thought through in advance: how to get the specimens to the various participating laboratories and, conversely, how to get the results back to the central registry. Specimens may need prompt or special handling (e.g., chemicals added, centrifugation, or freezing), or transportation (e.g., by hand, automobile, or mail). Thus, the collection and delivery system needs to be organized and coordinated so that everyone involved knows what to expect, when to expect it, and what to do with it after it arrives.

PUBLICATION DELAYS

Once the data have been collected, more work and great effort are still needed to get the whole project completely finished. "Finished" means published in a reputable, peer-reviewed medical journal. Many investigators, particularly inexperienced research fellows, make the error of assuming that writing a paper is simple and can easily be done in a matter of weeks; 4 to 6 months is a better estimate. Failure to allow sufficient time to finish the entire manuscript—including text, tables, figures, and references—before the responsible research fellow moves on to his or her next position is ruinous; the pressures of the new job invariably mean long delays before work on the manuscript resumes.

Junior investigators, and sometimes even senior scientists, can also cause long delays in preparing work for publication, but the reason in these instances is different: these investigators prefer doing new experiments to writing up the results of old ones. This illustrates the simple fact that preparing a scientific article is hard work, harder than performing research, and is a task that requires discipline and time. However, the facts are that aspiring academicians must "publish or perish," and old academicians must publish or risk not getting funded; these pressures have helped to keep the scientific presses rolling during the past few years.

There are other delays in the publication system that, for the most part, are not under the investigator's control. The first of these is the editorial review process, which may take from a few weeks to several months. (More than 2 months is unconscionable, yet quite common, and means that the editors or the reviewers—or both—should speed things up.) Then there is nearly always the need to revise the manuscript, which puts the ball back in the authors' court again. And finally there is acceptance and publication, involving editing, review of proofs, and printing; this usually requires from 2 to 4 months. Altogether, from the end of the experiments to the appearance of the printed article, the process takes from 18 months to 3 years.

This timetable assumes that the manuscript is accepted by the first journal to which it is submitted. If not, the duration to publication is greatly lengthened; extensive rewriting is usually required, which should always take into account the first reviewers' criticisms, and new experiments may need to be performed.

Writing in English, the most widely used language for scientific articles, presents special problems for authors from non-English-speaking countries. Even scientists who have trained in English-speaking countries for several years are unlikely to have acquired all the nuances necessary to write an articulate, easily understood manuscript. This problem can be overcome only by having someone fluent in English—preferably an investigator who is familiar with the subject of the study—review and correct the paper before it is submitted to a journal for consideration. This, of course, adds another delay, but will greatly increase the chances of the manuscript's being accepted.

The Future of Clinical Research in Critical Care

It should be obvious to the reader that we believe that carefully planned, thoughtfully executed studies of critically ill patients are important, challenging, and rewarding. But there are some serious problems impeding the full development of clinical investigation in this field, and they are likely to worsen in the future.

ACADEMIC BASE

Critical care medicine has come of age during the past decade, and is now a designated field of special competence of the American Board of Internal Medicine and its counterparts in the fields of surgery, anesthesiology, pediatrics, obstetrics, and neurology. Moreover, the concept of the "intensivist," which has long been accepted in Europe, is now taking hold in the United States. However, critical care medicine in this country is still languishing as an academic discipline, because responsibility for patient care, teaching, and research is fragmented among the different departments and subspecialty divisions that control most of the ICUs in hospitals. Each of these units is a direct extension of a department's or division's other activities, and as such does not constitute a unique academic entity. The advantage of this system is high-quality clinical input; the disadvantage is a "Tower of Babel" research enterprise. Part of the resulting problem in research communication is alleviated by the availability of professional societies that deal with the broad field of critical care medicine. However, it seems to us that American, and some European, chest physicians concerned with critical care save their best work for presentation at the American Thoracic Society; likewise, surgeons like to present their work before surgical societies; and so on. New and important advances are seldom heard first at critical care meetings. It is unlikely that the present haphazard organization of ICUs within the majority of academic institutions in the United States is going to change soon; until it does, clinical investigation of critically ill patients will not reach its full potential.

MANPOWER

Major medical centers with academic commitments need to have sufficient manpower in their ICUs to meet their obligations for patient care, teaching, and research. At present, it is not clear where all this manpower is going to come from—especially for carrying out research.

The physicians who do clinical research—clinical investigators—are diminishing in number and have been called "an endangered species."[27] There are many reasons for the decline in appeal of clinical investigation for young physician-academicians (e.g., salaries, the seduction of clinical practice, uncertainties of funding, etc.); probably the most important is the realization, reinforced by available research dollars, that molecular biology and other basic-science disciplines offer the fastest track to academic stardom. What is less well known is that it is extremely difficult, if not impossible, for a physician to maintain reasonably adequate clinical skills—which does take time—and compete successfully against PhDs and other full-time investigators in one of the fast-moving fields of basic science. To avoid this kind of academic schizophrenia, Mason[28] has argued persuasively that one can be both a productive scientist and an effective clinician, provided he or she has had suitable training, seeks an academic position with adequate protected research time (75 percent), and focuses on a research topic of clinical interest. If one's chosen specialty is critical care medicine, clinical investigation in the ICU makes the other component of a perfect partnership. There is much more to learn about the scientific basis of intensive care medicine, enough for generations of academicians.

FUNDING

The problem of manpower aside, another limiting factor in clinical investigation of critically ill patients is the unavailability of research funds. We have already commented on the difficulties of obtaining support for clinical investigation in general, and for studies of seriously ill patients in particular—problems that are not easily solved. What is needed is more money for clinical investigation or a reallocation of funds from basic research to clinical research. Neither seems likely in the foreseeable future.

Nevertheless, some research support is available, so the enterprise limps on. We believe it is a system worth investing in and preserving, not only because of discoveries that can be made with existing technology, but to prepare for new advances. No matter what miraculous medical breakthroughs are generated by cell biologists or molecular geneticists, sooner or later they have to be evaluated in patients. That is called *clinical investigation.*

WHY ENCOURAGE CLINICAL RESEARCH?

The main reason for doing clinical research in critically ill patients was pointed out in the introduction to this chapter: to provide new knowledge that leads to improvements in patient care. But there are additional reasons that go far beyond this tangible scientific goal; two of the most important are the following.

INTELLECTUAL ENVIRONMENT

There is no doubt that having an active clinical research program in an ICU enriches the intellectual ambience of the service. We have already pointed out that the nurses, attending physicians, and house staff who care for seriously ill patients must be fully informed about the questions being asked and the methods being used; they should also be brought up to date about the results of the study as these are obtained. In this way, the clinical research activities will contribute to the on-going education of all the professional personnel of the acute care unit.

We also believe that the meticulous approach and rigorous discipline that contribute to a successful research project will spin off to the medical and nursing staff and enhance their performance. We know from personal experience that the presence of a clinical investigation program in a critical care unit improves morale and generates an attitude of pride and excitement in the entire staff.

TRAINING

Training young physician-scientists to do clinical investigation of seriously ill patients is an obligation of the senior medical staff of academically oriented ICUs. We have mentioned previously that an active research program in a critical care unit provides an intellectual boost to everyone concerned, and is a powerful educational factor. The presence of a research training program centered in the unit has the same beneficial effects. Knowledge and attitudes spread, and having a few eager and active research fellows constantly on the scene is a good way to impart a critical and scientific manner of thinking that gradually takes hold throughout the unit. Thus, research and training are complementary educational influences that lead to improvements in patient care.

References

1. Pingleton SK: State of the Art: Complications of acute respiratory failure. Am Rev Respir Dis 137:1463, 1988.
2. Seidenfeld JJ, Pohl DF, Bell RC, et al: Incidence, site and outcome of infections in patients with adult respiratory distress syndrome. Am Rev Respir Dis 134:12, 1986.
3. Wemberly N, Faling LJ, Bartlett JG: A fiberoptic bronchoscopy technique to obtain lower respiratory secretions for bacterial culture. Am Rev Respir Dis 119:337, 1979.
4. Torres A, Puig de la Bellacasa J, Rodriguez-Roisin R, et al: Diagnostic value of telescoping plugged catheters in mechanically ventilated patients with bacterial pneumonia using the Métras catheter. Am Rev Respir Dis 138:117, 1988.
5. Torres A, Puig de la Bellacasa J, Xaubet A, et al: Diagnostic value of quantitative cultures of bronchoalveolar lavage and telescoping plugged catheters in mechanically ventilated patients. Am Rev Respir Dis 140:306, 1989.
6. Fagon J-Y, Chastre J, Hance AJ, et al: Detection of nosocomial lung infection in ventilated patients. Use of a protected specimen brush and quantitative culture techniques in 147 patients. Am Rev Respir Dis 138:110, 1988.
7. Murray JF, Matthay MA, Luce JM, Flick MR: An expanded definition of the adult respiratory distress syndrome. Am Rev Respir Dis 138:720, 1988.
8. Knaus WA, Draper EA, Wagner DP, et al: APACHE II: A severity of disease classification system. Crit Care Med 13:818, 1985.
9. Cohen J: *Statistical Power Analysis for the Behavioral Sciences.* New York Academic Press, 1977, pp 1–474.
10. Matthay MA: New modes of mechanical ventilation for ARDS. How should they be evaluated? Chest 95:1175, 1989.
11. Hill JD, O'Brien TG, Murray JJ, et al: Prolonged extracorporeal oxygenation for acute post-traumatic respiratory failure (shock-lung syndrome). Use of the Bramson membrane lung. N Engl J Med 286:629, 1972.

12. Zapol WM, Snider MT, Hill JD, et al: Extracorporeal membrane oxygenation in severe acute respiratory failure. JAMA 242:2193, 1979.
13. Wallenstein S, Zucker CL, Fleiss JL: Some statistical methods useful in circulation research. Circ Res 47:1, 1980.
14. Boyd KD, Thomas SJ, Gold J. Boyd AD: A prospective study of complications of pulmonary artery catheterizations in 500 consecutive patients. Chest 84:245, 1983.
15. Hallman M, Spragg R, Harrell JH, et al: Evidence of lung surfactant abnormality in respiratory failure. Study of bronchoalveolar lavage phospholipids, surface activity, phospholipase activity and plasma myoinositol. J Clin Invest 70:673, 1982.
16. Jeffery PK, Wardlaw AJ, Nelson FC, et al: Bronchial biopsy in asthma. An ultrastructural, quantitative study and correlation with hyperreactivity. Am Rev Respir Dis 140:1745, 1989.
17. The HIFI study group: High-frequency oscillatory ventilation compared with conventional mechanical ventilation in the treatment of respiratory failure in preterm infants. N Engl J Med 320:88, 1989.
18. Federal Register, May 30, 1974
19. Stossel TP, Stossel SC: Declining American representation in leading clinical-research journals. N Engl J Med 322:739, 1990.
20. Lind SE: Sounding Board: Finder's fees for research subjects. N Engl J Med 323:192, 1990.
21. Roca J, Ramis LI, Rodriguez-Roisin R, et al: Serial relationships between ventilation-perfusion inequality and spirometry in acute severe asthma requiring hospitalization. Am Rev Respir Dis 137:1055, 1988.
22. Luce JM, Montgomery AB, Marks JD, et al: Ineffectiveness of high-dose methylprednisolone in preventing parenchymal lung injury and improving mortality in patients with septic shock. Am Rev Respir Dis 138:62, 1988.
23. Beauchamp TL, Childress JF (eds): *Principles of Biomedical Ethics*, 2d ed. Oxford, Oxford University Press, 1983, pp 338–343.
24. Barry M: Sounding Board. Ethical considerations of human investigation in developing countries. The AIDS dilemma. N Engl J Med 319:1083, 1988.
25. Angell M: Ethics in international collaborative clinical research (editorial). N Engl J Med 319:1081, 1988.
26. Rodriguez-Roisin R, Ballester E. Roca J, et al: Mechanisms of hypoxemia in patients with status asthmaticus requiring mechanical ventilation. Am Rev Respir Dis 139:732, 1989.
27. Wyngaarden JB: The clinical investigator as an endangered species. N. Engl J Med 301:1254, 1979.
28. Mason RJ: The academic pulmonary physician: Can one be both a productive scientist and an effective clinician? Am Rev Respir Dis 139:1551, 1989.

Chapter 189

INTERNATIONAL PERSPECTIVES ON CRITICAL CARE

JEAN-LOUIS VINCENT

Introduction

Academic critical care programs now exist in many countries around the world. Much of this growth has been a shared and common experience, facilitated and somewhat homogenized by the scientific literature, international conferences, visiting professorships, and trainees traveling abroad to gain expertise that is then brought home. Some aspects of critical care, however, have evolved uniquely, determined by the historical, cultural, and sociopolitical contexts of a given nation or region. To offer the student of critical care a perspective on some of these differences in approach, the editors invited Dr. Jean-Louis Vincent to gather overviews from leaders of critical care drawn broadly from the international community. This chapter includes commentary on the critical care environment in Australasia, China and Hong Kong, Israel, Japan, South Africa, South America, the former German Democratic Republic (GDR), and Western Europe. We have chosen to include the review of critical care in the GDR understanding the likelihood of rapid change in Eastern Europe, all the more to highlight the way in which health care systems may respond quickly to changes in the larger environment in which they arose.

189A/Critical Care in Australasia

MALCOLM McD. FISHER

GEOGRAPHIC FEATURES

The countries of New Zealand and Australia are geographically unique. The population of New Zealand is 3,250,000, and the country is relatively small and consists of two major islands with the majority of industry and people in the North Island. There are seven major intensive care units (ICUs), although only four offer access to cardiac surgery and neurosurgery. Australia is an island the size of mainland United States with a population of 15 million. The majority of the population lives near the coast and over half the population lives in five cities.

In both countries the provision of retrieval services has thus been a major priority in critical care. Thus the development of such services has paralleled that of critical care. In Australia, travel by retrieval teams of distances of 600 miles is common.

HISTORY

The initial development of ICUs in both countries was largely based on the enthusiasm of individuals who gradually obtained recognition and developed teams of doctors whose major specialist interest was critical care.[1] The first recognized unit was founded in Auckland, New Zealand, by Dr. Mathew Spence in 1955, and in the late 1950s Dr. John Forbes of Fairfield Infectious Diseases Hospital in Melbourne installed a respiratory unit with tank ventilators. In most other hospitals, critical care was practiced by enthusiasts in the recovery ward areas. The first respiratory unit with mechanical ventilators was established at Prince Henry Hospital in Sydney in 1961, and the first general ICU was established in St. Vincent's Hospital, Melbourne, in the same year.

The increasing interest in critical care led to a portion of the Australian Society of Anaesthetists meeting being devoted to critical care. In 1974 the Society of Critical Care Medicine was formed in Melbourne, and in 1975 the Australian and New Zealand Society of Intensive Care (ANZICS) was formed with Dr. Mathew Spence as its first president. In 1978 the societies amalgamated.

In 1975 the Royal Australasian College of Physicians and the Faculty of Anaesthetists of the Royal Australasian College of Surgeons commenced discussion on training in critical care. In spite of strong lobbying by ANZICS, it was not possible to create a single diploma due to the difference in structures of training systems and examinations. At present critical care is a recognized subspecialty of internal medicine and/or anaesthesia. Close cooperation between the Faculty of Anaesthetists and the College of Physicians has been maintained by including members of each college on training committees. The first postgraduate examination in critical care in the world was held by the Faculty in 1979, and over 50 graduates have now passed this examination. The majority of large units are now staffed by graduates of both internal medicine and anaesthesia training programs. Although most major units are staffed by doctors whose primary interest is critical care, the poor financial rewards for critical care in Australia have led to many intensivists having other interests such as intensive care in private hospitals, perfusion for cardiopulmonary bypass, general or respiratory medicine, and anaesthesia.

RESEARCH

Research has not been a strong point in Australasian critical care. There are only three academic departments of anaesthesia and critical care and no independent chairs in critical care. Only eight intensivists have postgraduate research diplomas. This is probably related to the major time commitment to clinical medicine required of intensivists. Also, that status among peers in Australasia is related more to clinical than to academic ability and achievements. Support from industry for research has occurred with increasing frequency over the past few years. The development of research in critical care is a major goal of ANZICS, which has recently established a research foundation to fund and foster research among intensivists.

FINANCIAL ASPECTS

In New Zealand all public and university hospitals take nonpaying patients; private health insurance is optional (these aspects began to change with a new government in 1991). Few private hospitals provide intensive care facilities apart from postcardiac surgical intensive care. In Australia private insurance is also optional but is held by a higher percentage of the population (45 percent). Patients with private insurance may opt for care in private or public hospitals, and uninsured patients receive free health care in public (government) and teaching hospitals. Larger private hospitals generally provide intensive care facilities, particularly postoperatively, although many insurance companies only support such care for limited time periods.

CRITICAL CARE IN AUSTRALIA COMPARED WITH THE UNITED STATES

There are major differences between ICUs in Australasia and those in the United States.

First, in Australasia there have been surprisingly few "turf wars" over control of ICUs. Surgeons have shown little inclination to become intensivists or play a major role in critical care, although postoperative neurosurgical and cardiac surgical ICUs have traditionally been run by surgeons. In most units the patient remains under the referring doctor, although the majority of care is provided by the critical care team.

Second, medical care in Australasia is delivered largely by a senior fellow or specialist, including both technical aspects of care (such as placement of lines) and clinical aspects. Intensivists there have a much greater commitment to bedside delivery of care than their American counterparts.

Both countries are less litigious than the United States, and legal action against intensivists or units is almost unheard of. Indeed, in New Zealand the no-fault automatic compensation for people involved in "accidents" makes the possibility of litigation almost impossible. A further advantage of this social difference is that ethical matters such as withdrawal of treatment are decided at the bedside rather than in the committee room or courtroom.

Respiratory technicians do not exist, and their work is divided between doctors, nurses, and physiotherapists.

A comparative study of New Zealand and U.S. ICUs[2] showed similar mortality figures, but in the New Zealand hospitals there were less postoperative patients, the patients were younger, they had less chronic disease, and half the admissions were due to trauma, drug overdose, or asthma, which only provide 11 percent of admissions in the United States. Comparative figures for Australia do not exist.

NURSING

In the past five years, a shortage of nurses in Australasia has become the limiting factor in the availability of intensive care beds. Training for postgraduate nurses in critical care occurs in hospitals and through nursing colleges. Recently, undergraduate nursing training has been shifted from hospitals to universities, and there is much debate about the merits or drawbacks of this shift. Hospitals are restricted in their ability to offer financial or educational incentives to attract nurses from other hospitals. The situation is compounded by active recruitment of Australian nurses by American organizations and has been alleviated to a degree by active recruitment of nurses from the United Kingdom. The American concepts of primary care nursing, collaborative practice, and nursing diagnosis are not in general use. The shortage of nurses in Australia has led to improvement in salaries, career structure, and more flexible rostering.

OVERSEAS TRAINEES

The clinical strengths of critical care in Australasia have led to increasing demand for training from physicians in the United States and the United Kingdom. As specialist positions in Australia have been filled with relatively young specialists, there has been a reduction in the number of Australian postgraduate doctors wishing to train in critical care, and positions for overseas graduates are increasingly becoming available.

CONCLUSION

Because the populations in both Australia and New Zealand are small, the number of full-time intensivists is also small. They are nevertheless an extremely united, enthusiastic, and active group. Consequently, the concept that critically ill patients should be cared for primarily by doctors trained specifically in the care of the critically ill is well established in both countries.

In organization, training, and status, the specialty of critical care is accepted and strong.

REFERENCES

1. Byth P: The history of the Australian and New Zealand intensive care Society, in Wiseman J (ed): *To Follow Knowledge.* Royal Australasian College of Physicians, Melbourne, 1988, p 9569.
2. Zimmerman JP, Knaus WA, Judson JA, Havill JH, Truhubovich RV, Draper EA, Wagner DP: Patient selection for intensive care: A comparison of New Zealand and United States hospitals. Crit Care Med 16:318, 1988.

189B/China and Hong Kong

T. MICHAEL MOLES

In China and Hong Kong, health services and their intrinsic specialties including critical care have developed in a rather sporadic and fragmentary fashion that has been dictated, to a significant extent, by the demographic and sociopolitical turbulence that has beset these two countries. This section will briefly review the relevant demography and outline the development and current status of health care systems and, in particular, critical care in these disparate communities.

THE CHANGING POLITICAL SCENE

The conclusion of World War II brought only momentary respite for China and Hong Kong, both of which were promptly engulfed once more in turmoil. China, already debilitated by the protracted war that had begun with the Japanese occupation of industrial Manchuria, plunged into a devastating civil war that only ended in 1949 with the Communist victory and the establishment of the People's Republic. The flight to Formosa of the defeated Kuomintang deprived China not only of the vast monetary assets that were to serve as the financial foundation for present-day Taiwan but also of the axis of its intelligentsia, leaving the country destitute and devoid of administrative, professional, and educational expertise, with adverse consequences for a population approaching 1 billion.

Hong Kong, also recovering from Japanese occupation but too accessible to escape the impact of the civil war in China, was subjected to a staggering refugee influx from China, the population of this small territory exploding in just four years from 3.5 to 5.5 million.

The primitive and poverty-stricken health resources of both communities were thus at once confronted with health care demands of unprecedented magnitude. Two years later, the Korean War sealed the frontier and effectively separated the two countries. Each, with their different economic systems, then set about the attainment of their own divergent sociopolitical objectives with characteristically imaginative and energetic pragmatism.

In 1997 the two countries will be reunited under the *one country–two systems* accord between Britain and Beijing. Hong Kong will then revert to the suzerainty of the People's Republic of China, retaining for the first 50 years a measure of autonomy, the guarantee of which, however, is a matter of deep distrust, which presently overshadows the future of the territory, its people, and indeed, its health services.

CRITICAL CARE IN CHINA

In the 1950s, initial health development strategies were directed toward the establishment of a nationwide system of primary health care, and almost all available resources were empirically invested into a program of preventive medicine; these were the days of the barefoot doctors. Specialist services, providing interventive medicine, were accorded only a deferred development priority, although at this time the Soviet Union, in parallel with the program of military and industrial technology transfer, did provide a significant contribution to both system and hospital development and to early specialist training programs, an influence still clearly visible today.

In the 1960s and early 1970s specialist training and the corresponding quality of clinical care made only slow progress, impeded by continuing austerity and the impact of two extraordinary political discontinuities: first, the ideological rift with the Soviet Union in 1960, which resulted in an almost complete severance of all connections with Western-style medical education, technique, and technology and, second, the cultural revolution of 1966 and the ensuing decade of deportation of specialist teachers to forced labor or political rehabilitation, which cut the continuum of intrinsic medical education.

During these years, although remarkable independent advances in specialist fields were achieved, many of these were unfortunately discredited through distortion and exaggeration by the Maoist propaganda machine. By the 1980s China had begun to relax its political and economic stance and both intellectual exchange and technology transfer flourished, although exchange programs in intensive and critical care were not highly coordinated. However, in 1986, following the 7th Asian Australasian Congress of Anaesthesiologists in Hong Kong, an authoritative international delegation of over 100 academics participated in the first national-international Symposium on Anaesthesia and Critical Care, held in Beijing in collaboration with the Chinese Society of Anaesthesiologists. This symposium was specifically orchestrated, first, to provide opportunities for a strategic review of the current critical care options available to China[1] and, second, to create initiatives for the development of coordinated postgraduate training programs in anaesthesia and critical care for Chinese specialists overseas, an exercise that brought about the almost immediate establishment of new programs sponsored by the United Kingdom, the United States, France, and West Germany, complementing the organized exchanges already underway with Japan.

In this same period of economic expansion, inward technology transfer gathered momentum. Japan and Italy sponsored the construction of lavish ultramodern hospitals in Beijing, the Italian project being the Beijing Emergency Medical Centre, featuring the first de novo purpose-built intensive care facility in China. Through other aid programs, ICUs were established and provided with contemporary equipment in numerous district hospitals throughout the country, although in a rather random manner.

Current strategies have shown a shift of emphasis toward interventive medicine with aggressive development of hospital-based services and specialties. The present 5-year plan, outlined recently by Cui Yue Li, Minister of Public Health, proposes a massive hospital development program, increasing the present hospital bed facilities of 2.8 million by over 250,000 to 3.3 million, accompanied by the establishment of 10 more medical schools to meet a production target of 60,000 high-level medical graduates by 1992. These ambitious projects imply a substantially increased resource allocation for surgical interventive programs; however, there is no apparent proposal or provision for a concurrent increase in manpower or material for either anaesthesia or critical care, an oversight that may eventually curtail development of the surgical programs.

In September 1989, following the Sixth World Congress in Hong Kong, a remarkable Symposium in Emergency Medicine was conducted in Beijing in collaboration with the Chinese Association for Emergency Medicine. However, it has not proved possible in the present political climate to develop complementary exchange programs in the field of critical care.

The metamorphosis of China, in just 50 years, from a medieval agrarian economy to the threshold of industrialization is undoubtedly a remarkable accomplishment. In terms of social, health, and welfare services, however, China has progressed and modernized very little. The executive structure is gerontocratic, the administration is incapable of delivering what it promises, and the bureaucracy is suspicious enough to be inefficient and ineffective. Furthermore, infrastructural resources and management skills are outdated, and both capital and currency are in chronic deficit. Such deficiencies, in combination with China's recent isolation, have encouraged consistently punitive production technology joint-ventures; a resolute refusal to become signatory to patent and copyright conventions has further conspired against internal developments in sophisticated medicine, particularly in a technology-dependent specialty such as critical care.

From a western perspective, hospitals, still mostly dating from earlier than 1950, are overcrowded and in need of maintenance and repair. Intensive care and support diagnostic and service units, still by no means universal, are not current, are often inappropriately located and accommodated, and are almost invariably undersupervised and understaffed. Furthermore, with the exception of those units funded by overseas charities or donations, most hospitals are equipped with obsolete or poorly maintained hardware (such as ventilators and monitors) and are frequently short of disposables.

These appearances are, however, in some measure deceptive. Specialist medical staff, considering the relatively poor access to current overseas journals, are impressively literate and versed in the content and critique of contemporary literature and clinical practice; above all, they are exceedingly imaginative and ingenious in adapting local resources to meet the demands of such a sophisticated specialty, something of an object lesson for the profligacy and wastefulness of Western medicine.

Specialist training is almost universally perfunctory, a situation deriving partly from lack of a formal type of accreditation system and partly from the absence of a professional organization to initiate, develop, or operate a program of structured postgraduate training. Such defects, however, are intrinsic to all specialties in China.

Research is presently inadequately supported and coordinated. Indeed, the discipline and rigor of the Western scientific method is often lacking, even at the professorial level. As such, publications often tend to be pragmatic and profusely anecdotal. Currently there are no epidemiologic or clinical databases established, nor is there use of international scoring systems such as APACHE, information that enables any critical comparison of the quality of care either within or without a country.[2] Salaries and promotional incentives are below most Western standards, a senior resident earning the equivalent of about U.S. $1600 per annum, and research and conference funding is very austere. Overall, these factors further conspire against the bright young men willing to enter this challenging field.

To these general observations there are however notable exceptions, mostly the result of dedicated initiatives taken by individuals of imagination, resource, and tenacity. At the Second University Hospital in Shanghai and at the Peking Union Medical College in Beijing, impressive critical care units have been established with a measure of support and encouragement from overseas; in Nanjing and Wuhan, independent units, providing both clinical service and centers for regional training programs, have been in operation for several years.

Within China, our colleagues from emerging specialties such as critical care face an uncertain future. Internally, the euphemistic "normalization," imposed by the government since the dalliance with democracy in 1989, has been achieved only at the cost of widespread political persecution and censorship.

Externally, the recent extraordinary events in Eastern Europe pose a serious threat to investment in China and the prospect of a return to economic privation and zero growth.

If the momentum of development in intensive care is to be sustained, renewed commitment and enlightened collaboration from the specialty elsewhere may have a crucial contribution to make, particularly during the coming decade.

CRITICAL CARE IN HONG KONG

Since 1960 Hong Kong, apart from the occasional episode of economic vertigo, has roared with unencumbered entrepreneurial elan from postwar poverty to unparalleled prosperity. Throughout this period, the government health services administration and to a considerable extent the profession have singularly and persistently failed to harness this opportune prosperity to any complementary strategic developments in primary, secondary, or tertiary care. In the interim, therefore, tertiary superspecialty development, for example in critical care, has been by crisis management, sporadic and often anachronistic.

The mid-1960s saw the establishment, nevertheless, of the first ICU as a special project, located in Queen Mary Hospital, then the sole university medical center. Intensive care units have been incorporated into hospitals commissioned since then, although often in fragmentary fashion, and older hospitals have been modified to provide similar units, although some would have to be described as rather rudimentary.

By the 1980s the eight district general hospitals, each with 1000 to 2000 acute beds, all had small ICUs with bed establishment ratios at around 1 percent or less. Commonly, so-called high dependency care, including ventilatory and other life support, was provided in satellite areas scattered among the specialist wards, a practice persisting today. In 1984 the second university hospital came on stream; the intensive care services were provided by the inaugural professorial department of anaesthesia and intensive care, a singular precedent for Hong Kong, particularly since at that time the overall establishment of consultant staff anaesthesiologists for the territory was only one tenth of that for a comparable demographic unit in the United Kingdom.

In 1991 all the major hospitals, whether government managed or sponsored, are being incorporated into a single coordinating directorate, the Hospital Authority, presenting a unique opportunity for review and rationalization of intensive care services.

Staffing for the secondary and tertiary specialties of anaesthesia and critical care has been chronically neglected by a myopic administration and a professional autocracy. Despite the availability of accredited specialists in critical care, the majority of these units have been, and indeed continue to be, operated under the direction and management of middle echelon physicians and surgeons with only incidental superspecialty involvement, the lamentable provision of anaesthesiology staff mandating a prior commitment to that service. Rotational training programs are, however, established, and anaesthesiology remains the only source of accredited specialists.

In 1983, with the support of the Western Pacific Association for Critical Care Medicine and on the initiative of Professor Nishimura, a Critical Care Society was formed. The Society provides active continuing education services for nursing staff but has been less successful at a medical level.

The ICU at the Prince of Wales Chinese University Hospital is outstanding from all other facilities in China or Hong Kong and merits attention as an example of what can be achieved in consequence of enlightenment and commitment. The unit is operated under the aegis of the Department of Anaesthesia and Intensive Care, whose chairman is Professor T. E. Oh. The unit has, in addition to the professor, a director and a consultant, all of them being accredited, diplomate specialists in critical care. The unit functions as a 12-bed, 24-h, dedicated specialist coverage, general intensive care facility. Coronary and neonatal/pediatric intensive care are provided by the respective specialties. There is no policy for subordinate high dependency care to be provided outside the unit.

The service is supervised by consultant staff, augmented by postfellowship anesthesiologists and medical officers attached to a 3-month rotational training program that is internationally accredited. Nursing staff, under the supervision of a senior nursing manager, are provided to meet staffing rations of 1:1 by day and 1:1 to 1:2 by night.

Admission policy provides for open access, caring for some 800 to 900 broad spectrum patients per annum; the generous flexibility of admission policy, substantively at the dictate of cultural considerations, results in a high mean APACHE admission score, around 23, with medical-surgical distribution at 40:60. Epidemiologic and clinical audit, analysis protocols, and research programs are fully established and operational; the mortality figures, at 20 to 30 percent, compare favorably with equivalent APACHE subsets in other countries.[3]

The immediate future for Hong Kong is uncertain. Treachery in Whitehall and truculence in Beijing concerning guarantees of civil liberty in Hong Kong after 1997 have seriously eroded confidence. The territory as a whole and the professions and their specialties in particular are now seriously sapped by a brain-drain, initially insidious but now threatening to become torrential. Anaesthesia and critical care are transferrable skills; government must now, at last, realistically confront the long-predicted manpower crisis in these specialties.

SUMMARY

In both China and Hong Kong, perhaps in common with elsewhere, the hospital specialists who most use, and abuse, intensive care are those who exhibit both a resistance to comparative audit and a reluctance to recognize or accord a remit to critical care as an autonomous specialty.

Intensive care units have been developed therefore from crude concepts which lack strategy or rationale and often extend no further than a primitive logistic necessity. Almost no units have been allocated sufficient resources to provide for accredited specialists as directors or consultants; lack of supervision and staff is endemic at both medical and paramedic levels. Structured postgraduate training and career incentives are practically nonexistent.

Operational protocols and procedures are poorly formulated and admission criteria rarely defined or applied, although there is some cultural mitigation. Furthermore, processes of epidemiologic and clinical audit and cost-benefit analysis are hardly perceptible. Nevertheless, to these generalities there are visionary and vigorous exceptions that have created promising precedents for improvements in clinical intensive care services in the next few years.

These clinical developments will soon be augmented by complementary academic and continuing education initiatives. In the next year or so Hong Kong will establish an Academy of Medicine charged with the future custody of postgraduate training of specialists in the territory. The recently incorporated Hong Kong College of Anaesthesiologists will be affiliated to the academy and has made an unequivocal commitment to assume a leading role within the academy with regard to the training and accreditation of specialists in intensive care.

On March 3 to 8, 1993 Hong Kong will host the Asia Pacific Congress on Critical Care Medicine under the chairmanship of Professor Teik Oh. This congress will present a unique opportunity not only to take a perspective view of intensive care, both Asian and global, but also to establish and enhance regional initiatives, perhaps collaborative, for the future development of critical care.

REFERENCES

1. Moles TM; Strategic options for the development of anaesthesia services in China. Med China (1):79, 1987.
2. Knaus WA, Draper EA, Wagnor DP, Zimmerman JE: APACHE II. A severity of disease classification system. Crit Care Med 13:816, 1985.
3. Fergnaow MR, Oh TE: Pattern and severity of intensive care admissions in Hong Kong. J Hong Kong Med Assoc 10(4):273, 1988.

189C/Israel

SIMON BURSZTEIN

Although critical care medicine is well developed in Israel, it is not a recognized subspecialty, probably due to opposition from the Society of Anesthesia to dissociation of this field from the specialty of anesthesia.

Since Israel is a country unfortunately living under conditions of war, critical care has evolved under this condition. During the Six Day War in 1967, several physicians from the United States and Europe, volunteering to provide critical care, highlighted the deficiency in this subspecialty. The concept of continuous monitoring of severely ill patients, routine use of mechanical ventilators, massive fluid resuscitation for traumatic shock, and routine blood gas analysis all gained wide recognition and application at the time.

By the time of the Yom Kippur war in 1973, aggressive volume administration in the management of shock in the field was routine, and many cases of adult respiratory distress syndrome (ARDS) were encountered, likely related to this treatment. Most of these victims responded to support with mechanical ventilation and establishment of a negative fluid balance. At this time enteral and parenteral nutrition was also introduced to the management of multiple trauma and severely burned patients. Early nutritional support was likely excessive (with patients sometimes receiving more than 6000 kcal). Adverse effects were not encountered, however. In South Lebanon several instances of mass injury after bombings or explosions were encountered. The resulting rhabdomyolysis and complicating acute renal failure were largely prevented by early aggressive fluid therapy, an intervention now routinely employed in disaster medicine.

Since Israel is a country of immigrants, the pioneers of critical care medicine often came with different concepts concerning how, by whom, and where ICUs should be established. There was also a diversity of opinion as to the use of multidisciplinary versus specialty units. This controversy, existing in many other countries, was particularly intense in Israel, where discussion was held by people trained in Western and Eastern Europe, the United States, South Africa, South America, and elsewhere. As critical care has gained recognition and even prestige, most physicians are now interested in playing a key role during the acute phase of their patient's disease. Accordingly, many specialties have their own ICUs, including neurosurgery, cardiac and thoracic surgery, internal medicine, pneumonology, and pediatrics. This is not really unique to Israel, and indeed, the number of multipurpose units is relatively greater than in other Western countries, mainly for economic reasons.

The Society of Critical Care was established in 1973, at which time there were four adult ICUs and one pediatric ICU. Today most of the hospitals have ICUs directed by anesthesiologists, surgeons, chest physicians, cardiologists, internists, or pediatricians. All major hospitals have training programs for intensive care nurses and respiratory therapists. Furthermore, most of the medical students from the four medical schools in the country will have some kind of exposure to the specialty before ending their studies.

The scientific council of the Israel Medical Association has been considering for the past 10 years the recognition of critical care as a separate specialty. Hopefully this process will come to a conclusion shortly. In order to be eligible for board specialization in critical care, specialists in internal medicine, surgery, anesthesia, and pediatrics will be required to pass a board examination after 2 years of training in a recognized ICU.

It should also be noted that the Society of Critical Care Medicine in Israel is very active, organizing four to five national scientific meetings per year. This group organized its first international symposium in 1980 and in 1985 was the host of the Fourth World Congress on Intensive and Critical Care Medicine held in Jerusalem.

189D/Japan

NAOKI AIKAWA

Since World War II, Japan has achieved rapid industrialization; economic growth and cultural development have resulted in a leadership role for the country in health care, education, and research. With an increase in the critically ill elderly population, advances in surgical therapies, and recognition of needs to improve care following industrial and traffic injuries, the importance of critical care medicine has been well recognized in the past two decades.

BACKGROUND*

The population of Japan was 122.7 million in 1988, 99 percent of the people being of Japanese descent and living in a land area of 143 thousand square miles. The majority live in an urban area, and the Tokyo metropolitan area contains 10 percent of the population. Of the total population, 11.2 percent are 65 years or older as compared with the figures (in 1985) of 11.7 percent for the United States, 12.4 percent for France, 15.1 percent for the United Kingdom, and 16.9 percent for Sweden. Children (ages 0 to 14) constitute 19.5 percent.

Japan had achieved a unique indigenous culture and national identity by the time of the Meiji restoration in the mid-nineteenth century. European influences changed the country into a modern industrialized nation by the mid-twentieth century. After World War II, American culture had the greatest influence on our society, which enjoys a high standard of living in the 1990s.

As a result of an educational system established about a century ago and modeled after that of Germany, Japan is one of the most literate nations in the world. However, the language used is Japanese. English, which is the most popular foreign language, is not used in clinical settings. Although doctors can read English, bilingual doctors are few, and the majority of Japanese nurses do not speak foreign languages. As for religious groups, 96 million are Shintoists, 87 million are Buddhists (note that one can be both Shintoist and Buddhist), and 896,000 are Christians (45 percent Catholic, 55 percent Protestant).

HEALTH STATISTICS AND THE HEALTH CARE SYSTEM

There were 1.469 million inpatients on one day of a survey in 1987 of hospitals all over Japan, the ratio of inpatients being 1197 per day per 100,000 population. Of these, cerebrovascular diseases accounted for 14.3 percent; malignancies for 9.4 percent; trauma and intoxication for 8.0 percent; benign gastrointestinal, bilary, and pancreatic diseases for 7.6 percent; and cardiovascular diseases for 6.9 percent.[1] The figures for the number of patients requiring critical care is not available from this survey. However, because the number of beds in the ICUs was 14,786,[2] and the occupancy by critical care patients was 82.5 percent,[3] we can estimate the number of critical care patients nationwide to be 12,200 per day.

The death rates per 1000 population were 6.8 for males and 5.6 for females, and the average life expectancies were 75.61 years for males and 81.39 years for females. The death rates are the lowest and the life expectancies the longest in the world, and this has been attributed to the advanced public health system and well-organized delivery of medical care as well as to the high level of critical care medical services including neonatal intensive care, which contributes to the neonatal mortality rate being the lowest (2.7 per 10^3 births in 1988) in the world. The leading cause of death in Japan is malignant disease followed by cardiovascular disease, cerebrovascular disease, and respiratory infection. Deaths from traffic accidents had increased in 1988 to 10,344 per year, which is 8.4 per year per 10^5 population.

Medical practice is only allowed by physicians who have passed a national examination. As of December 1989, there were 201,658 active licensed physicians, or 164.2 per 100,000 population. Of these 56.2 percent are employees of hospitals and 32.4 percent are in private practice. As for the medical specialties related to critical care, there were 131,747 internists, 33,284 general surgeons, 4508 neurosurgeons, 1461 cardiac surgeons, 874 chest surgeons, and 4883 anesthetists.[4] The actual number of physicians actively involved in critical care is not known. However, there are 409 physicians who are certified for the board from the Japanese Society for Acute Medicine (Emergency and Critical Care Medicine).[5] There are 373,000 registered nurses and 322,000 licensed practical nurses as of 1988, 79.1 percent of them actively working in the hospitals.[4]

As of October 1987, there were 137,275 hospitals, asylums, and clinics, private or public.[2] Of these 8749 were general hospitals. The total number of beds in general hospitals was 1.312 million (1069 beds per 10^5 population). Of the hospitals 1772 (20.3 percent of general hospitals) had ICUs and 570 had coronary care units (CCUs) (Table 189-1).

All Japanese citizens are covered by a medical insurance system. Employees of companies or government and their dependents are covered by the Hiyohsha Hoken (employee's insurance) system, while others (37.2 percent of the population) are covered by the Kokumin Hoken (people's insurance) system. Depending on the policy, 70 to 90 percent of the medical cost is covered by insurance, and for elderly patients (70 years or older) most of the medical cost is paid by the government. Also, workmen's compensation and liability insurance policies cover costs for labor-related diseases or injuries and injuries caused by accidents, re-

TABLE 189-1 Number of Intensive Care Units and Beds in Japan

	1984		1987	
	Units	Beds	Units	Beds
ICU	1,604	8,348	1,772	9,683
CCU	498	1,826	570	2,180
Neonatal ICU	343	2,586	361	2,736
Pediatric ICU	—	—	28	190
Total	2,445	12,760	2,731	14,789

Number of hospitals: 8500 in 1984, 8749 in 1987.
Abbreviations: ICU—intensive care unit (includes respiratory, surgical, and general intensive care units). CCU—coronary care unit.
SOURCE: Adapted and translated with permission from Sanagi S et al: Medical facilities. J Health Welfare Statist 36:191, 1989 (in Japanese).

*All statistics are figures in 1987 unless otherwise stated.

spectively. Medical charges including the price of drugs are under government regulation for reimbursement through the insurance system. For example, in the author's hospital (a 1071-bed university hospital in the center of Tokyo) the average bill is 315,000 yen (140 yen = U.S. $1) per day for general surgical patients and 875,000 yen per day for emergency patients treated in the ICU.

The national medical care expenses in 1987 were 18.076 trillion yen, which accounted for 5.23 percent of the gross national product and 6.68 percent of the national income.

EVOLUTION OF CRITICAL CARE

PRE-ICU ERA

The first ICU was opened in Japan in 1964. Until the mid-1970s, when many hospitals became equipped with ICUs, critically ill or injured patients were cared for by physicians with specialties such as cardiology, pulmonology, general surgery, thoracic surgery, or neurosurgery depending on the disease or injury causing the critical illness. With the rapid increase in traffic injuries in the mid-1960s, several hospitals including Osaka University Hospital and Saiseikai Kanagawa Hospital opened trauma units where surgeons with various surgical specialties worked together in the intensive treatment of severely injured patients. The management of hemorrhagic shock and respiratory failure in polytrauma or extensive burns received major attention.

Another stream in the development of critical care was through the postoperative management of patients after extensive surgery for carcinoma of the esophagus or stomach, pancreatic surgery, or hepatic surgery. Early on, general surgeons had to spend days in the surgical ward with these postoperative patients monitoring and titrating cardiopulmonary supportive therapies. To treat acute respiratory failure, anesthetists were invited for consultation and various modalities of ventilatory support such as positive end-expiratory pressure (PEEP) became popularized. Similar developments occurred on cardiac surgical services with the management of complex postoperative patients and in the cardiology departments in the treatment of critically ill patients with acute myocardial infarction, a disease that was increasing in the urban areas of Japan.

DEVELOPMENT OF THE ICU

Recognizing the need for systematic management of critically ill patients, major hospitals (particularly hospitals attached to medical schools with a heavy surgical load) started to construct ICUs in the mid-1960s. Anesthetists took a leading role in the development of these units because the majority of patients were postoperative with respiratory failure and hemodynamic derangement as the major problems. Many anesthetists returned to Japan after several years of training in the United States to join these newly established units. They brought new knowledge and the technology of critical care medicine developed in the United States.

CRITICAL CARE CENTER SYSTEM

In 1977 the Japanese government established a nationwide system for the treatment of critical diseases and injuries. The plan was to establish critical care centers (Kyumei Kyukyu Center in the Japanese language) at a ratio of one center per one million population with at least one center per prefecture. The centers are currently designed to be capable of treating any critically ill patient on a 24-h basis and to be staffed with 14 or more full-time specialists to cover more than 20 intensive care beds. The government subsidizes the construction, equipment, and staffing of the center. This means that the government has recognized the need to maintain the level of critical care as well as the high medical costs involved in the delivery of critical care, which cannot be covered by the ordinary health insurance system. By the end of 1989, there were 99 centers in active operation throughout the country. Clinical activities in these centers have become the source of tremendous advances in critical care medicine in the last decade.

DELIVERY OF CRITICAL CARE

PREHOSPITAL EMERGENCY CARE

The transportation of critically ill patients is provided by the fire departments of the local governments. Ambulances are operated by three-men teams trained in the assessment of vital signs and the procedures of cardiopulmonary resuscitation using a bag-mask. Unlike North America, however, present law does not allow them to give any medical treatment other than oxygen or clearing the airway.

In Tokyo, for example, 13 million people are covered by 162 ambulances and 1470 full-time personnel. An average of 997 emergency transportations per day was recorded in 1988; 58.2 percent were for illness, 21.10 percent for traffic accidents, and 13.2 percent for other injuries. There were 3102 patients who were dead on arrival and 7740 patients in critical condition. Owing to a well-organized dispatch system, an ambulance took an average of 4 min 48 s to arrive after a telephone request and 8 min 6 s to transport the patients to an appropriate hospital.[6] During transport primary cardiopulmonary resuscitation (CPR) is carried out if necessary, and this efficient prehospital care system contributes to the survival of critically ill patients.

Because of the high density of population and hospitals, air transport of critically ill patients is not popular except from some islands. Helicopter transport systems are operating in three locations in Japan, and the Tokyo Fire Department transported only 25 patients by air in 1988.[6]

ORGANIZATION OF CRITICAL CARE FACILITIES

In addition to the 99 critical care centers, there are 4130 hospitals in the country, which are approved by the local governments to receive ambulances. Patients in critical condition, however, are primarily transported to one of the centers or a university hospital where a high level of care is available. Also, these high-level facilities receive critically ill patients from ordinary hospitals for further advanced treatment.

TABLE 189-2 Survey of Intensive Care Units in Japan

Year opened (n = 119)	1977, 45	1978–1979, 11	1980–1984, 40	1987, 23
Number of beds (n = 126)	<5, 34	6–10, 68	≥11, 24	Average 8.3 beds
Space (m^2) (n = 109)	<99, 6	100–399, 52	>400, 51	Average 417.8 m^2
Occupancy (%) (n = 100)	<49, 3	50–89, 54	90–100, 43	Average 82.5%
Days in ICU (n = 110)	<4, 37	5–9, 61	≥10, 12	Average 12.6 days
Nurses per bed (n = 99)	−1.4 20	1.5–2.9, 36	≥3.0, 43	Average 2.5 nurses per bed
Central monitoring (n = 125)		Yes, 119	No, 6	
BGA apparatus in ICU (n = 126)		Yes, 98	No, 28	
Pacemaker (n = 126)		Yes, 119	No, 7	
IABP (n = 126)		Yes, 87	No, 39	

NOTE: Data are from the survey of 126 ICUs in 1988 by the Japanese Society of Intensive Care Medicine. Abbreviations: n, number of ICUs answered to each item; BGA, blood gas analysis; IABP, intraarterial balloon pumping.
SOURCE: Adapted and translated with permission from Japanese Society of Intensive Care Medicine.[3]

DELIVERY OF CRITICAL CARE IN THE ICU

The delivery of critical care is not too different from the United States or Canada, and the design of the ICU and equipment used in the unit are similar to those in North American hospitals (Table 189-2). Most of the ICUs are attached to anesthesia departments and run by physicians with anesthesiology training. Residents may rotate from surgical departments. Nurses in the units are specially trained for the fundamental pathophysiology, monitoring, and nursing of critically ill patients. Most respiratory therapy is given by anesthetists because there are no approved respiratory therapists in Japan. In addition to the ICU, some hospitals have a cardiac care unit and a neonatal ICU that is separate from the adult ICU (Table 189-1).

Almost all machines and equipment used in North American ICUs are available in Japan. Although ventilators are mostly imported from the United States, reliable cardiovascular monitors, pacemakers, endoscopes, echographs, and computed tomographs are domestically made, and domestic computers are widely used for data processing. Also, domestic supplies of disposable catheters, tubes, syringes, gowns, and drapes are available. As for pharmaceutical products, essentially all drugs used in North American ICUs are available, although they may carry different brand names. In addition, some products such as protease inhibitors, thromboxane synthetase inhibitor, antithrombin III, and haptoglobin preparation are approved in Japan for clinical use.

CRITICAL CONDITIONS AND DISEASES

The most frequent critical condition in ICU patients is acute respiratory failure. Of the patients in the ICU from the author's department, 68 percent required ventilatory support. Septic shock, heart failure, disseminated intravascular coagulation (DIC), acute renal failure, and multisystem organ failure (MSOF) are other common conditions.[7] These conditions develop mostly in patients with cerebrovascular diseases, postoperative sepsis, myocardial infarction, polytrauma, and extensive burns.[8] Penetrating injuries such as gunshot or knife wounds, narcotics or cocaine overdose, and alcohol-related disease are relatively rare in Japan, although an increase in benzodiazepine and antidepressant overdoses has been noted in urban areas. As for infectious diseases, nosocomial infection with methicillin-resistant *Staphylococcus aureus* is a major problem. Most ICU personnel are vaccinated against hepatitis B, and acquired immunodeficiency syndrome (AIDS) patients are still few in number in Japan.

ACADEMIC ASPECTS

MEDICAL EDUCATION

Education in a medical school lasts 6 years after the completion of a high school education. There are 80 medical schools (43 national, 8 public, and 29 private institutions) producing 7880 graduates a year. Education in critical care and emergency medicine had been carried out through lectures in anesthesiology, surgery, or internal medicine in most schools until the end of the 1970s. In 1977, a department of emergency medicine was opened in Kawasaki Medical College, where a formal program in critical care medicine has been started. By the end of 1989, 39 medical schools had established departments for education in critical care, and there are 11 professorships of emergency and critical care medicine.

POSTGRADUATE TRAINING AND SPECIALTY BOARDS

Most of the 39 medical schools with emergency and critical care departments and critical care centers have residency training programs for physicians carrying a Japanese medical license. The training is for 4 to 6 years depending on the program. The Japanese Association for Acute Medicine has a program for board certification that requires 3 years of training in one of the 156 approved institutions and the mastering of basic procedures and knowledge of critical care (Table 189-3). There were 409 board-certified physicians as of 1989.

MEDICAL SOCIETIES AND PUBLICATIONS

Medical societies related to critical care medicine are listed in Table 189-4. There are more than 120 textbooks, handbooks, and manuals on critical care and related medical sciences available. In addition to the journals published by the medical societies, there are several journals such as *Kyukyu Igaku (Emergency Medicine)* and *Shuchu Chiryo (Intensive Care),* which have a substantial number of subscribers. All of the publications are in the Japanese language although some journals include English papers and English abstracts of Japanese articles.

REFERENCES

1. Sanagi S, Hasegawa T, Ushio M, et al: Injuries, diseases, and delivery of health care. J Health Welf Statist 36(9):87, 1989 (in Japanese).
2. Sanagi S, Hasegawa T, Ushio M, et al: Medical facilities. J Health Welfare Statist 36(9):191, 1989 (in Japanese).
3. Japanese Society of Intensive Care Medicine: 1988 survey of intensive care units in Japan. J Intens Care Med 13(Suppl):10, 1989 (in Japanese).
4. Sanagi S, Hasegawa T, Ushio M, et al: Personnel in health care. J Health Welfare Statist 36(9):179, 1989 (in Japanese).
5. Japanese Association for Acute Medicine: List of the board certified physicians of the association. Jpn J Acute Med, March (Suppl):S-544, 1989.
6. Tokyo Metropolitan Fire Department: Activities of emergency transportation and care: Report of emergency activities in 1988. Tokyo, Tokyo Metropolitan Fire Department, 1989, p 13.
7. Aikawa N, Abe O: Multiple organ failure in surgical patients. Surg Diag Treat (Geka Shinryo; Tokyo) 29:715, 1987 (in Japanese).
8. Aikawa N, Shinozawa Y, Ishibiki K, et al: Clinical analysis of multiple organ failure in burned patients. Burns 13:26, 1987.

TABLE 189-3 Minimum Experiences and Knowledge Required for the Board of Japanese Association for Acute Medicine (Emergency and Critical Care Medicine)

Essential experiences
Insertion of an airway
Jaw lifting
Tracheal intubation
Cricothyroid puncture
Suction of tracheal fluid
Mouth-to-mouth breathing
Use of a bag mask
External cardiac massage
Direct current (DC) defibrillation
Thoracentesis
Stomach tube insertion
Gastric lavage
Balloon catheter insertion
Paracentesis
Phlebotomy
Arterial puncture
Spinal tap
Use of splints for fractures
Management of bleeding by direct compression
Use of tourniquet
Suturing techniques
Management of epistaxis
Use of ventilators
Essential knowledge
Reading Emergency x-rays and electrocardiograms
Indications for emergency operations
Assessment of emergency laboratory data
Differential diagnosis of coma
Management of shock
Use of drugs for critical care
Indication for DC defibrillation
Other experiences (preferable)
Tracheostomy
Open cardiac massage
Pericardiocentesis
Insertion of chest drain
Intercostal nerve block
Use of Sengstaken tube
Subclavian vein puncture
Insertion of central venous pressure (CVP) catheter
Removal of foreign bodies from the eye, ear, and nose
Local treatment of burns
Puncture of the urinary bladder
Other knowledge (preferable)
Differential diagnosis of respiratory distress
Abdominal pain
Gastrointestinal bleeding and arrhythmias
Systemic care of burns
Indications for acute hemodialysis and peritoneal dialysis
Management of electrolyte and acid-base imbalances
Management of poisonings and intoxications
Additional preferable experiences
General anesthesia
Traction of fractures

TABLE 189-4 Medical Societies and Associations in Critical Care Medicine in Japan

Society or Association	Year Established	Active Members	Publication
Japanese Association for Acute Medicine	1973	6855	*J Jpn Assoc Acute Med*
Japanese Society of Intensive Care Medicine	1974	4664	*J Intens Care Med*
Japanese Society of Reanimatology	1982	1225	*Jpn J Reanimatol*
Japan Shock Society	1986	823	*Shock*

NOTE: Societies such as the Japan Surgical Society and Japan Society of Anesthesiology are excluded. Publications are in the Japanese language with English abstracts.

189E/South Africa

PETER D. POTGIETER

HISTORICAL PERSPECTIVE

Critical care in Southern Africa had its origin in the late 1950s with pioneering work in the management of neonatal tetanus commencing in 1957 in Cape Town by A. B. Bull and P. M. Sykes in Durban. The introduction of tetanus units at the Red Cross Children's Hospital and use of curare and intermittent positive-pressure ventilation (IPPV) with East Radcliffe ventilators significantly reduced the mortality in this almost universally fatal disease.[1] Although a small number of patients with poliomyelitis had been treated previously by cuirass, tank, and East Radcliffe ventilators at the City Hospital, an infectious diseases hospital, the tetanus units were the forerunners of modern critical care. Adult ICUs were soon to follow in all the major teaching hospitals when the value of critical care for treating patients with tetanus, polyneuropathy, and asthma and following major surgery was recognized.

These early beginnings were further stimulated by the first heart transplant performed by Christian Barnard in 1967. Thus, ICUs started with specialized units that were to set the pattern for subsequent development in critical care in this region. Although many units are staffed medically by anesthetists, the concept of multidisciplinary units has failed to develop. Most units are specialized and remain under the umbrella of the major disciplines. A multidisciplinary approach is unusual in all but a few major teaching hospitals.

South Africa has a dual health care system.[2] A state-funded system exists that incorporates the teaching hospitals and provides care for all patients irrespective of income. The fee structure is based on income, and patients unable to pay receive free treatment. The second, or private, fee-paying system is largely supported by numerous medical insurances.

Over the past 5 years this group of private hospitals has established ICUs that provide acceptable routine postsurgical and medical intensive care. Legislation does not allow these hospitals to employ doctors, and consequently, the medical care is reliant on doctors who may not be in the hospital at all times. This private system unfortunately cannot provide the same degree of critical care found in the teaching hospitals yet poses a threat to academic critical care because of competition for well-trained nurses to whom they offer a much more attractive salary.

Apartheid, or separate development, a policy that encouraged racial segregation, has been enforced in South Africa by the ruling government since 1948. Over the past few years, however, there have been major changes, and the apartheid system is rapidly being dismantled. Integration first started in medicine, particularly in the ICUs, and medical staff was fully integrated as early as 1972. Integration of other staff and patients followed shortly thereafter. Currently, most ICUs are open to patients of all races, and hospitals are rapidly following this trend.

ORGANIZATION AND TRAINING IN CRITICAL CARE

In 1976 the Critical Care Society of Southern Africa was established allowing full membership from all disciplines in medicine as well as professions allied to medicine (nurses, physiotherapists, and medical technologists), with an interest in critical care. The current society membership is 510. The objective of this society is to promote the discipline of critical care by education, encouraging research and ensuring the maintenance of a high standard of intensive care. This group has been strongly supported by other disciplines, particularly anesthesia. The concept of acceptable standards for critical care was established when the Society of Anaesthetists of South Africa produced a document on standards for anesthesia in South Africa that included a section on critical care. This was formulated by members of both the critical care society and the South African Society of Anaesthetists. The publication of an official biannual peer-reviewed journal, *The Southern African Journal of Critical Care Medicine,* since 1983 has also helped to establish firm links within the society as well as to provide an avenue for education and publication of scientific papers.

The recognition of formal medical specialization in critical care has fallen on stony ground despite active lobbying for more than 10 years by the Critical Care Medicine Society and the South African Society of Anaesthetists. The College of Medicine of South Africa, the recognized specialist training body, has debated the subject of accreditation repeatedly and heatedly, though little concensus has been reached between the different faculties within the college. Two universities have, however, recognized the need for postgraduate training in critical care. The University of the Orange Free State offers a bachelor degree in critical care, and the University of Cape Town offers a master of philosophy (critical care). The requirements of the latter are similar to critical care postfellowship requirements in Australia and the United States (viz. 2 years experience in an accredited critical care unit with an examination and thesis to be completed following a specialist fellowship in either internal medicine, anesthesia, surgery, or a related specialty). More recently, the South African Medical and Dental Council, our registering body, has accepted that subspecialty recognition is acceptable in certain disciplines such as cardiology; critical care may well soon follow this route.

Nursing training in intensive care is far advanced, with 12 nursing colleges offering a diploma in critical care nursing. This was first established in 1965, and approximately 170 intensive care nurses are trained annually and contribute to the pool of 2099 ICU registered nurses. All the training courses are similar and can be completed over a 14-month period. Requirements include in-service training in all fields of intensive care as well as formal lectures.

Critical care technology has recently been introduced into medical technology, and currently two centers have started training students. The trained technologist will bridge the gap between technology and the patient, and they will be involved with patient monitoring, ventilator care, side-room laboratory operations, and the maintenance of equipment.

CONTEMPORARY PRACTICE OF CRITICAL CARE

Eight major teaching hospitals all have active specialist ICUs within major disciplines including neonatal, pediatric, coronary care, respiratory, surgical, neurosurgical, cardiothoracic, and multidisciplinary ICUs in different combinations. The majority of these major units have independent direction by physicians who have been trained in critical care. Smaller hospitals usually have ICUs that are more multidisciplinary in nature, but many have dedicated staff usually with an anesthesia background. By contrast, in the private sector, patients are admitted by their primary physicians who maintain full control of their management since there are no dedicated intensive care physician staff. Not unexpectedly, the standard of critical care varies, though in general all units are well equipped with modern and sophisticated equipment that includes electrocardiographic (ECG), pressure, and pulse oximetry monitors. Specialized therapeutic modalities such as plasmapheresis and hemodialysis are only practiced in the teaching hospital units and in major state hospitals.

The patient population in Southern Africa differs significantly from the Western world in that the ages are much younger, and diseases differ widely and include tropical diseases and infectious diseases, usually poorly controlled by primary care and immunization; this lack of primary care is also seen in late and delayed presentations in many patients. Patients are thus frequently young and previously fit, with a catastrophic illness precipitating ICU admission. Such illnesses include infective diseases, toxic envenomation, tetanus, major trauma (usually as a pedestrian), and delayed surgical abdomen as well as many common diseases such as asthma and drug overdose. Tuberculosis is endemic, and a large number of patients are admitted with disseminated disease, pulmonary disease, or even tuberculosis associated with another primary cause for admission. Thus, a spectrum of Third World diseases are treated in hospitals where active transplant programs including kidney, heart, heart-lung, and liver transplants may also be performed. The spectrum of diseases, APACHE II, scores and results of 3 years of admissions to the 10-bed respiratory ICU at Groote Schuur Hospital, Cape Town (an 1800-bed teaching hospital attached to the University of Cape Town), are shown in Table 189-5. During 1989 there were 374 admissions, including 79 black, 221 of mixed origin, and 74 white patients. The mean APACHE II score was 14.06 with a predicted mortality of 17.58 percent and an actual mortality of 13.4 percent. This gives a mortality ratio of 0.776, which places the results between the top 2 of 13 U.S. hospital results reported by Knaus.[3] The overall admissions and results in two other teaching hospitals and two private hospitals are shown in Table 189-6.

Research has been neglected because of a shortage of medical staff and excessive patient loads. Virtually no basic research exists. Many units are however actively participating in clinical research that has provided significant insight into the management of many diseases including tetanus, tuberculosis, and others.[4–6]

RELATIONSHIPS TO OTHER SOUTHERN AFRICAN STATES

The Critical Care Society of Southern Africa has members from many Southern African states. Since its main objective is education, much encouragement is given to these other states. The newly independent Namibia has ICUs staffed by personnel trained in major teaching centers in South Africa, and there is a constant interplay between different areas with academic visits and consultations over difficult problems. This includes a fixed wing jet rescue service that provides intensive care facilities while transporting critically ill patients over thousands of kilometers to centers where they can be more adequately handled.[7] Anesthetists from Harare participate in scientific meetings and continue the maintenance of appropriate critical care in Zimbabwe. Critical care links with Malawi are maintained, and regular contact has been established by the Critical Care Department of the University of the Orange Free State.

TABLE 189-5 Annual Admissions to the Respiratory ICU at Groote Schuur Hospital, Cape Town

Diagnosis	1987			1988			1989		
	NO.	APACHE II	MORTALITY (%)	NO.	APACHE II	MORTALITY (%)	NO.	APACHE II	MORTALITY (%)
Asthma	38	13	0	46	12	2	49	10.4	0
Pneumonia	65	17	42	58	18	26	37	16	16
ARDS	30	14	27	21	15	14	29	15.3	20
COAD	18	19	17	18	18	6	16	16.7	0
Other lung disease*	35	13	14	35	16	20	34	13	20
Neurologic disease†	15	13	20	28	10	4	26	14.9	12
Overdose	22	14	14	28	12	7	25	12.9	0
Poisoning	7	12	0	6	8	0	8	12.1	25
Cardiac arrest	11	26	64	9	29	78	4	28.5	75
Other disease	64	20	31	89	19	25	75	18.1	22
Elective surgery	48	10	4	32	11	0	21	12.6	9
Blunt chest trauma	38	8	5	36	9	0	50	9.2	2
TOTAL	391	15	19.9	406	14.75	15.1	374	14.06	13.6

*Includes pulmonary tuberculosis (12 cases, 33% mortality) and disseminated tuberculosis (6 cases, 33% mortality).
†Includes tetanus (7 severe cases, 0 mortality).

FUTURE OF CRITICAL CARE IN SOUTHERN AFRICA

Economic pressures in developing countries have led to greater emphasis being placed on preventative rather than interventional medicine. Critical care is regarded by many as excessive expenditure for little reward, and current feeling exists that this type of expenditure would be better utilized to prevent rather than treat diseases. Even more so in this climate than in the context of the Western world, we should be looking toward careful audit and accounting of patient care, benefits, and costs. It is encumbent upon every practicing intensive care physician to show the value of critical care; not only the benefit to the individual patient but, of more importance, the value of providing training for medical, nursing, and other staff and the spin-off of better care in other areas in the hospital. Entwined in the economics of the overall pattern of medical care is the value of the well-trained intensive care nurse. Currently a major nursing crisis exists, and many well-trained ICU nurses leave teaching hospitals for more profitable pursuits. This may mean leaving the profession completely or a move to the private sector. This creates a major shortage in the teaching centers essential for the training of new staff as well as for advancing the frontiers of critical care medicine.

REFERENCES

1. Smythe PM, Bull AB: Treatment of tetanus neonatorum with IPPR. Br Med J 2:107, 1959.
2. Benatar SR: Medicine and health care in South Africa. New Engl J Med 315(8):527, 1986.
3. Knaus WA, Draper EA, Wagner DP, Zimmerman JE: An evaluation of outcome from intensive care in major medical centres. Ann Int Med 104:410, 1986.

TABLE 189-6 Types of Admissions and Outcome of Four South African ICUs

Hospital No.* Year	ADMISSIONS							
	No. of beds	Total	Medical (Mort., %)	Surgical (Mort., %)	Trauma (Mort., %)	Paeds (Mort., %)	Ventilated, %	Mortality, %
1 (1989)	8	653	2 (0)	369 (22)	286 (29)	—	42†	25
2 (1988) 6 months	7	271	40 (38)	150 (13)	65 (25)	16 (25)	82	20
3 (1988) 6 months	15	477	33 (20)	414 (3)	30 (10)	—	12	4
4 (1989)	4	491	260 (NA)	231 (NA)	22 (NA)	9 (NA)	9.2	4.9

*Hospital: **1.** Surgical ICU, King Edward VIII Hospital, Durban, University of Natal (Dr. J. Aitchison, personal communication). **2.** Addington Hospital, General ICU, University of Natal, Durban (Dr. D. Burrows, personal communication). **3.** St Augustines, Entabeni, Parklands and Westville Private Hospitals, Durban (Dr. R. McGillivray, personal communication). **4.** Medi City Private Hospital, Somerset West (Dr. E. Blaine, personal communication).
†Ventilated for ≥24 hours.

4. James MFM, Manson EDM: The use of magnesium sulphate infusions in the management of very severe tetanus. Intens Care Med 11:5, 1985.
5. Levy H, Kallenbach JM, Feldman C, Thorburn SR, Abramowitz JA: Acute respiratory failure in active tuberculosis. Crit Care Med 15:221, 1987.
6. Westerman DE, Benatar SR, Potgieter PD, Ferguson AD: Identification of the high risk asthmatic patient. Experience with 39 patients subjected to ventilation for status asthmaticus. Am J Med 66:565, 1979.
7. Linton DM, La Grange SAB, Van Wyk EA: Monitoring in motion: An update on the Air Ambulance Service of the South African Red Cross Society (Cape Region). S Afr Med J 77(7):365, 1990.

189F/South America

HERNAN ARTUCIO
NORMA MAZZA

The development of medical science and the delivery of medical care in South America is highly related to the physical, demographic, and social environment. Knowledge of these factors is a necessary prerequisite to understand and evaluate the quality of medical care. It is probable that most readers are not acquainted with South America. In fact, there are great regional differences among countries and even regions. A description of critical care throughout the continent is beyond the scope of this article. Rather, we will focus on our own country, Uruguay, and compare it to other South American countries whenever pertinent and provided that data are available.

Uruguay is a small country by Latin American standards (187,000 km^2) with a population of about 3 million inhabitants. The native population largely disappeared at the turn of the century, and most inhabitants are of European descent. The landscape is flat, without mountains or deserts. Land is fertile; agriculture and cattle breeding are the main economic activities. Industrialization is developing rapidly and communications are good, although there are still some isolated areas beyond the reach of medical care. The cultural level is acceptable with an illiteracy rate below 5 percent. Uruguay differs from other South American countries where the territorial extensions are enormous, large native groups have different life styles and languages, and illiteracy is high.

The Uruguayan population is mainly urban, 45 percent living in the capital city and 31 percent in other cities. Only 14 percent live in rural areas. Life expectancy is 69.8 years (67 for males and 73 for females). There is an abundance of doctors (8000, one for every 346 inhabitants) and a shortage of professional nurses (one for every 2900 inhabitants). Medical care is delivered through a prepaid system that covers about two-thirds of the total population (2 million people). One-third is delivered directly through the hospital system of the Ministry of Health. Private practice is negligible. This system provides acceptable but uneven medical care to the whole population. There are about 6000 beds for acute patients, with 110 intensive care beds in the capital city. In the rest of the country, 4000 acute care beds are available with 40 intensive care beds.[1]

ORGANIZATION

Critical care was started at the University Hospital in 1971. From the very beginning, it was considered that care of critically ill patients was a difficult and trying task best accomplished by a multidisciplinary team. Team work was accepted as a method, and the initial organization was based on this concept.

The first ICU was organized at the University Hospital with a permanent staff made up of doctors and nurses that were exclusively devoted to the care of critically ill patients. The ICUs of other hospitals were organized under the same model. All are run by a permanent staff. The referring physician shares the responsibility of major decisions, such as reoperations or treatment withdrawal, but primary care responsibility lies with the members of the permanent staff.

The size of the units varies widely, from 4 to 30 beds. One or more intensivists are available to the unit on a 24-h basis. As a rule, one intensivist takes care of 4 to 5 beds. The nurse-patient ratio is 1:1.5 to 1:2. A major advance in the past decade has been the development of intermediate care areas closely connected to the ICU and run by the same staff of physicians and nurses. This allows a very fluid relationship between both areas, thus facilitating rational use of the available beds and resources.

Although the organization of North American units was the model we used, the initial organization of the ICU with closed staff introduced a variation that was not widely accepted at the time. Objective evidence favoring this system as opposed to the open staff has only recently become available.[2]

The organization of the ICUs with permanent staff was part of early recognition of the fact that critical care was more than a place delivering specialized care. The concept evolved from this primitive view to one of titrated, uptempo differential diagnosis and management of the critically ill patient. Very soon the idea of a definitely new specialty was considered. It was not an easy task to convince other colleagues, but by the end of the decade a consensus was reached to accept the new specialty. Critical care has been recognized by the Uruguayan health authorities as an independent specialty since 1980. As far as we know, even today it has not been recognized as such in most of the Latin American countries.

The transfer of knowledge and skills to the younger generations is a real challenge. It has been very encouraging that young physicians are extremely interested in this discipline. A training program was designed with the aim of preparing specialists in critical care on the basis of a 3-year-long course covered through different types of teaching sessions. Evaluation every 6 months is mandatory.

The certificate of specialist in critical care is given by the Department of Postgraduate Education, belonging to the School of Medicine. This certificate is required to staff any ICU in the country. Three hundred physicians have received the certificate of specialist in critical care since 1980, and about 200 are currently taking courses at different stages of the training program.

CRITICAL CARE AND THE MEDICAL COMMUNITY

The development of a new specialty represented an intellectual challenge to the traditional internist. The characteristic physiologic point of view of intensivists in their obstinate search for the pathophysiologic mechanisms underlying each disease was interpreted on occasion as antithetical to standard approaches. Intensivists were often identified by internists as doctors with machines rather than clinicians with a new useful approach. In fact, we have gone a long way in better defining the interface between intensivists and internists. The result was a sharing of language and methodology by which internal medicine has been enriched.

Progress was often easier with surgeons, who promptly realized that critical care allowed them to perform more complicated operations at less risk for the patient and also offered a better understanding and treatment of systemic postoperative complications. As a matter of fact, once they became convinced that critical care was indeed a new and necessary specialty, relationships were rapidly established.

We believe that critical care offers a new intellectual approach that yields improved care for surgical and medical patients. It also provides a framework for advances in other specialties. The strong influence of critical care on North American general hospitals has been recently acknowledged.[3]

ACADEMIC CRITICAL CARE

Critical care at the University Hospital offered a model for patient care. Since this model was appropriate and effective, it served as a guide for the organization of most of the units in the country, and trainees provided by the University Hospital Critical Care Department now manage such units.

Clinical research is severely limited by lack of financial resources. In the past it was extremely difficult to obtain support for research projects from either private or public organizations. The situation is currently changing, and the university and other public entities are encouraging research through special grants for specific projects. Despite these limitations, clinical research has always been performed at the University Hospital, positively influencing the quality of care delivered.

FUTURE DIRECTIONS

Critical care is a strong and growing specialty in Uruguay and in most South American countries. The Society of Intensive Care Medicine is vigorous, and almost all subspecialists participate in its activities. An intensive care journal has been established, one of only three in South America (Argentina, Chile, and Uruguay). Frequent domestic and regional scientific meetings are the result of the interest of these specialists in exchanging knowledge, sharing problems, and finding common guidelines for the development of the specialty.

In our country, we view the future with optimism. Young intensivists are extremely enthusiastic and encourage their institutions to invest in critical care. Since the technical level is more than acceptable, the benefits in terms of survival and quality of life for our patients are likely substantial, although a nationwide objective evaluation of results has not been done. Another stimulus for development has been the demand for critical care by the general population. Lay interest in critical care, likely stimulated by personal encounters with this subspecialty, has led to a strong demand for intensive care whenever the patients or their families feel that benefits may be obtained. Thus, health administrators are apt to divert resources to critical care because of pressures exerted by physicians and the public. In addition, the presence of an ICU in a hospital is often seen as a means of enhancing and ensuring quality of care.

Critical care in this and other Latin American countries must face and solve many problems. Delivery of care is sufficient in most of the urban areas, at least in Uruguay, but a regionalized system must be developed to provide care more widely. The needs of each particular country or region should be established and the optimal geographic location of such centers determined.

The future of the specialty seems encouraging since there are still available positions in a country where the number of doctors is too high and many of them are jobless. A different problem is the future of young doctors that have become specialists. It is clear for many of them that they cannot be intensivists forever. Conviction is growing that intensivists must have a second specialty that will provide some balance for the "burn-out" of managing the critically ill. We think that this belief is threatening the future of the specialty, and creative solutions to this problem have yet to be devised.

The specialty has had an astonishing development in the past decade. However, it is imperative that ethical and economic limits be delineated if conflicts in the next decade are to be avoided. The economic future for the developing countries of the Southern Hemisphere is likely to include many constraints, and health resources should be optimally apportioned.

In a country where life expectancy is increasing and the population aging, the ICUs very often receive old, severely diseased patients in whom the benefits of intensive care are doubtful and probably do not affect the outcome. Despite this observation, the decision of whether to continue or withhold care must be considered on an individual basis, with guidelines for decision making supported by scientific knowledge.[4,5]

We believe special areas should be developed where patients whose survival is unprecedented but whose care requirements are nonetheless extensive can be managed.[6] Treatment in these areas would focus upon comfort and relief of pain without interfering with the process of dying.[5,6] This approach has deep philosophic and ethical roots, implies active therapy (comfort) for dying patients and their families, and allows a rational use of high-technology resources of the critical care environment.

REFERENCES

1. Margolis E, Piazza de Silva N: *Organización de la Atención Médica en el Uruguay*. Montevideo, Nordan Comunidad, 1989, p 365.
2. Knaus WA, Draper EA, Wagner DP, Zimmerman JE: Evaluation of outcome from intensive care in major medical centers. Ann Intern Med 104:410, 1986.
3. NIH Consensus Development Conference on Critical Care Medicine. Crit Care Med 11:466, 1983.
4. Ruark JE, Raffin TA: Stanford University Medical Center Committee on Ethics: Initiating and withdrawing life support: principles and practice in adult medicine. N Engl J Med 318:25, 1988.
5. Weil MH, Weil CJ, Rackow EC: Guide to ethical decision making for the critically ill: The three R's and Q.C. Crit Care Med 16:636, 1988.
6. Field BE, Devich LE, Carlson RW: Impact of a comprehensive supportive care team on management of hopelessly ill patients with multiple organ failure. Chest 96:353, 1989.

189G/The Former German Democratic Republic

MANFRED MEYER

The German Democratic Republic (GDR), one of the two German states now unified as one, can serve as an example of the organization of critical care medicine in a socialist country. Multidisciplinary Intensive Care Medicine (MICM) in the GDR is managed mainly by a specialist who is the holder of a state certificate in anesthesiology and intensive therapy, one of the 32 specialties officially recognized in this country. Today, MICM is learned within an integrated system of teaching, training, and continuing education.

TRAINING IN CRITICAL CARE MEDICINE

UNDERGRADUATE TEACHING

The teaching of essentials begins at the universities. In a nationwide program, undergraduates in medicine and dentistry are instructed in the pathophysiology of life-threatening diseases, complications of critical illness, and resuscitation measures. This knowledge is conveyed in an interdisciplinary series of lectures and seminars. In the fourth and fifth year of studies the students become conversant with monitoring systems and life support and learn to apply the principles of fluid balance and parenteral nutrition. These specific information bases are communicated within the larger context of care conducted in an interdisciplinary fashion.

POSTGRADUATE TRAINING

Postgraduate training in critical care starts immediately after the completion of university studies and follows a nationwide fellowship program, the standards of which have been established by close cooperation between the Chair of Anesthesiology and Intensive Care Medicine of the Academy of Postgraduate Medical Education and the Board of the Society of Anesthesiology and Intensive Therapy of the GDR.[1] This program is subject to final approval by the Ministry of Health.

Training takes place at 21 designated hospitals and departments and lasts 5 years. Depending on the extent to which the respective departments meet the standards of the program, the time permitted for training is fixed at 2 to 5 years. If any limitation exists, the trainee has to be delegated for the rest of the time to a fully authorized department. The knowledge required covers conditions and treatments common among critically ill patients. The following organ or system failures can be considered the core of the program: cardiovascular, pulmonary, metabolic, nephrourologic, gastrointestinal, neurologic, infectious diseases, overdose and/or intoxications, trauma, pediatric life-threatening conditions, and resuscitation. The program, furthermore, aims at special knowledge and perfection in other medical disciplines related to critical care and emergency medicine so as to guarantee a greater versatility.

Certification as a specialist in anesthesiology and intensive therapy is granted only after a final examination before a special examiner's board of the Academy of Postgraduate Medical Education, consisting of 11 members of academic rank appointed by the Ministry of Health. If the exam is passed successfully, the relevant report is forwarded to the central medical authorities and a state certificate in the applicant's specialty is issued.

CONTINUING EDUCATION

After qualification, continuing education helps to maintain skills and knowledge. The Chair of Anesthesiology and Intensive Care Medicine of the academy organizes joint studies so as to achieve a group approach to new techniques. Courses are organized for those senior staff members of the 21 departments recognized for training who work as tutors, providing lectures in pedagogics, psychology of motivation, and team leadership, the latest development in the specialty and related fields, medical opinions, and legal aspects. Such courses must be taken every 5 years by every senior staff member.

POLITICAL AND ECONOMIC ASPECTS OF HEALTH CARE

Along with other basic human rights, every citizen has the right to comprehensive health care irrespective of job and income.[2] The entire health service is run and developed by the government on planned lines. Hospitals, health centers, and clinics are for the most part publicly owned and financed by the national treasury. The vast majority of doctors, nurses, laboratory technicians, and other paramedical staff receive their salaries from the government. All medical services (preventive, therapeutic, or follow-up), regardless of value or duration, are provided free of charge and are available to everyone regardless of social status, place of residence, or other circumstances. Everyone is financially secure in illness, disablement, and old age. The monthly contribution to the social security program by all employees amounts to 10 percent of their earnings up to a maximum of 60 marks (equivalent to about $32). In the context of this subsection, the expenses of critical care medicine are also covered by the social security program.

THE PRACTICE OF CRITICAL CARE

There are 127 clinics or departments of anesthesiology and intensive therapy in the GDR responsible for and providing MICM.[3] By the definition provided by the Ministry of Health, only a multidisciplinary approach to this kind of highly specialized treatment may be called *intensive care medicine*. All other specialty-oriented departments or wards bear the name *intensive observation department* regardless of the special treatment provided (e.g., coronary care unit, dialysis unit). The only exceptions are specialty-oriented university departments providing highly specialized diagnostics, treatment, and research.

As of May 31, 1988, the 127 MICM clinics provided 1429 beds and were served by approximately 420 full-time intensivists (290 specialists and 130 trainees). An additional number of the 1690 doctors working in anesthesiology and intensive therapy serve part time in MICM. On the basis of a population of 16.6 million, there is one ICU bed per 11,600 people. Whereas the goal of one ICU bed per 10,000 people[4] has nearly been achieved, the desired key relation of one intensivist per two ICU beds is attained on the average only to a level of 58 percent. This is due to a shortage of doctors in this specialty or to a lofty goal.

General intensive care is provided in a graduated system of different hospitals from the district to the provincial level and up to university hospitals or health centers. If there are any limitations in treatment at one level, a patient can be taken to a more specialized department by means of a doctor-assisted ambulance, even when continuous controlled ventilation is required.

In the GDR there are 55 departments for hemodialysis (3 especially for children), 3 clinics for kidney transplantation, 28 departments for obstetrical-neonatologic intensive therapy, 5 cardiosurgical clinics where interventions including heart transplants are performed, and 1 highly specialized surgical university clinic at the famous Charité Hospital of Humboldt University, where liver and combined kidney-pancreas transplantation have been performed. Two centers for bone marrow transplantation complete the wide range of special treatment and intensive care.

RESOURCE ALLOCATION TOWARD CRITICAL CARE

In comparison with the critical care currently practiced in North America, there is no difference with respect to the kind of clientele. Everyday critical care in the GDR is provided according to international standards to patients suffering from life-threatening organ system failure or who are at markedly increased risk of complications.

Referring to the classes of the *Manual of the International Classification of Diseases, Injuries and Causes of Death* (MISCD),[5] patients treated belong to all classes, though with different distributions.

In 1987, 46,059 patients were treated, or approximately 2.77 patients per 10,000 citizens.[6] Of these 6210 patients died, yielding an overall death rate of 13.48 percent. In contrast to North America, modern electronic equipment for bedside diagnostics and/or monitoring is less available, a result of the shortage in foreign currency for imports. While there is a supply of GDR-made monitors, pacemakers, and ventilators for short-term application, the majority of sophisticated electronic equipment must be imported from Western countries. Leading critical care units are still able to acquire Servo ventilators for adults and babies, invasive and/or noninvasive cardiac output computers, hemodialysis and hemoperfusion devices, defibrillators and/or pacemakers, and automatic blood gas and/or acid-base analyzers. Sufficient basic therapeutic agents are available, but drugs produced outside the GDR can be received from the pharmacy only after special application. All expenses for critical care, even for imported items, are covered by the Social Security Program (vide supra).

RELATIONSHIP OF CRITICAL CARE PHYSICIANS TO ALLIED HEALTH PERSONNEL

Though MICM is mainly managed by the anesthesiologist and/or Intensivist, the multidisciplinary approach to critical care requires close cooperation with the specialists from other medical disciplines. In many intensive care departments these physicians are fully integrated into the staff. Surgeons, urologists, gynecologists, and neurologists are part-time members of the team and cooperate on call. Smaller departments operate exclusively on the basis of specialist's consultation if additional support is needed.

Experienced nurses in intensive care bear a state certificate as specialist in anesthesiology and intensive care nursing. This certificate can be acquired by fully licensed nurses after additional coursework and training in intensive care. The nursing staff consists of such specialist nurses, fully licensed nurses, and trainees. As in other countries, a shortage of nurses exists in the GDR.

Respiratory therapists are not available in this country. Supportive respiratory therapy is supplied by physiotherapists who take care of spontaneous breathing patients. Ventilator therapy is the doctor's responsibility alone.

RESEARCH

In 1971, the Ministry of Health and the Municipal Council of the GDR capital, Berlin, jointly began the Research Department of Intensive Care Medicine at Friedrichshain Hospital of Berlin, the leading emergency hospital in the GDR. The staff of this research department is organized on a multidisciplinary basis and consists of 12 full-time researchers including anesthesiologists with additional pharmacologic as well as physiologic education, biochemists, a bioengineer, and a biomathematician. The clinical basis for the research projects forms a 15-bed interdisciplinary ICU. There is very close cooperation with the clinical intensivists who take part on a joint basis in the projects. The results obtained are of immediate benefit for the diagnosis and/or treatment of patients.

ANTICIPATED CHANGES AFTER UNIFICATION OF BOTH GERMAN STATES

The unification ahead gives hope for better economic situation for hospitals and, therefore, critical care departments. Not only will unification ideally improve resources for equipment and staffing, but it is hoped that it will also facilitate international exchange with fellow specialists in Western countries. This will provide invaluable support for the further development of critical care medicine in this country after 40 years of isolation.

REFERENCES

1. Bildungsprogramm "Facharzt für Anästhesiologie und Intensiv therapie." Anaesthesiol Reanimat (Berlin) 13:245, 1988.
2. *First-hand Information "Health Care in the GDR."* Berlin, Panorama DDR Auslandspresseagentur, 1983.
3. Presseinformation Nr. 145, vom 13.12.1988 des Ministerrates der Deutschen Demokratischen Republik.
4. Scheidler K and Wolf E. (Hersg.): *Notfallmedizin—Organisation und Praxis 2. überarbeitete und erweiterte Aufl.* Berlin, VEB Verlag Volk u. Gesundheit, 1981.
5. World Health Organization: *Manual of the International Statistical Classification of Diseases, Injuries and Causes of Death,* 1975 Revision, Vol 1. Geneva, WHO, 1977.
6. Mitteilungen, Institut für Medizinische Statisik und Datenverarbeitung, Berlin (DDR), Jahrgang XXV, Heft 1, 1989, pp 48–50.

189H/Academic Aspects of Critical Care in Europe

PETER M. SUTER

The academic activity of critical care medicine has developed in European countries in a way similar to other parts of the world. The old continent has participated actively in the technical innovations, the establishment of a scientific basis for practice, and the development of appropriate pre- and postgraduate teaching and training programs over the past 30 years. However, important differences still exist between the different countries in Europe, and the concept of the ICU physician's specific academic role is not understood in the same way by the specialty branches of medicine such as anesthesia, surgery, internal medicine, or pediatrics. Only very recently has the idea of uniform postgraduate training and certification resulted in the creation of a European Diploma of Critical Care Medicine, defining a core curriculum with a written and oral examination.

ACADEMIC ACTIVITY DURING THE EARLY STAGES OF CRITICAL CARE MEDICINE

The late 1940s and early 1950s mark the beginning of critical care in Europe as prolonged ventilatory support was applied to polio victims.[1,2] Anesthesiologists and pneumologists were the first to introduce teaching and research programs in this new field. They were later joined by internists, cardiologists, and surgeons, when acute phases and complications of drug intoxications, severe infections such as pneumonia or meningitis, myocardial infarction, trauma, and postoperative therapy were seen to benefit from the knowledge and technologic innovation developed for respiratory intensive care.[3]

Anesthesiologists such as Norlander and internists such as Dönhart and Aschenbrenner were instrumental in developing teaching and research in this new field. From these early days up until the present, the bulk of teaching is directed at postgraduate students and residents. However, some aspects of critical care medicine have been included in pregraduate education in the programs of surgery, internal medicine, emergency medicine, and cardiology.

The research during the early stages of critical care medicine focused mainly on the pathophysiology of acute respiratory failure and mechanical ventilatory support. Soon investigations of cardiac failure and arrhythmias after myocardial infarction and circulatory shock developed.

TEACHING OF CRITICAL CARE MEDICINE IN EUROPE

The academic aspect of critical care that has resulted in the most immediate direct benefits for patients has been the teaching of medical students, residents, and nurses.

PREGRADUATE LEVEL

As in other young specialties, the major part of teaching critical care during medical school (the pregraduate level) is provided within the envelope of more established medical fields such as anesthesiology, internal medicine, pediatrics, and surgery. Table 189-7 summarizes some important topics and their curriculum location in a number of medical schools in Europe. However, the content as well as the number of hours devoted to these topics vary widely within

TABLE 189-7 Teaching Critical Care during Medical School (Pregraduate)

Rotation	Includes
Emergency medicine	Diagnosis and management of shock, cardiac arrest, and respiratory arrest
Trauma	Initial approach—evaluation and first steps, cardiocirculatory and respiratory management, complications, early and late
Burns	Approach and evaluation; volume resuscitation
Cardiac emergencies	Myocardial infarction, pulmonary embolism, acute cardiac failure
Respiratory emergencies	Status asthmaticus, acute pulmonary failure, acute on chronic respiratory failure

TABLE 189-8 Critical Care Teaching Provided during Postgraduate Training

Specialty	Topics
Anesthesiology	Cardiopulmonary resuscitation, management of hypovolemia and shock states, respiratory emergencies Practical teaching in the ICU for residents doing a full-time rotation (valid for all specialty training programs)
Internal medicine	Cardiopulmonary resuscitation, management of hypovolemia and shock states, cardiac decompensation—acute cardiac failure, respiratory emergencies, sepsis and septic shock
Pediatrics	Cardiopulmonary resuscitation, management of hypovolemia and shock states, cardiocirculatory failure, respiratory emergencies, acute upper airway obstruction, sepsis and septic shock Neonatal resuscitation and other emergency situations in perinatal medicine
Surgery	Cardiopulmonary resuscitation, acute cardiac or respiratory failure in surgical patients, management of the trauma patient, postoperative intensive care
Cardiology	Cardiopulmonary resuscitation, acute myocardial infarction, acute heart failure
Pneumology	Cardiopulmonary resuscitation, acute respiratory failure, status asthmaticus

one country and even more so between different countries in Europe. Similarly, the basic medical speciality of the teacher can be different from one medical school to another. The historical strong role of anesthesiologists in teaching critical care remains particularly strong in Great Britain, Scandinavia, and Italy. Internal medicine and surgery contribute more to this task in Germany, France, Belgium, Holland, and Switzerland. Only Spain, and France to a certain extent, have a separate postgraduate training track for critical care. Physicians trained in this area participate in a variable but sometimes important way to pregraduate teaching in this field. Didactic pregraduate education is complemented by a clinical rotation in the ICU for medical students in many countries. This training period usually lasts several months but is not compulsory in most countries.

Theoretical and practical knowledge in critical care can be tested at the final examinations of the medical school within the branches of anesthesiology, internal medicine, or surgery. This seems to be done quite frequently throughout Europe for the more basic topics or emergency medicine but less for topics related to more involved critical care problems and therapies.

POSTGRADUATE LEVEL

Training in critical care in the postgraduate phase should be progressive for residents in anesthesia, internal medicine, pediatrics, surgery, cardiology, and pneumology. However, training programs vary widely among institutions, and many residents in certain programs have no access to the care of critically ill patients in the ICU.[4] In addition, only a very few ICUs have well-structured training programs. It is therefore not surprising that even in 1991 additional postgraduate experience in centers abroad with recognized teaching programs must be recommended for physicians planning a full-time career in intensive care medicine (vide infra). The minimum content of a curriculum in critical care at the postgraduate level is shown in Table 189-8. As mentioned above for pregraduate teaching, a number of topics listed may be provided by teachers with only limited experience in clinical care in the ICU. However, this shortcoming has improved significantly in recent years.

The clinical training for the subspecialty of critical care includes 2 years full time in the ICU in addition to the theoretic background. Activity without direct supervision or on-call duties alone do not count toward this requirement. An examination at the end of the training program has been recommended.[5]

The national committees responsible for postgraduate medical education in several European countries have recently adopted standards for certification in critical care as an independent medical subspecialty according to the principles described above.[6] These standards are similar to those applied in the United States and Canada.[7,8] Critical care will only be able to fulfill its academic role with competence when teaching and training of high quality can be provided.

TEACHING AND TRAINING OF INTENSIVE CARE NURSES

A number of European countries have longstanding full-time training programs for ICU nurses, while others are in the process of developing such programs. A short description of such programs will be given here to allow a better understanding of academic aspects of critical care and because these teaching duties are fulfilled by ICU physicians.

Nurses can qualify for entry in an official training program after fulfilling the following conditions:

- Completion of a recognized nursing school program of at least 4 years duration.
- Two years of subsequent professional activity.

An ICU can be recognized for postgraduate training program for nurses when the following conditions are satisfied.

- A minimum number of beds, patients, admissions, and days of mechanical ventilation are demonstrated.
- An ICU physician is present.
- At least 25 percent of the nursing personnel must be certified, i.e., have successfully completed the critical care training program.

The introduction of well-structured educational programs for ICU nurses has increased their competence and the quality of care. Concomitantly, it has increased the pressure on physicians to improve their training and has stimulated academic activities in critical care.

CRITICAL CARE RESEARCH IN EUROPE

After the early years of active innovation and research, scientific contributions from Europe arguably declined in the 1950s and 1960s. During the past 15 to 20 years, however, a resurgence has been noted. A number of research groups have expanded both basic and clinical investigations from this continent, and several journals devoted to critical care have been founded. A number of the most active scientists, but not all of them, did benefit from additional research training in the United States or Canada. On the other hand, an active collaboration on a local level with the basic medical sciences and other specialties has provided interesting opportunities to explore and to benefit from mutual interest and expertise. The foundation of the European Society of Intensive Care Medicine by scientifically oriented physicians in 1982 was a major stimulus to research activities. A continuing exchange with colleagues and groups in North America, presentation of data at international congresses, and publication in both North American and European journals were other important factors ensuring high-quality research.

The importance of research for the professional and academic future of critical care is certainly recognized today. However, as only a very few specific academic positions have been created, the majority of full-time critical care physicians with ambition for an academic career are forced to keep one foot in a traditional medical specialty (vide infra). This activity in two fields is certainly not ideal to promote high standards in clinical work and research in critical care medicine. Such imperfect academic career possibilities are, however, not unique to Europe.

AN ACADEMIC CAREER IN CRITICAL CARE MEDICINE IN EUROPE

At this time and for the next 5 to 10 years, many more clinical than academic positions are and will be available in Europe. Despite this, how should an academic career be planned today? In the majority of medical schools of Europe, the "primary clinician but also scientist" corresponds best to the profile requested for a lecturer and professor in clinical medicine. As the two parts of this job description cannot be easily prepared for simultaneously, it seems important to fix priorities during one's training. In Table 189-9 two possible schedules for training are proposed. The most important features are certainly not the precise timing but rather an early involvement in research and teaching activities. This will be decisive for future career development because the passion for this part of the profession will ensure long-term satisfaction and success. Part of the postgraduate training and an additional period of preparation could be done abroad with substantial benefits of widening one's perspective and creating wider contacts with colleagues. As indicated in Table 189-9, complete training in a classical medical specialty is recommended because of the candidate searching for an academic position has more options, and in the event of job dissatisfaction or other adverse events, alternative professional pathways can be chosen.

ACADEMIC POSITIONS IN CRITICAL CARE IN EUROPE

Over the past 10 years, an impressive number of posts of lecturer, associate, and full professor have been created in Europe. In addition, dozens of critical care physicians have been elected to chairs of anesthesiology and internal medicine and a few also to chairs in surgery and pediatrics. Comparison between countries and medical schools are however difficult, and precise figures cannot be given.

TABLE 189-9 Examples for Planning an Academic Career in Critical Care

Option 1	Option 2
Clinical training until specialty certification (not more than 6 years)	Research, e.g., in basic medical science (2–3 years)
Clinical or experimental research (2–3 years)	Clinical training until specialty certification (not more than 6 years)
Critical care medicine (2 years)	Research and teaching as part-time activity (2 years)
Research and teaching as part-time activity (2 years)	Critical care medicine (2 years)
Additional training in research and/or clinical practice abroad	Special competence training in cardiology, pneumology, infectious diseases, pathophysiology, or others

What is the likely future evolution of these positions? Looking at past developments and future needs in this field, the number of academic positions will certainly increase over the next years. Given the ever-present budget restrictions, the problem of funding remains important. However, nobody can seriously argue that the costs of creating this position for teaching and research will not be outweighed by the benefits for the training of doctors and nurses in critical care.[9]

REFERENCES

1. Aschenbrenner R, Dönhardt A: Klinik und Therapie der Atemstörungen bei der Poliomyelitis. Dtsch Med Wschr 508, 1948.
2. Lassen HCA: A preliminary report on the 1952 epidemic of poliomyelitis in Copenhagen. Lancet 1:37, 1953.
3. Björk VO, Engström CG, Friberg O, Feychting H, Swensson A: Ventilatory problems in thoracic anaesthesia. A volume cycling device for controlled respiration. J Thor Surg 31:117, 1956.
4. Li TCM, Philips MC, Shaw L, Cook EF, Natanson C, Goldman L: On-site physician staffing in a community hospital intensive care unit. JAMA 252:2023, 1984.
5. Safar P, Grenvik A: Organization and physician education in critical care medicine. Anesthesiology 47:82, 1977.
6. Publikation des Zentralvorstandes der Verbindung der Schweizer Ärzte. Publication du Comité central de la Fédération des Médecins Suisses (FMH): Untertitel Intensivmedizin zum Haupttitel Spezialarzt FMH für Anästhesiologie, Chirurgie, Innere Medizin oder Pädiatrie. Sous-spécialité "médecine intensive" à adjoindre au titre de spécialiste FMH en anesthésiologie, chirurgie, médecine interne ou pédiatrie. Schweizerische Ärztezeitung/Bulletin des médecins suisses 71:2059, 1990.
7. Kelley MA: Critical care medicine—A new specialty? N Engl J Med 318:1613, 1988.
8. Meyer AA, Fakhry SM, Sheldon GF: Critical care education in general surgery residencies. Surgery 106:392, 1989.
9. Brown JJ, Sullivan G: Effect on ICU mortality of a full-time critical care specialist. Chest 96:127, 1989.

189I/Aspects of Critical Care Organization in Europe

DINIS REIS MIRANDA
JOHN F.A. SPANGENBERG

HISTORICAL BACKGROUND

Critical care in Europe began over 40 years ago when ventilatory assistance was extended to victims of a polio epidemic. Since mechanical ventilation was the main treatment necessary, anaesthetists usually cared for these patients in the recovery room. The success of these interventions stimulated the creation of facilities for treating a wider range of critically ill patients. These patients were gathered in special ICUs, and many medical specialties became involved in critical care.

From the beginning, the proliferation of ICUs in Europe has not followed specific criteria or guidelines. A new ICU is most often created based on local needs and availability of finances. Consequently, the expansion of ICUs in Europe is not necessarily directly related to the broader planning of health care.

CURRENT ICU RESOURCES

There is an enormous diversity of ICUs across Europe, even inside each country. In Table 189-10, the analysis of 307 answers to a questionnaire distributed among hospitals larger than 400 beds in 11 European countries[1] illustrates this point. The percentage of total hospital beds allocated to ICUs is smallest in the United Kingdom (2.6 percent) and largest in Denmark (4.1 percent), and the number of beds per ICU varies from 6 beds per ICU in the United Kingdom up to 19 beds per ICU in Belgium. There were also significant differences in utilization of ICU facilities with widely different occupancies and length of stay (Table 189-11). Short length of stay is explained in part by the recovery room function of ICUs in some European countries.

It was also apparent from this survey that university hospitals have almost two times as many beds (1229 ± 754) as nonuniversity hospitals (657 ± 365). The number of ICU beds (including coronary care unit beds) in each hospital was also different: 46.3 ± 35 (or 4.2 ± 2.7 percent of hospital beds) in university hospitals and 17.3 ± 11 (or 2.9 ± 1.6 percent of hospital beds) in nonuniversity hospitals.

In 63 percent of the hospitals with more than 400 beds, a general ICU is the type of unit found.[1] Fifty percent of these units are operating independently from other departments, with the department of anesthesia having the predominant role in the management of ICU patients. The frequency of general ICUs is higher in nonuniversity hospitals (72 percent) than in university hospitals (46 percent).

A medical director or similar position exists in 95 percent of the university hospitals and in 88 percent of the nonuniversity hospitals. The referring physician is responsible for the clinical management of the ICU patient in 5 percent of

TABLE 189-10 Percentage of Beds Allocated to ICUs in European Hospitals

Country	ICU beds (%)	Beds per ICU
Austria	2.8 ± 1.3	10 ± 3
Belgium	3.7 ± 2.0	19 ± 16
Denmark	4.1 ± 2.0	14 ± 4
France	3.3 ± 2.9	11 ± 6
Germany	3.4 ± 1.6	12 ± 5
Holland	3.6 ± 1.3	10 ± 7
Spain	3.0 ± 1.5	14 ± 11
Sweden	3.3 ± 1.8	13 ± 5
Switzerland	3.8 ± 1.4	14 ± 8
United Kingdom	2.6 ± 2.0	6 ± 2

TABLE 189-11 Utilization of ICU Facilities in European Hospitals

Country	Admissions per Bed per Year	No. Days per Patient	Occupancy Rate (%)	No. Nurses per Bed
Austria	46 ± 10	5.3	67.6	2.2
Belgium	67 ± 18	4.6	88.6	2.4
Denmark	74 ± 07	2.9	59.0	1.2
France	58 ± 35	5.6	83.3	1.9
Germany	83 ± 38	4.4	94.8	2.1
Holland	93 ± 40	3.5	78.0	3.0
Spain	50 ± 17	5.9	72.6	2.2
Sweden	124 ± 54	3.0	99.0	1.9
Switzerland	74 ± 21	3.0	60.2	3.1
United Kingdom	65 ± 47	3.5	67.6	4.2

university hospitals and in 12 percent of the nonuniversity hospitals.[1]

ECONOMICS OF CRITICAL CARE

ICU costs are not known precisely. We estimate that in the Netherlands they are 10 to 15 percent of the total health care costs, and this probably is true of other European countries. Generally speaking, health care costs increased sharply until the seventies. Since then the observed increase of these costs is fairly consistent with the increase of the gross national product, and the projections for 1989 and 1990 even show a decrease in relative costs.

Health care is undergoing a fundamental technologic, economic, demographic, and regulatory transformation. This transformation, which is more evident in some countries (such as in the Netherlands), is characterized by the following trends:

- Declining fertility rates with an "aged" population
- Intense focus on cost control and productivity
- Medical technology assessment with consequent preference for cost-effectiveness rather than "high" technology
- Focus on accreditation and quality assurance
- Substitution of standardized high-cost care by tailor-made (lower cost) care
- Increased competition (focus on specialties, quality, and costs)
- Large number of hospital managers
- Standardization of health care norms in European Economic Community countries (1992)
- Joint professional bureaucracy in hospitals (more cooperation between hospital managers and physicians)

PLANNING FOR CRITICAL CARE IN EUROPE

In order to encourage the different European countries to join in standardization and improvement of critical care, helping at the same time to control the increasing costs of health care, the European Society of Intensive Care Medicine (ESICM) created an international multidisciplinary task force for defining the guidelines for better use of resources. This task force produced an extensive document, recently published, entitled *Management of Intensive Care*.[2] The guidelines concentrated in four major points of action: regionalization, quantification, professionalization, and levels of decision making.

REGIONALIZATION

Regionalization aims at the appropriate match between the organization of each facility and the need for intensive care. The rationales for optimal distribution of ICUs are as follows:

1. Not all patients, or groups of patients, need the same intensity of care. The severity of illness of intensive care patients is usually related to the hospital and the levels of medical activity practiced there.
2. More severely ill patients do require a higher level of ICU organization (personnel, equipment, etc.) and, therefore, a higher investment of resources.
3. The minimal requirements of an ICU require it to be prepared for acute resuscitation and for temporary support of vital functions.

Such services should be available at an effective time and distance from any portion of the population.

The ESICM task force proposed the regionalization of ICUs into three levels of care (Table 189-12), and the interested reader is referred to the published report.[2] In practice, the levels of care are established according to local and regional needs. The allocation of resources takes place after needs are inventoried. Every ICU should be prepared to take care of the most critically ill patient even if only for that short period of time required for stabilizing vital functions before transferring the patient to another ICU at a higher level of organization. Therefore, adequate regionalization of critical care means centralization of the facilities together with decentralization of knowledge. Consequently, teaching and training of intensive care has to be organized and implemented at a national level.

QUANTIFICATION

Quantification is necessary for defining patients needing critical care, for regionalizing the ICUs, for the organization of the facilities, and for the objective evaluation of the per-

TABLE 189-12 Proposed ESICM Levels of ICU Care

	Level I	Level II	Level III
Physicians per patients	1 per unit	1/6.5	1/5
Nurses per patients	1/4	1/2.5	1/1
SAPS/Points*	5–10	8–15	> 13
TISS points†	3–15	14–35	> 30
Calculated cost per bed per day (U.S.A. dollars)	100	550	1000

*Simplified Acute Physiologic Score.
†Therapeutic Intervention Score System.

formance of each ICU. Severity of illness, manpower required for the effective treatment of each category of disease, and the results (output) of each ICU are very essential information to be quantified. Severity of illness and manpower are the two important elements for defining the three levels of care.[2]

PROFESSIONALIZATION

Professionalization of health care workers involved in critical care requires identification of necessary knowledge and skills, implementation of training programs, certification procedures, and then the means of continuing education. In addition, because this field is multidisciplinary, guidelines that define individual responsibilities but promote a team approach to care are desirable.

LEVELS OF DECISION MAKING

Although the production of outputs is proportionally related to the consumption of resources, the level of production is generated outside the critical care organization. In other words, critical care will have difficulty in efficiently controlling its participation in the use of resources without the assistance of policymakers of other medical activities. When planning for organ transplantation, cardiac surgery, radical cancer surgery, etc., one should also augment ICU resources in the area where these new activities will be implemented.

MANAGEMENT OF ICUS

The quality and efficiency of the ICU can only be assured when the ICU is conceived as a responsibility center in which the management and the staff are held accountable for the ICU outcomes. Figure 189-1 presents a model including the main determinants of ICU performance.

ICU performance is defined as reductions in avoidable mortality or morbidity. Inputs include the size of the unit (number of beds), the capacity of the unit (staff and equipment), the design of the unit (square feet per bed), and the layout of the unit (integration within the hospital).

ICU throughputs include organizational structure, quality of the management, working climate, and communication between staff members. Each ICU has an entry and an exit barrier.

Intensive care involves strategic choices about the conditions under which it is appropriate to treat and the degree of severity justifying intervention or discharge. For individual patients, tactical decisions have to be made as to when to initiate intensive therapy and when to discontinue support at an intensive level. These matters bear on issues of medical ethics and costs.

There is a need for improved criteria for admission and discharge since there are many sources of misuse of ICU facilities. The use is inappropriate in the case of low-risk admission or when the patient is too ill to benefit. When the risks of complications outweigh the expected benefit, treatment will be unsafe. Perhaps the greatest waste of resources is the overtreatment of the hopelessly ill patient.

DETERMINANTS OF ICU OUTCOME

The purpose of intensive care is to reduce avoidable mortality in patients who are critically ill. The multicenter prospective methodology of Knaus[3] enables a ranking of ICUs on the basis of standardized mortality ratios. In a 13-center

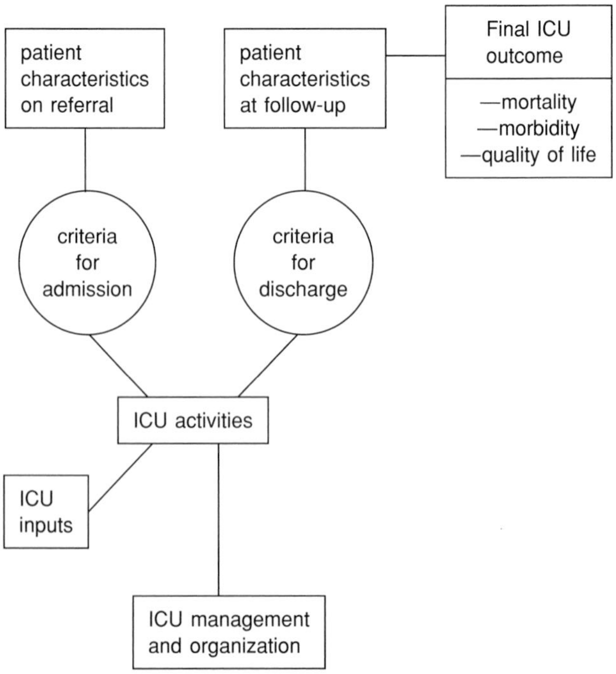

FIGURE 189-1 Flow of ICU patients.

study he found that one hospital (1) had significantly better results with 69 deaths predicted and 41 observed, whereas another hospital (13) had significantly inferior results with 58 percent more deaths than expected. These differences occurred within specific diagnostic criteria, for medical patients alone, and for medical and surgical patients combined. Relating this outcome to the characteristics of the ICU organization, evidence for the impact of structure and process of service given in the ICU was found. For example, the best ICU had a full-time director, a 24 hour-in-unit physician coverage, and no problems with adequate nurse staff. In addition, directors and staff jointly control decisions for admission and discharge and for therapy. Obviously, more evidence is needed to determine the impact of organization and management on ICU effectiveness. This evidence may be provided by a recent 40-center study conducted by the ICU research center in the United States and by a 40-center study conducted by the Foundation for Research on Intensive Care in Europe (FRICE) in the Netherlands, since both large-scale studies include assessment of outcome and of the inputs and throughputs of intensive care.

REFERENCES

1. Miranda DR, Langrehr D (eds): *The ICU: A Cost-Benefit Analysis.* Excerpta Medica, International Congress Series 709, 1986.
2. Miranda DR, Williams A, Loirat Ph (eds): *Management of Intensive Care: Guidelines for Better Resource Use.* Kluwer Academic Publishers, 1990.
3. Knaus WA, et al: An evaluation of outcome from intensive care in major medical centers. Ann Intern Med 104:410, 1986.

Limiting Therapy in the Hopelessly Ill Patient: European Attitudes

JEAN-LOUIS VINCENT

CONSIDERATIONS IN LIMITING THERAPY

It has become well recognized that some limitation should be brought to the intensive care therapy of hopelessly ill patients to avoid futile therapy. It has also been accepted that there is no real ethical difference between withholding and withdrawing therapy. The possibility of withdrawal should be defended to limit the risk of excessive "withholding" decisions. It rather provides all patients with maximal therapy unless the situation really becomes hopeless.[1]

The view held in various European institutions, including ours at the Free University of Brussels (a nonreligious institution), is that there is no real difference between withdrawal of life-supporting measures and administration of agents that will result in the cessation of all organ function. Both attitudes will most often lead to the patient's death. However, withdrawal of life support might bring discomfort to the patient and prolong an arguably useless agony. On the other hand, a pharmacologic intervention that can hasten an ongoing dying process will avoid suffering, indignity, and the costs associated with a prolonged terminal phase.

Ethical objections have been that there is a fundamental difference between the two attitudes since one can be seen as "killing" and the other "letting die." This difference, however, becomes meaningless in a particular environment where something can still be done to support the failing body. In his book *The End of Life,* James Rachels[2] took the example of an individual whose intention was to kill a child by drowning him in a swimming pool, so as to simulate an accident. Before any murder was performed, the child unexpectedly slipped in the pool and fell unconscious. According to his plans, the adult did not intervene and the child did drown. Is there really a fundamental ethical difference between killing and letting die in this particular criminal circumstance? The difference might exist legally, but not ethically.

Nobody could argue that withdrawal of minimal support (i.e., fluids and nutrition) will result in death, exactly as increasing doses of sedating drugs will. In most European institutions, starving someone to death is felt to be unacceptable by physicians and nurses as well as the public (patients and families). In the context of a dying patient in the intensive care unit, the precise definition of the means used to shorten the dying process is irrelevant provided the patient does not suffer. Withdrawal of mechanical ventilation is seldom performed because it might bring discomfort to the patient. It could be argued that sedatives could be simultaneously administered to ensure patient comfort. Why then should the mechanical support be discontinued? Sometimes, mechanical ventilation could even be started in a dyspneic patient before sedation is applied once the patient is relieved of dyspnea (this latter attitude might not always be logical but is sometimes requested by the nursing personnel in our institution).

According to a recent survey of the European Society of Intensive Care Medicine,[3] withdrawing therapy was applied by 63 percent and euthanasia by 36 percent of European intensivists. Withdrawal of therapy was usually preferred to euthanasia. Both withdrawal of life support and euthanasia were less common in Italy, Spain, and Portugal.

The word *euthanasia* has various meanings and sometimes frightening connotations. If it refers to active killing of a patient at his or her request by a physician, as it is a present topic of debate in the Netherlands,[4] it hardly applies to the patient in the ICU. Discontinuation of care is only seldom considered in critically ill patients who are conscious. To the contrary, it is not uncommon that intensive care is continued in competent patients who request its discontinuation. The respect for patient autonomy is then outweighed by the duty of the physician to support the patient when there are reasonable chances of improvement. The underlying concept is that the patient is likely to change his or her mind when he or she improves. Indeed, in these circumstances, it is not uncommon for the patient to later acknowledge that he or she went through a depressive phase.

The ethical dilemma is in part related to the definition of death. Today more than ever, death cannot be defined by the cessation of respiration or cardiac activity. Death can be defined by a permanent cessation of brain function.[5] Even in the absence of brain death criteria, the permanent cessation of a cognitive life has already occurred in many hopelessly ill patients with postanoxic coma, cerebrovascular accident, or multiple organ failure.

Therefore, this decision about termination of care generally concerns patients with an impaired mental status who cannot participate in the decision. In our department, the decision is always made by the entire ICU staff (including nurses) during rounds and after the relatives' opinion has been expressed. This is not the case throughout Europe. Most European intensivists consider that the nurses, like the patient and his or her family, should be involved in these decisions, but they simultaneously acknowledge that this is not widely done in practice.[3] The attitude of the nursing personnel can vary geographically. Sometimes the nurses would not consider the cessation of treatment as a possible option. In other institutions such as ours, the nurse is usually the person who first raises the issue of futile therapy.

An obstacle to the discontinuation of care can be the hesitation of the primary physician (e.g., oncologist, surgeon) who always finds arguments suggesting that the situation might not be irremediably fatal. If this occurs in our institution, this primary physician is invited to discuss this point with the ICU staff. The presentation of a consensus opinion by the ICU staff can be a convincing argument to the primary physician that treatment has become futile and stubborn (what is called *acharnement therapeutique* in French).

Finally, the vast majority of European intensivists consider that these decisions are ethical and not legal. The problems are related to everyone's health as defined by physical and mental well-being. Therefore, by definition, they are primarily medical. The laws prohibiting killing should be maintained to defend everyone's right to life. Nevertheless, limitations to intensive care therapy in hopelessly ill patients have become sometimes inescapable. Judges and lawyers are not better than doctors to decide upon these delicate matters. Therefore, the procedures should not be complicated by elaborate discussions before committees including nonmedical professionals. Death, like birth, should remain a natural event of our everyday life. The right to die with dignity must remain a fundamental ethical principle.

REFERENCES

1. Sprung CL: Changing attitudes and practices in foregoing life-sustaining treatments. JAMA 263:2211, 1990.
2. Rachels J: *The End of Life.* Oxford University Press, New York, 1986.
3. Vincent JL: European attitudes towards ethical problems in intensive care medicine: Results of an ethical questionnaire. Intensive Care Med 16:256, 1990.
4. de Wachter MAM: Active euthanasia in the Netherlands. JAMA 262:3316, 1989.
5. Schaffner KF, Snyder JV, Abramson NS, et al: Philosophical, ethical, and legal aspects of resuscitation medicine, III: Discussion. Crit Care Med 16:1069, 1988.

INDEX

The letters f or t following a page number indicate that either a figure or a table is being referenced.